HENRY'S
Clinical Diagnosis and Management by Laboratory Methods

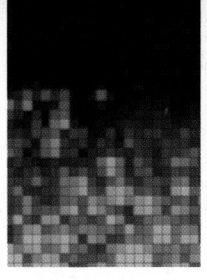

ASSOCIATE EDITORS

Naif Z. Abraham Jr., MD, PhD
Director, Division of Clinical Pathology
Assistant Professor of Pathology
State University of New York Upstate Medical University
Syracuse, New York

Martin H. Bluth, MD, PhD
Associate Professor of Pathology
Director of Translational Research
Associate Director, Transfusion Service
Wayne State University School of Medicine
Detroit Medical Center
Karmanos Cancer Institute
Detroit, Michigan

Jay L. Bock, MD, PhD
Professor and Vice Chair of Pathology
Director of Clinical Pathology
University Hospital and Medical Center
State University of New York at Stony Brook
Stony Brook, New York

Robert E. Hutchison, MD
Professor of Pathology
Director of Clinical Pathology
Director of Hematopathology
State University of New York Upstate Medical University
Syracuse, New York

H. Davis Massey, MD, PhD
Associate Professor of Pathology
Director of Surgical Pathology
Virginia Commonwealth University
Richmond, Virginia

Jonathan L. Miller, MD, PhD
Director of Medical Center Clinical Laboratories
Professor and Vice Chairman, Department of Pathology
University of Chicago
Chicago, Illinois

Katherine I. Schexneider, MD
Associate Professor, Department of Pathology
Uniformed Services University
Medical Director, Blood Bank
Staff Pathologist, Department of Laboratory Medicine
National Naval Medical Center
Bethesda, Maryland

Gregory A. Threatte, MD
Professor and Chairman
Department of Pathology
State University of New York Upstate Medical University
Syracuse, New York

Elizabeth R. Unger, MD, PhD
Acting Chief, Chronic Viral Diseases Branch
Division of High-Consequence Pathogens and Pathology
National Center for Emerging and Zoonotic Infectious Diseases
Centers for Disease Control and Prevention
Atlanta, Georgia

Gail L. Woods, MD
Chief, Pathology and Laboratory Medicine
Central Arkansas Veterans Healthcare System
Professor of Pathology
Department of Pathology
University of Arkansas for Medical Sciences
Little Rock, Arkansas

22nd EDITION

HENRY'S
Clinical Diagnosis and Management by Laboratory Methods

Richard A. McPherson, MD

Harry B. Dalton Professor and Chairman
Division of Clinical Pathology
Virginia Commonwealth University
Director
Clinical Pathology
Medical College of Virginia Hospitals
Richmond, Virginia

Matthew R. Pincus, MD, PhD

Professor
Department of Pathology
State University of New York Downstate Medical Center
Brooklyn, New York
Chairman
Department of Pathology and Laboratory Medicine
Veterans Affairs New York Harbor Healthcare System
New York, New York

ELSEVIER
SAUNDERS

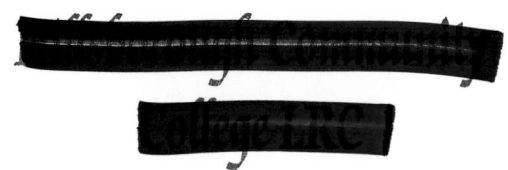

ELSEVIER
SAUNDERS

1600 John F. Kennedy Blvd.
Ste 1800
Philadelphia, PA 19103-2899

HENRY'S CLINICAL DIAGNOSIS AND MANAGEMENT ISBN: 978-1-4377-0974-2
By Laboratory Methods, Twenty-Second Edition

Notices

Knowledge and best practice in this field are constantly changing. As new research and experience broaden our understanding, changes in research methods, professional practices, or medical treatment may become necessary.

Practitioners and researchers must always rely on their own experience and knowledge in evaluating and using any information, methods, compounds, or experiments described herein. In using such information or methods they should be mindful of their own safety and the safety of others, including parties for whom they have a professional responsibility.

With respect to any drug or pharmaceutical products identified, readers are advised to check the most current information provided (i) on procedures featured or (ii) by the manufacturer of each product to be administered, to verify the recommended dose or formula, the method and duration of administration, and contraindications. It is the responsibility of practitioners, relying on their own experience and knowledge of their patients, to make diagnoses, to determine dosages and the best treatment for each individual patient, and to take all appropriate safety precautions.

To the fullest extent of the law, neither the Publisher nor the authors, contributors, or editors assume any liability for any injury and/or damage to persons or property as a matter of products liability, negligence or otherwise, or from any use or operation of any methods, products, instructions, or ideas contained in the material herein.

Library of Congress Cataloging-in-Publication Data
Henry's clinical diagnosis and management by laboratory methods.—22nd ed. / [edited by] Richard A. McPherson, Matthew R. Pincus.
p. ; cm.
Clinical diagnosis and management by laboratory methods
Includes bibliographical references and index.
ISBN 978-1-4377-0974-2 (hardcover : alk. paper) 1. Diagnosis, Laboratory. I. McPherson, Richard A. II. Pincus, Matthew R. III. Henry, John Bernard, 1928– IV. Title: Clinical diagnosis and management by laboratory methods.
[DNLM: 1. Clinical Laboratory Techniques. QY 25]
RB37.C54 2011
616.07′56—dc22

2011004091

Acquisitions Editor: William R. Schmitt
Developmental Editor: Kathryn DeFrancesco
Publishing Services Manager: Anne Altepeter
Project Manager: Louise King
Designer: Ellen Zanolle

Printed in China

Last digit is the print number: 9 8 7 6 5 4 3 2 1

CONTENTS

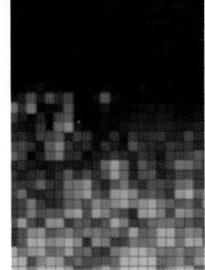

PART 8 Molecular Pathology

EDITED BY Martin H. Bluth, Elizabeth R. Unger, Matthew R. Pincus

PART 9 Clinical Pathology of Cancer

EDITED BY Matthew R. Pincus, Martin H. Bluth, Richard A. McPherson

APPENDIXES

EDITED BY Richard A. McPherson, Matthew R. Pincus, Naif Z. Abraham Jr.

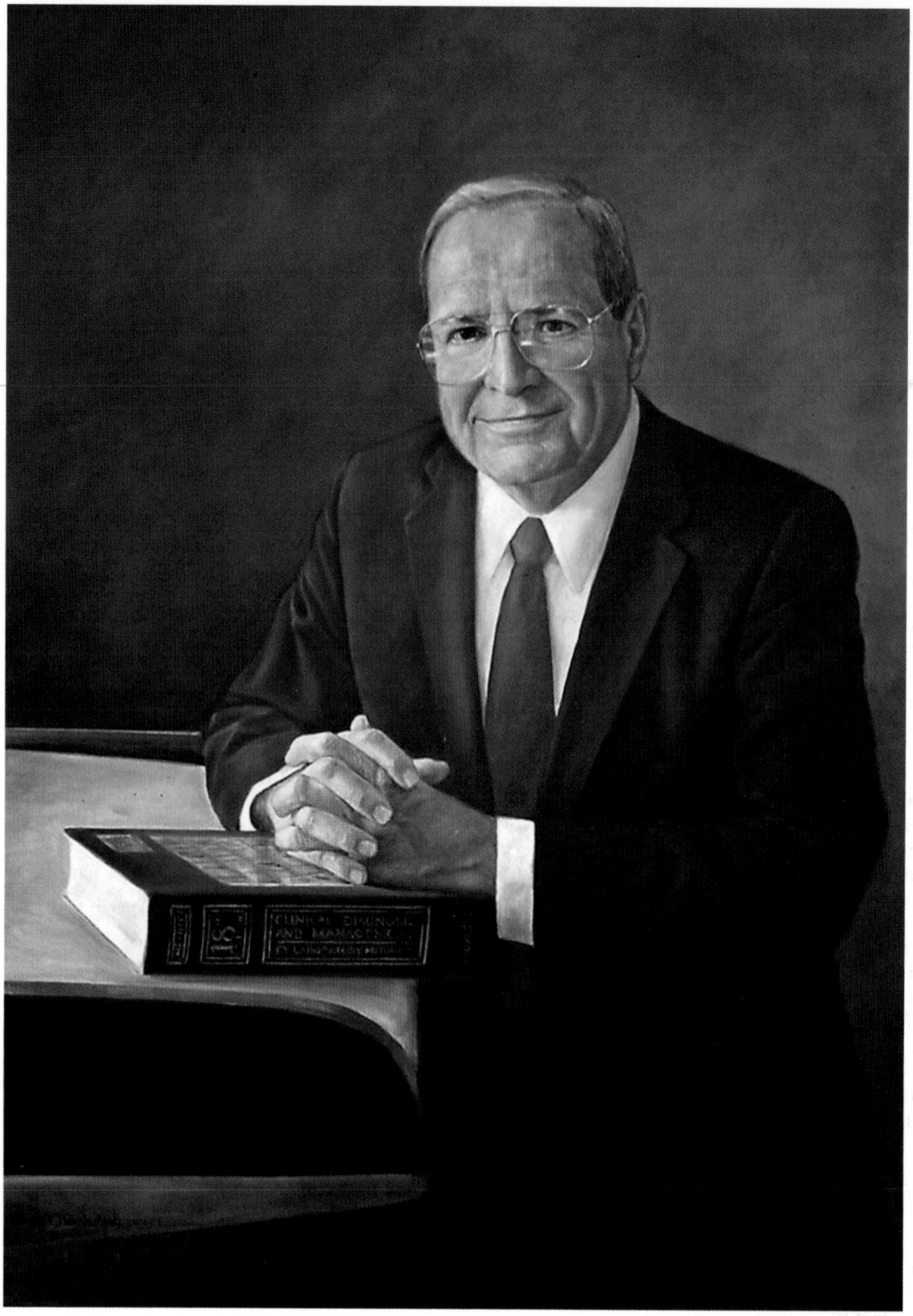

Detail of Brian O'Toole Makepeace's 1992 painting of John Bernard Henry, MD. Courtesy the Medical Photography Department and the Historical Collections, Health Sciences Library, State University of New York Upstate Medical University, Syracuse, N.Y.

In Memoriam

John Bernard Henry, MD

1928–2009

It was with a profound sense of sadness and loss that we learned of the passing of Dr. John Bernard Henry, editor of seven editions of this textbook from 1969 to 2001. Dr. Henry, who died in Skaneateles, New York, on April 10, 2009, was a superb academic physician who made immense contributions to medicine, especially to the development of the medical laboratory in both the diagnosis and treatment of human disease.

John grew up in Elmira, New York, where he graduated from Elmira Catholic High School. He enlisted in the United States Navy just after World War II where he served as a corpsman. He then attended Cornell University on a New York State Scholarship and graduated with a Bachelor of Arts degree in 1951. Using his GI Bill, John went on to the University of Rochester School of Medicine and Dentistry where he was elected to the Alpha Omega Alpha Medical Honor Society and received his Doctor of Medicine degree in 1955. Also while at Rochester, he married Georgette Boughton, his wife of 56 years.

John interned at Barnes Hospital in St. Louis, Missouri, and began his pathology training at Columbia Presbyterian Medical Center in New York City. He finished his residency at the New England Deaconess Hospital in Boston as a National Cancer Institute Trainee. While a resident, he also received training in forensic pathology at the City of New York Medical Examiner's Office and training in the clinical use of radioisotopes at the Cancer Research Institute of the New England Deaconess Hospital.

He joined the faculty of the University of Florida at Gainesville in 1960 as an assistant professor and rose to the rank of associate professor while directing the Blood Bank. In 1964, he relocated to Syracuse to become Professor of Pathology and the Director of Clinical Pathology in what was then the new University Hospital of the State University of New York (SUNY) Upstate Medical Center. There John started the Clinical Pathology Residency program and the Medical Technology School at a time when clinical pathology was a rapidly growing field.

Starting as an inspector for the National Committee on Inspection and Accreditation, John went on to serve as president (1970–1971) and member of the board of directors of the American Association of Blood Banks. He served as president (1976–1978) and trustee of the American Board of Pathology. He served as president (1980–1981) and member of the board of directors of the American Society of Clinical Pathologists. In addition, he served on the Scientific Advisory Board of the Armed Forces Institute of Pathology as well as the Pathology Advisory Council for the Veterans Administration.

For the College of American Pathologists, he served in numerous roles, including chairperson of the Future Technology Committee, the Section of Academic Pathology, the Committee on the Teaching of Pathology, and the Joint Policy Committee of the American Society of Clinical Pathology and College of American Pathologists, and as a member of the Board of Governors.

Awards given to Dr. Henry include the American Association for Clinical Chemistry's Gerald B. Lambert Award (1972) and its General Diagnostics Award in Clinical Chemistry (1982), the Royal Society of Medicine's S.C. Dyke Founder Award (1979), the Distinguished Service Award of the American Society of Clinical Pathologists (1979) and its H.P. Smith Memorial Award (1984), and the ASCP/CAP Joint Distinguished Service Award (1997). In 1997, the State University of New York Board of Trustees named him a Distinguished Service Professor.

Parallel with his career in pathology, Dr. Henry began a career as an executive in 1971 when he became the first dean of the SUNY Upstate Medical Center's College of Health Related Professions. He left Syracuse to serve as the dean of the Georgetown University School of Medicine in Washington, DC, from 1979 to 1984. The seventeenth edition of this textbook adopted the blue and gray colors of Georgetown University during this period. Finally, John returned to Syracuse in 1985 as president of the Upstate Medical Center, which became the SUNY Health Science Center at Syracuse, and is now the SUNY Upstate Medical University. While president, he secured the construction of a new library, the Institute for Human Performance, and the first six floors of the east wing of the hospital. A state-of-the-art children's hospital has now been added to that east wing. A quote from John frequently heard by friends, family, and colleagues was, "Good decisions and a sustained focus in pursuit of excellence in patient care with goals and objectives will serve you well."

A man of tremendous energy, John also served as a captain in the U.S. Navy Reserves from 1979 until his retirement. In 1990, he was awarded the Navy Commendation Medal for Meritorious Achievement by the Secretary of the Navy. For much of this era, John could be found on his sailboat on Skaneateles Lake where he was a member of the Skaneateles Country Club and directed the Junior Sailing program for 13 years. He was also an avid skier, served on the Greek Peek Ski Patrol for 30 years, and taught skiing at the Skaneateles Ski Hill Ski Club for 13 years.

John was an inspirational leader and role model for generations of medical students, residents in training, and pathologists in practice. He was a strong advocate for promoting academic pathology, with special interests in the advancement and adoption of new technologies in the clinical laboratory. He had a particular interest in medical education and, upon stepping down from the presidency of SUNY Upstate Medical University, John became intensively involved with development of medical school course content emphasizing the spectrum of the understanding of diseases, from the molecular level to their manifestations as organ injury. He served on editorial boards of several journals in pathology and health care, and on numerous committees and advisory groups for universities, hospitals, government, and industry. His enthusiasm and determination to improve the teaching and practice of pathology were infectious to everyone around him. He will be remembered for always encouraging his colleagues to strive to achieve their best and to maintain the highest of professional standards, and particularly for advancing the careers of junior faculty members.

His work on this textbook began as co-editor with Israel Davisohn for the fourteenth edition in 1969; he then was the principal editor through the twentieth edition in 2001. Among John's contributions to this book were sections on the use of organ panels, automated instrumentation, laboratory management, and information systems. He had a knack for recruiting top authors in every field to prepare original chapters on topics such as histocompatibility, microbiology, molecular diagnostics, blood banking, hematology, clinical chemistry, and immunology. To honor John's consummate leadership of this book and his vision that shaped it for seven editions, it has been renamed *Henry's Clinical Diagnosis and Management by Laboratory Methods* beginning with the twenty-first edition.

John Bernard Henry will be missed by his wife, Georgette, and their six children: Maureen A. Mayer, Julie P. Henry, MD, William B. Henry, Paul B. Henry, John B. Henry Jr., and T. David Henry, SJ. He will also be missed by the countless pathologists and laboratory scientists whose lives he either shaped or touched.

Richard A. McPherson, MD

Matthew R. Pincus, MD, PhD

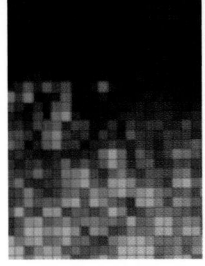

CONTRIBUTORS

Naif Z. Abraham Jr., MD, PhD
Director, Division of Clinical Pathology
Assistant Professor of Pathology
State University of New York Upstate Medical University
Syracuse, New York

Yoshihiro Ashihara, PhD
Managing Director, Board Member
Research and Development Division
Fujirebio Inc.
Tokyo, Japan

Katalin Banki, MD
Associate Professor of Pathology
Director of Special Hematology
Department of Pathology
State University of New York Upstate Medical University
Syracuse, New York

Sylva Bem, MD
Assistant Professor of Pathology
Upstate University Hospital
State University of New York
Syracuse, New York

Jonathan Ben-Ezra, MD
Department of Pathology
Tel Aviv Sourasky Medical Center
Tel Aviv, Israel

Martin H. Bluth, MD, PhD
Associate Professor of Pathology
Director of Translational Research
Associate Director, Transfusion Service
Wayne State University School of Medicine
Detroit Medical Center
Karmanos Cancer Institute
Detroit, Michigan

Jay L. Bock, MD, PhD
Professor and Vice Chair of Pathology
Director of Clinical Pathology
University Hospital and Medical Center
State University of New York at Stony Brook
Stony Brook, New York

Dorota Borawski, MD
Clinical Assistant Professor
Department of Obstetrics and Gynecology
State University of New York Downstate Medical Center
Attending Physician, Department of Obstetrics and Gynecology
University Hospital of Brooklyn
Brooklyn, New York

Michael J. Borowitz, MD, PhD
Professor
Division of Hematologic Pathology
Department of Pathology
The Johns Hopkins Medical Institutions
Baltimore, Maryland

Wilbur B. Bowne, MD
Assistant Professor of Surgery
Division of Surgical Oncology
State University of New York Downstate Medical Center
Brooklyn, New York

Paul W. Brandt-Rauf, MD, ScD, DrPH
Dean
School of Public Health
University of Illinois at Chicago
Chicago, Illinois

David J. Bylund, MD
Staff Pathologist
Department of Pathology
Scripps Mercy Hospital
Staff Pathologist
San Diego Pathologists Medical Group
San Diego, California

Donghong Cai, MD
Clinical Assistant Instructor
Department of Pathology
State University of New York Health Sciences Center at Brooklyn
Brooklyn, New York

Robert P. Carty, PhD
Associate Professor
Department of Biochemistry
State University of New York Downstate Medical Center
Brooklyn, New York

Laura Cooling, MD
Associate Professor of Pathology
Department of Pathology
Associate Director, Blood Bank and Transfusion Service
Director, Cell Therapy Laboratory
University of Michigan Hospitals
Ann Arbor, Michigan

Michael Costello, PhD
Technical Director—Microbiology
ACL Laboratories
Rosemont, Illinois

Ann C. Croft, MT(ASCP)
Supervisor, Bacteriology Laboratory
ARUP Laboratories
Salt Lake City, Utah

David R. Czuchlewski, MD
Assistant Professor
Department of Pathology
University of New Mexico Health Sciences Center
Albuquerque, New Mexico

Robertson D. Davenport, MD
Associate Professor of Pathology
Medical Director, Blood Bank and Transfusion Service
Department of Pathology
University of Michigan Health System
Ann Arbor, Michigan

Julio C. Delgado, MD, MS
Assistant Professor of Pathology
University of Utah School of Medicine
Medical Director, Laboratory of Immunology, ARUP Laboratories
Associate Medical Director, Histocompatibility and Immunogenetics Laboratory
University of Utah Health Care
Salt Lake City, Utah

Thomas J. Dilts, MT(ASCP), MBPA
Associate Professor
Vice Chair of Administration and Operations
Department of Pathology
Virginia Commonwealth University Medical Center
Richmond, Virginia

Theresa Downs, MT(ASCP)SBB, CQA(ASQ)
Laboratory Supervisor
Department of Pathology—Blood Bank
University of Michigan Hospital and Health Centers
Ann Arbor, Michigan

M. Tarek Elghetany, MD
Professor of Pathology
Baylor College of Medicine
Texas Children's Hospital
Houston, Texas

Omar R. Fagoaga, PhD
Associate Professor
Department of Pathology
Wayne State University, School of Medicine
Technical Director
HLA Laboratory
Harper University Hospital
Detroit Medical Center
Detroit, Michigan

Amal F. Farag, MD
Chief
Department of Endocrinology
Veterans Affairs New York Harbor Healthcare System
Brooklyn, New York

Maly Fenelus, MD
Clinical Assistant
Department of Surgery
State University of New York Downstate Medical Center
Brooklyn, New York

Andrea Ferreira-Gonzalez, PhD
Professor and Chair
Division of Molecular Diagnostics
Department of Pathology
Virginia Commonwealth University
Director, Molecular Diagnostics Laboratory
Virginia Commonwealth University Health System
Richmond, Virginia

Louis M. Fink, MD
Director, Core Laboratory Services
Division of Laboratory Medicine
Nevada Cancer Institute
Las Vegas, Nevada

Thomas R. Fritsche, MS, MD, PhD
Head, Clinical Microbiology Section
Marshfield Clinic
Marshfield, Wisconsin
Adjunct Professor of Microbiology
University of Wisconsin
La Crosse, Wisconsin

Susan S. Graham, MS, MT(ASCP)SH
Associate Professor and Chair
Department of Clinical Laboratory Science
State University of New York Upstate Medical University
Syracuse, New York

Frank G. Gress, MD
Professor of Medicine
Chief, Division of Gastroenterology and Hepatology
Department of Medicine
State University of New York Downstate Medical Center
Brooklyn, New York

Wayne W. Grody, MD, PhD
Professor
Divisions of Molecular Pathology and Medical Genetics
Director
Diagnostic Molecular Pathology Laboratory
Departments of Pathology and Laboratory Medicine, Pediatrics, and Human Genetics
University of California–Los Angeles School of Medicine
Los Angeles, California

Helena A. Guber, MD
Assistant Professor of Medicine
Department of Endocrinology
Veterans Affairs New York Harbor Healthcare System
Attending Endocrinologist
Veterans Affairs New York Harbor Medical Center
Brooklyn, New York

Geraldine S. Hall, PhD
Medical Director
Bacteriology, Mycobacteriology, and Specimen Processing
Clinical Microbiology
Department of Clinical Pathology
Cleveland Clinic
Professor of Pathology
Cleveland Clinic Lerner College of Medicine of Case Western Reserve University
Cleveland, Ohio

Charles E. Hill, MD, PhD
Assistant Professor of Pathology
Department of Pathology and Laboratory Medicine
Emory University School of Medicine
Director, Molecular Diagnostics Laboratory
Department of Pathology and Laboratory Medicine
Emory University Hospital
Atlanta, Georgia

Henry A. Homburger, MD
Professor Emeritus
Department of Laboratory Medicine and Pathology
Mayo Clinic and Mayo College of Medicine
Rochester, Minnesota
Medical Laboratory Director
Phadia Immunology Reference Laboratory
Phadia US
Kalamazoo, Michigan

Charlene A. Hubbell, BS, MT(ASCP)SBB
Adjunct Associate Professor
Clinical Laboratory Science
College of Health Professions
Supervisor, Histocompatibility, Immunogenetics, and Progenitor Cell Bank
State University of New York Upstate Medical University
Syracuse, New York

M. Mahmood Hussain, PhD
Professor
Department of Cell Biology and Pediatrics
State University of New York Downstate Medical Center
Brooklyn, New York

Robert E. Hutchison, MD
Professor of Pathology
Director of Clinical Pathology
Director of Hematopathology
State University of New York Upstate Medical University
Syracuse, New York

Peter C. Iwen, MS, PhD, D(ABMM)
Professor of Microbiology
Department of Pathology and Microbiology
Associate Director
Nebraska Public Health Laboratory
University of Nebraska Medical Center
Omaha, Nebraska

Shilpa Jain, MD
Fellow
Department of Pathology
New York University School of Medicine
New York, New York

Jeffrey S. Jhang, MD
Assistant Professor of Clinical Pathology
Department of Pathology and Cell Biology
College of Physicians and Surgeons of Columbia University
Director, Special Hematology and Coagulation Laboratory
Clinical Laboratory Service
New York-Presbyterian Hospital
New York, New York

Joby Josekutty
Graduate Assistant
Department of Cell Biology
State University of New York Downstate Medical Center
Brooklyn, New York

Donald S. Karcher, MD
Professor and Chair
Department of Pathology
George Washington University Medical Center
Director of Laboratories
Department of Pathology
George Washington University Hospital
Washington, DC

Yasushi Kasahara, PhD, DMSc
Visiting Professor
Department of Clinical Pathology
Showa University
Department of Public Health
Kyorin University
Tokyo, Japan

Mukhtar I. Khan, MD
Associate Professor
State University of New York Upstate Medical University
Syracuse, New York

Michael J. Klein, MD
Professor of Pathology and Laboratory Medicine
Weill Medical College of Cornell University
Pathologist-in-Chief and Director
Department of Pathology and Laboratory Medicine
Hospital for Special Surgery
Consultant in Pathology
Memorial Sloan-Kettering Cancer Center
New York, New York

Katrin M. Klemm, MD
Staff Pathologist
East Alabama Medical Center
Opelika, Alabama
Gadsden Regional Medical Center
Gadsden, Alabama

Alexander Kratz, MD, PhD
Associate Professor of Clinical Pathology
Department of Pathology and Cell Biology
College of Physicians and Surgeons of Columbia University
Director, Core Laboratory
Clinical Laboratory Service
New York-Presbyterian Hospital
New York, New York

Anthony S. Kurec, MS, H(ASCP)DLM
Clinical Associate Professor
Department of Clinical Laboratory Science
Administrator
Department of Pathology
State University of New York Upstate Medical University
Syracuse, New York

Richard S. Larson, MD, PhD
Vice President for Research, Health Sciences Center
Senior Associate Dean for Research, School of Medicine
Department of Pathology
University of New Mexico
Albuquerque, New Mexico

P. Rocco LaSala, MD
Assistant Professor
Department of Pathology
West Virginia University
Robert C. Byrd Health Sciences Center
Director, Clinical Microbiology
Department of Pathology
Ruby Memorial Hospital
Morgantown, West Virginia

Peng Lee, MD
Associate Professor of Pathology and Urology
New York University School of Medicine
Staff Pathologist
Veterans Affairs New York Harbor Healthcare System
New York, New York

Jing Li, PhD
Assistant Professor
Department of Oncology
Wayne State University School of Medicine
Director, Pharmacology Core Laboratory
Karmanos Cancer Institute
Detroit, Michigan

Mark S. Lifshitz, MD
Director, Clinical Laboratories
New York University Langone Medical Center
Clinical Professor
Department of Pathology
New York University School of Medicine
New York, New York

Ronald Mageau, MD
Hematopathology Fellow
Department of Pathology
Virginia Commonwealth University
Richmond, Virginia

Richard A. Marlar, PhD
Professor of Pathology
The University of Oklahoma Health Sciences Center
Chief, Clinical Pathology
Oklahoma City Veterans Affairs Medical Center
Oklahoma City, Oklahoma

H. Davis Massey, MD, PhD
Associate Professor of Pathology
Director of Surgical Pathology
Virginia Commonwealth University
Richmond, Virginia

Sharad C. Mathur, MD
Associate Professor
Department of Pathology and Laboratory Medicine
University of Kansas Medical Center
Chief, Pathology and Laboratory Medicine Service
Kansas City Veterans Affairs Medical Center
Kansas City, Missouri

Rex M. McCallum, MD, FACP, FACR
Vice President, Chief Physician Executive
Professor of Medicine/Rheumatology
University of Texas Medical Branch
Galveston, Texas

Richard A. McPherson, MD
Harry B. Dalton Professor and Chairman
Division of Clinical Pathology
Virginia Commonwealth University
Director
Clinical Pathology
Medical College of Virginia Hospitals
Richmond, Virginia

W. Greg Miller, PhD, DABCC, FACB
Professor
Department of Pathology
Director of Clinical Chemistry and Pathology Information Systems
Virginia Commonwealth University
Richmond, Virginia

Jonathan L. Miller, MD, PhD
Director of Medical Center Clinical Laboratories
Professor and Vice Chairman, Department of Pathology
University of Chicago
Chicago, Illinois

Paul D. Mintz, MD
Professor of Pathology and Medicine
Chief
Division of Clinical Pathology
Director of Clinical Laboratories and Transfusion Medicine Services
University of Virginia Health System
Charlottesville, Virginia
Co-Medical Director
Virginia Blood Services
Richmond, Virginia

†Robert M. Nakamura, MD
Chairman Emeritus
Department of Pathology
Scripps Clinic
La Jolla, California

Frederick S. Nolte, PhD, D(ABMM), F(AAM)
Professor of Pathology and Laboratory Medicine
Vice-Chair, Laboratory Medicine
Director, Clinical Laboratories
Medical University of South Carolina
Charleston, South Carolina

Man S. Oh, MD
Professor of Medicine
State University of New York Downstate Medical Center
Brooklyn, New York

Matthew R. Pincus, MD, PhD
Professor
Department of Pathology
State University of New York Downstate Medical Center
Brooklyn, New York
Chairman
Department of Pathology and Laboratory Medicine
Veterans Affairs New York Harbor Healthcare System
New York, New York

Margaret A. Piper, PhD, MPH
Director, Genomics Resources
Technology Evaluation Center
Blue Cross Blue Shield Association
Chicago, Illinois

Herbert F. Polesky, MD
Professor Emeritus
Department of Laboratory Medicine and Pathology
University of Minnesota School of Medicine
Minneapolis, Minnesota

A. Koneti Rao, MBBS
Director, Sol Sherry Thrombosis Research Center
Chief, Hematology Section
Sol Sherry Professor, Medicine
Professor, Thrombosis Research Center
Professor, Pathology and Laboratory Medicine
Professor, Pharmacology
Temple University School of Medicine
Philadelphia, Pennsylvania

Roger S. Riley, MD, PhD
Director of Coagulation and Professor of Pathology
Department of Pathology
Virginia Commonwealth University
Richmond, Virginia

Rhonda K. Roby, PhD, MPH
Associate Professor
Department of Forensic and Investigative Genetics
Project Coordinator
Center for Human Identification
Institute of Investigative Genetics
University of North Texas Health Science Center
Fort Worth, Texas

Lazaro Rosales, MD
Associate Professor of Pathology
Director of Hemapheresis and Deputy Director of Transfusion Medicine
Department of Pathology
State University of New York Upstate Medical University
Syracuse, New York

Susan D. Roseff, MD
Professor and Associate Director of Clinical Laboratories
Medical Director, Transfusion Medicine
Department of Pathology
Virginia Commonwealth University Health System
Richmond, Virginia

Ralph Rossi, PhD
Director
Division of Clinical Chemistry
Veterans Affairs New York Harbor Healthcare System
Brooklyn, New York

Linda M. Sabatini, PhD
Department of Pathology and Laboratory Medicine
Roswell Park Cancer Institute
Buffalo, New York

†Deceased

Martin J. Salwen, MD
Distinguished Service Professor
Department of Pathology
State University of New York Downstate Medical Center
Brooklyn, New York

Kimberly W. Sanford, MD, MT(ASCP)
Assistant Professor
Department of Pathology
Associate Medical Director, Transfusion Medicine
Medical Director of Stony Point Laboratory
Virginia Commonwealth University Health System
Richmond, Virginia

Katherine I. Schexneider, MD
Associate Professor, Department of Pathology
Uniformed Services University
Medical Director, Blood Bank
Staff Pathologist, Department of Laboratory Medicine
National Naval Medical Center
Bethesda, Maryland

Alvin H. Schmaier, MD
Robert W. Kellermeyer Professor of Hematology/Oncology
Director, ICC Laboratory and Adult Hemophilia Program
Case Western Reserve University
University Hospitals Case Medical Center
Cleveland, Ohio

Rangaraj Selvarangan, BVSc, PhD
Associate Professor of Pediatrics
University of Missouri School of Medicine
Director of Clinical Microbiology and Virology Laboratories
Children's Mercy Hospital
Kansas City, Missouri

Ankoor Shah, MD
Fellow
Division of Rheumatology and Immunology
Duke University Medical Center
Durham, North Carolina

Haseeb A. Siddiqi, PhD
Associate Professor
Departments of Cell Biology, Medicine, and Pathology
State University of New York Downstate Medical Center
Brooklyn, New York

Anthony N. Sireci, MD
PGY-3, Clinical Pathology
Department of Pathology and Cell Biology
College of Physicians and Surgeons of Columbia University
New York, New York

Michael B. Smith, MD
Terminology Manager
SNOMED Terminology Solutions
College of American Pathologists
Northfield, Illinois

James Soh
Graduate Assistant
Department of Cell Biology
State University of New York Downstate Medical Center
Brooklyn, New York

Constance K. Stein, PhD
Professor
Department of Pathology
Director of Cytogenetics
Associate Director of Molecular Diagnostics
State University of New York Upstate Medical University
Syracuse, New York

Martin Steinau, PhD
Chronic Viral Diseases Branch
Division of High-Consequence Pathogens and Pathology
National Center for Emerging Zoonotic and Infectious Diseases
Centers for Disease Control and Prevention
Atlanta, Georgia

Robert L. Sunheimer, MSMT(ASCP)SC, SLS
Professor
Department of Clinical Laboratory Science
State University of New York Upstate Medical University
Syracuse, New York

Gregory A. Threatte, MD
Professor and Chairman
Department of Pathology
State University of New York Upstate Medical University
Syracuse, New York

Philip M. Tierno Jr., PhD
Clinical Professor
Departments of Microbiology and Pathology
New York University School of Medicine
Director
Clinical Microbiology and Diagnostic Immunology
New York University Langone Medical Center
New York, New York

Paul Tranchida, MD
Assistant Professor
Department of Pathology
Detroit Medical Center
Detroit, Michigan

Elizabeth R. Unger, MD, PhD
Acting Chief, Chronic Viral Diseases Branch
Division of High-Consequence Pathogens and Pathology
National Center for Emerging and Zoonotic Infectious Diseases
Centers for Disease Control and Prevention
Atlanta, Georgia

Neerja Vajpayee, MD
Associate Professor of Pathology
Department of Pathology
State University of New York Upstate Medical University
Syracuse, New York

David S. Viswanatha, MD
Consultant and Associate Professor
Division of Hematopathology
Mayo Clinic
Rochester, Minnesota

Carlos Alberto von Mühlen, MD, PhD
Full Professor of Rheumatology and Internal Medicine
Pontifical Catholic University School of Medicine
Porto Alegre, Brazil

David H. Walker, MD
The Carmage and Martha Walls Distinguished University Chair in Tropical Diseases
Professor and Chairman
Department of Pathology
Executive Director
Center for Biodefense and Emerging Infectious Disease
University of Texas Medical Branch
Galveston, Texas

Ruth S. Weinstock, MD, PhD
Professor of Medicine and Chief, Endocrinology, Diabetes, and Metabolism
State University of New York Upstate Medical University
Endocrinologist
Department of Medicine
Veterans Affairs Medical Center
Syracuse, New York

David S. Wilkinson, MD, PhD
Professor and Chair
Department of Pathology
Virginia Commonwealth University
Laboratory Director
Department of Pathology
Virginia Commonwealth University Health System
Richmond, Virginia

Jeffrey L. Winters, MD
Associate Professor
Department of Laboratory Medicine and Pathology
Mayo Clinic College of Medicine
Medical Director
Therapeutic Apheresis Unit
Department of Laboratory Medicine and Pathology
Mayo Clinic
Rochester, Minnesota

Brent L. Wood, MD, PhD
Professor of Laboratory Medicine
Department of Laboratory Medicine
University of Washington
Seattle, Washington

Gail L. Woods, MD
Chief, Pathology and Laboratory Medicine
Central Arkansas Veterans Healthcare System
Professor of Pathology
Department of Pathology
University of Arkansas for Medical Sciences
Little Rock, Arkansas

William Woolf
Financial Administrator
Department of Pathology
Virginia Commonwealth University Health System
Richmond, Virginia

Ruliang Xu, MD, PhD
Associate Professor of Pathology
New York University School of Medicine
New York, New York

Margaret Yungbluth, MD
Staff Pathologist
Department of Pathology
St. Francis Hospital
Evanston, Illinois

PREFACE

Clinical laboratory measurements form the scientific basis upon which medical diagnosis and management of patients is established. These results constitute the largest section of the medical record of patients, and laboratory examinations will only continue to grow in number as new procedures are offered and well established ones are ordered more frequently in the future. The modern concept of an electronic health record encompasses information from a patient's birth through that individual's entire life, and laboratory testing is a significant component of that record from prenatal and newborn screening through childhood, adulthood, and geriatric years. Traditional areas of testing are well established in clinical chemistry, hematology, coagulation, microbiology, immunology, and transfusion medicine. Genetic testing for hereditary disease risk assessment is becoming a reality beginning with individual disease testing that is expected to be followed by whole genome screening for a multitude of conditions. The rapid pace in the introduction of new testing procedures demands that laboratory practitioners be expert in several divergent aspects of this profession. The environment of clinical laboratories is extremely well suited for translation of research procedures into diagnostic assays because of their traditional involvement in basic analysis, quality control, professional competencies, and cost-effective strategies of operation. All of these applications are made stronger for occurring under regulations of federal and state governments as well as the standards of accreditation of professional pathology organizations. Clinical laboratories excel in these tasks, and they are now responding to pressures for even greater accomplishments in areas of informatics, advanced analytic methods, interpretation of complex data, and communication of medical information in a meaningful way to physician colleagues. The most successful practitioners of laboratory medicine will incorporate all of these approaches into their daily lives and will be leaders in their institutions for developing initiatives to promote outstanding health care in a fiscally responsible endeavor. This textbook strives to provide the background knowledge by which trainees can be introduced to these practices and to serve as a resource for pathologists and other laboratory personnel to update their knowledge to solve problems they encounter daily.

This twenty-second edition marks more than 100 years since *A Manual of Clinical Diagnosis*, authored by James Campbell Todd, was introduced in 1908. In its current format as *Henry's Clinical Diagnosis and Management by Laboratory Methods*, this textbook remains the authoritative source of information for residents, students, and other trainees in the discipline of clinical pathology and laboratory medicine, and for physicians and laboratory practitioners. The current edition continues the tradition of partnership between laboratory examinations and the formulation and confirmation of clinical diagnoses followed by monitoring of body functions, therapeutic drug levels, and other results of medical treatments. Beginning with the twenty-first edition, color illustrations have been used throughout the book to accurately and realistically depict clinical laboratory test findings and their analysis. The overriding mission of this book is to incorporate new discoveries and their clinical diagnostic applications alongside the wealth of information that forms the core knowledge base of clinical pathology and laboratory medicine. Our contributing authors, who are experts in their specialties, present to the reader the essential basic and new information that is central to clinical laboratory practice.

Part 1, The Clinical Laboratory, covers the organization, purposes, and practices of analysis, interpretation of results, and management of the clinical laboratory from quality control through informatics and finances. The general structure of this section includes general management principles with emphasis on preanalytic, analytic, and postanalytic components of laboratory analysis as well as oversight functions. Administrative concepts for the laboratory are considered in Chapter 1, with optimization of workflow presented in Chapter 2. Preanalytic factors such as variations arising from specimen collection, transport, and handling and other variables are discussed in Chapter 3. The principles of analysis, instrumentation, and automation are presented in Chapters 4 and 5. The growing arena of near-patient laboratory services beyond central hospital laboratories in the format of point-of-care testing is presented in Chapter 6 along with a new section on this application in the military. Postanalysis processes of result reporting, medical decision making, and interpretation of results are presented in Chapter 7, while selection of laboratory testing and interpretation for most cost-effective and efficient information gathering for medical problem solving by clinical laboratory testing is discussed in Chapter 8. A key component to all phases of laboratory processes, interpretation of results, and decision making is statistical analysis, which is introduced in Chapter 9. Explicit applications of statistics are in quality control (Chapter 10). Maintaining order for the complexities of laboratory test result ordering and reporting and the management of clinical information are possible only through sophisticated information systems that are essential to all clinical laboratories (Chapter 11). Management decisions in the clinical laboratory involve choice of analytic instrumentation, automation to process and deliver specimens to analytic stations, and computer systems to coordinate all of the preanalytic, analytic, and postanalytic processes to meet the mission of the institution. These choices determine the productivity that a laboratory can achieve (especially its ability to respond to increased volumes of testing and complexity of measurements and examinations as the standards of practice advance). Paramount is the manner in which the laboratory can muster its resources in equipment, personnel, reagent supplies, and ingenuity of its leadership to respond to the needs of health care providers and patients in terms of access, timeliness, cost, and quality of test results. New challenges continue to emerge for the laboratory to provide excellent quality services at fiscally responsible expense; the changing models of reimbursement for medical and laboratory services demand that pathologists and laboratory leaders develop and maintain a strong understanding of the principles of financial management and are well aware of mechanisms that laboratories can utilize for responding to these new approaches to reimbursement (Chapter 12). Laboratory organization should also include preparedness for threats to our security through bioterrorism and related activities (Chapter 13).

Part 2, Clinical Chemistry, is organized to present laboratory examinations according to organ systems and their disorders. Some of the most commonly ordered laboratory tests are directed at the evaluation of renal function, water, electrolytes, metabolic intermediates and nitrogenous wastes, and acid-base balance, all of which are critically important for monitoring acutely ill patients and in the management of patients with kidney and pulmonary disorders (Chapter 14). The important field of bone metabolism and bone diseases, stemming from the enormous public interest in osteoporosis of our aging population, is covered in Chapter 15. The significance of carbohydrate measurements with particular emphasis on diabetes mellitus, the overall hormonal regulation of glucose metabolism, and disorders of other sugars are reviewed in Chapter 16. Chapter 17 covers the extremely important topic of lipids and disorders in their metabolism and highlights the critical patterns in lipoprotein profiles that indicate disposition to cardiac malfunction, especially myocardial infarction. In Chapter 18, the serodiagnostic markers for cardiac injury evaluation and the related disorders of stroke are elaborated. The clinical significance of specific proteins and their analysis with emphasis on electrophoresis of blood and body fluids is covered in Chapter 19. The field of clinical enzymology with applications to assessment of organ injury is covered in Chapter 20. The principles of enzymology (e.g., transition state theory) have been used directly in the design of new effective drugs against specific diseases such as hypertension and AIDS. Therefore, these applications are now also discussed in this chapter. Laboratory assessment of liver function is presented in Chapter 21 and that of gastrointestinal and pancreatic disorders in Chapter 22. Toxicological analysis and therapeutic drug monitoring are covered in Chapter 23, with applications of both immunoassays and mass spectroscopy emerging in endocrinology (Chapter

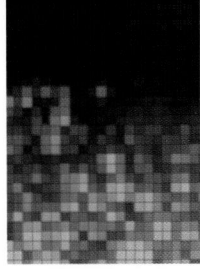

24) and pregnancy and perinatal testing as well (Chapter 25). Nutritional analysis with examination of vitamins and trace metals is presented in Chapter 26. A new presentation on the chemical basis for analysis covers this topic, which is crucial to the understanding of virtually all laboratory measurements (Chapter 27).

Part 3, Urine and Other Body Fluids, reviews the utility and methods for examining fluids other than blood. Chapter 28 presents the basic examination of urine, with extensive discussions of both chemical testing and microscopic examination of urine sediment. A special area for consideration is body fluid analysis, which has received national attention recently in terms of standardizing the approach to testing of typical fluids and other alternative specimens (Chapter 29). A large range of specimen types is considered in this discussion.

Part 4, Hematology, Coagulation, and Transfusion Medicine, introduces techniques for the basic examination of blood and bone marrow (Chapter 30) and provides a wealth of background on the physiologic processes involved in hematopoiesis (Chapter 31). Erythrocytic disorders and leukocytic disorders and their diagnosis are covered in Chapters 32 and 33, respectively. Modern techniques for use of flow cytometry for diagnosis of hematopoietic neoplasias are presented in Chapter 34 to round out the approaches to diagnosis in this rapidly changing field. Immunohematology, which is so important for the understanding of erythrocyte antibodies and their impact on transfusion, is covered in Chapter 35. Blood component manufacture and utilization are covered in Chapter 36 along with transfusion reactions. Chapters 37 and 38 deal with the rapidly expanding areas of apheresis with its applications to therapy of multiple blood disorders as well as the collection, processing, and dispensing of hematopoietic progenitor cells (adult stem cells) from bone marrow, peripheral blood, and cord blood for treatment of both malignant and non-malignant diseases.

Part 5, Hemostasis and Thrombosis, was first introduced in the last edition of this textbook, and is based on the vast increase in our knowledge of the pathways involved in clotting and in fibrinolysis and the panoply of new testing and therapeutic modalities that have evolved as a result. This section continues to reflect the impact of our growing knowledge of coagulation and fibrinolysis (Chapter 39) plus that of platelet function disorders with emphasis on von Willebrand disease (Chapter 40). Advances in the diagnosis and monitoring of thrombotic disorders are covered extensively in Chapter 41, with particular interest in the prediction of thromboembolic risk. Along with our better understanding of thrombosis have come new drugs for treatment of patients with vascular occlusive disorders, particularly ischemic events in the heart or the brain. Principles of antithrombotic therapy and the laboratory's role in its monitoring is covered in Chapter 42. Also discussed in this section is the major advance in pharmacogenomics (fully discussed in Chapter 72) that now allows determination of the optimal anticoagulant therapies for individual patients.

Part 6, Immunology and Immunopathology, presents a framework both for classifying disorders of the immune system and for the role of laboratory testing in diagnosing those diseases (Chapter 43). Measurements based on immunoassays have long been the essential components of understanding a multitude of disorders; an excellent account of the principles of immunoassay and immunochemistry is included in Chapter 44. Evaluation of the cellular immune system is described in Chapter 45, which is newly updated. Humoral immunity and the examination of immunoglobulins in disease are covered in Chapter 46, with particular emphasis on the evaluation of monoclonal disorders in the blood. The material on complement and other mediators of inflammation (Chapter 47) is also newly updated and reorganized. Also brought up to date are Chapter 48 on the major histocompatibility complex (MHC), with its significant applications to organ transplantation, and Chapter 49, which looks at MHC and disease associations. The evaluation of immunodeficiency disorders includes many standard examinations for protein and cellular functions plus new genetic tests for specific abnormalities (Chapter 50). The assessment of autoimmune diseases is presented for the systemic rheumatic diseases (Chapter 51), the vasculitides (Chapter 52), and organ-specific diseases (Chapter 53). Allergic diseases, with their ever-increasing laboratory evaluations, are presented in Chapter 54.

Part 7, Medical Microbiology, covers an enormous spectrum of infectious diseases and related topics that includes viral infections (Chapter 55); chlamydial, rickettsial, and mycoplasmal infections (Chapter 56); classical medical bacteriology (Chapter 57); and susceptibility testing of antimicrobial agents (Chapter 58). Other major topics and infectious organisms of special note are spirochete infections (Chapter 59); mycobacteria (Chapter 60), with immense concern about emergence of resistant strains; mycotic diseases (Chapter 61), with a wide array of photographs of cultures and photomicrographs; and medical parasitology (Chapter 62), with worldwide significance that is growing as large numbers of people move between countries and continents. In line with the importance of achieving maximum diagnostic benefit from the laboratory, specimen collection and handling for diagnosis of infectious disease are detailed in Chapter 63. Although the classic techniques in microbiology have consisted of culturing microbiology organisms with identification and antimicrobial susceptibility testing through functional bioassays, modern methods of nucleic acid amplification and detection are now becoming widespread for each type of microbiologic organism; these applications are described in each chapter about the various organisms.

Part 8, Molecular Pathology, covers some of the most rapidly changing and exciting areas of clinical laboratory testing. Chapter 64 provides an introduction to the role of molecular diagnostics, with an updated discussion of the principles and techniques of the field in Chapter 65. Similar updates are provided for the vital molecular diagnostic techniques of polymerase chain reaction and other amplification methods (Chapter 66) and newer approaches to nucleic acid hybridization (Chapter 67). The application of cytogenetics with modern methods of karyotyping, including fluorescent in situ hybridization and examination for chromosomal abnormalities, is covered in Chapter 68. Translation of research techniques to the molecular diagnostic laboratory is presented in Chapter 69, which also deals with procedures for establishing a molecular diagnostics laboratory that follows all the expectations for well-standardized testing and is fully compliant with regulations and good laboratory practices. This section is rounded out with excellent presentations on the application of molecular diagnostics to genetic diseases for which screening is becoming more important (Chapter 70) and to identity testing as used in parentage testing and forensic analysis (Chapter 71). Finally, an entirely new presentation on pharmacogenomics (Chapter 72) provides an understanding of how molecular analysis of selected genes crucial for response to therapeutic drugs or for the metabolism of drugs can be used to optimize individualized treatment plans, also known as *personalized medicine*.

Part 9, Clinical Pathology of Cancer, is a further outgrowth of this section that was new in the twenty-first edition. Because of the explosion of new diagnostic information as a result of the successful sequencing of the human genome, genetic profiles of different forms of cancers have now become available. Specific forms of cancer are beginning to be diagnosed using microchips containing gene arrays in which patterns of gene expression and mutation are evaluated. In addition, new methods of proteomics (i.e., determination of expression of multiple proteins in patients' body fluids and tissues) allow for cancer detection, monitoring, and treatment. Thus there has been a vast increase in information about the principles and applications of laboratory methods for diagnosis and monitoring of malignancies in just the past few years. Chapter 73 deals with the important protein markers for cancer in blood and tissues that are commonly used for the diagnosis and management of malignant diseases. Chapter 74 extends this discussion with exciting new applications of oncoproteins and growth factors and their receptors in the assessment of malignancies and modification of therapies. A broad spectrum of molecular and cytogenetic markers is now commonly used for the initial evaluation of hematopoietic neoplasms (Chapter 75) that could well become a model for assessment of most, if not all, malignancies. Because the methods in molecular pathology used in diagnosing cancer in body fluids are the same as in solid-tissue diagnosis, breaking down the barriers between anatomic and clinical pathology, we have now included a new chapter on the evaluation of solid tumors by these methods in Chapter 76.

The prospects for early detection, prognosis, and implementation of treatment regimens for cancer based on specific alterations in the genome have never been more apparent. These chapters in cancer diagnostics emphasize the genome-based approaches and other new methods such as proteomics, which has the potential to identify patterns of protein alterations that can be used both for discovery of new targets for examination and for direct detection of clinical abnormalities. Many of these technologies have been developed in the past few years and many more versions of them are sure to appear as the competitive advantage of rapid and inexpensive genomic analysis emerges. We think it is vital for pathologists to understand the bases of molecular diagnostics, the power of this type of analysis for clinical decision making, and the paths such testing is likely to take in the future. To this end, the final chapter (77) presents the diagnostic and prognostic impact of high-throughput genomic and proteomic technologies and the role they can play in the present and future practice of pathology.

The fundamental task for trainees in laboratory medicine is to achieve a sound understanding of analytic principles and the power and limitations of laboratory examinations so that they can interpret whether abnormal results are due to a patient's physical condition or to other potential interferences such as altered physiologic state, drug interactions, or abnormalities introduced by specimen mishandling. Based on mastery of these technical aspects of test performance and interpretation, pathologists should be able to recommend strategies to provide the appropriate level of care for multiple purposes: to screen for disease, to confirm a diagnosis, to establish a prognosis, and to monitor the effects of treatment. National practice recommendations from the American Medical Association and the U.S. Department of Health and Human Services have led to the formulation of standardized panels of multiple individual tests that are targeted to several organ systems such as through the basic metabolic panel and comprehensive metabolic panel (Appendix 7). These panels consist of individual tests that are highly automated and can be conveniently and inexpensively delivered through most hospital laboratories. Such convenience was not always the case when these assays for basic constituents such as potassium, sodium, chloride, bicarbonate, calcium, bilirubin, and all the various metabolites, proteins, and enzyme activities were performed manually, as documented in previous editions of this textbook. Beyond those relatively simple tests, immunoassays, too, have undergone similar transformation: A mere 30 years ago the rapid assay for thyroid-stimulating hormone (TSH) required 2 days, whereas today a third-generation TSH measurement can be completed in 20 minutes or less. Conversion from highly complex and operator-interactive testing to immediately available and inexpensive assays will almost certainly occur with procedures that are now at the cutting edge of technology and require elaborate instrumentation and special expertise to perform. These include tandem mass spectrometry for small molecules such as hormones, vitamins, and drugs; whole genome sequencing for assessing risk of developing hereditary disorders and diagnosing malignancies; and proteomics for screening a wide array of proteins in blood, body fluids, and tissues for disease detection and evidence of progression. The configuration of these assays will consolidate multiple analyses onto miniature platforms such as chip technologies. Although these new technologies will likely be expensive to implement initially, the hope is that they will reduce costs in other parts of the health care system through initiating prevention or treatment earlier than would be possible without such complex and intimate information about a patient's disease state or propensity to develop a disease.

Within this context, it is clear that the role of the clinical laboratory in the future will involve more than simply providing numeric results for physicians to glance at during rounds or after clinic duty. The complexity and the enormity of the test results that will be routinely available will require entirely new approaches to data presentation and interpretation to provide useful information for clinical diagnosis and management. The challenge to laboratories and clinicians alike is to develop "meaningful uses" in which electronic health records can store and present all of this information about a patient—from cradle through an entire life—in which several segments are integrated: genetic background, environmental factors, previous diagnostic and monitoring tests, and contemporaneous monitoring tests. All of these aspects of a patient's history have the potential to be meaningful in the most rigorous sense to provide personalized medical treatments.

This textbook provides grounding in the practice of modern laboratory medicine, and it points the way to new disciplines that will contribute to the evolution of strategies for creating, analyzing, and presenting medical information in the future. We hope that the discussions in this textbook will stimulate our colleagues at all levels to embrace new diagnostic laboratory technologies, in addition to those that are now standard, and to retain the most valuable from each into practices of the future. The legacy of this book over the past century has been to provide a clear and useful account of laboratory tests that generate the solid scientific information upon which medical decisions are based. Building on that foundation, we enthusiastically anticipate new diagnostic capabilities, and we hope that this textbook will be a stimulus to their development.

It is a privilege and an honor to serve as editors for this twenty-second edition.

Richard A. McPherson, MD

Matthew R. Pincus, MD, PhD

April 2011

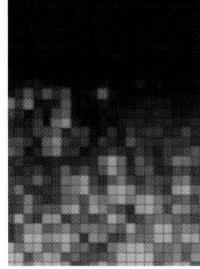

ACKNOWLEDGMENTS

We gratefully acknowledge the outstanding contributions made by our expert colleagues and collaborators who served as associate editors: Jay L. Bock, MD, PhD; Martin H. Bluth, MD, PhD; Robert E. Hutchison, MD; H. Davis Massey, MD, PhD; Jonathan L. Miller, MD, PhD; Gregory A. Threatte, MD; Katherine I. Schexneider, MD; Elizabeth R. Unger, MD, PhD; and Gail L. Woods, MD. They all have made extensive contributions to the quality of this book both through development of textual matter and through the exercise of practiced review of the chapters under their guidance. We deeply appreciate their efforts in this edition.

We gratefully acknowledge the participation in previous editions of Robert P. DeCresce, MD, MBA, MPH; D. Robert Dufour, MD; Timothy Hilbert, MD, PhD, JD; Mark L. Jaros, MBA, MT(ASCP), SM(AAM); Irina Lutinger, MPH, DLM(ASCP); Herb Miller, PhD, MT(ASCP), CLS (NCA); Robert A. Webster, PhD; and Edmond J. Yunis, MD. We also acknowledge our gratitude to them for the opportunity to revise their prior chapters from the twenty-first edition for this, the twenty-second one.

It is with sadness that we note the passing of Robert M. Nakamura, MD, an outstanding immunologist, who co-authored three chapters in this edition and served as author and associate editor in other editions. We will greatly miss his leadership, expertise, and strength of character in the pursuit of academic excellence.

All of our students, residents, and colleagues have for decades contributed enormously to the development of our knowledge in human disease and in the use of laboratories for diagnosis and patient management. We are grateful for all their questions and the stimulus they have provided to our professional growth. We are especially grateful for the mentorship and encouragement provided in our careers by Alfred Zettner, MD; Cecil Hougie, MD; Abraham Braude, MD; Charles Davis, MD; James A. Rose, MD; Robert P. Carty, PhD; Donald West King, MD; George Teebor, MD; Phillip Prose, MD; Fred Davey, MD; and Gerald Gordon, MD. We will remember them always and the standards for excellence they set.

The development of this edition, with its myriad details, would not have been possible without the outstanding professional efforts of our editors at Elsevier: William R. Schmitt, Kathryn DeFrancesco, and Louise King, each of whom added tremendously to this enterprise. We are sincerely grateful to them and to all the staff of Elsevier. They have made this endeavor a happy one. We also send very special thanks to Anne Erickson, who has drawn many of the illustrations in both the twenty-first and twenty-second editions with a fine eye to beauty in presentation and ease of comprehension.

We are grateful to all the authors for accepting the challenge to participate in the education of future and present laboratorians and physicians in all fields of medicine by distilling the essential information from each of their fields of expertise and creating readable and authoritative text for our audience. Special thanks to the authors, who have created wholly new chapters on molecular pathology and cancer diagnostics for this edition.

We also remember with perpetual gratitude the inspiration provided to us by John Bernard Henry, MD. He provided leadership for seven editions of this book. Moreover, he encouraged us, guided us, and demanded excellence from us in our profession.

Upon the completion of this twenty-second edition, we humbly thank all the individuals who have played roles in making it possible. It is not possible to name all of the individuals who have contributed to this textbook. To those mentioned here and to those not explicitly named, we thank you for your prodigious efforts and support.

Richard A. McPherson, MD

Matthew R. Pincus, MD, PhD

PART 1

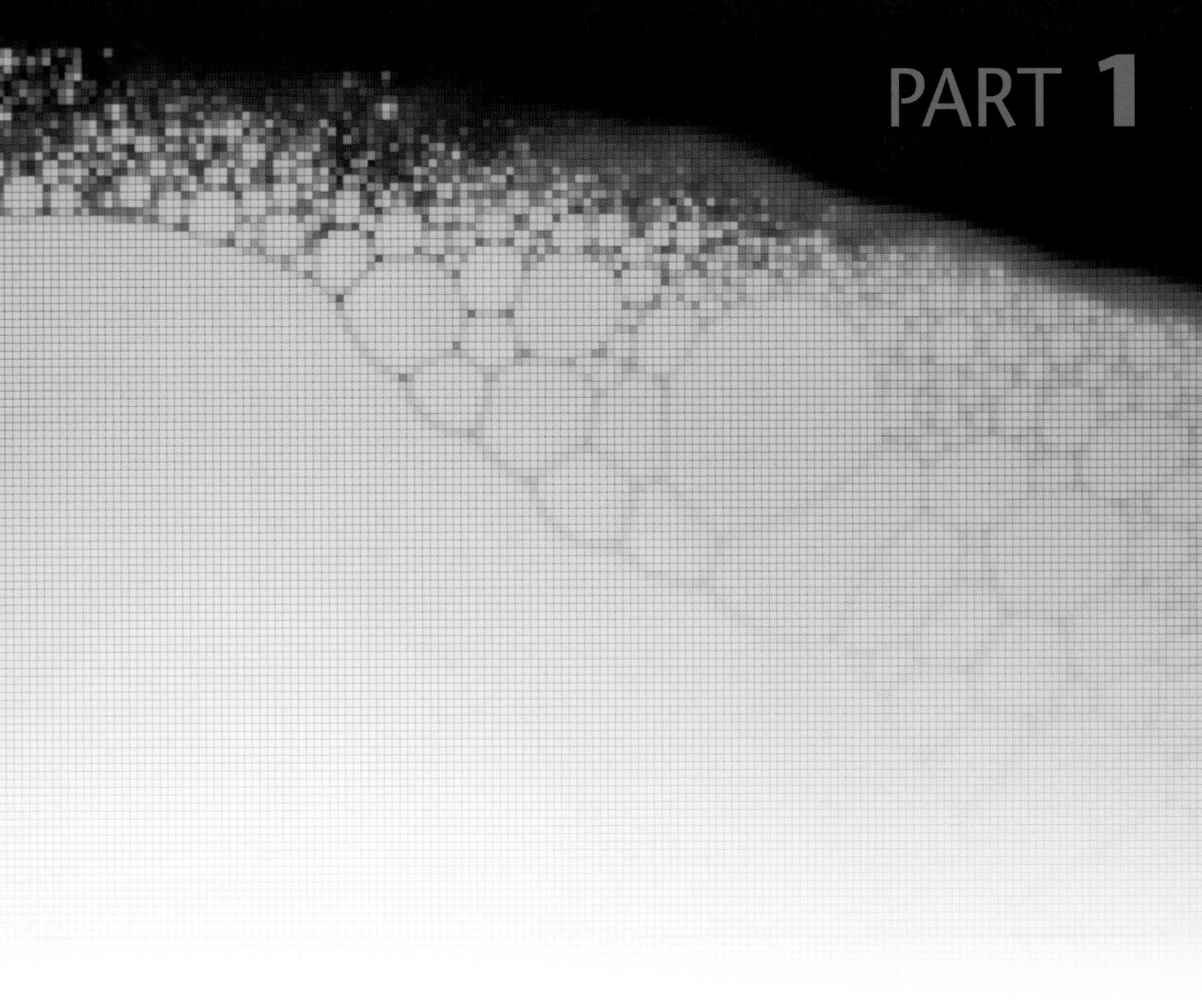

The Clinical Laboratory

EDITED BY
Jay L. Bock
Matthew R. Pincus
Gregory A. Threatte

CHAPTER 1

GENERAL CONCEPTS AND ADMINISTRATIVE ISSUES

Anthony S. Kurec, Mark S. Lifshitz

KEY POINTS

- Effective laboratory management requires leaders to provide direction and managers to get things done. Strategic planning, marketing, human resource management, and quality management are all key elements of a laboratory organization.
- Most laboratory errors occur in the preanalytic and postanalytic stages. Six Sigma and Lean are tools that can be used to reduce laboratory errors and increase productivity.
- Laboratory services are provided in many different ways and can be thought of as placed on a continuum from point-of-care tests producing immediate answers to highly complex laboratory tests that require sophisticated technology and skilled staff.
- Clinical laboratories are highly regulated; many laboratory practices are the direct result of federal or state/local legislation. At the federal level, laboratory activities are regulated through the Clinical Laboratory Improvement Acts of 1988.
- Biological, chemical, ergonomic, and fire hazards cannot be completely eliminated from the laboratory, but can be minimized through the use of engineering controls (i.e., safety features built into the overall design of equipment and supplies), personal protective equipment, and work practice controls (such as hand washing).

The laboratory plays a central role in health care. How critical is the laboratory? By one estimate, 70% of all medical decisions are based on laboratory results (Silverstein, 2003), although laboratory costs account for only 2.3% of total health care dollars (Terry, 2009). The laboratory is a $55.1 billion industry that offers high clinical value at relatively low cost.

The purpose of the laboratory is to provide physicians and other health care professionals with information to: (1) detect disease or predisposition to disease; (2) confirm or reject a diagnosis; (3) establish prognosis; (4) guide patient management; and (5) monitor efficacy of therapy (Kurec, 2000). The laboratory also plays a leading role in education and research, information technology design and implementation, and quality improvement. To successfully achieve its goal, a laboratory must use (1) medical, scientific, and technical expertise; (2) resources such as personnel, laboratory and data processing equipment, supplies, and facilities; and (3) organization, management, and communication skills. The goal of this chapter is to provide a fundamental understanding of general administrative concepts and issues that are the basis of sound laboratory practices. Crucial to a well-managed laboratory that generates accurate and timely laboratory reports is sound leadership with skills to guide staff in performing their daily tasks. A more detailed discussion of these topics is available elsewhere (Nigon, 2000; Snyder, 1998).

LEADERSHIP AND MANAGEMENT

An organization is only as good as its people, and people are guided by leaders and managers. The terms leadership and management are often used interchangeably but represent different qualities (Table 1-1). Leadership provides the direction of where one (or an organization) is going, whereas management provides the "road" to get there. The adage, "If you don't know where you are going, any road will get you there," illustrates why leadership must be visionary and must set clear goals with strategic objectives. Effective management uses certain talents to work with people to get things done. It requires an optimal mix of skilled personnel, dedicated people, and task-oriented leaders to achieve these goals. These skills fall under four primary management functions: (1) planning and prompt decision-making, (2) organizing, (3) leading, and (4) controlling.

Leadership is a pattern of behaviors used to engage others to complete tasks in a timely and productive manner. One model of leadership describes four key leadership styles: supporting, directing, delegating, and coaching. A supportive leader provides physical and personal resources so that an individual can accomplish his or her duties. A directive leader presents rules, orders, or other defined instructions to the individual. The former approach offers flexibility and encourages creative problem-solving, whereas the latter approach offers concise and detailed instructions on how to complete a task. Other styles are also defined by these qualities: A delegating leader provides low support and direction, whereas a coaching leader provides high support and direction. A leader may adopt any behavior style periodically to suit a situation, but in general, one style usually dominates.

Good management uses, in the most efficient and effective manner, the human, financial, physical, and information resources available to an organization. Some basic managerial responsibilities are listed in Table 1-2. Managers can be stratified as first-line managers (supervisors, team leaders, chief technologists), middle managers (operations managers, division heads), and top managers (laboratory directors, chief executive officers [CEOs], chief financial officers [CFOs], chief information officers [CIOs]). Each managerial level dictates the daily activities and skill sets required for that position. Top-level managers concentrate on strategizing and planning for the next 1–5 years, while first-line managers are more concerned about completing the day's work. A top-level manager may or may not possess technical skills that a first-line manager uses every day. Middle managers may straddle both areas to some degree by engaging in a variety of activities that may be strategic as well as tactical.

STRATEGIC PLANNING

Technology has moved the science of laboratory medicine from using numerous manual methods to applying highly automated ones. This has leveled the playing field of laboratory science to a point where testing can be done in the clinic, in the physician's office, and even in the home by nontraditional laboratorians. This makes the laboratory a commodity that must engage in competitive business practices. To survive and even thrive in a competitive environment, a laboratory must constantly reevaluate its goals and services and adapt to market forces (e.g., fewer qualified laboratory personnel, reduced budgets, stricter regulatory mandates, lower reimbursements, new sophisticated technologies). This requires a leader to

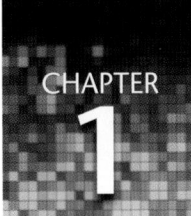

TABLE 1-1
Leader versus Manager Traits

Leader	Manager
Administrator	Implementer
Organizer and developer	Maintains control
Risk taker	Thinks short term
Inspiration	Asks how and when
Thinks long term	Watches bottom line
Asks what and why	Accepts status quo
Challenges status quo	Is a good soldier
Does the right thing	Does things right

Adapted from Ali M, Brookson S, Bruce A, et al. Managing for excellence. London: DK Publishing; 2001, pp 86–149.

TABLE 1-2
Basic Management Responsibilities

Operations Management
Quality assurance
Policies and procedures
Strategic planning
Benchmarking
Productivity assessment
Legislation/regulations/HIPAA compliance
Medicolegal concerns
Continuing education
Staff meetings
Human Resource Management
Job descriptions
Recruitment and staffing
Orientation
Competency assessment
Personnel records
Performance evaluation/appraisals
Discipline and dismissal
Financial Management
Departmental budgets
Billing
CPT coding
ICD-10 coding
Compliance regulations
Test cost analysis
Fee schedule maintenance
Marketing Management
Customer service
Outreach marketing
Advertising
Website development
Client education

CPT, Current Procedural Terminology; *HIPAA,* Health Insurance Portability and Accountability Act; *ICD-10,* International Classification of Diseases, Tenth Revision.

carefully make strategic decisions that can have an impact on the laboratory for years.

The process by which high level decisions are made is called strategic planning and can be defined as (1) deciding on the objectives of the organization and the need to modify existing objectives if appropriate; (2) allocating resources to attain these objectives; and (3) establishing policies that govern the acquisition, use, and disposition of these resources (Lifshitz, 1996). Strategic planning is usually based on long-term projections and a global view that can have an impact on all levels of a laboratory's operations. It is different from tactical planning, which consists of the detailed, day-to-day operations needed to meet the immediate needs of the laboratory and works toward meeting the long-term strategic goals that have been set. For example, a global strategy to develop an outreach business may prompt addressing issues such as bringing more reference work in-house; the need for additional instrumentation and/or automation; enhancing information technology tools; and adequate staffing to satisfy service expectations. Risk can be involved in initiating a specific strategy. A wrong decision may burden a laboratory with unnecessary costs, unused equipment, and/or overstaffing, making it that much harder to change course in response to future market forces or new organizational strategies. Yet not taking a risk may result in loss of opportunities to grow business and/or improve services.

TABLE 1-3
SWOT Analysis for a New Hospital Outreach Program

Strengths
1. Use current technology/instrumentation
2. Have excess technical capacity
3. Increased test volume will decrease cost per test
4. Strong leadership support
5. Financial resources available

Opportunities
1. Opening of a new physician health care facility
2. Department of Health mandates lead testing on all children younger than 2 years old
3. Have access to hospital marketing department
4. Hospital X is bankrupt; laboratory will close

Weaknesses
1. Staffing shortage
2. Morale issues
3. Inadequate courier system
4. Need to hire additional pathologist
5. Limited experience in providing multihospital/client LIS services
6. Turnaround times are marginal

Threats
1. Competition from other local hospital laboratories
2. Competition from national reference laboratories
3. Reimbursement decreasing
4. Three local hospitals have consolidated their services, including laboratory
5. Several new patient service centers (phlebotomy stations) already opened

LIS, Laboratory information system.

Strategic planning generally is not the result of a single individual's creation but rather is derived from a committee. Managers spend a significant amount of time in meetings that often are nonproductive if not organized efficiently. A variety of techniques can be used to facilitate the strategic planning process; these include histograms/graphs/scattergrams, brainstorming, fishbone diagrams, storyboarding, Pareto analyses, and Delphi analyses (Kurec, 2004a). Another way to evaluate the risks associated with new strategies is the Strengths, Weaknesses, Opportunities, and Threats (SWOT) analysis. Generally, environmental factors internal to the laboratory are classified as strengths and weaknesses, and external environmental factors are opportunities and threats. This process is a particularly useful tool for guiding a marketing strategy (Table 1-3) and can be used in developing such a program (Table 1-4). Successful strategic planning requires preplanning, organization, well-defined goals, communication, and a firm belief in what is to be accomplished.

QUALITY SYSTEMS MANAGEMENT

A key management goal is to ensure that quality laboratory services are provided. To accomplish this, every laboratory should strive to obtain modern equipment, to hire well-trained staff, to ensure a well-designed and safe physical environment, and to create a good management team. A key study from 1999 by the IOM (Institute of Medicine, 2000) is often referred to when quality health care issues and medical error rates are addressed. This study concluded that 44,000 to as many as 98,000 Americans die each year because of medical errors (Silverstein, 2003; Kohn, 1999). Among those errors, 50% were failure to use appropriate tests, and of those, 32% were failure to act on test findings and 55% were due to

TABLE 1-4
Issues to Consider When Establishing a Marketing Program

Environmental assessment	Remember the four Ps of marketing: • Product • Price • Place • Promotion What are the customer needs? Who is the competition? Do you have the right testing menu, equipment, and facilities? Do you have enough personnel? Do you have adequate financial resources? Do you know what it costs to do a laboratory test (test cost analysis)?
Define your customer segments	Physicians, nurses, dentists, other health care providers Other hospital laboratories, physician office laboratories (POLs) Insurance companies Colleges, universities, and other schools Nursing homes, home health agencies, and clinics Veterinarians and other animal health care facilities Researchers, pharmaceutical companies, clinical trials Identify unique socioeconomic and/or ethnic groups. Look for population shifts and location (urban, rural, suburban).
Process	Develop a sales/marketing plan and team. Set goals. Ensure infrastructure (courier service, LIS capabilities, customer service personnel, etc.) is adequate. Develop additional test menu items. Educate laboratory personnel in customer service. Support and maintain existing client services. Find advertising/public relations resources.
How to market	Review test menu for comprehensive services (niche testing, esoteric testing, other unique services that could be provided to an eclectic group). Place advertisements. Develop brochures, specimen collection manuals, and other customer-related material. Develop website. Attend/participate in community health forums. Identify specific target customers: • Other hospital laboratories, independent laboratories, reference laboratories • College/school infirmaries, health clinics, county laboratory facilities (preemployment, drug screening) • Nursing homes, extended care facilities, drug/alcohol rehabilitation centers, correctional facilities • Physician offices, groups, and specialties (pediatrics, dermatology, family medicine, etc.)

LIS, Laboratory information system.

avoidable delays in rendering a diagnosis. The frequency of laboratory error varies across the vast number of laboratory tests performed annually. In one study, error rates were reported to range from 0.05%–0.61%; and the distribution of errors among the testing stages was similar, with most (32%–75%) occurring in the preanalytic stage and far fewer (13%–32%) in the analytic stage (Bonini, 2002). Preanalytic errors included hemolyzed, clotted, or insufficient samples; incorrectly identified or unlabeled samples; and wrong collection tube drawn and improper specimen storage. Analytic errors included calibration error and instrument malfunction. Postanalytic errors included reports sent to the wrong physician, long turnaround time, and missing reports. Concerted efforts by various governmental regulatory agencies and professional associations have resulted in mandated programs that focus on ways to identify errors and to prevent them.

Total quality management (TQM) and *continuous quality improvement* (CQI) have been standard approaches to quality leadership and management for over 30 years (Juran, 1988; Deming, 1986). TQM is a systems approach that focuses on teams, processes, statistics, and delivery of services/products that meet or exceed customer expectations (Brue, 2002). CQI is an element of TQM that strives to continually improve practices and not just meet established quality standards. Table 1-5 compares traditional quality thinking versus TQM. TQM thinking strives to continually look for ways to reduce errors ("defect prevention") by empowering employees to assist in solving problems and getting them to understand their integral role within the greater system ("universal responsibility").

Two other quality tools often used are Six Sigma and Lean. Six Sigma is a process improvement program that is a hands-on process with the single mantra of "improvement": improved performance, improved quality, improved bottom line, improved customer satisfaction, and improved employee satisfaction. Six Sigma is a structured process that is based on statistics and quantitative measurements. Through this process, the number of defects per million opportunities (DPMO) is measured. A defect is anything that does not meet customer requirements, for example,

TABLE 1-5
Quality Management: Traditional Versus TQM Thinking

Traditional thinking	TQM thinking
Acceptable quality	Error-free quality
Department focused	Organization focused
Quality as expense	Quality as means to lower costs
Defects by workers	Defects by system
Management-controlled worker	Empowered worker
Status quo	Continuous quality improvement
Manage by intuition	Manage by fact
Intangible quality	Quality defined
We versus they relationship	Us relationship
End-process focus	System process
Reactive systems	Proactive systems

TABLE 1-6
Six Sigma Steps

Six Sigma step	Example
Define project goal or other deliverable that is critical to quality.	Emergency department results in less than 30 minutes from order
Measure baseline performance and related variables.	Baseline performance: 50% of time results are within 30 minutes, 70% within 1 hour, 80% within 2 hours, etc. Variables: Staffing on each shift, order-to-laboratory receipt time, receipt-to-result time, etc.
Analyze data using statistics and graphs to identify and quantify root cause.	Order-to-receipt time is highly variable because samples are not placed in sample transport system immediately and samples delivered to laboratory are not clearly flagged as emergency.
Improve performance by developing and implementing a solution.	Samples from emergency department are uniquely colored to make them easier to spot among routine samples.
Control factors related to the improvement, verify impact, validate benefits, and monitor over time.	New performance: Results available 90% of time within 30 minutes

a laboratory result error, a delay in reporting, or a quality control problem. So, if a laboratory sends out 1000 reports and finds that 10 are reported late, it has a 1% defect rate; this is equivalent to 10,000 DPMO. The goal of Six Sigma is to reduce the number of defects to near zero. The sigma (σ), or standard deviation, expresses how much variability exists in products or services. By reducing variability, one also reduces defects. Thus, one sigma represents 691,463 DPMO, or a yield (i.e., percentage of products without defects) of only 30.854%, whereas the goal of Six Sigma is to reach 3.4 DPMO, or a 99.9997% yield (Brue, 2002). Most organizations operate at or near four sigma (6210 DPMO). To put this in perspective, per Clinical Laboratory Improvement Act (CLIA) '88 guidelines, most proficiency testing (PT) requires an 80% accuracy rate. This translates to 200,000 defects per million tests, or 2.4 sigma. The reported PT accuracy rate for CLIA participating laboratories was 97%, or 3.4 sigma (Garber, 2004). Six Sigma practices can be applied to patient care and safety, providing a tool for meeting process improvement needs (Riebling, 2008). Examples, based on College of American Pathologists (CAP) Q-Probes and Q-Tracks programs, show the outcomes of applying Six Sigma to some common performance quality indicators. In these studies, the median variance (50th percentile) for test order accuracy was 2.3%, or 23,000 DPMO; patient wristband error was 3.13%, or 31,000 DPMO; blood culture contamination was 2.83%, or 28,300 DPMO; and the pathology discrepancy rate was 5.1%, or 51,000 DPMO (Berte, 2004). By lowering defects, quality of care is improved and cost savings are realized by eliminating waste (e.g., supplies and materials for reruns), unnecessary steps, and/or staff time (Sunyog, 2004). By some estimates, the cost of doing business is reduced by 25%–40% in moving from 3 sigma to 6 sigma performance. An example of the Six Sigma process is provided in Table 1-6.

The Lean process, first implemented in Japan by Toyota, was ultimately designed to reduce waste ("nonvalued activities") (Blaha and White, 2009). The intent of Lean is to reduce costs by identifying daily work activities that do not directly add to the delivery of laboratory services in the most efficient or cost-effective ways. A Lean laboratory utilizes fewer resources, reduces costs, enhances productivity, promotes staff morale, and improves the quality of patient care. Lean directly addresses the age-old concept of "that's the way we always did it" and looks for ways to improve the process. Lean practices can be very broad in nature or unique to a single laboratory work area by focusing on work flow actions in performing specific tasks, procedures, or other activities accomplished by critically reviewing each step in the process to determine where inefficiencies can be eliminated. Some changes require minimal resources and can be accomplished relatively quickly. Examples include relocating analytic equipment to an area that would require fewer steps, thus improving turnaround time; consolidating test menus to fewer instruments, eliminating the expense of maintaining multiple instruments and supplies; placing pipettes, culture plates, etc., in easy to access areas; and reallocating staff to maximize use and minimize wasteful downtime.

TABLE 1-7
Quality System Essentials (CLSI)

1. Organization
2. Personnel
3. Documents and records
4. Facilities and safety
5. Equipment
6. Purchasing and inventory
7. Information management
8. Occurrence management
9. Assessments—internal/external
10. Process improvement
11. Customer service
12. Process control

CLSI, Clinical and Laboratory Standards Institute.

Many laboratories are taking a more focused and stringent approach to quality system management. In a cooperative effort, the International Organization for Standardization (ISO) established guidelines that reflect the highest level of quality. The ISO 15189:2007 has been adopted by CAP in an effort to improve patient care through quality laboratory practices. A laboratory that meets or exceeds these guidelines can be CAP-certified, indicating a high level of confidence in the quality of services provided by that laboratory. In a similar fashion, the CLSI has created 12 Quality System Essentials (Table 1-7) based on ISO standards. Each of these 12 areas serves as a starting point in establishing a quality system that covers pretesting, testing, and posttesting operations. Quality Systems Management ultimately dispels the concept of "good enough" and promotes one of "it can always be done better."

HUMAN RESOURCE (HR) MANAGEMENT

Recruiting, hiring, training, and retaining qualified personnel have become major challenges for today's manager. Over the past 20–30 years, almost 70% of accredited Medical Technology programs have closed, resulting in a 22% reduction in the number of graduating students. In a recent survey, the average vacancy rate for staff medical technologists was 10% (Bennett, 2009) with an anticipated employment growth rate of 14% (U.S. Bureau of Labor Statistics, 2009). The need to compete with other professions has necessitated implementation of more creative recruitment incentives such as offering competitive salaries and comprehensive benefits and ensuring a nonhostile work environment. Today's job market is volatile and draws from around the world; thus a greater understanding of cultural, ethnic, and gender-related traits is necessary to properly evaluate and attract a pool of competent employees who will meet the needs of the laboratory and contribute to accomplishing anticipated goals (Kurec, 2004b).

Labor accounts for 50%–70% of a laboratory's costs; thus any new or replacement position must be justified. It is appropriate to review the authority level, experience and education required, and responsibilities of a position and compare them with any related changes in technology, required skills, or other factors. To ensure that the position is still necessary and covers responsibilities at an appropriate level, ask the question, "If the position remained unfilled or downgraded, how would that impact the department or the hospital?" For example, could a particular position be refilled by an entry-level technologist or a laboratory aide without compromising patient care or creating other staffing hardships?

Once the justification review is complete, a criterion-based job description should be developed (Kurec, 2004b). The criterion-based job description should focus on roles and not on specific tasks, as the latter may require frequent changes depending on operations. A criterion-based job description includes title, grade, and qualifications (including certification or licensure) and clearly identifies responsibilities, accountability, and internal and external organizational relationships. This provides a clear guide to expectations for both employee and employer.

The recruiting and hiring process requires understanding current and potential future needs of the laboratory, finding a qualified individual, and being aware of current local and federal hiring guidelines. During the interview process, an employer must restrict questions to what can be legally asked, yet still be able to gain insight as to whether the position is the right fit for both parties. Also important is developing a sensitivity toward gender and generational or cultural differences that may be misinterpreted or misunderstood during the selection process (Kurec, 2005).

Laboratory Design and Service Models

Laboratory services are provided in many different ways and can be thought of as a continuum from point-of-care tests producing immediate answers to highly sophisticated laboratory tests that may take days to complete. Ease of Internet access has added a level of transparency to how health care is provided to the public and, in particular, provides a better understanding of laboratory testing through websites such as www.webmd.com and www.labtestsonline.org. This has increased awareness of what tests are available and what they mean, and has increased the expectancy that laboratories will provide high quality and timely services. To meet this demand, laboratories have been redesigned for efficiency, accessibility, safety, and reliability. Laboratories have changed their internal design from a very compartmentalized environment to a more centralized one, where traditional laboratory sections have been consolidated. When appropriate, regionalized laboratories have been developed to perform specialty or complex testing, thus capitalizing on expertise, equipment, and materials. In many institutions, laboratory testing has been pushed out to point-of-care testing (POCT) to shorten turnaround time for critical results and enhance convenience for both patients and caregivers. These internal and external organizational changes have fostered a greater awareness of the importance of laboratory services and how they contribute to the continuum of care.

The *functional design of a laboratory* and its relationship to other testing sites within a facility have evolved from one with discrete hematology, chemistry, microbiology, and blood bank sections to one where boundaries have been obscured. In an effort to lower costs and respond more rapidly to clinical needs, laboratories have employed both highly automated "core" facilities and distributed testing at peripheral stat laboratories and/or POCT sites. Based on current technology, tests that once were performed in separate laboratory sections are now performed on a single testing platform (single analyzer), on a workcell (two or more linked instruments), or with the use of total laboratory automation (workcell with preanalytic and postanalytic processing). In conjunction with improved preanalytic sample handling (e.g., bar coding, automated centrifuges, decapper), use of highly accurate analyzers and timely postanalytic activities (e.g., reporting laboratory results via networked computer systems, the Internet, autofaxing) further contributes to enhancing the quality of services provided. These configurations will be discussed further in Chapters 2 and 5.

Regionalization is a consolidation process on a grand scale. In the "hub and spoke" model, a single, core laboratory serves as the hub, providing high volume, routine testing. One or more other laboratories act as the spokes, thus consolidating certain functions into one highly specialized laboratory. For example, a single laboratory may focus on providing just microbiology, virology, parasitology, mycology, or other related services. In constructing such a unique site, the redundancy of procuring technical expertise, expensive biohazard hoods, negative pressure rooms, clinical and molecular testing equipment, and other materials can be minimized. Similar opportunities may exist for other laboratory sections such as cytogenetics, molecular diagnostics, cytology, or histocompatibility. Establishing regionalized laboratory systems can require significant up-front resources, appropriate space requirements, and commitment from senior personnel from all institutions involved to make this work. In hospital settings, a Stat or rapid-response laboratory would be necessary to handle urgent test requests. Challenges to consider in implementing and succeeding with this model include timely specimen transportation, resistance to change, personnel issues, morale issues, "lost identity" of the laboratory, and union problems.

The design of facilities is important regardless of the type of laboratory and may best be accomplished by implementing Six Sigma/Lean techniques to ensure the highest level of productivity. Location of the specimen processing area, patient registration and data entry, specimen testing workflow, short- and long-term storage, and laboratory information system (LIS) connectivity requirements must be considered. Spatial requirements in relationship to other hospital services (proximity to emergency department, intensive care units, and surgical operating suite) should be viewed as a multidisciplinary process. Robotics, pneumatic tubes, computers, hand-held devices, and facsimile machines are the new tools used in modern laboratories and must be accounted for in the design plans. Electrical power, temperature/humidity controls, access to water (distilled/deionized), drainage sources, and air circulation/ventilation issues must be considered for access and adequate quantity. Regulatory compliance codes must be reviewed carefully and implemented appropriately to ensure that safety, ergonomic, and comfort needs are met (Table 1-8). Recently, concerns of reducing environmental impact have come into play (Kurec, 2009). Many municipalities and hospitals offer strong incentives, or even mandates, to "go green" by purchasing alternative, nontoxic chemicals, recycling used electronic products, integrating paperless reporting, and generally raising staff awareness of energy-wasting practices. To ensure that one meets local, state, and federal codes, a qualified architect who has had experience in designing clinical laboratories should be consulted at the beginning of relocation or renovation designs. This minimizes costly change orders and maximizes on-time start-up of the new facility.

TABLE 1-8
Laboratory Physical Design Considerations

In developing a needs assessment, identify space for offices, personal facilities, storage, conference/library area, and students.
Routinely review all floor plans and elevations for appropriate usage, and ensure space and function are related; handicapped accessibility may be required.
Develop and use a project scheduler to ensure on-time progress.
Fume hoods and biological safety cabinets must be located away from high traffic areas and doorways that might cause unwanted air current drafts.
Modular furniture allows for flexibility in moving or reconfiguration of the laboratory according to current and anticipated needs; conventional laboratory fixtures may be considered in building depreciation, whereas modular furniture may not.
Consider HVAC requirements to ensure proper temperature (68° F–76° F), humidity (20%–60%), air flow (12 air exchanges/hour); extremes in any one area can adversely affect patients, staff, and equipment.
Base cabinets (under laboratory counters) provide 20%–30% more storage space than suspended cabinets.
Noise control in open laboratories may be obtained by installing a drop ceiling. Installation of utilities above a drop ceiling adds to flexibility in their placement.
In general, space requirements are 150–200 net square feet (excludes hallways, walls, custodial closets, etc.) per FTE, or 27–40 net square feet per hospital bed.
Rooms larger than 100 square feet must have two exits; corridors used for patients must be 8 feet wide, and those not used for patients must be 3 feet 8 inches wide.
An eyewash unit must be within 100 feet of work areas; hands-free units are preferred.
Suggested standard dimensions in planning and designing a laboratory: • Laboratory counter width: 2 feet 6 inches • Laboratory counter-to-wall clearance: 4 feet • Laboratory counter-to-counter clearance: 7 feet • Desk height: 30 inches • Keyboard drawer height: 25–27 inches • Human body standing: 4 square feet • Human body sitting: 6 square feet • Desk space: 3 square feet

Painter, 1993; Mortland, 1997.
FTE, Full-time equivalent; *HVAC,* heating, ventilating, and air conditioning.

Regulation, Accreditation, and Legislation

Clinical laboratories are among the most highly regulated health care entities (Table 1-9). Understanding these laws is necessary to avoid legal or administrative repercussions that may limit a laboratory's operations or shut it down completely. To operate (and receive reimbursement for services), laboratories must be licensed and often accredited under federal and/or state requirements. Although all pathologists must be state-licensed physicians, 13 states currently require laboratory personnel licensure—a key consideration when attempting to hire technical staff (Table 1-10).

At the federal level, laboratory activities are regulated through CLIA '88 (*Federal Register* 55, 1990; *Federal Register* 57, 1992; http://

TABLE 1-9
Laboratory Regulations and Their Significance

1983	**Prospective Payment System** for Medicare patients established payment based on diagnosis-related groups (DRGs). Hospitals are paid a fixed amount per DRG, regardless of actual cost, thereby creating an incentive to discharge patients as soon as medically possible. For inpatients, laboratories become cost centers instead of revenue centers (Social Security Amendments P.L. 98-21).
1984	**Deficit Reduction Act** (P.L. 93-369): Established outpatient laboratory fee schedule to control costs; froze Part B fee schedule.
1988	**Clinical Laboratory Improvement Act of 1988 (CLIA '88)** (amended 1990, 1992): Established that all laboratories must be certified by the federal government with mandated quality assurance, personnel, and proficiency testing standards based on test complexity. Until this time, the federal government regulated only the few laboratories conducting interstate commerce or independent or hospital laboratories that wanted Medicare reimbursement. CLIA applies to all sites where testing is done, including physician's offices and clinics.
1989	**Physician Self-referral Ban** (Stark I; PL 101-239): Prevents physicians from referring Medicare patients to self-owned laboratories. **Ergonomic Safety and Health Program Management Guidelines:** Establish OSHA guidelines for employee safety.
1990	**Three-Day Rule** initiated by CMS: Payment for any laboratory testing done 3 calendar days before admission as an inpatient is not reimbursed because testing is considered to be part of the hospital stay (Omnibus Reconciliation Act); directs HHS to develop an outpatient DRG system. **Occupational Exposure to Hazardous Chemicals in Laboratories:** Establishes OSHA guidelines to limit unnecessary exposure to hazardous chemicals.
1992	**Occupational Exposure to Blood-Borne Pathogens:** Establishes OSHA guidelines to limit unnecessary exposure to biological hazards.
1996	**Health Insurance Portability and Accountability Act:** Directs how health care information is managed. This law protects patients from inappropriate dispersion (oral, written, or electronic) of personal information and is the basis for many of the privacy standards currently in place.
1997	**OIG Compliance Guidelines** for clinical laboratories: Help laboratories develop programs that promote high ethical and lawful conduct, especially regarding billing practices and fraud and abuse.
2001	**CMS National Coverage Determinations:** Replaced most local medical review policies used to determine whether certain laboratory tests are medically necessary and therefore reimbursable. Before this, each Medicare intermediary had its own medical necessity guidelines.
2003	**Hazardous Material Regulations:** Deal with shipment of blood and other potentially biohazardous products (DOT).

CMS, Centers for Medicare and Medicaid Services; *DOT,* U.S. Department of Transportation; *HHS,* U.S. Department of Health and Human Services; *OIG,* Office of Inspector General; *OSHA,* Occupational Safety and Health Administration.

TABLE 1-10
States Requiring Laboratory Personnel Licensure

California	Hawaii
Georgia	Montana
Louisiana	New York
Nevada	Puerto Rico
North Dakota	Tennessee
Rhode Island	West Virginia
Florida	

TABLE 1-11
CLIA Categories Included and Excluded

Test categories (based on analyst/operator and complexity to run test)
- Waived (e.g., blood glucose, urine pregnancy)
- Moderate complexity
- High complexity

Not categorized (because they do not produce a result)
- Quality control materials
- Calibrators
- Collection kits (for HIV, drugs of abuse, etc.)

Not currently regulated (by CLIA)
- Noninvasive testing (e.g., bilirubin)
- Breath tests (e.g., alcohol, *Helicobacter pylori*)
- Drugs of abuse testing in the workplace
- Continuous monitoring/infusion devices (e.g., glucose/insulin)

Data from Sliva C. Update 2003: FDA and CLIA. IND roundtable 510(k) workshop, April 22, 2003.
CLIA, Clinical Laboratory Improvement Act; *HIV,* human immunodeficiency virus.

www.cms.hhs.gov/clia/). Before CLIA '88, no consistent federal regulatory standards had been provided for most laboratories, only sporadic state initiatives that carried various levels of authority and oversight of laboratory activities. CLIA '88 was enacted in response to concerns about the lack of national laboratory quality standards. Minimum standards are enforced by the federal government or by their designees that have received "deemed status," reflecting standards equivalent to or stricter than those put forth by CLIA '88. Most of the clinical laboratories in the United States are CLIA-certified to perform testing on human samples, indicating that the laboratory meets personnel, operational, safety, and quality standards based on test complexity (Table 1-11). Detailed, current guidelines may be found at http://wwwn.cdc.gov/clia/regs/toc.aspx.

The Laboratory Compliance Program was mandated by Congress (*Federal Register* 63[163], Aug 24, 1998) in response to concerns from the Centers for Medicare and Medicaid Services (CMS) about fraud and abuse of payments. This program requires that laboratories that receive payment for services from any federal agency must have policies addressing the medical necessity for tests ordered, ensuring accurate billing for testing, and promoting a standard of conduct to be adopted by laboratory employees. Failure to have an active program could cause a laboratory to be excluded from participating with CMS and could lead to significant financial and legal penalties. Consider, for example, the patient mix that may be encountered over the next decade or so. The largest population segment at this time will be the baby boomer generation (about 78 million). It has been estimated that those 65 years and older will utilize five times as many laboratory tests per year as are currently used (Terry, 2009). This will have an impact not only on test volume requirements, but also on the kind of testing appropriate for this age set. Physicians must now select the most appropriate tests and avoid the "shotgun" approach to test ordering practices. Ordering the right tests must be justified as medically necessary and must meet evidence-based medicine protocols (Wians, 2009).

The Health Insurance Portability and Accountability Act (HIPAA) was enacted in 1996, providing standards that protect the confidentiality of health information while allowing interchange of information in appropriate circumstances (*Federal Register* 63, 1998). Various rules have been implemented that have a direct impact on the laboratory and include the use and disclosure of protected health information (PHI). PHI includes any oral, written, electronic, or recorded information such as date of birth, social security number, address, phone number, or other patient identifier. Access to this information is restricted on a "need-to-know" basis as described within an employee's job description/title. Failure to adhere to these rules can result in significant fines, and in blatant cases of abuse, prison time.

A variety of other government agencies and nongovernment organizations directly or indirectly influence laboratory operations. These agencies address laboratory issues and other business practices and provide

TABLE 1-12
Laboratory-Related Governmental Agencies

CDC	**Centers for Disease Control and Prevention** is under the U.S. Department of Health and Human Services (HHS) and provides oversight of public health and safety, including the laboratory (www.cdc.gov).
CMS	**Centers for Medicare and Medicaid Services** (formerly known as HCFA) oversees the largest health care program in the United States, processing more than 1 billion claims per year. Medicare (see Chapter 12) provides coverage to approximately 40 million Americans over the age of 65, some people with disabilities, and patients with end-stage renal disease, with a budget of $309 billion (2004). Medicaid provides coverage to approximately 50 million low-income individuals through a state–federal partnership that costs $277 billion (2004). CMS sets quality standards and reimbursement rates that apply to the laboratory and are often used by other third-party payers (www.cms.hhs.gov).
DOT	**U.S. Department of Transportation** has the responsibility of regulating biohazardous materials that include blood and other human products. Laboratory specimens sent to reference laboratories must be packaged per guidelines set by this agency (www.dot.gov).
EPA	**Environmental Protection Agency** sets and enforces standards for disposal of hazardous laboratory materials, such as formalin, xylene, and other potential carcinogens (www.epa.gov).
EEOC	**Equal Employment Opportunity Commission** oversees and enforces Title VIII dealing with fair employment practices related to the Civil Rights Act of 1964 and the Equal Employment Opportunity Act of 1972. Hiring of laboratory staff falls under the same rules as most businesses (www.eeoc.gov).
FDA	**U.S. Food and Drug Administration** is part of HHS and regulates the manufacture of biologics (such as blood donor testing and component preparation) and medical devices (such as laboratory analyzers) and test kits through its Office of In-Vitro Diagnostic Device Evaluation and Safety. FDA inspects blood donor and/or component manufacturing facilities irrespective of other regulatory agencies and/or accrediting organizations (www.fda.gov).
HHS	**U.S. Department of Health and Human Services** oversees CMS, OIG, and FDA.
NARA	**National Archives and Records Administration** provides a number of databases, including access to the *Federal Register,* where laboratory and other regulations are published (www.gpoaccess.gov/fr/index.html).
NRC	**Nuclear Regulatory Commission** develops and enforces federal guidelines that ensure the proper use and operation of nonmilitary nuclear facilities. Laboratory tests that use radioactive materials (like radioimmunoassays) must adhere to guidelines set by this agency (www.nrc.gov).
NIDA	**National Institute on Drug Abuse** regulates standards for performing and maintaining appropriate quality control for drugs of abuse testing (www.nida.nih.gov).
NIOSH	**National Institute of Occupational Safety and Health** is a part of HHS and provides research, information, education, and training in the field of occupational safety and health. NIOSH makes recommendations regarding safety hazards but has no authority to enforce them (www.cdc.gov/niosh/homepage.html).
NIH	**National Institutes of Health** is an agency of HHS and is a world leader in medical research. It publishes a variety of clinical practice guidelines, some of which are applicable to the laboratory, such as those for diabetes and lipid testing (www.nih.gov).
NIST	**National Institute of Standards and Technology** is a branch of the Commerce Department and has contributed to the development of many health care products. In addition, it has developed standards for calibration, weights and measures, and the International System of Units (www.nist.gov).
OIG	**Office of the Inspector General** is part of HHS and is responsible for auditing, inspecting, and identifying fraud and abuse in CMS programs such as laboratory testing. The focus of OIG is usually noncompliance with reimbursement regulations such as medical necessity (www.oig.hhs.gov).
OSHA	**Occupational Safety and Health Administration** is part of the U.S. Department of Labor and develops and enforces workplace standards to protect employees' safety and health. Recommendations from OSHA include guidelines addressing blood-borne pathogens, chemical safety, phlebotomies, latex gloves, ergonomics, and any other potentially hazardous situation that may be found in the workplace (www.osha.gov).
State Department of Health	**State Departments of Health** vary in the extent to which they regulate laboratories. Some states, like New York, license all laboratories and oversee mandatory proficiency testing and laboratory inspection programs; others do neither. New York and Washington have Clinical Laboratory Improvement Act "deemed status."

regulations concerning human resource practices, transportation of specimens, environmental protection, and interstate commerce, to name just a few (Tables 1-12 and 1-13). The responsibilities assumed by these agencies represent federal, state, and professional guidelines that are designed to protect the public and employees from shoddy laboratory testing practices or unnecessary exposure to biological, chemical, or radioactive hazards. These guidelines also ensure the availability of quality blood products, access to laboratory testing as needed, and a safe work environment for employees. Professional associations play an important part in establishing guidelines and often lobby for their acceptance as standard of care practice by governmental agencies. For example, Table 1-14 provides suggested time limits for record and specimen retention based on CAP guidelines.

SAFETY

The clinical laboratory exposes staff, and potentially the public, to a variety of hazards, including infectious patients, infectious patient specimens, and potentially hazardous chemicals and equipment. All health care facilities should have policies that address routine job-related exposures to biological, chemical, and radiation hazards, as well as ergonomic/environmental hazards, fire safety, act-of-God occurrences (tornadoes, hurricanes, floods, etc.), and epidemic emergency preparedness plans. Laboratories are obligated to identify hazards, implement safety strategies to contain the hazards, and continually audit existing practices to determine whether new ones are needed. Situations such as the H1N1 flu outbreak of 2009 required plans to meet staffing shortages and to manage the infected patient population (Satyadi, 2009). Frequent safety reviews and disaster drills and general employee awareness help maintain a safe work environment.

Good safety practices benefit patients and employees and the bottom line of the laboratory. Injuries and harmful exposures can negatively affect the laboratory financially, by reputation due to bad press, and through potential lawsuits, lost workdays and wages, damage to equipment, and poor staff morale. An injured person may be absent for an indefinite period and often cannot work at peak efficiency upon return. During this time off, the workload has to be absorbed by existing staff or through additional temporary services. Careful planning and compliance with the laws will minimize undesired outcomes. Although inexperience may be a cause for some accidents, others result from ignoring known risks, pressure to do more, carelessness, fatigue, or mental preoccupation (failure to focus

TABLE 1-13
Laboratory-Related, Nongovernmental Organizations

AABB	Formerly known as American Association of Blood Banks, AABB is a peer professional group that offers a blood bank accreditation program that can substitute for (but coordinate with) a CAP inspection. It has CLIA deemed status (www.aabb.org).
ASCP	American Society for Clinical Pathology is the largest organization for laboratory professionals and offers certification for various specialties (www.ascp.org).
CAP	College of American Pathologists offers the largest proficiency survey program in the United States and has a peer-surveyed laboratory accreditation program that has CLIA deemed status. CAP accreditation is recognized by The Joint Commission as meeting its laboratory standards (www.cap.org).
CLSI	Clinical and Laboratory Standards Institute (formerly NCCLS) is a peer professional group that develops standardized criteria regarding laboratory practices; accrediting and licensing entities often adopt these as standards (e.g., procedure manual format) (www.clsi.org).
COLA	COLA (originally the Commission on Office Laboratory Accreditation) is a nonprofit organization sponsored by the American Academy of Family Physicians, the American College of Physicians, the American Medical Association, the American Osteopathic Association, and CAP. It has CLIA deemed status, and its accreditation is recognized by The Joint Commission. It was originally organized to provide assistance to physician office laboratories (POLs), but has recently expanded its product line to other services (www.cola.org).
TJC	The Joint Commission (formerly known as Joint Commission on Accreditation of Healthcare Organizations) is an independent, not-for-profit entity that accredits nearly 17,000 health care organizations and programs in the United States based on a comprehensive set of quality standards. It has CLIA deemed status and may substitute for federal Medicare and Medicaid surveys; it also fulfills licensure requirements in some states and general requirements of many insurers. TJC usually surveys the laboratory as part of an overall health care facility survey (www.jointcommission.org/).

CLIA, Clinical Laboratory Improvement Act.

TABLE 1-14
Suggested Guidelines for Record and Specimen Retention*

Record/specimen type	Retention
Requisitions	2 years
Accession logs	2 years
Maintenance/instrument logs	2 years
Quality control records	2 years
Blood bank donor/receipt records	10 years
Blood bank patient records	10 years
Blood bank employee signatures/initials	10 years
Blood bank QC records	5 years
Clinical pathology test records	2 years
Serum/CSF/body fluids	48 hours
Urine	24 hours
Blood/fluid smears	7 days
Microbiology stained slides	7 days
Wet tissue	2 weeks
Surgical pathology (bone marrows) slides	10 years
Paraffin blocks/slides	10 years
Cytology slides	5 years
FNA slides	10 years
Reports (surgical/cytology/nonforensic)	10 years
Cytogenetic slides	3 years
Cytogenetic reports/images	20 years
Flow cytometry plots/histograms	10 years

*College of American Pathologists, Northfield, Ill. (March 2009) and/or CLIA '88 guidelines (*Federal Register* 55, 1990; 57, 1992); check with other organizations (like AABB) or local regulatory agencies for current requirements that may differ from those above.

attention or to concentrate on what is at hand). A number of strategies may be used to contain hazards, including the use of work practice controls, engineering controls, and personal protective equipment (Table 1-15). The most effective safety programs use all three strategies.

BIOLOGICAL HAZARDS

Biological hazards expose an unprotected individual to bacteria, viruses, parasites, or other biological entities that can result in injury. Exposure occurs from ingestion, inoculation, tactile contamination, or inhalation of infectious material from patients or their body fluids/tissues, supplies or materials they have been in contact with, or contaminated needles, or by aerosol dispersion. The potential also exists for inadvertent exposure to the public through direct contact with aerosolized infectious materials, improperly processed blood products, and inappropriately disposed of waste products.

The spread of hepatitis B virus (HBV), hepatitis C virus (HCV), human immunodeficiency virus (HIV), and tuberculosis (TB) has focused the responsibility on each health care organization to protect its employees, patients, and the general public from infection. The Centers for Disease Control and Prevention (CDC) and the Occupational Safety and Health Administration (OSHA) have provided guidelines (Universal Precautions) that recommend precautions in handling body fluids and human tissues for all patients regardless of their blood-borne infection status (CDC Recommendations and Reports, 1989). OSHA defines occupational exposure as "reasonably anticipated skin, eye, mucous membrane, or percutaneous contact with blood or other potentially infectious materials that may result from the performance of an employee's duties" (*Federal Register* 29CFR, 1910.1030, 1992). Blood, all other body fluids, and any unfixed tissue samples are considered potentially infectious for various blood-borne pathogens. In the laboratory, individuals should avoid mouth pipetting; consumption of food; smoking; applying cosmetics; potential needlestick situations; and leaving unprotected any skin, membranes, or open cuts. Aerosol contamination may be due to inoculating loops (flaming a loop), spills on laboratory counters, expelling a spray from needles, and centrifugation of infected fluids.

Although many laboratories require wearing of gloves when performing phlebotomies, OSHA strongly recommends that gloves be used routinely as a barrier protection, especially when the health care worker has cuts or other open wounds on the skin, anticipates hand contamination (biological or chemical), performs skin punctures; or during phlebotomy training (OSHA, 1991). All other phlebotomy access procedures may require use of gloves as determined by local or institutional policy. Employees must wash their hands after removal of gloves, after any contact with blood or body fluids, and between patients. Gloves should not be washed and reused because microorganisms that adhere to gloves are difficult to remove (Doebbeling, 1988). Masks, protective eyewear, or face shields must be worn to prevent exposure from splashes to the mouth, eyes, or nose. All protective equipment that has the potential for coming into contact with infectious material, including laboratory coats, must be removed before leaving the laboratory area and must never be taken home or outside the laboratory (such as during lunch or personal breaks). Laboratory coats must be cleaned onsite or by a professional. It is helpful for all employees to know what areas (offices, conference rooms, lounges, etc.) and equipment (telephones, keyboards, copy machines, etc.) are designated as laboratory work areas because they can be potentially contaminated. Avoid contamination by not wearing soiled gloves when in these areas or when using nonlaboratory equipment. Use of medical safety devices will help reduce the 600,000 to 800,000 needlestick injuries each year (Sharma, 2009; NIOSH; The Needlestick Safety and Prevention Act of 2000, Pub. L. 106-430, 2000; Bloodborne Pathogens Standard, *Federal Register* 29CFR 1910.1030, 1992). Table 1-16 outlines some common materials that may be used for decontamination (CLSI M29-A3, 2005).

CHEMICAL HAZARDS

All clinical laboratories are mandated by OSHA to develop and actively follow plans that protect laboratory workers from potential exposure to

TABLE 1-15
Laboratory Hazard Prevention Strategies

Work practice controls (general procedures/policies that mandate measures to reduce or eliminate exposure to hazard)	Hand washing after each patient contact Cleaning surfaces with disinfectants Avoiding unnecessary use of needles and sharps and not recapping Red bag waste disposal Immunization for hepatitis Job rotation to minimize repetitive tasks Orientation, training, and continuing education No eating, drinking, or smoking in laboratory Warning signage
Engineering controls (safety features built into the overall design of a product)	Puncture-resistant containers for disposal and transport of needles and sharps Safety needles that automatically retract after removal Biohazard bags Splash guards Volatile liquid carriers Centrifuge safety buckets Biological safety cabinets and fume hoods Mechanical pipetting devices Computer wrist/arm pads Sensor-controlled sinks or foot/knee/elbow-controlled faucets
Personal protective equipment (PPE; barriers that physically separate the user from a hazard)	Nonlatex gloves Gowns and laboratory coats Masks, including particulate respirators Face shields Protective eyewear (goggles, safety glasses) Eyewash station Chemical-resistant gloves; subzero (freezer) gloves; thermal gloves

TABLE 1-16
Common Decontamination Agents

Heat (250° C for 15 minutes)
Ethylene oxide (450–500 mg/L @ 55° C–60° C)
2% Glutaraldehyde
10% Hydrogen peroxide
10% Formalin
5.25% Hypochlorite (10% bleach)
Formaldehyde
Detergents
Phenols
Ultraviolet radiation
Ionizing radiation
Photo-oxidation

TABLE 1-17
Chemical Hazard Communications Plan

1. Develop written hazard communication program.
2. Maintain inventory of all chemicals with chemical and common names, if appropriate.
3. Manufacturer must assess and supply information about chemical or physical hazards (flammability, explosive, aerosol, flashpoint, etc.).
4. Employers must maintain Material Safety Data Sheets (MSDS) in English.
5. MSDS must list all ingredients of a substance greater than 1%, except for known carcinogens if greater than 0.1%.
6. Employers must make MSDS available to employees upon request.
7. Employers must ensure that labels are not defaced or removed and must post appropriate warnings.
8. Employers must provide information and training ("right-to-know").
9. Employers must adhere to Occupational Safety and Health Administration permissible exposure limit, threshold limit, or other exposure limit value.
10. Designate responsible person(s) for the program.

hazardous chemicals. To minimize the incidence of chemically related occupational illnesses and injuries in the workplace, OSHA published its "Hazard Communication Standard" (*Federal Register* 29CFR 1910.1200; 1983) and "Chemical Hygiene Plan" (*Federal Register* 29CFR 1910.1450; 1993), requiring the manufacturers of chemicals to evaluate the hazards of the chemicals they produce and to develop hazard communication programs for employees and other users who are exposed to hazardous chemicals (Table 1-17). These OSHA standards are based on the premise that employees have the right to know what chemical hazards they are potentially exposed to and what protective measures the employer needs to take to minimize hazardous exposure. Many states have developed individual guidelines and regulations mandating that employers develop and implement safety and toxic chemical information programs for their workers that are reviewed with all employees each year (e.g., the Right-to-Know Law in New York State [Chap. 551, Art. 48, 12 NYCRR Part 820]).

ERGONOMIC HAZARDS

OSHA presented guidelines (*Federal Register* 54, 29CFR 1910, 1989) to address ergonomic hazards in the workplace and to assist employers in developing a program to prevent work-related problems that primarily include cumulative trauma disorders. This is a collective group of injuries involving the musculoskeletal and/or nervous system in response to long-term repetitive twisting, bending, lifting, or assuming static postures for an extended period of time. These injuries may evolve from environmental factors such as constant or excessive repetitive actions, mechanical pressure, vibrations, or compressive forces on the arms, hands, wrists, neck, or back. Human error may also be a causative factor when individuals push themselves beyond their limits, or when productivity limits are set too high.

Among laboratory personnel, cumulative trauma disorders are usually related to repetitive pipetting, keyboard use, or resting their wrists/arms on sharp edges, such as a laboratory counter. These actions can cause carpal tunnel syndrome (compression and entrapment of nerve from wrist to hand), tendonitis (inflammation of tendon), or tenosynovitis (inflammation or injury to synovial sheath) (Gile, 2004). Awareness and prevention are essential in managing these disorders. Work practice and engineering controls, in addition to various hand, arm, leg, back, and neck exercises, may reduce these problems (Prinz-Lubbert, 1996). The costs of implementing programs to help employees understand and avoid ergonomic hazards can be financially justified. Back injuries are the second most common cause for employee absenteeism after the common cold and can cost employers up to $16,000 per episode (Prinz-Lubbert, 1996).

SELECTED REFERENCES

Bonini P, Plebani M, Ceriotti F, et al. Errors in laboratory medicine. Clin Chem 2002;48:691–8.

A review on the literature on laboratory errors, including an analysis of the types and/or volume of preanalytic, analytic, and postanalytic errors, as well as transfusion errors.

Lifshitz MS, De Cresce RP. Strategic planning for automation. In: Kost GJ, editor. Clinical automation, robotics, and optimization. New York: John Wiley & Sons; 1996. p. 471–96.

An overview of the laboratory strategic planning process with special emphasis on how to assess the environment, define objectives, and audit operations and technology.

Nigon DL. Clinical laboratory management. New York: McGraw-Hill; 2000.

Covers fundamental principles of laboratory management and provides many practical examples and case studies that help illustrate concepts.

Snyder J, Wilkinson DS. Management in laboratory medicine. 3rd ed. Philadelphia: Lippincott; 1998.

Comprehensive reference dealing with all aspects of laboratory management, including leadership, human resource management, marketing, safety, etc.

REFERENCES

Access the complete reference list online at http://www.expertconsult.com

CHAPTER 2

OPTIMIZING LABORATORY WORKFLOW AND PERFORMANCE

Thomas J. Dilts, Richard A. McPherson

KEY POINTS

- An effective testing process requires integration of preanalytic, analytic, and postanalytic steps.
- An understanding of workflow is a fundamental prerequisite to any performance optimization strategy.
- A variety of techniques should be used to collect workflow data. These include sample and test mapping, tube analysis, workstation analysis, staff interviews, and task (process) mapping.
- Though technology is a critical component of every laboratory, it is only a tool to reach a goal. Technology alone does not improve performance and workflow; its success or failure depends on how it is implemented and whether it was truly needed.
- Consolidation, standardization, and integration are key strategies that can optimize workflow using concepts such as Six Sigma to achieve Lean processes. Managing test utilization may also change overall operational needs and workflow patterns.
- Assessment of excess capacity is useful in establishing the feasibility of increasing testing workload, especially in outreach programs.

The clinical laboratory is a complex operation that must smoothly integrate all three phases of the testing process: preanalysis, analysis, and postanalysis. Preanalysis refers to all the activities that take place before testing, such as test ordering and sample collection. The analysis stage consists of the laboratory activities that actually produce a result, such as running a sample on an automated analyzer. Postanalysis comprises patient reporting and result interpretation. Collectively, all of the interrelated laboratory steps in the testing process describe its workflow; this, in turn, occurs within the overall design of a laboratory operation as described in its policies and procedures.

The steps in the testing process can be generally categorized according to testing phase, role (responsibility), or laboratory technology (Fig. 2-1). Note that the testing process and the grouping of steps vary somewhat from one facility to another. Depending on the laboratory service model and technology used, some steps may fall into one category or another. For example, centrifugation may be performed in a physician office (preanalysis) or in the laboratory as part of a total automation workcell (analysis). Depending on the technology selected, a laboratory may automate some or many of the steps identified in Figure 2-1. Information technology is the essential "glue" that binds these steps. A more detailed discussion of each testing phase is presented in Chapters 3–8. This chapter will explore the interrelationship of laboratory workflow, technology, and performance.

UNDERSTANDING WORKFLOW

To fully understand a laboratory's workflow, one must audit all phases of the testing process. Only then can one determine how to optimize performance and to what degree technologic or nontechnologic solutions are needed. Table 2-1 provides some of the issues to consider.

Data are of paramount importance in any workflow analysis. Although laboratory data are rather easy to produce because they are readily available from automated analyzers and information systems, they may not be complete, valid, or in the format required. Because laboratory data play a central role in laboratory decision-making (e.g., determining which analyzer to acquire), they have to be accurate; otherwise, one may make wrong downstream decisions that can have a negative impact on operations. One must understand how data are collected by each of these systems and whether they are valid. For instance, do the test statistics pulled from an analyzer provide information on how many patient reportable tests are done, or do they count how many total tests are done (with quality control, repeats, etc.)? Are panel constituents counted individually, is only the panel counted, or are both counted? Are the "collect" times accurate on turnaround time reports that measure "collect to result"? Or are samples indicated as "collected" on a patient floor before they are actually collected, thereby making the turnaround time appear longer than actual? Ultimately, there is no substitute for carefully reviewing data to determine whether they make sense. Sometimes, this requires manually verifying data collected electronically or directly observing a work area. For example, it may be necessary to observe when samples arrive in the laboratory to determine how long a delay exists before staff assign a receipt time in the computer. By doing so, one can determine the accuracy of the sample receipt time.

DATA COLLECTION TECHNIQUES

Many types of data can be used to assess workflow. Although some of the fundamental data analysis techniques are described in this chapter, they may have to be supplemented with additional data collection to analyze unique characteristics of a laboratory's operation. It is always useful (some would say imperative) to check that the data collected reflect actual laboratory experience rather than anomalies created by unusual workflow patterns or laboratory information system (LIS) programs or definitions.

Sample and Test Mapping

One fundamental data collection technique is to analyze the distribution of samples and tests over time (Fig. 2-2). Depending on what is mapped, the time interval can be a day (e.g., hour increments for frequently ordered tests like those in general chemistry) or a week (e.g., daily increments for tests batched several times a week). The goal is to identify overall workload patterns to assess whether resources are appropriately matched to needs, and whether turnaround time or other performance indicators can be

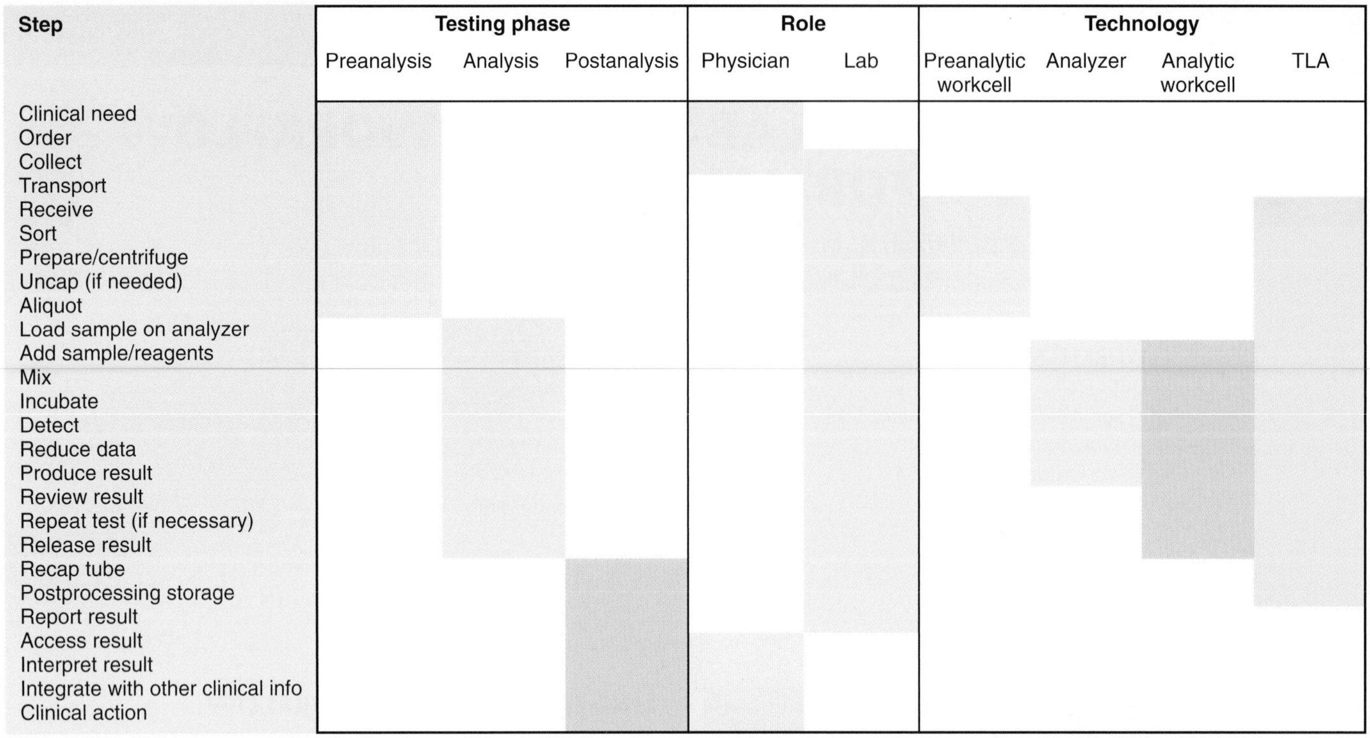

Step
Testing phase
Preanalysis
Analysis
Postanalysis
Role
Physician
Lab
Technology
Preanalytic workcell
Analyzer
Analytic workcell
TLA
Clinical need
Order
Collect
Transport
Receive
Sort
Prepare/centrifuge
Uncap (if needed)
Aliquot
Load sample on analyzer
Add sample/reagents
Mix
Incubate
Detect
Reduce data
Produce result
Review result
Repeat test (if necessary)
Release result
Recap tube
Postprocessing storage
Report result
Access result
Interpret result
Integrate with other clinical info
Clinical action

Figure 2-1 Laboratory testing process. Note that the steps can be categorized according to testing phase, role (responsibility), or laboratory technology, as indicated by the shading. *TLA,* Total laboratory automation.

TABLE 2-1
Issues to Consider When Auditing Operations

Test ordering	Where are orders placed—in the laboratory, patient unit, or office? Are inpatient orders handled differently than outpatient ones? Is there a paper or electronic requisition?
Sample collection	Who collects the samples—laboratory or physician? When are they collected—all hours or just in the AM? Are samples bar coded at the site of collection or in the laboratory? How are the labels generated? Is there a positive patient ID system? Does the label contain all the information needed to process the sample?
Transportation	How are samples delivered—by messenger, automatic carrier transport, or a combination? Do all laboratories participate? Are all patient care areas served? How are stats handled? What is their impact? Is there a separate system for emergency department and intensive care units?
Sample receipt	Is there a central receiving area? How are samples distributed to each laboratory? Does physical layout promote efficient sample flow? How are stat samples distinguished from routine ones? How are problem samples handled? Are samples sorted by workstation or department?
Sample processing	Are samples centrifuged centrally or in distributed locations? Are stats handled differently? Are samples aliquoted? If so, where? Is a separate sample drawn for each workstation?
Testing	How many workstations are used? How does capacity relate to need? How are samples stored and retrieved? How long are samples kept? When and why are samples repeated? Are repeat criteria appropriate?
Reporting	How are results reported? Electronically? By remote printer? How are stat and critical values reported, and are criteria appropriate? How many calls for reports does the laboratory receive, and why? How are point-of-care tests reported?

improved. It is important that the workload measured reflects actual experience. For example, if phlebotomists remotely mark specimens "received" or the laboratory actually orders tests in the LIS, the measured workload distribution may not accurately reflect the underlying processes. As part of the exercise, it is also important to map routine samples versus stat ones and to map locations that may have special needs such as the emergency department. In addition to sample mapping, one should map key tests and the number or "density" of tests per sample. This is of special interest in the chemistry section. Outpatient samples typically have greater test density than inpatient ones, so an equal number of inpatient and outpatient samples may be associated with different inpatient and outpatient workloads. In automated chemistry, sample mapping more closely reflects staffing needs in that much of the labor is associated with handling and processing tubes rather than actually performing the assays. In contrast, test mapping more closely reflects instrument needs (i.e., the test throughput it needs to complete its workload in a timely manner). By mapping samples and tests and relating them to turnaround time and staffing, a laboratory can identify production bottlenecks and alter workflow to achieve better outcomes. Very frequently, laboratories discover that delays are less the result of instrument issues per se, and are more the result of workflow patterns that are not matched to instrument capabilities.

Tube Analysis

Part of the laboratory's daily work is related to processing collection tubes or containers. "Tube labor" includes sorting and centrifuging; aliquoting; racking, unracking, loading, and unloading samples on analyzers; retrieving tubes for add-on tests; performing manual dilutions or reruns (depending on instrument); and storing tubes. Although the time needed to perform a tube task may seem insignificant, it has to be repeated many times per day, and this can add up to a substantial amount of time. For example, at an average of 10 seconds per tube, it will take a laboratory 3.3 hours to sort 1200 tubes per day. Automation can often reduce this labor, but redesigning the workflow may be a less expensive and more efficient alternative. To the extent that a laboratory reduces the number of tubes and/or the number of tasks associated with each tube, it can reduce tube labor and positively influence workflow and staffing needs.

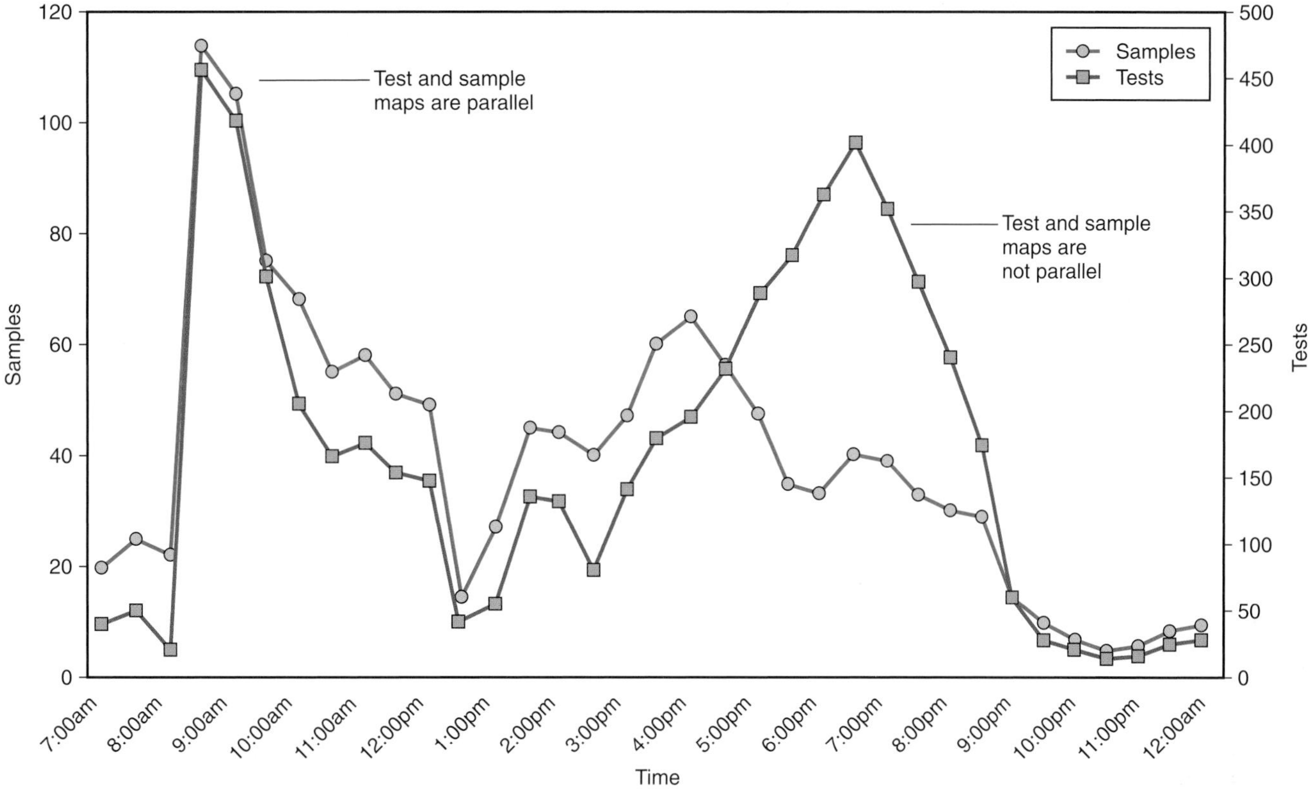

Figure 2-2 Sample and test mapping. Note that the morning volume peak is due to inpatients, and the density is roughly four tests per sample. The evening peak is largely due to outpatients and density is far greater, about 10 tests per sample. Test density fluctuates during the day; thus both sample mapping and test mapping are necessary to accurately evaluate workload.

TABLE 2-2
Chemistry Tube Analysis

	Analyzer A	Analyzer B
Total tubes run	500	500
Mechanical error	13	15
Dilution	7	20
Clot/low volume	20	30
Total instrument-related reruns	40 (32% of total reruns)	65 (65% of total reruns)
Delta check	62	21
Panic value	23	14
Total laboratory criteria–related reruns	85 (68% of total reruns)	35 (35% of total reruns)
Total reruns	125	100
% reruns	25%	20%

Chemistry "reruns" are caused by different factors and can be a source of nonproductive technologist time and/or turnaround time delays. Most Analyzer A reruns are related to overly tight limits for delta checks and panic values that flag too many test results for technologist review and rerun. Most Analyzer B reruns are related to instrument flags caused by a narrow linear range for many methods and a large sample volume requirement per test. A nontechnologic solution (i.e., altering laboratory rerun/review criteria to reduce the number of tubes flagged for rerun) benefits Analyzer A; however, only a technologic solution (i.e., a new analyzer) can lower the number of reruns in Analyzer B.

Reducing tube labor is one of the main goals of consolidating chemistry and immunodiagnostic tests into a single analyzer or workcell. Sample mapping provides information about how many containers are received within a specified interval; tube analysis helps to analyze how many additional "tube-related" tasks have to be done. Tube analysis includes the number of containers other than tubes (e.g., fingerstick collections that may require special processing or aliquoting) and the number of reruns (i.e., repeats) needed as the result of instrument flags and/or laboratory policies (Table 2-2).

Workstation Analysis

A typical laboratory is divided into stations for allocating work and scheduling staff. Some workstations consist of a variety of tasks or tests that are grouped together for purposes of organizing work for one or more staff. For example, all manual or semiautomated chemistry tests may be grouped into a workstation, even though testing might actually be performed at different sites or using different equipment around the laboratory. More typically, a workstation is one physical location (e.g., a fully automated analyzer or group of analyzers such as hematology cell counters or a chemistry workcell). Regardless of how a laboratory is organized, it is important to understand where, when, and how the work is performed. This is the goal of a workstation analysis.

Instrument Audit

A key component of any workstation is equipment. By performing an instrument audit (Table 2-3), one can better understand how each analyzer is used, its associated costs, and what potential opportunities might exist to improve performance. The operating characteristics of each instrument should be detailed as part of this process. Examples include the maximum number of samples that can be processed per hour, the number of samples that can be loaded at a single time, and the numbers of reagent containers and assays that can be stored onboard. Instrument throughput (tests/hour) should also be studied by conducting timing studies and reviewing various statistical reports that can be extracted from the instrument and the LIS. Most chemistry analyzers are test-based systems, that is, they perform a specific number of tests per hour, irrespective of how many tests are ordered on each sample. On the other hand, some of these systems are affected by test mix (e.g., the relative proportion of electrolytes, general chemistries, and immunoassays), and this is the major reason that actual throughput experienced in the laboratory may be lower than what is claimed by the vendor. The latter may assume an ideal test mix that cannot be achieved in a given laboratory. It is important to understand how test mix affects an analyzer's throughput, and whether work can be redistributed in a way that enhances throughput. An instrument that was well suited for the laboratory's test mix and volume when initially acquired may no longer provide adequate throughput given a change in test mix. It is important to ensure that a vendor's throughput analysis is based on the laboratory's actual test mix, and not on a standard used by the vendor.

TABLE 2-3
Instrument Audit

Instrument model
Vendor
Date acquired
Method of acquisition
Purchased
Leased
Reagent rental
Service cost per year
Supplies cost per year
Reagents
Controls, calibrators
Consumables
Total test volume per year
Patient samples
Controls and calibrators
Test menu
Hours of operation
Days
Shifts
Number of staff trained
Operating mode
Batch versus continuous
Primary system versus backup

It may turn out that the number of instruments proposed may not meet the laboratory's needs.

It is equally important to receive a clear and concise definition of up-time from the vendor for the instrument(s). This definition should be simple. If the laboratory cannot report patient results, the instrument is down. Some vendors consider an instrument down only if the vendor is called for service. This may mean the percent of up-time by the vendor may be valued higher than the actual up-time experienced by the laboratory. It is important to include this definition in a contract if a laboratory expects a vendor to uphold desired operational performance levels necessary to consistently maintain patient care support.

Last, labor considerations should not be ignored. Must the instrument be attended at all times, or does it have walkaway capability? This information can be very useful in identifying processing bottlenecks and redesigning workflow.

Test Menu

A careful review of the laboratory's test offerings should be done during a workstation analysis. Are the tests performed appropriate for the facility, given the volume and frequency of test analysis? Just because a laboratory can perform a test does not mean that it should. For example, if a test is performed only once a week but requires considerable equipment, training, or labor input, it may make more sense to send it to a reference laboratory where it is performed more frequently. Sometimes the best way to improve turnaround time and lower the cost of a test is not to perform it. Unfortunately, this option can be easily overlooked if one focuses only on how to improve the way existing tests are performed, instead of analyzing how to best meet clinician needs.

Processing Mode and Load Balancing. These can affect both the cost and the timeliness of testing. Samples can be processed in batches or run continuously as they arrive in the laboratory. When grouped into batches, samples are run at specific intervals (e.g., once a shift, once a day, every other day) or whenever the batch grows to a certain size (e.g., every 20 samples). Batch processing is often less expensive than continuous processing because the setup costs (quality control, labor, etc.) are spread over many specimens (see Table 12-2); however, batch processing produces less timely results. Sometimes batch processing is a limitation of the instrument that is used. A batch analyzer cannot be interrupted during operation; thus, a newly arrived sample cannot be processed immediately if the instrument is already in use. Most currently available general chemistry and immunoassay analyzers are random access analyzers that continuously process samples. These analyzers can randomly access sample and reagents and can accommodate an emergency sample at any time. The characteristics of these analyzers are discussed more fully in Chapter 5. Continuous processing is facilitated by load balancing, a technique of spreading testing over a longer period to better match instrumentation throughput. For example, outpatient work, which does not require a rapid turnaround time, can be sequenced into the workflow during off hours. This improves testing efficiency, reduces the labor content of individual tests, and reduces throughput requirements (and capital cost) of instruments. In addition, if significant outreach testing (which does not typically require a rapid turnaround) is performed, some or all of this volume can be shifted to times that the laboratory is not as busy. The feasibility of load balancing can be evaluated only if accurate test mapping and tube analysis are performed.

Interviews

Data collection is not complete without interviewing staff. This exercise provides an opportunity for staff to participate in analyzing workflow and improving performance. It also identifies issues that would not be readily apparent from data collection alone. For example, many hospitals require electronic order entry on patient care units. Although this practice may eliminate paper requisitions, laboratory staff members may still be placing orders for "add-on" tests that are called into the laboratory (or added electronically), processing special requests, and troubleshooting incorrect orders, unacceptable samples, or misaligned bar code labels applied by nonlaboratory staff during sample collection. This residual work is likely to be transparent because it probably will not appear on reports, logs, or computer printouts. Thus, "computer-generated orders" may still be associated with considerable manual laboratory labor that may be identified only through interviews.

Interviews are particularly valuable in understanding what occurs outside the laboratory. Test ordering patterns or habits can have a significant impact on a laboratory's ability to meet clinician needs. Visits to patient care units and discussions with nursing unit staff can identify preprocessing improvements that cost little to implement but save considerable money downstream.

Early patient discharge can be a challenging task for hospitals trying to shorten length of stay. A full understanding of the discharge process requires interviewing all related staff. One issue that sometimes emerges is the sample collection time for patients awaiting discharge pending a laboratory result. To avoid delays in providing results for discharge patients, some facilities develop elaborate "stat" systems to collect, identify, and process these samples, as well as report results, during the busiest time of the day—the early morning. Sometimes, dedicated (stat instrument) or new technology (point-of-care device) is used for this purpose. However, one can ensure that results are available in the chart during early morning clinical rounds by simply collecting laboratory samples from patients on the evening before discharge. Thus, not all solutions require technology. A careful mix of workflow restructuring and appropriate technology is usually the correct approach and the most cost-effective solution.

Task Mapping

No workflow study is complete without mapping of the tasks or processes involved in performing a test (Middleton, 1996). A rigorous review will detail every specimen-handling step, each decision point, and redundant activities. Task mapping can be applied to any segment of a laboratory's workflow, whether technical or clerical. A full understanding of the tasks involved usually requires thorough staff interviews, as discussed previously. Task mapping should be an ongoing activity and should also be undertaken whenever one contemplates adding a workstation, test, new technology, or any significant change to a laboratory process. When implementing change, it is important to avoid unnecessary or additional steps that are inadvertently added in the name of "efficiency"; task mapping helps identify these steps. Mapping also helps compare processes before and after change (Fig. 2-3, *A* and *B*).

WORKFLOW ANALYSIS

Workflow analysis assimilates all of the previously discussed data and transforms them into valuable information. This step can be done manually or, as will be described later, using commercially available software for part of the analysis. A comprehensive workstation analysis should identify bottlenecks and highlight areas where improvements are necessary.

How is this done? The easiest way, and one that does not require computer support, is to follow the path of a specimen or group of specimens through the entire process. This should begin at or near the bedside to see how physicians are ordering tests and should proceed to specimen acquisition and delivery to the laboratory. A flow sheet, which follows the sample from initial order to arrival in the laboratory, should be created.

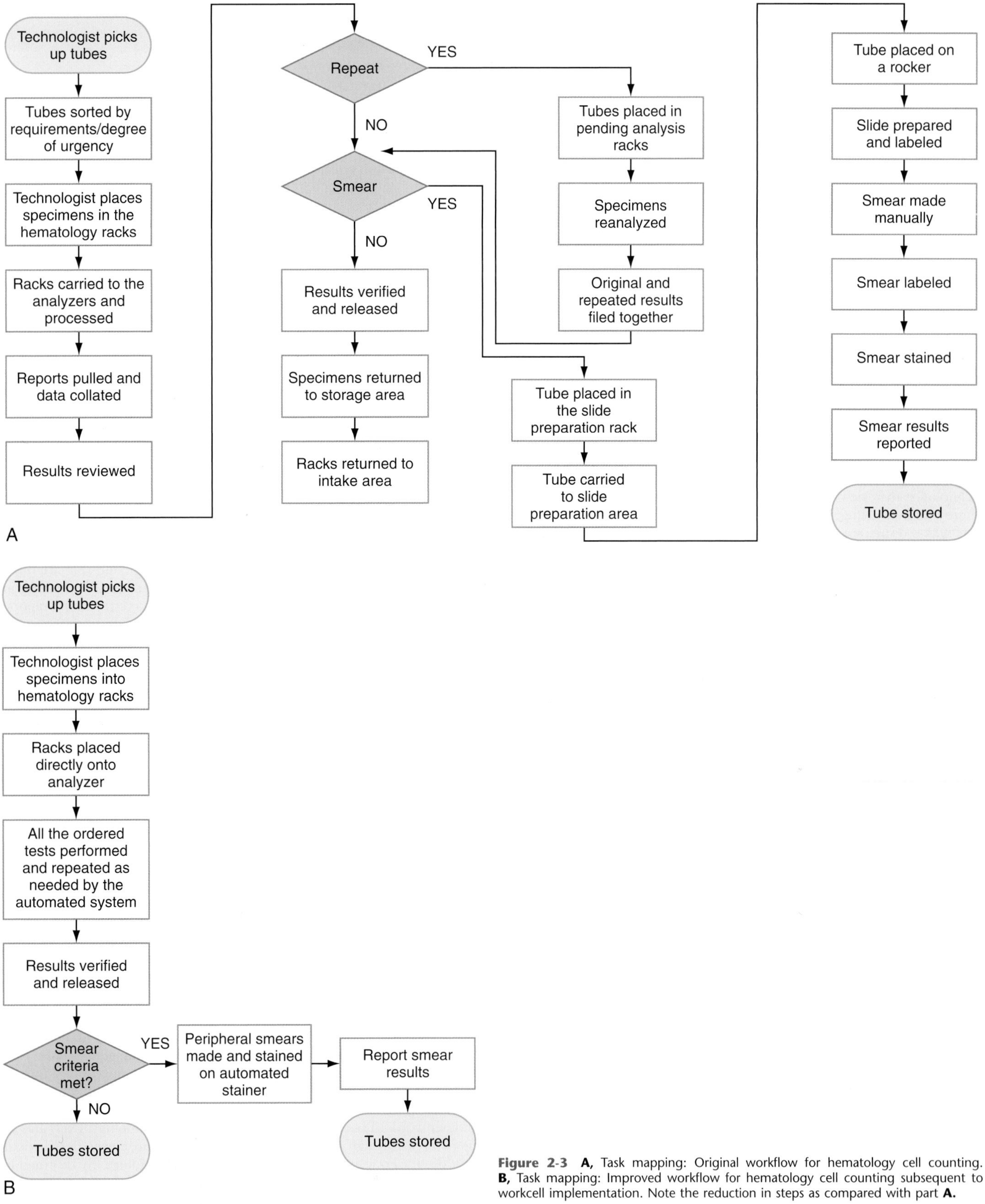

Figure 2-3 **A,** Task mapping: Original workflow for hematology cell counting. **B,** Task mapping: Improved workflow for hematology cell counting subsequent to workcell implementation. Note the reduction in steps as compared with part **A.**

A separate task force is usually assigned to the prelaboratory phase because multiple departments and staff are usually involved; the laboratory often has little or no direct control over this critical portion of workflow, especially when nonlaboratory staff collect samples.

Specimen transit through the laboratory should then be documented, noting areas where batch processing occurs. For example, one should identify minimum and maximum centrifugation times for applicable specimens (such as those that have to be aliquoted). If specimens require 10 minutes for loading and spinning, this should not be assumed to be the average time because a sample queue may form during peak periods. Using the sample arrival mapping done in data collection, an average time can be assigned by time of day. If this is done manually, it is best to select a

TABLE 2-4
Interrelated Variables Simulated by Workflow Software Models

Equipment configuration
Facility design
Labor by shift and day
Throughput
Routine maintenance
Downtime
Sample volume (distribution and peak demand)
Sample container type
Review policy and rerun rates
Batch size

number of key times and average them, if possible. Similarly, one should note whether loading specimens on the analyzer is delayed. Many other examples of physical bottlenecks need to be identified and quantified. It is not always possible to completely eliminate bottlenecks; however, it is possible to mitigate their impact through new technology, alternative processing modes (e.g., random access vs. batch processing), and workflow redesign.

Nonphysical bottlenecks should also be identified and quantified. A classic example is the mode of result verification. Batching results for a technologist to review and accept is every bit as much a bottleneck as is waiting for a centrifuge to process a sample. In contrast, LIS autoverification (where results are automatically released on the basis of preset criteria) can reduce test turnaround time without requiring a major reorganization of the laboratory. However, the degree to which autoverification enhances workflow depends on the manner in which it is implemented and the algorithms defined to qualify a result for this feature. This, in turn, may depend on the LIS used. These issues are discussed further in Chapter 11.

Many vendors who want to sell automated equipment systems to the laboratory will provide free workflow analysis. They usually have experienced technical staff who do this, and the information can be very helpful. The laboratory will need to provide the necessary data or access to the laboratory for data collection. Together the vendor and laboratory leadership need to analyze the workflow to identify opportunities to improve operations, which may well involve the vendor's automated system.

Workflow Modeling

Although the analyses discussed earlier are critical to understanding current and proposed workflow designs, they usually provide a somewhat static picture (i.e., each describes a single data element and often how it changes over time). In practice, however, workflow consists of many interrelated variables, and it is difficult to understand (or to evaluate in the laboratory) how a change in one variable affects another. Further, although workflow studies can be very beneficial, they consume resources that may not be available in every laboratory. To address this need, technology vendors have developed workflow simulations. By using sophisticated workflow modeling software, one can analyze these complex interrelationships to better predict the outcome of a given workflow design (Table 2-4). Workflow modeling can help identify bottlenecks and the impact of staffing changes or different equipment configurations on cost and turnaround time. It can also be used to gain a better understanding of how a given analyzer responds to changes in test volume and test mix. For example, one can simulate the impact of increasing routine test volume on an instrument's turnaround time for stat samples (Mohammad, 2004). As with all workflow analyses, however, software modeling must be based on accurate data collection techniques.

Because most simulation programs are proprietary products, they may not allow modeling of all available instruments. Workflow simulation is still a powerful tool, and inferences can be drawn about more efficient processing and testing regardless of the model instrument involved. More important, these programs readily highlight deficiencies in a laboratory's current operations and can point to specific areas where the greatest improvements are achievable.

Pneumatic Tube Transport of Specimens

Many laboratories, especially those in large hospital facilities, use pneumatic tube systems for specimen transport to the laboratory. They can greatly decrease transport time and thus total turnaround time for test results. Some of these systems can be extensive, especially the branching systems that can reach most parts of a hospital. Once a laboratory has a tube system, it becomes very dependent on it, requiring a good service and support system to maintain it. Usually the plant operations or engineering department of the hospital maintains the system on a daily basis. In addition, enough specimen carriers must be available to supply all areas of the hospital in need of specimen transport to the laboratory. It is important to monitor the number of carriers in the system and to order new carriers when existing supplies wear out or "disappear" (it is not uncommon for locations to "stockpile" carriers, at the expense of other locations, to ensure their availability).

TABLE 2-5
Breakthrough Technology

Changes fundamental workflow
Consolidates workstations
Saves labor
Improves service
Sets new performance standard
Leads to premium pricing

UNDERSTANDING TECHNOLOGY

No discussion of workflow is complete without examining the role of technology (De Cresce, 1988). Laboratory technology refers largely to three functional areas: testing equipment (i.e., analyzers), preanalytic processors, and information technology (IT). Although the former two areas are specific to the laboratory, IT is not, and its design and role are often determined by factors outside the laboratory. For example, the manner in which a laboratory information system is used for data retrieval and reporting (i.e., whether or not physicians directly access the LIS to view results) depends on whether a hospital information system is available to serve this purpose (see Chapter 11). In the latter case, laboratory data are accessed and reported through a secondary system. Also, the laboratory system may be part of a broader approach or a single IT vendor solution within the health care center and not a standalone product to be selected by the laboratory. Under these circumstances, the technology selected, although optimal for the general institution, may not be optimal for the laboratory. Changes in hospital-wide systems are rarely made to accommodate efficiencies in ancillary services like the laboratory. These systems are primarily geared toward easy access to clinical information by caregivers and accurate billing by the hospital finance department.

THE ROLE OF TECHNOLOGY: PRINCIPLES AND PITFALLS

Technology has radically changed the clinical laboratory over the past 30 years and continues to be the driving force behind many new developments. Periodically, a breakthrough technology is introduced that revolutionizes laboratory medicine (Table 2-5). Examples include the random access chemistry analyzer, the automated immunodiagnostics system, the chemistry and immunodiagnostics integrated workcell, and molecular diagnostics. Each change profoundly alters how a laboratory functions and the type of information it provides clinicians. Although breakthrough technologies offer a large potential benefit, they cost more. Over time, a breakthrough technology is adopted by multiple vendors, competition develops, prices fall, and its use becomes widespread among laboratories; in other words, it becomes a current or derivative technology. Early adopters of breakthrough technology often pay more and receive less benefit than those who wait until it becomes a current technology. By thoroughly understanding the role of technology one can determine how to best use it in the clinical laboratory. The following issues should be considered when evaluating technology.

Is technology needed? Technology is an integral part of a modern laboratory; however, it is not the solution to every problem. Often a nontechnologic solution provides a faster, better, and less expensive workflow approach than a technologic one. Knowing when to introduce a nontechnologic solution instead of a technologic one can mean the difference between a targeted, cost-effective solution and an expensive one that does

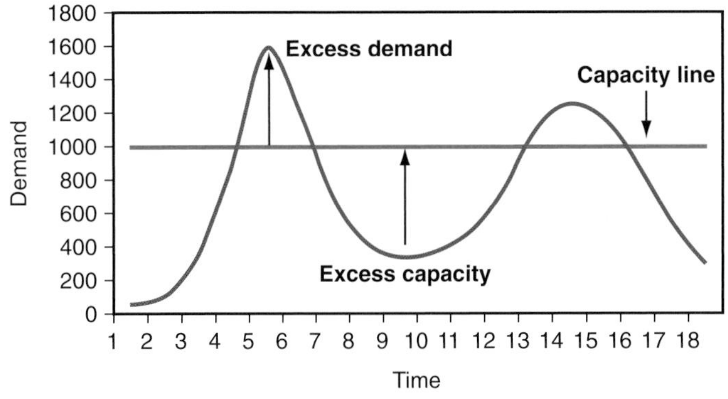

Figure 2-4 Test demand versus instrument capacity. Note that demand exceeds capacity during peak periods, thereby creating backlogs. In many facilities, short backlogs are acceptable. If they are not clinically acceptable, the laboratory should explore ways to more evenly match capacity and demand, for example, by altering blood collection schedules or introducing new work from additional clients. New technology should be the last approach that is considered.

not fully address the initial problem, provides unnecessary functionality, or provides necessary functionality but at an unnecessary cost. For example, a laboratory may experience a sharp morning spike in samples, thereby creating workflow backlogs (Fig. 2-4). Instead of purchasing more equipment to provide additional capacity during peak periods, the laboratory should look for ways to distribute work more evenly during the shift. The key is to avoid delivering large sample batches to the laboratory. Outreach samples can be more evenly distributed because the turnaround time is usually not critical. One approach might be to rearrange phlebotomy draw schedules so that blood draws begin earlier and are spread out over a longer period (Sunyog, 2004). Another approach is to have phlebotomists send samples to the laboratory after every few patients instead of waiting to collect a large batch from an entire floor. One consideration is to have the inpatient nursing unit staff perform specimen collection. This may control the number of inappropriate stat orders because nursing units are more familiar than a laboratory phlebotomist with the status of the patient. This requires consistent phlebotomy training for all nursing unit staff that collect specimens to prevent specimen integrity problems. Thus one should analyze and reengineer processes to the greatest possible degree before embarking on a technology solution; this approach may yield an inexpensive solution that is quicker and easier to implement. Sometimes, nontechnologic solutions, although preferable, are out of the direct control of the laboratory staff and consequently do not receive the attention they deserve. Thus, a technology solution is selected because it can be implemented without the support of other departments.

Technology is a means to an end, not an end. Technology alone does not improve performance and workflow; it is only a tool to reach a goal. Ultimately, new technology succeeds or fails according to how it is implemented. This, in turn, depends on people and their ability to clearly analyze how technology and workflow can be optimally integrated into their setting. What works for one location may not work for another. Sometimes this means changing long-standing practices or staff schedules. For example, if four chemistry analyzers are consolidated into two, staff need to be reallocated to take into account fewer workstations and/or peak testing needs. Similarly, batching certain tests on a new high throughput analyzer does not take full advantage of its continuous processing capabilities and in some instances may yield a lower throughput than the analyzer it replaces. Last, manually transcribing physician orders from paper requisitions into a hospital or laboratory information system provides far less functionality and error reduction capability than is provided by direct electronic order entry by physicians. Because technology has to be "customized" for each site, laboratories implement the same technology in different ways and experience different outcomes. It should never be assumed that improvements and results seen at another facility will automatically occur in one's own facility. The most successful implementations require a total workflow reassessment to evaluate how best to integrate technology. By critically evaluating existing practices, one can avoid perpetuating inefficient processes even with new equipment.

Overbuying—the cardinal sin. More than anything else, overbuying increases costs that burden an operation over the life of the technology. Although it is tempting to overbuy "just in case" capacity needs grow (such as with new outreach work), these needs may not materialize or may occur slowly over time, allowing for an incremental and more cost-effective approach. A new instrument in the laboratory rarely, if ever, directly translates into new testing volume. The market demand for testing is generally independent of the laboratory's capacity to test, although greater capacity may allow the laboratory to more aggressively market services. Different types of overbuying may occur. For example, one may buy three analyzers instead of two or an analyzer that performs 1000 tests per hour instead of a device that runs 500 tests per hour. Alternatively, a total laboratory automation solution may be implemented instead of one based on several smaller workcells or standalone analyzers. In all instances, overbuying increases costs. All of the previous examples increase depreciation costs, require more service and maintenance, and can lead to ineffective labor utilization and suboptimal workflow. Buying more analyzers than necessary can also increase reagent costs in that each instrument has to be calibrated, controlled, and cross-correlated with other devices running the same test. Reagent waste (due to outdating) may also increase if low volume tests are set up on all of the analyzers.

Overbuying should not be confused with excess capacity that is sometimes unavoidable when necessary backup systems are implemented. Ultimately, it is the laboratory service model that determines whether backup is needed. For some tests (e.g., cardiac markers), the laboratory may need a backup system; for others (e.g., tumor markers), it may not. Also, a stat laboratory's backup needs will differ from those of a reference laboratory. A well-designed workflow can balance a laboratory's need for some backup without unnecessary overbuying. For a laboratory that needs a 1000 test/hour capacity, this may mean selecting two 500 test/hour analyzers instead of two running 1000 tests/hour. Alternatively, it may mean selecting one 1000 test/hour analyzer and using a laboratory nearby (that is interfaced to the first laboratory's information system) for backup. Last, it may mean selecting two 1000 test/hour analyzers but running one at a time. This last solution is rarely successful because it duplicates expensive technology and increases maintenance costs. A simple analogy to the family car is often instructive—people rarely buy two automobiles to do what one can do most of the time. Instead, they rely on alternative sources such as renting, public transportation, or taxis to fill occasional needs. One must be sure not to underbuy as well. Many times the number of analyzers is dependent not only on volume throughput but also on stability (up time). If instrumentation is down a significant amount of time, and the effort to bring it back online will take hours or days, a backup instrument is critical for continued testing support. Many large laboratory operations have extensive automation in chemistry and hematology that require constant availability of service support by the vendor to make sure the instrumentation is always in working order. In some cases, a vendor will actually have a service engineer routinely present onsite during weekday hours to maintain the automation system and to help train staff to do the same. Because of staffing shortages on a national level, automation has helped laboratories do more with less, but only if the automation stays consistently functional. Ultimately, the goal is to "right buy," that is, to avoid overbuying or underbuying technology.

Do you understand what you are buying? There is a difference between "buying" technology and being "sold" technology by vendors. The former approach requires an analysis by the laboratory to identify what it needs and a thorough understanding of the technology under consideration, whereas the latter relies more heavily on the vendor to provide a solution to the laboratory. The risk of being "sold" a technology is that it might not be the optimal solution. Most instruments work and do what they are advertised to do. Unfortunately, "what they do" may not be what one needs.

The type of technology is also important. Current technology is generally easier to understand and offers a less risky strategy than breakthrough technology, although it might also provide less reward. Breakthrough technology is, by definition, a new technology, and it may be difficult to fully understand whether it is appropriate in a given laboratory setting, how best to implement it, or how significant a financial impact it will make.

Other issues to consider relate to the technology itself and whether it currently offers all the features required by a laboratory. A vendor may promote certain enhancements or capabilities scheduled for the future, especially when marketing analyzers. These may include tests in development, instrument or computer hardware improvements, new versions of software, or automatic upgrades to a next-generation system. Although

TABLE 2-6
Workflow Metric Examples

Metric	Comments
Turnaround Time (TAT) Studies	
Collection to receipt	Is collection time correct? How long does it take for samples to reach laboratory? Is tube transport system functioning properly? Are messenger pickups reliable?
Receipt to result	How long does testing take once the laboratory receives a sample? Is it held in a central receiving area before it is brought to the technologist?
Order (or collection) to result	This is what the physician perceives as total turnaround time. Is it accurate? How long does it take for a released laboratory result to appear in the hospital information system? Do networking issues external to the laboratory delay the appearance of results?
Stat and routine TAT by hour	Is stat TAT longer in AM when routine samples from morning collection arrive? What is the difference in TAT for routine and stats? Are some tests affected more than others?
Monthly Volume Statistics	
"Billable" tests	How many orderable tests are performed? What is the trend? Has total volume or a specific test's volume changed enough to warrant a reevaluation of workflow or testing capacity? Should any tests be sent to a reference laboratory rather than performed in-house?
"Exploded" tests	Exploding chemistry panels into individual components provides a more accurate assessment of general testing "load" on analyzers and reagent usage than orderable tests alone. Has volume changed? Is it related to a specific location or a new service?
By location	Has testing volume changed in specific nursing units or outpatient settings? Has the volume of inpatient and outpatient testing changed?
Reference laboratory tests	Are certain tests increasing in volume; if so, why and at what cost? Are total monthly costs changing? (Tests with the highest cost/year are not always the highest volume ones.) Should certain tests be screened for appropriateness? Does it make sense to perform any of these tests in-house ("buy versus make" decision)?
Sample and Test Mapping	
Tubes per hour	Tube handling in chemistry has a direct impact on staff and includes centrifugation, aliquoting, and storage.
Tests per hour by department or workstation	This is needed to compare "testing demand" versus "instrument capacity" and can help determine optimal instrument configuration.

these future enhancements may seem attractive, they may not materialize, so they should not be a primary reason for choosing technology. A better approach is to delay purchasing the system until it can offer the laboratory the capabilities it needs. Another potential mistake is overestimating a technology's lifetime or usefulness because this will underestimate its true cost. In the end, the question each laboratorian should ask is not "Does this technology work?" but rather "Does this technology work for me?"

Optimizing Performance

Optimizing performance refers to the process by which workflow (including laboratory design) and technology are integrated to yield an operation that best meets the clinical needs and financial goals of the organization: high quality at low cost. In practice, there are times when workflow changes improve service levels and reduce cost. For example, consolidating chemistry systems may lower capital and operating costs and may improve turnaround time. At other times, there is a tradeoff between cost and quality. For example, a phlebotomy staff reduction, while lowering costs, may lengthen the time necessary to complete morning blood collection. This, in turn, may delay when test results become available, but this may not be significant if results are not needed until later in the day. On the other hand, if a patient's discharge is contingent on reviewing the result in the morning, a testing delay could increase length of stay. Ultimately, these decisions need to be analyzed within the framework of the overall institution, taking into account the downstream impact of these actions and their effects on other departments.

Optimizing performance is an ongoing process that requires one to constantly assess and reassess workflow and needs. This requires periodic data collection and analysis. Table 2-6 provides examples of workflow metrics that are useful to monitor. Ultimately, the degree to which any of these reports is useful depends on the accuracy of the data. Many different approaches may be taken to optimizing performance; some of the more common ones are discussed here and in Table 2-7.

Consolidation, integration, and standardization are three key interrelated strategies that have assumed increasing importance in recent years as laboratories have become affiliated with one another through large health care networks. These concepts are also relevant to a single facility.

Consolidation. Testing can be consolidated from multiple sites or workstations in a single facility, or selected tests from many facilities can be centralized in one or more locations. Consolidation creates larger sample batches or runs; this improves testing efficiency in that fixed quality control and calibration costs are distributed over more samples. This, in turn, lowers per unit costs. Consolidation may yield larger reference laboratory test volume. A "make versus buy" analysis can determine whether it is economically feasible to insource tests previously sent to a reference laboratory (Kisner, 2003). Consolidation may also improve turnaround time by making it cost-effective to perform tests more frequently or to use a more automated technology. Some tests may not be appropriate to consolidate. For example, blood gases and other point-of-care tests may have to be performed at multiple sites in a hospital to provide the necessary turnaround time demanded by clinicians. Similarly, little benefit may be derived from performing routine hospital complete blood counts (CBCs) at a central off-site location instead of at the main hospital rapid response laboratory. In contrast, it may be beneficial to consolidate across facilities those tests that are less time-sensitive (e.g., tumor markers) or that require special skills and/or dedicated equipment at each site (e.g., microbiology services). To successfully consolidate tests from multiple facilities, a central site must control new costs (by minimizing additional staff or equipment to perform the tests) and provide better or comparable quality and service to what had been provided (Carter, 2004). It must also foster a collaborative approach to ensure that all of the sending facility's needs are met, including common physician concerns such as longer turnaround time and limited ability to access information or interact with a remote laboratory. A successful consolidation should be transparent to the clinician.

Standardization. Standardized policies, methods, and equipment benefit laboratories in several ways. Direct benefits, like lower costs, can be realized when the laboratory aggressively negotiates with one vendor to supply all chemistry or hematology equipment and reagents. Indirect benefits are due to the simplified operations that result from standardization and make it easier to cross-train staff or implement policies and procedures. Standardization is a gradual process that can take several years to complete. Rapid transition usually is not possible because of vendor contract lock-ins; a buyout of an existing contract is usually too expensive and can partially

TABLE 2-7
Strategies to Optimize Performance

Strategy	Example
Consolidate	One facility: Run stat and routine samples together on the same analyzer; run routine and specialty tests on the same platform; collapse number of analyzers and workstations and use workcell, if applicable. Consolidation can reduce "tube labor." Multiple facilities: Centralize selected low volume, high cost tests/services at a single location (e.g., molecular diagnostics [HIV viral load], blood donor collection).
Standardize	Equipment: All equipment purchased from one vendor yields larger volume discounts and lower costs for reagents and analyzers, especially in chemistry and immunodiagnostics. Method: Uniform reference range for all laboratories promotes seamless testing environment for inpatients and outpatients with data comparability and trending results across laboratories; it also provides system backup without excess redundancy. Policies: Simplify procedure manuals and compliance documents so they can be shared. Staff: Standardized operations make it easier to share staff among facilities. LIS: Database management is simplified.
Integrate	Computer: Network LIS system with other data systems to promote seamless flow (e.g., sending point-of-care results into the LIS). Courier: Use single service to deliver samples among multiple sites.
Strategic sourcing	Long-term strategy: Competitively bid equipment, supplies, reference laboratory services, etc., taking into account payment terms, delivery charges, value-added services, and product costs.
Rapid repricing	Short-term strategy: Renegotiate pricing with existing vendors.
"Make versus buy"	Review all send-out tests and low volume in-house tests to identify which tests to "buy" (i.e., send out or outsource) and which to "make" (i.e., do in-house) based on cost and turnaround time. Also, review services such as couriers.
Review laboratory policies and tasks	Critically review laboratory policies and procedures to determine their relevance and appropriateness: Can delta check limits be narrowed or eliminated to reduce the numbers of test repeats and verifications without compromising quality? Are critical call values clinically appropriate, or do they generate unnecessary calls to physicians? Can nonurgent expensive tests be batched twice weekly instead of every day? Do clinicians need certain tests daily that are available only several times a week? Are quality control and maintenance procedures excessive?
Make maximum use of simple and/or existing IT solutions	Rule-based autoverification process eliminates need for technologist to manually release each result (Crolla, 2003); sample racking storage system eliminates most of the time spent looking for samples.
Cross-train staff	Train technologists to perform automated chemistry and hematology tests instead of chemistry or hematology alone.
Adjust skill mix	Adjust skill level (and compensation) of staff to match task performed: Use laboratory helpers instead of technologists to centrifuge samples or load samples on analyzers.
Adjust staff scheduling	Use part-time phlebotomists to supplement peak blood collection periods instead of full-time phlebotomists who are underutilized once morning collection is finished.
Change laboratory layout	Design open laboratory that allows all automated testing to run in the same location and promotes cross-training of staff.
Manage utilization	Require pathologist or director approval to order select costly reference laboratory tests, and/or restrict usage of various tests to specialists.

HIV, Human immunodeficiency virus; *IT,* information technology; *LIS,* laboratory information system.

or completely offset any intended savings from a new contract. Sometimes, the unique needs of a location may preclude standardization with other laboratories, or a single vendor may not offer a product line that is suitable for each facility. In these instances, it is still possible to significantly lower costs and/or improve performance albeit using a more varied or limited approach.

Integration. Integration is the process by which services at one location are coordinated, shared, and/or connected to those at another to provide a seamless operation. Although integration is often a byproduct of consolidation and standardization, the latter two strategies are not a prerequisite to successful integration. For example, consider a laboratory information system that links several facilities. Although a single seamless operation can be created with a single vendor's system, it is also possible to network systems from different vendors, albeit with greater difficulty and possibly less functionality. Other integration examples include cross-training staff among different laboratory sections or facilities and interfacing point-of-care laboratory data to the main laboratory system.

Six Sigma and Lean. Six Sigma is a management concept that was first introduced by Motorola in 1979 (Gras, 2007). The ultimate goal is to reduce defects to fewer than 3.4 per million procedures. Lean is a management concept that reduces waste and streamlines an operation (Sunyog, 2004). It was used to describe the automaker Toyota's business process in the 1980s. (See Chapter 1 for a complete discussion of Six Sigma and Lean).

Managing Utilization. Thus far, strategies to optimize performance have focused on ways to do work better and at lower cost. Although this is important, it does not address the most basic question—Is the work, that is, the test, necessary? After all, the least expensive test is the test that is not done. Lowering test volume may change overall operational needs and workflow patterns. Keep in mind that inpatient laboratory work generally is not reimbursed (see Chapter 12), so each laboratory test is an added cost for the hospital. Thus, lowering inpatient utilization has a direct impact on costs. In contrast, outpatient testing generally is reimbursed by a third-party payer or by the patient. Despite this, the amount reimbursed may not be sufficient to cover the cost of the test. This is especially true for expensive new reference laboratory tests for which the laboratory may receive only $0.20–0.30 for each dollar spent. So, selectively controlling outpatient utilization can be financially beneficial. Appropriate utilization of tests does not only mean lowering utilization. In some instances, tests that should be ordered may not be ordered; this could potentially have an impact on patient care and could lengthen stay.

A laboratory may use different strategies to manage utilization depending on the type of test (Lewandrowski, 2003). Over the years, laboratories have realized large cost savings through productivity improvements. As a result, it is far easier and less costly to run a $0.10 test than to determine whether each one is appropriate. Although this is true for many high-volume tests (like CBCs and basic metabolic panels) it is not true for many new, complex, and costly reference laboratory tests such as cancer diagnostics and viral genotyping. Thus, a different strategy is needed to manage utilization of costly reference laboratory tests than to manage CBCs. For example, reference laboratory utilization can be managed by reviewing each order (for certain tests) and its cost with the clinician according to guidelines developed with the clinical services. This cost avoidance strategy not only ensures that clinical indications are met; it also educates physicians about the costs and challenges each one to evaluate the cost-benefit of using it. In contrast, high-volume tests such as a CBC require a broader strategy that restricts or guides ordering frequency electronically through various clinical pathways or guideline-based decision support systems (van Wijk, 2002). For example, a comprehensive or basic metabolic panel might be limited to one order per admission if the patient is stable. Little can be saved by eliminating one low-cost laboratory test from a panel of five other tests. The most significant cost savings is realized when a phlebotomy is eliminated. This usually requires rethinking the frequency of laboratory orders across all clinical services and changing practice patterns to reduce the number of times a patient's blood is collected. Test repetition is a common component of overall test utilization and is costly (van Walraven, 2003).

A laboratory-based diagnostic algorithm can assist with medical decision-making and reduce test utilization. With this approach, a physician requests the laboratory to perform a diagnostic workup (e.g., thyroid function evaluation) instead of ordering specific tests. Thus, the laboratory determines the appropriate tests to run and in what order (Yang, 1996).

EVALUATING EXCESS CAPACITY

Multiple factors are involved in the assessment of whether a laboratory has excess capacity that will allow it to accept additional specimens for testing (Table 2-8).

Philosophy and Mission. Before embarking on a program of expansion in testing, it is essential to establish whether additional work brought into a laboratory is consistent with the role of that laboratory and its parent institution. A privately constituted laboratory without direct affiliation to a medical center might look at the situation simply as a business decision with a potential for profit. In contrast, a laboratory that is part of a hospital would have to consider whether additional testing efforts such as outreach specimens from external clients might interfere with delivery of laboratory services to patients being cared for by that health system. Once a statement of purpose has laid out the overall expectations consistent with the philosophy and mission of the organization, a business plan can be developed to decide the resources needed to achieve expansion of laboratory testing.

TABLE 2-8
Factors for Assessing Excess Capacity

Philosophy and mission of laboratory/health system
Maintained service level for existing patients
Revenue enhancement
Business plan
Physical resources
Instrument testing capacity
Periods of peak and slack activity each day
Measurement of actual throughput
Information system enhancements to connect with new clients
Personnel and activities
Preanalytic phase (usually greatly expanded over existing activities within a medical center)
Specimen transport by couriers
Client service representatives/sales persons
Collection of billing and insurance information
Analytic phase
Time and effort study for available time
Specimen receiving, processing, testing, storing, retrieval
Postanalytic phase
Reporting of results by paper, facsimile, computer interface
Economy of scale
Fixed costs of reagents and labor spread over larger number of test specimens
Incremental cost of additional testing

Physical Resource Assessment. Strictly speaking, there would be no sense in growing business by bringing in more specimens for testing if the analytic capability of available laboratory instruments is not sufficient to perform it. In practice, most laboratories have slack periods every day when relatively low numbers of specimens arrive, thereby lending credibility to the idea of excess testing capacity. In addition, it is a generally accepted principle that redundancy of essential analyzers should be maintained, further increasing excess capacity.

Most automated instruments have a product claim of numbers of specimens tested per hour; however, this number could actually be lower than claimed, depending on how many different tests of varying complexity are ordered on each specimen. In addition, it is necessary to take into account both scheduled and actual downtimes for daily and periodic preventive maintenance, for quality control and proficiency specimens, for repeat testing of problem specimens, and for general troubleshooting of unanticipated problems. A review of turnaround times and numbers of specimens tested at peak hours of specimen arrival could yield a reasonable estimate of throughput capacity at greatest efficiency with all instruments fully functional and with a steady supply of specimens to test. Other factors such as speed of delivery of specimens manually or on an automated track system, capacity to process specimens by batching for centrifugation, and time for each batch to be readied for analysis must also be taken into account. Of course, an assessment that comes up short on analytic capacity might be justification for acquisition of additional analyzers to handle increased test volumes.

A particular concern with accepting testing from new clients is the connectivity of information systems and what might need to be done to facilitate direct interface between physician office computers and the computer of a laboratory in a hospital for purposes of ordering and reporting of results and correct billing and insurance information. The costs of computers, interface devices, and software must be taken into account for new client sites.

Personnel. A key question on expansion of testing is whether existing personnel will be sufficient to perform not only additional analytic tasks but also other activities associated with the acquisition and handling of specimens from other sites. A time and effort study can reveal how much time each employee spends receiving, processing, testing, and storing specimens, and retrieving specimens for tests added later. The effort involved in other tasks must also be accounted for; these include instrument calibrations, quality control, proficiency testing, troubleshooting, review of results for repeat testing, proportion of repeat testing, preventive maintenance, and interactions with other personnel both within and outside the laboratory. Factors for vacation and sick leave as well as work breaks and lunch must be included. This type of analysis can measure the amount of time available to perform more testing without increasing the number of employees.

In reality, increasing the number of specimens from new sources and sites such as physician offices will require new tasks to be performed, such as specimen transport and delivery by couriers, account acquisition and maintenance by client service representatives/sales personnel, entry of correct billing and insurance information, and reporting of test results by various means such as paper copy, facsimile transmission, computer interface between laboratory and physician office information systems, and even telephoning of critical results.

Expansion and Economy of Scale. The simplest way to estimate the costs of reagents and other consumable supplies for increased testing volumes is to use the existing rate of such expenses for existing volumes. In fact, whenever an increase in volume can be managed without performing additional calibrations or quality control testing, then this economy of scale allows the additional work to be done at an incremental cost consisting of only the additional reagents and consumables. This economy of scale also extends to labor costs whenever excess capacity exists and no additional personnel are needed to perform more tests. Thus fixed costs become a smaller percentage of operating expenses as the volume of test specimens increases.

Most laboratories at some point will have the need to assess the feasibility of adding testing to enhance revenues. For this reason and also simply to be prepared for expansion of testing requirements from existing clients, it is good practice to periodically update the laboratory's capacity to expand delivery of services.

SELECTED REFERENCES

De Cresce RP, Lifshitz MS. Integrating automation into the clinical laboratory. In: Lifshitz MS, De Cresce RP, editors. Perspectives on clinical laboratory automation. New York: WB Saunders; 1988. p. 759–74.

General overview of how to analyze workflow and evaluate technology, including many practical considerations.

Middleton S, Mountain P. Process control and on-line optimization. In: Kost GJ, editor. Handbook of clinical automation, robotics and optimization. New York: John Wiley & Sons; 1996. p. 515–40.

Provides an overview of task and process mapping using flow diagrams. Also discusses how to integrate automation, information systems, and staff to optimize performance.

REFERENCES

Access the complete reference list online at http://www.expertconsult.com

CHAPTER 3

PREANALYSIS

Kimberly W. Sanford, Richard A. McPherson

KEY POINTS

- Errors and variables in the preanalysis stage can affect test results.
- Patient variables include physical activity, diet, age, sex, circadian variations, posture, stress, obesity, smoking, and medication.
- Strict adherence to proper technique and site selection can minimize collection variables such as hemolysis, hemoconcentration, clots, and other causes for sample rejection or erroneous results.
- Blood collection containers are color-coded based on additive or preservative, and each is suitable only for specific tests. Failure to use the proper tubes or filling tubes in the wrong sequence can produce erroneous results.
- Blood collection staff must be adequately trained in safety and confidentiality issues.
- Blood, urine, and other body fluid constituents can change during transport and storage. The extent of these changes varies by analyte.
- The most common reasons for specimen rejection are clotted blood for hematology or coagulation tests; insufficient volume in a tube for coagulation tests; and hemolysis, icterus, and lipemia in serum or plasma that can cause interferences in chemistry testing.

Preanalysis refers to all the complex steps that must take place before a sample can be analyzed. Over the years, a series of studies identified that 32%–75% of all testing errors occur in the preanalytic phase (Bonini, 2002; Hofgartner, 1999; Lapworth, 1994; Plebani, 2010; Stahl, 1998), and technologic advances and quality assurance procedures have significantly reduced the number of analytic-based errors. This has exposed the preanalysis stage as a major source of residual "error" and/or variables that can affect test results. Preanalytic factors include patient-related variables (diet, age, sex, etc.), specimen collection and labeling techniques, specimen preservatives and anticoagulants, specimen transport, and processing and storage. Potential sources of error or failure in this process include improperly ordered tests, sample misidentification, improper timing, improper fasting, improper anticoagulant/blood ratio, improper mixing, incorrect order of draw, and hemolyzed or lipemic specimens. The most frequent preanalytic errors include improperly filling the sample tube, placing specimens in the wrong containers or preservatives, and selecting the incorrect test (Plebani, 2010). Table 3-1 lists 10 of the most common errors associated with specimen collection.

Errors in the preanalytic stage create rework or additional investigation that may cause unnecessary procedures for patients and costs to the health care system (Stankovic, 2010). Preanalytic issues have downstream impact on the use of laboratory resources, hospital costs, and overall quality of care. By some estimates, specimen collection errors cost the average 400-bed hospital about $200,000/year in re-collection costs. Proper collection technique is also essential to minimize injury to the phlebotomist and the patient. Treatment for an injury related to a traumatic needlestick can cost $500–$3000, and poor technique can result in patient injury such as nerve and arterial damage, subcutaneous hemorrhage, infection, and even death. The Centers for Disease Control and Prevention (CDC) estimates that 385,000 needlestick injuries occur per year (CDC, 2008). Many go unreported. This chapter discusses the preanalytic process with special emphasis on the clinical impact of variables and sources of failure.

PRECOLLECTION VARIABLES

In preparing a patient for phlebotomy, care should be taken to minimize physiologic factors related to activities that might influence laboratory determinations. These include diurnal variation, exercise, fasting, diet, ethanol consumption, tobacco smoking, drug ingestion, and posture.

PHYSIOLOGIC FACTORS

Diurnal variation. This may be encountered when testing for hormones, iron, acid phosphatase, and urinary excretion of most electrolytes such as sodium, potassium, and phosphate (Dufour, 2003). Table 3-2 presents several tests affected by diurnal variations, posture, and stress.

Exercise. Physical activity has transient and long-term effects on laboratory determinations. Transient changes may include an initial decrease

TABLE 3-1
Ten Common Errors in Specimen Collection

1. Misidentification of patient
2. Mislabeling of specimen
3. Short draws/wrong anticoagulant/blood ratio
4. Mixing problems/clots
5. Wrong tubes/wrong anticoagulant
6. Hemolysis/lipemia
7. Hemoconcentration from prolonged tourniquet time
8. Exposure to light/extreme temperatures
9. Improperly timed specimens/delayed delivery to laboratory
10. Processing errors: Incomplete centrifugation, incorrect log-in, improper storage

followed by an increase in free fatty acids, and lactate may increase by as much as 300%. Exercise may elevate creatine phosphokinase (CK), aspartate aminotransferase (AST), and lactate dehydrogenase (LD), and may activate coagulation, fibrinolysis, and platelets (Garza, 1989). These changes are related to increased metabolic activities for energy purposes and usually return to preexercise levels soon after exercise cessation. Long-term effects of exercise may increase CK, aldolase, AST, and LD values. Chronic aerobic exercise is associated with lesser increases in plasma concentration of muscle enzymes such as CK, AST, alanine aminotransferase (ALT), and LD. Decreased levels of serum gonadotropin and sex steroid concentrations are seen in long-distance athletes while prolactin levels are elevated (Dufour, 2003).

Diet. An individual's diet can greatly affect laboratory test results. The effect is transient and is easily controlled. Glucose and triglycerides, absorbed from food, increase after eating (Dufour, 2003). After 48 hours of fasting, serum bilirubin concentrations may increase. Fasting for 72 hours decreases plasma glucose levels in healthy women to 45 mg/dL (2.5 mmol/L), while men show an increase in plasma triglycerides, glycerol, and free fatty acids, with no significant change in plasma cholesterol. When determining blood constituents such as glucose, triglycerides, cholesterol, and electrolytes, collection should be done in the basal state (Garza, 1989). Eating a meal, depending on fat content, may elevate plasma potassium, triglycerides, alkaline phosphatase, and 5-hydroxyindoleacetic acid (5-HIAA). Stool occult blood tests, which detect heme, are affected by the intake of meat, fish, iron, and horseradish, a source of peroxidase, causing a false-positive occult blood reaction (Dufour, 2003). Physiologic changes may include hyperchylomicronemia, thus increasing turbidity of the serum or plasma and potentially interfering with instrument readings.

Certain foods or diet regimens may affect serum or urine constituents. Long-time vegetarian diets are reported to cause decreased concentrations of low-density lipoproteins (LDLs), very-low-density lipoproteins (VLDLs), total lipids, phospholipids, cholesterol, and triglycerides. Vitamin B_{12} deficiency can also occur, unless supplements are taken (Young, 2001). A high meat or other protein-rich diet may increase serum urea, ammonia, and urate levels. High protein, low carbohydrate diets, such as the Atkins diet, greatly increase ketones in the urine and increase the serum blood urea nitrogen (BUN). Foods with a high unsaturated-to-saturated fatty acid ratio may show decreased serum cholesterol, while a diet rich in purines will show an increased urate value. Foods such as bananas, pineapples, tomatoes, and avocados are rich in serotonin. When ingested, elevated urine excretion of 5-HIAA may be observed. Beverages rich in caffeine elevate plasma free fatty acids and cause catecholamine release from the adrenal medulla and brain tissue. Ethanol ingestion increases plasma lactate, urate, and triglyceride concentrations. Elevated high-density lipoprotein (HDL) cholesterol, γ-glutamyl transferase (GGT), urate, and mean corpuscular volume (MCV) have been associated with chronic alcohol abuse.

Serum concentrations of cholesterol, triglycerides, and apoB lipoproteins are correlated with obesity. Serum LD activity, cortisol production, and glucose increase in obesity. Plasma insulin concentration is also increased, but glucose tolerance is impaired. In obese men, testosterone concentration is reduced (Young, 2001).

Stress. Mental and physical stresses induce the production of adrenocorticotropic hormone (ACTH), cortisol, and catecholamines. Total cholesterol has been reported to increase with mild stress, and HDL cholesterol

TABLE 3-2
Tests Affected by Diurnal Variation, Posture, and Stress

Cortisol	Peaks 4–6 AM; lowest 8 PM–12 AM; 50% lower at 8 PM than at 8 AM; increased with stress
Adrenocorticotropic hormone	Lower at night; increased with stress
Plasma renin activity	Lower at night; higher standing than supine
Aldosterone	Lower at night
Insulin	Lower at night
Growth hormone	Higher in afternoon and evening
Acid phosphatase	Higher in afternoon and evening
Thyroxine	Increases with exercise
Prolactin	Higher with stress; higher levels at 4 and 8 AM and at 8 and 10 PM
Iron	Peaks early to late morning; decreases up to 30% during the day
Calcium	4% decrease supine

to decrease by as much as 15% (Dufour, 2003). Hyperventilation affects acid-base balance and elevates leukocyte counts, serum lactate, or free fatty acids.

Posture. Posture of the patient during phlebotomy can have an effect on various laboratory results. An upright position increases hydrostatic pressure, causing a reduction of plasma volume and increased concentration of proteins. Albumin and calcium levels may become elevated as one changes position from supine to upright. Elements that are affected by postural changes are albumin, total protein, enzymes, calcium, bilirubin, cholesterol, triglycerides, and drugs bound to proteins. Incorrect application of the tourniquet and fist exercise can result in erroneous test results. Using a tourniquet to collect blood to determine lactate concentration may result in falsely increased values. Prolonged tourniquet application may also increase serum enzymes, proteins, and protein-bound substances, including cholesterol, calcium, and triglycerides, as the result of hemoconcentration when plasma water leaves the vein because of back pressure. After bed rest in the hospital, a patient's hemoglobin (Hb) can decrease from the original admitting value enough to falsely lead a physician to suspect internal hemorrhage or hemolysis (Dufour, 2003). This effect can be amplified by intravenous fluid administration. Patients should be advised to avoid changes in their diet, consumption of alcohol, and strenuous exercise 24 hours before having their blood drawn for laboratory testing.

Age. Age of the patient has an effect on serum constituents. Young defines four age groups: newborn, childhood to puberty, adult, and elderly adult (Young, 2001). In the newborn, much of the Hb is Hb F, not Hb A, as seen in the adult. Bilirubin concentration rises after birth and peaks at about 5 days. In cases of hemolytic disease of the fetus and newborn (HDFN), bilirubin levels continue to rise. This often causes difficulty in distinguishing between physiologic jaundice and HDFN. Infants have a lower glucose level than adults because of their low glycogen reserve. With skeletal growth and muscle development, serum alkaline phosphatase and creatinine levels, respectively, also increase. The high uric acid level seen in a newborn decreases for the first 10 years of life, then increases, especially in boys, until the age of 16 (Young, 2001). Most serum constituents remain constant during adult life until the onset of menopause in women and middle age in men. Increases of about 2 mg/dL (0.05 mmol/L) per year in total cholesterol and 2 mg/dL (0.02 mmol/L) per year in triglycerides until midlife have been reported. The increase in cholesterol seen in postmenopausal women has been attributed to a decrease in estrogen levels. Uric acid levels peak in men in their 20s but do not peak in women until middle age. The elderly secrete less triiodothyronine, parathyroid hormone, aldosterone, and cortisol. After age 50, men experience a decrease in secretion rate and concentration of testosterone and women have an increase in pituitary gonadotropins, especially follicle-stimulating hormone (FSH) (Young, 2001).

Gender. After puberty, men generally have higher alkaline phosphatase, aminotransferase, creatine kinase, and aldolase levels than women; this is due to the larger muscle mass of men. Women have lower levels of magnesium, calcium, albumin, Hb, serum iron, and ferritin. Menstrual blood loss contributes to the lower iron values (Young, 2001).

TABLE 3-3

Changes in Serum Concentration (or Activities) of Selected Constituents Due to Lysis of Erythrocytes (RBCs)

Constituent	Ratio of concentration (or activity) in RBC to concentration (or activity) in serum	Percent change of concentration (or activity) in serum after lysis of 1% RBC, assuming a hematocrit of 0.50
Lactate dehydrogenase	16:1	+272.0
Aspartate aminotransferase	4:1	+220.0
Potassium	23:1	+24.4
Alanine aminotransferase	6.7:1	+55.0
Glucose	0.82:1	−5.0
Inorganic phosphate	0.78:1	+9.1
Sodium	0.11:1	−1.0
Calcium	0.10:1	+2.9

Modified from Caraway WT, Kammeyer CW. Chemical interference by drug and other substances with clinical laboratory test procedures. Clin Chem Acta 1972; 41:395; and Laessig RH, Hassermer DJ, Paskay TA, et al. The effects of 0.1 and 1.0 percent erythrocytes and hemolysis on serum chemistry values. Am J Clin Pathol 1976; 66:639–644, with permission.

COMMON INTERFERENCES

In Vivo

Tobacco Smoking

Tobacco smokers have high blood carboxyhemoglobin levels, plasma catecholamines, and serum cortisol. Changes in these hormones often result in decreased numbers of eosinophils, while neutrophils, monocytes, and plasma fatty free acids increase. Chronic effects of smoking lead to increased Hb concentration, erythrocyte (RBC) count, MCV, and leukocyte (WBC) count. Increased plasma levels of lactate, insulin, epinephrine, and growth hormone and urinary secretion of 5-HIAA are also seen. Vitamin B_{12} levels may be substantially decreased and have been reported to be inversely proportional to serum thiocyanate levels. Smoking also affects the body's immune response. Immunoglobulin (Ig)A, IgG, and IgM are lower in smokers, and IgE levels are higher. Decreased sperm counts and motility and increased abnormal morphology have been reported in male smokers when compared with nonsmokers (Young, 2001).

In Vitro

Collection-Associated Variables

On occasion, when there is a problem finding a vein for phlebotomy, the specimen may be hemolyzed as the result of sheer forces on the red blood cells. Hemolysis can also be caused by using a needle that is too small, pulling a syringe plunger back too fast, expelling the blood vigorously into a tube, shaking or mixing the tubes vigorously, or performing blood collection before the alcohol has dried at the collection site. Hemolysis is present when the serum or plasma layer is pink. Hemolysis can falsely increase blood constituents such as potassium, magnesium, iron, LD, phosphorus, ammonium, and total protein (Garza, 2002). Table 3-3 shows changes in serum concentrations (or activities) of selected constituents caused by lysis of RBCs.

Because of the extremely important role of potassium in cardiac excitation, elevations due to hemolysis can be problematic, especially for emergency room patients who are at risk of hemolysis during frantic blood collection. The relationship between level of hemolysis and potassium (as determined on a Siemens ADVIA 1650 chemistry analyzer [Siemens Healthcare Diagnostics, Deerfield, Ill.]) in serum and plasma specimens is shown in Figure 3-1. Even with no hemolysis, the range of potassium concentrations can be broad in a combination of healthy and sick individuals. Low levels of hemolysis cause only minor elevations, but very strong hemolysis can raise the potassium level by 2 to 3 mEq/L into a critical range.

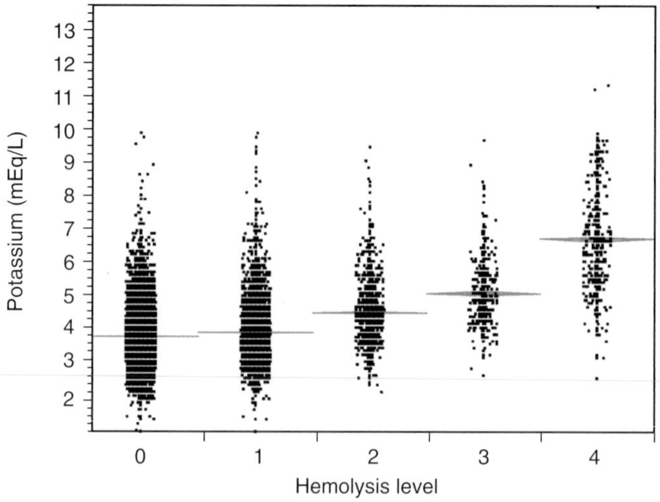

Figure 3-1 Relationship between hemolysis and potassium in 60,989 serum and plasma specimens grouped according to level of hemolysis. The mean values of potassium were 4.12, 4.23, 4.80, 5.36, and 6.93 mEq/L for levels of hemolysis from 0 through 4, respectively.

Another special case where pseudohyperkalemia can occur is in patients with extremely high blast counts in acute or accelerated phase leukemias. Those blasts can be fragile and may lyse during standard phlebotomy, releasing potassium. In contrast, specimens with very high WBC counts that are collected gently can show pseudohypokalemia when potassium is taken up by highly metabolically active leukemic cells along with glucose; such specimens can be transported on ice to slow this enzymatically mediated uptake.

Normally platelets release potassium during clotting, so serum has a slightly higher value of potassium than plasma from the same individual; this difference is accentuated when the platelet count is extremely elevated.

To avoid problems with hemoconcentration and hemodilution, the patient should be seated in a supine position for 15 to 20 minutes before the blood is drawn (Young, 2001). Extended application of the tourniquet can cause hemoconcentration, which increases the concentrations of analytes and cellular components. When blood collection tubes that contain various anticoagulants/additives are used, it is important to follow the proper order of draw and to thoroughly mix an anticoagulated tube of blood after it has been filled. Failure to mix a tube containing an anticoagulant will result in failure to anticoagulate the entire blood specimen, and small clots may be formed. Erroneous cell counts can result. If a clot is present, it may also occlude or otherwise interfere with an automated analyzer. It is very important that the proper anticoagulant be used for the test ordered. Using the wrong anticoagulant will greatly affect the test results.

Each collection tube containing an anticoagulant has a specific manufacturer's color code. Icteric or lipemic serum provides additional challenges in laboratory analysis. When serum bilirubin approaches 430 mmol/L (25 mg/L), interference may be observed in assays for albumin (4-hydroxyazobenzene-2-carboxylic acid [HABA] procedure), cholesterol (using ferric chloride reagents), and total protein (Biuret procedure). Artifactually induced values in some laboratory determinations result when triglyceride levels are elevated (turbidity) on the basis of absorbance of light of various lipid particles. Lipemia occurs when serum triglyceride levels exceed 4.6 mmol/L (400 mg/dL). Inhibition of assays for amylase, urate, urea, CK, bilirubin, and total protein may be observed. To correct for artifactual absorbance readings, "blanking" procedures (the blank contains serum, but lacks a crucial element to complete the assay) or dual-wavelength methods may be used. A blanking process may not be effective in some cases of turbidity, and ultracentrifugation may be necessary to clear the serum or plasma of chylomicrons.

SPECIMEN COLLECTION

THE TEST ORDER

One of the most frequent preanalytic errors involves selecting the wrong laboratory test or panel of tests, leading to inappropriate interpretation of results (Bonini, 2002). Laboratory tests are usually ordered electronically (e.g., computer) or in writing (e.g., paper requisition). This information is conveyed through written or computer order entry. Online computer input is the most error-free means of requesting laboratory tests. The clinician initiates the request for a laboratory measurement or examination by completing a written order for desired laboratory measurements or examinations in the patient's medical record or chart. Verbal requests are made in emergency situations and should be documented on a standard form; after the blood is drawn, an official laboratory request or computerized order should be placed (Garza, 2002). Physician direct order entry and result acquisition through user-friendly networked computers are realistic approaches to providing prompt and accurate patient care. Patient demographics include the patient's name, sex, age, date of birth (DOB), date of admission, date on which measurement or examination was ordered, hospital number, room number, physician, and physician's pharmacy code number. Computerized laboratory information systems (LISs), common in today's laboratories, are used to generate requisitions and specimen labels. Some systems also generate requisitions with the number of tubes and the types of tubes required for collection.

Most laboratories facilitate test ordering by providing a written or computerized medical information system, which lists available tests, types of specimens required, collection methods, color of blood collection tubes used, amounts of blood/body fluid required, turnaround time, reference intervals, test codes, costs, diagnostic information, etc. All specimens must be clearly labeled. Preprinted bar code labels applied after proper patient identification, and after the specimen is collected, avoid preanalytic transcription errors. Frequently, the laboratory receives requests for "add-ons." These are additional tests requested to be performed on a specimen that has previously been collected. Problems are encountered when the specimen is not the proper type for the add-on requested test, the residual volume is not sufficient to perform the test, or storage conditions result in deterioration of the analyte (e.g., bicarbonate). This is usually due to the presence or absence of a particular anticoagulant or additive. All add-on requests must be documented.

Medicolegal concerns include proper identification of the patient, proper labeling of the specimen, patient consent issues, patient privacy issues, and chain of custody. Laboratories should have clearly written policies for these issues. In addition, policies should describe what to do when a patient refuses to have blood drawn, what to do if the patient was unable to be drawn, what to do if a patient is unavailable, and how to deal with a combative patient, as well as emergency measures for patients who become ill or faint during phlebotomy. The Health Insurance Portability and Accountability Act (HIPAA) ensures the security and privacy of health data and protects the confidentiality of all patient record information, including all laboratory data. Employees must be trained to comply with HIPAA.

TIME OF COLLECTION

Sometimes, samples have to be collected at a specific time. Failure to follow the planned time schedule can lead to erroneous results and misinterpretation of a patient's condition. The most common tests in this category are the ASAP and stat collections. ASAP means "as soon as possible" and stat is an American medical term meaning "immediately" (from the Latin "statim"). The exact definitions of these terms vary from one laboratory to another. Stat specimens are collected and analyzed immediately. They are given the highest priority and are usually ordered from the emergency department and critical care units (Strasinger, 2003). Timed specimens are ordered for a variety of reasons, usually to monitor changes in a patient's condition, to determine the level of a medication, or to measure how well a substance is metabolized. For example, a physician may want to monitor a cardiac marker to determine if it is rising or decreasing. In therapeutic drug monitoring, trough and peak levels of a drug may be ordered. Trough specimens reflect the lowest level in the blood and are generally drawn 30 minutes before the drug is administered. The peak specimen is drawn shortly after the medication is given; the actual collection time varies by medication. Drug manufacturers specify the length of time that must pass between trough and peak collection times. Measuring how well the body metabolizes glucose involves a 2-hour postprandial specimen and/or a glucose tolerance test. Two-hour postprandial specimens are drawn 2 hours after the patient eats a meal. Results are compared with those of the fasting level. In a glucose tolerance test, multiple samples are drawn over time—one sample before and one or more after the administration of a standardized glucose solution. This test is used to diagnose diabetes mellitus by determining how well the body metabolizes glucose over a given time period.

TABLE 3-4
Reasons for Specimen Rejection

Hemolysis/lipemia
Clots present in an anticoagulated specimen
Nonfasting specimen when test requires fasting
Improper blood collection tube
Short draws, wrong volume
Improper transport conditions (ice for blood gases)
Discrepancies between requisition and specimen label
Unlabeled or mislabeled specimen
Contaminated specimen/leaking container

SPECIMEN REJECTION

All specimens must be collected, labeled, transported, and processed according to established procedures that include sample volume, special handling needs, and container type. Failure to follow specific procedures can result in specimen rejection. Inappropriate specimen type, wrong preservative, hemolysis, lipemia, clots, etc., are reasons for rejection. Not only is specimen rejection costly and time-consuming, it may cause harm to the patient, especially when the blood sample in the tube is mislabeled. The first goal of The Joint Commission 2008 National Patient Safety Goals for Laboratories is to improve "the accuracy of patient identification" (www.jointcommission.org/PatientSafety/NationalPatientSafetyGoals). Misidentification of patients during sample collection for transfusion or at the time of transfusion can be a life-threatening medical error. The incidence of patient misidentification at the time of specimen collection is approximately 1 in 1000, and 1 in 12,000 patients receives a unit of blood that was not intended for that individual (Dzik, 2003; Linden, 2000). As a result, the College of American Pathologists requires laboratories to have a plan to reduce the risk of mistransfusion and suggests as options collecting two samples at separate phlebotomy events, or utilizing an electronic identification verification system such as an electronic bar code reader for patient identification wrist bands (CAP TRM.30575). It is therefore essential to thoroughly train all medical staff in all aspects of patient identification, specimen collection, transportation, and processing. Table 3-4 lists various reasons for specimen rejection.

BLOOD COLLECTION OVERVIEW

Venipuncture is accomplished using a needle/adapter assembly attached to an evacuated glass/plastic test tube with a rubber/plastic stopper. Blood may also be collected in a syringe and transferred to the appropriate specimen container (evacuated tube system). A syringe may be helpful when procuring a specimen from the hand or ankle, or from small children. In addition, patients with small or poor veins may experience collapse of veins with use of an evacuated tube system. AccuVein (AccuVein LLC, Huntington, N.Y.) is a newly marketed hand-held medical device that helps medical staff visualize veins before phlebotomy. The device emits infrared light and is held about 7 inches over the potential phlebotomy site. Hb in the blood absorbs infrared light and projects an image map of the veins onto the patient's overlying skin. The device is able to distinguish between Hb in the veins and surrounding tissue. This device assists the phlebotomist in determining the best site for needle placement, especially for challenging patients such as the elderly, the obese, burn victims, oncology patients, and patients with other chronic diseases requiring many diagnostic or therapeutic procedures (http://www.accuvein.com).

Blood collection tubes have color-coded stoppers that distinguish the presence of a specific anticoagulant or additive, how the tube is chemically cleaned (e.g., for lead or iron determinations), or if the tube does not contain any additives. Table 3-5 lists the most frequently used anticoagulants/additives based on color-coded tube stoppers. Tubes also come in various sizes for adult and pediatric patient populations. Draw volume is determined by the internal vacuum within the sealed tubes (e.g., 3.5, 4.0, 4.5, or 8.5 mL). The use of anticoagulants allows for analysis of whole blood specimens or plasma constituents obtained by centrifugation and separation of the plasma. Plasma contains fibrinogen, which is missing from serum. Many laboratories have converted from glass to plastic collection tubes to minimize exposure to biohazardous material (e.g., blood) and broken glass; to lower biohazard waste disposal costs; and to comply with Occupational Safety and Health Administration (OSHA) guidelines

TABLE 3-5
Tube Color and Anticoagulant/Additive

Stopper color	Anticoagulant/additive	Specimen type/use	Mechanism of action
Red (glass)	None	Serum/chemistry and serology	N/A
Red (plastic/Hemogard)	Clot activator	Serum/chemistry and serology	Silica clot activator
Lavender (glass)	K_3EDTA in liquid form	Whole blood/hematology	Chelates (binds) calcium
Lavender (plastic)	K_2EDTA/spray-dried	Whole blood/hematology	Chelates (binds) calcium
Pink	Spray-dried K_2EDTA	Whole blood/blood bank and molecular diagnostics	Chelates (binds) calcium
White	EDTA and gel	Plasma/molecular diagnostics	Chelates (binds) calcium
Light blue	Sodium citrate	Plasma/coagulation	Chelates (binds) calcium
Light blue	Thrombin and soybean trypsin inhibitor	Plasma/coagulation	Fibrin degradation products
Black	Sodium citrate	Plasma/sed rates—hematology	Chelates (binds) calcium
Light green/black	Lithium heparin and gel	Plasma/chemistry	Inhibits thrombin formation
Green	Sodium heparin, lithium heparin	Plasma/chemistry	Inhibits thrombin formation
Royal blue	Sodium heparin, K_2EDTA	Plasma/chemistry/toxicology	Heparin inhibits thrombin formation Na_2EDTA binds calcium
Gray	Sodium fluoride/potassium oxalate	Plasma/glucose testing	Inhibits glycolysis
Yellow	Sterile containing sodium polyanetholesulfonate	Serum/microbiology culture	Aids in bacterial recovery by inhibiting complement, phagocytes, and certain antibiotics
Yellow	Acid citrate dextrose	Plasma/blood bank, HLA phenotyping, and paternity testing	WBC preservative
Tan (glass)	Sodium heparin	Plasma/lead testing	Inhibits thrombin formation
Tan (plastic)	K_2EDTA	Plasma/lead testing	Chelates (binds) calcium
Yellow/gray and orange	Thrombin	Serum/chemistry	Clot activator
Red/gray and gold	Clot activator separation gel	Serum/chemistry	Silica clot activator

EDTA, Ethylenediaminetetraacetic acid; *HLA,* human leukocyte antigen; *K_2EDTA,* dipotassium form of EDTA; *K_3EDTA,* tripotassium form of EDTA; *N/A,* not applicable; *Na_2EDTA,* disodium EDTA; *WBC,* white blood cell.

TABLE 3-6
Order of Draw: Evacuated Tube and Syringe

1. Blood-culture tubes (yellow)
2. Coagulation sodium citrate tube (blue stopper)
3. Serum tubes with or without clot activator or gel separator
4. Heparin tubes with or without gel (green stopper)
5. Ethylenediaminetetraacetic acid tubes (lavender stopper)
6. Glycolytic inhibitor tubes (gray stopper)

mandating substitution. This change from glass to plastic has required a modification in the order of draw. Glass or plastic tubes with additives, including gel tubes, are drawn after the citrate tube (blue top) to avoid interference with coagulation measurements (Table 3-6). Glass or plastic serum tubes, without a clot activator or gel separator, may be drawn before the coagulation tubes are drawn, consistent with National Committee on Clinical Laboratory Standards (NCCLS) guidelines (H3-A6) (Ernst, 2004).

ANTICOAGULANTS AND ADDITIVES

Ethylenediaminetetraacetic acid (EDTA) is the anticoagulant of choice for hematology cell counts and cell morphology. It is available in lavender-top tubes as a liquid or is spray-dried in the dipotassium or tripotassium salt form (K_2EDTA in plastic, spray-dried, and K_3EDTA in liquid form in glass tubes). K_3EDTA is a liquid and will dilute the sample ≈ 1%–2%. K_2EDTA is spray-dried on the walls of the tube and will not dilute the sample. Pink-top tubes also contain EDTA. The EDTA is spray-dried K_2EDTA. Pink tubes are used in immunohematology for ABO grouping, Rh typing, and antibody screening. These tubes have a special cross-match label for information required by the American Association of Blood Banks (AABB) and approved by the U.S. Food and Drug Administration (FDA) for blood bank collections. White-top tubes also contain EDTA and gel. They are used most often for molecular diagnostic testing of plasma. For coagulation testing, a light blue–top tube containing 0.105 M or 0.129 M (3.2% and 3.8%) sodium citrate is commonly used because it preserves the labile coagulation factors. Black-top tubes also contain buffered sodium citrate and are generally used for Westergren sedimentation rates, as are lavender-top tubes. They differ from light blue–top tubes in that the ratio of blood to anticoagulant is 4:1 in the black-top tubes and 9:1 in the light blue–top tubes.

Heparin, a mucoitin polysulfuric acid, is an effective anticoagulant in small quantities without significant effect on many determinations. Heparin was originally isolated from liver cells by scientists looking for an anticoagulant that could work safely in humans. Heparin is available as lithium heparin (LiHep) and sodium heparin (NaHep) in green-top tubes. Heparin accelerates the action of antithrombin III, neutralizing thrombin and preventing the formation of fibrin. Heparin has an advantage over EDTA as an anticoagulant, as it does not affect levels of ions such as calcium. However, heparin can interfere with some immunoassays. Heparin should not be used for coagulation or hematology testing. Heparinized plasma is preferred for potassium measurements to avoid an elevation due to the release of potassium from platelets as the blood clots (Garza, 2002). Lithium heparin may be used for most chemistry tests except for lithium and folate levels; for lithium, a serum specimen can be used instead. Sodium heparin cannot be used for assays measuring sodium levels, but it is recommended for trace elements, leads, and toxicology. Sodium heparin is the injectable form used for anticoagulant therapy.

Gray-top tubes are generally used for glucose measurements because they contain a preservative or antiglycolytic agent, such as sodium fluoride, which prevents glycolysis for 3 days (Strasinger, 2003). In bacterial septicemia, fluoride inhibition of glycolysis is neither adequate nor effective in preserving glucose concentration. Red-top tubes have no additive, so blood collected in these tubes clots.

Red-top tubes are used for most chemistry, blood bank, and immunology assays. Integrated serum separator tubes are available for isolating serum from whole blood. During centrifugation, blood is forced into a thixotropic gel material located at the base of the tube. The gel undergoes a temporary change in viscosity during centrifugation and lodges between the packed cells and the top serum layer (Strasinger, 2003). Pediatric-sized tubes are also available. Advantages of serum separator tubes include (1) ease of use, (2) shorter processing time through clot activation, (3) higher serum yield, (4) minimal liberation of potentially hazardous aerosols, (5) only one centrifugation step, (6) use of single tube (same one as patient specimen), and (7) ease of a single label. A unique advantage is that centrifuged specimens can be transported without disturbing the separation.

TABLE 3-7
Anticoagulant/Additive Effect on Blood Tests

Additive	Test	Effect
EDTA	Alkaline phosphatase	Inhibits
	Creatine kinase	Inhibits
	Leucine aminopeptidase	Inhibits
	Calcium and iron	Decrease
	PT and PTT	Increase
	Sodium and potassium	Increase
	Platelet aggregation	Prevents
Oxalate	Acid phosphatase	Inhibits
	Alkaline phosphatase	Inhibits
	Amylase	Inhibits
	LD	Inhibits
	Calcium	Decreases
	Sodium and potassium	Increase
	Cell morphology	Distorts
Citrate	ALT and AST	Inhibit
	Alkaline phosphatase	Inhibits
	Acid phosphatase	Stimulates
	Amylase	Decreases
	Calcium	Decreases
	Sodium and potassium	Increase
	Labile coagulation factors	Preserve
Heparin	Triiodothyronine	Increases
	Thyroxine	Increases
	PT and PTT	Increase
	Wright's stain	Causes blue background
	Lithium (LiHep tubes only)	Increases
	Sodium (NaHep tubes only)	Increases
Fluorides	Acid phosphatase	Decreases
	Alkaline phosphatase	Decreases
	Amylase	Decreases
	Creatine kinase	Decreases
	ALT and AST	Decrease
	Cell morphology	Distorts

ALT, Alanine aminotransferase; *AST,* aspartate aminotransferase; *EDTA,* ethylenediaminetetraacetic acid; *LD,* lactate dehydrogenase; *LiHep,* lithium heparin; *NaHep,* sodium heparin; *PT,* prothrombin time; *PTT,* partial thromboplastin time.

Some silica gel serum separation tubes may give rise to minute particles that can cause flow problems during analysis. Filtering the serum solves the problem.

A few specialized tubes exist. Red/gray- and gold-top tubes contain a clot activator and a separation gel. These tubes are referred to as serum separator tubes (SSTs) and are used most often for chemistry tests. Therapeutic drug monitoring specimens should not be collected in tubes that contain gel separators, as some gels absorb certain drugs, causing a falsely lowered result. Significant decreases in phenytoin, phenobarbital, lidocaine, quinidine, and carbamazepine have been reported when stored in Vacutainer SST tubes (Becton, Dickinson, and Company [BD], Franklin Lakes, N.J.), while no changes were noted in theophylline and salicylate levels. Storage in standard red-top Vacutainer collection tubes without barrier gels did not affect measured levels of the above therapeutic drugs (Dasgupta, 1994). Studies indicate that this absorption is time dependent, and therefore speed in processing minimizes absorption. Acrylic-based gels do not exhibit the absorption problems associated with silicone and polyester gels (Garza, 2002).

Tubes containing gels are not used in the blood bank or for immunologic testing, as the gel may interfere with the immunologic reactions (Strasinger, 2003). Clotting time for tubes using gel separators is approximately 30 minutes, and tubes that have clot activators, such as thrombin, will clot in 5 minutes. Plain red-stoppered tubes with no additives take about 60 minutes to clot completely (Strasinger, 2003).

Anticoagulants may affect the transport of water between cell and plasma, thereby altering cell size and constituent plasma concentration. Oxalate anticoagulants may shrink red cells; thus blood anticoagulated with oxalate cannot be used to measure hematocrit. Combined ammonium/potassium oxalate does not have the same effect of shrinking cells.

EDTA, citrate, and oxalate chelate calcium, thereby lowering calcium levels. Fluoride, used for glucose determinations, prevents glycolysis by forming an ionic complex with Mg^{++}, thereby inhibiting the Mg^{++}-dependent enzyme, enolase (Young, 2001). Table 3-7 lists anticoagulants/additives and their effects on various blood tests.

BLOOD COLLECTION DEVICES

The most common blood collection system uses a vacuum to pull blood into a container; it consists of a color-coded evacuated collection tube, a double-headed needle, and an adapter/holder. Small tubes are available for pediatric and geriatric collections. The blood collection holder accommodates various sizes (gauge) of blood collection needles. Needles vary from large (16 gauge) to small (23 gauge). Several types of holders have been designed to eject the needle after use. Recent OSHA policies require that the adapters be discarded with the used needle (OSHA, Needlestick Safety Prevention Act, 2002). Pediatric inserts are available for adapters and accommodate the smaller-diameter pediatric blood collection tubes. Also available are a variety of safety needles that cover the needle after use, or retract the needle before it is discarded.

Winged infusion sets (butterfly needles) can be used when blood has to be collected from a very small vein. Butterfly needles come in 21, 23, and 25 gauge. These needles have plastic wings attached to the end of the needle that aid in insertion of the needle into the small vein. Tubing is attached to the back end of the needle, which terminates with an adapter for attachment to a syringe or evacuated collection holder. Every effort must be made to protect the phlebotomist from being stuck with a used needle when a butterfly infusion set is used.

Blood collected in a syringe can be transferred to an evacuated tube. Special syringe safety shield devices are available to avoid unnecessary contact with the blood sample. If blood requires anticoagulation, speed becomes an important factor, and the blood must be transferred before clot formation begins. Once the blood has been transferred, the anticoagulated tube must be thoroughly mixed to avoid small clot formation.

Several additional pieces of phlebotomy equipment are necessary. A tourniquet, usually a flat latex strip or piece of tubing, is wrapped around the arm to occlude the vein before blood collection and is discarded after each phlebotomy. OSHA guidelines state that gloves should be worn when performing phlebotomy and should be changed between patients. Gloves are available in various sizes and are made of various materials to avoid latex sensitivity as experienced by some individuals. Other supplies include gauze pads, alcohol or iodine wipes for disinfection of the puncture site, and a Band-Aid (Johnson & Johnson, New Brunswick, N.J.) to prevent bleeding after completion of the phlebotomy.

BLOOD STORAGE AND PRESERVATION

During storage, the concentration of a blood constituent in the specimen may change as a result of various processes, including adsorption to glass or plastic tubes, protein denaturation, evaporation of volatile compounds, water movement into cells resulting in hemoconcentration of serum and plasma, and continuing metabolic activities of leukocytes and erythrocytes. These changes occur, although to varying degrees, at ambient temperature and during refrigeration or freezing. Storage requirements vary widely by analyte.

Stability studies have shown that clinically significant analyte changes occur if serum or plasma remains in prolonged contact with blood cells. After separation from blood cells, analytes have the same stability in plasma and serum when stored under the same conditions. Glucose concentration in unseparated serum and plasma decreases rapidly in the first 24 hours and more slowly thereafter. This decrease is more pronounced in plasma. Two approaches have been used to minimize this effect. First, the serum or plasma may be rapidly separated from the red cells, or the specimen may be collected in a fluoride tube to inhibit glycolysis of the red blood cells, thereby stabilizing the glucose level during transport and storage. Fluoride has little effect on reducing glycolysis within the first hour of storage and may not reach complete inhibition until 4 hours of storage. One study has demonstrated a reduction in glucose concentration by 0.39 mmol/L in specimens collected in fluoride that are not immediately separated. These authors suggest that specimens collected in fluoride have a negative bias in blood glucose levels (Shi, 2009). Lactate levels increase, and a greater rise is seen in plasma than in serum. Chloride and total carbon dioxide (CO_2) show a steady decrease over 56 hours, with the degree of change more pronounced in plasma. K^+ is reported to be stable for up to 24 hours, after which a rapid increase takes place. The degree of change is slightly more pronounced in plasma. Unseparated serum and plasma yield clinically significant increases in total bilirubin, sodium, urea, nitrogen, albumin, calcium, magnesium, and total protein. These changes are attributed to movement of water into cells after 24 hours, resulting in hemoconcentration (Boyanton, 2002). Other studies found potassium, phosphorus, and glucose to be the analytes that were least stable in serum not removed from the clot within 30 minutes. Albumin, bicarbonate, chloride, C-peptide, HDL-cholesterol, iron, LDL-cholesterol, and total protein were found to be unstable after 6 hours when the serum was not separated from the clot (Zhang, 1998).

When serum and plasma are not removed from the cells, lipids (such as cholesterol) and some enzymes increase over time, with the change more pronounced in plasma than in serum. LD activity continuously increases over 56 hours. AST, ALT, and CK were found to be stable over 56 hours. GGT activity in plasma, with and without prolonged contact with cells, was found to be 27% lower than in serum at 0.5 hours; however, plasma GGT activity steadily increases with prolonged exposure to cells. Creatinine can increase by 110% in plasma and by 60% in serum after 48 to 56 hours (Boyanton, 2002).

Serum and plasma may yield significantly different results for an analyte. For example, when serum and EDTA plasma results for parathyroid hormone (PTH) are compared from specimens frozen within 30 minutes of collection, EDTA plasma results are significantly higher (>19%) than those obtained from serum (Omar, 2001). The effect of freeze–thaw cycles on constituent stability is an important consideration. In plasma or serum specimens, the ice crystals formed cause shear effects that are disruptive to molecular structure(s), particularly to large protein molecules. Slow freezing allows larger crystals to form, causing more serious degradative effects. Thus, quick freezing is recommended for optimal stability.

IMPORTANCE OF POLICIES AND PROCEDURES

It is essential to establish institution-specific phlebotomy policies and procedures that include personnel standards with qualifications; dress code and evaluation procedures; safety protocols including immunization recommendations; universal precautions; needlestick and sharps information; personal protective equipment; test order procedures; patient identification; confidentiality and preparation; documentation of problems encountered during blood collection; needlestick site selection and areas to be avoided (mastectomy side, edematous area, burned/scarred areas, etc.); anticoagulants required and tube color; order of draw; special requirements for patient isolation units; and specimen transport. The laboratory should have available all CDC, College of American Pathologists (CAP), Clinical and Laboratory Standards Institute (CLSI), OSHA, and The Joint Commission (TJC) guidelines, as well as other government regulations pertaining to laboratory testing. All employees must be trained about safety procedures, and a written blood-borne pathogen exposure control plan must be available. See Chapter 1 for a more complete discussion of safety.

The OSHA Bloodborne Pathogens Standard concluded that the best practice for prevention of needlestick injury following phlebotomy is the use of a sharp with engineered sharps injury protection (SESIP) attached to the blood tube holder and immediate disposal of the entire unit after each patient's blood is drawn (OSHA, 2001). Information on exposure prevention can be found on the Exposure Prevention Information Network (EPINet), a database coordinated by the International Healthcare Worker Safety Center at the University of Virginia (http://www.healthsystem.virginia.edu/internet/epinet/). OSHA further mandates that employers make available closable, puncture-resistant, leak-proof sharps containers that are labeled and color-coded. The containers must have an opening that is large enough to accommodate disposal of the entire blood collection assembly (i.e., blood tube, holder, and needle). These containers must be easily accessible to employees in the immediate area of use, and if employees travel from one location to another (one patient room to another), they must be provided with a sharps container that is conveniently placed at each location/facility. Employers must maintain a sharps injury log to record percutaneous injuries from contaminated sharps while at the same time protecting the confidentiality of the injured employee.

BLOOD COLLECTION TECHNIQUES

Table 3-8 summarizes the technique for obtaining blood from a vein (CLSI H3-A6, 2007).

TABLE 3-8
Venous Puncture Technique

1. Verify that computer-printed labels match requisitions. Check patient identification band against labels and requisition forms. Ask the patient for his or her full name, address, identification number, and/or date of birth.
2. If a fasting specimen or a dietary restriction is required, confirm patient has fasted or eliminated foods from diet as ordered by physician.
3. Position the patient properly. Assemble equipment and supplies.
4. Apply a tourniquet and ask the patient to make a fist without vigorous hand pumping. Select a suitable vein for puncture.
5. Put on gloves with consideration of latex allergy for the patient.
6. Cleanse the venipuncture site with 70% isopropyl alcohol. Allow the area to dry.
7. Anchor the vein firmly.
8. Enter the skin with the needle at approximately a 30-degree angle or less to the arm, with the bevel of the needle up:
   a. Follow the geography of the vein with the needle.
   b. Insert the needle smoothly and fairly rapidly to minimize patient discomfort.
   c. If using a syringe, pull back on the barrel with a slow, even tension as blood flows into the syringe. Do not pull back too quickly to avoid hemolysis or collapsing the vein.
   d. If using an evacuated system, as soon as the needle is in the vein, ease the tube forward in the holder as far as it will go, firmly securing the needle holder in place. When the tube has filled, remove it by grasping the end of the tube and pulling gently to withdraw, and gently invert tubes containing additives.
9. Release the tourniquet when blood begins to flow. Never withdraw the needle without removing the tourniquet.
10. Withdraw the needle, and then apply pressure to the site. Apply adhesive bandage strip over a cotton ball or gauze to adequately stop bleeding and to avoid a hematoma.
11. Mix and invert tubes with anticoagulant; do not shake the tubes. Check condition of the patient. Dispose of contaminated material in designated containers (sharps container) using Universal Precautions.
12. Label the tubes before leaving patient's side with:
    a. patient's first and last name
    b. identification number
    c. date of collection
    d. time of collection
    e. identification of person collecting specimen
13. Deliver tubes of blood for testing to appropriate laboratory section or central receiving and processing area.

ARTERIAL PUNCTURE

Arterial punctures are technically more difficult to perform than venous punctures. Increased pressure in the arteries makes it more difficult to stop bleeding, with the undesired development of a hematoma. In order of preference, the radial, brachial, and femoral arteries can be selected.

Before blood is collected from the radial artery in the wrist, one should do a modified Allen test (Table 3-9) to determine whether the ulnar artery can provide collateral circulation to the hand after the radial artery puncture. The femoral artery is relatively large and easy to puncture, but one must be especially careful in older individuals because the femoral artery can bleed more than the radial or brachial. Because the bleeding site is hidden by bedcovers, it may not be noticed until bleeding is massive. The radial artery is more difficult to puncture, but complications occur less frequently. The major complications of arterial puncture include thrombosis, hemorrhage, and possible infection. When performed correctly, no significant complications are reported except for possible hematomas.

Unacceptable sites are those that are irritated, edematous, near a wound, or in an area of an arteriovenous (AV) shunt or fistula (McCall, 1993). Arterial spasm is a reflex constriction that restricts blood flow with possible severe consequences for circulation and tissue perfusion. Radial artery puncture can be painful and is associated with symptoms such as aching, throbbing, tenderness, sharp sensation, and cramping. At times, it may be impractical or impossible to obtain arterial blood from a patient for blood gas analysis. Under these circumstances, another source of blood can be used, with the recognition that arterial blood provides a more accurate result. Although venous blood is more readily obtained, it usually reflects the acid-base status of an extremity—not the body as a whole.

TABLE 3-9
Modified Allen Test

1. Have the patient make a fist and occlude both the ulnar (opposite the thumb side) and the radial arteries (closest to the thumb) by compressing with two fingers over each artery.
2. Have the patient open his or her fist, and observe if the patient's palm has become bleached of blood.
3. Release the pressure on the ulnar artery (farthest from the thumb) only, and note if blood return is present. The palm should become perfused with blood. Adequate perfusion is a positive test indicating that arterial blood may be drawn from the radial artery. Blood should not be taken if the test is negative. Serious consequences may occur if this procedure is not followed, which may result in loss of the hand or its function.

TABLE 3-10
Arterial Puncture Procedure

1. Prepare the arterial blood gas syringe according to established procedures. The needle (18–20 gauge for brachial artery) should pierce the skin at an angle of approximately 45–60 degrees (90 degrees for femoral artery) in a slow and deliberate manner. Some degree of dorsiflexion of the wrist is necessary with the radial artery, for which a 23–25 gauge needle is used. The pulsations of blood into the syringe confirm that it will fill by arterial pressure alone.
2. After the required blood is collected, place dry gauze over the puncture site while quickly withdrawing the needle and the collection device.
3. Compress the puncture site quickly, expel air from the syringe, and activate the needle safety feature; discard into sharps container.
4. Mix specimen thoroughly by gently rotating or inverting the syringe to ensure anticoagulation.
5. Place in ice water (or other coolant that will maintain a temperature of 1°–5° C) to minimize leukocyte consumption of oxygen.
6. Continue compression with a sterile gauze pad for a minimum of 3 to 5 minutes (timed). Apply an adhesive bandage.

TABLE 3-11
Skin Puncture Technique

1. Select an appropriate puncture site.
   a. For infants younger than 12 months old, this is most usually the lateral or medial plantar heel surface.
   b. For infants older than 12 months, children, and adults, the palmar surface of the last digit of the second, third, or fourth finger may be used.
   c. The thumb and fifth finger must not be used, and the site of puncture must not be edematous or a previous puncture site because of accumulated tissue fluid.
2. Warm the puncture site with a warm, moist towel no hotter than 42° C; this increases the blood flow through arterioles and capillaries and results in arterial-enriched blood.
3. Cleanse the puncture site with 70% aqueous isopropanol solution. Allow the area to dry. Do not touch the swabbed area with any nonsterile object.
4. Make the puncture with a sterile lancet or other skin-puncturing device, using a single deliberate motion nearly perpendicular to the skin surface. For a heel puncture, hold the heel with the forefinger at the arch and the thumb proximal to the puncture site at the ankle. If using a lancet, the blade should not be longer than 2 mm to avoid injury to the calcaneus (heel bone).
5. Discard the first drop of blood by wiping it away with a sterile pad. Regulate further blood flow by gentle thumb pressure. Do not milk the site, as this may cause hemolysis and introduce excess tissue fluid.
6. Collect the specimen in a suitable container by capillary action. Closed systems are available for collection of nonanticoagulated blood and with additives for whole blood analysis. Open-ended, narrow-bore disposable glass micropipets are most often used up to volumes of 200 µL. Both heparinized and nonheparinized micropipets are available. Use the appropriate anticoagulant for the test ordered. Mix the specimen as necessary.
7. Apply pressure and dispose of the puncture device.
8. Label the specimen container with date and time of collection and patient demographics.
9. Indicate in the report that test results are from skin puncture.

Arterial Puncture Technique

The artery to be punctured is identified by its pulsations, and the overlying skin is cleansed with 70% aqueous isopropanol solution followed by iodine. A nonanesthetized arterial puncture provides an accurate measurement of resting pH and partial pressure of carbon dioxide (pCO_2) in spite of possible theoretical error caused by patient hyperventilation resulting from the pain of the arterial puncture. The use of butterfly infusion sets is not recommended. Using 19-gauge versus 25-gauge needles does not vary the pCO_2 or the partial pressure of oxygen (pO_2) by more than 1 mm Hg. The amount of anticoagulant should be 0.05 mL liquid heparin (1000 IU/mL) for each milliliter of blood. Using too much heparin is probably the most common preanalytic error in blood gas measurement (Garza, 2002). Table 3-10 lists the procedure for arterial puncture (CLSI H11-A4, 2004).

FINGER OR HEEL SKIN PUNCTURE

For routine assays requiring small amounts of blood, skin puncture is a simple method by which to collect blood samples in pediatric patients. In the neonate, skin puncture of the heel is the preferred site to collect a blood sample; in older children, the finger is the preferred site. The large amount of blood required for repeated venipunctures may cause iatrogenic anemia, especially in premature infants. Venipuncture of deep veins in pediatric patients may rarely cause (1) cardiac arrest, (2) hemorrhage, (3) venous thrombosis, (4) reflex arteriospasm followed by gangrene of an extremity, (5) damage to organs or tissues accidentally punctured, (6) infection, and (7) injury caused by restraining an infant or child during collection. Accessible veins in sick infants must be reserved exclusively for parenteral therapy. Skin puncture is useful in adults with (1) extreme obesity, (2) severe burns, and (3) thrombotic tendencies, with point-of-care testing or with patients performing tests at home (blood glucose). Skin puncture is often preferred in geriatric patients because the skin is thinner and less elastic; thus a hematoma is more likely to occur from a venipuncture.

In newborns, skin puncture of the heel is frequently used to collect a sample for bilirubin testing and for newborn screening tests for inherited metabolic disorders. A deep heel prick is made at the distal edge of the calcaneal protuberance following a 5- to 10-minute exposure period to prewarmed water. The best method for blood gas collection in the newborn remains the indwelling umbilical artery catheter. Table 3-11 lists the steps for a skin puncture (CLSI H4-A6, 2008).

CENTRAL VENOUS ACCESS DEVICES

Central venous access devices (CVADs) provide ready access to the patient's circulation, eliminating multiple phlebotomies, and are especially useful in critical care and surgical situations. Indwelling catheters are surgically inserted into the cephalic vein, or into the internal jugular, subclavian, or femoral vein and can be used to draw blood, administer drugs or blood products, and provide total parenteral nutrition. Continuous, real-time, intraarterial monitoring of blood gases and acid-base status has been accomplished with fiberoptic channels containing fluorescent and absorbent chemical analytes (Smith, 1992).

CVA Collection Technique

Blood specimens drawn from catheters may be contaminated with whatever was administered or infused via the catheter. The solution (usually heparin) used to maintain patency of the vein must be cleared before blood for analysis is collected. Sufficient blood (minimum of 2–5 mL) must be withdrawn to clear the line, so laboratory data are reliable. Specialized training is therefore necessary before a catheter line is used to collect blood specimens. To obtain a blood specimen from the indwelling catheter, 5 mL of intravenous fluid is first drawn and discarded. In a separate syringe, the amount of blood required for the requested laboratory procedure(s) is then drawn. Strict aseptic technique must be followed to avoid site and/or catheter contamination. Coagulation measurements such as prothrombin time (PT), activated partial thromboplastin time (APTT), and thrombin time (TT) are extremely sensitive to heparin interference, so that even larger volumes of presample blood must be withdrawn before laboratory

TABLE 3-12
Order of Draw From Catheter Lines

1. Draw 3–5 mL in a syringe and discard.
2. Blood for blood culture
3. Blood for anticoagulated tubes (lavender, green, light blue, etc.)
4. Blood for clot tubes (red, SST, etc.)

SST, Serum separator tube.

results are acceptable for these tests. The appropriate volume to be discarded should be established by each laboratory.

The laboratory is sometimes asked to perform blood culture studies on blood drawn from indwelling catheters. Because the indwelling catheters are in place for a few days, this procedure is not recommended because organisms that grow on the walls of the catheter can contaminate the blood specimen. Lines, such as central venous pressure (CVP) lines, are specifically inserted and used for immediate blood product infusion and are less likely to become contaminated. Determination of catheter contamination requires special handling and careful analysis of multiple samples from the catheter and peripheral blood. Table 3-12 lists the order of draw from catheter lines.

URINE AND OTHER BODY FLUIDS COLLECTION

URINE

Collection and preservation of urine for analytic testing must follow a carefully prescribed procedure to ensure valid results. Laboratory testing of urine generally falls into three categories: chemical, bacteriologic, and microscopic examinations. Several kinds of collection are used for urine specimens: random, clean-catch, timed, 24 hour, and catheterized. Random specimens may be collected at any time, but a first-morning-voided aliquot is optimal for constituent concentration, as it is usually the most concentrated and has a lower pH caused by decreased respiration during sleep. Random urine specimens should be collected in a chemically clean receptacle, either glass or plastic. A clean-catch midstream specimen is most desirable for bacteriologic examinations. Proper collection of a clean-catch specimen requires that the patient first clean the external genitalia with an antiseptic wipe; the patient next begins urination, stops midstream, and discards this first portion of urine, then collects the remaining urine in a sterile container. The vessel is tightly sealed, is labeled with the patient's name and date of collection, and is submitted for analysis. A urine transfer straw kit for midstream specimens (BD Vacutainer) can be used to remove an aliquot from the sterile collection container, which then can be transported to the laboratory. The system consists of an adapter that attaches to a yellow evacuated sterile tube. The vacuum draws the urine into the sterile tube. The adapter assembly must be treated like a needle assembly system and be discarded into a biohazard container. A similar product is available for cultures; it uses a sterile, gray-top tube containing 6.7 mg/L of boric acid and 3.335 mg/L of sodium formate, along with the adapter device described previously (BD Vacutainer).

Timed specimens are obtained at designated intervals, starting from "time zero." Collection time is noted on each subsequent container. Urine specimens for a 24-hour total volume collection are most difficult to obtain and require patient cooperation. Incomplete collection is the most frequent problem. In some instances, too much sample is collected. In-hospital collection is usually supervised by nurses and generally is more reliable than outpatient collection. Pediatric collections require special attention to avoid stool contamination. One can avoid problems in collecting 24-hour specimens by giving patients complete written and verbal instructions with a warning that the test can be invalidated by incorrect collection technique. The preferred container is unbreakable, measures 4 L (approximately), is plastic, and is chemically clean, with the correct preservative already added. One should remind the patient to discard the first morning specimen, record the time, and collect every subsequent voiding for the next 24 hours. An easy approach is to instruct the patient to start with an empty bladder and to end with an empty bladder. Overcollection occurs if the first morning specimen is included in this routine. The total volume collected is measured and recorded on the request form, the entire 24-hour specimen is thoroughly mixed, and a 40 mL aliquot is submitted for analysis.

It is difficult to determine whether a collection is complete. If results appear clinically invalid, this is cause for suspicion. Because creatinine excretion is based on muscle mass, and because a patient's muscle mass is relatively constant, creatinine excretion is also reasonably constant. Therefore, one can measure creatinine on several 24-hour collections to assess the completeness of the specimen and keep this as part of the patient's record. One- and 2-hour timed collection specimens may suffice in some instances, depending on the analyte being measured. Urobilinogen is subject to diurnal variation, with the highest levels reached in the afternoon. Commonly, urine is collected from 2–4 PM, when a quantification of urobilinogen is requested.

TABLE 3-13
Changes in Urine With Delayed Testing

Result	Reason
Changes in color	Breakdown or alteration of chromogen or other urine constituent (e.g., hemoglobin, melanin, homogentisic acid, porphyrins)
Changes in odor	Bacterial growth, decomposition
Increased turbidity	Increased bacteria, crystal formation, precipitation of amorphous material
Falsely low pH	Glucose converted to acids and alcohols by bacteria producing ammonia. Carbon dioxide (CO_2) lost
Falsely elevated pH	Breakdown of urea by bacteria, forming ammonia
False-negative glucose	Utilization by bacteria (glycolysis)
False-negative ketone	Volatilization of acetone; breakdown of acetoacetate by bacteria
False-negative bilirubin	Destroyed by light; oxidation to biliverdin
False-negative urobilinogen	Destroyed by light
False-positive nitrite	Nitrite produced by bacteria after specimen is voided
False-negative nitrite	Nitrite converts to nitrogen and evaporates.
Increased bacteriuria	Bacteria multiply in specimen before analysis.
Disintegration of cells/casts	Unstable environment, especially in alkaline urine, hypotonic urine, or both

Special Urine Collection Techniques

Catheterization of the urethra and bladder may cause infection but is necessary in some patients (e.g., for urine collection when patients are unable to void or control micturition). Ureteral catheters can also be inserted via a cystoscope into the ureter. Bladder urine is collected first, followed by a bladder washing. Ureteral urine specimens are useful in differentiating bladder from kidney infection, or for differential ureteral analysis, and may be obtained separately from each kidney pelvis (labeled left and right). First morning urine is optimal for cytologic examination.

Urine Storage and Preservation

Preservation of a urine specimen is essential to maintain its integrity. Unpreserved urine specimens are subject both to microbiologic decomposition and to inherent chemical changes. Table 3-13 lists common changes that occur as urine decomposes. To prevent growth of microbes, the specimen should be refrigerated promptly after collection and, when necessary, should contain the indicated chemical preservative. For some determinations, addition of a chemical preservative may be best to maintain analytes when performing 24-hour urine collections. If a preservative is added to the empty collection bottle, particularly if acid preservatives are used, a warning label is placed on the bottle. The concentrated acid adds a risk of potential chemical burns; the patient should be warned about this potential danger, and the container labeled accordingly. In this scenario, the clinician must assess the patient's risk of exposure to the preservative; therefore, refrigeration may be more appropriate, and the preservative may be added upon submission to the laboratory. Light-sensitive compounds, such as bilirubin, are protected in amber plastic bottles. Precipitation of calcium and phosphates occurs unless the urine is acidified adequately before analysis.

It is particularly important to use freshly voided and concentrated urine to identify casts and red and white blood cells, as these undergo decomposition upon storage at room temperature or with decreased concentration (<1.015 specific gravity). They disappear rapidly

TABLE 3-14

24 Hour Urine Collection Preservatives

Preservative	Tests
None (refrigerate)	Amino acids, amylase, calcium, citrate, chloride, copper, creatinine, delta ALA, glucose, 5-HIAA, heavy metals (arsenic, lead, mercury), histamine, immunoelectrophoresis, lysozyme, magnesium, methylmalonic acid, microalbumin, mucopolysaccharides, phosphorus, porphobilinogen, porphyrins, potassium, protein, protein electrophoresis, sodium, urea, uric acid, xylose tolerance
10 g boric acid	Aldosterone, cortisol
10 mL 6N HCl	Catecholamines, cystine, homovanillic acid, hydroxyproline, metanephrines, oxalate, VMA
0.5 g sodium fluoride	Glucose
If processing delayed longer than 24 hours: equal amounts of 50% alcohol, Saccomanno's fixative, and SurePath or Preserve CT	Cytologic examination

ALA, Alanine aminotransferase; *5-HIAA,* 5-hydroxyindoleacetic acid; *VMA,* vanillylmandelic acid.

in hypotonic and alkaline urine. Bilirubin and urobilinogen decrease, especially after exposure to light. Glucose and ketones may be consumed, while bacterial contamination and loss of CO_2 lead to increase of pH, formation of turbidity with precipitates, and change in color. Ideally specimens should be delivered to the laboratory and analyzed within 1 hour of collection.

Urine may be frozen in aliquots to be assayed at a later date for chemical analysis only. When repeat testing is expected, the specimen should be stored in multiple aliquots to circumvent specimen degradation as a result of repeated freeze–thawing of a single specimen. Preservatives may also be added, depending on the substance to be tested. Sodium fluoride can be added to 24-hour urine for glucose determinations to inhibit bacterial growth and cell glycolysis, but not growth of yeast. About 0.5 g of sodium fluoride is added to a 3 to 4 L container. Sodium fluoride may inhibit reagent (enzyme-embedded) glucose strip tests. Tablets containing formaldehyde, mercury, and benzoate (95 mg tablet/20 mL urine) have also been used; however these preservatives elevate specific gravity (0.002/one tablet/20 mL). Boric acid in a concentration of 1 g/dL preserves urine elements such as estriol and estrogen for up to 7 days. Boric acid maintains the pH at about 6.0 and preserves protein and formed elements well without interfering with routine testing except for pH. Boric acid is a bacteriostatic preservative, not a bactericidal, and it does not inhibit the growth of yeasts. Boric acid has been reported to interfere with drug and hormone analysis (Strasinger, 2001). For catecholamines, vanillylmandelic acid (VMA), or 5-hydroxyindoleacetic acid (5-HIAA) collections, 10 mL of 6N HCl is added to a 3 to 4 L container. The HCl establishes a pH of approximately <3.0 that is good for chemical testing. However, the low pH destroys formed elements and enhances uric acid precipitation. Table 3-14 lists preservatives commonly used for 24-hour urine specimens. The NCCLS approved guidelines for urinalysis and collection, transportation, and preservation of urine specimens provide useful information on various preservatives recommended for 24-hour urine collections (NCCLS, 2001).

OTHER BODY FLUIDS

Cerebrospinal Fluid

Lumbar punctures (LPs) are performed to collect cerebrospinal fluid (CSF) for laboratory evaluation to establish a diagnosis of infection (bacterial, fungal, mycobacterial, or amebic meningitis), malignancy, subarachnoid hemorrhage, multiple sclerosis, or demyelinating disorders. The most common site for lumbar puncture is between the third and fourth lumbar vertebrae, or between the fourth and fifth lumbar vertebrae. A serious complication of an LP is cerebellar tonsillar herniation in patients with elevated intracranial pressure, and it should be avoided unless CSF findings are expected to improve treatment or outcome. Patients with spinal cord tumors with paresis may progress to paralysis following LP. Patients with sepsis in the lumbar region (skin infection, cellulitis, or epidural abscess) should not have an LP performed, to avoid introduction of infection. Other complications of LP include asphyxiation in infants due to hyperextending the head forward, thus occluding the trachea, paresthesia, headache, and, rarely, hematomas. CSF is also collected by cisternal puncture. A needle is inserted into the cisternal subarachnoidea, or small space, that serves as a reservoir for CSF between the atlas and the occipital bone in the back of the head, or by lateral cervical puncture (Kjeldsberg, 1993). Specimens can also be collected from ventricular cannulas (shunts) when present.

Before CSF is collected, the pressure should be between 90 and 180 mm Hg; this is measured by allowing fluid to rise in a sterile, graduated manometer. Holding one's breath, abdominal compression, congestive heart failure, inflammation of the meninges, obstruction of intracranial venous sinuses, mass lesions, or cerebral edema may cause the pressure to be elevated (>180 mm Hg). When pressure is normal, 20 mL of specimen may be removed. On closing, the pressure should be between 10 and 30 mm Hg. A marked decrease in pressure following this procedure suggests cerebellar herniation or spinal cord compression; thus, no additional CSF should be collected. Patients with partial or complete spinal block may have low pressure (<80 mm Hg), falling to zero after removal of only 1 mL. Again, no additional fluid should be removed. Not more than 2 mL can be removed when the pressure is greater than 200 mm Hg. Three aliquots are generally collected in separate, sterile tubes labeled appropriately with name, date, and sequential tube collection number, and distributed. Hospital policies differ as to which tube is distributed to which laboratory for analysis. It is generally recommended that Tube #1 goes to chemistry for glucose and protein analysis, or to immunology/serology; Tube #2 goes to microbiology for culture and Gram stain; Tube #3 goes to hematology for cell counts. Tube #3 is the least likely to be contaminated by a bloody tap at collection. Expansion of tests ordered on CSF to include molecular diagnostic procedures has placed even greater demand on proper utilization of the entire volume of CSF collected, with special efforts to conserve specimens in each laboratory section so that additional tests may be performed.

Synovial Fluid

Synovial fluid found in the joint cavities is an ultrafiltrate of plasma that is passed through fenestrations of the subsynovial capillary endothelium into the synovial cavity. Once in the cavity, it is combined with hyaluronic acid, a glycosaminoglycan secreted by the synovial lining cells. Synovial fluid differs from the other serous fluids in that it contains hyaluronic acid (mucin) and may contain crystals. Synovial fluid is collected by arthrocentesis, an aspiration of the joint using a syringe, moistened with an anticoagulant, usually 25 units of sodium heparin per mL of synovial fluid. Oxalate, powdered EDTA, and lithium heparin should not be used, as they can produce crystalline structures similar to monosodium urate (MSU) crystals. Once removed, the synovial fluid is usually transferred to three tubes—one sterile, one containing EDTA or heparin, and one red-top tube; 5–10 mL of fluid is added to each. The sterile tube is sent to microbiology, the anticoagulated tube is sent to hematology, and the red-top tube, after centrifugation, is used for chemical analysis. Some hospitals transfer synovial fluid to aerobic and anaerobic blood culture bottles for microbiologic culture.

Pleural Fluid, Pericardial Fluid, and Peritoneal Fluid

Pleural fluid is an ultrafiltrate of the blood plasma. It is formed continuously in the pleural cavity. This cavity, normally containing 1–10 mL of fluid, is formed by the parietal pleura, lining the chest wall, and the visceral pleura, covering the lung. Each lung is enveloped by this double membrane of contiguous mesothelial layers. Pleural fluid acts as a natural lubricant for contraction and expansion of the lungs during respiration. It is reabsorbed by the lymphatics and the venules in the pleura (Miller, 1999).

Thoracentesis is a surgical procedure to drain fluid (effusions) from the thoracic cavity and is helpful in diagnosing inflammation or neoplastic disease in the lung or pleura. Pericardiocentesis and peritoneocentesis refer to the collection of fluid from the pericardium (effusion) and the peritoneal cavities (ascites), respectively. These cavities normally contain less than 50 mL of fluid.

The patient, sitting in an upright position, with arms and head extended on an overbed table, is prepared with a local anesthetic after appropriate cleansing of the site. A 50 mL syringe is fitted with a stopcock and rubber tubing to assist in the aseptic collection process. Specimens are obtained for chemical, microbiologic, and cytologic examination and are transferred to collection tubes with appropriate additive(s). For most chemical evaluations, no additive is used and the specimen is allowed to clot. Bacteriologic and cytologic specimens may be collected in EDTA or sterile sodium heparin (without preservatives). Special studies for *Mycobacterium*, anaerobic bacteria, or viruses may require special handling procedures. Special handling procedures must be reviewed before collection is begun.

Specimen Transport

Transport of blood, urine, body fluids, and tissue specimens from the collection site to the laboratory is an important component of processing. For blood samples, it accounts for approximately one third of the total turnaround time (TAT) (Howanitz, 1992). Excessive agitation of blood specimens must be avoided to minimize hemolysis. Specimens should be protected from direct exposure to light, which causes breakdown of certain analytes (e.g., bilirubin). For analysis of unstable constituents such as ammonia, plasma renin activity, and acid phosphatase, specimens must be kept at 4° C immediately after collection and transported on ice. Routine urine is collected in a sterile, disposable, 200 mL plastic container. Pediatric urine collectors are flexible polyethylene bags, which may be sealed for transportation. All laboratory specimens must be transported in a safe and convenient manner to prevent biohazard exposure or contamination of the specimen. Broken or leaking specimens are a biohazard to those who may come in contact with them and require collection of a new specimen; this can delay treatment of the patient and add to the cost.

The stability of the constituents must be determined before specimens are transported. The laboratory usually provides this information along with instructions for specimen preparation and shipping. Polystyrene or other high-impact plastic-type containers are commonly used. Specimens requiring refrigeration must be maintained at between 2° C and 10° C and can be appropriately carried in an insulated container. Large-volume urine specimens should be collected in a leak-proof, 3 to 4 L container. Stool specimens are transported in a cardboard container and placed in a polyethylene bag. To mail a specimen in the frozen state, solid carbon dioxide (dry ice) may be packed in a polystyrene container with the specimen, which can be kept frozen at temperatures as low as −70° C.

The OSHA Bloodborne Pathogens Standard (OSHA: 1910.1030) requires specimens of blood or other potentially infectious materials (OPIM) to be placed in a container that prevents leakage during collection, handling, processing, storage, transport, and/or shipping. This container must be labeled or color-coded according to specific standards (OSHA: 1910.1030[g][1][i]). Furthermore, according to the standard, if contamination of the outside of the primary container occurs, or if the specimen could puncture the primary container, the primary container must be placed in a secondary container that is puncture-resistant in addition to having the previous characteristics (OSHA: 1910.1030[d][2][xiii]).

Labeling is required on all containers used to store, transport, ship, or dispose of blood or other potentially infectious materials, except as noted in the OSHA standard. For example, if individual containers of blood or OPIM are placed in a larger container during storage, transport, shipment, or disposal, and that larger container is labeled with the OSHA "BIOHAZARD" label or is color-coded, the individual containers are exempt from the labeling requirement. OSHA accepts the Department of Transportation's (DOT's) "INFECTIOUS SUBSTANCE" label in lieu of the "BIOHAZARD" label on packages where the DOT requires its label on shipped containers, but requires the "BIOHAZARD" label where OSHA regulates a material but DOT does not. If the DOT-required label is the only label used on the outside of the transport container, the OSHA-mandated label must be applied to any internal containers containing blood or OPIM. The accepted "BIOHAZARD" label is fluorescent orange.

For local, onsite transport, pneumatic tube systems provide a rapid, efficient, and cost-effective way of transporting laboratory specimens to a specific location. For laboratory use, blood specimens are placed in a carrier with liners to prevent leakage and padding to ensure that specimen containers remain intact. The advantages of a pneumatic tube system are improved TAT, reliability, minimal training, low maintenance, availability 24 hours/day, 7 days/week, and improved staff utilization. Studies have shown that most routine chemical and hematologic evaluations, including blood gases, red cell packs, coagulation tests, and LD values, are not substantially affected by rapid transport (Hardin, 1990; Keshgegian, 1992).

Specimen Processing

Processing of specimens includes three distinct phases: precentrifugation, centrifugation, and postcentrifugation. Continuing appraisal of all specimen handling activities is an important preanalytic component of total quality control. Appropriate guidelines must be established and adhered to by laboratory personnel in each phase of specimen handling to ensure the generation of reliable and medically meaningful measurement and examination results.

PRECENTRIFUGATION PHASE

Ideally, all measurements should be performed within 45 minutes to 1 hour after collection. Whenever this is not practical, the specimen should be processed to a point at which it can be properly stored to preclude alteration of constituents to be measured. With the exception of blood gases and ammonia determinations, plasma or serum is preferred for most biochemical determinations. In clinical chemistry, serum and plasma are interchangeable except for a few measurements. Serum is required for protein electrophoresis and immunofixation assays, just as plasma is necessary for fibrinogen and other coagulation measurements. Serum is most commonly the specimen of choice, owing to its simplicity in collection and handling. Additionally, interference from anticoagulants is obviated. Plasma may be used in medical emergencies because samples do not have to clot before centrifugation. Usually, a greater volume of plasma than serum is obtained from a given volume of whole blood owing to the clot formation process. Hospitalized patients are likely to be receiving heparin (especially under critical care), which can delay clotting in blood collection tubes even with activators and lead to fibrin strands that can clog up aspiration probes on instrumentation. Accordingly it is good practice to collect blood from hospitalized patients into tubes with heparin anticoagulant to obtain plasma for chemical tests.

Blood should be stoppered in the original container until ready for separation. For plasma preparation, centrifuge blood within 1 hour after collection, for 10 minutes at a relative centrifugal force (RCF) of 850–1000× gravity (g), keeping the container stoppered to prevent evaporation of plasma or serum water. Adequate time for clotting must be allowed to prevent latent fibrin formation, which may cause undesirable clogging of automated chemistry analyzers. Loosening the clot by "trimming" or "ringing" the tube may cause some hemolysis and should be avoided. When glass tubes are used, they should be centrifuged in an aerosol-contained vessel. Serum or plasma must be stored at 4° C to 6° C if analysis is to be delayed for longer than 4 hours. One study suggests that this may not be necessary (Melanson, 2004). Many laboratories store samples for 7 days in case a test is added.

CENTRIFUGATION PHASE

A centrifuge uses centrifugal force to separate phases of suspensions by different densities. It is most frequently used in processing blood to derive plasma or serum fractions. Urine and other body fluids may be centrifuged to concentrate particulate matter as sediment to be examined and to minimize interference with other determinations from the same material. Conditions for centrifugation should specify both the time and the centrifugal force. In selecting a centrifuge, one should look for the highest possible centrifugal force and not the rotational speed. The RCF in g units, that is, multiples of the gravitational force, may be calculated by using the following formula:

$$RCF = 1.118 \times 10^{-5} \times r \times (rpm)^2$$

where 1.118×10^{-5} is a constant; r is the radius, expressed in centimeters, between the axis of rotation and the center of the centrifuge tube; and rpm is the speed in revolutions per minute. The RCF can also be obtained from a nomogram that gives the RCF without the need to calculate it from the previous formula.

Several principles must be observed to avoid damage to the centrifuge, or the specimen, and danger to personnel. Tubes, carriers, or shields of equal weight, shape, and size should be placed in opposing positions in the centrifuge head to achieve appropriate balance. Tubes must be balanced across the center of rotation, and each bucket must be balanced with respect to its pivotal axis (Seamonds, 2001). Specimens must be placed with regard for a geometrically symmetrical arrangement, using water-filled tubes to attain balance.

Recentrifugation of gel separator tubes has been associated with pseudohyperkalemia. One study demonstrated that after initial centrifugation, a new serum layer will develop under the gel within the cellular layer. During storage, potassium leaks from the cellular layer into the new serum layer, creating hyperkalemia in this layer. When the tube is recentrifuged, the new serum layer will move above the gel layer and cause a pseudohyperkalemia in the serum for analysis. The same authors also demonstrated that a pseudonormokalemia in patients with true hypokalemia may be erroneously reported after recentrifugation (Hira, 2001; Hira, 2004).

Equipment

A wide variety of centrifuges and accessories are available to meet specific needs in the clinical laboratory. These include tabletop, general laboratory centrifuges; horizontal head, fixed-angle, or angle-head; high-speed centrifuges; portable floor models, undercounter models; microcentrifuges; refrigerated and unrefrigerated types; and ultracentrifuge models. Ultracentrifuges are high speed and capable of reaching a centrifugal force of 165,000 times gravity. These centrifuges require refrigeration chambers to compensate for the considerable heat produced. Ultracentrifuges are used to clear serum of chylomicrons, which is necessary to avoid interference with clinical testing (Bermes, 2001). An example of a centrifuge designed for fast speed and quick turnaround time is the StatSpin Express 3 (StatSpin, 2005), a microprocessor-controlled, high-speed bench-top centrifuge designed to rapidly separate blood in evacuated tubes. This centrifuge accelerates rapidly and brakes very fast, decreasing specimen processing time. The centrifuge operates at a fixed speed of 8500 rpm, produces a RCF of 4440 × (g), and can be operated with a 120- or 180-second spin cycle.

Centrifuge capacities vary with model type and centrifuge head. Specimen volume (per tube), number of tubes to be centrifuged, speed required for adequate separation, and durability of equipment should be considered. For every laboratory procedure requiring centrifuge operation, a written specification identifying centrifuge type, temperature, g forces, and length of centrifugation time is required. Calibration of the centrifuge must be part of the quality assurance process. Speed settings must be calibrated using rpm, and RCFs must be calculated using the earlier formula or a nomogram. Any significant changes will indicate deterioration effects, such as wearing of brushes or bearing problems. Timers must be checked for accuracy.

INTERFERENCES

One of the main concerns in the preanalysis phase is whether any substance or artifact is introduced as the result of specimen handling or other patient-related factors that lead to alterations in the technical measurement of clinical specimens in the analysis. The patient's medical condition might cause abnormalities that can be evaluated by measurement of various analytes, and some of those abnormally elevated substances can markedly interfere with some basic modes of analysis.

SPECIMEN COLLECTION

The appropriate tube should always be used for collection of blood specimens because of interferences from some anticoagulants such as EDTA, which chelates both calcium and magnesium, thereby lowering the measurement of those ions and inhibiting some enzymes that require divalent cations (e.g., alkaline phosphatase by also chelating zinc). Plasma separator tubes containing lithium heparin should not be used for lithium measurements, and electrolyte measurements are not valid in tubes with potassium EDTA or sodium citrate. Proper collection technique avoids hemolysis (release of potassium; introduction of spectral interference) and contamination of blood with tissue fluid using fingersticks or heelsticks.

Small volumes of blood may be acceptable for some chemistry tests or cell counts; however, coagulation tests require a minimal volume of blood in the collection tube to achieve correct balance with citrate anticoagulant, which also chelates calcium. Excess citrate in plasma from insufficient blood volume leads to falsely elevated clotting times. This interference is also important in polycythemia, when the hematocrit is abnormally high and plasma volume in which the citrate distributes is small. Thus, even in an apparently correctly filled tube, polycythemia can lead to falsely prolonged PT and PTT unless the amount of citrate anticoagulant in the tube is reduced proportionally to the decrease in plasma volume in that patient.

OPTICAL INTERFERENCES

The most common interfering conditions are hemolysis and icterus, which strongly absorb particular wavelengths of light, and also lipemia, which scatters light and so blocks its transmission. All three of these interferents can have severe effects on spectrophotometric methods of analysis (Grafmeyer, 1995). Lipemia can potentially be cleared from a serum or plasma specimen by ultracentrifugation, and hemolysis that occurs at the time of blood collection can be eliminated by re-collection of the specimen; however, bilirubin in a specimen is not readily removed and so may cause spectral interference through its high absorbance at wavelengths between 340 and 500 nm. Bilirubin can also interfere chemically, particularly in peroxidase-coupled assays such as those for uric acid, cholesterol, and triglycerides (Spain, 1986). Result reporting should include a statement about the appearance of a specimen if it is particularly abnormal and a qualification about the validity of the results for the physician to use in interpreting any abnormal findings (e.g., elevated potassium in hemolyzed specimens).

IMMUNOASSAYS

Most modern immunoassays utilize mouse monoclonal antibodies in various configurations, often with separate solid phase capture antibody and signal antibody that detect specific antigens through molecular sandwich formation (see Chapter 44). The signal antibody is typically conjugated with an enzyme of other substance such as a chemiluminescent tag. In many enzyme immunoassays (EIAs), the label is peroxidase, which converts a colorless substrate to a colored product in solution whose optical absorbance is proportional to the concentration of the analyte. Although bilirubin and lipemia can interfere in principle with EIAs, wash steps may remove significant amounts of them and so minimize their effects from spectral interference. In contrast, Hb from a heavily hemolyzed specimen can have marked interference in peroxidase-based EIAs even after the prescribed number of wash steps because of the pseudoperoxidase activity of Hb in the residue remaining in the assay well. This effect is especially problematic for severely hemolyzed specimens such as blood collected postmortem. Consequently such hemolyzed specimens may not be at all suitable for analysis by peroxidase-based EIAs. Other EIAs that use alkaline phosphatase or β-galactosidase on the signal antibody or those that employ chemiluminescence as a tag do not have as much interference from hemolysis (Demuth, 2004).

Another problem sometimes encountered in immunoassays with mouse monoclonal antibody reagents is the presence of human anti-mouse antibodies (HAMAs) or heterophile antibodies in patients. HAMAs can arise following antigenic stimulation from therapeutic mouse monoclonal antibodies that are administered to alter immune responses (e.g., anti–T cell antibody), to bind and remove toxic levels of drugs (e.g., digoxin), or to attack tumors. Some individuals with HAMAs have no history of therapeutic exposures but could conceivably have had incidental exposure to mouse proteins through contaminated food or other environmental sources. The effect of HAMAs in immunoassays can be to cross-link capture and signal antibodies in a sandwich that mimics true antigen (Klee, 2000). For example, an immunoassay for thyroid-stimulating hormone (TSH) that has separate antibodies against α and β subunits might yield an astonishingly high false-positive result in a euthyroid person with HAMA; in this case, the other thyroid function tests could be completely normal. The presence of HAMA can be confirmed by direct measurement (usually sent to a reference laboratory) and can also be inferred by adsorption of the HAMA onto special tubes coated with mouse antibodies, followed by repeat measurement of the analyte to look for reduction in signal strength in the treated specimen (Madry, 1997).

SPECIMEN MATRIX EFFECTS

Common biochemical analytes such as electrolytes, small molecules, enzymes, etc., are generally distributed in the water phase of plasma or serum. Consequently, specimens with reduced water phase due to hyperproteinemia (e.g., from very high concentrations of a myeloma protein) or hyperlipidemia (e.g., high chylomicron content) can have reduced content of those solvent analytes even though other properties such as ionic activities in those specimens may be within normal physiologic range. This phenomenon is termed the *solvent exclusion effect*, referring to the exclusion of water and small molecules in the aqueous phase when more volume within a specimen is occupied by protein or lipid that excludes water. The content of small molecules per volume is the osmolarity (which is the measurement that can be erroneous), whereas the physiologically important aspect such as ionic activities is the osmolality. If excess lipids are the cause, they may be removed by ultracentrifugation. If interference is due to excess protein, an alternative mode of analysis such as ion-selective electrode in undiluted specimen can be employed to yield correct electrolyte activity (i.e., equivalent of osmolality).

Matrix effects from very high or very low concentrations of proteins and other constituents may be problematic when dealing with other body fluids, especially when the specimens are highly viscous or otherwise atypical (see Chapter 29). In those situations, it may be necessary to qualify results in the report to indicate the site of the body fluid and possible limitations in accuracy of measurement.

MOLECULAR DIAGNOSTICS

Laboratory manipulations of nucleic acids are susceptible to interferences at various stages, including specimen collection and processing. Introduction of inhibitory substances and contamination with false-positive signals are among the significant interferences. Blood specimens for nucleic acid testing are generally collected into EDTA anticoagulant to inhibit enzymes that might break them down. Heparin is a poor choice for anticoagulant in this application because it can be coextracted with DNA and inhibits DNA polymerase in polymerase chain reactions (PCRs). Hemin from hemolysis in plasma or serum can also inhibit DNA polymerase. RNA is labile in blood or tissues, and so these specimens must be stored appropriately by rapid freezing in liquid nitrogen if the extraction will be delayed.

Extraction of nucleic acids from clinical specimens such as plasma (e.g., for viral load measurement), blood cells (e.g., for genetic testing), or tissues (e.g., for analyzing mutations in tumors) entails lysing cells and separating nucleic acids from proteins and lipids. Reagents for extraction include salts, proteases, and phenol-chloroform to denature the substances complexed with nucleic acids. This process must be optimized for specimen type to recover high quality nucleic acids with good quantitative yield (see Chapter 65). Care must be taken to avoid contamination of specimens with target nucleic acids from other specimens or with amplified targets from specimens that have been analyzed previously in that vicinity. Accordingly, laboratories practicing nucleic acid amplification should have separate preamplification, amplification, and postamplification areas with strict rules about personnel movements between them (see Chapters 65 and 69).

EFFECTS OF DRUGS

Analytic methods that are based on oxidation–reduction reactions may be influenced positively or negatively by ingested substances such as ascorbic acid (vitamin C). This interference is observed in chemical testing of serum on automated analyzers (Meng, 2005), and it can also occur in urine testing for glucose (positive interference for reducing substance method; negative interference with enzymatic method). In stool testing for occult blood, peroxidases from meats (myoglobin) or vegetables (horseradish) in the diet can yield a false-positive result with guaiac-based methods, as can topical iodine or chlorine used as a disinfectant.

Drugs can have unanticipated reactions with the reagents intended for specific chemical tests. The list of potential interfering drugs is extremely long, and some methods for a particular analyte may be strongly affected, whereas other methods may not be affected. A voluminous compendium of drug interactions has been developed by Dr. Donald S. Young (Young, 2007). In addition to assisting with recognition of potential interferences, this source can be used to evaluate a different method that is unaffected by a particular drug to confirm the accuracy of measurement in cases of suspected interference. These interferences are separated into those whose effects are manifested directly in the assay in vitro and those that are due to drug actions in vivo, whereby physiologic functions are changed (e.g., prolonged prothrombin time with Coumadin; lower potassium in blood with some diuretics).

SELECTED REFERENCES

Boyanton L, Blick K. Stability studies of twenty-four analytes in human plasma and serum. Clin Chem 2002;48(12):2242–7.

This article studies plasma and serum analyte stability over 56 hours in samples removed from cells and allowed to remain on cells. No significant changes were found in the serum and plasma specimens removed from the cells within 30 minutes of collection. The article provides an excellent historical bibliography of the major studies performed on this topic.

Centers for Disease Control and Prevention. Workbook for designing, implementing, and evaluating a sharps injury prevention program, introduction. Division of Healthcare Quality Promotion—(DHQP Home) privacy policy—Accessibility. Published date: June 4, 2004; Reviewed date: July 28, 2004. Online. Available at: http://www.cdc.gov/sharpssafety/pdf/sharpsworkbook_2008.pdf.

This excellent Internet publication available for free download includes an overview of sharps risks and prevention, organizational steps for development of prevention programs, recommendations for selection of sharps injury prevention devices, and education and training materials. The appendices contain useful worksheets for all aspects of sharps injury and prevention documentation.

Garza D, Becan-McBride K. Phlebotomy handbook: blood collection essentials. 6th ed. Upper Saddle River N.J.: Prentice Hall; 2002, p. 163, 205, 263, 341.

This handbook presents a complete discussion of all aspects related to phlebotomy. Included are safety procedures, equipment, step-by-step procedures, and management and legal issues. It contains an excellent, basic discussion of the circulatory system with colored diagrams.

Strasinger SK, DiLorenzo MS. The phlebotomy workbook. 2nd ed. Philadelphia: FA Davis; 2003, p. 115, 164, 95, 96.

This text contains a comprehensive presentation of all aspects of phlebotomy. It is an excellent teaching guide and discusses state-of-the-art equipment and techniques. The book is divided into three parts: general phlebotomy, safety and health care information; techniques for blood collection; and medical terminology, anatomy, and physiology. Contained within the various chapters are excellent summary tables and quick reference charts. It also provides an extensive description of the various blood collection tubes and anticoagulants/additives they contain and information on preanalytic factors affecting laboratory results.

Young DS. Effects of preanalytic variables on clinical laboratory tests. 3rd ed. Washington, DC: AACC Press; 2007.

This is the preeminent resource for interferences in laboratory tests that covers the effects of drugs, as well as other contributing conditions.

Young MB, Bermes EW. Specimen collection and other preanalytical variables. In: Burtis CA, Ashwood ER, editors. Tietz fundamentals of clinical chemistry. 5th ed. Philadelphia: WB Saunders; 2001, p. 30–54.

This chapter contains many of the most important preanalysis factors that affect laboratory results. Dr. Young has also written a series of reference books that contain peer-reviewed information regarding test interactions; they are published by AACC Press, Washington, DC, and include the following: Young DS, Friedman RG. Effects of disease on clinical laboratory tests, 4th ed, 2001; Young DS. Effects of drugs on clinical laboratory tests, 5th ed, 2000; and Young DS. Effects of preanalytical variables on clinical laboratory tests, 2nd ed, 1997.

REFERENCES

Access the complete reference list online at http://www.expertconsult.com

PART 1

CHAPTER 4

ANALYSIS: PRINCIPLES OF INSTRUMENTATION

Robert L. Sunheimer, Gregory A. Threatte, Matthew R. Pincus, Mark S. Lifshitz

KEY POINTS

- Many analytic determinations made in clinical laboratories are based on measurements of radiant energy that is absorbed or transmitted. The devices used to measure absorbed or transmitted light energy are photometers and spectrophotometers.
- The basic components of spectrophotometers include radiant energy source, wavelength selector, cuvet holder, photodetector, signal processors, and readout devices.
- A reflectometer is used to measure analytes by measuring the quantity of light reflected by a liquid sample that has been dispensed onto a grainy or fibrous solid support.
- Nephelometers are used to detect light that is scattered at various angles, whereas turbidimetry measures a reduction in light transmission due to particle formation.
- A flow cytometer measures light patterns produced as particles pass single-file through a laser light beam. The flow cytometer is used to count and sort cells. It is also a key component of hematology analyzers and a technology used to differentiate white blood cells.
- Electrochemical principles are used to measure numerous analytes in biologic fluids. Specific electrochemical techniques include potentiometry, amperometry, coulometry, conductivity, and anodic stripping voltammetry.
- Analytes measured by electrochemical techniques include electrolytes, blood gases, pH, metabolites (e.g., glucose, urea nitrogen), ionized calcium, lead, and chloride in sweat.
- Chromatography is a separation technique based on the different interactions of specimen compounds with a mobile phase and a stationary phase, as the compound travels through a support medium.
- Mass spectrometers have become increasingly important clinical instruments, especially in emerging fields such as proteomics. Mass spectrometry is based on fragmentation and ionization of molecules. The relative abundance of each of the ions yields a characteristic mass spectrum of the parent molecule. The basic components of a mass spectrometer include an ion source, a mass analyzer, and an ion detector.

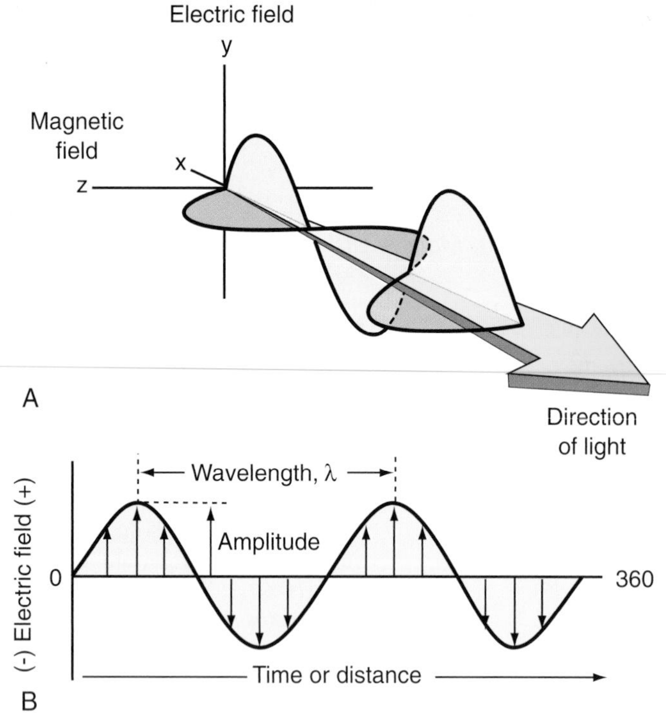

Figure 4-1 Diagram of a beam of monochromatic, plane-polarized light. **A,** Magnetic (y-axis) and electrical (x-axis) field vectors at right angles to one another. **B,** Two-dimensional view of the electrical vector.

A fundamental understanding of the principles of instrumentation used in clinical laboratories is essential. These instruments must provide the clinician with the best possible data to be of value to the patient. Without a thorough understanding of the necessary principles associated with an analyzer, operators will be ill equipped to perform maintenance procedures and calibrations, and to troubleshoot problems that may arise.

The goal of this chapter is to provide the reader with a brief and broad description of the essential principles of analytic instruments in the clinical laboratory. For a more comprehensive review of this topic, the reader is referred to references on clinical instrumentation at the end of this chapter.

PRINCIPLES OF INSTRUMENTATION

SPECTROPHOTOMETRY

Absorption spectroscopy has provided scientists with a means to use both qualitative and quantitative methods of measuring analytes in body fluids. Bouguer initially developed the principles of absorption spectroscopy in the early 1700s. Two other scientists, Lambert and Beer, continued to develop the fundamental principles of absorption spectroscopy, commonly known as Beer's law. Before reviewing the laws of spectroscopy, it is prudent to gain an understanding of light and the effects of its interactions with matter.

Diverse spectrophotometric methods use electromagnetic radiation (EMR), which can take several forms, the most recognizable being light and radiant heat. Other types of EMR include gamma (γ) rays and x-rays, as well as microwaves, radiofrequency radiation, and ultraviolet radiation. The energies involved with specific regions of the electromagnetic spectrum (EMS) and their corresponding wavelengths change dramatically from radio waves to γ radiation.

Some properties of EMR can be described by means of a classical sinusoidal wave model. Parameters associated with this waveform include wavelength, frequency, velocity, and amplitude, as shown in Figure 4-1, *B*. EMR requires no supporting medium for its transmission and passes readily through a vacuum.

The sine wave model does not provide the total picture when discussing the absorption and emission of radiant energy. EMR also exists as a stream of discrete particles, or packets, of energy called photons. The energy of the photons is proportional to the frequency of the radiation. This dual nature of EMR is considered complementary and applies to the behavior of streams of electrons, protons, and other elementary particles.

The wave model allows us to represent EMR as both an electrical and a magnetic field that can undergo in-phase, sinusoidal oscillation at right angles both to each other and to the direction of propagation. The electrical and magnetic fields for a monochromatic beam of plane-polarized light (with oscillation of either the electric or magnetic fields within a single plane)* in a specific direction of propagation are shown in Figure 4-1, *A* (Skoog, 1998).

The electrical vector or component of the waveform is shown in two-dimensional format. Remember that a vector has both magnitude and direction. The electrical field vector at a certain point in time and space is proportional to its own magnitude.

Time or distance of wave propagation is plotted on the abscissa. Most of the instrument principles widely used in the laboratory involve the electrical component of radiation and will represent the focus of discussion throughout this chapter. An exception will be nuclear magnetic resonance (NMR). With this technique, the magnetic component produces the desired effect.

Several wave parameters will be described. *Amplitude* of the sine wave is shown as the length of the electronic vector at maximum peak height. A *period*, *p*, is defined as the time in seconds required for the passage of successive maxima or minima through a fixed point in space. The number of oscillations of the waveform in a second is called *frequency*, v. The unit of frequency is hertz (Hz), which corresponds to one cycle per second. Frequency is also equal to $1/p$. A *wavelength*, λ, is the linear distance between any two equivalent points on a successive wave. A widely used unit for wavelength in the visible spectrum is the nanometer, nm (10^{-9} m). Electromagnetic radiation in the x-rays or gamma region may be expressed in terms of angstrom units, Å (10^{-10} m). Finally, because of its much longer wavelength, EMR in the infrared region may have units corresponding to the micrometer, µm (10^{-6} m).

Example 4-1. 1 nm = 10^{-9} m = 10^{-7} cm; other units sometimes used include the following:

1 µm = 10^{-6} m = 10^{-4} cm

1 Å = 10^{-10} m = 10^{-8} cm

Velocity of Propagation

Velocity of propagation, v_i in meters per second, is determined by multiplying frequency by wavelength. Thus:

$$v_i = v\lambda_i \quad \textbf{(4-1)}$$

The frequency of light is determined by the source and does not change, whereas the velocity depends upon the composition of the medium through which it passes. Therefore, Equation 4-1 implies that the wavelength of radiation is also dependent upon the medium.

The velocity of light traveling through a vacuum is independent of wavelength and is at its maximum. This velocity is represented by the symbol c, and is equivalent to 2.99792×10^8 m/s. Equation 4-1 can then be rewritten as follows:

$$c = v\lambda = 3.00\times10^8 \text{ m/s} = 3.00\times10^8 \text{ m/s}^{-1} = 3.00\times10^{10} \text{ cm/s} \quad \textbf{(4-2)}$$

Example 4-2. What is the wavelength in nm for EMR having a frequency of 1.58×10^{15} Hz?

SOLUTION

$\lambda = c/v$

$$\lambda \text{ (nm)} = \frac{3.00\times10^8 \text{ m/s}}{1.58\times10^{15} \text{ Hz}}$$

λ (nm) = 190

In any medium containing matter, the propagation of radiation is slowed by the interaction between the EMR field of the radiation and the electrons bound in the atoms of that matter. Because the radiant frequency does not vary and is fixed by the source, the wavelength must decrease as radiation passes from air to a slower medium.

Energy of EMR

One should note the following safety concern: optical devices that emit high frequency EMR generate very high energies and can damage the eyes. Examples include deuterium and xenon lamps.

*Unpolarized radiation has waves in many planes.

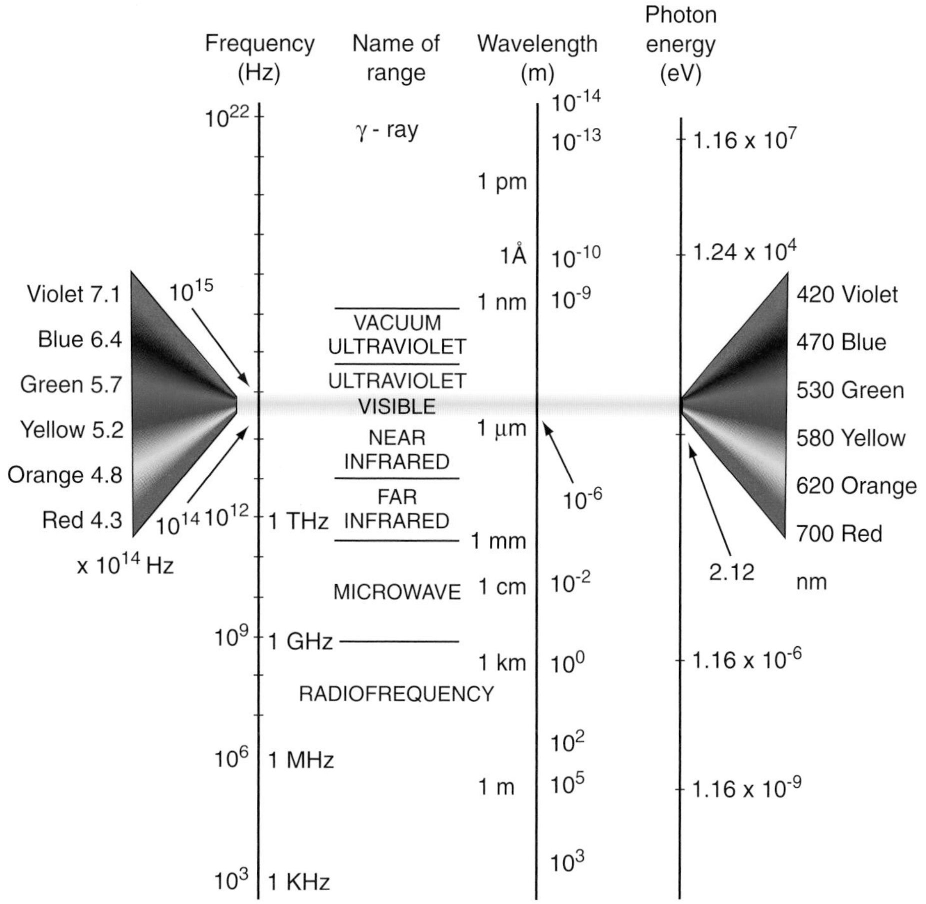

Figure 4-2 A diagram of the names, frequencies, wavelengths, and photon energies of electromagnetic radiation (EMR). Visible and ultraviolet light are widely used in analytic methods.

Wavelength and frequency are related to the energy of a photon, E, by Planck's* constant h, 6.626×10^{-34} J s, and c, the velocity of light in a vacuum (3.00×10^8 ms^{-1}):

$$E = hv = hc/\lambda \qquad \textbf{(4-3)}$$

where:

E is the energy of a photon in Joules or eV
h is Planck's constant (6.626×10^{-34} J s)
v is frequency in Hz (cycles/s).

Quite often the energies of photons are stated in terms of an electron volt (eV). An eV is defined as the energy acquired by an electron that has been accelerated through a potential of 1 volt. The conversion factors between Joules and eV are as follows:

$$1\ \text{J} = 6.24 \times 10^{18}\ \text{eV}$$
$$1\ \text{eV} = 1.602 \times 10^{-19}\ \text{J}$$

To illustrate the difference in energies of photons in the EMS, compare the energy of photons in the ultraviolet (UV) region versus the visible region of the EMS.

Example 4-3. What is the energy in Joules and eV of EMR equivalent to (a) 190 nm? (b) 520 nm?

SOLUTION

(a)

$E = hc/v$

$$E = \frac{(6.626 \times 10^{-34}\ \text{J s})(3.0 \times 10^8\ \text{m/s})}{190\ \text{nm}\,(10^{-9}\ \text{m/nm})}$$

$E = 1.046 \times 10^{-18}$ J

Or to convert to eV, use the conversion of 1 J = 6.24×10^{18} eV. Therefore the number of eVs is 6.53.

(b)

$E = hc/v$

$$E = \frac{(6.626 \times 10^{-34}\ \text{J s})(3.0 \times 10^8\ \text{m/s})}{520\ \text{nm}\,(10^{-9}\ \text{m/nm})}$$

$E = 3.82 \times 10^{-19}$ J or 2.38 eV

The relationship of frequency, wavelength, and photon energy throughout the EMS can be seen in Figure 4-2. This graphic illustrates for example that very-high-energy gamma photons have extremely short wavelengths and very high frequencies (Rubinson, 2000). The converse is true for television and radio wave parameters.

Scattering of Radiation

Transmission of radiation in matter can be viewed as a momentary retention of the radiant energy by atoms, ions, or molecules followed by re-emission of the radiation in all directions as particles return to their original state. Destructive interference removes most but not all of the re-emitted radiation involving atomic or molecular particles that are small relative to the wavelength of the radiation. The exception is radiation that travels in the original direction of the beam; the path of the beam appears to be unaltered because of the interaction. It has been shown that a very small fraction of the radiation is transmitted at all angles from the original path, and that the intensity of this scattered radiation increases with particle size.

Rayleigh Scattering

Scattering by molecules or aggregates of molecules with dimensions significantly smaller than the wavelength of the radiation is referred to as *Rayleigh scattering*. The intensity is proportional to the inverse fourth power of the wavelength, the square of the polarizability of the particles, and the dimensions of the scattering particles. In Rayleigh scattering, the wavelengths of absorbed and emitted photons are the same. An example of Rayleigh scattering is the blue color of the sky, which results from increased scattering of the shorter wavelength of the visible spectrum.

*Also expressed in units 6.626×10^{-27} erg s.

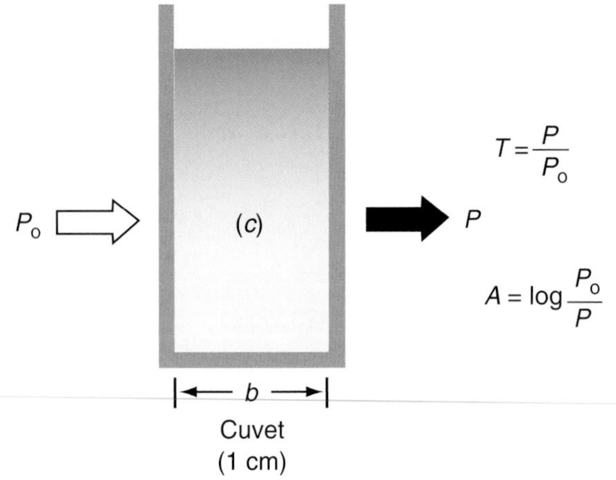

Figure 4-3 Attenuation of monochromatic light by an absorbing solution.

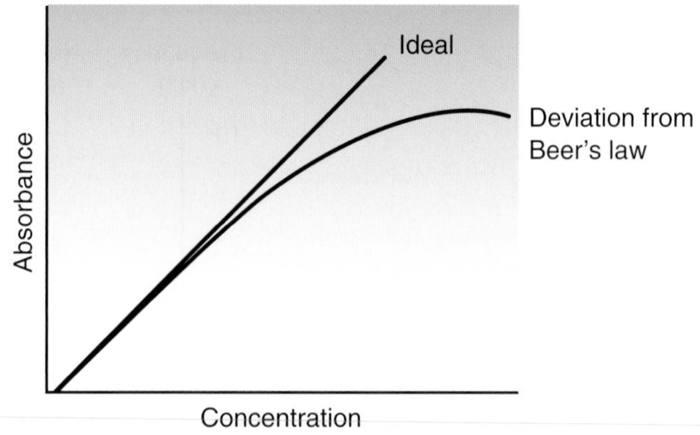

Figure 4-4 A plot of absorbance versus concentration illustrating deviation from Beer's law.

Tyndall Effect

The Tyndall effect occurs with particles of colloidal dimensions and can be seen with the naked eye. Measurements of scattered radiation are used to determine the size and shape of polymer molecules and colloidal particles.

Raman Scattering

Raman scatter involves absorption of photons producing vibrational excitation. Emission or scatter occurs at longer wavelengths. Raman scatter always varies from the excitation energy by a constant energy difference.

Beer–Lambert Law

If monochromatic EMR (P_o) is directed toward a cuvet containing an absorbing species, the amount of light (P) transmitted (T) is equal to:

$$T = P/P_o \tag{4-4}$$

and percent transmittance is equal to $100T$.

Lambert proved that for monochromatic radiation that passes through an absorber of constant concentration, a logarithmic decrease is seen in the radiant power as the path length increases arithmetically. The absorbance (A) of a solution was determined to be equivalent to:

$$A = \log P_o/P \tag{4-5}$$

The relationship between transmittance, T, or percent transmittance ($P/P_o \times 100$), and absorbance is shown in Figure 4-3. Absorbance and percent transmittance are inversely related as given by the following:

$$A = 2 - \log \%T \tag{4-6}$$

Example 4-4. What is the absorbance of a solution whose transmittance is 10%?

SOLUTION

$A = 2 - \log \%T$

$A = 2 - \log 10\%T = 2 - 1 = 1$

Beer followed with studies on the relationship between radiant power and concentration. His approach was to keep the path length and wavelength constant while determining the relationship of radiant power, P, and concentrations of the absorbing species. Based on previous work by Lambert, Beer discovered that for monochromatic radiation, absorbance is directly proportional to the path length, b, through the medium and the concentration, c, of the absorbing species. The work culminated in the Beer–Lambert law, or simply Beer's law.

The principles established are represented by the following:

$$A = -\log T = \log P_o/P = abc \tag{4-7}$$

where:

a is absorptivity in L g^{-1} cm^{-1}
b is path length of 1 cm
c is concentration in units of g/L.

When the concentration in Equation 4-7 is expressed in moles per liter and the path length in centimeters, the term applied is *molar absorptivity*, given the symbol ε, epsilon, and is equivalent to the extinction coefficient ("a") times gram molecular weight of the absorbing species.

$$A = \varepsilon bc \tag{4-8}$$

where units for ε are L mol^{-1} cm^{-1}.

The graph of absorbance versus concentration shows the intercept at zero and a linear plot with a slope equivalent to "ab." Absorption spectroscopy is used best for solutions whose absorbance values are less than 2.0. Absorbance values greater than 2.0 may yield erroneous results because of other interactions of light with matter (e.g., variations in the refractive index of a solution). This may cause a deviation from Beer's law, resulting in bending of the linear plot as shown in Figure 4-4.

Deviations from Beer's law may be caused by changes in instrument functions or chemical reactions. Instrument deviation is commonly a result of the finite band pass of the filter or monochromator. Beer's law assumes monochromatic radiation, but truly monochromatic radiation is best achieved using only unique line emission sources. If absorptivity is constant over the instrument band pass, then Beer's law is followed within close limits.

Deviations from Beer's law become apparent at higher concentration (i.e., higher absorbance). In Figure 4-4, the curved line bends toward the concentration axis as opacity is approached. This lack of adherence to Beer's law in a negative direction is undesirable because of the somewhat large increase in the relative concentration error.

Deviation from Beer's law can occur with shifts or changes in chemical or physical equilibrium involving the absorbing species. Changes in solution pH, ionic strength, and temperature can result in such deviations.

Components of a Spectrophotometer

A typical photometer or spectrophotometer contains six basic components in a single or double-beam configuration. These components include (1) a stable source of radiant energy; (2) a filter that isolates a specific region of the electromagnetic spectrum; (3) a sample holder; (4) a radiation detector; (5) a signal processor, and (6) a readout device. Each component of a typical photometer is shown in Figure 4-5.

The following steps outline the function of each component in any absorption-type photometer as it detects light and provides information to the operator:

1. The light source provides the energy that the sample will modify or attenuate by absorption. The light is polychromatic (i.e., all visible wavelengths are present).
2. A wavelength selector or filter isolates a portion of the spectrum emitted by the source and focuses it on the sample.
3. The sample in a suitable container (e.g., a cuvet) absorbs a fraction of the incident light and transmits the remainder.
4. The light that passes through the cuvet and sample strikes the cathode of a photodetector and generates an electrical signal.
5. The electrical signal is processed electronically (e.g., amplified, digitized).
6. The processed signal is electronically coupled to the display unit (e.g., light-emitting diode [LED], X-Y strip chart recorder, meter).

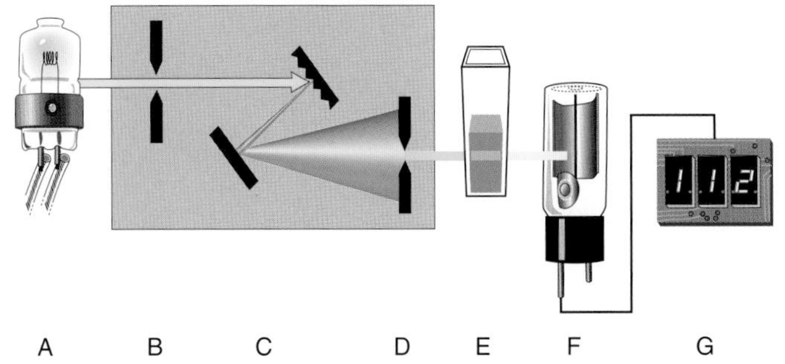

Figure 4-5 Components of a single-beam spectrophotometer. **A,** Exciter lamp; **B,** entrance slit; **C,** monochromator; **D,** exit slit; **E,** cuvet; **F,** photodetector; **G,** light-emitting diode (LED) display.

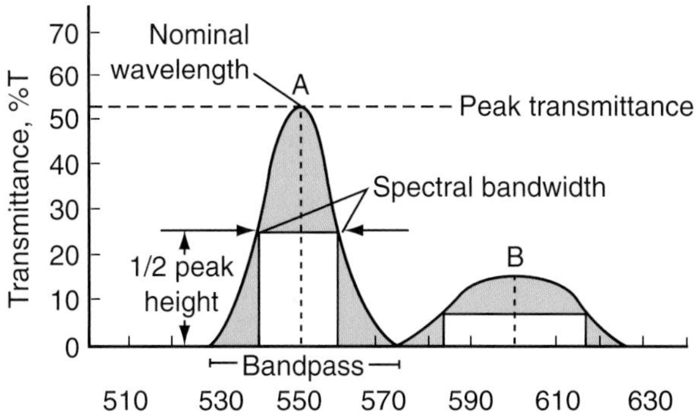

Figure 4-6 Comparison of spectral characteristics of two types of filters: **A,** Interference filter; **B,** absorption filter. The spectral bandwidth of filter A is much less than filter B and therefore allows fewer wavelengths of light through.

Radiant Energy Sources

Radiant energy sources or lamps provide polychromatic light and must generate sufficient radiant energy or power to measure the analyte of interest. A regulated power supply is required to provide a stable and constant source of voltage for the lamp. Radiant energy sources are of two types: *continuum* and *line*. A continuum source emits radiation that changes in intensity very slowly as a function of wavelength. Line sources emit a limited number of discrete lines or bands of radiation, each of which spans a limited range of wavelengths.

Continuum sources find wide applications in the laboratory. Examples of continuum sources include tungsten, deuterium, and xenon. For testing in the visible region of the EMS, tungsten or tungsten–halogen lamps are widely used. The filament in the tungsten–halogen lamp is maintained at a higher temperature than in the normal tungsten lamp. This takes advantage of the Wien and Sefan relationship to provide a source with a maximum wavelength near the center of the visible spectrum (whiter), and with a greater energy output (brighter). Introducing a halogen gas into the lamp envelope counteracts the problem of increased atom vaporization from the high temperature filament.

The deuterium lamp is routinely used to provide UV radiation in analytic spectrometers. The voltage applied is typically about 100 volts, which gives the electrons enough energy to excite the deuterium atoms in a low pressure gas to emit photons across the full UV range.

The strong atomic interaction in a high pressure xenon discharge lamp produces a continuous source of radiation, which covers both the UV and the visible range. The discharge light is normally pulsed for short periods with a frequency that determines the average intensity of the light from the source and also its lifetime.

In atomic emission line sources, electrons move between atomic energy levels. If the atom is free of any interaction with other atoms, the amount of energy liberated can be very precise, and all of the photons share a very clearly defined wavelength. This is the characteristic sharp "line" emission from an electronic discharge in a low pressure gas. Line sources that emit a few discrete lines find wide use in atomic absorption, molecular, and fluorescent spectroscopy. Mercury and sodium vapor lamps provide sharp lines in the ultraviolet and visible regions and are used in several spectrophotometers. For atomic absorption spectroscopy applications, the hollow cathode lamp provides atomic emission from free metal atoms by using the heat of a gaseous discharge (e.g., in neon) to vaporize metal atoms into the discharge. Typically, each lamp is specific to a particular metal. However, some lamps use two, three, or more metals, although the emission from each of these is reduced.

A laser source is very useful in analytic instrumentation because of its high intensity and narrow bandwidth, and the coherent nature of its outputs. Several specific uses of lasers include high resolution spectroscopy, kinetic studies of processes with lifetimes in the range of 10^{-9} to 10^{-12} s, as light sources for nephelometers, and as ionization inducers in the MALDI and SELDI mass spectrometric techniques (see later).

Wavelength Selectors

A critical component of all spectrometers is the device used to select the appropriate wavelength. Several types of wavelength selectors are available, including filters, prisms, grating monochromators, and, recently, holographic gratings. The quality of these selectors is described by their nominal wavelengths, spectral bandwidths, and bandpass. *Nominal wavelength* represents the wavelength in nanometers at peak transmittance. Spectral bandwidth is the range of wavelengths above one-half peak transmittance. It is sometimes called the half power point or full width at half peak maximum (FWHM). The total range of wavelengths transmitted is the *bandpass*. Figure 4-6 summarizes these characteristics of wavelength selectors. This figure also summarizes the difference in wavelength selectivity between interference (*A*, left) and absorbance filters (*B*, right) as we now discuss.

Filters

An important component of the spectrophotometer is the wavelength filter. Its purpose is to isolate monochromatic light, or at least as narrow a range of wavelengths of light as possible, and direct it to the sample or to the photodetector. Remember, the purpose of absorption spectroscopy is to detect how much light is absorbed by the sample. This is a measure of the absorbance of an analyte in a sample that is directly proportional to concentration (see Beer's law above). The percent transmittance is the ratio of the amount of light transmitted through the sample to the amount of light transmitted in the absence of the sample (e.g., buffer or solvent without the sample). Theoretically, it should be possible to determine this ratio without any filter at all. However, under these circumstances, most of the light that enters the sample in the cuvet will not be absorbed, so that, to determine absorbance, it would be necessary to measure a small difference between two large numbers (i.e., the amount of light transmitted in the absence [control] and the presence of the sample). Therefore, to obviate this condition, it becomes necessary to filter out as much "extraneous" light as possible to enable accurate measurements of absorbance.

Two approaches may be taken to filtering light waves. The first is to limit the wavelengths of light that enter the sample with appropriate filters, so-called pre-sample filters. The second is to allow multiwavelength light to pass through the sample and then to break up this light into its component wavelengths using a high resolution prism, and focus each of these component wavelengths on specific detectors, essentially one for each of the component wavelengths. If a sample absorbs light at one wavelength, then the ratio of the light transmittance of this wavelength of the sample to that for the control can be used to compute the percent transmittance and absorbance. This arrangement is termed post-sample filtering.

Pre-Sample Filters (Bender, 1987). Fundamentally, two types of these filters are used: absorption and interference filters. Absorption filters simply absorb regions of the electromagnetic spectrum and allow only a limited domain of this spectrum to pass through to the sample cuvet. The simplest sort of absorption filters consist of different forms of glass. One form of glass allows transmission only of wavelengths of light greater than 400 nm, while a second form allows transmission only of wavelengths of light less than 600 nm. If both glasses are arranged serially, they allow for transmission of light of wavelengths of only between 400 and 600 nm, with a peak at 500 nm. As a refinement of this approach, the older spectrophotometers utilize colored glass or transparent plastic materials. These colors are arranged in a circle or wheel so that light of a relatively narrow range of wavelengths is transmitted when each colored sector is in the light path. For example, if light in the green portion of the visible spectrum is desired, the wheel is turned so that the green filter is placed in the light path. The spectral bandwidth of these absorption filters ranges from about 30–50 nm (see Fig. 4-6).

This bandwidth is rather large but is adequate for determining the concentration of compounds in solution; absorbance filters are less adequate for scanning the absorption spectra of individual compounds and macromolecules or for accurately determining low concentrations of molecules. To achieve the latter goals, it becomes necessary to use interference filters.

In the simplest interference filter, light on the path to the sample cuvet enters a magnesium fluoride chamber that is coated with micro-mirrors on the interior. As shown in Figure 4-7, *A*, light enters evenly spaced ports or slits on the left. Only light that enters each slit can continue; the rest is absorbed by the chamber. Light entering a slit, at an angle to the horizontal, travels across the chamber and is reflected back to the opposite wall. In Figure 4-7, *A*, if the path length ab equals bc, and the path length equals the desired wavelength of light, it can be shown from the theory of optics that the light whose wavelength equals that of the path length or integral multiples of this path length will undergo constructive interference (i.e., the waves will add to one another exactly) with incoming light at slits above it. For example, in Figure 4-7, *A*, light of wavelength $L = ab$, reflected from *b* to *c*, will be exactly in phase with light of wavelength *L* or integral multiples of *L*, entering the slit at *c*; all other wavelengths will destructively interfere with light entering slit *c*. The light is then reflected again at *c* to *d* and back again to *e*, where, again, it will add to (constructively interfere with) only light waves of the same wavelength or integral multiples of it. Eventually, only light at the desired wavelength will be transmitted through the opposite wall at slits *f* and *h*.

It is important to note that, because integral multiples of the wavelengths of incident light will constructively interfere with transmitted light in the chamber, more than one wavelength of light can be transmitted from the chamber. The actual quantitative relationship between the wavelengths (*L*) transmitted by the chamber, the angle of incidence, *q*, of the light entering a slit, the refractive index, *R*, of MgF_2 (1.38), and the distance, *d*, across the chamber, is as follows:

$$ML = 2dR\sin(q) \tag{4-9A}$$

where *M* is any integer. Note that this equation predicts that for any given distance, *d*, many wavelengths of integral multiples to the fundamental wavelength where $M = 1$ can be transmitted. In practice, many of these other wavelengths can be excluded by using such techniques as placing appropriate glass filters in series with the interference chamber.

The above arrangement successfully transmits (close to) monochromatic light at a particular wavelength. However, it does not allow for scanning of wavelengths to obtain the absorption spectra of different samples. To accomplish this, another, similar arrangement is used. In this case, however, advantage is taken of another principle from the theory of optics—the principle of light diffraction. As shown in Figure 4-7, *B*, when monochromatic light is allowed to enter two slits on one surface of a chamber, very much like the one shown in Figure 4-7, *A*, except that there is no material (MgF_2) in the chamber, the two light waves interfere with one another such that if a screen is placed on the opposite surface of the chamber, discrete regions of light and dark bands will be seen (Bender, 1987). The light bands are from light waves that have added constructively to one another and are transmitted; the dark bands result from destructive interference of the light waves, and no light waves are transmitted. The position of the bands and the distance between the bands depend on the wavelength of light that enters the two apertures and on the angle of incidence of both beams. Because, for a given angle of incidence, the position of the light bands for transmitted monochromatic light depends exclusively on the wavelength of light, if exit apertures are placed on the opposite surface only where the light bands occur for light of a desired wavelength, only light of that wavelength will be emitted from the chamber. This effect can be enhanced by placing multiple entry apertures next to one another in a sawtooth or grating pattern, such that adjacent apertures are at a fixed distance, *d*, from one another, as shown in Figure 4-7, *B*.

Now, polychromatic light is composed of multiple different monochromatic wavelengths of light. When polychromatic light is allowed to pass through the two apertures, as in Figure 4-7, *B*, each of the wavelengths will constructively and destructively interfere with itself, as described earlier. Two different wavelengths of light will interfere only destructively with one another unless they are integral multiples of one another, as discussed in the case of the MgF_2 chamber described previously. This allows us to "trap" the light of the desired wavelength by placing the exit apertures where the light bands are known to occur on the opposite surface for that monochromatic wavelength. A limiting factor for selecting truly monochromatic light is the size of the aperture that can allow some "stray" light from adjacent light bands for very close wavelengths to exit.

As with the MgF_2 interference chamber described previously, another source of contaminating light can occur from light of wavelengths that are integral multiples of the desired wavelength. The relationship that

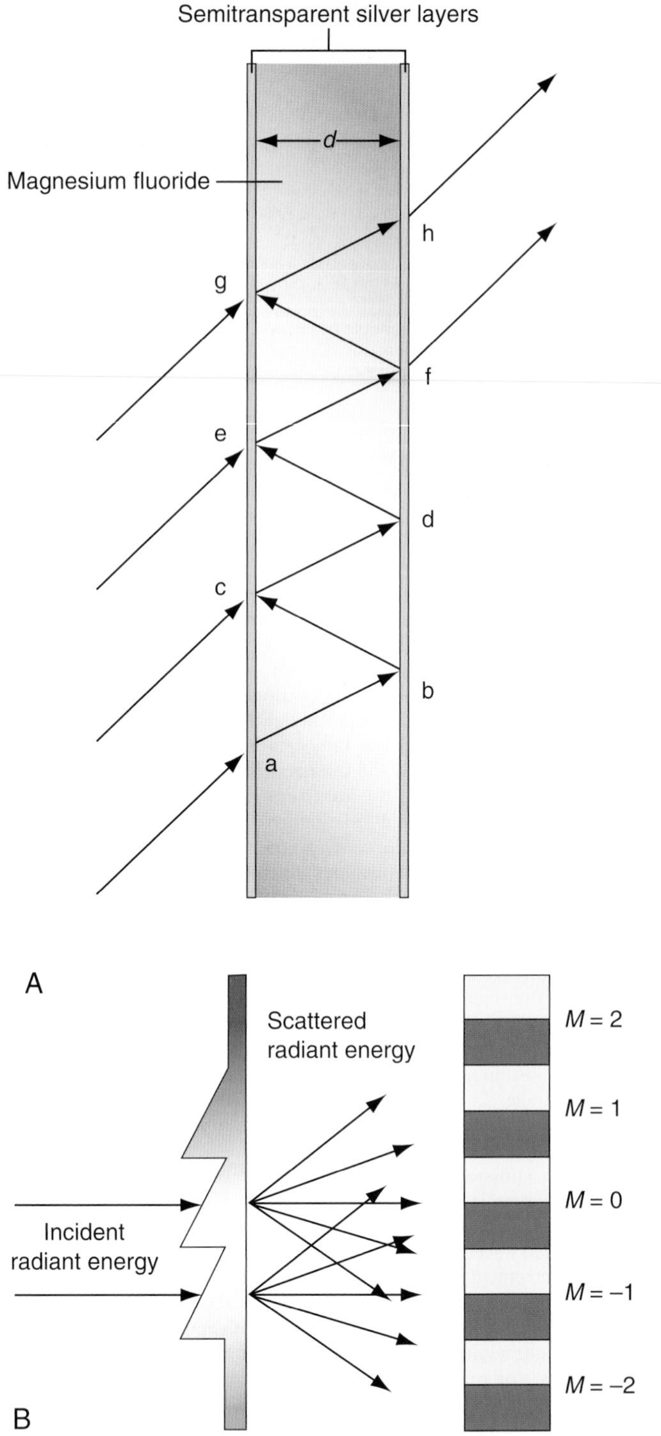

Figure 4-7 **A,** An interference MgF_2 filter. Light enters the filter at regularly spaced apertures at the same angle of incidence at each aperture. Going from the bottom of the figure, the light entering at *a* travels to *b*, where a mirror is reflecting it to *c*. Path lengths $ab = bc$. If these, in turn, are equal to the desired wavelength (or integral multiples of it), light of the desired wavelength arriving at *c* will be exactly in phase with light from the light source of that wavelength, and this will result in constructive interference. It will be out of phase with all other wavelengths and will therefore destructively interact with them. This summation process takes place multiple times until only light of the desired wavelength escapes through exit apertures such as at *f* and *h* (after Bender, 1987). **B,** A diffraction filter. When light enters multiple apertures, as in part **A,** each of which is equidistant from its two neighbors, light of each of the wavelengths interferes both constructively and destructively with itself, giving rise to light *(yellow)* and dark *(blue)* bands or fringes that can be observed on a screen. The position and spacing of these bands depend only on the wavelength and the angle of incidence. As shown in this figure, if apertures are placed only at the points where light *(yellow)* fringes occur in the figure, only light of a specific wavelength will pass through this exit aperture.

describes the wavelength as a function of the distance is similar to that for the MgF_2 chamber, that is,

$$ML = d\sin(q) \tag{4-9B}$$

Here, however, *d* is the distance between two adjacent entry slits on the near surface (toward the light source), *not* the distance across chamber as with the MgF_2 chamber. Note that for a given distance, *d*, and angle of incidence, *q*, this equation has multiple solutions. For example, if the desired wavelength is 800 nm, $d\sin(q) = 800$. But this is for $M = 1$, $L = 800$ nm. Another solution is $M = 2$, $L = 400$ nm, and another $M = 3$, $L = 266.67$ nm, etc. As discussed for the MgF_2 chamber, these other wavelengths can be filtered out by the use of appropriate glass or other filters.

Note that the system shown in Figure 4-7, *B*, allows for continuous scanning of the absorption spectrum for any analyte. Wavelengths can be continuously changed, most often using electronic devices, by changing the position of the aperture on the exit side of the chamber or by changing the angle of incidence of the entering light by altering the angle of the near surface of the chamber. Filters that have this capacity are called monochromators. Both interference systems in Figure 4-7 have spectral bandwidths of approximately 1.5% of the wavelength at peak transmittance, much lower than the absorption filters illustrated in Figure 4-6.

Post-Sample Filters. A different approach to obtaining monochromatic light and an accurate determination of absorbance is simply to allow the light to pass through the sample unfiltered. The light is then passed through a prism, where it is broken into its constituent wavelengths. The action of a prism depends on refraction of radiation by the prism material. The dispersive power depends on the variation of the refractive index with wavelength. A ray of radiation that enters a prism at an angle of incidence is bent toward the normal (vertical to the prism face), and at the prism–air interface, it is bent away from the vertical. As we describe in the section on photomultipliers that follows, each wavelength is focused onto a photodiode array such that each photodiode responds to only a specific set of wavelengths. The amount of transmitted light in the presence of the sample is compared with that in the absence of the sample. Photodiode arrays are examples of devices that convert photon energy into electrical currents in a system where photons excite the outer electrons in metal to move in the so-called conduction band, generating a current.

Sample Containers (Cuvets)

Sample containers (i.e., cells or cuvets) are used to hold samples and must be made of material that is transparent to radiation in the spectral region of interest. In the ultraviolet region of the electromagnetic spectrum (below 350 nm), cuvets are made from fused silica or quartz. Silicate glasses can be used in the region between 350 and 2000 nm. Plastic containers have also found application in the visible region. Generally, the path length of cuvets is 1 cm, although much smaller path lengths are used in automated systems. However, to increase sensitivity, some cuvets are designed to have path lengths of 10 cm, increasing the absorbance for a given solution by a factor of 10 (Beer's law; Equation 4-7).

Many double-beam spectrophotometers are designed with two cuvet holders: one for the sample and the other for the solvent. If two cuvets are used, they should be optically matched for more accurate results. Matched pairs of cuvets are obtainable from a manufacturer, but their optical performance should be verified before use by measuring the absorbance of identical solutions and comparing their values. One cell should then be reserved for the sample solution, and the other for solvent. Cells should be scrupulously cleaned before and after each use.

Photodetectors

It is necessary to determine how much light passes through the sample in the cuvet. To accomplish this task, advantage is taken of the photoelectric effect that forms the basis of the quantum theory. Photons of specific wavelength excite the outer shell electrons of metals at their resonance frequencies to high energy states in which they move through the so-called "conduction band," in which electrons move through the outer shells of the metal, thereby causing a current. This current, the magnitude of which is directly related to the intensity of the incident light, can then be detected and digitized.

Photomultiplier Tubes (PMTs). Perhaps the most common type of photon detector is the photomultiplier. Photomultiplier tubes are commonly used when radiant power is very low, which is characteristic of very low analyte concentrations. The operating principle is similar to the phototube with one significant difference. Some PMTs are designed to provide

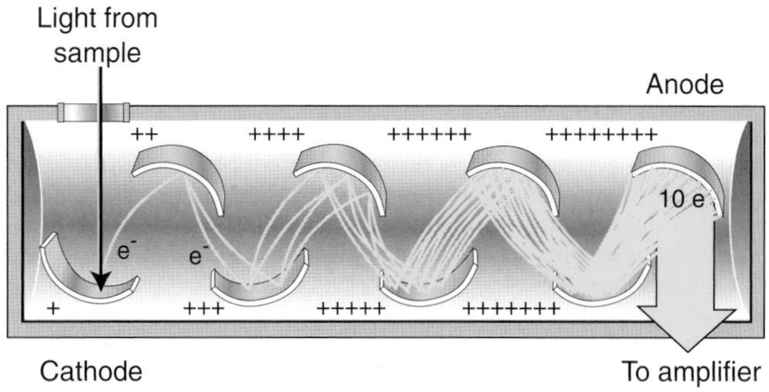

Figure 4-8 Schematic of a photomultiplier tube. In this diagram, a tenfold amplification of the initial signal is produced at the anode. *(Redrawn from Simonson MG. In Kaplan LA, Pesce AJ, editors. Nonisotopic alternatives to radioimmunoassay. New York: Marcel Dekker; 1981.)*

an amplified signal nearly one million times larger than their phototube counterparts. This is accomplished by using multiple dynodes positioned throughout the PMT. The response of the PMT begins when incoming photons strike a photocathode. Electrons are ejected from the surface of the photocathode. A PMT has several additional electrodes called dynodes, each having a potential that is approximately 90 V higher than the previous one. Upon striking a dynode, each photoelectron causes emission of several additional electrons; these, in turn, are accelerated toward a second dynode, which is 90 V more positive than the previous dynode, which further amplifies the incident signal. This process, shown in Figure 4-8, continues within the PMT until all electrons are collected at the anode, where the resulting current is passed to an electronic amplifier.

Photomultiplier tubes are highly sensitive to ultraviolet and visible radiation. They also have very fast response times. These tubes are limited to measuring low power radiation because intense light causes irreversible damage to the photoelectric surface.

Photovoltaic or Barrier Layer Cell. A variant method of detecting photon-induced current is the photovoltaic cell. This is a basic phototransducer that is used for detecting and measuring radiation in the visible region. This cell typically has a maximum sensitivity at about 550 nm and the response falls off to about 10% of the maximum at 350 and 750 nm. It consists of a flat copper or iron electrode upon which is deposited a layer of semiconductor material, such as selenium. The outer surface of the semiconductor is coated with a thin transparent metallic film of gold or silver, which serves as the second or collector electrode. When radiation of sufficient energy reaches the semiconductor, covalent bonds are broken, with the result that conduction electrons and holes are formed. The electrons migrate toward the metallic film and the holes toward the base upon which the semiconductor is deposited. The liberated electrons are free to migrate through the external circuit to interact with these holes. The result is an electrical current of a magnitude that is proportional to the number of photons that strike the semiconductor surface and a photocurrent that is directly proportional to the intensity of the radiation that strikes the cells.

These types of photodetectors are rugged and low cost, and require no external source of electrical energy. Low sensitivity and fatigue are two distinct disadvantages of these cells. For routine analyses at optimum wavelengths, these photocells provide reliable analytic data.

Vacuum Phototubes. A vacuum phototube has a semicylindrical cathode and a wire anode sealed inside an evacuated transparent envelope. The concave surface of the electrode supports a layer of photoemissive material that tends to emit electrons when it is irradiated. When a potential is applied across the electrode, the emitted electrons flow to the wire anode, generating a photocurrent that is generally about one-tenth as great as the photocurrent associated with photovoltaic cells for a given radiant intensity. The number of electrons ejected from a photoemissive surface is directly proportional to the radiant power of the beam that strikes the surface. All of the electrons are collected at the anode. Several types of photoemissive surfaces are used in commercial phototubes. These include (1) highly sensitive bi-alkali materials made up of potassium, cesium, and antimony, (2) red sensitive material using multialkalis, for example, Na/K/Cs/Sb, (3) ultraviolet sensitive with UV transparent windows, and (4) flat response-type substances using Ga/As compositions.

Silicon Diode Transducers. Silicon diode transducers are more sensitive than vacuum phototubes but less sensitive than the PMTs described above.

Photodiodes have spectral ranges from about 190–1100 nm. These devices contain positively (p) and negatively (n) charged semiconductive materials adjoining one another embedded on a silicon chip. A power supply is attached to this arrangement so that its positive pole connects to the *n*-type, and its negative pole to the *p*-type material. This arrangement results in a depletion layer that reduces the conductance of the junction to nearly zero. If radiation is allowed to impinge on the chip, holes and electrons formed in the depletion layer are swept through the device to produce a current that is proportional to radiant power (Skoog, 1998). This process is shown in Figure 4-9.

Multichannel Photon Transducers. In the discussion of post-sample filters, it was noted that unfiltered light emerging from the sample could be broken up into its constituent wavelengths using prisms; these different wavelengths are then directed to electronic detectors such that the intensity of light of each of the constituent wavelengths can be quantitated. Here, we describe some of these multiwavelength photodetectors.

A multichannel transducer consists of an array of small photoelectric-sensitive elements arranged linearly or in a two-dimensional pattern on a single semiconductor chip. The chip, which is usually silicon and typically has dimensions of a few millimeters on a side, also contains electronic circuitry that makes it possible to determine the electrical output signal from each of the photosensitive elements sequentially or simultaneously. The alignment of a multichannel transducer is generally in the focal plane of a spectrometer, so that various elements of the dispersed spectrum can be converted and measured simultaneously. Several types of multichannel transducers currently are used; they may include (1) photodiode arrays (PDAs), (2) charge-injection devices (CIDs), and (3) charge-coupled devices (CCDs).

Photodiode Arrays. By using the modern fabrication techniques of microelectronics, it is now possible to produce a linear (one-dimensional) array of several hundred photodiodes set side-by-side on a single integrated circuit (IC), or "chip" (Fig. 4-10). Each diode is capable of recording the intensity at one point along the line, and together they provide a linear profile of the light variation along the array.

A multiplex method is used to sort all of the signals received from the PDA. It records each signal individually, and then feeds the signals sequentially to a single amplifier. The output of the PDA is a histogram profile, along the array, of the charge leaked by each photodiode. This mirrors the variation of light intensity across the array. Thus, the PDA detection occurs in three main stages:

1. initialization
2. accumulation of charge at each pixel-integration time
3. read-out signals

In comparison with the PMT, the PDA has a lower dynamic range and higher noise. It is most useful as a simultaneous multichannel detector (Skoog, 1998).

Charge-Transfer Devices. Recent developments in solid-state detection techniques have now produced very effective two-dimensional array detectors that operate on a charge-transfer process, as an alternative to photodiodes. The term "charge-transfer device" (CTD) is a generic term that describes a detection system in which a photon, striking the IC semiconductor material, releases electrons from their bound state into a mobile state. The released charge, consisting of negative electrons and positive holes, then drifts to, and accumulates at, surface electrodes. An array of these surface electrodes divides the detector into separate, light-sensitive "pixels." The charge that accumulated at each electrode is proportional to the integrated light intensity falling on that particular pixel.

Two distinct classes of CTDs are known: charge-injection devices (CIDs) and charge-coupled devices (CCDs). In a CCD, all of the charge packets are moved "in-step" along the array row from one pixel to the next, as in a "bucket chain." At the end of the row, the charge packets are fed sequentially into an *on-chip* low noise amplifier, which then converts the charge into a voltage signal. The overall signal profile across the two-dimensional array is recorded one row at a time, thus giving a series of voltage signals corresponding to all of the pixels in the detection area.

In a CID, the charge accumulated in each pixel can be measured independently and nondestructively by using a network of "sensing" electrodes, which can monitor the presence of the accumulated charge. This is an important factor that differentiates CID systems from CCD and PDA systems, in which the whole of the detection area is "read" destructively in a single process.

Signal Processors and Readout

The processing of an electrical signal received from a transducer is accomplished by a device that amplifies, rectifies AC to DC (or the reverse), alters the phase of the signal, and filters it to remove unwanted components. In addition, the signal processor may need to perform mathematical operations on the signal such as differential calculations, integration, or conversion to a logarithm. Several readout devices have been used and include digital meters, d'Arsonval meters, recorders, light-emitting diodes (LEDs), cathode-ray tubes (CRTs), and liquid crystal displays (LCDs).

Quality Assurance in Spectrophotometry

Several photometric parameters must be monitored periodically by users. Monitoring these parameters is recommended by most regulatory agencies and accrediting organizations. The parameters routinely monitored include the following:

- wavelength or photometric accuracy
- absorbance check
- linearity
- stray light

Accuracy is the closeness of a measurement to its true value. Wavelength accuracy implies that a photometer is measuring at the wavelength that it is set to. Photometric accuracy can be assessed easily using special glass-type optical filters. Two examples of commonly used filters include didymium and holmium oxide. Didymium glass has a broad absorption peak around 600 nm, and holmium oxide has multiple absorption peaks with a sharp peak occurring at 360 nm.

An absorbance check is performed using glass filters or solutions that have known absorbance values for a specific wavelength. The operator simply measures the absorbance of each solution at a specified wavelength and compares the results with the stated values. Each user should establish a tolerance for the measurements based on accepted criteria.

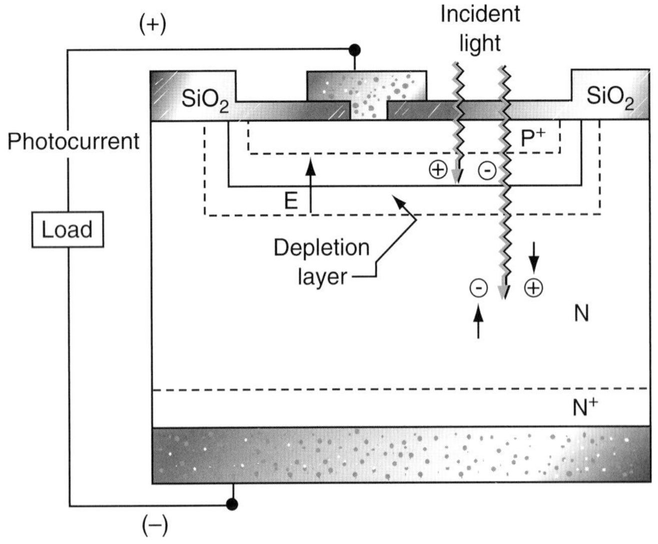

Figure 4-9 Schematic of a semiconductor photodiode used as a detector in many spectrometers.

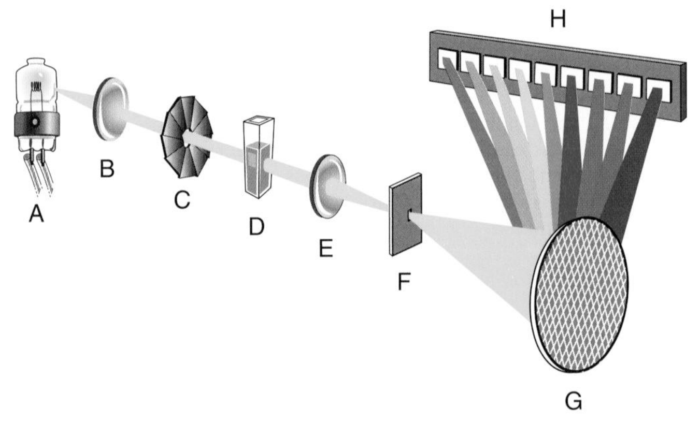

Figure 4-10 Photodiode array. **A,** Lamp; **B,** lens; **C,** shutter; **D,** cell; **E,** lens; **F,** slit; **G,** grating; **H,** photodiode array.

Linearity is defined as the ability of a photometric system to yield a linear relationship between the radiant power incident upon its detector and the concentration (i.e., Beer's law). The linearity of a spectrometer can be determined using optical filters or solutions that have known absorbance values for a given wavelength. Linearity measurements should be evaluated for both slope and intercept.

Stray light is described as any light that impinges upon the detector that does not originate from a polychromatic light source. Stray light can have a significant impact on any measurement made. Stray light effect can be evaluated by using special cutoff filters.

Types of Photometric Instruments

Several instrument designs and configurations may be used for absorption photometry. Each has unique terminology associated with its design. The terminology is not universal among users but is presented here as a guide. A *spectroscope* is an optical instrument used for visual identification of atomic emission lines. It has a monochromator, usually a prism or diffraction grating, in which the exit slit is replaced by an eyepiece that can be moved along the focal plane. The wavelength of an emission line can then be determined from the angle between the incident and dispersed beam when the line is centered on the eyepiece.

A *colorimeter* uses the human eye as the detector. The user compares the observed color of the unknown sample against a standard or a series of colored standards of known concentrations. *Photometers* consist of a light source, a filter, and a photoelectric transducer as well as a signal processor and readout. Some manufacturers use the term colorimeter or photoelectric colorimeters for photometers. These photometers use filters for isolation of specific wavelengths—not gratings or prisms.

A *spectrometer* is an instrument that provides information about the intensity of radiation as a function of wavelength or frequency. Spectrophotometers are spectrometers equipped with one or more exit slits and photoelectron transducers that permit determination of the ratio of the power of two beams as a function of wavelength, as in absorption spectroscopy. Most spectrophotometers use a grating monochromator to break up the light into a spectrum, as discussed earlier in the section on presample filters.

Single-beam spectrophotometers are the simplest types of absorption spectrometers. These instruments are designed to make one measurement at a time at one specified wavelength. The absorption maximum of the analyte must be known in advance when a single-beam instrument is used. The wavelength is then set to this value. The reference material (solvent blank) is transferred into a suitable cuvet and is placed in the path of the monochromatic light. The spectrometer is adjusted to read 0%T when a shutter is placed, so as to block all radiation from the detector, and to read 100%T when the shutter is removed. After these adjustments have been made, the sample is placed in the light path, the absorbance is measured, and the concentration is determined using calculations based on Beer's law or by constructing a calibration curve for the analyte.

A double-beam spectrophotometer splits or chops the monochromatic beam of radiation into two components. One beam passes through the sample, and the other through a reference solution or blank. In this design, the radiant power in the reference beam varies with the source energy, monochromator transmission, reference material transmission, and detector response, making the difference between the sample and the reference beam largely a function of the sample. The output of the reference beam can be kept constant, and the absorbance of the sample can be recorded directly as the electrical output of the sample beam.

Two fundamental instrument designs are used for double-beam spectrophotometers: (1) double beam in space and (2) double beam in time. A double beam in space design uses two photodetectors: one for the sample beam and the other for the reference beam. The two signals generated are directed to a differential amplifier, which then passes on the difference between the signals to the readout device. A schematic of the double beam in space system is shown in Figure 4-11.

A double beam in time instrument uses one photodetector and alternately passes the monochromatic radiation through the sample cuvet and then to the reference cuvet using a *chopper*. A chopper is the term used for a device such as a rotating sector mirror that breaks up or rotates radiation beams. Each beam, consisting of a pulse of radiation separated in time by a dark interval, is then directed onto an appropriate detector. A schematic of the double-beam in time system is shown in Figure 4-12.

A scanning double-beam system includes a double-beam spectrophotometer and a recorder that can provide an X-Y plot of absorbance versus wavelength for a given test sample. This type of configuration is ideal for determining the wavelength spectrum of an analyte in solution. The spectrophotometer has an automatically driven wavelength cam that can rotate at a predetermined speed. The recorder can be calibrated to the

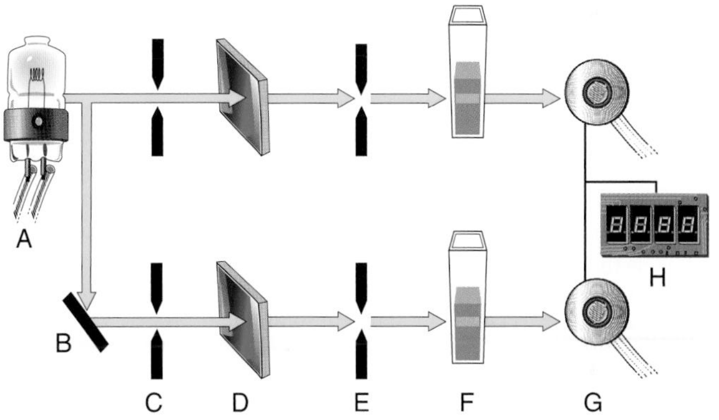

Figure 4-11 Double beam in space design of spectrophotometer. **A,** Exciter lamp; **B,** mirror; **C,** entrance slits; **D,** monochromators; **E,** exit slits; **F,** cuvets; **G,** photodetectors; **H,** light-emitting diode (LED).

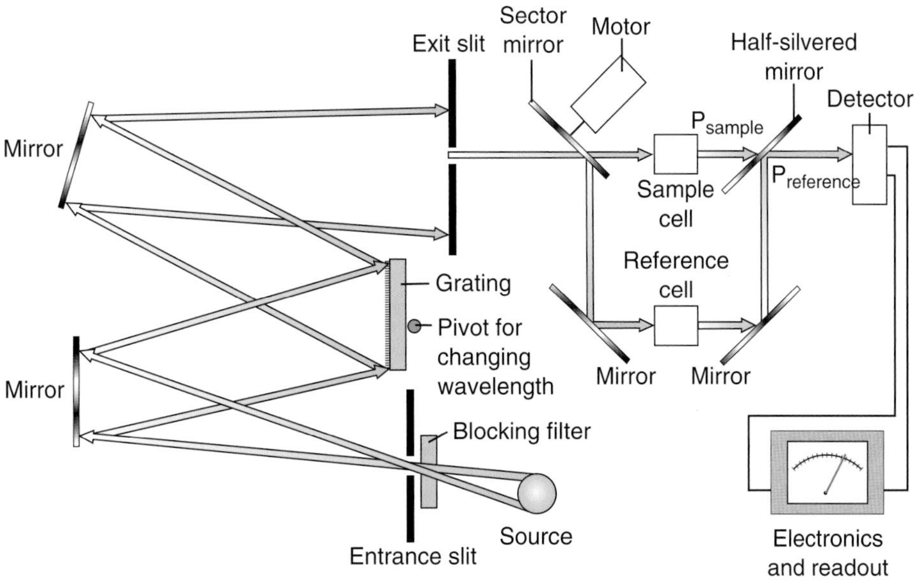

Figure 4-12 Double beam in time design of spectrophotometer.

wavelength of the monochromator to facilitate the identification of each peak maxima.

REFLECTOMETRY

Measurement of analytes in biologic fluids using reflectometry has been used for decades. Two clinical applications include urine dipstick analysis and dry slide chemical analysis. The instruments used for these applications include a reflectometer. A reflectometer is a filter photometer that measures the quantity of light reflected by a liquid sample that has been dispensed onto a grainy or fibrous solid support.

Two types of reflectance are known: (1) specular, and (2) diffuse. Specular reflectance occurs on a polished surface where the angle of incidence of the radiant energy is equal to the angle of reflection. Polished surfaces, for example, a mirror, may be used to direct and manage radiant energy but are not used to determine concentration. Diffuse reflectance occurs on nonpolished surfaces (i.e., a grainy or fibrous surface), as noted earlier. The reflected radiant energy tends to go in many directions. Diffuse reflection occurs within the layers and depends on the properties and characteristics of the layers themselves. A colored substance absorbs the wavelength of its color and reflects all other wavelengths at many different angles. Therefore the amount of a substance present can be measured as an indirect function of the reflected light.

A typical reflectometer used in a clinical laboratory detects only a constant fraction of the diffuse reflected light. Thus the reflectance of a sample is represented by the following:

$$R_{(\text{diffuse reflectance})} = \frac{R'_{(\text{fraction of diffuse reflectance of sample})}}{R'_{(\text{fraction of diffuse reflectance of a standard})}} \qquad \textbf{(4-10A)}$$

The amount of light reflected by a solution dispensed onto a white granular or grainy surface is inversely related to the concentration of the sample, as given by the following:

$$R_{\text{density}} = -\log\left(\frac{R_{\text{sample}} - R_{\text{black}}}{R_{\text{standard}}}\right) \times R_{\text{white}} \qquad \textbf{(4-10B)}$$

where:

R_{density} is the corrected reflectance density of the sample
R_{sample} is the measured reflectance of the sample
R_{black} is the reflectance of a black reference
R_{white} is the reflectance of a white reference
R_{standard} is the reflectance of a standard solution.

The ideal reflectance value of a pure white standard of ceramic material is *one* (i.e., all light is reflected), and conversely, the ideal reflectance value of pure black material is *zero* (i.e., all light is absorbed).

The relationship of percent reflectance and concentration of an analyte is nonlinear. Several algorithms have been developed for linearizing this relationship. The specific algorithm used depends upon the reflection characteristics of the composition material of the pad or film, the nature of the illumination, and the geometry of the instrument.

Reflectometers

The components of a reflectometer are very similar to those of a photometer, as shown in Figure 4-13. A tungsten–quartz halide lamp serves as a source of polychromatic radiation. A monochromator (e.g., stationary filter or filter wheel for multiple analytes) is used to isolate the wavelength of interest. Next, the monochromatic light passes through a slit and is directed onto the surface of a urine dipstick pad or dry slide, depending upon the instrumentation used. Solid-state photodiodes are typically used to detect reflected radiant energy. Special optical devices, for example, fiberoptics or ellipsoidal mirrors, may be used to direct radiant energy onto the detector. A computer or microprocessor is used to convert nonlinear reflectance signals into direct readout concentration units.

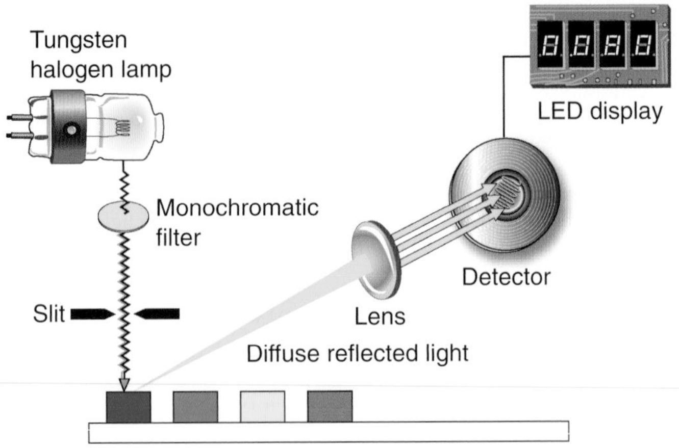

Figure 4-13 Components in a typical reflectometer used to measure analytes on urine dipstick. The different colored blocks represent different tests performed in urinalysis; the *blue* represents the quantitation of analyte using reflectance (i.e., the reflectance of light focused on the sample and reflected at an angle *[yellow beam]*, where it is detected).

MOLECULAR LUMINESCENCE SPECTROSCOPY (FLUOROMETRY)

Principle

Luminescence is based on an energy exchange process that occurs when certain compounds absorb electromagnetic radiation, become excited, and return to an energy level lower than or equal to their original level. Because some energy is lost before emission from the excited state by collision with the solvent or other molecules, the wavelength of the emitted light is longer than that of the exciting light. Most uncharged molecules contain even numbers of electrons in the ground state. These electrons fill molecular orbits in pairs with their spins in opposite directions. No electron energies can be detected by application of a magnetic field to such spin patterns, and this electronic state is called the singlet state. Similarly, if an electron becomes excited by electromagnetic radiation and its spin remains paired with the ground state, this creates a singlet excited state. The lifetime of the excited state is the average length of time the molecule remains excited before emission of light. For a singlet excited state, the lifetime of the excited state is on the order of 10^{-9} to 10^{-6} s. The light emission from a singlet excited state is called *fluorescence*. When the spins of the electrons in the excited state are unpaired, the electron energy levels will be split if a magnetic field is applied, and this electronic state is called a triplet state. Triplet state lifetimes range from 10^{-4} to 10 s (Willard, 1988). Light emission from an excited triplet state is called *phosphorescence*.

Luminescence is widely used because of its high sensitivity—the signal/noise ratio is very high, because light is measured against a nearly dark background. High specificity is a function of using two spectra, the excitation and emission spectra, and the possibility of measuring the lifetime of the fluorescent state. Two compounds that are excited at the same wavelength but emit at different wavelengths are readily differentiated with this technique.

Components of Fluorometers and Spectrophotofluorometers

Instruments designed for fluorescence measurement have the following basic components: a light source, an excitation (primary) monochromator, a cuvet, an emission (secondary) monochromator, and a photodetector (Fig. 4-14). The exciter lamp is a high-intensity light source such as a mercury vapor lamp or a xenon arc lamp. Simple instruments use mercury vapor lamps that do not require any special power supply. Mercury vapor lamps produce discrete and intense resonance lines that are not ideal for compounds with absorption bands at wavelengths not coinciding with these emission bands. For such compounds, xenon arc lamps producing an intense continuous spectrum between 300 and 1300 nm are appropriate. These lamps are used in nearly all commercial spectrophotofluorometers. In fluorescence measurements, the emitted light is detected at a right angle to the incident light to eliminate potential interference by the excitation signal. Phototubes or photomultiplier tubes (PMTs) are required for fluorescence measurements because the signals are generally of low intensity. Newer fluorometers on the market today use diode array and CTDs, which allow the rapid recording of both excitation and emission spectra and are particularly useful in chromatography and electrophoresis.

Time-resolved fluorescence assays minimize problems inherent in other fluorescent assays such as overlapping excitation or emission spectra of compounds present in the sample with the fluorophore. The label most commonly used is a chelate of europium (Eu^{3+}). Energy is absorbed by the organic ligand, leading to an excited state as the electrons migrate from the ground state singlet to the excited singlet state. The excitation may

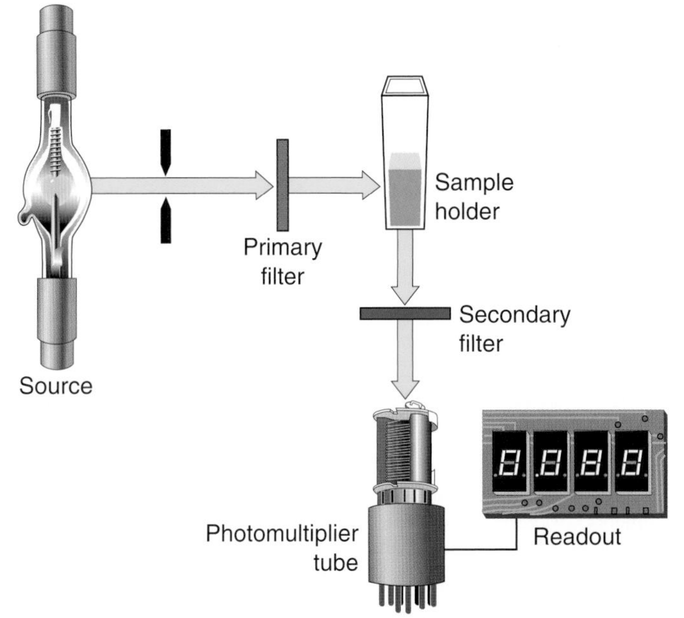

Figure 4-14 Components of a fluorometer. *(From Bishop ML, Duben-Engelkirk JL, Fody EP. Clinical chemistry: principles, procedures, correlations. Philadelphia: JB Lippincott Company; 1992, with permission.)*

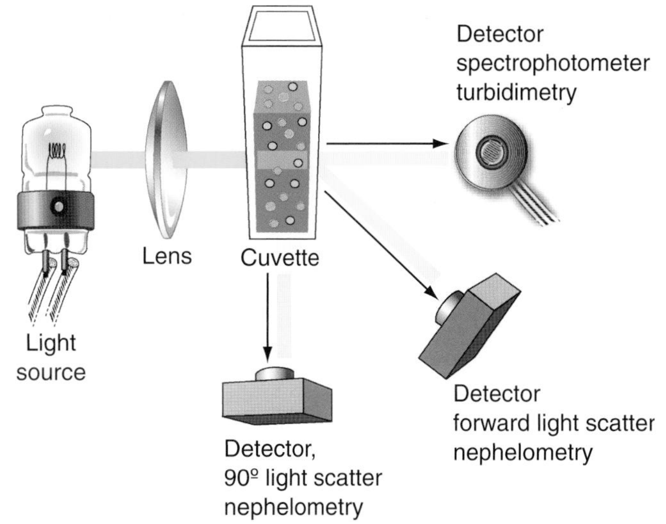

Figure 4-15 Optical arrangements of nephelometry and turbidimetry. Note that nephelometry detects (right-angle or forward) scattered light, and turbidimetry measures a reduction of light transmitted in the forward direction. *(Modified from Bishop ML, Duben-Engelkirk JL, Fody EP. Clinical chemistry: principles, procedures, correlations. Philadelphia: JB Lippincott Company; 1992, with permission.)*

lead to any vibrational multiplet of the excited state S_1. The molecule rapidly returns to the lowest energy levels in S_1 by a nonradiative process. The energy is transferred to the metal ion, which becomes excited and subsequently emits characteristic radiation. The radiative transition of excited Eu^{3+} after an energy transfer from triplet state results in an emission wavelength of 613 nm. The fluorescence lifetime of Eu^{3+} chelate is 10–1000 μs compared with nanoseconds for the most commonly used fluorophore. Therefore, Eu^{3+} with its longer emission lifetime makes it more attractive to use over a fluorophore like fluorescein with a lifetime of 4.5 ns. Time-resolved fluorescence instruments are similar to a typical fluorometer, except that time-resolved fluorometers use a time-gated measure on only a portion of the total emission spectra.

Chemiluminescence applications have increased dramatically owing to the increased sensitivity over fluorescence. (In chemiluminescence, the light signal is measured against a completely dark background because no excitation light is required.) The primary application has been in the area of immunoassays where several chemiluminescence compounds have been used as antigen labels. Chemiluminescence differs from fluorescence and phosphorescence in that the emission of light is created from a chemical or electrochemical reaction, and not from absorption of electromagnetic energy. The chemical reaction yields an electronically excited compound that emits light as it returns to its ground state, or that transfers its energy to another compound, which then produces emission. Chemiluminescence involves the oxidation of an organic compound (e.g., dioxetane, luminol, acridinium ester) by an oxidant (hydrogen peroxide, hypochlorite, or oxygen). These oxidation reactions may occur in the presence of catalysts, such as enzymes (alkaline phosphatase, horseradish peroxidase, or microperoxidase), metal ions (Cu^{2+} or Fe^{3+} phthalocyanine complex), and hemin. The excited products formed in the oxidation reaction produce chemiluminescence on return to the singlet state. A luminometer is used to detect chemiluminescence; it contains a PMT that provides a very strong electrical output signal. A typical signal from a chemiluminescent compound rises rapidly with time and reaches a maximum when reagent and analyte are completely mixed. An exponential decay of the signal follows until baseline is reached.

NEPHELOMETRY AND TURBIDIMETRY

Nephelometry and turbidimetry are used to measure the concentrations of large particles (such as antigen–antibody complexes, prealbumin, and other serum proteins) that because of their size cannot be measured by absorption spectroscopy. Nephelometry detects light that is scattered at various angles; scattered light yields a small signal that must be amplified. In contrast, turbidimetry measures a reduction in light transmission due to particle formation; thus, it detects a small decrease in a large signal (Fig. 4-15).

Principle

Nephelometry and turbidimetry are based on the scattering of radiation by particles in suspension. When a collimated light beam strikes a particle in suspension, portions of the light are absorbed, reflected, scattered, and transmitted. Nephelometry is the measurement of the light scattered by a particulate solution. Three types of light scatters occur according to the relative size of the light wavelength (Gauldie, 1981). If the wavelength (λ) of light is much larger than the diameter (*d*) of the particle ($d < 0.1\lambda$), the light scatter is symmetrical around the particle. Minimum light scatter occurs at 90 degrees to the incident beam and was described by Rayleigh (Rayleigh, 1885). If the wavelength of light is much smaller than the particle diameter ($d > 0.1\lambda$), then the light scatters forward owing to destructive out-of-phase backscatter, as described by the Mie theory. If the wavelength of light is approximately the same as the particle size, more light scatters in the forward direction than in other directions, as defined by the Rayleigh–Debye theory. A common application of nephelometry is the measurement of antigen–antibody reactions. Because most antigen–antibody complexes have a diameter of 250–1500 nm, and the wavelengths used are 320–650 nm, light is scattered forward (Rayleigh–Debye type).

Nephelometer

A typical nephelometer consists of a light source, a collimator, a monochromator, a sample cuvet, a stray light trap, and a photodetector. Light scattered by particles is measured at an angle, typically 15–90 degrees to the beam incident on the cuvet (see Fig. 4–15). Light scattering depends on the wavelength of incident light and particle size. For macromolecules with size close to or larger than the light wavelength, measurement of forward light scatter increases the sensitivity of nephelometry. Light sources include a mercury-arc lamp, a tungsten–filament lamp, a light-emitting diode, and a laser.

Lasers produce stable, nearly ideal monochromatic light of narrow bandwidth and emit radiant energy that is coherent, parallel, and polarized. A laser beam can be maintained as a very slim cylinder only a few micrometers in cross-section. A typical helium–neon laser lamp consists of a helium-pumping electrode (cathode) and a hollow glass laser core surrounded by a laser plasma tube (anode). Both the plasma tube and the core are filled with free helium and neon gases. The electrical discharge between the cathode and the anode is confined to the hollow glass core to keep it concentrated for maximum energy transfer. Two mirrors are positioned at the ends of the laser tube. One of them is fully reflective, and the other partially transparent. When the electrode is charged, the helium atoms are excited to a higher energy state and then transfer this energy to the neon atoms by collision. In turn, the excited neon atoms emit photons. Photons bounce back and forth between the two end mirrors, stimulating other atoms to emit additional photons, resulting in an amplification process. The amplified light eventually emerges as a laser beam through the partially transparent mirror. With the high intensity monochromatic beam, a substantial increase in sensitivity has been seen with lasers over conventional light sources. Disadvantages of laser sources include cost, safety and cooling requirements, and limited availability of wavelengths.

Turbidimetry

The measurement of the reduction in light transmission caused by particle formation is termed turbidimetry. Light transmitted in the forward direction is detected. The amount of light absorbed by a suspension of particles depends on the specimen concentration and on the particle size. Solutions requiring quantitation by turbidimetry are measured using visible photometers or visible spectrophotometers. Higher sensitivity has been achieved using photodetectors that can detect small changes in photon signals. Sensitivity comparable with nephelometry can be attained using low wavelengths and high quality spectrophotometers. Many clinical applications exist for turbidimetry. Various microbiology analyzers measure turbidity of samples to detect bacterial growth in broth cultures. Turbidimetry is routinely used to measure the antibiotic sensitivities from such cultures. In coagulation analyzers, turbidimetric measurements detect clot formation in the sample cuvets. Turbidimetric assays have long been available in clinical chemistry to quantify protein concentration in biologic fluids, such as urine and cerebrospinal fluid (CSF).

REFRACTOMETRY

Refractometry is based on light refraction. When light passes from one medium into another, the light beam changes its direction at the boundary surface if its speed in the second medium is different from that in the first. The angle created by the bending of the light is called the *critical angle*. The ability of a substance to bend light is called *refractivity*. The refractivity of a liquid depends on the wavelength of the incident light, the temperature, the nature of the liquid medium, and the concentration of the solute dissolved in the medium. If the first three factors are held constant, the refractivity of a solution is an indirect measurement of total solute concentration. Refractometry can be used to measure protein concentration, specific gravity of urine, and column effluent of high-performance liquid chromatography analysis.

OSMOMETRY

Osmometry is the measurement of the osmolality of an aqueous solution such as serum, plasma, or urine. As osmotically active particles (e.g., glucose, urea nitrogen, sodium) are added to a solution, causing its osmolality to increase, four other properties of the solution are also affected. These properties are osmotic pressure, boiling point, freezing point, and vapor pressure. They are called colligative properties of the solution because they can be related to each other and to the osmolality. As the osmolality of a solution increases, (1) the osmotic pressure increases, (2) the boiling point is elevated, (3) the freezing point is depressed, and (4) the vapor pressure is depressed. Osmometry is based on measuring changes in the colligative properties of solutions that occur owing to variations in particle concentration. Freezing-point depression osmometry is the most commonly used method for measuring the changes in colligative properties of a solution. It is based on the principle that addition of solute molecules lowers the temperature at which a solution freezes.

Principle of Freezing-Point Osmometry

The freezing point is the temperature at which water and ice are in equilibrium and is related to solute concentration. It is described by the following equation:

$$\rho T_f = K_f\, m \qquad \textbf{(4-11)}$$

where:

ρT_f = the change in freezing–point temperature
K_f = the freezing point constant of the solvent
m = the molality

A 1.0 mOsm/kg solution has a freezing point depression of 0.00186° C when compared with pure solvent (usually water). Thus blood plasma, with an osmolality of about 285 mOsm/kg, has a freezing point of about −0.53° C.

Freezing-Point Osmometer

A freezing-point osmometer consists of a sample chamber containing a stirrer and a thermistor (temperature-sensing device) connected to a readout device. The sample is rapidly supercooled to several degrees below its freezing point in a refrigeration chamber containing, for example, ethylene glycol. The sample is then agitated with the stirrer to initiate freezing. As ice crystals form, heat is released from the solution; this raises the temperature of the sample. The rate at which this heat of fusion is released from the ice being rapidly formed reaches equilibrium with the rate of heat removed by the colder temperature of the sample chamber. This equilibrium temperature, known as the freezing point of the solution, stays constant for several minutes once it is reached. This freezing point is detected by the thermistor, and the osmolality of the sample is converted to units of milliosmoles per kilogram of water.

FLOW CYTOMETRY

A flow cytometer measures multiple properties of cells suspended in a moving fluid medium. As each particle passes single-file through a laser light source, it produces a characteristic light pattern that is measured by multiple detectors for scattered light (forward and 90 degrees) and fluorescent light (if the cell is stained with a fluorochrome). Flow cytometry is used to count and sort cells, as well as viral particles, DNA fragments, bacteria, and latex beads. It is a core component of hematology cell counters and the technology used to differentiate white blood cells.

In flow cytometry, the term *particle* describes any object flowing through the instrument. An *event* is anything that is interpreted by the instrument to be a single particle. An *event* may be determined correctly or incorrectly by a flow cytometer. Methods have been developed to compensate for measurement of unwanted *events*. An example is the correction for measuring the simultaneous passing of two particles. Particles must be in suspension as single cells to be analyzed. If not, they can be made suitable for flow cytometry by the use of mechanical disruption or enzymatic digestion. Size restrictions also apply; cells or particles must be from 1–30 μm in diameter. Specialized flow cytometers are designed to handle smaller particles such as DNA fragments or bacteria.

Instrument Components

The system shown in Figure 4-16 has all of the design features of a flow cytometer with cell sorting capabilities. The cell suspension aliquots are introduced into the flow chamber using air pressure. As cells pass through the flow chamber, a low-pressure sheath fluid surrounds them. This outer fluid stream creates a laminar flow forcing the specimen to the center, and results in a single-file alignment of the individual cells. This process is called *hydrodynamic focusing*. A laser beam passes through each cell as it flows through the chamber. Forward light scatter is proportional to cell size, and 90-degree or right-angle scatter is related to cell granularity and nuclear irregularity. If the cells are labeled with appropriate fluorochromes, fluorescent signals proportional to the amount of bound label can be measured. Green fluorescence usually means that the dye fluorescein was used as a marker; red fluorescence usually means that a dye such as phycoerythrin was used as the contrasting marker. These dyes are usually attached to antibodies to specifically target selective antigens on cells or particles.

Forward light scatter is directed to the forward scatter photodetector. At right angles to the laser beam are mirrors that divide the right-angle light scatter among the remaining photodetectors (e.g., a right-angle scatter detector and two fluorescence detectors). Across the forward lens is an obscuration bar that blocks the laser beam after it passes through the stream. Only light from the laser that has been refracted or scattered as it strikes a particle in the stream is diverted enough from its original direction to avoid the obscuration bar and strike the forward positioned lens and the photodiode behind it. Granulocytes, monocytes, and lymphocytes are separated on the basis of size and granularity patterns, as determined by simultaneously analyzing forward and right-angle light scatter. For example, granulocytes with irregular nuclei scatter more light to the side than do lymphocytes with their spherical nuclei. Cell subpopulations can be identified by using electronic gating and analyzing fluorescence patterns (based on labels used for specific cells).

FACS, an acronym for *fluorescence-activated cell sorter*, describes the ability of a flow cytometer to physically sort cells in a liquid suspension. To do so, the instrument design has to be modified to electrically charge cells of interest. This is done by first vibrating the sheath stream to break it into drops. The stream of drops flows past two charge (high-voltage) plates where cells of interest are electrically charged with a voltage pulse.

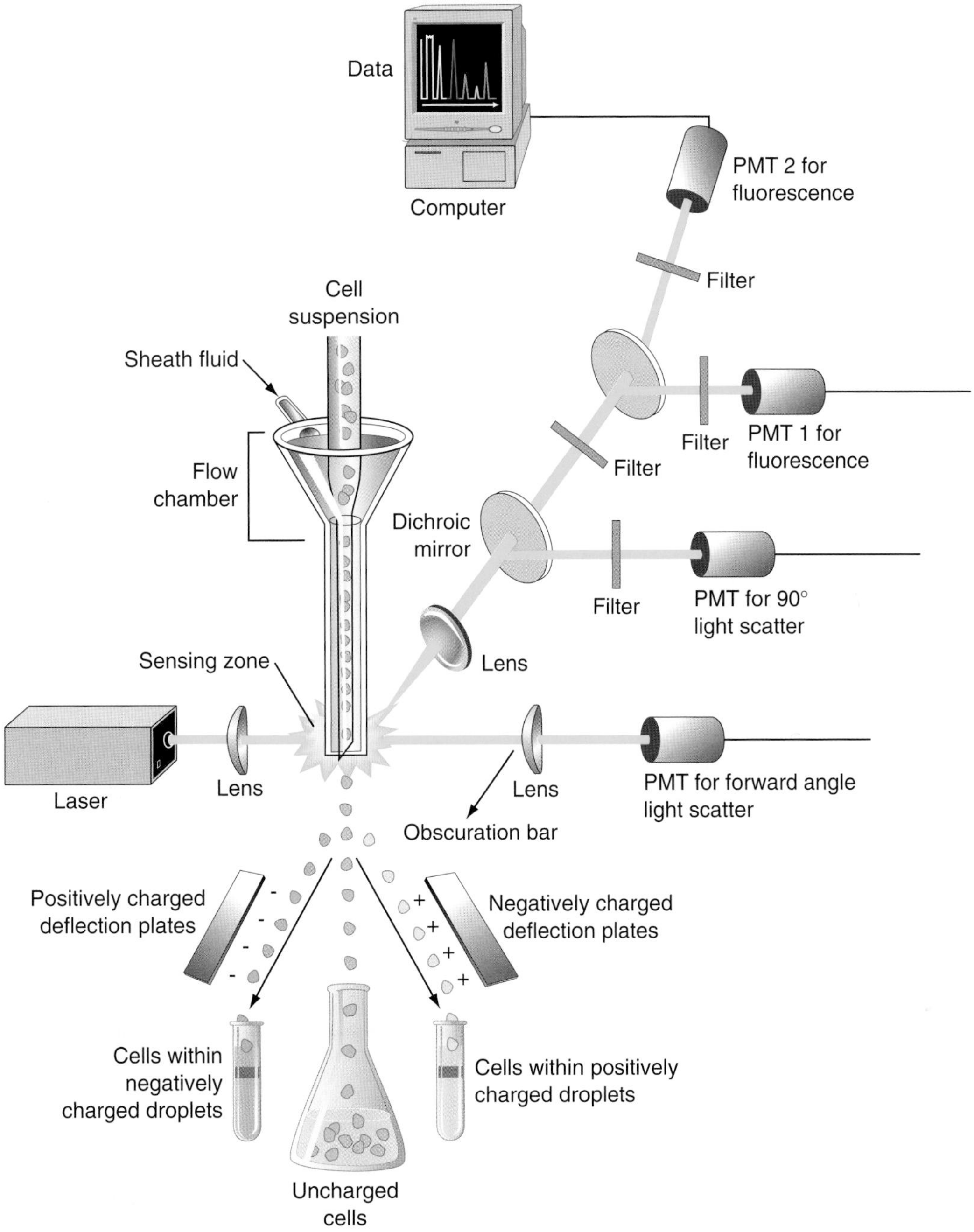

Figure 4-16 Components of a flow cytometer and a cell sorter. *(Redrawn from Ward KM, Lehmann CA, Leiken AM. Clinical laboratory instrumentation and automation; principles, applications, and selection. Philadelphia: WB Saunders; 1994, with permission.)*

Then the flow stream enters an electrical field where charged cells are deflected into suitable collection containers. Unwanted cells are not charged and are not deflected upon passing through the field.

ELECTROCHEMISTRY

Electrochemistry involves measurement of the current or voltage generated by the activity of specific ions. Analytic techniques include potentiometry, coulometry, voltammetry, and amperometry.

Potentiometry

The measurement of potential (voltage) between two electrodes in a solution forms the basis for a variety of procedures for measuring analyte concentration. Electrical potentials are produced at the interface between a metal and ions of that metal in a solution. Such potentials also exist when a membrane semipermeable to that ion separates different concentrations of an ion. To measure the electrode potential, a constant-voltage source is needed as the reference potential. The electrode with a constant voltage is called the reference electrode, whereas the measuring electrode is termed the indicator electrode. Concentration of ions in a solution can be calculated from the measured potential difference between the two electrodes. The measured cell potential is related to the molar concentration by the Nernst equation:

$$E = E^{\circ} - RT/nF \ln a_{red}/a_{ox} = E^{\circ} - 2.302\,RT/nF \log a_{red}/a_{ox} \quad \textbf{(4-12)}$$

where:

E = the cell potential measured
E° = the standard reduction potential
n = the number of electrons involved in the reaction
a_{red} = activity of the reduced species
a_{ox} = activity of the oxidized species
F = faraday (96,485 C/mol)
T = absolute temperature
R = molar gas constant

Substituting molar concentration for activity and common logarithm for natural log:

$$E = E^{o} - (0.0592/n)\log C_{red}/C_{ox} \quad \textbf{(4-13)}$$

where:

C_{red} = concentration of reduced species
C_{ox} = concentration of oxidized species

The Nernst equation is useful for predicting the electrochemical cell potential given the concentrations of oxidized and reduced species for a given electrode system.

Reference Electrodes

In many electroanalytic applications (e.g., measuring pH), it is desirable that the half-cell potential of one electrode be known, constant, and completely insensitive to the composition of the solution under study. An electrode that fits this description is called a reference electrode.

An ideal reference electrode should (1) conform to the Nernst equation, (2) exhibit a potential that is constant with time, (3) return to its original potential after being subjected to small currents, and (4) exhibit little hysteresis (i.e., lags with temperature cycling). The standard hydrogen electrode (SHE) exhibits many of these qualities but is not practical to use in clinical laboratory instrumentation. Thus, the calomel and silver/silver chloride reference electrodes are widely used for clinical measurements.

The calomel electrode (saturated calomel electrode [SCE]) consists of mercury in contact with a solution that is saturated with mercury (I) chloride (calomel) and that also contains a known concentration of potassium chloride. The silver/silver chloride electrode consists of a silver electrode immersed in a solution of potassium chloride that has been saturated with silver chloride. Silver/silver chloride electrodes have the advantage in that they can be used at temperatures greater than 60° C, whereas calomel electrodes cannot. On the other hand, mercury (II) ions react with fewer sample components than do silver ions (which can react with proteins, for example); such reactions can lead to plugging of the junction between the electrode and the analyte solution.

Ion-Selective Electrode

An ion-selective electrode (ISE) is an electrochemical transducer capable of responding to one specific ion. An ISE is very sensitive and selective for the ion it measures. It consists of a membrane or other barrier separating a reference solution and a reference electrode from the solution to be analyzed. The complexity of ion-selective electrode design depends on the membrane/barrier composition that determines its ionic selectivity. Many types of ISEs are available, including glass electrodes, liquid membrane electrodes, precipitate-impregnated membrane electrodes, solid-state electrodes, gas electrodes, and enzyme electrodes.

pH Electrode

Glass electrodes were the first and are still the most common electrodes for measuring hydrogen ion activity (pH or negative log of the hydrogen ion concentration). A pH electrode consists of a small bulb made of layers of hydrated and nonhydrated glass, which contains a chloride ion buffer solution. The buffer has a known hydrogen ion concentration. An internal electrode, usually silver/silver chloride, serves as an internal reference electrode. A saturated calomel electrode is used as an external reference electrode. One theory suggests that the sodium ions in the hydrated glass layer drift out. Sodium ions have a large ionic radius. Specimens containing hydrogen ions, which have a smaller ionic radius, replace the sodium ions. The result is a net increase in the external membrane potential. This potential propagates through the thin, dry membrane to the inner hydrated surface of the glass. Chloride ions in the inner buffer solution respond by migrating to the internal glass layer. Potentials generated at the pH electrode are referenced to the external reference electrode (saturated calomel), and the difference or change is displayed as pH units.

pCO_2 Electrode

The pCO_2 electrode is a pH electrode contained within a plastic jacket. This plastic jacket is filled with a sodium bicarbonate buffer and has a gas-permeable membrane (Teflon or silicone) across its opening. When whole blood containing dissolved carbon dioxide (CO_2) contacts the Teflon membrane, CO_2 from the blood passes through and mixes with the buffer. The equilibrium reaction shown in Equation 4-14 shifts depending upon the number of carbon dioxide molecules in a sample. The hydrogen ion activity is measured by a potentiometric pH indicator system.

$$CO_2 + H_2O \rightleftharpoons HCO_3^- + H^+ \quad \textbf{(4-14)}$$

Coulometry

Coulometry measures the quantity of electricity (in coulombs) needed to convert an analyte to a different oxidation state. By definition, a coulomb is the quantity of electricity or charge that is transported in 1 second by a constant current of 1 ampere. For a constant current of 1 ampere for t seconds, the number of coulombs (Q) is given by the expression:

$$Q = It \quad \textbf{(4-15)}$$

A Faraday is the charge in coulombs associated with one mole of electrons. The charge of the electron is 1.6018×10^{-19} C, thus 1 Faraday is equal to 96,485 C/mol.

Coulometry is used to measure chloride ion in serum, plasma, CSF, and sweat samples. In measuring chloride with coulometry, a constant current is applied across the two silver electrodes, which liberate silver ions into the specimen at a constant rate. Chloride ions in the sample combine with released silver ions to produce insoluble silver chloride. A pair of indicator and reference electrodes senses the excess silver ions and stops the titration. The number of silver ions released by ionization, which is exactly equal to that of chloride ions in the sample, can be calculated from Faraday's law:

$$Q = It = znF \quad \textbf{(4-16)}$$

where:

z = the number of electrons involved in the reaction
n = the number of moles of analyte in the sample
F = Faraday's constant (96,485 C/mol of electrons)

Amperometry

Amperometry is the measurement of the current flow produced by an oxidation–reduction reaction. Several immobilized enzyme electrodes use this principle, as do pO_2 electrodes (discussed later) and chloride titrators. The measurement of chloride in samples involves the use of two electrochemical methods: coulometry (discussed earlier) and amperometry. In the chloride titrator, a pair of silver electrodes serves as the indicator electrodes. When all of the chloride has been consumed, the silver appears in excess, causing an increase in current. This signals the endpoint of the reaction.

pO_2 Gas-Sensing Electrode

A widely used oxygen-sensing electrode (to determine partial pressure of oxygen in blood) incorporated in blood gas analyzers uses an amperometric or current-sensing electrolytic cell as the indicator electrode.

The pO_2 electrode uses a gas-permeable membrane, usually polypropylene, which allows dissolved oxygen to pass through. This membrane also prevents other blood constituents (that may interfere with the electrode) from passing through. Once the oxygen permeates the membrane, it reacts with a polarized platinum cathode according to the following reaction:

$$\begin{aligned} &O_2 + 4e' \rightarrow 2O^- \\ &2O^- + 2H_2O \rightarrow 4OH^- \end{aligned} \quad \textbf{(4-17)}$$

This, in turn, produces a change in the current through the cell, and the change is directly proportional to the partial pressure of oxygen present in the specimen.

Voltammetry

Voltammetry is a method in which a potential is applied to an electrochemical cell and the resulting current is measured. The most important advantages of voltammetry are sensitivity and the capability for multielement measurements. Analytes can be detected in the parts-per-billion range. With careful selection of testing conditions and methods, several analytes can be measured simultaneously in a single voltammetric study. Voltammetry consumes minimal analyte, unlike coulometry, which converts all of the analyte to another state. *Anodic stripping voltammetry* is an electrochemical technique used to measure heavy metals such as lead. The measurement of lead in blood occurs in basically two steps. First, free lead is electroplated (deposited) onto the platinum cathodes at a characteristic voltage. Second, the lead is stripped off of the platinum cathode, and the current is monitored over time. The current value is proportional to the amount of lead in the blood sample. This technique allows the sample to be preconcentrated at the electrode, which enables the method to detect very low analyte levels.

CONDUCTANCE

The principles of conductance have several applications associated with clinical laboratory procedures. Examples include monitoring water purity, measuring analytes in blood such as urea, and serving as components of detectors used in high-performance liquid chromatography (HPLC), gas chromatography (GC), cell counters, and capillary electrophoresis.

Electrolytic conductivity is a measure of the ability of a solution to carry an electrical current. Solutions of electrolytes conduct an electrical current by migration of ions under the influence of a potential gradient. The ions move at a rate dependent on their charge and size, the microscopic viscosity of the medium, and the magnitude of the potential gradient. Thus, for an applied potential, E, maintained constant but at a value that exceeds the deposition potential of the electrolyte, the current, I, that flows between the electrodes immersed in the electrolyte, varies inversely with the resistance of the electrolytic solution, R. The reciprocal of resistance, $1/R$, is called the conductance, G, and is expressed in reciprocal ohms, or mhos.

IMPEDANCE

Electrical impedance measurement is based on the change in electrical resistance across an aperture when a particle in conductive liquid passes through this aperture. Electrical impedance is used primarily in the hematology laboratory to enumerate leukocytes, erythrocytes, and platelets. In a typical electrical impedance instrument by Coulter, aspirated blood is divided into two separate volumes for measurements. One volume is mixed with diluent and is delivered to the cell bath, where erythrocyte and platelet counts are performed. As a cell passes through the aperture, partially occluding it, the electrical impedance increases, producing a voltage pulse, the size of which is proportional to the cell size. The number of pulses is directly related to the cell count. Particles measuring between 2 and 20 fL are counted as platelets, whereas those measuring greater than 36 fL are counted as erythrocytes. The other blood volume is mixed with diluent and a cytochemical-lytic reagent that lyses only the red blood cells. A leukocyte count is performed as the remaining cells pass through an aperture. Particles greater than 35 fL are recorded as leukocytes.

ELECTROPHORESIS AND DENSITOMETRY

Electrophoresis is the separation of charged compounds based on their electrical charge. When a voltage is applied to a salt solution (usually sodium chloride), an electrical current is produced by the flow of ions: cations toward the cathode, and anions toward the anode. Conductivity of a solution increases with its total ionic concentration. The greater the net charges of a dissolved compound, the faster it moves through the solution toward the oppositely charged electrode. The net charge of a compound, in turn, depends on the solution pH. Electrophoresis separations often require high voltages (50–200 V DC); therefore, the power supply should supply a constant DC voltage at these levels. The buffer solution must have a carefully controlled ionic strength. A dilute buffer causes heat to be generated in the cell, and a high ionic strength does not allow good separation of the fractions. Common support media for electrophoresis in clinical work include cellulose acetate, agarose, and polyacrylamide gels. Total volume of specimen applied depends on the sensitivity of the detection method. For clinical work, 1 μL of serum may be applied. Once the electrophoresis is completed, the support medium is treated with a dye to identify the separated fractions. The most common dyes used for the visualization step include Amido Black, Ponceau S, Fat Red 7B, and Sudan Black B. To obtain a quantitative profile of the separated fractions, densitometry is performed on the stained support medium.

A densitometer measures the absorbance of the stain on a support medium. The basic components of a densitometer include a light source, a monochromator and a movable carriage to scan the medium over the entire area, an optical system, and a photodetector. Signals detected by the photodetector are related to the absorbance of the sample stain on the support, which is proportional to the specimen concentration. The support medium is moved through the light beam at a fixed rate, so that a graph may be constructed that represents multiple density readings taken at different points. Most densitometers have a built-in integrator to find the area under the curve, so that all sample fractions can be quantified.

ISOELECTRIC FOCUSING

Proteins are polymers of amino acids that can be anions or cations depending on the pH environment. At a specific pH, a protein will have a net charge of zero when the positive charge and the negative charge of its amino acids cancel each other out. At this pH value, known as the protein's isoelectric point (pI), the protein is isoelectric. Isoelectric focusing (IEF) techniques are performed similarly to other electrophoresis methods, except that the separating molecules migrate through a pH gradient. This pH gradient is created by adding acid to the anodic area of the electrolyte cell and adding base to the cathode area (Fig. 4-17). A solution of ampholytes (mixtures of small amphoteric ions with different pIs) is placed between the two electrodes. These ampholytes have high buffering capacity at their respective isoelectric points. The ampholytes close to the anode carry a net positive charge, and those close to the cathode carry a net negative charge. When an electrical voltage is applied, each ampholyte will rapidly migrate to the area where the pH is equal to its isoelectric point. With their high buffering capacity, the ampholytes create stable pH zones for the more slowly migrating proteins. The advantage of isoelectric focusing techniques lies in their ability to resolve mixtures of proteins. Using narrow-range ampholytes, macromolecules differing in isoelectric point by only 0.02 pH units can be identified. Isoelectric focusing has been useful in measuring serum acid phosphatase isoenzymes. Its application has also been extended to detect oligoclonal immunoglobulin bands in CSF and isoenzymes of creatine kinase and alkaline phosphatase in serum.

CHROMATOGRAPHY

Chromatography is a separation method based on different interactions of the specimen compounds with the mobile phase and with the stationary phase as the compounds travel through a support medium. Compounds interacting more strongly with the stationary phase are retained longer in the medium than those that favor the mobile phase. Chromatographic techniques may be classified according to their mobile phase: gas chromatography and liquid chromatography. Figure 4-18 shows a typical chromatogram representing the concentration of each detectable compound eluting from the column as a function of time. Retention time (t_R) is the time it takes a compound to elute. This value is characteristic of a compound and is related to the strength of its interaction with the stationary phase and the mobile phase. The retention time therefore can be used to determine a compound's identity. In this example, two compounds are separated, and their retention times are represented by (t_{R1}) and (t_{R2}). These are uncorrected retention times and are measured from the injection time, $t = 0$. A column's ability to separate two compounds depends on several factors, which include (1) the difference in retention of the compounds or capacity factor, k', (2) the selectivity factor, α, and (3) the number of theoretical plates.

The value of k' can be calculated by the following equation:

$$k' = (t_{R1} - t_m)/t_m \text{ or } t_{R1'}/t_m \qquad \textbf{(4-18)}$$

where:

t_m is the retention time of a unretained compound

$t_{R1'}$ is the corrected retention time.

Another measurement derived from the calculated capacity factor is the selectivity factor (α) or relative retention of two solutes. A ratio of both capacity factors is used to calculate the selectivity factor. To measure the width of each peak, draw tangents along the sides of the peak to the baseline. W_b represents the distance between the two intersected lines. Another useful concept is theoretical plates. This describes the process by which the sample is transported down the column. In each "plate," the sample equilibrates between stationary and mobile phases. The analyte moves down the column as the equilibrated mobile phase transfers sample from one plate to another. To calculate the number of theoretical plates (N), use the following equation:

$$N = 16(t_R/W_b)^2 \qquad \textbf{(4-19)}$$

A plate number has no units, and the larger the value of N for a column, the greater is its separation efficiency. The combined effects of solvent efficiency and column efficiency are expressed in the resolution (R_s) of the column:

$$R_s = (t_{R2} - t_{R1})/0.5(W_{b1} + W_{b2}) \qquad \textbf{(4-20)}$$

The concentration of unknown compound can be derived by integration of peak areas or by using the method of internal standardization.

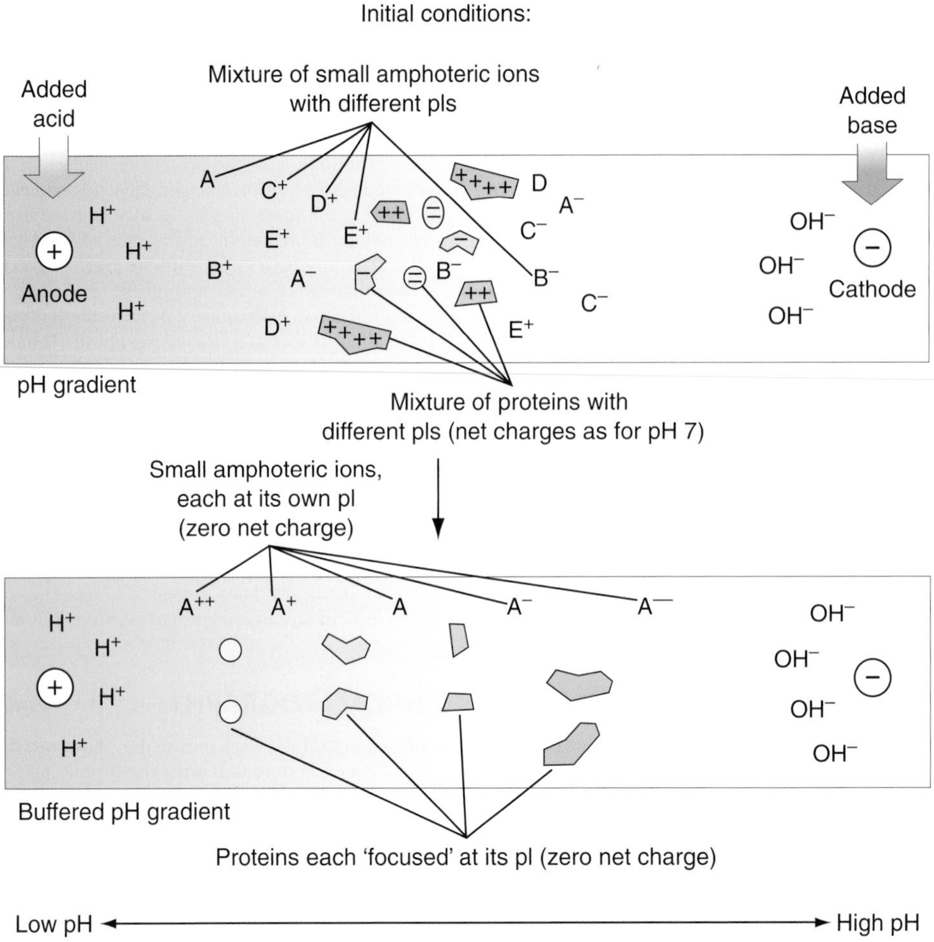

Figure 4-17 Isoelectric focusing (see text). *(Redrawn from Schoeff LE, Williams RH. Principles of laboratory instruments. St Louis: Mosby; 1993, with permission.)*

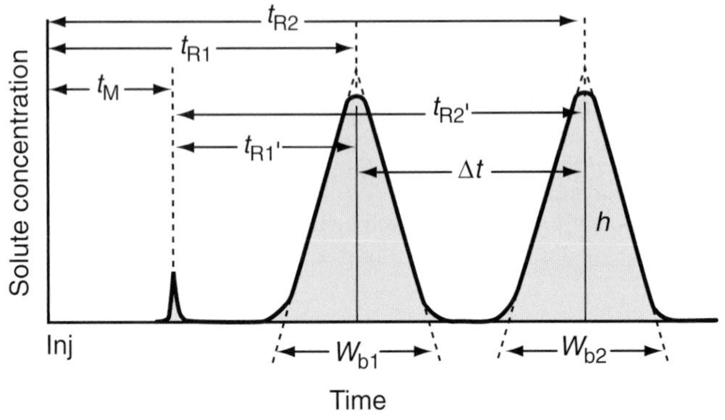

Figure 4-18 Chromatogram for the separation of two compounds. Note that the uncorrected retention time (t_{R1} and t_{R2}) is from injection (Inj) to peak; the corrected time ($t_{R1'}$ and $t_{R2'}$) takes into account the retention time of a nonretained compound (tM). *(Redrawn from Ravindranath B. Principles and practice of chromatography. New York: John Wiley & Sons; 1989, with permission.)*

Gas Chromatography

Gas chromatography (GC) is useful for compounds that are naturally volatile or can be easily converted into a volatile form. GC has been a widely used method for decades owing to its high resolution, low detection limits, accuracy, and short analytic time. Applications involve various organic molecules, including many drugs (see Chapter 23). Retention of a compound in GC is determined by its vapor pressure and volatility, which, in turn, depends on its interaction with the stationary phase. Two types of stationary phases commonly used in GC are solid absorbent (gas–solid chromatography [GSC]) and liquids coated on solid supports (gas–liquid chromatography [GLC]). In GSC, the same material (usually alumina, silica, or activated carbon) acts as both the stationary phase and the support phase. Although this was the first type of stationary phase developed, it is not as widely used as other types, primarily because of the strong retention of polar and low volatile solutes by the column (Ravindranath, 1989). GLC uses liquid phases such as polymers, hydrocarbons, fluorocarbons, liquid crystals, and molten organic salts to coat the solid support material. Calcine diatomaceous earth graded into appropriate size ranges is often used as a stationary phase because it is a stable inorganic substance. The use of fused silica capillary columns in which the stationary phase is chemically bonded onto the inner surface of the column has become very popular with chromatographers. The advantage of this type of column is that the stationary phase does not leave the solid support and bleed into the detector, and a uniform monomolecular layer of the stationary phase is obtained through the bonding procedure.

Components of a typical GC system are illustrated in Figure 4-19. Its basic design consists of five components: a gas cylinder as a mobile phase source, a sample injector, a column, a detector, and a computer for data acquisition. These systems may be automated to provide the user with a more precise and efficient separation. Carrier gases (mobile phase), which must be chemically inert, include helium, hydrogen, and nitrogen. Other substances used as mobile phases include steam and supercritical fluids. Examples of these are carbon dioxide, nitrous oxide, and ammonia. The carrier gas should be of high purity, and the flow must be tightly controlled to ensure optimum column efficiency and reproducibility of test results. Samples are manually introduced into the GC using a syringe pipet or an automated syringe pipet system. A pipet tip pierces a plastic septum located in the injector port. Each injection port is heated to very high temperatures. Samples are vaporized and swept onto the column. If the molecule of interest is not volatile enough for direct injection, it is necessary to derivatize it into a more volatile form. Most derivatization reactions belong to one of three groups: silylation, alkylation, and acylation. Silylation is the most common technique that replaces active hydrogens on the compounds with alkylsilyl groups. This substitution results in a more volatile form that is also less polar and more thermally stable.

Retention of compounds in a GC column can also be adjusted by changing the column temperature. The column temperature affects the

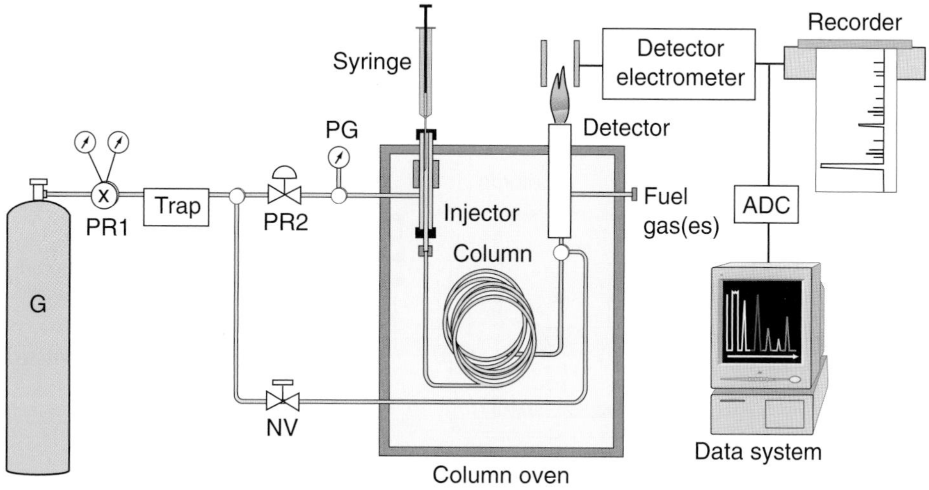

Figure 4-19 Components of a gas chromatographic system. *(Redrawn from Ravindranath B. Principles and practice of chromatography. New York: John Wiley & Sons; 1989, with permission.) G,* Gas cylinder; *NV,* valve for adjusting the gas flow rate; *PG,* pressure gauge; *PR1* and *PR2,* regulators.

volatility of the compounds and thus the degree of their interaction with the stationary phase. By proper selection of the starting temperature and temperature gradient during the procedure, good resolution of both weakly and strongly retained compounds may be achieved. The GC column, enclosed in a temperature-controlled oven, can be a packed column or a capillary column. Packed columns are usually 1–5 m long and 2–4 mm in diameter, and are filled with a stationary phase. Capillary columns range from 5–100 m in length and from 0.1–0.8 mm in diameter, and have a stationary phase located on their interior surface (Bartle, 1993). Capillary columns generally have higher efficiency and better detection limits. However, packed columns have a larger specimen or sample capacity, making them more useful in purification work. Examples of detectors used in GC include a flame ionization detector, a thermal conductivity detector, a nitrogen–phosphorus detector, an electron capture detector, a flame photometric detector, and a mass spectrometric detector. Flame ionization detectors (FIDs) are commonly used and are capable of detecting a wide variety of organic compounds and many inorganic compounds. This type of detector measures the ions produced by the compounds when burned in a hydrogen–air flame. An electrode collects the ions, and the magnitude of the resulting electrical current is proportional to the amount of substance (Tipler, 1993). FIDs can be modified to make them especially sensitive to molecules, including many drugs that contain either nitrogen or phosphorus (the so-called nitrogen–phosphorus detector, or NPD).

Liquid Chromatography

GC as a separation technique has some restrictions that make liquid chromatography a suitable alternative. Many organic compounds are too unstable or are insufficiently volatile to be assayed by GC without prior chemical derivatization. Liquid chromatography techniques use lower temperatures for separation, thereby achieving better separation of thermolabile compounds. These two factors allow liquid chromatography to separate compounds that cannot be separated by GC. Finally, it is easier to recover a sample in liquid chromatography than in gas chromatography. The mobile phase can be removed, and the sample can be processed further or reanalyzed under different conditions.

Many forms of liquid chromatography are available, and the selection of an appropriate form depends on a variety of factors. These factors include analysis time, type of compound, and detection limits. Paper, thin-layer, ion-exchange, and exclusion liquid chromatography often result in poor efficiency and a very long analysis time owing to low mobile phase flow rates. High-performance liquid chromatography (HPLC) emerged in the late 1960s as a viable form of liquid chromatography that provided advantages over other forms of liquid chromatography and gas chromatography. HPLC uses small, rigid supports and special mechanical pumps, producing high pressure to pass the mobile phase through the column. HPLC columns can be used many times without regeneration. The resolution achieved with HPLC columns is superior to that of other forms of liquid chromatography, analysis times are usually much shorter, and reproducibility is greatly improved. All of these attributes of HPLC render it a better method of separation over other forms of liquid chromatography.

Five separation techniques are commonly used in liquid chromatography. They include adsorption, partition, ion-exchange, affinity, and size exclusion. Each is characterized by a unique combination of stationary phase and mobile phase. In *adsorption (liquid–solid) chromatography*, the compounds are adsorbed to a solid support such as silica or alumina. Although this was the first type of column liquid chromatography developed, it is not widely used owing to the strong retention of many compounds by the supports, making them difficult to elute from the column. *Partition (liquid–liquid) chromatography* separates compounds based on their partition between a liquid mobile phase and a liquid stationary phase coated on a solid support. Partition chromatography includes normal-phase liquid chromatography, which uses a polar liquid stationary phase, and reverse-phase liquid chromatography, which uses a nonpolar stationary phase. *Ion-exchange chromatography* uses column packing material that has charge-bearing functional groups attached to a polymer matrix. The mechanism in this type of chromatography is the exchange of sample ions and mobile-phase ions with the charged group of the stationary phase. *Affinity chromatography* uses immobilized biochemical ligands as the stationary phase to separate a few solutes from other unretained solutes. This type of separation uses the so-called lock-and-key binding that is widely present in biologic systems. *Size-exclusion* chromatography separates molecules according to differences in their size. The support material has a certain range of pore sizes. As solutes travel through, the small molecules can enter the pores, whereas the larger ones cannot and will elute first from the column.

Liquid chromatography is similar in many aspects to GC, and therefore, the instrumentation is similar. A typical liquid chromatography system consists of a liquid mobile phase, a sample injector (manual or automatic), a mechanical pump, a column, a detector, and a data recorder (Fig. 4-20). The liquid mobile phase is pumped from a solvent reservoir through the column. A mechanical pump must provide precise and accurate flow, often working at high pressures (typically up to 6000 PSI). The pump must have low internal volume and be constructed of material that does not react with the solvent. Sample injection is achieved using a syringe and depositing the sample into a loop. The injection may be performed manually or automatically using a microprocessor control autosampler. Most analytic separations are performed using packed columns. Many types of packing material are available. Selection of the appropriate packing material is largely dependent on the type of compound(s) to be separated. In liquid chromatography, the physical properties of the sample and the mobile phase are often very similar. Two basic types of detectors have been developed. One is based on the differential measurement of a physical property common to both the sample and the mobile phase; examples include refractive index, conductivity, and electrochemical detectors. The other is based on the measurement of a physical property that is specific to the sample, either with or without the mobile phase; examples include absorbance and fluorescent detectors.

A widely used clinical application of HPLC is the separation and quantitation of various hemoglobins associated with specific diseases (e.g., thalassemia). Whole blood measurement of glycosylated hemoglobin (HbA_{1c}) can be accomplished using HPLC with complete analysis within 5 minutes.

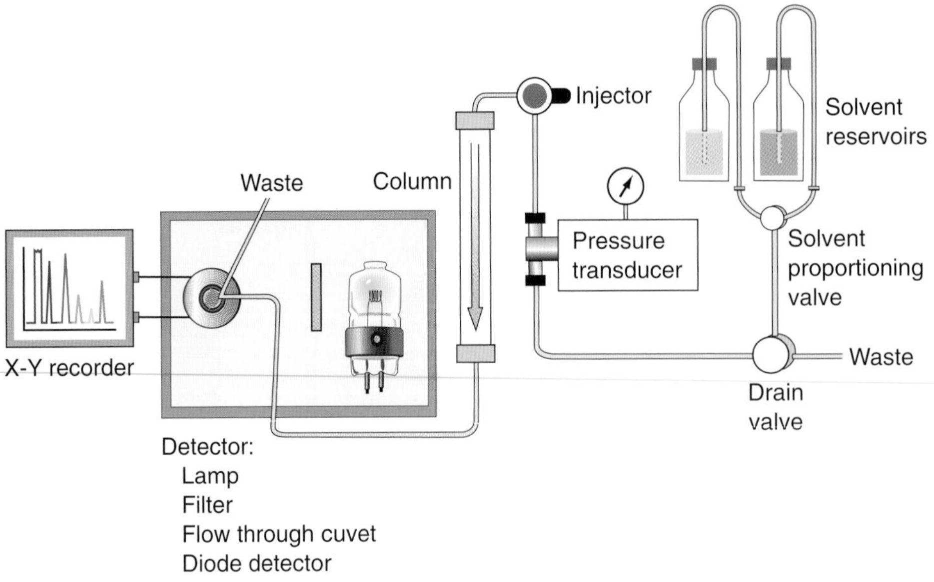

Figure 4-20 Components of a high-performance liquid chromatograph.

MASS SPECTROMETRY

Mass spectrometry (MS) is based on fragmentation and ionization of molecules using a suitable source of energy. The resulting fragment masses and their relative abundance yield a characteristic mass spectrum of the parent molecule. Before a compound can be detected and quantified by mass spectrometry, it must be isolated by another method: GC or HPLC. Mass spectrometry typically involves the following major steps: (1) conversion of the parent molecule into a stream of ions (usually singly charged positive ions); (2) separation of the ions by mass/charge ratio (m/z), where m is the mass of the ion in atomic mass units and z is its charge; and (3) counting of the number of ions of each type or measurement of current produced when the ions strike a transducer. Because most of the ions formed are singly charged, the m/z is usually simply the mass of the ion. MS is also described in Chapter 23 (see especially Figs. 23-5 and 23-6) as a technique for drugs of abuse testing. MS techniques are available for proteomics, which is discussed in Chapter 77.

Atomic Weights (amu and Da)

Atomic and molecular weight are generally expressed in terms of atomic mass units (amu) or daltons (Da). The amu or Da is based upon a relative scale in which the reference is the carbon isotope $^{12}_{6}C$, which is assigned a mass of exactly 12 amu. Therefore the amu or Da is defined as $\frac{1}{12}$ of the mass of one neutral $^{12}_{6}C$ atom. From this definition, we derive the following equality:

$$1\ \text{amu} = 1\ \text{Da} = 1.66054 \times 10^{-27}\ \text{kg/atom}\ ^{12}\text{C}$$

Also, 1 mole of $^{12}_{6}C$ weight 12.0000 g

Example 4-5. What are the masses in Da for $^{12}C^1H_4$ and $^{13}C^1H_4$?

SOLUTION

$^{12}C^1H_4$

$m = 12.000 \times 1 + 1.007825 \times 4 = 16.031$ Da

$^{13}C^1H_4$

$m = 13.00335 \times 1 + 1.007825 \times 4 = 17.035$ Da

Mass/Charge Ratio

Mass/charge ratio (m/z) is obtained by dividing the atomic or molecular mass of anion m by the number of charges z that the ion bears.

Example 4-6.

$^{12}C^1H_4^{+}$

$m/z = 16.035/1 = 16.035$

$^{13}C^1H_4^{2+}$

$m/z = 17.035/2 = 8.518$

Many ions produced in mass spectrometers are singly charged; thus the term mass/charge ratio is often shortened to the more convenient term mass. Strictly speaking, this abbreviation is incorrect, but it is widely used in mass spectrometry literature. This term also represents the x-axis for MS spectrums of molecules plotted against their relative abundance (y-axis).

Basic Components

All mass spectrometers have three basic components: an ion source, a mass analyzer, and an ion detector. The inlet unit admits samples to the mass spectrometer. When the instrument is part of a GC/MS arrangement, the inlet unit must be heated to maintain the volatile compounds in the vapor state upon coming into the ion source unit. It must also strip away most of the carrier gas to adapt to the high-vacuum condition required for mass spectrometry operation.

Ion Source Unit

The ion source unit is maintained at high temperature and vacuum to provide adequate conditions for ionizing the vaporized sample molecules. Several types of energy sources are available to ionize the sample molecules in mass spectrometry. One commonly used source is a beam of electrons produced by a heated filament. The process of bombarding the sample with electrons is called *electron-impact ionization*. Other processes of ionization include *chemical ionization*, in which the sample molecules are ionized by a reagent gas that has been ionized by an electron beam, and *fast atom bombardment*, in which a solid sample is ionized by a beam of atoms such as argon.

Most laboratorians are familiar with the use of mass spectrometers for drug and other low molecular weight compound analysis. Two examples are confirmation of positive drug screens (see Chapter 23) and amino acid analysis. These techniques conventionally couple a gas chromatograph and a mass spectrometer (GC/MS). This conventional approach had several limiting factors, including the need to separate analyte from specimen matrix and the need to make stable volatile derivatives, amenable to ionization by electron impact (EI) or chemical ionization (CI). Although these conventional techniques produced highly specific and sensitive analyses, they were also technically demanding and lacked the ruggedness required for the clinical laboratory. However, the increased focus on protein analysis, molecular diagnostics, and genetic-related testing has ushered in a new wave of mass spectrometers possessing the capabilities of evaluating complex compounds such as proteins.

The *matrix-assisted laser desorption ionization (MALDI)* source consists of a solid mixture of analyte and matrix (including organic chromophore) on a sample plate, along with a laser light and ion optics (Fig. 4-21, *A*). (This technique is further described in Chapter 76.) When the chromophore absorbs the laser light, it vaporizes and lifts the analyte ions from the surface into a gas phase directly above the target plate and into the analyzer. The MALDI technique is considered an offline ionization technique because the sample is purified, deposited, and dried on the sample plate before analysis (Skoog, 1998). *Surface-enhanced laser desorption ionization (SELDI)* is a technique that measures proteins from complex biologic

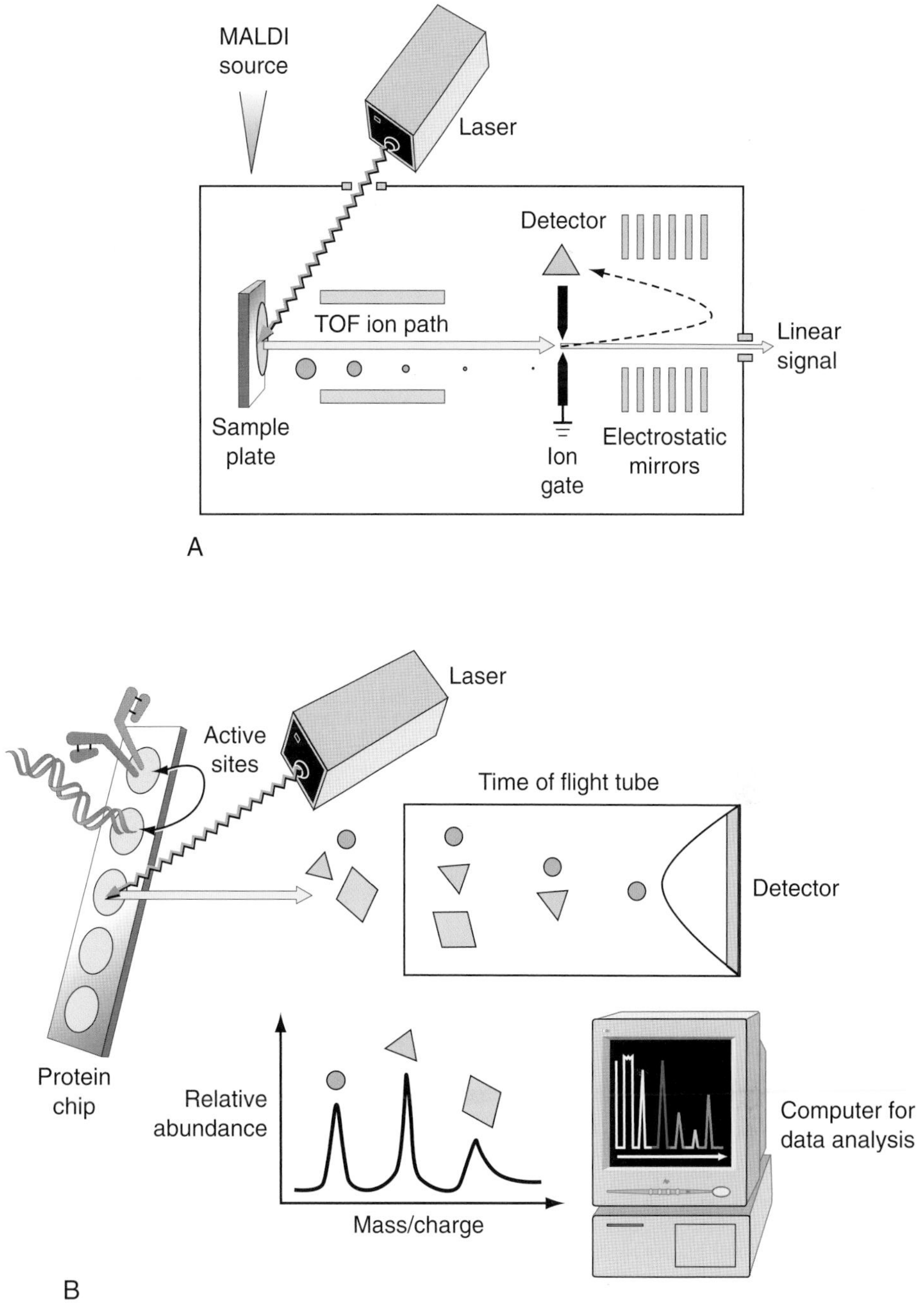

Figure 4-21 Diagrams of two systems widely used for proteomic research. **A,** Matrix-assisted laser desorption ionization (MALDI) time-of-flight mass spectrometer. **B,** Surface-enhanced laser desorption ionization (SELDI) time-of-flight mass spectrometer.

specimens such as serum, plasma, intestinal fluids, urine, cell lysates, and cellular secretion products (see also Chapter 76). Proteins are captured by adsorption, partition, electrostatic interaction, or affinity chromatography on a solid-phase protein chip surface. A laser ionizes samples that have been co-crystallized with a matrix on a target surface. The protein chip chromatographic surfaces in SELDI are uniquely designed to retain proteins from complex mixtures according to their specific properties. After the addition of a matrix solution, proteins can be ionized with a nitrogen laser and their molecular masses measured by time-of-flight (TOF) MS (Fig. 4-21, *B*) (see also Fig. 23-5). The protein chip arrays are the heart of the SELDI-TOF MS technology and distinguish it from other MS-based systems. Each array is composed of different chromatographic surfaces that, unlike HPLC or GC, are designed to retain, not elute, proteins of interest. The protein chip arrays have an aluminum base with several spots composed of a chemical (anionic, cationic, hydrophobic, hydrophilic, or metal ion) or biochemical (immobilized antibody, receptor, DNA, enzymes, etc.) active surface. Each surface is designed to retain proteins according to a general or specific physicochemical property of the proteins. Chemically active surfaces retain whole classes of proteins, and surfaces to which a biochemical agent, such as an antibody or other type of affinity reagent, is coupled are designed to interact specifically with a single target protein (Skoog, 1998).

Mass Spectrometer Analyzer Unit

The output of the ion source is a stream of positive or negative gaseous ions that are then accelerated into the mass analyzer, which sorts the parent molecular ions and their fragment ions according to their mass/charge ratio. This is accomplished in several different ways. *Time-of-flight* (*TOF*) analyzer consists of a metal flight tube, and the m/z ratios of the ions are determined by accurately and precisely measuring the time it takes the ions to travel from the MALDI or SELDI sources to the detector. Given that all ions of different m/z receive the same kinetic energy, low m/z ions will reach the detector sooner than high m/z ions. In the *quadrupole mass spectrometer* (Fig. 4-22, *A*, and Fig. 23-5), direct electrical current and radiofrequency voltages of selected magnitudes are applied to two pairs of metallic rods. Only ions of specific mass/charge ratio can pass undeflected to the end of the rods, where they are detected. All other ions have unstable trajectories along the path and are deflected toward the rods, never reaching the detector. An advantage of this design is that this system can perform tandem mass spectrometry scan modes in the same analyzer. The *ion-trap*

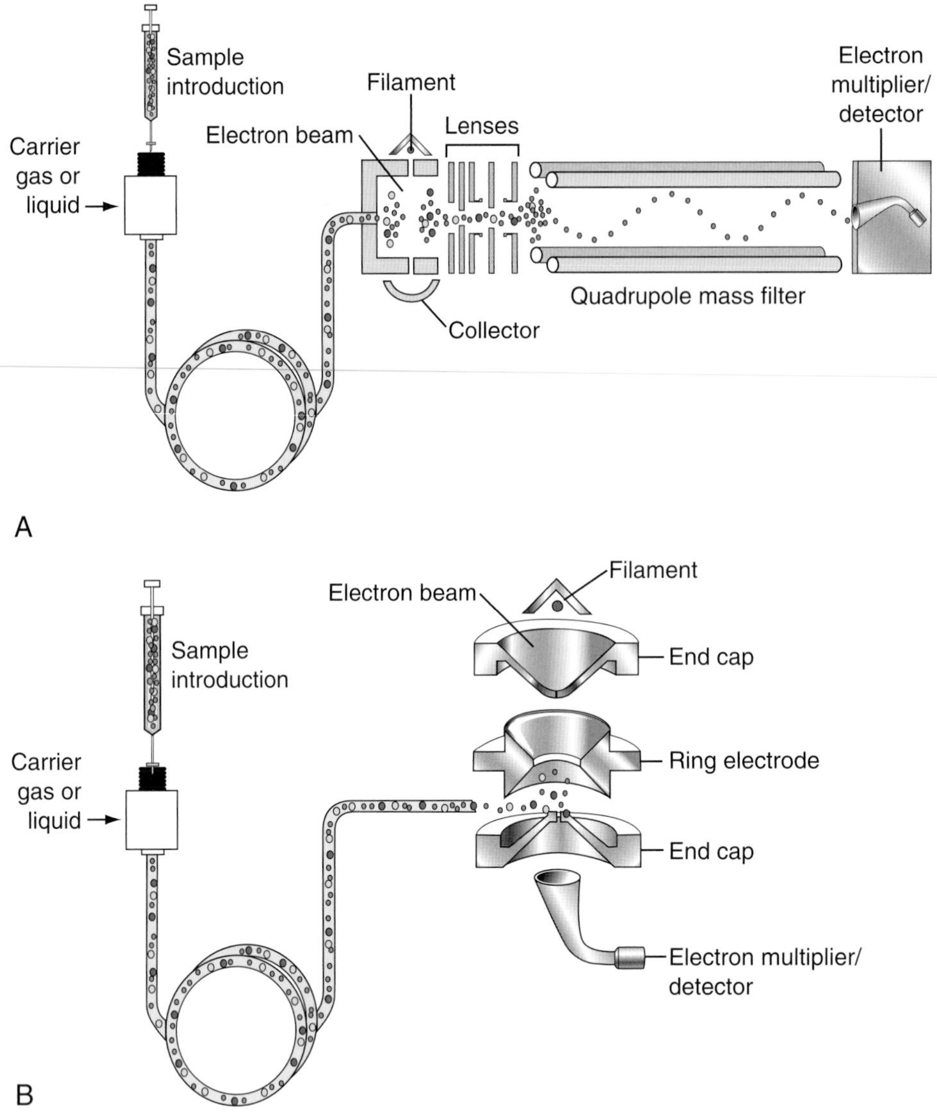

Figure 4-22 Mass spectrometer: **A,** Quadrupole type; **B,** ion-trap type. *(Redrawn from Schoeff LE, Williams RH. Principles of laboratory instruments. St Louis: Mosby; 1993, with permission.)*

mass spectrometer (Fig. 4-22, *B*) functions as a mass analyzer and as an ion source unit. Three electrodes, in a ring shape and two end caps, produce ions in the cavity until selectively ejected to the ion detector as the scanning radiofrequency voltage on the ring electrode varies. A major advantage of the ion-trap analyzer is its ability to get full mass spectra at very low sample concentrations (Karasek, 1988). In the *magnetic sector mass spectrometer*, a very high voltage accelerates the ions out of the ion source unit onto a magnetic field. The exiting path curvature of an ion depends on its mass/charge ratio, magnetic field strength, and applied voltage. The magnetic field or the voltage can be varied to allow selective ions to exit the magnetic field.

Ion Detector

The ion detector in a mass spectrometer is usually an electron multiplier or an ion–photon conversion detector. In an *electron multiplier*, the ions strike the detector's first dynode, which triggers the release of secondary electrons. A cascade of electrons occurs similarly to that in a photomultiplier tube, resulting in amplification of about a millionfold. In an *ion–photon conversion detector*, the ions strike a phosphor that emits a photon for each corresponding ion. A conventional photomultiplier tube then amplifies the signal in the usual fashion. The computerized data unit controls the multiple operating parameters of the instrument components and stores and analyzes a vast quantity of acquired data. The built-in libraries of reference mass spectra for known compounds can be searched by computer and compared with the sample spectrum for identification. As emphasized in Chapter 23, each compound or macromolecule has a unique mass spectrum—a "fingerprint" of the molecule. A typical mass spectrum is shown in Figure 23-6.

Modern mass spectrometers are extremely powerful and versatile instruments that can be interfaced to liquid chromatographs (LC) (eliminating the need to make volatile derivatives) and can perform separations in tandem (i.e., a gentle ionization step allows separation of parent ions, which can then be identified by their individual fragmentation patterns). Such LC/MS/MS techniques are finding increased application in the clinical laboratory, although mainly in reference laboratories.

SCINTILLATION COUNTER

Scintillations are flashes of light that occur when gamma rays or charged particles interact with matter. Chemicals used to convert their energy into light energy are called scintillators. If gamma rays or ionizing particles are absorbed in a scintillator, some energy absorbed by the scintillator is emitted as a pulse of visible light or near-UV radiation. A photomultiplier tube detects light directly or through an internally reflecting optic fiber. A scintillation counter is an instrument that detects scintillations using a photomultiplier tube and counts the electrical impulses produced by the scintillations. An application for scintillation counting is radioimmunoassay (RIA). Two types of scintillation methods exist: crystal scintillation and liquid scintillation.

Crystal scintillation generally is used to detect gamma radiation. When a gamma ray penetrates the sodium iodide (NaI) crystal, which contains 1% thallium, it excites the electrons of iodide atoms and raises them to higher energy states. When the electrons return to ground state, energy is emitted as UV radiation. The UV radiation is promptly absorbed by the thallium atoms and emitted as photons in the visible or near-UV range.

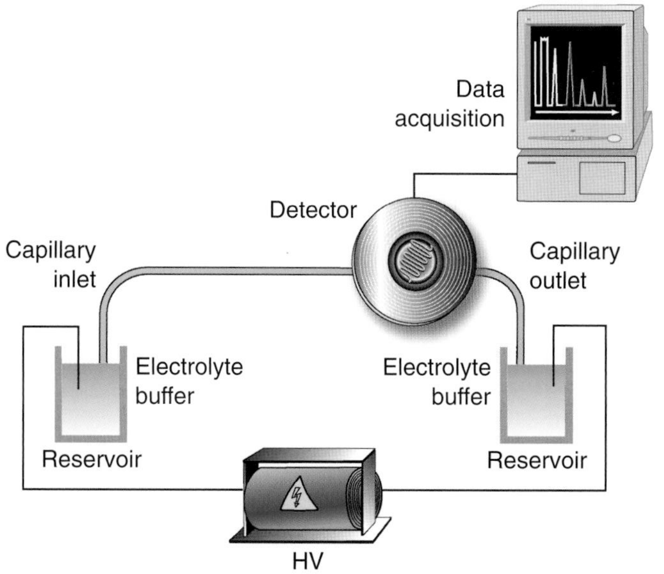

Figure 4-23 Capillary electrophoresis system. *(Redrawn from Ward KM, Lehmann CA, Leiken AM. Clinical laboratory instrumentation and automation; principles, applications, and selection. Philadelphia: WB Saunders; 1994, with permission.) HV,* High-voltage source.

The photons pass through the crystal and are detected by a photomultiplier tube. A pulse-height analyzer sorts out the pulse signals from the photomultiplier tube according to their pulse height and allows only those within a restricted range to reach the rate meter for counting.

Liquid scintillation is primarily used to count radionuclides that emit beta particles. A sample is suspended in a solution or "cocktail" consisting of a solvent such as toluene, a primary scintillator such as 2,5-diphenyloxazole (PPO), and a secondary scintillator such as 2,2′-p-phenylenebis (5-phenyloxazole) (POPOP). Beta particles from the radioactive sample ionize the primary scintillator of the solvent. A secondary scintillator absorbs the photons emitted by the primary scintillator and re-emits them at a longer wavelength. The secondary scintillator facilitates more effective energy transmission from the beta particles, especially when a large amount of quenching is present. Quenching is a process that results in a reduction of the photon output from the sample. This phenomenon may be due to chemical quenching, in which impurities in the sample compete with the scintillators for energy transfer, or color quenching, in which colored substances such as hemoglobin absorb the light photons produced by scintillation. The light photons produced in the sample are detected and amplified by the photomultiplier tubes in the same manner as for the crystal scintillation counter.

CAPILLARY ELECTROPHORESIS

Capillary electrophoresis (CE) represents another alternative in separation techniques. A typical capillary electrophoresis system, as shown in Figure 4-23, consists of a fused silica capillary, two electrolyte buffer reservoirs, a high-voltage power supply, and a detector linked to a data acquisition unit. The sample is introduced into the capillary inlet. When a high voltage is applied across the capillary ends, the sample molecules are separated by electro-osmotic flow, a bulk flow resulting from excess positive ions at the inner capillary surface moving toward the cathode. The positive ions in the specimen emerge early at the capillary outlet because the electro-osmotic flow and the ion movement are in the same direction. Negative ions in the specimen also move toward the capillary outlet but at a slower rate. As the sample ions migrate toward the capillary outlet, different types of detectors, including optical, conductivity, electrochemical, mass spectroscopy, or radioactivity detectors, are used to detect and measure them. Advantages of CE over conventional electrophoresis and HPLC are its short analytic time, improved resolving power, and microsample volumes (Love, 1994). Using nanoliter quantities of specimen, complex mixtures of molecules can be separated with a theoretical plate number approaching one million. Separations may be completed in less than 10 minutes by applying very high voltage. The application of high voltage is made possible by the capillary's high surface/volume ratio, which allows for efficient heat transfer through the capillary wall. Applications of capillary electrophoresis include separation of serum proteins and hemoglobin variants.

NUCLEAR MAGNETIC RESONANCE SPECTROSCOPY

Nuclear magnetic resonance spectroscopy (NMR) is a technique for determining the structure of organic compounds. Unlike mass spectroscopy (MS), NMR is nondestructive, although it does require a larger sample volume than MS. Although NMR is widely used as a diagnostic imaging technique, it has been adapted for only a limited number of clinical laboratory analyses, the most popular being lipoprotein particle measurements (see Chapter 17). It also has the unique capability of performing chemical analysis in vivo.

Nuclear magnetic resonance is a phenomenon that occurs when the nuclei of certain atoms are immersed in a static magnetic field and are exposed to a second oscillating magnetic field (i.e., the magnetic component of electromagnetic radiation [EMR]). Some nuclei experience this phenomenon and others do not, depending upon whether they possess a property called spin. A single proton, or hydrogen nucleus, possesses spin, and because hydrogen atoms occur very frequently, they are useful in determining structure.

When EMR is used to bombard molecules, the hydrogen atoms present will absorb photons of different energies depending upon the location of the hydrogen atom. For example, in compounds containing hydrogen and chloride, the proton near two chloride atoms produces a different NMR than the proton located near a single chloride and a single hydrogen. The energy absorbed by the spinning nuclei can be plotted versus the frequency of the applied EMR to obtain an NMR spectrum of the molecule.

In lipoprotein subclass measurements, the NMR signal originates in the protons of the terminal methyl groups of the lipid carried in the particles (primarily the cholesterol ester and triglyceride of the particle core, and the phospholipids of the particle shell). Signals from these different lipids combine to produce one signal with a characteristic frequency and shape related to particle size (i.e., the diameter of the phospholipids shell), excluding the influence of the apolipoprotein attached to the particle.

Basic components of an automated NMR spectrometer designed to provide fast, simultaneous subclass quantitative analysis of VLDL, LDL, and HDL are presented in Figure 4-24.

The automated sampler provides a micro sample probe that aspirates an aliquot of serum or plasma from a tray and transfers it to the NMR probe in a flow injection mode. Each sample passes through the 400 MHz magnet. The magnetic property of lipoproteins that gives them a characteristic resonance is a difference in their magnetic behavior induced by the degree of orientation of phospholipids in the shell surrounding the neutral lipid core. The equation describing this effect reveals that all lipoprotein particles of different diameters should have a different lipid NMR signature. This is displayed on the NMR processor.

The signature patterns are relayed to a networked PC, which provides access to high quality spectral data from isolated subclasses of lipoproteins incorporated into proprietary analysis software. The information is contained in a reference library that is accessible with permission from the vendor.

GENERAL ANALYTIC METHODS AND ISSUES

Perhaps the most fundamental aspect of the analytic process is the preparation of high quality reagents that will be used in the analytic procedure. In this process, the quality of water, the purity of the chemical, the selection of correct glassware or plasticware, and the correct preparations of reagents are all important for the proper operation of laboratory equipment and the performance of testing procedures. In this section, several topics will be presented that relate to analytic process and will ultimately have an impact on the results of a test performed on a patient's specimen.

CHEMICALS

The chemicals used to prepare reagents for chemical testing exist in varying degrees of purity. Proper selection of chemicals is important, so that the desired results may be attained. Chemicals acquired for reagent preparation are characterized by a grading system. The grading of any chemical is greatly influenced by its purity. The type and quantity of

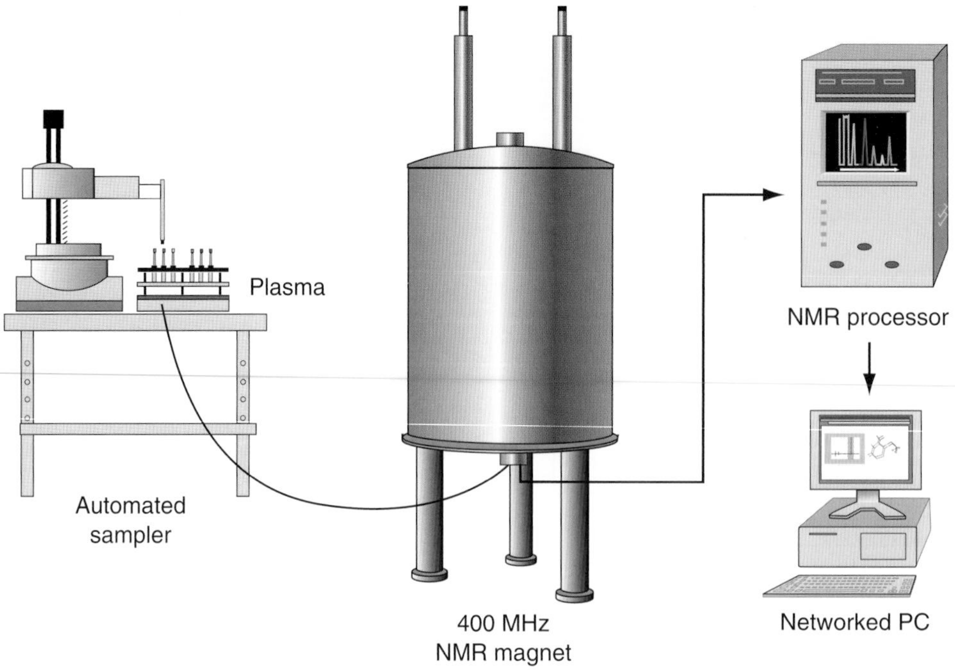

Figure 4-24 Schematic of an automated nuclear magnetic resonance (NMR) system using an automated flow-injector sampler.

impurities are usually stated on the label affixed to the chemical container. Less pure grades of chemicals include practical grade, technical grade, and commercial grade. These grades of chemicals are unsuitable for use in most quantitative assays performed in a clinical laboratory.

Most qualitative and quantitative procedures performed in the clinical laboratory require the use of chemicals that meet the specifications of the American Chemical Society (ACS). These chemicals are classified as analytic grade or reagent grade. Examples of other designations of chemicals that meet high standards of purity include spectrograde, nanograde, and HPLC grade. These are often referred to as ultrapure chemicals.

Pharmaceutical chemicals are produced to meet the specifications defined in *The United States Pharmacopoeia* (USP), *The National Formulary*, and *The Food Chemical Index*. These specifications define impurity tolerances that are not injurious to health.

The International Union for Pure and Applied Chemistry (IUPAC) has developed standards and purity levels for certain chemicals. These include atomic weight standard (grade A), ultimate standard (grade B), primary standard (grade C), working standard (grade D), and secondary substances (grade E).

A very good source of highly purified chemicals, especially reference materials, is the National Institute of Standards and Testing (NIST) (Gaithersburg, Md.). NIST defines its chemical and physical properties for each compound and provides a certificate documenting their measurements. NIST also provides Standard Reference Materials (SRMs) in solid, liquid, or gaseous form. The solids may be crystalline, powder, or lyophilized.

Two professional organizations can provide laboratory staff with guidelines for proper chemical selection and reagent preparation. They are the College of American Pathologists (CAP; Northfield, Ill.) and the Clinical and Laboratory Standards Institute (CLSI), formerly the National Committee for Clinical Laboratory Standards (NCCLS) (Wayne, Pa.).

WATER

Water has numerous uses in the clinical laboratory. Water is used to prepare reagents, as diluent for controls and calibrators, to flush and clean internal components of analyzers, to serve as a heating bath for cuvets, and to wash and rinse laboratory glassware. For most of these uses, the water must be of the highest purity, whereas the water required for rinsing glassware may be of a lesser purity.

Types of Water Purity

CLSI and CAP have defined three grades of water purity. They are types I, II, and III. The criteria for each type are outlined in the CLSI guidelines (NCCLS, 1997). When selecting a water purification system, the purchaser must pay strict attention to these criteria, so that all of the appropriate filters and components necessary to produce type I water are included. Also, special attention must be given to the "feed-water," which is usually the laboratory tap water. The feed-water may contain unique contaminants or may have a high mineral content (hardness), which will often require the inclusion of additional components in the water processing system.

Purification

Many laboratories produce or purify their own water. Several means are available by which to produce reagent-grade water. Most water filtration systems use a prefilter to begin the process. This prefilter has feed-water running through it to trap any particulates before sending it on to the next component. At this point in the water filtration process, water may be distilled or passed through a reverse osmosis filter. Distillation is the process by which a liquid is vaporized and condensed and is used to purify or concentrate a substance or separate a volatile substance from a less volatile substance. Water that has been distilled does not meet the specific resistivity requirements of CAP type I water. Reverse osmosis (RO) is a process by which water is forced through a semipermeable membrane that acts as a molecular filter. The RO filter removes 95%–99% of organic compounds, bacteria, and other particulate matter, and about 95% of all ionized and dissolved minerals, but not as many gaseous impurities. Reverse osmosis alone does not produce type I water, but like distillation, if additional filters such as ion-exchange and carbon particulate filters are added to the system, type I water may be produced.

Ion-exchange filters remove ions to produce mineral-free deionized water. Deionization is accomplished by passing water through insoluble resin polymers that contain anion- or cation-exchange resins. These exchange resins replace H^+ and OH^- ions for impurities present in ionized form in the water. Another type of material used is a mixed bed resin that contains both anion and cation-exchange materials. Deionizers are capable of producing water that has specific resistance exceeding 1–10 Mohm·cm (MΩ·cm).

Carbon filters containing activated charcoal may be added to the water purification system to help remove several types of organic compounds that may still be in the water. When these filters are used, CLSI/CAP considers the end-product to contain minimal organic material.

A particulate filter may be added to the end of the system. This filter with a mean pore size down to about 0.22 μm will serve to trap any remaining particulates as large as or larger than the pore size.

Monitoring Water Purity

Because water is such an integral part of laboratory analysis, its purity must be monitored on a consistent basis. The frequency of water testing is dependent on many factors, including the composition of the feed-water, the availability of staff to perform water testing, and the amount of water the laboratory uses during a given period of time. At the very least, resistivity and bacterial content of the water should be monitored on a regular basis. In addition, pH, silica content, and organic contaminants may be determined. Depending on the laboratory's resources, some or all of these parameters should be checked on a periodic basis.

Most water filtration systems will have an in-line resistivity meter available. Resistivity measurements are used to assess the ionic content of purified water. The higher the ion concentration in water, the lower the resistivity value will be. CLSI/CAP requires that type I water have a resistivity greater than 10 MΩ·cm.

Bacterial contamination can be monitored easily. The water should be allowed to run for at least 1 minute to flush the system. Next an aliquot of water is taken, depending on the procedure used, and is plated on appropriate media. After an appropriate incubation time, the number of colony-forming units on the agar plate is determined. The most commonly found organisms in water after the purification process is complete are gram-negative rods.

Once Your System Has Been Installed

Most water purification systems are designed for easy access to end-product type I water. Therefore it is advisable to use only type I water for most applications in the laboratory. Type II or III water could be used for rinsing glassware and cleaning exterior surfaces. If a procedure, for example, heavy metal testing or HPLC, requires the use of specially prepared water, then type I water should not be used. Ultra pure water can be purchased from NERL Diagnostics Corporation (East Providence, RI).

MEASUREMENT OF MASS

Mass is the quantity of matter contained within an object. The weight of a body is the gravitational acceleration exerted on it, and unlike mass, it varies with altitude. The weight is equal to mass times gravity. In the laboratory, we are measuring the mass of an object.

Types of Balances

Several different types of balances are available, depending on what needs to be weighed. For example, to weigh a fecal fat specimen, an appropriate balance to use would be a top-loading precision balance capable of accurately weighing kilogram amounts. Preparation of standards for toxicology assays requires microgram quantities, thus a single-pan microbalance would be appropriate.

Unequal-Arm Substitution Balances

Unequal-arm substitution balances are typically single-pan types and are commonly used in laboratories, although almost all of these balances are being replaced by electronic-type balances. The single-pan, mechanical, unequal-arm balance operates on the principle of removing weights rather than adding them. A fixed mass counterweight is used to balance the combined mass of the pan and the removable weights across two arms of unequal weight. When a sample is placed on the weighing pan, internal weights in 1 g or 10 g increments are moved one at a time by the operator turning a set of knobs. This is continued until the system returns to equilibrium, at which time the sum of the weights removed is equal to the weight of the object.

Magnetic Force Restoration Balance

Another widely used balance is the single-pan balance that relies on magnetic force restoration. The restoring force is the force required to put the balance back into equilibrium. The unknown mass is placed on the pan, and this system goes out of equilibrium. The operator who adjusts the internal weights restores partial equilibrium. The null detector optics circuit senses when equilibrium is near and provides a signal to the sensor motor to generate a restoring current until equilibrium is reached. At this time, the unknown mass is equal to the mass of the weights removed plus the value of the restoring current.

Top-Loading Balances

Single-pan top-loading balances operate on the same principle as single-pan analytic balances (i.e., weighing by substitution). Damping is accomplished by magnetic rather than an air-release mechanism. These balances are especially suitable for rapidly weighing larger masses (up to 10,000 g) that do not require as much analytic precision, such as large-volume reagent preparation.

Electronic Balances

Several electronic balance designs are available. One design uses a strain gauge load cell. This is a small, thin device, which changes electrical resistance when it is stretched or compressed. Typically, several strain gauges are used in a Wheatstone bridge arrangement, and they are glued onto the load cell in a protected location. A load cell is usually in the shape of a beam or plate. When the beam or plate is displaced, it bends a tiny amount, and this tiny bending is detected by the strain gauges. The amount of bending might be only a thousandth of an inch, but that is enough for a strain gauge to measure.

Another electronic balance design operates on the principle of electromagnetic force (EMF) compensation. A coil, placed between the poles of a cylindrical electromagnet, is mechanically connected to a weighing pan. Mass placed on the pan produces a force that displaces the coil within the magnetic field. A regulator generates a compensation current just sufficient to return the coil to its original position. The more mass that is placed on the pan, the larger is the deflecting force, and the stronger is the current required to correct the deflection of the coil. The measuring principle is based on a strict linear relationship between compensation current and force produced by the load placed on the pan.

Several additional features may be available on some models of electronic balances. For example, some electronic balances include an electronic vibration damper. Any excess vibration can be detected when variation of the pointer or oscillation of the number in the last decimal place of the digital display is observed. Another feature available in some models is built-in taring. This allows the weight of the weighing container to be "zeroed." Also electronic balances can be interfaced with computers to provide calculations such as weight averaging and statistical analysis of multiple weighing. The fundamental design of electronic balances allows for faster weighing, which is advantageous when doing multiple readings (e.g., pipet calibrations).

Calibration

Laboratory balances require calibration at regular intervals. The NIST states that there is no fixed calibration interval for scientific applications. Calibration intervals should coincide with the requirements of the laboratory's licensing and accrediting organizations.

The mass standard and test weight accuracy classes for weights used in calibrating balances have been updated and replace the older requirements specified by National Bureau of Standards (NBS) class S and class S1 weights. The new mass standards and test weight accuracy classes appropriate for laboratory balances include the American Society for Testing and Materials (ASTM) classes 1 and 2. Reference should also be made to ASTM E617-97 for specific information regarding range, readability, and best uncertainty applicable to these classes.

NIST class 1 weights (extra-fine accuracy) are available up to 250 mg and may be used for high-precision (e.g., single-pan and electronic) balances that are precise to four decimal places. The range of weight for class 2 balances may be in excess of 1000 g.

Handling Weights Used for Testing Accuracy

Meticulous care must be used when handling class 1 or 2 weights. The operator must avoid direct contact with the weights by using clean gloves or special lifting tools (e.g., forceps). Hand contact with the weights can cause corrosion. The weights should not be dragged across any surface, including the stainless steel weighing pan. Usually the weights are sent in a covered box and should always be stored in that box.

Environmental Concerns for Best Weighing Accuracy

Several aspects of the environment may have an impact on the performance of a laboratory balance. They include temperature, air drafts, floor vibrations, table instability, and static electricity. The effects of the environment on your weighing procedures can often be minimized easily. For example, if air drafts are present in the room, a shroud or enclosure can be placed around the balance. A marble table can be used to reduce table vibrations or instability.

Balance Specifications

An operator should be knowledgeable about several important specifications related to balances. They include the following:

- capacity—which represents the maximum load one can weigh
- accuracy—which is dependent on the smallest mass one will be weighing
- linearity—the ability of a balance to provide accurate output over its full range
- resolution (readability)—the smallest increment of weight that may be discernible

Laboratory accrediting agencies require verification of accuracy of balances at various time intervals. Several sources are available to guide the laboratory through this requirement.

LABORATORY GLASSWARE AND PLASTICWARE

Types of Glassware

The most common type of glassware encountered in volume measurements is borosilicate glass. This glass is characterized by a high degree of thermal resistance, has low alkali content, and is free from the magnesium-lime-zinc group of elements, heavy metals, arsenic, and antimony. Commercial brands are known as Pyrex (Corning, Corning, N.Y.) and Kimax (Kimble, Vineland, N.J.). The caustic conditions involved in storing concentrated alkaline solutions in borosilicate glass will etch or dissolve the glass and destroy the calibration. Borosilicate glassware with heavy walls, such as bottles, jars, and even larger beakers, should not be heated with a direct flame or hotplate. Glass should not be heated above its strain point (for Pyrex, 515° C) because rapid cooling strains and cracks glass easily when heated again. In the case of volumetric glassware, heating can destroy the calibration.

Corex (Corning, N.Y.) brand glassware is a special alumina-silicate glass strengthened chemically rather than thermally. Corex is six times stronger than borosilicate glass (e.g., Corex pipets have a typical strength of 30,000 psi, compared with 2000–5000 psi for borosilicate pipets) and will outlast conventional glassware by tenfold. Corex also resists clouding and scratching better.

Low actinic glassware is a glass of high thermal resistance with an amber or red color added as an integral part of the glass. The density of the red color is adjusted to permit adequate visibility of the contents, yet give maximum protection to light-sensitive materials, such as bilirubin standards. Low actinic glass is commonly used in containers used to store control material and reagents.

Types of Plasticware

Several types of plasticware are used in clinical laboratories, for example, pipet tips, beakers, flasks, cylinders, and cuvets. Polypropylene, polyethylene, Teflon, polycarbonate, and polystyrene are all examples of types of plastics used for laboratory plasticware.

Plastic pipet tips are made primarily of polypropylene. This type of plastic may be flexible or rigid, is chemically resistant, and can be autoclaved. These pipet tips are translucent and come in a variety of sizes. Polypropylene is also used in several tube designs, including specimen tubes and test tubes. Specially formulated polypropylene is used for cryogenic procedures and can withstand temperatures down to −190° C.

Polyethylene is widely used in plasticware too, including test tubes, bottles, graduated tubes, stoppers, disposable transfer pipets, volumetric pipets, and test tube racks. Polyethylene may bind or absorb proteins, dyes, stains, and picric acid.

Polycarbonate is used in tubes for centrifugation, graduated cylinders, and flasks. The usable temperature range is broad: −100° C to +160° C. It is a very strong plastic but is not suitable for use with strong acids, bases, and oxidizing agents. Polycarbonate may be autoclaved but with limitations (refer to furnished instructions).

Polystyrene is a rigid, clear type of plastic that should not be autoclaved. It is used in an assortment of tubes, including capped graduated tubes and test tubes. Polystyrene tubes will crack and splinter when crushed. This type of plastic is not resistant to most hydrocarbons, ketones, and alcohols.

Teflon is widely used for manufacturing stirring bars, tubing, cryogenic vials, and bottle cap liners. Teflon is almost chemically inert and is suitable for use at temperatures ranging from −270° C to +255° C. This type of plastic is resistant to a wide range of chemical classes, including acids, bases, alcohol, and hydrocarbons.

VOLUMETRIC LABORATORYWARE

Pipets

Many kinds of pipets are available for use in a clinical laboratory, each intended to serve a specific function. They are used for reconstituting controls and calibrators, preparing serum or plasma dilutions, and aliquoting specimens. Thus, a high degree of accuracy and precision is required. Manual pipets fall into two general categories: transfer (volumetric) and measuring. Three subclassifications include to contain (TC), to deliver (TD), and to deliver/blow-out (TD/blow-out).

Class A Designation

Class A glassware, including pipets, is manufactured and calibrated to deliver the most accurate volume of liquid. Class A specifications are defined by NIST. The College of American Pathologists (CAP) specifies that volumetric pipets must be of certified accuracy (Class A), or the volumes of the pipets must be verified by calibration techniques (e.g., gravimetric, photometric). The letter "A" appears on all pipets that conform to the standards of Class A glassware. Volumetric glassware designated as Class A has been manufactured to Class A tolerances as established by the American Society for Testing and Materials (ASTM) E694 (West Conshohocken, PA) for volumetric apparatus. Other standards include ASTME 542 for calibration of volumetric apparatus and ASTME 288 for volumetric flasks.

Types of Pipets

TC pipets are often referred to as rinse-out pipets because they must be refilled or rinsed out with the appropriate solvent after the initial liquid has been drained from the pipet. TC pipets contain an exact amount of liquid that must be completely transferred for accurate measurement. Examples of TC pipets are Sahli hemoglobin and Long-Levy pipets. These pipets do not meet Class A certification criteria.

TD pipets are designed to drain by gravity. They must be held vertically with the tip placed against the side of the container and must not touch the liquid in it. The stated volume is obtained when draining stops. This type of pipet should not be blown out. Examples of TD pipets include Mohr, serologic, and volumetric transfer pipets. These pipets are designed to meet the requirements of Class A type pipets.

Volumetric TD pipets have an open-ended bulb, which holds the bulk of the liquid. On one side of the pipet is a long glass tube with a line indicating the extent to which the pipet is to be filled. The other end is tapered for smooth delivery of liquid. These pipets should be allowed to drain freely and should not be shaken, or hit against the container. Any disruption of the free-flowing liquid may result in inaccurate delivery of the liquid.

Some TD pipets are designed so that most of the contents are allowed to drain freely, after which the remaining fluid in the tip is blown out. These pipets are not rinsed out. Examples of pipets designed to be blow-out–type pipets include Ostwald-Folin and serologic pipets. TD/blow-out pipets are identified by the presence of one or two frosted bands near the mouthpiece of the pipet. It is vital to remember that one should never pipet or blow out solutions by mouth. It is always necessary to use an appropriate pipetting aid (e.g., bulb).

Serologic glass or plastic pipets are long tubes with uniform diameters. They have volume graduations extending to the delivery tip of the pipet. The last volume of liquid blown out is included in the delivery volume. The design of the Mohr TD pipet is different from that of the serologic pipet. Mohr pipets are not graduated to the tip. The accuracy of the Mohr pipets is valid only when the pipet is filled. If smaller volumes are dispensed, accuracy decreases proportionately.

Micropipets

The two most widely used types of micropipets are air displacement and positive displacement. These pipets are capable of delivering liquid volumes from 1–1000 μL. Some micropipets are designed to deliver a fixed volume, and others can deliver variable amounts of sample.

Air-displacement pipets are piston-operated devices. A disposable, one-time use polypropylene tip is attached to the pipet barrel. The pipet tip is placed into the liquid to be aspirated and is drawn into and dispensed from this tip.

Positive-displacement pipets use a capillary tip that may be siliconized glass, glass, or plastic. This type of pipet is useful if a reagent reacts to plastics. Positive-displacement pipets use a Teflon-tipped plunger that fits tightly inside the capillary. These capillary tips are reusable, and carry-over is negligible if the pipet is properly maintained. Some procedures require a washing or flushing step between samples.

Pipet Calibration

Not only is monitoring the performance of pipetting devices mandatory in most states that issue licenses to laboratories that perform diagnostic testing, it is also very wise. Micropipets should be verified for accuracy and precision before they are put into use and monitored during the course of the year. The frequency of verification depends in part on the amount of use and the requirements put forth by the licensing and/or accrediting agency. Proper maintenance of air-displacement pipets is very important. This type of pipet has a fixed stroke length that must be maintained. It also has seals to prevent air from leaking into the pipet when the piston is moved. These seals require periodic greasing to maintain their integrity.

Positive-displacement micropipets need to have their springs checked and Teflon tips replaced periodically. A slide wire is used to quickly check the plunger setting. This check does not replace scheduled precision and accuracy checks.

Several procedures are used by laboratories to verify the precision and accuracy of micropipets. Most of these procedures are time-consuming, especially those that require the weighing of water. No matter, this verification procedure must be done to ensure proper performance of the laboratory micropipets.

CLSI has provided an acceptable procedure for determining pipet accuracy and precision (I8-P; NCCLS, 1984). This gravimetric procedure is labor intensive but does provide a low-cost means of complying with the regulations set forth by the various accrediting agencies.

More expensive procedures for calibrating micropipets include the following:

- commercial photometric pipet calibration products
- calibration services providers
- Pipet Tracker (Labtronics Inc., Ontario, Canada)

One of the major concerns when considering the costs attributed to pipet calibration procedures is technologist time. The technologist time required for the photometric procedures is often 50%–60% less than for the inexpensive manual weighing techniques.

Volumetric Flasks

Volumetric flasks represent a special type of glassware in the laboratory. These flasks are often used to prepare standards for quantitative procedures. Therefore, their accuracy must be optimal. Volumetric flasks used for the preparation of standards and other solutions requiring optimal accuracy must meet Class A specifications as defined by NIST. These specifications are imprinted on the flasks. Volumetric flasks are used to contain an exact volume when the flask is filled to the *mark*. A Teflon or ground-glass stopper should be used to seal the flask. Volumetric flasks should not be used for reagent storage.

Calibration of Volumetric Glassware

According to the strictest of standards, every piece of volumetric glassware in the clinical laboratory should be coded, and a record kept of its calibration. Any piece of glassware that does not meet Class A tolerance should be rejected. To prepare a piece of glassware for calibration, thoroughly wash and dry it using appropriate cleaning procedures. CLSI can provide the laboratory with an appropriate procedure to calibrate volumetric flasks.

THERMOMETRY

Thermometers and other types of temperature-sensing devices are used in the laboratory to monitor the temperature in refrigerators, freezers, water baths, heating blocks, and incubators. Special applications of thermometry include osmometry, refrigerated centrifuges, refrigerated reagent compartments of automated analyzers, warming compartments of automated analyzers, and circulating water baths for cuvet compartments in automated analyzers. All of these temperature-monitoring applications have the same requirements: accurate measurements and a constant temperature.

Appropriate quality control procedures must be carried out and documented routinely for all of these temperature-monitoring devices. Any temperature-sensitive device that fails to perform within established tolerances must be replaced. Because many assays performed in the laboratory are enzymatic in nature, even the slightest deviation from the optimal temperature required to perform the assay may cause an erroneous result.

Types of Thermometers

The two types of liquid-in-glass thermometers most widely used are total immersion and partial immersion. A total immersion thermometer requires that the bulb and the entire column of liquid be immersed into the medium measured. These thermometers are used to monitor freezers and refrigerators. Partial immersion thermometers must have the bulb and stem immersed to the immersion line or defined depth on the thermometer. This type of thermometer is often used for water baths and heating blocks.

Special Applications of Temperature-Sensing Devices

Thermistors are used in several types of instruments found in the laboratory, including freezing-point depression osmometers. A thermistor is a transducer that converts changes in temperature (heat) to resistance. It consists of a small bead constructed of a fused mixture of metal oxides, attached to two leads and encapsulated in glass. The metal oxide mixture has a large negative temperature coefficient of resistance. Thus a small decrease in temperature causes a relatively large increase in the resistance of the thermistor.

A thermocouple is a sensor that consists of two dissimilar metals, joined together at one end. When the junction of the two metals is heated or cooled, a voltage is produced that can be correlated back to the temperature. Thermocouples are available in several designs, including beaded wire, probes, and surface probes. An important feature of most thermocouples used in laboratory analyzers is their fast response time. The response time of a thermocouple is defined as the time required by a sensor to reach 63.2% of a step change in temperature under a specified set of conditions. Five time constants are required for the sensor to approach 100% of the step change value.

Laboratory applications for thermocouple use include gas and liquid chromatography, surface temperature measurements in heating compartments in automated analyzers, thermo-cuvets, and circulating water baths in chemistry analyzers

Mercury-Free Laboratories

Initiatives are under way nationwide to make laboratories mercury-free. For example, in June of 1998, a landmark agreement was put together between the American Hospital Association (AHA) and the U.S. Environmental Protection Agency (EPA) (JCAHO, 2002). A memo of understanding was signed between the two organizations in an effort to decrease and eventually eliminate hospital pollution practices over a 5 to 10 year period. One of the goals is to eliminate mercury waste.

Mercury is contained in numerous chemical reagents used by the laboratory and of course in mercury thermometers. The cost associated with proper disposal of mercury and the impact of mercury in the environment make replacing mercury thermometers a sound idea. Several alternatives exist for replacement thermometers that provide the necessary accuracy for laboratories procedures. They include the following:

- thermometers containing an organic red spirit and pressurized with nitrogen gas
- thermometers containing blue biodegradable liquid (isoamyl benzoate and dye)
- a red liquid thermometer filled with kerosene
- bimetal digital thermometers
- digital thermometers with stainless steel stems

Thermometer Calibration

Monitoring the temperature accuracy of thermometers is necessary to ensure the reliability of procedures requiring temperature regulation. Thermometers may be purchased with a certificate to indicate traceability to standards provided by NIST. Also, many commercially available thermometers meet or exceed NIST and American National Standards Institute (New York)/Scientific Apparatus Makers Association (UK) (ANSI/SAMA) tolerance for accuracy.

Noncertified thermometers can be calibrated by using an NIST SRM 934 thermometer or an NIST SRM 1968 gallium melting point cell. The SRM 934 clinical laboratory thermometer is calibrated per specifications by International Temperature Scale 1990 (ITS-90) at 0, 25, 30, and 37° C. A gallium melting point cell consists of about 25 g of very pure (99.99999%) gallium metal that has a single fixed melting point at 29.7646° C (as defined by ITS-90). The gallium is sealed in an inert plastic crucible and is surrounded by a stainless steel envelope (Strouse, 1997).

Temperature-monitoring devices should be verified for accuracy at 6 or 12 month intervals. Guidelines and procedures for proper monitoring and tolerances are available (NCCLS approved standard I2-A2, 1990).

WATER BATHS

For general clinical laboratory use, constant temperature water baths must offer variable temperature control from +5° C above ambient temperature to 100° C, with accurate control to ±0.2° C. Water baths can be circulating or noncirculating. Circulating water baths provide the best temperature control. Another important consideration in the selection of a constant temperature bath is that the model should be large enough to accommodate the desired working volume.

Maintenance

Maintenance of a constant temperature water bath is improved by filling it with type II (or type I) water. This prevents the accumulation of mineral deposits from regular tap water, which can affect the temperature-sensing elements and generally lead to poor heat transfer. However, if an accumulation of these minerals does occur, a weak hydrochloric acid solution will dissolve the deposits. Frequent cleaning and fresh water will prevent overgrowth of bacteria and algae. Also a 1:1000 dilution of thimerosal (Merthiolate) can be added to help prevent bacterial growth. Overheating and subsequent damage can occur if the bath goes dry. At higher temperatures, the bath should be covered, both to maintain proper temperature control and to prevent rapid evaporation to dryness.

Quality Control

A thermometer calibrated against another certified by NIST must be a component of any water bath. The temperature should be noted and recorded for each assay. This function by the operator ensures that indeed the temperature of the bath is the same as the reading of the thermometer.

HEATING BLOCKS, DRY-BATH INCUBATORS, AND OVENS

Heating blocks and dry-bath incubators are commonly used for incubating liquids at higher temperatures. Most incubators are constructed of an aluminum alloy that is capable of distributing the heat in a uniform manner. Their heating efficiency is less than that of a circulating water bath, but they will maintain a constant temperature within ±0.5° C. A certified thermometer or NIST calibrated thermometer must be present in the heating block to monitor the temperature.

Heating ovens are used in chromatography procedures, to dry chemicals, and to assist in extraction, and they are used to dry membranes or gels in electrophoresis. Several different designs are available, depending on the desired temperature and purpose. Oven designs include programmable, vacuum, and standard laboratory types. Temperature control is usually within ±1° C. The oven must have a certified thermometer or NIST calibrated thermometer available to monitor the interior temperature.

MIXING

Mixing is an operation intended to form a homogeneous mass or create a uniform heterogeneous system. Mixing is used to bring solids into solution; to bring phases into intimate contact, for instance, in extraction procedures; to wash suspended solids; to homogenize liquid phases; and to perform many other operations. A serious consequence of inadequate mixing can be failure to completely resuspend protein that settles out under long-term frozen storage of serum controls, resulting in invalid data. In some instances, excessive mixing may cause denaturation of protein or hemolysis. A phase separation occurs when serum (or plasma) specimens stand for a period of time and must be thoroughly mixed before analysis. The concentration of even small molecules in such a system will be heterogeneous as proteins settle and become more concentrated; thus effective water concentration decreases in this layer. This produces a water concentration gradient throughout the system and, consequently, a concentration gradient of all components.

Single-Tube Mixers

A vortex mixer is capable of a variable speed oscillation that results in a swirling motion to liquid contents of a test tube or other container. The angle of contact and the degree of pressure can be regulated for optimal mixing action. A very effective mixing action is created by a multiple-touch sequence (i.e., touching and withdrawing the tube from the neoprene oscillating cup of the mixer). The operator must be careful not to fill the container too full or to mix the liquid contents too fast, because spillage can occur.

Multiple-Tube Mixers

Various mixers are available that handle a number of tubes and tube sizes, and with different types of mixing motions. A Thermolyne Maxi-Mix (Sybron Corporation, Dubuque, Iowa) can conveniently be used for vortex mixing one tube or several tubes at the same time. Changing the pressure of the container against the replaceable foam rubber top varies mixing action. Circular motion on a tilted disk provides continuous inversion of contents in tubes, which are clip-mounted at the circumference of the rotating disk. Rotational speed can be varied to provide gentle or more vigorous mixing. Control sera are conveniently reconstituted on this type of mixer. Tube shakers that operate by tilting back and forth at variable speeds provide thorough mixing of whole blood samples.

AQUEOUS SOLUTION

The concentration of a solution may be expressed as molarity (M), normality (N), and, less frequently, molality (m). Accurate preparation of reagents requires fundamental knowledge of solution chemistry, basic mathematics, and basic techniques.

Molarity

Molarity (M) is equal to the number of moles of solute per liter of solution. A mole of a substance is the number of grams equal to the atomic or molecular weight of the substance. The atomic or molecular weight of a substance is the actual mass of the chemical particle (atom or molecule) relative to the mass of the carbon atom. One mole of any substance will contain approximately 6.02×10^{23} particles (Avogadro's number). Thus a one molar solution contains 1 mole of solute per liter of solution.

Example 4-7. How many grams of NaCl are required to prepare 1 liter of a 0.5 M solution? The gram molecular weight (GMW) of NaCl is 58.5?

SOLUTION
GMW × M = g/L
58.5 × 0.5 = 29.25 g/L

Therefore, weigh out 29.25 g of NaCl and transfer it to a 1 L volumetric flask. Add water to the 1 L mark on the flask.

Millimoles

When small concentrations are used, they are frequently expressed in millimoles per liter (1000 mmol = 1 mol). For example, to prepare 10 mL of a 10 mmol (0.01 mole) NaOH solution, 4 mg NaOH is diluted to 10 mL.

Normality

Normality (N) is equal to the number of gram equivalents of solute per liter of solution and is dependent on the type of reaction involved (e.g., acid-base, oxidation). One-gram equivalent weight of an element or compound equals the gram molecular weight divided by the number of replaceable hydrogens or hydroxyls (also valence):

$$\text{Gram equivalent weight} = \text{GMW}/\text{Number of replaceable hydrogens, hydroxyls, or valence}$$

$$1\text{ N} = \text{Number of gram equivalents of solute}/\text{L of solution}$$

Example 4-8. What is the gram equivalent weight of $Ca(OH)_2$ (GMW = 74)?

SOLUTION
Gram equivalent weight = 74/2 = 37
1 mole = 2 equivalents

Example 4-9. What is the gram equivalent weight of H_2SO_4 (GMW = 98)?

SOLUTION
Gram equivalent weight = 98/2 = 49
1 mole = 2 equivalents

Example 4-10. How many milliliters of concentrated H_2SO_4 (specific gravity, 1.84; percent purity, 96.2%) are required to prepare 1 liter of a 1 normal solution?

SOLUTION

Step 1: compute GEW H_2SO_4 = 98/2 = 49.

Step 2: compute the number of grams of H_2SO_4 in 1 liter = 98 g/L.

Step 3: compute the number of grams of H_2SO_4 per milliliter of solution = SG × % assay = 1.84 × 96.2 = 1.77.

Step 4: compute numbers of milliliters of concentrated H_2SO_4 required when preparing 1 liter of a 1 normal solution:

$$\frac{1.77\text{ g}}{1\text{ mL}} = \frac{49\text{ g}}{X\text{ mL}}$$

$X = 27.6$ mL

Molal

In the laboratory, we sometimes measure the physical properties of solutions, for example, when we measure the osmolality of serum or urine. The molality of the solution is determined instead of the molarity. A molal solution is 1 mole of solute in 1 kilogram of solvent. Molal solutions are based on weight, not volume. Because the density of water at room temperature is approximately 1 gram per milliliter, 1000 grams of water occupies about 1 liter. Therefore, a 1 molal aqueous solution is approximately the same as a 1 molar solution.

Example 4-11. How many grams of NaOH are needed to make a 2.00 molal solution?

SOLUTION

Step 1: determine the GMW of NaOH = 40 g.

Step 2: compute the number of grams of NaOH required to prepare the solution by using the following formula:

$$\text{Molality} = \frac{\text{Grams of solute/GMW of solute}}{1.0\text{ kg of solvent}}$$

$$2\text{ Molal} = \frac{X\text{ g of NaOH}/40.00\text{ g}}{1.0\text{ kg of solvent}}$$

$X = 80$ g of NaOH

Dilutions

Dilution procedures are not performed as frequently as in the past owing to improvements in computers and instruments whereby the system performs the dilution automatically. But, on occasion, a dilution has to be prepared. A brief review follows.

A laboratory procedure may involve the addition of one substance to another to reduce the concentration of one of the substances. This mixture is called a dilution. Laboratory staff often confuse the terminology associated with dilutions and ratios. The term ratio is more general and refers to an amount of one thing relative to an amount of something else with no other implications. Dilution, as the term is used in laboratories, is more specific. It refers to the number of parts of a substance in the total number of parts of mixture containing the substance. The implication is how the mixture was made or how it is to be made. The following are examples of ratios followed by dilutions:

Ratios

1. The serum/saline ratio is 1:9.
2. The saline/serum ratio is 9:1.
3. The serum/total volume ratio is 1:10.

Note that a colon is used as the ratio symbol.

Dilutions

1. Make a 1:10 dilution of serum in saline.
2. Make a 1:10 dilution of serum in saline.
3. Make a 1:10 dilution of serum with saline.

Example 4-12. Prepare a 1 mL/10 mL dilution of a serum sample.

SOLUTION

Pipet 1.0 mL of serum and add 9.0 mL of saline for a total volume of 10 mL.

A clinical application may involve the dilution of a patient serum sample because the bilirubin result exceeds the upper limit of linearity. The technologist decides to make a 1:2 dilution of the sample and assay the diluted sample. To prepare the dilution, the technologist pipets 100 μL of patient serum and adds 100 μL of water, for a total volume of 200 μL. The sample is assayed for bilirubin, and the analyzer prints out a value 12 mg/dL. Before reporting the patient's bilirubin result, the technologist must multiply the analyzer value times 2 (the dilution factor) and then report the value of 24 mg/dL.

Acids, Alkalis, and pH

An acid molecule yields hydrogen ions (protons) in aqueous solutions; an alkali accepts these. At room temperature in pure water:

$$[H^+] = [OH^-] = 1 \times 10^{-7}\text{ molar}$$

In all aqueous solutions, both acid and alkaline:

$$Kw = [H^+] \times [OH^-] = 10^{-14}$$

In an acid solution, $[H^+]$ is greater than 1010^{-7} mol. In an alkaline solution, $[H^+]$ is less than 1010^{-7} mol. pH is the exponent that must be applied to 10 to give the value of $1/H^+$, that is,

$$pH = \log_{10} 1/H^+$$

When pH is	1	H^+ is	10^{-1}	and OH^- is	10^{-13}
	2		10^{-2}		10^{-12}
	4		10^{-4}		10^{-10}
	6		10^{-6}		10^{-8}
	10		10^{-10}		10^{-4}
	13		10^{-13}		10^{-1}

A change of one pH unit indicates a tenfold change in H^+ concentration.

Buffer Solution

The theory of buffers and their preparation can be found in Appendix 1. For most commonly used buffers, the quantities of salts of the acids and bases have been predetermined and may be found in reference books (e.g., Bates, 1973, which contains a very good discussion of the theoretical aspects of buffers and extensive information on how to prepare several buffer solutions).

SELECTED REFERENCES

ASTM. E288-03 Standard specification for laboratory glass volumetric flasks. ASTM International. Online. Available at: http://www.astm.org.

ASTM. E542-01 Standard practice for calibration of laboratory volumetric apparatus. ASTM International. Online. Available at: http://www.astm.org.

ASTM. E694-99 Standard specification for laboratory glass volumetric apparatus. ASTM International. Online. Available at: http://www.astm.org.

For referenced ASTM standards, visit the ASTM website, or contact ASTM Customer Service at service@astm.org. For annual book of ASTM standards volume information, refer to the standard's document summary page on the ASTM website.

Clinical and Laboratory Standards Institute (CLSI), formerly the National Committee for Clinical Laboratory Standards (NCCLS) (Wayne, Pa.).

Provides comprehensive guidelines and procedures for basic laboratory methods.

Skoog DA, Holler FJ, Nieman TA. Principles of instrumental analysis. 5th ed. Philadelphia: Harcourt Brace; 1998.

Provides a comprehensive explanation of instrument principles for nearly all clinical laboratory equipment.

REFERENCES

Access the complete reference list online at http://www.expertconsult.com

CHAPTER 5

ANALYSIS: CLINICAL LABORATORY AUTOMATION

Robert L. Sunheimer, Mark S. Lifshitz, Gregory A. Threatte

KEY POINTS

- Laboratory testing has undergone revolutionary changes over the past decade so that all routine chemistry and hematology testing is completely automated.
- This includes specimen processing; all tubes are initially bar coded; they can be directly placed on autoanalyzers, which not only read which tests to perform but can directly sample from tubes and enter all results in the laboratory computer system, which is linked directly to the hospital information system.
- The three stages of laboratory testing are pre-analytic, analytic, and post-analytic. Several examples of how these stages have been automated are presented in this chapter.
- Instrument manufacturers are attempting to design systems that will offset staff shortages, provide a safer working environment for technologists, and provide the test menus and throughputs being demanded by clinicians.

Automation in clinical laboratories has been available since the mid-1950s with the introduction of the Technicon AutoAnalyzer (Pulse Instrumentation Ltd., Saskatoon, Saskatchewan, Canada) for laboratory use. The primary driver of automation has been the need to reduce or eliminate the many manual tasks required to perform analytic procedures. Continued development has led to, at first, the consolidation of most high-volume chemistry measurements onto a single platform and, more recently, the consolidation of chemistry and immunoassay systems onto a single platform. By eliminating manual steps, error due to analyst fatigue or erroneous sample identification is reduced. In parallel with automation in chemistry, the 1960s experienced remarkable growth in hematology laboratories with the introduction of automated electronic cell counting instruments that drastically changed measurements previously performed with pipets, hemocytometers, and microscopes. After initially improving accuracy and precision with red cell measurements, subsequent development and adaptations, including flow cytometric technology, have now allowed both the automation of most white blood cell differentials and a more flow cytometry–based classification of hematopoietic neoplasms.

During the 1970s, clinical laboratories were exposed to high-level computerization with the introduction and implementation of laboratory information systems (LISs), thus augmenting the flow of information throughout the clinical laboratory. Increased use of computers resulted in a significant reduction in errors, especially transcription errors. In the 1990s, giant leaps were made in technologies, which resulted in the introduction of intralaboratory transportation systems that used specimen carriers such as conveyors or transport tracks to move samples between analyzers, into and out of processing stations; these included centrifugation, decapping/capping, and storage and led to the design of total laboratory automation (TLA).

In the first decade of the new millennium, a significant amount of time and money has been dedicated by major vendors of laboratory automated systems, workcells, chemistry analyzers, immunoassay analyzers, and middleware systems to assemble an array of equipment that will meet the needs of small, medium, and high volume clinical laboratories. The diversity of platforms, footprints, detectors, and computer capabilities coincident with improved patient care, reduced error rates, and creation of quality laboratory results is unparalleled in any other decade in clinical laboratory technology.

Overall, the scope and magnitude of the drivers of automation have taken a direction similar to all other technologies. A list of factors that serve to drive automation is shown in Table 5-1. In this chapter, several of these drivers will be discussed in the context of how automation in the clinical laboratory has changed over time to become what it is today. Several analytic systems will be selected as examples of how manufacturers responded to the demands of the laboratory. The cause and impact of change on the three stages of laboratory testing will be presented, beginning with pre-analytic, then analytic, and finally post-analytic stages. The demands placed on the clinical laboratory are derived in part from the needs of clinicians and patients, and this has resulted in most of the drivers that push the changes seen in laboratory automation today.

AUTOMATED ANALYSIS

The measurement of samples using automated instrumentation has undergone an evolutionary process since the Technicon AutoAnalyzer. It began with a single-channel analyzer using continuous flow analysis that measured one analyte on a batch of samples (i.e., one sample, one test). These samples were measured in a sequential fashion (i.e., one sample after another). Specimen throughput rates were approximately 40–60 per hour. Technicon continued to develop and expand the capabilities of its continuous flow analyzers, and this resulted in the production of multiple-channel instruments (e.g., SMA 6-60, an SMAC II) that produced specimen throughput rates as high as 150 per hour with test throughput of

TABLE 5-1
Factors That Serve to Drive Laboratory Automation

Turnaround time (TAT) demands
Specimen integrity
Staff shortages
Economic factors
Less maintenance
Less calibration
Less downtime
Faster start-up times
24/7 uptime
Throughput
Computer and software technology
Primary tube sampling
Increasing the number of different analytes on one system
Increasing the number of different methods on one system
Reducing laboratory errors
Number of specimens
Types of fluids
Safety
Environmental concerns (i.e., biohazard risks)

approximately 3750 tests/hour depending on the test configuration. One significant disadvantage of continuous flow analysis is that all testing is performed in parallel fashion. This results in the measurement of every analyte configured on the system for every sample. This inflexibility in testing resulted in the development of analyzers that provide "discrete" testing (i.e., measured only the tests requested on a sample).

The next generation of automated analyzers included centrifugal analyzers and modular analyzer configurations. Centrifugal analyzers were discrete, batch-type systems. A significant limitation at the time was the throughput rates. Because the analyzers were configured to measure one analyte at a time, the only way to improve upon throughput was to purchase multiple systems so that several tests could be run simultaneously depending on how many systems the laboratory purchased.

A solution to the limitations associated with centrifugal analysis was to design a modular system that could be configured to measure multiple analytes on multiple samples with the process controlled by a computer rather than by humans. This is the essence of *random access testing*. Modular instruments allow the user to add on additional units (e.g., ion-selective electrodes [ISEs], immunoassay modules).

The ultimate result of combining modular design with random access testing was to increase specimen throughput rates to hundreds per hour and test throughput rates to thousands per hour. Patient care was improved by reduction in turnaround times. Also clinicians would request additional laboratory tests, knowing that they would receive quality patient results in a timely manner.

PREANALYTIC STAGE

The three stages of laboratory testing are preanalytic, analytic, and postanalytic. Improving efficiency and productivity during the preanalytic stage of laboratory testing was not the main focus of laboratory staff at the outset. Likewise, the postanalytic stage received very little attention. This lack of attention to improvements during these two stages was due in part to the lack of technologies that would later be developed and serve to change the scope of each of these stages. Also many of the drivers of automation that now exist were not a priority in the early days of clinical laboratories.

The preanalytic stage focuses on sample or specimen processing. For decades, specimens drawn within a facility were brought to the laboratory, usually by the blood drawers or "runners." If the specimens were obtained from outside the laboratory facility, a courier service was often used. Courier service is a batch process that requires scheduling from a given pick-up point. These individuals represented the first link between patient and laboratory, and were the source of problems that would result in some remarkable changes and innovations to the process of laboratory testing as a whole. One example of an early solution to replacing humans as specimen carriers was the introduction of pneumatic tubes.

TABLE 5-2
Examples of Sample Processing Tasks

ID/labeling
Sorting
Centrifuging
Decapping
Aliquoting
Recapping/storage/retrieval

Pneumatic tube delivery systems were installed to provide point-to-point delivery of specimens to the laboratory and offered several advantages over specimen transport by humans. Tubes are sent quickly in the pneumatic tube to the laboratory encased in a carrier lined with a foam-type material to reduce breakage. Pneumatic tube systems are designed to prevent hemolysis by avoiding significant elevation of *g* forces during acceleration and deceleration.

Electrical track vehicles can transport a larger number of specimens than pneumatic tubes. Electrical tracks require a station for loading and unloading specimens, and this may pose a problem in facilities with limited space. Similar to couriers, electrical tracks allow for batching of specimens.

Later, robots or mobile robots of many designs were used by laboratories to transport specimens from within and outside of the facility. Samples are usually batched for pick-up, and delays in the timing of pick-up notifications occurred.

Conveyors or track systems are used in some laboratory facilities, especially if the laboratory receives a very large number of samples. Conveyor or track systems are designed to transport specimens in a horizontal fashion and upward or vertically to another floor.

Once the specimens arrive at the laboratory processing workstation, several tasks need to be done. These tasks are listed in Table 5-2. Several novel approaches were used, and these culminated in what is termed "preanalytic modules," which are available from several instrument manufacturers. Many earlier attempts were made to process specimens with minimal human involvement before the development of preanalytic modules. Many of these devices are still used.

Labeling specimens by hand requires a substantial amount of time and proved to be a large source of laboratory error. Labeling went beyond the specimen tube and included pour-off tubes, sample cups, dilution cups, and send-out containers. The use of printed bar code labels facilitated this process tremendously. Later, as computers became more sophisticated and communication between computers improved, the bar code label system reduced processing time and pre-analytic errors.

Manual sorting or separating of samples was needed because of the diverse types of testing that most laboratories engaged in. Specimen tubes of all shapes and sizes would be received in the processing area of a clinical laboratory, and the technologist would have to sort tubes by stopper color, size, tests ordered, instrument design requirements, and tube destinations.

In the earlier days of clinical laboratories, each red-top tube was double-spun, so that clot removal was optimal. This step required manual decapping of the specimen tubes. The invention of the serum separator tube eliminated the need for this double-spin technique, and decapping at this stage was not necessary. A specimen would have to be decapped to process aliquots, poured off into sample cups, or be introduced into the analyzer. The decapping of tubes posed health hazards to the technologist via aerosol dispersal from the tubes and direct contact with blood.

Centrifugation of blood collection tubes required the technologist to manually load tube carriers and place them into the centrifuge. The tubes would then be removed from the centrifuge and re-sorted, aliquots would be processed, and the samples distributed to their destinations or target area. This whole process was fraught with potential safety hazards, opportunities for mistakes, and large increases in sample processing time.

Many specimens required aliquots to be poured off, also known as splitting of the samples. The aliquots were used by instrument operators, sent to other laboratory sections, sent out to reference laboratories, and used for dilutions. As with other manual processing steps, aliquoting blood specimens was a potential source of hazards for the laboratory staff and led to errors and increased processing time.

When the samples were no longer needed for testing, they were stored in a refrigerator or freezer. All of the samples were stored in an organized fashion in the event that they would be needed again for retesting. Manual

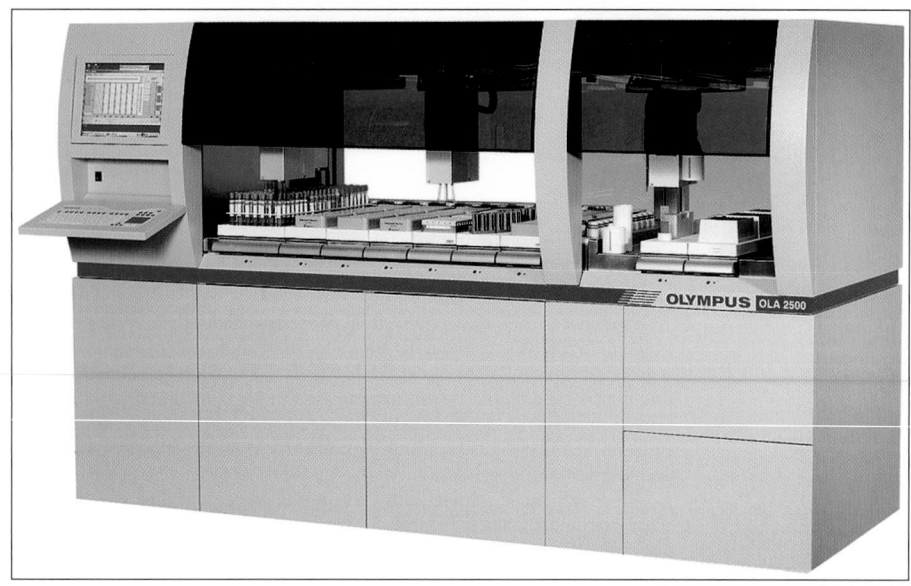

Figure 5-1 Beckman Coulter (formerly Olympus) OLA 2500 Lab Automation System. This system consists of a decapper, sorter, archiver, and aliquotter with throughput of 650 tubes/hour. *(From Beckman Coulter [formerly Olympus], with permission.)*

storage and retrieval of samples created problems for some laboratories. Samples were often lost, were not stored properly, and were difficult to locate.

AUTOMATED APPROACHES TO SPECIMEN PROCESSING

Two goals for automating specimen processing are (1) to minimize non–value-added steps in the laboratory process (e.g., sorting tubes), and (2) to increase available time for value-added steps in the tasks that technologists perform that help make a difference in the quality of the test result and, ultimately, in the diagnosis.

Advantages for automating laboratory testing include the following:
- increasing the quality of the pre-analytic steps
- reducing error rates
- reducing operator exposure to potentially hazardous biologic material
- eliminating repetitive stress injuries

Several front-end sample processing systems are available to improve upon all of the shortcomings associated with manual sample processing. The system designs may involve integrated specimen processing or modular processing. Some modular systems are designed to exist as standalone front-end processors.

Integrated specimen processing systems allow the user to perform some or all of the specimen handling tasks. These systems process only certain types of samples and specimen containers. This inflexibility with specimen containers caused many laboratories, especially hospital laboratories, to purchase modular specimen processing systems. Each module has its own on-board computer that is linked to a master controller computer system. Also, modular systems can accommodate several different specimen types (e.g., whole blood, serum, plasma) with their respective specimen containers.

Whatever the configuration, each automated pre-analytic system attempts to provide the user with some or all of the tasks necessary to prepare samples for testing. These tasks include the following:
- presorting
- centrifugation
- volume checks
- clot detection
- decapping
- secondary tube labeling
- aliquoting
- destination sorting into analyzer racks

The standalone system automates one portion of front-end processing, which includes sample sorting, sample uncapping, and aliquot functions. A centrifuge is not included in this design. If serum or plasma is required, the sample must be carried to the centrifuge by the technologist. One example of standalone automated units is the Roche Diagnostic Task Targeted RSD 800 PVT (Roche Diagnostics, Indianapolis, Ind.). These units are featured as task *targeted automation*, a concept that is characterized by state-of-the-art automation of preanalytic and postanalytic steps. Samples are processed by these units and then are hand carried to their respective workstation or targets. The RSD 800 PVT is designed to improve the quality of preanalytic steps, reduce operator exposure to hazardous biologic material, and eliminate repetitive stress injuries.

Archiving and retrieval of specimens in an automated fashion are also available in standalone designs. Automated sample archiving systems use bar-coded specimens that are scanned and placed in numbered positions in numbered racks. Retrieval of specimens is initiated by entering the patient's sample accession number or a medical record number into the archival system's database. The rack number and the position in the rack are determined and displayed for the user. Some systems include a refrigerator for sample storage and automatic disposal of samples at predetermined times.

Beckman Coulter Inc. (Brea, Calif.; formerly Olympus American Inc.) has designed a fully automated preanalytic and postanalytic sample handling system that can serve as a standalone unit or a modular unit to be utilized in configurations that match the laboratory's volume and workflow patterns. The OLA 2500 Lab Automation System (Fig. 5-1) has several unique features, including the following:
- A camera station that recognizes tube types and tube sizes and can be used for sample material recognition, as well as sample volume calculations
- The aliquoting unit, which uses disposable tips to eliminate carryover; it also can generate up to six daughter tubes from each mother tube
- Archiving, which can be performed in parallel with sorting or as a batch

Modular systems are designed to automate the entire process. The automated modular system decaps specimens, prepares aliquots, and sorts (mother and daughter samples) and transports specimens via a track system. A sample sensor or transducer senses liquid levels and separator gels and detects short samples. The Roche Modular Pre-Analytics (Roche Professional Diagnostics, Basel, Switzerland) (Fig. 5-2) combines many of the preanalytic steps that are coordinated using an intelligent process management component.

ANALYTIC STAGE

The analytic stage of testing has evolved to a very sophisticated level because of progress in technology and improvements in computer technology, and as a result of many of the drivers of automation listed earlier. Tasks in the analytic stage of laboratory testing are listed in Table 5-3.

SAMPLE INTRODUCTION

Automatic sampling may be accomplished using several different physical mechanisms. Peristaltic pumps and positive–liquid displacement pipets are two examples. Peristaltic pumps are an example of older technology but

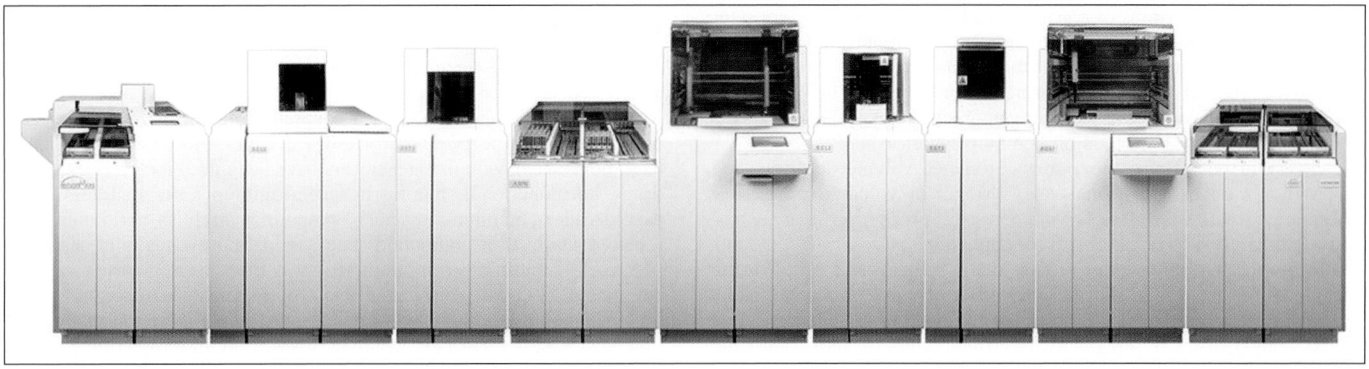

Figure 5-2 Roche Modular Pre-Analytics with "intelligent process management" and modules that provide bar code labels, centrifuge, destopper, aliquotter, restopper, and sorter. *(From Roche Diagnostics, with permission.)*

TABLE 5-3
Tasks Included in the Analytic Stage of Laboratory Testing

Sample introduction and transport to cuvet or dilution cup
Addition of reagent
Mixing of sample and reagent
Incubation
Detection
Calculations
Readout and result reporting

are still used in some instrument designs (e.g., electrolyte measurements). Positive–liquid displacement pipets are usually single pipets that transfer samples from cups or tubes to the next analytic process. Most positive-displacement pipets function in one of two ways. Either they dispense aspirated samples into the reaction container, or they flush out samples together with diluent.

Movement of the sample from the sample cup or tube to its destination via the sample probe is accomplished in several different ways. Some analyzers use a robotic-like arm that pivots back and forth, picking up a sample and depositing it into a reaction vessel or onto the surface of a porous pad. Other systems may use a worm gear device that pulls the sample probe from one point to another.

In most analyzers, samples are pipetted using a thin, stainless steel probe. The probe may be required to pierce a rubber stopper or may pass directly into a test tube or a cup. A given quantity of sample is aspirated into the probe, and the probe is moved toward an appropriate container for dispensing. A potential source of problems with this type of sample probe is the formation of a clot in a sample that subsequently attaches to the probe. These clots may plug the probe, making continued use impossible. Also, the clot may occupy sample volume and thus may cause an error in measurement. Because of the sticky nature of serum or plasma, the clot may adhere to the sample probe, and, as the sample probe swings toward its next destination, the whole clot and sample vessel may move along with it. This could result in an instrument malfunction and/or sample probe misalignment. Several sample probe designs have clot detector capability and reject a sample that is clotted. Another feature associated with sampling is the ability of the sample probe to detect the presence of a liquid by using liquid level sensors. These liquid level sensors detect the presence of an inadequate or short sample and will not allow the analyzer to continue processing this sample. The pipet and the liquid level sensor travel a specified distance into the sample container to determine if liquid is present or not.

Another problem associated with reusable pipet probes is carry-over. Carry-over is contamination of one sample by the previous sample. This contamination may cause serious variation in results for subsequent tests. Several instrument modifications have been used to reduce carry-over. One method used is to aspirate a wash solution between incidents of pipetting. Another technique is to back-flush the probe using a wash solution. The wash solution flows through the probe in a direction opposite to that of the aspiration, into a waste container. This technique tends to minimize the risk of pulling a small clot farther into the system.

Many samplers use disposable plastic pipet tips to transfer samples. This has the distinct advantage of eliminating carry-over associated with contamination within the sample probe and from sample to sample. A downside to the use of disposable tips is the increased cost associated with performing the assays.

REAGENTS

Reagents used in automated analyzers require attention to several concerns, which include the following:

- handling, preparation, and storage
- proportioning
- dispensing

Most laboratories use bulk reagents that are ready for use with little or no preparation. If the reagent is lyophilized, most analyzers will automatically dispense the proper diluent to dissolve the dried reagents. Chemistry analyzers that use unit test reagents (i.e., where sufficient reagent is present for the performance of a single test) may require some reagent preparation. For dry slide analysis, where a thin film is impregnated with the appropriate reagent, preparation consists of wetting the reagent with water, buffer, or sample. Another type of unit test reagent is a container or test tube consisting of premeasured liquid or powdered material to which water, buffer, or sample is added.

Reagents that come wet or dry are maintained within reagent compartments, and a complete inventory is established on a real-time basis within the computer. Most of the methods used in the laboratory require only a single reagent; some require two or more. When a reagent becomes depleted, the computer signals the operator that the reagent container is empty and a new one should be added. The quantity of reagents that should be available within the analyzer depends on the volume of testing done for any given analyte. On-board reagent storage compartments are refrigerated to maintain reagent stability.

Reagent identification and inventory processes are accomplished with the use of bar code labels. The bar code label may contain additional information such as expiration dates, lot numbers, and number of tests the contents of the container may provide. Some analyzers may couple a liquid level sensor onto the reagent probe, which is designed to alert the operator that an insufficient amount of reagent is available to complete the tests.

For all tests, the bar-coded reagent label stores critical information about calibrators. Examples of stored information include but are not limited to concentrations of calibrants, expected detector responses, calibration curve algorithms, and tolerances for acceptability of calibration. This information is often referred to as *master lot* or *master calibration*.

An important classification category for all automated analyzers is based on reagents. Automated analyzers are categorized as *open* or *closed* reagent systems. This distinction is often a key determinant used by laboratory staff to select and acquire an analyzer. An open reagent system is described as a system in which reagents other than the instrument manufacturer's reagents can be used. Also, in an *open* reagent system, the operator may change the parameters necessary to run the particular test. *Open* reagent systems provide users with greater flexibility and adapt easily to new methods and analytes. A *closed* reagent system is described as a system wherein the operator can use only the manufacturer's reagents. Usually the costs of reagents in a *closed* reagent systems tend to be more expensive, but *closed* reagent systems may save on expenses because reconstitution or preparation of the reagents for use does not require technologist time. Also the possibility of increased imprecision associated with the reconstitution of reagents in an *open* reagent system is negated by a *closed* reagent system. One problem with a closed system is that it may not be possible to introduce desired new tests that are not performed on the closed system.

The correct proportions of reagent(s) and sample(s) must be constant to achieve precise and accurate results. For unit test applications, reagents are already apportioned in appropriate amounts, thus only the sample needs to be added. Methods requiring the addition of bulk reagents provide an additional means of increasing imprecision. When bulk reagents are used, proportioning is accomplished by volumetric addition.

Delivery of bulk reagents requires automated volumetric dispensing devices. For random access analyzers, syringes or volumetric overflow devices are used. These devices volumetrically proportion reagent and sample into a test tube or other type of container.

Another mechanism used for proportioning reagents and sample is the continuous-flow technique. The sample and reagents are proportioned by their relative flow rates. Devices using continuous flow include peristaltic pumps. Many instrument designs use electronic valves to control the time reagents can flow. The flow rate is controlled by the air pressure applied to the reagent container and the flow resistance in the tubing connected to the reaction vessel.

Liquid reagents are aspirated, delivered, and dispensed into mixing chambers or reaction vessels by pumps or positive-displacement syringes. These pumps are connected to the reagent containers with the use of plastic tubing. On command from the computer, each pump draws a given amount of reagent or diluent out of the container and transports it via the tubing to its destination, where it is dispensed.

Syringe devices are widely used in automated systems for both reagent and sample delivery. Most are positive-displacement devices, and the volume of reagent delivered is computer controlled. If the reagent syringe is to be used for more than one reagent, adequate flushing between uses is essential to reduce carry-over of reagent.

MIXING

Many unique mixing devices and techniques are used in automated systems. They include the following:

- magnetic stirring
- rotating paddles
- forceful dispensing
- the use of ultrasonic energy
- vigorous lateral displacement

Dry slide analyzers do not require mixing of sample and reagents. The sample is allowed to flow through the layers containing the reagents.

INCUBATION

Warming components or solutions in automated analyzers is accomplished by heating air, water, or metal. The warming process must be constant and accurate. Electronic thermocouples and thermistors are used to monitor and maintain required temperatures within analyzers. Circulating water baths are used in several instruments as the warming mechanism. Thus these analyzers require a water purification and delivery system, which is usually external to the analyzer and is an additional cost to consider. With some analyzers, the cuvets or reaction vessels are allowed to incubate within a chamber containing circulating air. Heated metal blocks are a widely used device for incubating cuvets, test tubes, or plastic pouches containing solutions. The timing for each incubation period is monitored by the instrument's computer system and represents an extremely complex process, given the throughput for these systems.

Two novel approaches for incubating reaction mixtures have been developed and incorporated into automated chemistry analyzers. Siemens Healthcare Diagnostics (Deerfield, Ill.) uses an elongated cuvet path length and a fluorocarbon oil incubation bath to maximize result accuracy by enhancing absorbance values, while using microvolume technology for samples and reagents. This design feature is found in their model Advia chemistry systems.

Beckman Coulter uses a Peltier thermal electric module in the shape of a ring to maintain a constant temperature for analysis. Peltier modules are small solid-state devices that function as heat pumps. The Peltier thermal ring consisting of 125 quartz/glass cuvets is made of copper. Each cuvet is surrounded on three sides by copper. Temperature is maintained by the use of heating and sensing elements in physical contact with a copper core filled with Freon 134A, and this is controlled by the *reaction heat controller board* assembly, mounted in the wheel's handle. Calibration information is stored on two electrically erasable, programmable, read-only memory integrated circuits (ICs [electrically erasable programmable read-only memory]) on the *reaction heater controller board* and the *heater/sensor board*.

DETECTION

Absorption spectroscopy has been the principal means of measurement in automated analyzer design to measure a wide variety of compounds. Reflectance photometry has been adapted to dry slide analysis and has been used in chemistry laboratories for decades. Fluorescent compounds (e.g., fluorescein) as signal generators have been used for measurement of drugs, hormones, and vitamins in several immunoassay analyzers. In the past decade, chemiluminescence compounds such as acridinium have replaced fluorescent compounds because of improvements in sensitivity. Electrochemiluminescence methods have also been incorporated into automated systems. Automated electrolyte measurements have been accomplished using ion-selective electrodes. All of these means of detection have been discussed elsewhere in this edition. In this section, the focus will be on new approaches to measuring compounds with automated analyzers.

Novel approaches to measurement designs include not only addition of new measurement principles but also inclusion of two or more unique detectors in one analytic system. Most of the integrated chemistry analyzers being marketed today incorporate several measuring platforms. Each platform requires a distinct detector. The Roche Cobas Integra 800 incorporates a photometer, ISE, fluorescence polarization immunoassay (FPIA) optics, and turbidimetric optics.

The Beckman Coulter Synchron LXi725 Clinical System includes a luminometer, a photometer, electrochemical detectors, and a near infrared detector (Fig. 5-3). Infrared detection is used for the near infrared particle immunoassay (NIPIA) method to measure high-sensitivity C-reactive protein (hs-CRP). A 940 nm light-emitting diode produces light that is directed into a cuvet to measure hs-CRP.

OTHER UNIQUE FEATURES LOCATED IN NEW AUTOMATED INSTRUMENT DESIGNS

Most chemistry analyzers use a high intensity polychromatic light source, usually a quartz/halogen lamp. Some analyzers use a xenon light source; this lamp lasts longer (5-year life span) because its operating voltage is maintained at a lower level than in other lamps. The xenon lamp provides a very intense polychromatic light that is useful for many and varied analyses.

All fully automated general chemistry analyzers are capable of sampling directly from the collection tube. Direct tube sampling along with bar code reading has eliminated the need to transfer samples into another container, has reduced errors, and has minimized technologist exposure to potentially biohazardous material. Tubes are typically decapped before sampling; however, some chemistry systems such as the Beckman Coulter UniCell Dx analyzers offer cap-piercing technology. The analyzer uses a blade to slit the stopper, and the sample probe pierces the stopper to withdraw an aliquot of sample. Note that cap-piercing technology is available on all high throughput hematology analyzers.

Laboratory automation can consolidate multiple workstations into a single unit. The Siemens Dimension RXL integrated chemistry system combines comprehensive chemistry and stat immunoassay testing in a single, compact system with the smallest footprint for an instrument of its capabilities. The Dimension Xpand Plus features a large menu of varied assays, fast time for first results, stat interrupt capabilities, throughput of approximately 400 tests/hour, as well as reagent flexibility.

The Beckman Coulter Synchron LXi725 Clinical System is constructed differently from the Dimension Xpand Plus. The Synchron LXi725 system (see Fig. 5-3) is designed as a self-contained integrated modular system. Samples are placed in a load area and are shuttled to the *closed tube aliquot unit*, which is similar to a small track design. An aliquot of each sample is placed in the immunoassay analytic unit for processing; the rack and primary tubes are then released for general chemistry testing.

POSTANALYTIC STAGE

The electrical signal generated by the detector, representing analyte concentration, is directed into the analyzer's microprocessor or computer. The instrument computer represents a means to accomplish several tasks, which include signal processing, data handling, and process control.

Signal processing involves the conversion of an analog signal derived from the detector to a digital signal that is usable by all communication devices. The processing of data by computers has allowed automation of nonisotopic immunoassays, reflectance photometry, and other nonlinear

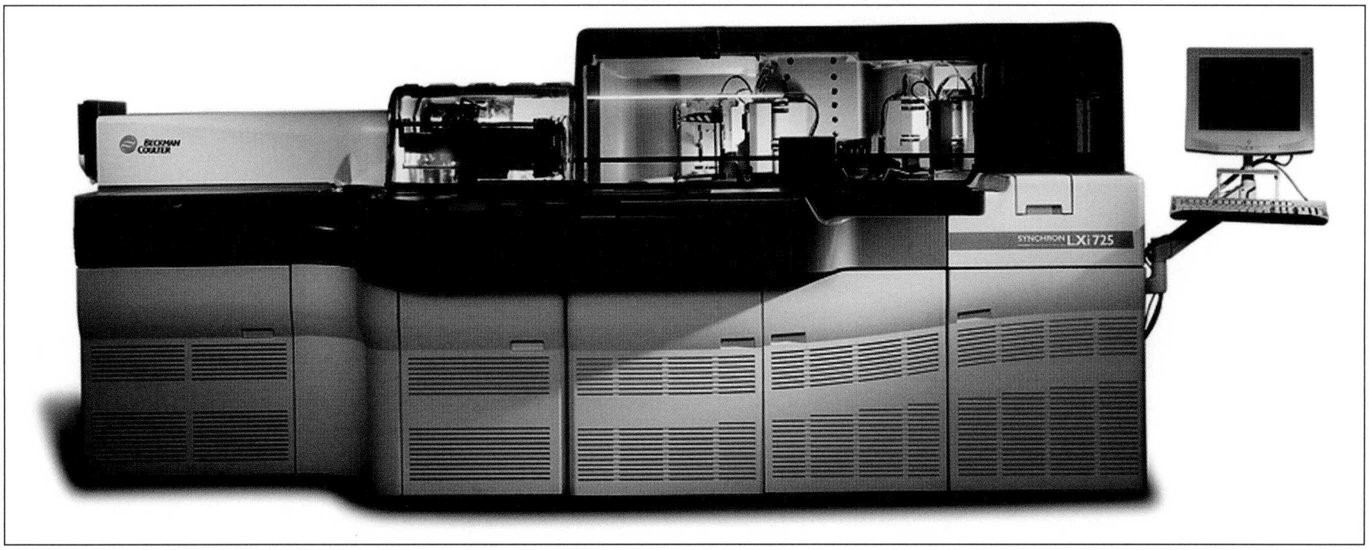

Figure 5-3 Beckman Coulter Synchron LXi725 Clinical System has a large test menu (146 assays) and will accept user-defined chemistries. *(From Beckman Coulter, Brea, Calif., with permission.)*

assays because computer algorithms can transform nonlinear standard input signals into linear calibration plots.

Data processing by computers includes data acquisition, calculations, monitoring, and displaying data. In addition to transforming data into linear calibration plots, computers can perform statistics on patient and control values. Computers can perform corrections on data, can subtract blank responses, and can determine first-order linear regression for slope and intercept. Computers can monitor patient results against reference values. They can also test control data against established quality control (QC) protocols. Computer monitors can display all types of information, including patient results, QC data, and maintenance and instrumentation operation checks.

The computer has a profound impact on the entire process of automated laboratory instruments. Within the analyzer, the computer commands and times electromechanical operations so they can be done in a uniform manner, in repeatable fashion, and in the correct sequence. These operations include activating pipetting devices, moving cuvets from one point to another, and moving sample tubes and dispensing reagents, to name a few.

A computer provides a means of communication between the analyzer and the operator. Instrument computers can display information usable by the operator, such as warnings that something may not be working properly, or that a specific reaction has exceeded method-defined parameters.

Chemistry analyzer computers can display graphic information such as Levey–Jennings QC charts and calibration curves. They also can be programmed to "flag" data that do not meet some predefined criteria. The operator can reprogram the computer to meet a specific need, such as adding a new test or changing an operating parameter.

A computer has the ability to be linked to other computers, and this has drastically improved automation efforts. Instrument computers can be linked via interfaces (e.g., RS232) to laboratory information systems (LISs) to provide a means of transmitting information in a unidirectional or bidirectional format. Instrument computers are now being equipped with the means to link to the internet via a transmission control protocol/Internet protocol (TCP/IP). Instrument manufacturers have designed analyzer computers that will link up from the laboratory's to the company's own manufacturing site. This link-up is done in real time and serves to monitor the instrument's performance at all times. If a problem with an analyzer does develop, the manufacturer can see real-time data to help the laboratory resolve the problem in the shortest time possible.

Several other features available in newer instrument designs are worth noting. On-board troubleshooting is available on many systems through the analyzer's computers. In the event a problem occurs, technologists may access the system's help protocols, which guide them through a step-by-step procedure in an effort to resolve the problem. Some of these on-board troubleshooting programs are sophisticated and include video and graphics. Another on-board feature available in some systems is a training program. This is an effective feature that serves to augment staff training of new users to the system.

Automated System Designs Available for Laboratories

TOTAL LABORATORY AUTOMATION

The idea of totally automating a clinical laboratory has its roots in Japan, and the process was first tried in the early 1980s. Early designs used one-arm robots, conveyor belts, and modifications to existing chemistry analyzers to perform as many preanalytic and analytic tasks as possible with no human intervention. Each laboratory workstation was coupled to the conveyor belts, so that samples could be moved from one workstation to another. Continued research and modifications to these earlier systems led to the development of commercial TLA systems designed for hospital-based laboratories.

A TLA approach can be described as the combination of several instruments, consolidated instruments, workcells, integrated workcells, or integrated modular workcells that are coupled to a specimen management and transportation system, as well as a process control software component, to automate a large percentage of laboratory work.

An example of a TLA is the Roche Diagnostics system that includes Modular Pre-Analytics (MPA) and platform C (i.e., the chemistry analyzer). The Roche TLA consists of an integrated tract device that connects all of the laboratory workstations, including front-end processing, instrumentation, and archiving, to create a continuous, inclusive network that serves to automate nearly every step involved in the testing of each sample. TLA can incorporate testing specimens for chemistry, hematology, coagulation, and immunochemistry.

Advantages of TLA include a decrease in labeling errors, reduced turnaround times, and a reduction in full-time equivalents (FTEs). Laboratories using a high degree of automation thus have the ability to bring new assays into the laboratory by using some of the staff no longer needed for automated testing.

Major limitations of TLA include the need for substantial financial investment and increased floor space (Wilson, 2003). Initial investment monies may reach millions of dollars, and floor space requirements may exceed 4000 square feet. Another factor that requires the attention of planners because of the complex nature of TLA is the need for highly technical personnel to operate and troubleshoot the system. Other challenges to TLA include infrastructure remodeling, personnel team building, and software interfacing. In addition, several of these systems do not allow interruption of the workflow to analyze emergency (stat) samples (Battisto, 2004).

MODULAR INTEGRATED SYSTEMS

In the United States, only about 7% of laboratories are considered able to benefit from TLA. A hospital with fewer than 600 beds may not be suitable for TLA. Therefore, modular automation provides a more attractive approach for hospital laboratories and physician group laboratories because

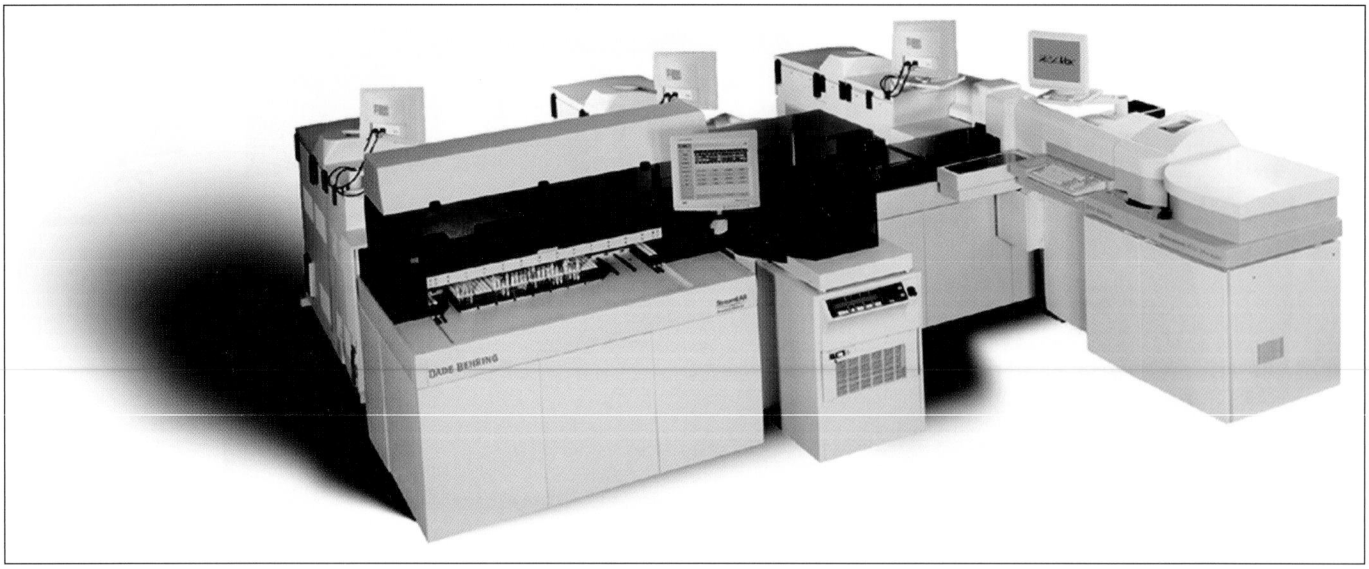

Figure 5-4 Siemens StreamLab Analytic Workcell links multiple-dimension systems via a single operator interface and features automated preanalytic and postanalytic functions. *(From Siemens, with permission.)*

the systems are smaller, and they require less initial capital investment and less planning than TLA (Sarkozi, 2003). Modular systems can be configured to include several different platforms (e.g., hematology, immunochemistry). Also, the combination of modules can include multiple identical models of analyzers, preanalytic models, and postanalytic modules. These modules are linked into a single testing platform that interconnects through a track or other "connector"-type device. Individual modules can be added to the entire system to reflect changes in workload or testing patterns.

Configuration of Automated Modules

WORKSTATION CONSOLIDATION

Workstations represent a unique environment within a laboratory facility dedicated to one type of testing (e.g., hematology, immunoassays). All stages of specimen testing are carried out for a particular discipline at its respective workstation. One approach to improving workflow has been to consolidate workstation data management. This design allows a technologist to monitor a variety of analyzers (typically from the same vendor) from a single workstation.

WORKCELLS

Workcells are configured in combination with a specimen manager and instruments or consolidated instruments, including, for example, both chemistry and immunochemistry systems that provide a broad spectrum of analytic tests. A specimen manager is a mechanical device that stores and buffers specimens before and after analysis. These devices may have pre-analytic and post-analytic specimen processing capabilities (e.g., centrifugation, decapping). Modular workcells are workcells in which the instruments used are configured to interface directly with the specimen manager. The Siemens StreamLAB analytic workcell (Fig. 5-4) is an example of this type of workcell. The StreamLAB integrates pre-analytic and multiple analytic components (e.g., Dimension Systems) via a single operator interface. Siemens offers an optional centrifugation module.

FULLY INTEGRATED SYSTEMS

The trend in automation design is to integrate several modules into one continuous system that will allow the user to assay photometric chemistry, immunoassay chemistries, both homogeneous and heterogeneous, and electrochemistries. The tests menu for fully integrated systems exceeds 125 tests and includes immunoassays, routine chemistries, and ion-selective electrodes. All modular integrated systems use random access technology that allows the analysis of different chemistry assay types.

Beckman Coulter (Olympus) integrated automation can incorporate analyzers, for example, the AU5400 Integrated Chemistry-Immunoassay Analyzer (Fig. 5-5), to provide the laboratory with a combination of instrument platforms. This system is a true random access analyzer with test throughput rates exceeding 3000 photometric tests/hour. For ISE measurements, the throughput rate is approximately 600 samples/hour. A distinct advantage of these modular systems is that they can be linked to two or more modules, thereby increasing throughput.

Siemens' modular automated Advia Solutions has a full track system integrated with other testing modules via the Advia WorkCell or the Advia LabCell automated sample transportation system. The processing system automatically sends general chemistry specimens to the Advia 1650 Chemistry Analyzer and immunoassay specimens to the Advia Centaur.

Another approach to modular integrated automation is exemplified by Roche Modular Analytics, shown in Figure 5-6. Modular Analytics incorporates most of the tests that other integrated systems offer but can increase the test menu by linking one more module (e.g., Roche Diagnostic E170). The E170 module offers 25 heterogeneous immunoassays. Therefore if the laboratory integrates all available modules, including the control unit and the core load unit, the Modular Analytic can provide a very large test menu and very high specimen and test throughput rates.

Ortho-Clinical Diagnostics (Raritan, N.J.) offers the Vitros 5600 Integrated System, which uses self-contained multiuse cartridges in dry slide format. Other technologies include potentiometry, enhanced chemiluminescence, and microparticle agglutination.

OTHER ENHANCEMENTS TO INTEGRATED AUTOMATED SYSTEMS

Middleware

New versions of middleware are being designed that are user friendly and entice even small and medium-sized clinical laboratories to incorporate them into their LIS. This trend has allowed these laboratories to take advantage of their sophisticated decision management and advanced rule-based intelligence.

Middleware allows laboratories to connect their existing LIS and instrumentation to facilitate automatic information processing and to performs tasks not currently done with laboratories' existing hardware and software. Middleware packages provide several features and functionality that includes the following:

- automatic verification of test results through rules-based decision processing
- automation and customization of work and information based on a laboratory's specific needs
- automatic tracking of data and location of samples requiring storage
- automatic sample interference testing and detection
- provision for real-time reflexive testing

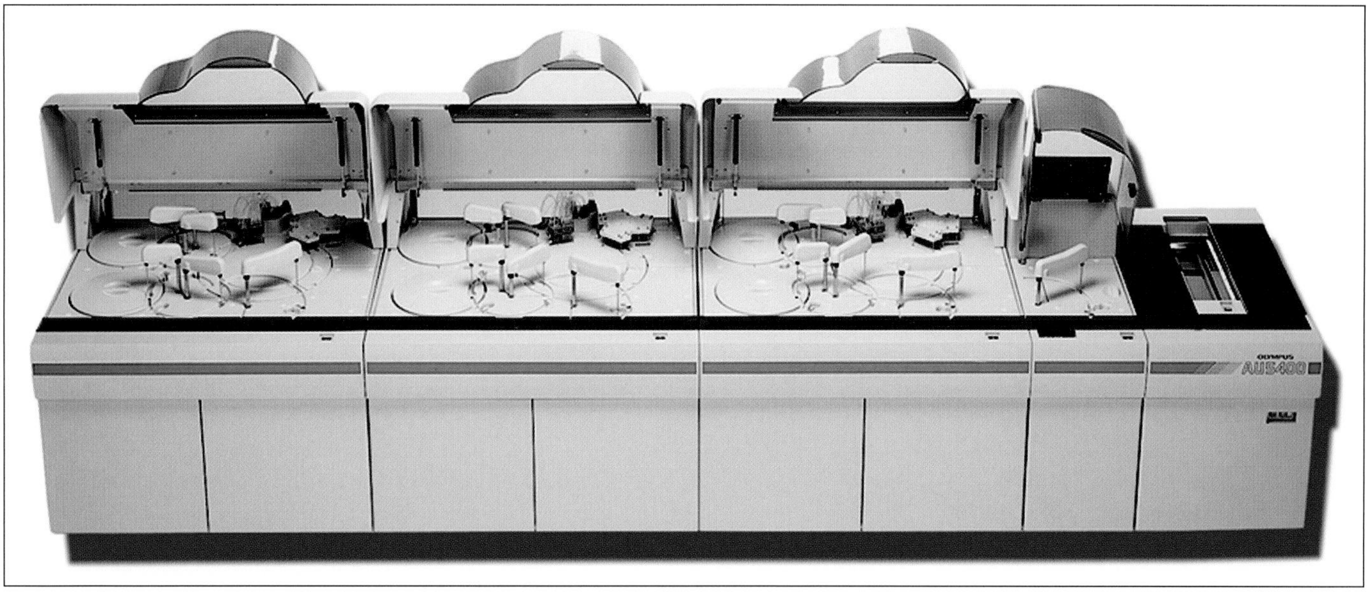

Figure 5-5 Beckman Coulter (formerly Olympus) AU5400 fully automated integrated system is available as a two or three photometric unit with versions including one single- or double-cell ion-selective electrode (ISE) unit. Throughput is 300–800 samples per hour, depending on analyzer configuration. *(From Beckman Coulter [formerly Olympus], with permission.)*

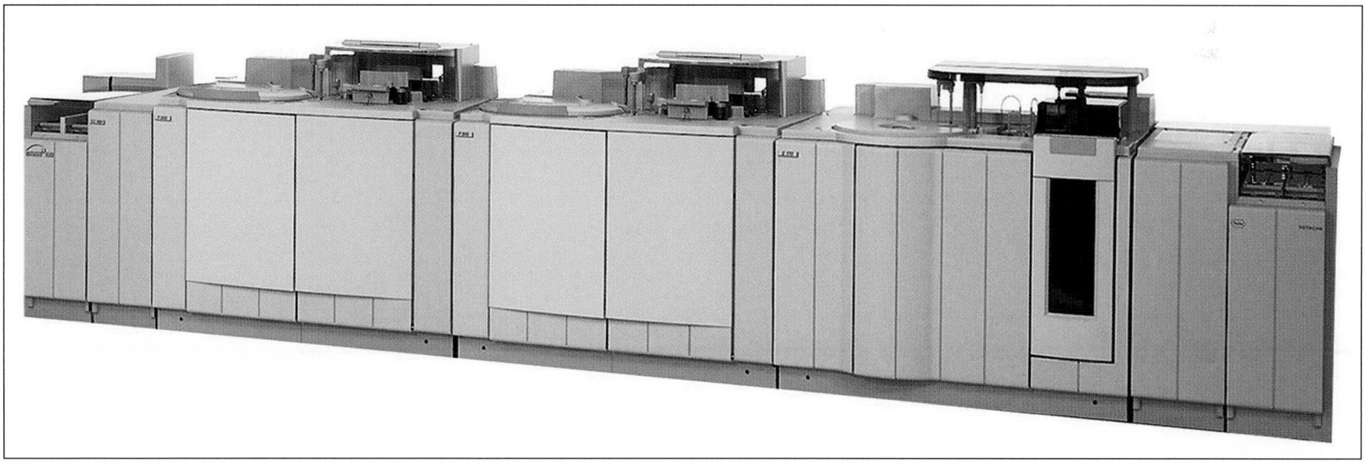

Figure 5-6 Roche Modular Analytics provides five different analyzer modules with 197 applications, producing throughput rates ranging from 170–10,000 tests/hour. *(From Roche Diagnostics, with permission.)*

- automatic comparison of current results with previous results on a patient's test (delta checking)

The following examples illustrate specific tasks that middleware can allow laboratories to complete, although most LISs are incapable of completing them:

1. Initiate a command that will not allow a calculated low-density lipoprotein (LDL) to be completed if the triglyceride is greater than 400 mg/dL.
2. Calculate serum indices for hemolysis, lipemia, and degree of icterus, and develop rules that will flag results that exceed their established limits.
3. Create a command that would remove an automated differential, and flag the result with a coded comment requiring that a manual differential needs to be done.
4. Implementation of autoverification protocols is gaining popularity throughout clinical laboratories in the United States. Middleware allows laboratory staff to develop their own results, guidelines, and tolerances for any analyte measured by the analyzer, whether chemistry or hematology.

Several hardware and software combinations are currently available. Software applications include the Windows-based Linux OS (Java-based embedded JResultNetSoftware), QNX (Ottawa, Ontario, Canada), and Compuware Uniface (Detroit, Mich.). Computer hardware to run these software operating systems and applications is primarily provided on PCs. The Linux OS uses Dawning JavaLin/PDI (Ft. Myers, Fla.), and the Linux operates using the Red Hat Linux (Rayleigh, N.C.) hardware platform.

On the Horizon

The drivers of automation listed above are continually changing and evolving, and this will lead to new approaches to the delivery of health care. Test menus will grow even larger, and new technologies will be needed to measure these analytes. These new technologies will have to be incorporated into existing systems. Another demand that systems manufacturers will need to address is the ability to link different instruments or modules to their systems. A standardized interface will be required to accomplish this, and LISs will need to adjust their processors as well. Increased emphasis on employee safety and support by legislative efforts will cause instrument manufacturers to continue to develop their products to reduce exposure to technologists. As the field of proteomics evolves, so will the methods and instruments required for measurement. Proteomic systems are currently coming to the marketplace, and in time, this type of testing will find a place in the clinical laboratory.

SELECTED REFERENCES

Battisto DG. Hospital clinical laboratories are in a constant state of change. Clin Leadersh Manag Rev 2004;18(2):86–99.

Provides valuable information that is current for laboratories contemplating changes in their facilities.

Kaplan L, Pesce A, Kazmierczak S. Clinical chemistry: theory, analysis and correlation. 4th ed. St Louis: Mosby; 2003.

Provides substantial amount of detailed information for all aspects of preanalytic, analytic, and postanalytic stages of laboratory testing.

Sarkozi L, Simson E, Ramanathan L. The effects of total laboratory automation on the management of a clinical chemistry laboratory: retrospective analysis of 36 years. Clin Chim Acta 2003;329(1–2):89–94.

Wilson LS. New benchmarks and design criteria for laboratory consolidations. Clin Leadersh Manag Rev 2003;17(2):90–8.

Shows the results of a consolidation project serving a multihospital system.

CHAPTER 6

POINT-OF-CARE AND PHYSICIAN OFFICE LABORATORIES

Gregory A. Threatte, Katherine I. Schexneider

KEY POINTS

- Point-of-care testing refers to the scope of laboratory tests that are performed where patient care is delivered. This includes physician office testing as well as various hospital locations outside the laboratory, such as the emergency department, operating room, and intensive care unit.
- When performed in a physician office, simple tests (such as urine dipstick and whole blood glucose meters) are exempt from most regulations involving personnel, proficiency testing, and rigorous quality assurance requirements. These are referred to as "waived" tests under the Clinical Laboratory Improvement Act. In hospitals, these tests fall under the laboratory certificate of the parent hospital or health care facility and generally are subject to stricter requirements.
- Special personnel requirements are necessary (including those for laboratory director) if a physician office laboratory performs moderate-complexity testing.
- Key components of a hospital point-of-care testing program include method validation, training of nonlaboratory staff, and clear policies and procedures to establish who is responsible for each part of the program. Laboratory oversight is mandatory.
- Current technology of select tests in hematology, chemistry, and microbiology is reviewed and limitations are discussed.
- Point-of-care technology in a military theater is reviewed as an example of the utility of good point-of-care implementation.

Point-of-care testing (POCT; also known as near-patient testing, alternative-site testing, or patient-focused testing) is used in a variety of settings such as the emergency department, operating suites, clinics, physician offices, nursing homes, community counseling centers, ambulances, pharmacies, and health fairs. POCT brings laboratory testing to the site of the patient encounter, rather than the traditional practice of obtaining a specimen and sending it to the laboratory. Real-time measurements of a patient's status may be obtained in a short period of time, allowing the health care provider to address acute patient needs. POCT is recognized by The Joint Commission (TJC) accreditation body and the Clinical Laboratory Improvement Act (CLIA) of 1988.

Until the 20th edition of this book, this chapter was devoted to physician office laboratories (POLs). As shown in Figure 6-1, the number of POLs grew from the 95,000 laboratories indicated in a similar figure in the 20th edition of this text to the 110,925 laboratories in October of 2009. However, the Centers for Medicare and Medicaid Services (CMS) CLIA database (at http://www.cms.gov/CLIA/downloads/statupda.pdf) shows that at present, only 59,790 of the 134,778 (or just 44%) registered Certificate of Waiver laboratories are POLs. This indicates that a large number of facilities that fall into the waived category are point-of-care facilities, such as emergency departments, operating suites, clinics, and nursing homes, as mentioned previously. This chapter will focus on the regulations and procedures recommended for small POLs and POCT sites where more of this waived testing is expected to occur.

Advances in medical technology, such as prepackaged reagent systems, microprocessor-controlled reactions and calibrations, and miniaturization of components, have led to a modern generation of laboratory instruments that require less technical skill on the part of the operator. Between 1992 and 2003, the U.S. Food and Drug Administration (FDA) rapidly granted waived status, described later, to 994 test systems ranging in scope from blood glucose to bladder tumor antigen cancer detection. Currently, more than 111 assays can be performed within this category. The global POCT market reached $6.7 billion in 2008 and is growing at a rate of approximately 7% per year and represents 15% of the U.S. market for clinical diagnostic testing reagents (Dooley, 2009).

An alphabetical list of currently waived tests can be found at http://www.accessdata.fda.gov/scripts/cdrh/cfdocs/cfClia/analyteswaived.cfm. As an example, a check on one of these assays at this FDA website reveals that more than 29 methods have been approved just for the measurement of high-density lipoprotein (HDL) cholesterol. New methods such as these will work their way into both POCT and POLs, blurring their technological differences. However, differences in regulatory requirements will remain and must be observed.

LABORATORY REGULATION

CLINICAL LABORATORY IMPROVEMENT ACT

Under CLIA, a laboratory is "A facility for the … examination of materials derived from the human body for the purpose of providing information for the diagnosis, prevention, or treatment of any disease or impairment

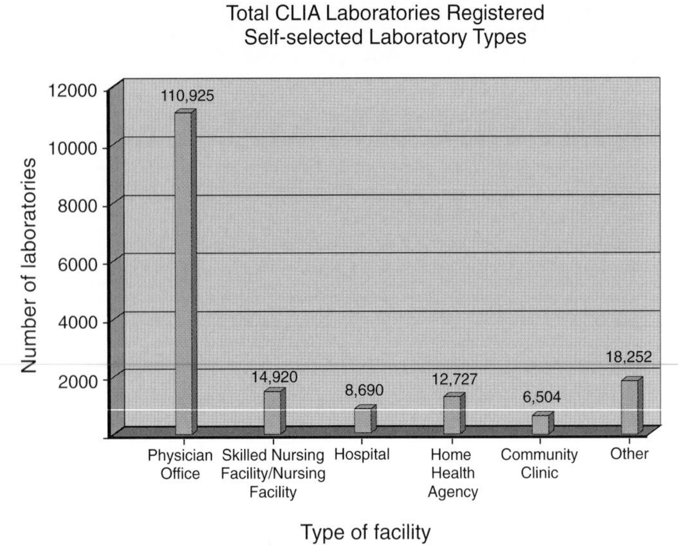

Figure 6-1 The number of physician office laboratories in October 2009 relative to hospitals, skilled nursing facilities, and independent laboratories *(from the CMS CLIA database, October 2009, at:* http://www.cms.gov/CLIA/downloads/statregi.pdf.*)*

TABLE 6-1
Types of CLIA Certificates

Certificate of Waiver
• Certificate issued to a laboratory to perform only waived tests
Certificate for Provider-Performed Microscopy Procedures (PPMPs)
• Certificate issued to a laboratory in which a physician, midlevel practitioner, or dentist performs no tests other than the microscopy procedures; permits the laboratory to also perform waived tests
Certificate of Registration
• Certificate issued to a laboratory that enables the entity to conduct moderate or high complexity laboratory testing or both until the entity is determined by survey to be in compliance with CLIA regulations
Certificate of Compliance
• Certificate issued to a laboratory after an inspection that finds the laboratory to be in compliance with all applicable CLIA requirements
Certificate of Accreditation
• Certificate issued to a laboratory on the basis of the laboratory's accreditation by an accreditation organization approved by the Health Care Finance Administration

Obtained at: http://www.cms.gov/CLIA/downloads/HowObtainCertificateofWaiver.pdf.
CLIA, Clinical Laboratory Improvement Act.

of, or the assessment of the health of, human beings. These examinations also include procedures to determine, measure, or otherwise describe the presence or absence of various substances or organisms in the body" (Federal Register, 1992). The idea behind CLIA is fairly straightforward: to ensure the accuracy of patient test results regardless of whether the test is performed in a large offsite lab or as self-testing in a patient's home. Currently, in vivo and externally attached patient-dedicated monitoring devices (e.g., pulse oximetry, mixed venous oxygen saturation [SvO_2] pulmonary artery catheters, capnographs) are not subject to CLIA. Should it be determined at a later date that they are subject to CLIA, proper notice and opportunity for public comment will be provided (general provisions, certificates, and proficiency testing sections of the CLIA regulations).

Under this definition, "laboratories" are prohibited from soliciting or accepting human specimens for analysis unless a certificate issued by the Secretary of the Department of Health and Human Services (HHS) is held for each procedure that is to be performed. All laboratories are required to be registered with the federal government and must pay biennial license fees to have a valid CLIA identification number before performing any laboratory analysis used in patient care. With evolving technology, the primary difference between the POL and POCT will be that in the POL, this certification will be held by the POL, while POCT will be performed under the laboratory certificate of the parent hospital or health care facility.

CERTIFICATION AND LICENSING REQUIREMENTS

CLIA certification relies on laboratory standards that vary according to the complexity of the measurements performed. Simple tests that the Centers for Disease Control and Prevention (CDC) has determined to have low patient risk even if performed incorrectly are waived from most regulations. These types of procedures include those that have been approved by the FDA for home use. All laboratories must be certified under one of the five types of CLIA certificates listed in Table 6-1.

A three-tiered approach was initially implemented to classify all laboratory tests on the basis of complexity of testing. The three categories are certificate of waiver or "waived" tests, moderate complexity tests, and high complexity tests. Laboratories performing only waived tests would be exempt from the personnel qualifications, proficiency testing, and the more rigorous quality assurance requirements associated with more complex testing. CMS retains the right to conduct spot checks to ensure that these laboratories are performing only waived tests. Original exempt tests included urinalysis dipstick or tablet reagent analysis of pH, specific gravity, glucose, protein, bilirubin, hemoglobin, ketone, leukocytes, nitrite, and urobilinogen. Laboratories performing only waived tests have to register and pay a biennial fee.

It is important to understand that the original list of waived tests specified by Congress included only the short list of generic tests provided earlier. In addition, provision was made so manufacturers could add specific methods to the waived list through a certification process maintained by both the CDC and the FDA. This incentive to manufacturers allowed them to appeal to a larger market and has led to a rapid influx of devices and methods that are now classified as waived. The list of approved waived tests is updated regularly and can be found at the FDA website given previously. Over the past decade, a majority of office laboratories began to shift from moderately complex testing to waived testing, most likely because of this rapidly broadening menu. These same measurements are appropriate for the POCT arena.

A fourth category, provider-performed microscopy procedures (PPMPs), was created in 1993 and expanded in 1995. This category consists of any test that involves a health care provider using a microscope and includes all of the following procedures: all urine sediment examinations; direct wet mount preparations for the presence or absence of bacteria, fungi, parasites, and human cellular elements; all potassium hydroxide preparations; pinworm examinations; fern tests; postcoital direct qualitative examinations of vaginal or cervical mucus; nasal smears for granulocytes; fecal leukocyte examinations; and qualitative semen analysis.

Only certain professionals are permitted to perform the procedures under this PPMP category if an exemption from the moderate complexity designation is to be retained. These include licensed physicians, dentists, and midlevel practitioners such as nurse practitioners, nurse midwives, and physician assistants under the supervision of a physician, only if authorized by the state in which the practice is located. With PPMP, the specimen must be examined during the patient visit; the specimen must be obtained from the provider's own patient or from a patient of a group medical practice of which the provider is a member or an employee.

The primary instrument for performing the test under the PPMP certificate is the microscope, limited to bright-field or phase-contrast microscopy. The specimen is usually labile, or a delay in performing the test could compromise the accuracy of the test result. In general, control materials are not available to monitor the entire testing process, and limited specimen handling or processing is required.

In moderately complex testing, a laboratory performs only waived tests and one or more tests designated as moderately complex by the FDA. To determine at which complexity level a particular method has been categorized, a searchable CLIA test complexity database is available at: http://www.accessdata.fda.gov/scripts/cdrh/cfdocs/cfCLIA/search.cfm. Manufacturers of moderately complex tests must submit their testing system to the FDA for classification. Therefore, this database will be continuously updated along with the waived test list.

Laboratories must submit an application to HHS or its designee on a form prescribed by HHS detailing the number, type, and methods employed for each measurement or examination, as well as the qualifications of the persons directing, supervising, and performing these

TABLE 6-2
Personnel Requirements for a Laboratory Performing Moderately Complex Testing

Director	The director is responsible for the overall management and direction of the laboratory but does not have to be onsite at all times. A broad range of experience and education is acceptable, for example, a physician with 1 year of experience directing/supervising a nonwaived laboratory with 20 continuing medical education credits (CMEs) in laboratory practice would qualify, as would a person with a bachelor's degree and 2 years' laboratory training/experience plus 2 years' supervisory experience in nonwaived testing. Depending on education and experience, the director could qualify for all other positions.
Testing personnel	These people are responsible for specimen processing, test performance, and test results reporting. The minimum requirement is a high school diploma or equivalent and training for the testing performed.
Technical consultant	These individuals are responsible for technical and scientific oversight of testing. The minimum requirement is a bachelor's degree with 2 years' laboratory training or experience in nonwaived testing.
Clinical consultant	These people provide clinical consultation. The minimum requirement is a doctoral degree with board certification.

From Centers for Disease Control and Prevention Moderate Complexity Testing Overview at: http://www.cdc.gov/clia/moderate.aspx.

procedures. Certificates may be valid for up to 2 years, and any changes in the information required in the application must be submitted to HHS or its designee within 30 days of any change in ownership, name, location, or director. Changes in method complexity require notification within 6 months of the change. This application may be submitted through an approved accrediting body or state agency if the accrediting standards of the agency are equal to or are more stringent than those of HHS, and if the agency is authorized to inspect the laboratory as frequently as required and submit to HHS required records and information.

Laboratory Directorship

Laboratories that perform under a Certificate of Waiver or with a certificate for PPMP can perform waived testing without the overhead of having personnel who meet established qualifications in training, experience, job performance, and competency. However, if any moderate complexity tests or measurements are performed, CLIA requires that the laboratory be directed by a laboratory director and/or a laboratory consultant with at least the directorship credentials listed in Table 6-2. This director is to be responsible for determining the qualifications of individuals performing and reporting test results, as well as ensuring compliance with all applicable regulations. The director is also responsible for the analytic performance of all assays, and must monitor ongoing proficiency, accuracy, and precision. If more than one individual in the practice qualifies as a laboratory director, the laboratory is required to designate one as being responsible. It must be demonstrated that the laboratory director is providing effective direction for the operation of the laboratory, and if he does not provide onsite direction, he must provide consultation by phone or delegate to qualified personnel with specific responsibility as required by regulation. Online courses are available that allow physicians to qualify as director of a moderately complex laboratory by obtaining 20 hours of continuing education credit. A list of courses can be found on the CMS website at: http://www.cms.gov/CLIA/15_CME_Courses_for_Laboratory_Directors_of_Moderate_Complexity_Laboratories.asp.

For POCT, a separate certification is usually not necessary when it is performed under the supervision of the laboratory director responsible for laboratory services in a health care facility. POCT that occurs within a health care facility, at sites that are located in contiguous buildings on the same campus, and under common direction can be performed under the certificate of the parent organization. When assays and procedures are performed in a situation such as this, the terms "waived" and "complexity" no longer have meaning. The test menu is no longer restricted to waived testing; however, more frequent inspections and higher scrutiny are received in return. Because the parent organization typically

TABLE 6-3
Point-of-Care Checklist

1. Equipment, if needed, must be evaluated.
2. A person of sufficient managerial authority is designated as being responsible for the site.
3. Persons performing the test must be trained and competency assessed, and this must be documented.
4. A written procedure must be available and followed.
5. Calibrations and quality control samples must be run at regular intervals.
6. All patient results must be documented, and the relationship to quality control measures must be clear.
7. Appropriate action must be taken and documented on all out-of-range quality control results.
8. Appropriate action must be documented on all abnormal patient results.

By congressional law, CLIA '88, a regulated test is any measurement used in the diagnosis, treatment, and management of a patient.
CLIA, Clinical Laboratory Improvement Act.

has a certificate that allows testing at all levels of complexity, it is the responsibility of the laboratory director to ensure that the test method used at the POCT site is appropriate for the skills and training of those performing the test. What inspectors do not tolerate could be called "rogue testing." This occurs when a clinic or service sets up a test without the knowledge and supervision of the laboratory director. With the new tracer method used by accrediting agencies such as TJC, if an inspector finds a lab result and traces it back to a laboratory that is not adequately supervised by the laboratory director, a citation may be issued to the discredit of the health care facility.

Compliance

In addition to CLIA, all laboratories must adhere to regulatory procedures, particularly in the outpatient setting. First, all testing for which Medicare is billed must be medically necessary. Screening tests and other measures of wellness generally are not covered. Medical necessity determination is implemented by Medicare, Medicaid, and other insurance carriers through Current Procedural Terminology (CPT) codes used in conjunction with International Classification of Disease (ICD) codes. When the ICD-10 code does not warrant the CPT-4 code, payment is rejected. Even worse, if it is determined that a laboratory deliberately added codes to obtain a higher payment than it deserves or payment for work that it has not done, it can be charged with fraud, which is a felony and the laboratory will be subjected to fines. Errors are assumed to be deliberate unless a compliance program is in place that actively seeks to uncover billing errors.

Another potential pitfall is Stark regulations. The Stark laws, which are named after their original sponsor Representative Fortney Pete Stark (D-CA), were intended to prevent unnecessary self-referrals intended to boost revenue. Under Stark, physicians are prohibited from referring Medicare patients to laboratories in which the physician (or a close family member) has a financial interest. Because this prohibition would be detrimental to most POLs, it is important to understand the "safe harbors" that allow legitimate self-referral.

CLIA '88 created standards for POL laboratories and POC testing in the United States that predated similar measures on the international scene. However, an international working group has proposed and adopted ISO 22870-2006 as an international standard for POCT testing. These standards are more extensive than current CLIA requirements; however, CLIA is a minimum federal requirement, and states and other accrediting agencies can impose standards that are more rigorous. An evolution of accreditation expectations may occur over the next few years to meet these international standards. Thomas has published a summary of these international standards with cross-referencing to current College of American Pathologists accreditation standards (Thomas, 2008).

Recommended Point-of-Care Protocol

Table 6-3 shows the recommended steps that should be taken when POCT tests are set up. In the first step, the equipment must be obtained and evaluated. Professional laboratorians usually have a good sense of what is available on the market. Point-of-care instrumentation tends to consist of handheld, durable units with easy analysis, simple quality control (QC), varied reporting methods, low throughput, and higher unit cost per test. Easy analysis and simple QC make these methods more likely to be classifiable as waived, allowing less well trained operators. At regular intervals, cross-correlation between POCT methods and central laboratory methods should be obtained to ensure that differences between POCT devices and central laboratory results are minimized and not mistaken for changes in a patient status.

Experience has shown that a POCT site operates far more efficiently when a person of sufficient authority is designated as being responsible for the site. With a responsible person in charge, reporting of suspected equipment malfunctions will be quicker, controls will be more reliably performed, and it is less likely that untrained individuals will attempt to perform testing.

In the third step, persons performing the test must be trained and their competency assessed, and this must be documented. Training documentation should include the date of initial training, as well as any additional in-services and competency assessments conducted. This documentation can include the performance of controls and/or proficiency samples as a measure of competency assessment.

Next, a written procedure must be available and followed. These procedures should adhere to the manufacturer's recommended steps and should be simple, easy to follow, and functional, rather than a collection of articles, package inserts, and instrument protocols that are too disorganized for the inexperienced operator to use. The procedure manual should include specimen requirements; procedures for specimen collection, identification, and processing; assay methods; reference intervals; and quality control and reporting methods. Because this is standard practice in laboratories, it should be fairly easy to have a procedure designed by the central laboratory staff.

Calibrations and quality control samples must be run at regular intervals. This is often the most difficult task to implement with nonlaboratory staff members who have not been indoctrinated in the importance of controls and calibrations. For this reason, many instruments designed for the POCT arena have features that block the reporting of results when appropriate calibrations and controls have not been performed. Some instruments can even lock out staff who have not been properly trained and issued a code recognizable to the machine.

All patient results must be documented, and their relationship to QC measures must be clear. Inspectors are not pleased when they find on tracers from medical records evidence of test results being used 7 days a week and controls being run Monday through Friday by only a small fraction of the users. In addition, if laboratory analyzers are in use, records of preventive maintenance and any corrective maintenance must be kept. Finally, if the POCT is being operated under the certificate of a central laboratory, it is a requirement that these POCT tests be enrolled in a proficiency testing program, such as that provided by the College of American Pathologists, in which results of proficiency samples are sent periodically to the proficiency testing service. These results are compared with those of a peer group to ascertain the accuracy of the specific tests.

Appropriate action must be taken and documented on all out-of-range QC results. Often it is best to have POCT staff call the central laboratory when controls fail because this creates the opportunity to review procedural steps and have a better-trained POCT staff. Quality has costs, but lack of quality can cost even more.

Appropriate action must be documented on all abnormal patient results. In this day of wireless networks, it is better to have POCT results transmitted to the computer and included with laboratory results generated centrally for comparison. If this option is not available, results should at least be written in the chart rather than being acted upon without proper documentation.

Selection of Measurements

With the explosion of waived methods coming onto the market, selection of POL/POCT lab measurements should begin with a check of available methods at the FDA website listed previously. The next, if not more important, consideration is the likelihood of reimbursement. Many insurance plans have agreements with national reference laboratories and require that lab tests be referred to the contracted lab. It may be necessary to prove the value of services rendered with patient satisfaction surveys, and the lab should be prepared to document better care and value to the managed care organization.

The next most important consideration in method selection is the volume of patient samples that will be measured and reimbursed. Infrequently performed assays are difficult to control for quality and can lead to expensive outdating of reagents. Some estimate of which measurements are most frequently ordered by the physician clientele is absolutely necessary. Ongoing monitoring of usage statistics in an established laboratory is also necessary. Even university hospitals, which generally attempt to provide full service, require special circumstances before providing an assay that is ordered fewer than 10 times per week. Low volume assays can easily degrade to a situation where controls, standards, calibrators, and repeats outnumber actual billable specimens at ratios greater than 2 : 1.

Point-of-care instrumentation tends to consist of hand-held, durable units with easy analysis, simple QC, varied reporting methods, low throughput, and higher unit cost. Easy analysis and simple QC make these methods more likely to be classifiable as waived, allowing less well trained operators. The menu of selectable tests can be limited, but the explosion of testing methods in the waived classification is changing this.

Central laboratory equipment tends to consist of desktop or floor standing units with high throughput and low cost per test, with full sample management and reporting capabilities if not connected to a laboratory information system. Here the intent is to perform moderate and high complexity testing. Greater technical skill is usually needed by the operator, and full proficiency assessment, including controls and regular proficiency testing, is required.

With POCT, the two most important considerations that must be taken into account are whether the testing is necessary for immediate decision-making, and whether staff members at the POCT site are sufficiently motivated to comply with testing procedures, including controls and competency maintenance. Examples of immediate decision-making include troponin testing as used in the emergency department (ED) to determine the disposition of the patient, and pregnancy testing administered before radiologic procedures. In these types of situations, the cost recovery in time savings and throughput to a health care system can be greater than the additional costs of maintaining the POCT site.

Maintenance of sufficient motivation by staff members at the POCT site to comply with testing procedures is critical for a successful POCT site. The first step should be to assign responsibility for all testing to someone at the site with sufficient managerial control over staff. Failure to do this usually results in the testing site staff failing to follow procedures because they do not directly report to laboratory staff, and hence perpetual arguments occur between laboratory QC staff and testing site staff.

Current Technology

The test menu is the greatest limitation in current POL/POCT technology. Although a large number of waived methods have been approved by the FDA, many are single test kits or single test strips, and separate devices may be needed at the POCT site to perform needed tests. With diabetes, which could be the largest market for POCT, as an example, where does one find a device that does both glucose and hemoglobin A1c (HbAlc)? This complicates staff training, method calibrations and controls, and reporting mechanisms. Incorporating results into the electronic medical record is hampered by this need for multiple devices, in that the cost of interfacing instruments that perform only one test can be prohibitive. For this reason, medical record interfaces tend to be limited to high volume tests such as bedside glucose testing or multitest platforms such as the I-Stat. The "art" of POL/POCT implementation and/or consultants is knowing how to craft the menu of POCT that would be most effective at a given location.

HEMATOLOGY

Hematology testing is somewhat limited in the POCT arena. Although hemoglobin or hematocrit is available on POCT blood gas or chemistry devices, no waived methods are available for the white blood cell count or differential. Therefore, a busy hematology/oncology service that is dependent on cell counts to decide whether to continue or change the dosage of therapy has to establish a moderate complexity lab with the associated regulatory and personnel requirements, or has to accept the delays of central lab testing.

Coagulation testing using POCT prothrombin time (PT) measurements has become a mature POCT area with the common establishment of "Coumadin clinics," where patients' anticoagulant therapy is monitored and regulated. This is advancing to self-testing with the use of waived devices, similar to home glucose monitoring, where patients monitor and alter dosage on the basis of home testing. Although this may seem dangerous, Mennemeyer and Winkelman have shown that switching from one laboratory to another between successive PT tests increased the odds of stroke and acute myocardial infarction by factors of 1.57 and 1.32, respectively (Mennemeyer, 1993). Therefore, the use of a consistent device in a POCT setting may be less dangerous than the changes that are seen in the PT and international normalized ratio (INR) when patients switch between laboratories.

CHEMISTRY

Glucose testing is clearly the industry leader in terms of volume of POCT testing, and hemoglobin A1c testing seems to be rapidly increasing. Concern has been expressed about using bedside glucose testing for tight glucose control in the intensive care unit setting because of potential episodes of hypoglycemia (Hoedemaekers, 2008), and Eastham has demonstrated that interfering substances can produce erroneous POCT measurements in 1.2% of patients admitted over a 12-month period (Eastham, 2009).

HbA1c measurements will be used more frequently in the future for the monitoring and diagnosis of diabetes. However, current POCT methods may not be up to the proposed task. Schwartz et al. described a multipractice study that compared a one-step POCT HbA1c instrument with central laboratory measurements; investigators found a bias that indicated that 18% of patients with laboratory HbA1c >7% would have been missed by the POCT test. And in a comparative study, Lenters-Westra and Slingerland found that six of eight available HbA1c POCT sites on the market failed to meet certification criteria of the National Glycohemoglobin Standardization Program (Lenters-Westra, 2010).

Intraoperative immunoassay of parathyroid hormone (PTH) measurements has revolutionized surgery for hormone-secreting tumors such as parathyroid adenomas (Sokoll, 2004). Although the cost of specialized testing in the operating suite using dedicated instrumentation, as well as frequent in-servicing of POCT staff, is high for the laboratory, when this is compared with the per minute cost of operating room time and the labor cost of physicians and staff involved in doing the surgery, the cost to the health care system is markedly reduced by POCT. Accuracy and comparison with the central laboratory PTH level are relatively unimportant because the values that are being compared involve large changes in PTH levels before and after an intervention.

Another area of chemistry that is rapidly changing involves creatinine and cardiac markers in EDs. Creatinine measurements and pregnancy tests are used to determine whether patients can be appropriately referred for radiologic procedures. Nichols et al. (2007) questioned the accuracy of two POCT creatinine assays. But in these situations, when values near the decision points for creatinine are obtained, the specimen can be referred to the central lab for confirmation, while the remaining patients can be moved on more rapidly increasing throughput. With pregnancy testing, an assay with high sensitivity should be selected to yield a high predictive value for a negative result.

In a review of the literature on the use of POCT for serum markers of cardiac necrosis in terms of the process and outcomes of patient care in the ED, Storrow (2009) found general agreement that POCT led to significantly decreased turnaround time for cardiac marker results reporting to the ordering physician. In addition, improvements in other ED efficiency measures (e.g., time to therapy and total ED length of stay) were seen. However, investigators could find no evidence that POCT for cardiac biomarkers has an effect on clinical outcomes of patients evaluated for acute coronary syndrome. In a multicenter, randomized, controlled study comparing laboratory and POCT cardiac marker testing strategies, Ryan et al. (2009) found similar reductions in turnaround time, but effects on ED length of stay varied between institutions. Across all sites, POCT testing did not decrease time to disposition for admitted or discharged patients (Ryan, 2009).

MICROBIOLOGY

Given the long turnaround times experienced with most microbiology testing, the availability of effective POCT could radically change practice in infectious disease. This can be seen quite clearly with the advent of effective POCT for human immunodeficiency virus (HIV). Performance characteristics of the available POCT HIV assays have been reviewed and were found to have comparable sensitivity and specificity to conventional enzyme immunoassays (Campbell, 2009). In early infection, however, these assays were found to be less sensitive than nucleic acid amplification testing. Appiah (2009) compared POCT HIV testing in a voluntary counseling and testing (VCT) clinic and in a tuberculosis (TB) clinic in Ghana and found that in both clinics, 100% of patients offered POCT accepted it, but only 93% of VCT clients and 40% of TB patients had accepted a standard HIV test offered 6 months earlier. Moreover, all patients attending the VCT or TB clinics who tested positive for HIV with the POCT test returned to the HIV clinic for care, but only 64% and 95%, respectively, of patients who tested positive in the previous cohort had returned for follow-up, indicating a strong change in patient behavior when access to POCT and immediate results is provided (Appiah, 2009).

Other infectious disease POCT is not quite so effective. Rapid group A streptococcal antigen testing is relatively insensitive, with sensitivity estimates ranging from 60% to 90%, making the recommendation necessary for backup blood agar culturing for all negative POCT antigen results. Waived testing for respiratory viruses is limited to respiratory syncytial viruses and influenza A and B viruses with similar sensitivities. Recent experience with the novel H1N1 outbreak, where all POCT tests indicating influenza A were assumed to be positive for H1N1, was less than satisfactory.

POCT in Military Operational Environments

BACKGROUND CONCEPTS

In the military operational environment, POCT utilizes hand-held testing devices to provide laboratory data on specific patient types in austere settings. Three concepts will help the reader grasp military operational POCT: the echelon of care system, planned evacuation of sick and injured patients, and hostile and/or spartan working conditions. Currently in the United States, theater medical care is organized into five ascending levels of capability (Stephenson, 2008). Echelon I, the lowest level, spans a range from "buddy" or self aid (such as placing a tourniquet on a wounded comrade in the field) to a makeshift medical tent, to a simple Troop Medical Clinic on a small base staffed by a physician and several trained assistants (called medics in the Army and corpsmen in the Navy). These small clinics will offer some POCT and are further discussed later. Echelon II sites are typically mobile facilities where emergent surgical stabilization can be performed. In the U.S. system, these are divided into forward resuscitative surgical suites (FRSSs) with two general surgeons and a few support staff, and forward surgical teams (FSTs) composed of four surgeons, including one orthopedic surgeon, and ancillary staff. The FST is a larger entity than the FRSS, but both can be transported on a few military vehicles and established and broken down in a matter of hours. Echelon II facilities include larger clinics than those in Echelon I, and some have limited in-patient capabilities. Echelon III is equivalent to a Level I trauma center in the United States. Such a facility may be a fixed structure, such as the Craig Joint Theater Hospital in Bagram, Afghanistan, or a series of tents, as in Balad, Iraq. Both offer trauma bays, surgical suites, intensive care unit patient care areas, and 24-hour physician and nurse coverage. The only theater Echelon IV facility is in Landstuhl, Germany. Echelon V centers include Walter Reed Army Medical Center in Washington, DC, the National Naval Medical Center in Bethesda, Md., and the Brooke Army Medical Center in San Antonio, Tex. Patients are successively evacuated to higher echelons, as indicated by their injury or illness, to a facility that can provide definitive treatment or rehabilitation. For the purposes of this discussion, POCT is considered in Echelons I, II, and III—those directly in the theater of operations.

UNIQUE ASPECTS OF MILITARY POCT

Three differences have been observed in military operational POCT compared with POCT in a stateside hospital or clinic: the patient population, the algorithm for decision-making, and the degree of flexibility that providers and technicians have in laboratory testing. First, patients differ in terms of demographic characteristics—most are young and healthy at baseline—and their presenting complaint. Obviously traumatic injury is the most serious complaint, and patients wounded by improvised explosive devices (IEDs) may present with massive tissue trauma and concomitant coagulopathy. Common illnesses include acute gastroenteritis, heat-related symptoms, and upper respiratory infections. Second, POCT is used to make the following decision: Treat the patient and release him to quarters

TABLE 6-4
Point-of-Care Testing (POCT) by Common Patient Type

	Goals	Data needed	POCT instrument
Trauma patient	Assess coagulopathy, anemia from blood loss	PT, PTT, Hb, Hct, electrolytes, blood gas	i-STAT or Hemochron Jr
Acute GI illness	Assess dehydration and electrolyte derangements	BUN, glucose, Hb, Hct, Na, K, Cl, HCO_3, anion gap, blood gas	i-STAT
Ward inpatient	Intervene as anemia, coagulopathy, electrolyte, or metabolic disturbances develop	Hb, Hct, PT, Na, K, Cl, HCO_3, Glucose	i-STAT, Precision Xtra

BUN, Blood urea nitrogen; *GI,* gastrointestinal; *Hb,* hemoglobin; *Hct,* hematocrit; *PT,* prothrombin time; *PTT,* partial thromboplastin time.

(and then have him return to duty), or stabilize the patient and evacuate him to the next echelon of care where more definitive treatment can be provided. Any patient who presents to a theater medical facility is evaluated using this algorithm, and laboratory data are an adjunct in making this decision. Third, laboratory testing in the austere setting of a military theater of operations enjoys flexibility not present in stateside facilities. Far from regulatory agencies, hospital and clinic laboratories have the option to streamline their testing as circumstances warrant. Thus, if quality control reagents cannot be delivered because the tactical environment so dictates, then tests are sometimes performed anyway. The justification is that it is more important to generate laboratory results on a wounded patient with a reasonable assumption that the data are accurate than it is to suspend testing until proper controls can be run. Laboratory staff members make great efforts to adhere to the standards in place in the United States, but do not hesitate to make well-informed adjustments to these standards when necessary.

KEY EXAMPLES OF POCT BY PATIENT TYPE

The Trauma Patient

The goals in this patient type are to stabilize the injured and then evacuate to the next appropriate echelon of care. (Table 6-4 summarizes the goals, necessary laboratory studies, and instruments in use in the theater.) Stabilization involves airway management, immediate wound care, and resuscitation with intravenous (IV) fluids and, as needed, blood products. Evacuation typically occurs within minutes to an Echelon II facility and within hours to an Echelon III hospital, although security and weather factor into this timeline. Patients may be held up to 6 hours at Echelon II and up to 3 days at Echelon III sites, but again, this is dependent on the ability of the patient to be safely evacuated if this is what is required for that individual's care. Key laboratory data in the trauma patient include Hb and hematocrit (Hct), PT, ionized calcium level, and arterial blood gases. The trauma patient with significant hemorrhage is in a dynamic state, and Hb and Hct must be interpreted accordingly; if the patient has been adequately volume resuscitated, then these data are useful. If not, then the ordering physician must integrate this fact into the assessment. A common platform in use in the theater is the i-STAT. The EG7+ cartridge provides Hb and Hct if the sample is anticoagulated with ethylenediaminetetraacetic acid (EDTA), and it provides Na, K, iCa, and blood gas parameters (pH, pCO_2, pO_2, TCO_2, HCO_3, BE, and SO_2) on whole blood samples with no anticoagulator with sodium heparin. Samples with no anticoagulant must be used for the i-STAT coagulation cartridge, which provides PT and INR. Another instrument used to assess coagulopathy is the Hemochron Jr Signature (International Technidyne Corporation, Piscataway, N.J.). It yields partial thromboplastin time (PTT) as well as PT and INR and uses citrated blood, which allows for a brief delay before the test must be performed. The i-STAT whole blood sample obviously must be run immediately, before the blood clots.

Acute Gastrointestinal Illness

The goals are to assess dehydration and the electrolyte disturbances that accompany it, and from there to determine if the patient can be managed with supportive care where he is, or if he requires evacuation to a higher echelon facility. Echelon I capabilities often include IV fluids and beds or stretchers for very short-term care; Echelon II sites may hold a patient for several hours. Necessary laboratory data include blood urea nitrogen (BUN), glucose, Cl, K, Na, Hb, Hct, anion gap, and blood gases. The i-STAT module EC8+ provides all of these and is a particularly useful cartridge for the patient with vomiting and/or diarrhea. If the laboratory data suggest severe dehydration and electrolyte derangement at an Echelon I facility, evacuation is probably indicated. Milder abnormalities are often managed with 1 to 2 liters of IV fluids, antiemetics, and a sick-in-quarters chit. Because acute gastroenteritis is a very common illness in the operational setting, physicians readily choose an i-STAT cartridge such as the EC8+ to capture just these data.

Ward Inpatients

The goal in the ward inpatient is to assess the patient's hemostatic and metabolic status, identifying any abrupt change that would require intervention. In select patients, blood glucose may be followed easily with POCT. In others, such as trauma victims or the critically ill, PT, Hb, and Hct may be performed immediately to assess a suspected change in hemostasis. Similarly, ionized calcium and electrolytes may be measured at the bedside in a patient with electrocardiogram or mental status changes with quick turnaround. For bedside glucose measurements, the Precision Xtra (Abbott Diabetes Care, Abbott Park, Ill.) is in use in at least one Echelon III center. The i-STAT fills the role of providing the other tests, using the EG7+ and PT/INR cartridges.

LIMITATIONS OF POCT IN OPERATIONAL ENVIRONMENTS

POCT has a few limitations in the operational environment. First, some smaller medical facilities, particularly at the lower echelons, utilize medics without extensive laboratory training to perform tests. Although the military has training programs specifically for laboratory technicians, the medic assigned to an Echelon I facility may be a generalist, or may have special training in some other allied health field but must fill the role of a generalist as operational requirements dictate. Thus, the medic's familiarity and skill in performing laboratory duties is not comparable to what one would see in a stateside hospital. Related to this is the risk that attention to QC and quality assurance (QA), record keeping, and supervisory review will be decreased compared with the norm in U.S. laboratories. This is the downside to increased flexibility. Smaller medical outposts do not willfully ignore the need for QA and documentation, but may of necessity give them lower priority than emergent treatment and evacuation of casualties. Finally, logistical backlogs hinder POCT as well. If controls or reagents cannot be adequately stocked, then technicians must choose between using expired reagents (if they have them) or not performing tests at all. Although the supply chain is an occasional obstacle in stateside laboratories, this is even more likely in a military theater.

CONCLUSIONS

POCT in a military theater of operations balances the limitations incurred in an austere setting with the flexibility inherent in hand-held testing instruments and unique to the field environment. Drawbacks to POCT exist both in the rigor of testing practice—less experienced staff and patchy quality assurance and supervisory oversight—and in the range of tests offered. Logistical considerations preclude the use of all testing panels available with the i-STAT instrument. A few select menus are utilized rather than all that are commercially available. Still, small, mobile platforms such as the i-STAT allow military corpsmen and medics to perform key tests on critically ill and injured patients and to assist in their treatment in a hostile setting, thus representing an extremely valuable adjunct to patient care.

SELECTED REFERENCES

Appiah LT, Havers F, Gibson J, et al. Efficacy and acceptability of rapid, point-of-care HIV testing in two clinical settings in Ghana. AIDS Patient Care STDs 2009;23:365–9.

Demonstrates improved patient behavior with immediacy of POCT.

Campbell S, Fedoriw Y. Point-of-care human immunodeficiency virus testing. Point of Care 2009;8:32–5.

Reviews sensitivities of POCT HIV assays.

Dooley JF. Point-of-care diagnostic testing markets. Point of Care 2009;8:154–6.

Reviews POCT market.

Eastham JH, Mason D, Barnes DL, et al. Prevalence of interfering substances with point-of-care glucose testing in a community hospital. Am J Health Syst Pharm 2009;66:167–70.

Reviews interfering substance effect on POCT glucose.

Federal Register, 57, 42CFR 493; Clinical Laboratory Improvement Act, 1992.

Hoedemaekers CW, Klein Gunnewiek JM, Prinsen MA, et al. Accuracy of bedside glucose measurement from three glucometers in critically ill patients. Crit Care Med 2008;36:3062–6.

Points out potential for error in critically ill patients.

Lenters-Westra1 E, Slingerland RJ. Six of eight hemoglobin A1c point-of-care instruments do not meet the general accepted analytical performance criteria. Clin Chem 2010;56:44–52.

Demonstrates variability in performance with hemoglobin A1c assays.

Mennemeyer ST, Winkelman JW. Searching for inaccuracy in clinical laboratory testing using Medicare data. JAMA 1993;269:1030–3.

Shows potential for patient injury when patients switch laboratories.

Nichols JH, Bartholomew C, Bonzagi A, Garb JL, Jin L. Evaluation of the IRMA TRUpoint and i-STAT creatinine assays. Clin Chim Acta 2007;377:201–5.

Ryan RJ, Lindsell CJ, Hollander JE, et al. A multicenter randomized controlled trial comparing central laboratory and point-of-care cardiac marker testing strategies: the disposition impacted by serial point of care markers in acute coronary syndromes (DISPO-ACS) trial. Ann Emerg Med 2009;53:321–8.

Analyzes outcomes when POCT is available.

Schwartz KL, Monsur J, Hammad A, Bartoces MG, Neale AV. Comparison of point of care and laboratory HbA1c analysis: a MetroNet study. J Am Board Fam Med 2009;22:461–3.

A multi center comparison of POCT and laboratory Hg A1C results showing errors with one POCT method.

Sokoll LJ, Wians FH, Remaley AT. Rapid intraoperative immunoassay of parathyroid hormone and other hormones: a new paradigm for point-of-care testing. Clin Chem 2004;50:1126–35.

Demonstrates potential for institutional savings using POCT.

Stephenson JC. Echelons of care and aeromedical evacuation from the Middle East area of operations. Australian Defense Forces Health 2008;9:9–14.

Storrow AB, Lyon JA, Porter MW, et al. A systematic review of emergency department point-of-care cardiac markers and efficiency measures. Point of Care 2009;8:121–5.

Thomas MA. Quality assurance and accreditation in point-of-care testing. Point of Care 2008;7:227–32.

Compares CLIA and international standards.

REFERENCES

Access the complete reference list online at http://www.expertconsult.com

CHAPTER 7

POSTANALYSIS: MEDICAL DECISION MAKING

Jeffrey S. Jhang, Anthony N. Sireci, Alexander Kratz

KEY POINTS

- Laboratory results must undergo a two-step postanalytic review for analytic correctness (using delta checks, linearity ranges, etc.) and for clinical significance for the patient (applying critical values, reference ranges, pretest and posttest probability, etc.)
- Reference intervals are most commonly defined as the range of values into which 95% of nondiseased individuals will fall; this definition implies that 5% of nondiseased individuals can have laboratory results outside the reference range.
- The ability of a test to discriminate disease from no disease is described by the sensitivity and specificity of the test. Sensitivity is the probability of a positive result in a person with the disease (true-positive rate). Specificity is the probability of a negative result in a person without disease (true-negative rate).
- Screening tests require high sensitivity so that no case is missed. Confirmatory tests require high specificity to be certain of the diagnosis.
- Altering a test cutoff has a reciprocal effect on sensitivity and specificity. A cutoff can be lowered to include all cases (100% sensitivity), but this reduces the specificity (i.e., increases false-positives).
- Receiver operator characteristic (ROC) curves plot the true-positive rate versus the false-positive rate and graphically present the range of sensitivities and specificities at all test cutoffs. If two tests are compared, the more accurate test is closer to the upper left-hand corner of the ROC curve.
- The likelihood ratio of a test refers to the ratio of the probability of a given test result in the disease state over the probability of the same result in the nondisease state. The likelihood ratio of a test changes as the cutoff value defining disease and nondisease is varied.
- Predictive value describes the probability of disease or no disease for a positive or negative result, respectively. The predictive value of a positive test increases with disease prevalence.
- Bayes' theorem uses information about test characteristics (sensitivity and specificity) and disease prevalence (pretest probability) to obtain the posttest probability of disease, given a positive test. Similarly, it can be used to determine the posttest probability of no disease, given a negative test.
- Evidence-based medicine is a process by which medical decisions can be made by using as many objective tools as possible; it integrates the most current and the best medical evidence with clinical expertise and patient preferences.

Every time a clinical laboratory produces a test result, the value must undergo a two-step postanalytic evaluation process. The result needs to be assessed for analytic correctness and for clinical significance. It is often assumed that these two tasks can be easily divided between the performing laboratory, which is responsible for determination of analytic correctness, and the clinical team, which is responsible for evaluation of the clinical meaning of the results. However, significant overlap is seen in the responsibilities for these tasks. Although the laboratory performs most of the review of laboratory results for analytic reliability by using techniques such as delta checks, flagging of questionable results, moving averages, and linear ranges, it is incumbent upon the clinician to review every laboratory result with regard to the patient's clinical situation and to question the analytic reliability of implausible results. On the other hand, one of the most important factors in the analysis of the clinical significance of a laboratory result is comparison of the reported value versus a reference range. In most settings, reference ranges are determined by the laboratory, with varying degrees of input from the clinical staff. Postanalytic decision-making is therefore a shared responsibility of the laboratory and the clinical staff, and it behooves both groups to maintain constant communications to optimize every part of the process. The purpose of this chapter is to discuss the process of postanalytic review of laboratory data and their use in medical decision making, and to provide general tools for the objective interpretation of laboratory results.

Assessment of Analytic Correctness of Results

ALARMS AND FLAGS

Modern diagnostic laboratories often analyze large numbers of samples with highly automated instruments. A majority of the results are never visually inspected by a human eye, and many results are released into patients' electronic medical records without prior review by a laboratory employee. To prevent the release of erroneous results, most laboratories utilize a variety of "flags" or alarms. The flagging of specimens or results that require additional analytic steps or review before they can be released can be performed by the automated instrument itself, by specialized middleware, or by the laboratory information system. Flags can indicate a problem with the specimen (e.g., the presence of an interfering substance) or an issue with the result (e.g., a numeric value outside the analytic range of the method, or the need for confirmation by an additional assay).

Flags for Problem Specimens

Many automated instruments can measure the amount of sample present in a collection tube and flag samples that contain amounts inadequate for a reliable analysis. The laboratory will have to identify another tube containing an adequate sample volume, or will request the collection of a new sample. Another frequent cause of inadequate samples is the presence of high concentrations of interfering substances in the specimen, most commonly lipids (lipemia), hemoglobin (Hb) (hemolysis), paraproteins (gammopathies), or bilirubin (icterus). The mechanism for this interference is dependent on the substance and the analytic method. For example, in spectrophotometric assays, lipids interfere mainly by increasing light scatter (turbidity); in assays using ion-specific electrodes for measurement, lipids will affect results by solvent exclusion. A more detailed discussion of interference mechanisms is provided elsewhere in this text. Most commercial assays will list concentrations of interfering substances, above which assay results are no longer valid. Visual inspection is often an adequate means of assessing the presence of unacceptable concentrations of interfering substances. Samples that are grossly hemolyzed or icteric, for example, may be immediately flagged by the technologist as inappropriate for analysis. However, automated analyzers are able to detect troublesome levels of interfering substances, even when they are not apparent to the laboratorian at the macroscopic level. Automated systems can measure the concentrations of bilirubin, lipid, and hemoglobin in samples and can present the degree of interference present as an index (Vermeer, 2005; Kroll, 1994). If the index exceeds a given threshold, then the sample is flagged as problematic and should be rerun after removal of the interfering substance, or it should be rejected. Serum bilirubin and Hb levels have been shown to correlate very tightly with interference indices, but because of the chemical heterogeneity of serum lipids, lipemia indices do not correlate as well (Fossati, 1982).

Flags for Specimens That Require Additional Analysis With Another Method

Some laboratory technologies are screening methods that allow for rapid analysis of large numbers of samples, almost instantaneous reporting of results on most samples, and identification of potentially abnormal samples, which requires follow-up with a more labor-intensive method. Automated cell counters are the paradigm of such instruments. These instruments can often analyze more than 100 samples per hour in a highly automated fashion; samples that are normal or that show only quantitative abnormalities (e.g., increased or decreased percentage of lymphocytes, low platelet counts, low red cell counts) can be reported immediately, and samples that could potentially contain qualitative abnormalities (e.g., atypical lymphocytes, platelet clumps, red cell fragments) are flagged for preparation of a blood smear and further evaluation. The flags are generally based on forward- and side-scatter and impedance measurements that provide information about size and nuclear complexity/granularity of the cells, and on special stains that help identify the potential presence of immature cells (Fujimoto, 1999). The sensitivities and specificities of these flags show poor discriminatory power, and clinical judgment is needed if suspicion of an underlying hematologic abnormality is high (Briggs, 1999; Ruzicka, 2001; Thalhammer-Scherrer, 1997).

Flags for Problematic Results

An analyte concentration outside the validated linear range is another common problem affecting samples. Generally, package inserts of commercial assays will provide end-users with an estimated range within which an increase in signal is linearly related to an increase in the analyte concentration. The laboratory may validate this range or may establish its own acceptable linear range when the assay is introduced. Analyzers, middleware, or the laboratory information system will identify and flag samples in which the measured analyte values falls outside the linear range. If the analyte falls above the linear range, many instruments can automatically dilute and reanalyze the sample. In some cases, a manual dilution may be necessary, or the information that the result is higher than a certain value may be sufficient for the requesting clinician. For example, patients in diabetic ketoacidosis will have glucose measurements >1000 mg/dL, far exceeding the linearity of most analyzers. These samples will be flagged, diluted by a predetermined factor, and then rerun before reporting. If an analyte concentration falls below the linear range, the sample is usually reported as "less than the limit of detection."

DELTA CHECKS

Advances in computer technology have facilitated the storage of data from large numbers of patients and increasingly complex calculations in laboratory information systems. This has made it possible to use patient data for quality control purposes in real time. For example, most laboratories routinely submit the results of certain laboratory assays to "delta checks" before releasing them into the patient record. Delta checks are defined as comparing a current laboratory result with results obtained on a previous specimen from the same patient. Parameters chosen for delta checks should not be subject to large intraindividual variations; for example, many laboratories have delta checks in place for the mean corpuscular volume of red cells. Suggested assays, thresholds, and time intervals between measurements can be found in the literature (Ladenson, 1975). Some studies have suggested the comparison of multiple test parameters to decrease the false-positive rate of the delta check; however, few laboratories have implemented such delta checks. Types of errors detected with delta checks include preanalytic (e.g., mislabeling of specimens) and analytic issues (e.g., aspiration of insufficient sample volume by the instrument sample probe) (Kazmierczak, 2003). Laboratories should define procedures for samples that have been flagged by delta checks; protocols usually incorporate repeating the assay, reviewing the specimen identification, and notifying the clinical staff of the possibility of a mislabeled specimen.

Assessment of Clinical Significance of Results

CRITICAL VALUES

A critical value (also known as a panic or alert value) is a laboratory result that may represent a life-threatening situation that may not otherwise be readily detectable and therefore requires rapid communication with a health care provider who can provide necessary medical interventions. The speedy communication of such results is required by federal law and regulatory agencies, and The Joint Commission has made it one of its National Patient Safety Goals. Regulations require that the critical value and the patient affected are read back by the health care provider to verify that the result was correctly communicated. The laboratory then has to document the communication of the critical value, the name and title of the caregiver who was notified, the time and date of notification, and the read-back by the care provider.

No universally accepted guidelines indicate which assays should have critical values, what the thresholds should be, whether critical values should be repeated before reporting, and what is an acceptable time from result availability to caregiver notification. Although it is generally established that critical values must be called to a caregiver who has the ability to act upon the information, there is no universal agreement regarding the types of caregiver (e.g., physician's assistant, registered nurse) who fulfill this definition. This has caused significant variation in procedures related to critical values at different institutions. It is ultimately the responsibility of the medical director of the laboratory to work with clinical colleagues to develop a critical values policy that meets the needs of patients and staff served by the laboratory.

REFERENCE RANGES

Definition of Reference Intervals

Comparison of a laboratory result versus a reference or "normal" range is often one of the most important aspects of medical decision making. Reference intervals are usually defined as the range of values into which 95% of nondiseased ("normal") individuals will fall; the corollary of this definition is that 2.5% of nondiseased individuals will have laboratory results below the reference range, and 2.5% of nondiseased individuals will have laboratory results above the reference range. For some analytes, the reference range is defined as "less than" or "greater than" a certain value; for example, a prostate-specific antigen (PSA) level of 4 ng/mL is often used to distinguish patients who require no further follow-up ("normal") from those who require a prostate biopsy ("abnormal"). Some reference ranges have been defined by professional organizations without adherence to the 95% rule. A paradigm of this is the recommendation of American and European cardiology associations that "an increased value for cardiac troponin should be defined as the measurement exceeding the 99th percentile of a reference control group" (Alpert, 2000). For other analytes (e.g., cholesterol/lipids), laboratories frequently provide therapeutic target ranges that represent recommendations based on clinical trials and/or epidemiologic studies (Grundy, 2004). Finally, it is common practice to provide therapeutic and/or toxic ranges for drug measurements.

Factors That Influence Reference Ranges

A variety of factors can influence reference ranges. Different laboratory methods often yield significantly different results and therefore require different reference ranges. This phenomenon is best documented and understood for methods in which measurement of the analyte is based on one or more antibody–antigen interactions, but it can affect all analytic methods. Because of differences in age, genetic background, or exposure to environmental factors, different populations may need different reference ranges for certain laboratory analytes. Many other factors such as the containers into which specimens were collected (e.g., glass vs. plastic tubes), the mode of transport to the laboratory (by messenger or by pneumatic tube system), the time between obtaining the specimen and analysis, and the storage conditions of the specimens before analysis can affect reference ranges.

Determination of Reference Ranges

Because many factors can affect reference ranges, laboratories are strongly encouraged to perform their own studies to establish reference ranges for all analytes they report, usually by testing at least 120 samples from nondiseased individuals in each "partition" (e.g., gender, age group). If this is not possible, the laboratory can verify a reference interval that it has previously established for a different method by transference (i.e., demonstrating that the new method yields identical results to the previous method). If the analyte was not previously tested for in the laboratory, the laboratory can verify another laboratory's or the manufacturer's reference interval (CLSI, 2008).

Variability of Laboratory Results

Interindividual variation of laboratory results often occurs because of factors specific to individual patients. For example, creatine kinase (CK) levels are proportional to muscle mass. Thus, a population of normal subjects will express a range of CK values according to each individual's muscle mass, but an individual patient will have a unique set value that is "normal" for that individual. In clinical practice, this unique value, if known, is the best "reference value" for a particular individual. Comparison of test results from a patient versus such an individualized reference value has to take into account random variability. Random variability is the sum of analytic and intraindividual variability. Analytic variability is the result of assay imprecision. It is usually determined during validation studies for a new method by running the same sample multiple times and is expressed quantitatively as the coefficient of variation (CV). Intraindividual variability is due to biologic changes that cause analyte levels to fluctuate over time. Well-known examples of this phenomenon include diurnal variations in cortisol levels, estrogen levels that vary with the menstrual cycle, and seasonal variations of vitamin D. Many other analytes show some biologic variability, including changes related to exercise or food intake. Table 7-1 provides estimates of interindividual and intraindividual biologic variation for common analytes. As expected, intraindividual variation is generally less than interindividual variation. The index of individuality is the ratio of intraindividual CV to interindividual CV. A low index (<0.6) means that results from a given individual fluctuate within a narrow range of the reference interval. In such instances, serial changes in an individual's analyte may be more useful in detecting disease than in comparing each of the measurements versus the reference interval (Lacher, 2005). Table 7-1 also shows that the method CV or degree of analytic variability is usually much lower than the biologic variability and hence is much less of a factor in affecting the overall random variability of measurements. For some analytes, guidelines have been published as to what constitutes a clinically significant difference between two consecutive patient sample results. As an example, Table 7-2 provides this information for various thyroid function tests (Baloch, 2003).

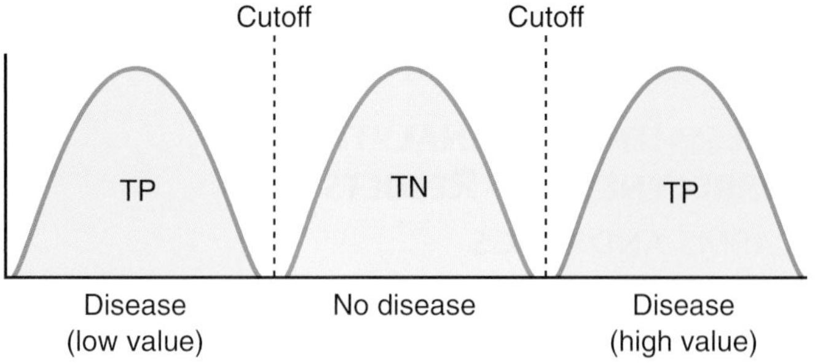

Figure 7-1 Distribution of test results from nonoverlapping populations of patients with and without disease (see Table 7-3). *TN*, True-negative; *TP*, true-positive.

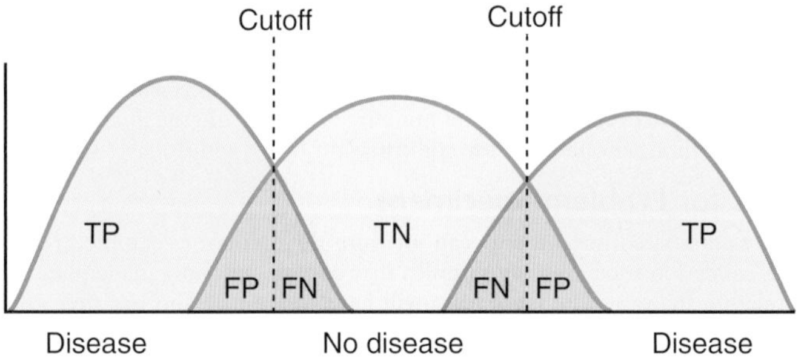

Figure 7-2 Distribution of test results from overlapping populations of patients with and without disease (see Table 7-3). *FN*, False-negative; *FP*, false-positive; *TN*, true-negative; *TP*, true-positive.

General Principles for the Interpretation of Laboratory Results

DIAGNOSTIC ACCURACY

Truth Table

Clinicians often find it helpful and intuitive to dichotomize a continuous test result into a binary one by applying a threshold value for the analyte. Although the reference range can be used to separate normal from abnormal values, clinically validated thresholds are also commonly used for disease classification. For example, the reference range for Hb A1c in a laboratory may be 4.0%–6.0%, but the clinically established threshold to classify a patient as diabetic is 6.5%. This means that a patient's result can be outside the reference range without meeting the threshold for diabetes.

A test with perfect diagnostic accuracy could determine the presence or absence of disease with certainty, and the established cutoff point would perfectly separate diseased from not diseased populations (Galen, 1975) (Fig. 7-1). However, nearly all laboratory tests are imperfect, and overlap is seen between populations at both low and high cutoffs (Fig. 7-2).

The diagnostic accuracy of a test is determined by comparing the test's ability to discern true disease from nondisease as determined by a diagnostic gold standard (i.e., truth). Based on results from the test and the gold standard, patients can be classified into four groups in a 2 × 2 table (see Fig. 7-2 and Table 7-3). Patients correctly classified as abnormal are called true-positives (TPs) and those correctly classified as normal are called true-negatives (TNs). These true results are the nonoverlapping areas of the two patient distributions. False results occur because the two populations overlap (i.e., because a test cannot completely discriminate all abnormal patients from normal ones). Patients incorrectly classified as

TABLE 7-1

Interindividual and Intraindividual Biologic Variability for Common Analytes

Analyte individual	Interindividual CV, %	Intraindividual CV, %	Index of CV, %	Method
Alanine aminotransferase	50.2	23.7	0.47	3.2
Albumin	8.9	2.8	0.31	3.4
Alkaline phosphatase	33.4	4.4	0.13	6.5
Apolipoprotein A	17.8	7.0	0.39	4.8
Apolipoprotein B	27.6	9.5	0.34	2.7
Aspartate aminotransferase	29.1	15.1	0.52	3.4
β-Carotene	67.4	24.2	0.36	7.4
Bicarbonate	13.3	11.0	0.83	2.4
Bilirubin, total	43.9	24.6	0.56	3.0
C-peptide	65.7	28.4	0.43	7.2
Calcium, ionized	3.6	2.4	0.67	1.4
Calcium, total	4.7	3.3	0.70	2.2
Chloride	3.1	1.9	0.61	1.0
Cholesterol, total	22.3	8.2	0.37	2.3
Creatinine	18.7	6.8	0.36	1.0
Creatinine, urine	61.3	43.0	0.70	2.2
Fibrinogen, plasma	25.6	16.2	0.63	3.9
Folate	64.3	22.6	0.35	3.6
γ-Glutamyl transferase	59.8	16.2	0.27	1.7
Glucose, plasma	12.5	8.3	0.66	1.7
Glycohemoglobin, blood	9.6	1.5	0.16	3.1
HDL cholesterol	28.3	12.4	0.44	2.5
Homocysteine	36.6	18.0	0.49	6.0
Iron	41.6	29.0	0.70	3.2
Iron binding capacity, total	15.5	6.9	0.45	3.3
Insulin, plasma	55.9	25.2	0.45	13.0
Lactate dehydrogenase	21.6	7.9	0.37	6.0
Phosphorus	15.8	9.2	0.58	2.0
Potassium	7.7	5.4	0.70	0.5
Protein, total	6.2	3.5	0.56	0.9
Selenium	13.2	5.1	0.39	4.8
Sodium	1.6	1.3	0.81	0.7
Triglycerides	56.8	28.8	0.51	4.7
Urea nitrogen	32.1	18.0	0.56	3.7
Uric acid	27.1	9.0	0.33	0.7
Varicella antibody	43.2	13.7	0.32	6.7
Vitamin A	30.7	9.5	0.31	2.5
Vitamin B_{12}	41.6	13.4	0.32	6.2
Vitamin E	35.1	11.3	0.32	2.9

Data from Lacher DA, Hughes JP, Carroll MD. Estimate of biologic variation of laboratory analytes based on the third national health and nutrition examination survey. Clin Chem 2005;51(2):450–452.

CV, Coefficient of variation; *HDL,* high-density lipoprotein.

TABLE 7-2

Clinically Significant Difference Between Two Consecutive Patient Results

Analyte	Change
Total T_4	2.2 μg/dL
Free T_4	0.5 ng/dL
Total T_3	35 ng/dL
Free T_3	0.1 ng/dL
TSH	0.75 mIU/L
Thyroglobulin	1.5 ng/mL

Data from Baloch Z, Carayon P, Conte-Devolx B, et al. Laboratory medicine practice guidelines: laboratory support for the diagnosis and monitoring of thyroid disease. Thyroid 2003;13(1):3–126.

T_3, Triiodothyronine; *T_4,* thyroxine; *TSH,* thyroid-stimulating hormone.

TABLE 7-3

Truth (2 × 2) Table: Classifying Patients

Result	Disease	No disease	Total
Positive	TP	FP	TP + FP
Negative	FN	TN	FN + TN
Total	TP + FN	FP + TN	TP + FP + FN + TN

$$\text{Sensitivity}\ (\%) = 100 \times \left(\frac{TP}{TP+FN}\right)$$

$$\text{Specificity}\ (\%) = 100 \times \left(\frac{TN}{TN+FP}\right)$$

$$\text{Positive predictive value}\ (\%) = 100 \times \left(\frac{TP}{TP+FP}\right)$$

$$\text{Negative predictive value}\ (\%) = 100 \times \left(\frac{TN}{TN+FN}\right)$$

FN, False-negative; *FP,* false-positive; *TN,* true-negative; *TP,* true-positive.

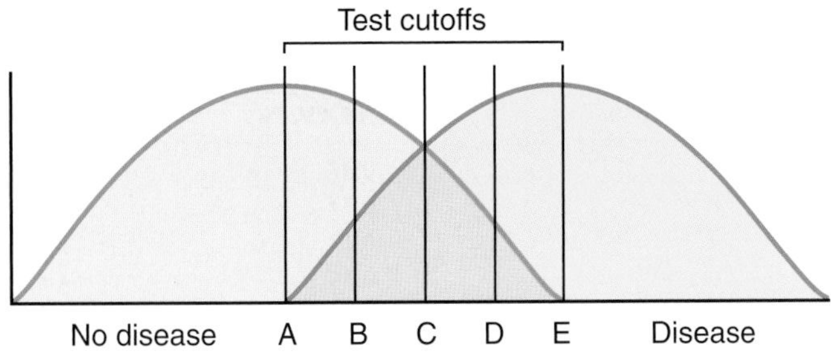

Figure 7-3 Effects of varying the test cutoff on overlapping populations of patients with and without disease.

TABLE 7-4
Example Truth (2 × 2) Table

Result	Disease	No disease	Total
Positive	196	20	116
Negative	4	180	184
Total	200	200	400

$$\text{Sensitivity (\%)} = 100 \times \left(\frac{196}{196+4}\right) = 98\%$$

$$\text{Specificity (\%)} = 100 \times \left(\frac{180}{180+20}\right) = 90\%$$

$$\text{Positive predictive value (\%)} = 100 \times \left(\frac{196}{196+20}\right) = 91\%$$

$$\text{Negative predictive value (\%)} = 100 \times \left(\frac{180}{180+4}\right) = 98\%$$

In this evaluation study of a hypothetical cardiac marker, 200 patients with acute myocardial infarction (AMI) and 200 healthy subjects are recruited for a study designed to mimic a prevalence of 50%. The assay is performed and is compared with a "gold standard" test for AMI, and the 2 × 2 truth table shown here is generated. Measures of diagnostic accuracy are determined according to the formulas outlined in Table 7-3.

normal are false-negatives (FNs), and those incorrectly classified as abnormal are false-positives (FPs). As seen in Figure 7-3, where for ease of illustration a single cutoff is used to discriminate disease from normal populations, varying the cutoff changes the numbers of true and false results in a given population. False results are produced when an analyte has two relevant cutoffs (e.g., thyroid-stimulating hormone), with overlapping populations at both the low end and the high end.

Sensitivity and Specificity

Sensitivity and specificity are measures of the diagnostic accuracy of a test; they are indicators of a test's ability to distinguish between disease and absence of disease at a chosen cutoff. Sensitivity and specificity therefore are not fixed characteristics of a test and must be calculated from a different 2 × 2 table for each cutoff chosen.

Sensitivity is the ability of a test to detect disease and is expressed as the proportion of persons with disease in whom the test is positive (see Tables 7-3 and 7-4). It may also be thought of as the probability of a positive test given a true disease state as defined by the gold standard. A test that is 90% sensitive will give positive results in 90% of diseased patients (TP) and negative results in 10% of diseased patients (FN). Specificity is the ability to detect the absence of disease and is expressed as the proportion of persons without disease in whom the test is negative (see Tables 7-3 and 7-4). It may be thought of as the probability of a negative test, given no disease as defined by the gold standard. Thus a test that is 90% specific will give negative results in 90% of patients without disease (TN) and positive results in 10% of patients without disease (FP). A test with a higher sensitivity identifies a greater proportion of persons with disease, and a test with a higher specificity excludes a greater proportion of persons without disease.

Sensitivity is also the TP rate, and the inverse (1 – sensitivity) is the FN rate. If the sensitivity is 95%, 5 of 100 individuals with the disease will test negative. Specificity is the TN rate, and the inverse (1 – specificity) is the FP rate. If the specificity is 95%, 5 of 100 individuals without disease will test positive.

Effect of Altering the Test Cutoff

When a test cutoff is altered, an inverse relationship between sensitivity and specificity is noted, and a trade-off between the numbers of FP and FN results can be seen. Altering a cutoff changes a test's sensitivity and specificity because it relates to overlapping normal and abnormal patient distributions along the test value continuum (see Fig. 7-3). For tests where high values indicate disease, lowering the cutoff (i.e., moving the cutoff line to the left) will lead to more diseased patients being classified as abnormal. Thus, in Figure 7-3, changing the cutoff from C to B increases sensitivity. If the cutoff is moved to A, then all diseased persons will have a positive test, and the sensitivity will be 100%. However, increased sensitivity is associated with decreased specificity, and the number of nondiseased persons with a positive test (FPs) increases as the cutoff is moved from C to B to A. If the cutoff is raised (i.e., the cutoff line is moved to the right), more nondiseased patients are classified correctly, and specificity increases. If the cutoff is moved to E, then all nondiseased persons will have a negative test, and the specificity will be 100%. However, this will be accompanied by concomitant decreased sensitivity and additional FN results.

The Need for High Sensitivity Versus High Specificity

FP and FN results can lead to misdiagnosis and inappropriate clinical management with adverse clinical and financial consequences. For example, a FP result may cause the unnecessary admission of a patient, needless additional testing, and invasive procedures. Similarly, a FN result may lead to a patient's release from the emergency department despite a life-threatening disorder. Enhanced assays that provide improved sensitivity and specificity and thereby allow better discrimination between diseased and nondiseased populations continue to be developed. However, it is nearly impossible to eliminate false results entirely because some overlap between diseased and nondiseased persons is always evident. In most situations, the cost of a FP or a FN result supersedes the other, and the cutoff that delineates normal from abnormal can be shifted to reduce the more significant of the two consequences.

In general, the sensitivity of a test used to screen a population for a serious disease should be high to capture the majority of cases for confirmation by a gold standard. When PSA is used to screen for prostate cancer, a low threshold is used to capture all potential cases. Many men without a malignancy (e.g., prostatitis, nodular hyperplasia) will also have a positive result and need to undergo an invasive procedure for a definitive diagnosis. These "unnecessary" prostate biopsies, which are performed to confirm the true cases of prostate cancer, are the FP cost of this sensitive, but not specific, screening test. In contrast, high specificity is required when the definitive diagnosis of a serious condition will be based on a positive result; initiation of toxic or costly therapy can be based only on a test with the ability to "rule in" the disease with high confidence. A highly specific test excludes persons without disease (eliminates FPs). In a test where higher values indicate disease, specificity can be increased by increasing the cutoff, thereby excluding all persons without the disease; however, this will also exclude some persons with the disease (see Fig. 7-3).

Less expensive and less labor-intensive screening procedures with high sensitivity are often used in combination with more complex, highly specific tests for confirmation. For example, an enzyme-linked immunosorbent assay (ELISA) is used as an initial test to screen for human immunodeficiency virus (HIV) infection by detecting broadly reacting antibodies against HIV antigens. However, some noninfected individuals with cross-reactive antibodies might test positive (FPs) with the highly sensitive ELISA screen. These FP individuals can be identified with a highly specific follow-up test, usually a Western blot. In many combinations of screening and confirmatory tests, the confirmatory test is both highly specific and highly sensitive, but is inappropriate to use as a screening test because of cost or test complexity.

Predictive Value and Prevalence of Disease

The predictive value of a positive test (sometimes referred to as positive predictive value) may be understood as the probability that a positive test indicates disease. It is the proportion of persons with a positive test who truly have the disease (see Tables 7-3 and 7-4). The predictive value of a negative test (sometimes referred to as negative predictive value) is the probability that a negative test indicates absence of disease. It is the proportion of persons with a negative test who are truly without disease (see Tables 7-3 and 7-4).

TABLE 7-5

Positive Predictive Value Decreases With Decreasing Disease Prevalence

Result	Disease	No disease	Total
Positive	49	95	144
Negative	1	855	856
Total	50	950	1000

$$\text{Positive predictive value (\%)} = 100 \times \left(\frac{49}{49+95}\right) = 34\%$$

$$\text{Negative predictive value (\%)} = 100 \times \left(\frac{855}{855+1}\right) = 100\%$$

In this study, a population of 1000 hospitalized patients is studied. Fifty (50) patients are determined to have an acute myocardial infarction (AMI), and 950 patients do not have an AMI according to a "gold standard" (prevalence = 5%). If the cardiac marker described in Table 7-4 is performed on this population, we would expect a TP rate of 49 (50 AMI patients × sensitivity = 50 × 0.98) and a FN rate of 1 (FN = total AMI − TP = 49-1); a TN rate of 855 (950 non-AMI × specificity = 950 × 0.90) and an FP rate of 95 (total non-AMI − TN = 950 − 855). The positive predictive value of the test decreases with a lower prevalence.

FN, False-negative; *FP,* false-positive; *TN,* true-negative, *TP,* true-positive.

The diagnostic accuracy of a test tends to diminish as the test becomes more widely used in a population. Initial validation studies are often performed on a small group of individuals in whom disease is clearly absent or present. Those who lack the disease are often selected from a population of subjects in overall good health. In practice, however, patients exhibit a spectrum of illness, including early or mild disease, which overlaps with nondiseased individuals, including those with other diseases, some cases of which might cause an abnormal test result. Thus, the proportion of false test results is often higher in clinical practice than is claimed by the manufacturer from more limited studies in healthy individuals.

The predictive value of a positive test is highly dependent on the prevalence of the disease being tested. The higher the prevalence, or pretest probability, the higher the posttest probability, or predictive value of a positive test. Consider a test with a sensitivity of 90% and a specificity of 90% for a disease with a prevalence of 0.1%. Based on the formula, the predictive value of a positive result (PV+) would be 0.9%. If the prevalence increases to 5.0%, the PV+ increases to 32%. Thus the predictive value of a positive test increases as the prevalence increases. This effect of prevalence on predictive value is shown in Table 7-5. Predictive value theory quantifies a concept that is intuitively obvious—a positive result is more likely to truly reflect disease if it comes from a population of patients with a high prevalence of disease.

The impact of prevalence on predictive value theory has a practical application in that it enables one to derive a higher predictive value from results of a test performed in a high prevalence setting as compared with a low prevalence setting. For example, consider serum creatine kinase-MB (CK-MB) measurement for a patient in the emergency department. The predictive value of an abnormal CK-MB might be only 10%. On the other hand, if cardiac damage is strongly suspected, the patient might be transferred to the cardiac care unit (CCU), where, on repeat testing, an elevated serum CK-MB will have a much higher predictive value. In the restricted setting of a CCU, the prevalence of acute myocardial infarction is higher. We can also examine this situation from a pretest probability point of view. For the patient to be in the CCU (instead of still in the emergency department), the clinical suspicion of myocardial damage must be significantly higher. Because pretest probability determines posttest probability, the stronger pretest suspicion translates into stronger prediction of disease (see Bayes' theorem later).

For a disease with low prevalence, even a test with high sensitivity and specificity will yield a low predictive value because most positive test results will be FPs. For example, consider a disease with a prevalence of 1 in 10,000 and a test that is 99% sensitive and 99% specific. The PV+ will be only about 1% because 99 of every 100 who test positive have a FP result. One can see that the accuracy of tests for rare conditions must be very high to reliably predict disease. Thus, besides requiring near perfect sensitivity, tests that are used to screen for rare diseases have greater utility in selected populations that offer a higher pretest probability.

On the other hand, the predictive value of a negative test decreases as the prevalence of disease increases. However, the effect is small, especially when sensitivity and specificity are high. Prevalence influences the

TABLE 7-6

Predictive Value of a Positive Test: The Effect of Prevalence and Accuracy

	PREDICTIVE VALUE OF A POSITIVE TEST	
Prevalence, %	**Sensitivity, 90% Specificity, 90%**	**Sensitivity, 99% Specificity, 99%**
0.01	0.09	0.9
0.1	0.9	9
5	32.1	83.9
50	90.0	99

predictive value of a negative test to a noticeable extent only when the starting prevalence is high.

Predictive Value and Accuracy

Improved accuracy (i.e., sensitivity and specificity) enhances the predictive value of a test. The formula for predictive value (see Table 7-3) from Bayes' theorem shows that sensitivity and specificity influence the predictive value. Further, Table 7-6 shows that the predictive value of a positive test increases with increasing prevalence and improved accuracy. Specificity has the biggest impact on the predictive value of a positive test, whereas sensitivity determines the predictive value of a negative test. This is also appreciated from Table 7-5, where the number of FPs directly influences the predictive value of a positive test, whereas the numbers of FNs have the same effect on a negative test.

When a test cutoff changes, its accuracy (sensitivity/specficity) and predictive value also change. As an example, D-dimer testing is used to exclude deep vein thrombosis in patients who present to the emergency department. In the reference population, a value greater than 400 U/mL is considered abnormal and indicative of thrombosis. For a patient in the emergency department with symptoms suggestive of thrombosis, an even lower D-dimer value will predict thrombosis to the same extent as the >400 U/mL value does in the general population. (Recall that posttest probability is dependent on pretest probability.) Because a cutoff of 400 U/mL is not 100% sensitive, it excludes some patients with thrombosis, thereby yielding FNs. Because one cannot risk neglecting a possible case of thrombosis, a lower value of 200 U/mL could be selected to improve sensitivity, decrease the proportion of FNs, and greatly improve the predictive value of a negative test. A negative test could then be used to exclude thrombosis and obviate the need for additional costly diagnostic studies such as radiologic scans or lower extremity Doppler.

BAYES' THEOREM

Clinical assessment and diagnostic tests are inherently flawed, and these uncertainties must be considered when medical decisions are made. Sensitivity and specificity represent a summary of the diagnostic accuracy of a test, but they do not indicate the probability that an individual patient has a disease after the test result is obtained. It would be useful to know how the test result changes the probability of disease (i.e., posttest probability), given certain assay characteristics and disease prevalence (i.e., pretest probability). Alternatively, it is useful to know that a condition can be ruled out given a negative test if the probability of disease after a negative test is very low. To determine this information, one must consider predictive value theory, also known as Bayes' theorem. Bayes' theorem describes the relationship between posttest and pretest probability of disease or no disease based on the sensitivity and specificity of the test. $P(D)$ is the probability of disease before the test result is obtained; this is also known as clinical suspicion, prevalence, or pretest probability. $P(D|T)$ is the probability of the disease after the test result is known; this is the posttest probability. $P(D|T)$ is the probability that the test is positive when the disease is present, or the TP rate. $P(\bar{D})$ is the probability of not having the disease. $P(T|\bar{D})$ is the FP rate. The probability (posttest) of disease or no disease is calculated; examples are shown in Table 7-7.

$$P(D|T) = \frac{P(T|D) \times P(D)}{P(T|D) \times P(D) + P(T|\bar{D}) \times P(\bar{D})}$$

$$\textit{Posttest probability} = \frac{\textit{sensitivity} \times \textit{pretest probability}}{(\textit{sensitivity} \times \textit{pretest probability}) + (FP \times [1 - \textit{pretest probability}])}$$

TABLE 7-7
Posttest Probability (Predictive Value) from Bayes' Theorem

Posttest probability of disease (predictive value) depends on diagnostic accuracy and disease prevalence. A test for rheumatoid factor is positive in 95 of 100 patients with rheumatoid arthritis (RA) (sensitivity of 95%), but is also positive in 10 of 100 non-RA patients (specificity of 90%). The RA pretest probability (prevalence) is 5% in a rheumatology practice.

$$\textbf{Posttest probability} = \frac{sensitivity \times pretest\ probability}{(sensitivity \times pretest\ probability) + ([1 - specificity] \times [1 - pretest\ probability])}$$

$$\textbf{Posttest probability} = \frac{0.95 \times 0.05}{(0.95 \times 0.05) + (0.1 \times 0.95)} = 33\%$$

Posttest probability of no disease for the same test characteristics.

$$\textbf{Posttest probability} = \frac{(1 - pretest\ probability) \times specificity}{([1 - pretest\ probability] \times specificity) + ([1 - sensitivity] \times [1 - pretest\ probability])}$$

$$\textbf{Posttest probability} = \frac{0.95 \times 0.9}{(0.95 \times 0.9) + (0.05 \times 0.05)} = 99.7\%$$

TABLE 7-8
Likelihood Ratio (LR)

Definition:

$$\mathrm{LR} = \frac{\text{probability of test result in persons with disease}}{\text{probability of same result in persons with no disease}}$$

Example

$$LR+ = \frac{sensitivity}{1 - specificity}$$

From Table 7-7, using the test for rheumatoid factor (RF) that is positive in 95 of 100 rheumatoid arthritis (RA) patients (sensitivity of 95%) but also positive in 10 of 100 non-RA patients (specificity of 90%)

$$LR+ = \frac{\frac{95}{100}}{\frac{10}{100}} = 9.5$$

$$LR- = \frac{1 - sensitivity}{specificity}$$

The same test for RF is negative in 90 of 100 non-RA patients but is also negative in 5 of 100 RA patients.

$$LR- = \frac{\left(\frac{5}{100}\right)}{\left(\frac{90}{100}\right)} = 0.06$$

The theorem applies population data and test characteristics directly to an individual subject, and calculates the probability of the presence of a disease for a particular patient after a positive test result is obtained and, alternatively, the probability of the absence of disease given a negative test. Although sensitivity and specificity describe a test at a particular cutoff value (e.g., what percent of diseased patients have abnormal results?), the predictive value describes the state of the patient (e.g., how likely is it that a given patient's positive result indicates disease?). The predictive value depends on sensitivity, specificity, and prevalence of the disease being tested. Table 7-6 illustrates how disease prevalence, test accuracy, and predictive value of a test are interrelated (Bayes' theorem).

This approach requires information about the individual patient and clinical suspicion of disease, which includes prevalence of the disease in different populations, to establish the pretest probability of a patient having a disease. For example, **if nothing is known about a patient other than the test result,** then the pretest probability of disease would be the prevalence of the disease in the population. Clinical suspicion may raise this pretest probability to 50% based on a thorough clinical history and physical examination, the clinician's personal experience, and knowledge of relevant literature. Pretest probability, or a priori probability, is the prevalence of disease in the patient's clinical setting. For example, the prevalence of myocardial damage among subjects with chest pain is higher in the CCU than it is in the emergency department.

The pretest probability is used in conjunction with the characteristics of diagnostic accuracy as summarized in the sensitivity and specificity of the test. Posttest probability, or a posteriori probability, is the probability of disease in the posttest situation and is commonly referred to as the predictive value of the test. As described earlier, pretest probability and posttest probability are related through Bayes' theorem (Table 7-7). Additionally, posttest probability = posttest odds/(posttest odds + 1). The value of posttest odds is equal to the pretest probability × the likelihood ratio (LR). The LR is used to change the probability based on test characteristics, as described later.

LIKELIHOOD RATIO

The LR is a convenient measure that combines sensitivity and specificity into a single number (Table 7-8). Similar to these other measures of test accuracy (sensitivity and specificity), the LR is an assessment of test performance, and not of disease status, in the patient being tested. Two likelihood ratios are known: the likelihood ratio of a positive test (LR+) and the likelihood ratio of a negative test (LR–) (see Table 7-8). The LR+ is the ratio of two probabilities: the probability of a positive test result when disease is present (TP) divided by the probability of the same test result when disease is absent (FP). In other words, the calculation gives the likelihood that a test result will occur in a diseased patient as opposed to a healthy one. For example, serum lipase is used to detect acute pancreatitis; it may be elevated (higher than the cutoff of 200 U/L) in 90 of 100 individuals with acute pancreatitis, but it may be similarly elevated in 10 of 100 individuals with other causes of abdominal pain. The LR+ at the 200 U/L cutoff is 9, which means that an abnormal lipase is nine times more likely in individuals with pancreatitis than in those without, or nine times as many patients with pancreatitis than with other abdominal diseases will have an elevated lipase. The LR refers to the likelihood of the test result, given the disease. This is not the same as the likelihood of pancreatitis being nine times greater, given an abnormal lipase. The latter would be the predictive value of a positive lipase. Alternatively, the LR– is the probability that an individual with the disease will have a negative test divided by the probability that an individual without the disease will have a negative test. Additional advantages of the LR are that it is not influenced by disease prevalence, and the LR can be calculated for multiple test cutoffs. Thus, a result's degree of abnormality can be taken into account and medical decisions can be made at a point where fewer FN and FP results are seen.

The LR may also be used, along with pretest probability (prevalence), to calculate posttest probability (predictive value). Although the concept is similar to Bayes' theorem, LR is used to calculate posterior probabilities in terms of odds and not direct probabilities, making it less intuitive than Bayes' method. This is illustrated in the examples in Table 7-9. For a positive test, an LR+ >1 will increase the posttest probability. The larger the LR, the greater is the difference between pretest and posttest probabilities. Regardless of prevalence, a high LR increases the probability that a positive test result predicts disease. The converse applies for a negative test result, for which any LR– <1 will decrease the posttest probability. Thus, tests likely to be useful in clinical practice are those for which a positive result has a high LR and a negative result has a low LR.

FAGAN NOMOGRAM

Table 7-9 shows two examples of how to calculate posttest probability, which can be very cumbersome. The Fagan nomogram is a convenient graphic tool that uses a logarithmic scale to determine posttest probability, given the LR at a specified cutoff and the pretest probability (Fagan, 1975). The pretest probability (e.g., clinical suspicion, prevalence) is plotted on the y-axis on the left-hand side, the posttest probability on the right-hand side, and the LR between them (Fig. 7-4, *A*). When the Fagan nomogram is used, the pretest probability is located on the left axis, and a line is drawn from that point to the LR+ value. Then this line is further extended until it intersects the right axis at the posttest probability. Online calculators are available to establish these values with a graphic representation (Schwartz, 2002). The example in Figure 7-4, *B*, is taken from the data in Example 1 in Table 7-8. In this example, a line is drawn from the pretest probability of 5% to the LR for a positive rheumatoid factor test (LR+ = 9.5) at a particular cutoff. The line is then extended and crosses the right axis to give a posttest probability of approximately 30%, which

TABLE 7-9

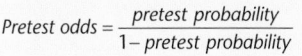

Likelihood Ratio (LR) and Probability of Disease

The LR and pretest probability (prevalence) can be used to calculate posttest probability (predictive value). This is best understood by expressing probability in terms of odds.

Definitions:

$\text{Pretest odds} = \dfrac{\text{pretest probability}}{1 - \text{pretest probability}}$	Step 1. Pretest probability is converted to pretest odds to calculate posttest odds of disease or no disease (see examples).
$\text{Posttest odds} = \text{pretest odds} \times LR$	Step 2. Posttest odds is calculated. Note: As LR of a positive or negative result increases, so do the odds that the result will predict disease or no disease, respectively.
$\text{Posttest probability} = \dfrac{\text{posttest odds}}{(1 + \text{posttest odds})}$	Step 3. Odds are converted back into probability to calculate the posttest probability (predictive value) of a positive or negative test.

Example 1

From Table 7-7, the rheumatoid arthritis pretest probability (prevalence) is 5% in a rheumatology practice. From Table 7-8, the LR of a positive rheumatoid factor test is 9.5. Note that the probability of disease increases from 5% (pretest) to 33% (posttest) because of the positive test result.

$$\text{Pretest odds} = \frac{\text{pretest probability}}{1 - \text{pretest probability}} = \frac{0.05}{1 - 0.05} = 0.053$$

$$\text{Posttest odds} = \text{pretest odds} \times LR+ = 0.053 \times 9.5 = 0.5$$

$$\text{Posttest probability} = \frac{\text{posttest odds}}{(1 + \text{posttest odds})} = \frac{0.5}{(1 + 0.5)} = 0.33 \text{ or } 33\%$$

Example 2

From Table 7-8, the LR of a negative rheumatoid factor test is 0.06. Although the probability of disease increases from 5% (pretest) to 33% (posttest) because of the positive test result (Example 1), the probability of disease decreases from 5% (pretest) to 0.3% (posttest) because of the negative test result.

$$\text{Pretest odds} = \frac{\text{pretest probability}}{1 - \text{pretest probability}} = \frac{0.05}{1 - 0.05} = 0.053$$

$$\text{Posttest odds} = \text{pretest odds} \times LR- = 0.053 \times 0.06 = 0.003$$

$$\text{Posttest probability} = \frac{\text{posttest odds}}{(1 + \text{posttest odds})} = \frac{.003}{1 + 0.003} = 0.3\%$$

is similar to the numeric calculation. In Example 2, the same pretest probability with a likelihood ratio of a negative rheumatoid factor test of 0.06 shows a posttest probability of approximately 0.3%, again similar to the manual calculation.

RECEIVER OPERATOR CHARACTERISTIC CURVES

Because diagnostic tests are not perfect, there is always a tradeoff between sensitivity and specificity, making it difficult to determine an optimal cutoff. The receiver operator characteristic (ROC) curve is a useful tool for identifying the optimal cutoff for a diagnostic test by calculating the sensitivity and specificity combinations across the entire range of cutoff values. In addition, the ROC curves of two or more tests can be compared to identify the one with the greatest discriminating ability (Zweig, 1993).

An ROC curve is constructed by calculating sensitivity and specificity across the entire range of cutoffs for the diagnostic test being evaluated. Sensitivity is plotted on the y-axis and 1− specificity (or the FP rate) on the x-axis; construction of the curve shows the tradeoff between sensitivity and specificity at each cutoff. The ROC curve for a test with no ability to

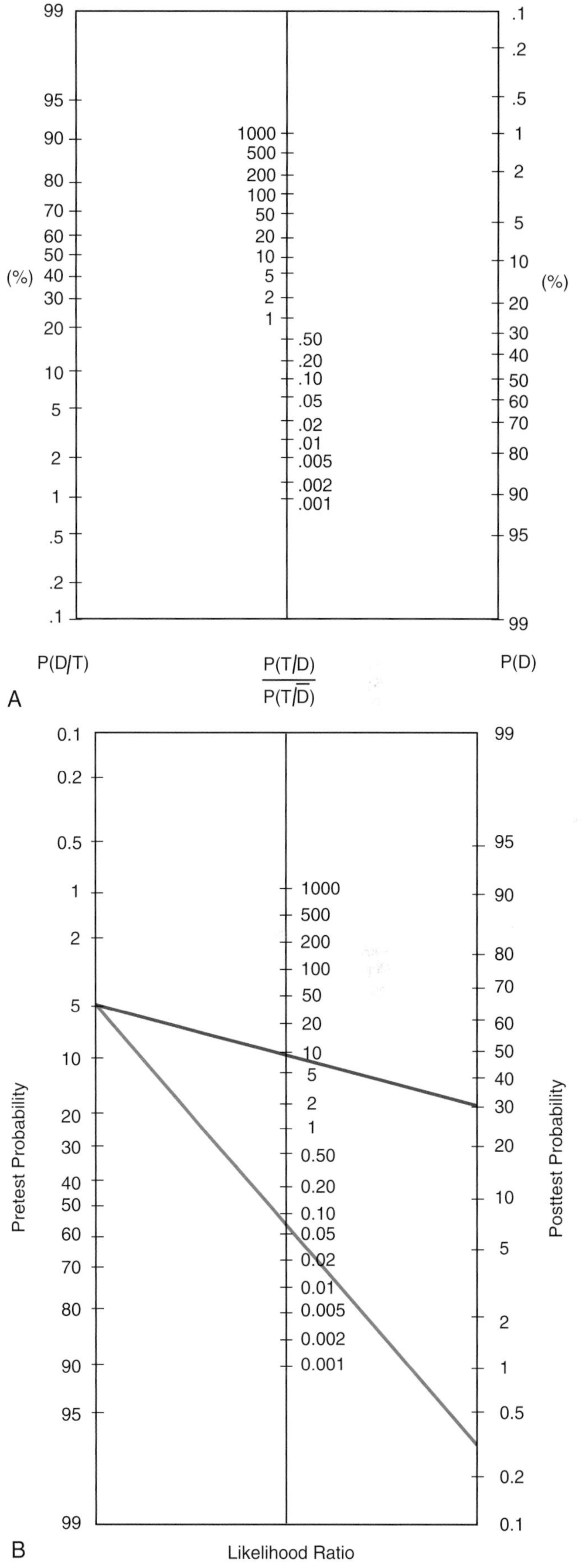

Figure 7-4 Fagan nomogram (see Table 7-9). (***A,*** *Modified from Fagan TJ. Letter. Nomogram for Bayes' theorem. N Engl J Med 1975;293(5):257.* ***B,*** *Modified from Schwartz A. Diagnostic test calculator, 2002. Available at:* http://araw.mede.uic.edu/cgi-bin/testcalc.pl.*)*

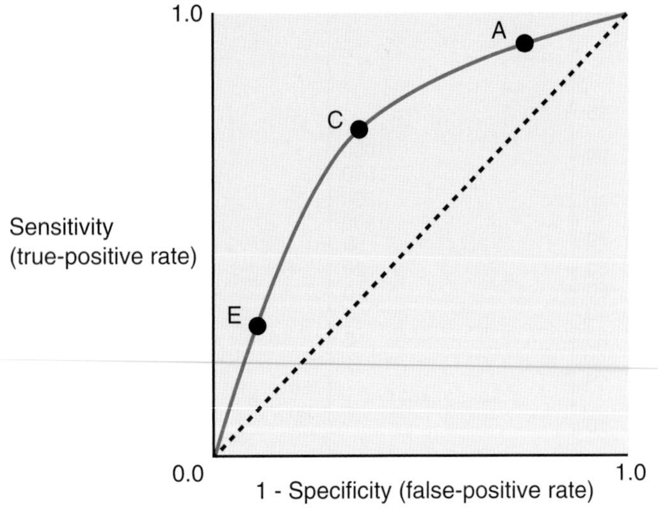

Figure 7-5 Receiver operator characteristics curve: effect of varying the cutoff value for separating disease from no disease (also see Fig. 7-3).

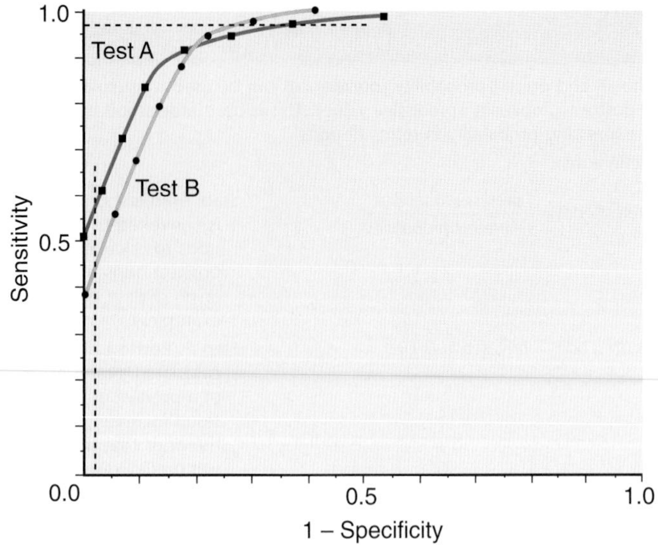

Figure 7-7 Receiver operator characteristic curves for two tests. Note that the curves cross. See text for interpretation.

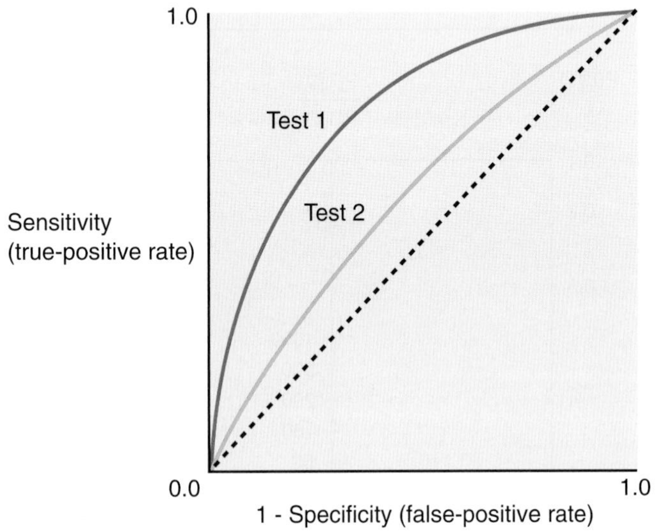

Figure 7-6 Receiver operator characteristic curves for two tests. Note that Test 1 is always superior to Test 2 because it has higher sensitivity than Test 2 (i.e., it is always above and to the left of Test 2).

predict disease (i.e., random chance) is a 45-degree line drawn through the origin. As the discriminatory ability of a test increases, the curve progresses outward toward the upper left-hand corner. The area under the ROC curve (AUC) is a single measure of the overall discriminating ability of a test; the minimum AUC is 0.5, which is the area under the 45-degree line, and the maximum AUC is 1.0 for a perfect diagnostic test. Because diagnostic tests are not absolutely perfect, the AUC will range from 0.5 to 1.0; the higher the AUC, the greater is the overall discriminating ability of the test. In general, an AUC that is greater than 0.8 suggests that the diagnostic test has good discriminatory power.

Point A on the ROC curve in Figure 7-5 has the highest sensitivity but has low specificity. Increasing the specificity to point B trades the higher specificity for lower sensitivity. The optimal cutoff is identified by the coordinate that maximizes discriminatory power, which, in this example, is point C. Point C is also the location on the ROC curve with the largest distance perpendicular from the 45-degree line. The second useful application for the ROC curve is to compare two or more diagnostic methods by calculating the area under the curve. If the area under the curve is similar, then no difference is observed between the two tests. However, if one ROC curve has a greater AUC than a comparison test, it has better sensitivity and specificity at all cutoffs. For example, in Figure 7-6, test 1 is better than test 2 at all cutoffs and therefore would be the better test. However, curves may cross, indicating that performance depends on the desired use of the test (i.e., whether a higher sensitivity or specificity is required for clinical use). In the example in Figure 7-7, test B has a lower FP rate than test A at high sensitivity, which makes it a better screening test; test A would be the better confirmatory test because it has greater sensitivity at high specificities.

POSITIVITY CRITERION

The LR may be used to select the optimal cutoff for an assay that best separates disease from nondisease. As was previously discussed, the LR, like sensitivity and specificity, varies with the cutoff. To select the optimal discriminatory cutoff, one might simply pick the cutoff resulting in the greatest LR for a positive test. However, this approach does not take into account the clinical impact of the test result. The clinical consequences of a FP test (e.g., unnecessary surgery) or a FN test (e.g., a missed chance to treat) need to be weighed when the optimal cutoff is determined. The *positivity criterion* is a method that allows one to assess the optimal cutoff with numeric estimates for clinical impact, or consequences, of test results.

In determining which cutoff will serve as the positivity criterion, a finite list of possible cutoffs is generated, and an LR for a positive test is calculated for each cutoff value. Next, the consequences of each of the four possible testing outcomes (TP, TN, FP, and FN) are assigned numeric estimates with respect to some outcome (e.g., morbidity, mortality, cost). For example, the clinical consequence of missing propionic acidemia on newborn screening by tandem mass spectroscopy is an increased risk of metabolic decompensation before diagnosis, with resultant developmental delay and long-term disability. One might estimate the consequence of this FN as 0.1; quality of life (QOL) lived in this state of misdiagnosis has 10% of the QOL lived without disease. It is important to note that the consequence of TP may not always be 100%, or equivalent to healthy life. Indeed, for propionic acidemia, even neonatal diagnosis may not completely alleviate the burden of disease. A possible estimate of the consequence of a TP on morbidity would be 80%. Similar estimates are determined for the remaining two outcomes. Values for the estimated consequences, as well as prevalence estimates of the disease, are then used in the equation that follows, where cTN, cFP, cTP, and cFN are the estimated consequences of each diagnostic category, and $P(D)$ is disease prevalence and $P(\bar{D})$ is 1-prevalance. The $LR_{threshold}$ is the optimal assay cutoff.

$$LR_{threshold} = \frac{P(\bar{D})}{P(D)} \times \frac{cTN - cFP}{cTP - cFN}$$

From the list of possible analyte concentrations, one can now select the cutoff that most closely approximates the $LR_{threshold}$. In this way, one may select a test cutoff that not only optimizes the discriminatory power of the assay, but also fits the clinical need that the test is meant to address.

TABLE 7-10
Positivity Criterion

Cutoff	% disease with this value or greater on assay	% without disease with this value or greater on assay	LR-positive test
R1—barely positive	5	30	0.17
R2—weakly positive	20	40	0.5
R3—intermediate positive	20	15	1.33
R4—strongly positive	25	10	2.50
R5—very strongly positive	30	5	6.00

The characteristics of a theoretical test for a disease with a prevalence of 10% are shown. Possible cutoff values for this assay ranging from a barely positive reading to a very strongly positive reading are denoted as R1 to R5, respectively. The percentage of patients with and without disease at or above each cutoff is also provided. The likelihood ratio (LR) for a positive test for R1–R5 is calculated from the information in the table (see explanation in text).

Consider a theoretical test for a disease shown in Table 7-10 with a prevalence (pretest probability) of 10%. R1–R5 represent possible assay cutoffs, where R1 represents a barely positive result and R5 a strong positive test result. Table 7-10 shows the percentage of diseased patients (defined by a gold standard) with a test result greater than the cutoffs defined as R1–R5. In addition, the percentage of patients without disease at each cutoff is shown. As the value for the cutoff increases from R1 to R5, the percentage of patients with disease increases. Using this information, an LR for a positive test can be calculated for each cutoff level.

Next we consider the consequences of an FN/FP and TP/TN result on the assay in terms of QOL. It is important to note that consequences can be estimated in terms of a variety of outcomes, including cost, excess mortality, or even cost-benefit, and each of these will result in a different positivity criterion. Assume that a missed diagnosis (FN) results in a QOL that is 70% that of a healthy person. Furthermore, assume that an FP result will lead to an unnecessary workup and anxiety, with a QOL that is 93% that of a healthy person. Finally, QOL for a TP living with a correctly diagnosed disease may be considered as 80% the QOL of a healthy person. Finally, a TN person experiences 95% the QOL as a fully healthy, untested person. Values for consequences are generally estimated from the literature or from expert opinion. By plugging the values for consequences into the above formula for $LR_{threshold}$, we obtain a value of 1.8. In other words, the assay is most efficient, in terms of maximized quality of life, at an LR+ of 1.8. From Table 7-10, the positivity criterion for this assay should be between R3 and R4, and closer to R3.

Evidence-Based Medicine

Historically, medical decisions have relied heavily on clinical experience, expert opinions, and other subjective or uncontrolled sources of information. This has also been true in laboratory medicine, where often an inadequate foundation of evidence is found to support existing practices (Price, 2000; Price, 2003). There may be no clear understanding of why a test is ordered, or what clinical question it is trying to answer. Alternatively, there may be no information on whether or how a test affects patient outcomes, such as morbidity, mortality, cost, patient satisfaction, risk, and discomfort (Bruns, 2001). For example, it is not clear whether point-of-care testing improves patient diagnosis and discharge in the emergency department (Price, 2003; Bruns, 2001; Kendall, 1998; Westgard, 2004; Trenti, 2003). Studies of clinical effectiveness in the clinical laboratory are hard to find because they are expensive and difficult to design (Price, 2000; McQueen, 2001). In addition, laboratory consultation is often based on the tradition of clinical and laboratory experience and less on a systematic approach to determining the current best evidence (Price, 2003). In contrast to traditional approaches, evidence-based medicine (EBM) is a process by which medical decisions can be made by using as many objective tools as possible. This, in turn, can help reduce the uncertainty of medical decision making. EBM is a systematic practice that integrates the most current and best evidence with clinical expertise and patient preferences when making medical decisions (Sackett, 2000). EBM places emphasis on critically analyzing information from the literature and developing knowledge for medical practice (Sackett, 1983; Elstein, 2004; Sackett, 1991; Ludmerer, 2004). EBM encourages the cultivation of continuous learning and sharing of medical knowledge at all levels of training from medical student to attending physician (Ludmerer, 2004). Since the time of its introduction, EBM has grown to become a key tool for all health care providers.

Practicing EBM consists of five steps (Price, 2000; Price, 2003; Sackett, 2000): (1) Ask a clinical question based on a patient encounter; (2) acquire information by searching resources; (3) analyze and critically evaluate the information, and reach a conclusion that answers the clinical question; (4) apply the information to individual patients; and (5) audit effectiveness and monitor the literature.

A clinical encounter of a patient with a health care provider generally results in a clinical question that necessitates one or more laboratory tests—whether for screening, diagnosis, prognosis, or monitoring of treatment. The question that is developed should be specific to a decision that must be made for that patient. The question compares an intervention such as ordering a diagnostic test versus accepted practice. The clinical question can be described in four parts and summarized with the acronym PICO (Sackett, 2000; Elstein, 2004): Problem (P): What is the problem of interest for the specific patient? Intervention (I): What intervention is being considered? Comparison (C): To what alternatives can the intervention be compared? Outcome (O): Is there a quantifiable clinical outcome that can be measured?

For example, a 55-year-old man, who recently returned from a trip to Europe, complains of swelling of the right leg, which upon examination is warm, red, and swollen. The clinical question can be summarized as follows: Problem: Is D-dimer a good "rule-out" test for deep vein thrombosis in a middle-aged man with a risk factor for thrombosis (such as lengthy travel)? Intervention: D-dimer test. Comparison: Venous ultrasound or venography as the reference method. Outcome: Predictive value of D-dimer in "ruling out" deep vein thrombosis.

A second example might be the following: A 58-year-old man with atrial fibrillation arrives in the emergency department with gastrointestinal bleeding due to a warfarin overdose. Problem: Is vitamin K effective in correcting coagulopathy caused by a warfarin overdose? Intervention: Vitamin K administration. Comparison: Fresh frozen plasma may be the alternative treatment. Outcome: Correction of bleeding and prothrombin time.

The strategy for answering these questions must be determined before searching the resources to prevent the introduction of selection bias. Information sources include textbooks, journals, electronic textbooks, and summary journals. Textbooks may provide an introduction to the pathophysiology of the disease, but they do not contain the current best evidence. Journal articles provide more up-to-date information than textbooks, but they too are outdated by the time the articles have been written, accepted, and published. Randomized clinical controlled trials (RCTs) that are double-blinded are the most valuable of the journal articles because they are the least biased. However, RCTs are highly dependent on the methods employed in the blinding and treatment of subjects (Lijmer, 1999).

Secondary articles and meta-analyses (a statistical technique to integrate results from multiple studies) summarize the best current evidence and provide practice guidelines. The Centre for Evidence-Based Medicine (http://www.cebm.net), the Cochrane Collaboration/Cochrane Library (http://www.cochrane.org), Up-to-Date (http://www.uptodate.com/), and Best Clinical Evidence (Godlee, 2004) are sources that present summarized information. The Evidence-Based Medicine (ebm.bmjjournals.com) series of journals are also an excellent resource for up-to-date summaries. Although convenient, a summary article should be evaluated with caution because an "expert" may introduce bias regarding which studies are assessed and the value applied to particular articles. Medical decision-making tools help the reader to critically analyze each step in the process and have been summarized (Guyatt, 2000).

SELECTED REFERENCES

Alpert JS, Thygesen K, Antman E, Bassand JP. Myocardial infarction redefined—a consensus document of The Joint European Society of Cardiology/American College of Cardiology Committee for the redefinition of myocardial infarction. J Am Coll Cardiol 2000;36(3):959–69.

Briggs CHP, Grant D, Staves J, Chavada N, Machin SJ. Performance evaluation of the Sysmex XE-2100TM, automated haematology analyser. Sysmex Journal International 1999;9:113–19.

Clinical and Laboratory Standards Institute (CLSI). Defining, establishing, and verifying reference intervals in the clinical laboratory: approved guideline. 3rd ed. Wayne, Pa.: Clinical and Laboratory Standards Institute; 2008. p. 59.

Fagan TJ. Letter. Nomogram for Bayes theorem. N Engl J Med 1975;293(5):257.

Fossati P, Prencipe L. Serum triglycerides determined colorimetrically with an enzyme that produces hydrogen peroxide. Clin Chem 1982;28(10):2077–80.

Fujimoto K. Principles of measurement in hematology analyzers manufactured by Sysmex Corporation. Sysmex Journal International 1999;9:31–40.

Galen RS, Gambino SR. Beyond normality: the predictive value and efficiency of medical diagnoses. New York: John Wiley & Sons; 1975.

This book serves as an introduction to understanding the interpretation of a laboratory test. The basics of diagnostic test accuracy and the predictive value of tests are well outlined.

Grundy SM, Cleeman JI, Merz CN, et al. Implications of recent clinical trials for the National Cholesterol Education Program Adult Treatment Panel III guidelines. Circulation 2004;110(2):227–39.

Kazmierczak SC. Laboratory quality control: using patient data to assess analytical performance. Clin Chem Lab Med 2003;41(5):617–27.

Kroll MH, Elin RJ. Interference with clinical laboratory analyses. Clin Chem 1994;40(11 Pt 1):1996–2005.

McQueen MJ. Overview of evidence-based medicine: challenges for evidence-based laboratory medicine. Clin Chem 2001;47(8):1536–46.

General overview of the practice of EBM as it relates to the laboratory, including examples and useful resources.

Ruzicka K, Veitl M, Thalhammer-Scherrer R, Schwarzinger I. The new hematology analyzer Sysmex XE-2100: performance evaluation of a novel white blood cell differential technology. Arch Pathol Lab Med 2001;125(3):391–6.

Sackett DL, Straus SE, Richardson WS, Rosenberg W, Haynes RB. Evidence-based medicine: how to practice and teach EBM. 2nd ed. London: Churchill Livingstone; 2000.

Comprehensive, easy-to-read primer on all facets of EBM that includes many examples.

Schwartz A. Diagnostic test calculator, 2002. Available at: http://araw.mede.uic.edu/cgi-bin/testcalc.pl.

Thalhammer-Scherrer R, Knobl P, Korninger L, Schwarzinger I. Automated five-part white blood cell differential counts: efficiency of software-generated white blood cell suspect flags of the hematology analyzers Sysmex SE-9000, Sysmex NE-8000, and Coulter STKS. Arch Pathol Lab Med 1997;121(6):573–7.

Vermeer HJ, Thomassen E, de Jonge N. Automated processing of serum indices used for interference detection by the laboratory information system. Clin Chem 2005;51(1):244–7.

Zweig MH, Campbell G. Receiver-operating characteristic (ROC) plots: a fundamental evaluation tool in clinical medicine. Clin Chem 1993;39(4):561–77.

An in-depth article on the concept, use, and application of ROC curves in clinical testing. A comparison with other measures of test accuracy is part of the discussion.

REFERENCES

Access the complete reference list online at http://www.expertconsult.com

CHAPTER 8

INTERPRETING LABORATORY RESULTS

Matthew R. Pincus, Naif Z. Abraham Jr.

KEY POINTS

- Accurate differential diagnoses can be made from a systematic study of the laboratory profiles of patients in a large majority of cases.
- Four basic types of anemia are known: Iron deficiency, anemia of chronic disease, hemolytic anemia, and macrocytic/nutritionally deficient anemia. These can be readily distinguished from one another by the hematologic profile and by simple laboratory testing.
- By examining the urinary sodium, potassium, and osmolarity, the causes of hyponatremia and hypernatremia can be readily determined.
- Liver function tests can distinguish among six different diseases of the liver: Hepatitis, cirrhosis, biliary disease, space-occupying lesions of the liver, passive congestion, and fulminant hepatic failure.
- Renal failure can be readily diagnosed by observing elevated blood urea nitrogen and creatinine; it is possible to pinpoint the site of renal failure (i.e., glomerular or tubular) from the ratio of serum to urine osmolality.
- Blood gas determinations allow determination of the causes of metabolic versus respiratory acidosis or alkalosis; a critical relationship exists between the partial pressure of oxygen and of carbon dioxide, such that in respiratory diseases, high levels of carbon dioxide block oxygenation of venous blood, leading to respiratory crisis.
- Elevation of cardiac troponin in serum, in the proper clinical context, is diagnostic of myocardial infarction.
- Elevations of serum C-reactive protein indicate inflammatory disease.
- Elevations of serum amylase and lipase point to acute pancreatitis.
- Two types of endocrine disease are discussed: Thyroid and adrenal. Serum levels of T_4 (or, better, free T_4) and thyroid-stimulating hormone can be used to diagnose primary or secondary hypothyroidism or hyperthyroidism; serum levels of cortisol and adrenocorticotropic hormone can be used to diagnose primary or secondary hypoadrenalism or hyperadrenalism.

INTERPRETING AND CORRELATING ABNORMAL LABORATORY VALUES

GENERAL CONSIDERATIONS

The major purpose of performing analyte determinations in the clinical laboratory is to aid in the diagnosis and management of disease and in health assessment. In this regard, the clinical pathologist is often called upon as a consultant to explain abnormal laboratory values, especially those that do not seem to correlate with one another, and to recommend or even to order laboratory tests that may lead to the correct diagnosis in the workup of patients for particular medical problems. In addition, evaluation of laboratory test results on individual patients by the clinical pathologist not only can reveal the (infrequent) occurrence of laboratory errors, but can help in the selection of appropriate, cost-effective tests from a wide variety of increasingly complex test choices (Witte, 1997; Dighe, 2001; Bonini, 2002).

For evaluation of test results, the laboratory computer is an invaluable aid. Virtually all such systems perform daily checks for patient values that lie significantly outside of their established reference intervals, or that have undergone large changes over a 24-hour period. These are often reported as "failed delta checks." Thus patients with significant laboratory findings can be identified.

This chapter presents an approach to interpretation of laboratory values that will enable laboratorians to aid in the establishment of clinical diagnoses and to assist in clinical management. This discussion is by no means comprehensive and cannot possibly cover every conceivable illness afflicting patients. Rather, this presentation is concerned with general approaches to interpreting abnormal values and discussion of the most common causes of such findings, so that the reader has a framework for interpreting abnormal values.

The reader may prefer to complete the Clinical Chemistry (Part 2) and Hematology, Coagulation, and Transfusion Medicine (Part 4) sections of this book before reading this section, which gives an overview of both of these vital diagnostic areas. Alternatively, the reader may decide to read this chapter to obtain the overview first before reading the chapters on chemistry and hematology.

FUNDAMENTAL PRINCIPLES IN INTERPRETATION OF VALUES

Before embarking on a discussion of specific conditions giving rise to abnormal values, certain precepts should always be followed, encapsulated as follows:

1. Never rely on a single out-of-reference range value to make a diagnosis. It is vital to establish a trend in values. A single sodium value of 130 mEq/L, for example, does not necessarily indicate hyponatremia. This single abnormal value may be spurious and may reflect such factors as improper phlebotomy technique, laboratory variability, etc. Rather, a series of low sodium values in successive serum samples from a given patient does indicate this condition. Thus it is vital to follow trends in particular values.
2. Osler's rule. Especially if the patient is younger than 60 years of age, try to attribute all abnormal laboratory findings to a single cause. Only if there is no possible way to correlate all abnormal findings should the possibility of multiple diagnoses be entertained.

ABNORMALITIES IN THE HEMATOLOGY PROFILE

Often in laboratory reports, the first section contains the hematology profile, including the CBC, or complete blood count. Comprehensive discussions of clinical hematopathology are given in Part 4. Here, we discuss very basic patterns of abnormalities to provide an overall frame of reference for interpreting values and for ordering further examinations. Although this part of the book is concerned with clinical chemistry or chemical pathology, we discuss the hematology profile because the interpretation of hematopathologic results often depends on the results of quantitative determinations performed in clinical chemistry.

ANEMIAS

Anemia, a common hematologic disorder, is defined pathophysiologically as a decrease in the oxygen-carrying capacity of the blood. All oxygen-carrying capacity of the blood is due to the binding of oxygen to hemoglobin (Hb) contained uniquely in red blood cells (RBCs). Because anemia can cause tissue hypoxia, it often produces such symptoms as fainting, fatigue, pallor, and difficulty in breathing.

Practically, the best indicator for this condition is a low RBC count or number of RBCs per volume of whole blood. Although the reference range for the red cell count varies with age, sex, and population, it encompasses values from around 4–6 × 10^6 RBCs per cubic millimeter (cu mm) or microliter. This range may change somewhat depending on the population. RBC counts below the lower limit of the reference range suggest the presence of anemia. In addition, RBCs occupy a well-defined range in terms of the percent of the volume of whole blood that they occupy, or the hematocrit (Hct). Generally, normal adult Hct values range from about 36%–45% (normal values for females are generally slightly lower than those for males). In addition, the concentration of Hb in whole blood is about 12–15 g/dL or approximately 33–36 g/dL in RBCs (i.e., the mean corpuscular Hb concentration). Normal values are also dependent on patient age and altitude of residence. Normally, the Hct is about three times the value of the Hb concentration, which, in turn, is about three times the value of the RBC count.

If anemia has been diagnosed, it is mandatory to determine the cause of the anemia. An excellent history and physical examination is required for appropriate test selection and diagnosis, and the best possible patient care and treatment. In addition, a review of the peripheral blood film with respect to red and white cell morphology is often helpful.

To narrow further the differential diagnosis and facilitate appropriate test selection, a number of classification schemes for anemia have been developed, with no single ideal scheme available. A particularly useful approach utilizes the common red cell indices of mean corpuscular volume (MCV), measured in femtoliters (fL), or 1 × 10^{-15} L, in conjunction with the red cell distribution width (RDW) and the reticulocyte count (percent reticulocytosis), or reticulocyte production index (RPI). A further aid in diagnosis is the chromicity of the red cells (i.e., the intensity of the red color of the cells due to intracellular Hb). The chromicity is measured quantitatively by the mean corpuscular hemoglobin concentration, or MCHC. Taken together, these indices help to form a working hypothesis for the underlying cause of the anemia.

Electronic determination of MCV directly from red cell distribution data allows for classification on the basis of RBC size as macrocytic (MCV generally >100 fL), microcytic (MCV generally <80 fL), or normocytic (MCV generally between 80 and 100 fL). The sizes (volumes) of red cells vary within a certain range in which the number of cells of particular volumes form a bell-shaped or Gaussian distribution (see Chapter 9); the standard deviation of the cell volumes divided by the mean cell volume gives the RDW, measured as a percent. As it happens, the RDW is a parameter that helps to further classify an anemia because it reflects the variation in RBC size. RDW generally varies between about 12 and 17, and is dependent on the patient's age, sex, and ethnic subgroup. It can be helpful in differentiating causes of microcytosis in that moderate to severe iron deficiency anemia (IDA) is associated with an increased RDW, while thalassemia and anemia of chronic disease (ACD) are associated with a normal RDW.

Peripheral blood reticulocytosis is a measure of bone marrow response in the face of anemia. A similar measure, RPI, corrects the reticulocyte count with respect to (1) the proportion of reticulocytes present in a patient without anemia, and (2) the premature release of reticulocytes into the peripheral circulation. Bone marrow response to anemia may be appropriate (hyperproliferative) with an RPI >3, generally indicating marrow red cell hyperproliferation; however, the anemia may be due to defective RBC production or marrow failure (hypoproliferative), which is generally indicated by an RPI <2. Thus, although these red cell indices are not pathognomonic of the cause of a particular type of anemia, the combination of MCV, RDW, and RPI examined together often will significantly narrow the differential diagnosis and facilitate further test selection. Table 8-1 illustrates common examples of anemia and their diagnostic workup using these red cell indices, as well as other helpful analytic abnormalities.

Microcytic Anemia

Common microcytic anemias include IDA and the thalassemias. Some hemoglobinopathies and ACD may also be microcytic. In our discussion, we will focus on IDA and ACD, a common differential diagnosis for patients with microcytic anemia. Both anemias appear to be disorders involving iron metabolism.

In IDA, there is a primary deficiency of iron available to the red cell (usually resulting from blood loss, but other causes include dietary deficiency, malabsorption, and pregnancy); chronic blood loss should always lead to further investigation because it is commonly associated with malignancy. ACD, however, appears to be due to defective iron utilization/metabolism and is associated with chronic nonhematologic disorders such as chronic infections, connective tissue disorders, malignancy, and renal, thyroid, and pituitary disorders. Because iron levels in red cells are low, Hb levels are also low in both of these conditions. Thus the MCHC

TABLE 8-1
Common Types of Anemia and Their Diagnostic Workups*

Anemia	Cause	Common analyte abnormality
1. Hypoproliferative, microcytic	Iron deficiency	Low ferritin Increased IBC Decreased serum iron Reduced Fe/IBC ratio Generally increased RDW
2. Hypoproliferative, microcytic	Anemia of chronic disease	Generally high ferritin Normal IBC Decreased serum iron Normal Fe/IBC ratio Generally normal RDW
3. Hyperproliferative, normocytic	Hemolytic anemia	Schistocytosis Increased reticulocytes Low haptoglobin Elevated carboxyhemoglobin Elevated LD Elevated indirect bilirubin Generally increased RDW
4. Hypoproliferative, normocytic	Aplastic anemia	Leukopenia Thrombocytopenia Hypocellular bone marrow Generally normal RDW
5. Hypoproliferative, normocytic	Renal failure	Elevated BUN and creatinine Low erythropoietin Burr cells may be present Generally normal RDW
6. Hypoproliferative, macrocytic		
A. Megaloblastic	B_{12} and/or folate deficiency	Low B_{12} and/or folate Hyperlobulated polymorphonuclear leukocytes Macroovalocytes Increased RDW
B. Nonmegaloblastic	Hypothyroidism	Elevated TSH Normal RDW

BUN, Blood urea nitrogen; *Fe,* iron; *IBC,* iron-binding capacity; *LD,* lactate dehydrogenase; *RDW,* red cell distribution width; *T_4,* thyroxine; *TSH,* thyroid-stimulating hormone.
*In this table, low is equivalent to depressed, and high is equivalent to elevated. Ferritin, haptoglobin, LD, bilirubin, BUN, creatinine, erythropoietin, TSH, and T_4 are all expressed as concentrations. All of these analytes are measured in serum.

mentioned earlier tends to be low, giving rise to what is termed a hypochromic (low red color in red cells or low MCHC), microcytic (low MCV) anemia.

To distinguish between IDA and ACD, a number of different laboratory measurements are very useful, in addition to the RDW. The diagnosis is typically made using additional serum or whole blood laboratory tests. However, because IDA is always accompanied by loss of iron that is stored bound to the protein ferritin in bone marrow macrophages, the diagnosis can always in principle be made with a bone marrow biopsy with an iron stain (e.g., nitroprusside) that shows the absence of marrow iron. This procedure is, of course, invasive and should be performed only as a last resort.

Serum Ferritin Levels

Normally, there is an equilibrium between intracellular and extracellular ferritin. The lower the stored iron becomes, the lower is the intracellular ferritin, and, consequently, the lower the extracellular ferritin becomes. The level of extracellular ferritin can be directly measured by determining the serum ferritin level, which is readily and accurately assessed on serum aliquots, using enzyme-linked immunosorbent assay (ELISA) techniques, as described in Chapter 44. Overall, therefore, serum ferritin levels give an excellent measure of available iron stores, noninvasively. Because iron stores in ACD are abundant, serum ferritin levels are characteristically normal to elevated. In contrast, in IDA, in which iron stores become depleted, serum ferritin levels are characteristically decreased. Thus serum ferritin level is one assay that can be used in differentiating IDA from ACD.

One caveat in using serum ferritin values to provide this distinction is the fact that ferritin also happens to be an acute phase reactant. Acute phase reactants are proteins (discussed in Chapter 19) that rise in response to an acute process, usually an acute inflammatory condition. So, if a patient has an acute infection, the serum ferritin level may be spuriously elevated. The net effect may be a ferritin in the reference interval. Usually, in IDA, accompanied by an acute process, this level is in the low reference range.

Use of Serum Iron and Iron-Binding Capacity

In addition to ferritin levels, serum iron and serum iron-binding capacity (IBC) can be measured. On average, serum iron is, of course, reduced in IDA and normal or sometimes low in ACD. The IBC is a direct measure of the protein transferrin, which transports iron from the gut to iron storage sites in bone marrow. In IDA, the serum iron is reduced, and the IBC is increased.

However, both serum iron and transferrin are subject to wide fluctuations because of such factors as diet and do not always reliably reflect iron stores. Also, transferrin is a β-protein (i.e., it migrates in the β-region in serum protein electrophoresis) and is an acute phase reactant (i.e., its serum levels change) (they usually decrease, as a so-called "negative acute phase reactant") in inflammatory conditions. Considerable overlap has been noted between serum levels of iron and iron-binding capacity in IDA and ACD. A somewhat more reliable discriminating measure of IDA is the ratio of serum iron to IBC, known as the transferrin saturation. This ratio is around 1 : 3 for normal individuals, and in IDA it is significantly reduced to values of around 1 : 5 or lower. Again, considerable overlap is seen even in this ratio for patients with IDA and ACD, so the values should always be interpreted with care.

Use of Red Blood Cell Distribution Width

Finally, use of automated procedures for determination of cell counts and indices enables us to obtain average erythrocyte sizes and size distributions. In IDA, a marked dispersion in cell volumes (sizes) occurs, so that the RDW increases, whereas it generally remains within normal limits in ACD. Normal RDWs occur in the range of 12%–17%. Unfortunately, standard deviations for normal individuals and for patients with IDA or ACD can overlap significantly, tending to limit the validity of using the RDW exclusively for distinguishing between these conditions.

The major laboratory findings that distinguish IDA from ACD are summarized as entries 1 and 2 in Table 8-1. Note that most of the major tests used to distinguish these two conditions are performed in the clinical chemistry laboratory. This emphasizes the strong interdependence of both of these services in obtaining definitive diagnoses through laboratory measurements.

Normocytic Anemia

In these anemias, the red cells show normal MCVs and MCHCs (i.e., they are normocytic and normochromic). Common causes of normocytic anemia include acute hemorrhage, hemolytic anemia, marrow hypoplasia, renal disease, and ACD. It may seem paradoxical that acute hemorrhage presents as normocytic anemia because it involves major blood loss that is associated with loss of iron stores. However, iron depletion requires time to develop; acutely, major blood loss presents as normocytic anemia.

Hyperproliferative Normocytic Anemias

Hyperproliferative normocytic anemias, associated with an increased reticulocyte count, include both hemolytic anemia and the anemia associated with acute blood loss; hypoproliferative anemias, associated with a decreased reticulocyte count, include such causes as bone marrow aplasia/hypoplasia, renal disease, and ACD. As mentioned earlier, a history and physical, as well as examination of the patient's peripheral blood film, are helpful in establishing a differential diagnosis. In this section, we will focus on the most common causes of normocytic anemia: Hemolytic anemia, aplastic anemia, and the anemia associated with renal disease.

Hemolytic Anemia. Hemolysis is defined as destruction of the red cell membrane, causing Hb release. This may occur slowly as a normal physiologic process or may be accelerated in pathologic states. Many different underlying causes are known for the decrease in survival/increase in destruction of RBCs. These include membrane defects (e.g., hereditary spherocytosis), enzyme defects (e.g., glucose-6-phosphate dehydrogenase [G6PD] deficiency), hemoglobinopathies (e.g., sickle cell disease or β-thalassemia), immune destruction (e.g., autoimmune hemolytic anemia or hemolytic transfusion reaction), and nonimmune destruction. The latter includes destruction due to infectious agents, toxic agents/drugs, physical agents, or hypersplenism, and those classified as microangiopathic hemolytic anemias—a group of anemias due to mechanical destruction of RBCs mainly in bone marrow where they are synthesized, caused by such factors as fibrin deposition within the blood vessels of the bone marrow microvasculature, fibrosis, or malignancies, including leukemia, lymphoma, and metastatic cancer. In addition, mechanical destruction can result from extramedullary causes such as prosthetic heart valves.

Hemolytic anemia can be recognized from Hb in plasma/serum and breakdown products of heme. Specific laboratory measurements that readily confirm the diagnosis of hemolytic anemia are based on the natural events that occur subsequent to hemolysis. After erythrocyte membrane breakdown, Hb is extruded. Thus plasma and urine may contain free Hb or its degradation products. Free Hb may be present acutely in the plasma (hemoglobinemia) or urine (hemoglobinuria), and hemosiderin may be present in the urine (hemosiderinuria) in more chronic episodes of hemolysis. Extruded Hb becomes bound to the α-2 fraction protein haptoglobin. The Hb–haptoglobin complex becomes catabolized by macrophages that engulf these complexes by receptor-mediated endocytosis. Thus an excellent laboratory test for hemolytic anemia is a *low haptoglobin value.* Extremely sensitive and rapid ELISA assays for haptoglobin are available for this purpose.

Because the red cell contents are extruded into the plasma, other indicators of red cell damage, besides Hb, are known: High serum potassium, because intracellular potassium concentration is much higher in red cells than in the extracellular fluid, and serum elevations of the enzyme lactate dehydrogenase (LD). As discussed in Chapters 18 and 20, there are five major isozymes of this enzyme, labeled LD1 through LD5. Peculiarly, the predominant isozyme of LD in red cells is LD1, which occurs predominantly in cardiac tissue.

Carbon monoxide (CO) and unconjugated bilirubin become elevated in blood in hemolytic anemia. When Hb is extruded, large amounts of it become oxidized to methemoglobin. The heme portion dissociates and then becomes oxidized ultimately to bilirubin. The first step in this process is the oxidative opening of the porphyrin ring of heme with attendant liberation of CO. CO may be measured easily by gas chromatographic techniques or even more conveniently by cooximetry, based on spectrophotometry (see Chapter 4), as carboxyhemoglobin (see Chapter 34). Elevated CO levels in normochromic, normocytic anemias are an excellent indicator of hemolytic anemia.

Because production of bilirubin, which is unconjugated, is increased (Chapter 21), at least a transient elevation of serum indirect bilirubin occurs. This elevation, in the presence of normal liver function, will be modest, usually in the range of about 2–2.5 mg/dL. (The upper limit of normal is around 1.2 mg/dL.)

Hemolytic anemia is almost always accompanied by an increased reticulocyte count and by evidence of red cell damage. As mentioned earlier, the reticulocyte count will be elevated (increase in polychromasia on the blood film), with erythroid hyperplasia present in the bone marrow, indicative of increased red cell production. In addition, the peripheral blood film may show evidence of the particular type of red cell damage associated with the particular type of hemolytic anemia (e.g., sickle cells in sickle cell disease, schistocytes/helmet cells in microangiopathic hemolytic anemia). A noticeable difference in red cell size (anisocytosis) and shape (poikilocytosis) is caused by the presence of damaged and/or young cells. Because of the often-marked changes in size and/or shape, the RDW is usually elevated. A number of nucleated RBCs may also be identified.

Other findings in hemolytic anemia can identify the cause. A direct antiglobulin test/direct Coombs' test can be used to detect immunoglobulin attached to the red cell surface that identifies immune hemolytic anemia as the cause of red cell destruction. A positive test suggests that an autoantibody or alloantibody may be responsible for the anemia. A positive G6PD screening test for G6PD deficiency will identify this enzyme deficiency as the cause of the hemolytic anemia. Selection of these tests will be dependent on the clinical evaluation and on the preliminary laboratory data.

Laboratory findings that are diagnostic of hemolytic anemia are summarized in entry 3 of Table 8-1. Note that virtually all of the quantitative diagnostic tests for hemolytic anemia (i.e., serum and urine Hb, haptoglobin, carboxyhemoglobin, indirect bilirubin, and LD) are performed in the clinical chemistry laboratory, again emphasizing the strong interdependence of the clinical chemistry and hematology laboratories.

Microangiopathic Hemolytic Anemia. As previously mentioned, red cell fragments (schistocytes) may be present on peripheral blood films as the result of mechanical (prosthetic heart valve) or thermal (severe burns) destruction. Mechanical rupture of red cells within the microvasculature may also occur by physical damage to red cells in the microvasculature of bone marrow. This may be due to space-occupying lesions, such as metastatic tumors or leukemia or lymphoma, to myelofibrosis, or to the intravascular deposition of fibrin strands upon endothelial cell surfaces. Because RBCs are damaged and destroyed, this process leads to so-called microangiopathic (i.e., lesions in the microvasculature) hemolytic anemia (MHA).

Besides space-occupying lesions, other causes of this type of anemia include disease states in which fibrin is deposited on endothelial surfaces, also resulting in shearing and fragmentation of newly synthesized red blood cells, as in disseminated intravascular coagulopathy (DIC), which is discussed later and in Chapter 38. In this condition, an abnormal activation of the coagulation process occurs, in which fibrin–platelet clots form intravascularly and embolize to virtually any tissue. These clots block the microvasculature of tissues, including that of bone marrow, resulting in the destruction of newly synthesized red cells. In addition, other disease states may give rise to MHA that may have an immunologic component (i.e., antibodies to determinants on endothelial cells or on other structures in the microvasculature), resulting in immune complex deposits with or without fibrin deposits. These states include thrombotic thrombocytopenic purpura (TTP) and the hemolytic anemic/uremic syndrome (HUS). Because these two conditions involve the microvasculature in general, other tissues are frequently affected. Thus, in both HUS and TTP, damage to the renal microvasculature occurs, resulting in renal failure, and is associated with elevated blood urea nitrogen (BUN) and creatinine, as described in Abnormalities in Clinical Chemistry later. In TTP, involvement of the cerebral circulation gives rise to behavioral changes and other neurologic sequelae. In addition, platelets are affected, giving rise to thrombocytopenia.

MHA may also occur with other immune-mediated disorders (e.g., connective tissue disorders such as disseminated lupus erythematosus), where, again, endothelial damage from the attachment of immune complexes and complement produces fibrin deposition on endothelial surfaces.

It is important to note that because MHA results from traumatic destruction of newly formed RBCs in the microvasculature, where both red and white blood cell (WBC) precursors are being formed, often both RBC and WBC precursors are released into the circulation. Thus, all findings of hemolytic anemia are present, in addition to which a significant number of precursor cells such as nucleated RBCs, myelocytes, and metamyelocytes are seen in the peripheral blood—a pattern termed the leukoerythroblastic picture.

As discussed later, in DIC and occasionally in TTP, laboratory findings include thrombocytopenia and increased prothrombin time, activated partial thromboplastin time, thrombin time, fibrin degradation products, and D-dimer levels (described later), but low fibrinogen levels. BUN and creatinine are also elevated.

Hypoproliferative Normocytic Anemias

Bone Marrow Hypoplasia/Aplastic Anemia. This is a hypoproliferative anemia, with MCV and RDW usually within normal limits, and typically affecting all peripheral blood elements (red cells, white cells, and platelets; see later). Immature white cells and red cells are not usually present on peripheral blood films. Bone marrow biopsy, which is commonly performed to obtain the diagnosis, typically shows severely hypoplastic/aplastic marrow with severe depletion of all hematopoietic marrow precursors. Aplastic anemia may be primary/inherited or secondary/acquired, with the latter due to chemical toxin, infection, radiation, or immune dysfunction. Serum iron may be elevated because of lack of erythropoiesis. Typical hematologic findings in this condition are summarized in entry 4 of Table 8-1. It is important to note that *none of the quantitative serum diagnostic tests for hemolytic anemia, such as haptoglobin, carboxyhemoglobin, and indirect bilirubin elevation, are positive in this condition.*

Myelodysplastic Syndrome. Another less common condition but nonetheless an important cause of hypoproliferative normocytic anemia is the myelodysplastic syndrome (MDS). This syndrome, which often presents as a normocytic anemia (although it can on occasion present as mildly macrocytic or as microcytic anemia), is refractory to treatment (e.g., transfusions of packed RBCs). It may present simply as a refractory anemia in its early stages and is thought to progress then to refractory anemia with ringed sideroblasts, and eventually to so-called preleukemic stages, in particular, refractory anemia with an excess of blasts (generally in the myeloid or lymphoid lines) and an excess of blasts in transformation. The condition may also present initially as a refractory cytopenia that involves all three (erythroid, granulocytic, megakaryocytic) hematopoietic cell lines. As might be surmised from this latter observation, MDS appears to be a clonal stem cell disorder that is characterized by ineffective hematopoiesis. Further discussion of this fascinating disease can be found in Chapter 33.

Anemia of Renal Failure. Another normocytic, hypoproliferative anemia is the anemia of chronic renal failure. Loss of the kidneys' excretory function produces an increase in BUN and creatinine, as discussed later, as well as a buildup of metabolic byproducts. The resulting uremia appears to be responsible for changes in red cell shape, with burr cells (echinocytes) and ellipsoidal cells commonly present on peripheral blood films. Identification of burr cells on peripheral blood films during the course of illness may signal the development of renal dysfunction. In addition to decreased excretory function, the kidneys' ability to produce erythropoietin is decreased, resulting in impaired erythropoiesis, such that the marrow's response to hypoxia becomes inadequate. In contrast to aplastic anemia (entry 4, Table 8-1), white cell and platelet counts usually remain within normal limits. Typical findings in this condition are summarized in entry 5 of Table 8-1. Again, as in bone marrow hypoplasia/aplastic anemia, none of the quantitative serum diagnostic tests for hemolytic anemia, such as haptoglobin, carboxyhemoglobin, and indirect bilirubin elevation, are positive in this condition.

Macrocytic Anemia

Macrocytic anemia can be diagnosed from the hemogram from a low RBC count and a high MCV, often exceeding 100 fL. By far the most common cause of macrocytic anemia is nutritional deficiency (i.e., vitamin B_{12} and/or folate deficiency). Lack of either factor is thought to disrupt DNA synthesis but not RNA synthesis, such that the nucleus and cytoplasm of the cell no longer mature in synchrony. Morphologically, the cell cytoplasm matures, while the nucleus remains immature, and the cell appears megaloblastic. This lack of synchrony produces hypersegmented neutrophils (five-lobed nuclei in more than 5% of neutrophils or any neutrophil with six or more lobes) and large, oval red cells termed macroovalocytes, both of which are present on the blood films of patients with megaloblastic anemia. In addition, the RDW is typically increased, and the reticulocyte count is decreased.

If macrocytic anemia is diagnosed, the first serum analytes whose concentrations should be determined are B_{12} and folate, for which rapid and accurate ELISA assays are performed. If these analytes are both found to be within the reference range, assays for thyroid function should be performed because hypothyroidism is a cause of macrocytosis. As discussed later in the endocrine function testing section, elevated thyroid-stimulating hormone (TSH) with low or normal thyroxine (T_4) serum levels confirms the diagnosis of primary hypothyroidism. Because certain therapeutic drugs, particularly azathymidine (AZT) used in the treatment of the acquired immune deficiency syndrome (AIDS), are known to induce macrocytic anemia, it is important to ascertain whether a patient is being treated with such drugs.

In this era of the automated CBC, it is possible also that red cell precursor forms, such as nucleated RBCs, may be counted as mature erythrocytes. Therefore, in a patient with a "macrocytic" anemia with normal B_{12}, folate, and thyroid hormone levels, it is important to check the reticulocyte and the nucleated RBC count to determine whether these are significantly elevated. If so, the possibility of a hemolytic anemia should be considered. Thus the diagnostic workup for hemolytic anemia described in the preceding section should be instituted.

Other possible causes of macrocytic anemia include posthemorrhagic states (differentiated by elevation of the reticulocyte count and polychromasia), alcoholism (associated with folate deficiency), liver disease, and myelodysplasia. Note again that the definitive tests for determining the cause of macrocytic anemia (i.e., B_{12}, folate, and thyroid function tests) are often performed in the Clinical Chemistry section.

The major clinical laboratory findings for macrocytic anemia are summarized as entries 6A and 6B in Table 8-1. Note that macrocytic anemias are divided into megaloblastic (entry 6A), typical of B_{12} and folate deficiency, and nonmegaloblastic (entry 6B), typical of hypothyroidism. Whether or not the macrocytic anemia is megaloblastic can be determined only by bone marrow biopsy. This procedure is not necessary in most cases because the cause of the macrocytosis can be determined by the assays described earlier.

Table 8-1 summarizes some of the pertinent findings and specific determinations used to distinguish and diagnose the common anemias previously discussed. Note that this table is a guide as to what specific tests should be ordered and, by implication, what tests need not be ordered. For example, a microcytic anemia should be worked up with orders for ferritin and Fe/IBC ratios, but generally there is no need to order B_{12} and folate levels. Conversely, there is no need to order ferritin, IBC, etc., for a macrocytic anemia, for which B_{12} and folate levels should be ordered.

QUANTITATIVE WHITE BLOOD CELL ABNORMALITIES

The WBC count encompasses several types of commonly circulating nucleated cells, including granulocytes (principally mature neutrophils, basophils, and eosinophils), lymphocytes, and monocytes. It should be noted that absolute concentrations (and not percentages) of these cells are significant in interpreting the WBC count. An increase to above the normal physiologic level in the WBC count, termed leukocytosis, may primarily involve any of these white cells, depending on which cell type is chiefly elevated (i.e., neutrophilia, basophilia, eosinophilia, monocytosis, and lymphocytosis). Occasionally, plasma cells may be found in the peripheral blood. Likewise, a decrease in the WBC count, termed leukopenia, may center on a single cell series (i.e., neutropenia, monocytopenia, and lymphocytopenia). Absolute decreases in eosinophils and basophils are difficult to identify because of the low numbers present normally. Certain differential diagnoses are commonly associated with certain WBC changes (e.g., infection and/or inflammation with neutrophilia, allergic reactions and parasitic infections with eosinophilia). In addition, elevations may be due to a benign process (e.g., infection) or a malignant process (e.g., leukemia). Here, we note several quantitative patterns and their associations that correlate with abnormal chemical findings.

Again, clinical history and physical findings are important in diagnosis and management of the patient. In addition, the CBC and white cell differential are important laboratory findings that are used, in conjunction with the clinical impression, to formulate the differential diagnosis. In adults, the reference range for the white count is approximately 4000–7000 white cells/μL; approximately two thirds of the white cells are neutrophils, and slightly less than one third are lymphocytes.

Infection: The Most Common Cause of Elevated WBC Count

An elevated WBC count between about 10,000 and 20,000/µL commonly points to an infectious/reactive process. In general, neutrophilia is associated with infection (bacterial, fungal, viral), inflammatory states (e.g., trauma, surgery), certain drugs (e.g., corticosteroids), and myeloproliferative conditions. Exceptions to the neutrophilia seen in bacterial infections include tuberculosis, brucellosis, pertussis, where the predominant cells are lymphocytes, and infections, mainly in newborns, with *Listeria monocytogenes*, for which a monocytic response is predominant.

Eosinophilia is commonly associated with allergic reactions, parasitic infections, and hematologic malignancies (Brito-Babapulle, 2003; Fischbach, 2008). Basophilia is commonly associated with hematologic malignancies (e.g., chronic myelogenous leukemia, or CML), but may be seen in some inflammatory states and allergic reactions. Lymphocytosis is commonly associated with acute viral infections, such as infectious mononucleosis (Epstein-Barr virus infection); chronic infections, such as tuberculosis, brucellosis, and pertussis; and hematologic disease and immune stimulation. Monocytosis is commonly associated with hematologic disease, such as chronic myelomonocytic leukemia, as well as with some infectious processes, such as tuberculosis, rickettsia, and *Listeria*.

Elevated WBC Count Due to Leukemoid Reaction

In patients who do not have leukemia, very high WBC counts (generally greater than $50 \times 10^3/\mu L$) may produce a peripheral blood film appearance similar to leukemia. This is termed a leukemoid reaction. The more common type of leukemoid reaction is granulocytic, although lymphocytic reactions may also occur. The granulocytic type usually reveals reactive neutrophils present in the peripheral blood film, with a left shift in the neutrophil series (i.e., immature forms such as bands, metamyelocytes, and myelocytes). Changes in the cytoplasmic appearance of cells, such as toxic granulation and Döhle body production (see Chapter 37), are commonly seen. Causes of the granulocytic type of reaction include bacterial infection (e.g., diphtheria), malignancy (Hodgkin disease), and reactive conditions such as rebound granulocytosis. Although these changes are helpful, C-reactive protein (CRP), an acute phase plasma protein, rapidly rises and falls with the onset and resolution of inflammation. CRP appears to be an earlier and more sensitive indicator of acute inflammation and infection (Seebach, 1997; Dantzer, 2008) and can be quickly measured using present-day analyzers. Leukemoid reaction must be distinguished from CML and other myeloproliferative conditions. It is important to note that the enzyme *neutrophil alkaline phosphatase* will be normal or elevated in a granulocytic leukemoid reaction, but is *decreased in CML*.

Elevated WBC Count Due to CML

At present, the definitive diagnosis of CML rests upon the demonstration of the Philadelphia chromosome (i.e., a translocation between chromosomes #9 and #22 resulting in the BCR-ABL fusion gene) by cytogenetics or by molecular techniques (e.g., see Silver, 2003; George, 2003; Sattler, 2003; Ross, 2008). Detection of molecular or cytogenetic abnormalities is of diagnostic (and possibly prognostic) significance in other hematologic diseases as well, including acute myeloid leukemia, acute lymphoblastic leukemia, T cell leukemia/lymphoma, and myelodysplasia (Swerdlow, 2008). Molecular techniques now are utilized to detect very early stages of disease, as well as to detect minimal residual disease, that is, disease that may be apparent only at the molecular level. For example, quantitative polymerase chain reaction can be used to monitor BCR-ABL translocation levels in CML patients being treated with the kinase inhibitor imatinib (Gleevec) (Ross, 2008).

Elevated WBC Count Due to Chronic Lymphocytic Leukemia

When the lymphocytes appear normal but are significantly increased in number in an older individual, the possibility of chronic lymphocytic leukemia (CLL) must be considered. Again, molecular techniques such as flow cytometric, immunophenotypic, and cytogenetic/fluorescence in situ hybridization analysis (Jaffe, 2001; Oscier, 2004; Shanafelt, 2004) can help establish the diagnosis. In CLL, the neoplastic B lymphocytes will be found to express an unusual (but characteristic) human leukocyte differentiation antigen designated CD5, which is typical for this disease. Other CD antigens can also be detected by flow cytometry and have become useful in resolving other hematologic diagnostic problems.

Leukocytosis Due to Acute Leukemias

Both acute myeloid and lymphoid leukemias present often as markedly elevated WBC counts. In lymphoblastic leukemia, numerous lymphoblasts are seen on the peripheral smear. Myeloid leukemias can present in a myriad of forms, including myeloblastic, promyelocytic, monoblastic/monocytic, myelomonocytic, erythroblastic, and megakaryoblastic. Again, flow cytometric, immunophenotypic, and karyotypic/molecular analyses can help establish the diagnosis and define prognosis (Winton, 2004). These are discussed fully in Chapter 33. Here, we point out that blast forms of any kind on a peripheral blood smear raise the strong diagnostic possibility of an acute leukemia.

Low White Cell Counts

Aplastic Anemia

Low WBC counts, if accompanied by marrow hypoplasia and two out of three of the following findings—anemia (with corrected reticulocyte count <1%), neutropenia (neutrophil count <500/µL), and thrombocytopenia (platelet count <20,000/µL)—may be part of a generalized pancytopenia secondary to marrow failure (Guinan, 1997; Marsh, 2003, 2005). Also known as aplastic anemia, this condition may be primary/inherited or acquired/secondary. Known causes of the acquired type include drugs/toxins, infections (including hepatitis), radiation, and immune dysfunction (Gordon-Smith, 2002). Cytogenetic study may be utilized to rule out myelodysplasia; if unsuccessful, molecular techniques such as fluorescent in situ hybridization may be necessary for chromosome analysis (Guinan, 1997). The primary/inherited types may not always be present at birth (i.e., congenital), and diagnosis of this type of marrow failure relies heavily on clinical assessment in conjunction with appropriate laboratory evaluation (Alter, 1999, 2002).

Gram Negative Sepsis as a Cause of Leukopenia

Leukopenia may also be seen in other conditions, including gram-negative sepsis. It is interesting to note that gram-negative sepsis with a low WBC count is often accompanied by a cholestatic pattern in the liver (i.e., a mild rise in bilirubin and alkaline phosphatase), as discussed later and in Chapter 21.

COAGULATION DISORDERS

This vast and complex topic is discussed in Part 5. For our review, we focus on four hematologic parameters that may be important in correlation with test results in chemistry determinations: The platelet count; the bleeding time; the activated partial thromboplastin time (APTT), reflecting the function of the intrinsic coagulation system; and the prothrombin time (PT), reflecting the function of the extrinsic coagulation system. Diminished values of the platelet count and/or abnormalities in platelet aggregation can lead to abnormal bleeding times. Elevated PTs and/or APTTs are not generally associated with abnormal bleeding times, except mainly in factor VIII deficiency with concomitant deficiency of von Willebrand factor. This latter factor is needed for platelet aggregation.

Bleeding Time Measures Platelet Function

Historically, the bleeding time (BT) was utilized as a screening test for platelet function. It should be noted that the BT is not believed to correlate accurately with or to predict bleeding (DeCaterina, 1994; Gerwirtz, 1996) and is now uncommonly used to screen for platelet function abnormalities (Kottke-Marchant, 2002).

Major Causes of Increased PT or APTT

The anticoagulant heparin, which accelerates the inactivation of thrombin and other coagulation factors (such as factor Xa), preferentially blocks the intrinsic system, leading to prolonged APTTs but not to significant elevations in PT. On the other hand, the vitamin K antagonist coumadin preferentially blocks factor VII in the extrinsic system, leading to prolonged PTs but not APTTs.

International Normalized Ratios for Patients Being Treated With Coumadin

The PTs of patients who are being anticoagulated on coumadin must be followed carefully to ensure that the therapeutic effect is occurring, but that the effective levels of coumadin are not sufficiently elevated to initiate hemorrhage. Thus it is important to establish a therapeutic range for PTs for patients on coumadin. Because different methods for determining PTs are available, somewhat different reference ranges for PTs among different laboratories have been developed, making it difficult on occasion to compare PT results from different laboratories for a given patient. To attempt to correct for these differences, the PT values are used in a formula that standardizes these "raw" values. This formula takes the ratio of the observed PT to the mean value for the PT reference range of the particular laboratory and then raises the resulting ratio to the power of what is termed the international standardized index, or ISI. This index is determined from the slope of a correlation plot of the logarithm of a laboratory's PTs for blood samples that contain different coumadin concentrations against the logarithm of the PTs determined by a reference ("gold standard") method. Thus the international normalized ratio (INR) is expressed as $(PTpat/PTmean)^{isi}$, where PTpat is the measured PT for the patient and PTmean is the mean value for the laboratory's reference range (Kamath, 2009). In most circumstances, INR values of 2–3 are considered to be therapeutic for patients who have atrial fibrillation, and 3–4 to be therapeutic for patients with prosthetic heart valves, but values over 4 are considered to require lowering of the coumadin dose or temporary cessation of treatment. Note that INRs are appropriate principally for patients who are being treated with coumadin.

The Other Cause of Isolated PT or APTT is Coagulation Factor Deficiency

If the PT or the APTT becomes elevated in the absence of treatment with heparin or coumadin, and the platelet count is normal, it is important to perform mixing studies of the patient's plasma with normal plasma to determine if the coagulation time normalizes (i.e., whether there is a factor deficiency). A not infrequent cause of factor deficiency is liver failure, discussed subsequently and in Chapter 21. Thus liver function measurements should also be checked in these instances. If mixing studies do not completely correct the prolonged coagulation times, the presence of coagulation inhibitors, such as *circulating lupus anticoagulant* or *antifactor antibodies*, should be suspected.

The Major Cause of Elevated PT and APTT is DIC

If the platelet count diminishes and the APTT and the PT both rise, the diagnosis of DIC should be entertained. This diagnosis is confirmed by the finding of elevated fibrin split products (FSPs) and, more specifically, the D-dimer, discussed in Chapter 40 as the D–D fragment of fibrin that results from the proteolytic action of plasmin upon the fibrin clot that forms during intravascular coagulation. D-Dimer is detected in an assay by utilizing a very specific monoclonal antibody to this cross-linked fibrin degradation product. This method has largely replaced the less specific assay for FSPs, which likewise are elevated in this condition. DIC is an extremely dangerous condition and must be diagnosed rapidly, as indicated earlier.

In this condition, abnormal activation of both coagulation cascades and consumption of platelets occur. This activation may be caused by gram-negative sepsis (activation of the cascades may result from bacterial endotoxins), cancer, chronic inflammatory states such as collagen vascular diseases, leukemia (especially acute promyelocytic leukemia), complications of pregnancy, blood transfusion complications, liver failure, and physical trauma such as burns, drowning, and central nervous system (CNS) injuries. DIC causes the formation of microemboli that can result in widespread tissue infarction or ischemia with attendant abnormal chemical values (e.g., elevated liver function enzymes; elevated BUN and creatinine, suggestive of renal failure; and even elevation of cardiac troponin, indicating myocardial damage). Thus low platelet counts and elevated APTT and PT, together with chemical abnormalities suggestive of multisystem dysfunction, strongly suggest DIC. Anticoagulant therapy must be instituted rapidly to block further embolization and tissue destruction.

Abnormalities in Clinical Chemistry: Chemical Pathology

ELECTROLYTE ABNORMALITIES

This topic is treated at length in Chapter 14 and in Oh (2003). Here we present an overview of the regulation of serum levels of critical electrolytes

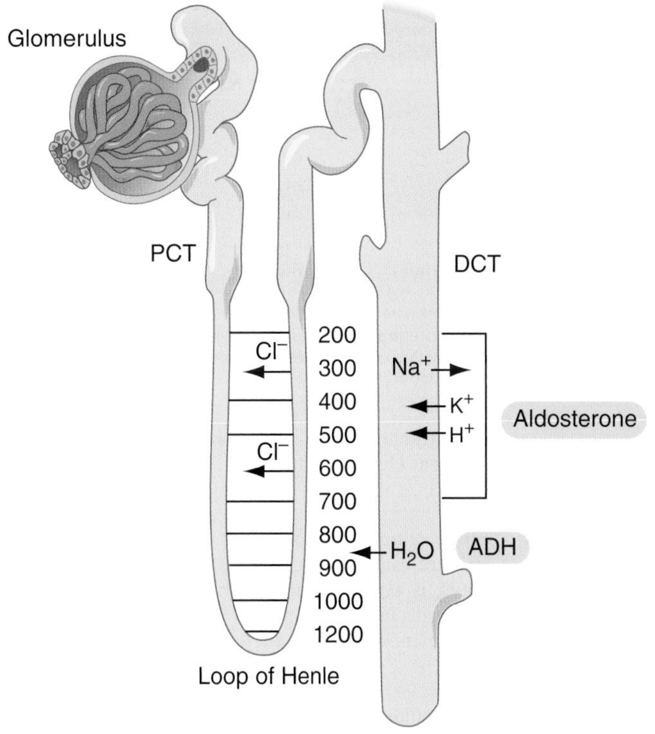

Figure 8-1 A schematic representation of a nephron showing the fundamental mechanism of water and salt conservation by the kidneys. Filtration occurs at the glomerulus *(upper left, showing capillaries in red)*, and the filtrate passes through the proximal convoluted tubule (PCT), where about 70% of the total filtered sodium is reabsorbed. In the loop of Henle, the countercurrent multiplier mechanism is operative. Chloride ion (Cl^-) is extruded from the ascending limb into the interstitial space *(shown in the upper middle part of the figure)*. Sodium ion passively follows. The cells of the ascending limb of the loop of Henle are impermeable to water, and the cells of the descending limb are impermeable to chloride ions. The result of this system is that high concentrations of NaCl are built up at the tip of the loop of Henle. The numbers beside the loop of Henle are osmolalities at different levels along the loop that, in humans, reach a maximum of 1200 mOsm/kg, as shown in the figure. At the top of the loop, the filtrate becomes isotonic (where the 300 mOsm/kg mark occurs) and then hypotonic because of the continuous extrusion of chloride ion. The hypertonic interstitium allows water to diffuse in from the collecting ducts (CDs), provided that antidiuretic hormone (ADH, *labeled and highlighted in color in the figure*) is secreted. More sodium ion can be conserved in the distal convoluted tubule (DCT), provided aldosterone *(labeled and highlighted in color)* is secreted, resulting in the one-to-one exchange of Na^+ for K^+ and H^+.

to enable accurate formulation of the possible causes of abnormalities in their serum levels. Figure 8-1 summarizes the basic mechanisms by which the kidneys control electrolyte and water balance. Functionally, keep in mind that the purpose of the kidneys is to conserve fluids or, tantamount to this, to concentrate the urine. The mechanism by which this conservation of fluids is effected is the building up of high sodium chloride gradients in the interstitial space between the descending and ascending limbs of the loop of Henle, using the countercurrent multiplier mechanism. By this mechanism, sodium chloride is extruded into the interstitial space such that sodium chloride (NaCl) concentrations become greater toward the tip of the loop of Henle. The ascending limb of the loop of Henle is impermeable to water, as are the distal convoluted tubules and collecting ducts. However, under the effect of antidiuretic hormone (ADH), the collecting ducts are made permeable to water, allowing it to flow into the interstitial space and to penetrate the vasa recta. The entire driving force for this process is the high concentrations of NaCl in the interstitium. Any interference with the countercurrent multiplier will block reabsorption of water because the ion gradients are eliminated.

As also shown in Figure 8-1, sodium ion, 70% of which is reabsorbed in the proximal convoluted tubule, can be further reabsorbed in the distal convoluted tubules and collecting ducts under the effect of aldosterone from the zona glomerulosa of the adrenal cortex. This hormone promotes the 1 : 1 exchange of sodium for potassium or hydrogen ion. Sodium levels in serum depend almost completely on the interplay between aldosterone and ADH. With these simple considerations in mind, the most common causes of hyponatremia and hypernatremia are now summarized with an explanation of how to identify them. It should be kept in mind that normal renal function is assumed. If renal failure occurs, the kidneys ultimately

TABLE 8-2
Common Causes of Hyponatremia and Electrolyte Patterns in Serum and Urine With Normal Renal Function*

Cause	Serum Na	Urine Na (UNa)	Urine osmolality	Serum K	24-hour UNa
1. Overhydration	Low	Low	Low	Normal or low	Low
2. Diuretics	Low	Low	Low	Low	High
3. SIADH†	Low	High	High	Normal or low	High
4. Adrenal failure	Low	Mildly elevated	Normal	High	High
5. Bartter's syndrome	Low	Low	Low	Low	High
6. Diabetic hyperosmolarity‡	Low	Normal	Normal	High	Normal

SIADH, Syndrome of inappropriate antidiuretic hormone.
*All Na and K values are concentrations except for 24-hour UNa, which is the total number of milliequivalents of Na excreted in 24 hours in the urine.
†Secretion of inappropriate levels of antidiuretic hormone.
‡In this condition, serum glucose is markedly elevated.

fail to be able to concentrate the urine, so that hyponatremia will result, as is discussed in the Renal Disease section later.

Hyponatremia

The four most common causes of hyponatremia are given in Table 8-2, together with a fifth, rare cause, Bartter's syndrome. A sixth, metabolic cause, diabetes mellitus, is also presented in this table. In all forms of hyponatremia, the chloride ion concentration is generally low because chloride is the chief counter-ion for sodium.

Basic Principle

All confirmed serum sodium abnormalities must be followed up with urinalysis on the patient, who should be fluid restricted. This urinalysis should include the urine sodium and urine osmolality. For conditions 1 and 2 in Table 8-2, the serum sodium tends to correct over a 24-hour period when the patient is fluid restricted.

Overhydration

In this condition, the most common cause of which is the consumption of large amounts of water or hypotonic fluids due to such causes as psychogenic polydipsia, serum sodium is reduced to below 135 mEq/L. Because the consumed water is excreted by the kidneys, the urine is also dilute in this ion. In fact, the osmolality of urine will be low (i.e., <300 mOsm/kg). Often accompanying hyponatremia in overhydration are low values of the Hct and low values of BUN, discussed subsequently. This triad of findings strongly suggests overhydration as the cause. Urinalysis in the fluid-restricted patient will reveal urinary sodium of <25 mEq/L and low osmolalities. Potassium may also be low, although it often remains within the reference range. Because mainly water is excreted in urine in this condition, the total 24-hour sodium excretion will be low (cause no. 1, Table 8-2).

Use and/or Abuse of Diuretics

Loop diuretics block the chloride pump in the loop of Henle, thereby blocking the formation of ion gradients via the countercurrent multiplier, which is necessary for water conservation. Thus water is lost. Also, because sodium is no longer retained because it follows chloride in the loop, it also is depleted from serum. Thus, unlike in overhydration, the total 24-hour sodium excretion is high (compare 24-hour urinary sodium [UNa] values for entries 1 and 2, Table 8-2). Except for this difference, the pattern for diuretics resembles overhydration (dilute serum and urine); however, loop diuretics cause severe potassium depletion unless the diuretic is combined with a potassium-sparing diuretic like triamterene. Combined hyponatremia and hypokalemia with a high urinary sodium and potassium 24-hour excretion point to diuretic use. Of course, a history will generally reveal use of diuretics.

Syndrome of Inappropriate ADH Secretion (Entry 3, Table 8-2)

In this condition, secondary to head trauma, seizures, other CNS diseases, and neoplastic conditions, especially lung, breast, and ovarian cancers that secrete ADH-like hormones, the serum sodium is depressed because of excessive retention of water in the collecting ducts. This results in depletion of water in the renal tubules, thereby concentrating the urine. Therefore, although the serum is dilute in sodium (hypotonic), the urine is concentrated to levels >40 mEq/L, and urine osmolality exceeds 300 mOsm/kg, while the serum osmolality is <280 mOsm/kg. This pattern clearly is diagnostic of syndrome of inappropriate antidiuretic hormone (SIADH).

Aldosterone Deficit (Entry 4, Table 8-2)

This condition occurs secondary to Addison's disease and AIDS-related hypoadrenalism. Without aldosterone, the Na^+-K^+ and Na^+-H^+ exchanges in the distal convoluted tubules and collecting ducts do not occur. Therefore, serum sodium concentration is reduced while serum potassium concentration increases, and mild metabolic acidosis is the result. Urinary sodium increases, but not to the high levels seen in SIADH, and the osmolality of urine also is not so elevated as in SIADH.

Bartter's Syndrome (Entry 5, Table 8-2)

This rare condition resembles diuretic use, except that the hyponatremia is not corrected with fluid restriction. Although the cause of this condition is not fully understood, it is known that the kidneys of these patients fail to retain potassium. This results in both hyponatremia and hypokalemia as in diuretic use/abuse. In addition, as in diuretic use, high 24-hour sodium and potassium excretion is noted.

Diabetic Hyperosmolar State (Entry 6, Table 8-2)

In patients with diabetes mellitus who are in a hyperosmolar state (i.e., where the serum glucose is markedly elevated, say around 700 mg/dL), the hyperosmolality of serum causes efflux of cellular water, with consequent osmotic dilution of serum sodium. Roughly, for each 100 mg/dL increase in serum glucose, a 1.6 mEq/L decrease in serum Na+ concentration is noted. Because transport of glucose into cells is accompanied by concurrent transport of potassium into cells, low insulin levels may also cause high serum potassium. So, the net effect of diabetic hyperosmolar states is a low serum sodium and a high serum potassium. This resembles hypoaldosteronism (entry 4, Table 8-1), but the presence of abnormally high glucose levels signals the possibility of diabetes mellitus as the cause.

Pseudohyponatremia

This condition is usually caused by the presence of excess lipids in serum. No sodium ions are dissolved in lipids, which can take up a considerable volume of serum. If the absolute amount of sodium in a given volume of serum is determined, as with such methods of sodium determination as flame photometry, this value is divided by the sample volume to get the concentration. But part of this volume is lipid that has no sodium. So a falsely low value of sodium can be obtained. This artifact is eliminated by the use of ion-selective electrodes that directly determine the concentration of sodium and do not depend upon knowledge of the volume of serum. Note that although most modern, high throughput chemistry analyzers measure serum sodium using ion-selective electrodes, they perform a predilution of the specimen (so-called *indirect* potentiometry), and hence the measurement is relative to volume and *is* susceptible to pseudohyponatremia.

Hypernatremia

Table 8-3 summarizes the three basic causes of hypernatremia. Note that each cause is the counterpart of a cause for hyponatremia. These causes are summarized as follows:

Dehydration (Entry 1, Table 8-3)

This can be caused by excess renal loss with high positive free water clearance (i.e., loss of water in excess of NaCl), excess sweating, and low water

TABLE 8-3

Common Causes of Hypernatremia and Electrolyte Patterns in Serum and Urine With Normal Renal Function*

Cause	Serum Na	Urine Na (UNa)	Urine osmolality	Serum K	24-hour UNa
1. Dehydration	High	High	High	Normal	Varies
2. Diabetes insipidus	High	Low	Low	Normal	Low
3. Cushing's disease or syndrome	High	Low	Normal	Low	Low

*All Na and K values are concentrations, except for 24-hour UNa, which is the total number of milliequivalents of Na excreted in 24 hours in the urine.

intake. The serum sodium is elevated, as is the Hct (possibly masking a true anemia), and the urine sodium is high as the result of increased renal excretion of NaCl.

Diabetes Insipidus (Entry 2, Table 8-3)

Diabetes insipidus (DI) may be central (neurogenic) (i.e., due to decreased vasopressin secretion) or nephrogenic (i.e., due to decreased renal response). Functionally, this condition is the reverse of SIADH (i.e., water retention in the tubules is not adequate). Although this condition is not completely understood and may be multifactorial, current research suggests that mutation and/or changes in protein expression of "water channel molecules" (renal aquaporins) and/or the vasopressin V2 renal collecting tubule cell receptor may play a role in both pathologic water loss, such as in nephrogenic DI, and pathologic water retention, such as SIADH (Oh, 2003; Schrier, 2003; Brown, 2003; Nguyen, 2003; Nielsen, 2002). The pattern shows elevated serum sodium but dilute urinary sodium caused by functionally inadequate levels of ADH.

Hyperaldosteronism (Entry 3, Table 8-3)

This condition may result from adrenal hyperplasia, Cushing's syndrome, and Cushing's disease. Levels of circulating aldosterone are inappropriately high, causing excessive reabsorption of Na and excretion of K^+ and H^+ ions. The patient will be hypernatremic and hypokalemic and will exhibit a mild metabolic alkalosis.

Hypokalemia

Many of the causes of hypokalemia, including overhydration, use of loop diuretics, SIADH, and Bartter's syndrome, overlap with those of hyponatremia, as discussed earlier. In addition to overlap of these causes with those of hyponatremia, the following states lead uniquely to hypokalemia.

1. *Infusion of insulin to diabetic individuals.* This results in rather large influxes of potassium into cells, which lower it in serum.
2. *Alkalosis.* RBCs are themselves excellent buffers. They are capable of exchanging potassium for hydrogen ions. Thus, in acidosis, H^+ ions enter red cells in exchange for K^+ ions. Conversely, in alkalosis, H^+ ions leave red cells (to neutralize excess base), and K^+ ions enter the red cells.
3. *Vomiting.* The major loss consists of both H^+ and K^+ from the stomach. Loss of K^+ in gastric fluid may be less important than the overall fluid loss, which causes activation of aldosterone and renal wasting of K^+.

Hyperkalemia

Among the major causes are those that also cause hypernatremia (e.g., dehydration, diabetes insipidus), as well as acidosis and diabetes mellitus (as discussed earlier), and hemolysis. Any kind of cell damage, such as rhabdomyolysis, and especially hemolysis of erythrocytes, can cause hyperkalemia. In hemolysis, all of the intracellular K^+ is extruded into plasma. Another analyte that is concentrated in red cells that rises with K^+ in hemolysis is LD. Concomitant elevations of potassium and LD in serum should be taken as indications of hemolysis that occurs artifactually after a blood sample has been taken from the patient or, less commonly, as hemolysis that results from an underlying hemolytic condition.

RENAL DISEASE (OH, 2003; SCHNERMANN, 1998)

Four analytes aid in the diagnosis of this condition: BUN, creatinine, calcium, and phosphate. It is amazing that neither BUN nor creatinine has an inherent relationship to kidney function, but both fortuitously are excellent indicators of renal condition.

BUN

Urea nitrogen is generally measured in plasma or serum but has historically been referred to as BUN. The formula for urea is $H_2N–CO–NH_2$. Two moles of nitrogen are present per mole of urea. This is the end product of NH_3 metabolism in the liver, as discussed in Chapter 21. Urea is excreted by the renal tubules at a rate that is roughly proportional to the glomerular filtration rate (GFR). Note, therefore, that the retained urea (i.e., plasma or serum urea or BUN) is approximately inversely proportional to the GFR, that is,

$$\mathrm{BUN} \propto 1/\mathrm{GFR} \qquad \textbf{(8-1)}$$

Creatinine

Creatinine is secreted but is also reabsorbed to an approximately equal extent, so that the net effect is that the amount filtered is the amount excreted. The total amount of creatinine filtered then is its urinary concentration, Ucr × volume of urine (V), over a given time. The total plasma that delivered this quantity of creatinine to the glomerulus is the total amount of creatinine filtered divided by the plasma concentration, Pcr. This quantity is also the creatinine clearance (Ccr). So the glomerular filtration rate is as follows:

$$\mathrm{GFR} = \mathrm{Ccr} = \mathrm{Ucr} \times \mathrm{V}/\mathrm{Pcr} \qquad \textbf{(8-2)}$$

Pre-Renal Disease

Suppose the BUN is abnormally high (reference range = 10–20 mg/mL). Two possible reasons for this are known. The first is pre-renal, where renal plasma flow is reduced from such lesions as renal artery stenosis, renal vein thrombosis, and the like. This causes a reduction in the GFR. From Equation 8-1, the BUN will then rise. However, the serum creatinine levels (Pcr in Equation 8-2), with a reference range of about 0.5–1.0 mg/dL, generally will remain within normal limits or may be mildly elevated because, from Equation 8-2, it can be seen that low GFR will result in lower urine flow (V in Equation 8-2). Pcr and Ucr generally will remain within normal limits. Thus a disproportionate rise in BUN over creatinine will be noted. The normal BUN/creatinine ratio is 10–20 : 1, and in pre-renal disease, it rises to well above 20 : 1.

Renal and Post-Renal Disease

The second cause of elevated BUN is true renal disease. Here again, there will be a rise in BUN due to low GFR. Now, however, creatinine filtration will be compromised, so that its serum level will rise correspondingly. Thus, in true renal disease, both BUN and creatinine rise together, maintaining the BUN/creatinine ratio at 10–20 : 1 (Oh, 2003). This pattern also occurs in so-called post-renal disease (i.e., obstructive uropathy due to renal or ureteral stones [nephrolithiasis or urolithiasis], prostatic enlargement from benign prostatic hyperplasia or prostatic carcinoma, urinary tract infection, bladder stasis, urothelial carcinoma, etc.

Pinpointing the Lesion

Suppose a patient is found to have a BUN of, say, 60 mg/dL and a creatinine of 3.5 mg/dL. True renal failure can therefore be diagnosed. Now, consider the kidney to be two compartments—one a filtration compartment (glomerulus), and the other a concentration compartment (renal tubules). If renal failure is present, where is the lesion—in the filtration or the concentration compartment? As discussed previously, the function of the kidneys is to conserve fluids or to concentrate the urine. Therefore, if a patient is on a fluid-restricted diet, the osmolality of urine (Uosm) should be significantly higher than the osmolality of plasma (Posm). In fact, Uosm/Posm is >1.2 for normal individuals. If a 24-hour urine specimen collection from the above patient on a fluid-restricted diet is measured for Uosm, we can determine where the lesion has occurred. If Uosm/Posm <1.2, then the urine is not being concentrated, so a tubular lesion must be present. On the other hand, if a normal ratio is found, then, by exclusion, the lesion must be glomerular. Causes of glomerular lesions are many and include glomerulonephritis, pyelonephritis, diabetes, and infarction among others; tubular lesions also have many causes, including pyelonephritis, diabetes, papillary necrosis, acute tubular necrosis, infarction, shock, ischemia, etc. It is remarkable that from a blood specimen of only 100 μL and several urine aliquots, not only can we determine the presence of renal failure, but we can localize the lesion and all of this virtually noninvasively.

Calcium and Phosphate

The kidneys play an important role in the regulation of calcium levels. In renal failure, calcium levels tend to fall, while phosphate levels correspondingly tend to rise. The topic of calcium and phosphorus metabolism is discussed in detail in the context of bone metabolism (see Chapter 15) and the endocrine system (see Chapter 24). Here, we discuss these two analytes for diagnostic purposes.

Remember that calcium is the most abundant cation in the body, and that most of it is stored in bone as a calcium hydroxyphosphate in hydroxyapatite crystal. Calcium complexes with phosphate in several different forms, depending on the ionization state of phosphate, that is,

$$H_3PO_4 \leftrightarrow H_2PO_4^- + H^+ \quad \textbf{(8-3)}$$

$$H_2PO_4^- \leftrightarrow HPO_4^{2-} + H^+ \quad \textbf{(8-4)}$$

$$HPO_4^{2-} \leftrightarrow PO_4^{3-} + H^+ \quad \textbf{(8-5)}$$

The most insoluble calcium phosphate forms are those with the most basic phosphates (i.e., those in Equation 8-5). Thus alkaline conditions promote calcium deposition in bone, while acidic conditions promote leaching of calcium from bone. Therefore, alkalosis promotes hypocalcemia, while acidosis promotes hypercalcemia.

Note also an equilibrium between soluble calcium phosphate and insoluble calcium phosphate in bone. We represent this equilibrium as follows:

$$Ca + P \leftrightarrow (CaP)\text{ insoluble} \quad \textbf{(8-6)}$$

where *P* represents all ionic phosphate forms, and where the left side is all soluble calcium phosphate salts and the right side is the insoluble salt forms. The equilibrium constant, Ksp, for this equilibrium is as follows:

$$Ksp = (Ca) \times (P)/(CaP)\text{ insoluble} \quad \textbf{(8-7)}$$

Because (CaP) insoluble is constant in concentration, the product of soluble Ca × soluble P is a constant, called the solubility constant, or Ksp. Thus there is an inverse relationship between Ca and P. Hypocalcemic states are almost always accompanied by hyperphosphatemic states, and vice versa. Of the soluble calcium, in the numerator of Equation 8-7 are two forms—calcium bound to albumin and globulin and small molecules in chelate form, and so-called ionized or nonchelated calcium. Biologically active calcium is present in the ionized form. Therefore, serum levels of ionized calcium are considered to be the best measure of hypocalcemia, normocalcemia, or hypercalcemia.

Causes of Hypocalcemia

The kidneys are vital in calcium metabolism and regulate calcium levels in two ways. First, parathyroid hormone stimulates the renal tubules to excrete phosphate. By Equation 8-7, the serum calcium level must then rise. Also, the kidneys are vital to the formation of active vitamin D in the synthesis of 1,25-dihydroxycholecalciferol, necessary for the absorption of calcium in the gut. In renal disease, where tubular failure occurs, phosphate excretion is inhibited by the nonresponsiveness of the tubules to parathyroid hormone. Therefore, phosphate levels rise, while calcium levels fall. In addition, active vitamin D production is reduced, lowering absorbed calcium. Hypocalcemia and hyperphosphatemia, in the face of elevated BUN and creatinine, indicative of renal disease, strongly suggest tubular failure.

Other Causes of Hypocalcemia

Besides alkalosis and renal failure, hypocalcemia may be caused by hypoparathyroidism, also leading to hyperphosphatemia. Rarely, as in medullary thyroid carcinoma and other amine precursor uptake and decarboxylase activity cell tumors, the elaboration of calcitonin, a well-known calcium-lowering hormone, may lead to decreased serum calcium levels. In addition, vitamin D levels may be low, resulting in diminished reabsorption of calcium for the gut. These causes may be encapsulated in the acronym, CHARD (Calcitonin, Hypoparathyroidism, Alkalosis, Renal failure, vitamin D deficit).

Causes of Hypercalcemia

Besides acidosis, possible causes of this condition may be summarized by Bakerman's "CHIMPS" mnemonic (Bakerman, 1994), or Cancer, Hyperthyroidism, Iatrogenic causes, Multiple myeloma, Hyperparathyroidism, and Sarcoidosis.

Calcium and Albumin

About half of the calcium circulating in blood is bound to serum protein, mainly albumin; the remainder may be chelated in tight complexes with ions such as citrate and oxalate or may be found in ionic complexes with counter-ions such as chloride—so-called free calcium. As is true for most hormones in the body, serum levels of parathyroid hormone (PTH) are determined by the levels of the free target of the hormone, in this case, free calcium. Also, virtually all of the effects of calcium in the body are induced by free calcium. Free or ionized calcium can be measured directly by an ion-selective electrode method. However, most laboratories measure total serum calcium using appropriate chelating dye methods; the concentrations of the calcium-dye complexes can be measured spectrophotometrically. Several formulas, none too reliable, have been developed to compute serum free calcium concentration from the total calcium ion concentration and serum albumin concentration (Larsson, 2003). More relevant is the computation of the "corrected" calcium concentration, most usually in hypocalcemia (Labriola, 2009). Generally, even if serum albumin concentrations fluctuate substantially, resulting in changes in total calcium levels, the ionized calcium levels in serum may remain relatively stable. If a patient has a total serum calcium that is lower than the lowest value for the reference range, and if the serum albumin level is concurrently low, a correction formula is used in which the total calcium is computed as the observed total calcium in mg/dL + a correction factor. Several different correction factors are known, perhaps the most commonly used of which is 0.8 × (4 g/dL – serum albumin concentration in g/dL). This correction is based on the ratio of bound calcium to albumin and the mean "normal" albumin value of 4 g/dL. If the corrected value results in total calcium in the reference range, it is assumed that the free calcium is in the normal range, that is, the "lost" calcium was all bound to albumin, and no free calcium was lost. Conversely, dehydration or hemoconcentration may elevate serum albumin, resulting in a falsely elevated total serum calcium. In this case, the correction will be a negative one because the albumin levels are elevated above 4 g/dL.

BLOOD GAS ABNORMALITIES

We have discussed the effects of acidosis and alkalosis on serum calcium levels. The actual diagnosis of acidosis or alkalosis, however, depends on measurement of the pH of arterial blood. This topic is discussed in depth in Chapter 14. Here we focus on how to interpret abnormal results and to correlate them with other laboratory findings.

Blood gas determinations refer to the quantitative measurement of the pH of arterial blood, the partial pressure of carbon dioxide (pCO_2), the bicarbonate, the partial pressure of oxygen (pO_2), oxygen saturation, and base excess. Three of these quantities are interdependent on one another, that is, the PCO_2, the bicarbonate, and the pH, by the Henderson-Hasselbalch equation as follows:

$$pH = 6.1 + \log[(HCO_3^-)/(H_2CO_3)] \quad \textbf{(8-8)}$$

Because the H_2CO_3 concentration in blood is directly proportional to the pCO_2 (i.e., at room temperature), H_2CO_3 = 0.03 = pCO_2, Equation 8-8 can be written as follows:

$$pH = 6.1 + \log[(HCO_3^-)/(0.03 \times pCO_2)] \quad \textbf{(8-9)}$$

Note that if bicarbonate, in the numerator of Equation 8-9, becomes consumed as in metabolic acidosis, the respiratory rate will increase, thereby decreasing the pCO_2, causing the denominator of this equation to fall, resulting in compensation. If the pCO_2 increases, as in respiratory acidosis, the kidneys retain bicarbonate, so that both numerator and denominator increase so as to maintain the ratio relatively constant.

In interpreting blood gas results, the first number to note is the pH. Regardless of the values of the bicarbonate and pCO_2, if the pH is less than 7.4, the patient is acidemic, that is, the hydrogen ion concentration in blood is elevated, which must reflect acidosis, that is, excessive production or retention of acid; if greater than 7.4, the patient is alkalemic, reflecting the process of alkalosis; if close or equal to 7.4, the patient is

TABLE 8-4
Patterns of pH, pCO_2, and Bicarbonate in Different Conditions

Condition	pH	Bicarbonate	pCO_2	Typical causes
1. Metabolic acidosis	<7.40	Low	Low	Diabetic ketoacidosis; lactic acidosis
2. Metabolic alkalosis	>7.40	High	High	Vomiting
3. Respiratory acidosis	<7.40	High	High	COPD; paralysis of respiratory muscles
4. Respiratory alkalosis	>7.40	Low	Low	Anxiety; acute pain

COPD, Chronic obstructive pulmonary disease; *pCO_2,* partial pressure of carbon dioxide.

neither acidemic nor alkalemic, but could still have compensating processes of acidosis and alkalosis. Once the diagnosis of acidosis or alkalosis is made, then the bicarbonate and the pCO_2 can be used to decide whether it is of metabolic or respiratory origin.

Table 8-4 summarizes the four basic abnormal states: Metabolic and respiratory acidosis and metabolic and respiratory alkalosis. In metabolic acidosis, the primary problem is production of acid, as in diabetic ketoacidosis, lactic acidosis (e.g., from gram-negative sepsis), and renal failure. This acid is buffered by bicarbonate, which is therefore consumed. To compensate for the bicarbonate loss, the breathing rate increases to lower the pCO_2. So a low pH combined with a low bicarbonate and a low pCO_2 point to metabolic acidosis, as shown in condition 1 of this table.

As shown in condition 2 of the table, the opposite condition, metabolic alkalosis, results in reversal of the levels shown in condition 1. The most common cause of metabolic alkalosis is vomiting with loss of HCl from the stomach and an attendant rise in bicarbonate.

When CO_2 is abnormally retained by the lungs, as in chronic obstructive pulmonary disease (COPD), the denominator of Equation 8-9 increases, causing the pH of blood to fall. To compensate, the kidneys retain bicarbonate, thus increasing the numerator of this equation. If the blood pH is below 7.4, and the CO_2 and bicarbonate are both increased (condition 3 in Table 8-4), the acidosis is of respiratory origin. Note the mirror image condition (opposite levels) for respiratory alkalosis in condition 4 of this table. Besides COPD, the major causes of respiratory acidosis include diseases such as myasthenia gravis, in which there is partial paralysis of the accessory muscles of breathing; pneumonia; and central nervous system diseases affecting the brainstem in areas involved in respiratory control. Respiratory alkalosis is due mainly to hyperventilation, often of psychogenic origin. Here, the pCO_2 is reduced because of the rapidity of breathing.

The pH of blood can affect the levels of electrolytes in serum. In acidosis, besides bicarbonate buffering, red cells also buffer excess H^+ ions by exchanging these for intracellular K^+ ions, the net effect being a mild hyperkalemia. An attendant hypokalemia occurs in alkalosis. Remember also that acidosis can cause a mild hypercalcemia; alkalosis can cause a mild hypocalcemia and can especially affect the ionized calcium moiety.

Anion Gap

All sodium ions must be neutralized by counter-ions, most of which, in blood, are constituted by chloride and bicarbonate ions, and, to a lesser degree, by phosphate, sulfate, and protein carboxylate groups. Normal serum sodium is about 140 mEq/L, chloride is usually around 100 mEq/L, and bicarbonate around 2 mEq/L. The anion gap is then defined as $Na^+ - (Cl^- + HCO_3^-)$, which for normal individuals is around 16. This 16 mEq/L really accounts for the other counter-ions that neutralize sodium but are not measured in serum.

If an individual has a metabolic acidosis, in which the rise in H^+ ion concentration is accompanied by a corresponding rise in Cl^- ions, the acid will be buffered by bicarbonate (converted to H_2CO_3). The bicarbonate value therefore will decrease, but a 1 : 1 increase in chloride ion will occur. Thus there will be no change in the anion gap. If the metabolic acidosis is due to the presence of an acid whose counter-ion is not Cl^-, such as acetoacetic acid (in diabetic acidosis) or lactic acid as in sepsis or hypoperfusion, then bicarbonate is reduced, as above, but no corresponding increase in Cl^- occurs. Therefore, there is an increase in the anion gap, which can reach values of 25–30 mEq/L. The presence of a widened anion gap signifies the presence of a metabolic acidosis due to a non–chloride-containing acid.

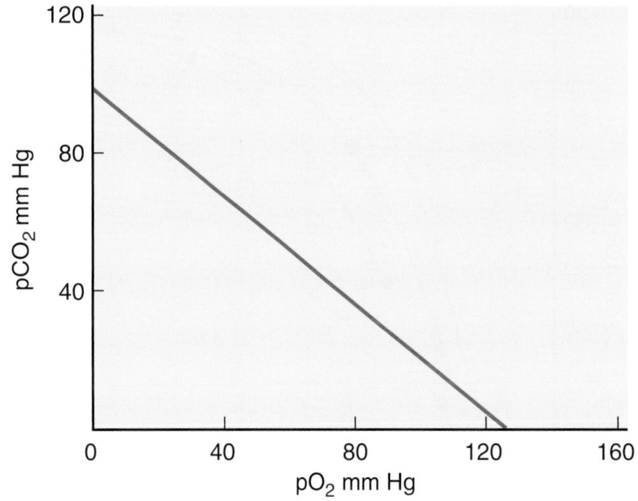

Figure 8-2 The effect of increased partial pressure of carbon dioxide (pCO_2) on the partial pressure of oxygen (pO_2) in the alveolus and in the arterial blood. This figure demonstrates that as pCO_2 increases, a greater than a one-to-one decrease in pO_2 occurs.

Low Anion Gaps

Consistently low anion gaps, typically in the range of 1–3 mEq/L, signify the presence of high levels of basic protein, often a monoclonal paraprotein as occurs in plasma cell dyscrasias. Basic protein contains ammonium ions, the counter-ions for which are chloride. Now the "invisible" ion is ammonium, and a measurable increase in chloride ion occurs. This tends to decrease the anion gap. Persistently low anion gaps are a serious sign of possible malignancy (e.g., multiple myeloma).

Oxygenation

Blood gases also give an excellent measurement of tissue perfusion through measurement of the pO_2 and the O_2 saturation of Hb. Normal pO_2 values should be between 90 and 100 mm Hg, while O_2 saturation should be 100%. Low values of either or both of these numbers flag underlying pathology. The major causes of low values for these measurements are myocardial infarction, pulmonary embolus, severe pulmonary interstitial disease (e.g., interstitial pneumonia), and tissue anoxic states secondary to hypoperfusion, as in septicemia and severe congestive heart failure. In pulmonary embolus, the pulmonary circulation is blocked by the embolus, despite adequate ventilation, giving rise to ventilation/perfusion inequalities. The hallmark of pulmonary embolus is a marked drop in the pO_2.

Hypercarbia as a Cause of Hypoxia

Another major cause of hypoxic states in arterial blood is CO_2 retentive states, as in severe COPD. This occurs because, as CO_2 builds up in alveoli, it reduces the volume of O_2 in the air space. At pCO_2 values of over 50 mm Hg, the effect on alveolar pO_2, represented as P_AO_2, becomes important, as illustrated in Figure 8-2. Oxygen, unlike CO_2, is not soluble in water or membranes, so that there is a difference of about 10–15 mm Hg pressure between alveolar and arterial O_2 (represented as P_aO_2), called the A–a gradient. Thus the P_aO_2 is even lower than the decreased P_AO_2. It is important to remember that the total oxygen breathed in, called the P_IO_2, is partitioned, therefore, between the alveolar sac and the arterial blood. This relationship may be written as follows:

$$P_IO_2 = P_AO_2 + P_aO_2 \quad \textbf{(8-10)}$$

For each mole of O_2 consumed, approximately 0.8 mole of CO_2 is produced. The ratio of CO_2 produced to O_2 consumed is called the respiratory quotient, or the RQ. The P_aO_2 may be written as P_aCO_2/RQ. Overall, Equation 8-10 can be rewritten as follows:

$$P_AO_2 = P_IO_2 - P_aCO_2/RQ \quad \textbf{(8-11)}$$

For an RQ of 0.8:

$$P_AO_2 = P_IO_2 - 1.25 \times P_aCO_2 \quad \textbf{(8-12)}$$

This equation states that, for each increment in the P_aCO_2, there will be a more than one-to-one decrease in the P_AO_2. This will result in severe O_2 deficits.

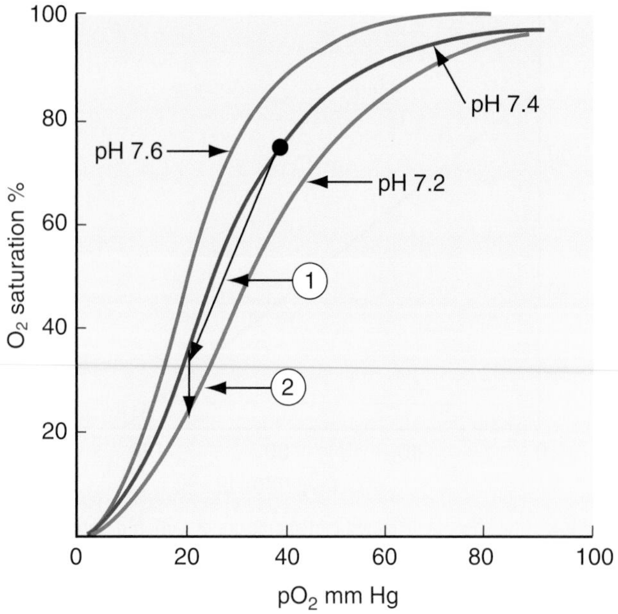

Figure 8-3 The effects of decreasing partial pressure of oxygen (pO_2) in the allosteric zone of the oxygen-hemoglobin dissociation curve. On the pH 7.4 *(middle)* curve, if the pO_2 drops from 80 to 60 mm Hg, little effect on oxygen saturation is seen. However, a drop from 40 to 20 mm Hg results in a large drop in oxygen saturation, from about 80% to 30% *(arrow 1 in the figure).* Combined with this low oxygen saturation is a marked tissue lactic acidosis from anaerobic metabolism. The increased acidosis results in a drop in blood pH to 7.2, shifting the oxygen-hemoglobin dissociation to the right (pH, 7.2 curve). Now, for a pO_2 of 20 mm Hg, the oxygen saturation drops even farther *(arrow 2 in the figure)* to about 20%, setting a vicious circle in motion.

Figure 8-3 is the oxygen-hemoglobin dissociation curve. Note that the curve is sigmoidal because of the allosteric nature of the binding of oxygen to hemoglobin. For pO_2 values between 70 and 100 mm Hg, the saturation of hemoglobin is close to 100%. But at pO_2 values <70 mm Hg, a steep drop in the saturation fraction is noted, so that small drops in pO_2 lead to large decreases in percent saturation. Compounding this effect is the disproportionate decrease in pO_2 whenever pCO_2 increases, as described previously. While these detrimental events transpire, tissue perfusion severely diminishes because of the diminished O_2 saturation of arterial blood. The result is tissue acidosis (mainly from lactic acid as a result of anaerobic metabolism). Acidosis shifts the oxygen-hemoglobin dissociation to the right, as in Figure 8-3, causing even lower saturation for a given pO_2, causing further diminished tissue perfusion and more tissue acidosis. This vicious cycle can be corrected by placing the patient on a respirator to cause increased expiration of CO_2.

The pattern of arterial blood gas determinations for this type of patient will be low arterial blood pH, low pO_2, low O_2 saturation, high pCO_2, and low bicarbonate. This pattern is not typical of the four basic patterns given in Table 8-4 because, on top of a fundamental respiratory acidosis (high pCO_2), there is a superimposed tissue metabolic lactic acidosis, causing low bicarbonate. These findings, together with the low pO_2, indicate the immediate need for ventilation of the patient on a respirator.

Unlike in myocardial infarction and pulmonary embolus, treatment of the acute hypercarbic state calls for not administering O_2 unless the patient is being adequately ventilated. Hypercarbia induces a CO_2-induced inhibition of the respiratory centers in the pons and the medulla oblongata in the brainstem. In fact, the only impetus to breathe is hypercarbia-induced hypoxia, which causes chemoreceptors in the aortic arch to send signals to the respiratory center in the brain to continue breathing. Administration of O_2 to patients with this condition without ventilation can cause cessation of respiration and the acute demise of the patient.

GLUCOSE ABNORMALITIES

The normal reference interval for fasting serum glucose is generally between 70 and 110 mg/dL. Recently, discussion has involved lowering the upper limit to 100 mg/dL (Nathan, 2009). As described in Chapter 16, the two basic abnormalities that occur with serum glucose levels are hyperglycemia, almost always associated with diabetes mellitus, and hypoglycemia due to iatrogenic (overdose with insulin in the diabetic patient) or to other underlying causes (such as reactive hypoglycemia due to "hypersensitivity" to insulin, insulinoma, etc.). To establish hyperglycemia, it is vital to determine whether the patient has (1) a fasting serum glucose level greater than or equal to 126 mg/dL, (2) a random serum glucose level greater than or equal to 200 mg/dL, or (3) a 2-hour postload plasma glucose concentration greater than or equal to 200 mg/dL during an oral glucose tolerance test (Nathan, 2009). Any one of these findings is diagnostic, if it can be confirmed by repeat testing on a subsequent day (Nathan, 2009).

In the glucose tolerance test, as described in Chapter 16, after giving the patient, who has not eaten for 12 hours overnight, a well-defined amount of glucose orally, blood and urine glucose levels are followed. Normally, serum glucose levels rise and then fall within about a 2-hour period. If the glucose levels remain elevated, however, the diagnosis of diabetes mellitus may again be made. If glucose is detected in the urine at any point, evidence for this condition is also obtained, although absence of urinary glucose does not in any way rule out diabetes mellitus.

High levels of serum glucose also result in the glycosylation of Hb. Glycosylated Hb levels change slowly over time and therefore constitute a stable and reliable indicator of serum glucose levels over the past 2–3 months. Glycosylated Hb levels that are greater than 6.5% are considered to be indicative of diabetes mellitus (Nathan, 2009), and efficacy of treatment is gauged by whether this serum level is reduced to less than 6.5%. Of all the methods for diagnosing and especially for monitoring the treatment of diabetes mellitus, measurement of glycosylated Hb levels is perhaps the most accurate and should be done in conjunction with blood glucose determinations (Blincko, 2001; Krishnamurti, 2001; Kilpatrick, 2004; Nathan, 2009).

Other Abnormal Laboratory Findings in Diabetes Mellitus

As discussed earlier in the electrolyte section, under the influence of insulin, whenever glucose is transported into the cell, it is accompanied by potassium. In diabetes, in the absence of insulin, blood glucose is elevated, as is potassium. Increased metabolism of fats leads to a buildup of acetoacetic acid, resulting in a metabolic acidosis. In diabetes where the blood glucose becomes exceptionally elevated (i.e., >300 mg/dL), serum osmolality becomes dangerously high and can cause nonketotic, hyperosmolar coma. In this condition, red (and white) cell water flows from the cells into the vascular volume, tending to dilute analytes such as sodium. Thus the nonketotic, hyperosmolar coma patient may have a hyperosmolar serum, hyperglycemia, hyperkalemia, and hyponatremia. In ketotic states, the patient will have, additionally, a metabolic acidosis and a large anion gap.

Hypoglycemia

Serum glucose levels of <60 mg/dL on a series of random fasting serum specimens strongly suggest hypoglycemia. The low glucose values should be associated with adrenergic and/or neuroglycopenic symptoms, which are relieved upon administration of glucose (Whipple's triad). Glucose tolerance tests show that after an initial sharp rise in serum glucose levels, an abnormally rapid drop occurs to levels substantially below 60 mg/dL. If hypoglycemia is suspected, it is advisable to give the patient a 5-hour glucose tolerance test because the hypoglycemic "dip" often is not seen until after 3 hours. Glucose tolerance tests should be performed with great caution in patients with suspected hypoglycemia because the procedure can induce severe reactive hypoglycemia, causing loss of consciousness and even shock.

LIVER FUNCTION TESTS

Liver function is discussed in depth in Chapter 21. In that chapter, a detailed breakdown is given of different patterns in abnormal liver function tests. The reader will find it difficult to retain these patterns without a basic understanding of the underlying principles. We can reduce the most common liver test abnormalities to a set of six conditions, which are summarized in Table 8-5. The principles for these patterns are explained as follows:

1. **Hepatitis and acute injuries and/or necrotic lesions** in the liver cause primarily a marked rise in the levels of aminotransferases, aspartate aminotransferase (AST) and alanine aminotransferase (ALT). Cell injury and necrosis also cause a rise in other enzymes such as LD. These include acute hepatitis (e.g., infectious,

TABLE 8-5
Six Fundamental Patterns of Liver Function Tests

Condition	AST	ALT	LD	AP	TP	Albumin	Bilirubin	Ammonia
1. Hepatitis	H	H	H	H	N	N	H	N
2. Cirrhosis	N	N	N	N–sl H	L	L	H	H
3. Biliary obstruction	N	N	N	H	N	N	H	N
4. Space-occupying lesion	N or H	N or H	H	H	N	N	N–H	N
5. Passive congestion	Sl H	sl H	sl H	N–sl H	N	N	N–sl H	N
6. Fulminant failure	Very H	H	H	H	L	L	H	H

ALT, Alanine aminotransferase; *AP,* alkaline phosphatase; *AST,* aspartate aminotransferase; *H,* high; *L,* low; *LD,* lactate dehydrogenase; *N,* normal; *sl,* slightly; *TP,* total protein.

chemically induced), infarction, and trauma. The biliary tract is always affected, so that direct bilirubin rises from interference with bile flow. Because of biliary tract injury, the enzyme alkaline phosphatase (AP) rises, along with γ-glutamyl transferase (GGT) and 5′-nucleotidase (5′-N). Hepatocyte injury causes loss of conjugation of transported bilirubin, so that indirect (unconjugated) bilirubin also rises. Because, generally, in hepatitis, much less than 80% of the liver is destroyed, total regeneration will occur, and enough tissue is present to enable adequate levels of protein synthesis and ammonia fixation as urea. Therefore, total protein and albumin and ammonia levels remain normal. These typical results are summarized in condition 1 of Table 8-5.

2. **Cirrhosis** of the liver is characterized by two cardinal features: Fibrosis, preventing regeneration of liver tissue wherever this has occurred, and nodules of regenerating liver tissue, which are the only source of any kind of hepatocytic function. Thus, in cirrhosis, as shown in condition 2 of Table 8-5, almost the reverse pattern occurs from the one seen in condition 1 in Table 8-5 for hepatitis. Because, in panhepatic cirrhosis, destruction of >80% of liver tissue occurs, with no regeneration of damaged liver tissue, the AST/ALT aminotransferases and LD levels (all from the regenerating nodules) tend to be normal or low or occasionally mildly elevated. However, total protein and albumin are both abnormally low. Because the liver is the sole site of ammonia detoxification via the urea cycle, and because, in this condition, loss of hepatocytic function occurs, serum ammonia levels are elevated. Because insufficient viable liver tissue remains, and because fibrosis destroys the cholangioles, both indirect and direct bilirubin tend to be elevated.
3. **Acute biliary obstruction** caused by stones in the biliary tree, or by neoplasms that block bile excretion, results in elevations in direct bilirubin and biliary tract AP, along with the enzymes GGT and 5′-N (see earlier). All other liver function test results are normal. For simple biliary obstruction, therefore, the pattern is as shown in condition 3 of Table 8-5.
4. **Space-occupying lesions** of the liver are characterized, for reasons that are not well understood, by isolated elevations of the enzymes AP and LD. This pattern is shown in condition 4 of Table 8-5. The most common cause of this condition is metastatic carcinoma to the liver.
5. **Passive congestion** of the liver is characterized by a mild elevation of aminotransferases (AST/ALT) and LD and, in more severe cases, by elevations of total bilirubin and AP. This pattern is also seen in infectious mononucleosis, where the rise in bilirubin may be marked. The general passive congestion pattern is shown in condition 5 of Table 8-5.
6. **Acute fulminant hepatic failure** from a variety of causes, which include Reye's syndrome and hepatitis C (Gill, 2001; Schiodt, 2003), is discussed in Chapter 21. This condition is total liver failure. The overall pattern (Sunheimer, 1994) is shown in condition 6 of Table 8-5. It appears as a combination of hepatitis and cirrhosis. Here AST and ALT reach exceptionally high values, often in excess of 10,000 IU/L. At the same time, total protein and albumin are markedly reduced, and ammonia levels are abnormally elevated, causing hepatic encephalopathy. LD, AP, and bilirubin are also elevated. Besides the marked rise in AST and ALT, combined with hyperammonemia, a characteristic disproportionate rise in AST over ALT occurs, further confirming the diagnosis. It is vital to recognize this pattern because the underlying condition is a medical emergency, which must be treated promptly.

Correlations of Liver Function Test Results With Other Laboratory Findings

In severe liver failure secondary to cirrhosis or to fulminant hepatic failure, it is not uncommon to find electrolyte abnormalities and abnormalities in renal function tests, and in the coagulation profile. Patients with condition 2 or 6 in Table 8-5 often have ascites, with marked third space fluid loss. This results in increased levels of both ADH and aldosterone to retain intravascular water. Depending on which levels "win out," the patient may become hyponatremic or hypernatremic.

Severe liver failure can also cause the hepatorenal syndrome (i.e., renal dysfunction secondary to hepatic failure). This disease is characterized by the typical patterns shown in conditions 2 and 6 in Table 8-5. As discussed earlier in the Renal section, renal failure results in elevations in BUN and creatinine, with a 10–20 : 1 ratio indicative of renal failure. The Uosm/Posm ratio is <1.2 : 1, indicating tubular dysfunction.

Severe coagulopathies with elevated APTTs and PTs may be seen because of the absence of production of coagulation factors. Not infrequently, DIC will accompany liver failure. This condition must be distinguished from low coagulation factor production combined with hepatosplenomegaly due to portal hypertension as in cirrhosis. The splenomegaly may result in sequestration of platelets, so that the overall pattern may resemble DIC but may not be true DIC. To clinch the diagnosis of DIC, elevations of D-dimer levels should be noted. Because in DIC, emboli occur in the microvasculature of different tissues, including bone marrow, bone marrow–induced hemolytic anemia may develop, in which schistocytes, burr cells, and fragmented forms appear in the peripheral blood smear; in addition, nucleated red cells and myeloid precursor cells such as myelocytes and metamyelocytes may be seen in the blood smear, the so-called leukoerythroblastic picture referred to earlier in the Coagulation section. Also, with severe liver failure, abnormal red cell forms, called target cells, may be seen in the peripheral blood smear.

Patients with cirrhosis and acute fulminant hepatic failure tend to be immunocompromised. Many of these patients have defective T cell function but produce an excess of (ineffective) immunoglobulin. Thus these patients tend to have low serum albumin levels from diminished albumin synthesis but elevated serum immunoglobulins.

CARDIAC FUNCTION TESTS

Diagnosis of Myocardial Infarction and Acute Coronary Syndrome

These are discussed at length in Chapter 18. Because acute myocardial infarction (AMI) requires rapid and accurate diagnosis, especially now that new treatment options with thrombolytic agents are available, the clinical laboratory has been called upon to provide serum diagnostic tests that can make this diagnosis at an early stage. Until recently, laboratory diagnosis was based on serial determinations of the MB fraction of creatine phosphokinase (CK-MB); confirmation of the diagnosis was provided by the so-called flipped ratio of the isozymes of LD 24–36 hours after the initial acute event and/or by observation of the characteristic time courses for elevations of the three enzymes CK, AST, and LD.

These approaches have been replaced mainly by two other analytes, myoglobin (MY) and especially cardiac troponin (cTn), which provide more rapid and specific diagnostic capabilities (Morrow, 2007). MY is an oxygen-binding/transport protein found in both cardiac and skeletal muscle. Its relatively small size and function allow for early release from irreversibly damaged cells. However, current methods of measurement cannot distinguish the tissue of origin of MY. Therefore, its use is confined to screening patients for possible AMI; positive results suggest the need for further workup for AMI.

Troponin is a regulatory protein complex in muscle tissue; it comprises three subunits designated troponin I (TnI), troponin T (TnT), and troponin C (TnC). Different genes encode TnI in skeletal and cardiac muscle, giving rise to isoforms that differ significantly in sequence. Cardiac TnI contains an additional 31 amino acid residues on its N-terminal. Rapid and accurate immunoassays for cardiac TnT and cardiac TnI have been developed. In AMI, cardiac TnI becomes elevated 4–8 hours after onset of chest pain, reaches a peak at about 12–16 hours, and remains elevated for 5–9 days. Values at or above 1.5 ng/mL are considered to be suggestive of AMI. However, because different assays (all immunoassays) measure different domains of TnT and TnI, reference ranges differ depending upon the antibodies used in the assays. Because cTn levels rise relatively rapidly and remain elevated for prolonged times, troponin determinations have replaced the so-called flipped ratio of the two isozymes of LD, LD1 and LD2 (LD2 : LD1 ratio rises to >0.75 and often exceeds 1.0), which occurs only about 36 hours after the onset of symptoms.

CK-MB is another biomarker that can be used in diagnosing AMI. CK-MB has three isozymes composed of two chains (called the M and B chains) which are MM, MB, and BB. The MB fraction is predominantly found in cardiac muscle (Roberts, 1997). To diagnose AMI from CK-MB serum levels, it is important to show a rise both in the concentration of CK-MB and in the ratio of CK-MB to total CK (also called the cardiac index) (Thompson, 1988; Woo, 1992). Because a small amount of CK-MB is found in skeletal muscle, diseases of skeletal muscle that cause the level of CK-MM to rise to high values will also cause the levels of CK-MB to rise to high absolute concentrations in serum, which can cause false-positive values for CK-MB. In addition, to increase both the sensitivity and the specificity of CK-MB in the diagnosis of acute AMI, it has been found necessary to perform serial determinations of MB fraction (at 3- to 4-hour intervals over a 12- to 16-hour period) that show a progressive rise that reaches a peak, followed by a fall to low levels. This pattern is virtually 100% diagnostic of myocardial infarction (Lott, 1984; Wu, 1999). It is important to note that CK-MB generally rises within 4–6 hours, and sometimes only 2 hours, after the onset of chest pain, and peaks within 12 hours. Therefore, MY and CK-MB were recommended (Wu, 1999; Alpert, 2000; Fromm, 2001; Lewandrowski, 2002) for use as early markers of AMI.

However, elevated TnT and TnI levels are more specific for cardiac injury than are elevated CK-MB levels. Similar to CK-MB, they rise within 4–6 hours, and sometimes within 2 hours, after the onset of chest pain.

Current protocols for the laboratory diagnosis of AMI vary and are evolving as assays for cTn improve (see Chapter 18). In some medical centers, TnI or TnT is used exclusively; in other centers, troponin and CK-MB are used together.

Diagnosis of Congestive Heart Failure

Until recently, this condition was diagnosed strictly on the basis of symptoms and/or as a result of procedures such as echocardiography. However, a new biomarker, B-type natriuretic peptide (BNP), has been discovered and approved as a definitive test for this condition and appears to be an excellent marker for early heart failure; this test may also be both diagnostically and prognostically significant in patients presenting with acute dyspnea and chest pain. The differential diagnosis in these patients includes dyspnea caused by chronic heart failure (signs and symptoms of which are typically nonspecific) versus other causes of acute dyspnea (e.g., pneumonia, carcinoma, effusion, asthma). Normal levels (i.e., a high negative predictive value for this test) appear useful in excluding a cardiac origin in these patients. Levels of BNP may also be an independent predictor of arrhythmia, stroke, and death (Clerico, 2004; Ishii, 2003; Mueller, 2004; Prahash, 2004; Wang, 2004; Winter, 2004; Novo, 2009). Studies suggest that serum BNP levels are useful in evaluating the efficacy of treatment of congestive heart failure (Novo, 2009).

PANCREATIC FUNCTION TESTS

Elevations in serum pancreatic amylase and lipase are definitive markers for pancreatic disease. The most common cause for such increases in the serum levels of these enzymes is pancreatitis. In acute pancreatitis, both enzymes are elevated. Because amylase can also be produced by the salivary glands, amylase is slightly less specific than lipase as a marker for pancreatitis. Elevations in the latter enzyme are definitive for pancreatic disease.

MARKERS FOR INFLAMMATORY CONDITIONS

As discussed previously in the Hematology section, increases in the WBC count, especially with a predominance of neutrophils, indicate acute infection. In most acute inflammatory conditions, as noted previously, acute phase reactant proteins are also found to be increased. These proteins occur in the α (including α-1-antitrypsin, α-2-macroglobulin) and β (including ferritin and C-reactive protein [CRP]) regions of the serum protein electrophoretogram, as discussed in Chapter 19 on serum protein electrophoresis. In this regard, quantitative determinations for serum CRP are very helpful in recognizing acute inflammatory states. Recently, specific antibodies to CRP have allowed for highly sensitive measurement of CRP (termed high-sensitivity CRP, or hs-CRP) at lower concentrations than were previously measurable (Roberts, 2000). Currently, elevated levels of hs-CRP appear to serve as an early marker of inflammation and may have utility in assessing cardiovascular risk for stroke and myocardial infarction (Abrams, 2003; Ridker, 2003; Libby, 2004).

Fibrinogen, also an acute phase reactant, may additionally increase. Often, the platelet count tends to rise, and platelets themselves have been considered as "acute phase reactants." In addition, in both acute and chronic inflammatory conditions, erythrocytes exhibit increased mobility. Thus there is an increase in the erythrocyte sedimentation rate. Recent studies suggest that the best marker for inflammation, especially as a guide to therapeutic efficacy, is CRP (Crowson, 2009).

Finally, one common cause of acute inflammation is gout (i.e., hyperuricemia), or elevations of uric acid in serum. Uric acid crystals cause a severe, acute arthritic condition (gout). Serum levels of uric acid >7.5 mg/dL are indicative of this condition. Less constant findings are the presence of uric acid crystals in the urinary sediment (see Chapter 32) or in joint fluid (see Chapter 33).

ENDOCRINE FUNCTION TESTING

We noted that abnormal functioning of the thyroid and adrenal cortex can give rise to important abnormal laboratory findings. Hypothyroidism, for example, can give rise to macrocytic anemia, while hypoadrenalism can give rise to electrolyte abnormalities (i.e., hyponatremia, hyperkalemia, and an acidosis); hyperadrenalism produces the opposite effect (i.e., hypernatremia, hypokalemia, and an alkalosis). It is therefore important to confirm that these endocrine glands are malfunctioning. The important topic of endocrine function testing is discussed in Chapter 24. Here we present simple principles for the laboratory diagnosis and identification of the site of origin of thyroid, adrenal, and parathyroid conditions.

Principle

All endocrine systems involve a stimulating hormone that is synthesized and secreted into the blood from one tissue such as the pituitary, the parathyroid glands, etc. These hormones are delivered to their targets, which may be the thyroid gland or the adrenal glands, or a nonendocrine target such as the renal tubules, in the case of the parathyroid glands. In all cases, for normally functioning endocrine systems, *elevations* of the hormones or products elaborated by the targets will result in *decreased* levels of the primary hormones. Conversely, *decreased levels* of the targets will result in *increased* levels of the primary hormones. For example, high levels of circulating T_4 will result in low levels of TSH, a condition called *primary hyperthyroidism*, and, conversely, low levels of T_4 will result in high levels of TSH, a condition called *primary hypothyroidism*. In contrast, if the pituitary gland secretes an excess of TSH because of an adenoma or other pathologic condition, this increase in TSH will result in elevated T_4. This condition is also referred to as *secondary hyperthyroidism*. Thus if *both* T_4 and TSH levels are elevated, a diagnosis of pituitary disease (e.g., pituitary adenoma) in which there is hypersecretion of TSH can be made. Conversely, decreases in both TSH and T_4 point to pituitary hyposecretive states also referred to as *secondary hypothyroidism*. Note that *changes in opposite directions of the stimulating and target hormones/effector molecules point to endocrine target gland (e.g., thyroid gland) disease, while changes in the two hormones in the same direction point to stimulating hormone gland (e.g., pituitary) disease.*

Thyroid Function

Thyroid function tests are the most commonly ordered tests for endocrine function. It is important to note that in a hospital population (as opposed to an ambulatory population), thyroid screening tests may be diagnostically misleading. This is due to endocrine stress responses (as well as medications) that may affect hormone levels (Van den Berghe, 2003). As discussed in Chapter 24, the thyroid gland synthesizes thyroid hormone, tetraiodothyronine, or T_4, with four iodines, which requires iodine uptake by the gland. This activity is strongly stimulated by the peptide hormone, TSH, from the pituitary. In the periphery, T_4 is converted to T_3 (three iodines). More than 99% of T_4 is bound to serum proteins (i.e., thyroid-binding globulin and albumin). However, it is the free T_4 (<1 percent of total T_4) that exerts all biological effects. Accurate methods exist that directly measure serum free T_4. Most commonly, total and free T_4 rise and fall together in serum; however, there are circumstances in which total T_4 may be elevated but T_4-binding proteins may also be elevated, so that free T_4 levels are normal. This may result in a euthyroid state in which TSH levels are also normal. Of prime importance, high T_4 (more correctly, high free T_4) causes inhibition of TSH secretion, and low T_4 (more correctly, low free T_4) causes elevation of TSH. In *primary hypothyroidism* (primary thyroid gland disease), T_4 is present at low serum levels while TSH becomes elevated. It is important to note that often in subclinical hypothyroidism, T_4 can be within the reference range, but TSH is elevated. In ambulatory patients, elevated TSH in the presence of low levels of T_4 is diagnostic of primary hypothyroidism. In *secondary hypothyroidism*, TSH is low because of pituitary failure, resulting in low T_4.

In *primary hyperthyroidism* (primary thyroid gland disease), excess T_4 is secreted by the thyroid gland, which is the source of the problem. As a result, TSH is decreased and T_4 is elevated. If, however, a primary lesion is present in the pituitary gland (e.g., hyperplasia, adenoma), TSH is oversecreted. Because TSH is elevated, T_4 secretion is elevated. This is known as secondary hyperthyroidism (secondary to pituitary disease).

These conditions and their patterns of T_4 and TSH levels are summarized in Table 8-6.

Adrenal Function

As discussed in depth in Chapter 24, the adrenal gland is divided anatomically into two endocrine glands: The adrenal cortex and the adrenal medulla. Adrenal cortical hormones are steroid hormones of three basic types: Mineralocorticoids, like aldosterone, that regulate sodium and potassium ions in the distal convoluted tubule, as discussed earlier; glucocorticoids, like cortisol, that are gluconeogenic; and the sex hormones (i.e., the estrogens and androgens). The adrenal medulla is a neuroendocrine gland that secretes epinephrine and norepinephrine, which act on the sympathetic nervous system. By far the most commonly ordered serum analyte used to measure adrenal cortical function is cortisol. Cortisol secretion by the adrenal cortex is stimulated by the pituitary hormone adrenocorticotropic hormone (ACTH). ACTH secretion, in turn, is stimulated by the hypothalamic hormone corticotropin-releasing hormone (CRH). Its serum levels are under diurnal control such that serum ACTH levels peak at about 200 pg/mL in the morning hours (about 7:00 AM), but they decline to their lowest values of around 100 pg/mL at midnight. Cortisol secretion follows ACTH secretion such that its serum levels are highest at 8:00–9:00 AM. Cortisol inhibits ACTH secretion by the pituitary gland both by directly blocking pituitary ACTH secretion and by inhibiting CRH secretion by the hypothalamus.

Therefore, if the adrenal cortex hypersecretes cortisol secondary to such conditions as adrenal hyperplasia, adenoma, or carcinoma, serum cortisol levels increase and block ACTH secretion. This condition is called primary hyperadrenalism. Serum cortisol levels are elevated (Cushing's syndrome), but ACTH levels decrease.

On the other hand, as with thyroid hormone secretion, if ACTH levels are elevated by an ACTH pituitary tumor (Cushing's disease) or as ectopic ACTH secretion (e.g., by a nonpituitary tumor), cortisol levels will also increase, giving rise to secondary hyperadrenalism. Both cortisol and ACTH are elevated in this condition. Here, note that both cortisol and ACTH change in the same direction (both are elevated), pointing to pituitary, not adrenal disease. In cases of Cushing's disease or syndrome, the diurnal variation in serum ACTH is absent.

In addition to measurements of serum cortisol, it is often desirable to measure urinary free cortisol in cases of hypercortisolemia. Normally, almost all cortisol is bound to serum protein, mainly transcortin, but, in hypercortisol states, cortisol exceeds the capacity of transcortin to bind to it and is consequently filtered by the kidneys. The reference range for morning serum cortisol is ≈ 10–25 μg/dL, and for urinary free cortisol, ≈ 24–108 μg/24 h for healthy males.

In cases of hypercortisolism, especially when ACTH levels may remain in the reference range or have "borderline" high or low values, it is often desirable to perform the dexamethasone suppression test. Dexamethasone is a potent glucocorticoid that strongly suppresses normal pituitary ACTH secretion. This can be accomplished with low-dose dexamethasone. If low-dose dexamethasone causes diminished serum cortisol levels and low values for urinary free cortisol, pituitary function is most likely normal while the adrenals are hypersecreting cortisol (i.e., primary hyperadrenalism). This test may be used further to distinguish the possible source of primary hyperadrenalism (i.e., hyperplasia vs. adenoma or carcinoma). High-dose dexamethasone will generally lower serum cortisol levels in adrenal hyperplasia, but it will have no effect in adrenal adenoma or carcinoma.

Conversely, in pituitary failure, serum ACTH levels decrease, as do serum cortisol levels, because ACTH stimulation of the adrenal gland decreases. This condition is referred to as secondary hypoadrenalism. If adrenal gland function is compromised (primary adrenal insufficiency), serum cortisol levels are decreased, resulting in less inhibition of pituitary secretion of ACTH and, consequently, in elevated serum levels of ACTH. This condition is referred to as primary hypoadrenalism, or Addison's disease. These conditions and the patterns of serum cortisol and ACTH levels in these conditions, including dexamethasone suppression test results where relevant, are summarized in Table 8-7.

Parathyroid Hormone and Vitamin D

In the previous Renal Disease section, it was noted that PTH induces elevated serum calcium levels by causing increased secretion of phosphate in the renal tubules and by promoting increased calcium ion absorption in the gut. Hypocalcemia with elevated PTH points to causes having to do with calcium metabolism (e.g., alkalotic states, decreased albumin, low dietary calcium and/or lack of absorption of calcium from the gut, low vitamin D levels). Hypocalcemia with low serum PTH levels points to parathyroid gland dysfunction. In rare instances, hypocalcemia that is not responsive to calcium infusions and vitamin D supplements can be caused by secretion of high levels of calcitonin, a serum calcium-lowering peptide that blocks osteoclastic resorption of bone (with attendant increases in serum calcium). Calcitonin is synthesized and secreted from the medullary cells of the thyroid. In medullary thyroid carcinoma, high levels of calcitonin are sometimes secreted. At high levels of calcitonin, hypocalcemia will result.

Hypercalcemia with low PTH again points to primary calcium metabolic causes, as in the "CHIMPS" mnemonic mentioned earlier, and acidotic states, while hypercalcemia with elevated PTH indicates parathyroid disease such as adenoma (most commonly) or carcinoma (uncommon). These conditions and the patterns of serum calcium and parathyroid hormone levels in serum in these conditions are summarized in Table 8-8.

Vitamin D

Vitamin D induces absorption of calcium from the gut by acting on vitamin D receptors in the cells lining the gut. It is produced from 7-dehydrocholesterol in skin by ultraviolet light that induces the synthesis of cholecalciferol. In the liver, cholecalciferol is converted to 25-hydroxycholecalciferol, which has a half-life of several weeks. This form is further hydroxylated in the kidneys to 1,25-dihydroxycholecalciferol, the active form of vitamin D. The half-life of active vitamin D is on the order of hours. Thus, in serum assays for vitamin D, the analyte whose serum level best reflects vitamin D levels is the precursor, 25-hydroxycholecalciferol (Zerwekh, 2008). This may give falsely elevated

TABLE 8-6

Patterns of Serum Levels of TSH and T_4 in Different Thyroid Gland Conditions

Condition	T_4 (most accurate, free T_4)	TSH	Site of disease
Euthyroid	Normal	Normal	None
Primary hypothyroidism	Low	High	Thyroid gland
Secondary hypothyroidism	Low	Low to normal	Pituitary
Primary hyperthyroidism	High	Low	Thyroid
Secondary hyperthyroidism	High	High	Pituitary

T_4, Thyroxine; *TSH,* thyroid-stimulating hormone.

TABLE 8-7
Patterns of Serum Levels of ACTH and Cortisol in Different Adrenal Gland Conditions

Condition	Cortisol	ACTH	Dexamethasone suppression, low dose	Dexamethasone suppression, high dose	Site of disease
Normal adrenal	Normal	Normal	N/A	N/A	None
Primary hypoadrenalism	Low	High	N/A	N/A	Adrenal gland
Secondary hypoadrenalism	Low	Low	N/A	N/A	Pituitary
Primary hyperadrenalism–high cortisol, low ACTH	High	Low	N/A	N/A	Adrenal
Primary hyperadrenalism–high cortisol, borderline low ACTH	High	Borderline low	Positive	N/A	Adrenal
Primary hyperadrenalism due to adrenal hyperplasia–high cortisol, borderline low ACTH	High	Borderline low	Negative	Positive	Adrenal
Primary hyperadrenalism due to adrenal adenoma/carcinoma–high cortisol, borderline low ACTH	High	Borderline low	Negative	Negative	Adrenal
Secondary hyperadrenalism	High	High	N/A	N/A	Pituitary

ACTH, Adrenocorticotropic hormone; *N/A,* not applicable.

TABLE 8-8
Patterns of Serum Levels of Calcium and PTH in Different Conditions

Condition*	Ionized calcium	PTH	Cause of disease
Normocalcemia	Normal	Normal	None
"Primary" hypocalcemia	Low	High	CHARD†
"Secondary" hypocalcemia	Low	Low	Parathyroid glands
"Primary" hypercalcemia	High	Low	Cancer, hyperthyroidism, iatrogenic causes, multiple myeloma, sarcoidosis
"Secondary" hypercalcemia	High	High	Parathyroid glands (e.g., adenoma, carcinoma)

PTH, Parathyroid hormone.
*The terms "primary" and "secondary" are not usually used for hypocalcemia and hypercalcemia. They are used here to emphasize the site of the disease to keep consistent with the conditions described in Tables 8-6 and 8-7.
†Mnemonic for **C**alcitonin, **H**ypoparathyroidism, **A**lkalosis, **R**enal failure, vitamin **D** deficit.

levels of vitamin D in cases of renal failure where conversion of the precursor to active vitamin D is impaired. However, 25-hydroxycholecalciferol itself has some effects on calcium reabsorption, although its affinity for the vitamin D receptor is only about one-one thousandth of that for the fully active form. The reference range for serum 25-hydroxycholecalciferol, also called 25-hydroxy vitamin D, is 30–100 ng/mL, although this is method dependent (Yates, 2008).

Over the past few years, requests for serum vitamin D levels, especially in the pediatric and geriatric populations, have greatly increased. This is due at least in part to the availability of reliable chromatographic, mass spectroscopic, and immunochemical methods that quantitate serum vitamin D levels. In the pediatric population, vitamin D levels are determined and followed for the diagnosis and treatment of vitamin D–dependent rickets. In the elderly, vitamin D levels are determined in the treatment of such diseases as osteoporosis and osteomalacia, because vitamin D supplements have been found to diminish the extent and severity of these diseases.

The discovery that many cells, besides epithelial cells of the gut, the principal site of vitamin D activity, have abundant receptors for vitamin D suggests that this vitamin has effects that go beyond regulation of calcium homeostasis (Bilke, 2009). Indeed, it has been found that vitamin D induces apoptosis in breast cancer and other malignant cells and has been used to treat such diseases as multiple sclerosis, heart failure, psoriasis, asthma, Crohn's disease, and many other conditions. Thus the demand for vitamin D levels has increased for patients with a wide variety of conditions.

Examples of Clinical Cases With Clinicopathologic Correlations

Given the previous overview of many salient features of the causes of the more common abnormal laboratory findings, laboratory results from a number of different patients are now presented to illustrate how analyte levels change in different disease states, and how these analyte concentrations are used to diagnose these conditions.

CASE A

A 64-year-old white male was found unconscious in his home after suffering a cerebrovascular accident (CVA) and was brought to the emergency medicine department. His Hct was 44%, but RBC count was 4.3 million/μL (lower limit of normal, 4.6 million/μL) with an MCV of 104 fL; a series of serum sodium values ranged from 164–175 mEq/L; admission BUN was 33 mg/dL; creatinine was 1.5 mg/dL. Total serum osmolality was 357 mOsm/kg (upper limit of normal, 290 mOsm/kg), and urine osmolality was 1008 mOsm/kg (upper limit of normal, 1000 mOsm/kg) and random urine sodium was 228 mEq/L.

A liver panel showed a marginally elevated AST at 41 IU/L (upper limit of normal, 39 IU/L), elevated but continually decreasing LD (admission value of 426 IU/L; upper limit of normal, 200 IU/L), GGT of 72 U/L (upper limit of normal, 43 IU/L), and total protein of 7.8 g/dL (normal), but a low albumin of 2.8 g/dL (normal 3.5–5.0 g/dL). Lipase was mildly elevated at 127 IU/L (upper limit of normal, 60 IU/L). Occult blood found in his stool was positive for *Clostridium difficile.* Urine was nitrite positive (indicative of bacteriuria) and was markedly positive for Hb, RBCs, and WBCs. After infusion of half-normal saline, the Hct was reduced to 34% but then rose to 38%, with a persistently elevated MCV. The sodium and the BUN were reduced to within the reference range.

Evaluation

The basic diagnosis of this patient's condition is hypernatremia. This patient was dehydrated as shown by the markedly elevated serum sodium (average value of 169 mEq/L), high normal Hct, and elevated BUN. Note that the diagnosis of dehydration was confirmed by the findings of high serum and urinary (228 mEq/L) sodium and high urinary osmolality of 1008 mOsm/kg (see Table 8-3). The RBC count was low, which seems to contradict the high normal Hct. This apparent discrepancy may be explained by the macrocytosis, causing each erythrocyte to occupy a greater than normal volume. Yet the total number of cells was reduced. The low red cell count indicates a true anemia. The macrocytosis was caused by a nutritional (vitamin B_{12}) deficiency. All of these findings may be attributed to malnutrition and insufficient fluid consumption, a not uncommon finding in the elderly, especially in this stroke victim.

Note that the BUN and creatinine were mildly elevated in a pattern with a ratio >20:1, suggesting a prerenal (low perfusion) origin. The renal tubules were evidently functioning well, as evidenced by the high urine/

serum osmolality ratio (1008/357 = 2.8, which is greater than 1.2 : 1). Hypoperfusion may have caused the mild abnormalities found in some of the liver function tests and the elevated pancreatic lipase.

Note also that the total protein was normal, even though the albumin, the most abundant serum protein, was low. Because of possibly two infectious diseases identified in urine and stool examinations, the patient may have produced elevated levels of immunoglobulins. Accompanying the CVA was a peptic ulcer, so-called Cushing's ulcer, known to be associated with this condition; hence the occult blood in this patient's stool. *C. difficile* is known to infect patients with chronic debilitating disease. The urinary tract infection was responsible for the high RBC count and Hb in this patient's urine. The next case illustrates a more complex electrolyte disorder.

CASE B

A 31-year-old white male patient with known type 1 diabetes mellitus, end-stage renal disease secondary to diabetic nephropathy, and a history of alcoholism was admitted with acute abdominal pain in the midepigastrium, with a serum glucose of 736 mg/dL that rose as high as 933 mg/dL; serum sodium of 134 mEq/L, which decreased to as low as 124 mEq/L; potassium of 7.1 mEq/L, BUN of 64 mg/dL, and creatinine of 18 mg/dL. These values were confirmed and were found to follow a consistent trend. Serum osmolality was 316 mOsm/kg. Blood gas values on admission were pH of 7.58, pO_2 of 121 mm Hg, O_2 saturation of 99%, pCO_2 of 20 mm Hg, and bicarbonate of 20 mEq/L. The anion gap rose in one day from 13 (high end of normal) to 20. Serum lipase was elevated at 469 IU/L (upper limit of normal is 60 IU/L). There was no urine output, and the patient was subjected to peritoneal dialysis.

Evaluation

This diabetic patient was evidently in a hyperosmolar state because of abnormally elevated glucose levels. The low serum sodium and high serum potassium might appear to be due to low circulating aldosterone or renal tubular failure. However, there was no urine output, so no filtration could occur. The end-stage renal disease is reflected in the BUN and especially in the creatinine value (18 mg/dL). The BUN/creatinine ratio of about 4 confirms the diagnosis of true renal failure.

As noted in the discussion on glucose, in diabetes mellitus with high serum glucose levels, an efflux of cell water causes dilution of serum analytes such as sodium. Whenever glucose is transported into cells under the influence of insulin, it is accompanied by potassium. Low insulin levels can therefore result in hyperkalemia. This mechanism was operative in this patient. Although the anion gap increased after admission, it was normal on admission. Thus this patient was in a nonketotic, hyperosmolar state but subsequently became ketotic. The admission blood gas picture suggests a respiratory alkalosis in that the arterial blood pH was 7.57 (alkalosis), but the pCO_2 was low at 20 mm Hg, and the bicarbonate was low at 20 mEq/L (condition 4 in Table 8-4). This is an unusual finding in a patient with diabetes mellitus in whom a finding of metabolic acidosis is more frequently encountered.

An explanation for this finding may be found in the serum lipase, which was markedly elevated, denoting pancreatitis, a common finding in patients with a history of alcoholism. The sharp epigastric pain caused increased respiration (respiratory rate on admission was 25/min), precipitating a lowering of the pCO_2, which was partially compensated for by lowering of the bicarbonate.

Treatment of this patient with dialysis, hydration, and insulin corrected the abnormal laboratory findings, and the patient was discharged on long-term dialysis.

The next case presents multiple disorders, including electrolyte disorders, all related to liver failure.

CASE C

A 38-year-old white female with a past medical history of multiple abdominal surgical procedures over a 7-year period, sporadic alcohol abuse, pancreatitis, and a 30 pack-year history of smoking, was brought to the emergency department in shock and acute abdominal distress. Significant laboratory values included WBC count of $12.1 \times 10^3/\mu L$, RBC count of $3.0 \times 10^6/\mu L$, Hct of 34.6%, and red cell indices that showed macrocytosis and hypochromia (low mean corpuscular Hb concentration). Vitamin B_{12} and folate levels were normal. The peripheral blood smear showed a leukoerythroblastic pattern. Serum glucose was low at 38 mg/dL; total protein was 4.3 g/dL, and albumin 1.5 g/dL. Lactate levels were elevated. The AP was elevated at 241 IU/L (upper limit of normal, 129 IU/L), and the bilirubin was mildly elevated at 1.6 mg/dL (upper limit of normal, 1.2 mg/dL). Serum ammonia was found to be elevated at 146 μmol/L (upper limit of normal, 30 μM). Screens for hepatitis A, B, and C were all negative. The patient was placed on broad-spectrum antibiotics. Multiple blood, urine, and throat cultures were negative. Exploratory laparotomy revealed abdominal adhesions and cholestasis. Postoperatively, the patient became encephalopathic; her liver function deteriorated, as evidenced by dramatic elevations of AST and ALT from normal levels to 1660 and 545 IU/L, respectively; of LD to 2190 IU/L; of bilirubin to 14.5 mg/dL; and of ammonia to 177 μM, despite lactulose administration. A liver–spleen scan performed on the fifth hospital day showed no dye uptake in the liver, consistent with functional liver failure. The serum sodium, normal on admission, increased within 5 days to 166 mEq/L, together with chloride levels that rose to 123 mEq/L—a pattern that persisted throughout the hospital course despite aggressive intravenous infusion of half-normal saline. Serum potassium was consistently <3.5 mEq/L. The BUN and creatinine both rose to abnormally high levels with a ratio of <20:1, suggesting renal failure. Plasma aldosterone was elevated at 13.2 ng/dL (upper limit of normal = 8.5 ng/dL). The platelet count dropped rapidly, while APTT and PT rose to values at least twice those of the corresponding normal controls, and her level of fibrin split products (FSPs) became abnormally elevated. Her condition worsened, and the patient expired on the eighth hospital day.

Evaluation

Although this is a complex patient presentation, the fundamental problem with this patient lay in the dramatically abnormal liver function test profile. Note the acute elevation in aminotransferases (transaminases), with AST/ALT ratios significantly greater than 1. Concurrent rapid elevations in bilirubin and in LD were noted. At the same time, the total protein and albumin were abnormally low. Ammonia levels rose rapidly (despite high doses of lactulose). The pattern is that of fulminant hepatic failure shown in condition 6 in Table 8-5. This condition is a medical emergency and is associated with fatal encephalopathy and severe DIC, as evidenced by the low platelet counts and elevated PT, APTT, and FSP levels. This condition can cause multiple system infarcts, resulting in multiple organ failure.

The patient's peripheral blood picture showed a macrocytosis but, concurrently, a leukoerythroblastic picture. This pattern suggests that the macrocytosis was caused by an increased number of erythrocyte precursor forms. This condition was most likely caused by DIC, which causes MHA with a leukoerythroblastic picture. It is also possible that, with the persistently elevated white cell count and the elevated lactate levels, gram-negative sepsis affecting bone marrow may have contributed to the leukoerythroblastic picture. Although cultures were consistently negative, the patient was being treated with broad-spectrum antibiotics, the effects of which may have blocked growth of the organism(s) in culture. As noted previously, patients with liver failure from cirrhosis or acute fulminant hepatic failure are generally immunocompromised. In both panhepatic cirrhosis and fulminant hepatic failure, severe third space fluid loss is associated with ascites, which invariably develops. We noted previously that, to retain vascular volume, both aldosterone and ADH rise. It appears that aldosterone became elevated to markedly high values, causing abnormal sodium retention and potassium loss in this patient. Almost always accompanying both cirrhosis and acute fulminant hepatic failure is renal failure, generally manifested by the hepatorenal syndrome. In fulminant hepatic failure, an additional possible cause is acute tubular necrosis (Sunheimer, 1994).

SELECTED REFERENCES

Bakerman S, Strausbauch P. ABC's of interpretive laboratory data. 2nd ed. Myrtle Beach, S.C.: Interpretive Laboratory Data; 1994.

This is an excellent review not only of the use of laboratory testing but also of the underlying methods.

Bonini P, Plebani M, Ceriotti F, Rubboli F. Errors in laboratory medicine. Clin Chem 2002;48:691–8.

This is an important review of laboratory errors and how to recognize them.

Nathan D (corresponding author for the International Expert Committee, American Diabetes Association). International Expert Committee report on the role of the A1C assay in the diagnosis of diabetes. Diabetes Care 2009;32:1327–34.

This summarizes the current standards for diagnosis of diabetes mellitus.

Oh M. Acid-base, electrolytes. Old Westbury, N.Y.: OHCO, LLC; 2003.

This is an excellent, concise discussion of renal physiology, electrolyte regulation, and acid-base balance.

Sunheimer R, Capaldo G, Kashanian F, et al. Serum analyte pattern characteristic of fulminant hepatic failure. Ann Clin Lab Sci 1994;24:101–9.

This paper summarizes serum liver function analyte patterns that have been found to occur in this uncommon but fatal disease. It correlates analyte patterns with tissue pathologic findings.

REFERENCES

Access the complete reference list online at http://www.expertconsult.com

CHAPTER 9

LABORATORY STATISTICS

Richard A. McPherson

KEY POINTS

- For statistical analyses, nominal variables can take on only a limited number of values (or categories), whereas continuous variables are used to report quantitative data.
- Independent variables are considered input (cause), and dependent variables are considered output (effect).
- Distributions of continuous data are described by a measure of central tendency (e.g., mean or median) and dispersion (standard deviation). Gaussian distributions derive from a mathematical formula and hence are parametric. A common application of descriptive statistics is to establish reference ranges.
- Statistical tests such as comparisons of different groups of data points may be parametric (i.e., assume Gaussian distributions; example is Student *t*-test) or nonparametric (i.e., make no assumption of distributions; example is test based on rank order).
- Confidence intervals are preferable over point estimates to express level of certainty in the calculation of any statistical parameter.
- Nominal data are conveniently analyzed with proportions using the chi-square test.
- The effects of multiple factors in a model system can be assessed through analysis of variance.
- Regression analysis between two continuous variables is usually done by least squares fit to a straight line. Applications of regression analysis are common when different analytic methods for validation are compared in clinical laboratories.

The quantification of information in meaningful summaries and comparisons is the domain of statistical analysis. The first task in analysis is to provide a description of the magnitude of the observations and how close the different measurements are to one another. Descriptive statistics provides a consistent framework for calculating or estimating the central tendency of continuous data in the familiar forms of mean, median, and mode. The variation in data is generally described by the mathematical calculations of variances and standard deviations, or by the simple allocation of data points into a range of percentiles (e.g., interquartile range). These approaches are everyday phenomena in clinical laboratories for the monitoring of all quantitative assays. Reference ranges are initially set up with these techniques. Methods of quality control for precision and proficiency testing for accuracy also are based on these principles. For data that are not continuous but take on only two or a few discrete values (e.g., positive or negative), the analysis might consist of counting the number in each category and looking at the proportions of all values by category.

Comparison of data typically asks the question whether one group is different from another group. These comparisons are usually done by *t*-test or by analysis of variance, depending on whether two or more groups of continuous data are compared. If the data are discrete, comparison is done by chi-square analysis. When data can take on a range of different values, it is convenient to do a correlation between two different data sets with a straight line fit. The newcomer to statistical analysis frequently poses the question: Which statistical test is best? The question of which test to use depends largely on whether the data are continuous or discrete, and whether continuous data follow particular distributions. However, statistics is based on convention, so that the investigator should try very diligently to understand the importance of differences between tests, and whether possible findings and conclusions are likely to reflect accurately the nature and significance of the question being asked. In contrast to the investigator who is interested in finding the right test for data already collected, the statistician is more interested in helping the investigator plan the experiment and collect data, so that statistical tests are most valid. This chapter relies heavily on common clinical laboratory examples for which specific statistical tests are applied to demonstrate some useful choices.

DEFINITIONS

- *Variables:* The things that we measure, count, or otherwise delineate are termed *variables* because the values they can assume vary. Variables are usually considered to fall into one of the following scales:
  - *Nominal scale* is where a variable can take on only a limited number of values, usually called categories (or characters). Examples of nominal variables are gender (male or female) and risk factors (e.g., smoker or nonsmoker).
  - *Ordinal scale* is where the variable takes on specific values that have some inherent order such as magnitude but without equivalent distances between categories (e.g., trace amount, 1+, 2+, etc. of protein in urine).
  - *Interval scale* is where a variable takes on values in a quantitative range with defined differences between points. It is conventional to treat most numeric laboratory measurements as continuous variables, even though they may be reported as discrete values (e.g., glucose values of 123 or 124 mg/dL, but not 123.857… mg/dL).

- *Coefficient of variation (CV)* is the standard deviation of a set of data points divided by the mean result expressed as a percentage or as a decimal fraction.
- *Confidence interval (CI)* is the interval that is computed to include a parameter such as the mean with a stated probability (e.g., commonly 90%, 95%, 99%) that the true value falls into that interval.
- *Degrees of freedom (df)* is a parameter related to the sample size (n). df indicates the number of quantities free to vary and is usually n–1 for applications such as the *t*-test. For the chi-square test, it is the number of rows minus one times the number of columns minus one. df is employed in calculating the *p* value for a statistical test.
- *Gaussian (normal) distribution* is a spread of data in which elements are distributed symmetrically around the mean with most values close to the center. It is explicitly described by a mathematical equation and so is a parametric distribution. Random scatter or random selection of a population often results in a Gaussian normal distribution. This type of distribution is often a criterion for completely valid application of many parametric tests.
- *Linear regression* is the mathematical process for calculating the best straight line to fit the relationship observed between two variables measured on the same items. *Simple* or *least squares linear regression* yields the best fit for x and y data sets by minimizing the sum of the squared *y*-axis (vertical distance) differences between each data point (*x,y*) and the line. This approach assumes the *x*-axis data to be nearly perfect or without error. Uneven distribution of data points across the entire range may significantly alter the reliability of linear regression. *Deming linear regression* does not assume the *x*-axis data to be free of error, but instead uses the weighted sum of squared *y*-axis and *x*-axis differences between the data points and the line. The *correlation coefficient (r)* describes how well the line fits the data (*r* ranges from −1 to 1).
- *Mean* is the sum of all results divided by the number of results. Also related are the *median*, which is the middle value that divides the distribution of data points into upper and lower halves (also called the 50th percentile); and the *mode*, which is the most common value. The mean, median, and mode are all measures of central tendency. The *geometric mean* is calculated as the *n*th root of the product of a distribution of *n* numbers; its use for estimating central tendency minimizes the effects from extreme values such as are found in a log-normal distribution.
- *Parametric statistics* are statistical measures that are calculated based on the assumption that the data points follow a Gaussian distribution and include parameters such as mean, variance, and standard deviation. *Nonparametric statistics* are based on rank or order of data.
- *Null hypothesis* (H_0) is the proposal that there is no difference in a comparison. The alternative hypothesis is that there is a difference. When the critical value of a statistic is exceeded, rejection of the null hypothesis occurs, thereby favoring the acceptability of the alternative hypothesis.
- *Significance level* (p *or* α) is the probability that a difference between groups occurred by chance alone, by convention set at less than .05.
- *Statistical power* ($1-\beta$) is the probability that a difference between groups will be detected by the study, generally set at least to 80%.
- *Standard deviation (SD)* is the square root of the sum of the squared differences of each data point from the mean divided by $n-1$ for samples (divided by n for populations). The SD is a predictable measure of dispersion from the mean in a Gaussian normal distribution.
- *Standard deviation index (SDI)* is the difference between the value of a data point and the mean value divided by the group's SD. The *z-transformation* is the expression of a result from the mean in SD units. The Z-value is the probability of a result being z SDs from the mean value. The SDI is commonly used in reporting performance in proficiency testing for an individual laboratory compared with peers.
- *Student* t*-test* is a statistical test for comparing means between two sample groups. The test can be paired (e.g., two separate measurements on the same individuals before and after some intervention) or unpaired. Values of *t* and *df* yield a level of statistical significance (*p* value).
- *Type I error (alpha error,* α*)* is incorrectly rejecting the null hypothesis and stating that two groups are statistically different when they really are not.
- *Type II error (beta error,* β*)* is incorrectly failing to reject the null hypothesis and stating that two groups are not statistically different when they really are.

Variables

Statistical questions are often posed in terms of input versus output, cause and effect, or correlation between two or more variables. The input or cause is considered an *independent variable* because it is already determined and so is not influenced by other factors. Examples of independent variables are age, gender, temperature, and time. In contrast, *dependent variables* are those things that might change in response to the independent variable. Examples of dependent variables are blood glucose concentration, enzyme activities, and the presence or absence of malignancy. Of course we can change our thinking and switch which is the independent and which is the dependent variable if the experimental question changes. For graphical display, the independent variable is plotted along the horizontal (*x*) axis or abscissa, while dependent variables are plotted along the vertical (*y*) axis or ordinate. With a single independent variable (e.g., time) on the *x*-axis, more than one dependent variable can be plotted on the *y*-axis to demonstrate different relationships simultaneously. The relationship observed between an independent variable and dependent variables is used to predict future outcomes of the dependent ones based on what values the independent variable assumes.

Preparing to Analyze Data

Most statistical calculations today are done automatically by computer with software programs that present multiple sophisticated options for analysis and even graphical displays of the data. To prepare data for these automated analyses, it is always necessary to enter them into readable format for the program. This process can entail automated transfer from one electronic data set to the statistical program or manual entry from printed sheets of data. Manual entry is obviously fraught with opportunity for typographic errors, but even automated transfer of data can result in erroneous entries, especially when translating older data sets that have been stored on media that might have been corrupted (e.g., magnetic tapes reexamined decades later). Even converting data strings to columns and rows of data points can leave some values in the wrong places. Consequently, it is always good practice to examine the data set for accuracy before performing the statistical analysis. This examination could be done by proofreading every entry or by double entry of each value and automatic comparison for discrepancies, although both of these approaches may be impractical when the data sets contain hundreds, thousands, or more values. At the very least, visual examination of the plotted values provides a quick idea of whether some serious data entry errors have occurred. For example, an incorrectly entered value of 50.0 for potassium (instead of 5.0) can be immediately identified by scanning all values on a graphical plot. The person preparing to perform statistical analyses should do this visual test to identify and correct the most obvious errors and to search for any systematic errors that might have arisen in data transfer and entry.

Descriptive Statistics

When multiple data points are collected, it is useful to provide a summary of those results that makes them easier to understand rather than simply listing all values. The methods used to summarize data are termed *descriptive statistics* because they describe what the magnitude of results is and how the data points differ from one another. In the case of categorical variables, this description can be a simple count of discrete values (e.g., how many men and how many women had blood drawn in a clinic). For continuous variables, it is conventional to use some measure of *central tendency* about which the data points cluster, and a measure of how far apart they are *dispersed* from one another (e.g., what are the ages of the patients who had blood drawn).

Central Tendency

The most widely recognized measure of central tendency is probably the mean or average value (also referred to as the *arithmetic mean*), which is calculated by adding the values of all the individual data points and dividing that sum by the total number of data points, expressed mathematically as follows:

$$Mean = \bar{x} = (x_1 + x_2 + \ldots x_n) \div n = \frac{1}{n}\sum_{i=1}^{n} x_i \qquad \textbf{(9-1)}$$

Because this technique derives the mean value from a defined formula, it is termed a *parametric method*. An alternative measure of central tendency is the *median*, which divides all data points exactly in half, with one half being higher and one half lower. The median is also called the 50th percentile. It is not calculated from a formula because it is taken from a straight count of the data points, so it is termed a *nonparametric method*. The third commonly used measure of central tendency is the *mode*, which is the most common value (i.e., the value of the variable that has the greatest number of data points). The mode is not a very useful measure for describing or comparing data sets, but it does have a role in understanding when a data set consists of two or more different populations that result in more than one mode. If two separate subpopulations are present, it is called a bimodal population.

Another measure of central tendency is the *geometric mean*, which has the feature of minimizing the influence from extreme values in a distribution. The geometric mean is calculated as the *n*th root of the product of all *n* values from a population, or

$$\text{Geometric mean} = \sqrt[n]{x_1 \times x_2 \times \cdots x_n} \quad \text{(9-2A)}$$

The following transformation is more convenient for calculating the geometric mean:

$$\log \textit{Geometric mean} = \sum_{i=1}^{n} \frac{\log x_i}{n} \quad \text{(9-2B)}$$

Thus the log of the geometric mean equals the mean of the logarithm of all observations, and taking the antilog of this summation yields the value of the geometric mean.

Consider the following distribution of values, which is heavily weighted toward the lower end but with some high values:

$$3, 3, 4, 4, 4, 5, 5, 5, 6, 6, 8, 9, 10, 15, 21$$

The arithmetic mean for these values is 7.2, whereas the geometric mean is 6.09, which better reflects the preponderance of values at the lower end than does the arithmetic mean.

In general, parametric methods allow numerous additional calculations for application of many different statistical tests that are based on specific formulas. The advantage of nonparametric methods is that they do not assume or require that the data points must follow any particular distribution for them to be applicable. Parametric methods can be applied to data sets that deviate from preferred distributions, but those calculations and conclusions may not be fully warranted if the deviations are extreme.

GAUSSIAN (NORMAL) DISTRIBUTION

The Gaussian (also called normal) distribution is a symmetrical, bell-shaped curve centered about the mean value (Fig. 9-1). It is described by the following mathematical formula:

$$P(x) = \frac{1}{\sigma\sqrt{2\pi}} e^{-\left(\frac{(x-\bar{x})^2}{2\sigma^2}\right)} \quad \text{(9-3)}$$

where σ is the standard deviation of the ideal Gaussian population (Dawson-Saunders, 1994). It corresponds to the distance from the mean to the x value at which the curve has an inflection point.

The area under this curve within $\pm 1\ \sigma$ from the mean is approximately 68.2% of the total area, meaning that 68.2% of data points from a Gaussian distribution should fall within $\pm 1\ \sigma$ of the mean. Similarly 95.5% of the data points will be within $\pm 2\ \sigma$ of the mean, and 99.7% will be within $\pm 3\ \sigma$ of the mean.

DISPERSION

A common parametric measure (based on the Gaussian distribution) of the dispersion of data points about the mean value of a population under examination is the standard deviation, mathematically calculated as:

$$SD = \sqrt{\frac{\sum_{i=1}^{n}(x_i - \bar{x})^2}{n-1}} \quad \text{(9-4)}$$

The quantity under the square root sign is termed *variance*. Use of the SD assumes that the data follow a bell-shaped curve that can be described mathematically by the formula for a normal or Gaussian distribution. To the extent that the data are normally distributed, the SD is a good estimate of the dispersion.

Two additional terms derive from the SD. One is the *coefficient of variation (CV)*, which is calculated as the SD divided by the mean. The CV is often expressed as a percentage, although it can also be expressed as a decimal fraction less than 1. For a situation where the mean = 25 and the SD = 5, the CV = 20%, or 0.20. The other term is the *standard deviation index (SDI)*, which is the distance that an individual data point is away from the mean value divided by the SD. The main use for the SDI is in such applications as proficiency testing, where performance of any one laboratory is standardized according to the dispersion of data in the performance by all laboratories.

A common clinical laboratory application of the normal distribution is to calculate the central 95% of values obtained from a healthy population when trying to establish the reference range for an analyte. This range of course is easily calculated as mean ± 2SD for a truly Gaussian normal population. An example of this application is calculation of the central 95% of values of the white blood cell (WBC) count in a group of 85 healthy medical students (Fig. 9-2). The bar graph plot is roughly bell shaped and symmetrical, although there is a slight asymmetry that can probably be ignored. The mean value is 6.60×10^9 cells/L, with an SD of 1.457×10^9 cells/L, and the calculated central 95% range is from $3.69–9.52 \times 10^9$ cells/L. This is a small group of individuals compared with what might be used for actual reference range calculations, but it does show a few persons with WBCs higher than this range and some lower, so this estimate of central 95% appears appropriate.

Another way of thinking about these calculations is that the persons tested represent only a sample of all persons to whom we are interested in generalizing these findings (Daniel, 1999). The mean value actually observed would probably be somewhat different if another group of 85 healthy people were tested. Based on the values observed and their spread, a confidence interval can be placed around the mean such that we can be certain by a desired percent that the true mean of WBCs from all healthy persons falls in that range. The confidence limit is calculated as follows:

$$\text{Confidence interval} = \bar{x} \pm z\frac{SD}{\sqrt{n}} \quad \text{(9-5)}$$

where the critical factor z derives from transformation of the problem to a standard normal distribution. The quantity $\sqrt{n}$ is termed the *standard*

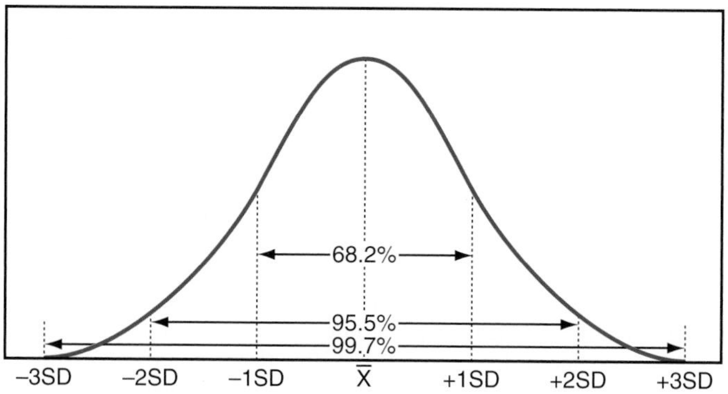

Figure 9-1 Idealized Gaussian (normal) distribution showing areas under the curve corresponding to mean ± 1, 2, and 3 standard deviations (SD).

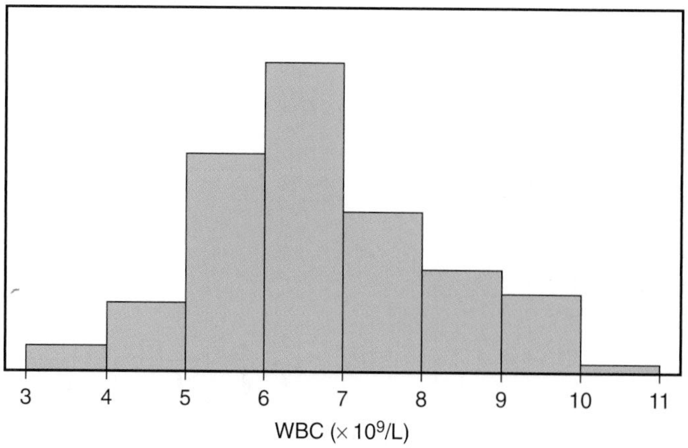

Figure 9-2 Distribution of white blood cells (WBCs) in the blood of 85 healthy individuals.

error of the mean. In this example, let the confidence interval be 95%, for which $z = 1.96$. The 95% confidence interval around the mean value is

$$6.60 \pm 1.96 \times \frac{1.457}{\sqrt{85}} \text{ or } 6.295\text{–}6.914 \times 10^9 \text{ cells/L}$$

Note that this range is the 95% confidence interval on the mean value alone, whereas the earlier calculations yielded the central 95% of all data points. Confidence intervals are used to give an idea of the broadness of the estimate of something. This can be made more certain by using 99% confidence intervals (i.e., 99% confident that the true mean falls in the interval), in which case $z = 2.575$ for the calculation, and the 99% confidence interval is broader at

$$6.60 \pm 2.575 \times \frac{1.457}{\sqrt{85}} \text{ or } 6.193\text{–}7.007 \times 10^9 \text{ cells/L}$$

NONPARAMETRIC MEASURES

The median value of WBC for this group of healthy persons is 6.4×10^9 cells/L, which is roughly the same as the mean value. For a perfectly Gaussian normal distribution, values of the mean, median, and mode are exactly the same. Delineation of the range from the 2.5-percentile to the 97.5-percentile also gives an estimate of the central 95% range (for the example of WBC, it is $3.94\text{–}9.89 \times 10^9$ cells/L, which is really the exact range for this specific population). This is a nonparametric estimate of the range because it does not use a calculation, but only divides the data points according to their order. Many applications of median use the central 50% of data points from the 25th percentile to the 75th percentile (also called interquartile range) to describe central tendency by the nonparametric method.

Sometimes the parametric method of mean ± 2 SD produces an erroneous estimate of the central 95% range. An example of this situation arises with the distribution of alanine aminotransferase (ALT) activities in the serum of apparently healthy individuals (Fig. 9-3). In this population, the mean value is 30.1 U, the SD is 12.69 U, and the calculated reference range (mean ± 2 SD) is 4.73–55.48 U. This range is not appropriate because the actual lowest value observed in the group was much higher (12 U). This estimate of the lower end of the range (4.73 U) is far too low. Similarly, the estimate of the upper end (55.48 U) is too low and excludes about 10% of the data points instead of only 2.5%. Another clue that the parametric method may not work here is that the median value is 27.0 U, which is somewhat different from the mean. The reason for this discrepancy is apparent upon looking at the distribution, which is skewed to the right with many values tailing off at the upper end. In this case, a much more useful estimate of the central 95% can be obtained simply from the 2.5-percentile to the 97.5-percentile range. It is 15.2–68.0 U. The form of this distribution for ALT is sometimes termed *log-normal*, because it can be converted to a normal distribution by using the values of log ALT instead.

Many laboratory measurements show distinctly non-Gaussian normal distributions. Values of 25-OH vitamin D in 12,434 serum specimens from 2000 through 2008 showed a skewed distribution, with lowest value 0.5 ng/mL and highest value 260.0 ng/mL (Fig. 9-4, *A*). The arithmetic mean of these values is 25.55 ng/mL, and the median is 20.90 ng/mL, reflecting the non-normal distribution. Plotting log 25-OH vitamin D

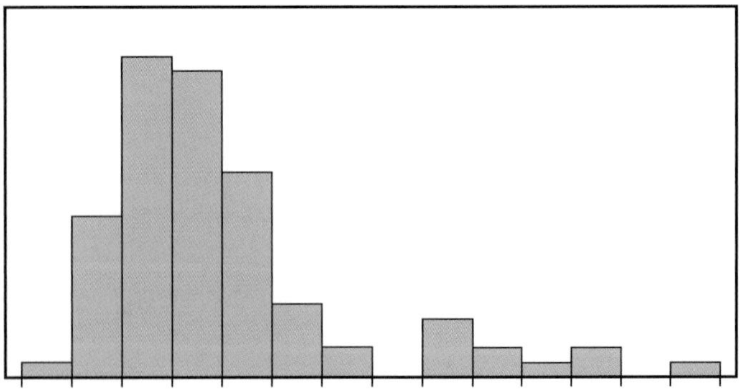

Figure 9-3 Distribution of alanine aminotransferase (ALT) in the serum of 86 healthy individuals.

shows a nearly normal distribution with mean value 1.3130 (Fig. 9-4, *B*). Then the geometric mean is $10^{1.3130} = 20.56$ ng/mL, which appears to be a better measure of central tendency for 25-OH vitamin D than the arithmetic mean.

COMPARATIVE STATISTICS

One of the questions frequently asked by statistical means is whether one group is different from another group in some characteristic. The question boils down to a comparison of the central tendency of one group versus that of the other and the scatter that each group exhibits about the central values. If the scatter of data is extreme, then calculated differences between mean values of two groups might not be important, but rather the result of adding in the extreme values. Another way to think about these comparisons is that of signal/noise ratio. If there is little noise (scatter of data), then the difference in the signal from each group is more believable.

STUDENT *t*-TEST

The most common method for comparison of a continuous variable between groups is probably the Student *t*-test (Dawson-Saunders, 1994). The pseudonym Student was used by William Gosset, a statistician working for the Guinness brewery, who wanted to keep his work for optimizing productivity unrecognized by competing companies. The *t*-test is based on a parametric calculation of the *t* statistic as follows:

$$t = \frac{\bar{x}_1 - \bar{x}_2}{SD_{12}\sqrt{\frac{1}{n_1} + \frac{1}{n_2}}} \quad \textbf{(9-6)}$$

where $\bar{x}_1$ is the mean value in group 1,
n_1 is the number of values in group 1,
$\bar{x}_2$ is the mean value in group 2,
n_2 is the number of values in group 2, and
SD_{12} is the standard deviation of groups 1 and 2 combined.

Fortunately, the calculation of *t* statistics is conveniently performed by computers in modern times, so the analyst now has the responsibility of vouching for the accuracy of data input and the correct choice of statistical tests and their validity for the situation.

Some specific assumptions about the data sets are also necessary for applicability. For example, it is necessary to have sufficient numbers of data points in each group to make a valid comparison with approximately equal numbers in each. The spread of the data points should be equivalent (usually assessed by whether the variances of the groups are equivalent). The selection of data points should be independent of one another; for example, it would be inappropriate to include the same patient twice in one group. The issue of independence is usually handled experimentally by a random selection of subjects or patients. Randomization of treatments is an exacting process for important research such as clinical trials. For laboratory use, it is more likely that data come from patients who present themselves to the hospital or clinic for testing, rather than being a random sample of all people in a city or from a country. The more random the selection process, the more likely it is that results can be generalized to a much larger target population for which inference is desired.

The statistical question for consideration is reduced to two mutually exclusive hypotheses that include all the possible situations. The null hypothesis (H_0) states that there is no difference between groups. The alternative hypothesis (H_{alt}) is that the difference between mean values is significant. If the *t* statistic has a sufficiently high value, we can reject the null hypothesis and consequently must accept the alternative hypothesis that there is a significant difference. If the *t* value is on the low side, we cannot reject the null hypothesis, but neither can we accept it. This decision is somewhat like that of the verdict from a trial in which the possible outcomes are "guilty" and "not guilty." The innocence of the defendant is never established, and similarly the null hypothesis is never proven. We could end up thinking that the null hypothesis is correct (particularly since the alternative hypothesis now seems unlikely), but the test we performed did not strictly lead to that conclusion.

Consider the distribution of hemoglobin (Hb) values in the whole blood of 36 healthy males and 49 healthy females (Fig. 9-5, *A* and *B*). Visual inspection of the bar graphs for Hb shows that the females generally have lower values (mean 13.2 g/dL, SD 0.80 g/dL) than the males (mean 15.1 g/dL, SD 0.96 g/dL). Only a portion of the males and females overlap one another in Hb values. In this example, the value of $t = 9.898$. One other factor must be taken into account, the degrees of freedom, which is

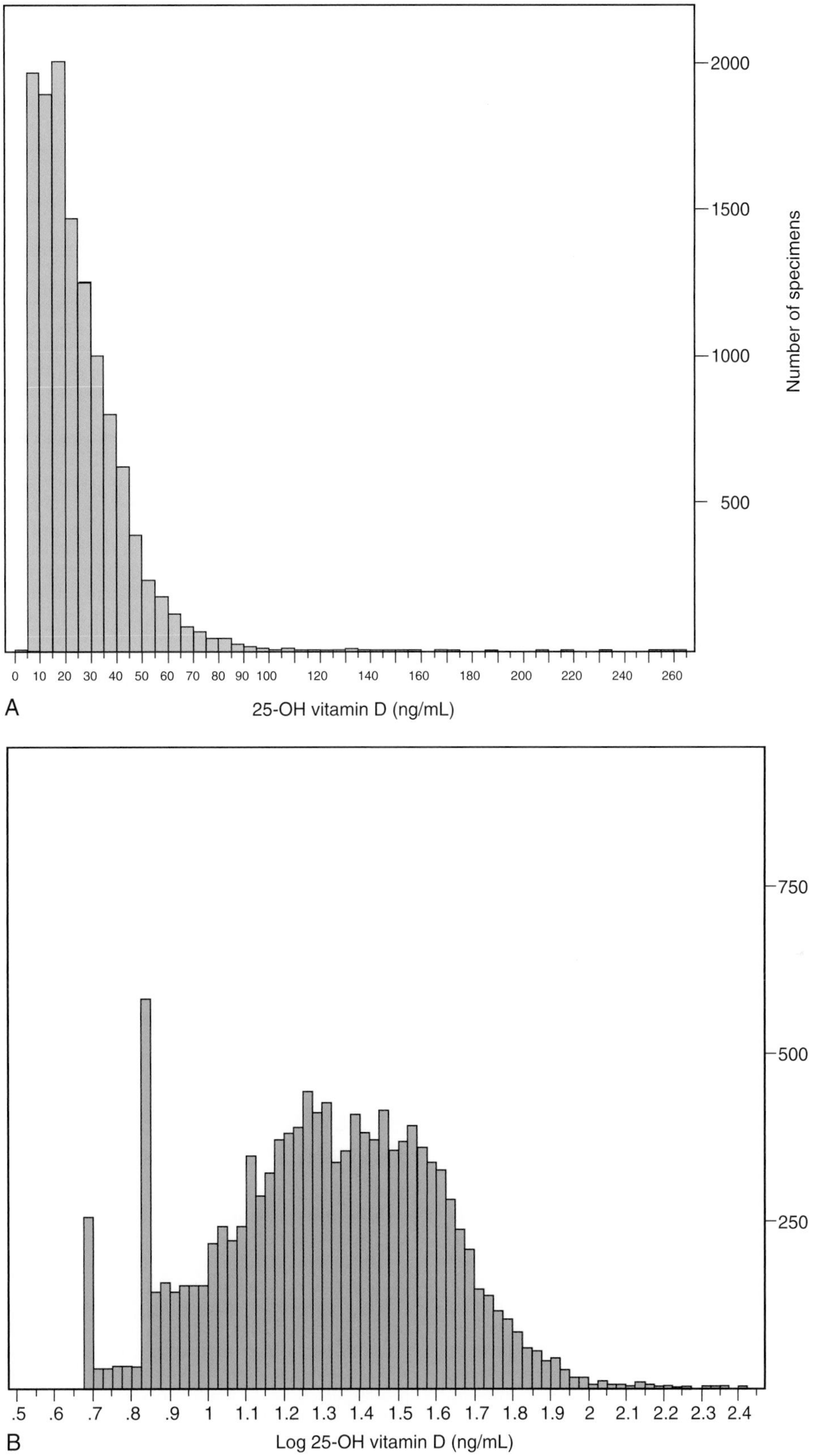

Figure 9-4 **A,** Distribution of 25-OH vitamin D in 12,434 serum specimens showing skewness to the right at higher values. **B,** Plotting log 25-OH vitamin D shows normal distribution following logarithmic transformation.

obtained from the total number of data points minus 2 or $df = n_1 + n_2 - 2 = 36 + 49 - 2 = 83$.

Significance

The value of the t statistic is assessed for significance according to the degrees of freedom. One way to approach the assessment is look up the value of t for which the degrees of freedom yield a probability (p) value that is to be applied for significance using a table of values. More often the software does this calculation automatically. Generally p values of 0.05 or less are required to claim statistical significance. A p value of 0.05 (also called alpha) means that the difference observed between the two groups could have occurred one time in 20 with the particular spread of data

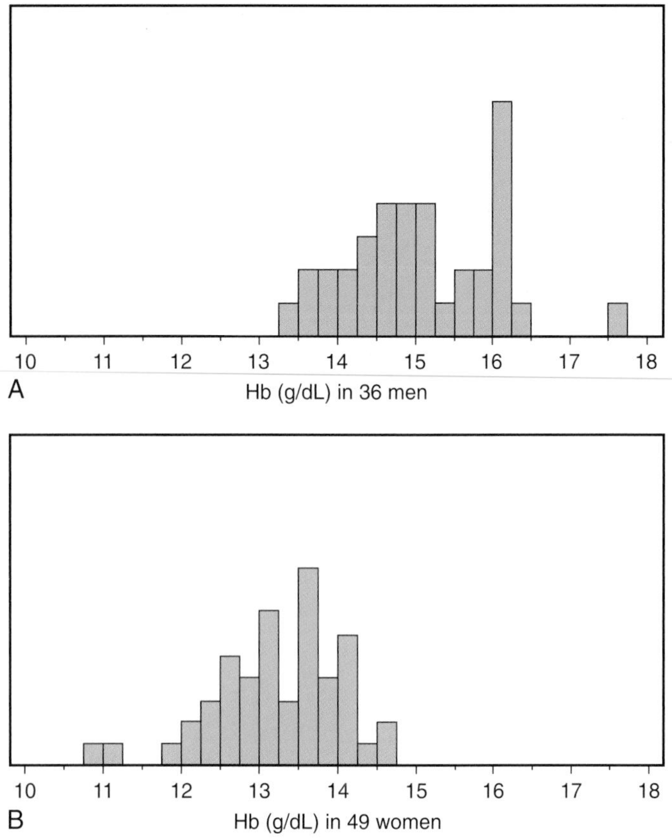

Figure 9-5 Distribution of hemoglobin (Hb) in the blood of **(A)** healthy men and **(B)** healthy women.

actually observed. The value of alpha is also thought of as the risk that we are willing to take to conclude falsely that there is a significant difference when in fact none exists (type I error). The use of alpha = 0.05 is merely an arbitrary convention, but it is ingrained in the minds of reviewers and protocols for evaluating studies. Of course, if the *p* value is much smaller, such as 0.01 or 0.001, then the statistical significance of a difference between group means is that much more credible.

Even though an observed difference between groups might have an extraordinarily impressive *p* value ($p = 0.001$ means that the result should happen by chance only 1 in 1000 times), it is incumbent upon the investigator to conclude whether the observation is clinically significant. The statistical significance of any difference can always be amplified, no matter how insignificant it is for decision-making, simply by increasing the number of data points (see the formula for calculating *t*, Equation 9-6).

A potential problem arises when a large number of comparisons are done in studies where no clear hypothesis is stated, but instead the data are mined for whatever might fall out upon examination. In this case, the minimal level of significance should be adjusted to reflect the large number of tests that could conceivably discover "significant results" by chance alone. After all, if a *p* value of 0.05 is used, then by doing 20 different comparisons, one ought to find on average some comparison with a statistically significant difference regularly. The Bonferroni correction is done to lower the risk of such false discovery. It consists of dividing the usually accepted *p* value by the number of comparisons. Thus for five different comparisons, the correction is *p* value = 0.05/5 = 0.01 as the acceptable threshold value for significance.

For this particular example, comparing Hb values between males and females, the *p* value is less than 0.0001, so we can reject the null hypothesis and can conclude that there is a significant difference between groups. Most statisticians would not report this level, but would be satisfied with saying that the *p* value was less than 0.001. Another condition to denote is whether this test is two-sided or one-sided, meaning that the question being asked is whether one group is simply different from the other (two-sided) as opposed to the question of whether one group is only higher than the other group (one-sided). Most journals require the use of two-sided *t*-tests because they are more demanding.

TABLE 9-1
Observed Values of Contamination in Blood Cultures

Result	Baseline period	Post training
Number of cultures contaminated	53	32
Number of cultures not contaminated	978	891

Sample Size

Suppose the two groups being compared showed a difference that was not quite statistically significant with a *p* value of .06. One way to achieve statistical significance is to increase the number of subjects studied. This will be the case if the difference remains the same, because the *t*-value will be increased by a greater *n*. A pilot study can be done in a clinical trial to establish roughly the difference between groups and the scatter of the data. These pieces of information are then used in a formula to calculate the sample size necessary to bring the results to statistical significance. Calculation of sample size also takes into account another factor called beta, which is the risk one has of missing a true effect by chance (type II error). The power of the study is 1 − beta. When beta is set to 0.20, the power of the study is 0.80, which says that the number of subjects calculated for use will yield a statistically significant result 80% of the time with the specified difference between groups and scatter of data.

The *t*-test used for this example was unpaired because the comparison was between different individuals. If the experimental design included a comparison of values on the same individuals before and after treatment, then it is appropriate to use a paired *t*-test. A paired test is potentially a more powerful mathematical tool because it looks only at the change between the values within each person and is not influenced by variation in background values between individuals.

NONPARAMETRIC TESTS

If the assumption about normality of the data is not valid, other nonparametric tests can be used to compare distributions between groups. The *Wilcoxon signed-ranks test* is such a technique. By this method, all values for both groups are given a numeric rank according to their magnitude. In the case of ties for the same value, both are assigned the intermediate rank (e.g., if 4th and 5th places are tied, then both are given the rank 4.5). All ranks are summed in each group and divided by the number of data points in each group. The difference between the rank scores is then given a probability. This technique is easily done by computer software and may be quite useful when assumptions required for a parametric method are not met by a data set.

ANALYZING DISCRETE DATA: TESTING PROPORTIONS

Analysis of discrete data takes on a different form from that of continuous variables that can be expressed as distributions. With discrete data, answers are typically dichotomous: Something is present or absent, patient gender is male or female, the patient lived or died. Consider the fictitious example of an intervention to lower contamination rates in blood culture collection. (This is a universal problem in all laboratories, but these data are only hypothetical.) Before the intervention, baseline information over a 2-month period showed that 53 cultures were considered contaminated and 978 were not. After training and implementation of the new collection process, a second 2-month period showed 32 contaminated cultures and 891 that were not. These nominal data are conveniently expressed in a 2 × 2 display termed a contingency table of observed values (Table 9-1). These data consist of simple counts in one category or another. The question to be asked is whether the proportion of contaminated cultures was significantly different in the two time periods.

CHI-SQUARE TEST

The statistical test to be used is the chi-square test. It is calculated as:

$$\chi^2 = \sum \frac{(observed - expected)^2}{expected} \qquad (9\text{-}7)$$

TABLE 9-2

Expected Values of Contamination in Blood Cultures

Result	Baseline period	Post training
Number of cultures contaminated	44.8	40.2
Number of cultures not contaminated	986.2	882.8

where the observed values are as listed earlier and the expected values are calculated from the overall assortment of counts (Dawson-Saunders, 1994). In this example, the expected number of contaminated cultures in the baseline period is the total number of cultures done in that period (53 + 978 = 1031) times the proportion of contaminated cultures in both time periods together (proportion calculated as [53 + 32]/[53 + 978 + 32 + 891] = 0.0435), or 1031 × 0.0435 = 44.8. Calculation of the other expected values follows similarly, resulting in a contingency table of expected values (Table 9-2). Then calculation of the χ^2 value is done by summing the squares of the differences (this converts all differences to positive values) between expected and observed values and dividing by the expected value in each cell of the table. In this example,

$$\chi^2 = \frac{(53-44.8)^2}{44.8} + \frac{(978-986.2)^2}{986.2} + \frac{(32-40.2)^2}{40.2} + \frac{(891-882.8)^2}{882.8} = 3.3 \quad \textbf{(9-7A)}$$

With one degree of freedom ([number of rows − 1][number of columns − 1]), the p value is 0.07, which does not meet the universal threshold of at least 0.05 for statistical significance. It is fair to say that a trend toward less contamination was observed after the intervention, but that it was not quite statistically significant. It is important to keep in mind that for χ^2 testing to be valid, each cell must have a minimum value of five observations.

TREND EVALUATION AND CORRELATIVE STATISTICS

The relationship between an independent variable and a dependent variable is demonstrated by plotting them on a scattergram or a plot with the independent (input) variable on the x-axis and the dependent (output) variable on the y-axis. If there is no relationship between the two variables, the data scatter randomly over the graph. If there is a relationship, it can be described mathematically by finding a line that is the best fit through all the data points. This line can be calculated by the least squares approach in which the vertical distances from each point to the calculated line are minimized for the entire population of values. This statistical method is referred to as *linear regression* (National Committee for Clinical Laboratory Standards, 2003).

LINEAR REGRESSION

The general form for the equation of a straight line is:

$$y = a + bx \quad \textbf{(9-8)}$$

in which the slope (b) indicates how the value of y changes when x changes. When $b = 1$, the relationship of change between x and y is one to one. The intercept (a) indicates how the relationship between x and y is offset or biased by a constant factor. The calculation is easily done by any of several statistical programs that also provide information about the goodness of fit of the line. This approach is commonly used when comparing an existing method (A) with a new method (B) for the same analyte (Fig. 9-6, *A*). This example shows a strong correlation between method A and method B because the data points fall very close to the line, which is described by the equation: *Method B* = 0.62 + 0.99 × *Method A*. The slope of 0.99 is almost perfect, and the intercept of 0.62 is quite small on the scale of possible values. In fact, the 95% confidence limits on b are −0.47 to 1.72, which includes the value 0, indicating that the intercept is not significantly different from 0.

The vertical (y axis) distances from each data point to the best fit line are termed the *residuals*. The most valid line fits are associated with relatively constant values of the residuals over the entire range of values. If the residuals grow larger at one end of the graph, then the line fit is less certain

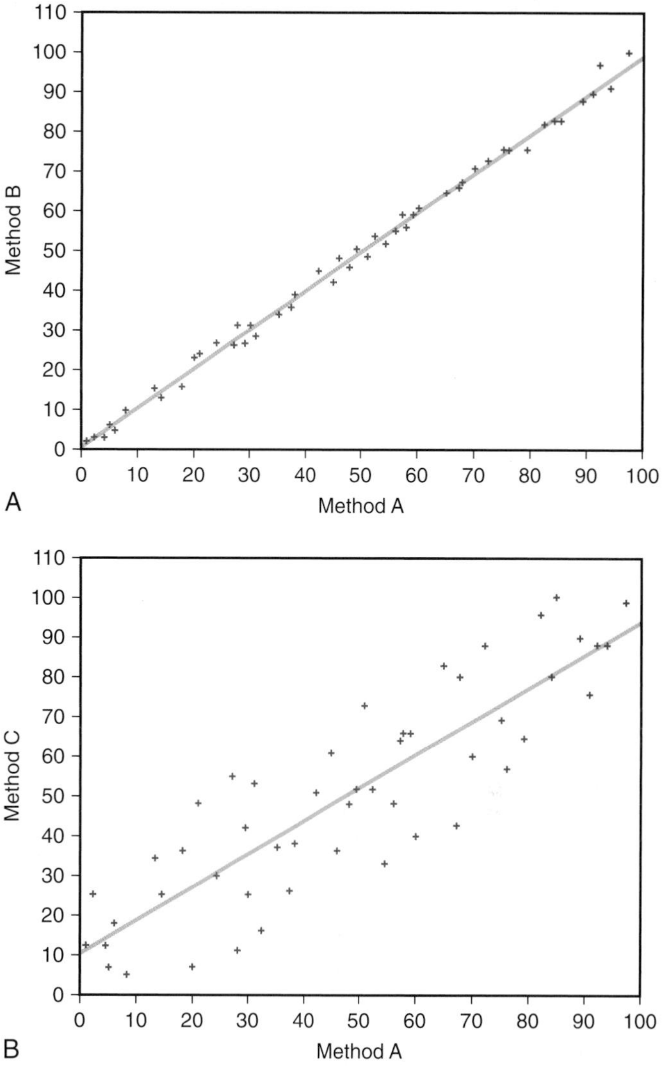

Figure 9-6 **A,** Regression analysis between method A and method B; strong correlation. **B,** Regression analysis between method A and method C; weaker correlation.

in that portion of the range. The *standard error of regression* (also called standard *error of the estimate*), denoted $S_{y.x}$, is used to estimate the variation that could be expected from doing the regression again with another sample of data points. The $S_{y.x}$ is calculated as the square root of the sum of residuals squared, divided by n − 2. It is important that data points from patient specimens be spread over the entire analytic range to yield the most valid comparison of methods unbiased by over-representation or under-representation of data in any region (National Committee for Clinical Laboratory Standards, 2002).

In laboratory practice, regression or correlation analysis is frequently used to compare the performance of a new method versus an old method. In this situation, the old method could have worse precision than the new one, and so it would not be appropriate to base a judgment just on how the new method compares with the old one as a "gold standard." A common approach to this issue is Deming regression analysis, named for W. Edwards Deming (1900–1993), a mathematician influential in principles of quality improvement. In Deming regression, the best line is obtained by minimizing the sum of squares of both x and y distances from the data points to the line (Cornbleet, 1979). In addition, Deming regression applies a weighting factor (λ) that incorporates the relative variances of both x and y data. The result is more heavily weighted in favor of the data set with better precision.

The relationship between method A and method B is further described by the *correlation coefficient (r)*, which can range in value from −1 to +1. A value of 0 indicates no relationship, and a value of 1 indicates a perfect relationship (−1 is also a perfect but inverse relationship). Other values between −1 and +1 indicate intermediate relationships. The square of the correlation coefficient is termed the coefficient of determination (r^2), which describes the amount of variation observed in the dependent variable that is due to the relationship between the two variables. In this example, $r = 0.9976$ and $r^2 = 0.9952$, both of which are very high values that show an extremely strong relationship between method A and method B that accounts for 99.52% of the variation. The p value on this correlation is less than 0.0001.

In contrast with the very good correlation between method A and method B, the performance of method C versus method A (Fig. 9-6, *B*) is not nearly as good. By simple visual examination, the data points are scattered farther from the line, and the line is shifted upward. The value of $r = 0.8757$ is somewhat less than between method A and method B, but still shows a strong correlation with p value less than 0.0001. The value of $r^2 = 0.7668$, so 76.68% of the variation can be accounted for by the relationship between method C and method A. The equation for this line is *Method C* = 10.2 + 0.84 × *Method A*, so the change in values using method C compared with method A is slightly less (slope of 0.84). A significant upward bias is seen by method C (intercept of 10.2 with 95% confidence limits of 2.8 to 17.6).

METHOD COMPARISONS

These two examples show somewhat different relationships, although both are statistically significant. It is up to the person assessing the performance to determine which is sufficient for the application. The comparison of method A versus method B is extraordinarily strong both by visual review and by statistical analysis, and so it can comfortably be said that these methods are equivalent for the purposes of replacing one with the other in clinical practice. On the other hand, the comparison of method A with method C is messier because of the larger amount of data scatter. The smaller slope suggests that the two methods do not react equivalently with the analyte, and furthermore there is a positive bias by method C. With expectations for excellent precision and accuracy on modern instrumentation, method C would probably be rejected if method B were a viable alternative. And yet the level of correlation observed between method A and method C might be very welcome to researchers trying to ask a different question related to cause and effect between biological processes that have inherently high levels of variation.

A special example of regression analysis termed *logistic regression* is employed when the outcome is a dichotomous or binary variable for continuous independent (predictor) variables.

ANALYSIS OF VARIANCE

When the mean values of more than two different groups are to be compared, the process is termed *analysis of variance (ANOVA)* (Dawson-Saunders, 1994). This analysis can be thought of as extending the t-test beyond two independent samples to three or more. The null hypothesis in this situation is that the mean values of all groups are the same. The alternative hypothesis is that not all the means are equal (some could be the same, but others different). The test statistic is the F-ratio of the mean squares among all groups (MS_A) to the error mean square (MS_E):

$$F\text{-ratio} = \frac{MS_A}{MS_E} \quad \textbf{(9-9)}$$

It compares the variance of the group means versus the mean of all the data (numerator) and the variance of individual data points within each group (denominator). If the group means differ from one another (signal) more than the variation within groups (noise), then the F-ratio will exceed a critical value for significance.

An example of ANOVA is the comparison of serum albumin values from patients at two inpatient sites, an outpatient clinic, and a student health clinic (Fig. 9-7). One hundred consecutive specimens from each site were recorded. The horizontal line shows the grand mean of all 400 values of 3.17 g/dL. Within each group, the diamonds indicate group means (midline) and 95% confidence intervals on those means (upper and lower vertices). The F-ratio = 279 for which the p value <0.0001, so the null hypothesis can be rejected with the conclusion that at least some of the means are different. This approach is more conservative and realistic than comparing each group with every other group using a series of different t-tests (with four groups, six comparisons could be made). The problem with too many comparisons is the possibility of "accidentally finding significance" that is not true. To extend ANOVA, comparisons of group means by such procedures as Tukey's honestly significant difference (HSD) can be done. In this example, Tukey's HSD indicates that IP1 and IP2 are

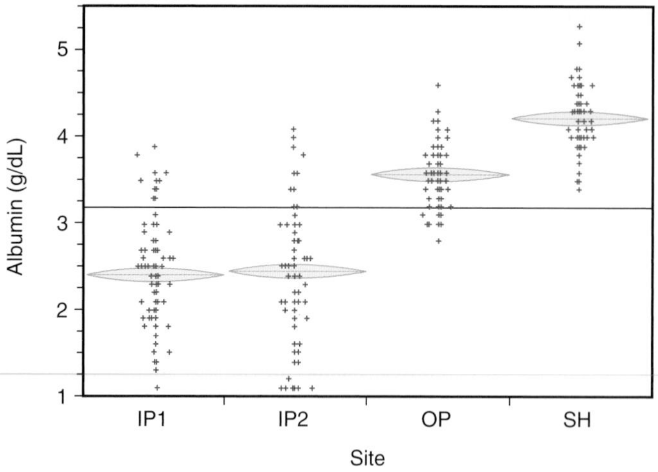

Figure 9-7 Analysis of variance. Serum albumin at different patient sites. *IP1, IP2,* Inpatient wards 1 and 2; *OP,* outpatient; *SH,* student health.

not different from one another, but that OP and SH are both different from all other groups. At this stage, the investigator is free to elaborate on potential reasons for these observed differences without putting further statistical significance on the individual differences.

Some conditions should be met for parametric ANOVA to be completely valid mathematically:

- The data were collected using random sampling where all observations are independent of one another.
- The data in each group are normally distributed.
- Each group has an equal number of data points.
- Each group has equal variances.

If this set of ideal criteria is not met, other methods are available for comparisons. The Mann-Whitney test can be used to compare medians. The Wilcoxon and Kruskal-Wallis tests for rank sums are nonparametric alternatives. This example of serum albumin shows greater variances for the inpatient groups than for the outpatients, so nonparametric analysis could be more appropriate. (The Wilcoxon test also showed significant differences among the groups of this example.) This case dealt with one variable, and so it was one-way ANOVA. To deal with two variables, the procedure can be extended to two-way ANOVA.

Linear regression might be used in error to analyze continuous outcome data when the independent variable has the appearance of being continuous but is actually categorical. Such a situation is seen with tumor grade (1 through 4) as an independent variable. Tumor grade is not continuous but rather consists of discrete categories that are not necessarily evenly spaced along a dimension. Although statistical programs would permit calculation of a regression on tumor grade, the proper approach would be one-way ANOVA to look for differences in the dependent variable (e.g., survival time) among groups (e.g., tumor grade).

ANALYSIS INVOLVING MULTIPLE VARIABLES

Two-way analysis of variance (two-way ANOVA) is used when the experimental design has two categorical independent variables (input) and a continuous dependent variable (output). An example is the effects of both gender and different (fixed) drug levels on a physiologic measurement such as blood pressure. In addition to the one-way effects of gender on blood pressure and of drug level on blood pressure, it is necessary to investigate a possible interaction of gender and drug level in two-way ANOVA. If such an interaction is significant, then response to drug level might be different in men versus women. These interactions are conveniently displayed graphically (e.g., a plot of response to drug in men and one for women; noninteraction results in parallel lines; intersection of the lines indicates an interaction).

Multiple analysis of variance (MANOVA) applies to a model with multiple categorical independent variables and two or more continuous dependent variables.

Sometimes the way a comparison is set up by selection of subjects into different groups can lead to a confounding effect from another variable besides the variable of primary interest. In this case, it is revealing to perform *analysis of covariance (ANCOVA)* to account for potential influence from the covariable. The intention of ANCOVA is to use statistical methods to eliminate effects arising from confounding variables that were not accounted for by random assignment in the original selection of subjects. Typically these effects might be due to an imbalance of subjects with certain characteristics in the experimental group compared with the control group (e.g., the treatment group might have 75% smokers and the control group only 25%; without adjusting for this potential confounding factor, one could not be certain that results from treatment were not in fact merely due to different proportions of smokers in each group).

As a laboratory example of ANCOVA, consider the comparison of serum calcium measurements in 61 male and 41 female healthy adults to establish whether different reference ranges of calcium would be necessary for males and females. Simple one-way ANOVA similar to that in Figure 9-7 yielded a statistically significant (p = 0.0045) difference between the group means of calcium (males 9.3 mg/dL, females 9.1 mg/dL). (Performing ANOVA with only two groups is equivalent to an unpaired t-test.) This finding was consistent with those of previous studies, so it probably is appropriate to have gender-specific reference ranges for serum calcium, but does this make sense from a physiologic view? It is also well recognized that serum albumin influences total calcium levels by binding some of the calcium. A linear regression for these subjects confirmed this relationship. The effects of gender and of the covariable albumin on calcium are sorted out by ANCOVA. In this example, the effect on calcium from gender was completely accounted for by the effect of albumin on calcium and the different distribution of albumin in males versus females. ANCOVA can be enlightening to discover and eliminate by statistical analysis those covariables that might not be known and planned for in the design of an experiment. Further discussion of ANCOVA can be found in more advanced texts on statistics (Matthews, 1988).

When multiple continuous independent variables (x_1, x_2, x_3, etc.) are tested to predict a continuous dependent variable (y) as outcome, *multiple regression analysis* is used to calculate the weighting factors (b_i) for a linear combination as follows:

$$y = a + b_1x_1 + b_2x_2 + b_3x_3 + \cdots \quad \textbf{(9-10)}$$

This analysis also allows use of nominal independent variables with so-called "dummy variables" that are arbitrarily given values of 1 or 0 (e.g., 1 for female and 0 for male). Thus if x_1 is gender, the coefficient b_1 is multiplied by 1 for females in calculating the values of y; however, for males, b_1 is multiplied by 0. This dummy coding permits convenient use of nominal variables in regression analysis.

Method Validation and Process Control

Statistical analysis is integral to the validation of new laboratory methods and to the monitoring of analytic and workflow processes in clinical laboratories (Lott, 1998).

REFERENCE RANGES

The examples depicted in Figures 9-2, 9-3, 9-4, and 9-5 demonstrate some of the issues encountered when reference ranges are established through application of descriptive statistics. The basic aim is to establish a range of values within which the majority of healthy people will fall, while excluding individuals with disease. The simplest approach is to use the central 95% of data points from healthy individuals by calculating mean ± 2 SD whenever the distribution is normal or bell-shaped, as for WBC in Figure 9-2. This parametric approach fails to provide a complete reference range when the data are skewed as for ALT in Figure 9-3. In this case, the central 95% can be determined nonparametrically by using the range 2.5-percentile to 97.5-percentile, which excludes 2.5% at both upper and lower ends. The distribution of ALT actually appears to have two subpopulations in these healthy people. Consequently, basing reference ranges solely on observed ranges in apparently healthy persons might not be the best approach. In fact, some new recommendations for ALT set the upper range much lower than wide-based population studies would suggest. The new guidelines try to eliminate persons who might have mild, asymptomatic liver changes such as steatosis (Prati, 2002). This approach is similar to the strategy used for setting desirable or healthy levels of cholesterol and lipid fractions (National Cholesterol Education Program, 2002) and of glucose (Report of the Expert Committee on the Diagnosis and Classification of Diabetes Mellitus, 2003). In the future, recommendations from other consensus groups or professional organizations will probably be even more useful in setting desirable ranges for other analytes in place of population-based reference ranges.

Finally, healthy subgroups of people should be recognized by separate reference ranges whenever major differences occur according to factors such as age or gender (see Fig. 9-5).

ACCURACY

The performance of a new method can be assessed for accuracy (e.g., the ability to correctly detect and quantify an analyte) by assaying patient specimens or interlaboratory survey materials with known values. The example of a strong correlation between methods in Figure 9-6, *A*, indicates that the analyte reacts in a nearly one-to-one manner by each method (slope ≈ 1) with essentially no bias (intercept ≈ 0). In contrast, the correlation depicted in Figure 9-6, *B*, has a slope different from 1, indicating that the analyte reacts differently with the two methods. One explanation for this type of discrepancy is found when tumor markers are measured by two immunoassays that employ different antibodies that potentially recognize different epitopes. A bias such as that shown by method C versus method A in Figure 9-6, *B*, also suggests a basic methodologic difference that has an impact on accuracy, albeit in a predictable way that could be compensated for with calibration adjustment.

The accuracy of any assay depends heavily on the calibrators, that is, how they are originally constituted, how they remain stable over time, and how they compare with calibrators from other vendors (see Chapter 10). The best situation is to have an assay calibrated against internationally distributed standards such as from the World Health Organization or other professional group. By using calibrators with such traceability and standardized units of measurement, it is feasible to use values from different assays interchangeably for the same patient, or to compare outcomes in different groups of patients being monitored with different methods.

After implementation of a method, periodic proficiency survey testing of unknown specimens is usually reported in terms of SDIs away from the mean of all laboratories. For example, if the mean of creatinine measurements is 11 mg/dL for all participants with SD of 2 mg/dL, then a laboratory reporting a value of 8 mg/dL would have SDI = (8 – 11)/2 = –1.5.

PRECISION

The reproducibility of an assay is conveniently expressed with the CV that allows the observed SD to be normalized by the magnitude of the signal being measured. It should be kept in mind that assays typically have different CVs for different ranges of analyte values. Therefore it is good practice to establish CVs for an assay at high, low, and mid-range values.

ANALYTIC SENSITIVITY

The lowest value that an assay can reliably detect is termed the analytic sensitivity. A common approach to making this judgment is to measure a zero standard multiple times (e.g., 10 times) and calculate the SD of the signal detected, which is noise. Then set the lowest reliable detection threshold at three or four times the value of the SD. This approach is often individualized within laboratories. This characteristic is also termed the detection limit. Another use of the term analytic sensitivity refers to the change in response of an assay for a given change in the amount or concentration of the analyte (Giacomo, 1984). In this respect, a highly sensitive assay has the characteristic of readily detecting small changes in analyte at concentrations in the mid-range of measurement.

ANALYTIC SPECIFICITY

The major interferents in laboratory measurements are hemolysis, icterus, and lipemia due either to interference with optical absorbances (or light scattering) or to actual chemical interactions (e.g., peroxidase activity of Hb in many immunoassays that use horseradish peroxidase as indicator). Beyond these endogenous interferents, drugs can also interact with various chemical or immunologic assays. The magnitude of these interactions (or lack thereof) is typically documented by the addition of known, large amounts of the substances to serum samples that are tested for recovery of the analyte in the serum.

ACCEPTABILITY OF A METHOD

The final decision of whether to accept a method as valid depends on a combination of factors. Do the statistical tests show a new method to perform analytically as it should with good accuracy and precision? Does the new method provide useful medical information that is not otherwise available? Is the method feasible to do (easy to perform, low cost, rapid)? Does the maximum error fall within medically acceptable limits? The final decision is a professional judgment based on all of these items.

RESOURCES FOR STATISTICAL ANALYSIS

Calculation of descriptive statistics and performance of statistical tests are now widely done using statistical software on computers. In the scientific realm, a few software packages are particularly popular, although applications from other vendors are also available. One of the most popular in the biomedical sciences is from the SAS (originally Statistical Analysis System) Institute, Inc., in Cary, N.C. SAS also provides JMP Software that has graphics linked to the statistics for ready visualization of results. Another well-established statistical software product is the Statistical Package for the Social Sciences (SPSS), which is now a part of IBM (SPSS Inc., Chicago). SPSS is still recognized for its prominence in the social sciences. Microsoft Excel also can provide statistical analyses along with expanded graphical capabilities.

Resources for performing statistical calculations directly online are available with simple searching. One such site is Martindale's Calculators On-Line Center at http://www.martindalecenter.com/Calculators2A_1_Cou.html#STAT-ALL.

A listing of similar sites is available on "Web Pages that Perform Statistical Calculations!" at http://www.statpages.org/.

When planning statistical analysis of data, in fact, even before planning the experimental design of a project, it is appropriate to consult with a biostatistician to ensure the most efficient design and one that is most likely to provide statistically sound results. A simple review of which statistical tests to employ for different combinations of categorical and continuous variables as independent (input) and dependent (output) variables can be found at The Decision Tree for Statistics at http://www.microsiris.com/Statistical%20Decision%20Tree/.

SELECTED REFERENCES

Daniel WW. Biostatistics: a foundation for analysis in the health sciences. 7th ed. New York: John Wiley & Sons; 1999.

This book is a more rigorous text on the use of statistical analysis in medicine and life sciences.

Dawson-Saunders B, Trapp RG. Basic & clinical biostatistics. 2nd ed. Norwalk, Conn.: Appleton & Lange; 1994.

This very readable book provides excellent descriptions of statistical procedures applied to multiple examples in the life sciences and medicine.

Lott JA. Process control and method evaluation. In: Snyder JR, Wilkinson DS, editors. Management in laboratory medicine. 3rd ed. Philadelphia: Lippincott; 1998. p. 293–325.

This book is a comprehensive source for all aspects of management in the clinical laboratory.

National Committee for Clinical Laboratory Standards. Evaluation of the linearity of quantitative measurement procedures: a statistical approach; approved guideline. Document EP6-A. Wayne, Pa.: NCCLS; 2003.

This and all the NCCLS guidelines have been developed through a consensus process involving international representatives from industry, government, and user laboratories to yield recommendations that can be applied worldwide. As of January 1, 2005, NCCLS has been renamed Clinical and Laboratory Standards Institute (CLSI).

REFERENCES

Access the complete reference list online at http://www.expertconsult.com

CHAPTER 10

QUALITY CONTROL

W. Greg Miller

KEY POINTS

- Quality control samples are assayed on a regular schedule to verify that a laboratory procedure is performing correctly.
- Interpretation of quality control results is based on acceptance criteria that will identify bias, trend in bias, or imprecision that exceeds expected method performance attributes.
- In the event of an unacceptable quality control result, corrective action is taken to fix the method problem, and all patient results from the time of the previous acceptable quality control result are repeated.
- Because of commutability limitations, quality control samples should not be used to verify that two methods, or two different lots of reagents, produce the same results for patient samples.
- Proficiency testing provides external evaluation that a laboratory is using a method correctly and in conformance to the manufacturer's specifications.

The purpose of a clinical laboratory test is to evaluate the pathophysiologic condition of an individual patient to assist with diagnosis and/or to monitor therapy. To have value for clinical decision-making, an individual laboratory test result must have total error small enough to reflect the biological condition being evaluated. The total error of a result is influenced by the following:

- Biological/physiologic variability within an individual
- Preanalytic variability in sample collection, transportation, processing, and storage
- Analytic variability in test performance
- Interfering substances such as drugs or metabolic components

Quality control (QC, also called statistical process control) is a process to periodically examine a measurement procedure to verify that it is performing according to preestablished specifications. This chapter addresses QC of an analytic measurement procedure using QC sample materials intended to simulate clinical samples from patients. Such QC sample materials are called surrogate samples. The QC samples are measured periodically in the same manner as clinical samples and their results examined to ensure that the measurement procedure meets performance requirements appropriate for patient care. Techniques for using results from patient samples in the QC program are also included. This chapter is organized as follows:

- Analytical accuracy and imprecision
- Calibration issues in quality control
- Overview of quality control procedures
- Implementing quality control procedures
- Reagent and calibrator lot changes
- Using patient data in quality control procedures
- Proficiency testing
- Quality management

Analytic Accuracy (Trueness) and Imprecision

Figures 10-1 and 10-2 illustrate the meaning of accuracy (trueness) and imprecision for a measurement. The relationship between the terms accuracy and trueness is clarified by following Figure 10-2. In Figure 10-1, the horizontal axis represents the numeric value for an individual result, and the vertical axis represents the number of repeated measurements with the same value made on aliquots of a sample. The red line shows the dispersion of results for repeated measurements of the same sample (e.g., a QC sample), which is the random imprecision of the measurement. The imprecision frequently follows a Gaussian (normal) distribution and is described by the standard deviation (SD). The SD is a measure of expected imprecision in a result when the method is performing correctly. Note that results near the average value (mean) occur more frequently than results farther

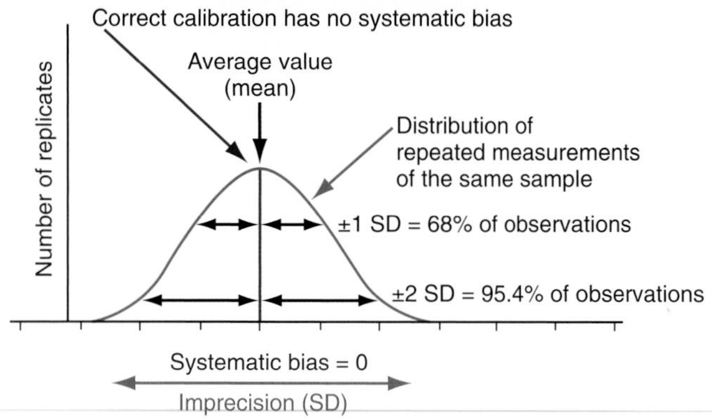

Figure 10-1 Illustration of results distribution showing expected imprecision for repeated measurements of a quality control sample.
SD, Standard deviation.

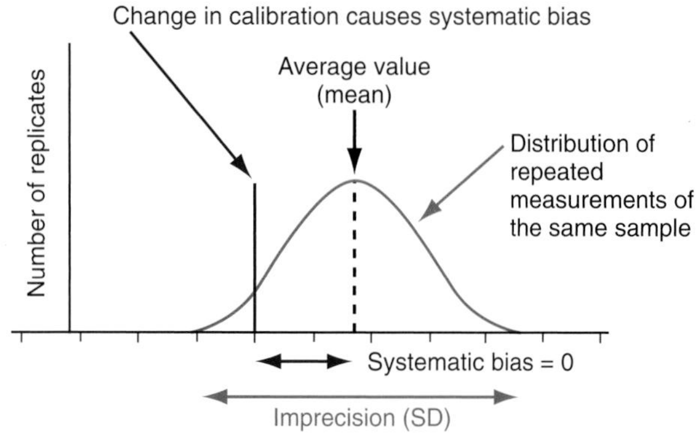

Figure 10-2 Illustration of systematic bias when a change in calibration has occurred.
SD, Standard deviation.

away from the mean. A result that is 2 SD from the mean is expected to occur 4.5% of the time (100%–95.4%) in a positive or a negative direction from the mean value. Correct calibration of a method eliminates systematic bias (within uncertainty limits), so the mean of repeated measurements of a sample becomes the expected value for that sample when the method is performing correctly.

Figure 10-2 illustrates that if the calibration changes for any reason, a systematic bias is introduced into the results. The systematic bias is the difference between the observed average value and the expected value for a sample. Note that the imprecision of an incorrectly calibrated method is the same as when correctly calibrated. All methods have an inherent imprecision. The primary purpose of measuring QC samples is to statistically evaluate the measurement process to verify that the method continues to perform within the specifications consistent with acceptable systematic bias and imprecision. QC result acceptance criteria, discussed in a later section, are based on the probability for an individual QC result to be different from the variability in results expected when the method is performing correctly.

The term accuracy is used for an individual result and is the combination of systematic bias and imprecision that occurred for that specific measurement. An individual QC sample result can evaluate the combined errors caused by systematic bias in calibration and imprecision of the measurement procedure. The result for an individual patient sample can also be influenced by interfering substances that may be present in that sample. Total error for a patient sample measurement is the sum of systematic bias, imprecision, and sample specific bias caused by any interfering substances that may be present. Statistical QC does not evaluate possible interfering substances that may affect results from patient samples. However, the imprecision observed in QC results provides a measure of the variability expected for individual patient results caused by the inherent imprecision of the method.

The term trueness is used to refer to an average systematic bias that may be present in a given method. Trueness is an attribute of a method that reflects how correctly the calibration of that method is traceable to a reference system and is discussed further in the next section.

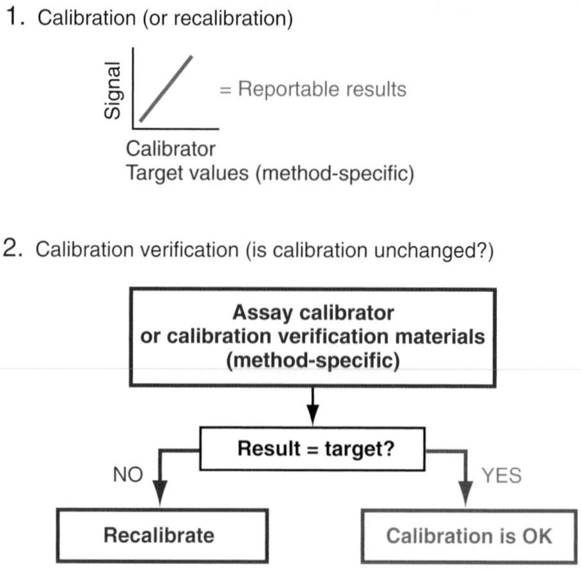

Figure 10-3 Calibration (1), and calibration verification (2) using method-specific calibrators (or other method-specific calibration verification materials).

Calibration Issues in Quality Control

Calibration of the analytic measurement procedure is a key component in achieving quality results. Figure 10-3 part 1 shows calibration of a method, which establishes the relationship between the signal measured and the quantitative value of analyte in the calibrator materials. This relationship is used to convert the measurement signal from a patient sample into a reportable concentration for the analyte. Specific techniques for calibration are unique to individual methods and will not be covered here. However, some general principles for implementing calibration procedures can contribute to the stability and clinical reliability of laboratory results.

CALIBRATION AND VERIFICATION OF CALIBRATION

Calibration of methods is most often performed by the laboratory using calibrator materials provided by the method or instrument manufacturer. In some cases (e.g., point-of-care devices), methods are calibrated during the manufacturing process, and the laboratory performs a verification of that calibration. In either situation, traceability of result accuracy to the highest-order reference system is provided by the method manufacturer. The method manufacturer's calibrator material(s) and assigned target value(s) are designed to produce accurate results with clinical patient samples assayed using that particular manufacturer's routine method. One manufacturer's product calibrator is not intended for use with other methods, and laboratories should not use calibrator materials intended for one method with any other method. Use of a calibrator with a method for which it was not specifically intended can produce miscalibration and erroneous patient results (see next section).

In principle, a measurement procedure should be calibrated only when evidence indicates that the current calibration is no longer valid. A recalibration event may introduce a small change in the relationship between analytic system response and sample concentration that contributes to overall long-term variability in method performance. Evidence that a recalibration is needed could come from QC sample results that demonstrate a shift or trend in bias over a time period. However, QC results are expected to have random variability that may make identification of a trend in bias difficult to detect. Consequently, it is common practice to recalibrate methods on a time schedule that is established based on experience with the sources of drift that are important for a given technology. In vitro device (IVD) manufacturers frequently specify calibration intervals.

The U.S. Clinical Laboratory Improvement Act (CLIA) regulations, section 493.1255, require calibration or calibration verification at least every 6 months, or more frequently if recommended by the method manufacturer (Department of Health and Human Services, 2003). When no change in method performance parameters has occurred, it is acceptable to verify that the current calibration has not changed (calibration verification), rather than perform a recalibration.

Figure 10-3 part 2 shows that a method's current calibration can be verified not to have changed rather than performing a recalibration. One common procedure to verify calibration is to assay the method calibrator materials as "unknowns." Recovery of target values for the calibrators indicates that the measurement system calibration has not changed (i.e., the current calibration is verified to be correct), and there is no reason to perform a recalibration to reestablish the same relationship between measurement signal and calibrator concentration that is already in use. The laboratory must establish criteria for agreement with the calibrator target value for calibration verification. Conservative criteria for agreement, such as ±1 SD from the target value, should be considered to avoid misinterpretation of calibration status.

CALIBRATION TRACEABILITY TO A REFERENCE SYSTEM AND COMMUTABILITY CONSIDERATIONS

Whenever possible, calibration of routine methods should be traceable to a higher-order reference measurement procedure or international reference material (Vesper, 2009). For commercially available methods cleared by the U.S. Food and Drug Administration (FDA), the IVD manufacturer provides product calibrators that have calibration traceable to the applicable reference system for an analyte (measureand in international terminology).

It is important to recognize that IVD manufacturer-provided calibrators typically have matrix characteristics and target values that are intended only for use with that specific method and cannot be used with any other manufacturer's methods. An IVD manufacturer can assign a target value to a method-specific calibrator that corrects for any matrix-related bias that may be present, so that results for clinical samples are correctly traceable to the reference system for an analyte. However, if such a method-specific calibrator is used with a different method, its target value will cause miscalibration, because it does not compensate for a different matrix-related bias with that different method (i.e., the calibrator is not commutable with clinical samples when used with a different method; see later).

A clinical laboratory may wish to verify that a method's calibration conforms to a method manufacturer's claim for traceability to the reference system used for a given analyte. Some method manufacturers provide calibration verification materials specifically intended for this purpose. Such materials may be provided as method-specific QC materials. As for method-specific calibrators, such method manufacturer–provided QC materials typically have matrix characteristics and target values that are intended only for use with the specific methods claimed in the instructions for use and cannot be used with any other manufacturer's methods. Such method-specific calibration verification materials may have target values that are specific for stated reagent lots, or may have values certified by the manufacturer to be suitable for all reagent lots. IVD manufacturer–supplied calibrators and calibration verification materials will not be commutable with clinical patient samples when used with a different method (see later).

National and international reference materials are available for some analytes. In most cases, these reference materials are intended for use with higher-order reference measurement procedures and may not be suitable for use with routine clinical laboratory methods. Laboratories should not use national or international reference materials to calibrate a routine method (or to verify calibration of a routine method) unless the reference material's commutability with patient samples has been verified for the specific routine method used by a laboratory. A commutable reference material has the same numeric relationship between two or more methods as is observed for a panel of clinical patient samples (Miller, 2006; CLSI, 2008; ISO, 2003). Consequently, a commutable reference material (or calibrator) reacts in a measurement system to give a numeric result that would be equivalent to that expected for a patient sample with the same amount of analyte. Differences in matrix-related bias between a reference material (or calibrator) and clinical patient samples cause a noncommutable relationship between the reference material (or calibrator) and the patient samples.

A reference material's certificate of analysis should be reviewed for commutability documentation. If a reference material is commutable with patient samples for a given method, it can be used for calibration or verification of calibration traceability to the reference system. Otherwise, its use for calibration or verification of calibration could cause the routine method to be miscalibrated and could produce erroneous patient results (Koch, 1988; Naito, 1993; Franzini, 1998; Thienpont, 2003; Miller, 2003, 2006). Most higher-order reference materials have not been evaluated for commutability with patient samples measured using clinical laboratory methods. If a reference material's commutability status is unknown, it must be assumed not to be commutable with patient samples.

Third-party QC materials (i.e., those provided by a manufacturer other than the routine method's manufacturer) are not suitable to verify calibration traceability. These materials are not validated for commutability with clinical samples for different routine methods, and they do not have target values that are traceable to higher-order reference measurement procedures. Such QC materials are designed to be used as QC samples for statistical process control, with target values and SD values assigned as described later in the Implementing Quality Control Procedures section. When third-party QC materials are used in an interlaboratory method comparison program with method-specific peer group mean values, these values can be used to confirm that a laboratory is using a specific method in conformance with other users of the same method (see Proficiency Testing section, later).

OVERVIEW OF QUALITY CONTROL PROCEDURES

Statistical QC evaluates the measurement procedure by periodically assaying QC materials for which the correct result is known in advance. If the result for a QC material is within acceptable limits of the known value, the measurement procedure is verified to be performing as expected, and results for patient samples can be reported with good probability that they are suitable for clinical use. If QC results are not within acceptable limits, patient results are not reported and corrective action is necessary. Good laboratory practice requires verification that a method is performing correctly at the time patient results are measured.

Figure 10-4 summarizes statistical QC and emphasizes its role as a component of an integrated quality management system. The key elements of statistical QC involve sampling the measurement system using QC samples for which the expected result is known. If the QC results indicate a stable measurement process (i.e., results are within acceptable limits, consistent with expected method performance), then the patient results have a high probability of being suitable for clinical use and can be reported. If the QC results fail evaluation criteria, then the patient results may not be reliable for clinical use. In the latter case, corrective action must be taken to fix the analytic process; this is followed by repeat assay of patient samples and QC samples to confirm that the defect was corrected.

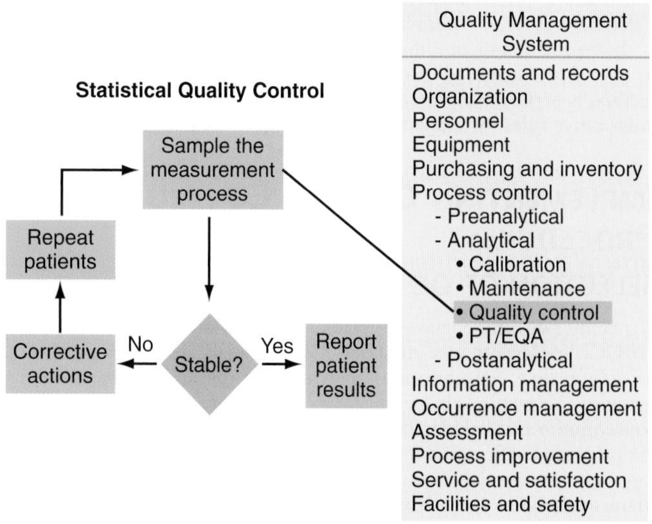

Figure 10-4 Overview of statistical quality control and its integration into a quality management system. *(Reprinted with permission from Miller WG, Nichols JH. Quality control. In: Clarke WA, editor. Contemporary practice in clinical chemistry, 2nd ed. Washington DC: AACC Press; 2010.)*
EQA, External quality assessment; *PT,* proficiency testing.

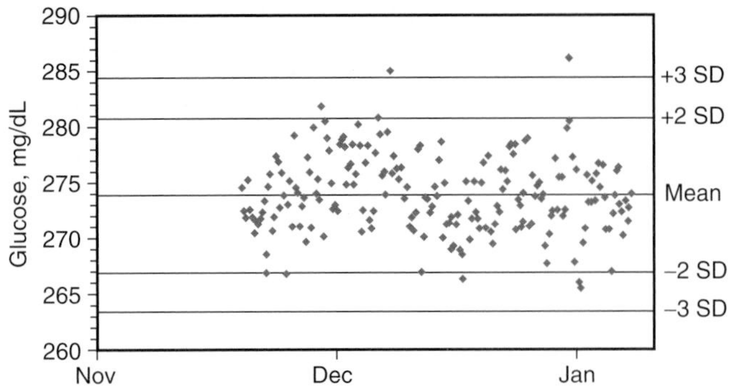

Figure 10-5 Levey-Jennings plot of quality control (QC) results (N = 199) for a single lot of QC material used for a 49-day period.
SD, Standard deviation.

Statistical QC is part of the analytic component of the overall quality management system. The quality management system integrates good laboratory practices to ensure correct results for patient care. Well-trained and competent personnel are critical for all aspects of laboratory medicine, including quality control. Written standard operating procedures (SOPs) are required for all aspects of laboratory operation, including preanalytic, analytic, and postanalytic components. For statistical process control, the SOP should include all aspects of the program, including the selection of QC materials, how frequently to sample the measurement process, how to determine statistical parameters to describe method performance, criteria for acceptability of QC results, corrective action when problems are identified, and documentation and review processes. The SOP should include who is authorized to establish acceptable control limits and interpretive rules for release of results, who should review performance parameters including statistical quality control results, and who can authorize exceptions to or modify an established QC policy or procedure.

Figure 10-5 shows a Levey-Jennings (Levey, 1950), also called Shewhart (Shewhart, 1931), plot, which is the most common presentation for evaluating QC results. This format shows each QC result sequentially over time and allows a quick visual assessment of method performance, including trend detection. The mean value represents the target (or expected) value for the result, and the SD lines represent the expected imprecision for the method. Assuming a Gaussian (normal) distribution of imprecision, the results are distributed as expected, with results scattered uniformly around the mean, and with results observed more frequently closer to the mean than near the extremes of the distribution. Note that a few results are greater than 2 SD, and two results slightly exceed 3 SD, which is expected on the basis of a Gaussian distribution of imprecision. For a large number of repeated assays, the number of results expected within the SD intervals is as follows:

- ±1 SD = 68.3% of observations
- ±2 SD = 95.4% of observations
- ±3 SD = 99.7% of observations

Interpretation of an individual QC result is based on its probability to be part of the expected distribution of results for the method when the method is performing correctly. A later section provides details regarding interpretive rules for evaluation of QC results.

IMPLEMENTING QUALITY CONTROL PROCEDURES

SELECTION OF QC MATERIALS

Generally, two different concentrations are necessary for adequate statistical QC. For quantitative methods, QC materials should be selected to provide analyte concentrations that monitor the analytic measurement range of the method. In practice, laboratories are frequently limited by concentrations available in commercial QC products. When possible, it is important to confirm that method performance is stable near the limits of the assay because defects may affect these concentrations before others. Many quantitative assays have a linear response over the analytic measurement range, and it is reasonable to assume that their performance over the range is acceptable if the results near the assay limits are acceptable. In the case of non–linear method response, it may be necessary to use additional controls at intermediate concentrations. Critical concentrations for clinical decisions (e.g., glucose, therapeutic drugs, thyroid-stimulating hormone, prostate-specific antigen, troponin) may also warrant QC monitoring. In the case of analytes that have poor precision at low concentrations, such as troponin or bilirubin, the concentration must be chosen to provide adequate SD for practical evaluation. For procedures with extraction or other pretreatment, controls must be used in the extraction or pretreatment step.

This chapter is primarily focused on QC procedures for quantitative methods. However, the principles can be adapted to most qualitative procedures with allowances for the lack of numeric results. For tests based on qualitative interpretation of quantitative measurements (e.g., drugs of abuse, human chorionic gonadotropin), negative and positive controls should be selected that have concentrations relatively near the threshold to adequately control for discrimination between negative and positive. For qualitative procedures with graded responses (e.g., dipstick urinalysis), negative, positive, and graded response controls are required. For qualitative tests based on other properties (e.g., electrophoretic procedures, stain adequacy, immunofluorescence, organism identification), it is necessary to ensure that the QC procedure will appropriately discriminate normal from pathologic conditions.

The QC materials selected must be manufactured to provide a stable product that can be used for an extended time period, preferably one or more years for stable analytes. Use of a single lot for an extended period allows reliable interpretive criteria to be established that will permit efficient identification of an assay problem, avoid false alerts due to poorly defined expected ranges for the QC results, and minimize limitations in interpreting values following reagent and calibrator lot changes.

Limitations of QC Materials

Limitations are inherent in currently available QC materials. One limitation is that the QC material is frequently noncommutable with clinical patient samples. A commutable QC material (or other reference material such as a method calibrator or proficiency testing [PT] material) is one that reacts in a measurement system to give a result that would be equivalent to that expected for an authentic patient sample with the same amount of analyte. QC and PT materials are typically noncommutable with clinical patient samples because the serum or other biological fluid matrix is usually altered from that of a patient sample (Franzini, 1998; Cattazzo, 2001; Thienpont, 2003; Miller, 2003, 2005, 2008). The matrix alteration is due to processing of the biological fluid during product manufacturing, use of partially purified human and nonhuman analyte additives to achieve desired concentrations, and various stabilization processes that alter proteins, cells, and other components. The impact of the matrix alteration on the recovery of an analyte in an assay system is not predictable and is frequently different for different lots of QC material, for different lots of reagent within a given analytic method, and for different analytic methods. Because of the noncommutability limitation, special procedures are required (discussed in later sections) when changing lots of reagent or comparing QC results among two or more methods.

A second limitation of QC materials is deterioration of the analyte during storage. Analyte stability during unopened storage is generally excellent, but slow deterioration eventually limits the shelf life of a product and can introduce a gradual drift into monitoring data. Analyte stability after reconstitution, thawing, or vial opening can be an important source of variability in QC results and can vary substantially among analytes in the same vial. User variables to be controlled are the time spent at room temperature and the time spent uncapped with the potential for evaporation. An expiration time after opening is provided by the product manufacturer but may need to be established by a laboratory for each QC material, and may be different for different analytes in the same control product. For QC materials reconstituted by adding a diluent, vial-to-vial variability can be minimized by standardizing the pipetting procedure (e.g., using the same pipet or filling device [preferably an automated device], having the same person prepare the controls) whenever practical.

Another limitation is that analyte concentrations in multiconstituent control materials may not be at levels optimal for all assays. This limitation may be caused by solubility considerations or potential interactions between different constituents, particularly at higher concentrations. It may be necessary to use supplementary QC materials to adequately monitor the analytic measurement range.

FREQUENCY TO ASSAY QC SAMPLES

The frequency to assay QC samples is a function of several parameters:

- Analytic stability of the method
- Risk of clinical action being taken before a significant error is detected

- Number of patient results produced in a period of time that may need to be repeated when an error condition is identified
- Need to verify a method's performance before recalibration or significant maintenance alters the condition of the measurement system
- Training and competency of the test operator, particularly for manual or semiautomated methods
- Residual risk of failure of the measuring device

Stability of the Measurement System

The stability of the measurement system is a fundamental determinant of how frequently a QC sample needs to be assayed. The more stable the system, the less frequently a statistical QC evaluation needs to be performed. Minimum laboratory practice, consistent with CLIA regulations, section 493.1256 (Department of Health and Human Services, 2003), is to assay controls at least once per 24 hours, or more frequently if specified by the method manufacturer, or if the laboratory determines that more frequent QC assays are necessary for the performance characteristics of a method. Some types of tests have more stringent requirements. For example, CLIA section 493.1267 requires that at least one control be assayed every 8 hours (including both high and low concentrations over a period of 24 hours) for blood gas measurements; in addition, a control must be run with each patient sample unless the instrument automatically calibrates at least every 30 minutes.

Risk of Harm to a Patient

The risk of clinical action being taken before a significant error is detected is an important consideration for more frequent QC sampling than one based strictly on method stability characteristics, or on regulatory minimum requirements. More frequent QC sampling is appropriate to avoid the situation of discovering a methodologic problem many hours after a physician has performed a clinical intervention based on an erroneous result. For example, QC sampling performed on a 24-hour cycle might be performed at 9 AM. If QC results indicate a method problem, the erroneous condition could have started at any time during the previous 24 hours. If the problem had occurred at 3 PM the previous day, erroneous results would have been reported for 18 hours.

The medical risk of harm to a patient from erroneous results must be considered and the frequency of QC testing established to minimize risk. From a practical perspective, the cost of a medical error, or simply the cost of repeating questionable patient samples since the last acceptable QC results, could be more expensive than a more frequent QC sampling schedule that would detect an error condition in a more timely manner.

CLSI has published a guideline addressing risk-based QC procedures. The document provides guidance to clinical laboratories on how to develop a QC plan based on evaluation of risk of harm to a patient and assessment of the effectiveness of risk mitigation procedures using information from the manufacturer and from other sources combined with the clinical requirements of the local health care setting and conditions in the laboratory (CLSI, 2010).

In general terms, the laboratory director is responsible to ensure that a result has a high probability to be correct at the time it is reported for clinical use. To make this judgment, the laboratory director needs to understand the risks that can cause a measurement technology to perform incorrectly, needs to evaluate the effectiveness of built-in control processes to mitigate those risks, and needs to ensure that adequate control procedures are in place to confirm that a result is correct at the time it is reported. A combination of built-in and external monitoring procedures using surrogate QC samples can be utilized to ensure that all risks have been appropriately mitigated and/or monitored at a frequency commensurate with the risk of malfunction and the risk of harm to a patient if an incorrect result was reported.

Equivalent Quality Control

The phrase "equivalent quality control" was introduced in the Survey Procedures and Interpretive Guidelines for Laboratories and Laboratory Services (Appendix C, 2003) of the CLIA quality control requirements (Department of Health and Human Services, 2003). "Equivalent quality control" was intended to justify less frequent assay of surrogate QC samples for measurement systems that utilized built-in control procedures to monitor various aspects of the measurement process. The survey procedures and interpretive guidelines defined three conditions to qualify a measurement system for less frequent assay of surrogate QC samples. No scientific evidence supports the validity of the arbitrarily defined options, and controversy surrounded their implementation (CLSI, 2005).

Some measurement systems have been designed with sophisticated built-in control procedures to mitigate the risk that an erroneous result may be produced. These control procedures have included electronic sensors, as well as liquid solutions integrated with reagent packaging, and measurement sensor devices with algorithms that prevent a result from being produced if any monitored conditions fail to meet criteria. Some of these measurement systems may be sufficiently stable and self-monitored to justify reduced frequency of surrogate QC sample testing. Because of the lack of scientific credibility for the three conditions used by the CLIA Survey Procedures and Interpretive Guidelines for Laboratories and Laboratory Services to qualify for reduced QC frequency, laboratory directors should use the risk assessment approach described in the CLSI (2010) document when evaluating the acceptability of manufacturers' claims.

QC Sample Assay Before Recalibration or Maintenance

It is necessary to assay QC samples before scheduled recalibration or maintenance. Each of these operations is intended to restore the measurement conditions to optimal specifications and to correct for any calibration drift or component deterioration that may have occurred. It is generally required to assay QC samples after these operations to verify correct method performance. It is also necessary to assay QC samples before these operations to verify that no significant errors in results have occurred since the last time QC samples were assayed, and before recalibration or maintenance alters the condition of the measurement system.

ESTABLISHING QC TARGET VALUE AND SD THAT REPRESENT A STABLE MEASUREMENT OPERATING CONDITION

QC target values and acceptable performance limits are established to optimize the probability to detect a measurement defect that is large enough to have an impact on clinical care, while minimizing the frequency of "false alerts" due to statistical limitations of the criteria used to evaluate QC results. The measurement system must be correctly calibrated and operating within acceptable performance specifications before the statistical parameters to establish QC interpretive rules can be established. Some sources of measurement variability are listed in Table 10-1. Measurement variability includes sources with short time interval frequencies, many of which can be described by Gaussian error distributions, and intermittent and longer time interval sources, which can cause cyclic fluctuations over several days or weeks, gradual drift over weeks or months, and more abrupt small shifts in results. QC interpretive rules need to be established that adequately account for all sources of variability in results that are consistent with the measurement system performing to specifications.

A QC material must have a reliable target value that represents the condition when systematic bias is as small as possible. This condition requires the method to be calibrated correctly and adequate replicate measurements to be obtained over a sufficient time interval to include the typical sources of measurement variability that will ensure that a representative mean value is calculated from the data. This objective is rarely met for longer-term variability components. The generally accepted minimum protocol for target value assignment is to use the mean value from assaying a QC material a minimum of 20 times, on 20 different days (CLSI, 2006). If a 20-day protocol is not practical, provisional target values can be established with fewer data but should be updated when additional replicate results are available. When applicable, more than one method of calibration should be represented in the 20-day period to adequately include the variability associated with the calibration process. If a QC material will be used for longer than 1 day, a single vial should be stored correctly and assayed on as many days as the material is planned to be used. This protocol will allow any variability caused by deterioration of the analyte to be averaged into the target value.

Some QC materials are provided by the method manufacturer with preassigned target values and ranges intended to confirm that the method meets the manufacturer's specifications. Such assigned values may be used initially by the laboratory. It is recommended that both the target value and the SD should be reevaluated and adjusted by the laboratory after adequate replicate results have been obtained because the QC interpretive rules used in a single laboratory should reflect performance for the method in that laboratory. The acceptability limits (product insert ranges) suggested by a manufacturer typically are based on data collected from several

TABLE 10-1
Common Sources of Measurement Variability

Source	Time interval for fluctuation	Likely statistical distribution
Pipet volume	Short	Gaussian
Instrument temperature control	Short or long	Gaussian or other
Electronic noise in the measuring system	Short	Gaussian
Calibration cycles	Short to long	Gaussian or shift (periodic step)
Reagent deterioration in storage	Long	Drift
Reagent deterioration after opening	Intermediate	Cyclic, periodic drift/step
Calibrator deterioration in storage	Long	Drift
Calibrator deterioration after opening	Intermediate	Cyclic, periodic drift/step
Control material deterioration in storage	Long	Drift
Control material deterioration after opening	Intermediate	Cyclic, periodic drift/step
Environmental temperature and humidity	Variable	Variable
Reagent lot changes	Long	Shift (random step)
Calibrator lot changes	Long	Shift (random step)
Instrument maintenance	Variable	Cyclic or shift (periodic step)
Deterioration of instrument components	Variable	Variable

laboratories. These data will inevitably account for sources of variability, such as between instruments, between reagent lots, and between calibrator lots, that will be greater than the variability expected for a method used in an individual laboratory. Use of product insert ranges that are too large will reduce a laboratory's ability to detect an erroneous measurement condition.

QC materials with assigned target values are also available from third-party manufacturers (i.e., manufacturers not affiliated with the method manufacturer). Caution should be used with third-party QC materials because the target values may have been assigned using inadequate statistical protocols. On the other hand, reliable peer group target values may be obtained from an interlaboratory comparison program with large numbers of laboratories using the same method.

Once a target value has been assigned to a QC material, a SD must be assigned that represents the typical imprecision of the method when it is performing according to its design specifications. SD is the conventional way to express method variability, even though non-Gaussian components of variability may influence QC results, because the statistical packages in instrument and laboratory computer systems are designed for QC data analysis that assumes only Gaussian uncertainty distribution. SD based on data from the 20-day target value assignment, or a 30-day monthly summary, has a large uncertainty (typically 30% for N = 20; CLSI, 2006) and is very unlikely to include all sources of variability expected over a longer time interval. It is recommended to determine the SD for stable measurement performance from the cumulative SD over a 6- to 12-month period for a single lot of QC material. This approach is likely to include all expected sources of variation. (See an important limitation when determining a cumulative SD, described later in the section Verifying QC Evaluation Parameters Following a Reagent Lot Change).

Figure 10-6 illustrates (with actual data for a glucose method) the fluctuation in SD that occurs when calculated for monthly intervals compared with the relatively stable value observed for the cumulative SD after a period of 6 months. Note that the cumulative SD is not the average of the monthly values but is the SD determined from all individual results obtained over a time interval since the lot of QC material was first used. Different sources of long-term variability occur at different times during the use of a method. The monthly SD does not adequately reflect the longer-term components of variability. However, the cumulative SD includes contributions from all sources of variability. Consequently, the cumulative SD will typically be larger than the monthly values, and will better represent the actual variability of the method. If the imprecision expected during normal stable operation is underestimated, the acceptable range for QC results will be too small, and the false alert rate will be unacceptably high. If imprecision for the stable condition is overestimated, the acceptable range will be too large, and a significant measurement error might go undetected.

It is important to include all valid QC results in the calculation of SD to ensure that the SD correctly represents expected method variability. A valid QC result is one that was, or would have been in the case of preliminary value assignment, used to verify acceptable assay performance and reporting of patient results. Only QC results that were, or would have been, responsible for not releasing patient results should be deleted (with documentation) from summary calculations. If inappropriate editing of QC results occurs, the method SD may be inappropriately small, which will produce inappropriately small evaluation limits and an increase in false QC alerts with concomitant reduction in the effectiveness of statistical QC evaluation.

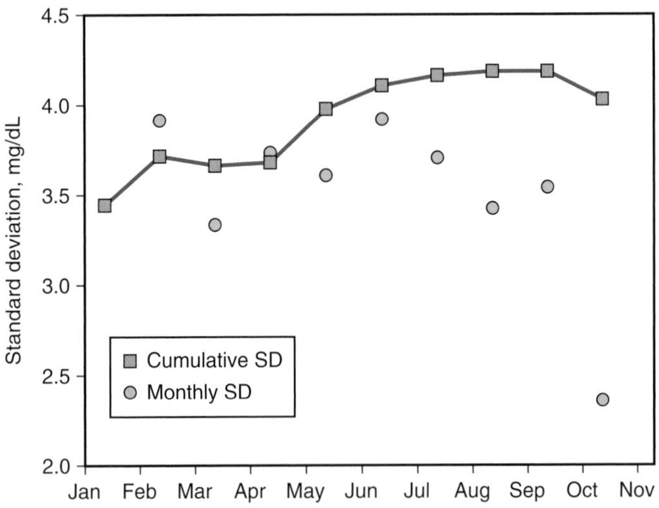

Figure 10-6 Cumulative standard deviation (SD) versus single monthly values calculated from the data in Figure 10-8.

When a method has been established in a laboratory, and a new lot of QC material is being introduced, the target value for the new lot is used along with the cumulative SD from the previous lot to establish acceptable ranges for the new lot of QC material. This practice is appropriate because in most cases measurement imprecision is a property of the method and equipment used and is unlikely to change with a different lot of QC material. If target values for the old and new lots are substantially different, a different imprecision may occur, and adjustment to the SD may be necessary as additional experience with the new lot is accumulated.

If a new method is introduced for which no historical performance information is available, the SD for stable performance must be established using data available from the method validation and target value assignment of the QC materials. In this case, the initial SD and evaluation criteria will need to be monitored closely and adjustments made as additional experience allows measurement imprecision from all sources to be reflected in the cumulative SD.

TABLE 10-2
Abbreviation Nomenclature for QC Evaluation Rules

Rule	Meaning	Detects
1_{2S}	One observation exceeds 2 SD from the target value. The 1_{2S} rule is not recommended because it has an excessive false alert rate.	Not recommended
1_{3S}	One observation exceeds 3 SD from the target value.	Imprecision or systematic bias
2_{2S} ($2_{2.5S}$)	Two sequential observations, or observations for two QC samples in the same run, exceed 2 SD (or 2.5 SD) from the target value in the same direction.	Bias
R_{4S}	Range between two observations in the same run exceeds 4 SD.	Imprecision
10_x or 10_m	Ten sequential observations for the same QC sample are on the same side of the target value (x or mean). The 10_x rule is not recommended because it has an excessive false alert rate.	Not recommended
8_{1S} ($8_{1.5S}$)	Eight sequential observations for the same QC sample exceed 1 SD (or 1.5 SD) in the same direction from the target value.	Bias trend
CUSUM	Cumulative sum of SDI for a specified number of previous results.	Bias trend
EWMA	Exponentially weighted moving average for a specified number of previous results with newer results having more influence (weight).	Bias trend

CUSUM, Cumulative sum; *EWMA*, exponentially weighted moving averages; *QC*, quality control; *SD*, standard deviation; *SDI*, standard deviation interval.

ESTABLISHING RULES TO EVALUATE QC RESULTS

The acceptable range and rules for interpretation of QC results are based on the probability of detecting a significant analytic error condition with an acceptably small false alert rate. The desired process control performance characteristics must be established for each analyte before the appropriate QC rules can be selected.

The conventional way to express QC interpretive rules is by using an abbreviation nomenclature popularized among clinical laboratories by Westgard (1981) and summarized in Table 10-2. Note that fractional standard deviation intervals are permissible as in the $2_{2.5S}$ example. Statistical procedures such as cumulative sum (CUSUM) or exponentially weighted moving averages (EWMA) are preferred to monitor for bias trends (Ryan, 1989). It is recommended to use one of these more advanced trend monitoring procedures if supported by an available computer system because they are more powerful than the 8_{1S} (or $8_{1.5S}$) approach for detecting trends. EWMA and CUSUM must be carefully implemented to avoid being too sensitive to small changes that may cause an excessive frequency of false alerts.

Power function graphs were developed (Westgard, 1979) to express the probability that a QC interpretive rule will detect an analytic error of a given magnitude. Westgard's statistical model assumed Gaussian (normal) error distributions and, despite the fact that non-Gaussian error distributions exist in measurement systems, has provided useful guidelines for selecting rules to interpret QC results. Other literature reports have addressed rule selection criteria using other statistical models and assumptions regarding distribution of errors (Parvin, 1997; Parvin and Gronowski, 1997; Westgard, 1992; Linnet, 1989).

Figure 10-7 shows a power function graph that plots the probability to detect a measurement error (*y*-axis), which is the probability that a result will exceed a particular interpretive rule, versus a systematic bias of known magnitude in a result (*x*-axis) with a fixed random imprecision of 1 SD. The three lines in Figure 10-7 represent the probabilities of different interpretive rules to detect systematic biases of various magnitudes. For example, for the 1_{2S} rule, a result with a systematic bias of 1 SD (*x*-axis) has a 0.35 (35%) probability (*y*-axis) of violating the rule (i.e., of having a result >2 SD from the target value). Note that this figure shows only systematic bias as SD on the *x*-axis, and a result with 1 SD systematic bias will also have imprecision that causes the 1_{2S} rule to be exceeded. Thus, a 1_{2S} interpretive rule has a 35% probability to detect a systematic error that is 1 SD in magnitude. Similar graphs can be created for other interpretive rules for both systematic bias and imprecision error conditions.

Note in Figure 10-7 that none of these interpretive rules has a 100% probability to detect a systematic bias until the error becomes relatively large. The 1_{2S} rule has a good probability of detecting errors (e.g. almost 90% probability of detecting a 2.5 SD bias) but has a high false alert rate as indicated by the *y*-intercept (note arrow showing that because of imprecision, the probability of indicating an error condition for zero bias is 10%). Because of this high false alert rate, it is not recommended to use a 1_{2S} rule. The 1_{3S} rule has a low false alert rate, but a lower probability to detect an error (e.g., a 55% probability to detect a 2.5 SD bias). It

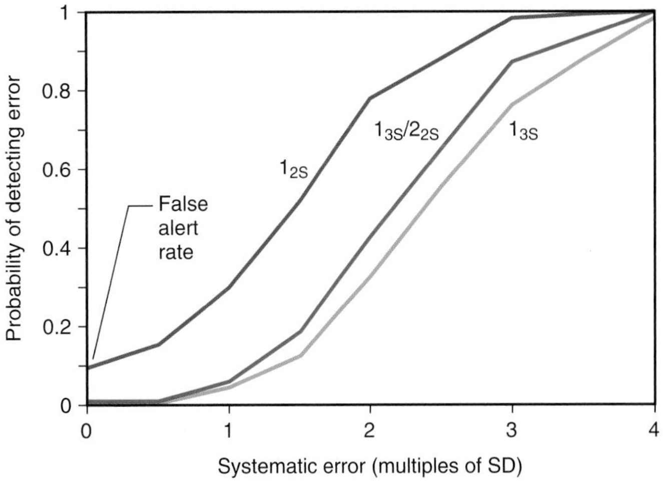

Figure 10-7 Power function graphs for the ability of different quality control interpretive rules to detect systematic error using two controls. Systematic error is expressed as number of standard deviations (SDs) from the target value. *(Adapted from Westgard JO, Smith FA, Mountain PJ, Boss S. Design and assessment of average of normals [AON] patient data algorithms to maximize run lengths for automatic process control. Clin Chem 1996;42:1683–1688, used with permission.)*

is recommended to improve the efficiency of QC interpretive rules by combining two or more rules and applying them simultaneously as multi-rule criteria. For example, the $1_{3S}/2_{2S}$ multi-rule identifies an error condition if one control exceeds ±3 SD from the target value, or if two controls exceed ±2 SD in the same direction from the target value. In Figure 10-7, the $1_{3S}/2_{2S}$ multi-rule has a low false alert rate similar to the 1_{3S} rule, but improved probability to detect an error (e.g., a 65% probability to detect a 2.5 SD bias and a 90% probability to detect a 3.2 SD bias). In this multi-rule example, the 1_{3S} component is sensitive to imprecision or large systematic bias, while the 2_{2S} component is sensitive to systematic bias.

A challenge in selecting interpretive rules for QC results is that the different sources of variation listed in Table 10-1 occur in most contemporary automated assay systems and introduce longer-term cyclic and step fluctuations in performance. These types of variability are not adequately described by Gaussian models for rules selection. Consequently, data acquired over a significant time period are necessary to determine an appropriately representative SD that represents typical variability when the method is stable and performing correctly. A representative SD is needed because essentially all commercially available QC computer systems use SD-based rules with an assumption of Gaussian error distributions. Laboratorians need to derive an SD that can be used in available computer algorithms and that reflects longer-term non-Gaussian contributions to imprecision. At certain periods of time, the short-term SD will be noticeably smaller than the long-term cumulative value (see Fig. 10-6). One must avoid concluding that the SD used for evaluation is too large because over

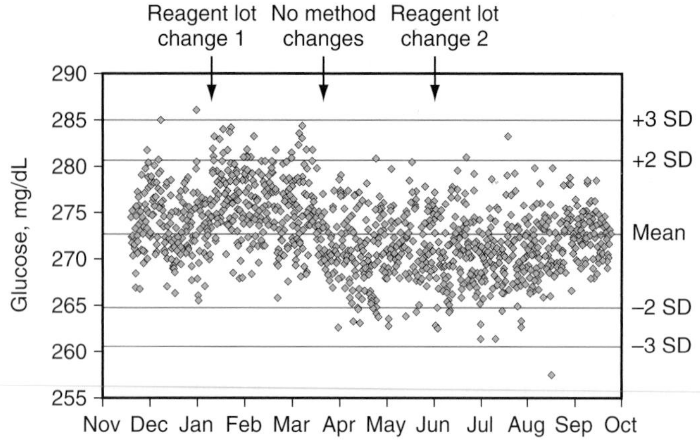

Figure 10-8 Levey-Jennings plot of quality control (QC) results (N = 1232) for a single lot of QC material used over a 10-month period. *(Reprinted with permission from Miller WG, Nichols JH. Quality control. In: Clarke WA, editor. Contemporary practice in clinical chemistry, 2nd ed. Washington DC: AACC Press; 2010.)*
SD, Standard deviation.

TABLE 10-3
Empirical Multi-rule for the QC Data in Figure 10-8

Multi-rule components	Type of variability detected
1_{3S}	Imprecision or bias
$2_{2.5S}$	Bias
R_{4S}	Imprecision
$8_{1.5S}$	Bias trend

QC, Quality control.

time the cumulative value will be more consistent with method performance, as periodic sources of variability are encountered.

Figure 10-8 shows how non-Gaussian error sources influenced results for a single lot of QC material used over a 10-month period for an automated glucose method. The glucose method stability and performance over the 10 months were considered acceptable for clinical use. Data for the first 49 days are the same as in Figure 10-5 and represent the initial experience with this lot of QC material. Examination of these data shows several fluctuations that cannot be described by a Gaussian statistical model. The first reagent lot change caused a step shift to higher values. The second reagent lot change had no effect on QC results. Between March and April, a transition to lower values occurred that did not correspond to any maintenance, reagent lot change, or calibration events. Throughout the 10-month period, intervals of several weeks' duration occurred when the imprecision was better or worse than at other time periods (also see Fig. 10-6 calculated from the same data).

In practice, empirical judgment is frequently used to establish acceptance criteria (rules) to evaluate QC results based on data acquired over a long enough time to adequately quantify the expected variability when a method is working correctly. It is not recommended to select QC rules based only on Gaussian models of imprecision because the rules will not correctly accommodate all the types of variability observed for many analytic systems.

Table 10-3 gives an example of an empirically developed multi-rule based on the data in Figure 10-8. This multi-rule had 0.6% false alerts when applied to the data in Figure 10-8, using the mean from the November–January (Fig. 10-4) period as the target value and the SD for the 10-month period to represent overall imprecision. If a 2_{2S} rule had been used instead of a $2_{2.5S}$ rule, the false alert rate would have increased by 1.2%, but the rule would detect slightly smaller biases. An $8_{1.5S}$ rule was used to provide detection of bias trends because it had a 0% false alert rate (compared with 0.5% for an 8_{1S} rule) and was adequate to detect a developing trend before it became clinically important because the SD was small, 4.0 mg/dL, at a concentration of 274 mg/dL. At other clinical concentration ranges, or for other analytes, an 8_{1S} or $6_{1.5S}$ rule may be more appropriate. A 10_x rule was not used because it would have increased the false alert rate by 10.6%. Many contemporary analyzers are very stable and may produce QC results with a small standard deviation interval (SDI) on one side of the target value for extended periods of time. Consequently, a 10_x rule generally is not recommended, as this condition does not infer a problem with clinical interpretation of patient results when the magnitude of the difference is small.

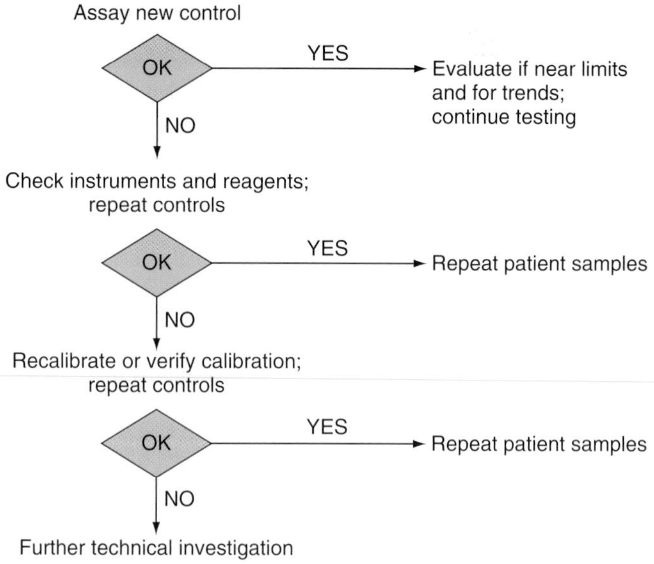

Figure 10-9 Generalized troubleshooting sequence following an unacceptable quality control result. *(Reprinted with permission from Miller WG, Nichols JH. Quality control. In: Clarke WA, editor. Contemporary practice in clinical chemistry, 2nd ed. Washington DC: AACC Press; 2010.)*

Whatever statistical approach is used, the balance between false alerts and the probability of detecting an error is improved when multiple rules are used in combination. When establishing rules to interpret QC results, it is important to remember that statistical process control can only verify that a measurement system is producing results that conform to the expected variability when the system is properly calibrated and in a stable operating condition. QC rules are chosen to detect changes in calibration and changes in imprecision that are significant enough to require correction before patient results are reported. Periodic measurement of QC samples does not identify random events (e.g., a temporary clot in a sample pipet, a random reagent pipet error) that do not persist until the next QC sample is measured.

It may be determined in the process of reviewing statistical parameters for QC data that a method's variability is too great to meet medical requirements. If the method is performing in a stable condition, the observed variability is an inherent limitation of the technology. In this case, the only solution is to improve the method or to use a different method. If the method performance cannot be improved and a better method is not available, the laboratory must accept the method limitations and communicate them to patient care providers. It is important in this circumstance not to make the QC limits or interpretive rules artificially stringent. This incorrect approach will not improve method performance, but will increase the QC false alert rate and will decrease the efficiency and practicality of the statistical QC process.

CORRECTIVE ACTION WHEN A QC RESULT INDICATES A MEASUREMENT PROBLEM

A QC alert occurs when a QC result fails an evaluation rule, which indicates that an analytic problem may exist. A QC alert means there is a high probability that the assay is producing results unreliable for patient care. When this condition occurs, it is necessary to take corrective action to investigate the cause of the QC alert. Figure 10-9 presents a generalized troubleshooting sequence. Repeating the QC measurement on the same QC sample is not recommended because, with properly designed control rules, it is more likely that a measurement system problem exists, than the QC result was a statistical outlier. However, QC materials can deteriorate after opening caused by improper handling and storage or because of unstable analytes. Thus, repeating the measurement on a new sample of the QC material is a useful step to determine if the alert was caused by deteriorated QC material rather than by a method problem. In this situation, if the result for the new QC sample is acceptable, testing of patient samples can resume. One caution, if the repeat result is near acceptability limits, is to consider that the repeat and original results may be essentially

TABLE 10-4
Example for Selected Chemistry Analytes of Empirical Criteria for Patient Test Result Agreement Between Repeated Assays; and for Agreement Among Results for a Single Patient Sample Measured on Multiple Instruments

Analyte	Acceptance criteria (difference between results)
Albumin	0.4 g/dL
ALP	10 U/L or 10%*
ALT	10 U/L or 10%*
Amylase	15 U/L or 10%
AST	10 U/L or 10%*
Bilirubin, total	0.3 or 10%*
Calcium, total	0.5 mg/dL
Chloride	4 mmol/L
Cholesterol	5%
CK	10 U/L or 10%
CO_2	4 mmol/L
Creatinine	0.2 mg/dL or 10%*
GGT	10 U/L or 10%
Glucose	6 mg/dL or 5%*
Iron	10 µg/dL or 10%
Lactate	0.32 mmol/L
LD	10 U/L or 10%
Lipase	10 U/L or 10%
Magnesium	0.3 mg/dL
Phosphorus	0.4 mg/dL
Potassium	0.3 mmol/L
Protein, total	0.4 g/dL
Sodium	4 mmol/L
Triglycerides	10%
Urea nitrogen (BUN)	3 mg/dL or 10%*
Uric acid	0.4 mg/dL

ALP, Alkaline phosphatase; *ALT,* alanine aminotransferase; *AST,* aspartate aminotransferase; *BUN,* blood urea nitrogen; *CK,* creatine kinase; *CO_2,* carbon dioxide; *GGT,* γ-glutamyl transferase; *LD,* lactate dehydrogenase.
*Whichever is greater.

of the same magnitude. In this situation, the probability is fairly high that a measurement problem exists, and this possibility should be investigated. In addition, current and preceding QC results should be examined for a trend in bias that indicates a measurement issue that needs to be corrected. These precautions in evaluating repeat results for a new QC sample can be challenging or impossible for automated evaluation by computer systems, thus requiring the laboratory technologist to be vigilant in reviewing results.

When repeat testing of a new QC sample does not resolve the alert situation, the instrument and reagents should be inspected for component deterioration, mechanical problems, etc. In many cases, it will be necessary to recalibrate (or verify calibration). When the problem is identified and corrected, QC samples should be assayed to verify the correction, and all patient samples since the time of the last acceptable QC results should be reassayed. The laboratory director must establish acceptable criteria to determine if the repeat results agree adequately to permit reporting of original results without issuing a corrected report. Otherwise, corrected results must be reported. As an example, Table 10-4 lists empirical criteria used in the author's laboratory for this purpose. The criteria for acceptability of repeated tests are based on method characteristics, population served, and clinical requirements of the medical services.

In some cases, sample volume may not be adequate (quantity not sufficient [QNS]) for repeat testing. In these situations, no results can be reported unless it is documented that the impact of the method defect on the original results was small enough to have minimal effect on clinical interpretation. A protocol to evaluate the clinical impact of the methodologic problem is to repeat those samples that have adequate volume. The repeated samples must represent the concentration range of the QNS samples, must represent the time span since the previous acceptable QC results, and should include a substantial proportion of the total samples

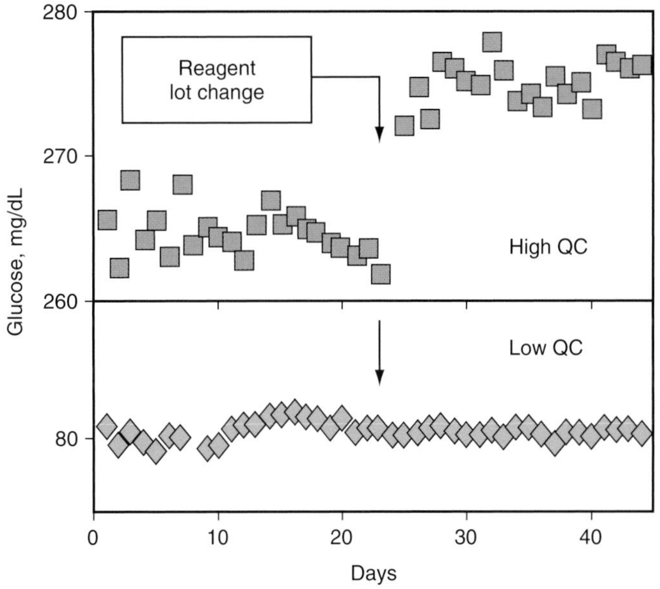

Figure 10-10 Levey-Jennings plot showing impact of a reagent lot change on matrix bias with quality control (QC) samples. *(Reprinted with permission from Miller WG, Nichols JH. Quality control. In: Clarke WA, editor. Contemporary practice in clinical chemistry, 2nd ed. Washington DC: AACC Press; 2010.)*

originally assayed while the method was in the unacceptable condition. If the repeat results for this sample group are within established criteria for repeat testing of patient samples, the original results for the QNS samples can be reported. Otherwise, the original results for the QNS samples are considered erroneous; no results can be reported, and the original results already reported need to be corrected to a "no result" condition.

Verifying QC Evaluation Parameters Following a Reagent Lot Change

Changing reagent lots can have an unexpected impact on QC results. Careful reagent lot crossover evaluation of QC target values is necessary. Because the matrix-related interaction between a QC material and a reagent can change with a different reagent lot, QC results may not be a reliable indicator of a method's performance for patient samples following a reagent lot change. In the example in Figure 10-10, QC values for the high concentration control shifted following the change to a new lot of reagents, but there was no change in results for the low control. A comparison of results for a panel of patient samples assayed using the new and old reagent lots, as shown in Figure 10-11, verified that patient results were the same when either lot of reagents was used. Patient results spanned the analytic measurement range and had nearly identical values, as indicated by the slope of 1.00 and the small intercept of −3 mg/dL. Consequently, the change in QC values for the high concentration material was due to a difference in matrix-related bias between the QC material and each of the reagent lots.

It is well documented that QC materials and PT materials, both of which are prepared similarly, have unpredictable matrix interactions when different methods and different reagent lots are used with the same method (Franzini, 1998; Cattazzo, 2001; Thienpont, 2003; Miller, 2003, 2005, 2008, 2011; Waymack, 1993). For this reason, it is necessary to use clinical patient samples to verify the consistency of results between old and new lots of reagents.

Figure 10-12 presents a procedure to verify or adjust QC material target values following a reagent lot change. The first step is to verify that calibration of the new reagent lot produces results for a group of patient samples that are consistent with results from the previous lot. The patient sample results, not the QC results, provide the basis for verifying that the method calibration is consistent with that of the previous reagent lot. If a problem is identified, the calibration of the new reagent lot must be investigated and corrected, or the new reagent lot may be defective and should not be used. When evaluating the patient results, keep in mind that the

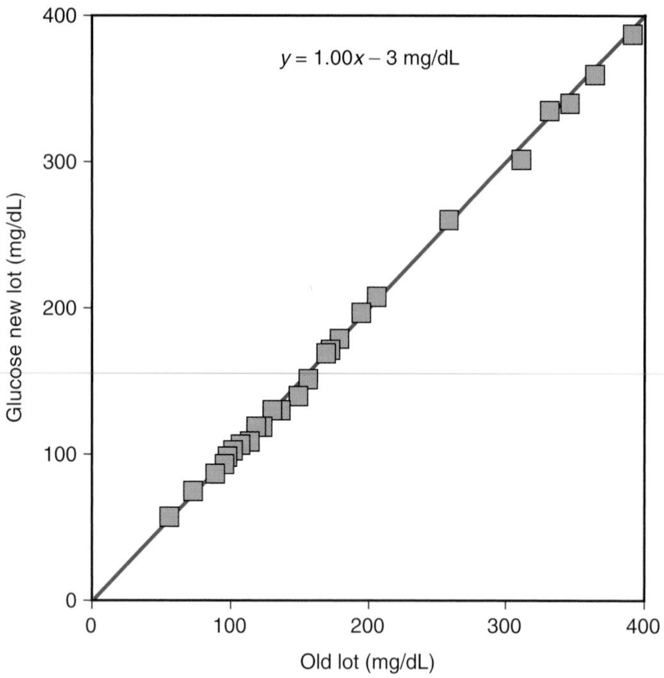

Figure 10-11 Deming regression analysis of results from a patient sample comparison between the same old and new lots of reagent shown in Figure 10-10 for quality control samples.

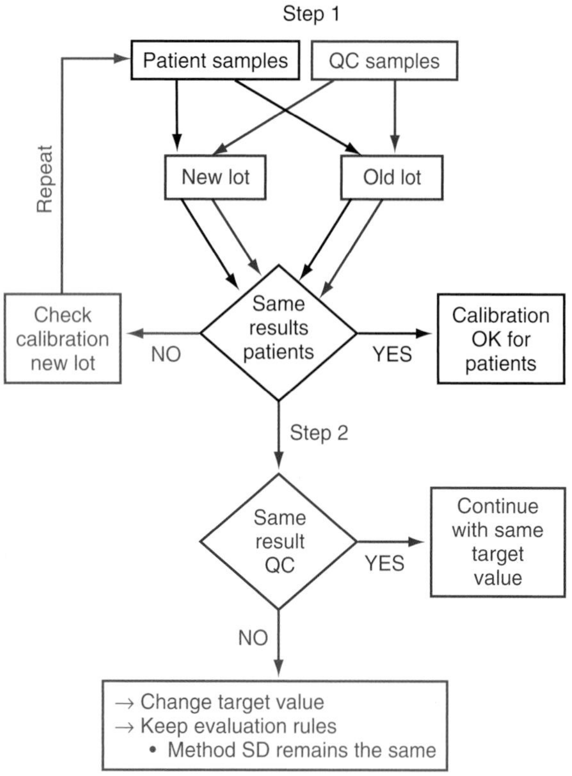

Figure 10-12 Process for assessment of potential matrix impact on quality control (QC) samples following a reagent lot change.
SD, Standard deviation.

calibration of the old reagent lot may have drifted and should be verified before concluding that the new reagent lot calibration is not correct.

There are no well established guidelines regarding the number of patient samples to use in this type of comparison when reagent lots are changed. It is recommended to select a group of patient samples that span the analytic measurement range to verify comparable results. A minimum of five samples is reasonable to cover the analytic measurement range. CLSI document C54, "Verification of Comparability of Patient Results Within One Healthcare System," includes a section on reagent lot changes and provides a statistical approach suitable for small sample sizes. Deming regression analysis (Cornbleet, 1979; Linnet, 1993) can be used with 10 or more patient samples and provides a more robust approach that allows assessment of average performance over the range of concentrations represented by the patient samples.

There are no well established clinical acceptance criteria for agreement between results; consequently, the laboratory must establish acceptance criteria consistent with the relatively small number of samples used, the analytic capability of a method, and the clinical requirements for interpreting results. As an example, empirical acceptance criteria used in the author's laboratory for assessment of individual results when five samples are used are provided in Table 10-4.

Once the results for patients are acceptable, the second step in Figure 10-12 evaluates results for each QC material to determine if its target value is correct for use with the new lot of reagent(s). If the target value has changed, it must be adjusted to correct for the change in matrix-related bias between old and new lots of reagent(s). This adjustment keeps the expected variability centered around the QC target value, so that QC interpretive rules will remain valid. Failure to make a target value adjustment will introduce an artifactual bias in subsequent QC results, causing an increased false alert rate. The SD used to evaluate QC results will not typically change when a new lot of reagent(s) is put into service. The SD represents expected variability when the method is stable and is performing according to specifications. In most cases, the variability of a method will be the same with any lot of reagent(s). However, occasional exceptions may occur, for example, if the new reagent lot is a reformulation, it may be necessary to adjust the SD after additional numbers of QC results are accumulated with the new reagent lot. A reagent lot verification typically is performed on a single day and will likely provide only a few QC results from which to evaluate if the target value has changed. Consequently, it is necessary to carefully monitor QC results as more data are acquired using the new reagent lot and, if needed, to further refine the new target value.

Note that a matrix-related bias can cause the numeric values for the QC results to shift, and this shift is an artifact of the interaction between the QC material and the reagent, not a property of the measurement system. The shift may cause an artifactual increase in the cumulative SD such that the cumulative SD may be larger than the inherent measurement variability. It is recommended to use cumulative SD from one or more single reagent lots when determining the SD to use for interpreting QC rules.

Verifying Method Performance Following Use of a New Lot of Method Calibrator

When a new lot of calibrator is used, with no change in reagents, there is no change in matrix interaction between the QC material and the reagents. In this situation, QC results provide a reliable indication of calibration status with the new lot of calibrator. If the QC results indicate a bias following use of a new lot of calibrator, the calibration has changed and needs to be corrected to ensure consistent results for patient samples.

Some methods are packaged as kits that include reagents, calibrators, and QC materials. In this case, QC results could fail to identify a calibration shift when a new kit lot is used, and it is necessary to assay clinical patient samples with the old and new kit lots to verify consistency of patient results. When possible, it is recommended to use QC materials that are independent of the kit lot, and to avoid changing lots of QC material at the same time as changing lots of reagent or calibrators. Assaying patient samples always provides a reliable approach to verify the consistency of results following changes in lots of reagents or calibrators.

Using Patient Data in Quality Control Procedures

Results from patient samples are used in four principal ways to support the QC processes in a laboratory.

- To verify consistency of patient results when changing lots of reagent or calibrators for a method (discussed in the previous section)
- To identify inconsistent results using a delta check with a previous result for a patient
- To verify consistency of patient results when an analyte is measured using more than one instrument or method in a health care system
- To verify method performance using results from patient samples in a statistical QC scheme

TABLE 10-5
Example Delta Check Criteria Intended to Identify Samples That Are Potentially Mislabeled or Contaminated With IV Fluids Due to Incorrect Collection

Test	Delta criteria
Sodium	5% change within previous 48 hours
Urea nitrogen	60% change within previous 48 hours
Creatinine	50% change within previous 48 hours
Calcium	25% change within previous 48 hours
Osmolality	5% change within previous 48 hours

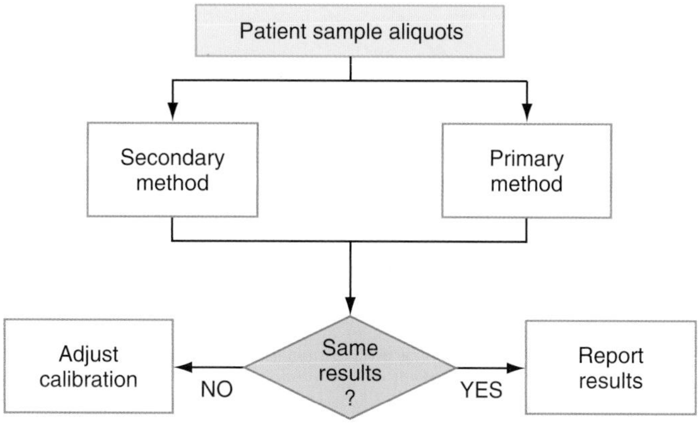

Figure 10-13 Process used to evaluate agreement between methods and to adjust calibration, if necessary, to achieve equivalent results from different methods.

DELTA CHECK WITH A PREVIOUS RESULT FOR A PATIENT

Some types of laboratory errors can be identified by comparing a patient's current test result against a previous result for the same analyte. This comparison is called a "delta check." The previous result is taken from a specified time interval in the past during which the result is not likely to have changed physiologically. This limitation restricts the analytes that can be effectively monitored with a delta check. Delta checks can detect analytic errors; however, their main purpose is to detect mislabeled samples and samples altered by dilution with IV fluid. Consequently, an effective delta check process can be established using a limited number of analytes. The difference between results that causes a delta check alert must be sufficiently large to avoid excessive numbers of false alerts and adequate to allow identification of samples that may be compromised and require follow-up investigation. Table 10-5 shows, as an example, the delta check parameters for automated chemistry used in the author's laboratory. Kazmierczak (2003) has reviewed and presented recommendations for using delta check and other patient data–based quality control procedures.

VERIFY CONSISTENCY OF RESULTS BETWEEN MORE THAN ONE INSTRUMENT OR METHOD

Another common use of patient results in a QC process is to verify consistency of patient results when an analyte is measured by using more than one instrument or method within the same health delivery system. Good laboratory medicine requires that multiple instruments or methods for the same analyte be calibrated to produce the same results for patient samples whenever possible. It may be necessary to modify the calibration settings of one measurement system to match another system's results. This strategy allows a common reference interval to be used, provides continuity in results between different laboratory testing locations, and avoids clinical confusion regarding interpretation of laboratory results. CLIA regulations, section 493.1281, require that the relationship between test results from different methods or from multiple locations should be evaluated at least twice a year (Department of Health and Human Services, 2003).

As illustrated in Figure 10-13, clinical patient sample aliquots are measured using each of two or more methods (or analyzers) to evaluate and if necessary adjust the calibration as needed to achieve agreement in results for patient samples. Such an analysis design is called a "round robin." One method/analyzer may be chosen to represent the primary method to which others will be adjusted to achieve equivalent results. The primary method should be chosen based on quality and reliability of results with consideration of its calibration traceability to national or international standards, its performance stability, its specificity for the analyte, and its susceptibility to interfering substances. An alternate approach is to evaluate each method for agreement with the mean of all methods and to adjust the calibration of any methods/analyzers as necessary to produce equivalent results among the group. When like analyzers in a group are compared, if results for one analyzer are different from results for the others, that analyzer's calibration is adjusted to conform to that of the group.

As mentioned previously, for evaluating consistency following reagent lot changes, there are no well established guidelines regarding the number of samples to use for a round robin exchange. The laboratory needs to establish the frequency of evaluation and the number of samples based on the stability of the methods, the frequency of reagent and calibrator lot changes, and the clinical requirements of the health delivery system. Common practices include a round robin exchange of one or more individual patient samples, or a pool prepared from several samples, on a weekly basis for high volume methods; or on a monthly or quarterly basis for lower volume or very stable methods; or the regulatory minimum of every 6 months. For frequent comparisons with one or two samples, concentrations should be chosen to evaluate the analytic measurement range over a period of several examinations. For less frequent comparisons, a larger number of samples is recommended to cover the analytic measurement range. When establishing interpretation criteria, the laboratory needs to consider the limited statistical power for the number of results available. CLSI document C54, "Verification of Comparability of Patient Results Within One Healthcare System," provides a statistical approach suitable for using 1–5 samples in a comparison.

Table 10-4 provides, as an example, empirical criteria used in the author's laboratory for evaluation of agreement among results for a single patient sample assayed weekly among multiple analyzers. These criteria were established based on the expected imprecision of the methods used and the clinical impact of discrepant results. To allow for the limitations of a single measurement of a single sample in a comparison, a result outside a criterion is typically not acted on unless the magnitude of a difference is much larger than the criterion, or the situation persists for 2 or more weeks.

It is recommended to use patient samples to verify agreement between multiple methods or analyzers. Results for QC materials should not be used for the purpose of verifying consistency of results for patient samples assayed using different methods or analyzers. As discussed in an earlier section, QC materials are not validated to be commutable with patient samples between different methods. Even when more than one method/analyzer from the same manufacturer is used, differences may be seen in the measured value for QC materials between different reagent lots. In principle, if more than one of the same model analyzer with the same reagent lots are used, all should have the same results for the same lot of QC material. In practice, differences in measurement details between different analyzers cause small differences in QC results. The acceptance criteria can be set to allow for such differences. However, more reliable conclusions will be drawn when patient samples are used to evaluate agreement among different analyzers.

USING PATIENT DATA FOR STATISTICAL QUALITY CONTROL

Patient results can be used in a statistical QC process to monitor method performance. For a sufficiently large number of results, the mean (or preferably median) value may be sufficiently stable to be used as an indicator of method consistency over time. This approach can be used on a periodic basis by extracting data for a specified time period (e.g., 1 month), calculating the mean and SD for the distribution of results, and comparing one time period versus another to determine whether any changes have occurred. This type of periodic evaluation can identify changes in calibration stability or in overall imprecision for a method. The mean and SD can also be compared for consistency between multiple methods for the same analyte.

Patient populations for sampling must be selected with consideration of the physiologic homogeneity of results. Important considerations include parameters likely to influence the reference interval, such as disease

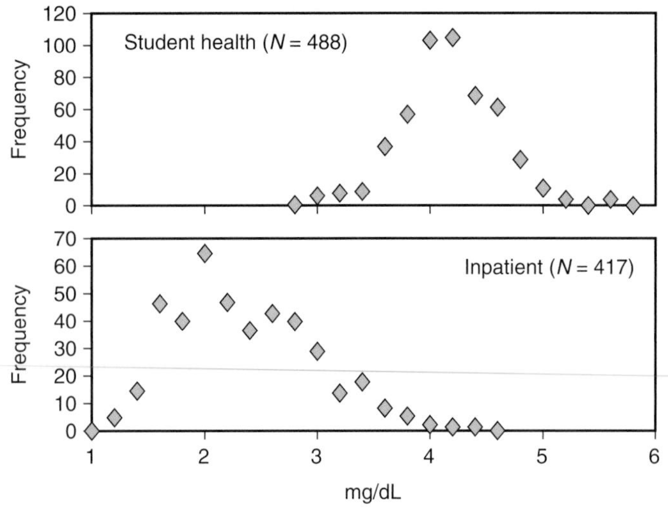

Figure 10-14 Histograms for distribution of sequential patient results for albumin from a student health outpatient clinic and a hospital general medicine inpatient unit.

status, pediatric versus adult, gender, and ethnic differences. Figure 10-14 shows an example of the potential impact of a nonhomogeneous sample of patients on distribution of albumin results for hospital general medicine inpatients compared with a student health outpatient clinic. The histograms are very different because the two patient groups differ in severity of disease, and in recumbent versus supine position for blood collection, which influences vascular water volume and the concentration of albumin.

Automated approaches to determine the mean (or median) for groups of sequential patient results used as a continuous process control parameter have been described. These methods are called "average of normals" (AON) or "moving average" techniques and are suitable for use in higher volume assays in chemistry and hematology (Westgard, 1996; Smith, 1996; Cembrowski, 1984; Ye, 2000; Kazmierczak, 2003). In general, these approaches evaluate sequential patient results over time intervals such as several hours to 1 or more days. For some analytes, patients may need to be partitioned to obtain subgroups whose results are expected to be homogeneous. Consideration of influences for partitioning includes age, gender, ethnicity, and disease conditions. Some approaches have arbitrarily trimmed abnormal results in an attempt to restrict results to more normal health conditions. Trimming approaches must be used with caution as excessive trimming will create an artificial subset of results that may not reflect a method's calibration condition.

The mean, median, or other statistical parameter for a group of results is tracked over time intervals to monitor method performance. Statistical procedures such as cumulative sum or exponentially weighted moving average are used to monitor trends in method calibration status. These approaches can be useful for supplementing traditional QC sampling techniques to monitor a method's calibration stability and to monitor calibration uniformity between multiple methods in higher volume settings. However, patient-based monitoring procedures have not been widely adopted because of lack of consensus guidelines for their use, and lack of computer support from instrument manufacturers and laboratory information system vendors.

Proficiency Testing

Proficiency testing (or external quality assessment) consists of evaluation of method performance by comparison of results versus those of other laboratories for the same set of samples. PT providers circulate a set of samples among a group of laboratories. Each laboratory includes the PT samples along with patient samples in the usual assay process. Results for the PT samples are reported to the PT provider for evaluation. PT allows a laboratory to verify that its results are consistent with those of other laboratories using the same or similar methods for an analyte, and to verify that it is using a method in conformance with the manufacturer's specifications.

PT is not available for some analytes because a particular test may be new to the clinical laboratory or is not commonly performed, or because analyte stability makes it difficult to include in PT material. In these situations, the laboratory should use an alternate approach to periodically

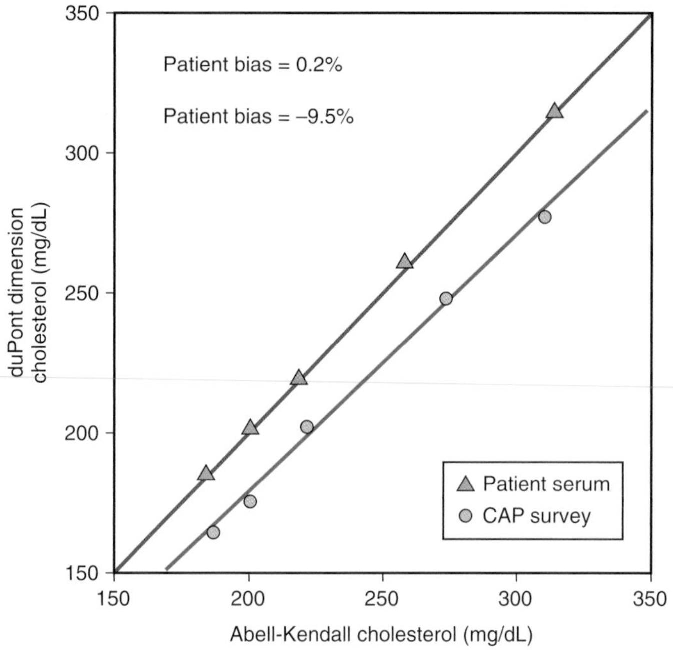

Figure 10-15 Example of noncommutable results between proficiency testing materials and pooled patient samples for a specific method. *(Adapted from Naito HK, Kwak YS, Hartfiel JL, et al. Matrix effects on proficiency testing materials: impact on accuracy of cholesterol measurement in laboratories in the nation's largest hospital system. Arch Pathol Lab Med 1993;117:345–351, used with permission.)*

verify acceptable performance of the method. CLSI has published a guideline document that provides several approaches for verifying method performance when formal PT is not available (CLSI, 2008).

QC material manufacturers may provide a data analysis service that uses peer groups for each method and calculates group statistics for performance evaluation. As with PT evaluation, this type of interlaboratory QC data analysis allows a laboratory to verify that it is producing QC results that are consistent with those of other laboratories using the same method.

NONCOMMUTABILITY OF PT MATERIALS AND PEER GROUP GRADING

It is a common practice for PT providers to organize results into "peer groups" of methods that represent similar technology expected to have the same result for a PT sample. The mean value of the peer group results is the target value. Peer group evaluation is used for PT because the materials typically used as PT samples are not commutable with native patient samples. As discussed earlier, matrix-related bias is unique to each combination of method and QC or PT material and can be quantitatively different for different method/material combinations for the same analyte. Several investigations have reported >50% incidence of noncommutable materials for many different analytes (Ross, 1998; Miller, 1993, 2003, 2005, 2008).

Figure 10-15 illustrates the effects of noncommutable materials on interpretation of PT results and demonstrates why "peer group" evaluation is used. In this example, pooled patient sera and PT samples were assayed by the duPont Dimension Analyzer (duPont, Wilmington, Del.) and by the Abell-Kendall reference method for cholesterol (Naito, 1993). The Abell-Kendall method is known to be unaffected by matrix-induced changes in PT samples (Ellerbe, 1990). The patient samples showed excellent agreement between the two methods (average bias = 0.2%). However, the PT samples had a large negative bias (–9.5%) between methods, caused by a matrix-related bias with the duPont method that was not present with the reference method (Kroll, 1990).

In this example, the routine method was correctly calibrated and produced results for patient samples that were traceable to the reference method. However, PT results gave an incorrect impression of the method's calibration relationship to the reference method. If the routine method's calibration had been erroneously adjusted on the basis of PT results, the results for patient samples would then be incorrect. PT results were useful for evaluating the performance of all laboratories using the duPont method, because the matrix-related bias was uniform within this peer

Proficiency Testing Participant Evaluation Report
Shipment date: 10/13/2003
Evaluation date: 11/21/2003

Test units method	Specimen	Reported result	Mean	SD	N labs	SDI	LIMITS OF ACCEPTABILITY Lower	Upper
Calcium	1	9.6	9.92	0.23	587	-1.4	8.9	11.0
mg/dL	2	8.8	8.86	0.26	592	-0.2	7.8	9.9
Arsenazo	3	7.5	7.65	0.23	587	-0.7	6.6	8.7
dye	4	8.2	8.43	0.23	590	-1.0	7.4	9.5
Vitros 950	5	10.8	10.87	0.25	589	-0.3	9.8	11.9
Iron	1	190	192.5	7.0	397	-0.4	154	232
mcg/dL	2	65	65.0	3.4	394	0.0	51	78
Pyridyl azo	3	74	69.2	3.2	395	+1.5	55	83
dye	4	124	107.9	4.6	395	+3.5	86	130
Vitros 950	5	277	260.9	8.8	396	+1.8	208	314

Figure 10-16 Example of an external proficiency testing evaluation report sent to a participating laboratory. *SD,* Standard deviation; *SDI,* standard deviation interval.

group. Consequently, if an individual laboratory's results agreed with those of the peer group, the individual laboratory could conclude that the method was performing in conformance with the manufacturer's specifications. In general, an individual laboratory depends on the manufacturer to correctly calibrate a clinical laboratory routine method to be traceable to the reference system for an analyte.

REPORTING PT RESULTS WHEN ONE METHOD IS ADJUSTED TO AGREE WITH ANOTHER METHOD

It is good laboratory practice (and consistent with CLIA regulations, section 493.1281) to adjust the calibration of different methods for the same analyte used within a health delivery system, so the results for patient samples are consistent, irrespective of which method is used. Such harmonization of results is important for uniform use of reference intervals and decision thresholds within a health delivery system. In this situation, it is important to report PT results such that they can be properly evaluated against the peer group target value. The peer group target value will reflect the method calibration established by the method manufacturer. For an individual laboratory's PT result to be evaluated against the peer group mean, that individual result must be reported to the PT provider after removing any calibration adjustments, so the reported result is consistent with the manufacturer's nonadjusted calibration. The most convenient way to remove a calibration adjustment is to first assay PT samples with the method calibration adjustment applied to the measurement system, as would be the usual assay process for patient samples. After the assay, adjust the PT results "in reverse" by mathematically removing the calibration adjustment factors, and report the results with any adjustment factors removed. One should not recalibrate the instrument with a new set of calibrators for the purpose of assaying PT samples, because this practice would violate regulations requiring the PT material to be assayed in the same manner as patient samples.

For example, a laboratory has performed a patient sample comparison between Method A used in the main laboratory and Method B used in a satellite laboratory. Method B consistently gave 10% higher results. Method B was adjusted to agree with Method A by putting the adjustment factor 0.9 in the Method B instrument to automatically multiply each measured result by 0.9 to lower the reported result by 10%. When PT results from Method B are reported, it is necessary to remove the 0.9 factor to allow the reported result to be compared with the peer group mean of measured results from all laboratories using Method B. Removing the 0.9 factor is accomplished by multiplying the reported PT result from Method B by the factor 1.10 to increase its numeric value by 10% to the nonadjusted value that was actually measured by the instrument according to the manufacturer's defined calibration procedure. This process allows the PT result measured by Method B to be appropriately evaluated in comparison with its peer group mean, which will reflect the manufacturer's established calibration. This process permits the PT sample to be assayed in the same manner as patient samples, and the numeric result reported to the PT provider to reflect the actual measured result using the manufacturer's recommended calibration settings.

INTERPRETATION OF PT RESULTS

Many countries have regulations (e.g., CLIA in the United States) requiring PT and specifying the evaluation criteria for acceptable performance. When criteria are not set by regulations, the PT provider sets evaluation criteria on the basis of clinically acceptable performance. PT evaluation criteria are designed to evaluate the total error of a single measurement. The acceptability limits for PT include bias and imprecision components considered clinically acceptable for an analyte plus other error components that are unique to PT samples, such as between-laboratories variation in calibration; homogeneity of the PT material vials; stability variability in the PT material both in storage/shipping and after reconstitution or opening in the laboratory; and variable matrix-related bias with different lots of reagent within a peer group. Consequently, the acceptability limits for PT samples are larger than what might be expected for clinically acceptable total error with patient samples.

Figure 10-16 is an example of a typical evaluation report sent to a participating laboratory. Each reported result is compared with the mean result for the peer group using the same method. The report also includes the SD for the peer group distribution of results, the number of laboratories in the peer group, and the SDI, which expresses the reported result as the number of SDs it is from the mean value [SDI = (result − mean)/SD)]. The limits of acceptability are shown. Acceptability criteria may be a number of standard deviations from the mean value, a fixed percent from the mean value, or a fixed concentration from the mean value. In Figure 10-16, calcium acceptability criteria are ±1 mg/dL from the mean value, and iron criteria are ±20% from the mean value.

Peer group evaluation allows a laboratory to verify that it is using a method according to the manufacturer's specifications and is producing patient results that are consistent with those of other laboratories using the same method (Miller, 2009). In Figure 10-16, the calcium results are in close agreement with the peer group mean (SDI ranges from −0.2 to −1.4). However, the iron results show greater variability, with one result +3.5 SDI. Although that iron result is within the acceptability criteria, it is recommended to investigate the method, as discussed in the next paragraph.

If an unacceptable PT result is identified, the method must be investigated for possible causes, and any necessary corrective action taken. Even when a PT result is within acceptability criteria, it is good laboratory practice to investigate PT results that are more than approximately 2.5 SDI from the peer group mean. When the SDI is 2.5, there is only a 0.6% probability that the result will be within the expected distribution for the peer group; consequently, the probability is reasonable that a method problem may need to be corrected. In addition, PT result(s) that have been near the failure limit for more than one PT event, even if the result(s) have passed the PT acceptance criteria, should initiate a review of systematic

TABLE 10-6
Examples of Causes of Proficiency Testing (PT) Failures

Condition	Examples
Technical problem with a method or equipment	• Calibration drift or incorrect calibrator target value • Deterioration of reagents or calibrators • Lot-to-lot variability in reagents or calibrators • Deterioration of other components (e.g., automated pipette system) • Method lacks adequate specificity for the analyte • Method lacks adequate sensitivity to measure the concentration • Inadequate SOP or QC procedures • Incorrect instrument settings or data processing procedures • Inadequate environmental control in the laboratory
Technical problem caused by laboratory personnel	• Failure to follow SOP • Incorrect instrument operation, maintenance, etc. • Incorrect preparation or handling of reagents, calibrators, or PT samples • Incorrect pipetting or dilution process • Incorrect calculation of result • Misinterpretation of result
Incorrect reporting of PT result (clerical errors)	• Failure to convert measurement units to those required for the PT report • Failure to identify correct method used • Transcription error on report form • PT sample was mislabeled in the laboratory.
Problem with the PT material	• Analyte not stable in PT material • Interfering substance in PT material • Sample deterioration in transit • Sample had weak or borderline reaction

QC, Quality control; *SOP,* standard operating procedure.

problems with the method. These practices support identification of potential problems before they progress to more serious situations. When results are investigated, a limitation of SD-based grading criteria should be considered. Very precise methods may have a very small SD, and a result may be outside an SD limit when the magnitude in reporting units is small and is not consistent with a clinical problem.

Common causes for PT failure are listed in Table 10-6 (based on Miller, 2009; CLSI, 2007). Incorrect handling and reporting are frequently unique to PT events and may not reflect the same process used in the laboratory for patient samples. Nonetheless, these situations reflect attention to detail, which is a necessary attribute for quality laboratory testing. Occasionally, the PT material may have a defect that causes it to perform inappropriately for all or a subgroup of methods. In this case, the PT provider will identify the situation and will not grade participants for that sample.

PT results are usually received several weeks after the date of testing. Consequently, investigation of unacceptable results requiring review of quality control, reagent, calibration, and maintenance records for the date of the test and the preceding several weeks or months is necessary. If review of these records suggests a stable operating condition, and review of the PT material handling and documentation does not identify a cause for the erroneous PT result, it may be concluded that the PT failure was a random event. Investigative steps, data reviewed, and conclusions from the review must be documented in a written report of the unacceptable PT result and reviewed by the laboratory director.

Limitations in Interpreting PT Results

PT providers also prepare a summary report, which includes the mean and SD for all peer groups represented by the participants' results. Similar reports are available from interlaboratory QC programs. Summary reports are very useful but must be interpreted with consideration of the limitations of noncommutable samples. The peer group mean and SD are useful for evaluating the uniformity of results between laboratories using the same method, to confirm that an individual laboratory is using the method correctly as designed by the manufacturer, and to evaluate the consistency of an individual laboratory's method performance relative to the peer group over time intervals from one PT event to the next (trend monitoring). Summary information also allows evaluation of the imprecision of various method groups, and the number of users in each method group reveals which methods are commonly used.

The frequent occurrence of noncommutability of PT materials makes it incorrect to use PT summary reports to compare an individual laboratory's result with the peer group mean for another method group, to compare method peer group mean values to each other, or to compare an individual method peer group value to a value from a reference measurement procedure. The noncommutability limitation prevents PT (or QC) results from being used to infer agreement, or lack of agreement, for patient results among different methods for the same analyte.

ACCURACY-BASED PT PROGRAMS

In special cases, PT providers have used commutable samples in PT programs. Commutable samples are typically prepared by pooling clinical patient samples with minimal processing or additives to avoid any alteration of the sample matrix. To achieve samples with abnormal values for analytes, donors are identified with known pathologic conditions, or blood and serum units from a general donor population can be prescreened for selected analytes. Supplementing patient samples or pools with purified analytes may be acceptable in some cases but has not been rigorously evaluated. When commutable PT samples can be prepared, the results reflect what would be expected if patient samples were sent to each of the different laboratories. Thus, agreement among different laboratories and methods (called harmonization) can be correctly evaluated. The agreement between an individual laboratory result and a reference measurement result (accuracy), and the agreement between a method group mean value and the reference measurement result (called trueness), can be evaluated when a reference measurement procedure is available for an analyte.

For example, the College of American Pathologists glycohemoglobin survey for many years has used pooled, freshly collected whole blood from both normal and diabetic donors. The target values for the pooled blood are assigned by reference measurement procedures for hemoglobin A1c. In this survey, the accuracy of individual laboratory results and the trueness of method group means versus the reference measurement procedure values can be evaluated because the PT samples are commutable with clinical patient samples. Method group trueness can be used by the respective method manufacturers to monitor the effectiveness of their calibration processes.

It has been challenging to prepare commutable materials for use in large PT programs. However, use of commutable materials adds substantial value to the information obtained from the results (Bock, 2005; Knight, 2005; Miller, 2003, 2005, 2008; Palmer-Toy, 2005; Schreiber, 2005; Steele, 2005). Procedures have been developed to validate the commutability of QC, PT, and reference materials (Vesper, 2007; CLSI, document C53-A, 2010).

QUALITY MANAGEMENT

Quality management (QM) refers to the overall process used to ensure that laboratory results meet the requirements for health care services to patients. The components of a QM system shown in Figure 10-4 were derived from the CLSI document GP26-A3, Application of a Quality Management System Model for Laboratory Services, and are consistent with the ISO document 15189:2007, Medical Laboratories—Particular Requirements for Quality and Competence. Laboratories are required to develop procedures to monitor and ensure quality in all aspects of laboratory services. A QM program is an accreditation requirement, and good documentation of the metrics, the review process, and the improvements made is necessary.

Statistical quality control and proficiency testing, covered in detail in this chapter, are two important components of a QM program that address measurement procedures. Metrics related to QC activities may be evaluated as part of monitoring the performance of a measurement system. The following may be useful indicators of method performance issues:

- Frequency of QC alerts
- Frequency of recalibration based on QC alerts
- Number of reagent changes due to QC alerts
- Number of times controls were repeated because of QC alerts
- Frequency of unscheduled maintenance due to QC alerts

Directly related to the quality of test results are preanalytic components such as patient preparation; sample collection, transportation, storage, and preparation for testing; and postanalytic components such as result reporting, critical value notification, and provision of interpretive information.

The other components listed in Figure 10-4 are also important to ensure that quality laboratory results are available for patient care. In some cases, the quality requirements extend outside the laboratory and require cooperation with health care partners who order laboratory tests and act on the results.

A QM program defines data-based metrics or indicators that are monitored at regular recurring intervals to provide information on the adequacy of all influences on laboratory quality. A QM committee oversees the development of metrics and their regular review, and initiates quality improvement actions in response to metrics that indicate a need for improved performance in a particular aspect of laboratory management. A QM committee is typically chaired by a laboratory director or section director and includes senior level representation from all service areas, including the laboratory information system. Monthly meetings are typical. The data collected are frequently from the previous month, so the review is retrospective. However, automation of data management can make some metrics available close to real time for more immediate monitoring and intervention. For example, turnaround time from specimen receipt to result reporting can be monitored continuously with a scrolling computer display report to assist medical technologists in tracking stat requests.

Table 10-7 provides a list of typical metrics that could be included in a QM program. In addition to the metrics, thresholds for acceptable values need to be defined for each metric. Metrics that exceed thresholds require analysis, and a plan is developed for corrective action. Thresholds are established on the basis of what is considered good laboratory practice and may be different in different situations. The example thresholds in Table 10-7 are illustrative and should not be taken as recommendations. It is not possible to have zero mistakes in laboratory service; consequently, thresholds need to be realistic and can be changed as quality improvement programs are applied. The total number of observations examined by a metric should be recorded, along with the data for a given reporting interval.

TABLE 10-7
Examples of Quality Management Metrics

Service monitor (metric)	Threshold	Total number reviewed	Example data	Analysis and action plan
Result Reporting				
Micro: Gram stain correlation with culture (% disagreement)	≤1%	1513	0%	
Micro: Blood culture contamination	≤3%	2468	2.7%	
Hematopathology consensus conference				
Percent bone marrow cases reviewed in consensus	≥10%	146	28.8%	
Number of cases with disagreements	2	146	0	
CAP survey exception reports; # flagged/total # results received from CAP (list by laboratory section)	0			
POCT: Glucose meters, QC failures	≤3%	9058	2.3%	
POCT: Glucose meter, critical value not confirmed by repeating on meter	≤5%	439	2.5%	
Turnaround times in minutes for 90% completed (in laboratory/total); examples shown				
Potassium, Stat, Chemistry, Day	45 min	1477	47/91	Reviewed, no action indicated
Troponin I, ED, Stat, Day	60 min	476	60/121	
Hb, Stat, Day	60 min	520	40/81	
PT, Stat, Day	60 min	528	41/94	
Urinalysis pH, Stat, Day	60 min	240	56/106	
Bacterial vaginosis, ED, Gram stains	60 min	231	40/91	
Critical call-back delay as (verified time – performed time); (minutes for 90% completed); examples shown				
Hb, inpatient	30 min	215	14	
Critical value delay, minutes				
Critical values not called Hematology	0	2474	4	SOP reviewed with medical technologist
Result corrections (list by laboratory sections)				
Specimens rejected/corrected at log-in (list by receiving location and type of problem; examples shown)				
Lost/not received				
Incomplete label or form				
Hemolyzed				
Clotted				
QNS				
Exceeds time limit				
Improper collection, container, specimen				
Improperly ordered				
Interfering substance				
Mislabeled specimens (identified by delta check or by notification from clinical staff) (list by receiving location)				
Blood bank: Emergency units not accounted for in ED and OR	0	35	0	
Sweat chloride QNS specimens, %	≤5%	18	0%	
Customer Satisfaction				
Client services: % calls lost	≤5%	5932	7%	
Client services: calls answered within 60 seconds	≥90%	5932	89%	
Service delivery reports from clinical units (# received/# laboratory responsible)	0		10/7	See attached report

Continued

TABLE 10-7
Examples of Quality Management Metrics—Cont'd

Service monitor (metric)	Threshold	Total number reviewed	Example data	Analysis and action plan
Personnel				
Safety (# incidents)				
Infectious agent exposure	0		1	See attached report
Chemical exposure	0		0	
Job-related injury/illness	0		2	See attached report
On-call utilization (# of instances a person was called in; list by laboratory section)				
Overtime utilization (hours paid; list by laboratory section)				
Vacancies and staff in training status (graph by laboratory section)				
Continuing education (total hours CE received/# staff receiving CE/total # staff); list by laboratory section				

CAP, College of American Pathologists; *CE,* continuing education; *ED,* emergency department; *Hb,* hemoglobin; *OR,* operating room; *POCT,* point-of-care testing; PT, prothrombin time; *QC,* quality control; *QNS,* quantity not sufficient; *SOP,* standard operating procedure.

It is recommended that the metrics are reported to allow trends to be identified, for example, by showing data for 6 or more months on a page. Graphical presentation is very effective to monitor trends and can easily include 1 or more years on a single graph. Many metrics are useful to track indefinitely to document that laboratory service continues to meet performance expectations, and to have an alert mechanism when a change in the environment has adversely affected laboratory service. However, data cannot be collected for all possible metrics, and the QM committee needs to determine which aspects of laboratory performance are most critical or in need of improvement and should develop suitable metrics to drive a quality improvement process. Specific interventions should be documented with a written report that describes the quality issue, the data used to understand the issue, the improvements made, and the data that document the effectiveness of the improvement.

SELECTED REFERENCES

CLSI. Statistical quality control for quantitative measurements: principles and definitions; approved guideline C24-A3. Wayne, Pa.: Clinical and Laboratory Standards Institute; 2006.

Consensus document describing the principles and implementation guidelines for a statistical quality control system.

Department of Health and Human Services. 42 CFR Part 493, Medicare, Medicaid, and CLIA programs: laboratory requirements relating to quality systems and certain personnel qualifications; final rule. Federal Register January 24, 2003;68:3639–714.

Clinical Laboratory Improvement Act of 1988; final rule containing the regulatory requirements for quality practices in laboratories in the United States.

Kazmierczak SC. Laboratory quality control: using patient data to assess analytical performance. Clin Chem Lab Med 2003;41:617–27.

Review of the strengths and limitations of patient sample–based QC, and the usefulness of several patient data–based QC practices.

Miller WG, Myers GL, Rej R. Why commutability matters. Clin Chem 2006;52:553–4.

Editorial describing the importance of commutable reference materials and the errors that can occur when commutability is ignored.

Miller WG, Myers GL, Ashwood ER, et al. State of the art in trueness and interlaboratory harmonization for 10 analytes in general clinical chemistry. Arch Pathol Lab Med 2008;132:838–46.

Report of the value added when a commutable PT material was used, and the impact of noncommutable materials on interpretation of PT results.

REFERENCES

Access the complete reference list online at http://www.expertconsult.com

CHAPTER 11

CLINICAL LABORATORY INFORMATICS

Paul Tranchida, Jay L. Bock, Martin H. Bluth

KEY POINTS

- Certain concepts and terms specific to informatics should be familiar to pathologists working in an ever-modernizing laboratory environment.
- The laboratory information system is typically part of a hospital or health care system network of clinical, registration, patient management, and financial systems that exchange information with one another.
- The laboratory information system supports workflow and information flow at all steps of the laboratory testing process, including patient registration, test ordering, sample collection, and testing and reporting.
- Informatics plays a key role in assisting physicians to manage laboratory orders (e.g., clinical pathways, decision support systems) and results (e.g., clinical alerts, interpretive reports, reflex tests). Together, these approaches maximize the usefulness of the laboratory to clinicians.
- Data exchange among diverse applications in health care depends on coding protocols for identifying procedures and medical conditions, as well as a communication language.

DEFINITION

The website (www.pathologyinformatics.org) for the Association for Pathology Informatics describes the field of pathology informatics as "[involving] collecting, examining, reporting, and storing large complex sets of data derived from tests performed in clinical laboratories, anatomic pathology laboratories, or research laboratories in order to improve patient care and enhance our understanding of disease-related processes." The high volume, detailed, and time-sensitive nature of the workflow in the clinical laboratory has helped push the implementation of computing technology to assist in information management.

BASIC INFORMATICS CONCEPTS AND TERMINOLOGY

Before the issues that pertain to each step in the information flow are addressed, certain basic definitions are warranted to facilitate comprehension of the technology on which this field is based. The following section is intended only to provide a brief summary of some pathology informatics concepts; readers interested in expanding their knowledge about this field are advised to refer to a more comprehensive list of relevant topics (Henricks, 2003).

HARDWARE AND SOFTWARE

A *computer* is a device that follows instructions to work with electronic data based on user input. *Hardware* refers to the physical components of an information system. *Software* refers to programs (which are essentially sets of instructions) that allow computers or other devices to perform tasks.

A *file* is a collection of data identified by a specific name and grouped in relation to a specific purpose. The two main types are *applications* (also referred to as "executable" files) and *data* files (e.g., image, text/document, sound). A *folder* (or *directory*) simply refers to a collection of files.

A *bit* (derived from "binary digit") is the basic unit of digital information, and a *byte*, the most common unit of measurement used, almost always refers to 8 bits. ASCII (American Standard Code for Information Interchange) is the standard dictionary for combinations of bits that represent the common letters, numbers, and symbols by which characters are represented on a computer screen or paper printout.

The *central processing unit* (CPU) refers to the circuitry that serves as the main information processor, and is driven by clock pulses; the speed is most commonly measured in Gigahertz (1 GHz = 1 billion clock pulses per second). *Memory* refers to the physical chips on the motherboard that hold programs and data for rapid access by the CPU. The two types are read only memory (ROM), which is permanent, and random access memory (RAM), which is volatile (i.e., the contents of these chips are lost when the computer is turned off).

Storage refers to the physical media that store data permanently. It can be internal (hard drive) or removable (CD-ROM, USB drive). Many labs utilize *drive arrays*, which are multiple hard drives configured to look like a single drive to the system. A common type of drive array is the redundant array of independent/inexpensive disks (RAID), in which two or more hard disk drives are used simultaneously to achieve greater levels of performance, reliability, and/or larger data volume sizes. *Mirrored drive arrays* refer to arrays where copies of files are written to each drive in array. Different parts of files are read simultaneously from different disks and "assembled" for delivery. This system is redundant: If one drive fails, files can be read from the other intact drive(s).

The *operating system* of a device, whether a computer or an analyzer, refers to a set of programs responsible for the management and coordination of activities and the sharing of resources. In the case of a computer, the operating system acts as a host for application programs. Applications are created within programming languages, which are artificial languages used to control the behavior of a computer. Programming languages can be specific for a hardware platform (e.g., BASIC, FORTRAN) or hardware-independent (e.g., Java). In addition, the computer needs small specialized files called *drivers* that are specific for an operating system and allow identification and utilization of various external peripherals and other devices. Ensuring hardware and software compatibility with all the different electronic components of a clinical laboratory can be an onerous task,

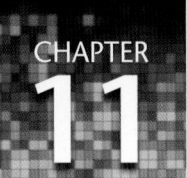

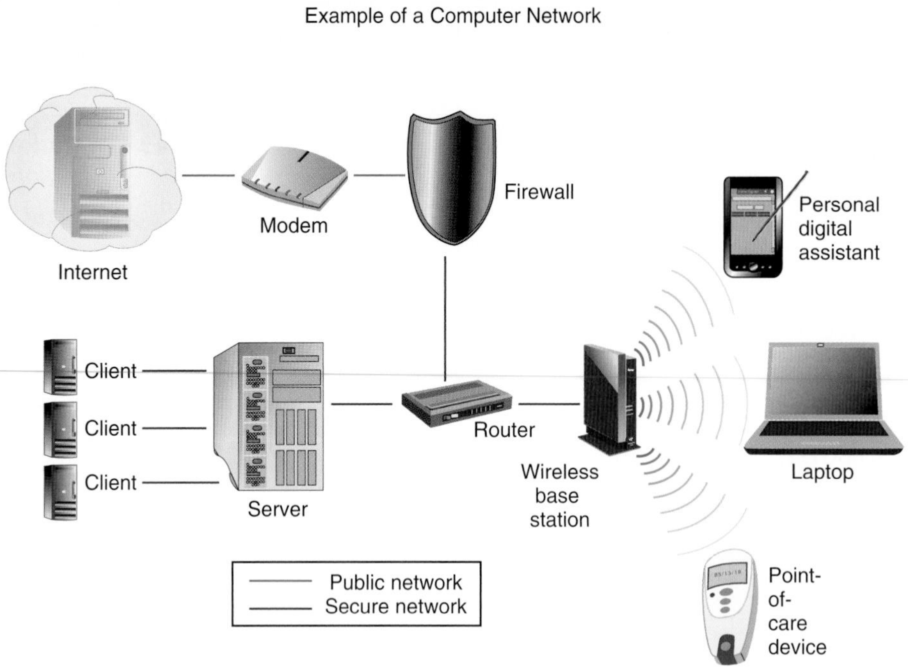

Figure 11-1 The red and green lines represent physically cabled connections (e.g., Ethernet), and the waves represent wireless connections.

TABLE 11-1
Common Network Components

Component	Function
Modem ("modulator-demodulator")	Modulates an analog carrier signal to encode digital information
Router	Routes and forwards information
Server	Accepts connections to service requests by sending back responses
Client	Application or system that accesses the server
Firewall	Device and/or software that inspects network traffic passing through it, and denies or permits passage based on a set of rules

especially if some of the equipment was introduced before an operating system upgrade of the predominant computing platform in the laboratory. As such, it often may be necessary to wrestle with compatibility issues when various software upgrades are introduced into a preexisting system.

NETWORKS AND SECURITY

A *network* is an interconnected group of computers that share information and resources, and as it pertains to the laboratory, the term refers to the ability to obtain orders from and send results to other information systems. Most computers need a card or adapter to connect to the network, and Ethernet is the most common type of networking standard. A variety of network types may be used: *Local area network*, which covers a small geographic area, and *wide area network*, which covers a broad area. The concept of *bandwidth* refers to the rate of data transmission. The different components of a network are listed in Table 11-1 and illustrated in Figure 11-1.

Networking often involves a *client* and a *server* environment. The client is the workstation with which the end user interacts and the server runs applications and maintains databases. The different client types are "thin" and "thick" or "fat"; the difference between the two is that in the former, all application logic executes on the client server, whereas in the latter, the client performs the bulk of any data processing operations itself. The traditional incarnation of the client-server relationship consisted of *mainframes* and *terminals* that fulfilled the roles of the servers and thin clients, respectively. An older laboratory information system (LIS) that still has this type of configuration generally cannot replace the old terminals once they begin to fail and therefore needs to run a program called a *terminal emulator*, which acts like a terminal but can be run on more modern hardware.

The *Internet* refers to a worldwide, publicly accessible series of interconnected computer networks. Data are transmitted by packet switching using the standard *Internet protocol (IP)*. The *World Wide Web* (WWW) refers to a hypertext-based data system that uses the Internet as its transportation (hypertext = text on a computer that will lead the user to other related information on demand). The language used is most commonly *hypertext markup language* (HTML), which specifies the appearance of a web page when interpreted by a web browser. An *intranet* refers to a private network that uses the aforementioned Internet protocols to share information within an organization as opposed to between separate entities.

Data security is of paramount importance for all networks, and particularly in health care, where patient privacy is a major concern. One way of ensuring secure data is *encryption*, which refers to the conversion of data via an algorithm that rearranges bits that cannot be deciphered without decryption. A common way of engaging in safe networking is through a *virtual private network*, which is a method by which a user can access an organization's internal network over the Internet in a secure manner. It provides users who are not on that internal network secure access to resources inside it. This is done by applying a software layer on top of an existing network, essentially creating virtual "tunnels" that wrap data packets destined for the internal network, and then encrypting those packets to send them across the Internet.

DATABASES

At their core, the building blocks of information systems are databases, which are structured collections of records comprising data fields. They need to be managed by a set of programs called a database management system. The two types of databases are *flat file* and *relational*. A flat file database is a single, two-dimensional array of data elements, similar to an electronic spreadsheet. In contrast, in a relational database, the data are organized in tables. In a table, each record (row) contains a unique instance of data for the fields (columns), and tables are related by a single field (the *primary key*) between common fields. Figure 11-2 gives a simplified example of a relational database for clinical laboratory data, comprising four linked tables: Patient Registration, Test Orders, Test Results, and Reference Ranges. The virtue of this structure is that redundancy is

Relational Database Structure

Patient Registration

Patient ID #	First Name	Last Name	Age	Sex
P1234	John	Smith	33	M
P3456	Mary	White	58	F

Test Order

Order #	Patient ID #	Date	Physician	Test
034782	P1234	04/12/2009	Jones	Hemoglobin
034783	P3456	04/12/2009	Chen	Hematocrit

Test Result

Order #	Test	Result
034782	Hemoglobin	15
034783	Hematocrit	33

Reference Range

Test	Adult Male	Adult Female	Child	Units
Hemoglobin	14-18	12-16	11-16	g/dL
Hematocrit	42-52	37-47	31-43	%

Figure 11-2 Sample relational database.

TABLE 11-2
Common Health Care Enterprise Information Systems

System	Functionality
Admission–discharge–transfer (ADT)	Runs the entire patient care workflow, from registration of patient information to bed tracking and discharge
Health information system (HIS)	Stores patient information generated by different departments during one or more visits
Laboratory information system (LIS)	Electronic data processing and information management functions necessary for laboratory operations
Electronic medical record (EMR)	A chronologically ordered paperless chart that summarizes the clinical history with diagnostic test results
Electronic data repository (EDR)	Contains patient information from all inpatient and outpatient systems in an enterprise, and is used for reviewing patient data
Electronic data warehouse (EDW)	Similar to the EDR, except the information is utilized for research by using databases and data analysis tools to uncover hidden patterns and relationships in data ("data mining")
Billing	Receives information on charges and/or tests performed to calculate charges to patient insurance

eliminated—a concept known as *normalization*. For example, demographic data about each patient are given only once, in the Patient Registration table. Other tables then link to that information using only the unique Patient ID identifier. If instead, other tables included both Patient ID and, for example, the patient's name, there would be an opportunity for inconsistencies to arise, and it would be more difficult to make updates such as a correction to the spelling of the name. The modest penalty for the normalized, relational architecture is that useful reports must typically integrate information from several tables, rather than simply printing records from a single table. However, this can be readily accomplished using a powerful, generic language known as Structured Query Language.

Laboratory Information Systems

An *information system (IS)* refers empirically to the hardware, software, and connectivity designed to perform data management functions. Different types of ISs are listed in Table 11-2. The LIS was classically a standalone insulated system that generated results for manual reporting by laboratory personnel or for viewing by the clinician. The LIS was used to communicate with analyzers and external systems such as the larger health information system (HIS) and/or billing systems. Today, it is frequently a major part of a health care system network with communication with the patient registration and billing systems and the electronic medical record (EMR). The LIS exchanges information with all these systems, and the effectiveness of this exchange is dependent on successful hardware and software implementation. Most LIS constructs have an interface, which is a combination of software and connections that translate electronic messages, so that data can be exchanged with different systems. The types of interfaces are instrument interfaces and application (other systems) interfaces. If the systems are not compatible, a laboratory may engage in ad hoc development of software known as *middleware* to enable communication between them. If multiple systems need to exchange information, an application known as an interface engine reduces the number of individual interfaces.

As well as the aforementioned interrelated programs and hardware that provide data management functions necessary for laboratory operations, the LIS often refers to the database that establishes and maintains standard definitions and information processing procedures. All LIS constructs utilize *dictionaries* (also referred to as *maintenance tables*), which provide a logical framework for laboratory operations and workflow. Dictionaries structure and standardize procedures and standardize laboratory and LIS terminology. They define allowable entries for data fields, in addition to the content and format of elements that appear on reports. The different worksheets and workstations that are available in the laboratory are specified in the LIS tables, and part of a test definition is assignment of the test to a laboratory workstation/instrument or laboratory location. Test orders are routed to LIS worksheets that are associated with given workstations; essentially, worksheets define the workflow in the laboratory because they define which tests are performed at different workstations. An emerging and popular feature of the LIS is its ability to perform *autoverification*, which refers to release of results from automated analyzers directly to LIS without prior human review. The autoverification criteria are defined and detailed in LIS tables and specify things such as allowable numeric result range and delta checks (in comparison with previous results).

Because of great variation in the types of data handled by different parts of the laboratory, LIS systems typically comprise several modules, which may even be entirely disparate systems from different vendors. A general laboratory module might include tests in the area of chemistry, hematology, and serology, where tests are usually relatively discrete, and results consist of a single number or a short string of text. The general LIS module serves many functions, some of which are listed in Table 11-3. Other areas of the lab may require very different functionality, as described later.

LEGAL REQUIREMENTS

A number of regulatory/accrediting bodies are pertinent to LIS constructs. In the U.S. government, these include the Centers for Medicare/Medicaid Services, the Food and Drug Administration, the College of American Pathologists (CAP), The Joint Commission, and the American Association of Blood Banks. The legal requirements for LISs involve issues such as unique specimen and patient identification, date of specimen collection, date and time of specimen receipt in the lab, records and dates of all specimen testing, personnel who performed the test(s), and the name and address of the laboratory where testing was performed, among others. The CAP Laboratory General Checklist requires periodic verification of data sent from the LIS to other computer systems.

The Health Insurance Portability and Accountability Act of 1996 (HIPAA) requires all health plans to accept electronically filed claims in a standard format (electronic data interchange). There must exist security measures to protect health information. There are limits on use/disclosure of health information. A requirement of reasonable safeguards to protect against incidental disclosure is also present. HIPAA addresses issues of consent with respect to protected health information (PHI), which refers to anything that could be used to identify an individual and is related to

TABLE 11-3
LIS Functions

Preanalysis	Patient registration (if not received from external system)
	Test ordering
	Customized requisitions (e.g., outreach clients)
	Phlebotomy draw lists
	Bar-coded collection labels and aliquot labels
	Specimen tracking/racking system
Analysis	Instrument worklist (via interface and automatic download)
	Manual worklist
	Manual results entry
	Automated results entry via interface
	Results validation and manual or automatic release
	Quality control
Postanalysis	Requisition-based patient reports (final, partial)
	Cumulative patient reports
	Corrected report
	Results inquiry
	Electronic reporting to external interfaced systems (e.g., HIS, billing)
Management	Pending (incomplete) list
	Turnaround time reports
	Workload statistics
	Ad hoc report writer
	HIS and instrument integrity monitoring tools

HIS, Health information system; *LIS,* laboratory information system.

health care or payment. The patient's consent is required to use or disclose PHI for treatment, payment, or health care operations. The law requires minimum necessary use or disclosure of PHI.

COMMUNICATION STANDARDS

The use of conventions and definitions to standardize information exchange between different systems is a less complex and time-consuming strategy than the traditional creation of custom interfaces between such applications. Originally, the major need for electronic transmission of these data was so that the Federal government (Medicare) and other payers could be billed for individual services provided. For this purpose, coding of laboratory procedures using Current Procedural Terminology (CPT) and coding of medical conditions using the International Classification of Diseases have been the norm. One example of a newer, and currently the most prevalent, standard developed by the health care industry is Health Level 7 (HL7) (www.hl7.org), which is a protocol for electronic data exchange that specifies syntax and rules for messaging. Another standard is Logical Observation Identifier Names and Codes (www.loinc.org), which is a set of universal identifiers for laboratory test code data fields within HL7 messages and in databases (McDonald, 2003). It provides a structured naming convention for describing laboratory tests and has fewer limitations than CPT. The American Society for Testing and Materials specifies protocols and formats for instrument interfaces, bar codes (e.g., Code 39, Code 128), other systems and components. The Systematic Nomenclature of Medicine—Clinical Terms system is a very elaborate nomenclature for medical conditions and related concepts, containing more than 300,000 unique clinical concepts. Originally developed by CAP, it is now maintained by the International Healthcare Terminology Standards Development Organisation, which was formed in 2006. A receiving system may not recognize certain codes as written, so the use of a *translation table* relates a code to its equivalent in the receiving system.

COMMON DATA ELEMENTS AND METADATA

The concept of a common data element (CDE) refers to the standardized component of a data set. CDEs are defined by metadata, which literally translate to "data about data," or a description and definition of data element attributes (e.g., type of data). CDEs have standardized, consistent metadata descriptions for discrete data elements. CDEs structure data in a way to facilitate reproducible capture at the time of entry and to ensure consistent data collection and categorization, while providing standard formatting for data exchange.

```
<Patients>

<Patient>
<PatientID>P1234</PatientID>
<FirstName>John</FirstName>
<LastName>Smith</LastName>
<Age>33</Age>
<Sex>M</Sex>
</Patient>

<Patient>
<PatientID>P3456</PatientID>
<FirstName>Mary</FirstName>
<LastName>White</LastName>
<Age>58</Age>
<Sex>F</Sex>
</Patient>

</Patients>
```

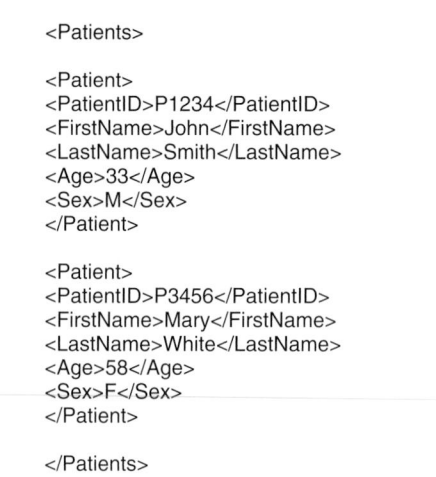

Figure 11-3 Example of an Extensible Markup Language (XML) database. This XML code contains the data from the Patients table shown in Figure 11-2. This text can be entered into Microsoft Excel, for example, which can then generate a spreadsheet to display the data.

A relatively new development in CDEs is the language XML, which stands for Extensible Markup Language. XML is a method to describe data, to structure information, and to format documents. The main purpose is to enable integration and sharing of information across disparate sources that otherwise have incompatible formats and data standards. XML markup tags describe the data marked by tag; thus XML tags are a type of CDE with specific metadata (an example is given in Figure 11-3). XML has great potential for becoming the standard by which textual information is encoded into a searchable format (Dolin, 1998; Sokolowski, 1999).

INFORMATION FLOW

The flow of information as it pertains to the LIS is generally uniform across different laboratories and is summarized in Table 11-4 and Figure 11-4, although obviously variations exist among different institutions. The critical issues of this workflow include patient safety and confidentiality, capture of clinically meaningful data, unambiguous identification of data elements, and synchronization of information among different systems within the health care institution (Aller, 2001). This section of the chapter will provide an overview of the information exchange steps as well as the key issues that pertain to each.

PATIENT REGISTRATION/IDENTIFICATION

The critically important initial step is registration of the patient with assignment of a unique patient identification number to the patient, often within the admission-discharge-transfer system. A unique laboratory encounter number may also be generated at this time, and again for subsequent encounters for the patient. No tests can be ordered until the patient record is created.

Patient identification information includes data such as name, birth date, sex, race, address, phone number, social security number, and medical record number, among others. Insurance and billing information generally is also included. Because the patient identification number needs to be unique, the social security number or an institution-generated number exclusive to the registration system should be utilized. Bar-coding may be utilized to ensure correct patient identification when obtaining samples. The radiofrequency identification (RFID) system is a new technology that provides hands-off, zero-error identification (Westra, 2009). It consists of a patient tag and a computerized scanner or reader. The "smart" label or tag contains human-readable information, a bar code, and an integrated circuit chip with memory. A small amount of radiofrequency energy ("excitation signal") is released from the scanner, energizing the RFID tag, which then emits a radiofrequency signal ("return signal") that transmits the patient's ID. Although several issues (e.g., data encryption, protocol standardization) are not completely resolved, RFID technology offers several benefits, including passive operation and dynamic data storage, features that favor its use in sample collection and tracking, bedside testing, drug management, and infection control.

TABLE 11-4
Key Steps in Laboratory Information Flow for a Hospital Patient

Step	Description
Register patient	Patient record (e.g., ID#, name, sex, age, location) must be created in LIS before tests can be ordered. LIS usually automatically receives these data from a hospital registration system (when the patient is admitted).
Order tests	Physician orders tests on a patient to be drawn as part of the laboratory's morning blood collection rounds. The order is entered into the HIS and is electronically sent to the LIS.
Collect sample	Before morning blood collection, the LIS prints a list of all patients whose blood is to be drawn and the appropriate number of sample bar code labels for each patient order. Each bar code has a patient ID, a sample container type (e.g., red-top tube), and a laboratory workstation (that can be used to sort the tube once it reaches the laboratory). Another and increasingly popular approach is for patient caregivers or nurses to collect the blood sample. Immediately before collection, sample bar code labels can be printed (on demand) at the nursing station on an LIS printer.
Receive sample	When samples arrive in the laboratory, their status has to be updated in the LIS from "collected" to "received." This can be done by scanning each sample container's bar code ID into the LIS. Once the sample is "received," the LIS transmits the test order to the analyzer that will perform the test.
Run sample	The sample is loaded onto the analyzer and the bar code is read. Having already received the test order from the LIS, the analyzer knows which tests to perform on the patient. No worklist is needed. For manually performed tests, the technologist prints a worklist from the LIS. The worklist contains a list of patients and the tests ordered on each. Next to each test is a space to record the result.
Review results	The analyzer produces the results and sends them to the LIS. These results are viewable only by technologists because they have not been released for general viewing. The LIS can be programmed to flag certain results (e.g., critical values) so a technologist can easily identify what needs to be repeated or further evaluated.
Release results	The technologist releases results (unflagged results are usually reviewed and released at the same time). The LIS can also be programmed to automatically review and release normal results or results that fall within a certain range. The latter approach reduces the number of tests that a technologist has to review. Upon release, results are automatically transmitted to the HIS.
Report results	Physician can view the results on the HIS screen. Reports are printed when needed from the LIS.

HIS, Health information system; *ID,* identification; *LIS,* laboratory information system.

TEST ORDERS

After the patient has been identified, tests are ordered manually with paper forms or electronically through the HIS, with orders then electronically sent to the LIS. Having the physician at the point of care directly enter laboratory orders electronically is an effective way to reduce the possibility of introducing error that is inherent in having to re-key requested tests from the paper form. Computerized pathology test order entry has also been shown to reduce laboratory turnaround time (Westbrook, 2006). Important data pertaining to the request (date/time/location of collection, storage medium, etc.) can be automatically generated at this time as well. The electronic nature of the patient's clinical data and the test ordering system allows the use of logic operations to ensure patient safety and optimal test utilization.

SAMPLE COLLECTION AND LABELING

A patient sample may be collected by the lab after an order is received or may be sent directly to the lab with a request. For inpatient samples, the LIS prints the list of patients who need to be drawn. At this point, labels can be printed identifying the necessary tubes and/or containers; this label printing can also take place at the patient's bedside using portable printers connected wirelessly to the LIS to confirm correct patient identification immediately after the patient's wristband has been scanned and read. When the sample is received, the LIS indicates receipt of the sample by changing its status from the previous value of "to be collected." The collected sample is then run on an analyzer.

PERFORMING TESTS

The analyzers of a clinical laboratory can communicate with the LIS unidirectionally or bidirectionally. Unidirectional analyzer communication typically refers to reporting of results to the LIS with no input from the latter during the testing process. Alternatively, analyzers that bidirectionally communicate with the LIS are able to receive orders from the LIS and then send results back. Many analyzers have the ability to read bar codes off specimen containers to identify which samples are about to be processed and send corresponding specimen status updates to the LIS.

RELEASING RESULTS

Regardless of whether the results are manually entered or automatically transferred, the computer performs a validity check on the results once they are received. Panic values can be flagged by the LIS once a valid result is determined to fall into a critical range. Autovalidation protocols can be used to automatically release results without review by the technologist or pathologist.

REPORTING RESULTS

Laboratory results can be electronically reported to a variety of clinical systems, including the HIS, the electronic data repository (EDR), the EMR, and state or federal public health agencies (White, 1999). The proliferation of different communication technologies allows a number of ways of reporting results to physicians, especially time-sensitive critical values. Computerized alerts can assist in improving the timeliness of reporting and clinicians' responses to laboratory values (Staes, 2008). For routine test results, the advent of the WWW allows a physician to review at his convenience the patient's results on the HIS screen and print as needed. The HTML code in web pages can generate new content automatically in response to user commands and therefore is well suited to automating report generation and facilitating custom data searches (Yearworth, 1998; Lowe, 1996). Data in the EDR can be transferred in batches to an electronic data warehouse, where algorithms can be performed to reveal general patterns and potentially assist in developing new knowledge about disease (Elevitch, 1999).

BIOINFORMATICS

Bioinformatics most commonly refers to the division of informatics that studies how information is stored in biological systems, from the molecular to the macromolecular level, with a large part of the focus being on DNA, RNA, and protein sequences (Sinard, 2006). As Batley and Edwards have noted, numerous improvements in DNA sequencing technology have led to a corresponding marked increase in the quantity of sequence data generated, which provides a challenge for bioinformatics in terms of management, storage, and visualization (Batley, 2009). Implemented properly, informatics can facilitate patient registration, specimen tracking, tissue cataloging, quality assurance, and specimen availability (Qualman, 2003). Research is currently under way that would eventually allow a patient's genetic profile to be handled by, or communicated to, the EMR. In turn, the EMR could then fulfill a valuable role by providing the information contained in the patient's bioinformatics profile to help pathologists and clinicians in determining the optimal diagnostic tests and/or therapeutic measures, respectively.

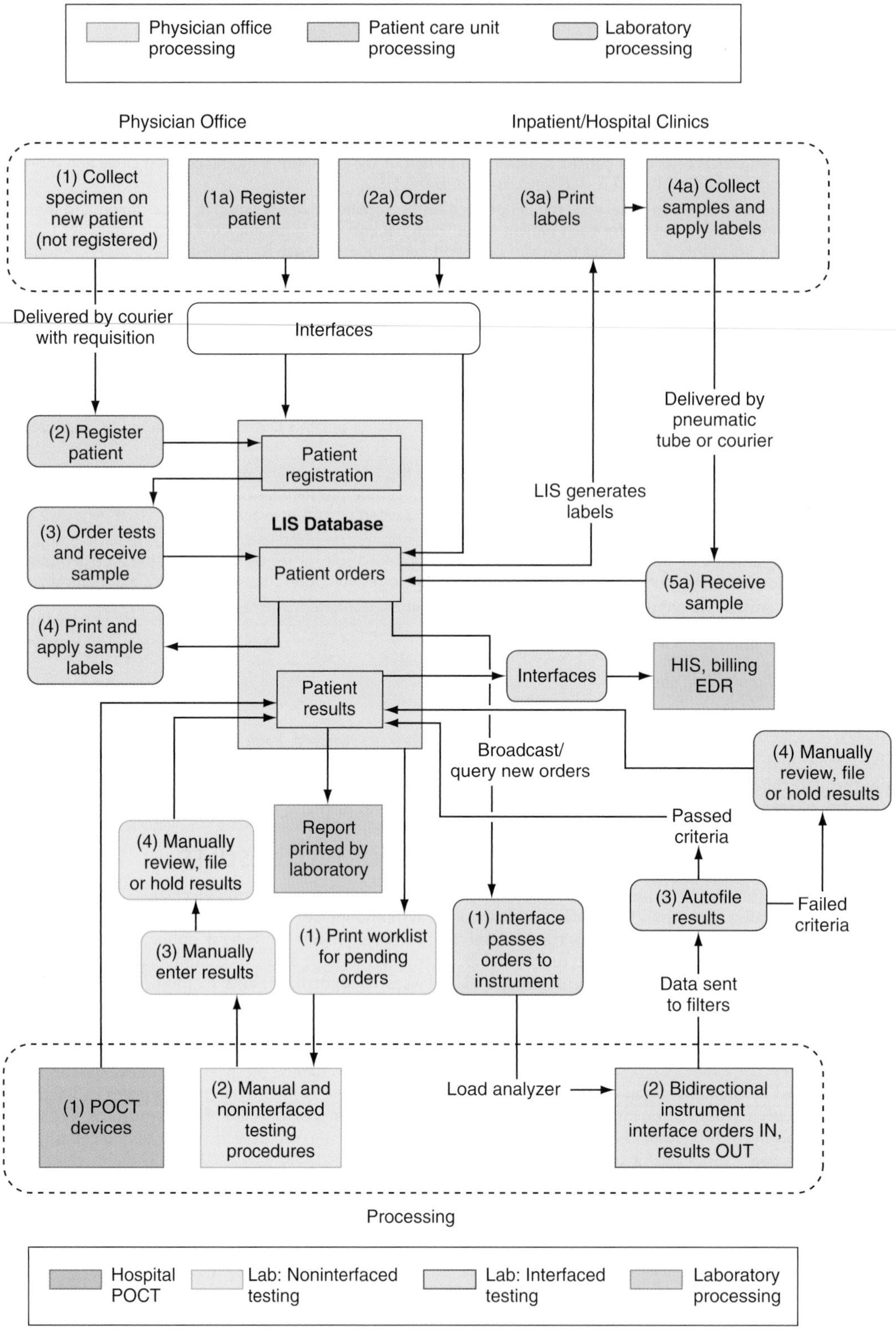

Figure 11-4 The role of the laboratory information system (LIS) in admission–discharge–transfer (ADT) and in processing orders and results. *(Adapted from Lifshitz MS, Blank GE, Schexneider KI. Clinical laboratory informatics. In: McPherson RA, Pincus MR, editors. Clinical Diagnosis and Management by Laboratory Methods, 21st ed. Philadelphia: WB Saunders; 2007.) EDR,* Electronic data repository; *HIS,* health information system; *POCT,* point-of-care testing.

Issues Regarding Implementation

Although the opportunities to streamline workflow offered by computing technology are numerous, there are also a number of potential pitfalls and opportunities for error of which diligent informaticians should be aware.

When deciding to purchase hardware or software for the laboratory, a request for proposal (RFP) should be submitted to the vendor. The main component of the RFP is a detailed listing of required functionality and features. The RFP asks the vendor to specify whether specified capabilities are present and to provide corporate information, pricing, and details of other attributes of the system. The RFP responses become part of the final contract. A different model is the application service provider (ASP) model, which is composed of a contractual agreement: The provider delivers service(s) remotely over a network, and the vendor manages everything (hardware, software, security, upgrades). Often there is a fixed subscription fee, which may be per transaction or a flat rate. Another type is the service level agreement (SLA), which is a contract that defines the technical and business parameters of the relationship between IT vendor and client, particularly for an ASP arrangement. The key terms of the SLA are *responsibility* (who does what), *performance*, and *remediation* for resolving problems. Quantifiable metrics such as system uptime (%), system response time, and time to address problem calls need to be specified. Lack of appropriate attention to these issues can cause considerable logistical and operational problems down the road.

One of the most critical features of an information system is the assurance that data that are transferred from one system to another are accurate and valid. The CAP Laboratory General Checklist Questionnaire requires periodic verification of data sent from the LIS to other computer systems. Absence of proof of fulfilling this requirement is a phase II violation.

Because many pathology practices evaluate patient samples from independent private physician offices, in addition to those from their own institutions, patients will need a unique identifier generated by the clinical information system (CIS); the CIS will also have to be able to store and link together all identifiers generated for this same patient if and when the patient ends up submitting additional specimens within the hosting institution.

Security is of paramount concern when it comes to transferring patient data many times over a network. To comply with HIPAA, all laboratories should have safeguards in place to ensure that patient data are accessed only by appropriate individuals in appropriate circumstances. This is essential not just with transfer of data between information systems, but also with electronic correspondence (e.g., e-mail), which laboratory personnel frequently use.

THE FUTURE OF INFORMATICS

With the emergence of new technologies, especially in the realm of bioinformatics, the roles of pathologists and of the laboratory will undoubtedly be redefined over time. Microfluidic instrumentation is being applied to common laboratory techniques, essentially providing a "lab-on-a-chip" solution that allows a patient-centric approach to testing, and may eventually perform at levels comparable to centralized analyzers (Yager, 2006). The efforts of Patel et al. (2007) in creating an informatics model for sharing information involving tissue banks from different institutions demonstrate how standardized communication protocols and shared common data elements allow free exchange of information to assist with research projects, thus enabling any laboratory to have a role in real-time collaboration in research. As society in general continues to become more knowledgeable about information technology, many patients may entrust private companies to safeguard their personalized health information; the laboratory will have to be able to communicate with those companies. Furthermore, as point-of-care (POC) instrumentation becomes more prevalent in the clinical marketplace, cross-talk between the clinical laboratory and POC centers (surgical suites, operating rooms, physicians' offices, etc.) may be warranted toward accessioning a patient's laboratory data set for efficient patient management and avoiding testing redundancy.

With all these developments taking place, the traditional role of the pathologist as one who provides data and interpretation to the clinician from which a therapeutic decision will be made will be expanded to include bioinformatics design and management. The pathologist will have to use informatics tools that span different diagnostic methods to integrate all available data and produce an outcomes-based treatment recommendation for optimal patient care.

SELECTED REFERENCES

McDonald CJ, Huff SM, Suico JG, et al. LOINC, a universal standard for identifying laboratory observations: a 5-year update. Clin Chem 2003;49:624–33.

A valuable summary of LOINC with a list of helpful resources for further education.

Sinard JH. Practical pathology informatics: demystifying informatics for the practicing anatomic pathologist. London: Springer-Verlag; 2006.

A comprehensive review of informatics with an emphasis on anatomic pathology, but useful for any branch of pathology.

Yager P, Edwards T, Fu E, et al. Microfluidic diagnostic technologies for global public health. Nature 2006;442:412–18.

Informative overview of "lab-on-a-chip"–type diagnostic systems and their potential benefit for developing countries.

REFERENCES

Access the complete reference list online at http://www.expertconsult.com

CHAPTER 12

FINANCIAL MANAGEMENT

David S. Wilkinson, Thomas J. Dilts, William Woolf, Mark S. Lifshitz

KEY POINTS

- Costs can be described in different ways, depending on how they relate to laboratory operations (direct/indirect), change with test volume (variable/fixed), pertain to staffing (salary/nonsalary), or are associated with the useful life of supplies or equipment (operating/capital). Cost per reportable result is a key indicator.
- Reimbursement for laboratory services comes mostly from third-party payers such as Medicare (government) and insurance companies (nongovernment/private insurance), and payments are almost always less than charges.
- Inpatient laboratory testing charges are usually not reimbursed directly; they are considered part of a per diem rate (i.e., general hospital daily room reimbursement rate) or a case rate, such as diagnosis-related group rate (i.e., set rate for the entire hospital stay, regardless of actual length of stay). Thus, inpatient laboratory testing is usually considered a "cost center." In contrast, outpatient laboratory charges are reimbursed directly; therefore, outpatient testing is usually considered a "revenue center."
- For reimbursement purposes, Current Procedural Terminology codes describe tests and International Classification of Diseases, Ninth Revision codes describe the diagnosis. Medical necessity requirements may limit reimbursement to those tests associated with specific predefined diagnoses.
- Budgeting is the process of planning, forecasting, controlling, and monitoring the financial resources of an organization.
- A variety of financial tools are used to evaluate a capital project, such as purchasing a chemistry analyzer. These measure how long it takes to recoup an investment (payback) and how much it generates in today's dollars (net present value) and its rate of return (internal rate of return).
- Laboratory equipment can be acquired in different ways, including purchase, lease, and per-test payment. Each has pros and cons.

Every organization, no matter the products or services it provides, must be concerned with the management, oversight, and accounting of its monetary resources. To sustain a viable, competitive entity, an organization not only must recoup the cost of operations, but must have a positive net income to reinvest in itself. The laboratory is no exception. To be successful in the financial management of the laboratory, the director/manager must be able to identify and categorize costs, understand the relationships between revenue and reimbursement, become familiar with the budget process, and use financial ratios and information to make sound decisions. Credibility with administrators and colleagues demands that the director/manager be comfortable and confident when explaining financial issues and when justifying the need for additional resources.

INDUSTRY OVERVIEW

Most industries in the United States are subject to traditional free-market competition. However, this principle does not fully apply to health care because relatively few people who use health care pay directly for it. Most people are beneficiaries of some form of health insurance. This, in combination with the increasing numbers of uninsured and underinsured, has led to a system that provides services even when no one pays adequately for them. Most medical claims are paid by a "third party" such as the government (Medicare, Medicaid) or a private insurance company. Thus, someone other than the patient usually pays the provider of health care services (Snyder, 1998).

The health care industry is one of the largest industries in the United States and continues to be a growing sector of the gross domestic product, having increased from 5.1% ($27 billion) in 1960 to 16.2% ($2.2 trillion) in 2007 (CMS, 2010a). Hospitals continue to be a driving force behind escalating health care costs. Most U.S. hospitals are tax exempt, not-for-profit entities. Though "not-for-profit" suggests that no profit is made, it actually means that profits are not distributed to owners or shareholders; instead, profits are reinvested in the organization. Historically, not-for-profit status led hospital administrators to be less profit conscious than counterparts in other businesses. However, today's hospitals are having a difficult time just covering operating costs, given dwindling reimbursement and increasing supply and labor costs. With scarce money left for capital reinvestment in equipment, buildings, facilities, and technology, hospitals are aggressively seeking new ways to produce a profit to invest for the future.

DEFINING AND IDENTIFYING COSTS

A cost (expense) is the supply, labor, and overhead money spent on a product or service (Travers, 1997). It is important to understand costs to accurately price tests and other services, to determine when and how to offer new tests, and to determine whether to acquire new outreach client

TABLE 12-1
Cost Classification

	Direct	Indirect	Variable	Fixed	Salary	Nonsalary	Operating	Capital
Reagents	■		■			■	■	
Proficiency testing		■		■		■	■	
Analyzer service		■		■		■	■	
Analyzer		■		■		■		■
Testing staff	■			■	■		■	
Management staff		■		■	■		■	
Rent		■		■		■	■	

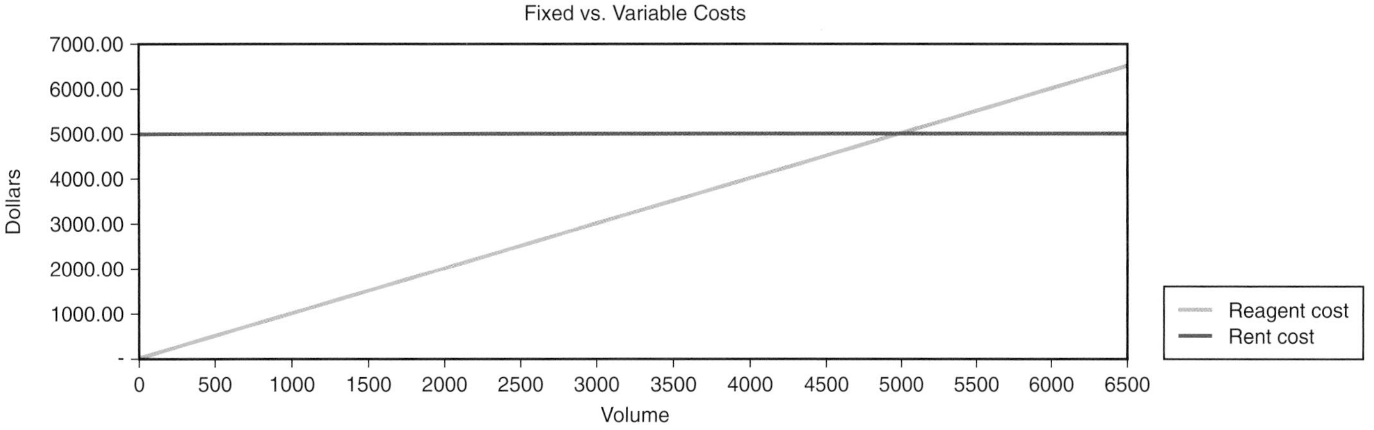

Figure 12-1 Fixed costs such as rent remain constant. Variable costs such as reagents are directly proportional to test volume.

business or a managed care contract. Costs can be classified in different ways (Table 12-1).

Direct costs are expenses that can easily be traced directly to an end product. In the laboratory setting, the end product is a billable test. Examples are reagents, consumables, and hands-on technologist time. In contrast, *indirect costs* are not directly related to a billable test, but are necessary for its production. Indirect costs are often referred to as overhead. Examples are proficiency testing and utility expenses.

Variable costs change proportionately with the volume of tests. As test volume grows, so do reagent costs. If the reagent cost per test is $1.00, when 1000 tests are performed, the reagent cost is $1000; when 20,000 tests are performed, the reagent cost is $20,000. *Fixed costs* do not change with the volume of tests performed. If a laboratory pays $5000 per month to rent its space, this expense remains the same if the laboratory produces 1000 or 20,000 tests per month (Fig. 12-1).

Because fixed costs do not vary with activity, the goal is to produce as much as possible from fixed costs to achieve economies of scale. The more that is produced, the lower is the *fixed cost per activity*. In the preceding scenario, if the laboratory produced 1000 tests, the fixed cost per test is $5.00; with 20,000 tests, the fixed cost per test falls to $0.25. Note that even some fixed costs have a variable component. For example, if an instrument's capacity is 20,000 tests per month and the volume increases beyond that, another instrument will have to be purchased, increasing the fixed costs per test. Fixed costs that change with increments of volume are called *step costs*.

Salary costs need to be looked at differently from *nonsalary costs* because salary costs have fringe benefits associated with them. Salary expenses account for approximately 60%–80% of the laboratory budget. Because salary expenses are generally fixed, it is important to strive for economies of scale. The hourly pay or salaried wage of an employee is not the entire cost of employment. Fringe benefits such as Social Security, health insurance, tuition reimbursement, pension plans, and life insurance can represent an additional 16%–28% expense above the base salary. Costs are also associated with the recruitment, interview, and selection process. Once an employee is hired, orientation, training, and ongoing growth and development costs are incurred.

Operating costs are the expenses incurred to produce a product or service. Many items have only a one-time use, and once used the item has no further value. Examples of one-time operating costs include reagents, electricity, disposable pipets, and the salary expense in the production of a test. Other items, such as analytic equipment, computers, and the physical plant, have a useful life greater than one production cycle. These items are capital items. To qualify as a *capital* item, the item must meet three criteria: Time, price, and purpose. To meet the time criterion, the item must have a useful life of longer than 1 year. The institution must designate a minimum dollar amount, usually $1000–$5000, that qualifies an item as capital. The purpose of acquiring capital items is usually to replace older equipment with safer and more efficient models, or to add new equipment to support new products or services. With time, capital equipment loses its value. The annual loss of a capital item's value is called *depreciation* and is an annual expense that is deducted from the revenue of a business. Depreciation is not a cash expense (i.e., you do not "pay it" each year), but it is a real expense in that it recognizes the "wearing out" of an asset that was acquired with cash and eventually will have to be replaced. If an analyzer has not yet been fully depreciated, it still has "book value." Note that operating and capital costs are budgeted separately (see later).

The cost of producing a test can be derived in different ways. *Microcosting* determines the total direct labor and supply costs of producing a test, and is the starting point for determining the fully loaded cost and ultimately the price for a test. Most testing in the clinical laboratory is performed in batches or continuous "runs" of many samples during one or more shifts. A run can be a group of tests that are performed once or many times during a shift or an entire 24-hour period. A run includes all quality control and calibration costs needed to produce patient results. When microcosting a test, it is important to consider how a test is performed because labor and supply costs vary according to workflow and laboratory policy for quality control and repeats. The *cost per reportable result* (CPRR) distributes the total direct costs of a run over the patient "reportable" results for that run. Testing efficiency is defined as the total reportable patient results/total test results. Thus, the more repeats and controls are performed, the lower is the efficiency, and the higher is the CPRR. As testing efficiency increases, the CPRR decreases. The *incremental cost* is the cost of producing one additional test that, typically, does not require additional salary or capital. For example, the incremental cost of running a chemistry test is usually the cost of dispensing reagent for one additional test, assuming there are no sample collection costs. Other associated costs, like technologist time, equipment, or quality control, are fixed costs that are incurred irrespective of the additional test. The incremental cost is usually the lowest possible cost incurred to produce a result. It is best used to assess how much it costs to produce small increments in test volume. As volume grows, a laboratory may need additional staff and equipment, and these costs would have to be included in the incremental costing analysis. Incremental costing is especially useful when one is trying to determine whether additional outreach work is profitable or not. The *fully loaded cost* for a test is the sum of direct and indirect costs. The allocation of indirect costs is usually done using a formula. The goal of allocating indirect costs is to apply the costs based on the strongest correlation between the indirect cost and to what it is being applied. For example, utilities could be based on departmental square footage, while human resources costs could be based on the number of employees in the department. *Make versus buy* decisions should be based on the fully loaded cost to produce the test compared with the price offered by a commercial or reference laboratory. If it costs more to produce a test than to buy it from another supplier, the test should be considered for outsourcing. However, when make versus buy decisions are made, cost is only one factor to consider. Medically necessary turnaround time, methods, and reliability of the potential alternative supplier should also be considered. The price charged for a test needs to be marked up (increased) from the fully loaded cost to realize a profit. One must also take into consideration the expected collection rate, relative to charge. The *contribution margin* is the balance remaining after the fully loaded costs are deducted from the price charged for a test. Table 12-2 demonstrates various ways to determine the cost of a test and how to establish its charge.

TABLE 12-2
Test Cost Analysis*

Test: Prostate-Specific Antigen

A. Microcosting: Instrument Run of One Reportable Test			
Direct Labor			
Determine the total "hands-on" time in minutes required to perform an instrument "run" of one patient test. Assume labor cost is $20 per hour.			
	Minutes	**Expense**	
Prepare specimen	5		
Prepare reagents	10		
Prepare instrument	10		
Computer and/or worksheet setup	5		
Documentation of results/quality control/maintenance	10		
Clean-up	10		
Total direct labor	50	$16.67	
Direct Supplies			
List all consumables needed to perform the test. Note 4 tests (1 sample and 3 controls) are needed to produce 1 patient reportable result. Calibration costs should be added if they are required with each run.			
	Unit cost	**Units**	**Expense**
Reagent ($700 kit/100 tests)	$7	4	$28.00
Disposable pipets ($10/100 pipets)	$0.10	4	$0.40
Disposable reagent cups ($10/200 cups)	$0.05	4	$0.20
Low, medium, and high control material (0.05 mL/test @ $20/mL)	$1	3	$3.00
Total direct supplies			$31.60
Total direct costs			$48.27
Cost per reportable (total direct cost/reportable results)	$48.27/1		$48.27
Testing efficiency (reportable patient results/tests)	1 result/4 tests		25%
B. Microcosting: Instrument Run of 15 Reportable Tests			
Direct Labor			
For a group of tests run on automated analyzers, use direct labor expense from microcosting. For manual batch testing, direct labor costs may apply to each batch; additional labor time studies may be necessary to derive accurate data.			
	Minutes	**Expense**	
Total direct labor per batch (same as microcosting in this example)	50	$16.67	
Direct Supplies			
Note: 18 tests (15 samples and 3 controls) are needed to produce 15 reportable results. Fixed costs (controls) are spread over more than 1 sample, in contrast to first example.			
	Unit cost	**Units**	**Expense**
Reagent ($700 kit/100 tests)	$7	18	$126.00
Disposable pipets ($10/100 pipets)	$0.10	18	$1.80
Disposable reagent cups ($10/200 cups)	$0.05	18	$0.90
Low, medium, and high control material (0.05 mL/test @ $20/mL)	$1	3	$3.00
Total direct supplies			$131.70
Total direct costs			$148.37
Cost per reportable (total direct cost/reportable results)	$148.37/15		$9.89
Testing efficiency (reportable patient results/tests)	15 results/18 tests	83%	

Continued

TABLE 12-2
Test Cost Analysis—Cont'd

C. Incremental Cost: Cost for One More Test			
	Units	Expense	
Reagent ($700 kit/100 tests)	1	$7	
Disposable pipets ($10/100 pipets)	1	$0.10	
Disposable reagent cups ($10/200 cups)	1	$0.05	
Total		$7.15	
	Unit cost	Units	Expense
D. Fully Loaded Cost			
Direct cost (cost per reportable result for typical size run) from Example B above	$9.89		
Indirect cost (estimated by typical hospital as 2.5 × direct costs)	$24.73		
Fully loaded cost			$34.62
E. Contribution Margin			
Example of Charging a 20% Mark-up for Laboratory Tests			
Fully loaded cost plus 20% mark-up (test charge at list price)	$34.62 × 1.2		$41.54
Fully loaded cost from Example D above			($34.62)
Contribution margin			$6.92

*This analysis is for illustration purposes only.

TABLE 12-3
Reimbursement Comparison for PSA* by Payer Type

	List price	Reimbursement terms	Amount paid	Contractual allowance
Inpatient				
Managed care (HMO)	$41.54	No separate reimbursement for laboratory tests because they are included in the contracted per diem rate	0	N/A
Medicare	$41.54	No separate reimbursement for laboratory tests because they are included in the DRG rate	0	N/A
Outpatient				
Indemnity insurance	$41.54	Usual and customary charge (UCC) is $38; insurance pays 80% of UCC.	$30.40	$11.14
Managed care (PPO)	$41.54	Contract pays 110% of Medicare fee schedule ($25.70 for PSA).	$28.27	$13.27
Managed care (HMO)	$41.54	No separate reimbursement for laboratory tests because of capitation arrangement: laboratory receives per member per month payment irrespective of usage	N/A	N/A
Medicare	$41.54	Medicare fee schedule	$25.70	$15.84

DRG, Diagnosis-related group; *HMO,* health maintenance organization; *N/A,* not applicable; *PPO,* preferred provider organization; *PSA,* prostate-specific antigen.
*Reimbursement amounts are for illustrative purposes only and may not accurately reflect current Medicare reimbursement.

The *total cost of ownership* (TCO) for a laboratory is the life cycle cost of its capital assets. It focuses attention on the sum of all costs of owning and maintaining all assets for a specific service or product, as opposed to the initial capital or operating costs. In the laboratory, TCO includes acquisition, setup (construction, training), support (ordering supplies, dealing with back orders), ongoing maintenance (scheduled and unscheduled downtime), service, and operating expenses (reagents, controls, repeat testing, inventory control, proficiency testing, testing personnel, supervisory personnel) of a specific workbench and its associated testing instrumentation. TCO is useful in considering make versus buy decisions, but determining an accurate TCO can be very difficult.

REVENUE

Revenue is the total price of services rendered or products sold (Harmening, 2007). It is the money a business is entitled to receive for the services and products it produces. In health care, revenue should not be confused with reimbursement or cash collected. *Gross patient revenue* consists of the total charges at a facility's full-established rates (list price) for provision of inpatient and outpatient care before deductions from revenue are applied. *Net patient revenue* is the gross inpatient and outpatient revenue minus all related deductions. *Deductions* from revenue include contractual adjustments, provision for bad debts, charity care, and other adjustments and allowances that reduce gross patient revenue. *Contractual adjustments* account for the difference between billings at full-established rates and amounts received or receivable from third-party payers under formal contract agreements. For example, if the list price of a test is $10 but the contracted payment from the insurance company is $6, the adjustment is $4. If all deductions and contractual allowances are correct, net patient revenue should equal cash collected, or $6 in the above example.

In health care, it is important to distinguish between inpatient and outpatient care because they are reimbursed differently. Inpatient laboratory testing charges usually are not reimbursed separately; they are considered to be part of a per diem rate (i.e., general hospital daily room reimbursement rate) or diagnosis-related group (DRG) rate (i.e., set rate for the entire hospital stay, regardless of actual length of stay). Thus, inpatient laboratory testing is considered a "cost center." The hospital is paid the same rate regardless of how many tests are provided. In contrast, outpatient laboratory testing is a revenue center because each test is separately reimbursed, usually by a third party (Table 12-3). Thus there is a financial disincentive to perform inpatient tests and an incentive to perform outpatient tests.

Payers and Reimbursement

Hospitals in early America served a different purpose from those of today. A visiting physician usually provided health care in the patient's home, and care was administered by family members, midwives, and servants. Early hospitals were founded to shelter older adults, the dying, orphans, those with mental illness, and vagrants, and to protect the citizens of a community from contagious diseases and the dangerously insane. Many of today's county, municipal, or religious order hospitals were originally a combination of these almshouses and isolation hospitals (Sultz, 2009).

The transformation of hospitals from charitable institutions to complex technical organizations came about with the passage of the Hill-Burton Hospital Construction Act of 1946 and the growth of private hospital insurance. The Hill-Burton Act provided federal money to the states to plan and construct new facilities. The first private health insurance policy was formed by a group of teachers and Baylor Hospital in Dallas, to provide coverage for certain hospital expenses. This arrangement created the model for the development of what was to become Blue Cross Insurance. The development of health insurance to provide reimbursement for routine medical care carried gigantic implications. The original concept of any insurance was to guard against the low risk of a rare occurrence such as premature death or accident. Today's health insurance provides for coverage of routine, predictable services, as well as unforeseen illnesses and injuries (Sultz, 2009).

PRIVATE INSURANCE

Private health insurance falls into two main categories: indemnity and managed care. Indemnity plans, also known as fee-for-service, are traditional insurance plans that give patients absolute freedom to choose their physicians and medical facilities. Insurance companies usually require the beneficiaries to fulfill a yearly deductible, usually between $300 and $500 per person per year. After the deductible is fulfilled, the insurance company pays a certain coinsurance rate of the usual and customary charge (UCC). The UCC (or fee schedule) is set by the payer and is usually less than the actual billed charge, in which case the patient may be responsible for the balance. Generally, the coinsurance is split 70%/30% or 80%/20%, where the insurance company pays the higher percentage and the insured the lower. Indemnity plans were the mainstay of the health insurance world before the 1980s. Today, managed care is the norm. Some employers still offer indemnity plans despite their high premium payments to allow their employees the freedom to choose medical services.

As an alternative to indemnity health insurance, managed care was introduced in 1973 with the passage of the Health Maintenance Organization Act. This Act encouraged and funded the development of health maintenance organizations (HMOs) as a strategy to contain the rising cost of health care (Sultz, 2009). HMOs utilized managed care features that coupled health care reimbursement with delivery of service and allowed payers significant economic control over how, where, and what services were delivered. Common features in managed care include the following: specific physicians and hospitals are selected to care for members; referrals from a case manager are usually necessary for specialty or inpatient services; and providers share in the financial risk through capitation agreements and per diem rates.

Capitation agreements pay the service provider (e.g., physician) a fixed dollar amount per member per month (PMPM). From this amount, the provider agrees to cover all care for plan members. For example, if a laboratory signs a capitation agreement to accept $1.50 PMPM for the outpatient testing needs of 2000 HMO members, the laboratory receives $3000 per month, and $36,000 per year. If it costs the laboratory more than $36,000/year to provide the services, it realizes a financial loss; if it costs less than $36,000, it realizes a profit. In a capitation testing agreement, a laboratory assumes the risk of spending more than it is paid. One key to managing this risk is gaining access to test utilization of plan members and accurately assessing laboratory costs.

Per diem rates are negotiated with hospitals to provide all necessary care and services for managed members requiring inpatient care. Reimbursement for any laboratory testing during the inpatient stay is included in the per diem amount. As with capitation, if it costs more to provide inpatient services than the per diem rate, the hospital is at financial risk.

Sometimes, a service is separately negotiated (i.e., it is not included as part of the capitation or per diem rate). This is called a "carve out." Esoteric and expensive tests (chromosome analysis, certain molecular testing) should be targeted as carve outs from capitation outpatient laboratory testing agreements. A negotiated fee-for-service price for these tests is appropriate. By excluding these tests from capitation, one can avoid huge financial losses due to unexpectedly high utilization of these costly services.

GOVERNMENT PAYERS

Medicare is federal health insurance for individuals age 65 and older, individuals who are permanently disabled, and those with end-stage renal disease who have met the specified waiting period. Medicare was established in 1965 by Title XVIII of the Social Security Act. It is administered by the Centers for Medicare and Medicaid Services (CMS), a division of the U.S. Department of Health and Human Services (HHS). Coverage is provided under Parts A, B, C, and D. Claims are processed by CMS-approved contractors. These contractors are usually private companies that serve as fiscal intermediaries (generally processing Part A claims) and carriers (generally processing Part B claims). However, CMS is moving to a new model, whereby the Medicare Administrative Contractor (MAC) will administer both Part A and Part B claims via 15 MAC jurisdictions. For a clinical laboratory to qualify for Medicare/Medicaid reimbursement, the laboratory must maintain Clinical Laboratory Improvement Act of 1988 certification (Washington G-2, 2009).

Medicare Part A covers inpatient hospitalization, hospice care, skilled nursing care, and home health care. Coverage is automatic for those who are eligible. Before the Tax Equity and Fiscal Responsibility Act of 1982 (TEFRA), inpatient hospitalization was reimbursed on a retrospective cost-based system. This system paid hospitals for all costs incurred during an inpatient stay. After TEFRA, the system switched to a prospective payment system (PPS), which reimbursed hospitals on the basis of preset payments for services provided to patients with similar diagnoses. With this DRG payment system, hospitals are reimbursed the same amount for a specific DRG no matter how many discreet units of services are provided. Thus, hospitals can earn a profit or realize a loss on each inpatient stay, depending on whether their costs are lower or higher than the DRG payment. The aim of the PPS, with its fixed DRG reimbursements, was to force hospitals to contain costs by reducing the length of stay and eliminating unnecessary and/or overutilized services (Sultz, 2009).

Medicare Part B covers outpatient laboratory tests, physician professional services, and other medical services and devices. Coverage is not automatic. Eligible beneficiaries must enroll for Part B coverage and pay premiums. Beneficiaries must pay an annual deductible and a 20% copayment for all Part B services, except for clinical laboratory testing, which is covered in full, provided certain conditions are met (see later).

The Part B fee schedule plays an important role in reimbursement because it is a baseline that nongovernment payers use to establish their own rates. For example, a private insurance company may set its fee schedule at 110% of the Part B fee schedule.

Medicare Part C (also known as Medicare Advantage) is an alternative to the traditional Part B fee-for-service program. It is designed to reduce patient "out of pocket" costs by providing services through health maintenance organizations and other managed care service models. *Medicare Part D* provides prescription drug coverage.

Medicaid is a Federal program that offers health care coverage for select low-income families. It was authorized in 1965 as a Federal/State-sponsored program designed to pay medical costs for certain families with low income or inadequate resources. Eligibility extends to people who are aged, blind, or disabled, and those in families with dependent children. Although Medicaid is a Federal program, it is under the jurisdiction of each individual state. This means that each state determines who is eligible, the range of health services offered, and how they are reimbursed. It is a common misconception that Medicaid covers health care costs for all low-income persons. Medicaid does not provide paid medical assistance to every single poor person. To receive medical assistance, a person must meet eligibility requirements.

Reimbursement Coding Systems

To be paid, a medical claim must document the patient's medical condition (or diagnosis) and must list the services (or tests) provided. This information is conveyed via a standardized coding system, recognized by all government and private payers: *H*ealthcare *C*ommon *P*rocedure *C*oding *S*ystem (*HCPCS*) codes describe the test or service (HCPCS 2010, 2009), and International Classification of Diseases, 9th Revision with Clinical Modification (ICD-9-CM), codes describe the patient's condition or diagnosis (ICD-9-CM 2010, 2009). These coding standards allow data to be accurately communicated among physicians, patients, and third-party payers.

HCPCS was developed in 1983 and consists of two levels of codes. Level I is the *C*urrent *P*rocedural *T*erminology (*CPT*) coding system and is used to identify nearly all clinical laboratory tests and most medical services (CPT, 2009, 2010). CPT codes are assigned by the American Medical Association (AMA) and are reviewed and updated annually to keep current with changes in technology and medical practice. Each CPT code consists of five digits and a description of the test or service. For example, the CPT code for a total prostate-specific antigen (PSA) test is 84153.

Level II HCPCS codes are assigned by CMS. CPT does not contain all the codes needed to report services or to describe special circumstances that may apply to Medicare. CMS developed this second level of codes to fill the gap. HCPCS Level II codes begin with a single letter (A through V) followed by four digits. These codes are updated annually by CMS. An example of Level II coding is prostate-specific antigen for cancer screening, G0103. Note that CMS treats this test differently than the PSA CPT code described earlier, even though the tests are identical to those of the laboratory. This allows CMS to assign different criteria for reimbursement, based on why a test is ordered.

The ICD-9 was originally developed by the World Health Organization (WHO) as a classification system for reporting of mortality and morbidity statistics by physicians throughout the world. The ICD-9-CM is a U.S. clinically modified revision of the WHO's ICD-9. This modification is maintained and updated by the National Center for Health Statistics. These modifications assist health care providers to index patient records, retrieve case data for clinical studies, and submit claims for health care services. It is worth noting that the WHO has already developed ICD-10, and HHS has set a deadline of October 1, 2013, for adoption of ICD-10 in the United States (Washingon G-2, 2009).

WHY ACCURATE CODING IS IMPORTANT

Correct coding is important for three reasons. First, one should be paid for services rendered. Insufficient or incorrect coding may yield lower reimbursement than is rightfully due. Second, one must not receive more reimbursement than is rightfully due. Coding for services not provided or assigning a code that recoups more reimbursement (this practice is known as "up-coding") is illegal and constitutes fraud. Third, one must comply with *medical necessity* requirements established by CMS for Medicare patients. These policies define under what conditions a test is considered "medically necessary" and thus reimbursable. Certain tests are considered "medically necessary" only if they are associated with specific diagnoses. Thus, reimbursement depends on whether the diagnosis or medical condition code (ICD-9 code) supports the test code (HCPCS code). For example, "malignant neoplasm of the prostate" supports the medical necessity of doing a PSA test, so Medicare would pay for the test; in contrast, "congestive heart failure" is not considered a medically necessary reason for a PSA test, so the test would not be reimbursed. Note that a physician (or other provider) can order any test on a patient, even if it is not "medically necessary," but it will not be reimbursed.

Most laboratory fee schedules are set by the local Medicare contractor (fiscal intermediary or carrier). Historically, each contractor established separate guidelines for determining which tests were subject to medically necessary diagnosis codes. *Local medical review policies* and local coverage decisions differ from one carrier to another, making it very difficult to submit and process claims. In some instances, a diagnosis code valid for a test from one carrier may not be considered medically necessary by another carrier. In an effort to standardize all carrier reimbursement guidelines for specific outpatient laboratory tests, 23 tests have been assigned *national coverage decisions* (*NCDs*); these medical necessity guidelines apply to all carriers in the country. See Table 12-4 for the list of NCD tests (CMS, 2010b).

Coding at any level should be as specific as possible. Medicare contractors employ the national Correct Coding Initiative to ensure correct coding practices based on the codes defined in the AMA's CPT code set (Washington G-2, 2009). These software edits flag inappropriate code combinations that should not be billed together for the same patient on the same day of service. Medicare has also added a system of medically unlikely edits (MUEs) that limit the units of service payable for a particular CPT code per patient, per provider, per day of service. Claims that exceed the MUE are rejected. Most analytes or tests have a specific CPT, similar to that of PSA. However, sometimes a new test does not have its own code. When that happens, the test must be identified by the method used to perform the analysis (e.g., 82486-Chromatography or 83519-Immunoassay, radioimmunoassay). A method code is usually reimbursed at a lower rate than a CPT code for a specific analyte.

TABLE 12-4
National Coverage Determinations for Laboratory Testing (CMS, 2010b)

General testing category	CPT codes included
Alpha-fetoprotein	82105
Blood counts	85004, 85007, 85008, 85013, 85014, 85018, 85025, 85027, 85032, 85045, 85049
Blood glucose testing	82947, 82948, 82962
Carcinoembryonic antigen	82378
Collagen crosslinks, any method	82523
Digoxin therapeutic drug assay	80162
Fecal occult blood test	82270
Gamma-glutamyl transferase	82977
Glycated hemoglobin/glycated protein	82985, 83036
Hepatitis panel/acute hepatitis panel	80074
Human chorionic gonadotropin	84702
Human immunodeficiency virus (HIV) testing (diagnosis)	86689, 86701, 86702, 86703, 87390, 87391, 87534, 87535, 87637, 87538
HIV testing (prognosis, including monitoring)	87536, 87539
Lipids	80061, 82465, 83715, 83716, 83718, 83721, 84478
Partial thromboplastin time	85730
Prostate-specific antigen	84153
Prothrombin time	85610
Serum iron studies	82728, 83540, 83550, 84466
Thyroid testing	84436, 84439, 84443, 84479
Tumor antigen by immunoassay CA 125	86304
Tumor antigen by immunoassay CA 15-3 (CA 27.29)	86300
Tumor antigen by immunoassay CA 19-9	86301
Urine culture, bacterial	87086, 87088, 87184, 87186

Certain tests that are performed together (i.e., as a panel) must be coded correctly. Ten panels have been approved by the AMA (Table 12-5). When these panels are performed, they must be coded with the unique panel code and not by each individual test's CPT code. Reimbursement is much lower for a panel than it is for the sum total reimbursement of each test. Coding for each individual test component as opposed to one panel code is considered "unbundling," which is a fraudulent billing practice.

Professional pathology physician services (e.g., test interpretation, slide review) are not included in the laboratory fee schedule. They are paid by the Medicare physician fee schedule, which uses a resource-based relative value scale to determine the payment based on a service's relative value unit. These amounts are adjusted to reflect local economic factors. Unlike the laboratory fee schedule, these professional services are subject to the annual deductible and the 20% copayment (Washington G-2, 2009).

MEDICARE REIMBURSEMENT

Medicare is the largest insurance program in the country. In many hospitals, it accounts for 25%–40% of all revenue. Outpatient services are reimbursed differently from inpatient ones.

Medicare Inpatients

DRGs make up a patient classification system that is used to reimburse inpatient (Part A) hospital costs for Medicare patients. Although the costs associated with inpatient clinical laboratory tests are included in the DRG, it does not cover physician services (Part B). After a Medicare patient has been discharged from the hospital, the patient's medical record is reviewed by health information management coders and is assigned appropriate ICD-9-CM and HCPCS codes for one or more diagnoses and procedures for the inpatient stay. These codes along with the patient's demographic

TABLE 12-5
AMA Organ or Disease-Oriented Panels (CPT, 2009)

CPT	Panel	Required components	
80047	Basic metabolic panel (calcium, ionized)	Calcium, ionized	(82330)
		Carbon dioxide	(82374)
		Chloride	(82435)
		Creatinine	(82565)
		Glucose	(82947)
		Potassium	(84132)
		Sodium	(84295)
		Urea nitrogen (BUN)	(84520)
80048	Basic metabolic panel (calcium, total)	Calcium, total	(82310)
		Carbon dioxide	(82374)
		Chloride	(82435)
		Creatinine	(82565)
		Glucose	(82947)
		Potassium	(84132)
		Sodium	(84295)
		BUN	(84520)
80050	General health panel	Comprehensive metabolic panel	(80053)
		Blood count, complete (CBC)	(85025) or (85027) and (85004)
		OR	
		CBC	(85027) and (85007) or (85009)
		Thyroid-stimulating hormone	(84443)
80051	Electrolyte panel	Carbon dioxide	(82374)
		Chloride	(82435)
		Potassium	(84132)
		Sodium	(84295)
80053	Comprehensive metabolic panel	Albumin	(82040)
		Bilirubin, total	(82247)
		Calcium	(82310)
		Carbon dioxide	(82374)
		Chloride	(82435)
		Creatinine	(82565)
		Glucose	(82947)
		Phosphatase, alkaline	(84075)
		Potassium	(84132)
		Protein, total	(84155)
		Sodium	(84295)
		Transferase, alanine amino	(84460)
		Transferase, aspartate amino	(84450)
		BUN	(84520)
80055	Obstetric panel	CBC	(85025) or (85027) and (85004)
		OR	
		CBC	(85027) and (85007) or (85009)
		Hepatitis B surface antigen	(87340)
		Antibody, rubella	(86762)
		Syphilis test, qualitative	(86592)
		Antibody screen, RBC	(86850)
		Blood typing, ABO	(86900)
		Blood typing, Rh	(86901)

Continued

TABLE 12-5
AMA Organ or Disease-Oriented Panels (CPT, 2009)—Cont'd

CPT	Panel	Required components	
80061	Lipid panel	Cholesterol, total HDL cholesterol Triglycerides	(85465) (83718) (84478)
80069	Renal function panel	Albumin Calcium Carbon dioxide Chloride Creatinine Glucose Phosphorus, inorganic Potassium Sodium BUN	(82040) (82310) (82374) (82435) (82565) (82947) (84100) (84132) (84295) (84520)
80074	Acute hepatitis panel	Hepatitis A antibody, IgM Hepatitis B core antibody, IgM Hepatitis B surface antigen Hepatitis C antibody	(86709) (86705) (87340) (86803)
80076	Hepatic function panel	Albumin Bilirubin, total Bilirubin, direct Phosphatase, alkaline Protein, total Transferase, alanine amino Transferase, aspartate amino	(82040) (82247) (82248) (84075) (84155) (84460) (84450)

ABO, Blood group; *HDL,* high-density lipoprotein; *IgM,* immunoglobulin M; *RBC,* red blood cell.

TABLE 12-6
National Coverage Determinations (NCDs) for Laboratory Testing (CMS, 2010)

Category	Medicare coverage	ABN necessary?
LMRP or NCD tests	Provider paid according to outpatient fee schedule, if medical necessity met	No, unless test is not "medically necessary"
FDA cleared or "homebrew" tests not included above	Provider paid according to outpatient fee schedule, if medical necessity met	No, unless test is not "medically necessary"
Investigational use only or research tests (i.e., not FDA cleared)	Not covered, no payment	Yes
Health and wellness screening	Not covered, with few exceptions: PAP smears covered every 2 years for all women and every year for those with high cancer risk or abnormal smear; PSA covered every year for men older than 50	Yes, unless it is one of the allowable exceptions

ABN, Advanced beneficiary nutrition; *FDA,* U.S. Food and Drug Administration; *LMRP,* local medical review policies; *PAP,* Papanicolaou smear; *PSA,* prostate-specific antigen.

information are grouped by decision trees (this process is computerized) into a specific DRG. Currently, more than 500 DRGs are used. CMS assigns a weight to each DRG based on the severity of the diagnoses, the types of procedures performed, the number of laboratory tests, the volume and type of drugs administered, and the presence of complications or comorbidity conditions. CMS assigns each hospital a specific rate that is calculated on the basis of the type of facility (community hospital vs. teaching hospital), the setting (urban vs. rural), and the location (West Coast vs. Midwest). The CMS-assigned rate for the DRG is multiplied by the hospital's assigned rate to determine reimbursement for the hospital stay. This amount is payment-in-full for the inpatient hospitalization. If it costs the hospital more than the reimbursed amount to treat the patient, the hospital must absorb the cost. The patient cannot be billed for any non-reimbursed Part A services (Sultz, 2009).

Medicare Outpatients

For many years after the enactment of DRGs, each outpatient service continued to be reimbursed individually (Harmening, 2007). However, the reimbursement system changed when CMS started to implement an outpatient prospective payment system with the introduction of the Ambulatory Payment Classification (APC) system in 2000. Under this system, virtually all hospital-based outpatient services (e.g., emergency department and clinic visits, oncology treatment and surgery) provided to Medicare patients are reimbursed on a prospective basis according to a preset rate, similar to DRGs. Clinical diagnostic laboratory tests are not currently included in the APC and are still reimbursed individually on the basis of the CMS fee schedule, with some exceptions.

Under certain conditions, Medicare does not pay for laboratory tests (Table 12-6). If a laboratory expects Medicare to deny payment because a test does not meet medical necessity requirements, it must inform the patient before the service is provided. An *advanced beneficiary notice (ABN)* is used to document that the beneficiary was told the test might not be covered by Medicare, the reason(s) for the possible denial, and the decision by the patient to pay for the test if Medicare does not reimburse or to refuse the test entirely (Washington G-2, 2009).

An important consideration for hospitals that have laboratories that perform outpatient testing on Medicare patients is the *72-hour rule* (CMS, 2010c). This rule states that a hospital cannot bill an outpatient (Part B) claim for laboratory tests performed within 72 hours of an inpatient admission. Outpatient testing that is performed 72 hours before the admission must be included with the inpatient claim and is reimbursed according to the assigned DRG for that stay. Hospital laboratories must identify outpatient Medicare services that are affected by this rule and must make sure they are not billed separately. A nonhospital independent laboratory is not subject to the 72-hour rule. Thus preadmission tests performed 3 days before hospitalization are not reimbursed if performed in the admitting hospital's laboratory but are reimbursed if done in an independent laboratory.

TABLE 12-7
Pro Forma Laboratory Budget

Category	Current year	Assumptions	Change	Projection for new year
Revenue	$3,000,000	4% growth	$120,000	$3,120,000
Total tests	370,000	4% growth	14,800	384,800
Revenue/test	$8.11			$8.11
Expenses				
Salaries	$950,000	3% cost of living increase	$28,500	$978,500
Laboratory supplies	$421,000	4% growth (no price increase)	$16,840	$437,840
Reference lab fees	$250,000	4% growth	$10,000	$262,600
		1% price increase (on projected $260,000)	$2600	
Phlebotomy supplies	$35,500	4% growth	$1420	$36,920
Maintenance contracts	$40,000	No change		$40,000
Total expense	$1,696,500		$59,360	$1,755,860
Cost per test	$4.59			$4.56

FINANCIAL PERFORMANCE AND MONITORING

BUDGETING

Budgeting is the process of planning, forecasting, controlling, and monitoring the financial resources of an organization (Garcia, 2004). The *operational budget provides a target* of day-to-day revenues and expenditures that are to be achieved in the forthcoming year.

Different budget-planning strategies are used based on the type and seasonality of the business; however, all use a method to forecast and project what will occur in the next budget cycle. Projections are made for the expected increases and decreases in revenues and expenses based on historical information and adjustments for inflation, loss of business, new business, and new product lines. The laboratory typically uses a *pro forma* budget. It provides in a pro forma or "predetermined set form" the expected annual revenue and expense based on various projections and assumptions, including test volume. It uses actual costs, ratios, and percent calculations to extrapolate from historical data what the new budget will be. Table 12-7 presents an example of a pro forma budget.

In contrast to the pro forma budget, which uses baseline data from 1 year to develop data for the next, a *zero-based budget* has no baseline. A zero-based budget requires management to annually evaluate all services and products to determine which should be funded or eliminated. Each department manager must justify its budget as if all of its activities are new. It assumes that no existing program is entitled to automatic budget approval, but rather must prove its financial merit when compared with the organization's other programs. Programs are ranked and funded by merit priority to the level of the organization's available funds. Laboratories use a zero-based approach to propose a new service (e.g., blood donor program, outpatient blood collection center) or laboratory section (e.g., mycology) or test (polymerase chain reaction assay) (Travers, 1997).

The *capital budget* is used to fund large capital projects such as acquiring an instrument or information system, or remodeling the laboratory (Garcia, 2004). These projects may cost thousands or millions of dollars and require several years to plan or implement. The laboratory's proposed projects must compete with those of other hospital departments for limited capital dollars. Each project is evaluated (see later) and ranked on the basis of a variety of financial and clinical factors. The operational budget must be linked to the capital budget, for it is the revenues generated by operations that are used to fund needed capital items and projects. Operational budgets must generate surplus revenue to fund capital projects; a business must reinvest in itself to remain competitive.

VARIANCE ANALYSIS

The operational budget should be reviewed periodically, usually monthly, to determine how closely the projected budget matches actual revenues and expenses (Garcia, 2004). A variance is the difference between the projected budget and the actual revenue and expenses (Budget − Actual = Variance). Both favorable variances (more than expected revenue or less than expected expenses) and unfavorable variances (less than expected revenue or more than expected expenses) need to be analyzed. By analyzing a variance, one can identify whether it can be controlled or not. Once the cause is determined, one can take necessary action to improve performance and more accurately prepare future budgets.

If revenues (and expected test volume) are within budget, but laboratory supplies show an unfavorable variance, one must investigate the reason for the discrepancy. For example, technologists may be repeating tests too frequently, running too many controls, or scheduling work inefficiently, in many small batches. This is an example of a variance that can be controlled by the laboratory if it changes its practices. Actions to consider include increasing the frequency of instrument maintenance to reduce problems that require repeats and controls, providing staff education to reinforce policies on when repeats and controls are needed, and rescheduling work into more efficient batch sizes.

An example of an uncontrollable variance occurs if a hospital decides to eliminate the cardiac chest pain service. In this scenario, a favorable reagent expense variance (i.e., less money spent on reagents than expected) would be related to doing fewer cardiac marker tests. A laboratory manager can do nothing to correct this variance. However, this does not absolve the manager from a duty to review it. One must verify the amount of the variance and must determine if it is appropriate for the amount of lost business. When forecasting for the next budget cycle, one should decrease projected revenues and expenses attributed to the loss of cardiac services.

FINANCIAL REPORTING AND STATEMENTS

Managerial accounting is used to prepare and monitor budgets. Revenue and expenses are organized into logical groupings known as cost centers that represent a laboratory section (such as microbiology, core lab, blood bank) or function (phlebotomy). Each cost center is subdivided into a variety of expense and revenue categories. Salary and nonsalary expense categories are grouped separately. Periodic review, at least monthly, of the cost center's accounts is needed to monitor the variances and put corrective action in place to keep the organization on its expected financial plan. Table 12-8 provides an example of a laboratory cost center's accounts.

Financial accounting is a system used to report business information to external entities such as the Internal Revenue Service or its stockholders. Generally accepted accounting principles are used to standardize this information. Balance sheet, income statement, and statement of cash flows are the financial statements most commonly used to assess an organization's financial position. Banks and investors rely heavily on these statements to determine whether to lend money to a business or to purchase shares of stock.

The *balance sheet* is the statement of an organization's financial position at a specific point in time. This statement is usually generated at the end of an organization's fiscal year or at the end of the calendar year. It records the organization's assets (what it owns), its liabilities (what it owes), and its equity or net worth (what is left after subtracting what it owes from what it owns). From this statement is derived the fundamental accounting equation: Assets = Liabilities + Equity (net worth). This statement is used to assess an organization's level of indebtedness to what it owns.

The *income statement*, also known as the statement of profit and loss, summarizes the organization's revenues and expenses over an accounting period, usually quarterly or annually. The income statement records all of

TABLE 12-8
Cost Center: Microbiology

Account number	Account name	Current month Actual	Current month Budget	Current month Variance	Year to date Actual	Year to date Budget	Year to date Variance
		REVENUE					
20100	Inpatient revenue	$1,414,245	$1,403,172	$11,073	$2,892,427	$2,764,597	$127,830
20200	Outpatient revenue	$906,343	$894,405	$11,938	$1,699,418	$1,748,169	$(48,751)
Total revenue		$2,320,588	$2,297,577	$23,011	$4,591,845	$4,512,766	$79,079
		EXPENSES					
40100	Salary, management	$22,045	$21,811	$234	$43,310	$43,622	$(312)
40200	Salary, technical	$85,161	$105,410	$(20,249)	$170,437	$210,820	$(40,383)
40201	Overtime	$3385	$3907	$(522)	$6713	$7814	$(1101)
Total salary expense		$110,591	$131,128	$(20,537)	$220,460	$262,256	$(41,796)
41580	Laboratory supplies	$109,961	$96,114	$13,847	$193,102	$188,461	$4641
41590	Medical surgical supplies	$1682	$1715	$(33)	$3964	$3362	$602
41890	Service contracts	$75	$355	$(280)	$150	$710	$(560)
42010	Minor equipment	$1112	$1083	$29	$2568	$2166	$402
45300	Sendout test expense	$14,973	$13,750	$1223	$28,812	$27,500	$1312
46300	Accreditation expense	$—	$100	$(100)	$—	$200	$(200)
Total nonsalary expense		$127,803	$113,117	$14,686	$228,596	$222,399	$6197
Total expense		$238,394	$244,245	$(5851)	$449,056	$484,655	$(35,599)

a laboratory's gross patient revenue, less allowances for a given period, and deducts the expenses for that same period to arrive at net income before taxes. Taxes are paid only if the organization is for-profit. Net income is realized when net revenues exceed expenses. A net loss is realized when expenses exceed net revenues. Note that revenue does not necessarily equate to cash generated. Many times a test is performed and recorded as income, although the payment (cash) may not be received for several months. The income statement records the organization's ability to make a profit; it does not reflect its cash position.

The *statement of cash flows* shows the amount of cash generated by an organization over a period of time, usually a calendar or fiscal year. Cash outflows (cash paid out) are subtracted from cash inflows (cash received) to calculate the net change in cash for the period. Excess cash in a given period can be reinvested in the organization, used to make additional debt payments, or placed in easily liquidated securities for emergency use. If the net cash position for a period is negative, the organization must meet its cash obligations by using cash reserves from previous periods. If this trend is not reversed, the organization eventually will run out of cash.

BENCHMARKING AND PRODUCTIVITY MEASURES

Benchmarking and productivity measures go hand in hand. It does no good to collect productivity data if they are not compared with a standard or evaluated for trends over time. Benchmarking is the measurement of an organization's products or services against specific standards for comparison and improvement (Wallace, 1998). Benchmarking can be internal or external.

Internal benchmarking trends an organization's productivity over time. Productivity is the relationship between input (labor and supplies) and output (product or service) (Travers, 1997). It is usually expressed as a ratio of the product or service to the various inputs used for the production of the product or service. See Table 12-9 for common productivity ratios used in the laboratory. The purpose of trending internal productivity is to determine if internal standards are being met, exceeded, or not met. If adjustments to workflow or personnel are made, the next period's benchmarking data can be used to determine if the adjustments were the probable cause for improvements or for decreased productivity.

External benchmarking compares a laboratory's productivity with that of other laboratories. Its purpose is to identify top performers in a particular field. Top performers can be contacted to find out what processes or resources have been used to achieve high productivity. This information may guide a laboratory to make similar changes that could result in higher productivity. Professional organizations such as the College of American Pathologists or the University Healthsystem Consortium offer external laboratory specific benchmarking programs. Caution should always be used when interpreting external benchmarking information. Although clinical laboratories are similar, no two are exactly alike, and, despite best efforts, sometimes data are collected and reported differently. A laboratory may never be able to achieve productivity as high as its peers because of factors beyond the laboratory's control. Labor availability, the disease and acuity mix of patients, and access to technology and automation will each have an effect on how productive a laboratory is, and how much more productive it can become.

TABLE 12-9
Common Productivity Measures for Clinical Laboratories

Productivity measure	Target*	Quarter 1	Quarter 2
Billable tests/paid FTE	>3680	3798	3500
Billable tests/worked FTE	>4000	4128	4080
Worked FTE/paid FTE	>92%	95.2%	90%
Labor cost/billable test	<$5.00	$4.68	$5.01
Supply cost/billable test	<$1.00	$0.99	$1.01
Overtime/worked straight time	<3%	2.7%	3.5%

FTE, Full-time equivalent or 2080 paid hours in a year; *paid FTE,* all salaries paid (benefit time plus worked time).
*Target is for illustration purposes only. It should not be considered a laboratory standard.

EVALUATING A CAPITAL PROJECT

A hospital has limited capital; it cannot fund all requested projects, so it must prioritize them according to a variety of factors, including clinical need, patient or employee safety, and financial impact. Whether or not money is borrowed to finance these projects, it may be necessary for the project or investment to pay for itself and even generate excess cash to fund other projects. The following section discusses different ways to evaluate a capital project to answer the question, "Is it a good investment?" Table 12-10 compares these methods.

PAYBACK PERIOD

The payback period is commonly used to evaluate a capital project. The payback is the length of time required for an investment's net revenue to cover the cost of the initial investment (Brigham, 2009).

Because laboratory equipment or technology can become obsolete in a very short period of time, it is important to recover the investment cost as soon as possible. Many institutions want to see a payback in 3 years or

TABLE 12-10
Financial Evaluation of a New Automated Analyzer

GIVEN		
Investment (cost of analyzer)		$200,000
Discount rate (rate of inflation or interest rate of borrowed money)		10.00%
Useful life of analyzer	5 years	
Annual depreciation expense	$200,000/5 years	$40,000
Annual revenue	100,000 tests at $5.00/test	$500,000
Annual labor expense	100,000 tests at $2.50/test	$250,000
Annual supply expense	100,000 tests at $2.00/test	$200,000
Annual net revenue (annual revenue – annual expense)	$500,000 – ($250,000 + $200,000)	$50,000
Net revenue per test (test revenue – test expense)	$5.00 – ($2.50 + $2.00)	$0.50
CALCULATIONS		
PAYBACK PERIOD = Investment/Annual net revenue	$200,000/$50,000	4 years
BREAKEVEN		
Per year = Depreciation/Net revenue per test	$40,000/$0.50	80,000 tests
Life of analyzer = Investment/(net revenue per test)	$200,000/$0.50	400,000 tests
RETURN ON INVESTMENT (ROI) = Annual net revenue/Investment	$50,000/$200,000	25% per year
NET PRESENT VALUE (NPV) = Present value of the sum of future net revenue (cash flows) minus investment. *Note:* Present value interest factor (PVIF) for each year based on 10% discount rate is multiplied by net revenue to determine present value. PVIF is available from any financial data resource. NPV can also be calculated with financial calculator		
Today's investment	($200,000)	
Year 1 Net revenue × PVIF	$50,000 × 0.9091 = $45,455	
Year 2 Net revenue × PVIF	$50,000 × 0.8264 = $41,320	
Year 3 Net revenue × PVIF	$50,000 × 0.7513 = $37,565	
Year 4 Net revenue × PVIF	$50,000 × 0.6830 = $34,150	
Year 5 Net revenue × PVIF	$50,000 × 0.6209 = $31,045	
Present value of sum of future NPV net revenue	$189,535	$(10,465)
INTERNAL RATE OF RETURN (IRR) = Discounted interest rate at which NPV = 0. *Note:* Financial calculator is used to determine IRR by entering cash flow and discount rate.		
Today's investment	($200,000)	
Year 1 Net revenue × PVIF	$50,000 × 0.9265 = $46,326	
Year 2 Net revenue × PVIF	$50,000 × 0.8585 = $42,923	
Year 3 Net revenue × PVIF	$50,000 × 0.7954 = $39,769	
Year 4 Net revenue × PVIF	$50,000 × 0.7369 = $36,847	
Year 5 Net revenue × PVIF	$50,000 × 0.6828 = $34,140	
Present value of sum of future net revenue	$200,000	
NPV	$0	
IRR		8%

less. Once the initial investment is recovered, net revenue (Revenue – Expense) from this investment represents a profit to the organization. The sooner a capital project's payback period is reached, the sooner an organization can realize a profit from the investment.

BREAKEVEN POINT

The breakeven point of a capital project is reached when the volume of sales is such that total revenue equals total costs (fixed and variable), and therefore profit is zero. Before the breakeven point is reached, the project is operating at a loss; after it is reached, the project is realizing a profit (Brigham, 2009). As with the payback period, the sooner the breakeven point is reached, the better it is for the organization.

RETURN ON INVESTMENT*

The rate of return on an investment (ROI) for a capital project is the ratio of net income it generates to the total investment of the project (Travers, 1997). ROI is a standard for evaluating how wisely management uses its capital dollars, whether from its own cash reserves or from borrowing activities. The higher the rate of return is, the better the capital dollars are used. ROI is the formal means of expressing the phrase "better bang for your buck." Some institutions have automated the ROI process. Most information can be pulled from the financial data banks of the hospital computer system after a limited amount of information is provided by the laboratory. An ROI is pretty much a standard requirement of most facilities for any capital project.

NET PRESENT VALUE*

Money loses its value over time; $10,000 today is more valuable than $10,000 3 years from now. This concept is known as the time value of money. The payback period and return on investment calculations do not consider the time value of money. They assume that the value of future cash flows remains constant. To address this shortcoming, the net present value (NPV) calculation is used to determine whether a project's cash flows (i.e., cash it generates in the future) are sufficient to repay the original investment, taking into account that money loses value over time. Thus, cash received in the future has to be *discounted* (i.e., the value has to be reduced) to determine how much it is worth in today's dollars. The discount rate is usually the inflation rate (if no money was borrowed to finance

*Note: Financial calculators and financial software packages are programmed to calculate ROI, NPV, and IRR. The NPV and IRR are very tedious calculations requiring multiple steps and the use of discount tables. It is not recommended to do these calculations manually.

the project) or the interest rate on a loan used to fund the project. *Net present value (NPV)* is defined as the present value of future cash flows, which have been discounted at the interest rate used to fund the capital project (Brigham, 2009).

When the NPV is a positive number, the project will generate enough cash to pay for the original investment. When the NPV is a negative number, the project cost is not recouped and/or the future cash flows are not sufficient to cover the interest costs for borrowing the money.

INTERNAL RATE OF RETURN*

The internal rate of return (IRR) also discounts cash flow into today's value. It determines the actual rate of return that the investment earns. The IRR is the discount rate at which the present value of a capital project's expected cash inflows equals the present value of its costs, or in other words, when the NPV equals zero.

Identifying a project's IRR is necessary to ensure that its rate is higher than the cost of the capital borrowed for the project. The higher the IRR, the faster the project pays for itself. Hospitals and corporations use the IRR as one way to rank projects.

INTERPRETATION OF FINANCIAL CALCULATIONS

Although the preceding calculations are important tools, an organization should not make its capital decisions based strictly on the outcome of the equations. As with all budgeting activities, there is an element of the unknown in assumptions. Predicting future cash flows for replacement instrumentation is usually more reliable than predicting it for new product lines or technology. Assigning an expected life to a piece of capital equipment is also an educated estimate. Having a good sense of how reliable predictions are will determine how much credence should be given to the calculations.

If only the payback period, breakeven analysis, and ROI were considered when evaluating the example in Table 12-10, the project would look acceptable. However, when the NPV and IRR are also considered, it does not look as good. The NPV is unfavorable, and the IRR is much less than the ROI because the cost of capital is high (10%). Does this mean the project should not go forward? Not necessarily. Depending on other issues, it may be determined that this new chemistry analyzer is absolutely essential to support the mission of the organization.

These calculations have other inherent drawbacks. As mentioned earlier, some of the calculations take into account the time value of money, and others do not. The time value of money is a very important consideration when the cost of capital is high (as in the example in Table 12-10) or during periods of high inflation. The rate of return calculations yield a percentage, but the actual dollars they represent are not immediately apparent. A capital project that yields an ROI of 15% might look better initially than one that yields 10%. However, the size of the projects may differ considerably. For example, in the former, an initial investment of $10,000 could produce $1500 in net revenue, but in the latter project, an initial investment of $200,000 produces $20,000 in net revenue. None of these financial calculations should be considered in isolation, but they should be used in aggregate to assist in the analysis of capital projects.

CAPITAL ACQUISITION METHODS

When a capital project is evaluated, the method for acquiring the equipment is also an important consideration. Table 12-11 summarizes the advantages and disadvantages of acquisition methods: Purchase, leasing, and renting. Just as there is not a single best financial calculation when evaluating a project, there is not a single best acquisition method. The method selected depends on individual needs, characteristics and financial philosophy of the organization, and availability of capital dollars.

The concept of purchasing needed equipment is easy to understand, but is it the wisest use of an organization's money? If the capital (money) needed to fund the project is currently invested in a security that is earning a higher interest rate than the rate needed to borrow money, it makes financial sense to borrow the needed capital. Conversely, if capital earns a lower interest rate than the borrowing rate, it makes sense to use the organization's capital.

Once the equipment is purchased, it is an asset of the organization and is depreciated by a method appropriate for such a piece of equipment. Most laboratory equipment is depreciated over a 5-year period using the straight line depreciation method. The depreciation expense is noted in the income statement but probably will not be included in the monthly operational budget documents. It will depend on each organization as to whether depreciation is listed on the monthly budget reports. The operational expense for the equipment will consist of the supplies, maintenance, and labor needed to support it.

TABLE 12-11
Capital Acquisition Options

	Advantages	Disadvantages
Purchase	Ownership	Risk of obsolescence; opportunity cost
Operating (true) lease	Hedging obsolescence; flexibility in financing; cancelable	Nonownership; interest/financing cost
Financial lease	Ownership; flexibility in financing	Noncancelable; interest/financing cost
Rental	Hedging obsolescence; flexibility in length of use	High cost; nonownership

Many different variations and contract terms may be associated with a leasing agreement. Being certain to "read the fine print" never rings truer than when an equipment leasing arrangement is considered. Nonetheless, no matter how complicated the terms of a leasing contract are, there are only two types of leases.

An *operating lease* (also known as a "true" lease) allows an organization (lessee) full use of the equipment for a predetermined time. The time period is usually 1–3 years, but is always less than the useful life of the equipment. A termination clause could be included in the agreement. Equipment maintenance is included in an operating lease. The lessee has no right to ownership during or after the lease period. No equity is established during the term. The owner (lessor) retains full ownership of the equipment and full responsibility for it. The leasing agreement may or may not contain an option to allow the lessee to purchase the equipment at the end of the term. This is only an option, however, and should not be misinterpreted as established equity over the course of the agreement. If a purchase option is provided, it is usually for the equipment's fair market value at the end of the lease period. If the original lessee decides not to purchase the equipment at the end of the lease term, the lessor could re-lease it to the original lessee or to another organization, as the equipment still has useful life (Brigham, 2009).

The other lease type is a financial lease. With a *financial lease* (also known as a capital lease or lease-purchase), the lessee eventually gains ownership of the equipment. The lease period corresponds to the economic life of the equipment. Through lease payments, the lessor recovers the cost of the equipment plus an interest factor to ensure a return on its investment. A financial lease is not cancelable, and equipment maintenance is not included (Brigham, 2009).

Renting equipment is not the same as leasing it. The major differentiators include the following: Renting does not carry an option for later purchase, there is no predetermined specified length of time for renting, it can be terminated at any time, and maintenance and repair are the responsibility of the owner, not the renter (Travers, 1997). A reagent rental agreement is a misnomer; it is not a rental, but a lease. These agreements require the lessee to purchase reagents that are specific for a particular piece of equipment. The price of the reagents is marked up by a certain amount to cover the "rent" of the equipment. The mark-up is a lease payment to cover the cost of the capital. Whether or not the equipment will be owned at the end of the reagent rental agreement will determine if the agreement was a financial lease. Recent federal legislation requires vendors to clearly state the proportion of annual payments that are allocated to the capital portion of the lease. This simplifies the analysis of competing lease agreements.

Regardless of which method of capital acquisition is utilized, you should always have the vendor or lessor break out the agreement into cost of equipment, cost of service agreement, and costs of reagents and supplies. This way, you can see and negotiate the cost of each. It is prudent to include someone from the institution's purchasing department to help with negotiations.

Build in a Cap for Reagent/Supply Costs

Most equipment and instrumentation in laboratory medicine today are very complex, and because of industry competition, many "bells and whistles" have been added. At times, equipment can fail, and reagents and/or supplies can be a "bad lot" and not function correctly. This can result in a laboratory having to repeat patient testing over and over again. This repeating of tests and "getting the instrument to work properly" can result in a significant increase in costs for reagents and supplies beyond what you thought you needed based on the vendor recommendations.

One can protect the laboratory from the above costs by building a "cap" in any agreement for reagents and supplies as part of any equipment acquisition. One way to do this is to base the payment for reagents and supplies only on reportable patient results. If you need to repeat tests because of reagent or equipment failure, you do not pay for the increased reagent and supply usage.

Creating Financial Value/Conclusions

Financial oversight of any organization is not easy. For a clinical laboratory, this oversight is especially difficult because to remain competitive, it must offer state-of-the-art technologies that are often complex, expensive, and quick to become obsolete. This, combined with strict coding criteria for submitting claims that yield a predetermined fixed reimbursement rate, leaves little opportunity for the laboratory to cover costs, let alone make a profit.

The equation for net profit is defined as revenue minus expenses. Therefore the only way to increase net profit is to increase net revenue or to decrease expenses. In a managed care environment, increasing patient volume (and gross revenue) does little to increase net profit because variable expenses increase proportionately with the larger volume. For an increase in gross revenue to have a positive impact on net profit, the newly generated revenue must have a closer relationship to what is billed and to what is collected. The best way to achieve this is by providing testing to clients that is paid according to a fee schedule, instead of a DRG, APC, per diem, or capitation. Many laboratories attempt to do this by offering commercial or reference outreach programs. Target markets for outreach business include physician offices, clinics, and other laboratories or hospitals. Academic institutions also offer testing for grants, research, and clinical trials. If a laboratory has excess capacity for testing and can perform this additional testing without adding fixed costs, the increase in this revenue should increase the net profit. This of course also assumes that prices charged for the tests cover the expenses for this outreach testing. Once the increase in volume requires the addition of fixed costs (more labor, equipment, space, or other resources), careful evaluation of this new volume needs to be performed to ensure that the increase can cover the new costs.

Expense reduction seems to be the norm when one is trying to increase net profit in a managed care environment. Eliminating as much of the fixed cost as possible is the most effective way to accomplish this. Although it is very important to negotiate favorable pricing for supplies, reagents, and other variable cost items, reducing their unit cost by several cents or even several dollars will not have as great an impact as eliminating unneeded or underutilized fixed costs. Achieving economies of scale through maximum use and efficiency of an organization's fixed costs is critical in realizing substantial cost reductions.

Effective financial management requires careful planning, analysis, and critical thinking when decisions need to be made regarding how best to acquire capital equipment, assign pricing, and reduce costs. Keeping abreast of the various payer requirements ensures that the laboratory is reimbursed appropriately for services rendered. When applied with common sense, these tools and knowledge base will promote the financial success of a clinical laboratory operation.

SELECTED REFERENCES

Brigham EF, Houston JF. Fundamentals of Financial Management, 12th ed. Mason, Ohio: Cengage Learning; 2009.

An introduction to finance textbook written for the undergraduate business student.

Center for Medicare & Medicaid Services. National Health Expenditure Data. U.S. Department of Health & Human Services. Available at: http://www.cms.hhs.gov/nationalhealthexpenddata. Accessed September 2, 2010a.

This CMS web page contains an overview of health care spending in the United States.

Center for Medicare & Medicaid Services. Medicare Coverage Database, Lab NCDs. U.S. Department of Health & Human Services. Available at: http://www.cms.hhs.gov/mcd/index_section.asp?ncd_sections=40. Accessed September 2, 2010b.

This CMS web page lists the National Coverage Decisions for lab tests.

Center for Medicare & Medicaid Services. Medicare Claims Processing Manual, Inpatient Hospital Billing. U.S. Department of Health & Human Services. Available at: http://www.cms.hhs.gov/manuals/downloads/clm104c03.pdf. Accessed September 2, 2010c.

This CMS web page contains a copy of the Medicare Claims Processing Manual, Chapter 3, Inpatient Hospital Billing.

CPT 2010 Professional Edition. Chicago: American Medical Association; 2009.

This AMA publication is the authoritative listing of accepted CPT codes.

Garcia LS, editor. Clinical Laboratory Management. Washington, DC: ASM Press; 2004.

A multiauthored textbook with comprehensive coverage of all aspects of laboratory management.

Harmening DM. Laboratory Management: principles and processes. St. Petersburg, Fla.: D.H. Publishing & Consulting; 2007.

A textbook designed to balance theory and practical applications of laboratory management.

HCPCS 2010 Level II, Professional Edition. Chicago: American Medical Association; 2009.

This AMA publication is the authoritative listing of HCPCS 2010 Level II codes.

ICD-9-CM 2010. Chicago: American Medical Association; 2009.

This AMA publication is the authoritative listing of ICD-9-CM codes.

Snyder JS, Wilkinson DS. Management in Laboratory Medicine, 3rd ed. Philadelphia: Lippincott Williams & Wilkins; 1998.

A textbook developed to prepare medical technology students and pathology residents for the basic through intermediate levels of management.

Sultz HA, Young KM. Health Care USA: understanding its organization and delivery, 6th ed. Sudbury, Mass.: Jones & Bartlett; 2009.

A text describing the changing roles of the components of the health care system, in addition to the technical, economic, political, and social forces responsible for these changes.

Travers EM. Clinical Laboratory Management. Baltimore: Williams & Wilkins; 1997.

A comprehensive basic textbook for training health care professionals for clinical laboratory management roles.

Wallace MA, Klosinski DD. Clinical Laboratory Science Education & Management. Philadelphia: WB Saunders; 1998.

A textbook presenting the basic tenets of education and management for practical application in the field of laboratory medicine.

Washington G-2 Reports. Medicare Reimbursement Manual for Laboratory and Pathology Services, 2009.

This annual report provides updated and historical information on Medicare reimbursement.

REFERENCES

Access the complete reference list online at http://www.expertconsult.com

PART 1

CHAPTER 13

BIOLOGICAL, CHEMICAL, AND NUCLEAR TERRORISM: ROLE OF THE LABORATORY

Philip M. Tierno Jr., Mark S. Lifshitz

KEY POINTS

- Level A laboratories, also known as sentinel laboratories, may be the first to identify an unusual organism or cluster of isolates that may signal a bioterrorism event.
- The responsibility of a Level A laboratory is to "rule out" suspected biological agents rather than perform complete identification or highly complex analyses.
- Suspect samples must be handled safely and legally (using chain of custody).
- Specific protocols (and presumptive identification criteria) must be applied for each biological agent.
- Category A (highest priority) biological agents are easily disseminated, can cause high mortality, and can generate public panic. They include bacterial (anthrax, plague, tularemia), viral (smallpox, viral hemorrhagic fever) and toxin-mediated (botulism) agents.
- Level A laboratories play mostly a supportive role in the management of hospitalized patients who are victims of a chemical terror attack.

BIOTERRORISM

OVERVIEW

On September 11, 2001, following the unimaginable terrorist attacks on New York City and Washington, DC, the Centers for Disease Control and Prevention (CDC) recommended that health care professionals increase surveillance for any unusual disease occurrences, or clusters of disease, asserting that these may be sentinel indicators of bioterrorist attack. As predicted, anthrax cases were reported in several states, thereby justifying the CDC's suspicions that a bioterrorist was at large. Over the years, it has become clear that germ warfare is equally attractive to terrorist cells, organizations, and even disgruntled individuals as it is to countries. It delivers the greatest impact for the smallest amount of money, and it is relatively easy to carry out. It also comes with a big bonus—it has a dramatic psychological effect on the population. Compared with nuclear weapons or conventional armaments, biological weapons are relatively cheap and easy to make. For anyone with a rudimentary understanding of microbiology and the requisite materials, making biological agents of death in quantity is little more technically demanding than brewing beer. The microorganisms involved are often readily obtainable in nature, like the anthrax bacillus that abounds in soil throughout most of the world, or can be easily acquired from other sources such as a country's pharmaceutical and agricultural industries, or academic institutions. Toxic ricin, for example, which strikes at the central nervous system, can be extracted from the same castor beans that are the source of castor oil.

The U.S. Department of Defense and the CDC has published a list of the most likely biological weapons (NATO, 1996). They fall into three categories. The first includes deadly bacteria such as anthrax and plague. The second comprises viruses, such as those that cause smallpox, encephalitis, and hemorrhagic fevers like Ebola, Lassa, and Rift Valley fever. The last group is made up of toxins that attack the central nervous system, such as botulinum, fungal toxins, and ricin.

An effective national strategy to detect, prevent, and limit bioterrorism should consider the following:

- A coordinated plan is needed to network all federal, state, and municipal antibioterrorism programs. All first responders must be adequately educated and equipped to deal with any biowarfare or bioterrorism event.
- Military and law enforcement personnel and medical and health practitioners, especially first responders, should be vaccinated whenever possible so that they can more effectively carry out their respective missions.
- Research and development of new wave (subparticle) vaccines, blocking agents, and antibiotics are needed to prevent and treat disease caused by biological weapons.
- Vaccination programs for the general public should be instituted to protect against the likeliest biological weapons.
- The public should be kept informed about germ warfare and should be instructed to report unusual neighborhood activities to local authorities. "Bioterrorism watches" could be introduced on the model of "neighborhood crime watches."
- All physicians and health care providers should be familiar with the symptoms and treatment of diseases caused by the likeliest biological warfare agents. All hospitals and medical facilities should develop emergency preparedness plans and should establish disaster policies to deal with any bioterror event or other disaster. Included in such plans is the development of a clinical laboratory preparedness and response plan.

TABLE 13-1
Biological Safety Level (BSL) Practices

BSL-1 practices: For work with agents of minimal hazard
Restrict or limit access when working.
Prohibit eating, drinking, and smoking.
Prohibit mouth pipetting.
Needles and sharps precautions
BSL-2 practices: For agents of moderate hazard
BSL-1 practices plus:
Use Biological Safety Cabinet (BSC)-Class II
Type A1: 30% air exhausted to room
Type A2: 30% air exhausted to outside
Type B1: 70% air exhausted to outside
Type B2: 100% air exhausted to outside
Use leakproof containers.
BSL-3 practices: For agents of serious or potential lethal hazard
BSL-2 practices plus:
Use BSC-Class II 100% air exhausted to outside through double high-efficiency particulate air (HEPA) filtration or HEPA plus incineration. Cabinet is gas tight and sealed, with operation performed through rubber gloves.
Use PPE (personal protective equipment).

- A nationwide epidemiologic surveillance program should link all medical facilities with the CDC or another assigned federal, state, or local agency to identify clusters of cases (sentinel events). Small clusters may signal a terrorist practicing before a larger-scale act is carried out.

The keynote to all this is vigilance. Any complacency or overconfidence will surely prove fatal, sooner or later. The bottom line is that we must remain on alert for animal and human epidemics and must keep searching for better ways to respond to them, whether they are of natural or unnatural origin (Tierno, 2004).

This chapter explains how a Level A laboratory responds to a bioterror event as part of a health facility's larger emergency preparedness plan. This chapter excludes some common potential bioterror agents such as *Salmonella*, *Shigella*, *Escherichia coli* 0157, *Campylobacter*, *Vibrio*, etc., because they are well known and are routinely cultured by Level A laboratories (see Part 7, Medical Microbiology). Instead, it focuses on several more likely bioterror agents with which a Level A laboratory may be less familiar.

ROLE OF A LEVEL A LABORATORY

The Laboratory Response Network (LRN) is a new laboratory testing and referral system formed as an outgrowth of the CDC's Health Alert Network. Its purpose is to prepare for and provide a coordinated, rapid response to bioterrorism and other public health emergencies. The LRN consists of four types of laboratories, designated Levels A, B, C, and D.

Safety Issues

Level A laboratories must always operate in compliance with accepted biological safety level 2 (BSL-2) requirements, including regulations, policies, and procedures for handling blood-borne pathogens (Table 13-1). When handling any potential pathogen, all Level A laboratories should utilize BSL-3 practices for all culture manipulations that might produce aerosols. Level B laboratories operate in compliance with all BSL-2 requirements and always practice BSL-3 safety procedures. Level C laboratories operate in compliance with all BSL-3 safety requirements and are certified as BSL-3 facilities. Their staff is specially trained to handle highly pathogenic and potentially lethal agents.

It is of paramount importance to practice good laboratory safety. For example, staff that process viral cell cultures are at risk of contracting unsuspected bioterror agents, such as smallpox or hemorrhagic fever viruses (BSL-4 agents). To minimize exposure, staff must practice universal precautions and use biological safety cabinets to set up cultures (Gilchrist, 2000; NCCLS, 2001; CDC, 2001).

Laboratory Designations

Level A facilities are also known as sentinel laboratories, in that they may identify an unusual organism that may be highly suspect and therefore may be first to signal that a bioterrorism event has occurred. Alternatively, the Level A laboratory might report a cluster of isolates of the same organism for a number of patients that may be unusual and thus signal an event. Most clinical laboratories fall into this category. The cardinal responsibility of a Level A laboratory is to "rule out" suspected agents of bioterror rather than perform complete identification or highly complex analyses. Once a Level A laboratory reports a finding to a state or municipal public laboratory, it may be instructed to forward the microbe to a Level B or C laboratory, so that it can be "confirmed" using advanced methods. For example, if an agent is suspected of being *Bacillus anthracis*, but this cannot be ruled out by the Level A laboratory, it must be shipped out to a Level B or C facility.

Level D laboratories are even more advanced and may help develop and evaluate new tests for future use in Level B and C laboratories. They can usually type confirmed bioterror agents or may perform more sophisticated molecular testing on strains. Level D laboratories also archive organisms for future studies or reference (Gilchrist, 2000; CDC, 2001; NCCLS, 2001).

Once a Level A laboratory decides that it cannot "rule out" an agent, it is common policy for the laboratory to notify the infection control officer or hospital epidemiologist, who, in turn, notifies the local health department. The laboratory should be prepared to follow instructions for shipping the suspect agent according to the Infectious Substance Guidelines provided by the Department of Transportation or the International Air Transport Association. It is not the responsibility of the Level A laboratory to declare that a bioterrorist event has taken place. Such responsibility rests with the state and/or federal authorities.

Because environmental specimens usually become evidence in a legal case, these specimens require full chain of custody management that is the domain of Level B and C laboratories. Such *environmental* samples may also pose a hazard for patients in a hospital setting; therefore in no case should Level A laboratories accept or process environmental specimens. It is the FBI's responsibility to manage the investigation of environmental samples that are submitted to Level B and C laboratories.

Law Enforcement Issues

The Level A laboratory may play a role in a criminal investigation. If a specimen is suspected or known to possess a biological threat, it is important to preserve the original specimen, plates, cultures, etc. If the laboratory is contacted by the FBI or other law enforcement agencies, the Level A laboratory must notify state health authorities, as well as the hospital infection control officer or epidemiologist. Any information relevant to analysis of potential evidence cannot be released to the public and should be conveyed only to the appropriate law enforcement officials and health authorities.

Chain of custody is a legal document that describes how evidence is handled from the time it is acquired and through all subsequent examinations and storage. The laboratory should have a written chain of custody policy and should appoint one person to serve as an "evidence custodian," that is, the one who controls storage of evidence and documents access to it on a chain of custody form that is securely stored under lock and key. The LRN suggests completing a "receipt of property" form each time the laboratory receives evidence. This form should contain a unique identifier, the quality and quantity of each item, a description of each item, and as much information as possible regarding the submitter, etc. (Gilchrist, 2000; CDC/NIH, 2001; NCCLS, 2001).

BIOLOGICAL AGENTS/DISEASES

The CDC and other governmental agencies list biological agents/diseases in three categories (A, B, and C) according to priority of risk and ease of ability to disseminate to the population. Some representative examples in each category are listed in Tables 13-2, 13-3, and 13-4 (Gilchrist, 2000; USAMRIID, 2001; Tierno, 2002). Table 13-5 summarizes diagnosis and treatment issues related to the bioterror agents discussed later. The role of the Level A laboratory is described in Tables 13-6 through 13-14 for each agent discussed in this chapter.

Anthrax

(Table 13-6)

History and Background

Bacillus anthracis, the etiologic agent of anthrax, is a rod-shaped gram-positive bacterium that produces a spore. Ordinarily, these bacteria grow in a vegetative form, but when conditions are not ideal for growth, they sporulate. Thus, they can survive even under adverse conditions. The vegetative forms are relatively easy to kill with simple germicides, such as

TABLE 13-2
Category A Agents

HIGHEST PRIORITY OF AGENTS THAT POSE A NATIONAL SECURITY RISK	
Characteristics	**Agents**
Easily disseminated and/or transmitted from person to person Can result in high mortality rates with a major public health impact Might cause public panic	Anthrax (*Bacillus anthracis*) Botulism (*Clostridium botulinum*) Plague (*Yersinia pestis*) Smallpox (variola major) Tularemia (*Francisella tularensis*) Viral hemorrhagic fevers—filoviruses (i.e., Ebola, Marburg) and arenaviruses (i.e., Lassa, Machupo)

TABLE 13-3
Category B Agents

Characteristics	Agents
Moderately easy to disseminate Moderate morbidity and low mortality May require enhanced Centers for Disease Control and Prevention diagnostic capacity	Brucellosis (*Brucella* species) Epsilon toxin of *Clostridium perfringens* Food safety threats (i.e., *Salmonella* sp., *Escherichia coli* 0157:H7, *Shigella*) Glanders (*Burkholderia malleri*) Melioidosis (*Burkholderia pseudomallei*) Psittacosis (*Chlamydia psittaci*) Q fever (*Coxiella burnetii*) Ricin toxin from *Ricinus communis* (castor beans) Staphylococcal enterotoxin B Typhus fever (*Rickettsia prowazekii*) Viral encephalitis (alphaviruses: Venezuelan equine encephalitis, Eastern and Western equine encephalitis) Water safety threats (i.e., *Vibrio cholerae*, *Cryptosporidium parvum*)

TABLE 13-4
Category C Agents

Characteristics	Agents
Availability Ease of production and dissemination Potential for high morbidity and mortality Potential major health impact	Hantavirus Nipah virus Other emerging pathogens that could be engineered for mass dissemination

alcohol or peroxide, or even heat, but spores are very resistant to both chemicals and heat. *B. anthracis* spores survive for decades. This is a key point because spores cause infection. In nature, anthrax is usually associated with grazing animals such as sheep, goats, cattle, and wildlife that acquire spores as they feed on vegetation or meat from infected animals. *B. anthracis* is present in soil throughout the world; in the United States, it is found mostly along old cattle trails in Texas, Louisiana, Mississippi, Arkansas, New Mexico, Oklahoma, and some Midwestern states. However, anthrax is rare in the United States because it is controlled in animal populations by vaccination programs. Spores occur when the pH of a richly organic soil is higher than 6.0 and rainfall gives way to drought conditions. When herbivorous animals contract the infection, they can transmit the infection to humans by direct contact with animal products such as hair, wool, hides, bones, etc. Individuals in certain occupations, such as animal handlers, agricultural workers, and veterinarians, are at increased risk for contracting anthrax. About 90% of all human anthrax cases reportedly occur in millworkers handling imported goat hair. Humans can be infected three ways: (1) via the skin (cutaneous) through scratches or abrasions, (2) by inhalation of spores, or (3) by eating contaminated insufficiently cooked meat or meat products. The word *anthracis* comes from the Greek word meaning "coal," and the bacterium was so named because the microbe can cause a black scab (eschar) to form on the skin of cutaneous anthrax victims. For the same reason, it is sometimes called the "black carbuncle" (Tierno, 2002).

Anthrax is the single greatest biowarfare threat because it is easy to cultivate spores, although production of a weaponized spore is not so simple. The media sometimes refer to "weapons grade" anthrax versus "nonweapons grade." Criteria for weapons grade include small spore size, usually 1–3 microns; lack of clumping (usually accomplished by adding a polymer that prevents the natural tendency of spores to clump); the quantity of spores present; and an effective delivery system. By this description, the anthrax unleashed on the United States in the fall of 2001 was near weapons grade because it fulfilled two of the four criteria. The spores were small and dispersed well in the air, but particles were present in limited quantities and were delivered via the mail. If enough product had been made, and if it had been delivered effectively, it would have been considered weapons grade.

In nature, spores in soil tend to clump together, making it very difficult for a person to contract inhalation anthrax naturally. For a terrorist to weaponize anthrax spores, he must first prevent clumping of particles and then must deliver the weapon in sufficient quantity. Clearly, both of these tasks are very difficult. Even a crop-duster would have to be retrofitted quite extensively to deliver spores effectively. To be an effective weapon, the anthrax spores must remain airborne in a concentration that is high enough to be inhaled deep into the lungs. Based on available data, it appears that number varies from about 8000–40,000 spores. A few studies suggest that inhalation of small numbers of spores, around 500 over an 8 hour period, did not make goat mill workers develop disease. Although *B. anthracis* can cause three types of infection (skin, inhalation, and gastrointestinal) a bioterrorist would be most interested in causing inhalation anthrax because of the high mortality rate associated with it. In nature, however, approximately 95% of human cases of anthrax are cutaneous infections (Lew, 2000; Tierno, 2002).

Anthrax spores can survive inside macrophages, eventually vegetating and growing to such numbers that they cause the cells to burst and release bacilli into the bloodstream. These bacteria produce four virulence factors; three are toxins that cause systemic symptoms: protective antigen toxin, the lethal factor, and the edema factor. Last, anthrax produces a capsule that protects it from destruction by the body's leukocytes. Once systemic symptoms occur, antibiotics are useless because they have no effect on the circulating toxins (Tierno, 2002).

Clinical Features

Inhalation Anthrax. This form is a biphasic disease. The *initial* phase is characterized by mild flu-like symptoms (e.g., malaise, fatigue, low-grade fever) followed by a period of apparent wellness for about a day. This is immediately followed by the *acute* phase, which eventually leads to more serious symptoms (e.g., acute respiratory distress). The incubation period can vary from 1–5 days, depending on the number of spores inhaled, but can be as long as 60 days. Shock and death usually occur 24–36 hours after the onset of respiratory distress. The fatality rate of inhalation anthrax approaches 90%, even with antibiotic therapy. However, this figure will probably change for the better owing to the availability of newer antibiotics and superior intensive care treatment facilities. Inhalation anthrax is not spread via person-to-person transmission.

Cutaneous Anthrax. This skin form of anthrax occurs after spores are introduced beneath the skin by inoculation or contamination of a preexisting lesion or break in the skin. The incubation period is 2–7 days (rarely after 1 day) but more often lasts between 2 and 5 days. Lesions begin as small, painless pimples on exposed skin and progress to vesicles and eventually an ulceration that develops a black scab (eschar) at the center (within 2–6 days). Untreated cutaneous anthrax can have a fatality rate of up to 20%, but fatalities are rare (1%) with proper antibiotic treatment. Although anthrax is not transmitted person-to-person, secondary lesions can develop from direct exposure to vesicle secretions.

Gastrointestinal Anthrax. This form of anthrax occurs by ingesting contaminated meat, in particular raw or undercooked, from infected animals. It has recently been reported in association with animal-hide drumming events in New England (CDC, 2010).

The incubation period is 2–7 days. Two types of GI anthrax are characterized by different symptoms: intestinal (e.g., nausea, vomiting, diarrhea) and oropharyngeal (e.g., neck swelling, difficulty swallowing). Shock and toxemia can characterize both forms of the disease, especially in the terminal stages. The fatality rate is 25%–60%. Inhalation, cutaneous, and GI anthrax can be complicated by meningitis, which occurs in about 5% of cases (Lew, 2000).

TABLE 13-5
Bioterrorism Agents: Diagnosis and Treatment

Agent	Diagnosis	Tests and specimens	Treatment
Anthrax	Clinical evaluation and laboratory findings	*Culture:* Blood, CSF, wounds (definitive) *Nasal culture:* Determines extent of spore spread in population *Immunohistochemical (IHC):* Tissue *PCR*: Can confirm diagnosis if culture is negative *Serology:* ELISA, IFA	Antibiotics, including penicillin, quinolones, tetracycline. Treat inhalation anthrax for 60 days. Can combine antibiotics (30 days) and vaccine (3 doses at 0, 14, and 28 days). Full vaccination regimen is 6 doses at 0, 2, and 4 weeks and 6, 12, and 18 months followed by yearly boosters.
Plague	Clinical evaluation and laboratory findings	*Culture:* Sputum, blood, lymph *Direct FA:* Respiratory secretions *Serology:* F1–V antigen (fusion protein) assay	Antibiotics, including tetracycline; quinolones, streptomycin, gentamicin, and chloramphenicol for 10–14 days. *Prophylaxis:* Medication for 7 days. Formalin-killed vaccine given 0, 1, and 4–7 months Boosters every 1–2 years
Brucella	Difficult with many rule-outs; laboratory required	*Culture:* Nasal, sputum, respiratory specimens (can also use PCR); blood culture is definitive test *Serology:* IFA, ELISA, and microagglutination (gold standard) to detect antibodies	*Combination antibiotics (6 weeks):* Doxycycline and rifampin or quinolone and rifampin. Prophylaxis requires 3 weeks. Numerous vaccines (both killed or live attenuated) available with no proven success.
Tularemia	Difficult with many rule-outs; laboratory required *Key symptom:* Pneumonia with nonproductive cough	General laboratory tests not helpful *Culture:* Bacterium does not grow on ordinary media, needs cysteine blood or chocolate agar *Capsular AG detection or PCR:* Whole unclotted blood *Direct FA and PCR:* Nasal, induced respiratory specimens *IHC:* Tissue sometimes helpful *Serology:* ELISA AB	*Treatment:* Antibiotics like gentamicin, streptomycin, ciprofloxacin *Prophylaxis:* Doxycycline *Vaccine:* Live attenuated available
Botulism	Clinical evaluation; routine laboratory tests are of no value; toxin assay may be useful if toxin present in serum	*PCR and toxin assay:* Use nasal induced respiratory secretions and blood	*Supportive treatment:* Antitoxin can be administered up to 24 hours after exposure: two types, trivalent and pentavalent. Also available is a pentavalent toxoid vaccine.
Smallpox	Clinical findings (exanthems)	*Cell or chick embryo culture:* Skin lesions ideal; nasal swabs, respiratory secretions, serum specimens can also be cultured *Electron microscopy*: Identifies virus *PCR:* Use same specimens as earlier *Agar gel precipitation:* Skin lesions *Serology:* Tests are available	VIG must be used in conjunction with vaccinia vaccine if exposure occurs beyond a 3-day time frame. Within 3 days, only vaccinia vaccine need be given by scarification. Cidofovir offers promise.
VEE	Difficult with many rule-outs; laboratory required	*PCR or culture in cells/suckling mice:* Nasal, induced respiratory secretions and serum *Serology:* ELISA, IFA, and hemagglutination inhibition; detect AB	Some drugs show promise. At present, no specific therapy. Treatment geared toward relieving symptoms. Some vaccines show promise (i.e., TC-84).
VHF	Clinical evaluation; key finding is vascular involvement (i.e., petechiae, bleeding, postural hypotension, edema, etc.)	*General:* Leukopenia, thrombocytopenia; elevated AST *Serology:* ELISA, IFA, and PCR; detect different VHFs	Management of hypotension and fluid loss. Aggressive supportive care needed. Ribavirin and immune globulin therapy show some promise. Several vaccines under development.

AB, Antibody; *AG,* antigen; *AST,* aspartate aminotransferase; *CSF,* cerebrospinal fluid; *ELISA,* enzyme-linked immunosorbent assay; *FA,* fluorescent antibody; *IFA,* indirect fluorescent antibody; *PCR,* polymerase chain reaction; *VEE,* Venezuelan equine encephalitis; *VHF,* viral hemorrhagic fever, *VIG,* vaccinia immune globulin.

TABLE 13-6
Bacillus anthracis: Level A Laboratory Role

Presumptively identify based on criteria below, and then submit culture to a Level B or C laboratory for final identification.

Direct smears	Samples such as blood, CSF, and skin (eschar) show encapsulated gram-positive rods, single or in chains. Generally, spores not seen.
Culture smears	Large gram-positive bacilli (1–1.5 by 3–5 μm), which may be gram-variable after 72 hours; spores can be found in culture, especially under non-CO_2 atmosphere but are nonswollen and are terminal or subterminal.
Colonies on sheep blood agar plates	Rapidly growing 2–5 mm (overnight at 35° C), nonhemolytic, nonpigmented, dry "ground-glass" surface colonies with irregular edges having comma-shaped projections (Medusa head). The colony has a sticky (tenacious) consistency when teased with a loop.
Other criteria	Nonmotile, catalase-positive, urease-negative, nitrate-positive, encapsulated bacillus that can be lysed by gamma phage (gamma phage typing is usually performed by Level B or C laboratory).

CO_2, Carbon dioxide; *CSF,* cerebrospinal fluid.

Practical Considerations

- Hand washing is the single most important protective measure. Spores are effectively removed with soap and water.
- Any article suspected of being contaminated with spores should be sanitized with a 1:10 dilution of household bleach. Let bleach remain in contact for at least 30 minutes before rinsing. If heavy spore contamination is suspected, use concentrated bleach to decontaminate the article.
- N95 respirator masks are protective against spore aerosols.
- Any cut, scratch, or abrasion should be covered with a dressing that has been coated with 1% tincture of iodine. If the cut or abrasion is not too extensive, apply tincture of iodine to its surface. Iodine is an outstanding antiseptic and can be sporicidal. No contusion is too small to warrant attention.
- Homes that have central air conditioning fitted with high-efficiency particulate air (HEPA) will remove more than 99.97% of particles 0.3 microns or larger. Because anthrax spores tend to clump, they will be efficiently trapped by HEPA filters. Alternatively, an air purifier outfitted with a HEPA filter will serve to keep a "safe-room" free of spores.

Plague

(Table 13-7)

History and Background

"Black Death" or the "plague" that befell Europe in the 14th century killed more than 25 million people, or about 25% of the population. This period is called the "second" pandemic. The first of three pandemics started in 541 AD and continued through to the 8th century, with an estimated 40 million deaths. The third and last pandemic began in China in the 1860s and spread to Africa, Europe, and the Americas. The plague is a zoonotic disease that primarily infects rodents and is caused by the bacterium *Yersinia pestis*, transmitted by a rat flea (*Xenopsylla cheopis*, the oriental flea, or *Pulex irritans*, the human flea). In the past, human epidemics originated by contact with fleas of infected rodents. The great plagues spread from rats to man in crowded unsanitary urban areas. Man is only accidental to the usual cycle: rodent–flea–rodent. In the United States, most naturally occurring human cases of plague (about 12/year) are concentrated in the Southwest and Pacific states (Perry, 1997; Tierno, 2002).

In a biowarfare scenario, the plague bacillus could be delivered by contaminated fleas as vectors causing the bubonic plague, or could more likely be spread by an aerosol that would cause pneumonic plague. In nature, a rat flea regurgitates the bacterium upon biting its host. Cats are also susceptible and can transmit the pneumonic plague to humans. Unlike anthrax, which cannot be transmitted person-to-person, pneumonic plague can be transmitted via large aerosol droplets from a coughing patient.

Yersinia pestis can be killed by polymorphonuclear cells, but they can survive in monocytes, where they produce a capsule to resist phagocytosis. These bacteria can then rapidly reach the lymph system and bloodstream and be disseminated to all organs, causing hemorrhage and necrosis.

Fewer than 100 organisms are necessary to cause human infection. Studies have shown that the bacterium can remain alive for up to 1 year in soil and up to 270 days in live tissue. The bacterium is killed after heat exposure (15 minutes at 72° C/160° F) and within several hours of exposure to sunlight (Tierno, 2002).

TABLE 13-7
***Yersinia pestis*: Level A Laboratory Role**

Presumptively identify based on criteria below, and then submit culture to a Level B or C laboratory for final identification.

Direct smears	More likely to see bipolar staining ("safety pin") from clinical specimens (blood, sputum, aspirates, etc.) than from cultures. Bipolarity is better seen using Wayson or Wright-Giemsa stain. Beware that bipolar staining is not always observed and is not unique to *Y. pestis*.
Culture smears	Plump gram-negative rods (1–2 by 0.5 μm), single or in short chains.
Colonies on sheep blood agar plates	Grow at 35° C (faster at room temperature) as gray-white, nonhemolytic, translucent, pinpoint colonies at 24 hours, but by 48 hours, colonies are 1–2 mm in diameter, becoming yellowish with age. Growth occurs with or without carbon dioxide. Colonies can appear as "fried egg" or with "hammered copper" shiny surface. On MacConkey, grow as pinpoint non–lactose-fermenting colonies after 24 hours; slightly larger at 48 hours.
Other criteria	The bacterium is nonmotile at 35° C to 37° C and at room temperature (*Y. pestis* is the only *Yersinia* that is nonmotile at room temperature). It is oxidase and urease negative and catalase positive; growth in broth is flocculent and is described as "stalactite"; clumps at side and bottom of tube.

Clinical Features

Plague occurs in three clinical forms: Bubonic, characterized by swelling of the lymph nodes (buboes); pneumonic, in which the lungs are extensively involved; and septicemic, in which the bloodstream is infected with *Yersinia pestis*. The mortality rate of untreated pneumonic plague is 100%, and that of untreated bubonic plague is about 50%.

Bubonic Plague. The incubation period of 2–10 days is characterized by malaise, high fever, and tender lymph nodes (buboes) that enlarge and eventually necrose. Septicemia may occur, and bacteria can spread to the central nervous system, the lungs (this produces the pneumonic disease, which can then be spread person-to-person), and the rest of the body, eventually causing death.

Pneumonic Plague. The 1 to 3 day incubation period is shorter than that of bubonic plague. Symptoms include high fever, cough, chest pain, and bloody sputum; pneumonia can lead to respiratory and circulatory collapse (Perry, 1997).

Practical Considerations

- Pneumonic plague patients transmit infection through large particle droplets (greater than 5 microns) generated by coughing, talking, or sneezing. A simple surgical-type mask can protect workers or family members. "Droplet Precautions" should be maintained for 3 complete days of antibiotic therapy, after which a person is no longer contagious.
- Because "droplets" occur only within 3–5 feet of a patient, central air conditioning systems do not need to be fitted with HEPA filters (i.e., they do not need to provide bacteria- and particle-free air).
- If an outbreak occurs, it is important to control fleas, rats, and other animals such as cats. Insecticides and repellents are widely available.
- Hand washing is an essential prevention strategy.
- Because *Y. pestis* does not have a spore form, surfaces can be decontaminated with a simple germicide such as 10% bleach solution. Skin can be decontaminated by using any germicidal soap product. Alcohol-based hand sanitizers such as Purell can also be effective.
- Clothing should be washed with a germicidal detergent and hot water (155° F), even though exposure is unlikely to occur from re-aerosolization of bacteria from contaminated clothing.
- Stand clear (farther than 3–5 feet) of individuals taking a coughing fit or producing sputum with or without blood.

Brucellosis

(Table 13-8)

History and Background

Brucellosis is a systemic zoonotic disease caused by *Brucella melitensis*, *B. suis*, *B. abortus*, and *B. canis*. These bacteria ordinarily cause disease in domestic animals, such as goats, sheep, and camels (*B. melitensis*); cattle (*B. abortus*); and pigs (*B. suis*). The primary pathogen of dogs, *B. canis* rarely causes disease in humans. Natural infection in humans occurs when bacteria are inhaled as aerosols, ingested in raw unpasteurized infected milk or meat, or introduced into abrasions in skin or through contact with conjunctival surfaces. Human disease is called undulant fever, Malta fever, Bang's disease, Gibraltar fever, and Mediterranean fever and occurs worldwide. In developed countries, human infection is associated with the meat packing and dairy industries. Several studies report that human brucellosis is underdiagnosed and under-reported. By some estimates, 25–30 cases go unrecognized for every reported case. As a biological warfare agent, brucellae would likely be delivered via the aerosol route. Brucellae are intracellular bacteria; they are able to survive phagocytosis and thus can

TABLE 13-8
Brucella species: Level A Laboratory Role

Presumptively identify based on criteria below, and then submit culture to a Level B or C laboratory for final identification and/or confirmation, although most Level A laboratories are able to completely identify *Brucella*.

Direct smears	Blood and/or bone marrow most often submitted. *Brucella* appears as faintly staining, small gram-negative coccobacilli (0.5–0.7 by 0.6–1.5 μm), mostly seen as single cells appearing like "fine sand."
Culture smears	Similar to above.
Colonies on sheep blood (SBA) and chocolate (CA) agars	Usually not visible or are pinpoint at 24 hours; at 48 hours, colonies are tiny, nonpigmented, and smooth with an entire edge, and are nonhemolytic on SBA. Growth of some strains is enhanced by carbon dioxide tension. Some strains grow on MacConkey; Thayer-Martin can be used as a selective medium. Blood cultures are held for 21 days for suspect cases.
Other criteria	These coccobacilli are catalase, urease, and oxidase positive (*B. canis* is variable). They are nonmotile and do not require X and V factors. Brucellosis is one of the most commonly reported laboratory-acquired infections. Automated systems are not useful, nor are they recommended for identification. Remember that sniffing culture plates of *Brucella* can result in infection.

TABLE 13-9
Francisella tularensis: Level A Laboratory Role

Presumptively identify based on criteria below, and then submit culture to a Level B or C laboratory for final identification.

Direct smears	Gram stain of blood, biopsy material, scrapings, or aspirates may be difficult to interpret because bacteria are tiny, pleomorphic, poorly staining gram-negative coccobacilli seen mostly as single cells.
Culture smear	Very tiny (0.2–0.5 by 0.7–1.0 μm), poorly staining, pleomorphic, gram-negative coccobacilli. They are smaller than *Haemophilus influenzae* and *Brucella* spp. Their minuscule size should raise awareness.
Colonies on sheep blood (SBA), chocolate (CA), and blood cysteine (BCA) agars	Grow poorly and slowly on SBA as 1–2 mm gray-white, nonhemolytic colonies after 48–72 hours. On CA and BCA, colonies are slightly larger, 1–3 mm, gray-white to bluish-gray with an entire edge and smooth flat surface. Colonies do not subculture well to SBA (viability is usually lost). Subcultures should be made onto CA, BCA, or Thayer-Martin agar. Carbon dioxide is not required for growth. No growth occurs on MacConkey or eosin methylene blue agar.
Other criteria	*F. tularensis* is nonmotile and oxidase and urease negative; catalase can be weakly positive or negative. X and V factors are not required. Slow growth in thioglycollate broth with a dense band near top, which eventually diffuses downward with time.

be carried from lymph tissue to blood and deposited in numerous organs. Inside the phagocytes, the bacteria grow, and eventually their host cells are killed, and a new crop of bacteria is released. The "undulant" fever pattern observed with this disease corresponds to the release of bacteria into the blood, thereby causing fever. As these bacteria are eliminated, the fever subsides, only to recur when another crop of bacteria is released. Relapses are common. *Brucella* species have two morphologically different colony types: smooth and rough. The smooth form is more pathogenic because of the presence of a capsule that protects the bacterium from phagocytosis and destruction. *B. melitensis* and *B. suis* are more virulent than the other two species and have better intracellular survival. On the other hand, *B. abortus* and *B. canis* have an insidious onset but cause milder disease and fewer complications (Shapiro, 1998, 1999; Tierno, 2002).

Clinical Features

The incubation period can be 1–8 weeks but is usually 3–4 weeks. Onset is insidious, with malaise, fever, chills, sweats, headache, fatigue, myalgias, and arthralgias. Fever usually rises in the afternoon; it falls during the night and is accompanied by drenching sweat. Swollen lymph, spleen, and liver may also be present. The undulant fever can occur over weeks, months, or even years. Yet, there are many days when a patient has no fever and feels relatively well, only to experience another cycle of waxing and waning fever. Patients are often diagnosed with a fever of unknown origin. Cough occurs in about 20% of cases, but the radiograph appears normal. Mortality rate is about 6% for *B. melitensis* but 1% for the other species. Most deaths are associated with endocarditis or meningitis. Gastrointestinal symptoms occur in up to 70% of adult cases, although less frequently in children.

Practical Considerations

- Although *Brucella* species have a long incubation period and a slow onset, the characteristic undulant fever syndrome helps make a diagnosis, so that treatment can start.
- *Brucella* has such a low fatality rate (especially with proper antibiotic therapy) that it is not a very effective biological weapon.
- Brucellosis cannot be transmitted person-to-person, so that patient isolation is not required. However, contact precautions are indicated if a draining lesion is present.
- *Brucella* species have no spore form, so they are readily killed with any common germicide. Pasteurization (at 155° F) kills bacteria in contaminated food.
- Brucellosis is contracted through eye contact (i.e., rubbing or touching your eyes), so hand washing with germicidal soap or alcohol-based hand sanitizers is an important protective strategy.

Tularemia

(Table 13-9)

History and Background

The causative agent of tularemia (also known as "rabbit fever") is *Francisella tularensis*. These bacteria are gram-negative bacilli that are nonmotile and have no spore form. Humans acquire this zoonotic disease through contact with animals, usually through the inoculation of skin or their mucous membranes with blood or tissue fluids of infected animals or bites from infected ticks, mosquitoes, or flies. A less common method of acquiring infection is through inhalation of contaminated dusts or ingestion of contaminated foods or water. A bioterrorist would likely use an aerosol to deliver *Francisella* because it causes typhoidal (systemic) tularemia, a disease with a >10% fatality rate.

Because the bacterium is highly contagious, as few as 25 inhaled organisms or as few as 10 organisms administered subcutaneously can cause infection. The smallest break in the skin can serve as a portal of entry. The bacterium is so contagious that numerous cases of tularemia have resulted from laboratory accidents during processing of infected clinical or research samples. *Francisella* is distributed worldwide. In the United States, the disease has been reported primarily in Southern and South Central states.

F. tularensis produces a capsule that allows the organism to avoid immediate destruction by the body's phagocytes. It can survive as an intracellular parasite within cells of the lymph system.

Clinical Features

Six major syndromes are associated with tularemia; they differ by mode of infection.

1. *Ulceroglandular tularemia* (70%–85% of cases) typically presents with a skin ulcer, usually as the result of a tick bite, and swollen lymph nodes, fever, chills, headache, sweating, and coughing.
2. *Glandular tularemia* (5%–12% of cases) is characterized by fever and swollen lymph nodes but no obvious skin lesion.
3. *Typhoidal tularemia* (7%–14% cases) presents with acute onset of fever, chills, headache, vomiting, and diarrhea. Usually no skin lesions or swollen lymph nodes are present, but the condition is associated with primary or secondary pneumonia. This form has the highest mortality rate and is the most likely bioterror form.

TABLE 13-10

Botulinum Toxin Exposure: Level A Laboratory Role

Submit specimens immediately to public health laboratory for evaluation and referral, even if criminal activity is not suspected. Level A laboratories should not manipulate specimens, culture, identify, or perform toxin assays. Level A laboratory responsibility is limited to advising the medical staff on specimen selection, packing, shipping, and notifying the recipient laboratory about specimens from a suspected case.

	Specimen	Transport
Suspect food samples	25–50 g of food should be submitted in original containers that have been placed in a leakproof sealed system.	4° C
Nasal swabs	If aerosolized release is suspected, collect nasal swabs for toxin testing and/or polymerase chain reaction analysis.	Room temperature
Stool, enema fluid	Collect 25–50 g of stool into sterile leakproof containers.	4° C
Serum	Collect approximately 10 mL for serologic assays.	4° C
Other	Collect environmental and/or other samples on swabs.	4° C

Note: Level A laboratory responsibility for other suspected toxins such as staphylococcal toxins, mycotoxin, saxitoxin, ricin, etc., should be treated in a similar manner.

4. *Oculoglandular tularemia* (1%–2% cases) presents with severe conjunctivitis and swollen lymph nodes, usually as the result of self-inoculating the organism into the conjunctivae.
5. *Oropharyngeal tularemia* occurs in patients who have a primary lesion in the oropharynx. Patients present with severe headache and bilateral tonsillitis or severe streptococcal-type sore throat. Persistent swollen lymph nodes in the neck appear after 1–2 weeks.
6. *Pneumonic tularemia* (8%–13% cases) is primarily a complication of the other forms, especially typhoidal tularemia. It is also acquired by inhaling of infectious aerosols or as a result of blood-borne dissemination. Lymph nodes in the lungs are enlarged. Sometimes, the pneumonia is not evident (Wong, 1999).

In all tularemia syndromes, lymph nodes may remain enlarged for a long time and eventually may become necrotic and drain. Fever (usually low grade) is accompanied by malaise, headache, and pain in the regional lymph nodes.

Practical Considerations

- Hand washing with germicidal soap or alcohol-based hand sanitizers is the most important protective strategy. Any aerosolized bioterror attack would contaminate the surrounding environment and could lead to secondary exposure through direct contact with skin and mucous membranes. Simple germicides, such as bleach, destroy the bacterium on contaminated surfaces.
- Because there are no spore forms, only vegetative ones, bacteria are easily killed by heat (30 minutes at 145° F). The relatively low fatality rate does not make it a very effective biological weapon. Infected patients rapidly improve on adequate (10–14 days) antibiotic therapy.
- Because tularemia can be transmitted by contact with household pets such as cats and dogs, it is important to observe any changing habits and the health status of pets. They can be the sentinel event to warn you of an impending disaster, much like the "canary in the mine."
- *Francisella* is rarely transmitted by food or water; nevertheless, it is important to be alert to that possibility. Cooking food renders the bacterium harmless, as does filtering or heating water.

Botulinum Toxins

(Table 13-10)

History and Background

Clostridia are anaerobic, gram-positive, spore-forming bacilli that elaborate toxins. The most pathogenic species are *Clostridium perfringens* (agent of gas gangrene), *C. tetani* (agent of tetanus), and *C. botulinum* (agent of botulism). The aforementioned diseases are the result of exposure to the protein toxins that the bacteria produce, the most powerful of which is the botulinum toxin. Seven *C. botulinum* toxins are known: A, B, C, D, E, F, and G. Human illness is caused by four of the seven toxins: types A, B, E, and F. The toxins bind to synaptic vesicles of cholinergic nerves, preventing release of acetylcholinesterase at peripheral nerve endings (including neuromuscular junctions). Patients develop acute flaccid descending paralysis. By blocking neurotransmission, the toxins cause palsies and skeletal muscle weakness, which are common clinical features. *C. botulinum* toxins are among the most toxic substances known to man. A lethal human dose is only one-millionth of a gram (Tierno, 2002; Angulo, 1998).

Several forms of botulism occur in humans. The classic type is food-borne botulism, which typically occurs in adults and is caused by ingestion of toxins present in contaminated food. *C. botulinum* grows in food and produces its toxin. The usual foods involved are canned alkaline foods that are eaten without cooking, and smoked and vacuum-packed foods. Under anaerobic conditions, *C. botulinum* spores grow into vegetative forms that produce toxin. Wound botulism, the rarest form, occurs when bacteria gain access to a wound site and then produce toxins in vivo. Infant botulism, the most common type, occurs when a child consumes food contaminated with *C. botulinum* rather than consuming pre-formed toxins. Toxin is produced in the infant's gut, de novo, and poisons from within. Some botulism patients do not have an obvious food or wound source; they fall into the "classification undetermined" group.

As a bioterror weapon, botulinum toxin may be purified from large stores of toxin-producing *C. botulinum*. It then can be delivered as an aerosol that causes symptoms like those of food-borne botulism. Another approach might be to sabotage food supplies with toxin, although the latter is not an efficient delivery system (USAMRIID, 2001; Tierno, 2002). We know that botulinum toxins can be weaponized because the Iraqi government admitted to a United Nations inspection team in August 1991 that it had done research on these toxins before the Persian Gulf War. It is possible to weaponize any of the seven known botulinum toxins because they all would have the same effect.

Clinical Features

Symptoms usually begin 18–24 hours after ingestion or inhalation of toxin, although this may take several days. Initial symptoms include double vision, lack of coordination of eye muscles, inability to swallow, speech difficulty, generalized weakness, and dizziness. These are followed by descending progressive weakness of the extremities and weakness of the respiratory muscles. No fever is present, and the patient may be totally alert and oriented. Neurologic examination shows flaccid muscle weakness of the tongue, larynx, respiratory muscles, and extremities. A patient remains fully conscious until shortly before death from respiratory paralysis or cardiac arrest. Mortality rate is high. Patients who recover do not develop antitoxin in the blood. Suppression of antibody production is probably caused by the toxins, in much the same way that toxic shock syndrome toxin-1 produced by *Staphylococcus aureus* prevents antibody production. In infants, signs of paralysis are called "floppy baby" syndrome (Tierno, 2002).

Practical Considerations

- Antitoxins and vaccines are available for treatment and prophylaxis.
- Botulinum toxin is *less* toxic and lethal when delivered by inhalation than by a food-borne assault.
- Soap and water can be very effective at removing most toxins from skin, clothing, and equipment, so that decontamination of a toxin is *not* as critical as decontamination of an infectious microbe. A very mild bleach solution (1 part bleach in 9 parts water) effectively inactivates most protein toxins.
- A protective N95 mask if worn properly is effective against toxin aerosols. However, it is important that a tight fit is achieved because even a small leak could result in significant exposure. Bearded individuals would not be able to achieve a tight fit but nevertheless would reduce their exposure with a mask.
- Because botulinum toxin does not permeate the skin, special protective clothing is not as important as it would be for other agents, including chemical attacks.

Smallpox

(Table 13-11)

History and Background

Smallpox has the distinct honor of being the greatest single killer in recorded history; it is estimated that this virus has killed about 500 million people.

The smallpox virus, a.k.a. variola, is a member of the Orthopoxvirus group of viruses. Two variants of smallpox are known: variola major, which is associated with a higher mortality rate of 15%–40%, and variola minor, which causes a milder disease and is associated with a mortality rate of only 1%. Smallpox is the human type of poxvirus. Other poxviruses naturally infect animals but also can cause incidental infection in humans (zoonoses). These viruses share common antigens with smallpox, thus allowing them to be used as vaccines for humans. Thus, vaccinia virus has been the historically chosen animal virus for vaccine production. As the incidence of smallpox has waned, more complications related to the vaccinations have occurred than smallpox cases. Some of these complications were severe and included encephalitis and fatal reactions in immunocompromised patients who were vaccinated, sometimes inadvertently. Vaccinia viruses spread easily among unvaccinated immunocompromised patients in close contact. This still would be the case if a massive national vaccination program were to be considered. A large group of immunocompromised patients simply would not be candidates for the vaccine (Tierno, 2002).

In 1967, the World Health Organization introduced a worldwide campaign to eradicate smallpox. At the time, 33 countries had endemic smallpox, and about 15 million cases were reported per year. By 1979, smallpox was eradicated. Smallpox virus currently exists in only two laboratories: one in the United States and the other in Russia. The fate of these remaining stocks is debated. Destroying the stocks will preclude further research in the event of an outbreak. Similar to the plague, smallpox is very contagious from man to man. It is currently assumed that an aerosol infective dose is low and presumably ranges from 10–100 organisms (Tierno, 2002).

How would smallpox be weaponized? Smallpox can be spread in two ways: aerosol dispersal and contact. Because smallpox is highly contagious and is efficiently spread through air, an aerosol delivery system poses the greatest threat and exposes the greatest number of people. However, as learned with anthrax, this is not so easy to do. Smallpox can also be delivered by direct contact. One way would be to self-contaminate a group of volunteers, who would then interact with the general population, infecting people over days or weeks as they came in contact with them. If a smallpox outbreak is detected in an area, the CDC and other health authorities would be able to contain the outbreak by immediately vaccinating all individuals surrounding the index case or cases. Postexposure immunization with smallpox vaccine (vaccinia virus) is effective and is recommended if given within 3 days of exposure. However, even if more than 3 days elapse, vaccination and vaccinia immune globulin may provide protection. It is necessary to establish a ring of immunity around index cases. This is precisely the method used to eradicate smallpox worldwide and should be just cause for some optimism.

TABLE 13-11

Smallpox: Level A Laboratory Role

Smallpox is highest-level emergency; submit specimens immediately to public health laboratory. Virus is highly infectious; avoid manipulation; if necessary use Biological Safety Level-3 practices. Responsibility of Level A laboratories is limited to advising medical staff on specimen selection, packing and shipping sample, and communicating with reference laboratory. Level A laboratories should not culture, sample, or perform assays on specimens suspected of containing the virus. Clinical diagnosis is confirmed by Level D laboratory techniques.

	Specimen	Transport	Storage
Biopsy	Aseptically place two to four portions of tissue into sterile, leakproof, freezable container.	≤6 hours/4° C	−20° C to −70° C
Scabs	Aseptically place scrapings/material into sterile, leakproof freezable container.	≤6 hours/4° C	−20° C to −70° C
Vesicular fluid	Collect fluid from separate lesions onto separate sterile swabs. Always include material from base of each vesicle.	≤6 hours/4° C	−20° C to −70° C

Clinical Features

The entry portal for smallpox virus is the mucous membranes of the upper respiratory tract. Smallpox is transmitted by large or small respiratory droplets, and by contact with skin lesions or secretions. Patients are considered more infectious if they are actively coughing. The incubation period is typically 12 days, with a range of 10–12 days. Clinical illness begins with a 2 to 3 day period of vague symptoms such as malaise, fever, headache, chills, and backache. The fever can last as long as 5 days or may be as short as 1 day. After the fever, an exanthem (eruption of skin or rash) appears that undergoes papular, pustular, and crustular stages. The latter falls off 2–4 weeks after the initial lesion and leaves a pink scar. An important characteristic of smallpox is that lesions in affected areas appear in the same state. This differs from chickenpox, where lesions are not synchronous and occur in crops. Smallpox lesions are distributed centrifugally (more numerous on the face and extremities than on the trunk), unlike chickenpox. Hence, the smallpox exanthem is very characteristic and is a useful diagnostic tool. The fatality rate is 15%–40% in unvaccinated patients and <1% in those vaccinated.

Patients with smallpox are infectious as soon as a rash occurs and remain infectious until scabs fall off, approximately 3 weeks later. A rare form of smallpox called "hemorrhagic variola" is very pathogenic and has a very high mortality rate.

Practical Considerations

- If a major outbreak of smallpox occurs, prepare to stay indoors for a few days or weeks to reduce contact with those contaminated; this will contain the epidemic. Households should be stocked with adequate food supplies.
- Generally, respiratory droplets become infectious earlier than skin lesions. In hospitals, both airborne and contact precautions are required to prevent contagion. In contrast to plague precautions, a simple surgical mask is insufficient protection. A special respirator mask, N95 (certified to have at least 95% filter efficiency), is recommended and must be worn for such protection. Smallpox patients should be quarantined from the time the rash first appears until the scab finally falls off (about 3 weeks).
- If a household member contracts smallpox, all clothing, bed linens, or other materials that contacted the patient must be decontaminated with a germicide such as a 1:10 bleach solution, steam, or heat.
- Hand washing with germicidal soap is essential after any contact with a smallpox patient or his or her environment.

TABLE 13-12

VEE or Other Encephalitides: Level A Laboratory Role

Submit samples immediately to public health laboratory for evaluation and referral. Level A laboratory responsibility is limited to advising medical staff on specimen selection, packing and shipping sample, and communicating with reference laboratory.

	Specimen	Transport	Storage
Serum	For culture, PCR, or serologies (ELISA, FA, etc.)	<6 hours/4° C	−20° C to −70° C
CSF	For culture, PCR. or serologies	<6 hours/4° C	−20° C to −70° C
Nasal, respiratory (including induced samples)	For culture and PCR	<6 hours/4° C	−20° C to −70° C
Other	Biopsy, autopsy, stool, etc., for pathology, culture, hematology/chemistry analysis, etc.	<6 hours/4° C	−20° C to −70° C

CSF, Cerebrospinal fluid; *ELISA,* enzyme-linked immunosorbent assay; *FA,* fluorescent antibody (direct); *PCR,* polymerase chain reaction; *VEE,* Venezuelan equine encephalitis.

Venezuelan Equine Encephalitis

(Table 13-12)

History and Background

Venezuelan equine encephalitis (VEE) is clinically indistinguishable from other encephalitis viruses such as St Louis encephalitis, Eastern and Western equine encephalitis, Japanese B-type encephalitis, Russian Far East encephalitis, and even West Nile encephalitis virus. The first question to consider is why other such agents are not high on the list as potential bioterror weapons. Many can be, but the attack rate, that is, the number of people who would probably get the disease after being exposed to the agent, is much lower than for VEE. VEE has an attack rate of about 100% (pretty hard to beat). This is precisely the reason the U.S. government weaponized it in the 1950s and 1960s before terminating its offensive biowarfare program. However, it remains a potential weapon and one likely to serve as a surrogate virus to deliver more pathogens. Nevertheless, Level A laboratory responsibility is similar for all encephalitis viruses such as VEE (USAMRIID, 2001; Tierno, 2002). VEE can be weaponized in liquid or dry form for aerosol dispersal. It can be transmitted in three ways: (1) via mosquitoes, although the naturally occurring incidence of VEE is low; (2) via aerosol, either liquid or dry form; and (3) via secondary spread from person to person (although this has not yet been conclusively demonstrated).

In nature, VEE is a mosquito-borne viral disease that is neurotrophic, causing encephalitis in equine animals and an unremarkable febrile illness in humans. More than 50% of equines that become infected develop encephalitis, and among humans, almost 100% of those exposed develop an influenza-like illness. In naturally contracted disease, only 2%–4% of patients develop signs of central nervous system involvement, and less than 1% die (Tierno, 2002).

In the United States, VEE is a rare disease. The disease was first reported in Venezuela in 1936. VEE is prevalent in South and Central America, Trinidad, Mexico, and Panama. In the case of the West Nile encephalitis virus, a sentinel animal (birds) indicated the presence of disease before human infection occurred. In the case of VEE, that would have been horses, but because we vaccinate them, no sentinel animal system is available to warn us that a VEE virus attack has occurred. On the other hand, because we have eradicated VEE from the United States, any human with the disease would likely signal bioterrorism (Tierno, 2002).

VEE is an arthropod-borne alphavirus that has been incidentally associated with human disease. Eight serologically distinct viruses exist, but only two are important pathogens for humans: variants A/B and C (Tierno, 2002). Most encephalitis viruses are destroyed by heat and are easily killed by ordinary disinfectants.

Clinical Features

The incubation period is 1–5 days, after which there is rapid onset of fever (usually high), headache, dizziness, lethargy, depression, anorexia, chills, myalgia, photophobia, nausea, vomiting, cough, sore throat, and sometimes diarrhea. VEE is indistinguishable from other viruses that cause encephalitis. The acute phase of the disease lasts from 1–3 days and is followed by a prolonged period (up to 2 weeks) of lethargy. Full recovery usually occurs after 2 weeks. It is estimated that inoculation with 10–100 viruses can cause infection. In a naturally occurring epidemic, <5% of patients have a neurologic manifestation, one characterized by convulsions, coma, and paralysis.

Practical Considerations

- VEE has very low lethality and in most victims might manifest only as a flu-like disease. *Note:* Bioterrorists may use any encephalitis virus as a surrogate for a more pathogenic weapon via genetic engineering.
- If an outbreak occurs, the mosquito population must be controlled, similar to the approach used for West Nile virus.
- Hand washing can prevent the otherwise rare person-to-person transmission (via contact spread).
- Simple germicides such as a 10% bleach solution or Lysol and heat (165° F) easily destroy the VEE virus.
- Contaminated clothing can be washed with any detergent.

Crimean Congo and Other Hemorrhagic Fevers

(Table 13-13)

History and Background

Crimean Congo hemorrhagic fever (CCHF) is only one of many illnesses referred to as viral hemorrhagic fevers (VHFs). These agents and their natural mode of transmission are listed in Table 13-14. Any one of these hemorrhagic viruses, except dengue (which is transmissible only via mosquito), can be weaponized via aerosol delivery (USAMRIID, 2001; Tierno, 2002). In general, VHFs are very difficult to weaponize because there is no real carrier state.

TABLE 13-13
Crimean Congo and Other Hemorrhagic Fevers: Level A Laboratory Role

Submit samples immediately to public health laboratory for evaluation and referral. Some viruses are highly infectious; avoid manipulation; if necessary, use Biological Safety Level-3 practices. Level A laboratory responsibility is limited to advising medical staff on specimen selection, packing and shipping sample, and communicating with reference laboratory.

	Specimen	Transport	Storage
Serum	For culture, PCR, or serologies (ELISA, HI, FA, etc.)	<6 hours/4° C	−20° C to −70° C
Other	Biopsy, autopsy, etc., for pathology, culture, hematology/chemistry analysis, etc.	<6 hours/4° C	−20° C to −70° C

ELISA, Enzyme-linked immunosorbent assay; *FA,* fluorescent antibody (direct); *HI,* hemagglutination inhibition; *PCR,* polymerase chain reaction.

TABLE 13-14
Viral Hemorrhagic Fever Means of Transmission

VHF agent	Natural means of transmission
Ebola	Contact
Marburg	Contact
Lassa fever	Contact
Argentine (Junin)	Contact and aerosol
Bolivian (Machupo)	Contact and aerosol
Crimean Congo	Ticks and contact
Hantavirus	Contact and aerosol
Rift Valley fever	Mosquito and aerosol
Dengue	Mosquito
Yellow fever	Mosquito

CCHF is transmitted by ticks. Several reports describe person-to-person spread of CCHF in hospitals. As few as 1–10 viral particles can cause infection (USAMRIID, 2001). Rift Valley fever (RVF) is transmitted by mosquitoes as well as by aerosols; an inactivated vaccine is available for prevention, and RVF virus is susceptible to the antiviral drug ribavirin. The Ebola and Marburg viruses are transmitted by direct contact with blood, secretions, organs, or semen of infected patients. Argentine, Bolivian, and Hantavirus hemorrhagic fevers are also spread by dried rodent excreta (USAMRIID, 2001).

Clinical Features

The general clinical syndrome associated with all of the aforementioned viruses is similar and is called "viral hemorrhagic fever," or VHF. The most common presenting symptoms are fever, myalgia, low blood pressure, flushing, and ecchymoses anywhere on the body. Typically, the onset of CCHF occurs 3–12 days after tick exposure or inhalation of an aerosol. Extensive gastrointestinal bleeding and extensive ecchymoses may occur. Other symptoms include headache, back pain, nausea, vomiting, delirium, jaundice, and hepatomegaly. Mortality for CCHF is 15%–30%, but some hemorrhagic fevers, such as Ebola, can have a death rate near 90% (Tierno, 2002).

Practical Considerations

- Any individual who may have been exposed to blood, body fluids, secretions, or excretions from a patient with suspected VHF should immediately and thoroughly wash skin surfaces with soap and water; a shower is preferable.
- In hospitals, contact precautions should be instituted to prevent contagion. An N95 mask is recommended and should be worn for

protection. Infected patients should be quarantined for the duration of the illness.

- Anyone caring for (or visiting during convalescence) a patient who is stricken with VHF must practice strict "barrier nursing" techniques (in other words, must completely protect self from the infected patient by dressing in gown, gloves, mask, eye protection, hat, booties, etc.), because evidence indicates that large droplets or even fomites (inanimate objects) may act as mediators of virus transmission.
- Any contamination of mucous membranes must be immediately diluted with copious quantities of water. If contaminated, eyes can be irrigated with saline or products like Visine.
- Clorox (10% solution) can be used to decontaminate surfaces, equipment, or other articles.
- Deceased individuals should be sealed in leakproof material for prompt burial or cremation.
- Heavily soiled clothing should be discarded, or washed with bleach or a strong germicide-containing detergent.

CHEMICAL TERRORISM

HISTORY AND BACKGROUND

Chemical weapons were first used in modern warfare during World War I. On April 22, 1915, outside the Belgian village of Ypres, the German army released about 60 tons of chlorine gas from about 6000 pressurized gas cylinders into the winds, which carried clouds of chlorine gas over the Allied forces. A second attack using chlorine gas occurred 2 days later. The end result of both attacks was the grotesque choking death of approximately 10,000 troops. By the end of 1915, a more deadly gas agent, phosgene, was introduced by the Germans; it was 10 times more effective than chlorine. Both gases are considered chemical weapons that affect the lungs; thus they are called "pulmonary agents." They damage the membranes that separate air sacs (alveoli) from capillary blood vessels. Fluid (plasma) leaks into the air sacs, accumulates, and prevents air exchange. The victim is usually unable to get enough oxygen and eventually suffocates to death after an agonizing 2- to 24-hour period. Victims initially have shortness of breath with coughing fits, which can be quite severe. The production of large amounts of yellowish (chlorine) to clear (phosgene) frothy sputum occurs before death. Significant irritation of the eyes and nose and burning in the throat are reported (Byrnes, 2003).

By the time the Germans introduced phosgene, they were becoming very proficient at producing chemical weapons of various types and were equally proficient at delivering them. Great Britain quickly followed in kind with the use of chemical weapons against the German army. Great skill was needed to deliver gas weapons because if wind direction changed, or if the weapon was inappropriately delivered, poison gas could fall on one's own troops. This did happen often, especially during the early use of such chemical weapons. By the summer of 1917, the Germans introduced a new type of gas called mustard. Mustard gas is a chemical weapon that belongs to a group of agents called "blistering agents." As the name implies, one of the symptoms is a blistering of the skin and internal organs. The skin, eyes, and lungs, the gastrointestinal tract, the mucous membranes, bone marrow, and other organs can be severely damaged.

These early weapons forced armies to defend themselves by using gas masks, as well as protective suits or outer coverings, both of which hampered efficient fighting on the battlefield. Nevertheless, by the end of the war, more than 110,000 tons of chemical weapons were used by both sides, and the number of casualties measured over a million, including about 100,000 dead.

The Geneva Protocol

Because of the agonizing deaths and horrendous suffering that were inflicted by chemical weapons during World War I, an effort was made to ban their use after the war. The League of Nations met at Geneva and developed a protocol to eliminate chemical weapons during warfare. The "Protocol for the Prohibition of the Use in War of Asphyxiating, Poisonous, or Other Gases, and of Bacteriological Methods of Warfare" was signed by 38 nations in 1925 (Byrnes, 2003), although it had many loopholes and no provision to punish nations that violate the pact. During World War II, it was surprising that no chemical weapons were used in battle, even though the Germans had developed new chemical weapons, "nerve agents," including tabun, sarin, and soman. Nerve agents are a particularly potent class of chemical weapons that share some interesting properties. The mechanism of action of nerve agents such as sarin is that they disrupt nerve communication with the organs that they stimulate. In other words, the nerve is normal, but transmission of the nerve impulse to the muscle or other organ is faulty, usually causing overactivity. This interferes with basic bodily functions, and death can occur as soon as 1–10 minutes after inhalation. If a nerve agent is in liquid form, it is characteristically heavier than water. The vapors are also heavier than air, and they therefore tend to sink toward the ground or the basement of a building. Although nerve agent vapor affects victims within a very short period of time, the range of these effects will vary greatly, depending upon the degree of exposure. Exposure to nerve agents will initially affect airways and the portions of the face that come into contact with the agent: the eyes, nose, and mouth. The pupils become small (pinpoint), the eyes redden, and vision becomes blurred. Some patients also experience eye pain, headache, and nausea and vomiting. Rhinorrhea may be an important feature, as is excessive salivation. If a nerve agent is inhaled, airways can become constricted, and coughing fits or shortness of breath may be induced. If a sufficient quantity of the agent is inhaled, sudden loss of consciousness may be followed by convulsions. Within a few minutes, a victim stops breathing and becomes flaccid. Even a very small amount of a nerve agent like sarin can produce fasciculations (muscular twitching). Nausea and vomiting may accompany exposure. In cases of greater exposure, involuntary defecation and urination may also occur (Byrnes, 2003).

Many new "nerve agent" chemical weapons were developed from ordinary insecticides and/or pesticides. (People actually use weaker forms of nerve agents every time they tend their garden with insecticides. For example, insecticides such as malathion or carbaryl [Sevin] and dozens of others are actually nerve agents. They do the exact same thing to humans that sarin or other more potent nerve agents do, although they require much larger doses and longer contact time to have a similar effect.) In the early 1950s, Great Britain made what was considered a breakthrough discovery of a new nerve agent that was magnitudes greater in its lethal abilities than any other known substance at the time. The agent was called by its code name—VX. This agent not only was more lethal but also was more persistent (because it remains a liquid for longer than 24 hours) and could enter the body by inhalation or directly via the skin. Entry through the skin was possible because this agent is nonvolatile and is persistent. The United States cooperated with Great Britain on this project, eventually taking over the large-scale production of agent VX. Production and stockpiling of VX continued into the 1960s, until an accidental release of VX occurred at the manufacturing facility in Dugway, Utah, killing more than 6000 sheep. Probably the most infamous U.S. chemical agent, used primarily during the Vietnam War in the 1960s, was Agent Orange, an herbicide used to defoliate vegetation that offered cover to the enemy. Agent Orange contained varying quantities of dioxin (tetrachlorodibenzodioxin), which was later considered to be so dangerous that the Environmental Protection Agency, in 1986, prohibited its use anywhere. Animal studies have linked the chemical to non-Hodgkin's lymphomas, sarcomas, and carcinomas, as well as a host of other diseases (Byrnes, 2003).

Chemical weapons such as nerve agents and blistering agents are less convenient than toxins or poisons. For example, ricin is very convenient because it is a highly potent protein toxin derived from the mash left over from processing castor beans for their oil. Such processing is a worldwide activity, and the poison (toxin) is easily produced. The castor plant, *Ricinus communis*, received attention in the 1978 "umbrella murder case," when Bulgarian intelligence operations assassinated Bulgarian dissident George Markov in London, using an umbrella to deliver a ricin-containing pellet (Tierno, 2002). Mr. Markov died a day after the attack of ricin poisoning. Ricin blocks protein synthesis and is very toxic to cells, eventually killing them. Ricin can be delivered by aerosol, and within 8 hours after inhalation, severe respiratory symptoms occur, leading to respiratory failure. If the toxin is ingested (food or water), severe gastrointestinal symptoms will occur, followed by vascular collapse and death. If injected, ricin can cause multiorgan failure and death (Tierno, 2002). Numerous other toxic poisons such as mycotoxins and saxitoxins produce similar outcomes.

The 1972 Convention on Prohibition of Biological and Chemical Weapons

Throughout recent decades, efforts have been made to limit or ban the use of toxic weapons (both chemical and biological). In 1972, more than 140 countries, including the United States, signed the "Convention on the Prohibition of the Development, Production, and Stockpiling of Biologic and Toxic Weapons and Their Destruction," which theoretically limited further development and use of biological or chemical weapons (Byrnes, 2003). Unfortunately, numerous breaches have been made in that accord.

TABLE 13-15
Chemical Weapons

Category	Examples	Comments
Nerve agents	Sarin, tabun, soman, VX, malathion, carbaryl (Sevin)	Interfere with transmission of message from nerve to organ or muscle
Blood agents	Hydrogen cyanide, cyanogen chloride	Usually absorbed after inhalation; in the bloodstream cause lethal damage by acting on the cytochrome oxidase enzyme responsible for cellular respiration. Oxygen starvation occurs because cells are unable to use oxygen. (See Chapter 23.)
Blister agents	Nitrogen and sulfur mustards, lewisite	Cause blistering of skin as well as internal organs and tissues. This destroys the tissue and also causes massive numbers of mutations by crosslinking DNA and RNA.
Heavy metals	Arsenic	Metallic elements form poisonous compounds, disrupting cellular metabolic processes.
Pulmonary agents	Chlorine gas, phosgene	Damage the membranes of the lungs, causing fluid buildup and oxygen deprivation and eventually suffocation.
Dioxins	Tetrachlorodibenzodioxine	Associated with lymphomas, sarcomas, carcinomas, chloracne, and a host of other diseases. (A major long-term complication is type 2 diabetes.)
Incapacitating or psychotomimetic agents	Quinuclidinylbenzylate, phencyclidine	Cause pseudopsychotic disorders; affect ability to make decisions; cause disorientation, any of which could incapacitate an individual. Death due to respiratory arrest can occur with high doses.
Corrosive acids and bases	Sulfuric acid, sodium hydroxide	Cause severe burning and destruction of tissue in exposed areas.

To take two relatively recent examples of an ongoing trend, in 1988 Libya built a chemical weapons plant in the guise of a pharmaceutical factory. Often this occurs with the cooperation of companies that sell so-called dual-use technology to countries such as Iraq and Libya. A plant for making pesticides can readily be turned into one for making chemical weapons. Iraq used mustard gas in its long war with Iran and has used both mustard gas and toxic nerve agents against its own dissident Kurdish population. The 1980s saw the use of chemical warfare agents in Afghanistan, Cambodia, Iran, Iraq, and Laos (Tierno, 2002; Byrnes, 2003).

In March of 1995, a Japanese religious cult, Aum Shinriyko, released sarin nerve gas in the Tokyo subway system (Tierno, 2002). Thousands were injured, and 11 people were killed. This recent use of chemical weapons on the civilian population underscores the relative availability and ease of use of such weapons and raises public and governmental awareness.

Weaponization and Delivery of Chemical Agents

Any chemical agent must be weaponized before its delivery. In general, the process of weaponization involves numerous steps. First, an agent must be made in sufficient quantity and temporarily stored and stabilized to prevent evaporation or degradation. Thickeners are added to increase the viscosity of liquid agents, and a carrier agent is required to improve dispersion of the chemical. Next, the chemical agent must be inserted into an appropriate delivery device such as explosive, pneumatic, or mechanical munitions or a dissemination device. Regardless of approach, the goal is to aerosolize the chemical agent to a particulate size of 1–7 microns. This can be accomplished by using very sophisticated delivery systems such as munitions devices usually only available to governments, or unsophisticated devices like aerosol generators, such as underarm deodorants or garden sprayers, which can serve as an effective dissemination system. The important caveat here is that these unsophisticated devices are readily available to the masses. Numerous other factors might affect the weaponization and delivery of a chemical weapon, such as the following:

- *Temperature (air and ground):* Generally, higher temperatures cause faster evaporation.
- *Humidity:* High humidity may cause enlargement of particle size, reducing effectiveness.
- *Precipitation:* Heavy rain can dilute and disperse a chemical weapon; snow increases the persistence of a chemical weapon.
- *Wind speed:* Wind can disperse vapors, aerosols, and liquids, affecting the target area
- *Nature of buildings:* Buildings may absorb or adsorb agents; they can also offer protection.
- *Nature of terrain:* Woodlands and hills can create greater turbulence of low-lying clouds of the agent.

Categories of Chemical Weapons

Literally, hundreds of chemical agents and poisonous gases can be used in an attack, along with potentially new ones under development using newly described genetic engineering methods. Governmental agencies classify chemical weapons in various categories (Table 13-15).

ROLE OF LEVEL A LABORATORY: CHEMICAL TERRORISM

It goes without saying that timely detection of the relatively quick-acting chemical agents that a terrorist might use, such as nerve agents (i.e., sarin and VX), is critical not only for the patient (casualty) but also for the first responder or hazardous material (HAZMAT) unit member responding to an event. Rapid detection of the type of agent, as well as its concentration after a terror incident, can allow for effective treatment of the victim, including proper antidote selection, and can allow for an appropriate protective response to ensure the safety of the public at large. As such, it may be obvious, but the most appropriate entity to detect such agents is not the clinical laboratory; instead, it is the bailiwick of the first responder unit or HAZMAT team. These teams use a wide variety of commercially available equipment manufactured for the rapid detection of hazardous chemicals, including the agents of chemical terrorism. Likewise, the military has provided a number of devices that can be used to detect such chemical agents or their vapors. The most portable chemical vapor detector is the chemical agent monitor. It uses ion mobility spectroscopy to detect nerve, blister, and blood agents. The simplest and most rapid liquid detectors are also products of the military, namely, the M8 and M9 papers that can be used to detect mustard or nerve agents. These are mostly rapid screening devices that may show false-positive reactions (Byrnes, 2003). However, colorimetric tubes are the most common detection technology used by HAZMAT teams. Their analytic capabilities are broad and usually include tests for chlorine and phosgene gas (pulmonary agents), cyanide (blood agents), and organophosphates (nerve agents). In addition, HAZMAT teams possess a wide variety of some newer post-9/11 technologies, enabling their members to detect virtually ALL necessary chemical agents in a relatively rapid time frame (Byrnes, 2003).

Although the role of Level A clinical laboratories may be a secondary one, they nevertheless can still provide some support for detecting chemical agents used in an attack or their degradation products in victims, which can be useful for triage or treatment of incoming hospital patients. For practical purposes, we can divide the potential chemical agents that a clinical chemistry laboratory may offer in their analytic repertoire into four major categories: nerve agents, blood agents (cyanide), blister agents (vesicants), and pulmonary agents. The laboratory can also be useful in detecting toxins such as ricin or saxitoxins. These can be detected by specialized enzyme-linked immunosorbent assay methods, polymerase chain reaction assays that detect nucleic acid from the relevant plant source, or sensitive mass spectrometric methods.

Most modern clinical chemistry laboratories currently have the capacity to provide some specific and useful analytic data to support hospitalized victims of a chemical attack. For example, several automated chemistry analyzers can measure increased cholinesterase activity, which would be a hallmark of patients exposed to nerve agents. This information is used to measure progress and recovery of victims exposed to nerve agents. Gas chromatography–mass spectrometry has been used to detect metabolites of vesicants such as mustard gas or Lewisite (Byrnes, 2003), and is useful for measuring the progress of a patient's recovery post exposure. Unfortunately for patients exposed to pulmonary agents such as chlorine or phosgene, the laboratory's role is limited to supportive monitoring such as blood gas analysis (for measuring partial pressure of oxygen [pO_2]). This also applies to patients exposed to a blood agent such as cyanide. Gaseous cyanide is lethal in seconds, and patients who ingest cyanide need an antidote immediately to prevent anoxia and respiratory arrest. Therefore, the HAZMAT team may do the best job of analyzing and identifying such agents, and then providing antidotes to poisoned patients in the field, well before they reach a hospital.

In short, Level A laboratories play mostly a supportive role in the management of hospitalized patients who are victims of a chemical terror attack.

Nuclear Terrorism

HISTORY AND BACKGROUND OF NUCLEAR WEAPONS

In 1895, Ernest Roentgen discovered penetrating radiations that produced fluorescence; he named them X-rays. The following year, Henri Becquerel identified that these penetrating radiations (later classified as alpha, beta, and gamma rays) are emitted by uranium. In 1905, Albert Einstein formulated his now famous equation $E = mc^2$, which concluded that matter could be converted to energy. These discoveries provided the scientific framework used to eventually harness nuclear energy, although this did not occur until World War II. In 1942, Los Alamos, New Mexico, was selected as the central site for a laboratory to research the physics and design of atomic weapons. In approximately 30 months, the Manhattan Project (the name ascribed to the program that resulted in the production of the first atomic weapon) had achieved its goal of producing a nuclear weapon. By 1945, Germany had surrendered, but Japan continued its war effort. On July 26, 1945, the Potsdam Declaration was issued, wherein President Harry Truman, Chiang Kai-Shek of China, and Winston Churchill of Great Britain advised the Japanese government to proclaim an unconditional surrender of all Japanese armed forces, cautioning against the alternative. The Japanese government rejected the declaration on July 29, 1945 (Byrnes, 2003). On the morning of August 6, 1945, a U.S. aircraft named *Enola Gay* dropped *Little Boy*, an enriched uranium bomb, on Hiroshima, Japan (15 kilotons). Several days later, *Fat Man* was dropped on Nagasaki. The nuclear age had arrived.

The Potential Threat of Nuclear Terrorism

Since the end of World War II, the United States has manufactured more than 70,000 nuclear weapons, although many have since been retired. Today's weapons are larger (1000 kilotons, or 1 megaton) and far more destructive than the 15 kiloton Hiroshima bomb. Although the Cold War with Russia has officially ended, and efforts have been made to reduce the number of nuclear weapons, other countries possess or are trying to develop nuclear capabilities. There is concern that such weapons may fall into the hands of terrorists or might be used by rogue nations. Although it is possible that terrorists may gain access to nuclear weapons of mass destruction, it is much more likely that they will construct *dirty bombs*—a combination of conventional explosives and radioactive materials. Dirty bombs are relatively simple to build and detonate. The main purpose of a dirty bomb is not to kill people so much as it is to create widespread panic and psychological fear. The amount of radioactivity a dirty bomb yields depends on the radioactive material used in the device. However, even a small amount of radiation from such a device has the potential to cause a relatively large decontamination cost.

ROLE OF LEVEL A LABORATORY: NUCLEAR TERRORISM

The clinical laboratory is not actively involved in detecting radiation contamination. This is more likely done in a hospital emergency department with the use of one or more hand-held radiation survey instruments, such as the Ludlum Model 3/Model 44-9 combo Geiger-Mueller detector (Ludlam Measurements, Inc., Sweetwater, TX), which is able to detect alpha-, beta-, and gamma-emitting radionuclides. Routine HAZMAT and other first responder teams have such analytic capabilities and are the likely entity to first identify or detect a nuclear event. Clinical chemistry and hematology laboratories merely play a support role for any patients who may require hospitalization.

SELECTED REFERENCES

Byrnes ME, King DA, Tierno PM. Nuclear chemical and biological terrorism. Boca Raton, Fla.: CRC Press; 2003.

This text provides a comprehensive review of the various weapons of mass destruction, along with sound advice and simple actions that can be taken by emergency responders or the general public to reduce risks and avoid panic in the event of a terrorist attack.

CDC. Gastrointestinal anthrax after an animal-hide drumming event in New Hampshire and Massachusetts in 2009. Morbidity and Mortality Weekly Reports 2010;59:872–7.

Tierno PM. Protect yourself against bioterrorism. New York: Pocket Books; 2002.

This pocket guide to bioterrorism provides concise information on the 18 most common biological agents, including background, history, and clinical features. It discusses pre-exposure and postexposure management information, as well as numerous protective response strategies.

USAMRIID. Medical management of biological casualties handbook. 4th ed. Fort Detrick, Md.: United States Army Medical Research Institute for Infectious Diseases; 2001.

This is the U.S. Army's concise handbook on effective medical countermeasures against the likeliest bacterial, viral, and toxic agents to be used as bioterror weapons. It is designed as a quick ready reference and overview rather than a complete resource.

REFERENCES

Access the complete reference list online at http://www.expertconsult.com

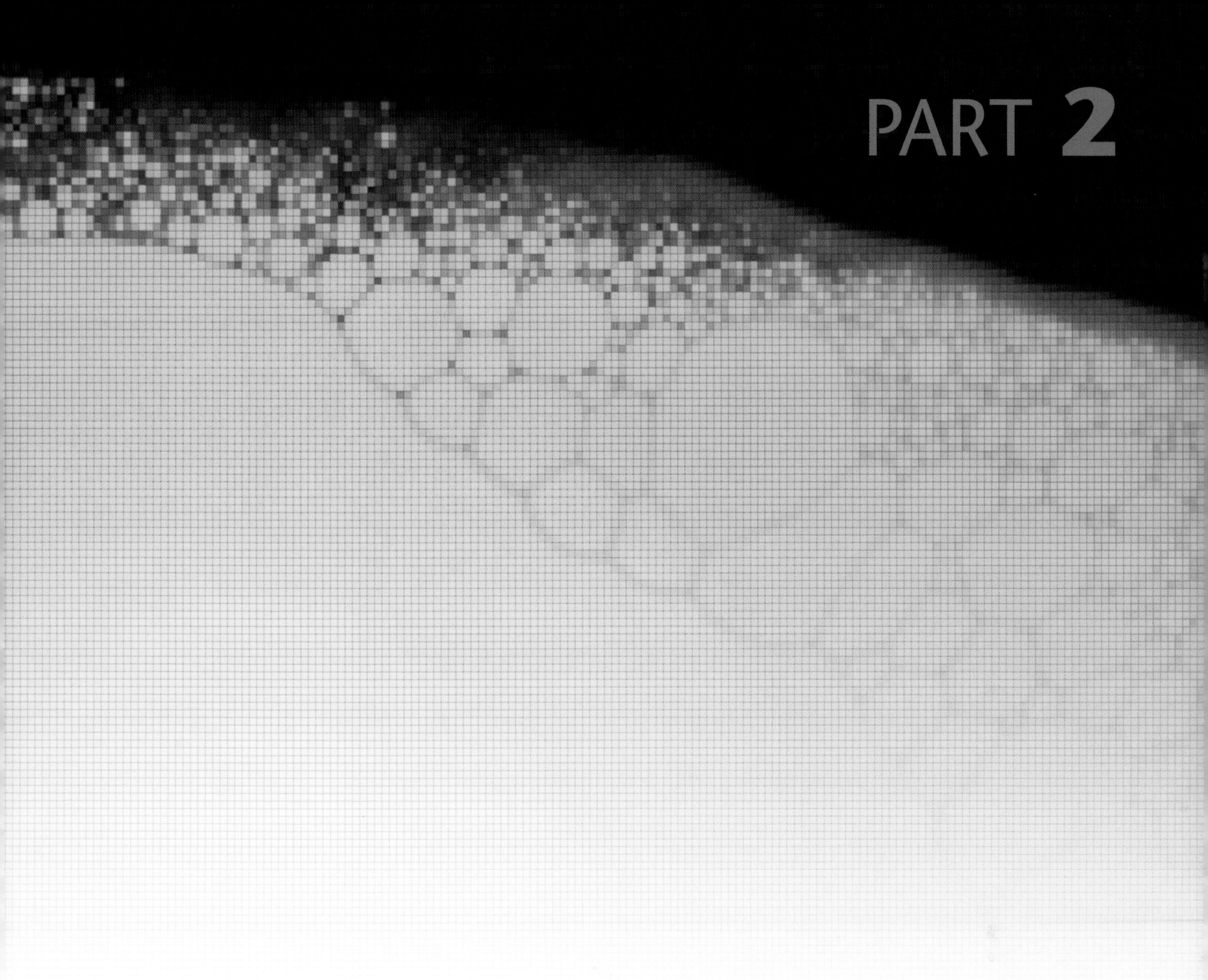

PART 2

Clinical Chemistry

EDITED BY

Martin H. Bluth
Jay L. Bock
Matthew R. Pincus

CHAPTER 14

EVALUATION OF RENAL FUNCTION, WATER, ELECTROLYTES, AND ACID-BASE BALANCE

Man S. Oh

KEY POINTS

- Normal volumes and composition of electrolytes in various body fluid compartments are essential for maintenance of life.
- The kidney is the most important organ in the maintenance of normal fluid volume and composition.
- The most important function of the kidney is elimination of the waste products of metabolism, and this function is best represented by the glomerular filtration rate.
- Glomerular filtration rate can be measured using exogenous or endogenous markers. The most important endogenous marker is creatinine. Glomerular filtration rate can be estimated from a determination of creatinine clearance, which requires measurement of creatinine in both plasma and a timed urine specimen. For many patients, however, a better estimate is obtained from an equation such as the Modification of Diet in Renal Disease, which requires only a measurement of plasma creatinine.

Continued

- Causes of abnormal potassium concentration include laboratory artifacts, cellular redistribution, renal failure, alterations in the renin-angiotensin-aldosterone axis drugs, poor intake, and various acquired or inherited disorders affecting renal excretion of potassium.
- Causes of abnormal sodium concentrations include laboratory artifacts, dehydration, disorders of thirst and antidiuretic hormone, renal disorders, water redistribution due to osmotically active substances such as glucose, drugs, and endocrine disorders.
- Causes of abnormal hydrogen ion concentration (i.e., acid-base disorders) include hypoventilation and hyperventilation, ketoacidosis, lactic acidosis, and toxic ingestions.

Laboratory tests for evaluation of disorders of renal, water, electrolyte, and acid-base status are the most common procedures performed in clinical chemistry laboratories; collectively, screening tests for these are often grouped together in a basic metabolic panel. Disorders of acid-base status and electrolytes are seen in a high percentage of hospitalized individuals, and electrolyte disorders are frequent complications of treatment for a variety of common conditions. Renal disease is one of the major sequelae of common disorders such as diabetes and hypertension. Proper interpretation of laboratory tests for renal, electrolyte, and acid-base disorders requires an understanding of the physiology and pathophysiology of these systems. Most central to an understanding of these disorders is knowledge of renal function and how the kidneys regulate extracellular volume.

VOLUME AND OSMOLALITY OF BODY FLUID

The body fluid is an aqueous solution containing electrolytes and nonelectrolytes, consisting of intracellular and extracellular compartments. The intracellular compartment is not a single compartment, but each cell has its own separate environment, communicating with other cells only via interstitial fluid and plasma. Consequently, differences exist among cells in various tissues in their solute composition and concentrations. Because cell membranes are permeable to water through the ubiquitous presence of aquaporins (water channels), osmotic equilibrium is maintained, so that the osmolality of all cells is the same and is in equilibrium with the extracellular osmolality (Agre, 2002; Nielsen, 2002; Frigeri, 2004).

Operation of normal metabolic functions of the body requires maintenance of optimal ionic strength in its environment, primarily the intracellular fluid (ICF), where most metabolic activities occur. The homeostatic mechanisms of the body are at work to provide such an environment. Because the extracellular fluid (ECF) is not the site of major metabolic activity, substantial alteration in its ionic strength may occur without adverse effects on body function. The main function of the ECF is to serve as a conduit among cells and organs. The plasma provides a route of rapid transit, and the interstitial fluid serves as a slow supply zone. The ability of the ECF to function efficiently as a conduit requires maintenance of optimal volume, particularly of vascular volume. An additional important function of the ECF is regulation of intracellular volume and its ionic strength. Because an osmotic equilibrium exists between the cells and the ECF, any alteration in extracellular osmolality is followed by an identical change in intracellular osmolality, which is accompanied by a reciprocal change in cell volume (Carroll, 1989).

Although cells and organs can be supplied with substrate and relieved of metabolic products with a much slower circulation, normal circulation is required to supply sufficient oxygen for the body's metabolic needs. Normal plasma volume is a prerequisite for maintenance of normal circulation. Because plasma is in equilibrium with the interstitial fluid, the maintenance of normal vascular volume requires normal extracellular volume. A low extracellular volume results in impaired organ perfusion, and an excessive extracellular volume leads to vascular congestion and pulmonary edema.

MEASUREMENT OF BODY FLUID VOLUMES

Total body water can be determined by dilution of various substances, including deuterium, tritium, and antipyrine. The gold standard of measurement is that using tritiated water or deuterium oxide (Lichtenbelt, 1994; Brans, 1990). The former is a radioactive isotope (Lister, 1962), and the latter requires a complicated method for its measurement. Both are very expensive. Antipyrine has been introduced as a cheap alternative, and was used extensively in the 1940s and 1950s (Axelrod, 1949). However, subsequent studies indicated that antipyrine is not a very reliable dilution marker (Brans, 1990; Garrett, 1959). It is metabolized in the liver; therefore, the equilibrium concentration at time zero must be obtained by interpolating the results.

Recently, the measurement of body fluid volumes by bioelectrical impedance analysis has become very popular. However, the results are not as accurate as those of dilution methods, and the technology is still evolving. The main advantages of this method include its easy applicability, noninvasiveness, and portability of measurements. The portability allows measurement of body fluid volumes in outpatient clinics and at the bedside (Woodrow, 2007).

The method is based on the principle that the body is an electrical conductor with a certain amount of resistance to flow (impedance), and resistance (R) is proportional to its length and inversely proportional to the cross-sectional area (A) (Kyle, 2004). Hence, $R = \rho L/A$, where ρ is the resistivity of the conducting material (i.e., the body). Because $V = AL$, $V = \rho L^2/R$. The body fluid offers two types of resistance to an electrical flow: resistive resistance and capacitative resistance. The former is simply called resistance, whereas the latter is called reactance. Impedance of the body to an electrical flow is a combination of these two types of resistance. The cell membrane, which is made of lipid, acts like capacitance, and is the cause of capacitative resistance. At zero or low frequency, the electrical current does not penetrate the cell membrane and therefore flows only through the ECF. At a very high frequency, the electrical current flows through both extracellular and ICF compartments (Kyle, 2004).

The term bioelectrical impedance analysis is used when a single or multiple frequencies of up to 8 frequencies are used, whereas the term bioelectrical spectroscopy is used when 256 or more multiple frequencies are used (Gudivaka, 1999). In bioelectrical spectroscopy, mathematical modeling and mixture equations are used to generate a relationship between R and body fluid volumes. Bioelectrical impedance analysis has been used to measure fat free mass, ECF volume, ICF volume, and total body water.

BODY FLUID VOLUMES

Total body water measured with antipyrine in hospitalized adults without fluid and electrolyte disorders is about 54% of body weight (Carroll, 1989). The fractional water content is higher in infants and children, and decreases progressively with aging. The water content also depends on the body content of fat; women and obese persons, because of their higher fat content, have less water for a given weight. A useful short cut for the calculation of total body water, using the fact that 54% of body weight in kg is body water, and 1 kg is 2.2 lb, is as follows:

$$\text{Total body water (L)} = \text{body weight (lb)}/4 \qquad \textbf{(14-1)}$$

For an obese subject, subtract 10% from the calculated body water, and for a lean person, add 10%. For a very obese person, subtract 20%. Women have about 10% less body water than men for the same body weight. Extracellular volume is measured directly, and intracellular volume is estimated as the difference between total body water and extracellular volume. The measurement of total body water is reliable, but the measurement of extracellular volume is not, because no ideal marker has been found. Markers such as sodium, chloride, and bromide are not located exclusively in the extracellular compartment, but they penetrate the cells to some extent, whereas other markers such as mannitol, inulin, and sucrose do not penetrate certain parts of the ECF. Thus, depending on the type of marker used, the ECF volume could vary from 27% to 53% of total body water (Carroll, 1989).

Extracellular volume measured with chloride and expressed as percent of total body water varies from 42% to 53%, greater in older subjects and women. Extracellular volume measured with inulin or sulfate is smaller, about 30% to 33% of total body water (Carroll, 1989). For discussion in this chapter, a value of 40% of total body water will be considered to represent extracellular volume. Extracellular volume is further divided into three fractions: interstitial (space between cells) volume (28% of total body water), plasma volume (8%), and transcellular water volume (4%) (Table 14-1). Transcellular water includes luminal fluid of the gastrointestinal tract, the fluids of the central nervous system, and the fluid in the eye, as well as lubricating fluids at the serous surface.

COMPOSITION OF THE BODY FLUID

Extracellular Composition

The concentrations of electrolytes in plasma are easily measured, and their values are well known. These concentrations increase by about 7% when expressed in plasma water because about 7% of plasma is solids (Nguyen, 2007). Thus, plasma sodium is 140 mmol/L, but the concentration in plasma water is about 150 mmol/L. The concentrations of electrolytes in interstitial fluid are different from those in the plasma because of differences in protein concentrations between plasma and interstitial fluid. Differences in electrolyte concentrations between plasma and interstitial fluid can be predicted by the Donnan equilibrium (Table 14-2) (Oh, 1995). With normal plasma protein concentrations, the concentrations of diffusible cations are higher in plasma water than in interstitial water by about 4%, while the concentrations of diffusible anions are lower in plasma than in interstitial fluid by about 4%. The concentrations of calcium and magnesium in the interstitial fluid are lower than the values predicted by the Donnan equilibrium because they are substantially protein-bound.

Part of the interstitial space is occupied by a ground substance consisting of glycosaminoglycans; the most abundant glycosaminoglycan is hyaluronan (hyaluronic acid) (Stern, 2004), and this space excludes the distribution of proteins. In the other part, proteins diffuse freely and communicate with lymphatics. The first part is a gel phase, and the second part a free phase. Interspersed within the interstitial space is elastin, which provides the elastic property of the interstitial tissue; this property is necessary for generation of a normal negative pressure of the interstitial space and a positive pressure with the development of edema (Reed, 1992; Aukland, 1993; Burton, 1988).

Intracellular Composition

Whereas sodium, chloride, and bicarbonate are the main solutes in the ECF, potassium, magnesium, phosphate, and proteins are the main solutes in the cell. Intracellular concentrations of sodium and chloride cannot be measured with accuracy and are estimated by subtracting the amount that is extracellular from the total tissue value. Because concentrations of electrolytes in the ECF are high, a small error in extracellular water volume measurement will cause a large error in the measurement of intracellular concentration of these ions.

TABLE 14-1
Volumes of Body Fluid Compartments*

Intracellular volume: 24 L (60%)	
Extracellular volume: 16 L (40%)	
Interstitial volume: 11.2 L (28%)	
Plasma volume: 3.2 L (8%)	
Transcellular volume: 1.6 L (4%)	

*A normal man weighing 73 kg (160 lb) with 40 L of total body water is used as a model.

The concentration of bicarbonate is calculated from cell pH, and the bicarbonate concentration shown in Table 14-2 is based on the assumption that average cell pH is 7.0.

The electrolyte composition of ICF is not identical throughout the tissues. For example, the concentration of chloride in muscle is very low, about 3 mmol/L, but it is about 75 mmol/L in erythrocytes. The concentration of potassium in the muscle cell is about 140 mmol/L, but in the platelets, it is only about 118 mmol/L. The concentration of sodium in the muscle and the red blood cell is about 13 mmol/L, but in the leukocytes about 34 mmol/L. The main phosphate in the red blood cell is 2,3-diphosphoglycerate, but in the muscle, adenosine triphosphate and creatinine phosphate are the main phosphates. Because the muscle represents the bulk of the body cell mass, it is customary to use the electrolyte concentration of the muscle cells as representative of the intracellular electrolyte concentration. A substantial portion of the anions inside the cell are polyvalent ions such as phosphate and protein, and consequently, the total ionic concentration in the cell in mmol/L is greater than that of the ECF to maintain osmotic equilibrium with the ECF.

MEASUREMENT OF PLASMA OSMOLALITY

Osmolarity refers to the number of moles of solute in a liter of solution, whereas osmolality refers to the number of moles of solute in a kg of water (solvent). Osmolality is the preferred term, because measurements of both osmolarity and osmolality are based on colligative properties, which are physical properties that are based on the number of particles dissolved in a given number of water molecules. Examples of colligative properties include freezing point, boiling point, and vapor pressure. The molecular mass of water represents the number of water molecules more accurately than the volume because water volume changes with temperature, but the molecular mass does not. However, the terms osmolality and osmolarity are often used interchangeably, because changes in the volume of liquid water with temperature change are negligible. One should note, however, that 1 kg of water occupies exactly 1 L at 4° C.

One mole of NaCl in solution contains 2 osmoles because NaCl is dissociated to Na^+ and Cl^-. One mole of D-glucose in solution contains 1 osmole because glucose does not dissociate. One mole of Na_3PO_4 in solution contains 4 osmoles, because it will dissociate into 3 Na^+ ions and one PO_4^{3-} ion. To calculate the osmolality of a solution whose solute dissociates into more than one particle, the following equation is used:

$$M \times a = Osm/L \tag{14-2}$$

where M is molarity, and a is the number of particles into which a molecule of the substance dissociates.

When the osmolal concentration of the ECF increases by accumulation of solutes that are restricted to the ECF (effective osmols) (e.g., glucose, mannitol, sodium), osmotic equilibrium is reestablished as water shifts from the cell to the ECF, increasing intracellular osmolality to the same level as the extracellular osmolality (Hill, 1990; Oh, 1995; Weisberg, 1978). When the extracellular osmolality increases by accumulation of solutes that can enter the cell freely (ineffective osmols) (e.g., urea, alcohol),

TABLE 14-2
Electrolyte Concentrations in Extracellular and Intracellular Fluids

	PLASMA		INTERSTITIAL FLUID		PLASMA WATER		CELL WATER (MUSCLE)	
	(mmol/L)	**(mmol/L)**	**(mmol/L)**	**(mmol/L)**	**(mmol/L)**	**(mmol/L)**	**(mmol/L)**	**(mmol/L)**
Na^+	140	140	145.3	145.3	149.8	149.8	13	13
K^+	4.5	4.5	4.7	4.7	4.8	4.8	140	140
Ca^{++}	5.0	2.5	2.8	2.8	5.3	5.3	10^{-7}	0.5×10^{-7}
Mg^{++}	1.7	0.85	1.0	0.5	1.8	0.9	7.0	3.5
Cl^-	104	104	114.7	114.7	111.4	111.4	3	3
HCO_3^-	24	24	26.5	26.5	25.7	25.7	10	10
SO_4^{2-}	1.0	0.5	1.2	0.6	1.1	0.55	–	–
P	2.1	1.2*	2.3	1.3*	2.2	1.2*	107	57†
Protein	15	1	8	0.5	16	1	40	2.5‡
Organic anion	5	5	5.6	5.6	5.3	5.3	–	–

*The calculation is based on the assumption that the pH of the extracellular fluid is 7.4, and the pK of inorganic $H_2PO_4^-$ is 6.8.
†The intracellular molal concentration of phosphate is calculated with the assumption that the pK of organic phosphates in the cells is 6.1, and the intracellular pH is 7.0.
‡The calculation is based on the assumption that each mmol of intracellular protein has on average 15 mEq.

osmotic equilibrium is achieved by entry of those solutes into the cell. Because most of the solutes normally present in the ECF are effective osmols, loss of extracellular water (e.g., insensible losses) will increase effective osmolality, and hence will cause shifting of water from the cells. Reduction in extracellular osmolality by loss of normal extracellular solutes or by retention of water reduces effective osmolality for the same reasons, and hence causes shifting of water into the cells.

Osmolality of serum or plasma can be measured directly with an osmometer, as described in Chapter 4 on the principles of instrumentation, or estimated as the sum of the concentration of all solutes in the plasma. Because an osmometer does not distinguish between effective and ineffective osmols, effective osmolality can only be estimated. As it happens, urea is the only ineffective osmol that has substantial concentration in the normal plasma, 5 mOsm/L. In the normal plasma, therefore, total osmolality is nearly equal to effective osmolality. Plasma osmolality is estimated as follows:

$$\text{Serum osmolality} = \{\text{serum Na}^+(\text{mmol/L}) \times 2\} + \{\text{glucose}(\text{mg/dL})/18\} + \{\text{urea}(\text{mg/dL})/2.8\} \quad \textbf{(14-3)}$$

With use of the above formula, osmolality of sodium and accompanying anions is overestimated by not considering the osmotic coefficient and assuming that all serum anions are univalent. On the other hand, osmolality is underestimated by ignoring nonsodium cations and their accompanying anions. At normal serum glucose and urea concentrations, osmolality almost equals serum $Na^+ \times 2$ because the opposing errors cancel each other. It should be noted that for the contributions of urea nitrogen and glucose for serum osmolality, their values in mg/dL are divided by one tenth of each (2.8 and 18) of their molecular weights (28 and 180), because osmolality is expressed as mOsm/L, not mOsm/dL.

Many of the solutes that may accumulate in the body in certain abnormal states are anions of an acid (e.g., salicylate, glycolate, formate, lactate, β-hydroxybutyrate). These substances should not be added in estimating plasma osmolality because they are largely balanced by sodium and therefore are already accounted for when plasma sodium is multiplied by 2. Non-electrolyte solutes that accumulate abnormally in the serum (e.g., ethanol, ethylene glycol, methanol, mannitol) will cause the measured osmolality to exceed the calculated osmolality, producing an osmolal gap (Gennari, 1984; Kruse, 1994). This osmolal gap is a useful clinical clue to the presence of the toxic substances listed previously. Accumulation of neutral and cationic amino acids also causes a serum osmolal gap.

Effect of Hyperglycemia on Serum Na$^+$

The permeability of a membrane for a given solute varies with the cell type. For example, glucose does not accumulate in the muscle. It does not enter the muscle cell freely, and when it enters the cell with the help of insulin, it is quickly metabolized. Thus, glucose is an effective osmol for the muscle cell (e.g., hyperglycemia will cause shift of water from the muscle cell). On the other hand, glucose is an ineffective osmol for red blood cells, liver, kidney cells, and most brain cells because it enters these cells freely. Glucose is generally categorized as an effective osmol mainly because the muscle cells represent the largest body cell mass, as noted previously in this chapter. Accumulation of glucose or mannitol in the ECF is a well-known cause of hyponatremia because, as discussed in Chapter 8, glucose is osmotically active and induces diffusion of water from the cells to the ECF, thus diluting its electrolytes. The fluid shift affects concentrations of all extracellular electrolytes, but its absolute effect is greatest on serum sodium because of its highest concentration. The relationship between change in serum sodium and change in glucose concentration in a normal adult is about 1.6 mmol/L of Na^+ for 100 mg/dL of glucose (Katz, 1973). However, the correction factor is not linear. When hyperglycemia is more severe, the change in serum sodium for a given change in glucose tends to be less, approaching 1.4 at serum glucose concentration of 1000 mg/dL (Moran, 1985). In sharp contrast, Hillier et al, on the basis of experiments on normal subjects, concluded that the correction factor was much larger—a 2.4 mmol/L change in serum sodium for every 100 mg/dL change in glucose (Hillier, 1999). A problem with this experiment and with the conclusion was that the authors disregarded the effects of water contained in intravenous glucose and urine output on serum sodium. Furthermore, infusion of somatostatin during induction of hyperglycemia would have increased serum potassium, and infusion of insulin during treatment of hyperglycemia would have had an opposite effect on serum potassium concentration. Changes in serum potassium would have the opposite effects on serum sodium concentration.

These figures suggested by various formulas are valid, however, only when the volume of distribution of glucose is between 40% and 50% of total body water. The volume of distribution of glucose refers to a theoretical volume into which glucose would be evenly distributed when none of the administered glucose is excreted and none is metabolized. For example, if 10 g (10,000 mg) of glucose is given to a person, and is the serum concentration increases by 1000 mg/L (100 mg/dL) (with the assumption that none was metabolized and none excreted), the volume of distribution would be 10 L. Normally, the volume of distribution of glucose is slightly greater than the extracellular volume because some cells allow free diffusion of glucose. As the volume of distribution of glucose in relation to total body water is increased, the effect of glucose on serum sodium decreases. Decreased volume of distribution of glucose has an opposite effect. The change in serum Na caused by hyperglycemia can be estimated with the following formula (Oh, 1995):

$$\Delta\text{Na}^+(\text{mmol/L}) = (5.6 - 5.6a)/2 \quad \textbf{(14-4)}$$

where ΔNa is a reduction in serum Na^+ in mmol/L for each 100 mg/dL increase in glucose, and a is the fraction of the volume of glucose distribution over total body water.

In conditions with marked expansion of extracellular volume (e.g., congestive heart failure, other edema-forming states), the volume of distribution of glucose represents a much greater fraction of total body water; hence a fall in serum sodium caused by hyperglycemia would be much less than usual. For example, when the volume of distribution of glucose is 80% of total body water (0.8), the decrease in serum Na^+ for a 100 mg/dL rise in glucose would be only 0.56 mmol/L: $(5.6 - 5.6 \times 0.8)/2 = 0.56$. When the volume of distribution of glucose is 20% of total body water, ΔNa^+ would be 2.2 mmol/L for a 100 mg/dL increase in glucose.

Tonicity

The concept of tonicity of a solution is based on the effect of a particular solution on the volume of cells. A hypertonic solution is one that shrinks the cells, and a hypotonic solution is one that causes swelling of the cells. An isotonic solution is one that does not induce any volume change in the cells. A solution of 0.9% saline (154 mM solution of sodium chloride) is isotonic in relation to normal body fluid. When the term tonicity is applied to a fluid in vitro, as in the urine, it is used almost interchangeably with total osmolality. Thus, urine with a high concentration of urea is called hypertonic (Pradella, 1988).

Osmolality and Specific Gravity

The specific gravity of a solution is the mass of the solution divided by the volume of the solution. Whereas the osmolality of fluid depends on the osmolal concentration of its solute, specific gravity is determined by the weight of the solute relative to the volume it displaces in solution. Plasma protein contributes little to osmolality because of its low molal concentration despite its great weight, but it is the major factor determining specific gravity of plasma. Urinary specific gravity and osmolality usually change in parallel, but discrepancy occurs between the two with heavy proteinuria and severe glycosuria (Carroll, 1989).

REGULATION OF EXTRACELLULAR VOLUME

As discussed below, the extracellular volume depends primarily on its sodium concentration, which is closely regulated by two hormones: Antidiuretic hormone (ADH) that promotes water retention, and aldosterone that promotes sodium retention, which in turn causes water to be retained with it, as discussed in Chapter 8. Because the extracellular sodium concentration is maintained within a fairly narrow range through the regulation of ADH release, the extracellular volume depends primarily on its sodium content. In most clinical situations, the extracellular volume correlates well with vascular volume, which in turn usually correlates positively with the effective vascular volume. Effective vascular volume is an imaginary volume that reflects cardiac output in relation to the tissue's demand for oxygen (Oh, 1995). Sometimes, effective vascular volume does not correlate well with vascular volume or extracellular volume.

Effective vascular volume, rather than extracellular volume or vascular volume, is the chief determinant of how much ECF is retained. The location and type of sensors that perceive changes in effective vascular volume are not well known. Most physiologists consider the baroreceptors, located in the atria of the heart and the aortic arch, likely candidates that send neural signals to the central nervous system, resulting in increases or decreases in ADH, and that alter sympathetic tone. However, a preponderance of evidence argues against the effectiveness of such receptors in chronic states of altered effective vascular volume. For example, in a hypertensive patient with congestive heart failure, both atrial low pressure and arterial high pressure baroreceptors would sense a higher than normal pressure. Yet, the neurohumoral responses (e.g., high ADH, high catecholamines, high renin and angiotensin concentrations) in such states suggest that the body senses low effective vascular volume. In such conditions, the kidney of course responds appropriately by reducing urinary excretion of sodium and chloride. These physiologic responses to low effective vascular volume sometimes lead to a pathologic retention of salt. For example, salt is retained in congestive heart failure despite markedly expanded extracellular volume and vascular volume, because effective vascular volume is decreased.

Theoretically, the salt content of the body can be altered in two ways: to alter the intake of salt, or to alter renal salt output. No well-developed mechanism influences salt intake in response to changes in effective vascular volume. Thus, alterations in salt content of the body are achieved primarily through changes in renal salt output. Changes in renal salt output can be achieved through physical and humoral factors. The physical factors for renal salt regulation work through changes in the glomerular filtration rate (GFR) and in peritubular capillary oncotic and hydrostatic pressures. When other factors that influence renal salt output are kept unchanged, the greater the GFR, the greater is the amount of sodium filtered, and the greater is the amount of sodium excreted. In general, however, tubular reabsorption rather than glomerular filtration plays a major role in the regulation of renal excretion of sodium. In advanced renal failure, GFR may be 10% of normal, but patients with renal failure excrete their usual amount of sodium intake, as do normal people.

Tubular reabsorption of sodium is regulated by humoral factors and physical factors. The influence of the latter on sodium reabsorption is limited mainly to the proximal tubule, where a great deal of sodium reabsorption occurs passively through the paracellular (between cells) pathway. Increased hydrostatic pressure on the peritubular capillary retards passive fluid reabsorption through the paracellular pathway, while it promotes passive back-diffusion of fluid into the tubular lumen. Increased oncotic pressure has the opposite effects. For example, in congestive heart failure, peritubular hydrostatic pressure is reduced by increased renal vascular resistance caused by constriction of both afferent and efferent arterioles. Constriction of afferent arterioles would tend to reduce glomerular capillary hydrostatic pressure. However, the glomerular pressure does not decrease much because the constriction of efferent arterioles is even greater than that of afferent arterioles. Maintenance of glomerular filtration pressure helps to minimize the fall in GFR in volume depletion states. The result is an increase in filtration fraction (the ratio of GFR to renal plasma flow), which increases to a greater extent than usual the concentration of plasma protein in the blood leaving the glomerular capillary through the efferent arterioles. Because the blood in the efferent arterioles flows into the peritubular capillaries, the oncotic pressure of the peritubular capillary would be higher than usual. A lower than usual hydrostatic pressure and a higher than usual oncotic pressure of the peritubular capillary blood in volume depletion states tend to favor reabsorption of salt and water through the paracellular pathway of the proximal tubule, the tubular segment, in which passive reabsorption of salt through the paracellular pathway plays a big role in overall renal tubular salt transport. Normally, the oncotic pressure of the peritubular capillary plasma in the proximal tubule is about 20% higher than the peripheral blood plasma because the filtration fraction is 0.25. In states of volume depletion, the value could be 30% or 40% higher than that of the peripheral plasma.

Humoral factors that influence tubular reabsorption of sodium include angiotensin II, aldosterone, and catecholamines. Angiotensin II directly increases proximal tubular sodium reabsorption through its effect on the sodium-hydrogen exchanger-3, and also indirectly by increasing aldosterone secretion, which, in turn, increases sodium reabsorption in the cortical collecting duct. Catecholamines influence sodium reabsorption mainly through their effects on renal blood flow, but they may have some direct tubular effect in the proximal nephron.

The role of ADH in the regulation of extracellular volume is modest because of the overwhelming importance of osmolality as the main regulator of ADH secretion. For this reason, *salt content of the body is the main determinant of the extracellular volume*. When sodium is retained, a proportionate amount of water is retained to maintain normal serum osmolality. Only when the effective vascular volume depletion is very great will ADH secretion occur despite hyponatremia.

In the presence of primary water retention, as in the syndrome of inappropriate ADH secretion, extracellular volume could theoretically increase in the absence of sodium retention. However, massive water retention without sodium retention will cause only a modest increase in extracellular volume. For example, if a person with 40 L of total body water gains 10 L of water without a change in sodium content, serum sodium would decrease from 140 mmol/L to 112 mmol/L ($140 \times 40/50 = 112$), a value that would cause severe morbidity or even death. This would increase the extracellular volume by only by 4 L, because the bulk (60%) of retained water would enter the cell. On the other hand, the same fluid volume retained with salt would remain almost exclusively in the extracellular space. In other words, the amount of water that can be retained without salt is limited by severe and fatal hyponatremia. This is the reason why a massive increase in extracellular volume as seen in severe congestive heart failure is possible only with massive sodium retention.

The ultimate source of energy for reabsorption of sodium at various nephron segments is Na^+-K^+-ATPase located on the basolateral membrane, which transports 3 Na^+ out of the cell in exchange for 2 K^+ transported into the cell. The resulting reduction in intracellular sodium concentration and the negative cellular electrical potential allow passive diffusion of Na^+ into the cell through the luminal membrane. Four major sites of sodium reabsorption in the nephron utilize four different mechanisms of luminal sodium entry (Fig. 14-1). A number of humoral factors have been proven or suggested to participate in the regulation of renal salt output. Those with well proven physiologic effects are aldosterone, catecholamines, angiotensin II, and perhaps ADH and prostaglandins (Oh, 1995; Biggi, 1995).

NONRENAL CONTROL OF WATER AND ELECTROLYTE BALANCE

1. *Insensible loss of water from the skin.* Water is lost from the skin primarily as a means of eliminating heat. Water loss from the skin without sweat is called insensible perspiration. Sweat contains about 50 mmol/L of sodium and 5 mmol/L of potassium. Because the main purpose of water loss from the skin is elimination of heat, water loss from the skin depends mainly on the amount of heat generated in the body:

$$\text{Water loss from the skin} = 30 \text{ mL per 100 calories} \qquad \textbf{(14-5)}$$

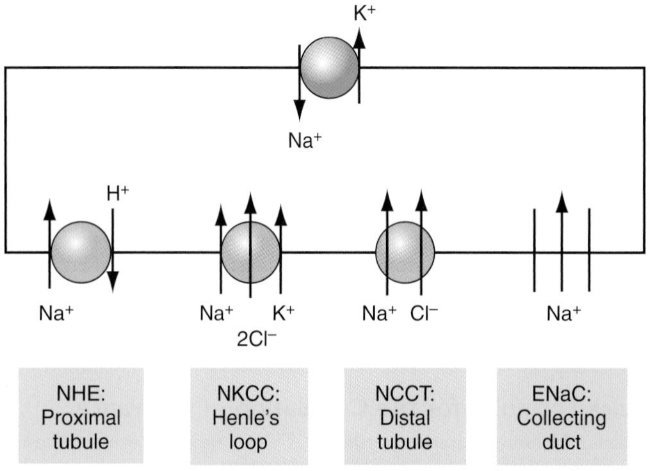

Figure 14-1 Mechanisms of sodium reabsorption at different nephron segments. The main source of energy for sodium reabsorption at all nephron segments is the basolateral Na^+-K^+-ATPase, which transports 3 Na^+ out of the cell in exchange for 2 K^+ into the cell. This pump creates a low intracellular sodium concentration and negative cellular potential, which allow passive diffusion of Na^+ into the cell through the luminal membrane. In the proximal tubule, Na^+ entry is accompanied by exit of H^+ through sodium-hydrogen exchanger type 3 (NHE-3). In the thick ascending limb of Henle, a Na^+ enters along with a K^+ and 2 Cl^- through the sodium-potassium-chloride co-transporter (NKCC). In the distal convoluted tubule, sodium enters with chloride through sodium chloride co-transporter (NCCT), and in the cortical collecting duct, sodium enters through the epithelial sodium channel (ENaC).

2. *Loss of respiratory water.* The water content of inspired air is less than that of expired air; hence water is lost during normal ventilation. Because the ventilatory volume is determined by the amount of carbon dioxise (CO_2) production, which in turn is determined by the caloric expenditure, ventilatory water loss in normal environmental conditions depends also on caloric expenditure:

$$\text{Respiratory water loss} = 13 \text{ mL per } 100 \text{ calories at normal } pCO_2 \quad \textbf{(14-6)}$$

By coincidence, the quantity of water lost during normal respiration is about equal to the metabolic water production. Hence, in calculating water balance, respiratory water loss may be ignored in the measurement of insensible water loss, provided that metabolic water gain is also ignored. Respiratory water loss increases with hyperventilation or fever disproportionately to metabolic water production (Carroll, 1989).

3. *Loss of water in the gastrointestinal tract.* The net activity of the gastrointestinal tract to the level of the jejunum consists of secretion of water and electrolytes. The net activity from jejunum to colon is reabsorption. Most of the fluid entering the small intestine is absorbed in the small intestine, and the remainder is absorbed by the colon, leaving only about 100 mL of water to be excreted daily in the feces. The contents of the gastrointestinal tract are isotonic with plasma, and any fluid that enters the gastrointestinal tract becomes isotonic. Thus, if water is ingested and vomited, solute is lost from the body.

MEASUREMENT OF RENAL FUNCTION

CONCEPT OF CLEARANCE

Renal clearance relates the rate of urinary excretion of material to the plasma concentration of that material. It is defined as the volume of plasma that would theoretically have to be "cleared" of the substance to account for the amount of the substance excreted in the urine during a given period. To calculate clearance, one first must know the amount of substance that is excreted in the urine, which is simply calculated from the urine concentration (U_x) and the volume (V). The next step is to know the plasma concentration of the substance (P_x) to determine the volume of plasma needed to account for the material excreted. For example, if a person excreted 1500 mg of creatinine in a day, he would need 150 L of plasma to account for that 1500 mg of creatinine if the plasma concentration were 10 mg/L (1 mg/dL); creatinine clearance (C_{creat}) then would be 150 L/day. At a plasma concentration of 100 mg/L (10 mg/dL), only 15 L of plasma would be needed to account for the same 1500 mg of creatinine; C_{creat} in this case would be 15 L/day. Customarily, clearance is expressed in mL/minute, but any volume and time units can be used. Thus, clearance of 150 L/day is equal to 6.25 L/hour and 104 mL/minute. The formal equation for clearance is as follows:

$$C_x = (U_x V)/P_x \quad \textbf{(14-7)}$$

where C_x is clearance of a substance x, U_x and P_x are concentrations of the substance in urine and plasma, respectively, and V is the volume of urine per unit time.

In estimating clearance, concentration and volume units must be consistent. For example, if urine creatinine concentration is 70 mg/dL and volume is 2000 mL/day, urine creatinine must also be expressed in mg/mL, not in mg/dL. So the total amount excreted is 0.7 mg/mL × 2000 mL/day = 1400 mg/day.

Clearance in mL/24 hours can be converted to clearance in mL/minute by dividing the value by 1440, because 24 hours equals 1440 minutes.

Quick Formulas for the Calculation of Clearance

When a 24 hour clearance is calculated in mL/minute, urine creatinine excretion may be expressed in g/24 hours instead of in mg/24 hours, while plasma creatinine is expressed as mg/dL instead of in mg/mL, as long as incorrect use of these units is corrected by multiplying the final result by 1000 (for using g instead of mg), and then by 100 (for using mg/dL instead of mg/mL). Further correction requires dividing the value by 1440 to convert a 24 hour clearance value to a value in mL/minute as follows (Carroll, 1989):

$$C_x = U_x V\,(\text{g}/24\text{ hours})/P_x(\text{mg/dL}) \times 100\,000 \times 1/1440 \quad \textbf{(14-8)}$$

Because 100 000/1440 = 70,

$$C_x(\text{mL/minute}) = 70 \times \{U_x(\text{g/day})/P_x(\text{mg/dL})\} \quad \textbf{(14-9)}$$

Conversion of Clearance in L/Week to mL/Minute

The conventional unit for clearance is mL/minute, but in certain situations, different units are more useful. For example, when one compares clearances of peritoneal dialysis in a patient on a continuous ambulatory peritoneal dialysis (CAPD) program versus hemodialysis, the clearance unit often used is L/week. A patient on CAPD treatment typically has 2 L of dialysate exchanged every 6 hours. Because the volume drained is usually about 2.5 L (a slightly higher volume because of transudation of fluid from the blood to peritoneal cavity), creatinine clearance is about 10 L/day or 70 L/week. In comparison, hemodialysis provides about 48 L of creatinine clearance with each treatment, or 144 L of clearance per week because usually three treatments are given each week. If weekly clearance in L/week is to be converted to mL/minute, the following shortcut may be useful.

$$\begin{aligned}\text{L/week} &= 1000 \text{ mL/week} = 1000 \text{ mL}/(7 \times 24 \times 60) \text{ minutes}\\ &= 1000/10\,080 = 0.1 \text{ mL/minute}\end{aligned} \quad \textbf{(14-10)}$$

In other words, (weekly clearance in L/week)/10 = minute clearance in mL/minute. For example, 70 L/week of clearance is equal to 7 mL/minute of clearance.

MEASUREMENT OF GLOMERULAR FILTRATION RATE

GFR is generally considered the best overall indicator of the level of kidney function (Smith, 1951). Two different approaches have been utilized for the measurement of GFR. One approach has been to use an endogenous substance, and the other has been to use an exogenous substance. It is important that whatever molecular marker is used to determine GFR, the substance is minimally reabsorbed and is minimally secreted by the renal tubules.

Measurement of GFR With Exogenous Substances

Clearance of inulin, a complex polysaccharide produced by certain plants, has been widely regarded as the gold standard for measuring GFR. Inulin clearance in healthy young adults has a mean value of 127 mL/min/1.73 m^2 in men and 118 mL/min/1.73 m^2 in women. GFR declines with age. After age 20 to 30 years, GFR decreases by approximately 1.0 mL/min/1.73 m^2 per year. The classic method of inulin clearance requires an intravenous infusion and timed urine collections over many hours. Determination of inulin clearance is not clinically practical at the present time. Consequently, a number of alternative measures for estimating GFR have been introduced (Price, 2000; Gaspari, 1997). The urinary clearance of exogenous radioactive markers such as ^{125}I-iothalamate and ^{99m}Tc-DTPA (metastable technetium^{99}-labeled diethylene triamine pentaacetic acid) provides good measures of GFR (Biggi, 1995; Brochner-Mortensen, 1969; Christensen, 1986; Fleming, 1991). Plasma disappearance of exogenous substances such as iohexol and chromium^{51}–labeled ethylenediaminetetraacetic acid (^{51}Cr-EDTA) has also been used to estimate GFR; an advantage of this method is that it does not require urine collection (Krutzen, 1984; Russel, 1985; Agarwal, 2003). However, plasma clearance methods are not as accurate as those that require urine collection. GFR has also been measured with nonradiolabeled iothalamate in blood and urine; an obvious advantage of this method is avoidance of radioactive materials (Rule, 2004).

Measurement of GFR With Endogenous Substances

Endogenous substances that are widely used to determine GFR include urea, creatinine, cystatin C, β trace protein [BTP], β-2 microglobulin, and tryptophan glycoconjugate. The first two are widely used in clinical practice, mainly because of their ready availability, but cystatin C is gaining popularity.

Creatinine as a Measure of Renal Function

Creatinine is an endogenous substance with a molecular weight of 113 Da. It is produced by the muscle from creatine and creatine phosphate through a nonenzymatic dehydration process. The rate of production of creatinine is proportionate to the creatine–creatine phosphate pool, which, in turn, is proportionate to the muscle mass (Oh, 1993). An additional source of creatinine is creatine contained in ingested meat or dietary supplements. The rate of in vitro conversion of creatine to creatinine in meat is dependent on temperature and acidity; high temperature and low pH increase conversion (Oh, 1993). Creatinine is the most widely used marker of GFR for several reasons. First, it is an endogenous substance with a fairly constant rate of production. Second, creatinine is not bound to plasma proteins; therefore it is filtered freely by the glomerulus. It is not reabsorbed by the renal tubules, and only a small amount is secreted by the tubules.

With the use of creatinine clearance, the inconvenience of urine collection and the uncertainty of its completeness can be avoided by estimating the excretion rate. When renal function is normal and stable, creatinine excretion is almost equal to its production, which depends primarily on muscle mass (Oh, 1993). Muscle mass varies with sex, age, and body weight. The creatinine production rate is estimated as follows (A = age):

$$\text{Creatinine production (mg/kg/day)}: 28 - 0.2A \text{ (men)} \quad \textbf{(14-11A)}$$

$$\text{Creatinine production (mg/kg/day)}: 23.8 - 0.17A \text{ (women)} \quad \textbf{(14-11B)}$$

In obese patients and wasted patients, the above formula will overestimate creatinine production. Normally, creatinine excretion in urine is slightly less than its production because some creatinine is broken down by colonic bacteria. The discrepancy increases progressively with decreasing renal function because of the nonrenal clearance of creatinine, which is about 0.04 L/kg/day (Oh, 1993). However, the metabolism of creatinine by colonic bacteria is inducible, and is increased more in chronic renal failure than in acute renal failure (Owen, 1979). Normally, a 70 kg man would have an extrarenal creatinine clearance of 2.8 L/day or 2 mL/minute, less than 2% of normal renal clearance. However, at a renal clearance of 4 mL/minute, 2 mL/minute of extrarenal clearance would represent one third of the total plasma clearance of creatinine.

However, several drawbacks to the use of creatinine as a measure of GFR have been identified. First, although the rate of production is fairly constant, it has substantial individual variation, depending mainly on the muscle mass (Oh, 1993). In the presence of severe muscle wasting, production of creatinine could be reduced to less than 25% of the amount predicted from the body weight (Kaizu, 2002). Second, creatinine is also derived from the dietary meat, and the quantity of meat ingestion can substantially influence total daily production. Third, creatinine measurement is made most commonly by the alkaline picrate method (see later for a more detailed discussion), and a number of chromogens, both endogenous and exogenous, interfere with its measurement by this technique. Finally, creatinine is partially secreted by the proximal tubules via the organic cation transport pathway, and tubular secretion is blocked by various drugs, including cimetidine, trimethoprim, pyrimethamine, and salicylate (Hilbrands, 1991; Van Acker, 1992). The extent of tubular secretion varies among individuals, and variation is much greater in the presence of renal dysfunction; tubular secretion could involve as much as 50% of the amount excreted in the urine in advanced renal failure. To obviate the errors due to tubular secretion, creatinine clearance has been obtained with the simultaneous administration of cimetidine, which inhibits tubular secretion of creatinine. However, suppression of creatinine secretion by cimetidine is not complete and demonstrates wide individual variation.

Creatinine Measurement

The most widely used method of creatinine measurement is based on the Jaffe reaction, described more than 100 years ago, which is based on the reaction of creatinine with trinitrophenol, an explosive compound also known as picric acid (Spencer, 1986; Weber, 1991). Alkaline conditions enhance the reaction, hence the term alkaline picrate method. Several substances such as ketones, glucose, fructose, protein, urea, and ascorbic acid also react with picrate and falsely increase creatinine concentration (Spencer, 1986; Weber, 1991; Kroll, 1983; Molitch, 1998; Watkins, 1967). Interference with creatinine measurement by glucose becomes significant when glucose concentration is very high, as in diabetic ketoacidosis or hyperglycemic coma (Sjoland, 2003). Glucose concentration is extremely high in dialysate fluid used in peritoneal dialysis, and a correction for the high glucose is needed when creatinine concentration is measured in the effluent of peritoneal dialysate. The magnitude of glucose interference with creatinine measurement has been shown not only in the glucose concentration but also in the creatinine concentration (Mak, 1997). Alterations in reaction and measurement conditions can minimize but not eliminate these interferences. The method of Hare involves isolating creatinine by absorption into Lloyd's reagent and discarding the plasma containing interfering chromogens (Abdul-Karim, 1986). Such pretreatment methods are cumbersome and are not suited to automation. Bilirubin and hemoglobin also interfere with the alkaline picrate method, resulting in falsely low values (Schoenmakers, 1993). Cephalosporin antibiotics also positively interfere with the alkaline picrate method, resulting in falsely elevated values (Swain, 1977; Kroll, 1983). Creatinine can alternatively be measured enzymatically with the use of creatinine amidohydrolase or creatinine iminohydrolase (Suzuki, 1984; Fossati, 1994). Creatinine is hydrolyzed by creatinine iminohydrolase to ammonia and N-methylhydantoin. The ammonia then combines with 2-oxoglutarate and nicotinamide adenine dinucleotide (NADH) in the presence of glutamate dehydrogenase to produce glutamate and NAD^+. Consumption of NADH measured as a decrease in absorbance at 340 nm is used to measure the concentration of creatinine. Creatinine can also be measured by converting creatinine to creatine by creatinine amidohydrolase. Creatine is then hydrolyzed by imidinohydrolase and sarcosine oxidase to produce hydrogen peroxide. In the presence of horseradish peroxidase, 2,4-dichlorophenolsulfonate is converted to a colorless polymer by hydrogen peroxide, and the concentration of the polymer is then measured at 510 nm. Interference by glucose and other Jaffe chromogens in creatinine measurement does not occur with enzymatic methods. However, enzymatic methods have certain interferences of their own (e.g., possible negative interference from bilirubin and catecholamines) (Peake, 2007; Saenger, 2009).

The ultimate reference standard for creatinine measurement is isotope dilution–mass spectrometry (IDMS) (Welch, 1986). Recent efforts are under way to make the calibration of routine creatinine measurements traceable to this standard, although this of course does not affect the problem of interference in individual samples.

Without removing noncreatinine chromogens, the upper limit of normal measured by the Jaffe reaction is 1.6–1.9 mg/dL for adults. The upper limit of normal for serum creatinine measured after removal of the chromogens is 1.2–1.4 mg/dL. Values for women are 0.1–0.2 mg/dL lower. When serum creatinine is very high, noncreatinine chromogens contribute proportionately less to the total reaction. With normal renal function, noncreatinine chromogens make up 14% (range, 4.5%–22.3%) of the total, but with advanced renal dysfunction, they contribute only about 5%.

Cimetidine-Enhanced Creatinine Clearance

Tubular secretion of creatinine results in falsely elevated values in creatinine clearance, especially in renal insufficiency; measurement of creatinine clearance with inhibition of tubular secretion with cimetidine substantially improves the creatinine clearance estimate of GFR in patients with mild to moderate renal impairment (Hilbrands, 1991; Van Acker, 1992; Hellerstein, 1998). However, tubular secretion of creatinine is not completely blocked by cimetidine; hence the method still overestimates glomerular filtration rate.

Formulas to Estimate Creatinine Clearance as an Estimate of GFR

With the realization that accurate urine collection is a major limitation of creatinine clearance as a measure of GFR, attempts have been made to mathematically transform serum creatinine to estimate glomerular filtration rate. In part because of the convenience, these methods are widely used in clinical practice. The two most widely used formulas are the Cockroft-Gault formula and the Modification of Diet in Renal Disease (MDRD) formula (Levey formula).

Cockroft-Gault formula (mL/minute) (Cockroft, 1976):

$$([140 - \text{Age}] \cdot [\text{IBW}])/(72 \times \text{SCr}); \text{ multiply by 0.85 if female} \quad \textbf{(14-12)}$$

where *IBW* is ideal body weight and *SCr* is serum creatinine concentration. IBW is calculated by the following formula:

$$\text{Males: IBW} = 50 \text{ kg} + 2.3 \text{ kg for each inch over 5 feet} \quad \textbf{(14-13A)}$$

$$\text{Females: IBW} = 45.5 \text{ kg} + 2.3 \text{ kg for each inch over 5 feet} \quad \textbf{(14-13B)}$$

The Cockroft-Gault formula reduces the variability of serum creatinine estimates of GFR caused by differences in creatinine production due to differences in muscle mass based on sex and age. However, because the formula does not take into account differences in creatinine production due to variation in muscle mass caused by disease states, it systematically overestimates GFR in individuals who have relatively low muscle mass in relation to their body weight such as obese, edematous, or chronically debilitated individuals. Moreover, it does not take into account variations caused by extrarenal elimination and tubular secretion.

In the MDRD study, Levey and coworkers measured GFR by I^{125}-iodothalamate to derive a formula for estimating GFR using six variables: age, sex, serum urea nitrogen, serum creatinine, race, and serum albumin concentration (Levey, 1999). In 2000, the same investigators produced a simplified MDRD formula based on four variables: serum creatinine, age, race, and sex. Few diabetic individuals were included in the original studies, and these formulas when tested in diabetic patients were found to be inaccurate.

$$\text{MDRD formula (mL/min/1.73 m}^3\text{): GFR} = 170 \cdot \text{Cr}^{-0.999} \cdot \text{Age}^{-0.176} \cdot (0.762 \text{ if female}) \cdot (1.180 \text{ if black}) \cdot \text{BUN}^{-0.170} \cdot \text{Alb}^{0.318} \quad \textbf{(14-14A)}$$

$$\text{The simplified MDRD formula (mL/min/1.73 m}^3\text{) based on four variables (serum creatinine, age, race, and sex): GFR} = 186 \cdot \text{Cr}^{-1.154} \cdot \text{Age}^{-0.203} \times 1.212 \text{ (for black)} \times 0.742 \text{ (for women)} \quad \textbf{(14-14B)}$$

where *Cr* is serum creatinine (mg/dL)
Wt is body weight (kg)
BUN is blood urea nitrogen (mg/dL)
Alb is serum albumin (g/dL).

The previous equation was derived before routine creatinine methods were commonly made traceable to the IDMS standard. For methods traceable to the IDMS standard, creatinine results tend to be lower, and the equation should be used with a smaller initial constant:

$$\text{GFR} = 175 \cdot \text{Cr}^{-1.154} \cdot \text{Age}^{-0.203} \times 1.212 \text{ (for black)} \times 0.742 \text{ (for women)} \quad \textbf{(14-14C)}$$

Whereas the Cockroft-Gault formula includes body weight, the MDRD formula does not include body weight, because the result of the latter is expressed in mL/min/1.73 m^3 rather than as an absolute value. The same errors resulting from variations in creatinine production rate caused by disease states are not eliminated by the Cockroft-Gault formula or by the MDRD formula. Both Cockroft-Gault formula and MDRD formula estimate GFR in adults and are not applicable to measurement of GFR in children. Following are the formulas used most often for estimating creatinine clearance for children (Schwartz, 1976; Counahan, 1976; Leger, 2002; Pierrat, 2003):

Schwartz Formula:

$$\text{GFR} = 0.55 \times \text{height (cm)/serum creatinine (mg/dL)} \quad \textbf{(14-15A)}$$

$$\text{GFR} = 48 \times \text{height (cm)/serum creatinine } (\mu\text{mol/L}) \quad \textbf{(14-15B)}$$

Counahan-Barrett Formula:

$$\text{GFR} = 40 \times \text{height (cm)/serum creatinine } (\mu\text{mol/L}) \quad \textbf{(14-16)}$$

In 2009, Schwartz et al further modified their formula to estimate GFR more accurately in children (Schwartz, 2009). The new formula is very similar to the MDRD equation in that it uses multiple exponential functions; use of the formula requires knowing values of serum creatinine, height, BUN, and serum cystatin C.

Modified Schwartz Formula:

$$\text{GFR (mL/min/1.73 m}^2\text{)} = 39.1[\text{height (m)/Cr (mg/dL)}]^{0.516} \times [1.8/\text{cystatin C (mg/L)}]^{0.294} [30/\text{BUN (mg/dL)}]^{0.169} [1.099]^{\text{male}} [\text{height (m)}/1.4]^{0.188} \quad \textbf{(14-17)}$$

It has been shown that GFR estimated from these various formulas is not very accurate. However, creatinine clearance values estimated from the formulas are still more accurate than those derived from direct measurements, mainly because of the inaccurate urine collections and variations in plasma creatinine concentration in the latter. Consequently, K/DOQI (Kidney Disease Outcomes Quality Initiative) guidelines have recommended the use of these formulas instead of direct measurements in calculating creatinine clearance (Levey, 1999).

All these formula are useful in the estimation of GFR in chronic states when creatinine production is assumed to be equal to the amount excreted in the urine. In acute renal failure, when serum creatinine rises rapidly during the development of renal failure and falls rapidly during the recovery phase, such an assumption is invalid; hence the estimation of GFR by either method is invalid. Measurement of creatinine in the urine with timed urine collection is more useful in determining creatinine clearance in acute renal failure.

Most recently, a new formula, known as the CKD-EPI (Chronic Kidney Disease Epidemiology Collaboration) equation, was reported to give improved performance over the widely used MDRD equation (Levey, 1999).

Urea as Measure of Renal Function

Urea is the main waste product of nitrogen-containing chemicals in the body. It has a molecular weight of 60 Da. However, by custom the concentration of urea is expressed only by the nitrogen content of urea. For this reason, the term serum or urine urea nitrogen is widely used in place of serum or urine urea. Because a molecule of urea contains 2 nitrogen atoms, the molecular weight of urea nitrogen is 28 Da.

Serum urea is widely used as a measure of renal dysfunction, but its value as a measure of GFR is not very good for several reasons. First, urea concentration in the serum depends not only on renal function but also on the rate of urea production, which depends largely on protein intake. The rate of protein intake varies widely from individual to individual.

Urea is freely filtered at the glomerulus but is reabsorbed substantially in the proximal convoluted tubule and the inner medullary collecting duct. Reabsorption of urea in the proximal tubule occurs passively through the lipid membrane without the help of urea transporters (Quigley, 2001), whereas in the inner medullary collecting duct, urea reabsorption is mediated by urea transporters (Pallone, 2007). Some of the urea reabsorbed from the inner medullary collecting duct then reenters the tubule in the thin descending limb of the cortical nephrons, which also express urea transporters (Pallone, 2007). The amount of urea reabsorbed in the proximal tubule varies greatly depending on the status of effective vascular volume; reabsorption is markedly increased in states of volume depletion because the luminal concentration of urea is high owing to the increased fractional reabsorption of salt and water. The amount reabsorbed in the inner medullary collecting duct is increased when urine osmolality is high because of the high urea concentration. For these reasons, urea clearance does not reflect GFR very accurately, but serum urea nitrogen is still widely used as a measure of renal dysfunction. In the presence of normal renal function without volume depletion, urea clearance is about 50% of creatinine clearance, but in the presence of severe volume depletion, its clearance could be as little as 10% of creatinine clearance. In advanced renal failure, urea clearance approaches unity with GFR, and is better than creatinine clearance as a measure of GFR (Schück, 1990).

Measurement of Urea

Essentially, three methods are available for the measurement of urea. The gold standard, which is used only as a reference method because of its high cost, is isotope dilution mass spectrometry (Kessler, 1999). In the clinical laboratory, urea is measured either by the colorimetric method based on a reaction of urea with diacetyl monoxime or by enzymatic methods (Barbour, 1992; Natelson, 1951; Passey, 1980). In the former, urea reacts directly with diacetyl monoxime under strong acidic conditions to give a yellow condensation product. The reaction is intensified by the presence of ferric ions and thiosemicarbazide. The intense red color formed is measured at 540 nm.

The initial reaction in all enzymatic methods is hydrolysis of urea by urease, which produces ammonia and CO_2. Ammonia and CO_2 produced are measured by various methods to calculate the concentration of urea in the original sample. Measurement of ammonia is most often used. In one of these methods, ammonia produced by urease converts glutamate and ATP to glutamine and adenosine diphosphate (ADP). The ADP so produced is consumed in reactions catalyzed sequentially by pyruvate kinase and pyruvate oxidase to generate hydrogen peroxide (Lespinas, 1989). The hydrogen peroxide is then measured as an indirect estimate of urea concentration. In another enzymatic method, as in the one used for creatinine described in the preceding section, ammonia produced from urea hydrolysis reacts with alpha-keto-glutarate and NADH to produce glutamic acid and NAD^+ by glutamate dehydrogenase (Fawcett, 1960). The amount of NADH consumed is measured photometrically to determine the urea concentration. Another urease method involves the indophenol method, in which ammonium produced by urease reacts with hypochlorite to form monochloramine (Higashi, 2000). In the presence of phenol and with an excess of hypochlorite, the monochloramine forms a blue compound, indophenol, the concentration of which is determined spectrophotometrically at 630 nm. Yet in another enzymatic method, CO_2 produced by urease is measured by thermal conductivity gas chromatography.

Other Measures of GFR

Cystatin C

Cystatin C is a 122 amino acid protein with a molecular weight of 13,000 Da; it is an inhibitor of cysteine proteinase. The substance is produced by all nucleated cells, and its production rate is relatively constant from age 4 months to 70 years (Massey, 2004; Laterza, 2002; Ylinen, 1999). The rate of production is not affected by muscle mass, sex, or race. Because of its small size (small for a protein) and a positive net charge, it is freely filtered at the glomerulus at the same concentration as in the plasma. The filtered peptide is completely reabsorbed by the proximal tubule, but then is destroyed rather than reentering the circulation. Because cystatin C has no extrarenal means of elimination, its plasma concentration is inversely related to GFR. Some evidence suggests that glucocorticoids reduce production of cystatin C (Risch, 2001), and this might result in overestimation of renal function in renal transplantation patients, who are regularly given glucocorticoids. A number of studies made comparison of serum creatinine versus serum cystatin C an indicator of renal function, and general consensus is that cystatin C is better than creatinine. However, cystatin C is not widely used clinically because measurements are difficult and expensive (Massey, 2004). It must be noted that cystatin C renal clearance cannot be measured because normally it is completely reabsorbed, and none is excreted in the urine. For this reason, changes in serum concentration of cystatin C are used as indirect estimates of GFR. A complex equation to estimate GFR using the exponential functions and plasma cystatin C concentrations has been developed, and the results were found to be better than those achieved by the MDRD equation and the Schwartz formula for estimation of GFR (Grubb, 2005).

$$\text{Modified cystatin C equation: GFR}\left[\text{mL}\cdot\text{min}^{-1}\cdot(1.73\ \text{m}^2)^{-1}\right]=84.69\times \text{cystatin C}\,(\text{mg/L})^{-1.680}\times 1.384\ (\text{if a child} <14\ \text{years}) \quad \textbf{(14-18)}$$

β-2-Microglobulin

β-2-microglobulin, a polypeptide with molecular weight of 11.6 kDa and length of 99 amino acids, is a component of the major histocompatibility complex class I molecule. It is present in all nucleated cells, and is needed for production of CD8 cells. Its production is increased in multiple myeloma and lymphoma. Because of the low molecular weight, β-2 microglobulin is freely filtered at the glomerulus, and then is reabsorbed and metabolized completely by the proximal tubule. Similar to cystatin C and BTP, the plasma level increases in renal failure. The protein appears in the urine when reabsorption is incomplete because of proximal tubular damage, as in acute kidney injury. The protein has a tendency to fold into a β-sheet configuration, resulting in amyloid formation; it is a common cause of dialysis-associated amyloidosis (Schwalbe, 1997; Bianchi, 2001).

β Trace Protein

BTP is a low molecular weight glycoprotein with 168 amino acids. The molecular weight varies between 23 000 and 29 000 Da, depending on the degree of glycosylation. BTP belongs to the lipocalin protein family and functions as prostaglandin D synthase. Because prostaglandin D is the major prostaglandin in the brain, BTP is isolated primarily from cerebrospinal fluid. Plasma BTP originates from the brain and is freely filtered at the glomerulus, then is reabsorbed completely by the proximal tubule and is catabolized there. The plasma level is increased in patients with renal disease because of reduced filtration in the presence of constant production. White et al (2007, 2009) and Pöge et al (2005, 2008) developed formulas to estimate GFR on the basis of plasma concentration of BTP and urea or creatinine. They claimed that the results were better than those obtained by the MDRD equation and serum cystatin C measurements. However, others showed that BTP was less sensitive than cystatin C (Abbink, 2008).

White Formula using *β* trace protein:

$$\text{GFR1}=112.1\times\text{BTP}^{-0.662}\times\text{urea}^{-0.280}\times(0.880\ \text{if female}) \quad \textbf{(14-19A)}$$

$$\text{GFR2}=167.8\times\text{BTP}^{-0.758}\times\text{creatinine}^{-0.204}\times(0.871\ \text{if female}) \quad \textbf{(14-19B)}$$

Poge Formula using BTP:

$$\text{GFR1}=89.85\times\text{BTP}^{-0.5541}\times\text{urea}^{-0.3018} \quad \textbf{(14-20A)}$$

$$\text{GFR2}=974.31\times\text{BTP}^{-0.2594}\times\text{creatinine}^{-0.647} \quad \textbf{(14-20B)}$$

GFR in mL/min/1.73 m^2; BTP in mg/dL; urea in mmol/L; creatinine in µmol/L.

Tryptophan Glycoconjugate

Mannopyranosyl-L-tryptophan (MPT) is a substance that is normally produced in the body by glycoconjugation of tryptophan; it is filtered at the glomerulus freely and is not reabsorbed. A strong linear correlation has been noted between clearances of MPT and inulin in rats (r = 0.97) and humans (r = 0.87), indicating that renal handling of MPT is similar to that of inulin. The current limitation for the use of MPT for renal function estimation is that it can be measured only by the high-performance liquid chromatography (HPLC) method, which is time consuming and expensive. Serum level of MPT increases progressively with declining renal function, but unlike creatinine, serum MPT concentration is not affected by muscle mass. It is not known whether dietary intake of tryptophan affects the serum concentration (Takahira, 2001).

UREA CLEARANCE AND UREA/CREATININE RATIO IN SERUM

In the absence of renal dysfunction and severe dehydration, urea clearance is about 50% of creatinine clearance, and hence about 50% of GFR, because about 50% of the filtered urea is reabsorbed. The bulk of urea reabsorption occurs in the proximal tubule, about 40% of the filtered load. Among the distal nephron sites, the inner medullary collecting duct reabsorbs urea extensively along a concentration gradient when urine is being concentrated. Most of the urea reabsorbed from the inner medulla reenters the tubule at the descending thin limb; this reentry represents intrarenal recycling of urea (Pallone, 2007). Urea reentry occurs mainly in the short loop of Henle. Some of the urea reabsorbed from the inner medullary collecting duet is carried away from the medulla by the ascending vasa recta; this amount represents about 10% of the filtered load with normal urine flow, but with marked urine concentration the amount can increase greatly (Lyman, 1986).

A marked reduction in urea clearance occurs when the proximal reabsorption of urea is greatly increased by a reduction in effective vascular volume. Reabsorption of urea in the proximal tubule is passive and depends on a favorable urea concentration gradient. This gradient is created by reabsorption of water in the proximal tubule. Normally, about 83% of the filtered water is reabsorbed in the proximal tubule as a result of reabsorption of salt (mainly sodium chloride). Loss of 83% of the water in the tubule increases urea concentration in the tubule six-fold, creating a favorable gradient for urea diffusion out of the tubule. When water reabsorption is 95% of the filtered load, the urea concentration would increase to 20 times the plasma concentration. Volume depletion and decreased renal plasma flow without volume depletion (e.g., renal artery stenosis) also reduce glomerular filtration rate, thereby reducing clearance of both creatinine and urea. Volume depletion decreases creatinine clearance only by reduced filtration, and urea clearance by both reduced filtration and increased reabsorption. Hence, in volume depletion, urea clearance decreases more than creatinine clearance does. Normally, the ratio of plasma urea nitrogen to plasma creatinine is about 10 : 1, but in volume depletion, the ratio is usually greater than 20 : 1.

Prediction of volume status by the urea/creatinine ratio is based on the assumption of constancy of urea and creatinine production, which often is not the case. Glucocorticoids and a high protein diet increase urea production, whereas chronic protein malnutrition decreases it. Creatinine production also varies considerably; marked muscle wasting may reduce its production to less than one fifth of the usual value. Nowadays, the main cause of a high BUN/creatinine ratio in the hospital is not dehydration, but adequate protein intake (often by a tube feeding) in a patient with severe muscle wasting. Thus, fractional excretion of urea (see below) would be a more reliable index of volume status than plasma urea/creatinine ratio (Carvounis, 2002). Mechanisms by which low effective vascular volume increases the proximal reabsorption of salt and water were explained earlier in the section on the control of extracellular volume.

As stated previously, because about 50% of filtered urea is reabsorbed, normal urea clearance underestimates GFR greatly, whereas creatinine clearance slightly overestimates GFR. As renal function declines, the fraction of urea reabsorbed declines progressively, whereas the tubular secretion of creatinine increases progressively (Herrera, 1998). As a result, in the presence of advanced renal dysfunction, urea clearance is a better predictor of GFR than is creatinine clearance (Schück, 1990).

GLOMERULAR FILTRATION RATE, RENAL PLASMA FLOW, AND FILTRATION FRACTION

As discussed in the preceding section, because inulin is filtered freely at the glomerulus but is neither reabsorbed nor secreted by the tubules, its clearance equals GFR, which is the rate (mL/minute) of plasma filtered by the glomerulus from the blood into the tubular system. The clearance of para-aminohippurate (PAH) measures another aspect of renal function. As it happens, whatever PAH is not filtered at the glomerulus is almost all secreted into the proximal tubule, thereby allowing PAH clearance to be a measure of renal plasma flow, which is the total quantity of plasma perfusing the glomerular capillary. The quantity of plasma filtered as a fraction of the total quantity perfusing the glomerular capillary is the filtration fraction (Smith, 1951). Because inulin clearance represents GFR and PAH clearance, the quantity of plasma perfusing the glomerulus,

$$\text{Filtration fraction (FF)} = C_{IN}/C_{PAH}, \quad \textbf{(14-21)}$$

where C_{IN} is inulin clearance, and C_{PAH} PAH clearance.

Filtration fraction in man is normally about 0.2. As was discussed earlier, low effective vascular volume as in heart failure decreases renal perfusion, but GFR decreases to a lesser degree because glomerular capillary pressure is maintained by increased efferent arteriolar tone. The result is an increase in filtration fraction. An increase in glomerular filtration for a given plasma flow (i.e., increased filtration fraction) increases the concentrations of plasma proteins by concentrating the nonfilterable plasma constituents. This increases the oncotic pressure of peritubular capillary blood, resulting in increased fluid movement from the tubular interstitium to the capillary. This in turn helps to increase fluid reabsorption from the proximal tubule into the interstitial space. Similarly, increased tone of efferent arterioles in an attempt to maintain a high glomerular capillary pressure tends to reduce the peritubular capillary hydrostatic pressure. This contributes to increased salt reabsorption by the proximal tubule.

The expanded effective vascular volume decreases filtration fraction because the increase in renal plasma flow is greater than the increase in GFR. Changes in oncotic pressure and hydrostatic pressure in the peritubular capillary blood and their effects on proximal salt and water reabsorption are the opposite of those encountered in conditions of reduced effective vascular volume (Oh, 1995).

FRACTIONAL EXCRETION

Fractional excretion (FE) is the quantity of a substance excreted in the urine expressed as a fraction of the filtered load of the same substance.

$$F_x = P_x \cdot GFR\ (16) \quad \textbf{(14-22)}$$

where F_x is the amount of a substance x filtered.

$$F_x = P_x \cdot C_{creat}\,(GFR = C_{creat}) = P_x \cdot (U_{creat}\ V/P_{creat})$$
$$E_x = V \cdot U_x \quad \textbf{(14-23)}$$

where E_x is the amount excreted in the urine, and U_x is the urine concentration of substance x.

$$\text{Hence, } FE = [(V \cdot U_x)]/[P_x \cdot (V \cdot Ucreat/Pcreat)] \quad \textbf{(14-24)}$$

When V is cancelled on both sides, the equation is simplified as follows:

$$FE = (U_x/P_x)/(U_{creat}/P_{creat})\ (20) \text{ or}$$
$$FE = (U_x/P_x) \cdot (P_{creat}/U_{creat}) \quad \textbf{(14-25)}$$

Thus, the measurement of fractional excretion can be obtained in a spot urine sample. When the substance excreted in the urine has a clearance less than the creatinine clearance, fractional excretion is less than 1. When FE is multiplied by 100, the result is %FE. FE of sodium is often used to distinguish between acute tubular necrosis (acute kidney injury) and prerenal azotemia. A value of FE of sodium of less than 0.01 (less than 1%) suggests prerenal azotemia, and a value greater than 0.01 suggests acute tubular necrosis (acute kidney injury).

RENAL FAILURE INDEX

Renal failure index (RFI) is another formula that is used for the differential diagnosis of acute renal failure. It is expressed as $U_{Na}{}^{+}/(U_{creat}/P_{creat})$. The renal failure index is different from fractional excretion of sodium by the exclusion of plasma Na^+ concentration in the formula. Hence, the value of the renal failure index will be 140 times the value of fractional excretion of Na^+ when the serum Na^+ concentration is 140 mmol/L. When fractional excretion of Na^+ is expressed as a % value,

$$\%FE_{Na}{}^{+} \times 1.4 = RFI \quad \textbf{(14-26)}$$

A word of caution: Both FE of Na^+ and the renal failure index are used only in the differential diagnosis of acute renal failure (acute kidney injury) with oliguria. For example, usual fractional excretion of Na^+ on regular salt intake in a normal person is usually less than 0.01, but this does not indicate the presence of prerenal azotemia.

FRACTIONAL REABSORPTION

Fractional reabsorption (FR) is the quantity of a substance reabsorbed expressed as a fraction of the filtered load. It is estimated from fractional excretion as follows:

$$FR = 1 - FE \quad \textbf{(14-27)}$$

FREE WATER CLEARANCE AND NEGATIVE FREE WATER CLEARANCE

Free water is the volume of water excreted in excess of the amount necessary to keep the urine isotonic to plasma. In other words, it is the volume of water that would have to be removed to make the urine isotonic. Free water clearance, like all other clearances, is expressed as volume per unit time, usually as mL/minute. To determine free water clearance, one first determines the total amount of solute in the urine (mOsm), which is measured from urine osmolality and urine volume ($U_{osm} \times V$), and then determines the amount of water required to hold that quantity of solute at the same osmolality as plasma, which is called osmolar clearance. Free water clearance is the difference between osmolar clearance and urine volume (Carroll, 1989).

$$\text{Osmolar clearance } (C_{osm}) = (U_{osm} \times V)/P_{osm} \quad \textbf{(14-28)}$$

$$\text{Free water clearance } (C_{H2O}) = V - C_{osm} \text{ or } C_{H2O}$$
$$= V - (U_{osm} \times V/P_{osm}) \quad \textbf{(14-29)}$$

If the urine is more concentrated than the plasma, then in a sense free water has been removed from isotonic urine, and the term negative free water clearance is used. In other words, it is the amount of water that would have to be added to make the urine isotonic.

$$\text{Negative free water clearance } (Tc_{H2O}) = C_{osm} - V \quad \textbf{(14-30)}$$

In the presence of normal renal function, the kidneys usually concentrate the urine, and therefore Uosm is greater than Posm, resulting in a negative value for C_{H2O}. On the other hand, loop diuretics block reabsorption of sodium chloride in the loop of Henle, interfering with both concentration and dilution of urine, and urine is approximately isotonic with little free water or negative free water.

BIOMARKERS OF ACUTE KIDNEY INJURY

Although many clinicians use acute kidney injury (AKI) and acute renal failure (ARF) almost interchangeably, the former term is used mainly when the actual injury occurs to the kidney, either biochemically or histologically, whereas the latter term encompasses all causes of acute renal failure, including prerenal azotemia and obstructive uropathy. This transition in terminology has called attention to the spectrum of disease much broader than previously emphasized with the realization that kidney injury exists along a continuum, ranging from minor injury with no change in serum creatinine or urine output to those who end up with end-stage renal disease requiring dialysis treatment (Honore, 2007). Furthermore, some authors use the term acute kidney injury to mean only acute tubular necrosis, which is a subset of causes of ARF, that includes all causes of intrinsic renal disease resulting in acute renal dysfunction, including acute glomerulonephritis and acute interstitial disease.

TABLE 14-3
RIFLE Criteria for Acute Kidney Injury

GFR and serum	Creatinine changes	Urine volume changes
R (Risk)	Increase in S-Creat >1.5×	Urine volume <0.5 mL/kg/hr >6 hr Decrease in GFR >25%
I (Injury)	Increase in S-Creat >2×	Urine volume <0.5 mL/kg/hr >12 hr Decrease in GFR >50%
F (Failure)	Increase in S-Creat >3× Decrease in GFR >75% S-Creat >4 mg/dL	Urine volume <0.3 mL/kg/hr >24 hr Anuria >12 hr
L (Loss)	Complete loss of kidney function >4 weeks	
E (ESRD)	End-stage kidney disease >3 months	

ESRD, End-stage renal disease; *GFR,* glomerular filtration rate; *S-Creat,* serum concentration of creatinine.

TABLE 14-4
New Classification for Acute Kidney Injury

Stage	Serum creatinine criteria	Urine output criteria
1	>0.3 mg/dL (26.4 μmol/L) or >150%–200%	<0.5 mL/kg for >6 hr
2	>200%–300%	<0.5 mL/kg for >12 hr
3	>300%, 4 mg/dL (354 μmol/L), or acute increase of >0.5 mg/dL	<0.3 mL/kg for >24 hr or anuria >12 hr

The Acute Kidney Injury Network was formed recently in an effort to improve the care of patients who are in AKI or at risk of developing AKI (Bellomo, 2004; Mehta, 2007). This group defined AKI as "functional or structural abnormalities or markers of kidney damage including abnormalities in blood, urine, or tissue tests or imaging studies present for less than three months." AKI is associated with retention of creatinine, urea, and other metabolic waste products that are normally excreted by the kidney. Although severe AKI may result in oliguria or even anuria, urine volume may be normal or even increased. Nevertheless, the committee defined AKI on the basis of increases in serum creatinine and changes in urine output. Initially, AKI was classified into five categories (Table 14-3); subsequently, this was simplified into three categories (Table 14-4).

Various biomarkers of AKI that are in clinical use include chemical components of serum or urine, imaging studies, and any other quantifiable parameter. The urine has yielded the most promising markers for the early detection of AKI. These urinary markers may be produced by the kidney as the result of kidney injury or may be filtered by the glomerulus but not well reabsorbed by the tubules because of injury to the tubules. Increased renal excretion is increased in part because some of these chemicals are produced in increasing amounts as the result of renal injury or conditions associated with renal injury. The advantage of these biomarkers over conventional markers of AKI such as serum creatinine and serum urea nitrogen is that the levels often increase long before any changes in serum creatinine or urea nitrogen or urine output occur (Lassning, 2004; Dennen, 2007). Earlier detection of renal injury can allow for better care of patients in anticipation of clinically overt AKI or perhaps can allow physicians to intervene by employing certain therapeutic measures, thereby preventing progression to overt AKI (Honore, 2007; Vaidya, 2008; Devarajan, 2008).

Thus, biomarkers of AKI help in diagnosing AKI before changes in serum creatinine are noted. These biomarkers also help to reveal the primary location of injury (i.e., proximal tubule, distal tubule, interstitium, or vasculature) to distinguish among different subtypes of AKI (e.g., prerenal, intrinsic renal, postrenal) and to delineate causes of AKI (e.g., ischemia, toxins, sepsis, or a combination) (Devarajan, 2008). Urine is likely to contain biomarkers of renal origin; therefore, urinary biomarkers are most widely used. On the other hand, urine samples are more prone to protein degradation, and their concentrations may be affected by urine flow rate. Serum samples are readily available and serum biomarkers are more stable, but serum biomarkers may reflect the systemic response to a disease process rather than specific organ involvement.

Conventional urinary biomarkers such as casts and fractional excretion of sodium are shown to be insensitive and nonspecific for the early recognition of AKI. Other traditional urinary biomarkers such as filtered high molecular mass proteins and tubular proteins or enzymes suffer from the lack of specificity. Application of innovative technologies has uncovered several new candidates that are promising biomarkers of AKI. Several of these candidates have now progressed through the first three stages of the biomarker development process and have entered phase IV drug trials. More than 20 biomarkers of AKI have been extensively studied; only the four most promising biomarkers are discussed here. These include neutrophil gelatinase–associated lipocalin (NGAL), interleukin (IL)-18, kidney injury molecule-1 (KIM-1), and liver-type fatty acid–binding protein (L-FABP). It seems that among these biomarkers, NGAL and L-FABP are likely the earliest biomarkers of AKI, and KIM-1 and IL-18 are later biomarkers that improve specificity (Honore, 2007).

KIDNEY INJURY MOLECULE-1

KIM-1 is a type I cell membrane glycoprotein that contains an immunoglobulin-like domain and a mucin domain in its extracellular region. KIM-1 mRNA levels increase more than any other known gene after kidney injury. The ectodomain of KIM-1 is shed into the urine after proximal tubular injury. In preclinical and clinical studies using several different models of kidney injury, urinary KIM-1 serves as an earlier diagnostic indicator of kidney injury when compared with any of the conventional biomarkers (e.g., plasma creatinine, BUN) (Han, 2008; Vaidya, 2008).

NGAL (to be discussed later) appears to be most sensitive at the earliest time points, but KIM-1 potentially adds specificity at later time points because expression of KIM-1 is limited to the kidney, and no systemic source of KIM-1 has been detected (Han, 2006; Ichimura, 2004). KIM-1 is induced in the kidney and is upregulated in the urine by a large number of nephrotoxins, including cyclosporine, cisplatin, cadmium, gentamicin, mercury, and chromium (Orfeas, 2009).

NEUTROPHIL GELATINASE–ASSOCIATED LIPOCALIN

NGAL is a 25 kDa protein initially identified bound to gelatinase in granules of the neutrophil. Other names for NGAL are lipocalin 2 and human neutrophil lipocalin.

NGAL is synthesized during a narrow window of granulocyte maturation in the bone marrow, but it also may be induced in epithelial cells in the setting of inflammation or malignancy. NGAL is upregulated and can be detected in the kidney and urine of mice 3 hours after cisplatin administration (Mishra, 2004; Mishra, 2006; Ronco, 2007); it has been proposed as an early biomarker for diagnosing AKI. A prospective study of pediatric and adult patients undergoing cardiopulmonary bypass for cardiac corrective surgery found urinary NGAL to be a powerful early marker of AKI, showing increased concentrations within 2–6 hours of the insult, preceding any increases in serum creatinine by 1–3 days (Bennet, 2008; Dent, 2007; Mishra, 2006; Devarajan, 2008). However, serum NGAL levels are known to increase in the setting of a number of inflammatory and infective conditions, and more studies are needed to determine the specificity of urinary NGAL for AKI in the setting of sepsis. NGAL has also been evaluated as a biomarker of AKI after contrast-induced nephropathy (Hirsch, 2007).

INTERLEUKIN-18

IL-18 is a cytokine, which is an interferon-γ-inducing factor. IL-18 activity has been described in a number of inflammatory diseases across a broad range of tissues. Renal IL-18 mRNA levels have been shown to be significantly upregulated in the proximal tubule following ischemia-reperfusion injury, inflammatory/autoimmune nephritis, and cisplatin-induced nephrotoxicity. Urinary IL-18 levels are elevated in patients with AKI and delayed graft function (Parikh, 2006), compared with normal subjects and patients with prerenal azotemia, urinary tract infection, chronic renal insufficiency, and nephrotic syndrome. Increased urinary IL-18 was found to be an early marker of AKI, preceding changes in serum creatinine by 1–2 days, and was an independent predictor of death (Washburn, 2008).

FATTY ACID–BINDING PROTEIN

FABPs are 14–15 kDa cytoplasmic proteins abundantly expressed in all tissues and particularly in the proximal convoluted and straight tubule of the kidney (Maatman, 1992; Negishi, 2009). Urinary L-FABP has been identified in preclinical and clinical models of AKI, and has been found to be a potential biomarker in a number of pathologic conditions, including chronic kidney disease, diabetic nephropathy, immunoglobulin A nephropathy, and contrast nephropathy. In a model of cisplatin-induced AKI, increased shedding of urinary L-FABP occurred within the first 24 hours, whereas a rise in serum creatinine was not detectable until after 72 hours of cisplatin treatment. Urinary L-FABP levels were significantly increased before the increase in serum creatinine only in those patients who developed AKI post contrast dye. In a recent study involving 12 living-related kidney transplant patients, a significant direct correlation was found between urinary L-FABP level and both peritubular capillary blood flow and ischemic time of the transplanted kidney. In AKI following cardiac surgery, increases in serum creatinine occurred 2–3 days post surgery, whereas urine L-FABP levels increased at 4 hours after surgery (Yamamoto, 2007; Portilla, 2008).

The previous discussion concerns the overall mechanisms by which the kidneys control extracellular volume and how measurements of specific chemicals, such as BUN and creatinine, in serum and urine are used to measure renal function. The kidneys regulate extracellular volume by regulating the concentrations of ions that are retained in blood. Disorders of renal function frequently result in electrolyte imbalances, and disorders of electrolytes often can be at least partially corrected by normally functioning kidneys.

In the following sections, three common disorders of electrolytes and acid-base balance, namely, disorders of potassium, disorders of sodium, water, and ADH, and finally disorders of acid-base equilibrium, are discussed.

Disorders of Potassium

Total body K^+ in hospitalized adults is about 43 mEq/kg of body weight, and only about 2% of this is found in the ECF. When potassium concentrations across the cell membrane are in electrochemical equilibrium, the gradient of K^+ is the main determinant of, and is also predicted by, the membrane potential (Em) according to the Nernst equation (Veech, 1995; Goldman, 1943):

$$\text{Em (mV)} = -61 \text{ Log}\left(\text{intracellular } K^+/\text{extracellular } K^+\right) \quad \textbf{(14-31)}$$

The normal ratio of (intracellular K^+/extracellular K^+) for the skeletal muscle is about 30; therefore, normal Em is −90 mV. The membrane potential tends to increase with hypokalemia and to decrease with hyperkalemia. In hypokalemia, both intracellular and extracellular K^+ tend to decrease, but the extracellular concentration tends to decrease proportionately more than the intracellular concentration. Hence, the ratio of (intracellular K^+/extracellular K^+) tends to increase. In hyperkalemia, the membrane potential tends to decrease because an increase in the extracellular K^+ is proportionately greater than that in the intracellular K^+. However, in dogs with severe hypokalemia, the resting membrane potential of the skeletal muscle is actually reduced rather than increased, indicating that the permeability of the membrane to potassium may change with severe hypokalemia (Bilbrey, 1973).

CONTROL OF TRANSCELLULAR FLUX OF POTASSIUM

Transmembrane electrical gradients cause diffusion of cellular K^+ out of cells and Na^+ into cells. Because the Na^+-K^+ pump, which reverses this process, is stimulated by insulin (Benziane, 2008) and catecholamines (through β-2-adrenergic receptors) (Putcha, 2007), alterations in levels of these hormones can affect K^+ transport and its serum levels (Meister, 1993; Feraille, 1999; Sweeney, 1998; Goguen, 1993; Putcha, 2007).

Cells can act as buffers. In acidosis, cells can take up H^+ ions in exchange for K^+ ions, and, in alkalosis, cells extrude H^+ ions in exchange for K^+ ions. These effects are summarized in Figure 14-2. The effects of acidosis and alkalosis on transcellular K^+ flux depend not only on the pH but also on the type of anion that accumulates. In general, metabolic acidosis causes greater K^+ efflux than respiratory acidosis. Metabolic acidosis due to inorganic acids (e.g., sulfuric acid, hydrochloric acid) causes greater K^+ efflux than that due to organic acids (e.g., lactic acid, keto acids). The reason is that organic anions accumulate substantially in the cell, as well as in the ECF, whereas inorganic anions accumulate mainly in the ECF. Acidosis causes efflux of K^+ from the cell because of the shift of H^+ into the cell in exchange for K^+. A modifying factor appears to be anion

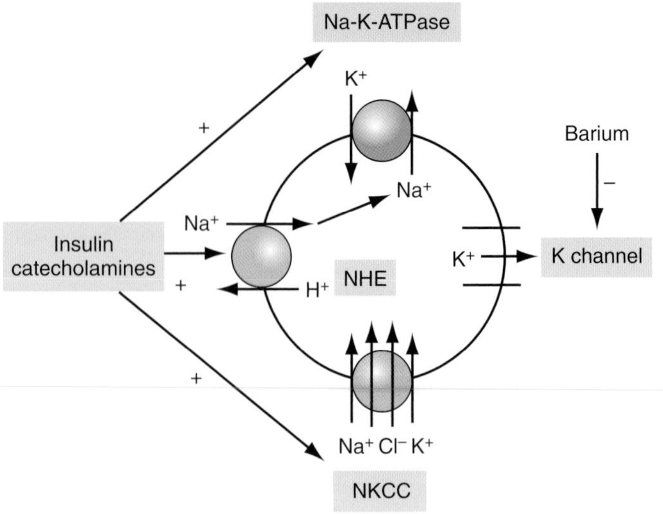

Figure 14-2 Control of transcellular movement of potassium. Potassium enters the cell through Na^+-K^+-ATPase (stimulated by beta-adrenergic agents or insulin) or through the sodium-potassium-chloride co-transporter (NKCC) (stimulated by insulin and catecholamines). Stimulation of the sodium-hydrogen exchanges (NHE) by high extracellular pH, catecholamines, or insulin increases intracellular sodium concentration, which in turn stimulates Na^+-K^+-ATPase and thereby increases intracellular movement of potassium.

accumulation in the cells. In organic acidosis, much of H^+ entering the cell is balanced by organic anions; therefore efflux of K^+ is prevented. In respiratory acidosis, the anion that accumulates in the cell to balance the incoming H^+ is bicarbonate (Perez, 1981). This explains why little K efflux from the cell occurs in respiratory acidosis. Alkalosis tends to lower serum K^+ because, as noted above, H^+ leaves cells in exchange for K^+, which enters the cells. As with acidosis, K^+ influx varies with the type of alkalosis. In respiratory alkalosis, with its lower partial pressure of carbon dioxide (pCO_2) and attendant lower intracellular bicarbonate by cellular buffering, K^+ influx is not as great as in metabolic alkalosis. When pH is kept normal with proportionately increased concentration of bicarbonate and pCO_2, K^+ tends to move into the cells; accumulation of bicarbonate in the cell must be accompanied by Na^+ and K^+. Similarly, when pH is kept normal with proportionately low bicarbonate and low pCO_2, K^+ tends to move out of the cells.

CONTROL OF RENAL EXCRETION OF POTASSIUM

About 90% of the daily K^+ intake (60–100 mEq) is excreted in the urine, and 10% in the stool. Potassium filtered at the glomerulus is mostly (70%–80%) reabsorbed by active and passive mechanisms in the proximal tubule. In the ascending limb of Henle's loop, K^+ is reabsorbed together with Na^+ and Cl^- by the sodium potassium chloride cotransporter. Because the quantities of Na^+ and Cl^- are far greater than K^+, most of the reabsorbed K^+ diffuses back to the lumen to maintain the reabsorption of Na^+ and Cl^-, but net reabsorption of K^+ still occurs in the thick ascending limb of Henle. The concentration of K^+ at the beginning of the distal convoluted tubule is about 1 mmol/L with fluid volume of about 25 L. Thus, K^+ excreted in the urine is largely what is secreted into the cortical collecting duct by mechanisms shown in Figure 14-3. Na^+-K^+-ATPase located on the basolateral side of the cortical collecting duct pumps K^+ into the cell, while it pumps Na^+ out of the cell. The luminal Na^+ enters the cell through the epithelial sodium channel (ENaC), providing a continuous supply of Na^+. The reabsorption of Na^+ through these steps is an absolute requirement of secretion of potassium in the cortical collecting duct. Aldosterone is the main regulator of the expression of ENaC on the luminal membrane through its genomic effect on the activity of serum and glucocorticoid-regulated kinase 1 (Fakitsas, 2007; Zhang, 2007, 2008), and therefore is the main determinant of renal excretion of potassium. The negative luminal potential that develops as a result of sodium reabsorption through ENaC causes reabsorption of Cl^- through the paracellular channels. Because Na^+ reabsorption is not followed one to one by Cl^- reabsorption, the charge imbalance occurs and is corrected by secretion of K^+ through a specialized K^+ channel, the renal outer medullary K (ROMK)

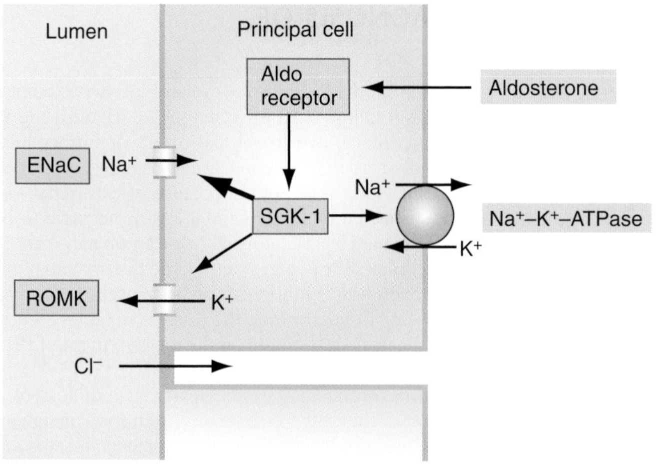

Figure 14-3 Control of potassium secretion at the cortical collecting duct. Sodium enters from the luminal fluid into the cell through the epithelial sodium channel (ENaC) and is transported out of the cell through the Na^+-K^+-ATPase on the basolateral membrane. These processes create the luminal electrical potential that is more negative than the electrical potential of the peritubular fluid. The electrical charge imbalance created by sodium reabsorption causes paracellular reabsorption of chloride, and allows entry of potassium into the lumen through the renal outer medullary K (ROMK), a potassium channel. Binding of aldosterone to its receptor results in upregulation of SGK-1 (serum- and glucocorticoid-regulated kinase-1), which, in turn, results in increased expression of ENaC on the luminal membrane. Upregulation of SGK-1 also stimulates ROMK and Na^+-K^+-ATPase. All three effects help to increase potassium secretion. (*ENaC,* Epithelial Na channel; *ROMK,* renal outer medulla K channel.)

channel (Yue, 2009; Wang, 2009). Thus, aldosterone increases K^+ secretion by increasing the passive entry of Na^+ from the lumen to the cell through increased expression of ENaC on the luminal membrane. The resulting increase in cellular concentration of sodium indirectly stimulates Na^+-K^+-ATPase, but aldosterone also directly stimulates Na^+-K^+-ATPase and ROMK activities (Yue, 2009). The peritubular K^+ concentration and the pH also influence K^+ secretion through their effects on Na^+-K^+-ATPase activity. High serum K^+ concentration and alkaline pH stimulate enzyme activity, and low serum K^+ and acidic pH inhibit this activity.

When Na^+ is accompanied by anions that are less permeable than Cl^-, luminal negativity is increased, resulting in enhanced K^+ secretion. Examples of such anions include sulfate, bicarbonate, and anionic antibiotics such as penicillin and carbenicillin. Bicarbonate in the tubular fluid enhances K^+ secretion, not only through its effect as a poorly reabsorbable anion, but also by enhancing ROMK activity. An increase in renal K^+ excretion in patients who vomit and develop metabolic alkalosis may be explained by this mechanism. ADH also increases the luminal K^+ channel activity. K^+ secretion is increased by rapid urine flow by maintaining a low luminal K^+ concentration. Renal K^+ wasting during osmotic diuresis could be explained by this mechanism. A high urine flow also activates another secretory K channel called maxi-K channel (Wang 2009). The more Na^+ is presented to the distal nephron, the more can be absorbed and the more K^+ can be secreted "in exchange." The increased Na^+ delivery to the collecting duct also increases renal K^+ excretion by its effect on urine flow (Giebisch, 1998; Halperin, 1998; Wang, 2009). A higher urine flow allows greater secretion of potassium into the luminal fluid, while reducing back-diffusion of potassium into the tubular cells, because the luminal concentration would be lower for a given amount of potassium secreted (Oh, 2003).

PLASMA RENIN ACTIVITY, PLASMA ALDOSTERONE CONCENTRATION, AND ABNORMALITIES IN POTASSIUM METABOLISM

Because abnormalities in plasma renin activity (PRA) and plasma aldosterone (PA) are frequently responsible for or are caused by abnormalities in K^+ metabolism, it is important to understand their relationships (Bock, 1992; Hollenberg, 2000; Laragh, 1995; Hall, 1991). The general principles are as follows: (1) Expansion of effective arterial volume caused by a primary increase in aldosterone (primary aldosteronism) or by other mineralocorticoids will cause suppression of PRA. When mineralocorticoids other than aldosterone are present in excess, they induce retention of salt and water, and the resulting volume expansion leads to suppression of both PRA and PA; and (2) a primary increase in PRA will always lead to an increase in PA (secondary aldosteronism). On the other hand, a primary defect in aldosterone secretion will cause volume depletion and will secondarily increase PRA. PRA may be high because of the following:

1. Volume depletion secondary to renal or extrarenal salt loss
2. Abnormality in renin secretion (e.g., reninoma [hemangiopericytoma of afferent arteriole], malignant hypertension, renal artery stenosis)
3. Increased renin substrate production (e.g., oral contraceptives)

Elevations in serum K^+ can directly stimulate the adrenal cortex to release aldosterone. When renin is deficient primarily, aldosterone is always low (e.g., hyporeninemic hypoaldosteronism).

TABLE 14-5
Causes of Hypokalemia

Intracellular Shift
Alkalosis
Hypokalemic periodic paralysis
Beta-2-adrenergic agonists
Barium poisoning
Insulin
Nutritional recovery state
Poor Intake
Gastrointestinal loss
Vomiting
Diarrhea
Intestinal drainage
Laxative abuse
Excessive Renal Loss
Primary aldosteronism (adrenal adenoma or hyperplasia); PRA is suppressed
Secondary aldosteronism (increase in aldosterone is secondary to increase in renin)
Malignant hypertension
Renal artery stenosis
Reninoma
Diuretics
Bartter's syndrome
Gitelman's syndrome
Excess mineralocorticoids other than aldosterone (e.g., Cushing's syndrome, ACTH-producing tumor, licorice)
Chronic metabolic acidosis
Delivery of poorly reabsorbed anions to the distal tubule (e.g., bicarbonate, ketone anions, carbenicillin)
Miscellaneous causes: Magnesium deficiency, acute leukemia, Liddle's syndrome

ACTH, Adrenocorticotropic hormone; *PRA,* plasma rennin activity.

CAUSES AND PATHOGENESIS OF HYPOKALEMIA

Hypokalemia occurs by one of three main mechanisms: intracellular shift, reduced intake, or increased loss (Table 14-5). Because the intracellular K^+ concentration greatly exceeds the extracellular concentration, the K^+ shift into the cell can cause severe hypokalemia with little change in its intracellular concentration (Clemessy, 1995; Matsumura, 2000; Rakhmanina, 1998; Jordan, 1999; Ogawa, 1999; Cannon, 2002; Jurkat-Rott, 2000; Bradberry, 1995; Steen, 1981). Alkalosis, insulin, and β-2-agonists can cause hypokalemia by stimulating Na^+-K^+-ATPase activity (Matsumura, 2000; Putcha, 2007). Defective activity of dihydropyridine-responsive Ca^{++} channels and potassium channels has been documented in some patients (Jurkat-Rott, 2000; Bradberry, 1995; Fontaine, 2008). A defect in the sodium channel is also known to cause hypokalemic periodic paralysis, but a defect in the sodium channel sometimes causes hyperkalemic or normokalemic paralysis (Fontaine, 2008). In barium poisoning, K^+ accumulates in the cell and hypokalemia develops because of inhibition of the K^+ channel by barium, resulting in inhibition of K^+ efflux from the cell (Bradberry, 1995), in the face of continuous cellular uptake of K^+ through the action of Na^+-K^+-ATPase. K^+ accumulates in the cell along with anions as the cell mass increases during nutritional recovery because K^+ is the main intracellular cation.

Poor intake of K^+ by itself is rarely a cause of hypokalemia because it is usually accompanied by poor caloric intake, which causes catabolism and release of K^+ from the tissues (Steen, 1981). Vomiting and diarrhea are common causes of hypokalemia (Steen, 1981). Diarrhea causes direct K^+ loss in the stool, but in vomiting, hypokalemia is mainly the result of K^+ loss in the urine rather than in the vomitus, because vomiting causes metabolic alkalosis, and the subsequent renal excretion of bicarbonate leads to renal K^+ wasting.

Renal loss of K^+ is by far the most common cause of hypokalemia. With rare exceptions, hypokalemia due to increased renal wasting of potassium can be attributed to increased activity of aldosterone or other mineralocorticoids. Increased aldosterone could be a primary disorder as in primary hyperaldosteronism, or it could be due to increased renin secretion as in secondary hyperaldosteronism. Even with increased aldosterone, renal K^+ wasting occurs only if it is accompanied by adequate distal delivery of Na^+ (Torpy, 1998; Stowasser, 1995; Abdelhamid, 1995; Litchfield, 1997; Vargas-Poussou, 2002; Finer, 2003; Kunchaparty, 1999; Seyberth, 1985; Krozowski, 1999; Heilmann, 1999). In primary aldosteronism, distal delivery of Na^+ is increased because increased NaCl reabsorption in the cortical collecting duct by the action of aldosterone inhibits salt reabsorption in the proximal tubule as the result of volume expansion. In secondary aldosteronism, hypokalemia occurs only in conditions that are accompanied by increased distal Na^+ delivery. Examples of secondary hyperaldosteronism that result in hypokalemia include renal artery stenosis, diuretic therapy, and malignant hypertension, and congenital defects in renal salt transport such as Bartter's syndrome and Gitelman's syndrome. It must be noted that, in the absence of extrarenal salt loss, renal salt excretion ultimately equals salt intake even in conditions of increased aldosterone or aldosterone deficiency, because prolonged imbalance between intake and output is impossible; without eventual balance, an individual could not survive volume excess or volume depletion, which would occur inevitably. However, when salt reabsorption is increased at the mineralocorticoid active site (i.e., cortical collecting duct), the amount of salt delivered to this site must be increased when the final salt output eventually equals the intake; when balance is achieved, an increased amount is delivered to the site, and an increased amount is reabsorbed, so that the normal amount equaling the intake is excreted; ultimate balance is possible only when the amount entering the body equals the amount leaving the body. This is the mechanism by which salt delivery to the aldosterone site is increased in primary hyperaldosteronism, as well as in all cases of secondary hyperaldosteronism that are associated with hypokalemia (Oh, 2003).

Bartter's syndrome, a rare potassium-losing autosomal recessive disorder, is caused by defective NaCl reabsorption in the thick ascending limb of Henle (Sakakida, 2003; Finer, 2003; Kunchaparty, 1999; Seyberth, 1985; Schultheis, 1998), whereas in Gitelman's syndrome, the defect in NaCl reabsorption occurs in the distal convoluted tubule (Schultheis, 1998). Defective Na^+ reabsorption proximal to the aldosterone effective site in these conditions results in increased delivery of Na^+ to the cortical collecting duct, and hence in hypokalemia. Heart failure does not lead to hypokalemia despite secondary hyperaldosteronism, unless distal delivery of Na^+ is increased by diuretic therapy.

Substances that are not aldosterone but have mineralocorticoid activity include corticosterone, deoxycorticosterone, and synthetic mineralocorticoid such as 9-α-fluodrocortisone (Florinef). With licorice intake, mineralocorticoid activity is increased, because cortisol, which is normally a potent mineralocorticoid but has a negligible concentration in the cortical collecting duct cells owing to rapid breakdown by the enzyme 11-β-hydroxy steroid dehydrogenase, maintains a high intracellular concentration, because compounds in licorice inhibit the enzyme (Krozowski, 1999; Heilmann, 1999).

Among rare causes of renal potassium wasting that are not accompanied by increased mineralocorticoid activity is Liddle's syndrome. Liddle's syndrome is a congenital disorder that is characterized by increased ENaC activity in the collecting duct in the absence of increased aldosterone, resulting in increased sodium reabsorption and enhanced potassium secretion; aldosterone secretion is reduced because salt retention due to increased ENaC activity leads to physiologic suppression of renin secretion (Warnock, 2001). In chronic metabolic acidosis, hypokalemia develops, probably because reduced proximal reabsorption of NaCl allows increased delivery of NaCl to the distal nephron. Direct stimulation of aldosterone secretion by metabolic acidosis (Gyorke, 1991) appears to be an additional mechanism that contributes to hypokalemia.

DIFFERENTIAL DIAGNOSIS OF HYPOKALEMIA

The first step in the differential diagnosis is to measure urinary excretion of K^+. If urinary K^+ excretion is low (<20 mEq/day or <0.01 mEq/mg of creatinine), the cause is low intake, extrarenal loss of K^+, or intracellular shift. Superacute development of hypokalemia usually suggests intracellular shift as the mechanism. The most common cause of extrarenal loss is diarrhea, which can be suspected by history and a low or negative urine anion gap (urine $Na^+ + K^+ -$ urine Cl^-); the normal urine anion gap is about 40 mmol/24 hours. Intracellular shift is suggested by the history and clinical findings. If urinary excretion is normal or increased (urine K^+ >30 mEq/day or 0.02 mEq/mg of creatinine), the cause is renal loss. Once a renal cause is suspected, the next step should be the measurement of PRA and plasma aldosterone.

High PRA and high aldosterone suggest secondary hyperaldosteronism, which includes diuretic therapy, renal artery stenosis, malignant hypertension, renin producing tumors, and hereditary defects in renal salt transport (Bartter's syndrome and Gitelman's syndrome). Blood pressure would be normal in subjects with Bartter's syndrome or Gitelman's syndrome, and in a normotensive person on diuretic therapy. Blood pressure would be high in all other conditions and in a hypertensive subject on diuretic therapy. Low PRA and high plasma aldosterone suggest primary hyperaldosteronism, which is caused by adrenal adenoma or bilateral hyperplasia. If PRA and plasma aldosterone are low, likely conditions include Liddle's syndrome, apparent mineralocorticoid excess states (both hereditary and drug- or licorice-induced), 11-hydroxylase deficiency, and 17-hydroxylase deficiency. Reduction in renal K^+ excretion will be achieved with spironolactone in all these conditions except for Liddle's syndrome, which will respond to ENaC blockers such as triamterene and amiloride (Oh, 2003).

CAUSES AND PATHOGENESIS OF HYPERKALEMIA

Hyperkalemia may be caused by one of three mechanisms: (1) shift of potassium from the cells to the ECF (Wasserman, 1997; Perazella, 1999; McIvor, 1985; McIvor, 1987; Emser, 1982), (2) increased potassium intake, or (3) reduced renal potassium excretion (Table 14-6). Hyperkalemic familial periodic paralysis, administration of succinylcholine in paralyzed patients (Fontaine, 2008; Delphin, 1987; Cooperman, 1970; Gronert, 1975; Larach, 1997), administration of cationic amino acids such as arginine and lysine, use of epsilon-aminocaproic acid (this chemical is neutral in its charge, but becomes a cationic amino acid in the cell),

TABLE 14-6
Causes of Hyperkalemia

Pseudohyperkalemia

Thrombocytosis, severe leukocytosis, use of tourniquet with fist exercise, in vitro hemolysis

True Hyperkalemia

Due to extracellular shift:
- Acute acidosis (more with inorganic acidosis)
- Catabolic states
- Periodic paralysis
- Succinylcholine (esp. in those with muscular dystrophy)
- Cationic amino acids
- Vigorous exercise
- Digitalis intoxication

Due to excessive ingestion: Rare if renal excretion of K^+ is normal

Decreased renal excretion:
- Hypoaldosteronism: Addison's disease; selective hypoaldosteronism (hyporeninemic hypoaldosteronism, heparin, congenital adrenal enzyme deficiencies, angiotensin-converting enzyme inhibitors)
- Tubular unresponsiveness to aldosterone (pseudohypoaldosteronism type I and II): Congenital, salt-losing nephropathy
- Potassium-sparing diuretics: Spironolactone, amiloride, triamterene
- Antibiotics with ENaC-blocking effects: Pentamidine, trimethoprim
- Antirejection medications: Cyclosporine, tacrolimus
- Severe dehydration

ENaC, Epithelial sodium channel.

rhabdomyolysis or hemolysis, and acute acidosis all cause hyperkalemia by extracellular potassium shift. Rhabdomyolysis and hemolysis cause hyperkalemia only when they are accompanied by renal failure. Although hyperkalemia is not as predictable with organic acidosis as with inorganic acidosis in experimental situations, hyperkalemia is common in diabetic ketoacidosis and phenformin-induced lactic acidosis. The more frequent occurrence of hyperkalemia in clinical organic acidosis may be explained by the longer duration of acidosis and the presence of other factors such as dehydration and renal failure and insulin deficiency in diabetic ketoacidosis (Perez, 1981).

Hyperkalemia can also occur in severe digitalis intoxication by extracellular shift of potassium as digitalis inhibits the Na^+-K^+ -ATPase pump. The ability of the kidney to excrete potassium is so great that hyperkalemia rarely occurs solely on the basis of increased intake of potassium. Thus, hyperkalemia is almost always due to impaired renal excretion. Three major mechanisms of diminished renal potassium excretion are known: reduced aldosterone or aldosterone responsiveness, renal failure, and reduced distal delivery of sodium. Aldosterone deficiency may be part of a generalized deficiency of adrenal hormones (e.g., Addison's disease), or it may represent a selective process (e.g., hyporeninemic hypoaldosteronism). Hyporeninemic hypoaldosteronism is the most common cause of all aldosterone deficiency states, and is by far the most common cause of chronic hyperkalemia among nondialysis patients (Oh, 1974; Phelps, 1980). Selective hypoaldosteronism can also occur with heparin therapy, which inhibits steroid production in the zona glomerulosa (Phelps, 1980). In patients with reduced aldosterone secretion, any agent that limits the supply of renin or angiotensin II may provoke hyperkalemia, for example, angiotensin-converting enzyme inhibitors, nonsteroidal anti-inflammatory agents, and beta blockers. The latter compound also interferes with potassium transport into cells. Renal tubular unresponsiveness to aldosterone (pseudohypoaldosteronism) may be congenital, but it is more often an acquired defect. This defect may involve only potassium secretion (pseudohypoaldosteronism type II), or sodium reabsorption and potassium secretion (pseudohypoaldosteronism type I) (Wilson, 2001; Wilson, 2003; Sebastian, 1981; Brautbar, 1978). Most cases of so-called "salt losing nephritis" appear to represent the latter defect. Severe volume depletion may cause hyperkalemia despite secondary hyperaldosteronism because volume depletion causes a marked reduction in delivery of sodium to the cortical collecting duct.

Pseudohyperkalemia is defined as an increase in potassium concentration only in the local blood vessel or in vitro, and has no physiologic consequences (Stewart, 1965; Stewart, 1979; Kim, 1990; Zaltzman, 1982; Bellevue, 1975; Iolascon, 1999; Hayward, 1999; Delaunay, 1999; Don, 1990). Prolonged use of a tourniquet with fist exercises can increase the serum potassium level by as much as l mmol/L. Thrombocytosis and severe leukocytosis cause pseudohyperkalemia through potassium release from the platelets and white blood cells, respectively, during blood clotting (see Table 14-6).

DIFFERENTIAL DIAGNOSIS OF HYPERKALEMIA

The first step in the differential diagnosis of hyperkalemia should be to rule out pseudohyperkalemia. Electrocardiographic (ECG) abnormalities of hyperkalemia are absent in pseudohyperkalemia, but the absence of ECG changes does not rule out true hyperkalemia because ECG changes are rare in chronic hyperkalemia. Pseudohyperkalemia should be suspected when conditions known to cause pseudohyperkalemia, such as thrombocytosis or in vitro hemolysis (pink serum), exist. In pseudohyperkalemia due to thrombocytosis, both serum and plasma K^+ should be obtained simultaneously. Once pseudohyperkalemia is ruled out, the next step is to differentiate among the three major causes of hyperkalemia: increased K^+ intake, shift of K^+ from the cell, and impaired renal excretion. Measurement of a 24 hour urine K^+ will distinguish increased intake from the other two causes. Although hyperkalemia due to a shift of K^+ from the cell would result in increased urinary excretion of K^+, renal excretion of K^+ is often not increased because conditions that impair renal excretion of K^+ often coexist. A careful dietary history will be sufficient to rule out hyperkalemia due to increased intake, unless the patient is deliberately trying to deceive the physician.

Chronic hyperkalemia is almost always due to impaired renal excretion, and a 24 hour urine K^+ measurement is rarely needed to prove impaired renal excretion of K^+ as the cause of hyperkalemia. Among the renal causes of hyperkalemia, acute renal failure is the most common cause of acute hyperkalemia, and this will be obvious from the serum creatinine and BUN. For differential diagnosis of chronic hyperkalemia of renal causes, the first step is to measure plasma renin activity, plasma aldosterone, and urinary excretion of Na^+ and K^+. A very low urinary Na^+ and a low K^+ in the absence of polyuria suggest that the aldosterone effect is normal; in this setting, K^+ excretion is impaired by the reduced availability of Na^+ and a marked reduction in collecting duct urine flow. Markedly increased proximal reabsorption of Na^+ due to low effective vascular volume, such as severe congestive heart failure, can cause hyperkalemia by such a mechanism. If urinary Na^+ is adequate (>20 mmol/L), plasma renin activity and aldosterone should be measured.

Low PRA and low aldosterone suggest hyporeninemic hypoaldosteronism, whereas high PRA and low aldosterone suggest a primary defect in aldosterone secretion such as Addison's disease, heparin therapy, and aldosterone biosynthetic defect. When PRA and aldosterone are both increased, the likely culprit is (1) pseudohypoaldosteronism, (2) very low Na^+ delivery to the cortical collecting duct, or (3) drugs that impair ENaC function or aldosterone action, such as potassium-sparing diuretics (e.g., amiloride, triamterene, spironolactone) and certain antibiotics (e.g., trimethoprim, pentamidine) (Oh, 2003). The presence of low PRA and high aldosterone in the setting of hyperkalemia is not a very likely combination, but it has been observed occasionally in a patient with a genetic defect of an enzyme WNK kinase, called pseudohypoaldosteronism type II (also known as Gordon's syndrome). The defect in WNK kinase causes increased NaCl transport in the distal convoluted tubule, resulting in hypertension and a defect in potassium secretion (Goldbang, 2005; Yang, 2007; San-Cristobal, 2008). The condition is a mirror image of Gitelman's syndrome, and is characterized by low PRA (due to hyperabsorption of NaCl) and low aldosterone, resulting in hyperkalemia; however, a variant of the condition is characterized by a separate severe defect in K secretion, resulting in hyperkalemia despite normal or sometimes high aldosterone. In such a patient, a high plasma aldosterone occurs in response to hyperkalemia, but renin is low because of volume expansion. By far, the most common cause of chronic hyperkalemia due to impaired renal excretion of potassium is hyporeninemic hypoaldosteronism, which is caused by chronic renal insufficiency of primarily tubulointerstitial disease (Phelps, 1980). The suggested mechanism is primary renal salt retention caused by renal disease, which leads to physiologic suppression of renin secretion and hence of aldosterone, ultimately resulting in hyperkalemia often accompanied by hypertension (Oh, 1974).

DISORDERS OF WATER, SODIUM, AND ANTIDIURETIC HORMONE METABOLISM

REGULATION OF THIRST AND ADH RELEASE

A rise in effective osmolality shrinks the hypothalamic osmoreceptor cells, which then stimulate the thirst center in the cerebral cortex and stimulate ADH production in the supraoptic and paraventricular nuclei. Conversely, a decline in effective osmolality causes swelling of the osmoreceptor cells, resulting in inhibition of ADH production. ADH produced in the hypothalamus is carried through long axons and is secreted from the posterior pituitary gland (McKinley, 1998; Ibata, 1999). Stimulation and inhibition of osmoreceptor cells affect both production by the hypothalamus and secretion of ADH by the pituitary.

Regulation of ADH secretion by a change in effective osmolality is extremely sensitive. It was thought that ADH secretion in response to a change in effective osmolality was so sensitive that a change of only 2%–3% would stimulate ADH secretion sufficiently to result in a maximally concentrated urine, and a decline in plasma osmolality of only 2%–3% would produce maximally dilute urine (<100 mOsm/L) (Bourque, 1997; Olsson, 1983). However, a more recent study has shown that changes in serum sodium concentration by 2%–3% in venous blood are accompanied by a much greater change in arterial serum sodium concentrations when oral intake of water is rapid. For example, drinking 20 mL/kg of water in 15 minutes reduced arterial serum sodium by about 8 mmol/L and resulted in rapid water diuresis, but the same amount given by slow sipping did not produce water diuresis. With rapid intake of water, venous sodium concentration was about 4 mmol/L higher than that of arterial blood. The osmoreceptors of course would respond to arterial, rather than venous, sodium concentration (Shafiee, 2005).

ADH release is also regulated by nonosmotic factors. Low effective vascular volume provokes thirst and ADH release, and high effective vascular volume has the reverse effects (Wells, 1998; Aguilera, 2000; Nielsen, 2002; Schrier, 1979). These effects are mediated through baroreceptors and some humoral factors. Alpha-catecholamines suppress and β-catecholamines enhance ADH output. Prostaglandins inhibit the effects of ADH on the kidney. Angiotensin II stimulates thirst and ADH release. Lack of glucocorticoid enhances ADH action on the kidney and increases ADH release. ADH in the pituitary gland acts similarly to corticotropin-releasing hormone and stimulates production of adrenocorticotropic hormone (ACTH). Cortisol in turn inhibits the release of ADH (Bahr, 2006). Physical and emotional stress (e.g., major surgery) increase ADH output, possibly in part through emetic stimuli, which are common complications of major surgery and are attributed to the effects of anesthesia and surgical trauma. Many drugs affect ADH release or its action; ethanol inhibits the output of ADH. Lithium and demeclocycline inhibit the effect of ADH on the kidney. Chlorpropamide increases the action of ADH on the kidney. Some drugs may operate through the emetic stimulus, which is one of the most potent physiologic stimuli to ADH release. The urine may become osmotically concentrated in the absence of ADH, if effective vascular volume is very low. The combination of reduced GFR and enhanced proximal reabsorption of filtrate reduces urine flow to the collecting duct so greatly that even the limited permeability of the membrane permits withdrawal of sufficient amounts of water to concentrate urine.

Three classes of ADH receptors are known: V1 receptors cause a rise in vasomotor tone and certain metabolic effects, V2 receptors are associated with antidiuresis, and V3 receptors cause stimulation of ACTH secretion in the anterior pituitary (Ma, 1999; Mouri, 1993; Bahr, 2006). The antidiuretic effect of ADH is mediated by promoting expression of aquaporin-2 on the luminal membrane of the collecting duct to make the tubule permeable to water, and by stimulating reabsorption of salt on the outer medullary thick ascending limb of Henle's loop (Knepper, 1997). Vasopressinase, which normally breaks down ADH, may be increased in pregnancy and may cause polyuria (Molitch, 1998). 1-Deamino-8-D-arginine vasopressin, a synthetic analog of arginine vasopressin, which resists vasopressinase, is useful in polyuria of pregnancy.

URINE CONCENTRATION AND DILUTION

About 180 L of water is filtered daily; 150 L is reabsorbed in the proximal tubule, and about 5 L in the descending limb of Henle of cortical nephrons. About 25 L of dilute urine is delivered to the ascending limb of Henle. Because the tubules from this point to the beginning of the cortical collecting duct are water impermeable, the volume remains unchanged at 25 L, but the osmolality decreases progressively to about 60–80 mOsm/L. Because of the conditional expression of aquaporin-2 on the luminal membrane of collecting ducts, which depends on the action of ADH, no water reabsorption occurs in the cortical and outer medullary collecting ducts when ADH is absent (Fig. 14-4). However, a small amount of water (about 5 L during water diuresis) is reabsorbed in the terminal portion of the inner medullary collecting duct, even when ADH is absent. Aquaporins may be present constitutively in this part of the nephron, or the membrane may be permeable to water without ADH. During maximal water diuresis, the combined effect of further salt reabsorption in the collecting duct and of small additional reabsorption of water in the inner medullary collecting duct allows final excretion of about 20 L of dilute urine at an osmolality of about 40 mOsm/L. It must be noted that maximal urine output during water diuresis depends greatly on salt intake, because the maximal urine output can never exceed the amount delivered into the ascending limb of Henle. Even with mild salt restriction (e.g., 2 g/day), the resulting mild volume depletion increases reabsorption of salt and water in the proximal tubule sufficiently to reduce volume delivery to the ascending limb of Henle's loop to 12–15 L/day, and final maximal urine output to 10–12 L/day.

In the presence of maximal ADH, urine can be concentrated to as high as 1200 mOsm/L as water is reabsorbed in the cortical and medullary collecting duct, with urine volume as low as 0.5 L/day (see Fig. 14-4). In the proximal tubule, water reabsorption passively follows salt reabsorption, whereas in the descending thin limb, water reabsorption is unaccompanied by salt reabsorption but occurs in response to salt reabsorption that takes place in the ascending limb. The osmolality of urine as it enters the ADH effective site (i.e., the cortical collecting duct) is the same during water diuresis and during antidiuresis, and the value is quite low, at about 60 mOsm/L. Urine osmolality is reduced by continuous salt reabsorption without water reabsorption in the ascending thin and thick limbs of Henle

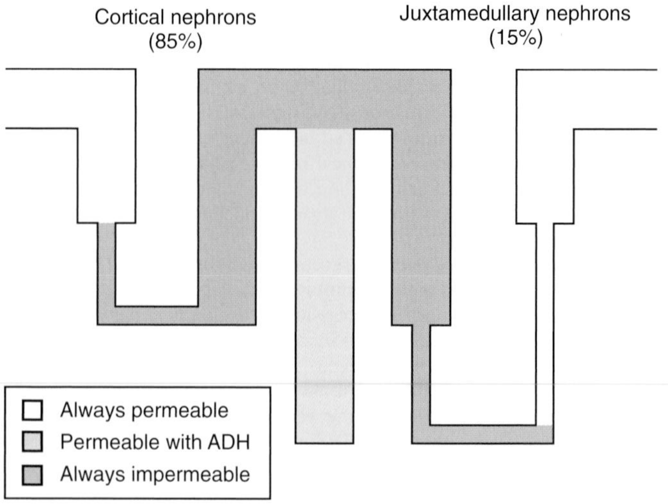

Figure 14-4 Transport of water at various nephron sites. The proximal tubules are always water permeable because aquaporins are constitutively expressed at these sites. The descending thin limbs of juxtamedullary nephrons (15% of all nephrons) also show expression of aquaporins and are therefore water permeable, but the descending thin limb of cortical nephrons (85%) lacks aquaporins and is water impermeable. The ascending thin limb and the ascending thick limb of Henle, the distal convoluted tubule, and the connecting tubule do not express aquaporins, and are always water impermeable. The collecting duct is water permeable when ADH action allows expression of aquaporins. *ADH,* Antidiuretic hormone.

and in the distal convoluted tubule and connecting tubule. Urine concentration is achieved by reabsorption of water in the collecting duct through transcellular reabsorption of water through the cells of the collecting duct; water first enters the cell through the luminal membrane, and then leaves the cell through the basolateral membranes. Diffusion of water through each membrane requires expression of aquaporins. Aquaporin-3 is constitutively expressed in the basolateral membrane of the cortical collecting duct, and aquaporin-4 is constitutively expressed in the basolateral membrane of the medullary collecting duct. Entry of water in the collecting duct, both cortical and medullary, from the lumen into the cell requires expression of aquaporin-2 on the luminal membrane; this is an ADH-mediated mechanism.

An increase in urine osmolality from a very low value at the beginning of the cortical collecting duct to an isotonic value at the corticomedullary junction requires only the presence of ADH and tubular responsiveness to ADH, because the interstitium of the cortex is always isotonic. However, the reabsorption of water in the medullary collecting duct requires not only the ADH action but also the hypertonicity of the medullary interstitium. Maintenance of medullary hypertonicity is achieved by the countercurrent multiplication mechanism. In short, the medullary interstitial fluid becomes progressively hypertonic, starting at the isotonic level at the corticomedullary junction and increasing to a level of about 1200 mOsm/L at the tip of the papilla. Medullary hypertonicity in the outer medullary area is achieved by active reabsorption of salt in the thick ascending limb of Henle that is not accompanied by water reabsorption. In the inner medulla, salt reabsorption in the thin ascending limb of Henle (the inner medulla lacks the thick ascending limb of Henle) is passive, and occurs with the help of urea that diffuses from the inner medullary collecting duct. The mechanism by which urea contributes to the concentration of urine is still hotly debated, and is beyond the scope of this discussion. Achievement of medullary hypertonicity is attributed to the countercurrent mechanism, which had been traditionally explained in the following manner: (1) selective reabsorption of salt from the ascending limbs of Henle without water reabsorption, (2) selective reabsorption of water from the descending limb of Henle, and (3) countercurrent arrangement of the descending and ascending limbs of Henle by bending of the tubule at the tip of Henle's loop (Hogg, 1986; Pallone, 2003; de Rouffignac, 1987; Oh, 1997; Sands, 1996; Burg, 1995; Schmidt-Nielson, 1977; Knepper, 1983; Hogg, 1978; Gregor, 1983).

It is now clear, however, that the previous sequence of events to achieve progressive hypertonicity of fluid in the descending thin limb of Henle is applicable to only a small fraction of nephrons, namely, the juxtamedullary nephrons, which represent only 15% of the total nephron population (Zhai, 2007). The cortical nephrons, representing 85% of the nephron population in humans, do not express aquaporins on the thin descending limb of Henle; therefore, those tubular segments are water impermeable. The progressive urine concentration that occurs along the descending limb of Henle occurs instead sodium and chloride entry (Halperin, 2008). This would create a wasted effort, in that sodium entering the descending limb will have to be reabsorbed again in the ascending limb, but the absence of water permeability of the descending limb of Henle allows relatively constant urine flow rates entering the distal convoluted tubule during water diuresis and antidiuresis (Halperin, 2008).

POLYURIA

Polyuria is arbitrarily defined as urine volume in excess of 2.5 L/day. Two types of polyuria are known: osmotic diuresis and water diuresis (Carroll, 1989).

Osmotic Diuresis

Osmotic diuresis is defined as increased urine output due to an excessive rate of solute excretion; the commonly accepted level of solute excretion for osmotic diuresis is a rate in excess of 60 mOsm/hour, or 1440 mOsm/day, in the adult (Carroll, 1989). Urine osmolality is usually greater than that of plasma, but it may be lower than plasma osmolality when it coexists with water diuresis. Solutes commonly responsible for osmotic diuresis include glucose, urea, mannitol, radiopaque media, and NaCl.

Water Diuresis

Water diuresis is characterized by excretion of a large volume of dilute urine. The polyuria is caused by reduced reabsorption of water in the collecting duct. Reasons for reduced water reabsorption in the collecting duct include lack of ADH (Vokes, 1988; Leggett, 1999; Siggaard, 1999; Rutishauser, 1999; Ito, 1997; Halperin, 2001) and unresponsiveness to ADH (nephrogenic diabetes insipidus). Nephrogenic diabetes insipidus (DI) can be congenital or acquired (Boone, 2009). Congenital nephrogenic DI may be due to a defective ADH receptor or to an aquaporin defect (Weir, 1992; Lam, 2000; Nielsen, 2002; Spruce, 1984; Li, 2001; Canada, 2003; Marples, 1995).

Lack of ADH, which may be congenital or acquired (Levine, 1987; Vokes, 1988; Arai, 1999; Leggett, 1999; Siggaard, 1999; Rutishauser, 1999; Ito, 1997), is due to primary deficiency (central diabetes insipidus) or to physiologic suppression by low serum osmolality (primary polydipsia, dipsogenic diabetes insipidus) (Levine, 1987; Rendell, 1978; Hariprassad, 1980). Deficiency of ADH can be mild, moderate, or severe. When ADH deficiency is partial, urine osmolality may be fairly close to normal. In rare instances, ADH is made but cannot be released in response to a rise in body fluid osmolality because of a defect involving osmoreceptor cells (e.g., hypothalamic lesions) (Leggett, 1999; Siggaard, 1999; Rutishauser, 1999; Ito, 1997; Loh, 2008). In such instances, ADH may be released in response to hypovolemia or to drugs. During pregnancy, ADH deficiency may be caused by excessive production of vasopressinase (gestational DI) (Molitch, 1998). Causes of polyuria, including central and nephrogenic DI, are listed in Table 14-7.

Primary polydipsia is defined as increased water drinking that is not caused by physiologically stimulated thirst (i.e., hyperosmolality or volume depletion) (Rendell, 1980; Hariprassad, 1980; Levine, 1987). Primary polydipsia is usually psychogenic in origin, hence the term psychogenic polydipsia. In contrast, polydipsia in patients with diabetes insipidus or in diabetic patients with severe glycosuria is secondary polydipsia, which is due to thirst stimulation in response to hyperosmolality. In primary polydipsia, increased urine output is due to physiologic suppression of ADH secretion; hence, serum Na^+ is usually in the low range of normal. In contrast, in central or nephrogenic DI, serum sodium is in the high normal range. Occasionally, serum sodium is frankly low in severe primary polydipsia, indicating that the capacity of the gastrointestinal (GI) tract to absorb water exceeds the capacity of the kidney to excrete water.

TABLE 14-7
Causes of Polyuria Due to Water Diuresis

Lack of ADH
Central DI: Congenital or acquired (idiopathic cell degeneration, tumors and granulomas, surgery, trauma, infarction, and infection of the pituitary or hypothalamus)
Dipsogenic: Psychogenic, organic brain disease, iatrogenic
Gestational DI: Excess vasopressinase
Failure of the Kidney to Respond to ADH (Nephrogenic DI)
Congenital nephrogenic DI: A defect in ADH receptor, a defect in aquaporin expression
Chronic renal failure
Acquired nephrogenic DI: Lithium toxicity, demeclocycline toxicity, methoxyflurane toxicity, amyloidosis, light-chain nephropathy, hypercalcemia, hypokalemia, obstructive uropathy

ADH, Antidiuretic hormone; *DI,* diabetes insipidus.

CAUSES AND PATHOGENESIS OF HYPONATREMIA (Table 14-8)

Hyponatremia, the most common electrolyte disorder, is defined as reduced plasma sodium concentration to a value less than 135 mmol/L. Generally, clinical concern arises when the concentration is less than 130 mmol/L.

The term pseudohyponatremia, as discussed in Chapter 8, is applied to a spurious reduction in serum sodium concentration caused by a systematic error in measurement. The most common, yet not widely known, cause of pseudohyponatremia is in vitro hemolysis, a well known cause of pseudohyperkalemia (Oh, 2003). Because cell lysis does not change osmolality of the plasma, any rise in serum potassium must be met by a reciprocal decrease in serum sodium. However, the reduction in serum Na^+ from hemolysis is somewhat greater than the increase in serum K^+, by a factor of 1.3, because hemoglobin released from the red cells cause additional reduction in serum Na^+, as in hyperproteinemia; this error occurs because hemoglobin is mostly a protein, and it has the same effect as hyperproteinemia in displacing plasma water. This additional error occurs only when samples are diluted before the measurement of serum sodium, just as pseudohyponatremia of hyperlipidemia and hyperproteinemia occurs only when samples are diluted before the measurement.

Other causes of pseudohyponatremia include hyperlipidemia, hyperproteinemia, and increased viscosity of the plasma (Weisberg, 1989; Milionis, 2002). The error in measurement in pseudohyponatremia due to hyperproteinemia and hyperlipidemia results from dilution of the sample, as occurs with the common technique of indirect ion–specific electrode measurement. In pseudohyponatremia, plasma osmolality, which is

TABLE 14-8
Classification of Hyponatremia by Pathogenesis

Due to Na^+ Loss
Thiazide diuretics in the presence of ADH
Saline infusion in the presence of ADH
Due to Water Retention
Excessive water intake: Primary polydipsia
Advanced renal failure
Appropriate ADH secretion: Edema-forming states (CHF, nephritic syndrome, ascites), salt depletion states (GI loss, diuretic therapy, aldosterone deficiency, hypothyroidism)
Inappropriate ADH secretion
Tumors: Cancers of the lung, pancreas, duodenum, ureter, bladder, prostate, lymphoma, thymoma, mesothelioma, Ewing's sarcoma
Intrathoracic causes: Bacterial and viral pneumonia, tuberculosis, lung abscess, aspergillosis, asthma, positive-pressure breathing, pneumothorax, cystic fibrosis
CNS abnormalities: Encephalitis, meningitis, brain tumors and abscess, head trauma, subdural hematoma, cerebrovascular accidents, Guillain-Barré syndrome, acute intermittent porphyria, brain atrophy, schizophrenia, hydrocephalus, acute psychosis, multiple sclerosis, cavernous vein thrombosis, lupus cerebritis, Shy-Drager syndrome, Rocky Mountain spotted fever, delirium tremens, seizure disorder
Drugs: Arginine vasopressin and its analogs, sulfonylureas, tricyclic antidepressants, clofibrate, carbamazepine, vinca alkaloids, cyclophosphamide, selective serotonin reuptake inhibitors, opiates, phenothiazines, haloperidol
Surgical and emotional stress
Emesis
Endocrine causes: Glucocorticoid deficiency, myxedema

ADH, Antidiuretic hormone; *CHF,* congestive heart failure; *CNS,* central nervous system; *GI,* gastrointestinal.

customarily measured without dilution, is normal. However, low plasma sodium concentration with normal plasma osmolality need not indicate the presence of pseudohyponatremia; true hyponatremia may be accompanied by a normal plasma osmolality because of the accumulation of some abnormal osmols or abnormal concentrations of normal nonsodium osmols such as urea and glucose. In hypergammaglobulinemic states, such as multiple myeloma, serum sodium may be falsely low because of displacement of serum water by gamma globulins, but the sodium concentration is also truly low because cationic charges of gamma globulins displace sodium to maintain electrical neutrality (Weisberg, 1978; Weisberg, 1989). Hyponatremia induced by acute hyperglycemia is not pseudohyponatremia because sodium concentration in the ECF is truly low; this occurs as a result of water shift from the cell caused by hyperglycemia. Serum sodium is decreased by 1.6 mmol/L for every 100 mg/dL rise in serum glucose, as discussed earlier (Katz, 1973).

The immediate mechanisms responsible for a reduction in extracellular sodium concentration are (1) shift of water from the cell caused by accumulation of extracellular solutes, such as glucose, other than sodium salts (Agraharkar, 1997; Akan, 1996; Agarwal, 1994); (2) retention of excess water in the body; (3) loss of sodium (Gowrishankar, 1998; Sonnenblick, 1993); and (4) shift of sodium into the cells. The appropriate physiologic response to hypotonicity is suppression of ADH release, which leads to rapid excretion of excess water and correction of hyponatremia. Persistence of hyponatremia therefore indicates the failure of this compensatory mechanism. In most instances, hyponatremia is maintained because the kidney fails to produce water diuresis, but sometimes ingestion of water in excess of the limits of normal renal excretion is responsible. Reasons for the inability of the kidney to excrete water include (1) renal failure, (2) reduced delivery of glomerular filtrate to the distal nephron, and (3) inappropriate presence of ADH.

The mechanism for impaired water excretion in renal failure is obvious and needs no further explanation. Reduced distal delivery of filtrate results from low glomerular filtration rate and enhanced proximal tubular reabsorption of salt and water when effective vascular volume is reduced.

In most cases of hyponatremia, the main reason for the fall of serum sodium is abnormal retention of water, which is ingested as such or is administered as hypotonic fluids. However, in certain clinical settings, reduction in serum sodium can occur without the administration or ingestion of hypoto nic fluid. The latter phenomenon occurs when urine is excreted with sodium and potassium at concentrations that exceed the sum of serum concentrations of the two ions, for example, if urine contains sodium at 140 mmol/L and potassium at 100 mmol/L, the combined concentration would be 240 mmol/L, which is far greater than the sum of serum sodium and potassium. Excretion of hypertonic urine with regard to sodium and chloride occurs in the setting of increased urinary sodium excretion in the presence of ADH, as occurs in patients with syndrome of inappropriate ADH (SIADH) who are given an infusion of normal saline, or in individuals who are given a thiazide diuretic. Excretion of such urine may cause hyponatremia without net water retention.

Loss of potassium has the same effect on serum sodium as loss of sodium. It must be noted that the development of hyponatremia with excretion of hypertonic urine occurs only when hypertonicity of urine is caused by increased excretion of sodium or potassium. Hypertonic urine by increased excretion of urea would not produce hyponatremia for obvious reasons.

The physiologic requirement for the excretion of hypertonic urine is an increased amount of ADH in the presence of marked sodium diuresis (Halperin, 2001; Halperin, 2008). Clinical examples include (1) the patient who receives a large amount of isotonic fluid in the immediate postoperative period, (2) the patient with SIADH who is treated with isotonic fluid, and (3) the patient who receives a thiazide diuretic (Gowrishankar, 1998; Sonnenblick, 1993). Normal dilution of urine requires delivery of adequate amounts of fluid to the diluting segment and reabsorption of solute without water at that segment. Increased body fluid tonicity causes release of ADH, which allows reabsorption of water in the collecting duct, helping to restore body fluid tonicity. The response is considered appropriate when ADH is released in response to hypertonicity of body fluid. However, release of ADH in the presence of hyponatremia is also considered appropriate if the effective vascular volume is reduced. The term syndrome of inappropriate ADH secretion, or SIADH, is therefore reserved for ADH secretion that occurs despite hyponatremia and normal or increased effective vascular volume.

Causes of SIADH include tumors, pulmonary diseases such as tuberculosis and pneumonia, central nervous system diseases, and drugs (Bartter, 1967; Ajaelo, 1998; Fallon, 1998; Gold, 1983; Hensen, 1995; North, 2000; Arlt, 1997; Johnson, 1997; Argani, 1997; Ferlito, 1997; Friedmann, 1994). Hyponatremia in clinical states associated with reduced effective vascular volume such as congestive heart failure and cirrhosis of the liver is caused by a combination of reduced delivery of fluid to the distal nephron and increased secretion of ADH. Salt restriction and diuretics increase the severity of hyponatremia. ADH secretion may be present despite hyponatremia in myxedema (Macaron, 1978) and glucocorticoid deficiency states. It is not clear, however, whether ADH secretion in these conditions is truly inappropriate or appropriate. Finally, mild hyponatremia may be caused by "resetting of the osmostat" at an osmolality lower than the usual level. In such cases, urine dilution occurs normally when the plasma osmolality is reduced below the reset level. Resetting of the osmostat is a form of SIADH (Robertson, 2006; Decaux, 2009), in that ADH secretion occurs inappropriately at hyponatremic levels in the absence of reduced effective vascular volume. Patients with chronic debilitating diseases such as pulmonary tuberculosis often manifest this phenomenon (Hill, 1990).

Some authorities believe the existence of a cerebral salt wasting syndrome, which is defined as renal loss of salt caused by humoral substances released in response to cerebral disorders such as acute subarachnoid hemorrhage. These patients are thought to manifest volume depletion that results in hyponatremia. However, careful analysis of existing data does not support the existence of such an entity, and those cases labeled as cerebral salt wasting syndrome probably represents cases of inappropriate ADH secretion (Oh, 2003).

CAUSES AND PATHOGENESIS OF HYPERNATREMIA

Hypernatremia is defined as an increased sodium concentration in plasma water, and is generally diagnosed at serum sodium levels >145 mmol/L. Whereas hyponatremia may not be accompanied by hypoosmolality, hypernatremia is always associated with an increased effective plasma osmolality, and hence with a reduced cell volume. However, the extracellular volume in hypernatremia may be normal, decreased, or increased.

Hypernatremia is caused by loss of water, gain of sodium, or both (Table 14-9). Loss of water may be due to increased loss or reduced intake, and gain of sodium may be due to increased intake or to reduced renal excretion. Increased loss of water can occur through the kidney (e.g., in diabetes insipidus, in osmotic diuresis), the gastrointestinal tract (e.g., gastric suction, osmotic diarrhea), or the skin. Reduced water intake occurs most commonly in comatose patients or in those with a defective thirst mechanism. Less frequent causes of reduced water intake include continuous vomiting, lack of access to water, and mechanical obstruction to the esophagus (e.g., esophageal tumor, stricture). Gain of sodium in a conscious person does not result in hypernatremia because a proportional amount of water is retained to maintain normal body fluid osmolality as long as the person has normal perception of thirst, is able to drink water, and water is available. Whereas the main physiologic defense against hyponatremia is increased renal water excretion, the most effective physiologic

TABLE 14-9
Causes of Hypernatremia

Reduced Water Intake
Defective thirst due to altered mental state or thirst center defect
Inability to drink water
Lack of access to water
Increased Water Loss (Water Intake Must Be Impaired)
Gastrointestinal loss: vomiting, osmotic diarrhea
Cutaneous loss: sweating and fever
Respiratory loss: hyperventilation and fever
Renal loss: diabetes insipidus, osmotic diuresis
Increased Sodium Content of the Body (Water Intake Must Be Impaired)
Increased oral or intravenous intake of sodium chloride
Hypertonic saline or sodium bicarbonate infusion
Ingestion of sea water
Renal salt retention, usually in response to primary water deficit

defense against hypernatremia is increased drinking of water in response to thirst. Because thirst is such an effective and sensitive defense mechanism against hypernatremia, it is virtually impossible to increase serum sodium by more than a few mmol/L if the water drinking mechanism is intact. Therefore, in a patient with hypernatremia, there will always be reasons for reduced water intake. These reasons include a defective thirst mechanism, inability to drink water, and unavailability of water (Marazuela, 2007). Excessive gain of sodium leading to hypernatremia is usually iatrogenic (e.g., from hypertonic saline infusion, accidental entry into maternal circulation during abortion with hypertonic saline, administration of hypertonic sodium bicarbonate during cardiopulmonary resuscitation, treatment of lactic acidosis). Reduced renal sodium excretion leading to sodium gain and hypernatremia usually occurs in response to dehydration caused by primary water deficit. Water depletion due to diabetes insipidus, osmotic diuresis, or insufficient water intake leads to secondary sodium retention through volume-mediated activation of sodium-retaining mechanisms. Consequently, in chronic hypernatremia, sodium retention plays a more important role than water loss (Carroll, 1989; Oh, 2003). Of course, net sodium retention is possible only if sodium is ingested or given.

Whether hypernatremia is due to sodium retention or to water loss can be determined by examination of the patient's volume status. For example, if a patient with a serum sodium concentration of 170 mmol/L has no obvious evidence of dehydration, one must conclude that hypernatremia is caused by water loss and by salt retention. Increasing the serum sodium to 170 mmol/L by water deficit alone would require loss of more than 20% of total body water.

Acid-Base Disorders

BICARBONATE AND CARBON DIOXIDE BUFFER SYSTEM

All body buffers are in equilibrium with protons (H^+) and therefore with pH, as is shown in the following equation (Ramsay 1965):

$$pH = pK + \log A^-/HA, \text{ where } A^- \text{ is a conjugate base of an acid HA} \quad \textbf{(14-32)}$$

Because HCO_3^- and CO_2 are the major buffers of the body, pH is typically expressed as a function of their ratio, as discussed in Chapter 8 and shown in the Henderson-Hasselbalch equation as follows:

$$pH = 6.1 + \log HCO_3^-/pCO_2 \times 0.03 \quad \textbf{(14-33)}$$

where 6.1 is the pK of the HCO_3^- and CO_2 buffer system, and 0.03 is the solubility coefficient of CO_2.

The equation can be further simplified by combining the two constants, pK and solubility coefficient of CO_2 (Carroll 1989):

$$pH = 6.1 + \log HCO_3^-/pCO_2 \times 0.03 = 6.1 + \log 1/0.03 + \log HCO_3^-/pCO_2 = 7.62 + \log HCO_3^-/pCO_2 = 7.62 + \log HCO_3^- - \log pCO_2 \quad \textbf{(14-34)}$$

When H^+ is expressed in nM instead of a negative log value (pH), pCO_2 can be related to HCO_3^- in an equation, such as the following:

$$H\,(nM) = 24 \times pCO_2(mmHg)/HCO_3^-(mM) \quad \textbf{(14-35)}$$

The Henderson-Hasselbalch equation indicates that pH depends on the ratio of HCO_3^-/pCO_2. pH increases when the ratio increases (alkalosis), and pH decreases when the ratio decreases (acidosis). The ratio may be increased by an increase in HCO_3^- (metabolic alkalosis) or by a decrease in pCO_2 (respiratory alkalosis). The ratio may be decreased by a decrease in HCO_3^- (metabolic acidosis) or by an increase in pCO_2 (respiratory acidosis).

DEFINITIONS OF ACID AND BASE

Arrhenius's definition: An acid is a substance that increases the concentration of hydrogen ion (H^+) when dissolved in water, and a base is a substance that increases the concentration of hydroxyl ion (OH^-) when dissolved in water.

Bronsted and Lowry's definition: An acid is a substance that donates a proton in a reaction, and a base is a substance that accepts a proton in a reaction.

Lewis's definition: An acid is a molecule or ion that accepts a pair of electrons to form a covalent bond, and a base is a molecule that donates a pair of electrons for a covalent bond. The definition of Bronsted-Lowry is the most widely accepted and most relevant clinically.

WHOLE BODY ACID-BASE BALANCE

Metabolic acidosis occurs because net acid production is increased, or because net acid excretion is reduced. Because a typical modern diet results in acid production, the normal function of the kidney is to excrete acid to remain in acid-base balance. For these reasons, proper understanding of disorders of acid-base balance requires knowledge of the sources of acid production and of the mechanisms by which acids are disposed of.

Net Acid Production

On a typical American diet, the daily production of nonvolatile acid is about 90 mmol/day. The main acids are sulfuric acid (about 40 mEq/day), which originates from the metabolism of sulfur-containing amino acids such as methionine and cysteine, and incompletely metabolized organic acids (about 50 mEq/day) (Oh, 1992). The source of sulfuric acid is protein, but the sulfur content varies greatly with the types of protein that are ingested (Lemann, 1959). In general, proteins of animal sources (meat, fish, milk, and egg) contain higher amounts of sulfur for a given amount of protein than proteins of plant origin (cereal, beans, and nuts). The sulfur content is much greater in fruits, vegetables, and potatoes, but these food groups are not important sources of protein in the amounts usually eaten. The total amount of acid/alkali content depends not only on the sulfur content but also on the alkali content of food, which is present mainly as salts of organic acids. When both factors are considered, milk has a net alkali value, whereas meat and fish have a net acid value. As a whole, fruits and vegetables contain a large quantity of net alkali because they contain large quantities of organic anions. The total quantity of organic acids normally produced is much more than 50 mEq/day, but the bulk of organic acids produced in the body is metabolized; only a small amount is lost in the urine as organic anions that escape metabolism (e.g., citrate) or as a metabolic end product (e.g., urate). On typical American diets, the amount of alkali absorbed from the GI tract is about 30 mEq/day (Lemann, 1959; Oh, 1992). Thus, the net amount of acid produced daily can be estimated as follows:

$$\text{Net acid production} = (\text{urine sulfate} + \text{urine organic anions}) - \text{Net alkali absorbed from GI tract} \quad \textbf{(14-36)}$$

Determination of the net alkali (or acid) content of diet is based on the metabolic fates of the chemicals in the diet after absorption into the body, rather than on its in vitro states. For example, citric acid in food is considered neutral because it would be metabolized to CO_2 and water in the body, whereas K^+ citrate is an alkali because it would be converted to K^+ bicarbonate after metabolism. Similarly, arginine Cl^- is an acid because metabolism of arginine in the body would result in the formation of HCl (Lemann, 1959). Thus, the net alkali value of a diet is best determined by the total number of noncombustible cations (Na^+, K^+, Ca^{++}, and Mg^{++}) in comparison with the total number of noncombustible anions (Cl^- and P):

$$\text{Net alkali content} = (Na^+ + K^+ + Ca^{++} + Mg^{++}) - (Cl^- + 1.8\ P) \quad \textbf{(14-37)}$$

All units are expressed as mEq/day, except for P, which is expressed as mmol/day multiplied by 1.8, because phosphate valence depends on pH, and at pH 7.4 the average valence of phosphate is 1.8. Only the above six ions are considered in the equation because other noncombustible ions are present in negligible amounts in normal food. Sulfate is not included here because sulfate is derived almost entirely from the metabolism of sulfur-containing amino acids, and is not ingested as such. The amount of alkali absorbed from the food is not equal to the amount present in the food because the absorption of divalent noncombustible ions, Ca^{++}, Mg^{++}, and P, is incomplete. Hence, traditionally, measurement of the net GI alkali absorption required analysis of the food, as well as the stool, which necessitated prolonged collection of stool (Oh, 1992; Relman, 1961). Thus, the net GI alkali absorption is expressed as follows:

$$\text{Net GI alkali absorbed} = \text{Net alkali of food} - \text{Net alkali of stool} \quad \textbf{(14-38)}$$

Analysis of the food for the measurement of net alkali content is cumbersome, and analysis of the stool is even more cumbersome. Such analyses typically require admitting the patient to a special metabolic unit. An alternative method has been developed to measure net GI alkali absorption. In this method, urine electrolytes, instead of diet and stool electrolytes, are measured. The method is based on the principle that noncombustible ions absorbed from the GI tract would eventually be excreted in the urine, and therefore, that the individual amounts of these electrolytes excreted in the urine would equal those absorbed from the GI tract. Hence,

$$\text{Net GI alkali absorption} = \text{urine}\left(Na^+ + K^+ + Ca^{++} + Mg^{++}\right) - \text{urine}\left(Cl^- + 1.8\ P\right) \quad \textbf{(14-39)}$$

Twenty-four hour urine can be collected in outpatient settings, while patients are eating their usual diets. The amount of net alkali absorbed on a typical American diet as stated earlier, 30 mEq/day, was measured by analysis of urine electrolytes using the above formula (Oh, 1992).

Net Acid Excretion

The most important function of the kidney in acid-base homeostasis is excretion of acid, which is tantamount to generation of alkali. Acid is excreted in the form of NH_4^+ and titratable acid. Another important function of the kidney is excretion of HCO_3^-. Usually, the main function of renal excretion of HCO_3^- is prevention of metabolic alkalosis, but a small amount of bicarbonate is normally excreted in the urine (about 10 mEq/day). Thus, net acid excretion, which is tantamount to net renal production of alkali, can be determined by subtracting HCO_3^- excretion from acid excretion (Lemann, 1959).

$$\begin{aligned}\text{Net acid excretion} &= \text{Acid excretion} - HCO_3^-\ \text{excretion}\\ &= NH_4^+ + \text{Titratable acid} - HCO_3^- \end{aligned} \quad \textbf{(14-40)}$$

Normally, about two thirds of acid excretion occurs in the form of NH_4^+, but in acidosis, NH_4^+excretion may increase by as much as 10-fold. Excretion of titratable acid is usually modest because of the limited amount of buffer that produces titratable acid (i.e., phosphate, creatinine, and urate) but may be increased markedly in disease states (e.g., BB in diabetic ketoacidosis). Maintenance of acid-base balance requires that net acid production equals net acid excretion. Metabolic acidosis develops when net acid production exceeds net acid excretion, and metabolic alkalosis develops when net acid excretion exceeds net acid production.

METABOLIC ACIDOSIS

Classification

All metabolic acidoses result from reduction in the bicarbonate content of the body, with two minor exceptions: acidosis resulting from dilution of body fluid by administration of a large amount of saline solution that does not contain alkali (dilution acidosis), and acidosis that results from shift of H^+ from the cell. Reduction in bicarbonate content may be due to a primary increase in acid production (*extrarenal acidosis*) or to a primary reduction in net acid excretion (*renal acidosis*) (Table 14-10). In this classification, nonrenal loss of bicarbonate or an alkali precursor is considered as part of increased acid production. In extrarenal acidosis, net acid excretion is markedly increased as the kidney compensates to correct the acidic pH. On the other hand, net acid excretion may be restored to normal in chronic renal acidosis as acidosis stimulates renal H^+ excretion. Normal net acid excretion in the presence of acidic pH suggests a defect in renal acid excretion, and therefore renal acidosis. If the renal acid excretion capacity is normal, net acid excretion should be markedly increased in the presence of extrarenal acidosis (Gennari, 2008, Goulet, 2009).

Renal Acidosis

Renal acidosis is further classified into two types: uremic acidosis and renal tubular acidosis (RTA). In uremic acidosis, reduced net acid excretion results from reduced nephron mass or generalized renal dysfunction (i.e., chronic or acute renal failure), whereas in RTA, reduction in net acid excretion results from a specific tubular dysfunction in acid excretory function. Because development of renal acidosis depends on the rate of net acid excretion, as well as the rate of net acid production, and the latter varies greatly according to the diet of individuals, the level of renal failure at which uremic acidosis develops depends on the dietary intake of acid. On a usual diet, uremic acidosis typically develops when GFR falls below 20% of normal (Bommer, 1996; Oh, 1992).

TABLE 14-10
Causes of Metabolic Acidosis According to Net Acid Excretion

Renal Acidosis: Absolute or Relative Reduction in Net Acid Excretion
Uremic acidosis
Renal tubular acidosis
Distal renal tubular acidosis (type I)
Proximal renal tubular acidosis (type II)
Aldosterone deficiency or unresponsiveness (type IV)
Extrarenal Acidosis: Increase in Net Acid Excretion
Gastrointestinal loss of bicarbonate
Ingestion of acids or acid precursors: Ammonium chloride, sulfur
Acid precursors or toxins: Salicylate, ethylene glycol, methanol, toluene, acetaminophen, paraldehyde
Organic acidosis
L-Lactic acidosis
D-Lactic acidosis
Ketoacidosis

Three types of RTA are known: Type I RTA, also called classical RTA or distal RTA, is characterized by an inability to reduce urine pH below 5.5. Because acidification of urine to a very low urine pH occurs at the collecting duct, the likely site of defect is the collecting duct, which is a part of the distal nephron, hence the term distal RTA. Because H^+ secretion in the collecting duct is also impaired in type IV RTA, some authors consider both type I and type IV RTA a form of distal RTA. However, the terms type I RTA and distal RTA are used synonymously. Type I RTA can develop as a primary disorder or secondary to drug toxicity, tubulointerstitial renal disease, or other renal disease (Rodriguez-Soriano, 2002).

Type II RTA, also called proximal RTA, has defective proximal bicarbonate reabsorption characterized by a reduced renal bicarbonate threshold. Urine can be made free of bicarbonate and acidified normally when serum bicarbonate decreases to a sufficiently low level. Most patients with proximal RTA have evidence of generalized proximal tubular dysfunction (i.e., Fanconi's syndrome) manifested by bicarbonaturia, aminoaciduria, glycosuria, phosphaturia, and uricosuria. Of these, renal glycosuria (glycosuria in the presence of normal blood glucose) is most useful in diagnosing Fanconi's syndrome. Type II RTA may be a primary disorder or may occur secondary to genetic or acquired renal dysfunction. Hypokalemia is a characteristic finding of both type I and type II RTA, but it tends to be more severe in type I than in type II. Type III RTA, a term used to describe a hybrid form of types I and II RTA, is no longer in use.

Type IV RTA is caused by aldosterone deficiency or tubular unresponsiveness to aldosterone, resulting in impaired renal tubular potassium secretion and hence hyperkalemia. Although reduced H^+ secretion in the collecting duct plays a role, the major mechanism of acidosis in type IV RTA is hyperkalemia-induced impairment in ammonia production in the proximal tubule. Type IV RTA is far more common than type I or type II RTA, and the most common cause of type IV RTA is hyporeninemic hypoaldosteronism. Diabetic nephropathy is the most common cause of hyporeninemic hypoaldosteronism leading to type IV RTA (Oh, 1974; Phelps, 1981).

Organic Acidosis

Among external causes of acidosis, overproduction of endogenous acids, especially lactic acid and ketoacid, is the most important mechanism. Only marked overproduction, well in excess of 1000 mmol/day of lactic acid, leads to acidosis because of the enormous capacity to metabolize organic acids. When organic acids react with bicarbonate, organic anions and CO_2 are formed. Retention of organic anions results in increased anion gap. Retained organic anions are potential bicarbonate; when they are metabolized, bicarbonate is regenerated. However, renal excretion of organic anions results in hyperchloremic acidosis with normal anion gap. Thus, loss of organic anions in the urine is tantamount to loss of bicarbonate. If an organic anion produced from organic acid is entirely retained, subsequent metabolism of the entire amount will result in complete recovery of the lost alkali. Characteristically, organic acidosis is rapid in onset and in recovery.

Lactic Acidosis. Lactic acid is produced from pyruvic acid by the action of the enzyme lactate dehydrogenase (LD) and the cofactor NADH.

TABLE 14-11
Causes of L-Lactic Acidosis

Type A Lactic Acidosis Due to Tissue Hypoxia
Circulatory shock
Severe hypoxemia
Heart failure
Severe anemia
Grand mal seizure
Type B Lactic Acidosis (No Tissue Hypoxia)
Acute alcoholism
Drugs and toxins (e.g., phenformin, antiretroviral drugs, salicylate intoxication)
Diabetes mellitus
Leukemia
Deficiency of thiamine or riboflavin
Idiopathic

Metabolism of lactic acid requires its conversion back to pyruvic acid, using the same enzyme and NAD^+ as a cofactor. For this reason, both production and metabolism of lactic acid are influenced by the same factors; increased concentrations of pyruvic acid and increased ratios of $NADH/NAD^+$ increase lactic acid production and reduce its metabolism. Consequently, in most cases of lactic acidosis, lactic acid production is increased, while its metabolism is reduced. By far the most common cause of lactic acidosis is tissue hypoxia, which results from circulatory shock, severe anemia, severe heart failure, acute pulmonary edema, cardiac arrest, carbon monoxide poisoning, seizures, vigorous muscular exercise, etc. (Carroll, 1989; Oh, 2003; Arenas-Pinto, 2003). Lactic acidosis in the absence of tissue hypoxia is called type B lactic acidosis, whereas that associated with tissue hypoxia is called type A lactic acidosis. In recent years, common causes of type B lactic acidosis include antiretroviral drugs and metformin (Strack, 2008; McGuire, 2006). Impaired metabolism of lactic acid is the cause of lactic acidosis in acute alcoholism and severe liver disease (Table 14-11).

D-Lactic Acidosis. Lactic acidosis, unless specified, refers to acidosis caused by L-lactic acid, which is the isomer produced in the human body, because the enzyme LD is an L-isomer. Accumulation of D-lactic acid causes D-lactic acidosis. The condition is characterized by severe acidosis accompanied by neurologic manifestations such as mental confusion and staggering gait, mimicking ethanol intoxication without elevated plasma levels of ethanol. The mechanism of D-lactic acidosis is the colonic overproduction of D-lactic acid by bacteria (Oh, 1979; Day, 1999). Requirements for overproduction of D-lactic acid in the colon include delivery of a large amount of carbohydrate to the colon (i.e., malabsorption syndrome) and proliferation of D-LD–forming bacteria in the colon (Uribarri, 1998; Oh, 1979). Treatment of D-lactic acidosis includes oral administration of poorly absorbable antibiotics such as neomycin and measures to alter the colonic bacterial flora (Uribarri, 1998).

Ketoacidosis. Keto acids, acetoacetic acid, and β-hydroxybutyric acid are produced in the liver from free fatty acids (FFAs) and are metabolized by extrahepatic tissues. Increased production of keto acids is the main mechanism for keto acid accumulation, although decreased utilization of keto acids by the brain with the patient in a coma may accelerate keto acid accumulation. Increased production requires a high concentration of FFA and its conversion to keto acids in the liver. Insulin deficiency is responsible for increased mobilization of FFA from the adipose tissue, and glucagon excess and insulin deficiency stimulate conversion of FFA to keto acids in the liver. The initial step in keto acid production from FFA is the entry of FFA into the mitochondria, which requires acyl-carnitine transferase. This step is stimulated by glucagon excess. The next step is metabolism of FFA to acetyl–coenzyme A (CoA), and then finally to keto acids. Diversion of acetyl-CoA to fatty acid resynthesis requires the enzyme acetyl-CoA caboxylase, and inhibition of this enzyme by insulin deficiency, glucagon excess, and an excess of stress-induced hormones such as catecholamines further contributes to increased keto acid synthesis.

The clinical diagnosis of ketoacidosis is usually made with Acetest, which detects acetoacetate (AA) but not BB. Although BB is the predominant acid in typical ketoacidosis (the usual ratio of BB/AA is about 2.5 : 3.0), the reaction to Acetest represents a fair estimate of the total concentration of keto acids as long as the ratio remains within the usual range. When the ratio of BB/AA is greatly increased, Acetest may be negative or only slightly positive, despite retention of a large quantity of total ketones in the form of BB. Such a condition is called BB acidosis, and it is commonly seen in alcoholic ketoacidosis (Delaney, 2000; Oh, 1977; Falco, 2003).

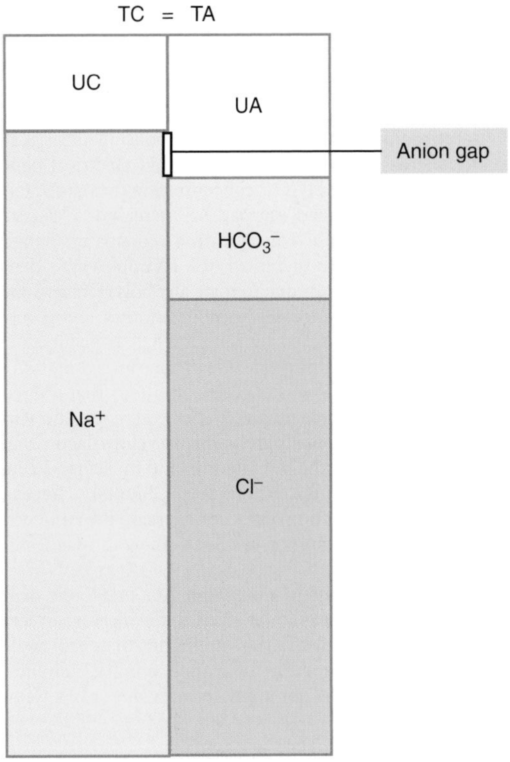

Figure 14-5 The anatomy of anion gap. When UC is defined as all serum cations other than Na, and UA as all serum anions other than Cl or bicarbonate, the serum anion gap can be stated as UA minus UC.

SERUM ANION GAP

Serum anion gap (AG) is estimated as follows: $Na^+ - (Cl^- + HCO_3^-)$ or $(Na^+ + K^+) - (Cl^- + HCO_3^-)$. Because normal serum potassium concentration is quantitatively a minor component of serum electrolytes, the fluctuation in its concentration affects the overall result very little; hence, the first of the two equations is more commonly used to estimate the AG. The normal value is about 12 mmol/L (8–16 mmol/L). Although the term anion gap implies that there is a gap between cation and anion concentrations, the total concentration of all cations in the serum is exactly equal to the total concentration of all anions. The anion gap, $Na^+ - (Cl^- + HCO_3^-)$, is 12 mmol/L because the total concentration of unmeasured anions (i.e., all anions other than chloride and bicarbonate) is about 23 mmol/L, and the total concentration of unmeasured cations (i.e., all cations other than sodium) is about 11 mmol/L.

Let us assume that total serum cations = Na^+ + unmeasured cations (UC), and that total serum anions = $Cl^- + HCO_3^-$ + unmeasured anions (UA). Because total serum cations = Total serum anions, $Na^+ + UC = (Cl^- + HCO_3^-) + UA$. Hence, $Na^+ - (Cl^- + HCO_3^-) = UA - UC$. Because the anion gap = $Na^+ - (Cl^- + HCO_3^-)$, the anion gap = UA − UC (Fig. 14-5; Oh, 1977).

It is apparent that a change in the anion gap must involve changes in unmeasured anions or unmeasured cations, unless a laboratory error involves the measurement of Na^+, Cl^-, or HCO_3^-. The anion gap can be increased by increased UA or decreased UC, or by a laboratory error resulting in a false increase in serum Na^+ or a false decrease in serum Cl^- or HCO_3^-. AG can be decreased by decreased UA or increased UC, or by a laboratory error resulting in a false decrease in serum Na^+ or a false increase in serum Cl^- or HCO_3^-. The equation also predicts that a change in UA may not change AG if UC is also changed to the same extent in the same direction.

Decreased AG is most commonly due to reduction in serum albumin concentration; increased AG is most often due to accumulation of anions of acids, such as sulfate, lactate, and ketone anions. Although bromide is an unmeasured anion, bromide intoxication is accompanied by low serum anion gap because bromide causes a false increase in serum Cl^-. A change in serum Na^+ usually does not cause a change in AG because serum Cl^- usually changes in the same direction. For the same reason, HCO_3^- concentrations cannot be used to predict a change in AG. For example, when serum HCO_3^- concentration increases in metabolic alkalosis, Cl^- concentration usually decreases reciprocally to maintain electrical neutrality, so the AG is unchanged. When HCO_3^- concentration decreases, Cl^- concentration may remain unchanged or may be increased. If bicarbonate is replaced by another anion, Cl^- concentration remains unchanged, hence normochloremic acidosis with increased AG. Examples are organic acidosis, uremic acidosis, and acidosis due to toxic alcohols (Kraut, 2008). When bicarbonate concentration decreases without another anion replacing it, electrical neutrality is maintained by a higher Cl^- concentration: hence, hyperchloremic acidosis with normal AG. Proper interpretation of serum AG requires knowledge of the existence of conditions that influence anion gap, even though they may have no direct effect on metabolic acidosis. For example, if a person with hypoalbuminemia develops lactic acidosis, the AG could be normal because the low albumin and the lactate accumulation have opposite effects on the AG (Kraut, 2007). Similarly, hypermagnesemia (increased unmeasured cation) does not decrease the AG if it is accompanied by increased sulfate (unmeasured anion), as in magnesium sulfate intoxication (Oh, 1977).

It has been suggested that in pure high AG metabolic acidosis, the decrease in serum bicarbonate is about equal to the increase in serum anion gap. A concentration of serum bicarbonate higher than expected has been taken as evidence for the presence of complicating metabolic alkalosis. However, this rule often does not apply in individual cases (Kraut, 2007; Rastegar, 2007).

Differential Diagnosis

One approach to the differential diagnosis of metabolic acidosis is to calculate the serum anion gap. The increased AG suggests organic acidosis, uremic acidosis, and acidosis due to various toxic alcohols (Kraut, 2008; Fenves, 2006; Judge, 2005; Schwerk, 2007; Zar, 2007) (Table 14-12). The normal AG suggests renal tubular acidosis and acidosis due to diarrheal loss of bicarbonate. Most cases of uremic acidosis are accompanied by normal AG; only in advanced chronic and acute renal failure is AG increased. Furthermore, a vast majority of patients with ketoacidosis pass through a phase of hyperchloremic acidosis (normal AG) during the recovery phase (Oh, 1990).

Another approach to the differential diagnosis of metabolic acidosis is to classify the acidosis into renal and extrarenal acidosis. Three major causes of extrarenal acidosis are organic acidosis, diarrheal loss of bicarbonate, and acidosis due to exogenous toxins. The presence of organic acidosis is usually obvious from clinical findings (e.g., evidence of tissue hypoxia in lactic acidosis, hyperglycemia and ketonemia in ketoacidosis). Diarrhea as the cause of metabolic acidosis is first suspected from history, but history is often misleading because the severity of diarrhea cannot be easily determined. The measurement of urine AG is useful in determining the severity of diarrhea. Urine AG, which is measured as urine ($Na^+ + K^+$) – urine Cl^-, is reduced or negative when diarrhea is severe. The low urine AG in diarrhea is explained by the preferential loss of $Na^+ + K^+$ in excess of Cl^- because diarrheal fluid contains more $Na^+ + K^+$ than Cl^-, as some of these cations are balanced by bicarbonate and organic anions. In other types of metabolic acidosis, urine AG is not altered as long as there is no extrarenal loss of electrolytes that are components of urine AG (Oh, 2002a). A history of drug ingestion and acute onset will suggest acidosis caused by exogenous toxins (Judge, 2005).

Once extrarenal acidosis is excluded, renal acidosis is the only alternative diagnosis. Of the two types of renal acidosis, uremic acidosis can be readily ruled out by normal values of serum creatinine and BUN. If renal acidosis is confirmed but uremic acidosis is ruled out, the diagnosis must be renal tubular acidosis. Among the three types of RTA, type IV RTA is suspected by the presence of hyperkalemia. Hypokalemia suggests type I or type II RTA. If spontaneous urine pH is below 5.5, type I RTA is ruled out. If urine pH is higher than 5.5, urine pH should be measured after oral administration of 40 mg of furosemide or 10 mg of torsemide (Han, 2005). The latter drug has higher sensitivity and specificity (Han, 2005). If the urine pH remains above 5.5, the likely diagnosis is type I RTA. Evidence of Fanconi's syndrome (the best evidence is renal glycosuria) suggests type II RTA.

Compensation of Metabolic Acidosis

Compensation of metabolic acidosis is achieved by hyperventilation, which results in decreased pCO_2. The compensation is moderately effective, and the maximal compensation is completed within 12 to 24 hours. The formula that predicts the expected decrease in pCO_2 (ΔpCO_2) is as follows:

$$\Delta pCO_2 = \Delta HCO_3^- \times 1.2 \pm 2 \; (\Delta HCO_3^- \text{ a given decrease in a serum } HCO_3^- \text{ concentration}) \quad \textbf{(14-41)}$$

METABOLIC ALKALOSIS

Causes and Pathogenesis

At normal serum bicarbonate concentrations, bicarbonate filtered at the glomerulus is almost completely reabsorbed. As serum bicarbonate concentrations rise above the normal level, bicarbonate reabsorption is incomplete, and bicarbonaturia begins. A slight increase in serum bicarbonate above 24 mmol/L causes marked bicarbonaturia. Hence, when renal tubular bicarbonate handling and GFR are normal, maintenance of a high plasma bicarbonate concentration is extremely difficult unless an enormous amount of bicarbonate is given. Therefore, maintenance of metabolic alkalosis requires two conditions: a mechanism to increase plasma bicarbonate and a mechanism to maintain an increased concentration. A bicarbonate concentration may be increased by administration of alkali, gastric loss of HCl through vomiting or nasogastric suction, or renal generation of bicarbonate (Table 14-13). Maintenance of high plasma bicarbonate concentration occurs in advanced renal failure, or when the renal threshold for bicarbonate is increased (Palmer, 1997). The two most common causes of increased renal bicarbonate threshold are volume depletion and K^+ depletion. Potassium deficiency reduces the intracellular pH of the proximal tubules, and this stimulates bicarbonate reabsorption. Increased reabsorption of potassium in exchange for proton by K^+-H^+-ATPase in the collecting duct appears to contribute to metabolic alkalosis in potassium deficiency states (Codina, 2006). Metabolic alkalosis corrected by administration of chloride-containing fluid (e.g., NaCl, KCl solution) is called chloride-responsive metabolic alkalosis (e.g., vomiting-induced alkalosis). Patients with chloride-responsive metabolic alkalosis are typically volume depleted (Oh, 2002b). However, in edema-forming

TABLE 14-12
Classification of Metabolic Acidosis by Anion Gap

Metabolic Acidosis with Increased Anion Gap (Normochloremic Acidosis)
Ketoacidosis
L-Lactic acidosis
D-Lactic acidosis
β-Hydroxybutyric acidosis
Uremic acidosis
Ingestion of toxins: Salicylate, methanol, ethylene glycol, toluene, acetaminophen
Metabolic Acidosis with Normal Anion Gap (Hyperchloremic Acidosis)
Renal tubular acidosis
Uremic acidosis (early)
Acidosis following respiratory alkalosis
Intestinal loss of bicarbonate
Administration of chloride-containing acid: HCl, NH_4Cl
Ketoacidosis during recovery phase

TABLE 14-13
Mechanisms and Causes to Increase Extracellular Bicarbonate Concentration

Loss of HCl from the stomach (e.g., gastric suction, vomiting)
Administration of bicarbonate or bicarbonate precursors (e.g., sodium lactate, sodium acetate, sodium citrate)
Shift of H^+ into the cell (e.g., K^+ depletion, refeeding alkalosis)
Rapid contraction of extracellular volume without loss of bicarbonate (e.g., contraction alkalosis by the use of loop diuretics)
Increased renal excretion of acid (e.g., diuretic therapy, high aldosterone state, potassium depletion, high pCO_2, secondary hypoparathyroidism)

pCO_2, Partial pressure of carbon dioxide.

conditions, administration of Cl^- may not improve metabolic alkalosis, even though the mechanism of a high renal bicarbonate threshold is volume depletion, because administered chloride is retained in the edema fluid. Parathyroid hormone normally interferes with bicarbonate reabsorption in the proximal tubule; therefore, the renal tubular bicarbonate threshold tends to be increased in hypoparathyroidism (Khanna, 2006).

Compensation of Metabolic Alkalosis

Compensation of metabolic alkalosis is achieved by hypoventilation that results in increased pCO_2. In part because hypoxemia occurs inevitably with hypoventilation in the absence of oxygen supplement, among the four types of acid-base disorders, compensation is least effective in metabolic alkalosis. The formula that predicts the expected increase in pCO_2 (ΔpCO_2) is as follows:

$$\Delta pCO_2 = \Delta HCO_3^- \times 0.7 \pm 5 \ (\Delta HCO_3^- \text{ is a given increase in serum } HCO_3^- \text{ concentration}) \quad \textbf{(14-42)}$$

The maximal compensation is completed within 12–24 hours. Observations have shown that no matter how severe the metabolic alkalosis, pCO_2 rarely exceeds 60 mmHg unless a complicating independent respiratory disorder that compromises ventilation coexists (Oh, 2003).

RESPIRATORY ACIDOSIS

Causes and Pathogenesis

Causes are usually apparent and include diseases of the lung (most common causes), respiratory muscle, respiratory nerve, thoracic cage, and airways, and suppression of the respiratory center by stroke, drugs such as phenobarbital, or severe hypothyroidism (Table 14-14).

Compensation of Respiratory Acidosis

The normal compensatory response to respiratory acidosis is to increase HCO_3^-concentration in an attempt to minimize the reduction in pH. This occurs in two distinct stages: first, by tissue buffering of CO_2, and second, by increased renal excretion of acid.

Tissue Buffering

This phase of compensation is extremely fast and occurs within a second. The chemical reaction is as follows:

$$CO_2 + H_2O \rightarrow H_2CO_3 \quad \textbf{(14-43)}$$

$$H_2CO_3 + KBuff \rightarrow HBuff + KHCO_3 \quad \textbf{(14-44)}$$

KBuff is a non-HCO_3^- buffer and HBuff is cellular acid buffers, and the reaction proceeds to the right because of the rising pCO_2. Because ECF has few non-HCO_3^- buffers, most of this buffering occurs in the cell. The increased concentration of cellular HCO_3^- causes an extracellular shift of HCO_3^- in exchange for Cl^- through the ubiquitous anion exchanger on the red blood cell membrane. The relationship between an increase in pCO_2 (ΔpCO_2) and the increase in serum levels of HCO_3^- (ΔHCO_3^-) in acute respiratory acidosis is shown in the following equation:

$$\Delta HCO_3^-(\text{mmol/L}) = \Delta pCO_2(\text{mmHg}) \times 0.07 \pm 1.5 \quad \textbf{(14-45)}$$

Renal Compensation

Renal compensation for respiratory acidosis is delayed, but it increases the HCO_3^- concentration to a much higher level. The increased concentration of HCO_3^- is achieved by increased net acid excretion, primarily in the form of NH_4^+. Maximal compensation requires 5 days but is 90% complete in 3 days. Increased excretion of NH_4^+ is accompanied by Cl^-. As new HCO_3^- is retained, Cl^- is lost. It follows therefore that when respiratory acidosis is corrected, excretion of HCO_3^- must be accompanied by retention of Cl^-, which is possible only if Cl^- is taken in. Restriction of NaCl intake during the recovery phase of chronic respiratory acidosis results in the maintenance of a high serum HCO_3^-. Such a condition is called posthypercapneic metabolic alkalosis.

The relationship between the increase in pCO_2 (ΔpCO_2) and the increase in HCO_3^- (ΔHCO_3^-) in chronic fully compensated respiratory acidosis is shown in the following equation:

$$\Delta HCO_3^-(\text{mmol/L}) = \Delta pCO_2(\text{mmHg}) \times 0.4 \pm 3 \quad \textbf{(14-46)}$$

TABLE 14-14
Causes of Respiratory Acidosis

Lung diseases: Chronic obstructive lung disease, advanced interstitial lung disease, acute asthma
Thoracic deformity or airway obstruction
Diseases of respiratory muscle and nerve: Myasthenia gravis, hypokalemia paralysis, botulism, amyotrophic lateral sclerosis, Guillain-Barré syndrome
Depression of the respiratory center: Barbiturate intoxication, stroke, myxedema

RESPIRATORY ALKALOSIS

Causes and Pathogenesis

With the exception of respirator-induced alkalosis and voluntary hyperventilation, respiratory alkalosis is the result of stimulation of the respiratory center. The two most common causes of respiratory alkalosis are hypoxic stimulation of the peripheral respiratory center and stimulation through pulmonary receptors caused by various disorders of the lung, such as pneumonia, pulmonary congestion, and pulmonary embolism. Certain drugs (e.g., salicylate, progesterone) stimulate the respiratory center directly (Saaresranta, 1999; Bayliss, 1992). High progesterone levels are responsible for chronic respiratory alkalosis of pregnancy (Wise, 2006). Respiratory alkalosis is also common in gram-negative sepsis and liver disease through unknown mechanisms (Ahya, 2006). Blood pH tends to be extremely high when respiratory alkalosis is caused by psychogenic stimulation of the respiratory center, because the condition is usually superacute, and therefore there is no time for compensation. Causes of respiratory alkalosis are listed in Table 14-15.

Compensation of Respiratory Alkalosis

Two types of compensation lower plasma HCO_3^- and minimize the increase in blood pH in respiratory alkalosis: tissue buffering and renal compensation.

Tissue Buffering

Compensation by buffering of HCO_3^- is completed within a second with the following reactions (Carroll, 1989):

$$HBuff + HCO_3^- \rightarrow H_2CO_3 + Buff \quad \textbf{(14-47)}$$

$$H_2CO_3 \rightarrow CO_2 + H_2O \quad \textbf{(14-48)}$$

The reactions proceed to the right because CO_2 is lost by hyperventilation. The magnitude of reduction in HCO_3^- content depends on the number of HBuff that react with HCO_3^-. As cellular HCO_3^- is consumed in the buffer reaction, extracellular HCO_3^- enters the cell in exchange for cellular Cl^- that enters the ECF. An additional mechanism of tissue buffering is increased production of lactic acid and other organic acids (Hood, 1998). Increased lactic acid production is explained in part by the stimulatory effect of alkaline pH on phosphofructokinase, a rate-limiting enzyme for glycolysis. The magnitude of reduction in plasma HCO_3^- concentration by acute compensation is predicted from the following equation:

$$\Delta HCO_3^-(\text{mmol/L}) = \Delta pCO_2(\text{mmHg}) \times 0.2 \pm 2.5 \quad \textbf{(14-49)}$$

(ΔHCO_3^- [mmol/L] is the expected decrease in plasma HCO_3^- for a given decrease in pCO_2 [ΔpCO_2] in mmHg.)

TABLE 14-15
Causes of Respiratory Alkalosis

Diseases of the lung: Any intrapulmonary pathology such as pneumonia, pulmonary fibrosis, pulmonary congestion, pulmonary embolism
Hypoxemia
CNS lesions
Gram-negative sepsis
Liver disease
Drugs: Salicylate, progesterone

CNS, Central nervous system.

Renal Compensation

Renal compensation of respiratory alkalosis is achieved by reduction in net acid excretion (Carroll, 1989; Oh, 2003). This is achieved initially by increased excretion of HCO_3^-, but later by reduced excretion of NH_4^+ and titratable acid. The magnitude of reduction in plasma HCO_3^- concentration due to renal compensation can be predicted from the following equation:

$$\Delta HCO_3^-(\text{mmol/L}) = \Delta pCO_2(\text{mmHg}) \times 0.5 \pm 2.5 \qquad \textbf{(14-50)}$$

(ΔHCO_3^- [mmol/L] is the expected decrease in plasma HCO_3^- for a given decrease in pCO_2 [ΔpCO_2] in mmHg.)

Among the four types of acid-base disorders, compensation is most effective in respiratory alkalosis; pH after compensation sometimes returns to normal levels. The process is completed within 2–3 days. When complete compensation does occur, one should look for evidence of complicating metabolic acidosis.

MIXED ACID-BASE DISORDERS

The term mixed acid-base disorder refers to a clinical condition in which two or more primary acid-base disorders coexist. They generally present with one obvious disturbance with what appears to be an inappropriate (excessive or inadequate) compensation. The "inappropriateness" of the compensatory process is probably the result of a separate primary disorder. Appropriate degrees of compensation for primary acid-base disorders have been determined by analysis of data from a large number of patients, and are expressed in the form of equations in the next table. When two disorders influence the blood pH in opposite directions, the blood pH will be determined by the dominant disorder. If disorders cancel out each other's effects, blood pH can be normal. When there is any degree of compensation for acid-base disorders, both pCO_2 and HCO_3^- change in the same direction (i.e., both are high or both are low). If pCO_2 and HCO_3^- have changed in opposite directions (e.g., pCO_2 is high and HCO_3^- is low, or pCO_2 is low and HCO_3^- is high), the presence of a mixed acid-base disorder is certain. Appropriateness of compensation can be determined by consulting Table 14-16. Compensation may be excessive, insufficient, or appropriate. One can also have an approximate idea about the appropriateness of compensation from the degree of pH deviation without consulting the formula for normal compensation.

In general, compensation is most effective in respiratory alkalosis (pH is often normalized); the next best is respiratory acidosis (pH may become normal), and the third best is metabolic acidosis. Compensation is least effective in metabolic alkalosis, probably because hypoxemia, an inevitable consequence of hypoventilation, stimulates ventilation. If a patient has low pCO_2 and low HCO_3^- with normal pH, the likely diagnosis is compensated respiratory alkalosis rather than compensated metabolic acidosis (Carroll, 1989; Oh, 2003).

TABLE 14-16
Formulas for Predicting Normal Acid-Base Compensation*

Metabolic acidosis: $\Delta pCO_2 = \Delta HCO_3^- \times 1.2 \pm 2$
Metabolic alkalosis†: $\Delta pCO_2 = \Delta HCO_3^- \times 0.7 \pm 5$
Acute respiratory acidosis: $\Delta HCO_3^- = \Delta pCO_2 \times 0.07 \pm 1.5$
Chronic respiratory acidosis: $\Delta HCO_3^- = \Delta pCO_2 \times 0.4 \pm 3$
Acute respiratory alkalosis: $\Delta HCO_3^- = \Delta pCO_2 \times 0.2 \pm 2.5$
Chronic respiratory alkalosis: $\Delta HCO_3^- = \Delta pCO_2 \times 0.5 \pm 2.5$

pCO_2, Partial pressure of carbon dioxide.
*ΔHCO_3^- and ΔpCO_2 represent the difference between normal and actual values.
†No matter how high the serum HCO_3^- rises, pCO_2 rarely rises above 60 mm Hg in metabolic alkalosis.

SELECTED REFERENCES

Aukland K, Reed RK. Interstitial lymphatic mechanisms in the control of extra cellular fluid volume. Physiol Rev 1993;73:1–78.
Carroll HJ, Oh MS. Water, electrolyte, and acid-base metabolism. Philadelphia: Lippincott; 1989.
Gennari FJ. Current concepts. Serum osmolality: uses and limitations. N Engl J Med 1984;310:102–5.
Giebisch GH. A trail of research on potassium. Kidney Int 2002;62:1498–512.
Halperin ML, Kamel KS, Oh MS. Mechanisms to concentrate the urine: an opinion. Curr Opin Nephrol Hypertens 2008;17:416–22.
Kraut JA, Madias NE. Serum anion gap: its uses and limitations in clinical medicine. Clin J Am Soc Nephrol 2007;2:162–74.
Kyle UG, Bosaeusb I, De Lorenzoc AD, et al. Bioelectrical impedance analysis–Part I: review of principles and methods. Clin Nutr 2004;23:1226–43.
Mehta R, Kellum JA, Shah S, et al. Acute kidney injury network: report of an initiative to improve outcomes in acute kidney injury. Crit Care 2007;11:R31.
Moore F. The body cell mass and its supporting environment. Philadelphia: WB Saunders; 1963.
Oh MS, Carroll HJ. The anion gap. N Engl J Med 1977;297:814–17.
Oh MS. Does serum creatinine rise faster in rhabdomyolysis? Nephron 1993;63:255–7.
Oh MS, Carroll HJ. Regulation of intracellular and extracellular volume. In: Arieff AI, DePronzo RA, editors. Fluid, electrolyte, and acid-base disorders. 2nd ed. New York: Churchill Livingstone; 1995.
Oh MS. Acid-base electrolytes. New York: Ohco; 2003.
Relman AS, Lennon EJ, Lemann J Jr. Endogenous production of fixed acid and the measurement of the net balance of acid in normal subjects. J Clin Invest 1961;40:1621–30.
Smith HW. Kidney: structure and function in health and disease. New York: Oxford University Press; 1951, p. 231–8.

REFERENCES

Access the complete reference list online at http://www.expertconsult.com

CHAPTER 15

BIOCHEMICAL MARKERS OF BONE METABOLISM

Katrin M. Klemm, Michael J. Klein

KEY POINTS

- The plasma concentration of calcium, phosphate, and magnesium is dependent on the net balance of bone mineral deposition and resorption, intestinal absorption, and renal excretion. The principal hormones regulating these processes are parathyroid hormone (PTH), calcitonin, and 1,25-dihydroxyvitamin D.
- The most common causes of hypercalcemia are primary hyperparathyroidism (elevated PTH) and malignant neoplasms (decreased PTH and usually elevated PTH-related peptide). They account for 80%–90% of all patients with hypercalcemia.
- The most common causes of hypocalcemia are chronic renal failure, hypomagnesemia, hypoparathyroidism, pseudohypoparathyroidism, vitamin D deficiency, and acute pancreatitis.
- Bio-intact PTH measures biologically active PTH; it is useful in patients with impaired renal function when various metabolites accumulate and interfere with traditional PTH assays.
- In patients undergoing surgery for primary hyperparathyroidism, intraoperative PTH measurements are useful in identifying whether the abnormal tissue is completely removed.
- Osteoporosis is the most common metabolic disease of bone and is characterized by decreased organic bone matrix. Serial bone resorption marker measurements can predict early response to therapy.
- Osteomalacia is failure to mineralize newly formed organic matrix (osteoid) in the mature skeleton.
- Phosphatonins comprise a newly described cascade of hormones, enzymes, and proteins related to phosphate metabolism.

MINERAL AND BONE METABOLISM

The skeleton is a metabolically active organ that undergoes continuous remodeling throughout life. This remodeling is necessary both to maintain the structural integrity of the skeleton and to fulfill its metabolic functions as a storehouse of calcium and phosphorus. Skeletal remodeling can be triggered by changes in mechanical forces or microdamage, and by hormonal response to changes in circulating calcium and phosphorus levels. The skeleton also serves as the second line of defense against acidosis, and it is able to liberate buffers in the form of inorganic phosphates (Raisz, 1999).

Bone can be classified into two types: cortical or compact bone, and cancellous or trabecular bone (Fig. 15-1, *A* and *B*). Cortical bone plays an important role in the supportive, protective, and mechanical functions of the skeleton; it comprises the shafts of long bones and the outer envelope of all bones. It constitutes approximately 80% of skeletal mass, and it is 90% bone and 10% space (vascular canals, osteocyte lacunae, and canaliculi) by volume. Cancellous bone, which constitutes the remaining 20% of skeletal mass, is 25% bone and 75% space by volume. It is present at the ends of long and short tubular bones, within carpal and tarsal bones, and in the medullary cavities of vertebral bodies and flat bones. It is arranged in highly perforated vertical plates interconnected by horizontal struts and has a honeycombed appearance. It serves as a repository for hematopoietic cells and provides a large surface area for short-term mineral exchange (Watts, 1999). Even though cancellous bone represents only 20% of the total skeletal mass, it provides such a large surface area—one that equals that of cortical bone because of its honeycombed structure—that it accounts for 50% of active bone turnover at any given time (Erikson, 1994). Both compact and cancellous bones are composed primarily of inorganic minerals (calcium and phosphorus) and an organic matrix. Approximately 90%–95% of this organic matrix is type I collagen, and the remaining 5%–10% consists of noncollagenous proteins, including osteocalcin, osteopontin, osteonectin, thrombospondin, sialoproteins, and other less well-characterized proteins. Osteoclasts actively resorb bone by producing hydrogen ions to mobilize the minerals and proteolytic enzymes to hydrolyze the organic matrix. Osteoblasts synthesize the organic matrix and control the mineralization of the newly synthesized matrix (Endres, 1999).

The plasma concentration of calcium, phosphate, and magnesium is dependent upon the net balance of bone mineral deposition and resorption, intestinal absorption, and renal excretion. The principal hormones regulating these processes are PTH, calcitonin, and 1,25-dihydroxyvitamin D. Much of bone metabolism reflects the body's effort to maintain serum calcium and phosphorus levels.

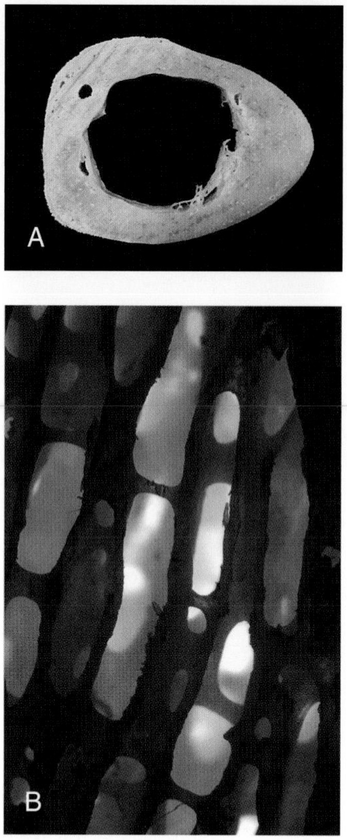

Figure 15-1 **A,** Compact bone, long bone, cross-section. The compact bone of the cortex of the femur in this 30-year-old male is continuous and solid, and the vascular spaces are not grossly visible. The hollow medullary cavity is filled with fatty marrow in vivo. **B,** Cancellous bone, longitudinal section. The cancellous bone is arranged in highly perforated vertical plates interconnected by delicate horizontal struts (braces). Most of its volume appears to be empty space once the marrow has been removed.

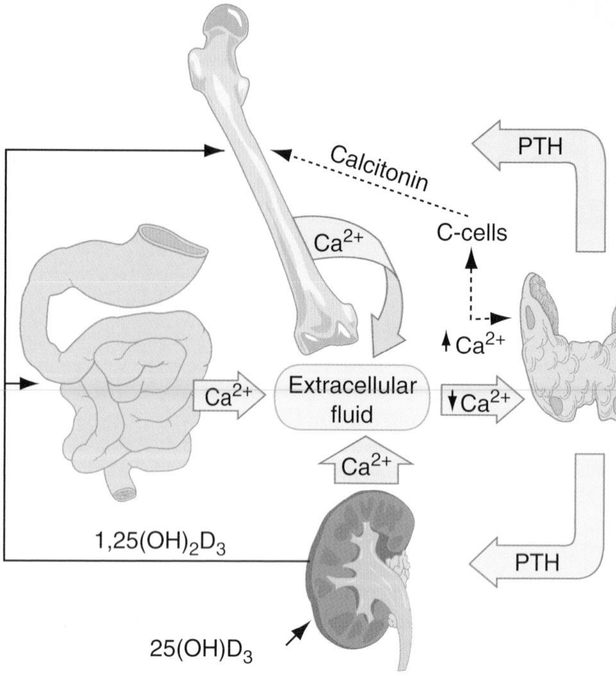

Figure 15-2 Calcium homeostasis. *Solid arrows* and *block arrows* indicate effects that increase serum calcium levels; *dashed arrows* indicate negative effects that decrease serum calcium.

CALCIUM

Physiology

Distribution

Calcium is the fifth most common element and is the most prevalent cation in the human body. A healthy adult contains approximately 1–1.3 kg of calcium, and 99% of this is in the form of hydroxyapatite in the skeleton. The remaining 1% is contained in the extracellular fluid (ECF) and soft tissues. Additionally, less than 1% of the skeletal content of calcium is in bone fluid and exchanges freely with the ECF (Mundy, 1999).

Serum (plasma) calcium exists in three distinct forms: (1) free or ionized calcium, which is the physiologically active form, accounting for approximately 50% of the total serum calcium; (2) complexed calcium, which is bound tightly to a variety of anions, including bicarbonate, lactate, phosphate, and citrate, accounting for approximately 10%; and (3) plasma protein-bound calcium, accounting for approximately 40%. Both ionized calcium and the calcium complexes are freely dialyzable. Approximately 80% of the protein-bound calcium fraction is associated with albumin.

Because ionized calcium binds to negatively charged sites on the protein molecules, there is competition with hydrogen ions for binding sites on albumin and other calcium-binding proteins, and its binding is pH dependent. Although total serum calcium levels may remain unchanged, the relative distribution of the three forms is altered as a result of pH changes in ECF. Alkalosis promotes increased protein binding, with a subsequent decrease in free calcium, whereas acidosis decreases protein binding, causing an increase in free calcium levels. Because calcium is bound to proteins, total calcium levels are also altered by plasma protein concentration.

Function

In addition to its obvious importance in skeletal mineralization, calcium plays a vital role in such basic physiologic processes as blood coagulation, neural transmission, plasma buffering capacity and enzyme activity, and in the maintenance of normal muscle tone and excitability of skeletal and cardiac muscle. It is an activator of intracellular signal transduction processes and is essential for DNA and RNA biosynthesis. Calcium is also involved in glandular synthesis and in regulation of exocrine and endocrine glands, as well as in the preservation of cell membrane integrity and permeability, particularly in terms of sodium and potassium exchange.

The average dietary intake of calcium for most adults in the United States is approximately 15–20 mmol/day (600–800 mg/day), most of which is derived from milk or other dairy products. The National Osteoporosis Foundation recommends that all adults have a daily intake of at least 1200 mg of elemental calcium with diet plus supplements. Lactating females and postmenopausal females not given exogenous estrogen therapy should probably have at least 1500 mg/day (Lewiecki, 2004).

Calcium is absorbed in the duodenum and upper jejunum via an active transport process. Less than half of dietary calcium is absorbed in adults. However, calcium absorption increases during periods of rapid growth in children, in pregnancy, and during lactation. It decreases with advancing age. The major stimulus to calcium absorption is vitamin D (see later). Calcium absorption is also enhanced by growth hormone, an acid medium in the intestines, and by increased dietary protein. The ratio of calcium to phosphorus in the intestinal contents is also important, because a ratio greater than 2 : 1 results in the formation of insoluble calcium phosphates and tends to inhibit calcium absorption. Phytic acid, derived from various cereal grains, can also form insoluble calcium compounds, as can dietary oxalate and fatty acids. Cortisol and excessive alkalinity of the intestinal contents are both inhibitory to calcium absorption.

Estimates of daily calcium excretion in sweat vary widely—from 15 mg to more than 100 mg. The loss can greatly exceed this range during extreme environmental conditions. The major net loss of calcium occurs via urinary excretion, and varies between 2.5 and 10 mmol/day (100–200 mg/day). In normal individuals, wide variations in dietary calcium intake have little effect on urinary calcium. Urinary calcium excretion is enhanced by hypercalcemia, phosphate deprivation, acidosis, and glucocorticoids. PTH, certain diuretics, and probably vitamin D diminish urinary calcium excretion. The physiology of calcium, its regulating hormones, and alterations of calcium homeostasis in disease have been extensively reviewed (Boden, 1990).

Calcium Homeostasis

Ionized calcium concentration of the ECF is kept constant within a narrow range of approximately 1.25µmol/L (Fig. 15-2). It is the ionized calcium concentration of the ECF that is the primary determinant of the hormonal influences that exert effects on ECF calcium levels. These effects are sometimes achieved at the expense of bone integrity. Adjustment of the ionized calcium concentration of the ECF is achieved mainly by the actions of PTH and active 1,25-dihydroxyvitamin D3 (1,25[OH]$_2$D$_3$), and calcitonin plays a smaller yet significant role. The principal target organs of these hormones are bone, kidney, and intestine. When plasma-ionized calcium concentration decreases, the parathyroid glands sense the change via membrane-bound calcium sensor protein and secrete PTH immediately. Although parathyroid hormone has no direct effect on osteoclasts, it stimulates osteoblasts and their precursors to produce RANKL (the receptor activator of nuclear factor κB ligand). This substance, a member of the tumor necrosis factor superfamily, activates its receptor, RANK, which is expressed on osteoclasts and their precursors. This, in turn, promotes osteoclast formation and activity, and prolongs osteoclast survival by suppressing apoptosis (Hsu, 1999). This explains why bone formation and bone resorption are coupled in normal bone physiology. The resorption of bone matrix releases calcium and phosphate into the ECF. At the same time, PTH also acts on the kidney to stimulate increased urine phosphate excretion and some calcium reabsorption in the distal nephron, returning the ionized calcium concentration to normal. It has been suggested that sufficient action of 1,25(OH)$_2$D$_3$ is mandatory for these steps to work appropriately. The kidney is almost exclusively responsible for this vitamin D activation (Kurokawa, 1999). Calcitonin may play a role in the regulating process, although its significance in humans is controversial. Other hormones that affect calcium metabolism but whose secretions are not primarily affected by changes in plasma calcium and phosphate include thyroid hormone, growth hormone, adrenal glucocorticoids, and gonadal steroids.

Analytic Techniques

Total calcium measurements include protein-bound calcium and ionized calcium; alternatively, ionized calcium alone can be measured. The total calcium measurement is easier to perform in the laboratory, but this result must be interpreted in clinical context. For example, patients with malignancies often exhibit hypoalbuminemia, a condition that may result in falsely low total calcium levels. When this occurs, the total calcium level (expressed in mg/dL) can be corrected with the following equation:

$$\text{Total calcium (mg/dL) corrected for hypoalbuminemia} = \text{Total calcium (measured)} + [(\text{Normal albumin} - \text{Patient's albumin}) \times 0.8] \quad \textbf{(15-1)}$$

An albumin of about 4.4 is typically used as the normal value in the previous formula. This corrected value is a more accurate assessment of the patient's calcium status. Because albumin is the primary protein that binds calcium, variations in this protein are clinically significant. Only a small percentage of calcium binds to other proteins such as γ-globulins. Therefore, clinical states such as hypogammaglobulinemia are unlikely to drastically alter the total calcium levels.

Total and Ionized Calcium

Although many total calcium procedures have been reported, only three methods are commonly used: (1) colorimetric analysis with metallochromic indicators; (2) atomic absorption spectrometry (AAS); and (3) indirect potentiometry.

Total calcium is most widely measured by spectrophotometric determination of the colored complex when various metallochromic indicators or dyes bind calcium. Orthocresolphthalein complexone (CPC) and arsenazo III are the most widely used indicators. The structures of both of these dyes are shown in Chapter 27. CPC reacts with calcium to form a red color in alkaline solution, which is measured at near 580 nm. Interference by magnesium ions is reduced by the addition of 8-hydroxyquinoline. Arsenazo III reacts with calcium to form a calcium-indicator complex usually measured at near 650 nm. The stable reagent exhibits high specificity for calcium at slightly acidic pH. These reactions are also discussed in Chapter 27.

Atomic absorption spectrophotometry is the reference method for determining calcium in serum. Despite its greater accuracy and precision compared with other methods, very few laboratories continue to use AAS for routine determination of total calcium. This may be because laboratories performing large numbers of sample determinations rely on automated methods that are not widely available for this technique. In addition, the level of equipment maintenance required in this technique is difficult for high-volume laboratories.

In indirect potentiometry, an electrode selective for calcium measures a sample that is also measured against a sodium-selective electrode, and calcium concentrations are proportional to the difference in potential between the electrodes.

Instruments with calcium-selective electrodes (see Chapter 27) provide accurate, precise, and automatic determinations of free (ionized) calcium. Calcium ion-selective electrodes (ISEs) consist of a calcium-selective membrane enclosing an inner reference solution of $CaCl_2$, AgCl, and other ions, as well as a reference electrode. Ion-selective electrodes are discussed in Chapters 4 and 27. In Chapter 27, use of ISEs to measure total calcium is also discussed.

Reference Interval

The reference interval for total calcium in normal adults ranges between 8.8 and 10.3 mg/dL (2.20–2.58 mmol/L). Serum is the preferred specimen for total calcium determination, although heparinized plasma is also acceptable. Citrate, oxalate, and ethylenediaminetetraacetic acid (EDTA) interfere with commonly used methods. Other factors that have been reported to interfere with the colorimetric methods include hemolysis, icterus, lipemia, paraproteins, and magnesium.

The reference interval for *ionized (free) calcium* in normal adults is 4.6–5.3 mg/dL (1.16–1.32 mmol/L). Whole blood, heparinized plasma, or serum may be used. Specimens should be collected anaerobically, transported on ice, and stored at 4° C to prevent loss of carbon dioxide (CO_2) and glycolysis, and to stabilize pH (because pH changes alter the ionized calcium fraction). Proper collection technique is important to ensure accurate ionized calcium results; a tourniquet left on too long can lower pH at the site of collection and falsely elevate levels.

The reference interval for *urinary calcium* varies with diet. Individuals on an average diet excrete up to 300 mg/day (7.49 mmol/day). Urine specimens should be collected with appropriate acidification to prevent calcium salt precipitation.

PHOSPHORUS

Physiology

Distribution

The total body phosphorus content in normal adults is around 700–800 g. Approximately 80%–85% is present in the skeleton; the remaining 15% is present in the ECF in the form of inorganic phosphate, and intracellularly in the soft tissues as organic phosphates such as phospholipids, nucleic acids, and adenosine triphosphate (ATP). The skeleton contains primarily inorganic phosphate, predominantly as hydroxyapatite and calcium phosphate.

In blood, organic phosphate is located primarily in erythrocytes, with the plasma containing mostly inorganic phosphate. Approximately two thirds of blood phosphorus is organic, while only about 3–4 mg/dL of the total of 12 mg/dL represents the inorganic form. Inorganic phosphate in serum exists as both divalent (HPO_4^{2-}) and monovalent ($H_2PO_4^-$) phosphate anions, both of which represent important buffers. The ratio of $H_2PO_4^-:HPO_4^{2-}$ is pH dependent and varies between 1:1 in acidosis, 1:4 at pH of 7.4, and 1:9 in alkalosis. Approximately 10% of the serum phosphorus is bound to proteins; 35% is complexed with sodium, calcium, and magnesium; and the remaining 55% is free. Only inorganic phosphorus is measured in routine clinical settings.

Function

In addition to its role in the skeleton, phosphate has important intracellular and extracellular functions. Phosphate is an important constituent of nucleic acids in that both RNA and DNA represent complex phosphodiesters. In addition, phosphorus is contained in phospholipids and phosphoproteins. It forms high-energy compounds (ATP) and cofactors (nicotinamide adenine dinucleotide phosphate [NADPH]) and is involved in intermediary metabolism and various enzyme systems (adenylate cyclase). Phosphorus is essential for normal muscle contractility, neurologic function, electrolyte transport, and oxygen carrying by hemoglobin (2,3-diphosphoglycerate).

Phosphorus Homeostasis

Most blood phosphate is derived from diet, but some is derived from bone metabolism. Phosphorus is present in virtually all foods. The average dietary intake for adults is about 800–1400 mg, most of which is derived from dairy products, cereals, eggs, and meat. About 60%–80% of ingested phosphate is absorbed in the gut, mainly by passive transport. However, there is also an active energy-dependent process, which is stimulated by $1,25(OH)_2D_3$. Serum calcium and phosphorus generally maintain a reciprocal relationship. Phosphorus is freely filtered in the glomerulus. More than 80% of the filtered phosphorus is reabsorbed in the proximal tubule, and a small amount in the distal tubule. Proximal reabsorption occurs by passive transport coupled to sodium (Na–P co-transport). Phosphorus intake and PTH mainly regulate this co-transport. Phosphorus restriction increases reabsorption, and intake decreases it. PTH induces phosphaturia by inhibition of Na–P co-transport. The effect is exerted mainly in the proximal tubule. The hormone binds to specific receptors in the basolateral membrane, resulting in the activation of two pathways—the adenylate cyclase/cyclic adenosine monophosphate/protein kinase A and the phospholipase C/calcium/protein kinase C systems, both of which are involved in inhibition of Na–P co-transport (Bellorin-Font, 1990).

Although PTH lowers serum phosphate, serum levels of phosphate are increased by administration of vitamin D and growth hormone. Vitamin D increases intestinal absorption and renal reabsorption of phosphorus. Growth hormone is a main regulator of skeletal growth. Its presence in the bloodstream reduces renal excretion of phosphates, thereby increasing serum levels.

Recently, a regulation cascade comprising a hormone, fibroblast growth factor 23 (FGF-23), an enzyme (phosphate-regulating gene with homologies to endopeptidases [PHEX]) thought to be involved in the metabolism of FGF-23, and a protein (matrix extracellular glycoprotein [MEPE]) has been elucidated (Quarles, 2003). This cascade is thought to be involved in phosphate homeostasis but remains only partially understood. FGF-23 is normally produced by osteocytes and osteoblasts, as well as in marrow pericytes, thymus, and lymph nodes; however, current data support that most of FGF-23 is derived from bone in response to phosphate levels (Lu, 2007) and provide the first evidence of an independent hormonal regulation of phosphate levels. Elevated levels of FGF-23 result in hyperphosphaturia, primarily by inhibiting sodium-dependent phosphate resorption channels; FGF-23 also inhibits intestinal phosphorus absorption by inhibiting 25OH-vitamin D 1-α-hydroxylase in the renal proximal tubules (Lu, 2007). Mutations involving FGF-23, PHEX, and MEPE have been implicated in phosphate wasting by the kidneys and have been associated with various mineralization abnormalities (Quarles, 2003).

Analytic Techniques

Most commonly used methods for determination of inorganic phosphate are based on the reaction of phosphate with ammonium molybdate to form phosphomolybdate complex (see Chapter 44). Direct ultraviolet (UV) measurement of the colorless unreduced complex by absorption at 340 nm, as originally described by Daly and Ertinghausen in 1972, has been adapted for use on most of the automated analyzers. Alternatively, the phosphomolybdate complex can be reduced by a wide variety of agents (e.g., aminonaphtholsulfonic acid, ascorbic acid, methyl-p-aminophenol sulfate, ferrous sulfate) to produce molybdenum blue, which can be measured at 600–700 nm. The formation of phosphomolybdate complex is pH dependent, and the rate of its formation is influenced by protein concentration. Measurements of unreduced complexes have the advantages of being simple, fast, and stable. An enzymatic method has also been described whereby phosphorus undergoes successive enzymatic reactions catalyzed by glycogen phosphorylase, phosphoglucomutase, and glucose-6-phosphate dehydrogenase. The NADPH produced can be quantitated fluorometrically or spectrophotometrically. The reaction takes place at neutral pH, thus permitting the measurement of inorganic phosphorus in the presence of unstable organic phosphate.

Serum is preferred because most anticoagulants, except heparin, interfere with results and yield falsely low values. Phosphorus levels are increased by prolonged storage with cells at room temperature. Hemolyzed specimens are unacceptable because erythrocytes contain high levels of organic esters, which are hydrolyzed to inorganic phosphate during storage, and thus yield elevated levels.

Reference Interval

In normal adults, serum phosphorus varies between 2.8 and 4.5 mg/dL (0.89–1.44 mmol/L). Higher phosphorus levels occur in growing children (4.0–7.0 mg/dL or 1.29–2.26 mmol/L). Serum phosphate is best measured in fasting morning specimens because of diurnal variation, with higher levels in the afternoon and evening, as well as a reduction in serum phosphate after meals. Levels are influenced by dietary intake, meals, and exercise.

MAGNESIUM

Physiology

Distribution

Magnesium is the fourth most abundant cation in the body after calcium, sodium, and potassium; it is the second most prevalent intracellular cation. The normal body magnesium content in an adult is approximately 1000 mmol, or 22.66 g, of which 50%–60% is in bone, and the remaining 40%–50% is in the soft tissues. One third of skeletal magnesium is exchangeable and probably serves as a reservoir for maintaining a normal extracellular magnesium concentration.

Only 1% of the total body magnesium (TBMg) is in extracellular fluid. In serum, about 55% of magnesium is ionized or free magnesium (Mg^{++}), 30% is associated with proteins (primarily albumin), and 15% is complexed with phosphate, citrate, and other anions. The interstitial fluid concentration is approximately 0.5 mmol/L. In cerebrospinal fluid (CSF), 55% of the magnesium is free or ionized, and the remaining 45% is complexed with other compounds (Elin, 1988).

Approximately 99% of the TBMg is in bone matrix or is intracellular. About 60% of this total is within bone matrix, and the other 40% is within skeletal muscle, within blood cells, or in the cells of other tissues. Intracellular magnesium concentration is approximately 1–3 mmol/L (2.4–7.3 mg/dL). Within the cell, magnesium is compartmentalized, and most of it is bound to proteins and negatively charged molecules; approximately 80% of cytosolic magnesium is bound to ATP. Significant amounts of magnesium are found in the nucleus, mitochondria, and endoplasmic reticulum. Free magnesium accounts for 0.5%–5.0% of the total cellular magnesium, and is the fraction that is probably important as a cofactor supporting enzyme activity.

Function

Magnesium is essential for the function of more than 300 cellular enzymes, including those related to the transfer of phosphate groups, all reactions that require ATP, and every step related to the replication and transcription of DNA and the translation of mRNA. This cation is also required for cellular energy metabolism and has an important role in membrane stabilization, nerve conduction, ion transport, and calcium channel activity. In addition, magnesium plays a critical role in the maintenance of intracellular potassium concentration by regulating potassium movement through the membranes of the myocardial cells. Thus, magnesium deficiency can result in a variety of metabolic abnormalities and clinical consequences, including refractory plasma electrolyte abnormalities (especially depressed potassium) and cardiac arrhythmias most often observed after stress such as cardiac surgery (Weisinger, 1998).

Magnesium Homeostasis

Total body magnesium depends mainly on gastrointestinal absorption and renal excretion. The average dietary intake of magnesium fluctuates between 300 and 350 mg/day, and intestinal absorption is inversely proportional to the ingested amount. The factors controlling the intestinal absorption of magnesium remain poorly understood.

The kidney is the principal organ involved in magnesium regulation. Renal excretion is about 120–140 mg/24 hours for a person on a normal diet. Approximately 70%–80% of the plasma magnesium is filtered through the glomerular membrane. Tubular reabsorption of Mg^{++} is different from that for other ions because the proximal tubule has a limited role, and 60%–70% of the reabsorption of Mg^{++} takes place within the thick ascending loop of Henle (Quamme, 1989). Even though the distal tubules reabsorb only 10% of the filtered Mg^{++}, they are the major sites of magnesium regulation. Many factors, both hormonal and nonhormonal (e.g., parathyroid hormone, calcitonin, glucagon, vasopressin, magnesium restriction, acid-base changes, potassium depletion), influence both Henle's loop and distal tubule reabsorption. However, the major regulator of reabsorption is the plasma concentration of Mg^{++} itself. Increased Mg^{++} concentration inhibits loop transport, whereas decreased concentration stimulates transport, regardless of whether or not there is magnesium depletion. The mechanisms appear to be regulated by the Ca^{++}/Mg^{++}-sensing receptor, located on the capillary side of the thick-ascending-limb cells, which senses the changes in Mg^{++} (Quamme, 1997). Other factors that may play a role in magnesium regulation include calcium concentration and rate of sodium chloride reabsorption.

In magnesium deficiency, serum levels decrease, and this leads to reduced urinary excretion. Later, bone stores of magnesium are affected as the process of equilibration with bone stores takes place over several weeks.

Because serum contains only about 1% of total body magnesium, it may not accurately reflect total stores. In general, a low serum level indicates deficiency, and a high level indicates adequate stores. However, the most common result—a normal level—should be interpreted with caution because it does not exclude an underlying deficiency. The most accurate assessment of magnesium status is generally considered to be the loading test, wherein magnesium is given intravenously. Magnesium-deficient individuals retain a greater proportion of the load and excrete less in the urine than normal individuals (Papazachariou, 2000). However, the test is not commonly used because it is difficult to administer.

Analytic Techniques

Total Magnesium

Serum is preferred over plasma for magnesium determination because anticoagulant interferes with most procedures. Serum magnesium is usually measured by photometry. The reference method for total magnesium is atomic absorption spectrophotometry. Most clinical laboratories use a photometric method on an automated analyzer. These methods use metallochromic indicators or dyes that change color upon selectively binding magnesium from the sample. Some of the chromophores used include calmagite, methylthymol blue, formazan dye, and magon (see Chapter 27). In the calmagite photometric method, which is the one most commonly used, calmagite, whose structure is shown in Chapter 27 (see Fig. 27-2), forms a colored complex with magnesium in alkaline solution. This complex is stable for over 30 minutes, and its absorbance at 520 nm is directly proportional to the magnesium concentration in the specimen aliquot. Some of these measurements are affected by increased serum bilirubin levels, which can result in a significant underestimation of Mg in the sample.

Ionized (Free) Magnesium. Ionized magnesium can be measured with magnesium ISEs that have been incorporated into several commercial clinical analyzers (Huijgen, 1999). These ISEs employ neutral carrier ionophores that are selective for Mg^{++}. However, in addition to Mg^{++}, these ISEs measure Ca^{++}, thus requiring a chemometric correction to calculate the true free magnesium levels in the sample. Studies have shown significant differences in the measured ionized magnesium on different analyzers that were attributed to interference from free calcium in the sample, as well as to insufficient specificity and lack of standardization of the calibrators (Hristova, 1995; Cecco, 1997). Further improvements in the method for ISEs for ionized magnesium will improve the performance and increase the availability of Mg^{++} determination in the clinical laboratory.

As with ionized calcium determinations, ionized magnesium measurements are affected by pH. The rate of change of ionized magnesium measurements is not as significant as that seen in ionized calcium determinations. Changes in magnesium in relation to alterations of pH are similar to those in ionized calcium, although less well characterized. With an increase in pH, ionized magnesium is decreased, and with a decrease in pH, it is increased (Wang, 2002).

Reference Interval

The reference interval for serum total magnesium in normal adults ranges between 0.75 and 0.95 mmol/L (1.7–2.2 mg/dL or 1.5–1.9 mEq/L). There appear to be no significant sex or age differences. Erythrocyte magnesium is about three times that of serum. The magnesium concentration in CSF is 2.0–2.7 mg/dL (1.0–1.4 mmol/L). The reference interval for ionized magnesium depends on the analyzer used for its measurement and varies from 0.44–0.60 mmol/L (Hristova, 1995).

HORMONES REGULATING MINERAL METABOLISM

The three principal hormones regulating mineral and bone metabolism are parathyroid hormone (PTH), 1,25-dihydroxyvitamin D_3 (1,25[OH]$_2D_3$), and calcitonin. PTH and 1,25(OH)$_2D_3$ are the primary hormones that exert an effect, while calcitonin is less prominent in the cycle that maintains mineral metabolism. In addition, the metabolic effects of calcitonin are less well understood.

Parathyroid Hormone

Physiology

Synthesis. PTH is synthesized and secreted by the chief cells of the parathyroid gland. Intact PTH is a single-chain polypeptide consisting of 84 amino acids with a molecular mass of 9500Da. It is derived from a larger precursor, pre-pro-PTH, of 115 amino acids, which undergoes two successive cleavages, both at the amino-terminal sequences. This yields, first, an intermediate precursor, pro-PTH, and then the hormone itself. Any pro-PTH that reaches the circulation is immediately converted to PTH and other products.

Secretion. Multiple factors control the release of PTH from the parathyroid glands, but only a small number are known to be physiologically important. PTH secretion is regulated on a time scale of seconds by extracellular ionized calcium and represents a simple negative-feedback loop. Extracellular signals are detected by a calcium-sensing receptor, located on the plasma membrane of the parathyroid chief cell. Stimulation of this receptor leads to suppression of the rate of PTH secretion via intracellular signals (inositol triphosphate and diacylglycerol) generated by the active receptor. The receptor is present in parathyroid glands, the calcitonin-secreting cells of the thyroid, brain, and kidney. This G-protein–linked receptor is mutated in the disorders of familial hypocalciuric hypercalcemia, neonatal severe hyperparathyroidism, and autosomal dominant hypocalcemia (Mundy, 1999).

Ionized magnesium has also been shown to influence the secretion of PTH. Hypocalcemic patients with low serum magnesium concentration often require administration of magnesium to increase serum PTH levels before the serum calcium concentration can be restored to the desired interval. Chronic severe hypomagnesemia such as that seen in alcoholism has been associated with impaired PTH secretion, whereas an acute decrease in the serum magnesium concentration can lead to an increased PTH.

Other levels of PTH control include regulation of PTH gene transcription and parathyroid chief cell mass by vitamin D and extracellular calcium. 1,25-Dihydroxyvitamin D_3 chronically suppresses the synthesis of PTH by interacting with vitamin D receptors in the parathyroid gland.

Function. The primary physiologic function of PTH is to maintain the concentration of ionized calcium in the ECF, which is achieved by the following mechanisms: (1) stimulation of osteoclastic bone resorption and release of calcium and phosphate from bone; (2) stimulation of calcium reabsorption and inhibition of phosphate reabsorption from the renal tubules; and (3) stimulation of renal production of 1,25-(OH)$_2D_3$, which increases intestinal absorption of calcium and phosphate. The amino-terminal end of the PTH molecule binds to the PTH receptor, which modulates adenylate cyclase and phospholipase C. Activating mutations in this receptor may cause the hypercalcemia and epiphyseal disorganization seen in Jansen's chondrodysplasia (Bastepe, 2004).

The net effects of PTH actions on bone, kidney, and indirectly on intestine include increased serum total and ionized calcium concentrations and decreased serum phosphate. Its immediate effects on the kidney are to increase renal plasma flow and cause a diuresis. At the level of the distal convoluted tubule, it causes increased reabsorption of calcium and chloride with the exchange of phosphate into the urine. These effects are mediated through its activation of renal adenyl cyclase. As a result, urinary cyclic adenosine monophosphate (cAMP) and urinary phosphate are increased with a mild secondary hyperchloremic acidosis. In the absence of disease, the increase in serum calcium reduces PTH secretion through a negative-feedback loop, thus maintaining calcium homeostasis. If this negative-feedback loop is sufficiently interrupted by an autonomously functioning parathyroid gland to increase resting calcium to abnormally high levels, the capacity of the distal tubules to reabsorb calcium is exceeded, and hypercalciuria results.

Heterogeneity. PTH metabolism is complex and produces several fragments of varying biological and immunologic reactivity. The intact PTH is the biologically active form and has a half-life in the circulation of less than 4 minutes. The kidney and liver clear intact PTH rapidly. In the liver, intact PTH is cleaved into discrete fragments and smaller peptides that are released into the circulation. The released inactive carboxy-terminal fragments circulate considerably longer than the intact hormone, mainly because they are cleared exclusively by glomerular filtration (Mundy, 1999).

Analytic Techniques

Historically, PTH immunoassays were developed to measure mid-region, N-terminal, and C-terminal regions. However, these assays cross-reacted with amino acid sequences present in both mid-region and carboxyl fragments of the intact hormone and measured mostly inactive fragments because they are present in greater concentration than the intact molecule. Because the kidney clears inactive PTH fragments, results from these assays were difficult to interpret, especially in patients with impaired renal function. PTH intact is measured by noncompetitive immunometric (sandwich) assays (see Chapter 44), which, depending on the type of detection system used, are divided into immunoradiometric assay (IRMA), when radiolabeled, and immunochemiluminometric assay, when labeled with a chemiluminescent compound. Most automated systems use immunochemiluminometric assays. These immunometric assays have several advantages over earlier assays: (1) increased sensitivity and specificity through the use of sequence-specific and affinity-purified antibodies, (2) extended assay concentration range, and (3) decreased incubation time, and (4) they do not utilize radioactive compounds.

Reference Interval

The reference interval for intact PTH in normal adults is 10–65 pg/mL (ng/L) when a two-site immunometric method is used. Studies have demonstrated that intact PTH is secreted in episodic or pulsatile fashion, with an overall circadian rhythm characterized by a nocturnal rise in intact PTH. Serum is the preferred specimen for measurement of PTH. Prolonged storage of the specimen aliquot causes falsely decreased levels.

Bio-Intact PTH

Physiology

Traditional tests for intact PTH detect and measure both the biologically intact 84 amino acid PTH molecule (1-84) and its minimally active to inactive metabolites. Recall that the intact, biologically active molecule is cleaved within minutes to the many metabolites that have a longer half-life, and of which there is a much higher concentration in the circulation at any given time. One of these cleavage products, the 7-84 PTH breakdown fragment, is a weak antagonist to PTH activity and may actually lower patient serum calcium levels. It is therefore important to distinguish between intact PTH and breakdown products in the setting of patients with chronic renal failure (Brossard, 2000). In uremic patients, the metabolites, including the 7-84 breakdown fragment, accumulate as the result of decreased renal clearance, and can therefore give the impression of an elevated PTH (Quarles, 1992).

Recent advances have made available a test for only the biologically active, intact PTH. This third-generation test eliminates interference by the metabolites and is of great clinical utility in patients with impaired renal function. The bio-intact PTH test specifically measures the (1-84) molecule via a two-site chemiluminescent assay. This assay yields a higher specificity than second-generation tests for the biologically active intact PTH, but cost and availability considerations make this a second-line test that is used primarily in following metabolic bone status in patients with renal insufficiency.

Normal ranges for this test show seasonal variation, in part because of lower serum 25(OH)D during the wintertime in the healthy population. Normal values for this test range from 8–50 pg/mL (Nichols Advantage, 2004).

Intraoperative PTH

Historically, parathyroid surgery has consisted of bilateral neck exploration in an attempt to identify enlarged parathyroid glands. In recent years, clinical practice has moved away from this costly and invasive procedure, which often requires an overnight hospital stay, to minimally invasive parathyroidectomy with or without the use of a hand-held gamma probe. This procedure consists of preoperative administration of technetium-99 m sestamibi 2 hours preoperatively followed by performance of a parathyroid scan. The parathyroid adenoma, with its increased numbers of cytoplasmic mitochondria, selectively absorbs large amounts of this radioactive substance, which then allows identification of the adenoma(s) with a hand-held gamma probe. This method of identifying the enlarged gland allows for removal of only the hyperfunctional parathyroid gland in cases of parathyroid adenoma. Cases of parathyroid hyperplasia still require bilateral neck exploration. Depending on the size of these enlarged glands, they may or may not be identified on the preoperative parathyroid scan (Goldstein, 2000; Sofferman, 1998; Sokoll, 2000).

Once the hyperfunctioning parathyroid gland is identified via sestamibi scan, and only a single parathyroid gland has been shown to be involved, patients are taken to surgery for minimally invasive parathyroidectomy. This approach has reduced surgical and hospital costs, as well as admission time (Goldstein, 1991).

Before surgery, a baseline PTH value is obtained. Following incision, dissection to the radioactive parathyroid gland is guided by the use of a gamma probe. Once identified, the parathyroid gland is removed. After removal, the surgeon waits about 10–20 minutes and obtains a post-removal PTH value. This post-removal PTH value should decrease to at least 50%–75% below the preoperative level or should have a "significant" trend toward normal in patients with markedly elevated preoperative PTH levels. The decrease in PTH levels reassures the surgeon that the adenomatous gland has been removed. If no or minimal decrease is noted in the intraoperative PTH level, the surgeon is obligated to resume neck exploration for additional abnormal glands, and multiple adenomas or hyperplasia is suggested as the underlying process. Intraoperative PTH testing is recommended for patients undergoing surgery for primary hyperparathyroidism, reoperative hyperparathyroidism, and venous/tumor localization presurgery in the angiography suite (Sokoll, 2004).

Analytic Techniques

The intraoperative technique for intact PTH customarily requires blood collected in an EDTA tube (plasma) or a red-top tube (serum). The sample is maintained at a cold temperature to minimize breakdown, and is submitted for rapid PTH testing. These immunochemiluminometric assays provide rapid results by modifying certain test parameters on the standard assay. Specifically, increased incubation temperature, continuous shaking of the reaction contents, and alterations in sample and reagent volumes are used to expedite antibody–antigen reactions. The end result is a more rapid assay, albeit one that is more costly, less sensitive, and more imprecise than the standard assay. These assays correlate well with standard assays and are totally acceptable for measuring large drops in PTH concentration during surgery.

Parathyroid Hormone–Related Peptide

Physiology

Parathyroid hormone–related peptide (PTH-rP) was first discovered in tumors derived from lung, breast, kidney, and other solid tissues. It has since been described as a hormone with paracrine and autocrine functions. PTH-rP is composed of 141 amino acids and shows significant homology with PTH in the first 13 amino acids. It is the product of a large gene on chromosome 12 that is syngeneic to the PTH gene on chromosome 11. This peptide shares the same receptor as PTH. Its actions include binding to and activating the PTH receptor, thus simulating the PTH biological effects on bone, kidney, and intestine. Similar to PTH, PTH-rP increases bone resorption by stimulating osteoclasts and promotes renal tubular reabsorption of calcium. The net effect is elevated serum calcium concentration. It is now known that PTH-rP is produced by approximately 50% of primary breast cancers, and its production may be enhanced by bone-derived factors such as transforming growth factor-β (Yin, 1999; see Chapter 74 for a description of this growth factor). Other malignant tumors also elaborate this peptide. PTH-rP has been implicated as the agent responsible for humoral hypercalcemia in patients with malignancy.

Elevation of PTH-rP has been observed in approximately 50%–90% of patients with malignancy-associated hypercalcemia. Increased PTH-rP is seen in squamous cell carcinomas of the lung, esophagus, cervix, and skin, as well as in other malignancies (e.g., islet cell carcinomas, T-cell and B-cell lymphomas, multiple myeloma). PTH-rP levels are normal in patients with primary hyperparathyroidism, hypoparathyroidism, chronic renal failure, and other conditions with hypercalcemia.

Some benign hyperplasias, including massive mammary hypertrophy, vasoactive intestinal peptide-secreting tumors, pheochromocytomas, and lactational changes of the breast, may elaborate this peptide (Strewler, 1997).

A recent study demonstrated that PTH-rP has therapeutic potential in the treatment of postmenopausal osteoporosis; PTH-rP increased bone mineral density by nearly 5%—a rate that exceeds those of current therapeutic approaches (Horwitz, 2003).

Analytic Technique and Reference Interval

PTH-rP is measured by immunometric assay (usually IRMA) in which antibodies to different sequences of the PTH-rP molecule are used as capture antibodies and radiolabeled signal antibodies. The limit of detection of these assays is between 0.1 and 1.0 pmol/L (Endres, 1999). The reference interval for PTH-rP is method-dependent. In normal individuals, PTH-rP levels range from undetectable to around 2 pmol/L, whereas the mean concentration of PTH-rP in patients with humoral hypercalcemia of malignancy has been reported to be 22.2 pmol/L. Recent studies have shown that most patients (95%) with a PTH level >26 ng/mL had no increased PTH-rP, a number that increased to 100% when only patients with hypercalcemia were evaluated. This study suggests that testing for PTH-rP in patients with low or low normal PTH may not be of clinical utility (Fritchie, 2009).

Calcitonin

Physiology

Synthesis and Metabolism. Calcitonin is synthesized and secreted by specialized C cells (parafollicular cells) of the thyroid gland and acts on the bones, kidneys, and gastrointestinal tract. Circulating immunoreactive calcitonin is derived from a larger precursor, and the monomeric form is the only biologically active entity. Calcitonin monomer is a 32 amino acid peptide with a molecular mass of 3500 Da. The ionized calcium concentration is the most important regulator of calcitonin secretion. Increases in ionized calcium lead to an increase in calcitonin secretion. Other potent calcitonin secretagogues include the gastrointestinal peptide hormones and gastrin in particular (Care, 1971). The latter could explain the presence of a mild postprandial increase in calcitonin concentration.

The calcitonin receptor is structurally similar to PTH/PTH-rP and secretin receptors; it exists in several isoforms, and its expression seems to be influenced by ambient concentrations of calcitonin itself (Mundy, 1999). Calcitonin is metabolized within minutes of secretion, primarily by the kidney.

Physiologic Role and Clinical Use. Although calcitonin has been viewed as a major calcium-regulating factor because of its calcium-lowering and phosphorus-lowering properties, its precise physiologic role is still unclear. Calcitonin directly inhibits osteoclastic bone resorption by directly binding to osteoclasts. The effect of this binding action is observed within minutes after calcitonin administration. This inhibition is transient and likely has little role in overall calcium homeostasis, although it may be important in the short-term control of calcium loads. Calcitonin also inhibits the action of PTH and vitamin D. Although some clinical studies suggest that serum calcium does not appear to be affected in patients with total thyroidectomy, other studies suggest that medullary thyroid carcinoma and an excess of calcitonin can give rise to marked hypocalcemia. In the kidney, calcitonin causes increased clearance of calcium and phosphate. The mechanisms of its action on the GI tract have not been elucidated entirely.

In addition to evaluation of calcitonin in the setting of bony abnormalities, testing for calcitonin is an important adjunct in the evaluation of the patient with nodular thyroid disease, and is often performed in the hope of identifying the patient with early medullary thyroid carcinoma, which may be seen in the setting of type II multiple endocrine adenomatosis (MEN II), as described in Chapter 24. Therapeutic success in medullary thyroid carcinoma hinges on its early identification, and slight elevations of calcitonin with subsequent surgical exploration of the thyroid may identify this lesion in its early, nonpalpable stage of development. It is well known that the therapeutic efficacy is poor in cases that are identified as well-developed palpable tumors because many such patients already have metastatic disease (Rieu, 1995; Horvit, 1997). Until recently, routine testing for calcitonin in patients with nodular thyroid disease was not considered cost-effective in the United States. Studies in Europe, however, have shown this to be cost-effective. A recent cost-effectiveness analysis performed in the United States concluded that routine calcitonin testing in patients with nodular thyroid disease is, in fact, of comparable cost-effectiveness as other screening tests, such as those for thyroid-stimulating hormone, breast cancer (mammography), and colon cancer (colonoscopy) (Cheung, 2008). Diagnostic sensitivity for medullary thyroid carcinoma is increased by pentagastrin stimulation before calcitonin level testing. A high index of suspicion for this aggressive neoplasm should exist in patients with plasma or serum calcitonin levels >100 pg/nL (Vierhapper, 1997).

Therapeutic applications of calcitonin have been explored and include its use in the treatment of osteoporosis and in the treatment of Paget's disease, the early stages of which are characterized by increased bone resorption.

Analytic Technique and Reference Interval

In the past, serum calcitonin was measured primarily by radioimmunoassay (RIA). However, differences in assay specificity and sensitivity, matrix and nonspecific serum effects, and heterogeneity of the circulating calcitonin have contributed to contradicting results and discrepancies in reference values for the hormone. At present, a number of highly sensitive (limit of detection as low as 2 pg/mL), two-site immunometric methods (electroimmunoassays and IRMAs) for serum calcitonin are available. These tests are now regarded as the most reliable methods of testing for serum calcitonin.

The reference interval for serum calcitonin in normal adults is less than 25 pg/mL for males, and less than 20 pg/mL for females. Gender, age, growth, pregnancy, lactation, and ingestion of food have been reported to affect the levels of calcitonin.

Vitamin D and Metabolites

Physiology

Synthesis and Metabolism. (See also Chapters 8 and 26.)

The steroid hormone $1,25(OH)_2D_3$ is the major biologically active metabolite of the vitamin D sterol family. The vitamin D precursor (cholecalciferol or vitamin D_3) may be ingested in the diet or synthesized in the skin from 7-dehydrocholesterol (provitamin D_3) through exposure to sunlight. The plant-derived form of vitamin D is called vitamin D_2 or ergosterol. Neither form of vitamin D has any significant biological activity; both must be metabolized to hormonally active forms. This activation occurs in two steps, the first of which takes place in the liver, and the second of which takes place in the kidney. Cholecalciferol is transported to the liver bound to a specific α_1-globulin. In the liver, vitamin D undergoes hydroxylation to produce 25-hydroxyvitamin D (calcidiol), a metabolite with limited biological activity. Because the liver only loosely regulates this step, circulating levels of 25-hydroxyvitamin D mirror the amounts of vitamin D that may be ingested or synthesized by the skin. The 25-hydroxyvitamin D is then bound by the vitamin D–binding protein and is transported to the kidney, where it undergoes further hydroxylation by 1-α-hydroxylase in the proximal tubular mitochondria to form the more potent metabolite $1,25(OH)_2D_3$ (calcitriol). Renal hydroxylation of 25-hydroxyvitamin D is the major controlling point in vitamin D metabolism—a step that is regulated by serum phosphate, calcium, and circulating PTH concentrations. PTH and phosphate depletion act independently to increase $1,25(OH)_2D_3$ production by inducing 1-α-hydroxylase activity, with PTH being the more potent stimulus. Decreased blood calcium stimulates the parathyroid glands to secrete PTH, which in turn increases production of $1,25(OH)_2D_3$ in the renal proximal tubules. Conversely, a rise in blood calcium suppresses PTH secretion, which lowers the production of $1,25(OH)_2D_3$. The only other known important extrarenal sites of $1,25(OH)_2D_3$ production are the placenta and the granulomatous tissue. In humans, the half-life of $1,25(OH)_2D_3$ in the circulation is approximately 5 hours. It is excreted as urinary and fecal metabolites (Mundy, 1999). Several other vitamin D metabolites are produced in the kidney; most of these have been shown to be biologically inert. The most notable of these is 24,25-dihydroxyvitamin D_3, produced by the action of 24-α-hydroxylase in the kidney; it is activated when PTH levels are low, or when inorganic phosphate levels are elevated (Fig. 15-3).

Physiologic Role. $1,25(OH)_2D_3$ bound to a vitamin D–binding protein is delivered to the intestine, where the free form is taken up by the cells and transported to a specific nuclear receptor protein. Although the receptor binds several forms of vitamin D, its affinity for 1,25-dihydroxyvitamin D_3 is about 1000 times that of 25-hydroxyvitamin D_3, thus accounting for why the former is so much more biologically active than the latter. As a result of this interaction in the intestine, calcium-binding protein is synthesized. In bone, osteocalcin, osteopontin, and alkaline phosphatase are produced. In the intestine, the net effect of $1,25(OH)_2D_3$ is to transport calcium and phosphate from the lumen of the small intestine into the circulation by stimulating the expression of calcium-carrying proteins, thus increasing plasma calcium and phosphate concentrations. It also increases bone resorption and enhances the effects of PTH in the nephron to promote renal tubular calcium reabsorption. $1,25(OH)_2D_3$ is a powerful differentiating agent for committed osteoclast precursors, causing their maturation to form multinucleated cells that are capable of resorbing bone. These pathways enable $1,25(OH)_2D_3$ to provide a supply of calcium and phosphate available at bone surfaces for the formation of normal mineralized bone (Mundy, 1999).

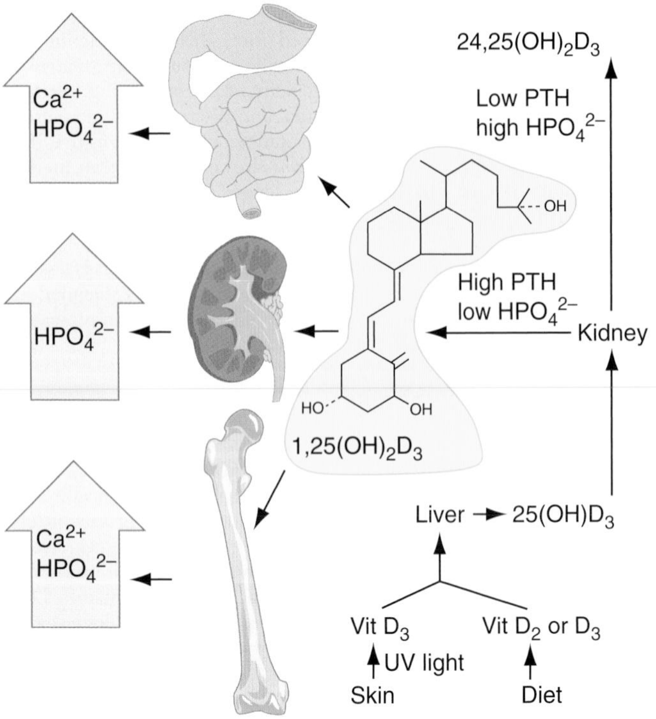

Figure 15-3 Pathways of vitamin D synthesis and their end-organ effects. The *large green arrows* indicate increases in calcium and phosphate induced by vitamin D (dihydroxycholecalciferol).

The demonstration that the sites of action of $1,25(OH)_2D_3$ are not limited to its target tissues, namely, the intestine, bone, and kidney, has expanded the therapeutic function of vitamin D. Administration of vitamin D hormone has been shown to be effective in the therapeutic management and prevention of postmenopausal and age-related osteoporosis. A recent study showed that higher-than-recommended (700–800 vs. recommended 600 IU) doses of vitamin D in nursing home residents reduced the number of patients with falls and the total number of falls in nursing home residents (Kerry, 2007). Another study showed that a similar dose acts to prevent fracture in a comparable population (Bischoff-Ferrari, 2005). Evidence suggests that, besides exhibiting calciotropic properties, vitamin D may be a developmental hormone. As discussed in Chapters 8 and 26, vitamin D has been found to exhibit antitumor growth activity.

Analytic Techniques

Of the more than 35 metabolites of vitamin D_2 and vitamin D_3, only 25(OH)D and $1,25(OH)_2D$ measurements are clinically important. 25(OH)D is a better marker than vitamin D for evaluation of vitamin D status because of its longer half-life (2–3 weeks vs. 5–8 hours) (Papapoulos, 1982), more limited fluctuation with exposure to sunlight and dietary intake, larger concentration, and ease of measurement. Measurement of $1,25(OH)_2D_3$ is useful in detecting certain states of inadequate or excessive hormone production in the evaluation of hypercalcemia, hypercalciuria, and hypocalcemia, as well as in bone and mineral disorders. Because both vitamin D_2 and vitamin D_3 are metabolized to compounds of similar if not equal biological activity, for clinical purposes the assays should measure $25(OH)D_2$ and $25(OH)D_3$ or $1,25(OH)_2D_2$ and $1,25(OH)_2D_3$, respectively. At present, the reference method for the assay of $25(OH)D_2$ and $25(OH)D_3$ is dual mass spectrometry. Most other assays for vitamin D metabolites are measured by RIA or chemiluminescent immunoassay.

Reference Interval

The reference interval for 25(OH)D in serum is approximately 10–50 ng/mL (25–125 nmol/L), and for $1,25(OH)_2D$ is 15–60 pg/mL (36–144 pmol/L) (Endres, 1999). Levels for 25(OH)D are influenced by sunlight exposure, latitude, skin pigmentation, sunscreen use, and hepatic function. 25(OH)D levels also exhibit seasonal variation. Winter values may be 40%–50% lower than summer values because of reduced UV radiation exposure. Concentrations of vitamin D metabolites vary with age and are increased in pregnancy.

Phosphatonins

Phosphatonins represent a new group of phosphate-regulating factors that remain incompletely understood, yet have thus far shed much light on the many disorders of phosphate and calcium metabolism. These factors include FGF-23, MEPE, and frizzled related protein 4. These substances act to reduce renal inorganic phosphate reabsorption both directly by their action on the renal tubules and indirectly through the inhibition of 25-hydroxyvitamin D_1 α-hydroxylase, causing a reduction in $1\alpha25(OH)_2D$ formation that results in decreased inorganic phosphate absorption and reduced calcium absorption. Both mechanisms produce decreased serum inorganic phosphate levels, resulting in rickets in children and osteomalacia in adults. Increased levels of these factors, as well as the previously discussed PHEX, have been causally implicated in tumor-induced osteomalacia, X-linked hypophosphatemic rickets, and autosomal dominant hypophosphatemic rickets (ADHR). X-linked hypophosphatemic rickets is associated with varied mutations of the *PHEX* gene, and ADHR is due to activating mutations of FGF-23 (Pettifor, 2008; Roetzer, 2007; Gaucher, 2009; Ichikawa, 2008; Schiavi, 2004). All of these entities are clinically characterized by reduced serum phosphate, increased urinary phosphate levels, and aberrant bone mineralization. In addition, these entities are customarily seen in the setting of normal serum calcium.

Although the previous entities result largely from increased FGF-23, mutations in FGF-23 resulting in a net reduced level of effective FGF-23 have also been described at multiple loci. They produce disease through a common mechanism of reduced phosphaturic activity, creating the clinical picture of hyperphosphatemic tumoral calcinosis (Araya, 2005; Larsson, 2005; Masi, 2009). Another factor implicated in the hyperphosphatemic form of this disease is UDP-N-acetyl-α-D galactosamine/polypeptide N-acetylgalactosaminyltransferase 3. Inactivating mutations of this gene result in accelerated degradation of FGF-23 into inactive metabolites (Jueppner, 2007).

Analytic Techniques

Thus far, there are no commercially available assays for these mutations. Currently, these growth factors have been evaluated experimentally via polymerase chain reaction (PCR) and more recently by enzyme-linked immunosorbent assay for intact FGF-23 and the processed fragments (18 and 12 kDa). In addition, reverse transcriptase-PCR (RT-PCR) for FGF-23 has been performed on formalin-fixed, paraffin-embedded tissue in the setting of phosphaturic mesenchymal tumors of the mixed connective tissue type with high sensitivity and specificity (Bahrami, 2009).

Disorders of Mineral Metabolism

HYPERCALCEMIA

Increased serum calcium is associated with anorexia, nausea, vomiting, constipation, hypotonia, depression, high-voltage T waves on electrocardiography, and occasionally lethargy and coma. Persistent hypercalcemia or persistently elevated calcium–phosphorus ionic activity product may cause ectopic depositions of calcium in tissues throughout the body. This may take the form of ectopically calcified blood vessel walls associated with necrotic skin lesions in calciphylaxis. It may also lead to calcifications in viable tissues (metastatic calcification/tumoral calcinosis), particularly those developing pH gradients with localized relative alkalosis (e.g., pulmonary alveolar walls, renal medullary pyramids, deep gastric mucosa). The most common causes of hypercalcemia are primary hyperparathyroidism and malignant neoplasms, which account for 80%–90% of all patients with hypercalcemia. Less frequent causes include renal failure, diuretics, vitamin A and D intoxication, lithium therapy, milk–alkali syndrome, immobilization, hyperthyroidism and other nonparathyroid endocrinopathies, and familial hypercalciuric hypercalcemia (Table 15-1). Recently, mutations in *FGF-23* and in another gene encoding the so-called N-terminal sterile α motif protein (*SAMD9* gene) have also been implicated in tumoral calcinosis. Mutations in *FGF-23* characteristically cause hyperphosphatemic tumoral calcinosis, while mutations in *SAMD9* cause normophosphatemic tumoral calcinosis. The tumoral calcinosis caused by both is familial (Araya, 2005; Larsson, 2005. Masi, 2009; Chefetz, 2005; Topaz, 2006; Chefetz, 2008). Disease due to *SAMD9* mutations appears to affect Yemenite Jews predominantly. *Primary hyperparathyroidism* (PHPT) is characterized by excessive secretion of PTH in the absence of an appropriate physiologic stimulus and with no response to the physiologic negative-feedback loop of hypercalcemia. This results in a generalized disorder of calcium, phosphate, and bone metabolism. Approximately

TABLE 15-1
Causes of Hypercalcemia

Parathyroid hormone (PTH) Mediated
Primary hyperparathyroidism (most common):
Sporadic
Multiple endocrine neoplasia (types 1 and 2)
Familial hypocalciuric hypercalcemia
Ectopic secretion of PTH by neoplasms (rare)?
Non–PTH Mediated
Malignancy associated (most common)
Vitamin D mediated
Vitamin D intoxication
Increased generation of 1,25$(OH)_2$D
Other endocrinopathies
Thyrotoxicosis
Hypoadrenalism
Immobilization with increased bone turnover
Milk–alkali syndrome
Sarcoidosis
Multiple myeloma

100,000 cases of PHPT occur each year in the United States, and the incidence increases with age. The disease affects women twice as frequently as it affects men. Most cases are caused by solitary parathyroid adenomas. Other causes include multiple parathyroid adenomas, hyperplasia, and, rarely, parathyroid carcinoma. Hypercalcemia in PHPT is characteristically associated with decreased serum phosphate due to PTH-induced phosphate diuresis and is frequently accompanied by mild acidosis from decreased renal reabsorption of bicarbonate. The hypercalcemia is attributed to (1) the direct action of PTH on bone, causing increased resorption; (2) PTH-activated renal tubular reabsorption; and (3) PTH-stimulated increased renal biosynthesis of 1,25$(OH)_2D_3$, which increases intestinal absorption of calcium (Boden, 1990). Half or more of patients with PHPT are asymptomatic. Symptomatic patients usually present with recurrent nephrolithiasis, chronic constipation, mental depression, neuromuscular dysfunction, recurrent chronic pancreatitis, or peptic ulcer, and less frequently with unexplained or premature osteopenia (Deftos, 1993).

The unique bone manifestation of PHPT is osteitis fibrosa cystica generalizata. This is characterized by diffuse skeletal radiolucency with focal cystic bone lesions, subperiosteal bone resorption most pronounced in the digits, and osseous deformities on routine radiographs. Histologically, paratrabecular fibrosis and marrow hypervascularity are accompanied by increased numbers of osteoclasts, causing trabecular scalloping (Howship's lacunae) as a result of accelerated bone resorption (Fig. 15-4, *A* and *B*). As the disease progresses, the marrow cavity is gradually replaced by fibrous tissue. The process is even more pronounced in compact bone, where large aggregates of osteoclasts demonstrate wedge-shaped resorption that enlarges Haversian canals (cutting cones). Fractures that develop through this altered bone tend to heal poorly and result in space-occupying lesions filled with fibrous tissue, multinucleated giant cells, hemorrhage, and hemosiderin; these are sometimes referred to as "brown tumors" even though they are not neoplastic. Generalized osteitis fibrosa cystica is now very uncommon because serum calcium and phosphate screening usually reveal early parathyroid hyperfunction long before signs or symptoms develop.

PHPT may be inherited as an autosomal dominant trait and may present as a part of MEN. MEN 1 consists of hyperparathyroidism and tumors of the pituitary gland and pancreas. It is often associated with Zollinger-Ellison syndrome, characterized by islet cell tumors with gastrin hypersecretion and peptic ulcer disease. MEN 2A consists of hyperparathyroidism, pheochromocytoma, and medullary carcinoma of the thyroid. Studies have identified the molecular defects in hyperparathyroidism. A gene locus on chromosome 11 has been associated with MEN 1. The same locus appears to be lost in approximately 25% of solitary parathyroid adenomas, implying that the defect responsible for MEN 1 can also cause the sporadic disease.

Secondary hyperparathyroidism is present when there is resistance to the metabolic actions of PTH, as occurs in patients with renal failure, vitamin D deficiency (osteomalacia), and pseudohypoparathyroidism. This leads to parathyroid gland hyperplasia and excessive production of PTH.

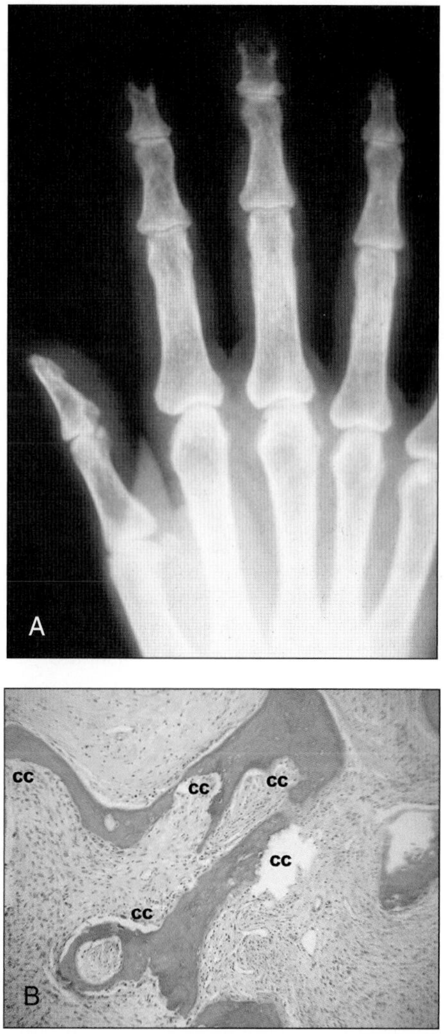

Figure 15-4 Hyperparathyroid bone disease (osteitis fibrosa cystica). **A,** The hand radiograph demonstrates scalloped cortical resorption on the radial *(left)* side of the phalanges and radiolucency of the terminal phalangeal tufts. **B,** Biopsy of compact bone with advanced hyperparathyroid disease demonstrates conversion of compact to cancellous bone with internal resorption of Haversian systems by osteoclastic cutting cones (CC) and paratrabecular fibrosis (100×).

The pathogenesis varies somewhat, depending on the nature and severity of renal disease. However, decreased renal excretion of phosphate as a consequence of impaired glomerular filtration is paramount. In such patients, there is an initial tendency toward hypocalcemia because as phosphate levels rise, calcium levels decrease, because their ionic activity product constant makes their serum concentrations inversely related (see Chapter 8 for a discussion of the solubility product constant). In addition, chronic renal failure includes reduced production of 1,25$(OH)_2$D by the kidney. Decreased 1,25$(OH)_2$D causes a reduced response of the skeleton to PTH and decreased calcium absorption from the intestine, contributing to hypocalcemia. Because of the decreased serum ionic calcium, there is positive feedback to increase parathyroid hormone secretion; this causes parathyroid gland hyperplasia. Initial clinical manifestations include low to normal serum calcium and hyperphosphatemia. Later, in cases with severe secondary hyperparathyroidism, both hypercalcemia and hyperphosphatemia develop. In addition, bone pain, ectopic calcifications, and pruritus may be seen. The complex bone disease occurring in secondary hyperparathyroidism and renal failure is usually termed renal osteodystrophy (Fig. 15-5) and is discussed in greater detail later. Autonomous hyperparathyroidism may sometimes supervene in the setting of chronic parathyroid stimulation. Typical patients are those with chronic renal failure or with some other disease that chronically lowers serum ionized calcium levels and stimulates long-term parathyroid hormone secretion. This chronic parathyroid stimulation results in increased parathyroid mass and diffuse parathyroid hyperplasia. If increased levels of parathyroid hormone are not diminished by hypercalcemia, whether it occurs in the setting of continued calcium wasting or if the calcium level is corrected

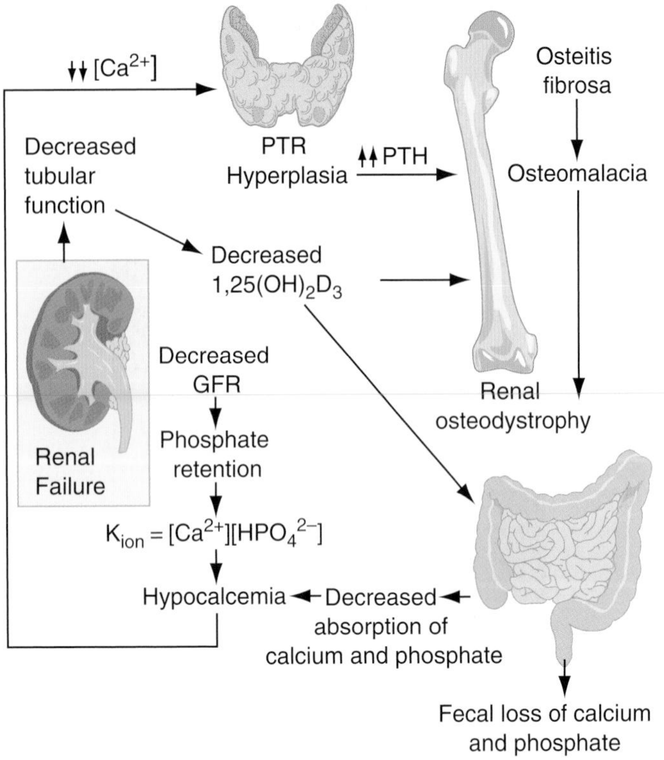

Figure 15-5 Relationships leading to renal osteodystrophy in chronic renal failure.

(e.g., after renal transplantation), the clinical syndrome is sometimes referred to as *tertiary hyperparathyroidism*. Patients with this syndrome may have parathyroid adenomas, parathyroid hyperplasia, and even parathyroid carcinomas. There is also a tendency for these patients to develop metastatic calcifications because their transiently increased calcium and phosphate levels may exceed the ionic activity product for these ions and cause precipitation of the excess.

Malignant tumors are the most frequent cause of hypercalcemia in the hospital inpatient population. *Malignancy-associated hypercalcemia* can be divided into cases with or without bony metastases. Radiolucent bone lesions indicative of metastatic disease are frequently seen in patients with hematologic malignancies (multiple myeloma, lymphomas, and leukemias), lung carcinoma, renal cell carcinoma, and thyroid carcinoma. Several possible mechanisms have been implicated in the development of malignancy-associated hypercalcemia, including direct tumor lysis, secretion of osteoclast-activating factor by tumor cells, and secretion of lymphokines with osteoclast potentiating activity such as interleukin-1 and tumor necrosis factor. Conventional bone radiographs and bone scanning can detect most bony metastases. Hypercalcemia without bony metastases is also known as *humoral hypercalcemia of malignancy* (HHM). Diagnosis in these cases, in general, is more difficult because the primary tumor may be occult. A variety of tumor types have been associated with this syndrome, including renal carcinoma, hepatocellular carcinoma, carcinomas of the head and neck, lung carcinomas, and islet cell tumors of the pancreas. The most common cause of HHM is secretion of PTH-rP by the tumor. The diagnosis is highly suggestive when urinary cAMP excretion (typically seen in hyperparathyroidism) is increased in the setting of reduced or normal PTH.

Vitamin D intoxication is another cause of hypercalcemia and is usually the result of excessive intake of vitamin supplements over a prolonged period of time. Excess vitamin D causes increased calcium absorption by the intestines, enhanced bone resorption, and hypercalciuria. PTH is suppressed, but the frequent development of renal failure may make it difficult to exclude hyperparathyroidism; 25(OH)D has been implicated as the major metabolite responsible for the syndrome. The diagnosis is supported by careful history taking, measurements of 25(OH)D, and a prompt response following steroid administration. Clinically, vitamin D intoxication is manifest by weakness, irritability, nausea, vomiting, and diarrhea. Soft tissue calcification is a common feature because serum phosphorus tends to be elevated. Intoxication may persist for months because of storage of vitamin D in adipose tissue.

TABLE 15-2
Causes of Hypocalcemia

Parathyroid hormone (PTH) Mediated
PTH deficiency
Permanent
Acquired
Postsurgical
Hereditary
Idiopathic hypoparathyroidism
DiGeorge syndrome (branchial dysgenesis)
Polyglandular autoimmune syndromes
Reversible
Severe hypomagnesemia
Long-standing hypercalcemia
PTH resistance
Pseudohypoparathyroidism
Vitamin D Mediated
Vitamin D deficiency
25(OH)D deficiency
$1,25(OH)_2$ deficiency
Reversible inhibition of 1-hydroxylase
Intrinsic renal defects (chronic renal failure, tubulopathies, Fanconi's syndrome)
Defective response to $1,25(OH)_2D$
Mutations of vitamin D receptor

Hypercalcemia associated with *granulomatous disorders* is seen commonly in patients with sarcoidosis and less frequently in patients with tuberculosis, silicone-induced granulomas, and fungal diseases such as coccidioidomycosis and candidiasis. Renal failure, soft tissue calcification, nephrolithiasis, and severe hypercalcemia are potential manifestations. Different mechanisms in the development of hypercalcemia have been implicated, including enhanced sensitivity to vitamin D, increased concentration of vitamin D metabolites, and unregulated generation of 1,25(OH)2D by macrophages in granulomatous tissue.

Milk–alkali syndrome was first reported in patients with peptic ulcer disease taking large amounts of milk and absorbable alkali (e.g., calcium carbonate). Recently, a rise in the incidence of the syndrome has been reported; this may be due to the widespread use of calcium carbonate preparations in the treatment and prophylaxis of osteoporosis. The syndrome is manifest by hypercalcemia, hypocalciuria, alkalosis, azotemia, and soft tissue calcifications.

Laboratory testing in the differential diagnosis of hypercalcemia includes measurements of serum total and ionized calcium, urine calcium, serum and urine phosphorus, alkaline phosphatase, albumin, intact PTH, PTH-rP, and urine cAMP. Determination of various other analytes (e.g., growth hormone, cortisol, cortisone suppression test, selective venous catheterization with measurement of local PTH concentration, measurements of vitamin D metabolites) can provide valuable information in selected cases. Meaningful interpretation of relevant laboratory data often requires various special studies, in addition to a complete history and physical examination. Renal function tests and studies of acid-base balance may be indicated. Histopathologic examination of bone biopsy specimens from appropriate sites can be of unique value in selected cases.

HYPOCALCEMIA

Chronic hypocalcemia presents with neuromuscular and neurologic manifestations, including muscle spasms, carpopedal spasm, peripheral and perioral paresthesias, cardiac arrhythmias, lengthening of the QT interval and low-voltage T waves on the electrocardiogram, and, in severe cases, laryngeal spasm and convulsions. Respiratory arrest may occur. Severe hypocalcemia will eventually result in tetany. Hypocalcemia has many causes, which can be divided into several major categories: (1) deficiencies in PTH production or secretion, (2) resistance to PTH action, (3) deficiency of vitamin D or vitamin D metabolites, and (4) deficiencies in bone mineralization with normal metabolism of PTH and vitamin D (Table 15-2). The most common causes of hypocalcemia are chronic renal failure, hypomagnesemia, hypoparathyroidism, pseudohypoparathyroidism, vitamin D deficiency, and acute pancreatitis. Less frequently, low plasma calcium may be seen in critically ill patients with sepsis, burns,

TABLE 15-3

Serum Calcium, Phosphate, and Vitamin D Levels in Various Disorders

Disorder	Calcium	25(OH)D	1,25(OH)D	Phosphate
25(OH)D intoxication	High	High	Low, normal	Normal, high
Primary hyperparathyroidism	High	Normal	Normal, high	Low
Secondary hyperparathyroidism	Low	Low, normal, high	Low, normal, high	Low, normal, high
Tertiary hyperparathyroidism	Normal, high*	Low, normal, high	Low, normal, high	Low, normal, high
Malignancy	High	Normal	Low, normal	Low
Vitamin D deficiency	Low	Low	Low, normal, high	Low
Renal failure	Low	Normal	Low	High
Hyperphosphatemia	Low	Normal	Low	High
Vitamin D rickets type I, II	Low	Normal, high	Low, normal, high	Low
Granulomatous diseases (sarcoid/TB)	High	Low, normal, high	High	Normal, high
Postmenopausal osteoporosis	Normal	Normal	Normal	Normal
Senile osteoporosis	Normal	Normal	Normal	Normal
Osteomalacia	Low, normal	Low, normal	Low	Low, normal, high

*Calcium may be normal in the setting of concurrent $1,25(OH)_2D_3$ deficiency.

and acute renal failure. Transient hypocalcemia can be observed after administration of a number of drugs, including heparin, glucagon, and protamine, as well as after massive transfusions of citrated blood products.

Hypoparathyroidism, hereditary or acquired, is characterized by diminished or absent PTH production by the parathyroid glands, which leads to a fall in plasma calcium and corresponding hyperphosphatemia. In addition, these patients have absent or low levels of $1,25(OH)_2D$. In the past, acquired hypoparathyroidism secondary to neck surgeries and thyroidectomies, in particular, was more common than hereditary hypoparathyroidism. With improvement in surgical techniques, however, its incidence has diminished dramatically. Hereditary hypoparathyroidism can occur as an isolated entity with a variable pattern of inheritance (idiopathic hypoparathyroidism), in association with defective development of both the thymus and the parathyroid glands (DiGeorge syndrome or branchial dysgenesis), or as part of a complex hereditary autoimmune syndrome involving failure of the adrenals, ovaries, and parathyroids, usually referred to as autoimmune polyglandular deficiency. Hereditary hypoparathyroidism is often manifested within the first decade of life. In addition to low or absent PTH and hypocalcemia, certain skin manifestations, such as alopecia and candidiasis, occur frequently.

Pseudohypoparathyroidism (PHP), also known as Albright's hereditary osteodystrophy, is a rare genetic disorder characterized by ineffective PTH action rather than failure of parathyroid gland hormone production. Clinically, PHP presents with some of the features of hypoparathyroidism, such as extraosseous calcifications, extrapyramidal symptoms and signs such as choreoathetotic movements and dystonia, chronic changes in fingernails and hair, lenticular cataracts, and increased intracranial pressure with papilledema. Serum calcium is depressed despite an increased concentration of PTH, suggesting resistance to PTH. Moreover, whereas infusion of PTH in patients with hypoparathyroidism generally results in a marked increase in both urinary cAMP and phosphaturia, patients with PHP usually respond with subnormal urinary phosphate excretion and cAMP production. This is due to a defect in the stimulatory G-protein of adenylate cyclase that is necessary for the action of PTH.

Hypocalcemia associated with hypomagnesemia is associated with both deficient PTH release from the parathyroid glands and impaired responsiveness to the hormone.

Hypocalcemia associated with hypovitaminosis D may occur as a result of inadequate production of vitamin D_3 in the skin, insufficient dietary supplementation, inability of the small intestine to absorb adequate amounts of the vitamin from the diet, and resistance to the effects of vitamin D. The latter may be due to deficient or defective receptors for $1,25(OH)_2D$ or to use of drugs that antagonize vitamin D action. Hypovitaminosis D is associated with disturbances in mineral metabolism and secretion of PTH and mineralization defects in the skeleton such as rickets in children and osteomalacia in adults (see later). Decreased levels of vitamin D lead to insufficient intestinal absorption of calcium and hypocalcemia, followed by increased secretion of PTH (secondary hyperparathyroidism). Increased PTH stimulates calcium release from bone and decreases calcium clearance by the kidney, thus increasing calcium levels in the circulation. If hypovitaminosis D persists, severe hypocalcemia may occur.

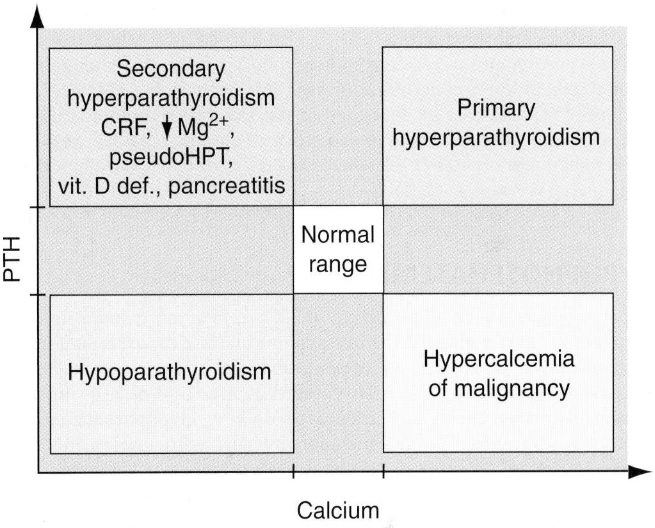

Figure 15-6 Graph correlating alterations in serum calcium levels and parathyroid hormone levels with the diseases most frequently causing these alterations.

An inherited disorder, characterized by defective production of $1,25(OH)_2D$ in the kidney, has been described. In this syndrome, known as pseudovitamin D–deficient rickets or vitamin D–dependent rickets type I, there is a deficiency in renal 25(OH)D-1α-hydroxylase activity, which results in low production of $1,25(OH)_2D$ and decreased levels in the circulation, but with a normal response to physiologic doses of calcitriol. In vitamin D–dependent rickets type II, mutations impair the function of the $1,25(OH)_2D$ receptor by altering the binding of the hormone to the receptor, causing elevated levels of circulating $1,25(OH)_2D$. Although administration of high doses of calcitriol produces further increases in the levels of $1,25(OH)_2D$, no physiologic response occurs. Another inherited disease associated with impaired vitamin D metabolism is X-linked hypophosphatemic rickets. This condition is characterized by a functional defect in 25(OH)D-1α-hydroxylase, hypophosphatemia, and normal or low serum levels of $1,25(OH)_2D$. Figure 15-6 summarizes the more common causes of abnormal calcium levels, along with their differential diagnoses.

Tables 15-3 and 15-4 summarize serum calcium, phosphate, vitamin D levels, and other laboratory values in altered metabolic states.

HYPERPHOSPHATEMIA

Hyperphosphatemia is usually caused by decreased renal excretion in acute and chronic renal failure; increased intake with excessive oral, rectal, or

TABLE 15-4
Laboratory Values in Various Altered States of Calcium Metabolism

	Primary hyperparathyroidism	Humoral hypercalcemia of malignancy	Secondary hyperparathyroidism	Tertiary hyperparathyroidism	Familial hypocalciuric hypercalcemia
Urine calcium	High	High	Normal, high	Normal, high	Low
Serum phosphate	Low	Low	Low, normal, high	Low, normal, high	Low
Urine phosphate	High	High	High	High	High
1,25(OH)D	Normal, high	Low, normal	Low, normal, high	Low, normal, high	Normal, high
PTH intact	High	Low	High	High	High
PTH-r protein	Normal	High	Normal	Normal	Normal

PTH, Parathyroid hormone; *PTH-r,* parathyroid hormone related.

intravenous administration; or an increased extracellular load due to a transcellular shift in acidosis. Less common causes include increased tubular reabsorption in hypoparathyroidism; pseudohypoparathyroidism; and increased extracellular load due to cell lysis in rhabdomyolysis, intravascular hemolysis, leukemia, lymphoma, and cytotoxic therapy. In addition, hyperphosphatemia may be seen secondary to overmedication with vitamin D and production of vitamin D by granulomatous diseases such as sarcoidosis and tuberculosis.

No direct symptoms result from hyperphosphatemia. When high levels are maintained for long periods, however, mineralization is enhanced, and calcium phosphate may be deposited in abnormal sites. Ectopic calcification is a frequent complication in patients with chronic renal failure receiving supplements of vitamin D when correction of hyperphosphatemia is inadequate (Weisinger, 1998).

TABLE 15-5
Causes of Abnormal Phosphate Levels

Elevated
Hypoparathyroidism and pseudohypoparathyroidism
Renal failure
Hypervitaminosis D
Cytolysis
Pyloric obstruction
Decreased
Alcohol abuse
Primary hyperparathyroidism
Acute respiratory alkalosis
Myxedema
Exogenous/endogenous steroids
Diuretic therapy
Renal tubular defects
Oncogenic phosphaturia
Diabetic coma

HYPOPHOSPHATEMIA

Hypophosphatemia is observed in 0.25%–2.15% of general hospital admissions. Alcohol abuse is the most common cause of severe hypophosphatemia, probably as the result of poor food intake, vomiting, antacid use, and marked phosphaturia. It is also caused by ingestion of large amounts of nonabsorbable antacids that bind phosphate. Hypophosphatemia is induced by several mechanisms, including internal redistribution, increased urinary excretion, decreased intestinal absorption, or a combination of these abnormalities. The most common cause is a shift of phosphorus from extracellular fluid into cells, which can be observed in acute respiratory alkalosis associated with sepsis, salicylate poisoning, alcohol withdrawal, heatstroke, hepatic coma, increased insulin during glucose administration, recovery from diabetic ketoacidosis, and refeeding of malnourished patients. Increased urinary excretion is usually secondary to hyperparathyroidism, renal tubular defects as in Fanconi's syndrome and familial hypophosphatemia, X-linked vitamin D–resistant rickets, aldosteronism, glucocorticoid and mineralocorticoid administration, and diuretic therapy. Hypophosphatemia due to urinary losses is observed in osmotic diuresis, acute volume expansion, and up to 30% of patients with malignant neoplasms such as certain leukemias and lymphomas. In oncogenic hypophosphatemia with osteomalacia, also referred to as tumor-induced osteomalacia, mesenchymal tumors, which are more often benign than malignant, produce hyperphosphaturia by a mechanism in which overproduction of FGF-23 has been implicated (Nelson, 2003; Folpe, 2004). Increased intestinal loss is due to vomiting, diarrhea, and use of phosphate-binding antacids. Decreased intestinal absorption is observed in malabsorption, vitamin D deficiency, and steatorrhea (Table 15-5).

Symptomatic hypophosphatemia is usually observed when plasma phosphorus falls below 0.32 mmol/L. Clinical manifestations include proximal weakness, anorexia, dizziness, myopathy, dysphagia, ileus, respiratory failure due to weakness of the respiratory muscles, impairment of cardiac contractility due to depletion of ATP in myocardial cells, and metabolic encephalopathy.

HYPERMAGNESEMIA

Hypermagnesemia (i.e., plasma Mg^{++} concentration >0.9 mmol/L) is rare and usually iatrogenic. Those most at risk are the elderly and patients with bowel disorders or renal insufficiency. Clinical manifestations of hypermagnesemia include hypotension, bradycardia, respiratory depression, depressed mental status, and electrocardiographic abnormalities (Weisinger, 1998).

HYPOMAGNESEMIA

Magnesium deficiency is found in approximately 11% of hospitalized patients. The usual reason is loss of magnesium from the gastrointestinal (GI) tract or the kidney. Depletion by GI tract occurs during acute and chronic diarrhea, malabsorption, and steatorrhea after extensive bowel resection, and in patients with the rare inborn error of metabolism, primary intestinal hypomagnesemia. Na^+ resorption may serve as the basis for magnesium depletion in the kidney because of a sodium-dependent magnesium efflux pathway in the same tubular segment (Ikari, 2003), or because of a primary defect in renal tubular reabsorption of Mg^{++}. Factors that can cause Mg^{++} losses from the urine include thiazide and loop diuretics, increased sodium excretion and volume expansion (parenteral fluid therapy), hypercalcemia and hypercalciuria (hyperthyroidism or malignancy), and nephrotoxic drugs (aminoglycoside antibiotics, cisplatin, amphotericin B, cyclosporine). Diabetes mellitus is a common cause of hypomagnesemia, probably secondary to glycosuria and osmotic diuresis. Another important and very common cause of magnesium deficiency is alcohol; this is found in approximately 30% of alcoholic patients admitted to hospital. Sustained and extensive stress, including that seen with varied surgical procedures and acute illnesses, may be associated with depressed serum magnesium levels (Table 15-6).

Signs and symptoms of magnesium depletion do not usually appear until extracellular levels have fallen to 0.5 mmol/L or less. Manifestations of significant magnesium depletion are largely due to the associated hypocalcemia and include neuromuscular hyperexcitability characterized by carpopedal spasm, seizures, muscular weakness, depression, and psychosis; metabolic abnormalities (carbohydrate intolerance, hyperinsulinism); and cardiac arrhythmias.

TABLE 15-6
Causes of Hypomagnesemia

Decreased Intake/Absorption
Protein-calorie malnutrition
Starvation
Alcoholism
Prolonged intravenous therapy
Inadequate parenteral supplementation
Malabsorption (e.g., celiac sprue)
Neonatal gut immaturity
Excessive GI losses
Prolonged gastric suction
Laxatives
Intestinal or biliary fistula
Severe diarrhea
Excessive Renal Losses
Diuretics
Acute tubular necrosis—diuretic phase
Acute renal failure—diuresis
Primary aldosteronism
Hypercalcemia
Renal tubular acidosis
Idiopathic renal wasting
Chronic renal failure with wasting
Miscellaneous
Idiopathic
Acute pancreatitis
Porphyria with syndrome of inappropriate antidiuretic hormone (SIADH)
Multiple transfusions with citrated blood
Endocrine
Hyperthyroidism
Hyperparathyroidism
Diabetes mellitus with diabetic ketoacidosis
Hyperaldosteronism
Medications (e.g., cisplatin, cyclosporine, gentamicin, ticarcillin)

Biochemical Markers of Bone Remodeling

The skeleton constantly undergoes a process of remodeling that is essential for bone health. Bone remodeling is a coupled process that begins with resorption of old bone by osteoclasts, a process that takes approximately 50 days, followed by formation of new bone by osteoblasts, which takes another 150 days, for a total turnover cycle lasting approximately 200 days (Erikson, 1994). Beginning at middle age or earlier, net bone loss occurs because resorption exceeds formation, a fact that was identified more than 50 years ago by Dr. Alton Fuller, the father of metabolic bone disease. He noted that postmenopausal women had elevated urinary calcium levels and deduced that this reflects a negative calcium balance that can result in osteoporotic fractures. Estrogen deficiency and many other diseases and conditions accentuate bone resorption (Watts, 1999).

Three major diagnostic procedures are available to monitor bone turnover and evaluate metabolic bone disease: bone imaging techniques, bone biopsy, and biochemical markers of bone turnover. Although bone density measurement is an important diagnostic tool in osteoporosis, it is difficult for the test to detect increased bone turnover in its early stages or to monitor acute changes. Also, bone densitometry gives a summated measure of mineralized bone matrix; it does not define abnormal distribution of bone loss. Bone biopsy can define the distribution of bone mass and can answer questions about bone mineralization that cannot be answered with bone densitometry. However, bone biopsy is invasive, and, in the absence of mineralization defects, it provides a relatively static glimpse into long and slowly developing processes; thus, it is not useful in routine clinical management of osteoporosis. In osteoporosis, net bone loss is caused by only a slight imbalance of bone resorption over formation, so conventional markers, such as calcium and PTH, are usually normal. In contrast, bone turnover markers are more sensitive to subtle change and can be used to noninvasively detect and monitor progression of metabolic bone disease. Laboratory assessment of these markers has been the focus of much attention in recent years (Ju, 1997; Souberbielle, 1999).

BONE RESORPTION MARKERS

Bone tissue has three components: an organic matrix (called osteoid), bone mineral, and bone cells. Bone resorption markers have included constituents of bone matrix such as calcium and collagen degradation products such as hydroxyproline, pyridinium crosslinks, and telopeptides, as well as cellular products involved with degradation of the mineralized matrix such as tartrate-resistant acid phosphatase (TRAP). Urinary calcium is affected by diet and renal function; thus, it is not sensitive or specific for assessment of bone remodeling (Watts, 1999). Tartrate-resistant acid phosphatase, a lysosomal enzyme found in osteoclasts, is not considered a useful test. Measurement of the amino acids hydroxyproline and glycosylated (galactosyl and glucosyl-galactosyl) hydroxylysine is not specific for skeletal collagen and has been found to correlate poorly with bone resorption, as determined by bone histomorphometry and calcium kinetics. The most useful tests measure pyridinium crosslinks and cross-linked telopeptides. Bone resorption markers have a diurnal rhythm, making the timing of sample collection critical, and serial samples that are to be utilized for monitoring response to antiresorptive medications should be collected at the same time of day. Values are highest in the mornings, thus collection of the sample during this time is indicated.

Recently, serum cathepsin K, the primary enzyme involved in proteolysis of bone type I collagen by osteoclasts, has been implicated as a possible valuable marker of bone resorption. However, the data are incomplete with respect to its efficacy as a useful clinical marker. Several other bone metabolism regulators, such as RANK, RANKL, and even osteoprotegerin, a decoy receptor of nuclear factor kappa, may be of interest. None of these have been evaluated to the extent where they have proven efficacy in following bone metabolism clinically. In fact, conflicting reports have described the utility of determining a osteoprotegerin/RANKL ratio, with some suggesting that this ratio in patients beginning therapy for rheumatoid arthritis was the single most important predictor of joint erosion measured 11 years later (van Tuyl, 2010). Another study with shorter follow-up did not show that this ratio predicted disease progression.

Pyridinium Crosslinks (Pyridinoline and Deoxypyridinoline)

Collagen fibrils consist of many cross-linked amino acids that effectively stabilize the mature collagen molecule. These include pyridinoline (Pyr), a cross-linked polymer formed from three hydroxylysine residues, and deoxypyridinoline (DPyr), which is formed from two hydroxylysine residues and one lysine residue. These crosslinks are found in collagen types I, II, and III. Although these crosslinks are not unique to bone, they are found in a unique ratio in the bone, a fact that makes these substances ideal candidates as markers for bone breakdown. In the collagen of most other tissues, the ratio of Pyr/DPyr is 10:1, while in bone it is 3–3.5:1. This difference means that DPyr is more pronounced in bone and metabolic bone disease. DPyr is essentially specific for bone, in that it is found in relatively significant amounts only in bone and has been shown to correlate well with bone turnover (Robins, 1995). An additional characteristic that makes evaluation of pyridinium crosslinks ideal is that they are neither metabolized upon their release nor absorbed from the diet. They are excreted in urine in free form (40%) and in peptide-bound form (60%). Because crosslink molecules are found only in mature collagen, their excretion in the urine reflects breakdown of mature collagen and is not an expression of newly synthesized bone collagen (Watts, 1999). Thus, their presence in urine suggests active bone resorption. Excretion of Pyd and DPyr is increased after menopause and can be utilized to study the effects of hormone replacement therapy on bone turnover (Fledelius, 1994). The clinical applications of measuring these substances include identification of individuals at risk for bone loss and fracture, assessment of metabolic bone disease, prediction of bone metastases, subsequent skeletal complications, and even outcome in cancer patients afflicted by solid tumors (prostate, breast, and lung most commonly) and primary bone tumors, as well as management of antiresorptive therapy. Pyr and Dpyr are measured in urine by high-pressure liquid chromatography (HPLC) (see Chapter 23 for a discussion of HPLC) or immunoassays. Care must be taken to account for the marked diurnal variation that is seen with urinary pyridinolines, with a peak late at night and early in the morning. Although a 24-hour urine collection avoids this issue and does not require correction for the creatinine concentration, an early morning fasting sample corrected for creatinine concentration is a more sensitive marker of bone turnover (Bettica, 1992).

Cross-linked Telopeptides

During bone resorption, only 40% of crosslinks are released as free pyridinium crosslinks; the remaining 60% are peptide-attached crosslinks (Risteli, 1993). Type I collagen has two sites with attached crosslinks. These are called telopeptides, and they occur in the amino-terminal and carboxy-terminal regions of the collagen molecule. These telopeptides are released into the circulation as collagen is degraded; they are then excreted into the urine. Amino-telopeptides (NTx) and carboxy-telopeptides (CTx) are excreted in the urine and can be measured by immunoassay. Testing for these crosslinks is widely available.

Cross-linked telopeptides have been utilized in estimating relative risks of hip fracture in postmenopausal women, and show promise in predicting such complications of osteoporosis (Chapurlat, 2000; Swaminathan, 2001).

Although baseline levels of cross-linked telopeptides do not necessarily correlate with baseline bone mineral density, their serial measurement has shown the capacity to predict early response to therapy (Fink, 2000). Studies have shown reductions of urinary CTx and NTx in the range of 50%–60% with 3–6 months of antiresorptive therapy (Eatell, 2003) and correlation of these reductions with the prediction of long-term bone mass response (Ravn, 2003).

BONE FORMATION MARKERS

Bone formation markers include alkaline phosphatase and three byproducts of bone matrix synthesis, including osteocalcin and amino- and carboxy-terminal procollagen I extension peptides.

Alkaline Phosphatase

(See Chapter 20.)

Bone alkaline phosphatase (ALP-B), an osteoblast membrane-bound enzyme, is released into the circulation by phosphatidylinositol glycanase activity and formation of membrane vesicles. Studies have shown that the amount of ALP-B activity in osteoblasts and in bone is proportional to collagen formation; thus, it can provide an index of the rate of bone formation. Human serum contains a variable mixture of ALP isoenzymes from liver, intestine, kidney, and bone. During pregnancy, alkaline phosphatase may be derived from the placenta (Farley, 1994). Certain malignant tumors may also produce a heat-stable ALP isoenzyme. The function of ALP is unknown; however, it has been postulated that ALP probably has a role in the mineralization of newly formed bone. Measurements of total serum ALP are useful to follow disease activity when the amount of bone isoenzyme is exceptionally high, as in Paget's disease or osteosarcoma.

The two major circulating ALP isoenzymes, bone and liver, are difficult to distinguish because they are the products of a single gene and differ only by post-translational glycosylation. Separation of the skeletal ALP can be achieved by heat inactivation, wheat germ agglutinin precipitation, electrophoresis, isoelectric focusing, and two-site immunoradiometric assays. At present, immunoassay is the method of choice because of high specificity and satisfactory precision.

Osteocalcin

Osteocalcin is the major noncollagenous protein of the bone matrix, and is produced by osteoblasts, odontoblasts, and even chondrocytes. It is a 49 amino acid polypeptide that is rich in glutamic acid. Its function is incompletely understood, but it may serve as a site of deposition for hydroxyapatite crystals. In addition, recent studies suggest that osteocalcin has effects on energy metabolism by affecting the production and even the action of insulin (Lee, 2007). During bone matrix synthesis, some osteocalcin is released into the circulation and is rapidly cleared by the kidneys. Osteocalcin can be measured by immunoassay in plasma or serum. However, assays for osteocalcin are not yet standardized because different antibodies recognize different fragments. Antibodies that recognize both the intact molecule and the large amino-terminal mid-molecule fragment appear to provide the best clinical information (Watts, 1999). Recent studies have shown that although vitamin K does not affect the amount of osteocalcin concentration, it does affect the amount of carboxylation. Undercarboxylated osteocalcin has been suggested to be a better predictor of certain outcomes such as fracture (Vergnaud, 1997). Osteocalcin is metabolized mainly in the kidneys and to a lesser extent in the liver; the half-life in the circulation is about 5 minutes. Osteocalcin is increased when there is high bone turnover, as occurs in hyperparathyroidism, acromegaly, and Paget's disease. It is decreased in hypoparathyroidism and hypothyroidism and in patients on glucocorticoid therapy. Osteocalcin reference intervals are approximately 1.1–11 ng/mL (adult male) and 0.7–6.5 ng/mL (adult female), and testing is not routinely available.

Procollagen Type I N-Terminal and C-Terminal Peptides

Procollagen type I N-terminal peptide and procollagen type I C-terminal peptide are the precursor peptides that are removed from procollagen type I to produce type I collagen. Upon cleavage, these peptides are released into the circulation, where they can be measured, thus serving as markers of collagen type I synthesis. Of the two markers, procollagen type I N-terminus is more stable and thus is a more reliable marker. Incidentally, the procollagen type I C-terminal peptide has also been implicated as a potentially useful marker in predicting the extent and severity of disease in systemic sclerosis (Kikuchi,1994).

METABOLIC BONE DISEASE

Metabolic bone disease may be defined as a general disease of metabolism that affects the entire skeleton. Because the disease is generalized, by definition every bone is involved. Consequently, a biopsy of any bone in the body should reflect these metabolic alterations to some extent. Although a very few metabolic disorders (e.g., fluorosis, vitamin A toxicity) may increase bone density, a vast majority of metabolic bone diseases are clinical problems resulting in decreased bone density. The result may be bones with decreased organic matrix with normal mineralization (e.g., osteoporosis), bones with decreased mineral content without a significant decrease in organic matrix (e.g., osteomalacia), or bones with both diminished organic matrix and decreased mineral content (e.g., renal osteodystrophy).

OSTEOPOROSIS

Osteoporosis is the most common metabolic disease of bone (Table 15-7). It is a systemic skeletal disorder characterized by decreased organic bone matrix and microarchitectural deterioration of bone tissue, with a subsequent increase in bone fragility and susceptibility to fracture (Ferrari, 1999). Although this may be expressed as low bone mineral density as measured by dual-energy x-ray absorptiometry (DEXA), the abnormality in no way reflects abnormal mineralization in that the mineral is normal in both structure and content. Rather, total bone mass is decreased in osteoporosis primarily because of a decrease in bone collagen.

Bone mass and strength are related to volumetric density, bone size, microarchitecture, and intrinsic tissue quality. These factors are likely to change during bone growth and bone loss, with selective modifications

TABLE 15-7
Deficiencies in Organic Bone Matrix

Primary Osteoporosis
Idiopathic (children and young adults)
Postmenopausal
Senile
Secondary Osteoporosis
Hyperparathyroidism
Hyperadrenocorticism
Hypogonadism
Thyrotoxicosis
Immobilization
Calcium deficiency
Prolonged heparin administration
Miscellaneous (alcoholism, malnutrition, liver disease, rheumatoid arthritis, malabsorption)
Disorders of Connective Tissue
Osteogenesis imperfecta
Ehlers-Danlos syndrome
Marfan syndrome

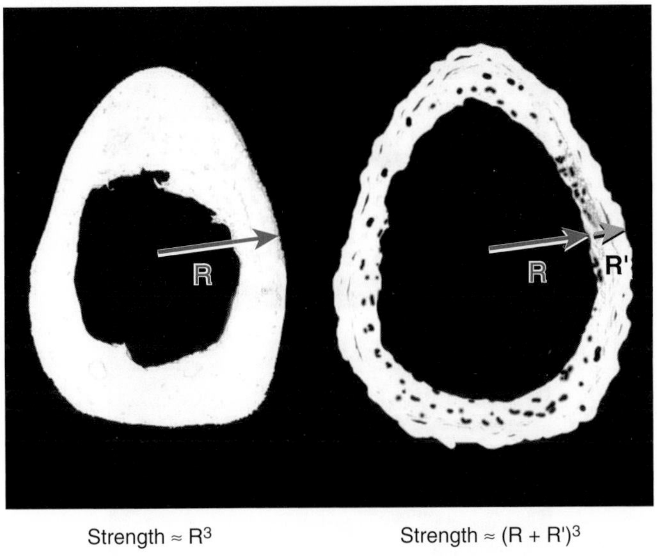

Figure 15-7 Schematic comparison of femoral cortex in a 30-year-old male *(left)* and a 75-year-old male *(right).* Note that the proportionate strength of the bone shaft on the right is greater than that on the left.

according to the skeletal site. Postmenopausal white and Asian women who are thin or small and have a positive family history are at greatest risk. Other risk factors include cigarette smoking, alcohol abuse, a sedentary lifestyle, and consumption of too little calcium. Strong evidence indicates that genetic and lifestyle factors are important determinants of peak bone mass.

As bone becomes less dense, it becomes more radiolucent; this appearance may be due to decreased collagen and/or decreased mineral. Collectively, this state is called *osteopenia*, a radiographic term that does not discriminate between the various sorts of metabolic bone disease. This term should not be confused with its use in bone densitometry studies, wherein osteopenia refers to a significant loss of bone density that is about one standard deviation less than is defined as osteoporosis. Radiologic loss of bone mass is due to loss of compact and cancellous bone, but the most common skeletal problems associated with osteoporosis arise from the loss of cancellous bone. This is as much due to the arrangement of each bone type as it is to actual decreased bone mass.

So long as the bony cortex forms a continuous ring, the strength of the shaft of a long bone is proportional to the distance from the center of the medullary cavity to the outside of the cortex raised to the third power; its stiffness is proportional to this distance raised to the fourth power. Because resorption of compact bone is primarily an endosteal event caused by osteoclasts, this means that as compact bones become more osteoporotic, their shafts become more hollow. Hollowing of the shafts is somewhat compensated for by intramembranous ossification on the cortical surface. Consequently, when the medullary cavity enlarges by endosteal osteoclasis, the diameter of the cortex also enlarges. This enlargement means that the radius from medullary midpoint to outer cortex increases. Because the strength of the intact bone is proportional to this distance raised to the third power, a small increase in appositional bone can biomechanically compensate for a relatively large loss of endosteal bone (Fig. 15-7).

Cancellous (trabecular) bone, on the other hand, is affected earlier by osteoporosis not only because it has less mass but because of its architecture. Cancellous bone is arranged in thin, highly perforated, vertically oriented parallel plates braced laterally by even thinner horizontal struts. Only 25% of the cancellous bone compartment is bone by volume; the remaining intertrabecular spaces are filled with fat and marrow (see Fig. 15-1, *B*). Compared with the cortex, the surface/volume ratio in the cancellous bone is very high, giving all bone cells free access to the delicate surfaces of the trabeculae; so cancellous bone is resorbed more rapidly than cortical bone. Furthermore, if osteoclastic resorption progresses at an equal rate in all parts of cancellous bone, the horizontal struts that serve to brace and reinforce the vertical plates are lost earlier because they began with significantly less bone mass than the vertical plates. Resorption of these horizontal braces contributes proportionately more to the morbidity of osteoporosis than the diffuse loss of bone mass. As these struts disappear, the vertical trabeculae form longer and longer vertical line segments that are subject to progressively increased bending forces (Fig. 15-8).

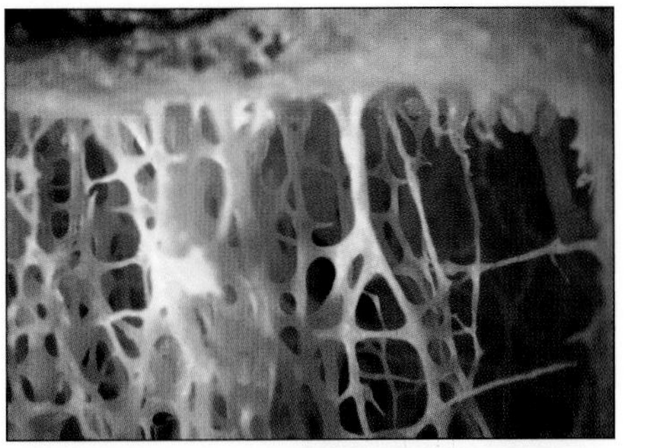

Figure 15-8 Osteoporosis of lumbar vertebra. There is generalized loss of bone. The vertical plates have become more perforated and the number of horizontal cross-braces is decreased markedly in proportion to the vertical plates (compare to Fig. 15-1, *B*).

Increasing the length of each of these vertical trabecular line segments increases their susceptibility to fatigue fracture by a factor of the incremental length squared. So if the unprotected length of a vertical plate is doubled, it is four times more likely to fracture. It is not surprising that pain, skeletal deformities, and fractures are common sequelae.

Osteoporosis may be divided etiologically into primary and secondary types. In primary osteoporosis, there are typical complex associations and patient ages, but the exact cause of bone loss in not known. The most common type of primary osteoporosis is postmenopausal osteoporosis, which occurs in the setting of hormonal decrease, has its maximal loss of bone mass in the first menopausal decade, and seems to be associated with increased osteoclastic activity. It is manifest mainly as a loss of cancellous bone. So-called senile osteoporosis manifests a decade or more later than the postmenopausal variety and is associated with a decline in osteoblast number proportionate to the demand for their activity; it affects mainly compact bone (Manolagas, 1995). Idiopathic juvenile osteoporosis occurs in the peripubertal period and is associated with increased osteoclastic activity. Unlike the postmenopausal and senile varieties, it is usually self-limited, and the skeleton may regain much of its bone mass.

In secondary osteoporosis, there is a known reason for the loss of bone mass, which may sometimes be preventable or even reversed. Etiologies include hyperparathyroidism and other endocrinopathies, space-occupying marrow lesions causing increased pressure in the marrow cavity, calcium deficiency, malabsorption, administration of steroids or heparin, and immobilization.

Certain connective tissue disorders such as osteogenesis imperfecta, Marfan syndrome, and Ehlers-Danlos syndrome also result in structural or functional osteoporosis.

Current treatment efforts are aimed at preventing resorption or stimulating new bone production. Current antiresorptive treatments include estrogens, selective estrogen receptor modulators (SERMs), vitamin D, calcitonin, and bisphosphonates, and the only anabolic agent is parathyroid hormone. Of these modalities, a more rapid effect is noted with antiresorptive medications; anabolic medications require a longer time to produce a measurable effect.

OSTEOMALACIA AND RICKETS

Osteomalacia and rickets are disorders of calcification. Osteomalacia is a failure to mineralize newly formed organic matrix (osteoid) in the mature skeleton. Osteoid formation continues, but the bones gradually become softer as the ratio of osteoid to mineralized bone increases over time. Weakness, skeletal pain and deformities, and fractures can occur as the disease progresses. Roentgenographic examination reveals a generalized decrease in skeletal radiodensity. Although the skeleton becomes less radiodense, this does not discriminate between absolute loss of mineralization and loss of mineralized organic matrix (osteoporosis).

Rickets, a disease of children, is the designation for osteomalacia that occurs before cessation of growth, that is, before closure of the epiphyseal plates of long bones. The skeletal deformities in rickets are accentuated as a consequence of compensatory overgrowth of epiphyseal cartilage, wide bands of which remain unmineralized and unresorbed. In severe cases of rickets, decreased growth can be associated with such evident deformities as swelling of the costochondral junctions of the ribs (rachitic rosary), a protuberant sternum, costodiaphragmatic depression (Harrison's sulcus), delayed closure of the anterior fontanelle with frontal bossing, and visibly widened metaphyses of the long bones.

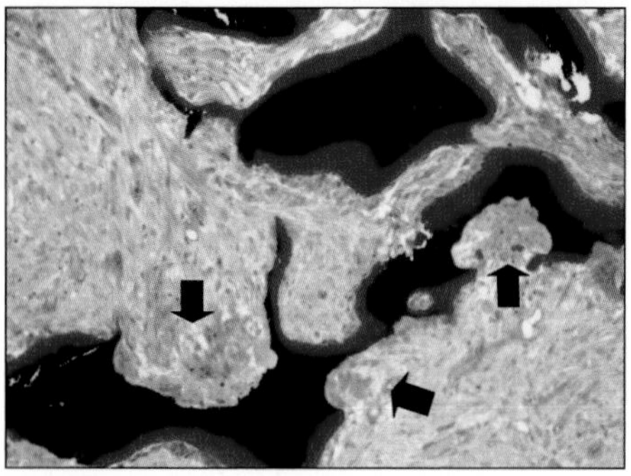

Figure 15-9 Renal osteodystrophy with hyperparathyroidism and osteomalacia. This undecalcified section is stained by the Von Kossa method, which stains mineralized bone black and osteoid with Alizarin red. The *thick red areas* represent seams of newly formed osteoid resulting from renal failure (see Fig. 15-10, *A*). The *solid black arrows* point to the cutting cones of osteoclasts tunneling into the mineralized substance of the bone trabeculae. Note that these scalloped resorption surfaces occur only in the black areas. The red areas are devoid of osteoclasts and are smooth (250×).

Optimal mineralization requires (1) an adequate supply of calcium and phosphate ions from the extracellular fluid, (2) an appropriate pH (≈7.6), (3) bone matrix of normal chemical composition and rate of synthesis, and (4) control of inhibitors of mineralization. The major categories of diseases that produce osteomalacia or rickets are vitamin D deficiency states, phosphate depletion, systemic acidosis, and inhibitors of mineralization.

Vitamin D deficiency is particularly important in childhood and may be caused by inadequate dietary intake, intestinal malabsorption, diminished synthesis of active metabolites, increased catabolism, or peripheral resistance to vitamin D action. Dietary deficiency is very uncommon in the United States because of the widespread use of fortified milk and bread and vitamin supplements. When vitamin D deficiency occurs in adults, it is usually a consequence of malabsorption. Because vitamin D is a fat-soluble vitamin, its absorption is impaired in celiac disease (nontropical sprue), biliary and pancreatic disease, or steatorrhea from other causes. Systemic resistance to vitamin D can be of major importance in the osteomalacia that accompanies chronic renal disease. On the other hand, hereditary resistance to $1,25(OH)_2D_3$, often called vitamin D–dependent rickets type II, is a rare disorder caused by a variety of defects in the vitamin D receptor.

RENAL OSTEODYSTROPHY

Renal osteodystrophy refers to the spectrum of bone abnormalities that occur in patients with end-stage renal disease (ESRD), predominantly osteitis fibrosa cystica, osteomalacia, or a combination of the two (see Fig. 15-5). Osteitis fibrosa cystica is characterized by increased bone turnover due to secondary hyperparathyroidism, a consequence of decreased levels of $1,25(OH)_2D_3$ and ionized calcium. (In general, bone dissolution is accelerated and bone formation decreased.) Osteomalacia is characterized by poor mineralization of bone resulting in the accumulation of surface osteoid (unmineralized bone). Osteoclasts cannot penetrate (resorb) these osteoid surfaces because they are attracted only to mineralized surfaces. Thus, osteoclasts dig cutting cones through the few remaining mineralized surfaces into the mineralized cores of old trabeculae. This phenomenon is histologically referred to as tunneling resorption because of the manner in which osteoclasts gain access to mineralized bone (Fig. 15-9).

The defective mineralization process in osteomalacia of ESRD patients can be attributed to low serum calcium levels, the accumulation of aluminum in bone, or other as yet unexplained factors. Renal failure patients who are treated orally with aluminum-containing phosphate binders to control hyperphosphatemia, or who undergo hemodialysis using aluminum-containing dialysates, can experience osteomalacia because aluminum ion can interfere with normal hydroxyapatite lattice formation. Undecalcified bone biopsies stained for aluminum can distinguish between this and the more usual types of osteomalacia (Fig. 15-10, *A* and *B*).

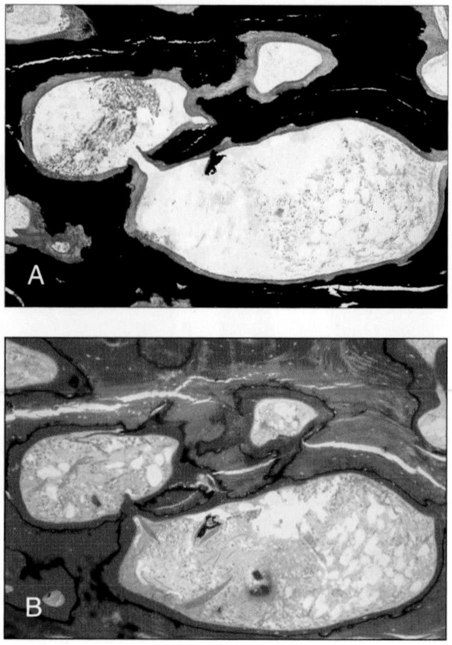

Figure 15-10 Osteomalacia in renal osteodystrophy. **A,** Von Kossa stain shows previously formed bone in black; newly synthesized, unmineralized osteoid stains magenta. Note that all surfaces are covered with thick magenta osteoid seams (125×). **B,** The same field of the same biopsy stained with solochrome azurine to detect aluminum. Note that the lines corresponding to the demarcation between black and magenta in the Von Kossa section are stained with a dark blue line. This corresponds to aluminum derived from dietary phosphate binders that has been incorporated into the hydroxyapatite matrix of the bone and interferes with further mineralization (125×).

PAGET'S DISEASE

Paget's disease of bone (osteitis deformans) is a chronic disorder of bone that may be unifocal or multifocal. Although it resembles a metabolic disease because involved bones are structurally and functionally abnormal, it is not a true metabolic disease because uninvolved bones are normal. The cause of Paget's disease is currently unknown; however, it has been suspected to be of viral origin because paramyxovirus-like particles have been identified in the nuclei of osteoclasts from affected bone. A family history of the disorder is sometimes identified. Regardless of its origin, the disease displays uncoupling of osteoclast and osteoblast function with osteoclastic activity predominating early in the disease and osteoblastic activity predominating late in the disease. The osteoclasts are often large and bizarre, with 50 or more nuclei; trabecular scalloping with multiple Howship's lacunae, paratrabecular fibrosis, and marrow hypervascularity may occur. The early histologic picture resembles osteitis fibrosa of hyperparathyroidism. As osteoblastic new bone production takes place, Howship's lacunae are filled in by irregular patches of mature and immature bone; the outlines of the original delimitations of osteoclast resorption are preserved as irregularly disposed reversal cement lines, and the resulting bone comes to resemble a tile mosaic. This results in structurally weak bone that is prone to both deformities and fractures. Patients with extensive bone lesions who have underlying heart disease may develop high output cardiac failure as a complication. Approximately 1% of patients eventually develop bone sarcomas, usually with osteosarcomatous differentiation. Laboratory findings are of some interest. Although serum calcium and inorganic phosphorus concentrations are typically normal, they may occasionally become elevated. Serum calcium levels may, in fact, become very elevated if an extensive area of Paget's disease is immobilized. Once osteoblast activity begins, serum alkaline phosphatase increases and may be used to follow the activity of the bone-synthesizing phase of the disease. Alkaline phosphatase levels rise further if a patient with Paget's disease develops osteosarcoma. Urinary excretion of calcium and phosphorus is normal or increased, whereas excretion of hydroxyproline is usually significantly increased. Paget's disease frequently responds both clinically and pathologically to therapeutic administration of calcitonin.

SELECTED REFERENCES

Mundy GR, Guise TA. Hormonal control of calcium homeostasis. Clin Chem 1999;45:1347–52.

Overview of calcium physiology and pathophysiology, including roles of PTH, vitamin D, PTH-related peptide, and calcitonin. Also presents physiologic defenses against hypercalcemia and hypocalcemia.

Sokoll L, Remaley A, Sena S, et al. National Academy of Clinical Biochemistry Laboratory Medicine Practice Guidelines: evidence-based practice for POCT. Intraoperative PTH. Draft 2, October 15, 2004.

This comprehensive evidence-based review proposes practice guidelines for all intraoperative PTH-related issues, including clinical indications, timing of draws, method, locations of testing, and financial impact. Guidelines are organized in clear question and answer format.

Watts NB. Clinical utility of biochemical markers of bone remodeling. Clin Chem 1999;45:1359–68.

This is a thorough overview of bone resorption and formation markers, including biological and assay variability issues and clinical uses. The latter are presented in a useful clinical question and answer format such as, "Is the patient responding to treatment?"

REFERENCES

Access the complete reference list online at http://www.expertconsult.com

CHAPTER 16

CARBOHYDRATES

Mukhtar I. Khan, Ruth S. Weinstock

KEY POINTS

- Normal fasting plasma glucose is <100 mg/dL (5.6 mmol/L), and normal glucose levels 2 hours post glucose load are <140 mg/dL (7.8 mmol/L).
- The diagnosis of diabetes requires a fasting plasma glucose ≥126 mg/dL (7.0 mmol/L) on at least two occasions or a casual plasma glucose level (or 2 hours post glucose load level) ≥200 mg/dL (11.1 mmol/L).
- Glycated hemoglobin (HbA_{1c}) ≥6.5% on at least two occasions can be used to diagnose diabetes using a method that is National Glycohemoglobin Standardization Program certified and standardized to the DCCT (Diabetes Control and Complications Trial) assay.
- Impaired fasting glucose (100–125 mg/dL), a 2-hour plasma glucose value 140–199 mg/dL after a 75-g glucose load, or HbA_{1c} 5.7%–6.4% indicates increased risk for diabetes.
- Oral glucose tolerance tests should be performed to diagnose gestational diabetes.
- Whole blood capillary glucose values obtained with point-of-care devices are useful for the detection of hyperglycemia and hypoglycemia in individuals with diabetes, and help to monitor and direct therapy. They should not be used to diagnose diabetes or hypoglycemic disorders. To establish these diagnoses, confirmation with laboratory measures of plasma glucose are essential because of their greater accuracy.
- HbA_{1c} levels should be performed every 3–6 months in individuals with diabetes to monitor glycemic control using a certified method, traceable to the DCCT reference method. Reliability and accuracy are diminished in the presence of shortened red blood cell survival, lower mean blood cell age, or need for transfusions, as seen with certain hemoglobinopathies and hemolytic conditions, as well as with uremia.
- Commonly used strips and tablets for ketone testing use sodium nitroprusside, which does not detect β-hydroxybutyrate. Because β-hydroxybutyrate levels are high in diabetic ketoacidosis (DKA) and fall with treatment, whereas acetoacetic acid and acetone levels rise with treatment, these strips are not useful for monitoring therapy. Calculation of the anion gap is commonly used to monitor recovery from DKA. Enzymatic methods for measuring β-hydroxybutyrate are also available.
- Circulating autoantibodies (GAD65, ICA512, IA-2, IAA) may be present before and at the onset of autoimmune type 1 diabetes. These tests should not be used for routine screening of asymptomatic nondiabetic individuals except in a research setting. When performed, assays should be used that have been shown by the Diabetes Antibody Standardization Program to have the best performance.
- Hypoglycemic symptoms with a plasma glucose level ≤55 mg/dL (3.0 mmol/L) in an individual who is not receiving medications for diabetes warrant further evaluation. A careful drug and medical history and measurements of insulin, C-peptide, proinsulin, insulin autoantibodies, β-hydroxybutyrate, and drug levels (sulfonylureas, repaglinide, nateglinide) during the hypoglycemic episode are recommended to determine the diagnosis.
- Glycogen storage diseases that primarily affect the liver usually manifest with hypoglycemia and hepatomegaly, whereas those affecting muscle commonly cause muscle cramps, weakness, fatigue, and exercise intolerance.

Carbohydrates are major constituents of physiologic systems. They are organic compounds composed of carbon, hydrogen, and oxygen [$C_x(H_2O)_y$], which, along with lipids and proteins, provide energy and contribute to the structure of organisms. Complex carbohydrates are digested into simple sugars, principally glucose, which is used primarily as an energy source or stored as glycogen. The most important dietary hexoses (six carbon-containing carbohydrates) are D-glucose, D-galactose, and D-fructose, but the principal sugar circulating in the bloodstream is glucose. Lactose (glucose and galactose) and sucrose (glucose and fructose) are important disaccharides. Carbohydrates are needed for specific cellular functions (such as ribose in nucleic acids) and can modify proteins and their function by glycosylation. Carbohydrates are measured in whole blood, serum, or plasma. In addition, measurements of glucose in urine, cerebrospinal fluid, and other body fluids are important clinically.

The concentration of glucose in blood is normally controlled within narrow limits by many hormones, the most significant of which, insulin, is produced by the endocrine pancreas. Diabetes mellitus is the most common disease of carbohydrate metabolism. Most individuals with diabetes have either type 1 (beta cell destruction with absolute insulin deficiency) or type 2 (insulin resistance and an insulin secretory defect). Measurements of glycemic control are increasingly important in diabetes, because the development and progression of microvascular and macrovascular complications are associated with glycemia. This chapter will review the aspects of carbohydrate metabolism most critical to the practice of medicine.

FUNCTION OF THE ENDOCRINE PANCREAS

The pancreas functions as both an endocrine and an exocrine organ in the control of carbohydrate metabolism. As an exocrine gland, it produces and secretes an amylase responsible for the breakdown of ingested complex carbohydrates. Further digestion leads to the production of monosaccharides, which can be absorbed. Once absorbed, the monosaccharides signal the endocrine pancreas, which regulates hormones involved in energy homeostasis. Enteroendocrine cells in the gastrointestinal tract are also stimulated by nutrients to secrete incretins, peptide hormones that affect pancreatic function, gastric emptying, and intestinal motility.

The endocrine pancreas secretes four hormones from different cells residing in the islets of Langerhans. Insulin is produced by the beta cells, glucagon by the alpha cells, somatostatin by the delta cells, and pancreatic polypeptide (PP) by the PP or F cells. In insulin-sensitive tissues such as skeletal muscle, fat, and liver, insulin stimulates glucose uptake and the formation of glycogen and inhibits glucose production. Glucagon acts primarily in the liver, where it stimulates glucose production and, over time, ketogenesis. Somatostatin, on the other hand, inhibits insulin and glucagon secretion, as well as the secretion of several other hormones. Nutrient ingestion is the major stimulus for PP secretion. The physiologic significance of PP is not clear, but it can reduce appetite and food intake. In the rare reported cases of islet cell tumors producing excess PP, or in PP hyperplasia, some patients have been asymptomatic, whereas other cases are associated with watery diarrhea syndrome (Bellows, 1998; Pasieka, 1999; Tomita, 1980).

The ratio of insulin to glucagon is important in the regulation of carbohydrate metabolism. Anabolism is favored when there is a relative increase in the insulin-to-glucagon ratio as in the postprandial state; catabolism is favored with a relative decrease in this ratio as in the fasting state. The ratio of insulin to glucagon is influenced by somatostatin, neural input, intestinal peptides, and the concentrations of glucose and other metabolites. The ratio of insulin to glucagon is tightly regulated to keep blood glucose concentrations within the normal range.

In addition to the hormones mentioned above, the pancreatic beta cell secretes a 37 amino acid protein called islet amyloid polypeptide (IAPP), or amylin. First discovered in 1987, amylin is colocalized and cosecreted with insulin in response to stimulation with nutrients. IAPP can inhibit insulin secretion, slow gastric emptying, and inhibit postprandial glucagon secretion. Oligomeric forms are associated with an increase in beta cell apoptosis. IAPP is first synthesized as a larger precursor peptide that is processed within the beta cell. High levels of IAPP have been observed in hyperinsulinemic, insulin-resistant states, such as impaired glucose tolerance and early type 2 diabetes, and low levels are seen in type 1 diabetes. Amyloid deposits, fibroid material derived from IAPP, are observed in islets in type 2 diabetes. IAPP levels can also be elevated in pancreatic cancer. Amylin assays are not used in clinical practice, but amylin analogs may be helpful in diabetes management by limiting postprandial glucose excursions. A synthetic analog of amylin, pramlintide acetate, is available for use by injection before major meals in patients with insulin-requiring diabetes.

INSULIN

Insulin is a peptide hormone with a mass of ≈5800 daltons (Da), secreted by the beta cells in the islets of Langerhans in the pancreas. It has a 21 amino acid A chain and a 30 amino acid B chain that are linked by two disulfide bonds. Insulin is synthesized initially as a longer single-chain peptide precursor hormone, pre-proinsulin. Proinsulin (≈9000 Da), the immediate precursor of insulin, is processed into insulin in the secretory granules of the beta cells by enzymatic removal of the 31 amino acid peptide segment that connects the A and B chains, known as C-peptide (Figs. 16-1 and 16-2). This proteolytic processing is catalyzed by proprotein convertases PC2 and PC1/PC3, which first convert proinsulin into the intermediate metabolites 32,33 split proinsulin and 65,66 split proinsulin, and then, after cleavage by carboxypeptidase H, to des-31,32 split proinsulin and des-64,65 split proinsulin. In adults, small amounts of intact proinsulin and these metabolically active conversion intermediates, especially des-31,32 split proinsulin, are cosecreted with insulin. Healthy infants and preterm neonates have higher proinsulin and 32,33 split proinsulin levels than adults. Proinsulin and its metabolites may cross-react with insulin in some insulin radioimmunoassays. This can be significant, especially because the half-life of proinsulin is at least three times as long as that of insulin. In vivo studies of proinsulin have shown that it has 10%–15% of the biological activity of insulin.

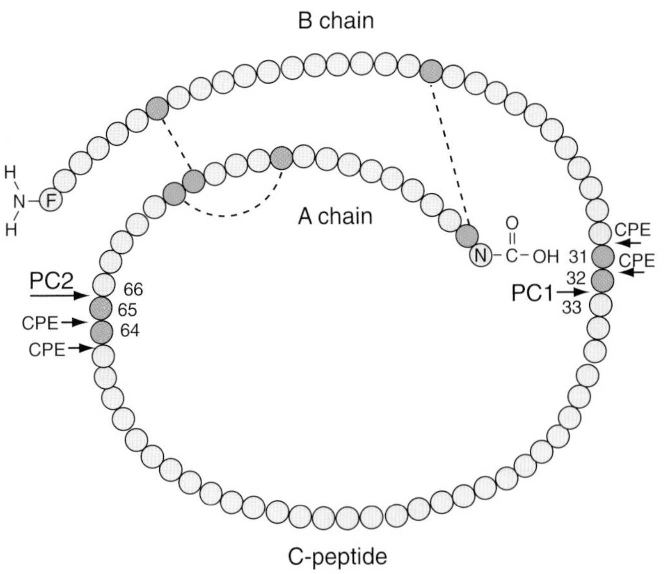

Figure 16-1 Human proinsulin, with cleavage sites for the proprotein convertases PC1 and PC2 and for carboxypeptidase H (CPE). *Orange circles* represent the two pairs of basic amino acids used for proteolytic processing, and *green circles* represent cysteine residues that participate in disulfide bonding. *(Diagnosis and classification of diabetes mellitus. Copyright © 2004 American Diabetes Association. From Mackin RB. Proinsulin: recent observations and controversies. Cell Mol Life Sci 1998;54:696–702, with permission.)*

Elevated proinsulin levels (intact and partially processed proinsulin) have been found in type 2 diabetes and are associated with decreased ability of the beta cells to secrete insulin (Roder, 1998). An increase in proinsulin levels has also been observed in pre-type 1 diabetes, where a reduction in beta cell function occurs, and may be the result of beta cell damage from cytokines produced by infiltrating immunocytes (Hostens, 1999). Less common conditions associated with high proinsulin levels include insulinomas. Familial hyperproinsulinemia is a rare condition caused by mutations in the proinsulin gene. In affected Japanese families, this genetic abnormality is associated with impaired glucose tolerance or type 2 diabetes, but in a three-generation Caucasian family with hyperproinsulinemia and mutant proinsulin (Arg65-His), glucose tolerance was normal (Roder, 1996).

C-peptide and insulin are secreted in equimolar amounts into the portal vein, but the ratio in serum is about 5:1 to 15:1. The molar concentration of C-peptide in blood is higher than that of insulin primarily because of the hepatic clearance of insulin. Approximately 50% of insulin is rapidly removed by its initial passage through the liver, but hepatic extraction of C-peptide is negligible. In cirrhosis, hyperinsulinemia is observed as the result of decreased hepatic insulin clearance. In healthy individuals, the half-life of both C-peptide and proinsulin is approximately 30 minutes, whereas it is only 4–9 minutes for insulin. In normal individuals, the molar ratio of C-peptide to insulin in the fasting state is 5:1. Whether C-peptide has any significant biological activity is unclear (Wojcikowski, 1990; Ido, 1997).

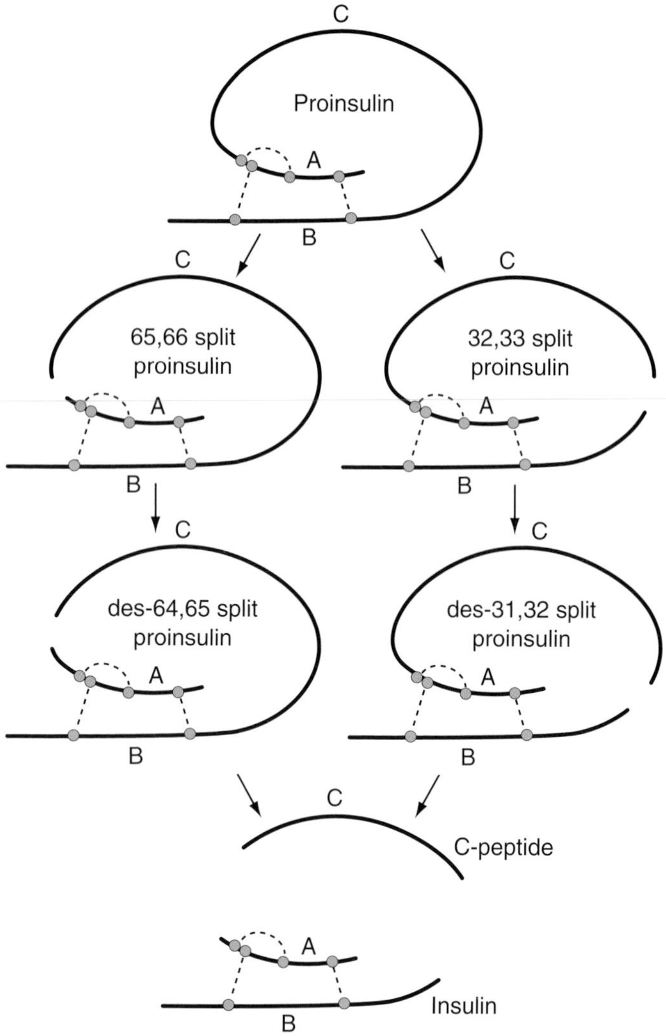

Figure 16-2 Processing of proinsulin to insulin. *Green circles* represent cysteine residues that participate in disulfide bonding. *(Copyright John Wiley and Sons Ltd; reproduced with permission from Temple R, Clark PM, Hales CN. Measurement of insulin secretion in type 2 diabetes: problems and pitfalls. Diabetic Med 1992;9:503–512.)*

Disease states occur when insulin concentrations are inappropriate for given blood glucose levels. Insulin deficiency, either absolute or relative, leads to diabetes mellitus. Serum insulin levels should be measured with a concomitant glucose level because insulin secretion is regulated primarily by glucose. Whereas a high insulin level in the presence of a low glucose level suggests inappropriate secretion or administration of insulin, high insulin levels can be observed in insulin-resistant individuals who need to secrete additional insulin to keep blood glucose levels normal.

Unregulated excess insulin secretion causes hypoglycemia. This is seen in insulin-secreting tumors, especially insulinomas, where patients have low serum glucose levels (<50 mg/dL), and elevated insulin and proinsulin levels with hypoglycemic symptoms (e.g., shakiness, palpitations, diaphoresis, confusion). C-peptide levels are measured in hypoglycemic states to help identify the cause of the hypoglycemia. Sera from insulinoma patients have high insulin and C-peptide levels, whereas hypoglycemia from injected or exogenous insulin is characterized by high insulin levels and low C-peptide levels. Commercially available insulin preparations are free of C-peptide and proinsulin. Because C-peptide is less stable than insulin, serum samples should be separated quickly and frozen.

In people with diabetes mellitus, C-peptide levels at baseline and after glucagon stimulation can be measured by immunoassay to help classify the cause of the diabetes and to provide information concerning beta cell secretory capacity. C-peptide and glucose can also be measured after an overnight 8-hour fast and 90 minutes after stimulation by an oral mixed meal. These tests usually are not performed in routine clinical practice, but they are used in research studies. Low C-peptide levels are characteristic of the absolute insulin deficiency of type 1 diabetes. C-peptide measurement can also be useful in follow-up evaluations after pancreatectomy and postpancreatic transplantation. Unlike insulin, both C-peptide and proinsulin are primarily degraded in the kidneys, and so levels are elevated in renal failure.

Many commercial immunoassays for insulin, C-peptide, and proinsulin are now available. The American Diabetes Association Task Force on Standardization of the Insulin Assay reviewed 17 insulin assays and found significant variability (Robbins, 1996). It was recommended that all assays be standardized to one reference method. Manufacturers were encouraged to publish data concerning the performance of their assays, including accuracy, recovery, precision, specificity, linearity, and lowest measurable concentration statistically different from zero/limits of quantitation. Laboratory certification was also encouraged. In the United States, an external quality assessment program for insulin and C-peptide measurements is available through the College of American Pathologists (Northfield, Ill).

Serum insulin measurements may be falsely low in the presence of hemolysis. An insulin-degrading enzyme found in red blood cells as well as in other tissues is responsible for this problem. C-peptide and proinsulin measurements appear to be less affected by hemolysis. Insulin antibodies will also interfere with insulin immunoassays, with both falsely elevated and suppressed levels reported.

GLUCAGON

Proglucagon is synthesized in the pancreatic alpha cells and the L cells of the distal small bowel. Through differential processing, the glucagon family of gene products is formed. Fasting plasma glucagon concentrations are normally 25–50 pg/mL. Pancreatic glucagon stimulates glucose production. It is an important regulator of hepatic glycogenolysis, gluconeogenesis, and ketogenesis. In type 1 diabetes, over time, progressive glucagon deficiency develops. This deficiency of glucagon results in increased glycemic fluctuations and difficulty recovering from hypoglycemia.

Serum glucagon levels are rarely measured in clinical practice. Glucagonomas are rare islet cell tumors that produce excessive glucagon. Clinically, glucagonomas present with a characteristic necrotizing migratory erythematous rash, stomatitis, glossitis, weight loss, anemia, and mild diabetes mellitus. These tumors are usually associated with fasting glucagon levels greater than 120 pg/mL, but levels can range from 900–7800 pg/mL. The processing of proglucagon is impaired, and large molecular weight forms can be seen. Mild elevations in blood glucagon levels are seen in patients with multifunctional neuroendocrine tumors. Glucagon levels can also be mildly elevated in cirrhosis, diabetes, Cushing's syndrome, pancreatitis, acromegaly, and renal insufficiency. In familial hyperglucagonemia, an autosomal dominant disorder, glucagon levels are high in the absence of tumor. Family history is helpful in making this diagnosis.

INCRETINS

Oral nutrients stimulate the release of incretins from the intestines. The incretin effect refers to the greater and earlier insulin response to the oral administration of glucose compared with intravenous glucose. The most important incretins in the regulation of insulin secretion are glucagon-like peptide 1 (GLP-1) and glucose-dependent insulinotropic peptide (GIP), both of which are members of the glucagon superfamily. GIP, originally called gastric inhibitory polypeptide, exerts some beta cell effects in animal models but does not affect glucagon release or gastric emptying in physiologic doses.

In the intestine, GLP-1 is formed from proglucagon and functions mostly as an incretin to rapidly stimulate insulin secretion in response to a meal. Other effects include suppression of glucagon secretion and inhibition of gastric emptying. GLP-1 may reduce appetite and promote weight loss (Flint, 1998). In vitro and animal studies indicate that GLP-1 can inhibit beta cell apoptosis and stimulate beta cell proliferation and neogenesis from precursor duct cells (Drucker, 2003a). Plasma meal-stimulated GLP-1 levels are decreased in type 2 diabetes mellitus (Toft-Nielsen, 2001). GLP-1 (7-37), the most common active form, has a half-life of only 2–3 minutes. It is rapidly cleaved by circulating aminopeptidases to the inactive GLP-1 (9-37). This inactive form represents 80% of the circulating GLP-1. Both forms of GLP-1 are short-lived and cleared by the kidney. Dipeptidyl peptidase-4 (DPP-4), a serine peptidase present on the surface of endothelial cells, inactivates GLP-1 by removing two N-terminal amino acids. Oral inhibitors of DPP-4 are used for the treatment of diabetes. Long-acting GLP-1 receptor agonists are available for use by injection in patients with type 2 diabetes.

SOMATOSTATIN

Somatostatin, a tetradecapeptide with a disulfide bond, was first isolated from the hypothalamus. Somatostatin was originally considered a hypothalamic hormone that inhibited growth hormone secretion, but the discovery of somatostatin in the islets of Langerhans prompted further investigation of its function in the endocrine pancreas. Subsequently, somatostatin was found in the gastrointestinal tract. It inhibits pituitary (growth hormone and thyrotropin), gastrointestinal (gastrin, secretin, vasointestinal peptide), and pancreatic (insulin, glucagon) hormones and possesses nonendocrine functions (e.g., inhibition of gastric acid secretion, gastric emptying time and, pancreatic enzyme release). The first isolated somatostatin peptide had 14 amino acids and is called somatostatin-14. Subsequently, somatostatin-28, which contains an N-terminal extension, was isolated and is a more potent inhibitor of other islet hormones.

In the pancreatic islets, somatostatin is produced in the delta cells, which make up 5%–10% of the islet cells. Rare islet cell tumors, somatostatinomas, secrete high levels of somatostatin. Elevated somatostatin levels can also be seen in small cell lung cancer, medullary thyroid cancer, and pheochromocytoma. Somatostatin has a very short half-life and is rarely measured in clinical practice. Two long-acting somatostatin analogs, octreotide and lanreotide, which bind primarily to the somatostatin receptor subtype 2 (SSTR2), are used to treat neuroendocrine tumors, as well as other disorders of the pancreas and gastrointestinal tract. Octreotide scintigraphy has also been used for tumor diagnosis, localization, and prediction for success of treatment with somatostatin analogs.

GLUCOSE MEASUREMENTS

SPECIMEN CONSIDERATIONS

Measurements of glucose are critical to the diagnosis and management of diseases affecting carbohydrate metabolism. Glucose is measured in whole blood, plasma, serum, cerebrospinal fluid, pleural fluid, and urine for a variety of diagnostic and management purposes. In addition, devices can measure glucose from interstitial fluid for continuous monitoring of glucose levels in people with diabetes. How and when specimens are collected and handled and the site of collection affect the clinical interpretation of the analytic result.

The standard clinical specimen is venous plasma glucose. Glucose is metabolized at room temperature at a rate of 7 mg/dL/hour (0.4 mmol/L/hour); at 4° C, the loss is approximately 2 mg/dL/hour (Weissman, 1958). The rate of metabolism is higher with bacterial contamination or leukocytosis. A serum specimen is appropriate for glucose analysis if serum is separated from the cells within 30 minutes, but if serum is in contact with cells for longer than 30 minutes, a preservative such as sodium fluoride that inhibits glycolysis should be added. However, in serum specimens without bacterial contamination or leukocytosis, results remain clinically acceptable even after a delay of up to 90 minutes before separation of serum and cells. If whole blood is refrigerated, 2 mg of sodium fluoride per milliliter of whole blood prevents glycolysis for up to 48 hours (Chan, 1989). When refrigerated, glucose is stable in serum or plasma for 48 hours. With long-term specimen storage, even at −20° C, glucose values decrease significantly and progressively.

GLUCOSE MEASUREMENT METHODS

Most measurements of glucose employ enzymatic methods. These enzymatic methods provide specificity and can be packaged to furnish point-of-care determinations. Three enzyme systems are commonly used to measure glucose: glucose dehydrogenase, glucose oxidase, and hexokinase. These reactions produce an electrical current that is proportional to the initial glucose concentration, or a product that measured spectrophotometrically is proportional to the initial glucose concentration. The assays can be initial rate-of-change assays, where the velocity of the reaction is dependent on the initial glucose, or end-point assays.

When glucose is measured using a glucose dehydrogenase method, glucose is reduced to produce a chromophore that is measured spectrophotometrically (Equation 16-1) or an electrical current (Equation 16-2) (Kost, 1998).

$$\alpha\text{-D-glucose} \rightarrow (\text{mutoarotase}) \rightarrow \beta\text{-D-glucose} \qquad \textbf{(16-1)}$$
$$\beta\text{-D-glucose} + \text{NAD} \rightarrow (\text{glucose dehydrogenase}) \rightarrow \text{D-gluconolactone} + \text{NADH}$$
$$\text{MTT} + \text{NADH} \rightarrow (\text{diaphorase}) \rightarrow \text{MTTH (blue color)} + \text{NAD}$$

$$\text{Glucose} + \text{Pyrroloquinoline quinone (PQQ)} \rightarrow (\text{glucose dehydrogenase}) \rightarrow \text{Gluconolactone} + \text{PQQH}_2 \qquad \textbf{(16-2)}$$
$$\text{PQQH}_2 + 2[\text{Fe(CN)}_6]^{3-} \rightarrow \text{PQQ} + 2[\text{Fe(CN)}_6]^{4-} + 2\text{H}^+$$
$$2[\text{Fe(CN)}_6]^{4-} \rightarrow 2[\text{Fe(CN)}_6]^{3-} + 2e^-$$

Glucose oxidase, a flavoenzyme, catalyzes the reactions shown in Equation 16-3. The peroxidase reaction can be measured spectrophotometrically and can be inhibited by high concentrations of uric acid, ascorbic acid, bilirubin, glutathione, creatinine, L-cysteine, L-dopa, dopamine, methyldopa, and citric acid (Zaloga, 1997). In addition, the glucose oxidase reaction can be coupled to the ferricyanide/ferricyanide couple to produce an electrical current, as shown in Equation 16-4. This system is dependent on the partial pressure of O_2 because oxygen will compete in the reaction to form hydrogen peroxide, so that the higher the partial pressure of O_2, the lower is the electrically measured glucose (Kurahashi, 1997). Glucose oxidase can be used in another electrical system, as shown in Equation 16-5.

$$\beta\text{-D-glucose} + \text{O}_2 \rightarrow (\text{glucose oxidase}) \qquad \textbf{(16-3)}$$
$$\text{D-gluconolactone} + \text{H}_2\text{O}_2$$
$$\text{gluconolactone} + \text{H}_2\text{O} \rightarrow \text{gluconic acid}$$
$$\text{H}_2\text{O}_2 + \text{chromogenic oxygen acceptor (ortho-diansidine, 4-aminophenazone, ortho-tolidine)} \rightarrow (\text{peroxidase}) \rightarrow \text{color chromogen} + \text{H}_2\text{O}$$
$$\beta\text{-D-glucose} + 2[\text{Fe(CN)}_6]^{3-} + \text{H}_2\text{O} \rightarrow (\text{glucose oxidase}) \rightarrow \text{D-gluconic acid} + 2[\text{Fe(CN)}_6]^{4-} + 2\text{H}^+ \qquad \textbf{(16-4)}$$
$$2[\text{Fe(CN)}_6]^{4-} \rightarrow 2[\text{Fe(CN)}_6]^{3-} + 2e^-$$
$$\beta\text{-D-glucose} + \text{O}_2 \rightarrow (\text{glucose oxidase}) \rightarrow \qquad \textbf{(16-5)}$$
$$\text{D-gluconolactone} + \text{H}_2\text{O}_2$$
$$\text{H}_2\text{O}_2 \rightarrow 2\text{H}^+ + \text{O}_2 + 2e^-$$

The hexokinase system assay is the generally accepted reference method for measuring glucose. The reaction is shown in Equation 16-6. The glucose concentration is proportional to the rate of production of nicotinamide adenine dinucleotide phosphate (NADPH), which is followed spectrophotometrically. Depending on the source of the glucose-6-phosphate dehydrogenase, the enzyme can require specificity for NADP, or from some sources, it can use NAD as well. Hemolyzed samples can be problematic in that contents released from the erythrocytes may interfere with the stoichiometric relationship between glucose and NAD(P)H accumulation.

$$\text{Glucose} + \text{MgATP} \rightarrow (\text{hexokinase}) \rightarrow \text{glucose-6-phosphate (G-6-P)} + \text{MgADP} \qquad \textbf{(16-6)}$$
$$\text{G-6-P} + \text{NA(P)}^+ \rightarrow (\text{glucose-6-phosphate dehydrogenase}) \rightarrow$$
$$\text{6-phosphogluconolactone} + \text{NADPH} + \text{H}^+$$

Whole blood glucose specimens can be analyzed with point-of-care devices. These monitoring devices are used in the home, in the physician's office, or at the bedside in the hospital to monitor for hypoglycemia and hyperglycemia. Most of these devices have been calibrated to give results similar to plasma levels and can report plasma or whole blood readings. Whole blood tends to give approximately 10%–15% lower glucose readings than plasma, but the percentage varies on the basis of hematocrit, analysis technique, and sample timing (fasting vs. postglucose load). Capillary blood is the source of most of these whole blood glucose measuring devices. Capillary blood glucose is similar to arterial glucose but can vary markedly from venous samples, depending on timing relative to food ingestion. For example, a postprandial specimen is higher in the capillary sample than in the venous sample. Capillary glucose tests, using point-of-care devices, should not be used to diagnose diabetes or hypoglycemic disorders. To establish these diagnoses, confirmation with laboratory measurements of plasma glucose is essential because of their greater accuracy.

Home blood glucose monitoring devices help people with diabetes better self-manage their disease. A wide variety of devices are available for home measurements. Proper training of patients in the use of individual meters is critical in avoiding operator errors, which, in one study, were reported in 12% of users (Schrot, 1999). Errors that may contribute to inaccurate readings in certain devices include the application of an insufficient volume of blood, milking the finger to acquire sufficient blood, the use of outdated test strips, environmental factors (humidity, heat, altitude), the use of a malfunctioning meter, the use of a dirty meter, hypertriglyceridemia, hypotension, and measurements outside of the hematocrit or temperature range. Some blood glucose monitoring devices are influenced by high levels of salicylate, acetaminophen, levodopa, uric acid, bilirubin, lipids, or low oxygen levels, and others are altered by touching the reaction area. Most are inaccurate at very high and low glucose values. The U.S. Food and Drug Administration has warned of the possibility of falsely elevated glucose readings using GDH-PQQ monitoring test strips with individuals who may have nonglucose sugars in their blood (i.e., use of Extraneal [icodextrin] peritoneal dialysis solution, maltose, and some immmunoglobulins; http://www.fda.gov/MedicalDevices/Safety/AlertsandNotices/PublicHealthNotifications/ucm176992.htm [accessed January 5, 2010]). Desirable features of home blood glucose monitoring devices, aside from performance characteristics (precision and accuracy), include the following: ease of use, requirement of a small volume of blood, low maintenance, large print readout, rapid testing, appropriate alarms, minimal interfering substances, and memory storage and download capabilities. Some meters permit alternative site testing (such as forearm, upper arm, thigh), but results from alternative sites may be less accurate when rapid changes in glucose levels occur. Others incorporate electronic logbooks for recording events, insulin doses, and carbohydrate intake. This information can be downloaded to a computer to present the data in several displays such as logbooks, graphs, charts, and summary statistics.

Interstitial glucose measuring devices have been developed for continuous monitoring of glucose levels in people with diabetes. Most of these devices use electrochemical methods to automatically and frequently measure glucose levels in the interstitial fluid of dermis or subcutaneous fat tissue, and require repeated calibration to plasma or whole blood glucose levels. Examination of these data provides information about glucose patterns over hours to days. This glucose "trend analysis" can reveal useful findings for modifying treatment, such as unsuspected nocturnal hypoglycemia or postprandial hyperglycemia (Kaufman, 2002).

Interstitial glucose is in slow (5–30 min) equilibrium with capillary blood glucose and therefore is not equal to blood glucose, except in stable systems (Zierler, 1999; Cheyne, 2002). Particularly during times when glucose levels are rapidly changing, such as after meal ingestion or recovery from hypoglycemia, interstitial fluid readings will lag behind fingerstick glucose levels. Because the precision and accuracy of currently available portable continuous glucose monitors are not as high as for conventional home blood glucose monitoring devices, they may supplement but cannot replace conventional home blood glucose monitoring. Individual glucose readings obtained by fingersticks should be used primarily to direct therapy. Technologies currently under development for noninvasive glucose monitoring include impedance spectroscopy, thermal emission spectroscopy, near infrared spectroscopy, far infrared spectroscopy, ellipsometry, magnetic resonance imaging, and methods using electromagnetic waves.

DIABETES MELLITUS

Diabetes mellitus is a group of diseases in which blood glucose levels are elevated. Diabetes is the most common set of disorders of carbohydrate metabolism, affecting approximately 24 million Americans in 2009 and projected to increase to 44 million in 2034 (Huang, 2009). The prevalence of diabetes is increasing, with the prediction of an estimated 33% of males and 39% females born in 2000 in the United States being diagnosed with diabetes during their lifetime (Narayan, 2003). This chronic disease is responsible for significant morbidity, mortality, and cost. Diabetes is the leading cause of treated end-stage renal disease, the most common cause of nontraumatic amputations, and the foremost cause of new blindness in adults ages 20–74 years. Nerve damage, known as diabetic neuropathy, occurs in 60%–70% of people with diabetes. Most diabetes-related deaths, however, are related to the increased risk of developing atherosclerotic disease. People with diabetes are at least two to four times more likely to have heart disease and cerebrovascular disease than those without diabetes. In 2007, it was estimated that diabetes in the United States cost $174 billion, representing $116 billion in direct costs and $58 billion in indirect costs (American Diabetes Association, 2008). Direct spending for diabetes was projected to increase from $113 billion to $336 billion from 2009 to 2034 (Huang, 2009).

The Expert Committee on the Diagnosis and Classification of Diabetes Mellitus revised the criteria for the diagnosis of diabetes in 1997, with recent modifications by the American Diabetes Association (2010a). A fasting plasma glucose level ≥126 mg/dL (7.0 mmol/L) on at least two occasions is diagnostic of diabetes (Table 16-1). The fasting glucose level should be obtained after an 8-hour fast. Symptoms of hyperglycemia (e.g., polyuria, polydipsia, polyphagia, unexplained weight loss) with a casual plasma glucose level ≥200 mg/dL (11.1 mmol/L) or HbA_{1c} ≥6.5% is sufficient to diagnose diabetes. Pre-diabetes designates conditions in which glucose homeostasis is abnormal, but serum glucose levels are not high enough to be classified as diabetes. This group includes individuals with impaired fasting glucose and impaired glucose tolerance (see Table 16-1). They are also at increased risk for cardiovascular and cerebrovascular diseases.

Formal oral glucose tolerance tests are not generally recommended for routine clinical use in the diagnosis of diabetes. If used, the procedure described by the World Health Organization (1985) utilizing a 75 g glucose load should be followed. For children, 1.75 g glucose/kg up to 75 g is recommended. The exception to these criteria is the diagnosis of gestational diabetes (Table 16-2), the glucose intolerance that develops during approximately 7% of all pregnancies (American Diabetes Association, 2004). To detect gestational diabetes in high-risk individuals, an oral glucose tolerance test (OGTT) should be performed (the "one-step"

TABLE 16-1
Diagnosis of Pre-Diabetes and Diabetes Mellitus

	Fasting plasma glucose		2-hour plasma glucose level (after 75 g glucose load)		HbA_{1c}
	mg/dL	*mmol/L*	*mg/dL*	*mmol/L*	%
Normal	<100	<5.6	<140	<7.8	
Pre-diabetes					5.7–6.4
Impaired fasting glucose	100–125	5.6–6.9			
Impaired glucose tolerance			140–199	7.8–11.0	
Diabetes mellitus	≥126	≥7.0	≥200	≥11.1	≥6.5

From American Diabetes Association. Diagnosis and classification of diabetes mellitus. Diabetes Care 2010a;33(suppl 1):S62–S69.
HbA_{1c}, Glycated hemoglobin.

TABLE 16-2
Diagnosis of Gestational Diabetes Mellitus

Initial Screening Test for Average-Risk Women

1-hour plasma glucose level (after 50 g glucose load)	Detection of gestational diabetes
≥130 mg/dL (7.2 mmol/L)	90%
≥140 mg/dL (7.8 mmol/L)	80%

Oral Glucose Tolerance Tests (OGTT) for High-Risk Women and Average-Risk Women With Abnormal Screening Test Results

	100 g OGTT plasma glucose		75 g OGTT plasma glucose	
	mg/dL	*mmol/L*	*mg/dL*	*mmol/L*
Fasting	≥95	≥5.3	≥95	≥5.3
1 hour	≥180	≥10.0	≥180	≥10.0
2 hour	≥155	≥8.6	≥155	≥8.6
3 hour	≥140	≥7.8		

Gestational diabetes mellitus diagnosed if ≥2 plasma glucose levels are exceeded (American Diabetes Association, 2004).

approach). The "two-step" approach is recommended for women with average risk. This approach uses an initial screening test, followed by an OGTT if the screening test glucose level is elevated.

Before an OGTT is performed, individuals should ingest at least 150 g/day of carbohydrates for the 3 days preceding the test without limitation in physical activity, and the test should be performed after an overnight 8- to 14-hour fast. The individual should not eat food, drink tea, coffee, or alcohol, or smoke cigarettes during the test, and should be seated. Venous glucose samples are preferably collected in gray-top tubes containing fluoride and an anticoagulant.

Approximately 64 million adults in the United States in 2000 had the metabolic syndrome, and this number is increasing (Ford, 2004). Of great concern is the increasing prevalence of the metabolic syndrome in U.S. adolescents, affecting more than 2 million, with more than 30% of overweight adolescents having the metabolic syndrome phenotype (Duncan, 2004). The metabolic syndrome is associated with increased risk of cardiovascular disease and of developing diabetes. Criteria defining the metabolic syndrome according to the Third Report of the National Cholesterol Education Program Expert Panel on Detection, Evaluation, and Treatment of High Blood Cholesterol in Adults include the presence of three or more of the following: (1) impaired fasting glucose, (2) blood pressure ≥30/85 mm Hg, (3) waist circumference >102 cm in men and >88 cm in women, (4) serum triglycerides ≥150 mg/dL (1.695 mmol/L), and (5) high-density lipoprotein (HDL) cholesterol <40 mg/dL (1.036 mmol/L) in men and <50 mg/dL (1.295 mmol/L) in women. Most commonly, these individuals are insulin resistant and have smaller, denser, more atherogenic low-density lipoprotein (LDL) cholesterol particles.

The classification of diabetes was revised in 1997 and is shown in Table 16-3 with recent minor modifications (American Diabetes Association, 2010a). The most common forms of diabetes are type 1 and type 2 diabetes (Table 16-4). Type 1 diabetes, characterized by absolute insulin deficiency and beta cell destruction, used to be called juvenile-onset diabetes or insulin-dependent diabetes, but these terms are no longer used. Although this disease is most commonly diagnosed in young people, its onset can occur at any age. Because people with other forms of diabetes also use insulin therapy, the term "insulin-dependent" is confusing and should not be utilized. Type 2 diabetes, characterized by insulin resistance and an insulin secretory defect, has been referred to in the past as adult-onset or non–insulin-dependent diabetes. These terms also are no longer used. Although the onset of type 2 diabetes is most common in older adults, it can occur at any age, including childhood. Many patients with type 2 diabetes use insulin therapy, so it is no longer referred to as non–insulin-dependent diabetes. Uncommon causes of diabetes include genetic defects of beta cell function and insulin action, pancreatic diseases, endocrinopathies such as Cushing's syndrome, acromegaly and pheochromocytoma, and certain drugs, chemicals, and infections (see Table 16-3).

TYPE 1 DIABETES

Type 1 diabetes mellitus represents approximately 10% of all cases of diabetes. There usually is an autoimmune destruction of insulin-producing beta cells in the islets of the pancreas, causing an absolute deficiency in insulin production. The genetic susceptibility to develop type 1 diabetes is related, at least in part, to the inheritance of specific immune response genes associated with HLA-DR/DQ on chromosome 6, as well as other genes and genetic markers. It is then hypothesized that a precipitating event occurs, such as a viral infection, toxin exposure, or other environmental influence, which triggers the autoimmune destruction of the beta

TABLE 16-3
Classification of Diabetes Mellitus

I. Type 1 diabetes (beta cell destruction, usually leading to absolute insulin deficiency)
   A. Immune mediated
   B. Idiopathic
II. Type 2 diabetes (may range from predominantly insulin resistance with relative insulin deficiency to a predominantly secretory defect with insulin resistance)
III. Other specific types
   A. Genetic defects of beta cell function
      1. Chromosome 12, HNF-1α (MODY3)
      2. Chromosome 7, glucokinase (MODY2)
      3. Chromosome 20, HNF-4α (MODY1)
      4. Chromosome 13, insulin promoter factor-1 (IPF-1; MODY4)
      5. Chromosome 17, HNF-1β (MODY5)
      6. Chromosome 2, NeuroD1 (MODY6)
      7. Mitochondrial DNA
      8. Others
   B. Genetic defects in insulin action
      1. Type A insulin resistance
      2. Leprechaunism
      3. Rabson-Mendenhall syndrome
      4. Lipoatrophic diabetes
      5. Others
   C. Diseases of the exocrine pancreas
      1. Pancreatitis
      2. Trauma/pancreatectomy
      3. Neoplasia
      4. Cystic fibrosis
      5. Hemochromatosis
      6. Fibrocalculous pancreatopathy
      7. Others
   D. Endocrinopathies
      1. Acromegaly
      2. Cushing's syndrome
      3. Glucagonoma
      4. Pheochromocytoma
      5. Hyperthyroidism
      6. Somatostatinoma
      7. Aldosteronoma
      8. Others
   E. Drug or chemical induced
      1. Vacor
      2. Pentamidine
      3. Nicotinic acid
      4. Glucocorticoids
      5. Thyroid hormone
      6. Diazoxide
      7. β-Adrenergic agonists
      8. Thiazides
      9. Dilantin
      10. γ-Interferon
      11. Others
   F. Infections
      1. Congenital rubella
      2. Cytomegalovirus
      3. Others
   G. Uncommon forms of immune-mediated diabetes
      1. "Stiff-man" syndrome
      2. Anti-insulin receptor antibodies
      3. Others
   H. Other genetic syndromes sometimes associated with diabetes
      1. Down syndrome
      2. Klinefelter's syndrome
      3. Turner's syndrome
      4. Wolfram's syndrome
      5. Friedreich's ataxia
      6. Huntington's chorea
      7. Laurence-Moon-Biedl syndrome
      8. Myotonic dystrophy
      9. Porphyria
      10. Prader-Willi syndrome
      11. Others
IV. Gestational diabetes mellitus

From American Diabetes Association. Diagnosis and classification of diabetes mellitus. Diabetes Care 2010a;33:S62–S69.

TABLE 16-4
Characteristics of Type 1 and Type 2 Diabetes Mellitus

	Type 1 diabetes	Type 2 diabetes
Frequency	5%–10%	90%–95%
Age of onset	Any, but most common in children and young adults	More common with advancing age, but can occur in children and adolescents
Risk factors	Genetic, autoimmune, environmental	Genetic, obesity, sedentary lifestyle, race/ ethnicity, hypertension, dyslipidemia, polycystic ovarian syndrome
Pathogenesis	Destruction of pancreatic beta cells, usually autoimmune	No autoimmunity Insulin resistance and progressive insulin deficiency
C-peptide levels	Very low or undetectable	Detectable
Pre-diabetes	Autoantibodies (GAD65, IA-2, IAA) may be present.	Autoantibodies absent
Medication therapy	Insulin absolutely necessary; multiple daily injections or insulin pump	Oral agents Insulin commonly needed
Therapy to prevent or delay onset of diabetes	None known Clinical trials in progress	Lifestyle (weight loss and increased physical activity) Oral medications (metformin, acarbose) may be helpful.

cells. It is only after most of the beta cells are destroyed that hyperglycemia develops. Antibody markers of beta cell destruction are commonly present before and at the time of onset of diabetes. These include antibodies to antigens for which recombinant autoantibody assays are available: Antibodies to the 65 kDa isoform of glutamic acid decarboxylase (GAD65), insulin autoantibodies (IAA), and islet cell antigen 512 autoantibodies (ICA512). ICA512 are autoantibodies to parts of the tyrosine phosphatase IA-2 antigen. The tyrosine phosphate IA-2β (phogrin) is a separate but partially homologous antigen to IA-2. ICA512 and IA-2 autoantibody assays are used more frequently than assays for IA-2β autoantibodies because IA-2β antibodies generally react with IA-2. Although the presence of antibodies may help in the differentiation of type 1 diabetes from other types of diabetes early in the course of the disease, the absence of antibodies does not exclude this diagnosis.

Those individuals at greatest risk of developing type 1 diabetes have high titers of multiple autoantibodies. In family, as well as in population studies, the detection of at least two autoantibodies is associated with increased risk of developing type 1 diabetes (Maclaren, 1999, 2003). GAD65 has the highest sensitivity (91%) as a single screening marker for detecting multiple antibody-positive individuals (Krischer, 2003). IAA are more common in young children who develop type 1 diabetes, whereas GAD65 is more common in adults. These antibody assays are being used in type 1 diabetes detection, treatment, and prevention research. Their use for routine screening of asymptomatic individuals is not recommended at the present time, in part because effective interventions have yet to be demonstrated (Verge, 1998).

In the past, the autoantibody assays have not been well standardized, and the cutoff values for these assays were not firmly established. Quality control programs are important, in that almost 50% of blinded samples that are considered “low positive” are found to be negative on repeat testing of a blinded duplicate aliquot (Eisenbarth, 2003). Fluid phase radioassays for GAD65 and IA-2 in general have better sensitivity and specificity than standard available enzyme-linked immunosorbent assays (Bingley, 2003). For IAA assays, the microradioassays perform best. These assays use a smaller volume of serum and utilize protein A precipitation (Williams, 1997). The Diabetes Antibody Standardization Program, a collaboration between the Immunology of Diabetes Society and the Centers for Disease Control and Prevention, has established a Proficiency Testing Service. This group has reported proficiency evaluations for different assays of GAD65, IA-2, and IAA (Bingley, 2003). Poorest performance (greatest variation) was observed in different IAA assays. In this study, GAD65 and IA-2 antibody values were expressed in common units, WHO units/mL, as suggested by the Immunology of Diabetes Society. Evaluation of assays for GAD and IA-2a in the Diabetes Antibody Standardization Program demonstrated improved performance from 2002–2005 (Torn, 2008).

The “pre-diabetes” period of gradual and progressive beta cell destruction can last for months, years, or decades. During this period, the acute insulin response to intravenous glucose, called the first-phase insulin release, becomes depressed or absent. The absence of first-phase insulin response is also found in other forms of diabetes. Eventually, in most people with type 1 diabetes, most or all of the beta cells are destroyed, resulting in inadequate or absent insulin secretion. C-peptide levels and endogenous insulin levels therefore are very low or undetectable. People with untreated type 1 diabetes develop diabetic ketoacidosis. Insulin therapy is required for all patients with type 1 diabetes.

TYPE 2 DIABETES

Type 2 diabetes is the most common type of diabetes, affecting approximately 90% of Americans with diabetes. This disease is familial, but the underlying genetic defects for most of those affected have yet to be determined. Risk factors include overweight (body mass index [BMI] ≥25 kg/m^2), sedentary lifestyle, family history of diabetes, advanced age (≥45 years), ethnicity (African Americans, Latinos, Native Americans, Asian Americans, and Pacific Islanders), and polycystic ovary disease, as well as history of gestational diabetes or delivery before diabetes of a baby weighing >9 lb, hypertension, vascular disease or dyslipidemia (HDL-cholesterol ≤35 mg/dL [0.90 mmol/L] and/or triglyceride level ≥250 mg/dL [2.82 mmol/L]), A1c ≥ 5.7%, impaired fasting glucose or impaired glucose tolerance, and other conditions associated with insulin resistance (i.e., acanthosis nigricans). This is not an autoimmune disease, so antibody testing is not worthwhile. C-peptide levels are measurable in type 2 diabetes. Of the estimated 24 million Americans with type 2 diabetes in 2009, 4–5 million are undiagnosed. Unlike undiagnosed type 1 diabetes, in which patients are usually symptomatic, people with new-onset type 2 diabetes can be free of symptoms. It is not unusual to diagnose type 2 diabetes after the onset of complications. Routine screening for high-risk individuals is therefore recommended.

The American Diabetes Association (2010b) recommends screening for type 2 diabetes by the individual’s health care provider if one or more risk factors are present. Testing for diabetes should be considered in any overweight or obese adult. In general, it is recommended that adults ages 45 and older be screened for diabetes every 3 years, but screening should be performed earlier and more frequently if the individual is at high risk. The preferred test is a fasting plasma glucose or HbA_{1c} level. If a random plasma glucose level is ≥160 mg/dL (8.9 mmol/L), a fasting plasma glucose, HbA_{1c}, or 2 hour 75 g OGTT should be performed (see Table 16-1). It should be remembered that whole blood glucose values, which are measured on some home blood glucose monitoring devices, are 10%–15% lower than plasma glucose values. These devices should not be used to diagnose diabetes. If, however, an individual does have a capillary glucose test on one of these machines that reads ≥140 mg/dL (7.8 mmol/L), he or she should be rescreened with a fasting plasma glucose, HbA_{1c}, or OGTT using venous samples (see Table 16-1). Point-of-care A_{1c} assays are not recommended for use for diagnosis at this time.

In recent years, type 2 diabetes has been diagnosed in younger individuals, including children. The American Diabetes Association (2010b) recommends screening children and adolescents, beginning at age 10 or at onset of puberty, who are overweight (BMI >85th percentile or weight >120% of ideal) with two of the following risk factors: Family history (type 2 diabetes in first- and second-degree relatives), high-risk race/ethnicity (Native Americans, African Americans, Hispanic Americans, Asians/South Pacific Islanders), signs of insulin resistance (acanthosis nigricans, hypertension, dyslipidemia, polycystic ovary syndrome, or small for gestational age birth weight), or maternal history of diabetes or gestational diabetes during the child’s gestation.

Most people with type 2 diabetes are insulin resistant and have a relative or absolute deficiency in insulin secretion. Most people with type 2 diabetes are also obese. Inappropriately high hepatic glucose production occurs, along with impaired glucose utilization peripherally. Decreased glucose transport can be demonstrated in muscle and adipose tissue. For glucose tolerance to remain normal, the pancreas has to secrete sufficient insulin. If the pancreas is unable to increase insulin secretion, impaired glucose homeostasis or type 2 diabetes results. Hyperglycemia is toxic to beta cell function and impairs insulin secretion. Over time, beta cell failure is usually progressive, and the beta cells produce lesser amounts of insulin, contributing to increasing insulin deficiency. Although many people with type 2 diabetes can be effectively treated with diet, exercise, and oral glycemic control agents, others require insulin therapy.

MEASURES OF GLYCEMIC CONTROL

It has been established that improved glycemic control is associated with preventing or delaying the progression of microvascular complications in diabetes. The Diabetes Control and Complications Trial (DCCT) demonstrated that lowering glucose levels in patients with type 1 diabetes slows or prevents the development of retinopathy, neuropathy, and nephropathy (DCCT Research Group, 1993). A 50%–75% decrease in complications was observed in the intensively treated group, in which a hemoglobin A_{1c} (HbA_{1c}) of 7.2% was achieved (compared with 9.0% in the conventionally treated group). In the DCCT follow-up Epidemiology of Diabetes Interventions and Complications study, reduction in cardiovascular disease was also found in the groups that had been intensively treated (Nathan, 2005). Reduction in microvascular complications in type 2 diabetes was reported in the United Kingdom Prospective Diabetes Study (UKPDS), as well as in a smaller Japanese study (UKPDS Study Group, 1998a,b; Ohkubo, 1995). In the UKPDS, microvascular complications were decreased by 25% in intensively treated patients by lowering the HbA_{1c} from 7.9% to 7.0%. In the UKPDS follow-up study, macrovascular disease was reduced as well. The standard of care is to measure HbA_{1c} levels every 3–6 months to monitor glycemic control (American Association of Clinical Endocrinologists, 2007; American Diabetes Association, 2010b). Glycemic goals are shown in Table 16-5.

Glycosylated hemoglobin (GHb) is formed nonenzymatically by the two-step reaction shown in Equation 16-7. The first reaction is rapid, reversible, and dependent on the ambient glucose concentration, and produces a labile aldimine or Schiff base. Over time, the aldimine slowly undergoes Amadori rearrangement and is converted to a stable ketoamine, glycosylated hemoglobin. Most HbA_{1c} assays measure this stable ketoamine, not the labile product, which is more prone to be influenced by recent dietary intake.

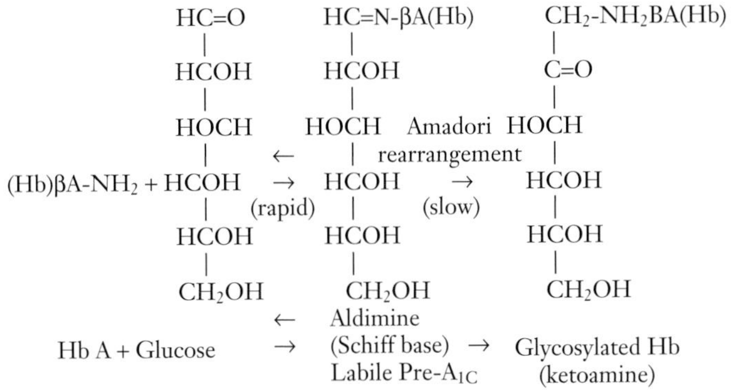

(16-7)

HbA_{1c} is now defined by the International Federation of Clinical Chemistry Working Group on HbA_{1c} as the hemoglobin A that is irreversibly glycosylated at one or both N-terminal valines of the β-chains of the tetrameric hemoglobin molecule, including hemoglobin that may also (but not solely) be glycosylated on lysine residues.

GHb testing provides an index of average blood glucose levels over the past 2–4 months. Although the life span of red blood cells is approximately 120 days, GHb levels represent a "weighted" average of glucose levels, with youngest erythrocytes contributing to a greater extent than older ones. Approximately 50% of the GHb level is determined by plasma glucose levels over the previous month, and 75% during the previous 2 months (Tahara, 1993). Testing methods have been standardized to the HbA_{1c} assay, which is now the preferred test to use to assess glycemic control. To avoid confusion for the general public, the American Diabetes Association, the American College of Endocrinology, and the National Diabetes Education Program recommend using the term "A_{1c}" testing when referring to HbA_{1c} equivalent (GHb) or HbA_{1c} results.

TABLE 16-5
Glycemic Goals

	Hemoglobin A_{1c} (%)	Preprandial glucose		Postprandial glucose*	
		mg/dL	*mmol/L*	*mg/dL*	*mmol/L*
ADA†	<7.0‡	70–130	3.9–7.2	<180	<10.0
AACE§	≤6.5	≤110	≤6.1	≤140	<7.8

*1–2 hours after beginning a meal.
†ADA, American Diabetes Association, 2010b.
‡Lower goals may be appropriate for selected individuals if this can be accomplished safely (without significant hypoglycemia). Higher goals may be appropriate in some individuals (e.g., with a history of severe hypoglycemia, limited life expectancy, advanced complications, extensive comorbid conditions, or long-standing diabetes in whom the goal is difficult to achieve with appropriate education, monitoring and therapies including insulin).
§AACE, American Association of Clinical Endocrinologists, 2007.

The National Glycohemoglobin Standardization Program (NGSP) began in 1996, with the goal of standardizing GHb tests to the high-performance liquid chromatography (HPLC) method reported as HbA_{1c} or HbA_{1c} equivalent, as used in the DCCT. Several types of certified methods are available for measuring hemoglobin A_{1c}: immunoassay, ion-exchange HPLC, electrophoresis, boronate affinity HPLC, and enzyme methods. Reliable bench-top point-of-care analyzers, such as one that uses a cassette-based immunoassay method, also are now available (Guerci, 1997). Most U.S. laboratories use a certified method and the College of American Pathologists' proficiency testing program, which utilizes whole blood and lyophilized samples (Little, 2001).

To obtain and retain a "Certificate of Traceability to the DCCT Reference Method" in the NGSP, the laboratory must annually satisfy precision criteria (CV ≤5%; ≤3% for Level 1 laboratories), bias criteria (95% confidence interval [CI] of differences between test method and Secondary Reference Laboratories [SRL] must fall within ±1% GHb of the SRL [±0.70% GHb for Level 1 laboratories]), and outlier criteria (greater than mean +3 standard deviation of absolute differences between pairs). Level 1 laboratories are usually large and involved in research studies. The NGSP website contains certification criteria and information on how to obtain certification and on assay interferences and hemoglobin variants (http://www.ngsp.org/prog/index3.html).

GHb assays vary in reliability in the presence of a variety of factors. Interference by carbamylated hemoglobin can occur with uremia, hypertriglyceridemia, and hyperbilirubinemia, and salicylates can cause interference by acetylated species. Hemoglobinopathies (HbSS, HbSC, HbCC) associated with high red blood cell turnover and the need for transfusions will adversely affect accuracy, as will chronic alcohol or opiate use, iron deficiency, and lead poisoning (Hoberman, 1982; Tarim, 1999). Vitamins C and E can falsely lower levels by inhibiting glycosylation, but vitamin C can also increase levels for some assays (Davie, 1992; Ceriello, 1991). Sample storage effects may occur. Any condition associated with shortened red blood cell survival or lower mean red blood cell age, such as hemolysis, recovery from acute blood loss, transfusions, or splenectomy, will lower the HbA_{1c} level as the result of reduced exposure to plasma glucose. Hyperglycemia has been associated with a decrease in erythrocyte survival, suggesting that HbA_{1c} levels in poorly controlled patients may underestimate their mean plasma glucose concentration (Virtue, 2004).

In 2007, a consensus statement on the international standardization of HbA_{1c} assays was issued by the American Diabetes Association, the European Association for the Study of Diabetes, the International Federation of Clinical and Laboratory Medicine, and the International Diabetes Federation (Consensus Committee, 2007). HbA_{1c} assays should be calibrated by a new reference measurement system (Weykamp, 2008). This reference method, developed by the International Federation of Clinical Chemistry and Laboratory Medicine, measures only HbA_{1c} (not non-A_{1c} components). The Consenus Committee also recommended that results be reported in a standardized manner (A_{1c} [%]; A_{1c} [mmol/mol], and estimated average glucose). The correlation between HbA_{1c} and estimated average plasma glucose levels for clinical use is shown in Table 16-6 (Nathan, 2008). HbA_{1c} levels used for the diagnosis of diabetes and increased

TABLE 16-6
Correlation Between Hemoglobin A1c and Plasma Glucose Levels

Hemoglobin A_{1c} (%)	Approximate mean plasma glucose	
	mg/dL	*mmol/L*
5	97	5.4
6	126	7.0
7	154	8.6
8	183	10.2
9	212	11.8
10	240	13.4
11	269	14.9
12	298	16.5

From Nathan DM, Kuenen J, Borg R, et al. Translating the A1C assay into estimated average glucose values. Diabetes Care 2008;31:1–6.

diabetes risk are shown in Table 16-1. HbA_{1c} goals for use in diabetes management are shown in Table 16-5.

The turnover time of serum proteins, primarily albumin, is much shorter than that of erythrocytes (14–20 days), so their glycosylation reflects glycemic control over narrower periods of time. The nonenzymatic glycation of these serum proteins occurs similarly to that of hemoglobin, with the formation of ketoamine-linked glucose protein. Several methods are available for measuring glycosylated proteins or glycosylated albumin, including affinity chromatography and immunoassays. These assays may be useful in patients for whom HbA_{1c} assays are inaccurate, such as those with hemoglobinopathies and hemolytic anemias, but unlike HbA_{1c} levels, their clinical utility has not been firmly established.

Fructosamine assays are the most widely used to assess short-term (3–6 week) glycemic control because the average half-life of the proteins is 2–3 weeks. These assays have the advantage of using serum samples and automated equipment, so are simple to perform and low in cost. They are more reliable than other glycosylated protein assays but can be affected by alterations in serum protein levels that are present during acute illnesses and liver disease. Whether fructosamine values should be corrected for serum protein or albumin concentrations is controversial. The assay should not be performed if the serum albumin level is ≤3.0 mg/dL. High uric acid, triglyceride and bilirubin levels, and the presence of heparin or hemolysis can also affect the assay.

KETONE TESTING

The ketone bodies β-hydroxybutyric acid, acetoacetic acid, and acetone are products of fatty acid degradation. β-Hydroxybutyric acid and acetoacetic acid are normally present in a 1:1 ratio at concentrations of 0.5–1.0 mmol/L each. Ketone testing, using urine or blood, is particularly important for individuals with type 1 diabetes mellitus to detect ketosis. Diabetic ketoacidosis (DKA) is a serious and potentially fatal hyperglycemic condition requiring urgent treatment. It is frequently associated with nausea, vomiting, abdominal pain, electrolyte disturbances, and severe dehydration. Type 2 diabetes patients who are poorly controlled, particularly in the presence of extreme stress or severe acute illness, can also develop DKA. Ketone testing may be useful in pregnancy and in determining the cause of hypoglycemic disorders.

The ratio of β-hydroxybutyric acid to acetoacetic acid is greatly increased in DKA as a result of the altered redox state and elevated levels of NADH in the hepatic mitochondria. The most commonly used strips and tablets use sodium nitroprusside (sodium nitroferricyanide) and turn purple in the presence of elevated levels of acetoacetic acid. Acetone is detected in the presence of glycine. False-negative results can occur with old strips and with strips that have had excessive contact with air, and after ingestion of large amounts of vitamin C. False-positive results have been observed with angiotensin-converting enzyme inhibitors and other sulfhydryl medications. β-Hydroxybutyric acid is not detected by these methods. Because β-hydroxybutyric acid levels fall and acetoacetic acid and acetone levels rise during the treatment of DKA, these tests are not useful for the monitoring of therapy.

To specifically quantitate β-hydroxybutyric acid, enzymatic methods are available for use by hospitals, as well as by individuals at home, using point-of-care devices. β-Hydroxybutyric acid can also be measured using electrochemical, chromatographic, electrophoretic, and colorimetric methods. For the monitoring of recovery from DKA in the hospital setting, serial measurements of β-hydroxybutyric acid can be followed, but more commonly, serum electrolytes, including bicarbonate with calculation of the anion gap, are used.

HYPOGLYCEMIA

Hypoglycemia results from an imbalance between glucose utilization (by brain, erythrocytes, muscle tissue, and kidneys) and production (endogenous glucose production by liver and kidneys and from ingestion of carbohydrates) in such a manner that the rate of glucose utilization exceeds the rate at which glucose is being produced (Guettier, 2006). The symptoms of hypoglycemia can be divided into two categories: neurogenic and neuroglycopenic. Neurogenic symptoms are triggered by the autonomic nervous system. Tremulousness, palpitations, and anxiety are catecholamine mediated, and diaphoresis, hunger, and paresthesias are related to acetylcholine release. The neuroglycopenic symptoms are due to diminished glucose supply to the central nervous system and include dizziness, tingling, difficulty concentrating, blurred vision, confusion, behavioral changes, seizure and coma (Towler, 1993; Schwartz, 1987; Mitrakou, 1991). Severe hypoglycemia if not corrected in a timely fashion can lead to brain death (Cryer, 2007).

Treatment of diabetes mellitus with insulin or agents that increase insulin secretion (insulin secretagogue drugs) such as sulfonylureas is the major cause of hypoglycemia. A number of drugs and medical conditions can also cause hypoglycemia (Table 16-7). Pancreatic hyperinsulinemic hypoglycemia can be diagnosed by demonstrating that insulin secretion is not suppressed normally when the individual develops hypoglycemia. Measurements of insulin, C-peptide, proinsulin, insulin and insulin receptor autoantibodies, β-hydroxybutyrate, and drugs (i.e., sulfonylurea/meglitinide levels) are recommended to determine the correct diagnosis. Insulin and proinsulin autoantibodies may interfere with the immunoassays for insulin, proinsulin, and C-peptide.

"Whipple's triad," initially proposed by Whipple for the diagnosis of hypoglycemic disorders, continues to be an important tool in assessing patients with episodes suggestive of low plasma glucose levels. Whipple's triad refers to symptoms consistent with hypoglycemia associated with a documented low plasma glucose level and relief of symptoms with correction of hypoglycemia (Whipple, 1938). Further evaluation is indicated if a person in good health presents with symptoms of hypoglycemia and a laboratory plasma glucose level ≤55 mg/dL (3.0 mmol/L) in the absence of treatment of diabetes mellitus (Cryer, 2009). A blood glucose level ≤50 mg/dL (2.8 mmol/L) in infants is considered abnormal and warrants diagnostic assessment (Sperling, 2004; Haymond, 1989).

HYPOGLYCEMIC DISORDERS

Drugs

Several drugs can cause hypoglycemia that may manifest as altered mental status. Most cases of drug-induced hypoglycemia have been described in patients with diabetes mellitus who are on glucose-lowering medication such as insulin and insulin secretagogue drugs (sulfonylureas, repaglinide, and nateglinide). Elevated insulin with low C-peptide levels is observed when exogenous insulin has been administered. High insulin and C-peptide levels with a positive drug screen for an insulin secretagogue would be expected when these oral agents have been used surreptitiously. It is important that these blood tests be drawn during the hypoglycemic episode. The assays for sulfonylureas and meglitinides should be sent to a laboratory that has the capability to measure very low levels of these drugs, as assays using higher detection limits can lead to an inaccurate diagnosis (Manning, 2003).

Pentamidine used for the treatment of *Pneumocystis* pneumonia causes hypoglycemia by damaging pancreatic beta cells. Hypoglycemia can occur within a few hours to days of administration of pentamidine. Plasma insulin levels are high despite low glucose concentrations, indicating excessive insulin leakage (Bouchard, 1982; Assan, 1995). Sulfonamide-induced hypoglycemia is also associated with increased insulin and C-peptide levels in susceptible individuals (Hekimsoy, 1997). Salicylate-induced hypoglycemia may be due to increased peripheral glucose utilization secondary to uncoupling of oxidative phosphorylation, decreased hepatic glyconeogenesis, and increased insulin release (Marks, 1999). Beta blockers, such as propranolol, can cause hypoglycemia by antagonizing catecholamine-mediated glycogenolysis (Chavez, 1999).

TABLE 16-7
Clinical Classification of Hypoglycemia

Drugs	Endogenous Hyperinsulinism
Insulin	Pancreatic beta cell disorders
Sulfonylureas	Tumor (insulinoma)
Benzoic acid derivatives (repaglinide)	Nontumor (nesidioblastosis or diffuse hyperplasia of the islets)
Nateglinide	**Autoimmune Hypoglycemia**
Alcohol	Insulin antibodies
Pentamidine	Insulin receptor antibodies
Beta-blockers	**Non–Beta Cell Tumors**
Quinine	Mesenchymal: Fibrosarcoma, mesothelioma, rhabdomyosarcoma, leiomyosarcoma, liposarcoma, lymphosarcoma, hemangiopericytoma
Salicylates	Carcinomas: Hepatomas, adrenocortical tumors, hypernephroma, Wilms' tumor
Sulfonamides	Neurologic and neuroendocrine tumors: Pheochromocytoma, carcinoid tumor, neurofibroma
Haloperidol	Hematologic: Leukemias, lymphoma, myeloma
Propoxyphene	**Hypoglycemia of Infancy and Childhood**
Para-aminobenzoic acid	Hyperinsulinism
Cibenzoline	Transient: Erythroblastosis fetalis, Beckwith-Wiedemann syndrome, uncontrolled diabetes (mother)
Gatifloxacin	Persistent: Hyperinsulinemic hypoglycemia of infancy
Indomethacin	Glycogen storage diseases
Lithium	Hereditary fructose intolerance
Clinafloxacin	Galactosemia
Glucagon	Defects in gluconeogenesis
Artesunate	Reye's syndrome
Artemisin	Deficiency of glucose transporters
Artemether	Impaired ketogenesis
Chloroquineoxaline sulfonamide	Carnitine deficiency
Insulin-like growth factor-1 (IGF-1)	Defects in mitochondrial function
Critical Illnesses	**Alimentary Hypoglycemia**
Hepatic failure	Postgastric bypass surgery
Renal failure	**Idiopathic (Functional) Postprandial Hypoglycemia**
Cardiac failure	
Sepsis	
Malnutrition	
Hormonal Deficiencies	
Glucagon	
Epinephrine	
Cortisol	
Growth hormone	

Adapted from Lteif AN, Schwenk WF. Hypoglycemia in infants and children. Endocrinol Metab Clin N Am 1999;28(3):619–646; Cryer PE, Axelrod L, Grossman AB, et al. Evaluation and management of adult hypoglycemic disorders: an Endocrine Society clinical practice guideline. J Clin Endocrinol Metab 2009;94(3):709–728; Murad HA, Coto-Yglesias F, Wang AT, et al. Drug-induced hypoglycemia: a systematic review. J Clin Endocrinol Metab 2009;94(3):741–745.

Adenosine triphosphate (ATP)–sensitive potassium (K_{ATP}) channels play a major role in the regulation of insulin secretion from pancreatic beta cells. Blockage of these channels causes depolarization of the beta cell membrane, opening of voltage-dependent calcium channels, and increased influx of calcium that causes release of insulin from the beta cell and lowering of blood glucose. Gatifloxacin, a fluoroquinolone, causes hypoglycemia by blocking the ATP-sensitive potassium channels of pancreatic islet cells, leading to increased insulin release. The K_{ATP} channel consists of eight subunits (four Kir6.0 and four SUR). Saraya et al. showed that the Kir6.2 subunit of the pancreatic beta cell is blocked by gatifloxacin and to a lesser extent by levofloxacin and temafloxacin (Saraya, 2004; Park-Wyllie, 2006). Gatifloxacin has been withdrawn (*Federal Register*, Vol. 73, No. 175/September 9, 2008/Notices accessed on June 21, 2009, at http://edocket.access.gpo.gov/2008/E8-20938.htm).

Alcohol consumption can inhibit hepatic gluconeogenesis and increase glycogen phosphorylase activity, depleting hepatic glycogen stores and resulting in hypoglycemia. Alcohol-induced hypoglycemia is usually seen in the setting of a history of alcohol intake of 50–300 g without food intake for the preceding 6 to greater than 36 hours. Alcohol can be detected in the blood or breath. Plasma β-hydroxybutyrate levels are elevated and plasma insulin and C-peptide levels are low during the hypoglycemic episode (Arky, 1989; Marks, 1999).

Severe Medical Illnesses

Widespread hepatic disease and severe cardiac failure can result in hypoglycemia. Pathogenic mechanisms can include impaired gluconeogenesis, hepatic congestion with decreased oxygen delivery to hepatocytes, impaired insulin degradation, and shunting of portal blood into the systemic circulation (Khoury, 1998). A decrease in glycogen reserves coupled with failure of gluconeogenesis and enhanced glucose utilization may be the cause of hypoglycemia in patients with severe sepsis (Miller, 1980). In addition, patients with very low muscle mass, such as those with spinal muscular atrophy and congenital myopathy, are at risk for hypoglycemia during prolonged fasting (23 hours), presumably related to poor availability of the gluconeogenic substrate alanine. Low plasma insulin and high plasma glucagon levels are observed during the hypoglycemia (Orngreen, 2003).

Hypoglycemia in end-stage renal disease (ESRD) can be related to defective gluconeogenesis, as well as impaired hepatic glycogenolysis due to poor nutritional status (Arem, 1989). Alcohol use, use of insulin or sulfonylurea drugs, sepsis, malnutrition, liver disease, and cardiac failure can increase the likelihood of hypoglycemic events in a patient with renal failure (Haviv, 2000). Gabapentin has been associated with hypoglycemia in a patient with ESRD on peritoneal dialysis. Plasma insulin and C-peptide levels were elevated during the hypoglycemic episode (Penumalee, 2003).

Hormone Deficiencies

Glucose counterregulation, mediated by glucagon, catecholamines, cortisol, and growth hormone, is important in preventing hypoglycemia. Glucagon initially stimulates glycogenolysis and later gluconeogenesis to increase plasma glucose levels. Catecholamines increase glycogenolysis, gluconeogenesis, and lipolysis, decrease insulin-mediated glucose uptake, and inhibit insulin release. Both growth hormone and cortisol decrease insulin-mediated tissue glucose uptake and increase release of glucose into the circulation. A deficiency in the secretion of these counterregulatory hormones can contribute to low blood glucose levels. Hypoglycemia in adults is rarely attributable to deficiencies of glucagon or catecholamines, but poor glucagon and epinephrine responses to hypoglycemia are common in patients with long-standing diabetes mellitus and are associated with prolonged hypoglycemic episodes. Infants and children with a deficiency of cortisol and growth hormone are prone to develop hypoglycemia, especially during an acute illness. Adults with glucocorticoid or growth hormone deficiency can also develop hypoglycemia, usually after a prolonged fast (Smallridge, 1980; Zuker, 1995; Bunch, 2002).

Non–Beta Cell Tumors

Non–islet cell tumor hypoglycemia (NICTH) originates from non–beta cell tumors, which cause hypoglycemia without producing insulin. Tumors of mesenchymal origin (mesothelioma, hemangiopericytoma, solitary fibrous tumors) and epithelial origin (hepatocellular, gastrointestinal stromal tumor) are commonly associated with NICTH. These tumors are associated with increased paraneoplastic production of insulin-like growth factor-II (IGF-II). Normally, IGF-II is produced by liver and is relatively independent of growth hormone (GH) action. The primary transcription product is pre-proIGF-II. Post-translational processing of pre-proIGF-II leads to the formation of proIGF-II that is cleaved to form IGF-II. The intermediate product proIGF-II may be secreted. Non–islet cell tumor hypoglycemia is associated with aberrant paraneoplastic production of proIGF-II, also known as "big" IGF-II (Fukuda, 2006; de Groot, 2007). It is believed that elevated levels of IGF-II increase glucose utilization and suppress endogenous glucose production (Chung, 1996; Daughaday, 1989). The diagnosis of NICTH can usually be made by the presence of fasting hypoglycemia, low insulin, proinsulin, and C-peptide levels, an elevated IGF-II–to–IGF-I ratio, and low growth hormone and β-hydroxybutyrate levels. The glucagon level is usually within the normal range despite hypoglycemia because of the suppressive effect of "big" IGF-II on glucagon secretion. Hypokalemia is frequently associated with hypoglycemia due to insulin-like activity of big IGF-II. Levels of "big" IGF-II and IGF-BP 2 (IGF binding protein 2) can be determined by immunometric assays and are usually elevated (van Doorn, 2002). Size-exclusion acid chromatography is considered the gold standard method for detecting "big" IGF-II in NICTH. However, this is a time-consuming procedure. Determination of "big" IGF-II by immunoblot analysis after 16.5% tricine sodium dodecyl sulphate-polyacrylamide gels is a rapid, reproducible, and sensitive method (Miraki-Moud, 2005). The tumor is usually detected on physical examination and is confirmed by radiologic diagnostic studies.

Endogenous Hyperinsulinism

Hypoglycemia from endogenous insulin secretion can be due to (1) insulin-secreting beta cell tumors (insulinomas), (2) congenital hyperinsulinism (also called nesidioblastosis/islet hypertrophy or noninsulinoma pancreatogenous hypoglycemia syndrome), and (3) autoantibodies to insulin in patients who have never been treated with insulin (Hirata, 1994). A supervised 72-hour fast is recommended for the diagnosis of insulinoma with frequent clinical and biochemical monitoring for signs of hypoglycemia. During the hypoglycemic episode, blood is drawn for glucose, insulin, proinsulin, C-peptide, and β-hydoxybutyrate levels. Blood or urine screening tests for sulfonylurea/meglitinide drugs are also performed.

Insulinomas are the most common tumors of islet cells, with an incidence of 2–4 patients per million of the population per year (Oberg, 2005). The diagnostic criteria for an insulinoma are as follows: Presence of signs and symptoms of hypoglycemia with plasma glucose level ≤55 mg/dL (3.0 mmol/L), insulin level ≥3 μU/mL (18 pmol/L) by immunochemiluminometric assay, C-peptide concentration ≥0.6 ng/mL (0.2 nmol/L), proinsulin concentration ≥5.0 pmol/L, β-hydroxybutyrate ≤2.7 mmol/L, an increase in the plasma glucose concentration of at least 25 mg/dL (1.4 mmol/L) in response to a 1 mg glucagon injection given intravenously, and a negative sulfonylurea/meglitinide blood/urine screen (Cryer, 2009). Those patients who are found to have endogenous hyperinsulinemic hypoglycemia with negative screening for oral antihyperglycemic agents and no evidence of insulin antibodies need further diagnostic tests to localize the insulinoma. These tests may include computed tomography (CT) or magnetic resonance imaging (MRI), as well as transabdominal and endoscopic ultrasonography (USG). Selective pancreatic arterial calcium injections with measurement of hepatic venous insulin levels can be used when conventional noninvasive means (CT, MRI, USG) have failed to localize the insulin-producing islet cell tumors (Guettier, 2009).

Autoimmune

Hypoglycemia can be due to antibodies directed against endogenous insulin or the insulin receptor. Hypoglycemia associated with autoantibodies to insulin in patients who have not received insulin injections is a rare condition called the autoimmune insulin syndrome (AIS). Individuals with autoimmune diseases or recent ingestion of sulfhydryl-containing medications (i.e., methimazole, penicillamine, captopril, imipenem, hydralazine, procainamide, isoniazid, penicillin G) are at increased risk for AIS. These patients commonly experience episodes of postprandial hypoglycemia. In some patients, fasting hypoglycemia, as well as hypoglycemia precipitated by increased physical activity, has been reported. Excessive amounts of insulin secreted after a meal are bound to antibodies, and as a result insulin becomes unavailable to target tissues. Hours later, insulin dissociates from the antibodies, resulting in hyperinsulinemia and hypoglycemia. Insulin levels are extremely elevated and distinctly higher than in insulinoma. C-peptide levels are incompletely suppressed, and a high insulin–to–C-peptide molar ratio is present. Serum insulin antibodies are elevated (Hirata, 1994; Dozio, 1998; Lidar, 1999; Cavaco, 2001; Vogeser, 2001; Yaturu, 2004; Lupsa, 2009).

Antibodies directed against the insulin receptor can cause hypoglycemia or hyperglycemia with extreme insulin resistance (type B insulin resistance). Type B insulin resistance is a rare condition that occurs in the third to fifth decades of life. It is more common in women and in persons of African heritage. Hyperglycemia may be the initial metabolic derangement in 80% of these patients; however, 20% may present with hypoglycemia. Hypoglycemia may develop some time later in 14% of patients who initially present with hyperglycemia (Fareau, 2007). Other autoimmune diseases, such as systemic lupus erythematosus and Hashimoto's thyroiditis, may also be present in these patients (Qing, 2009; Kato, 2008; Bao, 2007). In this condition, insulin receptor antibodies block insulin from attaching to the insulin receptor. In some patients, hyperglycemia is due to receptor degradation or downregulation leading to insulin resistance. Hyperglycemia and hypoglycemia sometimes can be seen in the same patient. Plasma glucose, β-hydroxybutyrate, and proinsulin levels are low, and insulin and the insulin–to–C-peptide ratio are inappropriately high. Insulin receptor antibodies can be detected by immunoprecipitation assays (Redmon, 1999; Taylor, 1989). Mutations in the insulin receptor gene are another rare cause of hypoglycemia.

Infancy and Childhood

Endocrine adaptive responses at birth help ensure neonatal nutrition. These include a decrease in insulin levels and an increase in glucagon and catecholamine levels. Glycogenolysis, gluconeogenesis, lipolysis, and beta-oxidation of fatty acids occur during this period of metabolic transition in early neonates. Blood glucose concentrations are usually lower than those observed in older infants and children. However, because of increased production and use of alternative fuels such as lactate and ketone bodies and differences in functional and metabolic requirements of neonatal brain, this "transitional hypoglycemia" is not associated with adverse effects. Hypoglycemia can be detrimental during the neonatal phase if the production of alternate fuels is impaired. Neonatal hyperinsulinism seen in infants of women with poorly controlled diabetes mellitus increases the risk of hypoglycemia during the few days after birth. A blunted glucagon surge (possibly mediated by intravenous glucose or formula feeds) or insufficient catecholamine release (due to maternal beta-blocker medication use) can lead to hypoglycemia requiring treatment (Hawdon, 2008). Other possible causes of hypoglycemia in infants include pituitary and adrenal disorders. Ketogenic hypoglycemia can be seen in children between 18 months and 5 years of age. Alanine, a gluconeogenic substrate, is found to be low in these patients. Usually, an episode of illness or prolonged fasting is associated with the hypoglycemia (Haymond, 1983).

Congenital Hyperinsulinism

Congenital hyperinsulinism (CHI) is associated with inappropriate secretion of insulin in relation to blood glucose concentration, leading to hyperinsulinemic hypoglycemia (HH). Genetic mutations in beta cells have been identified that result in dysregulated insulin release. Mutations in ATP-binding cassette, subfamily C, member 8; potassium inwardly rectifying channel, subfamily J, member 11; glutamate dehydrogenase; glucokinase; hydroxyacyl–coenzyme A dehydrogenase; solute carrier family 16, member 1; and hepatocyte nuclear factor 4 alpha have been linked to HH seen in CHI. Hyperinsulinemic hypoglycemia is characterized by a low blood glucose level with inappropriate insulin and C-peptide concentrations (Hussain, 2008; Kapoor, 2009).

The enzyme glucokinase (GCK) functions as a glucose sensor in the pancreatic beta cell and mediates glucose-stimulated insulin secretion. Activating mutations of GCK are inherited in an autosomal dominant manner and have been associated with familial hyperinsulinemic hypoglycemia. The hypoglycemia is usually mild (as compared with the autosomal recessive form) and is not limited to infancy. De novo mutations in the GCK gene resulting in hypoglycemia have also been described. In the hyperinsulinism hyperammonia syndrome, hypoglycemia is caused by an activating mutation of the glutamate dehydrogenase gene *(GLUD1)* located on chromosome 10. It is an autosomal dominant disorder characterized by hypoglycemia and elevated ammonia levels (three to eight times normal). Less severe hypoglycemia has been reported in sporadic cases (Sunehag, 2002; Straub, 2001; Cuesta-Munoz, 2004; Stanley, 1998). Hypoglycemia and lactic acidosis have been described in a child with mutation in a subunit of the mitochondrial respiratory chain complex III (Haut, 2003). In addition, mutations in enzymes involved in mitochondrial fatty acid oxidation can cause hyperinsulinemic hypoglycemia (Molven, 2004). Elevated plasma levels of hydroxybutrylcarnitine and urinary 3-hydroxyglutarate are seen in hydroxyacyl–coenzyme A dehydrogenase (HADH) deficiency (Clayton, 2001).

The noninsulinoma pancreatogenous hypoglycemia syndrome reported in adults is not associated with mutations in the *SUR1* or *Kir6.2* gene. These patients usually present with postprandial hypoglycemia. Serum insulin and C-peptide levels are elevated, and the drug screen for sulfonylureas and meglitinides is negative (Service, 1999).

Alimentary

Alimentary (reactive) hypoglycemia occurs usually within 4 hours after eating a meal. The OGTT is unreliable in diagnosing this condition. Individuals who have had gastric surgery are at risk. The dumping syndrome is characterized by vasomotor symptoms such as sweating, dizziness, and weakness, which usually occur less than an hour after ingestion of a meal. Hypoglycemia is not a characteristic of early dumping syndrome.

Hypoglycemia has been reported in patients who have undergone bariatric surgery for obesity. Hypoglycemia in the setting of gastric bypass surgery may be caused by trophic factors such as GLP-1 that cause endogenous hyperinsulinemia (Gebhard, 2001). These patients usually have a history of "spells" of postprandial hypoglycemia that fulfill Whipple's triad. An insulin level >3.0 μU/mL (18 pmol/L) with C-peptide >0.6 ng/mL (0.2 nmol/L) in the presence of plasma glucose <55 mg/dL (3.0 mmol/L) and negative sulfonylurea/meglinitide screen with normal adrenal, pituitary, and thyroid functions is important for diagnosis. Imaging studies are negative for pancreatic tumor.

Some individuals without gastrointestinal pathology report spontaneous symptoms suggestive of hypoglycemia 1–4 hours after intake of carbohydrate-rich meals but have a normal laboratory evaluation. These patients are believed to have idiopathic reactive hypoglycemia. The OGTT is also not useful for the diagnosis of this condition (Lefebvre, 1988). Increased insulin sensitivity has been seen in some patients exhibiting features of postprandial hypoglycemia (Tamburrano, 1989). Contributing factors may also include delayed release of insulin in response to a meal and concomitant alcohol ingestion (Flanagan, 1998).

Inborn Errors of Carbohydrate Metabolism

Normal plasma glucose levels are maintained by absorption of glucose from the diet, synthesis of glucose during gluconeogenesis, and the release of glucose from glycogen, the principal storage form of glucose. Glycogen storage diseases or glycogenoses result from defects in glycogen metabolism. These diseases are the consequence of inherited deficiencies of enzymes that control the synthesis or breakdown of glycogen. Abnormal quality or quantity of glycogen is found in these disorders. Liver and muscle are most commonly affected by defects in glycogen metabolism, as these tissues have abundant quantities of glycogen. Glycogen storage diseases that primarily affect the liver (hepatic glycogenoses) usually manifest with hypoglycemia and hepatomegaly. Muscle cramps, exercise intolerance, fatigue, and weakness are common complaints in glycogen storage diseases affecting muscles (muscle glycogenoses). Glycogen storage disease types I (glucose-6-phosphatase deficiency), III (debrancher deficiency), IV (brancher deficiency), VI (liver phosphorylase deficiency), IX (phosphorylase kinase deficiency), and 0 (glycogen synthase deficiency) and glucose transporter-2 (GLUT-2) deficiency mainly affect the liver. Table 16-8 shows the various characteristics of hepatic glycogenoses (Wolfsdorf, 1999; Chen, 2001). Muscle glycogenoses or glycogen storage diseases affecting the muscles (Table 16-9) include type V (muscle phosphorylase deficiency), type VII (muscle phosphofructokinase deficiency), and glycogen storage diseases secondary to defects in phosphoglycerate kinase, phosphoglycerate mutase, lactate dehydrogenase, fructose 1,6-biphosphate aldolase A, pyruvate kinase, muscle phosphorylase kinase, lysosomal acid

TABLE 16-8
Hepatic Glycogenoses

Type (GSD)	Defect	Clinical features	Laboratory findings	Treatment	Genetics
Ia/von Gierke disease	Glucose-6-phosphatase	• Thin extremities, short stature, protuberant abdomen, skin xanthomas, retinal changes, hepatomegaly, hypoglycemic seizures, growth retardation • Long-term complications: Growth failure, pulmonary hypertension, osteoporosis, renal disease, hepatic adenomas that can result in hepatocellular carcinoma (Franco, 2005)	• Hypoglycemia, lactic acidosis, hyperuricemia, dyslipidemia • Diagnosis: Liver biopsy to demonstrate glucose-6-phosphatase activity in both intact and fully disrupted microsomes • Targeted gene-based mutation analysis: Noninvasive method of diagnosis for most patients	• High complex carbohydrate feeds during the day, total parenteral nutrition, nocturnal nasogastric or gastrostomy tube infusion of glucose at night, uncooked starch • Restrict fructose and galactose • Treatment of other manifestations as and when indicated (e.g., gout, dyslipidemia etc.) • Liver transplantation may be considered in patients who do not respond to dietary therapy or in those who develop hepatic adenomas (Faivre,1999).	Autosomal recessive
Ib	Glucose-6-phosphatase translocase	• As for 1a, plus recurrent bacterial infections	• As for 1a, plus neutropenia and inflammatory bowel disease	• As for 1a, plus granulocyte and granulocyte/macrophage colony-stimulating factor for neutropenia	Autosomal recessive

Continued

TABLE 16-8
Hepatic Glycogenoses—*Cont'd*

Type (GSD)	Defect	Clinical features	Laboratory findings	Treatment	Genetics
IIIa (also called "Cori" or Forbes' disease)	Glycogen debranching enzyme (in both liver and muscle)	• Childhood: Hepatomegaly, hypoglycemia, growth retardation • Adult: Muscle atrophy, weakness, cardiomyopathy	• Childhood: Dyslipidemia, hypoglycemia, ↑ hepatic transaminases, fasting ketosis, normal lactate and uric acid • Adult: EMG shows myopathy • Diagnosis: Demonstration of abnormal glycogen and abnormal enzyme activity on liver and muscle biopsy • Gene-based mutation analysis is a noninvasive method of diagnosis.	• Childhood: Same as 1a, plus high-protein diet. No dietary restriction of fructose and galactose • Adult: No effective treatment of myopathy	Autosomal recessive
IIIb	Glycogen debranching enzyme in liver (normal muscle debranching enzyme)	• Same as in IIIa, with no muscle symptoms	• Same as in IIIa, with no muscle findings	• Same as in IIIa	Autosomal recessive

IV (also called Anderson's disease, amylopectinosis)	Glycogen branching enzyme	• Hepatosplenomegaly, failure to thrive, liver cirrhosis, portal hypertension, ascites, esophageal varices, and fatal by 5 years of age Hypoglycemia rare but may occur in liver cirrhosis
		• Neuromuscular form:
		  • Neonate: Hypotonia, muscle atrophy
		  • Childhood: Myopathy or cardiomyopathy
		  • Adulthood: Diffuse central and peripheral nervous system dysfunction (adult polyglucosan body disease)
			• Tissue deposition of amylopectin-like material
			• Deficiency of branching enzyme in liver
			• Adult polyglucosan body disease: Deficient branching enzyme in leukocytes or nerve biopsy
				• No specific treatment
				• Maintenance of normoglycemia
				• Liver transplantation in selected cases
					Autosomal recessive

VI (also called Hers disease)	Glycogen phosphorylase (in liver)	• Hepatomegaly, growth retardation in early childhood, benign course • Hepatomegaly improves with age.	• Mild hypoglycemia, dyslipidemia, ketosis • Normal uric acid and lactic acid • Diagnosis: Abnormal enzyme activity in biopsy of affected tissues • Molecular genetic testing: *PYGL* is the only gene associated with GSD VI and can be detected by sequence analysis.	• High-carbohydrate diet, frequent feedings • No specific treatment in most patients	Autosomal recessive
IXa	Phosphorylase kinase (in liver)	• Hepatomegaly, protuberant abdomen, growth retardation, delay in motor development	• Mild dyslipidemia, mildly elevated liver transaminases, fasting ketosis, mild hypoglycemia • Diagnosis: Abnormal enzyme activity in biopsy of affected tissues	• High-carbohydrate diet, frequent feeds • Course usually benign	X-linked
IXb	Phosphorylase deficiency (in liver and muscle)	• Hepatomegaly, growth retardation, muscle hypotonia (in some patients)	Same as in IXa	Same as in IXa	Autosomal recessive
0	Glycogen synthase	• Hypoglycemic symptoms in morning; no hepatomegaly • Mild growth delay (in few cases)	• Fasting hypoglycemia, hyperketonemia • Hyperglycemia and elevated lactate level after meals • Diagnosis: Mutation analysis of the hepatic glycogen synthase gene	• Uncooked starch feeding during night • Frequent feedings during day with high protein content	Autosomal recessive
XI (also called Fanconi-Bickel syndrome)	GLUT 2	• Protuberant abdomen due to hepatomegaly and renomegaly, rickets, failure to thrive	• Glucosuria, phosphaturia, aminoaciduria, bicarbonate wasting, hypophosphatemia, elevated alkaline phosphatase level • Mild fasting hypoglycemia and dyslipidemia • Rickets on radiologic studies	• No specific therapy • Symptomatic replacement of water, electrolytes, vitamin D • Restriction of galactose • Frequent small meals with corn starch supplement	Autosomal recessive

Adapted from Chen YT. Glycogen storage diseases. In: Scriver CR, Beaudet AL, Sly WS, Valle D, editors. The metabolic and molecular bases of inherited disease, 8th ed. New York, McGraw-Hill; 2001, p. 1521–1551; Wolfsdorf JI, Holm IA, Weinstein DA. Glycogen storage diseases: phenotypic, genetic, and biochemical characteristics, and therapy. Endocrinol Metab Clin N Am 1999;28(4):801–823; Weinstein DA, Wolfsdorf JI. Glycogen storage diseases: a primer for clinicians. Endocrinologist 2002;12:531–538.
GSD, Glycogen storage disease.

TABLE 16-9
Muscle Glycogenoses

Type	Defect	Clinical features	Laboratory findings	Treatment
V (McArdle disease)	Muscle phosphorylase	• Exercise intolerance, muscle cramps • Dark red urine after intense exercise • Usually presents in 2nd or 3rd decade	• Myoglobinuria, ↑ creatinine kinase at rest and increases after exercise, ↑ ammonia and ↑ uric acid with exercise • Diagnosis: enzymatic evaluation of muscle or mutation analysis	• ↑ Exercise tolerance by aerobic training, or by ingestion of sucrose, glucose, or fructose immediately prior to exercise. Low-dose creatine supplementation • (Quinlivan, 2008)
VII (Tarui disease)	Phosphofructokinase	• Same as in type V plus: • Severe exercise intolerance or myopathy in childhood, compensated hemolytic anemia, more hyperuricemia than type V, acute exercise intolerance post carbohydrate-rich meals	• ↑ Creatine kinase and ↑ bilirubin, reticulocytosis, hyperuricemia • Diagnosis: biochemical or histochemical demonstration of enzyme defect	• Avoid strenuous exercise for prevention of muscle cramps and myoglobinuria.
Phosphoglycerate kinase deficiency	Phosphoglycerate kinase	• Same as in type V plus hemolytic anemia, CNS dysfunction, and/or myopathy	• ↑ Creatine kinase (not always) • Abnormal enzyme assays in muscles	Same as in type VII
Phosphoglycerate mutase deficiency	Phosphoglycerate mutase M subunit	Same as in type V	↑ Serum creatine kinase level	Same as type VII
LD deficiency	Lactic acid dehydrogenase M subunit	Same as in type V plus erythematous rash, difficulties in childbirth (uterine stiffness)	↑ Creatine kinase level (not always)	Same as type VII
Fructose-1,6-biphosphate aldolase A deficiency	Fructose-1,6-biphosphate aldolase A	Same as type V plus muscle weakness, hemolytic anemia	↑ Creatine kinase (not always)	Same as type VII
Pyruvate kinase deficiency	Pyruvate kinase muscle isozyme	Muscle cramps, fixed muscle weakness	↑ Creatine kinase (not always)	Same as type VII
Muscle phosphorylase kinase deficiency	Muscle phosphorylase kinase (muscle specific)	Same as type V plus muscle weakness and atrophy	↑ Creatine kinase (not always)	Same as type VII
II/Pompe disease	Lysosomal acid alpha glucosidase (GAA) (acid maltase)	• Infant: Muscle weakness, feeding problems, macroglossia, hepatomegaly, cardiomyopathy • Late childhood: Proximal muscle weakness, swallowing difficulties, respiratory muscle weakness • Adult: Proximal muscle weakness with pelvic girdle, paraspinal and diaphragm muscles affected seriously	• ↑ Creatine kinase, ↑ aspartate transaminase, LD • Diagnosis: decreased or absent acid alpha-glucosidase (GAA) activity in muscle or cultured skin fibroblasts • Molecular genetic testing: GAA is the only gene associated with GSD11 and can be detected by sequence analysis or deletion/duplication analysis (Montalvo, 2006; Pittis, 2008).	• Infant: Enzyme replacement therapy with Myozyme (alglucosidase alfa) by slow intravenous infusion every 2 weeks should be initiated as soon as the diagnosis is established (Kishnani, 2007). • Late childhood and adult: High-protein diet • Ventilatory support

Adapted from Chen YT. Glycogen storage diseases. In: Scriver CR, Beaudet AL, Sly WS, Valle D, editors. The metabolic and molecular bases of inherited disease, 8th ed. New York, McGraw-Hill; 2001, p. 1521–1551; Tsujino S, Nonaka I, DiMauro S. Glycogen storage myopathies. Neurol Clin 2000;18(1):125–150.
LD, Lactate dehydrogenase.

alpha-glucosidase (type II, Pompe disease), and cardiac-specific phosphorylase kinase (Tsujino, 2000; Chen, 2001; Weinstein, 2002).

DEFECTS IN GALACTOSE METABOLISM

Galactose is a monosaccharide constituent, together with glucose, of the disaccharide lactose. Milk and milk products are the main sources of galactose. Enzymatic defects of galactokinase, galactose-1-phosphate uridyl transferase, and uridine diphosphate galactose-4-epimerase result in the defective metabolism and accumulation of galactose and its metabolites causing galactosemia (Holton, 2001).

Galactosemia with Uridyl Transferase Deficiency

Galactose-1-phosphate uridyl transferase (GALT) deficiency (classic galactosemia) has an autosomal recessive mode of inheritance. The most common mutation of the *GALT* gene is the *Q188R* mutation on chromosome 9. GALT deficiency presents early in infancy with symptoms of hypoglycemia, vomiting, diarrhea, irritability, feeding difficulties, and failure to thrive. These infants may have jaundice, hepatomegaly, and easy bruisability. Initial diagnostic tests may reveal hyperbilirubinemia, elevated liver transaminases, metabolic acidosis, galactosuria, glycosuria, hypoglycemia, and abnormal clotting measurements. These patients are at risk of developing cerebral edema. Vitreous hemorrhage and *Escherichia coli* sepsis have also been reported in affected individuals. Long-term complications in GALT deficiency include impaired cognition, ovarian failure in females, and ataxic neurologic disease. Microbiological and fluorometric assays are used in the screening of the newborn to detect galactosemia. A fluorescent spot screening test for GALT activity (Beutler test) is available. An abnormal test is followed by biochemical or molecular confirmation of the diagnosis. The quantitative assays can give false-negative results after blood transfusion. A milder form of galactosemia known as the "Duarte variant" is also caused by a mutation within the *GALT* gene and is characterized by decreased red cell enzyme activity, which generally is of no clinical significance. Treatment of GALT deficiency consists of restriction of galactose in the diet (Holton, 2001; Leslie, 2003).

Galactokinase Deficiency

In galactokinase (GALK) deficiency, galactose cannot be converted into galactose-1-phosphate, and this leads to cataract formation. Pseudotumor cerebri is another rare complication observed in this disorder. The diagnosis is made by demonstrating an elevated blood galactose level with normal uridyl transferase activity and absence of galactokinase activity in erythrocytes. A galactose-free diet can reverse cataracts if started in early infancy (Holton, 2001; Bosch, 2002).

Uridine Diphosphate Galactose-4-Epimerase Deficiency

The benign form is associated with enzyme deficiency limited to erythrocytes and leukocytes. These affected individuals are healthy, and no treatment is required. In the severe form, clinical findings are similar to those seen in GALT deficiency, with additional findings of hypotonia and sensorineural deafness. Treatment consists of dietary restriction of galactose (Walter, 1999; Holton, 2001).

DEFECTS IN FRUCTOSE METABOLISM

Essential fructosuria, hereditary fructose intolerance, and fructose-1,6-diphosphatase deficiency are the clinical conditions resulting from defects in fructose metabolism.

Essential Fructosuria

This autosomal recessive disorder results from fructokinase deficiency. Fructokinase catalyzes the conversion of fructose to fructose-1-phosphate. The condition is asymptomatic and usually is diagnosed incidentally by the detection of fructose in urine as a reducing substance. No treatment is necessary.

Hereditary Fructose Intolerance

A defect of fructose-1,6-biphosphate aldolase B activity in the liver, kidney, and intestine results in failure of conversion of fructose-1-phosphate and fructose-1,6-biphosphate into dihydroxyacetone phosphate, glyceraldehyde-3-phosphate, and glyceraldehydes. Fructose intake leads to accumulation of fructose-1-phosphate and causes symptoms of hypoglycemia and nausea followed by vomiting. Symptoms occur only when fructose-containing foods are ingested. Prolonged exposure to fructose-containing foods can cause frequent hypoglycemic episodes, hepatomegaly, irritability, lethargy, seizures, and proximal tubular dysfunction. Hepatic dysfunction can result in prolonged clotting time, elevated transaminases with elevated bilirubin levels, and hypoalbuminemia. The diagnosis is supported by clinical suspicion followed by an intravenous fructose tolerance test. Definitive diagnosis can be made by assay of aldolase B activity in a liver biopsy specimen.

Fructose-1,6-Biphosphatase Deficiency

This autosomal recessive defect in fructose-1,6-biphosphatase results in failure of hepatic glucose generation by gluconeogenic precursors such as lactate, glycerol, and alanine. Life-threatening episodes of hypoglycemia, hyperventilation, lactic acidosis, convulsions, and coma can be seen in affected patients. The diagnosis is established by demonstrating enzyme deficiency in a liver or intestinal biopsy specimen. Correction of hypoglycemia and acidosis by intravenous fluids is the treatment of choice during acute attacks. Prolonged fasting can cause symptoms in affected individuals if glycogen stores are depleted. Fructose and sucrose need to be limited in the diet (Steinman, 2001).

Lactic Acidosis

Lactic acid is a product of pyruvic acid metabolism. Approximately 1400 mmol of lactic acid is produced daily in healthy individuals, most of which is derived from glucose via the glycolytic pathway and deamination of alanine (Marko, 2004; Kreisberg, 1980). This enormous amount of lactic acid is eliminated by several mechanisms, including buffering by extracellular buffers and removal by the liver and kidneys. Under normal circumstances, the rates of lactate entry and exit from the blood are in equilibrium, and net lactate accumulation is zero. Excessive accumulation of L-lactic acid is caused by overproduction and/or underutilization of L-lactate (the levorotary form of lactic acid).

Selected causes of lactic acidosis are shown in Table 16-10. Lactic acid production increases during ischemia, seizures, vigorous exercise, and some leukemic conditions. High levels of lactic acid produced during strenuous exercise are rapidly cleared by both renal and hepatic mechanisms, as well as by aerobic metabolism in muscle (half-life approximately 60 minutes). A decrease in lactic acid utilization can also lead to accumulation of lactic acid. This is generally seen in diseases of the liver and kidneys. Defects in the removal of lactic acid have been associated with hepatic insufficiency, specific enzymatic defects, and severe acidosis. Metformin, which is widely prescribed for the treatment of type 2 diabetes, rarely causes lactic acidosis. Risk factors for metformin-related lactic acidosis include congestive heart failure, tissue hypoxia, renal insufficiency, and sepsis (Salpeter, 2003; Misbin, 2004). Nucleoside reverse transcriptase inhibitors used in the treatment of human immunodeficiency virus infection can also induce lactic acidosis (John, 2002; Ogedegbe, 2003).

TABLE 16-10
Selected Causes of L-Lactic Acidosis

Tissue Hypoxia
Septic shock
Cardiogenic shock
Hemorrhagic shock
Acute hypoxemia
Carbon monoxide poisoning
Metabolic/Medical Conditions
Uncontrolled diabetes mellitus
Hepatic insufficiency
Renal insufficiency
Tumors
Leukemia
Lymphoma
Drugs/Toxic Substances
Zidovudine
Metformin
Ethanol
Salicylates
Isoniazid
Cyanide
Methanol
Ethylene glycol
Inborn Errors of Metabolism
Type 1a glycogen storage disease (von Gierke disease)
Fructose-1,6-biphosphatase deficiency
Pyruvate dehydrogenase deficiency
Organic acidurias: propionic acidemia, methylmalonic acidemia
Mitochondrial diseases:
KSS (Kearns-Sayre syndrome)
PEO (progressive external ophthalmoplegia)
PS (Pearson's syndrome)
MERRF (myoclonic epilepsy with ragged-red fibers)
MELAS (mitochondrial encephalopathy, lactic acidosis, and stroke-like episodes)
MILS (maternally inherited Leigh's syndrome)

Lactic acidosis is diagnosed by the presence of high blood lactate levels (>45 mg/dL or >5.0 mmol/L), an elevated anion gap, and a low blood pH (<7.35). For accurate measurements of lactate, tourniquet use should be minimal, and the patient should not clench his or her fist at the time of the blood draw. A gray-top tube containing fluoride oxalate should be used for sample collection, as it blocks further glycolysis.

Treatment of lactic acidosis consists of correction of underlying conditions that initiated the disruption in normal lactate metabolism. Tissue oxygenation, improved fluid status, amplification of cardiac status, and treatment of sepsis play important roles in the treatment of lactic acidosis. Dialysis is sometimes necessary for removal of lactate. D-Lactic acidosis results from excessive accumulation of D-lactic acid (the dextrorotary form of lactic acid). It has been described in patients with jejunoileal bypass or small bowel resection. In these conditions, glucose and other carbohydrates are converted into D-lactic acid in the colon by bacteria. The D-lactic acid is absorbed into the systemic circulation and is slowly metabolized. Affected patients present with episodes of metabolic acidosis and encephalopathy. D-Lactate levels can be measured using D-lactate dehydrogenase enzymatic assays (Luft, 2001; Zhang, 2003).

SELECTED REFERENCES

American Association of Clinical Endocrinologists. Medical guidelines for clinical practice for management of diabetes mellitus. Endocr Pract 2007;13(suppl 1):3–68, 2007.

Describes the diabetes monitoring and management guidelines endorsed by the American College of Endocrinology.

American Diabetes Association. Standards of medical care in patients with diabetes 2010. Diabetes Care 2010b;33(suppl 1):S11–61.

Summarizes the criteria for the classification and diagnosis of diabetes, and provides recommendations for assessment of glycemic control, management goals, and strategies to prevent complications.

Bingley PJ, Bonifacio E, Mueller PW, and participating laboratories. Diabetes Antibody Standardization Program: first assay proficiency evaluation. Diabetes 2003;52:1128–36.

A report of the first proficiency evaluation of the Diabetes Antibody Standardization Program, which includes information concerning the performance of different assays for GAD, IA-2, and insulin autoantibodies.

Cryer PE, Axelrod L, Grossman AB, et al. Evaluation and management of adult hypoglycemic disorders: an Endocrine Society Clinical Practice Guideline. J Clin Endocrinol Metab 2009;94:709–28.

Reviews hypoglycemic disorders, with detailed clinical classification, a description of diagnostic testing, including a protocol for performing the 72-hour fast, mixed meal diagnostic tests, and management strategies.

Little RR, Rohlfing CL, Wiedmeyer H-M, et al. The National Glycohemoglobin Standardization Program: a five-year progress report. Clin Chem 2001;47(11): 1985–92.

Summarizes the National Glycohemoglobin Standardization Program, including descriptions of certification criteria and procedures, and progress in standardization nationally and internationally.

Weinstein DA, Wolfsdorf JI. Glycogen storage diseases: a primer for clinicians. Endocrinologist 2002;12: 531–8.

Reviews in detail the major glycogen storage diseases.

REFERENCES

Access the complete reference list online at http://www.expertconsult.com

CHAPTER 17

LIPIDS AND DYSLIPOPROTEINEMIA

James Soh, Joby Josekutty, M. Mahmood Hussain

KEY POINTS

- Although ultracentrifugation and electrophoretic techniques are of historical significance, most useful lipid and lipoprotein testing methods are now enzymatic.
- Low-density lipoprotein cholesterol can be measured directly but is usually calculated using the Friedewald formula. Calculated values require evaluation of fasting samples.
- Low-density lipoprotein cholesterol is currently considered the most important value in assessing cardiac risk and directing therapy.
- The profile currently recommended for initial screening in adults, age 20 or older, includes total cholesterol, low- and high-density lipoprotein cholesterol, and triglycerides. Testing should be repeated at least once every 5 years.
- Other tests, including apolipoprotein levels and lipoprotein subclasses, may prove valuable in fine-tuning risk assessment and evaluating response to therapy.
- New guidelines elevate the perceived atherosclerotic risk of diabetes and support aggressive intervention in diabetic patients and patients with metabolic syndrome.

Overview

Disorders of lipid metabolism play a major role in atherosclerosis and coronary heart disease (CHD). A clear-cut relationship is evident between elevated serum cholesterol and myocardial infarction. At the tissue level, cholesterol deposits occur in areas of endothelial cell damage and are a prominent part of atherosclerotic lesions. Although cholesterol may be considered "bad" because of the previous association, it is actually a vital structural component of cell membranes and a precursor of steroid hormones and bile acids. Another lipid, triglyceride, is a major source of energy for cells. Cholesterol and triglycerides are the most important lipids in the study and management of CHD risk.

Lipids are soluble in nonpolar organic solvents, such as chloroform and ether, but relatively insoluble in polar solvents such as water. Thus, cholesterol and triglycerides travel in plasma not as free-floating molecules, but as part of water-soluble complexes called *lipoproteins*. These particles contain cholesterol in two forms: free cholesterol, a polar nonesterified alcohol (about 30%), and cholesterol ester, a hydrophobic form wherein cholesterol is linked to a fatty acid (about 70%). The lipoprotein is arranged like a micelle (Fig. 17-1). The most hydrophobic lipids, such as cholesterol esters and triglycerides, are located in the core of the particle. Lipids with some hydrophilicity, such as free cholesterol and phospholipids, are arranged on the surface with polar groups pointing outward. *Apolipoproteins* (apo) the protein moiety of lipoproteins, are also arrayed on the surface. They show amphiphilic characteristics; hydrophobic residues interact with the hydrophobic core, whereas hydrophilic residues interact outside the aqueous environment.

Four major lipoprotein classes have been identified: Chylomicrons (CMs), very-low-density lipoprotein (VLDL), low-density lipoprotein (LDL), and high-density lipoprotein (HDL). The classification is based on the buoyant density of the particles (see later). Several minor lipoproteins have also been identified, including intermediate-density lipoprotein (IDL) and lipoprotein(a) (Lp[a]) (Tables 17-1 and 17-2). Lipoproteins can be differentiated by density, particle size, chemical composition, and electrophoretic mobility. These physical properties are due to differences in protein, triglyceride, and cholesterol content and reflect the role of each lipoprotein in lipid metabolism (see later). Each lipoprotein is associated with specific apos that play important roles in lipid transport, such as activating or inhibiting the enzymes involved in lipid metabolism, and binding lipoproteins to cell surface receptors. The apo composition of the lipoprotein classes is summarized in Table 17-1.

Lipoproteins are commonly differentiated from one another on the basis of their buoyant density and electrophoretic mobility (Fig. 17-2). Ultracentrifugation separates lipoproteins by buoyant density. Lipids and proteins have average densities of 1.0 and 1.4 g/mL, respectively. If centrifuged in solutions of different densities, these particles band at characteristic densities. The density of a lipoprotein particle is determined mostly by its protein and triglyceride content. As illustrated in the diagram, the higher the lipid content, the less dense is the lipoprotein particle; therefore, the closer they migrate to the top of the tube. Lipoproteins with high triglyceride and low protein content (CM and VLDL) are less dense than those with high protein and low triglyceride content (HDL). LDL and IDL are more dense than VLDL but less dense than HDL. When plasma lipoproteins are separated by agarose gel electrophoresis, CM remains at the origin and HDL migrates fastest in the α-region, followed by VLDL in the "pre-β" region and IDL and LDL in the β region.

Based on the presence and absence of apoB, lipoproteins can be classified as apoB-containing (CM, VLDL, IDL, LDL) and non–apoB-containing (HDL) lipoproteins. This classification is important because apoB is a nonexchangeable apolipoprotein, and only one molecule of apoB is present per lipoprotein. ApoB-containing lipoproteins may or may not contain additional apolipoproteins such as apoA1, apoC, and apoE. ApoB serves as a structural protein for these lipoproteins and is always associated with these particles. They are synthesized mainly by hepatocytes and enterocytes.

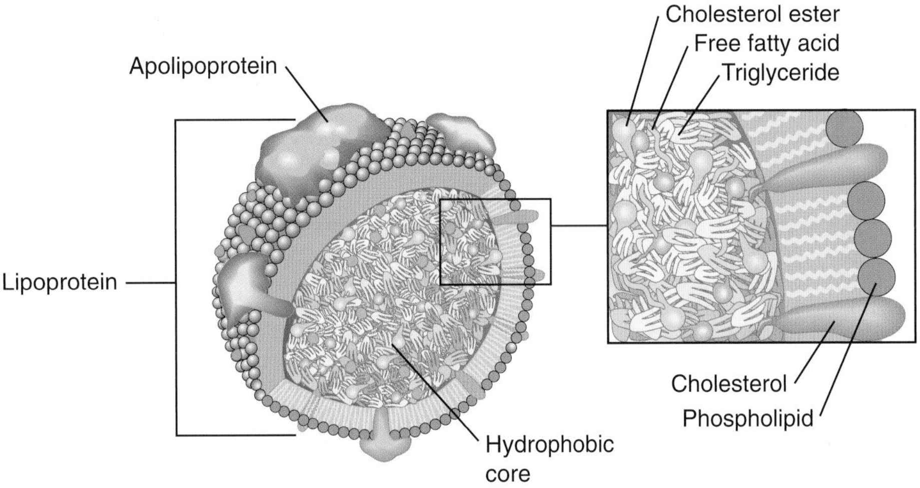

Figure 17-1 Lipoprotein structure. Lipoproteins are spherical particles with a hydrophobic core and an amphiphilic surface. The surface consists of a single layer of phospholipids. This surface layer also contains proteins and free cholesterol. The hydrophobic core mainly contains triglycerides and cholesterol esters.

TABLE 17-1
Major Classes of Human Plasma Lipoproteins: Physicochemical Characteristics

Particle	Electrophoretic mobility*	Major apolipoproteins	Diameter (Å)	Density (kg/L)	Sf†
Chylomicrons	Origin	ApoA-I, A-IV, B-48, C-I, C-II, C-III, E	750–12,000	<0.95	>400
VLDL	Pre-β	ApoB-100, C-I, C-II, C-III, E	300–700	0.95–1.006	20–400
IDL	β or pre-β	ApoB-100, E		1.006–1.019	12–20
LDL	β	ApoB-100	180–300	1.019–1.063	0–12
HDL_2	α	ApoA-I, A-II, E	50–120	1.063–1.125	
HDL_3	α	ApoA-II, A-I, E	50–120	1.125–1.210	
Lp(a)	Pre-β	ApoB-100, Apo(a)		1.045–1.080	

HDL_2, Ultracentrifugation subclass of high-density lipoprotein; *HDL_3,* ultracentrifugation subclass of high-density lipoprotein; *IDL,* intermediate-density lipoprotein; *LDL,* low-density lipoprotein; *Lp(a),* lipoprotein A; *VLDL,* very-low-density lipoprotein.
*Agarose gel electrophoresis.
†Svedberg flotation rate.

TABLE 17-2
Chemical Composition of Major Classes of Plasma Lipoproteins

	Protein (%)*	Free cholesterol (%)	Cholesterol esters (%)	Triglyceride (%)	Phospholipid (%)
Chylomicrons	1–2	1–3	2–4	80–95	3–6
VLDL	6–10	4–8	16–22	45–65	15–20
IDL	**Intermediate between VLDL and LDL**				
LDL	18–22	6–8	45–50	4–8	18–24
HDL	45–55	3–5	15–20	2–7	26–32

Data from Albers (1974), Fless (1984), Gaubatz (1983), Gotto (1986), Gries (1988), and Hegele (2009).
HDL, High-density lipoprotein; *IDL,* intermediate-density lipoprotein; *LDL,* low-density lipoprotein; *VLDL,* very-low-density lipoprotein.
*Percentage of dry weight.

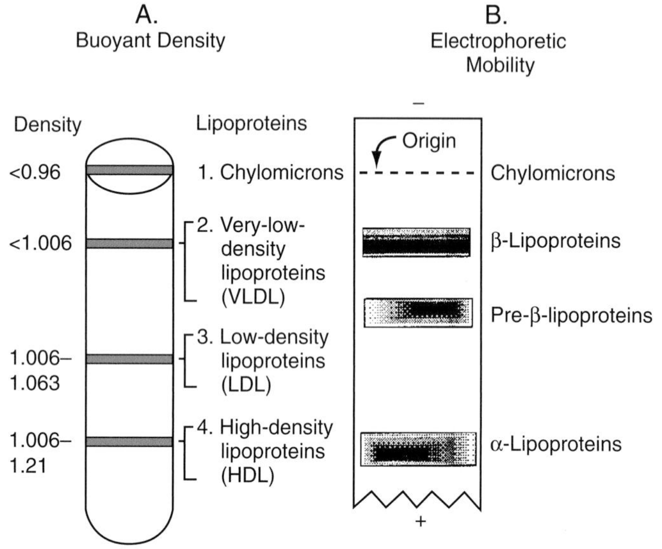

Figure 17-2 Lipoprotein classification. Lipoproteins are classified on the basis of buoyant density or electrophoretic mobility. Separation of lipoproteins based on buoyant density depends on the ratio between lipids and proteins present in them. Lipoproteins that contain higher amounts of lipids have lower buoyant density and are collected on top of the centrifuge tube. Separations based on electrophoretic mobility are based on the number of charges present on lipoproteins and are independent of their size and buoyant density.

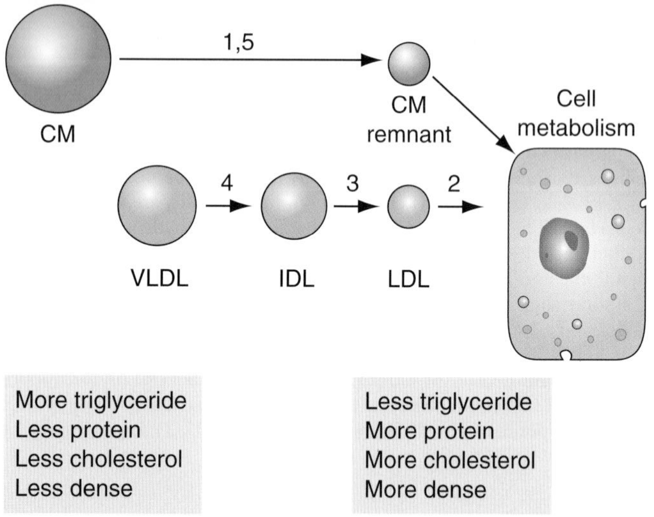

Figure 17-3 Metabolism of lipoprotein particles. The figure depicts successive shrinkage in the size of lipoproteins as a consequence of the lipolysis of triglycerides present in the particles. The number over each step in the pathway represents the functional hyperlipoproteinemia caused by a block between two intermediates (see Table 17-3). *CM,* Chylomicrons; *IDL,* intermediate-density lipoprotein; *LDL,* low-density lipoprotein; *VLDL,* very-low-density lipoprotein.

This group of lipoproteins is mainly involved in delivering lipids to tissues for storage or use in energy production. CM (formed in the intestine from dietary fat) and VLDL (formed in the liver) are triglyceride-rich particles that are metabolized after entering the circulation. Through the action of lipoprotein lipase (LPL), these particles shed triglycerides and cholesterol esters and are transformed into denser lipoproteins with a higher percentage of cholesterol. LDL is the densest of these particles, and elevated serum LDL-cholesterol (LDL-C) is a primary cardiac risk factor. Treatment of CHD-causing dyslipidemia is generally aimed at lowering LDL.

One way to understand heterogeneity in apoB-containing lipoproteins is to view them as a metabolic progression in which CM and VLDL release triglycerides to tissues via interaction with LPL. As a result of this interaction, CM and VLDL become triglyceride depleted, denser, and relatively protein and cholesterol rich, giving rise to CM remnants and LDL. These particles are internalized and metabolized by cells—CM by liver and bone marrow cells and LDL by liver cells and by cells throughout the body. LDL serves as the major source of cholesterol for tissues. This metabolic progression is presented in Figure 17-3.

A block in any step of the pathway leads to the accumulation of one or more lipoproteins. The number over each step in the pathway represents the functional hyperlipoproteinemia (originally described by Fredrickson [1967]) caused by a block between two intermediates. For example, a block in the progression from CM to CM remnants results in the accumulation of CM—Type 1 or 5 disease—and presents with high triglycerides and normal cholesterol. A block in the conversion of VLDL to IDL and LDL results in Type 4 disease (i.e., VLDL accumulation with elevated triglycerides and frequently elevated cholesterol). Often the cause of Types 1, 5, and 4 disease is LPL deficiency and the resulting inability to break down triglycerides. Type 2 disease results from a block in LDL metabolism and may have a genetic basis: a defective apoB protein that does not bind to the LDL receptor, or a mutant LDL receptor that does not recognize apoB. Type 2 is further subcategorized on the basis of triglyceride level. Note that other studies (see later) may be necessary to distinguish Type 2B and Type 3 because both present with elevated cholesterol and triglycerides. This functional classification is presented in Table 17-3. No ideal system is known for classifying lipid disorders. They can be categorized in many different ways: primary versus secondary, hereditary versus acquired, as well as by lipoprotein fraction phenotypes. In general, each category is heterogeneous with respect to genetic, clinical, and pathologic factors. These are discussed in greater detail at the end of the chapter.

The major protein present in non–apoB-containing HDL is apoA-I, which makes up about 70% of the HDL protein. HDL is formed in the liver and plays a key role in reverse cholesterol transport, the process by which excess cholesterol is returned from tissues to the liver, where it is reused or excreted in bile. Besides apoA-I, HDL contains several proteins. In addition to reverse cholesterol transport, other functions of HDL have been described on the basis of in vitro assays, including anti-inflammatory, antioxidant, antithrombotic, and nitric oxide–inducing mechanisms. Although the role of reverse cholesterol transport has been suggested as a protective mechanism against atherosclerosis, these other properties of HDL might also contribute to the "protective" effect. Consequently, such protection may stem from HDL function rather than from increased plasma levels of HDL. Nonetheless, therapies targeting increased HDL levels in plasma remain an active area of research.

LIPOPROTEINS, APOLIPOPROTEINS, AND RELATED PROTEINS

Lipoprotein particles are dynamic entities that acquire and shed protein and lipid components as they circulate in the body. As mentioned earlier,

TABLE 17-3
Classical Hyperlipidemia Phenotypes

WHO ICD and OMIM numbers	Type	Particle	Triglycerides	Cholesterol	Comments
E78.3 238600	1 (familial chylomicronemia or LPL deficiency)	CM	High	Normal	Low cardiac risk; hereditary, found mostly in pediatric patients and young adults; autosomal recessive mutation in *LPL* or *APOC2; APOA5, LMF-1,* and *GPIHBP1* mutations are linked to this phenotype.
E78.0 143890	2A (heterozygous and homozygous familial hypercholesterolemia)	LDL	Normal	High	High cardiac risk; mostly polygenic disease; about 10% are monogenic; heterozygous form is due to mutations in *LDLR, APOB,* or *PCSK9*; homozygous form is due to mutations in *LDLR* or *LDLRAP1* (ARH)
E78.4 144250	2B (combined hyperlipoproteinemia)	VLDL, LDL	High	High	High cardiac risk; polygenic disease; links to mutations in *USF1, APOB,* and *LPL*
E78.2 107741	3 (dysbetalipoproteinemia)	IDL	High	High	High cardiac risk; mutations in *APOE* gene or homozygous for E2 allele of *APOE*
E78.1 144600, 145750	4 (primary hypertriglyceridemia)	VLDL	High	Normal	Lower cardiac risk than type 2 or 3; polygenic disease
E78.3 144650	5 (mixed hyperlipidemia)	VLDL, CM	High	High	Low cardiac risk; polygenic disease; 10% of patients have mutations in *LPL, APOC2,* and *APOA5*; mutations in *APOE, TRIB1, CHREBP, GALNT2, GCKR,* and *ANGPTL3* are thought to contribute to this disease.

ANGPTL3, Angiopoietin-like 3; *APOA5,* apolipoprotein A-V; *APOB,* apolipoprotein B; *APOC2,* apolipoprotein C-II; *APOE,* apolipoprotein E; *CHREBP,* carbohydrate response element binding protein (or *MLXIPL*); *CM,* chylomicron; *GALNT2,* UDP-N′-acetyl-alpha-D-galactosamine-polypeptide N-acetylgalactosaminyltransferase 2; *GCKR,* glucokinase regulator; *ICD,* International Classification of Diseases; *IDL,* intermediate-density lipoprotein; *LDL,* low-density lipoprotein; *LDLRAP1,* LDL receptor adaptor protein 1 (also known as ARH); *OMIM,* Online Mendelian Inheritance in Man; *TRIB1,* tribbles homologue 1; *USF1,* upstream transcription factor 1; *VLDL,* very-low-density lipoprotein; *WHO,* World Health Organization.

CM and VLDL particles lose triglycerides and become smaller as they are metabolized. Thus, young VLDL and CM particles are larger and less dense than their more mature counterparts. For this reason, it is best to view each of the lipoprotein classes not as a collection of identical particles, but as a heterogeneous group. In fact, distinct lipoprotein subfractions or subclasses have been well described.

MAJOR LIPOPROTEINS

Chylomicrons

CMs are large particles produced by the intestine that transport lipids of dietary origin to the tissues of the body. They are very rich in triglycerides, but relatively poor in free cholesterol, phospholipids, and protein. These particles are secreted into mesenteric lymphatics and reach circulation at the thoracic duct. These lipoproteins acquire apoC-II, a cofactor for lipoprotein lipase, from plasma. The interaction of chylomicrons with lipoprotein lipase at the luminal surface of capillary endothelium results in the depletion of triglycerides and surface elements. The resulting smaller particles, called chylomicron remnants, are removed from circulation by the liver (Hussain, 1996), primarily through the interaction of apoE with receptors such as proteoglycans, the LDL receptor, and the LDL receptor–related protein (LRP). Because of the very high lipid/protein ratio, chylomicrons are considerably less dense than water and float without centrifugation. When present at high levels, chylomicrons result in "milky" plasma and accumulate as a floating creamy layer when left undisturbed for several hours. The apolipoproteins in chylomicrons include apoB-48, apoA-I, apoA-IV, apoC-I, apoC-II, apoC-III, and apoE.

Very-Low-Density Lipoproteins

VLDL particles are produced by the liver and supply the tissues of the body with triglycerides of endogenous, primarily hepatic, origin and cholesterol. As compared with chylomicrons, VLDL particles are smaller and produce turbid plasma when present in excessive amounts. They are rich in triglycerides, although to a lesser extent than chylomicrons, and have a higher buoyant density because of their lower lipid/protein ratio. By mass, VLDL particles contain approximately 50% triglyceride, 40% cholesterol and phospholipid, and 10% protein, mostly apoB-100 and apoC-I, apoC-II, and apoC-III, but also apoE. VLDL particles vary widely in size and chemical composition. Larger particles are rich in triglycerides and apoC. Smaller particles have less of these two components. Lipoprotein lipase hydrolyzes VLDL, and this produces highly atherogenic, smaller triglyceride and surface material–depleted particles called VLDL remnants and IDL. These particles can be removed from plasma by LDL receptors or further metabolized to LDL.

Low-Density Lipoproteins

LDL is produced through the metabolism of VLDL in circulation and constitutes about 50% of the total lipoprotein mass in human plasma. The particles are much smaller than the triglyceride-rich lipoproteins (VLDL and CM) and do not scatter light or alter the clarity of plasma even at greatly increased concentrations. LDL consists of approximately 50% cholesterol, mostly esterified, 25% protein, mostly apoB-100 with traces of apoC, 20% phospholipid, and some triglycerides. Although each VLDL and LDL particle is thought to contain only one apoB-100 molecule, the extraordinary size of this protein allows it to be the largest protein component of these particles. The liver takes up most of the LDL in circulation (approximately 75%), with apoB-100 serving as a ligand for the hepatic receptor. The remaining LDL is delivered to other tissues. Some LDL is modified and is removed from the circulation by scavenger cells such as those found in atheromatous plaque. Small LDL particles contain less cholesterol ester and have a lower cholesterol/apoB ratio. Increased amounts of the small particles have been found in patients with several common forms of dyslipoproteinemia that are associated with CHD.

High-Density Lipoprotein

HDL is a small particle, consisting mostly of protein, cholesterol, and phospholipids, with only traces of triglycerides. Produced by the liver and intestine, HDL is involved in reverse cholesterol transport. In vitro studies suggest that HDL is involved in anti-inflammatory, antioxidant, antithrombotic, and nitric oxide–inducing mechanisms. The major site for the clearance of HDL cholesterol is the liver, and the best understood mechanism is the selective uptake of cholesterol esters from HDL by the SR-B1 receptor expressed in the liver. In the selective uptake process, SR-B1 promotes cholesterol uptake without apolipoprotein degradation. Cholesterol esters are removed from the internalized HDL particles and cholesterol-depleted HDLs are re-secreted. Mouse models that lack SR-B1 exhibit increased plasma HDL, slower HDL uptake by the liver, and increased atherosclerosis. Reverse cholesterol transport is reduced. In contrast, mouse models overexpressing SR-B1 in the liver show increased reverse cholesterol transport with reduced HDL plasma levels; however, these same mice also exhibit reduced atherosclerosis. In studies done on humans who maintain normal lipid profiles, the contribution of SR-B1 to HDL uptake is minimal. The cholesterol ester transfer protein (CETP)

TABLE 17-4
Significant Human Apolipoproteins

Apolipoprotein	Major lipoproteins	Mr* (kDa)	Amino acids	Chromosome	PLASMA CONCENTRATION (mmol/L)	PLASMA CONCENTRATION (mg/dL)
A-I	HDL	29	243–245	11	32–46	90–130
A-II	HDL	17.4	154	1	18–29	30–50
A-IV	HDL, LDL	44.5	396	11		
(a)	Lp(a)	350–700	Variable	6		
B-100	VLDL, IDL, LDL	512.7	4536	2	1.5–1.8	80–100
B-48	CM	240.8	2152	2	<0.2	<5
C-I	CM, LDL	6.6	57	19	6.1–10.8	4–7
C-II	CM, LDL	8.9	78 or 79	19	3.4–9.1	3–8
C-III	CM	8.8	79	11	9.1–17.1	8–15
D	HDL	19	169	3		
E	CM, LDL, IDL	34.1	299	19	0.8–1.6	3–6
F	HDL, LDL, VLDL	29	162	12		8.35
H	VLDL	50	326	17		20
J	HDL	80	449	8		
L	HDL	39–42	383	22	Not present in plasma	
M	HDL, LDL, VLDL, CM	26	188	6		2–15
O	HDL, LDL, VLDL	22.3	198	X		

*Relative molecular mass.
CM, Chylomicron; *HDL,* high-density lipoprotein; *IDL,* intermediate-density lipoprotein; *LDL,* low-density lipoprotein; *Lp(a),* lipoprotein A; *VLDL,* very-low-density lipoprotein.

pathway is considered to be an alternative pathway for HDL metabolism. CETP transfers triglycerides from apoB lipoproteins in exchange for cholesterol esters in HDL. The result is an HDL particle depleted of cholesterol esters but enriched with triglycerides. Cholesterol transferred to apoB-lipoproteins is then cleared by LDL receptors.

HDLs are also heterogeneous particles. Discrete HDL particle subpopulations have been identified on the basis of differences in size or charge, including two major ultracentrifugation subclasses, HDL_2 and HDL_3 (Blanche, 1981; MacKenzie, 1973; Sundaram, 1974). The distinction is significant because HDL_2 is thought to be more cardioprotective than HDL_3, and people with low levels of HDL_2 are thought to be at increased risk for premature CHD. Additionally, HDL has been subfractionated into particles that contain apoA-I but not apoA-II, and those that contain both apoA-I and apoA-II (Fruchart, 1992; von Eckardstein, 1994). ApoA-I is present on virtually all HDL particles and makes up 70% of the protein content. ApoA-II makes up about 20% of the HDL lipoprotein and is present on about two thirds of all HDL particles in humans. The physiologic function of apoA-II is not fully understood; however, both apoA-I and apoA-II are required for normal HDL biosynthesis and metabolism. Studies have shown that apoA-II plays an important role in maintaining levels of HDL in plasma. A high percentage of HDL_2 particles fall into the apoA-I-only category. ApoE also associates with HDL particles. Laboratory measurement of such particles eventually may prove clinically useful.

MINOR AND ABNORMAL LIPOPROTEINS

Intermediate-Density Lipoproteins

Formed through the metabolism of VLDL in circulation, IDL can be removed from circulation quickly through interaction with the LDL receptor, or can be further metabolized to LDL. As expected, the lipid content, size, and density of IDL is intermediate between VLDL and LDL.

Lipoprotein(a)

Lp(a) is similar to LDL in terms of density and overall composition, and can be thought of as an LDL particle to which apo(a) has been added, linked to apoB-100 via a disulfide bond (Fless, 1984, 1985; Gaubatz, 1983). The electrophoretic mobility of Lp(a) is usually pre-β but can vary between that of LDL (β) and albumin (pre-α). Lp(a) is generally present in much lower concentrations than LDL; however, in normal subjects, values can range from <20–1500 mg/L or more. Increased levels can be familial, showing an autosomal dominant pattern of inheritance, and have been associated with an increased risk of CHD, cerebrovascular disease, and stroke. When concentrations in the plasma are increased to above 200–300 mg/L, Lp(a) appears electrophoretically as a lipid-staining pre-β band in the plasma fraction containing lipoproteins of density >1.006 g/mL.

Lp(a) is synthesized in the liver, but the details of its metabolism are not well understood. It binds to the LDL receptor by virtue of its apoB-100 component, albeit with lower affinity than LDL (Floren, 1981). The removal of apo(a) from Lp(a) increases the affinity of the residual apoB-containing particle for the LDL receptor (Armstrong, 1985), and it has been suggested that apo(a) may interfere with the uptake of apoB-100–containing particles (Scanu, 1988). At present, neither the function of Lp(a) nor its atherogenic properties are well understood. It has been speculated that Lp(a) or apo(a) might interfere with normal thrombolysis by virtue of their similarity to plasminogen.

LpX Lipoprotein

LpX is an abnormal lipoprotein found in patients with obstructive biliary disease, and in patients with familial lecithin/cholesterol acyltransferase (LCAT) deficiency. Lipids account for more than 90% of its weight (mostly phospholipids, unesterified cholesterol, and very little esterified cholesterol). Proteins, primarily apoC and smaller amounts of albumin, constitute <10% of LpX by weight.

β-VLDL ("Floating β" Lipoprotein)

β-VLDL ("floating β" lipoprotein) is an abnormal lipoprotein that accumulates in type 3 hyperlipoproteinemia. It is richer in cholesterol than VLDL and apparently results from the defective catabolism of VLDL. The particle is found in the VLDL density range but migrates electrophoretically with or near LDL.

IMPORTANT PROTEINS IN LIPOPROTEIN METABOLISM

Apolipoproteins

As mentioned previously, apos constitute the major protein component of lipoproteins. They are commonly referred to using the nomenclature introduced by Alaupovic (1971). Some significant properties of the apos are outlined in Tables 17-4 and 17-5.

Lipolytic Enzymes and Other Proteins

The major enzymatic systems that are known to participate in plasma lipoprotein metabolism are the LCAT and the lipolytic enzymes, lipoprotein lipase (LPL), hepatic triglyceride lipase (HL), and endothelial lipase (EL). Many other proteins are also involved in lipoprotein

TABLE 17-5

Apolipoprotein Functions and Significant Characteristics

Apolipoprotein	Main distribution	Function (if known)	Comments
A-I	HDL	Activates LCAT that esterifies cholesterol in plasma Ligand for *ABCA1*	Synthesized in liver and intestine; HDL biosynthesis
A-II	HDL		May inhibit lipoprotein and hepatic lipases and increases plasma triglyceride
A-IV	HDL, CM, and free in plasma		May be a cofactor for LCAT; increased during fat absorption; HDL biosynthesis
B-100	VLDL and LDL	Carboxy-terminal recognition signal targets LDL to the LDL (apoB, E) receptor	Very large structural protein, synthesized in liver with lipids of endogenous origin (i.e., not chylomicrons)
B-48	CM	Not recognized by LDL receptor	Synthesized in intestine, encoded by same gene and same amino terminus as apoB-100. Differential production of the two proteins involves RNA editing.
C-I	CM and VLDL		May inhibit hepatic uptake of VLDL and cholesterol ester transfer protein
C-II	CM and VLDL	Activates lipoprotein lipase	Deficiency causes reduced clearance of triglyceride-rich lipoproteins.
C-III	VLDL, HDL	Inhibits lipolysis of triglyceride-rich lipoproteins; decreases clearance rate of remnant particles	Deficiency causes reduced clearance of triglyceride-rich lipoproteins.
D	HDL	Activates LCAT	
E	CM, VLDL, IDL, remnants and HDL	Recognition factor that targets CM and VLDL remnants to hepatic receptor; also binds to cell surface LDL receptors and proteoglycans	E-2, E-3, and E-4 isoforms; E-4 is associated with high LDL-C, higher risk of CHD and Alzheimer's disease; E-2 associated with type 3 hyperlipoproteinemia
F	HDL, LDL, VLDL	Regulates CETP function	
H	VLDL	Related to activation of LPL; triglyceride metabolism	Antibodies against apoH or β_2-glycoprotein-I are a subset of antiphospholipid antibodies, and may be associated with hyperthrombosis and stroke.
J		Cell-aggregating factor in Sertoli cells; inhibitor of the C5b*7 complement complex; beta-amyloid clearance in glial cells; cholesterol trafficking in brain	Involved in apoptosis; linked to neurologic diseases like Pick's and Alzheimer's; also known as clusterin
L	HDL		May be linked to reverse cholesterol transport
M	HDL, CM, LDL, VLDL		May be linked to HDL remodeling
Apo(a)	Lp(a)		Homologous to plasminogen, may be prothrombotic; bound to apoB-100 by disulfide linkage

ABCA1, ATP-binding cassette transporter; *CETP*, cholesterol ester transfer protein pathway; *CHD*, congenital heart disease; *CM*, chylomicron; *HDL*, high-density lipoprotein; *IDL*, intermediate-density lipoprotein; *LCAT*, lecithin/cholesterol acyltransferase; *LDL*, low-density lipoprotein; *LDL-C*, low-density lipoprotein cholesterol; *Lp(a)*, lipoprotein A; *LPL*, lipoprotein lipase; *VLDL*, very-low-density lipoprotein.

metabolism. Some significant attributes of these proteins are summarized in Table 17-6.

Lipid Transport and Lipoprotein Metabolism

Triglycerides and cholesterol enter circulation as part of triglyceride-rich lipoprotein particles, CMs produced in the intestine, and VLDLs produced primarily by the liver. Their synthesis requires an intracellular chaperone microsomal triglyceride transfer protein (MTP) that transfers different lipids in in vitro systems (Hussain, 2003). In addition, MTP physically interacts with apoB. These two properties of MTP play a critical role in the biosynthesis of apoB-containing lipoproteins. It is believed that MTP physically associates with nascent apoB and lipidates it, forming a lipoprotein particle that is further matured and secreted. Enterocytes synthesize chylomicrons under postprandial conditions. In fasting conditions, they synthesize VLDL and smaller lipoproteins (Hussain, 1996). These lipoproteins are concentrated into mesenteric lymphatics and are delivered to blood at the thoracic duct. Hepatocytes synthesize VLDL and are directly secreted into the circulation. Their synthesis is also dependent on MTP activity. The main function of apoB-containing lipoproteins is to deliver cholesterol and triglyceride to different tissues. CMs are primarily involved in the absorption and delivery of dietary fat and fat-soluble vitamins, whereas VLDLs deliver endogenous lipids to other tissues.

Only one *APOB* gene is present in the human genome. Nevertheless, enterocytes and hepatocytes make two different forms of apoB to synthesize CMs and VLDL, respectively. In both tissues, the human *APOB* gene is transcribed into mRNA that is 15 kilobases long. This transcript is translated into a single polypeptide in the liver, called apoB-100. In the intestine, however, *APOB* mRNA undergoes a post-transcriptional change. One cytosine residue (at position 6666) is deaminated to a uracil. This changes a glutamine codon into a stop codon. Translation of the edited mRNA gives rise to a polypeptide of 2152 amino acids that is 48% of the apoB-100 (synthesized by the liver). This editing enzyme is not expressed in the liver; therefore, the liver synthesizes only full-length apoB-100.

These lipoprotein particles begin to undergo intravascular change almost immediately after entry into the circulation through the action of LPL. This enzyme hydrolyzes triglycerides and diglycerides, releasing fatty acids and monoglycerides, which are taken up by cells and used as a source of energy. ApoC-II stimulates the hydrolysis of triglycerides. In addition to losing triglycerides by LPL-mediated hydrolysis, CM lose surface lipids and apos by transfer of these components to HDL. Overall, CMs lose significant mass in the form of triglyceride and the A and C apolipoproteins. The depleted CM remnant particle contains apoB-48 and apoE as its major apolipoproteins. These particles are rapidly removed from plasma and are sequestered in the space of Disse by binding to proteoglycans. These particles can undergo further hydrolysis by hepatic lipase and are enriched with apoE. Eventually, they are internalized and degraded by means of a rapid and specific receptor-mediated endocytic process involving LDL receptors, LDL receptor–related protein, and proteoglycans. C apos inhibit the uptake of CMs, allowing them to remain in the circulation long enough to complete the hydrolysis of triglycerides. In the fasting state, the intestine continues to make apoB and secretes "intestinal VLDL" (small CMs). These particles may constitute up to 10%

TABLE 17-6
Enzymes and Other Proteins Important for Lipoprotein Metabolism

Enzyme	Gene location	Function	Deficiency	Tissue expression
ABCG5	2p21	Forms heterodimers with ABCG8 to pump out plant sterols back into the intestinal lumen	Increased plant sterol levels in plasma that can disrupt cell membranes and cause sitosterolemia; influences cholesterol levels in plasma	Tissue expression in liver, colon, and intestines
ABCG8	2p21	Forms heterodimers with ABCG5 to pump out plant sterols back into intestinal lumen; also associated with cholesterol and sterol excretion in bile	Increased plant sterol levels in plasma that can disrupt cell membranes and cause sitosterolemia; influences cholesterol levels in plasma	Tissue expression in the liver, intestines, and gallbladder
ABCA1	9q22-31	Efflux of cholesterol from peripheral cells into HDL	Tangier disease, with very low HDL and accumulation of lipids in peripheral cells	Many cell types, prominently in the liver, testis, and adrenal
CETP	16q21	Transfers CE, PL, and TG among lipoproteins, esp. the transfer of CE from HDL to apoB-100–containing lipoproteins in exchange for TG	Deficiency results in large cholesterol-laden HDL	Produced in liver and circulates with HDL
EL	18q21.1	Hydrolysis of PL and TG in lipoproteins, esp. PL in HDL. Homologous to LPL and EL and pancreatic lipase	Increased levels of HDL_2, and large buoyant LDL. Overexpression in mice, decreased TC, PL, and HDL-C	Expressed in many tissues, including liver. Synthesized by endothelium
HL	15q22-23	Hydrolysis of TG and PL, esp. from HDL_2, and may be necessary for HDL metabolism. Also active on lipids in VLDL remnants and IDL. Not very active on newly released VLDL or CM	Increased TC, TG, and HDL-C in deficiency	Associates with nonparenchymal liver cells
LCAT	16q22.1	Catalyzes the esterification of cholesterol, esp. in HDL, by promoting transfer of fatty acids from lecithin to cholesterol. Enables HDL to accumulate cholesterol as CE. Activated by apoA-I	Deficiency results in decreased HDL.	Produced in liver and circulates with HDL
LPL	8q22	Hydrolysis of TG in lipoproteins (esp. VLDL and CM), releasing free fatty acids and glycerol to tissues. ApoC-II are essential cofactors.	Large CM and VLDL with very high TG levels	Present on surface of capillary endothelial cells in adipose tissue and skeletal and heart muscle, but not produced by endothelial cells
LDLR	19p13.2	Binds apoE and apoB-100 and mediates endocytosis of lipoproteins, mostly LDL, but also VLDL, IDL, and CM remnants	Familial hypercholesterolemia results primarily in elevated LDL	Expressed on most cell types, but hepatic receptors clear 70% of LDL
MTP	4q24	Lipidates and regulates secretion of ApoB particles from the liver and intestines	Deficiency of MTP function leads to abetalipoproteinemia where ApoB lipoproteins are virtually undetectable in plasma.	Expression is seen in liver, intestines, heart, kidney, and eye.
PLTP	20q12	Transfer of PL to and from HDL. Important for HDL growth and remodeling	Deficiency in mice results in low HDL.	Expressed on many cell types
PCSK9	1p32.3	Influences the number of LDLRs expressed on cell surface	Depending on mutation—either gain of function or loss of function—the presence of PCSK9 affects availability of LDLR on cell surface and, consequently, the levels of LDL in plasma; gain of function leads to more LDL in plasma; loss of function associates with increased LDLR expression and thus less LDL in plasma.	Secreted protein by the liver cells; expressed in pancreatic islet beta cells and neuronal cells
SR-B1	12q24.31	Binds HDL on cell surface. Plays a role in selective uptake of CE from HDL in liver and steroidogenic tissues. May also enable macrophages to bind oxidized LDL	Accumulation of large CE-rich HDL, and accelerated atherosclerosis in mice	Macrophage, adrenal, liver and testis

ABCA1, ATP-binding cassette protein A1; *Apo,* apolipoprotein; *CE,* capillary electrophoresis; *CETP,* cholesterol ester transfer protein; *CM,* chylomicron; *EL,* endothelial lipase; *HDL,* high-density lipoprotein; *HDL_2,* ultracentrifugation subclass of HDL; *HDL-C,* high-density lipoprotein cholesterol; *HL,* hepatic lipase; *IDL,* intermediate-density lipoprotein; *LCAT,* lecithin cholesterol acyltransferase; *LDL,* low-density lipoprotein; *LDLR,* LDL receptor; *LPL,* lipoprotein lipase; *MTP,* microsomal triglyceride transfer protein; *PL,* phospholipid; *PLTP,* phospholipid transfer protein; *SR-B1,* scavenger receptor class B, member 1; *TC,* total cholesterol; *TG,* triglycerides; *VLDL,* very-low-density lipoprotein.

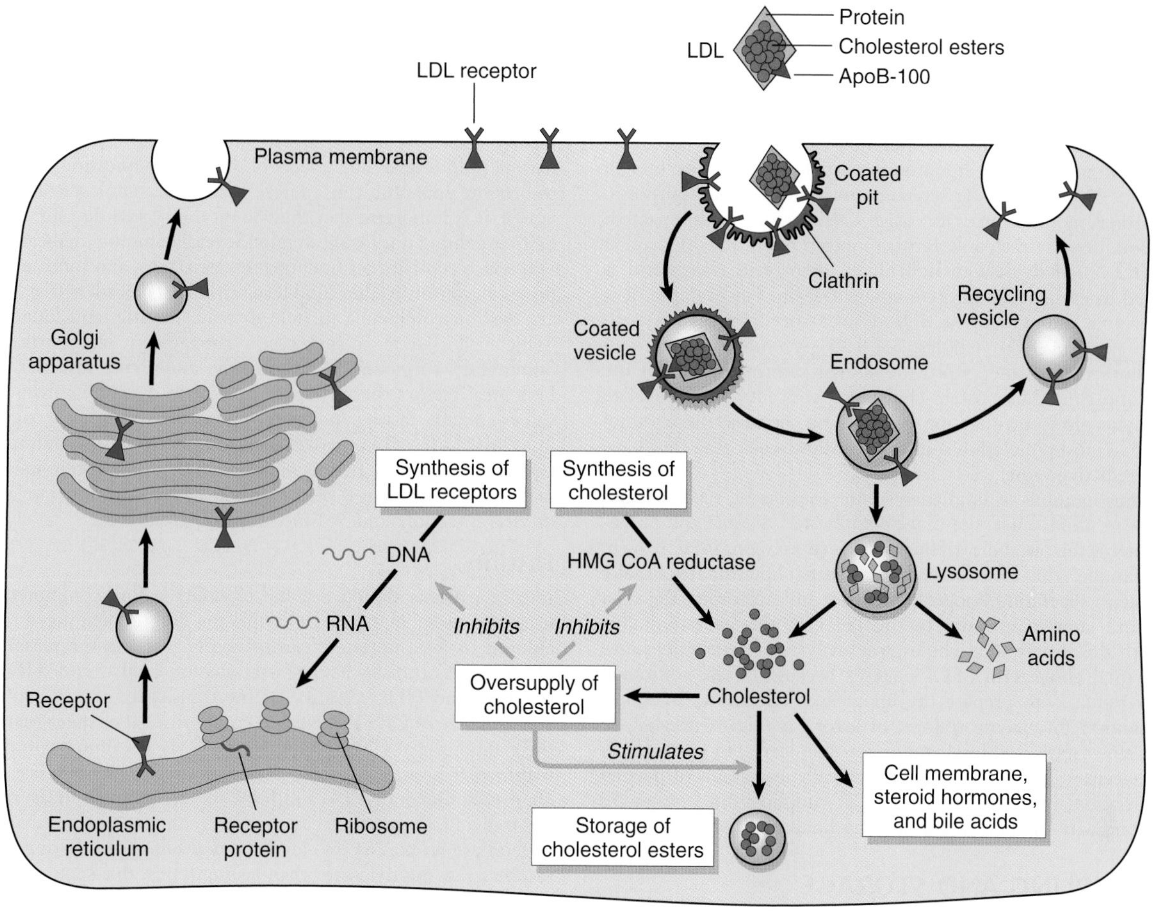

Figure 17-4 The low-density lipoprotein (LDL) receptor pathway and regulation of cholesterol metabolism.

or 20% of the circulating "VLDL," but are probably metabolized as CMs (Byers, 1960; Cenedella, 1974; Green, 1981; Risser, 1978).

VLDL is synthesized in the liver. Similar to CMs, VLDL is catabolized upon entry into the circulation, in part by lipoprotein lipase, and is converted to cholesterol-enriched VLDL remnants. Some of these remnants are removed from circulation by the liver via receptor-mediated endocytosis; others are further catabolized to LDL (Bachorik, 1988). LDL carries most of the circulating cholesterol and transports cholesterol to hepatic and extrahepatic tissues, where it is taken up by LDL-receptor–mediated endocytosis (Brown, 1981). LDL binds to the LDL receptor (i.e., via apoB-100) and is subsequently internalized and directed to the lysosome, where apoB-100 is degraded and cholesteryl ester and other lipids are hydrolyzed. LDL-receptors are recycled back to the cell membrane (Fig. 17-4).

The unesterified cholesterol produced via lysosomal hydrolysis becomes available for membrane, hormone, and bile acid synthesis. Excess cholesterol is re-esterified by the microsomal enzyme acyl : cholesterol acyl transferase (ACAT) and is stored until it is needed. Cellular cholesterol, when present in sufficient quantity, downregulates the LDL receptor, reducing the number of cell membrane receptors and consequently the uptake of LDL. About two thirds of LDL is removed from plasma via hepatic LDL receptors. Although most tissues use cholesterol only for membrane synthesis or store it as cholesteryl ester, the liver can utilize cholesterol in other ways. The liver excretes cholesterol into the bile both as unesterified cholesterol and after conversion to bile acids, and reuses cholesterol for lipoprotein synthesis, as when it secretes VLDL into the circulation. Steroid-secreting tissues use cholesterol as a precursor of the steroid hormones.

Although LDL and CM remnants deliver lipids to the tissues, HDL is thought to be the vehicle for reverse cholesterol transport, the process by which excess cholesterol is removed from peripheral tissues and transported back to the liver. HDL is secreted from both the liver and the intestine as nascent, disk-shaped particles that contain apos, cholesterol, and phospholipid (Havel, 1980; Oppenheimer, 1987; Oram, 1986; Scanu, 1982). The formation of nascent HDL particles is almost exclusively dependent on the synthesis and release of apoA-I. Some HDL also seems to arise de novo in circulation from excess surface material (e.g., free cholesterol, apoA-I, apoA-II, apoC, phospholipid) removed from the triglyceride-rich lipoproteins as they are catabolized. In peripheral tissues, excess cholesterol is exported from cells (including macrophages) in part through the action of the protein ABCA1. This free cholesterol is accumulated by nascent HDL particles and esterified by LCAT. As cholesterol esters move into the hydrophobic core, the particle becomes spherical and larger, developing eventually into HDL_3 and then HDL_2. Several plasma enzymes and proteins are involved in this remodeling process, including phospholipid transfer protein (PLTP) and cholesterol ester transfer protein (CETP). CETP catalyzes the transfer of cholesterol esters to apoB-100–containing particles in exchange for triglycerides (Tall, 1990). PLTP facilitates the transfer of phospholipids from other lipoproteins to HDL, allowing the particle to grow by acquiring surface phospholipid as it accumulates esterified cholesterol and triglyceride in its core. Once formed, HDL delivers excess lipids, especially cholesterol, to the liver and other tissues (Bachorik, 1987; Glass, 1983; Stein, 1984). This may occur directly when HDL is taken up by the hepatocytes via specific receptors or through the action of cell surface receptors and lipases (HL and EL) that deplete phospholipid and triglyceride without internalizing the HDL particles. Lipids may also return to the liver indirectly or be directed to peripheral tissues via apoB-lipoproteins to which they are transferred from HDL by CETP.

Although HDL particles may return to the liver soon after formation, the bulk of HDL seems to remain in circulation for several days, continuously exchanging lipids and apos with other lipoprotein particles, retrieving additional cholesterol from peripheral tissues, and delivering those lipids to the liver and steroid-producing tissues. This is supported by the fact that apoA-I has a half-life of several days in circulation. Eventually, HDL may be internalized by the liver (probably via the LDL receptor), or small lipid-depleted HDL may be catabolized in the kidney following filtration and cubulin-mediated reuptake in the proximal tubule.

Lipid and Lipoprotein Measurement

Lipoprotein concentrations have been measured and described in several ways. Some of these measurements, including particle mass and mass concentration (the mass of each lipoprotein particle as solute per liter of solution), are not easily applied for screening or routine clinical purposes. Fortunately, other methods may be used to describe the lipoprotein content of blood. Because the cholesterol composition of each lipoprotein class is similar from individual to individual, lipoprotein cholesterol is commonly used to evaluate lipoprotein concentration. For example, it is easier to determine the amount of LDL-C in a specimen than it is to determine the mass of LDL (cholesterol + triglyceride + protein) in solution, yet both measurements provide similar information about the LDL content of plasma. Lipoprotein-cholesterol concentrations correlate well with analytic ultracentrifugation values. Also, because these values have been used in most population studies of cardiovascular risk, they have documented predictive value.

When various methods of lipid analysis are considered, several issues should be kept in mind. First, the more complicated the analytic procedures, the greater is the variability of the analyses (Bookstein, 1990; Brown, 1990). For example, the measurement of plasma lipoproteins usually requires two steps: separating lipoprotein classes and measuring the class of interest. Both steps contribute to the error in the measurements. Consistent with this, lipoprotein cholesterol analyses are generally more variable than total cholesterol (TC) analyses because of the additional manipulations required to prepare the lipoprotein-containing fractions. Second, in addition to analytic sources of error, significant preanalytic variables may affect measured lipid and lipoprotein levels. In fact, plasma lipoprotein concentrations can change dramatically as a result of normal physiologic variation. In this section, issues of sampling and storage are considered, along with methods for measuring lipids and lipoproteins.

BLOOD SAMPLING AND STORAGE

Variation and error can be introduced before or during venipuncture, or when the samples are handled and stored before analysis. Therefore, it is important to standardize conditions under which blood specimens are drawn and prepared for analysis.

Biological Variation

Physiologic variations in cholesterol, triglyceride, and lipoproteins have been examined in a number of studies (Bookstein, 1990; Brown, 1990; Demacker, 1982; Kafonek, 1992; Warnick, 1979). For cholesterol, the coefficient of physiologic variation within an individual averages about 6.5%, but it can be higher in certain individuals (Table 17-7). When measured in serial samples from the same person, cholesterol levels in 95% of samples will vary by about 13% above or below that person's mean level. As a result, physiologic variation can be several times greater than analytic error, and measurements must be made in several blood samples taken at least a week apart to establish the individual's usual lipoprotein concentration.

A variety of biological factors can affect lipid and lipoprotein levels. Cholesterol levels rise with age, starting in early adulthood, in both sexes. Women have lower levels than men, except in childhood and after the early fifties. Age-related variation forms the basis for the National Cholesterol Education Program (NCEP) recommendation that cholesterol screening should be repeated every 5 years. Seasonal variation also occurs, such that cholesterol levels are slightly higher in the winter (Robinson, 1992). Also, dietary intake of saturated fat and cholesterol significantly influences plasma lipid levels. The effects of dietary modification take several weeks to become apparent; thus, before individuals' cholesterol levels are ascertained, it is important that they be on their usual diet for 2 weeks and are neither gaining nor losing weight. Several common medications, including oral contraceptives, postmenopausal estrogens, and some antihypertensive drugs, significantly alter lipid levels. Medical disorders that lead to secondary dyslipoproteinemia include thyroid, hepatic, and kidney disease (see Table 17-15, later). In such cases, management of hyperlipidemia is predominantly a function of treating the underlying disorder. Lifestyle and biological factors that produce short-term deviations from baseline lipid values include fasting, posture, venous occlusion, anticoagulants, recent myocardial infarction, stroke, cardiac catheterization, trauma, acute infection, and pregnancy. It is recommended that lipoprotein measurements be made no sooner than 8 weeks after any form of trauma or acute bacterial or viral infection, and 3–4 months after childbirth.

TABLE 17-7
Physiologic Variation of Plasma Lipids, Lipoproteins, and Apolipoproteins

Component	CVP (%)*	CVP (%)†
Total cholesterol	5.0	6.4
Triglycerides	17.8	23.7
LDL-cholesterol	7.8	8.2
HDL-cholesterol	7.1	7.5
ApoA-I	7.1	—
ApoB	6.4	—

CVP, Coefficient of physiologic variation; *HDL,* high-density lipoprotein; *LDL,* low-density lipoprotein.
*Data from patients of a lipid clinic (Kafonek, 1992).
†Data from the National Cholesterol Education Program 1995 Working Group on Lipoprotein Measurement.

Fasting

Ideally, patients should fast for 12 hours before venipuncture. CMs are usually present in postprandial plasma and, depending on the type and amount of food ingested, can markedly increase the plasma triglyceride (TG) concentration. Concentrations of LDL- and HDL-cholesterol (LDL-C and HDL-C) also decline transiently after eating, in part as a consequence of CETP-mediated compositional changes that occur during the catabolism of CMs (Cohn, 1988). CMs are almost completely cleared within 6–9 hours, and their presence after a 12-hour fast is considered abnormal. Generally, TC and HDL-C levels can be measured in nonfasting individuals, greatly facilitating screening and monitoring. Fasting has little effect on plasma TC levels, and although nonfasting HDL-C levels can be a few mg/dL lower than fasting levels, this should not lead to misclassification of patients with low HDL levels. When TG and LDL-C are being measured, fasting becomes a requirement. The postprandial appearance of CMs and compositional changes in LDL lead to the underestimation of LDL-C and can result in the misclassification of truly affected patients. The NCEP Adult Treatment Panel III (ATP III) (NCEP, 2002) has recommended that patients fast for at least 9 hours before blood specimens are taken for lipid and lipoprotein analysis. This is an accommodation for patients who may be unable or unwilling to fast for 12 hours. The shorter fasting period should produce only minor and clinically insignificant errors in the estimation of the patient's usual TG, LDL-C, and HDL-C levels. A 12-hour fasting period is still considered appropriate when lipoprotein measurements are made in clinical and epidemiologic studies.

Posture

When a standing patient reclines, extravascular water transfers to the vascular system and dilutes nondiffusible plasma constituents. Decreases of as much as 10% in the concentrations of TC, LDL-C, HDL-C, apoA-I, and apoB (Miller, 1992) have been observed after a 20-minute period of recumbence. The decrease in TG is about 50% greater, suggesting that factors other than simple hemodilution may also operate. These effects are about half as great in a standing subject who sits (Miller, 1992). Postural changes are reversible when the patient resumes the standing position. The position of the patient therefore should be standardized for venipuncture, preferably to the sitting position, which is most commonly used. Current NCEP guidelines recommend that patients be seated for 5 minutes before sampling to prevent hemoconcentration. If it is necessary to use the recumbent position, this position should be used each time the patient is sampled to minimize postural change. Prolonged venous occlusion can lead to hemoconcentration and cholesterol increases of 10%–15%. Tourniquets should not be applied for longer than a minute or two, if possible.

Venous vs. Capillary Samples

Although it is generally assumed that venous and capillary samples are equivalent, the available information at present is limited and somewhat contradictory. Some investigators have found that cholesterol measurements in the two kinds of samples agreed in about 4% (Koch, 1987) or less (Law, 1997; Lunz, 1987), but others have reported differences of 8%–12% (Bachorik, 1990). In general, measurements in capillary blood samples seem to be a little lower than in venous samples. Additionally, measurements in fingerstick samples tend to be more variable than in venous samples obtained at the same time, probably as the result of preanalytic sources of error. Estimates for the biological component of within-subject variations have been made for lipid and lipoprotein in venous and fingerstick samples, and are similar in both kinds of samples for cholesterol, TG, HDL, and LDL (Kafonek, 1996). Although the use of capillary samples may be unavoidable under some conditions, it is good to keep in mind first that the epidemiologic data from which risk levels for lipids and lipoproteins are derived are based on measurements in venous samples, and second, that for various physiologic and methodologic reasons, the measurements in the two kinds of samples may differ.

Plasma vs. Serum

Plasma or serum can be used when only cholesterol, TG, and HDL-C are measured, and LDL-C is calculated from these three measurements (see later); however, plasma is preferred when the lipoproteins are measured by ultracentrifugal or electrophoretic methods because the samples can be cooled to 4° C immediately to retard changes that can occur in the lipoproteins at room temperature. When plasma is to be used, blood is cooled in an ice bath as soon as it is drawn, and the cells are removed as soon as possible, generally within 3 hours. The plasma is then stored at 4° C until it is analyzed. Plasma should not remain in contact with the cells overnight. Even in the presence of the anticoagulant, protein aggregation can occur in plasma that is stored in the refrigerator for a few days or frozen for longer periods. This can make it difficult to obtain a homogeneous aliquot for analysis and can interfere with the flow of sample in automated analyzers, resulting in inaccurate or variable results. Protein aggregation occurs less frequently in serum.

The choice of anticoagulant is also important. Some anticoagulants, such as citrate, exert rather large osmotic effects that result in falsely low plasma lipid and lipoprotein concentrations. Heparin, because of its relatively high molecular weight, has little effect on plasma volume but can alter the electrophoretic mobilities of the lipoproteins. Ethylenediaminetetraacetic acid (EDTA) is the preferred anticoagulant even though cholesterol and triglyceride concentrations in EDTA plasma are about 3% lower than in serum (Laboratory Methods Committee of the Lipid Research Clinics Program, 1977). This anticoagulant retards certain kinds of oxidative and enzymatic alterations that occur in the lipoproteins during storage.

Storage

Generally, TC, triglycerides, and HDL-C can be satisfactorily analyzed in frozen samples, and LDL-C concentrations can be estimated with the Friedewald equation (Friedewald, 1972). Apolipoproteins can also be measured in frozen samples (see later). Frozen samples are not appropriate for ultracentrifugal analysis because the triglyceride-rich lipoproteins do not withstand freezing. When serum or plasma must be stored for long periods, it should be maintained at temperatures of −70° C or lower. For short-term storage (up to a month or two), the samples can be kept at −20° C, but they should not be stored in a self-defrosting freezer. The temperature in a self-defrosting freezer actually cycles between about −20° C and 2° C during the defrost cycle and effectively subjects the samples to daily freeze–thaw cycles, which can hasten their deterioration and cause the lipid and lipoprotein measurements to become variable (i.e., less reproducible).

ESTIMATION OF PLASMA LIPIDS

Cholesterol and triglycerides are the plasma lipids of greatest interest in the diagnosis and management of lipoprotein disorders. Phospholipid analyses generally provide little additional information and are seldom required. Occasionally, they may be requested in cases of obstructive liver disease or disorders associated with abnormally low lipoprotein levels.

Cholesterol

Cholesterol accounts for almost all of the sterol in plasma. It exists as a mixture of unesterified (30%–40%) and esterified (60%–70%) forms; the proportion of the two forms is fairly constant among normal individuals. TC and lipoprotein-cholesterol concentrations are usually expressed in terms of the sterol nucleus without distinguishing the esterified and unesterified fractions. In general, it is not necessary to distinguish the two forms, except in cases where the contribution of the fatty acid moiety to cholesteryl ester mass must be accounted for, or when the cholesterol/cholesteryl ester mass ratio is of interest.

This discussion considers primarily the enzymatic methods of cholesterol quantification, which have virtually replaced the chemical methods that were used for most clinical and research purposes (Bachorik, 1976; Lipid Research Clinics Program, 1982; Wood, 1980). However, one chemical method, a modification of the Abell-Kendall method (Abell, 1952), continues as the reference method for cholesterol used by the Centers for Disease Control and Prevention (CDC) and a network of secondary reference laboratories (Myers, 1989). In the Abell-Kendall method, cholesteryl esters are hydrolyzed with alcoholic potassium hydroxide (KOH), and the unesterified cholesterol is extracted with petroleum ether and measured with the Liebermann-Burchard reagent using purified cholesterol standards. This method can be accurate within about 0.5% of true value.

Enzymatic Methods

These methods measure TC directly in plasma or serum through a series of reactions in which cholesteryl esters are hydrolyzed. The 3-OH group of cholesterol is oxidized, and hydrogen peroxide, one of the reaction products, is quantified enzymatically:

$$\text{Cholesteryl ester} + H_2O \xrightarrow[\text{esterase}]{\text{Cholesteryl}} \text{Cholesterol} + \text{Free fatty acid} \qquad \textbf{(17-1)}$$

$$\text{Cholesterol} + O_2 \xrightarrow[\text{oxidase}]{\text{Cholesterol}} \text{Cholest-4-en-3-one} + H_2O_2 \qquad \textbf{(17-2)}$$

$$2H_2O_2 + \text{Phenol} + \text{4-aminoantipyrine} \xrightarrow{\text{Peroxidase}} \text{Quinoneimine dye} + 4H_2O \qquad \textbf{(17-3)}$$

To complete the enzymatic measurement of TC, there must be a way to quantify the byproducts of the reaction. One method is the measurement of oxygen consumption; a benefit of this method is that interference by some components within serum/plasma is minimized (Rifai, 2000). Interference will be discussed further later. However, oxygen consumption methods are not easily automated and generally require a lot of cholesterol oxidase. For this reason, this method has not been widely used.

Another approach is to measure cholest-4-en-3-one during the dehydrogenase reaction (Reaction 17-2). This compound can be measured at 240 nm. However, the procedure to measure the compound is time-consuming and very difficult to perform, and has thus fell out of favor for use clinically or in a purely research setting (Rifai, 2000). Currently, the most common method of quantifying the cholesterol oxidase reaction is to measure the amount of hydrogen peroxide produced (Reaction 17-3). The hydrogen peroxide produced in the cholesterol oxidase reaction can be oxidatively coupled to two chromogenic substrates by catalysis with a peroxidase, most commonly horseradish peroxidase (HRP). The chromogens used are usually phenol and 4-aminoantipyrine. When coupled with hydrogen peroxide, they produce a quinoneimine dye that can be read photometrically at 500 nm. The catalytic properties of HRP are very nonspecific; therefore, this step is most subject to interference from other components of serum/plasma.

Interfering Substances

Enzymatic methods are less subject to interference by nonsterol substances that react in the chemical methods; however, they are not absolutely specific for cholesterol. Cholesterol oxidase (Reaction 17-2) can react with sterols other than cholesterol that are present in plasma such as plant sterols, which are present in appreciable concentrations in the circulation of patients with β-sitosterolemia. These sterols also contribute to the cholesterol values measured via most chemical methods. Another type of interfering agent is ascorbic acid. Ascorbic acid is known for its properties as a reducing agent. These properties allow it to compete with the chromogenic substrates of Reaction 17-3 for hydrogen peroxide. Therefore, plasma/serum samples with elevated levels of ascorbic acid can result in lower measured levels of TC. It is currently accepted that ascorbic acid levels >30 mg/dL should be accounted for in TC measurements, although levels that high are infrequent (Rifai, 2000). Another interfering agent that acts in a similar manner is bilirubin. Bilirubin can interfere with TC measurements because of its own spectral properties; bilirubin absorbs light at 500 nm (Rifai, 2000). This tends to increase measured cholesterol values. However, bilirubin is also oxidized by H_2O_2, and as a result loses its absorbance at 500 nm. This complicates the application of a serum blank to correct for bilirubin absorbance. On the whole, interference by bilirubin seems to be significant only at concentrations exceeding 5 mg/dL, at which level it has been reported to decrease apparent cholesterol values by

5%–15% (Deacon, 1979; Naito, 1984; Pesce, 1977). Sample turbidity as a result of hypertriglyceridemia can also interfere with enzymatic methods (Pesce, 1977). Hemoglobin is another possible interfering agent in the measurement of TC. It has a pseudo-peroxidase activity that can consume the hydrogen peroxide produced in Reaction 17-2. More important, however, is that hemoglobin has an inherent color that can falsely elevate TC levels. Just as hemoglobin is a product of red blood cell hemolysis, other products of hemolysis such as catalase can compete with the peroxidase for hydrogen peroxide. However, hemolyzed products do not significantly affect cholesterol measurements even at abnormally high plasma concentrations (Deacon, 1979; Pesce, 1977).

In addition to their relative resistance to interference, enzymatic methods have other significant benefits. They consume only microliter quantities of sample and do not require a preliminary extraction step. They are rapid, and if the cholesteryl ester hydrolase step is omitted, they can be used to measure unesterified cholesterol. Finally, enzymatic methods are precise with coefficients of variation generally in the range of 1%–2%. For the most part, they use stabilized pure cholesterol standards or serum calibration standards for which the stated values are traceable to the CDC reference method for cholesterol (Pesce, 1977). Enzymatic values generally agree with reference values within 1%–2% when measured in a laboratory setting with modern equipment. Serum-based calibrators are inherently preferable to pure cholesterol, as they are subject to all analytic reactions undergone by patient samples.

Triglycerides

A wide variety of methods has been used to measure plasma triglycerides (Bachorik, 1977), but the methods most commonly used for clinical or epidemiologic purposes are based on the hydrolysis of triglycerides and the measurement of glycerol that is released in the reaction:

$$\text{Triglyceride} + 3H_2O \xrightarrow{\text{Lipase}} \text{Glycerol} + \text{Fatty acid} \qquad \textbf{(17-4)}$$

Because each glycerol molecule is calculated to represent a triglyceride molecule, TG concentrations are often overestimated if endogenous unesterified glycerol is not subtracted. Even so, TG levels will still remain an overestimation because of the presence of monoglyceride and diglyceride molecules. Despite this knowledge and the availability of reagents and methods to correct for endogenous glycerol, only about 5% of American clinical laboratories actually correct for endogenous glycerol. The reason for this is that in most normal individuals, endogenous glycerol levels are negligible.

TG measurements are almost universally performed enzymatically; as with cholesterol, the enzymatic methods have replaced earlier chemical methods (Kessler, 1966; Lipid Research Clinics Program, 1982).

One chemical method still used is the CDC reference method for triglycerides. The CDC-reference method uses a chloroform extraction procedure followed by silicic acid chromatography to isolate TG. Glycerol is released by saponification (alkaline hydrolysis of triglycerides) and is oxidized with sodium periodate:

$$\text{Glycerol} + NaIO_4 \rightarrow \text{Formaldehyde} + \text{Formic acid} \qquad \textbf{(17-5)}$$

The formaldehyde produced is measured by reaction with a sulfuric acid solution of chromotropic acid to produce a pink chromophore. This method is not specific for glycerol. Formaldehyde is also produced indirectly from glycerol-containing phospholipids; however, these and other interfering substances are removed during the extraction (with chloroform) and adsorption (silicic acid chromatography) steps and do not interfere with TG measurements made using the CDC reference method.

Enzymatic Methods

(Bucolo, 1973)

These are now universally used for TG analysis in the clinical laboratory. They are relatively specific, rapid, and easy to use. The analyses are performed directly in plasma or serum, and are not subject to interference by phospholipids or glucose.

Common to most enzymatic methods is the hydrolysis of triglycerides to free fatty acids and glycerol, followed by the phosphorylation of glycerol to glycerophosphate.

$$\text{Triglycerides} \xrightarrow{\text{Lipase}} \text{Glycerol} + \text{Fatty acids} \qquad \textbf{(17-6)}$$

$$\text{Glycerol} + \text{ATP} \xrightarrow{\text{Glycerokinase}} \text{Glycerophosphate} + \text{ADP} \qquad \textbf{(17-7)}$$

However, several methods may be used to quantify the amount of glycerol formed, and therefore the amount of triglyceride in plasma. In one approach, glycerophosphate reacts as follows:

$$\text{Glycerophosphate} + \text{NAD} \xrightarrow[\text{dehydrogenase}]{\text{Glycerophosphate}} \text{Dihydroxyacetone phosphate} + \text{NADH} + H_4 \qquad \textbf{(17-8)}$$

$$\text{NADH} + \text{Tetrazolium dye} \xrightarrow{\text{Diaphorase}} \text{Formazan} + \text{NAD}^+ \qquad \textbf{(17-9)}$$

NADH formation can be measured spectrophotometrically at 340 nm. In other methods, Reaction 17-9 has been added so that absorbance readings can be made in the 500 to 600 nm region of the spectrum, using instruments that are more commonly available in the clinical laboratory.

In a common variation, the glycerophosphate formed in Reaction 17-7 is oxidized by the action of glycerophosphate oxidase:

$$\text{Glycerophosphate} + O_2 \xrightarrow[\text{oxidase}]{\text{Glycerophosphate}} \text{Dihydroxyacetone} + H_2O_2 \qquad \textbf{(17-10)}$$

The resulting H_2O_2 is measured as described previously for cholesterol methods (Reaction 17-3).

In a third approach, adenosine diphosphate (ADP), rather than glycerophosphate is formed in Reaction 17-7, is quantified:

$$\text{ADP} + \text{Phosphoenol pyruvate} \xrightarrow[\text{kinase}]{\text{Pyruvate}} \text{ATP} + \text{Pyruvate} \qquad \textbf{(17-11)}$$

$$\text{Pyruvate} + \text{NADH} + H^+ \xrightarrow[\text{dehydrogenase}]{\text{Lactate}} \text{Lactate} + \text{NAD}^+ \qquad \textbf{(17-12)}$$

In this method, the disappearance of NADH is measured at 340 nm.

Enzymatic TG methods generally perform well. The reagents are available commercially as lyophilized preparations that need only be reconstituted before use. Based on recent College of American Pathologists (CAP) surveys, the interlaboratory coefficients of variation (CVs) for TG measurement using a variety of enzymatic methods were on the order of 5%–6%. It is prudent before selecting an enzymatic method to evaluate its accuracy and precision over the range of triglyceride concentrations likely to be encountered most frequently (1.299–12.987 mmol/L; 50–500 mg/dL).

Triglyceride Blanks

Enzymatic measurements of triglyceride involve the generation and measurement of glycerol. Although phospholipids and glucose do not interfere with enzymatic methods, free glycerol does. Glycerol is normally present in plasma in concentrations below 0.163 mmol/L (1.5 mg/dL), equivalent to a triglyceride concentration of about 14 mg/dL. However, concentrations can be higher in the following circumstances: after extremely vigorous exercise; in patients with uncontrolled diabetes; after chance contamination with the glycerol lubricant used on the stoppers of some blood collection tubes; after recent ingestion of glycerol-containing medications; or in a relatively rare disorder, hyperglycerolemia, which arises secondary to a mutation in the glycerol kinase gene on chromosome Xp21.3. A blank assay, without the addition of lipase, provides a measure of preexisting glycerol. Increased readings in the blank indicate the presence of glycerol, and measured TG values can be corrected accordingly. In an alternative procedure, free glycerol is consumed in a preliminary reaction before triglyceride hydrolysis is initiated. In this case, the measured value is the equivalent of a blanked triglyceride.

The blanking procedures described earlier are satisfactory for correcting spurious measurements that arise from many glycerol sources, but not for those that result from partial glycerides (diglycerides and monoglycerides). Partial glycerides are generally present at very low concentrations in fresh plasma or serum but can form through the slow hydrolysis of triglycerides when samples are stored. It is not clear whether partial glycerides in fresh plasma should be subtracted, but those that form during storage probably should not be subtracted because they arise from triglycerides that were originally present in the sample.

Fortunately, as complex as the blanking problem is, it is usually of little practical importance. Blanks are not determined routinely in many laboratories, and their use continues to be a matter of uncertainty. When measured, the magnitude of the blanks encountered in most fresh samples is on the order of 0.056–0.112 mmol/L (5–10 mg/dL), expressed as triglyceride, although they can be higher in samples with high triglyceride concentrations. However, blanks can assume importance in the standardization and quality control of triglyceride measurements because they can be on the order of 0.226–0.339 mmol/L (20–30 mg/dL) or greater in serum pools used for these purposes. This is probably a result of the partial hydrolysis of triglycerides during preparation of the pools.

Interfering Substances

As with cholesterol measurement interference, TG measurement is subjected to similar interference by the same substances. Plasma ascorbic acid is an antioxidant that can interfere with the oxidation/reduction reactions involved in the measurement of TG. Bilirubin can also cause interference, both spectrally and chemically. Significant plasma hemolysis can spectrally interfere with TG measurements and may cause the dilution of lipid constituents.

Phospholipids

Most of the phospholipid in human plasma is phosphatidylcholine (70%–75%) or sphingomyelin (18%–20%). Remaining phospholipids include phosphatidylserine, phosphatidylethanolamine (3%–6%), and lysophosphatidylcholine (4%–9%). Phospholipid measurement is not routinely performed in the clinical laboratory. The reason for this is that phospholipid analysis usually provides little additional information in cases of dyslipoproteinemia. Another reason is that the phospholipid concentration in plasma is not altered as markedly as that of cholesterol and TG in various pathologic conditions. However, estimation of lipoprotein phospholipids provides information that at times can be more important than cholesterol or TG concentrations. For example, only 10%–20% of the total weight of HDL is cholesterol, but almost 25%–30% of it is phospholipid, making it a far more accurate reflection of HDL content (Rifai, 2000). Furthermore, the phospholipid content of HDL is more important than cholesterol or even apolipoprotein A-I in reverse cholesterol transport; abnormalities in HDL phospholipid composition have been noted to have a greater effect on HDL function than cholesterol concentration. Phospholipids are also important substrates for a number of lipoprotein metabolizing enzymes (e.g., LCAT, LPL, HL); therefore changes in the composition could adversely affect the function of these enzymes. Most important, the dietary status of essential fatty acids is more accurately assessed by the fatty acid composition of phospholipids rather than total lipids. It has also been noted that the saturated fatty acid content of plasma phospholipids is reported to be an independent risk factor for atherosclerosis.

The only unique structural feature common to all phospholipids is the presence of lipid-bound phosphate. Therefore most of the methods originally designed to determine plasma phospholipids depend on the estimation of lipid phosphorus. Lipids are extracted from the sample and are oxidized completely to convert phospholipid phosphorus to inorganic phosphate, which is then determined colorimetrically. These procedures are reproducible and sensitive and can be adapted to measure total phospholipid phosphorus in 100 μL or less of plasma or serum. Each mole of phosphorus contributes about 4% to the total phospholipid mass; thus phospholipid mass can be determined by multiplying the phospholipid phosphorus concentration (expressed in mg/dL) by 25.

Serum or plasma phospholipids can also be measured enzymatically using commercially available methods. In the method available from WAKO Pure Chemical Industries, Ltd. (Osaka, Japan), lecithin (phosphatidylcholine), sphingomyelin, and lysolecithin are hydrolyzed using phospholipase D, and the choline liberated is oxidized.

$$\text{Phospholipid} \xrightarrow{\text{Phospholipase D}} \text{Choline} \quad \textbf{(17-13)}$$

$$\text{Choline} \xrightarrow[\text{oxidase}]{\text{Choline}} \text{Betaine} + H_2O_2 \quad \textbf{(17-14)}$$

The resulting H_2O_2 produced is measured in a manner similar to that shown in Reaction 17-3. Analysis of individual phospholipid classes is seldom required for evaluation of dyslipoproteinemia and is not discussed in this chapter.

ESTIMATION OF LIPOPROTEINS AND LIPOPROTEIN CHOLESTEROL

Because lipoproteins share common lipid and apolipoprotein components, the central problem in lipoprotein analysis is the separation of different lipoprotein classes from one another. Many methods have been applied to lipoprotein separation, including ultracentrifugation, adsorption, gel filtration, affinity chromatography, electrophoresis in various media, polyanion and alcohol precipitation, immunochemical procedures, and various combinations of methods. Some of these methods require special skills and equipment and are not easily adapted for clinical or epidemiologic purposes. This discussion is limited to several procedures that have been used by clinical laboratories.

Ultracentrifugation Methods

These take advantage of two properties of the lipoproteins. First, by virtue of their lipid content, lipoproteins have lower densities than the other plasma macromolecules. Second, each class of lipoproteins has a different density. Thus, lipoproteins can be readily separated on the basis of their densities by using ultracentrifugation techniques. The proportion of lipids, in particular TG, associated with appropriate proteins determines the density of a particular lipoprotein class. VLDL and chylomicrons are the most lipid-rich lipoprotein classes in human blood. This fact leaves them as the most buoyant in plasma. These lipoproteins have a density <1.006 kg/L (density measurement). LDL particles are smaller in size and in lipoprotein content, causing their density to range from 1.006–1.063 kg/L. HDL, the densest lipoprotein, ranges from 1.063–1.210 kg/L (Rifai, 2000). Ultracentrifugation methods are largely considered the best means to compare lipoprotein classes; however, the technique is difficult, time-consuming, and expensive, leaving it for research settings rather than clinical measurement.

Electrophoretic Methods

In the past, electrophoresis was widely used in the clinical laboratory to separate and measure lipoproteins. However, because the method has significant limitations (described later), it generally is not required for the diagnosis of dyslipoproteinemia, and its use in routine clinical practice has diminished in recent years. In general, the cost of the procedure, in terms of both time and money, is rarely justified by the information provided.

The most commonly used support medium for lipoprotein electrophoresis is agarose gel because of its speed, sensitivity, and ability to resolve the lipoprotein classes. Chylomicrons, if present, remain at the origin. Of the remaining major lipoproteins, HDL migrates the fastest, LDL the slowest, and VLDL at a rate intermediate between HDL and LDL. The electrophoretically separated lipoproteins have been named according to their mobilities: HDL (α-lipoprotein) moves with the α_1-globulins; LDL (β-lipoprotein) migrates with the β-globulins, and VLDL (pre-β lipoprotein) migrates with the β_2-globulins. Different properties of lipoproteins form the basis for electrophoretic and ultracentrifugal separation, and analogous fractions separated by the two techniques may not be identical. For example, β-VLDL (found in type 3 hyperlipidemia, see later) is isolated with VLDL by ultracentrifugation but moves electrophoretically with LDL. In the absence of additional information, a sample containing β-VLDL would appear to have an elevated VLDL concentration by ultracentrifugation and an increased LDL concentration by electrophoresis. Another example is that Lp(a) is isolated in the LDL–HDL density range by ultracentrifugation, but it has an electrophoretic mobility similar to that of VLDL. This dichotomy is responsible for naming Lp(a) "sinking pre-β-lipoprotein."

Electrophoresis can be performed using unfractionated plasma or in plasma fractions that contain other serum proteins. Lipoprotein electrophoretograms are usually visualized with a lipid-staining dye such as Oil Red O, Fat Red 7B, or Sudan Black B. These lipid stains react primarily with the ester bonds in triglycerides and cholesteryl esters. Lipoproteins rich in free cholesterol and phospholipids (such as LpX) stain very poorly and thus are grossly underestimated by electrophoretic techniques.

Attempts have been made to quantify the lipoproteins by densitometry. Lipoprotein levels have been expressed in terms of the percentage distribution of lipid-staining material in β-, pre-β-, and α-lipoproteins, or have been converted to lipoprotein–cholesterol concentrations according to calculations that incorporate assumptions about cholesterol content and dye uptake of the lipoproteins. In general, these approaches have not been successful for reasons that include incomplete resolution of β- and pre-β-lipoproteins, the presence of minor or unusual lipoproteins, and differences in the intensity of staining. Electrophoresis has been used most successfully in conjunction with other methods.

Polyanion Precipitation Methods

Some lipoproteins are precipitated with polyanions such as heparin sulfate, dextran sulfate, phosphotungstate, and others in the presence of divalent cations such as Ca^{++}, Mg^{++} and Mn^{++}. Conditions have been established in which the major classes of lipoproteins can be precipitated in stepwise fashion beginning with the lower-density, lipid-rich lipoproteins (Burstein, 1982). The more dissimilar the lipoproteins are from one another, the better is the separation. Thus, it is easier to separate apoB-containing lipoproteins from HDL than it is to separate VLDL from LDL or HDL_2 from HDL_3. Historically, polyanion precipitation was most commonly used to remove apoB-containing lipoproteins before analysis of HDL-C. This required a sample pretreatment and was not fully automated. Most clinical laboratories have replaced precipitation techniques with automated homogeneous assays for HDL-C and LDL-C.

Determining HDL-C Values

The NCEP recognizes HDL-C as an independent risk factor for CHD and recommends its measurement in conjunction with TC measurements. An HDL-C concentration of <35 mg/dL is considered high risk for CHD, while levels >60 mg/dL are considered protective. Historically, HDL-C has been measured in the supernatant of samples following the precipitation of apoB-containing lipoproteins by polyanion-divalent cations. Several combinations of polyanion-divalent cations have been used, and not all of them give precisely the same results. HDL-C values determined with heparan sulfate-Mn^{++} procedures agree closely with those obtained using analytic or preparative ultracentrifugation (Bachorik, 1976; Warnick, 1979). This method was widely used in epidemiologic studies. Dextran sulfate (relative molecular mass 50000 Da)-Mg^{++} and sodium phosphotungstate-Mg^{++} methods gained popularity because they do not interfere with enzymatic cholesterol studies. However, they give results about 5% lower than ultracentrifugation. Heparin-Ca^{++} appears to give results that are about 10% higher. These differences arise, in part, from the underprecipitation of apoB-containing lipoproteins, which leads to overestimation of HDL-C, or the overprecipitation of HDL, which can lead to underestimation of HDL-C. Increased triglycerides interfere with precipitation methods and overestimate HDL-C. Attempts were made to simplify precipitation methods by using dextran sulfate–coated magnetic beads to achieve selective separation of HDL from the apoB-containing lipoproteins (Naito, 1995).

Currently, homogeneous assays are the most popular method for measuring HDL-C. Unlike precipitation methods, these fully automated two-reagent procedures do not require off-line pretreatment and separation (hence the term "homogeneous") and can be adapted to most chemistry analyzers. Thus, they reduce hands-on time and overall assay costs. Test kits distributed in the United States are based on a variety of methods. Usually, the first reagent forms a stable complex with non-HDL lipoproteins, preventing them from participating in the reaction, and the second reagent releases HDL-C that is then measured enzymatically. According to CAP 2005 surveys, the most common method uses a synthetic polymer together with a polyanion to block non-HDL lipoproteins, followed by a selective detergent to release HDL-C (Genzyme Diagnostics, Cambridge, Mass.; Beckman Coulter, Inc). Other methods use polyethylene glycol–modified enzyme (Roche Diagnostics, Indianapolis), or immunoinhibition (Wako Chemicals USA, Inc, Richmond, Va.) to block non-HDL lipoproteins. A fourth method (Polymedco Inc, Cortlandt Manor, N.Y.) uses a special reagent to selectively eliminate cholesterol in non-HDL lipoproteins, followed by a second reagent that releases cholesterol from HDL (Denka Seiken Co, Niigata, Japan). These methods generally are not affected by high triglycerides, bilirubin, and globulins.

In a comprehensive review (Warnick, 2001), multiple HDL-C homogeneous assays were compared with traditional precipitation and ultracentrifugation procedures. The authors concluded that the new procedures simplify the determination of HDL-C and are accurate, precise, and meet NCEP criteria for total error. However, atypical lipoproteins evaluated by homogeneous assay may show discrepant results when compared with the established precipitation method. These differences are seen in patients with hyperlipidemia or liver or kidney disease when abnormal lipoprotein forms occur. Laboratories that encounter a high proportion of atypical lipoproteins (e.g., lipid clinics or research settings) should thoroughly validate a homogeneous assay for use with their patient population.

LDL-C Measurement

LDL cholesterol plays a causal role in the development of atherosclerosis. LDL-C >160 mg/dL with no risk factors is an indication for therapy (Rifai, 2000). With two or more CHD risk factors, the upper limit is lowered to 130 mg/dL for initiation of therapy. Several methods have been used to measure LDL-C. The first, a reference laboratory procedure, involves ultracentrifugation to separate LDL from other lipoproteins, followed by analysis as described previously to measure cholesterol. This method is not extensively discussed here. A much more common second method uses the Friedewald formula to calculate LDL-C. Finally, more recently developed homogeneous methods for measuring LDL-C are now available.

Friedewald Calculation

LDL-C can be determined by using the Friedewald formula, originally described by Friedewald, Levy, and Fredrickson (Friedewald, 1972). Generally, in fasting plasma samples, LDL contains the cholesterol that is not present in HDL or VLDL. Thus LDL-C can be determined by the following equation in which concentrations are expressed in mmol/L, and the term [Plasma TG]/2.175 is used to represent VLDL-C:

$$[\text{LDL-cholesterol}] = [\text{Total cholesterol}] - [\text{HDL-cholesterol}] - [\text{Plasma TG}]/2.175$$

The term [Plasma TG]/5 is used when concentrations are expressed in mg/dL. In this method, the plasma TC, TG, and HDL-C concentrations are determined as described. Because VLDL carries most plasma triglyceride, VLDL-C concentration is estimated from the ratio of triglyceride to cholesterol in VLDL:

$$\text{VLDL-C} = \text{Plasma TG}/2.175$$

It has been reported that the factor [Plasma TG]/2.825 gives a more accurate estimate of VLDL-C (DeLong, 1986). This is equivalent to Plasma TG/6.5, when concentrations are expressed in mg/dL. However, the factor that gives the best estimate of VLDL-C, and therefore the best estimate of LDL-C, varies among populations and depends on the triglyceride method used; the NCEP Working Group on Lipoprotein Measurement prefers the unmodified Friedewald equation (NCEP Working Group on Lipoprotein Measurement, 1995).

The Friedewald formula has significant limitations (Sniderman, 2003). These limitations arise largely from two assumptions on which the method is based. First, the calculation assumes that essentially all plasma triglycerides are carried in VLDL. Second, the method assumes that the triglyceride/cholesterol ratio of VLDL is invariant. Neither assumption is entirely true; as a result, this method is unsuitable for nonfasting samples that contain chylomicrons or samples that contain β-VLDL. As compared with VLDL, the ratio of triglycerides to cholesterol in chylomicrons is much higher. Thus, when CM is present, the use of the factor TG/2.175 to account for non-HDL, non-LDL cholesterol can overestimate the amount of cholesterol in VLDL, leading to underestimation of LDL-C. Similarly the ratio of triglyceride to cholesterol in β-VLDL is much lower than in VLDL; use of the factor TG/2.175 in the presence of β-VLDL can underestimate VLDL-C and thus overestimate LDL-C. A patient with type 3 hyperlipoproteinemia can be misclassified as having an elevated LDL-C. It is important to distinguish the two conditions because their treatments differ.

Even in CM-free samples, the ratio of VLDL-C to triglyceride changes as triglyceride levels increase, and this can lead to errors in estimates of VLDL-C. Because VLDL generally carries only about 25% of the TC in plasma, resulting errors in LDL-C are usually less than 5–10 mg/dL (0.130–0.260 mmol/L). However, the calculation is not suitable for samples with high triglyceride concentrations. Errors in LDL-C become noticeable at triglyceride levels >2.26 mmol/L (200 mg/dL) and become unacceptably large at triglyceride levels >4.52 mmol/L (400 mg/dL). The accuracy of LDL-C calculation also suffers at low LDL-C levels, indicating that calculated LDL-C values may not provide the best assessment of cardiac risk in patients who already are receiving cholesterol-lowering therapy (Sniderman, 2003). Provided that its limitations are appreciated, the Friedewald equation has broad utility, both as a screening tool and for following patients.

Another issue to consider is non-LDL lipoproteins. Generally, LDL contributes most of the cholesterol to the measurement, and IDL and Lp(a) contribute only a few mg/dL each. However, these lipoproteins can contribute significantly to cholesterol measurements in some hyperlipidemia patients. Because Lp(a) levels are not lowered by a number of treatments that effectively lower LDL levels, Lp(a) measurements can, in some circumstances, reveal why a patient does not respond well to LDL-lowering therapy.

Selective Chemical Precipitation

LDL-C is calculated as the difference between TC and the amount remaining after precipitation of LDL-C. Such methods are reasonably accurate if TG concentrations are low enough. However, this method allows only for the separation of apoB-containing lipoproteins, separating HDL from non-HDL particles.

Beta Quantification

Beta quantification assumes that virtually all cholesterol is contained in the three major lipoprotein classes (i.e., VLDL, LDL, and HDL). In this method, plasma is ultracentrifuged for at least 18 hours at 105 K × *g* VLDL and CMs accumulate as a floating layer, leaving predominantly LDL and HDL in solution (Rifai, 2000). The solution is measured for cholesterol and is precipitated for LDL lipoproteins. LDL-C is calculated according to the difference between these two measurements. Because TG-rich lipoproteins are removed from this sample, measurement of LDL-C is more reflective of actual concentration. The resulting difference also reflects contributions of IDL-C and Lp(a) cholesterol, both of which are considered pro-atherogenic. Therefore, measurement of LDL-C by this method represents the amount of cholesterol being transported in pro-atherogenic particles (Rifai, 2000).

Direct LDL-C Measurement

To a large extent, the ability to calculate LDL-C has eliminated the need for direct measurements. However, homogeneous direct LDL-C methods are useful when triglycerides are elevated because they are not subject to interference by triglycerides even at relatively high concentrations (600 mg/dL) (Bachorik, 2000). Direct assays have been adapted for use on a variety of analyzers and have been extensively reviewed elsewhere (Nauck, 2002; Miller, 2002). Although these methods differ significantly, in general, they use a combination of two reagents. The first reagent usually selectively removes non-LDL lipoproteins (and/or stabilizes or inhibits LDL from reacting with enzymes), and the second reagent releases cholesterol from LDL so that it can be measured enzymatically.

In one method (Equal Diagnostics, Exton, Pa.; Genzyme Diagnostics), the first reagent uses a detergent polymer mixture to disrupt non-LDL lipoproteins, releasing their cholesterol. The cholesterol is then de-esterified and reacts with cholesterol oxidase to generate hydrogen peroxide, which reacts to form a colorless compound. The second reagent contains a detergent that releases cholesterol from LDL. After de-esterification, the LDL-C proceeds through a similar set of reactions, except that the final step generates a colored compound. The intensity of the color is proportional to the concentration of LDL-C. Another method (Roche Diagnostics) is based on selective micellary solubilization of LDL by a nonionic detergent, as well as the interaction of a sugar compound with HDL, VLDL, and chylomicrons to inhibit participation in the measurement assay (Sugiuchi, 1998). A third method exploits the fact that reactivity of cholesterol in the different lipoproteins is affected by the hydrophile: lipophile balance (HLB) of solubilizing detergents. In this method, non–LDL-C is reacted with cholesterol esterase and cholesterol oxidase in conditions where LDL-C is inhibited, and the resulting peroxide is eliminated by catalase. A second reagent then alters the HLB of the detergent, creating conditions where LDL-C reacts. This reagent also contains an azide that inhibits catalase and allows the colorimetric detection of peroxide (see Reaction 17-3) (Polymedco Inc; Reference Diagnostics, Bedford, Mass.). In a fourth method, the first reagent contains amphoteric surfactants that protect LDL, allowing the elimination of non–LDL-C and resulting peroxide as described earlier. The second reagent contains nonionic surfactants that displace the protecting surfactants and allow measurement of LDL-C (Sigma Diagnostics, St Louis).

Although these methods are precise, they produce discrepancies in comparison with the reference ultracentrifugation procedures in a number of circumstances, including the presence of abnormal lipoproteins. When the triglyceride level is <400 mg/dL, homogeneous methods perform no better than the Friedewald calculation for classifying patients into treatment groups (Miller, 2002). However, unlike the calculation, homogeneous assays can provide clinically useful results when triglycerides >400 mg/dL. Another potential benefit is the convenience of measuring LDL-C in nonfasting individuals, although some have recommended against this practice (Miller, 2002). ATP III recommendations do not favor replacing calculated LDL-C with direct LDL-C because the constituents of the calculation have to be measured in any case. Running direct LDL-C would only add to the expense.

ADDITIONAL METHODS IN THE STUDY OF DYSLIPIDEMIA

Measurement of Lipoprotein Subclasses

Subpopulations or subclasses have been identified in VLDL, LDL, and HDL by techniques such as analytic ultracentrifugation, gradient gel electrophoresis, and nuclear magnetic resonance (NMR) spectroscopy (Krauss, 1992, 1987; Otvos, 1992). Some subclass distinctions are of clinical significance, yet the number of subclasses identified varies between methods of separation, and the nomenclature for subclasses is less than uniform. For example, when NMR technology is used to identify lipoprotein subclasses, particle subclass numbers tend to increase with increasing particle size; thus LDL particles of the L2 subclass are larger than L1 particles. When electrophoresis or ultracentrifugation is used, the opposite is true, and particles tend to decrease in size with higher numbers. Thus, in segmented gradient gel electrophoresis, LDL subclass IV (or LDL4) particles are smaller than subclass II (LDL2) particles; in gradient ultracentrifugation, subclass LDL4 particles are smaller than LDL3 particles.

Recent interest has focused on the role of subclasses in the development of atherosclerosis, specifically the smallest and least dense LDL particles. This fraction is thought to be more atherogenic than large LDL. Small HDL and large VLDL subclasses have also been associated with an increased incidence of atherosclerosis. The NMR Lipoprofile (LipoScience, Raleigh, NC) allows the quantification of lipoprotein particles by subclass based on their unique NMR-spectral characteristics. This profile provides information about CHD risk by quantifying the subclass distribution of lipoprotein particles (Otvos, 2002). At least partially, the appeal of this technique arises from the idea that the migration of LDL particles into the artery wall is gradient driven based on LDL particle number. When large numbers of small LDL particles are present, LDL-C measurements tend to underestimate the number of LDL particles, and thus the atherosclerotic effects of LDL. Triglyceride levels >100 mg/dL and HDL-C <60 mg/dL are associated with high levels of small LDL particles; when these conditions are present, NMR profiling may be a useful technique for assessing CHD risk. Sensitive electrophoretic methods should provide similar results. These methods are not currently viewed as screening tools. They are more appropriate for refining risk assessment and treatment in patients with previously identified CHD risk: those under treatment, and patients who have LDL-C values at or close to treatment goals. This is consistent with most accepted guidelines that stress the importance of LDL-C as the primary goal of therapy in most types of dyslipidemia.

Standing Plasma Test

Chylomicrons, if present in appreciable quantities, are detected using the "standing plasma" test. An aliquot of plasma (2 mL) is placed into a 10 × 75-mm test tube and allowed to stand in the refrigerator at 4° C undisturbed overnight. Chylomicrons accumulate as a floating "cream" layer and can be detected visually. The presence of chylomicrons in fasting plasma is considered to be abnormal. A plasma sample that remains turbid after standing overnight contains excessive amounts of VLDL; if a floating "cream" layer also forms, chylomicrons are present as well.

Detection of β-VLDL and Lp(a)

As mentioned earlier, the abnormal lipoprotein β-VLDL has the density of VLDL but migrates electrophoretically with LDL in the β-region. It can be detected when the ultracentrifugal fraction of d < 1.006 kg/L is examined electrophoretically. In practice, unfractionated plasma and both ultracentrifugal fractions (< and >1.006 kg/L) are examined at the same time; each sample thus serves as its own control to establish the relative migration of the lipoprotein bands. In normal plasma, the β (LDL and IDL), pre-β (VLDL), and α (HDL) lipoprotein bands are visible in unfractionated plasma; only the pre-β band is present in the d < 1.006 kg/L fraction, and the β- and α-lipoprotein bands are seen in the d > 1.006 kg/L fraction. When present, β-VLDL is observed as a band with β-mobility in the d < 1.006 kg/L fraction. Its presence is abnormal and is usually associated with dysbetalipoproteinemia (type 3 hyperlipoproteinemia), although occasionally it is seen in other disorders. Chylomicrons, which often are seen in type 3 patients, remain at the origin on agarose gel.

Lp(a) has a density similar to LDL but migrates similarly to VLDL on electrophoresis. Thus it can be detected when the d > 1.006 g/mL protein is examined electrophoretically. When Lp(a) is present in concentrations exceeding 20–30 mg/dL (i.e., when it contributes more than about 10 mg/dL to the LDL-C measurement), an additional band with pre-β mobility is observed in the d > 1.006 kg/L fraction (hence the name sinking pre-β-lipoprotein). Under these conditions, the physician may wish to request a quantitative Lp(a) measurement. Lp(a) can now be measured using immunoturbidimetric methods. When the Lp(a) level is very high, it may be necessary to correct LDL-C for the contribution of Lp(a)-cholesterol. The following relationship has been used to estimate the contribution of Lp(a)-cholesterol to the measured LDL-C value, where the values are given in mg/dL:

$$\text{Lp(a)-cholesterol} = 0.3 \times [\text{Lp(a) mass}]$$

$$\text{LDL-C} = \text{TC} - [\text{HDL-cholesterol}] - [\text{Plasma TG}]/5 - (0.3[\text{Lp(a) mass}])$$

VLDL-C/Plasma Triglyceride Ratio

The ratio of VLDL-C to plasma triglycerides may be useful in the evaluation of type 3 hyperlipoproteinemia. This ratio, expressed in mol/mol or

PART 2

(mass/mass), is generally in the range of 0.230–0.575 (0.1–0.25) in samples without β-VLDL, depending on the relative amounts of VLDL, LDL, and HDL present, and on the errors inherent in the VLDL-C and plasma triglyceride measurements. Type 3 subjects have ratios >0.689 (0.3), usually in the range of 0.689–0.919 (0.3–0.4), and higher ratios can be observed. Again, because of errors in the measurements, the observation of a ratio of 0.689 (0.3) on a single occasion may or may not be significant. Overt type 3 patients manifest both β-VLDL and a VLDL-C/plasma triglyceride ratio of 0.689 (0.3) or greater. Occasionally, a lipid disorder treatment clinic may request the assessment of apoE phenotype to supplement the diagnosis of type 3 hyperlipoproteinemia (see later), because homozygosity for apoE-2 is associated with this disorder. However, not all homozygous patients have type 3 hyperlipoproteinemia, and ultracentrifugation is still required for assessing the presence of β-VLDL.

Apolipoprotein Analysis

Studies have indicated that apoA-I and apoB may be better discriminators of atherosclerotic disease than lipid or lipoprotein determinations. Because apoA-I is present primarily in HDL, while apoB (in fasting samples) is present in VLDL, IDL, and LDL, it stands to reason that low apoB and high apoA-I levels, as well as a low apoB-to-apoA-I ratio would be a good thing. In general, the evidence for this has been more consistent for apoB than for apoA-I, but the reason for this is not clear. A large-scale, placebo-controlled intervention trial, AFCAPS (Gotto, 2000), found that apoB was the best single lipid, lipoprotein, or apolipoprotein measurement to predict both baseline and on-treatment CAD risk, followed by apoA-I. ApoB : A-I ratios may also be useful in assessing risk.

Apolipoproteins are usually measured by immunoassay or immunonephelometry. These techniques rely on measurement of the turbidity caused by apolipoprotein–antibody complexes (Lopes-Virella, 1980). A potential limitation of this method stems from the inherent turbidity of lipemic samples or even nonlipemic samples after repeated freezing and thawing. To some extent, automated systems can correct for such turbidity.

The NCEP Guidelines

The Third Report of the NCEP Expert Panel on Detection, Evaluation, and Treatment of High Blood Cholesterol in Adults (Adult Treatment Panel III, or ATP III) was published in 2002 (NCEP, 2002). It presents the updated NCEP evidence-based guidelines for cholesterol testing and management, and provides detailed information on other topics, including the classification of lipids and lipoprotein particles, CHD risk assessment, lifestyle intervention, drug treatment, specific dyslipidemias, and treatment adherence issues. More recently, the NCEP recommendations have been updated in consideration of new clinical trial data (Grundy, 2004).

RELIABILITY OF MEASUREMENTS

NCEP guidelines have shifted the focus from recognizing abnormal and normal cholesterol values to assessing overall cardiovascular risk based on cutoffs for cholesterol, triglycerides, HDL-C, and LDL-C. The adoption of a single set of cutoffs imposes a mandate on clinical laboratories to measure lipids and lipoproteins accurately and precisely. The Laboratory Standardization Panel of NCEP (NCEP, 1995) guidelines are presented in Table 17-8. Note that each test has a single maximum acceptable value for total error that includes assay bias (i.e., a measure of accuracy) and CV (i.e., a measure of imprecision). Total error is calculated as follows:

$$\% \text{ total error} = \% \text{ bias} + 1.96\ (\%\text{CV})$$

For each test, Table 17-8 provides an example of a target bias and CV that, when considered together, would yield the maximum acceptable total error. Note that by using total error, a laboratory can slightly exceed the limit for bias, provided that the CV is sufficiently small to maintain the total error within the guideline (the opposite is also true). For example, cholesterol has a target bias of 3% and a target CV of 3%. A laboratory with a bias of 3.5% and a CV of 2% exceeds the target for bias, even though it still meets the target for CV. However, the total error of 7.5% (i.e., 3.5% + 1.96 × 2%) is acceptable because it is less than the 9% target.

TESTING AND TREATMENT

ATP III introduced several new concepts for the evaluation of hyperlipidemia. Diabetes mellitus is now considered a risk equivalent because it confers a high risk of new CHD within 10 years. This means that for evaluation of elevated cholesterol levels, diabetic patients are treated like patients who already have CHD. Also, ATP III recognized patients with metabolic syndrome (described later) and patients with a high 10-year risk for CHD based on the Framingham risk projections as candidates for intensive intervention and therapy.

Cholesterol Goals

ATP III recommends a complete lipoprotein profile (TC, LDL-C, HDL-C, and triglycerides) as the initial test for evaluating blood cholesterol. Testing should be performed in all adults age 20 and older and should be repeated at least once every 5 years. If testing is performed in the nonfasting state, then only TC and HDL-C can be used. In such circumstances, if the TC is 200 mg/dL or the HDL is <40 mg/dL, then a follow-up profile should be performed. ATP III provides guidelines for acceptable test values and uses LDL-C as the primary target for cholesterol-lowering therapy (Table 17-9). Note that major risk factors (Table 17-10) can modify LDL cholesterol goals (Table 17-11). Therapeutic lifestyle change (TLC) and drug therapy are the two approaches used to reach the LDL-C goal. TLC involves dietary change and increased physical activity, combined with regular follow-up. Regardless of a patient's risk category or LDL goal, TLC represents the first line of therapy, although it may be combined initially with drug therapy when high-risk patients are treated. Note that patients in the moderate-risk category are further subdivided (for drug therapy) based on a Framingham Risk Score, which estimates the 10-year risk of cardiac events based on factors in Table 17-10, as well as

TABLE 17-8
NCEP Guidelines for Acceptable Measurement Error

Analyte	Total error	Bias	CV*
Cholesterol	≤9%	≤3%	≤3%
Triglyceride	≤15%	≤5%	≤5%
HDL-cholesterol	≤13%	≤5%	≤4%†
LDL-cholesterol	≤12%	≤4%	≤4%

HDL, High-density lipoprotein; *LDL,* low-density lipoprotein.
*Coefficient of variation defined as standard deviation/mean × 100.
†Precision criteria applied to HDL-cholesterol levels of 42 mg/dL (1.09 mmol/L) and higher. At lower levels, CV is not used; rather, standard deviation should not exceed 1.7 mg/dL (0.044 mmol/L).

TABLE 17-9
ATP III Classification for LDL, Total and HDL Cholesterol, and Triglyceride Values

LDL Cholesterol	
<100	Optimal
100–129	Near optimal/above optimal
130–159	Borderline high
160–189	High
≥190	Very high
Total Cholesterol	
<200	Desirable
200–239	Borderline high
≥240	High
HDL Cholesterol	
<40	Low
≥60	High
Triglycerides	
<150	Normal
150–199	Borderline high
200–499	High
≥500	Very high

Data from National Cholesterol Education Program Expert Panel: Third Report of the National Cholesterol Education Program Expert Panel on Detection, Evaluation, and Treatment of High Blood Cholesterol in Adults (Adult Treatment Panel III): final report. Circulation 2002;106:3143–3421.
HDL, High-density lipoprotein; *LDL,* low-density lipoprotein.

other factors such as TC and HDL-C (Wilson, 1998). Drug therapy for hyperlipidemia usually consists of four types of medications: statins, fibric acid derivatives, bile acid resins, and nicotinic acid. Some relevant characteristics of these medications are briefly summarized in Table 17-12.

Metabolic Syndrome

This physiologic syndrome is characterized by a constellation of known and emerging risk factors for CHD. Several organizations, including the World Health Organization (WHO) and NCEP, have proposed different definitions for this syndrome; however, risk factors generally include abdominal obesity, atherogenic dyslipidemia (elevated triglycerides, small LDL particles, and low HDL-C), raised blood pressure, insulin resistance (with or without glucose intolerance), and prothrombotic and proinflammatory states. First described as "syndrome X" in the late 1980s, this condition may be present in 20%–25% of adult Americans. In patients with metabolic syndrome, LDL-C is the primary target of therapy; however, patients are usually candidates for more intensive cholesterol-lowering therapy than might be suggested by their LDL-C alone. Other objectives include treatment of the underlying causes (i.e., obesity and physical inactivity) and treatment of associated nonlipid and lipid risk factors (Garber, 2004).

Hypertriglyceridemia

Supported by data from recent meta-analyses, ATP III identifies elevated triglycerides as an independent risk factor for CHD. Factors associated with a high triglyceride level include obesity, physical inactivity, cigarette smoking, excess alcohol intake, high-carbohydrate diets (>60% of energy intake), several diseases (e.g., type 2 diabetes, chronic renal failure, nephritic syndrome), certain drugs (e.g., corticosteroids, estrogens, retinoids, higher doses of β-adrenergic blocking agents), and genetic disorders (e.g., familial combined hyperlipidemia, familial hypertriglyceridemia, familial dysbetalipoproteinemia). In persons with elevated triglycerides, the primary aim of therapy is to achieve the target for LDL-C. In the fasting state, most circulating triglyceride is in VLDL remnant lipoproteins, so non-HDL cholesterol (TC-HDL cholesterol) can be used as a secondary target for therapy. Non-HDL cholesterol includes all apoB-containing lipoproteins but in the fasting state provides a combined assessment of LDL-C and VLDL-C. Treatment plans for hypertriglyceridemia emphasize weight reduction and increased physical activity with borderline high elevations, but include LDL-lowering medications and triglyceride-lowering drugs (nicotinic acid or fibrate) at higher levels. In rare patients with very high triglyceride levels (>500 mg/dL), the initial aim of therapy is to prevent acute pancreatitis.

Emerging Risk Factors

ATP III recognizes additional positive risk factors for CHD, including elevations in Lp(a), remnant lipoproteins, small LDL particles, fibrinogen,

TABLE 17-10
Major Risk Factors That Modify LDL Goals

Cigarette smoking
Hypertension (BP ≥140/190 or on antihypertensive medication)
Low HDL cholesterol (<40 mg/dL)
Family history of premature CHD (CHD in a male first-degree relative <55 years; CHD in a female first-degree relative <65 years)
Age (men ≥ 45; women ≥ 55)
Diabetes mellitus
Preexisting CHD

From National Cholesterol Education Program Expert Panel: Third Report of the National Cholesterol Education Program (NCEP) Expert Panel on Detection, Evaluation, and Treatment of High Blood Cholesterol in Adults (Adult Treatment Panel III): final report. Circulation 2002;106:3143–3421.
BP, Blood pressure; *CHD,* coronary heart disease; *HDL,* high-density lipoprotein.

TABLE 17-11
Risk-Based LDL-C Goals

Risk category	LDL goal (mg/dL)	Initiate TLC	Consider drug therapy
CHD and CHD risk equivalents	<100 *Optional:* <70	≥100	≥100 70–100
Moderately high risk (2+) risk factors* and a Framingham 10-year risk of 10%–20%	<130 *Optional:*	≥130 <100	≥130 100–129
Moderate risk (2+) risk factor* and a Framingham 10-year risk <10%	<130	≥130	≥160
Zero to one risk factor*	<160	≥160	≥190

Data from National Cholesterol Education Program Expert Panel: Third Report of the National Cholesterol Education Program (NCEP) Expert Panel on Detection, Evaluation, and Treatment of High Blood Cholesterol in Adults (Adult Treatment Panel III): final report. Circulation 2002;106:3143–3421; and Grundy SM, Cleeman JI, Merz CN, et al: Coordinating Committee of the National Cholesterol Education Program. Implications of recent clinical trials for the National Cholesterol Education Program Adult Treatment Panel III Guidelines. J Am Coll Cardiol 2004;4:44(3):720–732.
CHD, Coronary heart disease; *LDL,* low-density lipoprotein; *TLC,* therapeutic lifestyle changes.
*Note that modifying risk factors are listed in Table 17-10.

TABLE 17-12
Hyperlipidemia Drugs

Drug class	Primary effects	Secondary effects	Mechanism	Side effects	Examples
Statins	Lower LDL-cholesterol (20%–60%)	Small decreases in elevated triglyceride; modest increase in HDL-cholesterol	Inhibit HMG-CoA reductase	Rare GI disturbances, liver problems, rhabdomyolysis	Lovastatin Simvastatin Pravastatin Atorvastatin
Fibric acid derivatives	Lower triglycerides (20%–50%)	Small increases in HDL (10%–15%)	Not clearly defined; may decrease the catabolism of HDL, increase the activity of LPL, and inhibit the hepatic synthesis of VLDL	GI disturbances, increased likelihood of cholesterol gallstones, may increase effects of warfarin, and tendency of statins to cause rhabdomyolysis	Gemfibrozil Fenofibrate
Bile acid resins	Lower LDL-cholesterol (10%–20%)	Bind bile acids in intestine, leading to excretion	Mild GI disturbances	Cholestyramine	Colestipol Colesevelam
Niacin (nicotinic acid)	Lowers triglycerides (20%–50%)	Raises HDL-cholesterol (15%–35%)	May inhibit mobilization of fatty acids in adipocytes via G-protein–coupled receptor, HM74A, leading to decreased VLDL production by liver; reduce LDL-cholesterol (10%–20% decrease)	GI disturbances, flushing, chills, pruritus, liver problems, gout, elevated blood sugar	Niacin

GI, Gastrointestinal; *HDL,* high-density lipoprotein; *HmG-CoA,* 3-hydroxy-3-methylglutaryl-coenzyme A; *LDL,* low-density lipoprotein; *LPL,* lipoprotein lipase; *VLDL,* very-low-density lipoprotein.

homocysteine, high-sensitivity C-reactive protein (hs-CRP), impaired fasting plasma glucose (110–125 mg/dL), and preexisting subclinical atherosclerosis (as evidenced by myocardial ischemia on exercise testing, carotid intimal–medial thickening, and/or coronary artery calcium deposition). The links between some of these factors and CHD are obvious or are discussed elsewhere; however, others require expanded consideration. For example, elevated homocysteine levels have been linked to medications, as well as to genetic, disease and lifestyle conditions, and may contribute to CHD at least partially by exerting toxic effects on the endothelium. The links between hs-CRP (a marker of chronic inflammation) and fibrinogen (a marker of prothrombotic states) and CHD at this point remain largely statistical; clear mechanisms have not been established. Elevation of apoB (present in chylomicrons, VLDL, IDL, and LDL), decreases in apoA-I (present mostly in HDL), and increases in the apoB/apoA-I ratio have also been associated with increased risk of CHD (Walldius, 2004). Although these risk factors are not used widely for screening purposes, they may be useful in defining risk status and refining treatment in patients already known to be at risk.

Children

Current evidence indicates that atherosclerotic lesions can begin in childhood; children with high blood cholesterol levels typically maintain high blood cholesterol through adulthood. In an effort to intervene early in children with an atherosclerotic predisposition, guidelines for assessing CHD risk in children and adolescents have been promulgated by organizations such as the NCEP (NCEP Expert Panel on Children and Adolescents) (NCEP, 1992) and the American Heart Association (Kavey, 2003). Current recommendations support selective screening (starting at 2 years of age) of children and adolescents with a family history of premature cardiovascular disease or those with at least one parent with high blood cholesterol. Table 17-13 classifies these children by total and LDL-C levels. These recommendations do not support the universal laboratory screening of children and adolescents.

Intervention aimed at reducing risk is recommended when the averaged results of three fasting lipid profiles are above the cutoffs for TC and LDL described earlier, with elevated triglycerides (>150 mg/dL) or decreased HDL-C (<35 mg/dL). As in adults, intervention focuses on a search for medical causes of lipid abnormalities, TLC, and pharmacologic intervention when necessary.

Lipids, Lipoproteins, and Disease

Lipoprotein and lipid levels are used to predict CHD and form the basis of the NCEP guidelines discussed earlier. However, for many years, the Fredrickson Classification (alluded to in Table 17-3) was used to characterize lipid disorders (Hansen, 1998). The Fredrickson Classification used electrophoresis and a standing plasma test for CM to correlate clinical disease syndromes with laboratory phenotypes (Fredrickson, 1967). Note that each phenotype is not a specific disease but rather a variety of disorders that affect the same lipoproteins and therefore express the same lipid pattern. Thus treatment is usually the same for all disorders falling within the same phenotype. One limitation of this system is that it does not consider low HDL as a risk factor for CHD. In recent years, the Fredrickson Classification has proved less useful given modern analytic techniques and an evolving understanding of the genetics of these disorders. Nevertheless, the nomenclature for a few pathognomonic syndromes (e.g., Type 1 and Type 3 hyperlipidemias) has remained in use. Some pertinent details of the Fredrickson Classification are presented in Table 17-14.

As our understanding of lipids, lipoprotein metabolism, and genetics has evolved, far more complex systems for describing clinical lipid disorders have been conceived. Presently, no ideal scheme to categorize these disorders is available. They can arise from lifestyle or secondary causes, as

TABLE 17-13
Classification of Total and LDL-Cholesterol in Children: Targeted Fasting Screen in Children >2 Years of Age With Family History of Dyslipidemia or Premature CHD

Category	Total cholesterol (mg/dL)	LDL-cholesterol (mg/dL)
Acceptable	<170	<110
Borderline	171–199	111–129
High	≥200	≥130

From Kavey RE, Daniels SR, Lauer RM, et al: American Heart Association: American Heart Association guidelines for primary prevention of atherosclerotic cardiovascular disease beginning in childhood. J Pediatr 2003;142(4):368–372.
CHD, Coronary heart disease; *LDL,* low-density lipoprotein.

TABLE 17-14
Pertinent Details of the Fredrickson Classification

Type	Refrigerator test	Gel electrophoresis	Clinical presentation
1	Positive; clear plasma	Normal	Eruptive xanthoma; acute, recurrent pancreatitis in early childhood; lipids improve on low-fat diet
2a	Negative; clear plasma	Increased β band	Xanthelasma, tendon xanthoma; premature coronary disease; autosomal dominant familial inheritance; commonly known as familial hypercholesterolemia
2b	Negative; cloudy plasma; increased β and pre-β band	Isolated xanthelasma may be present; premature coronary disease; autosomal dominant pattern; affected family members must have varied patterns (e.g., isolated hypertriglyceridemia, isolated hypercholesterolemia, combined hyperlipidemia) to meet diagnostic criteria for familial combined hyperlipidemia	
3	Occasional cloudy plasma; increased pre-β band; eruptive xanthoma and palmar xanthoma; premature coronary disease; autosomal recessive pattern; a secondary cause of dyslipidemia, such as hypothyroidism, can unmask type 3, and treatment of the secondary condition can return lipids to normal		
4	Negative; cloudy plasma; increased α_2 band	May or may not be associated with premature coronary disease	
5	Positive; cloudy plasma; increased α_2 band	Eruptive xanthoma; may be associated with pancreatitis; may be associated with premature coronary disease	

well as from mutations in genes encoding apolipoproteins, apolipoprotein receptors, or enzymes of lipoprotein metabolism. Some genes (e.g., apoA-I, apoC-III, apoA-IV) are in close proximity and share similar response elements, allowing a single mutation to alter multiple aspects of lipoprotein metabolism. The following disorders of lipoprotein metabolism are categorized on the basis of laboratory findings. Lifestyle factors affecting lipid profiles and causes of secondary hyperlipidemia are listed in Table 17-15 in association with their most common laboratory presentation. As with the genetic dyslipidemias, these factors can produce overlapping and somewhat variable lipoprotein profiles. In Figures 17-5 and 17-6, some of the disorders described later are incorporated into the schemes of forward and reverse cholesterol transport, so that their cause and pathogenesis may be more readily understood.

HIGH CHOLESTEROL WITH HIGH LDL-C

These disorders share one feature—hyperbetalipoproteinemia (Fredrickson Type 2A), characterized by elevated LDL-C and normal triglycerides. It is associated with a high cardiac risk that is not surprising given the elevations in LDL, a highly atherogenic particle. This is a commonly encountered laboratory presentation.

Polygenic (Nonfamilial) Hypercholesterolemia

Polygenic (nonfamilial) hypercholesterolemia is a general term used to describe individuals for whom the cause of hypercholesterolemia is likely multifactorial (Soutar, 1998). Although some of the causative factors in this disease are thought to be genetic, before a patient's hypercholesterolemia

TABLE 17-15
Lifestyle Factors and Causes of Secondary Dyslipidemia

Lipoprotein profile	Secondary causes	Lifestyle factors
High cholesterol and high LDL-C with or without low HDL-C	Hypothyroidism and nephrotic syndrome Medications such as thiazide diuretics and steroids Chronic obstructive liver disease Cholestatic liver disease (primary biliary cirrhosis and related diseases)	Obesity Excess dietary cholesterol and/or saturated fat ApoE-4 may increase susceptibility
High triglycerides with normal total and LDL-C with or without low HDL-C	Medications such as thiazide diuretics, estrogens, corticosteroids, retinoids, cyclosporine, and beta-blockers (without intrinsic sympathomimetic) Insulin resistance/diabetes Chronic renal failure and nephrotic syndrome Antipsychotic drugs (clozapine/olanzapine)	Obesity Physical inactivity Cigarette smoking Excess alcohol intake High-carbohydrate diets
High cholesterol and high triglycerides with or without low HDL-C	Medications, notably high-dose steroids or cyclosporine Severe hypothyroidism, diabetes/insulin resistance, and nephrotic syndrome	Obesity HIV antiretroviral drugs
Isolated low HDL-C	Medications such as isotretinoin, probucol, anabolic steroids, beta blockers, and certain progestogens	Physical inactivity Increased body weight High-carbohydrate, low-fat diets
Isolated high HDL-C	Medications such as phenytoin, phenobarbital, rifampicin, griseofulvin, and estrogens	Alcohol intake

HDL-C, High-density lipoprotein cholesterol; *HIV,* human immunodeficiency virus; *LDL-C,* low-density lipoprotein cholesterol.

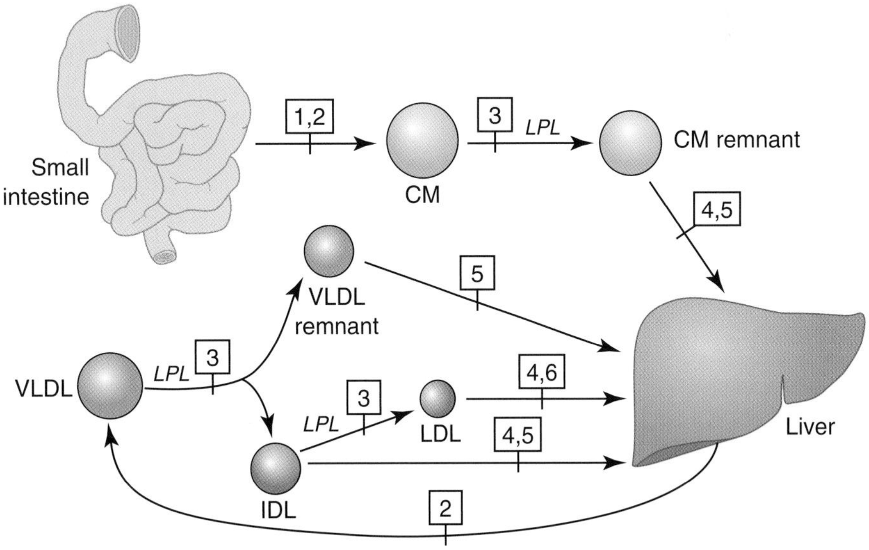

1 - Chylomicron retention (Apo B-48 defect)
2 - Hypobetalipoproteinemia/Abetalipoproteinemia
3 - LPL deficiency/Apo C II deficiency
4 - Familial hypercholesterolemia
5 - Dysbetalipoproteinemia (Type III hyperlipoproteinemia, associated with Apo-E-2)
6 - Familial defective Apo B

Figure 17-5 Disorders associated with the transport of lipids. *Apo,* Apolipoprotein; *CM,* chylomicron; *IDL,* intermediate-density lipoprotein; *LPL,* lipoprotein lipase; *VLDL,* very-low-density lipoprotein.

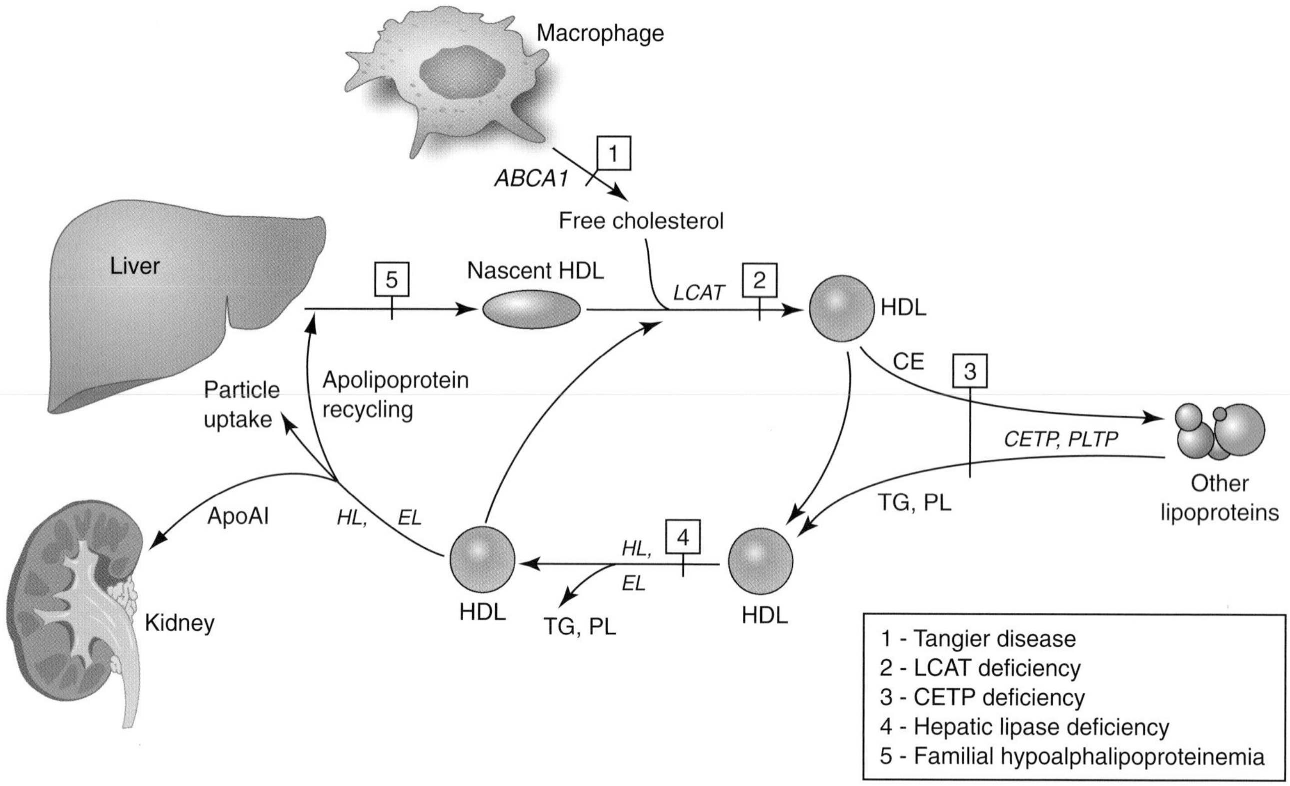

Figure 17-6 Disorders associated with the reverse transport of lipids. *ABCA1,* Adenosine triphosphate (ATP)-binding cassette protein A-1; *Apo,* apolipoprotein; *CE,* cholesterol ester; *CETP,* cholesterol ester transfer protein; *EL,* endothelial lipase; *HDL,* high-density lipoprotein; *HL,* hepatic lipase; *LCAT,* lecithin:cholesterol acyltransferase; *PL,* phospholipids; *PLTP,* phospholipid transfer protein; *TG,* triglycerides.

is labeled "polygenic," secondary and familial hypercholesterolemia (autosomal dominant) must be ruled out. Approximately 85% of the hypercholesterolemia in the population may fall into this category. Some clinicians use this term to describe patients who develop age-related increases in cholesterol that do not respond to lifestyle modification.

Familial Hypercholesterolemia

Familial hypercholesterolemia (FH) is an autosomal dominant disorder caused by one of several mutations in the LDL-receptor gene on chromosome 19. The resulting defective receptors cannot bind or clear LDL from the circulation (Hobbs, 1992). Several hundred mutations have been identified in the LDL receptor gene, and they affect most aspects of receptor synthesis, transport, and function (Fig. 17-7). This genetic heterogeneity has led to variability in presentation and responsiveness to therapy. Heterozygous FH occurs in 1 in 500 individuals and is associated with premature atherosclerotic disease. Affected heterozygous men usually present in their fourth decade and women 10–15 years later. Untreated LDL-C levels are typically >220 mg/dL. Further, FH heterozygotes exhibit LDL-C levels that vary with environmental factors and genetics. Homozygous FH presents in childhood with LDL levels >400 mg/dL. Vascular deposition of lipid results in premature symptomatic CHD. In addition, homozygotes are less affected by environmental factors in terms of LDL-C levels. Large valvular and supravalvular cholesterol deposits can produce symptomatic aortic stenosis. Other stigmata of the disease include corneal arcus, tendinous xanthomata, and xanthelasma. These stigmata generally develop in early childhood in homozygotes, and by adulthood in heterozygotes. Statins, which inhibit 3-hydroxy-3-methylglutaryl-CoA (HmG-CoA) reductase, may be effective; however, because these drugs may act indirectly by increasing LDL receptor activity, not all heterozygous patients will normalize their LDL-C despite receiving maximum doses of statins. Homozygous patients have two abnormal LDL receptor genes, making statin drugs ineffective unless combined with apheresis (Ose, 1999). Patients with homozygous FH are classified into two groups on the basis of tests for LDL receptor (LDLR) activity in skin fibroblasts: patients with less than 2% of normal LDLR activity are receptor-negative; patients with 2%–25% of normal LDLR activity are receptor-defective. Receptor-negative patients rarely live past the second decade; receptor-defective patients often develop significant atherosclerotic disease by the age of 30 years.

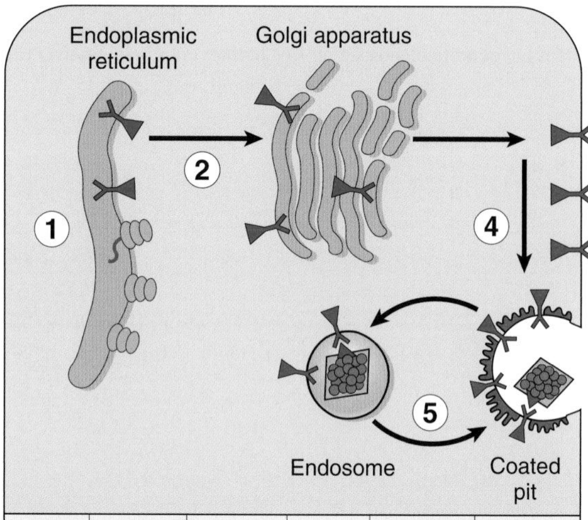

Mutation class	Synthesis	Transport	Binding	Clustering	Recycling
I	X				
II	———	→ X			
III	———	———	→ X		
IV	———	———	———	→ X	
V	———	———	———	———	→ X

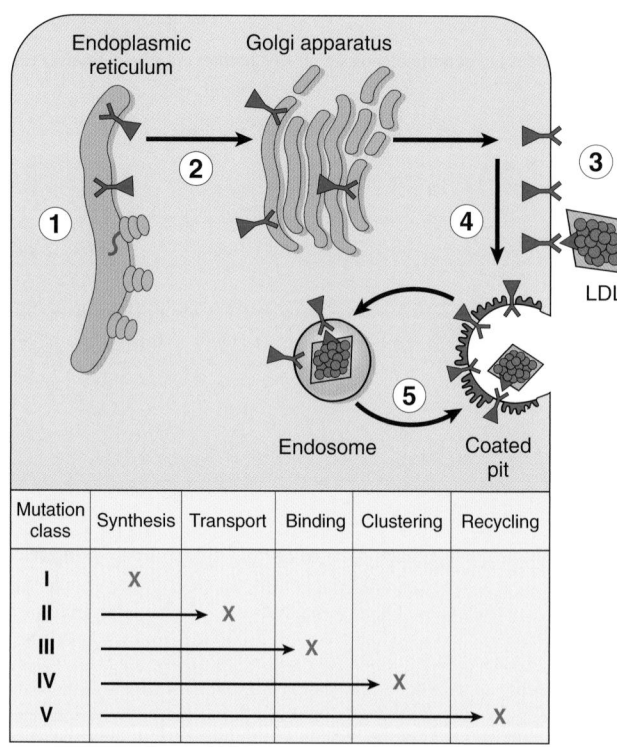

Figure 17-7 Classification of low-density lipoprotein (LDL) receptor mutations based on abnormal function of the mutant protein. These mutations disrupt the receptor's synthesis in the endoplasmic reticulum, transport to the Golgi complex, binding of apoprotein ligands, clustering in coated pits, and recycling in endosomes. Each class is heterogeneous at the DNA level. *(Modified with permission from Hobbs HH, Russell DW, Brown MS, Goldstein JL. The LDL receptor locus in familial hypercholesterolemia: mutational analysis of a membrane protein. Annu Rev Genet 1990;24:133–170. Copyright 1990 by Annual Reviews.)*

Familial Defective ApoB

Familial defective ApoB is an autosomal dominant disorder of the apoB gene on chromosome 2 that interferes with the recognition of apoB-100 by the LDL receptor (Hansen, 1998). The disease results from a missense mutation *(Arg3500Gln)* in the LDLR-binding domain of ApoB-100, although other mutations that occur less frequently can cause this disease. Estimated frequency in the population is 1 in 750. Patients with familial defective apoB have similar physical stigmata to those of FH: tendinous xanthomata, xanthelasma, and premature coronary disease. Untreated LDL-C levels can overlap those seen in FH but tend to be slightly lower. Further, patients with familial defective ApoB have levels of plasma LDL-C comparable with those in FH heterozygotes. Statin drugs are effective.

Sitosterolemia

Sitosterolemia is an extremely rare autosomal recessive disorder wherein phytosterols (plant sterols) are absorbed and accumulate in plasma and peripheral tissues. This disease results from mutations in the *ABCG8* or *ABCG5* gene, both of which are located at chromosome 2p21. Mutations in these genes disrupt the ABCG5 or 8 proteins from forming the proper channel to pump back absorbed plant sterols into the intestinal lumen, as well as the ability of liver to secrete absorbed phytosterols into bile. Most patients identified with sitosterolemia have had high plasma LDL-C levels during childhood. Children present with tendinous xanthomata and normal to high levels of LDL. Premature CHD is present. Cholesterol levels may be normal or elevated. Many common assays do not differentiate between cholesterol and plant sterols, and measurement of plasma phytosterols is necessary to confirm the diagnosis. Phytosterols are positively identified using gas–liquid chromatography in lipids extracted from plasma. A distinctive clinical presentation of sitosterolemia is the occurrence of low-level hemolysis. Red blood cells may be incorporating the plant sterols into their membranes. Diagnosis of sitosterolemia should be considered if the patient presents with xanthomatosis and hypercholesterolemia yet has parents who have normal levels of cholesterol. Treatment consists of restricting dietary phytosterol intake (Patel, 1998) and using ezetimibe and a bile acid sequestrant to limit sterol accumulation.

Autosomal Dominant Hypercholesterolemia

Autosomal dominant hypercholesterolemia (ADH) is an autosomal dominant disorder of the *PCSK9* gene on chromosome 1 that is involved in cholesterol homeostasis in the liver (Abifadel, 2003). Two known mutations of the gene may lead to gain of function of *PCSK9* (*S127R* and *F216L*). Individuals with gain-of-function mutations present clinically with increased plasma levels of LDL-C and exhibit higher risk of coronary heart disease. Relatively little is known about the frequency of ADH since the discovery of the mutation in three families in 2003. However, more gain-of-function *PCSK9* patients have been reported *(D374Y)*. *PCSK9* is a member of the proprotein convertase family of proteins. Although the mechanism of action is still unclear, it is known that *PCSK9* is secreted into plasma and binds to LDLR on the cell surface. This leads to endocytosis and intracellular degradation of the LDLR. Consequently, gain of function of *PCSK9* is thought be involved in decreasing levels of LDLR protein. In addition to the gain-of-function mutations, loss-of-function mutations have been found. These missense *(R46L)* and nonsense (*Y142X* and *C697X*) mutations have led to hypocholesterolemia in patients.

Autosomal Recessive Hypercholesterolemia

Autosomal recessive hypercholesterolemia (ARH) involves the ARH gene found on chromosome 1. ARH is also known as *LDLRAP1.* In these patients, LDLR expression is normal, but LDL clearance rates are low and comparable with those of patients with homozygous FH. ARH is thought to express a protein that is involved in internalization of the LDLR–LDL complex. Plasma levels of LDL-C in ARH patients tend to be between FH heterozygotes and FH homozygotes. The onset of atherosclerotic disease presents later than in homozygous FH patients. ARH patients can present with large, bulk xanthomas. Patients with ARH respond to lipid-lowering medications. However, most ARH patients are maintained on LDL apheresis as part of their treatment.

HIGH TRIGLYCERIDES WITH NORMAL CHOLESTEROL

These disorders are related to elevations of triglyceride-rich particles, namely, chylomicrons or VLDL (Fredrickson Types 1 and 4). This commonly encountered laboratory presentation is usually due to hyperprebetalipoproteinemia (VLDL) and may be due to secondary causes such as excess alcohol or a high-carbohydrate diet. LDL and LDL-C are typically normal.

Diabetic Dyslipidemia

Diabetic dyslipidemia consists of atherogenic dyslipidemia (high triglycerides, low HDL, and small dense LDL) in persons with type 2 diabetes. Current evidence supports the treatment of LDL-C as the primary target in patients with this disorder. Although cholesterol levels may be within the "normal" range, treatment is often directed at LDL-C because diabetes is viewed as a CHD risk equivalent and thus is associated with a lower than "normal" target cholesterol value (see Table 17-11).

Familial Hypertriglyceridemia

Familial hypertriglyceridemia occurs along with other lipoprotein abnormalities as part of a number of familial hyperlipidemia syndromes. Isolated hypertriglyceridemia (or Type 4 hyperlipidemia) is a relatively common autosomal dominant disorder, affecting approximately 1:300 to 1:50 people in the United States, depending on the criteria used for diagnosis. The disorder usually presents in adulthood with fasting triglyceride levels in the 200–500 mg/dL range. The pathophysiology remains elusive, but VLDL triglyceride production is increased in the setting of normal apoB production, resulting in the formation of "fluffy," triglyceride-rich VLDL particles. Some kindreds have premature CHD; however, it is unclear whether the CHD results from hypertriglyceridemia or from the frequently coexisting exacerbating factors, obesity and insulin resistance (Brunzell, 1983).

Lipoprotein Lipase Deficiency (Hyperlipoproteinemia Type 1 or Hyperchylomicronemia)

Lipoprotein lipase deficiency is a rare, autosomal recessive disorder that presents in childhood with abdominal pain and pancreatitis. Defective or absent LPL creates an inability to clear chylomicrons, creating the classic "type 1" chylomicronemia syndrome (see Tables 17-3 and 17-14). Fasting triglyceride levels may be >100 mg/dL and may rise to >10,000 mg/dL postprandially. Patients with LPL deficiency do not develop premature CHD, implying that chylomicrons themselves are not atherogenic. Treatment with a low fat diet to reduce chylomicron input is effective; fat-soluble vitamins should be supplemented, and drug therapy can be considered to lower endogenous VLDL production (Brunzell, 1995). Heterozygotes have half-normal LPL activity and occur in the general population at a frequency of 1 in 500. It has been speculated that heterozygous individuals with the defective *LPL* gene constitute a subset of families with familial combined hyperlipidemia (Babirak, 1989).

ApoC-II Deficiency

ApoC-II is an activating cofactor for LPL. Thus, the absence of apoC-II creates a functional LPL deficiency, which presents similarly to LPL deficiency as a rare autosomal recessive form of familial hyperchylomicronemia. The disorder presents in children and young adults as recurrent bouts of abdominal pain and pancreatitis. Several defects in the apoC-II gene have been described (Fojo, 1992). Patients can be treated with plasma transfusions during severe hypertriglyceridemia providing apoC-II, which will activate endogenous LPL.

ApoC-III Excess

ApoC-III excess interferes with the activity of lipoprotein lipase and binds to the carboxy-terminal portion of apolipoprotein B, preventing the binding of lipoproteins to the LDL receptor. Excess apoC-III, especially within the apoB-containing lipoproteins LDL and VLDL, may be an independent risk factor for CHD. ApoC-III levels can be increased in patients with diabetes type 2, hyperbilirubinemia, kidney deficiency, and thyroid dysfunction; further, genetic mutations in the apoC-III gene are known. In addition to genetic factors, serum apoC-III is affected by age and alcohol consumption in men and women; oral contraceptive use in women has also been associated with high levels of apoC-III. For males and females in their youth, post-pubescent status and oral contraceptive use have been shown to affect apoC-III levels. Several genetic polymorphisms of the apoC-III gene are known. They include point mutations at -641T/C, -482C/T, -455T/C, 1100C/T, 3175C/G, and 3026T/G of the start site of the apoC-III gene. The mutations at -455T/C and 1100C/T are more common in Caucasian males and boys. It is thought that the point mutation at -455T/C affects a transcription factor–binding site associated with insulin response. Consequently, lack of response to insulin at the apoC-III promoter, which downregulates apoC-III transcription, is thought to contribute to high levels of triglycerides in plasma. Genetic mutations at other genes such as *APOA4* or carrying APOE E4 alleles have been suggested to influence serum apoC-III levels as well.

ApoA-V

ApoA-V is a highly hydrophobic protein that has a preference for binding to lipids and HDL particles. The function of ApoA-V has been hypothesized as being involved in VLDL assembly; in addition, it has been postulated that ApoA-V may be involved in activation of LPL-mediated triglyceride hydrolysis. Consequently, low levels of ApoA-V may promote hypertriglyceridemia, whereas high levels of ApoA-V would have the opposite effect. One variant of ApoA-V has been found in humans that has a strong correlation with hypertriglyceridemic patients. The actual function of ApoA-V and its role in triglyceride metabolism require further investigation.

HIGH CHOLESTEROL WITH HIGH TRIGLYCERIDES

These disorders are related to elevations of LDL and triglycerides (Fredrickson Types 2B and 3). Familial combined hyperlipidemia (2B) is the most common primary hyperlipoproteinemia and presents with a variety of lipoprotein phenotypes within a family. The relatively rare dysbetalipoproteinemia (Type 3) is characterized by an abnormal LDL (IDL) that appears as a broad beta electrophoretic band and distinguishes it from familial combined hyperlipidemia. These disorders are associated with increased cardiac risk because of the elevated LDL.

Familial Combined Hyperlipidemia (Type 2B)

Familial combined hyperlipidemia (Type 2B) is a relatively common disorder wherein affected individuals may have simple hypercholesterolemia, simple hypertriglyceridemia, or a mixed defect. Because of the disorder's phenotypic heterogeneity and the lack of a definitive biochemical marker for the disorder, considerable overlap and confusion with other forms of hyperlipidemia have occurred. Estimated frequency in the population is 1 in 100. Affected families must have more than one pattern of lipid disorder to meet diagnostic criteria for familial combined. The genetic basis is unknown (deGraaf, 1998) and appears to be multifactorial, although inheritance was thought initially to be autosomal codominant. The specific gene or genes explaining the defect have not been fully elucidated.

Acquired Combined Hyperlipidemia

Acquired combined hyperlipidemia is common in patients who have metabolic syndrome. As the name suggests, the disease stems from a syndrome of conditions that include type 2 diabetes mellitus, hypertension, central obesity, and coronary heart disease. It is thought that the liver increases the production of VLDL through high levels of free fatty acids in plasma. As a result, the increased VLDL levels mature to LDL until this process is saturated. When LDL levels get high enough, VLDL levels follow, causing both hypercholesterolemia and hypertriglyceridemia.

Dysbetalipoproteinemia (Type 3)

ApoE is present on chylomicrons, VLDL, IDL, and chylomicron remnants. By binding to the LDL receptor, and probably other receptors, apoE helps to clear these lipoproteins from circulation. Three common electrophoretic isoforms of apoE are known, each form attributable to several different genetic mutations. The most common isoform is E-3, followed by E-4 and E-2. ApoE-2 has lower affinity for the LDL receptor (less than 2% of binding ability of E-3), thus lipoprotein particles accumulate in the blood of patients who are homozygous for E-2. However, although individuals with this genotype are relatively common in the Caucasian population (1 in 100), expression of an overt Type 3 phenotype occurs in 1 to 5 per 5000 individuals. Thus, the manifestation of the Type 3 hyperlipidemia phenotype is thought to contribute to the disease. Secondary factors implicated in the manifestation of disease include obesity, diabetes mellitus, hypothyroidism, and medications such as protease inhibitors.

Type 3 hyperlipidemia primarily affects adults and men more commonly than women. Symptomatic individuals typically have roughly equal elevations of cholesterol and triglycerides, presence of β-VLDL or cholesterol-enriched remnants of intestinal chylomicrons, and hepatic VLDL, xanthomas, and premature vascular disease such as coronary heart disease and peripheral artery disease. Type 3 has a pathognomonic feature: a broad abnormal band between VLDL and LDL known as "abnormally migrating beta lipoprotein," or β-VLDL. The cholesterol content in VLDL is also increased, and measurement of the VLDL-C/triglyceride ratio is a useful screen. Normally, the VLDL-C/triglyceride ratio is 0.2; typical Type 3 patients have a ratio >0.3. Day-to-day variation in lipid levels is more pronounced than usual. Other clinical stigmata include palmar xanthoma and tuberoeruptive xanthoma on elbows, knees, and buttocks. Premature atherosclerosis is highly prevalent and, unlike familial hypercholesterolemia, more often involves abdominal and femoral arteries. The atherosclerosis appears reversible with treatment of the lipid disorder (Kuo, 1988). Patients are responsive to low fat diets, weight loss, and most classes of lipid-lowering drugs.

Hepatic Lipase Deficiency

Generally resulting from mutations of the HL gene, this rare familial disorder is associated with combined hyperlipidemia characterized by TC levels of 250–1500 mg/dL and TG levels of 400–8000 mg/dL. Levels of HDL-C are normal or increased. Physical stigmata include palmar and tuberoeruptive xanthoma; the risk of atherosclerosis is thought to be increased. In contrast to Type 3 hyperlipidemia, although β-VLDL is increased, the TC/TG ratio is not increased. The triglyceride content of all lipoproteins is increased 3-fold to 5-fold. Families with compound heterozygous mutations have been described (Connelly, 1998). Patients with hepatic lipase deficiency are able to convert large VLDL to smaller VLDL particles; however, they are unable to convert VLDL to IDL and also LDL from IDL. HDL and LDL particles from hepatic lipase deficiency patients are large and enriched with triglycerides.

Cholesterol 7-Alpha-Hydroxylase Deficiency

Cholesterol 7-alpha-hydroxylase deficiency is a recessive disorder of the *CYP7A1* gene that encodes cholesterol 7-alpha-hydroxylase protein. *CYP7A1* encodes an enzyme that is involved in the first step of the classical pathway for bile acid biosynthesis. The few patients who present with this rare disease exhibit not only high cholesterol, but also high triglycerides in plasma. Very little is known about the disease. However, it has been reported that the few patients diagnosed with this disease are resistant to statin therapy, although the same patients managed to lower their plasma cholesterol with atorvastatin and niacin therapy. Lack of cholesterol 7-alpha-hydroxylase is thought to reduce hepatic LDLR activity; however, because so few patients have been identified with this condition, more information and patients will be necessary to confirm the relationship between the deficiency and its clinical presentation.

LOW TOTAL CHOLESTEROL AND TRIGLYCERIDE

These uncommon disorders are associated with defective apoB synthesis or metabolism, leading to low or nonexistent levels of apo-B lipoproteins such as CM, VLDL, and LDL. Triglycerides and cholesterol are low. Fat-soluble vitamin deficiencies are common. Low fat diet therapy is required.

Abetalipoproteinemia

Abetalipoproteinemia (also known as Bassen-Kornzweig syndrome) is a rare, autosomal recessive disorder involving mutations in the *MTTP* gene located on chromosome 4. *MTTP* encodes an 894 amino acid protein called MTP, or microsomal triglyceride transfer protein (MTP). MTP protein forms a heterodimer with a chaperone protein called protein disulfide isomerase (PDI) in the endoplasmic reticulum. Mutations in *MTTP* affect its binding to PDI and its ability to transfer lipids. Clinically, abetalipoproteinemia patients present with undetectable plasma apoB containing lipoproteins. During apoB translation, MTP incorporates lipids onto the nascent apoB protein and prevents it from proteasomal degradation. Consequently, the lack of functional MTP still allows for apoB protein production; however, the protein ends up misfolded and destroyed by endoplasmic reticulum (ER)-associated degradation mechanisms. Neither apoB-48 nor apoB-100 is present in plasma. Patients present in childhood or early adolescence with fat malabsorption, hypolipidemia, retinitis pigmentosa, cerebellar ataxia, and acanthocytosis. Laboratory testing usually shows decreased apoB, triglycerides, and TC (typically <50 mg/dL). Patients develop fat-soluble vitamin deficiencies caused by malabsorption of vitamins A, K, and E. Vitamin D does not require chylomicrons for absorption and therefore is typically not deficient. Because both vitamin A and vitamin K have transport systems independent of lipoproteins, clinical deficiency is not as severe as that seen with vitamin E, which not only depends upon chylomicrons for absorption but relies upon VLDL and LDL for delivery to tissues. Children with this disorder respond to a low-fat diet rich in medium-chain fatty acids and supplemented with high-dose fat-soluble vitamins, especially vitamin E. Replacing vitamin E stores improves the retinal and peripheral neuropathic symptoms. Heterozygotes have no symptoms and no evidence of abnormal plasma lipid levels.

Hypobetalipoproteinemia

Hypobetalipoproteinemia is an autosomal dominant disorder explained by nonsense or missense mutations in the *apoB* gene, leading to synthesis of various truncated forms of apoB. Severity of disease depends on the type of apoB synthesized. Generally, patients have very low LDL-C levels (Wu, 1999). The familial form is associated with a decreased risk for cardiovascular disease. Homozygous individuals have TC levels <50 mg/dL and present at an early age with fat malabsorption and low plasma cholesterol levels. Heterozygous individuals are usually asymptomatic and have low plasma LDL concentrations. They develop progressive neurologic degenerative disease, retinitis pigmentosa, and acanthocytosis, similar to patients with abetalipoproteinemia. Complications from vitamin E deficiency can be prevented by treatment with very high doses of vitamin E (100–300 mg/kg/day). Heterozygous individuals have LDL-C levels approximately half that of age- and sex-matched controls, but are otherwise asymptomatic.

Chylomicron Retention Disease

Chylomicron retention disease (Anderson's disease) presents in childhood with fat malabsorption and low levels of plasma lipids. This syndrome is distinct from abetalipoproteinemia, as only apoB-48 appears to be affected. Further, the disease is characterized by hypocholesterolemia, chronic diarrhea, failure to thrive, and deficiency of fat-soluble vitamins (vitamin E in particular); the latter can lead to neurologic deficits. The genetic abnormality associated with this disorder is linked to the *SARA2* gene on chromosome 5q3 that encodes the Sar1 GTPase protein. This protein belongs to a family of GTPases that govern the intracellular trafficking of proteins in protein-coated vesicles (Jones, 2003). Sar1 GTPase most likely plays a role in the steps involving intracellular trafficking of newly synthesized apoB-48–containing lipoproteins in the enterocytes. After proper folding and lipidation in the ER by the MTP, apoB-48 lipoproteins leave the ER through pre-chylomicron transfer vesicles (PCTVs). These vesicles fuse with a recipient Golgi membrane and are ultimately secreted. The precise role of Sar1 GTPase in intracellular trafficking has not been elucidated.

ISOLATED LOW HDL-C

Low HDL levels are associated with CHD, presumably because insufficient HDL is available to participate in reverse cholesterol transport, the process by which cholesterol is eliminated from peripheral tissues.

Familial Hypoalphalipoproteinemia

Familial hypoalphalipoproteinemia is a common autosomal dominant disorder that occurs in 1 in 400 people. Affected men have HDL-C levels <30 mg/dL, and women have HDL-C levels <40 mg/dL. The criteria for familial hypoalphalipoproteinemia include the following: (1) low HDL cholesterol in the presence of normal VLDL cholesterol and LDL cholesterol levels; (2) absence of diseases or factors that lead to secondary effects of hypoalphalipoproteinemia; and (3) the presence of a similar lipoprotein pattern in a first-degree relative. Half of affected families appear to have hepatic lipase or apoA-I/C-III/A-IV gene defects (Breslow, 1995). Mutations in the *ABCA1* gene, the same gene that is mutated in Tangier disease, have been associated with some cases of hypoalphalipoproteinemia. Premature CHD is typically present.

ApoA-I Deficiency and ApoC-III Deficiency

ApoA-I deficiency with ApoC-III deficiency is a rare autosomal recessive condition characterized by a reduction in the formation of HDL. It has been linked to point mutations in the *apoA-I* gene and to deletions/gene rearrangements at the *apoA-I/C-III/A-IV* gene locus on the long arm of chromosome 11 (Assman, 1995). HDL-C levels are <5 mg/dL; both corneal opacification and premature coronary disease are seen in some patients.

ApoA-I Variants

ApoA-I variants are rare, specific amino acid substitutions in the *apoA-I* gene. They have been shown to increase catabolism of HDL and apoA-I (Breslow, 1995). Homozygous patients generally present with autosomal recessive inheritance of low HDL-C levels (approximately 10 mg/dL), corneal opacifications, xanthomata, and premature coronary disease. Heterozygous individuals may present with low HDL-C. One mutation, *apoA-I-Milano*, shows autosomal dominant inheritance and is associated with low HDL-C levels but is not associated with premature coronary disease (Calabresi, 1997).

Tangier Disease

Tangier disease is a rare autosomal recessive disorder characterized by complete absence of HDL due to a mutation in the *ABCA1* gene on chromosome 9. The mutation leads to an inability to effectively transfer cholesterol and phospholipids from within the cell onto nascent apoA1 proteins in plasma. The resulting buildup of cholesterol within the cell becomes toxic. LDL cholesterol is reduced. In the homozygous state, patients present with low or undetectable HDL in plasma, hepatosplenomegaly, peripheral neuropathy, orange tonsils, and premature coronary disease (Rust, 1999). In normal cells, the ABCA1 protein enables cholesterol to exit the cell, upon which it combines with apoA-I to form the HDL. The small amount of HDL that is present in patients with this disorder differs qualitatively from normal HDL.

Lecithin : Cholesterol Acyltransferase Deficiency

Lecithin : cholesterol acyltransferase (LCAT) deficiency is characterized by corneal opacities, normochromic anemia, and renal failure in young adults. It is a very rare autosomal recessive disorder. The disease occurs in two forms: a classic (or complete) familial LCAT deficiency and a milder partial deficiency phenotype known as fish-eye disease (Peelman, 1999). In complete deficiency, HDL-C levels are typically <10 mg/dL, but total cholesterol levels are normal or high. Without LCAT, most cholesterol remains unesterified and HDL synthesis is impeded. Patients with complete LCAT deficiency have anemia, increased proteinuria, and renal failure. Diagnosis is made by LCAT quantification and cholesterol esterification activity in the plasma. Partial LCAT deficiency exhibits progressive corneal opacification, low plasma HDL levels (<10 mg/dL), and variable hypertriglyceridemia (also seen in complete LCAT deficiency). Premature CHD has been reported even in cases of partial LCAT deficiency (Kuivenhoven, 1997). No treatment can be given to raise LCAT levels; however, therapies for this condition involve dietary restriction of fat and management of complications from this disease.

ISOLATED HIGH HDL-C

Cholesteryl Ester Transfer Protein Gene Defects

HDL is involved in the reverse transport of cholesterol from peripheral tissues to the liver. An important step in this process involves CETP, the plasma protein that facilitates the transfer of cholesteryl esters from HDL to apoB-100–rich proteins (VLDL and LDL) in exchange for triglycerides. CETP deficiency is an autosomal recessive disorder in which the transfer of cholesterol esters is inhibited. As a result, HDL particles are large and laden with cholesterol ester, and apoA-I is increased, as is HDL-C (typically >100 mg/dL). The association of higher HDL-C plasma levels with risk of coronary heart disease is still unclear based on genetic studies of humans with *CETP* mutations. Heterozygotes have moderately increased HDL-C levels. Inhibition of CETP is an active area of research given the potential to raise HDL-C levels.

SELECTED REFERENCES

National Cholesterol Education Program Expert Panel: Third Report of the National Cholesterol Education Program (NCEP) Expert Panel on Detection, Evaluation, and Treatment of High Blood Cholesterol in Adults (Adult Treatment Panel III): final report. Circulation 2002;106:3143–421.

A comprehensive monograph that includes the latest recommendations for screening, evaluating, and treating hyperlipidemia.

Nauck M, Warnick GR, Rifai N. Methods for measurement of LDL-cholesterol: a critical assessment of direct measurement by homogenous assays versus calculation. Clin Chem 2002;48(2):236–54.

A comprehensive review of current LDL-C methods, including the advantages and disadvantages of each, performance characteristics, and an explanation of the chemistry and technology upon which the assay is based.

Warnick GR, Nauck M, Rifai N. Evolution of methods for measurement of HDL-cholesterol: from ultracentrifugation to homogeneous assays. Clin Chem 2001;47:1579–96.

A comprehensive review of all methods used to measure HDL-C, with particular emphasis on the new homogeneous assays. It discusses the pros and cons of each assay and its accuracy and precision and clinical usefulness, as well as the chemistry or technology upon which each is based.

REFERENCES

Access the complete reference list online at http://www.expertconsult.com

CHAPTER 18

CARDIAC INJURY, ATHEROSCLEROSIS, AND THROMBOTIC DISEASE

Jay L. Bock

PART 2

KEY POINTS

- The most important disease affecting the heart is coronary heart disease (CHD), which is atherosclerosis affecting the coronary arteries. CHD can lead to thrombotic occlusion of coronary blood flow, causing an acute coronary syndrome (ACS). ACS with frank necrosis of any amount of myocardium is known as myocardial infarction (MI).
- The primary tests for diagnosing ACS are electrocardiography and laboratory measurement of cardiac markers. Cardiac markers are proteins released into the circulation from damaged heart muscle. The most important cardiac marker today is cardiac troponin (cTn), which derives only from heart muscle.
- Troponin is a complex of three proteins, two of which are suitable as specific cardiac marker tests: cTnI and cTnT. These two proteins have different properties, but their clinical applications are similar. Clinically, MI is now essentially defined as an ACS that causes release of troponin.
- There is a delay of a few hours following MI before cTn is detected in the circulation; it peaks in about 24 hours and then declines over several days.
- Patients presenting to an emergency department with symptoms suggesting ACS must be processed rapidly and precisely to provide life-saving interventions as needed, yet avoid wasting resources. Rapid measurements of cTn, and possibly other laboratory markers, play a critical role.
- The clinical laboratory also measures risk factors associated with the development and progression of CHD. Significant laboratory markers of risk include lipids (cholesterol, triglycerides, and specific lipoprotein fractions—see Chapter 17), homocysteine (Hcy), and C-reactive protein (CRP). Hcy is an amino acid that exacerbates thrombosis. CRP is an inflammatory marker that appears to reflect the severity of CHD and may contribute to its pathogenesis.
- CHD and other heart diseases can impair the heart's ability to pump blood, causing the clinical syndrome of heart failure (HF). B-type natriuretic peptide (BNP), a 32 amino acid peptide secreted by the cardiac ventricles in response to wall-stretch stimuli, is a marker of the presence and severity of HF. BNP testing is particularly useful for aiding the differential diagnosis of patients who present to an emergency department with shortness of breath.
- Atherosclerosis affecting the carotid arteries or brain vasculature can lead to ischemic or hemorrhagic stroke. Some biomarkers show promise for the diagnosis or evaluation of stroke, but none are sufficiently discriminatory for routine use at present.
- Measurement of D-dimer, a degradation product of fibrin, has good sensitivity but poor specificity for the diagnosis of pulmonary embolism and venous thrombotic disease in general.

OVERVIEW

Heart disease is an affliction intimately tied to high technology. Technology has had a causal role, in part by allowing people to live longer, and in part by enabling a sedentary and overly consumptive lifestyle. During the twentieth century, heart disease rose from obscurity to become the leading cause of morbidity and mortality in developed nations (Table 18-1). Diagnosis and treatment of heart disease also depend heavily on advanced technology, including electrophysiologic, imaging, catheterization, surgical, and clinical laboratory modalities. The following major laboratory applications will be the subject of this chapter:

1. Measurement of proteins present in cardiac myocytes indicates recent damage to cardiac muscle. These tests are used mainly for the diagnosis and management of ischemic events (acute coronary syndromes). Although many different markers of ischemic damage have been used in the past, at the time of writing the most important markers by far are *cardiac troponin I* and *cardiac troponin T.*
2. Measurement of substances that are damaging to the coronary arteries, or at least have proven association with coronary heart disease, is used to assess risk and select appropriate preventive measures. The most important laboratory risk factors are lipids, which are discussed in Chapter 17. Of the many other substances that could be discussed, this chapter will focus on two: homocysteine (Hcy) and C-reactive protein (CRP).
3. Measurement of natriuretic peptides released from myocardium, particularly *B-type natriuretic peptide* (BNP) and the related inactive fragment, *NT-pro-BNP,* reflects the presence and severity of heart failure.
4. Laboratory testing has been less applicable to cerebrovascular disease, but some new biomarkers may be considered promising. Measurement of D-dimer is useful in ruling out pulmonary embolus.

TABLE 18-1
Heart Disease Statistics for the United States

- An estimated 80 million American adults, or about 1 in 3, has some form of cardiovascular disease (including hypertension).
- 16.8 million Americans have a history of CHD—of these, 7.9 million have had an MI and 9.8 million have had angina pectoris.
- 5.7 million Americans have HF.
- 6.5 million Americans have experienced a stroke.
- Cardiovascular disease is the underlying cause in 35.3% of all deaths in the United States, about 860,000 deaths per year. It claims about as many deaths as cancer, chronic lower respiratory diseases, accidents, and diabetes mellitus combined.
- The estimated annual direct and indirect cost of cardiovascular disease is $475 billion.
- Although some trends in cardiovascular disease are favorable, other factors, including an alarming increase in the prevalence of obesity and type 2 diabetes, will fuel the epidemic for many years to come.

From Lloyd-Jones D, Adams R, Carnethon M, et al. Heart disease and stroke statistics—2009 update: a report from the American Heart Association Statistics Committee and Stroke Statistics Subcommittee. Circulation 2009;119:e21–e181.
CHD, Coronary heart disease; *HF,* heart failure; *MI,* myocardial infarction.

TABLE 18-2
Clinical Abbreviations

ACS	Acute coronary syndrome
CHD	Coronary heart disease (also referred to as ischemic heart disease [IHD], atherosclerotic heart disease [ASHD])
HF	(Congestive) heart failure
MI	(Acute) myocardial infarction
NSTEMI	Non–ST-elevation myocardial infarction
STEMI	ST-elevation myocardial infarction
UA	Unstable angina

BACKGROUND (Table 18-2)

It is ironic that for the heart, an organ that pumps several liters of blood each minute, the most important disease process is ischemia—the lack of an adequate blood supply. This is so because heart muscle depends on constant nutrition through a system of coronary arteries, which are highly vulnerable to the process of atherosclerosis. Atherosclerosis is a chronic process involving damage to endothelium and the buildup of vessel-occluding lesions called plaque. In the early stages of atherosclerosis, as coronary blood flow is gradually reduced, there are typically no symptoms or laboratory evidence of cardiac injury. Once the diameter of a coronary artery is reduced to less than 10%–20% of its original size, chest pain (angina pectoris) often develops when demand for oxygen increases, particularly during exercise (exertional angina). More rapid reduction in blood flow can occur when plaque stimulates formation of a thrombus in a coronary artery, leading to an acute coronary syndrome (ACS). When a thrombus completely cuts off blood flow, the supplied muscle will develop irreversible ischemic damage, and the syndrome is a myocardial infarction (MI). When the blockage is not complete, irreversible muscle damage may be avoided, but the patient will experience severe angina, even at rest, and this syndrome is known as unstable angina. The broad spectrum of heart disease resulting from impaired coronary blood flow is referred to as coronary heart disease (CHD).

MIs can be categorized by whether they are accompanied by characteristic changes on the electrocardiogram (ECG). More severe MIs, generally involving transmural damage to the myocardium, typically cause the rapid appearance of ST-segment elevations and the later appearance of Q-waves. These are categorized as ST-elevation MIs (STEMIs). MIs without these changes (non–Q-wave MIs, or non-ST elevation MIs [NSTEMIs]) typically involve lesser degrees of muscle damage, possibly only to the subendocardium, but any ACS event carries serious risk for possibly lethal arrhythmias and for future events. Damage to a sizable quantity of cardiac muscle carries the additional risk of compromising the heart's ability to pump blood, leading to the clinical syndrome of heart failure (HF), which is discussed later.

Cardiac muscle is relatively resistant to ischemia, compared with other cells such as neurons and renal tubular epithelial cells, in which even short duration of ischemia can lead to cell death. In experimental animals, complete blockage of blood flow to an area of the heart does not cause cell death (MI) until after at least 20–30 minutes of ischemia; if blood flow had been previously restricted, cell death often is delayed for up to an hour. With complete coronary artery occlusion, there is typically a gradient of ischemia, with oxygen deprivation worst in areas receiving blood flow last (the subendocardial portions of the ventricular wall). Cells near the border between ischemic myocardium and normally perfused myocardium may receive some oxygen supply, and thus may remain viable for several hours. The longer the duration of ischemia, the higher is the percentage of cells at risk that will die; 3 hours of ischemia increases cell death to 80% of cells at risk, and 6 hours of ischemia causes the death of almost 100% of cells at risk. For this reason, early recognition of persistent ischemia and intervention to restore blood flow are needed to minimize cell death. Blood flow is most commonly restored by manipulating the plaque (usually by inflating a balloon) via a catheter inserted into a peripheral vein and then threaded into the coronary circulation (percutaneous coronary intervention). A mesh tube, or stent, may be inserted at the same time to maintain the patency of the coronary artery. When flow is blocked at multiple sites, it may be necessary to perform a coronary artery bypass graft.

The pathobiology of atherosclerosis and ACS remains incompletely understood. Formation of obstructive plaques probably begins with nonobstructive lesions known as fatty streaks, which have been observed in the coronary arteries of young individuals dying in combat or in accidents (Enos, 1953; Berenson, 1992; Strong, 1999). The lesions are likely triggered by uptake of oxidized low-density lipoprotein (LDL) particles by macrophages, which then invade the coronary endothelium (Ross, 1993; Witztum, 1994; Adams, 2000; Zaman, 2000). Inflammatory cells and mediators play a role in the evolution of the lesion, which eventually becomes a structure containing a lipid core (mainly cholesterol esters) surrounded by numerous macrophages and other inflammatory cells, and covered with a cap of endothelialized connective tissue (Davies, 2000; Weissberg, 2000; Hansson, 2005). Advanced lesions also contain new blood vessels and calcium deposits. Plaques in coronary arteries were formerly regarded as passive, physiologically irreversible barriers to blood flow. In recent years, their more dynamic role in ACS has been appreciated. A balance of inflammatory mediators, shear forces, and other factors can cause the fibrous cap of the plaque to strengthen or weaken. Erosion of the cap can expose thrombogenic material, leading to deposition of platelets and eventually enlargement of the lesion. More ominous is actual rupture of the plaque, causing thrombosis with sufficient occlusion to result in ACS. A major contributor to this concept of plaque vulnerability has been the finding that cholesterol-lowering statin drugs can diminish the risk of ACS substantially without causing appreciable diminution of the degree of stenosis caused by atherosclerotic lesions (see Chapter 17). Unfortunately, no good test is available at present to assess plaque vulnerability.

The severity of coronary atherosclerotic disease has traditionally been evaluated by coronary angiography, which uses a radiopaque "dye" to image blood flow through the coronary arteries. Besides being invasive, this test has the limitation that it can only identify restrictions to coronary blood flow; it says nothing about the biology of the plaque lesions. Electron beam computed tomography can noninvasively image the accumulation of calcium in atherosclerotic lesions, but ability to predict the future behavior of lesions is still limited (Fuseini, 2003). Blood tests that reflect the actual extent of atherosclerotic disease may be available in the future, for example, measurement of microparticles shed by plaque has been proposed (Heloire, 2003). At present, however, risk of CHD in individuals is mainly assessed indirectly through the measurement of risk factors, each of which appears to play a contributory but not necessarily definitive role (Stampfer, 2004). Several clinical parameters, summarized in Table 18-3, have been established as important risk factors. Additionally, hundreds of laboratory tests have been studied in relation to CHD risk. Of these, several lipid tests, as discussed in Chapter 17, have the best established role in risk assessment. Two newer markers, homocysteine and C-reactive protein, are discussed later.

Next to CHD, and often as a direct consequence of it, the most important heart disease is HF. HF is a clinical syndrome with prominent symptoms, including fatigue, shortness of breath, and pulmonary edema, resulting from impairment in the heart's pumping ability. It is most commonly caused by damage to the myocardium, as results from CHD. Because of the high incidence of CHD and the improving survival of people who suffer from it, HF is a rapidly increasing problem, especially

TABLE 18-3
Clinical (Nonlaboratory) Risk Factors for CHD

- Cigarette smoking (any smoking in the past month)
- Hypertension (blood pressure >140/90 mm Hg or on antihypertensive medication)
- Family history of premature CHD (CHD in male first-degree relative <55 years, or in female first-degree relative <65 years)
- Age (men >45 years; women >55 years)
- Obesity
- Diabetes mellitus
- Sedentary lifestyle

The definitions given in parentheses are used, along with the HDL-cholesterol level, in a risk estimate formula for targeting a desirable LDL-cholesterol level (National Cholesterol Education Program Expert Panel, 2002) (see Chapter 17).
CHD, Coronary heart disease; *HDL,* high-density lipoprotein; *LDL,* low-density lipoprotein.

in the elderly. HF can also be caused by mechanical problems, such as valvular disease, which interfere with the pump function of the heart. When the problem is related to filling of the left ventricle during diastole, it is often referred to as diastolic HF.

Diagnosing HF and monitoring its progression can be difficult. A defining parameter for systolic HF is the left ventricular ejection fraction (LVEF), which is the fraction of the left ventricle's blood volume that is ejected during systole. It can be measured by echocardiography or by radionuclide ventriculography. Symptomatic HF is usually associated with LVEF <40%, but correlation between LVEF and subjective symptoms is poor. Until recently, no clinical laboratory test had specific utility in disclosing the presence or severity of HF. This situation has changed with the introduction of testing for cardiac natriuretic peptides, which is discussed later.

Of the myriad other diseases that can affect the heart, brief mention should be made of genetic diseases that, although relatively uncommon, have disproportionate importance because of their potentially life-threatening consequences. The syndrome of hypertrophic cardiomyopathy, described more than a century ago, occurs in 1 in 500 individuals and is the most common cause of sudden death in the young (Taylor, 2004). More than 240 mutations have been tied to this disorder (Gomes, 2004); they affect various proteins of the contractile apparatus, including the troponins, actin, and myosin, and generally are inherited in autosomal dominant fashion. The long-QT syndrome, an abnormality in ventricular repolarization that can cause sudden death, has several distinct variants caused by both autosomal dominant and recessive mutations in ion channels and other proteins (Priori, 2004). Application of molecular diagnostics to these disorders is in its infancy, but evidence already indicates that identifying the genotype not only is useful for confirming the diagnosis but may play an important role in guiding specific therapy.

Markers of Myocardial Damage

HISTORICAL DEVELOPMENT

Biochemical markers of myocardial damage were essentially a serendipitous discovery in the early 1950s, when LaDue and coworkers were investigating the transaminase enzymes then known as glutamate-oxaloacetate transaminase; now aspartate transaminase, and glutamate-pyruvate transaminase; now alanine transaminase (LaDue, 1954). While surveying various hospital patients, investigators noted that serum transaminase levels rose sharply after an MI, and thus was born the era of "cardiac enzymes." The simple underlying principle, as with other organ markers, is that cell death will cause release of cellular proteins into the circulation. (A more difficult question, still not fully resolved, is the extent to which *reversible* cell damage can cause protein leakage.)

Transaminases have not endured as cardiac markers because of their abundance in liver, skeletal muscle, and other tissues. They were soon superseded for cardiac diagnosis by two other enzymes, lactate dehydrogenase (LD) and creatine kinase (CK) (Hess, 1963; Roe, 1977). LD is a zinc-containing enzyme that is part of the glycolytic pathway and is found in virtually all cells in the body. It utilizes reduced nicotinamide adenine dinucleotide (NADH) in catalyzing the reduction of pyruvate to lactate and nicotinamide adenine dinucleotide in catalyzing the reverse reaction, making it simple to assay this enzyme because the appearance or disappearance of NADH can be easily monitored at 340 nm (see Chapter 20). CK transfers high-energy phosphate between creatine and adenosine diphosphate, mainly in muscle cells, but it is found in all types of muscle and in brain and other tissues. With both of these enzymes, improved cardiac specificity was achieved through separation of isoenzymes. LD is a tetramer of two active subunits, H (for heart) and M (for muscle), with a molecular weight of 134 kDa. Combinations of subunits produce five isoenzymes ranging from LD_1 (HHHH) to LD_5 (MMMM); the intermediate isoenzymes contain differing combinations of H and M subunits (LD_2, HHHM; LD_3, HHMM; LD_4, HMMM). As the subunit names imply, LD_1 is relatively abundant in cardiac muscle, whereas LD_5 is more abundant in skeletal muscle. Patients with MI exhibit a characteristic pattern of "flipped" LD, where the normal finding LD2 > LD1 is reversed.

CK is predominantly found as a dimer of catalytic subunits, each with a molecular weight of about 40 kDa; the two subunits are termed M (for muscle) and B (for brain). The three resulting isoenzymes are CK_1 (BB), CK_2 (MB), and CK_3 (MM). CK is found in small amounts throughout the body, but is found in high concentrations only in muscle and brain, although CK from brain virtually never crosses the blood-brain barrier to reach plasma. In skeletal muscle, creatine kinase-MB fraction (CK-MB) accounts for 0% to 1% of the total CK in type 1 fibers and 2%–6% of CK in type 2 fibers. During regeneration of skeletal muscle, increased amounts of CK-MB are produced relative to CK-MM, similar to the pattern seen in fetal muscle (Tzvetanova, 1971). In the normal heart, an average of 15%–20% of the CK is CK-MB; its distribution is not uniform, with CK-MB percentage greater in the right heart than in the left heart (Marmor, 1980). A single study, however, suggests that CK-MB is not found in normal myocardium, but appears only when the muscle becomes diseased (Ingwall, 1985). CK-BB is the dominant isoenzyme of CK found in brain, intestine, and smooth muscle.

In the past, clinical laboratories would commonly analyze both CK and LD isoenzymes to improve overall diagnostic performance, especially because the two enzymes exhibit different kinetics, with changes in LD observable for a much longer time than changes in CK. Isoenzyme analyses were relatively lengthy and tedious, generally involving electrophoretic separation, followed by development of color or fluorescence using suitable substrates, followed by densitometric scanning. Hence these tests could be performed only about once per day—a situation that was acceptable at a time when "rule out MI" patients were generally admitted to hospital for at least a several-day period of observation. A major advance was the development of sensitive immunometric assays for proteins using monoclonal antibody technology (see Chapter 44). With this technology, it was possible to develop a CK-MB "mass assay" that did not depend on the protein's enzymatic activity (el Allaf, 1986; Mair, 1991). More important, it provided the opportunity to develop organ markers that were not traditional enzymes, leading to the advent of troponin testing.

High-resolution electrophoresis of serum CK discloses that the MM and MB isoenzymes are heterogeneous, with MB having two sub-bands, and MM three sub-bands. These species, known as isoforms, arise through the action of carboxypeptidase in serum cleaving the terminal lysine off of the M-subunit (Wevers, 1978; George, 1984). Thus the MB isoenzyme can be unmodified (MB_0) or can have one lysine cleaved (MB_1), whereas the MM isoenzyme can be unmodified (MM_0) or can have one (MM_1) or two (MM_2) lysines cleaved. Because enzymatic cleavage occurs over a period of hours following the release of unmodified enzyme into the blood, a relatively high fraction of the unmodified isoform can serve as an indicator of recent tissue damage, as in an acute MI. This test offers improved early sensitivity for detection of acute MI over CK-MB mass assay (Puleo, 1994; Bock, 1999), but it requires a dedicated electrophoresis workstation, and for this reason had somewhat limited use even before the troponin era.

CARDIAC TROPONIN

Troponin (Tn) is a regulatory complex of three proteins that resides at regular intervals in the thin filament of striated muscle. The three individual proteins are tropomyosin-binding subunit (TnT, 37 kDa), inhibitory subunit (TnI, 24 kDa), and calcium-binding subunit (TnC, 18 kDa). The Ca^{++} trigger for muscle contraction is transmitted via the Tn complex, which causes a conformational change in another thin-filament component, tropomyosin, allowing interaction between actin and myosin to proceed. In contrast to nearly all other muscle proteins, the forms of Tn found in skeletal and cardiac muscle differ. For TnC, the forms found in type 2 fibers and cardiac muscle are identical, obviating its use as a differential marker. TnI has a cardiospecific form (cTnI), as well as distinct forms in types 1 and 2 skeletal muscle fibers, each coded by a separate gene. The presence of the cardiospecific form in tissue other than cardiac muscle has never been documented (Bodor, 1995). TnT also has distinct forms in myocardium (cTnT) and in fast-twitch and slow-twitch skeletal muscle, but here the situation is more complicated, because cTnT has been detected in fetal skeletal muscle and diseased skeletal muscle. However, post-translational modifications cause detectable differences between cTnT produced in myocardium and cTnT produced in diseased skeletal muscle (Apple, 1998; Apple, 1999). Hence an immunochemical test for cTnT with carefully chosen antibodies, such as the current generation (but not earlier generations) of commercial cTnT assays, should have myocardial specificity approaching 100%. Nevertheless, small increases in circulating cTnT, even with newer assays, have been reported in patients with muscular dystrophy and renal failure who have no other evidence of cardiac disease (Muller-Bardorff, 1997; Hammerer-Lercher, 2001a).

Within the cardiac myocytes, cTnT and cTnI are bound predominantly to muscle fibers, as described earlier, and this bound form is released slowly over the course of 1 to 2 weeks following myocardial infarction. Thus, although cTnI and cTnT are relatively small proteins that are rapidly cleared, their plasma levels fall slowly after cardiac injury. A small fraction of cTn in the myocardial cell is free within the cytoplasm; this averages 6% for cTnT and slightly lower (2%–5%) for cTnI. The free fraction allows early leakage from injured myocardial cells and detection in a time frame similar to that of CK-MB, with cTn reaching a peak at about 24 hours after MI. Because of the slow release of fiber-bound cTn, the rapid decline in circulating cTn right after its peak is typically followed by a plateau or even a small secondary increase. It is important that such an increase *not* be interpreted as evidence of reinfarction. Circulating cTn declines to baseline levels in about 5–10 days, depending on infarct size (Mair, 1997) (Fig. 18-1).

In contrast to other cardiac markers, cTnT and cTnI are nearly absent from normal serum. With the best assays in wide use at present, which have detection limits around 0.01 ng/mL, many healthy individuals have undetectable levels, so the normal range is not well defined. The 99th percentile of the healthy population is around 0.04 ng/mL, depending on the assay. Levels above this threshold are almost certainly indicative of myocyte damage but possibly reveal a much lesser amount of damage than was detectable with earlier cardiac markers such as CK-MB. With the advent of cTn testing, it has become clear that myocyte damage can occur in many circumstances other than coronary artery obstruction: cTn elevations are observed in pericarditis, myocarditis, pulmonary embolism, renal failure, sepsis, and other critical illness (Roongsritong, 2004). Prolonged intense exercise, such as running a marathon, can cause small elevations (Mingels, 2009). Healthy newborns were found to have levels as high as 3.0 ng/mL (Araújo, 2004). Small measured elevations in cTn may also be analytic artifacts (see Assay Procedures later).

OTHER MARKERS

Myoglobin

Myoglobin is a heme-containing protein that binds oxygen within cardiac and skeletal muscle; only a single form is common to both muscle types. Having a molecular weight of only 18 kDa, myoglobin apparently leaks from damaged cells more rapidly than other proteins. Following MI, elevated myoglobin may be detectable in plasma before CK-MB or cTn. However, with the newest and most sensitive cTn assays, it is not clear how often this may occur. Typically, myoglobin peaks about 6 hours after MI and returns to baseline after 24 hours. Although myoglobin may offer some advantage in early detection of myocardial damage, its value is limited by its lack of specificity.

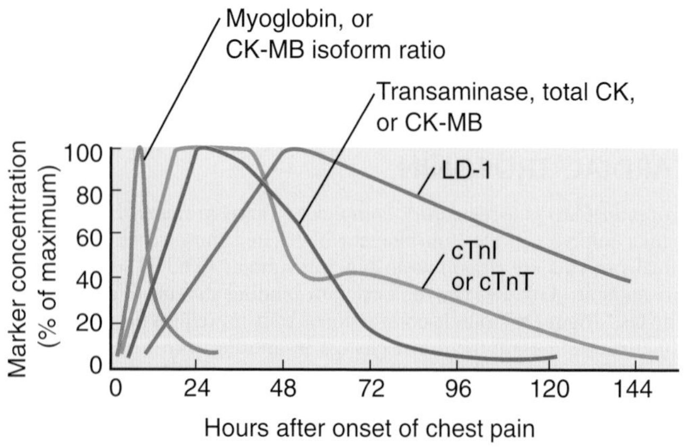

Figure 18-1 Schematic depiction of the kinetics of several cardiac markers following a myocardial infarction. *CK,* Creatine kinase; *CK-MB,* creatine kinase-MB fraction; *cTnI,* cardiospecific form of TnI; *cTnT,* myocardium form of TnT; *LD-1,* lactate dehydrogenase-1.

Carbonic Anhydrase III

Carbonic anhydrase III (CA III) is an enzyme present in skeletal but not in cardiac muscle, hence it can serve as a sort of "negative" cardiac marker. It is released from damaged muscle at a fairly fixed ratio to myoglobin. Thus myoglobin is a more specific indicator of myocardial damage when its ratio to CA III is also elevated (Väänänen, 1990; Brogan, 1996; Beuerle, 2000).

Glycogen Phosphorylase

Glycogen phosphorylase (GP) is a widely distributed enzyme that catalyzes the first step in glycogenolysis. A dimer of identical subunits, it has three characterized isoenzymes, named for the tissue in which they are most expressed: GPLL (liver), GPMM (muscle), and GPBB (brain). GPBB is also expressed in myocardium, as well as other tissues, but it is not found in skeletal muscle, which contains only GPMM. The potential usefulness of GPBB is that it appears to be released earlier than other markers, and may in fact be released under conditions of reversible ischemia that do not give rise to comparable elevations in other markers (Rabitzsch, 1995; Krause, 1996). However, comparisons with modern cTn assays have been limited and not particularly encouraging (Lang, 2000).

Heart Fatty Acid–Binding Protein

Heart fatty acid–binding protein (HFABP) is a low-molecular-weight (15 kDa) protein that is a relatively early marker of myocardial damage, with kinetics similar to that of myoglobin. It is not cardiac specific and therefore does not seem to offer advantages over myoglobin. However, the ratio of myoglobin to HFABP is much lower in heart than in skeletal muscle and may have diagnostic applicability (Van Nieuwenhoven, 1995; Zanotti, 1999).

Myosin

Myosin makes up the thick filament of the muscle contractile apparatus and is composed of a pair of heavy chains (200 kDa) and one pair each of type I and type II light chains (20–26 kDa). Several of these components have been examined as cardiac markers (Katus, 1988; Uji, 1991; Ravkilde, 1994; Ravkilde, 1995). It has not been possible to achieve complete cardiac specificity with myosin, and it is not clear that it would offer any important advantages.

Ischemia-Modified Albumin

Ischemia-modified albumin (IMA) is a unique type of cardiac marker (FDA approved in 2003) that is *not* a protein released from damaged myocytes (Bar-Or, 2000; Bar-Or, 2001; Christenson, 2001; Bhagavan, 2003). Rather, the test detects a variant form of albumin with a reduced affinity for metal ions near the N-terminus. The variant is measured by a spectrophotometric determination of Co^{++} binding. It is postulated to arise from interaction of albumin with free radicals at sites of tissue ischemia. The theoretical advantage of this test is that it detects ischemia before irreversible cell damage occurs. The change in albumin appears to occur within minutes of ischemia and lasts for about 6 hours. The test clearly is not specific for cardiac ischemia, but appears to have a clinical sensitivity of 80%–90% for ACS at the time of presentation—greater than that of the ECG (Roy, 2004; Sinha, 2004). Clinical specificity, in the context of emergency diagnosis of ACS, may be around 50%. Taking any one of elevated IMA, positive ECG, or elevated cTn as a positive result, a test for ACS with very high negative predictive value, but poor positive predictive value, is achieved. More prospective data will be needed to establish the clinical role of this unusual test.

ASSAY PROCEDURES

The measurement of cardiac markers has evolved from measurement of total enzyme activity, to electrophoretic or chromatographic isoenzyme separations, to the current era of sophisticated immunoassay technology. cTn and other protein markers are universally measured by sensitive immunometric assays employing monoclonal antibodies. These can be automated for high volume and round-the-clock availability, or alternatively adapted to point-of-care testing. In contrast, the IMA test is a colorimetric assay that is commercially available on high-throughput standard chemistry analyzers.

Despite the impressively high sensitivity and specificity of modern immunometric assays, they have intrinsic limitations that must be well recognized in the case of cTn. All proteins, because of post-translational modifications, are heterogeneous analytes, but cTn, which originates in a protein complex that degrades as it is released into the circulation, is especially so. Circulating forms that have been identified include a ternary cTnT-I-C complex, binary cTnI-C, free cTnT (but not free cTnI), oxidized forms (cTnI but not cTnT that contains cysteine residues that can be oxidized to form an intramolecular disulfide bond), phosphorylated forms, and degraded forms (Gao, 1997; Katrukha, 1998; Morjana, 1998; Wu, 1998b; Shi, 1999; Bunk, 2000; Labugger, 2000). Evidently certain epitopes are blocked or modified in some of these forms, because differences greater than 20-fold have been observed in their reactivity with different commercial assays for cTnI (Wu, 1998a; Datta, 1999; Newman, 1999; Shi, 1999; Tate, 1999; Kao, 2001). The problem does not arise in the same way for cTnT because assays are at this time marketed by only one manufacturer. A certified reference material for cTn has been prepared (Bunk, 2006), but it has demonstrated commutability only with plasma cTn specimens for half of the commercial assays (Christenson, 2006). cTn I results will always demonstrate some inconsistency among methods, unless manufacturers adopt the use of very similar antibodies.

Another problem is that because the normal level of plasma cTn is very low, even a minuscule degree of assay interference can elevate a result to the abnormal range, suggesting a strong possibility of ischemic disease to the caregiver. This may lead to unnecessary invasive procedures such as coronary angiography. Various cTnI assays have in fact been found susceptible to interferences from heterophilic antibodies, fibrin, and other substances (Roberts, 1997; Fitzmaurice, 1998; Dasgupta, 1999; Nosanchuk, 1999; Parry, 1999; Galambos, 2000; Dasgupta, 2001). Negative interference due to autoantibodies has also been reported (Eriksson, 2005).

Reference ranges and decision points have been a matter of some confusion (Jaffe, 2004), but in keeping with recent guidelines, there has been a general trend toward use of the 99th percentile of the healthy population as the cutpoint for elevated cTn. It is desirable that the precision of the assay be within a 10% coefficient of variation at this cutpoint, and this is achievable with the newest assays. As the low-end accuracy of cTn assays improves, it is becoming increasingly apparent that the 99th percentile can vary, depending on the reference population chosen, and that levels below the 99th percentile may have clinical significance (Latini, 2007; Eggers, 2009).

CLINICAL PROTOCOLS

Diagnosis of ACS

Diagnosis of MI has evolved from a somewhat leisurely process spanning several days of a hospital stay to an urgent task carried out largely in the emergency department (ED), sometimes within a specialized chest pain center (Zalenski, 1998). Approximately 8 million ED visits in the United States each year are related to chest pain or other symptoms, including shortness of breath, dizziness, or loss of consciousness, which may suggest ACS (Storrow, 2000; Fig. 18-2). Although diagnosis is often straightforward, the challenge is to achieve a very high level of accuracy. Missed diagnosis of ACS, which may occur in about 2% of cases, carries an increased risk of mortality and is the leading cause of malpractice payout for emergency physicians (Karcz, 1996; Pope, 2000). On the other hand, the conservative practice of hospital admission for most patients with suspected ACS spends billions of dollars unnecessarily, because two thirds of these patients turn out not to have ACS.

Biochemical markers play a secondary role in the initial management of patients with suspected ACS. The earliest decision-making, which ideally should take place within 10 minutes of the patient's arrival in the ED, is based on history, physical examination, and 12-lead ECG (Anderson, 2007) (Fig. 18-3). The ECG may establish the diagnosis of STEMI, at which point the patient is a candidate for immediate intervention to restore coronary blood flow (Antman, 2008). Biochemical marker results are not necessary before these interventions are provided, and in fact are likely to be negative at this early time.

If the initial ECG is negative for STEMI, biochemical markers assume increasing importance. Choice of markers and time points for testing has varied among institutions, but it is now generally agreed that cTn is the preferred marker, with little to choose between I and T (Anderson, 2007; Morrow, 2007). cTn does not rise until several hours after the onset of myocyte necrosis, so a specimen obtained at the time of presentation is likely to be negative, and an additional one or two specimens should be drawn at intervals of 6 to 9 hours. The diagnosis of NSTEMI is established by positive biomarker results with appropriate changes over time. Negative biomarker results with ischemic ECG changes (ST depression or T-wave inversions) or other evidence may establish the diagnosis of UA. These two diagnoses are managed similarly, possibly with invasive artery-opening therapy (Anderson, 2007).

If, after several hours, the patient's presenting symptoms have resolved, and ECG and biochemical findings have been consistently negative, then an ACS has been effectively ruled out. For increased safety, before such a

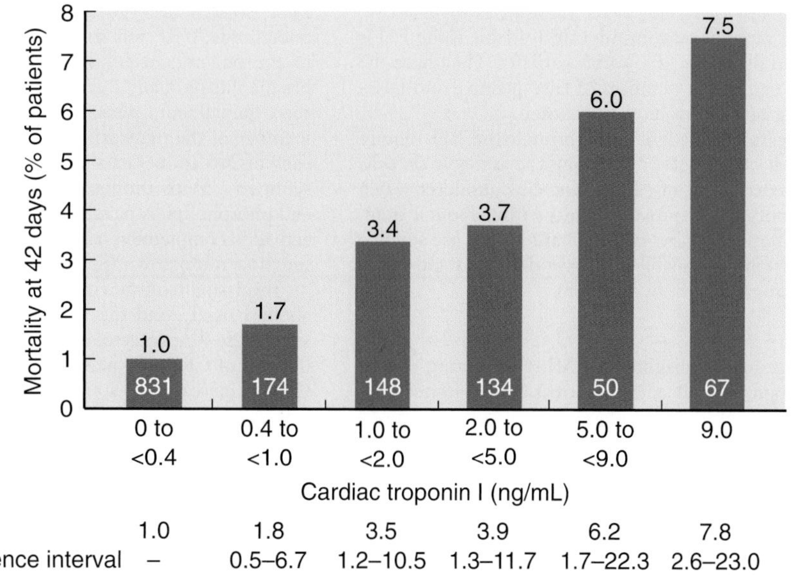

Risk ratio	1.0	1.8	3.5	3.9	6.2	7.8
95% confidence interval	–	0.5–6.7	1.2–10.5	1.3–11.7	1.7–22.3	2.6–23.0

Figure 18-2 Mortality rates of acute coronary syndrome patients as a function of cardiospecific troponin (cTnI) level. The 1441 patients in the TIMI IIIB study were from 21 to 76 years of age, had episodes of pain at rest that were presumed to be ischemic in origin and had lasted for at least 5 minutes (but less than 6 hours) within the preceding 24 hours, and had documented evidence of coronary heart disease. Patients were excluded from the study if left bundle-branch block was noted on presentation, a documented myocardial infarction had occurred within the previous 21 days, a treatable cause of angina was present, thrombolytic therapy had been administered within the previous 72 hours, or angioplasty had been performed in the previous 6 months. Mortality rates at 42 days are shown for ranges of cTnI measured at enrollment. The numbers at the bottom of each bar are the numbers of patients with cTnI in each range, and the numbers above the bars are percentages. $p < 0.001$ for the increase in mortality rate (and the risk ratio for mortality) with increasing levels of cTnI at enrollment. *(From Antman EM, Tanasijevic MJ, Thompson B, et al. Cardiac-specific troponin I levels to predict the risk of mortality in patients with acute coronary syndromes. N Engl J Med 1996;335:1342–1349, with permission).*

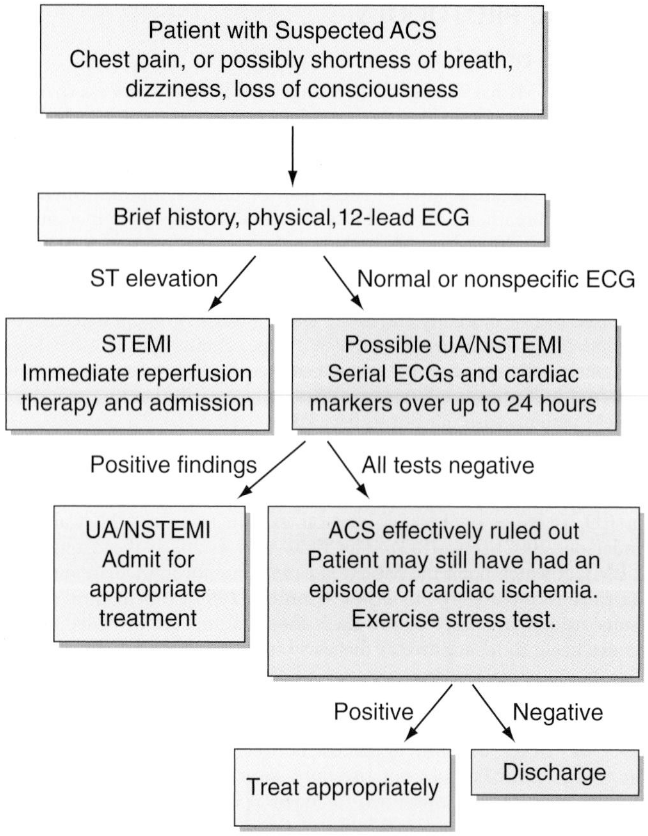

Figure 18-3 Outline of a clinical algorithm for treating patients presenting to an emergency department with symptoms suggesting acute coronary syndrome (ACS). The protocol is general and has to be customized to particular institutions and used with proper clinical judgment. *(Adapted from Pearson TA, Mensah GA, Alexander RW, et al. Markers of inflammation and cardiovascular disease: application to clinical and public health practice. A statement for healthcare professionals from the Centers for Disease Control and Prevention and the American Heart Association. Circulation 2003;107:499–511). ECG,* Electrocardiogram, *NSTEMI,* non-STelevation MI; *STEMI,* STelevation MI; *UA,* unstable angina.

patient is discharged, a provocative test for CHD is commonly performed, such as a simple exercise ECG test or a more elaborate nuclear imaging or echocardiography stress test (Farkouh, 1998; Lindsay, 1998; Storrow, 2000). These tests must be rapidly and continuously available if the ED is to achieve the desired rapid discharge of low-risk patients. They have the drawbacks of expense and significant numbers of false-positive and false-negative results, depending on the test modality chosen.

Because both clinical care and patient flow through the ED require rapid risk assessment, cardiac marker test results must be available quickly. It is commonly advocated that point-of-care testing be considered when the central laboratory cannot reliably provide results within about 1 hour. Both qualitative and quantitative tests for cardiac markers that are suitable for point-of-care testing are now available and have demonstrated effectiveness (Antman, 1997; Brogan, 1998; Bock, 2008).

Other Applications

Besides ruling in or ruling out the diagnosis of MI, cTn testing can be useful in determining prognosis and adjusting treatment. Higher cTn levels indicate a larger volume of infarcted muscle and a worse prognosis (Bøhmer, 2009; Kurz, 2009). A single specimen obtained 72 to 96 hours after the event appears to be most useful for assessment of infarct size (Younger, 2007; Giannitsis, 2008). Although more experience has been acquired in testing for reinfarction using CK-MB, which declines more rapidly after an uncomplicated MI than cTn, it appears that the latter can be equally effective in diagnosing reinfarction (Apple, 2005). When reinfarction is clinically suspected, a blood specimen should be drawn immediately and 3–6 hours later. An increase in cTn of >20%, with an absolute value exceeding the 99th percentile, confirms the diagnosis (Thygesen, 2007).

cTn measurements can usefully suggest adverse outcomes after procedures such as percutaneous coronary intervention (PCI) and cardiac surgery. Because these procedures may be intrinsically associated with some degree of myocyte damage, it is difficult to justify firm guidelines for defining periprocedural MI. General recommendations that have been advanced include the following: An increase of more than three times the 99th percentile indicates a PCI-related MI; and an increase of more than five times the 99th percentile during the first 72 hours following a coronary artery bypass graft, when associated with other clinical evidence, indicates a periprocedural MI (Thygesen, 2007). Cardioversion, whether external or internal, causes minimal to no elevation in cTn (Allan, 1997; Greaves, 1998; Rao, 1998; Gorenek, 2004).

Transaminases, LD, and LD isoenzymes are no longer recommended as cardiac markers (Apple, 2007). CK-MB testing has persisted to some degree in the troponin era, but because there are few if any situations where it clearly provides additional information, it generally is not regarded as a cost-effective addition to cTn testing (Saenger, 2008).

Markers of Coronary Risk

CHD is a chronic disease of aging, and obviously, the most desirable approach to management is to prevent or minimize its development. As summarized earlier in the Background section, our understanding of the causation of CHD is still incomplete, so definitive preventive measures are not foreseeable at this time. However, many lines of evidence, the most important being large epidemiology studies, have identified several risk factors associated with CHD. Most of these risk factors pertain not just to the heart but to the general processes of atherosclerosis and/or thrombosis. Hence they have important implications for stroke and peripheral vascular disease as well.

The major clinical risk factors for CHD (not related to laboratory tests) are summarized in Table 18-3. Of risk factors that can be identified by the clinical laboratory, the earliest identified, and still one of the most important, is serum cholesterol. It is actually the LDL fraction of cholesterol, which generally contains about 70% of the total circulating cholesterol, that is directly associated with risk; the high-density lipoprotein fraction is in fact a negative risk factor. The other major lipid class commonly measured in plasma, triglyceride, has been an issue of controversy but now is generally accepted as a significant risk factor. Lipid testing and its relationship to CHD risk assessment are discussed in Chapter 17.

Aside from the lipids, a wide array of plasma constituents have been related to CHD risk. These include various nutrients, hormones, clotting factors, drugs, toxins, oxidants, antioxidants, and markers of inflammation or infection. In this chapter, only two markers that appear to be relatively important will be discussed: CRP and Hcy.

C-REACTIVE PROTEIN

First isolated in 1930 from the plasma of patients with pneumococcal pneumonia, CRP was so named because it binds to the C-polysaccharide of the pneumococcus. It was later found that the protein appeared in plasma during many infectious or inflammatory conditions, and CRP was the original acute phase reactant. CRP has now been characterized as a member of the pentraxin family of proteins. It comprises five protomers, each of 206 amino acids and molecular weight 23 kDa, arranged in cyclic symmetry. With the participation of Ca^{++} ions, it binds various proteins and phospholipids, particularly phosphocholine. It opsonizes particles and activates complement via the classical pathway, but its actual biological function is unknown (Szalai, 1999; Black, 2004).

In plasma from normal individuals, the median CRP concentration is about 1 mg/L, and the 99th percentile is about 10 mg/L. In individuals with acute illness, cytokines, chiefly interleukin-6, stimulate hepatic production of CRP, and plasma levels increase to 300 mg/L or more. Plasma CRP is increased in a variety of disorders, including most bacterial (but usually not viral) infections. MI is among the acute illnesses associated with elevation of plasma CRP (de Beer, 1982).

Epidemiologic studies have established that individuals with higher baseline levels of plasma CRP are at increased risk for CHD and stroke. In the relatively early Physicians Health Study, which enrolled 22 000 male U.S. physicians to examine the cardioprotective effects of aspirin and beta-carotene, plasma CRP averaged 1.51 mg/L in participants who developed MI, 1.38 mg/L in those who developed stroke, and 1.13 mg/L in controls who did not suffer vascular events (Ridker, 1997). In the larger and more recent Reykjavik study, the average baseline CRP was 1.75 mg/L in participants who developed MI, versus 1.25 in those without vascular events (Danesh, 2004). Similar findings, as summarized in a 2004 meta-analysis, have been reported from some 20 other epidemiology studies, although the degree of independent risk associated with CRP has varied (Danesh,

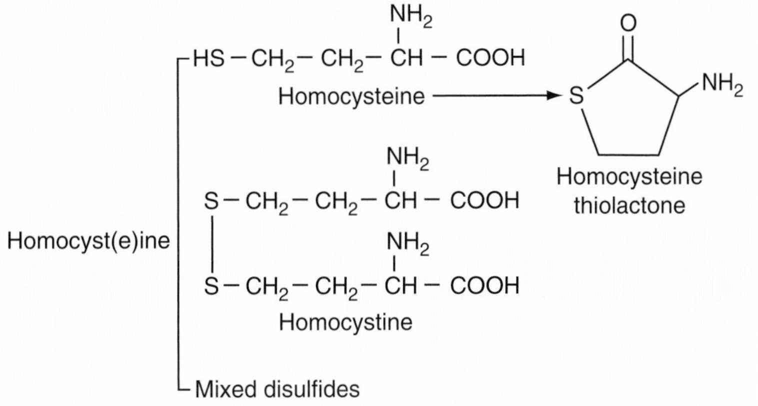

Figure 18-4 Chemical structure of homocysteine and related compounds.

2004). A report on the Women's Health Study suggested that CRP was actually more predictive than LDL cholesterol (Ridker, 2002), whereas investigators for the Reykjavik study reported that CRP is less predictive than total cholesterol, cigarette smoking, or systolic blood pressure. Differences may relate to the nature of the population studied and the means of correction used for traditional risk factors.

Elevation of plasma CRP (as indicated earlier) that confers excess coronary risk is minute compared with the hundred- to thousand-fold increases that occur with overt inflammatory or infectious diseases. For this reason, testing of CRP related to cardiac risk has been given the somewhat misleading name of high-sensitivity CRP (hs-CRP). Actually, even at concentrations around 1 mg/L or less, CRP is a relatively abundant plasma protein, which does not require the most sensitive (or expensive) techniques for accurate measurement. Methods such as nephelometry, which had been established for measuring CRP as an inflammatory marker, have been readily adapted to hs-CRP assays; the main differences involve degree of dilution and calibration. Commercial hs-CRP assays have adequate precision, and the long-term stability of hs-CRP in individual patients appears to be comparable with that of other risk factors, such as blood pressure and cholesterol (Danesh, 2004).

Although diverse evidence points to a role of inflammation in CHD (Paoletti, 2004; Hansson, 2005), a precise mechanism for the relationship of plasma CRP to CHD risk is lacking at this point. A key question still unresolved is whether the elevation in CRP is a cause or a consequence of the disease (or possibly both) (Hingorani, 2009). The inflammatory response associated with atheromatous lesions may trigger enough cytokine production to be associated with a measurable rise in plasma CRP. CRP may, in turn, through its proinflammatory effects, increase plaque vulnerability or have other effects that worsen the severity of CHD. The presence of CRP in human atheromatous lesions has been demonstrated (Reynolds, 1987), and in rats it has been shown that injection of human CRP after ligation of the coronary artery enhances infarct size (Griselli, 1999). Another intriguing possibility is that the risk associated with CRP relates to cytokine production by adipocytes, and that CRP is essentially a biochemical marker of the recently recognized metabolic syndrome (Yudkin, 1999; Ridker, 2004).

Given the variations in quantitative risk estimates, the unclear role of CRP in the pathogenesis of vascular disease, and the lack of specific treatment for high CRP, the usefulness of the hs-CRP test in individual patients has been controversial. A joint committee of the Centers for Disease Control and Prevention and the American Heart Association issued recommendations in 2003, some of which are listed in Table 18-4. Following a recent trial in which benefits of statin therapy were demonstrated in individuals with relatively low LDL cholesterol but high hs-CRP, it has been suggested that asymptomatic men older than 50 years and asymptomatic women older than 60 years be screened by hs-CRP when LDL cholesterol is not elevated and a decision to treat with statins is not otherwise clear (Ridker, 2008; Mora, 2009).

TABLE 18-4

Recommendations of a Joint Committee of the American Heart Association and the Centers for Disease Control and Prevention on CRP Testing to Assess CHD Risk

(Pearson, 2003)

- If inflammatory markers are to be used in assessment of CHD risk, hs-CRP is the current analyte of choice.
- Optimally, hs-CRP results should be averaged from two specimens drawn about 2 weeks apart. If a level >10 mg/L is identified, there should be a search for an obvious cause of infection or inflammation; this result should then be discarded, and another test done 2 weeks later.
- Decision intervals are as follows: <1 mg/L, low risk; 1–3 mg/L, intermediate risk; >3 mg/L, high risk (approximately corresponding to tertiles in the adult population).
- Patients most likely to benefit from an hs-CRP test would be those in whom the risk estimate from established factors is moderate (i.e., approximately 10%–20% risk of CHD in the next 10 years), and the physician desires additional information to guide preventive therapy.
- The role of hs-CRP in secondary prevention (i.e., prevention of disease progression in patients with established CHD) is limited, because it is not likely to alter management (which needs to be aggressive, regardless of additional information provided by CRP or other markers).
- Universal hs-CRP screening of the adult population is *not* warranted.

CHD, Coronary heart disease; *CRP,* C-reactive protein; *hs-CRP,* high-sensitivity C-reactive protein.

HOMOCYSTEINE

Hcy (Fig. 18-4) is a sulfur-containing amino acid that is not incorporated into protein but is a metabolic intermediate; it can be methylated to form methionine, or it can be converted through the transsulfuration pathway to cystathionine and then to cysteine. Hcy can exist in plasma as the species with a free sulfhydryl group, as a disulfide (homocystine), or as a mixed disulfide, linked to a plasma protein via one of its cysteine residues. It is the sum of these, which may be referred to as "total homocysteine," "homocyst(e)ine," or simply "homocysteine" that is generally measured.

Excessive levels of circulating Hcy generally reflect a diminished activity of one of the enzymes involved in its metabolism. The classical syndrome of homocystinuria, first described in 1962 (Carson, 1962; Gerritsen, 1962), is due to a homozygous defect in the enzyme cystathionine-β-synthase (CBS). It results in very high circulating levels of the various forms of Hcy and methionine. Clinical manifestations include dislocation of the optical lens, osteoporosis with associated skeletal abnormalities, mental retardation, psychiatric disturbance, and thromboembolic disease, such as CHD (Yap, 2003).

The basis of the damaging effects of Hcy is uncertain. At a biochemical level, oxidant stress and inhibition of transmethylation reactions are likely possibilities. Cellular effects that have been documented in experimental systems include endothelial injury, alteration of nitric oxide metabolism, platelet activation, and smooth muscle proliferation (Thambyrajah, 2000). Some of the toxicity of Hcy may derive from its enzymatic conversion to Hcy thiolactone (see Fig. 18-4), which can modify LDL and enhance its uptake by macrophages (McCully, 1993; Vignini, 2004).

The development of Hcy as a CHD risk marker in some ways parallels that of cholesterol: The regular occurrence of atherosclerosis in persons with massive elevation, due to an inborn error of metabolism, led to the hypothesis of increased risk in individuals with more moderate elevations. Experimentally induced hyperhomocysteinemia in animals lent support to the hypothesis (McCully, 1993). In humans, mild to moderate elevations in Hcy can have many causes. Genetic causes include a heterozygous defect in CBS, a defect in methionine synthase (rare), or a defect in 5,10-methylenetetrahydrofolate reductase (generally rare, except for a temperature-sensitive form that is relatively common). Nutritional causes include a deficiency of any of the vitamin cofactors involved in metabolism of Hcy: folate, B_{12}, or pyridoxine (B_6).

Many of the earlier epidemiology studies seemed to confirm a correlation between moderate Hcy levels and CHD. For example, in the Physicians Health Study, it was initially reported that having a Hcy level in the upper 5% of the population conferred a 3- to 4-fold higher risk (Stampfer, 1992). However, other studies, including a longer-term follow-up in the Physicians Health Study (Chasan-Taber, 1996) and many of the larger and more recent studies, have shown little or no association between moderate elevations of Hcy and CHD risk. A recent meta-analysis has supported a moderate association between Hcy and CHD risk (Humphrey, 2008). Widespread folate supplementation of food has probably tended to diminish average circulating Hcy in the U.S. population, and sparse data support the cardioprotective effects of Hcy-lowering therapy. For these reasons, no general advice regarding widespread Hcy screening is available (Kaul, 2006). However, measurement of Hcy may be warranted in individuals who develop CHD despite being at relatively low risk according to traditional risk factors.

Hcy has traditionally been measured by chromatographic techniques (Vester, 1991; Ubbink, 1999; Frick, 2003; Arndt, 2004). A method using enzymatic adenosylation followed by immunoassay has been automated on the Abbott IMx analyzer (Shipchandler, 1995), and purely enzymatic methods suitable for automation have also been introduced (Tan, 2000; Huijgen, 2004; Roberts, 2004). Attention must be paid to proper sample collection and storage to prevent an artifactual increase in measured Hcy (Willems, 2004).

MARKERS OF CONGESTIVE HEART FAILURE

CARDIAC NATRIURETIC PEPTIDES

The heretical concept that the heart could be an endocrine organ was enforced by two reports in 1956: (1) that inflating a balloon inside the left atrium of a dog caused an increase in urine flow (Henry, 1956); and (2) that structures resembling secretory granules were visible on electron micrographs of guinea pig atrial cells (Kisch, 1956). In 1981, extracts of rat heart atria (but not ventricles) were found to have a natriuretic effect (de Bold, 1981), and in 1984, a peptide named atrial natriuretic peptide (ANP) was isolated from human heart (Kangawa, 1984) A short time later, a similar peptide named brain natriuretic peptide (BNP) was isolated from porcine brain (Sudoh, 1988). It turns out that in humans, BNP is produced mainly in the cardiac ventricle (Mukoyama, 1991), so the hormone now is commonly referred to as B-type natriuretic peptide.

Members of the natriuretic peptide family are illustrated in Figure 18-5. Their notable common feature is a 17 amino acid ring structure, closed by a cystine bridge, with substantial homology among the family members. C-type natriuretic peptide (CNP), described in 1990, is produced not in the heart but rather in endothelial cells (Sudoh, 1990). D-type natriuretic peptide (DNP) was isolated in 1992 from the green mamba snake, *Dendroaspis angusticeps* (Schweitz, 1992). DNP immunoreactivity was later reported in human plasma (Schirger, 1999), but this peptide has not been definitively demonstrated in humans (Richards, 2002). Finally, urodilatin is a form of ANP with four additional amino acids at the N-terminus; it is likely produced in the kidney by alternative splicing of the same gene product (Schulz-Knappe, 1988). Both ANP and BNP have been investigated regarding testing for HF; the latter has proved more useful, so further discussion will be confined to the BNP system.

Circulating BNP derives from a 108 amino acid prohormone, proBNP, which is cleaved within the cardiac myocyte by the endoprotease furin to a 32 amino acid C-terminal fragment, the active BNP, and an inactive N-terminal fragment, N-BNP or NT-proBNP (Sawada, 1997). Secretion of both fragments is enhanced by ventricular wall stretch and volume overload, as occur in HF (Tabbibizar, 2002). BNP is removed from the circulation by binding to a clearance receptor and also through the action of endopeptidases; its circulating half-life is approximately 22 minutes. The circulating half-life of N-BNP is considerably longer (60–120 min), and its mechanism of clearance is not well understood.

BNP and the other natriuretic peptides exert their effects through two types of G-protein–coupled receptors, resulting in release of the second messenger cyclic guanosine monophosphate. They downregulate the renin-angiotensin-aldosterone system, decrease sympathetic nerve activity in the heart and kidney, increase renal blood flow, and increase sodium excretion via a direct effect on the renal collecting duct (Beltowski, 2002; Spevack, 2004).

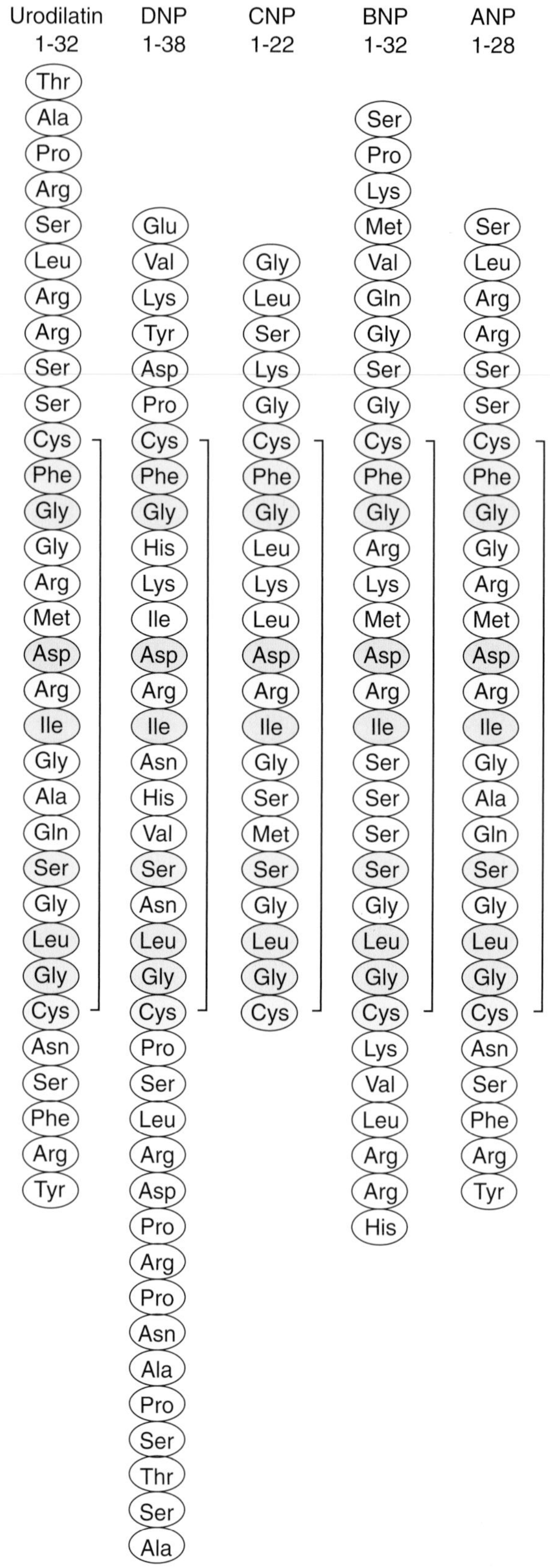

Figure 18-5 Amino acid sequences of the natriuretic peptides. Amino acids preserved through the family are indicated in color. *ANP,* Atrial natriuretic peptide; *BNP,* B-type natriuretic peptide; *CNP,* C-type natriuretic peptide; *DNP,* D-type natriuretic peptide.

Plasma levels of BNP are less than 100 pg/mL in most healthy individuals; reference ranges depend on age and gender. The best established application of BNP measurement is for diagnosing acutely ill patients presenting to emergency service with shortness of breath. Distinguishing HF from lung disease, such as emphysema, in these patients is occasionally difficult, and until now no laboratory test has been specifically applicable. The multinational Breathing Not Properly study enrolled patients who presented to emergency centers with dyspnea and used a point-of-care method for measurement of BNP. At a decision point of 100 pg/mL, the BNP test had the following characteristics for diagnosis of HF: sensitivity 90%, specificity 76%, positive predictive value 79%, and negative predictive value 89% (Maisel, 2002). Among patients with a history of ventricular dysfunction, BNP was higher in those whose current symptoms were thought to be caused by HF; it was also higher in patients with more severe failure (see http://www.americanheart.org/presenter.jhtml?identifier=4569) (Fig. 18-6).

BNP levels decline when effective therapy for HF is instituted, and so the test may be used to monitor the course of treatment (Cheng, 2001; Faggiano, 2009; Novo, 2009). Other proposed applications include risk stratification of patients with ACS (de Lemos, 2001; Omland, 2002; Jernberg, 2004; Wiviott, 2004); monitoring disease severity in patients with stable CHD (Weber, 2004); screening for ventricular dysfunction in selected populations (Bay, 2003; Nielsen, 2003); and testing for drug cardiotoxicity (Okumura, 2000). However, the test is relatively expensive, so routine application that leads to a large volume of testing needs to be carefully considered. Some medical centers have introduced restrictions to limit the use of BNP for monitoring inpatients (Lum, 2006).

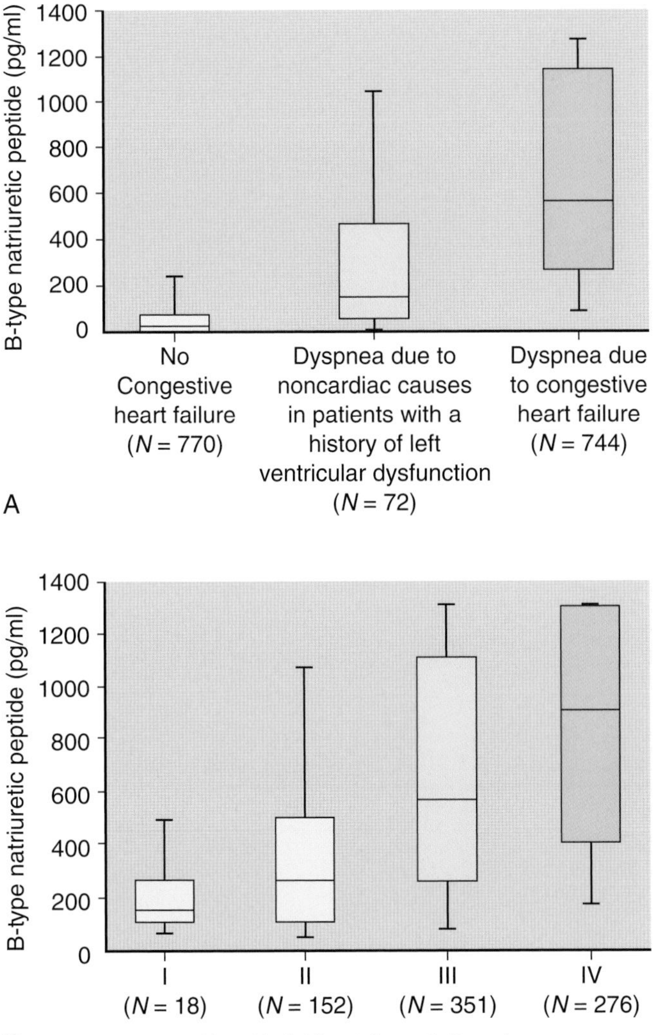

Figure 18-6 Box plots showing median levels of B-type natriuretic peptide in patients presenting to an emergency department with dyspnea, in the Breathing Not Properly study. **A,** Patients in different diagnostic categories. **B,** Patients with heart failure, classified according to the New York Heart Association criteria. A higher class indicates more severe disease, as evidenced by a lesser amount of activity needed to provoke symptoms. Boxes show interquartile ranges, and I bars represent highest and lowest values. *(From Maisel AS, Krishnaswamy P, Nowak RM, et al. Rapid measurement of B-type natriuretic peptide in the emergency diagnosis of heart failure. N Engl J Med 2002;347:161–167, with permission).*

A major limitation of BNP is that a wide range of values is observed in patients with and without HF, and all of the determinants of the circulating BNP level have not yet been well established. BNP is increased in conditions of fluid imbalance other than HF, particularly renal insufficiency, which commonly coexists with HF (McCullough, 2004). In individuals without HF, higher levels are associated with female gender, advanced age, and lower body mass index (Chiong, 2009). Also, patients with symptomatic HF, especially when it is chronic and stable, can have "normal" levels (Tang, 2003). Intraindividual variability is relatively high; in a group of patients with stable, chronic HF, week-to-week variability for BNP and N-BNP was 30%–40% (Bruins, 2004). At this time, it appears that the most appropriate use of the BNP test is as an adjunctive test to rule out HF in the acute setting; it must *not* be used as a sole criterion for establishing the diagnosis of HF (Jessup, 2009). In other contexts, it should be used judiciously as more information becomes available.

The earliest assay for BNP commercially available in the United States was an immunoassay using an instrument most suitable for point-of-care measurement. Recently, the test has become available on large, automated immunoassay platforms. Assays for both BNP and N-BNP are available; a clear advantage of one biomarker over the other for any particular application has not been established (Hammerer-Lercher, 2001b).

Besides being a biomarker for HF, BNP has natriuretic, vasodilatory, and other effects that are ameliorative for the syndrome, and in fact is available as the drug nesiritide (Natrecor) for the treatment of HF. Because of the short half-life of BNP, measured levels several hours after its administration would reflect endogenous secretion. However, the utility of BNP measurement in the context of its therapeutic administration has not been established at this time.

Other Conditions Associated With Atherosclerosis or Thrombosis

A cerebrovascular accident, or stroke, is another dreaded complication of atherosclerotic disease. About 795,000 Americans suffered a stroke in 2009, versus about 1,250,000 who suffered an ACS (Lloyd-Jones, 2009). Many strokes are presumably caused by a mechanism similar to the usual ACS, where atherosclerotic plaque eventually becomes unstable and ruptures, resulting in thrombotic occlusion. However, additional mechanisms can cause ischemic stroke, and 20% of strokes result from hemorrhage rather than from vascular occlusion. Considerable effort has been directed at finding biomarkers for stroke that might rival the utility of troponin and other markers for cardiac disease. Candidate markers have included neurotransmitters; proteins produced in neurons or glia such as tau, S100b, and neuron-specific enolase; inflammatory mediators such as CRP, interleukins, and matrix metalloproteinases; and others. At the time of writing, none has been shown to have sufficient sensitivity and specificity for incorporation into routine practice (Whiteley, 2009). Possibly a multiple marker approach will eventually be successful, but at present, the diagnosis and management of stroke rests on clinical findings and imaging studies.

Thrombosis in peripheral veins can result in dislodging of part of the thrombus—embolization—which, after passing through the right side of the heart, will lodge in the lung, causing the syndrome of a pulmonary embolus (PE). Depending on the size of the PE, consequences can range from minimal to sudden death. PE can cause chest pain, ECG abnormalities, and increased cTn levels, and thus may be confused with an ACS. Measurement of D-dimer, a specific degradation product of fibrin (see Chapter 39), has become a useful laboratory test for ruling out PE and venous thrombotic disease in general. Almost any activation of the coagulation cascade, anywhere in the body, leads to production of D-dimer; hence elevated levels are widespread, especially in hospitalized patients, and have little meaning. When pre-test probability of thrombotic disease is low, however, low levels of D-dimer have high negative predictive value in excluding the diagnosis of PE (as well as any venous thrombosis). Sensitive immunoassay measurements of D-dimer for this purpose are now available (Adam, 2009).

SELECTED REFERENCES

Adams MR, Kinlay S, Blake GJ, et al. Atherogenic lipids and endothelial dysfunction: mechanisms in the genesis of ischemic syndromes. Annu Rev Med 2000;51:149–67.

Reviews mechanisms involved in the genesis of CHD.

Danesh J, Wheeler JG, Hirschfield GM, et al. C-reactive protein and other circulating markers of inflammation in the prediction of coronary heart disease. N Engl J Med 2004;350:1387–97.

A relatively large study of coronary risk associated with CRP, along with a meta-analysis.

Mair J. Progress in myocardial damage detection: new biochemical markers for clinicians. Crit Rev Clin Lab Sci 1997;34:1–66.

Although some new information is missing, gives a relatively complete review of the biochemistry of cardiac markers.

Paoletti R, Gotto AM Jr, Hajjar DP. Inflammation in atherosclerosis and implications for therapy. Circulation 2004;109:III20–III6.

Discusses the role of inflammation in CHD.

Ridker PM, Cushman M, Stampfer MJ, et al. Inflammation, aspirin, and the risk of cardiovascular disease in apparently healthy men. N Engl J Med 1997;336:973–9.

One of the earlier major studies to establish CRP as a risk factor for CHD.

Ross R. The pathogenesis of atherosclerosis: a perspective for the 1990s. Nature 1993;362:801–9.

Discussion of the pathogenesis of CHD.

REFERENCES

Access the complete reference list online at http://www.expertconsult.com

CHAPTER 19

SPECIFIC PROTEINS

Richard A. McPherson

KEY POINTS

- The primary structure of a protein is its linear sequence of amino acids with different side groups, which determine how the protein folds on itself (secondary and tertiary structures) and how it reacts with other molecules and cells (i.e., its molecular identity).
- Methods to quantitate and fractionate proteins are based on turbidimetry, colorimetry, absorption spectrophotometry, dye binding, column chromatography, electrophoresis, and immunoassays.
- Protein electrophoresis separates proteins according to their electrical charges (usually at pH 8.6).
- The major proteins in plasma that contribute to the electrophoretic pattern are albumin, α_1-antitrypsin, α_2-macroglobulin, haptoglobin, β-lipoprotein, transferrin, complement C3, fibrinogen, and immunoglobulins.
- Several minor components of plasma proteins, such as ceruloplasmin, C-reactive protein, prealbumin, and protease inhibitors, have clinical utility in diagnosing and monitoring diseases and are quantitated by immunoassays.
- Patterns of protein electrophoresis in serum and urine are characteristic of specific diseases primarily involving changes in synthetic rates (liver), loss (renal), or inflammatory states.
- Hereditary deficiency of some plasma proteins leads to significant diseases (e.g., α_1-antitrypsin).
- Proteins in plasma play several roles, including maintaining oncotic pressure, transporting small molecules, and promoting or inhibiting inflammatory reactions.
- The major clinical use of serum and urine protein electrophoresis is to screen for monoclonal gammopathies.

Examination of the proteins in plasma can provide information reflecting disease states in many different organ systems. The most frequently performed measurement—that for total protein—is usually performed on serum, which has no fibrinogen and no anticoagulant that may slightly dilute proteins in plasma. Although total protein determination gives the physician some information as to a patient's general status regarding nutrition or severe organ disease (as in protein-losing states), further fractionations yield far more clinically useful information.

Additional quantitation of albumin, for example, is more informative regarding nutritional status, liver synthetic capacity, and protein-losing nephropathy or enteropathy. It allows the clinician to interpret high or low calcium and magnesium levels, because albumin binds about one half of each of those ions on a molar basis. Calculated differences between total protein and albumin represent the value of all globulins, a composite of the other fractions that individually may rise several-fold in severe disorders.

Protein electrophoresis separates the globulins from albumin and resolves the major proteins of serum into patterns that may be highly specific for some diseases. High-resolution techniques can provide a display of all components in concentrations down to about 1 g/L (0.1 g/dL in traditional units); however, at that level, quantitation by scanning of stained proteins is not highly reliable, and alternative methods should be employed. Such techniques, involving immunologic detection of individual proteins, have the dual advantages of specificity and sensitivity over electrophoresis (see Chapter 44).

Yet there is much to be appreciated from visual inspection of an electrophoretogram of proteins, because the human eye is highly efficient at detecting subtle variations in individual proteins, as well as alterations in protein patterns. Identification of these patterns is a useful screening method to be followed by more specific confirmatory procedures to identify and quantitate aberrant protein bands. Protein electrophoresis also can be a useful tool for monitoring patients over long periods of time when marked alterations are noted in levels of particular proteins, such as in myeloma, nephrotic syndrome, cirrhosis, or extensive body burn.

This chapter will review protein structure, methods of measurement and separation, the major plasma proteins (except coagulation factors, immunoglobulins, and the complement system, which are covered in Chapters 39, 46, and 47), and some of the patterns encountered in particular disease states.

PROTEIN STRUCTURE

The backbone of all protein molecules is a continuous chain of carbon and nitrogen atoms joined together through peptide bonds between adjacent amino acids. At one end (the amino-terminus) is a free amino group, and at the other end (the carboxy-terminus) is a free carboxyl group. Whereas the peptide backbone is qualitatively invariant between different proteins (its total length is equivalent to the total number of amino acids in a particular protein), proteins have structural identity by virtue of the side groups or residues of the constituent amino acids. The average molecular weight of an amino acid is 120 Da. Serum proteins range in size from roughly 66 kDa to over 700 kDa. These amino acid side chains are conventionally grouped according to chemical nature: hydrogen (glycine), aliphatic (alanine, valine, leucine, and isoleucine), hydroxymethylamino (serine and threonine), aromatic (tyrosine, phenylalanine, and tryptophan), imino (proline and hydroxyproline), acidic (aspartate and glutamate), basic (arginine, histidine, and lysine), amides (asparagine and glutamine), and sulfur-containing (cysteine and methionine). These different side chains may be charged, polar, or hydrophobic, resulting in the tendency for them to be relatively soluble or insoluble in water, respectively.

The linear sequence of amino acids in a protein is called its *primary structure*; this sequence of amino acids determines the identity of a protein, what its molecular structure is, what functions it can perform, how it can bind to other molecules, and how it can participate in the processes of recognition between molecules and cells. These biological interactions are guided by reactivities between charged groups on one molecule and those on another, and similarly by hydrophobic interactions between molecules. Analytic processes such as chromatography, electrophoresis, dye binding, light absorbance, and others also depend on the primary amino acid sequence.

The *secondary structure* refers to specific regular three-dimensional conformations into which portions of the polypeptide chain fold. Three such structures have been identified (Branden, 1991). First is the α-helix, in which the chain forms a regular helix such that the backbone C=O of the *i*th peptide group participates in a hydrogen bond with the N–H of the (*i*+4)th peptide unit. The second is β-pleated sheets in fully extended structures, in which the chain forms a flat structure such that the side chains of adjacent amino acids point in opposite directions; in this conformation, two or more extended chains can associate so that the maximum number of C=O•••H–N bonds form between them. β-Pleated sheets can have their individual β-strands in parallel or antiparallel orientations. Finally, a third grouping of structures is the bend conformation, in which the direction of the polypeptide chain reverses itself, thereby allowing long primary structures to bend back on themselves and assume compact conformations.

The core of a protein molecule typically consists of combinations of α-helices and β-strands linked by loops of various lengths and shape. This inner core generally contains hydrophobic amino acids, whereas the loops and other surface portions of the protein molecule are richer in polar and charged amino acids that are hydrophilic. Upon degradation, some proteins (e.g., serum amyloid-associated protein, immunoglobulin light chains, prealbumin) release fragments rich in β-regions. These fragments are capable of coming together spontaneously in vivo to form deposits of β-sheets in fibrils that constitute amyloid. Recent work has shown an association between the genotype of apolipoprotein E (especially the allele apoE-4) and the progression of late-onset Alzheimer's disease, in which cerebral plaques of amyloid form within the brain. These genetic findings suggest that Alzheimer's disease may be understood and treated as a disease that has a biochemical basis in β-pleated sheet generation (Roses, 1994; Hayashi, 2004).

Molecular regions with clusters of hydrophobic side groups tend to remain on the interior of a protein that is soluble in water, whereas those regions with clusters of charges or other hydrophilic moieties tend to appear on the protein's surface. Conversely, proteins that are membrane bound usually have a distinct hydrophobic segment that protrudes to anchor the protein molecule in the lipid phase of the membrane. The actual three-dimensional structure or folding pattern of the protein, uniquely determined by its amino acid sequence, is termed its *tertiary structure*. Individual proteins or monomeric subunits may form more stable complexes, such as dimers, trimers, and tetramers; this is termed *quaternary structure*.

The sulfhydryl group on a cysteine residue can form a disulfide (covalent) bond with another cysteine within the same protein to hold different segments tightly together. This action helps stabilize the whole structure from disruption by mechanical, thermal, or other forces. These intramolecular disulfide bonds most likely form after spontaneous protein folding along the linear amino acid sequence into most thermodynamically stable conformations. Disulfide bonds can also form between cysteine residues on different molecules, thereby stabilizing multimeric molecular structures (e.g., haptoglobin, von Willebrand antigen).

The acidic and basic amino acids determine the net charge on a protein and hence its electrophoretic mobility. The charge on carboxyl and amino groups is a function of pH (i.e., whether a hydrogen ion is bound to or dissociated from the group). Combining all the different side groups and their different degrees of dissociation, the pH at which a particular protein has net charge equal to zero is called its isoelectric point (pI). Proteins with pI less than 7 are acidic and tend to have carboxyl side groups exposed, whereas those with pI greater than 7 are basic (e.g., histones that, in turn, bind to the external helical structure of DNA that is negatively charged with phosphate groups).

Proteins are synthesized from the amino end to the carboxyl end by ribosomes translating from the information encoded in messenger RNA. The initial translation product of some proteins is acted on before secretion by proteolytic enzymes that convert a preform to the mature protein by removal of a signal peptide (generally hydrophobic) that otherwise holds the new protein molecule to the endoplasmic reticulum. Release of a preprotein from the endoplasmic reticulum entails passage through a membrane pore with the participation of various translocation factors (Brodsky, 1998). The correct assembly of a protein may critically depend on the function of so-called molecular chaperones, which are other proteins that guide the folding of nascent proteins in concert with proteases that remove selective segments to achieve functional conformations (Wickner, 1999). Many genetic diseases are due to harmful mutations in DNA, leading to alterations in the amino acid sequence of a protein that may block this complex assembly process or that may render any assembled protein molecules nonfunctional (Kuznetsov, 1998).

Additional modifications to protein structures occur post-translationally (i.e., after joining of the amino acids is complete) (Harding, 1985). Phosphorylation consists of the enzymatically regulated attachment of phosphate groups to serine and threonine groups as well as tyrosine (e.g., by tyrosine kinases) in the peptide backbone, thereby forming phosphoproteins with a more negative charge that can alter protein functions and state of activation. Glycosylation may occur spontaneously, in the presence of sugar molecules, or in a directed manner under enzymatic control, in which oligosaccharides, frequently terminating with sialic acid (which carries a negative charge), are attached to the protein (Van den Steen, 1998). These species of molecules are termed glycoproteins. Linkages are generally to asparagine residues through *N*-acetylglucosamine or to serine and threonine residues through *N*-acetylgalactosamine. Proteolysis results in the cleavage or removal of short segments of the peptide backbone that can open up catalytic sites of a zymogen (e.g., plasminogen to plasmin) or facilitate recognition by a receptor molecule (e.g., proinsulin to insulin). Many of these post-translational steps are unique to eukaryotic cells and do not occur in prokaryotic cells; this point is very important to the biotechnology industry, which uses cloned genes to produce human proteins in bacteria, yeast, or other artificial cell types, and so must take additional steps to synthesize accurate molecules (Jenkins, 1996). Post-translational changes in the structure of proteins influence their antigenicity, specific chemical or catalytic activities, abilities to bind to receptors, and electrophoretic mobilities.

TECHNIQUES OF PROTEIN SEPARATION

ELECTROPHORESIS

Modern understanding of the protein composition of serum and plasma derives from the electrophoretic techniques introduced by Tiselius. He separated proteins dissolved in an electrolyte solution by application of an electric current through a U-shaped quartz tube that held the protein solution. At pH 7.6, four serum protein fractions, designated albumin, α, β, and γ, were identified and quantified optically by change in refractive index at the boundaries among these bands. Because separation was achieved in a homogeneous solution without solid support medium, convective forces prevented resolution into distinct zones. Hence, this technique has been termed moving boundary or frontal electrophoresis. Introduction of filter paper as an anticonvection support medium permitted separation of the protein fractions into discrete bands or zones in a process termed *zonal electrophoresis*. On solid support medium and at pH 8.6, the α fraction further splits into two groups of proteins, α_1 and α_2. Other support media, such as cellulose acetate membrane, agarose gel, starch gel, and polyacrylamide gel, have been used. Cellulose acetate and agarose have predominated in the clinical laboratory because of ease of use, low cost, and commercial availability (Jeppsson, 1979).

Application of samples can be done in wells that are cut into the gel, but this process typically leaves an artifact that can interfere with the scan. A method to get around this problem involves soaking the sample into the gel by means of an overlying template. Each end of the gel is then immersed into separate buffer chambers in which electrodes are mounted. A voltage is applied between the electrodes, generating a current that passes through the gel, usually for a period of about 30 minutes, to achieve desired resolution. The ionic strength of the buffer determines the amount of current and the movement of the proteins for a fixed voltage. If ionic strength is low, relatively more current is carried by the charged proteins. If ionic strength is high, less current is carried by the proteins, which move a shorter distance. If the electrodes are not properly aligned, the current

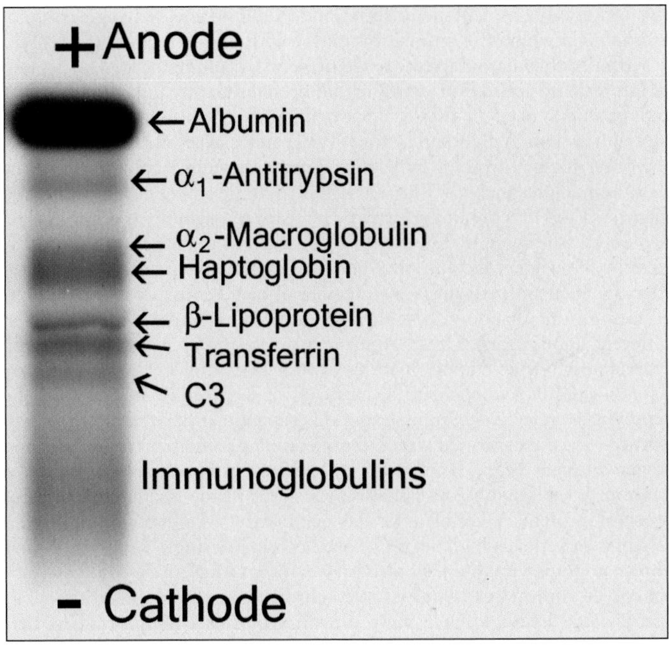

Figure 19-1 Positions of major serum proteins in a normal person using electrophoresis in agarose. Individual proteins separate according to their electrical charge between the anode (positive pole) and the cathode (negative pole).

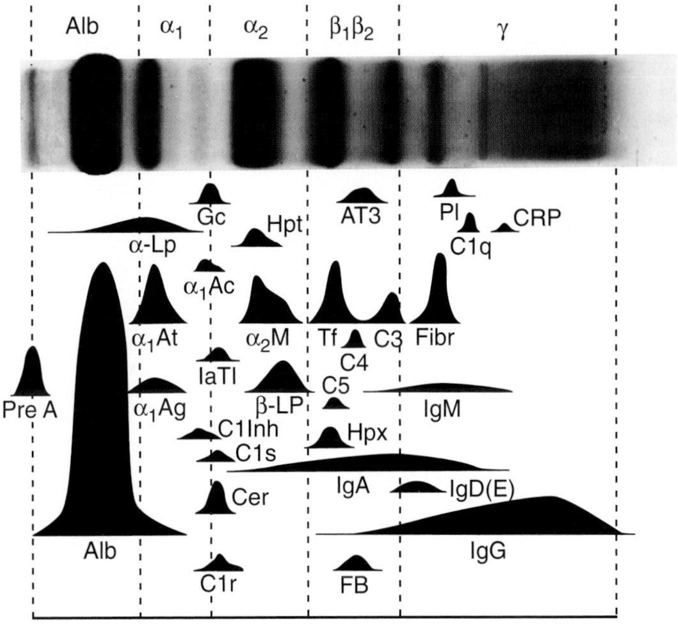

Figure 19-2 Plasma protein electrophoresis pattern in agarose gel is composed of five fractions, each composed of many individual species. Some of the major proteins are shown here in an artist's rendition for clarity. *(Adapted from Laurell CB. Electrophoresis, specific protein assays, or both in measurement of plasma proteins? Clin Chem 1973;19:99, with permission.)* *α_1Ac,* α_1-Antichymotrypsin; *α_1Ag,* α_1-acid glycoprotein; *α_1At,* α_1-antitrypsin; *α_2-M,* α_2-macroglobulin; *α-Lp,* α-lipoprotein; *Alb,* albumin; *AT3,* antithrombin III; *β-Lp,* β-lipoprotein; complement components *C1q, C1r, C1s, C3, C4, C5,* as designated; *C1Inh,* C1 esterase inhibitor; *Cer,* Ceruloplasmin; *CRP,* C-reactive protein; *Gc,* Gc-globulin (vitamin D–binding protein); *FB,* factor B; *Fibr,* fibrinogen; *Hpt,* haptoglobin; *Hpx,* hemopexin; immunoglobulins *IgA, IgD, IgE, IgG, IgM,* as designated; *IαTI,* Inter-α-trypsin inhibitor; *Pl,* plasminogen; *Pre A,* prealbumin; *Tf,* transferrin.

may be denser on one side of the gel than on the other; proteins will migrate farther on the side with more current. If electrophoresis proceeds too long, the proteins may migrate off the gel into the buffer. If there is a break in the electrical circuit and no current passes, the proteins will not move from the point of application. Frequently, gels show the "smile artifact," in which samples at the center of the gel migrate farther than those at the edges.

After electrophoresis, the gel is treated with a mild fixative, such as acetic acid, that precipitates the proteins at the positions to which they have migrated. They are then stained, and the gel is dried and cleared of excess stain. Protein patterns can be inspected visually for qualitative identification of abnormal proteins. Densitometric scanners are used to generate tracings and to quantitate the relative percentages of protein in each fraction. Those percentages are then multiplied by the total protein (separately measured) in the sample to yield the concentration of protein in each fraction.

When an electrophoretic support medium has a negative charge, the electromotive force to which it is subjected tends to move it toward the anode (positive pole; Fig. 19-1). However, the solid support medium is fixed, and so it cannot move. The complementary positively charged ions in the surrounding buffer are free to move under the electromotive force, and they carry with them molecules of the solvent water, which are clustered around their charges. The net result is flow of buffer toward the cathode. This buffer flow is termed electro-osmosis or endosmosis, which also carries the proteins with it to some extent by mechanical flow, not by charge. The actual distance traveled by a particular protein migrating in an electrical field is determined by the combined magnitudes of the electromotive force (a feature of the protein itself and the pH) and the electro-osmotic force (a function primarily of the support medium). When the electro-osmotic force is greater than the electrophoretic force acting on weakly anionic proteins (e.g., γ-globulins), those proteins move from the application point toward the cathode, even though their charge is slightly negative.

Through critical manipulations of buffer salt composition, endosmotic properties of the medium, and means of sample application, commercially available electrophoretic agarose plates now achieve consistently high-resolution quality that allows routine separation of all major serum protein species (Fig. 19-2). Because of variability in the chemical formulations of gels, it should not necessarily be expected that each manufacturer's electrophoretic system will yield identical protein separation patterns. Furthermore, optimal separation of isoenzymes generally requires different buffer and gel composition compared with the conditions for best resolution of serum proteins versus lipoproteins versus hemoglobins. A significant variation in conditions for protein electrophoresis is that for optimizing the separation of the γ-region to resolve and detect oligoclonal bands of immunoglobulin in cerebrospinal fluid (CSF). In this case, the endosmosis is set high to maximize the cathodal movement of immunoglobulins from the point of application over a span of the gel that is convenient for visual inspection.

Polyacrylamide is an inert support medium whose porosity is easily adjusted by changing the composition of acrylamide before polymerization. Although polyacrylamide gel electrophoresis (PAGE) is applicable to standard separation of native proteins, it can also be used for separating proteins according to molecular weight when they are denatured in the presence of sodium dodecyl sulfate (SDS). SDS-PAGE is at present the most widely used protein electrophoretic technique for research in molecular biology. However, its very power for resolving proteins and separating them into multitudinous subunits has virtually excluded it from routine use in the clinical laboratory. Nevertheless, there is promise for clinical application of two-dimensional electrophoresis (2-DE), which uses standard separation in one direction followed by SDS-PAGE in the perpendicular direction. 2-DE results in perhaps hundreds of identifiable protein peaks, from which it may be possible to obtain important diagnostic information by sophisticated pattern analysis.

Isoelectric focusing affords superior resolution of closely migrating proteins or various forms of a single protein that differ in charge owing to minor modification (e.g., post-translational) (see Chapter 4). By this technique, proteins migrate through a gel containing a gradient of pH established with a mixture of ampholytes. As each protein reaches the gel location where the pH is equal to its pI, the net charge on it becomes zero. It no longer has electromotive force acting on it, and it comes to rest. Thus the final pattern is strictly according to pI.

PRECIPITATION

Chemical precipitations of serum proteins have been devised to resolve albumin and the globulins into two or more fractions that can then be measured for protein content. With the addition of sodium sulfate, sodium sulfite, ammonium sulfate, or methanol, the globulins tend to precipitate, leaving albumin in solution. By measuring total protein in the original serum and protein in the precipitate or the supernatant, values for albumin and globulin can be derived. The ratio of these values (A/G ratio) has been used extensively because it accentuates abnormalities in serum protein composition, which in disease generally involve depression of albumin and elevation of one or more globulin fractions. Albumin may be depressed owing to decreased synthesis (malnutrition, malabsorption, liver failure, diversion to synthesis of other proteins) or increased loss (proteinuria, accumulation of ascites fluid, enteropathy). Globulins may be elevated owing to increased synthesis of many different proteins as part of acute or chronic reactions to disease. Lowering of albumin and elevation of globulins tend to occur simultaneously in disease, thus leading to exaggerated changes in the A/G ratio as the numerator and denominator move in opposite directions. Precipitation methods are not as accurate as zonal electrophoresis, because some α-globulins may fail to precipitate, thus leading to an overestimate of the albumin fraction.

Preparative procedures for the isolation of a single minor protein constituent usually begin with a precipitation step to remove the bulk of other undesired serum proteins. The next step in protein isolation typically involves a column that separates on the basis of molecular size (gel filtration) or charge (ion exchange).

COLUMN SEPARATIONS

Gel filtration media such as Sephadex or agarose beads are rated according to pore size, which in turn determines what size molecules can pass through the interior of each bead or particle of the column. After application of a sample composed of various-sized proteins in aqueous solvent containing buffer and salt, more of the buffer is applied to drive the sample through the column. Very large molecules tend to flow through interstices of the column without entering the beads and emerge first from the bottom of the column in the void volume. Slightly smaller molecules enter the largest pores before being washed through and so are slightly retarded in passing through the column. Small protein molecules pass into still smaller pores and are retained still longer. Finally, particles the size of dissolved salt penetrate farthest into the interior of gel filtration beads and come out after all the proteins have emerged in an amount of applied buffer called the salt volume. Thus, in gel filtration the order of protein elution is by molecular weight or size, from largest first to smallest last. Because all protein species continuously move through a gel filtration column all at the same time but at different rates, it is necessary to apply the sample in a small and uniform volume to optimize separation between peaks. Gel filtration requires that the medium be inert and not interact chemically or by charge with the proteins. It is not a method to be employed for high-resolution separation.

Ion-exchange chromatography, on the other hand, takes advantage of the charge on proteins to bind them to beads of a support medium with positively charged components such as diethylaminoethyl or quaternary aminoethyl. In anion-exchange chromatography, proteins are usually applied at a basic pH such as 8.6, at which they may be negatively charged (albumin and α_1-, α_2-, and β-globulins are anions) or may have no net charge (γ-globulins). The neutral proteins pass immediately through an anion-exchange column, whereas the anionic ones stick to the positively charged column matrix. If a buffer with a higher salt concentration is washed through, anions of the salt displace the anionic proteins and exchange for them by binding to the support medium. The proteins then elute from the column. By using a steadily increasing gradient of salt concentration in the eluting buffer, the proteins can be resolved according to charge. The ones with a small amount of charge will elute first, whereas those with the greatest charge (e.g., albumin) elute only when displaced by higher salt levels.

Alternatively, if pH is lowered while salt concentration is held low, anionic proteins acquire a net neutral or slightly positive charge and pass through the column. A gradient of falling pH can be used to resolve anionic proteins, with the order of elution being roughly β-, α_2-, and α_1-globulins, and albumin. Note that this order of elution is the reverse order of electrophoretic migration at pH 8.6, because in anion-exchange chromatography, mobility is retarded according to net negative charge, whereas in electrophoresis, mobility is enhanced by that charge.

Cation-exchange chromatography begins at an acid pH, with the proteins having positive charge (cations) and adhering to a negatively charged column matrix such as carboxymethylcellulose. They can be displaced by the cations of high salt in an eluting buffer or by increasing the pH, which will reverse the charge on the proteins to negative. By cation exchange, albumin should elute first, followed by α_1-, α_2-, β-, and γ-globulins.

Another separation modality by column is hydrophobic chromatography, in which samples are applied at high salt and are eluted with low salt. The support medium interacts with proteins with a hydrophobic nature; this is a good complementary technique to follow ion-exchange chromatography, in which the sample was eluted with high salt.

Affinity chromatography is based on specific binding between a protein of interest and another protein that has been covalently linked to the solid support medium of a column. For example, coagulation factor VIII complexed with von Willebrand factor (vWF) can be selectively removed from the other plasma proteins by passing plasma through a column that contains monoclonal anti-vWF antibody linked to the solid phase matrix. The factor VIII–vWF complex selectively binds to the column as other plasma proteins wash through. The factor VIII is then dissociated from the vWF, thereby allowing it to elute in a purified fraction suitable for transfusion therapy. Such antigen–antibody interactions may be disrupted by high salt concentration, change in pH, or a chemical denaturant, such as urea, in different applications. Other affinity chromatography gels use a binding phenomenon that mimics naturally occurring molecular interactions. Thus, some dyes coupled to agarose are able to bind albumin, thereby removing it selectively from serum. Therapeutic antibodies or their Fab portions are concentrated with affinity columns containing their intended target antigens (e.g., Digibind for digoxin, CroFab for crotalid snake venom). Immunoglobulins can also be absorbed from a sample by staphylococcal protein A coupled to the gel matrix. Many other separation schemes can effect a high degree of purification in a single step with affinity chromatography medium coupled to dyes, drugs, nucleotide cofactors, and sugars. A clinical test using affinity chromatography is quantitation of glycosylated hemoglobin using a dihydroxyboronate affinity matrix that selectively binds molecular species of hemoglobin to which glucose has been covalently attached, while allowing the nonglycosylated forms to pass through the column. The glycosylated hemoglobin is then separately eluted and quantitated.

Capillary electrophoresis is a separation method based on flow through a capillary tube that can be tailored to resolution of different molecules based on size, hydrophobicity, or stereospecificity. It is applicable to large molecules such as DNA or proteins, as well as to small ones such as hormones or therapeutic drugs. Physically, the method is similar to high-performance liquid chromatography (HPLC), in which solvent is pumped through a column that retains or passes solutes according to chemical interactions. Capillary electrophoresis for serum proteins employs a column with properties similar to agarose, so the separation of proteins is comparable with that from electrophoresis. This analysis can be automated with a detector at the effluent end that detects and quantitates protein bands without the need for staining and separate scanning. Although equipment costs are relatively high for capillary electrophoresis, reagent and labor costs are low and the procedure is fast and very quantitative, leading to the promise of more widespread clinical applications in the future (Chen, 1991; Brinkman, 2004).

PROTEIN DETECTION AND QUANTITATION

The ultimate reference method for determining concentration of protein is the analysis for nitrogen content. Nitrogen is present uniformly along the peptide bonds throughout the length of a protein and more irregularly in the side groups, wherever tryptophan, arginine, lysine, histidine, asparagine, or glutamine is present. The Kjeldahl technique consists of acid digestion to release ammonium ions from nitrogen-containing compounds. The ammonium can then be quantitated by conversion to ammonia gas and titration as a base, or by nesslerization, in which double iodides (potassium and mercuric) form a colored complex with ammonia in alkali. Although determination of nitrogen content can be extremely precise, its use for calculation of protein concentration depends on the exact protein composition of a sample, because each protein has a somewhat different nitrogen content according to amino acid composition. However, for a sample of a purified protein, nitrogen content is highly accurate for estimating protein concentration when the nitrogen content on a molar basis is already known for that purified protein. Knowledge of a protein's exact amino acid sequence allows an accurate calculation of what the nitrogen content should be. Because clinical samples consist of unpredictable mixtures of different proteins, and measurement of nitrogen content is not a simple procedure, it is not commonly used in clinical laboratories.

Refractive index can be accurate for measuring serum protein concentration as dissolved solute for levels above 2.5 g/dL. Hemolysis, lipemia, icterus, and azotemia produce erroneously high results. Refractive index cannot be used for urine protein measurements because of excess amounts of solutes in relation to the protein.

Specific gravity (and thus, by inference, protein content) can be estimated by pipetting drops of serum or blood into a graded series of copper sulfate solutions. A protein–copper shell forms about the drop to prevent dissolution for a short interval, during which time the drop falls to the bottom, remains stationary, or rises to the top. The protein concentration of a sample is estimated from the specific gravity of the copper sulfate solution in which the drop remains stationary. This technique is simple and has been used widely as a screening test for hemoglobin concentration in whole blood.

Proteins in solution absorb ultraviolet light at 280 nm (A_{280}), owing mostly to tryptophan but also to tyrosine and phenylalanine (Layne, 1957). For accurate conversion of A_{280} readings to protein concentration, the molar absorptivity must be used, because each protein contains a different amount of these three amino acids. However, the A_{280} of a mixture of proteins is not a perfect measure of protein content because molar absorptivities vary greatly between different proteins. Because nucleic acids (which absorb strongly at 260 nm and also somewhat at 280 nm) may be present in protein preparations, a better estimate of protein concentration in the presence of nucleic acids is given by the formula:

$$\text{Protein concentration (mg/mL)} = 1.55 \times A_{280} - 0.76 \times A_{260}$$

Direct measurements of absorbance can be used for quantitating proteins in the range of 0.05–1.5 mg/mL.

Turbidimetric methods are often used for a similar concentration range in CSF or urine. Protein forms precipitate on the addition of trichloroacetic acid, sulfosalicylic acid, or other acid reagent. The resulting turbidity can be used for protein quantitation by increment in optical density in comparison with similarly treated standards. However, these techniques are not specific to proteins, because other acid-insoluble substances such as nucleic acids can also precipitate.

A colorimetric technique highly specific for proteins and peptides is the Biuret method, by which copper salts in alkaline solution form a purple complex with substances containing two or more peptide bonds. Interferences are minimal, although ammonium ion may acidify the reaction, while hemoglobin and bilirubin absorb in the same region as the Biuret complex (540–560 nm). The Biuret method is extensively used in clinical laboratories, particularly in automated analyzers in which protein concentration can be measured down to 10 or 15 mg/dL.

Greater sensitivity can be obtained using the Folin-Ciocalteu reagent (or phenol reagent, phosphotungstomolybdic acid), which oxidizes phenolic compounds such as tyrosine and, in addition, tryptophan and histidine to give a deep blue color.

Lowry (1951) used the Biuret method followed by the phenol reagent, which greatly enhanced color formation, because the phenol reagent can react with Biuret complexes involving all peptide bonds. The Lowry assay has been extensively used for consistently accurate determinations of protein concentration.

Further sensitivity for detection down to 1 µg of protein can be obtained using Coomassie brilliant blue dye, which is free of interferences from a very wide range of substances.

Comparable sensitivity is obtained with ninhydrin, which develops a violet color by reacting with primary amines. This reagent is widely used for detection of peptides and amino acids after paper chromatography and amino acid analyses from ion-exchange columns, as well as for detection of drugs on toxicology screens using thin-layer chromatography (see Chapter 23).

Quantitation of albumin in the presence of other proteins is possible by virtue of the specific binding of albumin to certain dyes such as bromphenol blue, methyl orange, hydroxybenzeneazobenzoic acid, bromcresol purple, and bromcresol green (BCG). BCG is used extensively in automatic analyzers for determining serum albumin in parallel with Biuret reagent for total protein. Dyes bound to albumin absorb maximally at slightly different wavelengths, thus allowing direct spectrophotometric quantitation of the albumin.

The standard dyes used for staining electrophoresis are Coomassie brilliant blue, Ponceau S, and amido black. For detection of minor components in high-resolution gels, silver staining is very sensitive down to nanogram quantities (Merril, 1981).

In addition, special dyes, such as Oil Red O and Sudan black, stain lipoproteins, and periodic acid–Schiff stains glycoproteins separated in special electrophoretic applications.

Because electrophoresis followed by staining does not afford explicit identification of serum proteins, immunologic measurements have been instituted for quantitation of individual proteins (Laurell, 1966). Nephelometry detects the turbidity produced usually within minutes or less by the precipitation of a reagent antibody with its target protein in a serum sample (Maachi, 2004). The major serum proteins are now widely measured by this method on automated immunochemistry analyzers that have supplanted former measurements by radial immunodiffusion. Owing to the specificity of the antibody reagent, nephelometry has great specificity for quantitating individual proteins even in the presence of others. Proteins present in lower concentrations may be quantitated by immunologic methods, such as radioimmunoassay (RIA) or enzyme-linked immunosorbent assay.

SPECIFIC PLASMA PROTEINS

MAJOR COMPONENTS

The major serum proteins are those components that are readily resolved and detected on electrophoretic gels stained by conventional clinical laboratory techniques (Table 19-1 and Fig. 19-1).

Prealbumin

Prealbumin is defined electrophoretically as the fraction that migrates in a position faster than albumin toward the anode. Prealbumin has a tetrameric structure with a total molecular weight of 62,000 Da, making it one of the smaller serum proteins. Each monomer can bind a molecule of thyroxine. As such, it is also called thyroxine-binding prealbumin (TBPA) or transthyretin (TTR), although only a small fraction of thyroxine is

TABLE 19-1
Characteristics of Major Plasma Proteins

Protein	Concentration range (g/L)	Molecular weight	Actions
Prealbumin	0.15–0.36	62,000	Binds thyroxine; transports vitamin A
Albumin	39–51	66,000	Oncotic pressure; amino acid reservoir; carries small molecules
α_1-Antitrypsin	2.0–4.0	54,000	Protease inhibitor
α_2-Macroglobulin	1.5–3.5	725,000	Protease inhibitor
Haptoglobulin	0.4–2.9	100,000 (Type 1-1)	Binds hemoglobin
β-Lipoprotein	2.7–7.4	380,000	Lipid transport
Transferrin	2.0–4.0	80,000	Transports iron
C3	0.6–1.4	185,000	Component of complement system
Fibrinogen	1.0–4.0	340,000	Clot formation
Immunoglobulin A	0.4–3.5	160,000	Surface immunity
Immunoglobulin D	0.1–0.4	180,000	
Immunoglobulin E	50–600 (µg/L)	180,000	Binds to mast cells; hypersensitivity reactions
Immunoglobulin G	7–15	150,000	Humoral immunity
Immunoglobulin M	0.25–2.0	850,000	Humoral immunity primary response

actually bound to TBPA in normal individuals, because thyroxine-binding globulin has a 100-fold greater affinity for thyroxine (Oppenheimer, 1968). However, at least one molecular variant of prealbumin, inherited in a familial pattern, has a greatly increased affinity for thyroxine, resulting in elevated serum thyroxine content, although those individuals have normal free thyroxine concentrations and so are euthyroid (Moses, 1982).

Prealbumin plays a significant role in the metabolism of vitamin A by complexing with the retinol-binding protein (RBP), which, in turn, complexes with vitamin A to transport it through the body (Peterson, 1971). RBP is a small protein of only 182 amino acids, and so it would be rapidly removed from the circulation by filtration through the kidney if it were not held in the plasma by the larger protein prealbumin, which is not cleared into the glomerular filtrate. The complex of retinol, RBP, and transthyretin appears to be assembled in the endoplasmic reticulum of hepatocytes (Gaetani, 2002).

Prealbumin is rich in tryptophan (sometimes called tryptophan-rich prealbumin) and has considerable β-pleated sheet conformation. A portion of prealbumin is the source of the β-fibrillar amyloid component in type I familial amyloidotic polyneuropathy (Glenner, 1980). This hereditary amyloidosis derives from a mutation in the prealbumin gene that produces a protein (e.g., TTR Met 30 variant) susceptible to proteolytic cleavage to create the β-structured fragments that are the building blocks of amyloid in nerve fibers (Ii, 1991; Saraiva, 1989). More than 80 different mutations in transthyretin have been recognized, mostly affecting nerve or heart with amyloid. These pathogenetic variants of prealbumin cannot be distinguished from normal by standard protein electrophoresis. Current diagnosis is based on analysis at the DNA level.

Prealbumin has a relatively short half-life in the circulation (roughly 2 days) compared with other major serum proteins. Its synthetic rate is also exquisitely sensitive to intake of adequate nutrition and to alterations in hepatic function where it is produced. Therefore, prealbumin concentrations in serum fluctuate more rapidly in response to alterations in synthetic rate than do those of other proteins such as albumin. For this reason, quantitation of serum prealbumin has major clinical utility as a marker for nutritional status (Gofferje, 1978). Because of the rapid dynamics of its synthesis and clearance, prealbumin is considered to be a better early indicator of change in nutritional status than other commonly used markers, such as albumin and transferrin, which are more abundant, but whose levels respond to other factors as well and at slower time scales. In a study of 7815 hemodialysis patients, low levels of prealbumin were associated with greater risks of mortality and hospitalization for infection that were independent of other risk factors, including serum albumin (Chertow, 2005). Thus prealbumin measurements can be very important for planning patient management.

Because of its compactness, prealbumin crosses more easily into the CSF than do the other serum proteins. Therefore, concentrating CSF before electrophoresis allows visualization of a distinct prealbumin band in CSF. CSF normally contains a major peak of albumin plus prealbumin and a small amount of transferrin. Electrophoresis of CSF is usually requested for detection of oligoclonal bands of immunoglobulin, and the presence of a distinct band of prealbumin is used only as a landmark to confirm that the specimen was likely CSF. True prealbumin is generally below the level of detection by serum electrophoresis; instead it is best quantified by immunologic measurements such as nephelometry. A protein band frequently appears in the prealbumin position of of serum from patients who have had heparin therapy. In the circulation, heparin activates and releases lipoprotein lipase activity, which attacks triglycerides in lipoprotein fractions, thereby greatly enhancing their electrophoretic migration anodally. Protein stain reveals apolipoproteins in the prealbumin position but no β-lipoprotein fraction. This is an in vivo effect that does not occur if heparin is added to samples already collected.

Albumin

The single most abundant protein in normal plasma is albumin, usually constituting up to two thirds of total plasma protein (Peters, 1975). For this reason, depressions in albumin level due to impaired synthesis (e.g., malnutrition, malabsorption, hepatic dysfunction) (Rothschild, 1972) or to losses (e.g., ascites, protein-losing nephropathy or enteropathy) result in serious imbalance of intravascular oncotic pressure. This loss is manifested clinically by the development of peripheral edema (Slater, 1975). However, the congenital absence of albumin (analbuminemia) generally does not lead to such problems, presumably because of lifelong compensatory mechanisms that control hydrostatic pressures (Waldman, 1964). Albumin also serves as a mobile repository of amino acids for incorporation into other proteins. A third function ascribed to albumin is that of a general transport or carrier protein. Many organic and inorganic ligands (e.g., thyroxine, bilirubin, penicillin, cortisol, estrogen, free fatty acids, warfarin [Coumadin], calcium, magnesium, heme) are complexed with different regions of the albumin molecule in covalent (e.g., δ-bilirubin) (Lauff, 1982) or dissociable binding (Koch-Weser, 1976). These binding interactions with very different ligands are possible because of a wide variety of binding sites on the albumin molecule, which consists of 585 amino acids arranged in nine loops held together by the disulfide bonds between cysteine residues (Meloun, 1975). The primary sequence of albumin contains three major regions with three peptide loops each, suggesting that it arose from gene duplication of some ancestral gene in a tandem rearrangement process (Peters, 1977; Sevall, 1986). It is also interesting to note that α-fetoprotein has regions of homology with serum albumin, which may indicate a common ancestral gene origin for these two proteins.

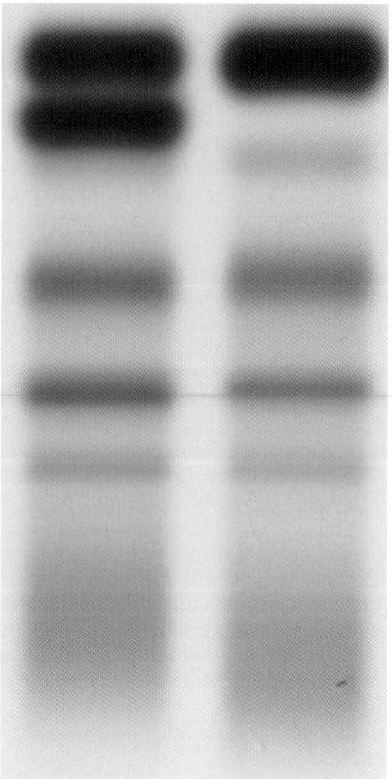

Figure 19-3 Bisalbuminemia. Serum protein electrophoresis with normal pattern in right lane and bisalbuminemia consisting of two equal intensity bands of albumin in left lane. The additional band of albumin in this patient migrated more slowly than normal albumin into the α_1-region.

In addition to the genetic abnormality of analbuminemia, many hereditary variants of albumin differ from the most common allotype, albumin A, by single amino acid substitutions. These variants can be rapid or slow migrating compared with albumin A, leading to two distinct albumin peaks (bisalbuminemia) in the heterozygous state (Fig. 19-3). None of the variant albumins appears to affect health, but one variant does have greatly enhanced affinity for thyroxine, which leads to elevated thyroxine content in the serum of such persons, who nevertheless remain euthyroid (Ruiz, 1982). At least 77 different mutations in albumin are recognized, 65 of which lead to bisalbuminemia; 12 cause analbuminemia, and 3 have strong binding of thyroid hormones, while others show variations due to frameshifts, with modifications near the carboxy terminus of the albumin molecule (Minchiotti, 2008).

Up to 8% of albumin circulating in normal persons becomes glycosylated nonenzymatically, whereas up to 25% becomes glycosylated during hyperglycemia in analogy with glycosylated hemoglobin (Guthrow, 1979). The half-life of circulating albumin is about 17 days, so that measurements of the glycosylated form may be useful in monitoring diabetic control during an interval of a few weeks. Measurement of glycosylated albumin (also called fructosamine) can be very useful for assessing diabetic control in patients with hemolytic anemias (e.g., sickle cell disease, thalassemia, autoimmune hemolysis), whose red cell survival is greatly shortened and in whom measurement of glycosylated hemoglobin is unreliable. Glycosylated albumin measurements may not be reliable for assessing diabetic control in patients with protein-losing nephropathy, in which albumin clearance is accelerated. Diabetic patients on hemodialysis can be monitored with glycosylated hemoglobin or glycosylated albumin (Ghacha, 2001).

Analysis of newly synthesized albumin from intracellular sites has revealed the existence of a precursor proalbumin, which has an additional hexapeptide at its amino-terminal end. The primary structure of albumin consists of 35 cysteine residues, of which 34 form intramolecular disulfide bonds and one remains free. On storage for many days, albumin forms covalently linked dimers through the free cysteines, resulting occasionally in an extra band of albumin on electrophoresis.

Clinical measurements of albumin are very frequent, with determinations of total protein and albumin often included in chemistry panel profiles. Organ- or disease-oriented panels of chemistry tests in current use include the following measurements: comprehensive metabolic panel has albumin and total protein; renal function panel has albumin; hepatic function panel has albumin and total protein.

Elevations of serum albumin concentration are infrequent, although they do occur in dehydration as the plasma water phase shrinks. Following rehydration, the albumin level should fall to within the normal reference range. Elevation of serum albumin may also occur artifactually as the result of prolonged application of a tourniquet for venipuncture. In this instance, increased hydrodynamic pressure from venous backup forces water and small solutes out of the intravascular space, thereby concentrating cellular elements, micellar forms of lipoproteins, and proteins such as albumin.

Depression of albumin concentrations is frequent in sick individuals, and a review of hospitalized patients reveals that a substantial proportion of albumin measurements are below healthy reference ranges (see Fig. 9-7). Although some of these decreases are likely dilutional, owing to the administration of intravenous fluids, others are caused by loss of albumin into urine, ascitic fluid, or the gastrointestinal tract in enteropathies, or by decreased synthesis in the liver caused by hepatic disease such as cirrhosis or by secondary effects on synthesis resulting from compromised nutrition or diversion of synthetic capacity to other proteins. This sensitive but nonspecific reduction of albumin in so many different conditions has led to its being termed a "negative acute phase reactant" (Post, 1991). Measurements of albumin concentrations are vital to the understanding and interpretation of calcium and magnesium levels because these ions are bound to albumin, and so decreases in albumin are directly responsible for depression of their concentrations, too. In some disease states, decreases in albumin are at least partially compensated for by increases in other serum proteins, thereby stabilizing oncotic pressures intravascularly. In particular, cirrhosis shows a major polyclonal increase of immunoglobulins in the γ-fraction (Fig. 19-4, *A*) and nephrotic syndrome shows high levels of α_2-macroglobulin (Fig. 19-4, *B*).

Body fluids that form normally, such as CSF, or pathologically, such as filtrates of plasma (e.g., ascites), contain albumin as the major component, with very little contribution from other plasma proteins. The presence of albumin in the urine is generally considered abnormal even in trace amounts, although some healthy individuals exhibit albuminuria following intense exercise. Progression of diabetic nephropathy can be assessed by the quantitative measurement of albuminuria, as it tends to appear ahead of the other serum proteins in urine during the course of renal glomerular damage. Immunologic measurement of microalbumin in urine is now considered a standard of care for management of diabetes mellitus and the early detection of diabetic complications. The nephrotic syndrome, which is marked by extensive hypoalbuminemia, is often due to diabetic nephropathy or one of several other primary glomerular diseases (Orth, 1998).

α_1-Antitrypsin

The major component of the α_1-globulins is the protease inhibitor α_1-antitrypsin (AAT), which has the capacity to combine with and inactivate trypsin (Eriksson, 1965; Berninger, 1985a). The first clue to this function came with the discovery that the serum of some young adults with pulmonary emphysema was deficient in α_1-globulin. Further investigation revealed a similar deficiency of AAT in children with cirrhosis (Sveger, 1976). Usually, no appreciable circulating levels of trypsin are found in blood, but other related proteases, such as elastase, are released from leukocytes responding to irritants or inflammation. AAT is able to neutralize the activity of these proteases, too, and hence is an intrinsic factor in the homeostatic mechanism modulating endogenous proteolysis within the body and preventing inappropriately severe biochemical response to inflammation (Cox, 1986).

AAT is coded for by the gene *SERPINA1* on chromosome 14. A majority of people are homozygous for the normal fully active *M* allele of AAT,

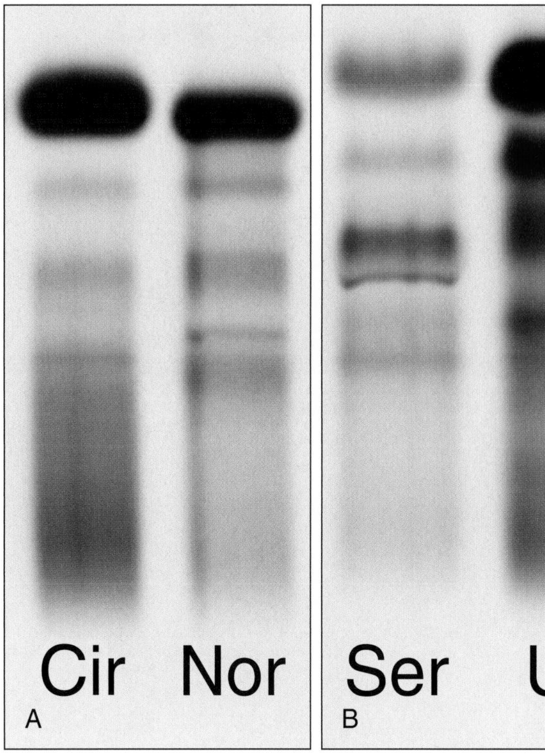

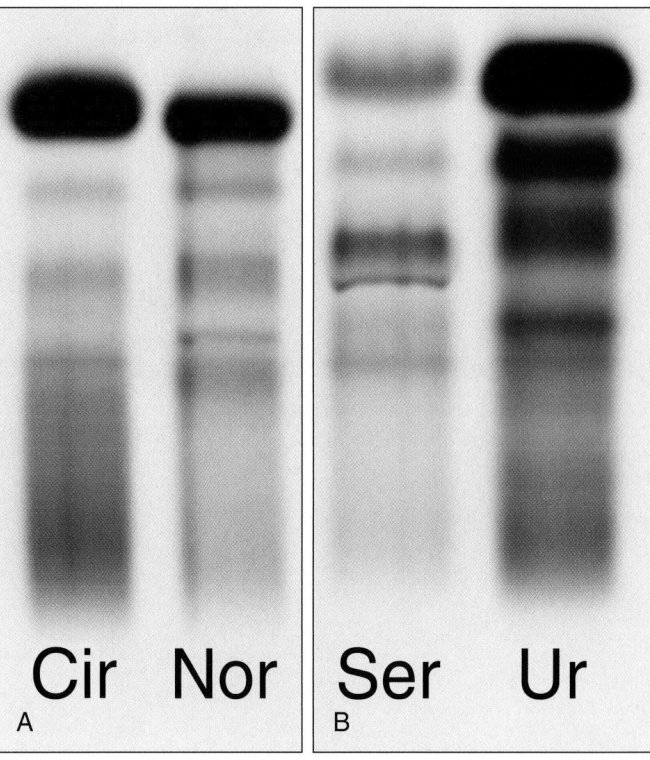

Figure 19-4 **A,** Serum protein electrophoresis in cirrhosis (Cir) shows more rapidly migrating albumin compared with normal serum (Nor) because of the additional negative charge from covalently linked conjugated bilirubin (i.e., δ-bilirubin). The γ-globulins are broadly increased in the polyclonal elevation characteristic of cirrhosis of the liver. **B,** Protein electrophoretic patterns of serum (Ser) and concentrated urine (Ur) in a patient with nephrotic syndrome. Smaller molecular-sized proteins such as albumin are preferentially lost from blood into urine. Larger proteins such as α_2-macroglobulin and β-lipoprotein are retained in the blood and constitute major bands in the serum pattern.

or phenotype MM (Lieberman, 1972). About 10% of white people (and fewer of other races) are heterozygous for *M* and some other allele of the protease inhibitor or Pi system. More than 2% carry the *PiZ* allele and exhibit the phenotype *MZ*. Although these individuals have somewhat reduced levels of trypsin inhibitory capacity in serum, they are generally asymptomatic; however, their homozygous ZZ offspring (who have very low levels of AAT) are susceptible to pulmonary or hepatic disease. The ZZ phenotype occurs in about 1 in 4000 individuals. Another common variant is the *PiS* allele, which shows moderate reduction in synthesis. Although the MS phenotype does not show related disease, both SS and SZ phenotypes are suspected to have increased risk of lung or liver disease. Another allele that may need special attention to detect is the null variant that produces no AAT protein.

Although AAT deficiency can be recognized on serum protein electrophoresis, an efficient diagnostic algorithm employs measurement of AAT concentration followed by phenotyping with isoelectric focusing electrophoresis and genotyping with molecular assays designed to detect specific mutations (Snyder, 2006; Bornhorst, 2007). Definitive typing may require analysis of the DNA sequence for the *AAT* gene. At least 75 different alleles exist for *AAT*. About 17 alleles have sufficiently low protein production to lead to pulmonary disease, and only a few are responsible for liver disease (Cox, 1986).

Therapy for pulmonary emphysema secondary to AAT deficiency has been greatly advanced by intravenous replacement of AAT, using concentrates or recombinant protein to bring circulating levels into ranges sufficient for antielastase protection to the lungs (Snider, 1989). Further replacement has also been successful with AAT inhalation for patients in whom pulmonary disease has not yet become extensive (Hubbard, 1989). Avoidance of cigarette smoking by homozygous individuals is essential, because cigarette smoke is a major source of irritants that trigger leukocytes in the lung to release proteases (Gelb, 1977). The cirrhosis in young children is treated by hepatic transplant, because the liver is the site of AAT synthesis. An interesting aspect of cirrhosis and the ZZ phenotype is the presence of unsialylated mutant-type AAT granules in the hepatocytes,

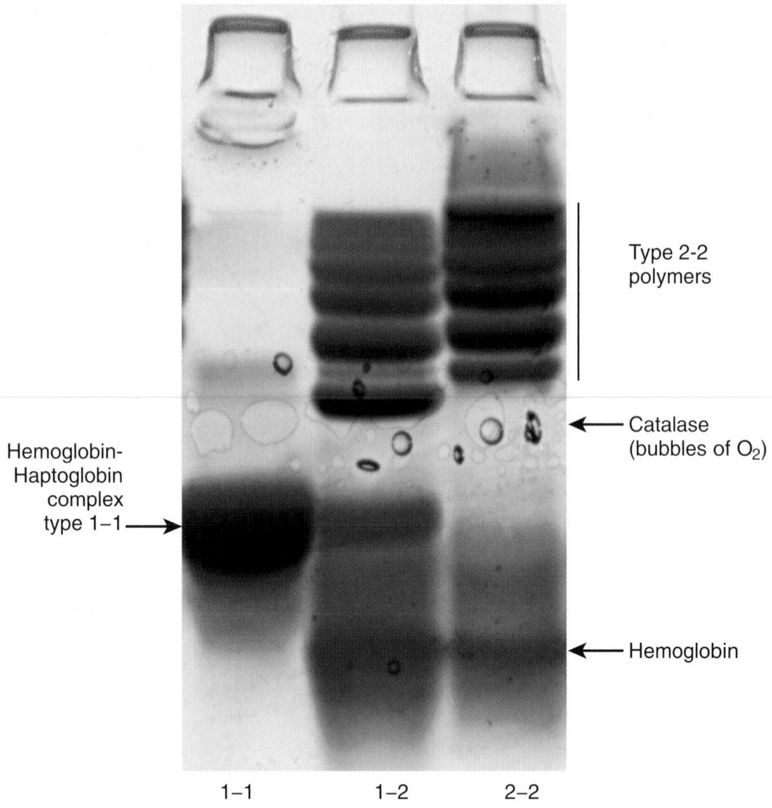

Figure 19-5 Phenotyping of haptoglobin. Patient serum specimens were mixed with free hemoglobin from erythrocytes lysed in vitro and electrophoresed in a polyacrylamide gel with high resolution of different molecular weight proteins. After electrophoresis, the gel was developed in a solution of substrate 3,3′,5,5′-tetramethylbenzidine and hydrogen peroxide. Hemoglobin exhibits pseudoperoxidase activity that converts substrate to a blue product wherever it has migrated including complexes with haptoglobin. Bubbles of oxygen formed in the gel at the location of catalase, which is also present in the lysate. Type 1-1 haptoglobin *(arrow in left lane)* migrated deeply into the gel *(from top to bottom)*, although unbound hemoglobin migrated even farther. Type 2-2 haptoglobin showed no band in the 1-1 position but migrated as a series of high molecular weight polymers, each binding hemoglobin *(bar next to right lane)*. Type 1-2 haptoglobin *(middle lane)* showed a minor band of 1-1 plus a series of high molecular weight polymers different from the bands observed with 2-2.

implying a defect of secretion in those alleles. Cirrhosis secondary to AAT abnormality has not been improved by replacement therapy. Children with this disorder can develop progressive, severe cholestasis, prompting liver transplantation. Following transplant, the recipient takes the AAT phenotype of the donor.

AAT is one of the serum glycoproteins that rise in response to acute inflammation, but such elevations lack clinical specificity. The α_1-fraction never appears completely empty in AAT deficiency, because other proteins (e.g., α-lipoprotein, α_1-acid glycoprotein) migrate there but do not resolve into distinct bands.

Genetic screening for AAT deficiency may be useful in targeted populations, resulting in early diagnosis, improved outcomes, and guidance for affected kindreds (Aboussouan, 2009).

α_2-Macroglobulin

α_2-Macroglobulin (AMG) is the largest major nonimmunoglobulin protein in plasma, with a molecular weight of 725,000 Da (Roberts, 1985). The serum concentration in normal individuals is comparable with that of the other major protease inhibitor, AAT, although women have higher levels than men in response to estrogen (Horne, 1970). The concentration of AMG rises 10-fold or more in the nephrotic syndrome when other lower molecular weight proteins are lost (Beetham, 1993). The loss of AMG into urine is prevented by its large size. The net result is that AMG reaches serum levels equal to or greater than those of albumin (≈2–3 g/dL) in the nephrotic syndrome, which has the effect of maintaining oncotic pressure (see Fig. 19-4, *B*). Synthesis of AMG in nephrotic syndrome may also be enhanced, which accounts for its absolute increase in concentration. AMG inactivates proteases by complexing with them and forming covalent bonds to them. Its own conformation is thereby altered, which enhances clearance by the reticuloendothelial system. At least four molecular forms of AMG differ in sialic acid, mannose, and galactose content and can be separated by isoelectric focusing. Other molecular variations probably are the result of proteases linked to AMG before removal from the circulation. The spectrum of inhibition by AMG is very wide, including virtually all types of serine, carboxyl, thiol, and metal proteases. AMG complexes with prostate-specific antigen (PSA) in a form that is not detected by immunoassay for PSA (see Chapter 73). Although AMG function is certainly important for maintaining balance in the ebb and flow of proteolysis, no specific deficiency with associated disease has been recognized, and no disease state is generally attributed to low concentrations of AMG. Mild but distinct elevations of AMG can be observed on serum protein electrophoresis early in the course of diabetic nephropathy.

AMG inactivates proteases through a molecular trap mechanism using a bait region to bind proteases that then are bound to AMG and cleared by macrophage receptors (Armstrong, 2006). AMG also has separate binding sites for β-amyloid peptide, transforming growth factor-β, nerve growth factor-β, and platelet-derived growth factor-BB. Polymorphisms of AMG may be important in the modulation and clearance of these substances, leading to varying risk for disorders such as Alzheimer's disease (Mettenburg, 2005).

Haptoglobin

The other major protein migrating in the α_2-region is haptoglobin, which has the function of combining with hemoglobin released by lysis of red cells to preserve body iron and protein stores. The circulating half-life of haptoglobin, free of hemoglobin, is roughly 4 days. Hemoglobin–haptoglobin complexes are removed from the circulation within minutes by the reticuloendothelial system, where the hemoglobin is broken down into globin and heme, which further degrades to iron and bilirubin. When the hemoglobin-binding capacity of haptoglobin is exceeded, free hemoglobin enters the glomerular filtrate as α-chain–β-chain dimers that are subsequently reabsorbed in the proximal renal tubules and converted to hemosiderin.

Haptoglobin has two heavy chains and two light chains linked by disulfide bonds in analogy to the basic structure of immunoglobulins. Some persons have a light chain gene that is duplicated in a head-to-tail arrangement (Type 2). Normal haptoglobin (Type 1-1) gives rise to a single molecular species of molecular weight 100,000. Heterozygous individuals (1-2) have, in addition to Type 1-1 haptoglobin, a series of multimers (e.g., dimers, trimers) by virtue of intermolecular disulfide linkages through the duplicated light chain. Type 2-2 haptoglobin consists of a different series of multimers, because the Type 2 light chain has a different molecular weight from the Type 1 light chain (Konigsberg, 1974). These different forms of haptoglobin can be distinguished by high-resolution electrophoresis (Fig. 19-5).

Haptoglobin can be quantitated in terms of its hemoglobin-binding capacity or by immunologic means, especially nephelometry. Owing to steric hindrance between molecular sites on the multimers, the different phenotypes of haptoglobin yield measurements of antigen- or hemoglobin-binding capacity that may be discrepant with the absolute amount of haptoglobin protein present in a sample. Accordingly, the reference range for haptoglobin is broader for an entire population of different phenotypes than within individual phenotypes. For this reason, interpretation of haptoglobin concentrations is soundest for serial measurements in the same individual. However, very high levels can readily be distinguished from very low ones, which can be important in the first-time evaluation of a patient for hemolysis. Congenital deficiency of haptoglobin appears not to have clinical consequences (Manoharan, 1997).

In diabetes mellitus, patients with Type 2-2 haptoglobin have shown higher risk for vascular complications, perhaps owing to different ability to clear hemoglobin, thus leading to altered iron handling and heightened oxidative load (Van Vlierberghe, 2004; Levy, 2010).

Serum haptoglobin rises in response to stress, infection, acute inflammation, or tissue necrosis, probably by stimulation of synthesis (see later under Acute Phase Reactants). After a hemolytic episode, haptoglobin concentrations fall as the complexes with hemoglobin are cleared from the circulation. This effect is dramatic following massive hemolysis in situations of hemolytic transfusion reaction, thermal burns, or autoimmune hemolytic anemia. It is also a useful measurement for serially monitoring patients who have a slow but steady rate of red cell breakdown such as by mechanical heart valves, hemoglobinopathies, or exercise-associated trauma. Low haptoglobin concentrations may accompany liver disease when hepatic synthetic capacity is impaired. There are also individuals with congenital deficiency of haptoglobin who apparently use other mechanisms to conserve body iron stores. Serum samples from blood hemolyzed in vitro during phlebotomy or processing show a displaced band of haptoglobin–hemoglobin complex on protein electrophoresis.

It should be noted that myoglobin does not bind to haptoglobin; therefore, release of large amounts of myoglobin by rhabdomyolysis does not diminish haptoglobin levels in serum. This difference can be useful in the workup of a positive dipstick test for blood (actually a test for pseudoperoxidase activity of heme in hemoglobin or myoglobin) in urine with no coexisting red cells. In this case, low serum haptoglobin suggests hemoglobinuria (hemolysis), whereas high serum haptoglobin suggests myoglobinuria. Lactate dehydrogenase (LD) isoenzyme 1 in serum is also associated with hemolysis, whereas LD5 and creatine kinase are released in rhabdomyolysis.

β-Lipoprotein

β-Lipoprotein (low-density lipoprotein [LDL]) migrates with a characteristic sharp leading cathodal edge and feathery trailing region more anodally. Although it is better quantitated by stains for lipid, apoprotein content is sufficient to be a distinct band on staining for protein. The exact position of the β-lipoprotein band is sensitive to recent ingestion of fatty foods; thus, samples from fasting versus postprandial collections will show the β-lipoprotein in slightly different positions. The other lipoproteins (very-low-density lipoprotein, high-density lipoprotein, and chylomicrons) are relatively small in intensity, and they occur in overlapping electrophoretic positions with other serum proteins, so that these fractions generally are not appreciated on protein stain. Administration of heparin activates post-heparin lipoprotein lipase, which degrades triglycerides in the circulating lipoprotein fractions. Consequently, heparinized patients transiently demonstrate an anomalous band of β-lipoprotein that can migrate very rapidly and unevenly across the electrophoretic path, even into the prealbumin region. Elevations of LDL, with greater staining intensity to the β-lipoprotein band, occur in hypercholesterolemia. Lipoproteins are discussed more thoroughly in Chapter 17.

Transferrin

The major β-globulin is transferrin (siderophilin), which transports ferric ions from the iron stores of intracellular or mucosal ferritin to bone marrow, where erythrocyte precursors and lymphocytes have transferrin receptors on their surfaces (Irie, 1987).

Transferrin consists of 687 amino acids with a calculated molecular weight of 79,550 Da (MacGillivray, 1982). Analysis of the amino acid sequence shows that transferrin has two homologous domains that may have arisen by contiguous duplication of an ancestral transferrin gene. Each domain has a binding site with very high affinity for iron. Transcription of mRNA for transferrin synthesis in the liver is regulated by the concentration of iron in the circulation and surrounding the hepatocytes.

In normal serum, transferrin ranges in concentration from 200–400 mg/dL, which is conveniently measured as iron-binding capacity (IBC) (Tsung, 1975). In response to short-term iron deficiency, transferrin levels rise markedly to twice normal levels or higher. Because transferrin is a single molecular species with a tight electrophoretic mobility, an elevated level can have the appearance of a paraprotein (pseudoparaproteinemia) in cases of severe iron deficiency (Zawadzki, 1970). At least some iron deficiency and elevation of transferrin should be expected with pregnancy (Mendenhall, 1970). Administration of iron to deficient patients increases saturation; this is followed by return of transferrin to normal.

Chronic saturation of transferrin occurs in idiopathic hemochromatosis and transfusional hemosiderosis. Because almost no unsaturated IBC is found in those syndromes, iron cannot be mobilized normally for excretion, resulting in excess deposition in tissues that is toxic. Current strategies to screen for hemochromatosis include measurement of serum iron and serum transferrin (usually by nephelometric immunoassay), with the calculation of percent saturation as the best index for identifying previously unrecognized cases. Hemochromatosis is a hereditary disorder that results in cirrhosis, diabetes, cardiomyopathy, arthritis, and other endocrine disorders owing to the toxic effects of excess free iron. Screening for hemochromatosis is desirable because disease progression can be halted by lowering the body burden of iron by such means as phlebotomy or chelation therapy.

Transferrin may also demonstrate an antibacterial effect by complexing iron and removing it from bacteria that require iron for growth (Reddy, 1970; Weinberg, 1978).

Congenital deficiency of transferrin (atransferrinemia) is a rare disorder characterized by microcytic anemia and iron overload (Aslan, 2007). In protein-losing nephropathy of sufficient severity, transferrin is lost from the circulation into the urine, carrying iron with it. This loss may contribute to the development of hypochromic anemia.

Electrophoretic variants of transferrin occur occasionally in serum owing to allotypic variation in the amino acid sequence, and hence have a different charge on the molecule. In this case, the heterozygous state shows a doublet in place of a single electrophoretic band for transferrin (Kamboh, 1987).

Transferrin is a glycoprotein in which various sugar molecules are added to newly synthesized protein molecules in the liver. Persons who engage in heavy alcohol consumption demonstrate abnormal carbohydrate-deficient transferrin (CDT) in their serum (Stibler, 1991). These aberrant molecules of disialo- and asialotransferrin as opposed to normally glycosylated tetrasialotransferrin may be due to failure of glycosyltransferases in hepatocytes, to increased sialidase activity in serum, or to a combination of the two (Xin, 1995). CDT can be detected by anion-exchange chromatography or isoelectric focusing of isoforms in serum followed by immunoblotting. Other methods include HPLC, capillary zone electrophoresis, mass spectrometry, and turbidimetric immunoassay (Bean, 2001). Although CDT is generally considered to be a highly specific marker for chronic alcohol abuse (Arndt, 2001), false negatives can occur in women, in nonsmokers, and in persons who have a high body mass index (both overweight and obese) (Whitfield, 2008).

A variant of transferrin has been recognized in CSF (Zaret, 1992), aqueous and vitreous humor of the eye (Tripathi, 1990), and perilymph of the ear (Thalmann, 1994). Chemically, it lacks sialic acid in glycosylation compared with the transferrin found in plasma (Hoffman, 1995); it is called asialotransferrin, τ protein, or β_2-transferrin because of slightly different electrophoretic migration (toward the cathode), because it carries less negative charge than plasma transferrin (Blennow, 1995). CSF contains both forms of plasma transferrin and asialotransferrin, whereas plasma contains only one form. Consequently, detection of asialotransferrin in fluid from a fistula or drainage is presumptive evidence for the presence of CSF in cases of skull fracture or other head trauma with nasal drainage (Solomon, 1999), or for the presence of perilymph in fistula fluid from otologic procedures such as cochlear implants (Delaroche, 1996). Asialotransferrin reacts immunologically as transferrin, and so it can be readily detected by immunoblotting following electrophoresis (Roelandse, 1998). This procedure is easily done by adapting commercially available agarose gel electrophoresis systems already used in many laboratories for direct immunofixation of immunoglobulins (Normansell, 1994); using an anti-transferrin antibody demonstrates a single band of transferrin in serum samples, but two bands if the specimen contains CSF (Fig. 19-6). It is necessary to include serum in addition to test fluid from the patient to rule out allelic variants of transferrin that could cause false positives if not recognized (Sloman, 1993). The presence of CSF in drainage fluid may require surgical repair or antibiotic therapy, so detection of asialotransferrin as a marker for CSF can have a substantial clinical impact.

Complement

A separate fraction of β-globulin consists of the C3 component of complement. Although this protein can be resolved easily with a fresh serum

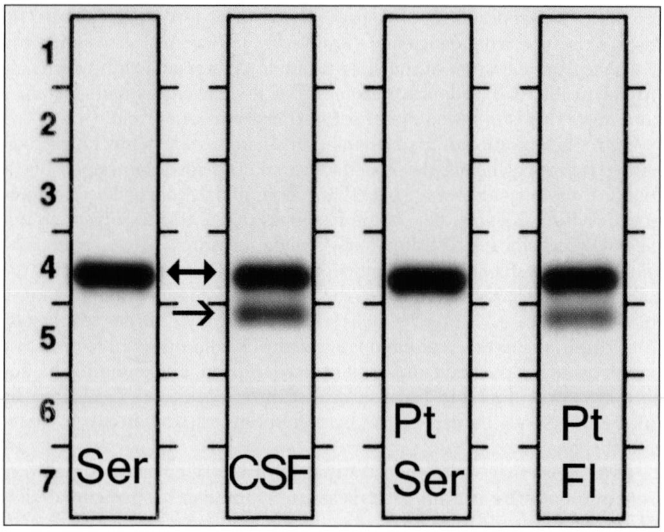

Figure 19-6 Immunofixation with transferrin antibody to test for presence of cerebrospinal fluid (CSF). *Ser,* Normal serum showing position of transferrin (Tf; *double-headed arrow*); *CSF,* normal position of Tf and asialotransferrin (aTf, *single-headed arrow*); *Pt Ser,* patient serum included to rule out electrophoretic variant of Tf; *Pt Fl,* unknown fluid from patient demonstrating bands of both Tf and aTf that confirm the presence of CSF in that fluid.

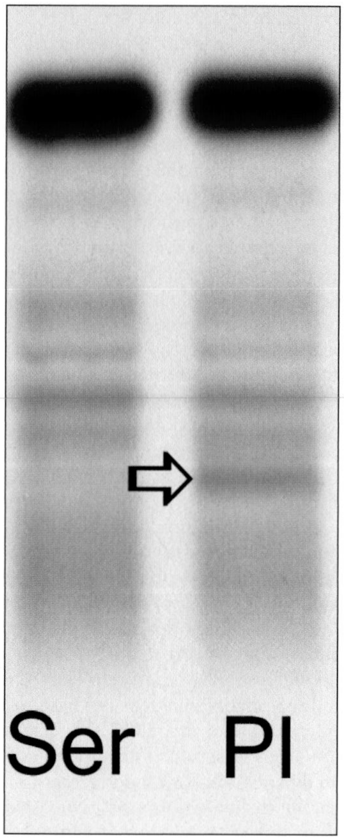

Figure 19-7 Comparison of serum (Ser) and citrated plasma (Pl) from the same individual demonstrates the position of fibrinogen *(arrow)* in plasma that should not be confused with a monoclonal immunoglobulin.

sample, in stored specimens and commercial control serum that has been lyophilized, C3 is cleaved to form C3c, which migrates anodally to native C3 as a band nondistinct from other β-globulins. Depression of C3 occurs in autoimmune disorders when the complement system is activated and C3 becomes bound to immune complexes deposited in tissues, thereby removing them from plasma. Thus, C3 (and also C4) concentration is a convenient marker for assessing disease activity in rheumatic disorders such as lupus erythematosus and rheumatoid arthritis. C4 is not appreciated on serum protein electrophoresis because its concentration is normally only about one-fifth that of C3. Both C3 and C4 are now easily quantitated by nephelometry for monitoring rheumatic disease activity. No particular diagnostic significance is ascribed to higher than normal levels of C3 or C4, except as mild indicators of an acute phase response. The complement system and its inhibitors are discussed further in Chapter 47.

Fibrinogen

Plasma contains 100–400 mg/dL of fibrinogen, which is the most abundant of the coagulation factors and which forms the fibrin clot. With an overall molecular weight of 340,000 Da, fibrinogen is a dimer consisting of three pairs of peptide chains (A-α, B-β, and γ) linked with multiple disulfide bonds near their amino-terminal ends (Doolittle, 1975, 2001). This region of the molecule is termed the E domain or disulfide knot. The chains extend outward into two other identical domains (D) at their carboxyl ends, where all three chains are intertwined. Thrombin cleaves fibrinopeptides A and B from the amino ends of the A-α and B-β chains, thereby resulting in a fibrin monomer that polymerizes into fibrils that macroscopically form a fibrin clot. Factor XIII then produces covalent bonds between lysine and glutamine residues on adjacent γ-chains of different fibrin molecules, making the fibrin clot essentially a single molecule. A cross-linked clot is refractory to dissolution by chemical denaturants and is mechanically very stable.

Numerous hereditary variants of fibrinogen (dysfibrinogenemias) have been identified, in which a functionally abnormal fibrinogen molecule is synthesized with altered amino acid sequence owing to genetic mutation. Some dysfibrinogenemias exhibit impairment of clotting and a hemorrhagic diathesis, whereas others show increased tendency to thrombosis (Menache, 1973). Congenital afibrinogenemia, in which essentially no fibrinogen is synthesized, results in a hemorrhagic disorder that paradoxically is not as severe as the hemophilias in terms of joint abnormalities secondary to hemorrhage (hemarthroses).

Fibrinogen levels become elevated with the other acute phase reactants, occasionally to over 1.0 g/L. In such instances, the erythrocyte sedimentation rate (ESR) is also markedly elevated owing to fibrinogen content directly. Fibrinogen levels also rise with pregnancy and use of contraceptive medications. Low levels generally indicate extensive activation of coagulation with consumption of fibrinogen. During this process, plasminogen is also activated into plasmin, which degrades fibrin and fibrinogen into split products that are measured for the assessment of intravascular coagulation. Normally, clots that form are removed by the action of plasmin, which, in turn, is inactivated by antiplasmin and the other protease inhibitors.

Fibrinogen is absent from normal serum but should appear in plasma electrophoresis as a distinct band between the β- and γ-globulins (Fig. 19-7). Not infrequently, blood drawn from heparinized patients does not fully clot, so that a fibrinogen band is present on electrophoresis. It can be distinguished by examining the specimen for a fine clot and by repeat electrophoresis of a thoroughly clotted sample. This maneuver is important to distinguish a residual fibrinogen band from a monoclonal spike of immunoglobulin that can migrate in the same electrophoretic position.

MINOR COMPONENTS

The next group of individual proteins are those not usually detected by standard protein electrophoresis owing to low levels in serum. Their quantitation is typically performed by immunologic methods.

Ceruloplasmin

Migrating with the α_2-globulins is a copper-binding protein, ceruloplasmin, which contains most of the copper in plasma and exhibits ferroxidase activity that is important in iron metabolism (Hellman, 2002). Synthesized in the liver, it has a molecular weight of 132,000 Da and consists of a single polypeptide chain. Although lower at birth (Al-Rashid, 1971), serum levels are 20–40 mg/dL in normal adults, with 2-fold elevations found in oral contraceptive therapy and pregnancy (Burrows, 1971), or as an acute phase reactant. Each molecule of ceruloplasmin can bind six atoms of copper, which imparts a blue color to the protein. The combination of this blue with the yellow from other chromogens of plasma imparts a greenish color to plasma with elevated ceruloplasmin concentrations (Schenker, 1971); this green appearance is frequently noted in bags of plasma donated for transfusions. Iron is oxidized from ferrous to ferric ions by ceruloplasmin, which may be a means of releasing iron from ferritin for binding to transferrin (Roeser, 1970).

Wilson's disease (hepatolenticular degeneration) results from disordered copper metabolism, in which hepatic excretion of copper into the bile is impaired, leading to toxic deposition of copper in tissues. Normal metabolism of copper includes incorporation by the liver into ceruloplasmin (about six to seven copper atoms per molecule), which is then secreted into the plasma. In Wilson's disease, this process is impaired, and copper that has been absorbed by the body and transported to the liver fails to re-enter the circulation as part of ceruloplasmin. Normal excretion of copper through the bile is diminished, with an overall increase in body copper deposits that are toxic to liver, brain, cornea, kidneys, bones, and parathyroids. Diagnosis is usually made in childhood or adolescence, when damage to the liver is first noticed. Other affected persons may present later in life when neurologic changes also occur. Treatment is long-term chelation with penicillamine or, in severe cases, liver transplantation, which may be curative.

Diagnosis of Wilson's disease is based on physical findings (liver disease, neurologic signs, Kayser-Fleischer ring in the cornea), measurement of low serum ceruloplasmin level, and increased copper concentrations in urine and on liver biopsy. The oxidase activity of ceruloplasmin can be used in a colorimetric assay, with *p*-phenylenediamine as substrate, for quantitation. Additionally, immunochemical methods are used, because the band is too faint to be used reliably on protein electrophoresis. Because no single clinical or laboratory finding is sufficient to make the diagnosis of Wilson's disease, a combination of them is necessary (Ferenci, 2004). Mutations in the ceruloplasmin gene leading to aceruloplasminemia result in iron overload affecting pancreas, liver, and brain with a spectrum of neurologic disease (McNeill, 2008).

Gc-Globulin

Vitamin D binds to the group-specific component (Gc) globulin (vitamin D–binding protein [DBP]) (Daiger, 1975; Bikle, 1986), which migrates as an α_1-globulin and has a molecular weight of about 51,000 Da. Normal serum concentration is 20–55 mg/dL. It may be decreased in severe liver disease. Gc-globulin has two autosomal codominant alleles expressed as three phenotypes: 1-1, 2-2, and 1-2 (Giblett, 1969). Congenital absence of this protein may be a lethal mutation, owing to impairment of vitamin D transport, because vitamin D has low solubility in aqueous media. Gc-globulin binds vitamin D and its metabolites on a mole-per-mole basis, but in plasma, it probably is not fully saturated. Nephrotic syndrome results in urinary loss of DBP, some of which is complexed with vitamin D. This loss of vitamin D may contribute to subsequent problems of calcium metabolism encountered in nephrotic syndrome (Goldstein, 1981). As a minor component of plasma proteins, Gc-globulin can be quantitated by radioimmunoassay, radioimmunodiffusion, or rocket immunoelectrophoresis (Walsh, 1982; Westwood, 1986). More recent studies with immunonephelometry have shown lower levels of Gc-globulin in trauma patients who develop organ dysfunction and sepsis (Dahl, 2003). Plasma concentrations of 25-hydroxyvitamin D are affected by polymorphisms of the vitamin D–binding protein (Sinotte, 2009) presumably caused by varying levels of this protein associated with the different phenotypes (Lauridsen, 2001).

Hemopexin

The β-migrating globulin hemopexin binds heme released by degradation of hemoglobin (Muller-Eberhard, 1970). By this means, this small porphyrin molecule with its iron atom is protected from excretion, thereby contributing to the preservation of body iron stores. Among plasma proteins, hemopexin has the strongest binding affinity for heme, which probably helps to limit the toxicity of free heme (Tolosano, 2002). Normal serum concentration is 50–120 mg/dL, so that it must be quantitated by immunologic means. It has a molecular weight of 70,000 Da, of which 20% is carbohydrate and consists of a single polypeptide chain. Although low levels of hemopexin can occur with nonspecific urinary loss or as the result of decreased synthesis in liver failure, the most profound decreases occur following intravascular hemolysis, when the amount of free hemoglobin exceeds the binding capacity of haptoglobin. The circulating plasma hemoglobin can then degrade to release heme, which is bound molecule per molecule by hemopexin. Heme–hemopexin complexes are cleared from the circulation by hepatocytes, which markedly lowers hemopexin concentration in serum. Excess heme then binds to albumin as methemalbumin. As more hemopexin is made available by new synthesis, heme passes from methemalbumin to hemopexin, which continues to depress the hemopexin level. As such, this can be an additional aid for diagnosing hemolysis at an earlier time, after haptoglobin levels have returned to normal but before full clearance of the heme (Wochner, 1974). Hemopexin can also be decreased in porphyrias and in rhabdomyolysis and chronic neuromuscular disease (Delanghe, 2001).

α_1-Acid Glycoprotein

This protein, also known as orosomucoid, has a very high carbohydrate content, which minimizes its visualization by standard protein stains (Alvan, 1986). With a molecular weight of roughly 44,000 Da, it passes into the glomerular filtrate to a large extent, resulting in a half-life of only about 5 days in the circulation. Serum levels are normally 40–105 mg/dL, with elevations during pregnancy (Schmid, 1975). It is an acute phase reactant, but its biological function is not known. As a binder of progesterone, it may be important in the transport or metabolism of that steroid hormone. It also binds some drugs (e.g., lidocaine) and keeps them in an inactive circulating pool. Measurements of this protein have clinical utility in interpreting levels of drugs, such as lidocaine, that may achieve high serum concentrations without expected therapeutic effect owing to being complexed in inactive form to higher than normal amounts of α_1-acid glycoprotein. Some genetic polymorphisms of this protein may be additionally complicated by isomorphic forms from specific tissue sources, although the primary site of its synthesis appears to be the liver. Although measurements of this protein have not been widely employed, its ability to bind various drugs such as the tyrosine kinase inhibitor STI571 (Gleevec, used in chronic myeloid leukemia) has led to concerns over possible drug-refractory states through binding and drug inactivation (Jorgensen, 2002; Le Coutre, 2002).

C-Reactive Protein

This serum constituent was discovered by mixing the serum of patients who had recovered from pneumococcal infections, with C-polysaccharide of that bacterium. Visible flocculates formed, which allowed extensive study and purification of the C-reactive protein (CRP) from serum in the 1940s. It was found that CRP is present in the serum of patients with disorders other than pneumococcal infection, but that it rises strikingly whenever there is tissue necrosis. Many other substances react with CRP, such as DNA, nucleotides, various lipids, and other polysaccharides (Hokama, 1982). Thus, it appears to serve as a general scavenger molecule. Its molecular weight is between 118,000 and 144,000 Da, with substantial carbohydrate content. The normal serum concentrations are about 100 ng/mL at birth, 170 ng/mL in children, and 470–1340 ng/mL in adults. Despite these low concentrations, CRP has major significance as a highly sensitive acute phase reactant (Deodhar, 1989). It is generally measured by its capacity to precipitate C-substance or by immunologic methods, including nephelometry, precipitations, RIA, and enzyme immunoassay (Saxstad, 1970; Claus, 1976). By electrophoresis, CRP is a γ-migrating protein that may form a minor but distinct monoclonal-appearing band in patients having a severe inflammatory response. CRP levels are sometimes used as a rapid test for presumptive diagnosis of bacterial infection (high CRP) versus viral infection (low CRP) (Clyne, 1999). CRP is often used by rheumatologists to monitor the progression or remission of autoimmune disease. The gene for CRP has been localized to human chromosome 1 (Whitehead, 1983). Recent epidemiologic studies have shown that a high-sensitivity assay for CRP can add to the predictive value of serum lipids for identifying individuals at risk of cardiovascular events, presumably owing to the role that inflammation plays in atherogenesis (Ridker, 2000). Persons with high normal CRP concentrations are at greater risk for stroke or myocardial infarction than those with low normal values (discussed in greater detail in Chapter 18).

PROTEASE INHIBITORS

In addition to α_1-antitrypsin and α_2-macroglobulin, which have already been considered, other distinct inhibitors of different proteases are present in plasma. They include α_1-antichymotrypsin (AAC) (Berninger, 1985b), inter-α-trypsin inhibitor (IATI) (Daniels, 1975), antithrombin III (AT3), antiplasmin, C1 esterase inhibitor (Prograis, 1985), protein C (Stenflo, 1984), and plasminogen activator inhibitor-1 (PAI-1) (Nilsson, 1984). None of these proteins attains plasma concentrations appreciable on stained protein electrophoresis. Whereas the other inhibitors show inhibition over a rather wide range of proteases, AAC is highly specific for neutralizing chymotrypsin, which cleaves peptide bonds at the carboxyl side of tyrosine and phenylalanine residues. AAC has a molecular weight of 68,000 Da with about 25% carbohydrate content. Normal serum concentration is 40–60 mg/dL, but AAC can rise rapidly to five times normal as an acute phase reactant that remains elevated throughout a period of inflammation (Kosaka, 1976). AAC complexes with prostate-specific antigen, measured as the bound form of PSA by immunoassay (see Chapter 73). It can be lost along with other low molecular weight serum proteins in the proteinuria of nephrotic syndrome.

IATI is a glycoprotein of molecular weight 160,000 Da. Its concentration normally is about 50 mg/dL. IATI does not rise appreciably as an acute phase reactant. Its role in disease states is probably similar to that of the major protease inhibitors in preventing autodigestion of tissues by endogenous cellular enzymes (Daniels, 1975).

AT3 is of special clinical interest because of the role it plays in neutralizing thrombin, which normally becomes activated intravascularly from prothrombin during clot formation. This 62,000-Da protein forms a covalently bonded complex with thrombin over a period of several minutes when mixed in solution. On addition of heparin, the complex formation occurs almost instantaneously (Rosenberg, 1975, 1985, 1987). Although AT3 is probably essential for successful therapeutic administration of heparin, only those rare individuals with marked deficiencies seem to have thrombotic disorders (Carvalho, 1976). The action of AT3 extends to other coagulation factors (IX, X, XI, XII, and kallikrein). Serum levels of AT3 may be depressed in severe liver disease or in protein-losing disorders when the similar-sized molecule albumin is lost, and also in disseminated intravascular coagulopathy (DIC). A new experimental protocol for treating DIC involves replacing AT3 by infusion of concentrates when the patient's AT3 level falls to very low concentrations as part of the consumptive coagulopathy. Presumably, return to normal levels of AT3 has the effect of blocking further thrombosis systemically. AT3 levels are lower in heparin therapy and slightly elevated in oral anticoagulant therapy owing to increased and reduced turnover, respectively.

Although AAT, AMG, and AT3 provide the bulk of plasmin-neutralizing activity in serum (Harpel, 1976), a distinct antiplasmin migrates as an α_2-globulin (Lijnen, 1985). This cross-reactivity of serum protease inhibitors for plasmin illustrates the difficulty in sorting out the precise physiologic function of each molecular species, because each one appears capable of substituting for another in different instances. However, antiplasmin binds quantitatively to the majority of plasmin that is generated from plasminogen in human plasma that undergoes clotting. Antiplasmin thus serves as one of the critical checks within the joint coagulation–fibrinolytic system, which maintains hemostasis by balancing clot formation against dissolution. By this mechanism, clot formation and breakdown are generally contained within local regions of the vasculature without extending to the entire circulation. Hereditary deficiency of antiplasmin results in a bleeding disorder due to relatively unlimited fibrinolysis.

PAI-1 acts to prevent activation of plasminogen, thereby blocking fibrinolysis at an early step. Deficiency of PAI-1 results in less inhibition, leading to greater fibrinolysis and potentially a bleeding disorder. Elevated levels of PAI-1 prevent fibrinolysis, leading to thrombotic disorders and to the progression of atherosclerosis. Protein C (with its cofactor protein S) inactivates activated coagulation factors V and VIII. Deficiency of protein C or S (Griffin, 1987) allows prolonged activity in vivo of procoagulant factors leading to thrombotic disorders.

The C1 esterase inhibitor is capable of inhibiting activated complement components C1r and C1s plus some other coagulation and fibrinolytic factors. It rises as an acute phase reactant. Hereditary deficiency of C1 esterase inhibitor allows activation of complement to proceed relatively unabated, a disorder termed hereditary angioedema. The complement system and its inhibitors are described in depth in Chapter 47.

ACUTE PHASE REACTANTS

The acute phase reactant proteins share the property of showing elevations in concentrations in response to stressful or inflammatory states that occur with infection, injury, surgery, trauma, or other tissue necrosis (Daniels, 1974; Laurell, 1975; Dowton, 1988). They include AAT, α_1-acid glycoprotein, haptoglobin, ceruloplasmin, fibrinogen, serum amyloid A protein, and CRP. Others are factor VIII, ferritin, lipoproteins, complement proteins, and immunoglobulins. It is easy to see how such a response of the plasma proteins would be advantageous to the body: Inflammation causes release from leukocytes of proteolytic enzymes in tissue that must be neutralized by enzyme inhibitors to limit their extent of destruction; scavenger proteins (haptoglobin, CRP) help collect and transport cellular debris and breakdown products to phagocytic cells (reticuloendothelial system) to process them and conserve vital substances (e.g., iron); and healing of wounds requires a large amount of fibrin, which arrives via the circulation as fibrinogen. Thus, the humoral response of the acute phase reactants can be viewed as a phenomenon that is geared to handle extensive insult each time it is triggered, even though not all components will be needed on every occasion. The elevation of acute phase reactants is likely a response to the cytokines, including interleukin-1, tumor necrosis factor, interferon-γ, and interleukin-6. The total physiologic response includes induction of fever, recruitment of leukocytes, catabolism of muscle, and a shift in protein synthesis patterns with reduction in albumin production.

For clinical use in diagnosis, other parameters in fact may be as sensitive as these and far easier to measure (e.g., fever, leukocytosis, ESR). However, these proteins provide another dimension of quantitation that can be useful for monitoring the course of a patient by serial determinations (van Oss, 1975). Of course, those patients with congenital deficiencies (Gitlin, 1975), those with other impairment of synthesis due to drugs or organ disease, and newborns who normally have lower levels of many constituents (Gitlin, 1969) may not show the dramatic increases expected. However, a generally useful acute phase reactant for monitoring response is CRP, which is the fastest rising acute phase reactant and one that returns to normal quickly following successful therapies (Fischer, 1976). CRP is frequently applied to the detection and preliminary classification of occult infections, because bacterial infections can stimulate much higher levels of CRP than viral ones. It is also widely used for assessing disease activity in autoimmune disorders, because it is rarely elevated persistently without continued inflammatory response. Elevations of CRP can be up to 1000 times normal levels, which greatly assists in detecting abnormal states compared with the other acute phase reactants, which may rise at most only several-fold in such responses, although ferritin levels may occasionally rise to values greater than 20,000 ng/mL.

PATTERNS OF PROTEIN ABNORMALITIES

Some of the most frequently encountered patterns of protein abnormalities in electrophoresis are shown as densitometric scans in Figure 19-8. Scanning allows quantitation of each fraction, but visual inspection of the electrophoretic strip provides more detailed information about individual proteins separated in high-resolution systems (Ritzman, 1975). Interpretation of electrophoretic results depends on visual inspection to identify abnormal patterns or aberrant bands, and on quantitation by scan to gauge the relative quantities of individual fractions.

Patterns of hypoproteinemia due to malnutrition or gross loss of protein show decreases in all fractions, but the most dramatic reduction is often seen in albumin compared with its normally high value as the most abundant serum protein (Fig. 19-9, lane 3). Severe starvation, malabsorption, or inanition associated with severe chronic disease will show marked reduction in albumin to levels below 20 g/L. The other serum proteins, including AAT, AMG, haptoglobin, transferrin, and C3, appear even fainter on electrophoresis. Reduction in staining intensity for the β-lipoprotein parallels a marked decrease in serum cholesterol concentration. The immune system is strongly affected by severe starvation, with decreased synthesis of immunoglobulins resulting in hypogammaglobulinemia and impaired resistance to bacterial and other infections. Protein-losing enteropathy (Fig. 19-8, *H*) shows a variation in the hypoproteinemia pattern, in which most fractions are diminished owing to the combination of decreased synthesis and increased loss, although α_2 may be relatively higher owing to a coexisting acute phase response (haptoglobin) or to preferential retention of larger molecules (α_2-macroglobulin).

Specific loss of proteins into the urine as in nephrotic syndrome occurs on a molecular weight basis, with smaller proteins being lost more rapidly than larger ones. Accordingly, albumin appears early in the course of protein-losing nephropathies, followed by smaller quantities of AAT, transferrin, and, ultimately, immunoglobulins (Fig. 19-10, lanes 1 and 2). The very large molecule AMG is retained, as are the large micelles of β-lipoprotein. The result is complementary patterns of proteins in the serum (decreases in albumin and α_1-, β-, and γ-globulins; increased α_2-macroglobulin and elevated β-lipoprotein) versus those in urine (see Fig. 19-4, *B*) (glomerular proteinuria with albumin, α_1-, β-, and γ-fractions present but without α_2-macroglobulin in the urine sample). Tubular proteinuria that is due to impaired renal tubular reabsorption of small proteins shows a pattern of α, β, and γ in the urine with only minimal albumin loss into the urine (Killingsworth, 1982) (see Fig. 19-10, lane 4). In addition to glomerular and tubular patterns of proteinuria (Maachi, 2004), it is important to recognize the important pattern of a monoclonal gammopathy in urine (see Fig. 19-10, lane 3, and Fig. 19-11). A similar pattern of a single large band occurs in hemoglobinuria (see Fig. 19-10, lane 5), which must be distinguished from a monoclonal immunoglobulin or free light chains.

Acute phase or immediate response patterns have greatest effect on serum protein electrophoresis by increasing the amount of haptoglobin while slightly decreasing the concentration of albumin. Increases in haptoglobin usually indicate some form of response, whether acute or chronic,

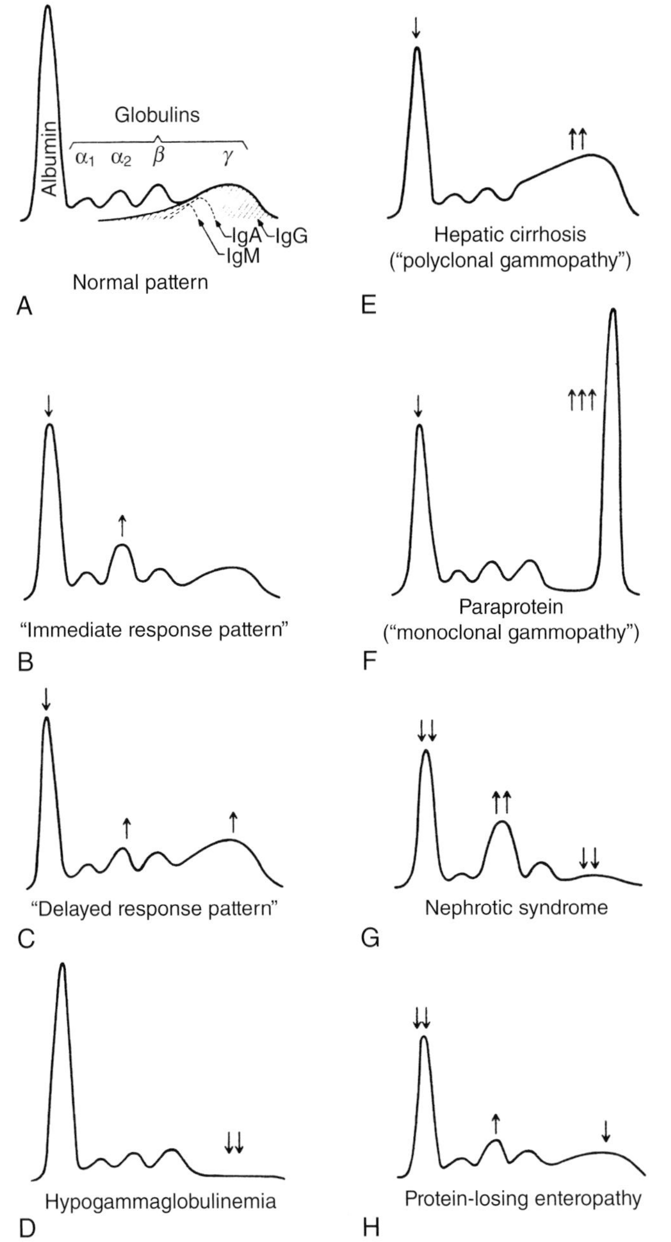

Figure 19-8 Serum protein electrophoresis: clinicopathalogic correlations. *(Courtesy of Dr. A. E. Krieg.)*

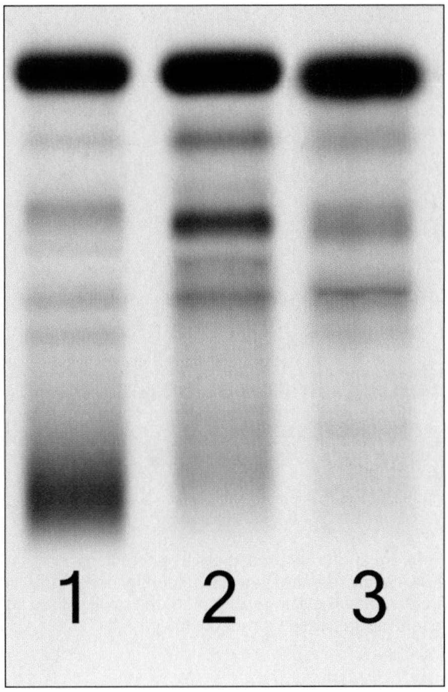

Figure 19-9 Serum protein patterns in (1) chronic inflammation with decreased albumin and increased γ-globulins; (2) acute inflammation with increased α_2-fraction (haptoglobin) and decreased C3 due to activation and consumption of complement; (3) inanition post–spinal cord injury with hypoproteinemia of several fractions.

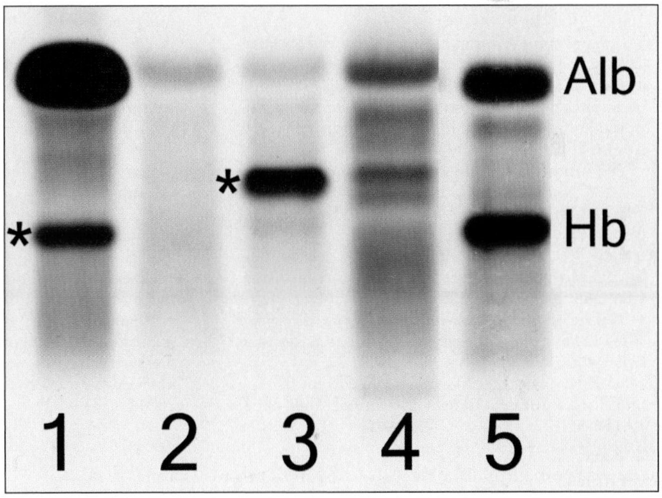

Figure 19-10 Patterns of urine protein electrophoresis in different disorders. (1) Severe glomerular proteinuria with a major band of albumin plus a secondary one of transferrin (*). (2) Trace proteinuria with a faint band of albumin and other diffuse proteins. (3) Immunoglobulin light chains (*). (4) Tubular proteinuria with multiple bands that do not correspond to major serum proteins. (5) Hematuria with a major band of hemoglobin (not to be confused with monoclonal gammopathy), in addition to albumin.

to stressful stimuli (Fig. 19-9). Other proteins such as AAT can contribute to this response; minor components such as CRP do not contribute significantly to this protein stain pattern, although immunologic measurement of CRP may show up to 1000-fold elevations. If the haptoglobin has been depleted in a patient as a result of active hemolysis, an independent band of hemoglobin may be migrating in the β- or α_2-region. Hemolysis of a sample in vitro may show a red band (on the unstained gel) of the haptoglobin–hemoglobin complex that migrates differently from hemoglobin alone. The pattern of delayed response or chronic pattern is an extension of the acute phase response (high haptoglobin, slight reduction in albumin) with greater decrease in albumin and polyclonal increase in immunoglobulins broadening the γ-region.

A striking elevation of transferrin in the β-region sometimes occurs in patients suffering from iron deficiency anemia. The increase in transferrin corresponds to increased IBC, and the percent saturation is low (Koerper, 1977). This variation may be confused with a myeloma protein because the transferrin band forms a narrow, clonal-appearing band.

Cirrhosis of the liver creates a protein pattern that is recognizable (Fig. 19-4, *A*). Hepatocellular damage from cirrhosis results in diminished capacity to synthesize albumin. Furthermore, the imbalance of hemodynamic pressures in portal hypertension secondary to cirrhosis leads to the formation of ascitic fluid, which contains almost exclusively albumin. This decreased synthesis, coupled with increased loss, greatly reduces serum albumin concentrations. The loss of albumin is balanced to some extent by marked polyclonal increase in immunoglobulins with a γ-fraction that may contribute significantly to oncotic pressures. The increase in γ-globulin involves all immunoglobulins; the increase in immunoglobulin A (IgA) in the slow β-region shows a continuum with the γ (also termed β–γ bridging).

In contrast to polyclonal increases, oligoclonal bands consist of only a few clones of distinct immunoglobulins that migrate in defined positions. This pattern is seen in serum in cases in which an immunologic disorder is present, or in some patients treated with chronic immunosuppression for organ transplantation (Myara, 1991). Oligoclonal bands in the CSF are used to indicate immunologic activity in the central nervous system and occur in infectious diseases or autoimmune or demyelinating disorders (see Chapter 46).

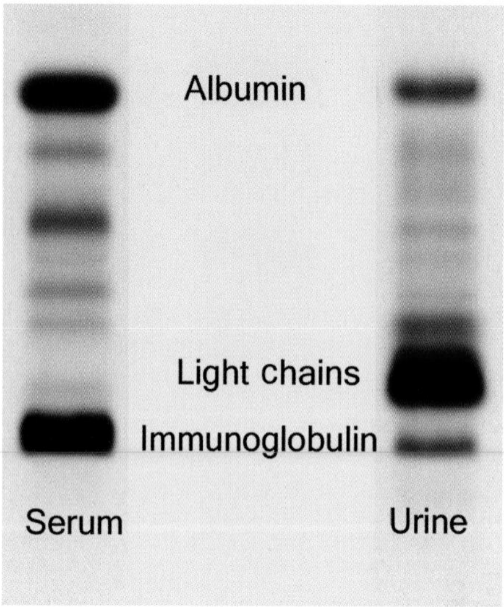

Figure 19-11 Serum and urine protein electrophoretic patterns in a patient with multiple myeloma. Serum demonstrates a predominance of the larger complete immunoglobulin; the urine has a large amount of the smaller-sized light chains with only a small amount of the whole immunoglobulin.

Hypogammaglobulinemia is manifested as a nearly to completely absent γ-fraction. It occurs normally in neonates before maturation of the immune system. It also occurs in some congenital immunodeficiency states such as Bruton's agammaglobulinemia and other states involving B cell function. Perhaps more commonly, this pattern is seen in adults with lymphoreticular disorders in whom normal plasma cells have been displaced by lymphocytic proliferations, and to some extent after chemotherapy for eradication of malignancies, as well as in hypoproteinemic states (see Fig. 19-9, lane 3).

The single most important and widespread clinical application of serum protein electrophoresis is used for the detection of monoclonal gammopathies. This very explicit pattern comes from a paraprotein (immunoglobulin) secreted by a monoclonal proliferation of plasma cells and is generally found without normal amounts of polyclonal γ as normal plasma cells are replaced by the malignant clone (see Fig. 19-11). The presence of a paraprotein with normal polyclonal γ suggests a possible plasmacytoma that has not yet spread throughout the bone marrow. Laboratory evaluation of myeloma should include serum and urine protein electrophoreses to detect aberrant clonal bands, immunoelectrophoresis or immunofixation to type the heavy and light chains of the paraprotein, and quantitation of immunoglobulins to provide a baseline for monitoring the patient's response to therapy or disease progression. Other proteins that may sometimes be mistaken for monoclonal bands of immunoglobulin on serum protein electrophoresis include haptoglobin–hemoglobin complexes, C3 and its variants, β-lipoprotein, transferrin, fibrinogen, immune complexes, CRP, and occasionally, α_2-macroglobulin.

Immunoglobulins, disorders of the immune system, and abnormalities of complement are discussed further in Chapters 46, 47, and 50.

SELECTED REFERENCES

Bean P, Harasymiw J, Peterson CM, Javors M. Innovative technologies for the diagnosis of alcohol abuse and monitoring abstinence. Alcohol Clin Exp Res 2001;25:309–16.

Comprehensive review of assays for carbohydrate-deficient transferrin and strategies for their use.

Bornhorst JA, Procter M, Meadows C, et al. Evaluation of an integrative diagnostic algorithm for the identification of people at risk for α_1-antitrypsin deficiency. Am J Clin Pathol 2007;128:482–90.

This article describes the modern approach to diagnosis of AAT deficiency using the combined modalities of immunoassay, phenotyping by isoelectric focusing, and genotyping.

Delanghe JR, Langlois MR. Hemopexin: a review of biological aspects and the role in laboratory medicine. Clin Chim Acta 2001;312:12–23.

This review article provides a comprehensive description of the biochemistry of hemopexin and how it fluctuates in different disease states.

Ferenci P. Review article: diagnosis and current therapy of Wilson's disease. Aliment Pharmacol Ther 2004; 19:157–65.

Up-to-date account of the role of laboratory testing in diagnosing Wilson's disease.

Hellman NE, Gitlin JD. Ceruloplasmin metabolism and function. Annu Rev Nutr 2002;22:439–58.

This article is an excellent summary of ceruloplasmin chemistry and its clinical importance.

Lauff JJ, Kasper ME, Wu TW, Ambrose RT. Isolation and preliminary characterization of a fraction of bilirubin in serum that is firmly bound to protein. Clin Chem 1982;28:629–37.

Early account of δ-bilirubin and its relationship to albumin.

Layne E. Spectrophotometric and turbidimetric methods for measuring proteins. Meth Enzymol 1957;3:447–55.

Classical paper on protein measurements.

Maachi M, Felahi S, Regeniter A, et al. Patterns of proteinuria: urinary sodium dodecyl sulfate electrophoresis versus immunonephelometric protein marker measurement followed by interpretation with the knowledge-based system MDI-LabLink. Clin Chem 2004;50:1834–7.

This paper presents patterns of proteinuria and new methods for their discrimination.

Minchiotti L, Galliano M, Kragh-Hansen U, Peters T. Mutations and polymorphisms of the gene of the major human blood protein serum albumin. Hum Mutat 2008;29:1007–16.

This article provides a comprehensive listing of known genetic mutations in the human albumin gene.

Peters T. Serum albumin: recent progress in the understanding of its structure and biosynthesis. Clin Chem 1977;23:5–12.

Comprehensive review of clinically important structure–function relationships of albumin.

Tolosano E, Altruda F. Hemopexin: structure, function, and regulation. DNA Cell Biol 2002;21:297–306.

Comprehensive discussion of the chemistry and roles of hemopexin.

Zaret DL, Morrison N, Gulbranson R, Keren DF. Immunofixation to quantify beta 2-transferrin in cerebrospinal fluid to detect leakage of cerebrospinal fluid from skull injury. Clin Chem 1992;38:1908–12.

Description of assay for a specific marker for CSF in unknown fluid.

REFERENCES

Access the complete reference list online at http://www.expertconsult.com

CHAPTER 20

CLINICAL ENZYMOLOGY

Matthew R. Pincus, Naif Z. Abraham Jr., Robert P. Carty

KEY POINTS

- Enzymes are protein catalysts utilized by essentially all mammalian cells in specific biochemical reactions in different organs of the body, which may also be physically located in different organelles and structures within a cell.
- Enzymes lower the activation energies of the chemical reactions that they catalyze, so as to cause greatly enhanced rates of reaction. They do not become modified in these reactions and do not affect the equilibrium between reactants and products in the reaction.
- Most enzymes have a practical or trivial name as well as a name based on standardized nomenclature of the International Union of Biochemistry; the latter is based on the type of reaction catalyzed by the enzyme.
- Along with certain narrow ranges of pH, temperature, and protein and salt concentrations, most enzymes require additional organic molecules and/or inorganic ions for optimal enzyme function.
- An understanding of enzyme kinetics allows for laboratory measurement of serum and other body fluid enzyme levels, as well as determination of possible enzyme inhibition.
- Transition state theory of enzyme action has resulted in major breakthroughs in drug design.
- Damaged or dying cells within organs can release enzymes into the circulation; these plasma enzyme levels can be used clinically to develop a differential diagnosis of a patient with respect to specific organ disease and dysfunction.
- In addition, many enzymes have isozymes (i.e., polypeptide chains that differ in sequence but have similar enzymatic activity). Some enzymes are composed of two or more different polypeptide chains, such as the M and B chains of creatine phosphokinase, giving rise to isozymes that differ in chain composition (e.g., the MM, MB, and BB forms of creatine phosphokinase). In a number of diseases, specific isozymes become elevated in serum, facilitating diagnosis.

GENERAL PROPERTIES OF ENZYMES

All enzymes are proteins and function as catalysts. This means that they accelerate the rates of chemical reactions in the body but do not become chemically altered themselves in these reactions. Virtually every reaction that occurs in the body, both intracellularly and extracellularly, is catalyzed by an enzyme. The molecule for which a particular enzyme catalyzes a reaction is called the substrate. As will be explained further later, enzymes interact very specifically with their substrates and, with the possible exceptions of closely related molecules, do not interact with any molecules other than their substrates. The concentrations and/or activities of different enzymes in blood give vital information about the functioning of specific tissues. Furthermore, many enzymes exist predominantly in specific tissues and not in other tissues. Thus certain enzymes can serve as biomarkers for diseases in specific tissues. Therefore, a vital focus of the medical laboratory is determination of the concentrations and/or activities of specific enzymes in blood and other body fluids. The fact that an enzyme interacts selectively with only specific substrates facilitates determination of enzyme concentrations. Simply by adding a specific substrate to serum or other body fluid and observing the rate at which the substrate disappears, or the product of the reaction forms, the concentration of an enzyme can be determined. This chapter is concerned with the principles of how enzyme concentrations are determined.

CATALYSIS

A catalyst accelerates the rate of a chemical reaction. The acceleration may occur in solution, and the process is called homogeneous catalysis. Catalysis on an insoluble surface is termed heterogeneous catalysis. Biological catalysts are called enzymes and for the most part are proteins that exhibit homogeneous catalysis. However, some enzymes are embedded in membrane structures and should be considered insoluble, heterogeneous catalysts.

ENZYME SPECIFICITY

Enzyme specificity defines the capacity of protein catalysts to recognize and bind only one or a few molecules, the substrate(s), excluding all others,

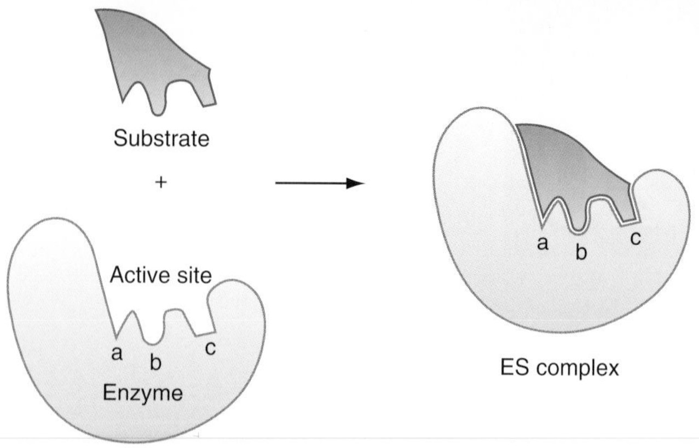

Figure 20-1 The **lock and key** model of substrate binding to the enzyme active site. The enzyme exhibits preformed steric and electronic complementarity to the shape and charge distribution of the substrate. No shape changes or electronic redistributions in the enzyme or the substrate are necessary for optimal binding. *(By permission of W.H. Freeman and Company, San Francisco; Stryer L. Biochemistry. 2nd ed. Stanford, Calif.: Stanford University; 1981.)*

a process referred to as binding specificity. An enzyme catalyzes a unique chemical process (i.e., a solitary type of covalent bond is broken or formed). This is called reaction specificity. Most enzymes exhibit absolute reaction specificity, that is, no minor byproducts are formed. Binding specificity permits many biochemical reactions to occur simultaneously within the same biological space. Absolute reaction specificity saves energy because it reduces the pool of unwanted metabolites.

Enzymes are stereoselective because of the asymmetry of their active sites. They recognize only one enantiomeric form (i.e., one of a pair of compounds having a mirror image relationship) of a chiral substrate. Hence, proteases exclusively bind polypeptides made up of L-amino acids (and not D-amino acids) and catalyze their hydrolysis. Enzymes exhibit geometric specificity exemplified by the fumarase reaction, in which the Krebs cycle intermediate, fumarate (the *trans* isomer), but not maleate (the *cis* isomer), undergoes hydration.

ENZYME CONCENTRATION AND ACTIVITY

The concentration of enzyme molecules within a given intracellular or extracellular space depends on their rate of synthesis and degradation. Control of enzyme synthesis occurs at both transcriptional and translational levels. In eukaryotes, cells of different organs express different isoforms, called isozymes (discussed later), of the same enzyme, which alters rates and specificity suitable for selective cellular homeostasis. The presence of substrate, or other inducing molecule, can cause a sudden increase in enzyme levels.

Enzymatic activity is also subject to control through the binding of small molecules that produce conformational changes in the structure of the enzyme. This binding can alter substrate affinity for the enzyme, or change the enzyme's catalytic activity, or both. Generally, enzymes that catalyze rate-determining steps in metabolic pathways are subject to this type of regulation.

Enzymes do not affect the value of the equilibrium constant between reactants and products. In a reversible reaction, they accelerate forward and reverse reactions by the same relative amount. The equilibrium distribution of reactants and products is unchanged whether the equilibrium state has been achieved in the presence or absence of an enzyme.

As noted previously, almost all known enzymes are proteins or conjugated proteins. A few enzymes are nucleoproteins, which are ribonucleic acid (RNA) molecules complexed to proteins. Enzymes contain a surface region referred to as the active site, where binding and catalysis occur. It is a cleft or crevice in which are embedded specific groups, suitably oriented, which carry out the roles of binding and bond-making, or bond cleavage. The three-dimensional shape of the active site is a vital determinant in the recognition and specificity process. The enzyme–substrate complex is the adduct formed by the physical adsorption of the substrate to the active site. Enzyme–substrate complex formation requires specific alignment of atoms in the active site with atoms in the substrate molecule. This complementary arrangement is referred to as the lock-and-key fit of the substrate in the active site and is illustrated in Figure 20-1. Sometimes the shape of the substrate molecule does not exactly match the contour of

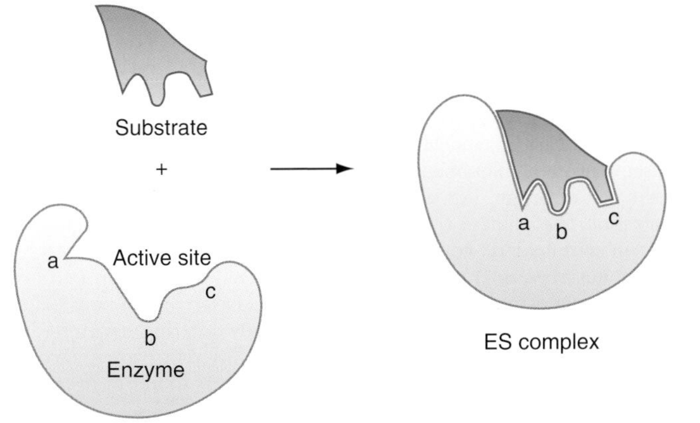

Figure 20-2 The **induced fit** model of substrate binding to the enzyme active site. The induced fit model postulates an initial weak, flexible interaction of the substrate with groups in the enzyme's substrate (ES) binding site. This is sufficient to trigger a conformational rearrangement of the enzyme's surface that exposes additional ligand binding groups that enhance the binding affinity of the substrate for the enzyme. *(By permission of W.H. Freeman and Company, San Franscisco; Stryer L. Biochemistry. 2nd ed. Stanford, Calif.: Stanford University; 1981.)*

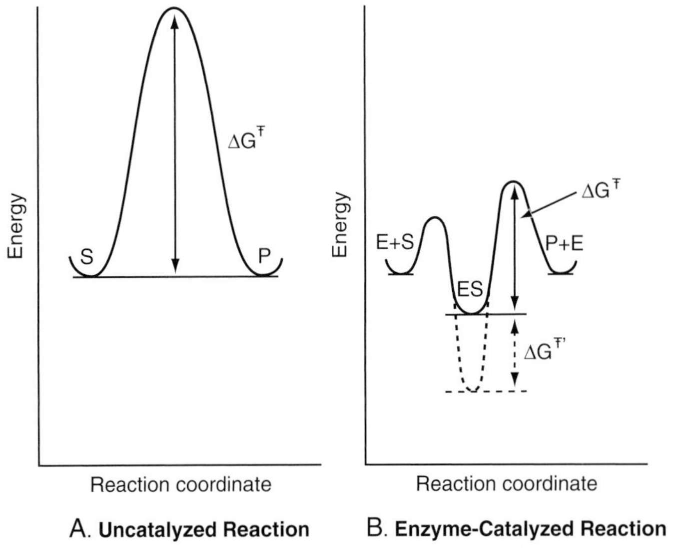

Figure 20-3 The free energy path of a reactant molecule through its transition state on its way to becoming a product molecule. The energy trajectory followed by a molecule undergoing a chemical reaction is the minimum free energy pathway known as the **reaction coordinate.** The transition state, the state of highest free energy, is the point where there is an equal probability that a reaction will take place, or that the **activated complex** will decompose back to the reactant. The free energy change, ΔG‡, is the energy that the substrate molecule must acquire to reach the activated complex, also called the activation energy barrier. **A,** The uncatalyzed reaction. The reactant, called S, must acquire the necessary energy, ΔG‡, to become converted into the product, P. This energy is the difference between the energy of the transition state and the ground-state energy of S. **B,** The enzyme-catalyzed reaction. In this case, the enzyme binds noncovalently to the substrate, resulting in a stable enzyme–substrate (ES) complex. In most textbooks, the ES complex is shown as having slightly higher energy than that for free E and S. This is because the energy of the substrate increases when it binds to the enzyme because the enzyme recognizes the transition state of the substrate (discussed later), which is a higher energy form for the substrate. However, overall, the energy of the ES complex is lower than for the free enzyme and free substrate, as reflected in the favorable affinity constant (usually measured as $1/K_M$) for the binding of S to E. This is why the energy of ES is shown as lower than for the two isolated species. However, although this complex has a lower free energy than that for the two separated species (S and E), it should not be too much lower, as discussed later. The energy of activation, ΔG‡, now becomes the difference in energy between that of the transition state in the ES complex, and not for S alone, and that of the ground state ES complex. This energy is less than that for the uncatalyzed reaction. A major reason why ΔG‡ for the enzyme-catalyzed reaction is less than for the uncatalyzed reaction in **A** is that the enzyme has a high affinity for the transition state, lowering its energy relative to that for the ground state ES complex. Note in **B** what would happen if the enzyme had a very high affinity for **ground state** ES *(broken line).* If the same transition state is assumed, the energy barrier to reach this transition state, instead of just being ΔG‡, will now be ΔG‡ + ΔG‡′, resulting in a slower rate of reaction.

the active site. Yet the substrate binds tightly because of its capacity to reshape the active site to a conformation that binds the substrate with high affinity. This type of substrate adsorption is described as **induced fit.** It is illustrated in Figure 20-2. Active sites of induced fit enzymes become complementary only after the substrate is bound. Some of the favorable binding energy is used in reorganizing the shape of the active site.

MOLECULAR BASIS FOR ENZYME CATALYSIS

The free energy of activation is the energy absorbed by reactant molecules before they have a chance to convert to products. The free energy of activation is a barrier to chemical reactivity. When this barrier is large, the rate of a chemical reaction is very slow. The lower the barrier, the faster is the reaction rate. The barrier exists for almost all chemical reactions because, for bonds to be broken, they must be stretched and sometimes bent away from their equilibrium positions. These deformations require energy. Enzymes lower the free energy of activation. Most metabolic reactions have very high activation barriers, and in the absence of enzymes, reaction rates are imperceptibly slow. Cells can selectively reduce metabolic reaction rates to near zero by abolishing enzyme activity. This feature of metabolism allows cells to "turn on" and "turn off" metabolic pathways during different stages of the cell cycle. Enzymes lower the free energy of activation in various ways. Binding and appropriate orientation of the substrate in the active site increase its proximity to the catalytic groups. Various types of catalysis are used by enzymes. The major types of catalysis are acid-base, electrophilic, nucleophilic, elimination reactions, decarboxylation reactions, and metal ion and electrostatic catalysis. Reductions in the free energy of activation occur through preferential binding of the transition state (or intermediate enzyme–substrate complex) to active site groups. The side chains of different amino acids participate in catalysis. The side chain of histidine is an effective acid-base catalyst, and the side chains of serine, cysteine, lysine, histidine, and aspartic acid participate in covalent catalysis. The side chains of lysine and arginine, as well as metal ions, can act as electrostatic catalysts by stabilizing negative charges that develop during catalysis. Conversely, the side chains of aspartate and glutamate residues can stabilize the positive charges that develop during catalysis.

The rate of the reaction is proportional to the concentration of molecules that have attained energy equal to the free energy of activation, ΔG‡. This energy is higher for the uncatalyzed reaction. The idea that enzymes accelerate chemical reactions by lowering G‡ is illustrated in Figure 20-3, where the free energy needed for a productive reaction is compared for an uncatalyzed and an enzyme-catalyzed reaction. As shown in this figure, enzymes lower the activation energy. As explained later, an enzyme binds to its substrate to form an enzyme–substrate complex in an initial recognition step. In the subsequent step, the substrate is converted to product. The enzyme–substrate complex is more stable than the two separated species (i.e., has a lower free energy). However, this energy cannot be too low, as in the case of the dotted lines in Figure 20-3, because in this case, the activation energy would be raised, and the reaction rate would be slower. As explained later, an enzyme binds to what is called the transition state on the reaction pathway. This is the reactive form of the substrate that is of relatively high free energy compared with the free energy of the ground state of the substrate. Thus, although the energy of the substrate is raised in the transition state complex, the enzyme provides stabilizing interactions with the transition state that result in overall stabilization of the complex and in an enhanced rate of reaction.

Enzymes have developed as extremely efficient catalysts because their active sites have evolved to bind transition states very tightly. It is this tight binding that stabilizes the transition state and lowers the free energy of activation. Enzymes do not alter the ground state energies of reactants and products of a chemical reaction. The equilibrium state is characterized as a state of lowest energy, and the composition of the reactant and product mixture at equilibrium is a reflection of these ground state energies. Enzymes emerge from the catalytic process unaltered, although some undergo transient chemical modification during the reaction.

NOMENCLATURE OF ENZYMES

The nomenclature of commonly measured enzymes was standardized by the Enzyme Commission (EC) of the International Union of Biochemistry

(1979, 1992). Each enzyme has two names: a practical or trivial name, and a systematic name. The latter consists of a unique numeric code designation and the nature of the catalytic reaction, as follows: Enzymes are named by citing the name of the substrate molecule and by following that with the suffix, -ase; sometimes the name also includes a designation of the type of reaction catalyzed.

Examples

1. RNA is hydrolyzed by an enzyme called ribonuclease.
2. Lactic acid is oxidized to pyruvic acid by an enzyme called lactic acid dehydrogenase.

Older trivial names persist in the literature. Examples are trypsin, a protein-hydrolyzing enzyme secreted into the gut, and papain, a plant enzyme that also hydrolyzes proteins. A more systematic classification of enzymes has been implemented in the biochemical literature (International Union of Biochemistry, 1979, 1992). Enzymes have been organized by reaction type into six major classes, as shown in Table 20-1.

ISOZYMES

Many enzymes have isoenzymes, called isozymes, of different forms that catalyze the same reaction. These different forms occur because of differences in the amino acid sequences of enzymes. Despite these differences in sequence, the enzymes fold to the same three-dimensional structures and frequently exhibit similar affinities for and catalytic rates with substrates. Often, isozymes occur as the result of differences in the chain composition of enzymes, as discussed later. Most commonly, different isoenzymes are found in specific organs or tissues; determination of the type of isoenzyme present can then be of use in identifying the damaged tissue and releasing the enzyme. The standard nomenclature of isoenzymes is based on their electrophoretic migration, with the isoenzyme migrating farthest toward the anode designated **isoenzyme 1.** The most widely recognized isoenzymes are those that are composed of varying combinations of subunits; common examples are creatine kinase (CK), a dimer of muscle (M) and brain (B) subunits, and lactate dehydrogenase (LD), a tetramer of heart (H) and M subunits. In other cases, isoenzymes may have the same protein component but may differ based on modifications made by the cell of origin. For example, the bone, renal, and liver isoenzymes of alkaline phosphatase (ALP) have identical amino acid sequences but differ in carbohydrate composition.

In some cases, isoenzymes may have completely different protein structures. Distinct cytoplasmic and mitochondrial isoenzymes of both CK and aspartate aminotransferase (AST) have markedly differing structures. Placental and intestinal ALP isoenzymes have a different protein structure compared with that of the tissue-nonspecific forms found in liver, bone, and other organs.

Finally, enzymes can be modified by proteases present in serum to produce forms that differ slightly from each other; these are termed isoforms. As an example, CK-M subunits are partially metabolized by carboxypeptidase N, removing a lysine residue from the carboxy-terminal end of the molecule and converting the tissue isoform to a differently charged plasma isoform. The relative amounts of the tissue and plasma isoforms can be used as a marker of duration of injury to CK-containing cells. The official names and EC numbers of the commonly measured, clinically useful enzymes are given in Table 20-2 (Zollner, 1989).

ENZYME COFACTORS

Two thirds of all enzymes contain cofactors that are a group of heat-stable substances required for catalysis. They are low molecular weight organic molecules and inorganic ions. The combination of cofactor plus the protein portion, the apoenzyme, forms the complete catalytic entity and is known as the holoenzyme. Organic cofactors are bound covalently or noncovalently to the apoenzyme. Covalently bound cofactors are sometimes referred to as prosthetic groups. Cofactors are observed in oxidation–reduction, group transfer, and isomerization reactions, and in reactions that form covalent bonds. Hydrolytic reactions generally do not require cofactors. Organic cofactors are listed in Table 20-3. Inorganic cofactors that include mainly metal ions are listed in Table 20-4. A cosubstrate is an organic cofactor that behaves as a second substrate in an enzyme-catalyzed reaction. Cofactors such as nicotinamide adenine dinucleotide (NAD^+) can serve as cosubstrates for many oxidoreductases. A single molecule of NAD^+ may act as a cosubstrate many thousands of times. The product, NADH (reducing agent derived from NAD^+), must first be oxidized back to NAD^+ before it can participate again as an electron and H atom acceptor. The recycling of the NAD-NADH oxidation–reduction couple depends on the ready availability of a chemical system capable of regenerating NAD^+ from

TABLE 20-1
Enzyme Classification

Class	Type of reaction catalyzed
1. Oxidoreductases	Oxidation–reduction reactions
2. Transferases	Transfer of functional groups
3. Hydrolases	Hydrolysis reactions
4. Lyases	Group elimination to form double bonds
5. Isomerases	Isomerizations
6. Ligases	Bond formation coupled with ATP hydrolysis

ATP, Adenosine triphosphate.

TABLE 20-2
Names, Enzyme Numbers, Substrates for Enzymes

Enzyme (IUB group, EC number)	Substrate	Comments
AChE (hydrolase, EC 3.1.1.7)	Acetylcholine, acetyl thiocholine; hydrolyzes acetyl-β-methylcholine	Choline is HO-CH_2-CH_2-N^+-$(CH_3)_3$, a quaternary amine; many esters with the OH group are substrates. Critical in regulating acetylcholine neurotransmission
PChE (hydrolase, EC 3.1.1.8)	Many aliphatic esters of choline; unlike AChE, does not hydrolyze acetyl-β-methylcholine but, also unlike AChE, does hydrolyze butyryl- and benzoylcholine	Largely unknown function; it is critical in hydrolyzing the muscle relaxant, succinyl choline
ACP (hydrolase, EC 3.1.3.2)	G6P, phenyl-P, 3-glycerophosphate, phenolphthalein-P, thymolphthalein-P, naphthol-P	Cleaves phosphate esters like ALP (see next entry) but at pH values around 5.0
ALP (hydrolase, EC 3.1.3.1)	See ACP	ALP has unusual pH optimum of about 9. Optimum pH varies with substrate and buffer
ACE (bradykinin, hydrolase, EC 3.4.15.1)	Splits C-terminal His-Leu dipeptide of angiotensin 1 to yield angiotensin 2; also splits hippuryl-His-Leu to hippurate + His-Leu	Considered a nonspecific hydrolase; acts on Met- and Leu-enkephalin
LD (oxido reductase, 1.1.1.27)	Pyruvate and other keto acids + NADH Also lactate and other 2-hydroxy acids + NAD^+	Moderately specific
5′-Nucleotidase (hydrolase, EC 3.1.3.5)	5′-Monoribonucleotides	Wide specificity for 5′-monoribonucleotides

ACE, Angiotensin-converting enzyme; *AChE,* acetylcholinesterase; *ACP,* acid phosphatase; *ADP,* adenosine diphosphate; *ALP,* alkaline phosphatase; *ATP,* adenosine triphosphate; *EC,* Enzyme Commission; *G6P,* glucose-6-phosphate; *IUB,* International Union of Biochemistry; *LD,* lactate dehydrogenase; *NAD⁺,* nicotinamide-adenine dinucleotide; *NADH,* the reduced form of NAD^+, *P,* phosphate; *PChE,* pseudocholinesterase; *pNPP,* *p*-nitrophenylphosphate.

NADH. A substrate molecule is usually irreversibly changed in a reaction. In contrast, cosubstrate molecules are recycled.

FACTORS AFFECTING PLASMA ENZYME ACTIVITIES

Plasma levels of enzymes may be increased by several mechanisms. Because enzymes are high molecular weight compounds, the most common cause for increased plasma enzymes is death of enzyme-containing cells. As cells die, activation of phospholipases leads to development of holes in the plasma membrane, allowing leakage of cytoplasmic macromolecules such as proteins. Enzymes are also released in the process of normal cell turnover; this is thought to be the source of normal plasma levels of various enzymes. Increased synthesis of enzymes by cells also leads to increased plasma enzyme levels. With increased activity of osteoblasts, plasma levels of the bone isoenzyme of ALP increase. This may be responsible for the increase in muscle-related enzymes seen with increased exercise (Dickerman, 1999). Many drugs that stimulate microsomal enzymes, including ethanol and antiepileptic agents, lead to increased plasma γ-glutamyl transferase (GGT). In some cases, release of enzyme from cells occurs without cell death or increased synthesis.

As discussed in Chapter 21 on liver function, ethanol causes expression of the mitochondrial isoenzyme of AST on the surface of hepatocytes and increased plasma levels. Ischemia of myocardial cells leads to loss of glycogen phosphorylase BB isoenzyme and the MB isozyme of CK into plasma. Ingestion of food leads to release of intestinal ALP into lymphatic fluid, and may transiently increase plasma levels of ALP. A number of liver enzymes (ALP, GGT, leucine aminopeptidase, 5′-nucleotidase [5′-NT]) are bound to the canalicular surface of the hepatocyte. Increased concentrations of bile salts with canalicular obstruction may release fragments of membrane with enzyme attached into the circulation, or may solubilize the membrane-binding domain (Van Hoof, 1997). Finally, increased plasma enzyme levels may be due to decreased clearance of enzymes from the circulation. Some smaller enzymes, such as amylase and lipase, are partially cleared by glomerular filtration; renal failure increases their plasma levels. For many enzymes, autoantibodies against one or more isoenzymes may cause the development of enzyme–antibody complexes (often termed macroenzymes) (Sosolick, 1997), which result in enzyme half-lives similar to the 3-week half-life of immunoglobulin G (Remaley, 1989). Most commonly, no specific clinical feature is associated with such macroenzymes; however, it is common to see antibodies against the intestinal isoenzyme of ALP in persons with bacterial infection (Mader, 1994). A similar phenomenon can occur when enzymes are bound to antibodies directed against other antigens, such as LD complexes with antibodies to streptokinase (Podlasek, 1989).

TABLE 20-3
Enzyme Cofactors

Coenzyme	Reaction type	Deficiency
Coenzyme A	Acyl transfer	
Thiamine pyrophosphate	Aldehyde transfer	Beriberi
Folic acid coenzymes	One-carbon transfer	Megaloblastic anemia
Cobamide (B_{12}) coenzymes	Alkylation	Pernicious anemia
Nicotinamide coenzymes	Oxidation–reduction	Pellagra
Flavin coenzymes	Oxidation–reduction	
Biotin	Carboxylation	
Lipoic acid	Acyl transfer	
Pyridoxal phosphate	Amino group transfer	
Coenzyme Q	Electron transfer	

TABLE 20-4
Inorganic Cofactors for Enzymes

Mg^{++}	Ca^{++}
Fe^{++}/Fe^{+++}	Mn^{++}
Zn^{++}	Co^{++}
Cu^{+}/Cu^{++}	

FACTORS AFFECTING THE LIFETIME OF ENZYMES IN BLOOD

The time course of appearance and disappearance of enzymes with cell injury is dependent on a number of factors. With cell death, defects in cellular membranes enlarge gradually over time; thus, smaller cytoplasmic enzymes will leak from damaged cells sooner than larger ones. For example, with myocardial injury, CK and AST are smaller than LD and appear in plasma sooner. Some enzymes are not cytoplasmic, but may be within mitochondria (isoenzymes of CK and AST) or bound to plasma membranes (such as ALP and GGT); cell death typically does not lead to release of such enzymes. If cell death is due to infarction caused by interruption of blood flow to a portion of an organ, enzymes released from damaged cells must diffuse away from the nonperfused region before appearing in the circulation. For example, in myocardial infarction, CK peaks later in persons whose coronary arteries are not successfully reperfused by the use of thrombolytic agents. The degree of elevation of an enzyme is related to the number of cells injured, the gradient in concentration between cell and plasma, and the rates of enzyme entry into and clearance from plasma. In myocardial infarction, the amount of CK released is strongly correlated to size of infarction; thus, enzyme levels with one-time injury are related to the amount of cell injury occurring. If injury is ongoing, plasma enzyme levels will continue to be elevated for a longer time period. For example, in acute hepatic injury, the time course of enzyme changes can be used to differentiate viral hepatitis, in which immunologic damage causes ongoing cell death and prolonged enzyme elevation, from ischemic and toxic injury, in which damage is immediate but short-lived and enzyme elevations rapidly return to normal.

Other important determinants of the time course of enzyme changes include the relative gradient in enzyme levels between cells and serum and the rate of clearance of enzyme from plasma. For any given amount of cell damage, the enzyme with the higher gradient between cells and serum will show greater elevation of plasma levels. For example, with hepatocyte injury, AST levels in hepatocytes are higher than those of alanine aminotransferase (ALT), and both are many times higher than levels of LD. Immediately after injury, therefore, AST will show a greater degree of elevation than will ALT, and LD will show the least degree of increase. In cardiac tissue, the gradient of CK between myocardial cells and plasma is several times higher than that for LD, leading to higher peak CK than LD levels. Once enzyme reaches plasma, the rate of clearance also becomes important; for example, the half-life of AST is much shorter than that of ALT, and the half-life of CK is shorter than that of the cardiac isoenzymes of LD. With hepatic injury, therefore, plasma ALT often becomes higher than AST within a short time after injury. Following myocardial infarction, CK returns to normal several days earlier than does LD.

ENZYME KINETICS: DETERMINATION OF TOTAL ENZYME CONCENTRATIONS IN SERUM AND OTHER BODY FLUIDS

The basic objective of clinical enzymology is the determination of the total concentrations of specific enzymes in serum and other body fluids. Qualitatively, detecting the presence of enzymes in body fluids is fortunately quite simple because each enzyme has almost total specificity for one or at most a few substrate(s). By adding the substrate, say, to serum, and observing either its disappearance or the appearance of the product, the presence of the enzyme can be ascertained. As is now explained, the rate at which substrate disappears or product appears can be directly used to determine the concentration of enzyme present (Cleland, 1970, 1990; Dixon, 1979; Cornish-Bowden, 1995; Fersht, 1999; Segel, 2009).

THE MICHAELIS-MENTEN EQUATION GIVES THE MEANS TO DETERMINE TOTAL ENZYME CONCENTRATION IN SERUM AND OTHER BODY FLUIDS

Enzymes exhibit saturation, which occurs when the rate becomes unresponsive to further increases in substrate concentration. Ordinary chemical reactions occur with rates proportional to the entire range of reactant concentrations. In an enzyme-catalyzed reaction, at low substrate concentrations rates are proportional to substrate concentration. At higher concentrations, the rate does not increase in direct proportion. At still higher substrate concentrations, the rate becomes constant and unresponsive to any further change in substrate concentration. This led to the proposal that enzyme catalysis is a two-step process that consists of an initial adsorption whereby the substrate combines with the enzyme to form a noncovalent enzyme–substrate (ES) complex, followed by a second step in which the ES complex decomposes into product (P) and free enzyme (E).

$$E + S \underset{k_{-1}}{\overset{k_1}{\rightleftharpoons}} ES \xrightarrow{k_2} P + E \qquad \textbf{(20-1)}$$

The formation of enzyme–substrate may be regarded as the step in which the enzyme recognizes the substrate. This process involves the formation of specific *noncovalent* interactions between enzyme and substrate. These interactions include ionic interactions, hydrophobic interactions, hydrogen bonding, and van der Waals interactions.

The physical explanation for saturation is that binding reduces the number of active sites available to form the enzyme–substrate complex. When all sites are filled, no further binding can occur until an active site discharges its contents. The step that determines the overall rate is the k_2 step. Adding additional substrate molecules under saturating conditions does not change the rate because all unbound substrate molecules must wait until an active site becomes vacant. This kinetic model is now used to derive the Michaelis-Menten equation that enables direct determination of total enzyme concentration or activity.

Derivation of the Michaelis-Menten Equation

The velocity, v, the rate at which product forms, of an enzyme-catalyzed reaction is defined as:

$$v = v_0 = d[P]/dt = k_2[ES] \qquad \textbf{(20-2)}$$

where *t* is time. Note that *v* is the *initial* velocity of the reaction, referred to as v_0, where we know the concentration of the substrate. It is important to measure initial velocities to ensure the absence of product inhibition (when time [t] = 0, [P] = 0) and the loss of enzyme due to proteolysis, denaturation, or time-dependent adsorption onto glass or plastic surfaces.

The differential rate law, which gives the rate of change of [ES] with time, is the difference between the rate of the k_1 step leading to formation of the complex and the rates of the steps leading to the disappearance of [ES] and k_1 and k_2 steps.

$$d[ES]/dt = k_1[E][S] - k_{-1}[ES] - k_2[ES] \qquad \textbf{(20-3)}$$

For a wide variety of enzyme-catalyzed reactions, it has been found that, over long periods of time, after an initial transient phase lasting a few milliseconds, the concentration of the ES complex remains constant (i.e., does not change in time), especially when S >> E. This is the steady-state assumption. Therefore,

$$d[ES]/dt = 0 = k_1[E][S] - k_{-1}[ES] - k_2[ES] = k_1[E][S] - (k_1 + k_2)[ES] \qquad \textbf{(20-4)}$$

and

$$[ES] = k_1[E][S]/(k_{-1} + k_2) = [E][S]/K_M \qquad \textbf{(20-5)}$$

where the ratio of the rate constants $k_1/(k_{-1} + k_2)$ is defined as $1/K_M$. K_M is termed the Michaelis constant, whose significance is discussed later.

If E_T is the total concentration of enzyme, it is equal to free enzyme plus enzyme bound to substrate, that is,

$$[E_T] = [E] + [ES] \qquad \textbf{(20-6)}$$

Then, using Equation 20-5,

$$[E_T] = [E] + [E][S]/K_M \qquad \textbf{(20-7)}$$

and

$$[E] = [E_T]/(1 + [S]/K_M) \qquad \textbf{(20-8)}$$

and substituting for [E] in Equation 20-5,

$$\begin{aligned}[ES] &= [E][S]/K_M \\ &= [E_T]/(1 + [S]/K_M) \times [S]/K_M \\ &= [E_T][S]/(K_M + [S])\end{aligned} \qquad \textbf{(20-9)}$$

Combining Equation 20-9 with Equation 20-2, we have

$$\frac{d[P]}{dt} = V_0 = k_2[ES] = \frac{k_2[E_T][S]}{(K_M + S)} \qquad \textbf{(20-10)}$$

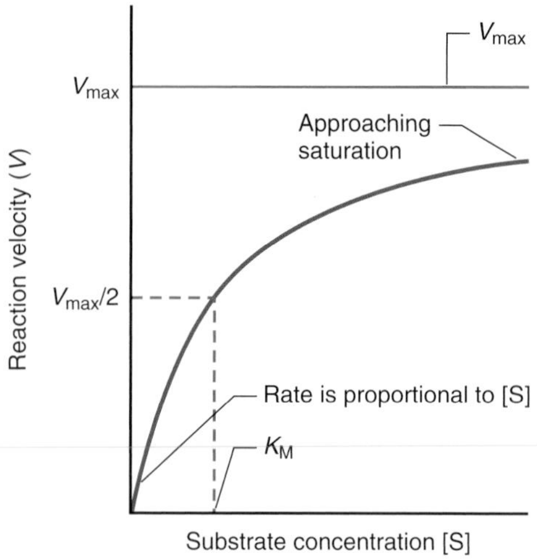

Figure 20-4 The effect of substrate concentration [S] on the velocity (V) of an enzyme-catalyzed reaction. The plot is for an enzyme that obeys Michaelis-Menten kinetics, where the maximal velocity is V_{max} and [S] equals K_M where (v) equals $V_{max}/2$.

Equation 20-10, termed the **Michaelis-Menten equation,** accurately describes virtually all single-substrate enzyme-catalyzed reactions and many bisubstrate reactions in which the concentration of one substrate is constant throughout the course of the reaction.

Total Enzyme Concentration Can Be Determined From the Initial Rate at Saturation

A typical plot of v_0 versus initial substrate concentration is shown in Figure 20-4. The curve is a rectangular hyperbola, and the initial rate increases up to a particular substrate concentration beyond which the rate remains constant. This occurs on the curve where $[S] >> K_M$. This is referred to as saturation, where all of the enzyme molecules are bound to substrate, making it impossible to increase the rate any further by increasing [S]. Note that, where saturation occurs, that is, where $[S] >> K_M$, Equation 20-10 reduces to

$$d[P]/dt = v_0 = k_2[E_T] \qquad \textbf{(20-11)}$$

Because the rate is constant at saturation, the rate is zero order with respect to substrate; the rate does not depend on the concentration of reactants. There is a dependence on E_T, which, however, is not consumed in the reaction. At saturation, the initial velocity of the reaction is referred to as the maximal velocity, or $V_{max} = k_2E_T$. Under this saturating condition, the initial rate of the reaction is directly proportional to the total enzyme concentration. If k_2 is known, then E_T can be directly computed as the observed initial rate divided by k_2. This equation solves the problem of determining the total enzyme concentration from measurements of the rate of the enzyme-catalyzed reaction where $[S] >> K_M$.

Knowledge of k_2 and K_M Allows Determination of [S] Values That Will Saturate the Enzyme

To fulfill the conditions of Equation 20-11, it is necessary to know both K_M and k_2. These can be estimated from plots similar to the one shown in Figure 20-4. To generate these plots, the purified enzyme is dissolved in aqueous solution in a series of tubes at the same concentration. To each of these tubes, a different concentration of substrate is added, and the initial rate of reaction for each tube is determined using a suitable (mostly spectrophotometric) technique. The value of v_0 vs initial substrate concentration [S] can be plotted; the value of S at which the rate levels off (i.e., becomes constant) can be estimated from the plot.

The Lineweaver-Burk Plot Gives k_2 and K_M

The problem with this approach is that, in the v_0 versus [S] plot, the rate approaches V_{max} asymptotically. Therefore, V_{max} can only be estimated, often inaccurately, from such a plot. A more accurate method by which to accomplish this goal is to linearize the Michaelis-Menten equation (20-10) by taking the reciprocal of both sides of the equation and rearranging the terms, that is,

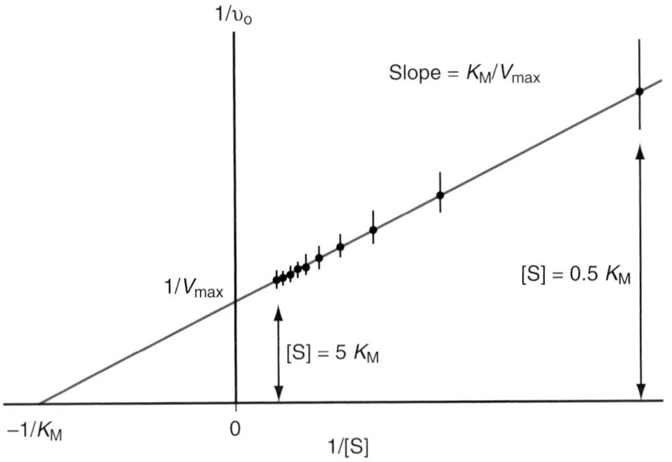

Figure 20-5 A typical Lineweaver-Burk ($1/v_o$ vs. 1/[S]) plot, from Equation 20-12, for an enzyme-catalyzed reaction. v_0 is the initial velocity of the reaction at time t = 0, where the substrate concentration, [S], is known. The figure shows that [S] must cover a range from where it is significantly less than K_M (0.5 K_M) to where it is significantly greater than K_M (5 K_M) to obtain reliable values for K_M and V_{max}. The Y-intercept is $1/V_{max}$, and the X-intercept is $-1/K_M$. The slope is K_M/V_{max}.

$$\frac{1}{V_0} = \frac{K_M}{V_{MAX}} \bullet \frac{1}{[S]} + \frac{1}{V_{MAX}} \qquad \textbf{(20-12)}$$

As can be seen from Equation 20-12, a plot of $1/v_0$ versus 1/[S], called the double reciprocal plot, also called the Lineweaver-Burk plot, should be linear; the Y-intercept should be $1/V_{max}$, and the slope should be K_M/V_{max}. Because $1/V_{max}$ is the intercept, K_M can be computed as the slope/Y-intercept. Because from Equation 20-12, the X-intercept is $-1/K_M$, K_M can also be computed directly from this relationship. K_M can be computed directly from the Michaelis-Menten equation (20-10) from V_{max}. When [S] = K_M, from Equation 20-10, $v_0 = V_{max}/2$. Thus the K_M is the substrate concentration necessary to reach $V_{max}/2$. A typical Lineweaver-Burk plot is shown in Figure 20-5.

Practically, after the points are obtained from the double reciprocal plot, the least squares best line is drawn through the points from which the slope and X- and Y-intercepts are directly determined. The correlation coefficient, which is a measure of the closeness-of-fit of the experimental points to the best line, is also calculated and should be greater than 0.9, that is, a high correlation.

Note in the above procedure and as is illustrated in Figure 20-5 that substrate concentrations must span a range that brackets K_M. Measurements of v_0 at low [S] have relatively large errors, as illustrated in the upper right portion of the line in Figure 20-5, yet it is these estimates which are critical in determining accurate values of K_M and V_{max}. Modern computer programs provide reasonably accurate values for K_M and V_{max} based on weighted values of the initial velocities. Weights are assigned based on the magnitude of v_0. In addition, other computer programs use nonlinear regression analysis to fit the weighted data to a hyperbolic v_0 versus [S] curve, as in Equation 20-10, and a Lineweaver-Burk plot is used only for visual display of the kinetic data.

Once K_M is known, saturating concentrations of substrate can be used such that [S] > > K_M. So, for example, if $K_M = 1 \times 10^{-5}$ M for a certain enzyme for which an assay is desired, we can use a substrate concentration of 1×10^{-3} M (1 mM) and be assured that [S] > > K_M, here by a factor of 100, so that Equation 20-11 applies. The substrate at this concentration is added to a patient sample (most often, serum), and the rate is observed and then divided by k_2 to obtain the total concentration of enzyme. As discussed later, because many enzymes exist as different isozymes with different k_2 and K_M values, division by k_2 is not performed, and the results are reported directly as k_2E_T, referred to as total activity units.

A Word About K_M

Equation 20-1 shows that the ES complex is in equilibrium with free E and free S. We can write an equilibrium constant for this process as a dissociation constant, K_s, as k_{-1}/k_1, which is equal to [E][S]/[ES]. The reciprocal of this constant, or the association constant, K_A, is k_1/k_{-1} = [ES]/[E][S]. From Equation 20-5, K_M is defined as $(k_{-1} + k_2)/k_1$. Note that when $k_{-1} > > k_2$, K_M is the same as K_S. This condition actually pertains to most enzyme-catalyzed reactions; k_{-1} is the rate of dissociation for the enzyme–substrate complex that almost always involves the breaking of noncovalent bonds, and k_2 is the rate for the breaking and/or making of covalent bonds. Usually, the energy necessary for the former process is much less than for the latter; therefore, the rate of dissociation, k_{-1}, of the noncovalent ES complex is higher than the rate, k_2, for the covalent catalysis step. Thus K_M is the dissociation constant for the ES complex. The reciprocal of this is K_A, the association constant, and it is the affinity of the substrate for the enzyme.

However, in some cases, the rate for the covalent catalytic step is greatly enhanced. Examples include carbonic anhydrase ($k_2 = 10^6$ sec^{-1}; carbon dioxide is the substrate) and catalase ($k_2 = 10^7$ sec^{-1}; hydrogen peroxide is the substrate). For these enzymes, because k_2 is large, K_M is not a dissociation constant, but rather a steady-state constant, equal to k_2/k_1.

Enzyme Activity

As noted previously, computation of total enzyme concentration using Equation 20-11 is often not performed because many enzymes have multiple isozymes. For example, at least five isozymes of LD are known, each having a different set of values for K_M and k_2. In this case, the total enzyme activity of LD is given, that is, $k_2 \times [E_T]$. In these cases, enzyme activities are all reported in units called international units, defined originally in 1964 by the International Commission on Enzymes. One international unit (IU) is the amount of enzyme that catalyzes the formation of one micromole of product (or the disappearance of 1 micromole of substrate) in 1 minute. It applies only under specified conditions of pH, temperature, and ionic strength, all factors which influence enzyme activity, as discussed later.

With development of the Système International d'Unités system and the use of moles and seconds as base units, a second definition for the unit of enzyme activity was developed, the katal: 1 katal is defined as the amount of enzyme that catalyzes the conversion of 1 mol of substrate to product in 1 second, under the conditions used in the assay. One IU is equal to 16.7 nanokatal (nkat), and 1 katal is equal to 6×10^7 IU. Both definitions unfortunately omit volume. Generally, 1 IU is reported per liter (L); the right side of Equation 20-11 has the units of concentration per time so that IU/L conforms to these units. It is vital that, if total enzyme activity is reported, the substrate used in the assay for the enzyme also be reported because the k_2 value differs for different substrates.

As discussed later, many factors affect enzymatic activity, including pH, temperature, ionic strength, concentration of cofactors of an enzyme, presence of inhibitors, use of other enzyme reactions as indicators, and whether the forward or backward reaction is used to measure the enzyme concentration. For example, LD measured using the forward reaction has approximately one third the activity of LD measured using the reverse reaction, and lipase measured with colipase present has 5 to 10 times the activity of lipase measured without its cofactor.

Therefore, even if the same substrate is used by different laboratories, the reference ranges of enzymes may differ dramatically among these laboratories. Furthermore, differences in reference ranges between two different laboratories can still exist even if the above factors are the same for both, because of different assay conditions.

To attempt to standardize enzyme activities, one approach is to have each laboratory set the upper boundary of the reference range to 100 (Langdon, 1994). Then all other values are expressed as percentages or ratios. A result indicating that an enzyme level was 10 times normal is useful to a physician. If the result is 10X U/L, then the physician must hunt the value of X and calculate the ratio. As long as the assays are performed with internal consistency in a highly reproducible manner, quantitative results are comparable between one laboratory and another if relative activities are reported. More commonly, the results of enzyme assays are now expressed in IU along with the reference ranges for each enzyme, allowing for evaluation of the patient's condition, progression of disease, or efficacy of therapy.

Measuring Enzyme Activity

In principle, in the measurement of enzyme activity, either the rate of disappearance of substrate or the rate of appearance of product can be measured. In general, it is easier to measure small increases in product than to measure small decreases in a relatively high concentration of substrate often needed to achieve saturation. As discussed previously, to measure enzyme activity in a sample, it is most common to use substrates at saturating concentrations where zero-order kinetics with respect to [S] occur. Under these conditions, the reaction rate is directly proportional to the total amount of enzyme present.

Equation 20-11 states that, at saturation, the rate of product formation with time is constant. This implies that the concentration of product increases linearly with time. Experimentally, P is determined at different time points, and a least-squares best-fit line through the points is determined. If the correlation coefficient is high, [P] increases linearly with t, confirming saturation of the enzyme by substrate. The slope of this line is V_{max}, which may be reported directly as activity or divided by k_2 to give enzyme concentration.

The most common cause of a *non*linear relationship between P and t is the presence of an inhibitor that will be discussed later. In cases such as these, dilution of the serum or other body fluid sample is warranted because this will dilute the concentration of the inhibitor, although it will also dilute the total enzyme concentration. However, as long as [S] is present at saturating conditions, and [P] can be measured, valid total enzyme concentrations or activities can be measured.

Typically, in enzyme assays, a lag phase follows mixture of the specimen and reagents, when preliminary reactions and mixing of sample occur. The initial absorbance of the sample is based on the absorbance due to the reagents and the sample, and is considered to be zero in terms of making an interpretation of enzyme activity. Once the reaction begins, the graph will follow a straight line for a period of time; at this point, the reaction is zero-order and enzyme activity can be determined. If the reaction is allowed to proceed, substrate is consumed and [S] falls toward K_M. If [S] falls substantially below K_M, the reaction will then be first-order, and v_0 will be affected both by the amount of substrate (which is not a constant) and by the enzyme activity.

Spectrophotometric Assays

In most cases, enzyme activity is measured spectrophotometrically. In addition, other detection methods are used as appropriate, depending on the product being measured. For example, lipase acts on emulsions of lipid; these are often turbid, so that measurement of the rate of clearance of turbidity could be used to determine lipase activity. Glucose oxidase, widely used to measure glucose concentration, is a flavoprotein that uses oxygen as an electron acceptor. The change in potential due to alteration in charge on the acceptor can be measured to determine the reaction rate. Urease is widely used to measure urea concentration; urease splits urea into bicarbonate and ammonium ions. The change in conductance of the specimen due to the appearance of the ions in the sample can be used to determine the rate of reaction.

Because assay methods based on spectrophotometry are the most common, we will focus on these in describing how enzyme assays are performed. In the simplest case, the substrate does not absorb light at a particular wavelength at which the product absorbs strongly. An excellent example of this is LD, which catalyzes reversibly the oxidation of lactate to pyruvate. Because lactate is a unique substrate for LD, it is preferred. Pyruvate can be used as the substrate, except that it is also the substrate for several other enzymes such as pyruvate dehydrogenase and ALT, among others.

When lactate is oxidized to pyruvate, the cofactor, NAD^+, becomes reduced to NADH. For each mole of lactate oxidized to pyruvate, 1 mole of NADH forms. NADH absorbs strongly at 340 nm, and NAD^+ does not absorb light at this wavelength. Therefore, the addition of saturating concentrations of both lactate and NAD^+ to a patient's serum will result in a linear increase in absorbance at 340 nm over a given period, from which total enzyme activity is directly determined as described earlier. In this case, the increase in concentration of NADH, ΔP, over the time period, Δt, is proportional to the increase in absorbance, ΔA, at 340 nm, by Beer's Law, as described in Chapter 4, that is,

$$\Delta P/\Delta t = \varepsilon \times (\Delta A/\Delta t) \times L \qquad \textbf{(20-13)}$$

L in Equation 20-13 is the pathlength of the reaction vessel or cuvette, almost always equal to 1 cm. ε is a proportionality constant (most often, the molar extinction coefficient) in Beer's Law, which is 6.22×10^3 L mol^{-1} cm^{-1} for NADH at 340 nm. On most current chemistry analyzers, a volume of a patient's serum sample is added to the reaction cuvette containing the reaction components (lactate and NAD^+), and ΔA is observed. This results in dilution of the volume (Vp) of the patient's serum to the total volume of the reaction mixture (Vo), so that

$$\text{Enzyme activity} = \Delta P/\Delta t = \varepsilon \cdot (\Delta A/\Delta t) \cdot L \cdot (Vo/Vp) \qquad \textbf{(20-14)}$$

One caveat in the previous assay is that LD also catalyzes the reverse reaction (i.e., pyruvate to lactate). Therefore, as pyruvate forms, it can serve as an end-product competitive inhibitor (see Enzyme Inhibition section later) and can drive the reaction back to lactate. Therefore, it is important to be able to take the measurements in Equation 20-14 over a short time before pyruvate builds up to significant levels.

Coupled Enzymatic Reactions

In many instances, however, neither the product nor the substrate of a chemical reaction can be measured conveniently. In such instances, the enzymatic reaction can be "coupled" to another reaction that uses the product of the enzyme-catalyzed reaction to produce an indicator substance. An example of a typical coupled enzymatic reaction is the Oliver-Rosalki method for measurement of CK activity, illustrated in Equations 20-15 through 20-17, later. The reverse reaction of CK is used, producing adenosine triphosphate (ATP), which is used in a second reaction to produce glucose-6-phosphate (G6P) from glucose + ATP. The third reaction in the sequence results in the reduction of nicotinamide adenine dinucleotide phosphate, or $NADP^+$, to NADPH, the indicator of the reaction. In these coupled reactions, it is critical that the rate-limiting step in the overall reaction is the CK-mediated step that generates ATP. This can be achieved by using high concentrations of the indicator enzymes to ensure rapid conversion of the substrates of the subsequent reactions.

One potential problem with CK measurements when this reaction scheme is used is the presence of other enzymes that can generate ATP. Adenylate kinase, an enzyme found in red blood cells and liver, converts adenosine diphosphate (ADP) to ATP (see Equation 20-34); specimens with high adenylate kinase activity will have falsely elevated values for CK activity.

$$\text{Creatine phosphate} + \text{ADP} \rightarrow \text{Creatine} + \text{ATP (catalyzed by CK)} \qquad \textbf{(20-15)}$$

$$\text{Glucose} + \text{ATP} \rightarrow \text{G6P} + \text{ADP (catalyzed by hexokinase)} \qquad \textbf{(20-16)}$$

$$\text{G6P} + \text{NADP}^+ \rightarrow \text{6-Phosphogluconate} + \text{NADPH (catalyzed by glucose-6-phosphate dehydrogenase, or G6PD)} \qquad \textbf{(20-17)}$$

Complication:

$$2\ \text{ADP} \rightarrow \text{ATP} + \text{AMP (catalyzed by adenylate kinase)} \qquad \textbf{(20-18)}$$

The absorbance increase at 340 nm due to NADPH is proportional to the [ATP] generated as the end-product of the CK reaction, as expressed in Equation 20-15.

In assays of enzyme activity, some methods use **endpoint** measurements, determining the concentration of substrate or product at a specific time after addition of the sample. Endpoint methods are typically used in simple methods, such as bedside glucose testing or dipstick reactions, as for glucose or leukocyte esterase in urine. Endpoint methods may give erroneously low results in situations where enzyme activity is very high. Most enzymatic assays use **kinetic** methods of measurement (as discussed earlier), whereby the rate of change in concentration of substrate or product is determined. (For the sake of simplicity, throughout the rest of this section, only measurement systems that detect appearance of product will be described; the same principles, however, would apply to situations where rate of disappearance of substrate is being monitored.) Kinetic methods are more accurate and make it easier to detect changes in reaction conditions and samples requiring dilution. In a time-course study, the rate of reaction can be expressed as ΔP/Δt, the change in amount of product per unit time. Because the IU and the katal represent the amount of enzyme producing a specific amount of product in a given time period, this approach allows direct reporting of enzyme activity in either IU or katal, as desired.

Enzyme Assays Under Nonsaturating Conditions: First-Order Rate Processes

As discussed later, there are circumstances under which it may not be possible to perform an enzyme assay under saturating conditions where Equation 20-11 applies. In these circumstances, assay conditions may be used in which $S < K_M$. The Michaelis-Menten equation (20-10) then becomes

$$v_0 = d[P]/dt = k_2E_T \cdot [S]/K_M \qquad \textbf{(20-19)}$$

Because E_T is constant, the initial rate of the reaction depends only on the concentration of S. When S decreases, ES and P increase so that $-d[S]/dt$

$= d[ES]/dt + d[P]/dt$. But, under the reaction condition that $[S] >> [E]$, the steady-state assumption, $d[ES]/dt = 0$, is valid. Therefore, the rate of product formation equals the rate of substrate depletion, that is,

$$v_0 = d[P]/dt = -d[S]/dt = k_2E_T \cdot [S]/K_M \quad \textbf{(20-20)}$$

This is the equation for a first-order process, that is, the rate depends only on the concentration of a single species, in this case the substrate. Because the rate also formally depends on E_T, it is properly called a second-order reaction, but in this case, E_T is constant and does not change during the reaction. It is therefore referred to as a *pseudo-first*-order reaction. E_T can be determined from determination of the initial rate of the reaction where the initial substrate concentration, S_0, is known. Because K_M and k_2 are known,

$$E_T = (v_0/[S_0]) \times (K_M/k_2) \quad \textbf{(20-21)}$$

If only total enzyme activity is to be reported, then v_0/S_0, which is equal to $(k_2/K_M)[E_T]$, is reported because this quantity is directly proportional to E_T. Note though that these are not the same activity units as are used under saturating conditions because the total enzyme concentration in that case is multiplied only by k_2, and in the current circumstance, it is multiplied by k_2/K_M because of the fact that saturation has not occurred.

Another approach to determination of E_T under nonsaturating conditions is to integrate Equation 20-20 for S in terms of t. This results in the following relationship:

$$\ln([S]/[S_0]) = 2.303\log([S]/[S_o]) = -(k_2E_T/K_M) \cdot t \quad \textbf{(20-22)}$$

where ln is the natural logarithm to the base e and $[S_0]$ is the initial substrate concentration. If the substrate concentration is determined at specific times, a plot of the log (S/S_0) versus time should give a straight line whose slope is $-(k_2E_T/K_M)/2.303$. Because both k_2 and K_M are known, E_T can be directly evaluated. This method eliminates the need to measure initial velocities involving small changes in [S]. This method is advantageous when the substrate solubility does not permit saturating substrate concentrations to be reached.

The above first-order rate equation is the general equation for all first-order rate processes that abound in biology. Many reactions in the body occur either by first-order processes or by pseudo-first-order processes in which the rate depends only on the concentration of one species. As is discussed in Chapter 23, when drugs are administered to the body, they decay very often by a first-order process, where the rate of disappearance of the drug depends only on the concentration of the drug. One important feature of this process is the so-called **half-time.** Note, from Equation 20-22, that the half-time, or the time required for half of S_0 to be consumed, that is, when $[S] = [S_0]/2$, is a constant that depends only on the rate constant in the equation. The nondependence of $t_{1/2}$ on concentration is a cardinal feature of first-order rate processes.

Because log (2) = 0.3, the above equation reduces to

$$t_{1/2} = 0.69/k \quad \textbf{(20-23)}$$

where, in this case, $k = K_M/k_2E_T$ and $t_{1/2}$ is the half-time, that is, the time required for half of the substrate to be consumed. Thus, if the half-time for substrate consumption is known, E_T can also be directly computed from Equation 20-23, provided that K_M and k_2 are known.

OTHER FACTORS AFFECTING ENZYME ACTIVITY

Temperature

Enzyme-catalyzed reaction rates are extremely sensitive to temperature changes; to ensure accuracy, the temperature of the reaction mixture must not deviate by more than ±0.1° C from the assigned temperature. In general, every 10° C increase in the temperature leads to an approximate doubling of enzyme activity, although this varies slightly from one enzyme to another. The use of higher temperatures gives faster reaction rates and improves sensitivity—an advantage when enzyme activities are low. Lower temperatures increase the linear limit of an assay, requiring fewer dilutions. The choice of temperature with most modern instruments is governed by the capabilities of the instrument. There is a limit to the amount of temperature increase that can be used; most enzymes start to denature and become inactive as the temperature is increased. For example, CK starts to denature at 37° C, and amylase begins to denature at 45° C. On the other hand, some enzymes remain stable at extremely high temperatures. As an extreme case, the Taq polymerase used in the polymerase chain reaction is stable at 95° C. Taq polymerase and the polymerase chain reaction are discussed in Chapter 66.

pH

Enzymes have a pH optimum for maximal activity; usually, the pH of the reaction conditions is chosen to be that at which the enzyme exhibits the greatest activity. Selection of pH is not always critical; some enzymes have a very broad pH maximum, so that small changes in pH do not appreciably change activity. For example, ALP has maximum activity at pH values between 9 and 10. In some cases, particularly for enzymes with multiple isoenzymes, selection of pH represents a compromise, as different isoenzymes may have maximum activity at differing pH values. In this situation, the pH for the reaction is selected to allow measurement of the activities of all isozymes.

Salt and Protein Concentrations

The ionic strength of solutions affects enzyme activity; if ionic strength is too high, enzyme activity drops. The activity of many enzymes is also affected by protein concentration. When enzyme activity is over the linear limits of the assay, dilution of plasma typically requires use of **enzyme diluents** containing plasma proteins. Human plasma contains about 70 g protein/L, but normal urine has almost no protein; use of proteins such as albumin increases the activity of urinary amylase and standardizes its measurement. In protein-free solutions, enzymes lose activity rapidly either by denaturation or by adsorption to the walls of the container.

Inhibitors and Interferences

Typically, enzymes are measured in serum samples. Heparinized plasma is generally considered an equivalent sample to serum for most routine analytes, but this may not be the case for enzymes. Heparin may inhibit the activity of some enzymes, notably amylase and AST (using some, but not all, methods). Citrate, used in evacuated collection tubes for coagulation testing and as a preservative in blood products, complexes divalent cations; citrate-containing specimens may cause falsely low results for enzymes such as CK and ALP. Ethylenediaminetetraacetic acid (EDTA) and fluoride inhibit the activity of many enzymes and should almost never be used for specimens for enzyme analysis. An exception is in measurement of renin, where EDTA inhibits the action of enzymes that convert prorenin to the active enzyme renin and prevents artifactual increase in renin activity.

CAVEATS IN ENZYME ASSAYS

Some of the causes of errors in enzyme assays, such as the presence of inhibitors, have been mentioned previously. Here, we summarize the most common problems that can be encountered.

K_M-Type Mutations

In certain deficiency states, the conditions of the in vitro assay may not mirror the in vivo conditions that give rise to the deficiency state. In cases where a genetic defect does not alter normal protein levels of enzyme, and the k_{cat} value is unchanged, by applying the principle that the assay should be carried out at saturating substrate concentration, it is possible that a K_M-type mutation may go undetected because the enzyme, inactive at low substrate levels, exhibits full or nearly full activity at the higher [S] used in the assay. For example, a variant erythrocyte hypoxanthine-guanine-phosphoribosyltransferase is inactive in assays at low [S], but full activity is restored by increasing the substrate concentration. To guard against such a false positive, a clinical evaluation should include a determination of the K_M for the mutant enzyme.

One technique that can be employed to detect enzyme mutations that affect activity is the use of monoclonal antibodies directed against the enzyme of interest. Immunoassays for enzymes are discussed later. Correspondence between measurement of enzyme activity and the protein (enzyme) concentration from immunoassays will pertain as long as the enzyme antigen is fully active. Such is not always the case when inherited deficiencies associated with point mutations are involved. In these instances, estimates of enzyme concentration based on immunoassays can exceed those based on measurements of enzyme activity, indicating a defect in the enzyme. If the underlying basis of disease is genetic, it is best to estimate enzyme activity from kinetic measurements and compare these with normal values. Some mutations destabilize protein structure, leading to rapid intracellular proteolysis of the enzyme. In this instance, the result derived from immunologic methods and enzyme activity measurements can concur. The presence of inhibitors in the source biological fluid may lead to underestimation of the amount of enzyme present based on activity, but not immunologic measurements. Usually, reversible enzyme inhibitors will not interfere with immunologic estimates of enzyme concentration.

Cyclic Enzyme Instability

In some cases, an enzyme defect may go undetected because the clinical evaluation occurs at an inappropriate time. Administration of the antimalarial primaquine to a G6PD-deficient individual carrying the common type **A–** variant (G6PD **A–**) causes transient hemolytic anemia. Patients can recover completely from the anemia despite continued drug treatment. The type **A–** variant has normal kinetic parameters but reduced thermal stability. The initial episode clears older erythrocytes that have reduced G6PD activity. The older cells are replaced by new cells that have higher amounts of enzyme. The quantity of G6PD molecules in erythrocytes is a function of erythrocyte age, and the rate of loss of enzyme molecules in type **A–** variant cells exceeds that in normal cells by a significant margin. Levels of G6PD activity following recovery from anemia will be substantially higher than if assays are performed before or during the hemolytic episode, because hemolysis selectively destroys older cells containing smaller amounts of enzyme. Recovery results in the replacement of these older cells with new cells with higher levels of G6PD **A–** molecules. During and following recovery, the younger set of cells is able to cope with the primaquine treatment because of the presence of higher levels of enzyme activity.

Presence of Enzyme Inhibitors

As is discussed later, enzyme inhibitors present in biological fluids may permit underestimation of the amount of enzyme present. It is important to note that if the presence of an inhibitor is suspected, the most effective procedure is to dilute the sample, so that the effect of the inhibitor will be minimal. In case of the possibility of end-product inhibition, initial velocity determinations eliminate this effect because, initially, at $t = 0$, $[P] = 0$, where there will be no inhibitory effect. In rare cases, in enzyme-catalyzed reactions in which the product binds to the enzyme with a much higher affinity than the substrate, $\Delta P/\Delta t$ or $-\Delta S/\Delta t$ may be curvilinear, and estimates of the initial velocity are best made from tangents drawn to the substrate or product time-course curves at $t = 0$. These tangents are best determined from continuous traces of substrate disappearance or product formation.

Protease Degradation of Unstable Enzymes

Proteases in plasma may attack the enzyme while the velocity estimate is being made. This is especially true for enzymes that may have reduced thermal stability as discussed earlier. If the enzymes become unfolded, they are subject to attack by serum proteases, including trypsin and chymotrypsin and a number of other proteases. Enzyme damage through proteolysis, and substrate decomposition, may be corrected by the use of suitable blanks and preincubation studies.

Thermal Instability

The stability of the enzyme under evaluation must be known, and sample storage conditions must be determined. For example, LD cannot be stored at temperatures <0° C without significant loss of activity.

Presence of Inhibitory Compounds in Blood Collection Tubes

As discussed previously, in many cases serum or plasma and not whole blood must be used for the determination of enzyme activity in whole blood samples collected in anticoagulant-containing tubes. Polyanionic anticoagulants, such as citrate, heparin, and EDTA, inactivate metal-containing enzymes. For example, EDTA inactivates the zinc-containing enzyme ALP, an enzyme that is commonly assayed.

Competing Reactions in an Enzyme Assay

As noted in the preceding section, substrates used to assay specific enzymes may be subject to attack by other enzymes normally present in biological fluids. Assays for LD using pyruvate as the substrate can be complicated by the presence of other enzymes such as pyruvate dehydrogenase and ALT that react with this substrate. The coupled assay system for CK activity can be complicated by the presence in serum of the enzyme adenylate kinase, which can consume the substrate ADP. (See Equation 20-18.) This problem cannot be corrected by using saturating concentrations of ADP because the product of the adenylate kinase reaction is also ATP, and the ATP produced in the CK reaction has to be used to determine the amount of G6P produced to determine accurately the CK level.

Time-Dependent Inactivation of Certain Enzymes

Sample age may be important in determining enzyme activity. Enzymes whose activity depends on active-site sulfhydryl groups may suffer slow inactivation through oxidation and/or disulfide exchange reactions. In many instances, these processes are irreversible and lead to underestimation of the enzyme concentration by activity measurements.

ANTIBODY-BASED TECHNIQUES FOR MEASURING ENZYMES

As mentioned earlier, immunoassays can be used to measure the mass of enzyme protein. These assays are described at length in Chapter 23 and in Part 5. Immunoassays are the method of choice when it is desired to quantitate one or more isoenzymes of an enzyme in a sample because specific antibodies raised against each individual isoenzyme will identify and quantitate each of the variants present in the sample.

Immunoassays are, in general, less affected by factors that affect enzyme activity and are often more precise. As with enzyme activity, however, the determination of enzyme mass may vary depending on the reagents used; calibrators often lead to different results for mass activity between different methods. Examples include the MB isoenzyme of CK, the pancreatic isoenzymes of amylase, the prostatic and bone isoenzymes of acid phosphatase (ACP), and the bone isoenzyme of ALP. Antibodies can also be used to selectively inhibit or bind particular enzyme subunits. This approach allows the total and isoenzyme measurements to be expressed in the same units. For example, antibodies to CK-M subunits inhibit half of CK-MB isoenzyme and all of CK-MM isoenzyme. Measurement of CK activity of a sample after incubation with an anti-M antibody can be used to determine the activity of non-M subunits of CK.

Antibodies can also be used as **capture** antibodies to separate a particular isoenzyme from other forms of the same enzyme, followed by measurement of enzymatic activity. Examples of such capture assays include tests for the bone isoenzyme of ALP and the bone and prostate isoenzymes of ACP . Some enzymes circulate bound to antiproteases, such as prostate-specific antigen (PSA) (see Chapter 73) and α-1-antichymotrypsin or trypsin and α-1-antitrypsin. Antibodies may differ in their ability to measure free and bound forms. Some enzymes are also bound to β-2-macroglobulin, such as PSA (Otto, 1998) and ACP (Brehme, 1999); enzyme bound to this antiprotease usually is not enzymatically active and cannot be measured by most immunoassays, because the binding site is hidden from antibody recognition. Finally, in common with other immunoassays, measurement of enzymes by immunoassay can show interferences from substances that bind to reagent antibodies, such as heterophile antibodies (Sosolik, 1997) and rheumatoid factor (Dasgupta, 1999).

INHIBITION OF ENZYMES

The inhibition of enzymes may be reversible or irreversible. In irreversible inhibition, a covalent bond is formed between the inhibitor and the enzyme, and enzyme activity cannot be restored by dissociation of the inhibitor. Examples include the inhibition of acetylcholinesterase (AChE) and pseudocholinesterase (PChE) by chemical warfare agents such as sarin and tabun that irreversibly phosphorylate the side chain **OH** group of the active-site serine residue. The first fluorinated anesthetic, fluroxene (**$CF_3CH_2OCH{=}CH_2$**) proved to be too toxic for use as a general anesthetic because it irreversibly alkylated a heme ring N atom in the cytochrome P450 monooxygenase responsible for its detoxification. This alkylation led to complete loss of enzyme activity.

Reversible inhibition is one of three types: competitive, uncompetitive, and noncompetitive. As noted earlier, if the presence of an inhibitor is suspected in an enzyme assay of a patient's sample, such as by observation of a nonlinear [P] versus time curve, an effective strategy is to dilute the sample, so that the effect of the inhibitor is reduced. Even if this procedure concurrently dilutes the enzyme, the enzyme assay can still be effectively performed, especially if the substrate is present at saturating conditions.

COMPETITIVE INHIBITION

Competitive inhibition occurs when the inhibitor binds at the same site as the substrate. The molecular basis for the binding of competitive inhibitors at the active site is that the substrate and the inhibitor are structurally

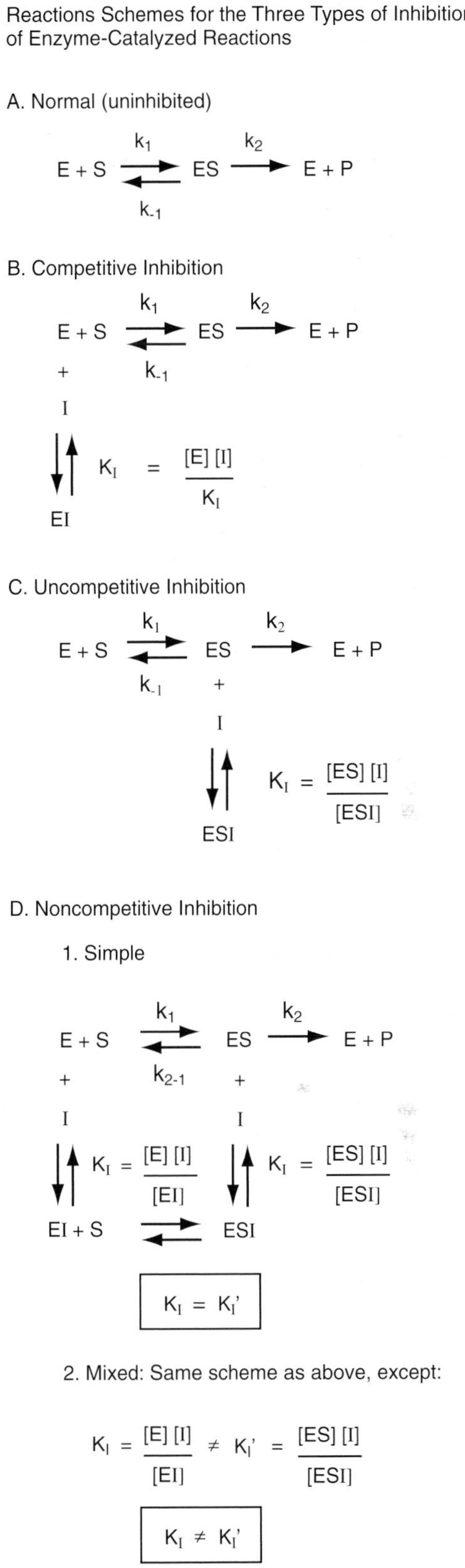

Figure 20-6 Schemes for all types of inhibition of enzyme activity. **A,** The scheme for an uninhibited reaction. **B,** The scheme for competitive inhibition, showing that the inhibitor binds competitively to free enzyme, decreasing the binding of the substrate to the free enzyme. This results in a lower apparent affinity of the substrate for the enzyme, making the apparent K_M higher than the true K_M. However, this inhibition does not affect the catalytic rate, V_{max}. K_I is the dissociation constant for the enzyme–inhibitor complex ([EI]). **C,** The scheme for uncompetitive inhibition, showing that the inhibitor binds only to the enzyme–substrate complex such that it blocks catalysis but not the binding of the substrate to the enzyme and therefore affects V_{max} but not K_M. K_I in this case is the dissociation constant for the enzyme–substrate–inhibitor ternary complex ([ESI]). **D,** The scheme for noncompetitive inhibition, which is of two types: (1) simple and (2) mixed. In both cases, the inhibitor binds both to the free enzyme *and* to the enzyme–substrate complex, affecting both V_{max} and K_M. In simple noncompetitive inhibition *(1),* the affinity of the inhibitor both for the free enzyme and for the enzyme–substrate complex is the same, making the two respective dissociation constants, K_I and K_I', equal. In mixed noncompetitive inhibition *(2),* K_I and K_I' are not equal.

similar, with the result that the enzyme is "deceived" into recognizing and binding the inhibitor. Examples of competitive inhibition include the inhibition of trypsin by α-1-antitrypsin, chymotrypsin by α-1-antichymotrypsin, dihydrofolate reductase by the chemotherapeutic agent methotrexate, and the Krebs cycle enzyme succinic dehydrogenase by malonate. In some reactions, the product of the reaction, which may be structurally similar to the substrate, may competitively inhibit the reaction, a phenomenon known as **end-product inhibition.** A variation of this phenomenon can occur occasionally in which the buildup of the end-product can reverse the forward reaction, regenerating the substrate. Not infrequently, drugs are used as competitive inhibitors of targeted enzymes. For example, as discussed later, a major target of antihypertensive drugs is angiotensin-converting enzyme (ACE).

HOW COMPETITIVE INHIBITORS AFFECT THE MICHAELIS-MENTEN EQUATION

The kinetic mechanism for **competitive inhibition** is shown in Figure 20-6, *B.* The inhibitor is assumed to be in rapid equilibrium with free **E** and the **EI** complex. Kinetically, the inhibitor reduces the concentration of free **E** available to combine with **S**. The equation of conservation of enzyme now reads

$$[E_T] = [E] + [EI] + [ES] \tag{20-24}$$

[EI] is defined in terms of the equilibrium constant, $\mathbf{K_I}$, for the dissociation of the inhibitor from the **EI** complex, and

$$[EI] = [E][I]/K_I \tag{20-25}$$

Because the steady-state equation for ES (Equations 20-3, 20-4, and 20-5) remains the same, Equation 20-24 becomes

$$E_T = E + [E][S]/K_M + [E][I]/K_I \tag{20-26}$$

and

$$[E] = \frac{[E_T]}{\left(1 + \frac{[S]}{K_M} + \frac{[I]}{K_I}\right)} \tag{20-27}$$

Because, as in Equation 20-2,

$$d[P]/dt = k_2[ES] = [E][S]/K_M \tag{20-28}$$

$$\frac{dP}{dt} = \frac{k_2[S]}{K_M} \bullet \frac{[E_T]}{\left(1 + \frac{[S]}{K_M} + \frac{[I]}{K_I}\right)} \tag{20-29}$$

and

$$\frac{d[P]}{dt} = k_2[ES] = \frac{k_2[E_T][S]}{K_M\left(1 + \frac{[I]}{K_I}\right) + [S]} \tag{20-30}$$

Note from this equation that the factor $(1 + [I]/K_I)$ multiplies K_M in the denominator. This means that K_M is multiplied by a number ≥1. Thus, if a competitive inhibitor is present at an appreciable concentration so that this factor >> 1, concentrations of S that would have saturated the enzyme will now no longer be able to do so. If a competitive inhibitor is present, its effect can be eliminated by increasing the substrate concentration such that $S >> K_M(1+[I]/K_I)$.

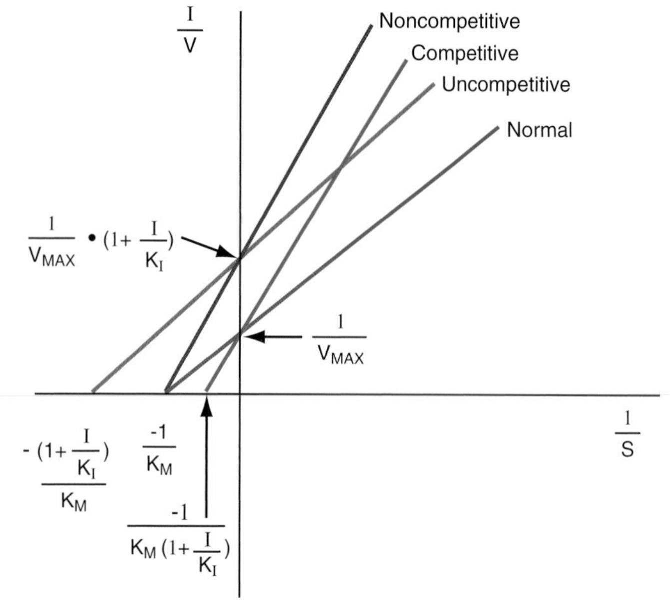

Figure 20-7 Lineweaver-Burk plots for each type of inhibition shown in Figure 20-6, showing Y- and X-intercepts. To avoid cluttering, the slopes are not shown. The slopes of the lines for uninhibited reaction *(blue)* and uncompetitive inhibition *(green)* are K_M/V_{max}. The slopes of the lines for competitive *(red)* and noncompetitive *(purple)* inhibitions are K_M (1 + I/K_I).

Inversion of Equation 20-30 gives the Lineweaver-Burk linear transform as follows:

$$\frac{I}{V_0}=\frac{K_M\left(1+\frac{[I]}{K_I}\right)}{V_{MAX}}\bullet\frac{1}{[S]}+\frac{1}{V_{MAX}} \qquad \textbf{(20-31)}$$

Plots of 1/v_o versus 1/[S] at different inhibitor concentrations give linear traces in which the slope, but not the intercept, is altered in the presence of a competitive inhibitor. V_{max} is unchanged, and only K_M is altered. K_M is modified by the coefficient (1 + [I]/K_I). The X-intercept of this equation (where 1/v_o is 0) is −1/[(1 + I/K_I)K_M]. The effect of competitive inhibitors on enzyme-catalyzed reactions is summarized in Figure 20-7.

UNCOMPETITIVE INHIBITION

As shown in Figure 20-6, *C*, **u**ncompetitive inhibition occurs when the inhibitor binds only to the ES complex, and not to free E. Therefore, no EI complex forms. Binding of the substrate causes a conformational change, creating a site for binding of the inhibitor.

EFFECT OF UNCOMPETITIVE INHIBITORS ON THE MICHAELIS-MENTEN EQUATION

In keeping with a similar procedure that was used for deriving Equation 20-30 above, we obtain the following expression:

$$V_0=\frac{V_{MAX}[S]}{K_M+[S]\left(1+\frac{[I]}{K_I}\right)} \qquad \textbf{(20-32)}$$

Note here that the same factor, (1 + [I]/K_I), now multiplies S, rather than K_M, in the denominator of the Michaelis-Menten equation, as in the case of competitive inhibition discussed previously. This has the paradoxical effect of causing saturation to be reached at *lower* values of S than for the normal, uninhibited case (see Fig. 20-6) because S is multiplied by a factor that is >1. However, the *rate* of the uncompetitively inhibited enzyme-catalyzed reaction at saturation is *lower* than it normally should be; the maximal rate at saturation is V_{max}/(1 + I/K_I). No matter how high the substrate concentration is in this case, the normal rate at saturation, that is, V_{max}, cannot be reached, unlike in the case of competitive inhibition discussed in the preceding section.

At low **[S]** values, v_o approaches V_{max}/K_M[S], as for the uninhibited case, and the uncompetitive inhibitor is without effect. This suggests that dilution of the specimen will remove the effect of the inhibitor and will enable the uninhibited rate of the reaction to be determined. Under these conditions, E_T or activity can be directly computed from the first-order kinetic analysis (Equation 20-19) at low substrate concentration.

The double reciprocal form of Equation 20-32 above is as follows:

$$\frac{1}{V_0}=\frac{K_M}{V_{MAX}}\bullet\frac{1}{[S]}+\left(1+\frac{[I]}{K_I}\right)\bullet\frac{1}{V_{MAX}} \qquad \textbf{(20-33)}$$

The Lineweaver-Burk plot of this equation has a slope that is the same as for the uninhibited (normal) reaction, but the intercept, (1/V_{max}) (1 + [I]/K_I), will be higher for uncompetitive inhibition than for the normal case, that is, 1/V_{max}, as shown in Figure 20-6, *C*. The X-intercept (where 1/v_o = 0) is −(1 + [I]/K_I)/K_M. If [I] is known, either intercept can be used to compute K_I. The effect of uncompetitive inhibitors on enzyme-catalyzed reactions is summarized in Figure 20-7.

SIMPLE AND MIXED NONCOMPETITIVE INHIBITION

Noncompetitive inhibition occurs when the inhibitor, similar to the uncompetitive inhibitor, binds at a site distinct from the substrate-binding site. Both the inhibitor and the substrate are capable of binding the enzyme simultaneously. Binding of the inhibitor to this second site may completely abolish enzyme activity or may only partially reduce it. Hence, noncompetitive inhibition may be **full** or **partial**. Unlike uncompetitive inhibitors, noncompetitive inhibitors bind both to free E and to ES. If the binding of the inhibitor and of the substrate occurs independently of each other, **simple noncompetitive inhibition** exists. If bound substrate alters the affinity of the enzyme for the inhibitor, a condition of **mixed competitive inhibition** exists. Binding of the noncompetitive inhibitor alters the conformation of the substrate-binding site. The substrate can still bind; however, the binding affinity and/or the catalytic activity is/are reduced.

EFFECTS OF NONCOMPETITIVE INHIBITORS ON THE MICHAELIS-MENTEN EQUATION

The kinetic scheme for this type of inhibition is shown in Figure 20-6, *D*. Here, the inhibitor can bind *both* to the free enzyme *and* to the enzyme–substrate complex. If the affinity or dissociation constants for each of these processes are the same, as shown in Figure 20-6, then the pattern appears to be a combination of competitive and uncompetitive inhibition and is termed simple noncompetitive inhibition. Thus, in this case, the term (1 + [I]/K_I) multiplies both terms in the denominator of the Michaelis-Menten equation (see Equation 20-10), or

$$V_0=\frac{V_{MAX}\bullet[S]}{\left(1+\frac{[I]}{K_I}\right)\bullet K_M+\left(1+\frac{[I]}{K_I}\right)\bullet[S]} \qquad \textbf{(20-34)}$$

If the two K_I constants differ, the inhibition is termed **mixed** noncompetitive inhibition. For this latter case, if K_I is the dissociation constant for the inhibitor when it binds to free enzyme, and if K_I' is the dissociation constant for the inhibitor when it binds to the enzyme–substrate complex, then the Michaelis-Menten rate law for noncompetitive inhibition is

$$V_0=\frac{V_{MAX}\bullet[S]}{\left(1+\frac{[I]}{K_I}\right)\bullet K_M+\left(1+\frac{[I]}{K_I'}\right)\bullet[S]} \qquad \textbf{(20-35)}$$

The Lineweaver-Burk equation for simple noncompetitive inhibition is

$$\frac{1}{V_0}=\frac{K_M}{V_{MAX}}\bullet\left(1+\frac{[I]}{K_I}\right)\bullet\frac{1}{[S]}+\frac{1}{V_{MAX}}\bullet\left(1+\frac{[I]}{K_I}\right) \qquad \textbf{(20-36)}$$

And, for mixed inhibition,

$$\frac{1}{V_0}=\frac{K_M}{V_{MAX}}\bullet\left(1+\frac{[I]}{K_I}\right)\bullet\frac{1}{[S]}+\frac{1}{V_{MAX}}+\left(1+\frac{[I]}{K_I'}\right) \qquad \textbf{(20-37)}$$

As can be seen from Equation 20-35, for simple noncompetitive inhibition, in the presence of inhibitor, both the slope and the intercept increase in value by the factor (1 + [I]/K_I). This result is based on the assumption that the substrate does not modify the affinity of the enzyme for the inhibitor, and vice versa. Note that, because the inhibitor binds to the enzyme–substrate complex, thereby inactivating it, the maximal velocity is lowered as was the case for uncompetitive inhibition as discussed earlier. Therefore, the intercept for this condition is 1/V_{max} (1 + [I]/K_I), that is, instead of 1/V_{max} as in the normal case. Likewise, K_M is increased by the same factor.

TABLE 20-5

Slopes and Intercepts From Double Reciprocal Plots and Computed Values of Vmax and KM From These Plots for Various Types of Reversible Inhibitors

Type of inhibition	Slope	Y-intercept	X-intercept	V_{max} (apparent)*	K_M (apparent)*
None	K_M/V_{max}	$1/V_{max}$	$-1/K_M$	V_{max}	K_M
Competitive	$(K_M/V_M)(1 + I/K_I)$	$1/V_{max}$	$-1/[K_M(1 + I/K_I)]$	V_{max}	$K_M(1 + I/K_I)$
Uncompetitive	K_M/V_{max}	$(1/V_{max}) \bullet (1 + I/K_I)$	$-(1 + I/K_I)/K_M$	$V_{max}/(1 + I/K_I)$	K_M
Noncompetitive (simple)	$K_M/V_{max} \bullet (1 + I/K_I)$	$(1/V_{max}) \bullet (1 + I/K_I)$	$-1/K_M$	$V_{max}/(1 + I/K_I)$	K_M

*The observed value that equals the derived expression from the double reciprocal plots shown for each condition.

However, as discussed previously, K_M is computed as the **ratio** of the slope of the Lineweaver-Burk plot to the intercept. Because both of these terms contain the factor $(1 + [I]/K_I)$, this factor cancels, and the computation yields the value of the actual K_M. This, of course, does not happen in mixed noncompetitive inhibition where the two constants for inhibitor binding differ from one another. In this case, K_M^{app} is $K_M \bullet (1 + [I]/K_I)/(1 + [I]/K_I')$. The X-intercept for simple noncompetitive inhibition from Equation 20-36 above is $-1/K_M$, and, for mixed noncompetitive inhibition, it is $-(1 + [I]/K_I')/(1 + [I]/K_I)K_M$. The effect of simple noncompetitive inhibitors (that have the same K_I value for free enzyme and enzyme–substrate complex) on enzyme-catalyzed reactions is summarized in Figure 20-7.

Table 20-5 summarizes changes in the apparent values of V_{max} and K_M derived from the intercepts and slopes of double reciprocal Lineweaver-Burk plots for competitive, uncompetitive, and simple noncompetitive inhibition. Figure 20-7 summarizes the Lineweaver-Burk plots for a normal enzyme-catalyzed reaction and for the three types of inhibition of enzyme-catalyzed reactions and the values of the Y- and X-intercepts in each condition.

Catalytic Efficiency: Transition State Theory and Drug Design

Equation 20-19 applies to circumstances where the substrate concentration is present at concentrations below the value of K_M for an enzyme. The rate constant for this reaction is k_2/K_M, which is formally a second-order rate constant because this reaction depends on the concentrations of both the substrate and the enzyme. (As noted previously, the reaction is actually pseudo-first-order in that the total enzyme concentration, E_T, is constant, and only the substrate concentration, [S], changes.) Catalytic efficiency is assessed in terms of the rate constants of the catalyzed reaction. The constant k_2/K_M, often written as k_{cat}/K_M, is a reflection of the frequency of productive encounters of enzyme and substrate molecules in solution.

ENZYMES ACHIEVE HIGH RATES OF REACTION THAT GREATLY EXCEED THOSE FOR UNCATALYZED REACTIONS

An upper boundary to the frequency of encounters is determined by the temperature and the diffusion coefficients of the substrate and enzyme. This limiting value is on the order of 10^8 to 10^9 $M^{-1}sec^{-1}$, called the diffusion-controlled limit. If the value of k_{cat}/K_M is at the diffusion-controlled limit, every encounter of the enzyme and substrate leads to product formation, and the enzyme has achieved what may be termed **catalytic perfection.** Some enzymes have actually approached this state. These include superoxide dismutase ($k_{cat}/K_M = 2.8 \times 10^9$ $M^{-1}sec^{-1}$), AChE ($k_{cat}/K_M = 1.5 \times 10^8$ $M^{-1}sec^{-1}$), and catalase ($k_{cat}/K_M = 4.0 \times 10^8$ $M^{-1}sec^{-1}$). Most other enzymes do not have constants that are of this magnitude but have values that vastly exceed those for the corresponding uncatalyzed reactions, the second-order rate constants which are termed k_{uncat} (*uncat*alyzed).

The ratio k_{cat}/k_{uncat} gives the rate enhancement, which is often difficult to obtain because most cellular reactions occur very slowly in the absence of enzymes. For enzymes, rates are in the range of 10^8 to 10^{12}, but some are even higher. For example, the rate acceleration for adenosine deaminase, which catalyzes the deamination of adenosine to inosine, is 10^{14}, and the rate acceleration of ALP is 10^{17}. Both adenosine deaminase and ALP have modest k_{cat} values, 10^2 sec^{-1}. Their unusually large rate accelerations stem from the stability of their substrates at pH 7.0 and 25° C. For example, the half-time for the deamination of adenosine to inosine at 20° C and pH 7.0 is approximately 20,000 years, and k_{uncat} is10^{-12} sec^{-1}! The nonenzymatic rate constant for the hydrolysis of phosphate esters under neutral, room temperature conditions is estimated to be on the order of 10^{-15} sec^{-1}. The question arises as to how enzymes can induce such large rate enhancements and in some instances attain rates that are the highest that can physically be achieved.

ENZYMES ACHIEVE HIGH RATE ENHANCEMENTS BY BINDING TO THE TRANSITION STATE ON THE REACTION PATHWAY

From Figure 20-3, it can be seen that when the enzyme binds noncovalently to the substrate, if the energy of the resulting enzyme–substrate complex is lowered significantly relative to the energies of the separated species, this would lead to an increased activation energy. However, if the enzyme rather stabilizes the transition state leading to the formation of products, then the activation energy would be greatly lowered, as indicated in Figure 20-3. Considerable accumulating evidence suggests that enzymes have high affinities for **transition states.** Because, in the transition state, the substrate is somewhat distorted from its ground state structure by the incipient breaking and making of covalent bonds, the resulting increase in energy of the substrate is greater than that compensated by favorable interactions of the distorted substrate with the enzyme. It should be realized that transition states in reactions are not stable structures but rather are inferred from knowledge of the reaction path. However, substrate molecules have been designed that have critical features of inferred transition states, and these modified substrates have been found to bind to the enzymes with enhanced affinities (Fersht, 1999).

These considerations have direct clinical applicability in two areas: drug design and the advent of so-called catalytic antibodies, that is, antibodies that have been designed to have strong and specific enzyme activity. We give one example of each of these applications to illustrate the importance of transition state theory to practical clinical problems.

TRANSITION STATE THEORY IN DRUG DESIGN

HIV Protease Inhibitors in Treating HIV-AIDS

A host of new drugs have been developed as protease inhibitors that block the protease enzymes of the human immunodeficiency virus (HIV) involved in viral replication of the acquired immunodeficiency syndrome (AIDS) virus (Vance, 1997). Proteases catalyze hydrolytic reactions in which peptide or amide bonds are cleaved by water into a carboxylic acid and a primary (or, in the case of proline, a secondary) amine. HIV proteases are vital for cleaving large protein precursors into gag and pol proteins that enable viral replication. Absence of this protease activity results in inability of the virus to replicate. Thus this protease has become the target for the design of inhibitory compounds (Vance, 1997).

HIV protease functions as a homodimer, that is, two subunits having the exact same sequence. It catalyzes the hydrolysis of X-Pro (proline) peptide bonds where X is an aromatic amino acid, such as phenylalanine (Phe) or tyrosine (Swain, 1990; Vance, 1997). Two critical aspartic acid residues (25 and 125) are known to be the actual catalytic residues effecting peptide bond cleavage (Swain, 1990). Thus HIV protease, similar to a number of other proteases such as angiotensin-converting enzyme, discussed in the next section, is an aspartic acid peptidase. It has been known for many years that the hydrolysis of peptide (and ester) bonds involves

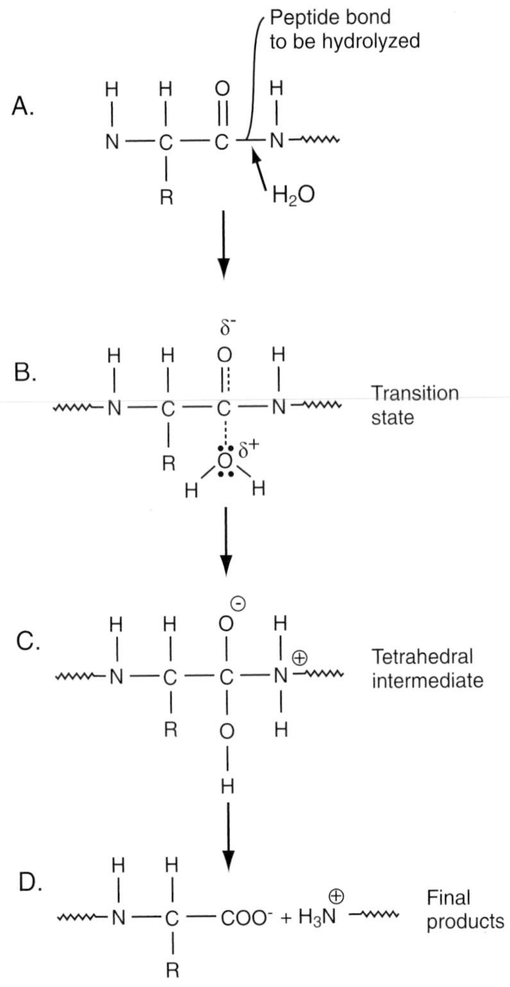

Figure 20-8 Steps in the hydrolysis of a peptide bond. **A,** A typical peptide bond for two amino acids in a peptide bond link. R is the side chain of the first amino acid. This bond will be cleaved by addition of water to the carbonyl group, as shown by the arrow. **B,** The transition state on the way to the addition of water to the carbonyl group. The carbonyl oxygen takes on a partial negative charge (δ^-). **C,** The tetrahedral intermediate that results from the addition of water. Note that an oxyanion forms on the former carbonyl oxygen. The attacking water molecule has given up a proton that can add to the amino nitrogen of the leaving group, that is, the amino acid on the right of the peptide bond, or to the oxyanion of the former carbonyl group. **D,** The final products, that is, a carboxylate from the left amino acid and an amine (ammonium ion) from the right amino acid.

the formation of a so-called tetrahedral intermediate, as illustrated for a peptide bond in Figure 20-8. This intermediate results from the addition of water to the unsaturated carbonyl carbon on the reaction pathway. The carbonyl carbon and the three atoms to which it is attached all lie in the same plane, the so-called planar configuration. Attack by the oxygen atom of water on the carbonyl carbon results in the addition of a fourth atom attached to the carbonyl carbon, causing replacement of the planar arrangement of the atoms by a tetrahedral arrangement of these atoms. Note that the transition state leading to this intermediate is inferred also to have tetrahedral features and a partially negatively charged oxygen. Thus, substrates have been designed that have, in place of the normally occurring amide bond, a tetrahedral structure with an oxy anion or a hydroxyl group at this position that resembles the transition state.

An example of an inhibitory transition state analog of HIV protease is shown in Figure 20-9. For comparison, a typical substrate of HIV protease is also shown (Matayoshi, 1990). As can be seen in Figure 20-9, in the Phe residue in the transition state analog, the normally occurring planar C=O group in the peptide backbone is replaced with a tetrahedral C(H)–OH group, giving rise to the so-called Phe-Psi residue. This occurs at the normal peptide cleavage site. This analog binds to HIV protease with a K_I (dissociation constant) of 0.24 nM (Swain, 1990). The substrate has a K_M on the order of 103 μM (Matayoshi, 1990). This K_M is a true dissociation constant in that the k_2 is much lower than the noncovalent dissociation constant. Therefore the ratio of the affinity constant (reciprocal of the dissociation constant) for the transition state analog to that of the substrate is on the order of 400,000! Thus, the application of transition state theory has resulted in the design of a very potent HIV protease inhibitor. Newer HIV protease transition state inhibitors, such as the modified peptide KNI-272, that have substantially lower K_I values have been designed (Adachia, 2009). The X-ray crystal structures of the transition state analogs bound to HIV protease have been determined (Swain, 1990; Adachia, 2009). The two critical Asp residues interact strongly with the tetrahedral atoms of the modified Phe residue and are clearly involved in stabilization of the tetrahedral transition state (Swain, 1990; Adachia, 2009).

One drawback to the HIV protease inhibitors currently being used clinically in the treatment of AIDS is that viral mutations result in HIV proteases that have lower affinities for these inhibitors. More recently, therefore, new transition state analogs have been designed such that they interact with amino acid residues that surround the active site and actually bind to critical backbone atoms of sections of the polypeptide chain that have well-defined secondary structures (such as α-helices and β-sheets), greatly increasing their affinities (K_I's in the picomolar range) (Ghosh, 2008). In this case, because mutations of constant structural residues would be expected to decrease the stability of the protease greatly, it is hoped that viral mutations will have much less effect on their efficacies.

Design of New Catalytic Antibodies With Predetermined Enzyme Activity

Antibodies generally bind to antigens with high affinities. If antibodies can be raised to transition state analogs of compounds that undergo specific chemical reactions, by stabilizing the transition state for these specific chemical reactions they might themselves serve as enzymes that catalyze these reactions. Although still in its infancy, this area of enzymology has achieved some notable success, providing, in turn, further support for the transition state theory of enzyme action. As an example, a clinically important finding using this approach is seen in the design of antibodies that induce hydrolysis of cocaine. Hydrolysis of the benzoate and acetyl esters results in effective inactivation of this drug of abuse, as discussed in Chapter 23. The structure of cocaine and a tetrahedral transition state analog are shown in Figure 20-10 (Cashman, 2000). This analog has a tetrahedral structure for the benzoyl moiety in which a nonhydrolyzable phenyl phosphonate ester replaces the normally occurring carbonyl group. Antibodies have been raised to a thiol derivative of cocaine and then assayed for their abilities to bind to the transition state analog. Several antibodies have been isolated that bind strongly to the transition state analog and also catalyze, with large rate enhancements over the uncatalyzed reaction, the hydrolysis of the benzoyl ester of cocaine, resulting in a cocaine derivative of much lower potency. It is of considerable interest that, using another approach, the serum enzyme, butyrylcholinesterase, discussed in the next section, has been modified, based on the X-ray crystal structure of this enzyme bound to inhibitors, using site-specific mutagenesis techniques, so that it is active in the de-benzoylation of cocaine leading to its inactivation. The rates of catalysis of the catalytic antibodies and the engineered butyrylcholinesterase are similar to one another. Both approaches may provide rational treatment modalities for detoxification of harmful substances, in this case, drugs of abuse.

SPECIFIC ENZYMES

Numerous enzymes are clinically useful in recognition and monitoring of particular disease processes. In all but a few circumstances, abnormal conditions in specific tissues are recognized by *elevations* of one or more enzymatic activities or enzyme concentrations. For example, elevations of the activity of serum CK suggest the presence of muscle disease. The reason for elevation of specific enzymes in blood and other body fluids as the result of disease processes in specific tissues is not completely understood. One explanation for this occurrence is that disease processes that cause cell injury or death result in damage to the cell membrane, leading to the release of specific intracellular enzymes into tissue spaces and the microvasculature, causing increased enzymatic activity in serum or other body fluids. On occasion, mutant forms of enzymes occur, resulting in *lowering* of their activities, although, generally, not of their concentrations. One prominent example of this phenomenon is butyrylcholinesterase (discussed later).

Several enzymes are distributed predominantly in a single tissue, so that damage to this tissue results in elevations of the enzyme in serum. For example, as discussed in Chapter 21 on liver function, elevation of the level of the enzyme ALT, which is distributed predominantly in the liver, indicates acute hepatic injury, often as a result of hepatitis. Although measured

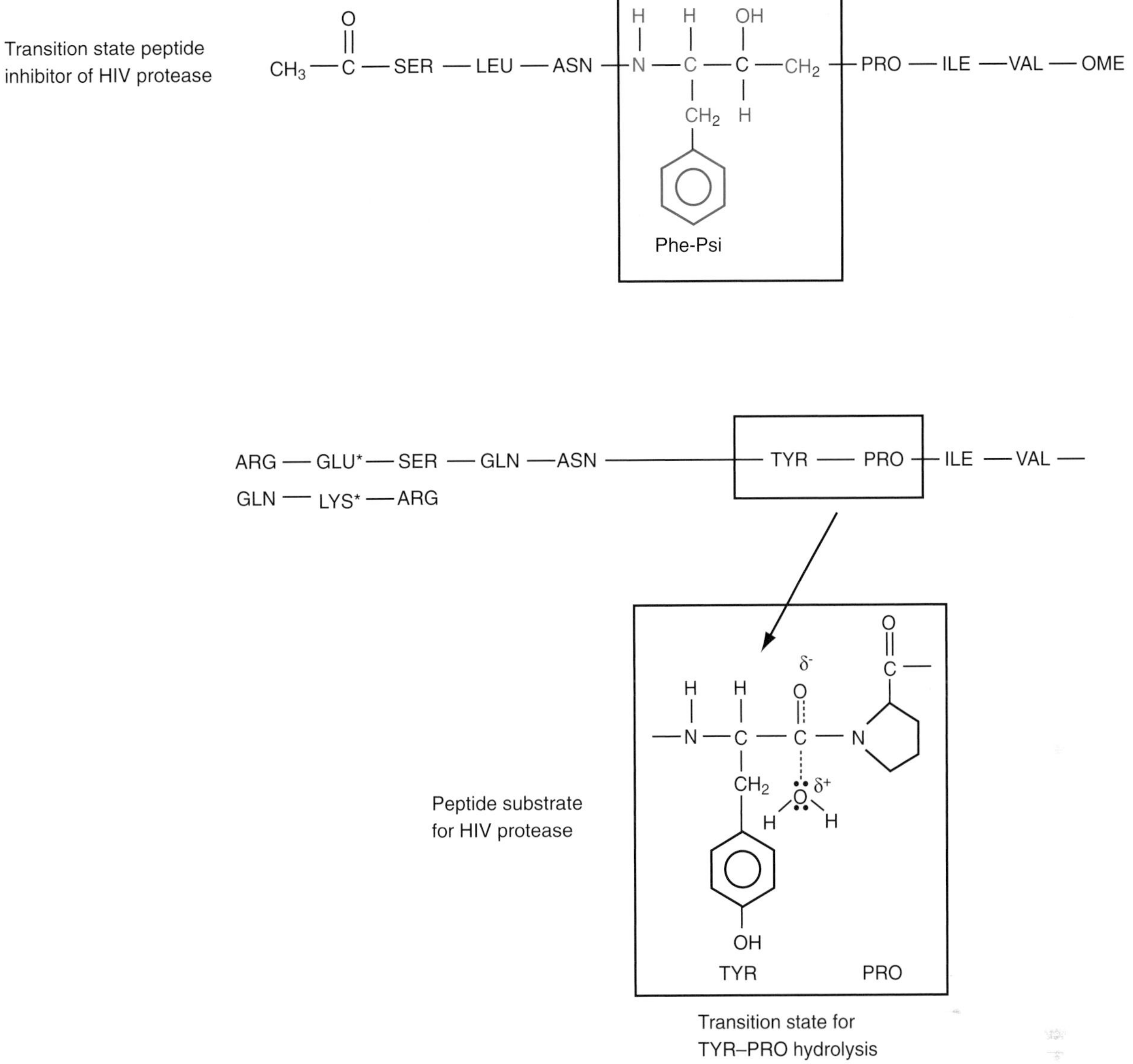

Figure 20-9 Human immunodeficiency virus (HIV) protease transition state analog peptide inhibitor. HIV protease cleaves at X-Pro bonds, where X is an aromatic amino acid like Tyr and Phe. In this case, X is a modified Phe residue, labeled Phe-Psi, most of whose atoms are colored red such that, in place of the normally occurring C=O (carbonyl) group, a tetrahedral carbon is present attached to an OH group. The tetrahedral atoms are shown in blue. This mimics the transition state shown for a substrate of HIV protease whose amino acid sequence is shown below that for the transition state analog. This sequence contains the bond cleavage site, TYR-PRO, as shown in the small box. The tetrahedral transition state for this cleavage is shown in the larger box. The asterisks on the two substrate residues denote that these residues can be attached to fluorescent probes in an enzyme assay for this protease using this substrate. Because the transition state analog resembles the transition state in the hydrolysis of the Tyr-Pro peptide bond, it is a strong and specific inhibitor of the protease.

by immunoassay, PSA is a form of chymotrypsin and occurs almost exclusively in the prostate gland. Serum elevations of PSA, therefore, suggest prostate pathology, often prostate cancer. Other enzymes do not have selective tissue distributions but have isozymes that do have selective distributions, making elevations of these isozymes valuable in diagnosing specific tissue pathology. For example, as discussed in Chapter 18, elevation of serum levels of CK-MB (also, see previous discussion) points to myocardial disease, most often infarction. As discussed later, elevations of specific isozymes of ALP point to specific tissue disease. The biliary tract form is elevated in biliary disease, and the bone form is elevated in diseases of bone.

For enzymes with no tissue-specific isozymes, the relative amounts of different enzymes in plasma provide a clue as to the type of organ injured. For example, LD, AST, and ALT are found in many organs, but the relative amounts in each differ (Table 20-6). If LD is markedly elevated, while AST and ALT are only slightly elevated, this would suggest damage to an organ or tissue (such as red blood cells, white blood cells, or tumors) with a high LD/AST ratio. On the other hand, if AST and ALT are elevated, but LD is only slightly elevated, this suggests damage to liver, which has a low LD/AST ratio.

Many other enzymes, elevations of which denote damage to specific tissues, are discussed in other chapters of this book. Discussion of enzymes and enzyme inhibitors in serum and urine for recognition of renal disease is found in Chapter 14; enzymes of bone metabolism are presented in Chapter 15; enzymes and other proteins utilized for the diagnosis of myocardial infarction are discussed in Chapter 18; enzymes useful in recognition of liver and biliary tract disease are discussed in Chapter 21; pancreatic enzymes are covered in Chapter 22; and enzyme deficiencies that produce hemolytic anemia are discussed in Part 4.

The remainder of this chapter is concerned with a discussion of enzymes, each of whose isozymes is specific for a different tissue (e.g., acid and alkaline phosphatases, 5′-NT, LD), and two enzymes that are not tissue specific but whose activities have major systemic effects: angiotensin-converting enzyme, vital for control of blood pressure, and AChE, which is critical in neuromuscular transmission.

ACID PHOSPHATASE (EC 3.1.3.2)

Biochemistry and Physiology

ACPs belong to the hydrolase class of enzymes (see Table 20-1) and occur as several isoenzymes with a common enzymatic function (the hydrolytic breakdown of phosphate monoesters). They all show optimal enzyme

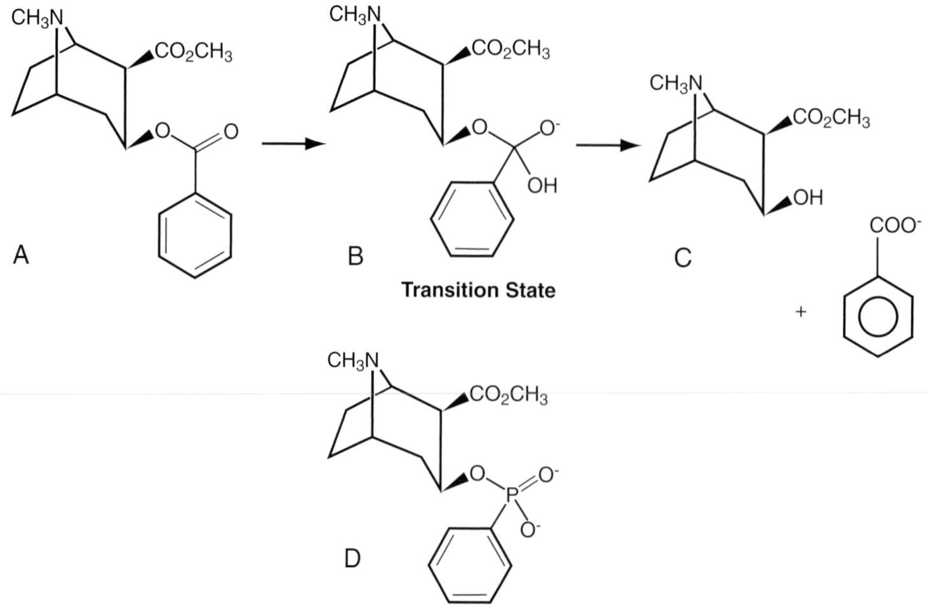

Figure 20-10 Hydrolysis of the benzoate ester moiety of cocaine **(A)** an ecgonine derivative, occurs via a tetrahedral intermediate **(B)** containing an oxyanion, and, presumably, a tetrahedral transition state resulting in the free –OH group of an ecgonine derivative shown in **C** and benzoic acid. This results in a cocaine derivative that is much less active. **D,** A nonhydrolyzable benzyl phosphonate ester transition state analogue which has a tetrahedral structure that likewise contains an oxyanion. An antibody that binds with high affinity to this analogue has been found to catalyze the hydrolysis of cocaine with a greatly enhanced rate over that for the noncatalyzed reaction.

TABLE 20-6
Relative Amounts of Enzymes in Various Organs (Relative to Serum)*

Tissue	AST†	ALT	LD	CK
Liver	7000	3000	7000	
Kidney	4500	1200	500	10
Brain				1700
Spleen	700	150		
Heart	8000	500	600	5000–8000
Skeletal muscle	5000	300	700	20,000–30,000
Smooth muscle				300–600
Red cells	15	7	500	0

ALT, Alanine aminotransferase; *AST,* aspartate transaminase; *CK,* creatine kinase; *IU,* international unit; *LD,* lactate dehydrogenase.
*Relative amount is calculated by dividing the activity of enzyme in tissue (in IU/kg of tissue) by the upper reference limit of plasma activity of the enzyme (in IU/L), assuming that 1 L of plasma = 1 kg. Because the data are derived from multiple publications, the relative amounts among enzymes may be approximate, but the relative amount of a single enzyme in each tissue is accurate.
†Total amount in cells; varying amounts represent mitochondrial isoenzyme, which reaches serum in only small amounts.

activity below a pH of 7.0. They possess some tissue specificity (greatest concentrations occur in prostate, liver, spleen, erythrocytes, and bone). The major forms are coded for by different genes and possess different molecular weights and structures, as well as differences in sensitivity to tartrate inhibition. Lysosomal, prostatic, erythrocyte, macrophage, and osteoclastic ACPs are five important types found in humans. Normally, concentrations in serum are low (Moss, 1999; Bull, 2002). The activity of erythrocyte ACP can be distinguished from that of the other ACP isoenzymes in that it is inhibited by 2% formaldehyde solution and 1 mM cupric sulfate solution. This is in contrast to the other isoenzymes, which are not inhibited by these agents. In addition, erythrocyte ACP is not inhibited by 20 mM tartrate solution, which does inhibit the other isoenzymes. It is important to note that tartrate-resistant acid phosphatase (TRAP) is present in certain chronic leukemias and some lymphomas, most notably in hairy cell leukemia, as described in the section on leukocytic disorders. In addition, a particular isoform of TRAP, called TRAP-5b, occurs predominantly in osteoclasts in bone marrow and is used as a marker for bone remodeling (Lu, 2006); it has also been proposed as a marker for metastatic cancer (e.g., breast cancer) in bone marrow (Chao, 2005).

Reference Ranges and Preanalytic Variation

Reference values depend on age, gender, and hormonal status (in women). Total and tartrate-resistant ACP values are high in children, rising through the first decade to peak at three to four times adult levels in adolescence, paralleling changes in ALP (Chen, 1979). In the late teen years, levels decline to adult values that are constant to approximately 80 years in both genders. Normal men and women up to about age 55 have the same reference ranges for ACP. In women, total and tartrate-resistant ACPs increase after menopause (Schiele, 1988) and increase with the use of depot medroxyprogesterone acetate in premenopausal women (Mukherjea, 1981).

The enzymatic activity of ACP is unstable at normal plasma pH; specimens must be acidified to prevent loss of ACP activity (Theodorsen, 1985). The effect of specimen pH is not as consistently seen with immunoassays for prostatic ACP; some studies have recommended routine use of acidification for all ACP specimens, but it is not clear that this is essential (Panteghini, 1992).

The half-life of prostatic ACP is about 1 to 3 hours (Wadstrom, 1985). Day-to-day variation in ACP is relatively high; average variation of the prostatic isoenzyme is 30% (Maatman, 1993), although it may be as high as 100% in patients with prostatic carcinoma (Brenckman, 1981), and bone isoenzyme variation averages about 35% (Panteghini, 1995).

Measurement

Assays for all phosphatases utilize the strategy that phosphate esters, which have no visible light absorbance, are hydrolyzed to inorganic phosphate and a strongly visible light-absorbing alcohol or alcohol anion. Total ACP is typically measured by its ability to cleave phosphate groups at an acid pH. Usually the test is utilized for the measurement of prostatic serum ACP in the diagnosis or monitoring of prostatic adenocarcinoma. A variety of substrates and conditions have been used to measure enzymatic activity with increased specificity; these include thymolphthalein monophosphate and α-naphthyl phosphate, both of which give rise to strongly absorbing products, α-naphthol and thymophthalein. *High bilirubin causes falsely low values for TRAP activity*, but not for total ACP (Alvarez, 1999).

Isozymes of ACP can be separated by electrophoresis (Moss, 1986); however, there is usually little interest in isoenzymes other than prostate and bone. Immunoassays (Bull, 2002) for both prostatic and bone isoenzymes of ACP have been developed; the former are widely available.

TABLE 20-7
Relative Levels of Enzymes, by Gender, Relative to Young Adult Males (1.0)*

Enzyme	Gender	AGE, YEARS 8	12	16	22	30	40	50	60
Aspartate aminotransferase	Male	0.75	0.86	0.82	1.00	1.16	1.26	1.21	1.11
	Female	0.73	0.80	0.69	0.89	0.89	1.01	0.77	0.96
Alanine aminotransferase	Male	1.14	1.09	0.89	1.00	1.03	1.11	1.06	0.83
	Female	0.11	0.89	0.83	0.75	0.75	0.75	0.72	0.83
Alkaline phosphatase	Male	3.61	4.76	4.48	1.52	1.00	1.00	0.95	0.95
	Female	0.14	4.10	2.52	0.81	0.86	0.76	1.00	1.38
γ-glutamyl transferase	Male	0.25	0.29	0.37	0.62	1.00	1.07	1.16	0.99
	Female	0.24	0.28	0.33	0.38	0.52	0.58	0.9	1.09

Data from Siest G, Henry J, Schiele F, Young DS. Interpretation of clinical laboratory tests: reference values and their biological variation. Foster City, Calif.: Biomedical Publications; 1985.
*Results expressed as upper reference limits as a fraction of the upper reference limits for healthy young males.

Causes of Abnormal Results

The main cause of increased ACP is prostate disease; with development of PSA as the major serum test for prostate (see Chapter 73), ACP has become less popular for use in prostate cancer, although, with the availability of newer immunochemical methods, its use in the diagnosis of prostate cancer is being reevaluated (Pontes, 2006). In early prostate cancer, the sensitivity of ACP is inferior to that of PSA (Burnett, 1992), although ACP, similar to PSA, is elevated in a significant percentage of patients with benign prostatic hyperplasia (Salo, 1990) or prostatic infarction, making ACP of little use for prostate cancer screening (Kaplan, 1985). Almost all patients with prostate cancer and elevated ACP have extracapsular extension or metastases (Salo, 1990; Burnett 1992), so that an elevated ACP may provide useful information in staging of patients. Occasionally, elevated prostatic ACP may be due to other causes. Urinary tract obstruction and acute urinary retention may cause elevated ACP (Collier, 1986). Extensive prostatic massage, prostatic inflammation, infarction/ischemia, and prostatic manipulations such as needle biopsy and cystoscopy may also cause a transient increase in serum ACP; testing should be done before any procedures are performed.

After surgical treatment of prostate cancer, ACP falls faster than PSA (Price, 1991), and levels should become undetectable after complete tumor resection. Because PSA is an androgen-dependent protein, androgen deprivation therapy decreases PSA production but has no effect on ACP (Price, 1991; Narayan, 1995), suggesting that ACP may be of use in monitoring patients treated in this fashion.

ACP has been used for many years in cases of suspected rape. Fluid collected from the vagina on a cotton swab will give a positive test for ACP if semen is present, provided a stabilizing fluid with an acidic pH is used (Ricci, 1982). Peak values are generally present in the first 12 hours, and values remain elevated for up to 4 days.

ALKALINE PHOSPHATASE (EC 3.1.3.1)

Biochemistry and Physiology

Similar to ACP , ALPs are a type of hydrolase (see Table 20-1). Discussion of ALP in the canalicular (biliary) system can be found in Chapter 21 on liver function. Alkaline phosphatases represent a family of enzymes coded for by different genes. Their physiologic role is not completely understood. The most abundant plasma ALP isoforms are coded for by a single gene on chromosome 1, producing the tissue-nonspecific isozyme found in kidney, liver, and bone. However, in different tissues, this **parent** isozyme is subjected to different posttranslational modifications, resulting in differences in their carbohydrate side chains. Two other genes on chromosome 2 code for ALP of placental and intestinal origin; another gene on chromosome 2 codes for the so-called germ cell or placental-like isoenzyme, which has some antigenic and physical similarities to the placental isozyme.

In cells, ALP is primarily bound to cell membranes, where it appears to be involved in cleavage of phosphate-containing compounds and may facilitate movement of substances across cell membranes. Hepatocytes produce ALP in the liver, where it is found attached to the canalicular surface of the cells (see Chapter 21). Osteoblasts produce bone ALP, which appears to be involved in cleavage of pyrophosphate, an inhibitor of bone mineralization. Intestinal epithelial cells produce intestinal ALP, which is released into the intestine following ingestion of fatty foods.

There appear to be different mechanisms for release of ALP from cells, leading to varying forms of ALP in plasma. With liver injury, ALP synthesis increases, but bile acids dissolve fragments of canalicular cell membranes with attached enzymes (including ALP, GGT, leucine aminopeptidase, and 5′-NT [Moss, 1997]). In normal serum, a single form (of liver or bone origin) of ALP is typically seen; however, with hepatobiliary disease, both the normal product and the membrane-attachment form (high molecular weight) bound to lipoproteins can be seen (Wolf, 1994). The intestinal isoenzyme of ALP is released in large amounts into duodenal fluid (Deng, 1992), and large amounts enter lymphatic fluid, draining the intestinal tract following a meal (Reynoso, 1971). However, much of the isoenzyme apparently becomes bound to red blood cell (RBC) ABO antigens (Bayer, 1980), so that only small amounts reach the plasma, except in individuals who possess both the secretor gene and a large amount of H substance (group O or B), where ALP may increase by up to 30 IU/L following a meal (Domar, 1993). ALP is also higher in individuals of group O or B than in A and AB individuals (Agbedana, 1996) because of differences in intestinal ALP levels (Domar, 1993). It is curious that placental ALP is also lower in pregnant women of groups A and AB (Ind, 1994).

The half-lives of isoenzymes of ALP differ significantly, so it is necessary to know the isoenzyme that is elevated before rate of clearance can be evaluated: intestine, minutes; bone, 1 day; liver, 3 days; and placenta, 7 days. Day-to-day variation in total ALP is 5% to 10%, although the bone isozyme shows 20% day-to-day variability.

Reference Ranges and Preanalytic Variation

Reference ranges for ALP are highly dependent on age and gender (Table 20-7). During childhood, levels gradually rise throughout the first decade, reaching peak values three to four times normal adult levels, and are higher in boys than in girls. The higher values in children are due to the bone isoenzyme. After a peak in the early teens, values gradually decrease to adult levels by the early 20s, and are similar in men and women until age 50. After menopause, the bone isoenzyme increases slightly in women, causing a rise in reference limits after age 50. Reference limits are 15% higher in African American men and 10% higher in African American women (Manolio, 1992). Pregnancy causes a two- to threefold increase in ALP, mainly due to the placental isoenzyme, but also because of an increase in bone isoenzyme (Valenzuela, 1987).

A number of other factors affect ALP levels as well. High body mass index is associated with a 10% average increase in ALP (Salvaggio, 1991). Oral contraceptives decrease ALP by an average of 20% (Schiele, 1988; Dufour, 1998a); fibric acid derivatives decrease total ALP by 25% and the liver isoenzyme by 40% (Day, 1993). Antiepileptic agents commonly cause increased total ALP, mainly because of increases in the liver isoenzyme; however, in some cases, the bone isozyme may also be elevated (Nijhawan, 1990). Smoking causes an average 10% increase in total ALP as the result of pulmonary production of placental-like ALP (Kallioniemi, 1987). Blood transfusion and cardiopulmonary bypass decrease alkaline phosphatase, often causing low levels (Kyd, 1998); this may be due to chelation of necessary cations by citrate.

Measurement

Although numerous methods are known, ALP activity is usually measured using *p*-nitrophenyl phosphate as the substrate at alkaline pH. Hydrolysis of this phosphate ester yields inorganic phosphate plus the highly colored (and, therefore, easily measured) *para*-nitrophenoxide anion. A variety of buffers are used to bind phosphate groups; this increases activity, because inorganic phosphate (as well as some other anions) inhibits ALP (competitive end-product inhibition). Zinc is a component of the enzyme, and magnesium and other cations activate the enzyme. Chelators present in collection tubes (such as EDTA, citrate, and oxalate) falsely lower ALP activity; in the case of EDTA, activity is often too low to measure. The activity of the enzyme increases slowly on storage because of loss of inhibitors, but specimens are relatively stable at 4° C for up to 1 week.

Isoforms

High-performance liquid chromatography (see Chapter 23) using weak anion-exchange columns has been able to separate at least six different isoforms of ALP in the sera of healthy individuals (Haarhaus, 2009). These are bone/intestinal (B/I), two bone isoforms, called B1 and B2, and three liver isoforms termed L1, L2, and L3. Recently, another bone isoform was isolated, termed B1x, that appears in the serum of dialysis patients (Swolin-Eide, 2006). These bone isoforms have been used to study low bone mineral disease (BMD) in patients with chronic kidney disease and have been found to rise in BMD of the hip, which is predominantly made up of trabecular bone. It is interesting to note that acid phosphatase TRAP-5b, discussed in the preceding section, was also found to be a marker for this condition (Haarhaus, 2009).

In addition, several other methods have been used to separate ALP isoenzymes. Inhibition by phenylalanine reduces reactivity of intestinal and placental isoenzymes, and levamisole inhibits bone and liver isoenzymes; inhibition assays are poorly reproducible and are seldom used. Heat fractionation has been used for many years to determine the source of an elevated total ALP. The most heat-stable isoenzyme is placental (and germ cell) ALP; the liver isoenzyme is moderately stable, and the bone isoenzyme is the most heat-labile. To achieve reliable results, use of standards of known composition and careful control of both temperature and time are essential. For these reasons, electrophoretic separation has been used for a number of years. Standard cellulose acetate and agarose gel electrophoresis cannot completely resolve bone and liver isoenzymes, making them unsuitable for other than qualitative studies. Because the difference between these isoenzymes is seen in their carbohydrate side chains, use of neuraminidase (to remove sialic acid) and wheat germ lectin (to bind to other isoenzymes) improves separation of bone and liver forms, allowing their quantitation. High-resolution electrophoresis using polyacrylamide gel and isoelectric focusing are capable of resolving multiple bands of ALP. Immunoassays for bone and placental isoenzymes of ALP are available commercially. Bone isoenzyme assays typically show some degree of cross-reactivity with the liver isoenzyme, and placental isoenzyme assays have varying cross-reactivity with the germ cell isoenzyme.

Causes of Abnormal Results

The most common causes of increased ALP are liver and bone disease. Hepatic causes of elevated ALP are discussed in greater detail in Chapter 21; disorders causing cholestasis more frequently cause elevation of ALP than do hepatocellular disorders. Increased osteoblastic activity in Paget's disease, osteosarcoma, tumor metastatic to bone, and metabolic bone disease are the most common causes of elevated bone isoenzyme. It appears that acid phosphatase TRAP-5b is associated with bone resorption conditions, and that the three major isoforms of bone ALP (B/I, B1, and B2) are associated with conditions involving bone deposition. Occasionally, patients will have elevations of both bone and liver isoenzymes, especially in metastatic carcinoma. Rarely, marked transient elevations of ALP occur, usually in children and often following trivial illness; these may reach several thousand IU/L and may persist for weeks to months before resolving (Steinherz, 1984).

Increases in intestinal ALP may occur in patients with intestinal infarction, inflammation, and ulceration. Increases in placenta-like isoenzymes, such as Regan and Nagao, are commonly found in patients with malignancies (ovary, cervix, lung, breast, colon, pancreas) and are due to ectopic production by the neoplasm.

As mentioned before, low ALP may occur transiently after blood transfusion or cardiopulmonary bypass. Prolonged, severely low levels of ALP occur in hypophosphatasia, a rare inherited disorder of bone metabolism (Whyte, 1996) as the result of missense mutations of tissue-nonspecific ALP (Haarhaus, 2009). Decreased ALP can also occur in zinc deficiency because zinc is a necessary cofactor for ALP activity, as well as other conditions.

Placental alkaline phosphatase (PLAP) is a useful tumor marker in serum and cerebrospinal fluid (CSF) for most germ cell tumors. In the latter case, CSF levels of PLAP are of diagnostic value in discerning whether a tumor in the pineal body is a pinealoma or a germ cell tumor. Because most germ cell tumors are radiosensitive, elevated CSF levels of PLAP suggest radiation treatment for this condition, allowing circumvention of surgical removal.

ANGIOTENSIN-CONVERTING ENZYME (EC 3.4.15.1)

Biochemistry and Physiology

ACE, also known as kininase II and peptidyl-dipeptidase A, belongs to the hydrolase class of enzymes (see Table 20-1) and is usually involved in the hydrolysis of peptide bonds at a free C-terminus, releasing the dipeptide His-Leu in the reaction. However, it may also act as an endopeptidase or an aminopeptidase. Its chief function is to cleave the His-Leu sequence from a decapeptide called angiotensin 1, whose sequence is Asp-Arg-Val-Tyr-Ile-His-Pro-Phe-His-Leu. This peptide, in turn, is cleaved from an α 2-macroglobulin called angiotensinogen, produced predominantly in the liver. Angiotensin I travels to the lungs, where ACE cleaves its carboxyl-terminal His-Leu peptide to produce angiotensin 2. The latter peptide has two major activities: It is a potent vasoconstrictor in arterioles, and it induces the secretion of aldosterone from the zona glomerulosa of the adrenals. As discussed in both Chapters 8 and 24, aldosterone induces sodium retention in the collecting ducts in the kidneys, resulting in conservation of water. This action results in an increase in vascular volume. Therefore, by increasing arteriolar resistance via vasoconstriction and by increasing vascular volume, thereby increasing flow, angiotensin 2 induces higher arteriolar pressures. The renin-angiotensin system is summarized below:

$$\text{Angiotensinogen} \xrightarrow{\text{Renin}} \text{Angiotensin 1} \xrightarrow{\text{ACE}} \text{Angiotensin 2} \rightarrow \text{Vasoconstriction}$$
$$\downarrow$$
$$\text{Aldosterone} \rightarrow \text{Renal Na retention} \qquad \textbf{(20-38)}$$

It is interesting to note that ACE also inactivates bradykinin (in the kallikrein-kinin system) by cleaving a dipeptide from its carboxyl terminus. Although the catalytic action of ACE is somewhat nonspecific in vitro, only angiotensin 1, bradykinin, and the hemoregulatory peptide Ac-DSKP are definite in vivo substrates (Macours, 2004). Because angiotensin 2 induces increased blood pressure, and because it is produced uniquely by the activity of ACE, the latter enzyme is a major target of competitively inhibiting drugs in the treatment of hypertension.

ACE consists of a single polypeptide chain, with two homologous, zinc-binding catalytic sites (ACE is a zinc-metalloprotease). Enzyme activity is lost if zinc is bound to a chelating agent, such as EDTA, or is replaced by a different cation. It is important to note that ACE, similar to HIV protease as discussed earlier, is an aspartic acid protease, that is, two Asp residues are involved in catalysis at each active site. In cells, ACE is a transmembrane protein with a large amino-terminal extracellular domain, a very short hydrophobic transmembrane domain, and a small intracellular carboxyl-terminal domain; the cell-bound molecule is referred to as tissue ACE. The two catalytic sites are present in the extracellular domain: one near the amino terminus and one nearer the carboxyl terminus. The carboxyl-terminal active site is thought to harbor the predominant angiotensin 1 hydrolytic activity, and the amino-terminal active site has activity against bradykinin. Proteolytic cleavage releases the functional enzyme from the cell membrane into the extracellular environment, producing circulating ACE.

The majority of ACE is tissue bound (>90%), with much lower levels circulating in plasma. ACE is found predominantly in endothelial cell membranes throughout the body. The lungs and the testes are particularly rich in ACE. Information on the molecular biology and structure of ACE is available (Dzau, 2002; Macours, 2004). There appear to be two distinct forms of ACE: a somatic form (sACE) and a smaller isoform found in testes (tACE). A single gene encodes both forms by utilizing alternative promoters. sACE is found in many tissues and contains two active sites (as described previously); tACE contains only the C-terminal active site and is exclusively found in testes. Although both active sites of sACE require zinc ion, their biochemical properties are not identical (Dzau, 2002; Macours, 2004).

The Design of ACE Inhibitors

As mentioned earlier, ACE is a critical target for inhibitory drugs designed to lower blood pressure. Because ACE and HIV protease are Asp proteases, many of the considerations used for the design of these inhibitors were subsequently used in the design of HIV protease inhibitors, as discussed earlier. It was known that the nonapeptide teprotide, from the snake *Bothrops jararaca* whose sequence is Glu-Trp-Pro-Arg-Pro-Gln-Ile-Pro-Pro, was a potent antihypertensive that acted by competitively inhibiting ACE (Crantz, 1980). This was the first effective therapeutic ACE inhibitor, but it could not be given orally because of its hydrolysis in the stomach and the gut. Because it was known that there was a critical positively charged Arg residue in the active site, in addition to the positively charged Zn ion, and that the enzyme had a high affinity for Phe and Pro residues, the inhibitor succinyl proline was developed. The affinity of this inhibitor was greatly enhanced if the carboxylate of the succinic acid moiety was replaced with a thiol that had a high affinity for the bound Zn ions. This resulted in the synthesis of 3-mercapto-2-methylpropanoyl-L-proline, also called captopril, a highly effective agent that, however, had several undesirable side effects such as skin rash and loss of taste (Cushman, 1991). In addition, Phe-containing tripeptides that contained carboxylate groups were synthesized, allowing for tight binding to the active site and to Zn concurrently (i.e., enalapril and lisinopril—both effective agents). In addition, transition state analog inhibitors, such as the ones discussed for HIV protease, have been developed (Dive, 2004; Gerogiadis, 2004; Redelinghuys, 2006). Several contain modified Phe as seen in the HIV protease inhibitors, except that they also contain nonhydrolyzable tetrahedral phosphinic acid in place of the normally occurring backbone carbonyl group. Several of these inhibitors inhibit the carboxyl-terminal active site preferentially, making them good antihypertensive agents, because it is this active site that predominantly hydrolyzes angiotensin 1. At the same time, considerable bradykinin hydrolytic activity still occurs in the amino-terminal active site; this is considered desirable in that bradykinin itself induces vasodilatation and angioedema and can compound the lowering of blood pressure so as to induce hypotension, an undesirable side effect.

Reference Ranges and Preanalytic Variation

ACE activity is higher in children than in adults; during adolescence, values are higher in boys than in girls (Beneteau-Burnat, 1990), gradually falling to adult levels by 18 years. Men and women have the same values, although not all studies show this pattern. ACE appears to be cleared by the liver; the half-life in plasma is roughly 48 hours. Average day-to-day variation is less than 10%, with no diurnal variation (Thompson, 1986).

A number of other factors affect ACE levels. Smokers have ACE activities about 30% lower than in nonsmokers or former smokers who have stopped smoking for at least 10 years (Ninomiya, 1987). Thyroid hormone stimulates ACE synthesis. Postmenopausal estrogen replacement causes a 20% fall in ACE activity in serum (Proudler, 1995). Rare families lack an endogenous inhibitor of ACE activity and, consequently, have markedly elevated serum ACE levels (Luisetti, 1990).

Measurement

ACE is typically measured by its ability to cleave synthetic peptides, releasing hippuric acid (Hip) or other indicator molecules as in the following reaction:

$$\text{Hip-L-His-L-Leu} + H_2O \rightarrow \text{Hip} + \text{L-His-L-Leu} \quad \textbf{(20-39)}$$

Hip is then extracted, and its absorption is measured at 228 nm. A modification of the assay is required in CSF samples because of their much lower ACE activity (Oksanen, 1985).

Causes of Abnormal Results

The most common reason for ordering ACE levels involves the diagnosis and monitoring of sarcoidosis. In general, ACE levels are directly related to the number of organs affected (Muthuswamy, 1987) and the activity of granulomas; mature granulomas tend to produce less ACE than developing ones (Mimori, 1998). In sarcoidosis, a general correlation has been noted between disease activity and ACE levels (Gupta, 1992); as disease progresses to fibrosis, ACE levels decline. ACE is more likely to be elevated with pulmonary involvement than with purely hilar adenopathy. ACE is also increased in many other granulomatous diseases, although not as frequently as in sarcoidosis. Although most individuals with sarcoidosis have elevated ACE, the frequency of elevation of other granulomatous disorders is 10% (Studdy, 1978). For this reason, ACE is not usually considered a diagnostic test, although it may be helpful in patients with primarily ocular involvement, in whom biopsy cannot be readily performed (Power, 1995).

ACE is frequently elevated in a number of other disorders, including multiple sclerosis (Constantinescu, 1997), Addison's disease (Falezza, 1985), hyperthyroidism (Reiners, 1988), diabetes mellitus (Schernthaner, 1984), alcoholic hepatitis (Borowsky, 1982), peptic ulcer (D'Onofrio, 1984), and nephrotic syndrome (Huskic, 1996), and at various stages in patients with bacterial (Kerttula, 1986) or *Pneumocystis* pneumonitis (Singer, 1989). Other pulmonary disorders with a significantly increased ACE are emphysema, asthma, small cell carcinoma, and squamous cell carcinoma (Ucar, 1997). In chronic renal failure, it is increased only in those on hemodialysis and rises during the course of a dialysis procedure (Docci, 1988); it is decreased in those with chronic renal failure who are not on dialysis (Le Treut, 1983). In HIV infection, the frequency and degree of elevation correlate with stage of disease (Ouellette, 1992). Decreased ACE levels are seen in various malignancies (Romer, 1980; Schweisfurth 1985), in chronic liver disease (Sakata, 1991), in anorexia nervosa (Matsubayashi, 1988), and in hypothyroidism (Reiners, 1988).

Use of CSF ACE levels for diagnosis and monitoring of neurosarcoidosis has been criticized (Dale, 1999). A number of other diseases cause elevated CSF ACE, among them viral encephalitis, multiple sclerosis, and central nervous system (CNS) syphilis (Schweisfurth, 1987).

In all cases of assays for ACE, attention should be paid to the possible use of ACE inhibitors in hypertensive patients. Because virtually all ACE inhibitors are competitive inhibitors, if competitive inhibition is suspected, use of higher concentrations of Hip-His-Leu substrate in the ACE assay can be used to overcome the inhibition. Alternatively, the sample can be diluted to remove the effect of the inhibitor. Assays for the levels of ACE inhibitors such as captopril have been developed (Prior, 2007).

ACETYLCHOLINESTERASE (EC 3.1.1.7) AND BUTYRYLCHOLINESTERASE (EC 3.1.1.8)

Biochemistry and Physiology

AChE (true cholinesterase or choline esterase I) and PChE (or choline esterase II) are carboxylic ester hydrolases (class 3; see Table 20-1) that have different specificities (Abdallah, 2007). AChE catalyzes the following reaction:

$$\text{Acetylcholine} + H_2O \rightarrow \text{Choline} + \text{Acetate} \quad \textbf{(20-40)}$$

PChE catalyzes this reaction:

$$\text{Acylcholine} + H_2O \rightarrow \text{Choline} + \text{Carboxylate} \quad \textbf{(20-41)}$$

AChE and PChE are two different enzymes produced by different tissues that are able to cleave acetylcholine, one of the body's major neurotransmitters. True cholinesterase has acetylcholine (ACh) as its primary natural substrate and is also inhibited by it at approximately 10^{-2} mole/L; it is found in high activity in the CNS, RBCs, lung, and spleen. ACh is a primary neurotransmitter at various sites in the CNS, and AChE rapidly hydrolyzes ACh, producing rapid termination of neurotransmission. AChE is not normally found in amniotic fluid.

The normal function of the enzyme found in serum, PChE (also called acetylcholine acylhydrolase), is not known, but it is important in the cleavage of acetylcholine antagonists such as succinylcholine and mivacurium, muscle relaxants used during surgery. Serum PChE is not subject to substrate inhibition by high levels of ACh. PChE production occurs primarily in the liver, although other tissues, such as myocardium and pancreas, can also produce it. Although both enzymes hydrolyze acetylcholine, AChE, but not PChE, hydrolyzes acetyl-β-methylcholine; conversely, PChE, but not AChE, hydrolyzes butyryl- and benzoylcholine.

A number of genetic variants of PChE have reduced affinity (higher K_M) for acetylcholine, as well as for competitive inhibitors such as dibucaine and fluoride, when compared with the common U (usual) form; these are termed A (for atypical), F (for fluoride resistant), and S (for silent). The S variant actually represents a number of mutations that may cause absence of enzymatic activity or absence of PChE synthesis. Heterozygous deficiency is found in about 4% of the population, and homozygous deficiency affects 0.3% to 0.5% of individuals. These variants cause decreased (or, in the case of the *S* variant, absent) PChE activity when present in homozygous or mixed heterozygous forms (AA, AF, AS, FF, FS, SS). Because of the broad range of normal values, reduced PChE activity is not usually found in U form heterozygotes.

Another way to detect such variants is to measure the percent of enzyme activity remaining after in vitro incubation of serum enzyme with dibucaine or fluoride (termed dibucaine number, or DN, and fluoride number, respectively). As mentioned previously, increased K_M of variants produces less effective catalysis than normal; decreased affinity thus exists for dibucaine and fluoride, making these variants more resistant to inhibition than normal. In general, dibucaine inhibits U plasma cholinesterase activity by approximately 70% to 90%. Variant cholinesterase activity is more resistant to inhibition, such that heterozygote activity is inhibited by approximately 50% to 70%, and homozygous variant activity is inhibited by approximately 10% to 30%. The DN will then reflect percentage inhibition of enzyme activity and will give a rough measure of the enzyme's activity; this in turn will indicate the presence or the absence of a variant form of the enzyme. The DN is calculated using the formula in Equation 20-42. For example, the UU form may show 85% inhibition, or 15% remaining activity, and may yield a DN of 85.

$$\text{Dibucaine (fluoride) number} = 100\text{X}$$
$$(1 - \text{Enzyme activity with inhibitor/Enzyme activity without inhibitor}) \quad \textbf{(20-42)}$$

Newer molecular biology techniques, such as the use of polymerase chain amplification with separation of the reaction products by gel electrophoresis (Cerf, 2002), allow much more accurate identification of variants, as compared with traditional biochemical analysis.

Pseudocholinesterase as an Antixenobiotic Enzyme

In addition to its involvement in the metabolism of anticholinergic drugs, PChE has been found to catalyze the debenzoylation of cocaine (Duysen, 2008; Yang, 2009) and the hydrolysis of procaine (Duysen, 2008). Although catalysis by PChE of debenzoylation of cocaine is inefficient, absence of this enzyme or mutations that reduce its activity, discussed in the preceding section, can prolong and exacerbate the negative effects of cocaine such as its cardiotoxicity (Duyson, 2008). It is interesting to note that recently, based on transition state theory analysis and molecular modeling of this enzyme bound to cocaine, site-specific mutagenesis of the gene encoding this enzyme has resulted in a form of PChE that efficiently debenzoylates cocaine (Yang, 2009). Humanized forms of this engineered enzyme may prove to have significant therapeutic value.

Reference Ranges and Preanalytic Variation

PChE values are low in infants and gradually rise to adult levels by 4 months of age (Karlsen, 1981). Values in men do not change after this point until age 45; in women, they fall by about 10% at menarche and increase by 15% after menopause. A recent study (Abou-Hatab, 2001) found no significant correlation between older patient age and changes in plasma enzyme activities of AChE and PChE; healthy young and older individuals (study age range, 18–85 years) showed similar enzyme activities. Values in men are about 15% to 20% higher than in women until age 45, when values in women become equal. Oral contraceptives cause a decrease of about 15% in PChE activity (Lepage, 1985). About a fourfold range of values is seen in normal individuals. Increased body mass index is associated with an increase in PChE, and low protein intake leads to decreased PChE.

The half-life of PChE has been estimated at between 2 and 10 days. Average day-to-day variation is about 7% (Moses, 1986)—much smaller than that for most other enzymes.

Measurement

Enzyme activity is typically measured using an acylthiocholine ester as a substrate; released thiocholine reacts with Ellman's reagent (dithiobisnitrobenzoic acid), releasing 5-mercapto-2-nitrobenzoic acid, which is measured spectrophotometrically. Pseudocholinesterase activity is measured in serum, and AChE activity is measured in a hemolysate of washed RBCs. AChE may also be determined in amniotic fluid by gel electrophoresis. To measure dibucaine or fluoride numbers, serum is incubated with dibucaine (30 µmol/L) or fluoride (4 mmol/L) in the assay reaction mixture.

Causes of Abnormal Results

The main reasons for measuring PChE are (1) to monitor exposure to cholinesterase inhibitors, (2) for use as a liver function test, or (3) for diagnosis of genetic variants. Organophosphate insecticides are irreversible inhibitors of both AChE and PChE, although typically PChE plasma activity falls before AChE activity in RBCs with poisoning (Areekul, 1981). Because of small individual variation and large interindividual variation in PChE values, it is advisable to obtain baseline values for PChE before individuals are exposed to organophosphates (Trundle, 1988). A decrease of 40% from baseline is needed before symptoms develop, and severe symptoms typically occur with falls in values greater than 80%; thus, symptoms often occur with PChE values within the reference range. If no baseline values are present, serial determinations are helpful. In one study, 90% of symptomatic organophosphate poisonings were associated with PChE values within the reference range, and postexposure levels showed a rise, confirming toxicity (Coye, 1987). Although PChE reflects acute toxicity, AChE (RBCs) better reflects chronic exposure.

In contrast to other hepatocyte enzymes, PChE production by the liver appears to reflect synthetic function rather than hepatocyte injury. Levels of PChE are decreased in acute hepatitis, cirrhosis, and carcinoma metastatic to liver. PChE is decreased in malnutrition but is normal or increased in nephrotic syndrome. As is the case when monitoring organophosphate exposure, changes in values compared with baseline are more useful than single values, limiting the diagnostic usefulness of PChE as a nutritional or liver injury monitor.

The other common use of PChE measurements is in recognizing the presence of genetic variants. Most commonly, such testing involves family members of individuals who have prolonged apnea after use of succinylcholine or mivacurium (neuromuscular blocking agents/muscle relaxants) during anesthesia. Testing typically involves both total PChE and determination of fluoride and dibucaine numbers to recognize homozygous or compound heterozygous variants that put an individual at risk from exposure to cholinesterase inhibitors. Patients at risk (with variant cholinesterase forms) may more slowly hydrolyze the neuromuscular blocking agent, unexpectedly increasing the duration of respiratory muscle relaxation and prolonging apnea. This is in contrast to the usual rapid drug hydrolysis seen with the U forms, leading to rapid recovery of the patient.

As mentioned previously, measurement of RBC AChE is useful in organophosphate exposure and poisoning. In addition, qualitative analysis of AChE in amniotic fluid may be useful in the diagnosis of neural tube defects, especially in high-risk groups (Muller, 2003). AChE can be identified in amniotic fluid from pregnancies with neural tube defects, as well as some other types of birth defects. AChE is absent in amniotic fluid from normal pregnancies.

LACTATE DEHYDROGENASE (EC 1.1.1.27)

Biochemistry and Physiology

LD is a class 1 enzyme (oxidoreductase; see Table 20-1) that acts on a CH–OH group of donors with NAD^+ as acceptor and catalyzes the transfer of hydrogen in the form of a hydride ion:

$$\text{(L)-Lactate} + \text{NAD}^+ \leftrightarrow \text{Pyruvate} + \text{NADH} + \text{H}^+ \quad \textbf{(20-43)}$$

The enzyme is also capable of oxidizing other (L)-2-hydroxymonocarboxylic acids.

LD is a zinc-containing enzyme that is part of the glycolytic pathway; it is found in the cytoplasm of all cells and tissues in the body. LD is a tetramer of two active subunits: H and M with a molecular weight of 134 kDa. Combinations of subunits produce five isoenzymes ranging from LD_1 (HHHH) to LD_5 (MMMM); the intermediate isoenzymes contain differing combinations of H and M subunits (LD_2, HHHM; LD_3, HHMM; LD_4, HMMM). Inherited forms of deficiency of H (Joukyuu, 1989) and M (Kanno, 1980), subunits of LD, are associated with low LD levels in plasma and only one isoenzyme on electrophoresis. Another form of LD composed of four C subunits is found in spermatozoa and in semen but has never been detected in serum, even in individuals with seminoma (Vogelzang, 1982). Rarely, another band detected in electrophoresis and termed **LD_6** can be seen; this probably represents alcohol dehydrogenase, which can also metabolize lactate (Kato, 1984). LD_1 and LD_2 have lower K_Ms (higher affinities) for lactate than for pyruvate, and the reverse is true for LD_4 and LD_5.

The tissue distribution of LD varies primarily in its isoenzyme composition, not in its content of LD (see Table 20-6). It is important to note that LD_1 and LD_2 are expressed at high levels in myocardial tissue and in erythrocytes and at much lower levels in tissues such as liver and muscle; the reverse is true for LD_4 and LD_5. In myocardial damage, the predominant isozymes that become elevated in serum are LD_1 and LD_2; in liver

TABLE 20-8
Relative Percentage of LD Isoenzymes in Various Tissues

Tissue	LD_1	LD_2	LD_3	LD_4	LD_5
Serum	25	35	20	15	5
Heart	45	40	10	5	0
Red cells	40	35	15	10	0
Renal cortex	35	30	25	20	0
Lung	10	15	40	30	5
Skeletal muscle	0	0	10	30	60
Liver	0	5	10	15	70

LD, Lactate dehydrogenase.

or skeletal muscle disease, the LD_4 and LD_5 isozymes become elevated predominantly in serum. In contrast to enzymes such as AST, ALT, and CK, which show marked variation in enzyme activity between tissues, the range in values for LD is only about 1.5-fold between those with the highest amounts (such as liver) and those with lower amounts (such as kidney); most tissues have LD activities that are 500 to 1000 times greater in tissue than those found in normal serum (see Table 20-6). Thus, significant elevation of plasma levels occurs with a small amount of tissue damage/breakdown. The tissue distribution of LD isoenzymes is shown in Table 20-8. The specific composition of elevated isoenzyme levels found in plasma will reflect tissue origin. In plasma, the majority of LD comes from breakdown of erythrocytes and platelets, with varying contributions from other organs. LD is apparently eliminated in bile, as injection of radiolabeled LD results in radioactivity in the gallbladder and small intestine (Smith, 1988).

Reference Ranges and Preanalytic Variation

LD values are highest in newborns and infants; values do not change with age in adults, and there is no gender difference. Persons over age 65 tend to have slightly higher values. Exercise causes, at most, slight increases in total LD; even strenuous exercise causes only a 25% rise in average values (Tanada, 1993). Even trace to slight hemolysis invalidates LD and LD isoenzyme analyses. Contact with the clot increases LD, and physical agitation of specimens, as occurs in most pneumatic tube systems, tends to cause some hemolysis and increased LD. Hemolysis affects both total LD and the LD_1/LD_2 ratio. Exercise has little effect on LD or its isoenzymes. Extreme exercise can cause LD_1 to become greater than LD_2. Total LD increases transiently after blood transfusion but returns to baseline within 24 hours (Wiesen, 1998). Delayed separation of red cells from serum does not affect LD values for 1 to 2 days. Few drugs directly affect LD activity, but granulocyte-macrophage colony-stimulating factor appears to increase LD in parallel to the increase in white blood cell (WBC) count (Sarris, 1995).

The half-life of LD isoenzymes varies greatly, from approximately 4 to 4 ½ days for LD_1 to 4 to 6 hours for LD_5. Day-to-day variation of LD is only 5% to 10%.

Measurement

LD activity can be measured using either the forward (lactate-to-pyruvate) or the reverse (pyruvate-to-lactate) direction of the reaction. A vast majority of laboratories use the forward reaction; the reverse reaction, predominantly used in the dry slide method for LD, produces activities that have good correlation with the forward reaction but at measured activities approximately threefold higher. This underscores the point made earlier—if total activity units are reported, it is vital to list the substrate and to provide the reference range for that substrate.

The reverse (pyruvate-to-lactate) reaction is used in a few laboratories currently because of faster reaction kinetics, the less costly cofactor (NADH) needed, and the smaller specimen volume requirement. Disadvantages of the pyruvate-to-lactate reaction include early loss of linearity of reaction kinetics, the effect of potent LD inhibitors in some NADH preparations, and use of suboptimal concentrations of pyruvate because of substrate inhibition. Also, lactate is a more specific substrate for this enzyme; pyruvate is less specific and serves as a substrate for such enzymes as pyruvate dehydrogenase.

Electrophoretic separation of LD isoenzymes is typically used when quantitation of different isoenzymes is required; agarose gel is most commonly used. Quantitation usually uses the forward reaction, allowing detection of fluorescent NADH or a reduced formazan dye in a colorimetric development step. The electrophoretic support and developing agent affect the results, and the reference ranges for the different methods are not the same. Inhibition methods for LD_1 are also available but allow quantitation only of this isoenzyme; results are often expressed as the ratio of LD_1 to total LD. Hydroxybutyrate is preferentially cleaved by the LD_1 isoenzyme; until the early 1970s, measurement of **hydroxybutyrate dehydrogenase** was used as a diagnostic test for myocardial infarction.

Serum LD is, on average, 30 IU/L higher than plasma LD, owing to release of LD from platelets. With prolonged incubation of plasma containing platelets (separated at <1200 *g* centrifugation), LD can leak from damaged platelets, increasing plasma LD as well (Hollaar, 1979). LD is not stable on storage at 4° C because of cold lability of LD_5. Specimens can be stored for up to 24 hours at room temperature with little change. Three days of storage at room temperature decreases total LD by about 20%, increases apparent LD_1 by 20%, and decreases apparent LD_5 by 18%. If specimens are frozen, LD_5 decreases significantly and the isoenzyme pattern shifts with an artifactual increase in LD_1 and decrease in LD_5. Serum should not be frozen for assay of LD or for its isoenzymes.

Causes of Abnormal Results

LD is a highly nonspecific test; an abnormal value is not specific for damage to any particular organ. Relative amounts of LD, AST, and ALT (along with CK) may provide clues to the source of LD elevation. If LD is markedly elevated, but AST, ALT, and CK are normal or minimally increased, this suggests damage to cells such as red or white blood cells, kidney, lung, lymph nodes, or tumors. Increases in both CK and LD, with greater increases in AST than ALT, occur with cardiac or skeletal muscle injury. Increases in LD occur in liver disease, and LD can be elevated in hepatitis, although these increases by themselves are not specific to liver injury (Cassidy, 1994). Recently, it was found that in fulminant hepatic failure (see Chapters 8 and 21), the serum levels of ALT and LD both increase such that LD increases more rapidly initially. An ALT-LD index has been computed in these patients and was found to be a reliable predictor of survival in patients with this condition (Kotoh, 2008). As discussed in Chapters 8 and 21, serum elevations of LD and ALP frequently occur in space-occupying lesions of the liver; most cases are identified as metastatic carcinoma or primary hepatocellular carcinoma.

In many conditions, such as shock and metastatic carcinoma, LD is increased because of damage to multiple organs, so that mixed patterns can be seen. Marked elevations of LD (>5 to 10 times normal) are seen in megaloblastic anemia, hemolytic anemias, advanced malignancies (particularly lymphoma and leukemia), sepsis or other causes of shock, and cardiopulmonary arrest. LD is often moderately elevated in *Pneumocystis carinii* pneumonia (Smith, 1988) but is often normal in most other forms of pneumonia (Rotenberg, 1988). Although LD is highly sensitive (so that normal values make the diagnosis unlikely) (Quist, 1995), the predictive value of LD is not adequate to establish a diagnosis in an HIV patient (Grover, 1992). In patients with biliary pancreatitis (inflammation due to gallstones impacted in the bile duct), the LD/AST ratio is elevated, which appears to indicate the presence of pancreatic necrosis (Isogai, 1998). Note that 10% to 20% of patients with biliary pancreatitis may present with normal liver function tests (Dholakia, 2004).

In cases where the cause of elevated LD cannot be determined by other means, LD isoenzymes may be useful in determining the source of injury. In normal serum, the LD isoenzymes, in decreasing order of activity, are 2 > 1 > 3 > 4 > 5. In germ cell tumors (particularly seminoma and dysgerminoma), LD_1 is increased and can serve as a tumor marker (von Eyben, 2000, 2001).

As noted in Chapter 18 on cardiac function, LD increases in serum over about a 36-hour period, during which time the LD_1/LD_2 ratio, which is normally less than 1, increases to values of 1 or above, the so-called flipped ratio. This confirmed the diagnosis of myocardial infarction (MI) but could not be used to make acute diagnoses of MI because of the prolonged time (36 hours) required for the flipped ratio to develop. As discussed in Chapter 18, better biomarkers, specifically the inhibitory subunit of troponin, are available for the acute diagnosis of MI and for confirmation of the diagnosis (serum troponin levels remain elevated for longer than 1 week after the acute event). Also, hemolytic anemia, megaloblastic anemia, and renal cortical diseases such as renal infarcts and renal cell carcinoma cause increases in LD_1 and, often, a flipped LD_1/LD_2 ratio. In tumors of WBCs (leukemia, lymphoma, multiple myeloma) LD_3 and often LD_4 are typically increased, whereas the relative amounts of LD_1 and LD_2

are decreased (Ricerca, 1988; Copur, 1989; Pandit 1990). Pulmonary disease can produce a similar pattern. Increases in LD_5 and sometimes LD_4 are typically seen with skeletal muscle injury or with ischemic or toxic hepatic injury. The presence of LD_6 is associated with a poor prognosis (Ketchum, 1984). An isomorphic pattern, in which total LD is increased but isoenzymes are present in normal proportions, and a **tombstone** pattern, seen when the relative amount of each isoenzyme is roughly the same, are typically noted in persons with diffuse tissue damage, often accompanied by shock or hypoxemia.

5′-NUCLEOTIDASE (EC 3.1.3.5)

Biochemistry and Physiology

5′-NT is a phosphoric monoester hydrolase (class 3 enzyme; see Table 20-1), also known as 5′-ribonucleotide phosphohydrolase, which catalyzes the following reaction:

$$\text{5′-Ribonucleotide} + H_2O \rightarrow \text{Ribonucleoside} + \text{Phosphate} \quad \textbf{(20-44)}$$

It is a cytoplasmic membrane–bound phosphatase with a wide specificity for 5′-ribonucleotides and a molecular weight of about 70 kDa. It acts only on nucleotides (such as adenosine 5′-monophosphate and guanosine 5′-monophosphate) and is believed to function in extracellular adenosine production, nutrient absorption, and cell proliferation. 5′-NT is a metalloprotein, and zinc is believed to be an integral part of the enzyme. It is widely distributed in the body, predominantly attached to cell membranes (similar to ALP and GGT). Plasma 5′-NT is derived predominantly from the liver. A detailed review of 5′-NT is available (Sunderman, 1990).

Reference Ranges and Preanalytic Variation

5′-NT is normally present at low activities in children, rises in adolescence, and plateaus until age 40, when levels increase significantly (Moses, 1986); reference values are independent of gender and race. A slight increase in 5′-NT is seen during the second and third trimesters of pregnancy (Bacq, 1996). Similar to ALP and GGT, antiepileptic drugs can increase 5′-NT activity; however, values are usually less than twice the reference limits, and less than 25% of those taking such agents show elevated 5′-NT activity (Fortman, 1985).

Measurement

Measurement of 5′-NT is difficult because other phosphatases, notably ALP, are capable of cleaving the substrate used to measure the lower activity of 5′-NT present in the sample. Approaches usually utilize large quantities of other, nonnucleoside substrates to "competitively inhibit" ALP (although they are actually undergoing reactions catalyzed by ALP, they prevent ALP from acting on nucleotide phosphates). Although it would be simplest to measure generated phosphate, this cannot be done because cleavage of other phosphates by ALP would produce incorrect results. Therefore, measurement of the nucleoside released by the action of 5′-NT is required. Most chelating agents such as EDTA inhibit enzyme activity, presumably by making zinc unavailable.

Causes of Abnormal Results

Similar to GGT, 5′-NT is most commonly used to determine whether the source of an elevated ALP is liver or bone. Although 5′-NT is more commonly elevated in cholestatic disorders, acute hepatitis causes an increase in 5′-NT synthesis by the liver and a slight elevation in 5′-NT in plasma (Fukano, 1990). 5′-NT is increased in ovarian carcinoma (Chatterjee, 1981) and in rheumatoid arthritis, where levels correlate with extent of inflammation as reflected by erythrocyte sedimentation rate (Johnson, 1999). Sapey et al (2000) prospectively studied ALP, GGT, and 5′-NT in 80 cholestatic patients, correlating intrahepatic (i.e., secondary to intrahepatic parenchymal disease) and extrahepatic (i.e., secondary to biliary tree obstruction) causes with enzyme changes. They found markedly increased levels with extrahepatic causes (compared with intrahepatic disease) and noted that elevations in GGT and 5′-NT levels were independently linked to cause. The GGT/5′-NT ratio differed significantly between the two groups, with a ratio <1.9 highly suggestive of (but insensitive to) intrahepatic disease (Sapey, 2000).

SKELETAL MUSCLE INJURY: CREATINE PHOSPHOKINASE

The basic assay for this enzyme was discussed earlier (see Equations 20-15 to 20-17). This enzyme has two major isoenzymes, M and B, each of which has the same activity. CK is composed of three types of dimers: MM (mainly in skeletal muscle), MB (found mainly in cardiac tissue), and BB (found predominantly in brain and intestine). As discussed at length in Chapter 18, because CK-MB is found mainly in myocardial tissue, CK-MB is used as a serodiagnostic test for MI. In this section, CK is discussed as a biomarker for skeletal muscle injury.

Skeletal muscle injury can occur from a variety of sources. Direct trauma, as occurs with physical injury (including contact sports), surgery, strenuous exercise, and intramuscular injection, are common causes of mild elevations of CK (up to about five to six times reference limits). In these situations, CK typically increases rapidly and then falls quickly, returning to baseline with a half-life of approximately 24 hours. An important clinical disorder associated with acute muscle injury is neuroleptic malignant syndrome, a rare complication of treatment with phenothiazines or other psychotropic agents. Typically, affected individuals present with muscle rigidity, fever, and elevated WBC counts; CK is considered a diagnostic test for this disorder. Prompt recognition and treatment are necessary to prevent death from this syndrome; discontinuation of medications and use of the muscle-stabilizing agent dantrolene are the cornerstones of treatment (Pelonero, 1998).

Chronic damage to muscle causes more persistent elevation of CK, which may be mild or more extensive. The broad range of normal values and the preanalytic variation seen in total CK values can hamper recognition of mild, ongoing muscle injury. Generally, persistent elevation above the reference limits for an appropriate comparison group despite cessation of any other factors known to affect CK is needed to diagnose muscle injury in asymptomatic individuals. Common causes of chronic muscle injury include medications (particularly 3-hydroxy-3-methylglutaryl-coenzyme A reductase inhibitors and glucocorticoids), congenital myopathies (such as Duchenne's muscular dystrophy), inflammatory disorders (such as polymyositis and dermatomyositis), hypothyroidism, and alcohol abuse. In chronic myopathies, CK-MB is often increased, reflecting its production by regenerating muscle.

With severe acute damage to muscle, a clinical picture termed rhabdomyolysis may develop. In such situations, CK-MB/total CK may be elevated above normal, in the absence of myocardial infarction (cardiac troponin levels are normal); this is commonly seen in patients with inflammatory muscle disease (Kiely, 2000). In addition to normal cardiac troponin levels with elevated CK levels, two distinct isoforms (representing fast or slow skeletal fiber types) of serum skeletal troponin I may be identified (Simpson, 2002).

No specific criteria are known for differentiating rhabdomyolysis from lesser degrees of muscle injury; among the more important features are the higher total CK (one suggested diagnostic level is CK >20 times upper reference limits), the rapid rise and fall of CK, and the appearance of myoglobinuria. Many assays for myoglobin (found in skeletal, smooth, and cardiac muscle) are relatively insensitive, and myoglobin has a short half-life; thus, CK is a more reliable test for establishing the diagnosis. As a form of **cell lysis syndrome,** rhabdomyolysis is associated with the release of other cell contents, such as potassium, phosphate, and nucleotides that can be converted to uric acid. Qualitative testing for myoglobin in the urine is important because myoglobin is potentially toxic to the kidneys, and the patient is at risk for acute renal failure. Myoglobinuria may lead to the development of acute tubular necrosis, with the appearance of pigmented casts in the urine sediment. If renal failure develops, hyperkalemia, hyperphosphatemia, and hyperuricemia typically also will be present. No direct relationship has been discerned between the degree of elevation of CK and the likelihood of development of renal failure (Gabow, 1982; Ward, 1988). Common causes of rhabdomyolysis include drugs (particularly ethanol and cocaine), viral infection, extreme exertion, hyperthermia, trauma including crush injuries, ischemia of the lower extremities, and inflammatory myopathy. In addition, strenuous exercise in individuals with sickle trait can result in massive rhabdomyolysis, leading to myoglobin-induced renal failure and the other sequelae discussed previously (Mitchell, 2007; Ouyang, 2008).

SELECTED REFERENCES

Bull H, Murray PG, Thomas D, Fraser AM, Nelson PN. Acid phosphatases. J Clin Pathol Mol Pathol 2002;55:65–72.

Recent review of acid phosphatases, with emphasis on tartrate-resistant acid phosphatase and its function and clinical usefulness in processes involving bone resorption.

Dzau VJ, Bernstein K, Celermajer D, et al. Pathophysiologic and therapeutic importance of tissue ACE: a consensus report. Cardiovasc Drugs Ther 2002;16:149–60.

Report from a recent consensus conference examining the actions of angiotensin-converting enzymes (ACEs) in the pathology of cardiovascular disease and the use of tissue ACE inhibitors as antihypertensive agents in these patients.

Macours N, Poels J, Hens K, Francis C, Huybrechts R. Structure, evolutionary conservation, and functions of angiotensin- and endothelin-converting enzymes. Int Rev Cytol 2004;239:47–97.

Recent overview of both angiotensin-converting enzymes and endothelin-converting enzymes examining the structure and biological roles of these molecules.

von Eyben FE. A systematic review of lactate dehydrogenase isoenzyme 1 and germ cell tumors. Clin Biochem 2001;34:441–54.

Review of lactate dehydrogenase isoenzyme 1 as a possible serum marker in patients with germ cell tumors.

REFERENCES

Access the complete reference list online at http://www.expertconsult.com

CHAPTER 21

EVALUATION OF LIVER FUNCTION

Matthew R. Pincus, Philip M. Tierno Jr., Maly Fenelus, Wilbur B. Bowne, Martin H. Bluth

KEY POINTS

- The liver is composed of three systems: the hepatocyte, concerned with metabolic reactions, macromolecular (especially protein) synthesis, and degradation and metabolism of xenobiotics (e.g., drugs); the biliary system, involved with the metabolism of bilirubin and bile salts; and the reticuloendothelial system, concerned with the immune system and the production of heme and globin metabolites (e.g., bilirubin).
- The function of each of these systems can be measured conveniently and virtually noninvasively by determining the serum levels of specific analytes, in the so-called **liver function test profile.**
- One of the most common causes of acute liver injury is viral hepatitis, mainly hepatitis A, B, and C, all of which induce acute elevations of serum alanine and aspartate aminotransferase.
- Diagnosis of viral hepatitis can be made by screening for viral antigens, especially in hepatitis B, and for immunoglobulin M and G directed against specific viral antigens. Confirmation of the diagnosis of a particular form of viral hepatitis is carried out using suitable molecular diagnostic techniques such as real-time PCR using primers encoding specific viral gene sequences.
- The diagnosis of specific liver diseases, including hepatitis, cirrhosis, chronic passive congestion, acute biliary obstruction, space-occupying lesions, autoimmune diseases, and fulminant hepatic failure, can be made from specific patterns of serum liver function tests and from the presence of specific antibodies in serum.

Normal Liver Function

The liver is the largest and most complex organ of the gastrointestinal tract. Overall, it comprises three systems: first, the biochemical hepatocytic system, which is responsible for the vast majority of all metabolic activities in the body, including protein synthesis; aerobic and anaerobic metabolism of glucose and other sugars; glycogen synthesis and breakdown; amino acid and nucleic acid metabolism; amino acid and dicarboxylic acid interconversions via transaminases (aminotransferases); lipoprotein synthesis and metabolism; xenobiotic metabolism (e.g., drug metabolism), usually involving the cytochrome P450 oxidation system; storage of iron and vitamins such as A, D, and B_{12}; and synthesis of hormones such as angiotensinogen, insulin-like growth factor I, and triiodothyronine. It is also the site of clearance of many other hormones such as insulin, parathyroid hormone, estrogens, and cortisol. Uniquely, the liver is the site of metabolism of ammonia to urea.

Albumin in the body is synthesized in the liver, as are all coagulation factor proteins, with the exception of von Willebrand factor, which is synthesized in endothelial cells and megakaryocytes. Patients with liver disease may have signs or symptoms related to disturbance of any of the above functions.

The second major hepatic system is the hepatobiliary system, which is concerned with the metabolism of bilirubin, a process that involves transport of bilirubin into the hepatocyte and its conjugation to glucuronic acid and its secretion into bile canaliculi and the enterohepatic system. Last is the reticuloendothelial system, that is, Kupffer cells. These are a form of macrophage involved (a) with the immune system, including being a major site of defense against intestinal bacteria and the primary location for removal of antigen–antibody complexes from the circulation, and (b) with the breakdown of hemoglobin from dead erythrocytes, giving rise to bilirubin, which, together with bilirubin from the spleen, enters the hepatocyte.

Because clinical symptoms in liver disease often lag behind the progression of disease, it is important to detect the presence and even the onset of these conditions. Fortunately, evaluation of liver function can often be achieved by determination of serum analytes in a test profile known as **liver function tests,** many of whose components are not unique to liver but, when evaluated together, allow for accurate diagnosis of abnormalities of liver function. An outline of liver function tests and their interpretation has been presented in Chapter 8.

This chapter reviews the most common laboratory tests for evaluation of liver function and injury, methods used for their measurement, testing for causes of liver injury, and patterns of laboratory abnormalities seen in specific liver diseases.

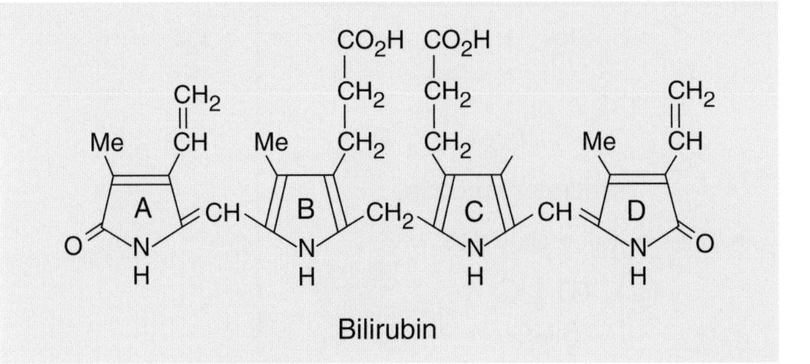

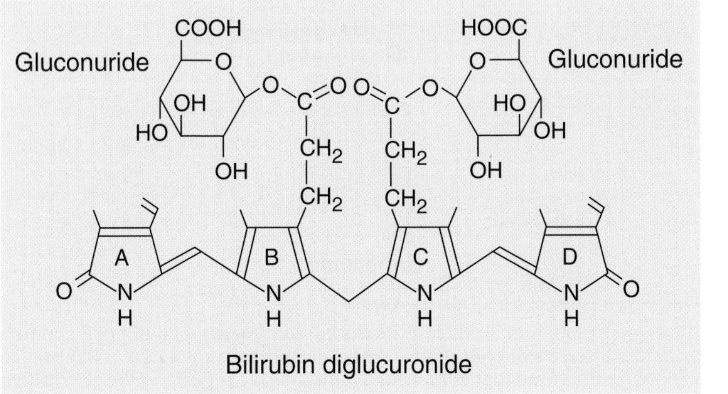

Figure 21-1 Structures of critical molecules in the metabolism of bilirubin to its diglucuronide. Bilirubin is transported into the hepatocyte, where it is converted into the diglucuronide form and secreted into canaliculi. *(From Crawford JM, Hauser SC, Gollan JL. Formation, hepatic metabolism, and transport of bile pigments: a status report. Semin Liver Dis 1988b;8:105–18.)*

METABOLIC FUNCTIONS

Bilirubin

Normal Bilirubin Metabolism

Bilirubin is the major metabolite of heme, the iron-binding tetrapyrrole ring found in hemoglobin, myoglobin, and cytochromes. Approximately 250–350 mg of bilirubin is produced daily in healthy adults, about 85% of which is derived from turnover of senescent red blood cells (Berlin, 1981; Chowdhury, 1988; Berk, 1994a). In macrophages mainly in the spleen, methemoglobin from red cells is split to give free globin chains and heme. The porphyrin ring of heme is oxidized by microsomal heme oxygenase, producing the straight-chain compound biliverdin and releasing iron. In this ring-opening reaction, 1 mole of carbon monoxide is released, which is transported ultimately as carboxyhemoglobin, whose serum levels can be useful in the diagnosis of hemolytic anemia, as discussed in Chapter 8. Biliverdin is then reduced to bilirubin (Fig. 21-1) by the nicotinamide adenine dinucleotide phosphate (NADPH)-dependent enzyme, biliverdin reductase. Bilirubin, bound mainly to albumin, is then transported mainly in the portal system to the liver, where it enters the hepatocyte through its membrane surface in contact with the sinusoids, as shown in Figure 21-2.

As free bilirubin enters hepatocytes, additional bilirubin dissociates from albumin. This process is highly efficient; clearance of unconjugated bilirubin at normal values is about 5 mg/kg/day or, for a 75-kg individual, about 400 mg/day (Berk, 1994b). The half-life of unconjugated bilirubin is short; 60% of labeled bilirubin appears within hepatocytes within 5 minutes of injection (Bloomer, 1973). Clearance rate increases with an increasing concentration of unconjugated bilirubin up to at least 4 mg/dL (Berk, 1994b).

In its most common isomeric *(trans-)* form, bilirubin is highly insoluble in water, and most of it is transported bound to albumin, with only a small fraction of free bilirubin. Light can cause photoisomerization of bilirubin, from a *trans-* form to a more compact *cis-* form, making it much more water soluble and allowing it to be excreted in urine (Onishi, 1986); this forms the basis for phototherapy in the treatment of neonatal (unconjugated) hyperbilirubinemia. The pathway for clearance of bilirubin by the liver is illustrated in Figure 21-2. Note that unconjugated bilirubin enters the hepatocyte at the membrane surface adjacent to the sinusoids, opposite the face that is in contact with bile canaliculi.

Bilirubin enters hepatocytes by two mechanisms: one is passive diffusion, and the other is receptor-mediated endocytosis. As summarized in Figure 21-2, once in the hepatocyte, bilirubin is "handed-off" from one protein complex to another in a chain. First, it complexes with the so-called **Y and Z proteins,** and then it binds sequentially to a protein complex called **ligandin.** From this complex, it is transported to the smooth endoplasmic reticulum (SER). In the SER, bilirubin becomes the substrate of the enzyme, glucuronyl transferase, which catalyzes the esterification of the propionic acid side chains of bilirubin with glucuronic acid (present as uridine diphosphoglucuronic acid) to form mainly the diglucuronide conjugate shown in Figure 21-1 (Chowdhury, 1988). Some monoglucuronide and a small amount of triglucuronide also form. The ratio of monoconjugated to diconjugated pigment in bile is 1:4, whereas the ratio is nearly 1:1 in plasma, suggesting that monoconjugates reflux into plasma more readily.

As schematized in Figure 21-2, conjugated bilirubin is then transported to the canalicular face of the hepatocyte at which it is directly secreted, by an energy-dependent mechanism, into the canaliculi; only conjugated bilirubin can be directly excreted into the canaliculi, and unconjugated bilirubin cannot traverse this membrane.

Once bilirubin is excreted into the canaliculi and ultimately into the intestinal tract, it is further metabolized by intestinal bacteria, which affect its deconjugation and oxidation or reduction with the formation of compounds collectively called **urobilinogen** and **urobilin,** which can then be reabsorbed from the gut. Most urobilinogen absorbed is reexcreted by the liver. A minor fraction may be excreted in the urine. Larger quantities are found in the urine in conditions leading to hyperbilirubinemia, or in conditions in which the liver cannot readily secrete urobilinogen absorbed from the gut. Ultimately, intestinal urobilinogen is converted to stool pigments such as stercobilin; their absence leads to clay-colored stools, often an early sign of impaired bilirubin metabolism.

When conjugated bilirubin is present in serum, it can become covalently bound to albumin, producing biliprotein or delta-bilirubin (Lauff, 1982; McDonagh, 1984). Although conjugated bilirubin has a half-life of less than 24 hours, delta-bilirubin has a half-life similar to that for albumin at 17 days (Fevery, 1986), causing prolonged jaundice during recovery from hepatocellular injury (Van Hootegem, 1985) or biliary obstruction (Kozaki, 1998). Conjugated bilirubin, being water soluble, can be filtered by the glomerulus and can appear in urine, where it may be detected by dipstick examination; urobilinogen measurement adds little to standard tests of liver function or injury, however (Binder, 1989). Urinary bilirubin is elevated in most patients with increased serum conjugated bilirubin (Binder, 1989).

Derangements of Bilirubin Metabolism

As shown in Figure 21-2, in each step in the processing of bilirubin a possible lesion leads to elevated serum levels of unconjugated or conjugated bilirubin. Each of these is discussed in turn.

Causes of Elevated Serum Levels of Unconjugated Bilirubin

Hemolysis. As discussed in Chapter 8, in hemolytic anemias unconjugated bilirubin rises as a result of abnormally high levels of hemoglobin released from erythrocytes. If the rate of bilirubin formation exceeds the rate of liver clearance (i.e., a state of overproduction of bilirubin) there will be a rise in the bilirubin level in serum. Virtually all of this bilirubin will be unconjugated bilirubin. This is particularly likely to occur in neonates, whose glucuronyl transferase activity is low. Thus, one manner of confirming a diagnosis of hemolytic anemia is the finding, in adults, of elevated indirect bilirubin levels in serum. Usually, these levels are not dramatically elevated and are generally in the 1.5–3.0 mg/dL range.

Gilbert's Syndrome and the Crigler-Najjar Syndrome Are Caused by Gene Mutations and Deletions. In Gilbert's syndrome, characterized by a mild unconjugated hyperbilirubinemia, the most common genetic lesion appears to be the insertion of two bases into the promoter region of the *UGT1A1* gene, resulting in lower transcriptional rates (Kraemer, 2002; Maruo, 2004) and overall lower enzymatic activity (reduced to about 30% of normal). In the more serious Crigler-Najjar syndrome, frequently characterized by high serum levels of unconjugated bilirubin, multiple mutations are found to occur in this gene, including shifts in the reading frames, stop codons, and critical amino acid substitutions, all of which give rise to a spectrum of dysfunctional proteins from mildly dysfunctional to completely nonfunctional proteins (Kraemer, 2002).

In Gilbert's syndrome, which occurs in a significant fraction (3%–5%) of the population, the genetic defect may be necessary but not sufficient because, in an earlier study (Persico, 1999), a significant percentage of

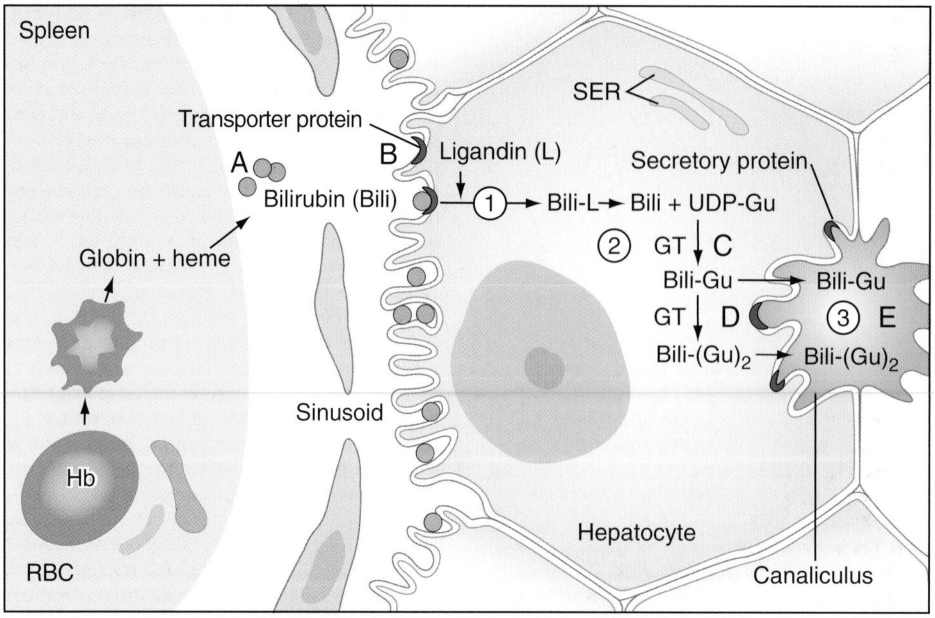

Figure 21-2 Schematic summary of the pathway of bilirubin *(Bili, in brown circles)* transport and metabolism. Bilirubin is produced from metabolism of heme, primarily in the spleen, and is transported to the liver bound to albumin. It enters the hepatocyte by binding to a transporter protein *(red crescents)* and crosses the cell membrane *(circled 1),* thus entering the cell. It binds to Y and Z proteins *(not shown)* and then to ligandin for transport to the smooth endoplasmic reticulum (SER). In the SER, bilirubin is conjugated to glucuronic acid by UDP-glucuronyl transferase 1 *(circled 2 and labeled GT),* producing monoglucuronides and diglucuronides of bilirubin—Bili-Gu and Bili-$(Gu)_2$. Conjugated bilirubin is then secreted into the canaliculi *(circled 3)* by the adenosine triphosphate-binding cassette transporter protein MRP2/cMOAT/ABCC2 *(shown as blue crescents).* In overproduction disease **(A),** such as hemolytic anemia, unconjugated bilirubin is produced at rates that exceed the ability of the liver to clear it, leading to a usually transient increase in unconjugated bilirubin in serum. In both Gilbert's and Crigler-Najjar syndromes, mutations in the gene encoding UDP glucuronyl transferase *(UDPGT1A1),* shown at **C** in the figure, result in buildup of unconjugated bilirubin in hepatocytes and ultimately in serum. In Gilbert's syndrome, there may also be a defect in the bilirubin transporter protein, shown at **B** in the figure. Mutations in the *MRP2/cMOAT/ABCC2* gene result in defective secretory proteins, causing buildup of conjugated bilirubin in hepatocytes and, ultimately, in serum, resulting in the Dubin-Johnson syndrome **(D),** an autosomal recessive disease. Conjugated hyperbilirubinemia is also found in the Rotor syndrome, possibly virus induced. In adults, blockade of any of the major bile ducts, especially the common bile duct, by stones or space-occupying lesions such as tumors **(E),** is the most common cause of conjugated hyperbilirubinemia.
Hb, Hemoglobin; *RBC,* red blood cell.

males with this defect were found to have hyperbilirubinemia, but no females with this enzyme deficit were found to have elevated serum bilirubin levels (Bosma, 1995). In some patients with Gilbert's syndrome, the rate of organic anion uptake has been found to correlate negatively with serum bilirubin (Persico, 1999), suggesting that an additional defect may be present to cause hyperbilirubinemia that may be related to a transport deficit in the sinusoidal membrane of the hepatocyte. In this condition, total bilirubin, virtually all of which is unconjugated, is typically elevated to 2–3 mg/dL; levels can increase further with fasting but seldom exceed 5 mg/dL. Because passive diffusion of bilirubin into hepatocytes occurs, this condition is rarely serious and may result in mild elevations of bilirubin such as those seen in hemolytic anemia as described previously.

Gilbert's syndrome has perhaps been overdiagnosed; it is most frequently diagnosed in young adults ranging in age from 20–30 years. However, normal bilirubin ranges are age dependent and actually reach their highest levels in adolescents and young adults (Rosenthal, 1984), as discussed further later.

In the more serious or type I form of the Crigler-Najjar syndrome (i.e., homozygously nonfunctioning proteins), the unconjugated hyperbilirubinemia becomes marked, almost always exceeding 5 mg/dL and causing jaundice, and sometimes exceeding 20 mg/dL. Affected infants develop severe unconjugated hyperbilirubinemia, which typically leads to kernicterus, deposition of bilirubin in the brain, particularly affecting the basal ganglia, mainly the lenticular nucleus, causing severe motor dysfunction and retardation. In the less severe type II form, enzyme activity is approximately 10% of normal, and survival to adulthood is possible (Berk, 1994c). The danger of kernicterus is a certainty at levels exceeding 20 mg/dL. It is vital to treat these infants with phototherapy, as discussed earlier, to cause excretion of the unconjugated bilirubin.

Causes of Elevated Serum Levels of Conjugated Bilirubin

Excretion Deficits: Dubin-Johnson Syndrome. In another inborn error of metabolism, called **the Dubin-Johnson syndrome,** there is a blockade of the excretion of bilirubin into the canaliculi, caused by defects in the adenosine triphosphate (ATP)-binding cassette (ABC) canalicular multispecific organic anion transporter, MRP2/cMOAT/ABCC2 (Paulusma, 1997; Tsujii, 1999; Gottesman, 2001). This protein is a member of a family of approximately 100 different transporter proteins that share homology within the ABC region and contain transmembrane domains involved in recognition of substrates, which are transported across, into, and out of cell membranes and include proteins involved in multiple drug resistance to chemotherapeutic agents in cancer treatment. Some protein members utilize ABCs to regulate ion channels. Several genetic diseases result from transporter mutations, including the Dubin-Johnson syndrome, cystic fibrosis, age-related macular degeneration, Tangier disease, and progressive familial intrahepatic cholestasis (Gottesman, 2001).

Dubin-Johnson syndrome is associated with increased plasma conjugated bilirubin, typically with mild jaundice (total bilirubin, 2–5 mg/dL), and intense dark pigmentation of the liver due to accumulation of lipofuscin pigment. Thus conjugated bilirubin accumulates within the hepatocyte and eventually back-diffuses into the circulation, where it is detected in serum. This inborn error can sometimes be confused with the Rotor syndrome, possibly of viral origin, where there is also a block in the excretion of conjugated bilirubin but without liver pigmentation (Berk, 1994d). In these cases, liver biopsy often will reveal cytosolic inclusion bodies within hepatocytes.

Biliary Obstruction. In adults, cholelithiasis is the most common cause of hyperbilirubinemia. This condition results from the presence of bile stones (that are composed of bilirubin or cholesterol) most commonly in the common bile duct (choledocholithiasis). Most frequently, patients presenting with this condition are parous white females in early middle age (giving rise to the semi-mnemonic, "fair, fecund, fortyish female"). Biliary obstruction due to cholelithiasis results in elevation of total bilirubin, with >90% being direct bilirubin. In more than 90% of such patients, a concomitant rise in alkaline phosphatase occurs. The levels of this enzyme are variable but are frequently above 300 international units (IU)/L.

Inflammatory conditions of the biliary tract, such as ascending cholangitis, also give rise to elevated serum levels of direct bilirubin and alkaline phosphatase, as discussed later in this chapter. The rise in direct bilirubin often exceeds 5 mg/dL. In gram-negative sepsis, there can be what appears to be a mild inflammation of the biliary tract, resulting in mild elevation of direct bilirubin to levels of 2–3 mg/dL. A concomitant elevation of alkaline phosphatase to levels of 200–300 IU/L is also observed.

In hepatitis, in which toxic destruction of hepatocytes is due to viral, chemical, or traumatic causes, focal necrosis and/or cellular injury results both in blocking conjugation of bilirubin and in excretion of conjugated bilirubin. Thus elevation of both direct and indirect bilirubin occurs. Serum levels of bilirubin are variable, depending on the severity of infection and the extent of disease. In viral hepatitis, such as hepatitis B, as discussed subsequently, serum bilirubin levels often reach levels of 5–10 mg/dL or greater.

Aside from liver disease, elevations of conjugated bilirubin may occur with a few other disorders. Septicemia (as noted previously), total parenteral nutrition, and certain drugs such as androgens commonly cause increased conjugated bilirubin, but the mechanism is not understood (Zimmerman, 1979). Fasting causes increases in unconjugated bilirubin in normal individuals, but to a lesser degree than is seen in Gilbert's syndrome.

Laboratory Tests for Bilirubin

Bilirubin is typically measured using diazotized sulfanilic acid, which forms a conjugated azo compound with the porphyrin rings of bilirubin, resulting in reaction products that absorb strongly at 540 nm. Because unconjugated bilirubin reacts slowly, accelerants such as caffeine or methanol are used to measure total bilirubin. Deletion of these accelerants allows determination of direct-reacting, or direct, bilirubin.

Until the early 1980s, it was accepted that direct bilirubin was equal to conjugated bilirubin. The introduction of dry slide technology, using differential spectrophotometry to measure conjugated and unconjugated bilirubin separately, led to the observation that the sum of these two entities did not equal total bilirubin and to the characterization of delta-bilirubin. Approximately 70%–80% of conjugated bilirubin and delta-bilirubin and a small percentage of unconjugated bilirubin are measured in the direct bilirubin assay (Lo, 1983; Doumas, 1991). Although good data support the measurement of conjugated bilirubin instead of estimating it from direct bilirubin (Arvan, 1985; Doumas, 1987), the direct bilirubin assay is still widely used. The accuracy of direct bilirubin assays is dependent on sample handling and reagent composition. Prolonged exposure to light causes photoisomerization, increasing direct-reacting bilirubin (Ihara, 1997). Use of wetting agents or incorrect pH buffers increases the amount of unconjugated bilirubin measured as direct bilirubin (Doumas, 1991). Typically, direct bilirubin should measure 0–0.1 mg/dL in normal individuals, with rare values of 0.2 mg/dL in the absence of liver or biliary tract disease.

Reference values for total bilirubin are both age and gender dependent. Bilirubin levels typically reach peak values at around ages 14–18, falling to stable adult levels by age 25 (Rosenthal, 1984; Notter, 1985; Zucker, 2004). Values are higher in males than in females at all ages (Rosenthal, 1983; Carmel, 1985; Notter, 1985; Dufour, 1998a; Zucker, 2004). Strenuous exercise causes a significant increase in bilirubin values compared with those seen in sedentary individuals or those with chronic exercise (Dufour, 1998b). African Americans have bilirubin levels significantly lower than those of other ethnic groups.

Other Metabolic Tests

Ammonia

This critical and toxic compound is metabolized exclusively in the liver. Ammonia is derived mainly from amino acid and nucleic acid metabolism. Some ammonia is also produced from metabolic reactions such as the action of the enzyme glutaminase on glutamine, resulting in the production of glutamic acid and ammonia. As it happens, ammonia can be metabolized only in the liver because the liver uniquely contains the critical enzymes for the Krebs-Henseleit or urea cycle, in which ammonia, a toxic substance, is ultimately converted into urea, a nontoxic compound that is readily excreted. In this cycle, ammonia, with the enzyme carbamoyl phosphate synthetase, is condensed with carbon dioxide (CO_2) and ATP to form carbamoyl phosphate that then, in the rate-determining step, carboxamidates the delta-amino group of ornithine to form citrulline using the enzyme ornithine carbamoyltransferase (OCT), an enzyme that is unique to the liver. Congenital deficiency of this or other urea cycle enzymes leads to increased levels of ammonia in serum and in cerebrospinal fluid (Batshaw, 1994).

A unique feature of liver tissue is its ability to regenerate. To abolish liver tissue function, more than 80% of the liver must be destroyed. If most of the liver is destroyed as a result of such conditions as cirrhosis (Stahl, 1963) or, less commonly, acute fulminant hepatic failure, including Reye's syndrome (Heubi, 1984; Sunheimer, 1994), urea cycle enzymes are no longer present, resulting in the toxic buildup of ammonia and some of the amino acid intermediates in the urea cycle, such as arginine, which has known neurotoxic effects. The result is an increase in ammonia and these amino acid intermediates in the circulation and in the central nervous system (CNS), giving rise to hepatic encephalopathy. In addition, in most cirrhotics, intrahepatic portal-systemic shunting occurs, thereby causing ammonia to bypass the liver and resulting in elevated serum ammonia concentrations. Elevated serum levels of ammonia therefore often indicate some form of liver failure, although other conditions can also induce increases in serum ammonia levels.

In patients with cirrhosis or fulminant hepatic failure, there has been some dispute as to whether ammonia itself is the cause of the observed metabolic encephalopathy; possibly other toxins that accumulate as a result of absent hepatic detoxification are the cause. One of the arguments often used is that there is no clear correlation between the severity of the encephalopathy and serum ammonia concentrations (Lewis, 2003). Countering this argument is the finding that, although venous ammonia levels do not correlate with degree of encephalopathy (Stahl, 1963), arterial levels of ammonia do generally correlate with degree of encephalopathy. Furthermore, in patients with cirrhosis or fulminant hepatic failure, lowering the serum ammonia invariably diminishes the severity of the encephalopathy (Pincus, 1991). Furthermore, idiopathic hyperammonemia, not related to liver disease, also induces lethal encephalopathy (Shepard, 1987; Davies, 1996). An important mechanism by which ammonia can cause toxicity to the CNS is its ability to lower the concentration of γ-aminobutyric acid (GABA), a critically important neurotransmitter in the central nervous system, by reacting with glutamic acid to form glutamine via reversal of the glutaminase-catalyzed reaction (Butterworth, 1987). This depletes glutamic acid in the CNS. However, GABA is formed directly from the decarboxylation of glutamic acid, so that GABA levels consequently decrease, with potentially serious effects on neurotransmission (see Chapter 23). Because ammonia causes accumulation of glutamine in the CNS, there is the suggestion that, at least in valproic acid–induced hyperammonemia, cerebrospinal fluid levels of glutamine can be used in the diagnosis and management of hepatic encephalopathy (Vossler, 2002). More recently, besides evidence that ammonia in the CNS is directly toxic to astrocytes, other evidence indicates that ammonia induces neutrophil dysfunction that results in the generation of reactive oxygen species contributing to oxidative stress and inflammation, with lowered ability of the CNS to block infectious agents (Shawcross, 2010). One major new finding put forth by these studies is that treatment of hepatic encephalopathy with suitable antiinflammatory agents may be effective.

At present, most commonly, elevated serum ammonia concentrations in hepatic encephalopathy are reduced by the agent lactulose, which is metabolized by specific gut bacteria to lactic acid. The acid so produced in the intestinal lumen traps ammonia as ammonium ion, which can no longer diffuse across the intestinal membrane and is thus excreted. Ammonia-producing bacteria in the intestine are removed by treatment with antibiotics such as neomycin.

Assays for Ammonia. Ammonia is typically measured by enzymatic assays using glutamate dehydrogenase, which catalyzes the reaction of α-ketoglutarate and ammonia to form glutamate, with oxidation of NADPH to NADP as the indicator (decrease in absorbance at 340 nm, as described in Chapter 20). Ammonia is also measured via a dry slide method (e.g., on the Johnson and Johnson Vitros systems) using alkaline pH buffers to convert all ammonium ions to ammonia gas, with bromphenol blue as the indicator (Huizenga, 1994). Because ammonia is a product of cellular metabolism, methods used in specimen collection and transportation are critical in preventing artifactually increased levels. Arterial blood is the preferred specimen for measurement of ammonia. Although venous blood is not recommended, if used, tourniquets should be used minimally, and fist clenching and relaxing avoided during collection. Specimens should be kept in ice water until separation of cells from plasma occurs (Howanitz, 1984; da Fonseca-Wollheim, 1990).

Lipids

Cholesterol and Other Lipids

(See Chapter 17.)

Because the liver is vital in lipoprotein synthesis and interconversions, hepatic disorders often cause derangements in lipoprotein metabolism. Although none of these abnormalities is used to diagnose liver pathology, it is important to recognize that they may result from liver disease. In severe liver injury, including cirrhosis, these abnormalities include a decrease in high-density lipoprotein (HDL), particularly the HDL_3 (but often not the HDL_2) subfraction, and in other altered lipoprotein distributions, caused in part by deficiencies of lecithin/cholesterol acyltransferase (the enzyme that esterifies cholesterol) and lipoprotein lipases, resulting in hypertriglyceridemia (triglyceride levels ranging from 250–500 mg/dL). In addition, decreased synthesis of LCAT and lipoprotein lipases causes increases in blood and in the HDL fraction of unesterified cholesterol, as well as increased levels of phospholipids, including lecithins, in blood and in the very-low-density lipoprotein fraction, along with increased serum triglycerides. Overall, the resulting lipoprotein pattern is that of the so-called **abnormally migrating β-lipoprotein,** typical of type III hyperlipoproteinemia (see Chapter 17). However, in cirrhotics with poor nutrition, despite critical enzyme deficiencies, low levels of cholesterol (<100 mg/dL) may be found.

In contrast, in alcohol-induced liver injury, alcohol induces increased expression of apolipoprotein (apo)A-I protein. Thus, HDL, especially HDL_3, may be elevated if alcohol ingestion continues. Because, in cirrhosis, apoA-I protein decreases, serum levels of this protein have been used to diagnose this disease using the so-called **PGA index** (Teare, 1993)—a combination of prothrombin time (PT), which increases, with γ-glutamyl transferase activity (discussed later), which also increases, and apoA-I protein. This index differs for alcoholic hepatitis, enabling the distinction to be made between these two conditions without the necessity of liver biopsy (Mun, 2003).

In cholestasis, regurgitation of biliary contents into the bloodstream results in the buildup of lipoprotein X (LpX) (discussed in Chapter 17) and elevation of biliary lipids. Because LpX carries high levels of unesterified cholesterol, cholesterol levels in serum can become markedly elevated (Turchin, 2005).

Bile Salts

Bile salts, which are products of cholesterol metabolism, facilitate absorption of fat from the intestine. They are stored in the gallbladder and released to the intestine after meals through gallbladder contraction mediated by cholecystokinin. They are not usually used in the diagnosis of abnormal liver function but are important in that they constitute a substantial amount of bile in bilirubin excretion and can therefore be of use in diagnosing cholestasis. Also, in severe biliary obstruction, the buildup of bile salts in serum causes symptomatic illness in the form of intractable itching, although this has been disputed (Jones, 1999). The primary bile salts, cholate and chenodeoxycholate, are produced in the liver; they are excreted into the biliary and enterohepatic systems, and, in the intestinal tract, they are metabolized by bacteria, producing secondary bile salts (i.e., lithocholate, deoxycholate, and ursodeoxycholate) (Carey, 1988) by bacterial 7-α-dehydroxylation in the intestinal lumen. Ursodeoxycholate, an end-product of bile salt metabolism in man, is produced by isomerization of secondary bile salts and has been found to be therapeutic in cholestatic diseases (Rost, 2004). These bile salts are conjugated, in the microsomal system discussed later, to glycine and taurine and are also sulfated and glucuronidated. Conjugation of bile salts to taurine and sulfates increases with the severity of cholestasis in conditions causing obstruction to bile outflow. Recirculation of bile salts to the liver occurs by reabsorption from the terminal ileum, where deoxycholate is almost completely reabsorbed, and chenodeoxycholate is about 75% reabsorbed. In cirrhosis, a disproportionate decrease in cholic acid is seen, along with a reduced ratio of primary to secondary bile salts. With cholestasis, secondary bile salts are not formed; thus, the ratio of primary to secondary bile salts is markedly increased.

Renal clearance of bile salts is negligible in normal patients, but in cholestasis, renal excretion of bile salts, mainly in the form of sulfates and glucuronides, is enhanced. Fasting bile salts, when normal, can exclude the presence of parenchymal liver disease in patients with Gilbert's syndrome (Vierling, 1982), as discussed previously. It should also be recognized that defective production of bile salts, which helps solubilize the contents of bile, in the liver may predispose to the formation of bilirubinate or cholesterol stones and posthepatic biliary obstruction.

Analysis of bile salts must be performed on serum taken from patients who are in the fasting state, or on serum taken at a specified time after meals, because food ingestion causes a significant increase in bile acid levels. Bile salts can be measured by many techniques, but chromatographic methods, particularly high-performance liquid chromatography, as discussed in Chapter 23, are most widely used and allow separation of different bile salts.

Drug Metabolism

Many xenobiotics, such as drugs, are metabolized in the liver, mainly in the microsomes of hepatocytes. Complex series of reactions occur, many of which are dependent on cytochrome P450, which is involved in the oxidation of these compounds. Whether or not specific exogenous compounds are converted to metabolites depends on the isoforms of cytochrome P450, such as CYP1A and CYP2B (cytochrome P450 1A and 2B, respectively). Often, the conversion of xenobiotics into metabolites using this system involves two phases: phase I reactions involve oxidations/hydroxylations, and phase II reactions conjugate the metabolite (or parent compound) to polar compounds, such as glucuronic acid, glycine, taurine, and sulfate. In more severe liver disease, which involves microsomal damage, this ability to metabolize xenobiotics is compromised. Thus the ability of hepatocytes to metabolize drugs can be used to measure liver damage.

This is generally accomplished by administering a known dose of radiolabeled (usually ^{13}C-labeled) drug and measuring the $^{13}CO_2$ exhaled over time in a patient's breath. Two categories of breath tests have been developed based on the rate-limiting step in metabolism. The first group includes drugs such as aminopyrine, caffeine, and diazepam, which are metabolized at rates that are independent of hepatic blood flow to the liver and depend only on the enzymatic activity of different cytochromes P450 (e.g., CYP1A). The second group is composed of drugs such as methacetin, phenacetin, and erythromycin, whose rates of metabolism depend on the rate of blood flow (i.e., their rates of metabolism are fast compared with their rates of delivery to the liver). These types of dynamic tests appear not to be so useful in the initial diagnosis of hepatic disease; rather, they are more useful in estimating the extent of liver damage in known liver disease (Nista, 2004).

Some interferences that complicate interpretation of the results of these tests include dependence of the demethylation of aminopyrine (the methyl group is oxidized to CO_2) on vitamin B_{12}; in cases of vitamin B_{12} deficiency, less than normal amounts of $^{13}CO_2$ will be exhaled because of low B_{12} levels, not necessarily because of liver damage. Rates of caffeine metabolism generally decrease with increasing age but are increased by smoking; these findings can complicate interpretation of test results.

SYNTHETIC FUNCTIONS

Protein Synthesis

The liver is the site of synthesis for most plasma proteins. Major exceptions include immunoglobulins (Igs) and von Willebrand factor. Synthesis of more than 90% of all protein and 100% of albumin occurs in the liver. Thus extensive destruction of liver tissue will result in **low serum levels** of total protein and albumin. In cirrhosis, besides hepatocyte destruction, another cause of diminished protein production is portal hypertension, which decreases delivery of amino acids to the liver. Two vital measurements of liver function, therefore, are total protein and albumin levels in serum. However, it should always be kept in mind that other major causes of low serum total protein and albumin have been identified; these include renal disease, malnutrition, protein-losing enteropathy, and, less commonly, chronic inflammatory disease. These alternative causes must always be considered when liver function status is evaluated.

In liver disease with widespread injury or necrosis, such as fulminant hepatic failure and cirrhosis, plasma levels of liver-synthesized proteins fall, such that proteins with longer half-lives tend to decrease more slowly. Albumin has a half-life of about 20 days, so that decreases in its serum levels occur more slowly than those of proteins with shorter half-lives. Among the liver-produced proteins with short half-lives are factor VII (4–6 hours), transthyretin (1–2 days), and transferrin (6 days).

Determination of Serum Protein Levels

This is based usually on the Biuret method. This method reflects the ability of the peptide backbone C=O groups of proteins to form color complexes with copper that absorb strongly at 540 nm. Some methods utilize a dye-binding method in which the proteins form a complex with the dye Coomassie blue. Albumin forms a unique color complex with the dyes bromcresol green and bromcresol purple, such that they absorb maximally at slightly different wavelengths, thus allowing direct spectrophotometric quantitation (Ihara, 1991). Bromcresol purple tends to react more exclusively with albumin than does bromcresol green (which reacts to a minor extent with some globulins), so that serum albumin levels may be slightly lower when determined with bromcresol purple. The reference range for total serum protein levels is generally in the 6–7.8 g/dL range. At least 60% of this should be albumin, the normal range for which is about 3.5–5 g/dL.

Serum protein electrophoresis and quantitative Igs may reveal characteristic changes in liver disease, as discussed in Chapter 19. Typically, in cirrhosis, albumin is significantly decreased, as are the α-1, α-2, and β (principally transferrin) bands. However, a polyclonal increase in Igs, which is seen frequently, produces the characteristic β-γ **bridging** pattern, as discussed in Chapter 19. In autoimmune hepatitis, albumin is typically decreased; this is accompanied by a marked polyclonal increase in IgG. Primary biliary cirrhosis is accompanied by a polyclonal increase in IgM.

Albumin

Albumin is the major protein produced by the liver; liver synthesis is increased by low plasma oncotic pressure and is decreased by cytokines, particularly interleukin-6. Although normal albumin synthesis occurs at about 120 mg/kg/day, the rate of synthesis can approximately double with low oncotic pressure. A decrease in albumin is one of the major prognostic features in patients with cirrhosis. Albumin measurements were discussed previously and more fully in Chapter 19.

Albumin is a transport protein for many substances, both endogenous (e.g., bilirubin, thyroid hormone) and exogenous (e.g., drugs). Low serum albumin levels due to liver disease are almost always caused by massive destruction of liver tissue and are seen primarily in cirrhosis, most often secondary to alcoholism. The diminution in albumin is paralleled by a fall in total serum protein. Because albumin is the osmotically active intravascular colloid, hypoalbuminemia often results in edema. In cirrhosis, where increased resistance to blood flow in the sinusoids causes portal hypertension, the combined effect of elevated hydrostatic pressure in the portal system and low colloid osmotic pressure results in ascites, a frequent finding in cirrhosis. These same changes may also be seen acutely in fulminant hepatic failure (Sunheimer, 1994).

Other Serum Proteins

Although most of the proteins discussed in Chapter 19 are produced by the liver, two bear special importance in the detection of congenital liver disorders.

α-1-Antitrypsin. α-1-antitrypsin (AAT), the most abundant α-1-globulin, is the most important protease inhibitor in plasma. Although its name indicates that it inhibits trypsin, it also is an inhibitor of other serine proteases, such as elastin. AAT is coded for by the *Pi* gene on chromosome 14; several genetic variants are due to point mutations, leading to single amino acid substitutions (Chappell, 2004). The most common variant, M, is associated with normal serum AAT levels. The mutations present in the S and Z variants prevent normal protein glycation, leading to accumulation of AAT within hepatocytes and reduced plasma AAT levels (Propst, 1994). In the United States, the overwhelming genotype is PiMM, where Pi is the protease inhibitor. The other genotypes—PiZZ, PiSS, PiSZ, PiMZ, and PiMS—all contain measurable activity of antiprotease, except a rare null genotype Pi^{-}. If the antiprotease activity of the MM phenotype is used as the reference, then the activity in phenotype ZZ is 15%, SS is 60%, MZ is 57.5%, and MS is 80%. Adults with PiZZ are most prone to develop emphysema relatively early in life as a result of uninhibited trypsin activity on alveolar wall elastin. Patients with PiZZ tend to accumulate the Z protein in periportal hepatocytes, where it forms discrete cytoplasmic bodies and may also develop neonatal hepatitis. Curiously, although infants may die of hepatic injury, it resolves in most infants and progresses to cirrhosis in only about 3% (Sveger, 1988). In adults, the likelihood of liver injury is increased in patients heterozygous or homozygous for the Z variant of AAT; this may be due to accumulation of AAT in the endoplasmic reticulum that induces autophagy and apoptosis of hepatocytes (Teckman, 2004). AAT phenotyping can be performed using isoelectric focusing (Propst, 1994). Because AAT is an acute phase reactant, its serum levels can be normal in MZ heterozygotes.

Ceruloplasmin. The major copper-containing protein in serum, ceruloplasmin, is also the enzyme present in highest circulating concentration. Ceruloplasmin is a ferroxidase, essential for converting iron to the ferric state to allow binding to transferrin. Low levels of ceruloplasmin are found in Wilson's disease, a rare congenital disorder (1 in 30,000 individuals) associated with one of many mutations in the gene on chromosome 13 coding for a cellular adenosine triphosphatase (ATPase), ATP7B, a new member of the cation-transporting p-type ATPase family (Bull, 1993). This protein is principally expressed in the liver and promotes copper secretion into plasma, coupled with ceruloplasmin synthesis, and into the biliary tract. More than 200 mutations of this Wilson's disease gene have been detected, resulting in impairment of ATP7B function and intracellular copper accumulation (Langner, 2004). Excess intracellular copper is deposited in lysozomes in hepatocytes; it induces free-radical reactions such as lipid peroxidation and membrane instability. Resultant liver damage can lead to chronic active hepatitis, cirrhosis, or, uncommonly, fulminant hepatic failure. In addition, steatosis and inflammation can result in this condition. Copper becomes deposited in the CNS, especially in the lenticular nucleus of the basal ganglia, causing neuropsychiatric disease; it can also be deposited at the edge of the iris, forming the observed Keyser-Fleischer rings.

The diagnosis of Wilson's disease is made on the basis of typical clinical and laboratory findings, including low serum ceruloplasmin, which can be measured by immunoassay or by enzymatic assay, increased urinary copper excretion, and increased hepatic copper content. Although ceruloplasmin is characteristically low in Wilson's disease, factors that increase ceruloplasmin synthesis (e.g., cytokines, pregnancy, estrogens) may cause normal ceruloplasmin levels in up to 15% of patients overall, and in as many as 35% with hepatic manifestations of Wilson's disease (Dufour, 1997), particularly acute Wilsonian hepatitis (Berman, 1991). Genetic testing is the most reliable means to establish the diagnosis, but it is difficult because more than 200 mutations have been shown to cause disease.

Clotting Factors

As mentioned earlier, except for the von Willebrand factor, which is made by endothelial cells and megakaryocytes, coagulation proteins are synthesized in the liver. In addition, inhibitors of coagulation, such as antithrombin III, α-2-macroglobulin, α-1-antitrypsin, C1 esterase inhibitor, and protein C, are synthesized in the liver. In addition, fibrin degradation products are catabolized in the liver. Low levels of antithrombin III in patients with cirrhosis and hepatitis may be caused by decreased synthesis, increased consumption, or alteration in the transcapillary flux ratio (Kelly, 1987). The most common coagulopathy seen in liver failure (i.e., cirrhosis and acute fulminant hepatic failure) is disseminated intravascular coagulopathy (DIC), as discussed in Chapter 8 and extensively throughout Part 5 of this book. This condition is characterized by increased consumption of clotting factors and platelets, causing thrombocytopenia and elevations of both prothrombin (PT) and partial thromboplastin (PTT) times. The mechanism has been postulated to be decreased synthesis of clotting inhibitory factors, decreased clearance of activated clotting factors, or release of tissue thromboplastin from hepatocytes (Kelly, 1986). D-Dimer and fibrin split products, detected in DIC, have been found in up to 80% of patients with liver disease without evidence of fibrinolysis (Van de Water, 1986). It is important that the diagnosis of DIC be made certain by determination of elevated blood D-dimer levels, as described in Part 5 on hemostasis and thrombosis. In some cases of liver failure, platelet counts are decreased because of sequestration in an enlarged spleen due to hepatosplenomegaly. This condition combined with elevated levels of PT and PTT caused by low levels of synthesis of coagulation factors can masquerade as DIC. In these cases, D-dimer levels are not elevated, excluding this diagnosis.

Perhaps the most frequently ordered laboratory test for detecting liver-associated coagulation abnormalities is PT and its associated measurement, the international sensitivity ratio, as described in Part 5. The PT measures the efficacy of the extrinsic clotting system in which factor VII is activated by tissue factor, as discussed in Part 5; because factor VII is uniquely synthesized in the liver, its measurement can be used to evaluate liver function status. Often, PT is computed as the international normalized ratio (INR), which attempts to standardize all PT measurements relative to a "gold standard" PT-measuring method, using the international sensitivity index (ISI), as described in Part 5.

Some Caveats in Using PT and INR to Evaluate Liver Function. Because PT and PTT measure the status of the coagulation cascades (extrinsic and intrinsic, respectively), any coagulation disorder will give rise to abnormal PT and/or PTT, independent of liver function. In addition, in patients with cholestasis (i.e., disease of the biliary tract) with no hepatocytic dysfunction (e.g., cirrhosis, fulminant hepatic failure), absorption of fat-soluble vitamin K from the gut may be impaired because of low levels of bile salts that allow membrane transport of this vitamin. Because factors II, VII, IX, and X depend on vitamin K for biosynthesis via carboxylation, coagulation abnormalities often result. Therefore, in patients with cholestasis, normal serum levels of inactive precursor forms of these four coagulation factors can be detected, as discussed later. Correction of prothrombin time by the administration of vitamin K is usually possible when factor V is normal in patients with cholestatic liver disease.

Also, use of the INR in evaluating liver function can provide misleading results. As discussed in Part 5, the INR is based on PT values for patients treated with Coumadin (warfarin, which blocks mainly the extrinsic system). Thus its appropriateness for evaluating non–Coumadin-induced coagulopathies has been questioned, especially in view of the finding that PT increases much less with lower ISI in patients with liver disease than in patients being treated with Coumadin (Kovacs, 1994; Ts'ao, 1994; Johnston, 1996; Robert, 1996).

Prothrombin Times Are Used to Compute the MELD Score. The PT is an integral part of the model for end-stage liver disease (MELD) score in evaluating priority for liver transplantation in liver disease (Trotter, 2004). This score is a computed number based on the values of bilirubin, creatinine, and INR and is applied in categories of 10 (i.e., scores of 40 or higher predict 100% mortality [30–39, 83%; 20–29, 76%; 10–19, 27%; <10, 4%]). Although this score appears to predict accurately the 3-month mortality for cirrhotic patients awaiting liver transplantation (Farnsworth, 2004), it must be used with caution both because reference ranges of these analytes differ among different laboratories, making standardization difficult, and because caveats are associated with using INR values, as described earlier.

Des-γ-Carboxy Prothrombin

The vitamin K–dependent coagulation factors (II, VII, IX, X) are synthesized in the liver and require a vitamin K–mediated posttranslational modification (γ-carboxylation of a number of terminal glutamic acid residues to γ-carboxyglutamic acid) to occur before secretion into the blood, which is necessary for functional activity of these factors in the coagulation cascade. The unmodified precursor of prothrombin, des-γ-carboxy prothrombin (DCP), has been found to be elevated in the sera of patients with hepatocellular carcinoma. DCP is measured using two monoclonal antibodies, 19B7 and MU-3. Recently, a new rapid immunoassay for DCP has been developed (Yamaguchi, 2008). Increases of DCP in patients with hepatocellular carcinoma predict decreased survival times (Nagaoka, 2003). However, assays for DCP do not have the same general use as α-fetoprotein, discussed later, for diagnosing and following this disease, although both analytes are sometimes assayed together in screening for and following this disease.

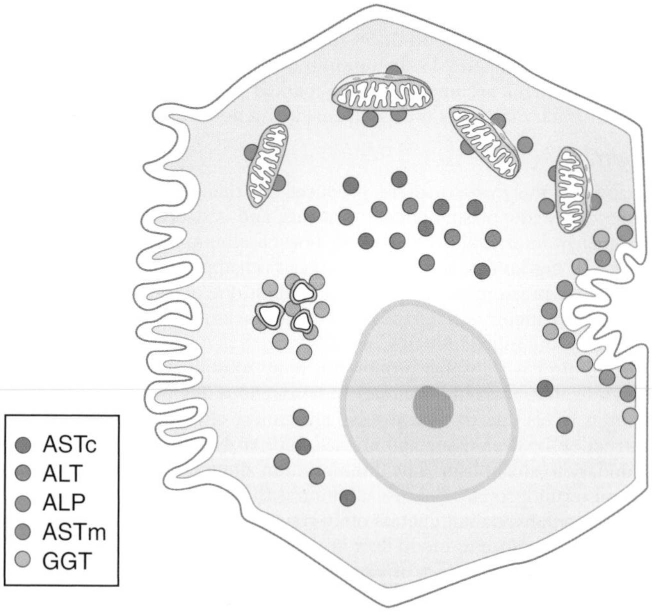

Figure 21-3 Location of hepatocellular enzymes. The major diagnostic hepatocellular enzymes are located at various sites in the hepatocyte, giving rise to different patterns of enzyme release with different causes of injury. Alanine aminotransferase (ALT) and the cytoplasmic isoenzyme of aspartate aminotransferase (ASTc) are found primarily in the cytosol. With membrane injury as in viral or chemically induced hepatitis, these enzymes are released and enter the sinusoids, raising plasma AST and ALT activities. Mitochondrial aspartate aminotransferase (ASTm) is released primarily with mitochondrial injury, as caused by ethanol as in alcoholic hepatitis. Alkaline phosphatase (ALP) and γ-glutamyl transferase (GGT) are found primarily on the canalicular surface of the hepatocyte. Bile acids accumulate in cholestasis and dissolve membrane fragments, releasing bound enzymes into plasma. GGT is also found in the microsomes, represented as pink rings in the figure; microsomal enzyme-inducing drugs, such as phenobarbital and Dilantin, can also increase GGT synthesis and raise plasma GGT activity.

Tests of Liver Injury

PLASMA ENZYME LEVELS

As metabolically complex cells, hepatocytes contain high levels of a number of enzymes. With liver injury, these enzymes may leak into plasma and can be useful for diagnosis and monitoring of liver injury. Although enzymes were discussed in Chapter 20, an understanding of the cellular locations of enzymes and patterns of enzyme change is critical in understanding the findings in various types of liver disease.

Cellular Locations of Enzymes

Within the hepatocyte, the commonly measured enzymes are found in specific locations; the type of liver injury will determine the pattern of enzyme change. Figure 21-3 illustrates the locations of the most important hepatocytic enzymes. Cytoplasmic enzymes include lactate dehydrogenase (LD), aspartate aminotransferase (AST), and alanine aminotransferase (ALT). Mitochondrial enzymes, such as the mitochondrial isoenzyme of AST, are released with mitochondrial damage. Canalicular enzymes, such as alkaline phosphatase and γ-glutamyl transferase (GGT), are increased by obstructive processes.

Mechanisms of Enzyme Release

Enzymes are released from hepatocytes as a result of injury to the cell membrane that directly causes extrusion of the cytosolic contents. In addition, agents like ethanol cause release of mitochondrial AST from hepatocytes and its expression on cell surfaces (Zhou, 1998a). Accumulation of bile salts with canalicular obstruction causes release of membrane fragments with attached canalicular enzymes (Schlaeger, 1982; Moss, 1997). Increased synthesis of GGT, and to a lesser extent alkaline phosphatase, can occur with medications that induce microsomal enzyme synthesis, notably ethanol, phenytoin, and carbamazepine (Aldenhovel, 1988).

Aminotransferases (Transaminases)

Two diagnostically very useful enzymes in this category are AST, also known as serum glutamate oxaloacetate transaminase, and ALT, formerly called **serum glutamate pyruvate transaminase.** These enzymes catalyze reversibly the transfer of an amino group of AST or ALT to α-ketoglutarate to yield glutamate plus the corresponding ketoacid of the starting amino acid (i.e., oxaloacetate or pyruvate, respectively). Both enzymes require pyridoxal phosphate (vitamin B_6) as a cofactor. Using ALT as an example, alanine reacts with pyridoxal phosphate to yield pyruvate plus pyridoxine. Pyridoxine then reacts with α-ketoglutarate to yield glutamate plus regenerated pyridoxal phosphate.

At the core of these reactions is the cofactor, pyridoxal phosphate (vitamin B_6). In many of the serum assays for ALT and AST, it is assumed that the patient's serum provides a sufficient complement of pyridoxal phosphate, a circumstance that does not always apply. In a most poignant case illustrating this point, a patient, a known alcoholic, was admitted to a hospital with a presumptive diagnosis of alcoholic hepatitis, a condition described at length later. His admission clinical chemistry profile showed normal to low serum levels of ALT and AST. This finding is unusual in alcoholic hepatitis because, as we discuss later, both enzymes become significantly elevated such that AST levels are higher than those for ALT. During the course of the next 24 hours, he was treated for his condition, with apparent clinical improvement. However, a repeat liver function profile showed marked elevations of both enzymes to levels greater than 200 IU/L. This presented a diagnostic dilemma, which was resolved when it was realized that, as part of the protocol for treatment of alcoholic hepatitis, the patient had received vitamin supplements, including vitamins B_6 and B_{12}. Because the serum assays for both ALT and AST required vitamin B_6 supplied by the patient's serum, and the patient, an alcoholic, was vitamin B_6 deficient (common in alcoholics), the assays for both enzymes showed normal to low levels caused by the absence of vitamin B_6. Upon therapeutic intervention, when vitamins were administered, sufficient serum levels of vitamin B_6 were present to allow full enzyme activities. This clinical history illustrates the central role of pyridoxal phosphate in enzyme catalysis by AST and ALT, and the importance of understanding the chemical basis for enzyme assays.

AST and ALT have respective blood half-lives of 17 and 47 hours, respectively, and have upper reference range limits of around 40 IU/L. (See Chapter 20 for the definition of international units, or IU.) AST is both intramitochondrial and extramitochondrial, but ALT is completely extramitochondrial. Mitochondrial AST isoenzyme has a half-life of 87 hours (Panteghini, 1990). AST is ubiquitously distributed in the body tissues, including the heart and muscle, whereas ALT is found primarily in the liver, although significant amounts are also present in the kidney.

Total cytoplasmic AST is present in highest activity in hepatocytes, with cell AST level approximately 7000 times that in plasma. ALT is also present in highest activity in hepatocytes, with cell ALT level approximately 3000 times that in plasma. With pyridoxine deficiency, hepatic synthesis of ALT is impaired; a similar phenomenon occurs in hepatic fibrosis and cirrhosis. The enzyme changes seen in hepatic injury can be readily explained by differing hepatic activity levels and half-lives of enzymes. With most forms of acute hepatocellular injury, such as hepatitis, AST will be higher than ALT initially because of the higher activity of AST in hepatocytes. Within 24–48 hours, particularly if ongoing damage occurs, ALT will become higher than AST, based on its longer half-life.

An exception to these observations is seen in acute alcohol-induced hepatocyte injury, as in alcoholic hepatitis. Studies suggest that alcohol induces mitochondrial damage, resulting in the release of mitochondrial AST, which, besides being the predominant form of AST in hepatocytes, has a significantly longer half-life than do extramitochondrial AST and ALT. This frequently results in the disproportionate elevation of AST over ALT, yielding an AST/ALT quotient, also called the **DeRitis ratio,** of 3–4 : 1 in alcohol-induced liver disease. Whether cessation of alcohol consumption reduces this ratio is a topic of disagreement. In one early study, serum mitochondrial AST was measured in cirrhotic and noncirrhotic patients who abused alcohol (Nalpas, 1986). Patients with chronic alcohol abuse, regardless of the extent of their underlying liver disease, had more consistent mitochondrial AST elevations than other patients; values dropped by more than 50% with abstinence for longer than 1 week. On the other hand, in more recent studies, involving more than 300 patients, it was found that high AST/ALT ratios suggest advanced alcoholic liver disease (Nyblom, 2004). It should also be noted that many alcoholics are vitamin B_6 deficient, causing lower rates of synthesis of ALT and suppression of existing ALT activity.

In chronic hepatocyte injury, mainly in cirrhosis, ALT is more commonly elevated than AST; however, as fibrosis progresses, ALT activities typically decline, and the ratio of AST to ALT gradually increases, so that by the time cirrhosis is present, AST is often higher than ALT (Williams, 1988; Sheth, 1998). However, in end-stage cirrhosis, the levels of both enzymes generally are not elevated and may be low as the result of massive tissue destruction. In acute fulminant hepatic failure, as discussed later and in Chapter 8, the serum levels of both aminotransferases are markedly increased and are such that the AST/ALT ratio is often significantly greater than 1 (Sunheimer, 1994).

Overall, ALT activity is more specific for detecting liver disease in nonalcoholic, asymptomatic patients. Mild elevations are often seen in hepatitis C infection. AST is used for monitoring therapy with potentially hepatotoxic drugs; a result more than three times the upper border of normal should signal stopping of therapy. Chronic elevation of aminotransferase activities in asymptomatic patients may have several causes, including alcohol or medication use, chronic viral hepatitis, or nonalcoholic fatty liver disease. Weight reduction may lower ALT in overweight patients whose ALT is elevated (Palmer, 1990). Ursodeoxycholic acid lowers ALT as well as GGT (see later) when these are found to be elevated in blood donors (Bellentani, 1989).

Assays for AST and ALT

Several variants of assays can be used with these enzymes. In one, alanine for ALT or aspartate for AST is added to force the reaction to the right, yielding glutamate. Production of the latter is then coupled to the enzyme glutamate dehydrogenase, in the so-called **indicator reaction,** yielding α-ketoglutarate. In this reaction, nicotinamide adenine dinucleotide (NAD) is converted to NADH (reducing agent derived from NAD), which can be measured as an increase in absorbance at 340 nm. These reactions must be evaluated over short periods because one of the substrates for these enzymes, α-ketoglutarate, is regenerated by the indicator reaction. Another variant for AST involves coupling the oxaloacetate (OAA) that is formed from aspartate in the reaction to malate dehydrogenase, which converts OAA to malate, and in which NADH is converted to NAD that is measured by a decrease in absorbance at 340 nm. For ALT, conversion of alanine to pyruvate allows coupling to the pyruvate dehydrogenase complex in which pyruvate is converted to acetyl coenzyme A, and in which NAD is converted to NADH that can be directly measured by an increase in absorbance at 340 nm. As noted earlier, it is vital that pyridoxal phosphate be present in sufficient quantity to allow these reactions to proceed.

Lactate Dehydrogenase

As described in Chapter 20, this cytosolic glycolytic enzyme catalyzes the reversible oxidation of lactate to pyruvate. As discussed in Chapter 18, five major LD isozymes exist, consisting of tetramers of two forms, H and M, the former having high affinity for lactate, the latter for pyruvate. Progressing from HHHH to MMMM, the five possible isozymes are labeled LD_1–LD_5. LD_1 and LD_2 predominate in cardiac muscle, kidney, and erythrocytes. LD_4 and LD_5 are the major isoenzymes in liver and skeletal muscle. The upper reference range limit for total LD activity in serum is around 150 IU/L (see Chapter 20 for the definition of international units, or IU). Serum LD levels become elevated in hepatitis; often, these increases are transient and return to normal by the time of clinical presentation (Dufour, 1988c; Singer, 1995; Fuchs, 1998) because LD isozymes originating in liver (LD_4 and LD_5) have relatively low activity in hepatocytes relative to plasma (about 500 times) and a half-life of approximately 4–6 hours.

More important is the large increase in total LD to levels of 500 IU/L or more, combined with a significant increase in alkaline phosphatase (ALP), discussed later and in Chapter 20, to levels >250 IU/L, in the absence of other dramatic abnormalities in liver function enzyme levels, especially AST and ALT. These selective increases often accompany space-occupying lesions of the liver, such as metastatic carcinoma and primary hepatocellular carcinoma or, rarely, benign lesions, such as hemangiomata and adenomas. The source of the LD, most often the LD_5 isozyme, is not clear because it can originate from hepatocytes, from the tumor, or from both. The rise in ALP is due to blockage of local canaliculi and ductules by the masses in the liver, as discussed later. Assays for LD are described in Chapter 20.

Enzymes Primarily Reflecting Canalicular Injury

As shown in Figure 21-3, these enzymes are located predominantly on the canalicular membrane of the hepatocyte and include alkaline phosphatase, γ-glutamyl transferase, and 5′-nucleotidase. In contrast to cytoplasmic enzyme activities, canalicular enzyme activities within hepatocytes are typically quite low; focal hepatocyte injury seldom causes significant increases in canalicular enzyme levels.

Alkaline Phosphatase

As discussed at length in Chapter 20, ALP is present in a number of tissues, including liver, bone, kidney, intestine, and placenta, each of which contains distinct isozymes that can be separated from one another by electrophoresis. Total ALP in serum is mainly present in the unbound form and, to a lesser extent, is complexed with lipoproteins or rarely with Igs.

ALP in the liver, which has a half-life of about 3 days, is a hepatocytic enzyme that is found on the canalicular surface and is therefore a marker for biliary dysfunction. The bone isozyme is particularly heat labile, allowing it to be distinguished from the other major forms. In addition, small intestinal and placental ALP is antigenically distinct from liver, bone, and kidney ALP. The bulk of ALP in the serum of normal patients is made up of liver and bone ALP.

In obstruction of the biliary tract by stones in the ducts or ductules, or by infectious processes resulting in ascending cholangitis, or by space-occupying lesions, biliary tract ALP rises rapidly to values sometimes in excess of 10 times the upper limit of normal. The reasons for this increase probably include a combination of increased synthesis and decreased excretion of ALP. In obstructive cholestasis, ALP most commonly rises to twice the upper limit of normal or greater, roughly paralleling the rate of rise in serum bilirubin. If obstruction is partial, ALP usually increases as much as with complete obstruction, often out of proportion to the increase in conjugated bilirubin (dissociated jaundice). Passive congestion of the liver can occasionally result in moderate ALP elevations, more so than abnormal bilirubin levels. ALP is also moderately elevated in most instances of jaundice resulting from hepatic injury. When the resulting cholestasis is relieved, serum ALP levels fall to normal more slowly than bilirubin.

A high molecular weight ALP appears in serum in cholestasis. This ALP is attached to fragments of canalicular membrane. Bile salts solubilize the enzymes from the sinusoidal and canalicular membranes. In serum, the membrane-bound enzymes aggregate with lipids and lipoproteins. This may explain the relationship that has been observed, for instance, with LpX (see Chapter 17). Another form of high molecular weight ALP, which migrates differently on electrophoresis from the isozyme just described, has been found in malignant disease involving the liver (Viot, 1983).

Intestinal ALP is increased in a variety of disorders of the intestinal tract and in cirrhosis. Serum intestinal ALP is detected in more than 80% of cirrhotic patients as compared with 10% of normal controls. Measurement of this enzyme activity was suggested as one method of discriminating intrahepatic from extrahepatic jaundice, because intestinal

ALP may be absent in extrahepatic obstruction, but it lacks adequate sensitivity and specificity (Collins, 1987). Assays for ALP are described in Chapter 20.

γ-Glutamyl Transferase

This enzyme regulates the transport of amino acids across cell membranes by catalyzing the transfer of a glutamyl group from glutathione to a free amino acid. Its major use is to discriminate the source of elevated ALP (i.e., if ALP is elevated and GGT is correspondingly elevated, then the source of the elevated ALP is most likely the biliary tract). The highest values, often greater than 10 times the upper limit of normal, may be found in chronic cholestasis due to primary biliary cirrhosis or sclerosing cholangitis. This enzyme is also elevated in about 60%–70% of those who chronically abuse alcohol, with a rough correlation between amount of alcohol intake and GGT activity (Whitehead, 1978). Levels often decline slowly with abstention from alcohol and remain elevated for at least 1 month after abstinence begins (Belfrage, 1977; Moussavian, 1985). GGT has a half-life of 10 days, but, in recovery from alcohol abuse, the half-life may be as long as 28 days. It tends to be higher in obstructive disorders and with space-occupying lesions in the liver than with hepatocyte injury (Kim, 1977).

The gene for human GGT has been cloned and the nucleotide sequence identified (Rajpert-De Meyts, 1988). GGT can be detected in three major forms in serum (Wenham, 1985), but such determinations are not readily available. A high molecular mass form is present in normal serum, as well as in biliary obstruction, and more frequently in malignant infiltration of the liver. An intermediate molecular mass form consists of two fractions—the major one detected in liver disease and the other one found in biliary obstruction. Determination of these fractions lacks sufficient sensitivity and specificity to be worthwhile (Collins, 1987). The third form is a low molecular mass compound of uncertain importance.

Serum levels of GGT differ from those of ALP during pregnancy, in which GGT remains normal even during cholestasis in pregnancy. GGT is often increased in alcoholics even without liver disease; in some obese people; and in the presence of high concentrations of therapeutic drugs, such as acetaminophen and phenytoin and carbamazepine (increased up to five times the reference limits), even in the absence of any apparent liver injury. Possibly, increases in GGT occur to restore glutathione used in the metabolism of these drugs, which may account for the elevated GGT activities assayed. Glutathione is conjugated to these drugs via the glutathione S-transferase system, and the complex is then excreted.

Most assays for GGT utilize the substrate γ-glutamyl–p-nitroanilide. In the reaction catalyzed by GGT, p-nitroaniline is liberated and is chromogenic, enabling this colored product to be measured spectrophotometrically.

Other Enzymes

5′-Nucleotidase activity is increased in cholestatic disorders with virtually no increase in activity in patients with bone disease. This enzyme is discussed further in Chapter 20. Measurement of 5′-nucleotidase can corroborate the elevation of ALP from a hepatic source. Other enzymes, such as **leucine aminopeptidase (LAP),** can be used for the same purpose but virtually never are. **Isocitrate dehydrogenase** and **OCT** (the latter unique to the liver) activities are elevated in hepatocellular injury and parallel ALT and AST. Again, as with LAP, they are virtually never used in routine laboratory assays.

α-FETOPROTEIN

α-Fetoprotein (AFP) is synthesized by embryonic hepatocytes and fetal yolk sac cells and peaks in the second trimester of pregnancy, reaching levels that constitute up to one third of fetal serum protein. The function of AFP is not known. It may be immunosuppressive, preventing fetal destruction by circulating maternal antibodies.

As discussed in Chapter 25, AFP becomes elevated to abnormal levels in fetal neural tube deficits. The reasons for this correlation are unclear. It is important to note that normal AFP levels vary considerably with gestational age. Therefore, the decision that the serum level of this protein is abnormally high will depend on the reference interval for the gestational age of the patient. Shortly after birth, AFP levels fall, reaching the adult normal range at around 1 year of age. After acute hepatic injury, a rise in AFP (typically 100–200 ng/dL) from regenerating hepatocytes usually occurs. Often, however, these typical elevations after acute hepatic insults do not occur after surgical resection of the liver. Regeneration is therefore not a sufficient impetus for the occurrence of elevated AFP levels.

As discussed in Chapter 73, AFP has been found to be an important marker for hepatocellular carcinoma (HCC) (Zhou, 2006). Elevated levels occur in more than 90% of patients with this disease. As noted previously, elevated levels can also occur after acute liver disease and fibrosis, making this marker somewhat nonspecific. However, at levels >400 ng/dL, there is a high probability of HCC, but at these levels of AFP the tumor is widespread, so its use as an early detector of HCC is limited. Recent studies have shown that serial measurements of AFP in those with HCC receiving chemotherapy may serve as a good prognostic tool (Chan, 2009). Serum levels of AFP in HCC are also dependent on the extent and degree of differentiation of the tumor and the age of the patient. In addition, α-fetoprotein has been used as a marker for rare germ cell tumors, especially yolk sac (endodermal sinus) tumors of infants, and other even rarer tumors such as Sertoli–Leydig cell tumors (Watanabe, 2008).

AUTOIMMUNE MARKERS

Antimitochondrial Antibody Is a Marker for Primary Biliary Cirrhosis

Occasionally, autoimmune disease may be the primary cause of liver injury. The most common autoimmune liver disease is primary biliary cirrhosis (PBC), which occurs primarily in women, usually in the fifth decade, often accompanied by other autoimmune diseases (especially Sjögren's syndrome). There is a strong association of occurrence of this disease among siblings. This condition, which is discussed at length in Chapter 53, causes fibrosis of the bile canaliculi in the portal triads. Bile eventually seeps into hepatocytes, causing necrosis. Granulation tissue replaces hepatocytes, so that fibrosis eventually spreads into the liver parenchyma, giving rise to the pattern of fibrosis and regenerating nodules. A similar course occurs in secondary biliary cirrhosis as a result of other underlying conditions such as choledocholithiasis, carcinoma of the head of the pancreas, and, occasionally, hepatitis and sepsis.

A vital difference between primary and secondary biliary cirrhosis is that the former uniquely appears to be part of a generalized autoimmune condition. More than 90% of patients with primary biliary cirrhosis are found by immunofluorescence to have serum antibodies that react with liver, kidney, stomach, and thyroid tissue. These circulating antibodies, which can be detected in serum using an enzyme-linked immunosorbent assay, are directed against mitochondrial antigens (anti–mitochondrial antigen [AMA]) from the inner mitochondrial membrane, called **M2**, which has been found to be dihydrolipoamide acetyltransferase, a component of the pyruvate dehydrogenase multienzyme complex (Kaplan, 1984; Coppel, 1988; Krams, 1989). Antimitochondrial antibodies have been found in a variety of disease states, but two anti-M2 antibodies in primary biliary cirrhosis uniquely react either with a protein of molecular mass 62 kilodalton (kDa)—the E2 subunit of pyruvate dehydrogenase (Manns, 1987; Fussey, 1988), the predominant autoantibody—or with a 48-kDa E2 subunit of branched-chain oxo-keto-acid dehydrogenase. In other disorders, AMA against M1 antigen has been found in syphilis, anti-M5 in collagen vascular disease, anti-M6 in iproniazid-induced hepatitis, and anti-M7 in cardiomyopathy (Berg, 1986). AMA with anti-M2 specificity is 100% specific for primary biliary cirrhosis.

In a recent human genome–wide study (see Chapter 77), DNA samples from more than 500 patients with this condition and a control group were genotyped for more than 300,000 single-nucleotide polymorphisms (SNPs). This analysis revealed that PBC has a strong association with two SNPs in the HLA-2 region, particularly in the gene encoding interleukin (IL)-12, and a more modest but significant association with SNPs at the signal transducer and activator of transcription 4 (STAT4) locus and the CTLA4 locus, encoding cytotoxic T lymphocyte–associated protein 4. These results now implicate IL-12 signaling and CD4-positive helper T cells in the pathogenesis of this condition (Hirschfield, 2009).

ANCA Is a Marker for Primary Sclerosing Cholangitis

Primary sclerosing cholangitis (PSC) is an autoimmune disease associated with destruction of extrahepatic and intrahepatic bile ducts. More than 80% of patients with this disease have circulating perinuclear antineutrophil cytoplasmic antibodies (p-ANCAs) (Chapman, 2005) with specificities against antigens such as bactericidal/permeability-increasing protein, cathepsin G, and/or lactoferrin (Mulder, 1993; Roozendaal, 1998). Up to

75% also have other autoantibodies such as antinuclear antibodies (ANAs) or anti–smooth muscle antibodies (ASMAs) (Chapman, 1986). There is some question as to whether pANCA, which is a reliable indicator of large cholangiole disease, can likewise serve as a reliable biomarker for PSC involving small cholangioles (Tervaert, 2009). Unlike primary biliary cirrhosis, PSC occurs primarily in young to middle-aged men and is often associated with inflammatory bowel disease, particularly ulcerative colitis.

Serum Markers for Autoimmune Hepatitis

Autoimmune hepatitis is responsible for as much as 3%–5% of chronic hepatitis and occasionally may present as acute hepatitis. Several variants of autoimmune hepatitis are associated with various markers (Czaja, 1995a,b). In the United States, the most common variant, type 1, is associated with ANAs most commonly, and also with antibodies to actin (often detected as ASMAs). Titers of AMAs and/or ASMAs greater than 1:80 support the diagnosis in patients with hepatitis (Johnson, 1993). Type 2 autoimmune hepatitis typically affects children and is much more common in Europe than in the United States, where it is rarely encountered. ANAs and ASMAs are often negative in type 2, and antibodies to liver–kidney microsomal antigens are positive in most cases. Lower-level titers of ANAs or ASMAs are commonly seen in other forms of liver disease, particularly hepatitis C, in which they may be found in up to 40% of cases (Czaja, 1995a,b). Both types of autoimmune hepatitis affect females predominantly.

TESTING FOR VIRAL-INDUCED HEPATITIS

Numerous viruses cause liver damage. Some, such as hepatitis A, B, and C viruses and the arboviruses, are hepatotoxic, but others, such as Epstein-Barr virus, cytomegalovirus, varicella zoster virus, herpes simplex virus, human herpesvirus 6, human immunodeficiency virus (HIV), adenovirus, and echovirus, induce transient to moderately aggressive hepatitis. Even newly identified hepatitis G causes only a self-limited form of hepatitis. In actuality, viruses are the cause of 80%–90% of acute and chronic hepatitis. Although a variety of such viruses can affect the liver, most viral-induced liver pathology is caused by five viruses that are known to cause hepatocyte injury and are termed **hepatitis viruses,** namely, hepatitis A, B, C, D, and E.

Hepatitis A

Hepatitis A virus (HAV) is a member of the picornavirus family of RNA viruses. It is transmitted by the fecal–oral route and typically has an incubation period of 15–50 days with a mean time of about a month, dependent upon the inoculum (Brown, 2003). Epidemics or clusters of HAV infection often occur with conditions of poor sanitation, in day care centers, with military actions, and from contaminated food. Epidemics of HAV occur generally in crowded urban areas, especially where there is a preponderance of uncooked food. Infection with HAV is almost always self-limiting, although in 5%–10% of cases a secondary rise in enzymes occurs. The time course of markers of HAV infection is shown in Figure 21-4.

During the incubation period, HAV RNA is present in stool and in plasma and remains detectable for an average of 18 days after clinical onset of hepatitis (Fujiwara, 1997). The initial immune response to the virus is IgM anti-HAV, which typically develops about 2–3 weeks after infection; increasing AST and ALT develop after antibody development. IgM antibodies typically persist for 3–6 months after infection. The presence of elevated titers of IgM anti-HAV is considered to be diagnostic of acute infection, although some apparently false-positive results have been found (Funk, 2005), resulting in the recommendation that only symptomatic individuals be screened for acute infection using IgM titers. IgG antibodies develop within 1–2 weeks of IgM antibodies and typically remain positive for life (Skinhoj, 1977).

"Total" anti-HAV assays detect both IgM and IgG antibodies. The prevalence of total anti-HAV varies, ranging from 5%–10% in children younger than 5 years to 75% in those older than 50 years of age (Koff, 1995). Following HAV immunization, using attenuated hepatitis A virus, detectable antibody develops in 2–4 weeks and persists to 5 years in 99% of responders (Totos, 1997). Similar protection from the use of Igs in passive immunization seems to occur, although this conclusion is tentative (Liu, 2009). If necessary for epidemiologic purposes, polymerase chain reaction (PCR) assays are available to identify HAV RNA in plasma and stool. There is no need, however, to incorporate the use of PCR for routine diagnostic purposes.

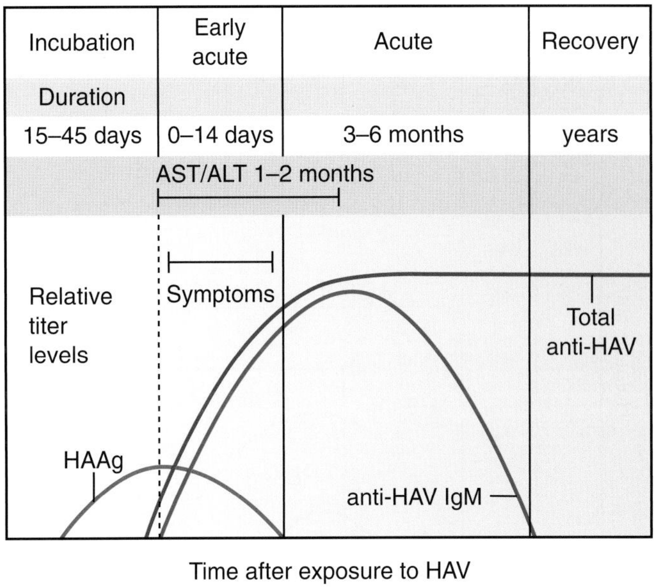

Figure 21-4 Typical time course for appearance of viral antigens and antiviral antibodies in hepatitis A viral (HAV) infection. The appearance of the hepatitis A antigen, HAAg, occurs early on; it is no longer present during the acute phase, during which time jaundice may develop. During the incubation period (which averages 2–3 weeks), HAV RNA is replicating, and viral particles can be detected in stool by immune electron microscopy. Viral RNA is also detectable during this time by real-time polymerase chain reaction (PCR). The most effective diagnostic determination of hepatitis A acute infection is the detection of anti-HAV immunoglobulin (Ig)M. Also shown in this figure is the rise of the aminotransferases, aspartate aminotransferase (AST) and alanine aminotransferase (ALT), which occurs at the beginning of the early acute phase and lasts for several weeks to 1–2 months. The patient ceases to be infectious after anti-HAV IgM falls to undetectable levels in 3–6 months post early phase. Permanent anti-HAV IgG rises over several months and lasts for many years, conferring immunity on the exposed or infected individual. *(Adapted from Abbott Laboratories Diagnostic Educational Services. Hepatitis A diagnostic profile. North Chicago, Ill.: Abbott Labs; 1994, with permission.)*

Hepatitis B

Hepatitis B virus (HBV) is a member of the hepadnavirus (i.e., hepato-DNA virus) family, a group of related DNA viruses that cause hepatitis in various animal species. This virus causes infection of the liver with clinical features that are extremely variable, ranging from absent or mild disease to severe liver failure (Horvat, 2003). Viral particles attach to host cells by an unknown receptor, where they enter the cell by receptor-mediated endocytosis and are transferred to the nucleus by so-called **chaperone proteins.**

Once in the nucleus, HBV replicates by an unusual mechanism (Beck, 2007; Kay, 2007). The viral DNA is partially duplex and consists of a shorter plus strand and a longer minus strand. It consists of four known genes: **C,** that encodes the core protein; X, whose protein product is unknown; P, that encodes DNA polymerase; and S, that encodes the surface protein, also called the **surface antigen.** The latter consists of three open reading frames, giving rise to three types of surface proteins—large, middle, and small. During viral replication, the two unequal strands elongate and become circular. Several messenger RNAs (mRNAs) are transcribed, and the longest is longer than the original coding DNA. This mRNA is secreted into the cytosol, where it is involved in the replication of more virions, requiring the use of **reverse transcriptase,** as in retroviruses. Thus HBV replication requires reverse transcriptase, making it susceptible to reverse transcriptase inhibitors. Four serotypes of HBV (adr, adw, ayr, ayw) and eight genotypes, some of which occur in geographically different regions, have different virulences and may respond differently to different treatment modalities (Kramvis, 2007).

Hepatitis B is transmitted primarily by body fluids, especially serum; however, it is also spread effectively by sex and can be transmitted from mother to baby. Hepatitis B produces several protein antigens that can be detected in serum: a core antigen (HBcAg), a surface antigen (HBsAg or HBs), and e antigen (HBeAg), related to the core antigen; commercial assays are available for HBsAg and HBeAg. Antibodies to each of these antigens can also be measured, and commercial assays for each are available. The time course of self-limited infection with HBV is illustrated in

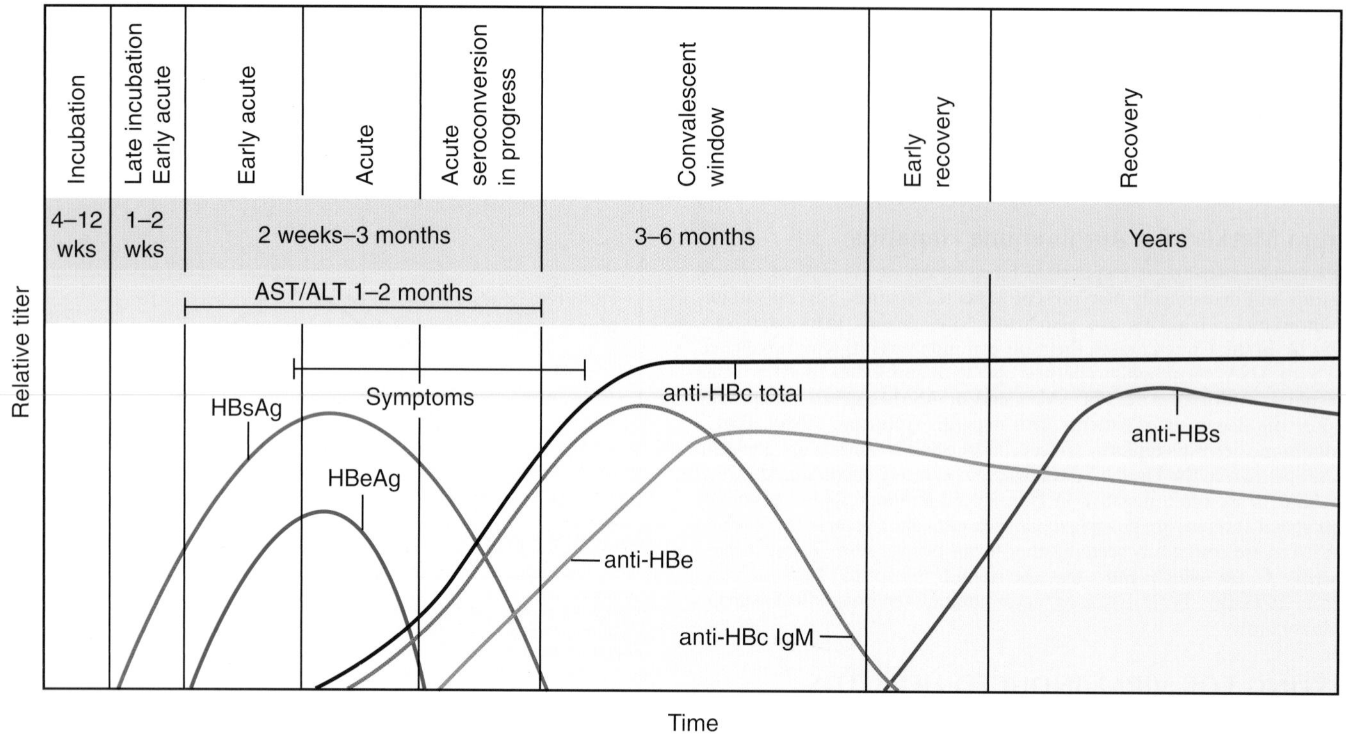

Figure 21-5 Typical time course for appearance of viral antigens and antiviral antibodies in hepatitis B viral (HBV) infection. In the early acute phase, the HBV surface antigen (HBsAg) *(red curve)* appears and lasts for several months. Detection of this antigen signifies acute HBV infection. Between the time the titer of HBsAg falls and the titer of anti-HBV immunoglobulin (Ig)G *(dark blue curve),* which confers immunity, rises, there is a gap of about 6 months. In this time period, the titers of anti-HBV core antigen (anti-HBc) IgM *(purple curve)* and IgG *(black curve)* rise, indicating acute HBV infection. This is the so-called **core window.** IgG anti-HBV e antigen (anti-HBe) *(cyan or light blue curve)* also rises during this core window period. Permanent immunity is conferred by anti-HBsAg IgG (anti-HBs) *(dark blue curve).* It is difficult to determine the time at which the patient is no longer infectious. Generally, an individual is considered noninfectious when no HBsAg or HBeAg, and no anti-HBcAg IgM, can be detected, and the anti-HBsAg IgG has plateaued. Also shown in this figure is the pattern of aspartate aminotransferase (AST) and alanine aminotransferase (ALT) elevations. These occur in the early acute phase, slightly after HBsAg rises. AST and ALT levels may remain elevated for several weeks to several months, after which time they decline. In HBV chronic active hepatitis, HBsAg is present continuously. AST and ALT generally remain elevated, although they can oscillate throughout the course of the disease. *(Adapted from Abbott Laboratories Diagnostic Educational Services. Hepatitis B diagnostic profile. North Chicago, Ill.: Abbott Labs; 1994, with permission.)*

Figure 21-5. Different groups of tests are recommended for three different clinical situations as follows:

1. Acute HBV hepatitis: HBsAg, IgM anti-HBc.
2. Chronic HBV hepatitis: HBsAg, IgG anti-HBc, IgG anti-HBs
3. Monitoring chronic HBV infection: HBs, HBeAg, IgG anti-HBs, IgG anti-HBe, and ultrasensitive quantitative PCR.

The initial serologic marker of acute infection is HBsAg, which typically becomes detectable 2–3 months after infection. After another 4–6 weeks, IgM anti-HBc appears, accompanied by increases in AST and ALT. When symptoms of hepatitis appear, most patients still have detectable HBsAg, although a few patients have neither detectable HBs nor anti-HBs, leaving anti-HBc the only marker of infection **(core window).** IgM anti-HBc typically persists for 4–6 months; however, it may be intermittently present in patients with chronic HBV infection (Czaja, 1988).

In most individuals, HBV hepatitis is self-limited, and the patient recovers; about 1%–2% of normal adolescents and adults have persistent viral replication, which causes chronic hepatitis. The frequency of chronic HBV infection is 5%–10% in immunocompromised patients and 80% in neonates, with the likelihood of chronic infection declining gradually during the first decade of life. With recovery from acute infection, HBsAg and HBcAg disappear, and IgG anti-HBs and IgG anti-HBe appear; development of anti-HBs is typically the last marker in recovery and is thought to indicate clearance of virus. Anti-HBs and anti-HBc are believed to persist for life, although in about 5%–10% of cases anti-HBs ultimately disappears (Seeff, 1987). Isolated anti-HBc can also occur during periods of viral clearance in acute and chronic hepatitis, and as a false-positive result. The titer of anti-HBc is important in determining its significance; low titers are typically false-positive results, and high titers almost always (50%–80% of cases) indicate immunity to HBV infection, as demonstrated by an anamnestic response to hepatitis B vaccine (Aoki, 1993).

The newest assay to assess HBV infection is the ultrasensitive quantitative real-time PCR technology, which is discussed extensively in Part 8. This quantitative HBV DNA PCR detects a highly conserved region of the surface gene at a level as low as 200 copies of viral genome per mL (0.001 pg/mL) with a range up to 2×10^8 copies/mL. Its primary use is to monitor therapeutic responsiveness in clinically infected patients.

Also available is the quantitative digene hybrid capture assay, which employs a signal amplification antibody capture microplate test that utilizes chemiluminescent detection. But this quantitative HBV PCR technique utilizes an RNA probe and has detection limits of 5000 copies/mL (0.02 pg/mL), making it less sensitive than the ultraquantitative assay, although branched-DNA assays, discussed in Chapter 66, are also used widely, with detection limits of 2000 copies/mL. Patients who have clinically recovered from HBV infection and are anti–HBs positive have no detectable HBV DNA using most assays.

Using sensitive PCR assays, circulating HBV DNA can be found in a high percentage of anti–HBs-positive patients who have clinically recovered from HBV infection (Cabrerizo, 1997; Yotsuyanagi, 1998), as well as in patients with hepatitis C and isolated anti-HBc (Cacciola, 1999). The significance of finding low levels of HBV DNA is not known, although in patients with concurrent hepatitis C viral infection this finding may be associated with more severe liver damage. The e antigen has historically been used to detect the presence of circulating viral particles; a good correlation has been noted between levels of HBeAg and amount of HBV DNA (Hayashi, 1996). In chronic HBV infection, approximately 1%–1.5% of patients will spontaneously clear HBeAg each year; some will recover, but others enter a nonreplicative phase in which HBV DNA integrates into the cell genome. This transition phase is often associated with a rise in AST and ALT and, occasionally, jaundice. Rarely, HBeAg may again be detectable in plasma in such patients. Patterns of HBV markers and their interpretation are shown in Table 21-1.

Hepatitis C

Hepatitis C (HCV) is an RNA virus of the flavivirus group consisting of an icosahedral viral protein coat, embedded in cellular lipid and surrounding RNA. The viral RNA encodes a single protein with more than 3000 amino acids that is then processed into individual proteins using viral and host cellular proteases. These include two core proteins, E1 and E2, and

TABLE 21-1
Interpretations of Patterns of HBV Markers

Interpretation	IgM Anti-HBc	Total Anti-HBc	HBsAg	Anti-HBs	HBeAg	Anti-HBe
Incubation period of HBV infection	–	–	+	–	–	–
Acute HBV infection	+	+	+	–	+	–
Recent, resolving HBV infection	+	+	–	+	–	+
Acute HBV infection in core window	+	+	–	–	–	–
Active chronic HBV infection	–	+	+	–	+	–
Chronic HBV carrier state	–	+	+	–	–	+
Resolved HBV infection	–	+	–	+	–	+
HBV immunity after vaccination	–	–	–	+	–	–

HBV, Hepatitis B virus; *HBc,* hepatitis B core; *HBeAg,* hepatitis B e antigen; *HBsAg,* hepatitis B surface antigen; *IgM,* Immunoglobulin M.

TABLE 21-2
Interpretation of Patterns of HCV Markers

Interpretation	Anti-HCV	RIBA	HCV RNA
Acute HCV infection	–	–	+
Active HCV infection	+	+	+
Possible HCV clearance	+	+	–
False-positive HCV test	+	–	–
Requires further study	+	Indeterminate*	–

HCV, Hepatitis C; *RIBA,* recombinant immunoassay.
*Indeterminate result: only one band positive, or more than one band and nonspecific reactivity.

a series of proteins labeled as NS1–5. NS2 is a transmembrane protein, NS3 contains protease and RNA helicase activities, and NS4A and B proteins are known cofactors; NS5A is an interferon-resisting protein, and NS5B is RNA polymerase. The virus has a tropism for hepatocytes that it enters via specific receptors, including CD 81 protein. Once inside the hepatocyte, HCV initiates the lytic cycle utilizing the intracellular translational machinery required for its replication (Lindenbach, 2005). Replication using NS5B RNA polymerase produces a negative-strand RNA intermediate, which then serves as a template for the production of new positive-strand viral genomes. Because viral replication does not involve proofreading, the mutation rate for HCV is high. On the basis of sequencing studies, six genotypes, labeled 1–6, that have been further divided into subgroups (e.g., 1a, 1b, 2a, 2b) have been recognized. Genotype 1a predominates in North America, and 1b predominates in Europe. Genotypes 4 and 5 are unique to Africa. It is important to note that genotypes 1 and 4 are more resistant to interferon therapy than are the other genotypes, resulting in longer treatment times (48 vs. 24 weeks). Thus genotyping has therapeutic implications.

HCV, formerly known as non-A, non-B hepatitis, is the primary etiologic agent, transmitted via blood transfusions and transplantation before 1990. At present, 60% of all new cases occur in injection drug users, but other serum modes of transmission are also seen, such as accidental needle punctures in health care workers, dialysis procedures in patients, and, rarely, transmission from mother to infant. Although sexual transmission is thought to be an inefficient means of transmitting infection, it nevertheless accounts for at least 10% of new cases. Monogamous sexual partners of HCV-infected patients rarely become infected, although a history of multiple sexual partners has been recognized as a risk factor. In contrast to HAV and HBV, chronic infection with HCV occurs in about 85% of infected individuals, with an estimated 4 million individuals chronically infected in the United States alone (Alter, 1999). About half of HCV chronically infected individuals with persistent viremia will have elevated ALT levels. Physical symptoms are absent for the first two decades after infection. As the disease progresses, inflammation and liver cell death can lead to fibrosis, and in about 20% of patients, fibrosis will advance to cirrhosis. The risk for HCC in a patient with chronic HCV is about 1%–5% after 20 years. HCC is seen only in patients with cirrhosis (Shuhart, 2003). Laboratory tests for HCV infection and their common uses are summarized in Table 21-2.

HCV has not been grown in culture; however, HCV genomes can be amplified by recombinant technology. A number of structural and nonstructural antigens have been identified. An immunoassay for the core antigen of HCV has been developed (Aoyagi, 2001) but has been found to be less sensitive than HCV RNA assays (Krajden, 2004). The major diagnostic test for HCV infection has been the second-generation anti-HCV, which detects the presence of antibody to one of four different viral antigens at an average of 10–12 weeks after infection (Alter, 1992a). A third-generation anti-HCV assay detects antibody at an average of 7–9 weeks after infection (Barrera, 1995). IgM anti-HCV is present in both acute and chronic HCV infection and is therefore not helpful diagnostically (Brillanti, 1993). Total anti-HCV typically persists for life, although it may disappear with recovery from HCV infection (Seeff, 1994; Beld, 1999).

In high-risk populations, the predictive value of anti-HCV for HCV infection is over 99%, so that further testing is not typically needed to prove viral exposure (Pawlotsky, 1998). In low-risk populations, such as blood donors, the predictive value of positive anti-HCV is only 25%. In low-risk patients, or when needed to confirm HCV exposure, supplemental tests for anti-HCV should be used. The HCV recombinant immunoassay test uses recombinant HCV proteins isolated in a dot or strip blot assay; this is analogous to Western blot tests used to confirm positivity in other types of infectious disease. Using the second-generation RIBA-2 assay, the presence of antibodies to two (of four) or more HCV antigens is considered a positive result, and the absence of antibodies is considered negative; an antibody to one antigen or an antibody to more than one antigen and the nonspecific marker superoxide dismutase are considered indeterminate results. In the third-generation RIBA assay, isolated antibody to the NS5 antigen is virtually never associated with HCV viremia, suggesting that it may indicate a false-positive result (Vernelen, 1994; LaPerche, 1999).

The primary test for confirming persistence of HCV infection is HCV RNA, detected by a variety of amplification techniques. Quantitative assays can typically detect as few as 1000 copies/mL; however, results from different assays are not interchangeable, and detection limits vary between methods (Ravaggi, 1997; Lunel, 1999). Qualitative HCV RNA assays generally have lower limits of detection compared with quantitative methods using the same amplification technique, are less expensive, and are more useful for detecting the presence or absence of infection.

A World Health Organization standard has been developed to improve comparability between methods (Saldanha, 1999) and is based on an international unit or IU/mL of serum or plasma and on recently developed real-time PCR techniques, which have a detection range of 5–200,000,000 IU/mL, thereby eliminating the need to obtain qualitative and quantitative levels. In a recent study (Shiffman, 2003), it was found, using the international standard, that approximately 90% of serum values for HCV RNA were within 1 log unit, irrespective of which virologic assay was used. However, significant differences in results have been found, a few samples giving a maximum of 2 log unit differences (factor of 100). Such discrepant results may have an impact on the management of patients receiving interferon therapy. These findings suggest that it is important to obtain more than one HCV RNA determination before making treatment decisions (Shiffman, 2003).

With acute infection, HCV RNA is typically present within 2 weeks of infection but falls with development of antibody; as many as 15% of those with acute HCV infection have negative HCV RNA (Alter, 1992b; Villano, 1999). Viral RNA may be intermittently present for the first year of infection, but then becomes persistently present (Villano, 1999). In later stages of infection, HCV RNA levels generally fluctuate by no more than 0.5–1.0 log around mean values (Nguyen, 1996). HCV has a high rate of mutation, similar to that of other reverse transcriptase viruses such as HIV. This produces a number of "quasispecies" of HCV that may emerge, often associated with fluctuating ALT levels (Yuki, 1997). Unique species of

HCV are termed genotypes. In the United States, the most common is genotype 1, divided into subtypes 1a and 1b; these together cause about 65% of HCV infections in Caucasians, but 90%–95% of infections in African Americans (McHutchison, 1999; Reddy, 1999). Genotypes 2 and 3 are generally more responsive to treatment (McHutchison, 1998; Poynard, 1998); other strains are responsible for 1%–2% of infections. Detection of the unique nucleic acid sequences of each strain by one of several nucleic acid methods (Lau, 1995), discussed at length in Part 8, is the most reliable means to identify the responsible genotype in an individual.

Hepatitis D

Hepatitis D (delta-agent; HDV) is an RNA virus that can replicate only in the presence of HBsAg; circulating viral particles have viral RNA inside a shell of HBsAg. Although HDV is rare in the United States, occurring primarily in injecting drug users and hemophiliacs, it is endemic in some parts of the world (London, 1996). Overall, about 20 million individuals may be infected with HDV (Taylor, 2006). In patients with HBV infection, HDV may occur in two forms. If infection with both viruses occurs at about the same time (coinfection), the course of infection is more severe, often follows an atypical course, is a cause of acute fulminant hepatic failure (Sunheimer, 1994), and has a higher fatality rate than HBV infection alone. If HDV infection occurs in the presence of persistent HBV infection (superinfection), progression of disease may be faster. The major diagnostic test is the presence of anti-HDV; both total and IgM antibody tests are available. Both antibodies may eventually disappear following convalescence. The simultaneous assessment of anti-HBc IgM will help differentiate coinfections (present) from superinfections (absent).

Hepatitis E

Hepatitis E (HEV), an RNA virus, now classified as a Hepevirus, with a clinical course similar to that of HAV infection, is common in parts of Asia, Africa, and Mexico, but is rarely seen in the United States, except in individuals who have traveled to endemic areas (Erker, 1999). Similar to HAV, it is spread by the fecal–oral route. Person-to-person transmission of HEV appears to be uncommon. For travelers to endemic areas, the usual food and water hygiene precautions are recommended. Evidence suggests that humans can contract this virus from animal reservoirs (e.g., from uncooked boar and deer meat), but this route of transmission has not been fully verified (Kuniholm, 2008). When infection occurs in pregnancy, there is an increased fatality rate of about 20%, although in general the fatality rate is between 0.5% and 4%. HEV infections range from inapparent illness to severe acute hepatitis, sometimes leading to fulminant hepatitis and death. The signs and symptoms cannot be distinguished from those associated with cases of acute hepatitis caused by other hepatotropic viruses (Schlauder, 2003).

The viral genome encodes at least six proteins, including a capsid protein, whose X-ray structure has recently been determined (Guu, 2009). There are presumed to be five genotypes: 1 and 2 are from humans, 3 and 4 from humans and swine, and a fifth genotype is an avian HEV found in chickens that represents a branch distinct from human and swine HEVs. Genotypes 1 and 2 occur in younger populations, whereas genotypes 3 and 4 occur in older age groups that may be immunocompromised. Antibody tests for HEV are available but appear to have frequent false-positive results, depending on the antigens used to detect reactivity (Mast, 1998). Two serologic tests are available: anti-HEV IgM, which detects recent or current infection, and anti-HEV IgG, which detects current or past infection. Because of the current questionable specificity of serologic assays, a confirmatory test is required. A PCR amplification of an HEV RNA-specific product using serum, plasma, bile, or feces becomes the definitive indicator of acute infection. However, the PCR test window of detection is from 2–7 weeks after infection.

Hepatitis G

Two other viruses have been suspected, but have not been proven, to cause posttransfusion hepatitis: hepatitis G virus (HGV, sometimes called **G-B**) (Laskus, 1997), and transfusion-transmitted virus (Matsumoto, 1999). Although both viruses can be isolated from a high percentage of persons with posttransfusion hepatitis, and viremia is found in at least 1% of blood donors, they do not seem to cause liver disease in these cases. To date, no serologic or PCR assays that can detect these agents are commercially available. Although acute and chronic HGV can be detected at some research centers with a qualitative PCR assay for HGV RNA, no routine testing is recommended because the clinical significance of HGV remains unknown (Shuhart, 2003). Several other viruses, including herpes viruses, can cause hepatitis, but they typically affect other organs as well. These viruses are discussed in Chapter 55.

Diagnosis of Liver Diseases

In Chapter 8, the fundamental patterns of laboratory findings in liver function abnormalities are summarized and are encapsulated in Table 8-5. In this section, the major hepatic disorders are discussed with emphasis on laboratory evaluations that enable diagnoses to be made, often without the need to perform invasive procedures such as liver biopsies.

It is important to remember that in acute hepatitis, the principal changes include significant elevations of aminotransferases; in cirrhosis, these tend to remain normal or become slightly elevated while total protein and albumin are depressed, and ammonia concentrations in serum are elevated. In posthepatic biliary obstruction, bilirubin and alkaline phosphatase become elevated; in space-occupying diseases of the liver, alkaline phosphatase and lactate dehydrogenase are elevated. In fulminant hepatic failure, the aminotransferases and ammonia are elevated, but total protein and albumin are depressed.

HEPATITIS

Hepatitis usually first manifests clinically with the symptoms of fatigue and anorexia. Microscopically, cell injury and generally minimal necrosis are caused both by direct virus (or toxic agent)–induced cell damage and by the immune response to the virus. Jaundice may be present. By far, the most common cause (>90% of cases) of hepatitis is viral, with about 50% of cases due to hepatitis B, 25% to hepatitis A, and 20% to hepatitis C. Jaundice is often initially seen as scleral icterus when the patient has total serum bilirubin concentrations above 2 mg/dL. The cause of *acute* hepatitis is likewise almost always (>90% of cases) viral, although chemical exposure such as to carbon tetrachloride or chloroform or to drugs such as acetaminophen, especially in children, should be considered. A special category of toxin-induced hepatitis is that induced by alcohol, discussed later.

The cardinal finding in hepatitis is a rise in the aminotransferases to values greater than 200 IU/L and often to 500 or even 1000 IU/L. An exception to this finding is seen in hepatitis C, in which only modest elevations of ALT (but not AST) can occur. The AST/ALT ratio generally favors ALT. The bilirubin is frequently elevated and is composed of both direct and indirect types. Frank jaundice occurs in about 70% of cases of acute hepatitis A (Lednar, 1985), 33% of cases of hepatitis B (McMahon, 1985), and about 20% of acute hepatitis C cases (Hoofnagle, 1997). Elevations of indirect bilirubin are due to the inability of injured hepatocytes to conjugate bilirubin, and the rise in direct bilirubin is due to the blockage of compromised canaliculi secondary to the inflammatory process that occurs in the acute phase. Because of hepatocyte damage, LD levels are mildly elevated to values typically around 300–500 IU/L. Because of inflammation and/or necrosis or apoptosis of canalicular and ductular lining cells, the alkaline phosphatase may also be elevated typically to values of 200–350 IU/L. Unless the hepatitis is severe and involves the whole liver, progressing to fulminant hepatic failure, total protein and albumin are within their normal ranges. The γ-globulin fractions may be elevated as a result of infection (Lotfy, 2006).

Given the pattern of the analytes suggestive of hepatitis as previously discussed, screens for specific causes should be made (i.e., determination of serologic markers for hepatitis A, B, and C). Screening for anti–hepatitis A IgM and for HBsAg can be performed within 1 day. If either of these is positive, the diagnosis is established. If negative, further screening for hepatitis B should be undertaken (i.e., determination of serum titers of anti-HBcAg IgM and IgG [core window] and anti-HBsAg IgG, as already described). If only the latter is positive, it may be difficult to establish whether hepatitis B is the cause of the infection, or whether the patient has had past exposure to the virus. Unless the patient has chronic active or persistent hepatitis, in which case HBsAG is continuously present, elevated titers of anti-HBsAg IgG occur long after the aminotransferases return to normal levels. Screens for hepatitis C should also be performed. If these are negative, other viral causes should be sought (e.g., cytomegalovirus, Epstein-Barr virus). Especially in the event that a viral hepatitis screen is negative, nonviral causes, such as chemical toxins, should be considered. In addition, less common causes of hepatitis such as Wilson's disease (see earlier), in which decreased serum ceruloplasmin and increased urinary copper are found, and autoimmune hepatitis should be considered. Both conditions can present as acute or chronic disease; in chronic forms, both can give rise to chronic active hepatitis and, less commonly, cirrhosis. In the chronic form of autoimmune hepatitis (often accompanied by elevations in ANA titers), polyclonal increases in the γ-globulins can usually be detected.

Alcoholic Hepatitis

In alcoholic hepatitis, the previously described pattern of abnormal analyte concentrations holds, except that AST, much of it mitochondrial AST, often becomes disproportionately elevated over ALT. In addition, marked elevations of the enzyme GGT are often out of proportion to elevations in alkaline phosphatase. Unless malnutrition exists in the alcoholic patient, total protein and albumin are found to be within their reference ranges.

Chronic Hepatitis

In chronic hepatitis, hepatocyte damage is ongoing, and chronic inflammation is seen in hepatocytes on biopsy. This condition is caused mainly by chronic hepatitis B or C infection, detected by persisting HBsAg or real-time PCR for hepatitis C sequences, respectively, and is a major predisposing factor for cirrhosis and hepatocellular carcinoma, the two leading causes of death from liver disease. Chronic hepatitis may be asymptomatic or mildly symptomatic. A mild elevation of AST and ALT is seen, and, more commonly in hepatitis C, a mild elevation of only ALT may be noted.

CHRONIC PASSIVE CONGESTION

In chronic passive congestion of the liver, most often secondary to congestive heart failure, back pressure from the right heart is transmitted to the hepatic sinusoids from the inferior vena cava and the hepatic veins. Increased pressure causes sinusoidal dilation, which may cause physical damage to hepatocytes. The result is a mild increase in aminotransferases and occasionally mild hyperbilirubinemia. Other analytes that measure liver function are usually within their reference ranges.

CIRRHOSIS

Cirrhosis of the liver is a condition that results in parenchymal fibrosis and hepatocytic nodular regeneration and can be caused by alcoholism (macronodular or Laennec's cirrhosis), panhepatic hepatitis, chronic active hepatitis, toxins and drugs, and diseases of the biliary tract, such as primary and secondary biliary cirrhosis as discussed previously.

In addition, systemic disease can predispose to cirrhosis. In hemochromatosis, for example, excess iron becomes deposited in a variety of tissues, including liver, and becomes toxic to hepatocytes, predisposing to cirrhosis. As discussed in Chapter 23, this disease is caused by single amino acid substitutions, most commonly tyrosine for cysteine 282 (C282Y), in the protein product of the *HFE* gene on chromosome 6 (Feder, 1996; Crawford, 1998a). This protein is thought to be involved in the interaction of transferrin with the transferrin receptor (Zhou, 1998b), and in amino acid substitutions such as C282Y, which induce protein malfunction, resulting in abnormal iron deposition in tissues, including liver. More recent work suggests that the HFE protein can regulate intracellular iron storage independently of its interaction with transferrin receptor-1 (Carlson, 2005).

Testing for this condition involves determination of the serum iron-binding saturation, discussed in Chapter 23, which is greater than or equal to 45%. This test has high sensitivity but low specificity, diminishing its screening value. Other tests for this condition include determination of iron content of liver biopsy samples and genetic analysis.

As discussed previously, in Wilson's disease, copper deposits in liver are also toxic and can likewise lead to a form of chronic active hepatitis and cirrhosis. In α-1-antitrypsin deficiency, because of continuing proteolysis in hepatocytes, patients have a significantly increased propensity to develop cirrhosis. Chronic hepatitis due to persistent circulating hepatitis B or C virus and autoimmune disease with elevated ANA or ASMA also predispose to cirrhosis.

In general, irrespective of the cause, cirrhosis is a chronic but gradually worsening condition that can occasionally progress to fulminant hepatic failure, as discussed later (Sunheimer, 1994). At its inception, it is often focal and may not be evident clinically.

Diagnosing and Following Cirrhosis, Fibrosis, and Necroinflammation of the Liver Noninvasively Using Serum Analytes

The definitive diagnosis of fibrosis and/or necrosis and inflammation of the liver is attained by liver biopsy. Because this invasive procedure carries with it morbidity such as bleeding and pneumothorax, and because the liver biopsy itself has the confounding problem of sampling errors, a search is under way to devise methods to diagnose and follow these disease processes noninvasively using the levels of serum analytes that measure liver function. The first of these was the **PGA index** (Poynard, 1991), computed from the PT and from serum levels of γ-glutamyl transferase and apolipoprotein A-I. Ranges of values for each of these analytes are divided into four categories, numbered 0–4, in increasing order of severity. For example, GGT values between 20 and 49 are scored as 1, values between 50 and 99 are scored 2, etc. For apoA-I, increasing severity of disease correlates with decreasing concentration of this protein in serum. The prothrombin time increases with severity of disease because the liver is the sole site for synthesis of coagulation factors. These scores are then summed to give the PGA index. Higher PGA scores have been found to correlate with the degree of hepatic fibrosis and with the severity of cirrhosis as judged both by clinical grading and from liver biopsies (Teare, 1993). This index also has a good correlation with the level of procollagen type III propeptide in serum, also used to follow active cirrhosis.

More recently, other indices have been developed that appear to be more effective. These include the Fibrotest and the Actitest index (Poynard, 2004), which utilize the measurement of six analyte levels (i.e., apolipoprotein A1, GGT [these two analytes also being in the PGA index], haptoglobin, total bilirubin, α-2-macroglobulin, and ALT) and also include the patient's age and gender. Correlations with liver biopsy results are then performed based on an artificial intelligence algorithm, resulting in an equation that computes the score on a scale of 0 to 1.0. These scores correspond to the scores of one or more histopathologic staging systems, the most commonly used one of which is called **METAVIR** (METAVIR Cooperative Group, 1994; Bedossa, 1996), as follows: F0, no fibrosis; F1, portal fibrosis; F2, bridging fibrosis with few septa; F3, bridging fibrosis with many septa; and F4, frank cirrhosis. Actitest scores are computed likewise on a scale of 0–1.0, using the same parameters, except that they are correlated with necroinflammatory activity using a METAVIR grading system (Bedossa, 1996) as follows: A0, no activity; A1, minimal activity; A2, moderate activity; and A3, severe activity. These indices are widely used in Europe but thus far not in the United States. Some disagreement has been seen as to the efficacy of these indices in diagnosing and following liver fibrosis and necrosis/inflammatory activity. For example, in one study (Rossi, 2003) on 125 patients with hepatitis C, serum samples were obtained and assayed for the six analytes in the Fibrotest and the Actitest. Using cutoffs of <0.1 to signify minimal fibrosis and >0.6 to indicate severe fibrosis, of 33 patients with a score of <0.1, 6 (18%) were found to have significant fibrosis, and of 24 patients with scores >0.6, 5 (21%) were found to have mild fibrosis on biopsy. On the other hand, in another similar study of more than 300 patients with hepatitis C, for whom analyses were performed before and after a treatment regimen using antiviral agents, high values (almost 0.8) for the areas under the receiver-operator curves (see Chapter 7) were found at pretreatment and posttreatment. The overall sensitivity (see Chapter 7) of the method was 90%, and the positive predictive value was 88%. These values indicate that the index is of value in detecting fibrosis.

It has been pointed out that false-positive results may occur as the result of treatment for hepatitis C with ribavirin because this drug can induce hemolysis, thereby reducing haptoglobin and increasing unconjugated bilirubin, both of which will change the index in a manner unrelated to increasing liver fibrosis (Halfon, 2008). Other conditions that are unrelated to liver fibrosis and can change the index are acute hepatitides, extrahepatic cholestasis (as from choledocholithiasis), Gilbert's disease, acute inflammatory conditions, and severe hemolysis (Halfon, 2008) as mentioned previously. With these caveats, Poynard has estimated that 18% of discordances between liver biopsy and Fibrotest and Actitest results are due to sampling errors on liver biopsy, a known problem with this procedure, especially for small biopsy sample sizes of <15 mm, and that 2% were due to the test (Poynard, 2004). For biopsy sizes of >15 mm, correlation of Fibrotest scores with biopsies resulted in an area of 0.88 under the receiver-operator curve (see Chapter 7). Other investigators have concluded from studies that there is a need for standardization of methods, so that all testing laboratories obtain similar values for individual test results (Rosenthal-Allieri, 2005), as well as a need for large prospective studies (Afdhal, 2004). More recently, it has been found that, overall, Fibrotest, which is now commercially available from the Laboratory Corporation of America (LabCorp, Philadelphia) under the title "Fibrosure," has a similar prognostic value to that obtained from liver biopsy and appears to be the most accurate of the noninvasive biomarker indices (Naveau, 2009).

These other indices (reviewed and evaluated in Parkes, 2006) include the FIBROSpect II index based on tissue inhibitors of metalloproteinases, α-2-macroglobulin, and hyaluronic acid, the latter appearing to give better correlations with liver fibrosis than procollagen type III peptide, as mentioned earlier; the INR; platelet count; ratio of AST to ALT; AST/platelet ratio index, and the Forns index, which correlates age, platelet count, GGT, and cholesterol with extent of liver fibrosis (Forns, 2002). These appear to have similar although somewhat lower sensitivities and/or specificities than the Fibrotest and the Actitest (Thabut, 2003; Naveau, 2009).

Biochemical and Clinical Correlations of Cirrhosis

As cirrhosis progresses to involve most (>80%) of the liver parenchyma, liver function becomes compromised. Total protein synthesis drops to low levels, as does synthesis of albumin. Portal hypertension, together with the drop in colloid osmotic pressure, results in ascites and even anasarca. Compression of the intrahepatic bile ductules and cholangioles results in diminished excretion of bilirubin and bile salts, causing hyperbilirubinemia and a rise in alkaline phosphatase, GGT, and 5′-nucleotidase. The serum concentrations of hepatocyte enzymes such as AST, ALT, and LD may be normal or diminished. If injury to viable hepatocytes is ongoing, the levels of these enzymes in serum may become mildly elevated. In more advanced stages of cirrhosis, serum ammonia levels become significantly elevated and correlate roughly with the degree of encephalopathy.

Four clinically graded levels of hepatic encephalopathy have been identified: motor tremors detected as asterixis, in which the hands of the patient, when pressed back and are then released, move back and forth in a flapping motion; a lethargic, stuporous state; severe obtundation; and frank coma. Lowering ammonia levels reduces the degree of encephalopathy. More recently, earlier signs of encephalopathy have been observed, including sleep disturbance and abnormal results on neuropsychiatric tests.

Because the liver is the site of synthesis of all of the coagulation factors except von Willebrand factor, and because synthesis of these factors is markedly diminished in cirrhosis, coagulation disorders may result, as discussed previously. Accelerated partial thromboplastin and prothrombin times become prolonged, often accompanied by diminished platelet counts. The latter may be caused by splenic sequestration due to splenomegaly caused by portal hypertension. However, disseminated intravascular coagulopathy may occur in cirrhosis, as evidenced by high levels of D-dimer and fibrin split products in serum, and may be the cause of the diminished platelet count. Because of derangements in lipid metabolism in the liver, fats enter the circulation and become deposited in erythrocyte membranes, causing these cells to appear as target cells.

Loss of vascular volume from ascites and anasarca can cause low tissue perfusion and lactic acidosis. Volume receptors, sensitive to volume loss, stimulate the secretion of antidiuretic hormone. The retained water causes serodilution, leading to hyponatremia.

Cirrhosis of the liver is often associated with renal failure as a result of the hepatorenal syndrome. In this condition, which is not well understood, renal tubular function is compromised. Serum blood urea nitrogen and creatinine rise to markedly elevated levels, indicating renal failure. Low tissue perfusion may also cause acute tubular necrosis. In hepatorenal syndrome, restoration of liver function generally reverses the renal failure.

Primary and secondary types of biliary cirrhosis have been discussed previously in this chapter. The diagnosis of these conditions is made difficult by the changing pattern of serum analyte concentrations used to evaluate liver status. Usually beginning as an obstructive pattern, in which alkaline phosphatase and sometimes bilirubin are elevated, the pattern progresses to one that resembles hepatitis because of the toxic effects of bile salts on hepatocytic function. With time, this pattern gives way to a cirrhotic pattern in which the aminotransferases decrease, total protein and albumin decrease, and ammonia rises. In patients with a persistent obstructive pattern indicated by laboratory results, with no evidence of mass lesions or stones causing blockage of bile flow, the presence of anti-M2 antimitochondrial antibody should be ascertained. Increased titers of this antibody are virtually 100% diagnostic of primary biliary cirrhosis. In addition, assays for serum p-ANCA antibodies should be performed to detect secondary biliary cirrhosis, which can also produce a cholestatic pattern.

Survival for patients with primary biliary cirrhosis may be computed using an empirical formula, analogous to the MELD score discussed earlier, that utilizes the age of the patient, the serum albumin and bilirubin, the prothrombin time (as in the MELD score), and the extent of edema (Dickson, 1989). This formula gives an estimate of the time within which the patient may undergo liver transplantation.

POSTHEPATIC BILIARY OBSTRUCTION

Posthepatic biliary obstruction refers to blockage of the intrahepatic and extrahepatic ducts and/or to blockage of bilirubin excretion from the hepatocyte into the canaliculi, leading to backflow of bile into the hepatocyte and ultimately into the circulation. The most common cause of this condition is cholelithiasis. Other causes include primary biliary cirrhosis and primary sclerosing cholangitis, as discussed earlier, and inflammation of the biliary tract, as occurs in ascending cholangitis and in gram-negative sepsis. Drugs such as the neuroleptics, like chlorpromazine, can cause cholestatic jaundice. Mass lesions such as carcinoma of the head of the pancreas or lymphoma can also cause posthepatic biliary obstruction by blocking the common bile duct at the porta hepatis. These conditions cause elevated bilirubin (most of it direct), ALP, and GGT. Often, however, especially in inflammatory conditions in the biliary tract, obstruction to bile flow is incomplete, resulting in partial flow of bile. Under these conditions, bilirubin remains normal or is only mildly increased. However, alkaline phosphatase, GGT, and 5′-nucleotidase become significantly elevated.

Occasionally, hyperbilirubinemia may be observed in patients who are otherwise normal. The bilirubin is of the indirect type and most often results from hemolysis, usually in hemolytic anemia. Hemolytic anemias may be triggered by hepatic disease. For example, viral hepatitis may precipitate hemolysis in patients with glucose-6-phosphate dehydrogenase deficiency. In Zieve's syndrome, hemolysis occurs in conjunction with alcoholic hepatitis and hyperlipidemia. Wilson's disease is sometimes associated with acute hemolysis. Patients with chronic hepatitis secondary to autoimmune disease may develop severe hemolytic disease, sometimes requiring splenectomy.

SPACE-OCCUPYING LESIONS

In space-occupying lesions of the liver, a high percentage of which are due to metastatic cancer; a smaller percentage to lymphoma, primary hepatocellular carcinoma, and angiosarcoma of the liver; and a small percentage to benign lesions such as hemangioma of the liver, the cardinal finding is isolated increases in the two enzymes LD and alkaline phosphatase. Increases in the latter are caused by encroachments of the mass(es) on canaliculi and cholangioles and even on the main bile ducts. The reasons for increases in LD are not clear. Most commonly, it is the LD_5 fraction that is responsible for the increase. This fraction may be produced by the liver but also may be produced by tumors. Typically, the values for LD are 500–1000 IU/L or more, and for alkaline phosphatase, >500 IU/L. If a malignant tumor spreads widely through the liver, mild elevation in the aminotransferases may be seen, along with hyperbilirubinemia due to bile duct obstruction, and low protein and albumin. The latter findings may not be caused as much by liver dysfunction as by generalized cachexia associated with tumor spread. A number of cancers that originate in the liver can be identified using serodiagnostic tests. For example, as discussed earlier in this chapter, serum levels of AFP are elevated in hepatocellular carcinoma. As discussed in Part 9 of this book, angiosarcomas can be diagnosed using specific antibodies to mutated ras-p21 protein.

FULMINANT HEPATIC FAILURE

In acute fulminant hepatic failure, an uncommon but highly fatal condition, massive destruction of liver tissue results in complete liver failure. Depending on the nature and extent of the destruction, ultimate liver regeneration frequently does not occur, although if cell death is limited, and if hepatocytes can recover from the acute injury, normal liver function may return. The causes of this condition are largely unknown. Reye's syndrome is an example of this condition, in which a child has an acute viral infection with fever and is treated with aspirin. Within 1–2 weeks after the infection and fever have dissipated, the child suddenly becomes encephalopathic secondary to hyperammonemia caused by acute hepatic failure. An adult form of Reye's syndrome has also been described. Other possible causes of fulminant hepatic failure include acute hepatitis B with hepatitis D superinfection, Budd-Chiari syndrome and other hepatic vein thrombotic conditions, vascular hypoperfusion of the liver, ileojejunal bypass for obesity, Tylenol intoxication, alcoholism, and cirrhosis. Another significant predisposing condition is the fatty liver of pregnancy (Sunheimer, 1994).

Two histopathologic forms of fulminant hepatic failure are known: panhepatic necrosis, in which all hepatocytes have become necrotic, and microvesicular steatosis, in which sinusoidal enlargement and cholestasis are present. The latter is most commonly observed in Reye's syndrome and the fatty liver of pregnancy. It is important to note that, because the microvesicular steatosis pattern often shows only minimal changes histologically, liver biopsy is unrevealing. It is necessary to rely on laboratory analysis of liver function for a definitive diagnosis, as described later.

Many of the pathophysiologic sequelae of cirrhosis also occur in fulminant hepatic failure (Sunheimer, 1994). Patients develop ascites and become encephalopathic as the result of hyperammonemia. Total serum protein and serum albumin are depressed. Virtually all patients with fulminant hepatic failure exhibit severe coagulopathy, particularly disseminated intravascular coagulopathy, and virtually all are anemic. All develop renal failure as a result of the hepatorenal syndrome and acute tubular necrosis.

In addition, many patients become hypoglycemic, possibly because of the absence of enzymes involved in glycogenolysis. Lactic acidosis also develops as the result of poor tissue perfusion. It is interesting to note that, unlike in cirrhosis, in which patients become hyponatremic, patients with fulminant hepatic failure may become hypernatremic and hypokalemic. This observation may be explained by the finding that circulating levels of aldosterone in the serum of some of these patients are quite high (Sunheimer, 1994). Perhaps failure of the liver to clear aldosterone from the circulation results in the observed high levels of this hormone.

Diagnostic laboratory findings for fulminant hepatic failure include rapid increases in serum levels of the aminotransferases to markedly elevated levels, such that AST, which can reach levels greater than 20,000 IU/L, may be at least 1.5 times greater in value than ALT because of acute release of mitochondrial AST, as discussed previously. Although these enzymes rise in value, the total protein and albumin become markedly depressed. Overall, this pattern resembles hepatitis and end-stage cirrhosis combined, except that usually in acute hepatitis, save alcoholic hepatitis, AST and ALT rise in a ratio of about 1 : 1, or in a ratio that favors ALT. Shortly after these patterns occur, serum ammonia increases rapidly, leading to encephalopathy. LD, alkaline phosphatase, and bilirubin all increase markedly. All of the changes described previously occur over a period of about 1 week. After another week, the serum AST and ALT return to low, sometimes undetectable, levels. This finding signifies complete destruction of all viable liver tissue (Sunheimer, 1994).

Patients whose AST and ALT undergo the stereotypic changes described should be observed closely for fulminant hepatic failure, especially if there is any indication of encephalopathy. Although supportive therapy can sometimes result in restoration of normal liver function, for most patients in fulminant hepatic failure the only ultimate cure is liver transplantation. The MELD score, as discussed earlier, has been shown to have prognostic value in patients with hepatic failure, in particular those with alcoholic hepatitis, and serves as a predictor of patient survival among liver transplant candidates (Dunn, 2005; Srikureja, 2005).

SELECTED REFERENCES

Farnsworth N, Fagan SP, Berger DH, Awad SS. Child-Turcotte-Pugh versus MELD score as a predictor of outcome after elective and emergent surgery in cirrhotic patients. Am J Surg 2004;188:580–3.

This is an excellent survey of the efficacy of different predictive methods for patients with cirrhosis.

Gottesman MM, Ambudkar SV. Overview: ABC transporters and human disease. J Bioenerg Biomembr 2001;33:453–8.

This is a succinct discussion of the family of transporter proteins that share homology within the ATP-binding cassette (ABC) region and contain transmembrane domains involved in recognition of substrates, which are transported across, into, and out of cell membranes, including the bilirubin glucuronides that are secreted by an ABC protein in the canaliculi.

Shiffman ML, Ferreira-Gonzalez A, Reddy KR, et al. Comparison of three commercially available assays for HCV RNA using the international unit standard: implications for management of patients with chronic hepatitis C virus infection in clinical practice. Am J Gastroenterol 2003;98:1159–66.

This is an important summary of the issues concerning standardized international units for assays for hepatitis C.

Sunheimer R, Capaldo G, Kashanian F, et al. Serum analyte pattern characteristic of fulminant hepatic failure. Ann Clin Lab Sci 1994;24:101–9.

This describes the major pathophysiologic aspects of fulminant hepatic failure and gives a summary of liver function profiles in different liver disease states.

REFERENCES

Access the complete reference list online at http://www.expertconsult.com

CHAPTER 22

LABORATORY DIAGNOSIS OF GASTROINTESTINAL AND PANCREATIC DISORDERS

Martin J. Salwen, Haseeb A. Siddiqi, Frank G. Gress, Wilbur B. Bowne[1]

KEY POINTS

- Almost all patients with duodenal ulcers and most with chronic gastritis have demonstrable *Helicobacter pylori* infection. *H. pylori* stool antigen assays and urea breath tests are useful in diagnosis and in monitoring for eradication after treatment.
- Acute pancreatitis presents with abdominal pain and elevated levels of serum amylase or lipase. Reversible causes must be excluded in patients with recurrent episodes of acute pancreatitis. Routine laboratory testing is of limited value in diagnosing chronic pancreatitis.
- Sweat chloride determination is the necessary initial test in the workup for cystic fibrosis. Genetic testing can be used to identify the mutations associated with this disease.
- Patients with chronic diarrhea should be evaluated for fecal blood, fat, leukocytes, and stool pathogens (bacterial culture on routine media, ova and parasite examination).
- *Clostridium difficile* should be considered a cause of diarrhea in patients on antibiotic therapy or hospitalized for more than 3 days.
- Diagnostic evaluation of a patient suspected of celiac disease should be initiated with anti–tissue transglutaminase immunoglobulin A and total serum immunoglobulin A before placing the patient on a gluten-free diet.
- Primary lactose intolerance is common in adults, and secondary lactose intolerance may occur in infection and in inflammatory bowel disease.
- Positivity of perinuclear antineutrophil cytoplasmic antibody is most often associated with ulcerative colitis, and that of anti–*Saccharomyces cerevisiae* antibody with Crohn's disease.
- Endoscopy has replaced gastric acid aspiration for diagnosis. Gastric acid output testing is useful when acid levels are very high or very low.
- Gastrin, the most powerful gastric acid stimulator, varies inversely with gastric acid secretion. Serum gastrin levels are elevated in gastric atrophy, and gastric acid levels are reduced.
- Secretin stimulates gastrin production in patients with a gastrinoma but not in patients with other causes of hypergastrinemia.
- Intraoperative gastrin measurements are useful in identifying whether the abnormal tissue is completely removed in patients undergoing surgery for gastrinomas.
- Fecal occult blood test is used to screen for colon cancer.

Diagnosis of gastrointestinal disease is guided by the patient's history and the significant signs and symptoms. Findings with strong negative predictive values exclude some possible causes and focus the differential diagnosis. Initially, noninvasive procedures are preferentially performed. Patient preparation is as important as correct selection of the diagnostic tests or procedures indicated. Endoscopy, when warranted, can provide direct visualization of the entire gastrointestinal lumen and permits biopsy. Imaging-assisted invasive techniques may be required in the critically ill with gastrointestinal bleeding or obstruction. To ensure interpretable endoscopic results, and to avoid false-positive and false-negative results, stringent patient preparation is required. Similarly, testing requires appropriately collected specimens. Emphasis is given in this chapter to frequently used diagnostic tests.

Pancreatic Disorders

MACROAMYLASEMIA

Macroamylasemia is not a disease, but an acquired benign condition that is more frequent in men and is usually discovered incidentally in the fifth through seventh decades (Remaley, 1989). A persistent increase in serum amylase is seen without clinical symptoms. Urine amylase is normal or low.

[1]The authors gratefully acknowledge the original contributions of Martin H. Bluth, Rosemarie E. Hardin, Scott Tenner, Michael E. Zenilman, and Gregory A. Threatte to Laboratory diagnosis of gastrointestinal and pancreatic disorders. In: McPherson RA, Pincus MR, editors. Henry's Clinical Diagnosis and Management by Laboratory Methods. 21st ed. Philadelphia: WB Saunders; 2007, upon which portions of this chapter are based.

TABLE 22-1
Differential Diagnosis of Hyperamylasemia and Macroamylasemia

Condition	Serum amylase	Serum lipase	Urinary amylase	$C_{am}:C_{cr}$	Serum macroamylase
Pancreatic hyperamylasemia	High	High	High	High	Absent
Salivary hyperamylasemia	High	Normal	Low or normal	Low or normal	Absent
Macroamylasemia	High	Normal	Low	Low	High

Adapted from Kleinman DS, O'Brien JF. Macroamylase. Mayo Clin Proc 1986;61:669–70.
$C_{am}:C_{cr}$, Amylase clearance:creatinine clearance ratio = (urinary amylase/serum amylase) × (serum creatinine/urinary creatinine).

Macroamylases are heterogeneous complexes of normal amylase (usually salivary isoenzyme) with immunoglobulin (Ig)G, IgA, or polysaccharide (Van Deun, 1989). Because of their large size, macroamylases cannot be filtered through the glomerulus and are retained in the plasma; they are not present in urine. Plasma amylase activity is often increased two- to eightfold. Serum lipase is normal. Macroamylasemia is found in about 1% of randomly selected patients. Renal function is normal, and the amylase/creatinine clearance ratio is low (Table 22-1).

PANCREAS IN SYSTEMIC DISEASE

Cystic Fibrosis

Cystic fibrosis (CF) is the most common genetic disorder in Caucasian North Americans and is often fatal in childhood. Some Native American tribes (Pueblo) have a similar incidence. It is also frequent in Hispanics but is uncommon in Asians and blacks. More than 25,000 Americans have CF, and almost 1000 new cases are diagnosed each year. The incidence is 1 in 1600 Caucasian births and 1 in 17,000 African American births in the United States.

CF of the pancreas is an autosomal recessive disease of ion transport affecting the CF transmembrane conductance regulator (CFTR) gene on chromosome 7 that encodes an epithelial chloride channel protein. Approximately 1 in every 20 Caucasians is a carrier of one of the alleles. More than 1300 nonfunctional mutations of the CFTR gene have been identified. Available probes can be used to test for 70 mutations that account for >90% of cases of CF. Genetic testing can identify the mutations associated with CF (Weiss, 2005).

The degree of the defect depends on the nature of the mutation. Several characterized mutations lead to a milder form of the disease. The classic δ *F508* mutation leads to CF when two copies of the gene are inherited. Persons heterozygous for the *R117H* mutation may develop pancreatic insufficiency as the result of plugging of ducts, causing idiopathic chronic pancreatitis (Durie, 2000).

CF is characterized by abnormally viscous mucous secretions from the various exocrine glands of the body, including the pancreas, salivary glands, and peritracheal, peribronchial, and sweat glands. Involvement of the intestinal glands may result in the presence of meconium ileus at birth. Two thirds of cases are diagnosed before 1 year of age. Chronic lung disease and malabsorption resulting from pancreatic insufficiency are the major clinical problems of those who survive beyond infancy, but intelligence and cognitive functions are unaffected and are normal (Cheng, 1990).

Because of multiple alleles at the cystic fibrosis gene, the demonstration of increased chloride in the sweat is a necessary initial test in the workup. More than 99% of children with CF have concentrations of sweat chloride greater than 60 mmol/L. The sweat chloride may not be as dramatically increased in adolescent or adult patients. The test needs to be performed with care (LeGrys, 2007).

In children, chloride concentrations greater than 60 mmol/L in sweat on at least two occasions are diagnostic. Levels of between 50 and 60 mmol/L are suggestive in the absence of adrenal insufficiency. Patients in whom cystic fibrosis is suspected on the basis of indeterminate sweat electrolyte results may undergo confirmatory testing following administration of a mineralocorticoid such as fludrocortisone. In those patients with CF, electrolyte values would remain unchanged, whereas normal controls would show a decrease in sweat electrolytes. Sodium concentrations in sweat tend to be slightly lower than those of chloride in patients with cystic fibrosis, but the reverse is true in normal subjects. Sweat chloride concentrations greater than 60 mmol/L may be found in some patients with malnutrition, hyperhidrotic ectodermal dysplasia, nephrogenic diabetes insipidus, renal insufficiency, glucose-6-phosphatase deficiency, hypothyroidism, mucopolysaccharidosis, and fucosidosis. These disorders usually can be easily differentiated from cystic fibrosis by their clinical symptoms. False-negative sweat test results have been seen in patients with cystic fibrosis in the presence of hypoproteinemic edema.

Sweat electrolytes in about half of a group of premenopausal adult women were shown to undergo cyclic fluctuation, reaching a peak chloride concentration most commonly 5–10 days before the onset of menses. Peak values were slightly less than 65 mmol/L. Men showed random fluctuations up to 70 mEq/L. For this reason, interpretation of sweat electrolyte values in adults must be approached with caution (Rosenstein, 1998; NCCLS, 2000).

Sweat Chloride

Pilocarpine is introduced into the skin by iontophoresis to stimulate locally increased sweat gland secretion. The resulting sweat is absorbed by filter paper or gauze and is weighed, diluted with water, and analyzed for sodium and chloride concentrations. Total body sweating in patients with cystic fibrosis is hazardous, and a number of deaths from the procedure have been reported.

When performed properly in duplicate, the sweat test has a sensitivity of 90%–99%. High rates of incorrect results have been attributed to problems associated with sweat specimen sample collection and test analysis (NCCLS, 2000; LeGrys, 2007).

Heterozygotes have no recognizable clinical symptoms. Homozygotes fully express the syndrome of recurrent pulmonary infection, pancreatic insufficiency, steatorrhea, and malnutrition. CF is due to defective epithelial chloride transport across membranes, which causes abnormally dehydrated tenacious secretions of all exocrine glands. The viscid inspissated mucous plug ducts cause chronic inflammation with atrophy of acini, fibrosis, dilation, and cystic duct changes.

Pancreatic abnormalities occur in >80%. The clinical manifestations are varied. Islets of Langerhans are usually spared. No cure is available. Median survival has increased, in the past 25 years, from 18 to 36 years of age because of advances in treatment. Ninety percent die from pulmonary complications.

Resultant pancreatic lipase deficiency causes maldigestion of fat and steatorrhea. Pulmonary changes are the most serious in cystic fibrosis. Thick intestinal mucus may cause intestinal obstruction in the neonate as the result of meconium ileus. Most CF men are infertile with azoospermia due to duct obstruction.

Hemochromatosis

Excessive body iron accumulation from any source is directly toxic to cells and causes fibrosis. Symptoms include the triad of bronze coloration of the skin, cirrhosis, and diabetes. Humans have no major iron excretory pathway. The screening test consists of transferrin saturation (TS) = serum iron ÷ total iron binding capacity × 100. Results are interpreted as abnormal if >60% in women and >50% in men. Confirm with fasting TS and ferritin levels. Liver biopsy with assay for iron is used to confirm and assess the extent of tissue iron load (Powell, 2002).

Early diagnosis and chelation therapy and/or phlebotomies are effective in preventing tissue damage. In disease, the pancreas is slightly enlarged and deep brown as the result of accumulated hemosiderin, the iron-containing pigment. When untreated, progressive fibrosis of the pancreas with atrophy occurs. Iron is deposited in the acinar and duct cells and in the β cells of the islets. Other cells of the islets appear spared. Similar pigments are noted in the skin. β-cell loss results in **bronze diabetes.** Hypogonadism with pituitary dysfunction is present in half of cases, and cardiomegaly and osteoarthritis are present in most cases. Cirrhosis is seen in 70% of cases. Hepatocellular carcinoma occurs in 30% of cases, and this tumor has become a chief cause of death in hereditary hemochromatosis (HH) (Barton, 1998).

Secondary hemochromatosis is typically seen in anemia caused by multiple blood transfusions, hemolytic anemias, or increased oral iron intake, which result in excess iron storage.

TABLE 22-2
Laboratory Tests in Acute Pancreatitis

Laboratory test	Purpose	Usage and limitations
Amylase	Diagnosis	Accurate over 3× the upper normal limit; decreased specificity in renal failure; normally elevated in macroamylasemia; test interference in hypertriglyceridemia; elevated from other sources such as salivary gland and/or intraabdominal inflammation (not above 3×); can be normal in alcohol-induced pancreatitis
Lipase	Diagnosis	Decreased specificity in renal failure; immune complex creates false positives; elevated from salivary gland and intraabdominal inflammation
Trypsinogen 2	Diagnosis	Limited use; unclear if superior to amylase/lipase
AST/ALT	Etiology	If greater than 3× upper normal limit; gallstones present as cause in 95% of cases; low sensitivity
Lipase/amylase ratio	Etiology	>5 is diagnostic for alcohol-induced acute pancreatitis; low sensitivity
CDT	Etiology	Useful in patients who deny alcohol; remains elevated for weeks after binge drinking
TAP	Severity	>30 mmol/L in 6- to 12-hour urine; 100% negative predictive value
Hematocrit	Severity	>44 on admission, or rising over initial 24 hours; associated with pancreatic necrosis
C-reactive protein	Severity	>200 IU/L associated with pancreatic necrosis; useful after first 36–48 hours

ALT, Alanine aminotransferase; *AST,* aspartate aminotransferase; *CDT,* carbohydrate-deficient transferrin; *TAP,* trypsinogen activation peptide.

Hereditary Hemochromatosis

HH is a human leukocyte antigen (HLA)-linked autosomal recessive defect in duodenal iron absorption regulation. The *HFE* gene is on the short arm of chromosome 6. In this common genetic disease, the homozygosity frequency is 1 in 220. When hereditary hemochromatosis is diagnosed, other family members should be screened; one quarter of siblings will test positive (Powell, 1996; Bulaj, 2000; Beutler, 2002).

INFLAMMATORY DISEASES OF THE PANCREAS

Pancreatitis is an inflammation of the pancreas caused by injury to acinar cells due to activation of digestive enzymes within the pancreatic parenchyma; it is characterized by significant morbidity and mortality. Clinical manifestations of pancreatitis are highly variable.

Acute Pancreatitis

Acute reversible inflammation is due to enzymatic necrosis. Acute pancreatitis occurs at any age—usually 30 to 70 years—but is rare in children. Diagnosis is based on compatible clinical features such as abdominal pain, nausea, and vomiting. Clinical suspicion is supported by findings of elevated serum amylase and/or lipase (Table 22-2). The pancreas contributes 40% of the total serum amylase; the rest comes mostly from the salivary glands (Halangk, 2005).

In 30% of patients, the diagnosis of acute pancreatitis was not suspected and was made only at autopsy (Wilson, 1985). Many causes have been identified. Gallstones continue to be the leading cause (30%–60%), and alcohol is the second most common cause (responsible for 15%–30%). Other causes include duct obstruction due to tumors or parasites, duct anomalies such as pancreas divisum, infections (mumps, coxsackievirus A), blunt trauma or post endoscopic retrograde cholangiopancreatography (ERCP), many drugs (diuretics, sulfonamides), organophosphates, methyl alcohol, nitrosamines, hypertriglyceridemia, and hypercalcemia.

Amylase

Amylase in serum and urine is stable for 1 week at ambient temperature and for at least 6 months under refrigeration in well-sealed containers. Plasma specimens that have been anticoagulated with citrate or oxalate should be avoided for amylase determination because amylase is a calcium-containing enzyme. Heparinized plasma specimens do not interfere with the amylase assay.

Diagnosis is confirmed by detection of elevated serum amylase threefold above normal. It peaks in 20–30 hours, often at 10–20 times the upper reference limit (Papachristou, 2005). Amylase returns to normal in 48–72 hours. Elevated values persisting longer than this suggest continuing necrosis or possible pseudocyst formation. Serum amylase sensitivity is 72%, and specificity is 99% (Treacy, 2001). Serum amylase has poor sensitivity for pancreatitis; it is not increased in about 20% of patients with pancreatitis. Serum amylase increases nonspecifically in many acute abdominal conditions. In hyperlipidemic patients with pancreatitis, normal serum and urine amylase levels are frequently encountered. The spuriously normal levels are believed to be the result of suppression of amylase activity by triglyceride or by a circulating inhibitor in serum. Serum amylase levels do not correlate with cause or severity of pancreatitis. Amylase is also produced by the salivary glands.

Although a variety of reliable amylase methods are available, care is required in specimen handling. Caution must be exercised to avoid contamination of specimens with saliva, because its amylase content is approximately 700 times that of serum. Red cells contain no amylase, so hemolysis does not affect most methods, except those coupled-enzyme methods in which the released peroxide is determined by a coupled-peroxidase reaction.

The urine amylase activity rises promptly, often within several hours of the rise in serum activity, and may remain elevated after the serum level has returned to the normal range. Values greater than 1000 Somogyi units/hour are seen almost exclusively in patients with acute pancreatitis. In a majority of patients with acute pancreatitis, serum amylase activity is elevated, and a concomitant increase in urine amylase activity occurs. Increased renal clearance of amylase can be used in the diagnosis of acute and relapsing pancreatitis, but the ratio of amylase clearance to creatinine clearance expressed as a percentage adds little to the diagnosis, because elevated ratios may be found in unrelated conditions.

Lower than normal serum amylase activity may be found in patients with chronic pancreatitis and has been seen in such diverse conditions as congestive heart failure, pregnancy (during the second and third trimesters), gastrointestinal (GI) cancer, bone fracture, and pleurisy.

Serum amylase may be elevated in patients with pancreatic carcinoma, but often too late to be diagnostically useful. Serum amylase activity may also be elevated in patients with cholecystitis, peptic ulcer, renal transplant, viral hepatitis, or ruptured ectopic pregnancy, or post gastrectomy.

Increased ascites fluid amylase levels have been seen in patients with pancreatitis, a leaking pancreatic pseudocyst, pancreatic duct rupture, pancreatic cancer, abdominal tumors that secrete amylase, and perforation of a hollow viscus. Fractionation of amylase in serum, urine, and other body fluids can be done by physical means, such as electrophoresis, chromatography, or isoelectric focusing; each isoenzyme is then quantitated by direct densitometry.

Lipase

The pancreas is the major and primary source of serum lipase. Human pancreatic lipase is a glycoprotein with a molecular weight of 45,000 Da. Lipase is not present in the salivary glands. Lipases are defined as enzymes that hydrolyze preferentially glycerol esters of long-chain fatty acids at the carbon 1 and 3 ester bonds, producing 2 moles of fatty acid and 1 mole of β-monoglyceride per mole of triglyceride. After isomerization, the third fatty acid can be split off at a slower rate. Lipolysis increases in proportion to the surface area of the lipid droplets, and the absence of bile salts in duodenal fluid with resultant lack of emulsification renders lipase ineffective.

Serum lipase is more specific for the diagnosis of acute pancreatitis. Serum lipase increases in 4–8 hours and remains elevated for 8–14 days. Increased lipase activity rarely lasts longer than 14 days; prolonged increases suggest a poor prognosis or the presence of a pancreatic cyst. Hyperglycemia and elevated bilirubin concentrations may be present, and leukocytosis is frequently reported.

Pancreatic lipase must be differentiated from lipoprotein lipase, aliesterase, and arylester hydrolase, which are related but different enzymes. The activities of these enzymes may be included in the measurement of lipase activity unless suitable assay conditions for **pancreatic lipase** are adapted. Lipase is also present in liver, stomach, intestine, white blood cells, fat cells, and milk.

Calcium is necessary for maximal lipase activity, but at higher concentrations it has an inhibitory effect. It is speculated that the inhibitory effect is due to its interference with the action of bile salts at the water/substrate interface. Similar to serum albumin, bile salts prevent the denaturation of lipase at the interface. Heavy metals and quinine inhibit lipase activity.

Lipase is filtered by the glomeruli owing to its low molecular weight; it is normally completely reabsorbed by the proximal tubules and is absent from normal urine. In patients with failure of renal tubular reabsorption caused by renal disorders, lipase is found in the urine. Urine lipase activity in the absence of pancreatic disease is inversely related to creatinine clearance.

Serum lipase is stable up to 1 week at room temperature and may be kept stable longer if it is refrigerated or frozen. The optimal reaction temperature is about 40° C. The optimal pH is 8.8, but other values ranging from 7.0–9.0 have been reported. This difference probably is due to the effects of differences in types of substrate, buffer, incubation temperature, and concentrations of reagents used. Serum is the specimen of choice for blood lipase assays. Icterus, lipemia, and hemolysis do not interfere with turbidimetric lipase assays.

Both serum lipase and amylase are useful in ruling out acute pancreatitis. Although determination of serum lipase has diagnostic advantages over serum amylase for acute pancreatitis, this value is not specific for acute pancreatitis. Serum lipase may also be elevated in patients with chronic pancreatitis, obstruction of the pancreatic duct, and nonpancreatic conditions, including renal disease, acute cholecystitis, intestinal obstruction or infarction, duodenal ulcer, and liver disease, as well as alcoholism and diabetic ketoacidosis, and in patients who have undergone ERCP. Patients with trauma to the abdomen uniformly have increases in both serum amylase and lipase. Elevation of serum lipase activity in patients with mumps strongly suggests significant pancreatic involvement by the disease.

Trypsinogen

Trypsin is produced in the exocrine pancreas as two proenzymes, known as trypsinogen 1 and trypsinogen 2. These proenzymes are activated in the duodenum by an enterokinase that yields trypsin 1 and trypsin 2, respectively. Trypsin present within the peripheral circulation is inactivated by complexing with α-2-macroglobulin or α-1-antitrypsin (AAT). Trypsin, unlike amylase, is produced solely by the pancreatic acinar cells, and therefore is a specific indicator of pancreatic damage. Premature activation of the proenzyme to active trypsin within the pancreatic parenchyma is thought to be a key mechanism in the development of acute pancreatitis (Andersen, 2001). Currently, levels of all forms of trypsin are determined by specific immunoassays.

Trypsin assays are currently used to differentiate the cause of an acute episode of pancreatitis. One study demonstrated that trypsinogen 2 and trypsin-2-AAT are increased in all forms of acute pancreatitis but are more elevated in alcohol-associated pancreatitis than in biliary pancreatitis. Trypsinogen 1, amylase, and lipase were found to be more elevated in patients with biliary pancreatitis. Furthermore, the ratio of serum trypsin-2-AAT to trypsinogen 1 was determined to be the best discriminator between biliary and alcoholic pancreatitis (Andersen, 2001). Another study supported the use of trypsin assays for the diagnosis of acute pancreatitis, because the determined time course profile of trypsinogen 2 and trypsin-2-AAT is appropriate for diagnostic purposes. These enzymes are elevated within hours of onset of the acute episode and therefore are already elevated upon admission; this is followed by a rapid rise. Both enzyme levels remain elevated longer than amylase, and the magnitude of elevation corresponds to the severity of pancreatic inflammation, which is extremely useful for diagnosing acute pancreatitis upon admission, for predicting severity of illness, and for monitoring disease progression (Kemppainen, 2000). Elevated trypsin-1-ATT has also been demonstrated in patients with biliary tract cancer (Andersen, 2001).

Serum trypsinogen 2 levels rise rapidly, showing a ten-fold to twenty-fold increase. Urinary concentrations are even more steeply elevated. A urinary strip test is available. The limitation is the frequent false-positive elevations seen in cases of nonpancreatic abdominal pain. However, a negative trypsinogen 2 urinary test strip can exclude acute pancreatitis with a high degree of probability. Irrespective of the cause, all origins allow activation of the inactive proenzyme trypsinogen to trypsin, which then activates most of the other digestive enzymes and produces tissue damage and necrosis of the pancreas, surrounding fat, and adjacent structures.

TABLE 22-3
Laboratory Findings in Acute Pancreatitis

At onset		At 48 hours	
Age	>55	Hematocrit	Fall by ≥10%
Leukocyte count	>16,000/mm^3	BUN	Increase by ≥5 mg/dL (1.8 mmol/L) despite fluids
Blood glucose	>200 mg/dL (11.1 mmol/L)	Serum calcium	<8 mg/dL (2 mmol/L)
LD	350 U/L	pO_2	<60 mm Hg
AST	>250 U/L	Base deficit	>4 mEq/L
		Fluid sequestration	>6000 mL

AST, Aspartate aminotransferase; *BUN*, blood urea nitrogen; *LD*, lactate dehydrogenase; *pO_2*, partial pressure of oxygen.

Other enzymes that have been proposed as diagnostic tools include pancreatic isoamylase, phospholipase A, elastase 1, and trypsinogen 2 (Forsmark, 2007). Other tests (aspartate aminotransferase, alanine aminotransferase, C-reactive protein [CRP], hematocrit, carbohydrate-deficient transferrin [CDT], trypsinogen activation peptide [TAP]) have shown low sensitivity for diagnosing acute pancreatitis. CDT is a marker for chronic alcoholism. Urinary TAP is a valuable marker for severity of pancreatitis. Markers of inflammatory response (e.g., CRP) peak, following interleukin (IL)-1 and IL-6 increases, on day 3 after onset of abdominal pain; this is useful in predicting the severity of pancreatitis (Smotkin, 2002).

Computed tomography (CT) scan is the most useful test to establish the diagnosis, with characteristic radiologic findings of enlarged edematous and inflamed pancreas with or without surrounding fluid collection, with or without necrosis. An ultrasonogram may be useful in showing a diffusely enlarged, hypoechoic pancreas, and may show the presence of gallstones in the gallbladder, indicating a possible cause. A CT severity score (the Balthazar score) is based on the degree of necrosis, inflammation, and fluid collection. A 23% mortality rate is associated with any degree of pancreatic necrosis, and a strong association has been noted between necrosis and morbidity and mortality. After initial assessment, a CT scan need not be repeated unless one suspects development of a complication such as pancreatic necrosis. Magnetic resonance imaging (MRI) is being used increasingly to detect pancreatitis, and to characterize the **pancreatic necrosis** seen on CT into peripancreatic necrotic fluid collection, necrotic pancreatic parenchyma, and hemorrhagic foci. MRI can also detect pancreatic duct disruption, seen early in the course of acute pancreatitis.

Serum and urine amylase elevations occur in many conditions other than pancreatitis, such as renal failure, parotitis, and diabetic ketoacidosis. Patients with acidemia may have spurious elevations of serum amylase. This explains why patients with diabetic ketoacidosis may have marked elevations of serum amylase without evidence of acute pancreatitis. No data indicate that measuring both amylase and lipase adds significant diagnostic accuracy. Once the diagnosis is established, daily measurement of amylase or lipase provides little value in gauging the clinical course or the prognosis.

Predictors of severe acute pancreatitis include hematocrit >44% with failure to decrease at 24 hours (this is indicative of pancreatic necrosis and is predictive of organ failure) and C-reactive protein >150 mg/L. Serum creatinine >2.0 mg/dL or marked hyperglycemia (>150 mg/dL) is predictive of mortality (Lankisch, 2001). A strong association has been found between the extent of blood urea nitrogen (BUN) increase and mortality at 24 hours. Each increase in BUN of 5 mg/dL was associated with a corresponding increase in mortality. A reduction in blood urea was associated with significantly improved survival (Wu, 2009) (Table 22-3).

Hemorrhagic pancreatitis, a severe form of acute pancreatitis, results from necrosis within and around the pancreas with hemorrhage that may cause shock and death. Initially, necrosis is coagulative, but necrotic cells rapidly undergo liquefaction. Biliary tract disease with gallstones or inflammation of the gallbladder or bile ducts, or alcoholism, is present in about 80% of patients. The male/female ratio is 1:3 in acute pancreatitis associated with biliary tract disease, and 6:1 in alcoholism. Pancreatic microlithiasis may be responsible for many cases.

The sequence of changes following release of activated intrapancreatic enzymes in acute pancreatitis consists of microvascular leakage causing edema, necrosis of fats, and acute inflammatory reaction. Proteolytic destruction of pancreatic tissue and blood vessels causes edema and focal dilation of acini with variable amounts of hemorrhage. In fat necrosis, neutral fats are broken down, glycerol is reabsorbed, and fatty acids combine with calcium salts to form soaps (saponification) with a zone of acute inflammation around the foci of necrosis. After a few days, secondary infection with suppuration and abscesses may occur.

In 15%–30% of those with pancreatic necrosis, poorly defined areas of acute fluid collection occur, along with fibrosis. The liquefied areas are walled off, and pseudocysts form. Pseudocysts contain pancreatic fluid enclosed in fibrous tissue with no epithelial lining; they often communicate with a pancreatic duct and continue to increase in mass.

Complications of Acute Pancreatitis

Hypocalcemia and mild jaundice may appear after 24 hours as the result of biliary obstruction. A sepsis-like syndrome due to digestive enzymes in the systemic circulation may cause the release of inflammatory cytokines, a systemic immune response syndrome with severe systemic complications. About 75% of patients with acute pancreatitis have a benign course and recover rapidly. No treatment has proven to interrupt the inflammatory process effectively.

Idiopathic acute pancreatitis occurs in about 10%–20% of patients with pancreatitis. It is believed that many cases are germline mutations of cationic trypsinogen *(PRSS1)* or serine protease inhibitor, kazal type 1 *(SPINK1)*. There is high risk for development of endocrine or exocrine insufficiency and pancreatic adenocarcinoma. These mutations can cause an autosomal recessive hereditary acute or chronic pancreatitis with onset in childhood or early adulthood. *PRSS1* abrogates the inactivation of trypsinogen for cleavage of trypsin. *SPINK1* mutation inactivates pancreatic secretory trypsin inhibitor (Howes, 2005; Schneider, 2005).

Patients with these disorders typically have recurrent acute pancreatitis sometime between infancy and the fourth decade. Chronic pancreatitis and pancreatic cancer develop at a relatively young age. No specific treatment is known for the prevention or treatment of hereditary pancreatitis. Clinical testing is available for the disorders described (Etemad, 2001).

Chronic Pancreatitis

It is the irreversible damage and often progressive inflammation with irregular fibrosis, duct dilation, and loss of pancreatic parenchyma that characterize chronic pancreatitis. This occurs after repeated bouts of acute pancreatitis, obstruction of pancreatic duct by mechanical blockage or congenital defect or by neoplasm, gallstone duct obstruction, or alcoholism. Early in the course, the pancreas becomes enlarged. Some cases develop pseudotumor mass lesions. Subsequently, as the result of scarring, the gland usually shrinks with loss of acini and still later loss of ductules. Preserved or even increased islets are seen in the fibrous scar. Patients seek medical attention for abdominal pain or maldigestion.

Maldigestion/malabsorption and steatorrhea are due to pancreatic insufficiency with loss of enzymes; glucose intolerance or diabetes, and islet damage. A low level of fecal elastase is diagnostic. Clinically, recurrent or chronic pain is reported at a lower incidence than in acute pancreatitis, but this is now increasing in frequency. The incidence is greater in males than in females, and the average age of onset is 40 years. It is more prevalent in tropical countries, and the main form is chronic calcifying pancreatitis with duct calcifications. In temperate areas, chronic alcoholism is reported in more than half of cases. No causative factor is apparent in 40% of cases.

The central enzyme involved in activation of all digestive proenzymes is trypsin, which is synthesized and maintained as inactive trypsinogen in secretory granules in the pancreatic acinar cell. After release into the pancreatic duct, trypsinogen is cleaved by enterokinase on the brush border of the duodenum to active trypsin. Trypsin is stabilized in the pancreatic acini by a serine protease inhibitor, *SPINK1*. Mutations in *SPINK1* increase the risk of chronic pancreatitis almost 12-fold by impairing the ability of acinar cells to counteract and inhibit the damaging effects of intracellular trypsin (Schneider, 2004; DiMagno, 2005). *PRSS1* mutations involving codons 29 and 122 cause autosomal dominant forms of hereditary pancreatitis (Whitcomb, 2000; Cohn, 2005).

Gastroenterologic Disorders

PEPTIC ULCERATION

Helicobacter pylori has been recognized as the principal cause of duodenitis and duodenal ulcers, and has been strongly associated with chronic antral gastritis, gastric ulcer, nonulcer dyspepsia, gastric carcinoma, and mucosa-associated lymphatic tissue lymphoma (Peterson, 1991; Veldhuyzen, 1994; Thiede, 1997; Wotherspoon, 1998). The use of nonsteroidal anti-inflammatory drugs (NSAIDs) causes or aggravates peptic and gastric inflammation and ulceration. Hypersecretory states are a much rarer cause of peptic ulcer disease. Data gathered by history and physical examination may initially suggest peptic ulcer disease. Radiologic and/or endoscopic techniques are employed to confirm the diagnoses. Testing for *H. pylori* and hypersecretory states involves laboratory analysis.

Because *H. pylori* has been shown to be the most important cause of peptic ulcer disease and is significantly associated with multiple other types of upper GI pathology, a great deal of research has focused on its detection and treatment, and on confirmation of pathogen eradication. Within the last decade, numerous products used for the detection of this bacterium have become commercially available. A cogent argument has been made that all patients found to harbor this organism should be treated (Graham, 1997). Although the numbers and types of tests will likely continue to grow, tissue sampling, breath tests, and fecal antigen detection are currently the mainstay in the diagnostic armamentarium.

Testing for *H. pylori* often utilizes the organism's ability to produce urease. Radioactive and nonradioactive hydrogen breath tests are examples of noninvasive means for detecting active *H. pylori* infection. Each is sensitive and specific before therapy. The incidental use of proton pump inhibitors (PPIs), antibiotics, or bismuth-containing antacids may lead to false-negative tests. Treatment of *H. pylori* may not lead to complete eradication of the organism. Hydrogen breath tests may be falsely negative if they are performed too soon after treatment, before the bacterial load is great enough to be detected (Atherton, 1994).

Serum antibodies directed against *H. pylori* can be used to detect exposure to *H. pylori*. Enzyme immunoassay (EIA) tests are available and reliable (Feldman, 1995; Feldman & Evans, 1995; van de Wouw, 1996). Although quantitative levels of these antibodies are not currently routinely utilized in the clinical setting to determine whether there is current or past infection, they have been reported to be highly accurate (Lerang, 1998). At present, serology is generally used to screen for *H. pylori*, and breath tests are used to confirm eradication after treatment. Alternatively, endoscopy allows collection of tissue for rapid urease testing or histologic examination (Megraud, 1997).

Urease-based chemical tests are used routinely to detect *H. pylori* in biopsy specimens obtained via endoscopy. Fresh biopsy specimens obtained via endoscopy are placed into fluids or gels containing urea. The bacterial urease splits the urea, producing ammonia. The change in pH affects a color indicator, thus providing the basis for detection. Bacterial load will determine the amount of urease present and can affect the rapidity of the response. If the load is too low, the test can be falsely negative (Xia, 1994).

Office-based serologic quick-test kits are available. The accuracy of these kits has been shown to be dependent on the antibody preparations used. IgG preparations perform most consistently. Other test qualities such as reproducibility, cost, and ease of utilization are factors to be considered when reviewing each of the many available brands marketed today (Laheij, 1998). Histologic review of biopsy specimens stained with Warthin-Starry or Giemsa stain remains one of the most frequently employed techniques to detect active infection. Culture of the organism may be inconsistent and usually is not done in routine clinical settings. If endoscopy must be performed for other reasons, a rapid urease test is the least expensive means of documenting the presence of *H. pylori*.

Hypersecretory states are suggested by extensive peptic ulcer disease, especially in the absence of *H. pylori*, and by the use of NSAIDs. Failure to respond to the usual doses of histamine-2 (H_2)-receptor blocking agents and PPIs also suggests oversecretion of hydrochloric acid. Although gastric analysis remains the "gold standard" with regard to the amount of acid secreted, it is invasive and is used much less frequently. Care must be taken to avoid the use of antisecretory medications for the appropriate time intervals before such testing. H_2-receptor blockers should be held for 48 hours, and PPIs should be avoided for 7 days. H_2-receptor blockers are available without a prescription, so patient education is important, and clinicians must remember to review all of the medications utilized by their patients.

ZOLLINGER-ELLISON SYNDROME

This syndrome is defined by the triad of peptic ulceration, hyperchlorhydria, and non–β islet cell tumors (gastrinomas). Duodenal ulcers do not occur in achlorhydric individuals but are present in those with extreme hyperchlorhydria. Gastrinomas may occur in the body or tail of the pancreas or in the upper duodenum; they may be multiple and malignant.

About 25% of Zollinger-Ellison (ZE) patients have multiple endocrine neoplasia (MEN) 1 with hyperparathyroidism (Hung, 2003).

Gastrin levels, with and without secretin stimulation, can be used to diagnose ZE syndrome. Serum gastrin levels greater than 150 ng/L (reference, <100 ng/L), especially with simultaneous gastric pH values of <3, are highly suggestive of a gastrinoma. For equivocal results, secretin (2 U/kg in 10 mL 0.9% sodium chloride) can be given intravenously in 30 seconds, and serial gastrin levels can be drawn at 0, 2, 5, 10, 15, 20, and 30 minutes. An increase in gastrin of ≥200 ng/L within 15 minutes of injection is considered a positive test result. Octreotide, a synthetic form of somatostatin, has been used for localization of tumors. Radiolabeled octreotide binds to somatostatin receptors and can be subsequently localized by scintigraphy (Zimmer, 1995). If such tumors are surgically removed, gastrin levels can be used to assess potential success or future recurrence (see Gastrinoma in the Neuroendocrine Tumors section).

Gastrin is a primary GI hormone that is produced mainly by the antral G cells; it regulates gastric acid secretion and stimulates growth of the gastric mucosa, among other functions. To a lesser extent, gastrin is produced by G cells of the proximal small intestine and δ cells of the pancreas. Gastrin acts on the parietal cells located in the fundus of the stomach, stimulating the secretion of gastric acid. Gastrin also increases blood flow to the stomach and is responsible for increased gastric and intestinal motility. Other functions include stimulation of gastric pepsinogens and intrinsic factor secretion, release of secretin from the small intestine, and secretion of pancreatic enzymes as well as bicarbonate (Hill, 2006). This hormone is secreted from antral distention mainly after the detection of digested protein products. Maximal stimulation of gastrin secretion occurs within a pH range of 5–7. An acid environment serves as a negative feedback mechanism for the release of gastrin, with 80% reduction in secretion at a pH of 2.5 (Hill, 2006). This serves to protect the stomach from overacidification caused by excess stimulation of gastrin. For this reason, individuals on acid suppression therapy for peptic ulcer disease may have elevated gastrin levels.

Three main forms of gastrin are found in human blood and tissues: G34, G17, and G14, known as big gastrin, little gastrin, and mini gastrin, respectively. There are different assay sensitivities to these forms. All gastrins originate from a single precursor, preprogastrin, which is cleaved by the action of trypsin. It is interesting to note that in pathologic cases of increased gastrin production, as with achlorhydric gastritis or gastrinomas, larger molecular forms of gastrin and incompletely processed precursors are present and are beyond the scope of detection by conventional assays. In such cases, only little gastrin would be detectable in serum (Goetze, 2003).

Laboratory determination of gastrin levels with radioimmunoassay (RIA) or EIA is indicated for the confirmation of suspected gastrin-secreting tumors, namely, gastrinomas or ZE syndrome. The antibodies present in these assays are specific for the biologically active C-terminal of the gastrin molecule, and they have minimal cross-reactivity with cholecystokinin (CCK) peptides. Before determination of gastrin levels, a patient must be fasting for 12 hours because the concentration of G34 doubles and the concentration of G17 quadruples following a meal, altering the results of the assay. Specimens must be frozen immediately because gastrin is unstable in serum. Because of the action of proteolytic enzymes, 50% of the specimen's immunoreactivity may be lost within 48 hours at a temperature of 4° C. It is recommended that specimens should be kept in a freezer at a temperature of −70° C without a self-defrosting cycle, if long-term storage is required. Specimens must be analyzed immediately after thawing, while avoiding refreezing and thawing.

Fasting serum gastrin levels are increased with increasing age, especially in patients older than 60 years, in part because of gastric mucosal atrophy. Approximately 15% of individuals older than 60 years may have gastrin levels between 100 and 800 ng/L (Hill, 2006). Reference intervals for infants and children differ from those for adults; interpretation should use age-specific reference ranges. Gastrin concentration greater than 1000 ng/L with gastric acid hypersecretion (basal acid secretion >15 mmol/hour) is diagnostic of gastrinoma. The secretin stimulation test is a provocative biochemical test that can help confirm the diagnosis of ZE in questionable cases. Infused secretin should cause a drop in gastrin levels in normal individuals. However, in patients with ZE, a dramatic increase in gastrin level is seen after secretin infusion. The mechanism by which secretin stimulates an increase in gastrin levels in these patients is poorly understood; however, it is thought to be due to a direct local effect on blood flow to the tumor (Ashley, 1999). Limitations include altered results from conditions that may lead to elevated gastrin levels such as gastric ulcer disease, chronic renal failure, hyperparathyroidism, pyloric obstruction, vagotomy, retained gastric antrum, short bowel syndrome, and pernicious anemia. Certain medications, such as antacids, H_2-blocking agents, and proton pump inhibitors, can also increase gastrin measurements; all of these agents are commonly used in the treatment of patients with peptic ulcer disease. However, the elevations are moderate and certainly are not as high as in a patient with a gastrin-secreting tumor.

Intraoperative testing for gastrin is of potential use because gastrinomas can be multiple and are often difficult to locate, because they can be distributed widely in the stomach, pancreas, and duodenum or periaortic lymph nodes. Intraoperative gastrin measurement is of potential use because gastrin has a short half-life of approximately 10 minutes. The catabolic breakdown of most peptide hormones follows first-order exponential decay. Therefore, if the entire hormone-secreting tissue is surgically resected, only approximately 12.5% of the baseline concentration would be present in serum after three half-lives. When patients with ZE or gastrinoma were evaluated with intraoperative gastrin assays, a drop in gastrin levels to within reference values within 20 minutes of resection was indicative of cure (Sokoll, 2004).

Pepsin and Pepsinogen

Pepsinogens are the biologically inactive proenzymes of pepsins that are produced by chief cells and other cells in the gastric mucosa and are found in two distinct types: pepsinogen I (PGI), also known as pepsinogen A, and pepsinogen II (PGII), also known as pepsinogen C. Pepsinogen secretion is stimulated by the vagus nerve, gastrin, secretin, and CCK, and is inhibited by gastric inhibitory peptide (GIP), anticholinergics, histamine H_2-receptor antagonists, and vagotomy (Hill, 2006). PGI is produced in the chief cells and mucous cells of oxyntic glands; PGII is produced in mucous cells in oxyntic and pyloric regions and in the duodenum. The ratio of concentration of PGI to PGII in the serum or plasma of healthy individuals is approximately 4:1 (Samloff, 1982). Pepsinogen is converted to the active form, pepsin, by gastric acid that can activate additional pepsinogen autocatalytically. Both groups of pepsinogens are activated at an acid pH below 5 and are destroyed by alkaline pH. Both types can be detected in blood. Only type I pepsinogens are present in the urine. Pepsins are responsible for the hydrolysis of proteins to polypeptides. The pepsinogen released from the gastric mucosa constitutes a major component of gastric fluid. Only approximately 1% gets into the peripheral blood. Active pepsin is rapidly inactivated in the bloodstream, whereas pepsinogen is stable in the blood. Pepsinogen is then filtered by the kidneys and is excreted in the urine, where the slightly acidic pH converts the pepsinogen, now called **uropepsinogen,** to uropepsin (Hill, 2006). Immunoassay is the method used to detect serum pepsinogen. However, the PGI isoform is commonly analyzed in the clinical laboratory because it is the isoform commonly associated with disease.

Serum levels of pepsinogen I provide an accurate estimate of parietal cell mass and correlate with the acid-secretory capacity of the stomach. Increased pepsinogen levels and associated activity are observed in patients with disease states that lead to increased gastric output or with increased parietal cell mass, namely, gastrinoma, ZE syndrome, duodenal ulcer disease, and acute and chronic gastritis. Decreased levels of pepsinogen are associated with decreased parietal cell mass, atrophic gastritis, and gastric carcinoma, as well as with myxedema, Addison's disease, and hypopituitarism (Hill, 2006). The PGI/PGII ratio decreases linearly with worsening atrophic gastritis. Absence of pepsinogen is noted in patients with achlorhydria. PGI levels measured by immunoassay usually range from 20–107 μg/L, and PGII levels usually range from 3–19 μg/L.

Pepsinogen assays are being explored for their utility in the noninvasive identification of patients with chronic atrophic gastritis and to obtain an estimate of the extent of atrophic gastritis, a known precursor of gastric carcinoma. Severe atrophic body gastritis causes a four- to fivefold increase in the risk of gastric carcinoma compared with healthy individuals (Miki, 2003). It is hoped that this finding will help to identify a subgroup of individuals with chronic atrophic gastritis who would benefit from endoscopic evaluation for detection of early-stage gastric tumor. These assays are currently utilized in Japan, an area marked by high prevalence of gastric cancer, as a potential method for widespread screening of high-risk individuals (Miki, 2003). These authors recommended that criteria for diagnosing chronic atrophic gastritis should include persons with PGI <70 μg/L and a PGI/PGII ratio <3.0. In Japan, the pepsinogen serum screening test has been demonstrated to detect a higher percentage of early cancers compared with conventional methods, and a considerable number of patients have subsequently been candidates for treatments with endoscopic surgery (Miki, 2003). The most sensitive test for fundic atrophic gastritis is considered to be the PGI/II serum ratio, with 99% sensitivity and 94% specificity (Hill, 2006). Furthermore, PGII levels may be a useful marker of prognosis, serving as an independent predictor of tumor biology and survival in patients with gastric carcinoma. The absence of PGII production has been associated with aggressive tumor behavior and shorter overall survival in gastric cancer patients (Fernandez, 2000). Pepsinogen assays therefore may prove useful as a serum screening method for detection of gastric carcinoma among high-risk individuals.

DIARRHEA AND MALABSORPTION

Diarrhea

About 8–10 L of fluid enters the duodenum every 24 hours. Much of this fluid is absorbed in the small intestine, and about 1.5 L enters the large intestine, but only 100–150 mL is voided in stools. Increased fluid secretion or decreased fluid absorption in the small or large intestine may result in diarrhea. One of the most important parameters defining diarrhea in an individual patient is a change in the usual bowel habit to more frequent looser stools. Diarrhea is the passage of three or more loose or liquid stools per day, or more frequently than is normal for the individual (WHO, 2009). A decrease in fecal consistency (i.e., increased fluidity) is difficult to measure, thus increased stool weight, frequency, and duration are used in defining diarrhea.

The diagnosis of diarrhea starts with a thorough history to characterize the condition: Is the diarrhea bland or bloody (dysentery); are there constitutional symptoms; what is the duration of the illness? Self-limited, acute diarrhea (<2 weeks in duration) without bleeding or constitutional symptoms rarely requires diagnostic testing. Chronic diarrhea, the passage of blood, and constitutional symptoms all suggest the need for a specific diagnosis. History is the key to developing the differential diagnosis and guiding the laboratory evaluation (Table 22-4). The physical examination, although usually less helpful than the history, must be comprehensive.

Acute diarrheas of <4 weeks generally have an infectious origin. Those with a course of >4 weeks are considered chronic diarrheas (Fine, 1999) and are categorized as osmotic, secretory, or inflammatory. Hypermotility or shortened gut may reduce the transit time and absorptive surface, resulting in diarrhea and/or some degree of malabsorption.

Osmotic diarrhea results from unabsorbable or poorly absorbed solutes. These include polyethylene glycol in colon-cleansing solutions, magnesium salts (magnesium citrate in cathartics, magnesium hydroxide in some antacids), sorbitol in chewing gum, lactulose in the treatment of hepatic encephalopathy, and lactose in lactase-deficient individuals. These osmotically active substances in the lumen alter the osmotic gradient that normally favors Na^+ absorption, drawing fluid into the lumen.

Fasting or cessation of consumption of the suspected solute stops osmotic diarrhea. Stool pH values of <5.6 are consistent with carbohydrate malabsorption (Fine, 1999). Sodium and potassium concentrations in stool water are measured to calculate the fecal osmotic gap, which estimates the contributions of electrolytes and nonelectrolytes to water retention in the gut lumen. Osmotic gap is useful in differentiating osmotic from secretory diarrhea; it is best calculated as $290 - 2 \times ([Na^+] + [K^+])$, where 290 represents the stool osmolality that approximates plasma osmolality, and a factor of 2 is used to account for associated anions. Osmotic gaps of >125 mOsm/kg characterize osmotic diarrhea, and those of <50 mOsm/kg are seen in secretory diarrhea (Fine, 1999).

Stool osmolality must be measured on a freshly collected specimen. Because of continued degradation of stool carbohydrates, osmolality of the specimen increases over hours. Continued diarrhea during a 48-hour fast is suggestive of a secretory process, although fecal weight may decrease because of increasing dehydration (Fordtran, 1967; Fine, 1999).

Disaccharidase Deficiency

Many of the previously listed conditions causing malabsorption may also be associated with intolerance to disaccharides. Disaccharide absorption may be diminished from primary disaccharidase deficiencies such as sucrase-isomaltase deficiency, lactase deficiency, primary alactasia, or primary trehalase deficiency; or from secondary disaccharidase deficiencies due to celiac disease, tropical sprue, acute viral gastroenteritis, or drugs such as orally administered neomycin, kanamycin, and methotrexate. These secondary disaccharidase deficiencies are usually transient and involve more than one enzyme. Although the incidence of lactose intolerance due to congenital lactase deficiency is low, the prevalence of lactose intolerance in adults is quite high. About 10% of Caucasians, 70% to 80% of African Americans, and an even greater percentage of Asians manifest some degree of lactose intolerance, even though they were able to digest lactose well as infants. In these disorders, intestinal bacteria ferment unhydrolyzed and unabsorbed carbohydrates, producing gas, lactic acid, or other organic acids. Normally, absorption of digested carbohydrates is rapid and fairly complete in the proximal small intestine. Unhydrolyzed disaccharides or monosaccharides unabsorbed because of deficiencies in transport are osmotically active and hence cause secretion of water and electrolytes into the small and large intestines. This can result in protracted diarrhea, as well as complaints of bloating and flatulence.

Screening tests for disaccharidase deficiencies include oral challenge of suspected disaccharides to reproduce the abdominal symptoms, followed by stool analysis. The stools are usually watery, acidic, explosive, and fermentative. Stool pH of less than 5.5 is suggestive, but the measurement of pH is not valid if the patient is taking oral antibiotics. High pH does not exclude the diagnosis. Normal infants between 3 and 7 days of age commonly have high stool pH. Stools can be analyzed for sugars by chromatography or by one of the semiquantitative nonspecific tests for urinary sugar adapted for stool analysis. The Clinitest tablet (Bayer Diagnostics, Australia) is suitable for this purpose. The presence of 0.25 g/dL reducing substances is considered normal; from 0.25–0.5 g/dL is regarded as suspicious; and more than 0.5 g/dL is considered abnormal. In patients with intolerance to sugar, the amount of total reducing substance in the stool usually exceeds 0.25 g/dL feces.

An oral tolerance test using a specific sugar such as lactose or sucrose can be used to establish a specific carbohydrate intolerance. Although the oral tolerance test is fairly specific and sensitive, in some instances 23%–30% false-positive results were noted following administration of lactose, that is, a flat tolerance curve and less than 20 mg/dL (1.1 mmol/L) increase in blood sugar (Krasilnikoff, 1975). Delayed gastric emptying appears to be the cause of the false-positive result because duodenal instillation of lactose eliminates the flat tolerance curve.

Definitive diagnosis of disaccharidase deficiency depends on the demonstration of low specific enzyme activity in the mucosa of small intestinal biopsy material. An assay for disaccharidase has been published (Dahlqvist, 1968).

Lactose Tolerance Test

A lactose tolerance test provides a presumptive diagnosis of lactase deficiency. In patients with alactasia or hypolactasia, whether primary or secondary to mucosal disease, oral lactose results in an insignificant rise in blood glucose. Following an overnight fast, a blood sample is drawn, and 50 g of lactose dissolved in 400 mL of water is orally administered. A 100 g lactose dose has been reported to yield more definitive results. Blood samples are collected at 30, 60, and 120 minutes after lactose ingestion. An optional 5-hour stool specimen can be collected, and its appearance, consistency, and pH noted.

Patients with lactase deficiency exhibit a peak rise of <20 mg/dL of reducing substances, expressed as glucose. In individuals with flat tolerance curves, the test should be repeated in 2 days and the less abnormal of the two curves used for interpretation. In patients with lactase deficiency, the nonabsorbed lactose, upon reaching the colon, is degraded to gas and lactic acid, which inhibits salt and water absorption, resulting in abdominal discomfort and diarrhea. In children, the oral dose of lactose or other sugars is 2 g/kg body weight. Lactase can also be detected in a mucosal biopsy specimen.

Secretory diarrhea is evoked by a variety of exogenous and endogenous secretagogues. The hypersecretion of isotonic fluid exceeds the absorptive capacity of the colon. Cholera toxin activates mucosal cyclic adenosine monophosphate (cAMP) that results in outpouring of vast quantities of salt and water in jejunum with normal structure. In Verner-Morrison syndrome (pancreatic cholera), vasoactive intestinal peptide also activates cAMP. Thus, secretory diarrhea remains unrelieved despite fasting.

Diarrhea also occurs in hypergastrinemic states (e.g., ZE syndrome). Sustained hypersecretion of acid lowers intestinal pH, denatures pancreatic enzymes (causing steatorrhea), and precipitates bile salts (causing bile salt malabsorption); the latter induces water secretion in the colon. In patients with mastocytosis, excessive histamine release stimulates acid hypersecretion, but plasma gastrin concentrations remain low or normal. Gastrointestinal dysfunction caused by release of mast cell mediators can be observed in both cutaneous and systemic mastocytosis (Liu, 2010). Signs and symptoms include abdominal pain, diarrhea, nausea, vomiting, peptic ulcer disease, and GI bleeding. Diarrhea can result from increased motility induced by prostaglandin D_2 secretion or from decreased rectal compliance and overactive rectal contractility (Jensen, 2000).

Drug-Induced Diarrhea

Prokinetic agents (metoclopramide, domperidone, cisapride), proton pump inhibitors, and antibiotics (erythromycin and other macrolides)

TABLE 22-4
Laboratory Tests in the Differential Diagnosis of Diarrhea

Test	Method	Use
Initial Screening Tests		
Fecal leukocytes	Wright's stain or methylene blue	Identify inflammatory diarrhea
Fecal occult blood test	Peroxidase reaction for hemoglobin	Identify hemorrhagic diarrhea
Fecal osmotic gap	$290 - 2 \times (\text{fecal } Na^+ + K^+)$	Distinguish secretory vs. osmotic diarrhea
Stool alkalinization	Color change after adding NaOH to stool/urine	Phenolphthalein laxative ingestion
Infectious Causes		
Stool bacterial culture	Routine culture and sensitivity	Identify *Shigella, Salmonella*
Stool special culture	Specialized culture and serotyping	Identify *Escherichia coli* 0157:H7, *Yersinia, Campylobacter*
Stool *Clostridium difficile* toxin assay	EIA for toxins A and B	Pseudomembranous colitis
HIV serology	EIA, Western blot	HIV enteritis
Stool rotavirus screen	EIA for antigen	Rotavirus enteritis
Stool ova and parasites	Concentration and stains	Enteric parasitic infection
Stool mycobacteria	Acid-fast stain and culture, PCR	*M. tuberculosis,* MAI complex
Stool *Entamoeba histolytica* antigen (Ag)	EIA for antigen	*E. histolytica*
Stool *Giardia* Ag	EIA for antigen	*Giardia lamblia*
Stool *Cryptosporidium* Ag	EIA for antigen	*Cryptosporidium parvum*
Endocrine Causes		
Urine 5-HIAA or blood serotonin	HPLC	Carcinoid syndrome
Serum VIP	RIA	VIPoma
Serum TSH, free thyroxine (T_4)	Immunoassay	Hyperthyroidism
Serum gastrin	RIA	Zollinger-Ellison syndrome
Serum calcitonin	RIA	Hypocalcemia-related diarrhea
Serum somatostatin	RIA	Somatostatinoma
Malabsorption		
Lactose tolerance test	See text	Lactase deficiency
Stool-reducing sugars	Clinitest tablets	Carbohydrate intolerance
Sweat chloride	See text	Cystic fibrosis
D-Xylose absorption test	See text	Evaluate jejunal function
Fecal fat stain	Sudan stain for globules	Lipid malabsorption
Serum carotene	Spectrophotometry	Lipid malabsorption
^{14}C-glyceryl trioleate test malabsorption	See text	Lipid malabsorption
Serum IgA	Nephelometry	Rule out IgA deficiency
Anti–tissue transglutaminase antibody	EIA	Celiac disease
Hydrogen breath test	Gas chromatography	Carbohydrate malabsorption
Bacterial colony count	Small bowel aspirate and quantitative culture	Bacterial overgrowth
Other		
Serum ionized calcium	Ion-specific electrode	Hypocalcemia-related diarrhea
Serum protein and albumin	Nephelometry, turbidimetry	IBD, protein-losing enteropathy
Stool α-1-antitrypsin	See text	Protein-losing enteropathy
Quantitative immunoglobulins	Nephelometry	Agammaglobulinemia
7-α-hydroxy-4-cholestin-3-one	HPLC	Bile salt malabsorption
Fecal elastase or pancreolauryl test	EIA	Pancreatic insufficiency
Intestinal biopsy	Endoscopic or open biopsy	Whipple's disease, MAI, abetalipoproteinemia, neoplasia, lymphoma, amyloidosis, eosinophilic gastroenteritis, agammaglobulinemia, intestinal lymphangiectasia, Crohn's disease, tuberculosis, graft-versus-host disease, *Giardia,* other parasitic infections, collagenous colitis, microscopic colitis
Extraintestinal causes	See text	Hyperthyroidism, diabetes, hypoparathyroidism, adrenal cortical insufficiency, hormone-secreting tumors

5-HIAA, 5-hydroxyindoleacetic acid; *Ab,* antibody; *Ag,* antigen; *EIA,* enzyme immunoassay; *HIV,* human immunodeficiency virus; *HPLC,* high-performance liquid chromatography; *IBD,* inflammatory bowel disease; *Ig,* immunoglobulin; *MAI, Mycobacterium avium-intracellulare; PCR,* polymerase chain reaction; *RIA,* radioimmunoassay; *TSH,* thyroid-stimulating hormone; *VIP,* vasoactive intestinal polypeptide.

produce loose stools or diarrhea. Erythromycin binds motilin receptors on the GI smooth muscle membranes (motilin agonist). When used as a prokinetic agent, intravenous administration is more effective than oral dosage, and long-term use downregulates motilin receptors.

Other Causes of Diarrhea

Diarrhea may occur in patients with hypothyroidism and hyperthyroidism, diabetes and adrenal insufficiency, tumors (villous adenoma, small bowel carcinoid), and infiltrative disorders (scleroderma, reactive amyloidosis, gut lymphoma). Ethanol abuse, ischemic bowel disease, and radiation enteritis also produce diarrhea. Heat-labile enterotoxin of *Escherichia coli* and toxins of *Staphylococcus aureus* and *Clostridium perfringens* activate biochemical events that induce a secretory response.

Gut Peptides in Diarrhea

In acute infectious diarrheas, the plasma concentrations of glucagon, PYY, and motilin may be increased, contributing most likely to altered gut motility and promoting mucosal repair. Patients with Crohn's disease have an elevated pancreatic polypeptide, GIP, motilin, and glucagon, and in ulcerative colitis, a modest elevation is observed in pancreatic polypeptide, GIP, motilin, and gastrin, the last in response to the associated hypochlorhydria. No demonstrable abnormalities in gut peptides account for disordered motility in the irritable bowel syndrome.

Vasoactive Intestinal Peptide

VIPomas are rare tumors that secrete vasoactive intestinal polypeptide (VIP). VIP suppresses gastric acid secretion, resulting in secretory diarrhea with stool volume exceeding 700 mL/day in all patients (even during fasting) and 3 L/day in approximately 70%. The stools are tea-colored and odorless, with features of a secretory diarrhea such as persistence with fasting, high sodium concentration, and a low stool osmotic gap. Most patients with VIPoma have the watery diarrhea–hypokalemia–hypochlorhydria (WDHA) syndrome. The diagnosis of VIPoma is established by the presence of an otherwise unexplained high-volume secretory diarrhea and a serum VIP concentration in excess of 75 pg/mL. It is important to replace fluid losses in these patients, and octreotide may be used to control diarrhea.

Patients usually present between 30 and 50 years of age; 90% of cases are primary pancreatic tumors, most commonly arising in the body or tail. Metastatic spread has already occurred in 60%–70% at presentation. Long-acting somatostatin analogs control symptoms in >90% (Kapoor, 2009).

Vasoactive intestinal peptide, released in response to gut distention, is a potent vasodilator and is responsible for the relaxation of vascular and nonvascular smooth muscle of the intestinal tract. It is also a potent stimulator of water and electrolyte secretion, acting through stimulation of cAMP. Similar to glucagons, VIP stimulates breakdown of glycogen and lipid stores and inhibits histamine-stimulated acid secretion in the stomach, resulting in hypochlorhydria or achlorhydria.

Laboratory evaluations for determination of VIP levels are clinically relevant for diagnosis of VIPomas. These VIP-secreting tumors, most commonly of pancreatic origin, account for 10% of neuroendocrine tumors of the gastrointestinal tract. Approximately 60% of VIPomas are malignant, and 6% are associated with MEN type 1. This syndrome was first described in 1958 by Verner and Morrison, and is characterized by WDHA.

VIPomas produce a severe, secretory diarrhea that has been termed pancreatic cholera. Diarrhea may be present for several years before the diagnosis of VIPoma. Patients typically produce more than 3 L of watery stools per day, although volume can be as high as 30 L/day. Diarrhea is not controlled with fasting, and an average secretion of 300 mmol of potassium per 24 hours occurs (Vinik, 2004). Stool volume of less than 700 mL/day excludes the diagnosis of VIPoma. If the diagnosis is missed or delayed, as is often the case, chronic diarrhea results in severe fluid and electrolyte imbalances that produce a myriad of clinical symptoms, the most severe of which is sudden death from cardiac arrhythmias resulting from electrolyte disturbances with potassium depletion and acidosis. The typical metabolic profile seen in these patients is hypokalemia with hyperchloremic metabolic acidosis. The diagnosis of VIPoma is made with confirmation of raised fasting VIP levels in association with secretory diarrhea and the presence of a lesion, most commonly located in the pancreas and associated with VIP production.

The biochemical assay of VIP is sensitive and specific. The normal value for circulating VIP levels is <170 pg/mL. For patients with functional VIP-secreting tumors, values range from 675–965 pg/mL (Thomas, 2003). Appropriate handling of the serum sample is critical for the accuracy of the VIP assay because VIP has a half-life of 1 minute. The serum must be added immediately to aprotinin, a protease inhibitor that prevents breakdown of VIP. The sample must be separated within 10 minutes and frozen to −20° C. Some of the non-VIP products of the precursor molecule are secreted at higher levels than VIP; however, commercially available assays are not available, and clinical utility has not been established. False-positive elevations of VIP can be observed in patients with small bowel ischemia or severe low-flow states resulting from diarrhea and subsequent dehydration not associated with VIP-producing lesions. In addition, serum pancreatic polypeptide level should be determined at the time of the VIP assay; this value will be elevated if the VIPoma is located within the pancreas.

CT scan, MRI, and abdominal ultrasound are useful imaging modalities for VIPoma tumor localization. Angiography can be used to localize smaller tumors. Various nuclear scans have been utilized for localization of VIPomas, including ^{123}I VIP receptor scintigraphy, which is currently under investigation.

Antibiotic-Associated Diarrhea

This term is typically reserved for *Clostridium difficile*, a gram-positive, spore-forming anaerobic bacillus that is the most important cause of nosocomial diarrhea in adults; more than 300,000 cases are reported per year in the United States. It is thought to be associated with approximately 25% of all antibiotic-associated cases of diarrhea and 50%–75% of cases involving antibiotic-associated colitis (Malnick, 2000). It may present clinically, from a mild watery diarrhea to life-threatening pseudomembranous colitis and toxic megacolon. This can lead to colonic perforation and peritonitis, with a mortality rate as high as 38% (Poutanen, 2004). Patients can present with watery diarrhea, lower abdominal pain/cramping, or systemic symptoms such as fever and malaise, or can have occult gastrointestinal bleeding. The pathogenesis of this disease entity usually involves disruption of the normal colonic flora, typically following a course of antibiotic therapy in hospitalized patients, followed by exposure to a toxigenic strain of *C. difficile*. Broad-spectrum antibiotics such as penicillin, clindamycin, and cephalosporins have been particularly implicated; however, any antibiotic can lead to development of *C. difficile* colitis (Malnick, 2000). Clinical suspicion of the disease is confirmed with detection of *C. difficile* toxin A or B virulence factors in stool samples. Toxins A and B lead to increased vascular permeability and have the potential to cause hemorrhage. They induce the production of tumor necrosis factor-α and inflammatory interleukins that are responsible for the inflammatory response and pseudomembrane formation (Poutanen, 2004).

Endoscopic visualization of the colonic mucosa is required for diagnosis of pseudomembranous colitis associated with *C. difficile*. However, endoscopy should be avoided in cases of suspected fulminant colitis because of the risk of perforation. Laboratory methods are available for confirmation of *C. difficile* infection. Tissue culture cytotoxicity assays, which take at least 48 hours to complete, are considered the “gold standard” for the detection of *C. difficile* cytotoxin B in stool specimens, with a sensitivity ranging between 94% and 100% and a specificity of approximately 99%. This tissue culture assay can detect as little as 10 pg of toxin in stool specimens. Rapid EIAs, which can be completed within several hours, have been developed for the detection of toxin A or B from stool specimens. However, the sensitivity and specificity of these immunoassays are 65%–85% and 95%–100%, respectively, compared with cytotoxic assays. The EIA can detect 100–1000 pg of toxin in stool specimens. In hospitalized patients with more than six stools per day, EIA is the optimal diagnostic test (Malnick, 2000). Stool cultures can also be performed but require up to 96 hours for completion. Polymerase chain reaction (PCR) methods for detection of *C. difficile* toxin A or B are currently being developed with similar sensitivity and specificity profiles compared with cytotoxic assays (Poutanen, 2004). However, PCR is unable to distinguish between asymptomatic carriage and symptomatic infection. It is currently recommended that these tests be performed on diarrheal stools; in most cases, one stool sample is sufficient for the diagnosis of *C. difficile* infection (Poutanen, 2004). However, multiple samples may be required for confirmation, and empirical treatment with oral antibiotics may be indicated in patients with clinical evidence of *C. difficile* infection. Diarrheic stools can also be screened by an immunoassay for glutamate dehydrogenase antigen, a *C. difficile*–specific antigen, and those positive should be tested for toxins A and B (Fenner, 2008). Refer to Table 22-5 for laboratory tests available for the diagnosis of *C. difficile*–associated diarrhea.

HIV-Related Diarrhea

Diarrheal disease in human immunodeficiency virus (HIV)-infected individuals is frequently caused by infectious agents but may also be due to infiltrative diseases, such as lymphoma or Kaposi's sarcoma. Common enteric pathogens with sufficient virulence that cause disease in healthy hosts can also cause diarrheal disease in HIV-infected individuals with intact or compromised immunologic function. Less virulent pathogens such as *Cryptosporidium parvum*, which appear to require some immune compromise to establish disease, are more common in patients with more advanced HIV infection or acquired immunodeficiency syndrome (AIDS).

Mycobacterium avium-intracellulare complex (MAC) is predominantly associated with lung infection in immunocompetent patients. MAC may also produce disseminated disease with bowel infiltration and malabsorption in patients with severe immune compromise and should be considered in the differential diagnosis. In these cases, blood should also be obtained in fungal isolator tubes for culture.

In patients with HIV, it is important to ascertain the nature and chronicity of symptoms and the CD4 cell count. Patients with CD4 cell counts <100 cells per microliter are at risk for opportunistic infections that are

TABLE 22-5
Laboratory Tests for the Diagnosis of *Clostridium difficile*–Associated Diarrhea

Test	Advantages	Disadvantages
Clostridium difficile cytotoxin assay	Excellent specificity (99%–100%)	Decreased diagnostic sensitivity (80%–90%); test results not available until after 48 hours; requires tissue culture facility; detects toxin B only
Immunoassay for glutamate dehydrogenase antigen (GDA) of *C. difficile*	High negative predictive value without additional tests	Toxin assay required because GDA does not distinguish toxigenic and nontoxigenic strains
Immunoassay for detection of toxin A or toxins A and B	Good specificity (95%–100%); test results available within 4 hours; technically simple	Reduced sensitivity as compared with cytotoxin assay
Stool culture to isolate *C. difficile* with subsequent cytotoxin assay of isolate	Excellent sensitivity (>90%) and specificity (>98%); enables typing of strain for outbreak investigation	Results not available for at least 72–96 hours; labor intensive; requires tissue culture facility

Adapted from Poutanen SM, Simor AE. *Clostridium difficile*-associated diarrhea in adults. Can Med Assoc J 2004;171:51–8; Fenner L, et al. Rapid and reliable diagnostic algorithm for detection of *Clostridium difficile*. J Clin Microbiol 2008;46:328–30.

typically chronic, such as *C. parvum*, MAC, cytomegalovirus, *Isospora belli*, or microsporidia.

An epidemiologic history with focus on travel history *(Entamoeba histolytica, Giardia lamblia)*, sexual exposure (history of unprotected anal intercourse suggesting transmission of herpes simplex virus, *Neisseria gonorrhoeae*, *Chlamydia trachomatis*, or, occasionally, *E. histolytica*), and food associations (lactose intolerance) should be sought. In patients who are taking highly active antiretroviral therapy, medication-induced diarrhea (nelfinavir, ritonavir) should be considered, particularly when diarrhea is the sole presenting symptom. *Clostridium difficile* should be considered because most patients with HIV are given antibiotics for the treatment of various infection (Sanchez, 2005).

Malabsorption Syndromes

Malabsorption is the pathologic state of impaired nutrient absorption in the gastrointestinal tract. Normal nutrient absorption occurs in three steps: luminal and brush border processing, absorption into the intestinal mucosa, and transport into the circulation. Disruption in any one or a combination of these steps can result in inadequate mucosal absorption of carbohydrates, proteins, fats, vitamins, or minerals. Malabsorption can also result from the presence of substances in the bowel that cannot be absorbed (e.g., lactulose, sorbitol). Maldigestion results from an intraluminal defect that leads to the incomplete breakdown of nutrients into their absorbable substrates. This can occur with pancreatic insufficiency and loss of exocrine function, resulting in increased osmotic load of the colon and diarrhea. In addition, patients can have selective malabsorption/maldigestion of specific nutrients, resulting in associated clinical sequelae. Irrespective of the cause, diarrhea, especially steatorrhea, is the most common feature of malabsorption.

Hepatic maldigestion results from interference or obstruction of bile flow. Loss of bile salts interferes with fat emulsification, diminishing the surface area available for lipolytic action. In addition, bile salt activation of lipase activity is lost. Patients are usually jaundiced, pass dark urine, and have other signs of liver disease. Hepatic steatorrhea may coexist with pancreatic steatorrhea, as in patients with a neoplasm obstructing the ampulla of Vater. The inability to assimilate fats and proteins due to maldigestion also occurs in patients with vasculitis, diabetes mellitus, carcinoid syndrome, hypogammaglobulinemia, and relative vitamin B_6 or B_{12} deficiency.

Enteric malabsorption comprises a variety of conditions that have in common normal digestion but inadequate net assimilation of nutrients. This may result from competition by bacteria or altered bacterial flora, as in the blind loop syndrome or diverticulosis of the small bowel, or from obstruction to the flow of lymph. It may also result from diseases affecting the small bowel mucosa, such as amyloidosis, inflammation following irradiation (radiation enteritis), diminished mucosal surface area as in gastroileostomy (gastric bypass), or small bowel resection. Depending on the location within the intestinal tract of such pathology, preferential loss of specific substrates may occur. One of the most common clinical scenarios encountered is regional enteritis localized to the distal ileum, the site of vitamin B_{12} and bile salt absorption, which will result in vitamin B_{12} deficiency, as well as a decreased pool of circulating bile salts for metabolism.

Steatorrhea is a hallmark finding in patients with malabsorption, resulting in fluid, semifluid, or soft and pasty, pale, bulky, and foul-smelling stools. These stools may be foamy because of the high fat content and may float on water. However, the latter may occur with stools from healthy individuals and therefore is a nonspecific sign of malabsorption.

In patients with steatorrhea, unabsorbed fecal dietary fat is passed in stools above and beyond the normal 1%–9%, along with as much as 40% of ingested fat. The quantity of fecal fat depends on the dietary fat intake. Thus, dietary fat intake must be known for proper interpretation of fecal fat, which is expressed as percentage of dietary fat, allowing assessment of variation in an individual patient. Normally, >93% of dietary fat is absorbed, but diarrhea of any cause may lead to a slight increase in fecal fat content.

Another clinical presentation of malabsorption is the development of fat-soluble vitamin (A, D, E, and K) deficiencies. Primary and secondary alterations of the bowel mucosa may also result in deficiencies of water-soluble vitamins. Other evidence of nutritional deficiencies, such as hypoprothrombinemia, glossitis, anemia, edema, ascites, and osteomalacia, may be evident in these individuals. These patients may experience significant weight loss due to diarrhea, leading to cachexia in severe cases.

Quantitative fecal fat measurement has many limitations and should be abandoned (Holmes, 1988; Hill, 2001). Sample collection is known to be incomplete (Ditchburn, 1971; West, 1981). Also, there is poor precision in the analytic performance, making interpretation uncertain (Duncan, 1998). Newer tests provide improved sensitivity and specificity for the diagnosis of malabsorption (Hill, 2001): ^{14}C-glycerol trioleate breath test (Turner, 1987) and mixed-chain triglyceride breath test are widely available (Vantrappen, 1989; Amarri, 1997). However, these tests have limited reliability in diabetes, obesity, hyperthyroidism and hypothyroidism, and chronic respiratory insufficiency, and should not be performed in pregnancy.

The test is based on the measurement of $^{14}CO_2$ in expired air following the ingestion of various ^{14}C-labeled triglycerides (triolein, tripalmitin, and trioctanoin). Steatorrhea from pancreatic insufficiency or other causes results in decreased absorption of triglycerides. This in turn results in a decrease in expired carbon dioxide (CO_2) derived through the metabolism of triglyceride fatty acids.

After an overnight fast, the patient consumes ^{14}C-labeled triglyceride. Periodically, breath CO_2 is collected in a trapping solution containing an indicator that changes color when a predetermined amount of CO_2 is in solution. The radioactivity of the $^{14}CO_2$ is then measured in a liquid scintillation counter, and the results are reported as a percentage of the dose of $^{14}CO_2$ excreted per hour.

To distinguish pancreatic insufficiency from other causes of steatorrhea, some investigators have developed a two-stage breath test (Goff, 1982). In the first stage of the test, the patient consumes a ^{14}C-labeled triglyceride, and $^{14}CO_2$ is measured as previously described. The second stage of the test is performed 5–7 days later and is the same as the first stage, except that the patient is given an oral dose of pancreatic enzymes along with the dose of ^{14}C-labeled triglyceride. In patients with steatorrhea due to pancreatic insufficiency, the amount of $^{14}CO_2$ expired should increase relative to the amount of $^{14}CO_2$ expired in the first stage of the test. Patients with steatorrhea from other causes should show no significant change in the amount of $^{14}CO_2$ expired following the oral administration of pancreatic enzymes.

Agammaglobulinemia

X-linked agammaglobulinemia is a primary humoral immunodeficiency characterized by recurrent bacterial infection of the respiratory tract and increased susceptibility to enteroviral infection. Absence of humoral immunity makes the patient susceptible to bacterial gastroenteritis.

Abetalipoproteinemia

Abetalipoproteinemia is a rare autosomal recessive disorder that is characterized by defective assembly and secretion of apolipoprotein B (apoB) and apoB-containing lipoproteins, resulting from mutations in the gene encoding the microsomal triglyceride transfer protein; the serum β lipoprotein is absent. Abetalipoproteinemia causes defective absorption of lipids. Patients may have neurologic manifestations, acanthocytes, fat malabsorption, steatorrhea, and associated fat-soluble vitamin deficiencies (Gregg, 1994).

Tests for Steatorrhea

Screening tests for detection of steatorrhea include microscopic examination of feces for fat globules and determination of serum carotenoid. Carotenoids are a group of compounds that are the major precursors of vitamin A in humans. Absorption of carotenoids in the intestines depends on the presence of dietary fat. Because carotenoids are not stored in the body to any appreciable degree, lack of carotenoids in the diet or disturbances in absorption of lipids from the intestine can result in decreasing levels of serum carotenoid. This is a simple and useful screening test for steatorrhea. In addition to steatorrhea and poor dietary intake, liver disease and high fever may cause a low level of serum carotenoid. Elevated serum carotenoid levels are seen in patients with hypothyroidism, diabetes, hyperlipidemia, and excessive intake of carotene.

Tests for Malabsorption

When a diagnosis of malabsorption is being entertained, it is important to distinguish pancreatic maldigestion from enteric malabsorption. In children, the main cause of pancreatic malabsorption is CF, and the sweat chloride determination should be used when clinical evidence warrants it. Screening tests based on absent stool trypsin have also been used. One of the most valuable differential diagnostic tests, especially in adults, is the D-xylose absorption test.

The cellobiose-mannitol sugar permeability test and the lactulose-mannitol test have been used in the diagnosis of celiac disease. Modern evaluation of this disorder has been described earlier. Isotopic techniques and the starch tolerance test have been used as alternatives to the D-xylose test. Quantitative specific fecal trypsin and chymotrypsin assays may be helpful, as may the Schilling test for vitamin B_{12} absorption, which tends to be abnormal in patients with enteric steatorrhea in whom the abnormality is not correctable with intrinsic factor. Endoscopy, radiologic studies, and biopsy have replaced these methods in many cases.

Fecal Elastase. Elastase-1 is a proteolytic enzyme produced by the pancreas. Pancreatic elastase survives intestinal transit intact and is five- to sixfold concentrated in the feces (Lankisch, 2004). Reduced pancreatic elastase-1 in feces indicates pancreatic insufficiency in infants older than 2 weeks of age with CF and in older children with the disorder (Phillips, 1999; Cade, 2000; Leus, 2000).

This EIA is unaffected by pancreatic enzyme replacement therapy. Although sensitive for detection of severe pancreatic insufficiency, it lacks sensitivity for detection of milder forms. Fecal elastase is better than fecal chymotrypsin, para-aminobenzoic acid, bentiromide, and pancreolauryl tests (Lankisch, 2004). Single analysis of a 100 mg stool sample is adequate for determination of fecal elastase levels. If borderline values are detected, a repeat sample may be useful. This test should be performed only on formed stool. With a cutoff of 200 μg/g stool, the positive predictive value of fecal elastase determination is estimated to be approximately 50% (Lüth, 2001).

Xylose Absorption Test. The D-xylose absorption test is a valuable test for the differential diagnosis of malabsorption. In this procedure, a 25-g dose of pentose sugar in water is administered orally, and the amount excreted in urine over a 5-hour period is determined. If the amount excreted is less than 3 g, the diagnosis is most likely enterogenous malabsorption, because pancreatic enzymes are not required for absorption of D-xylose. D-Xylose is passively absorbed in the small intestine and is not metabolized by the liver, although a portion of an orally or intravenously administered dose is destroyed. The accuracy of the method depends not only on the rate of absorption of D-xylose but also on the rate of renal excretion. Therefore, in patients with renal disease, xylose should be quantified in blood 2 hours after its oral administration because urine values are difficult to interpret in the absence of reference values.

Isotopic techniques and the starch tolerance test have been used as alternatives to the D-xylose test. Quantitative specific fecal trypsin and chymotrypsin assays may be helpful, as may the Schilling test, which is used to assess the function of the terminal ileum. An oral dose of radioactive vitamin B_{12} is followed by an intramuscular large dose of nonradioactive vitamin B_{12}, and radioactivity in urine is measured. Urinary radioactivity reflects the absorbed amount of vitamin B_{12}. A repeat test to diagnose pernicious anemia or gastric pathology in a patient with steatorrhea involves coadministration of intrinsic factor and vitamin B_{12}. An abnormal result indicates ileal disease.

Laxative Abuse

Surreptitious laxative abuse is a frequently overlooked cause of chronic diarrhea and is the final diagnosis for chronic diarrhea in 15%–26% of patients at referral centers (Bytzer, 1989; Duncan, 1992). In Munchausen's syndrome by proxy, adults administered laxatives surreptitiously to young children (Duncan, 2000). The main prerequisite for making the diagnosis of surreptitious laxative abuse is clinical suspicion. Analysis of urine and fecal samples taken during diarrhea is necessary. Phenolphthalein is less frequently found since over-the-counter sales were banned. Senna, aloin, and cascara are colonic stimulants that are abused and can be detected by thin-layer chromatography.

Celiac Disease

Celiac disease (gluten-sensitive enteropathy) is a disorder precipitated, in genetically predisposed individuals, by the ingestion of gluten, the major storage protein of wheat and similar grains, characterized by intestinal malabsorption of nutrients due to sensitivity to the alcohol-soluble portion of gluten known as gliadin. Wheat, rye, and barley contain this protein and can induce mucosal damage in the gut, causing nonspecific villous atrophy of the small intestinal mucosa. Celiac disease does not develop unless a person has alleles that encode for HLA-DQ2 or HLA-DQ8 proteins, products of two of the human leukocyte antigen genes. This genetic predisposition is most common in Caucasians of Northern European descent. The prevalence is not clear but is estimated to be as high as 1% in some countries, and the condition is being increasingly recognized (Green, 2007; Sabatino, 2009).

Some patients remain asymptomatic, but an astute clinician may suspect this disorder when patients present with thin stature, iron deficiency anemia, weight loss, chronic bloating, and/or diarrhea. In severe cases, one may see malabsorption, steatorrhea, and wasting. Associations have been noted between celiac disease and type 1 diabetes mellitus, Down syndrome, dermatitis herpetiformis, IgA deficiency, autoimmune thyroid disease, and other disorders (Barr, 1998). Because of enteropathy associated with the disorder, multiple hematologic and biochemical abnormalities may be found in persons with untreated celiac disease, including deficiencies of iron, folate, or vitamin D. The peripheral blood film may reveal nonspecific target cells, siderocytes, crenated red cells, Howell-Jolly bodies, and Heinz bodies. Similarly, small bowel absorptive testing will be abnormal, including oral D-xylose testing and fecal fat evaluation.

The gold standard for diagnosis remains histologic examination of multiple biopsies of the affected small bowel mucosa for the identification of villous atrophy and crypt hyperplasia. The lesions may be patchy, and sampling errors can occur (Green, 2007; Ensari, 2010). Biopsy is reserved for patients in whom the diagnosis is suspected on the basis of signs or symptoms of the disease, especially in higher-risk populations with supporting serologic findings. These patients must be maintained on a gluten-free diet for the rest of their lives to control symptoms and mitigate cancer risk.

In current clinical practice, four serologic studies are used to assist in the diagnosis of celiac disease. These include testing for antibodies to gliadin (AGA-IgA and AGA-IgG), endomysium (EMA-IgA), reticulin (ARA-IgA), and transglutaminase (tTG-IgA), all of which are commercially available. Results of serologic testing for celiac disease must be analyzed with caution because this disease is associated with selective IgA deficiency that will give rise to false-negative serum IgA antibody tests (Thomas, 2003). Transient IgA deficiency may be seen in patients on phenytoin, penicillamine, or sulfasalazine. Therefore, total IgA levels should be checked or specific IgG serology performed if there is a high clinical suspicion of celiac disease. The sensitivity and specificity of these tests are extremely high when compared with a gold standard of flattened small bowel villi responding to dietary changes (Farrell, 2001). Endomysial antibodies have the best sensitivity and specificity, but they are currently detected via immunofluorescence of sections of monkey esophagus or human umbilical cord and are costly, cumbersome, and subject to interobserver interpretive variability.

Wheat storage protein, gliadin, is available to be used as an antigen in an EIA. Although serum IgA and IgG AGA levels are frequently elevated in untreated celiac disease, these tests are of only moderate sensitivity and specificity. IgG AGA testing is particularly useful in the 2% of patients with celiac disease who appear to be IgA deficient. However, these tests have largely been replaced by EMA. EMA binds to connective tissue surrounding smooth muscle cells. Most laboratories use sections of human umbilical cord. Serum IgA EMA binds to the endomysium to produce a characteristic staining pattern seen on indirect immunofluorescence. The antibody is highly sensitive and specific. However, after treatment, the titers fall quickly to undetectable levels (Volta, 1995). The epitope against which EMA is directed has been shown to be tissue transglutaminase. Use of IgA anti-tTG assays has been shown to be highly sensitive and specific for the diagnosis of celiac disease (Dieterich, 1998). An EIA for IgA anti-tTG is widely available, less costly, and easier to perform than the older immunofluorescence assays for IgA EMA.

Antigliadin antibody serology is best avoided in the diagnosis of celiac disease because of frequent false positives. A second generation of antigliadin antibody test based on the potentiation of toxic gliadin peptides by tTG enzymatic activity is used to monitor dietary compliance. These IgA and IgG deamidated gliadin peptide (DGP) assays appear similar to tTG IgA or IgG in diagnostic accuracy, leading to the belief that strongly positive tTG IgA in conjunction with positive DGP serology may be used as confirmation of celiac disease without the need for biopsy histology.

Although IgG endomysium and IgG tTG antibodies may be suitable for serologic diagnosis of celiac disease, they cannot be used to monitor the response to dietary modification. Endomysium IgA antibodies disappear following treatment of celiac sprue with a gluten-free diet.

The HLA-DQ2 allele is identified in 90%–95% of patients with celiac disease, and HLA-DQ8 in most of the remaining patients. These alleles occur in 30%–40% of the general population, and the absence of these alleles is important for its high negative predictive value. Thus, the presence of HLA-DQ2 and HLA-DQ8 is important for determining which family members should be screened with serologic testing (Kaukinen, 2002).

Uncontrolled celiac disease appears to predispose patients to intestinal carcinomas and lymphomas (Nehra, 1998).

Whipple's Disease

It is a rare multisystem disease that often presents with arthralgias, diarrhea, malabsorption, and weight loss. It is predominantly found in males, and about 15% of patients do not present with classical signs and symptoms of this disease (Fenollar, 2007). It is caused by *Tropheryma whipplei*, a bacillus that does not stain well with Gram stain, although it is classified with gram-positive bacteria based on 16S rRNA sequencing (Marth, 2003). This disorder can affect the central nervous system and cause endocarditis. Demonstration of periodic acid-Schiff (PAS)–positive material in the lamina propria and villous atrophy of the small intestine is diagnostic. A prothrombin time should be checked before biopsy because of the frequent occurrence of vitamin K malabsorption.

T. whipplei has been cultured from the stools of a patient with Whipple's disease using a specific axenic medium and specific techniques (Raoult, 2006). PCR testing of infected tissue or cerebrospinal fluid has been used to confirm the diagnosis and monitor treatment (von Herbay, 1997). Biopsy of the duodenum with PAS staining had been considered pathognomonic for Whipple's disease. It is now recognized that PAS-positive macrophages may be seen in AIDS patients with *Mycobacterium avium-intracellulare* complex. Thus, PCR has gained even more importance in the management of this entity. Long-term antibiotic therapy with central nervous system penetration is used to treat patients with Whipple's disease (Ramzan, 1997; Singer, 1998).

Inflammatory Bowel Disease

Immunologic mechanisms within the colon are involved in the pathogenesis of inflammatory bowel disease. The underlying antigenic challenge to the immunologic response is not clearly understood. Over the past decade, two antibody tests have become available that assist in the laboratory evaluation of patients with inflammatory bowel disease (Rutgeerts, 2000). The combination of clinical findings, endoscopy, radiologic imaging, and blood work may help differentiate the subtypes of inflammatory bowel disease. Perinuclear-antineutrophil cytoplasmic antibody (p-ANCA) and anti–*Saccharomyces cerevisiae* antibody (ASCA) can be used to help distinguish abdominal pain seen in irritable bowel syndrome from inflammatory bowel disease, and can help distinguish ulcerative colitis from Crohn's disease

TABLE 22-6
Markers for Inflammatory Bowel Disease

	FREQUENCY, %	
	p-ANCA	**ASCA**
Irritable bowel syndrome (normal patients)	<5	<5
Ulcerative colitis	70	15
Crohn's disease	20	65

ASCA, Anti-*Saccharomyces cerevisiae* antibody; *p-ANCA,* perinuclear antineutrophil cytoplasmic antibody.

(Sendid, 1998; Shanahan, 1994) (Table 22-6). These tests have limitations, and interpretation requires careful understanding of the tests. Whereas few normal persons with irritable bowel syndrome will have ANCA, 70% of persons with ulcerative colitis and 20% of persons with Crohn's disease will have significant titers. Among patients with inflammatory bowel disease, 65% of those with Crohn's disease will have ASCA, whereas only 20% of patients with ulcerative colitis will have significant titers. Given their low sensitivity and specificity, use of these tests should be dependent upon the clinical circumstance. For example, a person with diarrhea and equivocal biopsy findings found to have a positive ANCA is more likely to have inflammatory bowel disease than irritable bowel syndrome. Likewise, if a person with what appears to be ulcerative colitis is found to have a positive ASCA, Crohn's colitis may be present.

GASTROINTESTINAL TUMORS

Pancreatic Adenocarcinoma

Ductal adenocarcinomas of the exocrine pancreas are malignant epithelial tumors composed of mucin-producing glandular structures. They constitute 85% of all pancreatic tumors and are the fourth most frequent cause of death from cancer. They originate in small ducts and progress from noninvasive pancreatic intraepithelial lesions to invasive cancers. Little change in their incidence or survival rate has been seen in the past 20 years; 5-year survival is <5%. A slight male predominance has been noted, especially in younger age groups. This is a disease mostly of late life; 80% of patients are 60–80 years of age, although cases in the third decade are not uncommon. This cancer is more common in African Americans and Native Americans. A two- to threefold greater risk has been reported among cigarette smokers. Patients with chronic pancreatitis and diabetes mellitus are at increased risk. High intake of meat and fat appears to be a risk factor, as well as intake of nitrosamines and polycyclic hydrocarbons. The neoplastic mechanism remains obscure.

Clinical presentation depends largely on the location of the tumor: 60% arise in the head, often with painless jaundice; 10% in the body and 10% in the tail are often silent until quite large or widely disseminated; 20% are diffuse at presentation. Familial clusters have been reported, but no distinct genetic abnormality has been described.

The ampullary region is invaded by carcinomas of the head of the pancreas, causing bile duct obstruction. Acute painless dilation of the gallbladder (Courvoisier's sign) and jaundice occur as the result of common bile duct obstruction by tumor in most cases. Carcinomas of the body and tail do not impinge on the biliary tract. Migratory thrombophlebitis (Trousseau's sign) develops in 10% of patients with pancreatic cancer, especially those with tumors of the body and tail, probably because of platelet-aggregating factors and procoagulants from the tumor. Anorexia, conspicuous weight loss, and gnawing epigastric pain that radiates to the back are frequent clinical features.

Early diagnosis of pancreatic carcinoma is unusual. These tumors are typically silent until they impinge on a vital structure or on the posterior wall of the abdomen and then cause severe pain. Pain is usually the first symptom. Less than 20% of the tumors are resectable at the time of presentation.

No morphologic difference is known between carcinomas of the head of the pancreas and those of the body and tail. These tumors are usually moderately or poorly differentiated mucin-producing adenocarcinomas. They have abortive tubular structures and dense stromal fibrosis and aggressive infiltrative growth, often with perineural invasion. Tumor cells are cuboidal or columnar and are usually poorly differentiated. The adjacent pancreatic parenchyma often demonstrates foci of ductal dysplasia and intraductal tumor growth.

TABLE 22-7
Pancreatic Cancer–Associated Genetic Syndromes

Genetic syndrome	Gene(s)	Pancreatic cancer risk increase	Histopathologic features
Hereditary breast and ovarian cancer syndrome	*BRCA2* *BRCA1*	3.5- to 10-fold 2-fold	Ductal adenocarcinoma
Peutz-Jeghers syndrome	*STK11/LKB1*	132-fold	Intraductal papillary mucinous neoplasm
Familial adenomatous polyposis	*APC*	Up to 4-fold	Ductal adenocarcinoma, intraductal papillary neoplasm, pancreatoblastoma
Familial atypical multiple melanoma	*CDKN2A*	13- to 22-fold	Ductal adenocarcinoma
Hereditary nonpolyposis colorectal cancer syndrome	Mismatch repair genes	Increased	Medullary carcinoma
Hereditary pancreatitis	*PRSS1* *SPINK1*	53-fold	Ductal adenocarcinoma
Familial pancreatic cancer	Unknown	9- to 32-fold	

Adapted from Shi C, Hruban RH, Klein AP. Familial pancreatic cancer. Arch Pathol Lab Med 2009;133:365–74.

Point mutations in *KRAS* and in *p16* are found in >90% of cases, and mutations in *p53* cause inactivation in 50%–70% of cases. Both carcinoembryonic antigen (CEA) and CA 19-9 (tumor marker for pancreatic cancer) are elevated in some pancreatic adenocarcinomas. The serum markers *KRAS*, CEA, and CA19-9 have not been useful in case finding for early diagnosis. However, their increases can be used to monitor for recurrence (Table 22-7).

Neuroendocrine Tumors

Gastroenteropathic neuroendocrine tumors (GEP-NET) are relatively rare neoplasms with varied clinical manifestations. Abdominal pain and diarrhea are two of the more common clinical symptoms. Carcinoid tumor was the term chosen, more than 100 years ago, to distinguish these tumors from carcinomas of the GI tract. Because these tumors are rare, they were lumped together. Recently, with greater knowledge of their development and biological behavior, the World Health Organization classification of GEP-NET was published in 2000. Specific markers of normal and neoplastic neuroendocrine cells are the hormones that occur in the GEP system. The organ in which a certain hormone-producing tumor develops appears to make a difference (e.g., the differing malignant potential of duodenal compared with pancreatic gastrinoma) (Klöppel, 2004). These tumors exhibit amine precursor uptake and decarboxylation (APUD) and are therefore known as APUDomas. Cells of the GEP-NET belong to the system of disseminated neuroendocrine cells called **APUD cells.** These cells are scattered throughout the mucosa of the GI tract and the islets of the pancreas. Insulinomas and gastrinomas are the most common pancreatic endocrine tumors. Glucagonomas are rare and make up 2%–5% of series. Other even rarer types, such as somatostatinomas and VIPomas, have been identified (Perry, 1996). Chemical measurement of the secretagogues of these tumors generally suggests the diagnosis in the right clinical setting.

Localizing these tumors can be challenging. Ultrasonography, CT scanning, MRI, endoscopy, angiography, and octreotide scanning all have significant technical limitations. With the exception of ultrasonography and MRI, potential morbidity can result from the testing as well. Although it was initially hoped that octreotide scanning would replace other modes of localization, recent data suggest that it is useful in determining the extent of carcinoids and gastrinomas, although of little use in finding insulinomas or nonfunctional tumors (Kisker, 1997). These tumors are often small, frequently are multifocal, and can be located in a variety of organs. They can be malignant or benign. They are similar on histologic examination, so histologic staining is used to distinguish the types (Perry, 1996). As with all neoplastic lesions, biopsy is essential to confirm the diagnosis.

GEP-NET make up about 10% of pancreatic neoplasms and are classified as functioning or nonfunctioning tumors. These tumors are single or multiple, and benign or malignant. They are often solitary, circumscribed lesions, amenable to surgical resection. Immunohistochemistry is needed for demonstration of endocrine activity. Hormone assays are useful for the diagnosis of pancreatic endocrine tumors (Modlin, 1997; Eriksson, 2000; Barakat, 2004).

Cytologic criteria are unreliable in diagnosis. The diagnosis of malignancy requires demonstration of metastases and vascular or tissue invasion. These tumors are often slow growing. Functioning tumors cause recognizable clinical syndromes due to excess peptide hormone secretion. Nonfunctioning tumors have a worse prognosis and typically present with metastases or local symptoms.

GI endocrine tumors may be part of the syndrome of MEN 1 with parathyroid disease and pituitary and pancreatic tumors. Islet cell tumors may secrete various normal hormones that are not ordinarily produced in the pancreas, including adrenocorticotropic hormone (ACTH), parathyroid hormone, calcitonin, and vasopressin.

Insulinoma

Insulinomas are derived from β cells and produce insulin that induces clinically significant hypoglycemia. Factitious disease due to exogenous insulin is part of the differential diagnosis. Insulinomas are usually found in the pancreas and are typically small and solitary and often contain amyloid; 10% are malignant. Diagnosis is made by demonstrating elevated plasma insulin associated with hypoglycemia and measurement of C-peptide. C-peptide is equimolar to insulin and is needed to exclude increases in insulin from exogenous sources.

Gastrinoma

Gastrinomas are gastrin-secreting non–β cell pancreatic tumors that cause a syndrome of intractable peptic ulcer disease and gastric acid hypersecretion. Gastrin binds cholecystokinin-B receptors on parietal cells of the stomach to stimulate acid secretion and also has a trophic effect on gastric mucosal parietal and enterochromaffin-like cells, causing mucosal hypertrophy (McIntyre, 2002). The mean age of onset is 50 years, with male preponderance. At the time of diagnosis, 70%–90% of the tumors are malignant with metastases or local invasion. Up to 60% of gastrinomas are associated with MEN 1, and about one half of MEN 1 patients develop gastrinomas. Most gastrinomas arise in the gastrinoma triangle: duodenum, pancreatic head, hepatoduodenal ligament.

Gastrin is not usually detected in the adult pancreas, but is present in the fetal pancreas. Gastrinomas induce peptic ulcer disease refractory to treatment, esophagitis, and diarrhea. High levels of plasma gastrin are noted with high basal gastric acid secretion. Increased gastrin levels are also caused by gastric atrophy and by acid antisecretory drugs such as H_2 blockers. Some gastrinoma patients are hypercalcemic because of PTH-related protein production, or because patients with MEN 1 may develop hyperparathyroidism. About 50% of patients with gastrinomas have metastases, mainly to the liver and nodes. The 5-year survival is 20% with liver metastases, and without metastases, 80% will survive for 5 years.

Gastrinomas can cause high-volume diarrhea through an increased rate of gastric acid secretion, resulting in a volume that cannot be fully reabsorbed. The acid exceeds the neutralizing capacity of the pancreatic bicarbonate and inactivates the pancreatic digestive enzymes; this interferes with the emulsification of fat by bile salts, resulting in steatorrhea. A secretory component to the diarrhea has also been observed. Diagnosis is established by measuring serum gastrin levels; a level greater than 1000 pg/mL is virtually diagnostic. The secretin stimulation test can differentiate patients with gastrinomas from those with the many other causes of hypergastrinemia; this test should be performed in every patient suspected to have the ZE syndrome who has a nondiagnostic fasting serum gastrin concentration (Berna, 2006).

Glucagonoma

This is a rare tumor, mostly of pancreatic origin, that secretes glucagon (α cells), which induces glycogenolysis and gluconeogenesis in the liver and raises blood glucose levels. It causes a syndrome of mild diabetes, necrotizing migratory erythematous rash, anemia, and venous thrombosis, and is associated with severe infection. Onset occurs at 40–70 years of age, with slight female predominance (Bloom, 1987). These are large, locally invasive tumors that histologically resemble trabecular and solid patterns of insulinomas; two thirds are malignant. Plasma glucagon levels are elevated up to 30 times above normal.

Somatostatinoma

These usually solitary tumors are derived from δ cells that produce somatostatin, which inhibits pituitary release of growth hormone and secretion by α, β, and δ cells. This peptide also regulates glucose homeostasis and causes a syndrome of mild diabetes, gallstones, steatorrhea, and hypochlorhydria, due to the inhibitory effect of somatostatin on the other islet and gastrointestinal neuroendocrine cells (Krejs, 1979). Somatostatin measurement in a fasting serum specimen may aid diagnosis; patients with somatostatinomas may have 1000-fold elevated concentrations. These tumors may also secrete calcitonin or ACTH, and most are malignant with metastases at diagnosis.

VIPoma

These tumors are presented in the previous section on diarrhea and malabsorption.

Carcinoid Syndrome

Pancreatic carcinoids are rare malignant neoplasms resembling intestinal carcinoids. They synthesize serotonin and motilin. When confined to the pancreas, these tumors may induce an atypical carcinoid syndrome that consists of facial flush, hypotension, periorbital edema, and lacrimation. Cases with liver metastases cause a classical carcinoid syndrome. Diagnosis is aided by demonstration of increased 5-hydroxyindoleacetic acid (5-HIAA) levels in 24-hour urine specimens.

Amyloidosis

GI amyloidosis is mainly of the reactive type (secondary or amyloid-associated [AA] amyloidosis) and results from mucosal or neuromuscular infiltration. It may result in GI bleeding from vascular friability. The patient may also have diarrhea from a combination of altered intestinal motility, bacterial overgrowth, and protein-losing enteropathy. Liver involvement can be seen in primary (amyloid light chain) or AA amyloidosis. Common symptoms include involuntary weight loss, fatigue, and abdominal pain. Common physical findings consist of hepatomegaly, ascites, purpura, and splenomegaly. The most common laboratory abnormality is an elevated alkaline phosphatase. The diagnosis of multiple myeloma should be confirmed by tissue biopsy of duodenal or colorectal mucosa. Although GI complications can result in significant morbidity, they usually are not the cause of death, which is most often caused by renal failure, restrictive cardiomyopathy, or ischemic heart disease (Ebert, 2008).

GASTROINTESTINAL BLEEDING

Throughout most of the GI tract, the lumen of the gut is separated from the capillary blood supply by only a single layer of epithelial cells. Thus even minor injury to the epithelial lining may result in GI bleeding. Occult GI bleeding is bleeding unknown to the patient. Iron deficiency anemia should be considered to be the result of GI bleeding until excluded (Rockey, 2010).

Hemoglobin and hematocrit are usually low, and their levels may have some relation to blood loss. A low mean cell volume (MCV) may indicate that the patient is iron deficient, and that chronic blood loss has occurred. An elevated MCV may indicate a folate or vitamin B_{12} deficiency with macrocytosis and raises the possibility of ethanol abuse, chronic liver disease, gastric cancer in association with pernicious anemia, or regional enteritis involving the terminal ileum.

If a clotting defect exists, prompt correction of the deficiency is crucial. Extensive transfusion dilutes platelets and clotting factors, particularly factors V and VII. Also, a high proportion of patients who bleed while taking therapeutic anticoagulants do so from a clinically significant lesion. It is important to evaluate these patients for a GI pathologic condition and to correct their clotting status. Leukocytosis may accompany acute GI bleeding, but it is usually not in excess of 15,000 white blood cells/mm^3. Leukocytosis should not be attributed to acute blood loss without completion of a search for sources of infection.

Elevated BUN in a patient whose BUN was recently normal, or whose serum creatinine concentration is normal, suggests an upper GI bleed. The BUN rise may be due to the hypovolemia of acute blood loss, but digestion of blood proteins in the small intestine and absorption of nitrogenous products may be the cause.

Fecal Occult Blood Testing

The fecal occult blood test (FOBT) depends on the peroxidase activity of hemoglobin. Reagents used include guaiac (Hemoccult), benzidine (marketing restricted by federal regulation because of its carcinogenicity), orthotoluidine (Hematest), and ortho-dianisidine. The reagents differ in sensitivity, although all are associated with frequent false-positive and false-negative results, mostly due to the specimen tested. Specimens collected by digital rectal examination have a high frequency of false positives caused by injury to the rectal mucosa.

The normal person loses 0.5–1.5 mL of blood into the GI tract daily in association with the normal shedding of epithelial cells. Commercial tests are designed to turn positive with blood loss greater than 5–10 mL per day. This corresponds to 5–10 mg of hemoglobin/gram of feces, assuming a blood hemoglobin of 15 g/dL and an average daily 150-g stool.

In addition to sample handling and testing, diet is very important in compromising these tests. The high rate of false positives is due to the lack of specificity of the reagents and the presence of peroxidase activity in other fecal constituents, as well as the sensitivity of the different chromogens to peroxidase activity. The myoglobin and hemoglobin of ingested meat and fish have peroxidase activity that may falsely indicate the presence of occult blood. Bacteria in the bowel, as well as ingested vegetables and fruits, such as horseradish, turnips, bananas, black grapes, pears, and plums, have peroxidase and can falsely elevate fecal peroxidase activity. False-negative tests occur in the presence of large amounts of vitamin C and other antioxidants.

Patient preparation and specimen collection are important in ensuring valid test results. For 72 hours prior, patients should be on a diet free of exogenous peroxide activity (meat, fish, turnips, horseradish), GI irritants (aspirin, nonsteroidal antiinflammatory drugs), and vitamin C. Variations in testing technique produce errors due to stool consistency, the application of large aliquots of stool, and, particularly, inaccurate timing of the reaction.

Immunochemical tests for hemoglobin are more sensitive and specific and yield fewer false negatives. They are not affected by diet, animal hemoglobin, or human myoglobin. Dietary peroxidases do not affect immunochemical test results. They are useful only for screening blood of the lower intestinal tract and are insensitive to upper GI bleeding because globin is destroyed in the small intestine. Immunochemical tests are expensive and are not done at the point-of-care.

Fecal immunochemical testing for human hemoglobin, such as HemeSelect or InSure, has been developed to improve the sensitivity and specificity of guaiac testing to detect colonic neoplasia. HemeSelect testing is based on an antigen–antibody reaction involving fixed chicken red blood cells coated with anti–human hemoglobin antibody (Allison, 1996). Samples demonstrating agglutination are interpreted as positive for occult human blood. InSure is a test that uses monoclonal mouse anti–human hemoglobin antibody with subsequent colorimetric detection; it is sensitive enough to detect 50 µg hemoglobin/g feces (Quest Diagnostics). These tests do not react with nonhuman hemoglobin or peroxidase, so food restrictions are not necessary. Immunochemical InSure tests target the globin portion of hemoglobin, which does not survive passage through the upper GI tract. Therefore, these tests are more specific for lower gastrointestinal colonic bleeding (Quest Diagnostics).

Colon cancer is a leading cause of cancer-related deaths in the United States, accounting for approximately 55,000 deaths annually. According to recent cancer statistics, approximately 150,000 new colon cancer cases were diagnosed in 2003. Evidence has demonstrated the clinical usefulness of FOBT to detect these cancers at an earlier stage, potentially resulting in decreased mortality. Because of the generally favorable clinical biology of these tumors when detected earlier (with an 80%–90% survival rate with local confined disease) (Helm, 2003) and the relatively inexpensive, noninvasive nature of FOBT, this may serve as a useful screening technique. Several professional organizations recommend annual or biennial FOBT, but universally accepted screening protocols have not been established. The American Cancer Society guidelines for colorectal cancer screening, the most widely utilized, recommend annual FOBT and flexible sigmoidoscopy every 3–5 years, beginning at age 50, in asymptomatic, average-risk individuals (Marshall, 1996). Limitations of this testing include the high numbers of false-positive and false-negative results. The sensitivity of FOBT has been estimated at between 30% and 50%. The true sensitivity of FOBT is difficult to determine because individuals who test negative do not undergo further colonoscopic evaluation to determine whether the FOBT is a true negative. Only approximately 5%–10% of positive reactions prove to be caused by an occult malignancy (Simon, 1998). However, following a stepwise approach to colon cancer screening should minimize the clinical effects of limited sensitivity and specificity and offer valuable information nonetheless.

Occult blood can be detected by chemical (guaiac), hemoporphyrin, or immunologic methods. Occult blood may arise anywhere along the intestinal tract and is often the first warning sign of GI malignancy. Other potential sources of occult blood may arise from bleeding esophageal varices, polyps, esophageal or gastric inflammation, hemorrhoids or fissures, inflammatory bowel disease, peptic ulcer disease, or angiodysplasias of the colon. Laboratory diagnosis of the presence of fecal occult blood generally involves a guaiac-smear test (Hemoccult, Seracult, Coloscreen), the most commonly used method at present. Guaiac is a naturally occurring phenolic compound that is oxidized to quinone by hydrogen peroxidase, resulting in a detectable color change. These tests detect the pseudoperoxidase activity of heme as intact hemoglobin or as free heme (Allison, 1996). These tests are not specific for human hemoglobin, and hemoglobin from red meat, peroxidase from fruits and vegetables, and certain medications can lead to false-positive results. The presence of more than 5–10 mL/day of blood in the stool results in a positive guaiac smear. Stool specimens should be received from three consecutive stools. Two slides should be prepared for each stool sample. Slides should not be rehydrated and should be developed within 7 days of collection. To ensure quality testing, some medical institutions now require that stool samples be sent to the laboratory for guaiac testing, rather than having residents or nurses perform tests on the ward. In addition, the test must be performed under appropriate conditions that serve to limit its sensitivity. Factors that can cause inaccuracies in the results include the presence of bleeding gums, for example, or ingestion of large amounts of red meat before testing. In addition, patients may be using certain medications that will influence the results of FOBT. For example, drugs that can cause GI irritation and subsequent bleeding, such as anticoagulants, aspirin, NSAIDs, or colchicines, may lead to false-positive results. Other drugs that have been implicated include reserpine and oxidizing drugs such as iodine. Ingestion of large amounts of vitamin C can cause false-negative results. Patients should avoid such medications or food products before FOBT. A positive FOBT prompts further evaluation for a GI lesion. Additional evaluations usually include sigmoidoscopy with barium enema or full colonoscopy, the latter being the preferred modality. A negative FOBT, however, cannot definitely rule out the presence of colonic neoplasia. If a patient is presenting with signs and symptoms suggestive of colon cancer, further evaluation is warranted, even in the presence of negative FOBT.

Fecal DNA testing is a promising technique for colorectal cancer screening. This test involves the collection of a single stool specimen, which is then screened for DNA markers. PCR is used to amplify the fecal DNA. These tests are useful because DNA is shed continuously and remains stable in stool, and minute amounts are detectable. Clinical studies have shown that fecal DNA testing has high specificity and sensitivity for cancer detection, considerably more than chemical guaiac testing. Several markers have been investigated; however, further evaluation and improved specificity and sensitivity are needed for their widespread use (Itzkowitz, 2008; Mandel, 2008; Lieberman, 2009).

Blood in Newborn Feces (Apt Test for Swallowed Blood)

When blood is found in the GI tract or stool of neonates, usually on the second or third day of life, a determination must be made of whether it is swallowed blood of maternal origin or is secondary to disease in the newborn (Guritzky, 1996). The Apt test is a qualitative test that is used to make this determination in grossly bloody stools or vomitus (hematemesis) from a newborn. Infants may ingest maternal blood during birth, or from a fissured or bleeding nipple. The sample first is mixed with water and then is centrifuged. The supernatant, which should be pink, is then mixed with 1% sodium hydroxide in a 5:1 ratio. If the blood is of maternal origin, the mixture turns yellow-brown after several minutes. Fetal blood remains pink because fetal hemoglobin is more resistant to alkali denaturation than adult hemoglobin. The test has relatively low sensitivity, and the result must be interpreted with caution (McRury, 1994).

MARKERS FOR GASTROINTESTINAL AND PANCREATIC TUMORS

Tumor markers are substances produced by tumor cells or other body cells in response to neoplastic or certain nonneoplastic conditions; they are found in tissues or body fluids. Different tumor markers are found in different types of cancers, and the same tumor marker may be found in more than one type of cancer. Tumor markers are not expressed in all people with cancer, and some are expressed in patients with benign conditions. Identification or measurement of tumor markers is used in detection, diagnosis, or management of some types of cancer. Although an abnormal tumor marker level may suggest cancer or limited efficacy of therapy, this alone is not enough to establish diagnosis and is usually combined with other tests such as biopsy (Bigbee, 2003; Chan, 2006; Locker, 2006).

Enzymes

Enzymes were one of the first groups of tumor markers identified, and their elevated levels were linked with cancer. Most changes in enzyme levels are not specific or sensitive enough to be used to identify the cancer type or the specific organ involved. Lactate dehydrogenase, a glycolytic pathway enzyme, is released as a result of cell damage, and its elevation in malignancy is nonspecific (Schwartz, 1982). Neuron-specific enolase (NSE) is found in neural tissue and in cells of the diffuse neuroendocrine system. NSE is found in association with tumors of neuroendocrine origin, and its serum levels are of prognostic significance (Zeltzer, 1986). Urokinase-plasminogen activator, a serine protease system, is a prognostic marker in colorectal cancer (Duffy, 1999). Tumor-associated trypsin inhibitor (TATI) is identical to pancreatic secretory trypsin inhibitor, also known as the kazal inhibitor. It is strongly expressed in pancreatic cells and in low concentrations in normal GI and urogenital tissues. TATI is a useful marker for GI, urologic, and pancreatic cancers (Stenman, 2002).

Hormones

Hormones are normally produced in endocrine organs but may also be produced in nonendocrine tissue. They are assayed by EIA using monoclonal antibodies, or by RIA. Multiple endocrine neoplasia (MEN 2A and MEN 2B) syndromes synthesize several polypeptide hormones such as ACTH, calcitonin, gastrin, glucagon, and insulin. Vasoactive intestinal peptide is produced by some endocrine tumors (Perry, 1996).

ACTH may be the result of pituitary or ectopic production. Elevated ACTH levels have been reported from pancreatic, gastric, and colonic carcinomas. Patients with serotonin-producing carcinoid tumors often have marked ten-fold increases in urinary 5-HIAA excretion. Ingestion of serotonin-rich foods, such as bananas, chocolate, plums, or walnuts, or medications containing guaifenesin may produce false-positive elevations (Kema, 1992).

Other Protein Markers

Oncofetal antigens are proteins produced in fetal life that decrease to low levels or disappear after birth but reappear in cancer patients. The discoveries of α-fetoprotein (AFP) and carcinoembryonic antigen (CEA) in the 1960s had a profound effect on the use of tumor markers. AFP is a marker for hepatocellular and germ cell (nonseminomatous) carcinomas. CEA, a glycoprotein, is a marker for colorectal, GI, lung, and breast carcinomas. CEA testing may be useful as an adjunct to clinical staging (Sikorska, 1992). Amplification of Her2/neu, a tyrosine kinase receptor of the epidermal growth factor family, is seen in GI, breast, and ovarian tumors. bcl-2, a protein known to inhibit apoptosis, appears early in colorectal cancer. C-peptide is a marker for insulin production.

Blood Group Antigens

Some of the blood group carbohydrates are tumor markers with elevated levels in specific types of cancer. CA19-9, a sialylated Lewis antigen, is elevated in patients with colorectal and pancreatic carcinomas (Lamerz, 1992). Its levels are elevated in benign conditions such as Mirizzi's syndrome (Robertson, 2007). It is absent in individuals with pancreatic tumors who are Lewis negative. Another related Lewis antigen, C50, is used as a pancreatic tumor marker but is considered less sensitive than CA19-9. CA 242 and CA 72-4 are markers for GI and pancreatic tumors, but CA 72-4 is considered of greater prognostic value in pancreatic cancer (Louhimo, 2004).

Genetic Markers

Two classes of genes are implicated in cancer: cell activator genes and cell suppressor genes. Most oncogenes code for proteins that activate cell proliferation. Mutated K-*ras* is present in 95% of pancreatic cancers, in 40% of colon cancers, and in lower percentages of other tumors (Chan, 2006). Mutations of *ras* oncogenes have been detected in the stools of 9 of 15 patients with curable colorectal tumors (Sidransky, 1992).

Any genetic testing requires that the physician clearly understand how to interpret the results and how the results may affect patient management; patients and their family members must be counseled appropriately (Grody, 2001; LeGrys, 2007).

Tumor Suppressor Genes

Oncogenicity derives from loss of the gene, rather than its activation, as with the *p53* gene. Three fourths of colon carcinomas show deletion in one *p53* allele and a point mutation in the other allele.

STOOL COLLECTION AND EXAMINATION

COLLECTION

Uninstructed patients sometimes exhibit considerable ingenuity in collecting stool specimens, but a few simple instructions are likely to produce more satisfactory specimens. A scoured, well-rinsed bedpan is a convenient collection container. If the patient does not own one, a carefully cleaned, rinsed, and boiled glass jar of suitable size is a satisfactory alternative. Patients should be warned against passing urine at the same time into the bedpan or container because, among other things, urine has a harmful effect on protozoa. Tongue depressors or pieces of cardboard are reasonably convenient instruments for transferring the stool from bedpan to transport vessel, for which plastic, cardboard, and glass containers are available. We prefer to use two 2-oz ointment jars with screw caps for small stool samples because they are odor free, leakproof, and easy to transport. Patients should be instructed not to contaminate the outside of the container and not to overfill the container. Gas, which frequently accumulates, should be released gradually by carefully loosening the cap. Failure to observe this simple precaution, especially in the case of an overfilled container, can result in an explosive release of contents. Fecal specimen collection at home is by no means simple and easy unless the patient has been instructed properly.

MACROSCOPIC EXAMINATION

The quantity, form, consistency, and color of the stool should be noted. Normally, 100–200 g of stool is passed per day. Diarrheic stool is watery. Passage of large amounts of mushy, foul-smelling, gray stool that floats on the water is characteristic of steatorrhea. Constipation may be associated with passage of small, firm, spherical masses of stool (scybala). Clay color suggests diminution or absence of bile or the presence of barium sulfate. Blood, especially blood originating from the lower gut, may cause the stool to be red; beets in the diet may mimic this. Bleeding from the upper GI tract is more likely to cause the stool to be black and have a tarry consistency. Bismuth, iron, and charcoal may also cause a black color. Stool that is allowed to stand in the air for a time may darken on the surface.

Mucus

The presence of recognizable mucus in a stool specimen is abnormal and should be reported. Translucent gelatinous mucus clinging to the surface of the formed stool suggests spastic constipation or mucous colitis. It is seen in stools of emotionally disturbed patients and may result from excessive straining. Bloody mucus clinging to the fecal mass suggests neoplasm or inflammatory processes of the rectal canal. Mucus associated with pus and blood is found in stools of patients with ulcerative colitis, bacillary dysentery, ulcerating diverticulitis, and intestinal tuberculosis. Patients with villous adenoma of the colon may pass copious quantities of mucus, amounting to 3–4 L in 24 hours. They frequently develop severe dehydration and electrolyte disturbances, especially hypokalemia.

Pus

Patients with chronic ulcerative colitis and chronic bacillary dysentery frequently pass large quantities of pus with the stool, the recognition of which requires microscopic examination. This also occurs in patients with localized abscesses or fistulas communicating with the sigmoid colon, rectum, or anus. Large amounts of pus seldom accompany the stools of patients with amebic colitis, and its presence is evidence against this diagnosis. No inflammatory exudate is seen in the watery stools of patients with viral gastroenteritis.

MICROSCOPIC EXAMINATION

Fat

The simplest technique is microscopic examination using one of the Sudan stains. This procedure has been widely employed for screening because of its simplicity. In our experience, results have correlated well with quantitative measurements when aliquots of the same homogenized stool have been analyzed. For this purpose, a small aliquot of stool suspension is placed on a slide and is mixed with two drops of 95% ethanol; then two drops of saturated ethanolic solution of Sudan III are added, with further mixing. A coverslip is applied. Under these conditions, fatty acids are present as lightly stained flakes or as needle-like crystals that do not stain and therefore may be missed. Soaps also do not stain but appear as well-defined amorphous flakes or as rounded masses or coarse crystals. Neutral fats, however, appear as large orange or red droplets. When 60 or more stained droplets of neutral fats per high-power field are seen, one may be reasonably certain that the patient has steatorrhea. Caution is advisable in interpretation, however, because mineral oil or castor oil may mimic neutral fat. The procedure is then repeated by adding several drops of 36% (v/v) acetic acid to the stool mixture and warming the slide several times over a flame until slight boiling occurs. This converts neutral fats and soaps to fatty acids and melts the fatty acids, causing them to form droplets that stain strongly with Sudan III. The slide is then examined while warm. After this procedure has been performed, the presence of up to 100 stained droplets per high-power field is considered normal. Patients with steatorrhea of pancreatic origin are likely to have greater increases in fatty acids and soaps.

Meat Fiber

The technique for sampling is identical to that used for Sudan preparations for detection of fecal fat. The stool is mixed thoroughly on a slide with a solution of eosin in 10% ethanol; it is then allowed to stain for 3 minutes and is examined for muscle fibers. The entire area under the coverslip is examined, and only rectangular fibers with clearly evident cross-striations are counted. More than 10 fibers/high-power field suggests maldigestion and/or hypermotility. It appears that examination for meat fibers correlates well with chemical determination of fat excretion (Moore, 1971).

Leukocytes

A small fleck of mucus or a drop of liquid stool is placed on a glass microscopic slide with a wooden applicator stick. Two drops of methylene blue are added and mixed thoroughly and carefully. A coverslip is placed on the mixture, which is allowed to stand for 2–3 minutes for good nuclear staining. Using low-power scanning, rough quantitative counts are made by approximating the average numbers of leukocytes and erythrocytes. All differential counts should be made under high power, counting 200 cells when possible. Only those cells clearly identified as either mononuclear or polymorphonuclear are included in the differential count. Macrophages and epithelial cells that cannot be clearly identified are ignored. The initial cell counts should be performed at the time of presentation of the specimen.

SELECTED REFERENCES

Allison JE, Tekawa IS, Ransom LJ, et al. A comparison of fecal occult-blood tests for colorectal-cancer screening. N Engl J Med 1996;334:155–60.

Evaluation of three commonly used screening tests for fecal occult blood with regard to sensitivity, specificity, and predictive value related to colonoscopy and biopsy findings.

NCCLS—National Committee for Clinical Laboratory Standards. Sweat testing: sample collection and quantitative analysis: approved guidelines. Wayne, Pa.: National Committee for Clinical Laboratory Standards (now Clinical and Laboratory Standards Institute); 2000. NCCLS Document C34-A2.

Guideline for the performance of the sweat test for the diagnosis of cystic fibrosis. This document addresses issues pertaining to collecting, analyzing, reporting, and evaluating sweat test results. Sweat stimulation and collection and quantitative measurement of sweat chloride are described, along with quality assurance and result evaluation.

Sokoll LJ, Wians FH, Remaley AT. Rapid intraoperative immunoassay of parathyroid hormone and other hormones: a new paradigm for point-of-care testing. Clin Chem 2004;50:1126–35.

This study reviews the use of hormone-related intraoperative testing approaches, including parathyroid hormone, cortisol, gastrin, insulin, adrenocorticotropic hormone, and testosterone, regarding preoperative localization studies and/or assessment of the effectiveness of tumor resection during surgery.

Thomas PD, Forbes A, Green J, et al. Guidelines for the investigation of chronic diarrhea, 2nd ed. Gut 2003;52(suppl V):v1.

Provides guidelines to establish an optimal investigative scheme for patients presenting with chronic diarrhea to maximize positive diagnoses while minimizing the number and invasiveness of investigations. Also features summary/recommendation tables with sections devoted to noninvasive testing.

REFERENCES

Access the complete reference list online at http://www.expertconsult.com

CHAPTER 23

TOXICOLOGY AND THERAPEUTIC DRUG MONITORING

Matthew R. Pincus, Naif Z. Abraham Jr.

KEY POINTS

- Testing for the presence of drugs in the blood and other body fluids of patients has undergone a vast increase over the past 20 years.
- Testing for the presence of drugs of abuse and/or poisons in patients has become mandatory both in the emergency room and in employment screening.
- Most drugs for which monitoring is standard can be assayed using homogeneous immunologic techniques.
- Gas chromatography–mass spectroscopy, which involves separation and identification of compounds in the gas phase from their mass/charge ratios and fragmentation patterns, is the "gold standard" for detection and quantitation of drugs in body fluids.
- The mechanisms of action of many therapeutic drugs have been at least partially elucidated. Many of these, such as the antiinflammatory, antiasthmatic, and immunosuppressive drugs, block specific points in signal transduction pathways.
- Ingestion of poisons causes life-threatening illness; poisons include cyanide, carbon monoxide, and a number of metals, such as lead, mercury, iron, and arsenic. If detected, the effects of these poisons can often be reversed.

Toxicology is the study of substances introduced exogenously into the body. Elsewhere in this textbook, the analytic methods presented are concerned with determining the presence and levels of natural substances involved in normal body function. In this chapter, we discuss the biological effects and methods for detection of exogenous chemical compounds that profoundly influence bodily functions, often in a deleterious way but also for therapeutic benefit.

Toxicology has become divided into four areas. The first two areas are the detection of drugs of abuse and the determination of levels of therapeutic drugs being administered to patients. Also, it has been recognized that certain environmental compounds that are mutagens and carcinogens such as benzpyrene and acetylaminofluorene cause mutations in critical sequences of human DNA, leading to the frank development of cancer. In the ongoing revolution in molecular biology, this field has now expanded into the detection of certain markers such as abnormal DNA sequences or the presence of mutated proteins or the presence of carcinogens bound to DNA. This rapidly expanding field is the subject of discussion in Parts 8 and 9, especially in the chapters concerning serum and solid tissue diagnostic markers for cancer and pharmacogenomics. Finally, there are numerous toxins to which individuals become exposed, such as carbon monoxide, cyanide, metals, and so forth, for which detection is vital if physicians are to be able to reverse the adverse acute physiologic effects. In this chapter, we discuss each of these divisions of toxicology with special reference to the detection of drugs and toxins in body fluids.

Basic Techniques for Detecting Drugs in Serum and Urine

The techniques involved in detecting the presence and/or the level of particular drugs, whether they are drugs of abuse or therapeutic drugs, are of two basic types: immunochemical and chromatographic.

IMMUNOCHEMICAL METHODS

Much drug testing today is performed using the so-called **homogeneous immunoassay.** The term homogeneous refers to the fact that these assays are all performed in solution, without any requirement for a phase separation that is traditionally used to separate bound from free ligand. This technology has revolutionized toxicology because it allows performance of rapid, stat analyses of blood and urine constituents. The technique is shown schematically in Figure 23-1. Here we show examples of two types of assays. In the first, the enzyme-mediated (or multiplied) immunologic technique (EMIT), the drug itself is covalently attached to an enzyme such as glucose-6-phosphate dehydrogenase (Fig. 23-1, *A-1*). When the drug–enzyme complex is incubated with an antibody to the drug, enzyme activity is markedly decreased as a result of blocking of the active site of the enzyme by the antibody. When, as in Figure 23-1, *A-2*, exogenous drug (such as in serum) is added to the immune complex, this exogenous drug competes with the drug–enzyme complex for the antibody. Liberated drug–enzyme results in increased enzymatic activity. Increasing concentrations of drug in serum result in increased observed enzymatic activity. This method was pioneered largely by the Syva Corporation (now part of Siemens, Palo Alto, CA) and has been applied both to therapeutic drug monitoring and to detection of drugs of abuse.

Fluorescence polarization immunoassay (FPIA) is the second type of homogeneous drug assay, as shown in Figure 23-1, *B*. Rather than being linked to an enzyme, as in Figure 23-1, *A*, the drug is covalently attached to a fluorescent probe molecule. If a fluorescent molecule is excited with polarized light and is stationary (i.e., it does not "tumble" in solution), it will emit polarized light as a fluorophore. This emitted light has the same polarization as the exciting light. So, for example, if the exciting light is polarized to the left, the emitted light will also be polarized to the left. If a fluorophore tumbles freely in solution, however, the polarization is lost; that is, the emitted light is now polarized equally to the left and right. However, if the fluorophore is bound to a macromolecule such as an antibody, the polarization is strong, because attached to the nontumbling antibody it remains relatively stationary. In these assays, the probe-labeled drug is incubated with the antibody. The fluorescence polarization of the probe-labeled drug is, of course, high because the fluorescence probe is relatively immobilized when bound to the antibody directed against it (Fig. 23-1, *B-1*). Addition of exogenous drug, as in serum, to the incubated mixture results in displacement, by the exogenous drug, of some of the fluorescent probe-labeled drug molecules, as shown in Figure 23-1, *B-2*. These displaced molecules can now tumble freely in solution. The result is a decrease in fluorescence polarization. This decrease is directly related to the concentration of drug in serum.

This assay can detect drug levels in the nanomolar range and is both highly sensitive and specific. Both Abbott Laboratories (Chicago), on the TDX, IMX, and AXSYM analyzers, and Roche Diagnostic Laboratories (Nutley, N.J.), on the COBAS and INTEGRA analyzers, have pioneered this effective technique in monitoring a wide variety of therapeutic drugs and drugs of abuse.

DRUG BINDING TO ANTIBODIES

In both of the homogeneous methods discussed previously, a nonlinear relationship exists between the concentration of drug in serum and the response of the system—that is, the color that results from the enzymatic reaction (see Fig. 23-1, *A*) or the decrease in fluorescence polarization (see Fig. 23-1, *B*). This nonlinearity in response is due to the phenomenon of binding (i.e., the drug must bind to antibody before it is detected). This phenomenon may be expressed by the following equilibrium:

$$D + D^* - Ab \leftrightarrow D - Ab + D^* \qquad \textbf{(23-1)}$$

where D is the drug concentration in serum, D* is the "marker" drug (i.e., drug labeled with an enzyme or a fluorescent probe), and Ab is the antibody. The concentration of free D* is a measure of D–Ab, because both are equimolar. The concentration of D–Ab is, in turn, related to D; the more D is present, the more D–Ab is formed. However, because the concentration of Ab is fixed in a given experiment, at sufficiently high concentrations of D, all of the Ab will be saturated, so that at higher concentrations of D, no further D–Ab can form. The relationship between D and D–Ab is given by the Langmuir expression:

$$r = (D - Ab)/(Ab_0) = nkD/(kD + 1) \qquad \textbf{(23-2)}$$

where (Ab_0) is the total concentration of antibody, k is the equilibrium constant for formation of the D–Ab complex, n is the number of antibody-binding sites per molecule of antibody, and D is free drug concentration as defined above. Equation 23-2 is very similar to the Michaelis-Menten equation discussed in Chapter 20 (Equation 20-10), except that there is no catalytic step here. This equation shows that the concentration of D–Ab is nonlinear in D, except where Kd << 1. Where kD >> 1, saturation is achieved. This equation can be linearized in the form used for a Scatchard plot, that is,

$$r/D = kn - kr \qquad \textbf{(23-3)}$$

where r/D is plotted versus r. Given the results for a set of experiments, a least-squares-best-fit line is drawn through the points. The slope of the line is −k, and the intercept is nk, so that n (the number of sites on the antibody) is equal to the intercept/slope. Thus the values of n and k are readily determined. Once values for n and k are known, the value of D for any measured value of r can be directly computed from Equation 23-3.

Two problems that arise in using Equation 23-3 are that often the antibodies are nonhomogeneous, so that the Scatchard plot is nonlinear, and possible blockage of free antibody sites by drug molecules is seen in solid-phase immunoassays. The first problem was solved by Rodbard (1971), wherein the analysis mentioned previously was applied to multiple-binding equilibria. This analysis is used commonly in microprocessors that analyze the calibration curves in immunoassays. The second problem has been analyzed using a different theoretical approach (Pincus, 1981). Equation 23-3 illustrates the basic principle of how the results of the drug immunoassay on serum are converted into drug concentrations in serum.

CHROMATOGRAPHIC TECHNIQUES

Chromatographic procedures (see Engelhardt, 2004, for an excellent brief history of liquid chromatography) have been applied mainly to the qualitative detection of drugs of abuse and toxins, and less to the determination of levels of therapeutic drugs. The three major methods are thin-layer chromatography (TLC), high-performance liquid chromatography (HPLC), and gas chromatography–mass spectroscopy (GC-MS). Although GC-MS is considered the "gold standard" for detection and quantitation of volatile drugs and poisons, newer analytic techniques such as capillary electrophoresis (CE) and liquid chromatography–mass spectroscopy (LC-MS) are available. These techniques are all discussed in turn.

Thin-Layer Chromatography

Many compounds can be separated from one another with this method, based on their relative affinities for a polar solid stationary phase (usually

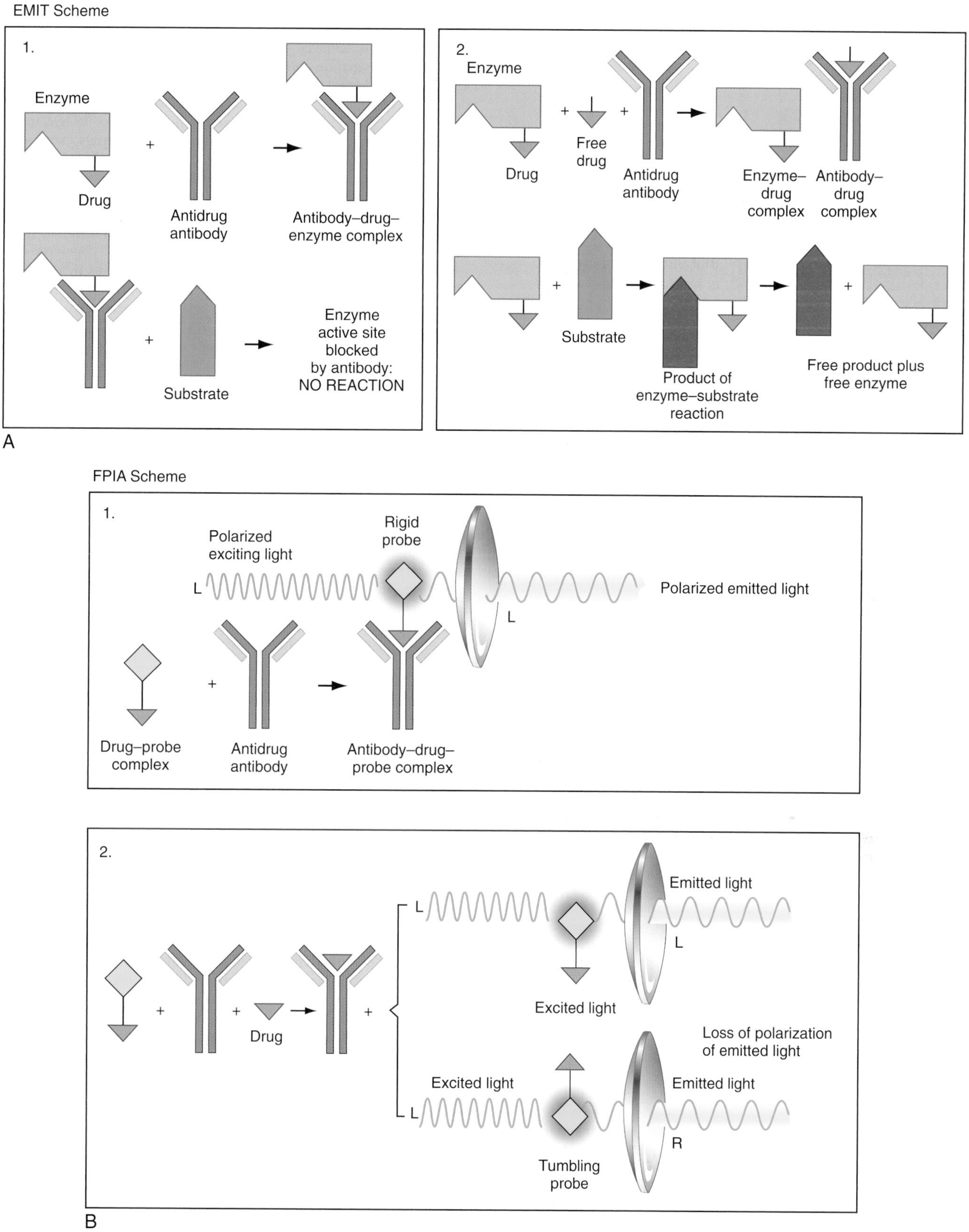

Figure 23-1 Homogeneous methods for detecting qualitatively or quantitatively the levels of drugs in body fluids. **A,** In the enzyme-mediated immunologic technique (EMIT), a drug–enzyme complex is used as the marker. When bound to the antidrug antibody, the active site of the enzyme (linked to the drug) is blocked. Therefore, when substrate is added, no reaction will occur, as is shown in Part 1. However, if free drug (as in serum) is present, some or most of the enzyme–drug complex is displaced from the antidrug antibody. Now the active sites of the liberated enzyme–drug complexes are free, and the substrate undergoes reactions as indicated in Part 2. **B,** In the fluorescence polarization immunoassay assay (FPIA), the same general approach is used as in **A,** except that, in this method, the drug is attached to a fluorescent label or fluorophore. As shown in the upper scheme, Part 1, when the drug–label complex is bound to the antidrug antibody, it becomes immobilized *("rigid probe")*. When excited with polarized light *(shown as polarized to the left or "L")*, the fluorophore emits light, which is likewise polarized to the left *(also seen as "L" in the figure)*. As shown in the lower scheme, Part 2, when displaced by free drug, as in serum or urine, the drug–probe complex is displaced from the antidrug antibody. It is no longer immobilized and therefore tumbles freely in solution. This results in loss of polarization of the emitted light ("L" and "R," for left and right polarization), that is, in diminished fluorescence polarization.

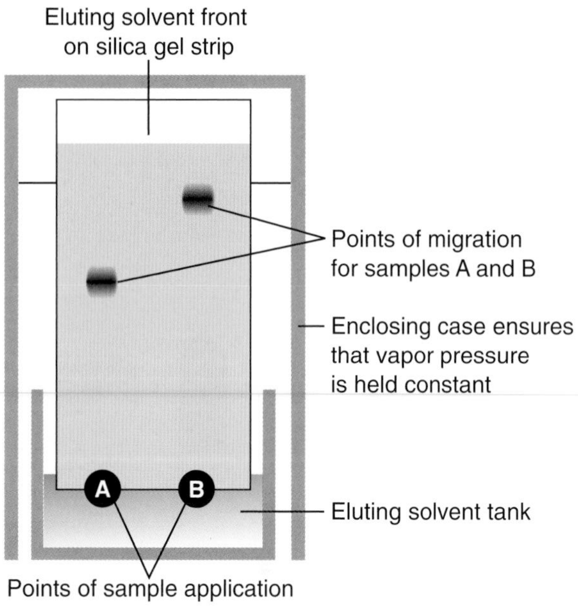

Figure 23-2 Illustration of the principle of thin-layer chromatography (TLC). Two solutes, **A** and **B,** are applied to the polar silicate strip. **A** is more polar than **B** and has a higher affinity, therefore, for the polar stationary phase than for the nonpolar mobile phase (usually methanol in chloroform). Moreover, this relative affinity of **A** is higher than the affinity of **B** for the polar phase. Therefore, **A** separates out first on the strip, and **B** migrates further on the strip.

a hydrated silicate) and a mobile liquid phase that is nonpolar (such as 10% methanol in chloroform). Depending on these affinities, different compounds adsorb to the hydrated silicate at different positions as the nonpolar solvent migrates up the stationary hydrated silicate. The principle is illustrated in Figure 23-2. For a given solvent system, the ratio of the distance traversed by the compound to the distance traversed by the solvent front is a constant for the compound and can be used to identify the compound in a mixture. This ratio is called the $\mathbf{r_f}$. This technique is central to identifying different drugs of abuse, many of which can be separated from one another using TLC. The method has been packaged in the form of Toxi-Lab (Irvine, Calif.) kits in which the user is supplied with discrete strips of silicate, extraction solvents, and color-developing solutions.

Toxi-Lab Procedures

The best specimen for drug detection, by chromatography, is urine because large quantities can be collected noninvasively. Once a urine specimen is collected, it is subjected to concentration and extraction procedures. In extraction procedures, acidic drugs are separated from basic ones. Almost all drugs of abuse are basic drugs, all of which are amine derivatives. The important **acid drugs** comprise almost exclusively the barbiturates. In aqueous solution, the basic drugs are charged because of the equilibrium in Equation 23-4, *A:*

$$R-NH_2 + H^+ \leftrightarrow R-NH_3^+ \quad \textbf{(23-4A)}$$

$$R-NH_3^+ + OH^- \leftrightarrow R-NH_2 + H_2O \quad \textbf{(23-4B)}$$

in which a primary amine (secondary and tertiary amines exhibit the same equilibrium) is represented by RNH_2. The ammonium ion form (right side of Equation 23-4A) is soluble in water but not in nonpolar organic solvents. However, the amine-free base (left side of Equation 23-4A) is soluble in nonpolar organic solvents. Extraction procedures to isolate the basic drugs are aimed at treating the urine with base, so that significant amounts of the basic drugs will be uncharged as the amine-free base (Equation 23-4B). This form can then be extracted into a nonpolar organic phase and applied to the silicate strip. The reverse process is carried out for acidic drugs (i.e., these are treated with acid and are extracted into nonpolar solvents). In practice, a small paper disk is added to the organic extraction mixture, and the solvent is then evaporated so that all basic drugs adsorb onto the paper disk. This disk is then applied to one end of the silicate strip, and the strip is placed in the migrating nonpolar solvent. A separate strip is used for each extraction; the A strip is used for basic drugs, and the B strip for acidic drugs. The chief utility of the B strip is in identifying the barbiturates, as is discussed subsequently.

Identification of Specific Drugs

After separation of the drugs on the plate, it is necessary to identify them. This objective is achieved by subjecting the drugs to standard color reactions for each separate compound. In this procedure for basic drugs, the strip is simply dipped successively in three different solvents, which results in characteristic color patterns for each drug. The strip is also subjected to ultraviolet (UV) light, which excites fluorescence in selected compounds. Similar procedures are used for the acidic drugs extracted onto the B strip. As shown in Figure 23-3, which is from the Toxi-Lab reference pattern book, each drug can be identified not only by its r_f but also by its color and characteristic color change in different reagents. These patterns are reinforced by the fluorescence characteristics. As an example, notice in Figure 23-3, *A,* on the Toxi-Lab A worksheet that morphine, the main metabolite of heroin, has a characteristic r_f of 0.14 and a characteristic dark red or purple color in the first solvent that diminishes in intensity and changes color in the second solvent, water. It is nonfluorescent. If one or more of these characteristics differ(s) from this pattern, strong doubt about identification of the spot as morphine would exist. If all criteria are met, the sensitivity and specificity of the method are increased.

Reliability of the Method

Because the identification of each drug depends on the use of qualitative color changes and/or the presence of fluorescence, the sensitivity of the method is limited by the ability of the naked eye to detect these changes. Practically, the level of detection is on the order of 1 μg/mL of compound present on the strip. The chief value of the chromatographic method is confirmatory (i.e., confirmation of a positive immunoassay test result). The two methods are often performed together on a single specimen.

The major problems that occur with this method are that extraction procedures are occasionally inefficient, so that insufficient amounts of drug are absorbed onto the disk. Also, the extraction and evaporation procedures are somewhat time consuming, requiring approximately a half-hour for full processing. Furthermore, cocaine has a number of metabolites that are polar (e.g., ecgonine), and that barely migrate from the origin, so that it is sometimes difficult to detect the presence of this drug of abuse because it has been converted completely to the polar metabolites before excretion. Some difficulty may also be encountered in distinguishing among various opiates, such as between morphine and other opiates, because the r_f values of these drugs can be close to one another (see Fig. 23-3 Toxi-Lab A worksheet). However, experienced personnel can make this distinction in most cases. Also, some nontoxic drugs may give characteristic color changes, and r_f values that are similar to those for the drug of abuse. A case in point is that certain antihistamines appear on the A strip to be very similar to amphetamines.

High-Performance Liquid Chromatography

TLC allows direct qualitative detection of drugs in a panoramic way. HPLC allows quantitative detection of drugs and allows sharper separation of these same drugs. In HPLC, the stationary phase, which can be either polar (silicic acid) or nonpolar (such as the C-18 columns), in reverse-phase chromatography is composed of uniform, ultrafine particles that vastly increase its adsorptive surface area. This stationary phase is packed into a column. The resistance to flow in this column is high, so that large pressures are required to deliver constant reasonable flow rates. In the Waters HPLC instrument (Waters Corporation, Milford, Mass.), a constant pressure head is delivered to the column by the use of two pumps that operate so that as one withdraws, the other pushes forward (i.e., the two operate 180 degrees out of phase). The eluate from the column is monitored by a variety of detectors ranging from UV multiwavelength detectors to redox potential electrode detectors. It is the usual practice in performance of quantitative HPLC to use an internal standard—that is, a compound similar in structure to the drug(s) of interest, which is added to the specimen to be analyzed in a known concentration. By knowing how much of this marker compound or internal standard is placed on the column and how much is recovered from the column in the eluate, the percentage recovery from the column can be calculated for this compound and, by extrapolation, for all of the drugs of interest for which concentrations are being quantitated. Thus, losses due to the column (in addition to losses in extraction procedures) can be corrected for using this technique. Generally, HPLC has been used for the quantitation of specific therapeutic drugs but has found use in detection of cocaine and heroin in urine. The sensitivity of the method is in the nanomolar to micromolar range.

One of the greatest uses of HPLC is in the separation and quantitation of the tricyclic antidepressants and their metabolites. These are among the most commonly prescribed drugs and are also used in excess as drugs of

Toxi-lab A Worksheet

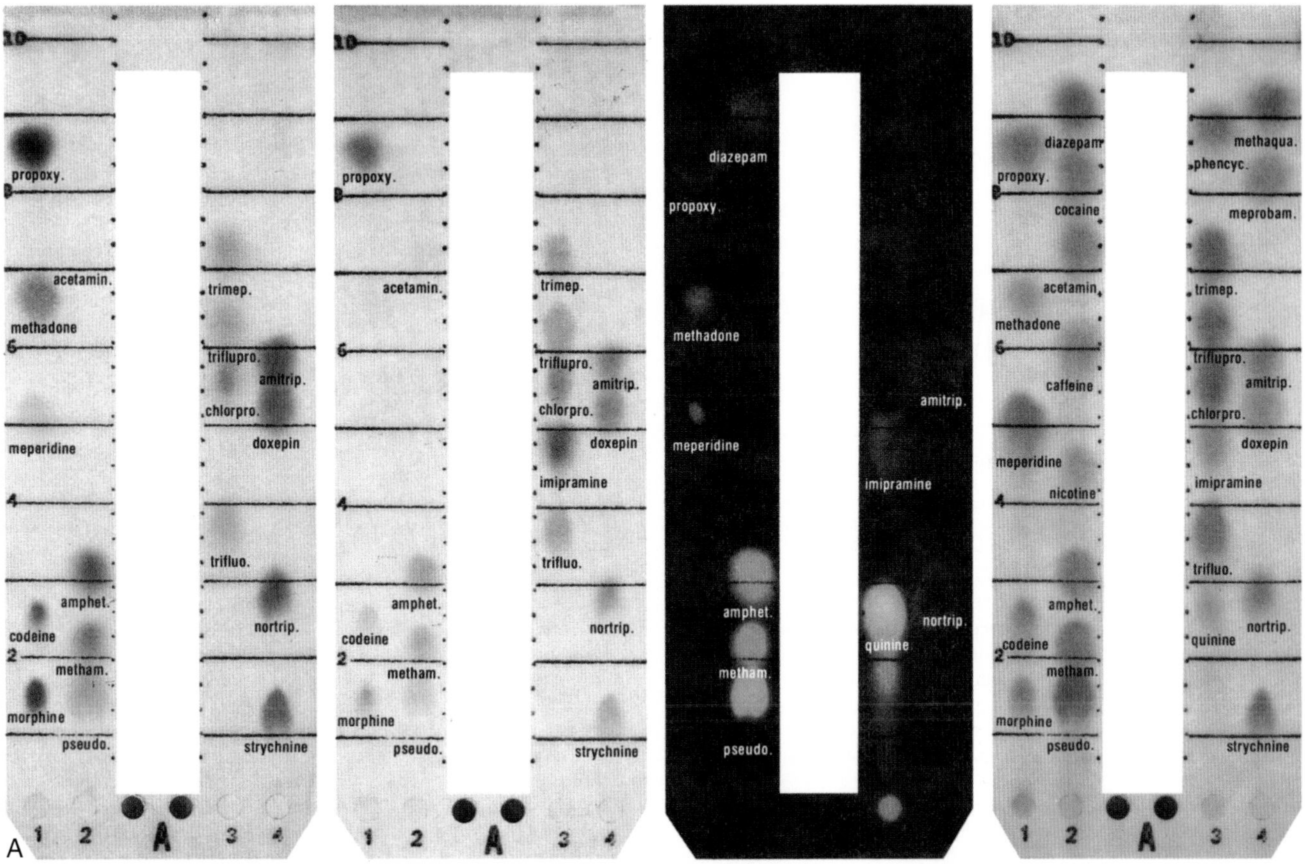

Toxi-lab B Worksheet

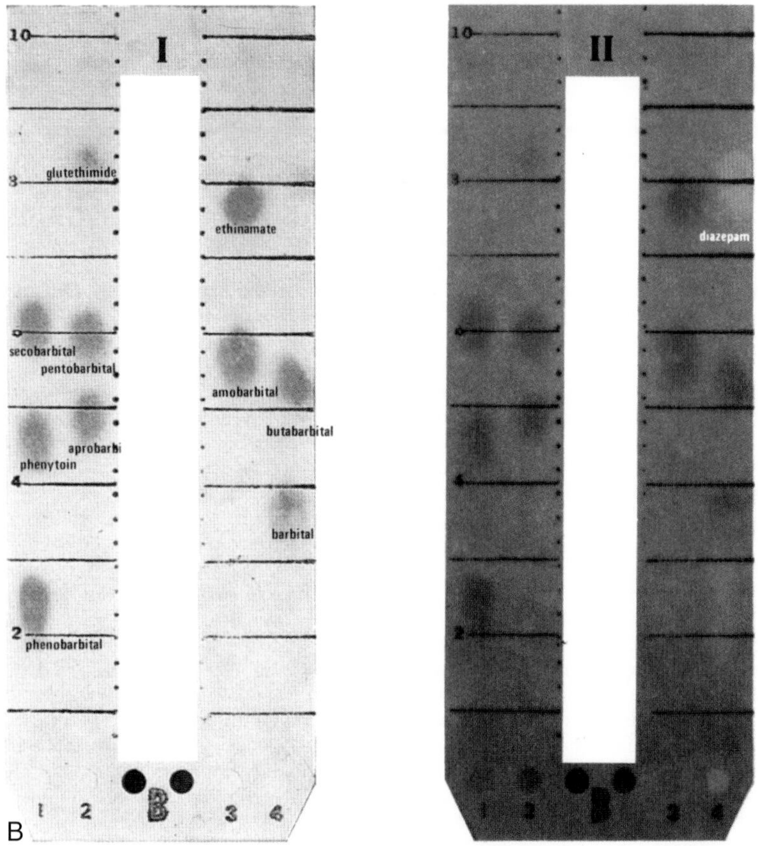

Figure 23-3 A set of typical separations of the major drugs of abuse (and some therapeutic drugs) on Toxi-Lab thin-layer chromatography. Toxi-Lab **A** worksheet: Typical separation of basic drugs on the **A** strip, together with characteristic color changes. The third Toxi-Lab **A** strip shows characteristic fluorescence of different drugs. Note that amphetamine and methamphetamine on the lower left are both fluorescent. Toxi-Lab **B** worksheet: *Left:* Typical separation of the more acidic drugs on the **B** strip with characteristic color changes. The major use of the **B** strip is to identify the presence of the barbiturates. *Right:* Fluorescence patterns of drugs on the **B** strip.

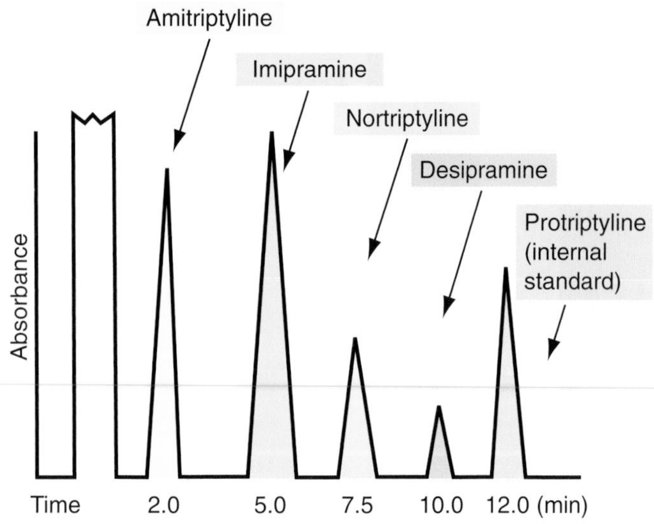

Figure 23-4 Sketch of a typical separation of the major tricyclic antidepressants on high-performance liquid chromatography. A complete separation can be effected in 12 minutes. The concentration of each drug is on the order of 100 mcg/mL.

abuse in suicide attempts. It is often necessary to determine the levels not only of the parent tricyclic antidepressant but also of its active and inactive metabolites reviewed subsequently. Figure 23-4 shows a typical separation on a silicate column. Protriptyline, a less inactive tricyclic compound, is the internal standard. It is clear that the separation among the metabolites and parent compounds is quite sharp. This separation is completely reproducible.

A recent variant of TLC that includes the advantages of HPLC is CE (Tagliaro, 1998; Shihabi, 1993). In this method, a capillary tube, lined with silicate, 10–100 μm in internal diameter and 100–1000 mm in length, is used as the solid support in an electrophoresis apparatus. Here, the driving force for separation is the voltage (on the order of 25 kV) rather than pressure, as in HPLC. Because of the vast surface area, separations are quite sharp. The system is highly versatile and can be used to separate serum proteins and small molecules. CE possesses a wide analytic spectrum (including biopolymers, pesticides, aromatic compounds, drugs, inorganic ions, etc.) because of high versatility in terms of separation modes. Different analyte selectivity is based on different physicochemical principles of separation without changes in instrumental hardware—a distinct advantage of this technique. Capillary zone electrophoresis, micellar electrokinetic capillary chromatography (MECK), capillary isotachophoresis, capillary isoelectric focusing, capillary electrochromatography, and capillary gel electrophoresis are different separation modes utilized in CE separations. For example, by adding a detergent to the buffer system, as with MECK, micelles will form. A neutral compound (such as a pesticide) will partition into the detergent, forming micelles, and the complex will separate out based on the mobility/charge of the micelle. In addition, new platforms such as chip-based CE and immunoaffinity CE are currently being developed. CE has not yet enjoyed as widespread use as the immunoassay techniques (discussed previously) in clinical toxicology but is commonly utilized in analytic forensic toxicologic studies, as well as in molecular diagnostic studies, and can easily be extended to other uses in clinical laboratory medicine (Boone, 2003; Petersen, 2003).

GAS CHROMATOGRAPHY–MASS SPECTROSCOPY

Testing for drugs of abuse has become one of the most rapidly developing areas in the clinical laboratory in view of the widespread and ever-expanding use of these drugs among large segments of the working population. In view of the increasing requirements for routine drug screening, it is necessary to have "gold standard" techniques to confirm the results obtained using screening methods such as EMIT and TLC.

GC-MS has proved to be such a gold standard because of its great sensitivity and its reliability. This method, as its name implies, involves two techniques: gas–liquid chromatography and mass spectroscopy. In the former, compounds are directly heated into the gas phase or are derivatized to make them labile to facilitate heating them into the gas phase. They are then passed over a column containing the stationary phase, which often consists of a liquid, usually a hydrocarbon or silicone oil, that coats a solid support in the column and offers a large surface area for adsorption. Separation is based, much as in TLC, on the ability of each compound to adsorb to the stationary phase, which partially depends on the relative solubilities of the compound in the gas versus the liquid phase. Normally, the compounds eluting from the column could be detected by conventional techniques, as discussed previously, except that once the compounds are in the gas phase, where they are heated, advantage can be taken of another feature of the system—the ability of compounds that are heated to high temperatures to lose or gain electrons.

At high temperatures, the highest energy electrons of a compound (i.e., the ones of lowest ionization potential) can be excited, such that the molecule can lose electrons and become charged. This process may be aided by such techniques as electron bombardment in a specially designed chamber that directly creates molecule-ions. Most of these resulting molecule-ions are single cations. Different molecule-ions in general have different sizes and different molecular weights. These molecule-ions decompose into characteristic fragments whose ratios with respect to one another and whose positions of migration relative to one another are also constant. The molecule-ions are then passed through an electric field generated by four rods that are subjected to rapidly alternating currents, the so-called **quadrupole detector.** Depending on the frequency of the alternating current, certain molecule-ions with specific mass/charge ratios can pass through the field to a detector. Thus, the molecule-ions can be separated on the basis of molecular weight or, more exactly, on their mass/charge ratios. The overall design of GC-MS is shown in Figure 23-5.

The presence of the molecule-ion on the plate is detected by a charge multiplier detector system. The technique of GC-MS has become highly refined. Each molecule-ion created in the gas phase can undergo further changes, such as elimination reactions and rearrangements, and further degradation to small fragments that, in turn, ionize and give characteristic decomposition patterns. The patterns of thousands of compounds have now been determined. The position of the parent molecule-ion of the compound and the decomposition fragments give rise to a **fingerprint pattern** unique to the compound. These patterns are stored in a computer so that when a pattern for an unknown compound or group of compounds is obtained, the pattern is compared with the stored patterns to identify the compound(s) of interest. The entire method has been highly successful in detecting even low levels of cocaine and/or its metabolites in body fluids. A typical cocaine pattern is shown in Figure 23-6. Because single molecule-ion species give rise to significant currents in the detector, it is possible to detect very low levels of drugs, making this technique the ultimate reference method and the best confirmatory testing procedure available at present.

LIQUID CHROMATOGRAPHY–MASS SPECTROSCOPY

(Davis, 1989; Maurer, 1998; Marquet, 2002; Niessen, 1995, 2003).

As discussed previously, GC-MS is the gold standard for the identification of volatile compounds. Nonvolatile compounds, however, can be detected utilizing LC-MS. Unlike GC-MS, however, the coupling of LC with MS requires sophisticated interfaces between the LC and MS components. The interface must volatilize nonvolatile compounds that have been separated on the LC; must remove the liquid solvent from the LC; and must correct flow-rate incompatibility between the LC and MS. Two interface methods, electrospray (ES) and atmospheric pressure chemical ionization (APCI), appear to have become the gold standards for LC-MS. Both interface methods are utilized with atmospheric pressure ionization devices to facilitate removal of the mobile phase. They differ primarily in the range of analytes that can be accommodated and in how the solvent phase is nebulized.

Ionizable analytes of high molecular weight and/or high polarity can be accommodated with ES, and APCI can be used for analytes of less polarity and lower molecular weight. At present, ES appears to have more clinical and forensic applications than APCI in toxicology. LC-MS can be used to confirm positive test results from a screening assay and has been used for confirmation of drugs-of-abuse assays, poisoning detection in acute or chronic intoxication, therapeutic drug identification and quantitation, and pharmacokinetic and drug metabolism studies. Although LC-MS has limitations when compared with GC-MS, it has become a powerful "mature and validated" (Marquet, 2002) technique in analytic toxicology and a complementary method to GC-MS.

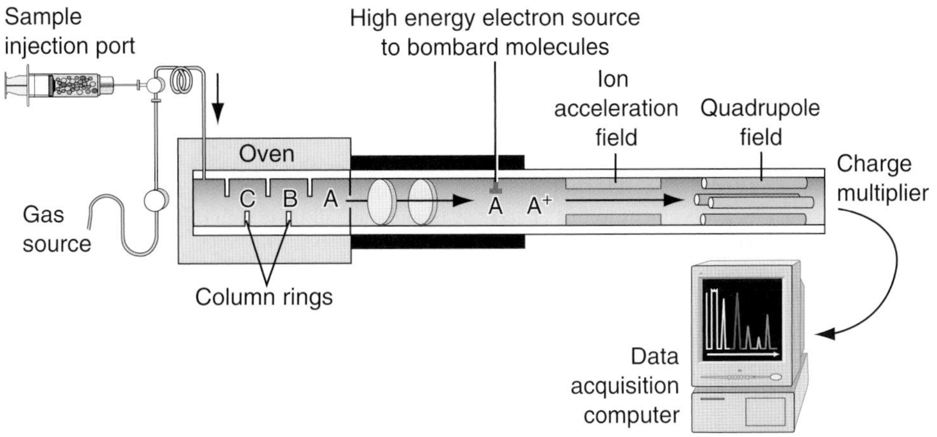

Figure 23-5 A schematic view of the components of gas chromatography–mass spectroscopy instrumentation. On the left of the figure is the gas chromatographic system, where a volatilized compound is moved by an inert gas over a column consisting of rings coated with a liquid. Compounds C, B, and A separate on this column and are maintained in the gas phase by the oven that surrounds the column. The separated compounds then enter the mass spectrometer on the right side of the figure, where they are subjected to bombardment by electrons, resulting in molecule ion species. These ionic species then are accelerated in a field and are passed through an electric quadrupole field. Only those ions with a narrow range of mass/charge ratios (m/e ratios) will pass through the tuned field so that they strike the detector. The electric currents that result are digitalized and stored in a computer that analyzes the data (Davis, 1989).

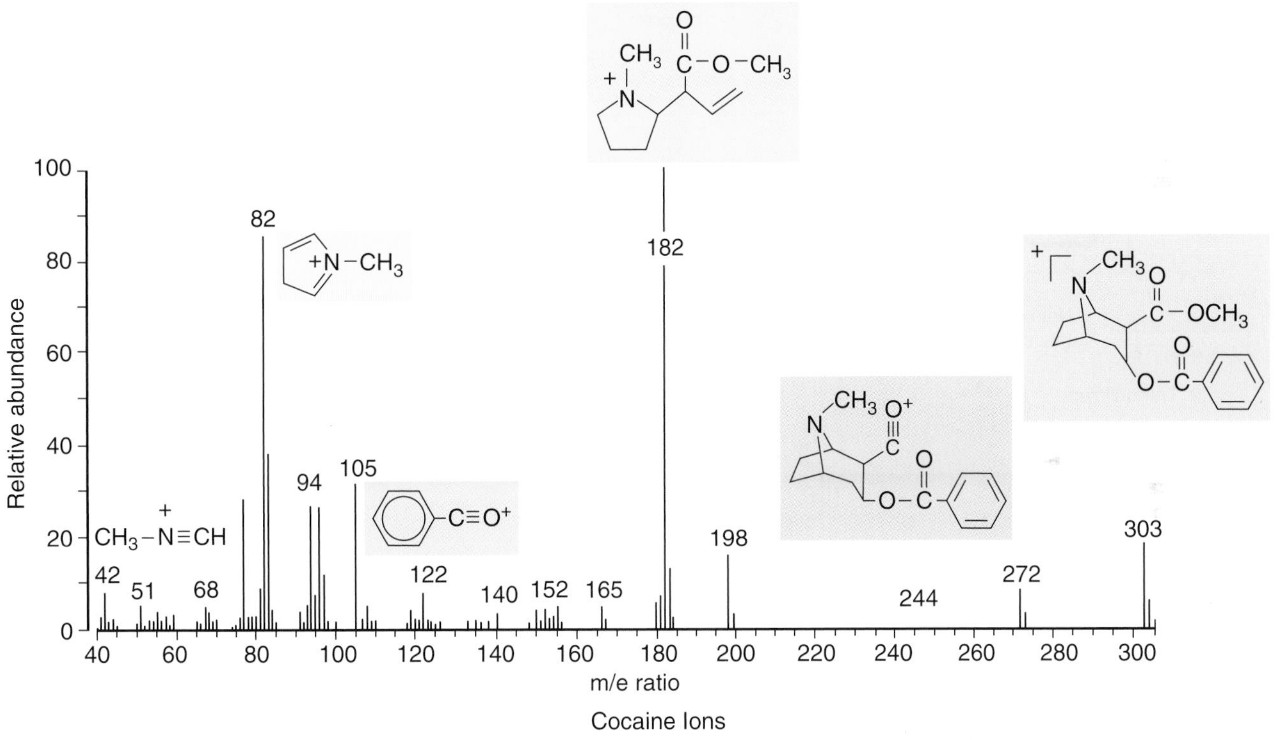

Figure 23-6 Fragmentogram for cocaine using gas chromatography–mass spectroscopy. The specimen is urine. This figure shows the characteristic peaks for cocaine metabolites. m/e is the mass to charge ratio, which for most ions is a measure of the molecular mass. *(Courtesy of Dr. Chip Walls, Onondaga County, N.Y., Medical Examiners Office.)*

GAS CHROMATOGRAPHY COUPLED WITH INFRARED SPECTROSCOPY

Infrared (IR), or Fourier-transformed infrared, spectroscopy (FTIR) utilizes light of high wavelength (low frequency), which excites vibronic states of molecules involved in bond stretching and bond angle bending. Every compound has a characteristic IR "fingerprint," that is, IR absorption pattern, so that even closely related compounds can be distinguished readily from one another by gas phase IR. Thus the fractions of patients' samples that elute from a GC or liquid chromatography column can be analyzed using this technique. As with mass spectroscopy, the FTIR spectra for different compounds can stored in a computer attached to the GC-FTIR system; the spectra obtained from the eluates from the column are then analyzed for the presence of specific drugs of abuse. This method is particularly well suited for the detection of amphetamines (Belal, 2009).

SCREENING FOR DRUGS OF ABUSE

In most states of the United States, two levels of testing for drugs of abuse have become recognized: emergency room testing and employment screening/forensic testing. The former involves rapid, stat screening methods, in particular, EMIT (or FPIA) and TLC. The purpose of this type of screening test is to detect the presence of a drug or several drugs of abuse in the patient's urine. Rarely are the more sophisticated chromatographic procedures such as HPLC and GC-MS used for this purpose. Forensic testing, on the other hand, requires not only a screen but also an independent confirmatory method, which is almost always chosen to be GC-MS or, less commonly, HPLC. It should be noted that, strictly by law, any confirmatory method is valid, provided it is a completely different method from the primary one. Thus, TLC can confirm EMIT, whereas FPIA cannot confirm it because both EMIT and FPIA are immunochemical methods. Another important legalistic consideration in forensic testing is the so-called **chain of custody** (DeCresce, 1989; Poklis, 2001). This process is used in the collection of urine from the individual from whom the specimen is taken. It may begin by observation of specimen collection by one person. Then, that person or another specifically designated individual, usually a police officer (in the case of prisoners or suspects) or some other designated official, accompanies the messenger, who brings the specimen from the individual to the laboratory. This individual is a witness to the testing (and must sign a legal document to this effect) of the specific urine sample collected. More than one designated individual may be involved as the witness in this chain.

The Drugs of Abuse

GENERAL ASPECTS OF THE MECHANISMS OF ACTION

The major drugs of abuse (Flomenbaum, 2006; Sweetman, 2002) are shown in Figure 23-7 (O'Neil, 2001; Haroz, 2006). As may be seen in this figure, these drugs, with the exception of the barbiturates and the cannabinoids, are all basic amino group–containing compounds, most of which also contain benzene rings. The steric relationship of the amino group with respect to the aromatic benzene rings is rather similar, especially in

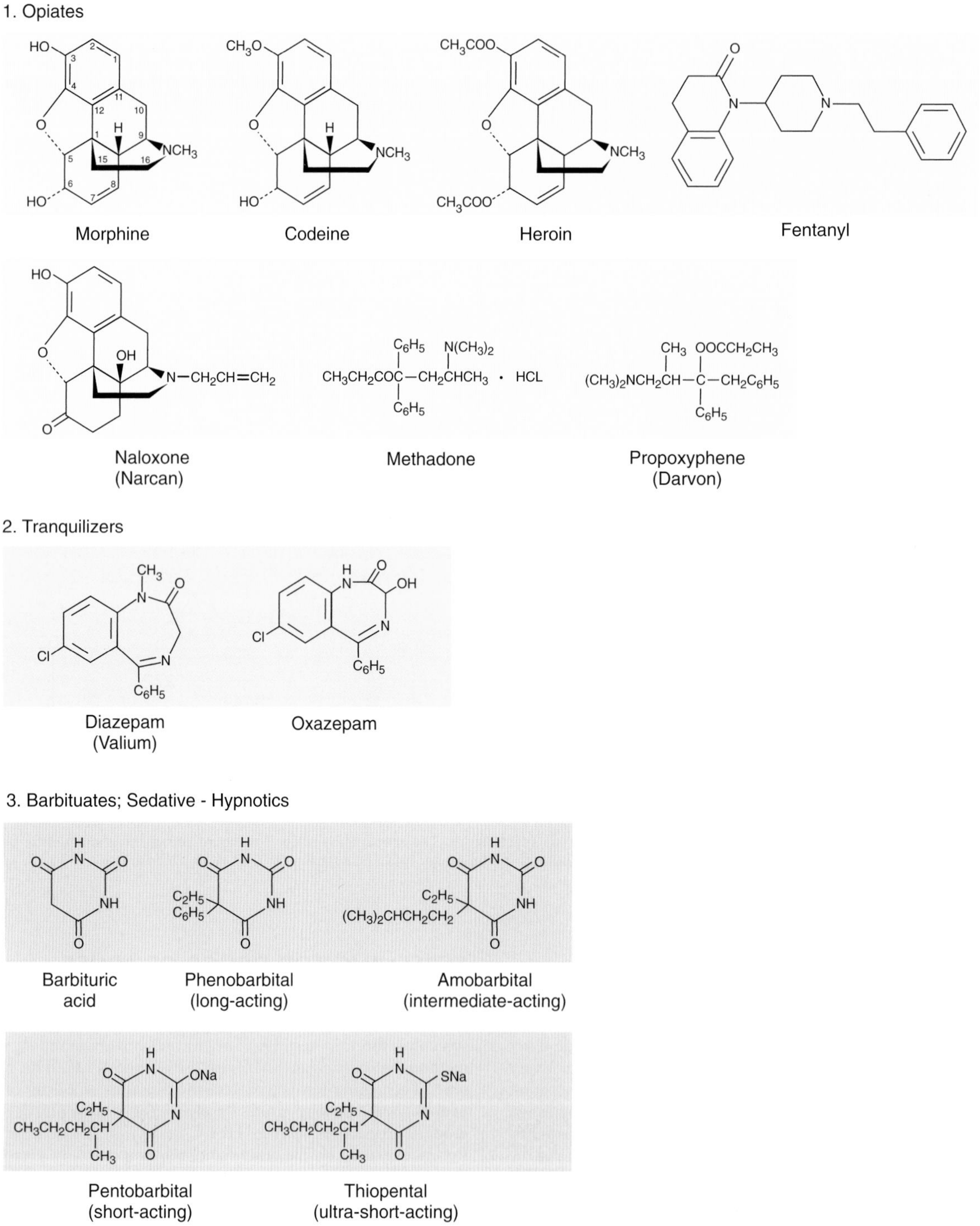

Figure 23-7 Chemical structures for the major drugs of abuse. All of the opiates are seen to be basic compounds that are tertiary amines and that contain benzene rings. Notice that, in the barbiturate series, barbituric acid may be considered as a condensation product of urea and malonic acid.

4. Dopaminergic Pathway Stimulants

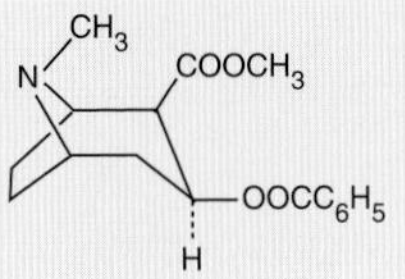

Cocaine

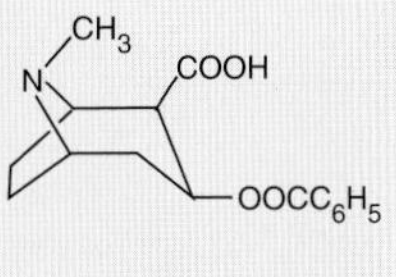

Benzoylecgonine
(less active metabolite)

Amphetamines

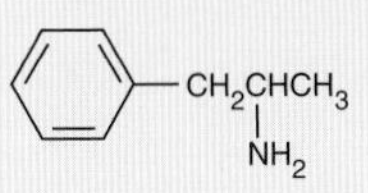

Amphetamine

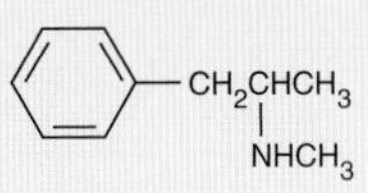

Methamphetamine

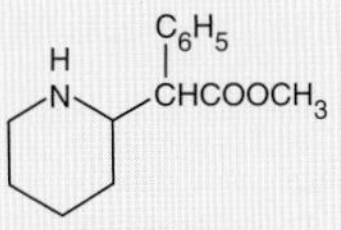

Methylphenidate
(Ritalin - used to treat hyperactive children)

4A. "Designer" Amphetamines/Phenylethylamines

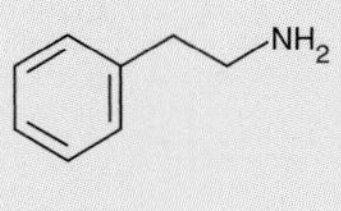

Phenylethylamine-base compound

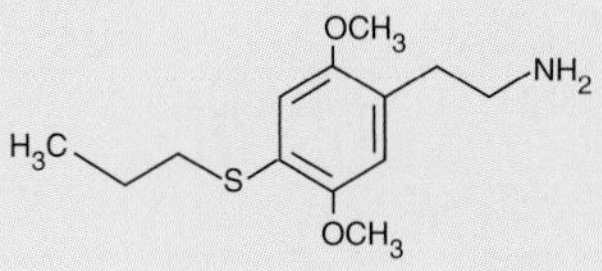

2,5-dimethyoxy-4(n)-propyl-thiophenethylamine (2C-T-7)

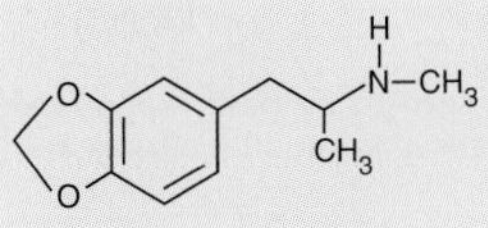

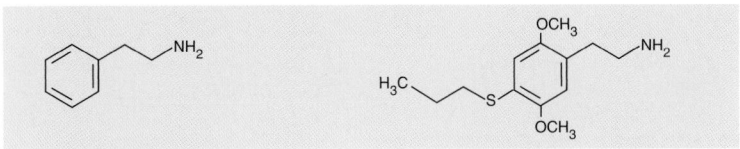

3,4-dimethyleneoxy-methamphetamine
(MDMA or "Ecstasy")

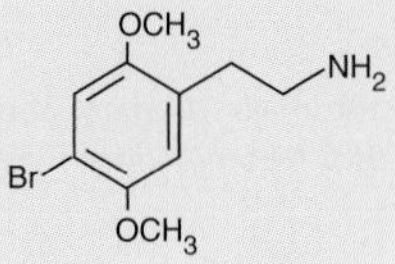

4-Bromo-2,5-methoxy-phenylethylamine (2CB)

5. Hallucinogens

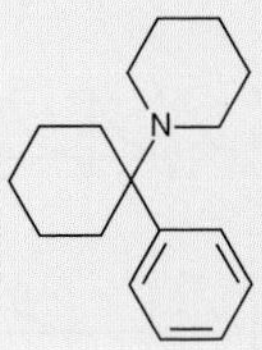

Phencyclidine

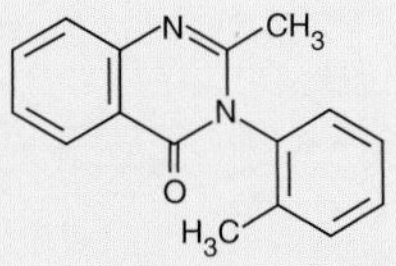

Methaquaalone

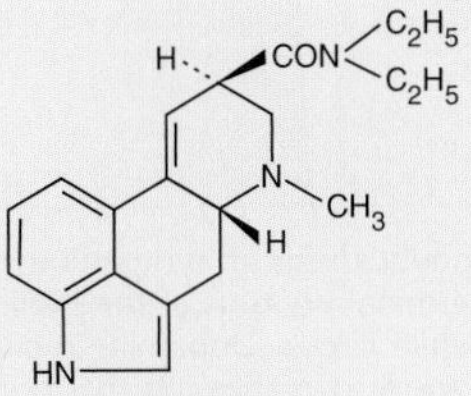

Lysergic acid diethylamide
(LSD)

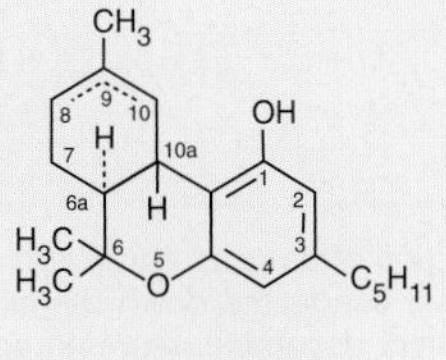

Tetrahydro cannabinol

Figure 23-7, cont'd For legend, see opposite page.

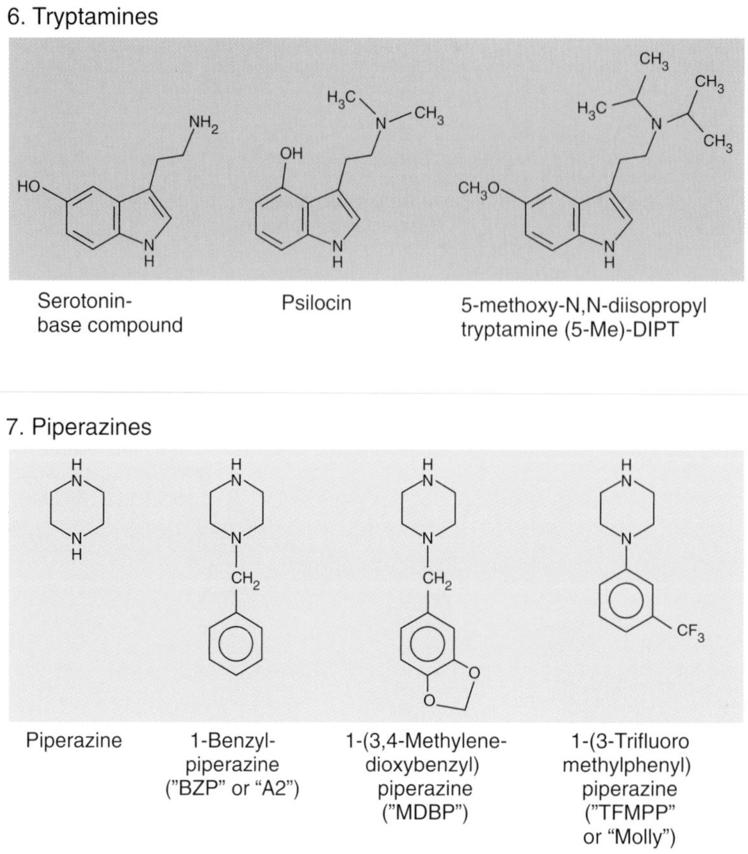

Figure 23-7, cont'd Chemical structures for the major drugs of abuse. All of the opiates are seen to be basic compounds that are tertiary amines and that contain benzene rings. Notice that, in the barbiturate series, barbituric acid may be considered as a condensation product of urea and malonic acid.

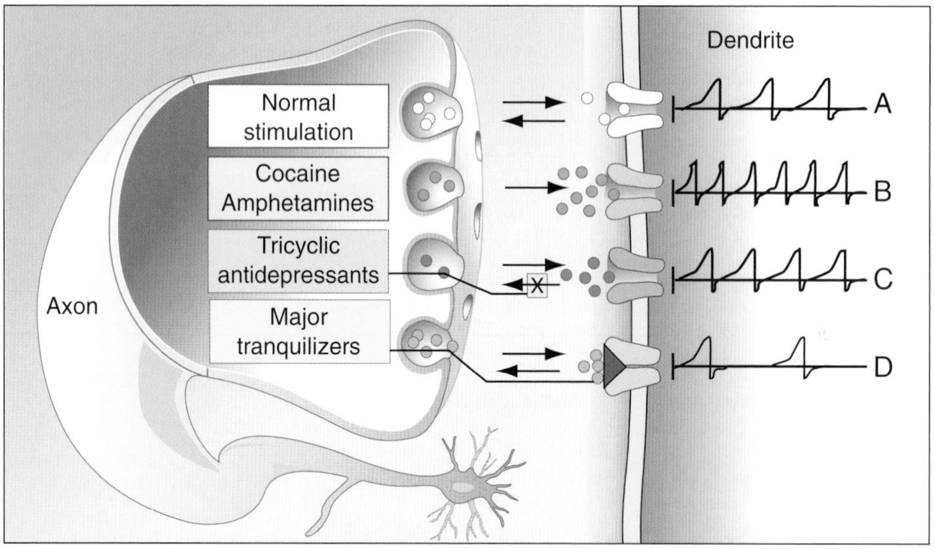

Figure 23-8 Illustration of the possible mechanisms of action of drugs of abuse and some therapeutic drugs on sympathomimetic amine (dopamine and norepinephrine) pathways. *A,* Normal neural transmission. A nerve impulse is conducted down the axon to the terminal boutons at the nerve ending. Vesicles, represented by the round gray structure, release their contents of neurotransmitter, here dopamine, represented by small white circles. Dopamine molecules traverse the synaptic cleft and bind to dendritic receptors, initiating action potentials *(at right under "dendrite")* in the dendrites. Notice the arrows showing that dopamine is both released and taken up by the vesicles. *B,* In the presence of cocaine and amphetamines, enhanced release of neurotransmitter *(red circles)* from vesicles occurs, increasing the rate of firing in the dendrites. *C,* Tricyclic antidepressants block (arrow with "X" in yellow box) reuptake of the neurotransmitter *(purple circles),* in this case norepinephrine and, less specifically, dopamine, causing more neurotransmitter to "recycle" to the dendritic receptors, resulting in increased firing. *D,* Some of the neuroleptics act by blocking *(gray wedge)* postsynaptic dendritic receptors for dopamine *(blue circles),* causing decreased firing.

cocaine, the opiates, and methadone. As might be expected, these compounds can cross-react with each other's target receptors. The primary physiologic mechanisms of action of these drugs are not well understood, but some rudimentary knowledge has been gained as to some of the main targets of these drugs. Many of these drugs act directly on dopaminergic and norepinephrinergic neurotransmitter systems, especially the limbic system (sometimes referred to as the **smell brain**). This system is a more primitive one associated with pleasure seeking and is discussed further later.

In Figure 23-8, possible effects of several of the most important drugs on this system are shown. It appears that the amphetamines, closely related structurally to dopamine and the catecholamines, and cocaine cause release of dopamine from the vesicles at the axonal side of the synapse, which may partially be responsible for their producing a pleasant sensation (so-called

high) in many individuals (Hurd, 1988). The tricyclic antidepressants stimulate pathways that utilize norepinephrine as the neurotransmitter. These pathways, like the dopaminergic pathways, are involved in arousal and pleasure seeking. In this case, the tricyclic antidepressants, rather than promoting release of the neurotransmitters, block the reuptake of norepinephrine into the vesicles on the axonal side of the synapse. They also may exert nonspecific reuptake blockade of dopamine in the dopaminergic pathways (Baldessarini, 2006a). It is of great interest that, paradoxically, the tricyclic antidepressants such as imipramine (Tofranil) have been used successfully to treat the effects of cocaine, although, as described later, benzodiazepine tranquilizers are now preferred. The major tranquilizers such as haloperidol (Haldol) and chlorpromazine, used to treat psychotic states such as schizophrenia, appear to block attachment of dopamine to the dendritic receptors in the synapse, thereby blocking the stimulatory effects of dopamine. Associated with many dopaminergic neurons are inhibitory neurons that use γ-aminobutyric acid (GABA) as their neurotransmitter. It appears that many benzodiazepine receptors exist on these neurons, causing potentiation of GABA at the synapses in this system, reducing the dopaminergic effects of the stimulatory pathways on the limbic system. Thus, some of the tranquilizing effects of diazepam (Valium) and other benzodiazepines can be explained.

Widely distributed throughout the central nervous system and periphery are a variety of opioid receptors classified mainly as μ-, δ-, κ- (the three classic opioid receptor types), and ε- (not well characterized; see Tseng, 2001; Snyder, 2003) receptors. The μ-receptors appear to be highly specific for morphine and heroin, both of which produce a general analgesic state. At the moment, there appears to be no direct relationship between these receptors and the dopaminergic pathways.

It is interesting to note that the naturally produced opiate peptide, metenkephalin, whose amino acid sequence is Tyr-Gly-Gly-Phe-Met, cross-reacts significantly with μ-receptors, although its primary "target" is ε-receptors. It has been shown that the benzodiazepines may be structurally related to enkephalin, which, in turn, may be structurally related to morphine (Pincus, 1987; Murphy, 1992). It is therefore possible that these compounds have similar effects, at least indirectly, on the dopaminergic pathways.

Many of the drugs of abuse also act on two other major pathways in the brain: those using serotonin (serotonergic) and those utilizing *N*-methyl-D-aspartate (NMDA) as their neurotransmitter. Neurotranmission by serotonin occurs by its binding to the 5-hydroxytryptamine (5-HT) receptor on the dendritic side of the synapse. There is a rather wide range of 5-HT receptors, not all of which produce the same physiologic effects. The major ones appear to be 5-HT_1 and 5-HT_2 receptors. The serotonin pathways encompass a rather wide swath of the brain and even the spinal cord. This neurotransmitter is the principal one for the limbic system and, in addition, the basal ganglia, especially the amygdala that is involved in aggressive behavior. As mentioned earlier, the limbic system is involved in pleasure seeking and pleasure reinforcement. Serotonergic pathways also extend to the hippocampus and are involved in memory. As a neurotransmitter in the spinal cord, serotonin induces muscle contraction. NMDA pathways are more involved in nociceptive (pain) pathways and are involved in memory and neuronal plasticity (Zhuo, 2009). They have been found to be involved in chronic pain reinforcement. Blockade of NMDA pathways by drugs of abuse can therefore remove this perceived undesirable effect.

COCAINE

Cocaine is derived from the coca plant and has enjoyed much popularity as an additive to certain foods. At the beginning of the 20th century, it was used in Coca-Cola, but owing to its addictive effects, this practice was discontinued. Cocaine is a derivative of the alkaloid ecgonine (i.e., the methyl ester of benzoylecgonine), as shown in Figure 23-7 (Group 4 drugs). The normal route of administration of cocaine is nasal (i.e., inhalation, called **snorting**), such that the drug passes through the nasal membranes. A particularly potent form of cocaine, called **crack,** is the free-base form that passes rapidly across the nasal membranes such that, for a given dose, most or all of it enters the bloodstream rapidly. The half-life of cocaine is 1–2 hours, and the parent compound and its metabolites are usually cleared from the body within 2 days.

It is estimated that as many as 25 million people in the United States have used cocaine at least once (Jones, 2006). As of 2008, it was estimated that 5.3 million Americans 12 years of age and older actually abused this drug (National Institute of Drug Abuse, 2009). Fatalities from cocaine abuse are of two types: direct toxicity of the drug (Johanson, 1989), and crime related to the illicit acquisition of the drug. Up to 25% of myocardial infarctions in patients between the ages of 18 and 45 have been attributed to cocaine abuse (Jones, 2006).

Cocaine is used medically to induce local anesthesia during nasopharyngeal surgery. However, in large doses, it induces a euphoric state (the "high" experienced by the user) and may also induce hallucinatory states. It can also promote violent behavior (Flomenbaum, 2006; Hoffman, 2006). Many of these results can be explained by cocaine's dopaminergic effects. One study (Azmitia, 1990) suggests that cocaine induces increased calcium ion influx in dopaminergic neurons. The increased intracellular calcium activates phospholipases that possibly act as second messengers in causing ultimate release of dopamine in synapses. Prolonged action of phospholipases, however, ultimately causes cell death. In the previously mentioned study, in fact, cocaine was found to be neurotoxic. It also has a general cytotoxic effect from formation of an *N*-oxide free-radical produced in the metabolism of this compound in the liver. It appears then that, over time, cocaine induces neuronal loss. In addition, binding of cocaine to cell receptors in the limbic system induces synthesis of cyclic adenosine monophosphate (cAMP) that appears to be critical in activating cell processes involved in dopamine release (Cami, 2003). Cocaine may also block the reuptake of dopamine at the axonal side of the synapse. As if becoming toxic from cocaine abuse was not sufficient, many cocaine abusers consume this drug together with alcohol. Ethanol becomes esterified to cocaine in the liver to form cocaethylene, which blocks reuptake of dopamine in dopaminergic pathways more effectively than does cocaine and causes pronounced vasoconstriction of the coronary arteries and induces increased myocardial oxygen demand. This cocaine derivative is deadlier than either cocaine or ethanol alone (Jones, 2006).

Studies (Lange, 1989, 2001; Frishman, 2003; Jones, 2006) further indicate that prolonged use of cocaine results in cardiotoxicity—that is, cocaine can cause progressive atherosclerosis and causes constriction of the coronary arteries that can, in turn, induce myocardial ischemia and sometimes frank infarction. Cocaine has been found to induce sympathomimetic effects on the myocardium by increasing heart rate. At the same time, it induces increased vasoconstriction. The net effect is increased chronotropy and afterload, resulting in increased oxygen demand by the myocardium. At the same time, cocaine induces platelet aggregation and stimulates production of plasminogen activator inhibitor (Jones, 2006). These events all predispose to development of myocardial infarction.

One highly disturbing aspect of cocaine abuse is the fact that cocaine passes readily across the placenta and also into the lactating mammary gland and is readily passed from mothers to nursing infants. Often in the hospital setting, mothers receive the drug from dealers and breastfeed their newborn babies, who are therefore maintained on this drug. Cocaine causes mental retardation, delayed development, and strong drug dependence in newborns. It can also produce malformations in utero.

Cocaine has not been considered classically to be an addictive drug, as it does not cause the true physical dependence typical of abusers of barbiturates and opiates. However, the high produced by the drug is extraordinarily reinforcing, so that the drug-seeking behavior of the cocaine and opiate abuser is similar. Evidence in experimental animals suggests that cocaine can induce the release of β-endorphins that bind to μ-receptors in the limbic system (Gianoulakis, 2004). This induces a pleasant and positive feeling of reinforcement. Clinically, patients who are overdosed with cocaine may become violent and irrational, requiring sedation. The treatment of choice for patients in hyperexcitable states with cardiac symptoms such as palpitations is one of the benzodiazepines. Thus, it is not uncommon to find cocaine and Valium in the urine of cocaine addicts. Occasionally, overdosed patients will become obtunded or comatose. The treatment for these patients is usually supportive. As noted in the previous section, antidepressants, including the tricyclics, and selective serotonin reuptake inhibitors (SSRIs), like fluoxetine (Prozac), have been found to inhibit some of the undesirable effects of cocaine and have been used in the treatment of cocaine abuse.

Metabolism

The half-life of cocaine, as stated previously, is approximately 1–2 hours. It is metabolized to more polar compounds that have significantly less potency than the parent compound. These metabolites have longer half-lives and, with techniques such as GC-MS, can be detected up to 48 hours after administration of the drug. The immunoassay methods can detect the drug for about 24–36 hours after administration. If a patient has inhaled cocaine free-base ("crack"), it is possible to detect the parent compound, cocaine, by TLC up to several hours after administration, owing to the high doses of drug present.

THE OPIATES (HEROIN, MORPHINE, CODEINE, FENTANYL)

The structures for these drugs are shown in Figure 23-7. As can be seen in this figure, the first three drugs of abuse—morphine, codeine, and heroin—have quite similar structures. In fact morphine is a metabolite of heroin. Morphine itself is used as a powerful analgesic and acts by binding to μ-receptors in the limbic system (central nervous system [CNS]), mainly in the nucleus accumbens and the ventral tegmental area, resulting in an analgesic state. Binding of each agent to the μ-receptor inhibits the release of GABA from the nerve terminal, reducing the inhibitory effect of GABA on dopaminergic neurons. The resulting increased activation of dopaminergic neurons results in sustained activation of the postsynaptic membrane, causing a sense of euphoria. On the molecular level, binding of morphine to these receptors activates a cell signaling cascade via G-protein activation that results in elevated expression of many transcriptionally active proteins such as ERK, jun, and fos, and superactivation of adenyl cyclase resulting in high intracellular levels of cAMP (Tso, 2003). Besides being used as a major analgesic, morphine (Dilaudid) is important in treating acute congestive heart failure by lowering venous return to the heart (i.e., it is a powerful preload reducer by causing increased splanchnic pooling of blood). Codeine is used as a mild analgesic and as an antitussive. The codeine analog dextromethorphan (D-3-methoxy-*N*-methylmorphine), is an antitussive agent that is a component of cough suppressive medications.

Heroin induces a pleasant, euphoric state and is highly addictive both physically and psychologically. As can be seen in Figure 23-7, heroin is a diacetyl form of morphine. This characteristic facilitates heroin's crossing the blood-brain barrier, allowing it to reach higher concentrations in the CNS. Withdrawal from this drug is exceedingly difficult, with a myriad of symptoms such as hypothermia, palpitations, cold sweats, and nightmares. This is a true physical dependence, the molecular basis for which is not fully understood. It appears that the dependence is strongly linked to the number of cell surface μ-receptors (Tso, 2003).

This class of compounds exhibits certain important paradoxical effects on the parasympathetic nervous system. These drugs exert a procholinergic effect on the eyes and on blood vessels in the periphery (i.e., they cause constriction of pupils [**pin-point pupils**] and peripheral vasodilation). In contrast, in the gut they lower gastrointestinal (GI) motility (i.e., they exhibit anticholinergic effects in the GI tract). This fact enables rapid diagnosis of heroin or, in general, opiate abuse in a patient brought to the emergency room in an obtunded or comatose state. These patients typically have severe miosis (pupillary constriction). Although the sign is not useful in acute diagnosis, constipation commonly occurs.

Administration of heroin occurs via the intravenous route. Addicts are readily recognized by the presence of needle tracks on their arms and hands and by extensive thrombosis of their peripheral veins. The half-life of heroin via the intravenous route is about 3 minutes, and the effects of the drug last approximately 3 hours. The major metabolites are *N*-acetylmorphine and morphine. The half-life of morphine is about 3 hours. Overdoses of heroin are extremely dangerous and can cause severe obtundation, coma, respiratory arrest, hypotension (secondary to histamine release), and cardiac arrhythmias. One of the most common therapeutic modalities for heroin overdose is intravenous treatment with naloxone (Narcan) (see Fig. 23-7), a strong competitive antagonist to the action of heroin. Heroin addiction, as a chronic problem, is treated pharmacologically with a partial agonist of heroin—methadone, which is discussed later.

Codeine and Analogs

The structure of codeine is similar to that of morphine and heroin (Group 1 structures in Fig. 23-7). Codeine, like morphine, has a strong analgesic effect, is a potent antitussive agent, and acts in a manner similar to that of morphine. Dextromethorphan (D-3-methoxy-*N*-methylmorphine), an analog of codeine, is the active component of cough syrups because of its antitussive effects. Recently, there has been a "run" on cough medicines by addicts, who can obtain them legally and then consume quantities sufficient to reach their desired euphoric state. Unlike codeine, dextromethorphan is believed generally not to be addictive, although cases of drug dependency have been documented. For therapeutic use, the recommended dose of dextromethorphan is 15–30 mg given three to four times per day. **Light intoxication** is achieved at about 100–200 mg, and **heavy intoxication** is reached at around 1500 mg (Haroz, 2006). It is surprising to note that dextromethorphan does not have analgesic properties because of its lack of affinity for μ-, κ-, and δ-receptors. It has been found to induce the release and to block the reuptake of serotonin. Similar to the action of phencyclidine (PCP), discussed later, dextromethorphan has also been found to block NMDA receptors that are critical for neuronal plasticity and memory and are involved in central pain pathways in the brain, as discussed earlier (Zhuo, 2009). Dextromorphan is readily absorbed from the GI tract and, in about 85% of individuals, is rapidly metabolized to dextrophan, an active metabolite, and D-hydroxymorphinane via the 2D6 cytochrome P450 isozyme (Haroz, 2006). It is dextrophan that has a high affinity for NMDA receptors, so that most individuals experience PCP-like effects (i.e., euphoria; tactile, auditory, and visual hallucinations; paranoia, altered time perception; and general disorientation). For the 15% of individuals who are slow metabolizers of dextromethorphan, these effects are much less pronounced and are replaced by sedation and dysphoria (Haroz, 2006). Overdoses of dextromethorphan can result in mainly neurologic effects, such as lethargy, or, conversely, hyperexcitability; ataxia; slurred speech; tremors and fasciculations; hypertonia and hyperreflexia; and nystagmus, as well as either pupillodilation or pupilloconstriction. Diaphoresis may also occur. In addition, cardiovascular sequelae include tachycardia and hypertension. Unfortunately, a number of antitussives contain, in addition to dextromethorphan, anticholinergic agents such as chlorpheniramine. Thus, abuse of antitussive medication can give rise to such symptoms as tachycardia, mydriasis, flushed skin, urinary retention, and constipation.

Fentanyl

This opiate analgesic (Group 1 drugs in Fig. 23-7), is about 80 times more potent than morphine in blocking pain. It can be taken orally as so-called **fentanyl lollipops**, smoked, inhaled, or administered by transdermal fentanyl patches (Haroz, 2006). Overdose effects of this drug are the usual ones seen for opiate abuse and include respiratory depression and miosis. Treatment may involve irrigation of the bowel, and antiopiates such as naloxone may be administered. Hypotension is less common than with other opiates like morphine, because of the lack of histamine release.

METHADONE

This interesting compound, whose structure is shown in the Group 1 drugs in Figure 23-7, is a nonbicyclic drug that binds competitively with morphine to μ-receptors in the brain. However, although it can become addictive, the addictive effects are less than those of equivalent concentrations of heroin, possibly because its binding affinity is lower, so that it induces less of an effect than heroin. Thus, administration of methadone to heroin addicts allows them to experience the effects of heroin but in a modulated manner. By gradually lowering the methadone dose, physical dependence becomes reduced, and it appears that a trough serum methadone level greater than 100 ng/mL is adequate for effective methadone maintenance (Bell, 1988). However, it should be noted that addiction to methadone can also occur. In toxicology laboratories, the most common request received for methadone screens comes from methadone clinics to test whether a patient is administering methadone or has relapsed into taking heroin. As can be seen in Figure 23-3, it is a simple matter to distinguish methadone from the opiates by TLC. Similarly, EMIT or FPIA detects each drug with high specificity.

AMPHETAMINES

These compounds, as can be seen in Figure 23-7 (Group 4 drugs), bear a close resemblance to the adrenergic amines such as epinephrine and norepinephrine and may be expected to exert sympathomimetic effects. They also resemble dopamine and may be expected to have effects on dopaminergic pathways. The amphetamines cause euphoria and increased mental alertness that may be attributed to their effects on these pathways. This group of drugs, however, also exerts pronounced stimulatory effects on γ- and β-receptors in the cardiovascular system and in the kidney to cause pronounced adrenergic effects such as increased heart rate, increased blood pressure, palpitations, bronchodilation, anxiety, pallor, and tremulousness. Studies indicate that amphetamines are also competitive inhibitors of the enzyme monoamine oxidase, which inactivates adrenergic neurotransmitters by oxidatively removing their amino groups. Blockage of this enzyme prolongs the effects of epinephrine and norepinephrine, with the attendant neurologic and cardiovascular sequelae. One particular amphetamine,

3,4-methylenedioxymethamphetamine (MDMA or **ecstasy**), a derivative of methamphetamine (see Group 4A drugs in Fig. 23-7), has become popular as a recreational drug of abuse because it has euphoric and psychedelic effects but minimal hallucinogenic effects (Gill, 2002; Haroz, 2006).

Clinical Symptoms

The pharmacologic action of amphetamines includes CNS and respiratory stimulation and sympathomimetic activity (e.g., bronchodilation, pressor response, mydriasis). Loss of weight may also occur as the result of an anorectic effect. Psychic stimulation and excitability, leading to a temporary increase in mental and physical activity, can occur; anxiety and nervousness can also be produced.

Acute Toxicity

Initial manifestations of an overdose may be cardiovascular in nature; symptoms may include flushing or pallor, tachypnea, palpitation, tremor, labile pulse rate and blood pressure (hypertension and hypotension), cardiac arrhythmia, heart block, circulatory collapse, and angina. Mental disturbances such as delirium, confusion, delusions, disorientation, and hallucinations may occur. Acute psychotic syndromes may be characterized by vivid auditory and visual hallucinations, restlessness, homicidal or suicidal tendencies, panic state, paranoid ideation, loosening of associations, combativeness, and changes in affect. A frequent and potential sign of acute intoxication is hyperpyrexia; rhabdomyolysis has also been associated with acute amphetamine overdose. Cardiovascular collapse is the usual cause of death.

Chronic Usage

Tolerance may be produced within a few weeks, and physical or psychic dependence may occur with prolonged usage. Symptoms of chronic abuse include emotional lability, somnolence, loss of appetite, occupational deterioration, mental impairment, and social withdrawal. Trauma and ulcer of the tongue and lip may occur as a result of continuing chewing or teeth-grinding movements. A syndrome with the characteristics of paranoid schizophrenia can occur with prolonged high-dosage use. Aplastic anemia and fatal pancytopenia are rare complications.

Treatment

No specific antidote for amphetamine overdose is known, and treatment of overdose is symptomatic with general physiologic supportive measures immediately implemented. When cardiovascular symptoms are noted, propranolol (Inderal), discussed subsequently under therapeutic drugs, can be used as an antidote.

Detection

Both Toxi-Lab (Irvine, Calif.) and EMIT (Syva, San Jose, Calif.) procedures are effective in detecting these drugs of abuse. Occasionally, on the Toxi-Lab A strip, amphetamines may be confused with antihistamines like diphenhydramine.

"Designer" Amphetamines and Related Drugs of Abuse

The quest for euphoria-producing drugs has resulted in the advent of synthetic phenylethylamines, so-called **designer drugs,** like MDMA, several further examples of which are shown in category 4A of Figure 23-7. With all of these drugs, the price for the sought-after effects of euphoria and hallucinations consists of headaches, nausea, vomiting, anxiety, agitation, violent behavior, tachycardia, hypertension, respiratory depression, and seizures, as discussed previously in the case of **standard** amphetamines.

Other phenylethylamine derivatives shown in Figure 23-7, especially 2C-T-7 and 2CB, bind to 5-HT_2 receptors and induce hallucinogenic effects (Haroz, 2006). These drugs have been taken orally or have been insufflated, smoked, administered intravenously, and even taken rectally. Death from overdose of these designer drugs has been reported but is uncommon. Unfortunately thus far, no specific assays are available for most of these drugs in urine. Their presence must be ascertained by history and/or symptoms reported in the absence of positive urine tests for standard amphetamines. On occasion, GC-MS is used to detect their presence.

TRYPTAMINES

These drugs are derivatives of serotonin whose structure is shown in Figure 23-7—Group 6 drugs. These tryptamines, some of which occur in plants, are relatively simple to obtain and were not proscribed until relatively recently. An example is *N,N*-dimethyltryptamine (DMT), which has strong hallucinogenic properties. Smoking DMT results in the rapid onset of hallucinogenic effects that are short-lived, giving rise to the term, **businessman's lunch.** Other tryptamines contain modifications of the indole ring, as shown in the Group 6 drugs in Figure 23-7. These also allow them to interact with 5-HT receptors (Haroz, 2006), and this interaction is thought to result in their hallucinogenic effects. However, the mechanism of action of this class of drugs is not well understood. Psilocin shown in this figure is a component of the so-called **Psilocybe,** called **magic mushrooms** because of their hallucinogenic effects. The hallucinogenic effects of these drugs are enhanced by the presence of monoamine oxidase inhibitors such as β-carbolines (Haroz, 2006). The mixture of these two compounds is present in a South American tea called **ayahuasca,** which combines two plants—one containing DMT and the other carbolines, which themselves can induce nausea and vomiting. Like the amphetamines and other phenylethylamine derivatives, the tryptamines cause, in addition to the "desired" effects of euphoria and empathy, auditory and visual hallucinations, nausea, vomiting, diarrhea, and emotional distress. Symptoms further include agitation, tachycardia, hypertension, diaphoresis, salivation, dystonia, mydriasis, tremors, confusion, seizures, and, in a few cases, rhabdomyolysis and paralysis. Currently, no routine assays are available for these compounds. As with the amphetamines, many of the psychogenic and physiologic effects of the tryptamines can be countered with supportive therapy and the administration of benzodiazepines.

PIPERAZINES

The structure of the parent compound, piperazine, is shown in Group 7 of Figure 23-7. Several of the derivatives of piperazine are also shown in this figure. Many of these piperazines were used as antihelminthics during the 1950s but were subsequently discontinued. However, their euphoria-producing effects were discovered, leading to a "legal" way of obtaining drugs of abuse. Two classes of piperazine derivatives have been identified: *N*-benzylpiperazines, the parent compound of which is *N*-benzylpiperazine (BZP), and phenylpiperazines. The former group includes 1-(3,4-methylenedioxybenzyl)piperazine, and the latter group includes 1-(3-chlorophenyl)piperazine, 1-(4-methoxyphenyl)piperazine, and 1-(3-trifluoromethylphenyl)piperazine (TFMPP). BZP (known as **A2**) and TFMPP (known as **Molly**) are among the most popular piperazines. Studies have shown that these piperazines produced effects that were similar to those of the amphetamines, suggesting that the target receptors of these drugs are the same. Both classes of piperazines have been found to increase dopamine and serotonin levels. TFMPP has been found to act as a partial agonist at 5-HT_{2A} receptors and is a full agonist at other 5-HT receptors. Although TFMPP is three times less potent than MDMA, it produces a full MDMA effect when combined with BZP, with which it is synergistic (Haroz, 2006). The TFMPP-BZP combination at low doses induces euphoria with decreased motor action, making the euphoric "experience" more pleasurable. The acute undesirable effects of piperazines are similar to those of the amphetamines and MDMA (i.e., hallucinations, psychomotor agitation, increased heart rate and blood pressure, and increased body temperature). Two deaths from BZP have been reported when combined with another drug like MDMA (Haroz, 2006). Both TFMPP and BZP have skin-irritant properties, causing sore nasal passages and throats. As with the tryptamines and designer amphetamines, currently no standard assay method detects these drugs in urine; treatment is supportive, as described in the preceding section.

BENZODIAZEPINES

Among this group of drugs, shown in Figure 23-7 (Group 2), the most prominent is Valium; they are used therapeutically, as so-called **minor tranquilizers.** Their mechanisms of action appear to be potentiation of GABA, a neurotransmitter that *inhibits* conduction in dopaminergic neurons, and facilitation of its binding to GABA receptors (Campo-Soria, 2006). Benzodiazepines bind to the α subunit of the so-called **$GABA_A$ receptor** at a site that is distinct from that for GABA itself and cause an increase in the frequency of chloride ion channel opening at the $GABA_A$ receptor. Usually used as a therapeutic drug to produce calming effects at doses between 2.5 and 10 mg and to produce muscle-relaxing effects at higher doses, Valium has been used by drug addicts in high dosage to counter the excitatory effects of other drugs of abuse or as a means of inducing tranquil states. Among some drug abusers, benzodiazepines are used to potentiate the effects of heroin (Fraser, 1998). A number of drug abusers have become addicted to Valium when using high doses several times each day. Acutely, benzodiazepine overdose may produce somnolence, confusion, seizures, and coma. Rarely, hypotension, respiratory depression, and cardiac arrest may occur. Chronically, physical and psychological dependence occur. Sudden discontinuance of the drug may lead to anxiety, sweating, irritability, hallucinations, diarrhea, and seizures. Treatment is supportive. Gradual diminution of the benzodiazepine removes physical dependence. The half-life for Valium is 20–70 hours, but the half-life of one of its active metabolites is 50–100 hours.

PHENCYCLIDINE

This interesting tricyclic compound, shown in Figure 23-7 (Group 5), has numerous effects on a variety of different neural pathways. Used almost exclusively as a drug of abuse, this drug is traded on the streets under the name of **angel dust** or **angel hair.** It is peculiar that the use of this drug appears to be periodic. The physiologic effects of PCP appear to be analgesic and anesthetic and, paradoxically, stimulatory. This drug has been found to interact with cholinergic, adrenergic, GABA-secreting, serotonergic, and opiate neuronal receptors. It has also been found to block NMDA receptors (Hevers, 2008). Thus, a wide variety of bizarre and apparently paradoxical symptoms can be seen in the same patient. This drug has been shown to bind to specific regions of the inner chloride channels of neurons, apparently profoundly affecting chloride transport. It has also been found to bind strongly to a class of neural receptors called **sigma-receptors** (Schuster, 1994). This receptor binds strongly to the neuroleptic, antipsychotic drug haloperidol (Haldol)—a finding that may implicate the sigma-receptor in some of the clinical findings of severe psychosis in patients suffering from overdose with PCP.

Because of its varied actions, clinically acute manifestations vary from depression to euphoria and can involve catatonia, violence, rage, and auditory and visual hallucinations. Vomiting, hyperventilation, tachycardia, shivering, seizures, coma, and death are among the common occurrences that result from abuse of this drug. Most fatalities occur from the hypertensive effects of the drug, especially on the large cerebral arteries (Bayorh, 1984). As can be inferred from this spectrum of possible symptoms, diagnosis based on clinical findings is impossible. Only the results of a drug screen can be diagnostic. Treatment of drug abuse with PCP is supportive, with the patient kept in isolation in a darkened, quiet room. Acidification of the urine increases the rate of PCP excretion. As might be expected from findings regarding the sigma-receptor, treatment with Haldol results in sedation of the violent, hallucinating patient.

BARBITURATES: SEDATIVE-HYPNOTICS

An almost bewildering variety of these major sedative drugs is available. However, all are derivatives of barbituric acid, which may be regarded as the condensation product of urea and malonic acid, as indicated in Figure 23-7 (Group 3 drugs). Depending on the substituents of the $–CH_2$ group of the malonic acid portion, the particular drug may be long acting, as is phenobarbital, with a benzene ring and ethyl group substituents on this carbon; short acting, as is pentobarbital, with neopentyl and ethyl groups at this position; or ultra-short acting, as is the case with thiopental. The long-acting barbiturate phenobarbital is a therapeutic drug that is used as an anticonvulsant, unlike the short- and ultra–short-acting drugs, and is discussed subsequently under therapeutic drugs. All of the barbiturates are fat soluble and therefore pass easily across the blood-brain barrier. All of them seem to stabilize membranes such that depolarization of the membranes becomes more difficult.

As with the benzodiazepines, the barbiturates are known to interact with GABA receptors. In particular, they bind to the α subunit of the $GABA_A$ receptor at a site that is distinct both from the GABA binding site and from the benzodiazepine binding site. Their effect is to increase the *duration* of chloride ion channel opening at the $GABA_A$ receptor, potentiating the GABA effect (i.e., inhibition of dopamine-dependent nerve conduction). It is thought that this action of chloride channel opening, called **direct gating** of the chloride channel, is the basis for barbiturate toxicity, which is greater than for the benzodiazepines, which do not increase the **duration** of chloride channel opening but rather increase the **frequency** of channel opening, as discussed previously in the benzodiazepine section. In addition, at higher doses, barbiturates have been found to inhibit a subtype of glutamate receptors, called **AMPA receptors.** Glutamate is a major excitatory neurotransmitter. More generally, barbiturates have been found to block calcium ion–induced release of neurotransmitters.

For unknown reasons, the short-acting and ultra–short-acting barbiturates seem to inhibit selectively the reticular activating system, involved with arousal—hence their sedative and hypnotic effects. The ultra–short-acting barbiturates rapidly diffuse out of the CNS, accounting for their rapid action. Phenobarbital, however, selectively reduces the excitability of rapidly firing neurons and is therefore a highly effective anticonvulsant. It may be more than coincidental that phenobarbital and the equally effective anticonvulsant phenytoin (Dilantin) bear structural resemblance to one another and may exert similar effects on rapidly firing neurons. The mechanism of action of phenytoin is discussed subsequently.

Clinically, at low doses, the short-acting and ultra–short-acting barbiturates produce sedation, drowsiness, and sleep. They also impair judgment. At higher doses, anesthesia is produced. At very high dose, these drugs can cause stupor, coma, and death. The toxic manifestations of these drugs are depression, Cheyne-Stokes respiration, cyanosis, hypothermia, hypotension, tachycardia, areflexia, and pupillary constriction. Treatment of drug overdose is supportive and includes the standard treatment for shock. When administered within 30 minutes of drug ingestion, activated charcoal is an effective barbiturate chemoadsorbent.

Diagnosis of drug abuse with short- and ultra-short-acting barbiturates is done by immunoassay and TLC screening procedures. HPLC has found some use in this regard but is not a standard method. The barbiturates are weak acids, the N-H protons being somewhat acidic, so they are acid extracted and placed on the B strip in Toxi-Lab (Irvine, Calif.) procedures. Their presence is easily detected by Toxi-Lab TLC, as shown in Figure 23-3, Worksheet B. Immunoassays for those drugs are also excellent, the one caveat being that high levels of phenobarbital in urine cross-react with antibodies against the short-acting barbiturates. Thus, it is important that TLC confirms a positive immunoassay result for sedative-hypnotic barbiturates.

PROPOXYPHENE (DARVON)

This analgesic drug, whose structure is shown in the Group 1 drugs in Figure 23-7, has pharmacologic properties very similar to those of the opiates, like morphine. As can be seen in Figure 23-1 (drug Group 1), the structure of propoxyphene is quite similar to that of methadone. This drug can be taken orally, so that the sedated, good feelings induced by opiates can be induced without the need to have recourse to the intravenous apparatus needed for infusion of heroin. A major cause of drug-related death is propoxyphene overdose alone or in combination with CNS depressants like barbiturates and alcohol. Toxic symptoms are similar to those seen with overdoses of opiates (namely, respiratory depression, cardiac arrhythmias, seizures, pulmonary edema, and coma). Nephrogenic diabetes insipidus may also occur. In addition, propoxyphene has been found to cause cardiac arrhythmias (Barkin, 2006). Treatment for propoxyphene overdose is mainly supportive. Administration of naloxone (Narcan) reverses the toxic effect of the drug.

METHAQUALONE (QUAALUDE)

Methaqualone is a 2,3-disubstituted quinazoline (Group 5 drugs in Fig. 23-7). Although not structurally similar to the barbiturates, it has many of the same sedative-hypnotic properties as the barbiturates. This compound also possesses anticonvulsant, antispasmodic, local anesthetic, antitussive, and weak antihistamine actions. Oral administration leads to rapid and complete absorption of the drug, with approximately 80% bound to plasma protein. Peak plasma concentrations are reached in approximately 2–3 hours, and almost all of the drug appears to be metabolized by the hepatic cytochrome P450 microsomal enzyme system, with only a small percentage (<5%) excreted unchanged in the urine. The serum half-life ranges from 20–60 hours. The dosages used for its hypnotic-sedative actions range from 150–300 mg daily. Toxic serum concentrations are generally reached at 10 μg/mL. Tolerance to some of its actions, as well as dependence, occurs, such that abusive dosages can be up to six to seven times greater than those employed therapeutically. Symptoms of overdose can be similar to barbiturate toxicity and produce CNS depression with lethargy, respiratory depression, coma, and death. However, unlike barbiturate overdose, muscle spasms, convulsions, and pyramidal signs (hypertonicity, hyperreflexia, and myoclonus) can result from severe methaqualone intoxication. Treatment for overdose includes supportive therapy, as well as delaying absorption of remaining drug with activated charcoal and drug removal by gastric lavage.

MARIJUANA (CANNABIS)

This is one of the oldest and most widely used of the mind-altering drugs. Marijuana is a mixture of cut, dried, and ground portions of the hemp plant *Cannabis sativa*. Hashish refers to a more potent product produced by extraction of the resin from the plant. The principal psychoactive agent in marijuana is considered to be δ-9-tetrahydrocannabinol (δ-9-THC) (Group 5 drugs in Fig. 23-7), a lipid-soluble compound that readily enters the brain and may act by producing cell membrane changes. δ-9-THC binds to the presynaptic neural cannabinoid receptor CB1, which releases the inhibitory neurotransmitter GABA in the hippocampus, amygdale, and cerebral cortex (Iversen, 2003). Different forms of THC have been found to cause distinctly different physiologic effects (Fusar-Poli, 2009). δ-9-THC induces an increase in anxiogenic effects, and cannabidiol produces a diminution in anxiety. The latter derivative was found to attenuate blood oxygenation levels in the amygdala and the anterior and posterior cingulate cortex; δ-9-THC was found to modulate activation in frontal and parietal regions of the brain.

Marijuana may be introduced through the lungs by smoking or through the gastrointestinal tract by oral ingestion in food. Once THC enters the body, it is readily stored in body fat and has a half-life of approximately 1 week. Biotransformation is complex and extensive, and less than 1% of a dose is excreted unchanged. About one third is excreted in the urine as, primarily, δ-9-carboxy-THC and 11-hydroxy-δ-9-THC. These metabolites may be detected in the urine from 1–4 weeks after the last ingestion, depending on both dosage and frequency of ingestion.

Marijuana does not appear, in general, to cause physiologic dependence, but tolerance (Martin, 2004) and psychological dependence do seem to occur, although a proportion of chronic users of this drug can develop physiologic dependence on it (Iversen, 2003). Two major physiologic effects of marijuana are reddening of the conjunctivae and increased pulse rate. Muscle weakness and deterioration in motor coordination can also occur. The preponderant changes seen with cannabis intoxication are perceptual and psychic changes. These range from euphoria, relaxation, passiveness, and altered time perception, seen at low doses, to adverse reactions such as paranoia, delusions, and disorientation, which can be seen at high doses in psychologically susceptible individuals.

The dosage, the route of administration, the individual's psychological makeup, and the setting are important determinants in each individual's reaction to cannabis intoxication. Thus, high doses in an individual unprepared or unaware of drug consumption may produce a disturbing experience. More commonly, experienced users report mild euphoria, enhancement or alteration of the physical senses, introspection with altered emphasis or importance of ideas, and heightening of subjective experiences. Heavy chronic use may produce bronchopulmonary disorders; although the relative safety of chronic use is controversial, acute panic reactions, delirium, and psychoses occur rarely (Bryson, 1989). Few users seek treatment, and when this occurs in a distressed patient, medical intervention is generally conservative. However, following an acute episode, psychological evaluation may be necessary in an individual with an underlying psychiatric disturbance. Rarely, marijuana may be ingested by intravenous infusion of a boiled concentrate. Severe multisystem toxicity may be produced by this route of administration. Symptoms may include acute renal failure, gastroenteritis, hepatitis, anemia, and thrombocytopenia.

LYSERGIC ACID DIETHYLAMIDE (LYSERGIDE)

Lysergic acid diethylamide (LSD) (Group 5; see Fig. 23-7) is a semisynthetic indolalkylamine and a hallucinogen. It is one of the most potent pharmacologic materials known, producing effects at doses as low as 20 mcg, and is equally effective by injection or oral administration. Comparison of the structure of LSD with that of 5-hydroxytrptamine (serotonin), as shown in the Group 6 drugs in Figure 23-7, reveals that LSD has a tryptamine-like nucleus, but it lacks the 5-hydroxyl group of serotonin. LSD has multiple complex effects in the CNS. In the locus coeruleus and the median raphe of the midbrain, which utilize serotonergic pathways, it has the paradoxical effect of **inhibiting** both the firing of neurons in these structures and the release of serotonin at the axonal sides of synapses (Passie, 2008). This process, in turn, may produce a state of CNS hyperarousal. On the other hand, it actually acts as a serotonin **agonist** on postsynaptic HT_{1A} receptors. It is a pure agonist on 5-HT_2 receptors in other serotonergic pathways. Recently, it has been found that the hallucinogenic effect of LSD is due to its agonistic effect on 5-HT_2 receptors, and that it behaves very much like the tryptamines (Group 6 drugs; see Fig. 23-7) and phenylethylamines (Groups 4 and 4A drugs; see Fig. 23-7), discussed previously, in producing this effect. In addition, it has been found to have both agonistic *and* antagonistic effects on dopaminergic pathways. Thus it acts at multiple sites in the CNS in complex ways. LSD further affects both the sympathetic and parasympathetic nervous systems. However, the sympathetic effect appears to be greater, and initial symptoms include hypertension, tachycardia, mydriasis, and piloerection.

The usual dosage of LSD is 1–2 mcg/kg; LSD produces an experience that begins within an hour of ingestion, usually peaks at 2–3 hours, and generally lasts 8–12 hours, after ingestion. Metabolism occurs in the liver, whereas excretion occurs mainly in the bile.

LSD is the most commonly abused drug in its class and is believed by its users to provide insights and new ways of solving problems. The psychic effects are usually intense and vary, depending on the user's personality, expectations, and circumstances. LSD acts on all body senses, but visual effects are most intense. Common perceptual abnormalities include changes in the sense of time, organized visual illusions or hallucinations, blurred or **undulating** vision, and synesthesias. Mood may become very labile, and dissolution and detachment of ego may occur. LSD toxicity levels are low, and deaths are generally due to trauma secondary to errors in the user's judgment. Panic reactions—a **bad trip**—are the most common adverse reactions. These may occur in any user and cannot be reliably predicted or prevented. Borderline psychotic and depressed individuals are at risk for the precipitation of suicide or a prolonged psychotic episode by the usage of LSD. Flashbacks, which are poorly understood, occur days to months after ingestion. This occurs when the user experiences recurrences of a previous hallucinogenic experience in the absence of drug ingestion.

Acute panic reactions may be treated by frequent reassurance and a quiet and calm environment; diazepam may also be effective. However, except for treating specific complications, LSD abuse has no systematic program of treatment.

THERAPEUTIC DRUG MONITORING

It has now become recognized that serum levels of many of the therapeutic drugs administered to patients must be frequently determined, both because of the possible toxic side effects of many of these medications and because, often, lack of patient compliance results in subtherapeutic levels of the drug, requiring intervention. Furthermore, it is important for the physician, when initiating drug therapy, to ascertain when the serum levels of the drug have achieved a stable therapeutic level. It becomes important, therefore, to understand the principles, called **pharmacokinetics,** on which drug therapy is based. Some of the basic principles of pharmacokinetics and then the physiologic effects of specific classes of therapeutic drugs are presented in this section. The ones discussed are those whose specific levels are most commonly followed by clinicians and are most commonly assayed for in clinical laboratories. It should be noted that virtually all therapeutic drugs are assayed from specimens of serum, not urine, most commonly using immunoassay techniques such as FPIA.

PHARMACOKINETICS

Figure 23-9 summarizes the two ways in which a therapeutic drug is administered to a patient: discontinuously or continuously (Gerson, 1987a,b). The former method is the most common. Most patients are treated with medications taken orally at fixed periods. For example, to achieve antiinflammatory effects, two aspirin tablets of 350 mg each are taken every 4–6 hours. In this case, the aspirin is taken at discrete times, between which a certain amount will be metabolized and/or excreted before the next dose is given. Sometimes, a patient will be infused with a drug intravenously such as with lidocaine (Xylocaine) in the intensive care unit for a cardiac arrhythmia, or with heparin to prevent thromboembolic events. In this case, while the drug is metabolized, a constant amount of the drug is being infused continuously. Eventually, with continuous infusion of a drug, a steady-state concentration of the drug is reached once the amount of drug infused in a unit of time equals the amount of drug eliminated in the same unit of time. A steady-state concentration of a drug that is discontinuously infused is also reached. However, repeated dosing (equal doses spaced equally apart) produces peak and trough serum concentrations that vary around a steady-state or average concentration.

For both discontinuous and continuous infusions, the ultimate drug level is determined by a battle between the amount infused and the amount

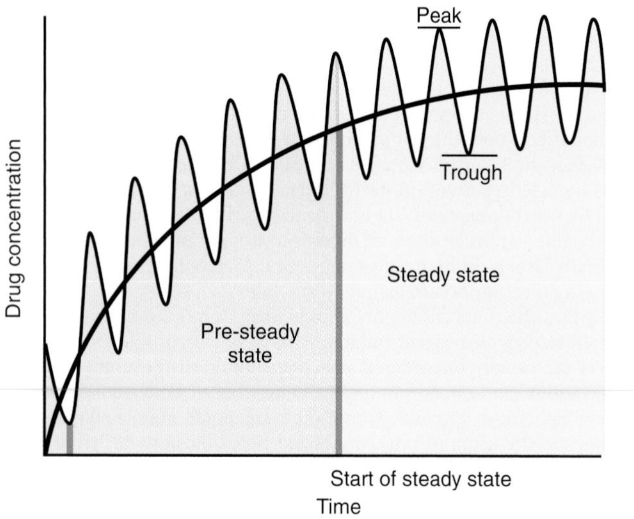

Figure 23-9 Illustration of the time course of drug levels as a function of method of administration. In the discontinuous method, represented by the curve showing peaks and troughs, a constant dose of a drug is administered at regular intervals. After each drug dose, the drug level increases to a peak value, followed by a fall that continues to a trough level, at which time the next regular drug dose is given, resulting in another peak level. After approximately 4 half-times ($4\,t_{1/2}$), the drug levels achieve the steady state, as labeled in the figure, when constant peak and trough levels occur. Note that, if a loading dose can be given to the patient, equal to the peak steady-state value, the entire left portion (pre–steady-state) of the curve is eliminated. After the loading dose, the steady state is maintained by giving periodic maintenance doses. The black smooth curve shows a typical time course for drugs that are administered continuously, mainly by the intravenous route. The steady state is achieved as a continuing constant value rather than as peaks and troughs, as in the discontinuous method.

excreted. All drugs are eventually excreted. They can be excreted unchanged in urine, or may be excreted in urine as metabolites of the parent drug. These metabolic conversions occur predominantly in the liver. Occasionally, some drugs enter the enterohepatic circulation and are excreted in stool. Regardless of their mode of excretion, many but not all drugs have a half-life that is more or less independent of their concentrations. The half-life of a drug is the time taken for half the drug that was initially present in serum to be excreted. The reason that the half-life of a drug is independent of its concentration is that many drugs are excreted according to so-called **first-order kinetics,** as discussed in Chapter 20 (Equations 20-22 and 20-23). This process may be summarized as follows:

$$D \xrightarrow{k} E \qquad (23\text{-}5)$$

where D is the drug concentration, and E is the excreted and/or inactivated form of the drug. The constant, k, is the rate constant for the disappearance of D. The half-life, called $t_{1/2}$, is related to the rate constant, k, by the following relationship:

$$t_{1/2} = 0.693/k \qquad (23\text{-}6)$$

As can be seen from this equation, $t_{1/2}$ is a constant and does not depend on drug concentration. Thus, the half-life of the drug determines the time to reach the steady-state or average concentration.

The object of all drug therapy is to achieve a constant serum level of the drug that will be therapeutic. If the half-life for a drug is known, it is possible to compute the divided dose of the drug that should be given and the time interval between doses so that this level will be achieved. As can be seen in Figure 23-9, at the beginning of drug administration, wide fluctuations in the drug level occur until, after a given period, the fluctuations give the same maxima (peaks) and the same minima (troughs), and the mean level of the drug becomes constant. The problem in dosing is to ensure that the maximum level of the drug will be in the therapeutic range and will not reach toxic levels and, at the same time, to ensure that the minimum level of the drug will remain in the therapeutic range and will not be subtherapeutic.

In general, for discontinuous doses, the drug level at the end of the nth dosing period can be expressed as the sum of a geometric series:

$$D = (D_0 r^N - D_0)/(r - 1) \qquad (23\text{-}7)$$

where D_0 is the constant dose given at each regular time period; r is the fraction of drug remaining after the constant time interval between doses; and n is the number of the dose (e.g., the second dose, the third dose). Note that, because r is a fraction less than 1, as N becomes large, the first term in Equation 23-7, D_0r^N, becomes small, so that

$$D = D_0/(1 - r) \qquad (23\text{-}8)$$

For example, if the time interval between doses is chosen as the $t_{1/2}$, then r = ½. If the time interval is chosen to be that for ¾ of the drug to remain, then r = ¾. (This time can be calculated directly from the $t_{1/2}$ as $\frac{1}{2} \times t_{1/2}$.) Suppose we take r = ½. Then after four timed doses, the first term in the numerator of Equation 23-7 is $D_0 \times (\frac{1}{2})^4 = D_0/16$ or approximately $0.06 \times D_0$, which is small compared with D_0, and, in effect,

$$D = 2D_0 \qquad (23\text{-}9)$$

This level is the maximum (peak) level shown in Figure 23-9. It is the level achieved just after the dose, D_0, is given. Note that, at the end of the dosing period, just before the next dose, D_0, is given, the drug level decreases to $r \times (2D_0)$. If r = ½, then this level becomes D_0. The problem then in pharmacokinetics is to determine what dose, D_0, and what period, r, to choose, such that the peak and trough values lie within the therapeutic range for the drug. Frequently it is found that, to achieve the right peak and trough levels, the time required to achieve the steady state is too long, especially where the need for drug therapy is urgent. In these cases, a **loading dose** can be administered. Here, the peak level is administered; for the above example, this level would be $2D_0$. Then, after the usual time period, defined by r, elapses, a **maintenance dose,** D_0, is given. This process is repeated every r-defined time period so that the peaks and troughs are maintained. This process obviates the entire dosing schedule shown in Figure 23-9 (i.e., the entire left side of the curve is eliminated, leaving only the steady-state portion). The reason that this process is not performed uniformly is that not all patients can tolerate large initial doses of specific drugs. Therefore, giving loading doses may not always be possible.

For continuous infusions (Fig. 23-9), for the simplest case where drug distribution is instantaneous, the rate of drug infusion is constant, and the drug is excreted in a first-order manner, the rate law is

$$dD/dt = k_1 - k_2 D \qquad (23\text{-}10)$$

where D is the drug concentration, k_1 is the constant rate of infusion, and k_2 is the first-order rate constant for excretion/inactivation of D. This equation can be solved for D:

$$D = (k_1/k_2)(1 - e^{-k_2 t}) \qquad (23\text{-}11)$$

From Equation 23-11, if t is large, the term $e^{-k_2 t}$ becomes small, and D approaches its steady state value, k_1/k_2. This value is approached when the rate of drug infusion equals the rate of drug disappearance. Another way to obtain this value is to note that, at steady state, as in the formation and disappearance of the enzyme–substrate complex in Michaelis-Menten kinetics (see Chapter 20, Equation 20-4), dD/dt must = 0. Then, from Equation 23-10,

$$dD/dt = k_1 - k_2 D = 0 \qquad (23\text{-}12)$$

so that

$$D_{\text{steady state}} = k_1/k_2 \qquad (23\text{-}13)$$

As in the case of periodic drug administration at constant intervals, 4 half-lives are sufficient to reach the steady-state condition. Because, as shown previously in Equation 23-6, $k_2 = 0.693/(t_{1/2})$, after 4 half-lives when $t = 4t_{1/2}$,

$$D = (k_1/k_2) \cdot (1 - e^{-2.772}) \qquad (23\text{-}14)$$

where, in effect, D is close to k_1/k_2. Thus, for continuous infusions, the ratio of k_1 (the rate of drug infused per unit of time) to k_2 (the rate constant for the first-order disappearance of the drug) is the desired steady-state level of the drug (i.e., where the amount of drug delivered equals the amount of drug eliminated over the same unit of time). Unlike the situation with discontinuous infusion, the only parameter that is needed to achieve the steady-state level in a given time is k_1, which includes drug concentration and infusion rates, whereas with discontinuous administration of the drug, both D_0 and r are needed.

There are two major points from this presentation. First, it is a good rule of thumb to wait for 4 or more half-lives to achieve the steady-state level of a drug. Second, results of an assay for a drug level in the time period during which this steady state is being achieved should be interpreted with extreme caution—a rule often forgotten in clinical practice. Notice from Figure 23-9 that if assays are performed in the pre–steady-state period (before achievement of 4 or more half-lives), erratic results are obtained owing to fluctuations in drug concentrations for the discontinuous case, and rising but persistently low values for the continuous case.

Volume of Distribution

When one is administering drugs, it is of vital importance to know whether the drug is stored in fat or other tissue, or whether it is all present in serum. Because a given dose of a drug is known and the concentration of the drug in serum can be determined, one can measure the total volume of body fluid in which the drug is dissolved by the following relation:

$$D = D0/V_d, \text{ or } V_d = D0/D \qquad \textbf{(23-15)}$$

where D is the concentration of drug in serum, D0 is the amount of drug administered, and V_d is the volume in which D0 must be dissolved to give the concentration D. This volume, V_d, is referred to as the volume of distribution. If all of the drug is present in serum, V_d is the blood volume that can be determined from conversion tables relating body weight to blood volume. If, however, some of the drug is stored in body tissue, a smaller amount is present in serum, so that the denominator in Equation 23-15 ($V_d = D0/D$) is reduced and V_d will be larger than the expected blood volume, indicating that some drug is being stored in tissue. If this result occurs, it means that the drug will very likely be released continuously from storage depots (i.e., tissues), which can raise anomalously the level of drug in serum, potentially to toxic levels. Thus, before any drug is administered, the volume of distribution should be known.

Metabolism in the Liver

Many drugs are converted to metabolites, some of which are pharmacologically active and some inactive. Much of this conversion occurs in the extramitochondrial, microsomal system present in hepatocytes. This metabolic system is mainly an oxidative one that utilizes a series of oxidative enzymes that, in turn, utilize a special cytochrome system: cytochrome P450 (Gonzalez, 2006). This extremely critical cytochrome system has now been strongly implicated as predisposing particular individuals to develop cancer by metabolizing certain environmental compounds, such as benzopyrene, into frank carcinogens (see later). In addition, genetic polymorphism of the cytochrome P450 enzymes affects an individual's particular response to a drug, including toxicity and an adverse drug reaction (Ingelman-Sundberg, 2004). As is described in Chapter 72, it is now possible to test individuals for their abilities to metabolize specific drugs by amplification of their genes encoding cytochrome P450. Certain amino acid substitutions in this protein cause it to be very active in drug metabolism (i.e., rapid inactivation of the drug). This implies that the patient may need substantially higher doses to achieve a therapeutic level, or that it may be necessary to use another less rapidly metabolized drug.

Because the excretion of many drugs depends on the integrity of the liver and the cytochrome P450 system, in patients with liver failure due to passive congestion, hepatitis, cirrhosis, and the like, the effective half-life of the drug is increased, making it necessary to lower the divided dose of the drug. Conversely, some drugs induce the intracellular synthesis of the microsomal enzymes, leading to diminished half-life values, so that it may be necessary to raise the divided dose.

One example of drug induction of microsomal enzymes is phenobarbital. (Dilantin is another example of this phenomenon.) This drug induces its own metabolism (so that its concentration levels do not obey first-order kinetics). In instances in which the levels of a drug metabolized in the liver are higher than the highest therapeutic value, reductions in the levels may be induced by administering low levels of phenobarbital to induce the microsomal system.

This summary of some of the general principles of drug administration should be helpful in the interpretation of values clinically and should permit a better understanding of the subsequent discussion of specific therapeutic drugs, most commonly measured or determined in the laboratory. Tables 23-1 to 23-7 summarize the critical pharmacologic data for a number of commonly assayed drugs.

In the following presentation, seven classes of the drugs most commonly assayed for are discussed: cardiotropic, anticonvulsant, anti-asthmatic, anti-inflammatory, immunosuppressive, psychotropic, and chemotherapeutic. (Antibiotics are discussed in Part 7.) The emphasis in this discussion is on the mechanisms of action of these drugs. Common to most of these drugs is the fact that they interfere with specific steps in signal transduction pathways in cells, which are often remarkably similar to one another. Despite these similarities, specific drugs block signal transduction pathway steps that affect only specific cells and seem not to affect signal transduction in other cells.

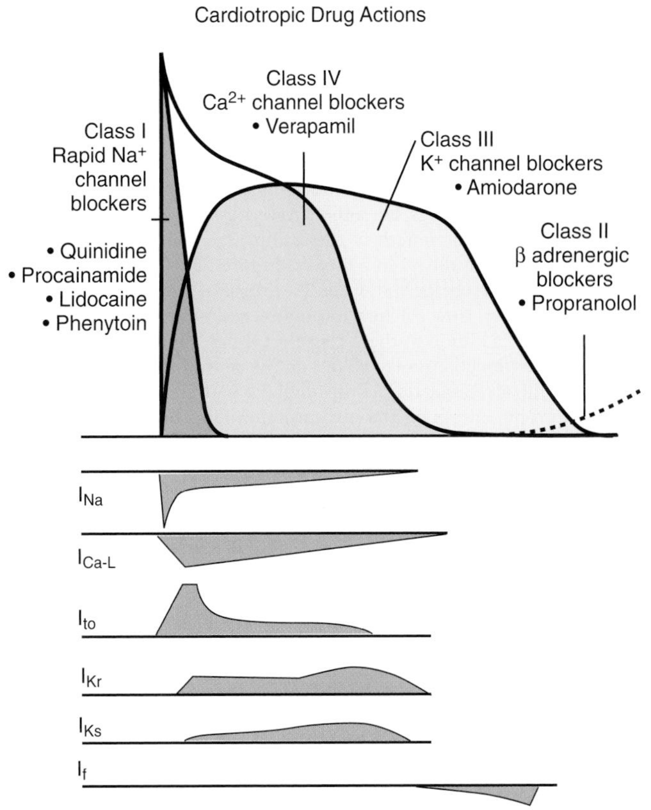

Figure 23-10 Overview of the effects of different antiarrhythmic agents on the myocardial conduction system. The normal action potential is shown as the *black line* that first spikes to a high voltage, mainly because of a rapid sodium influx into cells in the conduction system. This component of the action potential, caused by sodium ion influx, is shown enclosed in the *red area*. The actual action potential is prolonged by a succeeding influx of calcium ions shown enclosed under the *blue area* that overlaps somewhat with the red (sodium influx) area. Termination of the calcium ion influx and efflux of potassium ions results in repolarization, shown by the *curve bordered by the blue area*. Class I channel blockers, as listed in the figure, block sodium influx, thereby diminishing the rate of depolarization. Class II blockers, like propranolol, block β-adrenergic (epinephrine and norepinephrine) stimuli, diminishing the rate of diastolic depolarization. Class III blockers, like amiodarone, block potassium channels, resulting in reduction in potassium efflux and slowing down repolarization. This results in prolongation of the action potential, as shown by continuation of the voltage curve over the *yellow area*. Class IV blockers, like verapamil, block calcium channels, again prolonging the action potential (*blue*), although this prolongation is not explicitly shown. By prolonging the action potential, Class III and IV agents slow down nodal conduction through prolonged refractoriness of the affected cells. Various ion currents induce the action potentials. *(Redrawn from Opie LH, Gersh BJ. Drugs for the heart. 5th ed. Philadelphia: WB Saunders; 2001.)*

CARDIOTROPICS

(Opie and Gersh, 2001; Roden, 2006).

These drugs are the ones most commonly used to treat congestive heart failure and cardiac arrhythmias. Despite differences in the structures and properties of the drugs and their specific uses, all of them act on one or another phase of the action potentials in cells that are in the conduction system and in myocytes. Their net effect is to slow down electrical conduction. In addition, it is important to remember that the conduction tissue is innervated by both sympathetic and parasympathetic (mainly vagal) nervous systems. The former increases the conduction rate, and the latter tends to slow conduction. The actions of each of the cardiotropic drugs are summarized in Figure 23-10. As shown in this figure, several major ion currents control the action potentials of the cells making up the pacemaker tissue of the atrioventricular (AV) node and the ventricular conduction bands (composed of Purkinje cells): first, rapid sodium influx current, and then decreased flux (shutoff of sodium conductance channels), as outlined in the red area in Figure 23-10; second, a calcium ion influx that prolongs the action potential and then calcium channel shutoff, as outlined in the blue area in Figure 23-10; and third, potassium ion efflux that promotes repolarization of the cell. As shown in Figure 23-10, there are four classes of drugs that act on one or more of these phases of the action potential, resulting in its prolongation. Class I drugs block sodium influx in phase I and include quinidine, procainamide, and lidocaine. These agents, especially lidocaine, act by blocking the rapid sodium influx of phase I, decreasing the rate of ventricular diastolic depolarization. Class II drugs include the β-receptor blockers, like propranolol (Inderal), that inhibit the chronotropic effects of adrenergic neurotransmitters like epinephrine and norepinephrine. Class III drugs, like amiodarone, block repolarizing potassium currents, increasing the length of the action potential, as represented by the black curve over the yellow area in Figure 23-10, and increase the length of the refractory period. Class IV drugs, of which verapamil is an important member, slow calcium ion influx, resulting in action potential prolongation. In addition to these classes of drugs, digitalis cardiac glycosides have parasympathetic-like effects on the cells of the AV node, resulting in slowing of conduction. Both digitalis and amiodarone also have marked inotropic effects on the myocardium. Thus both are used in the treatment of congestive heart failure. In damaged myocardium, digitalis blocks sodium-potassium adenosine triphosphatase (ATPase), resulting in transient increases in sodium ion around the sarcolemma, which leads to the release of cytosolic calcium ion to the T-system. This allows increased myocardial contractility. We now discuss the key properties and actions of these cardiotropic drugs.

Cardiac Glycosides (Digitalis and Its Derivatives)

Digoxin

Because they slow conduction in the AV node, digoxin and the other cardiac glycosides are used to treat atrial arrhythmias, in particular atrial flutter and atrial fibrillation. Their main antiarrhythmic effect is to block rapid atrial conduction signals to the ventricles, thereby slowing ventricular response. This is due to their proparasympathetic effects, which include enhancement of blockade of depolarizing calcium currents and increased hyperpolarizing potassium currents in the AV node. These effects result in shortening action potential duration and increasing AV nodal refractoriness (Roden, 2006).

Their direct positive inotropic effect increases cardiac output in cardiac failure. This effect has been found to be due to increased intrasarcolemmal concentration of calcium, allowing it to activate proteins such as troponin C that are important in the contractile apparatus (Rocco, 2006). This increase in calcium concentration is due to the binding of digoxin to the α subunit of sodium-potassium–activated ATPase, causing its inhibition and the consequent reduction of sodium efflux and diminution of the trans-membrane potential; as this potential increases, more calcium efflux occurs, resulting in less activation of muscle contraction. Blockade of sodium efflux therefore allows accumulation of intrasarcolemmal calcium and increased activation of contractile proteins (Rocco, 2006).

Digoxin (Table 23-1) has a rapid onset of action (within 1–2 hours when given orally) and a relatively short half-life (35–40 hours). Most patients will excrete approximately 50%–75% of a dose unchanged in the urine. The general range of therapeutic serum levels is from 0.5–2 ng/mL. High concentrations of the drug are found in skeletal and cardiac muscle, as well as in liver, brain, and kidneys.

Digitoxin

In contrast, digitoxin has a longer half-life (4–6 days) with a relatively slower onset of action (within 1–4 hours when given orally, with maximal effect in 8 hours); 90%–100% of a dose is absorbed, with approximately 95% bound to plasma protein. The general range of therapeutic serum levels is from 9–25 ng/mL. The drug is extensively metabolized in the liver (90%), with digoxin being the active metabolite.

Toxic side effects of the digitalis glycosides include gastric disturbances, nausea, vomiting, and atrial and ventricular arrhythmias. It is crucial that levels of digoxin (or digitoxin) be monitored closely and accurately while the patient is initially being given this drug. As mentioned previously, the therapeutic range for digoxin is from 0.5–2 ng/mL (i.e., the range is narrow). Toxic levels exceed 2 ng/mL, so the difference between therapeutic and toxic doses is small. This difference necessitates careful digoxin assay.

Digoxin toxicity is often treated with Digibind (GlaxoSmithKline, Research Triangle Park, N.C.), consisting of ovine Fab fragments. This antidote can interfere with determination of digoxin serum levels (Valdes, 1998). Some assays have been reported to determine only the "free" digoxin level (i.e., that not bound to Digibind Fab), which inactivates digoxin. For other assays that determine total digoxin (i.e., free plus Fab-bound digoxin), it is recommended that an ultrafiltrate of serum be employed to determine the level of free or active digoxin. Alternatively, given that Digibind can cause spurious and erroneous results, it has been recommended that, because the half-life of Digibind is 15–20 hours, therapeutic levels of digoxin should be determined 2–4 days after the last Digibind dose.

TABLE 23-1
Digoxin

Purpose	Treatment of congestive heart failure and atrial fibrillation-flutter
General adult dose	Oral: 0.75–1.5 mg for digitalization, 0.125–0.5 mg/day for maintenance
Usual bioavailability	Approximately 60%–85% for tablet or elixir; 90%–100% for liquid-filled capsules
Half-life	Approximately 35–40 hours; however, prolonged in patients with decreased renal function
General therapeutic range	0.5–2 ng/mL
General toxic level	>2 ng/mL, but somewhat variable
Transport	Approximately 20%–25% plasma protein bound
Metabolism	Generally, only small amounts are metabolized (liver, lumen of large intestine)
Elimination	Approximately 50%–75% unchanged in urine
Steady state	Approximately 7 days in undigitalized patients with normal renal function
Mechanism of action	Causes release of calcium ions in T-system of myocardium; slows AV node conduction
Toxic effects	Gastric disturbances, nausea, vomiting, atrial and ventricular arrhythmias; irregular pulse

AV, Atrioventricular.

TABLE 23-2
Procainamide

Purpose	Treatment of supraventricular or ventricular arrhythmias
General adult dose	Oral: 4 g/day, in divided doses, for maintenance therapy
Usual bioavailability	75%–95%
Half-life	Approximately 3.5 hours in patients with normal renal function
General therapeutic range	4–10 mcg/mL
General toxic level	>12 mcg/mL
Transport	Approximately 15% plasma protein bound
Metabolism	Hepatic: *N*-acetylprocainamide (active), with $t_{1/2}$ approximately 7 hours in patients with normal renal function
Elimination	Approximately 50%–60% unchanged in urine
Steady state	Minimum of 12 hours
Mechanism of action	Prolongation of atrial refractory period and decreased myocardial excitability
Toxic effects	Reversible lupus erythematosus-like syndrome, irregular pulse, hypotension, rash, agranulocytosis

Procainamide (Pronestyl)

Procainamide (Table 23-2) is a class I antiarrhythmic drug that is useful in treating supraventricular or ventricular arrhythmias. One of its major effects includes increased refractoriness of the atrium and decreased myocardial excitability by blocking open sodium channels and outward potassium currents, both of which prolong action potentials and increase refractoriness (Roden, 2006). Because there is an effect on potassium currents, some of its effects resemble those of the Class III potassium current blockers. The bioavailability of procainamide is 75%–95%. Approximately 15% is bound to plasma protein, and approximately 50% is excreted by the kidneys. The half-life is approximately 3.5 hours, with a general range of therapeutic serum level of 4–10 μg/mL. *N*-acetylation to the major active metabolite *N*-acetylprocainamide (NAPA) is the major metabolic pathway of biotransformation. NAPA, however, does not block open sodium channels but effectively prolongs action potentials (Roden, 2006). Both drugs prolong the QRS and Q-T intervals on electrocardiography over time.

Toxic side effects include a reversible lupus-like syndrome with elevated antinuclear antibody titers, urticaria, rash, agranulocytosis, and nephrotic syndrome. The lupus-like syndrome may be initiated by leukocyte metabolism of procainamide to a chemically reactive metabolite that could then covalently bind to monocyte/macrophage membrane proteins to stimulate production of autoantibodies. In addition, the tertiary amino moiety of the covalently bound procainamide metabolite might mimic a portion of histone protein, resulting in the production of antihistone antinuclear antibody (Uetrecht, 1988).

Quinidine

Quinidine, also a class I antiarrhythmic, like procainamide, is used to treat supraventricular and ventricular arrhythmias and tachyarrhythmias. The prevention of ventricular tachycardia or frequent premature ventricular contractions and the maintenance of sinus rhythm after the conversion of atrial flutter or atrial fibrillation are its two major uses (Valdes, 1998). Like procainamide, quinidine blocks sodium channels and outward potassium currents, especially the I_{Kr} rectifier current, resulting in prolongation of action potentials and increased refractoriness, leading to prolongation of both the QRS complex and the Q-T interval (Roden, 2006).

The bioavailability of quinidine is 90%–100%, with approximately 85% of the drug bound to plasma protein. Quinidine is 60%–85% metabolized in the liver via hydroxylation reactions, with some metabolites being active. Urinary excretion is approximately 20%. The half-life of quinidine is 5–12 hours, and the general therapeutic range is 2.3–5 mcg/mL. Maximal serum levels are reached in 1–3 hours. Toxic side effects of quinidine include cinchonism (vertigo, tinnitus, headache, visual disturbances, and disorientation), fever, hepatitis, and blood dyscrasia. Ventricular arrhythmias, AV block, and ventricular fibrillation leading to syncope and sudden death can occur.

Lidocaine

Lidocaine (Xylocaine), another class I antiarrhythmic, can also be used as a local anesthetic. Its major use as an antiarrhythmic is in the acute control and prevention of ventricular arrhythmias after acute myocardial infarction. Its effect is to block sodium channels mainly in ventricular but not atrial tissue. Unlike procainamide and quinidine, lidocaine does not cause QRS and Q-T prolongation (Roden, 2006). A loading intravenous dose of 50–100 mg is given over 2–3 minutes to treat ventricular arrhythmias in adults. These dosages may be repeated in 5- to 10-minute intervals of 25–50 mg, up to a maximum of 300 mg in a 1-hour period. Following loading, infusion is then continued at a rate of 1.4–3.5 mg/min for a 70-kg man. In children, 0.5–1 mg/kg can be given every 5 minutes for a maximum of three doses. Unfortunately, lidocaine can cause heart block and congestive heart failure, limiting its use in critical care patients (Roden, 2006).

Lidocaine is neither highly protein bound nor appreciably stored in body tissues; it has a half-life of approximately 2 hours and a therapeutic serum range of 1.2–5.5 mcg/mL. The time to reach a maximum serum level is generally 5–8 hours. Ninety percent of a dose of lidocaine is metabolized in the liver via *N*-dealkylation. Urinary excretion is 10%. Toxic side effects include convulsions, coma, and respiratory depression (CNS effects), as well as bradycardia and hypotension.

Propranolol

Propranolol, a class II antiarrhythmic β receptor–blocking drug that antagonizes the effects of epinephrine on the heart, on the arteries and arterioles of skeletal muscles, and on the bronchus, exerts its effects largely on the AV node and is used to treat sinus tachycardia, atrial tachycardia, and ventricular arrhythmias. Overall, blockade of β-1-receptors increases AV conduction time and reduces heart rate, myocardial contractility and output, and cardiac automaticity. Because it is a vasodilator, it is also used in the treatment of angina pectoris; hypertension; and symptomatic coronary artery disease, particularly after an acute myocardial infarction. Oral dosages vary from 40–320 mg daily in adults for antiarrhythmic activity, to as high as 480 mg daily in the control of hypertension. Both supine and standing blood pressures are also reduced. Bioavailability of propranolol is approximately 30%. The half-life of propranolol is 3 hours, with a therapeutic serum range of 50–100 ng/mL, and with maximum serum levels reached in approximately 6 hours. Approximately 93% is protein bound. Propranolol is metabolized in the liver, with 0.5% excreted in the urine unchanged. Toxic effects include bradycardia, arterial insufficiency (Raynaud's type), hypotension, AV block, nausea, vomiting, pharyngitis, bronchospasm, and thrombotic thrombocytopenic purpura. Marrow suppression occurs rarely.

Amiodarone

Amiodarone, a structural analog of thyroid hormone, is chiefly a class III antiarrhythmic drug, which markedly prolongs the action potential mainly by blocking potassium channels in cardiac muscle (see Fig. 23-10). Its activity is complex in that it significantly blocks inactivated sodium channels by a poorly understood mechanism, thus exhibiting class I action, and also exhibits weak adrenergic- and calcium channel–blocking effects (Roden, 2006). All of these actions prolong the effective refractory period along the conduction bands. Its indication for use is with life-threatening ventricular arrhythmias. The oral loading dose is 1200–1600 mg/day with a maintenance dose of 200–400 mg/day. Bioavailability is ≈35%–65%. Amiodarone has two components in its half-life: a rapid component of 3–10 days (involving ≈50% of the drug) and a slow component of 25–110 days. The general therapeutic range is 1–2.5 mcg/mL, although this is not well defined, and the toxic level is >2.5 mcg/mL, again not well defined. Approximately 96% is plasma protein bound; the drug undergoes liver metabolism and shows extensive body distribution because of its hydrophobic (lipid soluble) structure. Excretion is very slow by skin, biliary tract, and lacrimal glands. Toxic effects can be profound and include symptomatic bradycardia, heart block, fatal pulmonary fibrosis, hepatitis, visual field disturbances, photodermatitis, and mainly hypothyroidism but sometimes hyperthyroidism.

Verapamil

Verapamil is a class IV antiarrhythmic drug that blocks activated and inactivated calcium channels that are especially prominent in nodal tissue (particularly the AV node). Indications include angina, hypertension, and supraventricular arrhythmias. Unlike β-adrenergic receptor blockers, calcium channel blockers have not been found to reduce mortality after a myocardial infarction (Roden, 2006). The oral dose is 120–480 mg/day in three to four divided doses. Bioavailability is ≈10%–20%. The half-life is 2–8 hours but increases to 4.5–12 hours after repeated oral doses. The general therapeutic range is 80–400 ng/mL, although this is not well defined. Approximately 90% is plasma protein bound, and the drug undergoes extensive metabolism in the liver, where norverapamil, an active metabolite, is produced. Approximately 75% of the active components are eliminated by the kidney and ≈25% through the GI tract. Toxic effects include hypotension, ventricular fibrillation, constipation, and peripheral edema.

ANTICONVULSANTS

Anticonvulsants are used in the treatment of seizure disorders, in particular grand mal, petit mal, and psychomotor seizures and other specialized seizure disorders such as tic douloureux (trigeminal neuralgia). Although the mechanisms of action of these drugs are incompletely understood, it appears that all of these agents, with the possible exception of phenobarbital, block sodium influx into neurons that have damaged membranes, as schematized in Figure 23-11. In addition, several of these agents, especially phenytoin, block secondary calcium influxes into such cells, which also seems to inhibit the rapid firing of these cells. Another effect of phenobarbital, and possibly also of phenytoin, is membrane stabilization through intercalation, as is shown in Figure 23-11. Many of the anticonvulsants are effective against grand mal seizures but have no effects or adverse ones on petit mal seizures. Only drugs like ethosuximide (Zarontin) and valproic acid (Depakote) are effective against this condition. Thus, although the mechanism of action of these drugs appears to be similar, they differ in specificities.

Phenobarbital

Phenobarbital (Table 23-3), a long-acting barbiturate, is used in the treatment of generalized grand mal tonic-clonic seizures and simple partial seizures with motor or somatosensory symptoms, as well as for anxiety and insomnia. It is not used in the treatment of absence seizure (i.e., petit mal), which may be exacerbated by phenobarbital, nor for complex partial seizures, which do not respond well. As discussed previously in the barbiturates section under The Drugs of Abuse, phenobarbital increases the duration of chloride ion channel opening at the $GABA_A$ receptor, thereby potentiating the GABA effect and raising the threshold for neuronal

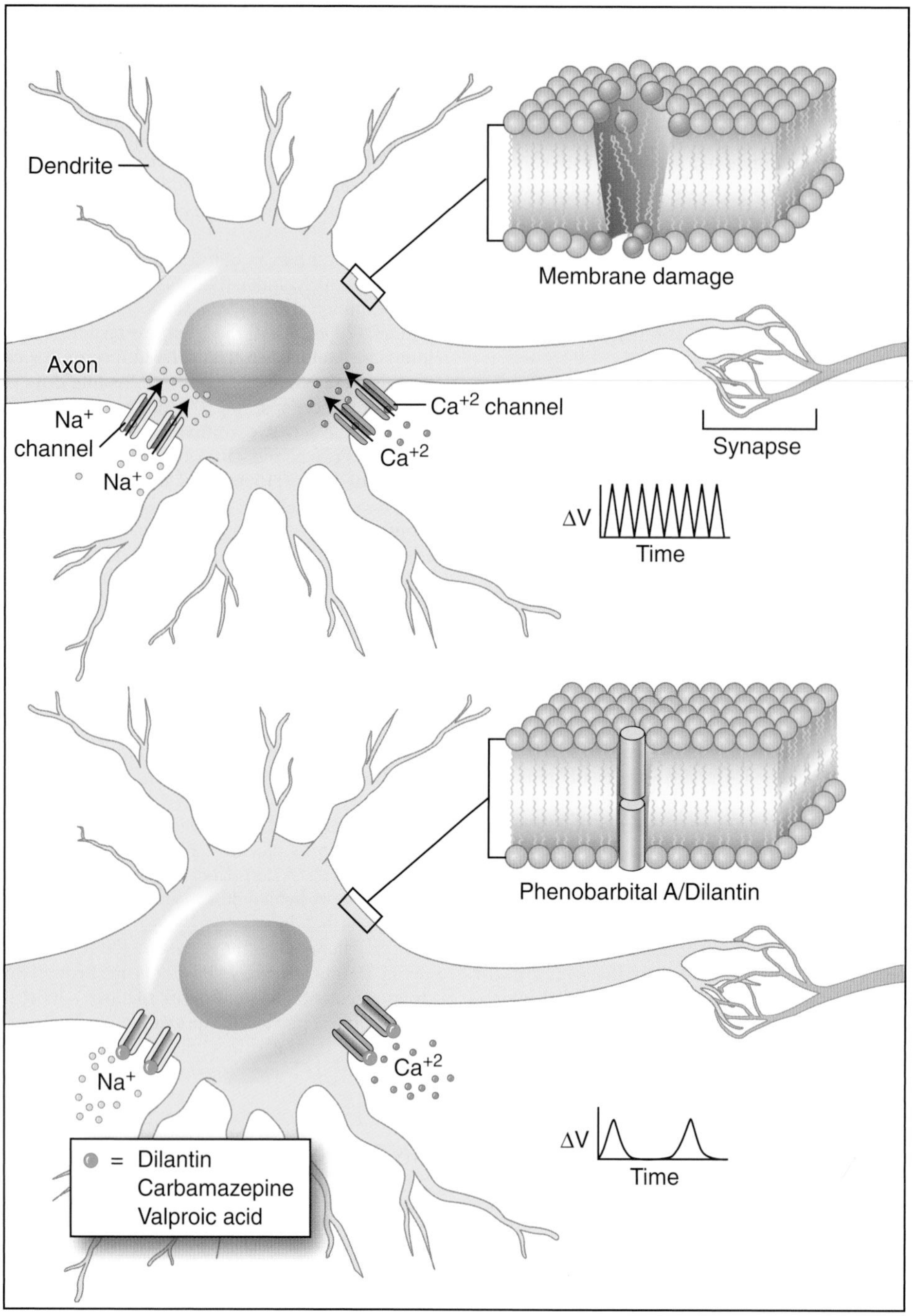

Figure 23-11 Effects of anticonvulsants on neurons. *Top:* Damaged neuronal membranes, as shown in the section in the upper right of the figure, result in sodium *(yellow circles)* and calcium *(red circles)* influxes via their respective channels that cause repeated firing, as shown in the voltage–time curve to the right of the figure. *Bottom:* Anticonvulsants like phenytoin (Dilantin), carbamazepine (Tegretol), and valproic acid (Depakote; *represented by small blue circles*) block sodium and calcium channels, resulting in a substantially diminished rate of firing, as shown in the voltage–time curve to the right of the figure. Both phenytoin and phenobarbital, shown as blue cylinders, are also thought to stabilize the damaged neuronal membrane, as shown in the membrane section schematized in the upper right drawing.

membrane depolarization, resulting in the diminished frequency of firing of action potentials. In addition, it can stabilize damaged neuronal membranes (see Fig. 23-11).

Phenobarbital is also given for withdrawal symptoms in infants born to opiate- or barbiturate-addicted mothers. Because phenobarbital enhances the metabolism of bilirubin by induction of cytochrome P450–dependent enzymes in the hepatic microsomal system, it has been used to treat patients with congenital hyperbilirubinemia (familial nonhemolytic, nonobstructive jaundice). The oral dose of phenobarbital for anxiety in adults is 30–120 mg daily in divided doses; for sleep induction in adults, 100–320 mg daily is generally used. For seizure control, divided doses of 100–200 mg/day in adults or 30–100 mg/day in children are generally used.

Phenobarbital has a long half-life of 4–6 days. Oral doses are almost completely absorbed (90%–100% bioavailability), and the optimal serum concentration for seizure control is generally 15–30 μg/mL; 40%–60% is metabolized in the liver, whereas 10%–40% may be eliminated unchanged in the urine. Approximately 40%–60% is plasma protein bound, and the main site of storage is the brain. A steady state is reached in 14–21 days. Toxic side effects include nystagmus, ataxia, stupor, respiratory depression, coma, and hypotension. Barbiturates are contraindicated in patients with acute intermittent porphyria (i.e., partial porphobilinogen deaminase deficiency), because barbiturates enhance the synthesis of δ-aminolevulinic acid synthetase and thus the synthesis of heme pathway intermediates in the liver.

Phenytoin (Dilantin)

Phenytoin is used to treat generalized tonic-clonic, simple partial, and complex partial seizures (Table 23-4). It is ineffective in treating myoclonus, absence (petit mal), and atonic seizures. It is usually given intravenously in addition to intravenous diazepam to terminate status epilepticus.

TABLE 23-3
Phenobarbital

Purpose	Treatment of generalized tonic-clonic seizures, simple partial seizures, anxiety, insomnia
General adult dose	Oral: 100–200 mg/day for seizure control; 30–120 mg/day for anxiety; 100–320 mg for sleep induction
Usual bioavailability	Approximately 90%–100%
Half-life	Approximately 5–6 days in adults; approximately 3–4 days in children
General therapeutic range	15–30 mcg/mL for epilepsy control
General toxic level	>40 mcg/mL, although tolerance may develop
Transport	Approximately 40%–60% plasma protein bound
Metabolism	Approximately 75% hepatic: *p*-hydroxyphenobarbital, inactive
Elimination	Approximately 25% unchanged in urine
Steady state	Approximately 14–21 days
Mechanism of action	Stabilizes damaged membranes and raises threshold for neuronal membrane depolarization
Toxic effects	Drowsiness, depression, respiratory depression, coma, sedation, hypotension. Respiratory depression may be caused by rapid intravenous administration.

TABLE 23-4
Phenytoin (Dilantin)

Purpose	Treatment of generalized tonic-clonic seizures, simple partial seizures, complex partial seizures
General adult dose	Oral: 300–400 mg/day maintenance dose
Usual bioavailability	Variable: 30%–95%
Half-life	24 ± 12 hours, and dose dependent
General therapeutic range	10–20 µmcg/mL
General toxic level	>20 µmcg/mL
Transport	Approximately 90%–95% plasma protein bound
Metabolism	Hepatic: 5-(*p*-hydroxyphenyl)5-phenylhydantoin, inactive
Elimination	Approximately 5% unchanged in urine
Steady state	Approximately 7–8 days
Mechanism of action	Appears to block sodium and calcium ion influxes into repeatedly depolarizing CNS neurons
Toxic effects	Nystagmus, ataxia, diplopia, drowsiness, coma; rapid intravenous administration may produce cardiovascular collapse and/or CNS depression

CNS, Central nervous system.

Remarkably, phenytoin has no apparent effects on resting neurons or on normally firing neurons. It is thus specific for epileptogenic foci in the CNS (Yaari, 1986). It is interesting to note that carbamazepine (Tegretol) exerts similar effects, as discussed later. Data on the mechanism of action of this drug strongly suggest that phenytoin blocks sodium and calcium influxes into repeatedly depolarizing neurons in the CNS and also into neurons that are partially depolarized. Reducing sodium and calcium influx into these cells reduces their excitability and prolongs their refractory period (Yaari, 1986). In fact, phenytoin appears to bind selectively to fast-firing sodium channels in their refractory states, thereby prolonging their refractory periods (Bazil, 1998) (i.e., it slows the rate of recovery of inactivated sodium channels) (McNamara, 2006). This finding helps explain the ability of phenytoin to block only neurons that are firing rapidly and repetitively.

Although the average daily maintenance dose in adults is 300–400 mg, dosage must be tailored to the patient's response and serum drug concentrations. The usual therapeutic serum concentration is 10–20 µg/mL, with a steady state reached in 5–10 days (for plateau; see Figure 23-9). The serum half-life is generally 24 hours, but it is dose dependent. Thus, its excretion is not a first-order process. Phenytoin is stored in the brain, is metabolized in the liver (95%), and is approximately 90%–95% bound to plasma protein. Both aspirin and phenylbutazone can displace phenytoin from serum albumin and can significantly increase the serum concentration of phenytoin. Because phenytoin, like phenobarbital, is a relatively potent hepatic microsomal enzyme inducer, certain antibiotics, oral anticoagulants, quinidine, and oral contraceptives may be more rapidly metabolized, thus decreasing their effectiveness.

Because the relationship between serum concentrations and daily dosage is not linear, small increases in dosage can greatly increase therapeutic serum concentrations. Symptoms of toxicity generally occur at serum concentrations greater than 20 µg/mL. Toxic side effects include nystagmus, ataxia, stupor, and coma. Arrhythmias can be produced by rapid intravenous administration.

Fosphenytoin is a water-soluble parenteral formulation of phenytoin that is rapidly converted (half-life of 8–15 minutes) in vivo to phenytoin. The half-life is independent of plasma concentration, and it has identical pharmacodynamic, pharmacokinetic, and clinical properties to phenytoin. This prodrug offers improved flexibility and tolerability for the patient, as compared with intravenous phenytoin, and is indicated for the treatment of partial and generalized seizures in adults in whom intravenous administration is indicated (Bazil, 1998).

Primidone (Mysoline)

Primidone is used to treat generalized tonic-clonic, simple partial, and complex partial seizures. Its chemical structure is closely related to the basic structure of the barbiturates, and it is metabolized in the liver into two active metabolites: phenobarbital and phenylethylmalonamide. Thus some of its anticonvulsant effects are due to phenobarbital activity. Unlike phenobarbital, however, primidone may increase the threshold of membrane depolarization within the CNS.

Oral doses range from 250 mg daily to 2 g/day in divided doses. Absorption is rapid and complete (100%), with a usual therapeutic serum concentration of 5–21 µg/mL. A steady state is reached in 4–7 days, and the half-life is approximately 12 hours. Plasma protein binding is relatively low (20%), with most of the drug remaining free in the serum, and with little drug being stored in body tissues.

Sedation is a common toxic side effect. Dizziness, ataxia, and skin rashes have also been observed. Primidone, like phenobarbital, is contraindicated in patients with acute intermittent porphyria.

Ethosuximide (Zarontin)

Ethosuximide is the drug of choice for absence (petit mal) seizures unaccompanied by other types of seizures. It is preferred over valproic acid (see later), at least initially, because hepatotoxicity is a rare but serious side effect of valproic acid. Ethosuximide may depress the motor cortex and may reduce the frequency of neuronal firing. It also inhibits T-current spikes on the electroencephalogram that underlie bursts of action potentials in the thalamus but does not affect normal electrical conduction (McNamara, 2006). The basis for its specificity, however, is not well understood.

The oral dosage in adults is generally 500–1000 mg daily. Absorption is fairly rapid and complete (100%), with peak serum concentrations occurring in 1–4 hours. A steady state is reached in 8–10 days. The usual therapeutic serum concentration is 40–100 µg/mL, but it can be as high as 170–190 µg/mL in children. The serum half-life is generally 60 hours in adults and 30 hours in children. Ethosuximide is essentially free in serum and not protein bound. It is mainly metabolized in the liver (60%–90%) to desmethylmethsuximide. Gastrointestinal disturbances are among the most common toxic effects and include nausea, vomiting, and gastric distress. Other effects include drowsiness and ataxia. Rare serious side effects, such as systemic lupus erythematosus, aplastic anemia, and pancytopenia have been reported.

Carbamazepine (Tegretol)

Carbamazepine (Table 23-5) is a primary antiepileptic drug that is used in the treatment of generalized tonic-clonic seizures and simple partial and complex partial seizures, as well as in combinations of these seizure types. Absence (petit mal), myoclonic, and atonic seizures may be exacerbated by this drug. This drug is also used to treat tic douloureux (trigeminal neuralgia) and glossopharyngeal neuralgia, and is, in fact, the drug of choice in the treatment of these neuralgias.

Carbamazepine is a tricyclic compound (i.e., iminostilbene) that is chemically related to imipramine, a tricyclic antidepressant. It is believed that a reduction in excitatory synaptic transmission in the spinal trigeminal nucleus is the basis for this drug's antineuralgic action. Its antiepileptic

TABLE 23-5
Carbamazepine (Tegretol)

Purpose	Treatment of generalized tonic-clonic seizures, simple partial seizures, complex partial seizures; trigeminal neuralgia and glossopharyngeal neuralgia
General adult dose	Oral: 0.8–1.2 g/day maintenance for seizure control; 0.2–1.2 g/day for neuralgia
Usual bioavailability	70%
Half-life	Initially approximately 35 hours; approximately 8–20 hours after 3–4 weeks of administration
General therapeutic range	4–12 mcg/mL
General toxic level	>12 mcg/mL
Transport	60%–70% plasma protein bound
Metabolism	Hepatic: carbamazepine-10,11-epoxide (active); carbamazepine-10,11-transdihydrodiol (inactive)
Elimination	1%–2% unchanged in urine
Steady state	3–7 days
Mechanism of action	Decreases sodium and calcium ion influx into repeatedly depolarizing CNS neurons; reduces excitatory synaptic transmission in the spinal trigeminal nucleus
Toxic effects	Drowsiness, ataxia, dizziness, nausea, vomiting, involuntary movements, abnormal reflexes, irregular pulse

CNS, Central nervous system.

action is quite similar to that of phenytoin, that is, it decreases sodium and calcium influx into hyperexcitable neurons (Yaari, 1986; Bazil, 1998). Like phenytoin, carbamazepine slows the rate of recovery of voltage-activated sodium channels from inactivation (McNamara, 2006).

Oral doses of carbamazepine are completely absorbed, and the usual adult maintenance dose is 0.8–1.2 g/day. Ninety-eight percent is biotransformed in the liver into two active metabolites: a 10,11-epoxide form, which is active (McNamara, 2006), and a 10,11-dihydroxy form of carbamazepine. The usual therapeutic serum concentration is 4–12 μg/mL, and steady state is reached in 3–4 days. The serum half-life of Tegretol is 8–20 hours (after 3–4 weeks of administration), and 60%–70% is plasma protein bound. The more common toxic reactions seen with this drug include drowsiness, ataxia, dizziness, nausea and vomiting, and light-headedness. Rare hematologic reactions may occur and can be quite serious; they include aplastic anemia, thrombocytopenia, and agranulocytosis.

Valproic Acid (Depakene)

Valproic acid is commonly used in the treatment of generalized tonic-clonic seizures, absence seizures, myoclonic seizures, and atonic seizures. It is not effective for the treatment of infantile spasms. Although the mechanism of action is not definitely known, valproic acid is thought to enhance the activity of the GABA-mediated inhibitory system. In addition, its action is similar to that of phenytoin and carbamazepine in that it inhibits sustained, repetitive firing of depolarized neurons by prolongation of the refractory state of sodium channels (Hardman, 2001; McNamara, 2006). Like ethosuximide, it decreases T-current–induced action potentials (McNamara, 2006). Absorption of valproic acid is rapid and complete. The average daily maintenance dose of valproic acid in adults is 15–30 mg/kg, when utilized alone, and 30–45 mg/kg in combination with other antiepileptic drugs. The usual therapeutic serum concentration is 50–100 μg/mL, and a steady state is reached in 1–4 days. Most (90%–100%) of the drug is metabolized in the liver, and a high percentage (90%) is plasma protein bound. The serum half-life is 8–15 hours.

Valproic acid has been shown to produce teratogenic effects in experimental animals; these included developmental abnormalities and skeletal defects. Thus, valproic acid should be used with caution in pregnant women. Toxic side effects include sedation, gastric disturbances, hematologic reactions, ataxia, somnolence, and coma. Rare fatal hepatotoxicity has occurred, and severe or fatal pancreatitis has been reported (Sztajnkrycer, 2002).

Newer Anticonvulsants

Topiramate, lamotrigine (Lamictal), gabapentin (Neurontin), and felbamate are four anticonvulsant agents that have been approved recently for use in this country for patients whose response to the more established anticonvulsants is less than optimal. Therapeutic ranges and toxic concentrations for these drugs have not been determined. Topiramate and lamotrigine are utilized as adjunctive treatment for partial seizures in adults. Topiramate is a substituted sulfamate monosaccharide that induces hyperpolarizing potassium currents and enhances $GABA_A$ receptor currents at synapses (McNamara, 2006). Lamotrigine is a triazine derivative that acts much in the same manner as phenytoin and carbamazepine. However, because it has broader antiseizure activity than either of these other two anticonvulsants, other mechanisms may be involved, one of which appears to be blockade of glutamate release at synapses using this amino acid as a neurotransmitter (McNamara, 2006).

Topiramate has a half-life of approximately 21 hours, with approximately 15% of the drug bound to protein. Lamotrigine has a variable half-life, depending on whether the drug is used as monotherapy or with an inducer. Approximately 55% of lamotrigine is protein bound.

Gabapentin is also utilized as adjunctive treatment for partial seizures and for migraines, chronic pain, and bipolar disorder (McNamara, 2006). As its name suggests, it was designed to act as a GABA-like drug, but it has been found that it does not have this effect but rather seems to induce cortical release of GABA from synaptic vesicles by a poorly understood mechanism (McNamara, 2006). It has a half-life of 5–7 hours with less than 3% protein binding.

Felbamate is a phenyl-substituted dicarbamate that not only inhibits NMDA-evoked responses but also enhances GABA-evoked responses (McNamara, 2006).

Common side effects of topiramate include fatigue, psychomotor slowing, somnolence, and difficulty with concentration and speech. Acute-angle glaucoma can also occur (Asconape, 2002). Common side effects of lamotrigine include ataxia, CNS depression, diplopia, dizziness, abnormal thinking, nausea, nervousness, rash, and somnolence. An additional major toxic effect reported for lamotrigine is Stevens-Johnson syndrome (Brodtkorb, 1998; Warner, 1998). Common side effects of gabapentin include ataxia, dizziness, fatigue, and somnolence. Felbamate has been found to produce a relatively high incidence of aplastic anemia and hepatic failure (Asconape, 2002). Thus, the drug is utilized in patients failing other treatments only when the potential clinical benefits outweigh the potential clinical risks (Bazil, 1998; Brodtkorb, 1998; Asconape, 2002; McNamara, 2006).

ANTIASTHMATICS

Asthma is a form of chronic obstructive pulmonary disease that has a variety of causes, some of them allergenic in nature. As indicated in Figure 23-12, at the heart of asthma is bronchoconstriction due to contraction of smooth muscle fibers in bronchioles. This may be induced by allergenic causes that trigger inflammatory processes that, in turn, result in the release of histamine from mast cells. Histamine, when it binds to H_1-receptors in smooth muscle cells, induces second messengers such as inositol triphosphate and diacylglycerol that ultimately stimulate muscle contraction (see Fig. 23-12). Opposing this process is the binding of epinephrine to β-2-receptors, resulting in stimulation of adenylate cyclase that induces synthesis of cAMP, a second messenger molecule that induces blockade of muscle contraction. As part of a regulatory process, phosphodiesterase induces hydrolysis of cAMP and thus helps to remove inhibition of smooth muscle contraction.

As indicated in Figure 23-12, there are at least three different therapeutic strategies for blocking bronchiolar smooth muscle contraction. The first is blockade of release of histamine from mast cells by drugs such as cromolyn. This is not the only inflammatory process that can induce the bronchoconstriction of asthma. Other components of the inflammatory process may also be active in provoking bronchoconstriction. These are summarized in Figure 23-13, which shows that, among the agents promoting bronchoconstriction, the leukotrienes and the prostaglandins are quite prominent. To counter these effects, oral anti-inflammatory agents, such as the leukotriene inhibitors zileuton and zafirlukast, have been found to be effective in asthma because they interrupt the leukotriene/arachidonic acid pathways involved in inflammation and bronchial reactivity. It is important to note that steroids have been found to be highly effective in blocking inflammation-induced bronchospasm. As indicated in Figure 23-13, these agents potently inhibit leukotriene, prostaglandin, and platelet-activating factor production (not shown in Fig. 23-13) by inhibiting phospholipase A2 and the inducible cyclo-oxygenase-2 isoform. Lipid-soluble steroids, especially in aerosolized form, avoiding adverse systemic effects, have been found to be among the most effective agents against

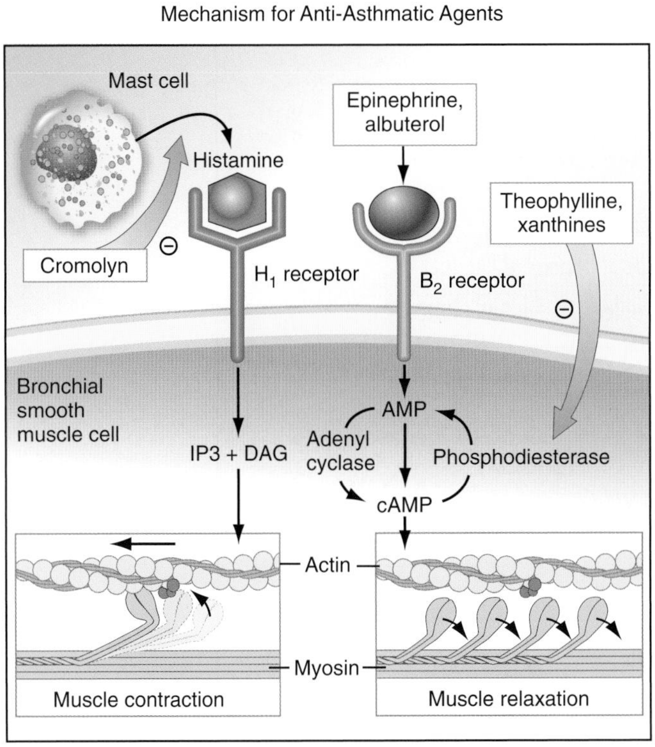

Figure 23-12 Summary of the mechanisms of action of antiasthmatic agents. Three basic mechanisms are shown. Note that all three mechanisms result in promotion of smooth muscle relaxation in the small airways (i.e., fewer actin–myosin cross-bridges) *(arrows show loss of cross-bridges),* as shown at the bottom of the figure. On the left, release of histamine from mast cells in response to allergenic stimulation results in histamine–H_1-receptor complexes that promote a signal transduction pathway in which inositol triphosphate (IP_3) and diacylglycerol (DAG), both second messengers, are induced and promote smooth muscle contraction. Histamine release is blocked *(minus sign in circle, next to green arrow)* by the drug, cromolyn. In the middle of the figure, epinephrine and albuterol are shown to form complexes with β-receptors; these complexes induce adenyl cyclase activity such that cyclic adenosine monophosphate (cAMP) is synthesized; this second messenger blocks smooth muscle contraction. On the right, xanthines, such as theophylline, are shown to block the enzyme phosphodiesterase, resulting in prolonged lifetimes of cAMP, allowing it to function for prolonged periods in blocking smooth muscle contraction.

asthma. These agents include beclomethasone, flunisolide, and triamcinolone. Longer-acting lipid-soluble β-2-agonists, such as formoterol and salmeterol, are also available and appear to be long acting because of their ability to dissolve into the bronchial smooth muscle membrane.

Second, for severe asthmatic attacks, subcutaneous injection of epinephrine is effective in relieving bronchoconstriction on an acute basis via the mechanism shown in Figure 23-12. For more long-term treatment, β-2-receptor–binding agonist drugs, including albuterol (Proventil, Ventolin) and terbutaline (Brethine), are effective in reversing this process by the same mechanism. Both of these agents stimulate production of cAMP, as shown in the central pathway of Figure 23-12. Third, as shown in Figure 23-12, blockade of phosphodiesterase by such drugs as theophylline and the xanthines prevents hydrolysis of cAMP, allowing for continuous inhibition of bronchoconstriction.

Although still a commonly prescribed antiasthmatic drug, theophylline is being replaced with other antiasthmatics such as steroid and β-adrenergic bronchial inhalers, used mainly for acute and subacute asthmatic attacks in adults. These latter agents have fewer toxic side effects (Pesce, 1998). However, laboratory assays for therapeutic levels of antiasthmatics have been performed only for theophylline, predominantly because its therapeutic range is narrow, and potential side effects are serious, as is now discussed.

Theophylline

Theophylline (Table 23-6) is used as a bronchodilator for the treatment of moderate or severe asthma, both for the prevention of attacks and for the treatment of symptomatic exacerbations. Besides its main effect of inhibiting a variety of phosphodiesterases, theophylline also inhibits the bronchoconstrictive action of adenosine and activates histone deacetylases. The latter action may result in decreases in the transcription of

TABLE 23-6
Theophylline

Purpose	Treatment and prevention of moderate to severe asthma
General adult dose	Depends on body weight, route of administration, and age and condition of patient
Usual bioavailability	Varies according to form, with about 100% for oral liquids and uncoated tablets
Half-life	Varies: 8–9 hours in nonsmoking adults, 5–6 hours in adults who smoke, and 3–4 hours in children, but may vary widely
General therapeutic range	10–20 mcg/mL
General toxic level	>20 mcg/mL
Transport	60% plasma protein bound
Metabolism	Hepatic: caffeine; 1,3-dimethyluric acid; 1-methyluric acid; 3-methylxanthine
Elimination	10% unchanged in urine
Steady state	5 half-lives; 90% of steady state reached in 3 half-lives
Mechanism of action	Increases intracellular cAMP by inhibiting phosphodiesterase; this causes the smooth muscle of the bronchial airways and pulmonary blood vessels to relax
Toxic effects	Hypotension, syncope, tachycardia, arrhythmias, seizures, gastrointestinal bleeding

cAMP, Cyclic adenosine monophosphate.

proinflammatory genes. It also inhibits the release of proinflammatory agents, like histamine, from a variety of inflammatory cells (Undem, 2006).

Theophylline exerts additional actions such as vasodilation, diuresis, positive cardiac inotropic effects, and stimulation of diaphragmatic contraction. Owing to the latter stimulating effect, theophylline may be of benefit to some patients with emphysema. Theophylline has also been effective in the treatment of primary apnea of prematurity, in which the absence of respiratory effort lasts longer than 20 seconds in newborn infants. This latter effect is thought to be due to medullary stimulation by the drug. It has been found that caffeine is more effective for this purpose because it has diminished toxicity (Pesce, 1998).

In the treatment of asthma, dosage is calculated on the basis of body weight and depends on the route of administration and the age of the patient. Because the therapeutic index (i.e., the closeness of toxic levels to therapeutic levels) of theophylline is low, cautious dosage determination is essential. Careful monitoring of patient response and serum theophylline levels is required because theophylline is metabolized at different rates for each patient. Theophylline levels can be estimated 1 hour after intravenous administration, 1–2 hours after oral administration, or generally 3–8 hours after extended-release administration from appropriately drawn blood samples.

The therapeutic serum level is 10–20 mcg/mL, and the mean half-life is approximately 8.7 hours in nonsmoking adults (5.5 hours in smoking adults). However, the half-life may vary widely among individuals, again indicating the need for close supervision of the patient and appropriate monitoring of serum concentrations in each patient. Approximately 60% of the drug is protein bound, and about 90% is metabolized in the liver, with caffeine being one of the metabolites produced. Theophylline crosses the placenta and may be teratogenic in pregnant females. Other common side effects include tachycardia, arrhythmias, seizures, and gastrointestinal bleeding.

ANTIINFLAMMATORY AND ANALGESIC DRUGS

As noted in the preceding section, and as shown in Figure 23-13, membrane damage, resulting from immune complexes, trauma, or other stress, induces, among other events, the release of phospholipids. These, in turn, become substrates for phospholipase A_2, which results in the production of arachidonic acid. This centrally important compound may be converted into leukotrienes via lipooxygenase, or thromboxanes and prostaglandins via cyclooxygenase (COX). All of these agents provoke chemotaxis of neutrophils, resulting in their activation and, ultimately, in inflammation.

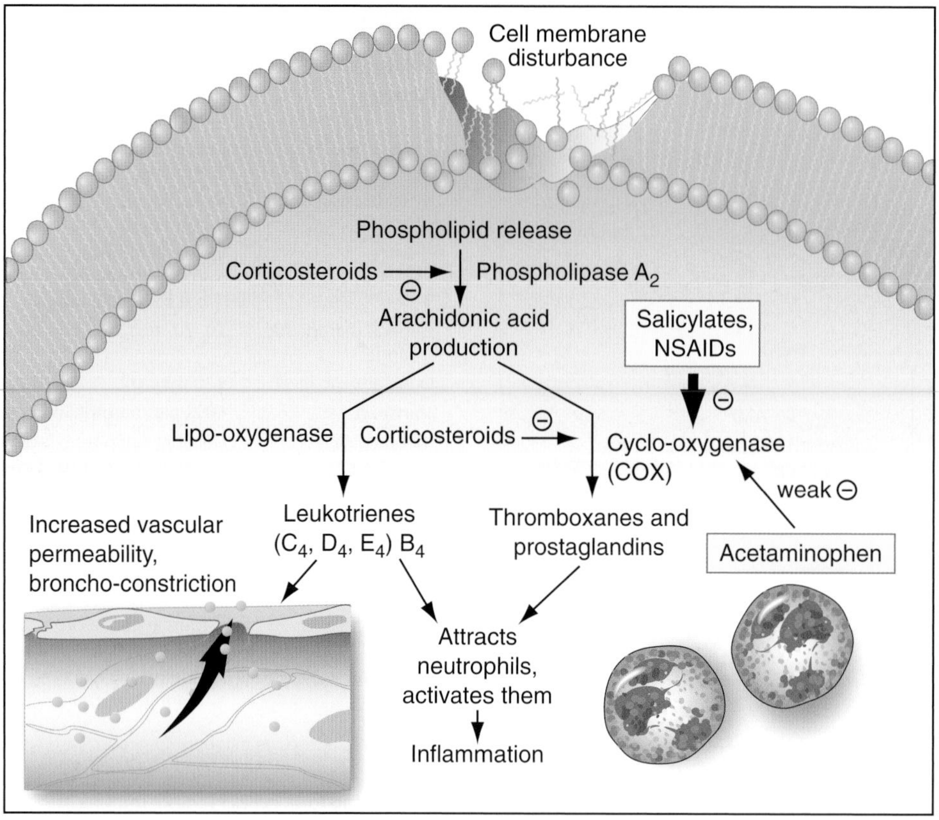

Figure 23-13 Mechanisms of action of antiinflammatory drugs. The figure shows that the fundamental event in inflammation-induced cell death is membrane damage in cells that results in activation of phospholipase A_2. This enzyme promotes the synthesis of arachidonic acid. This is a substrate for two critical enzymes: lipooxygenase, which promotes synthesis of leukotrienes, and cyclooxygenase (COX), which promotes synthesis of thromboxanes and prostaglandins. Both classes of compounds promote neutrophil chemotaxis *(lower right)* with resulting phagocytosis of damaged cells and a further destructive inflammatory response. Leukotrienes themselves promote increased vascular permeability, causing increased migration of neutrophils to damaged cells, and smooth muscle contraction *(lower left)*. In this figure, corticosteroids such as prednisone and cortisone are shown to block *(black minus signs in circles, next to arrows)* two key enzymes in this signal transduction inflammatory cascade: phospholipase A_2 and cyclooxygenase. Corticosteroids are also thought to stabilize damaged membranes. Nonsteroidal antiinflammatory drugs (NSAIDs) block predominantly cyclooxygenase; acetaminophen (Tylenol) blocks mainly COX in the central nervous system and only weakly blocks peripheral COX and is therefore more of an antipyretic than an antiinflammatory drug.

In addition, they increase vascular permeability (inducing more influx of neutrophils) and smooth muscle contraction. As noted in the preceding section, and as shown in Figure 23-13, corticosteroids are powerful antiinflammatory agents that work through the blockade of cyclooxygenase, in addition to their blocking the formation of arachidonic acid.

Although steroids are highly effective antiinflammatory agents, they provoke a number of undesirable side effects, including fluid retention, weight gain, osteoporosis, gastrointestinal bleeding, and mental changes. Other nonsteroidal drugs, including **nonsteroidal antiinflammatory drugs,** have been found to be effective in blocking inflammation by similar mechanisms, as shown in Figure 23-13, without the undesirable side effects of the corticosteroids. These agents, most of which block COX specifically, include such drugs as naproxen (Naprosyn), ibuprofen (Advil, Motrin), and piroxicam (Feldene). These agents inhibit two forms of COX: COX-1 and COX-2. The former is involved in maintaining membrane integrity of mucosal cells in the gastrointestinal tract, and the latter is involved in the inflammatory process. Because all of these agents inhibit both forms of COX, they have the undesirable side effect of gastrointestinal tract toxicity and induce GI bleeding. Newer agents that more selectively inhibit COX-2 have recently become available, including celecoxib (Celebrex) and rofecoxib (Vioxx). Because some patients treated with Vioxx have been diagnosed with myocardial infarction, this drug was withdrawn.

Aspirin, a potent cyclooxygenase inhibitor, is an effective antiinflammatory agent and has, in addition, antipyretic and analgesic effects, which also result from cyclooxygenase inhibition. The latter two effects are thought possibly to be due to inhibition of COX in the CNS (so-called **COX-3**), mainly in the hypothalamus, although this is not certain (Burke, 2006).

Acetaminophen (Tylenol) inhibits COX-3 but exerts little effect on COX-1 and COX-2. Thus it is non-antiinflammatory, does not result in gastrointestinal tract bleeding, and is an effective analgesic and antipyretic.

Of all of these drugs, therapeutic drug monitoring is performed only with aspirin and Tylenol. We therefore discuss these two drugs further.

Aspirin

Acetylsalicylic acid (aspirin) is a nonsteroidal antiinflammatory compound that is used as an analgesic, an antipyretic, and, in larger doses, an antiinflammatory agent. In lower doses, it exhibits its anticoagulant activity due to its antiplatelet activity through inhibition of COX in platelets, resulting in blockade of platelet plug formation. It can be effective in the treatment of fever, neuralgia, headache, myalgia, and arthralgia, and in the management of some rheumatic diseases.

Oral dosages of aspirin that are generally used for analgesia and antipyresis in adults range from 500 mg as necessary, to a maximum of 4 g/day. Increased dosages (3.5–5.5 g/day) are used for rheumatoid arthritis and osteoarthritis in adults, and for juvenile arthritis (up to 3.5 g/day) in children.

The small intestine is the primary site of aspirin absorption, and absorption usually occurs rapidly following oral administration, with peak plasma levels established within 1–2 hours. Before entering the systemic circulation, aspirin is rapidly hydrolyzed to acetic acid and salicylic acid. Hydrolysis occurs partially by plasma esterase and partially by the liver. Both aspirin and salicylic acid enter the CNS.

Approximately 70%–90% of salicylic acid is plasma protein bound. The serum half-life is dose dependent and increases with the dose—from approximately 3 hours with 500 mg to approximately 15 hours with 4 g. Salicylic acid is cleared not only by metabolism but also by urinary excretion, and, as the half-life increases, the rate of urinary excretion decreases. This can produce toxic effects if the dosage interval is not increased appropriately. However, the rate of elimination can vary widely with the patient, necessitating individualization of dosage for large amounts of drug. Tinnitus, muffled hearing, and a sensation of fullness in the ears are the most common signs of chronic aspirin toxicity. In infants, young children, and

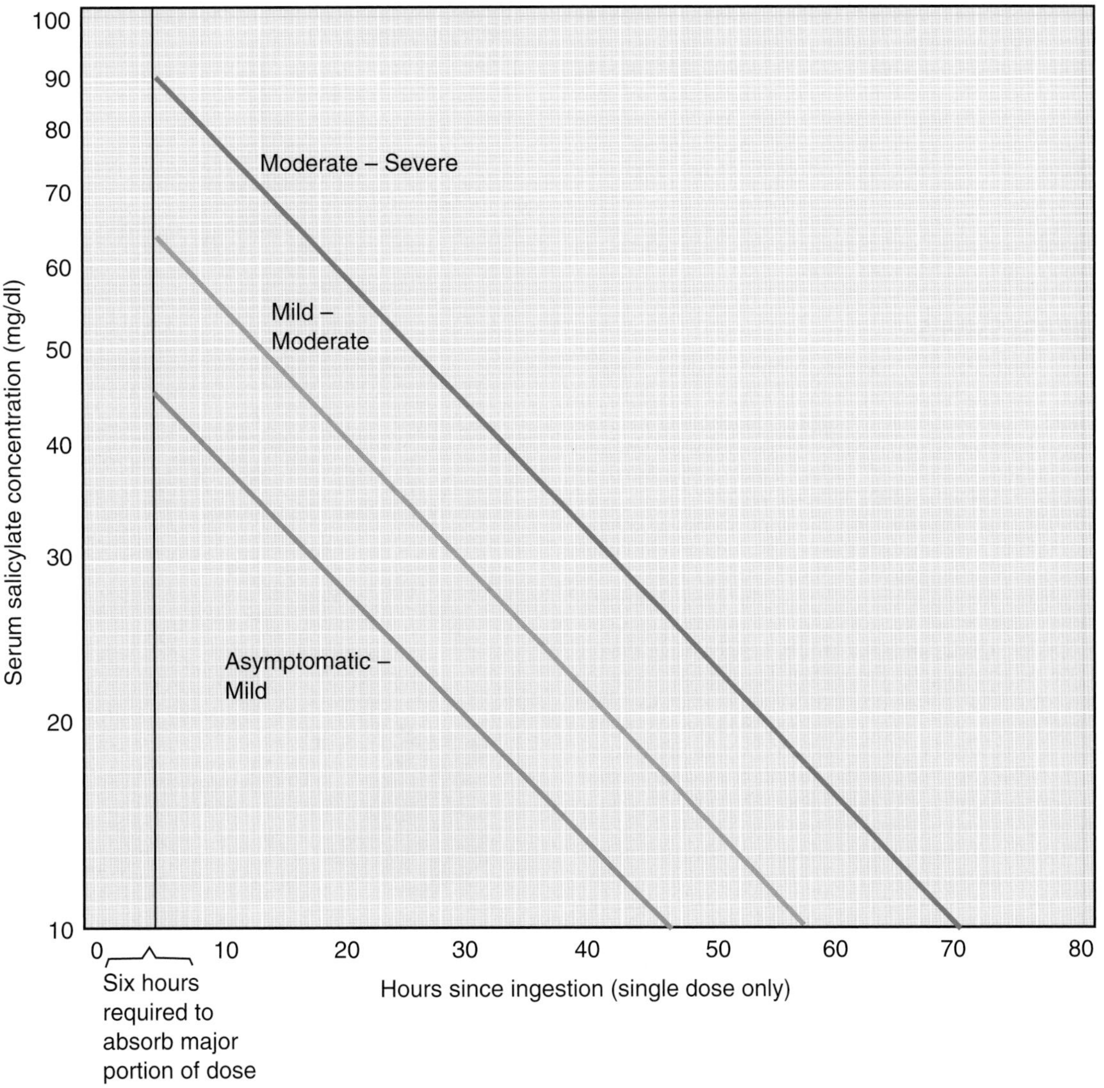

Figure 23-14 Aspirin toxicity levels in children as a function of time. (Howanitz, 1984; *modified with permission from Done AK. Pediatrics 1960;26:800.)*

patients with preexisting hearing loss, otic symptoms will not occur, and hyperventilation is the most common sign of overdose.

As discussed in Chapter 14, overdoses of aspirin can cause metabolic acidosis. Because salicylate itself stimulates central respiratory centers, overdose causes an increased breathing rate, leading to a respiratory alkalosis that can predominate, so that the patient exhibits respiratory alkalosis subsequent to initial metabolic acidosis. Acute aspirin intoxication is a common cause of fatal drug poisoning in children. Toxic doses produce acid-base disturbances, direct CNS stimulation of respiration, hyperpyrexia and hypoglycemia, gastrointestinal bleeding, and nausea and vomiting. Acute renal failure, CNS dysfunction with stupor and coma, and pulmonary edema may develop. Figure 23-14 summarizes the toxic levels of aspirin in children as a function of time after the toxic dose was taken.

A serious toxic effect of aspirin, mainly in children but also recognized in adults, is hepatotoxicity leading to fulminant hepatic failure (i.e., Reye's syndrome). This occurs when a patient is treated with aspirin for fever during a viral illness. After apparent recovery, the patient becomes seriously ill from hepatic failure with signs and symptoms, including hepatic encephalopathy, described in Chapters 8 and 21. Although once almost always fatal, newer supportive measures have resulted in a significant increase in survival from this life-threatening condition, the basic cause of which is as yet undetermined.

Acetaminophen

Acetaminophen (Tylenol), or *N*-acetyl-*p*-aminophenol, is used as an analgesic and antipyretic to treat fever, headache, and mild to moderate myalgia and arthralgia. Acetaminophen is as effective as aspirin in its analgesic and antipyretic actions and is preferred over aspirin in patients with a bleeding/coagulation disorder or in children requiring only antipyretics or analgesics, because no association between acetaminophen and Reye's syndrome has been demonstrated. Furthermore, an accidental overdose in children may be less toxic than with aspirin; hepatotoxicity is rarely associated with acetaminophen overdose in children younger than 6 years of age.

Oral doses of acetaminophen are rapidly and essentially completely absorbed from the GI tract. Generally, 325–650 mg at 4-hour intervals is prescribed for adults and children over the age of 12, with a maximum of 4 g daily. The plasma half-life is approximately 2 hours, with peak plasma levels of 5–20 μg/mL occurring in 30–60 minutes. Plasma protein binding is about 20% with therapeutic doses. The major metabolites of acetaminophen produced by the liver are glucuronide and sulfate conjugates, with minor metabolites being deacetylated and hydroxylated derivatives. The latter metabolite is thought to produce hepatotoxicity with overdose.

At therapeutic levels, about 90% of acetaminophen is conjugated as glucuronides or sulfates in the liver. About 5% is converted to a toxic metabolite, *N*-acetyl-*p*-aminobenzoquinoneimime (NAPQI), which is hepatotoxic at high concentrations (Rowden, 2006). It is this metabolite that causes toxic liver effects at high doses of acetaminophen in the liver by the cytochrome P450 mixed oxidase system. This metabolite is normally cleared by conjugation to glutathione (GSH) by glutathione-S-transferase (GST) in the liver. In cases of toxic levels of NAPQI, where the NAPQI levels overwhelm the GST system, acetylcysteine is administered. This compound conjugates to NAPQI, detoxifying it.

Toxic doses of acetaminophen occur at acute ingestion levels of 140 mg/kg (White, 1998). Acute manifestations of toxic doses generally occur within 2–3 hours after ingestion and include nausea, vomiting, and abdominal pain. A characteristic sign of toxicity is cyanosis of the skin, mucosa, and fingernails due to methemoglobinemia. However, this is seen more frequently with phenacetin poisoning. CNS stimulation followed by CNS depression may occur in severe poisoning, with vascular collapse, shock, and total seizures. Coma usually precedes death. At very high doses (as with suicide attempts), fulminant hepatic failure may occur, with maximum liver damage not becoming apparent until 2–4 days after drug ingestion (Sunheimer, 1994). Chronic acetaminophen abuse may produce chronic toxicity and death. Anemia, renal damage, and gastrointestinal disturbances are usually associated with chronic toxicity. Toxic effects can be treated effectively with NAC (Rowden, 2006).

IMMUNOSUPPRESSIVES

(Dunn, 2001; Dancey, 2002; Drosos, 2002; Scott, 2003; Mueller, 2004).

Although intact humoral and cell-mediated immunity is essential in preventing infection, it becomes vital to suppress functioning of these systems in some circumstances. These include aberrations of the immune system such as autoimmune disease (e.g., lupus erythematosus, Sjögren's syndrome) and normal functioning of the immune system (e.g., in tissue transplantation). In the latter circumstance, the most important component of the immune system is cell-mediated immunity. As shown in Figure 23-15, in host-versus-graft or in graft-versus-host disease, CD4+ T cells become activated when a foreign antigen binds to the major histocompatibility class (II) Ia protein on the surface of macrophages (antigen-presenting cells). Specific T cell clones bind to the antigen using their T cell receptors (CD3), which recognize the antigen–Ia complex. Activation of the T cell receptor results in a signal transduction cascade that ultimately ends in engulfment via receptor-mediated endocytosis of the antigen by the macrophage and destruction in lysosomes. In this cascade, calcium ions are mobilized, resulting in the activation of calcineurin, a phosphatase that forms a complex with calmodulin. Activated calcineurin dephosphorylates cytosolic nuclear factor of activated T cells $(NF\text{-}AT)^C$ resulting in its activation, whereupon it translocates to the nucleus and binds to NF-AT from the nucleus $(NF\text{-}AT)^N$. This transcriptionally active complex results in the synthesis of interleukin (IL)-2, which becomes secreted as an extracellular mitogen (i.e., an autocrine factor). It binds to the IL-2 receptor of the T cell, activating it toward the binding of a protein, called **target of rapamycin (TOR),** which serves to activate cyclin kinases that promote progression of the cell cycle from G1 to S and stimulate nucleotide synthesis. This ends in differentiation and proliferation of the T cell and ultimate antigen destruction.

As shown in Figure 23-15, there are specific agents (Hess, 1988; Kahan, 1989; Isoniemi, 1997; Braun, 1998; McEvoy, 2004: Krensky, 2006) that block one or more of these steps and, by so doing, inhibit antigen destruction. The drugs cyclosporine and tacrolimus are cyclic polypeptides that bind to intracellular proteins called **immunophilins.** Cyclosporine (CsA) binds to the immunophilin cyclophilin, while tacrolimus binds to the immunophilin called **FKBP12.** These complexes then block calcineurin-induced activation of NF-AT, and therefore block interleukin-2 synthesis, so that antigen destruction cannot occur. On the other hand, another immunosuppressive agent, rapamycin (Sirolimus), has no such effect on T cells, but rather binds to the critical TOR protein, disenabling activation of cyclin kinases so that T cell activation cannot proceed. Finally, mycophenolate mofetil, an antibiotic, is hydrolyzed to free mycophenolic acid in the cell. This agent is a powerful inhibitor of inosine monophosphate dehydrogenase and guanosine monophosphate synthetase, disenabling deoxypurine nucleotide synthesis, which, in turn, disables DNA synthesis uniquely in lymphocytes. Other cells have rescue pathways that circumvent this blockade, making the effects of this drug selective for lymphocytes (Krensky, 2006). In the same vein, some alkylating agents that are generally used as chemotherapeutic agents, such as cyclophosphamide (Cytoxan), can be used to suppress DNA synthesis in T cells, but these are not selective for lymphocytes.

It should be noted that the corticosteroids also have immunosuppressive effects on cell-mediated immunity but are much less specific and, as noted in the previous section, have multiple undesirable side effects. They are, therefore, not the drugs of choice for use in transplantation. In the following section, we discuss the properties of the more specific immunosuppressive drugs, most of which require monitoring of serum (plasma) levels.

Cyclosporine

CsA is a cyclic polypeptide containing 11 amino acids, five of which are methylated. Maximum suppression with CsA occurs during the first

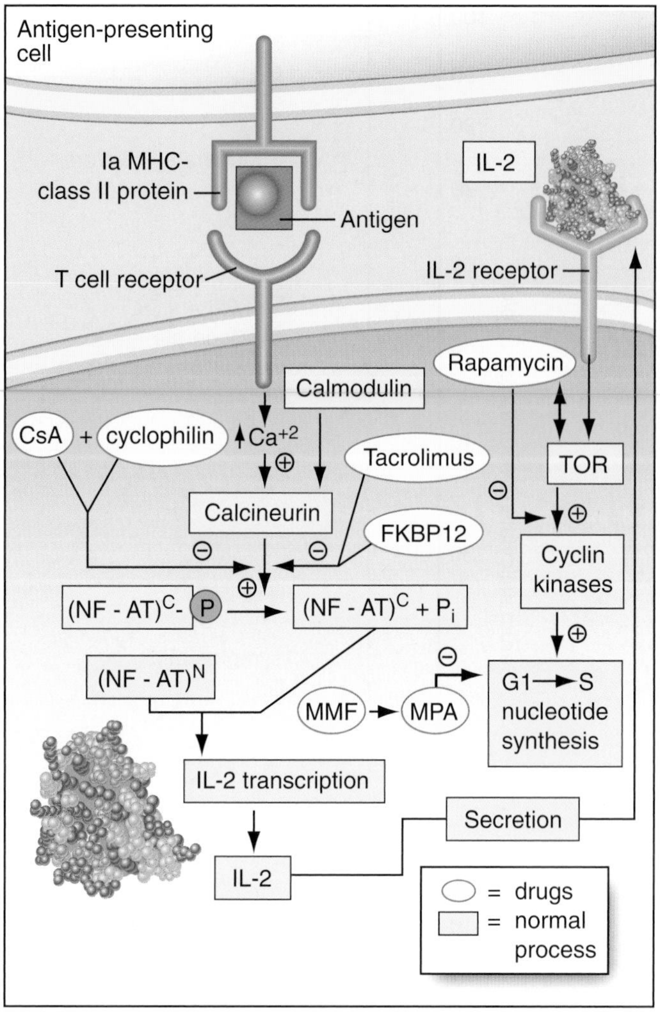

Figure 23-15 Mechanisms and sites of action of immunosuppressive drugs. This figure shows two linked, centrally important signal transduction pathways induced by antigen, in this case foreign transplanted cells, for activation of cell-mediated immunity. In the first pathway, antigen is "presented" to antigen-specific (clonal) T cells by attachment of the antigen to the Ia molecule (major histocompatibility class [MHC] II—or DR in humans—protein). The formation of a ternary complex of antigen *(red box),* Ia *(green receptor on the antigen presenting cell;* i.e., macrophage), and the T cell receptor *(purple receptor, upper left)* results in a signal transduction cascade that causes the synthesis of IL-2, shown as a space-filling model in the lower left part of the figure. Critical to this pathway is activation, by calcium-activated calmodulin, of the phosphatase, calcineurin, which dephosphorylates cytosolic nuclear factor of activated T cells $(NF\text{-}AT)^C$ resulting in its activation; whereupon it translocates to the nucleus and binds to NF-AT from the nucleus $(NF\text{-}AT)^N$, which directly promotes transcription of interleukin (IL)-2. In the second, linked, signal transduction pathway *(right side),* newly synthesized IL-2 is then secreted by the T cell and acts as an autocrine factor in binding to the extracellular domain of the IL-2 receptor of the T cell to form a complex as shown in the upper right part of the figure. This complex induces activation of a second signal transduction cascade in which target of rapamycin (TOR) protein is stimulated and, in turn, activates cyclin kinases that promote activation of cyclins, which, in turn, promote progression of the cell cycle from G1 to S necessary for blast transformation of clonal T cells that, with macrophages, engulf and destroy the antigen. All elements of the normal signal transduction pathways are shown as *pink boxes.* The immunosuppressive drugs and their target proteins block different parts of these two pathways and are shown as *yellow ellipses.* Cyclosporine (CsA) and tacrolimus complex, respectively, with cyclophilin and FKBP12 to form inhibitory complexes that block calcineurin in the first pathway. On the other hand, rapamycin blocks TOR, thereby blocking IL-2–induced blast transformation in the second pathway; mycophenolate mofetil (MMF) blocks nucleotide synthesis, thereby blocking G1-S progression in the second pathway.

24 hours of antigen stimulation by the allograft. Thus, CsA must be administered in the early phase of the immune response for optimal suppression of T cell function and increased success of transplantation (McEvoy, 2004).

CsA is indicated to prevent organ rejection in kidney, heart, and liver allogeneic transplants and is the drug of choice for maintenance of kidney, liver, heart, and heart–lung allografts. CsA may also be utilized as a first- or second-line drug in the treatment of acute graft-versus-host disease following bone marrow transplantation, in the active stage of severe rheumatoid arthritis, and for severe, recalcitrant plaque psoriasis. It may also be used in the treatment of other autoimmune diseases and in organ transplantation.

Because CsA is variably absorbed from the GI tract, the optimal dose must be carefully determined for each patient individually, and blood levels should be monitored frequently. It has been occasionally found that, although serum levels of the parent drug are low, the metabolites, some of which are active, maintain a therapeutic drug level. Therefore, in patients with apparently low levels of the parent drug, it is necessary to determine the levels of metabolites. Peak blood concentrations occur at approximately 3.5 hours after administration. About 20%–40% of a given dose of CsA is absorbed, and it is metabolized on the first pass through the liver. Human cytochrome P450 III A3 (CYP3A) of the P450 III gene family appears to be the primary enzyme responsible for CsA metabolism. Because a number of drugs may induce or may be metabolized by this cytochrome P450 isoenzyme, coadministration of these drugs may be responsible for alterations in CsA levels that can complicate CsA therapy (Kronbach, 1988). Agents that inhibit the CYP3A system include calcium channel blockers (e.g., verapamil, discussed earlier), antimicrobials, and HIV protease inhibitors. Grapefruit and grapefruit juice are also known to exert inhibitory effects on this system (Krensky, 2006). Trough whole blood or plasma concentrations, at 24 hours, of 250–800 ng/mL or 50–300 ng/mL, respectively (as determined by immunoassay), are believed to minimize graft rejection and, concurrently, toxic effects.

Adverse effects of CsA may occur in all organ systems of the body. Trough serum levels greater than 500 ng/mL are associated with CsA-induced nephrotoxicity, which is the most frequent toxic reaction seen with CsA. CsA-induced nephrotoxicity is accompanied by hyperkalemia and hyperuricemia, hypertension, and gingival hyperplasia.

Other toxic effects include neurologic effects (tremors, seizures, headache, paresthesia, flushing, confusion), dermatologic effects (hirsutism, hypertrichosis, rash), hepatotoxicity, GI effects (diarrhea, nausea, vomiting, anorexia, abdominal discomfort), infectious complications, hematologic effects (leukopenia, anemia, thrombocytopenia), and sensitivity reactions, including anaphylaxis (Philip, 1998). It is important to note that the risk of immunosuppressed states is increased, and the occurrence of lymphoma, especially CNS lymphoma, may be associated with immunosuppression by CsA. It has also been found that CsA induces immune system–independent increased invasiveness of adenocarcinoma cells in culture, apparently by activating transforming growth factor-β (TGF-β) (Hojo, 1999). This behavior is blocked by monoclonal antibodies to TGF-β.

Both oral and intravenous preparations of CsA are available. Interpatient and intrapatient absorption of the oral preparation is variable, and absorption can be affected by many factors. It is generally recommended that whole blood be used for drug level monitoring, and that an assay method with high specificity for unchanged drug (vs. metabolites) be used. Thus, the optimal dose must be carefully determined for each patient individually, and blood levels should be monitored frequently, with CsA blood concentrations qualified by biological fluid (whole blood vs. plasma vs. serum) and assay method (immunoassay vs. HPLC) used. At present, any currently available immunoassay (FPIA, EMIT) is acceptable for routine monitoring, although it is important that consistent laboratories and methods be used (McEvoy, 2004).

Neoral is a microemulsion formulation of CsA that is miscible in water; it increases the solubility of CsA in the small bowel (Miller, 1998). This preparation has shown superior pharmacokinetics with improved bioavailability and equivalent safety with no apparent increase in toxicity. It appears to offer advantages over oral solutions of CsA, by decreasing intrapatient and interpatient blood level variability. Intravenous CsA is reserved for patients unable to tolerate oral administration; this route of administration carries a low but definite (0.1%) risk of anaphylaxis, which does not occur following oral administration of the drug.

Tacrolimus (FK-506)

Tacrolimus is a macrolide lactone antibiotic with a mechanism of action similar to that of cyclosporine; it is more potent than CsA in its inhibitory effect (McEvoy, 2004). It is currently being utilized in transplant surgery to prevent organ rejection. As is the case with CsA, higher trough concentrations of tacrolimus appear to increase the relative risk of toxicity, and therapeutic drug monitoring is recommended. The same monoclonal antibody is used in the two methods available for monitoring. One method is a microparticle enzyme immunoassay, and the other method is an enzyme-linked immunosorbent assay. Whole blood is the specimen of choice. The toxic potential appears to be similar to the toxic effects of CsA. The most common include nephrotoxicity, neurotoxicity (such as tremor and headache), gastrointestinal effects such as diarrhea and nausea, hypertension, alterations in glucose metabolism (diabetes mellitus), hyperkalemia, and infectious complications. However, unlike with CsA, gingival hyperplasia and hirsutism do not occur. Anaphylaxis may occur with intravenous administration, and oral therapy is recommended whenever possible. Tacrolimus appears to be best suited for use in combination with other new immunosuppressive agents.

Rapamycin (Sirolimus)

Rapamycin is an antibiotic similar to tacrolimus. Peak concentrations are reached after about 1 hour after a single oral dose or after about 2 hours after multiple doses for patients who have undergone renal transplant (Krensky, 2006). The parent drug is the major active form, although several metabolites also have activity. About 40% of the drug is bound to serum proteins, especially albumin; it is metabolized predominantly in the liver by the CYP3A4 system (Krensky, 2006). Major side effects include GI symptoms, abnormalities in lipid levels, anemia, leukopenia, and thrombocytopenia. It can also cause delayed wound healing; however, it does not appear to be nephrotoxic. If used in combination with cyclosporine, because sirolimus aggravates CsA-induced renal dysfunction, administration of these two drugs must be separated in time (Krensky, 2006).

Mycophenolate Mofetil

Mycophenolate mofetil is a derivative of mycophenolate acid, a fungal antibiotic. The parent drug is metabolized to mycophenolic acid (MPA) within minutes of administration. The half-life of MPA is about 16 hours. Virtually all MPA is excreted in the urine as the glucuronide. This drug is used for prophylaxis of renal allograft rejection, usually in combination with a steroid or a calcineurin inhibitor (Krensky, 2006). Although this drug appears to decrease the rate of renal allograft rejection, differences in patient and allograft survival have not been demonstrated (Isoniemi, 1997). It may be of use in patients who do not tolerate CsA or tacrolimus (FK-506) well. Major side effects include GI symptoms such as diarrhea, nausea, and myelosuppression. Neither nephrotoxicity nor neurotoxicity has been demonstrated.

Leflunomide

Leflunomide (LFM), which inhibits lymphocyte proliferation by inhibiting dihydroorotic acid synthetase (Krensky, 2006), critical to deoxy pyrimidine nucleotide synthesis, is an isoxazole derivative. It is presently used in the treatment of rheumatoid arthritis, the only condition for which it has been approved for treatment, although it is being used increasingly for treatment of polyoma virus nephropathy seen in immunosuppressed renal transplant recipients (Krensky, 2006). LFM has not been demonstrated to cause nephrotoxicity or myelosuppression in humans.

DRUGS USED IN THE TREATMENT OF MANIA AND DEPRESSION

Both lithium and the antidepressants are used in the treatment of psychiatric affective disorders.

Lithium

Lithium is a monovalent cation, a member of the group of alkali metals, and is available commercially as citrate and carbonate salts. Lithium salts are considered to be antimanic agents and are used for the prophylaxis and treatment of bipolar disorder (manic–depressive psychosis) and as an adjunct to antidepressant therapy in melancholic depression (Baldessarini, 2006a). In addition, lithium is considered by some investigators to be the drug of choice for the prevention of chronic cluster headache, and it may be effective in episodic or periodic forms of cluster headache. Initial oral dosages of lithium for acute mania range from 0.6–1.8 g daily (maximum, 2.4 g) and produce a therapeutic serum level of 0.75–1.5 mEq/L. Once the attack subsides, the dose is reduced rapidly to produce a serum concentration of 0.4–1.0 mEq/L. Oral adult dosages for cluster headaches generally range from 0.6–1.2 g daily in divided doses. In cases of acute mania, especially in agitated, uncooperative patients, because of the relatively slow onset of action of lithium, a benzodiazepine sedative (e.g., lorazepam, clonazepam) or the anticonvulsant valproate (Depakote; see previous section) is administered until some stabilization of the agitated state is achieved. Then lithium is administered to achieve long-term stabilization. Alternatively, continuation of both drugs may be continued, or, in some cases, the patient can be maintained on Depakote alone (Baldessarini, 2006b).

In general, serum levels of and patient response to lithium are used to individualize dosage and must be monitored carefully. Complete absorption of lithium occurs 6–8 hours after oral administration. Plasma half-life varies from 17–36 hours, and onset of action is slow (5–10 days). Elimination occurs almost entirely by the kidneys, and about 80% of filtered lithium is reabsorbed. Lithium is not protein bound and is distributed in total body water, but it shows delayed and varied tissue distribution. Thus, symptoms of acute intoxication may not correlate well with serum levels, because the distribution of the drug into different organs may be slow and/or varied.

The exact mechanism of action of lithium is unknown, but lithium, as a monovalent cation, competes with other monovalent and divalent cations (such as sodium, potassium, calcium, and magnesium) at ion channels in cell membranes and at protein-binding sites such as membrane receptors and protein/peptide transport molecules and enzymes that are critical to the synthesis, storage, release, and uptake of central neurotransmitters. Lithium also has a marked inhibitory effect on inositol monophosphatase and on the synthesis of phosphatidylinositides, which are second messengers involved in neurotransmission, and on the synthesis of cAMP, also involved in neurotransmission (Phiel, 2001; Baldessarini, 2006a,b). These effects are exerted on the postsynaptic side of dopamine- and norepinephrine-utilizing tracts in the mesolimbic and mesocortical pathways that inhibit the mobilization of calcium ions required for postsynaptic depolarization. The effect, then, is to inhibit neurotransmission. In addition, lithium blocks release of dopamine from presynaptic vesicles, also resulting in diminished neurotransmission.

Toxicity may occur acutely, as the result of a single toxic dose, or chronically, from high and/or prolonged dosages or changes in lithium pharmacokinetics. Water loss (resulting from fever, decreased intake, abnormal gastrointestinal conditions such as diarrhea or vomiting, diuretics, or pyelonephritis) is the main contributing factor underlying chronic intoxication. Renal toxicity and hypothyroidism are also known possible side effects of lithium. Thus it is advisable to monitor creatinine and thyroid-stimulating hormone periodically in patients who are under continuing treatment with this drug. Severity of intoxication is not clearly related to serum lithium levels. However, an imprecise prediction of severity of intoxication may be attempted from serum lithium levels obtained 12 hours after the last dose: Slight to moderate intoxication with 1.5–2.5 mEq/L, severe intoxication with 2.5–3.5 mEq/L, and potentially lethal intoxication if greater than 3.5 mEq/L. Severity of lithium intoxication also depends on the length of time that the serum concentration remains toxic.

The most common symptoms of mild to moderate intoxication include nausea, malaise, diarrhea, and fine hand tremor. In addition, thirst, polydipsia, and polyuria, as well as drowsiness, muscle weakness, ataxia, and slurred speech, may occur. Symptoms of moderate to severe toxicity include hyperactive deep tendon reflexes, choreoathetoid movements, persistent nausea and vomiting, fasciculations, generalized seizures, and clonic movements of whole limbs. These may progress rapidly to generalized seizures, oliguria, circulatory failure, and death with serum levels greater than 3.5 mEq/L.

Antidepressants

Three classes of drugs are currently used in the treatment of clinical depression: classical tricyclic antidepressants (TCAs), SSRIs, and monoamine oxidase inhibitors (MAOIs) (Baldessarini, 2006a). The rationale for use of the first class of drugs is their ability to block the uptake of norepinephrine at the axonal side of synapses in neural tracts from the brainstem to the forebrain that utilize this neurotransmitter, as indicated in Figure 23-8. This blockade allows longer stimulation times and higher concentrations of norepinephrine at the dendritic side of the synapse, allowing them to bind to α-1-receptors in these tracts for prolonged times, resulting in prolonged and enhanced stimulation. Drugs in the second class produce the same effect in parallel neural pathways that utilize serotonin as the stimulatory neurotransmitter (see earlier in the The Drugs of Abuse, General Aspects of the Mechanisms of Action section). Finally, MAOIs block the inactivating metabolism of both norepinephrine and serotonin neurotransmitters by inhibiting their oxidation by the enzyme monoamine oxidase, present in the mitochondria of the presynaptic (axonal) terminal, wherein their amino groups are oxidized to the corresponding aldehydes. This inhibition results in increased concentrations of these neurotransmitters.

Tricyclic Antidepressants

The structures of these related compounds are shown in Figure 23-16. Also shown are two other effective antidepressant drugs: doxepin and Desyrel (trazodone), a second-generation, so-called **atypical antidepressant,** which does not contain the three fused ring system of the TCAs. Besides blocking reuptake of norepinephrine at the axonal side of synapses, the TCAs have been found to *bind directly* to two classes of norepinephrine receptors: α-1, which occur on the postsynaptic side of the synapse, and α-2, so-called **autoreceptors,** which occur on the presynaptic side of the synapse. The postsynaptic α-1-receptors are involved in postsynaptic membrane depolarization involving calcium ion fluxes resulting in nerve conduction. The presynaptic α-2-receptors, when bound to norepinephrine, induce its downregulation by causing decreased synthesis of tyrosine hydroxylase, the critical enzyme that catalyzes the rate-limiting step in norepinephrine biosynthesis (Baldessarini, 2006a). This results in decreased levels of norepinephrine and in decreased secretion of this neurotransmitter into the synaptic cleft.

When the TCAs bind to α-1-receptors, they cause temporary blockade of these receptors. This effect is thought to cause the **observed side effect of initial hypotensive episodes** in patients who are treated with these drugs. Over time, the binding of TCAs to these postsynaptic receptors apparently causes ***increased*** **sensitization** of the apha-1-receptors to norepinephrine, overcoming the initial inhibition, while the presynaptic reuptake blockade of norepinephrine continues unimpeded. Concurrently, binding of the TCAs to presynaptic α-2-receptors has the opposite effect from their binding to the postsynaptic α-1-receptors, that is, desensitization with resulting loss of inhibition of epinephrine biosynthesis. Thus the TCAs enhance norepinephrine-induced neurotransmission in the limbic system by blocking norepinephrine reuptake, sensitizing postsynaptic α-1-receptors, and desensitizing inhibitory presynaptic α-2-receptors. In addition, TCAs appear to block, in a nonspecific manner, the reuptake of dopamine in the dopaminergic pathways in the limbic system (Baldessarini, 2006a).

Besides stimulating dopaminergic pathways, the tricyclics, especially amitriptyline, have anticholinergic effects (Baldessarini, 2006a). The pharmacologic side effects of the tricyclic antidepressants, in fact, reflect their anticholinergic activities. These include dry mouth, constipation, blurred vision, hyperthermia, adynamic ileus, urinary retention, and delayed micturition. Other CNS effects include drowsiness, weakness, fatigue, and lethargy, which are most common, as well as agitation, restlessness, insomnia, and confusion. Seizures and coma can also occur. Extrapyramidal symptoms may occur and include a persistent fine tremor, rigidity, dystonia, and opisthotonos. It is important to note that TCAs unfortunately have been used in suicide attempts by some depressed individuals who are being treated with them. The cardinal signs of tricyclic antidepressant overdose are anticholinergic symptoms, such as dilated pupils and dry skin.

Toxicity. Overdose produces symptoms that are primarily extensions of common adverse reactions with excess CNS stimulation and anticholinergic activity. These include seizures, coma, hypotension, respiratory depression, areflexia, shock, and cardiorespiratory arrest. Agitation, confusion, hypertension, and the parkinsonian syndrome may also occur, as well as hallucinations and delirium. Occasional manifestations include ataxia, renal failure, dysarthria, and vomiting.

Treatment. Symptomatic and supportive care is the general mode of treatment. Gastric lavage, accompanied by instillation of activated charcoal, is usually recommended for removal of the tricyclic from the GI tract. Seizures are generally treated with intravenous diazepam. For overdoses with amitriptyline (see Fig. 23-16), use of cholinesterase inhibitors such as neostigmine has proved to be effective in reversing anticholinergic symptoms.

Selective Serotonin Reuptake Inhibitors

These are nontricyclic drugs with strong antidepressant activity that have been developed more recently. The most prominent of these is fluoxetine (Prozac), whose structure is shown in Figure 23-16. These drugs block the reuptake of serotonin in central serotonergic pathways as noted previously. Their effects on serotonin receptors parallel those of the TCAs on norepinephrine receptors, including ultimate downregulation of presynaptic autoreceptors. It is interesting to note that if the trifluromethyl group of fluoxetine is placed at the ortho rather than the para position, the

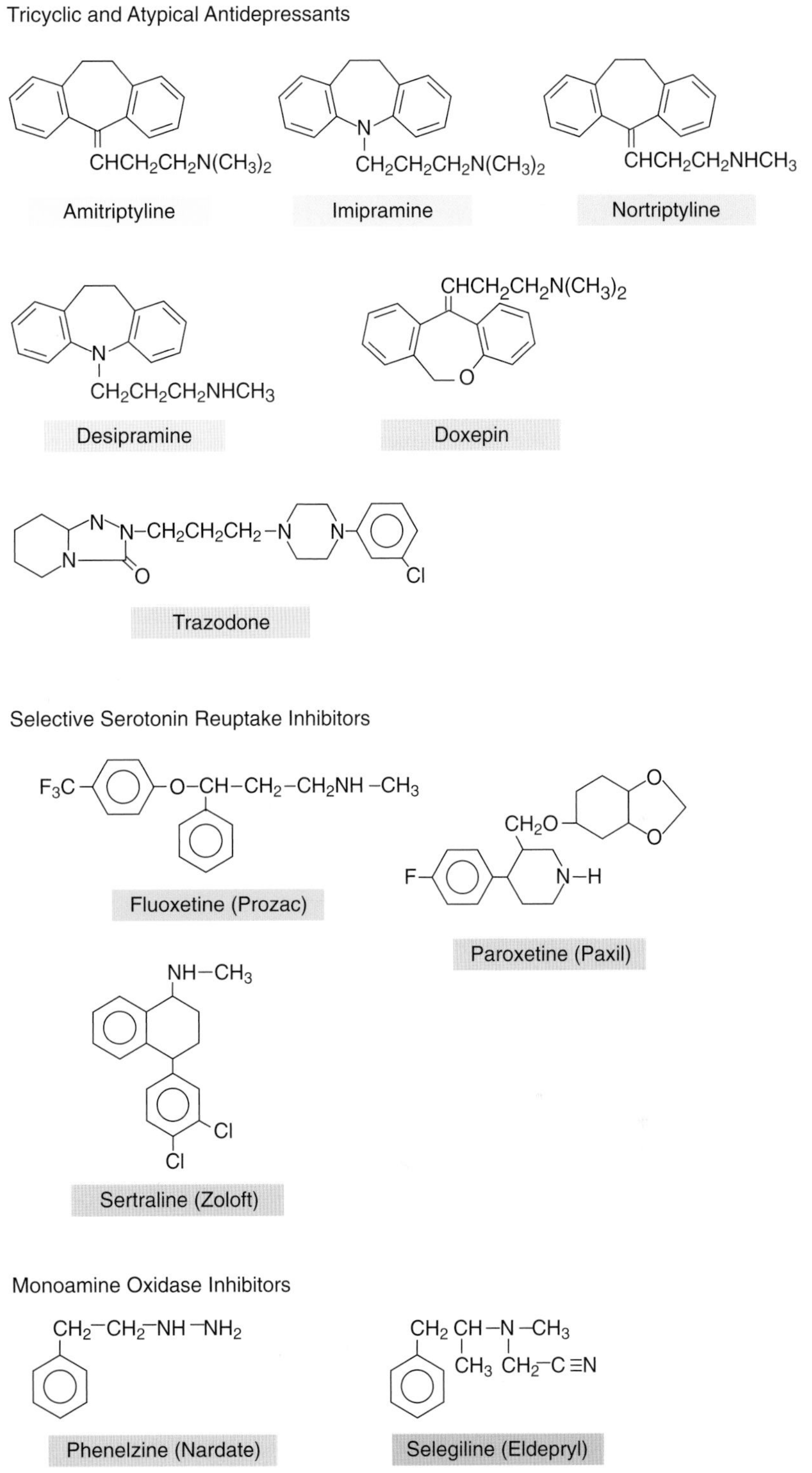

Figure 23-16 Structures of the most commonly used drugs in the three classes of antidepressants: tricyclic and atypical antidepressants, selective serotonin reuptake inhibitors, and monoamine oxidase inhibitors.

resulting drug behaves as a tricyclic antidepressant (Baldessarini, 2006a). It is an important note that Prozac and SSRIs in general do not appear to cause some of the side effects, such as the anticholinergic effects, associated with TCAs. For this reason, they have become the drugs of choice for treating clinical depression, although reports have described attempted suicide with some patients, especially adolescents, who are being treated with SSRIs. In addition, SSRIs have been reported to cause nausea and decreased libido and sexual function.

MAO Inhibitors

MAO is a flavin-containing oxidative enzyme that is encoded by two distinct genes. The two resulting enzymes, called **MAO-A** and **MAO-B,** have about 70% sequence identity. Each enzyme is found on the mitochondrial membrane. MAO-A deaminates epinephrine, norepinephrine, and serotonin, and MAO-B deaminates phenylethylamine. Both enzymes deaminate dopamine. Several MAOIs have been synthesized that inhibit either enzyme selectively. Thus, for example, MAO-A is inhibited selectively by clorgyline, and MAO-B is inhibited by selegiline (see Fig. 23-16).

MAOIs are not used as the "first line" of treatment for depression because of their potential toxic effects and unfavorable interactions with TCAs and SSRIs. Toxic effects from overdoses include hypertension and/or hypotension, agitation, hallucinations, hyperreflexia, fever, and seizures (Baldessarini, 2006a). The combination of an MAOI with an SSRI can lead to the so-called **serotonin syndrome,** which includes akathisia, myoclonus, hyperreflexia, diaphoresis, and shivering progressing to seizures and coma. In addition, MAOIs potentiate the action of over-the-counter anti-cold sympathomimetic amines such that they can cause hypertensive crises and intracerebral bleeding. Therefore, it is imperative to avoid use of these anticold medications in individuals treated with an MAOI. Their use is mostly for patients who do not respond to either SSRI or TCA therapy and who refuse electroconvulsant shock therapy.

Therapeutic Levels and Metabolism of Antidepressants

It is difficult to obtain reference ranges for the antidepressants because of their large numbers of metabolites, some of which may be active and others of which may be inactive, and which vary significantly in concentration from individual to individual—a problem that also exists for the neuroleptics discussed later. In addition, the volumes of distribution of these drugs are quite high because most are lipophilic and thus are stored in tissue and slowly released. For the TCAs, serum levels from 100–250 ng/mL generally are considered therapeutic; toxic effects may result at levels above 500 ng/mL and lethal doses above 1 µg/mL. Assays for the TCAs are performed by immunoassay (see Immunochemical Methods section earlier and Fig. 23-1) or by HPLC (see High-Performance Liquid Chromatography section earlier and Fig. 23-4).

Virtually all of these drugs are metabolized in the liver using the cytochrome P450–dependent oxidase system (Baldessarini, 2006a). Different antidepressants require different isoforms of cytochrome P450. These isoforms include CYP2D6, CYP2C19, CYP3A3/4, and CYP1A2. In general, for both TCAs and SSRIs, oxidation, a modification that often includes glucuronidation and elimination of these drugs, occurs over several days. Most tricyclics are completely eliminated within 10 days. Secondary amine TCAs and *N*-demethylated derivatives of SSRIs have about twice the half-lives of their parent compounds. The **atypical TCA,** trazodone, is metabolized to mCPP, a piperazine that is discussed earlier under the drugs of abuse section. MAOIs have much shorter half-lives than TCAs and SSRIs, requiring frequent dosing to maintain therapeutic levels.

THE NEUROLEPTICS, ANTIPSYCHOTIC MAJOR TRANQUILIZERS

These drugs are used mainly in the treatment of acute schizophrenia and result in suppression of the agitated state. All neuroleptics appear to block the actions of dopamine and serotonin postsynaptically in the limbic system and motor cortex (see Fig. 23-8). Specific dopaminergic pathways, called the **mesolimbic-mesocortical pathways,** connect the substantia nigra of the midbrain to the limbic system and motor cortex (Baldessarini, 2006b). In addition, the substantia nigra connects to the basal ganglia via the nigrostriatal pathway; depletion of dopamine in this pathway results in Parkinson's disease. Thus it may be expected that dopamine antagonists would affect the latter pathway, in addition to the mesolimbic-mesocortical pathways. Indeed many of the neuroleptics have, as side effects, dystonias, tardive dyskinesias, and frank parkinsonism, the latter fortunately being much less common. Originally, two classes of neuroleptics, the phenothiazines, typified by chlorpromazine, and the butyrophenones, typified by haloperidol (Haldol), were the drugs of choice. Besides postsynaptic blockade of dopamine, Haldol is known to bind with high affinity to sigma-receptors in the CNS, and this action may stimulate inhibitory pathways that modulate the activity of the dopaminergic pathways. All compounds in both classes have the undesired extrapyramidal side effects mentioned previously. In addition, the neuroleptics inhibit dopamine in the hypothalamic-pituitary tract, which inhibits release of prolactin by the pituitary. The effect of the neuroleptics therefore is to increase prolactin secretion by the pituitary, resulting in hyperprolactinemia. Treatment of patients with breast cancer with any neuroleptic that causes this effect is contraindicated (Baldessarini, 2006b).

Newer neuroleptics have been developed that affect the nigrostriatal pathway to a lesser extent but are potent postsynaptic dopamine blockers in the mesolimbic-mesocortical pathways and therefore are effective, with fewer of the extrapyramidal side effects of the older drugs. These newer drugs (Burns, 2001) include risperidone (Risperdal) (which does have some documented extrapyramidal side effects), olanzapine (Zyprexa), quetiapine (Seroquel), and aripiprazole (Abilify).

It has been difficult to monitor the levels of any of these drugs in serum because of the large number of metabolites for each drug resulting from extensive metabolism in the liver. Chlorpromazine, for example, has approximately 150 metabolites. The therapeutic efficacy of most of these metabolites is unknown. Reference ranges for serum levels therefore have not been established. Similar to the antidepressants, the neuroleptics, being lipophilic, have high volumes of distribution and are stored in tissues from which they are released over time.

Methods for assay include FPIA (see Immunochemical Methods section earlier and Fig. 23-1) and by HPLC (see High-Performance Liquid Chromatography section earlier and Fig. 23-4). It is not clear in FPIA which, if any, metabolites cross-react with the antibody. For chlorpromazine, the estimated therapeutic range is wide—between 50 and 300 ng/mL. The half-life of the drug is 16–30 hours, and its bioavailability is 25%–35%. Normal doses for chlorpromazine are 200–600 mg/day in divided doses. Other drugs in the phenothiazine series include thioridazine and fluphenazine (Prolixin).

Besides the extrapyramidal side effects, the phenothiazines can cause orthostatic hypotension, cholestasis, and, rarely, aplastic anemia. Occasionally, contact dermatitis has been reported to occur with phenothiazines. Of great importance is the subset of patients who have been chronically treated with these drugs and develop tardive dyskinesia. In most of these patients, the motor disturbances are irreversible.

Neuroleptics can cause a rare but important adverse reaction termed the neuroleptic malignant syndrome. This can occur in patients who are extremely sensitive to the extrapyramidal effects of these drugs, and it may be fatal. Marked muscle rigidity, the first symptom to occur, may be followed by high fever, altered pulse and blood pressure, and leukocytosis. An excessively rapid inhibition of postsynaptic dopamine receptors is believed to be responsible for this syndrome. Treatment is cessation of the drug.

CHEMOTHERAPEUTIC AGENTS: METHOTREXATE AND BUSULFAN

Serum levels of both of these agents are monitored to assess whether therapeutic serum levels are present. Both agents are used in the treatment of different forms of cancer.

Methotrexate

Methotrexate, an antimetabolite consisting of a mixture containing no less than 85% 4-amino-10-methylfolic acid and related compounds, is a folic acid antagonist (Table 23-7). It inhibits the enzyme dihydrofolate reductase (Chabner, 2006). This results in blockade of the synthesis of tetrahydrofolic acid, which is needed for the formation of *N*-5,10-methylene-tetrahydrofolate, an intermediate in the transfer of a methyl group to deoxyuridylate to form thymidylate, needed in DNA synthesis. It has also been suggested that methotrexate may cause a rise in the intracellular levels of adenosine triphosphate (ATP), which blocks ribonucleotide reduction, also resulting in blocking of DNA synthesis. Methotrexate appears to inhibit polynucleotide ligase involved in DNA synthesis and repair. Furthermore, methotrexate and its analogs, like pemetrexed, a pyrrolepyrimidine folate analog, accumulate in cells and are stored as polyglutamates, which allows them to inhibit other enzymes in DNA synthesis, including thymidylate synthase. Methotrexate polyglutamates also inhibit enzymes involved in purine nucleotide biosynthesis such as glycinamide

TABLE 23-7
Methotrexate

Condition	Usual dose	Serum level
Psoriasis	IM or IV: 7.5–50 mg/week Oral: 7.5–30 mg/week	<10 nM (Roenigk, 1998)
Refractory rheumatoid arthritis	IM: 5–25 mg/week Oral: 7.5–15 mg/week	(Tugwell, 1987a and b)*
Malignant neoplastic diseases†	IM or IV: 25 mg/m², 1–2 times/week Oral: 2.5–5 mg/day High-dose IV: 1.5 g/m² with rescue every 3 weeks (different regimens are available)	Approximately 50 nM

IM, Intramuscular; *IV,* intravenous.
*Baseline monitoring of patient parameters (hemoglobin; white blood cell count; mean corpuscular volume; platelet count; urinalysis; blood urea nitrogen; and serum creatinine, transaminase, and alkaline phosphatase levels) is advocated.
†With high-dose therapy, methotrexate levels are followed, and leucovorin doses are adjusted until serum methotrexate levels are less than 50 nM (Grem, 1995).

ribonucleotide transformylase, and aminoimidazole carboxamide transformylase in the synthesis of inosine monophosphate.

Methotrexate is used in the treatment of childhood acute lymphatic leukemia and a number of other hematologic malignancies, such as Hodgkin's lymphoma, usually in combination with other antineoplastic agents. It has also been used successfully in the treatment of choriocarcinoma (Chabner, 2006). Pemetrexed is used to treat mesothelioma and refractory non–small cell carcinoma of the lung.

Methotrexate is also an important immunosuppressive agent. Indications are severe, recalcitrant psoriasis and severe, active rheumatoid arthritis; in the latter, it may be used in combination with cyclosporine (Tugwell, 1995). Depending on the specific disease entity being treated, dosages given will vary, as will the therapeutic level of the drug. In Table 23-7, the doses and therapeutic drug levels for several different conditions are noted. The serum levels were determined by FPIA.

The kinetics of steady-state levels of this drug is triphasic: a rapid distribution phase followed first by a renal clearance phase with $t_{1/2}$ of 2–3 hours, and then by a slow phase with $t_{1/2}$ of 8–10 hours, in which methotrexate and its metabolites are filtered through the glomerulus and secreted in the renal tubules. If renal blood flow is compromised, the third phase is slowed, allowing toxic effects of the drug to occur. Excretion of the drug is biphasic: 92% is excreted within 24 hours, and the remainder over a period of days. Approximately 50% of the drug in blood is bound to serum proteins. Based on these considerations, it is important, when treating with methotrexate, not to administer drugs that compromise renal blood flow and not to modify the drug regimen to account for reduced renal blood flow. The same considerations apply to patients with renal insufficiency. In both circumstances, it is important to monitor blood levels of methotrexate. Treatment with high-dose methotrexate and leucovorin (see later) can itself be nephrotoxic because of the tendency of methotrexate to precipitate in acidic urine. Therefore, it is important to maintain high levels of hydration and to ensure alkalinization of the urine (Chabner, 2006).

As with most antineoplastic agents, methotrexate does not discriminate between transformed and normal cells. The rationale for using this drug is that it will kill rapidly dividing cancer cells that require rapid DNA synthesis but will not immediately affect normal cells, many of which are not dividing. Normal cells can be "rescued" from the effects of methotrexate and its analogs by treatment with *N*-5-formyltetrahydrofolate (called **leucovorin** or **citrovorum**), the product of dihydrofolate reductase. Leucovorin rescue is critical in cases where it is necessary to administer high doses of methotrexate to individuals with tumors that do not respond to normal doses of this drug. In such cases, leucovorin is given 18–36 hours after the initial methotrexate dose, while serum levels of methotrexate are monitored. In addition, leucovorin should immediately be administered to a patient receiving low-dose methotrexate when methotrexate overdose is suspected (Roenigk, 1998). Serum methotrexate levels should be monitored during this time (Grem, 1995; Chabner, 2006).

The methotrexate/leucovorin strategy is compromised by the existence of many fast-growing normal cells in bone marrow, the gastrointestinal tract, the skin, and other epithelial lining cells. These cells are as susceptible to the cell-killing effects of methotrexate as neoplastic cells. Thus, the toxic effects of methotrexate include hematologic effects (e.g., leukopenia, thrombocytopenia) from bone marrow suppression, gastrointestinal effects (e.g., ulceration, glossitis, stomatitis, nausea, vomiting), and dermatologic effects (e.g., urticaria, vasculitis). They further include hepatic lesions such as cirrhosis; pulmonary lesions such as pulmonary fibrosis; and CNS effects from intrathecal methotrexate, including arachnoiditis, leukoencephalopathy, and increased cerebrospinal fluid pressure.

Toxicity of methotrexate can be treated using continuous flow hemodialysis. Alternatively, intravenous infusion of carboxypeptidase G2, a methotrexate-cleaving enzyme, results in rapid clearing of the drug (Chabner, 2006).

Busulfan

Busulfan is an alkylating agent used to treat a variety of leukemias and lymphomas before bone marrow transplantation. It is cytotoxic to marrow cells and is used in combination with cyclophosphamide, which is cytotoxic to mature lymphocytes that may be involved in a graft-versus-host reaction (Slattery, 1998). The therapeutic index of the drug is narrow. High plasma levels increase the possibility of development of hepatic venoocclusive disease (VOD), a potentially fatal complication. Therefore, therapeutic monitoring of busulfan levels, using HPLC or GC-MS, with measurement of the dose interval of this drug, is now routinely performed at bone marrow transplant centers. This decreases the incidence of VOD in patients whose initial serum levels of busulfan are too high and allows increasing doses for patients with too low an initial level of busulfan, thus optimizing therapeutic levels for each patient.

Toxins and Acute Poisoning

In this section, agents that cause chronic or acute injury to the patient are discussed. This injury can be direct, as with poisons such as cyanide and carbon monoxide, or indirect, as with carcinogens that induce mutations in genes that encode proteins that are critical in controlling the cell cycle.

ENVIRONMENTAL CARCINOGENS

Over the past decade or so, attention has been focused on the effects of chemical agents in the environment—carcinogens, which predispose individuals exposed to them to develop tumors in various tissues where these agents accumulate. Many of the individuals who are exposed to these agents work in industries where these agents are produced. Benzpyrene, an aromatic compound produced in cigarettes and in the exhaust of engines, is a known potent carcinogen and has been implicated in causing lung cancer. Nitrites, used as preservatives in red meats, have been associated with colon cancer. Aflatoxin, produced by the fungus *Aspergillus*, has been implicated in causing hepatocellular carcinoma. Aromatic hydrocarbons such as benzene and ionizing radiation have been implicated in causing acute leukemias. Vinyl chloride and the formerly used dye Thorotrast have been linked to angiosarcoma. Benzidine dyes, β-naphthylamine, dimethylbenzanthracene, and other aromatic compounds have been linked to multiple malignancies occurring in humans. Exposure to asbestos has been strongly implicated as a carcinogen in lung cancer and mesothelioma. In animal studies, polychlorinated biphenyls (PCBs) and dioxin, the former produced in fires, have been strongly implicated as causing a variety of cancers.

A number of carcinogens, like benzpyrene, are inactive in their native forms but are transformed into carcinogens through oxidative reactions catalyzed by cytochrome P450–dependent systems. Thus, to be an active carcinogen, benzpyrene must be converted into benzpyrene diol epoxide. Because only particular isoforms of cytochrome P450 react with particular carcinogens, only those individuals carrying the genes that encode these forms are susceptible (Caraco, 1998). A major effort is now being devoted to identifying those individuals with phenotypes who would be at risk (Peto, 2001).

Much interest has been focused on workers in occupations where carcinogens are present in significant amounts. Steel foundries, shipbuilding and rubber plants, and other industrial plants may produce such carcinogens in significant amounts. In some of these industries, certain cancers occur at rates higher than in the general population (Brandt-Rauf, 1998; Pincus, 2003). Thus, in these exposed populations, it has become desirable to determine the levels of exposure to certain known carcinogens.

Carcinogens are thought to bind to DNA, leading ultimately to mutations in the genetic code, often resulting in synthesis of mutated proteins involved in control of the cell cycle (Brandt-Rauf, 1998; Pincus, 2003). These proteins are called **oncogene-encoded proteins or oncoproteins.** Mutagenesis, oncogenes, and oncoproteins are discussed in Chapter 74.

In populations with histories of exposure to carcinogens, assays have been developed to detect the presence of these carcinogens or of their DNA adducts. For detection of most unmodified carcinogens, the method of choice is currently GC-MS. For certain carcinogenic compounds like PCBs, the method of electron capture is used. Halogenated compounds like PCBs are separated on a GC column using an ionized gas as the carrier. Halogenated compounds "capture" electrons conducted through the carrier gas and thus are detected by the reduced currents.

Often, the presence of carcinogens in blood or urine is hard to detect directly. The carcinogens, however, may be bound to proteins or to DNA intracellularly. These adducts can be detected using Western blotting, which takes advantage of the existence of monoclonal antibodies to carcinogen–DNA adducts (Santella, 1987; Perera, 1988). This technique is sensitive to nanogram quantities of the nucleic acid adduct, which can be conveniently harvested from peripheral lymphocytes. It is also very useful in detecting oncoproteins in the body fluids of patients who have been exposed to carcinogens (De Vivo, 1994), as described in Chapter 74.

CYANIDE

The cyanide anion binds avidly to iron in the ferric or trivalent state. Because cyanide forms a relatively stable cyanoferric complex, it is able to inactivate iron-containing enzymes that cycle between the ferrous and ferric states in oxidation–reduction reactions. Cyanide produces tissue and cellular hypoxia primarily by reversibly binding to cytochrome A3 and by inhibiting its reoxidation. This inhibits the electron transport system and prevents cellular respiration and ATP (high-energy phosphate) formation. This blockade prevents the utilization of oxygen and aerobic metabolism, producing severe metabolic (lactic) acidosis. Although cyanide binds preferentially to the ferric form of iron, it can also bind to the ferrous iron of hemoglobin, producing cyanohemoglobin, which cannot transport oxygen. Cyanide will form complexes with other iron-containing enzymes, but its acute poisonous effect is attributable to the inhibition of electron transport and cell death, predominantly in the CNS.

The principal symptoms of cyanide overdose are tachypnea (initially), followed by respiratory depression and cyanosis, hypotension, convulsions, and coma. Death may occur in a matter of minutes because cyanide is a fast-acting toxin. Diagnosis may be difficult, and a high index of suspicion is needed to make the correct diagnosis. Clues include the odor of bitter almonds, the occurrence of an altered mental status and tachypnea in the absence of cyanosis, and an unexplained metabolic acidosis (with an increased anion gap).

Antidotal therapy has been based on a two-step strategy: First, to pull the CN^- ions away from cytochrome A3, hemoglobin is converted to methemoglobin ($Fe3+$ state) by using specific oxidants (i.e., amyl nitrite and sodium nitrite). The former is given first because it can be inhaled. Methemoglobin directly competes with ferricytochrome A3 to form a methemoglobin–CN^- complex. This cyanomethemoglobin complex is relatively nontoxic. In a second step, sodium thiosulfate is given intravenously. This reagent reacts with cyanomethemoglobin to form thiocyanate, which is harmless and is excreted in urine. The first step is necessary simply to remove CN^- from the respiratory chain. Approximately 25%–40% of the patient's total hemoglobin is converted to methemoglobin in this step; this methemoglobin is rapidly reconverted to oxyhemoglobin by red cell enzymes. The antidotes that are involved in each step are sold commercially as a cyanide antidote package by Eli Lilly and Company (Indianapolis). Cyanide also binds tightly to cobalt ions, and hydroxocobalamin (a form of vitamin B_{12}) has recently been U.S. Federal Drug Administration approved as a cyanide antidote (Cyanokit, King Pharmaceuticals, Bristol, Tenn). It has the advantages of rapid onset of action and low toxicity at antidotal doses, making it suitable for prehospital administration to firefighters and others (Hall, 2009). Unfortunately, hydroxocobalamin has a different type of side effect that laboratorians need to be aware of, namely, that its deep red color can interfere in certain assays (Beckerman, 2009).

CARBON MONOXIDE

Carbon monoxide (CO) intoxication produces tissue hypoxia as a result of decreased oxygen transport. CO disrupts oxygen transport by binding to hemoglobin to form a reversible complex, carboxyhemoglobin (CO-Hb). It produces toxicity by decreasing or inhibiting oxyhemoglobin saturation by inducing a leftward shift of the oxyhemoglobin dissociation curve, causing a decrease in oxygen delivery to tissues, and by binding to other heme-containing proteins such as myoglobin and cytochrome A3 (Kao, 2006). Binding to cytochrome A3 inhibits cellular respiration and electron transport, as occurs with cyanide poisoning (see earlier), and binding to hemoglobin decreases the oxygen reserve available to cardiac and skeletal muscle, with cardiac muscle being more severely affected.

However, binding of CO to hemoglobin cannot explain all of its toxic effects. Exchange transfusion into dogs of compatible blood that contained 57%–64% CO-Hb—levels that are fatal—failed to induce any effect on the recipients (Goldbaum, 1975; Kao, 2006). The role of CO in inducing toxicity is therefore more complicated. In fact, numerous studies suggest that CO, in addition to its binding to hemoglobin and cytochrome A3, is involved in multiple other toxicity-inducing pathways. These include direct cellular toxicity caused by its binding to myoglobin, resulting in direct damage to skeletal and cardiac muscle. Further, it has been found that CO activates guanylyl cyclase in the CNS; this results in increased cyclic guanosine monophosphate that induces cerebral vasodilatation and can cause loss of consciousness. CO also induces the synthesis of nitric oxide (NO), a potent vasodilator that causes large decreases in systemic blood pressure. CO-induced damage to CNS structures such as the basal ganglia, white matter, and hippocampus correlates with the degree of systemic hypotension that it induces. Abnormally elevated levels of NO appear also to cause oxidative damage to the brain, resulting in delayed neurologic sequelae (DNS). This effect may be due to the ability of NO to enhance the ability of neutrophils to adhere to the endothelium via specific adherence molecules, such as β-2-integrin, which results in free-radical formation via activation of such enzymes as xanthine oxidase (Kao, 2006). These free-radicals are thought to cause the oxidation of brain lipids that may serve as a basis for the observed DNS (Kao, 2006). Animal studies have further revealed that cerebrovascular vasodilation is inhibited by NO inhibitors. In addition, in several animal studies, it has been found that CO induces changes in myelin basic protein (MBP) that may cause an immunologic reaction. This effect is obviated in rats that have been made immunologically tolerant to MBP before exposure to CO (Kao, 2006).

Because the brain and the heart are most susceptible to carbon monoxide poisoning, CO intoxication is commonly manifested through respiratory, neurologic, and cardiac symptoms, with dyspnea being a principal symptom. Others include headache, visual disturbances, tachycardia, syncope, tachypnea, coma, convulsions, and death. However, diagnosis is difficult because no pathognomonic sign occurs, except for a cherry red color of the face that is a strong clue to acute CO poisoning. However, this sign is not common in CO poisoning (Kao, 2006). Another problem is delayed neurologic symptoms that develop from days to months after apparent recovery. These include mental deterioration, mutism, memory impairment, gait disturbance, and urinary and fecal incontinence, which may be caused by NO-induced damage to CNS membrane lipids and cerebral vasodilation as discussed previously (Kao, 2006).

CO poisoning should enter into the differential diagnosis of an acute encephalopathic state in the appropriate circumstances or setting. Car exhaust fumes cause more than 70% of known CO poisoning, including attempted suicides and chronic incidental exposure (e.g., auto repair). In addition, exposure to house fires, indoor heaters, and stoves predisposes to CO toxicity.

A cooximeter is utilized to make the definitive diagnosis by measuring the concentration of blood CO-Hb. This instrument is a dedicated spectrophotometer that measures total hemoglobin and the percentages of CO-Hb, oxyhemoglobin, and methemoglobin by screening at four different wavelengths simultaneously. This accurate and rapid analysis is mandatory to establish the diagnosis and should be performed with minimal delay after CO exposure. CO may also be quantitated by gas chromatography or GC-MS. Treatment is mainly with 100% oxygen, in some cases under hyperbaric conditions, with additional supportive treatment given as necessary.

ALCOHOLS AND GLYCOLS

Ethanol

Ethanol (Table 23-8) is probably the most common drug of abuse and is frequently responsible for the presentation of patients with altered mental

TABLE 23-8
Influence of Acute Ethanol Ingestion on Ethanol Levels and Behavior

Ounces	Blood concentration	Influence
1–2	10–50 mg/dL (2.2–10.9 mmol/L)	None to mild euphoria
3–4	50–100 mg/dL (10.9–21.7 mmol/L or greater)	Mild influence on stereoscopic vision and dark adaptation
	100 mg/dL (21.7 mmol/L)	Legally intoxicated
4–6	100–150 mg/dL (21.7–32.6 mmol/L)	Euphoria; disappearance of inhibition; prolonged reaction time
6–7	150–200 mg/dL (32.6–43.4 mmol/L)	Moderately severe poisoning; reaction time greatly prolonged; loss of inhibition and slight disturbances in equilibrium and coordination
8–9	200–250 mg/dL (43.4–54.3 mmol/L)	Severe degree of poisoning; disturbances of equilibrium and coordination; retardation of the thought processes and clouding of consciousness
10–15	250–400 mg/dL (54.3–86.8 mmol/L)	Deep, possibly fatal, coma

status to hospitals and emergency rooms. Ethanol is rapidly absorbed from the gastrointestinal tract, has a volume of distribution approximately equal to that of total body water, and diffuses freely in body tissues. It is predominantly metabolized by hepatic alcohol dehydrogenase to acetaldehyde and acetic acid/acetyl coenzyme A and then, by way of the Krebs cycle, to carbon dioxide and water. The fatal dose is generally 300–400 mL of pure ethanol (600–800 mL of 100 proof whiskey) consumed in less than 1 hour. Peak plasma concentrations are usually reached within 1 hour after ingestion. Table 23-8 summarizes the effects of different levels of ethanol in serum on human function.

Ethanol acts as a sedative-hypnotic and depresses the CNS irregularly in descending order from cortex to medulla. Acute intoxication may be manifested by decreased inhibitions, incoordination, blurred vision, slurred speech, stupor, coma, seizures, and death. Most fatal intoxications occur at blood concentrations greater than 400 mg/dL. Capillary and arterial blood samples most accurately reflect brain ethanol concentrations. Serum ethanol concentrations are usually determined by enzymatic, gas chromatographic, or electrochemical oxidation techniques. In the most accurate assays for ethanol, serum is incubated with alcohol dehydrogenase, which oxidizes ethanol to acetaldehyde, and nicotinamide adenine dinucleotide (NAD) is converted to NADH (reduced form of NAD). Thus, simple monitoring of the absorbance of the incubated serum at 340 nm gives a direct determination of alcohol present. Acute poisoning is generally treated by supportive therapy, gastric lavage with tap water, or hemodialysis, if indicated (>500 mg/dL). Symptoms of chronic intoxication, such as acute alcoholic mania, may be treated with diazepam. Phenytoin may be utilized in patients with a history of seizures.

Methanol

Methanol (wood alcohol) poisoning occurs in patients who ingest methylated spirits or methanol-containing antifreeze. It is rapidly absorbed from the gastrointestinal tract and is metabolized and excreted at approximately 20% of the rate of ethanol. The toxic range is thought to be 60–250 mL, although as little as 15 mL has caused death. Alcohol dehydrogenase metabolizes methanol to formaldehyde and formic acid, which is responsible for ocular toxicity (diminished light sensation or frank blindness), and anion gap metabolic acidosis; these are the principal symptoms of intoxication. Other symptoms include nausea, vomiting, headache, seizures, and coma. GC-MS is used to measure blood methanol levels, with a peak level greater than 50 mg/dL considered toxic. In addition, serum osmolality levels are increased to levels greater than 300 mOsm. Methanol (or ethylene glycol) poisoning should be considered in acutely ill patients with hyperosmolarity, metabolic acidosis, and increased anion gap.

Osmolal Gap

For methanol, ethylene glycol, and isopropyl alcohol poisoning, because the molecular masses of these simple compounds are low, relatively small quantities in serum give rise to high serum osmolalities. As discussed in Chapter 8, serum osmolality can be estimated as NaX2 + glucose/18 + blood urea nitrogen/2.8. This value should be close to the serum osmolality measured by freezing-point depression. If, however, any of these three compounds (or ethanol) is present in serum, the computed osmolality will be significantly less than the measured value (i.e., a so-called **osmolal gap** will exist), suggesting that a toxin is present. This is an effective screening method as a first step in detecting the presence of toxic compounds.

Ethylene Glycol

Ethylene glycol (1,2-ethanediol) is used in car radiator antifreeze. It has a half-life of around 3 hours and is metabolized to three major toxic compounds: glycolaldehyde, glycolic acid, and glyoxylic acid. The oxidation of ethylene glycol to glycolaldehyde is catalyzed by liver alcohol dehydrogenase. Both oxalic acid and formic acid are formed in smaller amounts. Oxalic acid itself is a highly toxic compound, which can rapidly precipitate as calcium oxalate crystals in various tissues as well as in urine. The formation of these crystals in urine, although not a constant finding, is an important diagnostic clue to ethylene glycol poisoning. The metabolite that accumulates in the highest concentrations in the blood is glycolic acid, and its concentration in blood and urine appears to correlate directly with symptoms and mortality. It is the major contributor to the high anion gap seen in metabolic acidosis. The fatal dose of ethylene glycol is around 100 g, and anuria and necrosis are the principal symptoms of acute poisoning. Other symptoms include nausea and vomiting, myoclonus, seizures, convulsions, depressed reflexes, and coma. Definitive diagnosis of ethylene glycol intoxication can be made by measuring serum ethylene glycol and glycolic acid by HPLC.

Treatment of ethylene glycol and methanol toxicity is similar and is based on symptoms and serum level. The mainstay of treatment is inhibition of the alcohol dehydrogenase enzyme, to minimize the formation of toxic metabolites, while the relatively nontoxic parent alcohol is eliminated renally. Although ethanol was originally used as a competitive inhibitor of alcohol dehydrogenase, the nonintoxicating agent fomepizole (4-methylpyrazole, Antizol, Paladin Labs, Montreal, Canada) is now generally preferred (Brent, 2009). Dialysis, either hemodialysis or peritoneal dialysis, is utilized to remove either parent compound and its corresponding toxic metabolic products.

Isopropyl alcohol has a half-life of approximately 3 hours and a volume of distribution similar to that of ethanol. It is readily absorbed through the GI tract and is metabolized at approximately 50% of the rate of ethanol. The metabolism of isopropanol occurs mainly by alcohol dehydrogenase to produce acetone, carbon dioxide, and water. The fatal dose of ingestion is 250 mL. Both isopropyl alcohol and its major metabolite, acetone, are CNS depressants.

CNS depression is the principal symptom of acute isopropanol intoxication. In addition, it produces significant GI irritation, which may be manifested by nausea and vomiting, including hematemesis and melena, abdominal pain, and gastritis. Other symptoms include confusion, coma, hypertension, respiratory failure, and death.

The diagnosis of isopropanol intoxication is difficult to make. Clues to the diagnosis include acetonuria, acetonemia and hyperosmolarity without glycosuria, hyperglycemia, or acidosis. Gas chromatography is generally considered to be the best technique to determine isopropanol blood concentrations. Treatment includes supportive care, activated charcoal with gastric lavage, and hemodialysis in severe poisoning.

ARSENIC

Arsenic is used in ant poisons, rodenticides, herbicides and weed killers, insecticides, paints, wood preservatives, and ceramics, in the production of various metal alloys and livestock feed, as a tanning agent, and in medicines. Inorganic arsenicals, including sodium arsenate and lead or copper arsenite; organic arsenicals, such as carbarsone and tryparsamide; and arsine gas are the major toxicologic forms of arsenic. Arsine gas poisoning generally occurs in the industrial setting, where its production arises from the action of acid or water on arsenic-bearing metals. Arsenic compounds occur in three oxidation states: elemental, trivalent arsenite, and pentavalent arsenate.

Arsenic is readily absorbed through the GI tract and lungs, whereas absorption through the skin occurs more slowly. Twenty-four hours after ingestion, arsenic is distributed to all body tissues. The major route of excretion is through the kidneys. Arsenic can cross the placenta. The major concern with arsenic ingestion is systemic poisoning, presumably through its reversible interaction with multiple enzyme sulfhydryl groups. This, in turn, leads to the disruption of multiple metabolic systems. This phenomenon suggests that effective treatment of arsenic poisoning would be provided through administration of sulhydryl-containing compounds that would compete with those of proteins for binding to the different forms of arsenic, as discussed later.

Arsine gas, the most dangerous of the three forms of arsenic, may irreversibly attach to sulfhydryl groups of hemoglobin, causing intravascular hemolysis, hemoglobinemia, and consequent acute renal failure, as well as direct nephrotoxicity. The acute fatal dosage of arsenic trioxide is approximately 120 mg, whereas less than 30 parts per million (ppm) of arsenic gas can produce poisoning. Organic arsenicals release arsenic slowly and have a fatal dose of approximately 0.1–0.5 g/kg.

Acute toxicity is usually manifested within the first hour of ingestion and generally reflects multiorgan involvement. Gastrointestinal symptoms are the most common presentation, with burning and dryness of the mouth and throat, difficulty in swallowing, vomiting, and watery or bloody diarrhea containing shreds of intestinal lining or mucus. The odor of garlic may be on the breath, and a metallic taste in the patient's mouth. Cyanosis, hypotension, tachycardia, and ventricular arrhythmias may develop. Neuropathy usually occurs late (approximately 1–2 weeks) after ingestion, or may become most intense during this time period. Severe volume depletion with resulting hypovolemic shock and acute renal tubular necrosis may occur, with death resulting from circulatory failure. Cutaneous manifestations of arsenic poisoning include hyperpigmentation of the skin and keratosis. The nail beds can show transverse white striations, called **Mees lines,** although this is not specific for arsenic poisoning (Ibrahim, 2006). Symptoms of poisoning with arsine gas usually manifest approximately 2–24 hours after exposure and may initially include nausea and vomiting, headache, anorexia, and paresthesias. Hematemesis and abdominal pain are also common, and acute renal failure, cardiac damage, anemia and hemolysis, or pulmonary edema may occur. The diagnosis of chronic intoxication is usually difficult and should be considered in patients with a combination of GI symptoms, neuropathy, and cutaneous, cardiovascular, and renal disturbances.

Analysis of urine, hair, and nails, using ion emission spectroscopy, is important for the diagnosis of chronic arsenic poisoning.

Treatment of acute poisoning includes removal of residual arsenic by gastric lavage or emesis, and treatment with dimercaprol, or British antilewisite (BAL), which combines with arsenic through its sulfhydryl groups to produce cyclic water-soluble complexes. However, the inherent toxicity of this compound limits its therapeutic usefulness. Less toxic derivatives of BAL are available, such as 2,3-dithioerythritol, which is less toxic in cell culture but shows greater efficacy than BAL at rescuing arsenic-poisoned cells in culture (Boyd, 1989). In severe poisoning, hemodialysis can be used to remove the arsenic–dimercaprol complexes.

MERCURY

Mercury compounds exist in four different forms with different toxicologic potential: elemental or metallic (Hg^o); mercurous (Hg+); mercuric (Hg2+); and alkyl mercury (i.e., organomercurials). Elemental mercury is poorly absorbed from the GI tract if mucosal integrity is preserved and shows no toxic effect unless it is converted to the divalent form. This may occur slowly by oxidation–reduction with water and chloride ion if a GI site for mercury stasis exists, but this is uncommon. Significant poisoning occurs with elemental mercury when it is inhaled or absorbed through the skin. It can pass through the blood-brain barrier and can accumulate in the CNS, where oxidation produces mercuric ion; thus, primarily pulmonary and CNS toxicities are produced.

Of the two inorganic salts of mercury, mercurous (Hg+) salts are poorly soluble and thus poorly absorbed. However, the mercuric (Hg2+) salt is readily soluble and is readily absorbed after oral ingestion or inhalation. Severe inflammation of the mouth and other GI symptoms can result. The kidney is a preferred site of accumulation of inorganic mercuric compounds, where acute renal tubular and glomerular damage can ensue. Both elemental mercury and the inorganic mercury compounds are excreted mainly in urine.

In contrast to elemental and inorganic mercury, organic mercury compounds, containing alkyl, aryl, and alkoxyalkyl moieties, are environmental pollutants. These compounds contain at least one covalent mercury–carbon bond. Both the alkoxyalkyl and aryl mercurial compounds undergo metabolic breakdown and biotransformation to produce inorganic mercury, which toxicologically acts and manifests intoxication as would the previously mentioned inorganic mercury compounds. In contrast, the mercury–carbon bonds that occur within the methyl and ethyl forms are extremely stable and produce greater toxicity than the aryl and alkoxyalkyl forms. The alkyl forms are more lipid soluble, pass readily through biological membranes, and, on ingestion, show generally greater absorption into the body. Their major chemical effect is on the CNS, and they show a biological half-life of 70–90 days. A devastating effect of methylmercury, known as congenital Minimata disease, has been described in Japan in the children of mothers who were exposed to methylmercury who were born with many of the stigmata of cerebral palsy (Ibrahim, 2006).

Because bile is the major route of excretion, methylmercury can be reabsorbed into the blood, via the enterohepatic system, accounting, in part, for its extended half-life. The major mechanism of action of mercury poisoning is through covalent bonding with protein sulfhydryl groups, producing widespread and nonspecific enzyme dysfunction, inactivation, and denaturation. Mercury inhibits the enzyme catecholamine-*O*-methyltransferase, a major enzyme in the metabolism of catecholamines, especially epinephrine and norepinephrine (see Chapter 24), resulting in hypertension, tachycardia, and sweating (Ibrahim, 2006). Thus mercury poisoning can masquerade as a pheochromocytoma, which should be ruled out by performing 24-hour urine catecholamine determination (see Chapter 24). At the same time, blood mercury levels should be determined (reference range <10 μg/L). Unfortunately, the usefulness of this testing is limited by the short half-life of mercury in the blood.

Mercury, depending on its form, may cause systemic toxicity or local skin and mucous membrane lesions. Both organic and elemental mercury can cause CNS effects, whereas GI symptoms primarily occur with inorganic salts. Elemental mercury may produce severe pulmonary reactions. Chronic exposure to elemental mercury can give rise to two syndromes: acrodynia and erethism (Ibrahim, 2006). Acrodynia, also called **pink disease, Feer-Swift disease,** and **Feer syndrome,** occurs mainly in children but can also occur in adults, and involves a complex of symptoms that include a desquamating, erythematous rash of the palms and soles, sweating, hypertension, tachycardia, pruritus, poor muscle tone, and weakness of the proximal pelvic girdle. Erethism is a complex of neurologic symptoms that include, most prominently, personality changes involving memory loss, drowsiness, withdrawal, depression, and irritability. A fine motor intention tremor of the hands also occurs. Inorganic mercury can induce severe renal tubular damage, especially in the proximal tubule; chronic exposure can cause membranous glomerulonephritis and nephrotic syndrome (Ibrahim, 2006).

In general, acute toxicity, with elemental, inorganic, or most organic forms, can be diagnosed from 24-hour urine levels. Blood levels may rise rapidly after acute exposure, but fall rapidly and may not reflect total body burden. In contrast, because the short-chain alkyl organic mercuric compounds are mainly excreted in the bile, blood levels are better indicators of tissue levels and significant acute exposure. Hair analysis for mercury may help identify chronic mercury exposure, especially with organic mercury.

Treatment includes gastric lavage or emesis to remove the ingested poison, as well as the use of dimercaprol and succimer. However, in methylmercury and alkylmercury poisoning, dimercaprol is contraindicated because it has been found to increase the concentrations of these compounds in the brain (Bryson, 1989). In these cases, treatment is symptomatic, although new agents are being evaluated clinically.

IRON

Acute iron poisoning is common in young children and is usually the result of ingestion of iron-containing products. Generally, iron overload that causes increased deposition of iron in tissues is termed hemosiderosis; if the excess iron induces tissue damage, the condition is termed hemochromatosis. Hemochromatosis can be inherited or acquired. Acquired hemochromatosis is caused by overingestion of iron or by leakage of iron from red blood cells, as may occur in a hemolytic crisis. Although ferric ions from food are usually reduced to ferrous ions and absorbed in the stomach, the large and small bowel can rapidly absorb toxic amounts (>30 mg/kg) of elemental iron. Once absorbed into the body, iron removal is difficult. Large doses of iron are thought to cause acute mucosal cell damage, and significant absorption of iron occurs once the binding capacity of transferrin is exceeded. Unbound iron in serum causes toxicity by hepatic cell damage, shock, and production of lactic acidosis. The hepatotoxicity seems to be dose related, occurs within 1–2 days of ingestion, and has been associated with levels equal to or greater than 1700 μg/dL (Tenenbein, 2001).

Iron absorption is tightly regulated by the HFE gene-encoded protein that is expressed mainly on hepatocytes and on epithelial cells in the gastrointestinal tract. This protein interacts with another protein synthesized in the liver called **hepcidin.** In addition, HFE protein interacts with transferrin receptors. In inherited or primary hemochromatosis, sometimes associated with other diseases such as type 2 diabetes (Davis, 2008), mutations in the *HFE* gene that result in single amino acid substitutions at critical positions in the amino acid sequence, such as cysteine-to-tyrosine 282 (C282Y) and histidine-to-aspartic acid 63 (H63D), cause this protein to fail to regulate iron absorption in the gut, resulting in iron overload. The occurrence of hereditary hemochromatosis is on the order of 1 per 200–300 individuals, making this condition important as a cause of iron overload. Recent studies have further determined that patients who have received more than 10 transfusions with packed red blood cells are at risk for developing acquired hemochromatosis (Takatoku, 2007).

Assays for Serum Iron

Iron can be determined by specialized techniques for trace elements such as atomic absorption spectrophotometry, but in the modern clinical laboratory setting, it is almost always measured using a colorimetric indicator such as ferrozine. The Fe^{2+}–ferrozine complex has an intense purple color (absorption maximum, 562 nm), and other metal ions generally do not interfere, with the possible exception of copper, whose effects can be minimized through addition of thiourea. It is necessary to use a reagent such as acid or detergent to release the serum iron from transferrin, and another reagent such as ascorbate to reduce iron to the ferrous state.

Iron-Binding Capacity

Normally all iron present in serum is bound to the iron-transporting protein, transferrin, which contains two iron-binding sites per transferrin molecule. In evaluating iron poisoning, it is important to measure iron-binding capacity, because toxicity will drastically increase as that capacity is exceeded. To obtain the total iron-binding capacity (TIBC), saturating concentrations of iron are added to a serum sample, excess iron is removed, for example, by adsorption with $MgCO_3$, and iron is remeasured. Alternatively, the amount of excess iron can be measured, and subtraction from the concentration of iron added gives the unsaturated iron-binding capacity.

Signs of Iron Intoxication

Vomiting appears to be an early manifestation of iron intoxication, along with severe gastroenteritis, melena, abdominal pain, and hematemesis. This occurs up to 6 hours after ingestion. For up to the next 10 hours, the patient may appear to improve. This is deceptive because manifestations of systemic toxicity (cyanosis, convulsions, shock, coagulopathy, renal and hepatic failure) may occur, producing death. Patients who develop severe systemic symptoms and those who do not may develop late complications, including GI obstruction or stricture.

Definitive diagnosis is made with measurements of serum iron concentration and TIBC. In addition to supportive treatment, emesis or gastric lavage is used to prevent iron absorption. Chelation therapy with deferoxamine is also utilized if the acute intoxication is severe.

LEAD

Both organic and inorganic compounds of lead may be highly toxic, with their most serious effects occurring in the central and peripheral nervous systems. Absorption may occur by inhalation or ingestion. If more than 0.5 mg of lead is absorbed per day, lead accumulation and toxicity are believed to occur, whereas 0.5 g of absorbed lead is considered a fatal dose. However, acute toxicity is uncommon and is generally observed in patients who have been exposed to high concentrations of lead dusts. Lead poisoning is seen in children in large cities who consume lead in the form of paint (pica). Acute manifestations are primarily CNS symptoms (encephalopathy, convulsions, stupor) and GI symptoms such as colic. Chronic toxicity with lead accumulating in blood, soft tissues, and bone is more common. The largest body compartment of lead is bone, which contains approximately 96% of the total body burden. The half-life of lead in bone is 32 years, and bone may act as a reservoir for endogenous intoxication. Chronic toxicity may be manifested by a wide range of systemic effects, including general malaise, weight loss, anorexia, and constipation; lead encephalopathy exhibited by malaise with apathy, drowsiness, stupor, and seizures; peripheral neuropathy with wrist drop or foot drop; and lead nephrosis with albuminuria, hematuria, and pyuria and anemia (hypochromic, microcytic, or normocytic) with basophilic stippling—the latter finding often a strong clue.

In addition, lead-induced pathologic changes may occur at even low levels of lead exposure. Needleman and Gatsonis (1990) reviewed 24 studies of childhood lead exposure to provide statistical evidence that low doses of lead may produce an intellectual deficit in children. However, the association of increased lead levels with decreased IQ has been called into question by the presence of confounding factors (Ibrahim, 2006). Schwartz and colleagues (1990) examined lead-induced anemia in children 1–5 years of age, using a cross-sectional epidemiologic study. They found a relationship between age, blood lead level, and hematocrit such that younger children had an increased risk of anemia at lower blood levels than children only a few years older. It thus appears that lead may produce deleterious effects, especially in children, at low levels of exposure. Generally, blood lead levels greater than or equal to 10 µg/dL indicate excessive lead absorption in children, and concentrations greater than 25 µg/dL indicate consideration of chelation therapy in the child. Several more recent studies suggest that no neurologic benefit is derived from chelation therapy among children with blood lead levels between 20 and 44 µg/dL (Ibrahim, 2006). The Centers for Disease Control and Prevention recommends universal screening of children, beginning at 6 months of age (Klaassen, 2001; Bernard, 2003).

Organolead compounds such as tetraethyl and tetramethyl lead are lipid soluble and, similar to the organomercurials discussed previously, produce their major toxic effects on the CNS. Lead encephalopathy may occur early in the onset of intoxication and does not correlate well with blood lead concentrations. Hyperactive deep tendon reflexes, intention tremor, abnormal jaw jerk, and abnormalities of stance and gait are the most consistently observed neurologic manifestations of organolead toxicity.

Lead appears to interact with thiol, carboxylic, and phosphate groups to form stable complexes with enzymes and proteins (Bryson, 1989). This is particularly well known for heme synthesis, in which lead blocks the action of δ-aminolevulinic acid (ALA) synthetase, δ-ALA dehydratase (ALAD), coproporphyrinogen decarboxylase, and ferrochelatase, producing anemia. In addition, lead blocks two other enzymes—pyrimidine-5′-nucleotidase and Na-K–dependent ATPase, resulting in diminished energy supply for red blood cells, leading to decreased cell membrane integrity. Because pyrimidine-5′-nucleotidase is required for removal of clumped intracellular RNA, lead inhibition of this enzyme results in clumping of RNA complexes, giving rise to the observed basophilic stippling of red blood cells (Ibrahim, 2006). Lead-induced disruptions in heme synthesis allow for objective testing for inorganic lead exposure. Increased amounts of ALA in urine, decreased ALAD activity in red blood cells, increased amounts of free erythrocyte protoporphyrin, and elevated amounts of zinc protoporphyrin are found with inorganic lead poisoning. The assay for zinc protoporphyrin is a particularly simple fluorometric one that is widely used and is an excellent screening test for frank lead toxicity, but the test is not sensitive to the low blood lead levels now regarded as harmful. The most sensitive screening test for organolead poisoning is decreased ALAD activity in urine because changes in the activities of other enzymes and in the levels of the products of heme synthesis are not consistent. Although whole blood lead concentrations are a reliable indicator of recent lead exposure, the short half-life of circulating lead in blood makes estimates of total body burden unreliable. However, use of in vivo X-ray fluorescence of bone allows determination of cumulative lead burden (Kosnett, 1994). Treatment of poisoning includes supportive therapy as well as removal of soluble lead compounds by gastric lavage. Dilute magnesium sulfate or sodium sulfate solutions are commonly used. In addition, chelating agents such as dimercaprol, calcium disodium edetate, and succimer may be utilized, if necessary.

Quantitation of Lead in Blood

Unlike many other toxins, lead is generally measured in whole blood rather than in serum or plasma, because most of the circulating lead is bound within the blood cells. Lead levels may be determined directly using atomic absorption spectroscopy, inductively coupled plasma/mass spectrometry (ICP/MS), or anode stripping voltammetry (ASV). In ICP/MS, a very hot source (the "inductively coupled plasma") atomizes the blood sample so that individual elements can be injected into and quantified by the mass spectrometer. In ASV, a voltaic cell is set up such that the anode consists of a mercury-coated graphite rod. When a negative potential is applied to this anode, cationic metals, such as lead, "plate out" in their metallic forms on the anode. The applied voltage is then stopped. Because an excess of electrons is present on the anode, current will flow to the cathode. Each of the metals plated on the anode therefore will become oxidized back to their respective ionic forms (i.e., be stripped from the anode). The metals with lowest oxidation potentials will strip first. Each metal will strip from the anode in the order of oxidation potential, recorded as the half-wave potential, which is a constant for a given metal. The total current associated with the stripping of each metal is proportional to the concentration of that metal.

ORGANOPHOSPHATES AND CARBAMATES

Pesticides generally contain organophosphates, which are esters of phosphoric acid or thiophosphoric acid, or carbamates, which are synthetic derivatives of carbamic acid. Although these are two distinctly different types of compounds, they both unfortunately interfere with neurotransmission. Both compounds inhibit the enzyme acetylcholinesterase (AChE), which normally hydrolyzes the neurotransmitter acetylcholine (ACh) after ACh has effected an action potential and has been released from its receptor site (see Chapter 20). Both compounds produce inhibition by reacting with the active site of AChE. This occurs by phosphorylation with the organophosphates to produce a relatively stable phosphate ester bond, and by carbamoylation with the carbamates to form a more labile, and hence more easily reversible, carbamate ester bond. Both compounds thus cause accumulation of ACh at neuronal synapses and myoneural junctions to produce toxicity.

ACh is an important neurotransmitter in both the peripheral and central nervous systems. It is located at a number of different synapses in the CNS, at ganglionic synapses between the sympathetic and parasympathetic preganglionic and postganglionic fibers, at junctions between parasympathetic postganglionic fibers and effector organs, and at junctions between somatic motor neurons and skeletal muscle cells. Thus, signs and symptoms of organophosphate poisoning include parasympathetic manifestations such as salivation, lacrimation, urination, and defecation;

pupillary constriction; bradycardia; and bronchoconstriction, which may predominate at low-dose poisoning. Autonomic ganglionic and somatic motor manifestations (such as muscular weakness, twitching, areflexia, tachycardia, and hypertension) and CNS manifestations (such as confusion, slurred speech, ataxia, convulsions, and respiratory and/or cardiovascular center depression) may predominate in severe intoxication. Death usually results from respiratory failure as the result of a combination of central depression, bronchospasm, excessive bronchial secretions, and respiratory muscle paralysis.

Morbidity and mortality due to carbamate poisoning are less severe because carbamates do not penetrate the CNS as effectively as organophosphates, and central cholinergic effects are thus minimal. In addition, the much greater lability of the carbamate ester bond allows spontaneous reactivation of AChE. This, in turn, decreases the slope of the toxicity dose–response curve, as compared with that of the curve for organophosphates, such that small increments in carbamate dose are less likely to produce severe increases in toxicity.

In addition to acute poisoning, organophosphates may produce an intermediate syndrome occurring 1–4 days after poisoning, and/or delayed neurotoxicity usually occurring 2–5 weeks after acute exposure. The former syndrome develops after acute cholinergic crisis and appears to involve cranial nerve palsies, proximal limb weakness, and respiratory paralysis, with the patient requiring ventilatory support (Senanayake, 1987, 1998). In contrast, delayed neurotoxicity, which is not seen with all organophosphate compounds, appears to be due to neurotoxic esterase inhibition and usually produces a distal and symmetric sensorimotor polyneuropathy of the extremities (Davies, 1987; Tafuri, 1987).

Diagnosis of organophosphate poisoning depends on a history of exposure shortly before the onset of illness, signs and symptoms of diffuse parasympathetic stimulation, and laboratory confirmation of exposure by measurement of erythrocyte acetylcholinesterase and plasma pseudocholinesterase activities (see Chapter 20). Whereas AChE is found primarily in nervous tissue and erythrocytes, pseudocholinesterase is found in plasma. The latter enzyme is much more nonspecific in its action than AChE, in that, in addition to hydrolysis of ACh, pseudocholinesterase can hydrolyze many other natural and synthetic esters, as described in Chapter 20. Both activities may be decreased, and both activities can be measured in the laboratory. However, only inhibition of AChE is considered specific for organophosphate poisoning because a number of conditions may produce a low plasma pseudocholinesterase level (Tafuri, 1987). Thus, the latter measurement is more sensitive but less specific than the red blood cell cholinesterase level for organophosphate poisoning. Generally, levels 30%–50% of normal indicate exposure, and toxic manifestations occur with greater than 50% inhibition; however, symptoms may not appear until levels are 20% or less of normal. In actuality, confirmation of poisoning, rather than diagnosis, occurs by laboratory determinations. Because baseline values of cholinesterase levels before exposure are unlikely to be available, sequential postexposure cholinesterase determinations appear to be the best way to confirm organophosphate poisoning (Coye, 1987).

Treatment of acute poisoning includes respiratory support and, if necessary, decontamination of the patient and gastric lavage or emesis. Administration of activated charcoal appears not to be effective in removing the toxic agent (Eddleston, 2008). In the presence of symptoms, atropine is given to ameliorate excessive parasympathetic stimulation by competitively blocking the action of ACh at muscarinic receptors. Pralidoxime is also given as a specific antidote for organophosphate poisoning. If pralidoxime is given within 24–48 hours of exposure, it may reactivate phosphorylated cholinesterase by removing the covalently bound phosphate group from the enzyme's active site. However, this time period is variable, and utilization of pralidoxime after 48 hours may be indicated (Clark, 2006; Howland, 2002). Chronic poisoning is usually treated by avoidance of further exposure until cholinesterase levels become normal.

SELECTED REFERENCES

Cami J, Farre M. Drug addiction. N Engl J Med 2003;349:975–86.

This is a discussion of drug addiction and the various factors involved in drug abuse, the molecular mechanism of action of various drugs, and the neurobiology and neuroadaptation of drug addiction.

Engelhardt H. One century of liquid chromatography: from Tswett's columns to modern high speed and high performance separations. J Chromatogr B 2004;800: 3–6.

This is an excellent overview of the development and history of liquid chromatography in the 20th century, describing early successes of "adsorption biochemical analysis," as well as the recent modern revolution in analysis.

Ingelman-Sundberg M. Pharmacogenetics of cytochrome P450 and its applications in drug therapy: the past, present and future. Trends Pharmacol Sci 2004;25:193–200.

An overview of cytochrome P450 pharmacogenetics, its clinical relevance, and possible future benefit for maximizing effective drug therapy.

Peto J. Cancer epidemiology in the last century and the next decade. Nature 2001;411:390–5.

Reviews the effective use of cancer epidemiology in the 20th century for identification of various causes of cancer in humans.

Senanayake N. Organophosphorus insecticide poisoning. Ceylon Med J 1998;43:22–9.

This is an excellent update on acute and chronic organophosphorous poisoning and the pathophysiology and behavioral effects of poisoning.

Snyder SH, Pasternak GE. Historical review: opioid receptors. Trends Pharmacol Sci 2003;24:198–205.

Early molecular biology of opioid receptors is historically reviewed, including receptor localization, identification, and cloning.

REFERENCES

Access the complete reference list online at http://www.expertconsult.com

CHAPTER 24

EVALUATION OF ENDOCRINE FUNCTION

Helena A. Guber, Amal F. Farag

KEY POINTS

- The endocrine system is a finely integrated system whereby the hypothalamus, the pituitary, and target glands continually communicate through feedback inhibition and stimulation to control all aspects of metabolism, growth, and reproduction. By understanding this interplay, and carefully manipulating these systems via provocative and suppressive stimuli, it is possible to characterize an underlying abnormality and provide directed treatment.
- Prolactin levels can be elevated as the result of a variety of pharmacologic and physiologic stimuli; however, values greater than 200 ng/mL are almost always associated with the presence of a pituitary tumor.
- The initial screen for someone suspected of having acromegaly should be a serum insulin-like growth factor-I.
- It is often unnecessary to perform provocative stimulation tests to document growth hormone deficiency in patients with a known history of pituitary disease or in those with evidence of three or more pituitary hormone deficiencies.
- Provided the hypothalamic-pituitary-thyroid axis is intact, the ultrasensitive thyroid-stimulating hormone test is the best method for detecting clinically significant thyroid dysfunction.
- When measuring thyroglobulin as a tumor marker for thyroid cancer, always check a simultaneous sample for thyroglobulin antibodies.
- The chromatographic measurement of plasma free metanephrines and normetanephrines is the best screening test for pheochromocytoma. The patient should avoid caffeine, alcohol and acetaminophen, monoamine oxidase inhibitors, and tricyclic antidepressants for at least 5 days before testing.
- It is frequently unnecessary to perform an adrenocorticotropic hormone stimulation test in critically ill patients. A random cortisol of greater than 25 μg/dL (700 nmol/L) during stress makes it highly unlikely that the patient is adrenally insufficient.
- The measurement of day 2–3 follicle-stimulating hormone is a good indicator of follicular reserve; a day 21–22 progesterone is used to assess whether cycles are ovulatory.

PITUITARY

The endocrine system is a finely tuned servo-system in which the hypothalamus, the pituitary, and various endocrine glands communicate through an intricate scheme of feedback inhibition and stimulation. In the classic sense, a hormone is defined as a substance that acts at a site distant from its place of origin. Under the rubric of hormones, we now include moieties that act in an autocrine (act directly upon themselves), paracrine (act adjacent to the cells of origin), or intracrine (act within the cells of origin without ever exiting the cells) fashion. It is through this intimate interplay of signals that the endocrine system serves to control metabolism, growth, fertility, and responses to stress.

The pituitary gland, also known as the hypophysis, is located within the confines of the sella turcica; it is connected by the infundibular stalk to the median eminence of the hypothalamus. It is divided into an anterior lobe (adenohypophysis) and a posterior lobe (neurohypophysis). It weighs about 0.6 g and measures about 12 mm in transverse and 8 mm in anteroposterior diameter. The anterior pituitary possesses five distinct hormone-synthesizing and -secreting populations of cells. These cell groups include somatotrophs, which secrete growth hormone (GH); lactotrophs, which secrete prolactin (PRL); thyrotrophs, which secrete thyroid-stimulating hormone (TSH); gonadotrophs, which secrete the α and β subunits of

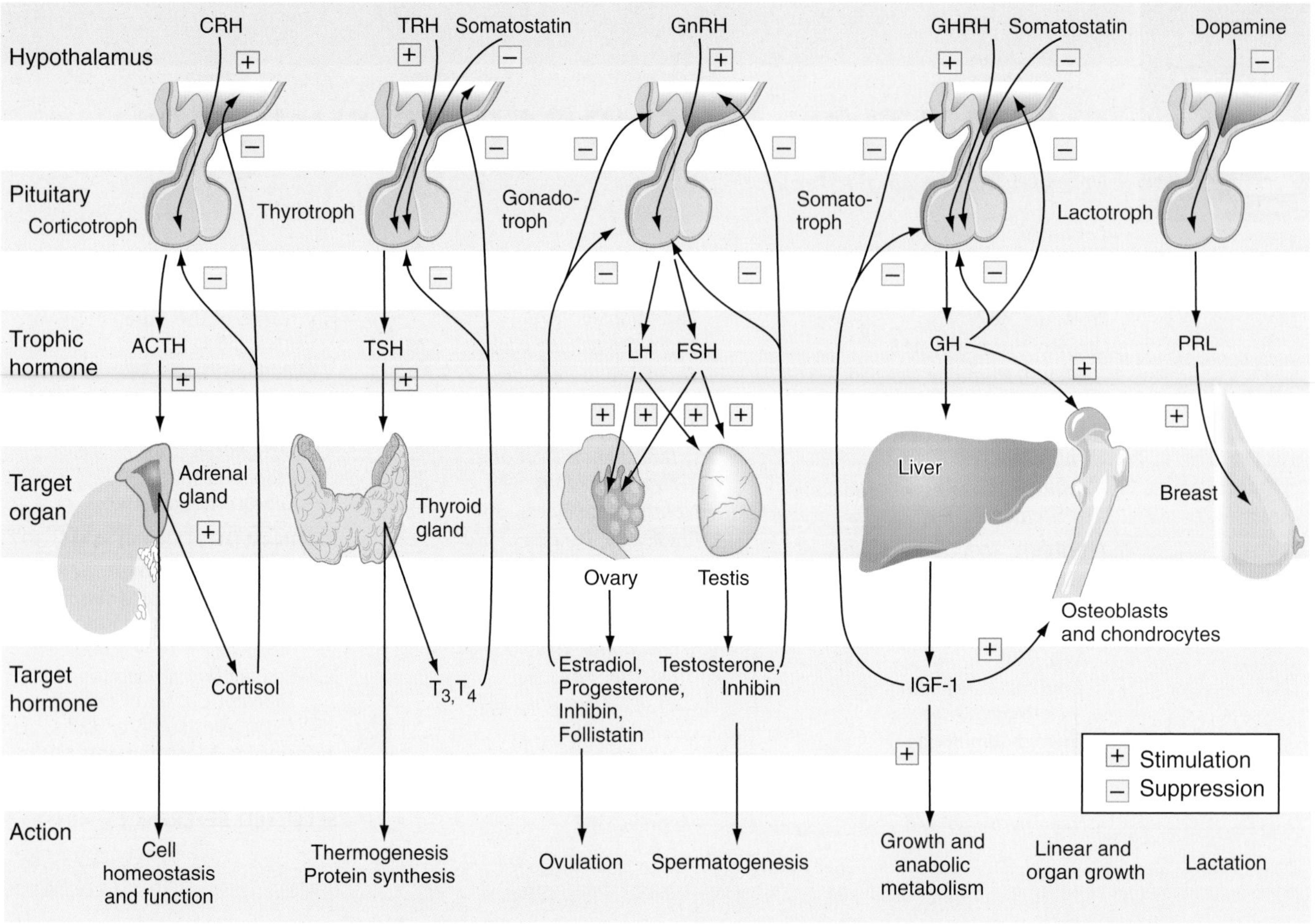

Figure 24-1 The hypothalamic-pituitary-target organ axis. *(Redrawn from Melmed S, Kleinberg D. Anterior pituitary. In: Larsen PR, Kronenberg HM, Melmed S, et al, editors. Williams textbook of endocrinology. 10th ed. Philadelphia: WB Saunders; 2003, p. 181, with permission.)* *ACTH,* Adrenocorticotropin; *CRH,* corticotropin-releasing hormone; *FSH,* follicle-stimulating hormone; *GHRH,* growth hormone–releasing hormone; *GnRH,* gonadotropin-releasing hormone; *IGF-1,* insulin-like growth factor; *LH,* luteinizing hormone; *PRL,* prolactin; T_3, 3,5,3′-triiodothyronine; T_4, thyroxine; *TRH,* thyrotropin-releasing hormone; *TSH,* thyroid-stimulating hormone.

follicle-stimulating hormone (FSH) and luteinizing hormone (LH); and corticotrophs, which secrete proopiomelanocortin (POMC). POMC is cleaved within the pituitary to form adrenocorticotropin (ACTH), β-endorphin, and β-lipotropin (β-LPH). The hypothalamus communicates with the anterior pituitary by secreting its own set of trophic hormones that are specific for each of the cell populations. (Fig. 24-1). These trophic hormones travel along the infundibular stalk to the adenohypophysis through a system of portal vessels.

In contrast to the anterior pituitary, the posterior pituitary (neurohypophysis) does not synthesize hormones. The hormones that it does secrete, arginine vasopressin (AVP; also known as antidiuretic hormone [ADH]) and oxytocin, are synthesized in the magnicellular neurons of the paraventricular and supraoptic nuclei of the hypothalamus, transported along the axons, and stored in the nerve terminals that end in the neurohypophysis. A summary of the different hormones secreted by the pituitary can be found in Table 24-1.

Abnormalities of pituitary function fall within two broad categories: hormonal excess and hormonal deficiency. Hormonal excess usually occurs as the result of clonal expansion of a distinct population of cells; however, it can result from an increase in trophic hormones from the hypothalamus or ectopic sites. The causes of hormonal deficiency are more varied (Table 24-2) and can result in the deficiency of one or more hormones, often with continued and progressive loss of other hormones over time.

TABLE 24-1
Hormones of the Pituitary

Anterior Pituitary—Adenohypophysis
Growth hormone (somatotropin) (GH)
Thyroid-stimulating hormone (thyrotropin) (TSH)
Gonadotropins
Follicle-stimulating hormone (FSH)
Luteinizing hormone (LH)
Proopiomelanocortin (POMC)
Adrenocorticotropin (ACTH)
β-lipotropin
β-endorphin
Prolactin (PRL)
Posterior Pituitary—Neurohypophysis
Arginine vasopressin (AVP) = Antidiuretic hormone (ADH)
Oxytocin

PITUITARY TUMORS

Pituitary tumors may be classified as microadenomas (<1 cm in greatest diameter and confined to the sella) or macroadenomas (≥1 cm in greatest diameter). They are further subcategorized into secretory and nonsecretory varieties (Table 24-3). All tumors have the potential to grow; in doing so, they can compress the optic chiasm, resulting in visual field defects, of which bitemporal hemianopia is the most frequent presentation. Invasion into the cavernous sinus can lead to compression of cranial nerves III, IV, VI, V1, and V2 and the intracavernous portion of the internal carotid artery. It can also lead to hydrocephalus caused by obstruction of the third ventricle. Aside from oversecretion of a particular hormone and extension

TABLE 24-2
Causes of Pituitary Hormonal Deficiency

Pituitary neoplasm
- Pituitary adenoma
- Craniopharyngioma
- Metastases or rarely primary carcinoma

Iatrogenic
- Radiation
- Hypophysectomy
- Stalk resection

Granulomatous disease
- Sarcoidosis

Infection
- Tuberculosis
- Syphilis
- Fungi

Hemorrhage and infarction
- Postpartum necrosis (Sheehan's syndrome)
- Head trauma
- Apoplexy

Aneurysms of the internal carotid artery

Autoimmune lymphocytic hypophysitis

Hemochromatosis

Primary hypothalamic disorders
- Tumor
- Granulomas

Idiopathic or genetic deficiencies of hormones within the pituitary or hypothalamus

TABLE 24-3
Relative Frequency of Occurrence of Pituitary Tumors

Lactotroph (PRL)	30%
Somatotroph (GH)	15%
Combined GH/PRL	8%
Corticotroph (ACTH)	15%
Thyrotroph (TRH)	1%
Pleurihormonal	4%
Nonfunctioning	27%

ACTH, Adrenocorticotropin; *GH,* growth hormone; *PRL,* prolactin; *TRH,* thyrotropin-releasing hormone.

into surrounding regions, these tumors can also cause hormonal deficiency due to compression of other cell lineages within the pituitary.

PROLACTIN

PRL is a polypeptide produced by the lactotrophs of the pituitary; it is responsible for the initiation and maintenance of lactation. Its secretion is normally kept at low levels by the inhibitory actions of dopamine produced by the hypothalamus. Similar to several pituitary hormones, PRL is secreted in a circadian fashion, with the highest levels attained during sleep and a nadir occurring between 10 AM and noon (Sassin, 1972). PRL is secreted in a pulsatile fashion, the amplitude and frequency of which not only vary throughout the day but are influenced by a variety of physiologic stimuli (e.g., stress, postprandially, exercise). Because of these factors and a serum half-life of 26–47 minutes, it is recommended that when a patient is screened for hyperprolactinemia, three specimens should be obtained at 20- to 30-minute intervals. These samples can be analyzed separately and their results averaged, or, alternatively, an equal aliquot from each sample can be pooled into one final sample that is then analyzed. PRL is measured by immunometric assay.

The major circulating form of PRL is the nonglycosylated monomer. A number of other forms can occur, including "big" PRL and macroprolactin ("big, big" PRL), which is considered to be PRL coupled with immunoglobulin (Yazigi, 1997; Conner, 1998). Because these forms all react with the immunoassays, they can produce falsely high PRL results in patients in whom pathologic elevation of PRL is not supported by computed tomography (CT) or magnetic resonance imaging (MRI). Various analytic methods have been developed to eliminate this confusion, including the performance of immunoassay following polyethylene glycol extraction and centrifugal ultrafiltration (Diver, 2001; Amadori, 2003; Fahie-Wilson, 2003; Prazeres, 2003; Suliman, 2003; Toldy, 2003).

TABLE 24-4
Causes of Hyperprolactinemia

Physiologic
- Sleep, stress, postprandially, pain
- Coitus, pregnancy, nipple stimulation or nursing

Systemic disorders
- Chest wall or thoracic spinal cord lesions
- Primary or secondary hypothyroidism
- Adrenal insufficiency
- Chronic renal failure
- Cirrhosis

Medications
- Psychiatric medications
  - Phenothiazines, haloperidol, thioxanthines, buspirone, olanzapine, risperidone, domperidone, monoamine oxidase inhibitors, fluoxetine, amitriptyline
- Metoclopramide
- Antihypertensives: labetalol, α-methyldopa, reserpine, verapamil
- Antihistamines H_2: cimetidine, ranitidine
- Estrogens, oral contraceptives, oral contraceptive withdrawal
- Opiates: heroin, methadone, morphine, apomorphine
- Thyrotroph (TRH)

Prolactin-secreting pituitary tumor: prolactinoma, acromegaly

Macroadenoma (compressing the pituitary stalk)

Macroprolactinemia

Pressure on or transection of the pituitary stalk, interrupting the transmission of dopamine to D_2 receptors on the lactotrophs
- Surgery, traumatic transection, granulomas, metastases, meningioma, irradiation, histiocytosis X

Ectopic secretion of prolactin by nonpituitary tumors

Idiopathic

Polycystic ovarian disease

Epileptic seizures

In some instances of prolactinoma, the values of PRL may be falsely low or minimally elevated considering the size of the tumor. Usually only a single dilution is performed when assaying for PRL, and extremely high concentrations can saturate the antibody binding sites, resulting in a falsely low result (Barkan, 1998; Petakov, 1998). This "hook" effect may result in misdiagnosis of the patient as having a nonfunctioning chromophobe adenoma. If the pretest probability of the patient having a macroprolactinoma is high, it is recommended that the serum sample be subjected to at least a 1 : 100 dilution.

PRL acts on breast tissue, where, in the setting of estrogen priming, it stimulates lactation. PRL also acts at the hypothalamus to inhibit the secretion of gonadotropin-releasing hormone (GnRH). Inhibition of GnRH results in a decrease in the release of LH and FSH from the anterior pituitary. In females, this leads to a decrease in estrogen and progesterone synthesis and secretion by the ovaries and failure of ovarian follicular maturation (ovulation). In males, a deficiency of FSH and LH causes a decrease in testicular production and synthesis of testosterone and a halt in spermatogenesis. In addition, it has been suggested that hyperprolactinemia may stimulate adrenal androgen production and may have an effect on immune responsiveness (Lobo, 1980; Walker, 1993).

The reference value for serum PRL is 1–25 ng/mL (1–25 μg/L) for women and 1–20 ng/mL (1–20 μg/L) for men. The higher PRL levels seen in females begin postpuberty and are presumably due to the stimulatory effect of estrogen (Eastman, 1996). During pregnancy, a progressive rise in serum PRL is observed, with levels reportedly reaching as high as 500 ng/mL by the third trimester (Rigg, 1977). This is largely due to an increase in the number of PRL-secreting cells and can be associated with a doubling or even greater increase in pituitary gland size (Scheithauer, 1990). PRL levels fall back to baseline about 3 weeks postpartum in women who are not breastfeeding. In nursing mothers, basal PRL levels remain moderately elevated, with episodic bursts in secretion in response to suckling.

PRL levels are increased by many physiologic and pathologic factors, as well as by a wide variety of medications (Table 24-4). Elevations in PRL resulting from physiologic and pharmacologic stimuli rarely exceed 200 ng/mL.

PRL deficiency can be seen with pituitary necrosis or infarction and in some cases of pseudohypoparathyroidism. In women with complete PRL deficiency, menstrual disorders and infertility have been found (Kauppila, 1997). It is PRL excess that is associated with clinical pathology. Hyperprolactinemia leads to inhibition of GnRH secretion, which typically manifests as sexual dysfunction and infertility in both men and women. Women may present with luteal phase abnormalities, oligomenorrhea, or frank amenorrhea, with or without galactorrhea. Men will present with hypoandrogenemia, decreased libido, and impotence. Pituitary adenomas are an important cause of hyperprolactinemia; however, any sellar or parasellar process that compresses the pituitary stalk and interrupts the tonic delivery of dopamine can lead to disinhibition of PRL secretion. Usually, the height of elevation of serum PRL levels correlates with the likelihood of the presence of a pituitary tumor, and levels of PRL in excess of 200 ng/mL almost always signify the presence of a prolactinoma (Kleinberg, 1977; Frantz, 1998; Freda, 1999). Unlike other functioning pituitary tumors, the degree of elevation of PRL correlates fairly well with the size of the tumor.

Hyperprolactinemia exists in 20%–40% of patients with acromegaly; this may be due to the presence of a mixed tumor (containing both lactotrophs and somatotrophs) or to interference with the normally active, PRL-inhibitory mechanisms (e.g., interruption of dopamine delivery owing to stalk compression by a tumor, resulting in disinhibition of prolactin secretion). Another important cause of hyperprolactinemia is hypothyroidism. Thyrotropin-releasing hormone (TRH) not only stimulates TSH secretion, but it also stimulates PRL secretion, thus explaining the mild hyperprolactinemia seen in both primary (thyroid) and secondary (pituitary) hypothyroidism. Therefore, thyroid function tests (free thyroxine [FT_4] and TSH) are always indicated to rule out hypothyroidism when a patient with hyperprolactinemia is evaluated. Thyroid hormone replacement therapy will usually return the PRL to normal.

It is important to evaluate all patients discovered to have an abnormally elevated PRL. Since hyperprolactinemia can be found in upward of 40% of cases of acromegaly, it is appropriate to measure insulin-like growth factor (IGF)-I. Other hormones that may be assayed include FSH, LH, free testosterone, estradiol, and, if clinically indicated, tests of adrenal axis function. Rarely, hyperprolactinemia may be caused by ectopic hormone production. All patients should undergo CT or MRI of the sella, performed with and without contrast. MRI provides better contrast and anatomic detail and is better for visualizing microadenomas. A formal visual field examination is also a key monitoring tool in managing patients with pituitary tumors and should be done at least yearly in patients with stable disease.

GROWTH HORMONE

GH is a single-chain polypeptide of 191 amino acids synthesized, stored, and secreted by the somatotrophs of the pituitary in response to the secretion of growth hormone–releasing hormone (GHRH) by the hypothalamus. Somatostatin, also produced by the hypothalamus, inhibits GH release. Although evidence exists for the direct action of GH on long bone growth in children, most of its anabolic and metabolic actions are mediated indirectly through an intermediary, IGF-I (also called **somatomedin C**). IGF-I is synthesized in the liver and in certain target tissues, in response to stimulation by GH. IGF-I circulates in the blood complexed to IGF-binding proteins (IGF-BPs); IGF-BP3 is the predominant circulating species. As with all hormones, it is the free, unbound form that is biologically active. Like somatostatin, IGF-I negatively feeds back on the pituitary to inhibit GH secretion.

GH is secreted in a pulsatile fashion; the frequency and amplitude of the peaks are greatest during puberty, exhibiting a steady decline with increasing age (Casanueva, 1992). As up to 70% of GH secretion occurs during stage 4 (slow wave) sleep, it has been suggested that the age-related decline in stage 4 sleep may account for the decline in GH seen with aging (Van Cauter, 1998, 2000). In addition to GHRH and somatostatin, several other factors regularly mediate GH secretion (Fig. 24-2). Major stress (e.g., surgery, sepsis), fasting, sex steroids, chronic malnutrition, apomorphine, levodopa, and high-protein meals all stimulate GH secretion. Women tend to have higher GH levels than men, perhaps because of estrogen sensitization of the hypothalamus to other GH stimuli (Eastman, 1996).

Serum GH is undetectable for most of the day in healthy, nonstressed individuals. This fact along with the episodic nature of GH secretion makes a single sampling difficult to interpret. As a result, the diagnosis of GH deficiency is made using GH measurements following pharmacologic stimulation, and GH excess is confirmed by failure of GH suppression following an oral glucose load. GH is commonly measured by chemiluminescent immunoassay.

Somatostatin is synthesized in the paraventricular and arcuate nuclei of the hypothalamus. It inhibits GH and TSH secretion. It also inhibits the secretion of insulin and several gut hormones (e.g., motilin, secretin, gastrin). Ghrelin, a 28 amino acid peptide produced by the gastric neuroendocrine cells and the hypothalamus, binds to the GH secretagogue receptor to stimulate the secretion of GHRH and GH.

Growth Hormone Deficiency

Idiopathic growth hormone deficiency is the most common cause of GH deficiency (GHD) in children, whereas a pituitary adenoma is the most common etiology in adult-onset GHD. No simple, reproducible method for determining abnormal GH secretory patterns exists. In healthy normal individuals, 70%–80% of GH results are below 1 ng/mL (<1 μg/L), and secretory peaks typically reach 20–40 ng/mL (20–40 g/L) (Baumann, 1987). Thus, in a child with decreased growth velocity, a low or nondetectable GH does not necessarily indicate GHD. Similar to GH, IGF-I declines with age. IGF-I is more diagnostically useful in patients younger than age 40; however, it is still not sensitive enough to be used as a stand-alone test to make the diagnosis of GHD (Almeretti, 2003). Manipulation of the endocrine system through stimulation and suppression of the various axes is often required for diagnosing conditions of hormonal deficiency and surfeit. In this vein, GHD is diagnosed by showing failure of GH to increase adequately in response to pharmacologic stimulation. Several endocrine organizations have published guidelines on GH deficiency, which patients to test, which test to utilize, and what cutoffs to apply (Ho, 2007; Casanueva, 2009). The insulin tolerance test (ITT) has long been considered the "gold standard" for diagnosing GHD; however, it is most unpleasant for the patient, requires the attendance of a physician throughout the testing period, and is contraindicated in those with a history of seizures or cardiac or cerebrovascular disease. Failure of GH to rise above 5 ng/mL in adults and above 10 ng/mL in children is considered to be abnormal. In patients unable to undergo an ITT and in those needing a second confirmatory test, arginine stimulation alone or in combination with GHRH is usually the next step. Combination testing with GHRH plus arginine is preferred, as many normal adults will fail stimulation with arginine alone (Biller, 2002). Failure of GH to rise above 4.1 carries a sensitivity of 95% and a specificity of 91% in diagnosing GH deficiency (Biller, 2002). Because body mass index (BMI) affects the GH response to stimulation with GHRH plus arginine, newer guidelines recommend the use of GH cutoffs based on BMI for interpretation of results (Cook, 2009). Other methods to assess for GHD include 24-hour or nighttime monitoring of GH and provocative tests using clonidine, L-dopa, or glucagon (following priming with propranolol). All of these tests carry significant individual variability and have not been systematically studied; they are used mainly in the pediatric population (Rose, 1988). The same normal ranges hold for these tests as described for the ITT. There are two settings in which an argument can be made against the need to test for GHD. The first is in patients with known pituitary disease who have a low IGF-I level. The other scenario is in patients with evidence of three or more pituitary hormone deficiencies; studies have shown these patients to have a >96% chance of being GHD (Hartman, 2002).

For children, it is common to use exercise testing in screening for GHD. Further testing is not indicated if the results are normal; however, if GH fails to increase adequately, pharmacologic testing is warranted (Eddy, 1974). Healthy children may not respond to any single GH provocative test; therefore, GHD in childhood is defined by failure of serum GH to reach defined levels when at least two different pharmacologic stimuli are used. IGF-I measurements have been used to screen for GHD in children; however, since a variety of factors can decrease IGF-I, it is not used to confirm the diagnosis of GHD. IGF-I levels decline in malnutrition, hypothyroidism, hepatic disease, uncontrolled diabetes mellitus, and with age. Levels of IGF-BP3 usually parallel those of IGF-I and are often low in GHD; however, results falling within the reference range do not exclude the diagnosis if GHD. Up to 18% of subjects with GHD may have normal IGF-I levels. Care should be taken when interpreting values for IGF-I, IGF-BP3, and GH because the assays themselves and the cutoffs used to define normal differ greatly between laboratories. To address these issues there is a move to have labs utilize a World Health Organization international standard for GH and IGF-I, and to create a normative range from a statistically valid control group (Giustina, 2010).

It is important to understand the difference in the physiology behind testing with GHRH as opposed to the other secretagogues. ITT and arginine stimulate the production of GHRH; clonidine inhibits somatostatin. For these stimuli to elicit a rise in GH, the hypothalamus must be intact. When GHRH is used, the hypothalamus is bypassed and the pituitary is directly stimulated. Therefore, it is possible to miss up to 50% of patients who have tertiary (hypothalamic) GHD. Individuals with

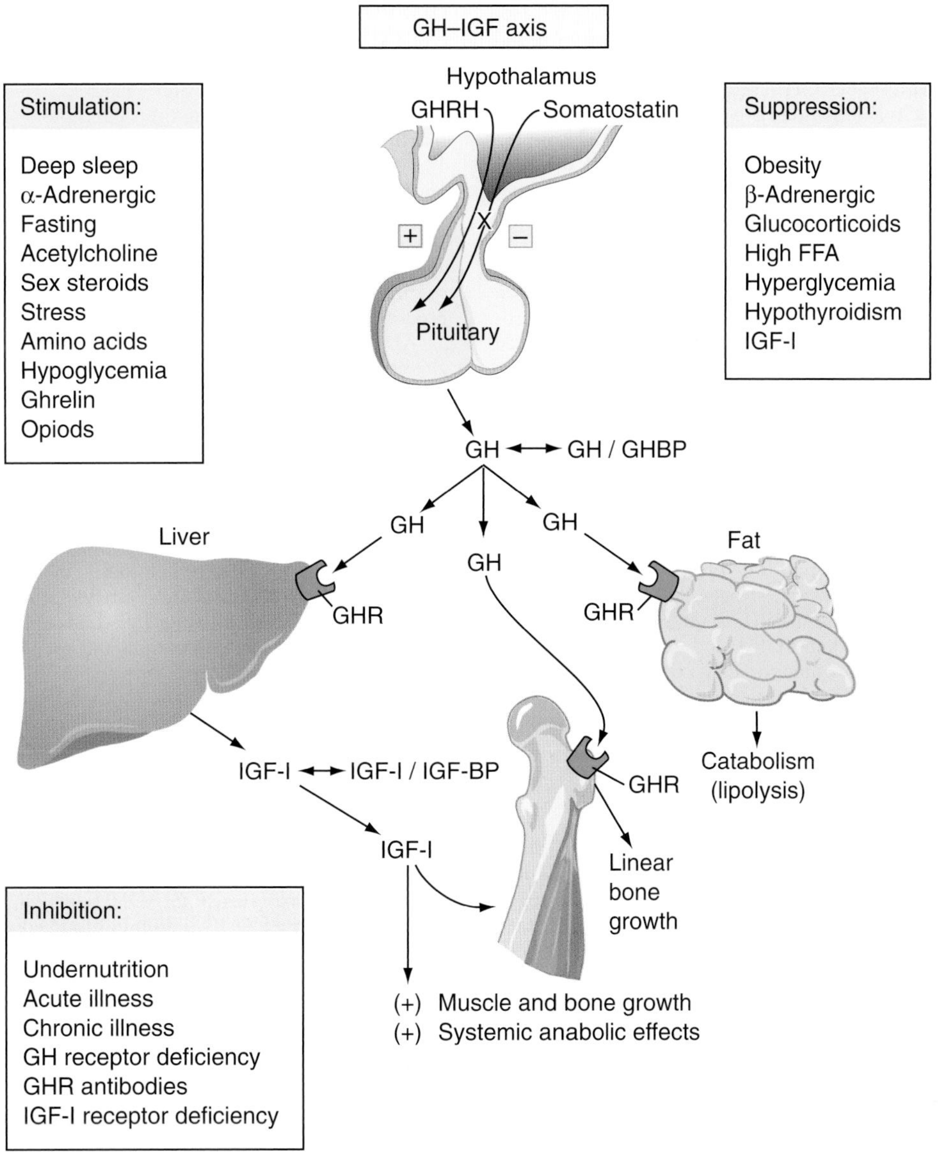

Figure 24-2 Hypothalamic-pituitary-growth hormone axis. Feedback loop influencing GH–IGF-I secretion and action. *(From Melmed S, Kleinberg D. Anterior pituitary. In: Larsen PR, Kronenberg HM, Melmed S, Polonsky KS, editors. Williams textbook of endocrinology. 10th ed. Philadelphia: WB Saunders; 2003, p. 221, with permission.) FFA,* Free fatty acid; *GH,* growth hormone; *GHBP,* growth hormone–binding protein; *GH-IGF,* growth hormone–insulin-like growth factor; *GHR,* growth hormone receptor; *GHRH,* growth hormone–releasing hormone; *IGF-I,* insulin-like growth factor I; *IGF-BP,* IGF-binding proteins.

childhood-onset idiopathic GHD are less likely to have permanent GHD. It is recommended that they be taken off GH replacement and retested when they reach early adulthood, unless they have a known genetic mutation, embryopathic lesion, or irreversible lesion/damage to the pituitary/hypothalamus (Molitch, 2006).

Growth Hormone Excess

Growth hormone overproduction can result in the condition called **acromegaly.** If the condition develops before closure of the epiphyses, these individuals may be exceedingly tall (**gigantism**). More commonly, it presents during adulthood, causing diffuse enlargement of soft tissues and organs throughout the body; characteristic features include prognathism, frontal bossing, and spade-like hands. The screening test for clinically suspected acromegaly is a randomly collected IGF-I. If the level of IGF-I is elevated with respect to the appropriate age- and gender-related reference range, then it is necessary to confirm the diagnosis using an oral glucose tolerance test (OGTT). The OGTT is performed by orally administering 75 g of glucose and obtaining blood samples at baseline and every 30 minutes over the next 2 hours for glucose and GH. A normal response is suppression of GH to <1 ng/mL (1 μg/L) at any time during the test. If GH fails to drop to below 1 ng/mL (1 μg/L), the patient is diagnosed as having acromegaly (American Association of Clinical Endocrinologists, 2004). The difficulty comes in diagnosing mild disease. Freda had studied 60 postoperative patients with acromegaly, 22 patients with active disease (elevated IGF-I), 38 patients in remission (normal IGF-I), and 25 healthy controls. The highest nadir GH was 0.13 μg/L in the controls and 0.3 μg/L in those with active disease. Fifty percent of those with active disease had GH values <1 μg/L, leading to misclassification of these individuals as being normal when the above stated criteria were applied (Freda 1998, Trainer 2002). In a more recent study of 16 patients with mild disease (the majority have microadenomas), Dimaraki (2002) found that 50% of patients with acromegaly were able to suppress their GH levels to <1 μg/L following an OGTT. A proposed reason for these patients with active disease showing normal suppression is that they may have subtle changes in GH secretion that are not elicitable with this short suppression test. To address this issue, the following suggestion has been proferred (Trainer, 2002). If an initial random IGF-I is normal and GH is <0.3 μg/L, then acromegaly is excluded. If either test is abnormal, repeat the IGF-I and proceed to an OGTT. Failure of GH to be suppressed below 0.3 μg/L, accompanied by an elevated IGF-I, is diagnostic of acromegaly. Suppression of GH below 0.3 μg/L with normal IGF-I excludes acromegaly. For those who adequately suppress their GH but have an elevated IGF-I, close follow-up is recommended (Trainer, 2002). Oral but not transdermal estrogen can reduce IGF-I concentrations (Giustina, 2010), therefore temporarily withholding oral estrogen therapy during testing may be prudent.

Acromegalic patients may show a paradoxical rise, an absent response, or a partial decline in GH in response to an OGTT (Ezzat, 1997). Random GH sampling is not adequate to establish the diagnosis of acromegaly because considerable overlap in GH exists between healthy persons and patients with the disease. In addition, GH can be increased in patients with a number of disorders, including renal disease, cirrhosis, malnutrition, and in patients under physical or emotional stress. Although larger adenomas are generally associated with higher GH levels, the correlation between GH levels and acromegalic manifestations is poor. In most patients with untreated acromegaly, GH levels remain above basal levels throughout the day, ranging from 10–100 ng/mL (10–100 μg/L). Serum GH levels in excess of 50–100 ng/mL (50–100 μg/L) are virtually never seen in nonacromegalic persons (Barkan, 1989). Other diagnostic maneuvers using TRH, GnRH, and GHRH yield discordant results in about 50% of patients with acromegaly; therefore, their use for diagnostic purposes or for monitoring disease activity is not recommended (American Association of Clinical Endocrinologists, 2004). In patients with documented acromegaly but no evidence of a pituitary tumor, GHRH should be measured to detect a hypothalamic or ectopic source for acromegaly.

Patients treated for acromegaly require lifelong monitoring for disease activity. Patients treated with surgery or radiation can be monitored by the GH response to OGTT and a random IGF-I measurement. The goal of therapy is to normalize IGF-I and suppress the GH response to OGTT to <1 ng/mL (<1 μg/L). Several studies have shown that when these goals are attained, mortality rates become comparable with those of the normal population (Swearingen, 1998; Holdaway, 2004; Rajasoorya, 1994; Orme, 1998). Caution is required in interpreting IGF-I levels in women on oral but not topical estrogen treatment, as oral estrogens lower IGF-I concentration (Giustina, 2010). For patients on somatostatin receptor analogues, monitoring is performed by random IGF-I and GH measurements. Patients on GH receptor blockers are monitored by a random IGF-I alone. In rare instances, acromegaly may be due to ectopic secretion of GHRH (e.g., bronchial carcinoid, pancreatic islet cell tumors, small cell lung cancer), in which case the measurement of GHRH may be useful.

POSTERIOR PITUITARY HORMONES

Oxytocin and vasopressin (see Chapters 8 and 14) are the two major hormones of the posterior pituitary. They each have distinct physiologic roles, with partially overlapping effects in stimulating smooth muscle contraction and in maintaining water homeostasis. They are small oligopeptides, each composed of nine amino acid residues with a total mass of about 1 kDa. They are synthesized in the nerve cell bodies within the hypothalamus and are transported along axons to the nerve terminals within the posterior pituitary, where they are stored in secretory granules. Neuronal action potentials originating in the hypothalamus are conducted along the axons, resulting in degranulation of the vesicles and release of oxytocin and vasopressin into the perivascular space and ultimately into the circulation. Unlike the anterior pituitary, the posterior pituitary is little more than a repository where hormones are held until they are secreted. Accordingly, disruption of the infundibular stalk or destruction or removal of the posterior pituitary does not necessarily result in complete loss of these hormones, as they are produced in the hypothalamus.

Oxytocin

Oxytocin secretion is stimulated by stretching of the cervix and vagina during parturition; this is known as the Fergusson reflex. Oxytocin contributes to uterine contractions late in labor both by direct action on the myometrium and by stimulation of prostaglandin secretion by the decidua (Fuchs, 1982). It also plays a role in hemostasis at the placental site following delivery. Throughout pregnancy, estrogen upregulates the numbers of oxytocin receptors on the uterus and decidua, resulting in increased sensitivity to oxytocin toward the end of term.

Oxytocin stimulates the myoepithelial cells surrounding the mammary glands and lactiferous ducts to contract, resulting in milk ejection. In response to suckling, neurogenic stimuli are transmitted from the nipple to the third, fourth, and fifth thoracic nerves, to the spinal cord, to the midbrain, and on to the hypothalamus, where oxytocin release is triggered. Psychological stimuli can bypass this pathway, with bursts of oxytocin secretion occurring with anticipation of nursing or on hearing a baby cry (Jenkins, 1991; Yokoyama, 1994). Stressful situations can inhibit its secretion, resulting in decreased milk ejection.

Pathologic conditions associated with oxytocin excess or deficiency are rare and are limited to case reports. Its function in males remains unknown. Clinical demand for the measurement of oxytocin levels is extremely rare. Because it has a half-life of 3–5 minutes and is subject to rapid degradation by oxytocinase, individual reference laboratory procedures for its collection must be strictly adhered to if meaningful results are to be obtained.

Arginine Vasopressin/Antidiuretic Hormone

AVP (ADH) is synthesized within the paraventricular and supraoptic nuclei of the hypothalamus. The major function of ADH is to maintain osmotic homeostasis by regulating water balance.

It does this by stimulating the V2 receptors on principal epithelial cells that line the cortical collecting ducts of the kidney. As discussed in Chapter 14, ADH induces an increase in the production of cyclic adenosine monophosphate (cAMP), which, in turn, causes the water channels (aquaporins) to fuse with the apical membrane of the principal cells, increasing water permeability and reabsorption. At much higher blood concentrations, AVP also acts as a potent pressor by causing vasoconstriction (V1 receptor), stimulates ACTH secretion from the anterior pituitary, and stimulates the production of clotting factor VIII.

ADH secretion is modulated by changes in serum osmolality and by alterations in intravascular volume. Changes in plasma osmolality are detected by osmoreceptors located within the anterior hypothalamus. Plasma ADH rises and falls in direct proportion to the serum osmolality. A concordantly linear relationship exists between ADH and the urine osmolality (Uosm). The Uosm is capped at about 1200 mOsm/kg, the maximum Uosm allowed by the renal medullary concentration gradient.

ADH secretion is maximally stimulated at a serum osmolality >295 mOsm/kg and is suppressed when the osmolality falls below 284 mOsm/kg. Thirst can be considered the fail-safe mechanism for fluid and osmotic homeostasis as it is initiated at a greater plasma osmolality (Posm) than is needed to stimulate ADH secretion. The thirst receptors are located within the hypothalamus and are distinct from the osmoreceptors that stimulate ADH secretion.

Changes in intravascular volume are detected by baroreceptors. There are two sets of baroreceptors: low-pressure volume receptors located in the right atrium and pulmonary venous system; and high-pressure arterial baroreceptors, located in the carotid sinus and aortic arch. These receptors are normally under tonic inhibition; a drop in intravascular volume removes the inhibition and results in a rise in ADH, leading to increased water reabsorption. ADH secretion is much more sensitive to changes in osmolality than to changes in intravascular volume. A 1%–2% increase in osmolality will cause a rise in ADH secretion, whereas a much greater stimulus, such as a 5%–10% drop in blood volume or blood pressure, is needed before the baroreceptors trigger the release of ADH.

In addition to changes in osmolality and intravascular volume, other physiologic factors that can stimulate ADH secretion include nausea, cytokine, interleukin (IL)-6, hypoglycemia, hypercarbia, and nicotine (Reihman, 1985; Masrorakos, 1994).

Basal plasma vasopressin normally ranges from 0.5–2 pg/μL. In concert with atrial natriuretic hormone, thirst, and the renin-angiotensin-aldosterone axis, ADH works to maintain blood pressure, volume, and tonicity. Accordingly, when a patient is evaluated for a disorder of water homeostasis, these multiple interactive factors must be taken into consideration. Normal plasma osmolality ranges from 280–295 mOsm/kg, and plasma sodium from 135–145 mmol/L. It can be determined directly by measuring the plasma freezing-point depression or the plasma vapor pressure. It can also be determined indirectly, by measuring the plasma sodium, blood urea nitrogen (BUN), and glucose, and applying the following formula:

$$\text{Plasma osmolality} = \{2 \times [\text{Na}]\,(\text{mmol/L})\} + \{\text{Glucose}\,(\text{mg/dL})/18\} + \{\text{BUN}\,(\text{mg/dL})/2.8\} \qquad \textbf{(24-1)}$$

This equation is discussed at length in Chapters 8 and 14.

Because sodium is the major plasma solute, hyponatremia is tantamount to hypoosmolality. There is usually excellent agreement between directly measured and calculated osmolality. However, there are two situations when this does not hold true: in pseudohyponatremia (also termed **factitious hyponatremia**), and in the presence of high concentrations of other effective solutes. In pseudohyponatremia, the plasma volume is displaced by the presence of high concentrations of lipids or proteins (e.g., hyperglobulinemia), resulting in a low plasma concentration of Na+, although the activity of Na+ in water is normal. If Na+ is directly measured with an ion-specific electrode (ISE) in this case, the activity reading is normal. However, high-throughput analyzers, in order to extend electrode life, generally perform ISE measurements on diluted plasma (so-called indirect ISE measurement), making the reading a plasma concentration measurement vulnerable to pseudohyponatremia. The measured Posm is unaffected by the presence of hyperlipidemia or paraproteinemia, as the concentration of solute particles per volume of fluid is unchanged.

The presence of high concentrations of osmotically active solutes such as glucose, radiographic contrast agents, mannitol, and ethylene glycol causes a shift of water from the intracellular to the extracellular compartment, leading to dilutional hyponatremia (this situation, though quite different from what was described in the preceding paragraph, is also sometimes referred to as pseudohyponatremia). Similar **translocational hyponatremia** occurs with the absorption of glycine during transurethral prostate resection, as well as in gynecologic and orthopedic procedures (Ayus, 1997; Hahn, 2001). The calculated Posm is unreliable in these situations; Posm must be measured directly instead. A difference between the calculated and measured Posm of >10 mOsm/kg supports the presence of pseudohyponatremia or other osmolar solutes (Kumar, 1998). The most common situation causing a large "osmolal gap" is ethanol intoxication.

In hyperglycemia, the measured Na^+ should be corrected by the addition of 1.6 mmol/L for each 100-mg/dL increase in serum glucose above normal (100 mg/dL). A more recent analysis suggested that this formula may underestimate the decrease in Na^+ caused by hyperglycemia, and supported the use of a 2.4-mmol/L correction factor (Hillier, 1999). True hyponatremia is present if, after the correction formula is applied, the serum Na^+ is still <135 mmol/L.

During pregnancy, there is a resetting of the osmostat with a drop in osmolality of approximately 10 mOsm/kg (Lindheimer, 1995). The precise mechanism for this is not known; however, studies have suggested a role for the hormone relaxin and for the enzyme oxytocinase. During pregnancy, there is a progressive increase in placental production of oxytocinase, which, in addition to breaking down oxytocin, breaks down vasopressin, possibly resulting in a change in the hypothalamic AVP osmolality feedback loop.

Diabetes Insipidus

Diabetes insipidus (DI) is classified as being either central (due to absent or decreased ADH secretion from the hypothalamus or neurohypophysis) or nephrogenic (due to renal resistance to the actions of ADH). Each is further subcategorized as being complete or partial. All variants are characterized by the passage of large volumes of dilute urine (>2.5 L/day) in the face of an inappropriately elevated plasma osmolality. Provided the thirst mechanism is intact and there is free access to water, most individuals can avoid dehydration and maintain normal plasma osmolality (Posm) and serum sodium levels.

The water deprivation test is the preferred diagnostic test for identifying the presence of DI (Table 24-5). Central and nephrogenic DI can be distinguished by the response to either endogenous or exogenous vasopressin (Table 24-6). In neurogenic DI, ADH levels are low and the kidney rapidly acts to conserve water in response to exogenous ADH administration. In contrast, nephrogenic DI is associated with normal or increased levels of ADH, and administration of additional ADH has little or no effect on renal water reabsorption. Differentiating partial nephrogenic DI from primary polydipsia can be more difficult. Unlike DI, where the underlying problem is difficulty in holding on to free water, in primary polydipsia the pathophysiology arises from increased intake of fluids. Primary polydipsia (PP) can be due to either dipsogenic DI or psychogenic polydipsia. In dipsogenic DI, the setpoint for ADH secretion is normal; however, a resetting of the thirst threshold occurs, so that it is now below the threshold for ADH secretion. In psychogenic polydipsia, the osmostat for ADH secretion is normal; however, because of underlying psychiatric illness, the subject has a compulsion to drink excessive volumes of liquid. This intake of copious volumes of fluid as seen in PP leads to a washout in the medullary concentrating gradient within the kidney, resulting in a decreased ability to concentrate the urine in response to dehydration. Differentiating between nephrogenic DI and PP, as well as among those who have an equivocal response to ADH, is best achieved by plotting the basal and postdehydration Uosm and plasma ADH on nomograms created by Zerbe and Robertson (Figs. 24-3 and 24-4) (Zerbe, 1981, 1987). Direct measurement of plasma ADH may be helpful in confirming the diagnosis of a pathologic ADH deficiency or excess in the presence of a known or

TABLE 24-5
Water Deprivation Test for Diagnosing and Classifying Diabetes Insipidus

Patients with mild polyuria may be instructed to withhold all fluid intake from 10 PM onward. For those with more severe polyuria (8–10 L/day), water deprivation should be started early in the morning under close observation.

1. During testing, the patient is forbidden to take in anything by mouth.
2. Obtain the following baseline parameters: urine volume (Uvol) and urinary osmolality (Uosm), plasma osmolality (Posm), and plasma sodium (PNa). Also record the weight and blood pressure (BP)/pulse (P) seated and standing.
3. Urine and plasma are collected hourly for Uvol, Uosm, and Posm. Weight, BP, and P are also recorded. Record requests for fluid.
4. When the Uosm has plateaued (e.g., hourly increase <30 mOsm/kg for 3 consecutive hours), or when body weight has decreased by 3%–5%, or the patient develops a >20 mm Hg drop in systolic BP, obtain samples for Uvol, Uosm, Posm, PNa, and AVP (plasma).
5. Administer 1 mcg of desmopressin IV or IM, or 5 mcg of AVP SC Uosm; urine output and Posm are recorded at 30, 60, and 120 minutes after the injection. The highest Uosm value is used to evaluate the patient's response to AVP.

Precautions

When possible, discontinue any medications that can influence ADH secretion. Observe for hypotension and nausea, which may stimulate ADH secretion. The patient should not be permitted to smoke during the test.

Interpretation

Normal	Final Uosm before AVP challenge is higher than Posm. Following AVP challenge, the Uosm is less than 10% higher than the maximal Uosm achieved with water restriction alone
Neurogenic DI	Final Uosm before AVP challenge is less than Posm. Following AVP administration, there is a greater than 50% increase in Uosm.
Nephrogenic DI	Final Uosm before AVP challenge is less than Posm. Following AVP administration, there is a less than 10% increase in Uosm.
Partial central DI	Uosm may be higher than Posm following dehydration; however, there is only a 10%–50% increase in Uosm following administration of AVP.
Partial nephrogenic DI	Uosm may be higher than Posm following dehydration; however, there is a greater than 10% increase in Uosm following administration of AVP.

Plotting basal and postdehydration Uosm and plasma ADH on the nomograms from Zerbe and Robertson will permit further distinction between partial nephrogenic DI, partial central DI, and primary polydipsia (see Figs. 24-3 and 24-4).

ADH, Antidiuretic hormone; *AVP,* arginine vasopressin; *DI,* diabetes insipidus; *IM,* intramuscular; *IV,* intravenous; *SC,* subcutaneous.

TABLE 24-6
Tests in the Differential Diagnosis of Disorders of Water Homeostasis

	BASELINE			AFTER 12-HOUR FLUID RESTRICTION			
Disorder	**Serum Na+ and osmolality**	**Urine Na+ and osmolality**	**Serum ADH**	**Serum Na+ and osmolality**	**Urine Na+ and osmolality**	**Serum ADH**	**Urine osmolality post-AVP challenge**
Normal control	N	N	N	N	High	High	Same
SIADH	Low	N–High	High	Low–N	High	High	—
Neurogenic DI	N–High	Low	Low	High	Low–N	Low	Increased
Nephrogenic DI	N–High	Low	N–High	High	Low–N	High	Same
Psychogenic polydipsia	Low–N	Low	Low	N	N–High	N–High	Same

ADH, Antidiuretic hormone; *AVP,* arginine vasopressin; *DI,* diabetes insipidus; *N,* normal; *SIADH,* syndrome of inappropriate secretion of ADH.

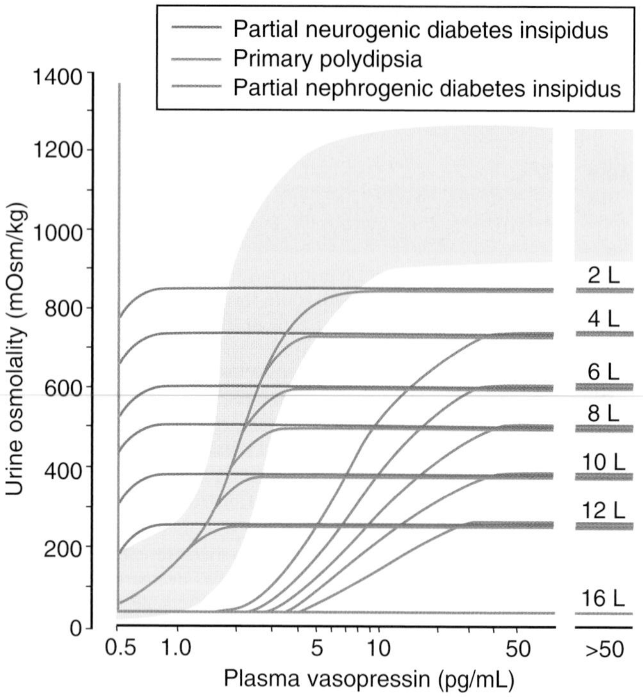

Figure 24-3 The relationship between urine osmolality (Uosm) and plasma arginine vasopressin (AVP/ADH) in patients with polyuria of diverse causes and severity. Each of the three categories of polyuria is described by its own family of sigmoid curves of differing heights. Differences in height within a family reflect differences in maximum concentrating capacity caused by "washout" of the medullary concentration gradient. They are proportional to the severity of the polyuria (indicated in liters per day at the right end of each plateau). The normal response is depicted in yellow. The three categories of polyuria differ principally in the ascending portion of the dose–response curve. In patients with partial neurogenic diabetes insipidus (DI), the curve lies to the left of normal, reflecting increased sensitivity to the antidiuretic effects of very low concentrations of plasma ADH. In contrast, in patients with partial nephrogenic DI, the curve lies to the right of normal, reflecting decreased sensitivity to ADH. In primary polydipsia, the relationship of Uosm to ADH remains relatively normal. *(Redrawn from Bichet DG. Diabetes insipidus and vasopressin. In: Moore WT, Eastman RC, editors. Diagnostic endocrinology. 2nd ed. St Louis: Mosby; 1996, p. 158, with permission.)*

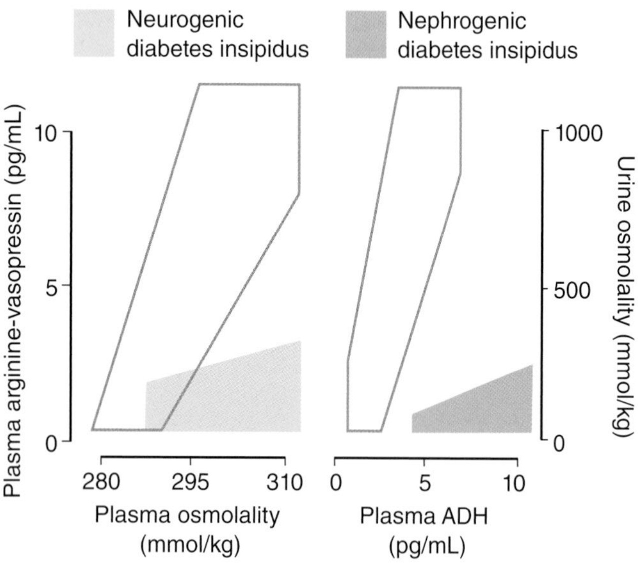

Figure 24-4 *Left:* Relationship between plasma arginine vasopressin (AVP/ADH) and plasma osmolality during the infusion of hypertonic saline. Patients with primary polydipsia and nephrogenic diabetes insipidus (DI) have values within the normal range *(open area),* in contrast to patients with neurogenic DI, who show a subnormal plasma ADH response to a rise in osmolality *(pink). Right:* Relationship between urine osmolality and plasma ADH during dehydration and water loading. Patients with primary polydipsia and neurogenic DI have values within the normal range *(open area),* in contrast to patients with nephrogenic DI, who have hypotonic urine despite high plasma ADH *(green). (Redrawn from Bichet DG. Diabetes insipidus and vasopressin. In: Moore TW, Eastman RC, editors. Diagnostic endocrinology. 2nd ed. St Louis: Mosby; 1996, p. 168, with permission.)*

TABLE 24-7
Causes of Diabetes Insipidus

Central
Primary
Familial
Idiopathic
Acquired
Tumors—craniopharyngioma, pituitary tumors, metastases (i.e., lung, breast), Rathke's cleft cyst, nonlymphocytic leukemia
Granulomatous disorders—sarcoidosis, Langerhans' cell histiocytosis, Wegener's granulomatosis
Traumatic—head trauma, surgery
Infectious—tuberculosis, meningitis, encephalitis
Vascular—cerebral aneurysm, sickle cell, Sheehan's syndrome
Drugs—alcohol, diphenylhydantoin, chlorpromazine, and β-adrenergic agonists
Other—lymphocytic hypophysitis, hypoxic encephalopathy
Nephrogenic
Hereditary
Mutation in the V2 receptor
Mutation in the aquaporin gene
Acquired
Drugs—lithium, phenytoin, demeclocycline, vinblastine, cisplatin, propoxyphene, colchicine, gentamicin, amphotericin, ethanol, atrial natriuretic hormone, norepinephrine, methoxyflurane anesthetics, furosemide
Electrolyte disorders—hypercalcemia, hypokalemia
Systemic illnesses—sickle cell, multiple myeloma, amyloidosis, sarcoidosis, Sjögren's syndrome, polycystic kidney disease
Other—low-protein diet, postobstructive uropathy

suspected disorder of renal function or fluid and electrolyte homeostasis, or when a patient is unable to tolerate physiologic testing. In cases of congenital DI, family members who are heterozygote carriers of ADH gene mutations may be identified by demonstrating decreased ADH levels, which may be the only subclinical manifestation of ADH deficiency.

Nephrogenic DI is either congenital or acquired. An X-linked receptor defect is the most common etiology for congenital nephrogenic DI; medications are the most common cause of acquired nephrogenic DI (Holtzman, 1994). Medications known to be associated with acquired nephrogenic DI include lithium, demeclocycline, and methoxyflurane anesthetics. Other causes of acquired nephrogenic DI include hypercalcemia, hypokalemia, sickle cell disease, and postobstructive uropathy (Table 24-7).

Neurogenic DI may be congenital, the result of an autosomal dominant mutation in the ADH signal peptide or in the exons that code for neurophysins (McLeod, 1993; Yuasa, 1993). More commonly, neurogenic DI is induced by lesions affecting the hypothalamus, (metastatic tumors, trauma, granulomatous disorders) or medications.. Drugs that may cause neurogenic DI by suppressing ADH release include phenytoin, chlorpromazine, and α-adrenergic agonists. It has been suspected that autoantibodies directed against the ADH-producing cells of the hypothalamus may be responsible for some cases of idiopathic neurogenic DI (De Bellis, 1994, 1999; Maghnie 2000). These antibodies are detectable by indirect immunofluorescence antibody.

Another common condition in which decreased ADH levels have been found is primary nocturnal enuresis in children. Although these patients have ADH levels only slightly lower than controls (2.9 ng/L vs. 3.6 ng/L), the clinical symptoms are reliably ameliorated by vasopressin therapy (Willie, 1994). The determination of ADH levels in diagnosing this condition is not always helpful because of moderate overlap between enuretic and normal children. Measuring the specific gravity in the first morning urine is more reliable for identifying children who may benefit from ADH supplementation; they will have a urine specific gravity below 1.015 (Mevorach, 1995).

Syndrome of Inappropriate Secretion of ADH

The syndrome of inappropriate secretion of ADH (SIADH) is characterized by a euvolemic hypoosmolar hyponatremia, associated with hyperosmolar urine (the result of continued inappropriate natriuresis). By definition, SIADH cannot be diagnosed until nonosmotic stimuli for ADH secretion and other pathologies that interfere with free water clearance have been excluded (Vistorina, 2002). Physiologic triggers of

TABLE 24-8
Water Load Test

1. Baseline: The patient must be euvolemic and have a serum Na+ between 125 and 150 mmol/L and Posm >275 mOsm/kg.
2. The patient is given 20 mL of water per kilogram of body weight (max = 1500 mL) to drink over 30 minutes.
3. With the patient maintained in the recumbent position, urine output is collected every hour for the next 5 hours. Record the volume and osmolality of each specimen.

Interpretation

Normals	Excrete 80%–90% of the administered water load within 4 hours, and suppress the Uosm to <100 mOsm/kg.
SIADH	Failure to meet these criteria in the absence of medications or other conditions that may impair diuresis is consistent with the diagnosis of SIADH.

SIADH, Syndrome of inappropriate secretion of ADH.

TABLE 24-9
Causes of SIADH

CNS disease
  Neoplasm, infection, trauma, cerebrovascular accident
Neoplasm
  Oat cell carcinoma and adenocarcinoma of the lung, pancreatic cancer, lymphoma
Pulmonary infection
  TB, pneumonia, positive-pressure ventilation
Idiopathic
  Medications
- Oral hypoglycemics—chlorpropamide, tolbutamide
- Antineoplastics—vincristine, cyclophosphamide
- Diuretics—hydrochlorothiazide
- Psychotropics—amitriptyline, phenothiazines, SSRIs, monoamine oxidase inhibitors
- Other—morphine, barbiturates, clofibrate, nicotine, acetylcholine, anesthetic agents, β-adrenergic stimulants, metoclopramide, desmopressin

CNS, Central nervous system; *SIADH,* syndrome of inappropriate secretion of ADH; *SSRIs,* selective serotonin reuptake inhibitors.

ADH secretion include nausea, pregnancy, hypoglycemia, intracranial hypertension, mechanical ventilation, and hypoxia. Hypothyroidism and glucocorticoid deficiency cause a decrease in free water clearance, leading to a dilutional hyponatremia. Mineralocorticoid deficiency can lead to hyponatremia caused by increased renal sodium loss. It is therefore extremely important to test for deficiencies of these axes and to institute appropriate hormonal replacement therapy before making a diagnosis of SIADH. Other confounding factors that can hamper the diagnosis of SIADH include renal disease, cardiac disease, and medications such as diuretics. In these situations, one can cautiously perform a water load test (Table 24-8). In the absence of medications or other conditions that may impair diuresis, failure to excrete 80%–90% of the administered water load within 4 hours and to suppress the Uosm to <100 mOsm/kg is consistent with the diagnosis of SIADH.

In the right clinical setting, the diagnosis of SIADH often can be confidently made on the basis of serum and urine electrolyte determinations alone. A spot urine Na^+ <30 mmol/L can generally distinguish those with hyponatremia due to volume depletion from those with SIADH, in whom urine Na^+ >30 mmol/L (Chung, 1987). In contrast, differentiating the patient with euvolemia and SIADH from the one with hypovolemia and concomitant renal salt-wasting (e.g., salt-losing nephropathy, diuretic use) can be much more difficult. In addition to hyponatremia, both have a spot UNa^+ >30 mmol/L and a fractional excretion of Na^+ >1. The fractional excretion of sodium (FENa [%]) is calculated as follows:

$$\frac{U_{[\mathrm{Na}^+]} \times P_{[\mathrm{Cr}]}}{P_{[\mathrm{Na}^+]} \times U_{[\mathrm{Cr}]}} \times 100 \qquad \textbf{(24-2)}$$

where $U[\mathrm{Na}^+]$ = urine sodium concentration; $P[\mathrm{Na}^+]$ = plasma sodium concentration; $U[\mathrm{Cr}]$ = urine creatinine concentration; and $P[\mathrm{Cr}]$ = plasma creatinine concentration.

One way to differentiate between the two is to administer 1 L of 0.9% NaCl intravenously over 24 hours for 2 days. A rise in serum Na^+ by more than 5 mmol/L is suggestive of hypovolemia. In SIADH, no change or an increase of less than 5 mmol/L occurs. Alternatively, fluid restriction to 600–800 mL/day for 2–3 days will lead to improvement in hyponatremia in SIADH but not in renal salt-wasting (see Table 24-6).

The cause of renal salt-wasting in SIADH is twofold. At the onset of the disease, there is volume expansion, which inhibits the renin-aldosterone axis and leads to greater improved delivery of sodium to the distal tubules. Continued sodium loss is due to secretion of atrial natriuretic protein (Kamoi, 1990).

Because of hyperfiltration and the local actions of ADH on the renal V2 receptor, SIADH is one of the two states in which some of the lowest uric acid levels occur; the other is pregnancy. In SIADH, the serum levels of ADH may be variably increased, usually out of proportion to Posm; however, approximately 20% of cases meeting the physiologic diagnosis of SIADH will not have detectable levels of ADH (Zerbe, 1980). This may be due to insensitivity of the assay to low levels of ADH, increased renal sensitivity to ADH, or perhaps the presence of another hormone with antidiuretic activity (Kamoi, 1997).

The diagnosis of SIADH is largely a diagnosis of exclusion, with the clinician having ruled out other causes of hyponatremia (Fig. 24-5). It most often occurs as a manifestation of the paraneoplastic syndrome; however, it may also occur in central nervous system trauma or infection, in lung disease, or as the result of medications (vinca alkaloids, tricyclic antidepressants, serotonin receptor uptake inhibitors) (Table 24-9).

THYROID

The normal thyroid gland weighs about 15–25 g. It is divided into lobules, each of which is composed of 20–40 follicles separated by highly vascular connective tissue. The follicles are ring-shaped structures, in which a single cell band of follicular cells surrounds a closed cavity containing colloid, thyroid hormone, thyroglobulin (Tg), and a variety of other glycoproteins. The follicular cells rest on a basement membrane that is rich in glycoprotein that separates the cells from surrounding capillaries. The apex of the follicular cells has microvilli that extend into the colloid, where iodination, exocytosis, and the initial phase of hormone secretion occur. The follicles are sites of thyroid hormone synthesis and storage. The thyroid gland also contains parafollicular cells, or C cells, which are responsible for the synthesis and secretion of calcitonin, a hormone important in calcium metabolism.

An intact hypothalamic-pituitary-thyroid (HPT) axis and a ready source of iodide are required for normal thyroid hormone synthesis. The hypothalamus secretes TRH, which, in turn, stimulates the thyrotrophs of the anterior pituitary to secrete TSH (thyrotropin). As implied by the name, TSH stimulates thyroid hormone synthesis and secretion by the thyroid gland. Thyroid hormone exerts negative feedback on both the hypothalamus and the pituitary gland to maintain a TSH concentration within narrow limits; it also acts peripherally to mediate numerous metabolic activities.

Under TSH stimulation, iodine enters the follicular cells as inorganic iodide and is transformed into thyroid hormones, thyroxine (T_4), and 3,5,3′-triiodothyronine (T_3) through a series of metabolic steps. The sequence of events as depicted in Figure 24-6 can be broken down into (1) active transport of iodide into the cell; (2) iodination of the tyrosyl residues on Tg; (3) coupling of iodotyrosine molecules within Tg to form T_4 and T_3; (4) proteolysis of Tg with release of free iodotyrosine, T_4, and T_3, and secretion of iodothyronine into the circulation; (5) deiodination of iodotyrosines within the thyroid and reuse of liberated iodide; and (6) deiodination of T_4 to T_3.

One hundred percent of circulating T_4 is of thyroidal origin, whereas only 20% of T_3 is of thyroidal origin; 80% is produced enzymatically in nonthyroidal tissues by 5′-monodeiodination of T_4 (Lum, 1984). Approximately 110 nmol (85 μg) of T_4 and 10 nmol (8.5 μg) of T_3 are produced daily by the thyroid. The thyroid hormones circulate while attached to plasma proteins. About 70% of T_4 is bound to thyroxine-binding globulin (TBG), 20% to transthyretin (formerly called **binding prealbumin**), and 10% to albumin. Although most of the circulating T_3 is bound to TBG; it does so with a 10-fold reduced affinity as compared with that of T_4 (Robbins, 1996; Braverman, 2000). Small percentages of T_4 and T_3 remain unbound to protein—about 0.03% and 0.3%, respectively. As with other hormones, it is the free component that is metabolically active.

Thyroid disease may be classified functionally into hyperthyroidism, hypothyroidism, and euthyroidism. Signs and symptoms of hyperthyroidism include heat intolerance, tachycardia, weight loss, weakness, emotional

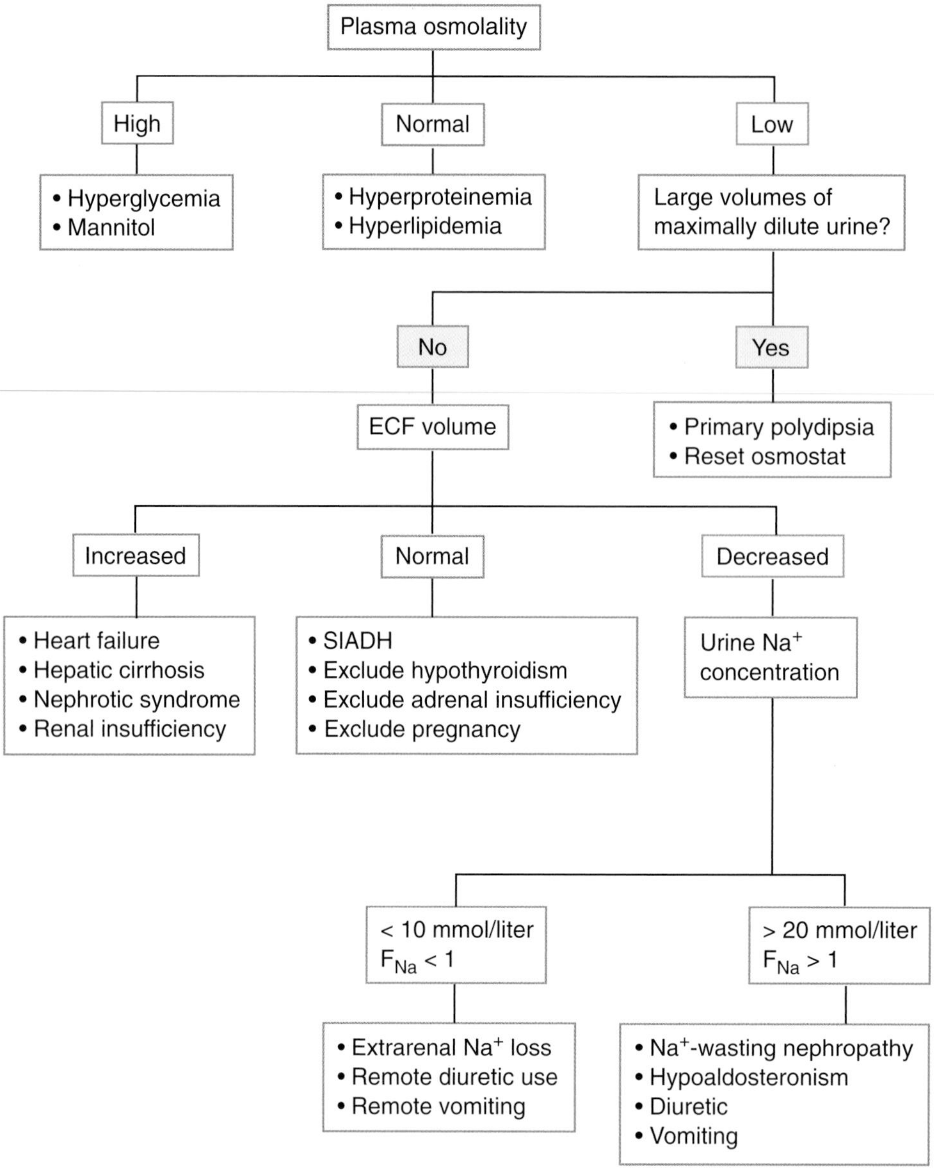

Figure 24-5 Algorithm for the evaluation of hyponatremia. *(From Singer GG. Fluid and electrolyte management. In: Carey CF, Lee HH, Woeltje KF, editors. The Washington manual of medical therapeutics. 29th ed. Philadelphia: Lippincott-Raven; 1998, p. 44, with permission.) ECF,* Extracellular fluid; *SIADH,* syndrome of inappropriate secretion of ADH.

lability, and tremor. The most common clinical syndrome associated with hyperthyroidism is Graves' disease, caused by circulating antibodies to the TSH receptor. Other disorders that lead to hyperthyroidism include toxic adenoma and, rarely, TSH-secreting pituitary tumors and thyroid carcinoma.

Hypothyroidism results in hoarseness, cold sensitivity, dry skin, constipation, bradycardia, and muscle weakness. Myxedema coma is an advanced stage of thyroid hormone deficiency characterized by progressive stupor, hypothermia, and hypoventilation. Failure of the thyroid itself to secrete an adequate amount of thyroid hormone is called **primary hypothyroidism** and is most commonly iatrogenic in origin, the result of either ablation with radioactive iodine or surgery to treat hyperthyroidism. Secondary hypothyroidism occurs when TSH secretion is decreased as a result of a pituitary disorder. Tertiary hypothyroidism is the result of hypothalamic dysfunction.

Thyroid diseases such as goiter, thyroid adenoma, and thyroid carcinoma typically occur in individuals who are euthyroid. Accurate TSH assays permit the diagnosis of subclinical hyperthyroidism and hypothyroidism. These patients appear clinically euthyroid; however, their TSH values are respectively suppressed or elevated. A number of clinical situations can lead to difficulties in the interpretation of thyroid function tests: The presence of abnormal protein–binding proteins (congenital or drug induced); alterations in thyroid hormone metabolism as seen in those hospitalized with acute psychiatric illness; alterations in thyroid hormone metabolism as seen in those on medications that affect thyroid hormone binding or the HPT axis directly. The most important and most common problem with thyroid function tests probably occurs in those patients with various illnesses that do not directly involve the thyroid, so-called **nonthyroidal illness.**

THYROID HORMONE SYNTHESIS AND METABOLISM

Iodine is a major component of thyroid hormone; the main source of iodine is dietary intake. Deiodination of organic iodine–containing moieties within the gland serves as another source. Inorganic iodide is transported into the follicular cell by the sodium–iodide symporter (NIS) located in the basolateral membrane (Chambard, 1983). TSH modulates NIS activity: An increase in TSH secretion augments the uptake of iodide into the follicular cell. Iodide transport into the thyroid gland is also influenced by the serum iodide level; iodide deficiency increases pump activity, and iodide excess inhibits iodide uptake.

Thyroglobulin is a glycoprotein synthesized by the rough endoplasmic reticulum in the basal and perinuclear regions of the follicular cell. It is acted upon by the Golgi apparatus in the apical portion of the follicular cell, where its tyrosyl residues are iodinated, leading to the formation of monoiodotyrosyls and diiodotyrosyls (MITs and DITs). Tg is then

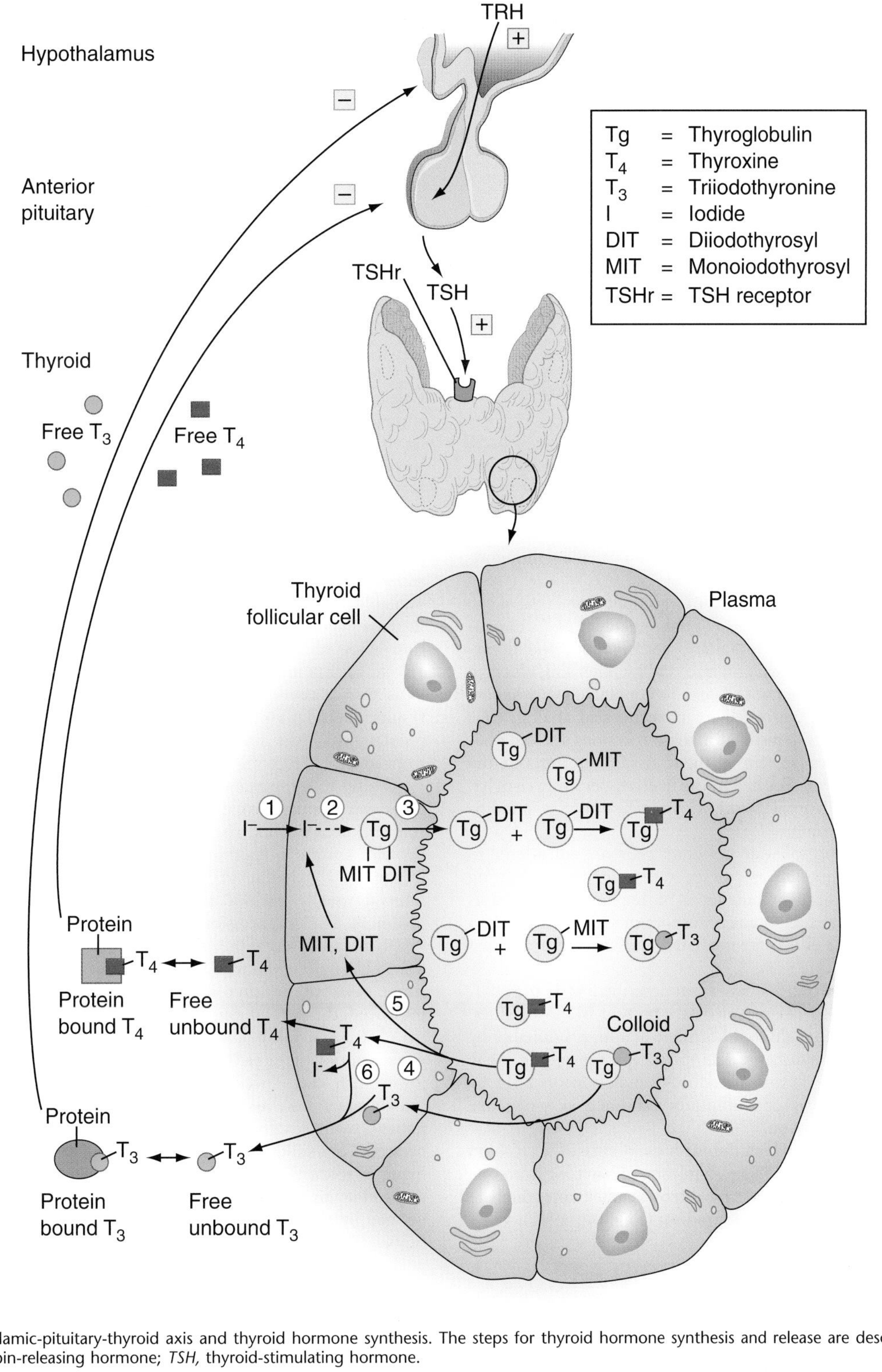

Figure 24-6 Hypothalamic-pituitary-thyroid axis and thyroid hormone synthesis. The steps for thyroid hormone synthesis and release are described in further detail in the text. *TRH,* Thyrotropin-releasing hormone; *TSH,* thyroid-stimulating hormone.

transferred into the colloid for storage (Vassart, 1973a; Roth, 1985). This transformation of thyroglobulin into thyroid hormone requires two separate oxidative reactions, both catalyzed by thyroid peroxidase (TPO): the binding of iodide to Tg tyrosyl residues to form the iodotyrosyls MIT and DIT, and the subsequent coupling of MIT and DIT to produce T_4 and T_3 (Deme, 1976; Bjorkman, 1981). T_4 is formed by the coupling of two molecules of DIT; T_3 results from the union of one MIT and one DIT. T_4 and T_3 are released from Tg via lysosomal degradation. They are then secreted into the circulation at the basal membrane. All of these reactions are under the control of TSH.

About half of all T_4 is monodeiodinated in the 5′ position to form T_3, and about 40% undergoes deiodination of the inner ring of T_4 to form reverse T_3 (rT_3). The formation of rT_3, the third major circulating form of thyroid hormone, is catalyzed by the enzyme 5-deiodinase. Reverse T_3 has no biological activity, has a short half-life of 4 hours, and circulates bound to TBG; its formation is considered a disposal pathway in the peripheral metabolism of T_4 (LoPresti, 1989).

The intake of iodide influences the DIT/MIT ratio in Tg. DIT is the preferential iodotyrosine formed; thus, when iodide is abundant, T_4 is the predominant form of hormone synthesized and secreted, but when iodide sources are diminished, MIT is produced in greater quantities, leading to increased T_3 formation and release. In addition, the thyroid gland has a 5′-deiodinase that converts T_4 to T_3. This process is under the control of TSH, so that T_3 secretion is enhanced during periods of TSH stimulation

TABLE 24-10
Metabolic Dynamics of T_4 and T_3

	T_4	T_3
Production rate, nmol/day	110	50
Fraction of circulating hormone of thyroid origin	100%	20%*
Serum concentration		
Total, nmol/L	100	1.8
Free, pmol/L	20	5
Fraction of total hormone in free form	0.0002	0.003
Half-life, days	≈7	0.75
Relative metabolic potency	0.3	1.0

From Larsen PR, Davies TF, Schlumberger MJ, Hay ID. Thyroid physiology and diagnostic evaluation of patients with thyroid disorders. In: Larsen PR, Kronenberg HM, Melmed S, Polonsky KS, editors. Williams textbook of endocrinology. 10th ed. Philadelphia: WB Saunders; 2003, p. 342.
T_3, 3,5,3′-triiodothyronine; *T_4*, thyroxine.
*80% of circulating T_3 comes from the peripheral deiodination of T_4. To convert total T_4 from nmol/L to μg/dL, or free T_4 from pmol/L to ng/dL, divide by 12.87. To convert total T_3 from nmol/L to ng/dL, or free T_3 from pmol/L to pg/dL, multiply by 65.1.

(i.e., primary hypothyroidism and cases with TSH-stimulating immunoglobulin [TSI]) (Ishii, 1983).

The monodeiodination of T_4 to T_3 and rT_3 accounts for 70% of the peripheral metabolism of T_4 (LoPresti, 1989); the remainder of T_4 metabolism occurs by conjugation of T_4 to sulfate, deamination, and decarboxylation to form the acetic acid analog tetrac, and by ether link cleavage (Engler, 1989) (Table 24-10). T_3 but not rT_3 can be conjugated with sulfate to form T_3-sulfate and can be converted to its acetic acid analog, triac (Engler, 1989). The enzymes responsible for these reactions are the phenolsulfotransferases, which are present in many tissues throughout the body, and the L-aminotransferase, located in the liver, respectively (Engler, 1984). After their formation from T_4, both T_3 and rT_3 undergo deiodination to form 3,3′-diiodothyronine (T_2).

Protein-bound thyroid hormones do not enter cells, are considered to be biologically inert, and function as storage reservoirs for circulating thyroid hormones. In contrast, the minute levels of free hormone fractions readily enter cells by specific membrane transport mechanisms to exert their biological effects. These effects are mediated by T_3 receptors located in the nucleus of the cell.

Four isoforms of the T_3 receptors have been described: α-1, α-2, β-1, and -β2 (Brent, 1991). -α1 and -β1 receptors are present in most tissues. Binding of T_3 to them promotes thyroid hormone action, presumably by increasing mRNA and protein synthesis. The -β2 receptor is unique to the pituitary and is central in the negative-feedback regulation of TSH by thyroid hormone. The -α2 receptor is inhibitory and acts as a negative regulator of thyroid hormone action.

Mutations in the β-receptors, which diminish the ability of T_3 to bind to the nucleus, have been described in the syndrome of thyroid hormone resistance. Individuals with this syndrome have growth and mental retardation of varying degrees, as well as hypothyroidism (Refetoff, 1991).

HYPOTHALAMIC-PITUITARY-THYROID AXIS

The physiologic regulators responsible for integrating the function of the thyroid gland and the periphery include the hypothalamic hormone, TRH; the pituitary hormone, TSH; and the serum free T_4 and free T_3 concentrations. TRH enhances TSH synthesis, stimulates the secretion of any preformed TSH from the thyrotrophs, and modulates the bioactivity of TSH, resulting in the secretion of bioactive TSH (Beck-Peccos, 1985; Shupnik, 1986). TRH itself is under the negative-feedback influence of circulating thyroid hormones (TRH mRNA levels are inversely related to the circulating T_3 values) (Kakucska, 1992). The same feedback inhibition occurs at the level of the thyrotrophs.

Thyrotropin-Releasing Hormone

TRH is a modified tripeptide (pyroglutamyl-histidyl-proline-amide) derived from a large prepro-TRH molecule. The TRH molecule is released from the prepro molecule by a peptidase (Yamada, 1990). TRH is found in the hypothalamus, the brain, the C cells of the thyroid gland, the β cells of the pancreas, the myocardium, and the prostate and testis, as well as in the spinal cord. The neuron bodies producing TRH are innervated by catecholamine, leptin, and somatostatin-containing axons; all these hormones can influence the rate of its synthesis.

Thyroid hormones regulate their own production by feedback inhibition to synthesis of TRH and TSH in the hypothalamus and pituitary, respectively. TRH acts also on the production of other pituitary hormones, especially prolactin. Leptin plays a significant role in the regulation of the TRH gene (Bjorbeck, 2004), affecting the individual's appetite for food intake. It is difficult to develop a specific antibody for TRH, and assays are not clinically useful.

Thyroid-Stimulating Hormone

TSH is a glycoprotein consisting of two monocovalently linked α and β subunits. The α subunit has the same amino acid sequences as LH, FSH, and human chorionic gonadotropin (hCG). It is the β subunit that carries specific information to the binding receptors for expression of hormonal activities.

The radioimmunoassay for measuring TSH was first developed by Odell and colleagues in 1965. This **first-generation assay** did not have sufficient sensitivity to distinguish normal TSH levels from the suppressed levels seen in primary hyperthyroidism. By the mid 1980s, a "sensitive" or second-generation immunometric TSH method using monoclonal or polyclonal antibodies was developed, which had an improved sensitivity to 0.1–0.2 mU/L. Refinements in the immunometric method led to the third-generation assays now in common use, which allow measurement down to about 0.005 mU/L. Although a fourth-generation TSH assay has recently been developed with a sensitivity of 0.0004 mU/L, it is not widely available, and the third-generation assays provide sufficient sensitivity for the vast majority of clinical applications. The American Thyroid Association (ATA) recommendations state that third-generation assays should be able to quantitate TSH in the 0.010–0.020-mU/L range on an interassay basis with a coefficient of variation of 20% or less. In reporting assay results, the ATA recommends using functional sensitivity, defined as the point at which the interassay precision has a coefficient of variation equal to or less than 20% (Spencer, 1996).

Owing to improvements in the sensitivity of the TSH assay, this test alone can identify virtually all instances of hyperthyroidism and hypothyroidism, except when there is damage to the hypothalamus or pituitary, thyroid hormone resistance, or interference with normal functioning of the HPT axis due to medication. TSH results within the reference interval usually exclude thyroid dysfunction and help distinguish the profound TSH suppression typical of frank Graves' thyrotoxicosis (TSH <0.01 mIU/L) from the modest degrees of TSH suppression (0.01–0.1 mIU/L) observed with mild (subclinical) primary hyperthyroidism and some cases of nonthyroidal illness. Of note, as assay sensitivity has improved, the normal range has not changed, remaining between approximately 0.5 and 5.0 mIU/L in most laboratories. However, the serum TSH concentration detected in patients with severe thyrotoxicosis has been lower with each successive improvement in the TSH assays: Using a fourth-generation assay, the serum TSH is less than 0.004 mIU/L in patients with severe hyperthyroidism. Hyperthyroid patients have suppressed TSH values, with the exception of those few individuals who have hyperthyroidism caused by a TSH-producing tumor or other diseases such as pituitary resistance to thyroid hormone. Subclinical hyperthyroidism is defined by the presence of a low TSH with normal levels of T_4 and T_3 (Table 24-11).

In most individuals with hypothyroidism, serum TSH results are clearly elevated, but results may be inappropriately normal for the levels of T_4 and T_3 in those with pituitary or hypothalamic disorders. The term *subclinical hypothyroidism* is used to describe patients with elevated TSH concentration but with normal levels of T_4, T_3, and FT_4. An important cause of both increased and decreased TSH results is nonthyroidal illness (NTI). Patients with NTI tend to have low TSH results during their acute illness, then TSH rises to within or above the reference range with resolution of the underlying illness, ultimately returning to normal once the acute illness has resolved. The situation is complicated because medications, including glucagons, opioids, glucocorticoids, and dopamine, suppress TSH. The sensitive TSH assays are helpful in evaluation of thyroid hormone treatment for both replacement therapy and suppressive therapy.

Despite the clinical sensitivity of TSH, a TSH-centered strategy has two primary limitations. First, it assumes that hypothalamic-pituitary function is intact and normal. Second, it assumes that the patient is stable (i.e., the patient had no recent therapy for hyperthyroidism or hypothyroidism) (Wardle, 2001). If either of these criteria is not met, the serum TSH result can be misleading (see Table 24-11). In these instances, to confirm the

TABLE 24-11
Characterization of Thyroid Disorders According to Results of Thyroid Function Tests

Disorder	TSH	T_4	T_3	FT_4	Tg	TBG	rT_3	aTPO	ATG	TBII	TSI	TBA
Primary hypothyroidism	↑	↓	N or ↓	↓	N or ↓	N	↓	N or ↑	N or ↑	N or ↑	n	n or ↑
Transient neonatal hypothyroidism	↑	↓	↓	↓	N or ↓	N	↓	N	N	↑	n	↑
Hashimoto's thyroiditis/hypothyroidism	↑	N or ↓	N or ↓	N or ↓	N or ↓	N	↓	↑	↑	n or ↑	n	n or ↑
Graves' disease	↓	↑	↑	↑	↑	N	↑	↑	↑	↑	↑	n or ↑
Neonatal Graves' disease	↓	↑	↑	↑	↑	N	↑	n or ↑	n or ↑	↑	↑	n or ↑
TSH deficiency	N or ↓	↓	↓	↓	↓	N	↓	n	n	n	n	n
Thyroid dyshormonogenesis	↑	↓	↓	↓	N, ↓ or ↑	N	↑	n	n	n	n	n
Thyroid hormone resistance	N or ↑	↑	↑	↑	↑	N	↑	n	n	n	n	n
TSH-dependent hyperthyroidism	↑	↑	↑	↑	↑	N	↑	n	n	n	n	n
T_4 protein-binding abnormalities*	N	V	V	N	N	V+	V	n	n	n	n	n
Nonthyroidal illness	V	N or ↓	↓	V	N	N	N or ↑	n	n	n	n	n
Subacute thyroiditis†	↓ or ↑	↑ or ↓	↑ or ↓	↑ or ↓	↑ or ↓	N	↑ or ↓	n	n	n	n	n

From Fisher DA, editor. Disorders of thyroid function, online version of the Quest diagnostic manual. 3rd ed. p. 268.
ATG, Antithyroglobulin; *aTPO*, anti-thyroid peroxidase; *FT_4*, free thyroxine; *N*, normal; *n*, negative; *rT_3*, reverse triiodothyronine; *TBA*, TSH receptor–blocking antibody; *TBII*, TSH-binding inhibiting immunoglobulin; *T_g*, thyroglobulin; *T_3*, triiodothyronine; *T_4*, thyroxine; *TBG*, thyroxine-binding globulin; *TSH*, thyroid-stimulating hormone; *TSI*, thyroid-stimulating immunoglobulin; *V*, variable.
*The spectrum of binding protein abnormalities includes increased or decreased TBG binding, increased or decreased transthyretin binding, and ↑ albumin binding.
†Subacute thyroiditis involves a transient period of hyperthyroidism followed by a transient hypothyroid state.

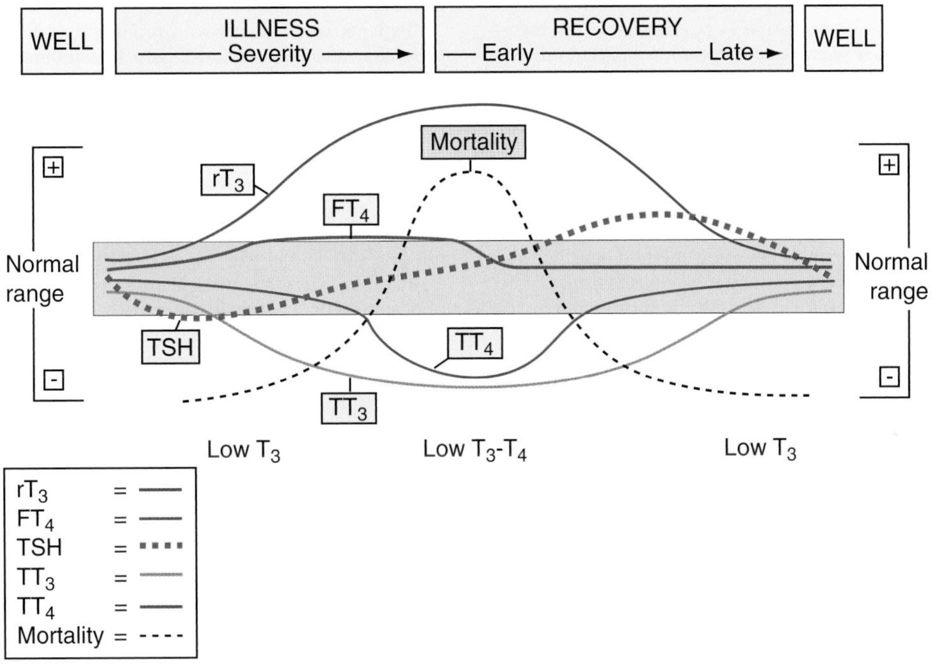

Figure 24-7 Changes in thyroid hormones during severe illness. *(Redrawn from Demers LM, Spencer CA. NACB: laboratory support for the diagnosis and monitoring of thyroid disease, 2003, p. 11, with permission. Available at: www.nacb.org.) FT_4*, Free thyroxine; *rT_3*, reverse triiodothyronine; *TSH*, thyroid-stimulating hormone; *TT_3*, total triiodothyronine; *TT_4*, total thyroxine.

presence of thyroid dysfunction, in addition to measuring TSH, measurement of FT_4 with or without total T_4 may prove helpful. Serum Free T_3 and serum TSH measurements are appropriate in patients suspected of hyperthyroidism, as they may have overproduction of T_3 with a normal to low-normal T_4 (**T_3 thyrotoxicosis**).

Thyroxine

After release from its thyroid follicles, thyroxine will bind to various proteins in the blood (thyroid-binding globulin, albumin, thyretin). Thyroxine can be measured by immunoassay after the hormone is separated from the carrier protein. The reference range is 5–12.5 µg/dL in adults, with slightly lower results for certain pediatric age groups. Although TSH is the most important test of thyroid function, thyroxine measurements are often used along with TSH and can be important in interpreting TSH results. The combination of a low T_4 and an increased TSH is indicative of primary hypothyroidism, whereas elevated T_4 and T_3 combined with decreased TSH are characteristic of primary hyperthyroidism. Hyperthyroidism, however, has been reported in patients with an elevated serum T_4 but with serum T_3 levels within the reference range or low. This so-called **T_4 thyrotoxicosis** can occur in patients with iodine-induced thyrotoxicosis; in patients on beta-blockers, amiodarone, or large doses of steroids; and in thyrotoxic patients with NTI. A suppressed TSH level associated with a normal to low-normal T_4 and a high T_3 characterizes T_3 thyrotoxicosis. This is more common in a toxic nodule (see Table 24-11).

Severe nonthyroidal illness is associated with low T_4 and low T_3; this so-called **low T_4 and T_3 syndrome** (an adaptive response to reduce metabolic demands and conserve protein stores) (LoPresti, 1995) is associated with a poor prognosis (Chopra, 1997). It is thought to arise from a maladjusted central inhibition of TRH (Van den Berghe, 1998, 2000) (Fig. 24-7).

Euthyroid hyperthyroxinemia is distinguished by the presence of an increased serum T_4 level in association with a normal TSH in an otherwise euthyroid individual. This entity has a variety of causes, including increased binding proteins as may be seen with certain drugs (e.g., estrogen) or medical conditions (e.g., liver disease). It is also seen in patients who are acutely hospitalized for psychiatric illness and in patients with familial dysalbuminemia. When medications or other factors cause increased protein binding, there is a consequent increase in the serum total T_4 level; conversely, a decrease in binding capacity leads to a decrease in serum total T_4. These perturbations do not have any physiologic effect, as it is the free hormone, not the protein-bound component, that is bioactive. In these situations, free T_4 correlates better with thyroid functional status than does serum total T_4.

The so-called **T_3 uptake (T_3-UP) test** is a classical method of adjusting a total T_4 measurement for alterations in binding protein. A T_3-UP result is a relative measurement of the unoccupied binding sites of all circulating proteins. It was originally performed by saturating available binding sites with radiolabeled T_3, then measuring the unbound T_3 by adsorbing it onto a resin (hence the term **T_3 resin uptake**). Methods giving analogous results can still be performed via nonisotopic methods on automated analyzers. The free thyroxine index (FTI) is then calculated as (T_3-UP of the patient)/(mean T_3-UP of the reference population) multiplied by the patient's total T_4. The FTI (reference range, 5.4–9.7) is only a relative estimate of the free T_4 concentration. In general, during thyrotoxicosis, both total T_4 and T_3-UP are elevated; conversely, in hypothyroidism, both total T_4 and T_3-UP are decreased, and when there is a binding globulin abnormality, these two values diverge (e.g., total T_4 is elevated and the T_3-UP is decreased, or the total T_4 is decreased and the T_3-UP is increased). The FTI has been largely replaced by the direct measurement of free T_4 by immunoassay, dialysis, or ultrafiltration.

Free Thyroxine

FT_4 is the biologically active fraction of thyroxine in circulating blood. In the past 10–15 years, direct measurement of FT_4 has increased in sensitivity and precision. The traditional reference method for FT_4 is equilibrium dialysis, a method that is not affected by changes in binding protein concentration. The sample is dialyzed against a nonprotein buffer, using a membrane impermeable to proteins, so that FT_4 will achieve equal concentrations on both sides of the membrane. Because bound T_4 vastly exceeds FT_4 in the plasma, their ratio is essentially unperturbed by this process. The protein-free solution is then collected and analyzed for T_4. This is a time-consuming method that cannot meet the high-volume demand of clinical laboratories. Even this laborious method does not give a true measure of FT_4 in all cases, because small molecules that may affect T_4 binding are diluted in the procedure. Theoretically more accurate are ultrafiltration (using pressure to push the plasma sample through a dialysis membrane) and **symmetrical dialysis** (where plasma is dialyzed against itself, using a radioactive tracer added on one side to measure the rate of diffusion of FT_4, which is proportional to its concentration). Mass spectrometry is well suited to measurement of thyroid hormone (De Brabandere, 1998), and a method using ultrafiltration followed by tandem mass spectrometry to simultaneously measure FT_4 and FT_3 has recently been published (Gu, 2007).

In common practice, FT_4 is usually measured by immunoassay techniques, which have employed different approaches over the years (Spencer, 1986; Hay, 1991). These methods can be performed on automated clinical chemistry platforms and provide appropriate results in most clinical circumstances. However, depending on the exact method, they can be unreliable in various circumstances and must be used with caution. For example, spurious results can occur with abnormal variants of any of the binding proteins (particularly familial dysalbuminemic hyperthyroxinemia, a condition with high T_4 but normal FT_4, caused by an albumin variant that binds T_4 abnormally) or in the presence of T_4 or T_3 autoantibodies (Langsteger, 1997). Increases or decreases in serum FT_4 without concomitant changes in metabolic state have been reported in pregnancy with NTI, and in patients being treated with certain drugs. For example, prolonged administration of phenytoin or carbamazepine results in a 15%–30% decrease in both serum T_4 and FT_4. In these circumstances, dialysis or ultrafiltration methods are indicated.

FT_4 can also be determined using mass spectroscopy, after the FT_4 is separated from the protein–hormone complex using ultrafiltration at 37° C and avoiding dilution effects.

Triiodothyronine

T_3, generally measured by immunoassay, has a reference interval typically in the range of 60–160 µg/dL (0.9–2.46 nmol/L). T_3 is much less bound to serum protein than T_4; thus a relatively greater proportion of T_3 than T_4 exists in the free, diffusible state. Serum total T_3 measurement is helpful in confirming the diagnosis of hyperthyroidism, especially in patients with no or minimally elevated T_4 or ambiguous clinical manifestation. In 90% of patients with hyperthyroidism, T_4 and T_3 values are increased, with the increase in T_3 usually greater than that in T_4. Serum T_3 levels, however, can be in the reference range or low in patients with hyperthyroidism if there is coexistent NTI, or if patients are on drugs that decrease the conversion of T_4 to T_3 (e.g., propranolol, amiodarone).

Hyperthyroidism with elevated serum T_3 but normal T_4 and free T_4 is termed T_3 thyrotoxicosis (Bitton, 1990). Patients with this syndrome are a heterogeneous group with no distinctive signs or symptoms. Although most patients have Graves' disease, T_3 thyrotoxicosis may occur in patients with other causes of hyperthyroidism such as toxic nodular goiter or toxic adenoma. About 1%–4% of thyrotoxic patients have T_3 thyrotoxicosis, except in regions of iodine deficiency, where it is more common.

Elevated serum T_3 levels with normal T_4 levels may also be seen in patients with hyperthyroidism early in the course of treatment with antithyroid drugs or during relapse after treatment. Elevated TBG will cause elevated T_3.

Generally, the measurement of serum T_3 is not useful in evaluating patients suspected of having hypothyroidism because serum T_3 levels are within the reference interval in 15%–30% of hypothyroid patients (Surks, 1990). However, decreased T_3 levels are seen in patients who have severe hypothyroidism, that is, those with serum T_4 levels less than about 2 µg/dL (32 nmol/L) (Bigos, 1978). Low serum T_3 may occur in patients with a wide variety of NTI. In patients with acute illness such as myocardial infarction, the decrease in serum T_3 occurs rapidly, declining to about 50% of the reference value within days (Utiger, 1980). Serum T_3 concentrations are also low in cord blood, but increase rapidly during the first few hours of life.

Patients receiving thyroid preparations containing T_3 such as desiccated thyroid and synthetic T_3 and T_4 combinations and those treated with T_3 will have uninterpretable serum T_3 results unless the time of hormone administration is known. Administration of T_3 (Ctyomel) results in a rapid rise in T_3 concentration that peaks within 2–4 hours and then begins to drop off. In contrast, the serum T_3 levels do not show a peak in patients treated daily with T_4 (levothyroxine); instead, stable levels of T_3, which is derived from the peripheral conversion of T_4, are reached after only a few weeks of therapy. A number of pharmacologic agents are associated with low levels of T_3 and free T_3, and with normal or even high levels of serum T_4 and FT_4. These include glucocorticoids, amiodarone, and large dosages of propranolol. These patients usually have normal TSH results; however, amiodarone can induce hyperthyroidism or hypothyroidism, in which case the TSH values will be suppressed or elevated respectively. Total T_3 concentrations are measured by competitive immunoassay methods that are now mostly nonisotopic and use enzymes, fluorescence, or chemiluminescence molecules as signals (Nelson, 1996).

Reverse Triiodothyronine

rT_3, a major metabolite of thyroxine, is produced by 5-deiodination of T_4.

In many clinical situations, serum T_3 and serum rT_3 have been found to vary reciprocally, but serum rT_3 measurements have found little clinical usefulness. Serum rT_3 is high in patients with NTI, whose serum total T_3 is decreased. Serum rT_3 is increased in healthy newborns, in patients with hyperthyroidism (including factitious hyperthyroidism), and in patients taking certain drugs, including amiodarone and propranolol.

Thyroglobulin

Tg is synthesized and secreted by the follicles. It is present in the serum of normal individuals in the range of up to about 30 ng/mL (45 pmol/L). The serum Tg concentration reflects thyroid mass, thyroid injury, and TSH receptor stimulation (Spencer, 1995). Tg is increased in a variety of disorders, including Graves' disease, thyroiditis, and nodular goiter. Patients with thyrotoxicosis factitia have undetectable levels of Tg in contrast to a high level found in patients with other causes of thyrotoxicosis. The routine measurement of Tg is never indicated. Its utility resides in the monitoring of recurrence of certain variants of thyroid cancer, in the diagnosis of thyroid dysgenesis in congenital hypothyroidism, and, as noted previously, in helping to distinguish subacute thyroiditis from thyrotoxicosis factitia.

The main value of Tg measurement is to follow patients with thyroid malignancy postoperatively (Ericsson, 1984). It is helpful in patients with well-differentiated thyroid carcinoma, but not in those who have undifferentiated tumors or medullary thyroid cancer. The clinical value of its measurement is limited by a number of technical problems, including the presence of antibodies, which are present in 20% of patients with thyroid carcinoma (Spencer, 1999). These antibodies interfere with Tg measurement, causing overestimation or underestimation of serum Tg levels. Therefore, whenever Tg level is drawn to monitor recurrence/persistence of thyroid cancer, it is extremely important to obtain a simultaneous sample for Tg antibodies (TgAb). In patients with positive TgAb, polymerase chain reaction (PCR) methods (using serum) used to amplify the Tg mRNA may eliminate this problem.

Recombinant human TSH (rhTSH) is commonly used to test patients with thyroid cancers for the presence of residual/recurrent disease. This is more practical, more convenient, and markedly less unpleasant for the patient than stopping thyroid hormone suppression over the span of several weeks to increase the TSH level; an elevated TSH is required for RAI (radioactive iodine) uptake to occur in any remaining remnant or recurrent tumor. Measurement of Tg 72 hours following the last dose of rhTSH correlates highly with the presence of recurrence, and some authorities support the use of this test alone without a concomitant whole body iodine scan for those with "low-risk" tumors (age <40, no distant metastases, size <1 cm, well differentiated). All other patients with thyroid cancer need to undergo whole body scanning, in addition to measurement of TSH; concomitant use of both equals the sensitivity of scanning performed after thyroid hormone withdrawal, which is about 97%. Any rise in post-rhTSH serum Tg above 2 ng/mL in patients with thyroid cancer who have undergone remnant ablation and are on hormone suppressive therapy is suspicious for recurrence/persistence of disease and needs to be worked up accordingly (i.e., full restaging while hypothyroid off of suppressive therapy).

Well-differentiated tumors typically display about a 10-fold increase in Tg in response to a high TSH (Spencer, 1999). Poorly differentiated tumors that do not concentrate iodide may display a blunted response to TSH stimulation (Schlumberger, 1980). In early weeks postthyroidectomy, serum Tg levels typically fall, with a half-life of 2–4 days. The pattern of change in serum Tg values on T_4 treatment is a better indicator of a change in tumor burden than any single serum Tg value (Spencer, 1995). Because of interassay variability, it is extremely important to use the same laboratory (TSH assay) for monitoring.

Thyroxine-Binding Globulin

TBG is the main serum carrier protein for both T_4 and T_3. Measurement of TBG may be helpful in patients who have serum T_4 and T_3 levels that do not agree with other laboratory parameters of thyroid function, or that are not compatible with clinical findings. TBG, which is measured by immunoassay, is in the range of 13–39 μg/dL (150–360 nmol/L) in healthy individuals. Inherited abnormalities in TBG include complete and partial deficiency, as well as TBG variants with decreased affinity for T_4 or T_3, and TBG excess (Langsteger, 1997). Among the acquired causes of abnormalities in the TBG concentration are a variety of medications and medical conditions (Table 24-12). Medications such as salicylates, phenytoin, penicillin, and heparin can displace T_4 from binding to TBG.

Thyroid Autoantibodies

Autoimmune thyroid disease causes cellular damage and alters thyroid gland function. Cellular damage occurs when the autoantibodies or the sensitized T lymphocytes bind to thyroid cell membranes, causing cell lysis and inflammatory reactions. Three thyroid autoantigens are responsible for the autoimmune thyroid disorders: TPO, Tg, and the TSH receptor. TPO antibodies (TPOAb) are involved in the tissue destructive process associated with hypothyroidism in Hashimoto's and atrophic thyroiditis. Some studies suggest that TPOAb may be cytotoxic to the thyroid (Chiovato, 1993; Guo, 1997). TgAb, if present even in low concentrations in serum, can interfere with the anti-Tg antibody used in the immunoassay for Tg measurement. Thus, the TgAb concentration should be measured in all patients before Tg analysis. In iodide-deficient areas, serum TgAb measurement can be used to detect autoimmune thyroid disease in patients with a goiter and to monitor iodide therapy in endemic areas.

TSH receptor antibodies (TRAbs) were previously known as thyroid-stimulating immunoglobulin or long-acting thyroid stimulators. TRAbs are classified as stimulating or blocking antibodies. Graves' disease (GD) is an autoimmune condition in which goiter and hyperthyroidism are induced by thyroid-stimulating antibodies that mimic the action of TSH. The target of the autoimmune response is the thyrotropin receptor. Although both stimulating and blocking antibodies are present in GD, the latter usually do not cause symptoms; however, in a few cases, they may lead to the development of hypothyroidism. TRAbs are positive in 85% of patients with GD. Measurement of TRAbs has been used to predict the outcome of Graves' patients treated with drug therapy; if the titer of the antibodies is low before therapy, patients have a better chance for remission after 6–12 months of therapy.

Measurement of TRAbs has also been used to predict the risk of thyroid dysfunction in newborns of mothers with GD as a result of transplacental passage of maternal TRAb (Heithorn, 1999; Radetti, 1999). In these patients, assays that distinguish blocking from stimulating antibodies are important clinically (Davies, 1998).

Longitudinal studies suggest that TPOAb may be a risk factor for future thyroid dysfunction, including postpartum thyroiditis and autoimmune complications from treatment with amiodarone, interferon-α, and lithium (Feldt-Rasmussen, 1994; Johnson, 1999; Martino, 2001).

Urinary Iodine Measurement

Iodine is required for normal thyroid hormone production. Iodine measurements are used mainly to assess the dietary iodine intake of certain populations. This is of great importance in that iodine deficiency disorders affect 2.2 billion persons throughout the world, including the United States (Delange, 1995; Dunn, 1998). Because most of the ingested iodine is excreted in the urine, measurement of urinary iodine (UI) excretion provides an accurate estimate of dietary iodine intake (Dunn, 1998). Suggested ranges for UI excretion are shown in Table 24-13.

Screening Programs for Detection of Neonatal Hypothyroidism

The prevalence of hypothyroidism in newborns is estimated from 1 in 3000 to 1 in 5000. It is higher in certain ethnic groups and is increased in iodine-deficient regions worldwide. Early detection of hypothyroidism in the neonatal period is critical to eliminate the severe mental retardation associated with thyroid hormone deficiency. Measurement of T_4 and TSH is used for screening, which is performed using dry blood spots or cord serum. The detection rate depends on the tests used and the timing of specimen collection. Measurement of only T_4 carries a high false-positive rate, necessitating recall of a large number of infants for retesting. Causes of false-positive results include low T_4 levels, which occur in both premature infants and those with congenital absence of TBG. Screening with only T_4 may miss infants with compensated or partial thyroid insufficiency. Because about 15% of infants with primary thyroid disorders have compensated hypothyroidism (normal serum T_4 levels in association with elevated TSH), an elevated TSH is the most sensitive test for the diagnosis of congenital hypothyroidism. However, false-positive results are occasionally seen, for example, in premature or severely stressed infants. In addition, by screening with TSH alone, those infants with hypothalamic

TABLE 24-12
Some Causes of Alterations in Thyroxine-Binding Globulin

Increases	Decreases
Drugs	Drugs
Clofibrate	Androgens
Estrogens, oral contraceptives	Glucocorticoids
5-Fluorouracil	Genetic
Heroin	Complete deficiency
Methadone	Partial deficiency
Genetic	Liver failure
Acute or chronic active hepatitis	Malnutrition
Pregnancy	Nephrotic syndrome
Idiopathic	Idiopathic

TABLE 24-13
Urinary Iodine Excretion and Iodine Deficiency

Urinary Iodine Excretion, μg/L	>100	50–99	20–49	<20
Degree of deficiency*	None	Mild	Moderate	Severe
Goiter prevalence	<5%	5%–19.9%	2%–29.9%	>30%

From Demers LM, Spencer CA, editors. NACB: laboratory support for the diagnosis and monitoring of thyroid disease, 2003, p. 75. Available from: www.nacb.org.
*IDD Newsletter, August 1999;15:33–48.

or pituitary disease will be missed. Very-low-birthweight infants should be retested at 2 and 4–6 weeks to detect late-onset transient hypothyroidism (Frank, 1996). For newborns, if the initial TSH value is <10 mIU/L, no further action need be taken; if it lies in the 10–20-mIU/L range, then a repeat test needs to be performed in 2–6 weeks. Finally, if the initial blood spot TSH >20 mIU/L, endocrinologic evaluation is necessary to make the diagnosis of hypothyroidism.

Nonthyroidal Illness

Seriously ill patients can have abnormal thyroid tests even without underlying thyroid pathology (DeGroot, 1992; Kaptein, 1996). A rapid decline in both total and free T_3 typically develops in the setting of severe illness (e.g., myocardial infarction, sepsis) (Piketty, 1996). As the severity of the illness increases, the serum total T_4 falls because of T_4-binding protein disruption by inhibitors in the circulation (Wartofsky, 1982; Docter, 1993; Wilcox, 1994). Patients with nonthyroidal illness (NTI) whose T_4 levels drop below 2 ng/dL carry an exceptionally poor prognosis. Alterations in thyroid function tests seen during NTI are termed the euthyroid sick syndrome or the low T_4 syndrome. Figure 24-7 shows the spectrum of changes in the thyroid tests as they relate to the severity and the stage of the illness. Patients with NTI tend to have low or low-normal TSH and normal or low-normal T_4 but very low T_3 during their acute illness; then TSH rises to within normal or above normal with resolution of the underlying illness and finally returns to the normal range (Faber, 1987). This situation can be complicated if certain drugs are used for this illness (e.g., glucagon, dopamine, and high doses of corticosteroids suppress TSH and can mask hypothyroid status during their use) (Kaptein, 1980; Skamene, 1984; Brabant, 1989; Samuels, 1990).

In uremia, there is accumulation of indoleacetic acid, which interferes with thyroid hormone binding (Iitaka, 1998).

Physiologic Variables

For practical purposes, variables such as age, gender, race, season, phase of menstrual cycle, cigarette smoking, exercise, fasting, and phlebotomy-induced stasis have minor effects on thyroid function tests in ambulatory adults (Hollowell, 2002). Studies have suggested that each individual has a genetically determined FT_4 setpoint (Meikle, 1988; Andersen, 2002); any deviation from this setpoint will be sensed by the pituitary and cause reciprocal change in TSH secretion. In the early stages of developing thyroid dysfunction, a serum TSH abnormality will precede the development of an abnormal FT_4 because TSH responds exponentially to subtle FT_4 changes as shown in Figure 24-8.

Despite the wider serum TSH variability seen in older individuals, there appears to be no justification for using a widened or age-adjusted reference range. This conservative approach is justified by reports that mildly suppressed or elevated TSH is associated with increased cardiovascular morbidity and mortality (Sawin, 1991; Parle, 2001). In children, the hypothalamic-pituitary-thyroid axis undergoes progressive maturation and modulation; there is a continuous decline in the TSH/FT_4 ratio from the time of midgestation until after puberty (Nilson, 1993; Adams, 1995; Lu, 1999; Zurakowski, 1999; Fisher, 2000a,b); as a result, higher TSH concentrations are typically seen in children.

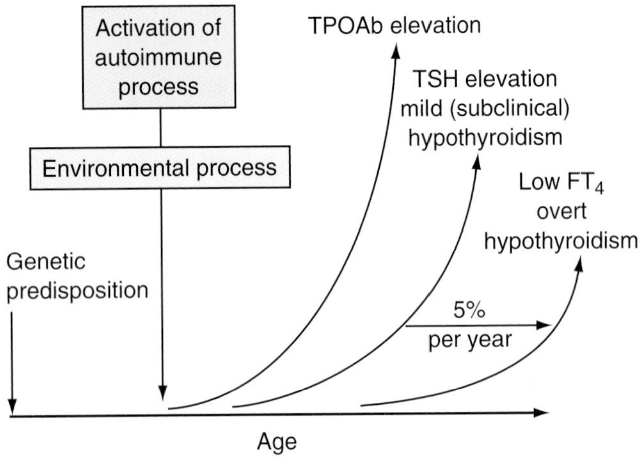

Figure 24-8 Depiction of the evolution of primary hypothyroidism of autoimmune origin. *(From Demers LM, Spencer CA. NACB: laboratory support for the diagnosis and monitoring of thyroid disease, 2003, p. 47. Available at: www.nacb.org.) FT_4,* Free thyroxine; *TPOAb,* thyroid peroxidase antibodies; *TSH,* thyroid-stimulating hormone.

During pregnancy, estrogen production increases, progressively elevating the TBG concentration and resulting in an increase in the total T_4 and T_3 reference range to approximately 1.5 times the nonpregnancy upper reference level by 16 weeks' gestation (Weeke, 1982; Pedersen, 1993; Nohr, 2000). Although TBG excess leads to an increase in both T_4 and T_3 concentrations, the serum FT_4 and T_3 concentrations remain unchanged.

Serum hCG, which has structural similarity to TSH, has weak thyroid-stimulating activity (Talbot, 2001). The increase in hCG soon after fertilization results in a small increase in FT_4 and T_3 concentrations, usually within the normal reference range. These changes result in a fall in serum TSH during the first trimester; a subnormal serum TSH may be seen in about 20% of mothers who have normal pregnancies (Glinoer, 1990, 1997; Panesar, 2001). The peak rise in hCG and the nadir of TSH occur together at about 10–12 weeks' gestation. In 2% of pregnancies, the increase in FT_4 reaches supranormal levels and, if prolonged, may lead to a syndrome referred to as gestational transient thyrotoxicosis, which is characterized by more pronounced symptoms and signs of thyrotoxicosis. This condition is frequently associated with first-trimester hyperemesis gravidarum (Goodwin, 1992; Hershman, 1999).

Medications and Thyroid Function Tests

Drugs can cause both in vitro and in vivo effects on thyroid tests. This can lead to the misinterpretation of test results, inaccurate diagnoses, and further unnecessary tests (Surks, 1995; Kailajarvi, 2000). Estrogen-induced TBG elevation causes abnormally high total T_4 and total T_3, but has no effect on TSH or FT_4 and free T_3. Glucocorticoids in large doses can suppress TSH and decrease the conversion of T_4 to T_3 (Samuels, 1997; Kaptein, 1980). Dopamine suppresses TSH and can temper the expected rise in TSH in hospitalized patients with primary hypothyroidism (Kaptein, 1980). Propranolol suppresses the conversion of T_4 to T_3 (this is one of the reasons it is used in the treatment of thyrotoxicosis).

Iodide, found in iodide-containing contrast media used in CT scans and coronary angiography or in solution to sterilize skin, and radiopaque dyes can cause both hyperthyroidism and hypothyroidism in susceptible patients (Meurisse, 2000). Iodine-containing drugs such as amiodarone (used as an antiarrhythmic agent) have complex effects on thyroid function and can cause hypothyroidism (10% of patients) or hyperthyroidism (1%–2%) in susceptible individuals with positive antibodies (TPOAb) (Martino, 1987, 2001; Caron, 1995; Harjai, 1997; Daniels, 2001).

Lithium inhibits thyroid hormone synthesis and release and can cause hypothyroidism in about 15%–50% of patients, especially those patients with positive TPOAb (Lazarus, 1998; Kusalic, 1999; Oakley, 2000). The mechanism of lithium action is similar to that of iodide. Lithium is concentrated by the thyroid and inhibits thyroidal iodine uptake. It also inhibits iodotyrosine coupling, alters thyroglobulin structure, and inhibits thyroid hormone secretion. The latter effect is critical to the development of hypothyroidism and goiter (Lazarus, 1998).

Drugs such as phenytoin, carbamazepine, salicylate, salsalate, and furosemide competitively inhibit thyroid binding to serum proteins. They therefore can cause total T_4 levels to be depressed (because the FT_4 is maintained at its normal level), and they can cause the FT_4 estimated by FTI or direct assays to be artifactually low. Therapeutic doses of phenytoin can induce acceleration of T_4 disposal and perhaps can directly suppress TSH centrally, all of these mechanisms being responsible for the reduced T_4 (Surks, 1995). Heparin can stimulate in vitro lipoprotein lipase and can liberate free fatty acids, which inhibit T_4 binding to serum proteins and falsely elevate FT_4 (Mendel, 1987).

Medications such as phenobarbital, phenytoin, rifampin, and carbamazepine increase the rate of thyroid hormone clearance by increasing the deiodination of T_4 and T_3. Hypothyroid patients treated with any of these medications need to have their hormone levels monitored closely, as an increase in levothyroxine (L-T_4) dose may be required. In turn, changes in thyroid hormone status affect the clearance of many medications, including those listed previously (e.g., hyperthyroidism can lead to increased clearance of phenobarbital, hypothyroidism to decreased clearance). Owing to these various alterations in thyroid hormone parameters, the best indicator of thyroid status is the measurement of TSH along with the FT_4. For those with pituitary disease or in those on Dilantin, T_4 by equilibrium dialysis should be used.

Somatostatin or its analog, octreotide, which is used to treat acromegaly (Itoh, 1988), and dopamine (Kaptein, 1980) inhibit TSH synthesis to undetectable levels in patients with severe NTI.

Thyroid Illness

Hyperthyroid patients may present with one or all of the following signs and symptoms: weight loss, sweating, heat intolerance, palpitations, insomnia, increased bowel movement, tremors, infertility, or amenorrhea. They have suppressed TSH values, with the exception of those few individuals who have secondary hyperthyroidism caused by TSH-producing pituitary tumors, or other rare disorders such as pituitary resistance to thyroid hormones. Subclinical hyperthyroidism is defined as low TSH (<0.1 μIU/mL) with levels of T_4 and T_3 within the reference values with no signs or symptoms of hyperthyroidism (Ross, 1991). Detection of subclinical hyperthyroidism is particularly important in patients who are over 60, as they have increased risk of atrial fibrillation, increased cardiovascular mortality (Sawin, 1994), and osteoporosis. Minimal thyroid hormone excess can cause atrial fibrillation and can stimulate osteoclastic activity in bone, causing osteoporosis.

Patients with primary hypothyroidism can present with one or all of the following signs and symptoms: cold intolerance, constipation, water retention, hypercholesterolemia, depression, pretibial myxedema, periorbital edema, and elevated TSH with low T_4 and T_3. TSH is low in patients with secondary hypothyroidism caused by pituitary or hypothalamic disorders. Patients with subclinical hypothyroidism have elevated TSH levels (>4.5 μU/mL), but both T_4 and T_3 are within the reference range. In 2004, an expert panel recommended TSH reference limits of 0.4–4.5 μU/mL, and that patients with TSH in the range of 4.5–10 mU/L, or 0.1–0.4, should not be routinely treated (Surks, 2004). The 2002 AACE guidelines (American Association of Clinical Endocrinologists, 2002) recommend treatment of those with TSH >10 μU/mL or those with goiter and positive TPOAb whose TSH is between 4.5 and 10 μU/mL. TPOAb measurement is useful for establishing the presence of autoimmunity; those with elevated antibodies have a greater probability of developing overt thyroid failure.

Screening for Thyroid Disease

The ATA guidelines recommend screening at age 35 and every 5 years thereafter (Ladenson, 2000). This appears to be a cost-effective strategy, especially for women (Parle, 2001) and the elderly (Vanderpump, 1995; Ladenson, 2000; Parle, 2001). Hashimoto's thyroiditis is an autoimmune disease of the thyroid caused when sensitized T lymphocytes and/or autoantibodies bind to cell membrane, causing cell lysis and an inflammatory reaction, resulting in cellular damage. This is associated with high TSH and positive TPOAb and is encountered with increasing prevalence with increasing age (Vanderpump, 1995). The incidence of low TSH is also increased in the elderly (Vanderpump, 1995).

Mounting evidence indicates that a persistent TSH abnormality may lead to major risks if left untreated. One study reported a higher cardiovascular mortality rate in patients with chronically low TSH (Parle, 2001), and numerous reports indicate that mild hypothyroidism in early pregnancy increases fetal loss and impairs the IQ of offspring (Pop, 1995, 1999; Haddow, 1999). It is important to always confirm any TSH abnormality in a fresh specimen drawn 3 weeks later before making the diagnosis of mild abnormalities.

Uses of L-Thyroxine

An average replacement dose is 1.6 μg/kg body weight/day for adults, up to 4.0 μg/kg body weight/day for children, and lower doses for older individuals (1.0 μg/kg body weight/day) (Sawin, 1983; Davis, 1984). The initial dose and the optimal time needed to establish the full replacement dose are dependent upon the age, weight, and cardiac status of each patient. The requirement might increase during pregnancy and in postmenopausal women starting hormonal replacement (Arafah, 2001). A serum TSH between 0.5 and 2.0 μU/mL is the therapeutic goal level for L-T_4 replacement in primary hypothyroidism. A serum FT_4 concentration in the upper third of the reference interval is the therapeutic target in central hypothyroidism.

TSH should be used to monitor patients receiving thyroid hormone replacement therapy, as well as those treated with hormone, to suppress malignant thyroid diseases (Spencer, 1990). Both TSH and FT_4 should be used to monitor hypothyroid patients suspected of intermittent noncompliance. At least 6 weeks is needed before retesting of TSH following a change in the dose of L-T_4. Annual TSH measurement is recommended in patients on a steady dose of T_4. If FT_4 is being assayed, patients should withhold their levothyroxine dose on the day of the test, as serum FT_4 will be increased (about 13%) above baseline for 9 hours after the last dose is ingested (Ain, 1993); the TSH, however, is unlikely to be affected. Ideally, L-T_4 should be taken before meals, at the same time every day and at least 4 hours from any other medications or vitamins/dietary supplements.

L-T_4 is used to suppress TSH in patients with well-differentiated thyroid carcinoma, for which thyrotropin is considered a trophic factor (Dulgeroff, 1994). It is recommended to use a TSH target of 0.05–0.1 μU/mL for low-risk patients and a TSH value <0.1 μU/mL for high-risk patients. If the thyroglobulin level is undetectable, and no evidence of recurrence is noted 5–10 years after thyroidectomy, the dose of L-T_4 can be reduced to give low-normal TSH values (<0.4 μU/mL).

Calcitonin

Medullary thyroid carcinoma (MTC) originates from the C cells of the thyroid. It accounts for 5%–8% of thyroid cancers and 0.57% of thyroid nodules (Pacini, 1994).

Among cases of MTC, 25% are hereditary (multiple endocrine neoplasia types 2A and 2B) (Dunn, 1994; Brandi, 2001; Cobin, 2001). These are autosomal dominant inherited multiglandular syndromes. An important, recurring MTC genetic mutation was found to be located on the chromosome subband 10q11.2 (Mulligan, 1993; Hofstra, 1994).

The C cell secretes calcitonin. An elevated level of calcitonin in circulating blood indicates the presence of MTC. Mature calcitonin results from posttranslational modification of a larger 141 amino acid precursor (preprocalcitonin) within the parafollicular C cells. Preprocalcitonin undergoes cleavage of a single peptide to form procalcitonin; the latter has 116 amino acid residues. The immature calcitonin peptide consisting of 33 amino acids is located centrally within the procalcitonin molecule. The mature, active, 32 amino acid calcitonin is produced from immature calcitonin by the enzyme peptidylglycine-amidating monooxidase. Measurement of calcitonin is done by two-site immunometric assays using monoclonal antibodies: One recognizes the N-terminal region, and the other the C-terminal region. This method is more sensitive and more specific (Motte, 1988; van Heyningen, 1994; Becker, 1996). The cutoff level in healthy adults is about 10 ng/L.

Serum calcitonin measurements are used as tumor markers for detecting residual thyroid tissue or metastasis in patients with MTC. It should be measured before and 6 months after surgery. The presence of residual tissue or a recurrence of MTC can be ruled out only if both basal and postpentagastrin or calcium-stimulated calcitonin are undetectable. Provocative stimuli, such as calcium and pentagastrin (Pg) or omeprazole, have been used to detect C cell abnormalities, as they increase calcitonin levels at all stages of MTC (Wells, 1978; Barbot, 1994; Gagel, 1996; Erdogan, 1997; Wion-Barbot, 1997; Vieira, 2002; Vitale, 2002).

In the Pg stimulation test for the diagnosis of MTC, an intravenous infusion of Pg (0.5 μg/kg body weight) is given over 5 seconds; blood samples are collected at baseline and 1, 2, 5, and 10 minutes after the start of the infusion. Interpretations of results are summarized in Table 24-14.

In the calcium stimulation test, intravenous injection of 2.5 mg/kg of calcium gluconate is given over 30 seconds; blood samples are then collected at baseline and at 1, 2, and 5 minutes. An increase in the plasma calcitonin level above 100 ng/L is an indication of C cell hyperplasia. The calcium infusion test has been reported to be less sensitive than the Pg test for the diagnosis of MTC, but, if combined with the Pg test, it enhances the sensitivity of the Pg test (Wells, 1978).

Calcitonin may also be elevated in other conditions unrelated to thyroid neoplastic conditions, as summarized in Table 24-15.

TABLE 24-14
Interpretation of the Pentagastrin (Pg) Test

Peak calcitonin (CT) ng/L (pg/mL)	Interpretation
<10	Normal (80% of adults)
>30 but <50	5% of normal adults
>50 but <100	Possible MTC or other thyroid pathology
>100	Probable MTC
Basal or post-Pg CT value >10 pg/mL	C cell pathology or residual tissue in MEN 2 patients and MTC patients after surgery

From Demers LM, Spencer CA, editors. NACB: laboratory support for the diagnosis and monitoring of thyroid disease, 2003, p. 69. Available from: www.nacb.org.
MEN, Multiple endocrine neoplasia; *MTC,* medullary thyroid carcinoma.

ADRENAL

The adrenal glands are pyramidal structures located above each kidney, each weighing approximately 4–6 g. Anatomically, the adrenal is divided into two distinct parts: The medulla (inner layer) and the cortex (outer layer). The medulla, which is of neural crest origin (ectoderm), stores and secretes catecholamines. The cortex is of mesenchymal origin and is further divided into three zones: The outermost zona glomerulosa, which produces mineralocorticoids; the zona fasciculata, which is responsible for glucocorticoid production; and the inner zona reticularis, which synthesizes androgens. The cortex makes up about 80%–90% of the adrenal gland. The glands have a very rich arterial supply that forms a subcapsular plexus and empties into a central vein. By weight, they have the highest perfusion of blood per gram of tissue—a feature that ensures rapid dissemination of hormones throughout the body in response to stress.

HORMONES OF THE ADRENAL MEDULLA

The adrenal medulla is part of the sympathoadrenal axis. Being of neural crest origin, it possesses the capability of synthesizing catecholamines through the process of amine precursor uptake and decarboxylation. The initial and rate-limiting step in catecholamine synthesis is the conversion of tyrosine to 3,4-dihydroxyphenylalanine (dopa) by the enzyme tyrosine hydoxylase. Through a series of steps, L-dopa is subsequently converted to dopamine (D), norepinephrine (NE), and epinephrine (E) (Fig. 24-9). Epinephrine is almost exclusively produced and secreted by the adrenal medulla, where the ratio of NE/E is about 1 : 4. However, because all three catecholamines are also synthesized within the central and sympathetic nervous systems, the peripheral NE/E ratio is more like 9 : 1.

The catecholamines are metabolized by either catechol-*O*-methyltransferase (COMT) or monoamine oxidase (MAO). COMT converts D to methoxytyramine, E to metanephrine, and NE to normetanephrine, all of which in turn can be oxidized to vanillylmandelic acid (VMA) by MAO. MAO can also convert E and NE to 3,4-dihydroxymandelic acid, which is acted upon by COMT to form VMA. 3-Methoxy-4-hydroxyphenylacetic acid (homovanillic acid [HVA]) is the final product of dopamine metabolism.

Pheochromocytoma

Pheochromocytomas are rare catecholamine-producing tumors, with an incidence of about 500–1600 per year (Pacak, 2001a). They account for <1% of all secondary causes of hypertension. Although 90% of pheochromocytomas are benign, they are almost invariably lethal if not diagnosed and properly treated (Pacak, 2001a). Approximately 90% of tumors arise within the adrenal medulla, and 10%–15% are of extraadrenal origin (paraganglioma). Most pheochromocytomas are sporadic; however, 10%–20% are familial, occurring as part of the multiple endocrine neoplasia type 2A or 2B (MEN 2A, MEN 2B), von Hippel–Lindau (VHL) disease, neurofibromatosis type 1 (NF-1), or familial paraganglioma (FP). The hereditary forms tend to present at a younger age, and except for FP, the tumors are usually intraadrenal and bilateral.

Sustained or paroxysmal hypertension is the most common manifestation of this disease and is present in about 90% of patients. Remarkably, 10% of patients are normotensive. More than 90% will present with paroxysmal attacks characterized by at least two of the three following symptoms: headache associated with palpitations and diaphoresis (Sheps, 1994). Other symptoms include orthostatic hypotension, labile blood pressure, excessive sweating, anxiety, nervousness, weight loss, fatigue, pallor, and tremor. These symptoms can last from a few seconds to several hours, with the interval between attacks being highly variable—from several times a day to once every few months. Indications for screening for pheochromocytoma are listed in Table 24-16.

There is ongoing debate as to which test is the best for diagnosing pheochromocytoma. With improvement in assay technique, evidence has come to support the measurement of plasma free metanephrine and normetanephrine levels via high-pressure liquid chromatography with tandem mass spectrometry as the initial test. The diagnosis of pheochromocytoma is made if the plasma concentration of either free metanephrine or normetanephrine is about four times the upper reference limit. Further testing is required in patients with high levels that are less than four times

TABLE 24-15
Conditions in Which Calcitonin May Be Elevated Other Than MTC

Neuroendocrine tumors	Small cell lung cancer, intestinal and bronchial carcinoid, all neuroendocrine tumors
Benign C cell hyperplasia (HCC)	Autoimmune thyroid disease, differentiated thyroid cancer
Other diseases	Kidney disease, hypergastrinemia, hypercalcemia

From Demers LM, Spencer CA, editors. NACB: laboratory support for the diagnosis and monitoring of thyroid disease, 2003, p. 70. Available from: www.nacb.org.
MTC, Medullary thyroid carcinoma.

TABLE 24-16
Indications for Screening for Pheochromocytoma

1. Hypertension with episodic features suggestive of pheochromocytoma.
2. Refractory hypertension.
3. Prominent lability of blood pressure.
4. Severe pressor response during anesthesia, parturition, surgery, or angiography.
5. Unexplained hypotension due to anesthesia, surgery, or pregnancy.
6. Family history of pheochromocytoma, MEN 2A or 2B, VHL disease, neurofibromatosis.
7. Incidentally discovered adrenal mass.
8. Idiopathic dilated cardiomyopathy.
9. Spells or attacks occurring during exertion, twisting and turning of the torso, straining, coitus, or micturition.

From Dluhy RG, Lawrence JE, Williams G. Endocrine hypertension. In: Larsen PR, Kronenberg HM, Melmed S, Polonsky KS, editors. Williams textbook of endocrinology. 10th ed. Philadelphia: WB Saunders; 2003, p. 557.
MEN, Multiple endocrine neoplasia; *VHL,* von Hippel–Lindau.

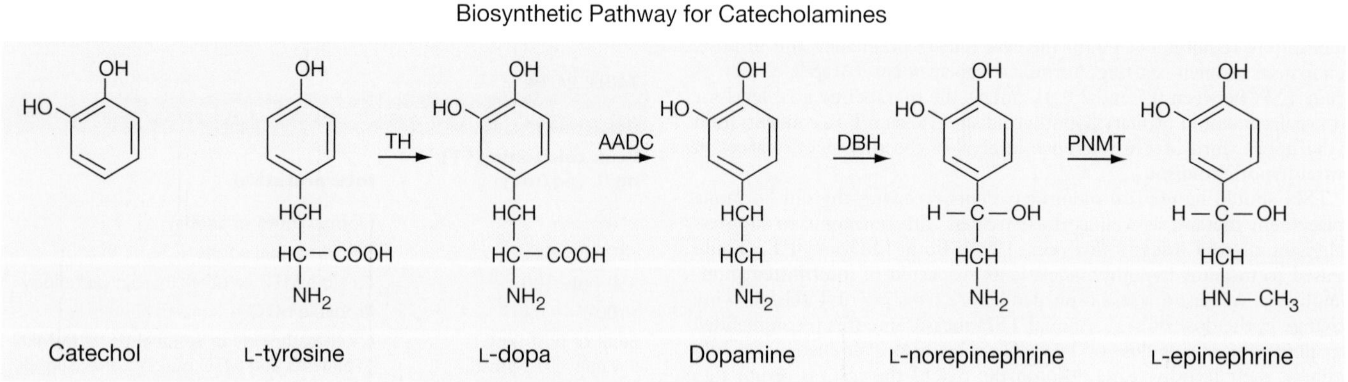

Figure 24-9 Catecholamines: biosynthetic pathway. The rate-limiting step is the conversion of L-tyrosine to L-3,4-dihydroxyphenylalanine (L-dopa) through the actions of tyrosine hydroxylase. *(Redrawn from Dluhy RG, Lawrence JE, Williams GH. Endocrine hypertension. In: Larsen PR, Kronenberg HM, Melmed S, Polansky KS, editors. Williams textbook of endocrinology. 10th ed. Philadelphia: WB Saunders; 2003, p. 555, with permission.)*

the upper reference limit (Sheps, 1994; Eisenhofer, 2004a,b). In centers where this assay is not available, the initial test should be the chromatographic measurement of a 24-hour urine collection for normetanephrine, metanephrine, fractionated free catecholamines (epinephrine, norepinephrine, dopamine), and creatinine (Lenders, 2002; Eisenhofer, 2004a,b). Metanephrine is the most sensitive and specific of these metabolites (Heron, 1996). The diagnosis of pheochromocytoma can also be made by measuring plasma catecholamines; however, given their short half-life and episodic secretion,, it is of use only if the sample is collected during a paroxysm. Values from the 24-hour urine collection or plasma catecholamines that are two to three times the upper limit of normal are usually diagnostic of pheochromocytoma.

In cases of **sporadic pheochromocytoma,** the choice and interpretation of diagnostic tests depend on the pretest level of suspicion for disease. In this setting, the 24-hour urinary fractionated metanephrine and fractionated catecholamine measurements provide clinically acceptable sensitivity and significantly better specificity than fractionated plasma free metanephrine values (Sawka, 2003). Given the difficulties in collecting a complete 24-hour urine sample from pediatric patients, fractionated plasma free metanephrines should be considered the biochemical test of choice in that population (Weise, 2002) (Table 24-17).

Several factors can cause false-positive test results, either by stimulating catecholamine secretion and/or by interfering with the assay (Table 24-18). When assaying for plasma free metanephrines, patients should abstain from caffeinated beverages and alcohol for 24 hours before testing. They should also avoid acetaminophen, tricyclic antidepressants, phenoxybenzamine, α-agonists (e.g., Aldomet), and monoamine oxidase inhibitors for at least 5 days before testing (Lenders, 1995). During testing for catecholamines, in addition to the list of items to avoid when testing for metanephrines, the patient should avoid nicotine, sympathomimetics (theophylline, pseudoephedrine), α-agonists (e.g., albuterol), and levodopa/carbidopa. If antihypertensive medications are needed, angiotensin-converting enzyme inhibitors (ACEIs), angiotensin receptor blockers, and selective α1-adrenoceptor blockers (e.g., prazosin) can be used without fear of causing false-positive results (Eisenhofer, 2003).

Although urinary catecholamine levels may be elevated in renal insufficiency and renal failure, the measurement of plasma free metanephrines can be used to reliably diagnose pheochromocytoma in both conditions (Eisenhofer, 2004b). Stressors such as an acute myocardial infarction, congestive heart failure, surgery, and acute cerebrovascular accident are all associated with elevated levels of catecholamines. In these situations, one can treat empirically and test once the patient has stabilized, or other diagnostic tests, including imaging studies, can be used. Plasma normetanephrine concentrations increase with age; as a result, elderly patients are particularly susceptible to having false-positive tests. The use of fractionated urinary metanephrines and catecholamines may be more suitable for this population (Sawka, 2003).

Plasma levels of normetanephrine less than 112 ng/L (0.61 nmol/L) and of metanephrine less than 61 ng/L (0.31 nmol/L) virtually exclude pheochromocytoma, so that no immediate further testing for the tumor should be necessary. With plasma concentrations of normetanephrine above 400 ng/L (2.19 nmol/L) or of metanephrine above 236 ng/L (1.20 nmol/L), the probability of pheochromocytoma is so high that the immediate task is to locate the tumor (Eisenhofer, 2003). More often than not, test results are returned as equivocal, requiring the need for confirmatory tests such as the clonidine suppression test or the glucagon stimulation test, or the measurement of urinary fractionated catecholamines. Clonidine is a centrally acting α-adrenergic agonist; it suppresses catecholamine release from the nervous system, but has no effect on its release by the tumor (Bravo, 1981). In those with pheochromocytoma, clonidine fails to adequately suppress plasma levels of norepinephrine. The clonidine suppression test is indicated only if the plasma catecholamines are greater than 1000 pg/mL (5.9 nmol/L). It is unreliable in those with normal or mildly elevated plasma catecholamines (Taylor, 1986; Elliott, 1988; Sjoberg, 1992). Eisenhofer (2003) showed that measuring plasma normetanephrines before and after clonidine testing increased the sensitivity and specificity of this test, especially in those who have only modest elevations of norepinephrine. The glucagon stimulation test can lead to dangerous rises in blood pressure and is rarely used. It should be performed only in patients whose blood pressure is well controlled, and a physician must be present throughout the test. A rise in plasma norepinephrine to greater than threefold, or greater than 2000 pg/mL, is diagnostic of pheochromocytoma (Table 24-19). The proposed mechanism of action is stimulation of glucagon-sensitive adenylate cyclase receptors expressed on these tumors.

TABLE 24-17

Sensitivity and Specificity of Hormone Levels for Diagnosing Pheochromocytoma

	SENSITIVITY		SPECIFICITY	
	Hereditary	**Sporadic**	**Hereditary**	**Sporadic**
Plasma				
Free metanephrines	97%	99%	96%	82%
Catecholamines	69%	92%	89%	72%
Urine				
Fractionated metanephrines	96%	97%	82%	45%
Catecholamines	79%	91%	96%	75%
Total metanephrines	60%	88%	97%	89%
Vanillylmandelic acid	46%	77%	99%	86%

Data from Pacak K, Eisenhofer G, Ilias I. Diagnostic imaging of pheochromocytoma. Front Horm Res 2004;31:76–106; Lenders JW, Pacak K, Walther MM, et al. Biochemical diagnosis of pheochromocytoma: which test is best? JAMA 2002;287:1427–34.

TABLE 24-18

Effects of Medications on Testing for Pheochromocytoma

	PLASMA				URINE			
Medication class	**NMN**	**NE**	**MN**	**E**	**NMN**	**NE**	**MN**	**E**
Tricyclics	+	+	−	−	+	+	−	−
Phenoxybenzamine	+	+	−	−	+	+	−	−
Buspirone	−	−	−	−	−	−	+	−
α-Adrenergic blockers	−	−	−	−	−	+	−	−
β-Adrenoceptor blockers	−	−	+	−	+	+	+	+
Calcium channel blockers	−	+	−	−	−	+	−	+
Sympathomimetics	+	+	−	−	+	+	−	−

Data from Eisenhofer G, Goldstein DS, Walther, et al. Biochemical diagnosis of pheochromocytoma: how to distinguish true from false-positive test results. J Clin Endocrinol Metab 2003;88:2656–66.

E, Epinephrine; *MN,* metanephrines; *NE,* norepinephrine; *NMN,* normetanephrine.

*Diuretics, angiotensin-converting enzyme inhibitors, and angiotensin II receptor blockers have little influence on the frequency of false-positive results.

TABLE 24-19

Pharmacologic Tests for Diagnosing Pheochromocytoma

Clonidine Suppression Test	
Indications	Patients with hypertension and clinical findings or family history that is highly suggestive of pheochromocytoma and the catecholamines are elevated but not to the extent that is diagnostic of pheochromocytoma.
Interpretation	Normal: Decrease in NE to below normal or a >50% decline from baseline. A decrease in normetanephrines to below normal or a 40% decline from baseline. Pheochromocytoma: Failure of NE to drop below normal or decrease by more than 50% from baseline. Failure of normetanephrines to drop below normal or decrease by more than 40% from baseline.
Glucagon Stimulation Test	
Indications	When clinical findings or family history is highly suggestive of pheochromocytoma but blood pressure is normal and catecholamines are only modestly elevated.
Interpretation	Pheochromocytoma: A threefold or greater increase in plasma NE, or a rise in the level to >2000 pg/mL.

NE, Norepinephrine.

Unless the history is compelling, or the patient falls into one of the categories of genetically inherited disorders, it is often unnecessary to repeat testing in those with slightly positive results.

Among catecholamine-secreting tumors, 10%–20% are familial. Genetic testing should be considered if the patient is younger than age 50 at presentation, has physical traits suggestive of one of the familial disorders, has multifocal disease, or has a positive family history. Tests include assaying for mutations in the gene for menin in MEN 1, the *RET* oncogene in MEN 2A (Sipple's disease) and MEN 2B, neurofibromin in NF-1, and *VHL* in von Hippel–Lindau syndrome. Familial paragangliomas are associated with various defects in the gene for succinate dehydrogenase. As with all genetic testing, pretest and posttest counseling is mandatory.

Chromogranin A (CgA) is a protein that is stored and secreted along with the catecholamines from the adrenal medulla and sympathetic nervous system. Although it is elevated in more than 80% of pheochromocytomas, it is not specific for this disorder, being secreted by other chromaffin tissues (Hsiao, 1991). CgA was initially thought to be useful in the diagnosis of pheochromocytoma, since medications typically used to treat it had no impact on CgA secretion or measurement. Despite a relatively high sensitivity of 86%, it has poor diagnostic specificity. This is due, in large part, to the fact that the kidneys play a major role in the clearance of CgA from the circulation, so that even mild degrees of renal impairment (e.g., creatinine clearance [CrCl] <80 mg/mL/min) can lead to significant increases in serum concentration of CgA (Bravo, 2003). Among hypertensive patients with CrCl less than 80 mL/min, overall sensitivity, specificity, and accuracy and positive and negative predictive values of serum CgA dropped to 85%, 50%, 59%, 38%, and 90%, respectively. However, when combined with elevated plasma catecholamines in patients with CrCl at least 80 mL/min, the diagnostic specificity and positive predictive values improved to 98% and 97%, respectively (Canale, 1994). Its major use is in postoperative monitoring for recurrence of these tumors.

Testing Procedures

For 24-hour urine collections, creatinine is measured to verify the adequacy of the collection. To preserve the specimen adequately, urine should be collected in a container to which 25 mL of 6 NHCl has been added.

Plasma catecholamines are collected after an overnight fast (water permitted). The patient is placed in a reclining position in a quiet environment, and a heparin lock is inserted intravenously. After 20–30 minutes, blood is collected in a prechilled ethylenediaminetetraacetic acid (EDTA) lavender-top tube. The whole blood sample should be kept in ice water until centrifuged (preferably at 4° C). Separation of plasma should take place within 2 hours of phlebotomy; the sample should then be frozen immediately.

Both urine and plasma specimens should be analyzed using high-performance liquid chromatography with tandem mass spectrometry, as this technique greatly eliminates problems caused by interfering substances (Taylor, 2002). For the urine metabolites, it is important to use age-appropriate reference ranges when interpreting the results. It is also important to be aware that reference ranges can vary widely not only from one laboratory to another, but even within the same laboratory, as newer methods are introduced.

Additional Follow-Up Testing

Once the diagnosis is confirmed biochemically, the tumor should be localized by a CT scan or MRI of the adrenals. If this is negative, imaging studies of the abdomen, chest, and pelvis should be performed. CT has greater sensitivity, and MRI, greater specificity. MRI is superior to CT in detecting extraadrenal lesions and has the advantage of not requiring ionizing radiation or needing ionic contrast. If a tumor cannot be located by CT or MRI, or if metastatic disease is suspected, scanning with ^{131}I- or ^{123}I-labeled meta-iodobenzylguanidine should be performed. Octreoscanning and positron emission tomography are reserved for when the other techniques have failed.

Following successful tumor resection, the prognosis is generally excellent. Urinary metanephrines should be retested several weeks after surgery to ensure that the resection was complete, and should be measured periodically thereafter as an early marker of disease recurrence (Werbel, 1995).

An algorithm to evaluate pheochromocytoma has been proposed by Eisenhofer (2003) (Fig. 24-10).

Neuroblastoma

Similarly to pheochromocytoma, neuroblastoma is of neural crest origin, arising within the adrenals or the sympathetic chain. It is the second most common solid malignant tumor in childhood, usually occurring before the age of 3. Symptoms relate primarily to tumor mass rather than to hypertension, which is often mild or absent. At the time of diagnosis, 70% of cases will have distant metastases. About 90% of patients have elevated urinary HVA levels at the time of diagnosis, whereas almost 75% have increased urinary VMA levels (Tuchman, 1985). Both tests should be ordered when screening for the disease. In healthy children, at least up until the age of about 15, urinary VMA and metanephrines tend to be higher (per milligram of creatinine) and more variable than in adults. Urinary metanephrines also can be elevated in neuroblastoma patients, but are not a sensitive measure of residual tumor. Urinary HVA is increased in familial dysautonomia (Riley-Day syndrome) and in some cases of pheochromocytoma.

HORMONES OF THE ADRENAL CORTEX

The adrenal cortex is composed of three distinct zones: The outermost zone, the zona glomerulosa, is followed by the intermediate zona fasciculata, which surrounds the innermost zona reticularis. In the broadest terms, each zone is responsible for the synthesis and secretion of a unique set of hormones: The zona glomerulosa—mineralocorticoids (aldosterone); the zona fasciculata—glucocorticoids (cortisol); and the zona reticularis—sex steroids (dehydroepiandrosterone sulfate and androgens). However, under certain pathologic and physiologic conditions, these distinctions become blurred.

Mineralocorticoid Axis

The chief mineralocorticoid is aldosterone, which promotes the reabsorption of sodium and water by the kidney to help maintain blood pressure and tonicity. Expression of the enzyme CYP11B2 (aldosterone synthetase) within the glomerulosa is site specific; as a result, the synthesis of aldosterone and its intermediary 18-hydroxylated metabolites is restricted to the zona glomerulosa. The precursor molecules to aldosterone, 11-deoxycorticosterone (DOC) and 11-deoxycortisol, similarly possess mineralocorticoid activity. However, unlike aldosterone, they can be synthesized within the zona fasciculata, as well as in the zona glomerulosa, which explains the hypertension and electrolyte disturbances seen in some forms of congenital adrenal hyperplasia. Although aldosterone will respond to acute changes in ACTH, it is mainly under the control of the renin-angiotensin system.

The zona fasciculata makes up 75% of the cortex, and is responsible for the synthesis and secretion of glucocorticoids and to a lesser extent androgens and estrogens. The glucocorticoids are 21-carbon steroid compounds with a hydroxyl group on carbon 17, hence the synonym 17-hydroxycorticosteroids (17-OHCS). Cortisol is the key glucocorticoid, regulating its own secretion through negative feedback on the hypothalamic-pituitary-adrenal (HPA) axis, inhibiting ACTH release from the pituitary and corticotropin-releasing hormone (CRH) from the hypothalamus. Both CRH and AVP (ADH) are produced by the parvocellular neurons of the paraventricular nuclei of the hypothalamus. ACTH secretion is stimulated by CRH and, to a much lesser extent, by AVP. ACTH in turn stimulates cortisol production by the adrenals. Cortisol is needed in times of stress to maintain blood pressure and blood sugar, and to prevent shock. Although cortisol is the most important glucocorticoid, corticosterone, which is a hormone of the mineralocorticoid pathway, also possesses glucocorticoid activity.

Androgens and estrogens are produced by the zona reticularis. The androgens are 18-carbon steroids with saturated A rings, in contrast to the estrogens, which are 17-carbon steroids with unsaturated A rings.

The functions of these hormones are summarized in Table 24-20.

Congenital Disorders of Adrenal Cortical Enzyme Deficiencies

The hormones of the adrenal cortex are steroid derivatives, synthesized from low-density lipoprotein (LDL) cholesterol. LDL is delivered to the adrenals where it is taken up by LDL receptors. Evidence also supports local synthesis of LDL from acetyl coenzyme A. Steroid acute regulatory protein (StAR) shuttles LDL across the mitochondrial membrane, where it begins its journey down the steroidogenic pathway (Fig. 24-11). The enzymes that catalyze these synthetic reactions are of four general types: hydroxylases, dehydrogenases, desmolases, and isomerases. Because most of the inborn errors of metabolism affecting steroid hormone synthesis in the adrenal cortex involve deficiencies of hydroxylases, they constitute the most clinically important group of enzymes.

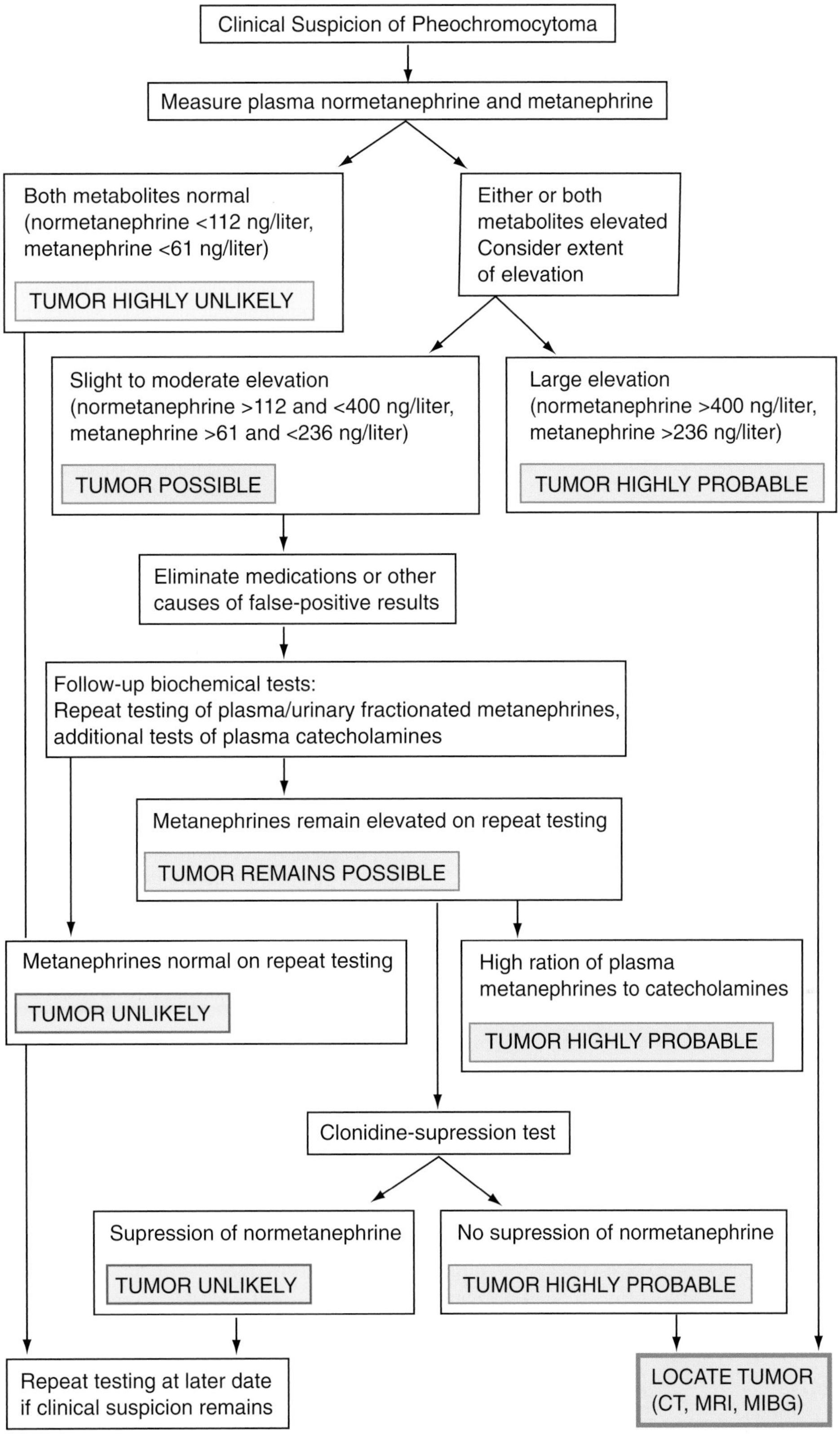

Figure 24-10 Algorithm for the evaluation of pheochromocytoma. *(Redrawn from Eisenhofer G, Goldstein DS, Walther MM, et al. Biochemical diagnosis of pheochromocytoma: how to distinguish true- from false-positive test results. J Clin Endocrinol Metab 2003;88:2656–66, with permission.) CT,* Computed tomography (scan); *MIBG,* metaiodobenzylguanidine (scan); *MRI,* magnetic resonance imaging.

At least eight different metabolic defects in the synthesis of cortisol and aldosterone have been described, each characterized by a deficiency of a specific adrenal enzyme. A vast majority of these enzymatic deficiencies are inherited as an autosomal recessive trait with variable degrees of penetrance. Those enzymatic defects that uniquely affect the biosynthesis of cortisol are grouped together under the rubric of congenital adrenal hyperplasia (CAH). These five enzymes are P450scc (defect in StAR), 3-β-hydroxysteroid dehydrogenase, 21-hydroxylase, 11-hydroxylase, and 17-hydroxylase. CRH and ACTH synthesis and secretion are normally under the negative-feedback control of cortisol. In CAH, defects in the enzymes necessary for cortisol production lead to cortisol deficiency; cortisol deficiency results in disinhibition of negative feedback on CRH and ACTH production. As a consequence, CRH and ACTH levels rise, inducing adrenal hyperplasia and a forward push in steroidogenesis, as the body tries to compensate and normalize cortisol production. Not only does this result in a buildup of hormonal precursors directly preceding the enzymatic defect, it also causes massive shunting of these precursors down the remaining functional pathways. The clinical manifestations of CAH are heterogeneous, depending on the severity and location of the enzymatic defects, which hormones are deficient, and which are produced in excess. Symptoms range from shock, salt-wasting, and anomalous sexual development in infancy, to hirsutism and infertility in the adult.

TABLE 24-20
Physiologic Effects of Steroids

Representative hormone	Biological effects
Cortisol (as a representative glucocorticoid)	Protein nitrogen catabolism increased
	Gluconeogenesis
	Increased blood glucose concentration
	Decreased glucose tolerance
	Increased liver glycogen
	Increased liver glycogenolysis
	Decreased peripheral uptake and utilization of glucose
	Decreased synthesis of acid-sulfated mucopolysaccharides
	Fat synthesis and redistribution
	Cellular or tissue effects
	Antiinflammatory
	Dissolution of lymphoid tissue
	Lymphopenia
	Eosinopenia
	Increased erythropoiesis
	Alteration of cellular permeability, especially decreased membrane permeability to water
	Increased gastric (HCl and pepsin) secretion
Aldosterone (as a representative mineralocorticoid)	Electrolyte regulation
	Sodium (Na+) retention
	Potassium (K+) excretion
	Retention of water and expansion of extracellular fluid volume
	Increases in blood pressure
Androgens (as representative sex hormones)	Protein nitrogen anabolism
	Growth and maturation—osseous and muscular
	Body hair (pubic and axillary)

Sometimes, as in partial enzymatic deficiencies of cortisol synthesis, near-adequate hormone synthesis is possible if hypersecretion of ACTH is able to stimulate adrenal hyperplasia to compensate for the deficiency. The clinical manifestations of various adrenal cortical enzyme deficiencies and their associated laboratory findings are summarized in Table 24-21.

The diagnosis is made by measuring the various serum hormone levels and assessing which steroids are produced in excess and which are deficient, and by calculating the precursor/product ratio and comparing these results to age- and sex-matched normative data. Levels of hormones distal to the block (product hormones) may be elevated as a result of peripheral conversion of the markedly elevated precursor hormones; the use of precursor/product ratios mitigates the risk of misdiagnosis due to misleading elevations of product hormones (Levine, 2002). If hormone levels return as borderline, but the clinical suspicion for CAH remains high, the steroid levels should be remeasured 60 minutes after intravenous administration of 0.25 mg of ACTH. ACTH drives steroidogenesis forward, accentuating the block. When there is a proband, the diagnosis can be more accurately determined by genotyping.

CAH is categorized according to severity of disease into classic (neonatal, severe) and nonclassic (late-onset, cryptogenic) forms. The classic form is further subdivided into salt-losing and non–salt-losing (simple virilizing) variants.

21-Hydroxylase Deficiency

The enzyme 21-hydroxylase (also referred to as CYP21, CYP21A2, and P450c21) is located within the mitochondrial endoplasmic reticulum. It is the most common cause of CAH, occurring in about 95% of all cases. Screening of newborns using capillary heel blood on paper filter disks has identified this disorder in about 1 in 14,000 persons in North America, and in as many as 1 in 300 Yupik Eskimos of Alaska (Pang, 1988, 1982). The classic form is detected in about 1 in 16,000 live births; the nonclassic form is seen in about 0.2% of the general Caucasian population, and in 1%–2% of those of Eastern European Jewish ancestry (Speiser, 1985; Therrell, 2001).

21-OH catalyzes the conversion of 17-hydroxyprogesterone (17-OHP) to 11-deoxycortisol (compound S), and progesterone to DOC. Thus, 21-OH deficiency leads to elevated levels of the steroid precursors 17-OHP and pregnanetriol in the urine and 17-OHP in the serum. These precursors are shunted toward the pathway, leading to excess androstenedione and testosterone production (Fig. 24-12). Clinical presentation often correlates with the severity of enzymatic dysfunction. The classic variety presents in the newborn period or in early childhood with adrenal insufficiency and virilization, with or without salt-wasting. The nonclassic form presents in late childhood as early adrenarche, or in young adulthood as

TABLE 24-21
Congenital Adrenal Hyperplasia: Clinical and Biochemical Features

Feature	21-Hydoxylase deficiency	11-β-hydoxylase deficiency	17-β-hydroxylase deficiency	3-β-hydroxysteroid deficiency	Lipoid hyperplasia	Aldosterone synthase deficiency
Defective gene	*CYP21*	*CYP11B1*	*CYP17*	*HSD3B2*	*StAR*	*CYP11B2*
Incidence	1:15,000	1:100,000	Rare	Rare	Rare	Rare
Ambiguous genitalia	+ (female)	+ (female)	+ (male) Absent puberty (female)	+ (male) Mild in female	+ (male) Absent puberty (female)	Normal
Acute adrenal insufficiency	+	Rare	No	+	++	Salt-wasting only
Laboratory findings	↑ plasma 17-OHP and pregnanetriol Greatly ↑ urinary pregnanetriol and 17-KS	↑ serum DOC and 11-deoxycortisol ↑ urinary 17-OHCS and 17-KS	↑ serum DOC, 18-OH DOC, B, and 18-OHB	↑ serum 17-OH-pregnenolone, pregnenolone and DHEA ↑ urinary 17-KS ↑ Δ5/Δ4 serum and urinary steroids	All serum and plasma steroids are decreased	↑ serum B, 11-DOC, and 18-OHB
Glucocorticoids	↓	↓	↓	↓	↓	Normal
Mineralocorticoids	↓	↑	↓	↓	↓	↓
Androgens	↑	↑	↓	↓ male, ↑ female	↓	Normal

From Stewart PM. The adrenal cortex. In: Larsen PR, Kronenberg HM, Melmed S, Polonsky KS, editors. Williams textbook of endocrinology. 10th ed. Philadelphia: WB Saunders; 2003, p. 533.

B, Corticosterone; *DHEA,* dihydroepiandosterone; *11-DOC,* 11-deoxycorticosterone; *17-KS,* 17-ketosteroids; *18-OHB,* 18-hydroxycorticosterone; *17-OHP,* 17-α-hydroxyprogesterone.

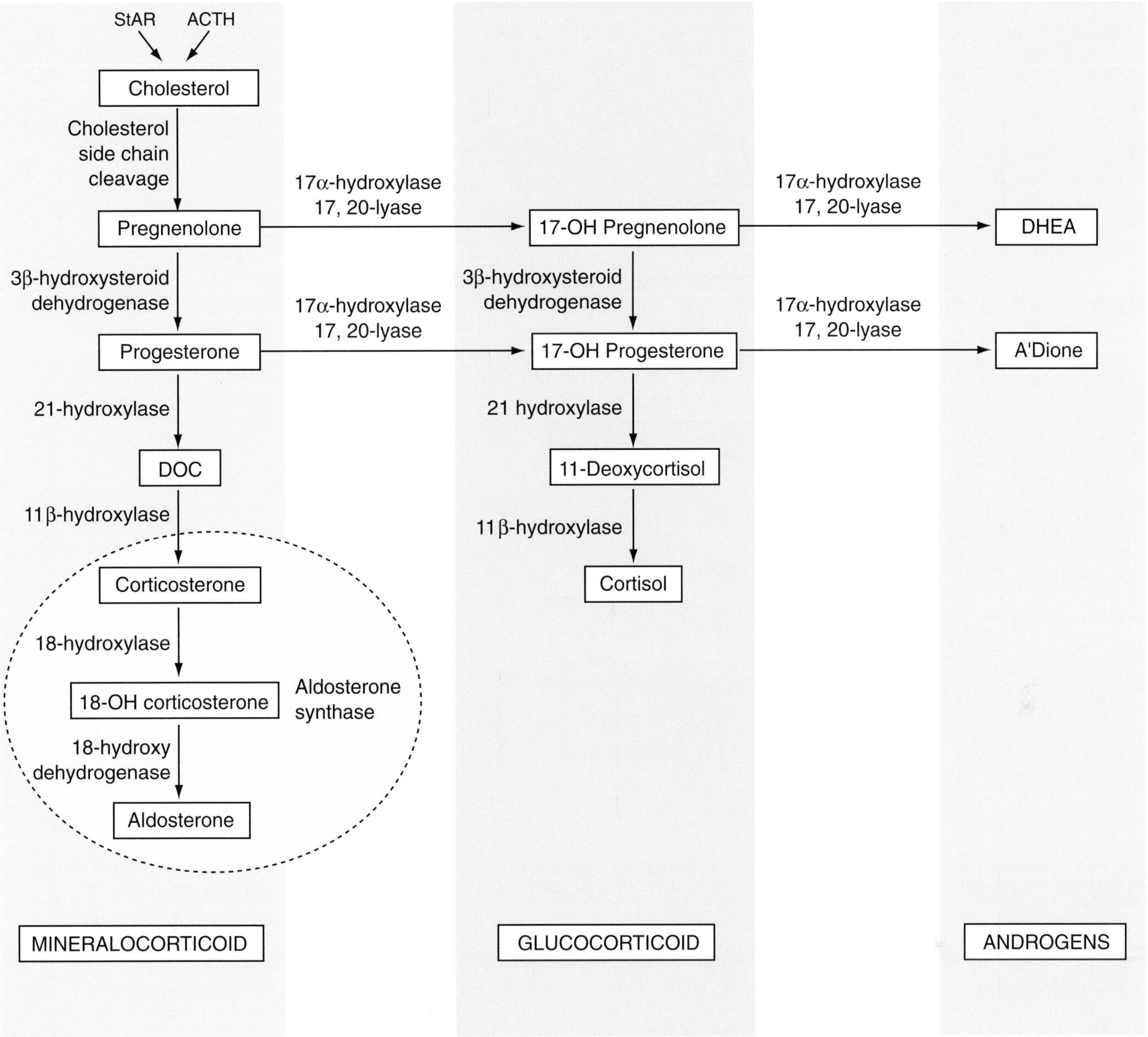

Figure 24-11 Steroidogeneic pathways of the adrenal cortex. The adrenal steroids are categorized according to mineralocorticoid, glucocorticoid, or androgenic activity. The chemical structures for these steroids are shown in Figure 25-1 in the succeeding chapter. *ACTH,* Adrenocorticotropin; *DHEA,* dehydroepiandrosterone; *DOC,* deoxycorticosterone; *StAR,* steroidogenic acute regulatory (protein).

hirsutism, amenorrhea, and infertility. The presentation in women is very similar to that of polycystic ovarian disease. Males may develop precocious puberty, adrenal rests within the testes, and infertility.

A close functional relationship exists between the adrenal cortex and the adrenal medulla. Dysplasia of the medulla and catecholamine hyposecretion have been described in classic 21-OH deficiency. In a study of 38 children with classic (CYP21A2) disease, levels of plasma epinephrine and metanephrine and urinary epinephrine were 40%–80% lower in affected individuals than in normal persons (Merke, 2000). In another study, those with CYP21A2 showed a significantly decreased catecholamine response to exercise that was unaffected by the administration of stress doses of glucocorticoids (Weise, 2004). It has been suggested that the degree of medullary impairment may be a biomarker for CAH severity (Merke, 2002).

Diagnosis. Prenatal diagnosis is important because suppressive treatment with steroids can abrogate the development of virilization of the female fetus. Diagnosis is made by measuring the level of 17-OHP in amniotic fluid or by genotyping cells obtained by chorionic villous sampling. The genes responsible for 21-OH deficiency, *CYP21* (CYP21A2) and *CYP21P* (CYP21A), are located on chromosome 6. Of these two homologous genes, only *CYP21* is active; deleterious mutations within *CYP21P* interfere with normal gene expression. These mutations can be identified by PCR and Southern blotting on chorionic villous samples (White, 1994a; New, 1995). The 2010 consensus statement on the management of CAH due to 21-OH deficiency recommends that prenatal treatment of CAH be regarded as experimental and that the diagnosis should rest on clinical and hormonal data, with genotyping being reserved for equivocal cases and genetic counseling (Speiser, 2010).

Neonatal screening, which is now mandatory in many states, is performed by measuring 17-OHP or by genotyping blood that has been obtained from a heelstick and collected on filter paper. Aside from genotyping being the most definitive test for diagnosing CAH, the fact that the genotype correlates fairly well with disease severity means that it can also be used as a prognostic tool (Nordenstrom, 1999).

In the newborn with salt-wasting, unstimulated 17-OHP levels are typically >8000 ng/dL, rising to 100,000 ng/dL (3000 nmol/L) following administration of ACTH. Levels in the simple virilizing variant range from 10,000–30,000 ng/dL (300–1000 nmol/L). Those with nonclassic disease typically have 17-OHP levels ranging from 1500–10,000 ng/dL (50–300 nmol/L) (New, 1983). It is of note that randomly drawn hormone levels may be normal in those with nonclassic disease; therefore it is important to test during the early morning. If the results are equivocal, the diagnosis can be confirmed by comparing serum 17-OHP levels before and 60 minutes after administration of 0.25 mg ACTH (Cortrosyn). ACTH acts to stimulate steroidogenesis, serving to dramatically increase

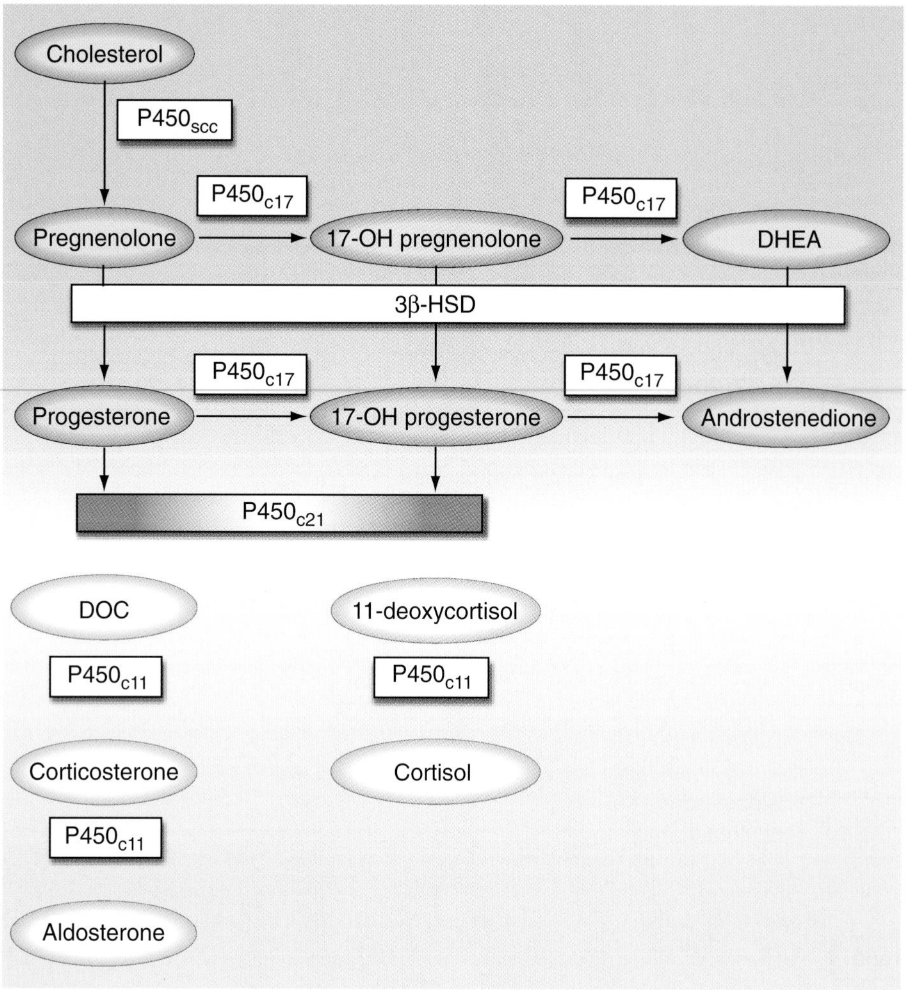

Figure 24-12 Defective steroidogenesis due to 21-hydroxylase deficiency. The relative increase in the hormones proximal to the block is depicted by more intense color. The more severe the enzymatic defect, the greater the concentration of the precursor hormones. *DHEA,* Dehydroepiandrosterone; *DOC,* deoxycorticosterone.

the bottleneck at the site of the enzymatic block, resulting in a dramatic increase in precursors, in this case, 17-OHP. Post-ACTH 17-OHP values <330 ng/dL are normal, 330–1000 ng/dL indicates a heterozygote carrier, and levels >2000 ng/dL are diagnostic for nonclassic CAH. If a proband is available, genotyping is superior to these older biochemical tests in identifying heterozygotes (Honour, 1993).

The goals of glucocorticoid and mineralocorticoid replacement therapy in children is the attainment of normal growth, weight, and pubertal development, and optimization of final adult height. On the other hand, major treatment goals in adults include lessening of signs of virilization and resumption of fertility. The objective of mineralocorticoid replacement is to normalize the plasma renin activity. The aim of glucocorticoid replacement is to keep the 17-OHP level partially suppressed to between 100 and 1000 ng/dL (3–30 nmol/L) and the ACTH under 100 ng/L, thereby preventing shunting toward testosterone synthesis, and normalizing levels of androstenedione and testosterone. Normalization of 17-OHP should not be attempted, because this requires supraphysiologic levels of glucocorticoids and may result in Cushing's syndrome (Speiser, 2003).

11-β-Hydroxylase Deficiency

The second most common enzyme deficiency of the adrenal cortex, accounting for about 7% of all cases of CAH, is the 11-β-hydroxylase (11-OH) deficiency. A defect in this enzyme blocks the final conversion of 11-deoxycortisol to cortisol and DOC to corticosterone. As with 21-OH deficiency, a compensatory increase in ACTH secretion leads to adrenal hyperplasia and a mass action shunting of precursor steroids toward testosterone synthesis, resulting in signs of virilization. This block also results in the accumulation of DOC; the mineralocorticoid activity of DOC leads to the development of hypertension and hypokalemia, similar to what is seen with hyperaldosteronism (Fig. 24-13).

11-OH deficiency is an autosomal recessive disorder caused by mutations of the genes *CYP11B1* and *CYP11B2,* located on chromosome 8q21-q22 (White, 1994b). Diagnosis in the neonate is established by the presence of a high basal and a high ACTH-stimulated 11-deoxycortisol. Concentrations of urinary tetrahydro-11-deoxycortisol in the urine are also elevated. During childhood and in young adults, the diagnosis of 11-OH deficiency is made by the presence of elevated early-morning and ACTH-stimulated serum levels of 11-deoxycortisol that are more than three times the upper limit for age-matched normals. Levels of DOC and adrenal androgens (androstenedione, dehydroepiandrosterone, and dehydroepiandrosterone sulfate) are also elevated. Plasma renin activity and aldosterone are often suppressed as a result of salt and water retention induced by elevations of DOC. Unlike the heterozygotes with 21-OH deficiency, those with 11-OH deficiency often fail to show a rise in precursors following ACTH stimulation (Pang, 1980). However, an exuberant response has been seen in those who had hirsutism (Gabrilove, 1965).

Prenatal diagnosis of 11-OH deficiency is made by measuring levels of tetrahydro-11-deoxycortisol (THS) in the maternal urine or amniotic fluid. These levels begin to rise in the first trimester. In addition to THS, elevation of levels of 11-deoxycortisol and of the THS to tetrahydrocortisol plus tetrahydrocortisone ratio is seen (Rosler, 1988).

Treatment consists of the replacement of glucocorticoids, causing normalization of DOC and plasma renin activity.

3-β-Hydroxysteroid Dehydrogenase Deficiency

3-β-hydroxysteroid dehydrogenase (3-β-HSD), which catalyzes the second enzymatic step in steroidogenesis, is coded by two genes, *HSD3BI* and *HSD3BII. HSD3BII* is expressed in the adrenals and gonads; *HSD3BI* is expressed in placenta, skin, and other peripheral tissues and usually remains functionally intact at these sites in CAH. A defect in 3-β-HSD leads to a

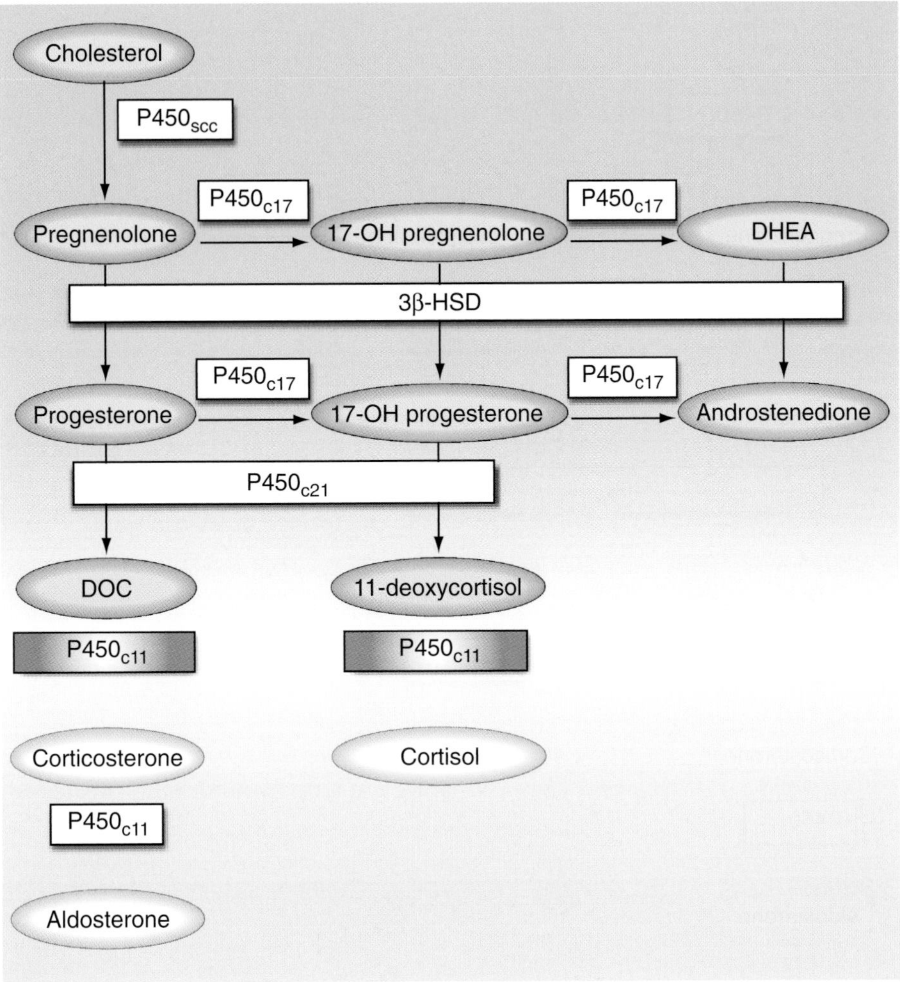

Figure 24-13 Defective steroidogenesis due to 11-β-hydroxylase deficiency. The relative increase in the hormones proximal to the block is depicted by more intense color. The more severe the enzymatic defect, the greater the concentration of the precursor hormones. High levels of 11-deoxycorticosterone (DOC) created by the block produce a state of mineralocorticoid excess. *DHEA,* Dehydroepiandrosterone.

block in the conversion of Δ5 steroids (pregnenolone, 17-OH pregnenolone, and dihydroepiandrosterone) to Δ4 steroids (progesterone, 17-OHP, androstenedione), resulting in an increase in circulating levels of Δ5 steroids (Fig. 24-14). However, because *HSD3BI* is usually intact, levels of the Δ4 steroids may be normal or even elevated.

Patients with classic disease will have manifestations of glucocorticoid deficiency, with or without the accompaniment of salt-wasting. Affected males have incomplete masculinization, and females may be normal or may have ambiguous genitalia. A late-onset variant has been described that is associated with features typical of polycystic ovary disease, such as hirsutism, oligomenorrhea, and infertility (Pang, 1985).

Previous criteria for the diagnosis of 3-β-HSD deficiency examined the basal and ACTH-stimulated Δ4/Δ5 steroid ratios, 17-OH-pregnenolone (17-OHP)/cortisol, and levels of pregnenolone, 17-OH-pregnenolone, and dehydroepiandrosterone in urine and blood. The standard for diagnosing this disorder has been recently revised to correlate more closely with genotypic studies. The ACTH-stimulated Δ5-17 P levels and Δ5-17 P/cortisol ratios have been shown to be the best indices for definitively diagnosing 3-β-HSD deficiency (Lutfallah, 2002). Applicability of these new criteria to patients with the nonclassic variant is still debatable.

Treatment consists of glucocorticoids and mineralocorticoids, as well as sex steroids, in accordance with normal growth and development.

17-Hydroxylase Deficiency

17-Hydroxylase (CYP17, $P450_{c17}$) is expressed in the adrenals and the gonads and encodes two enzymes—17-α-hydroxylase and 17,20-lyase. 17-α-hydroxylase catalyzes the conversion of pregnenolone and progesterone to their respective 17-OH derivatives. 17,20-Lyase converts 17-OH pregnenolone to dihydroepiandosterone, and 17-OH progesterone to androstenedione. CYP17 deficiency blocks the conversion of pregnenolone and progesterone to the 17-hydroxy derivatives, causing shunting from testosterone and cortisol synthesis to aldosterone (Fig. 24-15). Accordingly, these patients develop hypertension and hypokalemic alkalosis in association with incomplete masculinization (in the male) and decreased testosterone and cortisol levels. 17-OH deficiency is diagnosed by demonstrating high DOC, pregnenolone, and progesterone levels, along with decreased urinary 17-ketosteroids and 17-hydroxycorticosteroids. The gene associated with this condition (*CYP17*) has been located on chromosome 10q, the same gene as 17,20-desmolase (Kater, 1994).

Congenital Lipoid Adrenal Hyperplasia

Congenital lipoid adrenal hyperplasia (lipoid CAH) is the most severe form of CAH, in which the synthesis of all gonadal and adrenal cortical steroids is markedly impaired. Lipoid CAH may be caused by a defect in the StAR or the P450 side chain cleavage (scc) (Fujieda, 2003). StAR, located on chromosome 8p11, controls the rate-limiting step in steroidogenesis. It is responsible for the shuttling of cholesterol from the outer to the inner mitochondrial membrane. 20,22-Desmolase (CYP11A1, P450scc) converts cholesterol to pregnenolone (Fig. 24-16). Pathologically, the adrenal cortex shows marked accumulation of cholesterol and other lipids, which is the primary distinguishing feature from congenital adrenal hypoplasia.

The presentation of this extremely rare disorder is that of severe adrenal insufficiency with hypotension, salt-wasting, and feminization of external genitalia in males. Occasionally, females may not present until the onset of puberty. Diagnosis is made by the presence of extremely low cortisol and aldosterone concentrations and elevated ACTH and plasma renin activity.

Aldosterone Synthetase Deficiency

Aldosterone synthetase (CYP11B2) is the final step in the steroid synthetic pathway leading to the production of aldosterone. It stimulates a multistep

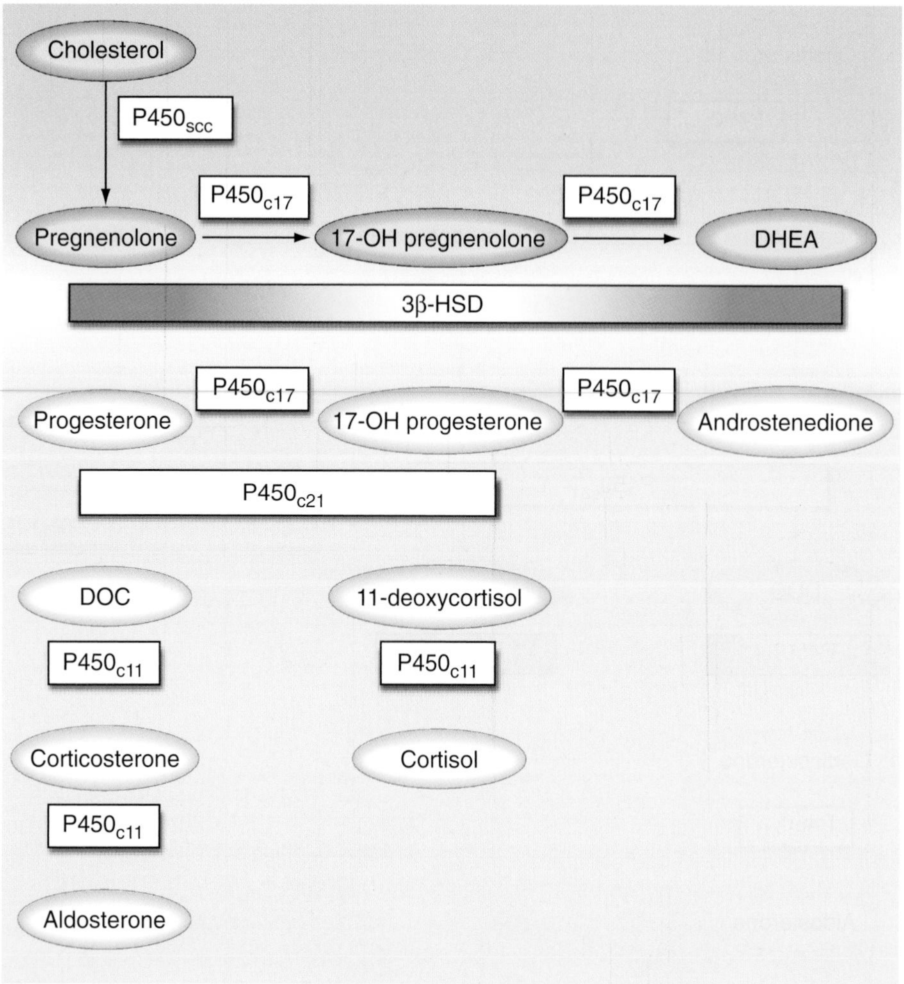

Figure 24-14 Defective steroidogenesis due to 3-β-hydroxysteroid dehydrogenase deficiency. The relative increase in the hormones proximal to the block is depicted by more intense color. The more severe the enzymatic defect, the greater the concentration of the precursor hormones. 17-α-hydroxyprogesterone levels may be elevated because of peripheral conversion of 17-α-hydroxy pregnenolone. *DHEA,* Dehydroepiandrosterone; *DOC,* deoxycorticosterone.

process: 11-hydroxylation of DOC to corticosterone, 18-hydroxylation of corticosterone to 18-hydroxycorticosterone, and finally, 18-dehydrogenation to aldosterone. Isolated enzyme deficiency leads to salt-wasting, hyperkalemia, and metabolic acidosis. This condition may be diagnosed by demonstrating the presence of metabolites of corticosterone and 11-deoxycorticosterone in the urine, elevated serum DOC, and deficiency of corticosterone, 18-hydroxycorticosterone, or aldosterone in the serum.

Cortisol and the Glucocorticoids

The adrenal cortex secretes cortisol in response to ACTH, a diurnal rhythm, and stress. ACTH, synthesized in the adenohypophysis, is formed from the cleavage of a much larger precursor molecule: POMC. In addition to ACTH, cleavage of POMC releases β-LPH, which in turn is cleaved to yield γ-LPH and β-endorphin. Within the ACTH sequence are α-MSH and the corticotropin-like intermediate lobe protein. Endorphins, which act on neurons in the brain, constitute a distinct peptidergic system related to pain perception. Although β-endorphin is secreted in parallel with ACTH, the significance of this remains unknown.

ACTH consists of 39 amino acid residues, of which residues 1–24 at the amino terminal possess full hormonal activity. Occasionally, POMC is incompletely processed; this leads to the formation of other forms of ACTH that usually have little biological activity, although they may retain immunoreactivity. These forms may predominate in malignant conditions such as ectopic production by primary or metastatic lung cancer, and in some patients with Nelson's syndrome, a disorder characterized by the occurrence of a pituitary tumor and skin hyperpigmentation following bilateral adrenalectomy. Defects in POMC cleavage enzymes may also be responsible for the formation of rare forms of isolated ACTH deficiency (Nussey, 1993).

ACTH is secreted in response to several factors, of which CRH and AVP are the most important. Among the other moieties reported to stimulate ACTH secretion are atrial natriuretic factor (ANF), angiotensin II, IL-6, IL-1, and tumor necrosis factor-α (Rivier, 1983; Chrousos, 1998).

CRH is synthesized and released from the hypothalamus; it acts to stimulate the synthesis and release of ACTH from the pituitary. CRH is released in a circadian pattern and in response to physiologic stimuli such as stress and hypoglycemia. The HPA axis consists of various feedback loops that control cortisol synthesis and secretion. When plasma cortisol increases, it suppresses the release of ACTH, CRH, and AVP, which, in turn, leads to lowering of the cortisol level. Conversely, when serum cortisol reaches a nadir, the hypothalamus and pituitary respond by increasing CRH and ACTH production, leading to stimulation of cortisol formation and secretion. By this mechanism, ACTH and cortisol control the concentration of each other within a very narrow range, and a small change in one results in a concomitant change in the other. When the adrenal is unable to respond to ACTH because of damage or disease, cortisol levels are low and ACTH levels are high. In those conditions in which the pituitary is destroyed, ACTH is not formed and cortisol levels are consequently low. Damage to the hypothalamus is also associated with low ACTH and cortisol levels; testing with CRH may permit the distinction between these two entities. Synthetic forms of CRH are used in testing the anterior pituitary reserve of ACTH by comparing plasma ACTH and cortisol before and 1 hour after CRH stimulation (Grodum, 1993). This test is useful in distinguishing between lesions affecting the hypothalamus, pituitary, and adrenal glands (Fukata, 1993). If the lesion is in the hypothalamus, after a time delay, ACTH levels rise following CRH administration. If it is in the pituitary, no significant ACTH response occurs. With primary adrenal insufficiency, administration of CRH causes a further rise in an already elevated ACTH level, but little or no rise in the level of cortisol.

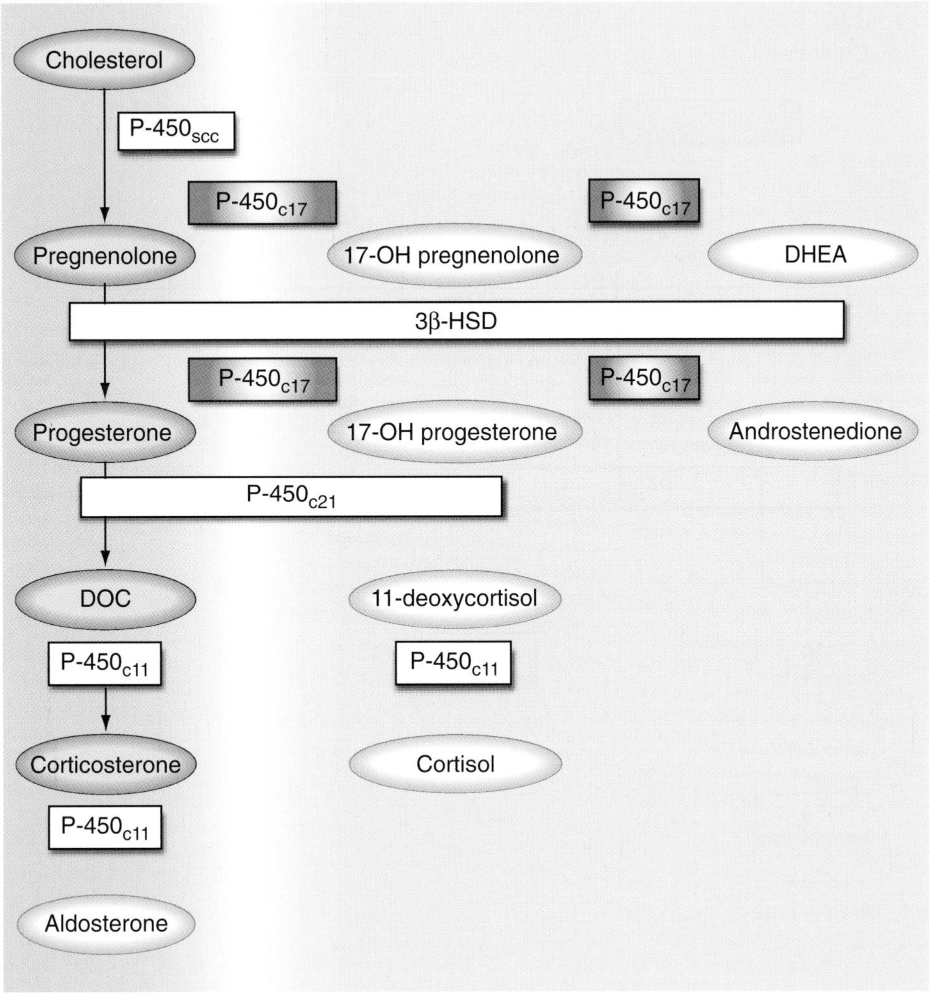

Figure 24-15 Defective steroidogenesis due to 17-hydroxylase deficiency. The relative increase in hormones proximal to the block is depicted by more intense color. The more severe the enzymatic defect, the greater the concentration of the precursor hormones. High levels of 11-deoxycorticosterone (DOC) and corticosterone created by the block produce a state of mineralocorticoid excess. *DHEA,* Dehydroepiandrosterone.

If the HPA axis is interrupted by the administration of large quantities of exogenous glucocorticoids, they will exert an inhibitory effect on the hypothalamus and pituitary, suppressing CRH and ACTH secretion. If this suppression continues over a period of weeks, it leads to atrophy of the adrenals; as a result, the HPA axis becomes unable to secrete cortisol in times of stress. The HPA axis can fully recover after tapering off of steroids.

The second influence on plasma cortisol levels is the diurnal pattern, which is due to the circadian pattern of ACTH release. Major increases in secretion occur at between 4 AM and 8 AM, followed by a decrease in ACTH during the rest of the day. In subjects with a normal sleep-wake cycle, the lowest ACTH concentrations are found shortly after midnight. Sudden changes in sleep-wake patterns have little effect on the diurnal pattern, but permanent changes in daily sleep habits result in a gradual change in diurnal secretory patterns. Superimposed on the circadian periodicity is an ultradian rhythm of 10–18 secretory bursts per 24 hours (Horrocks, 1990).

The third important influence on cortisol secretion is stress. Stimuli such as surgical trauma, pyrogens, hypoglycemia, and hemorrhage are capable of bringing about an acute increase in ACTH and cortisol secretion. This response to stress may be absent or decreased in magnitude in patients in whom large doses of steroids have been administered for some time. The initiation of any stress response is dependent on an intact nervous system. For example, trauma normally results in the acute release of ACTH and cortisol; however, in patients with spinal cord transections, the normal transmission of neurologic stimuli is interrupted, and as a result, the same trauma applied to an extremity will not elicit any ACTH or cortisol response. Evidence suggests that the stress response of cortisol is mediated through excitatory and inhibitory inputs that integrate at the level of the hypothalamus and modulate CRH secretion. Cortisol levels also rise after meals, especially those high in protein, and also in depression (Linkowski, 1987).

Most disorders of cortisol secretion can be classified by the patterns of response of the following three hormones to suppression and stimulation: ACTH, plasma cortisol, and urinary free cortisol (Snow, 1992).

Laboratory Measurement of ACTH

Plasma ACTH is measured using a two-site immunoradiometric assay or an immunochemiluminometric assay. To prevent degradation of ACTH, it is best to collect the sample in a prechilled EDTA lavender-top tube. The specimen should be kept in an ice bath and should be processed as soon as possible. Following centrifugation in a refrigerated centrifuge, the specimen should be separated, transferred to a plastic tube, and kept frozen at −20° C until time of analysis. The normal reference range is 2–12 pmol/L (9–52 pg/mL) between 7 AM and 10 AM. Plasma ACTH is a useful tool for distinguishing primary (adrenal) from secondary (pituitary) or tertiary (hypothalamic) adrenal insufficiency. In primary adrenal insufficiency, low cortisol concentrations are found, along with increased ACTH levels. In secondary or tertiary adrenal insufficiency, both ACTH and cortisol are expected to be low. ACTH levels best discriminate between healthy individuals and those with adrenal insufficiency when specimens for ACTH are collected between 8 AM and 10 AM.

ACTH is less useful in diseases of cortisol excess. Up to 50% of patients may have normal ACTH levels in Cushing's disease. Although the values tend to run higher (>20 pmol/L [>90 pg/mL]) in Cushing's syndrome due to ectopic ACTH production, the values overlap with those seen in Cushing's disease in 30% of cases (Findling, 1992). Because of the normal diurnal variation in ACTH and cortisol secretion, measurement of these values during their expected nadir, from 11 PM to 1 AM, is helpful in confirming the diagnosis of ACTH-dependent Cushing's disease. An elevated

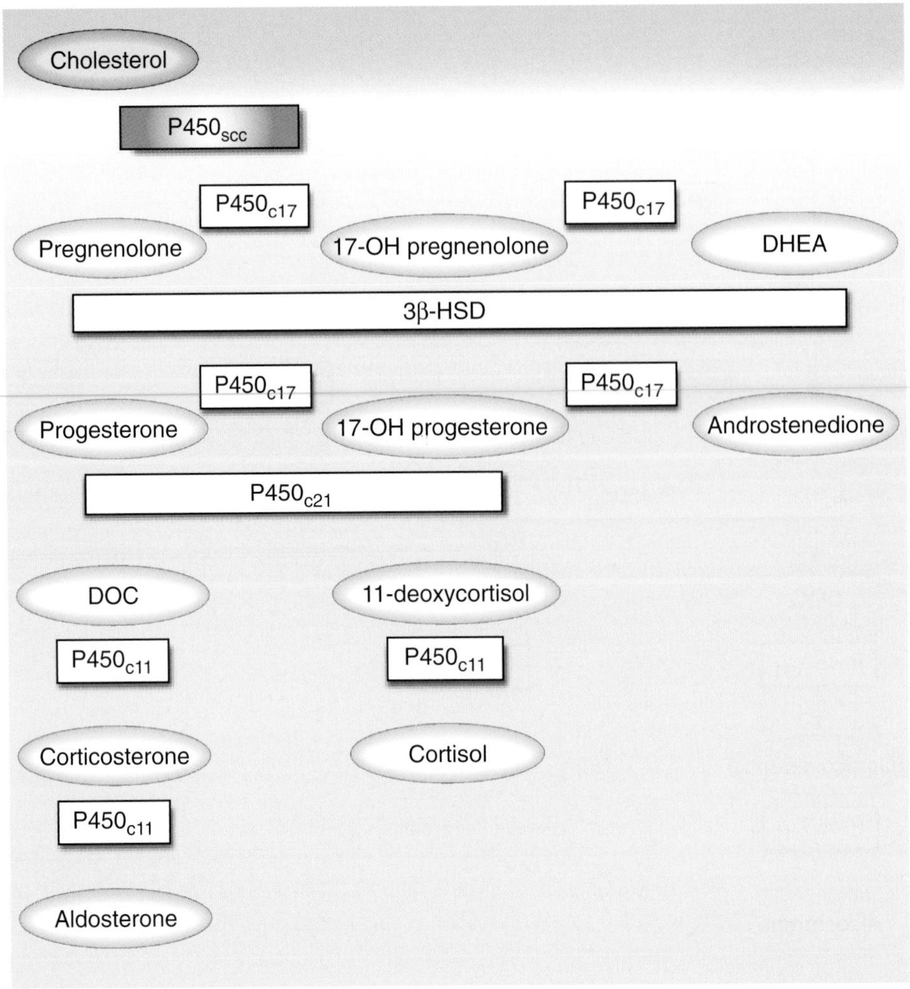

Figure 24-16 Defective steroidogenesis in congenital lipoid adrenal hyperplasia is due to a defect in steroidogenic acute regulatory protein or the side-chain cleavage enzyme (P450scc). The relative increase in hormones proximal to the block is depicted by more intense color. In this disorder, the synthesis of all classes of steroids is defective. *DHEA,* Dehydroepiandrosterone; *DOC,* deoxycorticosterone.

midnight ACTH of greater than 5 pmol/L (23 pg/mL) in the face of an elevated serum cortisol confirms the diagnosis of ACTH-dependent Cushing's disease. Those patients with ectopic ACTH-secreting tumors characteristically have markedly elevated plasma ACTH (usually >200 pg/mL) and elevated serum cortisol. Measurement of ACTH by plasma extraction, which detects ACTH precursors and fragments, may be useful in distinguishing patients with cancer-related syndromes or ACTH-secreting tumors from those with Cushing's disease, as the former entities are more likely to produce these other forms of ACTH (White, 1993). ACTH-secreting neoplasms may be occult, creating diagnostic difficulties; in this instance, ACTH measurement using selective venous sampling has proven useful in localization of the lesion.

In patients with increased levels of circulating glucocorticoids due to an adrenal adenoma or carcinoma, and those surreptitiously taking steroids, ACTH secretion is inhibited and levels are low or undetectable. In patients with pituitary-induced adrenal hyperplasia (Cushings' disease), plasma ACTH may be at or above the upper reference interval at 9 AM, and fail to show the expected fall after midnight. Another use of ACTH assays is in the determination of adequacy of cortisol replacement in congenital adrenal hyperplasia. When replacement therapy is optimal, ACTH values are similar to those seen in a reference population.

Plasma Corticotropin-Releasing Hormone

CRH measurements are performed by liquid chromatography and tandem mass spectrometry and remain largely a research tool.

CRH circulates in one of two forms—free or bound to CRH-binding protein. The level of CRH-binding protein increases during pregnancy. CRH is increased in patients with Cushing's syndrome due to ectopic production of CRH. The reference range for plasma CRH in men and nonpregnant women is <34 pg/mL. The normative range varies throughout pregnancy: first trimester <40 pg/mL; second trimester <153 pg/mL; and third trimester <847 pg/mL (Goland, 1986).

Serum Cortisol Measurements

About 90% of circulating cortisol is bound to serum protein, of which 10%–20% is loosely bound to albumin, and the remainder is bound to the glycoprotein transcortin (cortisol-binding globulin [CBG]). The remaining 10% of circulating cortisol is the unbound, free hormone. It is believed that only free cortisol is active, and that the protein-bound fraction is metabolically inert, probably serving as a reservoir for free cortisol. Protein binding also may protect cortisol from deactivation by the liver or filtration by the kidney.

One of the earliest and simplest methods used to determine serum cortisol was a fluorometric assay developed by Nelson and Samuels, which was based on a technique first developed by Porter and Silber (Porter, 1950; Nelson, 1952). A more specific method for cortisol estimation is immunoassay. Advantages include small specimen volume and rapid turnaround time. The problem was that some of the antibodies used showed a large degree of cross-reactivity with other steroid species, resulting in spuriously elevated cortisol concentrations. In chronic renal disease, various steroids and their glucuronides accumulate in the blood, and because these steroids and conjugates may cross-react with antibodies used in the cortisol assay, an interference that can be of the same magnitude as the actual cortisol concentration may result. In CAH, high concentrations of cortisol precursors are seen in the serum because of an enzyme defect. Because these precursors cross-react with assay antibodies, artificial elevations of cortisol are found. The degree of interference varies with the assay used and cannot be easily predicted. Nonisotopic immunoassay methods using organometallic tracers, fluorescence polarization, and enzyme immunoassay techniques have also been developed for cortisol determinations (Bacarese-Hamilton, 1992; Lentjes, 1993; Philomin, 1994). The major disadvantage of all of these cortisol assays continues to be lack of specificity.

The measurement of cortisol by radioimmunoassay (RIA) and chemiluminescent techniques has largely been supplanted by high-performance liquid chromatography (HPLC) with tandem mass spectrometry, which appears to offer the ultimate in specificity. Most HPLC systems for cortisol measurement use reverse-phase liquid chromatography with ultraviolet detection (Volin, 1992). This method is both highly sensitive and free from many of the sources of interference encountered in immunoassays (Samaan, 1993).

Serum cortisol is collected in a no-additive (red-top) tube. Reference values for serum cortisol for men and women roughly range from 5–25 μg/dL (140–690 nmol/L) at 8 AM to 10 AM, dropping to about 3–12 μg/dL (80–330 nmol/L) by 4 PM. Because of wide swings in basal cortisol levels resulting from its diurnal and ultradian pattern of secretion, serum cortisol assays are most useful when evaluated in the context of dynamic manipulation (i.e., adrenal stimulation or suppression).

Salivary Cortisol

Up to 30% of urinary free cortisol (UFC) and dexamethasone suppression screening tests may return an incorrect result. Recent studies have shown that the use of a midnight salivary cortisol (MSC) is a viable alternative. CBG is not present in saliva; therefore the results may be more useful in situations in which CBG concentration is altered. Salivary cortisol is highly stable and easy to collect, making it a useful tool for screening and for diagnosing instances of increased cortisol secretion. It does not appear to be affected by the rate of saliva production and can reflect a change in serum cortisol in as rapid as a few minutes (Read, 1990). Because of alterations in circadian rhythm, it may not be an appropriate test for shift workers or those with highly variable bed times. One study compared the sensitivity for the detection of Cushing's syndrome by nighttime salivary cortisol levels versus that for simultaneous inpatient serum cortisol levels and urine glucocorticoid excretion. It was found that the salivary cortisol measurements worked as well as plasma measurements and better than urine glucocorticoid excretion. The authors concluded that measurement of bedtime salivary cortisol was a practical and accurate screening test for the diagnosis of Cushing's syndrome (Papanicolaou, 2002). Another study compared the diagnostic performance of MSC measurement versus that of midnight serum cortisol (MNC) and UFC in differentiating 41 patients with Cushing's syndrome from 33 with pseudo-Cushing's states, 199 with simple obesity, and 27 healthy normal weight volunteers. In the whole study population, no statistically significant differences in terms of sensitivity, specificity, diagnostic accuracy, and predictive values were observed among tests. In particular, the overall diagnostic accuracy for MSC was similar to those of UFC and MNC (Putignano, 2003; Elamin, 2008). A recent review of the literature has shown that elevated late-night (11 PM–12 AM) salivary cortisol has greater than 90% sensitivity and specificity for the diagnosis of endogenous Cushing's syndrome (Raff, 2009). It is recommended to have the patient avoid tobacco on the day of specimen collection.

Urinary Free Cortisol Measurements

Only 1% of the total adrenal secretion appears in the urine as cortisol, but it is this fraction that provides valuable aid in the diagnosis of adrenal disease. In the kidney, glomerular filtration of free cortisol (unbound to CBG and albumin) is followed by passive tubular reabsorption without a demonstrable reabsorption maximum. At serum cortisol levels of about 20–25 μg/dL (the upper 8 AM reference value), the binding capacity of transcortin (CBG) is exceeded, leading to a very rapid and disproportionate increase in the unbound fraction compared with the total serum cortisol. Doubling of serum cortisol from 20–40 μg/dL results in at least a fivefold increase in unbound cortisol. At these levels, free cortisol clearance by the kidneys is directly proportional to the unbound serum cortisol concentration, and a steep rise in cortisol clearance is seen. Serum cortisol reflects the sum of free, CBG-bound and albumin-bound cortisol. Only free unbound cortisol is filtered by the kidneys; therefore unlike serum cortisol, UFC is not affected by conditions and medications that alter CBG and albumin concentrations. Thus, when UFC rather than serum cortisol is used, it is easier to differentiate patients with adrenal hyperfunction from a reference population.

UFC is the best specimen to submit because it provides an integrated profile of total cortisol secretion over a 24-hour period, which is most helpful in those with sporadic excess cortisol production. The collection should also be assayed for creatinine to ensure that an adequate specimen has been submitted. The reliability of the test may be further improved by submitting urine collected over 2 or 3 days because day-to-day fluctuations in cortisol excretion are known to occur. Urinary free cortisol levels are unaffected by alterations in hepatic metabolism of cortisol. Although total cortisol production and urinary 17-OHCS may be increased, serum cortisol and urinary free cortisol remain within the reference interval. Because renal clearance of cortisol is dependent on normal kidney function, it is not surprising that patients with renal disease have low UFC values. UFC is unreliable when CrCl is <20 mL/min, and is of reduced reliability when CrCl is <60 mL/min (Chan, 2004). Increased serum concentration of transcortin during pregnancy and with estrogen therapy results in increased serum cortisol levels. This increase is not reflected by an elevation of cortisol metabolites in urine, but urinary free cortisol may be increased. Conditions in which spuriously elevated levels occur include starvation, use of topical steroids, and perhaps hydration in the form of water loading.

Method. HPLC with mass spectrometry is considered the current reference method for measuring UFC; it has diagnostic sensitivity of 100% and specificity of 98% for distinguishing patients with Cushing's syndrome from normal individuals (Rudd, 1985). Prior assays (like RIA) were less specific with a tendency to overestimate the amount of cortisol present. When measuring free cortisol in the urine by RIA, reference intervals were found to vary with patient gender (men had higher reference intervals than women), use of an extraction procedure, and with the RIA test kit used (Lamb, 1994).

The normal range varies according to the assay technique used; however, values that are four times the upper reference limit are diagnostic for Cushing's syndrome. A low urinary free cortisol value is suggestive of adrenal hypofunction; however, because there is great overlap with the normal reference interval, this test is not used to make the diagnosis of adrenal insufficiency.

Hypercortisolism: Cushing's Syndrome

Cushing's syndrome is a group of clinical and metabolic disorders characterized by adrenocortical hyperfunction; it is associated with excess production of glucocorticoids, or glucocorticoids and androgens. Patients with severe forms of the syndrome are easily recognizable by their florid presentation. In less severely afflicted individuals, the vague signs and symptoms that occur may not be easily recognized as caused by hypercortisolism. Although patients with ectopic ACTH-producing tumors have elevated ACTH and glucocorticoid levels, because of the rapid growth of these tumors, the patients usually die before clinical signs of the syndrome can be manifest.

Laboratory findings in Cushing's syndrome include (1) excessive and persistent production of cortisol measured as elevated serum cortisol, urinary free cortisol, midnight salivary cortisol or 17-OHCS, (2) loss of circadian rhythm of ACTH and cortisol, (3) loss of suppression of cortisol production by administration of the synthetic glucocorticoid dexamethasone, and (4) hyperglycemia. Among the clinical findings in Cushing's syndrome, the most common are central obesity, hypertension, and hirsutism.

Cushing's disease is a state of glucocorticoid excess resulting from an ACTH-secreting pituitary adenoma. Cushing's syndrome is a more global term that encompasses a wide variety of entities associated with hypercortisolemia. Evaluation of a patient suspected of having Cushing's syndrome is best divided into two phases. The first phase is actual documentation of hypercortisolism; the second is identification of the pathophysiologic process behind the hypercortisolism. Cushing's syndrome is most commonly iatrogenic in origin; however, it may also be due to ectopic production of CRH or ACTH by a tumor or due to a primary adrenal malignancy. Adrenal Cushing's syndrome is a disorder of excess autonomous production of cortisol by the adrenals, resulting in suppression of the hypothalamic-pituitary axis. Adrenal Cushing's (adenoma or carcinoma) accounts for less than 20% of cases, whereas pituitary Cushing's accounts for about 68%, and ectopic production of ACTH (outside the pituitary-adrenal axis) is the cause of about 12% of cases (Orth, 1995). Because the treatment and prognosis differ depending on the cause, it is important that a specific diagnosis be reached.

Tests Used for the Diagnosis of Cushing's Syndrome

(Fig. 24-17)

Screening Tests. Three screening tests are used in the evaluation of a patient suspected of having Cushing's syndrome: the 24-hour urinary free cortisol, the overnight dexamethasone suppression test, and the plasma or salivary midnight cortisol level. The 24-hour urinary free cortisol is a reflection of the unbound circulating cortisol that is freely filtered by the glomerulus. Unlike serum cortisol, it is unaffected by the level of circulating CBG. HPLC or gas chromatography coupled with mass spectrometry

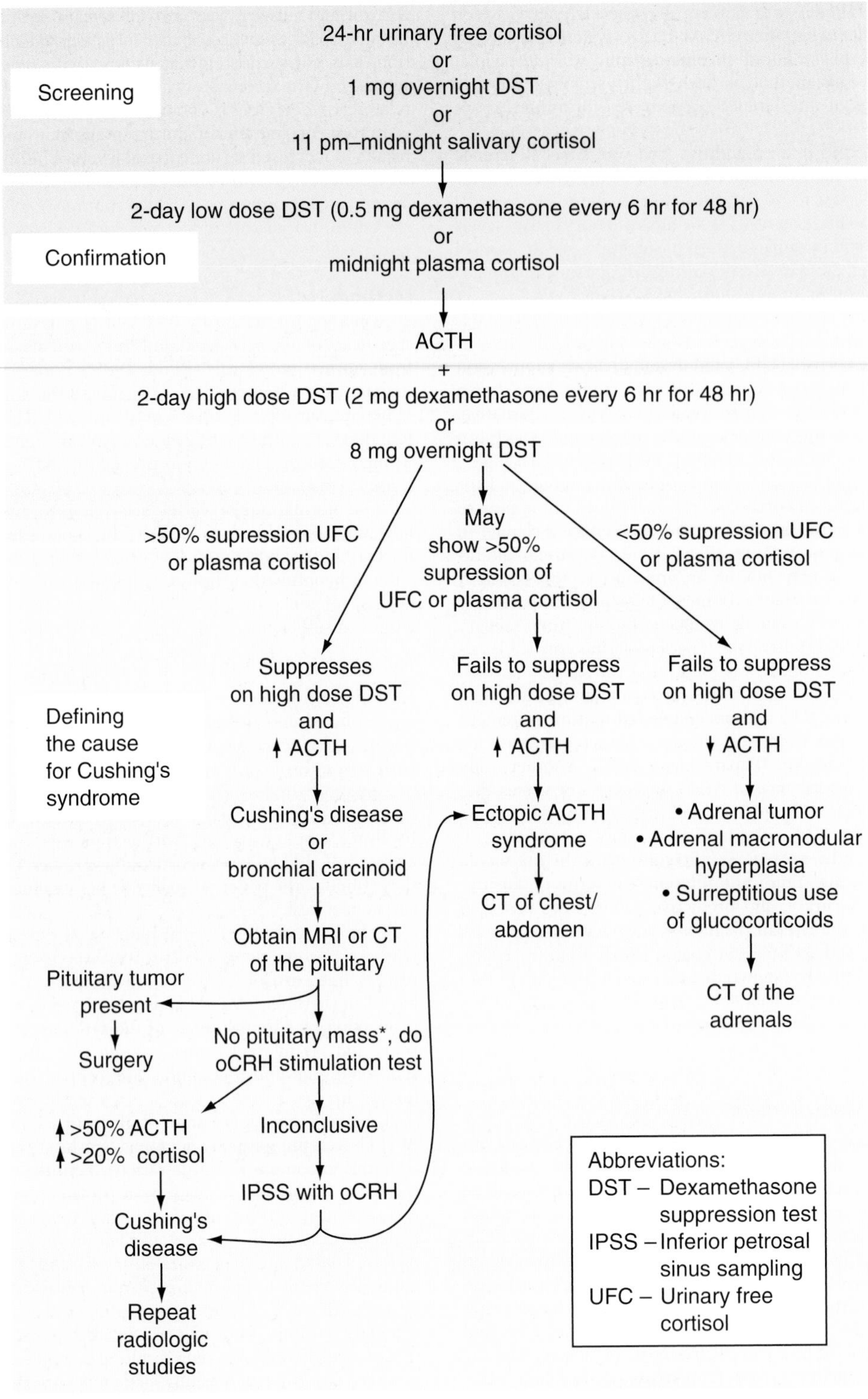

Figure 24-17 Algorithm for the evaluation of Cushing's syndrome. All screening tests must be followed by a confirmatory test. *ACTH,* Adrenocorticotropin; *CT,* computed tomography; *oCRH,* ovine corticotropin-releasing hormone; *MRI,* magnetic resonance imaging. *If there is no pituitary mass, obtain a chest radiograph and chest CT to rule out bronchial carcinoid before proceeding to IPSS.

provides the best specificity for measuring urinary free cortisol. Unlike RIA or enzyme-linked immunosorbent assay, these techniques are not affected by cross-reactivity with steroid metabolites or synthetic glucocorticoids. The upper range of normal with these methods is 110–138 nmol/24 hours (40–50 μg/hour) (Raff, 2003). The creatinine should be measured in all collections to ensure the adequacy of the specimen. Urinary cortisol excretion is decreased when the glomerular filtration rate is <30 mL/minute, and thus may be normal despite the presence of excessive cortisol production (Arnaldi, 2003). Values greater than four times the upper limit of normal are diagnostic of Cushing's syndrome. However, 10%–15% of patients with Cushing's syndrome will have at least one in four 24-hour urine collections for free cortisol return as normal (Nieman, 1990). If cortisol excretion is normal but clinical suspicion is high, the study should be repeated or a different screening method should be used. Milder elevations can be seen in pseudo-Cushing's and during normal pregnancy. Pseudo-Cushing's is an entity characterized by HPA axis overactivity but without true Cushing's syndrome. It has been described in depression, anxiety disorders, alcoholism, and morbid obesity. As per the latest guidelines for the diagnosis of Cushing's syndrome, any UFC concentration above the upper limit of normal for that particular assay should be considered a positive test (Neiman, 2008). Because most pediatric patients being evaluated for Cushing's are of adult weight (>45 kg), adult normal ranges may be used (Neiman, 2008).

The overnight dexamethasone suppression test is a much simpler test to perform. The patient takes 1 mg of dexamethasone orally between the hours of 11 PM and 12 midnight. The plasma cortisol is drawn the following morning between 8 AM and 9 AM. The original criterion for an abnormal response was failure to suppress the morning cortisol level to <5 µg/dL (138 nmol/L); however, this has been revised downward to <1.8 µg/dL (50 nmol/L) (Findling, 1999; Arnaldi, 2003; Neiman, 2008). Failure to suppress could be due to Cushing's syndrome or pseudo-Cushing's, and may even occur in some patients who are normal. The false-positive rate can be as high as 30% for a variety of reasons: Dexamethasone was taken too early; the patient was on phenobarbital, Dilantin, or another medication known to accelerate the metabolism of dexamethasone; malabsorption; alcoholism; or morbid obesity. Pregnancy and drugs such as estrogen, which increase serum transcortin (aka CBG), may also result in elevated cortisol levels. Because of these and possibly other factors, about 1% of healthy individuals, 13% of obese patients, and 25% of hospitalized and chronically ill patients show false-positive overnight dexamethasone suppression tests (DSTs). False-negative results, on the other hand, occur in less than 2% of patients.

The late-night (11 PM) salivary cortisol is a simple test that carries high diagnostic sensitivity and specificity. The patient can collect the sample at home. Two methods can be used to collect the sample: The patient can chew on a cotton pledget for 2–3 minutes and then place the pledget into a plastic tube; alternatively, the patient can passively drool directly into a test tube. The sample is then mailed to the reference laboratory; because salivary cortisol is very stable, there is little concern about degradation during transport. The sample is analyzed by immunoassay or by liquid chromatography-mass spectrometry (LC-MS/MS); normative values vary according to the reference laboratory.

Screening in Special Populations. The preferred screening test during pregnancy is the UFC. UFC levels normally rise during the second and third trimesters, therefore UFC values greater than three times the upper limit of normal are considered consistent with Cushing's syndrome (Neiman, 2008). Because of the decrease in cortisol filtration with declining renal function, the 1-mg DST is the recommended screen in patients with renal failure. For those suspected of having cyclic Cushing's, use of UFC or MSC is suggested. The diagnostic thresholds for MSC during pregnancy and in renal disease remain to be established. In instances of an incidentally discovered adrenal mass, the 1-mg DST or a late-night salivary cortisol are the screening tests of choice (Neiman, 2008).

Confirmatory Tests for the Diagnosis of Cushing's Syndrome. A positive screen for Cushing's syndrome is followed by confirmatory testing with a midnight plasma cortisol or low-dose DST performed alone or with the administration of CRH.

Midnight plasma cortisol requires hospital admission for at least 48 hours, insertion of a line for IV access before 10 PM, the patient sleeping at the time of the blood draw, and availability of staff to draw the blood at midnight. A midnight plasma cortisol greater than 7.5 µg/dL (207 nmol/L) is diagnostic of Cushing's; this has a 100% specificity for normals and those with pseudo-Cushing's (Papanicolaou, 1998). More recently, several authorities have suggested using 1.8 µg/dL (50 nmol/L) as the cutoff for normal. This value carries a very high degree of sensitivity (Newell-Price, 1995).

The low-dose (2-day 2 mg) dexamethasone suppression test (LDDST) requires the collection of two baseline 24-hour urines for UFC. The patient is then given 0.5 mg dexamethasone orally every 6 hours, starting at 9 AM for 2 days. On day 2 of dexamethasone, another 24-hour urine is collected for UFC. All 24-hour urine collections should include the measurement of creatinine to assay for adequacy of the collection. A normal response is a decrease in UFC to less than 10 µg (27 nmol) per 24 hours on the second day of dexamethasone. This has a sensitivity of 97%–100% for discriminating patients with Cushing's syndrome from normal individuals (Newell-Price, 1998). Instead of measuring UFC, serum cortisol can be measured at baseline (9 AM day 1) and at 48 hours following the first dose of dexamethasone. In this case, a normal response consists of suppression of the plasma cortisol to less than 1.8 µg/dL (50 nmol/L), which has a sensitivity and specificity of more than 95% (Newell-Price, 1998). Performance of the DST with CRH has been purported to better distinguish Cushing's syndrome from pseudo-Cushing's (Yanovski, 1993). For this 1-µg/kg ovine, CRH is administered IV 2 hours after the last dose of dexamethasone. Cortisol is measured 15 minutes later. A dexamethasone level should be measured at the time of CRH administration to exclude false-positive results. Adherence to the time schedule is important for both LDDST and LDDST with CRH. The normal response for both tests is a serum cortisol <1.8 µg/dL (<50 nmol/L).

TABLE 24-22
Differential Diagnosis of Hormonal Values Seen in Cushing's Syndrome

Cause	Plasma ACTH	Plasma cortisol (PM)	High-dose or overnight dexamethasone suppression
Pituitary-dependent	N–slightly ↑	↑	Yes
Adrenal disease	↓– undetectable	↑	No
Ectopic Cushing's*	↑↑↑	↑↑	Usually no
Pseudo-Cushing's	N–slightly ↑	N–↑	Usually yes

ACTH, Adrenocorticotropin; *N,* normal.
*ACTH levels may overlap with values seen in pituitary-dependent disease.

Tests for Defining the Cause of Cushing's. Once the diagnosis of Cushing's syndrome is established, the next step is to determine its cause. Cushing's is categorized as being ACTH dependent or ACTH independent; this is accomplished by measuring the plasma ACTH, or by performing a high-dose DST or a CRH stimulation test (Table 24-22).

ACTH-independent Cushing's syndrome results from autonomous production of cortisol, which would feed back on the hypothalamus and pituitary and cause suppression of CRH and ACTH secretion. The technique for measuring plasma ACTH has been described previously. Values below the level of detection or below 10 pg/mL (2 pmol/L) at 9 AM with concomitantly elevated cortisol support an ACTH-independent cause for Cushing's syndrome. Plasma levels greater than 20 pg/mL (4 pmol/L) in the face of hypercortisolism are strongly suggestive of an ACTH-dependent cause. A CRH stimulation test with measurement of ACTH is indicated for values between 10 and 20 pg/mL (2–4 pmol/L) (Orth, 1995). Although patients with ectopic ACTH production tend to have markedly elevated ACTH levels, there is great overlap with the levels seen in Cushing's disease; therefore, it cannot be used to reliably distinguish between these entities.

The high-dose (2-day 8 mg) DST is useful for distinguishing Cushing's disease from adrenal or ectopic Cushing's. It is of note that cortisol levels in neuroendocrine tumors such as bronchial carcinoid may also suppress on high-dose dexamethasone. For the high-dose DST, a baseline 24-hour urine for UFC is collected. Beginning on day 1, the patient receives 2 mg of dexamethasone orally every 6 hours for 48 hours; urine for UFC is collected on day 1 and on day 2. As an alternative to measuring UFC, plasma cortisol can be collected before, during, and after dexamethasone. Suppression of UFC or plasma cortisol by 50% or more from baseline is diagnostic of Cushing's disease. Most patients with adrenal adenomas, carcinomas, or ectopic ACTH syndromes do not show suppression. This test has a sensitivity and specificity of 60%–85%; the greater the degree of suppression, the greater the specificity.

The 8-mg overnight DST has been reported by several authors to share similar sensitivity and specificity to the high-dose DST (Dicheck, 1994). An 8 AM plasma cortisol is obtained, and 8 mg of dexamethasone is administered orally at 11PM. An 8 AM plasma cortisol is obtained the next morning. Reduction of cortisol to less than 5 µg/dL is strongly supportive of Cushing's disease (see Fig. 24-17).

Most pituitary tumors and a few ectopic ACTH-secreting tumors will respond to CRH stimulation with an increase in plasma ACTH and cortisol, whereas little response is noted in those with adrenal Cushing's. For the CRH stimulation test, two basal plasma cortisol and ACTH levels are collected about 5 minutes apart, then 1 µg/kg of body weight or a single dose of 100 µg of synthetic ovine CRH (oCRH) is injected intravenously. Blood is sampled every 15 minutes for 1–2 hours for cortisol and ACTH. Normal subjects will show a rise in ACTH and cortisol of approximately 15%–20%, while those with Cushing's disease typically show a greater than 50% rise in ACTH and a greater than 20% rise in cortisol above baseline (Kaye, 1990; Newell-Price, 2002; Stewart, 2003). Ovine CRH is superior to human CRH in distinguishing among the different causes of Cushing's syndrome (Nieman, 1989). Vasopressin stimulates ACTH release through the V3 receptors in the anterior pituitary. Administration of 10 units of vasopressin intramuscularly normally causes doubling of ACTH levels and an increase in serum cortisol of 150 µg/L over baseline. This offers no advantage over testing with CRH. It may prove useful, however, in differentiating Cushing's disease from pseudo-Cushing's syndrome and in the postoperative assessment of Cushing's disease (Newell-Price, 2002).

In rare instances, it may be necessary to use selective sampling of inferior petrosal sinus blood to document that the pituitary is the source of excess ACTH. This invasive, technically difficult procedure carries a relatively high cost and complication rate and should be performed only at a center well experienced with this technique. The ACTH concentration in the petrosal sinus blood should exceed twice that of peripheral venous blood to ensure diagnostic sensitivity and specificity of 100% (Orth, 1995). In those with ectopic production, the ratio is usually less than 1.4:1. Use of CRH during sampling increases the sensitivity and specificity.

Given that the incidence of **incidentaloma** of the adrenals and pituitary has been reported to be as high as 10%, imaging studies should be performed only after the hormonal diagnosis of Cushing's disease or syndrome has been made. In Cushing's disease, visualization of the sella is performed by MRI or CT, with and without contrast. For adrenal Cushing's, the test of choice is a CT of the abdomen; for ectopic disease, CT of the chest may also be needed.

Pseudo-Cushing's Syndrome

Excess activity of the hypothalamic-pituitary axis, similar to that seen in pituitary Cushing's syndrome, has been demonstrated in some patients with alcoholism, major depression, and obesity. Resolution of the underlying problem results in normalization of the HPA axis. These patients may not suppress on a low-dose DST and may have elevated UFC. Depressed patients who fail to suppress cortisol secretion in response to dexamethasone also show an impaired ACTH response to exogenous CRH, but will usually retain a normal cortisol response (Gold, 1986; Thalen, 1993). A single serum cortisol above 7.5 µg/dL at midnight has been shown to discriminate Cushing's syndrome from pseudo-Cushing's with 100% specificity (Papanicolaou, 1998). A more definitive test for distinguishing between these two entities is the combined dexamethasone-oCRH test. oCRH is infused 2 hours after a low-dose dexamethasone test. A plasma cortisol concentration greater than 38 nmol/L measured at 15 minutes following the administration of oCRH correctly identifies all cases of Cushing's syndrome and all cases of pseudo-Cushing's, with specificity, sensitivity, and diagnostic accuracy of 100% (Yanovski, 1993).

Adrenal Insufficiency

Adrenal insufficiency is categorized according to the key site of dysfunction within the HPA axis: primary (adrenal), secondary (pituitary), and tertiary (hypothalamic). A major distinction between primary adrenal insufficiency and either of the central causes is that primary disease is associated with mineralocorticoid deficiency. In the Western world, primary adrenal insufficiency, also known as Addison's disease, is most commonly due to autoimmune adrenalitis (70%–90% of all cases); other causes include tuberculosis (most common cause worldwide), granulomatous disorders, metastatic disease, hemorrhage, human immunodeficiency virus, acquired immunodeficiency syndrome, and infection. The most common cause of central adrenal insufficiency is HPA axis suppression due to prolonged treatment with pharmacologic doses of steroids.

Tests for the Diagnosis of Adrenal Insufficiency

Basal Hormone Measurements. An 8 AM to 9 AM plasma cortisol of <3 µg/dL (83 nmol/L) is indicative of adrenal insufficiency and obviates the need for further testing. Although most patients with hypocortisolism have low serum cortisol levels, a level drawn during a time of stress that falls within the reference range does not exclude the diagnosis. Rather, it may support this diagnosis, as a suboptimal cortisol level may have risen into the reference interval in response to a very high ACTH level induced by stress. A random cortisol of >25 µg/dL (700 nmol/L) during critical illness makes it unlikely that the patient is adrenally insufficient (Burke, 1985), whereas a random cortisol of <10 µg/dL is strongly suggestive of adrenal insufficiency (Fleseriu, 2009).

ACTH Stimulation Test. The most convenient procedure for studying patients suspected of having hypocortisolism is the ACTH stimulation test. This test, which can be performed at any time of day, consists of drawing a baseline serum cortisol and then administering 250 µg of Cosyntropin (commercially available ACTH analog) intravenously or intramuscularly. Serum for cortisol is again collected at 30 and 60 minutes post Cosyntropin. A normal response is a cortisol level greater than 18–20 µg/dL (500–550 nmol/L) at either time point (Speckart, 1971; Burke, 1985). Drawing an ACTH level at baseline may help in distinguishing primary adrenal insufficiency (associated with an elevated ACTH usually greater than 50–100 pg/mL) from secondary or tertiary forms (which would have a low ACTH level <10 pg/mL) (Oelkers, 1992) (refer to Laboratory Measurement of ACTH). The aldosterone response to ACTH may also help in making this distinction; failure of aldosterone to increase by more than 4 ng/dL over baseline suggests primary adrenal dysfunction.

Steroids should never be withheld from a critically ill patient suspected of having adrenal insufficiency; instead a random sample for cortisol and ACTH should be drawn and treatment initiated with dexamethasone, which does not interfere with the cortisol assay. Formal testing should take place within 72 hours, before HPA axis suppression occurs. About 90% of cortisol circulates bound to CBG and albumin, and approximately 10% circulates freely (unbound). CBG declines during critical illness, resulting in an increase in the fraction of unbound (free) cortisol compared with the bound fraction. Because the serum total cortisol concentration does not accurately reflect this alteration in free/bound cortisol, it is common to overdiagnose adrenal insufficiency in the critical care setting. Since access to laboratories that readily and reliably measure free cortisol is limited, some have advocated use of the free cortisol index (FCI) and calculated free cortisol (CFC) to better delineate those patients in true need of steroid replacement therapy (Hamrahian, 2004; Beishuizen, 2001; Ho, 2006). To obtain the FCI, it is necessary to measure the serum CBG. CFC is the total cortisol (nmol/L)/CBG (mg/L), with normal being a value above 12. Given that for the vast majority of institutions CBG determinations require the sample to be sent to a reference lab, it may be more prudent and certainly more direct to simply send aliquots from t-0, t-+30, and t-+60 minutes post ACTH stimulation for free cortisol and provide steroid coverage pending these results (Fleseriu, 2009). Salivary cortisol, which is unaffected by changes in CBG, may eventually prove useful in this setting (Raff, 2009).

Some have supported the use of a 1-µg dose of ACTH instead of the full 250-µg dose for diagnosing adrenal insufficiency. The premise is that the massively supraphysiologic dose of 250 µg will cause those with partial adrenal insufficiency to mount a normal response, and that these individuals will fail to show an adequate rise in cortisol in response to a 1-µg test dose. This procedure has not gained wide acceptance, nor has the normal range been standardized; more important, the diagnosis of **partial adrenal insufficiency** remains in contention.

The ITT has long been considered the gold standard for assessing the HPA axis. Unlike the ACTH stimulation test, the ITT assesses the integrity of the entire HPA axis. If the HPA axis is intact, insulin-induced hypoglycemia stimulates the hypothalamus and the pituitary to secrete CRH and ACTH, respectively, which, in turn, leads to a rise in cortisol. This test is contraindicated in individuals with ischemic heart disease, in the elderly (>age 70), during pregnancy, and in those with a history of seizures. Patients highly suspected of having central adrenal insufficiency (i.e., prior pituitary surgery or radiation therapy) should receive a lower dose (0.05 U/kg) of insulin, rather than 0.1–0.15 U/kg. Glucose and cortisol are measured at −15 mins, at baseline, and then at 15, 30, 45, 60, 90, and 120 minutes following insulin administration. For the test to be valid, adequate hypoglycemia must be attained (signs and symptoms of hypoglycemia and glucose <40 mg/dL [2.2 mmol/L]). A normal response is a rise in the cortisol level to greater than or equal to 18 µg/L or 20 µg/L at any time during the test (Nelson, 1978; Burke, 1985; Grinspoon, 1994). Preliminary work suggests there was no difference in peak GH or cortisol level attained when analog insulin was substituted for regular insulin for the ITT (Yuen, 2008).

The cortisol response to hypoglycemia can be predicted reliably by the response to acute ACTH stimulation—a safer, cheaper, and quicker test (Stewart, 2003). The ITT is used mainly as a second-line measure to further evaluate those patients who had a borderline response to the ACTH stimulation test.

In the days before the commercial availability of a reliable assay to measure ACTH, it was common to perform a prolonged ACTH stimulation test (ACTH infusion over a 2-day period) to distinguish central from primary adrenal insufficiency. In other hormone systems, lack of stimulation normally leads to upregulation of the end-organ receptors; however, the adrenals downregulate their ACTH receptors in response to lack of stimulation. A short ACTH stimulation test would typically produce an inadequate response. By priming the system with prolonged exposure to ACTH, those with hypothalamic disease display a delayed but normal rise in cortisol.

Overnight Metyrapone Test. Metyrapone has also been used to assess the integrity of the HPA axis. Metyrapone inhibits 11-β-hydroxylase, preventing the conversion of 11-deoxycortisol (compound S) to cortisol. Under normal circumstances, the metyrapone-induced drop in cortisol is detected at the level of the hypothalamus and pituitary; a compensatory increase in CRH and ACTH secretion occurs, stimulating steroidogenesis and leading to a buildup of 11-deoxycortisol, the hormone preceding the block. Patients with central adrenal insufficiency fail to increase CRH and/or ACTH, steroidogenesis is not stimulated, and 11-deoxycortisol fails to increase. Metyrapone 30 mg/kg is administered orally at midnight; blood for cortisol and 11-deoxycortisol is collected the following morning at 8 AM. A rise in 11-deoxycortisol to greater than 7 μg/dL (200 nmol/L) is normal (Fiad, 1994; Grinspoon, 1994). An abnormal response is defined by 11-deoxycortisol less than 7 μg/dL accompanied by cortisol less than 5 μg/dL. This test should be performed with caution as it may provoke an addisonian crisis in those with central hypocortisolism.

Corticotropin-Releasing Hormone Test. The oCRH test can be used not only to diagnose hypocortisolism, but to localize the site of damage (Schulte, 1984). It is a safe test; however, it is expensive. After blood is drawn for baseline ACTH and cortisol, 100 μg oCRH is administered intravenously. Blood is then collected for cortisol and ACTH every 15 minutes for 60–90 minutes. A normal response is seen as cortisol >20 μg/dL. Basal ACTH levels and their change in response to oCRH are used to localize the site of pathology. Plasma corticotropin usually peaks at 15–30 minutes and cortisol usually peaks at around 30–40 minutes post oCRH injection (Oelkers, 1996).

Antibodies against 21-hydroxylase antigen should be assayed in those whose Addison's disease (primary adrenal insufficiency) does not have an obvious explanation. Positive antibodies confirm autoimmune adrenalitis; these patients should be screened and monitored for the development of other autoimmune disorders.

The use of steroids in the treatment of malignant, inflammatory, and immunologic disorders is a common iatrogenic cause of adrenal insufficiency. The degree of adrenal suppression is dependent on the specific glucocorticoid dose, duration, frequency, and route of administration. Assessment of adrenal function in patients being tapered off of exogenous steroids can be performed once they are tapered to the equivalent of a daily dose of 10 mg hydrocortisone. Have them omit the morning glucocorticoid dose, and measure the 8 AM cortisol level. If it is greater than 10 μg/dL, routine supplementation of steroids can be ended. Because the adrenal cortex lags behind the pituitary in recovery from steroid suppression, complete adrenal recovery can also be demonstrated by an appropriate rise in serum cortisol following an 8 AM Cosyntropin infusion.

RENIN-ALDOSTERONE AXIS

At least 20 million people in the United States have hypertension, and 90%–98% of cases are classified as essential hypertension. The mortality and morbidity from associated myocardial, cerebrovascular, and renal complications necessitate aggressive treatment of this disorder. Investigation into the etiology of hypertension revealed the importance of the renin-angiotensin-aldosterone system, not only in the origin and persistence of hypertension but also as a guide to its treatment. The role of the renin-aldosterone axis is to maintain blood pressure within normal limits by sensing and responding to changes in plasma volume, salt balance, and renal perfusion pressure.

Renin is a proteolytic enzyme which, although formed by other tissues throughout the body, is mainly formed and stored by juxtaglomerular (JG) cells within the macula densa of the kidney. Renin is synthesized from a larger precursor protein, prorenin (big renin), and is converted to its active form within the JG cells. The release of renin into the circulation occurs in response to a variety of triggers: a drop in renal hydrostatic pressure, hyponatremia, hypokalemia, or a decrease in catecholamines, angiotensin II, or atrial natriuretic hormone. Both suppression of plasma renin activity induced by potassium administration and stimulation of renin activity following potassium depletion occur independently of changes in aldosterone secretion or in sodium balance (Brunner, 1970).

Several isoenzymes of rennin are known. Their release is regulated by cAMP. Renin acts on angiotensinogen (renin substrate), an -α2-globulin formed by the liver, converting angiotensinogen to angiotensin I. Angiotensin I in turn is converted into angiotensin II by the angiotensin-converting enzyme (ACE). ACE is found in the pulmonary and vascular endothelia, as well as in cell membranes of the kidney, heart, and brain (Brewster, 2004). It is believed that angiotensin II is the peptide responsible for the physiologic effects on target tissue. Angiotensin II not only stimulates the release of aldosterone, but it is also a very potent vasoconstrictor that can stimulate the release of catecholamines from the adrenals and norepinephrine from the sympathetic nervous system, and stimulate the release of vasopressin. The octapeptide angiotensin II is further split to a heptapeptide, angiotensin III; in addition, angiotensin I may be changed directly to angiotensin III without being converted to angiotensin II. Although speculation about the functions of angiotensin III is ongoing, it appears to modulate aldosterone secretion in a similar manner to angiotensin II. The active angiotensins are rapidly cleared by various aminopeptidases (angiotensinases) within the circulation and during transit through tissues. These relationships are shown in Figure 24-18.

Renin, through its product, angiotensin II, directly stimulates the synthesis and secretion of aldosterone by the adrenal zona glomerulosa. Renin release, the rate-limiting step in the renin-aldosterone axis, is dependent on changes in effective plasma volume, which, in turn, are dependent on tubular reabsorption of sodium by the kidney. Low plasma volume and low serum sodium stimulate the secretion of renin, resulting in aldosterone release, which, in turn, causes sodium retention along with an increase in plasma volume and blood pressure, and potassium loss. Conversely, an increase in effective blood volume or acute elevation in blood pressure results in low renin, low angiotensin, low aldosterone, and subsequent sodium loss. In contradistinction to aldosterone, renin secretion is inhibited by hyperkalemia (Fig. 24-19).

Aldosterone and glucocorticoids act at the mineralocorticoid receptor located in the cells lining the collecting ducts of the kidney to cause reabsorption of sodium, leading to an increase in intravascular volume. Aldosterone also causes renal potassium loss. Studies have suggested a role for aldosterone in the development and perpetuation of vasculopathy; it has been shown to stimulate genes for collagen synthesis, tissue growth factors, inflammatory factors, and plasminogen activator inhibitor type 1 (Brilla,

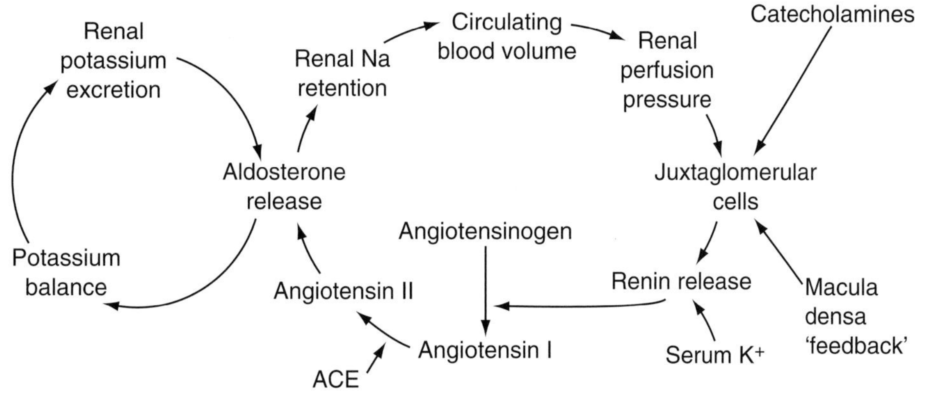

Figure 24-18 Renin-aldosterone axis. Elevated K^+ inhibits renin secretion but has a stimulatory effect on aldosterone. Catecholaminergic influence is variable; β-adrenergic activity stimulates and α-adrenergic activity inhibits renin secretion from the juxtaglomerular cells. *(Redrawn from Braunwald E, Fauci AD, Kasper D, et al, editors. Harrison's principles of internal medicine. 15th ed. New York: McGraw-Hill; 2001, p. 2087.)* *ACE,* Angiotensin-converting enzyme.

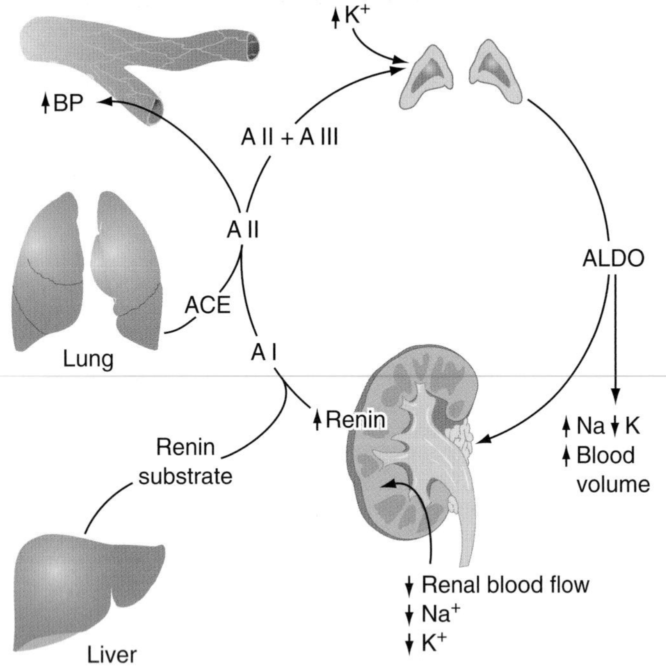

Figure 24-19 The normal renin-angiotensin-aldosterone axis. Renin, secreted by the kidney, cleaves angiotensin I from renin substrate (angiotensinogen) produced by the liver. Angiotensin I is converted to angiotensin II by angiotensin-converting enzyme (ACE), mainly in the lung. Angiotensin II increases peripheral vascular resistance and, together with angiotensin III, stimulates aldosterone (ALDO) secretion, which results in sodium retention and increased plasma volume. *(Adapted from Stewart PM. The adrenal cortex. In: Larsen PR, Kronenberg HM, Melmed S, Polansky KS, editors. Williams textbook of endocrinology. 10th ed. Philadelphia: WB Saunders; 2003, p. 499.)*

1994; Schunkert, 1997; Brown, 2000; Rocha, 2000; Luft, 2002). The synthesis of aldosterone is restricted to the zona glomerulosa; here the enzyme aldosterone synthetase (CYP11B2) converts corticosterone to aldosterone. The major stimuli for aldosterone secretion are angiotensin II and hyperkalemia. ACTH is a much weaker stimulus. Somatostatin, atrial natriuretic hormone, dopamine, and heparin directly inhibit aldosterone synthesis. Cortisol circulates at a much higher concentration than aldosterone, and although it binds with equal affinity to the mineralocorticoid receptor, it does not normally function as a major mineralocorticoid. The reason is that the enzyme 11-β-hydroxysteroid dehydrogenase II (11-HSD-2, also known as CYP11B2), expressed by the mineralocorticoid targets cells in the collecting tubules acts to convert cortisol to cortisone, an inactive metabolite.

RENIN AND HYPERTENSION

The work of Laragh has indicated that essential hypertension can be classified on the basis of renin measurements as high, low, or normal renin, and that drug selection can be based on this classification (Laragh, 1972; Laragh, 1993). About 15% of patients with essential hypertension have high-renin hypertension. Hyperreninemia resulting from renal parenchymal disease or renal vasculopathy leads to increased aldosterone production and the subsequent retention of sodium and enhanced potassium excretion. Patients with this condition are hypervolemic, intensely vasoconstrictive, and more prone to ischemic injury. Renin profiling has shown renin to be an independent risk factor for myocardial infarction. Even if pressures are controlled by antihypertensives, if they do not address plasma renin activity, such patients fare worse than individuals with lower renin levels (Alderman, 1991). Increased aldosterone (secondary aldosteronism) may contribute significantly to the symptoms and course of high-renin hypertension. Some of the causes of high-renin hypertension are listed in Table 24-23.

Renin-secreting tumors are extremely rare and can be difficult to diagnose. They can be benign or malignant, renal or extrarenal. The most common location is in the juxtaglomerular apparatus. A young patient with markedly elevated plasma renin activity, hyperaldosteronism, and hypokalemia in the absence of a renovascular lesion typifies the classic clinical presentation (Corvol, 1994). Malignant hypertension is also associated with high plasma renin activity and aldosterone. When such patients are

TABLE 24-23
Causes of Hypertension Associated With High Levels of Plasma Renin

Renin-secreting tumor	Cushing's syndrome
Malignant accelerated hypertension	Iatrogenic
Renovascular hypertension	Volume-depleting agents
Major arterial lesions	Vasodilating agents
Segmental lesions	Glucocorticoids
Chronic renal failure	Estrogens
End stage	
Transplant rejection	

given medications that interrupt the renin-aldosterone axis, such as ACEIs, blood pressure often normalizes. In renal vascular hypertension, the renin and aldosterone levels are also elevated. However, in contradistinction to malignant hypertension, treatment with ACEs usually results in further deterioration of renal function. Patients suspected of having renal artery stenosis should undergo further testing (e.g., captopril-induced renogram, renal duplex ultrasound, magnetic resonance angiography). A positive test leads to renal vein angiography and catheterization for selective blood sampling. In unilateral renal disease, both plasma renin and aldosterone are elevated. Asymmetry in the renin levels obtained during renal vein catheterization offers one of the best measurements to judge the likelihood of blood pressure response to corrective surgery. When the ratio of plasma renin in the renal vein of the affected to the nonaffected side is at least 1.5 : 1, surgery may lead to improvement. With suppression of renin release from the nonaffected side, renal vein renin levels approximating those found in blood specimens obtained from the inferior vena cava also indicate probable success of curative surgery. Almost 40% of these patients have peripheral blood plasma renin activity that is within the reference interval (Streeten, 1979); consequently, peripheral plasma renin is a poor predictor of response to surgery. Renin secretion can be found in lung cancer, hepatic hamartoma, and other rare conditions (Anderson, 1989).

When an acceleration of hypertension occurs, renin is usually markedly increased; however, with chronic renal failure, almost any renin level can be expected. A small number of hypertensive patients on dialysis have intractable, accelerated hypertension. In those patients in whom dialysis cannot control the hypertension, markedly elevated plasma renin levels can be lowered by nephrectomy or, in the case of renal artery stenosis, angioplasty or revascularization (Whitehouse, 1981; Sonkodi, 1990; Tullis, 1999). ACEIs can be used to mitigate the rise in aldosterone; however, in the setting of renal disease, they can precipitate or worsen hyperkalemia. In renal transplant patients, elevated plasma renin may be indicative of renal ischemia and rejection.

Systemic hypertension occurs in patients with Cushing's syndrome. Some of these patients have increased plasma renin and renin substrate. Other Cushing's syndrome patients have hypokalemia associated with secretion of a minor mineralocorticoid (such as DOC or corticosterone) that causes hypertension (Krakoff, 1975). In still other patients, severely elevated cortisol levels overwhelm the capacity of 11-hydroxysteroid dehydrogenase (11-HSD) to convert cortisol to its metabolically inactive form, cortisone, leading to a picture of excess mineralocorticoid activity with suppressed plasma renin activity. Other causes of high-renin hypertension include treatment with medications such as diuretics, vasodilators, or other antihypertensives. Hormonal agents such as glucocorticoids, as well as some estrogen-containing oral contraceptives, have been found to increase renin substrate activity.

Even though plasma renin activity, aldosterone, and urinary sodium excretion may be normal in 60% of hypertensive patients, evidence indicates that renin-angiotensin plays a significant part in normal-renin hypertension. The response of many hypertensive patients with normal renin to angiotensin-converting enzyme inhibitors or angiotensin II antagonists (saralasin) has implicated renin and angiotensin II in sustaining hypertension in these patients. Moreover, Ames showed that once blood pressure was increased by angiotensin infusion, it could be maintained with only one fifth of the original dose (Ames, 1965).

It was found that low-renin essential hypertension, which involves chronic expansion of plasma and extracellular fluid volume, is characterized by aldosterone oversecretion and responds to diuretic therapy. At least 25% of patients with essential hypertension are found to have low-renin hypertension. Most investigators have characterized this state as hyporesponsive, meaning that low-renin hypertensive patients fail to respond as well as healthy subjects do with upright posture, sodium restriction,

TABLE 24-24
Causes of Hypertension Associated With Low Levels of Plasma Renin

Primary Excess of Mineralocorticoids
Primary aldosteronism
Pseudoprimary (idiopathic) aldosteronism
Glucocorticoid-suppressible aldosteronism
11-Deoxycorticosterone excess (CAH due to 11-β-hydroxylase deficiency)
18-Hydroxy-11-deoxycorticosterone excess
Adrenal carcinoma (excess mineralocorticoids and/or glucocorticoids)
Secondary Excess of Mineralocorticoids
Licorice ingestion
Excess sodium intake
Hyporenin hypoaldosteronism
Long-standing essential hypertension
Diabetes mellitus

CAH, Congenital adrenal hyperplasia.

diuretics, vasodilators, or a combination of these. Atrial natriuretic peptide may be elevated in these patients, and the response of aldosterone to renin may be exaggerated (Sergev, 1990). Renin suppression increases with age and appears to be more common in women and in the black population.

Listed in Table 24-24 are a group of syndromes associated with low levels of plasma renin. These have been divided into a subgroup that is of adrenal origin (primary) and a subgroup that is nonadrenal or secondary in origin. Primary aldosteronism is uncommon compared with renin hypertension. It is characterized by (1) systolic and diastolic hypertension caused by oversecretion of aldosterone by an adrenal adenoma (aldosterone-producing adenoma [APA]) or hyperplasia (idiopathic hyperaldosteronism [IHA]), (2) low renin or a high aldosterone/renin ratio (>50), (3) renal potassium wasting, and (4) sodium retention. It should be suspected in patients with hypertension and spontaneous or diuretic-induced hypokalemia, resistant hypertension requiring more than three medications, onset younger than age 30, or an incidentally found adrenal mass. Several potential screening tests have been used to detect primary aldosteronism and to separate unilateral aldosterone-producing adenomas from other causes of primary aldosteronism. A low-salt diet (<2 g/day), stress, upright posture, and diuretics all increase plasma aldosterone, whereas a high-salt diet and lying in a supine position suppress aldosterone secretion in healthy subjects. Combinations of these maneuvers have been used in the diagnosis of excessive aldosterone secretion; however, they do not reliably distinguish APA from IHA. When healthy subjects are placed on a high-salt diet and lie in the supine position, they suppress their plasma aldosterone levels to less than 10 ng/dL (278 pmol/L).

Primary Hyperaldosteronism—Screening and Confirmation Tests

The algorithm proposed by Blumenfeld for evaluating hypertensive patients suspected of having primary hyperaldosteronism is to initially measure the serum potassium (Blumenfeld, 1994). If it is less than 3.6 mmol/L, then plasma renin activity is measured. Plasma renin activity of <1.0 ng/mL/hour leads to 24-hour urine collection for aldosterone and potassium excretion. Findings of 24-hour urinary potassium greater than 30 mmol/24 hours in the face of hypokalemia and of aldosterone greater than 15 mg/24 hours lead to the localization of the underlying pathology to the adrenal.

A more recent set of guidelines for the detection and diagnosis of primary hyperaldosteronism, as proferred by the Endocrine Society, include the following (Funder, 2008). Although patients with primary hyperaldosteronism classically present with spontaneous or easily provokable hypokalemia, many in fact will have serum potassium levels that are within the normal range. Thus, the preferred screening test is a plasma aldosterone concentration/plasma renin activity (PAC/PRA) ratio, PAC expressed in ng/dL, and PRA in ng/mL/hour. This is performed after the patient has remained upright for at least 2 hours. The patient should have stopped spironolactone and eplerenone for 4–6 weeks and other diuretics for at least 2 weeks before testing. Hypokalemia should be corrected (as it may suppress aldosterone secretion), and the patient should not be on a sodium-restricted diet. A PAC/PRA ratio greater than 30 is suggestive of primary hyperaldosteronism; a value greater than 50 is virtually diagnostic (Weinberger, 1993; Blumenfeld, 1994). It is of note that the lower limit of normal for the PRA assay varies by laboratory; therefore, the diagnosis is supported only when both the PAC/PRA ratio and the PAC are elevated. The preferred technique for measuring PRA is a validated immunometric assay. HPLC tandem mass spectrometry is preferred for measuring plasma and urine aldosterone (Funder, 2008). The PAC/PRA ratio is highly dependent on the renin concentration; as such, it is important to use an assay with sufficient sensitivity in the lower ranges (e.g., <0.2–0.3 ng/mL/hour).

The diagnosis of primary hyperaldosteronism is confirmed by performing one of the four following confirmatory tests: oral sodium loading test, saline infusion test, fludrocortisone suppression test, or the captopril challenge test (Funder, 2008). Saline suppression can be accomplished by infusing 2 L of 0.9% saline over 4 hours, or by administering sodium chloride tablets 10–12 g daily for 3 days. PAC at the end of the 4-hour infusion of less than 5 ng/dL (140 pmol/L) makes the diagnosis of hyperaldosteronism unlikely. A PAC greater than 10 ng/dL (280 pmol/L) strongly supports the diagnosis of primary hyperaldosteronism, whereas values greater than 5 ng/dL (140 pmol/L) but less than10 ng/dL (280 pmol/L) are considered indeterminate and may be seen with IHA. On the last day of oral sodium administration, a 24-hour urine is collected for aldosterone, creatinine (to assess for adequacy of the collection), and sodium (>200 mmol/day confirms adequate sodium intake). An aldosterone greater than 10 mg/24 hours (28 nmol/24 hours) following 3 days of sodium loading confirms the diagnosis (Bravo, 1983, 1994; Holland, 1984). For the fludrocortisone suppression test, 0.1 mg fludrocortisone is given orally every 6 hours for 4 days, together with slow-release potassium chloride supplements (in doses sufficient to maintain the plasma potassium close to 4.0 nmol/L) and slow-release sodium chloride (30 mmol three times a day) and liberalization of dietary sodium intake (enough to maintain a urinary sodium excretion of at least 3 mmol/kg). On day 4, an upright plasma cortisol is measured at 7 AM and 10 AM, and PAC and PRA are measured at 10 AM. A PAC greater than 6 ng/dL with a PRA less than 1 ng/mL/hour confirms the diagnosis, provided that the 10 AM cortisol is less than the 7 AM value. For the captopril challenge, baseline blood is collected for PRA, PAC, and cortisol; then 25–50 mg of captopril is administered orally. PRA, PAC, and cortisol are again collected at 1 and 2 hours post captopril. The patient is kept seated throughout the entire test. PAC is normally suppressed to greater than 30%; however in primary hyperaldosteronism, the PAC remains elevated and the PRA suppressed. The choice of test depends on several factors, including patient compliance, presence of uncontrolled hypertension, renal insufficiency, congestive heart failure, and local expertise.

Differentiating Among the Different Causes of Primary Hyperaldosteronism

APA differs from IHA by more extreme blood pressures, greater potassium wasting, and higher atrial natriuretic peptide levels. Also, urinary and serum levels of 18-oxocortisol, 18-hydroxycortisol (serum >300 ng/dL), and 18-hydroxycorticosterone (serum >100 ng/dL) tend to be higher. A positive postural stimulation test (plasma aldosterone: ambulating rising to <130% of the supine level) has a moderate sensitivity and specificity for adenoma, but not for hyperplasia. Once the diagnosis of primary hyperaldosteronism is confirmed, the next step is to image the adrenals by CT or MRI, looking for bilateral hyperplasia or a unilateral hypodense adenoma. The specificity of imaging to correctly categorize patients as having APA versus IHA varies from 67%–84% (Doppmann, 1992; Gleason, 1993; Harpe, 1999; Magill, 2001). Removal of the adenoma is curative in 35% of cases and leads to improvement in another 55% (Blumenfeld, 1994). Surgery can cure or improve hypertension in patients with unilateral disease. For those in whom the disease is bilateral, medical treatment with drugs such as spironolactone leads to improvement in 76% of cases. Hyperplasia is not always bilateral.

As a result of multiple factors, including the increased incidence of nonfunctioning adrenal adenoma after age 40, and the fact that hyperplasia may present as a unilateral adenoma on imaging, it is highly recommended that bilateral adrenal vein sampling be performed in individuals over age 40 who are contemplating surgery. Bilateral adrenal vein sampling is technically demanding and entails risk; however, as performed by an experienced radiologist, it is the gold standard for distinguishing adenoma from hyperplasia. An intravenous infusion of ACTH at 50 μg per hour is started 30 minutes before sampling and is continued throughout the procedure. This serves to mitigate any stress-induced fluctuations in aldosterone during the sampling, accentuate the gradient in cortisol from adrenal vein to inferior vena cava, and maximize the difference in secretion of aldosterone between the right and left adrenals in instances of APA. Samples for aldosterone and cortisol are obtained from each adrenal vein and from the periphery. An adrenal vein/peripheral vein cortisol of greater than 10:1 ensures that the samples are taken from the adrenal veins. There should be a <20% difference in cortisol measurements between both adrenals.

To correct for dilutional effects, the **cortisol-corrected aldosterone ratio** (i.e., aldosterone/cortisol) is utilized. In APA, the cortisol-corrected aldosterone ratio is usually at least fivefold higher on the side with the adenoma, and no gradient is seen in hyperplasia (Doppmann, 1996). As per the recent Endocrine Society guidelines, a cortisol-corrected aldosterone ratio from high side to low side of greater than 4:1 indicates APA, a ratio of less than 3:1 suggests IHA, and values between 4:1 and 3:1 are indeterminate and need to be interpreted in conjunction with imaging studies and clinical settings. Using these cutoffs, a sensitivity of 95% and a specificity of 100% are achieved (Funder, 2008).

Several studies have shown a discrepancy between radiologic findings and surgical findings in up to a third of all cases. Kempers found that when compared with adrenal vein sampling, CT and MRI misdiagnosed the cause of primary hyperaldosteronism in 37.8% of patients (Kempers, 2009). Given the increased prevalence (5%–10%) of adrenal incidentalomas (nonfunctioning adrenal tumors) with increasing age, many authorities are recommending adrenal vein sampling for those patients with hyperaldosteronism who are older than age 40 and have a unilateral hypodense adrenal nodule >1 cm on CT scan (Young, 1999). Based on the findings of large prospective studies, others have suggested that the major strength of this technique may be its use in evaluating those patients with a high probability of APA but with normal findings or bilateral nodular disease on CT. It should be stressed that this test is technically difficult, and even in the very best of hands is successful in only approximately 92%–96% of cases (Doppmann, 1992; Radin, 1992; Young, 1999).

The syndrome of **inapparent mineralocorticoid excess** is due to dysfunction of 11-β-hydroxysteroid dehydrogenase type 2 (11-β-HSD2). Cortisol can function as a potent mineralocoticoid, binding to the mineralocorticoid receptor in the kidney with the same affinity as aldosterone. 11-β-HSD2 mitigates the mineralocorticoid action of cortisol by converting it to the metabolically inactive form, cortisone. When activity of this enzyme is decreased because of hereditary factors, the ingestion of large quantities of licorice (which has a high content of glycyrrhizic acid) or chewing tobacco, hypertension, hypokalemia, low PRA, and low PAC may result. An elevated cortisol/cortisone concentration on a 24-hour urine collection confirms the diagnosis.

Renin may be suppressed by excessive sodium intake. It is also suppressed in the syndrome of hyporenin hypoaldosteronism, which is most commonly seen in patients with diabetes mellitus and renal disease. Secondary aldosteronism results from nonadrenal disease, in which both adrenal glands are stimulated (Table 24-25). Typically, these patients are not hypertensive.

Conditions such as nephrosis, cirrhosis, and heart failure are associated with decreased renal perfusion, causing a compensatory increase in renin and aldosterone levels (secondary hyperaldosteronism). The response of the renin-aldosterone system in pregnancy is especially complex; renin, renin substrate, angiotensin II, and aldosterone appear to be increased.

There are two variants of familial hyperaldosteronism (FH), FH-1, which is also known as glucocorticoid remedial hyperaldosteronism (GRA), and FH-2. GRA is an autosomal dominant inherited disorder characterized by hyperaldosteronism, hyporeninemia, and severe, usually refractory, hypertension, with onset typically occurring in those younger than age 20 with a positive family history of early hypertension and/or hemorrhagic stroke. It is the result of translocation of aldosterone synthetase (CYP18, CYP11B2) onto the ACTH-sensitive promoter sequence of the 11-β-hydroxylase *(CYP11B1)* gene within the zona fasciculata. Thus, aldosterone synthesis is stimulated by ACTH. In addition to increased aldosterone, these individuals produce excess 18-OH cortisol and 18-oxycortisol. Diagnosis can be confirmed by normalization of aldosterone following 4–6 weeks of steroid suppression, or by genetic testing using Southern blot or long polymerase chain reaction (Lifton, 1992; Kurtz, 1993). FH-2 is an autosomal dominant condition that is associated with APA, IHA, or both. Unlike FH-1, aldosterone does not suppress in response to glucocorticoid treatment.

Liddle syndrome is a rare autosomal dominant disorder characterized by hypertension and hypokalemia; however, unlike in primary hyperaldosteronism, PRA and PAC are both low. The defect is due to a mutation in the amiloride-sensitive sodium channel within the renal collecting ducts, leading to enhanced sodium reabsorption and increased potassium secretion. Liddle syndrome can be diagnosed by genetic testing or, if genetic testing is unavailable, by good clinical response to amiloride or triamterene, and by lack of response to dexamethasone or aldosterone antagonists.

ALDOSTERONE MEASUREMENTS

An isolated aldosterone measurement with no attention to patient preparation is of little clinical value. Even when time of sampling, posture, and dietary sodium and potassium are controlled, it is difficult to discriminate with certainty between primary aldosteronism and other forms of hypertension with the use of plasma aldosterone measurements alone. Interpretation of the aldosterone level must be done in the context of a simultaneously collected plasma renin and serum potassium.

Aldosterone assays are performed on plasma using extraction to remove aldosterone from plasma proteins, followed by chromatography and immunoassay or, preferably, LC-MS/MS. Urine is assayed following acid hydrolysis and extraction. Normative values exist for different age groups, postures, and sodium intakes (Table 24-26). HPLC with tandem mass spectrometry affords greater consistency and is gradually replacing older methods.

RENIN MEASUREMENTS

Important technical differences have been noted in assessment of renin using current methods. Renin measurements are of two types: PRA and PRC. The PRA is a bioassay wherein a plasma specimen containing renin is allowed to react with its substrate, angiotensinogen; after a specified period of time, the reaction is terminated, and generated angiotensin I is measured by RIA. For estimation of PRA, the endogenous substrate is not eliminated. Therefore, the rate of generation of angiotensin I is influenced by the concentrations of endogenous renin and its substrate. This type of assay is the most widely used method for the determination of renin. Comparison of results among laboratories is not possible because of procedural differences, such as variations in pH, ionic strength, length of the assay, the angiotensinase inhibitor, the conditions under which the specimen was obtained, and because of the lack of a specific reference preparation. In addition, the literature on renin assays reveals confusion regarding units of measurements employed; even when an attempt is made to express the many arbitrary units in the same terms (nanograms of angiotensin liberated per milliliter per hour), wide ranges are reported for human plasma renin activity in reference populations.

TABLE 24-25
Differentiating the Various Causes of Hyperaldosteronism

Disorder	Aldosterone	Renin	Serum K+
Primary hyperaldosteronism	↑	↓	↓
Renin-secreting tumor	↑	↑	↓–N
Dexamethasone-suppressible hyperaldosteronism	↑	↓	↓
Renovascular hypertension	N–↑	N–↑	↓–N
Bartter's syndrome	↑	↑	↓
Diuretics, congestive heart failure, cirrhosis, nephrotic syndrome	↑	↑	N–↓

N, Normal.

TABLE 24-26
Differentiating the Various Causes of Hypoaldosteronism

Disorder	Aldosterone	Renin	Serum K+
Addison's disease	↓	↑	↑
Cushing's syndrome	↓	↓	N or ↓
Liddle's syndrome	↓	↓	↓
Hyporenin hypoaldosteronism	↓	↓	↑
Apparent mineralocorticoid excess	↓	↓	↓
Isolated hypoaldosteronism	↓	↑	↑

N, Normal.

When PRC rather than PRA is measured, the effect of substrate is eliminated. The PRC assay is an immunoassay directed to the renin molecule itself.

Assays of PRA and PRC provide similar information, except in a few clinical situations. With oral contraceptive administration, PRC remains within the reference interval, whereas PRA increases owing to the increase in substrate. Other procedures such as freezing, thawing, and acidification have been found to convert prorenin to rennin, thereby increasing the values in PRC assays.

Because renin release is controlled by many physiologic and pharmacologic variables, it is extremely important to know the conditions under which the blood specimen was obtained. Such conditions as upright posture, the administration of diuretics, and low-sodium diets are potent stimuli of renin release and should be adequately controlled before plasma renin is measured. Renin also appears to be extremely labile, so the variables involved in specimen processing should be vigorously controlled. Blood should be drawn into an iced EDTA tube, which inactivates the enzymes (e.g., angiotensinases); it should be centrifuged at 4° C, and the plasma should be separated promptly from the cells, frozen immediately, and kept frozen until ready to be analyzed; with this technique, the specimen is stable for several months at −20° C.

Direct measurement of renin substrate, angiotensin I, or angiotensin II is not used widely in clinical practice because of tedious extraction or concentration steps, as well as difficulty in eliminating formation or degradation of these compounds by proteases and other enzymes involved in the renin system. Although ACE levels can be measured easily, they are of little use in the diagnosis of hypertensive disorders.

SELECTED REFERENCES

American Association of Clinical Endocrinologists. Medical guidelines for clinical practice for the evaluation and treatment of hyperthyroidism and hypothyroidism. Endocr Pract 2002;8:457–69.
An excellent reference for the diagnosis and treatment of commonly seen thyroid disorders, created by a consensus panel of experts in the field.

American Association of Clinical Endocrinologists. Medical guidelines for clinical practice for the diagnosis and treatment of acromegaly. Endocr Pract 2004;10:213–25.
An excellent reference for the diagnosis and treatment of acromegaly, created by a consensus panel of experts in the field of acromegaly.

Stewart PM. The adrenal cortex. In: Larsen PR, Kronenberg HM, Melmed S, Polonsky KS, editors. Williams textbook of endocrinology. 10th ed. Philadelphia: WB Saunders; 2003. p. 491–551.
One of the best written and most respected general endocrine reference textbooks; the chapter on the adrenals is concise, lucid, and well referenced.

REFERENCES

Access the complete reference list online at http://www.expertconsult.com

CHAPTER 25

REPRODUCTIVE FUNCTION AND PREGNANCY

Dorota Borawski, Martin H. Bluth

KEY POINTS

- Reproductive function and pregnancy are regulated by the complex interaction of a variety of hormones; they are synthesized and secreted by the testis (testosterone), ovary (estradiol and progesterone), pituitary (follicle-stimulating hormone [FSH] and luteinizing hormone [LH]), hypothalamus (gonadotropin-releasing hormone, and placenta (human chorionic gonadotropin [hCG], estrogens, and progesterone).
- Laboratory evaluation of reproductive function in the male typically begins with semen analysis. If the results are normal, further evaluation may be unnecessary. If the results are abnormal, then serum hormone measurements, particularly of testosterone, FSH, and LH, are important.
- Reproductive dysfunction in the female is often indicated by amenorrhea and/or infertility. Laboratory evaluation, as in the male, involves serum hormone measurements, particularly of hCG, prolactin, thyroid-stimulating hormone, free thyroxine, FSH, LH, and androgens.
- Infertility can be treated by several assisted reproductive technologies. These involve a variety of clinical manipulations, all of which are directed at externally controlling as much of the reproductive process as possible to achieve pregnancy and bring it to term. Laboratory monitoring of serum hormone levels (estradiol, progesterone, and hCG) plays an important role in these protocols.
- Early pregnancy is monitored by measuring serum hCG concentrations and determining that the pattern of dramatic increase during the first trimester is as expected.
- The risk for the most common birth defects, neural tube defects, and chromosomal aneuploidy is determined during the first- and second-trimester screenings.
- Fetal hemolytic disease is monitored by spectrophotometric estimation of the level of bilirubin in amniotic fluid or Doppler measurements of peak systolic velocity in the fetal middle cerebral artery.
- The status of fetal lung maturation is estimated from the evaluation of pulmonary surfactant in amniotic fluid. This can be accomplished by several methods, including determination of (1) the lecithin/sphingomyelin ratio and phosphatidyl glycerol by chromatography, or (2) microviscosity by fluorescence polarization.
- Toxemia of pregnancy, or preeclampsia, is characterized by hypertension and proteinuria, and consequently can be monitored by urine protein measurements.
- Risk for preterm delivery and the need for medical intervention can be evaluated by checking levels of fetal fibronectin in the cervical secretions.

NORMAL PHYSIOLOGY

Normal reproductive function is mediated by a variety of hormones synthesized and secreted by the gonads (testes and ovaries), adrenals, pituitary, hypothalamus, and placenta. In addition, peripheral nonglandular tissues can contribute to hormone synthesis. Paracrine and autocrine mediators are also involved, but in almost all cases their exact roles are not well understood.

SEX STEROIDS

The testes and ovaries synthesize sex steroids (androgens and estrogens) from cholesterol via the same initial pathway used in the adrenal glands to synthesize mineralocorticoids, glucocorticoids, and androgens (Fig. 25-1). The specific hormone secreted by an endocrine gland depends on the presence and relative activities of various enzymes in the steroid pathway. Whereas the adrenal synthesizes androgens like dehydroepiandrosterone (DHEA), DHEA-sulfate (DHEAS), and androstenedione, the testis metabolizes these steroids primarily to testosterone. The ovary converts testosterone to estradiol, and androstenedione to estrone. Peripheral tissues (including those targeted by androgens) reduce testosterone to dihydrotestosterone (DHT). Because DHT is two to three times more

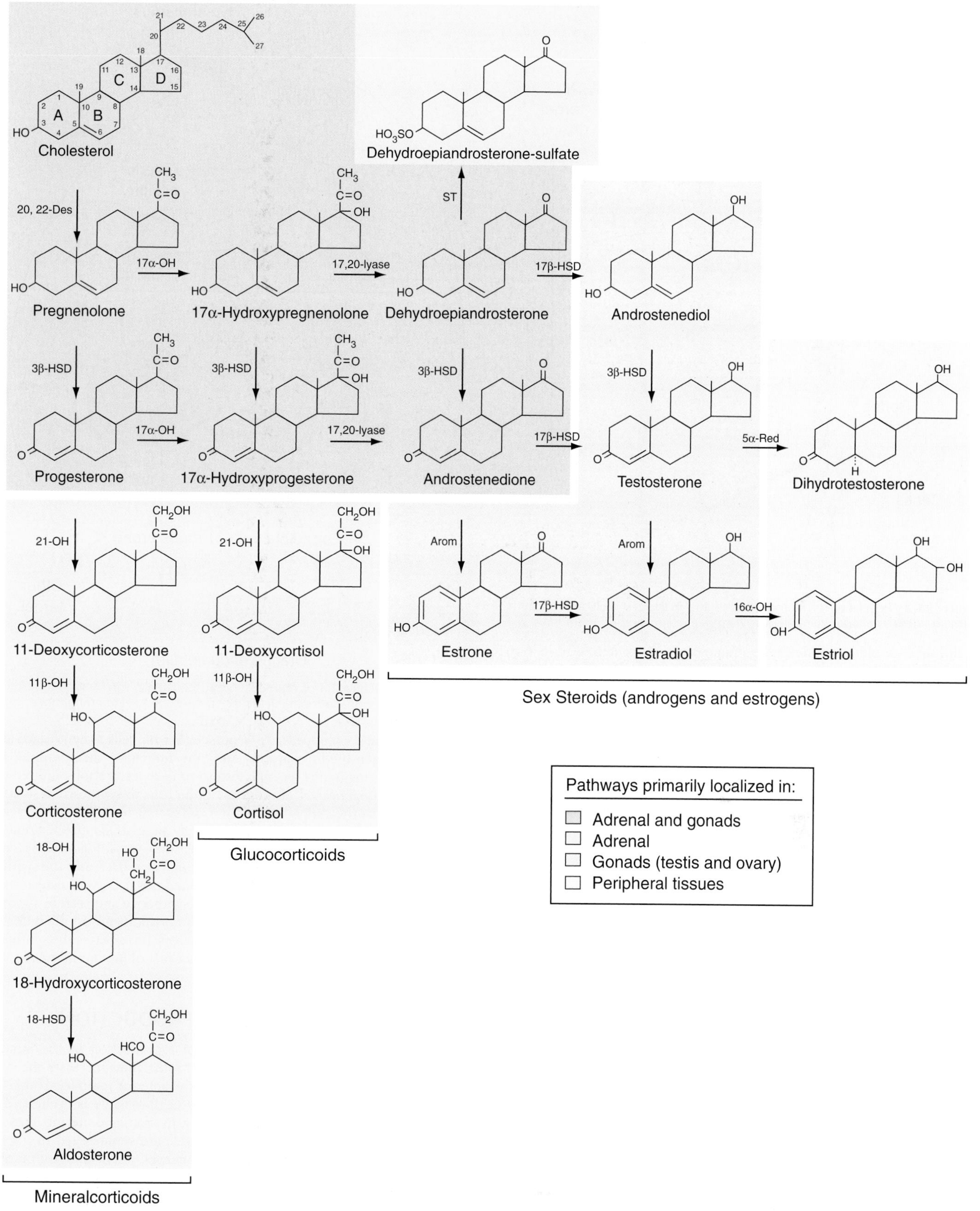

Figure 25-1 Steroid hormone synthesis. *Arom,* Aromatase; *16α-OH,* 16α-hydroxylase; *17-α-OH,* 17α-hydroxylase; *5α–Red,* 5α-reductase; *3β-HSD,* 3β-hydroxysteroid dehydrogenase; *17β–HSD,* 17β-hydroxysteroid dehydrogenase; *11-β–OH,* 11-β-hydroxylase; *20,22-Des,* 20,22 desmolase; *18-HSD,* 18-hydroxysteroid dehydrogenase; *18-OH,* 18-hydroxylase; *21-OH,* 21-hydroxylase; *ST,* sulfotransferase.

potent than testosterone, this process yields an enhanced or activated androgenic effect. Peripheral tissues, such as liver, also hydroxylate estradiol to estriol, a metabolite with only one-hundredth the estrogenic potency of its precursor. Thus, this conversion is an inactivation process. During pregnancy, estriol is synthesized via a different pathway, and it may play a different role than estradiol (see later). Peripheral tissues also convert adrenal androgens to testosterone and androgens to estrone and estradiol, the latter occurring in adipose tissue. Estrone is about one tenth as potent as estradiol, which likely further modulates estradiol potency. Note that, although progesterone serves as an intermediate in the synthesis

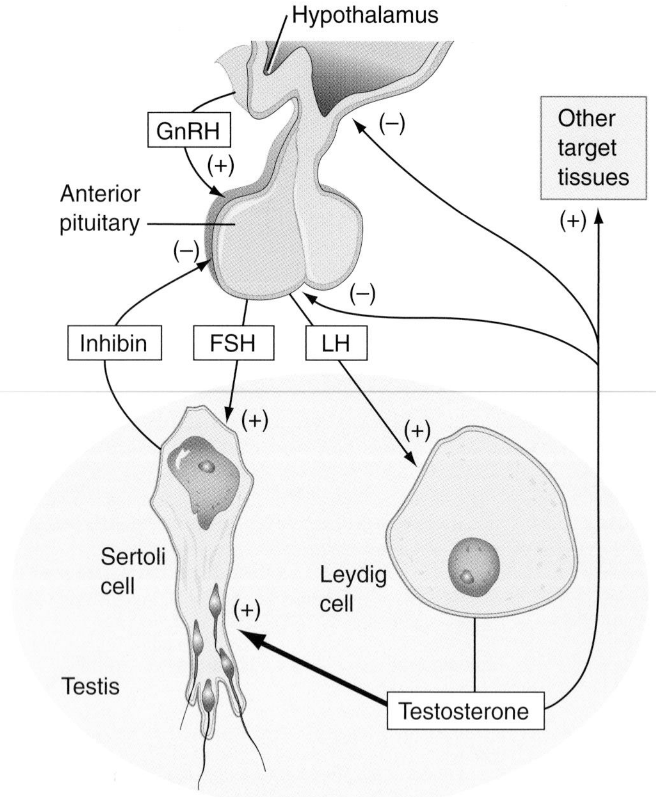

Figure 25-2 Regulation of reproduction in the male. *FSH,* Follicle-stimulating hormone; *GnRH,* gonadotropin-releasing hormone; *LH,* luteinizing hormone.

of all other steroid hormones, it also functions as a sex steroid in its own right in females.

As with any hormone, sex steroids act at tissue sites distant from their sites of synthesis and secretion. Once in the blood, most of the hydrophobic sex steroids become reversibly and noncovalently bound to plasma proteins. This interaction includes low-affinity, nonspecific binding to hydrophobic sites on albumin and high-affinity binding to specific transport proteins that are synthesized by the liver. Sex hormone–binding globulin (SHBG) transports androgens and estrogens, and corticosteroid-binding globulin (CBG) transports progesterone (as well as glucocorticoids). In blood, only about 1%–2% of the sex steroids are free (unbound). About half of the remainder are bound to SHBG or CBG, and about half are bound to albumin. Only the free fraction is biologically active, because only the free hormone can exit the vascular system (by diffusion) and interact with target cells.

Each steroid binds with high affinity to specific receptor proteins that activate or inactivate genes in the target cell. Thus, the same hormone can elicit a different response in each type of target cell. The potency of a steroid's hormonal effect (e.g., androgenic effect) is primarily a function of its affinity for the specific receptor protein and the affinity of that complex for the chromatin acceptor sites. Thus DHT is a more potent androgen than testosterone. DHEA and androstenedione bind only weakly, if at all, to the androgen receptor; hence their androgenic effect is low, and most if not all of their androgenic activity derives from their peripheral conversion to testosterone.

REGULATION OF MALE REPRODUCTION

Figure 25-2 summarizes the regulation of reproduction in the human male. Gonadotropin-releasing hormone (GnRH) is a decapeptide that is synthesized and secreted by neuroendocrine cells of the hypothalamus, primarily in the arcuate nucleus. GnRH binds to specific cell membrane receptors on gonadotrophs in the anterior pituitary, resulting in the synthesis and secretion of two protein hormones—FSH and LH—both named for their effects in females. Both FSH and LH are similar to thyroid-stimulating hormone (TSH), in that all three consist of two subunits and all of them share the same α subunit. Each has a different β subunit, however, which thus confers their functional specificity.

The seminiferous tubules of the testis contain cells in various stages of spermatogenesis (spermatogonia, spermatocytes, spermatids), along with Sertoli cells and Leydig cells. FSH induces Sertoli cells to synthesize and secrete androgen-binding protein into the lumen of the seminiferous tubule, and this maintains the high testosterone concentration required for normal spermatogenesis. LH induces Leydig cells to synthesize testosterone; some enters the general circulation and is transported to other target tissues, such as skeletal muscle, where it has an anabolic effect. Some is also transported to the hypothalamus and anterior pituitary, where the testosterone has a negative-feedback effect, that is, it decreases the synthesis and secretion of GnRH, FSH, and LH, and this decreases testosterone synthesis by Leydig cells. Sertoli cells also synthesize and secrete another protein hormone, inhibin. It interacts with gonadotrophs in the anterior pituitary, where it has a negative feedback effect: It decreases the synthesis and secretion of FSH, but not LH. The exact role of inhibin in the regulatory process is not understood.

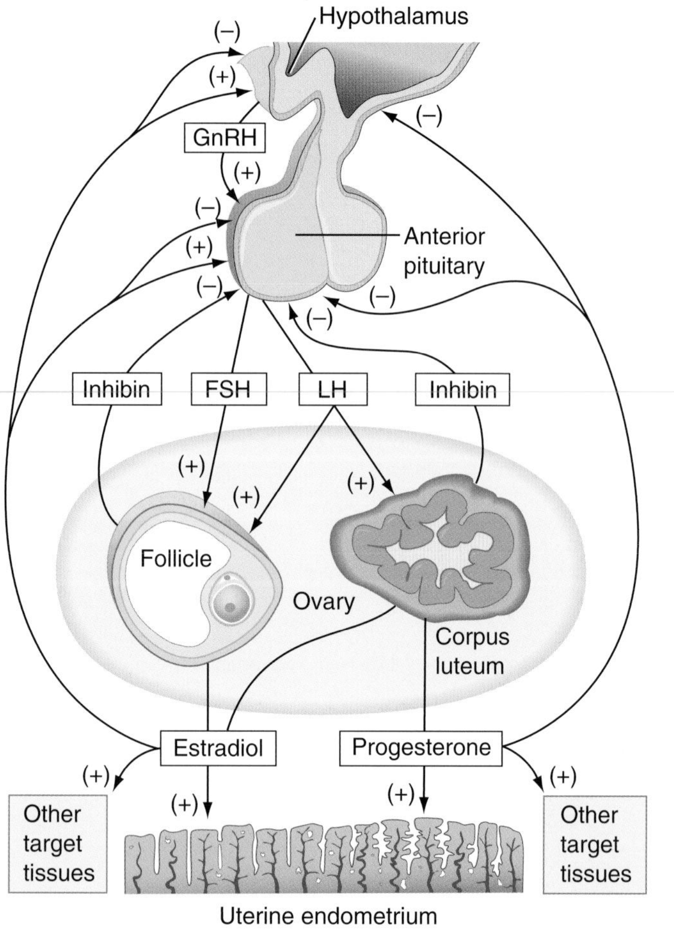

Figure 25-3 Regulation of reproduction in the female. *FSH,* Follicle-stimulating hormone; *GnRH,* gonadotropin-releasing hormone; *LH,* luteinizing hormone.

REGULATION OF FEMALE REPRODUCTION

Figure 25-3 summarizes the regulation of reproduction in the human female. As in the male, GnRH from the hypothalamus increases the synthesis and secretion of FSH and LH from the anterior pituitary. Unlike in the male, however, the regulatory process in the female is cyclic and is referred to as the menstrual cycle. Pituitary, ovarian, and uterine changes that occur during the 28-day menstrual cycle are summarized in Figure 25-4. As illustrated, the cycle begins with menses, or shedding of uterine endometrium. During this period in the ovary, a cohort of follicles is recruited to begin further growth and development. From this cohort, one follicle (usually) is selected to be the dominant follicle and to continue growth and development. The other recruited follicles undergo regression, or atresia. These processes occur during the follicular phase of the ovarian cycle, primarily as a result of the action of FSH. As the follicle grows, increasing amounts of estradiol are synthesized and secreted. Estradiol restores the endometrium via cell proliferation and growth; hence the proliferative phase of the uterine endometrial cycle. Estradiol also has a negative-feedback effect on the hypothalamus and the anterior pituitary, causing a decline in FSH levels during the latter part of the follicular phase.

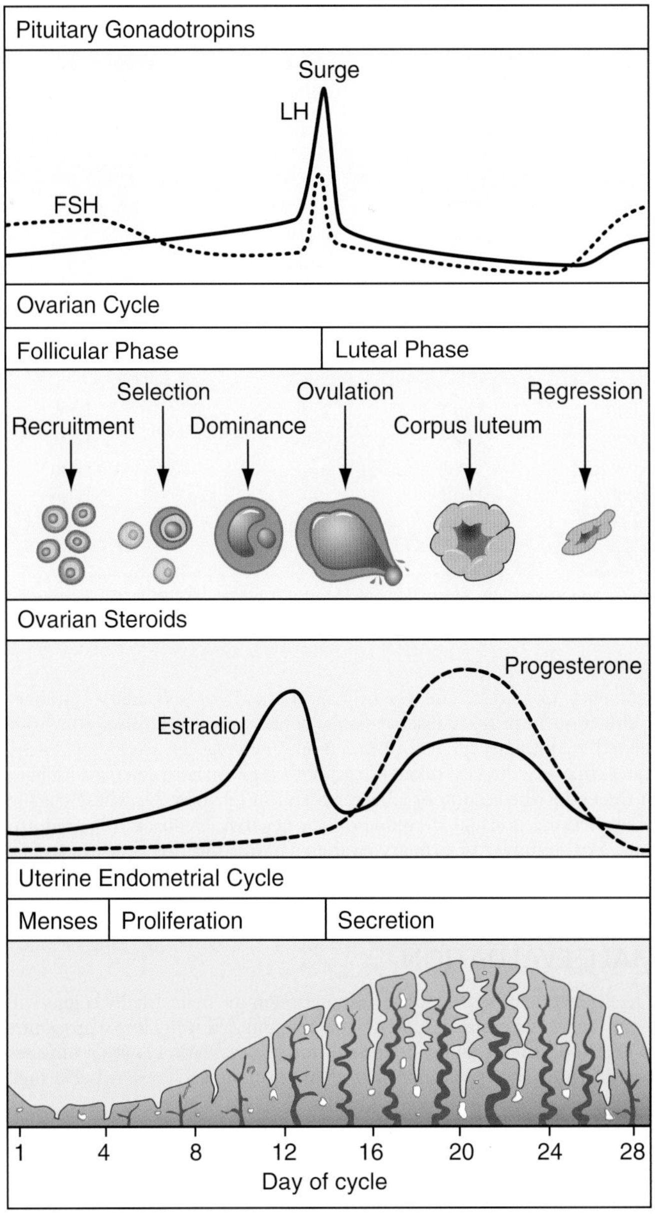

Figure 25-4 Pituitary, ovarian, and uterine changes during the human menstrual cycle. *FSH,* Follicle-stimulating hormone; *LH,* luteinizing hormone.

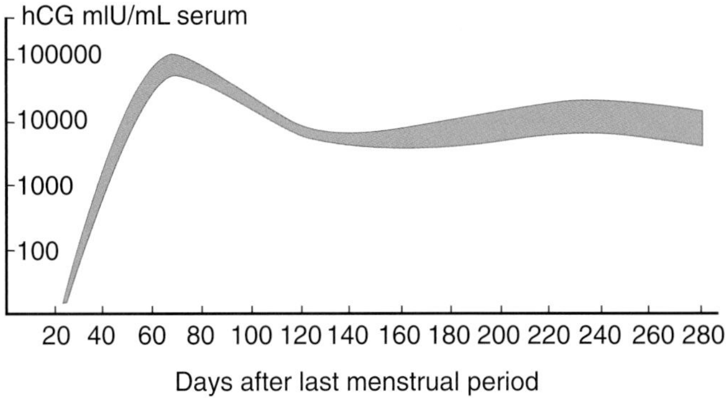

Figure 25-5 Serum hCG levels during normal pregnancy. *(From Lau HL. Testing for pregnancy. In: Practice of medicine, vol II. Hagerstown, Md.: Harper & Row; 1975, Chapter 29; and Braunstein GD, Rasor J, Adler D, Danzer H, Wade ME. Am J Obstet Gynecol 1976;126:678.) hCG,* Human chorionic gonadotropin.

Near the end of the follicular phase, when estradiol levels are at their highest, its feedback effect on the hypothalamus and anterior pituitary switches to positive. The mechanism for this change to positive feedback is not understood. Its effect, however, is dramatic. It causes a surge in the secretion of GnRH, FSH, and particularly LH, which culminates in ovulation. The oocyte enters the oviduct. Owing to disruption of the follicle, estradiol synthesis and secretion drop dramatically. The disrupted follicle begins to differentiate into the corpus luteum; thus begins the luteal phase of the ovarian cycle. The corpus luteum synthesizes estradiol and progesterone as a result of the action of LH. The combination of the two steroids acts on the uterine endometrium to cause development of numerous exocrine glands, producing the secretory phase of the uterine endometrial cycle. This phase prepares the endometrium for implantation, should fertilization and early development occur. LH levels decline gradually during the luteal phase, indicating restoration of negative-feedback regulation of the hypothalamus and anterior pituitary by estradiol and progesterone.

As in the male, inhibin has a selective negative-feedback effect on FSH. In the female, however, there are two different forms. One is synthesized and secreted by the developing follicles (inhibin B), and the other is from the corpus luteum (inhibin A) (Welt, 1999). Again, the exact regulatory roles they play are not understood.

In an infertile cycle, the corpus luteum begins to regress near the end of the luteal phase. This results in a decrease in estradiol and progesterone synthesis and secretion. Because these steroids are required for maintenance of the secretory endometrium, it begins to deteriorate and is ultimately shed during menstruation. With the drop in estradiol and progesterone, their negative-feedback effects decrease, and FSH and LH rise to begin another cycle.

PREGNANCY

If the oocyte is fertilized during its transit down the oviduct, it develops into a multicellular blastocyst by the time it reaches the uterus. Around the time of implantation (about 9 days after ovulation), and before the corpus luteum begins to regress, increasing amounts of an LH-like hormone, hCG, are found in maternal blood. hCG is synthesized and secreted by the trophoblast cells of the developing placenta. It is a dimeric protein hormone that has the same α subunit as LH, FSH, and TSH, but a different β subunit. The β subunit of hCG is very similar to that of LH, but larger. Hence, hCG can interact with LH receptors on luteal cells. This interaction prevents regression of the corpus luteum and allows it to continue synthesis and secretion of estradiol and progesterone, both of which are required for appropriate maintenance of the uterine endometrium throughout pregnancy.

During the first trimester of pregnancy, hCG increases from <5 mIU/mL serum to >100,000 mIU/mL (Fig. 25-5). This increase is responsible for the similarly dramatic increases in the levels of estradiol and progesterone. By the end of the first trimester, however, hCG levels begin to decline significantly. Estradiol and progesterone continue to increase, because, by this time, the placenta has assumed most steroid synthesis, including significant amounts of estrone and estriol. Unlike hCG, these steroid levels increase as placental mass grows. Steroid intermediates from the fetal adrenal gland and the fetal liver also contribute to this process. For example, estriol is synthesized not by hydroxylation of estradiol (see Fig. 25-1), but rather by conversion from fetal 16-hydroxy-DHEAS; this is why maternal estriol measurements were historically used to assess fetal well-being in late pregnancy (Carr, 2004). The estrogenic potency of estriol is only about one-hundredth that of estradiol and only one-tenth that of estrone. However, estriol promotes uteroplacental blood flow as potently as other estrogens, and this may be the reason for its dramatic increase during the last two trimesters (Resnik, 1974).

Another hormone synthesized in large quantities by the placenta during the last two trimesters is human placental lactogen (HPL). It is structurally similar to both prolactin and growth hormone and has both lactogenic and growth-promoting activities, although both are relatively weak. In addition, HPL is an insulin antagonist and thus may play a role in maternal glucose utilization. However, its exact role is unclear because apparently normal pregnancies have been described in which HPL is not detectable in maternal blood or placenta (Sideri, 1983). Unlike hCG, the increase in HPL also parallels the steady increase in placental mass (Carr, 2004).

The placenta also synthesizes inhibin. Whereas gonadal (testicular and ovarian) inhibin functions as an endocrine inhibitor of pituitary FSH secretion, placental inhibin may function as a paracrine or autocrine inhibitor of placental hCG secretion (Mesiano, 2004). Its exact regulatory role, however, has not been elucidated.

Parturition is the process by which the fetus is expelled from the internal environment of the maternal uterus to the external environment.

TABLE 25-1
Changes in Reproductive Hormone Levels in Different Disease States

DISEASE STATE		HORMONE LEVEL			
Classification	**Example**	**FSH**	**LH**	**Testosterone**	**Estradiol**
Male					
Primary deficiency	Klinefelter's syndrome	High	High	Low	–
Secondary deficiency	Panhypopituitarism	Low	Low	Low	–
Primary excess	Testicular tumor	Low	Low	High	–
Secondary excess	Precocious puberty	High	High	High	–
Other	Seminiferous tubule failure	High	Normal	Normal	–
Other	Partial androgen insensitivity	Normal	High	High	–
Female					
Primary deficiency	Menopause	High	High	–	Low
Secondary deficiency	Sheehan's syndrome	Low	Low	–	Low
Primary excess	Feminizing ovarian tumor	Low	Low	–	High
Secondary excess	Gonadotropin-producing tumor (rare)	High	High	–	High
Other	Polycystic ovarian syndrome	Normal	High	High	–
Other	Masculinizing ovarian tumor	Low	Low	High	–

From Nickel KL. The gonads. In: Kaplan LA, Pesce AJ, editors. Clinical chemistry—theory, analysis, and correlation. 3rd ed. St Louis: Mosby; 1996, p. 892–911, with permission.
FSH, Follicle-stimulating hormone; *LH,* luteinizing hormone.

This occurs as a result of a change in the activity of the uterine myometrium (smooth muscle), from irregular, long-lasting, low-frequency contractions to regular, high-intensity, high-frequency contractions. The initiation of this process in humans is not well understood and seems to differ from that in other mammals. For example, progesterone inhibits uterine contractions during gestation, and in most other mammals, the onset of parturition is preceded by a significant decrease in maternal plasma progesterone; in humans, however, this does not occur. A **parturition cascade** has been postulated for humans that involves multiple and redundant endocrine, paracrine, and autocrine mediators. These mediators are thought to include fetal cortisol and DHEAS; placental estriol, oxytocin, prostaglandins, and corticotropin-releasing hormone; and maternal oxytocin. The effects of these mediators may also be modulated by changes in their receptor levels (Norwitz, 2004).

Parturition is followed by lactation. Initial development of the mammary gland occurs at puberty, when estradiol causes growth and branching of the ducts, and progesterone causes formation of the alveoli. Similarly, during pregnancy, the high concentrations of estrogens and progesterone cause further branching of the ducts and growth of the alveoli. The secretory capability of the alveolar epithelial cells is induced by prolactin, which increases during pregnancy, and by HPL. At parturition, the decrease in estrogen and progesterone eliminates their inhibitory effects on milk secretion, which still requires prolactin. Milk ejection, however, requires oxytocin, acting as part of a neuroendocrine reflex. This reflex is initiated by the suckling stimulus, which generates nerve impulses that travel from the nipple to the hypothalamus. There they cause secretion of oxytocin from neuroendocrine cells in the posterior pituitary. The oxytocin travels to the mammary gland, where it stimulates the contraction of smooth muscle cells surrounding the alveoli, causing milk ejection. Prolactin also participates in this neuroendocrine reflex, in that nerve impulses reaching the hypothalamus also inhibit the synthesis and secretion of dopamine, which functions as a prolactin release-inhibiting hormone. This then promotes the release of prolactin from the anterior pituitary, which then travels to the mammary gland, where it stimulates milk secretion, to replace that lost by ejection. As long as lactation continues, plasma prolactin concentrations remain elevated. This postpartum hyperprolactinemia causes postpartum amenorrhea due to interference with normal regulation by GnRH of FSH and LH secretion. Although this hypogonadotropic state will prevent pregnancy, it is not considered a reliable means of contraception, particularly in modern societies where breastfeeding is variable.

LABORATORY EVALUATION OF REPRODUCTIVE FUNCTION

Table 25-1 describes laboratory findings in various male and female reproductive disease states typically categorized according to (1) hormone deficiency or excess, and (2) primary (gonad) or secondary (pituitary) dysfunction In primary disease states, gonadal steroid levels are inversely related to pituitary gonadotropin levels, whereas in secondary disease states, they are directly related (e.g., both high or both low), as discussed in the endocrine section of Chapter 8 and in Chapter 24. These changes occur because gonadal steroids provide negative feedback to gonadotropins. For example, in primary ovarian failure, the decrease in estradiol reduces its negative-feedback effect on the hypothalamic-pituitary axis, resulting in increases in FSH and LH.

MALE EVALUATION

The evaluation of reproductive dysfunction in the male usually begins with semen analysis, because it is a cost-effective and relatively simple procedure. In addition, if the results are normal, further evaluation is often unnecessary. If semen analysis is abnormal, then hormone analyses are performed.

Semen Analysis

In addition to its use in the evaluation of reproductive dysfunction, particularly infertility, semen analysis is used to select donors for therapeutic insemination and to monitor the success of surgical procedures, such as varicocelectomy and vasectomy. Semen analysis consists of microscopic and macroscopic components, and the latter include measuring physical (e.g., volume) and chemical (e.g., pH) properties. Useful guides and references for the procedure are available (Gilbert, 1992; Mortimer, 1994; Tomlinson, 1999; World Health Organization, 1999; Andrade-Rocha, 2003; Rylander, 2009).

Sample Collection

The patient should be instructed to collect semen after 3 days of sexual abstinence. Longer periods of abstinence usually result in a higher semen volume but reduced sperm motility. In such a case, a second semen specimen may be collected 2 hours after the first sample is collected. The bladder should be evacuated before ejaculation occurs. For semen collection, the laboratory should provide a preweighed sterile plastic (polypropylene) container with a screw top. The semen specimen should be delivered to the laboratory within 1 hour of collection and kept warm during transportation. A postejaculate urine sample may be collected at this time if retrograde ejaculation is suspected. Two specimens collected within 2- to 3-week intervals should be used for evaluation, and if they are markedly different, additional specimens should be collected. Ideally, semen specimens should be collected in the privacy of a room adjacent to the laboratory, because some samples require sperm to be separated from seminal plasma as soon as possible. Assisted reproductive technologies (ARTs; see later), such as in vitro fertilization (IVF), require that motile sperm be isolated from seminal plasma within 1 hour of ejaculation to protect sperm from the inhibitory effects of seminal plasma on fertilization. Semen should be obtained by masturbation, and if circumstances preclude such collection, special Silastic condoms should be made available for semen collection with intercourse. Incomplete semen specimens should not be analyzed.

Macroscopic examination should be performed after liquefaction, which usually occurs in less than 20 minutes at room temperature. Failure to liquefy may indicate inadequate prostate secretion. Semen should be thoroughly mixed before examination, and its viscosity recorded. The volume of ejaculate can be measured by weighing the collection cup before and after specimen collection. The appearance of a yellow hue in a semen specimen is associated with pyospermia, and a rust color with small bleedings in the seminal vesicle. The pH ranges from 7.2–7.8, but may be 8.0 or higher with acute infection in the prostate, seminal vesicle, or epididymis. The pH will be 7.0 or lower if there is contamination with urine or an obstruction in the ejaculatory ducts, or if the specimen consists of mainly prostatic fluid.

Microscopic examination should be performed to obtain estimates of sperm concentration, motility, and agglutination. Other cellular elements such as polygonal cells of the urethral tract and **round cells** such as spermatogenic cells and leukocytes can also be observed when sperm are counted in a hemocytometer. Because sperm motility and velocity are temperature dependent, these parameters must be assessed on a microscope with a warm stage. Typically, 8 μL of semen (of normal viscosity) placed under a 22 × 22-mm glass coverslip will yield a wet preparation that is 16.5 μm deep. Alternatively, 4 μL of sample added to disposable slides with two wells (used with thick glass coverslips) produces a 20-μm-deep preparation. A hemocytometer or microchamber may be used for the sperm count. At least four different fields in each of the two specimen aliquots should be counted, and the mean of the eight separate readings recorded. Total sperm count is then calculated by multiplying the dilution factor (normal concentration range, 20–50 million/mL) by its volume (normal range, 2–5 mL).

Motility (normal range 50% or above) is expressed as the percentage of sperm that move. In addition, forward movement is graded. Sperm moving rapidly in a straight line with little yaw and lateral movement are grade 4, or if they move more slowly, grade 3. Grade 2 sperm moves even more slowly and with substantial yaw. Grade 1 sperm has no forward progression. Zero progression denotes absence of any motility. If motility is less than 50%, a viability stain of eosin Y with nigrosin as a counterstain is done. In bright-field microscopy, dead sperm will stain red, whereas live sperm will exclude the dye and appear unstained. In samples with no visible sperm, such as postvasectomy semen, the entire sample should be centrifuged and the pellet examined for intact or damaged sperm fragments. The analysis should be repeated in 4–6 months.

Agglutination occurs when motile sperm stick to each other in an orientation that is reproducible within a given specimen, such as head to head, tail to tail, midpiece to midpiece, or mixed ways depending on the specificity of sperm antibodies. Agglutination suggests an immunologic cause of infertility, and a description of the type of agglutination should be recorded. This can usually be distinguished from clumping due to bacterial infection or tissue debris, which typically involves nonspecific orientation of the sperm.

Round cells should be differentiated into two classes: immature germ cells with a single or double highly condensed nucleus with a relatively large area of cytoplasm; and polymorphonuclear leukocytes, which are smaller than the germ cells and have a lower nuclear/cytoplasmic ratio. Peroxidase staining specifically identifies the polymorphonuclear leukocytes in the presence of lymphocytes and other cells that normally occur in semen. Bacterial contamination should be noted, as should the presence or absence of epithelial cells. If no sperm are seen in association with a low semen volume, a fructose test should be performed to confirm the presence of fluid from the seminal vesicle, and the same test should be performed on postejaculate urine to rule out retrograde ejaculation. However, the significance of a fructose test result has declined over the years because of the availability of more direct diagnostic tools such as transrectal ultrasonography.

Sperm morphology can predict fertility (Ombelet, 1997). Typically, >50% of the sperm in a semen specimen should exhibit normal morphology. Kruger and colleagues (1988) developed strict criteria for normal sperm morphology. Morphologically abnormal sperm usually have multiple defects, and the average number of defects per sperm, designated as the teratozoospermic index, is a significant predictor of sperm function both in vivo and in vitro. Strict morphology score greater than 14% of normal indicates excellent fertilizing capacity. Scores between 0 and 3% predict probable inability to fertilize. Wide variability in the size of the acrosomal cap is the most obvious characteristic of abnormal sperm. An acrosomal cap less than one third of the head surface is considered abnormal, as are retention of a cytoplasmic droplet greater than half of the head size and a tail less than 45 μm long. Of particular note is the direct relationship between acrosome size and the frequency of fertilization or pregnancy.

Immunologic Tests

Sperm antibody binding to head or tail antigens is considered specific for immunologic infertility. The antibodies are usually of the immunoglobulin (Ig)A or IgG class, and rarely, the IgM class; IgA antibodies are the most clinically significant. Current methods detect sperm-bound antibodies by direct or indirect mixed agglutination reaction (MAR) tests for IgG and IgA, or by immunobead assay, which detects all classes but with varying sensitivity. Both tests require motile sperm. The direct MAR test can be performed on fresh semen, and the result can be read within a few minutes with a light microscope.

Semen is mixed with latex particles coated with nonspecific human IgG, and then monospecific antisera to human IgG is added. The anti-IgG bridges the sperm-bound IgG, if present, and the particle-bound IgG to form mixed agglutinates. In the absence of sperm-bound IgG, the anti-IgG agglutinates only the latex particles. Under light microscopy, localized binding of the particles identifies the antibody as specific to head, tail, or any other region of the sperm structure. An indirect test can also be done with this reagent to detect the presence of sperm antibody in semen, cervical mucus, or serum.

The immunobead assay can detect all three immunoglobulin classes when beads are coated with monospecific antisera to each class. Therefore, sperm are washed to remove all free immunoglobulin before the beads are added. An indirect assay can also be designed with this reagent. The test is best read under phase microscopy. Increased risk of men developing sperm antibody is associated with vasectomy, repeat infections, obstruction of the ducts, cryptorchidism, varicocele, testicular biopsy, trauma, torsion, cancer, and genetic predisposition (Gilbert, 1992; Chamley, 2007). In women, sperm antibody is usually associated with intense mucosal inflammation of the genital tract.

Genital tract infections (see Part 7) may have significant adverse effects on male and female fertility (Pellati, 2008). For example, *Escherichia coli* can cause sperm agglutination and immobilization, and adherence of *E. coli* to sperm is mediated by mannose and mannose-binding cell surface structures present on both cell types (Sarkar, 1974; Wolff, 1993). Special precautions should be taken when collecting a semen specimen for detection of bacteria or yeast, to eliminate the possibility of external sources of contamination. Seminal plasma cultures may help diagnose male accessory gland infection, particularly of the prostate. If the concentration of bacteria exceeds 1000 colony-forming units per milliliter, the colonies should be identified and tested for antibiotic sensitivity.

Accessory Glands

Seminal vesicle, prostate, and epididymis function can be evaluated by analyzing unique constituents of each. Prostate secretions, for example, are acidic and contain acid phosphatase. Seminal fluid that is more alkaline than normal (pH >8.0) and that has reduced acid phosphatase suggests prostate dysfunction. Fructose is a measure of seminal vesicle secretory function. In azoospermia caused by the congenital absence of vasa deferentia, a low fructose level may indicate an associated dysgenesis of the seminal vesicles. Ejaculatory duct obstruction, or agenesis of the vasa deferentia and seminal vesicles, may result in the production of semen with low volume, low pH, lack of coagulation, and absence of characteristic semen odor. Neutral α-glucosidase originates solely from the epididymis, and its measurement is of diagnostic value for distal ductal obstruction when considered with hormonal and testicular findings.

Image Analysis

Routine semen evaluation can be carried out by an automated image analysis system that uses sperm head movement to derive the magnitude of various swimming parameters. However, human sperm are extremely heterogeneous with respect to morphology, swimming characteristics, and sperm DNA content. Thus no reference is made to evaluating specimens as normal or abnormal, fertile or infertile. Hence, semen evaluation by manual methods performed by trained technical staff remains a standard practice of andrology laboratories.

Hormone Analysis

If multiple semen analyses demonstrate azoospermia (no sperm), oligospermia (<20 million sperm per mL), or another abnormality, then

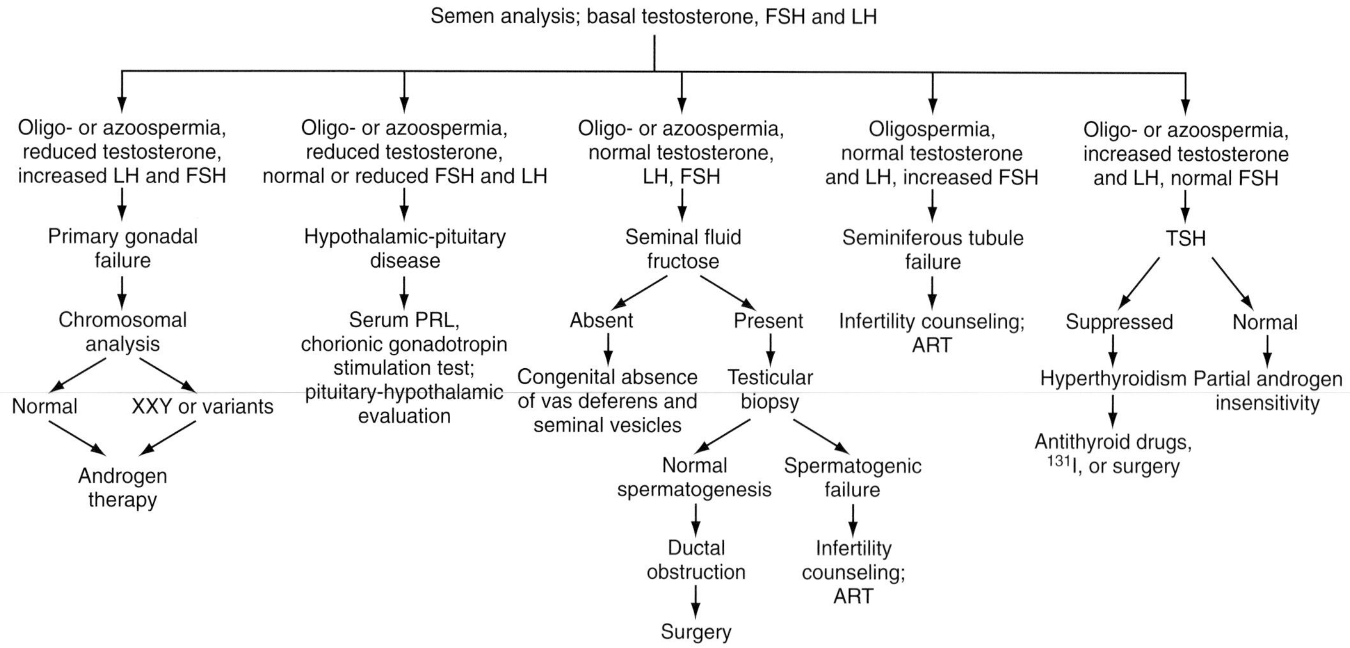

Figure 25-6 A diagnostic algorithm for male hypogonadism. *(From Braunstein GD. Testes. In: Greenspan FS, Gardner DG, editors. Basic and clinical endocrinology. 7th ed. New York: Lange Medical Books/McGraw-Hill; 2004, p. 478–510, with permission.) ART,* Assisted reproductive technology; *FSH,* follicle-stimulating hormone; *LH,* luteinizing hormone; *PRL,* prolactin; *TSH,* thyroid-stimulating hormone.

hormone analyses are performed to help identify the specific dysfunction. An example of a diagnostic algorithm is shown in Figure 25-6.

Decreased testosterone accompanied by increased LH and FSH indicates primary testicular failure. This can be an acquired or a genetic disease (Klinefelter's syndrome; see Chapter 68). Decreased testosterone accompanied by decreased or inappropriately normal LH and FSH indicates hypothalamic-pituitary disease, resulting in secondary testicular failure. When LH and FSH levels are normal, secondary disease can be confirmed with an hCG stimulation test. hCG interacts with LH receptors, and in the male, such interaction stimulates Leydig cells, if they are normal, to synthesize and secrete testosterone. Thus, administration of hCG should cause an increase in serum testosterone in secondary testicular failure, but not in primary testicular failure.

If hypothalamic-pituitary disease is suspected, then prolactin (PRL) should also be measured. Hyperprolactinemia interferes with the normal regulation of FSH and LH secretion by GnRH, and prolactinomas are the most common type of pituitary tumor. However, if prolactin is elevated, primary hypothyroidism must be excluded as a possible cause. In primary hypothyroidism, TSH and thyrotropin-releasing hormone (TRH) are elevated. Although the function of TRH is to stimulate the synthesis and secretion of TSH, TRH also stimulates the synthesis and secretion of prolactin. Thus, an elevated TSH suggests that primary hypothyroidism is the cause of the hyperprolactinemia, whereas a normal TSH suggests that a prolactinoma is the cause. If the latter were the case, then imaging techniques would be used to further evaluate the hypothalamic-pituitary axis.

If normal testosterone, LH, and FSH levels accompany oligospermia or azoospermia, then seminal fluid fructose should be evaluated. Its absence suggests the congenital absence of vasa deferentia and seminal vesicles. Its presence suggests ductal obstruction or spermatogenic failure, which can be distinguished using testicular biopsy. Oligospermia accompanied by normal testosterone and LH along with increased FSH suggests seminiferous tubule failure. The increase in FSH is likely due to reduced negative-feedback inhibition by decreased Sertoli cell inhibin. Increased testosterone and LH with normal/or elevated FSH suggest partial or complete androgen insensitivity. Testosterone provides negative feedback on GnRH secretion at the level of the hypothalamus through androgen receptors. Genetic mutations of androgen receptors in hypothalamic neurons result in increased pituitary release of LH, resistance to testosterone, hypogonadism, and oligospermia.

In evaluation protocols such as that shown in Figure 25-6, it is becoming more common to measure not just total testosterone, but also free and/or bioavailable testosterone. The latter represents the sum of free testosterone plus that bound weakly to albumin. The remaining testosterone is bound tightly to SHBG. Free or bioavailable testosterone more accurately represents the biologically active hormone in conditions where the concentration of SHBG is altered. For example, SHBG levels are increased with decreased testosterone, increased estrogen, hyperthyroidism, and liver disease, whereas they are decreased with increased testosterone, hypothyroidism, and acromegaly. Thus, if SHBG is high, total testosterone may be normal, but free or bioavailable hormone may be low. Conversely, if SHBG is low, total testosterone may be normal, but free or bioavailable hormone may be high (Ismail, 1986; Yeap, 2009). Methods for measuring total testosterone are readily available on automated immunoassay analyzers, but methods for measuring free and bioavailable testosterone are much more labor intensive. Consequently, free and bioavailable testosterone analyses are usually performed in a reference laboratory. The same considerations apply to testosterone measurements in females (see later).

Gynecomastia, or breast development in males, is thought to be due to a relative imbalance of androgen (decreased) and estrogen (increased) acting at the mammary gland. The decrease in androgen action can be due to a concentration deficiency and/or a receptor deficiency (insensitivity). The condition is not uncommon during the neonatal and pubertal periods. A variety of other causes have been identified, including endocrine abnormalities, tumors, systemic diseases, and many drugs. Discontinuing or changing medications can exclude drug-induced disease, and liver or kidney disease can be identified through biochemical blood screens. Measuring serum testosterone, estradiol, LH, hCG, prolactin, and TSH can reveal an endocrine abnormality or hormone-secreting tumor. Results from these tests together with imaging methods can help differentiate among the following as possible causes of gynecomastia: primary or secondary testicular failure, hyperthyroidism, androgen resistance, prolactinoma, testicular or extratesticular germ cell tumor, Leydig or Sertoli cell tumor, or adrenal tumor (Braunstein, 2004).

FEMALE EVALUATION

Evaluation of the female reproductive system can be simplified to confirmation of ovulation and normal female reproductive anatomy (Strauss, 2004). The abnormal menstrual cycle pattern is one of the best predictors of anovulation. Amenorrhea can be defined as the absence of menstrual flow by age 16, or by age 14 if no breast development occurs (Speroff, 2005). In patients who have not exhibited menses by age 16, this is often due to a genetic and/or anatomic abnormality. In such cases, however, an endocrine abnormality is still a possible cause, and the presence or absence of secondary sexual characteristics (e.g., breast development) is an important indicator in the evaluation. An endocrine abnormality is a more likely cause in patients who have a history of menstruation, but who have not experienced menses for >3 months. A stepwise approach to evaluating amenorrhea (Fig. 25-7) is based on measuring hCG, PRL, TSH, free

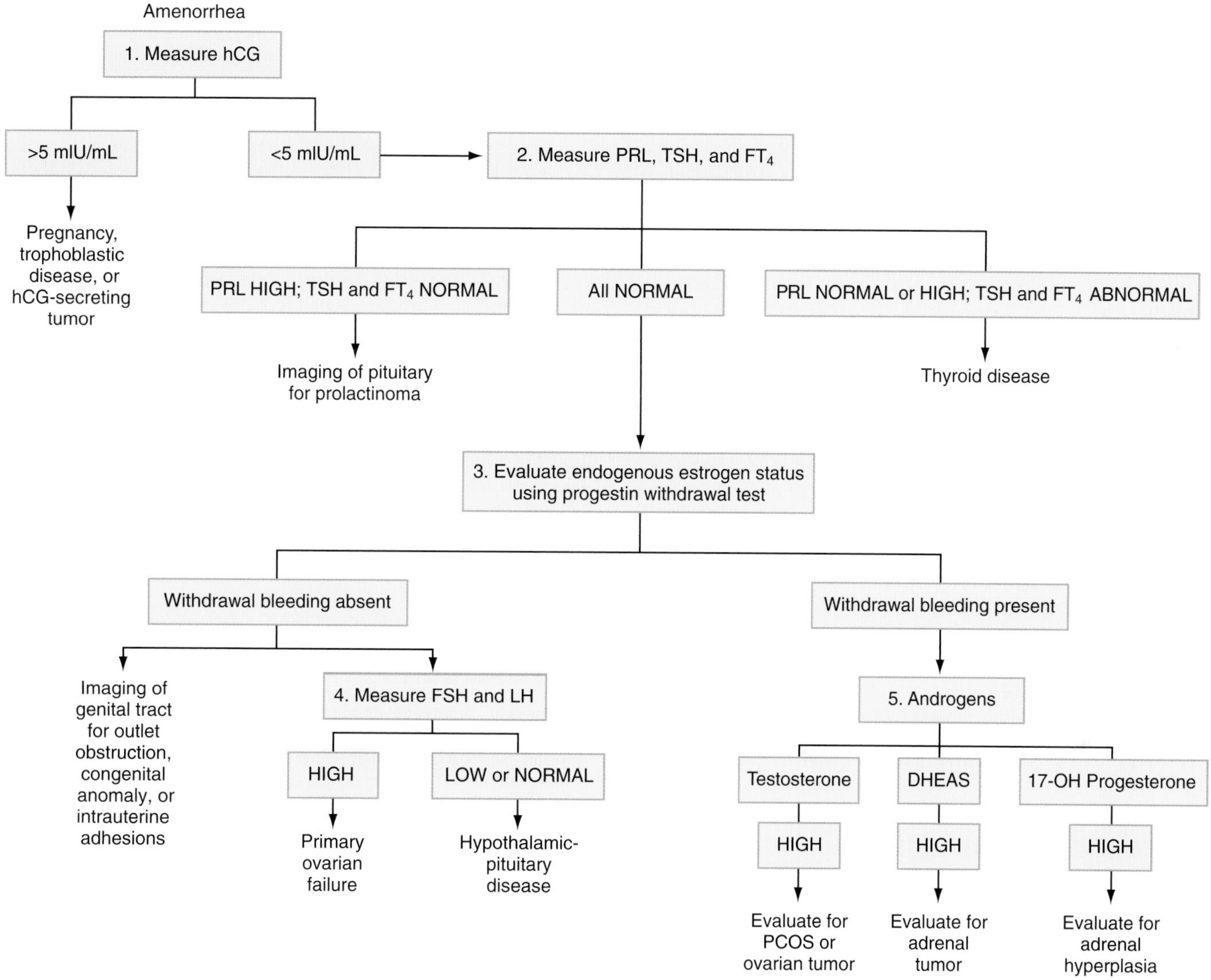

Figure 25-7 A diagnostic algorithm for amenorrhea. Sequential steps in the evaluation are numbered. *DHEAS,* Dehydroepiandrosterone-sulfate; *FSH,* follicle-stimulating hormone; *FT$_4$,* free thyroxine; *hCG,* human chorionic gonadotropin; *LH,* luteinizing hormone; *PCOS,* polycystic ovarian syndrome; *PRL,* prolactin; *TSH,* thyroid-stimulating hormone.

thyroxine (FT_4), FSH, LH, and androgen levels and assessing estrogen status.

Step 1: hCG is measured to exclude the most common cause of secondary amenorrhea—pregnancy. Although a result >5 mIU/mL is typically indicative of pregnancy, an elevated result can also be obtained with trophoblastic disease or an hCG-secreting tumor.

Step 2: PRL, TSH, and FT_4 are measured to exclude the endocrine disorders. Increased prolactin accompanied by normal TSH and FT_4 results suggests a prolactinoma, which would be further evaluated by imaging techniques. Hyperprolactinemia, however, can also be caused by primary hypothyroidism, as indicated by high TSH and low FT_4 (see Male Evaluation, earlier). The mechanism by which increased prolactin causes amenorrhea is the same as that discussed previously for postpartum amenorrhea in females and for hypogonadism in males. Low TSH and FT_4 suggest secondary hypothyroidism, in which case the patient should be evaluated for panhypopituitarism, a deficiency of all anterior pituitary hormones. Hyperthyroidism (increased FT_4) can also be associated with amenorrhea.

Step 3: If hCG, PRL, TSH, and FT_4 are all normal, then endogenous estrogen status is evaluated with the progestin withdrawal test. Progestin may be administered orally for 5–7 days or in one intramuscular injection (progestin dissolved in oil). The presence of withdrawal bleeding within 7 days after treatment indicates (1) that the outflow tract is intact, and (2) that sufficient estrogen was present at the outset to stimulate endometrial growth. If withdrawal bleeding is absent, the genital tract should be evaluated using imaging techniques.

Step 4: Serum FSH and LH levels should be determined. Elevated FSH and LH indicate primary ovarian failure, whereas low or inappropriately normal FSH and LH indicate secondary ovarian failure. The latter is of hypothalamic-pituitary origin and can result from a variety of clinical disorders, including Sheehan's syndrome, eating disorders, weight loss, and stress. If withdrawal bleeding is present, then Step 5 is followed.

Step 5: Androgen excess should be evaluated. Elevated testosterone (>150 ng/mL) indicates an ovarian tumor or polycystic ovarian syndrome. The latter is a clinical entity often associated with enlarged ovaries and infertility, as well as amenorrhea. Increased DHEAS suggests an adrenal tumor. 17-OH progesterone is an androgen precursor (see Fig. 25-1), and an increase in serum levels can indicate congenital or adult-onset adrenal hyperplasia due to 21-hydroxylase deficiency. These abnormalities may be accompanied by hirsutism (i.e., male pattern of hair growth in females).

The tests in Step 5 can also be used to evaluate hirsutism when it is the primary clinical presentation. Because amenorrhea or oligomenorrhea is often associated with infertility (Lobo, 1997), the latter can be evaluated with the type of diagnostic algorithm shown in Figure 25-7. Evaluation of the ovulatory function is a important step in the infertility workup. One of the methods used to confirm ovulation is monitoring the basal body temeperature. A rise in progesterone after ovulation increases basal body temperature by 0.4°–0.8° F. More reliable are urinary ovulation predictor kits, which measure urinary luteinizing hormone by colorimetric assay.

Testing should be started 2 to 3 days before the LH surge and should be continued daily. LH has a short half-life and is rapidly excreted in the urine. In most cases, the test will be positive for only 1 day of the menstrual cycle. Another method that is reliable and widely available involves measurement of midluteal phase serum progesterone levels on day 21 of the menstrual cycle. Values above 3 ng/mL indicate ovulation and production of progesterone by the corpus luteum (Besser, 2002). Inadequate progesterone levels result in luteal phase deficiency, in which maturation of the secretory endometrium is delayed so that implantation of the blastocyst does not occur. In many cases, but not all, such an **out-of-phase endometrium** can be demonstrated by histologic evaluation of an endometrial biopsy from the late luteal phase (Noyes, 1975). However, endometrial histologic dating is not a valid diagnostic tool and should not be considered in management of the infertile patient (Speroff, 2005). When the diagnosis of ovarian failure is suspected, levels of FSH in the early follicular phase (on day 3) should be determined. Concentrations greater than 10 mIU/mL are associated with diminished ovarian reserve, which is defined by low numbers of normal oocytes and the presence of poor quality oocytes. Diminished ovarian reserve is associated with decreased probability of live birth with a natural or IVF cycle (Scott, 1995). Additional information can be obtained by measurement of estradiol levels on the same day of each menstrual cycle (Buyalos, 1998). Levels greater than 80 pg/mL are considered abnormal and indicate ovarian stimulation of steroidogenesis by elevated FSH, which is typically seen in ovarian failure.

More extensive testing of ovarian reserve includes the clomiphene citrate challenge test. Clomiphene citrate, the nonsteroidal estrogen receptor modulator, is administered on day 5 through day 9 of the cycle; this is followed by measurements of estradiol and FSH on day 3 and on day 10. Women with a poor cohort and aging follicles cannot generate enough estradiol or inhibin B to suppress FSH. Therefore FSH remains high.

ASSISTED REPRODUCTIVE TECHNOLOGY

Infertility is defined as 1 year of unprotected intercourse without conception (Speroff, 2005). Initial treatments may include artificial insemination with washed and concentrated sperm and/or ovulation induction with clomiphene citrate. If these are unsuccessful, then one of several ARTs may be attempted. ARTs involve techniques of direct manipulation of oocytes that are performed to control as much of the reproductive process as possible to achieve pregnancy and bring it to term (Trounson, 2000). Much of this external control requires significant monitoring through laboratory analyses.

Indications for ART include male infertility, ovarian failure, unexplained infertility, and tubal disease and endometriosis. It is not uncommon for several causes of infertility to be present in one couple. ART can also be applied in infertile couples requiring oocyte donation. The latter involves two distinct groups of patients: (1) females without gonadal function because of gonadal dysgenesis, premature menopause (which may occur spontaneously or after surgical castration or castration induced by chemotherapy or radiotherapy), or resistant-ovary syndrome, and (2) women with functional ovaries who do not wish to use their own oocytes to become pregnant because of the risk of transmitting chromosomal abnormalities to the offspring (e.g., if there is a history of autosomal dominant disease or X-linked disease, or when both partners are carriers of an autosomal recessive disease) (Van Steirteghem, 1992; Pados, 1994). The most common form of ART is IVF; other forms involve gamete intrafallopian transfer, zygote intrafallopian transfer, or tubal embryo transfer, all performed with the use of laparoscopy.

A typical ART protocol has four steps: ovarian hyperstimulation with exogenous gonadotropins, retrieval of oocytes from ovaries, fertilization in the laboratory, and transfer of embryos into the uterus. Initially, a GnRH analog (Lupron) may be given to suppress normal FSH and LH synthesis and secretion, although this is not always necessary. Lupron downregulates FSH and LH secretion by paradoxically inducing initial hypersecretion of these two hormones, which, however, ultimately results in their depletion. The next step is to stimulate follicular growth using a human menopausal gonadotropin preparation, which will have FSH and LH activity, or predominantly FSH activity, depending on the specific material used. Unlike a normal reproductive cycle in which typically only one dominant follicle matures, in an ART cycle multiple follicles undergo growth and maturation. The number of follicles and their increase in size are monitored by regular ultrasound analysis. The function of the developing follicles is monitored by sequential serum estradiol measurements. When sufficient follicular maturation is achieved, according to ultrasound and estradiol analyses, a bolus of hCG is administered. This hCG functions as a surrogate LH surge, and the hCG interacts with follicular LH receptors to initiate the process of ovulation. This process is not allowed to progress to completion. Ovulation would normally occur approximately 48 hours after hCG administration. Therefore, 12 hours before induced ovulation, the oocytes are "retrieved" from the stimulated follicles. Each oocyte is then mixed with sperm. ART also includes methods for assisted fertilization by intracytoplasmic sperm injection obtained from ejaculate or extracted from epididymis or testis. Depending on the type of ART used, the gametes may be transferred immediately to the fallopian tube, or they may be incubated together for up to 48 hours; the resulting zygotes or embryos are transferred to the fallopian tube or uterus.

Oocyte retrieval disrupts the follicles, as does normal ovulation, and, as a consequence, estradiol levels drop immediately afterward. As the follicles differentiate into corpora lutea, however, estradiol levels rebound and serum progesterone increases. This process may require "boosting," however, with additional injections of hCG (lower dose than that used for oocyte retrieval) and/or injections of progesterone. As in a normal cycle, estradiol plus progesterone is required to prepare the uterine endometrium for implantation. Therefore, serum levels of the two steroids are monitored after transfer. Serum hCG measurements begin about 10 days after transfer to determine whether pregnancy has been achieved. About 20 days after transfer, ultrasound examination can be used to confirm the presence of a gestational sac.

ART may offer the preimplantation genetic diagnosis (PGD). PGD can be performed on polar bodies removed from oocytes before fertilization or on blastomeres removed from embryos before transfer. Preimplantation genetic testing may be indicated to detect chromosmal abnormalities and inherited single-gene disorders, as well as to determine gender. However, conventional prenatal diagnosis is still recommended later in pregnancy because of numerous potential errors associated with PGD (Speroff, 2005).

LABORATORY EVALUATION OF PREGNANCY

On a patient's first visit to an obstetrician, ideally early in the first trimester, a number of clinical laboratory tests are routinely ordered to identify disorders that can be treated or prevented (Willett, 1994). Simple, inexpensive blood and urine tests are carried out for anemia, red cell alloimmunization, and suspected viral or bacterial infection. Sometimes, the clinical history, physical examination, or test results indicate additional studies for genetic disease, disorders of coagulation or thrombosis, causes of spontaneous abortion, and other conditions. Laboratory procedures used routinely to monitor pregnancy are summarized in Figure 25-8.

hCG AND EARLY PREGNANCY

Elevated hCG in maternal serum and urine is a reliable indicator of pregnancy. The discovery of monoclonal antibodies in the late 1970s led to the development of simple and cheap immunoassays, such as agglutination-inhibition–based assays and sandwich enzyme-linked immunosorbent assay, used in home pregnancy tests.

Currently, most serum assays measure both the free β subunit and intact hCG (α-plus-β subunit), utilizing two different antibodies directed at different epitopes on the βsubunit. These assays can quantify hCG as low as 1–2 mIU/mL. Typically, urine assays use one antibody directed at the β subunit and the other directed at the α subunit, allowing these assays to measure intact hCG and fragments that appear in urine. Serum hCG increases above the reference interval (typically by 4–6 mIU/mL) by implantation, 6–12 (mean, 9.1) days after ovulation (Wilcox, 1999). Urine hCG levels are commonly measured by qualitative immunoassay test kits with detection limits of approximately 20 mIU/mL. These methods can detect elevated urine hCG 2–3 days later than serum methods. Qualitative assays meant for home use have detection limits of about 50 mIU/mL, and thus can detect elevated urine levels several days later, or shortly after the first missed menses.

Serum hCG increases dramatically during the first trimester, reaching a peak at about 10 weeks of gestation (see Fig. 25-5). Throughout pregnancy, intact hCG is the predominant form present. However, a small quantity of free β subunit is present in the first trimester. Free α subunit appears in the second trimester and steadily increases in the last trimester (Ozturk, 1987).

Some cancers and medical conditions may be associated with increased levels of hCG. These include germ cell tumors and gestational trophoblastic disease. Tumor production often includes significant amounts of free β subunit, in addition to intact hCG. The use of hCG as a tumor marker is discussed more fully in Chapter 73. False-positive β-hCG is usually due to interference by heterophilic Ig antibodies; it is characterized by large molecular weight and is not filtered by renal glomeruli. Serum

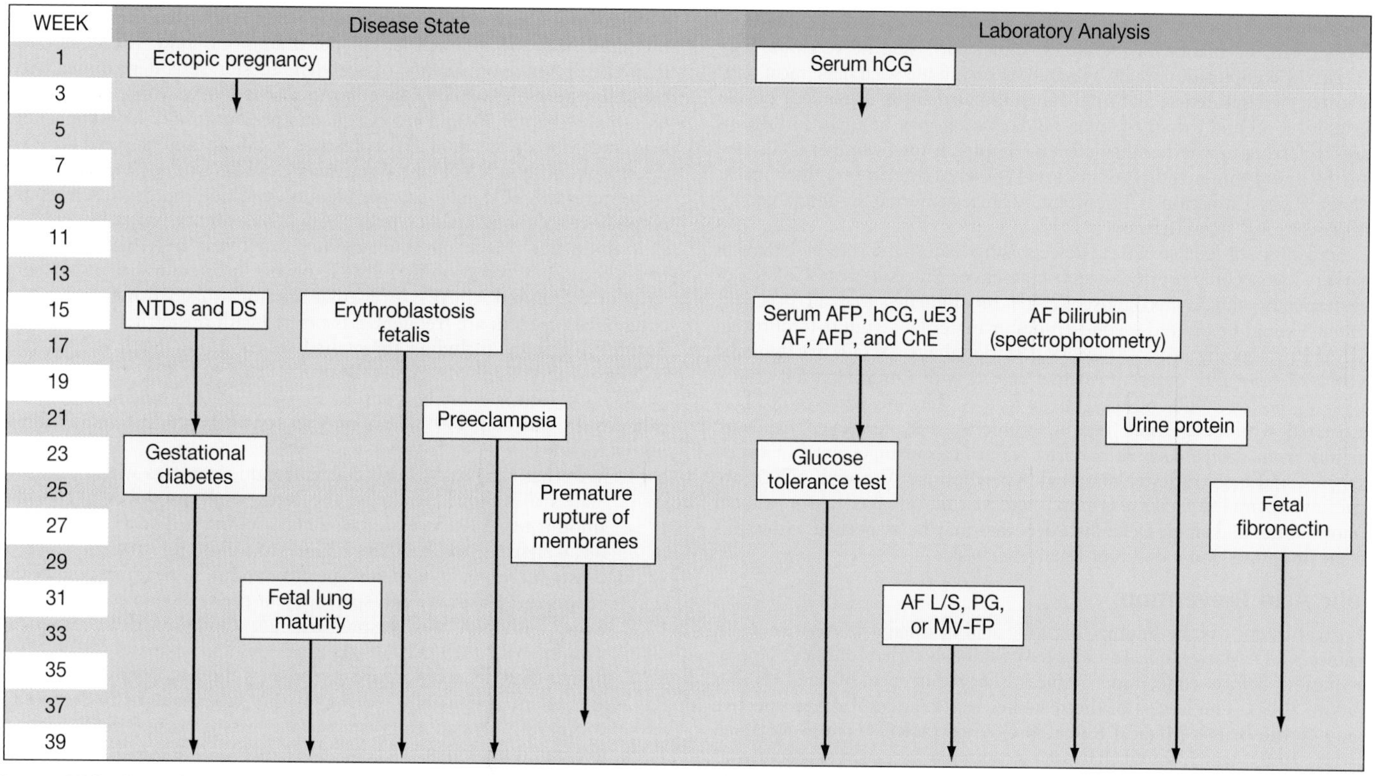

Figure 25-8 Approximate gestational weeks for laboratory evaluation of major disease states in pregnancy (when clinically indicated). *AChE*, Acetylcholinesterase; *AF*, amniotic fluid; *AFP*, α-fetoprotein; *ChE*, cholinesterase; *DS*, Down syndrome; *hCG*, human chorionic gonadotropin; *L/S*, lecithin/sphingomyelin ratio; *MV-FP*, microviscosity by fluorescence polarization; *NTDs*, neural tube defects; *PG*, phosphatidyl glycerol; and *uE3*, unconjugated estriol.

concentrations of β-hCG are typically less than 150 mIU/L with negative urine testing.

Quantitative measurements of hCG are indicated when a patient presents with early gestational vaginal bleeding or abdominal pain that may suggest the presence of ectopic pregnancy or spontaneous abortion. A simple protocol using only ultrasound and quantitative hCG examinations allows more accurate diagnosis and sound management than are obtained by clinical judgment alone (Koh, 1997). Because hCG concentrations rise quickly in normal early pregnancy, serial measurements can be used to ensure that an intrauterine implantation has occurred. Doubling of hCG in 2 days provides a greater than 80% probability of intrauterine implantation of the fertilized ovum. Increases in serum hCG of less than 53% in 2 days indicate abnormal pregnancy with 99% sensitivity (Barnhart, 2004).

Because circulating hCG increases very rapidly in the first days post-implantation, it is important to consider diverse causes of low-level quantitative results, including normal production of hCG in the pituitary, especially in post-menopausal females (Odell-Griffin, 1987); early abortion ("microabortion") (Wilcox, 1988); use of hCG as a drug; and assay interference, as mentioned previously.

When hCG concentrations exceed **discriminatory zone** values of 1500–2000 mIU/mL, an intrauterine gestational sac becomes visible on ultrasound examination in a normal singleton pregnancy (Kadar, 1994). Multiple gestations have higher hCG levels than singletons, and hCG levels may rise above 2000 mIU/mL before ultrasound findings of intrauterine gestational sac are obtained (Goldstein, 1988). Absence of an intrauterine gestational sac and failure to double the serum hCG or the presence of an adnexal mass indicates a possible ectopic pregnancy. Furthermore, failure to double the serum hCG suggests a loss of pregnancy.

Estradiol and progesterone measurements may provide additional information. Low serum progesterone (<15 ng/mL) or estradiol (<200 ng/mL) indicates a blighted ovum with 90% likelihood. If hCG is less than 1000 mIU/mL in a patient with vaginal bleeding, a progesterone value less than 5 ng/mL is 94% predictive of an abnormal pregnancy.

Progesterone measurements may provide additional information about abnormal pregnancy. Serum levels higher than 20 ng/mL usually are associated with normal intrauterine pregnancy. Low serum progesterone—less than 5 ng/mL—indicates an abnormal pregnancy with a specificity of 100% (Stovall, 1992). Serum progesterone levels are not helpful in assessment of the ectopic pregnancy, because most of the time values range between 10 and 20 ng/mL.

Medical intervention using intramuscular methotrexate for unruptured ectopic pregnancy is less costly than surgery, may be a less complicated procedure, and may improve the patient's fertility. Cases may be selected for methotrexate treatment by using ultrasound to ascertain a tubal implantation and differentiate it from an interstitial one, for which methotrexate is not indicated. Ultrasound also ensures a small volume (<3 cm) of conceptual tissue with absent fetal heart motion. A serum progesterone decrease to less than 1.5 ng/mL may be a better predictor of resolution because hCG concentrations do not decline as rapidly after surgery (and sometimes may increase) (Saraj, 1998).

The laboratory can provide testing to help determine why an early pregnancy aborted spontaneously. For example, recurrent abortion caused by the antiphospholipid syndrome can be diagnosed by the presence of anticardiolipin and specific phospholipid antibodies in the first trimester. Recurrent abortion due to inherited thrombophilia may be diagnosed by detection of factor V Leiden gene mutation, methylenetetrahydrofolate reductase gene mutation, prothrombin gene mutation, levels of proteins C and S, and activated protein C activity.

NEURAL TUBE DEFECTS

Neural tube defects (NTDs) are among the most common congenital malformations in the United States and worldwide. The incidence of NTDs in the United States has been reported at approximately 1 per 1000 pregnancies. Caucasians in the United States have an average occurrence of 0.96 per 1000, and Hispanics 1.2 per 1000; the lowest prevalence was reported in African Americans, with an incidence of 0.75 per 1000 (Feuchtbaum, 1999). An increased risk of recurrence has been noted in families. For example, when a couple has had one offspring with an NTD, the risk in each subsequent pregnancy for any type of NTD increases to approximately 1%–3% (Toriello, 1983). However, recent data suggests a decline in these rates due to increased education within the medical community and towards women of childbearing age regarding the benefits of folic acid consumption along with the mandated fortification of grain products in certain states (New York State Dept. of Health, 2005; for review see http://www.health.state.ny.us/diseases/congenital_malformations/docs/98report.pdf).

NTDs result from failure of the neural tube to close by the 27th day after conception. Anencephaly comprises 50% of NTDs and involves absence of the calvarium, cranial vault, and cerebral hemispheres; it is incompatible with life. Abnormalities of the caudal portion of the neural tube, known as spina bifida, present as a lumbar (or cervical) meningomyelocele, with herniation of meninges, spinal cord, and nerve roots. The severity of complications such as paralysis or muscle weakness, fecal and/or urinary incontinence, and intellectual impairment is dependent on the vertebral level and extent of spina bifida, which may be open in 80% of cases (referring to whether the defect is completely uncovered or is covered only by a very thin membrane) or closed (covered by skin or a thick membrane). This distinction is important because maternal serum screening will detect only open defects.

Screening for fetal structural defects using maternal serum biochemical markers has become routine obstetric practice. The American College of Obstetricians and Gynecologists (2003) recommends that all pregnant women should be offered second-trimester maternal serum α-fetoprotein (MSAFP) screening at 15–20 weeks gestational age. NTDs are sporadic in 90% of cases and represent isolated defects with a multifactorial origin, involving both genetic and nongenetic factors. The incidence of NTD is associated with geographic region, ethnicity, diet, teratogen exposure (mainly from drugs, such as maternal valproic acid ingestion), maternal diabetes, and first-trimester maternal hyperthermia. Although NTDs are typically isolated defects, it is important to rule out fetal chromosomal abnormalities and single-gene disorders that may be associated with a different prognosis and a different recurrence risk.

Folic Acid Prevention

Of great interest is the finding that folic acid is a major preventive agent against NTD. Many clinical studies have established that folic acid supplementation before conception reduces the recurrence of fetal NTDs (Pitkin, 2007). The largest of these studies was a randomized prospective study by the British Medical Research Council (MRC Vitamin Research Group, 1991), which found that preconceptional folic acid supplementation decreased the recurrence of NTDs by 72%.

Screening for NTD

The now well-established finding that AFP is a maternal serum marker for NTD was first reported in 1974 (Brock, 1974). AFP, produced initially by the fetal yolk sac and later by the fetal liver, is the most abundant protein in fetal serum. Its concentration increases in both fetal serum and amniotic fluid until about 13 weeks gestation, after which the liver gradually shifts to production of albumin. In NTDs, AFP becomes elevated because fetal serum from exposed neural membranes and blood vessels leaks into amniotic fluid (AF), producing a concentration in AF that is approximately 100-fold less than in fetal serum. Small amounts of AFP are also transferred across the placenta from fetal serum and across the amniotic membranes from AF to maternal serum (MS), where concentrations of AFP are nearly 1000-fold less than in AF. Amniotic fluid AFP peaks at 13–14 weeks and decreases in the second trimester by about 10% per week. Assays for AFP are based on immunochemical determinations using monoclonal antibodies against AFP and are available on autoanalyzers.

In the second trimester, when maternal screening is performed, MSAFP levels increase by approximately 15% per gestational week. This MSAFP increase, while AF levels are decreasing (see earlier), is due to combined changes in transfer to MS and maternal clearance (Ashwood, 1999). This measurable increase serves as the basis of midtrimester MSAFP screening for open NTDs (UK Collaborative Study, 1977).

MSAFP screening is based on comparison of serum AFP levels from pregnant women in the midtrimester of pregnancy versus median AFP values from women with normal fetuses at comparable gestational ages. These comparisons are subsequently expressed as multiples of the median (MoM). Median values are based on data from the reference population that is screened. Expressing patient results as MoMs normalizes the values, allows for direct comparison of results between laboratories, and adjusts for the large changes in expected values with increasing gestational age. The goal of any maternal serum-screening program is to identify those women at sufficient risk for a fetal disorder to warrant further evaluation and follow-up. Large prospective trials of MSAFP screening showed that most affected pregnancies can be identified by elevated MSAFP levels greater than 2.5 times the normal median for singleton pregnancies. Most laboratories set the cutoff at 2.0–2.5 MoM, such that the detection rate is about 85% of all NTDs with a false-positive rate less than 5% (Wald, 1977; Milunsky, 1980). Only 2% of all women with positive test results are carrying affected fetuses. Thus further evaluation with genetic counseling should be considered.

If MSAFP screening suggests an increased risk for an NTD, then a detailed fetal anatomic survey has to be performed. Normal findings on ultrasound results usually indicate the need for further evaluation, and the patient should be offered diagnostic amniocentesis to determine the amniotic fluid AFP and the fetal karyotype. If amniotic fluid AFP is elevated, then the presence or absence of acetylcholinesterase is determined. Acetylcholinesterase (AChE) is an enzyme that is derived only from neural tissue (see Chapter 20) and is consequently present in very high concentration in cerebrospinal fluid. The presence of AChE and elevated AFP are diagnostic for fetal NTDs and discriminate NTDs from other fetal defects with increased AFP, such as open ventral wall defects (gastroschisis and omphalocele), congenital nephrosis, benign obstructive uropathy, and fetal skin anomalies. Placental abnormalities can result in elevated MSAFP levels because of compromise in the fetomaternal membranes or placental structure. Elevated MSAFP levels that are not explained by a genetic or congenital problem are frequently associated with obstetric complications during pregnancy, including threatened abortion, low birth weight, preeclampsia, and oligohydramnios (Burton, 1988).

Clinical factors must be considered when patient-specific results are calculated (Ashwood, 1999). Laboratories routinely adjust for the following factors:

1. Maternal weight: MSAFP concentration decreases with increasing maternal weight. Although the fetus itself produces a constant amount of AFP, the maternal blood volume will vary according to the weight of the mother. Failure to adjust for maternal weight causes increases in both false-positive and false-negative results and affects the sensitivity and specificity of the test (Johnson, 1990a).
2. Race: Although the reasons are not known, African American women have MSAFP values that are approximately 10%–15% higher than those of Caucasian women (Johnson, 1990b). It is necessary to mathematically correct for this difference, or to correct by comparing African American patients versus normal median values generated from that reference population.
3. Insulin-dependent diabetes mellitus (IDDM): MSAFP levels in otherwise normal women with IDDM are approximately 20% lower than in the general population; therefore, the MoM values must be adjusted upward to reflect this phenomenon. This is typically accomplished by multiplying the initial MoM value by a factor, using a mathematical constant to increase the initial MoM result.
4. Multiple gestation: Multiple gestation (e.g., twins) will yield higher MSAFP levels because each fetus contributes its own AFP to the maternal blood. The MSAFP level is approximately proportional to the number of fetuses, and the effect can be factored into the laboratory calculation and interpretation of the results. Screening for fetal defects is not as reliable as for single pregnancies, in that one cannot determine the individual AFP contributions of each fetus. Therefore, the NTD detection rate is lower for multiple pregnancies than for single ones. The same principle applies to MoM adjustments for serum analytes in second-trimester screening for fetal chromosomal abnormalities (see later).
5. Gestational age determination: To establish a valid MoM value, a reliable estimate of gestational age is essential. The most common reason for abnormal MSAFP screening results is incorrect estimation of gestational age. Typically, laboratories follow specific protocols based on information obtained from the obstetric care provider to determine the most reliable gestational age. If pregnancy is initially dated using ultrasound, the sensitivity and specificity of the screening are accurate (Wald, 1994); however, ultrasound information frequently is not available at the time of MSAFP screening. Pregnancies with positive screening results that originally were dated by using the last menstrual period should have the gestational age verified by ultrasound. If the two estimated gestational ages differ by a defined amount (laboratory protocols vary, but usually by more than 9 days), then the results are recalculated based on the ultrasound results.
6. Fetal viability: Fetal demise raises the MSAFP levels. In cases of fetal demise, MSAFP does not have diagnostic value.

An algorithm for detection of NTD is summarized in Figure 25-9.

DOWN SYNDROME

All women should be offered screening for fetal chromosomal abnormalities before age 20 weeks, regardless of maternal age (ACOG, 2007). Many multicenter trials have evaluated the different approaches to screening for aneuploidy in the first and second trimesters. First-trimester screening, performed between 12 and 13 weeks, includes nuchal translucency measurement combined with two maternal serum analytes: β subunit of human chorionic gonadotropin with pregnancy-associated plasma protein A

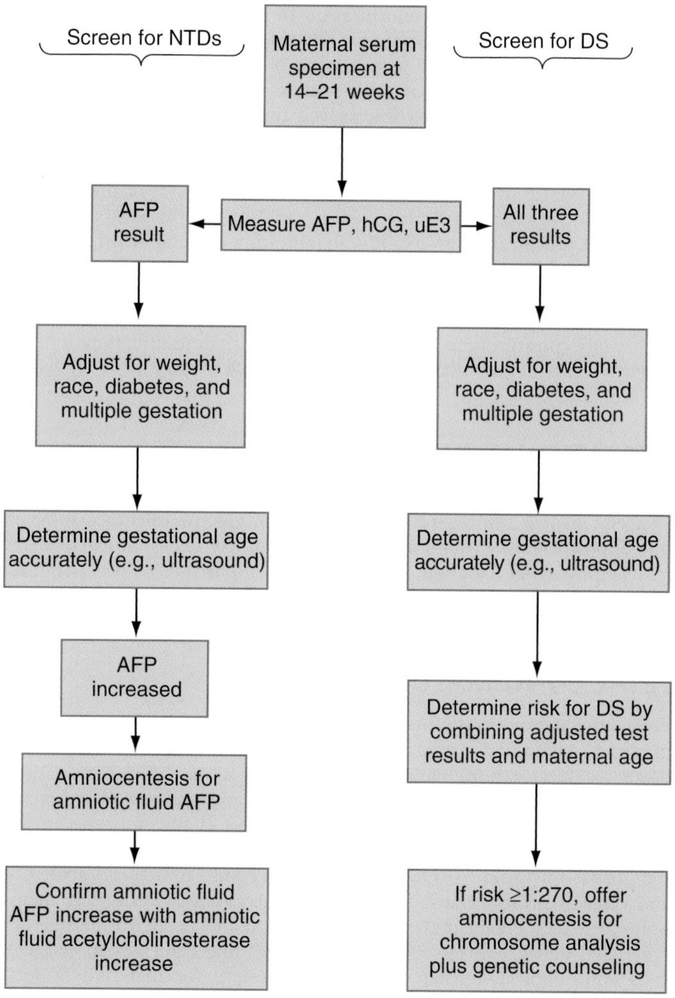

Figure 25-9 A diagnostic algorithm for the simultaneous screening of fetuses for neural tube defects (NTDs) and Down syndrome (DS). *AFP,* α-Fetoprotein; *hCG,* human chorionic gonadotropin; *uE3,* unconjugated estriol.

(PAPP-A), and maternal age. An increase in the size of nuchal translucency, which refers to a fluid collection at the back of the fetal neck in the first trimester, is characteristic of fetal chromosomal and structural abnormalities. Serum levels of analytes are changing with advancing maternal age. Patient data are converted to MoM based on population and gestational age. PAPP-A is a glycoprotein produced by the trophoblast; its levels are reduced to 0.48 MoM in affected pregnancies, whereas levels of β-hCG are elevated to 1.98 MoM in comparison with normal pregnancies (Spencer, 1999). Nuchal translucency, as a single ultrasonographic marker, has a detection rate of 64%–70% for Down syndrome, trisomy 18, trisomy 13, and Turner's syndrome. Adding the calculation of maternal serum PAPP-A and β-hCG improves the detection rate to 82%–87%. Women with increased risk of aneuploidy on first-trimester screening should be offered genetic counseling and the option of diagnostic testing, such as chorionic villous sampling or second-trimester amniocentesis (ACOG, 2007).

Other approaches to screening for fetal chromosomal abnormalities include the second-trimester triple screen with MSAFP, β-hCG, and unconjugated estriol performed between 15 and 20 weeks. The level of MSAFP in pregnancies with Down syndrome is reduced to 0.74 MoM and the uE3 level to 0.75 MoM, whereas β-hCG is increased to 2.06 MoM (Wald, 2003).

The detection rate of triple screen can be improved from 69% to 81% by adding the inhibin A (quadruple screen) dimeric protein produced by placenta and fetus. The level of inhibin A shows the same trend as β-hCG and is increased in pregnancies with Down syndrome at 1.77 MoM (Spencer, 1999).

Adjustments can be made to the multiple of median for special populations in which analytes are affected differently. For example, serum concentrations of each biomarker are approximately double in twin pregnancy but cannot be interpreted in higher-order multiples. In pregestational diabetes, MSAFP, E3, and inhibin A levels are reduced. As body weight increases, analyte levels decrease. In smokers, MSAFP and inhibin A levels are higher, while E3 and β-hCG levels are lower.

An algorithm for detecting Down syndrome is shown together with that for NTD in Figure 25-9.

Several strategies incorporating the results of first- and second-trimester screening have been proposed by American College of Obstetricians and Gynecologists (ACOG). The highest sensitivity rate with the lowest false-positive rates is achieved by using integrated first- and second-trimester screening with a detection rate of 94%–96% and a 5% false-positive rate (Malone, 2005). Results are reported to the patient after first- and second-trimester screening is completed. Those found to have increased risk of aneuploidy should be offered amniocentesis. With another approach, called **sequential screening,** the patient is informed about first-trimester results. Early diagnostic testing (chorionic villous sampling) is offered after a positive result, whereas patients with negative results may undergo additional second-trimester screening and may benefit from its higher sensitivity. The advantage of integrated and sequential screening is a lower false-positive rate that leads to fewer diagnostic procedures. Additionally, all patients who elected to have only first-trimester screening for chromosomal abnormalities should undergo neural tube defect screening in the second trimester (ACOG, 2007).

ERYTHROBLASTOSIS FETALIS

Severe hemolytic disease in a fetus is marked by anemia accompanied by normoblastic hyperplasia (erythroblastosis) and may be followed by congestive heart failure (hydrops) and intrauterine death. The role of transfusion medicine in the management of immunized (sensitized) RhO-negative mothers is reviewed in Chapter 36.

Hemoglobin (Hb), released by hemolysis, is catabolized to unconjugated bilirubin. A fetus with hemolytic disease does not develop hyperbilirubinemia or become jaundiced because the placenta normally removes the bilirubin. However, some bilirubin appears in the amniotic fluid. The measurement of amniotic fluid bilirubin levels using spectral analysis at 450 nm (ΔOD_{450}) was introduced to clinical practice by Liley in 1961 and has been the accepted method of assessing the severity of erythroblastosis in utero. Bilirubin absorbs light maximally at a wavelength of 450 nm and imparts a yellow color to AF. Some of the absorbance at this wavelength is due to Hb. Both bilirubin and Hb can be maternal and fetal in origin, so that pigmentation will not discriminate between a hemolytic process in the mother and one in the child.

In erythroblastosis, the net absorbance of light at 450 nm (A or ΔOD) due to bilirubin correlates with the severity of anemia (or hemolytic rate). Bilirubin is bound to albumin; its concentration is dependent on the turnover of the protein, and its concentration in AF does not change rapidly. To determine whether the net bilirubin concentration in amniotic fluid is elevated, a specimen of AF (5 mL) is collected, protected from light, and centrifuged or filtered. Light absorbance of the AF is scanned continuously between wavelengths 350 nm and 700 nm. The resulting spectrophotometric curve can be used to determine whether or not the fluid contains bilirubin and/or other pigmented products of hemolysis, and to quantify the bilirubin pigment that is present as follows.

Because the absorbance at 450 nm is due to both bilirubin and Hb, if hemolysis occurs, both of these molecules will be elevated in concentration above the background values for their combined absorbance at 450 nm. To determine whether the bilirubin in AF is elevated, both background absorbances at 450 nm must be determined, and the contribution of Hb must also be computed.

To determine the background absorbance of the AF (i.e., what the absorbance would have been with no hemolysis and hyperbilirubinemia), a straight line is drawn between the two absorbances from the scan—at 350 nm and 700 nm. Absorbances at these two wavelengths are not affected by bilirubin or Hb, and, in normal AF, absorbance changes linearly with wavelength between 350 and 700 nm. The absorbance from the straight line at 450 nm is therefore subtracted as the background value from the observed absorbance at 450 nm. This net absorbance still contains a contribution from Hb.

To correct for Hb absorbance, use is made of the fact that Hb uniquely absorbs at 410 nm—a wavelength at which bilirubin does not absorb. From scans of the absorbance of Hb versus wavelength, it is known that the absorbance of Hb at 450 nm is 0.05 of its absorbance at 410 nm. Thus by knowing the net absorbance of Hb at 410 nm, its absorbance at 450 nm can be calculated as 0.05 × absorbance at 410 nm. To obtain the net absorbance of Hb at 410 nm, the background absorbance at 410 nm must be

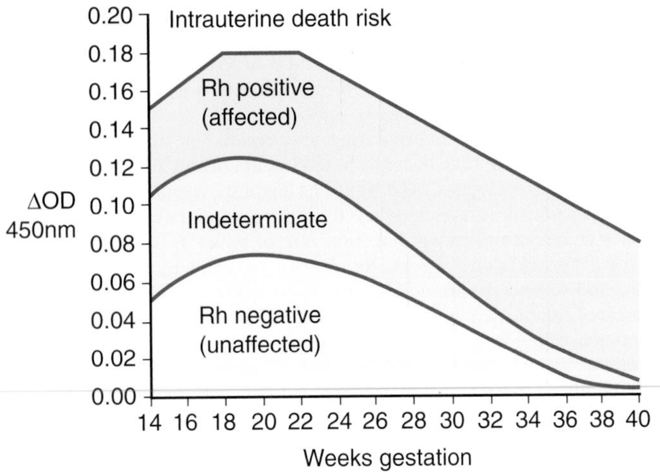

Figure 25-10 Graph for interpretation of net absorbance at 450 nm of amniotic fluid. The four zones are indicative of the relative level of fetal hemolytic disease. *(From Queenan JT, Tomai TP, Ural SH, et al. Deviation in amniotic fluid optical density [OD] at a wavelength of 450nm in Rh-immunized pregnancies from 14–40 weeks gestation: a proposal for clinical management. Am J Obstet Gynecol 1993;168:1370–6, with permission.)*

subtracted from the observed absorbance. This value, similar to the one at 450 nm, is obtained from the straight line drawn between the absorbances at 350 and 700 nm. The net absorbance at 410 nm is then multiplied by 0.05 to obtain the Hb contribution at 450 nm. The resulting value is subtracted from the net absorbance at 450 nm to obtain the net absorbance of bilirubin in AF. These computations may be summarized in the following equation:

$$A_{Bili450} = (A_{450} - A_{450background}) - 0.05(A_{410} - A_{410background}) \qquad \textbf{(25-1)}$$

where the background values are determined from the straight line between 350 nm and 700 nm as described previously.

The net bilirubin absorbance is recorded on a so-called **Liley graph,** an example of which is shown in Figure 25-10, which denotes weeks of gestation on the linear abscissa and net absorbance on the log scale ordinate (Ashwood, 1999). Spectrophotometry of aspirated fluid is most accurate after 26–28 weeks. Net absorbance at 450 nm decreases as the duration of an unaffected pregnancy increases after 28 weeks (before 26 weeks, background absorbance is relatively constant). Decreasing absorbance reflects fluid dilution by fetal urine and accounts for the negative slopes of lines demarcating Liley's prediction zones (lower = zone 1, mid = zone 2, upper = zone 3) for mild, moderate, and severe hemolysis, respectively, as shown in Figure 25-10. The greater the net absorbance at 450 nm, the greater is the hemolysis. Although Liley's method originally applied only to the third trimester of pregnancy, a modified curve for the second trimester has been proposed by Queenan (1993) and involves four zones instead of three (see Fig. 25-10). Serial testing (every 14 days or less often) allows for trending of net absorbance values.

Trends are usually unidirectional, either paralleling the negatively sloped lines on Liley's graph or showing a positive slope. A rising or plateauing trend of ΔOD_{450} values that reaches the 80th percentile of zone two on the Liley curve, or enters the intrauterine transfusion zone of the Queenan curve, necessitates investigation by fetal blood sampling. Cordocentesis is performed with blood readied for intrauterine transfusion if the fetal hematocrit is found to be less than 30%, or delivery is indicated if gestational age is 35 weeks or greater. If no rise in ΔOD_{450} values is detected, the last amniocentesis should be performed at 37 weeks with testing for fetal lung maturity and anticipated induction of labor (Moise, 2002).

Maternal and fetal acid-base imbalances can alter AF pH and shift the wavelengths of pigment absorbance maxima. Pigments that may be present other than bilirubin and that may affect the results include Hb, methemalbumin, and meconium. Each produces a characteristic spectrophotometric effect. Blood contamination (with interference by hemolysis) is encountered frequently. Less often, in vivo maternal jaundice or hemolysis can cause misinterpretation. The presence of fetal red cells in AF indicates worsening of anemia by blood loss, or may explain a rise in maternal antibody titer (anamnestic response to a new fetomaternal hemorrhage), development of new antibodies, and subsequent increase in the net absorbance of AF at 450 nm. Exposure of AF to light and maternal use of steroids, markedly increased AF Hb concentration, or poor calibration of a spectrophotometer may cause inaccurate net absorbance measurements.

The current trend in the management of Rh immunization is the use of Doppler measurements of peak systolic velocity in the fetal middle cerebral artery (MCA). This has proved to be an accurate noninvasive method of assessing and monitoring the degree of fetal anemia in pregnancies complicated by Rh immunization (ACOG, 2006). Based on one study, a value above 1.5 MoM for gestational age detects all cases of anemia, with a false-positive rate of only 12% (Mari, 2000). A rise in peak velocity of fetal MCA greater than 1.5 MoM is an indication for fetal blood sampling. If Doppler measurements were used as the method of fetal monitoring during pregnancy, ΔOD_{450} spectrophotometry with fetal lung maturity testing should be considered after 35 weeks to assess fetal status, because higher false-positive rates have been reported with determination of MCA after 35 weeks of gestation, followed by induction of labor at 37–38 weeks (Moise, 2002).

GESTATIONAL DIABETES

Any glucose intolerance in a pregnant woman is termed gestational diabetes (see Chapter 16), regardless of the state of glucose tolerance antepartum or postpartum. Prompt diagnosis and treatment of gestational diabetes may help to avoid maternal and fetal complications such as preeclampsia, fetal congenital malformation, fetal macrosomia (abnormally large body size), and fetal demise.

FETAL LUNG MATURITY

Fetal lung maturation is marked by production of surface-active phospholipid compounds called surfactant. The presence of surfactant decreases surface tension within the alveolar space during inspiration, allows continuous and effective gas exchange, and prevents alveolar collapse during expiration. It is produced by type II pneumocytes in the form of lamellar bodies. Deficiency of surfactant leads to neonatal respiratory distress syndrome (RDS), a disorder that results in hypoxia, acidemia, and vascular protein transudation into alveolar air spaces (hyaline membrane disease). Fetal lung maturity testing should be performed before scheduled delivery at less than 39 weeks and uncertain gestational age. It is contraindicated when delivery is necessary for maternal or fetal indications, or before 32 weeks, when most results show immaturity (ACOG, 2008). Although exogenous surfactant is available for prophylaxis and therapy in newborn RDS, the incidence and severity of the disease can be prevented by maternal antenatal steroid administration to enhance fetal lung maturity.

In the third trimester, fetal respiratory activity allows the passage of surfactant into amniotic fluid, and its quantity may be evaluated using tests of amniotic fluid samples. Before 35 weeks gestation, the major component of surfactant is α-palmitic β-myristic lecithin. After that time, dipalmitic lecithin predominates, and phosphatidyl glycerol (PG) appears about a week later. PG increases until term and maintains alveolar stability. Minor phospholipid components of surfactant include phosphatidyl inositol, phosphatidyl ethanolamine, phosphatidyl serine, and sphingomyelins. The concentrations of components of surfactant are determined by biochemical tests that measure the phosphatidyl glycerol presence and the lecithin/sphingomyelin ratio. Biophysical tests, like fluorescence polarization, lamellar body counts, foam stability index, and optical density, use the surface-active properties of the phospholipids. The lecithin/sphingomyelin ratio (L/S) test was the first practical chemical test to assess fetal pulmonary status (Gluck, 1971). It estimates the ratio of lecithin to sphingomyelin in amniotic fluid. Concentrations of sphingomyelin remain constant throughout the pregnancy, and levels of lecithin are increasing. Following extraction and purification with solvents, amniotic fluid surfactant lipids are chromatographed on thin-layer silica (see Chapter 23 for discussion of this technique). The phospholipids are made visible by heat charring or staining. Densitometric quantification determines the L/S ratio. L/S ratios >2.0 usually indicate maturity, and ratios <1.5 immaturity. In the presence of newer tests, assessment of L/S ratios becomes less cost effective with longer turnaround time. Some believe that the test is unsatisfactory in diabetic women, in whose neonates RDS can occur when L/S ratios are greater than 2.0 (Dubin, 1992).

The presence of phosphatidyl glycerol on the thin-layer chromatogram, in addition to an L/S ratio >2.0, indicates fetal pulmonary maturity with virtual certainty in any patient. The presence of phosphatidyl glycerol can be determined using a newer slide agglutination test with antisera specific to phosphatidylglycerol.

A test for fetal lung development using the principle of fluorescence polarization came into widespread use after it was automated on the Abbott TDx analyzer. The fluorescence polarization technique measures the tumbling rate of a fluorescent molecule (see Chapter 23). The tumbling rate of a fluorophore added to amniotic fluid will depend on how much of it binds to albumin (causing slow tumbling) versus dissolving in the surfactant produced by the fetal lungs (rapid tumbling). Values of surfactant greater than 55 mg per 1 g of albumin are consistent with fetal lung maturity, and values below 40 mg suggest immaturity. However, the manufacturer has announced the discontinuation of this methodology in 2011.

A recently developed method under investigation is the lamellar body count test, which uses the standard hematologic counter to establish lamellar body concentrations. Thresholds representing fetal lung maturity are still under investigation. The most common accepted cutoffs with high negative predictive value for RDS are between 30,000 and 40,000.

Overall, the following factors may affect fetal lung maturity tests:

1. Blood contamination appears to increase the number of false-positive test results (Carlan, 1997), except for those using phosphatidyl glycerol presence.
2. Meconium does not affect lamellar body counts and determination of phosphatidyl glycerol.
3. Amniotic fluid volumes: L/S ratios, lamellar body counts, and phosphatidyl gylcerol levels are lower in polyhydramnios (Piazze, 1998).
4. Diabetes mellitus: Studies have shown delayed production of phosphatidyl glycerol in the fetuses of pregnant women with diabetes; however, the same thresholds apply to pregnancies of diabetic and nondiabetic women (Melanson, 2007).
5. Method of collection of AF: Comparing the AF collected vaginally with that collected by amniocentesis shows whether results of fluid collected vaginally are mature. The test is more reliable (Edwards, 2000).

Comparison of previous tests in many studies has shown similar characteristics, with high sensitivity between 81% and 92%, and typical negative predictive value from 95%–100% (Neerhof, 2001; Winn-McMillan, 2005; Haymond, 2006).

TOXEMIA OF PREGNANCY (PREECLAMPSIA)

Preeclampsia is a syndrome characterized by hypertension of 140 mm Hg systolic or higher or 90 mm Hg diastolic or higher, with proteinuria greater than 0.3 g/L in a 24-hour urine specimen that occurs after 20 weeks of gestation in previously normotensive women (National High Blood Pressure Education Program Working Group Report on High Blood Pressure in Pregnancy, 2000). The incidence of preeclampsia is 5%–8% of all pregnant women. Preconceptional risk factors associated with preeclampsia include first pregnancy, chronic hypertension, renal disease, antiphospholipid syndrome, diabetes, obesity, advanced maternal age, thrombophilia, partner who fathered preeclamptic pregnancy in another woman, and history of preeclampsia in previous pregnancies.

Conditions that can mimic preeclampsia include systemic lupus erythematosus, idiopathic thrombocytopenic purpura, thrombotic thrombocytopenic purpura, hemolytic-uremic syndrome, cholestasis of pregnancy, and fatty liver disease (Sibai, 2004).

Life-threatening manifestations of preeclampsia that remain a cause of maternal mortality are eclampsia and HELLP syndrome (stands for **he**molytic anemia, **e**levated **l**iver enzymes, **l**ow **p**latelet count). Eclampsia, which is defined as new onset of grand mal seizures in women with preeclampsia, may result in intracranial hemorrhage.

The cause of preeclampsia remains unknown. Pathophysiologic abnormalities include abnormal trophoblastic invasion by placenta, resulting from imbalance between proangiogenic and angiogenic factors (Barton, 2008). Impaired uteroplacental flow causes intrauterine growth restriction, oligohydramnios, and placental abruption. The interaction of various vasoactive agents such as prostacyclin, thromboxane A_2, nitric oxide, and endothelins causes the vasospasm that leads to depleted intravascular volume and hepatic and renal changes. Hematologic changes usually are seen as hemoconcentration, thrombocytopenia, and hemolysis. Hepatic involvement manifests as elevation of aminotransferases, usually twice above normal limit. Lactate dehydrogenase (LD) is increased primarily because of hepatic disease (mostly LD_5) or as the result of hemolysis with increases in LD_1 and LD_2. Hyperbilirubinemia occurs in the presence of hemolysis as well. The proteinuria in preeclampsia is of a glomerular type (mostly albumin), and the urine sediment contains hyaline and finely granular casts. Mild to moderate increases in urea (>15 mg/dL) and creatinine (>0.8 mg/dL) are noted, as is a marked increase in uric acid.

Severe preeclampsia is diagnosed if one or more of these criteria are met: Blood pressure systolic of 160 or greater, diastolic of 110 or greater; proteinuria of 5 g or higher in 24-hour urine specimen; oliguria (<500 mL/24 hours); cerebral or visual disturbances; pulmonary edema; right upper quadrant pain; impaired liver function; thrombocytopenia (<100 K/μL); or fetal growth restriction (ACOG, 2002).

In the past decade, many biophysical and biochemical markers have been proposed to predict which women are likely to develop preeclampsia, but none of the screening tests has been found to be reliable and cost effective. Several studies have analyzed the levels of angiogenic factors in preeclampsia. Results revealed decreased levels of placental growth factor, placental protein-13, and pregnancy-associated plasma protein A, along with elevation of fms-like tyrosine kinase-1, endoglin (a transmembrane receptor that is vital for angiogenesis), and dimethylarginine (Levine, 2006) (a marker for atherosclerotic heart disease). However, because of differences in study design and methods of analysis, these markers have poor predictive value and specificity. A more promising test is Doppler velocimetry of the uterine arteries (Espinoza, 2007).

Mild preeclampsia can be managed expectantly and followed by delivery at term. Delivery at any gestational age is indicated for the following conditions: eclampsia, HELLP, placental abruption, non-reassuring fetal heart pattern, pulmonary edema, severe hypertension, worsening of renal function, persistent symptoms of headaches, visual disturbances, and epigastric pain.

PREMATURE RUPTURE OF MEMBRANES

Premature rupture of membranes is rupture of membranes before the onset of labor. It may be followed by a variety of complications, including chorioamnionitis, fetal pulmonary hypoplasia, placental abruption, and neonatal respiratory distress. The diagnosis of membrane rupture is made upon visualization of fluid passing from the cervical canal on the sterile speculum examination. Amniotic fluid constitutes part of the posterior vaginal fluid pool, and identification of the amniotic component is optimally carried out within 2 hours of membrane rupture. Unlike vaginal secretions, whose pH is acidic (pH, 4.5–5.5), amniotic fluid is alkaline, with pH of 7.0–7.5. The vaginal pool aspirate can be tested with nitrazine paper to estimate pH visually. A positive test is indicated by a blue color, and a negative one by a yellow-green color. Among false-positives, 5% are related to the presence of blood, mucus, semen, bacterial vaginosis, alkaline urine, or soap. False-negatives are less likely (1%) but may be seen with membrane rupture that occurred more than 24 hours earlier, or if sampling was inadequate. The nitrazine test is usually performed at the bedside and is said to have an overall accuracy of about 90% in the absence of bloody show, vaginal discharge, or prolonged membrane rupture (Friedman, 1969). An aliquot of the aspirated fluid can be applied to a glass microscope slide, dried for 5 minutes, and examined microscopically for arborization (ferning), which indicates the presence of amniotic fluid in the vaginal fluid pool. False-positive ferning occurs in less than 2% of cases and is associated with the presence of blood, urine, or cervical mucus. False-negatives occur in less than 5% of cases. An alternative method for detecting amniotic fluid in vaginal secretions is rapid immunoassay of placental alpha-1 microglobulin, currently marketed as the AmniSure test (N-Dia Inc., New York).

PRETERM LABOR

Numerous biochemical markers and biophysical tools have been evaluated for predicting preterm delivery. In 1991, Lockwood and colleagues discovered an association between the presence of fetal fibronectin (fFN) in cervical secretions and risk of preterm delivery. fFN is a glycoprotein produced by fetal membranes and found in the choriodecidual junction amniotic fluid; it is released as cervical secretions at up to 20 weeks of gestational age. It has been identified in malignant cell lines and is recognized by antibody FDC-6 (Lockwood, 1991). Fibronectin is responsible for the cellular adhesiveness of placenta and membranes to the decidua. Disruption of the chorion from the decidual layer of the uterus leads to the release of intact or degraded chorionic components of the extracellular matrix into the cervical and vaginal secretions. The fFN enzyme immunoassay is a U.S. Food and Drug Administration-approved test for assessment of the risk for preterm delivery in women between 24 and 35 weeks gestational age. The purposes of the test are to identify asymptomatic women who are at risk for preterm delivery and to predict the risk of delivery in symptomatic women with preterm contractions. The specimen is collected during sterile speculum examination with a swab from the posterior fornix of the vagina or the region of the external cervical os for 10 seconds. Concentrations of fFN in the cervicovaginal fluid greater than 50 ng/mL are considered positive (Garite, 1996). The swab should be performed before procedures that may disrupt the cervix, such as the digital examination, Papanicolaou smear, cervical culture, and vaginal ultrasound. The following criteria should be met: cervical dilation less than 3 cm, intact membranes, absence of uterine bleeding, sexual intercourse more than 24 hours before, and absence of cervical cerclage. A meta-analysis of many studies on patients with symptoms suggestive of preterm labor showed that cervicovaginal fFN is an effective predictor of preterm delivery (Leitich, 1999). Testing for fFN can reduce unnecessary hospitalization and avoid intervention in symptomatic pregnant women. Detection of fFN can also help in the management of pregnancy in asymptomatic women who have known risk factors for preterm labor, such as previous preterm delivery or short cervix.

It appears to be most valuable in ruling out imminent delivery in patients with symptoms with negative predictive values for delivery within 7, within 14, and at less than 37 weeks (99.5%, 99.2%, and 84.5%, respectively) (Peaceman, 1997). The test is often performed with sonographic assessment of cervical length. An fFN test has limited application for screening of asymptomatic women and those with no risk factors because of the low incidence of preterm labor in this population (Leitich, 1999). Future applications of fFN as a tool in predicting successful labor induction are under investigation.

INTRAPARTUM ASSESSMENT OF FETAL STATUS

The goal of intrapartum fetal surveillance is to recognize if the fetus with a nonreassuring fetal heart tracing on external monitoring is acidotic and at risk for neurologic impairment or death. Usually, episodes of hypoxemia are transient and well tolerated by the fetus. However, prolonged or repeat episodes may lead to hypoxic-ischemic encephalopathy. Available tests can help to ensure fetal well-being and reduce false-positive findings on external fetal heart monitoring. Noninvasive and preferred tests, such as digital scalp stimulation and vibroacoustic stimulation of the fetus, followed by the presence of reassuring fetal heart monitoring, indicate that the fetus is not acidotic. The direct method for evaluation of fetal acid-base status is fetal scalp blood sampling. This test is performed using the amnioscope with a light source; blood is collected from a punctured fetal scalp and is transferred in a heparinized capillary tube. A pH value less than 7.20 identifies fetal acidosis. However, the test has low sensitivity (36%) and poor predictive value (9%) in predicting fetal acidemia of pH less than 7.0 (Kruger, 1999). The use of fetal scalp pH assessment is decreasing in many institutions because of the difficulty involved in obtaining and processing samples and in obtaining standardized laboratory equipment.

Another method of predicting fetal acidosis involves the measurement of fetal lactate concentrations with the use of rapid enzymatic assays. Blood samples are collected by using techniques similar to those used in fetal scalp pH. Recently, a large, multicenter, randomized trial compared the effectiveness of pH analysis of fetal scalp blood versus use of lactate levels in identifying hypoxia at birth, and showed no differences between the two groups in obstetric and neonatal outcomes (Wiberg-Itzel, 2008).

The most objective tool for determining intrapartum fetal status and obtaining information related to obstetric management is umbilical cord sampling. Immediately after delivery, arterial blood is drawn from a segment of clamped umbilical cord to a heparinized capillary syringe and is analyzed for cord blood pH and blood gas values. ACOG (2006) recommends analysis of umbilical cord blood in neonates with low Apgar scores to differentiate hypoxia from metabolic acidemia and other causes of low Apgar scores. Significant metabolic acidosis is defined by umbilical cord blood pH values less than 7.0; base deficits of 12 mmol/L or greater are predictive of adverse neurologic outcomes and are included in the criteria for an acute intrapartum hypoxic event.

OTHER EVALUATIONS

Infection During Pregnancy

Viral, bacterial, and parasitic infections can have a significant impact on the mother, fetus, or both. Important examples are human immunodeficiency virus, hepatitis virus (A, B, and C), rubella virus, varicella virus, parvovirus B19, cytomegalovirus, *Chlamydia trachomatis*, group B *Streptococcus*, *Neisseria gonorrhoeae*, syphilis, tuberculosis, toxoplasmosis, and malaria. These are discussed in Part 7 of this text.

Hematologic and Coagulation Disorders

Various disorders can have a negative effect on mother, fetus, or both, including maternal anemias (nutritional, sickle cell), maternal and fetal thrombocytopenias (idiopathic thrombocytopenic purpura, fetal alloimmune thrombocytopenia, thrombotic thrombocytopenic purpura), maternal coagulopathies (acute disseminated intravascular coagulation, von Willebrand disease), and maternal thrombophilias. These are described in Parts 4 and 5.

SELECTED REFERENCES

Ashwood ER. Clinical chemistry of pregnancy. In: Burtis CA, Ashwood ER, editors. Tietz textbook of clinical chemistry. 3rd ed. Philadelphia: WB Saunders; 1999.
Overview includes detailed descriptions of amniotic fluid spectrophotometry of bilirubin for erythroblastosis fetalis (Liley's test).

Mortimer D. Practical laboratory andrology. New York: Oxford University Press; 1994.
Descriptive guide and reference for clinical evaluation of reproductive function in the male.

Speroff L, Fritz Marc A. Clinical gynecologic endocrinology and infertility. 7th ed. Philadelphia: Lippincott Williams & Wilkins; 2005.
General reference for female reproductive endocrinology and ART.

Strauss JF, Barbieri RL, editors. Yen and Jaffe's reproductive endocrinology. 5th ed. Philadelphia: WB Saunders; 2004.
Comprehensive reference for all aspects of reproductive function and pregnancy.

Trounson AO, Gardner DK. Handbook of in vitro fertilization. 2nd ed. Boca Raton, Fla.: CRC Press; 2000.
General reference for assisted reproductive technologies (ARTs).

Willett GD, editor. Laboratory testing in ob/gyn. Boston: Blackwell Scientific Publications; 1994.
Comprehensive and concise summary of laboratory evaluation of the female.

REFERENCES

Access the complete reference list online at http://www.expertconsult.com

CHAPTER 26

VITAMINS AND TRACE ELEMENTS

Martin J. Salwen

KEY POINTS

- Very small quantities of vitamins and trace elements are needed to satisfy metabolic requirements. Adequate supplies are essential for health.
- Vitamins and trace elements should be obtained from foods rather than from supplements.
- Vitamins are present in almost all foods, but no one food group is a good source of all vitamins.
- Several groups, including pregnant women, neonates and infants, the elderly, those receiving long-term parenteral nutrition or hyperalimentation, those on hemodialysis, and those with a disease causing malabsorption, warrant selective micronutrient supplementation.
- These heterogeneous essential micronutrients are unrelated organic catalysts and elements.
- Vitamins are essential organic substances that the body cannot synthesize, or does not sufficiently synthesize. This is species specific. Vitamins may function variously as enzymatic cofactors, antioxidants, or hormones and are active in energy metabolism, protein metabolism, blood cell maturation, and bone formation. Vitamins are unrelated chemically and have different physiologic activities and food sources.
- Vitamins may be single chemicals (e.g., ascorbic acid) or may include a family of closely related compounds (e.g., vitamins A, D, E, and K, cobalamin). They may be classified according to water or lipid solubility, which affects absorption and transport, storage, toxicity, excretion, and disease conditions that cause deficiencies, even when nutritional intake is sufficient.
- Deficiencies are most often due to malnutrition.
- Dietary reference intake includes reference values for each essential nutrient.
- The tolerable upper intake level is the maximum daily nutrient intake that is unlikely to have adverse affects for almost everybody.
- Assessment of both dietary intake and body stores requires different test strategies for diagnosis of deficiency or toxicity. Deficiencies are especially important at the age extremes of life and in malnutrition of whatever cause.
- A therapeutic trial of the nutrient considered deficient is the most reliable approach to diagnosis and treatment.
- Body stores of vitamins and minerals vary tremendously.
- Essential trace elements have specific metabolic functions that cannot be replaced by other minerals.
- Disease states significantly change the requirements for vitamins and trace elements.
- Deficiencies of trace elements may result from insufficient ingestion because soil, water, or plants in the region are inadequate in a specific element; other dietary substances interfere with absorption; or the protein needed for absorption or metabolism is lacking.
- Overt deficiencies of micronutrients are rare in Western countries, except in chronic illness or alcoholism.
- Immune function is adversely affected by poor intakes of almost all of the micronutrients.
- Micronutrients are often insufficient for displaced populations during violence or famine.
- Trace elements have structural, signal transduction, and catalytic functions. Some are components of metalloenzymes; they may function as enzyme cofactors or provide electron and oxygen transport, or they may be active in the maintenance of macromolecule conformation or vitamin or hormonal activity.
- To avoid contamination, trace elements must be analyzed with considerable care because they are widely distributed in the environment and are present in very minute concentrations in body fluids and tissues. Thus, techniques must be sensitive enough to analyze concentrations of μg/L or even ng/L.
- For most micronutrients, concentrations in body fluids indicate only the adequacy of recent intake because of lack of correlation with body tissue concentrations.
- Trace element concentrations in body fluids correlate poorly with amounts in body stores. Serum levels are unreliable because of the influence of unrelated conditions. No particularly good assays are available for trace element dietary status. Test results need be interpreted with caution.
- The only definitive test of human trace element deficiency is assessment of clinical response to controlled supplementation when the element is considered deficient.
- The intake required to cause toxicity is highly variable for the different trace elements.
- Toxicity rarely results from excessive dietary intake.
- Toxicity is usually due to overdoses of vitamin supplements.
- A poison is too much of anything. Toxicity is never a question of presence, only of amount.

Twenty-three vitamins and trace elements are collectively termed essential micronutrients. Adequate supplies of these heterogeneous nutrients are critical for health, development, and longevity. They are needed in small amounts for metabolism of proteins, carbohydrates, and fats, and for the body's structure (e.g., vitamin K in bone matrix). Many micronutrients are important antioxidants (e.g., vitamins C and E) or are cofactors for antioxidant enzymes (e.g., selenium in glutathione peroxidase). Recommended allowances reconcile optimum nutrition and the prevention of deficiency symptoms or diseases. The requirements for most essential nutrients to maintain health are now fairly well characterized.

Dietary reference intake (DRI) is an umbrella term that includes reference values or estimates of the dietary level for each essential nutrient. DRI was introduced by the Food and Nutrition Board, Institute of Medicine of the National Academy of Sciences (IOM, 1997, 1998, 2000, 2002), and provides four dietary reference values, primarily intended for nutritionists (Barr, 2002). **Recommended dietary allowance (RDA)** is the average daily dietary amount sufficient for the nutrient requirements of most (97%–98%) healthy people categorized by age, gender, and physiologic need. The RDA is derived from the **estimated average requirement,** that is, the average daily nutrient intake level estimated to meet the requirements of half the healthy individuals in a particular life stage and gender group. **Adequate intake** is an estimate of average recommended daily intake when the RDA cannot be determined. The **tolerable upper intake level (TUL)** is the maximum daily nutrient intake that is likely to pose no risk of adverse health effects for almost all individuals in the general population (IOM, 1998). As intake increases above the TUL, the potential risk of adverse effects increases. Also, the amounts recommended for enteral and intravenous nutritional support are available.

Because of a plentiful and inexpensive food supply, overt deficiencies of vitamins or trace elements (e.g., pellagra) are rare in Western countries, except in the chronically ill or alcoholic. Very small amounts of micronutrients are required to satisfy their diverse physiologic roles, and their functions are as varied as their compositions (Mason, 1996). They are usually ingested as foods and consumed in meals rather than as individual nutrients or molecules. Patients should obtain the vitamins and trace elements from foods rather than from supplements (Lichtenstein, 2005; Barnard, 2009). These essential nutrients are unrelated organic catalysts and elements that are not endogenously synthesized in sufficient amounts (Rubin, 2005). Insufficient micronutrient intake has short-term and long-term disease implications. For example, immune function is adversely affected by poor intakes of almost all of the micronutrients. Body stores of vitamins and minerals vary tremendously. Vitamin B_{12} and vitamin A stores are large, and an adult might not become deficient for 1 or more years after being on a depleted diet. However, folate and thiamine may become depleted within weeks when eating a deficient diet. Both deficiency and toxicity states are often insidious and may be attributable to inappropriate intake or defective utilization. Deficiencies are most often due to malnutrition (McLaren, 1994). Initial interest focused on the prevention of deficiency diseases and elucidation of the biochemical roles of these micronutrients as coenzymes and cofactors. Research on the assessment of vitamin and trace element nutriture has further identified their many other important functions, such as antioxidant activity and hormone-like stimulation, along with their regulatory roles (Machlin, 1992).

Micronutrients are often insufficient for displaced populations or refugees in instances of domestic upheaval, violence, or famine. Determination of the extent to which metabolic demands for micronutrients have been met is complex and very difficult. A clinical history obtained by an experienced practitioner or dietitian can provide only a crude assessment. Even a complete 3-day dietary diary is limited because of the problem of recording sizes of food portions and amounts consumed (Nelson, 2000).

Measurement of vitamin and trace element levels is sometimes helpful in nutritional assessment. Clinical assessment of their status is often poor. Disease conditions, infections, and trauma alter metabolism and significantly change the requirements for vitamins and trace elements in ways that are poorly understood (Shenken, 1997, 2000; Elia, 2001). Disease states may increase demand, but the effects of illness on the requirements are not well quantified. Laboratory studies improve the assessment of the balance of supply and demand but are limited (Gidden, 2000). Subclinical deficiencies are known to occur, but the extent of depletion that occurred before significant biochemical, physiologic, or histologic changes were noted can only be surmised. Analytic improvements in this field are greatly needed. Interpretation of tests of nutritional status requires reference intervals with provisions for relevant factors such as ethnicity, geographic variation, time of sampling, and development of functional tests. Subclinical vitamin and trace element deficiencies can be diagnosed by laboratory testing for some elements (e.g., zinc, folate, iron, vitamins B_6 and B_{12}), especially in geriatric age groups.

Concentrations of micronutrients are usually measured in plasma or serum, but these data provide a reliable indication of their status for only a few vitamins and trace elements. For most, concentrations in body fluids indicate only the adequacy of recent intake, because of lack of correlation with body tissue concentrations. For mobilization, binding proteins and concentrations in various body tissues (e.g., vitamin A in the liver) seem to be most significant. For some elements (e.g., manganese, chromium), the data permit assessment of toxicity. Tissue or blood cell concentrations can assess certain significant conditions (e.g., copper concentration in liver biopsy in suspected Wilson's disease; red cell folate or leukocyte vitamin C concentration for clinical evaluation). Urine measurements of the concentrations of most vitamins and trace elements are rarely helpful in that most are not under homeostatic control and indicate only the amount ingested. The time course for the development of a subclinical deficiency is variable for each vitamin and is affected by body stores. The extent of depletion and any subsequent progression to functional effects and clinical disease have been poorly characterized (Shenkin, 2006).

Vitamins and trace minerals have been invested with a magical aura. The misguided belief that megadoses can provide a panacea is widespread. Perhaps this reflects an awareness of the extraordinary physiologic prowess of these micronutrients, but they also pose a hazard. A risk of toxic overdose is present, although they are safe within TUL (IOM, 1998).

Several groups of people warrant selective micronutrient supplementation. These include pregnant women, neonates, and infants; elderly persons; patients receiving long-term parenteral nutrition or hyperalimentation; those with a disease causing malabsorption; and those with altered nutritional or metabolic states. Hemodialysis removes water-soluble vitamins. Poverty and food faddism are continued sources of deficiencies. Other at-risk groups likely to be deficient in micronutrients include alcohol-dependent patients with deficient vitamins C, E, and the B vitamins, particularly thiamine; and those following unsupplemented vegan diets.

Drug-Diet Interactions. Folic acid deficiency may result from anticonvulsant therapy (e.g., phenytoin, phenobarbital). Vitamin B_{12} absorption is decreased by acid suppression (e.g., proton pump inhibitors).

For the general population, with only certain exceptions, vitamin and trace element supplementation is not required and is unnecessary and even wasteful, because of their ubiquitous distribution and ready availability from a variety of food sources.

This section will review the micronutrients, which include vitamins and essential trace mineral elements. The thirteen vitamins are outlined in Table 26-1, along with their functions and summaries of deficiency and toxicity states. Table 26-2 lists RDAs and food sources for the vitamins, as well as laboratory assessments for subclinical deficiency states. Table 26-3 tabulates a classification of trace elements. Table 26-4 lists the 10 essential trace elements, along with their functions and summaries of the effects of deficiency and toxicity. Table 26-5 lists the properties of the essential trace elements.

VITAMINS

These organic molecules are required in trace amounts for health, growth, and reproduction (McCormick, 1994). Except for vitamin D, the body depends completely on dietary intake of vitamins, although some enteric bacterial production of vitamin K, nicotinic acid, riboflavin, biotin, cobalamin, and folic acid has been noted (Eastwood, 2003; Grodner, 2004). These syntheses occur mostly in the colon and are not nutritionally significant because these vitamins are poorly absorbed. The lack of each vitamin results in a clearly identifiable metabolic deficit, causing a clinical deficiency syndrome. This is species specific; differences in the synthesizing capabilities of different species have been observed. Many lower animals can produce their own ascorbic acid. Humans, however, cannot synthesize ascorbic acid and require ascorbate to prevent scurvy (Combs, 1998).

Vitamins may be classified according to their properties, such as function, nutritional source, or solubility in water (Table 26-1). Vitamins have been divided into two groups on the basis of solubility, which affects absorption and transport. Water-soluble vitamins are easily absorbed, which allows for minimal storage. However, deficiencies can develop quickly—within weeks (Grodner, 2004). Thiamine, riboflavin, niacin, pyridoxine, cobalamin, vitamin C, folate, pantothenic acid, and biotin are water

TABLE 26-1

Vitamins: Functions, Deficiency Syndromes, and Toxicity

Water-soluble vitamin	Functions	Deficiency syndromes	Toxicity
Ascorbate (vitamin C)	Many redox reactions Hydroxylation of collagen	Scurvy	Chronic megadoses of 10–150 times the RDA (1–15 g), cramps, diarrhea, nausea, kidney stones. With megadoses, body accelerates drug metabolism. Can produce scurvy if megadoses abruptly stop
Biotin	Cofactor in carboxylation reactions	Rare. Caused by lack of biotin in total parenteral nutrition. Also, avidin in raw egg whites binds biotin in gut, preventing absorption. Dermatitis, glossitis, hair loss, anorexia, depression, and hypercholesterolemia	No known toxicity
Cobalamin (vitamin B_{12})	Folate metabolism and DNA synthesis, maintenance of myelinization of spinal tracts	Megaloblastic anemia, peripheral neuropathy	No appreciable toxicity
Folate	Transfer and use one-carbon units in DNA and amino acid synthesis	Megaloblastic anemia, neural tube defects	Teratogenic effect in rodent model. No adverse effects at high oral doses
Niacin (nicotinic acid)	Incorporated into NAD and NAD phosphate, redox reactions	Pellagra: Dementia, dermatitis, diarrhea	Excess pre-formed niacin and nicotinic acid cause vascular dilation, "flushing"; hepatotoxic
Thiamine (vitamin B_1)	As pyrophosphate, is coenzyme in decarboxylation reactions	Dry (neuromuscular) and wet (cardiac failure) beriberi, Wernicke-Korsakoff syndrome	Only when given parenterally. Headache, muscle weakness, cardiac arrhythmia, convulsions
Pantothenic acid (vitamin B_3)	Incorporated in coenzyme A	No syndrome recognized	Very high doses: Diarrhea
Pyridoxine (vitamin B_6)	Derivatives are coenzymes in many intermediary reactions; amino acid, phospholipid, and glycogen metabolism	Cheilosis, glossitis, dermatitis, peripheral neuropathy, convulsions	Long-term megadose supplementation causes ataxia and sensory neuropathy. The UL is 100 mg/day
Riboflavin (vitamin B_2)	Converted to flavin coenzymes. Cofactor for many enzymes in intermediary metabolism	Ariboflavinosis, cheilosis, angular stomatitis, glossitis, dermatitis, corneal vascularization	Toxicity to riboflavin has not been reported. Absorption limited normally
Vitamin A (retinol)	A component of retinal rod pigment. Role in vision in dim light, growth; reproduction. Maintenance of resistance to infection	Squamous metaplasia, especially glandular, follicular hyperkeratosis; xerophthalmia; night blindness, reproductive disorders, vulnerability to infection	Livers of polar bears and large animals have very high levels of vitamin A. Acute: Can cause drowsiness, headache, vomiting, stupor, skin peeling, and papilledema. Chronic: Teratogenic, osteoporosis, hepatotoxicity. Carotenoids in excess, distinct orange-yellow skin color
Vitamin D (cholecalciferol)	Promotes absorption of calcium and phosphorus; mineralization of bones and teeth	Rickets in children; osteomalacia in adults; hypocalcemia, tetany	High intake of vitamin D: Hypercalcemia and hypercalciuria, toxicity above UL of 50 µg. Bone demineralization, constipation, muscle weakness, renal calculi
Vitamin E (tocopherol)	Antioxidant, scavenges free-radicals; cellular respiration, primarily in muscle, RBC integrity	Spinocerebellar degeneration, ataxia	Mild GI distress, nausea, coagulopathies in patients receiving anticonvulsants
Vitamin K (phytomenadione)	Cofactor of procoagulants—hepatic factors II (prothrombin), VII, and X, proteins C and S	Defective clotting, bleeding disorder	Foods containing vitamin K cause no toxicity problems. Excess amounts of vitamin K may decrease clotting time

Data from Berdanier, 1998; Combs, 1998; Eastwood, 2003; Grodner, 2004; Kane, 2005.
DNA, Deoxyribonucleic acid; *GI,* gastrointestinal; *NAD,* nicotinamide adenine dinucleotide; *RBC,* erythrocyte; *RDA,* recommended dietary allowance; *UL,* upper limit.

soluble. Vitamins A, D, E, and K are considered water insoluble or fat soluble, and they depend on normal lipid digestion and micellar solubilization, such as the presence of bile, for absorption. Malabsorption of fat may result in deficiencies of the fat-soluble vitamins, despite adequate dietary intake.

Vitamins are found in almost all foods, but no one food group is a good source for all vitamins (Table 26-2) (Grodner, 2004). The vitamin B complex includes thiamine, riboflavin, niacin, pyridoxine, and cobalamin. Cobalamin is present only in animal products, including meat, especially liver, milk, cheese, eggs, and other animal proteins. All of the other B complex vitamins are found in leafy green vegetables, milk, and liver. Vitamin A and niacin have precursor substances that can be converted to the active vitamin form in humans. Vitamin K and biotin are produced by the gut microflora, but in insufficient quantities to sustain metabolism. Niacin and vitamin D can be made in the human body. Both thiamine and biotin have natural antagonists.

Deficiencies are particularly important at the extremes of life. They are a matter of concern for the developing fetus and infant, and for the aged (Seymour, 2000). Deficiencies are also frequent among those with protein-energy malnutrition in developing nations. In developed countries, conditions resulting in vitamin deficiencies include decreased intake, absorption, or production. Decreased intake characteristically occurs in patients suffering from alcoholism (e.g., thiamine) or small bowel disease (e.g., folate and the fat-soluble vitamins; vitamins A, D, E, and K), as well as in vegans (vitamin D, cobalamin) and the elderly (e.g., vitamin D, folate). Conditions that result in decreased absorption in liver and in biliary tract disease (e.g., vitamins A, D, E, and K) are due to ileal disease or resection (e.g., cobalamin). Conditions that cause decreased production occur in renal disease (e.g., vitamin D) and with drugs such as methotrexate (e.g., folate). Deficiencies also occur in those with long-term chronic disease such as acquired immunodeficiency syndrome. Assessment of body stores and of the chronic nutritional state for micronutrients continues to present difficulties.

TABLE 26-2
Vitamins: RDA, Food Sources, and Analysis of Body Levels

Water-soluble vitamin	RDA	Food sources	Laboratory assessment for subclinical deficiency states
Ascorbic acid (vitamin C)	M: 90 mg F: 75 mg Smokers: 125 mg	Fruits and vegetables: Citrus fruits, red and green peppers, strawberries, tomatoes, broccoli, potatoes, green leafy vegetables	Fasting specimen required. S—ascorbic acid, deficient <11.4 μmol/L WBC—ascorbic acid by HPLC, reflects tissue stores, preparation and assay difficult. <11.4 nmol/10^8 cells associated with scurvy 24-hour U-ascorbic acid, reflects recent dietary intake Vitamin C load test U
Biotin	AI 30 μg	Liver, kidneys, peanut butter, egg yolks, yeast	Microbiological assay
Cobalamin (vitamin B_{12})	M/F: 2.4 μg	Meat, fish, poultry, eggs, and dairy products	S—vitamin B_{12} by CPBA, deficiency <200 ng/L U—methylmalonic acid
Folate	M/F: 400 μg Pregnancy: 600 μg Lactation: 500 μg	Leafy green vegetables, legumes, cereals, some fruits and juices	Hemolysis interferes. RBC—folate; S—folate S—methyltetrahydrofolate, reflects recent intake, not stores. Cutoff point, negative folate balance <6.8 nmol/L Polyglutamate forms of folate present, reflect body folate stores Folate (nmol/L): depleted <368 deficient <322 anemia <227 U—FIGLU Histidine load test U
Niacin (nicotinic acid)	NE = 1 mg niacin or 60 mg tryptophan M: 16 mg NE/day F: 14 mg NE/day	Protein-containing foods are good sources of both niacin and tryptophan. Meats, poultry, fish, legumes, enriched cereals, milk, coffee, and tea	Ratio of RBC—NAD and NADP nucleotide, <1 may indicate risk of niacin deficiency Ratio 2—pyridone (40%–60%): N′-Methyl nicotinamide (20%–30%), deficiency of niacin when ratio <1
Pantothenic acid	AI 5 mg	Whole grain cereals, legumes, meat, fish, poultry	Whole blood—pantothenic acid, inadequate intake <100 μg/dL 24-Hour U—pantothenic acid, abnormally low <1 mg/day
Pyridoxine (vitamin B_6)	M/F: 1.3 mg	Whole grains, cereals, legumes, chicken, fish, pork, and eggs	P-pyridoxal-5′-phosphate, cation exchange HPLC, assay by fluorometry B6 status: >30 nmol/L adequate ≥0.8 acceptable <0.5 marginal or inadequate RBC—aminotransferases, reflect long-term pyridoxine status; ALT more sensitive to B_6 deficiency than ALT U—4-pyridoxic acid, dietary intake of B_6 U—xanthenuric acid, tryptophan metabolite Tryptophan load test U
Riboflavin (vitamin B_2)	M: 1.3 mg F: 1.1 mg Riboflavin destroyed by light	Milk, enriched grains, broccoli, asparagus, dark leafy greens, whole grains, enriched breads, cereals. Also dairy products, meats, fish, poultry, and eggs	RBC—glutathione reductase, expressed as ratio of assays with and without flavin adenine dinucleotide 24-Hour U—riboflavin measures recent intake, not body stores, nonspecific; varies with physical activity
Thiamine (vitamin B_1)	M: 1.2 mg F: 1.1 mg	Whole or enriched grains and flour, lean pork, legumes, seeds, and nuts	RBC—transketolase activity, expressed as ratio of assays with and without thiamine pyrophosphate 24-Hour U—thiamine measures recent dietary intake, not body stores
Fat-soluble vitamin	**RDA**	**Food sources**	**Laboratory assessment for subclinical deficiencies**
Vitamin A (retinol)	M: 900 μg RAE F: 700 μg RAE	Natural pre-formed vitamin A only in fat of animal-related foods: Whole milk, butter, liver, egg yolks, and fatty fish Carotenoids are found in deep green, yellow, and orange fruits and vegetables (broccoli, cantaloupe, sweet potato, carrots, tomatoes, spinach)	Hemolysis interferes Liver retinol stores: S-retinol, insensitive test Dose response: S-retinol and dehydroretinol by HPLC 4–6 hours after oral 3,4-didehydroretinylacetate (100 μg/kg); more sensitive index than S-retinol of marginal retinol status RDR: Retinol-binding protein RBP, low specificity In Vitamin A deficiency, RBP accumulates in liver as apo-RBP (RBP not bound to retinol). After retinol dose, retinol binds to apo-RBP in liver, holo-RBP (RBP bound to retinol) released from liver, causing increased S-retinol. Blood sample at baseline and 5 hours after oral vitamin A. Calculate RDR (%), >14%–20%, marginal vitamin A status S—Carotenoids indicate current intake of carotenoids RDA for night blindness
Vitamin D	AI M/F: 5 μg Ages: 51–70 years, 10 μg >70 years, 15 μg	Butter, egg yolks, liver, and fatty fish Vitamin D–fortified milk Sunlight exposure converts precursor to active vitamin D	S—25-Hydroxy vitamin D: Deficiency <3 nmol/L Toxicity >500 nmol/L Separate S—25(OH)-D by HPLC, assay by CPBA, indicates total endogenous and exogenous vitamin D, reflects vitamin D content of liver

TABLE 26-2
Vitamins: RDA, Food Sources, and Analysis of Body Levels—*Cont'd*

Fat-soluble vitamin	RDA	Food sources	Laboratory assessment for subclinical deficiency states
Vitamin E (tocopherol)	α-tocopherol equivalents = α-TE M/F: 15 mg α-TE	Vegetable oils, corn, soy, safflower. Whole grains, seeds, nuts, wheat germ, green leafy vegetables	Ratio S—tocopherol: S—lipids; reverse-phase HPLC with high-sensitivity fluorescence detector; levels correlate with S—cholesterol deficiency when ratio <0.6 mg total tocopherol/g serum lipids
Vitamin K	AI M: 120 μg F: 90 μg	Vitamin K synthesized by bacteria in jejunum and ileum; dietary intake is still required. Dark green leafy vegetables	PT

Data from McCormick, 1994; Gibson, 2002; Grodner, 2004.
AI, Adequate intake; *ALT,* alanine aminotransferase; *CPBA,* competitive protein binding assay; *F,* female; *FIGLU,* formiminoglutamic acid; *HPLC,* high-performance liquid chromatography; *M,* male; *M/F,* male/female; *NAD,* nicotinamide adenine dinucleotide; *NE,* niacin equivalent; *P,* plasma; *PT,* prothrombin time; *RAE,* retinol activity equivalents; *RBC,* erythrocyte; *RBP,* index of retinol; *RDA,* recommended dietary allowance; *RDR,* relative dose response; *S,* serum; *U,* urine; *WBC,* leukocyte.

Concentrations in plasma often indicate only recent nutritional intake. A therapeutic replacement trial of the nutriment considered deficient is often the easiest and most reliable approach. Specific diagnostic strategies are helpful (see Table 26-2) (Feldman, 1994; Gibson, 2002). Mobilization into plasma is affected by the availability of appropriate binding proteins, irrespective of vitamin or trace element stores (Shenkin, 2006).

Toxicity rarely results from excessive dietary intake. Toxicity is usually due to overdoses of vitamin supplements. Single large doses of the water-soluble vitamins are rarely toxic because they are rapidly excreted, but repeated doses can cause toxicity. Vitamin A has a toxic potential greater than that of the other hypervitaminoses, although the actual incidence is low. Intakes as low as 25 times the RDA are considered potentially toxic for vitamin A. Carotenoids have low toxicity. Vitamin D is the other vitamin that has a relatively high potential for toxicity. Intakes of about 50 times the RDA have been reported as toxic in humans. Children have been particularly sensitive when large doses of vitamin D were used for prophylaxis or treatment of rickets, and hypervitaminosis D has been exacerbated by high intakes of calcium and phosphorus (Combs, 1998).

WATER-SOLUBLE VITAMINS

Thiamine (Vitamin B_1)

Thiamine pyrophosphate (TPP) is an essential cofactor of enzymes involved in carbohydrate amino acid intermediary metabolism, and is important in brain function. It is an essential cofactor in the decarboxylation of α-keto acids such as pyruvate in its conversion to acetyl coenzyme A. Good sources include yeast, legumes, enriched grain products, and pork. Early signs of deficiency include anorexia, weight loss, muscle weakness, apathy, confusion, and irritability. Later consequences include edema and high-output cardiac failure (wet beriberi), polyneuropathy with depressed reflexes, paresthesias, weakness and muscle atrophy (dry beriberi), and psychosis (Wernicke-Korsakoff syndrome) characterized by dementia, ataxia, and ophthalmoplegia. Lesions of the mamillary bodies and the area that abuts the third ventricle are distinctive findings (Rubin, 2005). The infantile form occurs in infants that are breastfed for months without supplementation. Cardiac failure in young infants may be sudden and rapidly fatal. Alcohol abuse in adults is often associated with deficiency, perhaps because alcohol interferes with thiamine uptake and metabolism. Thiamine deficiency is also seen in those with poor nutrition. No toxicity is described from high oral doses. Antithiamine factors are present in betel, tea, and some foods. In the United States, all breads and flours are enriched with thiamine. Significant loss of thiamine occurs when foods are cooked in water. Thiamine is unstable at high temperatures and is produced in the colon by normal enteric bacteria, but the contribution is apparently slight. Thiamine is absorbed throughout the small intestine and is bound to albumin in the plasma. At high thiamine intakes, the excess is excreted in the urine (Kohlmeier, 2003). Red blood cell transketolase activity with or without TPP added is a useful test for assessing thiamine deficiency. Heparinized whole blood is required, and the test is best run on a fresh specimen (Truswell, 2002a). The most reliable test for thiamine deficiency is the response to parenteral administration of thiamine (Rubin, 2005).

Riboflavin (Vitamin B_2)

Riboflavin normally forms two coenzymes: flavin mononucleotide and flavin adenine dinucleotide. These have an important role in electron transport in several oxidative systems. Dietary sources include milk and dairy products, meat, poultry, fish, and green vegetables. Breads and cereals are fortified with riboflavin. Absorption occurs mostly in the jejunum. In humans, riboflavin is so prevalent in the diet that deficiency severe enough to cause marked debilities is not known. Mild riboflavin deficiencies are probably commonplace. Deficiency frequently occurs in association with lack of thiamine and/or niacin (Guyton, 1997). With prolonged deficiency, cracking and swelling of the lips (cheilosis), cracking and inflammation of the angles of the mouth (angular stomatitis), deep-red smooth tongue (glossitis, atrophy), greasy scaling of the cheeks and the areas behind the ears (seborrheic dermatitis), and normocytic anemia (Kohlmeier, 2003) may occur. Interstitial keratitis of the cornea, the most troubling lesion, results in corneal opacification and ulceration (Rubin, 2005). Deficiencies during infancy and childhood impair growth. There is little danger of toxicity because excess riboflavin is rapidly lost. 24-hour urine indicates recent riboflavin intake (Kohlmeier, 2003).

Niacin (Nicotinic Acid)

Niacin has a major role in the formation of nicotinamide adenine dinucleotide and its phosphate, which are important in intermediary metabolism and in a large number of oxidation–reduction reactions. Animal proteins are foods high in tryptophan such as meat, eggs, and milk. They are good sources for endogenously synthesized niacin. Urine is the main excretory path for niacin metabolites. Niacin is found in many grains. Deficiency causes pellagra, which is now uncommon but is seen these days in malnourished alcoholics and in food faddists who do not eat sufficient protein, are tryptophan deficient, and are not taking exogenous niacin. Malabsorption of tryptophan, as seen in Hartnup disease, or the carcinoid syndrome, in which tryptophan is consumed to make serotonin, may produce mild symptoms of pellagra. Pyridoxine and riboflavin deficiencies increase the requirement for niacin because they are both cofactors required for the synthesis of niacin. Corn is a poor source of tryptophan, and the niacin in corn is bound and poorly available. Pellagra is prevalent in areas where corn (maize) is the staple food, as in certain parts of Africa (Guyton, 1997).

Pellagra is characterized by dermatitis, diarrhea, dementia, and, if untreated, death. It occurs as scaly dermatitis of those areas exposed to light or pressure, such as the knees and elbows. The hands show a rough scaly dermatitis with a glove-like distribution, along with a pattern of hyperkeratosis, vascularization, and chronic inflammation. Similar lesions are seen in the mouth and the vaginal mucous membranes (Rubin, 2005). Excessive intake of niacin causes flushing (burning and itching of the face, chest, and arms) and gastric irritation. Liver damage may result from continued, very high doses. Niacin has been used as a cholesterol-lowering drug.

Pyridoxine (Vitamin B_6)

Pyridoxine is a coenzyme that participates in more than 100 transaminations, decarboxylations, and other reactions, including the initial steps of porphyrin synthesis, glycogen mobilization, amino acid transsulfuration, and neurotransmitter synthesis. Good food sources include fortified cereals, organ meats, muscle foods, potatoes, and fruits other than citrus. Cooking results in leaching of pyridoxine into the discard water. Urine is the major excretory pathway. Deficiencies are usually seen with other vitamin or protein deficiencies that occur in alcoholics (see Chapter 21). Deficiency of pyridoxine is uncommon and may cause a microcytic hypochromic anemia in which iron stores are saturated, epileptic seizures, electroencephalographic abnormalities, depression, confusion, seborrheic dermatitis, and possibly platelet and clotting abnormalities. Several inborn errors of amino acid metabolism respond to very high doses of pyridoxine. Homocystinuria, which is associated with increased risk of cardiovascular disease, responds to supplements of folate, cobalamin, and sometimes pyridoxine. Tests include measurement of pyridoxal phosphate (normal >30 nmol/L); increased urinary xanthurenic acid after a tryptophan load; erythrocyte alanine aminotransferase; and urinary 4-pyridoxic acid (Truswell, 2002a). Very high doses of pyridoxine (>100 mg/day in adults) may cause a peripheral sensory neuropathy, possibly with skin lesions (Kohlmeier, 2003).

Cobalamin (Vitamin B_{12})

Cobalamin is a complex cobalt-containing molecule, synthesized only by bacteria. It comprises several "vitamers:" cyanocobalamin and hydorxycobalamin are pharmacologic forms, whereas adenosylcobalamin and methylcobalamin are the main biological forms. The main known cofactor roles of cobalamin are in the synthesis of succinate from methylmalonate and the synthesis of methionine from homocysteine. Hence cobalamin deficiency results in increased levels of methylmalonate and homocysteine. Clinically, many manifestations of deficiency are similar to those of folate deficiency and can be overcome by large amounts of folate. These include impaired deoxyribonucleic acid (DNA) synthesis, which results in megaloblastic anemia. Cobalamin deficiency also causes neuropsychiatric damage, largely related to demyelination in the posterior columns of the spinal cord, peripheral nerves, and even the cerebrum. Neurologic damage is not relieved, and may even be worsened, by treatment with folate.

Absorption of cobalamin is unique in that it requires formation of a complex between it and a glycoprotein called **intrinsic factor,** secreted by the parietal cells of the stomach. The complex is then absorbed in the terminal ileum. Inadequate dietary intake is not the usual cause of cobalamin deficiency. Most common is malabsorption due to atrophy of the gastric mucosa, so that inadequate intrinsic factor or disease of the terminal ileum may prevent absorption. It is important to note that any disease affecting the gastric epithelium can cause diminution of intrinsic factor release. One of these diseases is gastric cancer. The onset of sudden, unexplained macrocytic anemia caused by decreased vitamin B_{12} is therefore a serious finding in an adult and must be followed by appropriate examination of the stomach and the small bowel.

Normal body stores of cobalamin are sufficient to last for 3 to 6 years. Food sources include liver, shellfish, fish, meat, eggs, milk, cheeses, and yogurt. Vegans are at risk for cobalamin deficiency (Eastwood, 2003). Plasma cobalamin <80 pg/mL indicates a cobalamin deficiency. Elevated serum or urinary methylmalonate and raised plasma homocysteine also indicate that cobalamin is low. The classical Schilling test uses radiolabeled cobalamin to measure its absorption on different days, with and without intrinsic factor (West, 2002), but is not generally available today. Cobalamin has extremely low toxicity, and doses as large as 3 mg/day are tolerated without toxic effect. The average dietary intake of cobalamin is <1 μg/day (Eastwood, 2003).

Ascorbate (Vitamin C)

Ascorbate is a powerful reducing agent that is involved in many oxidation–reduction reactions and in the transfer of protons. Ascorbate participates in the synthesis of chondroitin sulfate and in formation of the hydroxyproline of collagen. It has an important role in wound healing, the biosynthesis of some neurotransmitters, and immune function (Rubin, 2005). It is essential for gums, arteries, and other soft tissues and bone (collagen synthesis), and for brain and nerve function (neurotransmitter and hormone synthesis), as well as for nutrient metabolism (especially iron, protein, and fat) and antioxidant defense and free-radical scavenging (directly and by vitamin E activation). Ascorbate is found in high concentrations in leukocytes, adrenal gland, pituitary, and brain. Food sources include citrus fruits, berries, tomatoes, and many fruits and vegetables. Prolonged storage and overcooking may cause significant vitamin loss. The RDA is 90 mg/day for men and 75 mg/day for women. Deficiency, termed scurvy, presents with symptoms of bleeding gums (if there are teeth), painful swollen joints, poor wound healing, confusion, fatigue, and diminished immune function. Now, scurvy is most often seen in alcoholics and in the aged poor living alone. The symptoms of scurvy have been described since antiquity. The disease was widespread among sailors in the 16th to 18th centuries, and the typical pattern consisted of bleeding gums, painful swollen joints, and muscle weakness. Onset occurred within months of the start of a voyage. British expeditions reported devastating losses of men due to scurvy. The carnage prompted the Admiralty to seek a cure, and in 1747, James Lind, a Scottish surgeon, performed a clinical nutrition experiment on board ship to test six different diet supplements given to six pairs of scorbutic sailors. Oranges and lemons cured scurvy, which he described in his 1753 *Treatise of the Scurvy* (Jacob, 1994). Lind believed that scurvy was caused by dampness and crowding. Only subsequently was it understood that scurvy was due to ascorbate deficiency. Daily ingestion of 2000 mg or more may cause gastric and intestinal irritation or kidney stones, and may interfere with copper metabolism. Unlike other vertebrates, humans are not able to complete the synthesis of ascorbate (Kohlmeier, 2003). Testing to assess ascorbate status can be done using serum or leukocytes. Both correlate well with dietary intake. Urine assays tend to reflect recent dietary intake (Skeaff, 2002).

Folate

Folate is the generic name for compounds related to folic acid (pteroylglutamic acid). Like cobalamin, it plays a coenzyme role in one-carbon transfer reactions, and deficiency leads to impaired synthesis of purines and pyrimidines and hence of DNA (Guyton, 1997). It is widely available from plants and, to a lesser extent, organ meats. More than half of the folate content of food is lost during cooking. Deficiency may result in megaloblastic anemia, similar to vitamin B_{12} deficiency, and leukopenia. In pregnancy, fetal neural tube defects are associated with low folate levels, and periconceptional supplementation has markedly reduced the incidence (Wildman, 2000).

Pantothenic Acid

Pantothenic acid is part of coenzyme A (CoA) and of acyl carrier protein (ACP). Both are carriers of acyl groups. Acetyl-CoA is involved in the tricarboxylic acid cycle, and CoA in the synthesis of lipids. Pantothenic acid is transported in erythrocytes as CoA. The highest tissue concentrations are found in liver, adrenals, kidneys, brain, heart, and testes. CoA and ACP are metabolized to free pantothenic acid and excreted in the urine. Urine levels indicate dietary intake and range from 2–7 mg/day. Pantothenic acid is widely present in foods, and dietary deficiency occurs only in severe malnutrition with other nutrient deficiencies. The **burning feet syndrome** that was seen in malnourished prisoners of war during World War II responded to large doses of Ca-pantothenate (Truswell, 2002a).

Biotin

Biotin is a coenzyme for several carboxylase enzymes: pyruvate carboxylase (provides oxaloacetate for tricarboxylic acid cycle), acetyl CoA (coenzyme A), and carboxylase (fatty acid synthesis). Biotin deficiency is rare because it is widely distributed in foods, and large intestine bacterial production supplements dietary intake. Avidin, an antivitamin, is found in uncooked egg white and can produce a deficiency of biotin when large amounts are ingested, because avidin binds biotin in the gut, preventing absorption. Biotin deficiency in humans has resulted from failure to include biotin in total parenteral nutrition; it is characterized by scaly dermatitis, glossitis, hair loss, anorexia, depression, and hypercholesterolemia (Truswell, 2002a).

FAT-SOLUBLE VITAMINS

Vitamin A (Retinol)

Vitamin A activity is derived from two compound classes: pre-formed vitamin A, retinol, and related compounds; and the precursors β-carotene and related carotenoids. The latter are the provitamins that are found in yellow and red vegetable pigments abundant in vegetables like carrots, and in some fruits. Retinol is the principal vitamin A vitamer. The term retinoids refers to retinol, its metabolites, and synthetic analogs with similar structure. Retinol is essential for vision at low light intensities, synthesis of **active sulfate,** and reproduction. Functions in which retinoic acid participates include cellular differentiation, involvement in morphogenesis, synthesis of glycoproteins, gene expression, immunity, growth, and prevention of cancer and heart disease (Semba, 1998; Truswell, 2002b). Vitamin A is needed to maintain certain specialized cell membranes, facilitate skeletal maturation, and participate in forming light-sensitive rods of the retina and the structure of cell membranes (IOM, 2002). Vitamin A deficiency is unusual in developed countries but continues to be a frequent cause of blindness due to corneal damage in the poorer regions of the world, particularly parts of Africa, the Middle East, and Southeast Asia. Retinol is present in high concentration in liver, and fish oil and leafy, green vegetables are rich sources of carotene (Rubin, 2005). Hippocrates (466–377 BCE) wrote that liver could cure night blindness (West, 2002). Vitamin A deficiency is seen when the diet has lacked dairy, produce, and vegetables for a long time, or with malabsorption syndromes (Eastwood, 2003) and with steatorrhea, as in celiac disease, chronic pancreatitis, and Crohn's disease. Because hepatic accumulation of vitamin A occurs during the last trimester of pregnancy, preterm infants are relatively vitamin A deficient. Deficiency results in squamous metaplasia; as a result, the sweat and tear ducts are blocked by squamous debris. The epithelia of the trachea, bronchi, renal pelvis, pancreatic ducts, uterus, and salivary glands are often affected. The earliest sign of vitamin A deficiency is vision loss in dim light (night blindness). Liver disease diminishes retinol binding protein (RBP) synthesis, as does severe zinc deficiency. Zinc is required for the production of RBP, which transports vitamin A from the liver to body tissues.

Toxicity is usually produced by excessive vitamin A supplements, especially in children (IOM, 2001). Vitamin A toxicity occurred in explorers who ate polar bear livers, which have an exceptionally high concentration of vitamin A. In toxicity, the liver and spleen are enlarged with lipid-laden macrophages. Vitamin A is in the hepatocytes, and prolonged toxicity causes cirrhosis. Headache, hyperexcitability, and bone pain are early symptoms (Bendich, 1989). The lesions are most often reversible, early in the course, upon discontinuation of excessive dosing. High doses of synthetic derivatives of retinoic acid are teratogenic. Excessive carotene is benign and causes a jaundice-like discoloration of the skin (Rubin, 2005).

Circulating retinol concentrations do not consistently correlate with retinol total body stores. The relative dose–response test (Loerch, 1979) indirectly assesses the stores. Two blood samples are collected—one before and one 5 hours after a physiologic dose of vitamin A. In vitamin A–depleted subjects, a rapid sustained rise in serum retinol concentration occurs, compared with a lower, shallow rise in those who are vitamin A sufficient (Loerch, 1979).

Vitamin D (Cholecalciferol)

Vitamin D plays an essential role as a hormone in the control of calcium and phosphorus metabolism. Ultraviolet light exposure of the skin converts naturally occurring 7-dehydrocholesterol to cholecalciferol or vitamin D_3. Because the body can produce vitamin D, some have termed this a hormone. It is a vitamin for those who are mostly indoors, especially in Northern latitudes, as well as those whose clothing completely covers their skin, blocking sunlight. Cholecalciferol is diet-derived from animal sources, particularly fish liver and oils. Ergocalciferol, or vitamin D_2, which is of equal potency in humans, is derived from its provitamin ergosterol, which occurs in fungi and plants and is the major synthetic form used to fortify milk and margarine. Both vitamins D_2 and D_3 require two hydroxylations to the active form. The first is a 25-hydroxylation in the liver, and the second is a 1-hydroxylation in the kidneys. The resulting active vitamin D is called **1,25-dihydroxycholecalciferol** or **calcitriol**. Fortified foods (milk, orange juice, yogurt, margarine) provide most of the dietary vitamin D in the American diet. Vitamin D promotes absorption of calcium and phosphate from the small intestine (Truswell, 2002b). Deficiency results from an inadequate diet; insufficient sunlight reaching the skin; inadequate absorption as occurs in fat malabsorption syndromes; or failure of conversion to the active metabolite due to chronic hepatic or renal disease. In children, before the epiphyses have closed, the bone lesion syndrome is called **rickets;** in the adult, osteomalacia. The incidence has declined with the addition of ergosterol to milk and other foods (Rubin, 2005). The major function of vitamin D is the homeostasis of Ca^{++} and phosphate (regulating intestinal adsorption), bone mineralization and mobilization, and renal excretion (Combs, 1998). Vitamin D is essential for promoting calcium absorption from the gut and for maintaining adequate serum calcium and phosphate concentrations to enable normal mineralization of bone and prevent hypocalcemic tetany. Sufficient vitamin D helps prevent rickets in children and osteomalacia in adults with calcium osteoporosis. Hypervitaminosis D is often due to ingestion of excessive vitamin D preparations. Abnormal conversion of active metabolites occurs sometimes in sarcoidosis. Hypervitaminosis D causes hypercalcemia. Early symptoms are weakness and headache. The sequelae of hypercalcemia include hypercalciuria, nephrocalcinosis, nephrolithiasis, and ectopic calcification of blood vessels, heart, and lungs (Rubin, 2005). Overexposure to ultraviolet light will result in sunburn of the skin but will not cause hypervitaminosis D. Plasma calcium and phosphate fall in vitamin D deficiency, and plasma alkaline phosphatase (bone isoenzyme) is increased in rickets and osteomalacia. As noted in Chapter 8, immunoassays for 25-hydroxy- and 1,25-dihydroxycholecalciferol are performed (Truswell, 2002b). However, because the half-life of the 1,25-dihydroxy vitamin D is brief (several hours) and the half-life of its 25-hydroxy vitamin D "parent" is much longer, most assays for vitamin D are used for the longer-lived 25-hydroxy vitamin D. As is also discussed in Chapter 8, vitamin D has now been implicated in a variety of important functions, in addition to calcium homeostasis. It induces apoptosis in breast cancer and in a variety of other malignancies and has been found to be effective in the treatment of a rather wide range of diseases such as heart failure, asthma, Crohn's disease, psoriasis, and multiple sclerosis. In view of these developments, monitoring of vitamin D serum levels has greatly increased over the past several years.

Vitamin E (Tocopherol)

This fat-soluble antioxidant, or free-radical scavenger, inactivates oxygen free-radicals. Eight naturally occurring forms have been identified. Vitamin E is the only known lipid-soluble antioxidant in plasma and red blood cell membranes. Fat-soluble antioxidant stops the production of reactive oxygen species formed when fat undergoes oxidation. The principal sources of vitamin E are oils and fats, particularly wheat germ oil and sunflower oil absorbed in the small intestine in the presence of bile. Deficiency is very uncommon but may occur as a result of malabsorption, in total parenteral nutrition, or in premature infants. Premature and low-birthweight infants are particularly susceptible to development of vitamin E deficiency. Signs of deficiency include irritability, edema, and hemolytic anemia. Vitamin E is necessary for neurologic and reproductive functions, for protecting red cells from hemolysis, and for prevention of retinopathy in premature infants (Brigelius-Flohe, 2002). The best defined role for vitamin E is inhibition of free-radical chain reactions of lipid peroxidation within polyunsaturated fatty acids of membrane phospholipids. No toxicity is known (Eastwood, 2003).

Vitamin K (Phytomenadione)

Vitamin K promotes clotting and is involved in the activation of important proteins in blood coagulation, prothrombin (II), factor VII, factor IX, and factor X, as well as protein C and protein S (see Chapter 42). Deficiency of the factors listed can result in defective clotting and a bleeding disorder. Prothrombin time (PT) functionally monitors vitamin K activity. Monitoring of vitamin K is discussed in Chapter 42. Vitamin K occurs in two forms. Vitamin K_1 is present in fresh green vegetables, for example, broccoli, cabbage, and spinach, and beef liver. Intestinal bacteria produce vitamin K_2. Dietary deficiency is uncommon. It does occur in fat malabsorption, as in sprue and biliary obstruction. Also, antibiotic sterilization of the intestinal flora may result in vitamin K deficiency. Use of high doses of naturally occurring vitamin K appears to have no untoward effect. No adverse effects are associated with vitamin K.

Because of low plasma concentration, vitamin K has been assessed by functional methods, using PT to determine its effect on clotting time.

TRACE ELEMENTS

Trace mineral elements consist of metals, except selenium, the halogens, fluoride, and iodine. Individually, these elements are found in tissue concentrations of <1 μg/g of wet tissue (Kane, 2005), and they constitute <0.01% of dry body weight (Gibson, 1990; Taylor, 1996). They were referred to as trace elements because quantitation using the analytic methods then available was not possible (O'Dell, 1997). Essential trace elements are those that result in impairment of normal health, function, or development when a deficiency is corrected by supplementation with physiologic levels of that element (Mertz, 1981a; Gibson, 1990). Trace elements have specific in vivo metabolic functions that cannot be effectively performed by other similar elements (Milne, 1994).

Various essential trace elements have been discovered by several different means. Deficiencies of some of these elements have been found in areas where the soil, water, or plants were inadequate in a specific element, such as iodine, fluorine, cobalt, or copper. Deficiencies were also identified when essential elements became biologically unavailable because of interference from other dietary ingestants, such as zinc deficiency, seen especially in males in the Middle East and in Hispanics in Denver, which results from eating unleavened bread high in phytate and is compounded by the high fiber content and low meat intake of their diets (Wildman, 2000) and the anemia of zinc-induced copper deficiency (Milne, 1994). Other deficiencies were caused by a mutation that resulted in the lack of a protein needed to absorb or metabolize the element. The symptoms of still other deficiencies were identified in patients on total parenteral nutrition not supplemented with an essential trace element (O'Dell, 1997).

Ten trace mineral elements have generally been recognized as essential in humans, as summarized in Table 26-3. Only copper, iodine, iron, selenium, and zinc are associated with well-characterized deficiency states

TABLE 26-3
Classification of Trace Mineral Elements

Essential in humans and animals	Essential in some animals and possibly in humans	Possibly essential in some animals	Not essential
Chromium	Arsenic	Bromine	Aluminum
Cobalt	Boron	Cadmium	Antimony
Copper	Lithium	Lead	Bismuth
Fluorine	Nickel	Strontium	Germanium
Iodine	Silicon	Tin	Mercury
Iron	Vanadium		Silver
Manganese			Thallium
Molybdenum			Titanium
Selenium			
Zinc			

Data from Gibson, 1990; O'Dell, 1997.

(Kane, 2005). A necessary biochemical role has not been conclusively demonstrated for fluorine or manganese, although signs of deficiency have been described (Mertz, 1981b). It is difficult to create a deficiency model because of the ubiquitous distribution of these elements in the environment and food supply, which frequently causes contamination of the testing system, and because only minute amounts are needed to support physiologic processes. It remains uncertain whether other trace mineral elements are essential in animals and humans. Some authors have concluded that arsenic, boron, lithium, nickel, silicon, and vanadium, which have been shown to have essential biochemical roles in some animal species, are presumptively essential in humans as well (Milne, 1994).

The roles of trace mineral elements include structural signal transduction and especially catalytic properties. These properties and the effects of deficiencies and toxicities of these trace elements are summarized in Tables 26-4 and 26-5. Some of the trace mineral elements are components of metalloenzymes, function as enzyme cofactors, provide electron and oxygen transport, and are active in the maintenance of macromolecule conformation, or vitamin and hormonal activity. These trace minerals are avidly accumulated by cells under the control of several families of proteins (Finney, 2003). Normally, homeostasis of these elements is tightly controlled. Only some of the biochemical mechanisms of the clinical effects of trace element deficiencies have been determined (Mertz, 1981b). Trace elements interact with available ligands, mainly the electron donors nitrogen, sulfur, and oxygen, to form a wide variety of compounds.

Deficiencies of trace elements are usually due to: nutritional deficiency; inadequate supplementation in total parenteral nutrition; or a disease state in which there is insufficient intestinal absorption, or increased excretion or utilization. Deficiencies can also be due to interactions between trace elements (e.g., zinc, copper) and with other nutrients (e.g., zinc, vitamin A), interfering with absorption or adversely affecting metabolic utilization. Large amounts of dietary zinc interfere with intestinal copper absorption, resulting in copper deficiency and anemia (Milne, 1994; Willis, 2005).

Genetic defects in trace element metabolism include Menkes' kinky hair syndrome (copper), congenital atransferrinemia (iron), acrodermatitis enteropathica (zinc), and xanthine and sulfite oxidase deficiencies (molybdenum) (Gibson, 1990).

Trace elements must be analyzed with considerable care because they are widely distributed in the environment (e.g., water, air), and the materials of biological devices (e.g., needles, syringes, stoppers) can readily contaminate a sample. Special collection and handling are necessary. Clean room techniques and ultra-pure reagents must be used. Reference materials and strict quality control are requisite with each assay run to ensure analytic accuracy. It is especially important that trained technical personnel perform the testing (Veillon, 1986). Improved materials are now available for collection, processing, and analysis of trace elements that reduce contamination. These include trace element–free syringes, evacuated tubes with fitted siliconized needles, acid-washed glassware, and standard reference materials with certified values (Casey, 1983; Gibson, 1990).

Major advances in understanding and managing the dynamics of trace mineral elements have been achieved during the past two decades by the extraordinary precision and sensitivity of the improved analytic instruments. Atomic absorption spectrometry (AAS) is the most widely used instrument for clinical trace element analysis in biological samples. Graphite furnace AAS has improved the limit of quantitation (LOQ) to parts per billion (ppb, μg/L) and permits the simultaneous measurement of multiple elements. Zeeman effect background correction improves element signal measurement when testing in complex specimens such as serum, plasma or blood, and other specimen handling enhancements have further improved sensitivity and precision. Flame AAS (FAAS) has an LOQ of parts per million (ppm, mg/L). Atomic emission spectrometry consists of FAAS and plasma source emission spectrometry, which measures photon output rather than photon absorption, as in AAS, and is supplanting AAS as the standard instrument for analysis. The emission lines of excited electrons are measured. The LOQ is ppm (mg/L) (Rahil-Khazen, 2000). The sample in neutron activation analysis (NAA) is irradiated with low-energy neutrons for the production of radioactive nuclides. In NAA, there is excitation of the atomic nucleus, so that the trace element is determined independent of its physical or chemical state. The newly formed radionuclide emits X-rays or γ rays. The LOQ is ppb (μg/L) to parts per trillion (ppt, ng/L) with multielement detection, but with a limited dynamic range. This technique is especially suited for in vitro trace element determination in biological matrices. In instrumental neutron activation analysis, there is direct measurement of the emitted X-ray or γ radiation. Inductively coupled plasma-mass spectroscopy (ICP-MS) is a highly sensitive and specific method for measurement of multiple trace elements in a single run over an especially broad dynamic range with low background interference and LOQs of ppb (μg/L) to ppt (ng/L). An internal standard is used for enhanced precision (Milne, 1994; Chan, 1998a).

Assessment of trace element status requires measurement of either the concentration in accessible tissues (hair, nails) and body fluids (serum, urine) or the activity of a trace element–dependent enzyme. There are no particularly good indicators for the determination of trace element dietary status because of poor correlation with total body stores. The only definitive test of human trace mineral element deficiency is the clinical response to controlled supplementation, with the element of concern followed by evaluation of improvement of an impaired function (Milne, 1994; Eastwood, 2003). Combination testing yields a more reliable interpretation, especially when the findings are concordant. Interpretation of plasma or serum levels can be deceptive because of the response to stress, or when expansion of blood volume or a decrease in serum albumin occurs, as, for example, in the third trimester of pregnancy. Also, hemolysis interferes with assays. Serum chromium, copper, manganese, molybdenum, and zinc levels are not reliable for assessing nutritional status or dietary intake because the results do not reflect body stores. Both serum and urine concentrations indicate recent dietary intake. Table 26-5 summarizes the primary tissue locations and metabolic properties of the major trace elements.

Hair and nail clippings should be collected with care and washed to avoid surface contamination.

Trace element assays in blood, serum, or urine usually reflect the current nutriture. The first morning void urine is less affected by recent dietary intake. Load tests measure the change in urine concentration following a loading dose of the mineral element. When tissue levels are low, the deficiency will cause retention of the element. Similarly, tolerance tests measure the change in plasma concentration following a challenge dose. Usually, the dose is in the pharmaceutical range rather than at the physiologic level normally experienced. Hair, fingernail, or toenail analyses provide a retrospective window or an assessment of chronic exposure for the period of hair or nail growth (Gibson, 2002). Because of the risk of environmental contamination, hair and nail clippings are of limited

TABLE 26-4
Function, Deficiency and Toxicity of Essential Trace Mineral Elements

Element	Function/enzyme component	Effects of deficiency	Effects of toxicity
Chromium (Cr)	Potentiates insulin action, glucose and lipid metabolism, Cr(III) low toxicity, poorly absorbed Component of glucose tolerance factor	No method to determine deficiency in humans; impaired glucose tolerance in type 2 diabetes, insulin resistance, hyperglycemia, peripheral neuropathy, hyperlipidemia	Cr(VI) toxic, oxidative damage, skin ulcers, contact dermatitis, asthma, renal and hepatic necrosis, lung cancer
Cobalt (Co)	Hemoglobin synthesis, Component of vitamin B_{12}	Cobalt deficiency, as such, not in humans; symptoms due to lack of vitamin B_{12}: Anemia, anorexia, growth depression	Cardiomyopathy, heart failure, goiter, hypothyroidism; warm sensation, vomiting, diarrhea
Copper (Cu)	Cellular respiration, neurotransmitter regulator, oxidation reaction, electron transport, collagen synthesis, development of vascular and skeletal structures and CNS, antioxidant Component of $CuZnSO_4$, metallothionein, cytochrome c, tyrosinase, dopamine β-hydroxylase, lysyl oxidase	Menkes' kinky hair syndrome, X-linked, congenital failure of Cu absorption; abnormal collagen cross-linking, muscle weakness Iron refractory hypochromic anemia, leukopenia, neurologic defects, hypopigmentation. In prematurity: Bone fractures, skeletal defects Occurs in malnourished children and premature infants not supplemented	Relatively nontoxic Wilson disease: Autosomal recessive, failure to excrete Cu in bile: Excess Cu in liver, kidneys, brain, eyes, hepatic necrosis, hypertension, Kayser-Fleischer rings in eyes Cu interferes with absorption of iron and zinc
Fluorine (F)	Prevents tooth decay.	Increased dental caries	Mottled enamel, fluorosis
Iodine (I)	Component of thyroid hormone	Goiter, hypothyroidism, cretinism in infants, myxedema in adults	Goiter, thyrotoxicosis
Iron (Fe)	Oxygen transport, respiration, amino acids and free-radical metabolism, lipids, oxidative phosphorylation Component of hemoglobin, metalloenzymes, vitamin A	Hypochromic microcytic anemia, glossitis, angular stomatitis, cheilosis, koilonychia Blood loss or inadequate iron intake; iron deficiency anemia: <7 g/100 mL blood	Hemochromatosis: Genetic, primary, autosomal recessive; acquired, secondary, iron overload Iron deposition in liver, pancreas, heart, and skin
Manganese (Mn)	Bone and connective tissue Component of metalloenzymes: Hydrolases, oxidoreductases and lipases, pyruvate carboxylase, superoxide dismutase, and arginase	Not well defined in humans; skeletal and cartilage defects	Least toxic of trace elements Psychiatric disorders: Memory, speech, hallucinations; syndrome resembles Parkinson's and Wilson's diseases
Molybdenum (Mo)	DNA metabolism, essential for uric acid production Component of sulfite and xanthine oxidase	Naturally occurring deficiency not known, growth depression, hypercuprinemia, defective keratin form, goiter, cretinism	Anemia, goiter, thyrotoxicosis, hypouricemia, hyperoxypurinemia
Selenium (Se)	Protects against oxidative damage of lipid, gene expression, thyroxine deiodinase Component of glutathione peroxidase	Keshan disease: Cardiomyopathy, cardiomegaly, heart failure, cataracts, osteoarthritis in children, myopathy, discolored/thickened nails, impaired growth	Hair and nail loss, selenosis, tooth decay, neuropathy, liver failure, garlic odor on breath
Zinc (Zn)	Protein synthesis, zinc finger proteins—gene expression, immunity, needed for normal skin, bones, and hair Component of metallothionein ≈300 enzymes	Acrodermatitis enteropathica; causes cardiomyopathy in children In children, low height, hypogeusia, growth retardation, infertility, immune deficits, delayed wound healing, glossitis, seborrheic-like dermatitis, osteoporosis	Relatively nontoxic: Nausea, vomiting, and GI irritation; causes copper deficiency

Data from da Silva, 1991; Kane, 2005; Alcock, 1996.
CNS, Central nervous system; *DNA*, deoxyribonucleic acid; *GI*, gastrointestinal.

use in determining dietary intake or body status, except when reduced (Eastwood, 2003).

"All substances are poisons … dose differentiates a poison."
Paracelsus (1493–1541)

Toxicity is never a question of presence, only of amount. Each of the essential and nonessential trace mineral elements can be toxic when present in high concentrations. A poison is too much of anything. Toxicity is quite variable for the different trace elements. Some have a high toxicity. The toxic effects of selenium are produced by intake of only 10 times the nutritional requirement. In contrast, chromium toxicity has never been reported after oral pharmacologic doses (Gibson, 1990).

CHROMIUM

Chromium (Cr) is known to enhance the action of insulin (Mertz, 1998). Absorption of chromium from the intestine is low. Chromium sources include meats, whole grains, green beans, broccoli, and some spices. After absorption, chromium binds to plasma transferrin and then concentrates in liver, spleen, heart, other soft tissues, and bone. Clinical signs of chromium deficiency were first described in patients receiving parenteral nutrition. Only a few cases have been reported in which absence of chromium was associated with insulin resistance, glucose intolerance, weight loss, and sometimes neurologic deficits that were reversed on chromium supplementation. Chromium depletion is thought to be associated with increased cardiovascular risk, and supplementation has demonstrated increased high-density lipoprotein cholesterol and decreased insulin.

Hexavalent chromium Cr^{6+} is a recognized carcinogen. Industrial exposure to metal fumes and dust is associated with lung cancer, dermatitis, and skin ulcers. Health risks are caused by soil contamination by Cr^{6+} waste disposal sites left by the leather tanning and dyestuff industries. Chromium is used extensively in the manufacture of stainless steel, in chrome plating, in tanning of leather, as a dye for printing, and as an anticorrosive in cooling systems. Air monitoring for Cr^{6+} is the usual way to test. Increased chromium in urine serves as confirmation of recent occupational or environmental exposure to excess chromium (Halls, 1988).

COBALT

Cobalt (Co) is essential for humans only as an integral part of vitamin B_{12} (cobalamin). Cobalt has no other known function in humans. Diet has to

TABLE 26-5
Properties of Essential Trace Mineral Elements

Element	Tissue distribution	Body content	Transport (reference value)	Excretion
Chromium (Cr)	Spleen, heart	4–6 mg Cr(III)	Transferrin-P 0.15 μg/mL Cr (0.12–2.1 μg/L)	Urine 100–200 ng/day
Cobalt	Muscle, liver, fat	1.1 mg	Albumin (0.11–0.45 μg/L)	Urine 80%
Copper (Cu)	Muscle and liver Liver 30–50 μg/g dry; 50%–70% of body Cu	50–80 mg (1.2–2.5 μg/g fat-free tissue)	Ceruloplasmin 60%–95%, albumin, transcuperin (Cu-S 70–140 μg/dL)	Feces includes bile and unabsorbed dietary Cu
Iodine (I)	Thyroid: 70%–80% of total body I in thyroxine bound to thyroglobulin	15–20 mg (11–15 mg in thyroid)	Thyroxine-binding protein 80% thyroxine-binding prealbumin (transthyretin)	Urine 100–150 μg/day
Iron (Fe)	RBC Hb 400–600 mg/L, liver, spleen, bone marrow 25%, myoglobin	4–5 g (¾ in Hb) 50 mg/kg 2.5 g in RBCs	Transferrin-P (2–2.5 g/L) Ferritin-S 1 μg/L = 10 mg tissue iron stores Hemosiderin 1 g iron	Bile 84 μg/kg, blood loss, menses, GI mucosal cells
Manganese (Mn)	Liver, bone, pancreas	12–20 mg	Mn-Blood 200 nmol/L	Bile and intestinal secretions
Molybdenum (Mo)	Liver, kidney, bone, adrenal	Blood 30–700 nmol/L	RBC protein, α-1-macroglobulin (S: 8–34 μg/L)	Urine 90%, bile 10%
Selenium (Se)	Liver, kidney, muscle	15 mg	Protein (Se-P: 7–30 μg/dL)	Urine 60%, feces 40%
Zinc (Zn)	Muscle 60%, bone 30%, liver, prostate, semen	1.2–2.3 g	Albumin 60%–70%, α-2-macroglobulin (Zn-P 11-22 μmol/L)	Feces, gut secretions, GI mucosal cells

Data from da Silva, 1991; Milne, 1994; O'Dell, 1997; Kohlmeier, 2003. *GI,* Gastrointestinal; *Hb,* hemoglobin; *RBC,* red blood cell.

supply human vitamin B_{12} needs. The microflora of the human intestine is not able to use cobalt to synthesize cobalamin; free cobalt does not interact with the body's vitamin B_{12} pool.

COPPER

Copper (Cu) is the third most abundant trace element in the human body, following zinc and iron. It is a very effective cation in reactions that involve electron transfer and binding to organic molecules (Samman, 2002). Copper is involved in electron transport and oxidation reactions and is essential for cellular respiration, neurotransmitter regulation, collagen synthesis, and nutrient metabolism, especially iron, and as an antioxidant against free radicals (Kohlmeier, 2003). Copper is present in all living cells (Marston, 1992) and functions mostly as a component of the cuproenzymes and copper-containing proteins. Copper-containing plasma amine oxidases catabolize some active amines such as tyramine, histidine, and polyamines, and inactivate the catecholamines (norepinephrine, tyramine, dopamine, and serotonin). Another cuproenzyme, **lysyl oxidase,** helps collagen proteins cross-link into larger fibers. This enzyme, which is encoded by the *ras*-recision gene *(rrg),* has also been found to have anticancer activity caused by its ability to block insertion of the *ras*-gene–encoded p21 protein into the cell membrane (Krzyzosiak, 1992).

Also, copper is a component of **cytochrome c oxidase,** which catalyzes the cellular utilization of oxygen (Wildman, 2000). Extracellular **superoxide dismutase** is present in high concentration in the lungs, thyroid, and uterus. Copper/zinc dismutases are in the cytosol of most cells, especially brain, thyroid, liver, pituitary, and erythrocytes. Both dismutases scavenge and reduce superoxide radicals. Copper-containing proteins include ceruloplasmin, albumin, and transcuperin, which transport copper; metallothionein, which sequesters and stores copper; and clotting factor V (Chan, 1998b).

Rich sources of copper include liver, shellfish, chocolate, nuts, and seeds. Copper pipes or vessels do not increase the copper content of water unless exposed to acids (Kohlmeier, 2003). The average daily copper intake of American adults is about 1.6 mg in males and 1.2 mg in females. Adults should get at least 0.9 mg/day (IOM, 2002). Smoking, strenuous exercise, infection, and injury increase the need for copper.

Copper absorption occurs in the stomach, especially in the small intestine (Wapnir, 1998). Bile adds about 5 mg/day to ingested copper. Absorption is decreased by excessive zinc or iron intake. Too much copper may cause iron deficiency. Histidine, as well as gluconate and citrate enhances copper absorption (Wildman, 2000). Ascorbate decreases copper absorption by reducing Cu^{++} to Cu^{+} (Kohlmeier, 2003).

Newly absorbed copper is transported bound to albumin and transcuperin and is rapidly cleared from the blood circulation by the liver. When copper reenters the circulation, it is bound to ceruloplasmin, which transports 65%–90% of the plasma copper, and metallothionein and other copper-containing proteins. Ceruloplasmin is not a transporter protein in that the copper is not exchangeable (Eastwood, 2003). Metallochaperones are specific binding proteins that provide targeted intracellular copper transport to shuttle copper for metabolic needs (Kohlmeier, 2003). Excess copper is bound to thionein, decreasing the potential for copper toxicity (Wildman, 2000). Free copper ions are a source of oxygen free-radicals, and intracellular free copper is kept at a very low concentration.

Total copper in an adult human measures 50–80 mg, mainly concentrated in muscle and liver. The liver has the highest copper concentration, averaging between 30 and 50 μg/g dry tissue. Reference ranges for serum copper concentration are age and sex dependent and are higher in pregnancy. Diurnal variation occurs with peak values in the morning. Copper as measured by ICP-MS is as follows: women: 49–184 μg/dL (7.7–29.0 μmol/L); men: 59–118 μg/dL (9.3–18.6 μmol/L) (Chan, 1998b). The most widely used clinical analytic method is FAAS. Serum and plasma copper levels are insensitive to the diagnosis of copper deficiency and are decreased only in severe deficiency (Gibson, 2002). Lower concentrations may indicate depleted copper stores. However, circulating copper levels are affected by factors unrelated to nutrition. Pregnancy, infection, inflammatory conditions, stress, and oral contraception increase the circulating copper level. Corticosteroids and corticotropin lower the circulating copper level (Jacob, 1993). Reduced serum proteins due to nephrosis, malabsorption, and malnutrition cause the serum copper to be low, without reflecting inadequate liver copper stores. Ceruloplasmin, a copper-containing protein, is a useful indicator of copper status. It is an α-2-globulin acute phase reactant. Ceruloplasmin is sensitive to the same factors that affect plasma copper and may be measured immunochemically or by its oxidase activity (Milne, 1994). It is increased in patients with infection, neoplasm, pregnancy, or hormonal contraception (Kohlmeier, 2003). Measurement of erythrocyte superoxide dismutase is useful for assessing copper status. The activity is reduced in copper-deficient states.

Excretion occurs primarily in the feces, which include unabsorbed dietary copper, and in biliary and gastrointestinal secretions, although small amounts are also lost in sweat, urine, and saliva.

Menkes' syndrome and Wilson's disease are genetic defects in copper metabolism. **Menkes' syndrome** is a rare X-linked recessive congenital defect of copper absorption that usually has clinical onset by 3 months of age. The condition is characterized by poor mental development, failure to keratinize hair, skeletal problems, and degenerative changes in the aorta. The brittle hair (steely) is kinky or twisted, and poor skin and hair pigmentation, hypothermia, and seizures have been reported. Hair resembles wool from sheep that graze in pastures lacking copper. Affected infants are copper deficient with decreased serum and liver copper. Red blood cell copper is normal (Wildman, 2000).

Wilson's disease (hepatolenticular degeneration) is an autosomal recessive disease that results from impaired biliary copper excretion. It presents in children and young adults between the ages of 6 and 40 years.

Excess copper is deposited in the liver and in the basal nuclei of the brain, causing sclerosis, and abnormalities of kidney, cornea, and brain may occur. Most often, the presenting disease pattern is that of acute, chronic, or fulminant hepatitis. Symptoms include neurologic disorders, cirrhosis of the liver, and Kayser-Fleischer rings caused by deposition of copper in the corneas. Urinary copper is increased to >100 μg/24 hours, and serum ceruloplasmin is usually decreased. Clinical severity of the disease correlates poorly with the ceruloplasmin level, because ceruloplasmin may be normal or increased in response to hepatic inflammation. Serum copper is generally decreased because of the low ceruloplasmin, and serum copper levels are not useful diagnostically. Serum ceruloplasmin <20 mg/dL with increased hepatic copper of >250 μg/g dry weight is diagnostic. Chelation is an effective treatment in promoting excretion of the copper (Milne, 1994).

Deficiency is unlikely except in people with rare genetic disorders or prolonged malnutrition or starvation. Deficiencies have been observed in premature babies, patients with malabsorption syndromes (celiac disease, tropical sprue, cystic fibrosis), malnourished infants and adults, those with long-term hyperalimentation with infusates deficient in copper, patients with sickle cell disease receiving zinc therapy, and those treated with copper-chelating agents like penicillamine (Milne, 1994). Excessive intake of oral zinc supplements causes induction of metallothionein in the intestinal mucosa, which then sequesters dietary copper, blocking absorption (Gyorffy, 1992; Igic, 2002). Reduced copper levels have been found in elderly patients with femoral neck fractures (Conlan, 1990). Symptoms of copper deficiency include hypochromic anemia, ataxia, neutropenia, osteoporosis and bone and joint abnormalities, decreased skin pigmentation, and neurologic abnormalities. Body stores last only a few weeks when intake is low.

Copper toxicity from food intake has not been reported. Doses in excess of 10 mg/day cause nausea, vomiting, abdominal cramps, and diarrhea, and can cause liver injury, especially in infants. Acute poisoning may present with hemolysis and brain and hepatic cellular damage (Eastwood, 2003). Higher doses can cause coma and death. Excess supplements and ingestion of contaminated water are the usual sources. Ingestion of fungicides containing copper sulfate or industrial exposure sometimes causes acute copper poisoning.

FLUORIDE

Fluoride (F^-) is used to prevent dental caries. Fluoridation of drinking water reduces the incidence of tooth decay now for more than 60% of the U.S. population and reduces the incidence of tooth decay by more than 60%. Dental fluorosis, the unsightly mottling of dental enamel, is seen in erupting teeth of children and is caused by excessive fluoride possibly from ingestion of fluoride-containing toothpaste. Occupational exposure to inhaled fluoride dust during aluminum refining causes severe bone abnormalities; safety equipment now limits such exposure. No cases are attributable to the controlled fluoridation of water supplies. A fluoride-specific electrode is used for water and urine analysis.

IODINE

Dietary iodine (I) is normally ingested as iodide and is the basic element in the synthesis of thyroid hormones, as described in detail in Chapter 24. It is transported to the thyroid follicles, where it is trapped and concentrated to several hundred-fold over its concentration in serum. The gland is stimulated by the pituitary hormone, thyroid-stimulating hormone, to incorporate iodide into tyrosine to form thyronines within the thyroglobulin in the follicular lumen. Proteolytic cleavage of thyroglobulin releases the iodothyronine hormones into the circulation. A tightly controlled feedback system between the thyroid, the hypothalamus, and the pituitary maintains the thyroid hormone concentration within physiologic limits.

Deficiency results in inadequate thyroid hormone and hypothyroidism. Depending on the patient's age, congenital hypothyroidism can cause mental retardation, cretinism, myxedema hypothyroidism in adults with mental status changes, and hypotension. Often, patients develop a goiter.

IRON

Body iron (Fe) is present in hemoglobin, myoglobin, storage iron, and tissue iron. Iron is stored as ferritin and hemosiderin. Normally, very small amounts of iron are present in most cells and in body fluids. No excretory system is used for excess iron. Rather, rigorous conservation of iron occurs. Ferritin is present in nearly all cells in the body. In hepatocytes and macrophages of the marrow, ferritin provides a reserve of iron for the formation of hemoglobin and other heme proteins. Hemosiderin is formed when ferritin is broken down. Iron is transported from one organ to another by the transport protein apotransferrin.

MANGANESE

Manganese (Mn) is associated with the formation of connective and bony tissue and carbohydrate and lipid metabolism. Food sources include whole grain foods, nuts, leafy vegetables, soy, and teas. Manganese is absorbed from the small intestines and transported to the liver, bound to albumin. Excretion occurs via bile into feces. Manganese is a constituent of many important metalloenzymes, including superoxide dismutase, pyruvate carboxylase, arginase, and glycosyl transferases. On a normal diet, deficiency has not been documented. Diet deficiency results in low plasma cholesterol, impaired glucose tolerance, skeletal abnormalities, dermatitis, color changes in hair, and reduced blood-clotting function not responsive to vitamin K.

Toxic exposure to manganese-containing dust produces neurologic symptoms resembling Parkinson's disease. Manganese deposition in the brain is seen with biliary atresia in children. Serum manganese and brain magnetic resonance imaging are used to detect excessive exposure. Plastic cannulas prevent sample contamination.

MOLYBDENUM

Molybdenum (Mo) is incorporated into metalloenzymes and several important enzymes, including sulfite oxidase and xanthine dehydrogenase. Grains, nuts, and legumes such as peas, lentils, and beans are good sources. Renal homeostatic regulation occurs, and urine output directly reflects dietary intake. Deficiency has not been observed in healthy people on a normal diet. Evidence suggests that for most patients, sufficient molybdenum acts as a contaminant in total parenteral nutrition fluids. A diagnosis of molybdenum deficiency is based on demonstration of excess sufite in the urine. Molybdenum compounds have low toxicity in humans. Excess intake induces copper deficiency, blocking copper absorption.

SELENIUM

Selenium (Se) is a constituent of glutathione peroxidase that is associated with vitamin E in its functions. It is a nonmetal and is important in defense against oxidative stress and regulation of thyroid hormone action. Deficiency in pediatric patients can cause endemic cardiomyopathy (Keshan disease) in areas with low soil selenium level, as well as skeletal muscle disorders with proximal weakness and serum creatinine elevation. Immunodeficiency can result from selenoprotein deficiency. Toxicity from selenium includes hair loss, garlic breath, irritability, mild nerve damage, and nail damage. Whole blood selenium can be quantitated by CFAAS.

ZINC

Zinc (Zn) is second to iron as the most abundant trace element in the body. It is the most common catalytic metal ion in the cytoplasm of cells. Total body stores of zinc in adult women are 1.5 g and in men 2.5 g, which is distributed in all tissues. It is almost entirely intracellular (King, 1994). Most zinc is found in skeletal muscle (≈60%) and in bone (≈30%) (Wildman, 2000). It is a cofactor for almost 300 enzymes and is involved in almost all aspects of metabolism. Zinc is important in protein and nucleic acid synthesis, and is essential for gene activation (Kohlmeier, 2003) and for the synthesis and action of insulin (Samman, 2002). Zinc is present only in the divalent state in biological systems, and oxidation–reduction functions are not possible. Important zinc-containing metalloenzymes include carbonic anhydrase, alkaline phosphatase, RNA and DNA polymerases, reverse transcriptase, thymidine kinase, caboxypeptidases, alcohol dehydrogenase, and superoxide dismutase.

Zinc is ubiquitous in food. Oysters are especially rich in zinc. Other shellfish and meats are also good sources. Plants have much lower concentrations. Phytate from whole grains and some vegetables interferes with zinc absorption (Kohlmeier, 2003). The estimated average requirement to maintain adequate stores is 8 mg/day for women eating a mixed diet and 11 mg/day for men (IOM, 2002). Vegetarians and pregnant or nursing woman need slightly more. Zinc is excreted primarily by the intestine.

Zinc is absorbed mainly from the duodenum, although some is absorbed from the small intestine. Some zinc enters the intestinal lumen with pancreatic secretions. Intraluminal digestion by proteases, DNAses, and

RNAses frees zinc so that complexes with histidine, cysteine, and nucleotides that improve absorption are formed. Phytate reduces absorption. High dietary calcium and low protein also reduce zinc absorption (Samman, 2002). Metallothionein regulates zinc transfer into the portal blood. In blood, zinc is bound to albumin and α-2-macroglobulin, with zinc blood concentrations of 10–17 μmol/L.

Muscle and bone, which contain most of the body's zinc stores, have a slow turnover and a half-life of 300 days (Wastney, 2000). The half-life of metallothionein-bound zinc in the liver is about 2 weeks; it can be readily mobilized to cover for an insufficient dietary intake. However, the liver pool is small and contains less than 170 mg. Zinc deficiency can become functionally significant within a week (Milne, 1994).

Almost all blood zinc is complexed to the large proteins, albumin and α-2-macroglobulin, so that little zinc is present in the glomerular filtrate. Urine losses total about 0.5 mg/day (Kohlmeier, 2003). About 1 mg/day is lost in sweat, skin, and hair. Fecal losses, which include diet and endogenous secretions, can be less than 1 mg/day (Sian, 1996). Each ejaculate contains about 0.5 mg, probably from prostatic secretions.

Inadequate zinc impairs DNA replication, food digestion and absorption, taste and appetite, growth and wound healing, synaptic transmission, gene expression, response to oxidant stress, immune function, and other functions.

Zinc fingers are looped sequence-specific DNA-binding proteins that act as transcriptional mediators for nucleic acids. Zinc chelates with cysteine and/or histidine that bind to a specific DNA region and control gene expression or repression, primarily by targeting promoter regions of the genes (Wildman, 2000).

Zinc deficiency is common in patients with diabetes mellitus, alcohol abuse, and malabsorption syndromes, as well as liver and kidney diseases. Symptoms are general because of the many enzymes and tissues affected. Severe deficiencies are characterized by hypogonadism, dwarfism, deformed bones, poor wound healing, abnormal hair and nails, loss of taste, gastrointestinal disturbances, poor chylomicron formation, central nervous system abnormalities, immunodeficiencies, and malabsorption. Zinc deficiency may cause teratogenicity during pregnancy, with congenital malformations, fetal dysmaturity, prematurity, neural tube defects, and spina bifida (Chan, 1998).

Nutritional zinc deficiency is fairly prevalent despite the wide availability of zinc in foods. Zinc deficiency produces a syndrome of growth retardation, male hypogonadism, skin changes, mental lethargy, hepatosplenomegaly, iron deficiency anemia, and geophagia (eating clay). It has been encountered most often in male children in Iran and Egypt as a result of a low-zinc diet and a high fiber content that decrease available zinc for absorption. Zinc deficiency has been reported from Turkey, Portugal, Morocco, and Yugoslavia (Milne, 1994). In some areas of the Middle East, people frequently eat unleavened bread that is high in phytate. Yeast contains phytase. However, the recipe for the dough of the unleavened bread does not include yeast. The high fiber content and the low meat and low protein intakes in this population result in zinc deficiency. Individuals respond well to dietary zinc sulfate supplementation (Eastwood, 2003). Growth failure, reduced taste acuity, and hypogonadism in young adults in New York and Tennessee and in school children in Colorado have been ascribed to zinc deficiency (Milne, 1994). Zinc deficiency has also been reported in old age, pregnancy, lactation, steatorrhea, extensive burns, renal disease, and diuretic and antimetabolite therapies. Zinc deficiency in alcoholic and cirrhotic individuals leads to low serum zinc concentrations and increased urinary excretion (Eastwood, 2003).

Acrodermatitis enteropathica is a rare autosomal recessive disorder with impaired intestinal absorption and transport of zinc. Symptoms include hyperpigmented skin lesions, pustular and bullous dermatitis, alopecia, growth retardation, diarrhea, secondary infection, irritability, lethargy, and depression. Plasma or serum zinc is below 40 μg/mL. Oral zinc therapy results in rapid and complete remission (Chan, 1998b).

A case of zinc deficiency called **acquired acrodermatitis enteropathica** was reported in a 41-year-old woman with alcohol abuse and type 1 diabetes mellitus, complicated by retinopathy, nephropathy, and end-stage renal disease. The case included a 5-month history of alopecia, brittle scalp hair, diarrhea, angular cheilitis, and a pruritic, scaly erythematous eruption involving the extremities, perineum, and buttocks. A skin biopsy disclosed confluent parakeratosis with absence of the granular layer. Serum zinc levels were markedly reduced at 0.35 μg/mL (normal, 0.66–1.10 μg/mL) 5.4 μmol/L (normal, 10.1–16.8 μmol/L). Oral zinc sulfate resolved her diarrhea and her skin eruption cleared and hair began to regrow (Wang, 2005).

Zinc toxicity is rare in humans. Animals given high levels of supplementation manifest dysphagia. Other effects, like weight loss, are attributed to reduced food intake. Inhalation of zinc oxide fumes is the most common cause of metal fume fever. Symptoms are of a flu-like illness with onset 4 to 6 hours after exposure to the fumes. Fatigue, chills, myalgias, cough, dyspnea, leukocytosis, thirst, metallic taste, and salivation characterize this self-limited illness, with resolution of symptoms in 36 hours.

No single test is definitive for the status of zinc stores. Two groups of tests are available: Analysis of zinc in a body tissue or body fluid, such as plasma, serum, blood cells, or urine; and testing of a zinc-dependent function, such as taste acuity, or measurement of the activity of zinc-containing enzymes. In most instances, assays will show a decrease with zinc deficiency. Test results should be interpreted with caution because levels may be affected by unrelated conditions. Diurnal variation in zinc levels has been noted. Zinc levels decrease after meals and are elevated after fasting. Albumin levels significantly affect the circulating zinc level. Also, many steroids, including adrenocortical and gonadal, depress the zinc level. Erythrocyte levels are 10 times that of serum, and hemolysis is a serious problem affecting the usefulness of the results.

FAAS is the method of choice for clinical testing for zinc in body fluids. ICP-MS is the reference testing method used for zinc testing in serum or plasma.

The zinc plasma level reference range is around 70–120 μg/dL (10.7–18.4 μmol/L), of which a third is bound to α-2-macroglobulin and the rest to albumin. Ten percent to 20% of blood zinc is present in the plasma. The remainder is associated with carbonic anhydrase in the erythrocytes. Hemolysis must be avoided. Fasting morning levels of zinc below 70 μg/dL (10.7 μmol/L) suggest marginal deficiency. Serum zinc values are 5%–10% higher than in plasma. Zinc levels are lower in nonfasting states, infection, inflammation, steroid administration, pregnancy, and hypoalbuminemia.

Zinc in erythrocytes and hair provides a long-term assessment of body zinc status. Lowered hair zinc has been demonstrated in several different zinc-deficient conditions. Care must be taken to avoid environmental contamination and to sample hair grown during the condition under study—not during the previous time period (Milne, 1994). Urinary zinc excretion reference values are around 0.15–1.00 mg/day (2.3–15.3 μmol/day). Urinary zinc excretion is usually decreased in zinc deficiency. In some conditions associated with zinc deficiency, such as cirrhosis, severe alcoholism, sickle cell anemia, postsurgical periods, and total parenteral nutrition, urinary zinc excretion is often increased (Jacob, 1993).

Hyperzincaemia is a familial disorder that results in elevated serum zinc levels but does not cause any apparent toxicity. In contrast, zinc overdoses that result in similar plasma zinc levels have been known to be fatal (Wildman, 2000).

SELECTED REFERENCES

Kohlmeier M. Nutrient metabolism. San Diego: Academic Press; 2003.

This text provides a systematic presentation of the metabolism of the vitamins and trace elements, with masterful integration of the vast subject of nutritional metabolism and biochemistry, in the context of normal human physiology. Extensive current references are provided.

Mann J, Truswell AS, editors. Essentials of human nutrition. 2nd ed. Oxford: Oxford University Press; 2002.

Covers the trace elements and vitamins with a focus on deficiencies, toxicity, and biochemical testing; and includes an appendix assessing numerous standard and newly introduced static and dynamic biochemical tests, as well as load and tolerance tests—their findings, utility, and interpretability.

Taylor A. Detection and monitoring of disorders of essential trace elements. Ann Clin Biochem 1996;33:486–510.

Presents the findings in deficiencies of essential trace elements due to metabolic disorders, with descriptions of clinical disorders; clinical signs and test results for the assessment of trace element status; findings, interpretability, and utility of the data; nonoccupational disorders associated with accumulation of essential trace elements; and protocols for testing in genetic, therapeutic, and disease states, including nonanalytic factors affecting interpretation and analytic techniques.

Wildman REC, Medeiros DM. Advanced human nutrition. Boca Raton, Fla.: CRC Press; 2000.

Presents the biochemistry and physiology of the vitamins and the essential trace elements, including tables of functions, tissue content and excretion, deficiency and toxicity symptoms, and food sources with their micronutrient content.

REFERENCES

Access the complete reference list online at http://www.expertconsult.com

CHAPTER 27

CHEMICAL BASIS FOR ANALYTE ASSAYS AND COMMON INTERFERENCES

Matthew R. Pincus, Jay L. Bock, Ralph Rossi, Donghong Cai

KEY POINTS

- The clinical chemistry metabolic profile gives important quantitative information for more than 25 serum analytes, often facilitating diagnosis of disease.
- Serum electrolyte concentrations for sodium, potassium, chloride, and sometimes calcium are most commonly assayed using ion-selective electrodes.
- Assays for other analytes, including total protein, albumin, bilirubin, creatinine, calcium, iron and iron-binding capacity, magnesium, and phosphate, are performed using spectrophotometry on complexes that are formed by each analyte with simple reagents. These complexes absorb light at wavelengths at which the analyte itself and the reagent have minimal absorbance. The concentration of the analyte is determined using Beer's Law.
- Assays for a number of serum analytes, including ammonia, bicarbonate, cholesterol, glucose, lactate, triglycerides, and urea and uric acid, utilize enzymes that catalyze reactions in which the analytes are converted into products whose concentrations can be measured conveniently.
- Spectrophotometric assays can be performed by waiting for the point at which the increase or decrease in absorbance of a complex at a particular wavelength ceases to change (endpoint method) or by determining the initial rates of complex formation (rate method).
- Assays for specific enzymes are performed using substrates that are specific for these enzymes. Concentrations of the products of the enzyme-catalyzed reactions are determined spectrophotometrically as described in Chapter 20, allowing for direct determination of enzyme activity.
- Often, the products of enzyme-catalyzed reactions are measured in coupled reactions in which the product of the enzyme-catalyzed reaction is the substrate for another enzyme added at high concentration, allowing for the rapid conversion of the product of the first reaction to another product whose concentration can be easily determined.

In many of the preceding chapters, we have discussed the chemical bases for the assays employed for the diagnosis of specific diseases. In this chapter, we present a consolidation of the methods used in the typical so-called **metabolic panel** in clinical chemistry, a panoply of chemical assays that are often requested for patients who are undergoing outpatient annual checkups or are being admitted to the hospital. We summarize and discuss the chemical bases for these assays in a concise manner, so that the reader can refer to these methods conveniently and can understand the assays and their limitations. Understanding of the assays contributes to an understanding of why certain substances interfere with particular assays and can give rise to misleading results. It should be kept in mind that, for many of the assays described here, more than one method can be used. Because it is impossible to cover all variations of methods used to quantitate each analyte, we describe the principles that underlie commonly employed methods and refer, where possible, to alternate approaches.

Metabolic panels consist of serum electrolytes (sodium, potassium, and chloride), bicarbonate, calcium, phosphate, magnesium, urea, creatinine, glucose, uric acid, total protein, albumin, total and direct bilirubin, cholesterol, high-density lipoprotein (HDL) and low-density lipoprotein (LDL), triglycerides, ammonia, iron and iron-binding capacity, and the enzymes, including: creatine kinase, aspartate aminotransferase, alanine aminotransferase (ALT), alkaline phosphatase, lactate dehydrogenase (LD), γ-glutamyl transferase (GGT), amylase, and lipase. The reader may recognize various panels that measure the functioning of specific tissues such as kidney (i.e., the renal **profile,** consisting of urea, creatinine, calcium, and phosphate). These panels are of great use in diagnosing disease states, as discussed in Chapter 8.

We divide the basic assays for these analytes functionally into four method-based groups:

1. Ion-selective electrodes.
2. Spectrophotometric assays based on color complexes for specific molecules (e.g., the color noncovalent complex of albumin with bromcresol green dye and bilirubin covalently reacted with diazotized sulfanilic acid to give azo-derivatized forms of the indole rings of bilirubin).

3. Analyte concentrations using enzymes as reagents. In Chapter 20, we discussed how small molecule substrates are used to determine serum enzyme concentrations. In a similar manner, this process can be reversed; enzymes can be used to determine the concentrations of small or large molecules (like proteins). If an analyte is a specific substrate for an enzyme, and if formation of the product or disappearance of the substrate can be conveniently followed, this method can be used effectively.
4. Enzyme assays (i.e., use of substrates to determine enzyme concentrations), as described in Chapter 20. Almost all of these assays are also based on spectrophotometric measurements, which depend on the substrates used in the assays and, in many cases, the need for the use of indicator enzymes in so-called **coupled reactions.**

ION-SELECTIVE ELECTRODES

As explained in Chapter 4, this technique is used to measure the concentrations of specific ions by an electrochemical method. This method is nonspecific in that it does not discriminate between ions in causing voltage differences between the measuring electrode and the standard electrode. It is the presence of an ion perm-selective membrane barrier on the measuring electrode that allows only a specific ion to pass through permitting contact with the measuring electrode. Each ion requires a different material that will be selectively permeable to this ion and to this ion only. Thus glass is perm-selective to hydrogen ion. A special polymer of the polyamino acid antibiotic valinomycin is perm-selective to potassium ions. A polymer resin of polyvinylchloride (PVC) is perm-selective to sodium ions. Recently, an anodized indium tin oxide membrane has been found to be even more perm-selective to sodium ions (Lin, 2010). Similarly, calcium-chelating organic molecules impregnated into PVC membranes serve as perm-selective membranes for calcium ions. In addition, dioctylphenyl phosphates, as shown in Figure 27-1, *C*, have been found to chelate calcium ions selectively and to serve as effective ion-selective electrodes.

Three basic causes of malfunctions of ion-selective electrodes have been identified. The first and most common consists of defects in the perm-selective membrane itself. This allows ions other than the one whose concentration is being measured to be present at the measuring electrode. The result is seen as ion concentrations that are falsely elevated. This defect is almost always detected in routine quality control that shows a strong upward drift in the controls despite frequent calibrations.

The second cause of inaccuracy in ion-selective electrodes is buildup of countervoltages from liquid junction potentials present at the salt bridge connecting the measuring electrode with the reference electrode. Because these voltages oppose the voltage between the two electrodes, the voltages are diminished, yielding lower than expected ion concentrations. Buildup of liquid junction potentials occurs over time and affects the lifetime of electrodes. It is therefore vital to change electrodes at the times specified by the manufacturer to avoid erroneous results.

The third cause of malfunctioning electrodes is buildup of proteins on the electrodes, resulting in alteration of the voltage between testing and reference electrodes. This phenomenon gives rise to erratic results and lack of reproducibility of ion concentrations in a single specimen. This problem can be avoided by performing washes of the electrodes at manufacturer-specified times.

SPECTROPHOTOMETRIC DETERMINATIONS

These are by far the most common types of assays. We discuss each analyte measured by this method.

BEER'S LAW

We remind the reader that all spectrophotometric determinations are made using the Beer-Lambert law (see Chapter 4), which states that the absorbance, A, of an analyte at a particular wavelength is proportional to its concentration, C, and the length of the light path, L, in the cuvette in which the analyte is dissolved in a solvent (usually water or aqueous buffer), that is,

$$A = \varepsilon \times C \times L \quad \textbf{(27-1)}$$

where ε is the proportionality constant, also called the extinction coefficient.

ENDPOINT VS. RATE METHOD

As we now describe, the spectrophotometric determination of the concentration of an analyte requires the addition of another compound or reagent

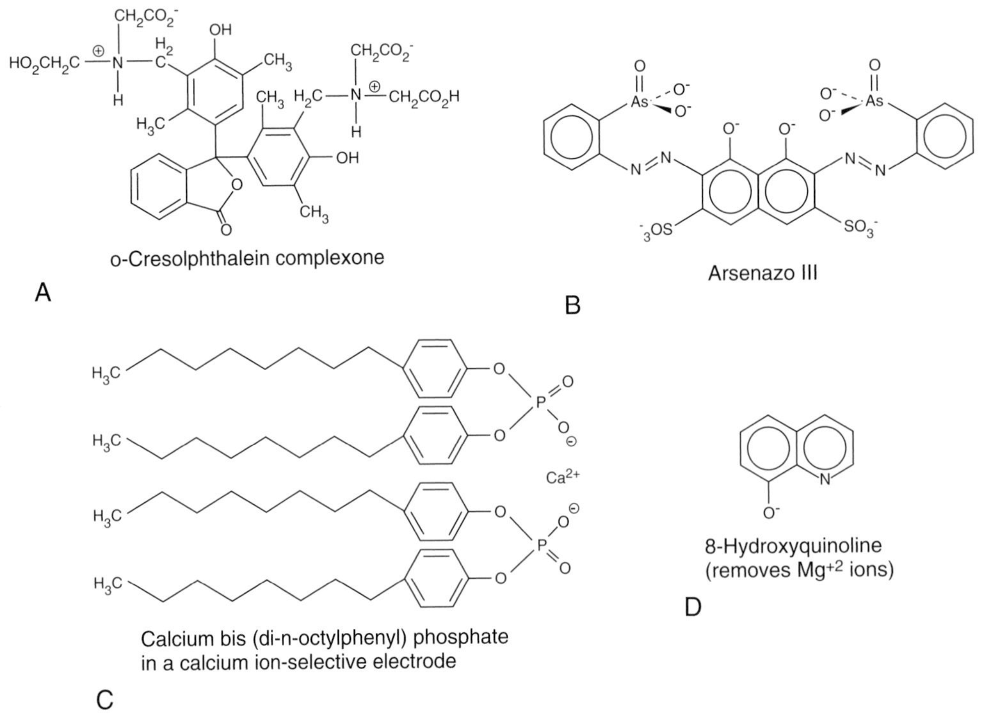

Figure 27-1 Structures of agents that bind selectively to Ca^{++} ions, with the exception of 8-hydroxyquinolone, which binds and precipitates Mg^{++} ions.

with which the analyte of interest reacts covalently or noncovalently. The reagent is always added in excess. The resulting complex absorbs light at a wavelength at which neither the free analyte nor the unbound reagent absorbs, or at which each species absorbs only minimally. If the reaction is allowed to proceed to completion and the absorbance is then determined, the method is referred to as an endpoint method. In some cases, the rate of formation of the complex is slow.

To avoid long waiting periods, the rate of the reaction over a short period is determined and is used to compute the concentration of the analyte. In Chapters 20 and 23, we discussed the order of reactions. In the case of formation of colored complexes, the analyte, A, reacts with the reagent, R, to form the measured product, that is, the color complex, or AR, as follows:

$$A + R \rightarrow AR \qquad \textbf{(27-2)}$$

The rate equation describing the rate of formation of AR, that is, d(AR)/dt, is

$$d(AR)/dt = k(A)(R) \qquad \textbf{(27-3)}$$

where k is the rate constant.

This is referred to as a *second-order rate process* because the rate depends on the concentrations of both A and R. However, because R is added in excess of A, at least initially, the concentration of R does not change appreciably, so that it may be considered constant. The reaction then becomes a *pseudo-first-order reaction*. In this case,

$$d(AR)/dt = kR_0(A) \qquad \textbf{(27-4)}$$

where R_0 is the defined added concentration of reagent, so that

$$d(AR)/dt = k'(A) \qquad \textbf{(27-5)}$$

where k′ is kR_0.

Thus the rate of formation of AR is proportional to the concentration of A. Plots of AR versus time should be linear for the initial time periods (which can range from seconds to minutes). The slope is $k' = kR_o$, whose value is known. Therefore, A must be equal to the slope of the initial straight line divided by k′. This process is similar to the one described in Chapter 20 for computing enzyme concentrations in serum at low substrate concentrations.

In the same manner in which we determine the concentrations of enzymes in serum by observing the *initial* rate of the enzyme-catalyzed reaction in the presence of saturating concentrations of substrate, where the concentration of the substrate is known, we can likewise determine the initial concentration of A by measuring the initial rate at which AR forms. This rate is proportional to the initial concentration of A, the desired quantity.

INTERFERENCES

Many color complex absorbances are determined at wavelengths higher than 500 nm, approaching the visible region of the electromagnetic spectrum, where most small molecules such as drugs and cofactors, such as nicotinamide adenine dinucleotide (NADH), flavine adenine dinucleotide, and pyridoxal phosphate, do not absorb. However, hemoglobin has strong absorbances in this range. Therefore, if hemolysis occurs, appreciable concentrations of hemoglobin may occur in serum, giving falsely elevated absorbances and hence analyte concentrations. In addition, the presence of lipids such as the triglycerides and cholesterol esters in appreciable concentrations in serum can cause falsely elevated concentrations of analytes at virtually any wavelength as the result of scattering of light, which leads to decreased transmittance and therefore increased absorbance. Although fortunately not common, the presence of certain drugs can interfere with spectrophotometric determination of the levels of some of the analytes.

QUANTITATION OF ANALYTES

We now discuss commonly used methods to determine the concentrations of analytes by formation of color complexes.

Albumin and Total Protein

Albumin

As noted in Chapter 19, albumin is the most anionic of the major serum proteins, and it migrates toward the anode on serum protein electrophoresis. It binds with high affinity to cationic dyes, among which are bromcresol green (BCG), a derivative of triphenyl methane, and bromcresol purple (BCP). The reaction with bromcresol green is as follows:

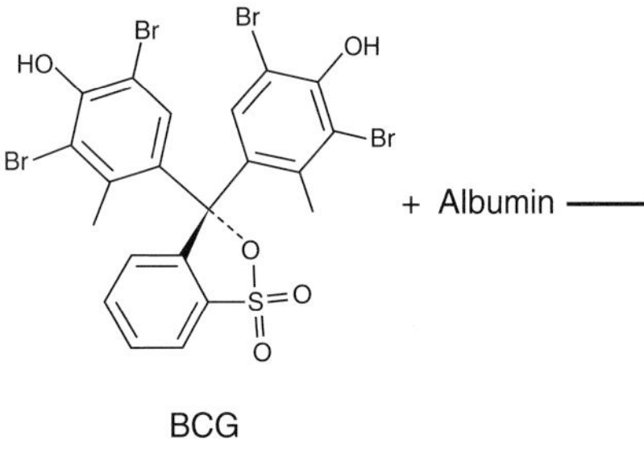

(27-6)

The amount of albumin present in the sample is measured as an endpoint reaction at 628 nm. A similar reaction with BCP yields a color complex whose absorbance is read at 603 nm. BCG reacts also to some extent with α_1- and α_2-proteins, sometimes tending to overestimate the concentration of albumin. BCP does not react with these proteins and so is considered to be more specific in quantitation of albumin. Interferences include hemolysis and lipemia.

Total Protein

From Chapter 19, it will be remembered that all proteins are polyamino acids linked together by peptide (CONH) bonds. These peptide bonds form complexes with cupric ions in cupric sulfate to form a color complex in alkaline solution, the so-called **Biuret reaction,** as shown below:

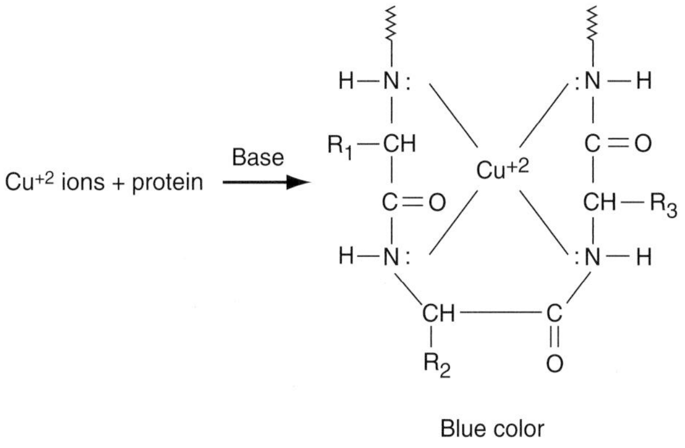

(27-7)

Note that this occurs for every four consecutive peptide units. Because most proteins contain at least 150–200 amino acid residues, and many of them more than 300 amino acid residues, many of these complexes are formed for each protein. Because large numbers of proteins are present in serum, this reaction is multiplied many-fold, making the Biuret method quite sensitive. The absorbance of the colored complex is determined at 540 nm. Major interferences with this reaction include hemolysis and lipemia.

Bilirubin

As discussed in Chapter 21, the most common method for measuring serum bilirubin is the Jendrassik-Grof method. In this method, diazotized sulfanilic acid reacts with two pyrole rings of bilirubin to give two phenylazo adducts, as shown in Equation 27-8 (Natelson, 1971):

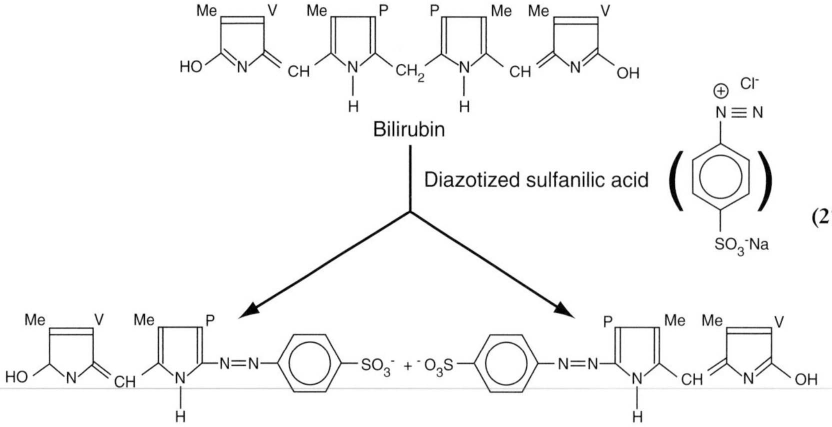

(27-8)

In this equation, Me is the methyl group, V is the vinyl group, and P is the 3-substituted propionic acid moiety. Note that electrophilic aromatic substitution occurs increasingly on the pyrole rings, such that the central methylene carbon is removed altogether, giving the two sets of phenylazo adducts.

As discussed in Chapter 21, bilirubin is conjugated to glucuronic acid at either or both propionic acid moieties. Unconjugated bilirubin is much less soluble than are the conjugated forms. Most of the unconjugated bilirubin is bound tightly to albumin, making it largely unavailable for reaction with the diazotized sulfanilic acid reagent. However, addition of agents such as ethanol, methanol, or caffeine-benzoate induces the dissociation of unconjugated bilirubin from albumin, allowing it to react with the reagent. Caffeine-benzoate is preferred because methanol and ethanol can induce protein precipitation and increased turbidity. Interference by hemoglobin as the result of hemolysis can also occur. The soluble bilirubins (mostly conjugated, but see later) that react in the absence of dissociating reagents are termed **direct bilirubin,** and the bilirubin that reacts in the presence of the dissociating agent is **total bilirubin.** So-called **indirect bilirubin** (mostly unconjugated bilirubin bound to albumin) is obtained by subtracting direct bilirubin from total bilirubin (Tolman, 1999). As noted in Chapter 21, not all conjugated bilirubin is detected as direct bilirubin, and a small amount of unconjugated bilrubin may be detected as direct bilirubin.

Calcium

Most methods rely on the formation of a color complex of Ca^{++} ions with an appropriate chelating agent with which it forms a color complex. Because approximately half of total calcium is bound to protein, mainly to albumin, lowering the pH of the sample liberates calcium ions. The calcium ions are then reacted with a strong chelating compound, with which they form a color complex. The two major calcium-chelating compounds currently used are ortho-cresolphthalein (forms a red complex) and arsenazo III (Rowatt, 1989; Morgan, 1993), whose structures are shown in Figures 27-1, *A* and *B*, respectively. The reaction is shown below:

$$\text{Dye} + \text{Ca}^{++} \rightarrow \text{Dye} - \text{Ca}^{++} \qquad \textbf{(27-9)}$$

where the dye may be ortho-cresolphthalein or arsenazo III.

Use of ortho-cresolphthalein is often accompanied by an additional step in which the reaction solution is treated with the compound 8-hydroxyquinoline, whose structure is shown in Figure 27-1, *D*, at alkaline pH, to prevent the formation of any possible complex with magnesium ion. The amount of complex that forms is rather strongly dependent on the temperature, which must therefore be carefully maintained. At low calcium concentrations, a one-to-one complex forms, whereas at higher calcium concentrations, 2 moles of calcium bind to 1 mole of dye. Because the extinction coefficients of monocalcium and dicalcium dye complexes differ, absorbance is nonlinear with respect to calcium concentration. However, a modified Beer's Law equation can be used to compute concentration from absorbance, or nonlinear methods can be used for this purpose.

Arseno III has a high affinity for calcium ions, but the amount of complex formed is strongly pH dependent. Usually, imidazole buffers at pH 6.0 are employed for this reaction. It is important to note that citrate, which is a tricarboxylic acid that can chelate calcium ions, has been found to interfere with this reaction. It has been observed that absorbance at 650 nm is the optimal wavelength for determination of the concentration of calcium ion complex with arseno III, at which little interference by other analytes is seen, other than in hemolyzed samples.

Ion-Selective Electrodes for Calcium Determinations

Because calcium can be released from its normally bound states by acidification, addition of acid to a serum sample will convert all calcium to readily measurable ionic forms. Thus total calcium can be measured voltametrically. The electrode is a specific calcium-ion exchanger, of which there are several types, including ETH 1001 and bis-di-(n-octylphenyl) phosphate. The structure of the latter is shown in Figure 27-1, *C* (Endres, 1999). Ionized calcium, that is, calcium that is not bound to protein or in complex formation with strong chelators, can be measured directly with ion-selective electrodes without the prior acid treatment step.

Creatinine

Creatinine has been found to form a complex with picric acid (2,4,6-trinitrophenol) under alkaline conditions, as shown below in the Jaffe reaction:

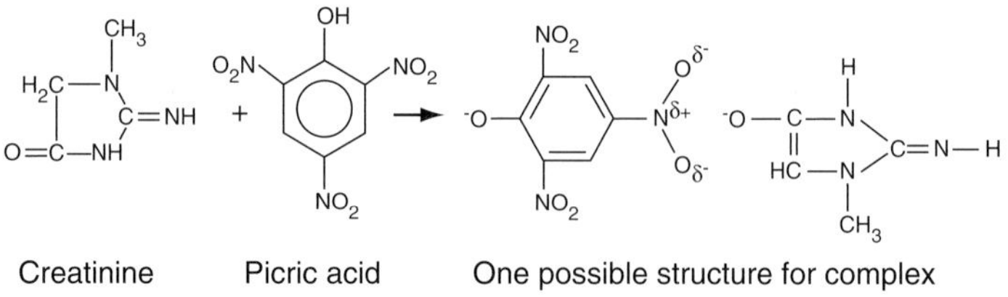

(27-10)

The actual structure of the complex is not completely known. Most studies suggest that it is a noncovalent ionic complex, as shown in Equation 27-10 (Vasillades, 1976). However, some evidence suggests that the carbonyl oxygen (in its enolate form) of creatinine can attack the 1-carbon of picric acid to form a covalent (so-called **Janovsky-like**) adduct (Kroli, 1987). Irrespective of the structure(s) of this complex, its absorbance is determined to be between 490 and 500 nm. The reaction is sensitive to temperature. Possible interferences include ketones, keto acids, and bilirubin. The enolate forms of ketones can react with picric acid much in the same manner as those of creatinine. The reaction of picric acid with bilirubin can be minimized by treatment with ferricyanide or small amounts of surfactant.

Iron

Serum iron levels can be readily determined by a specific reaction of ferrous iron (Fe^{++}) with the compound ferrozine, the structure of which is shown in Equation 27-11. The reaction is performed in an acid medium, so that ferrous ions can be dissociated from transferrin and maintained in the reduced state. Actually, each ferrous ion complexes with three ferrozine molecules to form a magenta-colored complex, remarkably insensitive to pH, whose absorbance can be determined at 562 nm. As might be expected, hemolysis can cause major interferences with this assay because of red cell iron and release of hemoglobin that can compete with ferrozine for binding to serum iron.

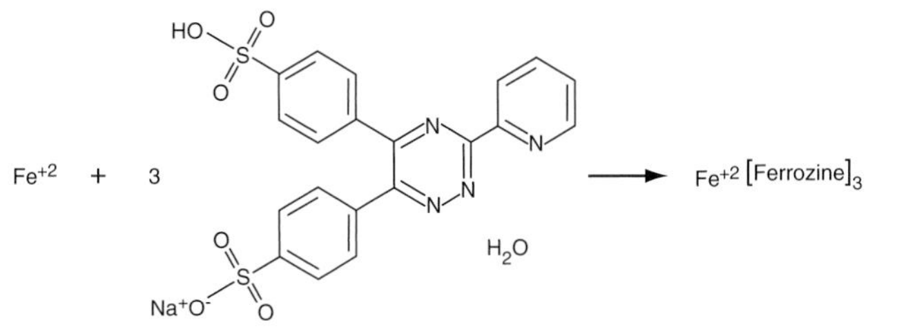

Ferrozine (27-11)

Total Iron-Binding Capacity

This is a measure of the total number of functional ferrous ion-binding sites in transferrin. As discussed in Chapter 23, the basic approach is to strip serum transferrin of all bound iron and then to add an excess of iron to the serum sample to determine the concentration of transferrin-bound iron. To accomplish this, the serum sample is added to an acidic buffer that dissociates all transferrin-bound iron and contains excess ferric chloride and ferrozine. All of the iron is now bound to ferrozine. The pH of the solution is raised into the neutral range, where the affinity of iron for transferrin is greatly increased over that for ferrozine. All iron that can bind to available sites on transferrin does so. This results in a decrease in the magenta color at 562 nm. This decrease is proportional to the total concentration of functional transferrin-binding sites. This set of reactions is summarized as follows:

$$\text{Iron-tranferrin} + \text{Buffer 1} \xrightarrow{\text{Low pH}} \text{Transferrin} + \text{Colored iron–dye complex} \quad \textbf{(27-12A)}$$

$$\text{Transferrin} + \text{Colored iron–dye complex} + \text{Buffer 2} \xrightarrow{\text{Increase pH}} \text{Iron-transferrin} + \text{Decreased colored iron–dye complex} \quad \textbf{(27-12B)}$$

Magnesium

Several dyes that form specific complexes with Mg^{++} ions are used to determine the serum concentrations of this metal ion. They include calmagite (530–550 nm), as shown in Figure 27-2, methylthymol blue (600 nm), and xylidyl blue (600 nm). The numbers in parentheses in the preceding sentence indicate the wavelengths at which complex concentrations are determined for each dye (Endres, 1999). In the case of calmagite, the calcium-chelating compound, ethylene glycol tetraacetic acid, can be used to remove interference from calcium ions, potassium cyanide can be added to remove interference from heavy metal ions, and polyvinylpyrrolidone can be added to the reaction solution to minimize interference from proteins.

Phosphate

Phosphate may be inorganic, mainly orthophosphate, or organic, such as glucose-6-phosphate, nucleic acids, phosphoproteins, and so forth. Most phosphate in serum is inorganic; organic phosphates are mainly intracellular. Phosphoric acid is a tribasic acid, and the main forms of phosphate at blood pH are $H_2PO_4^{-1}$ and HPO_4^{-2}. The most commonly used method to measure total serum inorganic phosphate is the phosphomolybdate method, in which ammonium molybdate is reacted with inorganic phosphate to form an ammonium–phosphomolybdate complex (Endres, 1999). The unreduced form of this complex can be determined readily by the increase in absorbance at 340 nm. The pH must be maintained in the acid range because alkaline conditions can result in reduction of the complex. In fact, reduction of this complex yields a blue product whose absorbance can be determined in the 600–700 nm range (the Fiske-Subbarow method). Reducing agents used include ascorbic acid, stannous chloride, ferrous

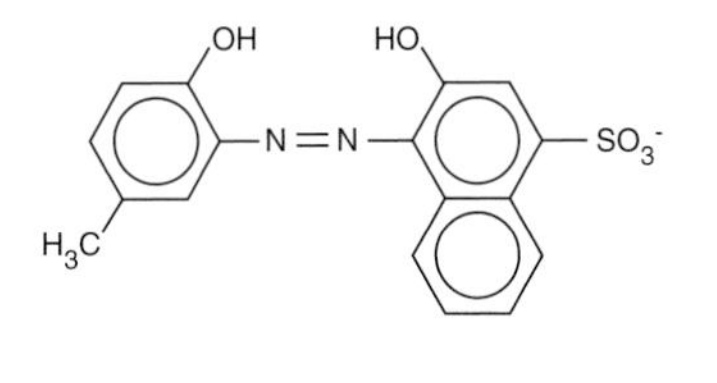

Calmagite for Mg^{+2} determination

Figure 27-2 Structure of calmagite, an agent that forms a selective color complex with Mg^{++} ions.

ammonium sulfate, 1-amino-2-naphthol-4-sulfonic acid (used originally), and many others. Most methods use the direct 340-nm determination because of its speed and the fact that it involves only one step.

Use of Enzymes as Reagents to Determine Analyte Concentrations

GENERAL FEATURES

Rate vs. Endpoint Methods

These are similar to the methods discussed earlier in the section on spectrophotometric determinations. For rate methods, the total amount of enzyme is added to the serum sample, so that, unlike in enzyme assays, total enzyme concentration is known. Note, though, that the substrate concentration is not known (we seek to determine this). It is not known whether or not saturation conditions prevail. Therefore, to compute the substrate concentration for an observed initial rate, the Michaelis-Menten equation is solved to determine substrate concentration. This is possible because K_m and V_{max} are known for the enzyme reagent used. As with dye-based methods, endpoint methods using enzymes are based on determination of the point at which the product concentration remains constant; this concentration is the total substrate or analyte concentration.

NADH and NADPH as Quantitative Indicators

In this section and in the following section, it will be seen that a common approach used in determining the serum concentrations of analytes and of enzymes is to follow the reduction of NAD or NADP to NADH or NADPH, respectively. NAD[P]H has strong absorbance at 340 nm, but the oxidized forms, that is, NAD[P], have no absorbance. Thus determination of the *increase* in absorbance at 340 nm for an enzyme-catalyzed reaction in which NAD[P] is converted to NAD[P]H, or of the *decrease* in absorbance at 340 nm for an enzyme-catalyzed reaction in which NAD[P]H is converted to NAD[P], is a very convenient means of measuring analyte concentration.

In some assays in which NAD[P]H is an end-product, the sensitivity of the level of NAD[P]H produced is enhanced by adding another step, wherein a dye reagent, a tetrazolium derivative, is reduced by NAD[P]H to yield a formazan that strongly absorbs at wavelengths around 500 nm. This reaction can be catalyzed by an electron transfer agent, such as the enzyme diaphorase (lipoamide dehydrogenase, EC 1.6.4.3) or phenazine methosulfate. A prototypical reaction is shown in Figure 27-3. This reaction can, in principle, be used for any reaction in which NAD[P]H is generated.

ANALYTES WHOSE CONCENTRATIONS ARE DETERMINED BY ENZYME REACTIONS

Ammonia

Ammonia is measured by using the versatile enzyme glutamate dehydrogenase (GLD). In this reaction, ammonia reacts with α-ketoglutarate to form glutamate in a reductive amination reaction. In the first step of this reaction, a Schiff base forms between ammonia and the α-keto group of α-ketoglutarate. In the second step, the resulting double bond is then reduced by NADPH, giving the primary amine in glutamate, plus NADP. The overall reaction is shown in Figure 27-4. Ammonia concentration can therefore be determined by the decrease in absorbance at 340 nm as NADPH is converted to NADP. This enzyme can be used in any reaction is which ammonia is generated.

Bicarbonate Ions

One of the glycolytic enzymes, phosphoenolpyruvate carboxy kinase (PEPK), utilizes bicarbonate ion (HCO_3^-) to carboxylate phosphoenolpyruvate to form oxaloacetate (OAA), a Krebs cycle intermediate, with attendant dephosphorylation (Equation 27-13). Thus, advantage can be taken of this reaction to consume serum bicarbonate in the reaction, thereby enabling us to determine its concentration. PEPK is added to the serum. The resulting OAA is then reduced by added malate dehydrogenase to form malate. In this second reaction, NADH is oxidized to NAD, so that the decrease in absorbance of NADH can be monitored at 340 nm. Often, an NAD analog is used, so that decreased absorbance at 410 nm, rather than at 340 nm, is monitored.

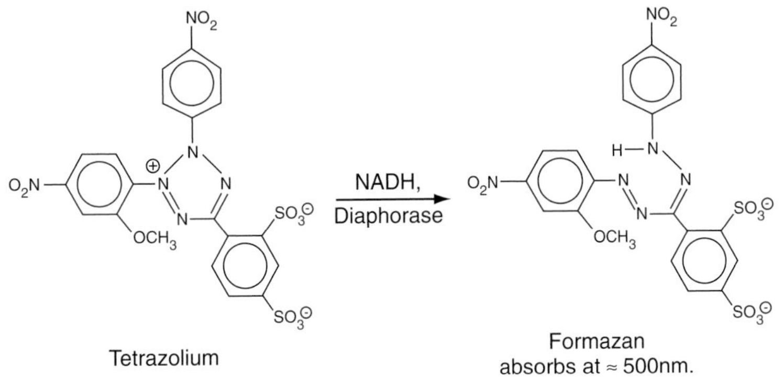

Figure 27-3 Reduction of a tetrazolium to a formazan in which NADH or NADPH is converted to NAD or NADP, respectively, in the presence of a catalyst, that is, the enzyme diaphorase, or phenazine methosulfate. The formazan strongly absorbs at 500 nm. This reaction can be used to enhance the sensitivity of reactions in which NADH or NADPH is generated. *NADH,* Nicotinamide adenine dinucleotide.

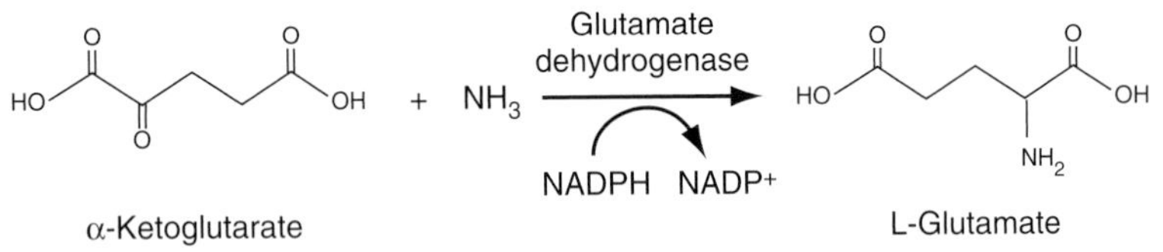

Figure 27-4 Reductive amination reaction, catalyzed by glutamate dehydrogenase, in which ammonia reacts with α-ketoglutarate to form the amino acid glutamic acid. In this reaction, NADH is converted to NAD, allowing the ammonia concentration to be determined by the total decrease in absorbance of light at 340 nm—the wavelength at which NADH absorbs. *NADH,* Nicotinamide adenine dinucleotide.

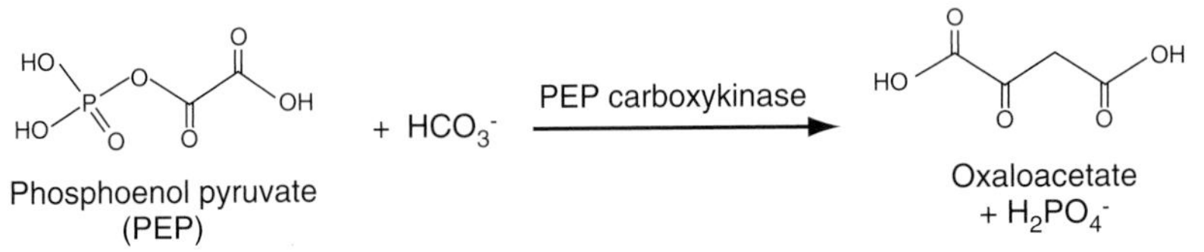

(27-13A)

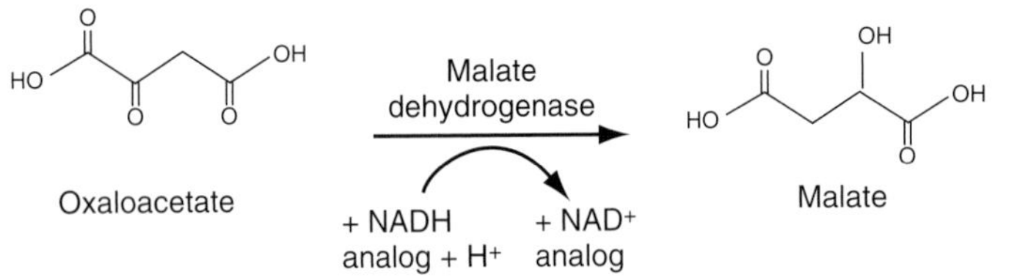

(27-13B)

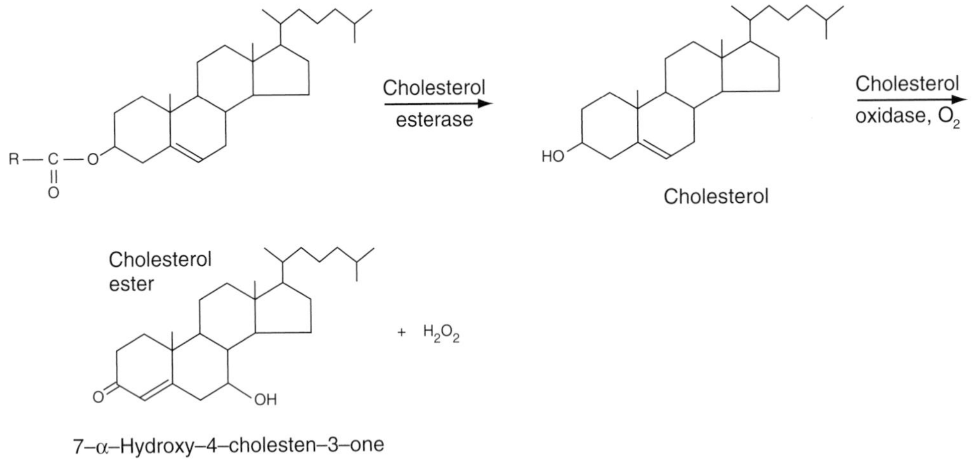

(27-14A)

Cholesterol

As discussed in Chapter 17, cholesterol circulates as both free (mainly in LDL particles) and cholesterol ester (mainly in HDL particles). To determine the serum concentration of total cholesterol, therefore, all cholesterol ester is first converted to free cholesterol using cholesterol esterase (Equation 27-14, *A*). The resulting total free cholesterol is then oxidized to 7-α-hydroxy-cholesten-3-one with cholesterol oxidase, as is shown in Equation 27-14, *A*. As can be seen, hydrogen peroxide (H_2O_2), a strong oxidizing agent, is generated in this reaction. Advantage can be taken of this property to generate strongly absorbing chromophores, as we now describe.

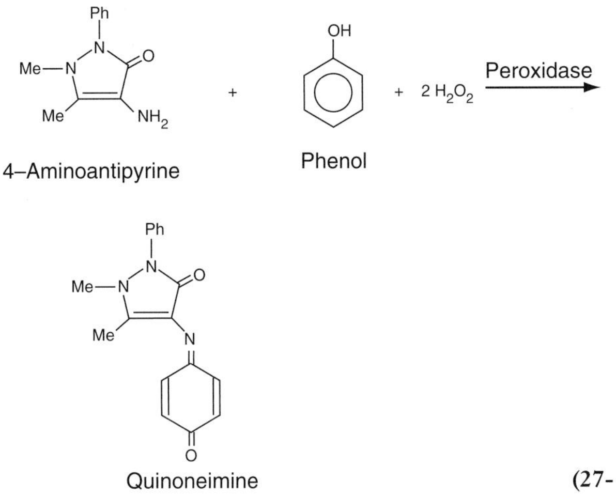

(27-14B)

The Quinoneimine Strategy

H_2O_2 can be reacted, in the presence of a peroxidase, with a phenazone, usually 4-aminoantipyrene, which forms a highly colored quinoneamine dye with phenol, as shown in Equation 27-14, *B*. This is a prototypical reaction in which the phenol is oxidized to the quinone, and in which the exocyclic $–NH_2$ group of 4-aminoantipyrene then adds to the quinone to form a strongly absorbing color complex. Phenol is one of many compounds that can be used to form a quinone or an oxidized aromatic ring, known collectively as Trinder reagents. Several of these are aniline derivatives and include *N*-ethyl-*N*-(2-hydroxy-3-sulfopropyl)-m-toluidine (absorbance is determined at 545 nm) and *N*-(2-hydroxy-3-sulfopropyl)-3,5-dimethoxyaniline, among other, similar compounds. We will have occasion to refer to this set of reactions in determining the concentrations of a number of analytes, in addition to cholesterol, as described in the following section.

For cholesterol determination, H_2O_2 is generated and is reacted with 4-aminoantipyrine and, generally, **phenol** in the presence of a peroxidase to yield the quinoneimine, shown in the previous equation, whose absorbance is determined at 505 nm.

HDL Cholesterol

(Jensen, 2002; Sugiuchi, 1995).

Until relatively recently, methods were used in which LDL or HDL fractions were selectively precipitated and centrifuged, and the cholesterol in the supernatant assayed. For example, to assay HDL cholesterol, fractions containing apo-B proteins as in LDL and very-low-density lipoprotein (VLDL) particles (see Chapter 17) were precipitated using a polyanion and a divalent cation, such as dextran sulfate–$MnCl_2$ or phosphotungstate–$MgCl_2$ combinations. The remaining cholesterol in the supernatant, presumably only HDL cholesterol, was then assayed using the method summarized previously in Equation 27-14. These methods are somewhat time consuming and require manual procedures that cannot be automated.

It was found that enzymes used in the two assays, as shown in Equation 27-14, could be made relatively specific for reacting with HDL cholesterol by the relatively simple expedient of adding polyethylene glycol (PEG 6000) to the free amino groups of basic amino acids of the polypeptide chains of these enzymes. Also, the addition of α-cyclodextran sulfate (average of 6 glucose units with an average of 2 sulfates per glucose unit) in the presence of Mn^{++} ions greatly reduces the reactivity of the cholesterol in LDL, VLDL, and chylomicron fractions. Thus addition of the two PEGylated enzymes with sulfated cyclodextran and $MnCl_2$ allows direct determination of HDL cholesterol. The indicator reaction with H_2O_2 is the same as in Equation 27-14, *B*. The overall method is summarized in Equation 27-15, *A* as follows:

LDL-C + Cyclodextran sulfate + $MnCl_2$ + PEG-cholesterol esterase/cholesterol oxidase → NR
HDL-C + Cyclodextran sulfate + $MnCl_2$ + PEG-cholesterol esterase/cholesterol oxidase → H_2O_2 + 7-α-Hydroxy-4-cholesten-3-one
$2H_2O_2$ + 4-Aminoantipyrene + Phenol or other Trinder reagent → Quinoneimine **(27-15A)**

where NR is no reaction.

LDL Cholesterol

(Nauck, 2002).

The basic strategy for direct determination of LDL cholesterol (LDL-C) is first to add a reagent that protects LDL-C from reacting with the two enzymes cholesterol esterase and cholesterol oxidase, then to react cholesterol from all of the other fractions, so that it is completely consumed, and finally to add a deprotecting agent that allows LDL-C to undergo reaction with the two enzymes. Charged surfactants have been found to block cholesterol in LDL from reacting with the two enzymes cholesterol esterase and oxidase. The release agent is also a surfactant that, in contradistinction to the protecting agent, is neutral.

In practice, two composite reagents are added to serum sequentially. The first contains protective surfactant and polyanions, which block the reaction of LDL-C with cholesterol esterase and oxidase, and catalase, which consumes the H_2O_2 generated in the reactions of all of the non–LDL-C, as summarized in Equation 27-15, *B*. Then a second reagent is added that consists of 4-aminoantipyrene, as described previously, sodium azide, which blocks catalase, peroxidase, the deprotecting surfactant that releases LDL-C, and an appropriate Trinder agent (i.e., chromophore-producing compound that reacts with the 4-aminoantipyrene to form the color complex). These reactions are summarized as follows in Equations 27-15, *B* and 27-15, *C*:

LDL-C + charged surfactant/polyanions + cholesterol esterase/cholesterol oxidase → NR
HDL-C + charged surfactant + cholesterol esterase/cholesterol oxidase → H_2O_2 + 7-α-hydroxy-4-cholesten-3-one
$2H_2O_2$ + catalase → $2H_2O + O_2$ **(27-15B)**

LDL-C/charged surfactant/polyanion + neutral releasing surfactant + cholesterol esterase/cholesterol oxidase + sodium azide-catalase → H_2O_2 + 7-α-hydroxy-4-cholesten-3-one
$2H_2O_2$ + 4-aminoantipyrene + phenol or other trinder reagent → quinoneimine **(27-15C)**

This set of reactions has multiple variations, all of which are based on the overall strategy described here.

Glucose

The most commonly used method to determine serum glucose levels is to induce phosphorylation of glucose, by hexokinase and adenosine triphosphate (ATP), to yield glucose-6-phosphate. By adding glucose-6-phosphate dehydrogenase, glucose-6-phosphate is converted into gluconolactone-6-phosphate (first step in the pentose phosphate pathway). This is an oxidation reaction. NADP is reduced to NADPH, whose absorbance can be determined directly at 340 nm. These reactions are summarized in Equation 27-16.

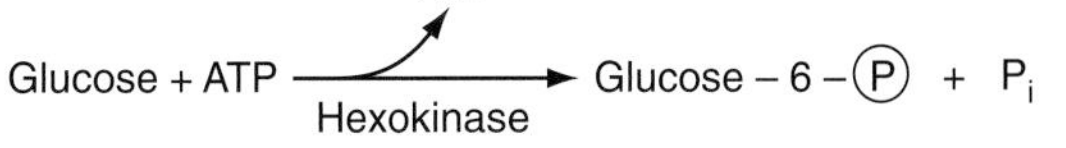

(27-16A)

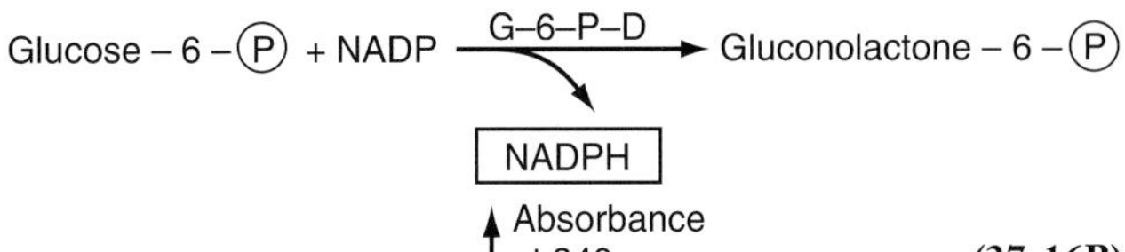

(27-16B)

In Equation 27-16, the circled P represents the phosphate moiety. This reaction sequence is perhaps the one most commonly used. Other methods for glucose determination are also available and are used most commonly in point-of-care testing (Yoo, 2010). In these reactions, glucose oxidase is used to convert glucose to gluconolactone. In this reaction, flavine adenine dinucleotide (FAD) is reduced to $FADH_2$. In the presence of oxygen, FAD is regenerated, and oxygen is reduced to H_2O_2. The latter is oxidized in the presence of a platinum electrode to yield $2H^+ + O_2 + 2e$ (electrons). The electrons flow through a circuit, giving rise to a current, which is proportional to the glucose concentration. Several variants of this strategy may be noted. In one of these, glucose dehydrogenase bound to the dye, pyrroquinolinequinone (PQQ), oxidizes glucose to gluconolactone plus the reduced form of PQQ, which has an intense red color that can be measured spectrophotometrically. Most commonly, the reduced dye is reoxidized and the released electrons measured as current electrochemically, as described earlier. Electrochemical methods for point-of-care testing use whole blood for glucose determination. Thus the hematocrit has an effect on the concentration of glucose that must be included in obtaining the whole blood glucose value (D'Orazio, 2009; Yoo, 2010).

Lactate

As discussed in Chapter 20, lactate reacts almost exclusively with LD, as shown:

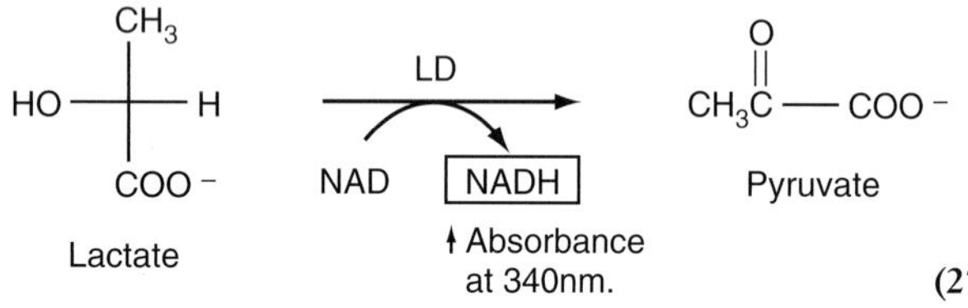

(27-17)

Because NAD is converted to NADH, as shown in the box, the increase in absorbance of NADH at 340 nm is followed until it becomes constant. After subtraction of a blank for background absorbance of the serum sample at 340 nm, the total absorbance is used to compute directly the increased concentration of NADH due to lactate oxidation.

Triglycerides

These are a heterogeneous group of triesters of fatty acids with glycerol (see Chapter 17). The nature of the fatty acid esters can differ widely in terms of chain length, presence and number of unsaturated bonds in the aliphatic chains, and chain arrangement. The strategy for determining triglyceride concentration is to hydrolyze all of the fatty acid esters of triglycerides to produce glycerol. The resulting total concentration of glycerol is taken as the total triglyceride concentration. Technically, this requires the use of a serum blank to determine the level of endogenous glycerol, but the level of glycerol in serum has been found to be quite low, so that these blank determinations are not usually performed (Rifai, 1999).

In the reference method for determining triglyceride concentration, the triglycerides are first extracted into chloroform; the extract is then treated with silicic acid to extract phospholipids from the chloroform extract. The chloroform extract is then treated with strong potassium hydroxide base to hydrolyze all of the fatty acid esters of glycerol in a process referred to as **saponification.** The resulting glycerol is treated with sodium periodate, resulting in the formation of 2 moles of formaldehyde and 1 mole of formic acid. The formaldehyde is then treated with chromotropic acid to obtain a chromogen whose structure has not been proved as yet, but that contains two chromotropic acid molecules linked together by a formaldehyde carbon bridge. This adduct absorbs strongly at 580 nm. Of course, this is a time-consuming, manual method that serves only as a reference method and cannot be automated.

In the automated methods performed directly on serum, triglycerides are hydrolyzed to glycerol plus free fatty acids using lipase. Here we point out that lipase cleaves the fatty acid esters of glycerol at positions 1 and 3 of glycerol but not at position 2. However, the two-acid esters of glycerol spontaneously rearrange to form the one– or three–fatty acid esters that are then hydrolyzed by lipase. This allows complete hydrolysis of the fatty acid esters of glycerol.

To determine the total glycerol concentration, the glycerol is converted by the enzyme α-glycerokinase to form 1-phosphoglycerol. This product is converted, in turn, to dihydroxyacetone by glycerophosphate oxidase in the presence of oxygen. This is an oxidation–reduction reaction that generates H_2O_2, which is used to oxidize phenol or *m*-chlorophenol in the presence of 4-aminoantipyrene to form a conjugated adduct, as described earlier. The absorbance (usually at 505 nm) of this adduct is proportional to the concentration of generated glycerol. These reactions are summarized here:

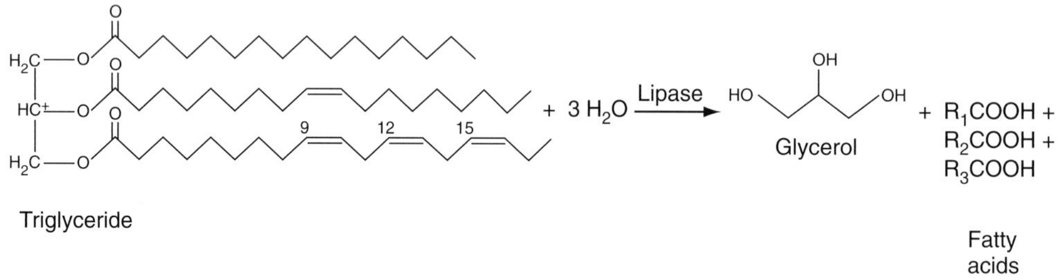

(27-18A)

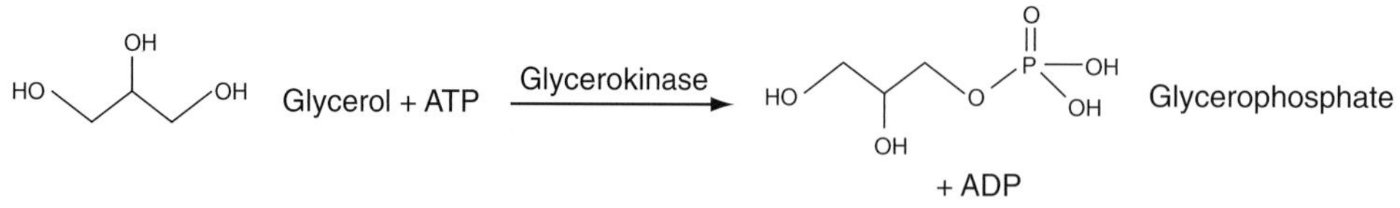

(27-18B)

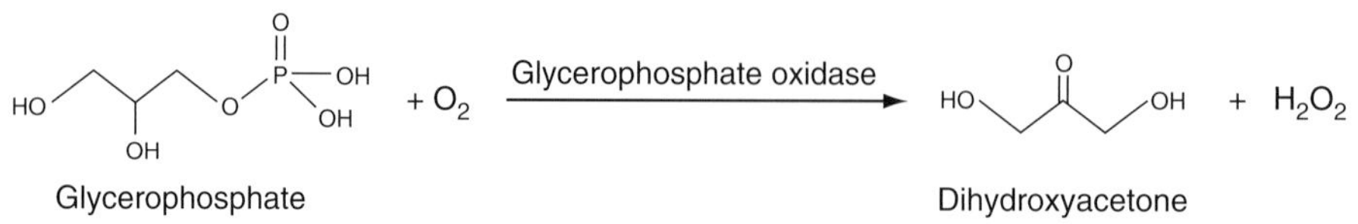

(27-18C)

$$H_2O_2 + \text{4-chlorophenol} + \text{4-aminophenazone} \xrightarrow{\text{Peroxidase}} \text{Colored quinoneimine adduct} \quad \textbf{(27-18D)}$$

Variants of this basic approach include subjecting the glycerophosphate shown in Equation 27-18, *B* to glycerophosphate dehydrogenase to produce dihydroxyacetone phosphate, in a reaction in which NAD is converted into NADH. The NADH can be directly determined at 340 nm.

Urea

The reactions here use ultimately the same GLD enzyme as was described previously for ammonia determination. Here, urea is hydrolyzed into carbon dioxide and ammonia in a reaction catalyzed by the enzyme urease. The resulting ammonia is then reacted with α-ketoglutarate to obtain glutamate in the reductive amination reaction shown in the following equations:

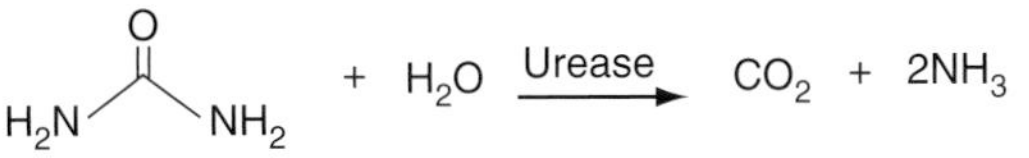

(27-19A)

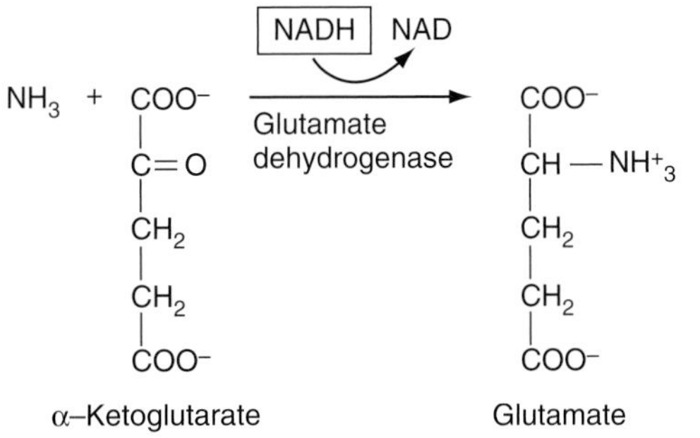

(27-19B)

The use of hemolyzed samples may cause significant interference with this method.

Uric Acid

As shown in Equation 27-20, *A*, uric acid is converted into allantoin by the enzyme uricase.

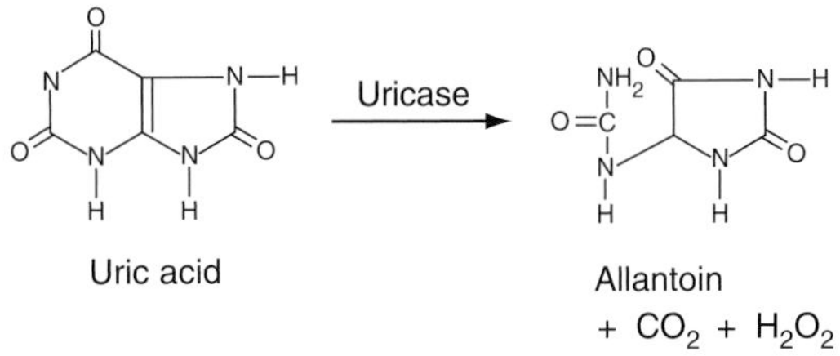

(27-20A)

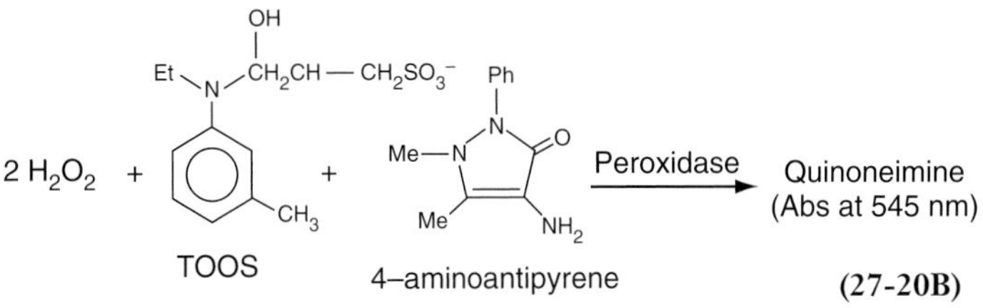

(27-20B)

In this reaction, H_2O_2 is generated. As shown in Equation 27-20, *B*, the resulting H_2O_2 can then be used to oxidize a Trinder reagent, in this case, TOOS (see earlier), which reacts with 4-aminoantipyrene to form a quinoneimine. Another approach is to use the resulting H_2O_2 to oxidize a convenient substrate such as ethyl alcohol to acetaldehyde by the enzyme catalase. The resulting acetaldehyde can then be further oxidized to acetate by the enzyme alcohol dehydrogenase. In this reaction, NADP is converted to NADPH, resulting in increased absorbance at 340 nm.

Assays for Enzymes

Enzyme assays are discussed in Chapter 20. As discussed in that chapter, most enzyme reactions are carried out under saturating conditions in which the substrate concentration is significantly greater than K_M. This ensures that the initial rate of the reaction is proportional to the total enzyme concentration. Most enzyme assay results are expressed in activities (i.e., international units [IU]), with slopes of the plots of product formed versus time, as described in Chapter 20.

ALANINE AMINOTRANSFERASE AND ASPARTATE AMINOTRANSFERASE

ALT

As described in Chapter 21, this enzyme, which is expressed mainly in liver, reversibly catalyzes the transamination reaction between alanine and α-ketoglutarate to obtain pyruvate and glutamate. It is vital that the cofactor B_6, pyridoxal phosphate, be present because it is the moiety that is involved in the actual reaction. As shown in Equation 27-21, *A*, the pyruvate that is produced is then reacted with LD in the presence of NADH to produce lactate. Because in this reaction NADH is converted to NAD, the decrease in absorbance of NADH at 340 nm is measured.

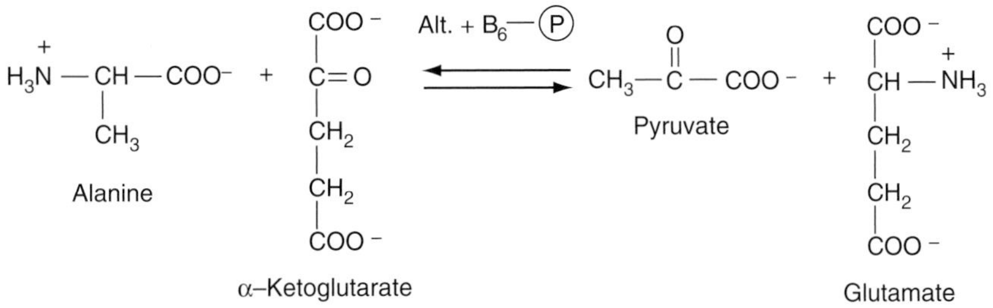

(27-21A)

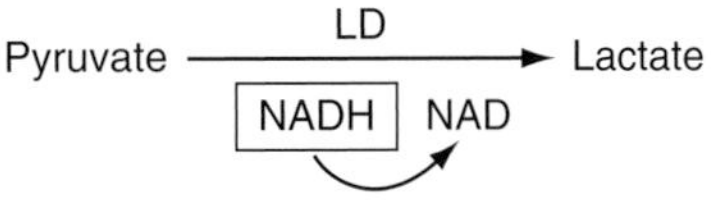

(27-21B)

The use of icteric and lipemic samples may cause significant interference with this method.

AST

As is also described in Chapter 21, this enzyme, which, similar to ALT, requires cofactor B_6 (pyridoxal phosphate), reversibly catalyzes the reaction of aspartic acid with α-ketoglutarate to yield OAA and glutamate. The resulting OAA is then reacted with malate dehydrogenase, which converts the OAA to malate. As in the detection reaction for ALT in the preceding paragraph, NADH is converted to NAD, resulting in decreased absorbance at 340 nm. These reactions are summarized in the following equations.

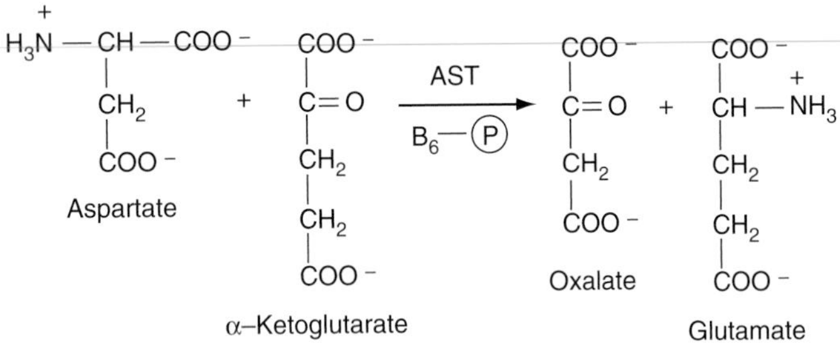

(27-22A)

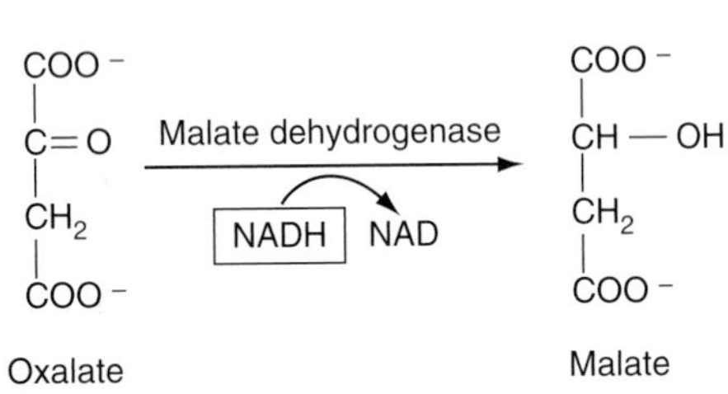

(27-22B)

ALKALINE PHOSPHATASE

As discussed in Chapter 20, the quantitative determination of serum alkaline phosphatase is based on the colorimetric measurement of the rate of formation of *p*-nitrophenol as the *p*-nitrophenoxide anion, a yellow compound, at 410 nm, from hydrolysis of para-nitrophenylphosphate by alkaline phosphatase, as shown in the following equation:

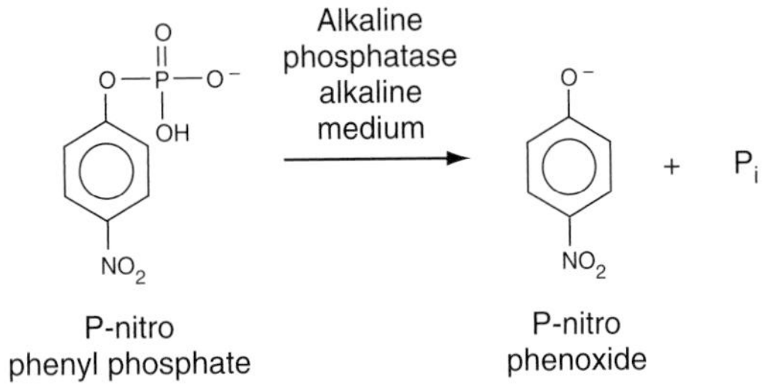

(27-23)

P_i represents inorganic phosphate cleaved from the substrate. The use of hemolyzed specimens may cause significant interference with this method.

AMYLASE

(Moss, 1999).

This enzyme hydrolyzes poly α-1,4-linked glucose polymers, as are found in starch, amylopectin, and glycogen, such that hydrolysis occurs at every second glucose residue. Two types of amylases are known: α and β. β-Amylase cleaves maltose units (glucosyl[α-1,4]glucose) from the reducing to the nonreducing end, as an exoamylase; α-amylase cleaves internally while cleaving from the reducing end of the α-1,4-linked glucose polymer. Serum amylase is of the α type. The two major sources of this enzyme are pancreas and salivary glands. Thus serum amylase levels can be used as markers for pancreatic and salivary gland function. Both strongly homologous isozymes are present in serum. More than 200 methods for assaying of these enzymes have been described. Older methods used starch as the substrate. The glucose polymer forms a well-defined helix in solution. Iodine can bind within this helical structure to form a colored complex. In the presence of amylase, the polymer is degraded, resulting in lower iodine binding and hence less color complex formation. This decrease in color over time can be followed. In addition, as starch is hydrolyzed by amylase, the turbidity of the solution decreases, allowing turbidimetry (see Chapter 4) to be used to measure amylase activity.

Chromogenic substrate polymers of glucose in which a dye is bound covalently to the polymer have been synthesized. In the presence of amylase, the polymer is hydrolyzed, releasing small dye-labeled oligosaccharides. In the Johnson and Johnson slide technology system, the oligosaccharide is bound to an anionic dye—drimarene red Z2B; the dye-labeled oligosaccharides from amylase cleavage diffuse into the reagent layer, where they are bound to a cationic polymer, so that their concentrations can be determined spectrophotometrically. The parent polysaccharide cannot diffuse into this layer and is thus excluded. On Abbott analyzers, the parent polymer is labeled with a fluorescent probe. Because the structure of the long polymer is rigid (a helical structure), the fluorescence is polarized when the probe is stimulated with polarized light. (See Chapter 23 for a description of fluorescence polarization.) When the polymer is hydrolyzed by amylase, probe-bound fragments are released that are much smaller than the parent polymer, and whose "tumbling times" are much faster, resulting in a major decrease in fluorescence polarization. Thus, decreased fluorescence polarization can be followed over time to determine the enzyme activity.

Digestion of glucose polymers by amylase results in the formation of oligosaccharides like maltose and maltotriose (three glucose units in α-1,4 linkage). Oligosaccharides with three or fewer glucose units can be hydrolyzed to glucose with α-glucosidase. The resulting glucose formed can be assayed as described earlier. A problem with this approach is the presence of endogenous glucose. This provides a high blank background. Endogenous glucose can be removed with a gel filtration column, although this does not lend the method to automation.

The methods already discussed use natural polymers of starch or amylopectin as substrates. This leads to the problem of standardization of the substrate material from lot to lot. In addition, the inhomogeneous substrate forms sols in aqueous solution that are easily contaminated. They are temperature sensitive and have limited stability. Newer methods involve the use of synthetic substrates.

In one such method, synthetic maltopentaose (5α-1,4-linked glucose residues) is hydrolyzed by amylase to yield maltotriose and maltose. These are directly hydrolyzed to glucose by α-glucosidase. Because the endogenous glucose background is high, this glucose is removed by a gel filtration column.

To obviate the endogenous glucose problem, synthetic maltotetraose (4α-1,4-linked glucose residues) is used as the substrate. Amylase cleaves this substrate into two maltose units. These are then treated with the enzymes maltose phosphorylase and inorganic phosphate to form glucose-1-phosphate + glucose. Glucose-1-phosphate is then converted to glucose-6-phosphate by phosphoglucomutase. The resulting glucose-6-phosphate is treated with glucose-6-phosphate dehydrogenase, so that the formation of NADPH at 340 nm can be followed over time. It may be noted that, because the glucose-6-phosphate is generated from maltose and not from any endogenous glucose, endogenous glucose does not interfere with this reaction. However, unfortunately, amylase is not completely specific for generating two maltose sugars from maltotetraose and also cleaves the substrate, to a more minor extent, to glucose and maltotriose. Thus for this reason, the assay somewhat underestimates the level of amylase.

Recently, chromogenic substrates have been synthesized. These contain oligo-α-1,4–linked glucose units with 4(or *p*)-nitrophenol (4-NP) in α-acetal linkage to the reducing sugar of the oligosaccharide. In one assay, maltoheptaose (seven glucose units in α-1,4 linkage), attached to 4-NP at its reducing end, is used as the substrate, as illustrated in Figure 27-5. Amylase hydrolyzes this substrate mainly into $(glucose)_4$-NP, $(glucose)_3$-NP, and $(glucose)_2$-NP plus $(glucose)_3$, $(glucose)_4$, and $(glucose)_5$, respectively. These reactions are summarized in the following equations:

$$\text{NP}-(\text{Glucose})_7 \xrightarrow{\text{Amylase}} \text{NP}-(\text{Glucose})_{4,3,2} + (\text{Glucose})_{3,4,5} \qquad \textbf{(27-24A)}$$

$$\text{NP}-(\text{Glucose})_{4,3,2} \xrightarrow{\alpha\text{-Glucosidase}} (4\ \text{glucose} + \text{NP}) + (3\ \text{glucose} + \text{NP}) + (2\ \text{glucose} + \text{NP}) \qquad \textbf{(27-24B)}$$

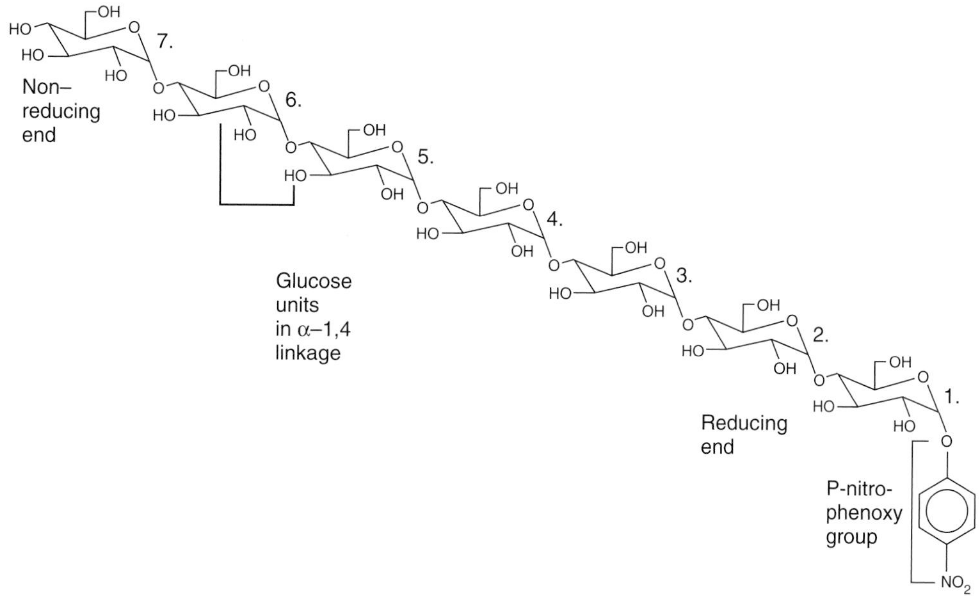

Figure 27-5 Structure of a synthetic substrate for amylase assays. This is the *p*-nitrophenyl glycoside of maltoheptaose. In practice, to enhance reaction specificity and to ensure more efficient cleavage by α-glucosidase, a protecting 4,6-ethylidene or benzylidene group is introduced on the seventh glucose unit on the nonreducing end.

As shown in Equation 27-24, *B*, the –NP-linked fragments are then further degraded with α-glucosidase to yield 4(or *p*)-nitrophenol, which, at alkaline pH, forms the *p*-nitrophenoxide anion that absorbs strongly at 405–410 nm, as discussed previously for alkaline phosphatase.

Note that Equation 27-24 assumes that a limit digest occurs for the tetra-, tri-, and disaccharides, always liberating 1 mole of *p*-nitrophenoxide anion per mole of each saccharide. In practice, this does not occur. In fact, hydrolysis of $(glucose)_4$-NP by α-glucosidase is slow, although the rate can be enhanced by blocking OH-groups of the terminal nonreducing glucose unit. Thus, 4,6-ethylidene, 4,6-benzylidene, and other blocking groups have been found to enhance α-glucosidase activity.

Other problems with this approach include the consideration that the pKa of nitrophenol is close to the pH of the assay reactions, so that only about half of the released *p*-nitrophenol will be present as the oxyanion. In addition, the method is sensitive to ionic strength effects and the concentration of protein present in the assay mixture, both of which affect the pKa of the *p*-nitrophenol. It may also be subjected to interference by hemoglobin.

It has been found that these problems are largely removed by the use of 2-chloro,4-nitrophenol, called **CNP,** in place of 4-NP. Because of the ortho electron-withdrawing property of the o-Cl group, the pKa of the liberated phenol is lowered, so that 100% of it exists as the colored phenoxide anion. It also minimizes the other complications listed above (except hemoglobin interference), and, because it is a better leaving group in the mechanism of α-glucosidase–induced hydrolysis, higher yields of the smaller saccharides, and thus of CNP, are obtained, allowing for higher yields of the colored final product.

CREATINE KINASE

As discussed in Chapter 20, creatine kinase reversibly catalyzes the reaction between creatine and ATP to yield creatine phosphate and adenosine diphosphate (ADP). This reaction occurs prominently in muscle tissue, allowing for storage of the so-called **high-energy phosphate bond** as creatine phosphate. For the purposes of the enzyme assay, the reaction is reversed (i.e., ADP and creatine phosphate are added to the sample to generate ATP + creatine). The product, ATP, is coupled into hexokinase–glucose-6-phosphate dehydrogenase reactions and generates NADPH, as shown in the equations that follow. The creatine kinase activity is proportional to the absorbance increase in NADPH at 340 nm.

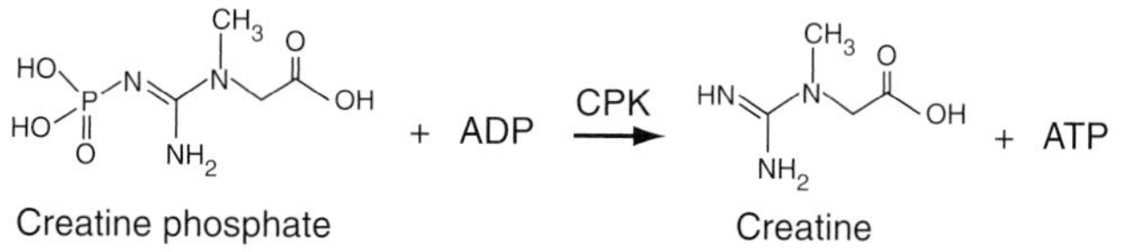

(27-25A)

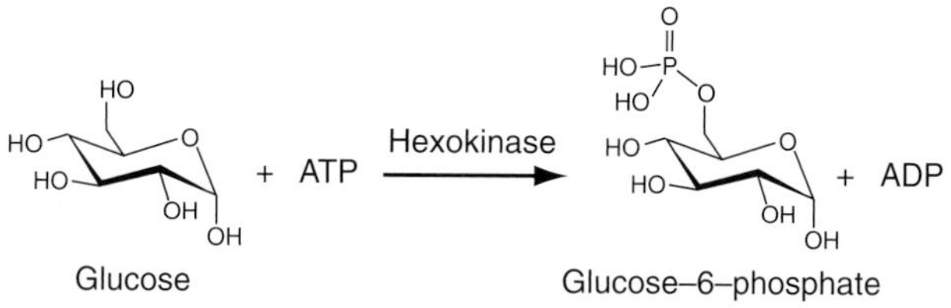

(27-25B)

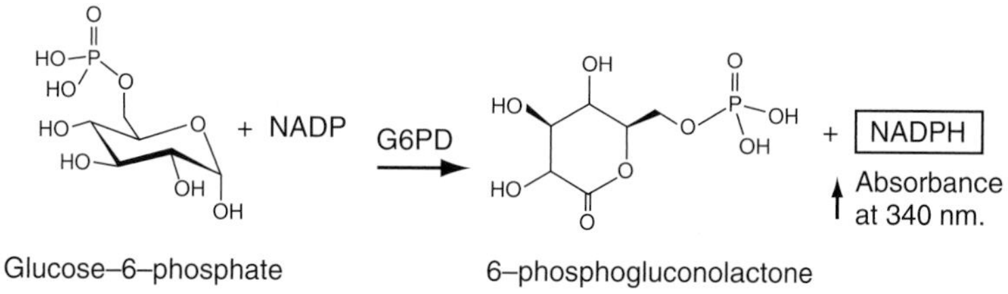

(27-25C)

The use of hemolyzed samples may cause significant interference with this method and should be avoided.

γ-GLUTAMYL TRANSFERASE

This enzyme occurs on the canalicular surface of the hepatocyte (see Fig. 21-3) and catalyzes the transfer of the γ-glutamyl residue of glutathione (γ-glutamyl-cysteinyl-glycine) to another amino acid, or to an exogenous agent such as a drug. As it happens, GGT transfers the γ-glutamyl residue from the synthetic substrate L-γ-glutamyl-3-carboxy-4-nitroanilide to glycylglycine to yield γ-glutamyl-glycylglycine and free 5-amino-2-nitrobenzoate (ANB), as shown in the equation below. Free ANB, which is a substituted aniline, absorbs at 410 nm. The rate of formation of ANB is measured as the increase in absorbance at 410 nm divided by the time interval over which it is measured, directly yielding GGT activity.

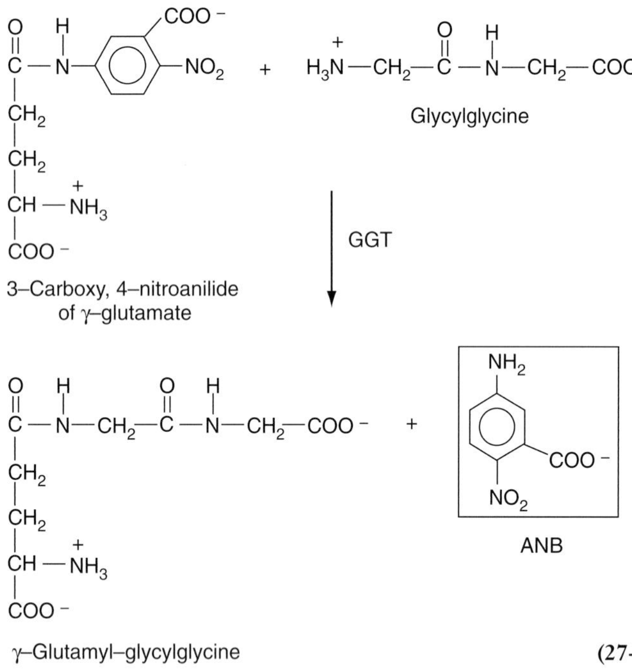

(27-26)

LACTATE DEHYDROGENASE

This enzyme, the reactions that it catalyzes, and assays for this enzyme are discussed in Chapter 20. Here we note that the reaction scheme shown in Equation 27-17 for the assay for lactate is the same scheme as for the assay for LD. In this case, lactate is added to the serum sample at a concentration above its K_M, and the activity is determined by the rate of increase of NADH absorbance at 340 nm.

LIPASE

As discussed previously, lipases cleave fatty esters of glycerol, and, as discussed in Chapters 17 and 22, there are several isozymes of lipase, including pancreatic lipase, intestinal lipase, lipoprotein lipase, and gastric lipase. The first three of these forms have strong homology to one another and significantly less homology to the gastric isozyme. These lipases hydrolyze triglycerides that are long-chain fatty acid esters of glycerol. In addition, aryl and aliesterases hydrolyze short-chain fatty acid esters and such simple esters as ethylacetate (aliesterase) and phenyl acetate (arylesterase) (Moss, 1999). In serum, pancreatic lipase is very much the predominant form. Thus, assays for lipase are used for the purpose of evaluating pancreatic function.

To be active, all lipases require a water–fat emulsion interface, the emulsion containing the substrate triglycerides. To attach to this interface, lipase requires the presence of a detergent, like cholate, and another protein to which it binds, colipase. The latter binds both to lipase and to the detergent–emulsion complex, allowing lipase to interact with the trigycerides. Thus, all assay mixtures for lipase must contain both the detergent and the colipase.

Assays for lipase can be performed by adding long-chain fatty acid esters to serum, and the reaction monitored titrimetrically. In this case, dilute sodium hydroxide solution is added to serum to neutralize the long-chain fatty acids that are released, but the pH of the reaction mixture is maintained constant. The amount of base added over a given time period is a measure of the increased concentration of fatty acids over the time period, yielding a rate that should be proportional to the total lipase concentration. The long-chain fatty acids used are contained in olive oil that has been treated to remove contaminating substances. This approach is also used with the pure triglyceride triolein as the substrate.

Although this is a reference method, it is difficult to adapt to continuously used autoanalyzers. Thus other approaches have been devised. In one of these, 1-oleoyl-2,3-diacetyl glycerol is hydrolyzed by lipase to yield oleic acid and diacetylglycerol. The latter is then reacted with an enzyme called *diacetinase* that hydrolyzes the two acetyl esters to yield glycerol and 2 moles of acetate. The glycerol generated in this reaction sequence is then treated with α-glycerol kinase + ATP, and the reaction sequences shown in Equations 27-18B through 27-18D are then carried out. In a variant of this sequence, a 1,2-diacylglycerol is used as the substrate to yield the 2-acylglycerol that is then hydrolyzed by monoglyceride lipase (to accelerate the reaction) to yield glycerol that is subjected to the reactions described earlier.

A recently developed assay for lipase that is being used successfully utilizes the artificial substrate for lipase,1,2-O-dilauryl-rac-glycero-3-glutaric acid-(6′-methylresorufin) ester, as shown in Figure 27-6. Lipase cleaves this substrate such that it generates 1,2-O-dilauryl-rac-glycerol and an unstable intermediate, the hemi-glutaric acid-(6′-methylresorufin) ester, which spontaneously degrades to glutaric acid and methylresorufin. The oxyanion of this dye that forms under basic conditions is red and strongly absorbs at 580 nm. Thus the absorbance increase in the red methylresorufin at 580 or 581 nm is proportional to the lipase activity. These reactions are summarized in Figure 27-6.

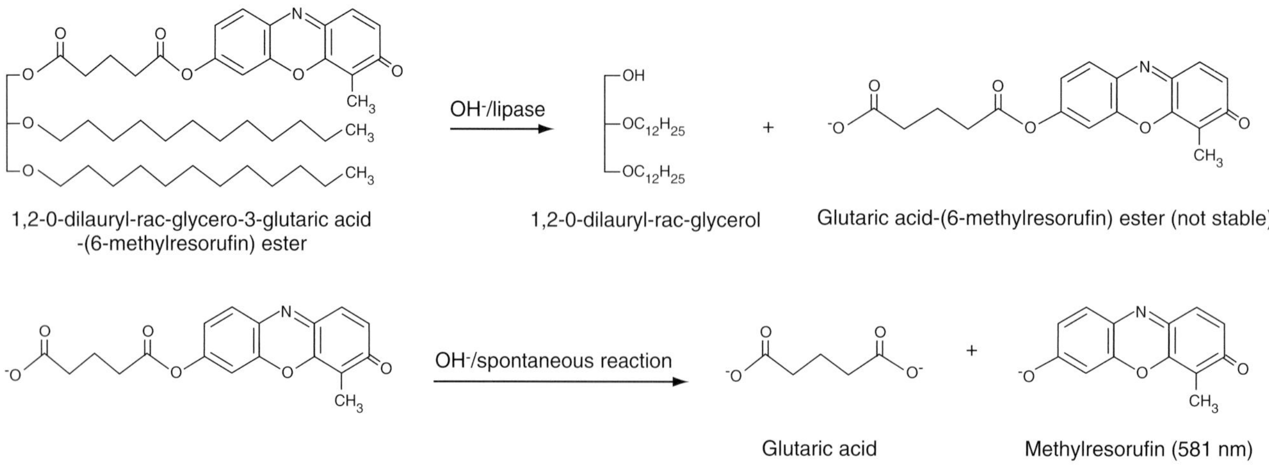

Figure 27-6 Artificial substrate for serum lipase resulting in liberation of methylresorufin, whose absorbance can be determined at 580 nm.

To obtain soluble substrates for lipase, artificial substrates with shorter-chain fatty acids are used. One of these is butyrin, the triester of *n*-butyric acid with glycerol. The glycerol generated by lipase is subjected to the reactions described previously. In a variant of this approach, the *n*-butyric acid ester of 2,3-dimercapto-1-ol, that is, a dithioester, is used. The limit digest of this substrate by lipase is 2,3-dimercapto-1-propanol. The two vicinal –SH groups can then be reacted with Ellman's reagent, 5,5′-dithio-bis-(2-nitrobenzoic acid), to form a color complex that absorbs strongly at 412 nm. A problem with the use of these shorter-chain substrates is that they are also substrates for the ali- and arylesterases in serum (Moss, 1999). To block the reaction of these enzymes, the covalent inhibitor phenylmethylsulfonylfluoride is added; this compound is a strong esterase (but not lipase) inhibitor.

PART 2

SELECTED REFERENCES

Jensen T, Truong, Q, Frandsen M, Dinesen B, Stender S. Comparison of a homogeneous assay with a precipitation method for the measurement of HDL cholesterol in diabetic patients. Diabetes Care 2002;25:1914–18.

This paper is an important study that compares a homogeneous method with an immunoprecipitation method for determination of LDL cholesterol.

Kroli MH, Roach NA, Poe B, Elln RJ. Mechanism of interference with the Jaffe reaction for creatinine. Clin Chem 1987;33:1129–32.

This is an interesting paper that presents possible structures for the creatinine–picrate complex and explains how ketones can interfere with this reaction.

Lin J-LJ, Hsu H-Y. Study of sodium ion selective electrodes and differential structures with anodized indium tin oxide. Sensors 2010;10:1798–809.

This paper presents a new, highly selective ion-selective electrode for sodium and illustrates how ion-selective electrodes are developed.

Nauck M, Warnick GR, Rifai N. Methods for measurement of LDL-cholesterol: a critical assessment of direct measurement by homogeneous assays versus calculation. Clin Chem 2002;48:236–54.

This paper is a concise summary of direct homogeneous methods for the quantitative determination of LDL cholesterol; it explains how results attained with these methods compare with those reported when the Friedwald calculation of LDL cholesterol is used.

Sugiuchi H, Uji Y, Okabe H, et al. Direct measurement of high-density lipoprotein cholesterol in serum with polyethylene glycol-modified enzymes and sulfated α-cyclodextrin. Clin Chem 1995;41:717–23.

This paper explains the basis for the homogeneous (direct) determination of HDL cholesterol.

REFERENCES

Access the complete reference list online at http://www.expertconsult.com

PART 3

Urine and Other Body Fluids

EDITED BY

Richard A. McPherson
Gregory A. Threatte
Matthew R. Pincus

CHAPTER 28

BASIC EXAMINATION OF URINE

Richard A. McPherson, Jonathan Ben-Ezra

KEY POINTS

- Many different diseases can display abnormalities in the urine. Therefore, examination of the urine is an important laboratory function.
- Basic urinalysis consists of gross examination of the urine, as well as a dipstick analysis for blood, white cells, sugar, and other substances. The dipstick may be read manually or by an automated instrument.
- A microscopic analysis of urine may be necessary in many cases. This is done to detect cellular elements, casts, and crystals. Each of these items can be caused by several different disease states.
- Although microscopic examination of the urine is usually performed manually, several automated instruments can perform this analysis.
- Red blood cells within the urine can come from any point along the urinary tract. Dysmorphic red blood cells are often a sign of glomerular disease.
- The first voided morning urine, because it is the most concentrated, is often the best specimen for analysis. Some procedures may require a 12- or 24-hour urine sample.
- Specific gravity and osmolality measurements reflect the concentrating ability of the kidneys. After a period of dehydration, the osmolality should be three to four times that of plasma.
- Proteinuria greater than 4 g/day is seen in the nephrotic syndrome. Although nephrotic syndrome is usually seen in primary renal disease, it is occasionally seen in a systemic disease that affects the kidneys.
- Ketonuria can be seen in diabetic individuals. It can also be seen in other states, such as febrile illness and cachexia.
- The dipstick nitrite and leukocyte esterase tests are used to help diagnose urinary tract infection. Positive results should be confirmed by microscopic analysis of the urine.
- Urinary calculi are most commonly formed from calcium. Workup of habitual stone formers should include analysis of both the urine and the stone.

A significant amount of information can be obtained through the examination of urine. Careful examination enables the detection of disease processes intrinsic to the urinary system, both functional (physiologic) and structural (anatomic), and sometimes unsuspected (Takemura, 2000). The progression or regression of various lesions can be monitored with only minimal distress to the patient. Furthermore, systemic disease processes, such as endocrine or metabolic abnormalities, can be detected through the recognition of abnormal quantities of disease-specific metabolites excreted in the urine. Laboratory urine tests will continue to play an essential role in clinical medicine.

The purpose of this chapter is to highlight the pertinent information that can be provided by the most common urine tests. Two main types of urinalysis are currently performed. These include (1) the dipstick (reagent strip) urinalysis, which is commonly performed in screening laboratories, in physician offices, and as patient home testing; and (2) the basic (routine) urinalysis, which adds a microscopic examination of urine sediment to the reagent strip urinalysis. These examinations utilize various laboratory disciplines, particularly chemistry and microscopy. In addition to these front-line diagnostic procedures, new technologies including immunocytochemistry, molecular diagnostics, DNA ploidy, and cell cycle analysis are constantly evolving to provide additional diagnostic and prognostic information. Urine microbiology studies, crucial to the diagnosis of infectious pathogens of the urinary tract, are addressed elsewhere in this text. It is important to remember that each of these modalities has a certain clinical utility. Table 28-1 lists the benefits of commonly ordered urine laboratory examinations.

Dipstick urinalysis provides information about multiple physicochemical properties of urine. Used predominantly in screening, dipstick testing requires less sophisticated training of personnel, and results are obtainable in only a few minutes. It has been shown that in certain situations, particularly when evaluating patients with signs or symptoms that prompt a urinalysis for the detection of blood or infection, urinalysis dipsticks can be substituted for a full routine urinalysis, with urine microscopy reserved for patients with discordance between clinical presentation and dipstick results (Jou, 1998). The routine urinalysis consists of two major components: (1) physicochemical determinations (appearance, specific

TABLE 28-1
Benefits of Common Urine Laboratory Tests

Type of test	Aims	CLINICAL UTILITY			
		Screen	Diagnosis	Monitor	Prognosis
Urine chemistry (reagent strip)	Glucosuria Proteinuria Hematuria Leukocyturia Infection	+++	+	+	+
Wet urinalysis (routine)	Diabetes Proteinuria Hematuria Leukocyturia Infections Cylindruria Crystalluria	++++	++	++	+
Urine microbiology	Infections	++	++++	++	+
Urine cytology (conventional)	Cancer Inflammation Viral infections	+	++	+	–
Cytodiagnostic urinalysis	Glomerular and renal tubular disorders LUT disorders Nonbacterial infections Lithiasis	+	++++	+++	++
Image cytometry and DNA analysis	Urothelial cancer	–	++	+++	+++
Flow cytometry	Urothelial cancer	–	+	+++	++

From Schumann GB, Schumann JL, Marcussen N. Cytodiagnostic urinalysis of renal and lower urinary tract disorders. New York: Igaku-Shoin Medical Publishers; 1995, with permission.
LUT, Lower urinary tract; –, negative; +, low positive; ++++, strongly positive.

gravity, and reagent strip measurements), and (2) a bright-field or phase-contrast microscopic examination of urine sediment for evidence of hematuria, pyuria, casts (cylindruria), and crystalluria. The latter examination is typically more time consuming and necessitates expertise in microscopy for an accurate interpretation; however, instrumentation is now available that automates routine urinalysis partially or completely. Cytopathologic urine sediment examination also requires special training and is the mainstay for diagnosis and follow-up of urinary tract neoplasms, as well as some nonneoplastic conditions, particularly renal allograft rejection.

We present in detail the pertinent components of the routine urinalysis. Various methods, including sample preparation, reagent strip reactions, confirmatory testing, and microscopic methods, are briefly reviewed. Major emphasis is given to clinicopathologic correlations related to the laboratory findings obtained from these urine tests.

Urine Formation

In the normal adult, approximately 1200 mL of blood perfuses the kidneys each minute, which accounts for about 25% of the cardiac output. The glomeruli (normally numbering at least 1 million per kidney) receive blood through afferent arterioles, and an ultrafiltrate of the plasma passes through each glomerulus into Bowman's space. From here, the filtrate is passed through the tubules and collecting ducts, where reabsorption or secretion of various substances and the concentration of urine can occur. Ultimately, the original glomerular filtrate volume of about 180 L in 24 hours is reduced to about 1–2 L, depending on the status of hydration. This urine formed in the kidneys passes from the collecting ducts into the renal pelvis, ureters, bladder, and urethra to be voided.

The kidneys take part in several regulatory functions. Through glomerular filtration and tubular secretion, numerous waste products, including nitrogenous products of protein catabolism, and both organic and inorganic acids and bases, are eliminated from the body. Fluid, electrolytes (including sodium, potassium, calcium, and magnesium), and acid-base status are regulated in homeostasis. Furthermore, the kidneys provide important hormonal regulation with erythropoietin and renin production, as well as vitamin D activation. Any derangement of these functions by renal or systemic disease can be reflected as chemically or cytologically altered urine.

Components of Basic (Routine) Urinalysis

The basic (routine) urinalysis consists of four parts: specimen evaluation, gross/physical examination, chemical screening, and sediment examination.

SPECIMEN EVALUATION

Before one proceeds with any examination, the urine specimen must be evaluated in terms of its acceptability. Considerations include proper labeling, proper specimen for the requested examination, proper preservative, visible signs of contamination, and whether any transportation delays may have caused significant deterioration. Each laboratory should have written and enforced guidelines for the acceptance or rejection of specimens. A properly labeled specimen must have the patient's full name and the date and time of collection. Additional information may be required by the institution, but these three essentials constitute minimum labeling requirements.

The first voided morning urine, which is the most concentrated, is best for routine urinalysis. At times, a catheterized specimen or suprapubic collected urine specimen is received. If a single specimen is submitted for multiple measurements, bacteriologic examination should be done first, provided that the urine has been properly collected. With pediatric patients and persons in acute renal failure, only a small volume of urine may be available for processing, and in such cases, a notation should be made and the measurements most pertinent to the diagnosis should be performed first. For quantitative measurements, timed (12- or 24-hour) urinary collection is preferred to random specimens.

GROSS/PHYSICAL EXAMINATION

Appearance

Some of the more important changes in the gross appearance of urine are described in this section. A comprehensive list is provided in Table 28-2.

Color

The yellow color of urine is due largely to the pigment urochrome, excretion of which is generally proportional to the metabolic rate. It is increased

TABLE 28-2
Appearance and Color of Urine

Appearance	Cause	Remarks
Colorless	Very dilute urine	Polyuria, diabetes insipidus
Cloudy	Phosphates, carbonates	Soluble in dilute acetic acid
	Urates, uric acid	Dissolve at 60° C and in alkali
	Leukocytes	Insoluble in dilute acetic acid
	Red cells ("smoky")	Lyse in dilute acetic acid
	Bacteria, yeasts	Insoluble in dilute acetic acid
	Spermatozoa	Insoluble in dilute acetic acid
	Prostatic fluid	
	Mucin, mucous threads	May be flocculent
	Calculi, "gravel"	Phosphates, oxalates
	Clumps, pus, tissue	
	Fecal contamination	Rectovesical fistula
	Radiographic dye	In acid urine
Milky	Many neutrophils (pyuria)	Insoluble in dilute acetic acid
	Fat	
	Lipiduria, opalescent	Nephrosis, crush injury—soluble in ether
	Chyluria, milky	Lymphatic obstruction—soluble in ether
	Emulsified paraffin	Vaginal creams
Yellow	Acriflavine	Green fluorescence
Yellow-orange	Concentrated urine	Dehydration, fever
	Urobilin in excess	No yellow foam
	Bilirubin	Yellow foam if sufficient bilirubin
Yellow-green	Bilirubin-biliverdin	Yellow foam
Yellow-brown	Bilirubin-biliverdin	"Beer" brown, yellow foam
Red	Hemoglobin	Positive } Reagent strip for blood
	Erythrocytes	Positive } Reagent strip for blood
	Myoglobin	Positive } Reagent strip for blood
	Porphyrin	May be colorless
	Fuscin, aniline dye	Foods, candy
	Beets	Yellow alkaline, genetic
	Menstrual contamination	Clots, mucus
Red-purple	Porphyrins	May be colorless
Red-brown	Erythrocytes	
	Hemoglobin on standing	
	Methemoglobin	Acid pH
	Myoglobin	Muscle injury
	Bilifuscin (dipyrrole)	Result of unstable hemoglobin
Brown-black	Methemoglobin	Blood, acid pH
	Homogentisic acid	On standing, alkaline; alkaptonuria
	Melanin	On standing, rare
Blue-green	Indicans	Small intestine infections
	Pseudomonas infections	
	Chlorophyll	Mouth deodorants

during fever, thyrotoxicosis, and starvation. Small quantities of urobilins and uroerythrin (pink pigment) also contribute to urine coloration. In normal individuals, both pale and dark yellow urine can be produced, and these differences are rough indicators of hydration and urine concentration. Pale urine, typically of low specific gravity, is excreted following high fluid intake; darker urine is seen when fluids are withheld. Note that pale urine of high specific gravity may be found in diabetes mellitus. For color changes of urine in pediatric patients, see Cone (1968). Table 28-3 lists the urine color changes associated with commonly used drugs.

Red Urine. The most common abnormal color is red or red-brown. When seen in females, menstrual flow contamination should be considered. Hematuria (presence of red blood cells [RBCs]), hemoglobinuria, and myoglobinuria may produce pink, red, or red-brown coloration. All three of these conditions are easily detectable on reagent strip testing; however, further evaluation is necessary for absolute differentiation (see later under Blood, Hemoglobin, Hemosiderin, and Myoglobin in Urine).

In the porphyrias, urine coloration is variable. It is usually red in congenital erythropoietic porphyria and porphyria cutanea tarda, but in lead porphyrinuria, the urine color is generally normal. In acute intermittent hepatic porphyria, it is normal but darkens on standing. Red urine also may be associated with the use of drugs and dyes in diagnostic tests, for example, phenolsulfonphthalein, which is sometimes used in assessing renal function, will cause a red color in alkaline urine. Patients with an unstable hemoglobin may produce urine with red-brown color that does not give a positive indication of hemoglobin or bilirubin. The pigment is probably a dipyrrole or bilifuscin. An innocuous red urine associated with ingestion of beets is seen in genetically susceptible persons.

Yellow-Brown or Green-Brown Urine. Yellow-brown or green-brown urine is generally associated with bile pigments, chiefly bilirubin. On shaking the urine specimen, a yellow foam may be seen, which distinguishes bilirubin from a normal, dark, concentrated urine, which will have white foam. In severe obstructive jaundice, the urine may be dark green.

Orange-Red or Orange-Brown Urine. Excreted urobilinogen is colorless but is converted in the presence of light and low pH to urobilin, which is dark yellow to orange. Urobilin will not color the foam on shaking, and in this way may be confused with a concentrated normal urine; reagent strip testing would be confirmatory in this situation.

Dark Brown or Black Urine. Acid urine containing hemoglobin will darken on standing because of the formation of methemoglobin. "Cola-colored" urine may be seen with rhabdomyolysis (Keverline, 1998) and in some patients taking L-dopa. Rarer causes of dark brown urine are homogentisic acid (alkaptonuria) and melanin. Urine-containing homogentisic acid will darken more rapidly when alkaline.

Clarity (Character)

Urine is normally clear, and the presence of particulate material in an unspun specimen warrants further investigation. The differential diagnosis for cloudy urine is broad and includes several nonpathologic entities. Turbidity may simply be due to the precipitation of crystals or nonpathologic salts referred to as amorphous. Phosphate, ammonium urate, and carbonate can precipitate in alkaline urine; these redissolve when acetic acid is added. Uric acid and urates cause a white, pink, or orange cloud in acid urine and redissolve on warming to 60° C.

Cloudy urine can be attributed to the presence of various cellular elements. Leukocytes may form a white cloud similar to that caused by phosphates, but the cloud remains after acidification. Likewise, bacterial growth may cause a uniform opalescence that is not removed by acidification or by filtration, and it has been suggested that turbidimetric assessment using a double-beam turbidimeter may be useful for urine infection screening (Livsey, 1995). Turbidity may also be due to RBCs, epithelial cells, spermatozoa, or prostatic fluid. Prostatic fluid normally contains a few leukocytes and other formed elements.

Miscellaneous causes for cloudy urine include mucus from the lower urinary tract or genital tract, blood clots, menstrual discharge, and other particulate material such as pieces of tissue, small calculi, clumps of pus, and fecal material. Fecal material in urine may occur with a fistulous connection between the colon or rectum and bladder. Contamination with powders or with antiseptics that become opaque with water (phenols) will also cause a turbid urine.

Chyluria. This is a rare condition in which the urine contains lymph. It is associated with obstruction to lymph flow and rupture of lymphatic vessels into the renal pelvis, ureters, bladder, or urethra. Although parasitic infection with *Wuchereria bancrofti* (filariasis) is the prevailing cause (Cortvriend, 1998), abdominal lymph node enlargement and tumors have also been associated with chyluria. Even with filariasis, this condition is rare.

The appearance of the urine varies with the amount of lymph present, ranging from clear to opalescent or milky. Clots may form, and if sufficient lymph is present, the urine may layer with the chylomicrons on top, and fibrin and cells beneath. Chylomicrons may not be apparent microscopically unless they have coalesced as microglobules. This fatty material can be extracted from urine using an equal volume of ether or chloroform. Urine phosphates, in contradistinction, will not clear with this method. Pseudochyluria occurs with the use of paraffin-based vaginal creams for the treatment of *Candida* infection.

Lipiduria. Fat globules appear in the urine most often with the nephrotic syndrome; these consist of neutral fats (triglycerides) and cholesterol. Lipiduria can also be present in patients who have sustained skeletal trauma with fractures to major long bones or the pelvis. Presumably, the source of lipid is exposed fatty marrow. Keep in mind that in addition to these endogenous lipids, oily contaminants such as paraffin may float on the

TABLE 28-3
Urine Color Changes with Commonly Used Drugs*

Drug	Color
Alcohol, ethyl	Pale, diuresis
Anthraquinone laxatives (senna, cascara)	Reddish, alkaline; yellow-brown, acid
Chlorzoxazone (Paraflex) (muscle relaxant)	Red
Deferoxamine mesylate (Desferal) (chelates iron)	Red
Ethoxazene (Serenium) (urinary analgesic)	Orange, red
Fluorescein sodium (given IV)	Yellow
Furazolidone (Furoxone) (Tricofuron) (an antibacterial, antiprotozoal nitrofuran)	Brown
Indigo carmine dye (renal function, cytoscopy)	Blue
Iron sorbitol (Jectofer) (possibly other iron compounds forming iron sulfide in urine)	Brown on standing
Levodopa (L-dopa) (for parkinsonism)	Red then brown, alkaline
Mepacrine (Atabrine) (antimalarial) (intestinal worms, *Giardia)*	Yellow
Methocarbamol (Robaxin) (muscle relaxant)	Green-brown
Methyldopa (Aldomet) (antihypertensive)	Darkens; if oxidizing agents present, red to brown
Methylene blue (used to delineate fistulas)	Blue, blue-green
Metronidazole (Flagyl) (for *Trichomonas* infection, amebiasis, *Giardia*)	Darkening, reddish brown
Nitrofurantoin (Furadantin) (antibacterial)	Brown-yellow
Phenazopyridine (Pyridium) (urinary analgesic), also compounded with sulfonamides (Azo Gantrisin, etc.)	Orange-red, acid pH
Phenindione (Hedulin) (anticoagulant) (important to distinguish from hematuria)	Orange, alkaline; color disappears on acidifying
Phenol poisoning	Brown; oxidized to quinones (green)
Phenolphthalein (purgative)	Red-purple, alkaline pH
Phenolsulfonphthalein (also sulfobromophthalein)	Pink-red, alkaline pH
Rifampin (Rifadin, Rimactane) (tuberculosis therapy)	Bright orange-red
Riboflavin (multivitamins)	Bright yellow
Sulfasalazine (Azulfidine) (for ulcerative colitis)	Orange-yellow, alkaline pH

*Other commonly used drugs have been noted to produce color change once or occasionally: amitriptyline (Elavil)—blue-green; phenothiazines—red; triamterene (Dyrenium)—pale blue (blue fluorescence in acid urine). An extensive list may be found in Young et al. Clin Chem 1975;21:379.

urine surface. Microscopic examination of the urine may be required to classify fatty materials as Oil Red O positive droplets or cholesterol esters with polarization.

Odor

Urine normally will have a faint, aromatic odor of undetermined source. Specimens with extensive bacterial overgrowth can be recognized by an ammoniacal, fetid odor. Additionally, ingestion of asparagus or thymol produces distinctive odors in urine.

Characteristic urine odors associated with amino acid disorders include the following:

Isovaleric acidemia and glutaric acidemia	Sweaty feet
Maple syrup urine disease (MSUD)	Maple syrup
Methionine malabsorption	Cabbage, hops
Phenylketonuria	Mousy
Trimethylaminuria	Rotting fish
Tyrosinemia	Rancid

Lack of odor in urine from patients with acute renal failure suggests acute tubular necrosis rather than prerenal failure.

Urine Volume

Under ordinary conditions, the main determinant of urine volume is water intake. The average adult produces from 600–2000 mL of urine per day, with night urine generally not in excess of 400 mL. In pregnancy, the usual diurnal variation may be reversed. Young children, compared with adults, may excrete about three to four times as much urine per kilogram of body weight. Measurement of urine output during timed intervals may be valuable in clinical diagnosis.

Increases in Urine Volume

Production of more than 2000 mL of urine in 24 hours is termed **polyuria; nocturia** is excretion of more than 500 mL of urine at night with a specific gravity of less than 1.018. In general, high volumes of urine tend to result in a low specific gravity.

Excessive intake of water (polydipsia) will result in polyuria, as will consumption of certain drugs with a diuretic effect, such as caffeine, alcohol, thiazides, and other diuretics. Intravenous solutions may increase the urine output. Increased salt intake and high-protein diets will require more water for excretion.

Pathologic states that result in excess renal fluid loss/urine excretion can be divided into three groups.

Defective Hormonal Regulation of Volume Homeostasis. Diabetes insipidus can be due to a deficiency (central/pituitary variety) of, or renal unresponsiveness (nephrogenic) to, antidiuretic hormone. In either situation, excessive thirst and water intake occur, together with marked polyuria and nocturia. Up to 15 L of urine per day may be produced.

Defective Renal Salt/Water Absorption. This can be due to the administration of diuretic agents, or an abnormality of the renal tubules, resulting in sodium wasting or impairment of the countercurrent mechanism. In progressive chronic renal failure, functioning renal tissue is diminished, and the ability to concentrate urine is gradually lost. To excrete the daily renal water and solute load, an increase in urine volume per residual nephron results, and the urine eventually becomes isoosmotic with the plasma ultrafiltrate.

Osmotic Diuresis. In diabetes mellitus with hyperglycemia, an excessive amount of glucose is excreted, causing a solute diuresis.

Decreases in Urine Volume

Oliguria is the excretion of less than 500 mL of urine per 24 hours, and anuria is the near-complete suppression of urine formation. Water deprivation will cause a decrease in urine volume even before signs of dehydration appear. Oliguria can be rather abrupt in onset, as can acute renal failure, or it may be due to a chronic progressive renal disease. In either case, retention of nitrogenous waste products (azotemia) can occur (see Chapter 14).

The causes of acute renal failure are classically categorized as follows.

Prerenal. Loss of intravascular volume may result from hemorrhage, or from dehydration associated with prolonged diarrhea, vomiting, excess sweating, or severe burns. So-called **third spacing** is the shifting of intravascular fluids to extracellular spaces. Additionally, conditions such as congestive heart failure, sepsis, anaphylaxis, or renal artery embolic occlusion may result in a decrease in renal blood flow.

Postrenal. Bilateral hydronephrosis, resulting from high-grade or long-standing obstruction of the urinary tract, may be associated with a marked decrease in urine flow and even anuria. This can occur with prostatic hyperplasia and carcinoma. Bilateral ureteral obstruction due to stones, clots, and sloughed tissue, and urethral obstruction due to stricture or valves, are other forms of obstruction. The anuria associated with sulfonamide therapy and dehydration is due to obstruction caused by the precipitation of crystals in the renal tubules when the urinary pH is acidic.

Renal Parenchymal Disease. This should be considered after other prerenal and postrenal causes of oliguria have been ruled out. The list of conditions is extensive and includes various vascular disorders, glomerulonephritis, interstitial nephritis, and acute tubular necrosis (ATN). A common cause of ATN is renal ischemia due to heart failure or hypotension. Numerous nephrotoxic agents may produce ATN, including several antibiotics, mercury, cadmium, carbon tetrachloride, and glycerol. Other causes include hemoglobinuria and myoglobinuria, associated with hemolysis and muscle damage, respectively, as well as excessive quantities of intratubular proteins or crystals.

Chronic renal failure, a progressive and irreversible loss of renal function, results from several disease entities. These include hypertensive and diabetes-associated nephrosclerosis, chronic glomerulonephritis, polycystic kidney disease, and other urologic disorders. Urinary specific gravity is low, and proteinuria, casts, and renal cells may be evident. Pyelonephritis or interstitial nephritis will cause predominantly tubular dysfunction with polyuria early in the disease, but later oliguria of chronic renal failure supervenes.

Specific Gravity and Osmolality

The volume of excreted urine and the concentrations of its solutes are varied by the kidney to maintain the homeostasis of body fluid and electrolytes. Specific gravity and osmolality measurements reflect the relative degree of concentration or dilution of a urine specimen. This in turn aids in evaluating the concentrating and diluting abilities of the kidneys. Both of these indices, as well as urine color, have been found to be reliable indicators of hydration status (Armstrong, 1998).

The specific gravity of a specimen indicates the relative proportions of dissolved solid components to total volume of the specimen; in other words, it reflects the density of the specimen. Osmolality, on the other hand, indicates the number of particles of solute per unit of solution. Larger particles, such as proteins and sugars, tend to elevate the specific gravity more than smaller electrolytes. In critical circumstances, the measurement of osmolality of urine (and plasma) is preferred to the measurement of specific gravity.

Specific Gravity

Urea (20%), sodium chloride (25%), sulfate, and phosphate contribute most of the specific gravity of normal urine. Normal adults with adequate fluid intake will produce urine of specific gravity 1.016–1.022 over a 24-hour period; however, normal kidneys have the ability to produce urine with specific gravity that ranges from 1.003–1.035. If a random specimen of urine has a specific gravity of 1.023 or more, concentrating ability can be considered normal. Minimum specific gravity after a standard water load should be less than 1.007.

Urines of low specific gravity are called hyposthenuric, with the specific gravity less than 1.007. In diabetes insipidus, loss of concentrating ability (as described earlier) results in production of large volumes of urine with specific gravity as low as 1.001 (specific gravity of water is 1.000). Prolonged excretion of urine with low specific gravity can also be seen with various renal abnormalities, including pyelonephritis and glomerulonephritis. High specific gravity can be seen after excess water loss/dehydration, adrenal insufficiency, hepatic disease, or congestive heart failure. When little or no variability is noted between several specimens from a patient, and the specific gravity is fixed at about 1.010, this is known as **isosthenuria.** This finding is indicative of severe renal damage with disruption of both concentrating and diluting abilities.

Methods. Several methods are available to measure specific gravity—reagent strip, refractometer, urinometer, and the falling drop method.

Reagent Strip. This is an indirect method for measuring specific gravity. The reagent area has three main ingredients present: polyelectrolyte, indicator substance, and buffer. The principle of this method is based on the pKa change of pretreated polyelectrolytes in relation to the ionic concentration of the urine. When the ionic concentration is high, the pKa (acid dissociation constant) is decreased, as is the pH. The indicator substance then changes color relative to ionic concentration, and this is translated to specific gravity values. This method is not affected by high amounts of glucose, protein, or radiographic contrast material, all of which tend to elevate the specific gravity readings obtained from refractometers and urinometers, described in the following sections.

Refractometer. This is also an indirect method. The refractive index of a solution is related to the content of dissolved solids present. The index is the ratio of the velocity of light in air to the velocity of light in a solution. It varies directly with the proportion of particles in solution and, therefore, with the specific gravity.

The clinical refractometer is a device that requires only a few drops of urine (unlike the 15 mL of urine necessary with the urinometer). Although the refractometer measures the refractive index of a solution, the scale used is valid only for urine and cannot be used to indicate the specific gravity of salt or sugar solutions. This should be kept in mind if salt solutions are to be used for calibration. Special graphs or tables are required to convert refractive index scale numbers to solute concentrations in aqueous solutions if this should be required (American Optical Catalog Number 10403). The specific gravity reading on the refractometer is generally slightly lower than a urinometer reading on the same urine specimen by about 0.002.

Procedure. A temperature-compensated hand model is available. The instrument is temperature compensated between 60° and 100° F (15° to 38° C). It is damaged by heat above 150° F (66° C) and by immersion of the eyepiece and focusing ring in water. It should read zero with distilled water; the zero reading can be reset if necessary by breaking the seal over the setscrew, turning it with a small screwdriver, and resealing. Check calibration daily. Copper sulfate solutions can be adjusted to monitor a high specific gravity level as an additional check.

To make a specific gravity determination of urine, clean the surfaces of the cover and prism with a drop of distilled water and a damp cloth, and allow them to dry. Close the cover. Hold horizontally, and apply a drop of urine at the notched bottom of the cover, so that it flows over the prism surface by capillary action. Point the instrument toward a light source at an angle that gives optimal contrast. Rotate the eyepiece until the scale is in focus. Read directly on the specific gravity scale the sharp dividing line between light and dark contrast. The entire procedure should be repeated with a second drop of urine from the same sample.

Urinometer. This is a hydrometer that is adapted to directly measure the specific gravity of urine at room temperature. It should be checked each day by measuring the specific gravity of distilled water. If the urinometer does not give a reading of 1.000, an appropriate correction must be applied to all readings taken with that urinometer. The accuracy of a urinometer may be further checked with solutions of known specific gravity.

Because temperature influences the specific gravity, urine samples should be allowed to come to room temperature before a reading is made, or a correction of 0.001 should be made for each 3° C above or below the calibration temperature indicated on the urinometer. Corrections must also be made for protein or glucose present; subtract 0.003 for every 1 g/dL of protein, and 0.004 for every 1 g/dL of glucose.

Procedure. The urinometer vessel is filled three-fourths full with urine (minimum volume required is about 15 mL). The urinometer is inserted with a spinning motion to make sure that it is floating freely. (When reading the urinometer, be sure that it is not touching the sides or the bottom of the cylinder. Avoid surface bubbles, which obscure the meniscus.) Read the bottom of the meniscus.

Falling Drop Method. This is a direct method for measuring specific gravity. It is more accurate than the refractometer, and is more precise than the urinometer. This method utilizes a specially designed column filled with water-immiscible oil. A measured drop of urine is introduced into the column, and as this drop falls, it encounters two beams of light; breaking the first beam starts a timer, and breaking the second turns it off. The falling time is measured electronically and is expressed as a specific gravity (Free, 1996).

Osmolality. The normal adult with a normal fluid intake will produce urine of about 500–850 mOsm/kg water. The normal kidney is able to produce a urine osmolality in the range of 800–1400 mOsm/kg water in dehydration, and a minimal osmolality of 40–80 mOsm/kg water during water diuresis. After a period of dehydration, the osmolality of the urine

TABLE 28-4
Recommendations for Reagent Strips

Storage

Protect from moisture and excessive heat.

Store in cool, dry area but not in a refrigerator.

Check for discoloration with each use; discoloration may indicate loss of reactivity.

Do not use discolored strips or tablets.

Keep container tightly stoppered.

Check manufacturer's directions with each new lot number for changes in procedure.

Testing

Test urine as soon as possible after receipt.

Remove only enough strips for immediate use; recap tightly.

Test a well-mixed, unspun urine sample.

Urine samples must be at room temperature before testing.

Do not touch the test area with fingers.

Do not use reagent strips in the presence of volatile acids or alkaline fumes.

Dip reagent strip into urine briefly—no longer than 1 second.

Drain excess urine off—run edge of strip along rim of tube, or blot edge on absorbent paper.

Do not allow reagents to run together.

Do not lay reagent strip directly on workbench surface.

Follow exact timing recommendations for each chemical test.

Hold reagent strip close to the color chart, and read under good lighting.

Know sources of error, sensitivity, and specificity of each test on the reagent strip.

Think! Make correlations between patient history and individual test, then follow through.

should be three to four times that of the plasma (e.g., with a plasma osmolality of 285 mOsm/kg water, the urine osmolality should be at least 855 mOsm/kg water).

Methods. The freezing-point depression method is commonly employed. A solution containing 1 osmol or 1000 mOsm/kg water depresses the freezing point 1.86° C below the freezing point of water. For methods, see Chapter 4.

CHEMICAL SCREENING

Reagent strips are the primary method used for the chemical examination of urine. Although easily used, they represent multiple complex, state-of-the-art chemical reactions. Table 28-4 lists recommendations for both storage and use of reagent strips. Although reading of the strips has traditionally been done manually, automated instruments, such as the Bayer Atlas (Siemens Medical Solutions Diagnostics, Tarrytown, NY), are now available that will aspirate a precise amount of urine, deposit it on the dipstick, and read the chemical reactions on the reagent strip by reflectance (Lyon, 2003; Penders, 2002). These systems provide excellent reproducibility of results and are not prone to some of the inconsistencies that occur when human hands try to time the reactions, and when human eyes attempt to discriminate different shades of color reactions.

It should be noted that reagent strip methods are changed periodically, sensitivities and color reactions altered, and new measurements added. Manufacturers supply tables of common interfering substances, and these should be consulted. Interference with ascorbic acid and drugs producing colored urines such as phenazopyridine (Pyridium) and other azo compounds, as well as methylthioninium chloride (methylene blue), may be encountered. More detailed information on drug interference is listed in Young (1990).

The chemical measures most commonly found on reagent strips will be discussed first, with less commonly measured chemical parameters following. A discussion on the clinical application of each analyte will precede reagent strip and other methods. Confirmatory methods will be included when available and necessary.

Urine pH

The kidneys and lungs normally work in concert to maintain acid-base equilibrium. The lung excretes carbon dioxide, whereas the renal contribution is that of reclaiming and generating bicarbonate and secreting ammonium ions. The proximal renal tubule is responsible for the bulk of the bicarbonate reabsorption/generation, and the distal tubule provides the remaining function.

The tubular cells exchange hydrogen ions for sodium of the glomerular filtrate. The metabolic activity of the body produces nonvolatile acids, principally sulfuric, phosphoric, and hydrochloric acids, but also small amounts of pyruvic, lactic, and citric acids and ketone bodies. These are excreted by the glomerulus as salts (sodium, potassium, calcium, and ammonium salts) and, together with ammonia produced by the proximal tubules, can then go on to trap secreted hydrogen ions for elimination in the urine (see Chapter 14).

Normal pH

The average adult on a normal diet excretes about 50–100 mEq of hydrogen ions in 24 hours to produce urine of about pH 6. In healthy individuals, urine pH may vary from 4.6–8.

Acid Urine

Acid urine may be produced by a diet high in meat protein and with some fruits such as cranberries. During the mild respiratory acidosis of sleep, a more acid urine may be formed. Also, therapeutic acidification of the urine by various pharmacologic agents, including ammonium chloride, methionine, and methenamine mandelate, is used in the treatment of some calculi. This would include phosphate and calcium carbonate stones, which tend to develop in alkaline urines.

In acid-base disturbances, the pH of the urine reflects attempts at compensation by the kidneys. Patients with metabolic or respiratory acidosis should produce acid urine with increased titratable acidity and ammonium ion concentration. In diabetic ketoacidosis, large quantities of hydrogen ions are excreted, much as ammonium ion. In potassium depletion, such as in hypokalemic alkalosis of prolonged vomiting or in hypercorticism, or with prolonged use of diuretics, paradoxical aciduria with slightly acid urine may occur in the presence of a metabolic alkalosis.

Alkaline Urine

Alkaline urine may be induced by a diet high in certain fruits and vegetables, especially citrus fruits. The urine tends to become less acid following a meal (the so-called **alkaline tide**). This was long believed to be a urinary compensation for gastric acid secretion; however, recent studies do not support this view (Johnson, 1995). Sodium bicarbonate, potassium citrate, and acetazolamide may be used to induce alkaline urine in the treatment of some calculi, particularly those composed of uric acid, cystine, or calcium oxalate. These agents may also be used in some urinary tract infections (the antibiotics neomycin, kanamycin, and streptomycin are more active in alkaline urine), in sulfonamide therapy, and in the treatment of salicylate poisoning.

The capacity to exchange hydrogen ion for cation and the formation of ammonia are decreased when tubular function is impaired. In classic renal tubular acidosis, glomerular filtration is normal, but the distal tubular ability to form ammonia and exchange hydrogen ions for cations is defective. Systemic acidosis results. The urine is relatively alkaline, and the pH cannot be lowered below 6–6.5, even with administration of an acid-loading substance. Additionally, titratable acidity and the concentration of ammonium are decreased (Singh, 1995). In proximal renal tubular acidosis, bicarbonate wasting occurs. This can also be seen in Fanconi's syndrome.

In metabolic alkalosis, an alkaline urine with higher levels of urinary bicarbonate is produced, and ammonia production is decreased. The kidney may produce urine with a pH as high as 7.8. In respiratory alkalosis, an alkaline urine is produced that is associated with increased excretion of bicarbonate.

Methods

Reagent Strip. Indicators methyl red and bromothymol blue give a range of orange, green, and blue colors as the pH rises, permitting estimation of pH values to within half a unit within the range of 5–9. It should be read immediately, but time is not critical. Care should be taken not to have excessively wet strips where acid buffer from the protein patch runs into the pH patch, causing it to become orange.

Measurement of urine pH and acidity must always be made on freshly voided specimens. If precise measurements are required, the container should be filled to minimize the amount of dead space, and the urine covered tightly. The container should be kept cold, preferably on ice, but not frozen. On standing, the pH tends to rise because of loss of carbon dioxide and because bacterial growth produces ammonia from urea.

pH Electrode. Although the estimate of the pH obtainable by indicator strip is usually sufficient, in patients with disturbances of acid-base balance, urinary pH may be accurately measured with a pH meter with a glass electrode. Because the pH meter may tend to drift, it must be standardized with three buffers of known pH immediately before use. After standardization, spray the electrodes with distilled water, clean, and dry with tissue. Immerse the electrode in the urine sample, and report the pH of urine at the temperature of measurement.

Titratable Acidity of Urine. The pH of the urine is largely dependent on the amounts of monobasic and dibasic phosphate present. Titratable acidity is measured by titrating an aliquot of 24-hour urine (collected on ice) with 0.1N NaOH with pH 7.4 as an endpoint. Measurement may be used, together with urinary ammonia determination, in patients with chronic acidosis of obscure origin. Normal titratable acidity is in the range of 200–500 mL 0.1N NaOH (or 6 mL 0.1N NaOH per kg body weight) or 20–40 mEq/24hours. This procedure is described in previous editions of this book (Henry, 1996).

Protein in Urine

Normally, up to 150 mg of protein is excreted in the urine daily, with the average urine protein concentration varying from 2–10 mg/dL, depending on urine volume. Anderson has demonstrated more than 200 urinary proteins, derived from both plasma and the urinary tract (Anderson, 1979). About one third is albumin, and the remaining plasma proteins include small globulins, such as α-, β-, and γ-globulins. Plasma proteins with molecular weight less than 50,000–60,000 pass through the glomerular basement membrane and are normally reabsorbed by proximal tubular cells. Albumin, molecular weight 69,000, is apparently filtered but only in very small amounts. Retinol binding, β_2-microglobulin, immunoglobulin light chains, and lysozyme are excreted in small amounts. Tamm-Horsfall glycoprotein (uromucoid), secreted by distal tubular cells and cells of the ascending loop of Henle, constitutes one third or more of the total normal protein loss. Immunoglobulin A (IgA) in secretions of the urinary tract, enzymes, and proteins from tubular epithelial cells, other desquamated cells, and leukocytes also contribute to urine protein.

Detection of an abnormal amount of protein in urine is an important indicator of renal disease because protein has a very low maximal tubular rate of reabsorption; increased filtration of protein quickly saturates the reabsorptive mechanism. Screening methods are routinely used to differentiate normal protein excretion from abnormal, and therefore should not detect less than about 8–10 mg/dL in a normal adult with a normal rate of urine flow. The reagent strip method is sensitive to albumin; acid precipitation methods detect all proteins and therefore will indicate the presence of globulins, as well as albumin. It should be noted that a very dilute random urine specimen may have a falsely low protein value. Because a positive result for protein is significant, it should be confirmed by a second method and on repeated specimens. Depending on the history and examination, confirmatory measurements for elevated protein should be accompanied by the evaluation of renal function, examination of the urine sediment, and urine culture.

Functional proteinuria is usually less than 0.5 g/day and can be seen in various situations in which dehydration contributes to the level of protein measured in urine. With strenuous exercise, a mixture of high and low molecular weight proteins appears in the urine, and many casts, both hyaline and granular, can be seen. Functional proteinuria may also accompany congestive heart failure, cold exposure, and fever. In any event, the proteinuria resolves with appropriate treatment or rest within 2–3 days.

Intermittent, transient proteinuria can occasionally be seen in patients with a normal history, normal physical examination findings, and otherwise normal renal function. Except for the occasional proteinuria, urinalysis is also normal. These patients are typically followed every 6 months to check for hypertension or other abnormalities, and the overall prognosis is good. A transient proteinuria may also occur in normal pregnancy, but any proteinuria in pregnancy is an important finding and requires investigation. Persistent proteinuria of 1–2 g/day in an asymptomatic person, or when accompanied by hematuria, has a poorer prognosis than intermittent (transient) or postural proteinuria.

Recent interest has focused on the importance of proteinuria in determining risk of adverse outcomes in chronic kidney disease (CKD). Current guidelines for classifying stages of CKD are based on estimated glomerular filtration rate; however, heavy proteinuria was found to be independently associated with a twofold or greater increase in all-cause mortality, myocardial infarction, and progression to renal failure (Hemmelgarn, 2010). A systematic review and meta-analysis of 26 cohort studies involving 169,949 individuals showed a strong and continuous association between proteinuria and risk of coronary artery disease, leading those authors to suggest the routine incorporation of testing for proteinuria into assessment of cardiovascular risk (Perkovic, 2008).

Hereditary proteinuria syndromes are rare and have heterogeneous forms ranging from congenital nephrotic syndrome with severe proteinuria to focal segmental glomerulosclerosis with moderate proteinuria. Progression to end-stage renal disease is a common outcome. Specific diagnosis is possible with genetic testing for mutations in the genes for various structural proteins of the glomerulus (Tryggvason, 2006).

Postural Proteinuria

Postural proteinuria (orthostatic) occurs in 3%–5% of apparently healthy young adults. In this condition, proteinuria is found during the day but not at night when a recumbent position is assumed. Persistent proteinuria may develop in some of these healthy subjects at a later date, and renal biopsies have shown abnormalities of the glomerulus in a few cases (Robinson, 1961). Proteinuria is apparently related to an exaggerated lordotic position and may result from renal congestion or ischemia. The total daily excretion of protein rarely exceeds 1 g, and in most instances, no other evidence of renal disease develops is apparent.

To evaluate the possibility of postural proteinuria, the patient is instructed to empty his or her bladder upon going to bed in the evening. Immediately upon arising in the morning, the patient voids and saves this specimen. After 2 hours of standing and walking about, the patient voids again and saves the specimen. The two urine specimens are assessed for protein, and if the first is negative and the second positive, the patient may have postural proteinuria. Frequent examination of the patient should be made to reevaluate this condition.

Proteinuria in the Elderly

The incidence of significant proteinuria found on urinalysis in the elderly population is substantially increased when compared with patients below age 60. It has been estimated that the elderly population in general has a threefold to fourfold greater incidence of glomerulonephritis, and approximately one quarter of those affected have a minimal change–like disorder that may respond to steroid therapy. Occult malignancies in this population may also give rise to membranous glomerulonephritis, with resultant proteinuria (Threatte, 1986).

Proteinuria Quantification

More useful information for the diagnosis of kidney disease and for following the response to treatment is obtained by quantitatively analyzing the amount of protein excreted over a 24-hour period. It should be noted that the accuracy of measurements of any quantitative urine determination depends on the adequacy and completeness of the urine collection. Erroneous results are often related to collection problems. Repeat measurements may be needed to decide whether the proteinuria is intermittent or persistent.

Heavy Proteinuria (>4 g/day). Heavy protein loss is characteristically seen with the nephrotic syndrome. Classically, a low serum albumin level, generalized edema, and increased serum lipids (cholesterol, triglycerides, and phosphatides) accompany this disorder. Lipoproteins, low-density and very-low-density, are increased in serum, whereas high-density lipoprotein, a smaller molecule, has been demonstrated in the urine (de Mendoza, 1976). It has been suggested that loss of lipoprotein lipase in urine contributes to the rise in serum lipid levels. γ-Globulin is also lost in the urine, and this may contribute to susceptibility to bacterial infections commonly found in nephrotic patients. When lipid is lost in urine, many granular casts, fatty casts, and fat-filled renal tubular epithelial cells (oval fat bodies) are found in the sediment. Cholesterol ester droplets may be demonstrable by polarization.

Nephrotic syndrome is principally associated with glomerular dysfunction/damage due to (1) primary renal diseases, including idiopathic disease, and (2) systemic diseases with renal involvement. Transient or mechanical causes include severe congestive heart failure, constrictive pericarditis, and renal vein thrombosis. The last can be a consequence of the nephrotic syndrome because of losses of anticlotting factors in urine and elevation of serum fibrinogen. In children, a common cause of nephrotic syndrome is minimal change disease (also known as nil lesion), a steroid-responsive glomerular disorder. Acute, rapidly progressive, and chronic types of glomerulonephritis are causes of heavy proteinuria and may be accompanied by urinary erythrocytes or erythrocyte casts. Diabetes mellitus and lupus erythematosus are systemic diseases that frequently cause glomerular injury and heavy proteinuria. Urine sediment may be "telescoped," that is, may display all types of cells and casts in lupus nephritis or with a hypersensitivity reaction. Malaria, malignant hypertension, toxemia of pregnancy, heavy metals (gold, mercury), drugs (penicillamine), neoplasia in general, amyloidosis, sickle cell disease, renal transplant rejection, and rarely primary antiphospholipid syndrome (Levy, 1998) are additional causes of heavy proteinuria.

Moderate Proteinuria (1.0–4.0 g/day). Moderate proteinuria may be found in the vast majority of renal diseases, including those mentioned previously, as well as nephrosclerosis, multiple myeloma, and toxic nephropathies. Also included are degenerative, malignant, and inflammatory conditions of the lower urinary tract, including irritative conditions such as the presence of calculi.

Minimal Proteinuria (<1.0 g/day). Minimal proteinuria may be noted in chronic pyelonephritis, in which case it may be intermittent, and in relatively inactive phases of glomerular diseases. It is also seen with nephrosclerosis, chronic interstitial nephritis, congenital diseases such as polycystic disease and medullary cystic disease, and renal tubular diseases. In tubular diseases, the urinary sediment usually is not abnormal, but erythrocytes, leukocytes, and tubular cells may be seen with interstitial nephritis. However, significant sediment findings may sometimes accompany trace protein results. Minimal proteinuria is also present in postural proteinurias and transient proteinuria.

Qualitative Categories of Proteinuria

Detection of the types of protein present in urine requires electrophoretic separation of urine proteins. Based on these and on clinical findings, proteinuria may be separated into a glomerular pattern and a tubular pattern, indicating which part of the nephron is primarily involved. However, these anatomic entities tend to merge as disease progresses.

Glomerular Pattern. Glomerular disease causes proteinuria, which may be heavy (>3–4 g/day). Loss or reduction of the fixed negative charge on the glomerular basement membrane allows albumin to permeate into Bowman's space in large quantities, more than can be reabsorbed by the proximal tubular cells. When serum albumin is lost in urine, other proteins of similar size or charge are also lost (e.g., antithrombin, transferrin, prealbumin, α_1-acid glycoprotein, α_1-antitrypsin). Because tubular function may still be normal, very small plasma proteins are largely reabsorbed. Large proteins, in contradistinction, are not seen in urine while the glomerulus is still selective (e.g., α_2-macroglobulin, β-lipoprotein). As larger proteins appear, the proteinuria is less selective, indicating greater damage to the glomerulus (e.g., with membranous nephropathy and proliferative glomerulonephritis).

Mechanisms of proteinuria in diabetic kidney disease with specific attention to glomerular damage were recently reviewed with special recognition that chronic kidney disease is actually a combination of both glomerular and tubulointerstitial scarring (Jefferson, 2008).

Tubular Pattern. This is associated with loss of a small amount of urinary protein that would otherwise be largely reabsorbed. These proteins most often are of low molecular weight (e.g., α_1-microglobulin, β-globulins such as β_2-microglobulin, light chain immunoglobulins, and lysozyme), usually without a clear predilection for albumin-sized molecules. By radioimmunoassay, β_2-microglobulin excretion has been measured in microgram amounts in urine as an indication of tubular damage; its normal excretion is about 100 μg/day. A tubular pattern proteinuria occurs with renal tubular diseases such as Fanconi's syndrome, cystinosis, Wilson's disease, and pyelonephritis, and with renal transplantation rejection. The amount of proteinuria is typically lower than that seen with glomerular disease, at about 1–2 g/day. Tubular proteinuria may be missed by the reagent strip test because of the absence or very low amounts of albumin, but it may be detected by an acid precipitation method.

Overflow Proteinuria. Overflow proteinuria is due to the overflow of excess levels of a protein in the circulation, and can be seen with hemoglobin, myoglobin, or immunoglobulin loss into the urine. These proteins are not initially associated with glomerular or tubular diseases, but may themselves cause renal damage. Myoglobin may cause acute tubular necrosis (see under Myoglobin). Hemoglobin in low amounts is not thought to be toxic unless hypovolemia is present.

Bence Jones Proteinuria. Bence Jones proteinuria is associated with multiple myeloma, macroglobulinemia, and malignant lymphomas. The incidence of Bence Jones proteinuria in multiple myeloma has been estimated as 50%–80%; however, its demonstration depends greatly on the technique used. Bence Jones protein may be missed altogether if only a reagent strip test for protein is used. Electrophoresis and immunofixation electrophoresis methods are the best detection and quantification methods, along with the immunoassay measurement of free light chains (see Chapter 46).

Excretion of Bence Jones protein in large amounts, sometimes several grams in 24 hours, causes the tubular cells to deteriorate because of the high levels of protein reabsorbed. Inclusions may form in the cells, and desquamated cells may form casts in the tubular lumen. Casts also form from immunoglobulin and Tamm-Horsfall protein mixtures. With renal failure, less protein is reabsorbed and more Bence Jones protein and other proteins appear in the urine. The damaged kidney is sometimes called a myeloma kidney, and the nephrotic syndrome may follow.

Microalbuminuria. Microalbuminuria is the presence of albumin in urine above the normal level but below the detectable range of conventional urine dipstick methods. Several authors have suggested that these lower urine albumin levels ranging from 20–200 mg/L (or an approximate rate of excretion of 20–200 μg/min) are an indicator of early and possibly reversible glomerular damage (Viberti, 1982; Mogensen, 1984). In diabetic patients, microalbuminuria is associated with a four- to sixfold increase in cardiovascular mortality, and is an independent risk factor for renal mortality (Bakris, 1996; Zelmanovitz, 1998). It is also more prevalent in hypertensive subjects (Gerber, 1998). Various methods have been introduced, including immunologic test systems and dye-binding chemical test strips, both of which are discussed in the next section.

Methods

Several screening methods and quantitative methods are available for the analysis of protein in urine. Because a positive screening test may have serious implications, it is important to be able to confirm results by a second, different method. Common screening tests include the qualitative/semiquantitative colorimetric reagent strip test and precipitation-based testing (Table 28-5).

Accurate results are obtained with reagent strips only when albumin is increased. Because of the lack of sensitivity of the reagent strip to globulins, it may be necessary to use an acid precipitation method for screening purposes. This will depend on the patient population and the diseases being screened. Reagent strips do have the advantage of avoiding false-positive reactions with organic iodides, such as those used for radiograph contrast, and tolbutamides or other drugs.

Most other qualitative screening methods rely on protein precipitation (e.g., with heat and acetic acid, with nitric acid, with sulfosalicylic [SSA] and trichloroacetic acids). These methods will precipitate globulins, as well as albumin. In practice, negative reagent strips with positive SSA methods in urine specimens are attributable to radiograph dye, to penicillins, and, rarely, to an isolated increase in globulins. Sulfosalicylic and trichloroacetic acids are used to precipitate protein in the cold and are used as a convenient screening method. The sensitivity may be as low as 0.25 mg/dL, depending on the technique used.

TABLE 28-5
Screening Test for Detection of Proteinuria

Urine constituents or condition	Reagent strip	Acid precipitation
Highly buffered alkaline urine	May cause FP	May cause FN
Drug metabolites	No effect	May cause FP
Radiocontrast media	No effect	May cause FP
Turbidity	No effect	May cause FP
Quarternary ammonium groups or chlorhexidine	May cause FP	No effect

FN, False negative; *FP*, false positive.

With the intense interest in utilizing proteinuria as a risk stratifier for both diabetic and nondiabetic nephropathy, as well as other conditions such as coronary artery disease, recommendations for measurement have centered on methods for urine albumin quantification rather than total protein (Lamb, 2009). Urine albumin measurements are considered much more standardized and reliable than total protein at low concentrations, where assessment of risk of progression in chromic kidney disease is important for diagnosis and planning therapy.

Reagent Strip. This method takes advantage of the protein error of pH indicators. Because proteins carry a charge at physiologic pH, their presence will elicit a pH change. The reagent strip is impregnated with tetrabromphenol blue buffered to an acid pH of 3, or tetrachlorophenol-tetrabromosulfophthalein. In the absence of protein, the strip is yellow; 30–60 seconds following urine application, variable shades of green develop, depending on the type and concentration of protein present. Results may be read in a "plus" system as negative, trace, and 1+ to 4+. Most methods will detect 5–20 mg of albumin per deciliter.

As stated previously, reagent strips tend to be more sensitive to albumin than to globulins, Bence Jones protein, or mucoprotein. "Trace" results may be seen with physiologic normal excretion of protein in concentrated urine specimens from healthy individuals. High salt levels will lower results. Exceptionally alkaline and/or highly buffered urine samples may give positive results in the absence of significant proteinuria (e.g., with a patient on alkaline medication or with bacterial contamination). False-positive results can occur with quaternary ammonium compounds, amido-amines in fabric softeners, and chlorhexidine, and with excessive leaching of the acid buffer of the test strip by excessive wetting. The method is unaffected by urine turbidity, radiographic media, and most drugs or their metabolites.

Sulfosalicylic Acid Method—Qualitative. This method depends on formation of a precipitate for determination of the presence of protein.

Procedure. Specimens should be centrifuged, and a clear supernatant used. To approximately 3 mL of supernatant urine in a clean test tube, aliquot an equal amount of 3% SSA. Invert to mix. Let stand exactly 10 minutes. Invert again twice. Using ordinary room light (not a lamp), observe the degree of turbidity and/or precipitation, and grade the results according to the following descriptions:

Negative—no turbidity (≈5 mg/dL or less)
Trace—perceptible turbidity (≈20 mg/dL)
1+—Distinct turbidity, but no discrete granulation (≈50 mg/dL)
2+—Turbidity with granulation, but no flocculation (≈200 mg/dL)
3+—Turbidity with granulation and flocculation (≈500 mg/dL)
4+—Clumps of precipitated protein, or solid precipitate (≈1.0 g/dL or more).

This method will detect about 5–10 mg/dL. Albumin, globulins, glycoproteins, and Bence Jones proteins are all detected. High levels of detergents may decrease the result. When radiographic dye is present, SSA precipitate will increase on standing, and typical crystals are seen on microscopic examination of the precipitate. In this situation, another urine specimen from the patient should be assayed. However, the effects of the radiographic media may persist for up to 3 days. A reagent strip test may be substituted, or heat and the acetic acid method may be used. In the acetic acid method, radiographic contrast media will clear with heat, whereas protein will increase.

Quantitative Protein Determinations and Confirmatory Methods. Quantitative measurements of urine protein are typically adaptations of one of the various precipitation methods, or are colorimetric in nature. SSA and trichloroacetic acid (TCA) are commonly used as precipitants; the resultant turbidity can be measured by a photometer or a nephelometer. If a visual interpretation is performed, a set of gelled commercial standards that correspond to 10, 20, 30, 40, 50, 75, and 100 mg/dL may be used, with results reported in milligrams per deciliter as opposed to the "plus" method of screening precipitation tests. With SSA, the turbidity produced with albumin is 2.4 times that produced with globulin; polypeptides, glycoproteins, and Bence Jones proteins are also precipitated with this method. Of historic note, Exton's reagent contains SSA, sodium sulfate, and an indicator—bromphenol blue. TCA, in contradistinction, will cause γ-globulin to be precipitated with greater turbidity than albumin; however, the difference is not marked.

More precise measurements suitable for smaller amounts of protein are available, and in these methods a TCA precipitate is dissolved in sodium hydroxide and measured by use of the biuret reaction. The quantitative TCA-biuret method is tedious but gives good precision. A color correction blank is used. For a comparison of biuret methods with the SSA turbidity method, see Lizana (1977).

Several dye-binding colorimetric methods are available to quantitate urine protein. These include Coomassie blue, Ponceau S, and benzethonium chloride turbidity methods (McElderry, 1982). Pyrogallol Red-Molybdate will also react with protein to form a bluish purple complex that absorbs at 600 nm.

Methods used to quantitate urinary protein have not been satisfactory. Participants in the College of American Pathologists proficiency testing surveys will be aware that the mean values reported vary twofold between methods, with the SSA method producing high values. Precision is poor, with the SSA turbidimetric method showing the poorest coefficient of variation. The TCA-biuret, Coomassie blue, and TCA turbidity methods show closer agreement and about half the coefficient of variation of the SSA method. Problems arise from nonstandardized methods. With turbidity methods, these include different acid concentrations and timing, along with variation in the protein standard.

Microalbuminuria Determination Methods. Very small amounts of proteins, such as albumin and β_2-microglobulin, are measured by immunologic means using antibodies to the proteins, nephelometric methods, or radioimmunoassay. The Micral II test strip (Boehringer Mannheim, Indianapolis) is an immunologic test system that gives an almost immediate, reliable semiquantitative determination of low urine albumin concentrations (Kutter, 1998). Oxytetracycline may interfere with this method, causing higher readings. There is no interference with pH. A newer method, the Clinitek microalbumin (Bayer Diagnostics, Tarrytown, N.Y.), is a highly sensitive dye-binding method. It has the further advantage of an additional test pad for simultaneous measurement of creatinine concentration. This method is not absolutely specific for albumin, for the dye compound also reacts with Tamm-Horsfall mucoprotein.

Bence Jones Proteinuria Determination Methods. Methods for detection of Bence Jones protein in urine include protein electrophoresis, immunofixation electrophoresis, and immunoassay for free light chains (see Chapter 46). The traditional electrophoretic procedure employs the Amido black stain on a 200-fold concentrated urine. Newer methods, performed on less concentrated urine, including a modified Coomassie brilliant blue stain, are comparably sensitive and specific (Wong, 1997). The presence of Bence Jones globulin or clonal production of immunoglobulin is indicated by a single sharp peak in the globulin region on protein electrophoresis. Bence Jones globulin represents either the κ or the λ immunoglobulin light chain.

Bence Jones protein precipitates at temperatures between 40° and 60° C, and redissolves at near 100° C. Other methods depend on precipitation in the cold with salts, ammonium sulfate, and acids. In the presence of marked Bence Jones proteinuria, most methods yield positive results. When only a small amount of Bence Jones protein is present, or when other globulins are present, results may be doubtful. False-positive reactions are seen when other globulins are precipitated by acetic acid in the heat precipitation method. A false-negative reaction may occur if the Bence Jones protein is too concentrated and the precipitate does not redissolve on boiling.

Glucose and Other Sugars in Urine

Various sugars may be found in the urine under certain circumstances, both pathologic and physiologic. These include glucose, fructose, galactose, lactose, maltose, pentose, and sucrose. Glucose is by far the most common and will be discussed in the next section.

Glucose

The presence of detectable amounts of glucose in urine is termed **glycosuria;** this condition occurs whenever the glucose level in the blood surpasses the renal tubule capacity for reabsorption. Glucose may appear in the urine at different blood glucose levels, and there is not always a concomitant hyperglycemia. Glomerular blood flow, tubular reabsorption rate, and urine flow also will influence its appearance. When hyperglycemia is present, however, glycosuria usually occurs when the blood level is greater than 180–200 mg/dL. Glycosuria may be seen in several different conditions described in the following sections.

Diabetes Mellitus. Although hyperglycemia alone is not necessarily indicative of diabetes mellitus, the appearance of glucose in the urine necessitates further workup. When glycosuria is present, it is typically accompanied by polyuria and thirst. Inadequate carbohydrate utilization in these patients results in elevated ketone levels in the blood and urine due to increased fat metabolism.

For diabetic individuals, the advantage of a urine method over a blood test for glucose is that it is painless and inexpensive. Urine glucose measurements are most useful for well-controlled diabetic individuals who do not have to make frequent adjustments in their insulin/hypoglycemic agents. In insulin-dependent diabetes, a negative urine measurement could correspond to a wide range of serum glucose levels; this is attributed to the great variation in renal threshold for glucose in diabetic patients. Therefore, urine measurements may be misleading, and home blood glucose monitoring is preferred.

Monitoring for glycosuria in diabetic patients is not without problems. Reagent strips may be difficult to interpret at the 1-g/dL (1%) and 2-g/dL (2%) glucose levels; copper reduction tests or newer, more sensitive reagent strips may be more efficacious. With the Clinitest tablet method, diabetic patients are able to estimate reducing substance levels in urine to about 10 g/dL, using one drop of specimen rather than two or five drops. In some clinics, the 24-hour urine glucose measurement is found to be useful for monitoring patients. It represents a defined longer time period, and, with blood levels of glycated hemoglobin, it contributes to the regular overall long-term management of the disease.

Several studies have looked at the usefulness of urine dipstick testing for glycosuria as a screening method for diabetes, and the results have been mixed. Bullimore (1997) concentrated on patients over 50 years old in a general practice setting and found this method to be practical and effective, whereas Friderichsen (1997) came to an opposing conclusion. He suggests that if diabetes screening is carried out in general practice, blood glucose measurements should be utilized for patients in selected risk groups. Routine dipstick glucose analysis can identify gravidas at increased risk for gestational diabetes (Gribble, 1995).

Other Causes of Glycosuria. Glycosuria with concomitant hyperglycemia is seen in several endocrine disorders (see Table 16-3). These include pituitary and adrenal disorders such as acromegaly, Cushing's syndrome, hyperadrenocorticism, functioning α- or β-cell pancreatic tumors, hyperthyroidism, and pheochromocytoma. Pancreatic disease with loss of functioning islet cells is also associated with glycosuria—for example, carcinoma, pancreatitis, and cystic fibrosis.

Numerous other causes of glycosuria with hyperglycemia have been recognized. These include central nervous system disorders, including brain tumor or hemorrhage, hypothalamic disease, and asphyxia. Disturbances of metabolism associated with burns, infection, fractures, myocardial infarction, and uremia, as well as liver disease, glycogen storage disease, obesity, and feeding after starvation, may all be associated with glycosuria, as are certain drugs (e.g., thiazides, corticosteroids and adrenocorticotropic hormone, birth control pills).

In pregnancy, an increase in glomerular filtration rate occurs, and all of the filtered glucose may not be reabsorbed. In this situation, glycosuria may appear at relatively low blood glucose levels. Persistent, or greater than trace amounts of, glycosuria should be investigated. In some patients, diabetes occurs only during pregnancy. Glucose tolerance may also be decreased in the aged, especially when patients have a poor intake of carbohydrate, but this is not necessarily accompanied by glycosuria.

Glycosuria without hyperglycemia is usually associated with renal tubular dysfunction. True inherited renal glycosuria is uncommon and is associated with reduced glucose reabsorption. In renal tubular transport diseases, glycosuria may be accompanied by impaired reabsorption of water, amino acid, bicarbonate, phosphate, and sodium—a pattern seen in Fanconi's syndrome. Galactosemia, cystinosis, lead poisoning, and myeloma are additional examples of conditions associated with renal tubular dysfunction and possible glycosuria.

Other Sugars in Urine

Small quantities of disaccharides are normally excreted in the urine—about 50 mg in 24 hours. With intestinal diseases such as severe sprue or acute enteritis, the level may rise to 250 mg or more. Fructose, galactose, lactose, maltose, and L-xylulose are found in urine in patients with inherited metabolic disorders (Scriver, 1989). If an inherited disorder is suspected, the sugar may be identified by thin-layer chromatography. Qualitative confirmatory tests generally are not satisfactory for sugars.

Fructose. Fructose appears in urine in association with inherited enzyme deficiencies that cause benign essential fructosuria and serious fructose intolerance associated with severe vomiting and liver and kidney disease. Fructosuria may also be seen with parenteral feedings that include fructose. Urinary fructose has been used as a marker of sucrose intake in dietary intervention studies (Luceri, 1996).

Galactose. Galactose is found in the urine in genetic disorders of galactose metabolism associated with a deficiency of galactose-1-phosphate uridyl transferase or galactokinase. In these diseases, galactose derived from dietary lactose is not converted to glucose, and early detection followed by dietary restriction may control the disease.

Lactose. Lactose may appear in the urine late in normal pregnancy or during lactation. In lactose intolerance, high levels of sugars accumulate in the gut, and lactose will be absorbed and excreted unchanged in the urine.

Pentose. Pentosuria may follow the ingestion of large amounts of fruit, causing the excretion of L-xylulose and L-arabinose in amounts up to 0.1 g/day. It may also be seen with certain drug therapies and with benign essential pentosuria.

Sucrose. Sucrose may appear in the urine after the ingestion of very large amounts of sucrose. Sucrase deficiency is associated with intestinal diseases such as sprue in the same manner as lactase deficiency. Sucrose intolerance is an inherited disorder associated with sucrase and α-dextrinase (isomaltase) deficiencies. Symptoms are similar to those seen with lactase deficiency and occur in the first few weeks of life when sweetened food is ingested. Tolerance may develop, but sucrose may have to be avoided permanently. Factitious sucrosuria may create a high specific-gravity urine with negative glucose oxidase and negative copper reduction tests.

Methods

Reagent Strip. This method is based on a specific glucose oxidase and peroxidase method, a double sequential enzyme reaction; reagent strips differ only in the chromogen used. The method is specific for glucose, and no reaction is seen with lactose, galactose, fructose, or reducing metabolites of drugs. The reagent strips may be used for semiquantitative results, and results should be reported as approximate grams per deciliter. Combination glucose and ketone reagent strips detect not only ketonuria, but also suppression of the glucose reaction by ketones seen with some reagent strips.

False-positive readings may be produced by strongly oxidizing cleaning agents in the urine container. Low specific gravity may falsely elevate results. Sodium fluoride used as a preservative will cause false-negative readings, as can high specific gravity and occasionally ascorbic acid. Glycolytic enzymes from cells and bacteria will reduce glucose levels in urine on standing; prompt refrigeration or testing is essential.

Chemistry

$$\text{Glucose} + O_2 \xrightarrow{\text{Glucose oxidase}} \text{Gluconic acid} + H_2O_2$$

$$H_2O_2 + \text{Chromogen} \xrightarrow{\text{peroxidase}} \text{Oxidized chromogen} + H_2O$$

Chromogens utilized in some common dipstick tests include the following:

Clinistix—o-toluidine chromogen. Color changes from pink to purple. This formulation detects 100 mg/dL of glucose and is more sensitive to interfering substances such as ascorbic acid than the following.

Multistix—potassium iodide chromogen. Color changes from blue to brown at 30 seconds.

Chemstrip—an aminopropyl-carbazol chromogen. Color changes from yellow to orange-brown at 60 seconds.

Copper Reduction Tests. As a screening test, the glucose oxidase method will not detect increased levels of galactose or other sugars in urine. It is therefore important that a copper reduction method be used, especially for young pediatric patients. A policy to screen for reducing sugars should be made by the individual laboratory, after consultation with its clinical staff. In many instances, policies related to performing this screening were instituted in the 1960s, before the widespread mandatory screening of newborns for inborn errors of metabolism became routine. With this state-mandated newborn screening, detection of an unsuspected reducing substance in the urine is rare, and the routine performance of this test, without a specific request by the patient's physician, may have outlived its usefulness (Naumova, 2006).

TABLE 28-6
Reactions of Substances to Test for Glucosuria

Constituent	Glucose oxidase reagent strip	Copper reduction tablet test
Glucose	Positive	Positive
Sugars other than glucose		
Fructose	No effect	Positive
Galactose	No effect	Positive
Lactose	No effect	Positive
Maltose	No effect	Positive
Pentose	No effect	Positive
Sucrose	No effect	Positive
Ketones (large quantities)	May depress color	No effect
Creatine	No effect	May cause false-positive
Uric acid		
Homogentisic acid (alkaptonuria)	No effect	Positive
Drugs*		
Ascorbic acid (large amounts)	May delay color	Trace positive
Cephalosporins (Keflin), etc.	No effect	Positive, brown color
L-Dopa (large amounts)	False-negative	No effect
Nalidixic acid glucuronide	No effect	Positive
Probenecid	No effect	Positive
Pyridium	Orange color may affect result	
Salicylate (large amounts)	May lower reading	No effect
X-ray dye (diatrizoates)	No effect	Black color
Contaminants		
Hydrogen peroxide	False-positive	May inhibit positive test
Hypochlorite (bleach)	False-positive	
Sodium fluoride	False-negative	No effect

Data from Caraway (1962), Wirth (1965), and Young (1975).
*Other drugs implicated in copper reduction are amino acids, caronamide, chloral, chloroform, chloramphenicol, formaldehyde, hippuric acid, isoniazid, thiazides, oxytetracycline, *p*-aminosalicylic acid, penicillin, phenols, streptomycin, phenothiazine, and sulfonamides.

The copper reduction method will detect sufficient quantities of any reducing substances in the urine, including reducing sugars such as lactose, fructose, galactose, maltose, and the pentoses. In those instances in which the copper method is positive and the glucose oxidase method is negative, glycosuria is ruled out; however, before investigation for other sugars is begun, the clinical findings and drug history should be evaluated. Although the copper reduction method will detect nonglucose reducing sugars, the yield for these sugars is extremely low.

Normal neonatal infants during the first 10–14 days of life may excrete urine that yields a positive reaction because of glucose, galactose, fructose, and lactose. Normal pregnant and postpartum women may also have positive reactions because of the presence of lactose.

Of the copper reduction methods used for screening purposes, the qualitative Benedict method is more sensitive to reducing substances in urine than is the single-tablet (Clinitest) copper reduction method. Many substances in urine, metabolites, and drug-related metabolites will influence urinary sugar methods (Table 28-6). Strong reducing substances such as ascorbic acid, gentisic acid, or homogentisic acid may inhibit the enzyme method while contributing to the positivity of the copper reduction method. The tablet method is not affected as much as the Benedict method. Very large doses of ascorbic acid do not affect the two-drop copper reduction method. Drugs, especially the cephalosporins, and radiographic media will give false-positive or unusual colors with Clinitest. Although large doses of ascorbic acid do not affect the two-drop Clinitest for sugars (i.e., do not cause false-positive results), delays in color development may be noted with the glucose oxidase method.

Chemistry. Copper sulfate, sodium hydroxide, sodium carbonate, and citric acid are incorporated into each Clinitest tablet. Copper sulfate reacts with reducing substances in the urine, converting cupric sulfate to cuprous oxide. Based on Benedict's copper reduction reaction,

$$Cu^{2+} \xrightarrow{\text{Hot alkaline solution}} Cu^{+}$$

$$Cu^{+} + OH^{-} \rightarrow CuOH\,(\text{yellow})$$

$$2CuOH \xrightarrow{\text{Heat}} Cu_2O\,(\text{red}) + H_2O$$

Heat is caused by the reaction of sodium hydroxide with water and citric acid.

Procedure. Clinitest reagent tablets will detect 250 mg of reducing substance per deciliter of urine. Both five-drop and two-drop Clinitest methods can be used, and corresponding color charts are available (Belmonte, 1967). The two-drop method was developed in response to a so-called **pass-through phenomenon** that may occur if more than 2 g/dL of sugar is present in the urine. In the pass-through phenomenon, the solution that results after addition of the Clinitest tablet goes through the entire range of colors and back to a dark greenish brown. This final color does not compare with any section of the color chart; however, it corresponds most closely to a significantly lower result. It is important to observe the entire reaction and to continue to oberve for 15 seconds after boiling inside the tube has stopped, so that reversion to a different color is not missed and a falsely low result reported.

Five-Drop Method. Place five drops of urine in a dry test tube and add 10 drops of water. Add one Clinitest tablet by easing it into the tube without touching it—it contains strong alkali. Watch while boiling takes place, but do not shake or touch the bottom of the tube—it is hot. Wait for 15 seconds after boiling stops, then shake the tube gently, and immediately compare the color of the solution with the color scale. Results correspond to the following approximate concentrations: Negative; 0.25 g/dL; 0.5 g/dL; 0.75 g/dL; 1.0 g/dL; 2.0 g/dL; and pass-through. It is important to watch the solution carefully while it is boiling. If the solution passes through orange to a dark shade of greenish brown, this indicates that more than 2 g/dL sugar is present; this should be recorded as greater than 2 g/dL without reference to the color scale. Urine samples showing this pass-through phenomenon should be retested with the two-drop method.

Two-Drop Method. Place two drops of urine in a test tube, and add 10 drops of water. Add one Clinitest tablet. Watch while boiling takes place, but do not shake. Wait 15 seconds after the boiling stops, then shake the tube gently; compare the color of the solution with the color scale supplied for the two-drop method. The pass-through phenomenon may also occur with the two-drop method with large concentrations of sugar—over 5 g/dL. Report results as 1 g/dL, 2 g/dL, 3 g/dL, 5 g/dL, and more than 5 g/dL if a pass-through reaction occurs. With negative or low-level results, the five-drop method should be performed.

Precautions. Observe the precautions in the literature supplied with the Clinitest tablets. The bottle must be kept tightly closed at all times to prevent absorption of moisture and kept away from direct heat and sunlight in a cool, dry place. The tablets normally have a spotted bluish white color. If not stored properly, they will absorb moisture or deteriorate from heat, turning dark blue or brown. In this condition, they will not give reliable results. They are also available individually packaged in aluminum foil to help prevent this absorption of moisture. Although more expensive, such packaging is useful when a limited number of measurements are performed.

Additional Tests for Sugars. As stated above, the copper reduction method will detect the majority of nonglucose sugars that might be present in urine, apart from sucrose, which is not a reducing sugar. It does not, however, differentiate between these sugars, therefore necessitating more complicated testing. Additional confirmatory testing will be discussed here.

Fructose. Fructose is identified by thin-layer chromatography. A qualitative measurement, a resorcinol test, is useful. Fructose will also reduce Benedict's reagent at low temperatures.

Galactose. Thin-layer chromatography is used to identify galactose in urine. However, the disease is usually identified by erythrocyte enzyme assay when suspected.

Lactose. Lactose is identified by thin-layer chromatography or a qualitative lactose test, such as described below.

Procedure. To 15 mL urine in a test tube, add 3 g lead acetate. Shake and filter. Boil filtrate, add 2 mL concentrated NH_4OH (ammonium hydroxide), and boil. Lactose will cause the formation of a brick-red solution and then a red precipitate with clear supernatant.

Pentose. At concentrations of 250–300 mg/dL, L-xylulose will reduce Benedict's qualitative reagent at 50° C (water bath) within 10 minutes or at room temperature in several hours. Generally, the pentoses are identified by thin-layer chromatography.

Sucrose. Sucrose will ferment yeast and can be separated by chromatography but needs to be stained with a substance not dependent on reducing properties.

Ketones in Urine

Whenever a defect in carbohydrate metabolism or absorption or an inadequate amount of carbohydrate is present in the diet, the body compensates by metabolizing increasing amounts of fatty acids. When this increase is large, ketone bodies, the products of incomplete fat metabolism, begin to appear in the blood and are consequently excreted in the urine. In ketonuria, the three ketone bodies present in the urine are acetoacetic (diacetic) acid (20%), acetone (2%), and 3-hydroxybutyrate (about 78%). Acetone is formed nonreversibly from acetoacetic acid; β-hydroxybutyric acid (3-hydroxybutyrate) forms reversibly from acetoacetic acid.

$$\text{Acetoacetic acid} \xrightarrow{-CO_2} \text{Acetone}$$

$$\text{Acetoacetic acid} \underset{-2H}{\overset{+2H}{\rightleftharpoons}} \text{3-Hydroxybutyrate}$$

Depending on the methods used, total ketone bodies (as acetone) can range as high as 17–42 mg/dL. According to Killander (1962), up to 2 mg acetoacetic acid per deciliter is normal. Ketonemia and ketonuria are commonly seen in uncontrolled diabetes mellitus, as well as several other conditions to be discussed here.

Diabetic Ketonuria

Ketonuria implies the presence of ketoacidosis (ketosis) and may provide a warning of impending coma. Up to 50 mg of acetoacetic acid per deciliter may be present without clinical evidence of ketosis. Type 1 diabetic patients are more prone to episodes of ketosis, often associated with infection, stress, or other problems in management. Whereas large amounts of ketones and glucose are present in urine in diabetic ketoacidosis, ketonuria is not found with the hyperosmolar hyperglycemic coma that sometimes occurs in type 2 diabetes.

Nondiabetic Ketonuria

In infants and children, ketonuria commonly occurs in a variety of conditions, such as acute febrile diseases and toxic states accompanied by vomiting or diarrhea. Inherited metabolic disease should be suspected when there is severe persistent neonatal ketosis. Ketonuria may be present in hyperemesis of pregnancy, in cachexia, and following anesthesia. In these cases, ketonuria is likely related to increased tissue (especially fat) catabolism in the face of limited food intake. In pregnancy, a normal patient may have a low fasting blood glucose level and mild ketonuria. Occasionally, ketonuria is seen following exposure to cold or severe exercise, or with a low-carbohydrate diet for weight reduction.

Lactic Acidosis

Lactic acidosis may coexist with many conditions, including shock, diabetes mellitus, renal failure, liver disease, and infection, and in response to certain drugs, especially phenformin and salicylate poisoning. Acetoacetate and 3-hydroxybutyrate may both be highly elevated, although usually the butyrate is high and acetoacetate low. Under these circumstances, ketonuria may not be detected by the usual nitroprusside test.

Methods. Because acetone, acetoacetic acid, and 3-hydroxybutyrate are all present in the urine with ketonuria, methods that indicate the presence of any one of these three ketone bodies are generally satisfactory to detect this condition. Commonly used nitroprusside strip and tablet tests based on the Rothera method detect acetoacetic acid and acetone. Different methods measure acetoacetic acid alone, or both acetone and acetoacetic acid. Ferric chloride (Gerhardt's test) detects acetoacetic acid. These methods do not measure 3-hydroxybutyrate, the predominant ketone body.

In urine and plasma, reagent strips and tablets react to 10 mg of acetoacetic acid per deciliter and are less sensitive to acetone. The blood level of ketone bodies may be estimated by the urine ketone dipstick at the bedside. This is especially helpful in determining the severity of ketosis for the treatment of diabetic acidosis.

When a patient is being followed with qualitative determinations of acetone and acetoacetic acid, repeated reports of marked elevations would not reflect the change that is actually taking place. In such an instance, semiquantitative results can be obtained with either the reagent strip or Rothera's tablet test by measuring several dilutions of each specimen.

Problems can occur with false-negative results because of unstable reagents and labile ketones. Bacterial action will cause loss of acetoacetic acid, which can happen in vivo as well as in vitro. Acetone is lost at room temperature but not if kept in a closed container in a refrigerator. Refrigerated samples should be brought to room temperature for testing. Preservatives do not prevent decay of ketones. If results are unexpected, fresh reagents, checked against known positive and negative controls, should be used.

Reagent Strip. This method is based on a nitroprusside (sodium nitroferricyanide) reaction for ketones. Different formulations are available. Reagent strips without alkali react to acetoacetic acid and not to acetone. With large (3+) results, urine may be diluted and remeasured, reporting a "moderate" result and the dilution factor.

Chemstrip reagent strips contain sodium nitroferricyanide and glycine, which react with acetoacetic acid and acetone in an alkaline medium to form a violet dye. A positive result is indicated by a color change from beige to violet, which is read at 60 seconds. The method detects about 10 mg/dL of acetoacetic acid and 70 mg/dL of acetone, and the sensitivity and reaction of the reagent strip are similar to those of the tablet (Acetest), described below.

Multistix contains buffers and sodium nitroferricyanide, which react with acetoacetic acid, producing a pink-maroon color in 15 seconds. The reagent area detects 5–10 mg acetoacetic acid per deciliter of urine. It does not react with acetone.

Reagent strips correlate only moderately well with quantitative acetoacetate in plasma and poorly with total blood ketones. Color reactions (false-positives) occur after the use of phthaleins (sulfobromophthalein [BSP] or phenolsulfonphthalein [PSP] dye) or in the presence of extremely large quantities of phenylketones and the preservative 8-hydroxyquinoline, or L-dopa metabolites. Acetylcysteine (aerosol) produces a strong red color. The antihypertensive drugs methyldopa and captopril give positive results. False-negative results occur because of loss of reagent reactivity.

Nitroprusside Tablet Test. A tablet test method may be useful if the urine has an interfering color. These tablets are very sensitive to humidity and will deteriorate if not stored properly. The Acetest tablet contains sodium nitroprusside, glycine, and a strongly alkaline buffer. It can be used to assay whole blood, plasma, serum, or urine.

Acetest will detect 5–10 mg acetoacetic acid per deciliter of urine and 20–25 mg acetone per deciliter of urine. Like the reagent strips, it does not react with 3-hydroxybutyrate. It will give positive results with L-dopa and large amounts of phenylketones and with BSP and PSP dyes, which react with the alkali in the tablets.

Procedure. Place the tablet on a clean surface, preferably a piece of white paper. Place one drop of urine, serum, plasma, or whole blood on the tablet. For urine measurements, compare the color of the tablet with a color chart at 30 seconds. For serum or plasma measurements, compare the color of the tablet with the color chart at 2 minutes. For whole blood measurements, remove clotted blood from the tablet and compare the color of the tablet with the color chart, 10 minutes after application of the specimen.

If acetone and acetoacetic acid are present, the tablet will show a color varying from lavender to deep purple. Report the results as negative, small, moderate, or large. If large, a dilution may be made. Report these analyses in a form such as this: Undiluted "large," 1 : 2 dilution "large," 1 : 4 dilution "moderate," and so forth.

Other Tests for Ketones. The Gerhardt ferric chloride test has been used for many years as a measurement for acetoacetic acid. However, ferric chloride methods are not very specific and the sensitivity is low, at about 25–50 mg/dL. The ferric chloride method gives positive results with salicylate and L-dopa. The test tube nitroprusside method of Rothera is sensitive to acetoacetic acid, at about 1–5 mg/dL, and to acetone with a sensitivity of 10–25 mg/dL.

Blood, Hemoglobin, Hemosiderin, and Myoglobin in Urine

The presence of an abnormal number of blood cells in urine is known as **hematuria,** whereas the term **hemoglobinuria** refers to the presence of free hemoglobin in solution in urine. Hematuria is relatively common, hemoglobinuria uncommon, and **myoglobinuria** rare.

Hematuria

Although asymptomatic microscopic hematuria may be detected by dipstick testing in up to 16% of screening populations (Rockall, 1997), many serious diseases of the urinary tract release red blood cells into the urine. A retrospective investigation of microscopic hematuria by renal biopsy disclosed several histopathologic findings, including membranous nephropathy, IgA nephropathy, non-IgA mesangioproliferative glomerulonephritis, focal glomerulosclerosis, and mild glomerular abnormalities. More than 15% of patients in this study showed normal histology (McGregor, 1998). Hematuria can occur with disease (neoplastic and non-neoplastic) or trauma (including calculi) anywhere in the kidneys or urinary tract, as well as with bleeding disorders and anticoagulant usage, and with the use of other drugs such as cyclophosphamide. A rare case of giant cell arteritis presenting with fever and hematuria has been reported (Govil, 1998). Hematuria may also be seen in healthy persons undertaking excessive exercise (marathon runners), in whom bleeding originates from the bladder mucosa.

Because of the diagnostic importance of small amounts of hematuria and because of the tendency of erythrocytes to undergo lysis in urine, a screening test for hemoglobin is a useful adjunct to microscopic examination of the sediment. In fact, some studies suggest that reagent strip hemoglobin screening may be more sensitive than urine microscopy in detecting hematuria (Ooi, 1998). However, a common problem with the method is the inhibition of the hemoglobin reagent strip by interfering substances, commonly ascorbic acid, and this problem emphasizes the need for a routine microscopic examination to screen for hematuria. A positive test for hemoglobin with a normal urinary sediment suggests that a fresh urine sample should be examined for erythrocytes, because an alkaline pH or urine specific gravity of less than 1.010 may cause lysis of erythrocytes.

Hemoglobinuria

Any cause of hemolysis has the potential of causing hemoglobinuria, but the presence of hemoglobinuria indicates significant intravascular hemolysis as opposed to extravascular hemolysis. Hemoglobin binds to plasma haptoglobin, and free hemoglobin will pass through the glomerulus as αβ dimers (molecular weight [MW], 32,000), once this binding capacity is saturated. Some hemoglobin is reabsorbed by proximal tubular cells, and the remaining hemoglobin is excreted.

Hemoglobinuria may follow severe exertion in which there is direct trauma to small blood vessels; many other causes of acute erythrocyte lysis are summarized in Table 28-7. Plasma appears pink at levels of about 50 mg/dL of hemoglobin, and with marked hemolysis, plasma levels may reach 1 g/dL. The plasma hemoglobin level is more often increased in severe acquired hemolytic anemias than in hereditary hemolytic anemias. However, moderately elevated levels occur with sickle cell disease and homozygous thalassemias. Note that unstable hemoglobins can cause a brown-pigmented urine; this is thought to be due to a dipyrrole or bilifuscin, and no reaction occurs with the reagent strip test for heme. A comparison of expected urine and plasma findings with moderate and marked hemolysis is shown in Table 28-8.

TABLE 28-7
Some Causes of Hemolysis and Hemoglobinuria

Erythrocyte trauma	Prosthetic cardiac valves (especially aortic)
	Ostium primum repair with patch causing turbulence
	Extensive burns
	Severe exercise
	Marching
	Severe trauma to muscle and other vascular tissues
Organisms	Malaria
	Bartonella
	Clostridium welchii toxin
	Brown recluse spider bite
Erythrocyte enzyme deficiencies	Glucose-6-phosphate dehydrogenase subjects in the following situations: Exposure to oxidant drugs (acetanilid, sulfamethoxazole, nitrofurantoin), antimalarials (primaquine, etc.), fava beans *(Vicia fava)* in susceptible groups, with diabetic acidosis, and with infection
Unstable hemoglobin diseases	With exposure to oxidant drugs
Immune-mediated (see Chapters 32 and 33)	Hemolytic-uremic syndrome
	Thrombotic thrombocytopenic purpura
	Incompatible blood transfusions
	Warm antibodies (autoimmune—transient after infection, drug-induced)
	Cold antibodies IgM—viral anti-i mycoplasma anti-I IgG—paroxysmal, Donath–Landsteiner anti-P
	Membrane sensitivity, complement-mediated (paroxysmal nocturnal hemoglobinuria)
	Drugs Acting as haptens (penicillins) Immune complex (quinidine, phenacetin) α-Methyldopa
Normal subjects	Oxidative hemolysis due to drugs, large doses or exposure to naphthalene (mothballs), some sulfonamides, sulfones, nitrofurantoin

TABLE 28-8
Urine and Plasma Findings with Intravascular Hemolysis

Test	Moderate hemolysis	Marked hemolysis
Urine		
Bilirubin (conjugated)	Absent	Absent
Urobilinogen	Normal or elevated	Elevated
Hemoglobin	Absent	Present
Hemosiderin	Absent	Present (late)
Plasma		
Bilirubin (conjugated)	Elevated	Elevated
Haptoglobin	Decreased	Absent
Hemoglobin	Elevated	Elevated (marked)

Hemosiderin in Urine

Free hemoglobin is readily filtered by the glomeruli and can be subsequently reabsorbed by proximal tubular cells, where it can be catabolized into ferritin and hemosiderin. Hemosiderin will be present 2–3 days after an acute hemolytic episode that caused hemoglobinuria. At this time, the reagent strip method for hemoglobin is often negative; however, hemosiderin can be found as yellow-brown granules that are free or in epithelial cells and occasionally in casts (Fig. 28-1). Hemosiderin also appears in the urine sediment in diseases with a true siderosis of kidney parenchyma (hemochromatosis). Although the existence of hemosiderinuria indicates a chronic hemolytic state, its presence is rarely needed to make the diagnosis of hemolysis; other tests, such as serum bilirubin, lactate dehydrogenase, and haptoglobin levels, will usually point to the correct diagnosis.

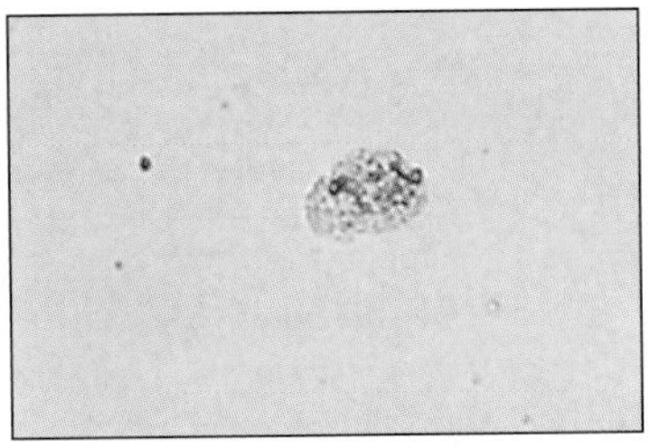

Figure 28-1 Renal tubular epithelial cell (unstained) containing brown pigment, iron (×260).

Because of the intermittent presence of hemosiderinuria, urinary iron levels may be quantitated to establish the presence of chronic intravascular hemolysis. Normal urinary iron excretion is about 0.1 mg/day, and this is increased with hemochromatosis and in association with erythrocytes traumatized by prosthetic heart valves. Urinary iron levels are normal with pernicious anemia and in hereditary spherocytosis.

Myoglobinuria

When acute destruction of muscle fibers (rhabdomyolysis) occurs, as with trauma, myoglobin is released, rapidly cleared from the blood, and excreted in the urine as a red-brown pigment. Free myoglobin, a monomer with MW of 17,000, is excreted quickly, whereas the hemoglobin–haptoglobin complex is more slowly removed. Myoglobinuria has been seen following a number of strenuous exercises, such as marathon running and karate. Other less common conditions associated with sustained or recurrent myoglobinuria include dermatomyositis (Rose, 1996), defects of muscle phosphofructokinase and adenosine monophosphate deaminase (Bruno, 1998), and mitochondrial trifunctional protein deficiency (Miyajima, 1997).

The diagnosis of rhabdomyolysis and myoglobinuria is usually made from the history and other laboratory findings as follows. Typically, the patient has muscle tenderness or cramps and voids red-brown urine within a day or two after exertion. The reagent strip urine test for hemoglobin is markedly positive, and protein and a few red blood cells are present. Serum is clear and has a markedly elevated creatine kinase (CK), aldolase, and a normal haptoglobin level. Serum creatinine may be increased. The urine usually clears in 2–3 days, and the serum CK level declines. The serum measurements and history help to distinguish myoglobinuria from hemoglobinuria.

The distinction between hematuria, hemoglobinuria, and myoglobinuria may be difficult to make on examination of the urine. In all three cases, the urine can be dark red to brown, and some erythrocytes are seen in the sediment (to a much greater degree with hematuria). The reagent strip test for blood is also positive in all three cases. If serum can be examined, it will often be pink with hemoglobinemia but a normal color with myoglobinemia because this pigment is cleared so rapidly. Accurate quantitative measurement of urine myoglobin can also be performed by immunoassay; although some slight interference by hemoglobin may occur, this is an excellent way to detect and quantify the presence of myoglobinuria (Loun, 1996). See Table 28-9, which compares hemoglobinuria, myoglobinuria, and hematuria.

Methods

Reagent Strip for Heme Compounds (Hemoglobin, Myoglobin). This method is based on the liberation of oxygen from peroxide in the reagent strip by the peroxidase-like activity of heme in free hemoglobin, lysed erythrocytes, or myoglobin. Intact erythrocytes are lysed on the strip, causing the hemoglobin to react. Therefore, well-mixed urine must be tested, as intact erythrocytes may be missed if only supernatant urine is used. The reagent area is impregnated with a buffered mixture of an organic peroxide and the chromogen tetramethylbenzidine.

$$H_2O_2 + \text{Chromogen} \xrightarrow{\text{Heme peroxidase activity}}$$
$$\text{Oxidized chromogen (color change)} + H_2O$$

Heme catalyzes the oxidation of tetramethylbenzidine to produce a green color. The strip is read at 60 seconds following sample application.

Multistix and Chemstrip detect 0.05–0.3 mg hemoglobin per deciliter urine. Note that 0.3 mg hemoglobin per deciliter is equivalent to that from 10 lysed erythrocytes per microliter. Normal erythrocytes contain approximately 30 pg of hemoglobin per cell.

TABLE 28-9
Differentiation of Hematuria, Hemoglobinuria, and Myoglobinuria

Condition	Plasma findings	Urine findings
Hematuria	Color—normal	Color—normal, smoky, pink, red, brown Erythrocytes—many Renal—red blood cell casts Protein—marked increase Lower urinary tract—no casts Protein—present or absent
Hemoglobinuria	Color—pink (early) Haptoglobin—low	Color—pink, red, brown Erythrocytes—occasional Pigment casts—occasional Protein—present or absent Hemosiderin—late
Myoglobinuria	Color—normal Haptoglobin—normal Creatine kinase—marked increase Aldolase—increased	Color—red, brown Erythrocytes—occasional Dense brown casts—occasional Protein—present or absent

Sensitivity is reduced in urine specimens with high specific gravity, in which erythrocyte lysis may not occur, and also when protein levels are high. Ascorbic acid in large concentrations may cause a false-negative result, as can formalin when used as a urine preservative. The presence of nitrite in large amounts will delay the reaction. Oxidizing contaminants such as hypochlorites (bleach) or iodine from skin-cleansing preparations may produce false-positive results. Microbial peroxidase, associated with urinary tract infection, potentially causes a false-positive reading.

Other Tests for Hemoglobin and Myoglobin. Qualitative tests have been generally unsatisfactory in separating myoglobin and hemoglobin, and both conditions may be present following crush injuries. Hemoglobin and myoglobin can be bound to proteins in urine, and this contributes to the difficulty of separating them by salt precipitation or electrophoresis. The salt precipitation method of Blondheim (1958) is described below.

Qualitative Test for Myoglobin.

1. Use a fresh urine specimen. Observe the color. Characteristically, urine with myoglobinuria is red when fresh and turns brown on standing, but some myoglobin may be present without color change. Myoglobin is less stable at an acid pH. Neutralize and refrigerate specimen pending testing.
2. Mix 1 mL of urine and 3 mL of 3% sulfosalicylic acid to assay for protein. If the pigment is precipitated, it is a protein. Filter. If the filtrate is a normal color, no abnormal nonprotein pigment is present. (Note: The heat and acetic acid test does not precipitate myoglobin or hemoglobin.)
3. To 5 mL of urine in a test tube, add 2.8 g of ammonium sulfate. Dissolve by mixing. The urine is now 80% saturated with ammonium sulfate. This is optimal for precipitation of hemoglobin. Filter or centrifuge. If the supernatant shows a normal color, the precipitated pigment is hemoglobin. If the supernatant fluid is colored, this is presumptive evidence of myoglobin.

This precipitation test has been largely replaced with specific immunoassays for myoglobin.

Capillary electrophoresis has been shown to successfully separate urinary hemoglobin from myoglobin based on differing electrophoretic mobility (Shihabi, 1995).

Detection of Hemosiderin in Urine. The Prussian blue reaction is used to demonstrate iron in hemosiderin (Fig. 28-2). A dry smear and an alternative wet preparation are described below.

Dry Procedure. When stained with Prussian blue reagent, hemosiderin appears as blue granules, 1–3 μm, singly or in groups, in renal tubular epithelial cells, as amorphous sediment, or as blue granules in casts. An iron stain used for the detection of siderocytes in blood or bone marrow is also suitable. Urine is collected in an iron-free glass container, overnight. Let stand for 2 hours. Decant three fourths of it, and centrifuge the

TABLE 28-10
Urine and Fecal Findings in Jaundice

Finding	Normal	Obstruction to bile flow	Hemolysis, hemolytic anemia	Liver damage, hepatitis, cholestasis
Urinary bilirubin	Absent	Increased, dark urine	Absent	Increased early
Urinary urobilinogen	Present	Neoplasm—low or absent; gallstones—variable	Increased	Decreased early; increased late
Fecal color	Dark	Pale; intermittent with gallstones in common bile duct; persistent with neoplasm in duct or pancreas	Dark	Pale early and dark late in hepatitis; pale with cholestasis

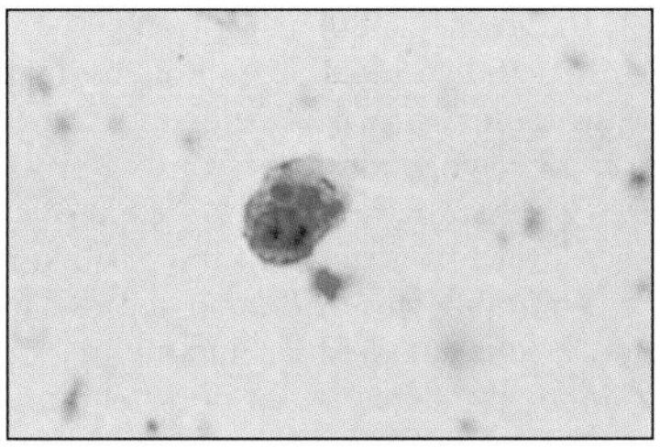

Figure 28-2 Renal tubular epithelial cell positive with Prussian blue stain, hemosiderin (×260).

remainder. Make a smear(s) of the sediment and allow to air dry. (Note: All glassware, slides, coverslips, etc., should be iron free. Water should be demineralized.)

Reagents. The Prussian blue reagent is made fresh.

Prussian blue stain: Add concentrated hydrochloric acid (HCl) to an aliquot of the potassium ferrocyanide solution (20% in demineralized water) until a white precipitate forms that remains stable on shaking. Filter through No. 5 filter paper.

Working counterstain: Dilute 1 mL safranin O stain (0.5 g in 100 mL distilled water) to 50 mL with phosphate buffer (pH, 6.4–4.7).

Procedure

1. Fix the smear in methyl alcohol for 10 minutes.
2. Rinse with iron-free water (demineralized) and air dry.
3. Stain with Prussian blue reagent for 30 minutes.
4. Wash gently for at least 4 minutes with iron-free water and air dry.
5. Counterstain with safranin O for 1–5 minutes.
6. Rinse with iron-free water. Air dry.
7. Mount coverslip.

Wet Procedure

1. Centrifuge a complete morning specimen or random urine sample for 5 minutes and pool the sediment. Examine several drops of sediment microscopically, searching for coarse yellow-brown granules, especially within renal tubular epithelial cells or casts.
2. If such granules are seen, suspend the rest of the sediment in a fresh mixture of 5 mL of 2% potassium ferrocyanide solution and 5 mL of 1% HCl, and allow to stand for 10 minutes.
3. Centrifuge, and discard the supernatant. Examine the sediment microscopically. Coarse granules of hemosiderin appear blue in this preparation in cells, casts, and amorphous material. If granules do not stain, reexamine after 30 minutes (occasionally the reaction is delayed).

Bilirubin in Urine

Bilirubin is a breakdown product of hemoglobin that is formed in the reticuloendothelial cells of the spleen, liver, and bone marrow. It is initially carried in the blood linked to albumin; this unconjugated bilirubin (or indirect bilirubin) is water insoluble and therefore is unable to pass through the glomerular barrier of the kidney. Unconjugated bilirubin is transported to the liver, where it is conjugated with glucuronic acid to form bilirubin glucuronide. This conjugated form of bilirubin (direct bilirubin) is water soluble and is able to pass through the glomerulus of the kidney into the urine. Conjugated bilirubin is normally excreted in the bile into the duodenum, and normal adult urine contains only 0.02 mg of bilirubin per deciliter. This small amount is not detected by the usual testing methods. Excretion of bilirubin is enhanced by alkalosis.

Conjugated bilirubin appearing in urine generally indicates that there is excess conjugated bilirubin in the bloodstream. This can occur when there is either (1) obstruction to bile outflow from the liver (intrahepatic or extrahepatic), or (2) hepatocellular disease with resultant inability of hepatocytes to sufficiently excrete conjugated bilirubin into the bile. For example, bilirubinuria may be present when intracanalicular pressure rises secondary to periportal inflammation, fibrosis, or hepatocyte swelling. Gallstones in the common bile duct and carcinoma of the head of the pancreas are possible sources of extrahepatic biliary obstruction leading to bilirubinuria. Bilirubinuria is often seen with acute viral hepatitis or drug-induced cholestasis before the appearance of jaundice; it typically accompanies jaundice of acute alcoholic hepatitis. In persons exposed to potentially hepatotoxic drugs or toxins, a positive test for bilirubinuria may be an early indication of cholestasis or liver damage. In congenital hyperbilirubinemias, bilirubin will appear in the urine in the Dubin-Johnson and Rotor types, and is not present with Gilbert's disease or Crigler-Najjar disease.

Bilirubinuria is associated with yellow-brown to greenish brown urine that may have a yellow foam, elevated serum bilirubin (conjugated), jaundice, and pale-colored feces. These acholic stools are so called because of the absence of bilirubin-derived pigment. A positive test for urinary bilirubin with a negative test for urobilinogen in urine is indicative of intrahepatic or extrahepatic biliary obstruction. This test is valuable in the differential diagnosis of jaundice, because bilirubinuria is not found with hemolytic jaundice. Table 28-10 summarizes typical urine and fecal findings in jaundice of various causes.

Methods

Reagent Strip. This test is based on the coupling reaction of bilirubin with a diazonium salt in acid medium. When this method is used, normal urine contains no detectable bilirubin. Specific tests differ in the diazonium salt utilized. Multistix uses diazotized 2,4-dichloroaniline as the diazo salt, with a color change from cream-buff to tan at 20 seconds. This system will detect 0.8 mg per deciliter urine; however, the color change may be difficult to read. Chemstrip uses 2,6-dichlorobenzene-diazonium tetrafluoroborate, and the color changes from pink to violet at 30–60 seconds. This test detects 0.5 mg per deciliter urine.

Urine must be fresh because bilirubin glucuronide in urine quickly hydrolyzes to less reactive free bilirubin. Oxidation of bilirubin in specimens that have stood too long, especially when exposed to light, will result in false-negative findings. Large amounts of ascorbic acid and nitrite can also lower bilirubin results. Metabolites of drugs such as phenazopyridine (Pyridium) give a reddish color at the low pH of the strip and mask the result. Rifampin and large amounts of chlorpromazine metabolites may cause false-positives, whereas salicylates do not interfere. Urobilinogen does not affect the result.

Confirmatory Bilirubin Tests. The diazo test method, in which bilirubin is coupled to *p*-nitrobenzene diazonium *p*-toluene sulfonate to form a blue or purple color (in the form of a tablet or reagent strip), is commonly used. The reagent strip test is much less reactive to free bilirubin than is the tablet test, so that a difference in results becomes more apparent as the urine ages. Another test employs a ferric chloride reagent to oxidize bilirubin to a green biliverdin. The diazo tablet method is described below.

Diazo Tablet Method. Tablets contain *p*-nitrobenzene diazonium *p*-toluene, as well as sulfosalicylic acid and sodium bicarbonate. The latter substances provide an acid medium for the reaction and an effervescent mixture that will ensure the solution of a portion of the tablet when water is added. (Ictotest kit, including absorbent mats and reagent tablets, is available through Bayer Corporation, Tarrytown, N.Y.)

Note: Reagent tablets are hygroscopic, and they should be protected from moisture or high humidity. The tablets are packed in a brown bottle because prolonged direct exposure to strong light results in decomposition of the stabilized diazonium compound. Prolonged exposure over several weeks to temperatures of 100° F or more may also result in deterioration of the tablets. A brown discoloration indicates deterioration, and when each new bottle is opened, tablets should be checked for positive and negative reactions.

Procedure

1. Place 10 drops of specimen on an asbestos-cellulose mat provided with the kit. Bilirubin, if present, will be adsorbed onto the mat surface.
2. Place a reagent tablet on the moistened area of the mat.
3. Place one drop of water onto the tablet. Wait 5 seconds, then place a second drop so that the water runs off the tablet onto the mat. If bilirubin is present, there will be a coupling of bilirubin with *p*-nitrobenzene diazonium *p*-toluene sulfonate from the tablet, as shown by the formation of a blue to purple color within 30 seconds. The tablet should be moved to reveal the purple color. A pink or red color is negative.

The diazo test reacts positively to bilirubin in amounts as low as 0.05–0.1 mg per deciliter. No purple reaction is seen with urobilin or other pigments, although high levels of urobilin or indican give a red color. Azo compounds (e.g., Pyridium) cause an atypical color. Rifampin may also interfere. Chlorpromazine metabolites in large amounts produce a purple color, and the metabolites of the antiinflammatory drugs mefenamic and flufenamic acid cause false-positive results.

Wash-Through Tablet Method. When false-positive reactions are suspected (e.g., with chlorpromazine), the contaminant can be diluted out with water in the mat.

Procedure. Prepare duplicate mats with 10 drops of urine on each. Add 10 drops of water to one mat. Place a reagent tablet on each mat and then two drops of water onto each tablet. Bilirubin, if present, is adsorbed into the mat fibers and will appear the same on each mat; an interfering substance produces a light color or no color on the mat with the extra water.

Urobilinogen in Urine

Conjugated bilirubin from the liver eventually reaches the duodenum, complexed with cholesterol, bile salts, and phospholipids within the bile. The conjugated bilirubin is not absorbed from the small intestine but instead passes on into the colon, where resident bacteria hydrolyze the conjugate. The free bilirubin is then reduced to urobilinogen, mesobilirubinogen, and stercobilinogen. Up to 50% of the urobilinogen is reabsorbed into the portal circulation and is reexcreted, unconjugated, into the bile. The vast majority of remaining urobilinogen is excreted in feces as colored urobilins or stercobilin, which are formed after further removal of hydrogen. A small amount is excreted in the urine.

Urobilinogen represents a group of closely related tetrapyrrole compounds, and because a mixture of substances is actually measured, the term **units** is frequently used instead of the more precise milligrams-per-deciliter terminology. These are roughly equivalent. Normal output of urobilinogen in the urine is 0.5–2.5 mg or units/24hours. These substances are colorless and labile, as opposed to the urobilins, the oxidation products of urobilinogen that impart a yellow-orange color to normal urine. Output of urobilinogen is increased in alkaline urine; the level is decreased in acid urine.

Whenever the liver is unable to efficiently remove the reabsorbed urobilinogen from the portal circulation, more urobilinogen than normal is routed through the kidney and hence is excreted in the urine. This can occur when there is hepatocellular damage due to viral hepatitis, drugs, or toxic substances, or in some cases of cirrhosis. With congestive heart failure, liver congestion prevents effective urobilinogen handling, and reexcretion into the bile is impaired. If an infection is present, such as cholangitis associated with obstruction, large amounts of urobilinogen are excreted in urine, together with bilirubin.

In contradistinction, an excess of urobilinogen in urine together with absent bilirubin is typically associated with hemolysis. This can be seen following acute lysis of erythrocytes, as well as with destruction of erythrocyte precursors in the bone marrow with megaloblastic anemias. Increased urobilinogen also accompanies bleeding into tissues and the subsequent formation of excess bilirubin. These jaundiced patients have dark-colored stools because excess urobilinogen is also excreted into the feces. Urinary urobilinogen may be increased when fever is associated with dehydration and concentrated urine.

Persistent absence of urinary urobilinogen occurs with complete obstruction of the outflow of bile into the intestine, accompanied by pale stools. Broad-spectrum antibiotics, which suppress the normal intestinal flora, may prevent the conversion of bilirubin to urobilinogen, and therefore may reduce its excretion in feces and urine.

The brown pigment mesobilifuscin is a dipyrrole that normally contributes to fecal and urine color. It does not react with tests for blood or bilirubin. Although it is not derived from bilirubin, as is urobilinogen, it is a likely byproduct of heme synthesis. Its excess causes a dark brown urine that can be seen with homozygous β-thalassemia, or whenever Heinz bodies form in erythrocytes (e.g., with the unstable hemoglobins).

Methods

Reagent Strip. Testing is based on the Ehrlich aldehyde reaction or on the formation of a red azo dye from a diazonium compound.

Multistix utilizes the former method; its test area is impregnated with an acid buffer solution and *p*-dimethylaminobenzaldehyde, which produces a reddish brown color with urobilinogen. Color varies from light yellow to shades of red-brown, and values from 0.2–1 mg per deciliter are considered normal. This test method is not specific for urobilinogen and will detect substances known to react with the Ehrlich reagent, including porphobilinogen, *p*-aminosalicylic acid metabolites, sulfonamides, procaine, 5-hydroxyindoleacetic acid, indole, and methyldopa (Aldomet). It is not a reliable method for the detection of porphobilinogen.

The Chemstrip urobilinogen test area is impregnated with 4-methoxybenzene-diazonium-tetrafluoroborate, which couples with urobilinogen in an acid medium to form a red azo dye. Results are read at 10–30 seconds, and the test can detect approximately 0.4 mg/dL. This test, unlike the Ehrlich reagent–based methods, is specific for urobilinogen.

A freshly voided sample is best for testing, given that urobilinogen is quite labile and will potentially form nonreactive urobilin in acid urine. Both reagent strips are affected by the metabolites of drugs such as phenazopyridine (Pyridium), which colors the urine orange-red in an acid medium, and other compounds such as Azo-Gantrisin. These may mask the reaction with urobilinogen or give a false-positive result. Bilirubin and blood do not usually affect the test, but bilirubin may occasionally cause a green color.

Other Urobilinogen and Porphobilinogen Tests. Qualitative testing for urobilinogen and porphobilinogen may be performed when reagent strip testing indicates more than 1 mg/dL of Ehrlich-reacting substance present in the urine (see later under Porphyrins for more information on these testing modalities).

Quantitative tests for urobilinogen in urine are seldom performed. Consult Henry (1979) for a 2-hour quantitative urobilinogen method, and Davidsohn (1974) or Schwartz (1944) for 24-hour quantitation. For quantitative comparative purposes in the same patient, a 2-hour test is used in which urine is collected from 2–4 PM after lunch. This period after the meal coincides with heightened excretion of urobilinogen, as the pH of the urine is more nearly neutral. Other 2-hour periods may be tested for comparison.

Indirect Tests for Urinary Tract Infection

It is not uncommon for significant urinary tract infections to be present in patients who do not experience typical symptoms. Given that these infections if untreated can cause severe renal damage, many physicians are finding it prudent to request tests for bacteriuria in high-risk individuals. These would include patients who are elderly, pregnant, or diabetic, and those with a previous history of urinary tract infections. The two most commonly utilized testing modalities for indirect assessment of bacteriuria and leukocyturia are the reagent strip nitrite and leukocyte esterase, respectively. These tests are best used to rule out urinary tract infections (St. John, 2006) and are discussed in the next sections. An immunochromatographic test strip for the measurement of urinary lactoferrin released from leukocytes may also prove useful for the rapid diagnosis of urinary tract infection (Arao, 1999). Microscopic urinalysis serves as a rapid confirmatory test for the presence of leukocytes and bacteria, with bacteriologic culture remaining the "gold standard" for detecting bacteriuria.

Nitrite

Many bacteria that are urinary tract pathogens are able to reduce nitrate to nitrite, and thus will generate a positive urine nitrite test when present in significant numbers ($>10^5$–10^6/mL bladder urine). Common organisms include *Escherichia coli*, *Klebsiella*, *Enterobacter*, *Proteus*, *Staphylococcus*, and *Pseudomonas* species; *Enterococcus* is unable to reduce nitrate to nitrite. If the nitrite test is positive, a culture should be considered, provided that the specimen was properly collected and stored prior to testing. A first morning clean-voided midstream specimen is best.

According to Kunin (1975), self-administered repeated nitrite tests (three tests) in a small group of patients revealed about 70% overall positive results when compared with cultures. When only *E. coli* was present, bacteriuria detected by a positive nitrite test in any of the three first morning specimens showed 93% agreement with culture results. No significant false-positive nitrite results were reported in his large test group. Other authors report more disappointing results with nitrite dipstick screening for urinary tract infection, particularly in hospital inpatients (Zaman, 1998).

Methods. The test depends on the conversion of nitrate to nitrite by bacterial action in the urine. Because overnight (minimum of 4 hours) bladder incubation is typically required for the infecting bacterial population to convert urinary nitrate to nitrite, a first morning specimen is best. A positive result is an indication for culture, unless the specimen has been improperly stored after collection, allowing contaminant bacterial growth.

Reagent Strip. The nitrite testing area of Multistix is impregnated with *p*-arsanilic acid, which forms a diazonium salt when it reacts with nitrite present in the urine. This compound is then able to couple with benzoquinoline to form a pink azo dye. This method detects 0.075 mg of nitrite per deciliter in solution and is read at 40 seconds. Chemstrip contains a benzoquinoline and sulfanilamide, which produce a pink azo dye with nitrite at 30 seconds, and is able to detect 0.05 mg of nitrite per deciliter. Note that pink spots or edges are interpreted as negative.

False-positive results most commonly occur with poorly collected/stored specimens as the result of contaminants and postcollection bacterial proliferation. False-positives may also be produced by medications that color the urine red or turn red in an acid medium (e.g., phenazopyridine).

False-negative nitrite results may be due to ascorbic acid, urobilinogen, or low pH (<6). Random specimens collected during the day and urine from patients with draining catheters do not show good correlation between the nitrite test and significant bacteriuria, presumably because of the time required for the chemical reduction to nitrite in the bladder urine. Additionally, some false-negative results occur because some nitrate-reducing organisms form compounds other than nitrite, such as ammonia, nitric and nitrous oxide, hydroxylamine, and nitrogen, and therefore give a negative nitrite test result. Lack of dietary nitrate may also produce false-negative results, even when a significant number of organisms are present.

Leukocyte Esterase

Extracts of human neutrophil azurophilic (primary) granules contain up to 10 proteins showing esterolytic activity, and this esterase activity is commonly used as a marker for these cells. Because neutrophils and other cells are labile in urine, leukocyte esterase activity can be indicative of remnants of cells that are not visible microscopically.

The presence of significant numbers of neutrophils in the urine suggests urinary tract infection; however, difficulty has arisen in determining suitable cutoff points for normal and abnormal numbers of these cells. Because quantitative counts are so low, precision is poor. Positive leukocyte esterase results correlate with "significant" numbers of neutrophils, either intact or lysed; with the use of a chamber count of about 10 neutrophils/µL of fresh urine as a cutoff point, the numbers of false-negative and false-positive results are low. Likewise, when a concentrated (10 : 1) urine sediment and a cytocentrifuged stained preparation are used, a negative reagent strip test is associated with fewer than 100 neutrophils in 10 high-power fields (hpf) (450×). The leukocyte esterase test may also be useful in the workup of suspected urethritis in male patients; it has a high negative predictive value in this diagnostic setting (Bowden, 1998).

Methods

Reagent Strip. This test is similar in principle to the naphthol chloroacetate reaction used for granulocyte esterase detection in hematology. Neutrophilic esterases catalyze the hydrolysis of esters to produce their respective alcohols and acids. For example, Multistix utilizes 3-hydroxy-5-phenyl-pyyrole-*N*-tosyl-L-alanine ester as a substrate, which reacts in the presence of leukocyte esterase to form pyrrole alcohol. The alcohol then reacts with a diazonium salt to produce a purple color. The intensity of the color produced is proportional to the amount of enzyme present, which is related to the number of neutrophils present.

Cells originating from the urinary tract (i.e., urothelium) and erythrocytes do not contribute to the esterase level. Elevated urine specific gravity, protein, and glucose may all decrease test results, as can the presence of boric acid and certain antibiotics such as tetracycline, cephalexin, and cephalothin. Very large amounts of ascorbic acid may inhibit the reaction.

Contamination of urine with vaginal fluid may give positive results, and large numbers of squamous epithelial cells and bacteria would be seen on microscopic evaluation. Also, *Trichomonas* and eosinophils may represent alternative cellular sources of esterases, causing false-positive results. Oxidizing agents and formalin may give false-positive colors, and nitrofurantoin and other strong colors may affect color interpretation.

Miscellaneous Chemical Screening Tests

Ascorbic Acid

Large quantities of ascorbic acid may occasionally be found in the urine of individuals taking therapeutic doses of vitamin C or other preparations containing abundant ascorbic acid. Because of its reducing properties, ascorbic acid may inhibit several reagent strip reactions (i.e., glucose, blood, bilirubin, nitrite, and leukocyte esterase). Reagent strips from various manufacturers differ in their susceptibility to this substance, and suspicious results should be investigated. For example, when the microscopic examination of urine sediment shows more than two erythrocytes per high power field, but heme is not detected by the reagent strip method, it may be useful to check for the presence of ascorbic acid.

Urine tests for ascorbic acid have also been used as an indication of adequate ascorbic acid therapy. With the usual Western diet, 2–10 mg/dL is excreted daily, but after ingestion of large amounts of ascorbic acid, levels in urine may rise to 200 mg/dL. Oxalate and sulfate are the metabolites of ascorbic acid, and with ingestion of large quantities (1 g or more per day), oxalate stones may form in susceptible persons.

Methods. Several manufacturers have developed reagent strip methods for detecting ascorbic acid, discussed below. Gas chromatographic/mass spectrometric measurement is a more accurate quantitative method (Deutsch, 1997).

Reagent Strip. The ascorbic acid testing area of C-Stix reagent strips is impregnated with phosphomolybdates buffered in an acid medium. The phosphomolybdates are reduced by ascorbic acid to molybdenum blue, and this test detects 5 mg/dL of ascorbic acid in urine after 10 seconds. Gentisic acid and L-dopa may cause false-positive results.

Stix reagent strips are not as sensitive as C-Stix; they can detect about 25 mg/dL of ascorbic acid at 60 seconds. The reagent in Stix is methylene green, which is reduced to its colorless form with ascorbic acid. Neutral red provides a background color, and the overall color changes from blue to purple at levels of 150 mg/dL. This same testing method is also incorporated into Multistix multiple reagent strips. Large amounts of bilirubin and pH greater than 7.5 interfere with the color. False-positive results are not seen with urates, salicylates, gentisic acid, or creatinine.

5-Hydroxyindoleacetic Acid

Serotonin (5-hydroxytryptamine) is produced by the argentaffin cells of the intestines from tryptophan, and is carried in the blood by platelets. Carcinoid tumors (argentaffinoma) can produce excessive amounts of serotonin, especially when metastatic. Characteristic symptoms include intestinal and vasomotor disturbances and bronchoconstriction; edema, right-sided valvular heart disease, and neurologic symptoms may also be present.

Although serotonin in the urine can be analyzed directly by high-performance liquid chromatographic methods (Panholzer, 1999), screening tests that detect the serotonin metabolite 5-hydroxyindoleacetic acid in the urine are more commonly used. The quantitative method is more sensitive because it eliminates the interfering keto acids and indoleacetic acid. The normal excretion of 5-hydroxyindoleacetic acid in 24 hours is 1–5 mg.

Screening Test. A random urine specimen is usually sufficient for screening purposes; if a 24-hour collection is made, it should be acidified with HCl. Boric acid may also be used as a preservative. Patients should be instructed not to take any drugs for 72 hours before the test; phenothiazines, acetanilid drugs, and mephenesin, a muscle relaxant, will interfere with this test.

The principle of the test is based on the development of a purple color specific for 5-hydroxyindoles with nitrous acid and 1-nitroso-2-naphthol. Ethylene dichloride is used to remove interfering chromogens. For the procedure, see Henry (1984).

Melanin

Normal melanocytes convert tyrosine to dihydroxyphenylalanine (DOPA), then to dopaquinone, and by oxidative steps to melanin. The enzyme tyrosinase is required for the first conversion step and is found in specific organelles in melanocytes called **melanosomes.** Its formation is increased by melanin-stimulating hormone. Melanosomes with pigment are normally transferred from melanocytes to skin and mucous membrane cells. Enlarged melanosomes are found in some neoplastic cells (e.g., nevus, melanoma).

Increased urinary excretion of melanin metabolites occurs as malignant melanoma metastasizes, although it is unusual to find dark-colored urine in these patients, even when the specimen stands at room temperature for 24 hours. These urinary melanogens include indoles, catechols, and catecholamines. DOPA does not appear in large amounts in urine from melanotic patients.

No simple specific test is available for melanuria. Screening tests for melanin should be made on fresh specimens of urine and include tests based on nonspecific color reactions produced with ferric chloride, Ehrlich's aldehyde reagent, and nitroferricyanide. Procedures for the ferric chloride and nitroferricyanide tests for melanin can be found in Henry (1984).

A column cation-exchange chromatographic method allows detection of melanin metabolites in urine. Another approach is to measure DOPA oxidase levels in urine. The enzyme is increased in the urine of patients with melanoma and is markedly increased with liver metastases.

Rarely, cells containing melanin pigment are seen in urine sediment when melanuria with pigment uptake by renal tubular cells or metastatic melanoma to the bladder is present. A ferrous ion uptake stain can be used to color the melanin in cells dark blue.

Porphyrins

The porphyrias are a group of diseases resulting from defects in the synthesis of heme. These are inherited enzyme deficiencies in which the enzyme substrate is usually excreted in excess in urine and/or feces. During the acute porphyric attack, high levels of porphobilinogen are excreted, but between attacks, levels of porphobilinogen may be increased or normal. The patterns of excretion of the various porphyrins vary with the different diseases, and together with the clinical findings help to establish the diagnosis.

The porphyrins are excreted in most of the porphyrias and in lead poisoning. Additionally, porphyrin metabolism may be abnormal in patients with established human immunodeficiency virus infection, particularly when there is a concomitant hepatitis C virus infection (O'Connor, 1996).

Skin photosensitivity and cutaneous lesions frequently accompany high levels of porphyrins. The one entity without skin lesions is acute intermittent porphyria. In patients presenting with neurologic disease and acute abdominal pain—the hepatic group—production and excretion of δ-aminolevulinic acid (ALA) and porphobilinogen are increased during the acute porphyric attack. This is likely due to increased activity of ALA synthase and subsequent increased production of the precursors. Exacerbations of the hepatic diseases are precipitated by drugs known to induce liver enzyme activity (e.g., barbiturates, certain steroids).

Methods. In patients suspected of having an acute porphyric attack, porphobilinogen is sought in urine specimens. The Watson-Schwartz test is used to separate causes of a positive Ehrlich-reacting test and to give an indication of large amounts of urobilinogen or the presence of porphobilinogen. A positive result for porphobilinogen in the Watson-Schwartz test can be further confirmed by the Hoesch test, because the former may show false-positive results for porphobilinogen as a result of drugs such as methyldopa. When a qualitative porphobilinogen test is specifically requested or a known porphyric patient is being followed, the simpler Hoesch test may be used instead of the Watson-Schwartz test.

Urine specimens for urobilinogen or porphobilinogen must be fresh. If testing will be delayed, the pH should be adjusted to near neutral (pH 7) and the specimen stored in a refrigerator, where it is stable for about 1 week. Urine may darken if the patient has porphyria, especially if left at room temperature.

Watson-Schwartz Test. Ehrlich's aldehyde reaction and Watson-Schwartz tests are based on solubility differences between urobilinogen and porphobilinogen. Urobilinogen can be extracted by chloroform and/or butanol, whereas porphobilinogen will remain in an aqueous phase.

Procedure

1. To 2.5 mL fresh urine, add 2.5 mL Ehrlich's reagent and mix.
2. Add 5 mL saturated sodium acetate and mix. Check with pH paper to confirm that the solution is in the pH range of 4–5. Adjust pH if necessary.
3. Add 5 mL chloroform; insert a stopper and shake vigorously for 1 minute. Permit the phases to separate.
4. Examine the upper (aqueous) phase. If the color is absent, consider the result of the screening test to be negative, and stop.
5. If color is present, separate the upper (aqueous) phase and add 5 mL of butanol. Insert a stopper and shake vigorously for 1 minute. Allow phases to separate.
6. A "pink to rose red" color in the lower aqueous layer indicates a positive result and suggests a concentration of porphobilinogen that is several times normal. A color in the upper butanol layer indicates an increase in urobilinogen concentration (Fig. 28-3).

Hoesch Test. The Hoesch test is based on the inverse Ehrlich's reaction (i.e., of maintaining an acid solution by adding a small urine volume to a relatively large reagent volume), eliminating the problem of urobilinogen reactivity. The sensitivity is similar to that of the Watson-Schwartz test, but the reaction is for porphobilinogen. This test will detect about 20–100 mg/L of porphobilinogen; urobilinogen in amounts up to 200 mg/L does not give a positive result (red color). A yellow color may be caused by urea.

The urorosein urinary pigment related to indoleacetic acid will produce a positive Hoesch test (in response to strong HCl), and the rose color may be confused with a positive porphobilinogen result. Some of the false-positive problems may be excluded by testing the specimen with concentrated HCl (6 mol/L) separately in conjunction with the Hoesch test. Urine from a patient having an acute porphyric attack may be dark red in color, necessitating a 1 : 10 dilution with water before testing.

The Watson-Schwartz test detects greater than 6 mg/L and the Hoesch test greater than 11 mg/L of porphobilinogen. The Watson-Schwartz test is more sensitive than the Hoesch test for porphobilinogen and may yield a positive result between attacks of acute intermittent porphyria. Large doses of methyldopa (Aldomet) gave positive results, as did indoles in some patients with intestinal ileus and the drug phenazopyridine (Pyridium), which becomes orange with HCl. A quantitative porphobilinogen test is necessary if the Watson-Schwartz test or the Hoesch test result is questionable; this situation may arise because of the instability of porphobilinogen.

Alternative urine screening tests for porphobilinogen have been described. These include a micellar electrokinetic capillary chromatographic method (Luo, 1996), as well as a semiquantitative kit in which urine is pretreated with ion-exchange resin, and the color of the Ehrlich–porphobilinogen adduct is compared to a set of standards (Deacon, 1998).

Uroporphyrin and coproporphyrin can be detected by fluorescence. An orange-red fluorescence is seen if a positive specimen is placed near an ultraviolet light source.

Fluorescence Screening Procedure for Porphyrin. In this method, the urine is acidified and the extracted porphyrin exposed to ultraviolet light.

1. Place 5 mL urine in a stoppered glass centrifuge tube. Add 3 mL of a mixture of one part glacial acetic acid with four parts ethyl acetate.
2. Shake and allow to separate. Centrifuging will accelerate the separation.
3. Using a Wood's lamp, observe the upper layer for fluorescence. Inspect the tube in a dark room with ultraviolet reflected light. A lavender to violet color indicates the presence of porphyrins; pink to red fluorescence indicates higher levels of porphyrin. Pale blue with no pink color is negative. Normal urine may fluoresce blue.

To increase the sensitivity of the test and remove interfering drug metabolites, transfer the upper layer to a glass tube and acidify with 0.5 mL of 3 M HCl (25 mL concentrated HCl diluted to 100 mL with water). Shake. Porphyrins are extracted into the lower aqueous layer and will produce a red-orange fluorescence.

An alternative screening method utilizes an anion-exchange resin column. Porphyrins are adsorbed, eluted, and exposed to fluorescent light. This method removes interfering substances and is similar in principle to the quantitative method for total porphyrins and for coproporphyrin and uroporphyrin.

Screening tests together with the clinical findings will indicate whether quantitative tests should be done. The latter are usually performed by reference or research laboratories.

Urine specimens for quantitative porphobilinogen should be kept at a near neutral pH (between 6 and 7) and protected from light. Frozen

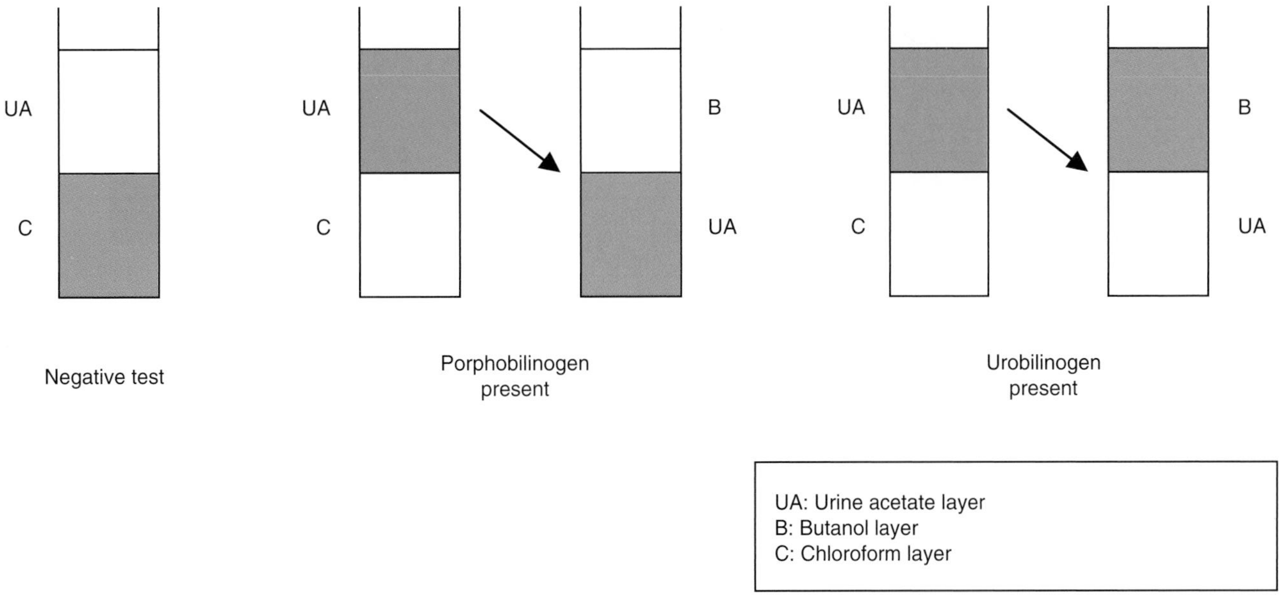

Figure 28-3 Watson-Schwartz test. Interpretation of screening method for urine urobilinogen and porphobilinogen.

specimens are fairly stable, although ALA is more stable if the urine is acidic. If the urine is to be tested for both substances, the near neutral pH is preferred and the urine aliquot is frozen. These substances are quantitated by eluting from different columns and reacting with Ehrlich's reagent. A micellar electrokinetic capillary chromatographic method has been described that allows separation of ALA and porphobilinogen (Luo, 1996).

Urine specimens for quantitative porphyrins are collected in a dark container containing 5 g sodium carbonate for a 24-hour specimen to give a concentration of 0.1% sodium carbonate or to produce urine of neutral pH. Coproporphyrin and uroporphyrin can be separated by thin-layer chromatography or by extraction and fluorometry and quantitated using ion-exchange columns. Additional methods include the Bio-Rad (porphyrin) column test, spectrophotometry (Zuijderhoudt, 1998), capillary electrophoresis (Chiang, 1997), fast atom bombardment mass spectrometry (Luo, 1997), and laser desorption/ionization time-of-flight mass spectrometry (Jones, 1995).

Fecal porphyrins can be qualitatively estimated using extraction and ultraviolet (UV) light, or quantitated. In some porphyrias, erythrocytes may show fluorescence when an unstained blood smear is examined microscopically. The nucleated bone marrow erythrocytes give greater fluorescence.

EXAMINATION OF URINE SEDIMENT

Microscopic examination of urine, in conjunction with dipstick chemical analysis, aids in the detection of renal and urinary tract disease processes. With microscopy, one can detect those cellular and noncellular elements of urine that do not give distinct chemical reactions. Microscopy can also serve as a confirmatory test in some circumstances (e.g., erythrocytes, leukocytes, bacteria) and yields new information 66% of the time (Tworek, 2008). In the routine laboratory, examination of the urine sediment is best reserved and most useful for those samples with abnormal dipstick results (European Urinalysis Guidelines, 2000).

To perform a microscopic evaluation of urine with competence, one must be knowledgeable of numerous morphologic entities (e.g., organisms, hematopoietic and epithelial cells, crystals, casts). Also, microscopists must be aware of the clinical relevance of urine findings, as well as the common chemical abnormalities associated with microscopic interpretations. Discrepancies should be investigated before a report is issued. The quality of the manual microscopic analysis of urine is dependent on the expertise and experience of the examiner (Tsai, 2005).

Centrifuged urine sediment should contain all the insoluble materials (commonly referred to as formed elements) that have accumulated in the urine following glomerular filtration and during passage of fluid through the renal tubules and lower urinary tract. Cellular elements are derived from two sources: (1) Desquamated/spontaneously exfoliated epithelial lining cells of the kidney and lower urinary tract, and (2) cells of hematogenous origin (leukocytes and erythrocytes). Cellular and noncellular casts may be seen; these are formed in the renal tubules and collecting ducts. Crystals of variable clinicopathologic significance may also be present. Organisms (bacteria, fungi, viral inclusion cells, parasites) and neoplastic cells represent elements that are typically foreign to urine; when detected, further investigation is required.

"Normal" or reference values for formed elements will vary from one laboratory to another because of (1) the variation in concentration of random urine specimens, and (2) the different methods used to concentrate the sediment by centrifugation. No specific standardized procedure is used. Individual laboratories have established their own reference values, often in conjunction with nephrologists and nephropathologists.

Methods for Examining Urine Sediment

In general, randomly collected urine specimens are satisfactory for microscopic evaluation; however, it is recommended that examination take place when the sample is fresh, particularly if no preservative has been added. Cells and casts begin to lyse within 2 hours of collection. Refrigeration (2°–8° C) helps prevent the lysis of pathologic entities; however, this may increase the precipitation of various amorphous and crystalline materials. Midstream collection is recommended for females to reduce contamination from vaginal elements.

Bright-field Microscopy

Although bright-field microscopy can be performed to a limited extent on unstained urine preparations, identification of leukocytes, histiocytes, epithelial cells, and cellular casts may be difficult. Subdued light is more effective in delineating translucent structures of the urine, such as hyaline casts, crystals, and mucous threads. A crystal-violet safranin stain is commonly used to aid in delineation of formed elements in urine.

Supravital Stain Reagents

Solution I:	Crystal violet	3.0 g
	Ethyl alcohol (95%)	20.0 mL
	Ammonium oxalate	0.8 g
Solution II:	Safranin O	1.0 g
	Ethyl alcohol (95%)	40.0 mL
	Distilled water	400.0 mL

Three parts of solution I and 97 parts of solution II are mixed and filtered. The mixture should be clarified by filtering every 2 weeks and discarded after 3 months. Separately, solutions I and II can be kept indefinitely at room temperature.

Several commercially available staining reagents are available. A 2% solution of methylene blue and toluidine blue may be used as a simple, quick supravital stain.

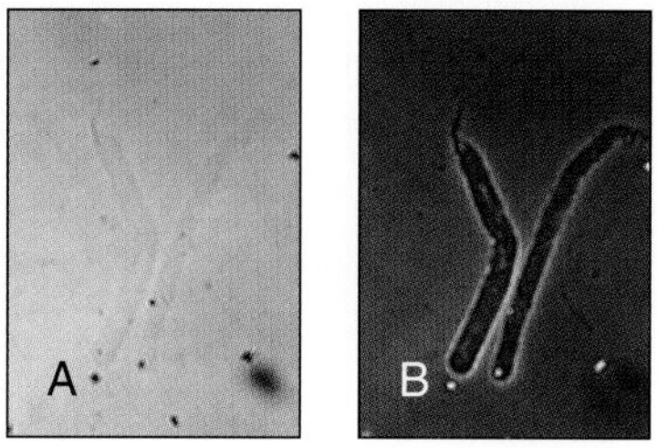

Figure 28-4 *A,* Hyaline casts. Bright-field (×100). *B,* Hyaline casts. Phase-contrast microscopy (×100).

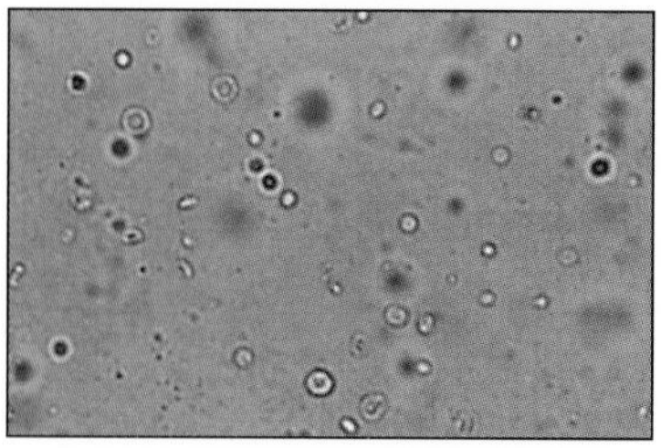

Figure 28-5 Dysmorphic erythrocytes (×160).

Procedure. Add one or two drops of stain to approximately 1 mL of concentrated urine sediment. Mix with a pipet, and place a drop of this suspension on a slide and coverslip.

Phase-Contrast Microscopy

Phase-contrast microscopy is beneficial for the detection of more translucent formed elements of the urinary sediment, notably casts that may escape detection under ordinary bright-field microscopy. Phase-contrast microscopy has the advantage of hardening the outlines of even the most transparent formed elements, making detection simple (Fig. 28-4, *A* and *B*). Scanning time is decreased, and the yield increased. Several microscopes have been designed to allow the operator to perform bright-field or phase-contrast examinations, depending on which objectives or condensors are utilized.

Polarized Microscopy

This is used to distinguish crystals and fibers from cellular or protein cast material. Lipid droplets or spherocrystals containing cholesterol esters are anisotropic in polarized light, show up brightly against a dark field, and form Maltese crosses with crossed polars. Visible evidence of anisotropy depends on the orientation of the crystal in the field; not all will be seen. If a red retardation plate is inserted, the cholesterol droplet will show typical blue and yellow quadrants against a red background. Starch granules will have a similar appearance when polarized but are much larger. Crystals, hair, and clothing fibers also show up brightly but do not exhibit Maltese cross forms. Fatty acids and triglycerides do not form liquid spherocrystals and do not show anisotropy, but glycosphingolipids in Fabry's disease are birefringent and may be seen in urinary sediments.

Quantitative Counts

The hemocytometer is used in many laboratories to quantify the elements of urine sediment. Cells and casts from undiluted well-mixed urine are counted and reported as the number of cells per microliter. Normal values for neutrophils vary from 5–30/μL according to different workers; upper limits for erythrocytes range from 3–20/μL and for casts as few as 1–2/μL. Counting cells from an unspun sample of urine in a hemocytometer has advantages over the examination of cytocentrifuged spun urine. These include decreased variability caused by centrifugation and suspension, a fixed volume of urine for examination, and a marked visual field for accurate counting. Kesson (1978) provided evidence that chamber counts on centrifuged urine sediments are more reliable in predicting renal functional abnormalities than is a conventional method using cells per high-power field. Recovery of cells may vary depending on centrifuge speed, specific gravity, and pH.

Microscopic Components in Urine Sediment

Cells

Erythrocytes. Under high power, unstained erythrocytes (RBCs) appear as pale biconcave disks that may vary somewhat in size but are usually about 7 μm in diameter. If the specimen is not fresh when it is examined, erythrocytes may appear as faint, colorless circles or "shadow cells," because the hemoglobin may dissolve out. They may become crenated in hypertonic urine and appear as small, rough cells with crinkled edges. In dilute urine, the cells will swell and rapidly lyse, releasing hemoglobin and leaving only empty cell membranes, referred to as **ghost cells.**

On occasion, erythrocytes may be confused with oil droplets or yeast cells. Oil droplets, however, exhibit greater variation in size and are highly refractile, and yeast cells usually show budding. If identification is difficult, two preparations may be made and a few drops of acetic acid added to one. Erythrocytes are lysed in the acidified preparation.

Erythrocytes are found in small numbers (0–2 cells/hpf) in normal urine; more than 3 cells/hpf is considered abnormal. The presence of increased numbers of erythrocytes in the urine may indicate a variety of urinary tract and systemic conditions. These include (1) renal disease—glomerulonephritis, lupus nephritis, interstitial nephritis associated with drug reactions, calculus, tumor, acute infection, tuberculosis, infarction, renal vein thrombosis, trauma (including renal biopsy), hydronephrosis, polycystic kidney, and occasionally acute tubular necrosis and malignant nephrosclerosis; (2) lower urinary tract disease—acute and chronic infection, calculus, tumor, stricture, and hemorrhagic cystitis following cyclophosphamide therapy; (3) extrarenal disease—acute appendicitis, salpingitis, diverticulitis, acute febrile episodes, malaria, subacute bacterial endocarditis, polyarteritis nodosa, malignant hypertension, blood dyscrasias, scurvy, and tumors of the colon, rectum, and pelvis; (4) toxic reactions due to drugs, such as sulfonamides, salicylates, methenamine, and anticoagulant therapy; and (5) physiologic causes, including exercise. When increased numbers of erythrocytes are found in the urine in conjunction with erythrocyte casts, bleeding may be assumed to be renal in origin.

Dysmorphic Erythrocytes. Numerous studies have concentrated on the variable morphology of urinary erythrocytes, attempting to localize the site of origin of hematuria. Red blood cells with cellular protrusions or fragmentation are termed dysmorphic (Fig. 28-5), and some authors have suggested that their presence in urine samples is strongly suggestive of renal glomerular bleeding (Fracchia, 1995). Others have not found dysmorphic morphology reliable in predicting primary renal hematuria (Favaro, 1997; Ward, 1998). The so-called "G1 cell," which has a doughnut shape with one or more membrane blebs, may be more specific than dysmorphic cells for diagnosing glomerular hematuria (Dinda, 1997). Another study describes immunocytochemical staining of urinary erythrocytes with Tamm-Horsfall protein in renal hematuria; this appears to be even more reliable than cellular morphology in terms of separating renal from nonrenal sources of erythrocytes (Fukuzaki, 1996). Normal persons may also have a mixture of distorted and undistorted erythrocytes in urine.

Leukocytes

Neutrophils. The polymorphonuclear leukocyte (neutrophil) is the predominant type of leukocyte (white blood cell [WBC]) that appears in the urine. Under high power, these cells appear as granular spheres about 12 μm in diameter with multilobated nuclei. Nuclear segments may sometimes appear as small, round, discrete nuclei. When cellular degeneration has begun, nuclear detail may be lost, and neutrophils may then become difficult to distinguish from renal tubular epithelial cells. Dilute acetic acid may enhance nuclear detail so that definition may still be possible (Fig. 28-6). Ultimately, however, with continued degeneration, neutrophilic nuclear segments fuse, making distinction from mononuclear cells difficult or impossible. Supravital staining may also be helpful in emphasizing nuclear detail. With crystal-violet safranin, neutrophilic nuclei appear reddish purple and cytoplasmic granules violet. The peroxidase cytochemical reaction is also useful in distinguishing neutrophils from tubular cells.

In dilute or hypotonic urine, neutrophils swell and their cytoplasmic granules exhibit brownian movement. Because of the refractility of the moving granules, neutrophils in this setting are known as **glitter cells.** These cells stain poorly with supravital stains and will show loss of nuclear segmentation. The leukocyte esterase reagent strip is valuable in the confirmation of pyuria in hypotonic urine specimens.

Additionally, leukocytes are rapidly lysed in hypotonic or alkaline urine. Approximately 50% are lost following 2–3 hours of standing at room

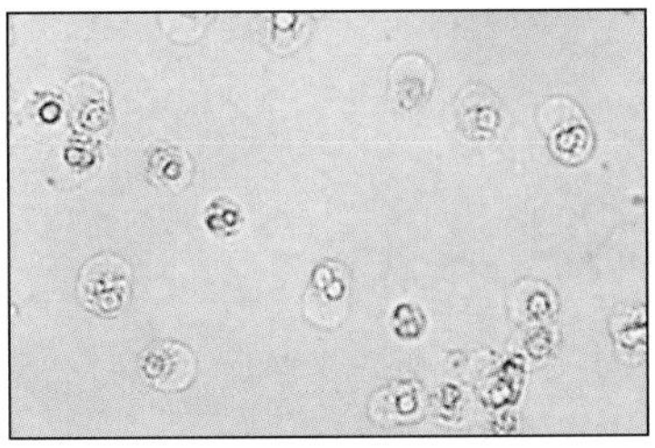

Figure 28-6 Neutrophils with dilute acetic acid (×100).

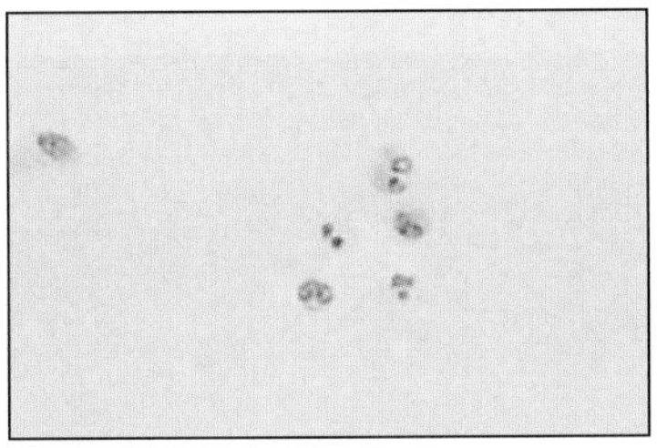

Figure 28-7 Eosinophils (×500).

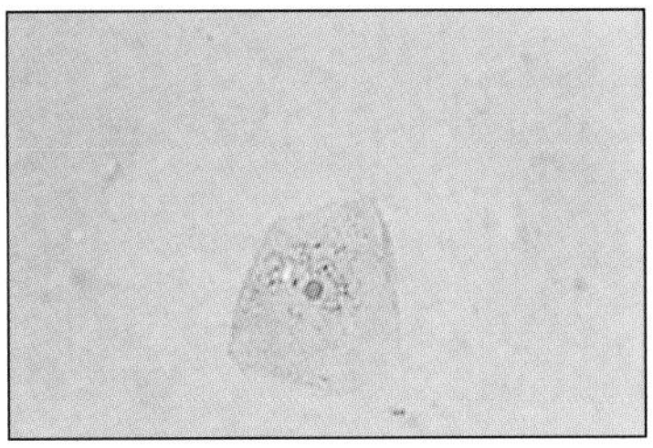

Figure 28-8 Squamous epithelial cell. Pyridium stained (×200).

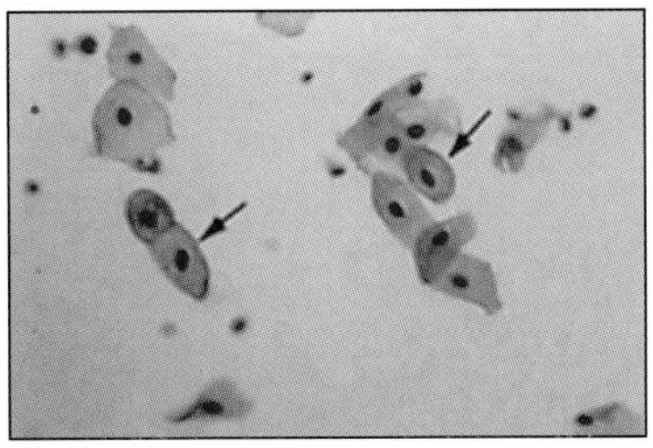

Figure 28-9 Transitional epithelial cells. Papanicolaou stained (×430).

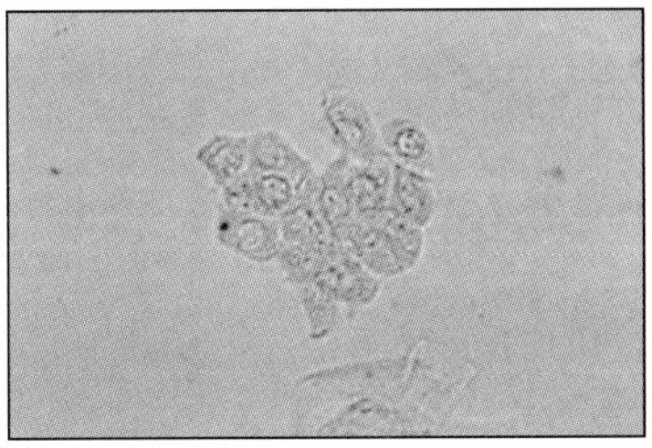

Figure 28-10 Renal tubular epithelial cells (×200).

temperature. This necessitates prompt examination of the urinary sediment following collection.

Pyuria. Typically, fewer than 5 leukocytes/hpf are seen in normal urine, although females not uncommonly will have somewhat higher quantities present. Increased numbers of leukocytes (principally neutrophils) in the urine constitute pyuria and indicate the presence of infection or inflammation in the urinary tract. When accompanied by leukocyte casts or mixed leukocyte–epithelial cell casts, increased urinary leukocytes are considered to be renal in origin.

Infection, either bacterial or nonbacterial, may be centered in the renal parenchyma (pyelonephritis) or may be localized as cystitis, prostatitis, urethritis, or balanitis. In women, the acute urethral syndrome (dysuria-pyuria syndrome) is regularly associated with greater than 8 neutrophils/μL in clean-catch urine specimens; however, bacterial colony counts are lower than expected. *Chlamydia trachomatis*, staphylococci, and coliforms are causative agents. Urinary neutrophil counts greater than 30 cells/hpf suggest acute infection, and repeated sterile cultures in this setting may indicate tuberculosis or a nephritis. Gross pyuria may reflect rupture of a renal or urinary tract abscess. It should be noted that the common finding of leukocytes in urine is not as reliable an indication of urinary tract infection as the detection of bacteriuria by Gram stain or culture of a fresh midstream specimen.

Increased leukocytes may be found in a variety of other urinary tract diseases, including glomerulonephritis, systemic lupus erythematosus (SLE), and interstitial nephritis. Calculous disease at any level may give rise to increased numbers of urinary leukocytes caused by stasis-induced ascending infection or localized mucosal inflammatory response. Bladder tumors, as well as a variety of acute or chronic localized inflammatory processes, may also cause leukocytes to be increased in the urine. Urine leukocytes may be transiently increased during fevers and following strenuous exercise.

Eosinophils. These cells are not normally seen in urine, and the finding of more than 1% eosinophils among the leukocyte population present is considered significant (Fig. 28-7). Evaluation of a concentrated stained urine is necessary for proper evaluation of urine for the presence of eosinophils. A cytocentrifuge preparation with Wright's, Diff-Quik, or Papanicolaou stain is commonly used, and the Hansel secretion stain (methylene blue and eosin-Y in methanol, Libe Labs, Florissant, MO) has been shown to be an excellent stain for recognition of eosinophiluria. Appropriately stained, bilobed eosinophils may be noted in patients with tubulointerstitial disease associated with hypersensitivity to drugs such as penicillin and its analogs. The cellular pattern in allergic interstitial nephritis typically includes many erythrocytes and some renal tubular epithelial cells. Eosinophiluria is also seen in other acute disorders of the genitourinary tract, with small numbers seen in urinary tract infections and renal transplant rejections.

Lymphocytes and Mononuclear Leukocytes. Small lymphocytes are normally present in urine and, along with histiocytes, are easily differentiated in stained smears. When mononuclear cells (histiocytes, lymphocytes, or plasma cells) constitute 30% or more of a differential count, chronic inflammation is indicated. Many small lymphocytes may be found in urine during renal transplant rejection. Plasma cells and atypical lymphocytes should be noted when present, and further investigation is warranted.

Epithelial Cells

Squamous Epithelial Cells. These cells are the most frequent epithelial cells seen in normal urine and the least significant. The distal one third of the urethra is lined by squamous epithelial cells, and in the urine, these cells are large and flat, with abundant cytoplasm and small round central nuclei (Fig. 28-8). Their margins are often folded. When stained with crystal-violet safranin, nuclei are purple and cytoplasm pink to violet. Many of the squamous cells present in female urine may be derived from the vagina or vulva.

Transitional (Urothelial) Epithelial Cells. Transitional epithelial cells line the urinary tract from the renal pelvis to the lower third of the urethra. These cells are smaller than squamous cells, their size ranging from 40–200 μm. They are round or pear shaped, with a round, centrally located nucleus. Occasional binucleate forms may be seen. When stained, transitional cells have dark blue nuclei with variable amounts of pale blue cytoplasm (Fig. 28-9). Another helpful clue to the proper identification of transitional cells is a characteristic **endo-ecto cytoplasmic rim.**

A few urothelial cells are present in normal urine, reflecting normal desquamation; similar to squamous cells, they are rarely of pathologic significance. The exception is the presence of large clumps or sheets of transitional cells in the absence of instrumentation (i.e., catheterization). This situation necessitates cytologic examination with the Papanicolaou stain to evaluate for possible transitional cell carcinoma.

Renal Tubular Epithelial Cells. These are the most significant types of epithelial cells found in urine because the finding of an increased number indicates tubular damage (Figs. 28-10 and 28-11). Small numbers of tubular cells may be seen in normal urine, reflecting the normal sloughing of aging cells. They may be present in somewhat larger numbers in the urine of normal newborns.

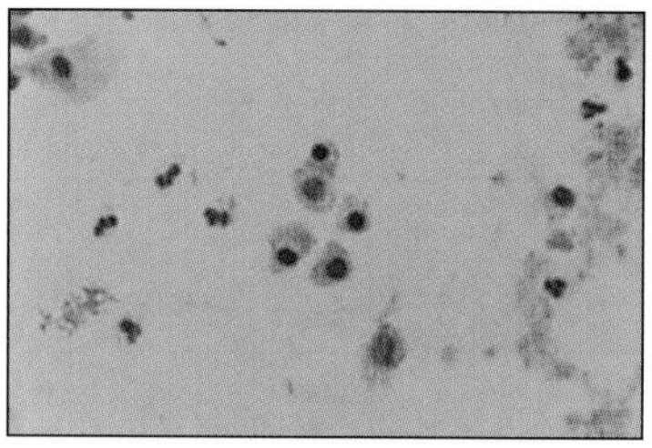

Figure 28-11 Renal tubular epithelial cells and neutrophils. Papanicolaou stained (×430).

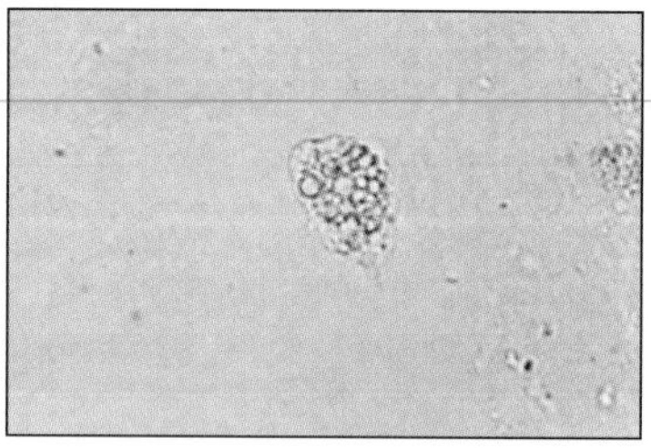

Figure 28-12 Oval fat body (×160).

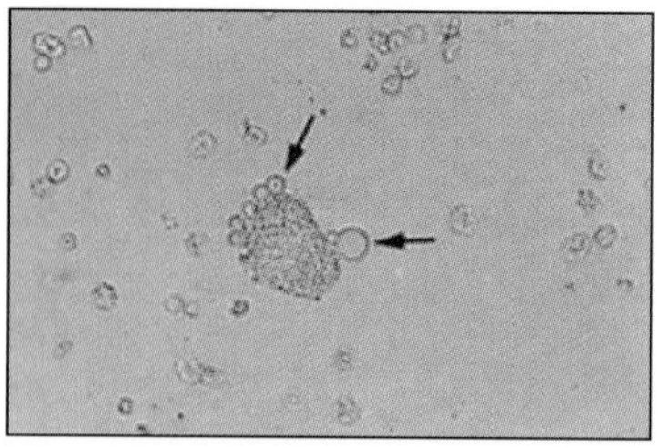

Figure 28-13 Oval fat body with attached fat droplets. Bright-field (×160).

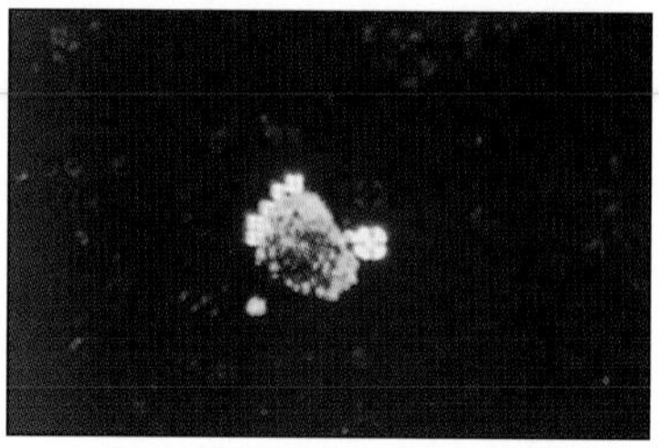

Figure 28-14 Oval fat body with attached fat droplets. Polarized (×160).

The Papanicolaou stain has been shown to be especially useful in distinguishing renal tubular cells from other mononuclear cells in urine. Renal epithelial cells from the proximal and distal convoluted tubules occur singly and are large (14–60 μm), oblong cells with characteristic coarsely granular eosinophilic cytoplasm. Nuclei may be multiple but are small with dense chromatin and rare nucleoli. Increased numbers of proximal and distal convoluted renal epithelial cells are seen in cases of acute tubular necrosis and with certain drug or heavy metal toxicities.

Epithelial cells from the collecting ducts measure 12–20 μm and are identified by their characteristic cuboidal or polygonal shape and large, usually slightly eccentric nucleus. Cytoplasmic properties include a basophilic endo-ecto cytoplasmic rim commonly found in transitional epithelial cells. Increased numbers of collecting duct epithelial cells are found in renal transplant rejection, acute tubular necrosis (diuretic phase), and other ischemic injuries to the kidney. They may also be found in increased numbers in malignant nephrosclerosis, as well as in cases of acute glomerulonephritis accompanied by tubular damage. Ingestion of various drugs and chemicals may cause significant tubular desquamation. Collecting duct tubular cells are easily found in the urine following salicylate intoxication.

Renal epithelial fragments of collecting duct origin have been described. Three or more renal cells of collecting duct origin constitute a renal epithelial fragment and indicate a more severe form of renal tubular injury with basement membrane disruption. Renal epithelial fragments are indicative of ischemic necrosis and are usually found accompanying varying degrees of renal tubular injury and pathologic casts. Proximal and distal convoluted tubular cells are not found in fragment form. Proper identification of renal epithelial fragments is essential, not only in diagnosing a more severe form of renal tubular injury, but also in avoiding a false-positive diagnosis of low-grade transitional cell carcinoma.

Lipids in Renal Tubular Epithelial Cells. Oval fat bodies are tubular cells that have absorbed lipoproteins with cholesterol and triglycerides leaked from nephrotic glomeruli (Fig. 28-12). Oval fat bodies therefore constitute one form of lipiduria. Lipids may also appear in the urine as free fatty droplets, or within histiocytes as ingested material. The presence of any or all of these lipid forms accompanied by marked proteinuria is characteristic of the nephrotic syndrome.

Positive identification of lipid is required before lipiduria is reported. When free or incorporated droplets contain large amounts of cholesterol, they exhibit Maltese cross formation under polarized light (Figs. 28-13 and 28-14). When they contain large quantities of triglycerides, fat stains (Oil Red O or Sudan III) are required for positive lipid identification.

Pigment in Renal Tubular Epithelial Cells. With hemoglobinuria or myoglobinuria, heme pigment is absorbed into the cells and is converted to hemosiderin. The iron-laden cells are desquamated and found in the urine sediment. The cytoplasmic granules appear yellow-brown and stain for iron with Prussian blue. These cells may also be incorporated into casts (see Figs. 28-1 and 28-2).

Melanin granules are absorbed into the tubular cells in rare cases of melanuria. The desquamated pigmented cells may be demonstrated in the sediment. Pigmented tumor cells are also found in cases of melanoma metastasis to the bladder.

Bilirubin pigment colors all of the elements of the sediment, including renal tubular epithelial cells and casts. Note that urobilin does not color cells and casts.

Casts

Casts are the only formed elements of urine that have the kidney as their sole site of origin. Tamm-Horsfall protein is the glycoprotein secreted by the thick part of the ascending loop of Henle (and possibly the distal tubule), which constitutes about one third of the total urinary protein in normal individuals. It is generally held that Tamm-Horsfall protein forms the matrix of all casts. The protein forms a meshwork of fibrils that can potentially trap any elements present in the tubular filtrate, including cells, cell fragments, or granular material.

Casts can be quite variable in their appearance, size, shape, and stability. Perhaps this variability is one factor in the apparent low precision of cast identification in some laboratories (Yoo, 1995; Rasoulpour, 1996). The width of a cast depends on the size of the tubule in which it was formed. Broad casts are seen in dilated tubules or with stasis in collecting ducts. Thin casts occur in tubules compressed by swollen interstitial tissue or as the result of disintegration. Casts may be short and stubby, or long and convoluted. The latter variety appears when diuresis occurs after urinary stasis. Casts typically have parallel sides and blunt ends, but with age they may begin to disintegrate and show thinning and irregularities. Fibrils may separate, causing a frayed appearance. Tails and tapering ends can be seen, and these disintegrating forms are referred to as **cylindroids.**

In the normal person, very few casts are seen in the urinary sediment. In kidney diseases, they may appear in large numbers and in many forms. Increased numbers of casts usually indicate that kidney disease is widespread, and that many nephrons are involved. Large numbers of casts may also be seen in healthy persons after strenuous exercise accompanied by proteinuria.

Cast formation increases with lower pH or increased ionic concentration and with stasis or obstruction of the nephron by cells or cell debris. It is increased when larger than normal quantities of plasma proteins enter the tubules. Usually the protein in excess is albumin, but globulins such as the Bence Jones immunoglobulin cause cast formation, as do hemoglobin and myoglobin. The plasma proteins possibly react or combine with Tamm-Horsfall protein to form less translucent casts and granular casts.

Casts may be classified according to their matrix, inclusions, pigments, and cells present, as shown in Table 28-11. A detailed discussion, including clinical significance, follows.

Cast Matrix

Hyaline Casts. These are the most frequently observed casts, consisting almost entirely of Tamm-Horsfall protein; zero to two hyaline casts per

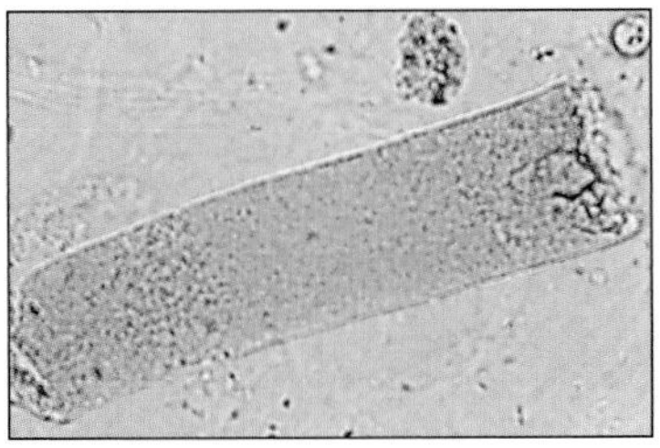

Figure 28-15 Waxy cast (×200).

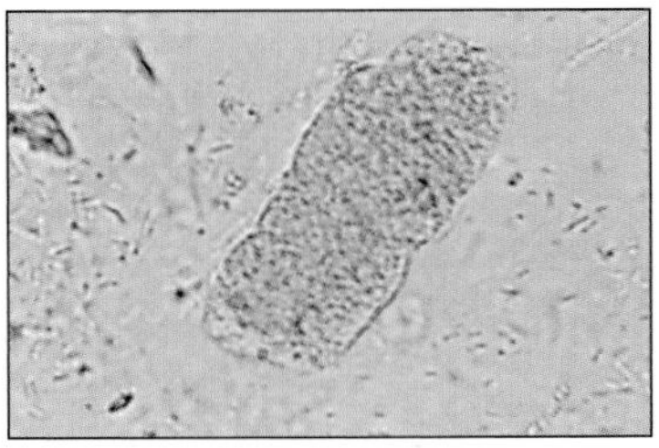

Figure 28-16 Fine granular cast becoming waxy (×200).

TABLE 28-11
Classification of Casts

Matrix	Pigments
Hyaline—variable size	Hemoglobin, myoglobin, bilirubin, drugs
Waxy—often broad in use	
Inclusions	Cells
Granules—proteins, cell debris	Erythrocytes and red blood cell remnants
Fat globules—triglycerides, cholesterol esters	Leukocytes—neutrophils, lymphocytes, monocytes, and histiocytes
Hemosiderin granules	Renal tubular epithelial cells
Crystals—uncommon	Mixed cells—erythrocytes, neutrophils, and renal tubular cells
Melanin granules—rare	Bacteria

low-power field (lpf) is considered normal. Hyaline casts are translucent with bright-field microscopy and pink with supravital staining, and are more easily visualized with phase-contrast microscopy (see Fig. 28-4, *A* and *B*). Increased numbers are seen with renal diseases and transiently with exercise, heat exposure, dehydration, fever, congestive heart failure, and diuretic therapy.

Waxy Casts. With chronic renal diseases, some casts become denser in appearance and are known as waxy. These differ from hyaline casts in that they are easily visualized because of their high refractive index. With bright-field microscopy, waxy casts are homogeneously smooth in appearance with sharp margins, blunted ends, and cracks or convolutions frequently seen along the lateral margins, indicating a measure of brittleness (Fig. 28-15).

Waxy casts are commonly associated with tubular inflammation and degeneration. They are observed most frequently in patients with chronic renal failure and are found during acute and chronic renal allograft rejection. Early waxy casts are believed by some investigators to reflect the final phase of dissolution of the fine granules of granular casts (Fig. 28-16). Because time is required for granules to undergo lysis, waxy casts imply localized nephron obstruction and oliguria. When waxy casts are unusually broad, they are known as **renal failure casts.** These casts imply advanced tubular atrophy and/or dilation, in turn reflecting end-stage renal disease and extreme stasis of urine flow.

Cellular Casts

Erythrocyte (Red Blood Cell) Casts. Finding these casts in the urine is significant because they are an indication of bleeding within the nephron. Glomerular damage allows erythrocytes to escape into the tubule; if there is concomitant proteinuria, and if conditions are optimal for cast formation, red cell casts form in the distal nephron. In urine, these casts appear yellow under low-power objectives. A prerequisite for the identification of an erythrocyte cast is that red blood cell outlines should be sharply defined in at least part of the cast (Fig. 28-17). The amount of matrix material that

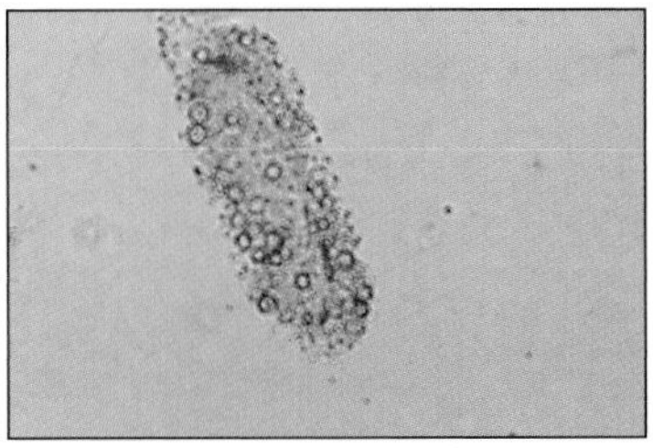

Figure 28-17 Erythrocyte cast (×200).

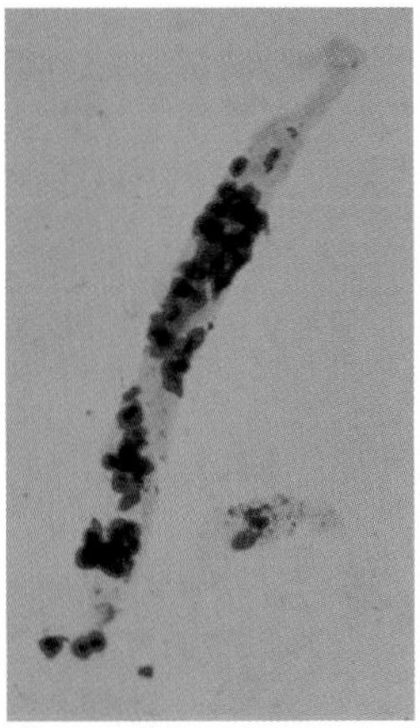

Figure 28-18 Leukocyte cast. IRIS urinalysis stain (×200).

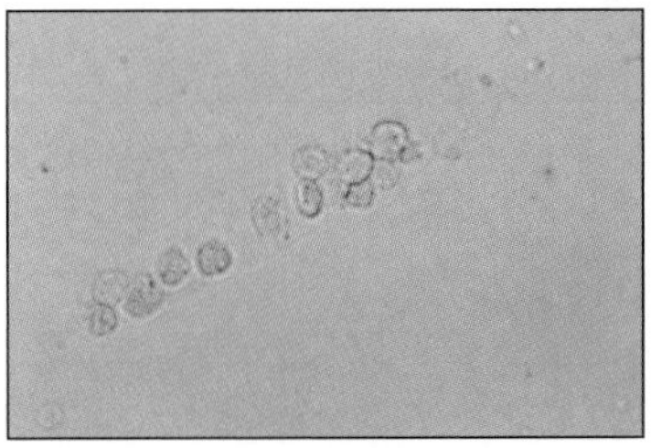

Figure 28-19 Cellular cast (×200).

may be visible ranges from scant to a prominent delicate hyaline matrix with only one or two visible red cells. These casts are better visualized with phase-contrast microscopy or with supravital staining, in which case the erythrocytes are colorless or lavender in a pink matrix. With prolonged stasis, red cell casts may degenerate and appear in the urine as reddish brown, coarsely granular hemoglobin (blood) casts.

Pathologic disorders in which erythrocyte casts appear in the sediment include many acute glomerulonephritides, IgA nephropathy, lupus nephritis, subacute bacterial endocarditis, and renal infarction. Rarely, tubulointerstitial disease may allow transtubular entry of erythrocytes with subsequent incorporation into a cast. This may occur in severe pyelonephritis. Additionally, the appearance of erythrocyte and leukocyte casts has been found to coincide with renal relapse in patients with SLE (Herbert, 1995).

Leukocyte (WBC) Casts. WBC casts are refractile and exhibit granules; frequently, multilobated nuclei will be visible (Fig. 28-18), unless disintegration has begun. Phase-contrast microscopy may be helpful in delineating nuclear segmentation. Supravital stains also enhance visualization.

Leukocytes usually enter tubular lumina from the interstitium, and for the most part, leukocyte casts (Fig. 28-19) reflect tubulointerstitial disease with neutrophilic exudates and interstitial inflammation. The most common disease of this category is pyelonephritis. Leukocyte casts may be present in glomerular disease owing to the chemotactic effect of complement. They are also seen in interstitial nephritis, lupus nephritis, and even the nephrotic syndrome.

Renal Tubular Epithelial Cell Casts. Renal tubular epithelial cell casts may be difficult to distinguish from leukocyte casts, particularly in unstained preparations viewed with bright-field microscopy. Supravital

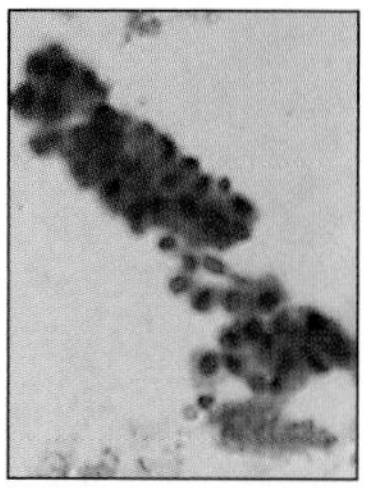

Figure 28-20 Renal tubular epithelial cell cast. Papanicolaou stained (×430).

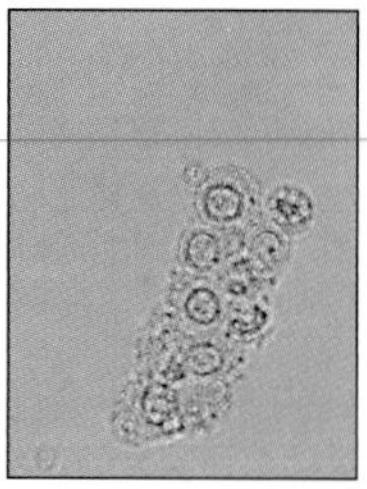

Figure 28-21 Mixed (leukocyte and renal epithelial tubular cell) cast (×200).

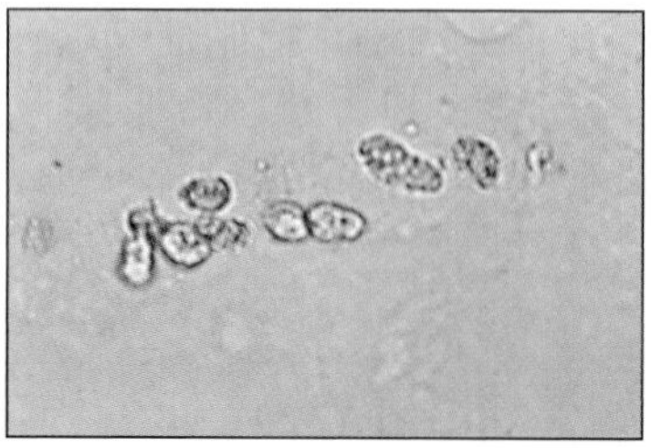

Figure 28-22 Cellular cast (×200).

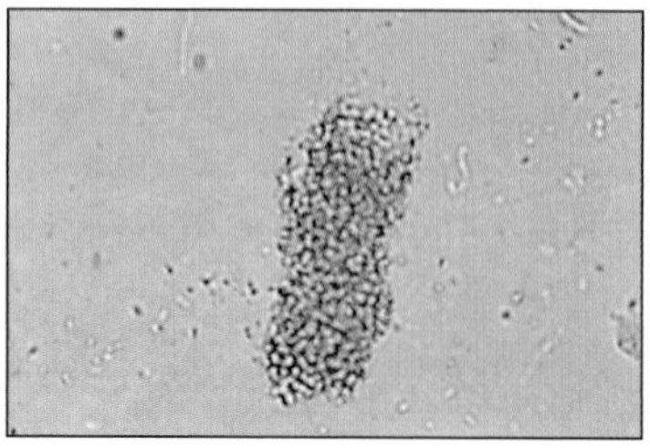

Figure 28-23 Granular cast (×200).

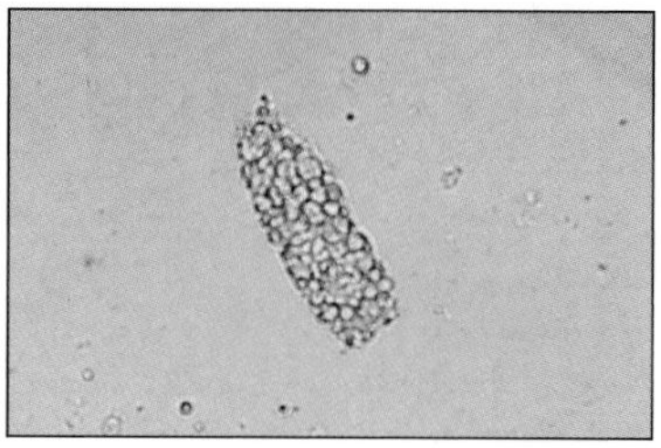

Figure 28-24 Fatty cast. Bright-field, nonpolarized (×160).

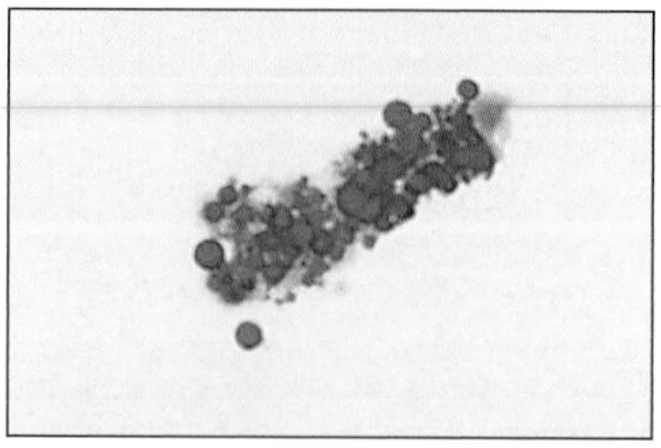

Figure 28-25 Fatty cast. Positive Oil Red O (×200).

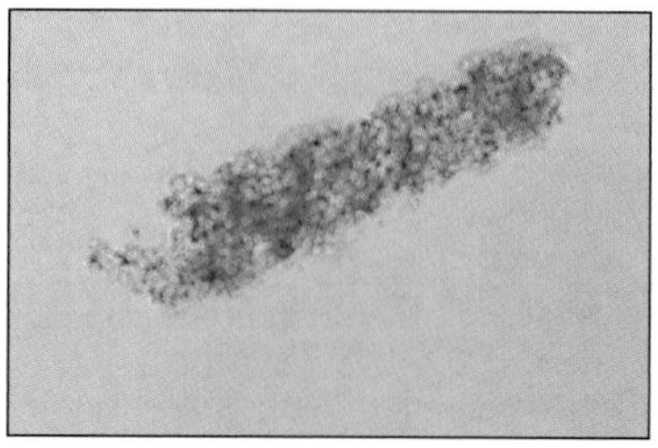

Figure 28-26 Hemoglobin cast (×200).

staining, phase-contrast microscopy, and Papanicolaou staining (see Figs. 28-19 and 28-20) are helpful in delineating between these two cast types. The most reliable distinguishing characteristic of renal tubular cells is their singular round nuclei.

Renal tubular epithelial cell casts are seen in urine with acute tubular necrosis, viral disease (e.g., cytomegalovirus disease), or exposure to a variety of drugs. Heavy metal poisoning and ethylene glycol and salicylate intoxication may cause tubular cells and casts to appear in the urine. In transplant units, these cells and casts constitute some of the more reliable criteria for detecting acute allograft rejection after the third postoperative day.

Mixed Cellular Casts. Not infrequently, two distinct cell types may be present within a single cast. This has been referred to as a **mixed cast,** and examples might include leukocyte/renal, erythrocyte/leukocyte, and eosinophil/renal (Fig. 28-21). When cell types cannot be established with certainty, the resulting cast is known as a **cellular cast** (Fig. 28-22). Some inferences as to cell type may be drawn from the dominant population of free cells in the surrounding sediment.

Inclusion Casts

Granular Casts. Granular casts are fairly common and may appear in both pathologic and nonpathologic conditions (Fig. 28-23). Granules may be small or large and may originate from plasma protein aggregates that pass into the tubules from damaged glomeruli, as well as from cellular remnants of leukocytes, erythrocytes, or damaged renal tubular cells. Fine salt precipitates and lysosomes may also be granular components. Protein aggregates include fibrinogen, immune complexes, and globulins. With prolonged stasis, large granules in casts may become smaller, and there appears to be no advantage to separating types of granular casts.

Granular casts appear with glomerular and tubular diseases but are also a feature of tubulointerstitial disease and renal allograft rejection. They may accompany pyelonephritis, viral infections, and chronic lead poisoning. Coarsely granular casts occur, with hematuria, in cases of renal papillary necrosis. It is possible that some fine granules represent calcium phosphate precipitants in hyperparathyroidism. Granular casts may also be seen following periods of extreme stress or strenuous exercise.

Fatty Casts. Fatty material is incorporated into the cast matrix from lipid-laden renal tubular cells. These are commonly seen when heavy proteinuria is present and are a feature of nephrotic syndrome (Figs. 28-24 and 28-25).

Crystal Casts. Casts containing urates, calcium oxalate, and sulfonamides (sulfamethoxazole) are occasionally seen. A matrix is visible in a true crystal cast, and the crystals may polarize. These casts indicate deposition of crystals in the tubule or collecting duct. Hematuria, possibly related to tubular damage, regularly accompanies crystal casts. These casts should be carefully distinguished from clumps of crystals forming at room or refrigerator temperatures.

Pigmented Casts

Hemoglobin (Blood) Casts. Hemoglobin casts typically appear yellow to red, although sometimes the color is pale (Fig. 28-26). Most often, hemoglobin casts, also known as blood casts, are seen with erythrocyte casts and glomerular disease. Less commonly, they are seen with tubular bleeding and rarely with hemoglobinuria.

Hemosiderin Casts. Hemosiderin granules in casts derive from pigment-laden renal tubular cells.

Myoglobin Casts. These casts are red-brown in color and occur with myoglobinuria following acute muscle damage. They may be associated with acute renal failure.

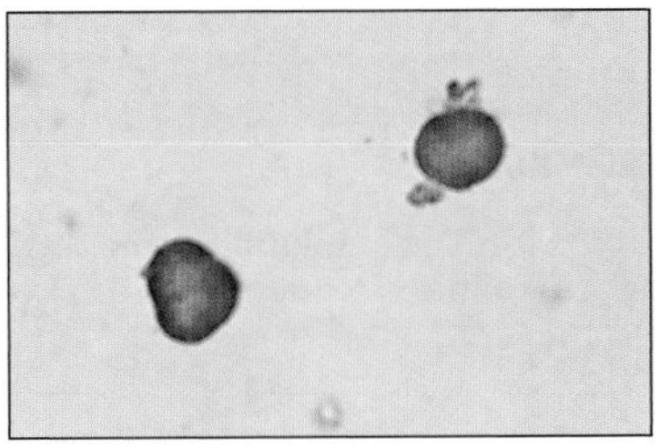

Figure 28-27 Acid urates (×160).

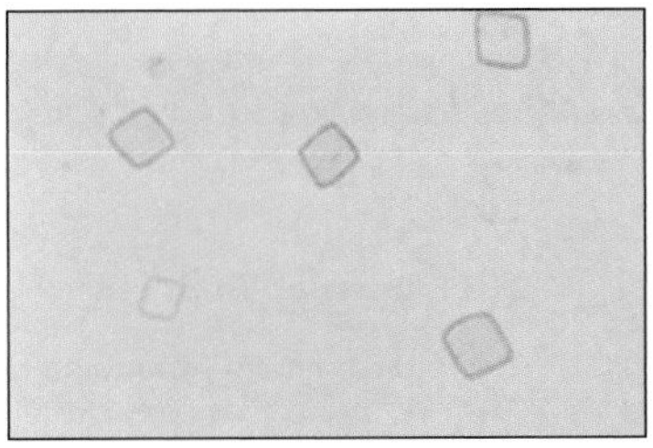

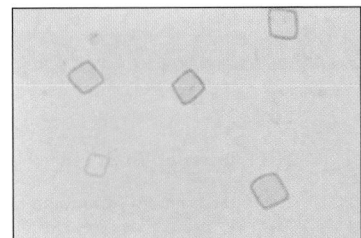

Figure 28-28 Uric acid crystals (×160).

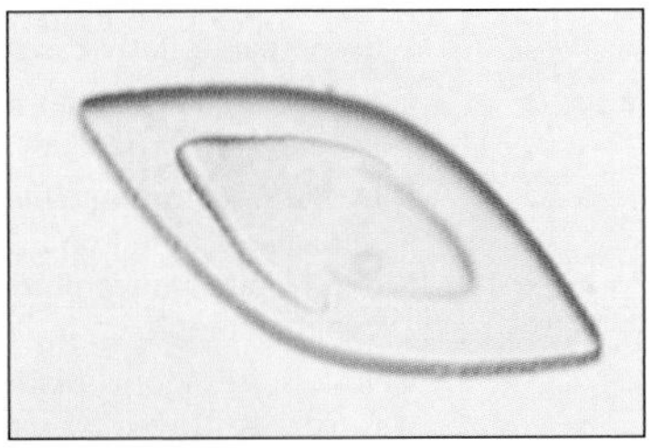

Figure 28-29 Large uric acid plate, laminated (×160).

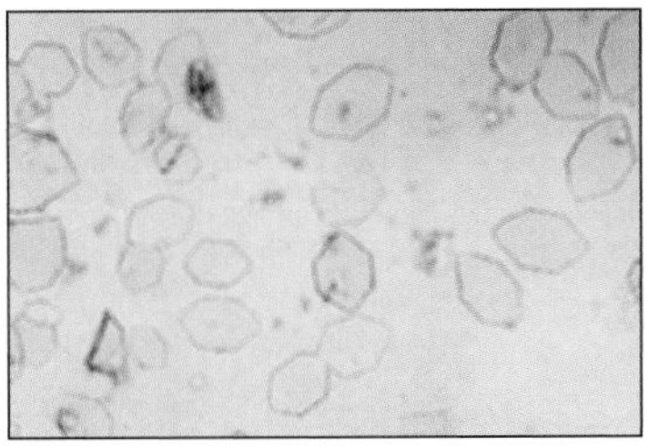

Figure 28-30 Hexagonal uric acid crystals. Bright-field (×50).

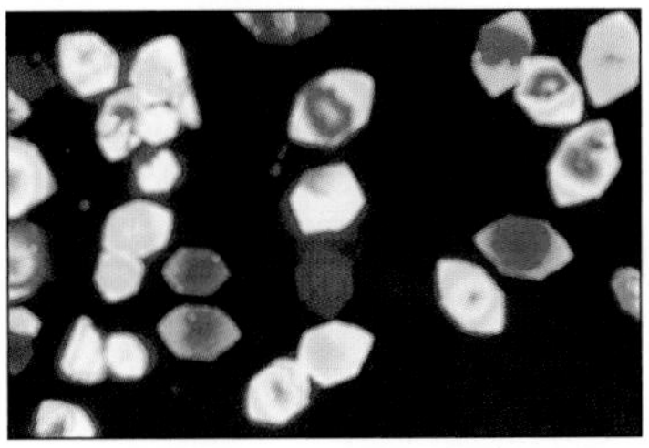

Figure 28-31 Hexagonal uric acid crystals. Polarized (×50).

Bilirubin and Other Drug Casts. Bilirubin is seen in urine when obstructive jaundice is present, and will color casts a deep yellow brown. Drugs such as phenazopyridine (Pyridium) cause a bright yellow to orange color in acid urine and color casts and cells as well.

Broad Casts. Broad casts are defined as those with a diameter two to six times that of normal casts. They indicate tubular dilation and/or stasis in the distal collecting duct. All types of casts may occur in broad forms, and they are typically seen in individuals with chronic renal failure. They portend a poor prognosis.

Other Miscellaneous Casts or Cast-like Structures. Bacteria may become embedded in cast matrices; on supravital staining, they appear dark purple with a pale pink matrix. Mucous threads are commonly confused with casts. However, these are larger, long, and ribbon-like, with poorly defined edges and pointed or split ends, in contradistinction to casts, which tend to have well-defined edges and blunt ends.

Telescoped Sediment. This term is used to describe the simultaneous occurrence of elements of glomerulonephritis and those of nephrotic syndrome in the same urine specimen. A telescoped sediment might therefore include red cells, red cell casts, cellular casts, broad waxy casts, lipid droplets, oval fat bodies, and fatty casts. Such sediment may be found in collagen vascular disease (notably lupus nephritis) and subacute bacterial endocarditis.

Crystals

Crystals form by the precipitation of urinary salts when alterations in multiple factors affect their solubilities. These include changes in pH, temperature, and concentration. Precipitates can appear in the urine in the form of true crystals or amorphous material. Most crystal formation takes place in refrigerated specimens and those allowed to sit at room temperature for several hours. Increased solute concentration is typically responsible for crystal formation.

Although most crystals in the urine are of limited clinical significance, proper identification is essential, so as not to miss the relatively few abnormal crystals that are associated with various pathologic conditions. Knowledge of urine pH is a valuable aid in crystal identification because it is the pH that determines which chemical will precipitate. Many of the commonly seen crystals have characteristic morphologies; however, variability does exist, sometimes leading to confusion between pathologic and nonpathologic crystal structures. For the purpose of separating abnormal from more commonly occurring **nuisance crystals,** a summary of crystal morphology is presented (Table 28-12).

Crystals Found in Normal Acid Urine

Amorphous Urates (Calcium, Magnesium, Sodium, and Potassium Urates). Amorphous urates will precipitate upon standing in concentrated urine of a slightly acid pH. When large quantities are present, the urine sediment may appear pink-orange to reddish brown on macroscopic examination; this appearance has been referred to as **brick dust.** Microscopically, this amorphous material appears as yellow-brown small granules that can form clumps and adhere to fibers and mucous threads. Amorphous urates will convert to uric acid crystals with acidification with acetic acid, and will dissolve with heat (60° C) and with dilute alkali.

Crystalline Urates (Sodium, Potassium, and Ammonium). These biurates and acid urates form small brown spheres (Fig. 28-27) or colorless needles in slightly acid urine. The spheres may cluster in pairs and triplets. Similar to amorphous urates, these crystalline forms will slowly revert to uric acid plates on acidification with acetic acid.

Crystalline Uric Acid. Uric acid crystals occur at low pH (5–5.5) and are seen in a variety of shapes, including rhombic or four-sided flat plates, prisms, oval forms with pointed ends (lemon-shaped), wedges, rosettes, and irregular plates (Figs. 28-28 and 28-29). Most are colored, typically yellow or reddish brown. Rarely, they are colorless and hexagonal, resembling cystine (Fig. 28-30). Unlike cystine, they show birefringence with polarized light (Fig. 28-31).

Large numbers of uric acid crystals and urates may reflect increased nucleoprotein turnover, especially during chemotherapy of leukemia or lymphoma. Increased quantities may be seen with Lesch-Nyhan syndrome and may provide circumstantial evidence of the nature of small stones lodged in the ureters, especially when radiolucent and found in conjunction with raised serum uric acid levels. They may also herald the urate nephropathy of gout.

Calcium Oxalates. Dihydrates may appear at pH 6 or in neutral urine. Their classic form is that of a small, colorless octahedron that resembles an envelope (Fig. 28-32). Dumbbell shapes and ovoid forms may occur (Fig. 28-33). Longer forms occur in calcium oxalate monohydrate. Oxalate crystals are insoluble in acetic acid.

Oxalate crystals in large numbers may reflect severe chronic renal disease or ethylene glycol or methoxyflurane toxicity. Oxaluria has come into prominence as a reflection of the increased absorption of oxalates from food following small bowel disease and resection, notably for Crohn's disease. Oxaluria may also be present in genetically susceptible persons following large doses of ascorbic acid.

TABLE 28-12
Characteristics of Amorphous and Crystalline Urinary Sediments

Substance	Description	URINE pH WHERE FOUND			Solubility characteristics and comments
		Acid	Neutral	Alkaline	
Ampicillin	Uncommon—from high dose; colorless; long prisms that form clusters, sheaves	+	–	–	
Bilirubin	Reddish brown; amorphous needles, rhombic plates, or cubes; may color uric acid crystals	+	–	–	Soluble in alkali, acid, acetone, and chloroform
Cholesterol	Rare; colorless; flat plate with corner notch; accompanies fatty casts and oval fat bodies	+	+	–	Very soluble in chloroform, ether, and hot alcohol
Calcium carbonate	Colorless; small granules in pairs, fours; spheres; rarely needles	–	+	+	Soluble in acetic acid with effervescence
Calcium oxalate	Dihydrate—common; colorless; small refractile octahedron Monohydrate—uncommon; dumbbell and ovoid rectangle	+	+	–	Soluble in dilute HCl
Cystine	Colorless; hexagonal plates, often laminated; rapidly destroyed by bacteria; may be confused with uric acid, but cystine is soluble in dilute hydrochloric acid	+	–	–	Soluble in alkali (especially ammonia) and dilute HCl; insoluble in boiling water, acetic acid, alcohol, ether; apply cyanide–nitroprusside reaction
Hematin	Small, biconvex "whetstone" seen with hemoglobinuria	+	–	–	
Hemosiderin	Golden brown; granules in clumps, in cells, casts	+	+	–	Blue with Prussian blue
Hippuric acid	Rare; colorless, needles, rhombic plates and four-sided prisms; distinguish from phosphates	+	+	+	Soluble with hot water and alkali; insoluble in acetic acid
Indigotin	Rare; blue; amorphous or small crystals; colors other crystals	+	+	+	Very soluble in chloroform; soluble in ether; insoluble in acetone
Phosphates					
Amorphous phosphate (magnesium, calcium)	Colorless; fine, granular precipitate	–	+	+	Insoluble with heat; soluble with acetic acid, dilute HCl
Calcium hydrogen phosphate	Less common; colorless, star-shaped or long, thin prisms or needles; form rosettes	sl	+	sl	Slightly soluble in dilute acetic acid, soluble in dilute HCl
Triple phosphate (ammonium, magnesium)	Common form: colorless; three- to six-sided prisms, "coffin lids" Less often: Flat, fern leaf form, sheets, flakes	–	+	+	Soluble in dilute acetic acid
Radiographic media (meglumine diatrizoate)	Intravenous: Colorless; thin, rhombic plates, some with notch, resemble cholesterol plates; elongated crystals Retrograde: Colorless; long, pointed crystals	+	–	–	Soluble in 10% NaOH: Insoluble in ether and chloroform; high specific gravity in urine: polarizes with interference colors
Sulfonamides					
Acetylsulfadiazine	Wheat sheaves with eccentric binding	+	–	–	
Acetylsulfamethoxazole	Brown; dense spheres or irregular divided spheres	+	–	–	
Sulfadiazine	Brown; dense globules	+	–	–	Soluble in acetone
Tyrosine	Rare; colorless or yellow, appears black with focusing; fine silky needles in sheaves or rosettes	+	–	–	Soluble in alkali, dilute mineral acid, relatively heat soluble; insoluble in alcohol, ether
Urates					
Amorphous (calcium, magnesium, sodium, potassium)	Common; colorless to yellow-brown; amorphous, granular precipitate	+	+	–	Soluble in dilute alkali; soluble at 60° C or lower; change to uric acid crystal with concentrated HCl or acetic acid
Monosodium urate	Colorless; needles or amorphous precipitate	+	–	–	
Urates (sodium, potassium, ammonium)	Brown; small, spherical; clusters resemble biurates	sl	+	–	Soluble at 60° C; change to uric acid with glacial acetic acid
Ammonium biurate	Common in "old" urine; dark yellow or brown; spheres or "thorn apples" (spheres with horns)	–	+	+	Soluble at 60° C with acetic acid; soluble strong alkali; change to uric acid with concentrated hydrochloric or acetic acid
Uric acid	Common; yellow, red-brown, brown; large variety of shapes—rhombic, four-sided plates, rosettes, "whetstones" lemon shapes; rarely, colorless hexagonals	+	–	–	Soluble in alkali: Insoluble in alcohol and acids; polarizes with interference colors
Xanthine	Rare; colorless; small, rhombic plates	+	+	–	Soluble in alkali; soluble with heat; insoluble in acetic acid

sl, Slight.

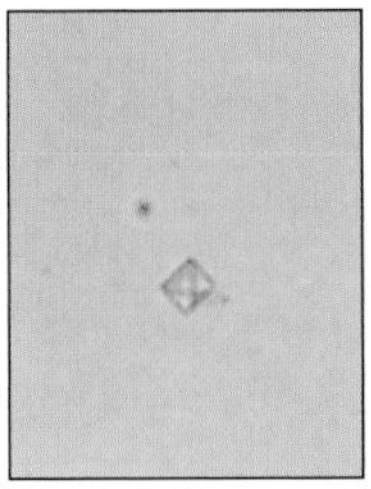

Figure 28-32 Calcium oxalate crystals (×200).

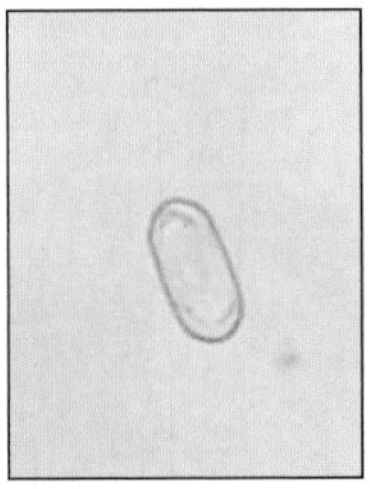

Figure 28-33 Calcium oxalate. Unusual oval form (×200).

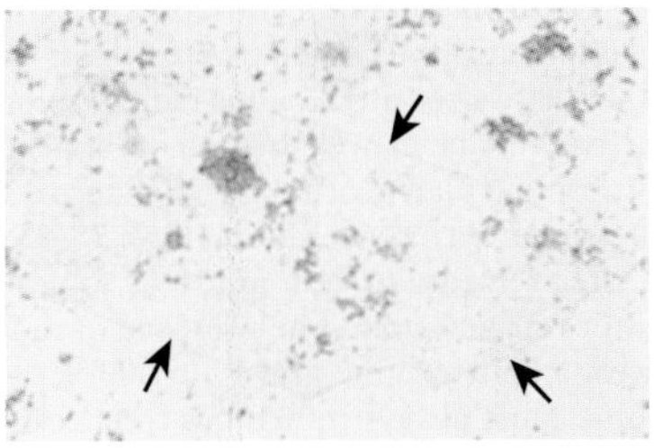

Figure 28-34 Calcium phosphate (large clear plate). Almost amorphous phosphates (×64).

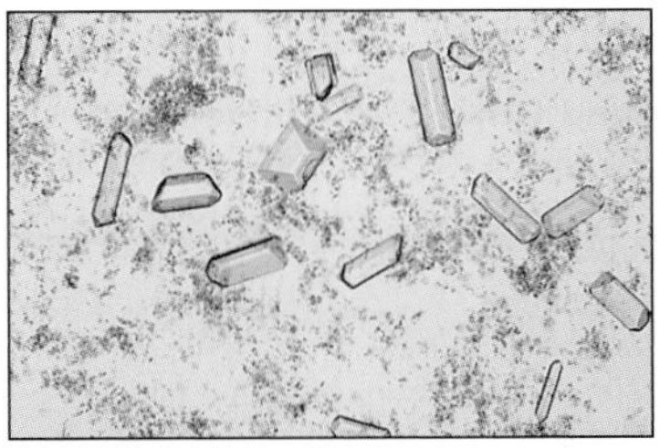

Figure 28-35 Triple phosphate (×50).

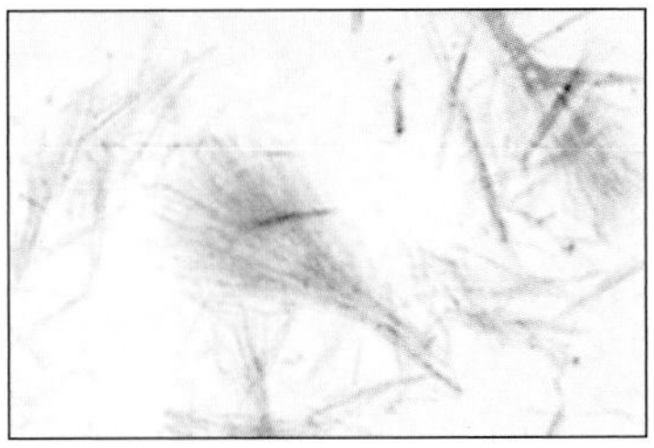

Figure 28-36 Calcium phosphate (fine sheaves) (×160).

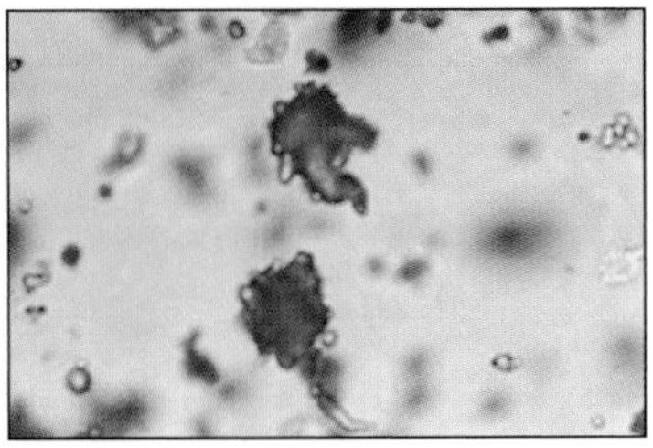

Figure 28-37 Ammonium biurate (×160).

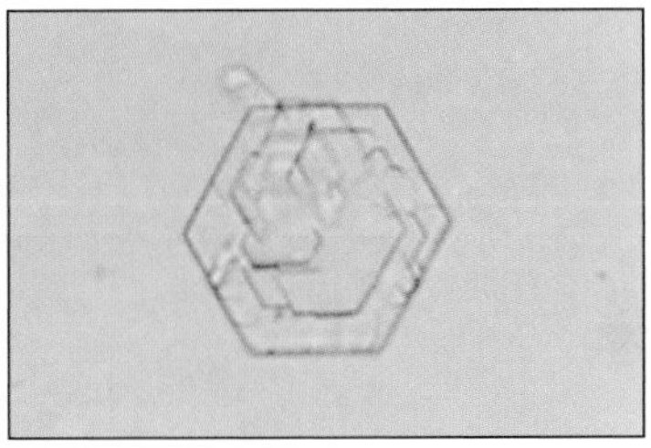

Figure 28-38 Cystine (hexagonal, laminated) (×200).

Crystals Found in Normal Alkaline Urine

Amorphous Phosphates (Calcium and Magnesium). Similar to amorphous urates, amorphous phosphates have a granular appearance microscopically; unlike the former, they tend to be colorless and will produce a fine or lacy white precipitate macroscopically. Clumps or masses can often be seen by light microscopy (Fig. 28-34). Large amounts of this material may precipitate out upon prolonged standing at room temperature or in a refrigerator.

Calcium and magnesium monohydrogen phosphates are the least soluble in alkaline urine, although the dihydrogen phosphates may be soluble at a similar pH. Phosphates, in general, will dissolve in acids such as dilute hydrochloric and nitric acids and vary in solubility in acetic acid. They do not dissolve in dilute sodium hydroxide solutions or alcohol.

Crystalline Phosphates. Triple phosphate (ammonium magnesium phosphate) crystals are one of the most easily identified urine crystals, although they commonly show variation in size. They are colorless, three- to six-sided prisms with oblique ends referred to as **coffin lids** (Fig. 28-35). They may form colorless sheets or flakes (Fig. 28-36). Magnesium phosphate forms colorless rhomboids, some with notched ends or corners. These are seldom recognized. Dicalcium hydrogen phosphate crystals, on the other hand, may be seen in neutral or slightly acidic urine, and are long, three-sided prisms with pointed ends. They may form clusters or rosettes. Overall, phosphate crystals have little if any clinical significance. They are often seen in infected urine of alkaline pH.

Calcium Carbonate. These uncommon crystals are small and colorless, with dumbbell or spherical shapes. They may form pairs, fours, or clumps. They are distinguished from other crystals/amorphous material by their production of carbon dioxide in the presence of acetic acid.

Ammonium Biurate. Similar to typical urate crystals, ammonium biurate crystals have a yellow-brown color and appear as spheres with radial or concentric striations and irregular projections or thorns (Fig. 28-37). Referred to as **thorn apples,** they may also be seen in neutral and occasionally in slightly acid urine. They dissolve with heat at 60° C and with acetic acid, reappearing as typical uric acid crystals after about 20 minutes.

Crystals Found in Abnormal Urine

Cystine. Cystine crystals are colorless, refractile, hexagonal plates (Fig. 28-38), which appear in acid urine. They are soluble in water at pH less than 2 or greater than 8, and they may be confused with hexagonal forms of uric acid (see Fig. 28-30). Whereas uric acid crystals polarize (see Fig. 28-31), thin cystine crystals do not, although thick laminated forms may polarize. Furthermore, both cystine and uric acid are soluble in ammonia water, but cystine will also dissolve in dilute hydrochloric acid, and uric acid will not.

Cystine crystals are among the most important crystals identified in urine sediment. They occur in patients with cystinuria and may be associated with cystine calculi. Confirmatory testing consists of the cyanide–nitroprusside reaction (see later under Cystinuria).

Tyrosine. In acidic urine, tyrosine forms fine silky needles that may be arranged in sheaves or clumps, especially after refrigeration. These may be colorless or yellow, appearing black as the microscope is focused (Fig. 28-39). They are soluble in alkali (ammonia and potassium hydroxide) and in dilute hydrochloric acid; they are not soluble in alcohol or ether.

These crystals, which are uncommon, are less soluble than leucine, and therefore are more often precipitated in urine (see later under Tyrosinuria). Tyrosine and leucine crystals are occasionally seen in the urine of patients with severe liver disease (see later under Urinary Screening for Inherited Metabolic Diseases).

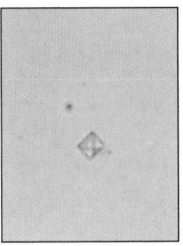

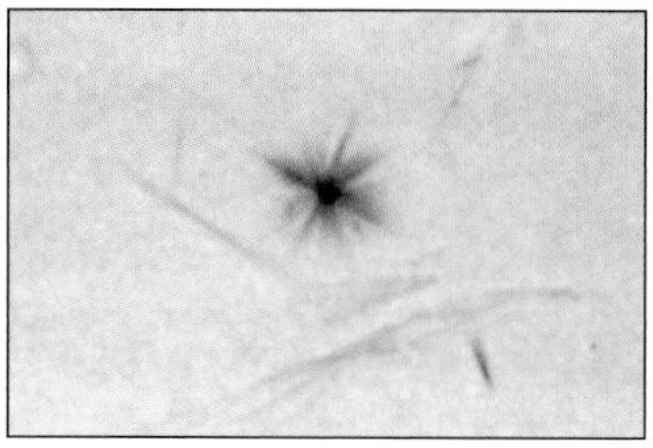

Figure 28-39 Tyrosine crystals (×160).

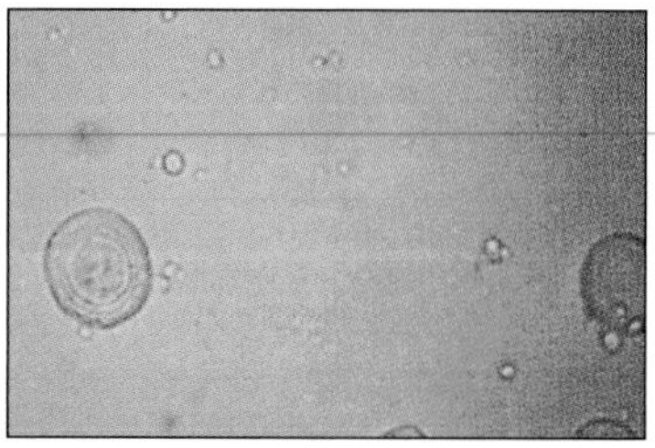

Figure 28-40 Leucine crystals (×160).

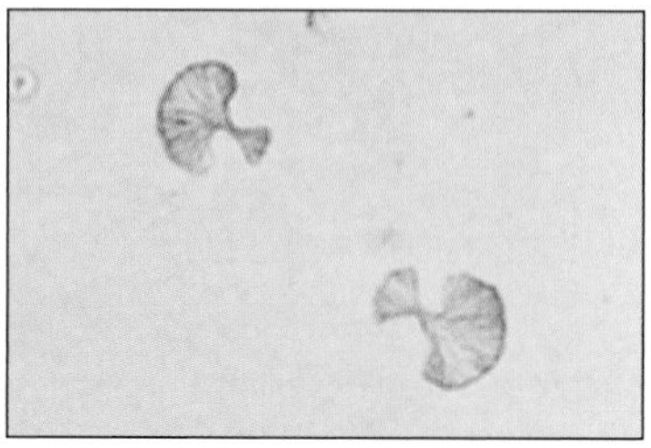

Figure 28-41 Sulfadiazine (×160).

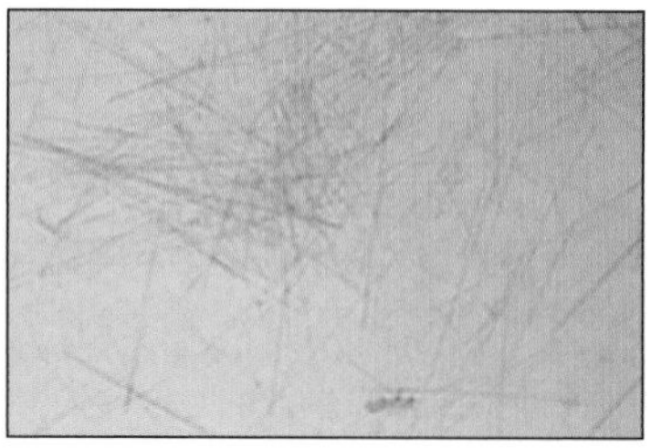

Figure 28-42 Ampicillin (×160).

Leucine. These crystals are also rare, occurring as yellow, oily-appearing spheres with radial and concentric striations (Fig. 28-40). They are soluble in both acids and alkalis. Leucine and tyrosine crystals may occur together; leucine may be precipitated with tyrosine crystals if alcohol is added to the urine.

Sulfonamide (Sulfadiazine) Crystals. These crystals may be seen in urine of acid pH and may take on various morphologies, depending on the form of drug involved. They may be seen as yellow-brown sheaves of wheat with central bindings, striated sheaves with eccentric bindings (Fig. 28-41), rosettes, arrowheads, petals, needles, and round forms with radial striations. They are occasionally colorless. Confirmatory testing is by the diazo reaction. High-performance liquid chromatographic and colorimetric methods have also been described (Simo-Alfonso, 1995; Mount, 1996).

With the advent of soluble sulfonamides, sulfa crystals are not as frequently found in urine, especially when urine is examined at 37° C. Before this development, these crystals could be seen in the urine of patients on sulfonamide therapy who were inadequately hydrated. This could result in renal tubular damage if crystal formation occurred within the nephron. Currently, sulfamethoxazole (Bactrim, Septra) is seen with some regularity.

Ampicillin (High Dosage). Ampicillin may crystallize in the urine under conditions of high dosage. These crystals appear in urine of acid pH as long, fine, colorless structures (Fig. 28-42). They may form coarse sheaves after refrigeration.

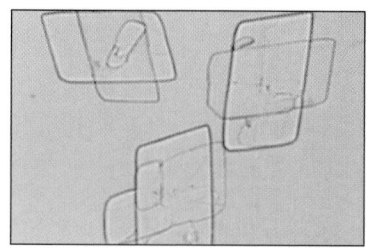

Figure 28-43 Renografin (meglumine diatrizoate). Bright-field (×160).

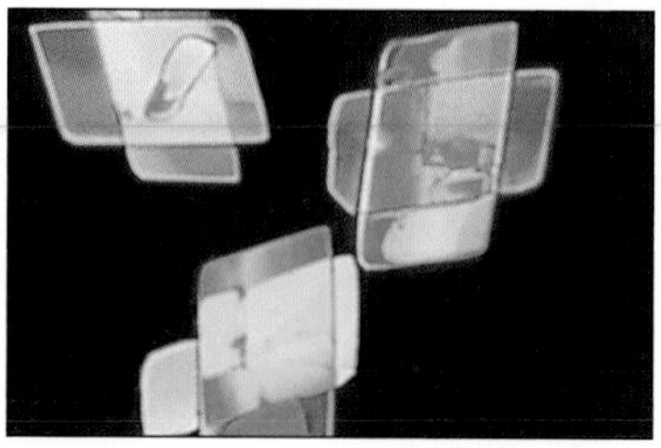

Figure 28-44 Renografin (meglumine diatrizoate). Polarized (×160).

Radiographic Media (Meglumine Diatrizoate). Urinary crystals form after radiographic examinations using diatrizoate dyes. They may be found in urine of acid pH shortly after intravenous radiographic studies (particularly if the patient has not been well hydrated), appearing as flat, clear, colorless, notched rhombic plates, or longer, slender rectangles. They are easily polarized, showing interference colors (Figs. 28-43 and 28-44). They may also be seen after retrograde cystograms as long, colorless needles, forming clusters after refrigeration. The presence of radiographic crystals should correlate with a high specific gravity (>1.040).

Other Drugs. One must always remember to check the patient's drug therapy when unusual crystals are found in the urine. Several drugs have been reported to cause crystalluria when administered in high-dosage schedules or following overdose. Examples include high-dosage 6-mercaptopurine therapy, primidone overdosage, and dihydroxyadenine from massive blood transfusion.

Abnormal Cells and Other Formed Elements

Tumor Cells. Malignant tumor cells exfoliated from the renal pelvis, ureter, bladder wall, and urethra are best identified using cytologic techniques. Myeloma cells have also been noted in urine, both with and without apparent renal involvement. For a comprehensive discussion of disease types and cytologic morphologies, the reader is directed to standard urinary cytology references (Bibbo, 1997).

Viral Inclusion Cells. Epithelial cells containing inclusion bodies may be found in the urine sediment in various viral infections involving the urinary tract. Syncytial giant cells containing eosinophilic, intranuclear inclusions are seen in patients during herpetic infections. In children or immunosuppressed patients with cytomegalovirus infection, affected cells are enlarged and contain basophilic intranuclear inclusions and/or cytoplasmic bodies. Polyomavirus (e.g., BK virus)-infected cells contain dense, basophilic, homogeneous intranuclear inclusions that often completely fill the nucleus. Cytologic techniques are far more sensitive in detecting all of the aforementioned viral cytopathic effects.

Platelets. These have been demonstrated in urine. Up to 30,000/μL have been demonstrated by phase-contrast microscopy and confirmed by electron microscopy in the urine of patients with hemolytic-uremic syndrome.

Bacteria. Finding bacteria in urine may or may not be significant, depending on the method of urine collection and how soon after collection of the specimen the examination takes place. If bacteria are identified with Gram stain in an uncentrifuged urine specimen under an oil-immersion lens, this suggests that more than 100,000 organisms/mL are present (i.e., significant bacteriuria). Most commonly, rod-shaped bacteria are seen because the enteric organisms are the causative agents in the majority of urinary tract infections (Fig. 28-45). Leukocytes will usually be seen in the sediment as well.

Acid-fast bacilli may be seen in urine sediment, but because the urethral flora may contain nonpathogenic acid-fast organisms, the presence of tuberculosis in urine must be substantiated by culture and/or polymerase chain reaction methods.

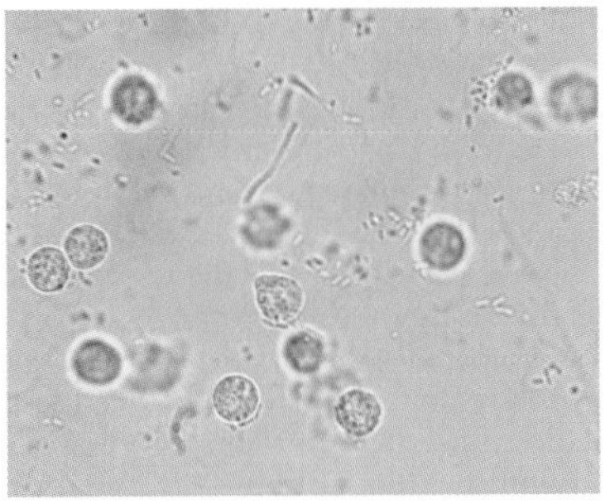

Figure 28-45 Bacteria and leukocytes (×600).

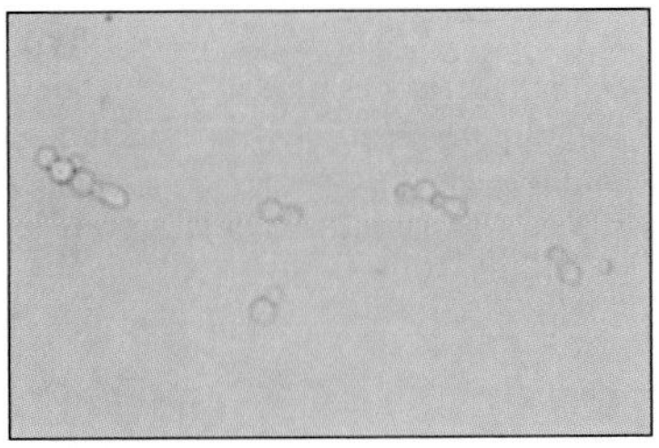

Figure 28-46 *Candida.* Budding yeasts (×200).

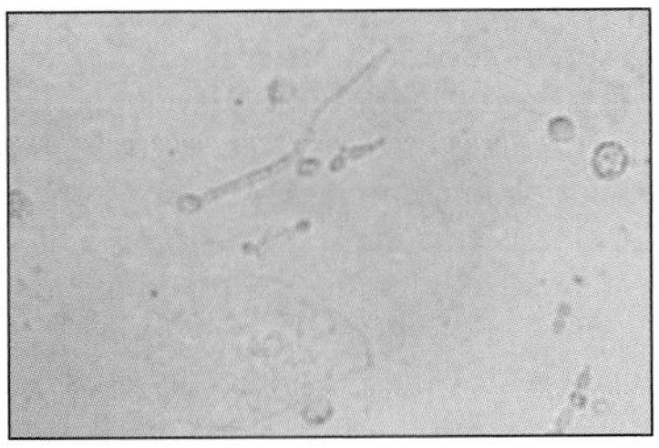

Figure 28-47 *Candida.* Pseudohyphae (×160).

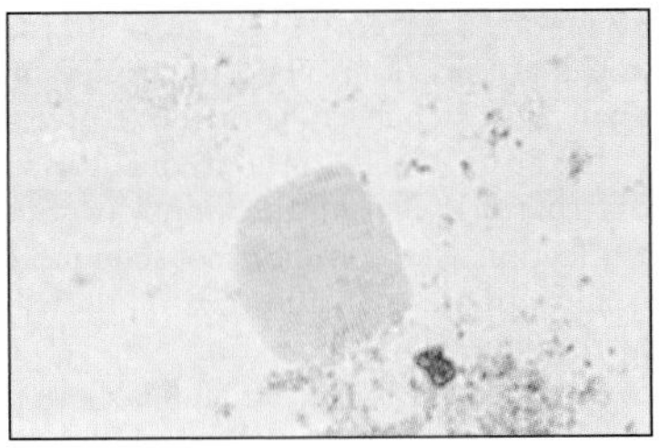

Figure 28-48 Muscle fiber (×200).

Fungi. Yeasts (most commonly *Candida* species) may be causative agents in urinary tract infection (e.g., in diabetes mellitus), but yeasts are also common contaminants from the skin, the female genital tract, and the air. On microscopic examination, they may be confused with erythrocytes; the presence of budding helps to identify them as yeast cells (Fig. 28-46). Pseudohyphae of *Candida* are occasionally found (Fig. 28-47).

Parasites. Parasites and parasitic ova may be seen in urine sediments as a result of fecal or vaginal contamination. When noted, repeat examination should be performed on a fresh, clean-voided urine specimen. Although *Trichomonas vaginalis* may be present in urine as a result of vaginal contamination, urethral or bladder infection can occur; when suspected, the protozoa should be searched for immediately in a wet preparation of the sediment. Motility of the organism is helpful in making the appropriate identification. In patients with schistosomiasis due to *Schistosoma haematobium*, typical ova are shed directly into the urine accompanied by erythrocytes from the urinary bladder. Amebae are rarely seen in the urine; they may reach the bladder from lymphatics or more likely from fecal contamination of the urethra. The pathogenic *Entamoeba histolytica* is usually accompanied by erythrocytes and leukocytes.

Contaminants and Artifacts. Partially digested muscle fibers or vegetable cells may be found when fecal contamination occurs (Fig. 28-48). Spermatozoa are occasionally present, and pollen grains contaminate

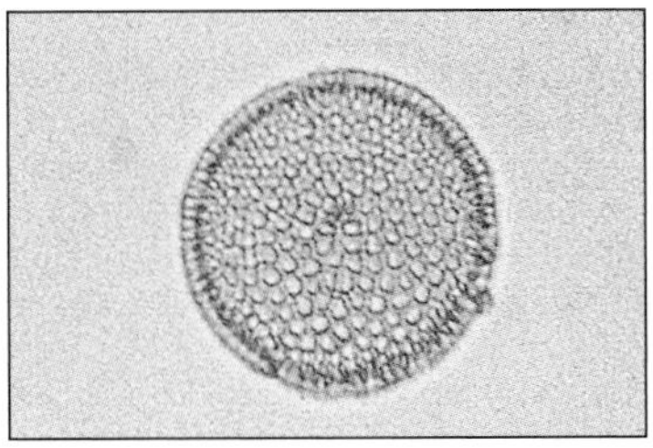

Figure 28-49 Pollen grain (×160).

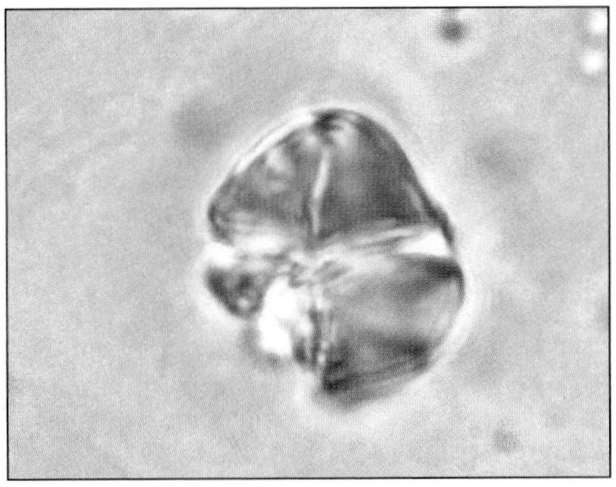

Figure 28-50 Starch granule (×160).

specimens seasonally (Fig. 28-49). Fibers from many different sources may be seen, including cotton, hair, wood fibers from applicator sticks, and synthetic fibers from disposable diapers. Unlike casts, these fibers polarize brightly.

Starch granules from surgical gloves are the most common contaminants of urine and other body fluids. Microscopically, they appear bright and faintly striated with an irregular outline and a central depression (Fig. 28-50). With crossed polarizing filters, starch granules exhibit a typical Maltese cross pattern, and because of their large size (several times larger than an erythrocyte), they are not likely to be confused with cholesterol droplets. Oil droplets from catheter lubricants may be confused with cells, especially red cells. Lipid material from vaginal creams also forms droplets in urine and may form large amorphous aggregates.

METHODS FOR URINALYSIS

BASIC (ROUTINE) URINALYSIS PROCEDURE

1. Pour 10–15 mL of a well-mixed urine specimen into a graduated disposable centrifuge tube. Perform physical examination and reagent strip chemical evaluations. Centrifuge at 450 g for 5 minutes.
2. Carefully remove and save the supernatant. The final volume used to resuspend the sediment may vary with the standardized system used but should remain constant within any given laboratory. Use a disposable pipet, specialized tube, or pipet system to concentrate the sediment.
3. Gently resuspend the sediment in the remaining supernatant, and add one drop of supravital stain if desired. Using an appropriate pipet, load/charge the examination chamber of a standardized slide. Allow the urine to settle for 30–60 seconds.
4. Examine with low- and high-power objectives. Subdued light or phase-contrast illumination will be required to detect sediment entities with a low refractive index. The fine focus should be varied continuously while scanning. Systematically progress around the entire examination chamber, being careful to examine along the edges for casts.
5. Count the number of casts in at least 10 lpf, average, and report the number of casts per lpf. A reasonable range may be used in reporting (e.g., 0–2, 2–5, 5–10). Use high power to identify casts by type. Casts will not be missed if phase-contrast microscopy is used (see Fig. 28-4, *A* and *B*).
6. Identify and count erythrocytes, leukocytes, and renal epithelial cells using the high-power objective. Count at least 10 hpf, average, and report as cells/hpf. A reasonable range may be used for reporting.

7. Comment on the following:
    a. Squamous and transitional cells if present in large numbers or as fragments (transitional cells).
    b. Bacteria, yeast, and microorganisms. Bacteriuria detectable on low power should be reported as at least 2+.
    c. Crystals (quantitated under low power). The presence of abnormal crystals should be confirmed chemically and correlated with the patient history.
    d. Large amounts of mucus.
8. The authors recommend confirming the following results with cytopathologic examination or specific chemical tests (crystals):
    a. More than two renal epithelial cells/hpf.
    b. Pathologic casts.
    c. Atypical mononuclear cells, particularly urothelial cells.
    d. Tissue fragments.
    e. Pathologic crystals.

Review the entire report, including physical, chemical, and microscopic data, and correlate with available clinical information. Discrepancies should be resolved before the report is released. Normal values for the procedure include the following: 0–10 RBCs/hpf, 0–10 WBCs/hpf, and 0–2 hyaline casts/lpf. Values will vary, depending on the standardized system used.

Routine urinalysis is a helpful diagnostic tool in the workup and follow-up of various urinary system disorders. Table 28-13 summarizes the macroscopic, reagent strip, and microscopic findings typical for the most commonly encountered entities.

AUTOMATED URINALYSIS

Several instruments have been developed to partially or completely automate routine urinalysis. In addition to enhancing workflow, automation can standardize some aspects of manual urinalysis. Most of these instruments can be interfaced with laboratory information systems, facilitating reporting and result retrieval.

Several instruments are available to automate the macroscopic/chemical analysis or the microscopic portions of the routine urinalysis. For example, fully automated urine chemistry reagent strip analyzers from several manufacturers are equipped to perform automatic pipetting or test strip dipping, as well as carry out photometric measurements of the reagent strip fields.

The IRIS Urinalysis workstations (now iQ200 series Automated Urinalysis System, Iris Diagnostics, Chatsworth, Calif.) (van den Broek, 2008) combine several automated subsystems to perform a complete urinalysis through a combination of dipstick chemistries and flow imaging technology. Specific gravity is measured by a mass gravity meter, urine chemistries are measured by a standard reflectance spectrophotometer, and microscopic analysis is facilitated with an automated intelligent microscopy system. No centrifugation is involved, and handling of the specimen is minimal. A touch-sensitive video screen eliminates keyboard entry. In the analysis, the urine specimen is poured into the instrument's entry port over a urine chemistry reagent strip. This reagent strip is then placed in the reflectance photometer reader platform. The urine chemistries are automatically timed, read, and collated by the internal computer. A portion of the specimen is diverted to the harmonic oscillator mass gravity meter for specific gravity determination; the rest of the specimen is then stained and passed into a laminar flow chamber, where the formed elements are detected and imaged by a video camera mounted to a microscope and a stroboscopic lamp that allows stop-motion images. Images of cells, casts, crystals, yeast, and bacteria found in the sediment are then sorted by size and presented to the operator on the touch-sensitive screen for identification. Because the volume of the laminar flow chamber is known, the images can be counted and related to a volume of urine with a precision that exceeds that which can be obtained with a centrifuged specimen, glass slide, and coverslip. The system can remove the need for microscopic analysis in most cases (Hughes, 2003). The computer then consolidates the report for printing or transmission to the laboratory information system.

The IRIS system bases its analysis on cell image analysis. Another way to analyze urinary cells and casts is by flow cytometry. These analyzers typically stain the DNA and membranes of the formed elements in native urine, pass the sample as a laminar flow through a laser beam, and measure the light scatter, fluorescence, and impedance. The UF-100 (Sysmex Corporation, Kobe, Japan) analyzes urine by flow cytometry and gives quantitative results for red and white blood cells, epithelial cells, casts, and bacteria (Fig. 28-51). It can detect yeast, crystals, dysmorphic red blood cells, and pathologic casts (Fig. 28-52) in the urine (Ben-Ezra, 1998; Ottinger, 2003). This technology may be useful in decreasing the number of urine specimens requiring routine microscopy (Fenili, 1998). Normal values are fewer than 20 RBCs/μL, fewer than 25 WBCs/μL, and fewer than 2000 bacteria/μL. Similar to the microscopic examination of urine on unspun specimens, the automated systems are not prone to the artifacts that characterize examination of spun urine sediment. A second generation of this machine, the UF-1000, provides better enumeration of bacteria with fewer artifacts due to interfering debris.

Although these automated sediment analysis machines are very useful in standardizing workflow and eliminating the need to perform a manual examination of the urine sediment in the routine clinical laboratory, they may not be that useful in a population with a high incidence of renal pathology (e.g., patients in a nephrology clinic) (Gai, 2003).

Automated urine sediment analyzers have the potential to add more quantitative information to the monitoring of abnormalities such as urinary tract infections by providing very exact counts of bacteria and cells in serial specimens while patients are under treatment. The clinical utility of this accurate information is yet to be determined. Its application would require a more comprehensive understanding of such counts by practicing physicians as opposed to the semiquantitative estimates now commonly in use.

SPECIAL TESTING AND MONITORING TECHNIQUES

URINARY CALCULI

Nephrolithiasis is a common condition, affecting nearly 5 in 1000 persons. It is a heterogeneous disorder, with stones developing from a wide variety of metabolic or environmental disturbances. Although most studies have concentrated on nonorganic components, many stones have been found to be associated with an organic matrix containing lipids and protein, suggesting the involvement of cellular membranes in the nucleation of crystals (Khan, 1996). One study showed that antisera raised against these stone matrix proteins had cross-reactivity between proteins isolated from different stones, irrespective of their mineral composition (Siddiqui, 1998). Many stone patients have been found to show elevation of interleukin-6, which may in the future be useful as a potential marker for stone disease (Rhee, 1998).

Upper (renal) stones are common in Western industrialized countries, whereas bladder stones are uncommon. The passage of stones down the ureter produces renal colic, which is characterized by severe pain in the flank radiating to the groin. Hematuria frequently accompanies stone passage. If stones obstruct the pelvis of the kidney or ureter, hydronephrosis can result, and infection is a common consequence. Recurrences are frequent, but with appropriate identification of the stones and the risk factors associated with them, stone formation may be greatly reduced.

Calcium oxalate or a mixture of oxalate and calcium phosphate is often found in stones (≈80%). Mixed calcium phosphate, magnesium ammonium phosphate, and uric acid are the next most common constituents (3%–10% each), and these are followed by cystine stones (1%–2%). Carbonate, which is frequently detected in chemical analysis, probably results from adsorption of carbon dioxide to the calcium phosphate crystal. Males are more often affected with calcium stones than females, and children are not often affected with calcium stones.

Calcium oxalate precipitates at an acid or neutral pH, and calcium phosphate—hydroxyapatite $Ca_{10}(PO)_6(OH)_2$—forms calculi at the normal urinary pH of 6.0–6.5. Uric acid, which is not very soluble, will crystallize at a low pH (5.3) and form stones. Magnesium ammonium phosphate (struvite) forms stones at alkaline pH, where the ammonium level is high. These tend to form in the pelvis of the kidney but apparently are not attached to papillae, as are the calcium stones. They may, however, develop on preexisting nuclei when infection from organisms such as *Proteus* causes alkalization of the urine. Struvite stones may become large, forming casts of the kidney pelvis and showing staghorns. Mixed stones may form when calcium or uric acid crystals (or stones) cause obstruction followed by infection and the subsequent deposition of ammonium salts.

Hypercalciuria and Calcium Stones

Calcium homeostasis is maintained by parathyroid hormone (PTH) and 1,25-dihydroxycholecalciferol (1,25[OH]$_2$D). Both affect bone resorption by osteoclasts. PTH causes a diminution of phosphorus reabsorption and an increase in calcium reabsorption by renal tubular cells. It also causes increased synthesis of 1,25(OH)$_2$D, which acts upon the small intestinal

TABLE 28-13

Various Urinary System Diseases and Corresponding Urinalysis Abnormalities

Diseases	Macroscopic urinalysis	Microscopic urinalysis
Acute glomerulonephritis	Gross hematuria "Smoky" turbidity Proteinuria	Erythrocyte and blood casts Epithelial casts Hyaline and granular casts Waxy casts Neutrophils Erythrocytes
Chronic glomerulonephritis	Hematuria Proteinuria	Granular and waxy casts Occasional blood casts Erythrocytes Leukocytes Epithelial casts Lipid droplets
Acute pyelonephritis	Turbid Occasional odor Occasional proteinuria	Numerous neutrophils (many in clumps) Few lymphocytes and histiocytes Leukocyte casts Epithelial casts Renal epithelial cells Erythrocytes Granular and waxy casts Bacteria
Chronic pyelonephritis	Occasional proteinuria	Leukocytes Broad waxy casts Granular and epithelial casts Occasional leukocyte casts Bacteria Erythrocytes
Nephrotic syndrome	Proteinuria Fat droplets	Fatty and waxy casts Cellular and granular casts Oval fat bodies and/or vacuolated renal epithelial cells occurring singly or as cellular clusters
Acute tubular necrosis	Hematuria Occasional proteinuria	Necrotic or degenerated renal epithelial cells Neutrophils and erythrocytes Granular and epithelial casts Waxy casts Broad casts Epithelial tissue fragments
Cystitis	Hematuria	Numerous leukocytes Erythrocytes Transitional epithelial cells occurring singly or as fragments Histiocytes and giant cells Bacteria Absence of casts
Dysuria-pyuria syndrome	Slightly turbid	Numerous leukocytes, bacteria Erythrocytes No casts
Acute renal allograft rejection (lower nephrosis)	Hematuria Occasional proteinuria	Renal epithelial cells Lymphocytes and plasma cells Neutrophils Renal epithelial casts Renal epithelial fragments Granular, bloody, and waxy casts
Urinary tract neoplasia	Hematuria	Atypical mononuclear cells with enlarged, irregular hyperchromatic nuclei and sometimes containing prominent nucleoli that occur singly or as tissue fragments
Diseases	Macroscopic urinalysis	Microscopic urinalysis Neutrophils Erythrocytes Transitional epithelial cells
Viral infection	Hematuria Occasional proteinuria	Enlarged mononuclear cells and/or multinucleated cells with prominent intranuclear and/or cytoplasmic inclusions Neutrophils Lymphocytes and plasma cells Erythrocytes

mucosa, causing increased absorption of calcium and phosphorus. Low serum ionized calcium levels cause increased PTH secretion, and low serum phosphorus stimulates 1,25$(OH)_2$D synthesis.

About 40% of patients with calcium stones will have hypercalciuria, defined as a daily urinary excretion of calcium in excess of 0.1 mmol/kg (Houillier, 1998). Increased calcium in urine may result from an increase in intestinal calcium absorption, lack of appropriate renal tubular reabsorption of calcium, resorption or loss of calcium from bone, or a combination of these factors. In a few instances of hypercalciuria, an underlying disease process can be identified. In most cases, however, it is primary, or idiopathic hypercalciuria (IH). Although the exact mechanism of hypercalciuria is still unknown in this disorder, it most likely includes a combination of factors, including those listed previously. Three hypotheses to account for IH pathophysiology have been proposed. These include

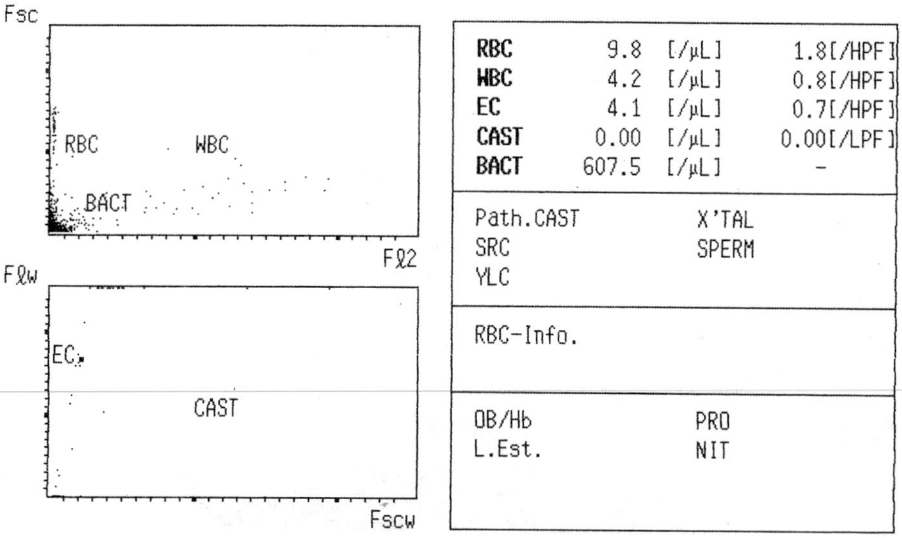

Figure 28-51 Printout from UF-100 automated urine analyzer, showing normal urine. Note the lack of RBCs, WBCs, bacteria, and casts. *RBCs,* Red blood cells; *WBCs,* white blood cells.

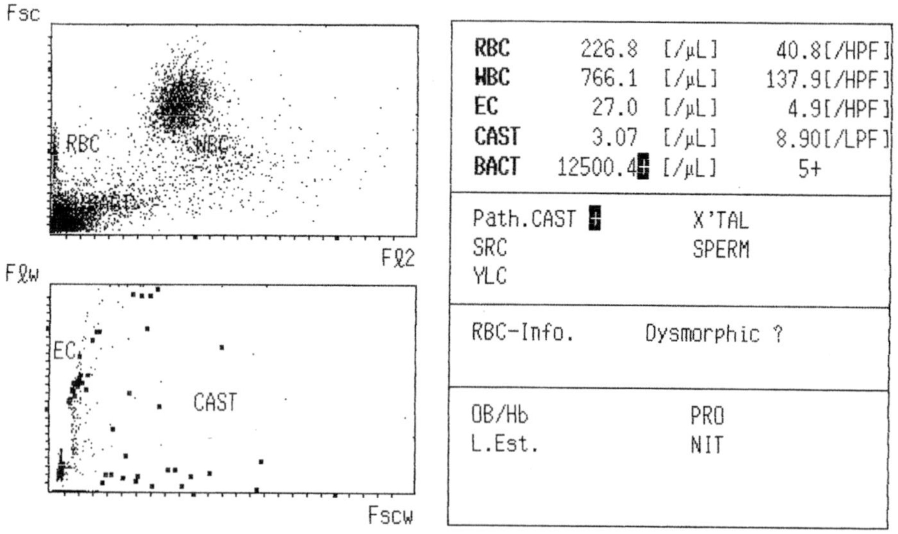

Figure 28-52 Printout from UF-100 automated urine analyzer, showing abnormal urine. Compare with Figure 28-51. Note the sizable numbers of RBCs, WBCs, bacteria, and casts. *ECs,* Squamous epithelial cells; *NIT,* nitrite; *PRO,* protein; *RBCs,* red blood cells; *SRC,* small round cells; *WBCs,* white blood cells; *X'TAL,* crystals; *YLC,* yeast-like cells.

possible defects in the fatty acid content of cell membranes, increased expression of the vitamin D or calcium receptors of the 25-hydroxyvitamin D_1 α-hydroxylase, or a disease of monocytes (Bataille, 1998).

Excess loss of calcium in urine and the possibility of stone formation may occur secondary to a variety of other conditions. For instance, hypercalciuria may result from increased absorption of calcium from the gut. This may occur following excessive loss of phosphorus from the kidney and low serum phosphorus levels, or when increased serum $1,25(OH)_2D$ is seen with normal serum phosphorus levels. Increased resorption of bone may occur with immobilization of the skeleton, rapidly progressive bone disease, thyrotoxicosis, and Cushing's disease, leading to hypercalciuria. Calcium may be lost from bone as a result of osteolytic tumors, as well as in the presence of renal disease such as distal renal tubular acidosis and medullary sponge kidney. Sarcoidosis, vitamin D excess, and furosemide may also cause renal hypercalciuria.

About 5%–10% of calcium stones are associated with primary hyperparathyroidism. In this disorder, increased mineral turnover in bone and hypercalcemia are important causes of hypercalciuria. Affected patients often present with stone symptoms, and calcium phosphate deposits may be found in the renal tissue, cornea, and other organs.

Dietary hypercalciuria is an uncommon cause of calcium stones; it is associated with a large calcium intake, on the order of 3–4 g/day, together with a high protein intake. About 800 mg/day is the normal recommended adult intake.

As stated previously, calcium oxalate stones are the most common. They may form with excess oxalate and uric acid in the urine, the latter sometimes providing a nidus for stone formation. Newly formed calcium oxalate aggregates are about 20–25 μm in diameter, much smaller than the outlet of the collecting ducts. Adherence to the epithelial surface apparently allows stones to continue growth rather than be excreted. Calcium phosphate stone formation is favored by a less acid urine, as is seen in renal tubular acidosis, with infection, and in persons consuming large amounts of alkali. These stones are also seen in primary hyperparathyroidism, although the urine is in the normal pH range. In a patient exposed to heat and dehydration, these may contribute to a rise in urinary solute levels, followed by crystallization and stone formation.

Hyperoxaluria

A majority of calcium stones (70%–80%) contain oxalate. Some of the oxalate in urine is dietary in origin from beverages (tea, cocoa, coffee, cola), vegetables (beans, rhubarb, spinach), nuts, berries, and citrus fruits. Oxalate is also derived from ascorbic acid.

The gastrointestinal system plays an important role in oxalate homeostasis. Oxalate absorption increases when calcium and magnesium intake decreases. Disorders of the small bowel such as Crohn's disease, ileal resection, and intestinal bypass surgery may result in excessive oxalate absorption, with subsequent excretion in the urine. Malabsorption with steatorrhea causes loss of calcium as soaps, and malabsorption with increased bile salts remaining in the gut is thought to promote oxalate absorption in the colon. Additionally, absence of *Oxalobacter formigenes* from the intestinal tract of patients with cystic fibrosis appears to lead to increased absorption of oxalate, thereby increasing the risk of hyperoxaluria (Sidhu, 1998).

Other causes of hyperoxaluria include pyridoxine deficiency and primary hyperoxaluria. The latter is a rare inherited autosomal recessive disease with oxoglutarate carboligase deficiency. Systemic oxalosis and renal failure may be seen in young adulthood. Renal transplantation and large doses of pyridoxine or nicotinamide have been tried for the treatment of these patients.

Hyperuricuria

Excessive excretion of uric acid may be due to excessive dietary intake of purines (liver, dried beans, some fish, meat) or various disease processes. Endogenous uric acid production is increased in gout, glycogen storage diseases, Lesch-Nyhan syndrome, many leukemias, and treated tumors with associated cell necrosis. Chemotherapy and irradiation can lead to increased breakdown of tumor cells (nucleotide/purine forms uric acid), which may cause acute renal failure secondary to tubular and ureteral obstruction by masses of uric acid crystals.

In gout, about 20% of patients form stones, most of which are pure uric acid or mixed uric acid and calcium. Heat, dehydration, and unusually acid urine contribute to stone formation. Gouty nephropathy occurs with sodium urate deposits in the medulla, even when stones are not present, and masses of crystals may cause obstruction of terminal collecting ducts in the kidney. Uricosuric drugs cause potential problems with massive uric acid output in the first 3–4 days of treatment.

Normally, about one third of the uric acid formed is degraded by bacteria in the colon. Absence of bacteria or intestinal diversion may cause increased absorption of uric acid from the gut. Because ileostomy patients lose large amounts of alkaline fluid from the intestine, they excrete concentrated acidic urine and are likely to produce uric acid stones.

The average uric acid excretion by adults is 500–600 mg/24hours. Solute concentration as well as pH appears to be important in the solubility of uric acid and urate. Uric acid, a weak acid, forms free, insoluble, undissociated uric acid and a urate (which is more soluble with some sodium and potassium present) at pH 5.5. The amount of free uric acid present in urine will decrease as the pH rises, and at pH 7, uric acid is more soluble as urate. With high salt concentrations, the urate becomes less soluble. If urine volume is low, the solubility of uric acid at acid pH will be exceeded.

Whereas large quantities of uric acid crystals are regularly seen in urinary sediment, uric acid stone formation is not common. Uric acid crystals form a sludge that may obstruct the nephron without forming a stone. On the other hand, uric acid and sodium acid urate crystals are found as nuclei for calcium stones. Most normal persons with a pH of 6 have urine saturated with uric acid but do not form stones. Further acidity or dehydration is apparently required to engender stone formation.

Cystine Stones

Cystine stones form in patients with an inherited amino acid transport disorder (see later under Cystinuria). Cystine, ornithine, lysine, and arginine are subsequently excreted in large amounts in the urine. Of these, only cystine forms crystals and stones. Cystine does not become soluble until the urine pH is 7.4, and stones form over a range of normal urinary pH values. Heterozygous carriers for the disease will have increased amounts of cystine in urine but do not form stones; homozygotes are stone formers. A 24-hour quantitative urine cystine measurement is needed to detect potential stone formers; this should always be done when cystine crystals are found in random specimens.

Rare Calculi

Calculi containing sulfonamides have been described, and silica calculi have been reported in patients ingesting silica gel over a long period of time. Triamterene (Dyazide, Dyrenium), a relatively insoluble diuretic, may contribute to stone formation. It can form 1- to 2-mm mustard-colored stones, giving a bright blue fluorescence when dissolved in butanol and with exposure to ultraviolet light. Rare adenine stones have been described in children with an inherited enzyme deficiency disorder and hyperuricemia. Xanthine stones are uncommon and may be associated with a genetic disorder with an absence of xanthine oxidase.

LABORATORY TESTS USED TO INVESTIGATE STONE FORMERS

Urine Examinations

1. Routine urinalysis, qualitative test for cystine, and urine culture. Hematuria is a constant finding when stones are present, even when they are asymptomatic. Proteinuria is usually not a feature of calculous disease, but with renal tubular damage, excretion of low molecular weight plasma proteins such as β_2-microglobulin, and some albumin, may be increased. Erythrocyte casts usually are not found, and other casts are unusual. Leukocytes are increased when infection is present, and the reagent strip nitrite and leukocyte esterase may be elevated. Multiple clusters of nonmalignant transitional cells may be found in urine of patients with calculous disease and may be helpful in the diagnosis of unsuspected calculi.
2. Twenty-four-hour urine specimen: Sodium, calcium, phosphorus, uric acid, oxalate, and creatinine clearance. Supersaturation values from 24-hour urine collections have been shown to accurately reflect stone composition (Asplin, 1998). Some authors suggest that spot urine samples are sufficient for the metabolic evaluation of stone formers, although because of day-to-day variation, three samples should be obtained to overcome the doubtful significance of a single result (Strohmaier, 1997).
3. Urine pH determination on a fresh specimen is important in determining the types of crystals likely to be precipitated, for example, uric acid with low pH (5–5.5), and triple phosphate with alkaline urine.

Serum Chemistry

Appropriate tests include calcium, phosphorus, uric acid, and electrolytes.

Stone Analysis

Calculi may be of various sizes, commonly described as sand, gravel, or stone. The physical characteristics of the various calculi rarely will suffice for their identification, but a few points are worth noting. Uric acid and urate stones are typically yellow to brownish red and are moderately hard. Phosphate stones are usually pale and friable. Calcium oxalate stones are very hard, often of a dark color, and typically have a rough surface. Cystine stones are yellow-brown and feel somewhat greasy.

Several methods are available for the analysis of calculi, such as optical crystallography, radiograph diffraction, and infrared spectroscopy. Electron beam analysis and mass spectroscopy are also used. A simplified method for analysis of renal calculi is presented by Farrington (1980). A quantitative method for five of eight frequently measured substances using available clinical chemistry methods has been described: calcium, phosphorus, magnesium, ammonium, and uric acid. Cystine, oxalate, and carbonate are detected by qualitative means and are interpreted with the quantitative results to characterize the stones. Most laboratories send calculi specimens out to more specialized laboratories for chemical analysis, where both chemical and specialized tests should be used to determine the composition of the stones.

Method for Gross Examination of Calculi

1. Wash the stone(s) free of blood, mucus, preservation solution, and so forth. Place stones in a beaker, cover with several thicknesses of gauze held firmly in place with rubber bands, and wash under cold running water. Drain, remove gauze carefully, and dry beaker and stones in an oven. Rinse tiny stones with water from a squeeze bottle (not running water).
2. Record the dimension of the stone.
3. Describe briefly the color and texture of the stone's exterior surface. The stone may be photographed for record purposes.
4. Cut, saw, or break the stone so as to examine the interior. Note whether a foreign body may have acted as a nucleus for its formation. Describe the color and texture of the interior and layers, if present.
5. Reduce small stones to a fine powder by pulverizing with a mortar and pestle.
6. If possible, when a stone is very large, it may be advisable to make separate analyses of layers that appear to have different constituents.

Because most small calculi consist of calcium oxalate, the best way to analyze them is to put all available powder in one test tube. (If the stone is very tiny, it may be placed directly in the test tube and crushed with a spatula.) Reagents used for the chemical determination of rare stones may be found in an earlier edition of this book (Henry, 1996). It is important to have known positive material to test the reagents.

Radiologic Examination

Asymptomatic stones are sometimes found. Most stones are radiopaque, except for pure uric acid and the rare xanthine; cystine stones are opaque because of their sulfur content.

URINARY SCREENING FOR INHERITED METABOLIC DISEASES

Urine has been used for many years to screen for metabolic diseases, particularly those resulting from a genetic predisposition. In many of these diseases, an abnormal metabolite or a larger than normal amount of a normal metabolite is excreted in the urine. Because these conditions are uncommon and their symptoms often nonspecific, and because some may be treatable if early diagnosis is confirmed, blood and urine should be analyzed using techniques that are highly selective and sensitive. Numerous inborn errors of metabolism have been identified, and this section will describe some of the more common disease entities.

Aminoacidurias

Excretion of one or more amino acids in the urine may be due to a block in a major metabolic pathway (overflow type) or a deficiency in renal tubular function (renal type). Phenylketonuria is an example of overflow aminoaciduria in which an enzyme substrate and other metabolites in the pathway accumulate, causing increased body fluid levels and increased substrate excretion in urine. Unlike the overflow-type diseases, renal-type aminoacidurias do not have high levels of the amino acid in the blood because the primary defect is in the renal tubular reabsorption mechanism. An example of renal transport aminoaciduria is cystinuria.

Phenylketonuria. Phenylketonuria is an autosomal recessive inherited disorder in which there is absence of the enzyme phenylalanine hydroxylase. Both sexes are affected equally, with an incidence of about 1 in 11,000. Allelic heterogeneity can be extensive, particularly in the United States (Guldberg, 1996). Mental retardation is the major clinical finding, and dietary restriction of phenylalanine has proven efficacious in these patients.

Because they are not converted to tyrosine in this disorder, phenylalanine and other normal metabolites accumulate in abnormal amounts. Plasma phenylalanine and phenylpyruvic acid levels are elevated; urinary phenylpyruvic acid (highest), phenylacetic acid, and phenylalanine are increased. Urinary indoleacetic acid and other indoles arising from altered tryptophan metabolism and indican (an indole) are also increased. The excretion of 5-hydroxyindoleacetic acid is diminished, paralleling the low level of serum 5-hydroxytryptamine. The urine and sweat of these patients have a characteristic mousy/musty odor due to phenylacetic acid.

Methods. Phenistix reagent strips contain ferric ammonium sulfate, magnesium sulfate, and cyclohexylsulfamic acid. At 30 seconds following immersion into urine, the color of the test area is compared with the color chart provided. A positive test result shows a gray to gray-green color. The test detects 5–10 mg/dL. Salicylates and metabolites of phenothiazine derivatives may cause a pink to purple color. Ion-exchange high-performance liquid chromatography has been found suitable for quantitative confirmatory testing of abnormal specimens (Reilly, 1998).

Alkaptonuria. Normally, phenylalanine and tyrosine are metabolized to homogentisic acid (dihydroxyphenylacetic acid), which is then oxidized to maleylacetoacetic acid. In alkaptonuria, the enzyme homogentisic acid oxidase is deficient, and homogentisic acid is excreted in urine in large quantities. The urine characteristically turns brown-black on standing or with alkaline pH. Patients with alkaptonuria develop dark blue to black pigmentation in cartilage and connective tissue; frequently, the disease is not diagnosed until arthritis has already developed.

Methods. Screening methods include ferric chloride and silver nitrate tests. A transient, dark blue color appears as two drops of 10% ferric chloride solution are added to about 2 mL urine containing homogentisic acid. The silver nitrate test involves adding 4 mL of 3% silver nitrate to 0.5 mL urine, mixing, and then adding several drops of 10% NH_4OH. Homogentisic acid will cause a black color to develop. Confirmatory methods include paper or thin-layer chromatography, as well as capillary electrophoresis. These methods should distinguish homogentisic acid from gentisic acid, an aspirin metabolite.

Tyrosinuria. Tyrosinemia with tyrosinuria occurs when the metabolism of tyrosine derived from the diet or from phenylalanine is abnormal. This may be part of a generalized amino acid disorder associated with liver disease, or it may represent one of the various genetic disorders involving tyrosine metabolism. Tyrosine crystals may appear in the urine as fine, silky crystals scattered singly or aggregated to form sheaves. They appear brown to black, precipitate at an acid pH, and are soluble in alkali. Small quantities of tyrosine may appear in the urine of normal individuals.

Transitory hypertyrosinemia may occur in low-birthweight and premature infants as a benign condition. Typically, these infants are asymptomatic, and no liver or renal disease is present. The elevated tyrosine levels may on occasion be accompanied by transiently elevated phenylalanine levels. Tyrosine and the phenolic acids *p*-hydroxyphenyllactic and *p*-hydroxyphenylpyruvic acids are excreted in larger than normal amounts in the urine. The nature of the enzymatic defect has not been well characterized, and the tyrosine level of these patients usually returns to normal within a few weeks to months.

Type I hereditary tyrosinemia (tyrosinosis) is an autosomal recessive disorder characterized by defects in fumarylacetoacetate hydrolase and maleylacetoacetate hydrolase. Succinylacetoacetone and succinylacetone accumulate and inhibit renal function, various hepatic enzymes, and porphobilinogen synthetase. Patients may experience liver failure, renal dysfunction, rickets, and acute intermittent porphyria–like symptoms. Hepatoma is a late complication. Generalized aminoaciduria, phosphaturia, glycosuria, and uricosuria may occur. A low-tyrosine/phenylalanine diet is the mainstay of therapy.

Type II tyrosinemia (Richner-Hanhart syndrome) is an autosomal recessive inherited deficiency of tyrosine aminotransferase. Patients will have tyrosinemia, tyrosinuria, and increased urinary phenolic acids. The metabolism of other amino acids, renal function, and hepatic function are otherwise normal. Erosions of the cornea, soles, and palms are common, and mental retardation sometimes occurs. Therapy centers on a low-tyrosine/phenlyalanine diet.

Methods. The nitrosonaphthol test for tyrosine is a nonspecific screening method and should be confirmed by chromatography or quantitative serum assay of tyrosine. Tyrosine and tyramine form soluble red complexes with nitrosonaphthol.

Maple Syrup Urine Disease. MSUD is one of a group of diseases associated with abnormal branched-chain amino acid metabolism. These include hypervalinemia, isovaleric acidemia causing "sweaty feet" odor, and other rare diseases. Several different clinical forms of MSUD have been described, together with various sites of biochemical derangement. The classic type of MSUD, inherited as an autosomal recessive trait, is marked by severe neonatal vomiting, seizures, stupor, irregular respirations, and often hypoglycemia. Left untreated, patients become rapidly comatose and die. Leucine, isoleucine, valine, and their corresponding keto acids are elevated in the plasma and excreted in the urine. Deficient decarboxylases and other enzymes are thought to prevent the conversion of keto acids to fatty acids. Intermittent, intermediate, thiamine-responsive, and dihydrolipoyl dehydrogenase (E3) deficiency forms of MSUD have been described (Holmes, 1997).

The urine of patients with MSUD has an odor resembling maple syrup, caramelized sugar, or curry, the source of which is not certain. The urinary keto acids are demonstrable by the first week of life.

Methods. The dinitrophenylhydrazine screening test indicates the presence of α-keto acids in the urine. Insoluble hydrazones are formed from the reaction of carbonyl groups with dinitrophenylhydrazine. A positive result is seen with MSUD and possibly in phenylketonuria (phenylpyruvic acid), histidinemia (imidazole pyruvic acid), and methionine malabsorption (oasthouse syndrome). The test is positive with ketonuria due to other inherited diseases and other causes. A preliminary screening test for ketones should be performed.

Procedure

1. Reagent and control (ketoglutaric acid, 25 mg in 100 mL normal urine) should be at room temperature.
2. Add 10 drops of reagent (100 mg of 2,4-dinitrophenylhydrazine in 100 mL of 2N HCl) to 1 mL of clear urine.
3. Within 10 minutes, a yellow or chalky white precipitate indicates a positive reaction. It should be the same as or greater than the control precipitate.

Gas or thin-layer chromatographic analysis and nuclear magnetic resonance spectroscopy of the urine may be used as confirmatory methods (Holmes, 1997).

Cystinuria. Cystinuria is a common amino acid disorder that occurs equally in both sexes, with an incidence estimated at about 1 per 10,000 (homozygous) (larger numbers for heterozygotes). In mass screening programs for infants, the homozygous form is detected at about the same rate as phenylketonuria. Defective transport of cystine by the epithelial cells of the renal tubules and gut is transmitted as an autosomal recessive trait. The basic defect is not known. Although large amounts of the dibasic acids ornithine, lysine, and arginine are also excreted in this disease, cystine is the only one that crystallizes out, with stone formation as a clinical manifestation.

Cystinosis, a recessively inherited disorder of unknown cause, is characterized by intracellular cystine crystal deposition within lysosomes. Crystals may accumulate in the kidney, eye, bone marrow, and spleen. The severe form of this disorder is characterized by photophobia, renal failure, rickets, and growth failure. With renal tubular involvement, Fanconi's syndrome develops with generalized aminoaciduria and glucosuria. Benign and intermediate varieties of cystinosis have been described. Unlike in cystinuria, the cystine loss in cystinosis parallels the loss of other amino acids in the urine.

Urinary cystine is sometimes detected in patients with various renal tubular diseases. Cystine is excreted with other amino acids in Wilson's disease, in Lowe's disease, and with the aminoaciduria of Hartnup's disease.

Methods. Examine a first morning urine specimen for colorless, hexagonal crystals of cystine. Cystine may not always crystallize in a concentrated urine, although it may be present in large amounts.

The cyanide-nitroprusside test used for the qualitative determination of urine cystine is Brand's modification of the Legal nitroprusside reaction. Cystine is reduced to cysteine by sodium cyanide, and the free sulfhydryl groups then react with nitroprusside to produce a red-purple color. Cysteine, cystine, homocystine, and ketones (dark red) all will give positive reactions. The qualitative test separates normal, heterozygote, and homozygote ranges of excretion. The lower limit of the test was 35–60 μmol of cystine per mole of creatinine, and this corresponded to the heterozygote range. Homozygous stone formers usually excrete more than 300 mg/g creatinine and are also detected by this test.

Procedure

1. Place 3–5 mL urine in a test tube and add 2.0 mL sodium cyanide solution (5 g/dL water); allow to stand for 10 minutes. Timing is important. Treat a control solution in the same way. For a positive control, use 5 mg cystine dissolved in 10 mL 0.1N HCl, diluted to 100 mL with normal urine.
2. Add fresh, aqueous sodium nitroprusside solution (5 g/dL) dropwise (about five drops), and mix.
3. Read immediately as positive or negative. A stable red-purple color will develop with cystine. "Trace" results may also be reported. A concentrated normal specimen could give a weakly positive "trace" result.

Further identification and quantification of cystine may be accomplished by thin-layer or quantitative ion-exchange chromatography, or high-voltage electrophoresis.

Homocystinuria. The classic form of homocystinuria is due to deficiency of cystathionine β-synthase, which catalyzes the formation of cystathionine from homocystine and serine in the methionine pathway. Homocysteine is rapidly oxidized to homocystine, which accumulates along with methionine and is excreted in the urine. Children with this disease may have seizures, thromboses, mental retardation, arachnodactyly, and kyphoscoliosis. Connective tissue manifestations are thought to result from accumulation of the intermediate homocysteine, which interferes with collagen cross-linking.

Urine for testing must be fresh because homocystine is labile. The cyanide-nitroprusside test, described earlier, is positive. Quantitative chemical analysis reveals high levels of homocystine, methionine, and cysteine-homocysteine disulfide. Urine levels are monitored to follow the effects of the methionine-restricted diet used to treat this disease.

ADDITIONAL URINE TESTING MODALITIES

A latex agglutination nephelometric immunoassay has been developed to measure urinary basic fetoprotein (BFP). Levels of this substance may be elevated with ureter stones, infection, and prostate and bladder cancers, making BFP a nonspecific marker of inflammation or tumor (Itoh, 1998).

The urine Trinder spot test, performed by emergency room physicians, is a sensitive screen for salicylates.

Rendl (1998) described a semiquantitative rapid urinary iodide test, suitable for epidemiologic surveys of iodine deficiency, particularly in developing countries.

Lastly, a monoclonal antibody assay for the detection of free urinary pyridinium cross-links can help to identify bone resorption in patients with osteoporosis, hyperthyroidism, hyperparathyroidism, and Paget's disease of bone (Gomez, 1996).

Cytopathologic examination of the urine is commonly performed to detect malignancies. Enzyme-linked immunosorbent assay and fluorescence in situ hybridization tests can be used to detect carcinoma of the urinary bladder. These tests are discussed in greater detail in Chapter 74.

SELECTED REFERENCES

Ben-Ezra J, Bork L, McPherson RA. Evaluation of the Sysmex UF-100 automated urinalysis analyzer. Clin Chem 1998;44:92–5.

In this study, the authors compare the Sysmex UF-100 automated urinalysis analyzer with manual microscopy. The UF-100 showed good correlation with microscopy for detection of cellular elements and casts in the urine.

Dinda AK, Saxena S, Guleria S, et al. Diagnosis of glomerular haematuria: role of dysmorphic red cell, G1 cell, and bright-field microscopy. Scand J Clin Lab Invest 1997;57:203–8.

This study shows that the presence of dysmorphic red blood cells in the urine has excellent sensitivity (82%) and specificity (100%) in the diagnosis of glomerular disease.

Gerber LM, Johnson K, Alderman MH. Assessment of a new dipstick test in the screening for microalbuminuria in patients with hypertension. Am J Hypertens 1998;11:1321–7.

The authors examined the applicability of a urine dipstick method in detecting microalbuminuria. Specificity with this test was 90%, with a negative predictive value of 93%–97%. Comparison between random and 24-hour urines showed good correlation.

Hemmelgarn BR, Manns BJ, Lloyd A, et al. Relation between kidney function, proteinuria, and adverse outcomes. J Am Med Assoc 2010;303:423–9.

This article shows a strong association between proteinuria and the adverse outcomes of mortality, myocardial infarction, and progression to kidney failure independent of the commonly used estimated glomerular filtration rate.

Jefferson JA, Shankland SJ, Pichler RH. Proteinuria in diabetic kidney disease: a mechanistic viewpoint. Kidney Int 2008;74:22–36.

This comprehensive review describes the pathophysiology of proteinuria through damage to the glomerulus with emphasis on the glomerular filtration barrier at the cellular level.

Lamb EJ, MacKenzie F, Stevens PE. How should proteinuria be detected and measured? Ann Clin Biochem 2009;46:205–17.

This review covers current guidelines for measurement of protein in urine, emphasizing the merits of assays for albumin over total protein to assess glomerular protein loss in chronic kidney disease but with consideration for loss of other proteins in tubular proteinuria.

Perkovic V, Verdon C, Ninomiya T, et al. The relationship between proteinuria and coronary risk: a systematic review and meta-analysis. PLoS Med 2008;5:e207.

This meta-analysis of 26 cohort studies demonstrated a strong and continuous association between proteinuria and risk for coronary artery disease, suggesting that proteinuria should be used in the risk assessment of cardiovascular disease.

Rockall AG, Newman-Sanders AP, al-Kutoubi MA, et al. Haematuria. Postgrad Med J 1997;73:129–36.

This is a review article on hematuria from a clinical perspective. It proposes a rational algorithm for the laboratory and clinical workup of patients with hematuria.

Strohmaier WL, Hoelz KJ, Bichler KH. Spot urine samples for the metabolic evaluation of urolithiasis patients. Eur Urol 1997;32:294–300.

This study describes the clinical and laboratory workup of urolithiasis patients. Spot urines were equally as informative as 24-hour urines in the evaluation of these patients.

Yoo YM, Tatsumi N, Kirihigashi K, et al. Inaccuracy and inefficiency of urinary sediment analysis. Osaka City Med J 1995;41:41–8.

In this study, the authors examined the laboratory characteristics of manual urine microscopy. Counts of cellular elements, but not casts, showed good reproducibility, even by inexperienced technologists. Most of the casts found were nonpathologic hyaline casts.

REFERENCES

Access the complete reference list online at http://www.expertconsult.com

CHAPTER 29

CEREBROSPINAL, SYNOVIAL, SEROUS BODY FLUIDS, AND ALTERNATIVE SPECIMENS

Donald S. Karcher, Richard A. McPherson

KEY POINTS

- Determining the etiologic cause of fluid accumulation in various body cavities (i.e., joints, chest, abdomen) is critical for proper treatment of these disorders.
- Appropriate laboratory examination of these fluids is therefore critical for the diagnosis of numerous diseases (i.e., bacterial, viral and fungal infections; distinction between various arthritides; primary [i.e., mesothelioma] and metastatic malignancies; among others).
- Accurate test interpretation depends on appropriate specimen collection, turnaround time, physician/laboratory communication, and reliable reference values.

CEREBROSPINAL FLUID

In adults, approximately 500 mL of cerebrospinal fluid (CSF) is produced each day (0.3–0.4 mL/min). The total adult volume varies from

90–150 mL, about 25 mL of which is in the ventricles and the remainder in the subarachnoid space. In neonates, the volume varies from 10–60 mL. Thus, the total CSF volume is replaced every 5–7 hours (Wood, 1980). An estimated 70% of CSF is derived by ultrafiltration and secretion through the choroid plexuses. The ventricular ependymal lining and the cerebral subarachnoid space account for the remainder. CSF leaves the ventricular system through the medial and lateral foramina, flowing over the brain and spinal cord surfaces within the subarachnoid space. CSF resorption occurs at the arachnoid villi, predominantly along the superior sagittal sinus.

The CSF has several major functions: (1) It provides physical support because the 1500-g brain weighs about 50 g when suspended in CSF; (2) it confers a protective effect against sudden changes in acute venous (respiratory and postural) and arterial blood pressure or impact pressure; (3) it provides an excretory waste function because the brain has no lymphatic system; (4) it is the pathway whereby hypothalamus releasing factors are transported to the cells of the median eminence; and (5) it maintains central nervous system ionic homeostasis.

The concept of the blood-brain barrier (BBB) is derived from dye-exclusion (tryphan blue) studies. It consists of two morphologically distinct components: A unique capillary endothelium held together by intercellular tight junctions; and the choroid plexus, where a single layer of specialized choroidal ependymal cells connected by tight junctions overlies fenestrated capillaries. The CSF ionic components (e.g., H^+, K^+, Ca^{++}, Mg^{++}, bicarbonate) are tightly regulated by specific transport systems, whereas glucose, urea, and creatinine diffuse freely but require 2 or more hours to equilibrate. Proteins cross by passive diffusion at a rate dependent on the plasma-to-CSF concentration gradient and inversely proportional to their molecular weight and hydrodynamic volume (Fishman, 1992). Thus, the BBB maintains the relative homeostasis of the central nervous system environment during acute perturbations of plasma components.

SPECIMEN COLLECTION AND OPENING PRESSURE

Cerebrospinal fluid may be obtained by lumbar, cisternal, or lateral cervical puncture or through ventricular cannulas or shunts. Details of the performance of lumbar puncture are described elsewhere (Herndon, 1989; Ward, 1992). Respiratory compromise may occur in infants if the head is flexed (Ward, 1992).

A manometer should be attached before fluid removal to record the opening pressure. CSF pressure varies with postural changes, blood pressure, venous return, Valsalva maneuvers, and factors that alter cerebral blood flow. The normal opening adult pressure is 90–180 mm of water in the lateral decubitus position with the legs and neck in a neutral position. It may be slightly higher if the patient is sitting up and varies up to 10 mm with respiration. However, the pressure may be as high as 250 mm of water in obese patients. In infants and young children, the normal range is 10–100 mm of water, with the adult range attained by age 6–8 years (Fishman, 1992). Opening pressures above 250 mm H_2O are diagnostic of intracranial hypertension, which may be due to meningitis, intracranial hemorrhage, and tumors (Seehusen, 2003). If the opening pressure is greater than 200 mm H_2O in a relaxed patient, no more than 2.0 mL should be withdrawn.

Idiopathic intracranial hypertension is most commonly seen in obese women during their childbearing years. When an elevated opening pressure is noted, CSF must be removed slowly and the pressure carefully monitored. Additional CSF should not be removed if the pressure reaches 50% of the opening pressure (Conly, 1983).

Elevated pressures may be present in patients who are tense or straining and in those with congestive heart failure, meningitis, superior vena cava syndrome, thrombosis of the venous sinuses, cerebral edema, mass lesions, hypoosmolality, or conditions inhibiting CSF absorption. Opening pressure elevation may be the only abnormality in cryptococcal meningitis and pseudotumor cerebri (Hayward, 1987). Decreased CSF pressure may be present in spinal-subarachnoid block, dehydration, circulatory collapse, and CSF leakage. A significant pressure drop after removal of 1–2 mL suggests herniation or spinal block above the puncture site, and no further fluid should be withdrawn.

Up to 20 mL of CSF may normally be removed. However, the clinician not only should be aware of the quantity of CSF required for the requested tests to ensure that a sufficient sample is submitted, but should also provide an appropriate clinical history to the laboratory. The sample site (i.e., lumbar, cisternal, etc.) should be noted because cytologic and chemical parameters vary at different sites. The necessity for a simultaneous serum glucose should also be considered. This is best obtained 2–4 hours before lumbar puncture because of the delay in serum–CSF equilibrium.

TABLE 29-1
Diseases Detected by Laboratory Examination of CSF

High sensitivity, high specificity*
Bacterial, tuberculous, and fungal meningitis
High sensitivity, moderate specificity
Viral meningitis
Subarachnoid hemorrhage
Multiple sclerosis
Central nervous system syphilis
Infectious polyneuritis
Paraspinal abscess
Moderate sensitivity, high specificity
Meningeal malignancy
Moderate sensitivity, moderate specificity
Intracranial hemorrhage
Viral encephalitis
Subdural hematoma

From American College of Physicians, Health and Public Policy Committee: The diagnostic spinal tap. Ann Intern Med 1986;104:880, with permission.
CSF, Cerebrospinal fluid.
*Sensitivity is the ability of a test to detect disease when it is present; specificity is the ability of a test to exclude disease when it is not present.

The CSF specimen is usually divided into three serially collected sterile tubes: Tube 1 for chemistry and immunology studies; tube 2 for microbiological examination; and tube 3 for cell count and differential. An additional tube may be inserted in the No. 3 position for cytology if a malignancy is suspected. However, under certain conditions, some variations are critical. For example, if tube 1 is hemorrhagic because of a traumatic puncture, it should not be used when protein studies are the most important aspect of the analysis (i.e., suspected multiple sclerosis). Indeed, tube 3 should be examined for the major purpose of CSF collection. Perhaps the only definite statement one can make is that tube 1 should never be used for microbiology because it may be contaminated with skin bacteria. If questions arise, communication between the laboratory and the clinician before CSF analysis is critical.

Glass tubes should be avoided because cell adhesion to glass affects the cell count and differential. Specimens should be delivered to the laboratory and processed quickly to minimize cellular degradation, which begins within 1 hour of collection. Refrigeration is contraindicated for culture specimens because fastidious organisms (e.g., *Haemophilus influenza*, *Neisseria meningitidis*) will not survive.

INDICATIONS AND RECOMMENDED TESTS

Indications for lumbar puncture can be divided into four major disease categories: meningeal infection, subarachnoid hemorrhage, primary or metastatic malignancy, and demyelinating diseases (American College of Physicians, 1986). Identification of infectious meningitis, particularly bacterial, is the most important indication for CSF examination (Table 29-1). Recommended laboratory tests are directed toward identification of these disorders (Table 29-2). CSF examination for other diseases is generally less helpful but often provides supportive evidence of a clinical diagnosis or helps to rule out other diseases (Irani, 2009). Limited routine studies followed by reflexive ordering of more focused tests (as needed) on the stored specimen have been advocated as a way of improving test efficiency (Albright, 1988).

GROSS EXAMINATION

Normal CSF is crystal clear and colorless and has a viscosity similar to that of water. Abnormal CSF may appear cloudy, frankly purulent, or pigment tinged. Turbidity or cloudiness begins to appear with leukocyte (white blood cell [WBC]) counts over 200 cells/μL or red blood cell (RBC) counts of 400/μL. However, grossly bloody fluids have RBC counts greater than 6000/μL. Microorganisms (bacteria, fungi, amebas), radiographic contrast material, aspirated epidural fat, and a protein level greater than 150 mg/dL (1.5 g/L) may also produce varying degrees of cloudiness. Experienced observers may be able to detect cell counts of less than 50 cells/μL with the unaided eye by observing for Tyndall's effect (Simon, 1978). Here,

TABLE 29-2
Recommended CSF Laboratory Tests

Routine
Opening CSF pressure
Total cell count (WBC and RBC)
Differential cell count (stained smear)
Glucose (CSF/plasma ratio)
Total protein
Useful under certain conditions
Cultures (bacteria, fungi, viruses, *Mycobacterium tuberculosis*)
Gram stain, acid-fast stain
Fungal and bacterial antigens
Enzymes (LD, ADA, CK-BB)
Lactate
Polymerase chain reaction (TB, viruses)
Cytology
Electrophoresis (protein, immunofixation)
Proteins (C-reactive, 14-3-3, τ, β-amyloid, transferrin)
VDRL test for syphilis
Fibrin-derivative D-dimer
Tuberculostearic acid

Modified from Kjeldsberg CR, Knight JA. Body fluids: laboratory examination of amniotic, cerebrospinal, seminal, serous, and synovial fluids. 3rd ed. Chicago: © American Society for Clinical Pathology; 1993, with permission.
ADA, Adenosine deaminase; *CK-BB,* creatine kinase-BB; *CSF,* cerebrospinal fluid; *LD,* lactate dehydrogenase; *RBC,* red blood cell; *TB,* tuberculosis; *VDRL,* Venereal Disease Research Laboratories; *WBC,* white blood cell.

direct sunlight directed on the tube at a 90-degree angle from the observer will impart a "sparkling" or "snowy" appearance as suspended particles scatter the light.

Clot formation may be present in patients with traumatic taps, complete spinal block (Froin's syndrome), or suppurative or tuberculous meningitis. It is not seen in patients with subarachnoid hemorrhage. Fine surface pellicles may be observed after refrigeration for 12–24 hours. Clots may interfere with cell count accuracy by entrapping inflammatory cells.

Viscous CSF may be encountered in patients with metastatic mucin-producing adenocarcinomas, cryptococcal meningitis due to capsular polysaccharide, or liquid nucleus pulposus resulting from needle injury to the annulus fibrosus.

Pink-red CSF usually indicates the presence of blood and is grossly bloody when the RBC count exceeds 6000/μL. It may originate from a subarachnoid hemorrhage, intracerebral hemorrhage, or cerebral infarct, or from a traumatic spinal tap.

Xanthochromia

Xanthochromia commonly refers to a pale pink to yellow color in the supernatant of centrifuged CSF, although other colors may be present (Table 29-3). To detect xanthochromia, the CSF should be centrifuged and the supernatant fluid compared with a tube of distilled water. Xanthochromic CSF is pink, orange, or yellow owing to RBC lysis and hemoglobin breakdown. Pale pink to orange xanthochromia from released oxyhemoglobin is usually detected by lumbar puncture performed 2–4 hours after the onset of subarachnoid hemorrhage, although it may take as long as 12 hours. Peak intensity occurs in about 24–36 hours and then gradually disappears over the next 4–8 days. Yellow xanthochromia is derived from bilirubin. It develops about 12 hours after a subarachnoid bleed and peaks at 2–4 days, but may persist for 2–4 weeks.

Visible CSF xanthochromia may also be due to the following: (1) oxyhemoglobin resulting from artifactual red cell lysis caused by detergent contamination of the needle or collecting tube, or a delay of longer than 1 hour without refrigeration before examination; (2) bilirubin (bilirhachia) in jaundiced patients; (3) CSF protein levels over 150 mg/dL, which are also present in bloody traumatic taps (>100,000 RBCs/μL) or in pathologic states such as complete spinal block, polyneuritis, and meningitis; (4) merthiolate disinfectant contamination; (5) carotenoids (orange) in people with dietary hypercarotenemia (i.e., hypervitaminosis A); (6) melanin (brownish) from meningeal metastatic melanoma; and (7) rifampin therapy (red-orange).

Although spectral absorbance scans provide an objective record of xanthochromia, careful gross CSF inspection has comparable sensitivity (Britton, 1983). Spectrophotometry can also help to differentiate hemoglobin-derived substances from other xanthochromic pigments with different maximal absorption peaks.

TABLE 29-3
Xanthochromia and Associated Diseases/Disorders

CSF supernatant color	Associated diseases/disorders
Pink	RBC lysis/hemoglobin breakdown products
Yellow	RBC lysis/hemoglobin breakdown products Hyperbilirubinemia CSF protein >150 mg/dL (1.5 g/L)
Orange	RBC lysis/hemoglobin breakdown products Hypervitaminosis A (carotenoids)
Yellow-green	Hyperbilirubinemia (biliverdin)
Brown	Meningeal metastatic melanoma

CSF, Cerebrospinal fluid; *RBC,* red blood cell.

Differential Diagnosis of Bloody CSF

A traumatic tap occurs in about 20% of lumbar punctures. Distinction of a traumatic puncture from a pathologic hemorrhage is, therefore, of vital importance. Although the presence of crenated RBCs is not useful, the following observations may be helpful in distinguishing the two forms of bleeding.

1. In a traumatic tap, the hemorrhagic fluid usually clears between the first and third collected tubes but remains relatively uniform in subarachnoid hemorrhage.
2. Xanthochromia, microscopic evidence of erythrophagocytosis, or hemosiderin-laden macrophages indicate a subarachnoid bleed in the absence of a prior traumatic tap. RBC lysis begins as early as 1–2 hours after a traumatic tap. Thus, rapid evaluation is necessary to avoid false-positive results.
3. A commercially available latex agglutination immunoassay test for cross-linked fibrin derivative D-dimer is specific for fibrin degradation and is negative in traumatic taps (Lang, 1990). However, false-positive results might be expected in disseminated intravascular coagulation, fibrinolysis, or trauma from repeated lumbar punctures.

MICROSCOPIC EXAMINATION

Total Cell Count

Although the traditional manual method for cell counting in CSF samples, using undiluted CSF in a manual counting chamber, continues to be a useful approach, because of the low cell counts frequently encountered in CSF, the precision of manual counting in these samples is inherently limited (Barnes, 2004). For example, using 18 large squares (1 mm^2 each) in a Fuchs-Rosenthal–type chamber with a depth of 0.2 mm, a total volume of 3.6 μL (18 × 0.2 μL/square) is examined. With 5 cells/μL, a total of 18 cells is counted. The coefficient of variation (CV), defined as 100 divided by the square root of the number of cells counted, is 24%; ±2 CV is about 48%. A Neubauer hemocytometer with nine 1-mm^2 squares with a depth of 0.1 mm has a CV of 45% (+90% for 2 CV) with the same cell concentration. Improvements in the hardware and software in flow cytometers now allow reliable use of these instruments in performing automated total WBC counts and WBC differential counts (Hoffman, 2002; Aune, 2004), and even in detecting bacteria (Nanos, 2008) in CSF samples; however, the low clinical decision levels for total WBC count and enumeration of some WBC types in CSF and limitations in detecting small numbers of RBCs continue to represent challenges in the use of these instruments with CSF (Hoffman, 2002; Andrews, 2005; Glasser, 2009; Kleine, 2009). Because of these limitations, laboratories should exercise caution in utilizing automated cell counters with CSF samples and should carefully follow manufacturer and Clinical and Laboratory Standards Institute guidelines (CLSI Approved Guideline H56-A, 2006) when implementing these automated methods.

The normal leukocyte cell count in adults is 0–5 cells/μL. It is higher in neonates, ranging from 0–30 cells/μL, with the upper limit of normal decreasing to adult values by adolescence. No RBCs should be present in normal CSF. If numerous (except a traumatic tap), a pathologic process is probable (e.g., trauma, malignancy, infarct, hemorrhage). Although red cell counts have limited diagnostic value, they may give a useful approximation of the true CSF WBC or total protein in the presence of a traumatic puncture by correcting for leukocytes or protein introduced by the traumatic puncture. To be valid, all measurements (WBC, RBC, protein)

TABLE 29-4
CSF Reference Values for Differential Cytocentrifuge Counts

Cell type	Adults, %	Neonates, %
Lymphocytes	62 ± 34	20 ± 18
Monocytes	36 ± 20	72 ± 22
Neutrophils	2 ± 5	3 ± 5
Histiocytes	Rare	5 ± 4
Ependymal cells	Rare	Rare
Eosinophils	Rare	Rare

CSF, Cerebrospinal fluid.

must be performed on the same tube. This procedure also assumes that the blood is derived exclusively from the traumatic tap. The corrected WBC count is as follows:

$$WBC_{corr} = WBC_{obs} - WBC_{added}$$

where

$$WBC_{added} = WBC_{BLD} \times RBC_{CSF}/RBC_{BLD}$$

and

WBC_{obs} = CSF leukocyte count
WBC_{added} = leukocytes added to CSF by traumatic tap
WBC_{BLD} = peripheral blood leukocyte count
RBC_{CSF} = CSF erythrocyte count
RBC_{BLD} = peripheral blood erythrocyte count.

An analogous formula may be used to correct for **added total protein** (TP):

$$TP_{added} = [TP_{serum} \times (1 - HCT)] \times RBC_{CSF}/RBC_{BLD}$$

In the presence of a normal peripheral blood RBC count and serum protein, these corrections amount to about 1 WBC for every 700 RBCs and 8 mg/dL protein for every 10,000 RBCs/µL. This latter RBC correction factor is reasonably accurate as long as the peripheral WBC count is not extremely high or low. Moreover, the accuracy of these corrections is limited by the precision of the CSF RBC count, which can significantly limit its value.

An observed/expected (added) WBC count ratio greater than 10 has a sensitivity of 88% and a specificity of 90% for bacterial meningitis. When the predicted WBC is below the observed count, the probability of bacterial meningitis appears to be low (Mayefsky, 1987; Bonadio, 1990).

Differential Cell Count

Suggested differential count reference ranges are presented in Table 29-4. A differential performed in a counting chamber is unsatisfactory because the low cell numbers give rise to poor precision, and identifying the cell type beyond granulocytes and "mononuclears" is difficult in a wet preparation. Direct smears of the centrifuged CSF sediment are also subject to significant error from cellular distortion and fragmentation.

The **cytocentrifuge method** is rapid, requires minimal training, and allows Wright's staining of air-dried cytospins. Indeed, it is the recommended method for differential cell counts in all body fluids (Rabinovitch, 1994). Cell yield and preservation are better than with simple centrifugation. From 30–50 cells can be concentrated from 0.5 mL of "normal" CSF. Variable artifactual distortions may be seen, but they are minimized when the specimen is fresh, albumin is added to the specimen (2 drops of 22% bovine serum albumin), and the cell concentration is adjusted to about 300 WBCs/L prior to centrifugation (Kjeldsberg, 1993). Manual differential cell counting on a cytocentrifuge preparation of CSF continues to be the most reliable method, even with low cell numbers. Although automated differential counts may be safely performed on CSF samples using flow cytometers (Hoffman, 2002; Aulesa, 2003), confirmation of the automated differential count by manual examination of a cytocentrifuged smear is recommended with some instruments (Aune, 2004) and is a requirement with specimens at risk of containing neoplastic cells.

Filtration and sedimentation methods are too cumbersome for routine use. Filtration does, however, allow concentration of large volumes of CSF for cytologic examination or culture, while retaining the fluid filtrate for additional studies.

In adults, normal CSF contains small numbers of **lymphocytes** and **monocytes** in an approximate 70 : 30 ratio (Fig. 29-1). A higher proportion of monocytes is present in young children, in whom up to 80% may be normal (Pappu, 1982). Erythrocytes due to minor traumatic bleeding are commonly seen, especially in infants. Small numbers of neutrophils (PMNs) may also be seen in "normal" CSF specimens, most likely as a result of minor hemorrhage (Hayward, 1988) and improved cell concentration methods. No general consensus regarding an upper limit of normal for PMNs has been established. We accept up to 7% neutrophils with a normal WBC count. Over 60% neutrophils has been reported in high-risk neonates without meningitis (Rodriguez, 1990). The number of PMNs may be decreased by as much as 68% within the first 2 hours after lumbar puncture owing to cell lysis (Steele, 1986).

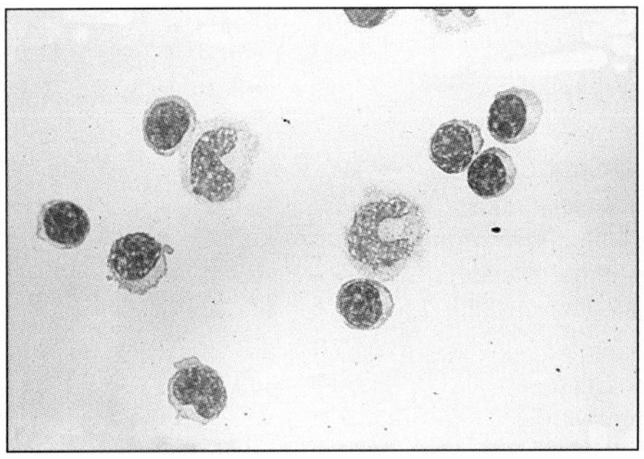

Figure 29-1 Cerebrospinal fluid cytology (lymphocyte to monocyte distribution ratio 70:30).

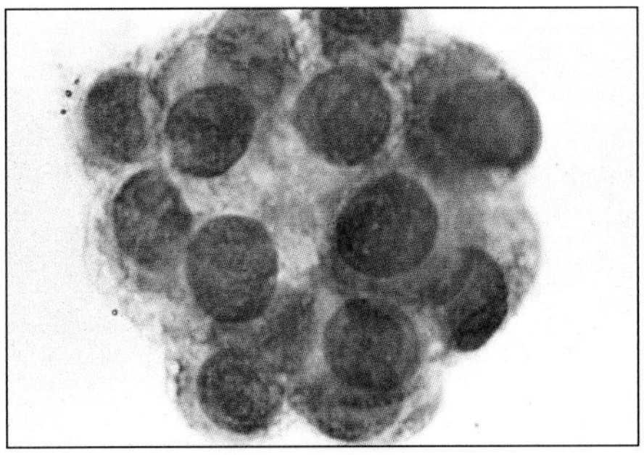

Figure 29-2 Choroid plexus cells in cerebrospinal fluid.

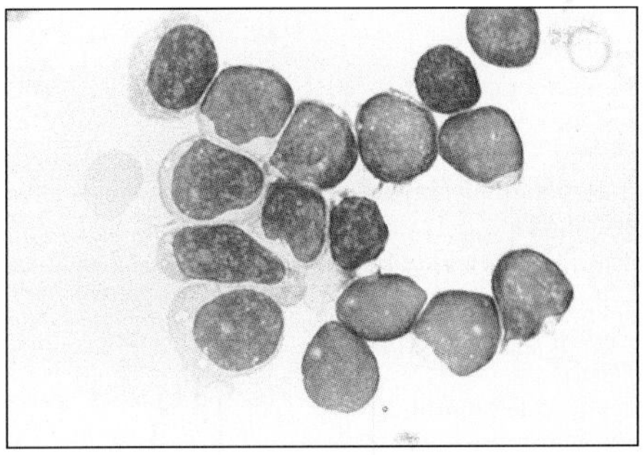

Figure 29-3 Cluster of blast-like cells in cerebrospinal fluid from premature newborn. *(From Kjeldsberg CR, Knight JA. Body fluids: laboratory examination of amniotic, cerebrospinal, seminal, serous and synovial fluids. 3rd ed. Chicago: © American Society for Clinical Pathology; 1993, with permission.)*

Traumatic puncture may result in the presence of bone marrow cells, cartilage cells, squamous cells, ganglion cells, and soft tissue elements. In addition, ependymal and choroid plexus cells may rarely be seen (Fig. 29-2). Moreover, blast-like primitive cell clusters, most likely of germinal matrix origin, are sometimes found in premature infants with intraventricular hemorrhage (Fig. 29-3).

Increased CSF **neutrophils** occur in numerous conditions (Table 29-5). In early bacterial meningitis, the proportion of PMNs usually exceeds 60%. However, in about one quarter of cases of early viral meningitis, the proportion of PMNs also exceeds 60%. Viral-induced neutrophilia usually changes to a lymphocytic pleocytosis within 2–3 days. A total PMN count of over 1180 cells/µL (or more than 2000 WBCs/µL) has a 99% predictive value for bacterial meningitis (Spanos, 1989). Persistent neutrophilic meningitis (over 1 week) may be noninfectious or due to less common pathogens such as *Nocardia*, *Actinomyces*, *Aspergillus*, and the zygomycetes (Peacock, 1984).

TABLE 29-5
Causes of Increased CSF Neutrophils

- Meningitis
  - Bacterial meningitis
  - Early viral meningoencephalitis
  - Early tuberculous meningitis
  - Early mycotic meningitis
  - Amebic encephalomyelitis
- Other infections
  - Cerebral abscess
  - Subdural empyema
  - AIDS-related CMV radiculopathy
- Following seizures
- Following CNS hemorrhage
  - Subarachnoid
  - Intracerebral
- Following CNS infarct
- Reaction to repeated lumbar punctures
- Injection of foreign material in subarachnoid space (e.g., methotrexate, contrast media)
- Metastatic tumor in contact with CSF

AIDS, Acquired immunodeficiency syndrome; *CMV*, cytomegalovirus; *CNS*, central nervous system; *CSF*, cerebrospinal fluid.

TABLE 29-6
Causes of CSF Lymphocytosis

- Meningitis
  - Viral meningitis
  - Tuberculous meningitis
  - Fungal meningitis
  - Syphilitic meningoencephalitis
  - Leptospiral meningitis
  - Bacterial due to uncommon organisms
  - Early bacterial meningitis where leukocyte counts are relatively low
  - Parasitic infestations (e.g., cysticercosis, trichinosis, toxoplasmosis)
  - Aseptic meningitis due to septic focus adjacent to meninges
- Degenerative disorders
  - Subacute sclerosing panencephalitis
  - Multiple sclerosis
  - Drug abuse encephalopathy
  - Guillain-Barré syndrome
  - Acute disseminated encephalomyelitis
- Other inflammatory disorders
  - Handl syndrome (headache with neurologic deficits and CSF lymphocytosis)
  - Sarcoidosis
  - Polyneuritis
  - CNS periarteritis

CNS, Central nervous system; *CSF*, cerebrospinal fluid.

TABLE 29-7
Inflammatory and Infectious Causes of CSF Plasmacytosis

• Acute viral infections	• Sarcoidosis
• Guillain-Barré syndrome	• Subacute sclerosing panencephalitis
• Multiple sclerosis	• Syphilitic meningoencephalitis
• Parasitic CNS infestations	• Tuberculous meningitis

CNS, Central nervous system; *CSF*, cerebrospinal fluid.

Increased CSF *lymphocytes* have been reported in various diseases/disorders (Table 29-6). Lymphocytosis (>50%) may occur in early acute bacterial meningitis when the CSF leukocyte count is under 1000/μL (Powers, 1985). Reactive lymphoplasmacytoid and immunoblastic variants may be present, particularly with viral meningoencephalitis. Blast-like lymphocytes may be seen admixed with small and large lymphocytes in the CSF of neonates.

Plasma cells, not normally present in CSF, may appear in a variety of inflammatory and infectious conditions (Table 29-7), along with large and small lymphocytes, and in association with malignant brain tumors (Fishman, 1992). Multiple myeloma may also rarely involve the meninges (Oda, 1991).

TABLE 29-8
Causes of CSF Eosinophilic Pleocytosis

Commonly associated with	Infrequently associated with
Acute polyneuritis	Bacterial meningitis
CNS reaction to foreign material (drugs, shunts)	Leukemia/lymphoma
Fungal infections	Myeloproliferative disorders
Idiopathic eosinophilic meningitis	Neurosarcoidosis
Idiopathic hypereosinophilic syndrome	Primary brain tumors
Parasitic infections	Tuberculous meningoencephalitis
	Viral meningitis

Modified with permission from Kjeldsberg CR, Knight JA. Body fluids: laboratory examination of amniotic, cerebrospinal, seminal, serous and synovial fluids. 3rd ed. Chicago: © American Society for Clinical Pathology; 1993.
CNS, Central nervous system; *CSF*, cerebrospinal fluid.

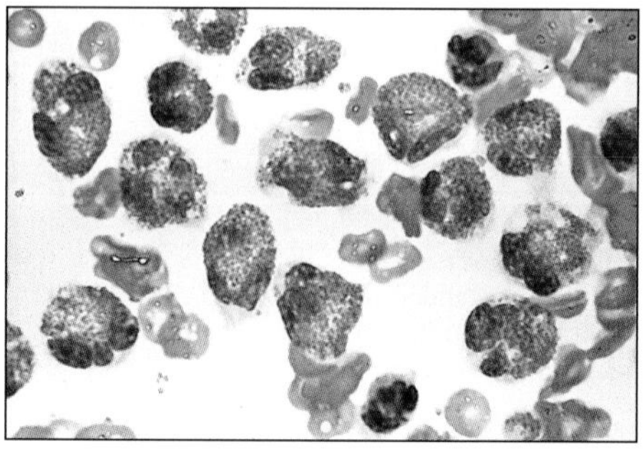

Figure 29-4 Eosinophils in cerebrospinal fluid from a child with malfunctioning ventricular shunt.

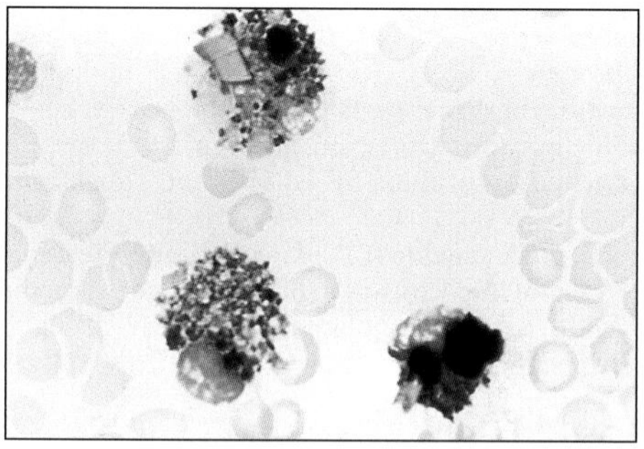

Figure 29-5 Hemosiderin-laden macrophages (siderophages) from the cerebrospinal fluid of a patient with subarachnoid hemorrhage. Hemosiderin crystals (golden-yellow) are also present. *(From Kjeldsberg CR, Knight JA. Body fluids: laboratory examination of amniotic, cerebrospinal, seminal, serous and synovial fluids. 3rd ed. Chicago: © American Society for Clinical Pathology; 1993, with permission.)*

Although **eosinophils** are rarely present in normal CSF, they may be increased in a variety of central nervous system (CNS) conditions (Table 29-8). For example, eosinophilia is frequently mild (1%–4%) in a general inflammatory response, but in children with malfunctioning ventricular shunts, it may be marked (Fig. 29-4). A suggested criterion for eosinophilic meningitis is 10% eosinophils (Kuberski, 1981); parasitic invasion of the CNS is the most common cause worldwide. *Coccidioides immitis* is a significant cause of CSF eosinophilia in endemic regions of the United States (Ragland, 1993).

Increased CSF **monocytes** lack diagnostic specificity and are usually part of a "mixed cell reaction" that includes neutrophils, lymphocytes, and plasma cells. This pattern is seen in tuberculous and fungal meningitis, chronic bacterial meningitis (i.e., *Listeria monocytogenes* and others), leptospiral meningitis, ruptured brain abscess, *Toxoplasma* meningitis, and amebic encephalomeningitis. A mixed cell pattern without neutrophils is characteristic of viral and syphilitic meningoencephalitis. **Macrophages** with phagocytosed erythrocytes **(erythrophages)** appear from 12–48 hours following a subarachnoid hemorrhage or traumatic tap. Hemosiderin-laden macrophages **(siderophages)** appear after about 48 hours and may persist for weeks (Fig. 29-5). Brownish yellow or red hematoidin crystals may form after a few days.

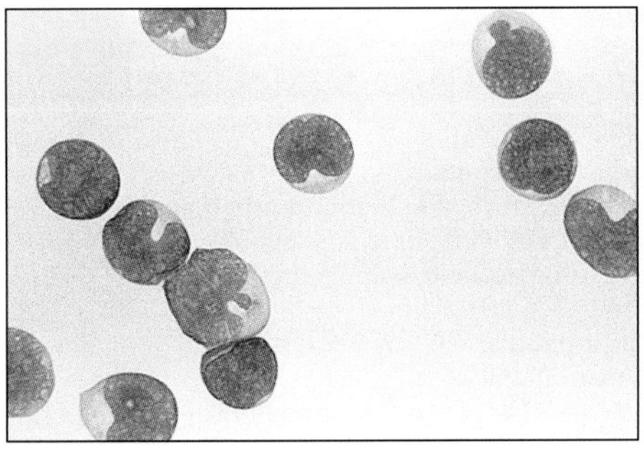

Figure 29-6 Acute lymphoblastic leukemia in cerebrospinal fluid. Note uniformity of the blast cells.

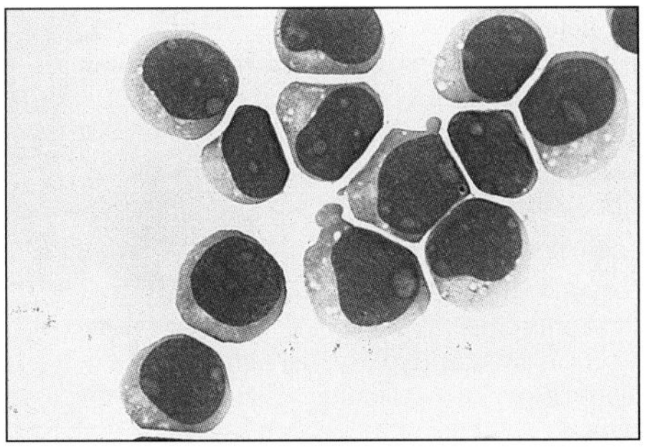

Figure 29-7 Acute myeloid leukemia in cerebrospinal fluid.

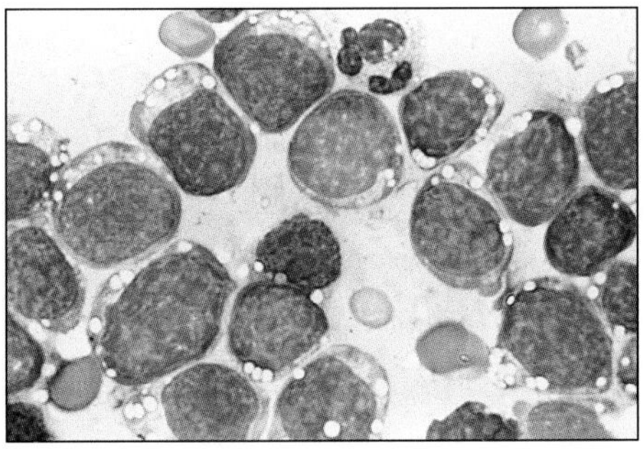

Figure 29-8 Burkitt's lymphoma in cerebrospinal fluid. The cells are characterized by blue cytoplasm with vacuoles and slightly clumped chromatin pattern. *(From Kjeldsberg CR, Knight JA. Body fluids: laboratory examination of amniotic, cerebrospinal, seminal, serous and synovial fluids. 3rd ed. Chicago: © American Society for Clinical Pathology; 1993, with permission.)*

TABLE 29-9
Adult Lumbar CSF Reference Values

Analyte	Conventional units	SI units
Protein	15–45 mg/dL	0.15–0.45 g/L
Prealbumin	2%–7%	
Albumin	56%–76%	
α_1-Globulin	2%–7%	
α_2-Globulin	4%–12%	
β-Globulin	8%–18%	
γ-Globulin	3%–12%	
Electrolytes		
Osmolality	280–300 mOsm/L	280–300 mmol/L
Sodium	135–150 mEq/L	135–150 mmol/L
Potassium	2.6–3.0 mEq/L	2.6–3.0 mmol/L
Chloride	115–130 mEq/L	115–130 mmol/L
Carbon dioxide	20–25 mEq/L	20–25 mmol/L
Calcium	2.0–2.8 mEq/L	1.0–1.4 mmol/L
Magnesium	2.4–3.0 mEq/L	1.2–1.5 mmol/L
Lactate	10–22 mg/dL	1.1–2.4 mmol/L
pH		
Lumbar fluid	7.28–7.32	
Cisternal fluid	7.32–7.34	
pCO_2		
Lumbar fluid	44–50 mm Hg	
Cisternal fluid	40–46 mm Hg	
pO_2	40–44 mm Hg	
Other Constituents		
Ammonia	10–35 μg/dL	6–20 μmol/L
Glutamine	5–20 mg/dL	0.3–1.4 mmol/L
Creatinine	0.6–1.2 mg/dL	45–92 μmol/L
Glucose	50–80 mg/dL	2.8–4.4 mmol/L
Iron	1–2 μg/dL	0.2–0.4 μmol/L
Phosphorus	1.2–2.0 mg/dL	0.4–0.7 mmol/L
Total lipid	1–2 mg/dL	0.01–0.02 g/L
Urea	6–16 mg/dL	2.0–5.7 mmol/L
Urate	0.5–3.0 mg/dL	30–180 μmol/L
Zinc	2–6 μg/dL	0.3–0.9 μmol/L

CSF, cerebrospinal fluid; *pCO_2,* partial pressure of carbon dioxide; *pO_2,* partial pressure of oxygen.

Morphologic cerebrospinal fluid examination for tumor cells has moderate sensitivity and high specificity (97%–98%) (Marton, 1986). Sensitivity depends on the type of neoplasm. CSF examination of leukemic patients has the highest sensitivity (about 70%), followed by metastatic carcinoma (20%–60%) and primary CNS malignancies (30%). Sensitivity may be optimized by using filtration methods with larger fluid volumes or by performing serial punctures in patients in whom a neoplasm is strongly suspected. Processing of CSF samples using liquid-based thin-layer methods also increases sensitivity in the detection of neoplastic cells and enhances preservation of these cells for potential immunocytochemical analysis (Sioutopoulou, 2008). These liquid-based methods are now commonly used for cytopathologic examination of CSF and other body cavity fluid specimens.

Leukemic involvement of the meninges is more frequent in patients with acute lymphoblastic leukemia (Fig. 29-6) than in those with acute myeloid leukemia (Fig. 29-7); both are significantly more common than CNS involvement in the chronic leukemias. A leukocyte count over 5 cells/μL with unequivocal lymphoblasts in cytocentrifuged preparations is commonly accepted as evidence of CSF involvement. The incidence of CNS relapse in children with lymphoblasts but cell counts lower than 6 cells/μL appears to be low and is not significantly different from cases in which no blasts are identified (Odom, 1990; Gilchrist, 1994; Tubergen, 1994).

Non-Hodgkin lymphomas involving the leptomeninges are usually high-grade tumors (lymphoblastic, large cell immunoblastic, and Burkitt's lymphomas) (Fig. 29-8); low-grade lymphomas and Hodgkin lymphoma are significantly less common (Bigner, 1992; Walts, 1992). T cells predominate in normal and inflammatory conditions, whereas most lymphomas, especially those occurring in immunocompromised hosts, are of B cell lineage. Lymphoblastic lymphoma, the most common T cell lymphoma, can be detected by terminal deoxynucleotidyl transferase stain.

Multiparameter flow cytometric immunophenotypic studies and/or molecular DNA analysis may significantly improve diagnostic sensitivity and specificity in CSF samples involved by leukemic or lymphoma cells (Rhodes, 1996; Finn, 1998; Scrideli, 2004; Bromberg, 2007; Quijano, 2009), and these are used increasingly as part of a complete evaluation in patients being worked up for these conditions.

Amebae, fungi (especially *Cryptococcus neoformans*), and *Toxoplasma gondii* organisms may be present on cytocentrifuge specimens but may be difficult to recognize without confirmatory stains.

CHEMICAL ANALYSIS

Reference values for lumbar cerebrospinal fluid in adults are listed in Table 29-9.

Proteins

Total Protein

More than 80% of the CSF protein content is derived from blood plasma, in concentrations of less than 1% of the plasma level (Table 29-10).

TABLE 29-10
Mean Concentrations of Plasma and CSF Proteins

Protein	CSF, mg/L	Plasma/CSF ratio
Prealbumin	17.3	14
Albumin	155.0	236
Transferrin	14.4	142
Ceruloplasmin	1.0	366
Immunoglobulin (Ig)G	12.3	802
IgA	1.3	1346
α_2-Microglobulin	2.0	1111
Fibrinogen	0.6	4940
IgM	0.6	1167
β-Lipoprotein	0.6	6213

Adapted from Felgenhauer K. Klin Wochenschr 1974;52:1158, with permission.
CSF, Cerebrospinal fluid.

Prealbumin (transthyretin), transferrin, and small quantities of nerve tissue–specific proteins are the major qualitative differences that normally exist between CSF and plasma proteins. Although some authors have argued against routine measurement of total protein (American College of Physicians, 1986), it is the most common abnormality found in CSF. Thus, an increased CSF protein serves as a useful, albeit nonspecific, indicator of meningeal or CNS disease.

Reference Values. CSF total protein reference values vary considerably between laboratories owing to differences in methods, instrumentation, and type of reference standard used (College of American Pathologists CSF Chemistry Survey, Set M-B, 1991*; Gerbaut, 1986). CSF protein levels of 15–45 mg/dL have long been accepted as the "normal" reference range (Silverman, 1994). Using the classic Lowry method, the reported adult range was 24.1–48.5 mg/dL (Tibbling, 1977). Others reported a reference range of 14–49 mg/dL using a trichloroacetic acid–Ponceau S method (Breebaart, 1978), and of 22.3–50.3 mg/dL with a biuret method (Ahonen, 1978). Reference levels were also compared using three different methods: (1) A modified biuret technique; (2) a Dupont aca method in which protein was precipitated and then reacted with trichloroacetic acid; and (3) a Kodak Ektachem colorimetric slide technique (Lott, 1989). All three methods gave similar, although significantly higher, levels than those previously reported (i.e., 14–62 mg/dL, 16–61 mg/dL, and 12–60 mg/dL, respectively).

Although discrepancies in gender and in those over the age of 60 years have been reported, the differences are probably not significant. However, infants have significantly higher CSF protein levels than older children and adults. Thus, mean levels of 90 mg/dL for term infants and 115 mg/dL for preterm infants were reported; the upper levels were 150 mg/dL and 170 mg/dL, respectively (Sarff, 1976). Similarly, others recently noted that the CSF protein concentration fell rapidly from birth to 6 months of age (mean levels, 108 mg/dL–40 mg/dL), plateaued between 3 and 10 years (mean, 32 mg/dL), and then rose slightly from 10–16 years (mean, 41 mg/dL) (Biou, 2000).

Elevated CSF protein levels may be caused by increased permeability of the blood-brain barrier, decreased resorption at the arachnoid villi, mechanical obstruction of CSF flow due to spinal block above the puncture site, or an increase in intrathecal immunoglobulin (Ig) synthesis. Common conditions associated with elevated lumbar CSF protein values (>65 mg/dL) are summarized in Table 29-11.

Low lumbar CSF total protein levels (<20 mg/dL) normally occur in some young children between 6 months and 2 years of age and in patients with conditions associated with increased CSF turnover. These include the following: (1) Removal of large CSF volumes; (2) CSF leaks induced by trauma or lumbar puncture; (3) increased intracranial pressure, probably due to an increased rate of protein resorption by the arachnoid villi; and (4) hyperthyroidism (Fishman, 1992).

Protein electrophoresis of concentrated normal CSF reveals two distinct differences from serum: A prominent transthyretin (prealbumin) band and two transferrin bands. Transthyretin is relatively high because of its dual synthesis by the liver and the choroid plexus. The second transferrin band, referred to as β_2-transferrin, migrates more slowly than its serum equivalent owing to cerebral neuraminidase digestion of sialic acid residues.

*College of American Pathologists, 325 Waukegan Road, Northfield, Ill.

TABLE 29-11
Conditions Associated With Increased CSF Total Protein

Traumatic spinal puncture
Increased blood–CSF permeability
Arachnoiditis (e.g., following methotrexate therapy)
Meningitis (bacterial, viral, fungal, tuberculous)
Hemorrhage (subarachnoid, intracerebral)
Endocrine/metabolic disorders
Milk–alkali syndrome with hypercalcemia
Diabetic neuropathy
Hereditary neuropathies and myelopathies
Decreased endocrine function (thyroid, parathyroid)
Other disorders (uremia, dehydration)
Drug toxicity
Ethanol, phenothiazines, phenytoin
CSF circulation defects
Mechanical obstruction (tumor, abscess, herniated disk)
Loculated CSF effusion
Increased immunoglobulin (Ig)G synthesis
Multiple sclerosis
Neurosyphilis
Subacute sclerosing panencephalitis
Increased IgG synthesis and blood–CSF permeability
Guillain-Barré syndrome
Collagen vascular diseases (e.g., lupus, periarteritis)
Chronic inflammatory demyelinating polyradiculopathy

CSF, Cerebrospinal fluid.

Methods. Turbidimetric methods, commonly based on trichloroacetic acid (TCA) or sulfosalicylic acid and sodium sulfate for protein precipitation, are popular because they are simple and rapid, and require no special instrumentation. However, they are temperature sensitive and require much larger specimen volumes (about 0.5 mL). Moreover, some methods are prone to significant variation from changes in the albumin/globulin ratio (Schriever, 1965). A false protein elevation may be observed using TCA methods in the presence of methotrexate (Kasper, 1988). Benzethonium chloride and benzalkonium chloride have been used as precipitating agents in automated methods and micromethods (Luxton, 1989; Shephard, 1992).

Colorimetric methods include the Lowry method, dye-binding, methods using Coomassie brilliant blue (CBB) or Ponceau S, and the modified Biuret method. The CBB method is rapid and highly sensitive, and can be used with small sample sizes. Immunologic methods measure specific proteins, require only 25–50 μL of CSF, and are relatively simple to perform once conditions and reagents have been standardized. Automated methods are also commonly used and usually show good correlation with standard methods (Lott, 1989).

Albumin and IgG Measurements

The permeability of the blood-brain barrier may be assessed by immunochemical quantification of the CSF albumin/serum albumin ratio in grams per deciliter (g/dL). The normal ratio of 1 : 230 (Tourtellotte, 1985) yields an unwieldy decimal of 0.004, which prompted the use of the **CSF/serum albumin index,** which is arbitrarily calculated as follows:

$$\text{CSF/Serum albumin index} = \frac{\text{CSF albumin (mg/dL)}}{\text{Serum albumin (g/dL)}} \quad \textbf{(29-1)}$$

An index value less than 9 is consistent with an intact barrier. Slight impairment is considered with index values of 9–14, moderate impairment with values of 14–30, and severe impairment with values greater than 30 (Silverman, 1994). The index is slightly elevated in infants up to 6 months of age, reflecting the immaturity of the blood-brain barrier, and increases gradually after age 40 years. A traumatic tap invalidates the index calculation.

Increased intrathecal IgG synthesis is reflected by an increase in the CSF/serum IgG ratio:

$$\text{CSF/Serum IgG ratio} = \frac{\text{CSF IgG (mg/dL)}}{\text{Serum IgG (g/dL)}} \quad \textbf{(29-2)}$$

The normal ratio is 1/390 or 0.003 (Tourtellotte, 1985). Similar to the albumin index, the CSF/serum IgG index may be obtained by using milligrams per deciliter for the CSF IgG value. The CSF/serum IgG index normal range is 3.0–8.7.

The **CSF/serum IgG index** can be elevated by intrathecal IgG synthesis or increased plasma IgG crossover from breakdown of the blood-brain barrier. Ig derived from plasma crossover may be corrected by dividing the CSF/serum IgG index by the CSF/albumin index to yield the CSF IgG index.

$$\text{CSF IgG index} = \frac{\text{CSF IgG (mg/dL)/Serum IgG (g/dL)}}{\text{CSF albumin (mg/dL)/Serum albumin (g/dL)}} \quad \textbf{(29-3)}$$

or

$$\text{CSF IgG index} = \frac{\text{CSF IgG (mg/dL)} \times \text{Serum albumin (g/dL)}}{\text{Serum IgG (g/dL)} \times \text{CSF albumin (mg/dL)}} \quad \textbf{(29-4)}$$

The normal reference range for the IgG index varies, reflecting variations in determination of the four index components. A reasonable normal upper limit is 0.8 (Souverijn, 1989). However, each laboratory should determine its own critical ratio.

The **IgG synthesis rate** is calculated by an empirical formula (Tourtellotte, 1985):

$$\begin{aligned}\text{IgG synthesis rate (mg/day)} = [&(\text{CSF IgG} - \text{Serum IgG/369}) - \\ &(\text{CSF albumin} - \text{Serum albumin/230}) \times \\ &(\text{Serum IgG/Serum albumin}) \times 0.43 \times 5\ \text{dL/day}]\end{aligned} \quad \textbf{(29-5)}$$

All protein concentrations are expressed in milligrams per deciliter. The first bracketed term represents the difference between measured CSF IgG and the IgG expected from diffusion across a normal blood-brain barrier; 369 is the normal serum/CSF ratio. The second bracketed term represents the difference between measured CSF albumin and expected albumin if the blood-brain barrier is intact; 230 is the normal serum/CSF albumin ratio. The CSF albumin excess is multiplied by the IgG/albumin ratio and the molecular weight ratio of IgG to albumin (0.43) to correct for changes in CSF IgG due to increased barrier permeability. The number 5 converts the result from a concentration to a daily amount, assuming an average daily CSF production of 500 mL (i.e., 5 dL). The formula does not consider variations in CSF production or Ig consumption. It assumes that the IgG/albumin ratio remains constant over various degrees of blood-brain barrier impairment—a concept that may lead to variable error (Lefvert, 1985). The normal reference interval for the synthesis rate is –9.9 to +3.3 mg/day. Values greater than 8.0 mg/day indicate an increased rate (Silverman, 1994).

CSF IgG is normally 3%–5% of total CSF protein, but in multiple sclerosis (MS), the concentration approaches that of plasma (15%–18%) (Hersey, 1980). The CSF IgG index and the IgG synthesis rate have a sensitivity of 90% in patients with definite MS, but the sensitivity is lower in patients with possible MS, in whom accuracy is most needed (Marton, 1986). In addition, the specificity for MS is only moderate because increased intrathecal IgG synthesis occurs in many other inflammatory neurologic diseases.

The Ig index and synthesis rate calculations may also be applied to IgM, IgA, Ig light chains, and specific antibodies to infectious microorganisms. For example, increased synthesis of IgM and free κ light chains have been suggested as markers for MS (Rudick, 1989; Lolli, 1991).

Electrophoretic Techniques. Although the diagnosis of MS is ultimately a clinical one, significant advances have been made in laboratory testing for this disorder. CSF total protein is increased in less than 50% of patients with MS. Indeed, if the CSF protein exceeds 100 mg/dL, the patient probably does not have MS. However, the γ-globulin fraction, as determined by CSF electrophoresis, is often increased in MS. Thus, the CSF total protein/γ-globulin ratio exceeds 0.12 in about 65% of cases (Johnson, 1977). Using **electroimmunodiffusion,** a CSF IgG/albumin ratio greater than 0.25 is present in about 75% of cases (Tourtellotte, 1971). Furthermore, levels greater than the mean CSF IgG index + 3SD are present in 80%–85% of MS cases. However, this upper reference level varies significantly between laboratories, and 0.58, 0.66, and 0.77 have been reported as cutoff values (Olsson, 1976; Tibbling, 1977; Markowitz, 1983, respectively). Therefore, laboratories should establish their own reference values.

High-resolution agarose gel electrophoresis of concentrated CSF from patients with MS often shows discrete populations of IgG, the **oligoclonal bands.** Although these discrete IgG populations are normally absent, two or more bands are necessary to support the diagnosis of MS; a single band is not considered a positive result. Using this technique, oligoclonal bands have been reported in 83%–94% of patients with definite MS, 40%–60% of those with probable MS, and 20%–30% of possible MS cases. However, they are also frequently present in patients with subacute sclerosing panencephalitis, various viral CNS infections, neurosyphilis, neuroborreliosis, cryptococcal meningitis, Guillain-Barré syndrome, transverse myelitis, meningeal carcinomatosis, glioblastoma multiforme, Burkitt's lymphoma, chronic relapsing polyneuropathy, Behçet's disease, cysticercosis, and trypanosomiasis, among others (Trotter, 1989; Chalmers, 1990; Fishman 1992; Hall, 1992). Subsequent studies indicate that agarose gel electrophoresis sensitivity for MS is less than previously reported (see later).

Oligoclonal light chains (both κ and λ) are present in about 90% of MS patients (Gallo, 1989; Sindie, 1991). They have also occasionally been identified in the CSF of those who are negative for IgG oligoclonal bands. However, because of their uncommon occurrence in the absence of IgG and cost-ineffectiveness, as well as the ready availability of magnetic resonance imaging, it is unlikely that this technique will become common.

Coomassie brilliant blue or paragon violet stains can resolve oligoclonal bands in only 5 µg of IgG (Silverman, 1994). However, **silver staining** is 20–50 times more sensitive than CBB and can be used on unconcentrated CSF. It is important to note that these electrophoretic techniques must be simultaneously carried out on the patient's serum to be certain that a polyclonal gammopathy is not present (e.g., liver disease, systemic lupus, rheumatoid arthritis, chronic granulomatous disease) because these disorders may be accompanied by Ig diffusion into the CSF, yielding false-positive results.

Immunofixation electrophoresis (IFE) is more sensitive than agarose gel electrophoresis and does not require CSF concentration (Cawley, 1976). A subsequent study reported a sensitivity of 74% using this technique compared with 57% for agarose gel electrophoresis (Cavuoti, 1998). More recently, using a semiautomated immunofixation-peroxidase technique, the sensitivity was 83% and the specificity was 79% in patients with clinically definite MS (Richard, 2002). However, IFE provides fewer bands than **isoelectric focusing and IgG immunoblotting** (IgG-IEF). Moreover, the bands obtained by IFE tend to be more diffuse.

IgG-IEF performed on paired CSF and serum samples is the most sensitive method for the detection of oligoclonal bands (Andersson, 1994). One study showed that IgG-IEF detected 100% of definite MS, but only about 50% were positive by agarose electrophoresis (Lunding, 2000). Others detected 91% of MS cases but only 68% with agarose (Seres, 1998). Similarly, a semiautomated IgG-IEF technique identified 90% of MS cases compared with 60% for agarose electrophoresis (Fortini, 2003). In 2005, an international consensus standard for the diagnosis of MS established IgG-IEF as the method of choice for qualitative detection of oligoclonal IgG bands as evidence of intrathecal synthesis of IgG (Freedman, 2005). This method is more sensitive and specific than quantitative methods.

In summary, the diagnosis of MS, as with many other neurologic disorders, is ultimately a clinical one based on neurologic history and physical examination. Nevertheless, advanced laboratory results in CSF, such as elevated IgG indices and particularly the detection of oligoclonal IgG bands, as well as neuroimaging techniques, have proved invaluable in the diagnosis of MS.

Other CSF Proteins

Approximately 300 different proteins have been identified in CSF using two-dimensional electrophoresis, the first dimension being isoelectric focusing and the second polyacrylamide gel in the presence of sodium dodecyl sulfate (Harrington, 1986). Using this technique, four abnormal proteins were identified in patients with Creutzfeldt-Jakob disease (CJD). Two of these proteins (molecular mass about 40 kilodaltons [kDa] each) were present in some, but not all, patients with herpes simplex encephalitis, Parkinson's disease, Guillain-Barré syndrome, and schizophrenia. They were not present in various other neurologic disorders, nor in 100 normal CSF control specimens. However, these and two other proteins (molecular masses about 26 and 29 kDa) were present in all cases of CJD and in 5 of 10 cases of herpes simplex encephalitis. Neither of these latter proteins was present in any other neurologic disease or in controls.

Increased concentrations of various specific CSF proteins have been associated with several CNS diseases (Table 29-12).

TABLE 29-12
CSF Proteins and Central Nervous System Diseases

Protein	Major diseases/disorders
α_2-Macroglobulin	Subdural hemorrhage, bacterial meningitis
β-Amyloid and τ proteins	Alzheimer's disease
β_2-Microglobulin	Leukemia/lymphoma, Behçet's syndrome
C-reactive protein	Bacterial and viral meningitis
Fibronectin	Lymphoblastic leukemia, AIDS, meningitis
Methemoglobin	Mild subarachnoid/subdural hemorrhage
Myelin basic protein	Multiple sclerosis, tumors, others
Protein 14-3-3	Creutzfeldt-Jakob disease
Transferrin	CSF leakage (otorrhea, rhinorrhea)

AIDS, Acquired immunodeficiency syndrome; *CSF*, cerebrospinal fluid.

Myelin Basic Protein. Myelin basic protein (MBP), a component of the myelin nerve sheath, is released during demyelination as a result of various neurologic disorders, especially MS. Thus, MBP has been shown to positively correlate with CSF leukocyte count, intrathecal IgG synthesis, and the CSF/serum albumin concentration quotient (Sellebjerg, 1998). These results support the use of MBP in CSF as a surrogate disease marker during acute MS exacerbations. Others have found that analysis of antibody against MBP in patients with a clinically isolated syndrome is a rapid and precise method for predicting early conversion to clinically definite MS (Berger, 2003). However, increased CSF levels have also been reported in Guillain-Barré syndrome, lupus erythematosus, subacute sclerosing panencephalitis, and various brain tumors, and following CNS irradiation and chemotherapy (Brooks, 1989; Mahoney, 1984). Measurement of CSF levels has also been proposed as a prognostic marker in patients with serious head injury (Noseworthy, 1985).

α_2-Macroglobulin. Except for a small amount transported across the BBB in pinocytic vesicles, α_2-macroglobulin (A2M) is normally excluded from the CSF because of its large size. The number of these vesicles is increased in certain polyneuropathies, resulting in an increased CSF A2M level. Significant elevation reflects subdural hemorrhage or breakdown of the BBB, as occurs in bacterial meningitis. A2M measurement alone, or in relationship to albumin and IgG, may assist in the evaluation of neurologic disorders and increased CSF protein, and in the rapid differentiation between bacterial and aseptic meningitis (Meucci, 1993; Kanoh, 1997).

β_2-Microglobulin. This protein is part of the human leukocyte antigen class I molecule on the surfaces of all nucleated cells. CSF levels above 1.8 mg/L are associated with leptomeningeal leukemia and lymphoma but are not highly specific (Weller, 1992), in that they have a maximal positive predictive value of 78% in cases with a positive cytology (Jeffrey, 1990). β_2-microglobulin (B2M) was also recently shown to be a marker for neuro-Behçet's syndrome (Kawai, 2000). Moreover, viral infections, including human immunodeficiency virus (HIV)-1, other inflammatory conditions, and various malignancies have also been associated with elevated levels. However, the measurement of B2M remains primarily investigational.

C-Reactive Protein. Early studies indicated that CSF C-reactive protein (CRP) is useful in differentiating viral (aseptic) meningitis from bacterial meningitis (Corral, 1981; Abramson, 1985; Stearman, 1994). Others have reported that CSF CRP is a more useful screening test for viral versus bacterial meningitis, especially in children (Sormunen, 1999). A meta-analysis of CRP studies since 1980 suggested that a normal CSF or serum CRP has a high probability of ruling out bacterial meningitis (i.e., negative predictive value about 97%) (Gerdes, 1998). Moreover, a recent study found not only that CSF CRP levels were increased in bacterial meningitis, but that these levels were significantly higher in patients with gram-negative bacterial meningitis than in those with gram-positive bacterial meningitis (Rajs, 2002).

Fibronectin. This large glycoprotein (molecular mass about 420 kDa) is normally present in essentially all tissues and body fluids. Its primary function is its role in cell adhesion and phagocytosis (Ruoslahti, 1981). Thus, cell adhesion allows leukocytes to adhere to and pass through the vascular endothelia and migrate to the inflammatory site.

In children with acute lymphoblastic leukemia, elevated CSF fibronectin levels are associated with a poor prognosis, presumably due to leukemic involvement of the CNS (Rautonen, 1989). Significant CSF elevations have also been reported in Burkitt's lymphoma (Rajantie, 1989), some metastatic solid tumors, astrocytomas, and bacterial meningitis (Weller, 1990; Torre, 1991). Decreased levels have been reported in viral meningitis and in the acquired immunodeficiency syndrome (AIDS)–dementia complex (Torre, 1991, 1993).

β-Amyloid Protein 42 and τ Protein. The diagnosis of Alzheimer's disease (AD) is based on the presence of dementia and a specific clinical profile (i.e., from medical history, clinical examination) suggestive of AD, together with the exclusion of other causes of dementia. Pathologically, the disease is characterized by the presence of neurofibrillary tangles and amyloid plaques.

Recent studies indicate that measurement of biochemical markers increases diagnostic accuracy, especially early in the course of the disease, when clinical symptoms are mild and vague and overlap with cognitive changes that accompany aging and ischemic dementia. Thus, increased CSF levels of microtubule-associated τ protein and decreased levels of β-amyloid protein ending at amino acid 42 have been shown to significantly increase the accuracy of AD diagnosis (Andreasen, 2001; Riemenschneider, 2002; Sunderland, 2003). Indeed, the predictive value for early AD is greater than 90% (Andreasen, 2001). Others have found that the calculated ratio of phosphorylated τ protein to β-amyloid peptide is superior to either measure alone (Maddalena, 2003). The results were as follows: Distinguishing patients with AD from healthy controls—sensitivity 96%, specificity 97%; patients with AD from those with non-AD dementia—sensitivity 80%, specificity 73%; and patients with AD from those with other neurologic disorders—sensitivity 80%, specificity 89%.

Protein 14-3-3. The transmissible spongiform encephalopathies constitute a group of uniformly fatal neurodegenerative diseases. Of these, CJD is the major spongiform disease in humans. Two proteins, designated 130 and 131, have been detected in low concentrations in CSF from CJD patients. These proteins have the same amino acid sequence as protein 14-3-3 (Hsich, 1996). Moreover, in patients with dementia, a positive immunoassay for the 14-3-3 protein in CSF strongly supports a diagnosis of CJD. In a subsequent study of patients with suspected CJD, the sensitivity of the 14-3-3 protein determined by immunoassay was 97%, and the specificity was 87% (Lemstra, 2000). False-positive results were seen primarily in patients with stroke and meningoencephalitis.

Others, using a modified Western blot technique, reported a 94.7% positive predictive value and a 92.4% negative predictive value for CJD (Zerr, 1998). False-positive results from a single CSF analysis were seen in patients with herpes simplex encephalitis, atypical encephalitis, metastatic lung cancer, and hypoxic brain damage.

Transferrin and CSF Leakage. Cerebrospinal fluid leakage usually presents as otorrhea or rhinorrhea following head trauma, in some cases beginning months to years after the injury. Recurrent meningitis is a serious complication, making accurate identification of the leaking fluid very important. In this regard, protein and glucose measurements are too nonspecific to be of value. Transferrin, an iron-binding glycoprotein with a molecular mass of about 77 kDa, is synthesized primarily in the liver. However, two transferrin isoforms are present in the CSF; the major isoform (β_1-transferrin) is present in all body fluids. The second isoform (β_2-transferrin), present only in the central nervous system, is produced in the central nervous system by the catalytic conversion of β-1-transferrin by neuraminidase. Immunofixation electrophoresis readily identifies both isoforms.

Protein electrophoresis with transferrin immunofixation is a noninvasive, rapid, and inexpensive test of high sensitivity and specificity that requires as little as 0.1 mL of fluid (Ryall, 1992; Normansell, 1994). Several reports have demonstrated the value of this technique in the diagnosis of CSF otorrhea and rhinorrhea—conditions in which both isoforms are readily identified (Irjala, 1979; Rouah, 1987; Zaret, 1992). Others have stressed the importance of β_2-transferrin identification in both CSF and inner ear perilymphatic leakage, as well as possible sources of error due to the presence of a transferrin allelic variant (Skedros, 1993a,b; Sloman, 1993).

Methemoglobin and Bilirubin. Although most cases of subarachnoid and intracerebral hemorrhage are readily identified by computed tomography (CT), patients with mild subarachnoid hemorrhage, small subdural or cerebral hematomas, and blood seepage from an aneurysm or neoplasm and from small cerebral infarcts often are not identified by this technique. In these cases, CSF spectrophotometric analysis has been shown to detect methemoglobin in colorless CSF (<0.3 μmol/L) (Trbojevic-Cepe, 1992). However, an increase in CSF bilirubin is now recognized as the key finding supporting the diagnosis of subarachnoid hemorrhage (UK National External Quality Assessment Scheme for Immunochemistry Working Group, 2003). Thus, a single net bilirubin absorbance cutoff point of >0.007 absorbance units is recommended in the decision tree for interpretation and reporting of results.

Glucose

Derived from blood glucose, fasting CSF glucose levels are normally 50–80 mg/dL (2.8–4.4 mmol/L)—about 60% of plasma values. Results should be compared with plasma levels, ideally following a 4-hour fast, for adequate clinical interpretation. The normal CSF/plasma glucose ratio varies from 0.3–0.9, with fluctuations in blood levels caused by the lag in CSF glucose equilibration time.

CSF values below 40 mg/dL (2.2 mmol/L) or ratios below 0.3 are considered to be abnormal. Hypoglycorrhachia is a characteristic finding of bacterial, tuberculous, and fungal meningitis. However, sensitivity can be as low as 55% for bacterial meningitis (Hayward, 1987), so a normal level does not exclude these conditions. Some cases of viral meningoencephalitis also have low glucose levels, but generally not to the degree seen in bacterial meningitis. Meningeal involvement by a malignant tumor, sarcoidosis, cysticercosis, trichinosis, ameba *(Naegleria)*, acute syphilitic meningitis, intrathecal administration of radioiodinated serum albumin, subarachnoid hemorrhage, symptomatic hypoglycemia, and rheumatoid meningitis may also produce low CSF glucose levels (Fishman, 1992).

Decreased CSF glucose results from increased anaerobic glycolysis in brain tissue and leukocytes and from impaired transport into the CSF. Bacteria are usually present in insufficient quantities to be a major contributor. CSF glucose levels normalize before protein levels and cell counts during recovery from meningitis, making it a useful parameter in assessing response to treatment.

Increased CSF glucose is of no clinical significance, reflecting increased blood glucose levels within 2 hours of lumbar puncture. A traumatic tap may also cause a spurious increase in CSF glucose.

Lactate

CSF and blood lactate levels are largely independent of each other. The reference interval for older children and adults is 9.0–26 mg/dL (1.0–2.9 mmol/L) (Knight, 1981). Newborns have higher levels, ranging from about 10–60 mg/dL (1.1–6.7 mmol/L) for the first 2 days, and from 10–40 mg/dL (1.1–4.4 mmol/L) for days 3 to 10 (McGuinness, 1983). Elevated CSF lactate levels reflect CNS anaerobic metabolism due to tissue hypoxia.

Lactate measurement has been used as an adjunctive test in differentiating viral meningitis from bacterial, mycoplasma, fungal, and tuberculous meningitis, in which routine parameters yield equivocal results. In patients with viral meningitis, lactate levels are usually below 25 mg/dL (2.8 mmol/L) and are almost always less than 35 mg/dL (3.9 mmol/L), whereas bacterial meningitis typically has levels above 35 mg/dL (Bailey, 1990; Cameron, 1993). Using 30–36 mg/dL as the cutoff value for bacterial meningitis, the sensitivity and specificity are about 80% and 90%, respectively. Viral meningitis, partially treated bacterial meningitis, and tuberculous meningitis often have intermediate lactate levels that overlap each other, limiting the use of lactate measurements in this differential diagnosis.

Persistently elevated ventricular CSF lactate levels are associated with a poor prognosis in patients with severe head injury (DeSalles, 1986).

F2-Isoprostanes

F2-isoprostanes are increased in diseased regions of the brain in patients with AD (Pratico, 1998). Compared with age-matched controls, CSF F2-isoprostanes are also elevated in patients with probable AD (Montine, 1999). Therefore, in conjunction with CSF τ and β-amyloid protein, the measurement of CSF F2-isoprostanes appears to enhance the accuracy of the laboratory diagnosis of AD (Montine, 2001).

Enzymes

A wide variety of enzymes derived from brain tissue, blood, or cellular elements have been described in the CSF. Although CSF enzyme assays are not commonly used in the diagnosis of CNS diseases, there are diseases/disorders in which they may prove useful.

Adenosine Deaminase

Adenosine deaminase (ADA) catalyzes the irreversible hydrolytic deamination of adenosine to produce inosine. Because ADA is particularly abundant in T lymphocytes, which are increased in tuberculosis, its measurement has been recommended in the diagnosis of pleural, peritoneal, and meningeal tuberculosis. Higher ADA levels are present in tuberculous infections than in viral, bacterial, and malignant diseases (Blake, 1982; Mann, 1982, Choi, 2002), although the degree of increase indicative of tuberculous infection varies depending on the specific assay used. ADA appears to have limited utility in HIV-associated neurologic disorders (Corral, 2004).

Creatine Kinase

Brain tissue is rich in creatine kinase (CK) because it participates in maintaining an adequate supply of adenosine triphosphate. Increased CSF CK activity has been reported in numerous CNS disorders, including hydrocephalus, cerebral infarction, various primary brain tumors, and subarachnoid hemorrhage, among others (Savory, 1979). In patients with head trauma, CSF CK levels correlate directly with the severity of the concussion (Florez, 1976).

CSF CK-MM and CK-MB are not normally present; when identified, they are due to blood contamination (CK-MM) and an equilibrium between CK-BB and CK-MM to produce CK-MB. Because the CK-BB isoenzyme accounts for about 90% of brain CK activity and mitochondrial CK (CKmt) the other 10%, CK isoenzyme measurements are more specific than total CK for CNS disorders (Chandler, 1984).

CSF CK-BB is increased about 6 hours following an ischemic or anoxic insult. Global brain ischemia following respiratory or cardiac arrest results in diffuse cerebral injury with peak CK-BB levels in about 48 hours (Chandler, 1986). Here, CSF CK-BB activity less than 5 U/L (upper normal level) indicates minimal neurologic damage; 5–20 U/L indicates mild to moderate CNS injury; and levels between 21 and 50 U/L are commonly correlated with death. Death occurs in essentially all patients with levels above 50 U/L.

Increased CSF CK-BB levels are also associated with the outcome following a subarachnoid hemorrhage (Coplin, 1999). Here, a CK-BB level greater than 40 U/L increased the chance of an unfavorable early or late outcome to 100%. The death rate was 13% when the CSF CK-BB level was less than 40 U/L.

Lactate Dehydrogenase

Lactate dehydrogenase (LD) activity is high in brain tissue, with a predominance of the electrophoretically fast-moving isoenzyme fractions LD_1 and LD_2. Total LD activity of 40 U/L is a reasonable upper limit of normal for adults and 70 U/L for neonates (Donald, 1986; Engelke, 1986). LD is useful in differentiating a traumatic tap from intracranial hemorrhage because a current traumatic tap with intact RBCs does not significantly elevate the LD level (Engelke, 1986). Sensitivity and specificity are about 70%–85% depending on the cutoff value. As with lactate, LD activity is significantly higher in bacterial meningitis than in aseptic meningitis (Donald, 1986; Engelke, 1986). Using a cutoff of 40 U/L, the sensitivity is about 86% and the specificity about 93%.

Total CSF LD levels are also increased in patients with CNS leukemia, lymphoma, metastatic carcinoma, bacterial meningitis, and subarachnoid hemorrhage (Kjeldsberg, 1993). CSF LD isoenzymes have been shown to add considerable specificity in the evaluation of various metastatic brain tumors (Fleisher, 1981). Thus, the LD_5/total LD ratio is increased (i.e., above 10%–15%) in patients with leptomeningeal metastases from carcinoma of the breast and lung and malignant melanoma. Isoenzyme analysis also shows a distinct pattern in young children with infantile spasms (Nussinovitch, 2003a) and febrile convulsions (Nussinovitch, 2003b). Compared with controls, both disorders are characterized by decreased LD_1, increased LD_2 and LD_3, and no changes in LD_4 and LD_5.

CT is of limited value in estimating recovery potential and neurologic outcome during the early stages of ischemic brain injury. However, compared with controls (mean LD, 11.2 U/L), patients with an early stroke had a mean level of 40.9 U/L, and those with a transient ischemic attack (TIA) had a mean value of 11.8 U/L (Lampl, 1990). Moreover, in patients with hypoxic brain injury, an increased LD level 72 hours following resuscitation indicates a poor prognosis (Karkela, 1992).

Lysozyme

Lysozyme (muramidase) catalyzes the depolymerization of mucopolysaccharides. Because the enzyme is particularly rich in neutrophil and macrophage lysosomes, its activity is very low in normal CSF. However, CSF lysozyme activity is significantly increased in patients with both bacterial and tuberculous meningitis. Thus, discriminant analysis demonstrated that 97% of patients with bacterial meningitis had increased lysozyme levels (Ribeiro, 1992). Others found that patients with tuberculous meningitis had significantly higher CSF lysozyme levels than those with bacterial meningitis, partially treated bacterial meningitis, and controls (Mishra, 2003). The diagnostic sensitivity and specificity for tuberculous meningitis were 93.7% and 84.1%, respectively. Increased levels are also present in cerebral atrophy, various CNS tumors, multiple sclerosis, intracranial hemorrhage, and epilepsy (Kjeldsberg, 1993).

Ammonia, Amines, and Amino Acids

CSF ammonia levels vary from 30%–50% of blood values. Elevated levels are generally proportional to the degree of existing hepatic encephalopathy but are difficult to quantify. Moreover, because hepatic encephalopathy generally correlates with blood ammonia levels, the measurement of CSF ammonia has little, if any, clinical value. However, cerebral glutamine, synthesized from ammonia and glutamic acid, serves as the means for CNS ammonia removal. Thus, CSF glutamine levels reflect the concentration of brain ammonia. Glutamine reference intervals are method dependent; the upper reference level is about 20 mg/dL. Values over 35 mg/dL are usually associated with hepatic encephalopathy (Fishman, 1992). Elevated CSF glutamine levels have also been reported in patients with encephalopathy secondary to hypercapnia and sepsis (Mizock, 1989).

A major etiologic theory of schizophrenia involves dopamine. The cornerstone for this theory is the fact that neuroleptic drugs that block dopamine receptors are effective in the treatment of this disorder. Thus, it has been reported that CSF levels of homovanillic acid (HVA), a metabolite of the biogenic amines, are related to the severity of schizophrenic psychosis (Maas, 1997). However, HVA concentration varied as a function of psychosis rather than being related to the diagnosis of schizophrenia per se. Others reported decreased CSF levels of 5-hydroxyindoleacetic acid, a metabolite of serotonin, in schizophrenic patients with suicidal behavior (Cooper, 1992). This report adds support for a possible relationship between suicide and CNS serotonin metabolism.

Although free CSF amino acids are relatively high in infants younger than 30 days of age, their concentration is further increased in those with febrile convulsions and bacterial meningitis. γ-Aminobutyric acid (GABA), a major inhibitory brain transmitter, is significantly decreased in basal ganglia neurons, and is very low or undetectable in the CSF of patients with Alzheimer's disease and Huntington's disease (Achar, 1976; Dubowitz, 1992). In addition, CSF GABA was detected in all patients with migraine attacks, but not in those with tension headaches or in the control group without headaches (Welch, 1975). Conversely, infants with startle disease, a rare inherited autosomal dominant disorder characterized by seizures or the so-called **stiff baby syndrome,** have significantly decreased CSF GABA levels (Dubowitz, 1992; Berthier, 1994).

Electrolytes and Acid-Base Balance

There are no clinically useful indications for the measurement of CSF sodium, potassium, chloride, calcium, or magnesium. Measurements of CSF pH, partial pressure of carbon dioxide (pCO_2), and bicarbonate are also not practical for patient care (Fishman, 1992).

Tumor Markers

Numerous studies have shown that various tumor markers are increased in the CSF of patients with both primary and metastatic tumors. However, the value of most of these tests in routine clinical practice has not been established.

Carcinoembryonic Antigen

Carcinoembryonic antigen (CEA) is an oncofetal protein produced by a variety of carcinomas. An early study found increased CEA levels in 44% of patients with metastatic brain tumors (Suzuki, 1980). Others reported that CSF levels of CEA have a sensitivity of only about 31%, although the specificity is about 90% for detecting metastatic carcinoma of the leptomeninges (Klee, 1986; Twijnstra, 1986). Recently, CSF levels of CEA in patients with benign, primary malignant, and metastatic brain tumors were 0.31 ng/mL, 0.92 ng/mL, and 6.3 ng/mL, respectively (Batabyal, 2003).

Other oncofetal proteins include **human chorionic gonadotropin** (hCG), produced by choriocarcinoma and malignant germ cell tumors with a trophoblastic component, and **α-fetoprotein,** a glycoprotein produced by yolk sac elements of germ cell tumors. Results of a recent study revealed that both β-hCG and α-fetoprotein may be useful in the diagnosis and monitoring of the response to therapy in patients with CNS germ cell tumors (Seregni, 2002).

Elevation of CSF **ferritin** is a sensitive indicator of CNS malignancy but has very low specificity because it is also increased in patients with inflammatory neurologic diseases (Zandman-Goddard, 1986).

MICROBIOLOGICAL EXAMINATION

A thorough and prompt examination of cerebrospinal fluid is essential for the diagnosis of CNS infection because an inaccurate or delayed report may result in significant mortality or morbidity. Although changes in opening pressure, total cell and differential counts, total protein, and glucose suggest an infectious origin (Table 29-13), Gram stain and culture are critical for a definitive diagnosis.

Bacterial Meningitis

The most common agents of bacterial meningitis are group B streptococcus (neonates), *Neisseria meningitidis* (3 months and older) (Fig. 29-9), *Streptococcus pneumoniae* (3 months and older), *Escherichia coli* and other gram-negative bacilli (newborn–1 month), *Haemophilus influenzae* (3 months–18 years), and *Listeria monocytogenes* (neonates, elderly, alcoholics, and immunosuppressed) (Graves, 1989; Wenger, 1990). *H. influenzae*, once

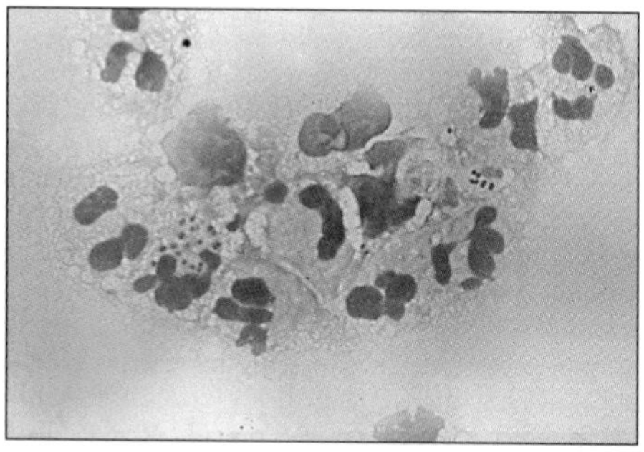

Figure 29-9 Cerebrospinal fluid Gram stain showing gram-negative diplococci characteristic of *N. meningitidis*.

TABLE 29-13
Typical Lumbar CSF Findings in Meningitis

Test	Bacterial	Viral	Fungal	Tuberculous
Opening pressure	Elevated	Usually normal	Variable	Variable
Leukocyte count	≥1000/μL	<100/μL	Variable	Variable
Cell differential	Mainly neutrophils*	Mainly lymphocytes†	Mainly lymphocytes	Mainly lymphocytes
Protein	Mild–marked increase	Normal–mild increase	Increased	Increased
Glucose	Usually ≤40 mg/dL	Normal	Decreased	Decreased: may be <45 mg/dL
CSF/serum glucose ratio	Normal–marked decrease	Usually normal	Low	Low
Lactic acid	Mild–marked increase	Normal–mild increase	Mild–moderate increase	Mild–moderate increase

Data from Body, 1987; Tang, 1988; Arevalo, 1989; Fishman, 1992; Wubbel, 1998; Zunt, 1999.
CSF, Cerebrospinal fluid.
*Lymphocytosis present in about 10% of cases.
†Neutrophils may predominate early in disease.

the most common bacterial cause of meningitis in young children, has decreased dramatically from widespread use of *H. influenzae* type b vaccine. Cerebrospinal fluid shunts, head trauma, and neurosurgery place patients at risk for CNS infections from *Staphylococcus* species, gram-negative bacilli, and *Propionibacterium* species.

The Gram stain remains an accurate, rapid method by which to diagnose CNS infection. All specimens should be concentrated by centrifugation before Gram stain and culture. Depending upon the type of infecting microorganism and its concentration in the cerebrospinal fluid, Gram stain sensitivity ranges from 60%–90%, with the greatest sensitivity corresponding to higher concentrations of bacteria (about 10^5 colony-forming units/mL). For example, the sensitivity of the Gram stain for detecting *Listeria monocytogenes* and gram-negative bacilli is 50% or less (Greenlee, 1990). For patients with many polymorphonuclear leukocytes but no organisms seen on Gram stain, the more sensitive acridine orange stain may be helpful. Cultures have a sensitivity of 80%–90%, but are about 30% less sensitive in partially treated cases (Greenlee, 1990).

Although standard culture-based methods remain the mainstay for diagnosis, the BinaxNOW *Streptococcus pneumoniae* antigen test, an immunochromatographic membrane assay that detects the presence of the C polysaccharide cell wall antigen common to all pneumococcal serotypes, has proved to be a valuable tool for the rapid diagnosis of pneumococcal meningitis from CSF. Latex agglutination bacterial antigen tests performed on CSF to detect *H. influenzae*, *N. meningitidis*, *S. pneumoniae*, and β-hemolytic group B streptococci historically were used as adjuncts to Gram stain and culture; however, the sensitivity is approximately the same as the Gram stain, and a negative test does not rule out the diagnosis of bacterial meningitis. Perhaps the best application of latex agglutination antigen tests is seen in partially treated, community-acquired meningitis that is negative for microorganisms by Gram stain (Perkins, 1995; Wilson, 1997).

The polymerase chain reaction (PCR) and sequencing of 16S ribosomal RNA in CSF have been shown to be very useful in the diagnosis of bacterial meningitis (Schuurman, 2004). Compared with bacterial culture, the assay shows a sensitivity of 86%, a specificity of 97%, a positive predictive value of 80%, and a negative predictive value of 98%. Nucleic acid amplification tests may also be helpful in patients already receiving antimicrobial therapy and in detecting more fastidious pathogens such as *N. meningitidis* (Porritt, 2000; Seward, 2000; Baethgen, 2003).

Spirochetal Meningitis

The incidence of neurosyphilis has increased in recent years, primarily in patients with HIV infection. In one report, 44% of patients with neurosyphilis had AIDS (Flood, 1998). Unfortunately, the remaining patients, who may have had HIV infection without AIDS, were not studied. The diagnosis of CNS infection in patients with syphilis relies primarily on CSF parameters and serologic testing, although molecular DNA testing may now represent a new approach. Abnormalities in CSF protein and cell counts are common in syphilitic meningitis, but are nonspecific. CSF serologic testing to diagnose neurosyphilis is difficult. The standard nontreponemal test performed on CSF is the Venereal Disease Research Laboratory (VDRL). If few erythrocytes are contaminating the CSF, the VDRL specificity is high, but its sensitivity is only 50%–60% (Davis, 1989). Treponemal tests, such as the treponemal antibody absorption (FTA-ABS), are both sensitive and specific for syphilis; however, their use in CSF for neurosyphilis is controversial. The CSF FTA-ABS is highly sensitive, but false-positive results may occur. Moreover, in the absence of CSF abnormalities or clinical suspicion, it should not be used as a screening test. Thus, the following generalizations have been proposed (Davis, 1989): (1) A nonreactive serum FTA-ABS test rules out neurosyphilis; (2) a reactive serum FTA-ABS test with a nonreactive CSF FTA-ABS test essentially rules out neurosyphilis; (3) a reactive CSF VDRL test makes a diagnosis of neurosyphilis likely; and (4) a reactive CSF FTA-ABS test may indicate active neurosyphilis, asymptomatic neurosyphilis, treated neurosyphilis, or a false-positive reaction. Recent studies have demonstrated the potential utility of a PCR-based assay as a sensitive and specific means of diagnosing neurosyphilis (Leslie, 2007).

Diagnosis of Lyme meningitis represents another challenge for the laboratory. The mainstay of diagnosis remains serologic analysis performed on a serum specimen, using an enzyme-linked immunosorbent assay (ELISA)-based screening assay followed by confirmation with Western blot. PCR-based analysis may be performed on CSF specimens; however, the sensitivity of this approach is low, particularly in patients with chronic neuroborreliosis (Steere, 2010).

Viral Meningitis

Enteroviruses (echoviruses, coxsackieviruses, polioviruses) and arboviruses are responsible for the majority of meningitis cases; a seasonal peak in spring to autumn has been noted for these agents. As an example, echoviruses 9 (E9) and 30 (E30) were found to be mainly responsible for an increase in cases of aseptic meningitis (Morbidity and Mortality Weekly Report, 2003). Most patients present with a CSF pleocytosis, and although neutrophils may be observed early in the infection, patients soon develop a predominance of lymphocytes.

Before molecular diagnostic testing, viral meningitis was a diagnosis of exclusion because the sensitivity of viral cultures can be low. Thus, in an early study, a specific etiologic diagnosis by viral cultures varied from 72% for enteroviruses to 5% for herpes simplex virus (HSV) (Marton, 1986).

Reverse transcriptase polymerase chain reaction (RT-PCR) is significantly more sensitive than cell culture (Dumler, 1999; Hausfater, 2004). Arguably, it has evolved as the "gold standard" for the diagnosis of viral meningitis secondary to enterovirus, herpes simplex virus, cytomegalovirus, varicella zoster, and JC virus. The use of RT-PCR may result in significant cost savings by shortening hospital stays and eliminating unnecessary diagnostic and therapeutic interventions (Ramers, 2000). For patients with arbovirus-associated meningitis, acute and convalescent serologic testing in serum remains the cornerstone for diagnosis, with CSF testing a possible adjunct. Presumptive diagnosis of West Nile viral meningitis may be made on a CSF specimen using an IgM antibody-capture ELISA assay. PCR testing for West Nile virus and other arboviruses may also be done on CSF specimens; however, these assays have low sensitivity because of the short-lived nature of the viremia in these diseases and are not recommended for routine use (Vaughn, 2010).

PCR amplification of HSV DNA has revolutionized the testing for HSV infection in CSF and has replaced brain biopsy as the primary method used in the early diagnosis of HSV meningoencephalitis (Tunkel, 2008). False negatives might occur in very early infections and with bloody taps, necessitating analysis of a second CSF specimen (Tyler, 2004).

Human Immunodeficiency Virus

A wide variety of CSF abnormalities may be found in HIV-positive patients with or without neurologic disease, including lymphocytic pleocytosis, elevated IgG indexes, and oligoclonal bands (Chalmers, 1990; Hall, 1992). Identifying opportunistic infection is the most important indication for examining the CSF. Serious fungal infections may exist in the presence of few or no CSF parameter abnormalities.

Fungal Meningitis

Cryptococcus neoformans is the most frequently isolated fungal pathogen from CSF. India ink or nigrosin stains for cryptococcus capsular halos have a sensitivity of about 25%, increasing to 53% with multiple lumbar punctures, and to greater than 90% in untreated HIV-infected patients (Marton, 1986). Detection of cryptococcal antigen from sera or CSF using latex agglutination has higher sensitivity, ranging from 60%–95%. False-negatives due to a prozone effect or low concentration of polysaccharide antigen may occur. Early disease, intraparenchymal infection, infection with nonencapsulated *C. neoformans* variants, and immune complexes (corrected with pronase treatment) may also produce false-negatives. Conversely, sera or CSF from patients with rheumatoid factor or *Trichosporon asahii* infection may be falsely positive. If clinical suspicion for dimorphic or filamentous fungi is high, large volumes of CSF (approximately 15–20 mL) are optimal for culture to improve the recovery of fungal organisms.

Tuberculous Meningitis

Abnormal CSF with elevated protein and lymphocytic predominance are the hallmark features of tuberculous meningitis. The sensitivity of CSF acid-fast stains for the diagnosis of tuberculous meningitis is highly variable, ranging from 10%–12% (Greenlee, 1990) to greater than 50% (Thwaites, 2004). Large volumes of CSF, often obtained from multiple lumbar punctures with the use of concentration techniques, are recommended to improve the sensitivity of both acid-fast stain and culture (Marton, 1986).

PCR nucleic acid amplification for detecting *Mycobacterium tuberculosis* DNA-specific sequences shows great promise in the rapid and accurate diagnosis of tuberculous meningitis (Lin, 1995; Desai, 2002). However, a negative PCR result does not exclude the diagnosis of tuberculous meningitis. Indeed, if high clinical suspicion remains, empirical therapy should be initiated.

DOT ELISA has been standardized to detect tuberculosis antigens and antibodies against *M. tuberculosis* in CSF. Using this technique, a positive reaction was present in 86% of cases with suspected tuberculous meningitis (Kashyap, 2003). Only 5% of patients with other disorders, mainly pyogenic meningitis, were positive.

Other tests have been shown to be useful in some cases of tuberculous meningitis. ADA levels are significantly higher in tuberculous meningitis than in other types of meningitis and CNS disorders (Pettersson, 1991; Choi, 2002), although the degree of increase indicative of tuberculous infection varies depending on the specific assay used.

Primary Amebic Meningoencephalitis

This rare disease is caused by the free-living ameba *Naegleria fowleri*, *Acanthamoeba* species, and *Balamuthia mandrillaris*. *Naegleria* and *Balamuthia* are more likely to cause an acute inflammatory response with a neutrophilic pleocytosis, a decreased glucose level, an elevated protein concentration, and the presence of erythrocytes. Gram stain is always negative. *Acanthamoeba* more often produces a granulomatous meningitis. Motile *Naegleria* trophozoites may be visualized by light or phase-contrast microscopy in direct wet mounts, allowing rapid diagnosis. Intact and degenerating organisms may be identified on Wright's- or Giemsa-stained cytospins but must be distinguished from macrophages (dos Santos, 1970; Benson, 1985). Acridine orange stain is useful in differentiating ameba (brick red) from leukocytes (bright green).

SYNOVIAL FLUID

Synovium refers to the tissue lining synovial tendon sheaths, bursae, and diarthrodial joints, except for the articular surface. It is composed of one to three cell layers that form a discontinuous surface overlying fatty, fibrous, or periosteal joint tissue.

Synovial fluid (synovia, SF) is an imperfect ultrafiltrate of blood plasma combined with hyaluronic acid produced by the synovial cells. Small ions and molecules (e.g., Na^+, K^+, glucose, urea) readily pass into the joint space and therefore are similar in concentration to plasma; large molecules are absent or present in trace amounts. Resorption of synovial molecules is by the lymphatics and is not size dependent. SF acts as a lubricant and adhesive and provides nutrients for the avascular articular cartilage.

Examination of the synovial fluid is essential to distinguish infectious from noninfectious arthritis. Results from gross and microscopic examination of synovial fluid have traditionally been divided into "reaction types," as depicted in Table 29-14. These groupings are largely descriptive, and considerable overlap between them is evident. Except for Gram stain, culture, and crystal examination, synovial fluid parameters can be nonspecific and must be integrated into the clinical context.

Noninflammatory effusions (Group I) typically have leukocyte counts less than 3000/µL, with a minority of neutrophils. Osteoarthritis, traumatic arthritis, neuropathic osteoarthropathy, pigmented villonodular synovitis, and early rheumatic fever usually present with little inflammatory response. Early rheumatoid arthritis, early bacterial infection, and viral arthritis may also present as noninflammatory effusions.

Inflammatory effusions (Group II) have leukocyte counts between 3000 and 75,000, with neutrophils accounting for more than 50% of the population. Rheumatoid arthritis, systemic lupus erythematosus (SLE), Reiter's syndrome, rheumatic fever, acute crystal-induced arthritis, arthritis associated with inflammatory bowel disease, psoriatic arthritis, and fat droplet synovitis are examples of this reaction group.

Purulent (infectious) effusions (Group III) typically have leukocyte counts greater than 50,000, of which 90% or more are neutrophils. Bacterial, fungal, and tuberculous joint infections constitute this group.

Hemorrhagic effusions (Group IV) may be seen in association with traumatic arthritis, pigmented villonodular synovitis, synovial hemangioma, neuropathic osteoarthropathy, joint prostheses, and hematologic disorders (hemophilia, thrombocytopenia, anticoagulant therapy, sickle cell disease or trait, myeloproliferative syndrome).

SPECIMEN COLLECTION

Joint fluid aspiration (arthrocentesis) should be confined to patients with an undiagnosed effusion or a significant clinical change related to a known effusion (Pal, 1999). It should be performed by an experienced operator using good sterile technique. Caution is necessary to avoid aspirating a sterile joint in someone with bacteremia or through a cutaneous or periarticular soft tissue infection into a sterile joint. Large joints such as the knee normally contain no more than 4.0 mL of synovial fluid, so small sample size is common unless an effusion is present.

Synovial fluid must be collected with sterile, disposable needles and plastic syringes to avoid contamination by birefringent particulates. The syringe may be heparinized with 25 U of sodium heparin/mL of SF in routine arthrocentesis. Oxalate, lithium heparin, and powdered ethylenediaminetetraacetic acid (EDTA) anticoagulants should be avoided because they form crystal artifacts that may be misleading during the microscopic examination. Before aspiration, turn or manipulate the joint to ensure mixing of its contents.

Ideally, the specimen should be separated into three parts: 3–10 mL into a sterile heparinized tube or syringe for microbiological studies; 2–5 mL in an anticoagulant tube (sodium heparin or liquid EDTA) for microscopic examination; and about 5 mL into a plain (no anticoagulant) tube for chemical analysis (normal synovial fluid does not clot because fibrinogen is absent). Heparin concentrations greater than 125 U/mL have an inhibitory effect on some pathogenic bacteria (Rosett, 1980). Specimens for culture, therefore, should be at least 1–2 mL in volume if they are submitted in green-top heparin tubes (Becton Dickinson, Rutherford, N.J.) containing 143 U/tube of heparin, or submitted in recapped syringes after removal of the needle and excess air.

Dry taps may still have fluid within the needle, which may be sufficient for the most critical tests. Such specimens should be submitted with the needle still on the syringe and its tip stuck into a sterile cork. Good communication with the laboratory is crucial to the appropriate processing of such specimens.

RECOMMENDED TESTS

Laboratory examination of synovial fluid is of major importance in the differential diagnosis of joint disease, especially in crystal-induced

TABLE 29-14
Synovial Fluid Findings by Disease Category

		CATEGORY			
Finding	**Normal**	**Group I noninflammatory**	**Group II inflammatory**	**Group III infectious**	**Group IV hemorrhagic**
Clarity	Transparent	Transparent	Transparent/opaque	Opaque	Opaque
Color	Clear to pale yellow	Xanthochromic	Xanthochromic to white/bloody	White	Red-brown or xanthochromic
WBCs/mL	0–150	<3000	3000–75,000	50,000–200,000	50–10,000
PMNs, %	<25	<30	>50	>90	<50
RBCs	No	No	No	Yes	Yes
Glucose (blood/SF difference, mg/dL)	0–10 (0–0.56 mmol/L)	0–10 (0–0.56 mmol/L)	0–40 (0–2.2 mmol/L)	20–100 (1.11–5.5 mmol/L)	0–20 (0–1.11 mmol/L)

Modified from Kjeldsberg CR, Knight JA. Body fluids: laboratory examination of amniotic, cerebrospinal, seminal, serous and synovial fluids. 3rd ed. Chicago: © American Society for Clinical Pathology; 1993, with permission.
PMNs, Polymorphonuclear cells, neutrophils; *RBCs,* red blood cells; *SF,* synovial fluid; *WBCs,* white blood cells.

TABLE 29-15
Recommended Synovial Fluid Tests

Routine tests
- Gross examination (color, clarity)
- Total and differential leukocyte counts
- Gram stain and bacterial culture (aerobic and anaerobic)
- Crystal examination with polarizing microscope and compensator

Useful tests in certain circumstances
- Fungal and acid-fast stains and cultures
- PCR for bacterial and mycobacterial DNA
- Serum–synovial fluid glucose differential
- Lactate and other organic acids
- Complement
- Enzymes
- Uric acid

Modified from Kjeldsberg CR, Knight JA. Body fluids: laboratory examination of amniotic, cerebrospinal, seminal, serous and synovial fluids. 3rd ed. Chicago: © American Society for Clinical Pathology; 1993, with permission.
DNA, Deoxyribonucleic acid; *PCR*, polymerase chain reaction.

and infectious arthritis. When either is suspected, arthrocentesis and a systematic examination of the synovial fluid are imperative, and when examination is carried out properly, it is usually diagnostic. In other joint diseases, a specific diagnosis may not be possible. Nevertheless, fluid examination is still important, if only to rule out infectious arthritis, which is a critical diagnosis to make in that a joint may be irreversibly damaged within a couple of days if not properly treated. This is especially true when *Staphylococcus aureus* is the infectious organism. Therefore, routine tests should be directed toward the diagnosis of these two disorders (Table 29-15). Although other tests are not of practical value for routine use, they may provide important diagnostic information under certain circumstances.

It is critical that these tests be performed well because they can provide highly specific diagnostic information. However, a major problem in the laboratory examination of synovial fluid is that, in contrast to CSF and amniotic fluid, in most laboratories no consensus exists as to what constitutes a "routine" analysis (Hasselbacher, 1987). Moreover, quality performance is not consistent, in part because of the fact that the average laboratory examines only one to two synovial fluids each month (Hasselbacher, 1987; Rabinovitch, 1994).

GROSS EXAMINATION

Total volume should be recorded at the bedside, especially if the sample is to be divided for submission to different laboratory sections.

Color should be evaluated in a clear glass tube against a white background. Normal SF is colorless but is often pale yellow because of diapedesis of a few RBCs associated with even mild trauma. Noninflammatory and inflammatory disorders are usually seen as straw- to yellow-colored (xanthochromia). Septic fluid may be yellow, brown, or green depending on the chromogens produced by the offending organism and the host response, including the presence of WBCs and RBCs.

A **traumatic tap** produces an uneven distribution of blood during arthrocentesis or streaking in the syringe. Although pale yellow xanthochromia is difficult to distinguish from normal, a red-brown color following centrifugation is good evidence of pathologic hemarthrosis.

Clarity relates to the number and type of particles within the synovia. Because normal SF is transparent, newsprint is easily read through the tube. Although translucent fluid obscures details, black and white areas can be distinguished, but opaque fluid completely obscures the background.

Leukocytes are most commonly responsible for changes in clarity. However, very large numbers of crystals may produce an opaque, milky opalescent fluid without leukocytes. A shimmering, oily-appearing specimen suggests an abundance of cholesterol crystals, which may grossly resemble pus.

Increased turbidity is less often due to concentrations of fibrin, free-floating **rice bodies** (fragments of degenerating proliferative synovial cells or microinfarcted synovium), metal and plastic particles from patients with joint prostheses, or cartilage fragments in osteoarthritis. A **ground pepper** appearance from pigmented cartilage fragments may be the result of a metabolic disorder (i.e., ochronosis).

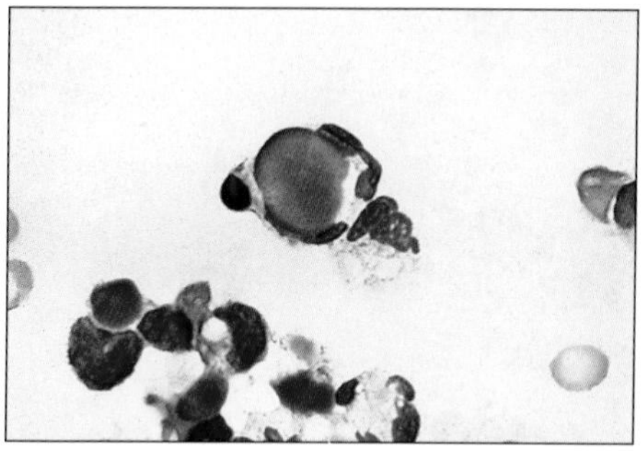

Figure 29-10 Lupus erythematosus cell in the synovial fluid from a patient with systemic lupus erythematosus.

MICROSCOPIC EXAMINATION

Total Cell Count

Total leukocyte counts should be performed promptly to avoid degenerative cell loss, which begins as soon as 1 hour following arthrocentesis. Tubes must be inverted before sampling to ensure uniform mixing. Cell counts are usually performed in a standard hemocytometer. Automated cell counters may be used, but their use risks clogging the machine aperture or obtaining spuriously high cell counts from non-WBC particles (e.g., crystals, fat globules), especially in multichannel machines. Pretreatment of highly viscous synovial fluid samples with hyaluronidase improves automated cell counting in these samples (Aulesa, 2003). A wet-prep slide count of 0–2 leukocytes per high-power field (hpf) (averaged over 10 fields) predicts fewer than 1300 WBCs by cell count (Clayburne, 1992). Leukocyte counts over 50,000/μL require dilution, which should be done with saline, not acetic acid, to avoid mucin clot formation and cell clumping.

Leukocyte counts greater than 10,000/μL, and often greater than 50,000/μL, are characteristic of crystal-induced arthritis (e.g., gout, pseudogout), chronic inflammatory arthritis (e.g., rheumatoid arthritis, systemic lupus erythematosus, ankylosing spondylitis), and septic arthritis (Kjeldsberg, 1993). Osteoarthritis, osteochondritis dissicans, trauma, and synovioma usually have total WBC counts less than 10,000/μL.

Erythrocytes should be routinely counted unless it is an obvious traumatic tap. If a large number of red cells interferes with the leukocyte count, they may be lysed by dilution with 0.3 normal saline or 1% saponin in saline.

The upper reference level for SF leukocytes is 150–200/μL (Kjeldsberg, 1993). Elevated cell counts are used to help divide findings into different disease categories but are nonspecific for any particular disease because of extensive overlap.

Differential Leukocyte Count

Cytospin preparations are preferred over smears from centrifuged SF because the cell morphology is significantly better preserved. Treatment with hyaluronidase may be necessary to produce thin smears in viscous specimens. Automated leukocyte differential counts utilizing flow cytometers may also be reliably peformed on synovial fluid samples (Aulesa, 2003); however, morphologic examination is still essential for identification of crystals, lipid droplets, etc.

Neutrophils normally account for about 20% of SF leukocytes. Neutrophils generally exceed 50% in urate gout, pseudogout, and rheumatoid arthritis (RA); they most often exceed 75% in acute bacterial arthritis. When 75% is used as a cutoff, the sensitivity for an inflammatory process is about 75% and the specificity is 92% (Shmerling, 1990). These cells frequently exhibit degenerative changes and may contain bacteria, crystals, lipid droplets, vacuoles, or dark blue to black granular inclusions (ragocytes, RA cells), which are similar to the toxic granulation occasionally seen in peripheral blood smears. The presence of ragocytes in patients with RA may indicate a poorer outcome (Davis, 1988).

Lupus erythematosus (LE) cells, not uncommonly present in patients with lupus arthritis, are most often neutrophils that have phagocytosed the nuclei of degenerating cells (Fig. 29-10). However, LE cells are not pathognomonic for SLE because they have also been identified in the synovial fluid of RA patients (Hunder, 1970).

Lymphocytes, normally constituting about 15% of SF cells, are prominent in early RA and other collagen disorders, as well as in chronic infections. Reactive forms, including immunoblasts, are occasionally present.

Monocytes and **macrophages** are the most common cells present in normal SF, accounting for approximately 65% of the cell count.

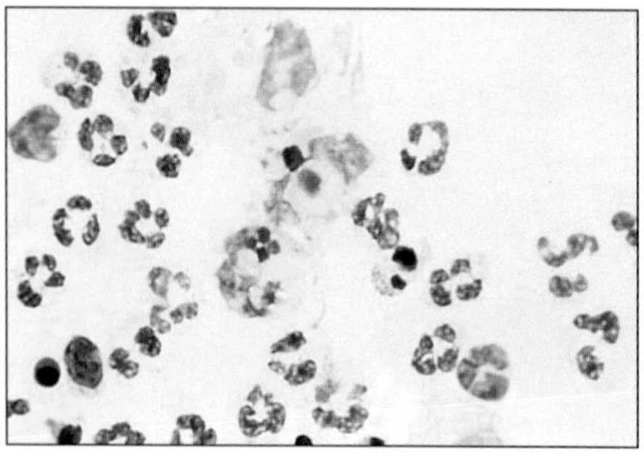

Figure 29-11 Reiter's cells in the synovial fluid from a patient with Reiter's syndrome.

Monocytosis may be self-limited in viral arthritis or serum sickness, or more chronic in SLE or undifferentiated connective tissue disorders. Reiter's cells, originally believed to be specific for Reiter's syndrome, are macrophages containing degenerating neutrophils (Fig. 29-11).

Eosinophilia, defined as more than 2% of the leukocyte count, has been reported in rheumatoid arthritis, rheumatic fever, metastatic carcinoma, Lyme disease, parasitic infection, chronic urticaria, and angioedema, and following arthrography (allergic reaction to dye) and irradiation (Podell, 1980; Kay, 1988).

Synovial cells have no pathologic significance. They appear similar to mesothelial cells and may be difficult to distinguish from monocytes and macrophages.

Lipid bodies are associated with trauma, aseptic necrosis, and RA. These droplets often form Maltese crosses under polarized light, can be associated with a leukocyte response, and may cause spurious elevations of the automated WBC count (Wise, 1987).

Crystal Examination

Crystals in synovial fluid lead to acute inflammation with increased WBC counts and a neutrophil-predominant infiltrate. Crystal identification, especially if intracellularly in neutrophils or macrophages, is pathognomonic for a crystal-induced arthritis (Judkins, 1997).

Gout refers to the process of crystal deposition in articular tissue. Common usage typically implies urate gout, and an inflammatory response to crystal deposition is referred to as gouty arthritis. The most common types of endogenous crystals responsible for gouty arthritis are **monosodium urate monohydrate** (urate gout), **calcium pyrophosphate dihydrate** (pyrophosphate gout, chondrocalcinosis, or "pseudogout"), apatite and other **basic calcium phosphates** (BCP; apatite gout), **calcium oxalate** (oxalate gout), and **lipids** (lipid gout).

Except for BCP, all of the above crystals can be detected by polarized light microscopy. A high-quality polarizing microscope with a first-order red plate compensator should be used. The **polarizer** filter is placed directly above the light source. The **analyzer** (another polarizing filter) is placed between the specimen slide and the microscope oculars, oriented 90 degrees from the polarizer to produce a dark background. The **compensator** is placed between the polarizer and the analyzer, usually oriented 45 degrees (halfway) between the planes of the two polarizing filters.

Initial examination should be performed on a wet preparation using polarized light. Phase-contrast microscopy enhances crystal detection. The slide and coverslip must be cleaned and carefully dried immediately before use to avoid birefringent dust particulate artifacts. The coverslip edges are sealed with nail polish, which retards but does not prevent evaporation. The coverslip edge is used to find the proper plane of focus. However, crystals in this location should be ignored because they are most likely artifacts. Most crystals are scanned with a 10× objective and are evaluated with at least a 40× objective, concentrating especially on cellular areas. Complete examination requires 100× oil immersion, however, because apparently negative fluids on scanning may contain a large population of small crystals (Gatter, 1991). Aligning the crystals' orientation to the compensator by rotating the microscope stage or the compensator facilitates recognition and identification. Crystal morphology, the extinction angle, strength, and signs of any birefringence (i.e., the ability to refract light and split the incident light into two rays: a fast ray and a slow ray) are noted. Nevertheless, the sensitivity and specificity of polarized microscopy for crystals are only 78% and 79%, respectively, for monosodium urate (Hasselbacher, 1987), and 12% and 67% for calcium pyrophosphate dihydrate (McGill, 1991). However, repeat examination following 24 hours of refrigeration at 4° C may result in a significant increase in the number of crystal-positive fluids (Yuan, 2003).

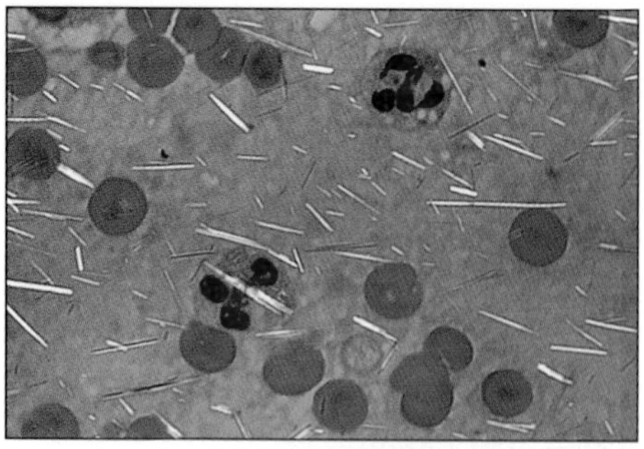

Figure 29-12 Monosodium urate crystals under polarized light from a patient with urate gout.

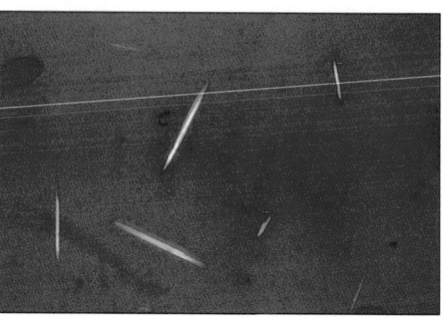

Figure 29-13 Monosodium urate crystals in synovial fluid. Compensated polarized light. *(From Kjeldsberg CR, Knight JA. Body fluids: laboratory examination of amniotic, cerebrospinal, seminal, serous and synovial fluids. 3rd ed. Chicago: © American Society for Clinical Pathology; 1993, with permission.)*

The Diff-Quik staining method may be a reliable alternative to polarized microscopy. Overall specificity, sensitivity, and accuracy were, respectively, 87.5%, 94.4%, and 91.9%. The overall positive predictive value was 92.7%; the negative predictive value was 90.3% (Selvi, 2001). Moreover, other more sophisticated and reliable methods, such as X-ray crystallography and Fourier transform infrared spectroscopy, have been described for identifying and characterizing crystals in biological specimens (Rosenthal, 2001).

Monosodium urate (MSU) crystals appear as needle-shaped rods 5–20 μm long, but they may be only 1–2 μm in length or, rarely, may appear as rounded spherolites. They are strongly birefringent (Fig. 29-12): Yellow when oriented parallel to the compensator and blue with perpendicular orientation (negative birefringence or elongation) (Fig. 29-13). A control slide of MSU crystals should always be used for comparison. Alternatively, betamethasone, a steroid that appears as a strongly negative birefringent rod, can be used to prepare a reference slide for the polarizing microscope (Judkins, 1997).

MSU crystals are found in 90% of acute urate gout and in about 75% of patients between attacks. Intracellular MSU crystals are characteristic of acute urate gout. They may occasionally be observed as a result of inflammation in septic arthritis (McCarty, 1988).

Calcium pyrophosphate dihydrate (CPPD) crystals are found in a group of conditions collectively known as CPPD crystal deposition disease. These crystals appear as rhomboids, rods, or rectangles 1–20 μm in length. CPPD crystals are weakly birefringent with positive elongation (blue when aligned with the compensator axis; Fig. 29-14). Many are too small to polarize the light, making them difficult to detect without phase-contrast microscopy. Extinction is incomplete and occurs between 20 and 30 degrees from the angle of the polarizer and analyzer (oblique or inclined extinction).

CPPD crystals are associated with degenerative arthritis and are seen in arthritides associated with hypomagnesemia, hemochromatosis, hyperparathyroidism, and hypothyroidism (Jones, 1992).

Calcium hydroxyapatite and the other BCP crystals are typically too small and nonbirefringent (isotropic) to see with light microscopy, unless they are clumped into 1- to 50-μm spherical microaggregates. **Alizarin red S dye** may be used to stain these and other calcium-containing crystals (Lazcano, 1993). At present, identification of BCP crystals is not important for diagnosis or prognosis, or as a guide in treatment.

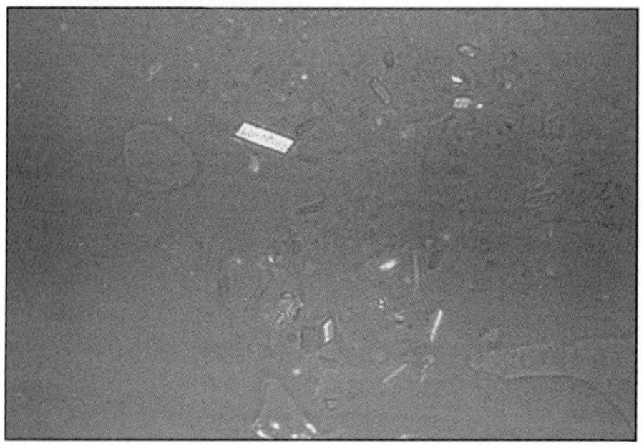

Figure 29-14 Calcium pyrophosphate dihydrate crystals in synovial fluid from a patient with pseudogout. Compensated polarized light. *(From Kjeldsberg CR, Knight JA. Body fluids: laboratory examination of amniotic, cerebrospinal, seminal, serous and synovial fluids. 3rd ed. Chicago: © American Society for Clinical Pathology; 1993, with permission.)*

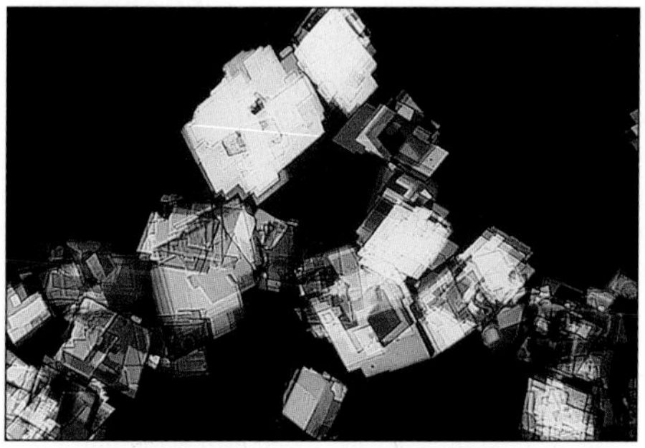

Figure 29-15 Cholesterol crystals in synovial fluid. Polarized light.

Calcium oxalate dihydrate crystals are 5- to 30-μm bipyramidal octahedral "envelopes" with variable birefringence and positive elongation. They are seen in arthropathy associated with chronic renal dialysis and primary oxalosis, a rare inborn error of metabolism. The monohydrate form is birefringent but nondescript in shape.

Lipid crystals are 1- to 20-μm spheres with a Maltese cross appearance and positive birefringence under compensated polarized light. They have been implicated as a cause of acute arthritis (McCarty, 1988).

Crystalline corticosteroids from intraarticular injection may have an appearance similar to MSU or CPPD crystals and persist up to a month following injection. Most often, they have blunt, jagged edges without clear crystal structure because they are prepared by grinding up larger crystalline forms. Triamcinolone hexacetonide is negatively birefringent, but most others show positive birefringence.

Cholesterol crystals typically appear as irregular birefringent plates, often with notched corners (Fig. 29-15). In chronic effusions (e.g., tuberculous arthritis, RA, SLE), needle- or rhomboid-shaped crystals similar to MSU or CPPD may be present (Ettlinger, 1979). Very small (1–5 microns) irregular, rod- and needle-shaped cholesterol crystals have been identified by X-ray diffraction analysis and by ultrastructural studies in osteoarthritis effusions (Fam, 1981). Cholesterol crystals are ethanol and ether soluble and are not phagocytosed by leukocytes. Moreover, if the crystals are cholesterol, quantitative analysis should show that the SF cholesterol level exceeds the plasma level.

Glove powder introduced during joint surgery appears as round, strongly birefringent particles 5–30 μm in diameter with a Maltese cross appearance when polarized.

A variety of other crystals or particulates may be present in synovial fluid. These include monoclonal Ig crystals or cryoglobulins, Charcot-Leyden crystals, amyloid fragments, cartilage fragments, collagen fibrils and fibrin strands, hematoidin crystals from prior hemorrhage, crystals from certain anticoagulants, nail polish, prosthetic fragments, and dust particles (Gatter, 1991).

CHEMICAL ANALYSIS

Chemical analyses of SF generally offer only supportive information to the routine tests. High viscosity may be remedied by dilution with normal saline, sonication, or hyaluronidase treatment. Reference intervals for the more important chemical analytes are shown in Table 29-16.

TABLE 29-16
Reference Intervals for Synovial Fluid Constituents

Constituent	Synovial fluid	Plasma
Total protein	1–3 g/dL	6–8 g/dL
Albumin	55%–70%	50%–65%
α_1-Globulin	6%–8%	3%–5%
α_2-Globulin	5%–7%	7%–13%
β-Globulin	8%–10%	8%–14%
γ-Globulin	10%–14%	12%–22%
Hyaluronic acid	0.3–0.4 g/dL	
Glucose	70–110 mg/dL	70–110 mg/dL
Uric acid	2–8 mg/dL	2–8 mg/dL
Lactate	9–29 mg/dL	9–29 mg/dL

Modified from Kjeldsberg CR, Knight JA. Body fluids: laboratory examination of amniotic, cerebrospinal, seminal, serous and synovial fluids. 3rd ed. Chicago: © American Society for Clinical Pathology; 1993, with permission.

Mucin Clot Test

Addition of acetic acid to SF precipitates hyaluronate into a mucin clot, which may be graded as good, fair, or poor. A fair to poor mucin clot test reflects dilution and depolymerization of hyaluronic acid—a nonspecific finding of several inflammatory arthritides. Although of historic interest, the mucin clot test has minimal clinical utility (Baker, 1991).

Glucose

Proper interpretation of SF glucose values requires comparison with serum levels, ideally preceded by a fast of 8 hours to allow glucose to equilibrate across the synovial membrane. The serum–synovia differential is less than 10 mg/dL in normal and many noninflammatory conditions. In septic arthritis, this difference ranges from 20–60 mg/dL but overlaps significantly with other inflammatory conditions, thereby limiting its clinical usefulness. When a cutoff value of 75 mg/dL is used, the sensitivity of low glucose for detecting an inflammatory joint disease is only 20%; the specificity is 84% (Shmerling, 1990).

In vitro glycolysis by large numbers of leukocytes may falsely reduce SF glucose values unless testing is performed within 1 hour of collection. However, tubes containing sodium fluoride, an inhibitor of glycolysis, prevent the loss of glucose.

Protein

The mean normal protein concentration is 1.38 g/dL in living volunteers (Weinburger, 1989) and 1.88 g/dL in cadavers. This difference most likely represents method variations. A reliable reference interval is 1.0–3.0 g/dL. With increasing inflammation, larger proteins (e.g., fibrinogen) enter the synovial space. Spontaneous clot formation may be detected in non-anticoagulated specimen tubes (fibrin clot test). Measurement of SF protein is highly nonspecific; the sensitivity is about 52% and the specificity 56% for inflammatory disorders. The total protein level generally is not useful in patient diagnosis, treatment, or outcome (Shmerling, 1990).

Enzymes

Numerous enzymes have been studied in SF, including lactate dehydrogenase, aspartate aminotransferase, adenosine deaminase, acid and alkaline phosphatase, and lysozyme, among others (Kjeldsberg, 1993). **Lactate dehydrogenase** is elevated in RA, gout, failed arthroplasties, and infectious arthritis. This increase most likely reflects the neutrophil infiltrate. Elevated **acid phosphatase** may have negative prognostic value in RA but is not specific (Luukkainen, 1989). Although enzyme analysis of SF is currently not clinically relevant, the measurement of various hydrolases may have significant predictive value in joint prognosis, especially RA.

Organic Acids

When compared with nonseptic monoarticular arthritis, SF **lactic acid** levels are usually increased in patients with septic arthritis (Kjeldsberg, 1993). Levels significantly greater than 30 mg/dL (3.7 mmol/L) are commonly associated with septic arthritis due to gram-positive cocci and gram-negative bacilli. Thus, the measurement of SF lactate may provide rapid provisional evidence for infection in specimens with negative Gram stains—a common occurrence, especially with gram-negative bacilli.

However, normal or intermediate levels neither rule in nor rule out infection. Moreover, gonococcal arthritis is notorious for having normal SF lactate levels (Curtis, 1983).

When gas–liquid chromatography is used, the presence of other organic acids not normally present in SF (e.g., **n-valeric, n-hexanoic,** and **succinic acids**) may be very helpful in differentiating septic from nonseptic arthritis (Brook, 1980; Borenstein, 1982).

Uric Acid

Synovial fluid uric acid levels generally, albeit not always, parallel serum levels in gout and noninflammatory arthropathies. An exception is inflammatory joint disorders other than gout, where SF urate levels may be significantly lower than in the paired serum (Beutler, 1996). It provides little clinical value in synovial fluid analysis except in some cases where gout is suspected but crystals are not identified (Reeves, 1965). Increased SF uric acid levels in these cases support a diagnosis of gout.

Lipids

In contrast to plasma, normal synovial fluid contains extremely low concentrations of lipids. Synovial fluid lipid abnormalities include (1) rare cholesterol-rich pseudochylous effusions typically associated with chronic RA; (2) lipid droplets, usually the result of trauma; and (3) extremely rare chylous effusions seen in association with RA, SLE, filariasis, pancreatitis, and trauma (Wise, 1987). These diseases can usually be differentiated clinically and by gross and microscopic examination; quantification of lipids currently has no clinical value in joint fluid analysis, except in cases where cholesterol crystals may resemble MSU or CPPD. In these cases, a cholesterol level that exceeds the plasma level supports the presence of cholesterol crystals.

IMMUNOLOGIC STUDIES

Rheumatoid factor (RF) is found in the synovia of about 60% of RA patients, usually at a titer equal to or slightly lower than the serum titer. **Antinuclear antibodies** (ANA) are found in the SF of about 70% of patients with SLE and 20% of patients with RA. Neither is specific enough for practical use. SF **complement** levels, normally about 10% of serum levels, increase to 40%–70% of serum activity with inflammation, proportional to the increase in protein exudation. Complement consumption in SLE and RA, in particular, results in levels less than 30% of serum complement. Complement is also decreased in some cases of bacterial and crystal-induced arthritis, so measurement is impractical for routine diagnosis.

MICROBIOLOGICAL EXAMINATION

Immediate transportation of joint fluid and good communication of clinical suspicions to the laboratory are extremely important in the rapid identification of an infectious agent.

Septic arthritis may be acute or chronic, and Gram stain and culture should be performed as part of the routine synovial fluid evaluation. Gram stain sensitivity varies from about 75% for staphylococcal infections and 50% for most gram-negative organisms, to less than 25% for gonococcal infections (Goldenberg, 1985). Concentration methods, including cytocentrifugation, may increase the sensitivity of the Gram stain.

Culture sensitivity ranges from 75%–95% for nongonococcal joint infections in patients who have not received antibiotics. For patients with gonorrhea, the sensitivity is only 10%–50% (Shmerling, 1994). In partially treated patients, the use of resin-containing blood culture bottles for culturing synovial fluid may improve isolation and identification of the responsible organism.

Although not yet in routine practice, the use of polymerase chain reaction with universal primers to detect bacterial DNA is helpful, particularly for the more fastidious, uncultivable pathogens (e.g., *Borrelia burgdorferi*, *Chlamydia* spp., *Mycoplasma* spp.) (Nocton, 1994; Li, 1996). Viruses are often associated with acute infectious arthritis, and, depending on the putative virus, serology, viral culture, and detection of viral DNA by nucleic acid amplification should be performed.

Depending on the clinical history, infectious arthritis may be associated with particular exposures and their associated pathogens. Arthritis develops in approximately 60% of patients with Lyme disease resulting from exposure to ticks infected with *Borrelia burgdorferi* (Golightly, 1993). The PCR test for detecting *B. burgdorferi* DNA in synovial fluid is positive in 96% of untreated cases (Nocton, 1994; Exner, 2003).

In patients with a travel history or outdoor occupations, synovial fluid/tissue should be examined for fungal pathogens by KOH/calcofluor white stain and cultured on selective fungal media. For example, a patient with a recent travel history to Arizona may present with a monoarticular arthritis secondary to *Coccidioides immitis*. Patients with chronic arthritis and risk factors for *Mycobacterium tuberculosis* or nontuberculous infections should undergo a synovial biopsy.

Ziehl-Neelsen or Kinyoun stains for acid-fast organisms have a sensitivity of about 20%. Cultures for *M. tuberculosis* are positive in about 80% of proven cases. Because conventional culture methods for *M. tuberculosis* are often very time consuming, applying PCR for the detection of *M. tuberculosis* is a novel and promising technique for more rapid diagnosis. Synovial biopsy is recommended for suspected tuberculous arthritis to provide a more rapid diagnosis (Verettas, 2003; Titov, 2004).

PLEURAL FLUID

The pleural cavity is a potential space lined by mesothelium of the visceral and parietal pleurae. The pleural cavity normally contains a small amount of fluid that facilitates movement of the two membranes against each other. This fluid is a plasma filtrate derived from capillaries of the parietal pleura. It is produced continuously at a rate dependent on capillary hydrostatic pressure, plasma oncotic pressure, and capillary permeability. Pleural fluid is reabsorbed through the lymphatics and venules of the visceral pleura.

An accumulation of fluid, called an **effusion,** results from an imbalance of fluid production and reabsorption. This fluid accumulation in the pleural, pericardial, and peritoneal cavities is known as a **serous effusion.**

SPECIMEN COLLECTION

Thoracentesis is indicated for any undiagnosed pleural effusion or for therapeutic purposes in patients with massive symptomatic effusions; however, pleural fluid samples are frequently collected, handled, and/or analyzed in a less than satisfactory manner. Indeed, improper collection/handling and undertesting or inappropriate testing are more common than with other body fluids. The laboratory often receives a large syringe or vacuum bottle, which must be circulated through the various laboratory sections. Moreover, a large blood or fibrin clot may be present as the result of inadequate anticoagulation or mixing.

Except for an EDTA tube for total and differential cell counts, the specimen should be collected in heparinized tubes to avoid clotting. Aliquots for aerobic and anaerobic bacterial cultures are best inoculated into blood culture media at the bedside. If malignancy, fungal infection, or mycobacterial infection is suspected, all remaining fluid (≥100 mL) should be submitted to maximize the yield of stains and culture. Because serous effusions are more forgiving than CSF in maintaining cellular integrity, fresh specimens for cytology may be stored up to 48 hours in the refrigerator with satisfactory results. For pH measurements, the fluid should be collected anaerobically in a heparinized syringe and submitted to the laboratory on ice. Grossly purulent specimens do not require pH measurement and may clog the analyzer.

TRANSUDATES AND EXUDATES

It has long been recognized that the initial classification of a pleural fluid as a **transudate** or an **exudate** greatly simplifies the process of arriving at a correct final diagnosis. Moreover, it determines whether further testing is needed.

Transudates are usually bilateral owing to systemic conditions leading to increased capillary hydrostatic pressure or decreased plasma oncotic pressure (Table 29-17). Malignant effusions may infrequently be transudative as the result of a simultaneous confounding clinical condition such as congestive heart failure (Ashchi, 1998). Exudates are more often unilateral, associated with localized disorders that increase vascular permeability or interfere with lymphatic resorption (see Table 29-17).

RECOMMENDED TESTS

The evaluation of serous body fluids (pleural, pericardial, peritoneal) is directed first toward differentiating transudative from exudative effusions. Transudates generally require no further workup. However, the fluid should be retained for 7–10 days in case further testing is needed. To separate the two, several chemical parameters have been proposed, although none is 100% accurate (Table 29-18).

TABLE 29-17
Classification of Pleural Effusions

Transudates: Increased Hydrostatic Pressure or Decreased Plasma Oncotic Pressure
Congestive heart failure
Hepatic cirrhosis
Hypoproteinemia (e.g., nephrotic syndrome)

Exudates: Increased Capillary Permeability or Decreased Lymphatic Resorption
Infections
- Bacterial pneumonia
- Tuberculosis, other granulomatous diseases (e.g., sarcoidosis, histoplasmosis)
- Viral or mycoplasma pneumonia

Neoplasms
- Bronchogenic carcinoma
- Metastatic carcinoma
- Lymphoma
- Mesothelioma (increased hyaluronate content of effusion fluid)

Noninfectious inflammatory disease involving pleura
- Rheumatoid disease (low pleural fluid glucose in most cases)
- Systemic lupus erythematosus (LE cells are occasionally present)

Pulmonary infarct (may be associated with hemorrhagic effusion)

Fluid From Extrapleural Sources
Pancreatitis (elevated amylase activity in effusion fluid)
Ruptured esophagus (elevated amylase activity and low pH)
Urinothorax (elevated creatinine and low pH)

LE, Lupus erythematosus.

TABLE 29-18
Laboratory Criteria for Pleural Fluid Exudate

Pleural fluid/serum protein ratio	≥0.50
Pleural fluid/serum LD ratio	≥0.60
Pleural fluid LD	≥ ⅔ upper limit of normal serum LD
Pleural fluid cholesterol	>45 mg/dL
Pleural fluid/serum cholesterol ratio	≥0.30
Serum–pleural fluid albumin gradient	≤1.2 g/dL
Pleural fluid/serum bilirubin ratio	≥0.60

LD, Lactate dehydrogenase.

Classical teaching stressed that exudates and transudates can be distinguished on the basis of total protein concentrations above (exudates) or below (transudates) 3.0 g/dL. However, using total protein alone misclassifies both exudates and transudates by about 30% (Melsom, 1979). It is now well accepted that test combinations increase sensitivity (any positive parameter indicates an exudate), improve accuracy, and serve as the basis for the well-established Light criteria (Light, 1972). Accordingly, an exudate meets one or more of the following criteria: (1) Pleural fluid/serum protein ratio greater than 0.5; (2) pleural fluid/serum LD ratio greater than 0.6; and (3) pleural fluid LD level greater than two thirds of the serum upper limit of normal. The sensitivity and specificity are about 98% and 80%, respectively.

Several subsequent reports support Light's criteria as the most reliable method to differentiate transudates from exudates (Peterman, 1984; Burgess, 1995; Assi, 1998; Gazquez, 1998).

Several alternative measurements have been proposed to differentiate exudates from transudates. Testing for total cholesterol, the albumin gradient, or a combination of LD and total cholesterol may discriminate effusions with equivocal Light's criteria results. For example, the albumin gradient is recommended to confirm a clinical transudate misclassified as an exudate by Light's criteria (Light, 1997), that is, a serum albumin level greater than 1.2 g/dL higher than the pleural fluid level indicates that the fluid is a transudate (Burgess, 1995). In many such cases, the patient is being diuresed. Other test combinations have equaled but not surpassed the performance of Light's criteria. A recent study indicated that in most cases the same categorization of pleural fluids as exudates or transudates was achieved using measurements of protein and LD alone without comparison with a blood sample, as was accomplished with application of Light's criteria (Murphy, 2008).

TABLE 29-19
Pleural Effusion: Recommended Tests

Routine tests
- Gross examination
- Pleural fluid/serum protein ratio
- Pleural fluid/serum LD ratio
- Examination of Romanowski-stained smear (malignant cells, LE cells)

Useful tests in most patients
- Stains and cultures for microorganisms
- Cytology

Useful tests in selected cases
- Pleural fluid cholesterol
- Pleural fluid/serum cholesterol ratio
- Albumin gradient
- pH
- Lactate
- Enzymes (ADA, amylase, LD)
- Interferon-γ
- C-reactive protein
- Lipid analysis
- Tumor markers
- Immunologic studies
- Tuberculostearic acid
- Pleural biopsy

Modified from Kjeldsberg CR, Knight JA. Body fluids: laboratory examination of amniotic, cerebrospinal, seminal, serous and synovial fluids. 3rd ed. Chicago: © American Society for Clinical Pathology; 1993, with permission.
ADA, Adenosine deaminase; *LD,* lactate dehydrogenase; *LE,* lupus erythematosus.

Some tests, such as the combination of pleural fluid LD and cholesterol, may be more convenient and cost-effective by avoiding the need for simultaneous blood tests (Costa, 1995). Bilirubin measurement is not a strong discriminator of effusions (Heffner, 1997).

Further analysis of exudates is directed toward ruling out malignancy and infection. Cytology and appropriate bacterial stains and cultures are the most useful tests in this regard. Moreover, given that pleural fluid DNA levels are significantly increased in exudates, quantitative analysis may be an effective new method to evaluate the causes of serous effusion (Chan, 2003). Recommended tests for the evaluation of pleural effusions are summarized in Table 29-19. The types of tests ordered and the interpretation of test results should always be correlated with clinical findings and differential diagnosis. Total leukocyte, differential, and red cell counts are of limited use in the evaluation of serous effusions.

GROSS EXAMINATION

Transudates are typically clear, pale yellow to straw-colored, and odorless, and do not clot. Approximately 15% of transudates are blood tinged. A bloody pleural effusion (hematocrit >1%) suggests trauma, malignancy, or pulmonary infarction (Jay, 1986). A traumatic tap is suggested by uneven blood distribution, fluid clearing with continued aspiration, or formation of small blood clots. A pleural fluid hematocrit greater than 50% of the blood hematocrit is good evidence for a hemothorax (Light, 1995).

Exudates may grossly resemble transudates, but most show variable degrees of cloudiness or turbidity, and they often clot if not heparinized. A feculent odor may be detected in anaerobic infections. Turbid, milky, and/or bloody specimens should be centrifuged and the supernatant examined. If the supernatant is clear, the turbidity is most likely due to cellular elements or debris. If the turbidity persists after centrifugation, a chylous or pseudochylous effusion is likely.

True chylous effusions are produced by leakage from the thoracic duct resulting from obstruction by lymphoma, carcinoma, or traumatic disruption. A creamy top layer of chylomicrons may form in the specimen on standing. Idiopathic congenital chylothorax is the most common form of pleural effusion in the newborn.

Pseudochylous or chyliform effusions may have a milky, greenish, or "gold paint" appearance. They accumulate gradually through the breakdown of cellular lipids in long-standing effusions such as rheumatoid pleuritis, tuberculosis, or myxedema. Features that distinguish true chylous from pseudochylous effusions are summarized in Table 29-20.

TABLE 29-20
Characteristic Features of Chylous and Pseudochylous Effusions

Feature	Chylous	Pseudochylous
Onset	Sudden	Gradual
Appearance	Milky-white, or yellow to bloody	Milky or greenish, metallic sheen
Microscopic examination	Lymphocytosis	Mixed cellular reaction, cholesterol crystals
Triglycerides*†	≥110 mg/dL (≥1.24 mmol/L)	<50 mg/dL (<0.56 mol/L)
Lipoprotein electrophoresis	Chylomicrons present	Chylomicrons absent

Modified from Kjeldsberg CR, Knight JA. Body fluids: laboratory examination of amniotic, cerebrospinal, seminal, serous and synovial fluids. 3rd ed. Chicago: © American Society for Clinical Pathology; 1993, with permission.
*Values in parentheses are SI units.
†Triglyceride levels between 50 mg/dL and 110 mg/dL are equivocal and require electrophoresis to confirm chylothorax.

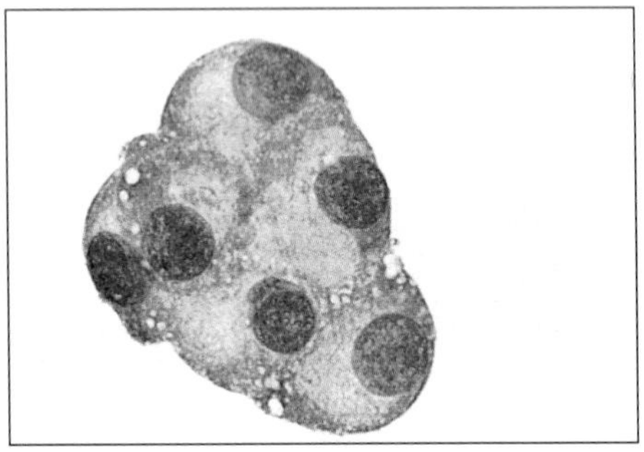

Figure 29-16 Mesothelial cells in pleural fluid.

MICROSCOPIC EXAMINATION

Cell Counts

Total cell counts may be performed using manual hemocytometer methods; however, automated cell counts are increasingly used with pleural fluid specimens (Conner, 2003). Leukocyte counts have limited utility in separating transudates (<1000/µL) from exudates (>1000/µL). Although red cell counts above 100,000/µL are highly suggestive of malignancy, trauma, or pulmonary infarction, they are not specific for these conditions.

Differential Leukocyte Count and Cytology

Examination is commonly performed on a stained smear, preferably prepared by cytocentrifugation and with the air-dried smear stained with a Romanowski stain. Indeed, examination by the hematology laboratory can be highly effective in the detection of malignant cells, especially hematologic malignancies (Kendall, 1997). Filtration or automated concentration methods with Papanicolaou stain may also be used, especially if cell loss is a matter of concern. Automated WBC differential counts may be done on pleural fluid samples; however, some variation in results from those of manual methods may be seen (Conner, 2003). Liquid-based thin-layer methods are increasingly used to prepare pleural and other serous fluid specimens for cytopathologic examination and show good performance in the detection of malignant cells (Moriarity, 2008).

Cytologic analysis will establish the diagnosis of metastatic carcinoma in 70% or more of cases when both smears and cell blocks are examined (Light, 2002). However, the sensitivity is significantly less efficient if the patient has mesothelioma (10%), squamous cell carcinoma (20%), lymphoma (25%–50%), or sarcoma (25%). Preparation of cell blocks is unnecessary, except for effusions in which malignancy is an important consideration (Jonasson, 1990).

Mesothelial cells are common in pleural fluids from inflammatory processes (Fig. 29-16). They are, however, conspicuously scarce in patients with tuberculous pleurisy, empyema, and rheumatoid pleuritis, and in patients who have had pleurodesis. Fibrin deposition and fibrosis occurring in these conditions prevent mesothelial cell exfoliation. Well-differentiated carcinoma cells may be easily recognized (Fig. 29-17) or may be highly undifferentiated (Fig. 29-18). A panel of immunocytochemical stains may be necessary for confirmation, and these studies are enhanced by the use of liquid-based preparation methods (Sioutopaulou, 2008).

Neutrophils predominate in pleural fluid from patients with pleural inflammation (Table 29-21). More than 10% of transudates will also have a predominance of neutrophils, but this has limited clinical significance.

Lymphocytes predominate in the disorders summarized in Table 29-21. Most are small, but medium, large, and reactive (transformed)

TABLE 29-21
Cellular Differential of Pleural Effusions

Neutrophilia (>50%)
Bacterial pneumonia (parapneumonic effusion)
Pulmonary infarction
Pancreatitis
Subphrenic abscess
Early tuberculosis
Transudates (>10%)
Lymphocytosis (>50%)
Tuberculosis
Viral infection
Malignancy (lymphoma, other neoplasms)
True chylothorax
Rheumatoid pleuritis
Systemic lupus erythematosus
Uremic effusions
Transudates (≈30%)
Eosinophilia (>10%)
Pneumothorax (air in pleural space)
Trauma
Pulmonary infarction
Congestive heart failure
Infection (especially parasitic, fungal)
Hypersensitivity syndromes
Drug reaction
Rheumatologic diseases
Hodgkin disease
Idiopathic

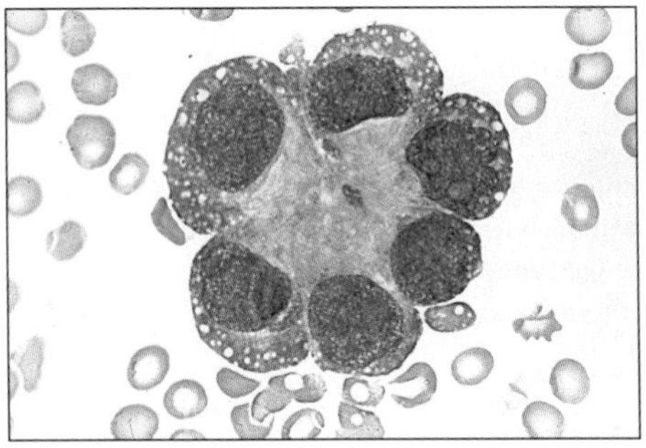

Figure 29-17 Well-differentiated breast carcinoma cells in pleural fluid.

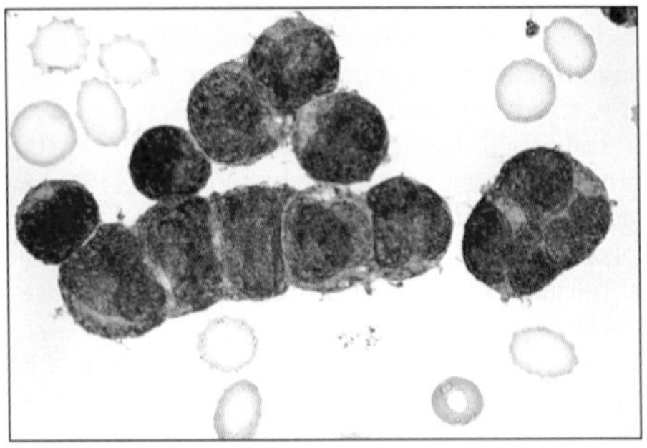

Figure 29-18 Small cell carcinoma of lung showing typical molding of nuclei.

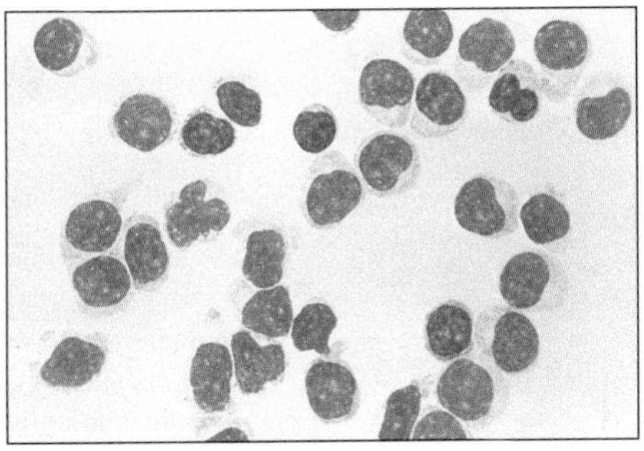

Figure 29-19 Pleural effusion in patient with non-Hodgkin lymphoma, small lymphocytic type. The cells are small round forms, difficult to distinguish from benign lymphocytes. *(From Kjeldsberg CR, Knight JA. Body fluids: laboratory examination of amniotic, cerebrospinal, seminal, serous and synovial fluids. 3rd ed. Chicago: © American Society for Clinical Pathology; 1993, with permission.)*

variants may be seen. Nucleoli and nuclear cleaving are more prominent in effusions than in the peripheral blood, and these features may be particularly prominent in cytocentrifuge preparations. **Plasma cells** may also be observed. Lymphocytosis associated with transudates is of limited clinical significance.

Low-grade non-Hodgkin lymphoma and chronic lymphocytic leukemia (CLL) may be difficult to distinguish from benign lymphocyte-rich serous effusion (Fig. 29-19).

Immunophenotyping by flow cytometry or immunocytochemistry, in conjunction with cellular morphology, is usually helpful in making a correct diagnosis. The relative proportions of T and B cells are, by themselves, not definitive for separating benign from malignant exudates (Ibrahim, 1989); however, the pattern of expression of Ig light chains and/or other distinctive cell marker combinations may allow specific diagnosis of lymphoproliferative disorders. Molecular DNA analysis may be another useful adjunct to morphologic analysis. An unusual form of high-grade B cell non-Hodgkin lymphoma, called **primary effusion lymphoma,** may be seen in pleural, peritoneal, and/or pericardial fluid specimens, typically from immunocompromised patients, with a characteristic highly anaplastic and immunoblastic morphologic appearance and without expression of most B cell–associated antigens (Karcher, 1997). The diagnosis is usually confirmed by demonstrating in the neoplastic cells the presence of human herpesvirus-8 (HHV-8) –associated antigens and/or DNA by immunophenotypic and/or molecular analysis.

An eosinophilic effusion is one that has 10% or more **eosinophils.** The most common causes are related to the presence of air or blood in the pleural cavity (see Table 29-21). Most of these are exudates; however, in about 35% of patients, the cause is unknown (Adelman, 1984). Although not of much assistance in diagnosing the cause of an effusion, eosinophilia appears to be independently associated with longer survival (Rubins, 1996). A small number of **mast cells** or **basophils** often accompany eosinophils. Eosinophil-derived **Charcot-Leyden crystals** may also be seen.

CHEMICAL ANALYSIS

Protein

The measurement of pleural fluid total protein or albumin has little clinical value except when combined with other parameters to differentiate exudates from transudates. Protein electrophoresis shows a pattern similar to serum, except for a higher proportion of albumin; it has little value for differential diagnosis (Light, 1995).

Glucose

The glucose level of normal pleural fluid, transudates, and most exudates is similar to serum levels. Decreased pleural fluid glucose, accepted as a level below 60 mg/dL (3.33 mmol/L) or a pleural fluid/serum glucose ratio less than 0.5, is most consistent and dramatic in rheumatoid pleuritis and grossly purulent parapneumonic exudates (Sahn, 1982). Low pleural fluid glucose may also be present in malignancy, tuberculosis, nonpurulent bacterial infection, lupus pleuritis, and esophageal rupture.

Lactate

Pleural fluid lactate levels can be a useful adjunct in the rapid diagnosis of infectious pleuritis. Levels are significantly higher in bacterial and tuberculous pleural infections than in other pleural effusions. Moderate elevations are generally observed in malignant effusions (Brook, 1980). Values greater than 90 mg/dL (10 mmol/L) have a positive predictive value for infectious pleuritis of 94% and a negative predictive value of 100% (Gastrin, 1988).

Enzymes

Amylase elevations above the serum level (usually 1.5–2.0 or more times greater) indicate the presence of pancreatitis, esophageal rupture, or malignant effusion (Light, 1973). Elevated amylase derived from esophageal rupture or malignancy is the salivary isoform, which differentiates it from pancreatic amylase (Kramer, 1989).

Pleural fluid LD levels rise in proportion to the degree of inflammation. In addition to their use in separating exudates from transudates, declining LD levels during the course of an effusion indicate that the inflammatory process is resolving. Conversely, increasing levels indicate a worsening condition requiring aggressive workup or treatment. LD isoenzyme analysis may be helpful in diagnosing problematic exudates but is not routinely recommended (Lossos, 1997).

ADA, which is particularly rich in T lymphocytes, is significantly increased in tuberculous pleuritis. At a level of 50 U/L, the sensitivity, specificity, positive predictive value, negative predictive value, and efficiency for tuberculosis are 91%, 81%, 84%, 89%, and 86%, respectively (Burgess, 1996). When the lymphocyte/neutrophil ratio is 0.75 or greater, the percentages are 88%, 95%, 95%, 88%, and 92%, respectively. ADA levels of 40 U/L or greater are present in about 99.6% of patients with verified tuberculous pleuritis (Lee, 2001). However, in patients with lymphocyte-rich pleural fluids from nontuberculous causes, ADA levels less than 40 U/L are present in 97.1% of cases.

Interferon-γ

Pleural fluid interferon (IFN)-γ levels are significantly increased in the pleural fluid of patients with tuberculous pleuritis. The sensitivity of levels of 3.7 IU/L or greater is 99%, and the specificity is 98% (Villena, 1996a). Test sensitivity does not differ in HIV-positive and HIV-negative patients. Only about 20% of patients with effusions due to hematologic malignancies have IFN-γ levels slightly above 3.7 IU/L (Villena, 2003a).

pH

Pleural fluid pH measurement has the highest diagnostic accuracy in assessing the prognosis of parapneumonic (pneumonia-related) effusions (Heffner, 1995). A parapneumonic exudate with a pH greater than 7.30 generally resolves with medical therapy alone. A pH less than 7.20 indicates a complicated parapneumonic effusion (loculated or associated with empyema), requiring surgical drainage.

Patients with borderline complicated exudates (pH 7.20–7.30) may be closely watched with repeat measurements. A concomitant pleural glucose level below 60 mg/dL (3.33 mmol/L), however, strongly suggests impending empyema. Rheumatoid pleuritis and malignant effusions with a poor response to pleurodesis also have pH values below 7.20 and a low glucose level (Rodriquez-Panadero, 1989). A pH below 6.0 is characteristic of **esophageal rupture,** although the pH in severe empyema may be 6.0 or less (Good, 1980).

Urinothorax, a collection of urine presumably produced by lymphatic drainage of perirenal accumulations into the pleural cavity, is also associated with a pleural fluid pH less than 7.30. These effusions are transudative because of their low protein content and smell of urine, and they have a creatinine level greater than in simultaneously drawn serum (Miller, 1988).

Lipids

Some serous effusions appear to be chylous (i.e., a milky appearance) but are not (pseudochylous), whereas others may not look chylous but are. Although pseudochylous fluids may be partially due to increased leukocytes and necrotic debris, they are primarily due to the presence of increased lecithin–globulin complexes. A true chylous effusion has chylomicrons at the origin on lipoprotein electrophoresis. Lipid measurements are also helpful in identifying chylous effusions (Staats, 1980). Thus, pleural fluid triglyceride levels above 110 mg/dL indicate a chylous effusion; values from 60–110 mg/dL (0.68–1.24 mmol/L) are less certain and require lipoprotein electrophoresis to confirm a chylothorax. Nonchylous and pseudochylous effusions generally have triglyceride levels below 50 mg/dL (0.56 mmol/L) and no chylomicrons on electrophoresis (see Table 29-20).

Cholesterol measurements may be useful in separating transudates from exudates, especially when there is a question regarding Light's criteria. A total cholesterol value of 54 mg/dL or more and a pleural fluid/serum cholesterol ratio of 0.32 or higher have sensitivity and specificity values similar to Light's criteria (Suay, 1995). Elevated levels and the presence of cholesterol crystals may be seen with pleural effusions that have been present for several years.

C-Reactive Protein

Pleural fluid CRP is often a clinically useful screening test for organ disease, index of disease activity, and measure of response to therapy (Castano, 1992). Pleural fluid CRP levels >30 mg/L reportedly have a sensitivity of 93.7%, a specificity of 76.5%, and a positive predictive value of 98.4% in parapneumonic infections (Turay, 2000). Mean CRP values are about 90 mg/L in parapneumonic infections compared with 26 mg/L and 23 mg/L for tuberculous and malignant effusions, respectively.

Tuberculostearic Acid (10-Methyloctadecanoic Acid)

Tuberculostearic acid (TSA) was first isolated from the bacillus *Mycobacterium tuberculosis*. This fatty acid is a structural component of mycobacteria and is not normally present in human tissue. Using gas chromatography/mass spectroscopy, TSA was measured in sputum, bronchial washings, and pleural fluid from patients with pulmonary tuberculosis (Muranishi, 1990). Here, pleural fluid TSA was identified in 24 of 32 (75%) patients with active tuberculosis; bronchial washings were positive for TSA in 15 of 22 cases. In patients with other pulmonary disorders, only 4 of 46 pleural fluids and 3 of 69 bronchial washings had detectable levels. A later smaller study reported the following for pleural fluid TSA: Sensitivity 54%, specificity 80%, positive predictive value 75%, negative predictive value 61%, and efficacy 66% (Yorgancioglu, 1996).

Tumor Markers

Although not recommended as a routine test, various tumor markers are often a useful adjunct in enigmatic noninflammatory exudates with negative cytology. Several tumor markers, especially CEA, CA 15-3, CA 549, CA 72-4, and CYFRA 21-1, among others, have been studied in pleural fluids. CEA is probably the most useful single marker for adenocarcinomas, but reported cutoff values vary considerably. The sensitivity of CEA for malignant effusions varies depending on tumor origin and is about 50% overall. Although complicated parapneumonic effusions may result in elevated CEA levels (Garcia-Pachon, 1997), they are usually not a problem to distinguish clinically.

A combination of tumor markers increases the accuracy of diagnosis. Thus, a combination of CEA, CA 15-3, and CA 72-4 had an accuracy of 90% with 78% sensitivity, 95% specificity, 88% positive predictive value, and 91% negative predictive value (Villena, 1996b). Similarly, CA 15-3 and CEA combined had an accuracy of 87% (Romero, 1996); a combination of CA 549, CEA, and CA 15-3 had a sensitivity of 65%, specificity 99%, and accuracy 85% (Villena, 2003b). The use of the cytokeratin 19 fragment (CYFRA 21-1) may also be useful in combination with other tumor markers.

Other tumor markers may also be useful in the diagnosis of unexplained effusions. For example, a marked increase in pleural fluid prostate-specific antigen (PSA) led to the correct diagnosis of a patient with metastatic prostate cancer who presented with severe anemia, peripheral edema, and pleural and pericardial effusions that were negative by cytologic examination (Chin, 1999).

IMMUNOLOGIC STUDIES

Approximately 5% of patients with RA and 50% with SLE develop pleural effusions sometime during the course of their disease.

RF is commonly present in pleural effusions associated with seropositive RA. Although a pleural fluid titer of 1:320 or greater in a patient with known RA is reasonable evidence of rheumatic pleuritis (Halla, 1980), elevated RF titers up to 1:1280 have been identified in 41% of patients with bacterial pneumonia, 20% of patients with malignant effusions, and 14% of patients with tuberculosis, making a routine test for RF of little value (Levine, 1968).

ANA titers may be useful in the diagnosis of effusion due to lupus pleuritis; the sensitivity is about 85% when a cutoff titer of 1:160 is used (Good, 1983). The specificity is not high, however, because elevated ANA titers also occur in various other conditions. Thus, pleural fluid ANA titers are not clinically useful.

Decreased **complement** levels (CH50 <10 U/mL or C4 level below 10×10^{-5} U/g protein) are present in most patients with rheumatoid or lupus pleuritis (Hunder, 1972; Halla, 1980). However, complement measurements are not highly specific and are of little value for routine diagnosis, although they may be helpful in the diagnosis of otherwise enigmatic effusions.

TABLE 29-22
Causes of Pericardial Effusions

Idiopathic (most often viral)	Renal failure
Infection	Hemorrhage
Bacteria	Trauma
Tuberculosis	Anticoagulant therapy
Fungi	Leakage of aortic aneurysm
Viruses	Autoimmune disorders
AIDS-related (usually viral)	Hypothyroidism
Neoplasm	Rheumatoid arthritis
Metastatic carcinoma	Systemic lupus erythematosus
Lymphoma	Inflammatory bowel disease
Drugs	Wegener's granulomatosis
Hydralazine	Acute myocardial infarction
Procainamide	Radiation therapy
Phenytoin	

AIDS, Acquired immunodeficiency syndrome.

MICROBIOLOGICAL EXAMINATION

Bacteria most commonly associated with parapneumonic effusions are *Staphylococcus aureus*, *Streptococcus pneumoniae*, β-hemolytic group A streptococci, enterococci, and some gram-negative bacilli. Anaerobic bacteria are isolated in a significant proportion of cases, so both anaerobic and aerobic cultures should be performed. The sensitivity of the Gram stain is approximately 50% (Ferrer, 1999), and concentration methods, such as cytocentrifugation, may increase the sensitivity. Use of resin-containing blood culture bottles may improve the isolation of certain bacteria in partially treated patients.

For patients with suspected *M. tuberculosis*, direct staining of tuberculous effusions for acid-fast bacteria has a sensitivity of 20%–30%, and positive cultures are found in 50%–70% of cases (Baer, 2001). Pleural biopsy yields the highest culture sensitivity (50%–75%) and may provide a rapid presumptive diagnosis of tuberculosis by histopathologic demonstration of granulomas or acid-fast bacteria. Combining culture and acid-fast stains with pleural biopsy increases the sensitivity to about 95% (Jay, 1986).

ADA can provide rapid chemical evidence for tuberculous effusions independent of HIV status (Burgess, 1996; Riantawan, 1999; Lee, 2001). Although the ADA-2 isoenzyme form is elaborated by activated lymphocytes in tuberculosis, only mild elevations occur in lymphocyte-rich pleural effusions from nontuberculous causes. However, the relatively low prevalence of tuberculous pleurisy in North America anticipates a lower positive predictive value rate compared with the excellent results reported in the Asian and European literature, where tuberculosis is more common. Moreover, the colorimetric Giusti method by which most ADA data were derived is, unfortunately, not widely available in the United States (Roth, 1999).

Pleural fluid interferon-γ is significantly increased in tuberculous pleuritis and may be helpful in some cases because it is independent of HIV status and is only modestly increased in about 20% of hematologic malignancies (Villena, 2003a).

PERICARDIAL FLUID

From 10–50 mL of fluid is normally present in the pericardial space, produced by a transudative process similar to pleural fluid. Pericardial effusions are most often caused by viral infection, and enterovirus is the most common etiologic agent. They may develop as a result of bacterial, tuberculous, or fungal infection, or in association with autoimmune disorders, renal failure, myocardial infarction, mediastinal injury, or the effects of various drugs; they may be idiopathic (Table 29-22). HIV-infected patients commonly have asymptomatic pericardial effusions, which may become large in more advanced disease (Silva-Cardosa, 1999) and/or with primary effusion lymphoma (Karcher, 1997). Many of the recommended laboratory tests described for pleural fluid also pertain to pericardial effusions (see Table 29-19).

SPECIMEN COLLECTION

Pericardial effusions of unknown origin or large effusions with signs of cardiac tamponade are generally submitted for laboratory examination. Fluid may be obtained by pericardiotomy following limited thoracotomy, or by pericardiocentesis (sterile needle aspiration).

Normal pericardial fluid is pale yellow and clear. Large effusions (>350 mL) are most often caused by malignancy or uremia, or they may be idiopathic. In HIV-associated cardiac tamponade, 45% of cases are idiopathic, and tuberculous and bacterial effusions each account for about 20% of cases (Chen, 1999). Infection or malignancy typically produces turbid effusions, whereas effusions due to uremia are usually clear and straw-colored. These and several other disorders may produce hemorrhagic effusions.

Blood-like fluid obtained by pericardiocentesis might represent a hemorrhagic effusion or inadvertent aspiration of blood from the heart. Blood obtained from the heart chamber will have a hematocrit comparable with that of peripheral blood, and blood gas analysis yields results similar to venous or arterial blood. In contrast, the hematocrit of a hemorrhagic effusion is usually lower than that of peripheral blood. The pH and partial pressure of oxygen are lower and the pCO_2 is higher than in venous or arterial blood (Mann, 1978). Blood from a cardiac puncture clots, but a hemorrhagic effusion usually does not.

A milky appearance suggests the presence of a chylous or pseudochylous effusion. Identification and differentiation of these effusions are discussed under Pleural Fluid.

GROSS EXAMINATION

The **postpericardiotomy syndrome** is a fairly common but nonspecific complication of cardiac surgery (or other cardiac damage) that develops days to weeks following the initial injury. It is hallmarked by the development of fever, pleuritic chest pain, and other signs of pleural, pericardial, and, less often, lung inflammation. Exudative pleural effusions develop in more than 80% of cases. These are often serosanguineous to hemorrhagic and typically have a pH greater than 7.4 and a normal glucose level (Stelzner, 1983). No specific tests are available for diagnosing this syndrome. Diagnosis, therefore, remains one of clinical exclusion. Although the cause is uncertain, the time course, presence of antimyocardial antibodies, and response to antiinflammatory therapy suggest an immune-mediated process. Increased levels of antimyocardial antibodies relative to serum, decreased complement levels, and immune complexes have been documented in pleural fluid from a single patient with the syndrome (Kim, 1996).

EXUDATES AND TRANSUDATES

Until recently, the criteria for differentiating exudates from transudates had not been carefully studied in pericardial effusions. According to Light's criteria, a pleural exudate has one or more of the following: pleural fluid/serum protein ratio >0.5; pleural fluid/serum LD ratio >0.6; and pleural fluid LD level >200 U/L. Light's criteria for pericardial fluid have now been shown to be the most reliable diagnostic tool for identifying pericardial exudates and transudates (Burgess, 2002a).

Routine testing of pericardial effusions should probably be limited to cell count, glucose, total protein, LD, bacterial culture, and cytology (Meyers, 1997). Other, more specific tests are appropriate for diseases of high clinical suspicion.

MICROSCOPIC EXAMINATION

The hematocrit and red cell count document the presence of a hemorrhagic effusion, but are of limited value for differential diagnosis. Total leukocyte counts over 10,000/μL suggest bacterial, tuberculous, or malignant pericarditis; however, low counts may be encountered in these conditions, limiting the value of this measurement (Agner, 1979). Although formal leukocyte differentials add little diagnostic information, a stained smear should always be examined.

Cytologic identification of malignant cells is usually not difficult. Metastatic carcinomas of the lung and breast are most frequently observed in malignant pericardial effusion. Cytology has a sensitivity of 95% and a specificity of 100% (Meyers, 1997).

CHEMICAL ANALYSIS

Chemical parameters for the diagnosis of pericardial effusions have not been studied to the same extent as in other body fluids. Although pericardial effusions are very similar to pleural fluids, routine application of these tests requires additional studies to fully appreciate their diagnostic importance.

Protein

A value greater than 3.0 g/dL has a sensitivity of 97% for exudative effusions, but a specificity of only 22%, which significantly limits its usefulness. Thus, total protein has no discriminating power in pericardial diagnosis (Meyers, 1997).

Glucose

Pericardial glucose levels less than 60 mg/dL have a diagnostic accuracy of only 36% in identifying pericardial exudates (Meyers, 1997). Values less than 40 mg/dL (<2.22 mmol/L) are common in bacterial, tuberculous, rheumatic, or malignant effusions.

pH

Pericardial fluid pH may be markedly decreased (<7.10) in rheumatic or purulent pericarditis. Malignancy, uremia, tuberculosis, and idiopathic disorders may have moderate decreases in the range of 7.20–7.30 (Kindig, 1983).

Lipids

Separation of true chylous from pseudochylous effusions may be facilitated by triglyceride and cholesterol measurements, as well as by lipoprotein electrophoresis for chylomicrons (see Table 29-20). See Lipids section in Pleural Fluids for further details on the diagnosis of chylous effusions.

Enzymes

A pericardial fluid LD level greater than 200 U/L has been suggested as a cutoff for pericardial exudates (Burgess, 2002a). Moreover, the measurement of LD and creatine kinase in postmortem pericardial fluid within 48 hours of death may be useful in establishing acute myocardial injury in cases where such injury is suspected but cannot be established by the usual histologic methods (Luna, 1982; Stewart, 1984). Pericardial fluid levels of CK-MB, myoglobin, and troponin I in postmortem pericardial fluid are significantly increased in patients with myocardial injury (Perez-Carceles, 2004).

ADA activity is a useful adjunctive test for tuberculous pericarditis in suspicious cases with negative acid-fast stains. The median ADA level in tuberculous pericarditis is significantly higher than in other pathologic effusions (Burgess, 2002b). Using a cutoff of 30 U/L, the sensitivity was 94%, specificity 68%, and positive predictive value 80%. Using a cutoff of 40 U/L, the sensitivity and specificity were 93% and 97%, respectively (Koh, 1994).

Interferon-γ

Increased IFN-γ levels have been reported in tuberculous serous effusions, including tuberculous pericarditis (Burgess, 2002b). Here, the IFN-γ level was greater than 1000 pg/L, which was significantly higher than in effusions from other pathologic conditions. A cutoff value of 200 pg/L resulted in a sensitivity and specificity of 100% for the diagnosis of tuberculous pericarditis.

Polymerase Chain Reaction

PCR is a sensitive technique and may be more specific than adenosine deaminase in the diagnosis of tuberculous pericarditis (Lee, 2002). However, a negative test does not rule out tuberculous pericarditis because some pericardial fluids from patients with large tuberculous effusions may not contain *M. tuberculosis*.

IMMUNOLOGIC STUDIES

A negative ANA test makes the diagnosis of lupus serositis highly unlikely. Conversely, high ANA titers in pericardial effusions lack specificity, even when they are as high as 1:5120 (Leventhal, 1990; Wang, 2000). If a high ANA titer is unexplained, malignancy should be considered.

MICROBIOLOGICAL EXAMINATION

The sensitivity of the Gram stain and culture for bacterial pericarditis is similar to other serous body fluids (i.e., about 50% and 80%, respectively). Important aerobic bacteria include *S. aureus*, *S. pneumoniae*, *S. pyogenes*, and gram-negative bacilli. Although infectious pericarditis due to anaerobic bacteria may be encountered rarely, the bacteria sometimes are not recognized because of inconsistent methods used for their isolation and identification (Brook, 2002). For this reason, proper laboratory technique is of particular importance when infection with an anaerobic organism is suspected. The major anaerobic organisms are the *Bacteroides fragilis* group, anaerobic streptococci, *Clostridium* species, *Fusobacterium* species, and *Bifidobacterium* species.

Identification of a specific etiologic agent in viral pericarditis is difficult because the viruses (e.g., coxsackieviruses, influenza virus, mumps) are rarely isolated from pericardial fluid. Obtaining acute and convalescent sera for antibody response to suspected viral pathogens may help support the diagnosis (Bellinger, 1987). Viral infection probably accounts for most idiopathic HIV-associated pericardial effusions.

The sensitivity of acid-fast stains and culture for tuberculous pericarditis is about 50% (Agner, 1979). PCR is a sensitive technique and may be more specific than the use of adenosine deaminase in the diagnosis of tuberculous pericarditis (Lee, 2002). However, a negative test does not exclude the diagnosis of tuberculous pericarditis.

PERITONEAL FLUID

Ascites is the pathologic accumulation of excess fluid in the peritoneal cavity. Up to 50 mL of fluid is normally present in this mesothelial-lined space. As with pleural and pericardial fluids, it is produced as an ultrafiltrate of plasma dependent on vascular permeability and on hydrostatic and oncotic Starling forces.

TRANSUDATES AND EXUDATES

Common causes of peritoneal effusion are listed in Table 29-23. The laboratory criteria for classifying ascitic fluid as a transudate or an exudate are not as well defined as they are for pleural and pericardial fluids. For example, infected or malignancy-related samples are not uncommonly reported with protein concentrations in the transudative range (i.e., <3.0 g/dL), and many patients with cirrhotic or heart failure ascites have protein values in the exudative range (>3.0 g/dL) (Runyon, 1992).

TABLE 29-23
Causes of Peritoneal Effusions

Transudates: Increased Hydrostatic Pressure or Decreased Plasma Oncotic Pressure
Congestive heart failure
Hepatic cirrhosis
Hypoproteinemia (e.g., nephrotic syndrome)
Exudates: Increased Capillary Permeability or Decreased Lymphatic Resorption
Infections
Primary bacterial peritonitis
Secondary bacterial peritonitis (e.g., appendicitis, bowel rupture)
Tuberculosis
Neoplasms
Hepatoma
Lymphoma
Mesothelioma
Metastatic carcinoma
Ovarian carcinoma
Prostate cancer
Trauma
Pancreatitis
Bile peritonitis (e.g., ruptured gallbladder)
Chylous Effusion
Damage to or obstruction of thoracic duct (e.g., trauma, lymphoma, carcinoma, tuberculosis and other granulomas [e.g., sarcoidosis, histoplasmosis], parasitic infestation)

The **serum–ascites albumin gradient,** defined as the serum albumin concentration minus the ascitic fluid albumin concentration, is widely considered as the most reliable method to differentiate peritoneal transudates from exudates (Runyon, 1992). Ascites caused by portal hypertension has a gradient of at least 1.1 g/dL (>11 g/L; transudate), whereas ascites produced by other causes has a gradient less than 1.1 g/dL (exudate) (Runyon, 1992). Indeed, the diagnostic accuracy was 98% for the serum–ascites albumin gradient compared with only 52%–80% for four other markers: Ascitic fluid total protein; ascites/serum total protein ratio; ascitic fluid LD concentration; and ascites/serum LD ratio (Akriviadis, 1996).

An ascitic fluid/serum bilirubin ratio of 0.6 or greater is also significantly associated with exudates (Elis, 1998). Indeed, the accuracies of the bilirubin ratio, the serum–ascites albumin gradient, and Light's criteria were 81.5%, 84%, and 80.2%, respectively. Others suggested that if the ascitic fluid LD is >130 U/L and the ascitic fluid/serum total protein ratio is >0.4, the fluid should be regarded as an exudate (Paramothayan, 2002).

Although the serum–ascites albumin gradient is probably the best single method to differentiate an ascitic exudate from a transudate, other methods compare favorably. Nevertheless, no ideal biochemical markers allow complete discrimination between ascitic fluid exudates and transudates.

SPECIMEN COLLECTION

Paracentesis

Diagnostic paracentesis is performed in most patients with new ascites, or if there is a change in the clinical picture of a patient with ascites, such as rapid fluid accumulation or fever development. A minimum of 30 mL is needed for complete evaluation. If possible, at least 100 mL should be provided for cytologic examination. Samples for cell counts should be placed in an EDTA-anticoagulated venipuncture tube. Culture specimens should include blood culture bottles that have been inoculated at the bedside with ascitic fluid (10 mL per culture bottle).

Diagnostic Peritoneal Lavage

This procedure is no longer recommended as a routine technique for the evaluation of abdominal trauma. Concerns of oversensitivity and nonspecificity, and improvements in noninvasive diagnostic procedures such as computed tomography and ultrasound, have limited its common use to (1) rapid screening for significant abdominal hemorrhage, and (2) evaluation of hollow viscous injuries.

A catheter is placed through a small incision into the abdominal cavity. If less than 15 mL of gross blood can be aspirated, diagnostic peritoneal lavage (DPL) is performed by infusing 1.0 L of saline or Ringer's solution (20 mg/kg in children) and retrieving the fluid by gravity drainage. At least 600 mL should be recovered to avoid falsely low counts (Sullivan, 1997). The catheter is sometimes left in place so that DPL may be repeated in 2–3 hours if initial results are negative or indeterminate.

Commonly accepted criteria for DPL interpretation after trauma are shown in Table 29-24. The positive predictive value is only 23% for an isolated (no other abnormal criteria) leukocyte count of 500/µL or greater (Soyka, 1990).

The conventional DPL criteria may be unreliable in detecting hollow viscous injury when blood is present from a simultaneous solid organ injury not requiring surgical repair, resulting in unnecessary exploratory laparotomies. Suggested modifications of DPL criteria to adjust for this source of bleeding include either of the following: (1) WBC count greater than or equal to RBC count divided by 150, where RBC is $10 \times 10^4/mm^3$ or greater (Otomo, 1998); or (2) cell count ratio greater than 1.0 (Fang, 1998). The cell count ratio is defined as the ratio between WBC and RBC counts in the lavage fluid divided by the WBC/RBC ratio in the peripheral blood. These new criteria have a reported specificity of 97% for hollow organ injury, especially if DPL is performed at least 3 hours following injury.

Other applications of DPL include the evaluation of patients with suspected acute peritonitis or pancreatitis. For example, a WBC count in the lavage fluid of 200 cells/mm^3 is associated with a 99% probability of acute peritonitis (Larson, 1992).

Peritoneal Dialysis

Dialysate fluid from renal patients undergoing chronic ambulatory peritoneal dialysis should be submitted to the laboratory to check for infection.

TABLE 29-24
Criteria for Evaluation of Peritoneal Lavage

Positive result	
	Aspiration of >15 mL gross blood on catheter placement
	Grossly bloody lavage fluid
	RBC >100,000/μL after blunt trauma
	RBC >50,000/μL after penetrating trauma
	WBC >500/μL
	Amylase >110 U/dL
Indeterminate result	
	Small amount of gross blood on catheter placement
	RBC 50,000–100,000/μL after blunt trauma
	RBC 1000–50,000/μL after penetrating trauma
	WBC 100–500/μL
Negative result	
	RBC <50,000/μL after blunt trauma
	RBC <1000/μL after penetrating trauma
	WBC <100/μL

Modified from Feied CF. Diagnostic peritoneal lavage. Postgrad Med 1989;85:40, with permission.
RBC, Red blood cells; *WBC,* white blood cells.

Peritoneal Washings

This procedure is performed intraoperatively to document early intraabdominal spread of gynecologic and gastric carcinomas. Samples are generally sent for cytologic examination only.

RECOMMENDED TESTS

The most important tests for the evaluation of ascitic fluid are listed in Table 29-25. Relative importance varies depending on the type of sample and the clinical findings. For example, RBC and WBC counts are more important than cytology or the serum–ascites albumin gradient in the evaluation of abdominal effects of trauma. Gross examination provides immediate information in the clinical and laboratory triage.

GROSS EXAMINATION

Whereas transudates are generally pale yellow and clear, exudates are cloudy or turbid because of the presence of leukocytes, tumor cells, or increased protein levels. The presence of food particles, foreign material, or green-yellow bile staining in a DPL specimen suggests perforation of the gastrointestinal or biliary tract. Acute pancreatitis and cholecystitis may also cause greenish discoloration.

Blood-tinged or grossly bloody fluid must be distinguished from a traumatic tap in which the blood usually clears with continued paracentesis. As little as 15 mL of blood per liter of fluid produces a bright red opaque color such that newsprint cannot be read through the lavage tubing. In most cases, the ability to read newsprint through the tubing results in a negative DPL. Opaque specimens require cell counts because newsprint readability is lost well below the 100,000 RBCs/μL criterion for a positive DPL (Bellows, 1998). Bloody ascites is also seen in malignancy and tuberculosis.

TABLE 29-25
Recommended Tests in Peritoneal Effusion

Useful in most patients	
	Gross examination
	Cytology
	Stains and culture for microorganisms
	Serum–ascites albumin concentration gradient
Useful in selected disorders	
	Total leukocyte and differential cell counts
	RBC count (lavage)
	Bilirubin
	Creatinine/urea nitrogen
	Enzymes (ADA, ALP, amylase, LD, telomerase)
	Lactate
	Cholesterol (malignant ascites)
	Fibronectin
	Tumor markers (CEA, PSA, CA 19-9, CA 15-3, CA-125)
	Immunocytology/flow cytometry
	Tuberculostearic acid

Modified from Kjeldsberg CR, Knight JA. Body fluids: laboratory examination of amniotic, cerebrospinal, seminal, serous and synovial fluids. 3rd ed. Chicago: © American Society for Clinical Pathology; 1993, with permission.
ADA, Adenosine deaminase; *ALP,* alkaline phosphatase; *CEA,* carcinoembryonic antigen; *LD,* lactate dehydrogenase; *PSA,* prostate-specific antigen; *RBC,* red blood cell.

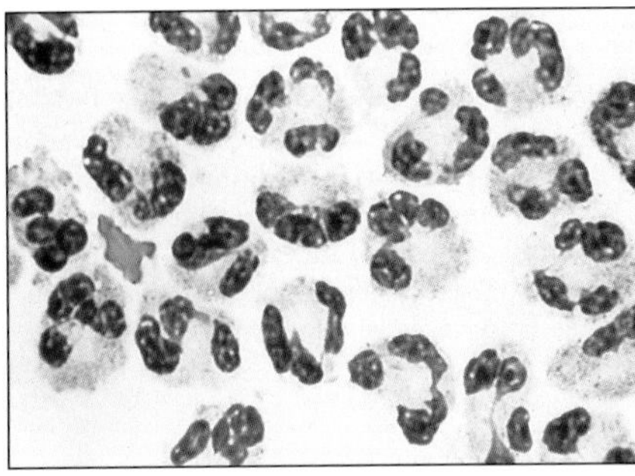

Figure 29-20 Neutrophils in a patient with bacterial peritonitis.

Milky fluid that does not clear with centrifugation suggests a chylous or pseudochylous effusion. True chylous peritoneal effusions are significantly less common than chylous pleural fluids. They are caused by disruption or blockage of lymphatic flow by trauma, lymphoma, carcinoma, tuberculosis, other granulomatous diseases (e.g., sarcoidosis), hepatic cirrhosis, adhesions, or parasitic infestation. Differentiation of true chylous and pseudochylous effusions is discussed under Pleural Fluid, Gross Examination.

MICROSCOPIC EXAMINATION

The total leukocyte count is useful in distinguishing ascites due to uncomplicated cirrhosis from spontaneous bacterial peritonitis (SBP), which is caused by migration of bacteria from the intestine into the ascitic fluid. Approximately 90% of patients with SBP will have leukocyte counts greater than 500/μL, more than 50% of which are neutrophils (Fig. 29-20) (Runyon, 1984; Stewart, 1986).

The ascitic fluid total neutrophil count is the preferred method for the diagnosis of SBP. Cutoff values of 250 and 500 neutrophils/μL have been recommended, with a diagnostic accuracy of about 94% for 500 neutrophils/μL and about 90% for 250 neutrophils/μL (Stassen, 1986; Albillos, 1990).

Cell counts, total protein, and albumin gradient values vary with fluid shifts associated with ascites formation and resolution. For example, diuresis may cause the WBC count to increase from 300/μL–1000/μL or more. When obtained by DPL, a leukocyte count of 200/μL or more is reported to be associated with a 99% probability of acute peritonitis (Alverdy, 1988; Larson, 1992).

Eosinophilia (>10%) is most commonly associated with the chronic inflammatory process associated with chronic peritoneal dialysis. It has also been reported in congestive heart failure, vasculitis, lymphoma, and ruptured hydatid cyst.

Cytology has an overall sensitivity of 40%–65% for malignant ascites. Peritoneal carcinomatosis accounts for only about two thirds of malignant effusions; however, cytology has a sensitivity of over 95% when confined to these cases (Runyon, 1988). Liquid-based thin-layer preparations of peritoneal effusions and pelvic washings have been shown to be superior to standard cytologic perparations in the detection of carcinoma (Moriarity, 2008). Immunocytochemical stains are useful in characterizing atypical cells in equivocal cases.

CHEMICAL ANALYSIS

Protein

The serum–ascites albumin gradient is superior to total protein content in differentiating cirrhosis from other causes of peritoneal effusion (Runyon, 1992). Spontaneous bacterial peritonitis is commonly associated with low total protein (<3.0 g/dL) and a high serum–ascites albumin gradient (>1.1 g/dL), making total protein measurements of little value in this disorder. Extracellular fluid shifts associated with ascites formation and resorption also cause variations in protein content.

Glucose

Early reports indicated that peritoneal fluid glucose levels of 50 mg/dL or less are present in 30%–60% of cases of tuberculous peritonitis and in about 50% of patients with abdominal carcinomatosis (Polak, 1973; Brown, 1976). However, a more recent study found decreased glucose levels in most cases of tuberculous ascites (Bansal, 1998). Nevertheless, glucose measurements are of little value because the sensitivity and specificity are generally too low to be of practical value.

Enzymes

Amylase activity in normal peritoneal fluid is similar to plasma levels. A level greater than three times the plasma value is good evidence of pancreas-related ascites, including acute pancreatitis and pancreatic pseudocyst (Runyon, 1987a). Amylase is not recommended in the routine evaluation of ascites, however, because the prevalence of pancreatic ascites is low. Retrospective amylase measurement on a stored specimen is indicated if initial studies are not diagnostic. However, amylase levels in peritoneal lavage fluid may be valuable in patients following blunt and penetrating abdominal trauma (McAnena, 1991). Here, amylase levels greater than or equal to 20 U/L had a sensitivity of 87%, a specificity of 75%, and a positive predictive value of 46% for significant intraabdominal injury. In these cases, laparotomy should be considered. Gastroduodenal perforation, acute mesenteric vein thrombosis, intestinal strangulation, or necrosis may also produce elevated amylase levels. Although various nonpancreatic malignancies may rarely produce amylase elevations, isoenzyme evaluation usually identifies the salivary isoform in these latter cases (Kosches, 1989).

Elevated **alkaline phosphatase** (ALP) levels greater than 10 U/L in diagnostic peritoneal lavage fluid are very useful in predicting hollow visceral injury in patients who would otherwise not undergo laparotomy (specificity 99.8%, sensitivity 94.7%) (Jaffin, 1993). Ascitic fluid ALP measurements may also be helpful in the differentiation of primary bacterial peritonitis from secondary bacterial peritonitis due to bowel perforation. Secondary peritonitis has significantly higher mean ALP levels than SBP. Thus, ALP levels >240 U/L were present in 92% of patients with secondary peritonitis versus 12% for SBP (Wu, 2001). The sensitivity and specificity for differentiating secondary peritonitis from SBP were 92% and 88%, respectively.

LD activity is often increased in malignant effusions (Gerbes, 1991). An ascitic fluid/serum LD ratio greater than 0.6 has a reported sensitivity of 80% (Boyer, 1978). Combined measurement of ascitic fluid LD and cholesterol totally discriminated peritoneal carcinomatosis from cirrhosis and hepatocarcinoma-related ascites (Castaldo, 1994; Halperin, 1999). Although both serum and peritoneal fluid LD levels are significantly higher in patients with ovarian cancer than in those with benign ovarian tumors or other gynecologic malignancies, peritoneal fluid LD has higher diagnostic sensitivity (87%) and diagnostic accuracy (90%) than serum LD (60% and 77%, respectively) (Schneider, 1997). LD has also been used for the early diagnosis of spontaneous bacterial peritonitis, in which it has a diagnostic accuracy of about 74% using an ascitic fluid/serum ratio cutoff of 0.4 (Lee, 1987).

The presence of **telomerase** is a specific discriminatory marker in malignant ascites (Tangkijvanich, 1999). Thus, telomerase activity was detected in 81% of malignant peritoneal effusions with a sensitivity of 76% and a specificity of 95.7%.

ADA is commonly used in endemic areas to identify patients with tuberculous peritonitis (Burgess, 2001). Using receiver operating characteristic curves and a cutoff value of 30 U/L, the sensitivity and specificity were 94% and 92%, respectively. Using a cutoff value of 33 U/L, the sensitivity, specificity, positive and negative predictive values, and overall diagnostic accuracy for diagnosing tuberculous peritonitis were 100%, 96.6%, 95%, 100%, and 98%, respectively (Dwivedi, 1990).

Fibronectin

Using a cutoff value of 85 μg/mL (85 mg/L), fibronectin was more reliable in differentiating malignant from sterile ascites (diagnostic accuracy, 79%) than were total protein, LD, γ-glutamyltransferase, pH, amylase, triglycerides, leukocyte count, and cytologic examination (Colli, 1986). In a subsequent study using a cutoff of 94.6 μg/mL, the sensitivity, specificity, positive accuracy, negative accuracy, and overall diagnostic accuracy in the diagnosis of malignant ascites were 100%, 95%, 93.8%, 100%, and 97.1%, respectively (Sood, 1997).

Lactate

Ascitic fluid lactate has been used with pH measurements to differentiate SBP from uncomplicated ascites. Sensitivity and specificity are approximately 90% using a cutoff of 40 mg/dL (4.44 mmol/L), with a positive predictive value of 62% (Stassen, 1986). Although not as accurate as leukocyte counts, the high specificity of lactate in hepatic ascites suggests that it has some value in the diagnosis of SBP in otherwise equivocal cases. Malignant and tuberculous ascites are also associated with elevated lactate levels.

Patients with hollow viscous perforation, gangrenous intestine, peritonitis, or intraabdominal abscess have a peritoneal fluid minus plasma lactate level of at least 13.5 mg/dL (1.5 mmol/L), which reportedly separates these patients completely from those with other conditions producing acute abdominal problems (DeLaurier, 1994). Additional studies are necessary to determine the utility of measuring ascitic fluid lactate in surgical decision making.

Creatinine and Urea

Measurement of creatinine and urea nitrogen is useful to differentiate between peritoneal fluid and urine. Elevated peritoneal fluid urea nitrogen and creatinine, in association with elevated serum urea but normal serum creatinine (due to back-diffusion of urea), suggest urinary bladder rupture.

Bilirubin

The mean (±SD) ascitic fluid bilirubin concentration in various types of ascites was reported as 0.7 ± 0.8 mg/dL, and the mean ascitic fluid/serum bilirubin ratio was 0.38 ± 0.44 (Runyon, 1987b). An ascitic fluid bilirubin greater than 6.0 mg/dL and an ascitic fluid/serum bilirubin ratio over 1.0 suggest choleperitoneum from a ruptured gallbladder. A ratio of 0.6 or greater has been advocated as an additional marker for an exudative process, although its accuracy is not as high as that of the serum–ascites albumin gradient (Elis, 1998).

pH

Ascitic fluid pH may be helpful in the diagnosis of SBP in patients with cirrhotic ascites, especially if it is used in conjunction with the leukocyte count (Attali, 1986; Stassen, 1986). A pH less than 7.32 or a blood–ascitic fluid pH difference of more than 0.1 has a reported sensitivity and specificity of about 90% for SBP, with the pH differential being slightly more accurate. Peritoneal fluid pH appears useless in detecting SBP, however, in the absence of neutrophils (Runyon, 1991). Patients with an ascitic fluid pH of less than 7.15 have a poor prognosis (Attali, 1986). Low pH is also found in patients with malignant and pancreatic ascites and tuberculous peritonitis.

Cholesterol

The ascitic fluid cholesterol level is a moderately useful index in separating malignant ascites (>45–48 mg/dL) from cirrhotic ascites (Mortensen, 1988; Castaldo, 1994). The sensitivity and specificity average just over 90% using a cutoff value of 45–48 mg/dL (1.2 mmol/L). Thus, using a cutoff value of 48 mg/dL, the sensitivity, specificity, positive and negative predictive value, and overall diagnostic accuracy for differentiating malignant from nonmalignant ascites were reported as 96.5%, 96.6%, 93.3%, 98.3%, and 96.6%, respectively (Garg, 1993).

Interleukin-8

Interleukin-8, a cytokine produced by a variety of cells in response to stimuli such as bacterial lipopolysaccharide, is significantly higher in spontaneous bacterial peritonitis compared with sterile ascites (Martinez-Bru, 1999). Using a cutoff value of 100 ng/L, the sensitivity and specificity were both 100% in cirrhotic patients.

Tuberculostearic Acid (10-Methyloctadecanoic Acid)

As noted in the Pleural Fluid section, TSA was detected in pleural fluid in 75% of patients with pulmonary tuberculosis using gas chromatography–mass spectroscopy (Muranishi, 1990). Using quantitative chemical ionization gas chromatography–mass spectrometry, the measurement of TSA is a valuable technique to identify tuberculous peritonitis, as well as tuberculous meningitis (spinal fluid) and pneumonia (pleural fluid) (Brooks, 1998).

Tumor Markers

Because of their reportedly low sensitivity and specificity, the measurement of tumor markers is generally considered to be of little value. They are often useful, however, in selected cases, such as in following a patient's response to therapy and in the early detection of tumor recurrence. They may also be very useful in cases where cytology is negative but suspicion of malignant ascites is high. Indeed, the poor sensitivity of cytologic examinations is disappointing. They were positive in only 40% (35 of 89 patients) of malignant cases, while tumor markers were positive in 80% (Cascinu, 1997). Moreover, excluding small cell lung and renal cancers, for which specific tumor markers are lacking, tumor markers (i.e., CEA, CA 19-9, CA 15-3, PSA) in ascitic fluid for other carcinomas were positive in 97% of cases. These tumor markers, as well as α-fetoprotein, were also found to be very specific (over 90%) for serous fluid malignancies, although their sensitivities were low (19%–38%) (Sari, 2001). The measurement of **PSA** may also be a valuable marker for the diagnosis of malignant effusions due to prostate cancer (Appalaneni, 2004).

CEA has a sensitivity of only 40%–50% and a specificity of about 90% using a cutoff value of 3.0 ng/mL (Mezger, 1988). Using a 5-mg/mL cutoff, the specificity is about 97% (Gulyas, 2001). Elevated CEA levels in peritoneal washings suggest a poor prognosis in gastric carcinoma (Irinoda, 1998).

Ascitic fluid **CA-125** is elevated to some degree in a variety of nonmalignant conditions. Indeed, cardiovascular and chronic liver disease may be the most frequent diagnoses in patients with increased CA-125 levels (Miralles, 2003), thereby supporting the general opinion that CA-125 lacks adequate specificity as a marker for malignancy. However, extremely high levels are more likely to be caused by epithelial carcinomas of the ovary, fallopian tubes, or endometrium.

The sensitivity for ovarian carcinoma depends on the tumor's stage (range, 40%–95%) and histologic subtype (mucinous adenocarcinomas have lower values) (Molina, 1998).

DNA ploidy analysis by flow cytometry or image analysis might provide useful complementary diagnostic information in cases with equivocal cytology results when the malignant cells carry an aneuploid karyotype. Image analysis appears to be more practical than flow cytometry when the tumor cells are scarce (Rijken, 1991).

MICROBIOLOGICAL EXAMINATION

Primary peritonitis occurs at any age and is seen in children with nephrotic syndrome and in adults with cirrhotic liver disease. Spontaneous bacterial peritonitis occurs in patients with ascites in the absence of recognized secondary causes such as bowel perforation or intraabdominal abscess. The bacteria in SBP are most often normal intestinal flora, and more than 92% are monomicrobial. Aerobic gram-negative bacilli (e.g., *E. coli, Klebsiella pneumoniae*) are responsible for two thirds or more of all cases (Gilbert, 1995), followed by *S. pneumoniae*, *Enterococcus* spp., and, rarely, anaerobes. The Gram stain has a sensitivity of 25% in SBP (Lee, 1987), and routine cultures are positive in only about 50% of cases (Castellote, 1990). Inoculation of blood culture bottles at the bedside and concentration of large volumes of fluid can improve sensitivity, but up to 35% of infected patients may still have negative ascitic fluid cultures (Marshall, 1988). Use of resin-containing blood culture bottles may improve the isolation of certain bacteria in partially treated patients.

Ascitic fluid total neutrophil count is the preferred method for the diagnosis of SBP (see under Microscopic Examination). However, as noted earlier, in difficult cases, several analytes may be useful in differentiating SBP from secondary bacterial or tuberculous peritonitis. More recently, PCR has been successfully used in the detection of bacterial DNA in culture-negative ascitic fluid (Such, 2002).

The sensitivity of acid-fast stains for *M. tuberculosis* is no more than 20%–30%, and cultures have a sensitivity of only 50%–70% (Reimer, 1985). Application of PCR to detect *M. tuberculosis* DNA has been studied, but a negative result does not exclude the diagnosis (Schwake, 2003). In a patient with a high clinical suspicion for tuberculous peritonitis, laparoscopic examination with biopsy may be indicated.

ALTERNATIVE SPECIMENS

SALIVA

Saliva is generally easily collected by noninvasive means, and so its acquisition is well accepted by patients. Because it is a filtrate of plasma, saliva has concentrations of some small molecules that are in equilibrium with the free (unbound) active fractions of those substances in plasma. This property has been especially useful for measuring free cortisol, which is the physiologically important fraction that reflects the secretion rate of cortisol and so is important for diagnosis. Salivary cortisol measurements have been used to assess adrenal function in critically ill subjects (Arafah, 2007) and in those with Cushing's syndrome and adrenal insufficiency (Raff, 2009), with late-night (or midnight) salivary cortisol being an effective screening test for Cushing's syndrome (Raff, 1998). Unfortunately, salivary concentrations of several other steroid hormones are not reliable measures of plasma free levels because of rapid fluctuations in their salivary concentrations (e.g., estradiol, progesterone, testosterone, dehydroepiandrosterone, aldosterone) (Wood, 2009).

Saliva also contains some antibody molecules that apparently derive from plasma. Thus measurements are sometime performed on saliva to detect antibodies against infectious agents in circumstances where collection of saliva is much more convenient or acceptable to patients. Testing of saliva for antibodies against human immunodeficiency virus has been practiced widely in sexually transmitted disease clinics, although episodes of false-positive results have diminished confidence in these point-of-care tests (MMWR, 2008).

Genetic testing requires DNA from the patient that can be obtained conveniently from leukocytes in blood specimens, or even more conveniently from buccal cells in saliva or from swabs of the interior of the mouth.

Drug testing has also been done in saliva to provide evidence of ingestion of illicit substances. Although drugs such as amphetamines, cocaine, and opioids are present in oral fluid at concentrations similar to those in plasma, local absorption of these drugs in the mouth can increase their concentration in saliva after use (Drummer, 2006).

HAIR AND NAILS

Drug testing has time limitations of detection in blood for periods of minutes to hours after ingestion. The need to detect illicit drug use over longer periods of time has prompted analysis of other body sources. Concentrations of drugs in saliva follow the same time course as blood of minutes to hours after ingestion. Detection in urine can be as soon as minutes up to many days after drug use. Sweat concentrations also rise in minutes but may persist for weeks. True long-term detection is possible in hair and nails, where drugs of abuse can be detected days to even years after ingestion. Although numerous companies offer drug testing of hair or nail specimens, there has not been official adoption of this strategy by government agencies, largely because of issues of uncertainty as to whether the substances detected from hair or nail specimens were actually "in" the hair following ingestion and incorporation into that tissue, or whether the detected drug was simply "on" the surface of the specimen because of incidental contact that did not involve ingestion (Curtis, 2008).

TISSUE ASPIRATES

Breast nipple aspirate fluid can be obtained by noninvasive means such as massage or with automated collection devices to yield material suitable for cytologic examination for early detection of breast cancer. This new collection approach may lead to other effective applications of cancer detection using modalities such as proteomics or still to be discovered biomarkers (Alexander, 2004).

Fine-needle aspiration for cytologic examination is frequently used to evaluate head and neck masses. Rapid identification of a mass of parathyroid tissue has been done by measuring parathyroid hormone (PTH) in saline, into which the needle aspirate is flushed (Conrad, 2006). This method was shown to be 99% accurate for diagnosis of parathyroid tissue because the measured values of PTH are orders of magnitude higher in parathyroid aspirates than in those from other tissues such as thyroid, adipose, or lymphatic. This type of specimen is truly unusual and would not likely be included in any manufacturer's claims for assay performance; however, this practice is well recognized by endocrine surgeons who now consider it a standard of practice.

BILLING FOR TESTS IN NONSTANDARD SPECIMENS

Although considerations of medical necessity provide strong motivation for performing tests in unusual specimen types to provide unique information that could not be obtained by other means, reporting of the results and subsequent billing may lead to confusion. Most laboratory computer systems have strictly defined specimen types, such as blood, serum, urine, and CSF. When dealing with an unusual specimen type that is not individually coded or recognized in a computer system, laboratories should take care not to enter these results as though they were serum or other commonly tested fluid. For both medical needs and reimbursement, some disclaimer should be included to indicate the specimen type, so that it is not confused with serum or other conventional fluid.

Chemical Measurements in Body Fluids

Plasma, serum, cerebrospinal fluid, and urine are standard fluids that are often submitted for chemical analysis. Manufacturers generally provide product claims for their assays in one or more of these body fluids, but they have not established assay behavior in other specimen types such as pleural fluid, peritoneal fluid, synovial fluid, and other accumulations of abnormal fluids such as drainage or lavage fluids. These types of fluids are not normally present in health but rather can form as the result of various pathologic processes, such as hemodynamic imbalance, infection, inflammation, malignancy, or other organ dysfunction. Consequently, the composition of these fluids can range widely, thereby leading to unpredictable effects on laboratory measurements. Matrix effects from variations in protein concentration can alter fluid surface tension, viscosity, and miscibility in a reaction mixture. All of these variations potentially might cause differences in measurements because of errors in pipetting fixed volumes or in speed and completeness of mixing with reagents in an assay. Other constituents present in these pathologic fluids (e.g., hyaluronic acid in synovial fluid) but not in serum also have the potential to alter measurements in assays intended for use in serum. This potential for erroneous measurements in body fluids due to matrix effects should be recognized when such requests for analysis are received.

A second issue concerning chemical measurements in pathologic fluids is what reference range to use for comparison in an interpretive report. Because abnormal fluid accumulations do not exist in a state of health, they cannot, of course, be collected from a normal healthy population to establish reference ranges.

These two issues of potential interferences and lack of reference ranges for analysis of body fluids fly in the face of Clinical Laboratory Improvement Act requirements for assay validation. In fact, the lack of manufacturers' claims for body fluid testing might actually place a greater burden on a laboratory to validate these assays than for use in serum for which manufacturer claims are typically cleared by the U.S. Food and Drug Administration. Without such validation, measuring chemical constituents in body fluids could be considered an off-label use of commercial assays.

In recognition of these difficulties faced by laboratories, the Clinical and Laboratory Standards Institute (CLSI) has developed the document C49A, Analysis of Body Fluids in Clinical Chemistry, to provide guidance in this situation (CLSI, 2007). The specific recommendations from CLSI are as follows:

1. Review performance claims of the manufacturer for the possibility of extending a commercial assay to body fluids with special attention to accuracy, precision, analytic measurement range, reference interval (usually in comparison with simultaneous measurement in serum, in addition to the patient's body fluid), and interferences from substances in the body fluid.
2. Existing methods may be suitably modified for body fluid analysis when necessary to obtain medically relevant information. Matrix effects that could alter the accuracy of measurement must be recognized. Furthermore, lack of a reference range for the analyte in body fluids should be compensated for by interpretation of results in comparison with a simultaneously collected serum specimen.
3. The preconditions for using a routine assay for an alternate body fluid are that the measurement system in another specimen type (serum plasma, urine)
   a. Has acceptable test characteristics.
   b. Has a reference method by which to ascertain bias.
   c. Has calibrators and controls.
   d. External proficiency testing should be done whenever available.
4. Specimen collection of body fluid and its handling, processing, and storage should follow guidelines for specimens of plasma or serum collected for that measurement. Special attention should be directed to the possibility of interference from anticoagulants into which a body fluid might be collected (e.g., heparin, EDTA, citrate).
5. Unusual properties of a body fluid such as high viscosity should be given consideration if they have the potential to alter the analyte concentration in the final solution of the reaction mixture (e.g., inaccurate pipetting, inadequate mixing).
6. The presence of an interferent in a body fluid can be assessed by testing the fluid neat and at 1:2 and 1:4 dilutions. Recovery of similar concentrations suggests lack of interference. Low concentrations can be checked for interference by mixing with a routine (serum) sample with a high measurable value to measure recoverability.
7. Result reporting should include the measured value and the type of fluid analyzed plus a statement that accuracy might be affected by sample type, and that results should be interpreted in the clinical context. The laboratory is urged to contact ordering physicians to explain these limitations.

A key point is that to be useful clinically, measurements in body fluids need not necessarily be highly accurate but instead must be within a clinically acceptable range of the true value. This CLSI document provides an extensive list of applications of many different chemical analytes that may provide medically unique information about the source of a body fluid (e.g., creatinine in peritoneal fluid to evaluate urinary tract injury; amylase in peritoneal fluid to evaluate for pancreatitis; triglycerides in pleural fluid as an indicator of chylous effusion from lymphatic damage).

SELECTED REFERENCES

Clinical and Laboratory Standards Instititute (CLSI). Analysis of body fluids in clinical chemistry: approved guideline. Wayne, Pa.: Clinical and Laboratory Standards Institute; 2007. CLSI Document C49-A.

The purpose of this document is to provide guidance on acceptable practices of chemical analysis in body fluids for which extensive method validation is not feasible, but that have the potential to contribute valuable or even unique diagnostic information.

Clinical and Laboratory Standards Instititute (CLSI). Body fluid analysis for cellular composition: approved guideline. Wayne, Pa.: Clinical and Laboratory Standards Institute; 2006. CLSI Document H56-A.

The purpose of this document is to provide guidance on the examination of cellular components of body fluids.

Conrad DN, Olson JE, Hartwig HM, et al. A prospective evaluation of novel methods to intraoperatively distinguish parathyroid tissue utilizing a parathyroid hormone assay. J Surg Res 2006;133:38.

This article provides a useful method to prepare fine-needle tissue aspirates for measurement of parathyroid hormone to assist in the rapid evaluation of tissue masses.

Curtis J, Greenberg M. Screening for drugs of abuse: hair as an alternative matrix: a review for the medical toxicologist. Clin Toxicol 2008;46:22.

This review article provides excellent background information regarding the physiology and toxicology of drug testing in hair, along with a description of many of the legal and practical issues surrounding this application.

Freedman MS, Thompson EJ, Deisenhammer F, et al. Recommended standard of cerebrospinal fluid analysis in the diagnosis of multiple sclerosis: a consensus statement. Arch Neurol 2005;62:865.

This article is a consensus statement commissioned by the Consortium of Multiple Sclerosis Clinics that establishes the "minimum standard" for evaluation of CSF in patients suspected of having multiple sclerosis.

Irani DN, editor. Cerebrospinal fluid in clinical practice. Philadelphia: WB Saunders; 2009.

This book provides a description of findings in CSF with different neurologic disorders.

Kjeldsberg CR, Knight JA. Body fluids: laboratory examination of amniotic, cerebrospinal, seminal, serous, and synovial fluids. 3rd ed. Chicago: American Society of Clinical Pathologists Press; 1993.

This classic book has served as the ultimate reference book for body fluid analysis with abundant photomicrographs of abnormal findings.

Light RW. Pleural effusions. N Engl J Med 2002;346:1971.

This article provides a step-by-step approach to the clinical evaluation of pleural fluids and the use of laboratory examinations in that process.

Raff H. Utility of salivary cortisol measurements in Cushing's syndrome and adrenal insufficiency. J Clin Endocrinol Metab 2009;94:3647.

This article is a comprehensive and useful review of the clinical applications of cortisol measurements in saliva.

Runyon BA, Montano AA, Evangelos A, et al. The serum–ascites albumin gradient is superior to the exudate–transudate concept in the differential diagnosis of ascites. Ann Intern Med 1992;117:215.

This study demonstrates the effectiveness of using the gradient of albumin from serum to ascites fluid over other markers in the diagnosis of exudate versus transudate.

REFERENCES

Access the complete reference list online at http://www.expertconsult.com

PART 4

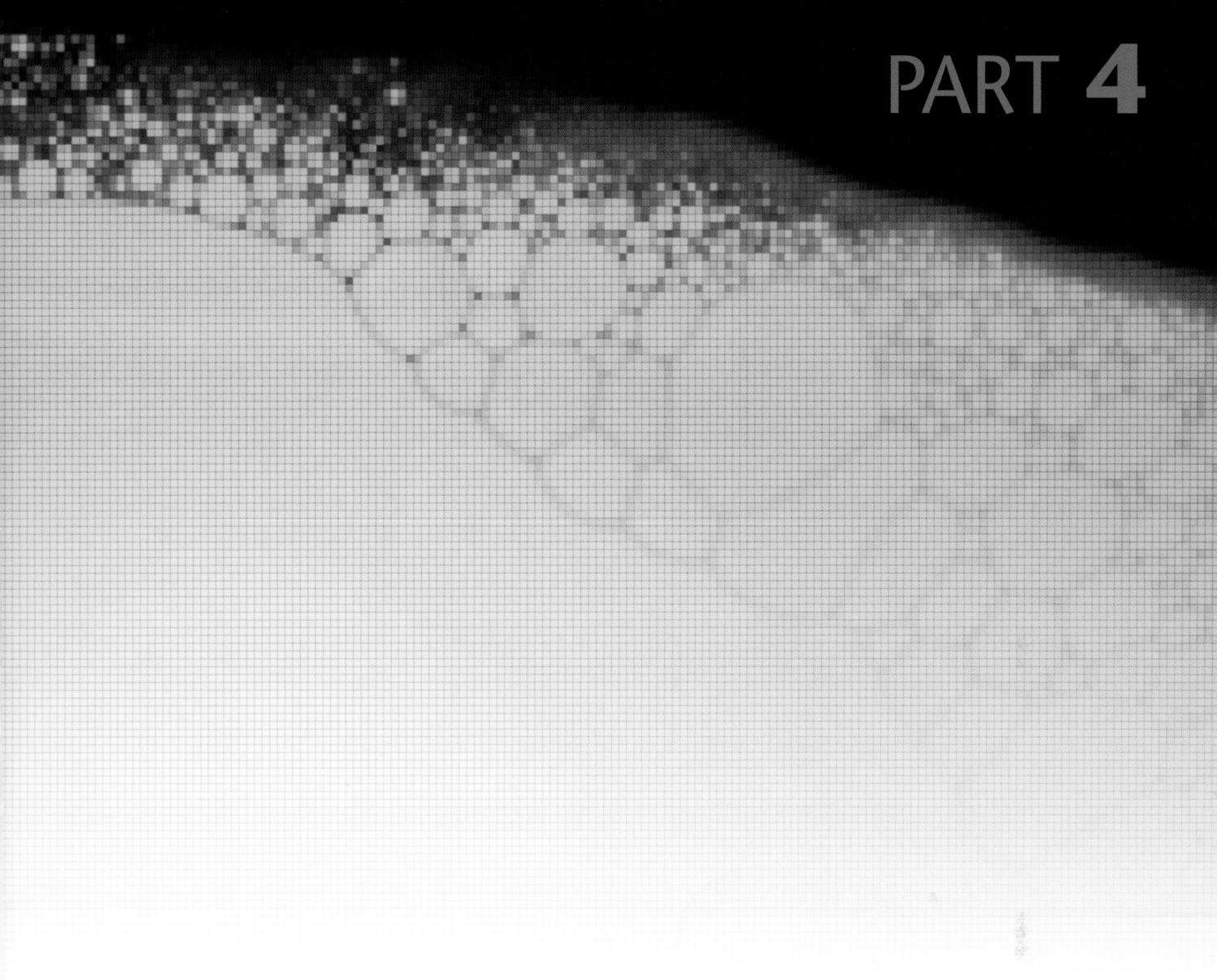

Hematology, Coagulation, and Transfusion Medicine

EDITED BY
Robert E. Hutchison
Richard A. McPherson
Katherine I. Schexneider

CHAPTER 30

BASIC EXAMINATION OF BLOOD AND BONE MARROW

Neerja Vajpayee, Susan S. Graham, Sylva Bem

PART 4

KEY POINTS

- Article I: Assessment of erythrocyte, leukocyte, and platelet counts from manual and automated particle counters is central to the diagnosis and management of hematologic disease.
- Article II: With few exceptions, manual methods have been replaced by automated hematology analyzers. The selection of analyzers is varied and voluminous enough to meet the needs of any hematology laboratory setting.
- Article III: Hematology automation combined with sophisticated algorithms for data interpretation has led to dramatic improvement in the utility of automated analyzers in patient care. Newer instrumentation has progressed far beyond the screening tool of the past.
- Article IV: Examination of peripheral blood with bone marrow smear/biopsy represents the cornerstone of hematologic diagnosis. The bone marrow examination provides a semiquantitative and qualitative assessment of the state of hematopoiesis, and aids in the diagnosis of several hereditary and acquired benign and malignant diseases.

Hematology includes the study of blood cells and coagulation. It encompasses analyses of the concentration, structure, and function of cells in blood; their precursors in the bone marrow; the chemical constituents of plasma or serum intimately linked with blood cell structure and function; and the function of platelets and proteins involved in blood coagulation. Advancement of molecular biological techniques and their increased use in hematology have led to detection of several genetic mutations underlying the altered structure and function of cells and proteins that may result in hematologic disease.

Hematology Principles and Procedures

HEMOGLOBIN

Hemoglobin (Hb), the main component of the red blood cell (RBC), is a conjugated protein that serves as the vehicle for the transportation of oxygen (O_2) and carbon dioxide (CO_2). When fully saturated, each gram of Hb holds 1.34 mL of O_2. The red cell mass of the adult contains approximately 600 g of Hb, capable of carrying 800 mL of O_2. A molecule of Hb consists of two pairs of polypeptide chains ("globins") and four prosthetic heme groups, each containing one atom of ferrous iron. Each heme group is precisely located in a pocket or fold of one of the polypeptide chains. Located near the surface of the molecule, the heme reversibly combines with one molecule of O_2 or CO_2. The main function of Hb is to transport O_2 from the lungs, where O_2 tension is high, to the tissues, where it is low. At an O_2 tension of 100 mm Hg in the pulmonary capillaries, 95%–98% of the Hb is combined with O_2. In the tissues, where O_2 tension may be as low as 20 mm Hg, the O_2 readily dissociates from Hb; in this instance, less than 30% of the O_2 would remain combined with Hb.

Reduced Hb is Hb with iron unassociated with O_2. When each heme group is associated with one molecule of O_2, the Hb is referred to as oxyhemoglobin (HbO_2). In both Hb and HbO_2, iron remains in the ferrous state. When iron is oxidized to the ferric state, methemoglobin (hemiglobin; Hi) is formed, and the molecule loses its capacity to carry O_2 or CO_2.

Anemia is a decrease to below normal Hb concentration, erythrocyte count, or hematocrit (Hct). It is a very common condition and is frequently a complication of other diseases. Clinical diagnosis of anemia or of high Hb based on estimation of the color of the skin and of visible mucous membranes is highly unreliable. The correct estimation of Hb is important and is one of the routine tests performed on practically every patient.

Hemoglobin Derivatives

Hemiglobin (Methemoglobin)

Methemoglobin (Hi) is a derivative of Hb in which the ferrous iron is oxidized to the ferric state, resulting in the inability of Hi to combine reversibly with O_2. The polypeptide chains are not altered. A normal individual has up to 1.5% methemoglobin. Methemoglobinemia will cause chocolate brown discoloration of blood, cyanosis, and functional "anemia" if present in high enough concentrations. Cyanosis becomes obvious at a concentration of about 1.5 g Hi/dL (i.e., 10% of Hb). Comparable degrees of cyanosis will be caused by 5 g Hb per deciliter of blood, 1.5 g Hi per deciliter of blood, and 0.5 g sulfhemoglobin (SHb) per deciliter of blood. The degree of cyanosis, however, is not necessarily correlated with the concentration of Hi. A small amount of Hi is always being formed but is reduced by enzyme systems within the erythrocyte. The most important is the NADH (reducing agent derived from nicotinamide adenine dinucleotide)-dependent methemoglobin reductase system (NADH-cytochrome-b_5 reductase). Others, which may function mainly as reserve systems, are ascorbic acid, reduced glutathione, and reduced nicotinamide adenine dinucleotide phosphate (NADPH)–methemoglobin reductase. The latter requires a natural cofactor or an auto-oxidizable dye such as methylene blue for activity.

Methemoglobinemia, an increased amount of Hi in the erythrocytes, may result from increased production of Hi or decreased NADH-cytochrome-b_5 reductase activity, and may be hereditary or acquired (Jaffé, 1989). The hereditary form is divided into two major categories. In the first, methemoglobinemia is due to a decrease in the capacity of the erythrocyte to reduce the Hi that is constantly being formed back to Hb. This is most often due to *NADH-cytochrome-b_5 reductase deficiency*, which is inherited as an autosomal recessive characteristic. The homozygote has methemoglobin levels of 10%–50% and is cyanotic. Only occasionally is polycythemia present as a compensating mechanism. Hi concentrations of 10%–25% may give no apparent symptoms; levels of 35%–50% result in mild symptoms, such as exertional dyspnea and headaches; and levels exceeding 70% are probably lethal. Therapy with ascorbic acid or methylthioninium chloride (methylene blue) in this form of hereditary methemoglobinemia will reduce the level of Hi, the latter apparently by activation of the NADPH–methemoglobin reductase system. Heterozygotes have intermediate levels of NADH-cytochrome-b_5 reductase activity and normal blood levels of Hi. They may become cyanotic because of methemoglobinemia after exposure to oxidizing chemicals or drugs in amounts that will not affect normal individuals.

In the second major category of hereditary methemoglobinemia, the reducing systems within the erythrocyte are intact, but the structure of the Hb molecule itself is abnormal. A genetically determined alteration in the amino acid composition of α- or β-globin chains may form a Hb molecule that has an enhanced tendency toward oxidation and a decreased propensity of the methemoglobin formed to be reduced back to Hb. Their principal consequence is asymptomatic cyanosis as a result of methemoglobinemia; they are designated as various forms of *hemoglobin M (Hb M)*. In six of the seven Hb M variants, tyrosine is substituted for histidine in the heme pocket of the proximal or distal globin chain. Nagai (1995) showed by spectroscopy that a considerable proportion of the mutant subunits of Hb M Saskatoon and Hb M Boston stay in the fully reduced form under circulation conditions. They are inherited as autosomal dominant traits (Lukens, 2004). Methylthioninium chloride therapy in these individuals is without effect, and treatment is not necessary.

Most cases of methemoglobinemia are classified as secondary or acquired, due mainly to exposure to drugs and chemicals that cause increased formation of Hi. Chemicals or drugs that directly oxidize HbO_2 to Hi include nitrites, nitrates, chlorates, and quinones. Other substances, which are aromatic amino and nitro compounds, probably act indirectly through a metabolite because they do not cause Hi formation in vitro. These include acetanilid, phenacetin, sulfonamides, and aniline dyes. Ferrous sulfate may produce methemoglobinemia after ingestion of very large doses. Levels of drugs or chemicals that would not cause significant methemoglobinemia in a normal individual may do so in someone with a mild reduction in NADH-cytochrome-b_5 reductase activity that, under ordinary circumstances, is not cyanotic. Such individuals are newborn infants and persons heterozygous for NADH-cytochrome-b_5 reductase deficiency (Bunn, 1986). Hi is reduced back to Hb by the erythrocyte enzyme systems. It can also be reduced (slowly) by the administration of reducing agents, such as ascorbic acid or sulfhydryl compounds (glutathione, cysteine); these, as well as methylthioninium chloride, are of value in cases of hereditary NADH-cytochrome-b_5 reductase deficiency. In cases of acquired or toxic methemoglobinemia, methylthioninium chloride is of great value; its rapid action is based not on its own reduction capacity but on its acceleration of the normally slow NADPH–methemoglobin reductase pathway. Hi can combine reversibly with various chemicals (e.g., cyanides, sulfides, peroxides, fluorides, azides). Because of the strong affinity of Hi for cyanide, the therapy of cyanide poisoning is to administer nitrites to form Hi, which then combines with the cyanide. Thus, the free cyanide (which is extremely poisonous to the cellular respiratory enzymes) becomes less toxic when changed to HiCN.

Hi is quantitated by spectrophotometry. If Hi is elevated, drugs or toxic substances must first be eliminated as a cause. Congenital methemoglobinemia due to NADH-cytochrome-b_5 reductase deficiency is determined by assay of the enzyme. An abnormal hemoglobin (Hb M) may also be responsible for methemoglobinemia noted at birth or in the first few months of life.

Sulfhemoglobin

SHb is a mixture of oxidized, partially denatured forms of Hb that form during oxidative hemolysis (Jandl, 1996). During oxidation of Hb, sulfur (from some source, which may vary) is incorporated into heme rings of Hb, resulting in a green hemochrome. Further oxidation usually results in the denaturation and precipitation of Hb as Heinz bodies (Fig. 30-1). SHb cannot transport O_2, but it can combine with carbon monoxide (CO) to form carboxysulfhemoglobin. Unlike methemoglobin, SHb cannot be reduced back to Hb, and it remains in the cells until they break down. The

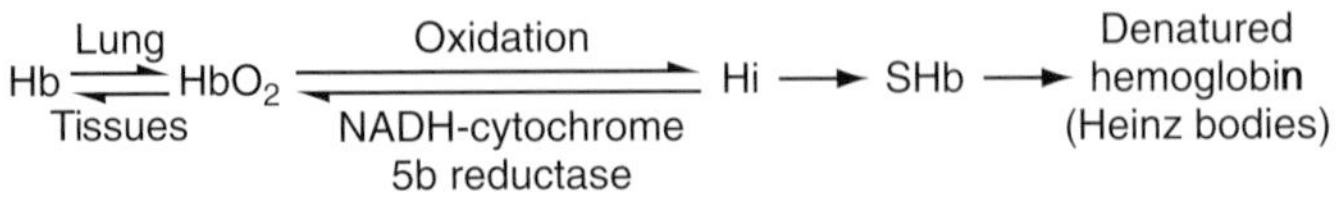

Figure 30-1 Simplified concept of oxidation of hemoglobin (Hb) to methemoglobin (Hi), as proposed by Jandl (1996). Reversible binding and release of oxygen occur in lungs and tissues; oxidation of ferrous ions and formation of Hb are reversible in the red cell to a limited extent; continued oxidation leads to irreversible conformational changes and sulfhemoglobin; still further oxidation results in denaturation of the Hb and precipitation within the erythrocyte as Heinz bodies. *HbO_2*, Oxyhemoglobin; *NADH*, reduced nicotinamide adenine dinucleotide; *SHb*, sulfhemoglobin.

blood is mauve-lavender in sulfhemoglobinemia. SHb has been reported in patients receiving treatment with sulfonamides or aromatic amine drugs (phenacetin, acetanilid), as well as in patients with severe constipation, in cases of bacteremia due to *Clostridium perfringens*, and in a condition known as enterogenous cyanosis. The concentration of SHb in vivo normally is less than 1%, and in these conditions it seldom exceeds 10% of the total Hb. It results in cyanosis and is usually asymptomatic. The reason why some patients develop methemoglobinemia, some sulfhemoglobinemia, and others Heinz bodies and hemolysis is not well understood. SHb is quantitated by spectrophotometry.

Carboxyhemoglobin

Endogenous CO produced in the degradation of heme to bilirubin normally accounts for about 0.5% of carboxyhemoglobin (HbCO) in the blood, and is increased in hemolytic anemia. Hb has the capacity to combine with CO with an affinity 210 times greater than for O_2. CO will bind with Hb even if its concentration in the air is extremely low (e.g., 0.02%–0.04%). In those cases, HbCO will build up until typical symptoms of poisoning appear. HbCO cannot bind and carry O_2. Furthermore, increasing concentrations of HbCO shift the Hb–O_2 dissociation curve increasingly to the left, thus adding to the anoxia. If a patient poisoned with CO receives pure O_2, the conversion of HbCO to HbO_2 is greatly enhanced. HbCO is light sensitive and has a typical, brilliant, cherry red color.

Acute CO poisoning is well known. It produces tissue hypoxia as a result of decreased O_2 transport. Chronic poisoning, a result of prolonged exposure to small amounts of CO, is less well recognized but is of increasing importance. The chief sources of the gas are gasoline motors, illuminating gas, gas heaters, defective stoves, and the smoking of tobacco. Exposure to CO is thus one of the hazards of modern civilization. The gas has even been found in the air of busy streets of large cities in sufficient concentration to cause mild symptoms in persons such as traffic police officers, who are exposed to it over long periods of time. Chronic exposure through tobacco smoking may lead to chronic elevation of HbCO and an associated left shift in the Hb-O_2 dissociation curve; smokers tend to have higher Hcts than nonsmokers and may have polycythemia. Healthy persons exposed to various concentrations of the gas for an hour do not experience definite symptoms (headache, dizziness, muscular weakness, and nausea) unless the concentration of gas in the blood reaches 20%–30% of saturation; however, it appears that in chronic poisoning, especially in children, serious symptoms may occur with lower concentrations. HbCO may be quantitated by differential spectrophotometry or by gas chromatography.

Measurement of Hb Concentration

The cyanmethemoglobin (hemiglobincyanide; HiCN) method has the advantages of convenience and a readily available, stable standard solution.

Hemiglobincyanide Method

Principle. Blood is diluted in a solution of potassium ferricyanide and potassium cyanide. The potassium ferricyanide oxidizes Hb to Hi (methemoglobin), and potassium cyanide provides cyanide ions (CN^-) to form HiCN, which has a broad absorption maximum at a wavelength of 540 nm (Fig. 30-2; Table 30-1). The absorbance of the solution is measured in a spectrophotometer at 540 nm and is compared with that of a standard HiCN solution.

Reagent. The diluent is detergent-modified Drabkin reagent:

0.20 g	Potassium ferricyanide ($K_3Fe[CN]_6$)
0.05 g	Potassium cyanide (KCN)
0.14 g	Dihydrogen potassium phosphate (anhydrous) (KH_2PO_4)
	Nonionic detergent, for example,
0.5 mL	Sterox S.E. (Harleco), *or*
1.0 mL	Triton X-100 (Rohm and Haas)
Distilled water to 1000 mL	

The solution should be clear and pale yellow, have a pH of 7.0–7.4, and give a reading of zero when measured in the photometer at 540 nm against a water blank.

Substituting dihydrogen potassium phosphate (KHP_2PO_4) in this reagent for sodium bicarbonate ($NaHCO_3$) in the original Drabkin reagent shortens the time needed for complete conversion of Hb to HiCN from 10 minutes to 3 minutes. The detergent enhances lysis of erythrocytes and decreases turbidity from protein precipitation.

Care must be taken with KCN in the preparation of the Drabkin solution, as salts or solutions of cyanide are poisonous. The diluent itself contains only 50 mg KCN per liter—less than the lethal dose for a 70-kg person. However, because hydrogen cyanide (HCN) is released by acidification, exposure of the diluent to acid must be avoided. Disposal of reagents and samples in running water in the sink is advised. The diluent keeps well in a dark bottle at room temperature but should be prepared fresh periodically.

Method. Twenty microliters of blood are added to 5.0 mL of diluent (1:251), mixed well, and allowed to stand at room temperature for at least 3 minutes (Dacie, 1991). The absorbance is measured against the reagent

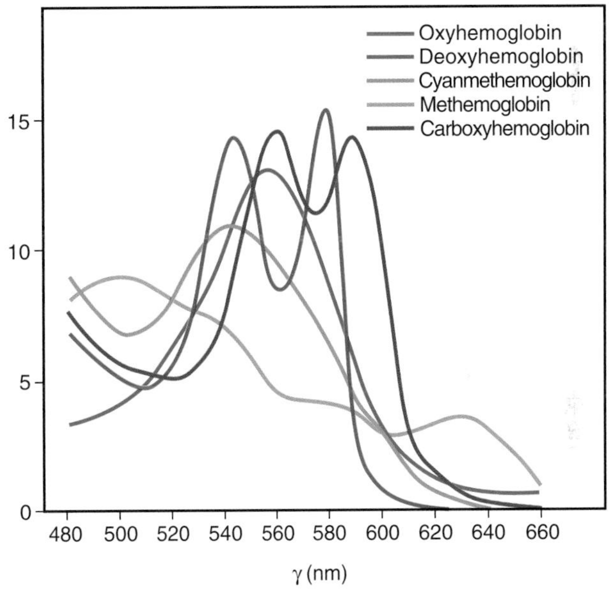

Figure 30-2 Absorption spectra of oxyhemoglobin (HbO_2), deoxyhemoglobin (Hb), methemoglobin (hemiglobin [Hi]), and cyanmethemoglobin (hemiglobincyanide [HiCN]). *(From Morris MW, Skrodzki Z, Nelson DA. Zeta sedimentation ratio [ZSR], a replacement for the erythrocyte sedimentation rate [ESR]. Am J Clin Pathol 1975;64:254–6. © 1975 American Society for Clinical Pathology.)*

TABLE 30-1
Nomenclature and Absorption Maxima of Hemoglobins

		Absorption peak 1		Absorption peak 2		Absorption peak 3	
Term	**Symbol**	λ	ε	λ	ε	λ	ε
Hemoglobin	Hb	431	(140)	555	(13.04)		
Oxyhemoglobin	HbO_2	415	(131)	542	(14.37)	577	(15.37)
Carboxyhemoglobin	HbCO	420	(192)	539	(14.36)	568.5	(14.31)
Hemiglobin (methemoglobin)	Hi	406	(162)	500	(9.04)	630	(3.70)
Hemiglobincyanide (cyanmet Hb)	HiCN	421	(122.5)	540	(10.99)		

Data from van Assendelft OW (1970).
The wavelength (λ) in nanometers for each maximum is followed by the extinction coefficient (ε) placed in parentheses.

blank in the photoelectric colorimeter at 540 nm or with an appropriate filter. A vial of HiCN standard is then opened and the absorbance measured, at room temperature, in the same instrument in a similar fashion. The test sample must be analyzed within a few hours of dilution. The standard must be kept in the dark when not in use and discarded at the end of the day.

$$\text{Hb (g/dL)} = [A^{540} \text{ test sample}/A^{540} \text{ standard}] \times [\text{Concentration of standard (mg/dL)}/100 \text{ mg/g}] \times 251$$

It is usually convenient to calibrate the photometer to be used for hemoglobinometry by preparing a standard curve or table that will relate absorbance to Hb concentration in grams per deciliter. The absorbance of fresh HiCN standard is measured against a reagent blank. Absorbance readings are made of fresh HiCN standard and of dilutions of this standard in the reagent (1 in 2, 1 in 3, and 1 in 4) against a reagent blank. Hb values in grams per deciliter are calculated for each solution as described previously. When the absorbance readings are plotted on linear graph paper as the ordinates against Hb concentration as the abscissa, the points should describe a straight line that passes through the origin. An advantage of the HiCN method is that most forms of hemoglobin (Hb, HbO_2, Hi, and HbCO, but not SHb) are measured.

The test sample can be directly compared with the HiCN standard, and the readings can be made at the convenience of the operator because of the stability of the diluted samples. Increased absorbance not due to Hb may be caused by turbidity due to abnormal plasma proteins, hyperlipemia, large numbers of leukocytes (counts $>30 \times 10^9$/L), or fatty droplets, any of which may lead to increased light scattering and apparent absorbance.

Errors in Hemoglobinometry

Sources of error may be those of the sample, the method, the equipment, or the operator.

Errors Inherent in the Sample. Improper venipuncture technique may introduce hemoconcentration, which will make Hb concentration and cell counts too high. Improper technique in fingerstick or capillary sampling can produce errors in either direction.

Errors Inherent in the Method. The HiCN method is the method of choice. Use of the HiCN standard for calibration of the instrument and for the test itself eliminates a major source of error. The broad absorption band of HiCN in the region of 540 nm makes it convenient to use both in filter-type photometers and in narrow-band spectrophotometers. With the exception of SHb, all other varieties of hemoglobin are converted to HiCN.

Errors Inherent in the Equipment. The accuracy of equipment is not uniform. A good grade of pipet with a guaranteed accuracy of greater than 99% is desirable. Calibration of pipets will lessen errors. Significant error can be introduced by the use of unmatched cuvets; therefore, flow-through cuvets are preferred. The wavelength settings, the filters, and the meter readings require checking. The photometer must be calibrated in the laboratory before its initial use and must be rechecked frequently to reduce the method's error to 2% (±CV).

Operator's Errors. Human errors can be reduced by good training, an understanding of the clinical significance of the test and the necessity for a dependable method, adherence to oral and written instructions, and familiarity with the equipment and with the sources of error. Errors increase with fatigue and tend to be greater near the end of the day. A technologist who is patient and critical by nature and by training and who is interested in the work is less prone to make errors.

The preceding discussion applies to manual techniques of hemoglobinometry. Automated equipment is widely used and eliminates most errors.

Spectrophotometric Identification of Hemoglobins

The various Hbs have characteristic absorption spectra, which can be determined easily with a spectrophotometer. Useful absorbance maxima are given in Table 30-1. The maxima for Hi vary considerably with pH. The maxima given in the two right-hand columns are useful for distinguishing among these forms of Hb. Absorbance between 405 and 435 nm (the Soret band) is considerably greater and may be used when small concentrations of Hb are to be measured.

HEMATOCRIT (PACKED CELL VOLUME)

The Hct of a sample of blood is the ratio of the volume of erythrocytes to that of the whole blood. It may be expressed as a percentage (conventional) or as a decimal fraction (SI units). The units L/L are implied. Dried heparin and ethylenediaminetetraacetic acid (EDTA) are satisfactory anticoagulants. Before taking a sample from a tube of venous blood for a hematologic determination, it is important to mix the blood thoroughly. If the tube has been standing, this requires at least 60 inversions of the tube, or 2 minutes on a mechanical rotator; less than this leads to unacceptable deterioration in precision (Fairbanks, 1971). The number of inversions required to achieve homogeneity of a specimen depends on the dimensions of the container. Standard 10–14 × 75-mm tubes, containing 5 mL of blood and an air bubble that constitutes at least 20% of the tube volume, require at least eight inversions (NCCLS, 1993). The venous Hct agrees closely with the Hct obtained from a skin puncture; both are greater than the total body Hct. The Hct may be measured directly by centrifugation with macromethods or micromethods, or indirectly as the product of the mean corpuscular volume (MCV) times RBC count in automated instruments. In blood kept at room temperature, swelling of erythrocytes between 6 and 24 hours raises Hct and MCV. Cell counts and indices are stable for 24 hours at 4° C (Brittin, 1969).

The Wintrobe macromethod Hct employs centrifugation of blood in a thick-walled glass tube with a uniform internal bore and a flattened bottom. It is no longer used.

Gross Examination

Hct determination is performed by centrifugation. Inspection of the specimen after spinning may furnish valuable information. The relative heights of the red cell column, buffy coat, and plasma column should be noted. The buffy coat is the red-gray layer between the red cells and the plasma; it includes platelets and leukocytes.

An orange or green color of the plasma suggests increased bilirubin, and pink or red suggests hemoglobinemia. Poor technique in collecting the blood specimen is the most frequent cause of hemolysis. If specimens are not obtained within an hour or two after a fat-rich meal, cloudy plasma may point to nephrosis or certain abnormal hyperglobulinemias, especially cryoglobulinemia.

Hematocrit Measurement by Micromethod

Equipment

A capillary Hct tube about 7 cm long with a uniform bore of about 1 mm is used. For blood collection directly from a skin puncture, heparinized capillary tubes are available.

Procedure

The microhematocrit tube is filled by capillary attraction from a free-flowing puncture wound or a well-mixed venous sample. The capillary tube should be filled to at least 5 cm. The empty end is sealed with modeling clay. The filled tube is placed in the radial grooves of the microhematocrit centrifuge head with the sealed end away from the center. Place the bottom of the tube against the rubber gasket to prevent breakage. Centrifugation for 5 minutes at 10,000–12,000 g is satisfactory unless the Hct exceeds 50%; in that case, an additional 5 minutes' centrifugation should be employed to ensure minimal plasma trapping. The capillary tubes are not graduated. The length of the blood column, including the plasma, and of the red cell column alone must be measured in each case with a millimeter rule and a magnifying lens, or with one of several commercially available measuring devices. The instructions of the manufacturer must be followed.

Interpretation of Results

Typical reference values for adult males are 0.41–0.51, and for females, 0.36–0.45. A value below an individual's normal value or below the reference interval for age and sex indicates anemia, and a higher value, polycythemia. The Hct reflects the concentration of red cells—not the total red cell mass. The Hct is low in hydremia of pregnancy, but the total number of circulating red cells is not reduced. The Hct may be normal or even high in shock accompanied by hemoconcentration, although the total red cell mass may be decreased considerably owing to blood loss. The Hct is unreliable as an estimate of anemia immediately after loss of blood or immediately following transfusions.

Sources of Error

Centrifugation. Adequate duration and speed of centrifugation are essential for a correct Hct. The red cells must be packed so that additional centrifugation does not further reduce the packed cell volume. In the course of centrifugation, small proportions of the leukocytes, platelets, and plasma are trapped between the red cells. The error resulting from the former is, as a rule, quite insignificant. The amount of trapped plasma is larger in high Hcts than in low Hcts. Trapped plasma accounts for about 1%–3% of the red cell column in normal blood (about 0.014 in a Hct of 0.47), slightly more in macrocytic anemia, spherocytosis, and hypochromic anemia (Dacie, 1991). Even greater amounts of trapped plasma are noted in the Hcts of patients with sickle cell anemia; these vary depending on the degree of sickling and consequent rigidity of the cells. In using the microhematocrit as a reference method for calibrating automated instruments, correction for trapped plasma is recommended (International Committee for Standardization in Hematology [ICSH], 1980).

Sample. Posture, muscular activity, and prolonged tourniquet-stasis can cause the same order of changes in Hct and cell concentrations as they do in nonfilterable soluble constituents. Unique to the Hct is error due to excess EDTA (inadequate blood for a fixed amount of EDTA): The Hct will be falsely low as a result of cell shrinkage, but the Hb and cell counts will not be affected. There is no uniformity as to which EDTA salt is used for anticoagulation (O'Broin, 1997). The tripotassium (K_3-EDTA) salt shrinks red cells about 2% and lowers packed cell volume compared with the dipotassium salt (K_2-EDTA) (Koepke, 1989). Also, because K_3-EDTA is a liquid, measured Hb and red and white cell counts are decreased by 1%–2%. Although the ICSH and the Clinical Laboratory Standards Institute recommend the K_2-EDTA salt (powder), the K_3-EDTA is more often used, perhaps because of its increased miscibility and fewer instances of specimen clotting (Geller, 1996).

Other Errors. Technical errors include failure to mix the blood adequately before sampling, improper reading of the levels of cells and plasma, and inclusion of the buffy coat as part of the erythrocyte volume. With good technique, the precision of the Hct, expressed as ±2 CV (coefficient of variation), is ±1%. With low Hct values, the CV is greater because of reading error.

ERYTHROCYTE INDICES

Wintrobe introduced calculations for determining the size, content, and Hb concentration of red cells; these erythrocyte indices have been useful in the morphologic characterization of anemias. They may be calculated from the red cell count, Hb concentration, and Hct.

Mean Cell Volume

The MCV, the average volume of red cells, is calculated from the Hct and the red cell count. MCV = Hct × 1000/RBC (in millions per μL), expressed in femtoliters or cubic micrometers. If the Hct = 0.45 and the red cell count = 5×10^{12}/L, 1 L will contain 5×10^{12} red cells, which occupy a volume of 0.45 L.

$$\text{MCV} = 0.45\ \text{L}/5 \times 10^{12} = 90 \times 10^{-15}\ \text{L}$$

$$\text{One femtoliter (fL)} = 10^{-15}\ \text{L} = 1\ \text{cubic micrometer}\ (\mu\text{m}^3).$$

Mean Cell Hemoglobin

The MCH is the content (weight) of Hb of the average red cell; it is calculated from the Hb concentration and the red cell count.

$$\text{MCH} = \text{Hb (in g/L)}/\text{RBC (in millions}/\mu\text{L)}$$

The value is expressed in picograms. If the Hb = 15 g/dL and the red cell count is 5×10^{12}/L, 1 L contains 150 g of Hb distributed in 5×10^{12} cells.

$$\text{MCH} = 150/(5 \times 10^{12}) = 30 \times 10^{12}\ \text{(pg)}$$

$$\text{One picogram (pg)} = 10^{-12}\ \text{g}$$

Mean Cell Hemoglobin Concentration

The mean cell hemoglobin concentration (MCHC) is the average concentration of Hb in a given volume of packed red cells. It is calculated from the Hb concentration and the Hct.

$$\text{MCHC} = \text{Hb (in g/dL)}/\text{Hct, expressed in g/dL}$$

If the Hb = 15 g/dL and the Hct = 0.45, the

$$\text{MCHC} = 15\ \text{g/dL}/0.45 = 33.3\ \text{g/dL}$$

Indices are determined in the electrical impedance instruments somewhat differently. The MCV is derived from the mean height of the voltage pulses formed during the red cell count, and the Hb is measured by optical density of HiCN. The other three values are calculated as follows:

$$\text{Hct} = \text{MCV} \times \text{RBC};\ \text{MCH} = \text{Hb/RBC};\ \text{MCHC} = (\text{Hb/Hct}) \times 100$$

The reference values for the indices will depend on whether they are determined from the centrifuged Hct or the cell counters. The values in normal individuals will be similar if both are corrected for trapped plasma. However, because of increased trapped plasma in hypochromic anemias and sickle cell anemia, the MCHC calculated from the microhematocrit will be significantly lower than the MCHC derived from the electrical impedance counters.

The 95% reference intervals for normal adults are as follows: MCV = 80–96 fL; MCH = 27–33 pg; and MCHC = 33–36 g/dL (Ryan, 2001a). In a healthy person, there is very little variation—no more than ±1 unit in any of the indices. Deviations from the reference value for an individual or outside the reference intervals for normal persons are useful, particularly in characterizing morphologic types of anemia.

In *microcytic anemias*, the indices may be as low as an MCV of 50 fL, an MCH of 15 pg, and an MCHC of 22 g/dL; rarely do any become lower.

In *macrocytic anemias*, the values may be as high as an MCV of 150 fL and an MCH of 50 pg, but the MCHC is normal or decreased (Dacie, 1991). The MCHC typically increases only in spherocytosis, and rarely is over 38 g/dL.

MANUAL BLOOD CELL COUNTS

Except for some platelet counts and low leukocyte counts, the hemocytometer is no longer used for routine blood cell counting. Yet it is still necessary for the technologist to be able to use this method effectively and to know its limitations. Any cell counting procedure includes three steps: dilution of the blood; sampling of the diluted suspension into a measured volume; and counting of the cells in that volume. Counts of erythrocytes, leukocytes, and platelets are each expressed as concentrations, that is, cells per unit volume of blood. The unit of volume was expressed as cubic millimeters (mm^3) because of the linear dimensions of the hemocytometer (cell counting) chamber.

$$1\ \text{mm}^3 = 1.00003\ \mu\text{L}$$

Although there is no consistency in the literature in the use of traditional/conventional units versus Système International d'Unites (SI) units, the ICSH recommends that the unit of volume be the liter (SI units), as on the right in the following examples:

Erythrocytes:

$$5.00 \times 10^6/\text{mm}^3 = 5.00 \times 10^6/\mu\text{L (conventional)} = 5.00 \times 10^{12}/\text{L (SI units)}$$

Leukocytes:

$$7.0 \times 10^3/\text{mm}^3 = 7.0 \times 10^3/\mu\text{L (conventional)} = 7.0 \times 10^9/\text{L (SI units)}$$

Platelets:

$$300 \times 10^3/\text{mm}^3 = 300 \times 10^3/\mu\text{L (conventional)} = 300 \times 10^9/\text{L (SI units)}$$

Erythrocyte Counts: Manual

Combining a microcapillary tube with a plastic vial containing a premeasured volume of diluent, the Unopette (Becton-Dickinson, Franklin Lakes, N.J.) is a valuable system for manual dilutions. After the capillary tube is filled, it is pushed into the container, and the sample is washed out by squeezing the soft plastic vial. This system is especially convenient for microsampling. Unopettes are available with diluents for counts of RBCs, white blood cells (WBCs), platelets, eosinophils, and reticulocytes.

Semiautomated Methods

Instruments are available for precise and convenient diluting which both aspirate the sample and wash it out with the diluent. The dilutor should perform a 1:250 or a 1:500 dilution with a coefficient of variation of less than 1%.

Reticulocyte Count: Manual

Principle

Reticulocytes are immature nonnucleated red cells that contain ribonucleic acid (RNA) and continue to synthesize Hb after loss of the nucleus. When blood is briefly incubated in a solution of new methylene blue or brilliant cresyl blue, the RNA is precipitated as a dye–ribonucleoprotein complex. Microscopically, the complex appears as a dark blue network (reticulum or filamentous strand) or at least two dark blue granules that allow reticulocytes to be identified and enumerated (ICSH, 1998). A proposed reference method for reticulocyte counting based on determination of the reticulocyte/red cell ratio has been published (ICSH, 1998), expanding on the 1994 ICSH red cell count reference method.

Reagent. One percent new methylene blue in a diluent of citrate/saline (one part 30 g/L sodium citrate plus four parts 9 g/L sodium chloride).

Controls. Although commercial controls are available, Ebrahim (1996) describes a method requiring about 2 hours that produces a multilevel control that is stable for several months. Hypotonic dialysis of RBCs in the presence of RNA followed by a short period of hypertonic dialysis to reseal the pores of the RBC membrane results in about 20% of the RBCs as "synthetic reticulocytes" with various amounts of encapsulated RNA.

Procedure

Three drops each of reagent and blood are mixed in a test tube, incubated 15 minutes at room temperature, and remixed. Two wedge films are made on glass slides and air dried.

Viewed microscopically with an oil immersion lens, reticulocytes are pale blue and contain dark blue reticular or granular material, and red cells stain pale blue or blue-green. The percentage of reticulocytes is determined in at least 1000 red cells. A Miller disk inserted into the eyepiece allows rapid estimation of large numbers of red cells by imposing two squares (one square is nine times the area of the other) onto the field of view (Brecher, 1950). Reticulocytes are counted in the large square and red cells in the small square in successive microscopic fields until at least 300 red cells are counted. This provides an estimate of reticulocytes among at least 2700 red cells, as follows:

$$\text{Reticulocytes (percent)} = [\text{No. reticulocytes in large squares}/(\text{No. red cells in small squares} \times 9)] \times 100$$

The absolute reticulocyte count is determined by multiplying the reticulocyte percentage by the red cell count.

Reference Values

Normal adults have a reticulocyte count of 0.5%–1.5%, or 24–84 × 10^9/L. In newborn infants, the percentage is 2.5%–6.5%; this falls to the adult range by the end of the second week of life.

Interpretation

Because reticulocytes are immature red cells that lose their RNA a day or so after reaching the blood from the marrow, a reticulocyte count provides an estimate of the rate of red cell production. An absolute reticulocyte count or reticulocyte production index is more helpful than the percentage (see Chapter 31).

Sources of Variation

Because such a small number of actual reticulocytes are counted, the sampling error in the manual reticulocyte count is relatively large. The 95% confidence limits may be expressed as follows:

$$R \pm 2\sqrt{[R(100 - R)/N]}$$

where R is the reticulocyte count in percent, and N is the number of erythrocytes examined. This means that if only 1000 erythrocytes are evaluated, the 95% confidence limits for a 1% count are 0.4%–1.6%; for a 5% count, 3.6%–6.4%; and for a 10% count, 8.1%–11.9%.

Leukocyte Counts: Manual

Specimen Collection

EDTA should be used; heparin is unsatisfactory as an anticoagulant.

Hemocytometer Method

Although this method is used only occasionally in leukocyte counting, the technologist should be able to perform it

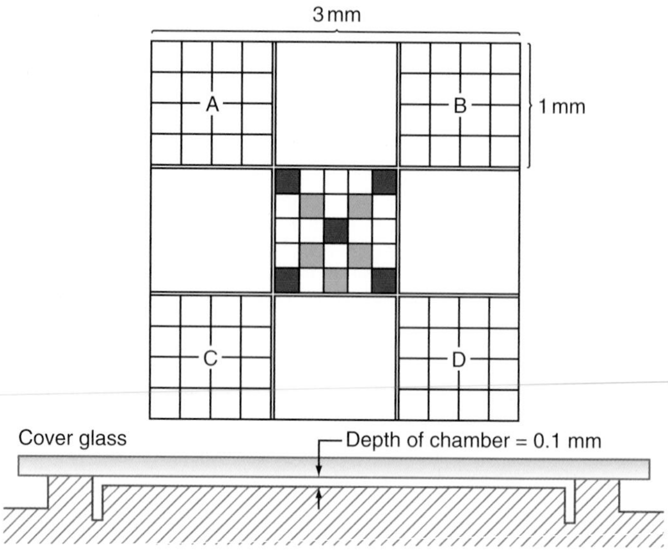

Figure 30-3 The upper figure is a diagram of the improved Neubauer ruling; this is etched on the surface of each side of the hemocytometer. The large corner squares, A, B, C, and D, are used for leukocyte counts. The five blue squares in the center are used for red cell counts or for platelet counts, and the 10 green plus blue squares for platelet counts. Actually, each of the 25 squares within the central sq mm has within it 16 smaller squares for convenience in counting. The lower figure is a side view of the chamber with the cover glass in place.

1. As a check on the validity of electronic methods for calibration purposes
2. As a check on the validity of electronic counts in patients with profound leukopenia or thrombocytopenia
3. For blood specimens with platelet counting interference (i.e., very microcytic RBCs), and
4. As a backup method.

It is also commonly used as a method for counting cells in cerebrospinal fluid (CSF).

Counting Chamber. The hemocytometer is a thick glass slide with inscribed platforms of known area and precisely controlled depth under the coverslip. Counting chambers and cover glasses should be rinsed in lukewarm water immediately after use; wiped with a clean, lint-free cloth; and allowed to air dry. The surfaces must not be touched with gauze or linen because these materials may scratch the ruled areas.

Diluting Fluid. The diluting fluid lyses the erythrocytes so that they will not obscure the leukocytes. The fluid must be refrigerated and filtered frequently to remove yeasts and molds.

Procedure.

1. Well-mixed blood is diluted 1:20 in diluting fluid and the vial rotated for about 5 minutes. The chamber is loaded with just enough fluid to fill the space beneath the cover glass.
2. The cells are permitted to settle for several minutes, and the chamber is surveyed with the low-power objective to verify uniform cell distribution.
3. Counting is performed. The condenser diaphragm of the microscope is partially closed to make the leukocytes stand out clearly under a low-power (10×) objective lens. The leukocytes are counted in each of the four large (1 mm^2) corner squares (A, B, C, and D in Fig. 30-3). A total of eight large corner squares from two sides of a chamber are counted.
4. Each large square encloses a volume of 1/10 mm^3, and the dilution is 1:20. A general formula is as follows:

$$\text{Leukocyte count (cells/mm}^3) = (cc/lsc) \times d \times 10$$

where cc is the total number of cells counted, d is the dilution factor, 10 is the factor transforming value over one large square (1/10 mm^3) to the volume in mm^3, and lsc is the number of large squares counted.

In leukopenia, with a total count below 2500, the blood is diluted 1:10. In leukocytosis, the dilution may be 1:100 or even 1:200.

Sources of Error. Errors may be due to the nature of the sample, to the operator's technique, and to inaccurate equipment. Errors that are inherent in the distribution of cells in the counting volume are called "field" errors and can be minimized only by counting more cells.

Hemocytometer leukocyte counts show a CV of about 6.5% for normal and increased counts, and about 15% in leukopenic blood. Utilizing electronic counters, on the other hand, results in CVs of approximately 1%–3%.

Errors Due to the Nature of the Sample. Partial coagulation of the venous blood causes changes in the distribution of the cells and/or decreases their number. Failure to mix the blood thoroughly and immediately before dilution introduces an error, which depends on the degree of sedimentation.

Operator's Errors. Errors caused by faulty technique may occur during dilution, when the chamber is loaded, and when the cells are counted.

Errors Due to Equipment. Equipment errors can be diminished by using pipets and hemocytometers certified by the U.S. Bureau of Standards.

Inherent or Field Errors. Even in a perfectly mixed sample, variation occurs in the numbers of suspended cells that are distributed in a given volume (i.e., come to rest over a given square). This "error of the field" is the minimal error. Another error is the "error of the chamber," which includes variations in separate fillings of a given chamber and in sizes of different chambers. Still another is the "error of the pipet," which includes variations in filling a given pipet and in the sizes of different pipets. In performing a WBC count, if 200 cells are counted using two chambers and one pipet, the CV = 9.1%, corresponding to 95% confidence limits of ±18.2% (twice the CV). Using four chambers and two pipets and counting twice as many cells reduces the 95% confidence limits to ±12.8%. This relatively large percentage error is of little practical consequence because of the physiologic variation of the leukocyte count.

Nucleated Red Blood Cells. Nucleated red blood cells (NRBCs) will be counted and cannot be distinguished from leukocytes with the magnification used. If their number is high, as seen on the stained smear, a correction should be made according to the following formula:

$$\text{True leukocyte count} = (\text{Total count} \times 100)/(100 + \text{No. of NRBCs})$$

where the *No. of NRBCs* is the number of nucleated red cells that are counted during the enumeration of 100 leukocytes in the differential count.

Example. The blood smear shows 25 NRBCs per 100 leukocytes. The total nucleated cell count is 10,000.

True leukocyte count = 10,000 × 100/125 = 8000/μL (8.0 × 10^9/L)

Reference Value. In the total leukocyte count, no distinction is made among the six normal cell types (neutrophils and bands, lymphocytes, monocytes, eosinophils, and basophils). The reference interval for adults is 4.5–11.0 × 10^9/L.

Platelet Counts

Platelets are thin disks, 2–4 μm in diameter and 5–7 fL in volume (in citrated blood). They function in hemostasis, in maintenance of vascular integrity, and in the process of blood coagulation.

In EDTA-blood, the mean platelet volume (MPV) increases with time up to 1 hour in vitro, is relatively stable between 1 and 3 hours, and then increases further with time. Change from a discoid to a spherical shape accounts for this increase in apparent volume in EDTA compared with citrate (Rowan, 1982). For reproducible results, platelet volume measurements obtained with multichannel instruments should be made between 1 and 3 hours after the blood is drawn. The frequency distribution of platelet volumes in an individual is log normal. However, a nonlinear, inverse relationship has been noted between the MPV and the platelet count within normal individuals (Fig. 30-4). Therefore, reference values for the MPV appear to vary with the platelet count (Bessman, 1981). The MPV is generally increased in hyperthyroidism (Ford, 1988) and myeloproliferative disease (Small, 1981). Platelets are more difficult to count because they are small (must be distinguished from debris) and have a tendency to adhere to glass, any foreign body, and particularly to one another. It is often possible to recognize a significant decrease in the number of platelets by careful inspection of stained films. With capillary blood, films must be made evenly and very quickly after the blood is obtained to avoid clumping and to minimize the decrease due to adhesion of platelets to the margins of the injured vessels. A better estimate is possible by examining stained films made from venous blood with EDTA as an anticoagulant (EDTA-blood), in which platelets are evenly distributed and where clumping normally does not occur. The visual method of choice employs the phase-contrast microscope. This is the reference method. Laboratories performing over five platelet counts per day can justify electronic platelet counting; both voltage pulse counting and electro-optical counting systems are satisfactory.

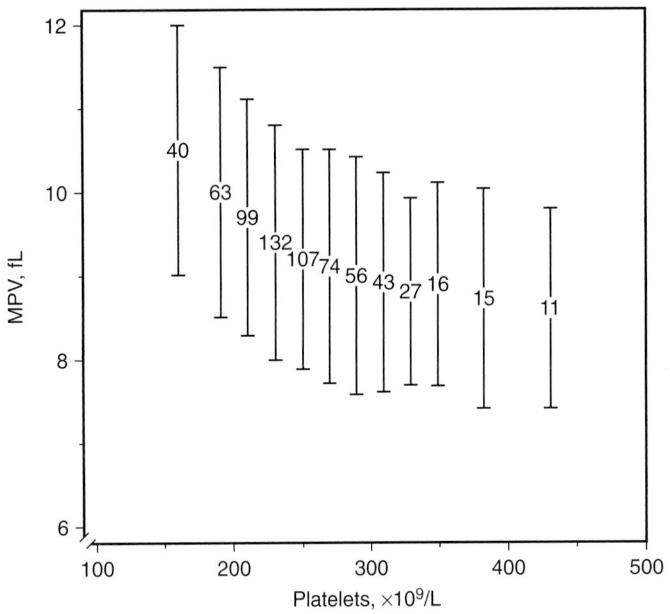

Figure 30-4 Mean platelet volume (MPV) related to platelet count in 683 normal subjects. Each group is shown as mean (number) ±2 SD (bar) of subjects grouped by platelet counts of 128–179, 180–199, 200–219, 220–239, 240–259, 260–279, 280–309, 310–319, 320–339, 340–359, 360–403, 404–462 × 10^9/L. The number of the mean position is the number of subjects in the group (Bessman, 1981).

Hemocytometer Method—Phase-Contrast Microscope

Specimen. Venous blood is collected with EDTA as the anticoagulant. Blood from skin puncture wounds gives more variable results but is satisfactory if the blood is flowing freely and if only the first few drops are used.

Diluent Solution. One percent ammonium oxalate is mixed in distilled water. The stock bottle is kept in the refrigerator. The amount needed for the day is filtered before use and the unused portion discarded at end of day.

Procedure

1. Well-mixed blood is diluted 1:100 in diluting fluid, and the vial containing the suspension is rotated on a mechanical mixer for 10–15 minutes.
2. The hemocytometer is filled in the usual fashion, using a separate capillary tube for each side.
3. The chamber is covered with a Petri dish for 15 minutes to allow settling of the platelets in one optical plane. A piece of wet cotton or filter paper is left beneath the dish to prevent evaporation.
4. The platelets appear round or oval and frequently have one or more dendritic processes. Their internal granular structure and a purple sheen allow the platelets to be distinguished from debris, which is often refractile. Ghosts of red cells that have been lysed by the ammonium oxalate are seen in the background.
5. Platelets are counted in 10 small squares (the black squares in Fig. 30-3), five on each side of the chamber. If the total number of platelets counted is less than 100, more small squares are counted until at least 100 platelets have been recorded—10 squares per side (black plus shaded squares; see Fig. 30-3) or all 25 squares in the large central square on each side of the hemocytometer, if necessary. If the total number of platelets in all 50 of these small squares is less than 50, the count should be repeated with a 1:20 or a 1:10 dilution of blood.

Calculation. Each of the 25 small squares defines a volume of 1/250 μL (1/25 mm^2 area × 1/10 mm depth): Platelet count (per μL) = (Number of cells counted/Number of squares counted) × Dilution × 250.

By adjusting the number of squares so that at least 100 platelets are counted, the field error (the statistical error caused by counting a limited number of platelets in the chamber) can be kept in the same range for low platelet counts as for high platelet counts. It has been shown that the CV due to combined field, pipet, and chamber errors is about 11% when at least 100 platelets are counted, and 15% when 40 platelets are counted.

Platelet counts tend to be the least reproducible of the blood cell counts, and the technologist must be vigilant to ensure their accuracy. This includes the readiness to confirm suspicious or abnormal results with a freshly drawn sample. Whenever the platelet count is in question, such as with an instrument flag, the blood film (prepared from EDTA-blood) must be checked to corroborate the count and to detect abnormalities in platelets or other blood elements that may give a false value. Further, because of the low number of platelets counted in the manual method and the high degree of imprecision with severe thrombocytopenia (CV >15%), 7×10^9 platelets/L is the lowest count that should be reported from manual quantitation (Hanseler, 1996).

Sources of Error. Blood in EDTA is satisfactory for 5 hours after collection at 20° C and for 24 hours at 4° C, provided that no difficulty was encountered in collection. Platelet clumps present in the chamber imply a maldistribution and negate the reliability of the count; a new sample of blood must be collected. The causes of platelet clumping are likely to be initiation of platelet aggregation and clotting before the blood reaches the anticoagulant; imperfect venipuncture; delay in the anticoagulant contacting the blood; or, in skin puncture technique, delay in sampling. Capillary blood gives similar mean values, but errors are about twice those with venous blood, probably because the platelet level varies in successive drops of blood from the skin puncture wound.

Falsely Elevated Counts. Fragments of leukocyte cytoplasm that are sometimes numerous in leukemias may falsely elevate the count. The phase-contrast hemocytometer method must be employed in these cases with a correction made based on the ratio of fragments to platelets determined from the blood film.

Falsely Low Counts. These can occur if platelets adhere to neutrophils (platelet satellitism) or if there is platelet clumping due to agglutinins (Lombarts, 1988), spontaneous aggregation, or incipient clotting due to faulty blood collection. The first two of these phenomena appear to depend on EDTA (Dacie, 1991). The reported incidence of EDTA-induced in vitro platelet clumping and pseudothrombocytopenia has ranged from 0.1% (Bartels, 1997) to 2% (Lippi, 1990). Alterations in platelet histograms or in quantitative cutoff measures derived from them should be used to screen for pseudothrombocytopenia (Bartels, 1997).

Variation In Automated Platelet Count

Standard guidelines with each instrument mandate performing manual platelet counts below and above the established reference ranges. For example, an automated platelet count below 30×10^9/L using Technicon HP 81 (Technicon Instruments Corporation, Tarrytown, N.Y.) should be replaced by the manual procedure (Hanseler, 1996).

Upon comparing the ADVIA 120 (Siemens Healthcare Diagnostics, Deerfield, Ill.) to Coulter STKS (Coulter, Hialeah, Fla.), Stanworth (1999) showed that in some cases of thrombocytopenia due to peripheral consumption, the ADVIA gave higher platelet counts and the blood film showed some large platelets. Further study with platelet-specific monoclonal antibodies such as CD61 will likely determine which count is more correct. Cantero (1996) showed that visibly turbid plasma in blood specimens resulted in, on average, a 47% increase in platelet count with the Technicon HP 83.

Reference values for platelet counts are 150–450 $\times 10^9$/L. Reference values for MPV are approximately 6.5–12 fL in adults.

Reticulated Platelets

Reticulated platelets are those newly released circulating platelets that have residual RNA. Reticulated platelet counts are an estimate of thrombopoiesis (Rapi, 1998), analogous to the use of reticulocyte count as an estimate of erythropoiesis. Matic (1998) describes an optimized flow cytometric analysis method after incubating whole blood with thiazole orange, which has a 3000-fold increase in fluorescence after binding to RNA. Phycoerythrin-labeled antibodies directed against GPIb on the surface of the platelet are also in the incubation mixture to distinguish platelets from other cells or debris. Recombinant human erythropoietin seems to improve platelet function in uremia not only by correcting the anemia, but also by increasing young platelets, detected as reticulated platelets (Tassies, 1998). Significantly lower median levels of reticulated platelets in frequent plateletpheresis donors than in new donors suggest that repeat platelet donation might lead to relative exhaustion of thrombopoiesis (Stohlawetz, 1998). Depending on the conditions of the measurement, published normal values for reticulated platelets vary tremendously from 3%–20% (Matic, 1998).

Increased reticulated platelet values have been reported in idiopathic thrombocytopenic purpura (Koike, 1998; Saxton, 1998), and hyperthyroidism (Stiegler, 1998). In neonates younger than 30 weeks' gestation, the reticulated platelet count was about twice that seen in full-term infants (Peterec, 1996). Bone marrow recovery after chemotherapy for acute myeloid leukemia (AML) showed an increase in reticulated platelets after about day 20 (Stohlawetz, 1999). *Decreased* reticulated platelet values have been reported in association with aplasia and liver cirrhosis (Koike, 1998; Saxton, 1998).

Electronic Counting

Because of the relatively low cost, reduced time (for labor and results), and increased accuracy of the automated analyzers, semiautomated instruments are rarely used in clinical practice these days. Speed of performance, elimination of visual fatigue of the technician, and improved precision are decisive advantages of the electronic cell counter over the hemocytometer/manual methods of performing blood cell counts. Electronic counting instruments are discussed in more detail in the next section, Instrument Technology.

INSTRUMENT TECHNOLOGY

The multichannel instruments used in the modern laboratory for performing cell counts are based on the principles of electrical impedance, light scattering, radiofrequency conductivity, and/or cytochemistry (Ward, 2000). The principles of these techniques are discussed in the following section. Combining hematology instrumentation with laboratory automation allows for reduction in preanalytic and postanalytic variables and positive identification of samples for processing and analysis, storage, and retrieval.

Electrical Impedance

Cells passing through an aperture through which a current is flowing cause changes in electrical resistance that are counted as voltage pulses. This principle, illustrated in Figure 30-5, is used in instruments marketed by Coulter (LH series, GEN-S, HmX, A-T, etc.; Beckman Coulter Inc., Brea, Calif.), Sysmex (XE and XT series, etc.; Sysmex America Inc., Mundelein, Ill.), Abbott (Cell-Dyn, 3700, Ruby, Sapphire, etc.; Abbott Diagnostics, Santa Clara, Calif.), ABX (Micros 60, Pentra series, etc.; ABX Diagnostics Inc., Irvine, Calif.), and others. An accurately diluted suspension of blood (CS) is made in an isotonic conductive solution that preserves the cell shape. The instrument has a glass cylinder (GC) that can be filled with the

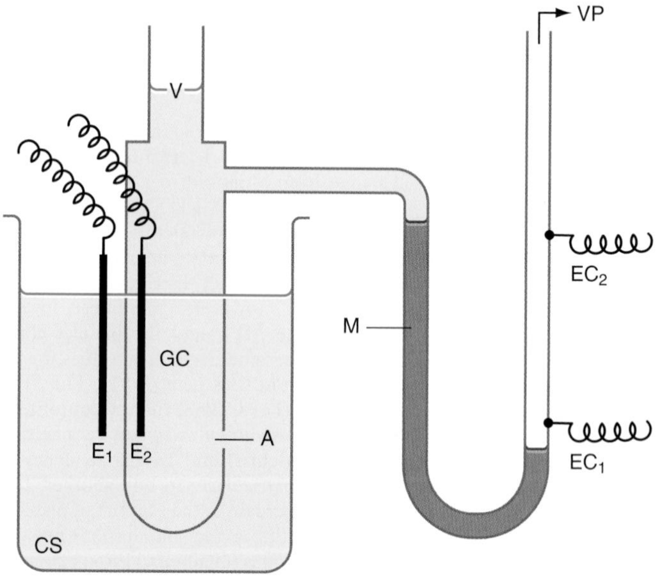

Figure 30-5 Schematic diagram of particle counter in which changes in electrical resistance are counted as voltage pulses. (Diagram adapted from Ackerman, 1972.) *A*, Aperture; *CS*, cell suspension; E_1 and E_2, platinum electrodes; EC_1 and EC_2, electrical contacts; *GC*, glass cylinder; *M*, mercury column; *V*, valve; *VP*, vacuum pump.

conducting fluid and has within it an electrode (E2) and an aperture (A) of 100 µm diameter in its wall. Just outside the glass cylinder is another electrode (E1). The cylinder is connected to a U-shaped glass tube that is partially filled with mercury (M), and that has two electrical contacts (EC1 and EC2). The glass cylinder is immersed in the suspension of cells to be counted (CS) and is filled with conductive solution and closed by a valve (V). A current now flows through the aperture between E1 and E2. As mercury moves up the tube, the cell suspension is drawn through the aperture into the cylinder. Each cell that passes through the aperture displaces an equal volume of conductive fluid, increasing the electrical resistance and creating a voltage pulse, because its resistance is much greater than that of the conductive solution. The pulses, which are proportional in height to the volume of the cells, are counted. This is the Coulter principle.

In the simplest system, the counting mechanism is started when the mercury contacts EC1 and stopped when it contacts EC2; during this time, the cells are counted in a volume of suspension exactly equal to the volume of the glass tubing between contact wires EC1 and EC2. If two or more cells enter the aperture simultaneously, they will be counted as one pulse; this produces a coincidence error for which corrections are now automatically made by analyzers. A threshold setting or pulse discriminator allows the exclusion of pulses below an adjustable height on certain counters. On others, a second threshold also excludes the counting of pulses above a certain height. One therefore counts only the cells in the "window" between the two settings. By systematically changing each threshold by given increments, one can determine a frequency distribution of relative cell volumes. Such cell size distributions can be automatically plotted and are valuable in the study of red cells, white cells, or platelets when two or more changing populations of cells are present. This is the basis for determination of the blood cell histograms, which are now routinely produced by the multichannel hematology analyzers.

Radiofrequency Conductivity

Conductivity is determined using a high-frequency electromagnetic probe that provides information on the cells' internal constituents (chemical composition, nuclear characteristics, and granular constituents) by permeating the lipid layer of a cell's membrane. Conductivity is especially helpful in differentiating between cells of like size such as small lymphocytes and basophils (Burns, 1992; Bentley, 1993). This principle is utilized in instruments marketed by Coulter (LH series, GENfi-S, HmX, A-T, etc.; Beckman Coulter Inc.) and Sysmex (XE-2100, XT 2000i, HST-N, etc.; Sysmex America Inc.).

Light Scattering

In the electro-optical analyzers (Fig. 30-6), a light-sensitive detector measures light scattering. All major multichannel analyzers now employ optical methods, at least to some extent. The size of the pulse detected is proportional to the size of the particle (WBC, RBC, or platelet). Although the precision of the instruments employing optical methods is equivalent to that of systems utilizing electrical impedance, some systems use a combination of the two methods to supply an internal comparison. Forward angle scatter of a laser-generated monochromatic light determines cell surface characteristics, morphology, and granulation. Measurement of light scatter at multiple angles allows enhanced differentiation of cell types. For example, in the Abbott Cell Dyn, four simultaneous light scattering measurements are made on each white cell. Zero-degree forward angle is primarily affected by and thus determines cell size. Ten-degree light scatter is an indicator of cell structure or complexity and is especially helpful in resolving basophils and separating all cell populations. Ninety-degree light scatter separates granulated cells and is termed **lobularity.** Depolarized 90-degree light scattering resolves eosinophils because of their large crystalline granularity. Abnormal cells can have distinctive locations in the size-versus-complexity scatterplot and help to determine WBC suspect flags (Cornbleet, 1992), such as for blasts, variant lymphs, bands, and immature granulocytes. Fluorescent deoxyribonucleic acid (DNA) dyes are used in the Abbott automated hematology systems to enumerate nucleated RBCs and identify populations of atypical lymphocytes and nonviable WBCs. Adaptive gating technology permits better separation of overlapping clusters of cell types. Suspect flags are generated when the distinction cannot be clearly delineated, as is often the case in the presence of abnormal WBC populations or interfering substances.

Cytochemistry

A method unique to the Siemens automated hematology series (Siemens Healthcare Diagnostics, Deerfield, Ill.) is the use of a cytochemical reaction to determine the peroxidase activity of white blood cells. The mean peroxidase index (MPXI), a measure of neutrophil-staining intensity, is determined for each specimen. The relative positivity seen in neutrophils, eosinophils, and monocytes is used in conjunction with data derived from light scatter to determine the WBC differential (Simson, 1986). ABX Diagnostics utilizes a cytochemical reagent that fixes the WBCs in their native state and subsequently stains their intracellular and plasmic membranes with chlorazol black E (Clinical Case Studies: Interpretation Guide for ABX 5-Part Diff Hematology Analyzers, ABX Horiba Diagnostics, Montpelier, France).

Reporting/Flagging

Each instrumentation system combines the data generated by these methods in their own configuration to provide a five- or six-part WBC differential along with RBC morphology and platelet parameters (Fig. 30-7). The principles of measurement specific to selected systems are detailed in Table 30-2. Data generated by the instrument that are not acceptable based on instrument- or user-defined criteria are flagged to alert the technologist that reporting the sample requires further investigation. Data management systems now include sophisticated programs that utilize user-defined criteria to determine reflex and repeat testing, including automated slide making and staining. Extreme care must be taken when defining these criteria, as the addition of each lessens the advantage provided by automating the process. The best configurations are developed with the patient population in mind. In addition, follow-up should be tailored to minimize the extended time necessary to derive the correct result.

Sources of Error

Table 30-3 lists various causes of erroneous results obtained from automated cell counters.

Automated Reticulocyte Counting

Many of the same principles applied in determination of the WBC differential may be utilized to determine reticulocyte counts, resulting in enhanced precision and increased accuracy in routine practice (Metzger, 1987). Depending on the specific model of analyzer, this process may be semiautomated or fully automated. All methods rely on the addition of a stain or dye to detect the RNA content of the RBC. Such stains include new methylene blue (NMB), oxazine, auramine O, polymethine, and thiazole orange. Methods of detection include impedance, light scatter, absorption, and fluorescence intensity. Reticulocyte fractions are separated based on RNA content, with the more immature cells containing the highest amount of reticulum. The immature reticulocyte fraction (IRF) quantitatively describes the youngest reticulocytes with the greatest staining intensity. This parameter allows early detection of an increased

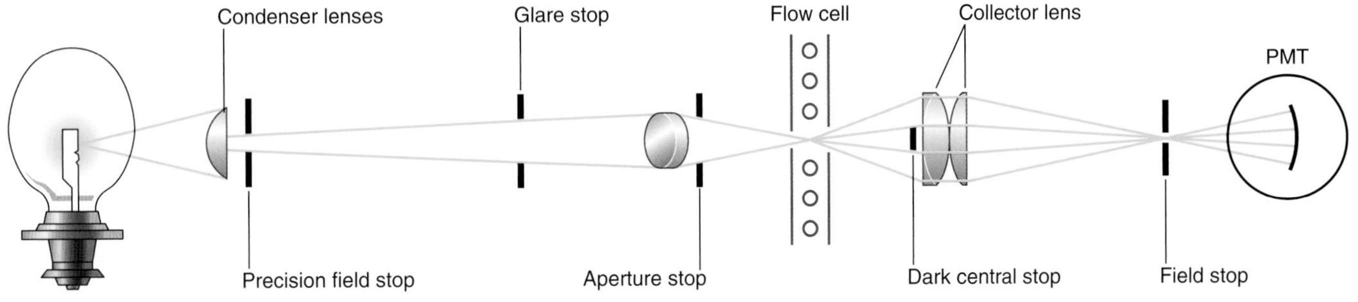

Figure 30-6 Schematic diagram of the electro-optical cell counter. Light is focused on the flow cell. Only light scattered by a cell reaches the photomultiplier tube (PMT), which converts to an electrical pulse. *(From Mansberg HP. Adv Autom Anal 1970;1:213, with permission. Reprinted courtesy of Technicon Instrument Corporation, Tarrytown, N.Y.)*

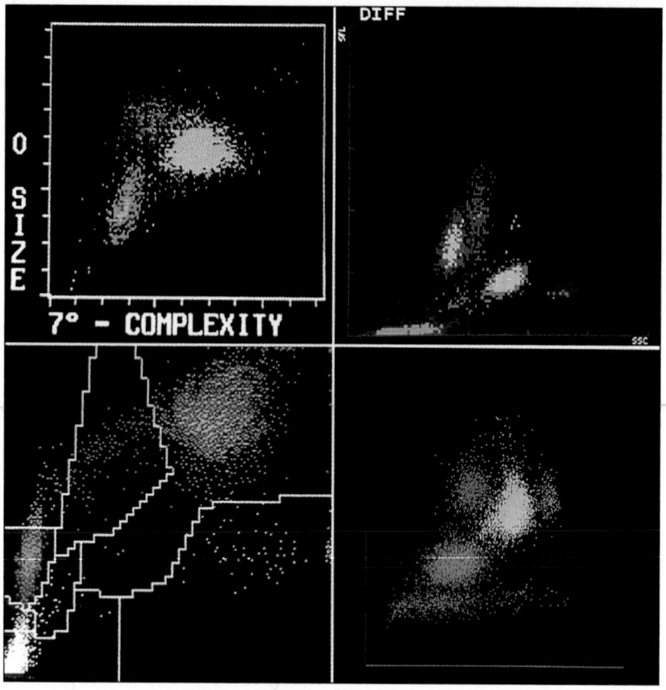

Figure 30-7 White blood cell (WBC) scattergrams/cytograms. *Top left,* Abbott CELL-DYN 4000 WBC scatterplot, light scatter vs. volume. *Top right,* Sysmex XT 2000i, WBC scattergram, side-scattered light vs. side fluorescence. *Bottom left,* Siemens Advia 120, WBC peroxidase cytogram. *Bottom right,* Coulter LH 750, WBC scattergram, light scatter vs. volume.

TABLE 30-2
Principles Used by Various Multichannel Instruments in the Clinical Laboratory

Method				
Instrument	**Impedance**	**Conductivity**	**Light scatter**	**Cytochemistry**
Abbott	x	x	x	
ABX	x		x	x
Siemens			x	x
Coulter	x	x	x	
Sysmex	x	x	x	

erythropoietic response, important in determining the response of the bone marrow recovering from chemotherapy or transplant or the response to erythropoietin therapy. It may also be used in conjunction with the absolute reticulocyte count to classify anemias (Davis, 1994, 1996; d'Onofrio, 1996). The reticulocyte Hb content (CHr) provides a sensitive index by which to identify hypochromic RBCs. This can be used to detect iron deficiency and evaluate patient response to iron therapy (Goodnough, 2000).

TABLE 30-3
Potential Causes of Erroneous Results With Automated Cell Counters

Parameter	Causes of spurious increase	Causes of spurious decrease
WBC	Cryoglobulin, cryofibrinogen Heparin Monoclonal proteins Nucleated red cells Platelet clumping Unlysed red cells	Clotting Smudge cells Uremia plus immunosuppressants
RBC	Cryoglobulin, cryofibrinogen Giant platelets High WBC (>50,000/mL)	Autoagglutination Clotting Hemolysis (in vitro) Microcytic red cells
Hb	Carboxyhemoglobin (>10%) Cryoglobulin, cryofibrinogen Hemolysis (in vitro) Heparin High WBC (>50,000/μL) Hyperbilirubinemia Lipemia Monoclonal proteins	Clotting Sulfhemoglobin
Hct (automated)	Cryoglobulin, cryofibrinogen Giant platelets High WBC (>50,000/μL) Hyperglycemia (>600 mg/dL)	Autoagglutination Clotting Hemolysis (in vitro) Microcytic red cells
Hct (microhematocrit)	Hyponatremia Plasma trapping	Excess EDTA Hemolysis (in vitro) Hypernatremia
MCV	Autoagglutination High WBC (>50,000/μL) Hyperglycemia Reduced red cell deformability	Cryoglobulin Cryofibrinogen Giant platelets Hemolysis (in vitro) Microcytic red cells Swollen red cells
MCH	High WBC (>50,000/μL) Spuriously high Hb Spuriously low RBC	Spuriously low Hb Spuriously high RBC
MCHC	Autoagglutination Clotting Hemolysis (in vitro) Hemolysis (in vivo) Spuriously high Hb Spuriously low Hct	High WBC (>50,000/μL) Spuriously low Hb Spuriously high Hct
Platelets	Cryoglobulin, cryofibrinogen Hemolysis (in vitro and in vivo) Microcytic red cells Red cell inclusions White cell fragments	Clotting Giant platelets Heparin Platelet clumping Platelet satellitosis

From Cornbleet J. Spurious results from automated hematology cell analyzers. Lab Med 1983;14:509.
EDTA, Ethylenediaminetetraacetic acid; *Hb,* hemoglobin; *Hct,* hematocrit; *MCH,* mean cell hemoglobin; *MCHC,* mean cell hemoglobin concentration; *MCV,* mean corpuscular volume; *RBC,* red blood cell; *WBC,* white blood cell.

PHYSIOLOGIC VARIATION

Physiologic Variation in Erythrocytes

Changes in red cell values are greatest during the first few weeks of life (Fig. 30-8). At the time of birth, as much as 100–125 mL of placental blood may be added to the newborn if tying the cord is postponed until its pulsation ceases. In a study of newborns whose cords had been clamped late, average capillary red cell counts were 0.4×10^{12}/L higher 1 hour after and 0.8×10^{12}/L higher 24 hours after birth compared with newborns whose cords had been clamped early. Capillary blood (obtained by skin puncture) gives higher RBC and Hb values than venous blood (cord). The differences may amount to about 0.5×10^{12} RBC/L and 3 g Hb/dL. Slowing of capillary circulation and the resulting loss of fluid may be the responsible factors. Examination of venous blood furnishes more consistent results than are obtained by examination of capillary blood.

In the full-term infant, nucleated red cells average about 0.5×10^9/L. The normoblast count declines to about 200/μL at 24 hours, 25/μL at 48 hours, and less than 5/μL at 72 hours. By 7 days, it is rare to find circulating normoblasts (Barone, 1999).

The normal reticulocyte count at birth ranges from 3%–7% during the first 48 hours, during which time it rises slightly. After the second day, it falls rather rapidly to 1%–3% by the seventh day of life. Hb concentration in capillary blood during the first day of life averages 19.0 g/dL, with 95% of normal values falling to between 14.6 and 23.4 g/dL. In cord blood the average is 16.8 g/dL, with 95% of normal between 13.5 and 20 g/dL. Frequently, an initial increase in the Hb level of venous blood is seen at

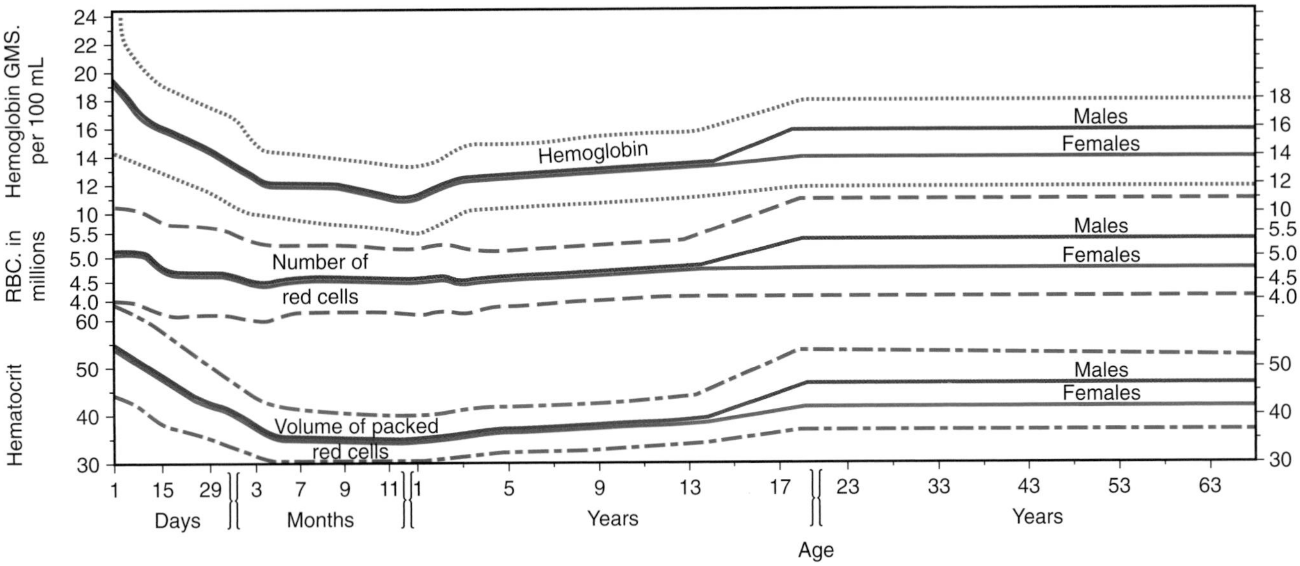

Figure 30-8 Values for hemoglobin (Hb), hematocrit (Hct; volume of packed red cells), and red cell count from birth to old age. Mean values are heavy lines. Reference interval for Hb is indicated by dotted lines, for red cell counts by dashed lines, and for Hct by dotted and dashed lines. The scales on the ordinate are similar, so that relative changes in Hb, red cell count, and Hct are apparent on inspection. The scale for age, however, is progressively altered (Wintrobe, 1974).

the end of 24 hours compared with that of cord blood. At the end of the first week, the level is about the same as in cord blood, and it does not begin to fall until after the second week. During the first 2 weeks, the lower limit of normal is 14.5 g/dL for capillary blood and 13.0 g/dL for venous blood. The Hct in capillary blood on the first day of life averages 0.61, with 95% of normal values between 0.46 and 0.76. In cord blood, the average is 0.53. Changes during the first few weeks parallel the Hb concentration. The Hb and Hct are highest at birth but fall rather steeply in the first days and weeks of life to a minimum at 2 months of age, at which time the lower limit of the 95% reference values and the mean value for the Hb are 9.4 and 11.2 g/dL, and for the Hct are 0.28 and 0.35, respectively. After the age of 4 months, the lower limit for the Hb is 11.2 g/dL and for the Hct is 0.32; these values rise gradually until about age 5 years, and somewhat more steeply in boys than in girls thereafter (Shannon, 2002). The normal MCV at birth ranges from 104–118 fL, compared with the adult reference interval of 80–96 fL. Because the RBC does not fall to the degree that the Hb and Hct do, the MCV decreases abruptly, then gradually, during the first few months of life. The lowest value is reached at about 1 year. In studies in which iron deficiency and thalassemia are excluded, the lower reference limit (95% reference values) for the MCV gradually rises between the ages of 1 year and 15 years—in boys from 70–76 fL, and in girls from 70–78 fL (Shannon, 1996). Reference intervals for RBC values in sexually mature adults are given in Table 30-4. The indices are similar in males and females, but the Hb is 1–2 g/dL higher in males, with commensurate increments in Hct and RBCs (see Fig. 30-8). This is believed to be mainly the effect of androgen in stimulating erythropoietin production and its effect on the marrow. In older men, the Hb tends to fall, and in older women, the Hb tends to fall to a lesser degree (in some studies) or even rise slightly (in other studies). In older individuals, therefore, the sex difference is less than 1 g Hb/dL (Dacie, 1991). Posture and muscular activity change the concentration of the formed elements. The Hb, Hct, and RBC increase by several percent when the change from recumbency to standing is made, and strenuous muscular activity causes a further increase, presumably owing primarily to loss of plasma water. Diurnal variation that is not related to exercise or to analytic variation also occurs. The Hb is highest in the morning, falls during the day, and is lowest in the evening, with a mean difference of 8%–9% (Dacie, 1991). In persons living at a higher altitude, the Hb, Hct, and RBC are elevated over what they would be at sea level. The difference is about 1 g Hb/dL at 2 km altitude and 2 g Hb/dL at 3 km. Increased erythropoiesis is secondary to anoxic stimulation of erythropoietin production. People who are smokers also tend to have a mild erythrocytosis.

Physiologic Variation in Leukocytes

The total white cell count at birth and during the first 24 hours varies within wide limits. Neutrophils are the predominant cell, varying from 6–28 × 10^9/L; about 15% of these are band forms (Altman, 1974), and a few myelocytes are present. Neutrophils drop to about 5 × 10^9/L during the first week and remain at about the same level thereafter. Lymphocytes are about 5.5 × 10^9/L at birth and change little during the first week. They become the predominant cell, on average, after the first week of life and remain so until about age 7, when neutrophils again predominate. The upper limit of the 95% reference interval for lymphocytes at age 6 months is 13.5, at 1 year 10.5, at 2 years 9.5, at 6 years 7.0, and at 12 years 6.0 × 10^9/L. For neutrophils at the same ages, the values are 8.5, 8.5, 8.5, 8.0, and 8.0 × 10^9/L, respectively—all somewhat higher than those for adults (Table 30-5).

Diurnal variation has been recognized in the neutrophil count, with highest levels in the afternoon and lowest levels in the morning at rest. Exercise produces leukocytosis, which includes an increased neutrophil concentration as a result of a shift of cells from the marginal to the circulating granulocyte pool. Increased lymphocyte drainage into the blood also appears to contribute to the total increase. Both average and lower reference values for neutrophil concentration in the black population are lower than in the Caucasian population; this difference must be taken into account in assessing neutropenia. Cigarette smokers have higher average leukocyte counts than nonsmokers. The increase is greatest (about 30%) in heavy smokers who inhale and affects neutrophils, lymphocytes, and monocytes.

Mild changes occur during the menstrual cycle. Neutrophils and monocytes fall and eosinophils tend to rise during menstruation. Basophils have been reported to fall during ovulation. The availability of precise automated leukocyte analyzers provides the potential for investigating physiologic sources of variation that have been obscured by statistical errors in traditional microscopic differential counts (Statland, 1978).

Physiologic Variation in Platelets

The average platelet count is slightly lower at birth than in older children and adults, and may vary from 84–478 × 10^9/L (Barone, 1999). After the first week of life, the reference intervals are those of the adult. In women, the platelet count may fall at the time of menstruation. Women have higher platelet (and WBC and neutrophil) counts than men, and Africans (and less so Afro-Caribbeans) have lower platelet, WBC, and neutrophil counts than Caucasians (Bain, 1996). Reported means (95% reference ranges) for platelet counts were 218 (143–332) for Caucasian men and 183 (115–290) for African men versus 246 (169–358) for Caucasian women and 207 (125–342) for African women. Among Australians west of Sydney and aged 49 or older, Tsang (1998) lists 247 (128–365) for mean platelet counts for men and 275 (147–403) for women.

ERYTHROCYTE SEDIMENTATION RATE

Erythrocyte sedimentation rate (ESR) is a useful but nonspecific marker of underlying inflammation. Recently, high-sensitivity C-reactive protein and other inflammatory markers have been used to detect or monitor disease, particularly cardiovascular disease and metabolic syndrome

TABLE 30-4
Typical Blood Cell Values in a Normal Population of Young Adults

	Men		Women
White cell count (×10⁹/L blood)		7.8 (4.4–11.3)	
Red cell count (×10¹²/L blood)	5.21 (4.52–5.90)		4.60 (4.10–5.10)
Hemoglobin (g/dL blood)	15.7 (14.0–17.5)		13.8 (12.3–15.3)
Hematocrit (percent)	46 (41.5–50.4)		40.2 (35.9–44.6)
Mean cell volume (fL/red cell)		88.0 (80.0–96.1)	
Mean cell hemoglobin (pg/red cell)		30.4 (27.5–33.2)	
Mean cell hemoglobin concentration (g/dL RBC)		34.4 (33.4–35.5)	
Red cell distribution width (CV, percent)		13.1 (11.6–14.6)	
Platelet count (×10⁹/L blood)		311 (172–450)	

The mean and reference intervals (normal range) are given. Because the distribution curves may be nongaussian, the reference interval is the nonparametric central 95% confidence interval. Results are based on 426 normal adult men and 212 normal adult women. Studies were performed on the Coulter model S-Plus IV (Morris, 1975).
CV, Cell values; *RBC,* bed blood cell.

TABLE 30-5
Normal Leukocyte Count, Differential Count, and Hemoglobin Concentration at Various Ages

	LEUKOCYTES*								
Age	**Total leukocytes**	**Total neutrophils**	**Band neutrophils**	**Segmented neutrophils**	**Eosinophils**	**Basophils**	**Lymphocytes**	**Monocytes**	**Hemoglobin (g/dL blood)**
12 months	11.4 (6.0–17.5)	3.5 (1.5–8.5) *31*	0.35 *3.1*	3.2 (1.0–8.5) *28*	0.30 (0.05–0.70) *2.6*	0.05 (0–0.20) *0.4*	7.0 (4.0–10.5) *61*	0.55 (0.05–1.1) *4.8*	12.6 (11.1–14.1)
4 years	9.1 (5.5–15.5)	3.8 (1.5–8.5) *42*	0.27 (0–1.0) *3.0*	3.5 (1.5–7.5) *39*	0.25 (0.02–0.65) *2.8*	0.05 (0–0.2) *0.6*	4.5 (2.0–8.0) *50*	0.45 (0–0.8) *5.0*	12.7 (11.2–14.3)
6 years	8.5 (5.0–14.5)	4.3 (1.5–8.0) *51*	0.25 (0–1.0) *3.0*	4.0 (1.5–7.0) *48*	0.23 (0–0.65) *2.7*	0.05 (0–0.2) *0.6*	3.5 (1.50–7.0) *42*	0.40 (0–0.8) *4.7*	13.0 (11.4–14.5)
10 years	8.1 (4.5–13.5)	4.4 (1.8–8.0) *54*	0.24 (0–1.0) *3.0*	4.2 (1.8–7.0) *51*	0.20 (0–0.60) *2.4*	0.04 (0–0.2) *0.5*	3.1 (1.5–6.5) *38*	0.35 (0–0.8) *4.3*	13.4 (11.8–15.0)
21 years	7.4 (4.5–11.0)	4.4 (1.8–7.7) *59*	0.22 (0–0.7) *3.0*	4.2 (1.8–7.0) *56*	0.20 (0–0.45) *2.7*	0.04 (0–0.2) *0.5*	2.5 (1.0–4.8) *34*	0.30 (0–0.8) *4.0*	15.5 (13.5–17.5) 13.8 (12.0–15.6)

Source: For leukocyte and differential count, Altman (1961); for hemoglobin concentrations, Dalman (1987).
*Values are expressed as mean (95% reference) values. For leukocytes and differential count cell types, the units are cells × 10⁹/μL; the numbers in italic type are mean percentages.

(Pearson, 2003; Rifai, 2005). When well-mixed venous blood is placed in a vertical tube, erythrocytes will tend to fall toward the bottom. The length of fall of the top of the column of erythrocytes over a given interval of time is called the ESR. Several factors are involved.

Plasma Factors

An accelerated ESR is favored by elevated levels of fibrinogen and, to a lesser extent, α_2-, β-, and γ-globulins. These asymmetric protein molecules have a greater effect than other proteins in decreasing the negative charge of erythrocytes (zeta potential) that tends to keep them apart. The decreased zeta potential promotes the formation of rouleaux, which sediment more rapidly than single cells. Removal of fibrinogen by defibrination lowers the ESR. No absolute correlation has been noted between the ESR and any of the plasma protein fractions. Albumin and lecithin retard sedimentation, and cholesterol accelerates the ESR.

Red Cell Factors

Anemia increases the ESR because the change in the erythrocyte/plasma ratio favors rouleaux formation, independently of changes in the concentrations of plasma proteins. By any method of measurement, ESR is most sensitive to altered plasma proteins in the Hct range of 0.30–0.40 (Bull, 1975). The sedimentation rate is directly proportional to the weight of the cell aggregate and inversely proportional to the surface area. Microcytes sediment slower than macrocytes, which have decreased surface area/volume ratios. Rouleaux also have a decreased surface area/volume ratio and accelerate the ESR. Red cells with an abnormal or irregular shape, such as sickle cells or spherocytes, hinder rouleaux formation and lower the ESR.

Stages in the ESR

Three stages can be observed: (1) In the initial 10 minutes, little sedimentation occurs as rouleaux forms; (2) for about 40 minutes, settling occurs at a constant rate; and (3) sedimentation slows in the final 10 minutes as cells pack at the bottom of the tube.

Methods

Westergren Method

Westergren method is widely used, as the method is very simple. The ICSH (1993) has recommended it as the reference method when undiluted whole blood is used. The ICSH states that the patient's Hct should not exceed 35% because reproducibility of sedimentation may be poorer in narrow tubes. A formula to convert between diluted blood ESR and undiluted is as follows:

$$\text{Diluted blood ESR} = (\text{Undiluted ESR} \times 0.86) - 12$$

Equipment. The Westergren tube is a straight pipet 30 cm long, 2.55 mm in internal diameter, and calibrated in millimeters from 0–200. It holds about 1 mL. The Westergren rack is also used, with levelers as needed for a vertical tube position.

Reagent. A 0.105 molar solution (range, 0.10–0.136) of sodium citrate is used as the anticoagulant–diluent solution (31 g of $Na_3C_6H_5O_7{\cdot}H_2O$ added to 1 L of distilled water in a sterile glass bottle). This is filtered and is kept refrigerated without preservatives.

Procedure

1. Two milliliters of whole blood are added to 0.5 mL of sodium citrate and mixed by inversion.
2. A Westergren pipet is filled to the 0 mark and is placed exactly vertical in the rack at room temperature without vibration or exposure to direct sunlight.
3. After exactly 60 minutes, the distance from the 0 mark to the top of the column of red cells is recorded in millimeters as the ESR value. If the demarcation between plasma and the red cell column is hazy, the level is taken where the full density is first apparent.

Modified Westergren Method

A modification of the Westergren method produces the same results but employs blood anticoagulated with EDTA rather than with citrate. This is more convenient because it allows the ESR to be performed from the same tube of blood as is used for other hematologic studies. Two milliliters of well-mixed EDTA-blood is diluted with 0.5 mL of 3.8% sodium citrate or with 0.5 mL of 0.85% sodium chloride. Undiluted blood anticoagulated with EDTA gives poor precision (ICSH, 1977). The ESR gradually increases with age. Westergren's original upper limits of normal (10 mm/hour for men and 20 mm/hour for women) appear to be too low. According to studies of Böttiger (1967) and Zauber (1987), upper limits of reference values for the Westergren method should be as follows:

	Men	Women
Below age 50 years	15 mm/hour	20 mm/hour
Above age 50 years	20 mm/hour	30 mm/hour
Above age 85 years	30 mm/hour	42 mm/hour

Smith (1994) states that the rise in ESR with age likely reflects higher disease prevalence in the elderly; therefore for practical purposes, it may be advisable to use the standard normal range in elderly patients.

Sources of Error

If the concentration of the anticoagulant is higher than recommended, the ESR may be elevated. Sodium citrate or EDTA does not affect the rate of sedimentation if used in the proper concentration. Heparin, however, alters the membrane zeta potential and cannot be used as an anticoagulant. It can also increase the ESR when used as a medication in vivo (Penchas, 1978). Bubbles left in the tube when it is filled will affect the ESR. Hemolysis may modify the sedimentation. The cleanliness of the tube is important. Tilting the tube accelerates the ESR. The red cells aggregate along the lower side while the plasma rises along the upper side. Consequently, the retarding influence of the rising plasma is less effective. An angle of even 3 degrees from the vertical may accelerate the ESR by as much as 30%. Plastic ESR pipets have slightly higher (1–2 mm/hour) values than glass pipets (Schneiderka, 1997).

Temperature should be within the range of 20°–25° C. Lower or higher temperatures in some cases alter the ESR. If the blood has been kept refrigerated, it should be permitted to reach room temperature and be mixed by inversion a minimum of eight times before the test is performed. The test should be set up within 2 hours after the blood sample is obtained (or within 12 hours if EDTA is used as the anticoagulant and the blood is kept at 4° C); otherwise, some samples with elevated ESRs will be falsely low (Morris, 1975). On standing, erythrocytes tend to become spherical and less readily form rouleaux.

No effective method is known for correcting for anemia in the Westergren method, although this can be done with the Wintrobe method.

Alternative Methods and Technologies to Measure ESR

The **VES-MATIC 20** instrument is a bench top analyzer designed to measure the ESR in 20 blood samples (Plebani, 1998; Caswell, 1991). It is completely automated. The blood is collected in special cuvets and is carefully mixed by the instrument; the samples are then left to sediment for a certain period. The 18-degree slant of the tubes with respect to the vertical axis causes acceleration of the sedimentation, allowing results comparable with those of Westergren at the first hour to be obtained in only 25 minutes; those comparable with Westergren at the second hour require only 45 minutes. The optoelectrical sensors automatically read the erythrocyte sedimentation level. The data are elaborated and then are printed or visualized on the display.

The **Micro-ESR method** has greater utility in pediatric patients. Barrett (1980) described a micro-ESR method using 0.2 mL blood to fill a plastic disposable tube 230 mm long with a 1-mm internal bore. Capillary blood values correlated well with venous blood micro-ESR and Westergren ESR values. Kumar (1994) refers to a micro-ESR (mESR) that utilizes whole blood to completely fill a 75-mm heparinized microhematocrit capillary tube.

Another instrument used to measure ESR is ESR STAT PLUS, which is a centrifugation-based method. The sample is placed in the centrifuge, and infrared laser tracks the erythrocyte-plasma interface and makes multiple measurements, from which the linear portion of the sedimentation curve is identified and is used by the software algorithm to determine the ESR result. This method requires smaller volumes of specimen than the Westergren method and is faster. The pitfall is correlation with the reference Westergren method, especially in the 0–20 mm/hour range. It can be also prone to human error because it requires a minimum of 15 mixing intervals, followed by a 5-minute limit before drawing into the capillary tube (Shelat, 2008).

Application

The ESR is one of the oldest laboratory tests still in use. Although some of its usefulness has decreased as more specific methods of evaluating disease (such as C-reactive protein [CRP]) have been developed (Zlonis, 1993), new clinical applications are being reported (Saadeh, 1998). Recently, the ESR has been reported to be of clinical significance in sickle cell disease (low value in the absence of painful crisis, moderately increased 1 week into the crisis), osteomyelitis (elevated, helpful in following therapy), stroke (ESR ≥28 mm/hour has poorer prognosis), prostate cancer (ESR ≥37 mm/hour has higher incidence of disease progression and death), and coronary artery disease (ESR >22 mm/hour in white men had high risk of coronary artery disease [CAD]) (Saadeh, 1998). In pregnancy, the ESR increases moderately, beginning at the 10th to the 12th week, and returns to normal about 1 month postpartum. The ESR tends to be markedly elevated in monoclonal blood protein disorders such as multiple myeloma or macroglobulinemia, in severe polyclonal hyperglobulinemia due to inflammatory disease, and in hyperfibrinogenemia.

Moderate elevations are common in active inflammatory disease such as rheumatoid arthritis, chronic infection, collagen disease, and neoplastic disease. The ESR has little diagnostic value in these disorders but can be useful in monitoring disease activity. It is simpler than measurement of serum proteins, which has tended to replace ESR. Because the test is often normal in patients with neoplasm, connective tissue disease, and infection, a normal ESR cannot be used to exclude these diagnostic possibilities. In patients with known cancer, however, when the value exceeds 100 mm/hour, metastases are usually present (Sox, 1986). The ESR is of little value in screening asymptomatic patients for disease; history and physical examination will usually disclose the cause of an elevated ESR (Sox, 1986). The ESR is useful and is indicated in establishing the diagnosis and in monitoring polymyalgia rheumatica and temporal arteritis, where the rate typically exceeds 90 mm/hour (Zlonis, 1993). Emergency physicians continue to use the ESR in evaluating temporal arteritis, septic arthritis, pelvic inflammatory disease, and appendicitis (Olshaker, 1997). Freeman (1997) urges immediate quick ESR estimation if giant cell arteritis is clinically indicated, as a delay of even a few hours in starting steroid therapy may result in irreversible visual failure. Harrow (1999) concludes that an ESR of 5 mm or less at 30 minutes correctly identifies most patients with normal ESR without misclassifying elevated ESRs.

In Hodgkin's disease, the ESR may be a very useful prognostic blood measurement in the absence of systemic ("B") symptoms (fever, weight loss, night sweats). In one study (Vaughan Hudson, 1987), one third of asymptomatic patients had both an ESR of less than 10 mm/hour and an excellent survival rate, regardless of age, stage, or histopathology. Asymptomatic patients with an ESR of 60 mm/hour or greater had a survival rate as poor as those with systemic symptoms.

Iversen (1996) reported that 70% of renal cell carcinoma patients had an increased ESR, which had been significantly rising for up to 6 years before diagnosis. They argued for a systematic graphing and baseline determination of the ESR over time, which showed a marked elevation in ESR a year before diagnosis. Such a trend of increasing ESR should lead to further investigation, as with renal ultrasound, which may then lead to curative nephrectomy before metastases occur.

BLOOD FILM EXAMINATION

Microscopic examination of the blood spread on a glass slide or coverslip yields useful information regarding all formed elements of the blood. The process of making thin blood film causes mechanical trauma to the cells. Also the cells flatten on the glass during drying, and fixation and staining involve exposure to methanol and water. Some artifacts are inevitably introduced, but these can be minimized by good technique.

EXAMINATION OF WET PREPARATIONS

It is sometimes advantageous to examine fresh blood under the microscope to avoid artifacts of fixation or staining. This is readily accomplished by sealing a small drop of blood diluted with isotonic sodium chloride beneath a coverslip on a glass slide. Buffered glutaraldehyde will preserve the cells for reexamination at a later time. Petroleum jelly or xipamide (Aquaphor) may be used to seal the edges of the coverslip to the slide. Wet preparations are used to detect sickling, and spherocytes may be readily detected in this manner. Wet preparations may be examined to ensure that the erythrocyte abnormalities seen on fixed films are not artifacts of drying or staining.

MAKING AND STAINING BLOOD FILMS

Examination of the blood film is an important part of the hematologic evaluation. The reliability of the information obtained depends heavily on well-made and well-stained films that are systematically examined. Blood films should be prepared immediately if possible. Three methods of making films are described: the two-slide or wedge method, the cover glass method, and the spinner method.

Wedge Method

Place a drop of blood 2–3 mm in diameter about 1 cm from the end of a clean, dust-free slide that is on a flat surface. With the thumb and forefinger of the right hand, hold the end of a second (spreader) slide against the surface of the first slide at an angle of 30–45 degrees, and draw it back to contact the drop of blood. Allow the blood to spread and form the angle between the two slides. Push the "spreader slide" at a moderate speed forward until all the blood has been spread into a moderately thin film. The spreader slide should be clean, dry, and slightly narrower than the first slide, so that the edges can be easily examined with the microscope.

The slides should be rapidly air dried by waving the slides or using an electrical fan. The thickness of the film can be adjusted by changing the angle of the spreader slide or the speed of spreading, or by using a smaller or larger drop of blood. At a given speed, increasing the angle of the spreader slide will increase the thickness of the film. At a given angle, increasing the speed with which the spreader slide is pushed will also increase the thickness of the film. The film should not cover the entire surface of the slide. A good film includes a thick portion and a thin portion and a gradual transition from one to the other. The film should have a smooth, even appearance and be free from ridges, waves, or holes. The edge of the spreader must be absolutely smooth. If it is rough, the film has ragged tails containing many leukocytes. In films of optimal thickness, some overlap of red cells is seen in much of the film, but with even distribution and separation of red cells toward the thin tail. The faster the film is air dried, the better is the spreading of individual cells on the slide. Slow drying (e.g., in humid weather) results in contraction artifacts of the cells. The slide may be labeled with a lead pencil on the frosted end or directly on the thicker end of the blood film.

Cover Glass Method

No. 1 or 1½ cover glasses 22 mm square are recommended.

Touch a cover glass to the top of a small drop of blood without touching the skin, and place it, blood side down, crosswise on another cover glass, so that the corners appear as an eight-pointed star. If the drop is not too large and the cover glasses are perfectly clean, the blood will spread out evenly and quickly in a thin layer between the two surfaces. Just as it stops spreading, pull the cover glasses quickly but firmly apart on a plane parallel to their surfaces. The blood usually is much more evenly spread on one of the cover glasses than it is on the other. Cover glasses should be placed film side up on clean paper and allowed to dry in the air, or they may be inserted back to back in slits made in a cardboard box. Films from venous blood may be prepared similarly by placing a drop of blood on a coverslip and proceeding as described.

Spinner Method

Blood films that combine the advantages of easy handling of the wedge slide and uniform distribution of cells of the cover glass preparation may be made with special types of centrifuges known as **spinners** (Rogers, 1973). The spinner slide produces a uniform blood film, in which all cells are separated (a monolayer) and randomly distributed. White cells can be easily identified at any spot in the film. On a wedge smear, disproportions (1) of monocytes occur at the tip of the feather edge, (2) of neutrophils are seen just in from the feather edge, and (3) of both occur at the lateral edges of the film (Rogers, 1973). This is of little practical significance, but it does result in slightly lower monocyte counts in wedge films.

Blood Stains

The aniline dyes used in blood work are of two general classes: basic dyes, such as methylene blue; and acid dyes, such as eosin. Nuclei and certain other structures in the blood are stained by the basic dyes and, hence, are called **basophilic.** Structures that take up only acid dyes are called **acidophilic,** or **eosinophilic.** Other structures stained by a combination of the two are called **neutrophilic.**

Polychrome methylene blue and **eosin stains** are the outgrowth of the original time-consuming Romanowsky's method and are widely used. They stain differentially most normal and abnormal structures in the blood. The basic components of thiazine include methylene blue (tetramethylthionine) and, in varying proportions, its analogs produced by oxidative demethylation: azure B (trimethylthionine); azure A (asymmetrical dimethylthionine); symmetrical dimethylthionine; and azure C (monomethylthionine) (Lillie, 1977). The acidic component eosin is derived from a xanthene skeleton. Most Romanowsky's stains are dissolved in methyl alcohol and combine fixation with staining. Among the best known methods are Giemsa and Wright's stains.

Wright's Stain

This is a methyl alcoholic solution of eosin and a complex mixture of thiazines, including methylene blue (usually 50%–75%), azure B (10%–25%), and other derivatives (Lubrano, 1977). Wright's stain certified by the Biological Stain Commission is commercially available as a solution ready for use or as a powder. The buffer solution (pH 6.4) contains primary (monobasic) potassium phosphate (KH_2PO_4), anhydrous 6.63 g; secondary (dibasic) sodium phosphate (Na_2HPO_4), anhydrous 2.56 g; and distilled water to make 1 L. A more alkaline buffer (pH 6.7) may be prepared by using 5.13 g of the potassium salt and 4.12 g of the sodium salt.

Procedure

1. To prevent the plasma background of the film from staining blue, blood films should be stained within a few hours of preparation or fixed if they must be kept without staining.
2. Fixation and staining may be accomplished by immersing the slides in reagent-filled jars or by covering horizontally supported slides or coverslips with the reagents. With the latter method, covering the film with copious stain avoids evaporation, which leads to precipitation.
3. Fixation is provided for 1–2 minutes with absolute methanol.
4. The slide is next exposed to undiluted stain solution for 2 minutes. Then, without removing the stain from the horizontal slide, an equal amount of buffer is carefully added and is mixed by blowing gently.
5. The stain is flushed from the horizontal slide with water. Washing for longer than 30 seconds reduces the blue staining. The back of the slide is cleaned with gauze.
6. The slide is allowed to air dry in a tilted position.
7. Cover glasses are mounted film side down on a slide with Canada balsam or other mounting medium.

Films stained well with Wright's stain have a pink color when viewed with the naked eye. Under low power, the cells should be evenly distributed. The red cells are pink, not lemon yellow or red. There should be a minimum of precipitate. The color of the film should be uniform. The blood cells should be free from artifacts, such as vacuoles. The nuclei of leukocytes are purple, the chromatin and parachromatin clearly differentiated, and the cytoplasmic neutrophilic granules tan in color. The eosinophilic granules are red-orange, and each is distinctly discernible. The basophil has dark purple granules. Platelets have dark lilac granules. Bacteria (if present) are blue. The cytoplasm of lymphocytes is generally light blue; that of monocytes has a faint blue-gray tinge. Malarial parasites have sky-blue cytoplasm and red-purple chromatin. The colors are prone to fade if the preparation is mounted in balsam of poor quality or is exposed to the light.

Staining Problems

Excessively Blue Stain. Thick films, prolonged staining time, inadequate washing, or too high an alkalinity of stain or diluent tends to cause excessive basophilia. In such films, the erythrocytes appear blue or green, the nuclear chromatin is deep blue to black, and the granules of the neutrophils are deeply overstained and appear large and prominent. The granules of the eosinophils are blue or gray. Staining for a shorter time or using less stain and more diluent may correct the problem. If these steps are ineffective, the buffer may be too alkaline, and a new one with a lower pH should be prepared.

Excessively Pink Stain. Insufficient staining, prolonged washing time, mounting the coverslips before they are dry, or too high an acidity of the stain or buffer may cause excessive acidophilia. In such films, the erythrocytes are bright red or orange, the nuclear chromatin is pale blue, and the granules of the eosinophils are sparkling brilliant red. One of the causes of the increased acidity is exposure of the stain or buffer to acid fumes. The problem may be a low pH of the buffer, or it may be the methyl alcohol, which is prone to develop formic acid as a result of oxidation on standing.

Other Staining Problems. Inadequately stained red cells, nuclei, or eosinophilic granules may be due to understaining or excessive washing. Prolonging the staining or reducing the washing may solve the problem.

Precipitate on the film may be due to unclean slides; drying during the period of staining; inadequate washing of the slide at the end of the staining period, especially failure to hold the slide horizontally during initial washing; inadequate filtration of the stain; or permitting dust to settle on the slide or smear.

Other Stains

Besides Wright's stain, Romanowsky-type stains include a number of others: Giemsa, Leishman's, Jenner's, May-Grünwald, MacNeal's, and various combinations. Some have been particularly recommended for certain purposes, such as Giemsa stain for excellence in staining malarial parasites and protozoa.

Reference Method

Studies have demonstrated the ability of the combination of just two dyes—azure B and eosin Y—to give the full range of colors provided by ideal Romanowsky's staining of blood and marrow cells. This is the reference method for Romanowsky's staining (ICSH, 1984a).

Automated Slide Stainer

Automated slide stainers are being used in several laboratories for routine hematology and microbiology slides. The stainer is a compact instrument with microprocessor control for flexibility in staining applications. Several slides can be stained uniformly in minutes. Typically, any automated stainer has several user-definable programs to choose from. Staining problems are encountered even with the use of automatic stainers and must be dealt with on an individual basis.

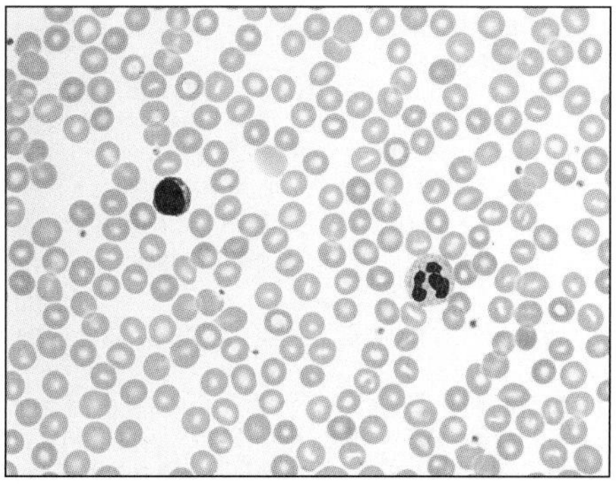

Figure 30-9 Normal peripheral smear. Erythrocytes appear as circular, homogeneous disks of nearly uniform size, ranging from 6–8 μm in diameter, with central pallor not exceeding more than one third of the cell. On average, the red cells are approximately the same size as the nucleus of a small lymphocyte (500×).

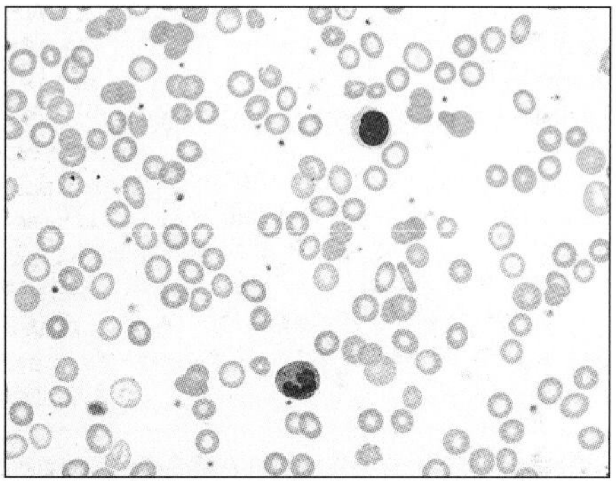

Figure 30-10 Microcytic hypochromic red cells in iron deficiency anemia. Red cells are hypochromic—the amount of hemoglobin per cell is decreased, and the central pale area becomes larger (more than one third) (500×).

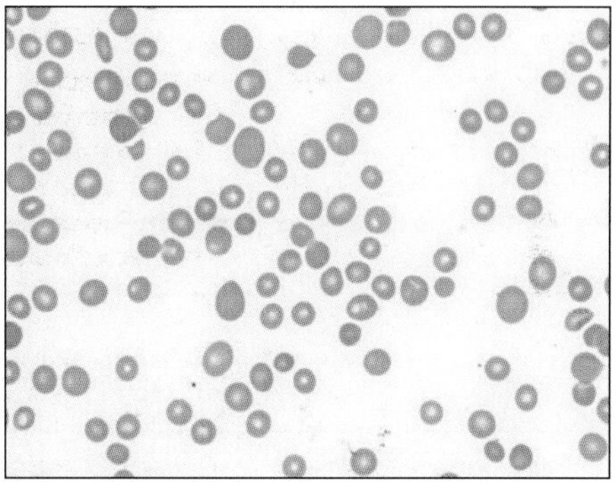

Figure 30-11 Macrocytes. Red cells are larger and thicker, stain deeply, and lack central pallor (500×).

ERYTHROCYTES

The practicing pathologist may be called upon to review peripheral blood smears, to confirm or compare his/her assessment with that of the technologist, and to review the findings with clinical colleagues at the multihead microscope. Although this is a daily task for the hematopathologist, the general pathologist examines the peripheral smear less frequently and the bone marrow preparation even less so. Following is a summary of the main features that he or she should evaluate. In the blood from a healthy person, the erythrocytes, when not crowded together, appear as circular, homogeneous disks of nearly uniform size, ranging from 6–8 μm in diameter (Fig. 30-9). However, even in normal blood, individual cells may be as small as 5.5 μm and as large as 9.5 μm. The center of each is somewhat paler than the periphery. In disease, erythrocytes vary in their Hb content, size, shape, staining properties, and structure.

Color

Hemoglobin Content

The depth of staining furnishes a rough guide to the amount of Hb in red cells, and the terms **normochromic, hypochromic,** and **hyperchromic** are used to describe this feature of red cells. Normochromic refers to normal intensity of staining (see Fig. 30-9). When the amount of Hb is diminished, the central pale area becomes larger and paler. This is known as **hypochromia.** The MCH and MCHC are usually decreased (Fig. 30-10). In megaloblastic anemia, because the red cells are larger and hence thicker, many stain deeply and have less central pallor (Fig. 30-11). These cells are hyperchromic because they have an increased MCH, but the MCHC is normal. In hereditary spherocytosis (Fig. 30-12), the cells are also hyperchromic; although the MCH is normal, the MCHC is usually increased because of a reduced surface/volume ratio. The presence of hypochromic cells and normochromic cells in the same film is called **anisochromia** or, sometimes, a **dimorphic anemia** (Fig. 30-13). This is characteristic of sideroblastic anemias but also is found some weeks after iron therapy for iron deficiency anemia, or in a hypochromic anemia after transfusion with normal cells.

Polychromatophilia

A blue-gray tint to the red cells (polychromatophilia or polychromasia) is a combination of the affinity of Hb for acid stains and the affinity of RNA for basic stains. The presence of residual RNA in the red cell indicates that

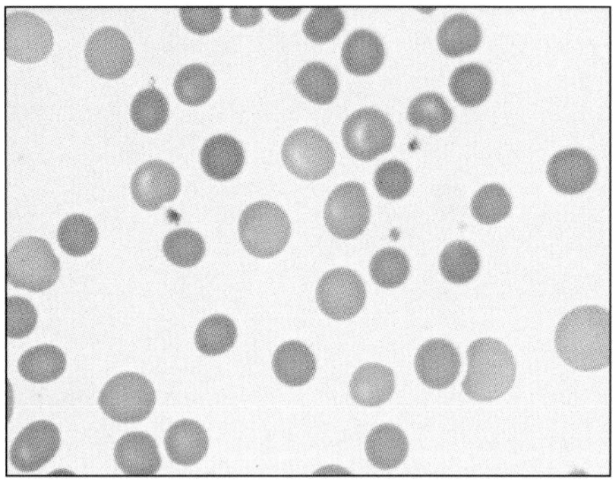

Figure 30-12 Hereditary spherocytosis. Spherocytes are nearly perfectly round in shape, smaller than normal red cells, and lack central pallor (hyperchromic) (1000×).

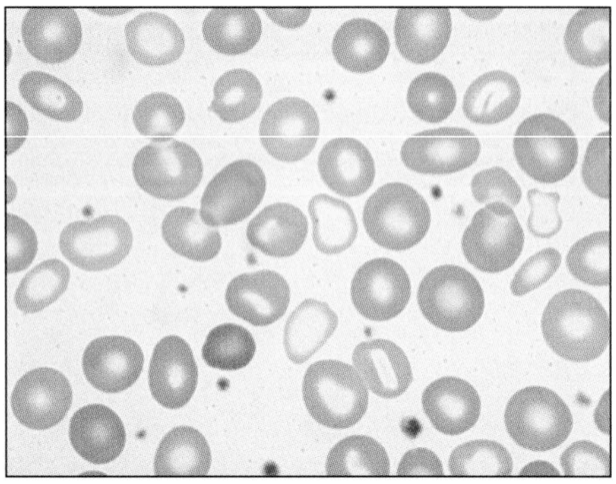

Figure 30-13 Dimorphic anemia. Anisocytosis and anisochromia characterized by the presence of microcytic hypochromic cells, normocytic cells, and few macrocytes (1000×).

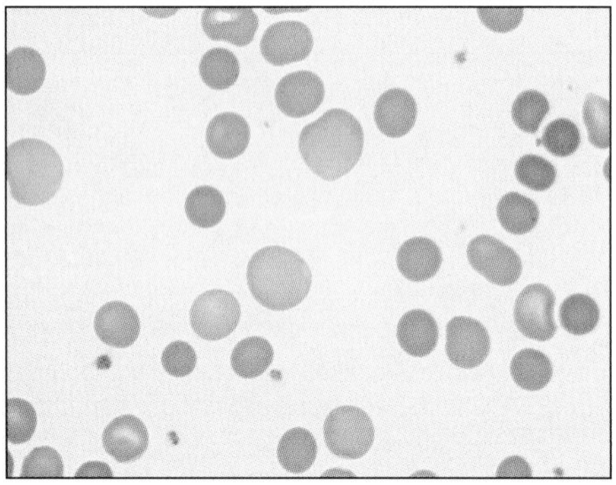

Figure 30-14 Polychromatophilia. Polychromatophilic red cells are young red cells, larger than mature red cells; they lack central pallor and appear slightly basophilic on Wright's stain. They are called reticulocytes when stained supravitally with brilliant cresyl blue (1000×).

it is a young red cell that has been in the blood for 1–2 days. These cells are larger than mature red cells and may lack central pallor (Fig. 30-14). Young cells with residual RNA are polychromatophilic red cells on air-dried films stained with Wright's stain but are reticulocytes when stained supravitally with brilliant cresyl blue. Therefore, increased polychromasia implies reticulocytosis; it is most marked in hemolysis and in acute blood loss.

Size

The red cells may be abnormally small, or microcytes (see Fig. 30-10), or abnormally large, or macrocytes (see Fig. 30-11), or they may show abnormal variation in size (anisocytosis) (see Fig. 30-13). Anisocytosis is a feature of most anemias; when it is marked in degree, both macrocytes and microcytes are usually present. In analyzing causes of anemia, the terms **microcytic** and **macrocytic** have greatest meaning when considered as cell volume rather than cell diameter. The mean cell volume is measured directly on a multichannel analyzer. We perceive the diameter directly from the blood film and infer volume (and the Hb content) from it. Thus, the red cells in Figure 30-10 are microcytic; because they are hypochromic,

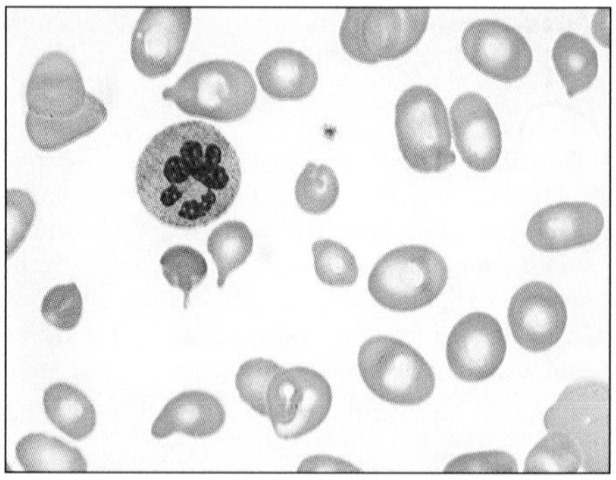

Figure 30-15 Poikilocytosis. Variation in shape of red cells. Abnormally shaped cells include oval, pear-shaped, and other irregularly shaped cells (1000×).

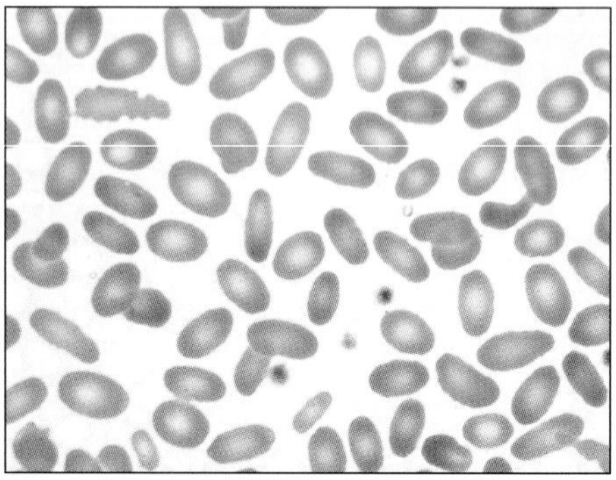

Figure 30-16 Hereditary elliptocytosis. Most cells are elliptocytes. They are seen in a normal person's blood, but usually account for less than 10% of cells. They are also common in iron deficiency anemia, myelofibrosis, megaloblastic anemia, and sickle cell anemia (1000×).

they are thinner than normal and the diameter is not decreased proportionately to the volume. Also, the mean cell volume in the blood of the patient with spherocytosis (see Fig. 30-12) is in the normal range; although many of the cells have a small diameter, their volume is not decreased because they are thicker than normal.

Shape

Variation in shape is called **poikilocytosis.** Any abnormally shaped cell is a poikilocyte. Oval, pear-shaped, teardrop-shaped, saddle-shaped, helmet-shaped, and irregularly shaped cells may be seen in a single case of anemia such as megaloblastic anemia (Fig. 30-15).

Elliptocytes are most abundant in hereditary elliptocytosis (Fig. 30-16), in which most cells are elliptical; this is a dominant condition that is only occasionally associated with hemolytic anemia. Elliptocytes are seen in normal persons' blood but account for less than 10% of the cells. They are more common, however, in iron deficiency anemia (see Fig. 30-10), myelofibrosis with myeloid metaplasia, megaloblastic anemia, and sickle cell anemia.

Spherocytes are nearly spherical erythrocytes, in contradistinction to normal biconcave disks. Their diameter is smaller than normal. They lack the central pale area or have a smaller, often eccentric, pale area (because the cell is thicker and can come to rest somewhat tilted instead of perfectly flattened on the slide). They are found in hereditary spherocytosis (HS) (see Fig. 30-12), in some cases of autoimmune hemolytic anemia (AHA), and in some conditions in which a direct physical or chemical injury has occurred to the cells, such as from heat (Fig. 30-17). In each of these three instances, tiny bits of membrane (in excess of Hb) are removed from the adult red cells, leaving the cells with a decreased surface/volume ratio. In HS and AHA, this occurs in the reticuloendothelial system; in other instances (e.g., in the patient with body burns), this may occur intravascularly.

Target cells are erythrocytes that are thinner than normal (leptocytes) and when stained show a peripheral rim of Hb with a dark, central, Hb-containing area. They are found in obstructive jaundice (Fig. 30-18), in which there appears to be an augmentation of the cell surface membrane; in the postsplenectomy state, in which there is a lack of normal reduction of surface membrane as the cell ages; in any hypochromic anemia, especially thalassemia; and in Hb C disease.

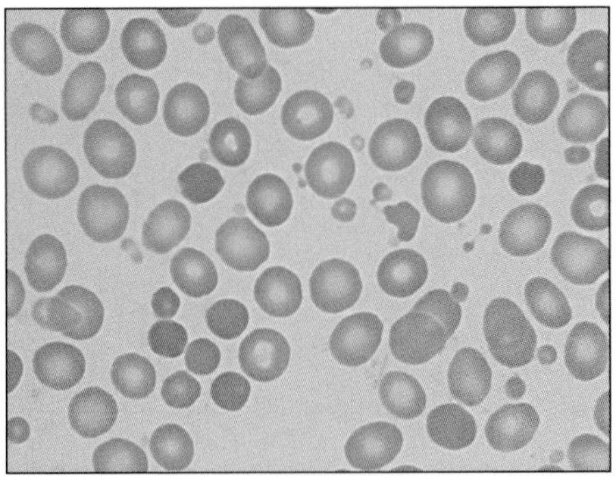

Figure 30-17 Thermal injury. Tiny bits of membrane (in excess of hemoglobin) are removed from the red cell surface, leading to formation of spherocytes (1000×).

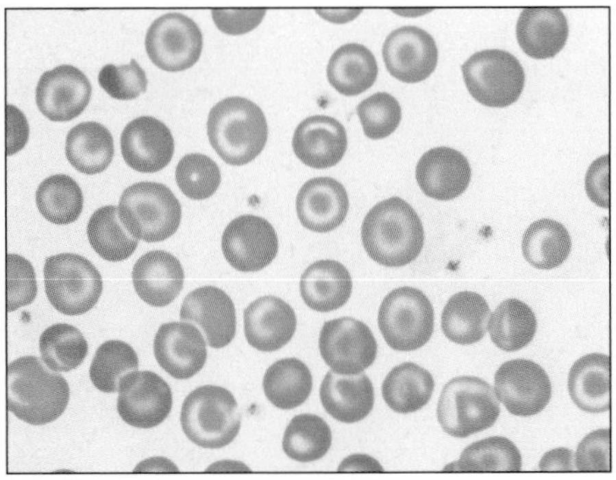

Figure 30-18 Target cells. Red cells with thin membrane, peripheral rim of hemoglobin (Hb), and dark, central, Hb-containing area. They are frequently seen in Hb C disease, in hypochromic anemia, and in liver disease (1000×).

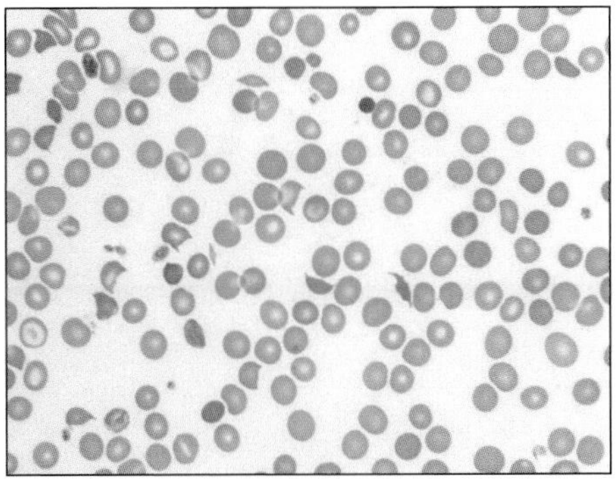

Figure 30-19 Schistocytes. Presence of cell fragments is indicative of hemolysis. Schistocytes can be seen in several conditions, including microangiopathic hemolytic anemia, megaloblastic anemia, burns, and disseminated intravascular coagulation (500×).

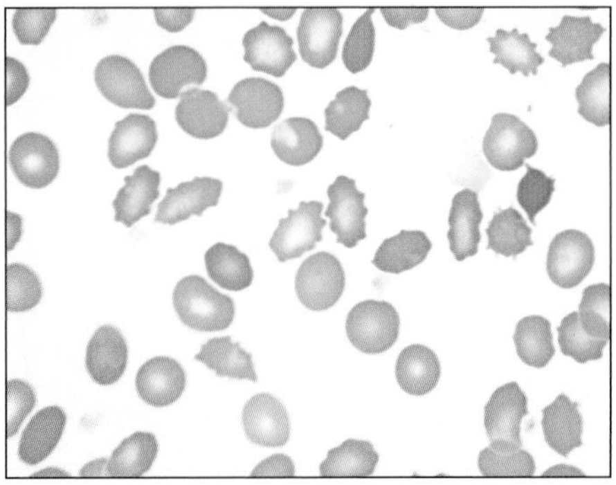

Figure 30-20 Acanthocytes. Irregularly spiculated cells with bulbous and rounded ends, frequently seen in abetalipoproteinemia or certain cases of liver disease (1000×).

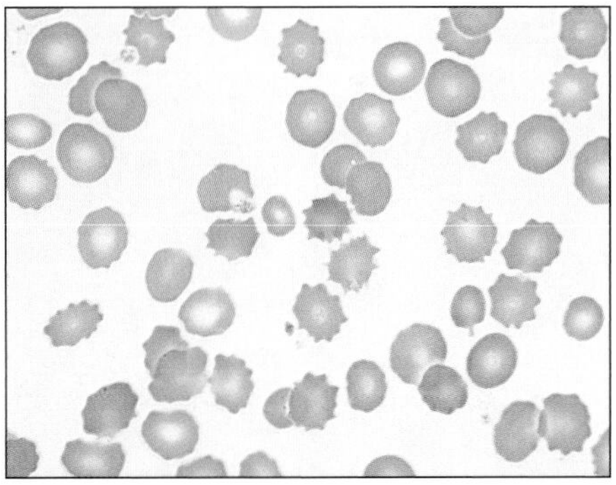

Figure 30-21 Echinocytes. Regularly contracted cells with sharp ends; may occur as an artifact during film preparation or as the result of hyperosmolarity or decreased adenosine triphosphate due to several causes (1000×).

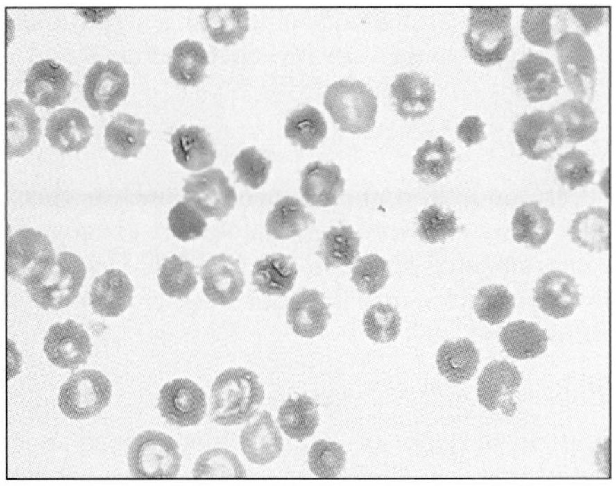

Figure 30-22 Artifact. Tiny pits or bubbles in the red cells. They can be caused by a small amount of water contaminating the Wright's stain or by insufficient slide drying (500×).

Schistocytes (cell fragments) indicate the presence of hemolysis, whether in megaloblastic anemia, severe burns (see Fig. 30-17), or microangiopathic hemolytic anemia (Fig. 30-19). The latter process may be associated with small blood vessel disease or with fibrin in small blood vessels and results in intravascular fragmentation; particularly characteristic are helmet cells and triangular cells. Burr cells are irregularly contracted red cells with prominent spicules and are seen in the same process; however, this term is used differently by different hematologists and therefore leads to confusion.

Acanthocytes are irregularly spiculated red cells in which the ends of the spicules are bulbous and rounded (Fig. 30-20); they are seen in abetalipoproteinemia, hereditary or acquired, and in certain cases of liver disease. Crenated cells or echinocytes (Fig. 30-21) are regularly contracted cells that may commonly occur as an artifact during preparation of films, or they may be due to hyperosmolarity, or to the discocyte–echinocyte transformation. In vivo, the latter may be associated with decreased red cell adenosine triphosphate (ATP) resulting from any of several causes. Artifacts resembling crenated cells consisting of tiny pits or bubbles indenting the red cells (Fig. 30-22) may be caused by a small amount of water contaminating the Wright's stain (or absolute methanol, if this is used first as a fixative).

Structure

Basophilic Stippling (Punctate Basophilia)

This is characterized by the presence, within the erythrocyte, of irregular basophilic granules, which vary from fine to coarse (Fig. 30-23). They stain deep blue with Wright's stain. The erythrocyte containing them may stain normally in other respects, or it may exhibit polychromatophilia. Fine stippling is commonly seen when there is increased polychromatophilia and, therefore, with increased production of red cells. Coarse stippling may be seen in lead poisoning or other diseases with impaired Hb synthesis, in megaloblastic anemia, and in other forms of severe anemia; it is attributed to an abnormal instability of the RNA in the young cell. Red cells with inorganic iron-containing granules (as demonstrated by stains for iron) are called **siderocytes.** Sometimes these granules stain with

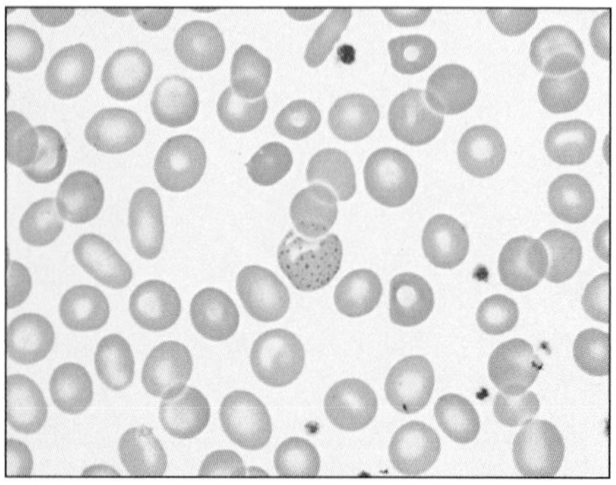

Figure 30-23 Basophilic stippling. Presence of irregular basophilic granules, either fine or coarse; commonly seen in increased red cell production. Coarse stippling is usually seen in lead poisoning, or other anemias due to impaired hemoglobin synthesis, such as megaloblastic anemia (1000×).

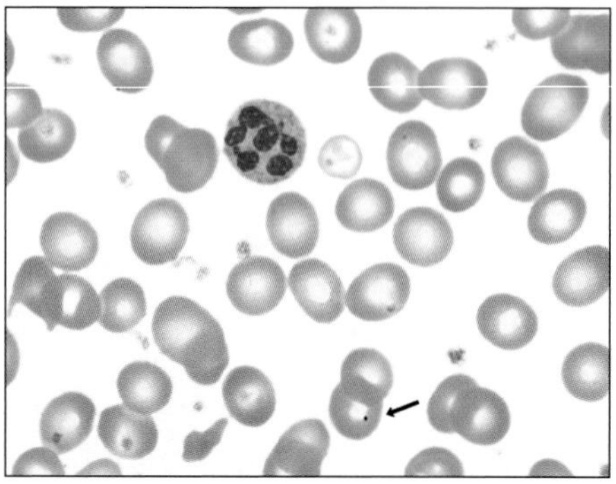

Figure 30-24 Howell-Jolly bodies. Smooth round remnants of nuclear chromatin. Seen in postsplenectomy states and hemolytic and megaloblastic anemias (a hypersegmented neutrophil is also seen) (1000×).

Wright's stain; if so, they are called **Pappenheimer bodies.** In contrast to basophilic stippling, Pappenheimer bodies are few in number in a given red cell and are rarely seen in the peripheral blood except after splenectomy.

Howell-Jolly Bodies

These particles are smooth, round remnants of nuclear chromatin. Single Howell-Jolly bodies may be seen in megaloblastic anemia (Fig. 30-24), in hemolytic anemia, and after splenectomy. Multiple Howell-Jolly bodies in a single cell usually indicate megaloblastic anemia or some other form of abnormal erythropoiesis.

Cabot Rings

These are ring-shaped, figure-of-eight, or loop-shaped structures. Occasionally, they are formed by double or several concentric lines. They are observed rarely in erythrocytes in pernicious anemia, lead poisoning, and certain other disorders of erythropoiesis. They stain red or reddish purple with Wright's stain and have no internal structure. The rings are probably microtubules remaining from a mitotic spindle (Bessis, 1977). They are interpreted as evidence of abnormal erythropoiesis.

Malarial Stippling

Fine granules may appear in erythrocytes that harbor *Plasmodium vivax*. With Wright's stain, the minute granules, "Schüffner's granules," stain purplish red. They are sometimes so numerous that they almost hide the parasites. These red cells are, as a rule, larger than normal.

Rouleaux Formation

This is the alignment of red cells one upon another so that they resemble stacks of coins. On air-dried films, rouleaux appear as in Figure 30-25. Elevated plasma fibrinogen or globulins cause rouleaux to form and also promote an increase in the erythrocyte sedimentation rate. Rouleaux formation is especially marked in paraproteinemia (monoclonal gammopathy). **Agglutination,** or clumping, of red cells is more surely separated from rouleaux in wet preparations, and on air-dried films tends to show more irregular and round clumps than linear rouleaux. Cold agglutinins are responsible for this appearance (Fig. 30-26).

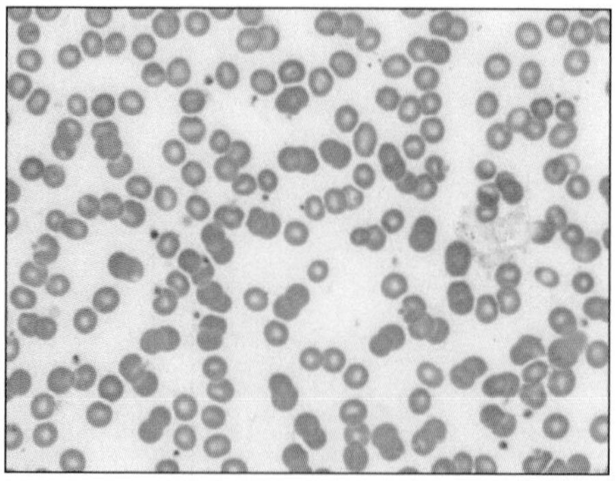

Figure 30-25 Rouleaux formation. Alignment of red cells one upon another, so that they resemble a stack of coins. It is usually caused by elevated plasma fibrinogen or globulins (500×).

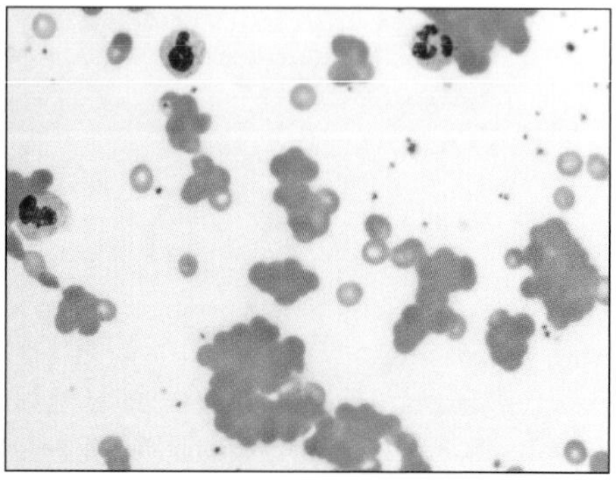

Figure 30-26 Agglutination. Clumping of red cells, which is more irregular than linear rouleaux formation. It is caused by cold agglutinins (500×).

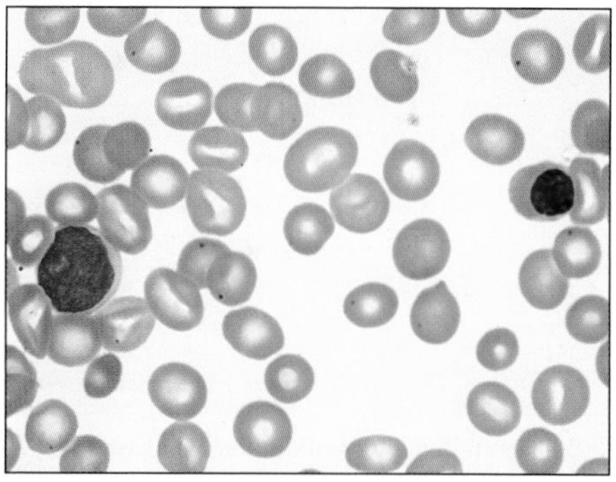

Figure 30-27 Nucleated red cell/normoblasts. Precursors of mature red cells, normoblasts are usually present only in the bone marrow. Their presence in blood is usually associated with increased red cell production or infiltrative bone marrow disorders (1000×).

Nucleated Red Cells

In contrast to erythrocytes of lower vertebrates and to most mammalian cells, the mammalian erythrocyte lacks a nucleus. Nucleated red cells (normoblasts; Figs. 30-27 and 30-48) are precursors of nonnucleated mature red cells in the blood. In the human, normoblasts are normally present only in the bone marrow. Stages in their production (see Chapter 31) from the earliest to the latest include pronormoblast, basophilic normoblast, polychromatophilic normoblast, and orthochromatic normoblast. In general, nucleated red cells that might appear in the blood in disease are polychromatic normoblasts. In some, however, the cytoplasm is so basophilic that it is difficult to recognize the cell as erythroid except by the character of the nucleus, intensely staining chromatin, and sharp separation of chromatin from parachromatin. Such erythroid cells are often mistaken for lymphocytes—an error that usually can be prevented by careful observation of the nucleus. The megaloblast (Fig. 30-28) is a distinct, nucleated erythroid cell—not merely a larger normoblast. It is characterized by large size and an abnormal "open" nuclear chromatin pattern. Cells of this series are not found in normal marrow but are

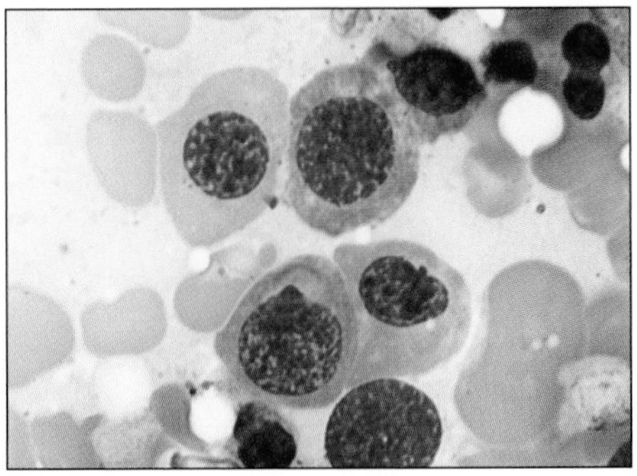

Figure 30-28 Megaloblast. Large nucleated red cell with abnormal "open" nuclear chromatin. They are frequently seen in the bone marrow in myelodysplastic syndrome or other megaloblastic anemia. Occasionally, these can also be seen in the peripheral blood (1000×).

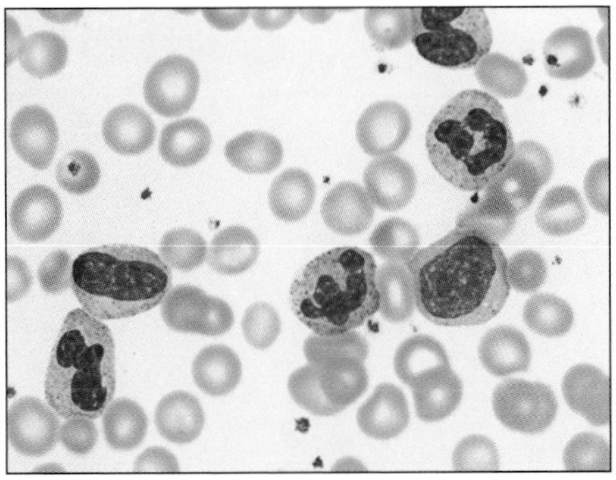

Figure 30-29 Leukemoid reaction. Left-shifted neutrophilic series with neutrophils, bands, and myelocytes. The neutrophils also show coarse toxic granulation (1000×).

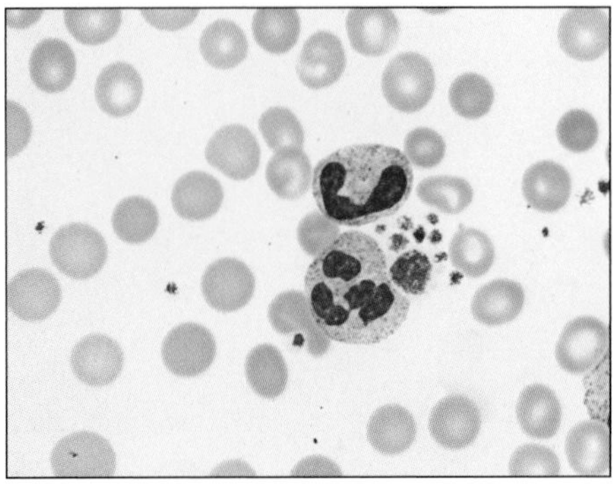

Figure 30-30 Neutrophil and band form. Neutrophil and band form depicting separation of nuclear lobes in the mature neutrophil vs. horseshoe-shaped nucleus in the band form. A giant platelet is also seen (1000×).

TABLE 30-6
Conditions Associated With Leukoerythroblastosis

0.63	0.26	Solid tumors and lymphomas
	0.24	Myeloproliferative disorders, including chronic myeloid leukemia (CML)
	0.13	Acute leukemias
0.37	0.03	Benign hematologic conditions
	0.08	Hemolysis
	0.26	Miscellaneous, including blood loss

Data are from Weick JK, Hagedorn AB, Linman JW. Leukoerythroblastosis: diagnostic and prognostic significance. Mayo Clin Proc 1974;49:110.
Proportions are based on a series of 215 cases discovered in a study of 50,277 blood film examinations in a 6-month period—a proportion of 0.004.

characteristically present in the marrow and sometimes in the blood of patients with pernicious anemia or other megaloblastic anemias.

Significance of Nucleated Red Cells

Normoblasts are present normally only in the blood of the fetus and of very young infants. In the healthy adult, they are confined to the bone marrow and appear in the circulating blood only in disease, in which their presence usually denotes an extreme demand made on the marrow, extramedullary hematopoiesis, or marrow replacement. Large numbers of circulating nucleated red cells are found particularly in hemolytic disease of the newborn (erythroblastosis fetalis) and thalassemia major.

Leukoerythroblastic Reaction

The presence of normoblasts and immature cells of the neutrophilic series in the blood is known as a **leukoerythroblastotic reaction** (Fig. 30-29). This often indicates space-occupying disturbances of the marrow, such as myelofibrosis with myeloid metaplasia, metastatic carcinoma, leukemias, multiple myeloma, Gaucher disease, and others. Nonetheless, in the study of Weick (1974), more than a third of patients with a leukoerythroblastotic reaction did not have malignant or potentially malignant disease (Table 30-6). In patients with metastatic malignancy, a leukoerythroblastotic reaction is good evidence for marrow involvement by tumor.

LEUKOCYTES ON PERIPHERAL BLOOD SMEAR EXAMINATION

Before evaluating leukocytes on the Romanowsky's-stained blood film, one should first determine that the film is well made, the distribution of the cells is uniform, and the staining of the cells is satisfactory. One first scans the counting area of the slide and, in wedge films, the lateral and feather edges, where monocytes, neutrophils, and large abnormal cells (if present) tend to be disproportionately represented. With coverslip preparations, this uneven distribution is less likely to occur. Suspicious cells are detected at 100× magnification and are confirmed at high power. Because nucleated red cells, macrophages, immature granulocytes, immature lymphoid cells, megakaryocytes, and abnormal cells are not normally found in blood, they should be recorded if present.

While scanning under low power, it is advisable to estimate the leukocyte count from the film. Even though it is a crude approximation, it sometimes enables one to detect errors in total count. One then proceeds to determine the percentage distribution of the different types of leukocytes, which is known as the differential leukocyte count. In patients with leukopenia, it may be necessary to concentrate the leukocytes by centrifuging blood anticoagulated with EDTA and preparing films from the top layer of the packed cells. This buffy coat contains primarily leukocytes and platelets. In the crenellation technique of counting, the field of view is moved from side to side across the width of the slide in the **counting area,** just behind the feather edge, where the red cells are separated from one another and are free of artifacts. As each leukocyte is encountered, it is classified, until 100, 200, 500, or 1000 leukocytes have been counted. The greater the number of cells counted, the greater is the precision, but for practical reasons, 100-cell counts are usually made. A record of the count may be kept by using a mechanical or electronic tabulator. Leukocytes that cannot be classified should be placed together in an unidentified group. In some conditions, notably leukemia, many of these unidentified leukocytes may be present. During the differential leukocyte counting procedure, the morphology of erythrocytes and platelets is examined, and the number of platelets is estimated. The absolute concentration of each variety of leukocyte is its percentage times the total leukocyte count. An increase in absolute concentration is an absolute increase; an increase in percentage only is a relative increase. Reference intervals are more useful if given as absolute concentrations rather than percentages (see Table 30-5).

Leukocytes Normally Present in Blood

Neutrophil (Polymorphonuclear Neutrophilic Leukocyte; Segmented Neutrophilic Granulocyte)

Neutrophils average 12 μm in diameter; they are smaller than monocytes and eosinophils and slightly larger than basophils. The nucleus stains deeply; it is irregular and often assumes shapes comparable to such letters as E, Z, and S. What appear to be separate nuclei normally are segments of nuclear material connected by delicate filaments.

A filament has length but no breadth as one focuses up and down. A **segmented neutrophil** (Figs. 30-30 and 30-49) has at least two of its lobes separated by a filament. A **band neutrophil** (see Figs. 30-30 and 30-49)

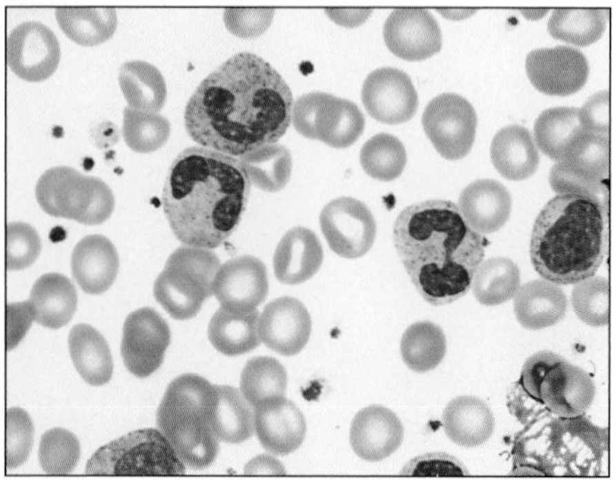

Figure 30-31 Neutrophilic granules. Cytoplasmic granules in myelocytes and mature neutrophils (1000×).

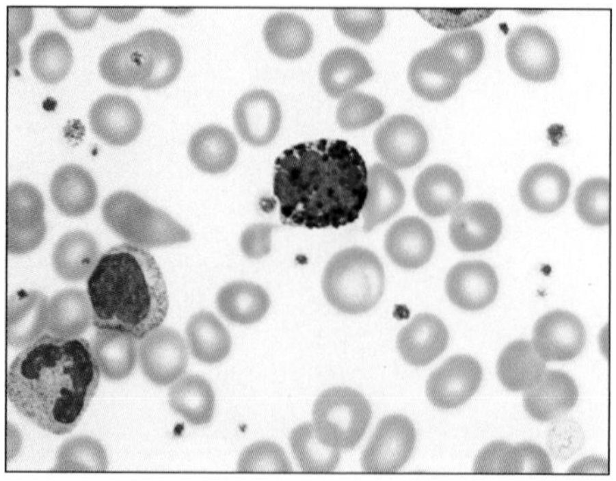

Figure 30-33 Basophil *(center)*, neutrophilic myelocyte and band *(left)*. The granules in the basophil are much bigger and coarser compared with the fine azurophilic granules of the neutrophil and precursors (1000×).

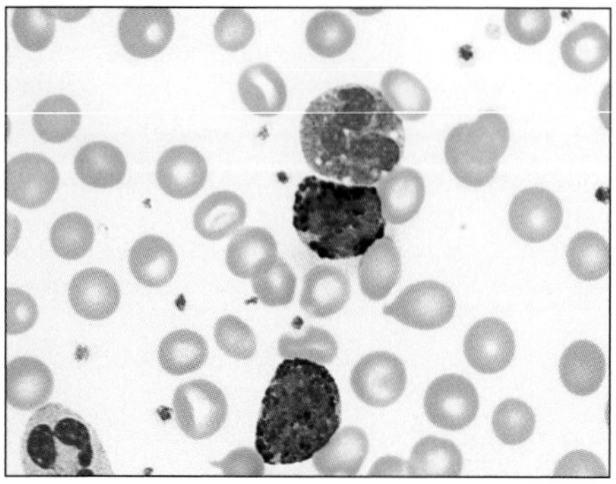

Figure 30-32 Basophil *(below)*, eosinophil *(above)*. Eosinophilic granules are coarser and bigger and often do not overlie the nucleus, unlike the basophil, which has large, deeply basophilic granules, often obscuring nuclear details (1000×).

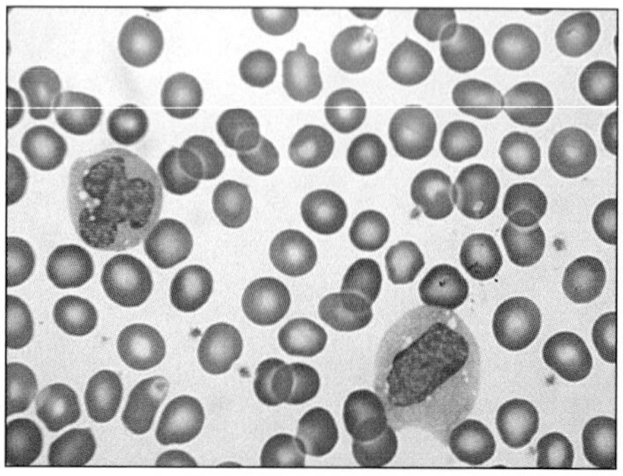

Figure 30-34 Monocyte. Among the normal blood cells, the monocyte is the largest and has the most delicate nuclear chromatin pattern. A moderate amount of light gray cytoplasm with fine granularity and vacuolation is noted (500×).

has either a strand of nuclear material thicker than a filament connecting the lobes, or a U-shaped nucleus of uniform thickness. The nucleus in both types of neutrophils has coarse blocks of chromatin and rather sharply defined parachromatin spaces. If, because of overlapping of nuclear material, it is not possible to be certain whether a filament is present, the cell should be placed in the segmented category (Mathy, 1974). The number of lobes in normal neutrophils ranges from two to five, with a median of three. The cytoplasm itself is colorless and has tiny granules (0.2–0.3 μm) that stain tan to pink with Wright's stain. About two thirds of these are specific granules, and one third azurophil granules. With light microscopy, the two types of granules often cannot be distinguished in the mature cell (Fig. 30-31). Segmented neutrophils average 56% of leukocytes; reference intervals are $1.8–7.0 \times 10^9/L$ in Caucasian adults but have a lower limit of about $1.1 \times 10^9/L$ in black adults. Band neutrophils average 3% of leukocytes; the upper reference value is about $0.7 \times 10^9/L$ in Caucasian people and slightly lower in black people (using the preceding definition and counting 100 cells in the differential) (see Table 30-5).

Normally, about 10%–30% of segmented neutrophils have two lobes, 40%–50% have three lobes, and 10%–20% four; no more than 5% have five lobes. A "shift to the left" occurs when increased bands and less mature neutrophils are present in the blood, along with a lower average number of lobes in segmented cells (see Figs. 30-29 and 30-31).

Neutrophil production and physiology are discussed in subsequent chapters. Neutrophilia or neutrophilic leukocytosis is an increase in the absolute count, and neutropenia is a decrease.

Eosinophil (Eosinophilic Granulocyte)

Eosinophils average 13 μm in diameter. The structure of these cells is similar to that of polymorphonuclear neutrophils, with the striking difference that, instead of neutrophilic granules, their cytoplasm contains larger round or oval granules that have a strong affinity for acid stains (Fig. 30-32). They are easily recognized by the size and color of the granules, which stain bright red with eosin. The cytoplasm is colorless. The nucleus stains somewhat less deeply than that of the neutrophils and usually has two connected segments (lobes), rarely more than three. Eosinophils average 3% of the leukocytes in adults, and the upper reference value is $0.6 \times 10^9/L$ when calculated from the differential count. If allergic individuals are excluded, the upper limit is probably $0.35 \times 10^9/L$ or 350/μL. The lower reference value is probably 40/μL; a decrease in eosinophils (eosinopenia) can be detected only by counting large numbers of cells as in direct hemocytometer counts (Dacie, 1991), or with a flow cytometer automated differential counter.

Basophil (Basophilic Granulocyte)

In general, basophils resemble neutrophils, except that the nucleus is less segmented (usually merely indented or partially lobulated), and granules are larger and have a strong affinity for basic stains (Figs. 30-32 and 30-33). In some basophils, most of the granules may be missing because they are soluble in water, leaving vacuoles or openings in the cytoplasm. The granules then are a mauve color. In a well-stained film, the granules are deep purple and the nucleus is somewhat paler and is often nearly hidden by the granules, so that its form is difficult to distinguish. Unevenly stained granules of basophils may be ring shaped and resemble *Histoplasma capsulatum* or protozoa.

Basophils are the least numerous of the leukocytes in normal blood and average 0.5%. The 95% reference values for adults are $0–0.2 - 10^9/L$ when derived from the differential count.

Monocyte

The monocyte is the largest cell of normal blood (Fig. 30-34). It generally has about two to three times the diameter of an erythrocyte (14–20 μm), although smaller monocytes sometimes are encountered. It contains a single nucleus, which is partially lobulated, deeply indented, or horseshoe shaped. Occasionally, the nucleus of a monocyte may appear round or oval. The cytoplasm is abundant. The nuclear chromatin often appears to be in fine, parallel strands separated by sharply defined parachromatin. The nucleus stains less densely than that of other leukocytes. The cytoplasm is blue-gray and has a ground-glass appearance and often contains fine red to purple granules that are less distinct and smaller than the granules of neutrophils. Occasionally, blue granules may be seen. When the monocyte transforms into a macrophage, it becomes larger (20–40 μm); the nucleus may become oval and the chromatin more reticular or dispersed, so that nucleoli may be visible. A perinuclear clear zone (Golgi) may be evident. The fine red or azurophil granules are variable in number or may have disappeared. The more abundant cytoplasm tends to be irregular at the cell margins and to contain vacuoles. These are phagocytic vacuoles, which

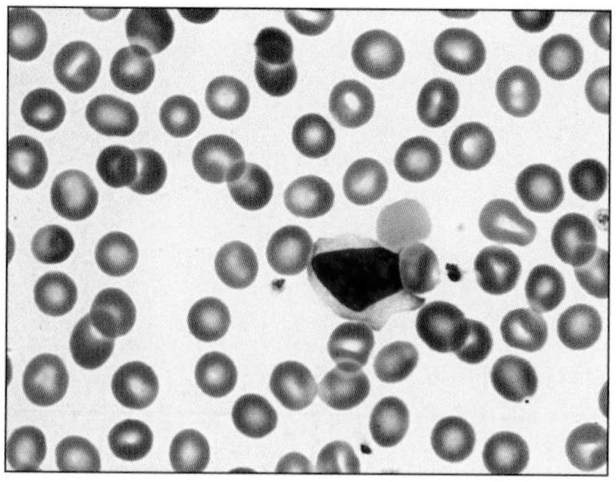

Figure 30-35 Lymphocyte. This is a benign reactive lymphocyte with moderately abundant pale gray cytoplasm hugging the surrounding red cells and distinct separation of chromatin/parachromatin (1000×).

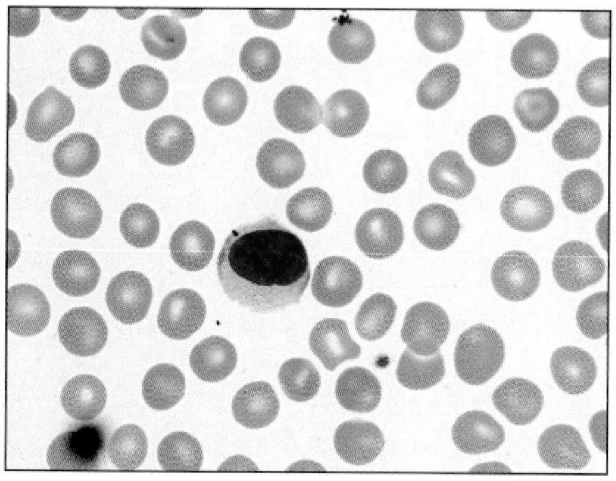

Figure 30-36 Reactive large lymphocyte with moderately abundant gray-blue cytoplasm (1000×).

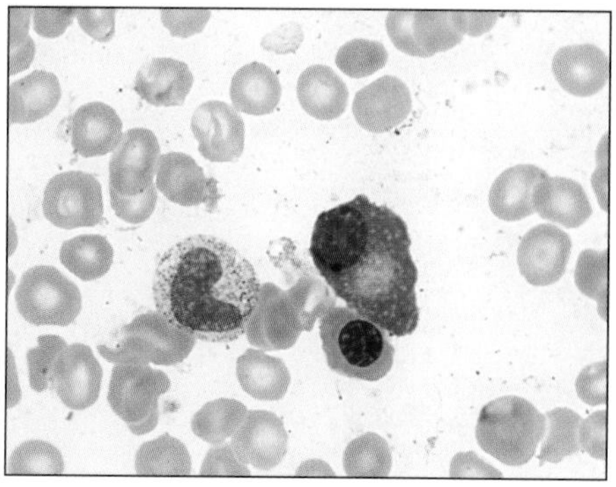

Figure 30-37 Plasma cell. Eccentric round nucleus with clumped nuclear chromatin and moderate amount of basophilic cytoplasm with prominent nuclear hof, or clear zone (1000×).

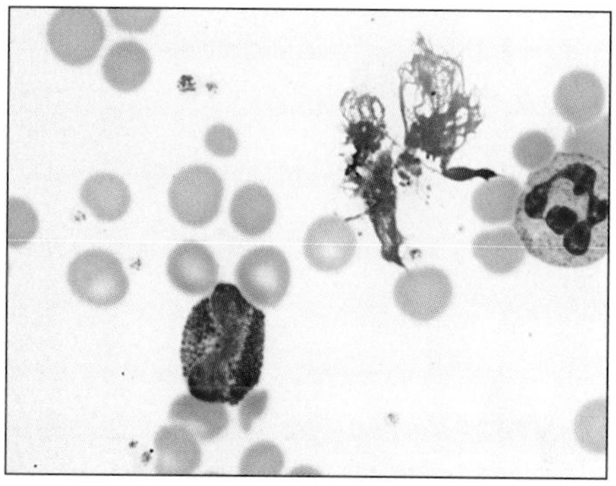

Figure 30-38 Broken cell. A broken cell of the myeloid series with ruptured cell membrane and disintegration of cytoplasmic contents (1000×).

may contain ingested red cells, debris, pigment, or bacteria. Evidence of phagocytosis in monocytes or the presence of macrophages in directly made blood films is pathologic and often indicates the presence of active infection.

Monocytes average 4% of leukocytes, and the reference interval for adults is approximately 0–0.8 × 10^9/L, depending on the method used to perform the differential count (see Table 30-5).

Lymphocyte

Lymphocytes are mononuclear cells without specific cytoplasmic granules. Small lymphocytes are about the size of an erythrocyte or slightly larger (6–10 μm) (see Fig. 30-9). The typical lymphocyte has a single, sharply defined nucleus containing heavy blocks of chromatin. The chromatin stains dark blue with Wright's stain, whereas the parachromatin stands out as lighter-stained streaks; at the periphery of the nucleus, the chromatin is condensed. Characteristically, a gradual transition or smudging is seen between the chromatin and the parachromatin. The nucleus is generally round but is sometimes indented at one side. The cytoplasm stains pale blue except for a clear perinuclear zone. Larger lymphocytes (Figs. 30-35 and 30-36), 12–15 μm in diameter, with less densely staining nuclei and more abundant cytoplasm, are frequently found, especially in the blood of children, and may be difficult to distinguish from monocytes. The misshapen, indented cytoplasmic margins of lymphocytes are due to pressure of neighboring cells. In the cytoplasm of about one third of large lymphocytes, a few round, red-purple granules are present. They are larger than the granules of neutrophilic leukocytes. There is a continuous spectrum of sizes between small and large lymphocytes and, indeed, there can be a transition from small to large to blast forms, as well as the reverse. It is not meaningful to classify small lymphocytes and large lymphocytes separately. The presence of significant proportions of atypical lymphocytes and blast forms (nonleukemic lymphoblasts, reticular lymphocytes) must be noted; these indicate transformation of lymphoid cells as a response to antigenic stimulation. Plasma cells have abundant blue cytoplasm, often with light streaks or vacuoles, an eccentric round nucleus, and a well-defined clear (Golgi) zone adjacent to the nucleus (Fig. 30-37). The nucleus of the plasma cell has heavily clumped chromatin, which is sharply defined from the parachromatin and is often arranged in a radial or wheel-like pattern. Plasma cells are not present normally in blood.

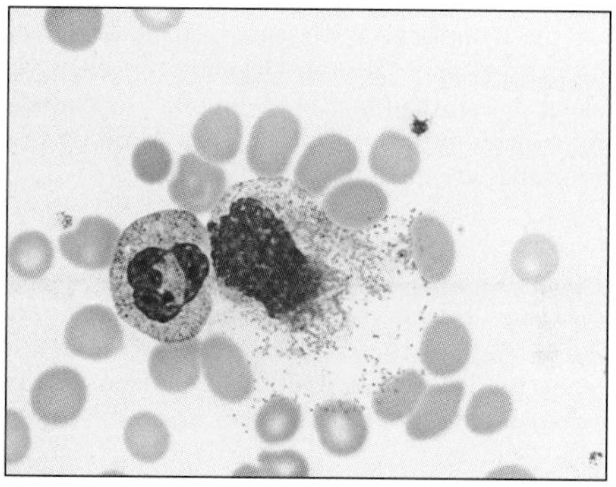

Figure 30-39 Ruptured cell. Ruptured/disintegrating leukocyte (1000×).

Lymphocytes average 34% of all leukocytes and range from 1.5–4 × 10^9/L in adults. The lymphocytes and their derivatives, the plasma cells, operate in the immune defenses of the body.

Artifacts

Broken Cells

Damaged or broken leukocytes (Figs. 30-38 and 30-39) constitute a small proportion of the nucleated cells in normal blood. Bare nuclei from ruptured cells (Figs. 30-40 and 30-41) vary from fairly well-preserved nuclei without cytoplasm to smudged nuclear material, sometimes with strands arranged in a coarse network, the so-called basket cells. They probably represent fragile cells, usually lymphocytes that have been broken in preparing the film. They are apt to be numerous when there is an atypical lymphocytosis, in chronic lymphocytic leukemia, and in acute leukemias.

Degenerative Changes

As EDTA-blood ages in the test tube, changes in leukocyte morphology begin to take place (Sacker, 1975). The degree of change varies among cells and in different individuals. Within a half hour, the nuclei of neutrophils may begin to swell, with some loss of chromatin structure. Cytoplasmic vacuoles appear, especially in monocytes and neutrophils. Nuclear

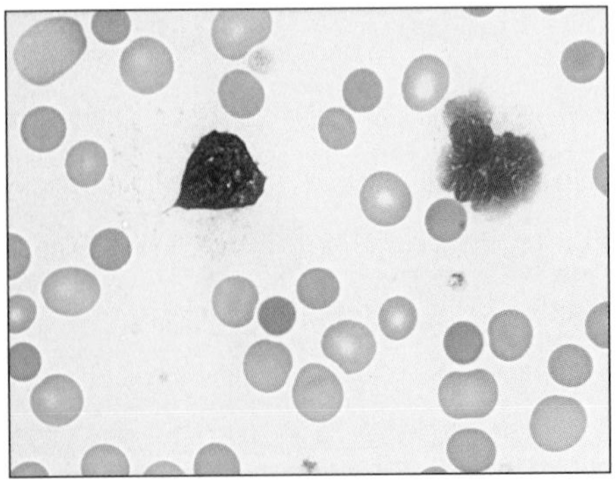

Figure 30-40 Smudge cell. Nuclear remnant from a damaged/broken white cell (1000×).

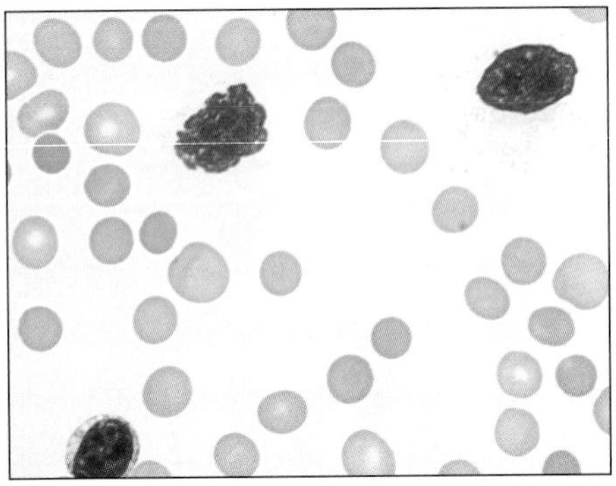

Figure 30-41 Basket cells (1000×).

lobulation appears in mononuclear cells; deep clefts may cause the nucleus to resemble a cloverleaf (radial segmentation of the nuclei; Rieder cells). Finally, loss of the cytoplasm and a smudged nucleus may be all that remains of the cell (see Fig. 30-40). Degenerative changes occur more rapidly in oxalated blood than in EDTA-blood. They arise more rapidly with increasing concentrations of EDTA, such as occur when evacuated blood collection tubes are incompletely filled.

Contracted Cells

In the thicker part of wedge films, drying is slow. Obvious changes in the film include rouleaux of the erythrocytes and shrinkage of the leukocytes. Because the leukocytes are contracted and heavily stained, mononuclear cells are difficult to distinguish. Optimal cell identification is usually impossible in these areas.

Endothelial Cells

Endothelial cells from the lining of the blood vessel may appear in the first drop of blood from a fingerstick specimen or, rarely, in venous blood. They have an immature reticular chromatin pattern and may be mistaken for histiocytes or for tumor cells.

Radial Segmentation of the Nuclei

Use of oxalated blood results in the appearance of abnormal segmentation of the nuclei of leukocytes on the blood film. This segmentation differs from that of the granulocytes in that the lobes appear to radiate from a single point, giving a cloverleaf or a cartwheel picture. Extensive changes can occur within an hour or two in oxalated blood. Less extensive changes occur with other anticoagulants, including EDTA.

Vacuolation

Vacuoles may develop in the nucleus and cytoplasm of leukocytes, especially monocytes and neutrophils from blood anticoagulated with EDTA. Vacuoles may be associated with swelling of the nuclei and loss of granules from the cytoplasm.

"Pseudophagocytosis"

Occasionally, a small lymphocyte, or more often an erythrocyte, will lie atop a granulocyte or a monocyte and thus will appear to have been ingested. The true positions of such cells can be suspected because they will come into sharp focus in a plane above that of the larger cell.

TABLE 30-7

Ninety-Five Percent Confidence Limits for Various Percentages of Blood Cells of a Given Type as Determined by Differential Counts*

a	n = 100	n = 200	n = 500	n = 1000	n = 10,000
0	0.0–3.6	0.0–1.8	0.0–0.7	0.0–0.4	0.0–0.1
1	0.0–5.4	0.1–3.6	0.3–2.3	0.5–1.8	0.8–1.3
2	0.0–7.0	0.6–5.0	1.0–3.6	1.2–3.1	1.7–2.3
3	0.6–8.5	1.1–6.4	1.7–4.9	2.0–4.3	2.6–3.4
4	1.1–9.9	1.7–7.7	2.5–6.1	2.9–5.4	3.6–4.5
5	1.6–11.3	2.4–9.0	3.3–7.3	3.7–6.5	4.5–5.5
6	2.2–12.6	3.1–10.2	4.1–8.5	4.6–7.7	5.5–6.5
7	2.9–13.9	3.9–11.5	4.9–9.6	5.5–8.8	6.5–7.6
8	3.5–15.2	4.6–12.7	5.8–10.7	6.4–9.9	7.4–8.6
9	4.2–16.4	5.4–13.9	6.6–11.9	7.3–10.9	8.4–9.6
10	4.9–17.6	6.2–15.0	7.5–13.0	8.2–12.0	9.4–10.7
15	8.6–23.5	10.4–20.7	12.0–18.4	12.8–17.4	14.3–15.8
20	12.7–29.2	14.7–26.2	16.6–23.8	17.6–22.6	19.2–20.8
25	16.9–34.7	19.2–31.6	21.3–29.0	22.3–27.8	24.1–25.9
30	21.2–40.0	23.7–36.9	26.0–34.2	27.2–32.9	29.1–31.0
35	25.7–45.2	28.4–42.0	30.8–39.4	32.0–38.0	34.0–36.0
40	30.3–50.3	33.2–47.1	35.7–44.4	36.9–43.1	39.0–41.0
45	35.0–55.3	38.0–52.2	40.6–49.5	41.9–48.1	44.0–46.0
50	39.8–60.2	42.9–57.1	45.5–54.5	46.9–53.1	49.0–51.0
55	44.7–65.0	47.8–62.0	50.5–59.4	51.9–58.1	54.0–56.0
60	49.7–69.7	52.9–66.8	55.6–64.3	56.9–63.1	59.0–61.0
65	54.8–74.3	58.0–71.6	60.6–69.2	62.0–68.0	64.0–66.0
70	60.0–78.8	63.1–76.3	65.8–74.0	67.1–72.8	69.0–70.9
75	65.3–83.1	68.4–80.8	71.0–78.7	72.2–77.7	74.1–75.9
80	70.8–87.3	73.8–85.3	76.2–83.4	77.4–82.4	79.2–80.8
85	76.5–91.4	79.3–89.6	81.6–88.0	82.6–87.2	84.2–85.7
90	82.4–95.1	85.0–93.8	87.0–92.5	88.0–91.8	89.3–90.6
91	83.6–95.8	86.1–94.6	88.1–93.4	89.1–92.7	90.4–91.6
92	84.8–96.5	87.3–95.4	89.3–94.2	90.1–93.6	91.4–92.6
93	86.1–97.1	88.5–96.1	90.4–95.1	91.2–94.5	92.4–93.5
94	87.4–97.8	89.8–96.9	91.5–95.9	92.3–95.4	93.5–94.5
95	88.7–98.4	91.0–97.6	92.7–96.7	93.5–96.3	94.5–95.5
96	90.1–98.9	92.3–98.3	93.9–97.5	94.6–97.1	95.5–96.4
97	91.5–99.4	93.6–98.9	95.1–98.3	95.7–98.0	96.6–97.4
98	93.0–99.9	95.0–99.4	96.4–99.0	96.9–98.8	97.7–98.3
99	94.6–99.9	96.4–99.9	97.7–99.7	98.2–99.5	98.7–99.2
100	96.4–100.0	98.2–100.0	99.3–100.0	99.6–100.0	99.9–100.0

Courtesy of Prof C.L. Rümke (1985).

*n is the number of cells counted; a, the observed percentage of cells of the given type. The limits for n = 100, 200, 500, and 1000 are exact; for n = 10,000, they have been determined with Freeman and Tukey's approximation, as described in the Geigy tables.

Sources of Error in the Differential Leukocyte Count

Even in perfectly made blood films, the differential count is subject to the same errors of random distribution. For interpretation of day-to-day or slide-to-slide differences in the same patient, it is helpful to know how much of the variation is ascribable to chance alone. Table 30-7 gives 95% confidence limits for different percentages of cells in differential counts performed, classifying a total of 100–10,000 leukocytes. In comparing the percentages from two separate counts, if one number lies outside the confidence limits of the other, it is probable that the difference is significant (i.e., not due to chance). Thus, on the basis of a 100-cell differential count, if the monocytes were 5% one day and 10% the next, it is probable that the difference is due solely to sampling error. Although the difference could be real, one cannot be sure of this because of the small number of cells counted. If, on the other hand, the differential count totaled 500 cells, the difference between 5% and 10% is significant; one can be reasonably certain (with a 5% chance of being wrong) that the difference is a real one and is not due to chance alone. Of course, this is a minimal estimate of the error involved in differential counts because it does not include mechanical errors (due to variations in collecting blood samples, inadequate mixing, irregularities in distribution depending on the type and quality of the blood films, and poor staining) or errors in cell identification, which depend on the judgment and experience of the observer. Meticulous technique, as well as accurate and consistent cell classification, is therefore required. The physician who interprets the results must be aware of possible sources of error, especially error due to chance in the distribution of cells. Table 30-5 shows the distribution of the various types of leukocytes in the blood of normal persons. Absolute concentrations are given, as these have considerably greater significance than percentages alone.

Automated Differential Leukocyte Counting

Because the differential leukocyte count is nonspecific, nonprecise, error-prone, usually labor intensive, expensive to perform, and of limited clinical significance as a screening test, some investigators have suggested that it may be prudent to discontinue use of the differential count as an inpatient screening test for adults (Connelly, 1982). Automation of the differential count eliminates some of the detractions. Ideally, requirements for the automated differential leukocyte counting system should include the following:

1. The distribution of cells analyzed should be identical to that in the blood.
2. All leukocytes usually found in blood diseases should be accurately identified, or detected and "flagged" in some way.
3. The speed of the process should enable a large number of cells to be counted to minimize statistical error.
4. The instrument should be cost-effective (Bentley, 1977).

Impedance counters and flow cytometer systems and their differential counts were discussed earlier under Instrument Technology.

The automated systems have the advantage of rapidly analyzing larger numbers of cells and significantly reducing the statistical error of counting.

Disadvantages include that the categories of cells are not completely consonant with those with which we are familiar on Romanowsky's-stained films. An "unclassified" category is difficult to interpret. When an abnormal result occurs, a film must be made and examined. Because of concern regarding the instrument flags, each laboratory should devise a policy for blood film examination and visual counting when indicated. Camden (1993) provides guiding questions to be asked in selecting a new hematology analyzer for your laboratory. The ICSH (1984b) also published a protocol for evaluation of automated blood cell counters.

Digital Image Processing

A uniformly made and stained blood film is placed on a motor-driven microscope stage. A computer controls scanning the slide and stopping it when leukocyte(s) are in the field. The optical details (e.g., nuclear and cytoplasmic size, density, shape, color) are recorded by a television camera, analyzed by computer, and converted to digital form; these characteristics are compared with a memory bank of such characteristics for the different cell types. If the pattern fits that of a normal cell type, it is identified as such; otherwise, the cell is classified as other or unknown. The coordinates of the unknown cells are kept by the instrument and relocated at the end of the count, so that the technologist can classify them (Lapen, 1982; Parthenis, 1992; Mukherjee, 2004).

PLATELETS ON PERIPHERAL BLOOD SMEAR EXAMINATION

In films made from EDTA-blood and stained with Romanowsky's stains, platelets are round or oval, 2–4 μm in diameter, and separated from one another (Fig. 30-42). The platelet count may be estimated from such films. On average, if the platelet count is normal, about one platelet is found per 10–30 red cells. At 1000× magnification, this is equivalent to about 7–20 platelets per oil immersion field in the areas where red cell morphology is optimal (Fig. 30-43). Platelets contain fine purple granules that usually fill the cytoplasm. Occasionally, granules are concentrated in the center (the "granulomere") and surrounded by a pale cytoplasm (the "hyalomere"); these are probably activated platelets, the appearance resulting from contraction of the microtubular band. A few platelets may have decreased concentrations of granules (hypogranular platelets). In EDTA-blood from normal individuals, the fraction of platelets that exceed 3 μm in diameter and the fraction of platelets that are hypogranular are both less than 5% if the films are made at 10 minutes or 60 minutes after the blood is drawn.

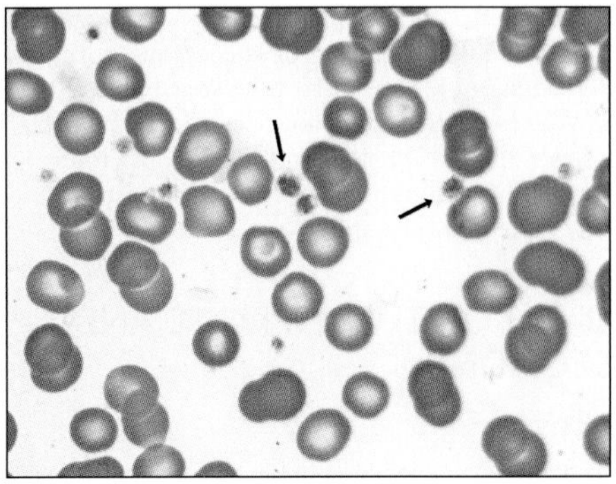

Figure 30-42 Platelet. Platelets are round to oval, 2–4 μm in diameter, and separated from one another (1000×).

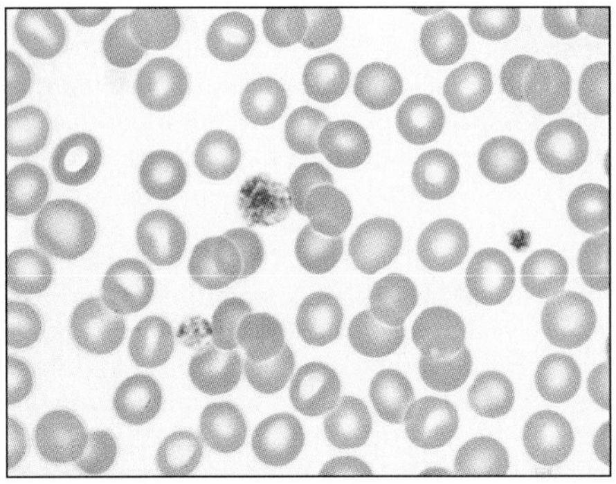

Figure 30-43 Platelet/giant platelet. Platelets show fine granularity; an occasional larger (giant) form is noted (1000×).

If films are made immediately or at 3 hours after blood drawing, the fraction of large platelets and the fraction of hypogranular or activated platelets are increased (Zeigler, 1978). These artifacts make it necessary to standardize time of film preparation when evaluating platelet size from films. In patients with immune thrombocytopenia, large platelets/giant platelets (see Fig. 30-30) are increased in number. They are also increased in patients with the rare Bernard-Soulier syndrome and in those with myelophthisis or myeloproliferative syndrome; in the latter, the platelets are frequently hypogranular or have a distinct granulomere and hyalomere. In blood films made from skin puncture wounds, platelets assume irregular shapes with sharp projections and tend to clump together.

BONE MARROW EXAMINATION

The bone marrow examination provides a semiquantitative and qualitative assessment of the state of hematopoiesis and aids in the diagnosis of several hereditary and acquired benign and malignant diseases. Marrow aspiration and biopsy can be carried out as an office procedure on ambulatory patients with minimal risk. It compares favorably with ordinary venipuncture and is less traumatizing than a lumbar puncture. As for any other special procedure, however, the clinical indications for marrow examination should be clear. In each instance, the physician should have in mind some reasonable prediction of its result and consequent benefit to the patient. Without exception, the peripheral blood should be examined carefully first. It is a relatively uncommon circumstance to find hematologic disease in the bone marrow without evidence of it in the peripheral blood. It is estimated that the weight of the marrow in the adult is 1300–1500 g. The marrow can undergo complete transformation in a few days and occasionally even in a few hours. As a rule, this rapid transformation involves the whole organ, as evidenced by the fact that a small sample represented by a biopsy or aspiration is usually fairly representative of the whole marrow. This conclusion is in accord with results of studies of biopsy samples simultaneously removed from several sites. According to these observations, the various sites chosen for removal of marrow for studies are in most instances equally good. Consequently, the difficulty of access, the risks involved, the ease of obtaining a good biopsy specimen, and discomfort to the patient are the main reasons for selection of a site in the particular patient. Within a given site, the cellular distribution may vary in apparently hyperplastic or hypoplastic areas. This is particularly the case immediately below the cortex.

Occasionally, failure to obtain quantitatively or qualitatively adequate material in one site may be followed by success in another location. Also, the need for repeated aspirations or biopsies may indicate the use of several different sites. We regard the posterior iliac crest as the preferred site. The large marrow space allows both aspiration and biopsy to be performed with ease at one time. The techniques of marrow aspiration and biopsy have been adequately reviewed (Hyun, 1988).

PREPARATION OF THE ASPIRATE AND BIOPSY SECTION

Marrow Films

Delay, no matter how brief, is undesirable. Films can be made in a manner similar to that used for ordinary blood counts. Gray particles of marrow are visible with the naked eye. They are the best material for the preparation of good films and serve as landmarks for the microscopic examination of stained smears.

Direct Films

A drop of marrow is placed on a slide a short distance away from one end. A film 3–5 cm long is made with a spreader, not wider than 2 cm, dragging the particles behind but not squashing them. A trail of cells is left behind each particle.

Imprints

Marrow particles can also be used for preparation of imprints. One or more visible particles are picked up with a capillary pipet, the broken end of a wooden applicator, or a toothpick, and are transferred immediately to a slide and made to stick to it by a gentle smearing motion. The slide is air dried rapidly by waving, and then it is stained.

Crush Preparations

Marrow particles in a small drop of aspirate may be placed on a slide near one end. Another slide is carefully placed over the first. Slight pressure is exerted to crush the particles, and the slides are separated by pulling them apart in a direction parallel to their surfaces. All films should be dried rapidly by whipping them through the air or by exposing them to a fan. As the aspirated material is being spread, the appearance of fat as irregular holes in the films gives assurance that marrow and not just blood has been obtained.

Special Studies

A sterile anticoagulated sample containing viable unfixed cells in single cell suspension is the best substrate for nearly all special studies that are likely to be required on a marrow sample. Specifically, flow cytometry is best performed on an EDTA or heparin anticoagulated aspirate specimen, which is stable for at least 24 hours at room temperature. For cytogenetic or cell culture analysis, anticoagulated marrow should be added to tissue culture medium and analyzed as soon as possible to maintain optimal cell viability. Cytogenetic specimens are generally not adversely affected by overnight incubation. DNA is relatively stable and can be extracted and analyzed from paraffin-embedded tissue sections. However, reverse transcriptase polymerase chain reaction (RT-PCR) assays, involving amplification of complementary DNA (cDNA) prepared from cellular messenger RNA (mRNA), are often needed for molecular diagnosis of translocations associated with leukemia and lymphoma. Messenger RNA has a variable half-life in an intact cell and is degraded rapidly (on the order of seconds to minutes) in a cell lysate by ubiquitous RNAses. For maximal mRNA recovery, cell suspensions, mostly buffy coat or mononuclear cell preparations, should be lysed in an appropriate RNAse inhibitor containing buffer as soon as possible after sampling. EDTA is the preferred anticoagulant, as heparin can interfere with some molecular assays (Ryan, 2001b).

Histologic Sections

The needle biopsy and clotted marrow particles (fragments) are fixed in Zenker's acetic solution (5% glacial acetic acid; 95% Zenker's) for 6–18 hours, or in B-5 fixative for 1–2 hours (Hyun, 1988). Excessive time in either fixative makes the tissue brittle. Although these fixatives, particularly B-5, provide the best histology, they contain toxic mercuric chloride and are gradually being replaced by fixatives such as zinc formalin and other preparations. The tissue is processed routinely for embedding in paraffin, cut at 4 μm, and stained routinely with hematoxylin and eosin (H&E). Giemsa and periodic acid–Schiff (PAS) stains are frequently useful. Embedding the tissue in plastic material allows thinner sections to be examined and better survival of protein structure, so that enzyme histochemistry and immunocytochemistry are practical for identification of cell lineages.

Sections provide the best estimate of cellularity and a picture of marrow architecture but are somewhat inferior for the study of cytologic details. Another disadvantage is that particles adequate for histologic sections are not always obtained, especially in conditions in which the diagnosis depends on marrow evidence (e.g., myelofibrosis, metastatic cancer).

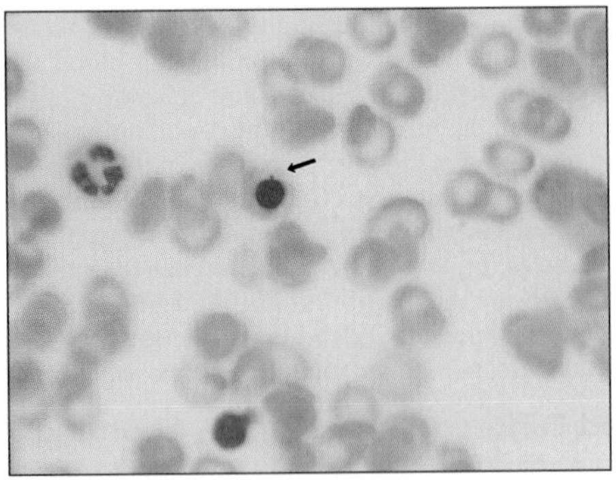

Figure 30-44 Normal sideroblast. Single iron granule seen in the cytoplasm of a maturing normoblast. Identification requires high magnification and bright illumination, while focusing up and down (1000×).

STAINING MARROW PREPARATIONS

Romanowsky's Stain

Marrow films should be stained with Romanowsky's stain (e.g., Wright-Giemsa) in a manner similar to that used for blood films. A longer staining time may be necessary for marrows with greater cellularity. Several special stains may be performed on peripheral blood smears, bone marrow aspirate, and touch imprint smears and bone marrow biopsy sections, besides the usual Romanowsky's and H&E stains. These include cytochemical stains (myeloperoxidase, Sudan black B, naphthol As-D chloroacetate esterase, nonspecific esterases, acid phosphatases, leukocyte alkaline phosphatase, periodic acid–Schiff stain, toluidine blue, and iron stain) and immunocytochemical stains, depending on the disease and the preliminary morphologic examination of the smear and/or section (Perkins, 2004). The procedure for the iron stain is discussed in the next section. The relevance of other stains is mentioned in subsequent chapters, along with the respective diseases.

Perls' Test for Iron

Procedure

One film containing marrow particles is fixed for 10 minutes in formalin vapor, immersed for 10 minutes in a freshly prepared solution that contains 0.5% potassium ferrocyanide and 0.75% hydrochloric acid, rinsed, dried, and counterstained with Nuclear Fast Red.

Interpretation

The Prussian blue reaction is produced when hemosiderin or ferritin is present; iron in Hb is not stained. It is reported as negative or 1+ to 5+. Storage iron, which is contained in macrophages, can be evaluated only in marrow particles on the film. In adults, 2+ is normal, 3+ slightly increased, 4+ moderately increased, and 5+ markedly increased. Storage iron in the marrow is located in macrophages. Normally, a small number of blue granules are seen. In iron deficiency, blue-staining granules are absent or extremely rare. Storage iron is increased in most other anemias, infections, hemochromatosis, hemosiderosis, hepatic cirrhosis, uremia, and cancer, and after repeated transfusions. Sideroblasts (Fig. 30-44) are normoblasts that contain one or more particles of stainable iron. Normally, from 20%–60% of late normoblasts are sideroblasts; in the remainder, no blue granules can be detected. The percentage of sideroblasts is decreased in iron deficiency anemia (in which storage iron is decreased) and also in the common anemias associated with infection, rheumatoid arthritis, and neoplastic disease (in which storage iron is normal or increased). The number of sideroblasts is increased when erythropoiesis is impaired for other reasons; it is roughly proportional to the degree of saturation of transferrin. The Prussian blue reaction can also be performed on slides previously stained with a Romanowsky's stain to identify sideroblasts or to determine

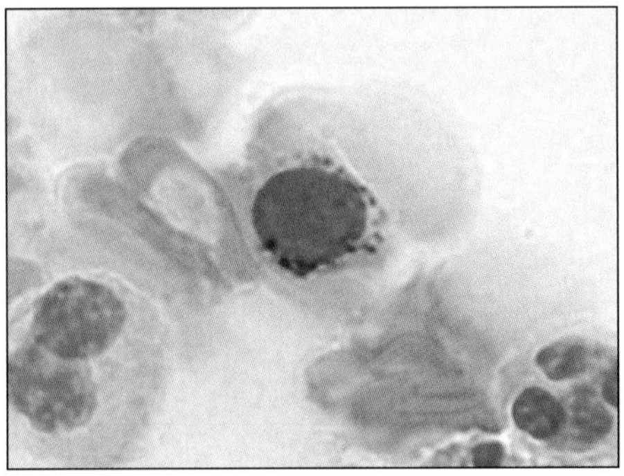

Figure 30-45 Ring sideroblast. Siderotic granules form a perinuclear ring spanning more than half of the nuclear diameter (Prussian blue stain, 1000×).

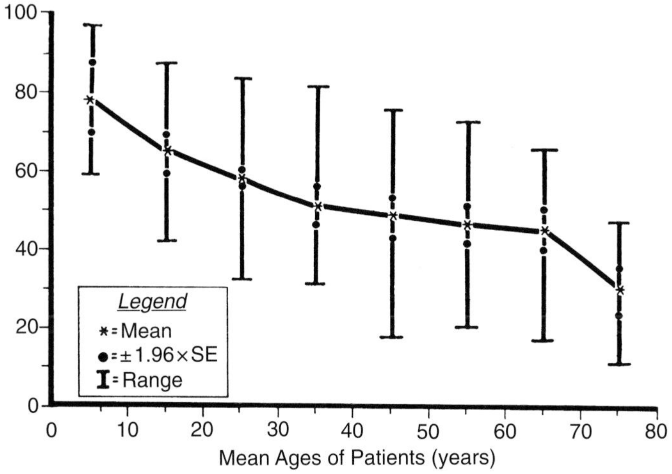

Figure 30-46 Marrow cellularity in hematologically normal individuals. Percent cellularity on the ordinate versus age, grouped by decade, on the abscissa. *(From Hartsock RJ, Smith EB, Petty CS. Am J Clin Pathol 1965;43:326, with permission.)*

whether iron is present in other cells of interest. Further, iron stain is used to evaluate for the presence of abnormal sideroblasts and ring sideroblasts (Fig. 30-45), as seen in various hematologic diseases.

Sections

Routine H&E stains are satisfactory for most purposes. Romanowsky's stains can be used to good advantage with fixed material. Iron stains are best performed on films that contain particulate marrow tissue. They are less sensitive in sections of marrow because some iron is lost in processing, and a lesser thickness of tissue is examined in sections.

EXAMINATION OF MARROW

It is desirable to establish a routine procedure to obtain maximum information from examination of the marrow.

Peripheral Blood

The complete blood cell count, including platelet count and reticulocyte count, should be performed on the day of the marrow study, and the results incorporated in the report. The pathologist or hematologist who examines the marrow should also carefully examine the blood film as previously described and should incorporate the observations in the marrow report.

Cellularity of the Marrow

Marrow cellularity is expressed as the ratio of the volume of hematopoietic cells to the total volume of the marrow space (cells plus fat and other stromal elements). Cellularity varies with the age of the subject and the site. For example, at age 50 years, the average cellularity in the vertebrae is 75%; sternum, 60%; iliac crest, 50%; and rib, 30%. Normal cellularity of the iliac bone at different ages has been well defined by Hartsock (1965), as summarized in Figure 30-46. If the percentage is increased for the patient's age, the marrow is hypercellular, or hyperplastic; if decreased, the marrow is hypocellular, or hypoplastic. Marrow cellularity is best judged by histologic sections of biopsy or aspirated particles (Fig. 30-47) but

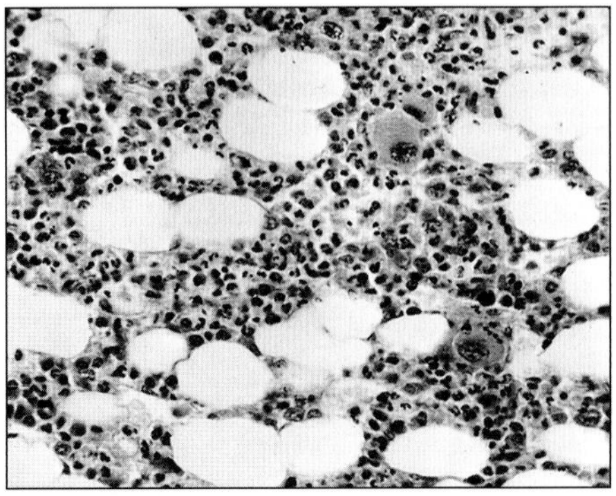

Figure 30-47 Marrow biopsy (1470×). Cellularity here is between 60% and 70%, which is normal for an adult. Three megakaryocytes are present, which is normal for this size of field. Granulocyte maturation appears normal, with all stages present. Very few normoblasts are noted. (Normoblasts have intensely staining nuclei and tend to occur in clusters.) The myeloid/erythroid (M/E) ratio is higher than 4:1, indicating erythroid hypoplasia. No other abnormalities are noted.

should also be estimated from the particles present in marrow films. This is done by comparing the areas occupied by fat spaces and by nucleated cells in the particles, as well as the density of nucleated cells in the "tail" or fallout of the particles. Comparison of films and sections on each marrow specimen will enable the observer to estimate cellularity reasonably well from films—a skill that is useful in the instances when sectioned material is unavailable.

Distribution of Cells

Distribution of various cell types can be ascertained in two ways. First, one scans several slides under low, then high, magnification; on the basis of previous experience, one then estimates the number and distribution of cells. Second, one actually makes a differential count of 300–1000 cells and calculates the percentage of each type of cell. A combination of both methods is preferred. The second of these methods, careful differential counting, is an essential part of training in this work, without which accuracy in the first method may be difficult to achieve. The differential count also affords an objective record from which future changes may be measured.

One first scans the marrow film under low power (100× or 200× magnification) while looking for irregularities in cell distribution, numbers of megakaryocytes, and the presence of abnormal cells. Then one selects areas on the film where marrow cells are both undiluted with blood cells and separated and spread out sufficiently to allow optimal identification. These areas are usually just behind marrow particles on direct films, or near the particles on crushed films. The differential count is performed at 400× or 1000× magnification. Examples of reference intervals for differential counts of marrow at selected different ages are given in Table 30-8.

Changes in the marrow cell distribution are most dramatic in the first month of life, during which a predominance of granulocytic cells at birth changes to a predominance of lymphocytes. This predominance of lymphocytes characterizes the bone marrow during infancy. A small proportion of "immature" or transitional lymphoid cells (fine nuclear chromatin, high nuclear/cytoplasmic ratio, small to intermediate cell size) is normally present; it may be that these cells include stem cells and progenitor cells. These cells probably include cells designated as "hematogones"; they may be increased in iron deficiency anemia, immune thrombocytopenic purpura, and other disorders, especially in infancy. Normoblasts fall after birth; rise to a maximum at 2 months; then fall to a stable, relatively low level by 4 months, and remain there during most of infancy. The myeloid/erythroid (M/E) ratio is the ratio of total granulocytes to total normoblasts. In newborns and infants, it is somewhat higher than in older children or adults (see Table 30-8). In adults, the range is broad, varying from about 1.2:1 to 4:1. Both the differential count and the M/E ratio are relative values and must be interpreted with respect to cellularity, or with respect to other evidence that one of the systems is normal. An **increased** M/E ratio (e.g., 6:1) may be found in infection, chronic myelogenous leukemia, or erythroid hypoplasia. A **decreased** M/E ratio (i.e., <1.2:1) may mean a depression of leukopoiesis or a normoblastic hyperplasia, depending on the marrow cellularity. The number of megakaryocytes is estimated more reliably in sections than in marrow films. In scanning areas of films with good cellularity under low power (100×), an average of one to three megakaryocytes should be found in each field in normal marrow.

TABLE 30-8
Differential Cell Counts of Bone Marrow in Percent of Total Nucleated Cells

	ROSSE (1977)			MAUER (1969)	JANDL (1987)
Cell types	**Birth (mean, SD)**	**1 month (mean, SD)**	**18 months (mean, SD)**	**Childhood (mean, range)**	**Adult (mean, range)**
Normoblasts, total	14.48 ± 7.24	8.04 ± 5.00	8.21 ± 3.71	23.1	21.5 (14.2–30.4)
Pronormoblasts	0.02 ± 0.06	0.10 ± 0.14	0.08 ± 0.13	0.5 (0.0–1.5)	0.6 (0.2–1.4)
Basophilic n.	0.24 ± 0.25	0.34 ± 0.33	0.50 ± 0.34	1.7 (0.2–4.8)	2.0 (0.7–3.7)
polychromatophilic n.	13.06 ± 6.78	6.90 ± 4.45	6.97 ± 3.56	18.2 (4.8–34.0)	12.4 (12.2–24.2)
Orthochromatic n.	0.69 ± 0.73	0.54 ± 1.88	0.44 ± 0.49	2.7 (0.0–7.8)	6.5 (2.0–22.7)
Neutrophils, total	60.37 ± 8.66	32.35 ± 7.68	36.06 ± 7.40	57.1	56.0 (45.1–66.5)
Myeloblasts	0.31 ± 0.31	0.62 ± 0.50	0.06 ± 0.08	1.2 (0.0–3.2)	1.0 (0.5–1.8)
Promyelocytes	0.79 ± 0.91	0.76 ± 0.65	0.64 ± 0.59	1.4 (0.0–4.0)	3.4 (2.6–4.6)
Myelocytes	3.95 ± 2.93	2.50 ± 1.48	2.49 ± 1.39	18.3 (8.5–29.7)	11.9 (8.1–16.9)
Metamyelocytes	19.37 ± 4.84	11.30 ± 3.59	12.42 ± 4.15	23.3 (14.0–34.2)	18.0 (9.8–25.3)
Bands	28.89 ± 7.56	14.10 ± 4.63	14.20 ± 5.23		11.0 (8.5–20.8)
Segmented	7.37 ± 4.64	3.64 ± 2.97	6.31 ± 3.91	12.9 (4.5–29.0)	10.7 (8.0–16.0)
Eosinophils	2.70 ± 1.27	2.61 ± 1.40	2.70 ± 2.16	3.6 (1.0–9.0)	3.2 (1.2–6.2)
Basophils	0.12 ± 0.20	0.07 ± 0.16	0.10 ± 0.12	0.06 (0.0–0.8)	<0.1 (0.0–0.2)
Lymphocytes, total	15.6	49.0	45.5	16.0 (4.8–35.8)	15.8 (10.8–22.7)
Transitional	1.18 ± 1.13	1.95 ± 0.94	1.99 ± 1.00		
Small	14.42 ± 5.54	47.05 ± 9.24	43.55 ± 8.56		
Plasma cells	0.00 ± 0.02	0.02 ± 0.06	0.06 ± 0.08	0.4 (0.2–0.6)	1.8 (0.2–2.2)
Monocytes	0.88 ± 0.85	1.01 ± 0.89	2.12 ± 1.59		1.8 (0.2–2.8)
Megakaryocytes	0.06 ± 0.15	0.05 ± 0.09	0.07 ± 0.12		<1.0 (0.0–0.2)
Reticulum cells					0.3 (0.0–0.5)
M/E ratio	4.2	4.0	4.4	2.9 (1.2–5.2)	2.5 (1.2–5.0)

Data are from Rosse (1977), Mauer (1969), and Jandl (1987).
M/E, Myeloid/erythroid ratio.

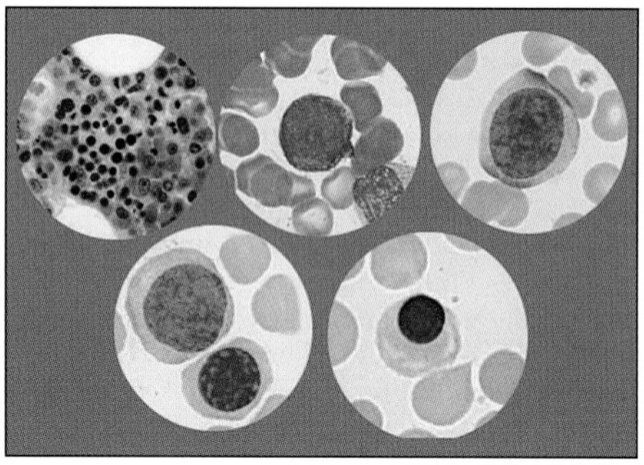

Figure 30-48 Normal erythroid maturation. Various stages of normoblastic erythroid maturation (1000×).

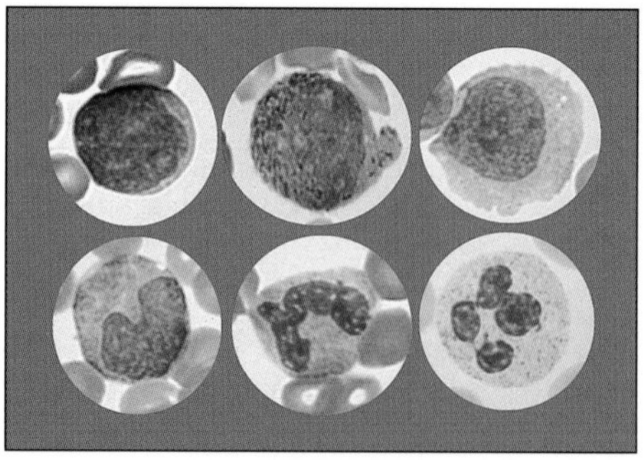

Figure 30-49 Normal myeloid (neutrophilic) maturation. Various stages of normal myeloid maturation from the blast to the mature neutrophil.

Maturation

While examining cells during the differential count, one should evaluate whether maturation is normal (Figs. 30-48 and 30-49), that is, whether nuclear and cytoplasmic development is in balance. Impaired cytoplasmic maturation in normoblasts, for example, occurs when Hb synthesis is impaired; impaired nuclear maturation occurs in megaloblastic anemias. Bizarre or dysplastic maturation occurs as a result of certain drugs, in some leukemias, and in dysmyelopoietic syndromes.

Presence of Rare Cell Types or Abnormal Cells

In scanning the marrow, one looks for the presence of rare or unexpected cell types.

Tissue mast cells (Fig. 30-50) are normally very infrequent. They are increased in number in aplastic or refractory anemias and in lymphoproliferative disorders.

Osteoblasts (Fig. 30-51) are cells that synthesize the collagen matrix of bone. **Osteoclasts** are cells that resorb bone and are thought to result from the fusion of histiocytes. Both cell types are normally present in small numbers in the aspirates of infants and children. They are uncommonly seen in adult marrow, except when bone destruction or repair is occurring, as in hyperparathyroidism, Paget's disease, metastatic tumor, or a recent biopsy at the same site.

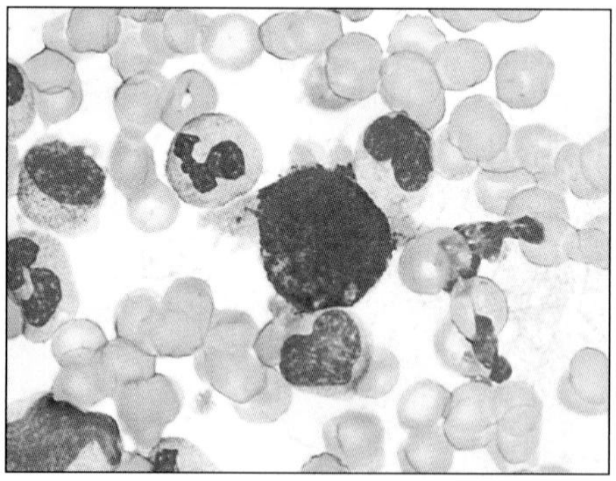

Figure 30-50 Tissue mast cell. Mast cells contain numerous dense dark-purple cytoplasmic granules that can completely cover the round nucleus (1000×).

Osteoblasts are large cells with a single eccentric nucleus that has reticular chromatin and a prominent nucleolus. The cytoplasm is moderately basophilic; a large pale Golgi zone is separated from the nucleus,

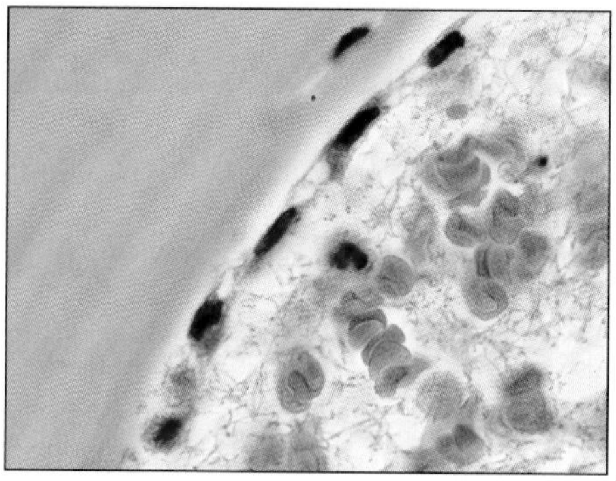

Figure 30-51 Osteoblast. Frequently found in pediatric patients, osteoblasts line the bone trabeculae. In smears, they appear as cells with eccentrically placed nuclei, resembling plasma cells, but the cytoplasmic clearing is more centrally located and is not found in the Golgi area, as in plasma cells (1000×).

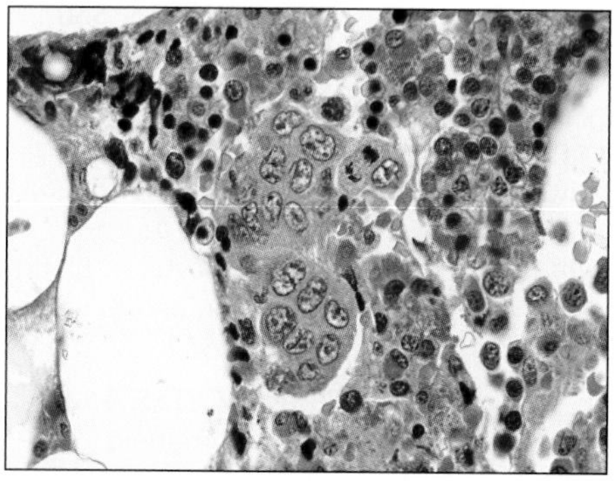

Figure 30-52 Metastatic tumor. Bone marrow biopsy with islands of metastatic gastric adenocarcinoma (1000×).

rather than abutting it as in plasma cells. Osteoblasts are often present in clusters and may be confused with immature plasma cells or myeloma cells. Osteoclasts are large, multinucleated cells up to 100 μm diameter that may be mistaken for megakaryocytes. They have multiple nuclei that are separate (not joined as in megakaryocytes). The chromatin is reticular, and a prominent nucleolus is usually present. The cytoplasm may be basophilic but usually has pink-purple granules that resemble megakaryocyte granules. Coarse fragments of purple-staining material are often present. Clusters of **metastatic neoplastic cells** (Fig. 30-52) may be found in one or more marrow films of patients with metastatic tumor in the bone sampled; they may be found in biopsy sections and not in films, in both, or, less commonly, in one or more films and not in the biopsy. Some metastatic neoplastic cells resemble myeloblasts or other primitive blasts. The clue to recognizing them is that they almost always appear in clusters or clumps of cells; this is not true of hematopoietic blast cells.

Evaluation of the Biopsy Specimen

Histologic sections allow better estimates of marrow cellularity and of the number of megakaryocytes than do marrow films (see Fig. 30-47). Normally, immature myeloid precursors lie along bone trabeculae, erythroid precursors are in discrete interstitial islands, and megakaryocytes are scattered in the interstitium. In good histologic preparations, cell distribution and maturation abnormalities can be quite reliably determined. In addition to more reliable detection of the presence of lymphomas or metastatic tumor, the histologic pattern can often be diagnostic of the type of neoplasm. Other focal lesions not found in films include granulomas, abscesses, and vascular lesions. In some conditions, such as myelofibrosis and hairy cell leukemia, the bone marrow cannot be aspirated, and biopsy is necessary to establish a diagnosis. Trabeculae should always be examined to detect bone abnormalities. Osteosclerosis with thickened bone trabeculae may accompany myelofibrosis or may be congenital. In osteoporosis, the bone trabeculae are thin. Osteomalacia is characterized by a recognizable osteoid seam. Osteitis fibrosa occurs in hyperparathyroidism and is characterized by irregular osteoclastic bone resorption, endosteal fibrosis, and some osteoblastic activity in areas of bone regeneration. Irregularly widened trabeculae with a "mosaic" pattern are typical findings in Paget's disease of bone.

Interpretation

The summary of the marrow report includes an estimate of cellularity, an estimate of the number of megakaryocytes, the M/E ratio, statements about any cytologic or maturation abnormalities, an estimate of the storage iron and proportion of sideroblasts, and statements about any other abnormal findings present. Abnormalities in blood cell counts and morphology are also summarized. An interpretation of observed findings is made, which of course includes a diagnosis if this is possible. In making such an **interpretation,** one should include an integration of marrow and blood observations with clinical findings and other laboratory data. Alterations in blood and marrow cells are discussed, with reference to the diseases and disorders considered in subsequent chapters.

INDICATIONS FOR MARROW STUDY

In microcytic anemia, evaluation of iron stores and sideroblasts allows categorization of the anemia (i.e., iron deficiency, anemia of chronic disease, sideroblastic).

In macrocytic anemia, marrow examination will confirm whether the process is megaloblastic or not; in some cases, changes in the blood are minimal, yet the marrow is megaloblastic. In normocytic anemia (or macrocytic anemia) without an increased reticulocyte production index, the marrow is evaluated for quantitative or qualitative abnormalities in erythropoiesis (e.g., pure red cell aplasia, myelodysplasia).

In neutropenia, thrombocytopenia, or pancytopenia, marrow study is helpful in assessing the presence and normality of the precursor cells in each series. This enables one to assess the probability of decreased production, impaired maturation, or increased destruction as the mechanism of the disorder. In cytopenias, marrow examination sometimes will reveal the presence of leukemia or another hematologic neoplasia.

In immunoglobulin abnormalities, the diagnosis of plasma cell myeloma or macroglobulinemia may be confirmed if infiltrations of abnormal plasma cells or lymphocytes are present. Marrow examination is essential for the diagnosis and classification of acute leukemia. It is frequently performed to assist in the diagnosis and staging of other neoplasms, including lymphomas and metastatic tumors, and to assess response to therapy for hematologic disorders. If the marrow cannot be aspirated ("dry tap"), biopsy is essential. Marrow biopsy should also be performed if blood changes suggest myelofibrosis with myeloid metaplasia, or if granulomatous disease or metastatic tumor is suspected.

SELECTED REFERENCES

Cornbleet J. Spurious results from automated hematology cell analyzers. Lab Med 1983;14:509.

Extremely useful reference for analysis of spurious results obtained from automated cell counters. It discusses reasons for spurious results with each parameter in a nicely tabulated format.

International Committee for Standardization in Haematology (ICSH). Protocol for evaluation of automated blood cell counters. Clin Lab Haematol 1984b;6:69–84.

This protocol evaluates automated blood cell counters to assess the performance, advantages, and limitations of such instruments.

Perkins SL. Examination of the blood and bone marrow. In: Wintrobe's clinical hematology. 11th ed. Philadelphia: Lippincott, Williams & Wilkins; 2004, p. 3–21.

Comprehensive review of blood and bone marrow examination, including detailed discussion of various ancillary studies that can be done for establishing the diagnosis of hematologic diseases.

Ryan DH. Examination of the blood. In: Williams hematology. 7th ed. New York: McGraw Hill; 2006a, p. 11–20.

Extensive review of bone marrow examination, including discussion of marrow aspiration technique.

Ryan DH, Felger RE. Examination of the marrow. In: Williams hematology. 7th ed. New York: McGraw Hill; 2006b, p. 21–31.

Extensive review of bone marrow examination.

Ward P. The CBC at the turn of the millennium: an overview. Clin Chem 2000;46:1215–20.

This review article effectively summarizes current methods utilized by automated hematology analyzers. It also offers comments on advantages and limitations of selected CBC and differential parameters.

REFERENCES

Access the complete reference list online at http://www.expertconsult.com

CHAPTER 31

HEMATOPOIESIS

Sharad C. Mathur, Katherine I. Schexneider, Robert E. Hutchison

KEY POINTS

- Hematopoietic tissue arises in the bone marrow from stem cells that differentiate into granulocytes, monocytes, lymphocytes, megakaryocytes, and erythroid cells.
- Differentiation and maturation of hematopoietic cells are influenced by soluble factors, including growth factors and cytokines, by interaction with the bone marrow stroma, and are mediated in part through interaction of adhesion molecules.
- The primary function of erythrocytes is delivery of oxygen from lungs to tissues. This is dependent on the particular properties and adequate production of hemoglobin and is regulated by oxygen tension in the kidneys, where erythropoietin is produced.
- Inherited or acquired abnormalities of heme biosynthesis, known as porphyrias because of abnormal accumulation of porphyrins and metabolites, primarily affect the nervous system.
- Neutrophils and monocytes are derived from a common progenitor cell under the influence of growth factors, and are the major phagocytic cells. They and the other granulocytic cells (eosinophils, basophils, and mast cells) respond to soluble factors, eliminate microorganisms, and modulate immunity.
- Megakaryocytes, stimulated by thrombopoietin, give rise to platelets and thus effect primary hemostasis.
- Lymphocytes arise in thymus and peripheral lymphoid tissue, as well as in bone marrow. They are made up of complex populations of genetically distinct individual B cells, T cells, natural killer (NK) cells, and related subtypes. These interact with other cells, secrete soluble factors including principally cytokines and immunoglobulins, and effect both humoral and cellular immunity.

STEM CELLS

In postnatal life in humans, erythrocytes, granulocytes, monocytes, and platelets are normally produced only in the bone marrow. Lymphocytes are produced in the secondary lymphoid organs, as well as in the bone marrow and thymus gland.

Most bone marrow cells are morphologically recognizable precursors of granulocytes or erythrocytes with smaller numbers of platelet precursors (megakaryocytes), lymphocytes, monocytes, macrophages, stromal cells (endothelial cells, fibroblasts, osteoblasts, and osteoclasts), eosinophils, plasma cells, basophils, mast cells, and blasts. The latter include hematopoietic stem cells (HSCs), which are capable of self-renewal and differentiation; and progenitors, which differentiate along a specific pathway.

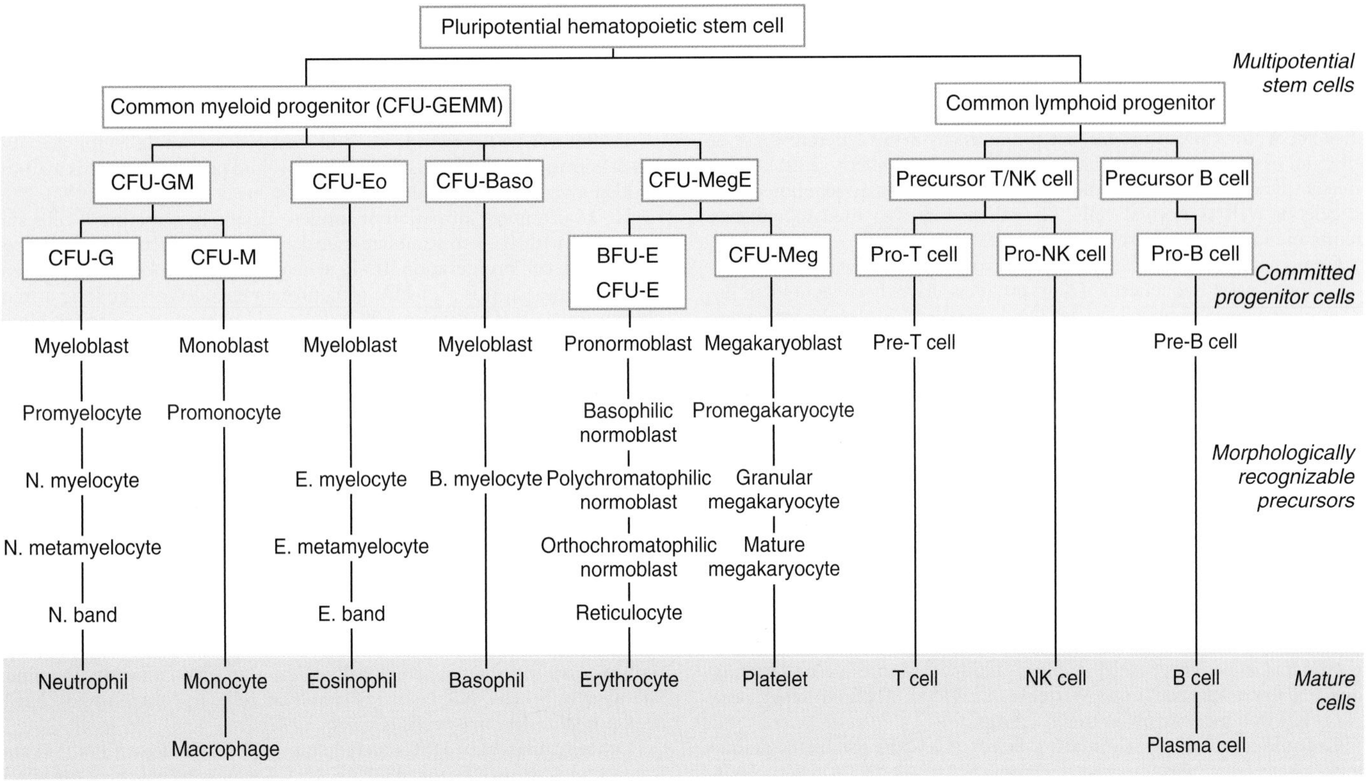

Figure 31-1 Hypothetical scheme of hematopoiesis. *B.,* Basophil; *BFU-E,* burst forming unit-erythrocyte; *CFU-Baso,* colony-forming unit-basophil; *CFU-E,* colony-forming unit-erythrocyte; *CFU-Eo,* colony-forming unit-eosinophil; *CFU-G,* colony-forming unit-granulocyte; *CFU-GEMM,* colony-forming unit-granulocyte/erythrocyte/macrophage/megakaryocyte; *CFU-GM,* colony-forming unit-granulocyte/macrophage; *CFU-M,* colony-forming unit-macrophage; *CFU-Meg,* colony-forming unit-megakaryocyte; *CFU-MegE,* colony-forming unit-megakaryocyte/erythroid; *E.,* eosinophil; *N.,* neutrophil.

HEMATOPOIETIC STEM CELLS AND PROGENITORS

Pluripotential hematopoietic stem cells give rise to multipotent progenitors, followed by lineage-committed progenitors. In the standard model of hematopoiesis, multipotent progenitors give rise to common myeloid progenitors and common lymphoid progenitors (Kondo, 1997; Akashi, 2000), although more recent work showing myeloid lineage potential in the earliest thymic T cell progenitors has raised questions about this binary split (Bell, 2008; Wada, 2008). Common myeloid progenitors give rise to granulocyte/macrophage lineage–restricted progenitors and megakaryocyte/erythrocyte lineage–restricted progenitors. These cells subsequently generate lineage-committed progenitors for the production of granulocytes, macrophages, platelets, and erythrocytes. Common lymphoid progenitors give rise to B lymphocytes, T lymphocytes, and natural killer cells. The capacity for self-renewal is progressively lost, and terminally differentiated cells cannot divide.

Human HSCs express CD34 but lack the major histocompatibility complex (MHC) class II antigen, HLA-DR (Quesenberry, 2001). CD34 is a glycoprotein that is encoded on chromosome 1q and is expressed by hematopoietic stem cells, as well as early progenitor cells. These cells also express high levels of multidrug-resistant (MDR1) protein and lack lineage-commitment markers such as CD38, CD33, thy-1, and CD71. These earliest known precursor cells constitute less than 1% of bone marrow cells and have the morphology of blasts. HSCs also occur in small numbers in the peripheral blood and are increased with administration of growth factors and/or some chemotherapeutic agents, allowing the use of peripheral blood, as well as bone marrow, to obtain stem cells used for bone marrow transplantation. Lineage commitment can be recognized by additional expression of CD38 antigen along with other antigens such as CD71 for erythroid differentiation, CD33 for myeloid differentiation, CD10 for B-lymphoid differentiation, and CD7/CD5 for T-lymphoid differentiation (Table 31-1). Selection and differentiation with progressively narrower lineage restriction are influenced by local effects in the bone marrow microenvironment and humoral factors and probably involve MHC class II molecule interactions.

TABLE 31-1
Lineage-Specific Markers

Erythroid—CD71
Myeloid—CD33
B-lymphoid—CD10
T-lymphoid—CD7/CD5

Based on in vitro culture studies and colony assays, multiple levels of progenitors with progressively limited differentiating capability are identified (Coulombel, 2004). The earliest myeloid progenitor is the colony-forming unit-granulocyte, erythrocyte, macrophage, megakaryocyte (CFU-GEMM) cell that expresses CD34 and CD33. Under the influence of different growth factors and cytokines, CFU-GEMM cells develop into colony-forming unit-granulocyte-macrophage (CFU-GM) cells and colony-forming unit-megakaryocyte-erythroid (CFU-MegE) cells. CFU-GM cells differentiate into colony-forming unit-granulocyte (CFU-G) cells, precursors of neutrophils, and colony-forming unit-macrophage (CFU-M) cells, precursors of monocytes, macrophages, and dendritic cells (Fig. 31-1). CFU-MegE cells give rise to burst-forming unit-erythrocyte (BFU-E) cells (and subsequently colony-forming unit-erythrocyte [CFU-E] cells) and colony-forming unit-megakaryocyte (CFU-Meg) cells. Progenitors committed to the development of eosinophils, basophils, and mast cells are also described (colony-forming unit-eosinophil [CFU-Eo] cells, colony-forming unit-basophil [CFU-Baso] cells, and colony-forming unit-mastocyte [CFU-Mast] cells). HSCs also give rise to osteoclasts, which are part of the monocytic and phagocytic system. In addition, evidence suggests that HSCs can transdifferentiate into nonhematopoietic cells (Zubair, 2002).

HEMATOPOIETIC GROWTH FACTORS

Soluble or membrane-bound biochemical factors contributing to control of hematopoiesis include hematopoietic growth factors and interleukins.

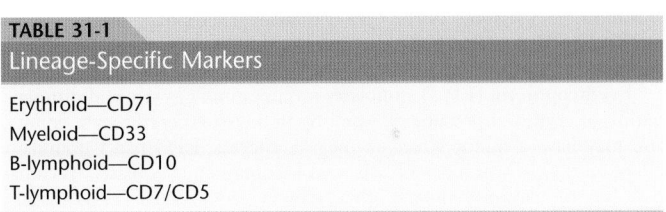

They consist of acidic glycoproteins, which are functionally diverse but structurally conserved (Kaushansky, 1993). They regulate the proliferation and differentiation of hematopoietic precursor cells and facilitate the function of mature blood cells. Hematopoietic growth factors may act locally near the site at which they are produced, or they may circulate in the blood. They act at low concentrations, are produced by many different types of cells, and usually affect more than one lineage (Quesenberry, 2001). They often act synergistically with other growth factors and may act on neoplastic cells as well as normal cells. Growth factors also tend to enhance membrane integrity and prevent apoptosis.

Genes associated with hematopoietic growth factors have been identified, cloned, and sequenced. Their products have been generated by recombinant deoxyribonucleic acid (DNA) methods. Molecular structures are frequently predicted using computer models from sequence data as well as analyzed directly by crystallography and magnetic resonance spectroscopy. Pure molecules are utilized experimentally, and several are now used therapeutically as drugs. The rapid growth in knowledge of hematopoietic growth factors and the complexity of their activities defies simple summation. Factors chiefly involved in hematopoiesis are briefly noted here.

Granulocyte/macrophage colony–stimulating factor (GM-CSF) is a pan-myeloid growth factor, stimulating erythroid, granulocyte, monocyte, megakaryocyte, and eosinophil progenitors, resulting primarily in increases of neutrophils, monocytes, and eosinophils, and in activation of phagocytic function. It is a 14- to 35-kDa glycoprotein encoded on the long arm of chromosome 5. GM-CSF is utilized clinically to combat neutropenia in patients receiving chemotherapy and in those undergoing bone marrow transplantation (Mertelsmann, 1993). Myeloid hyperplasia may result in bone marrow in these settings.

Granulocyte colony-stimulating factor (G-CSF) stimulates granulocyte production and functional activation. It is an 18-kDa protein encoded on the long arm of chromosome 17 (Bagby, 1991). G-CSF is frequently used to treat neutropenia and may induce less toxicity than GM-CSF (Root, 1999). It is also the growth factor most commonly used to mobilize CD34+ stem cells in the peripheral blood (Hübel, 2003).

Monocyte/macrophage colony-stimulating factor (M-CSF) (also known as colony-stimulating factor-1 [CSF-1]) stimulates monocyte–macrophage production and activity. It consists of two species of glycoprotein (40–50 and 70–90 kDa) that are encoded on the long arm of chromosome 5 (Bagby, 1991). CSF-1 induces macrophage production of interleukin (IL)-1. The CSF-1 receptor is the product of the FMS gene and acts as a tyrosine kinase to mediate cell activation.

Erythropoietin (EPO) stimulates proliferation, growth, and differentiation of erythroid precursors, resulting in increased erythrocyte counts, and may have a minor effect on megakaryocytes. EPO has a dominant effect on CFU-E, pronormoblasts, and basophilic normoblasts. Maximal BFU-E stimulation requires other growth factors such as IL-3 and GM-CSF. EPO, an 18-kDa protein (34–39 kDa when glycosylated) encoded on the long arm of chromosome 7, is primarily produced in the kidney in adult life and is induced by hypoxia (Bagby, 1991). Recombinant EPO is utilized clinically to treat anemia, particularly that associated with renal failure, chemotherapy, or bone marrow infiltration by cancer (Mertelsmann, 1993).

Thrombopoietin (TPO) is a 35-kDa polypeptide that is a ligand for the product of the proto-oncogene *c-mpl* (Kaushansky, 1994) and is the primary regulator of platelet production. It is produced by the liver, kidney, marrow stroma, and other tissues and stimulates both the production and differentiation of megakaryocytic precursor cells (Kaushansky, 2003). It is essential for the full maturation of megakaryocytes and enhances platelet production. TPO-mimetic drugs have been developed to speed the recovery of blood platelets after cytoreductive therapies.

IL-3 is a multipotential colony-stimulating factor that has activities analogous to GM-CSF but occurs at an earlier level. The 14- to 28-kDa protein is encoded near the GM-CSF gene on the long arm of chromosome 5, and is closely linked to the genes for GM-CSF, IL-4, and IL-5. IL-3 is produced by T cells, endothelial cells, fibroblasts, macrophages, and mast cells. It activates indirectly by stimulating other cytokines (Bagby, 1991).

IL-5 activates cytotoxic T cells, induces immunoglobulin (Ig) secretion, and stimulates eosinophils. It is a 50- to 60-kDa product of the long arm of chromosome 5 that is produced by activated T cells (Jandl, 1996).

IL-6 is a broad activating factor that appears to exert its influences indirectly through synergy with other factors. IL-6 facilitates B cell differentiation, promotes Ig secretion, and acts as a growth factor for malignant plasma cells (Teoh, 1997). It functions along with IL-3 to increase replication of myeloid precursors, synergizes with IL-2 and IL-4, and stimulates platelet production. It is a 26-kDa product of the short arm of chromosome 7 (Jandl, 1996) and is secreted by T cells, macrophages, and fibroblasts.

IL-9 is a T cell growth factor and mast cell–activating factor that also has effects in stimulating erythroid and myeloid proliferation. It is a 30- to 40-kDa glycoprotein encoded on chromosome 5 (Quesniaux, 1992).

IL-11 promotes formation of antigen-specific Ig-secreting B cells and synergizes with IL-3 to stimulate megakaryocyte production and pluripotential stem cell proliferation. IL-11 synergizes with IL-4 to promote stem cell proliferation. It is a 23-kDa glycoprotein encoded on the long arm of chromosome 19 (Quesniaux, 1992). It is used to speed recovery of blood platelets after cytoreductive therapies.

Stem cell factor (SCF) is the ligand for the tyrosine kinase receptor *c-kit* and is also referred to as kit ligand. It synergizes with most other growth factors, including GM-CSF and IL-3, to stimulate myeloid, erythroid, and lymphoid progenitors (Quesniaux, 1992). The SCF receptor is encoded on chromosome 4, whereas SCF is mapped to chromosome 12 (Broudy, 1997). SCF stimulates the growth, viability, and adhesion of primitive progenitor cells, erythroid precursors (BFU-E, CFU-E), myeloid precursors (CFU-GM), megakaryocytic precursors (CFU-Meg), and mast cells. It also stimulates the growth of B cells, T cells, NK cells, and dendritic cells.

Flt-3 ligand (FL) stimulates primitive progenitor cells, often in synergy with SCF. Similarly to the SCF receptor, the FL receptor is a tyrosine kinase. It acts synergistically with other growth factors to stimulate T cells, B cells, NK cells, and dendritic cells. In contrast to SCF, FL does not stimulate mast cells (Lyman, 1998).

Other regulators of HSCs include tumor necrosis factor (TNF)-α and transforming growth factor (TGF)-β. HSCs express receptors of the notch and Wnt families; these cytokine pathways are also likely important in self-renewal and differentiation (Ohishi, 2003; Sauvageau, 2004).

HSCs and the earliest myeloid progenitors (CFU-GEMM) require SCF, FL, IL-3, and IL-6 for duplication and differentiation into committed progenitors. Further development of myeloid progenitors (CFU-G and CFU-M) requires G-CSF and M-CSF, in addition to GM-CSF and IL-3. G-CSF is primarily responsible for neutrophil differentiation, M-CSF for monocyte/macrophage differentiation, IL-5 for eosinophil differentiation, IL-3 and SCF for basophil differentiation, and SCF for mast cell differentiation. Development of the earliest erythroid progenitor (BFU-E) is independent of EPO, but subsequent differentiation into CFU-E needs EPO, in addition to other growth factors such as GM-CSF, IL-3, and SCF. EPO is solely responsible for further maturation of the erythroid lineage. Megakaryocyte development is dependent on TPO, in concert with IL-3, IL-6, IL-11, and SCF.

In addition to growth factors, other families of cell surface molecules are involved in directional migration of developing hematopoietic cells. Adhesion molecules are required to modulate many interactions between hematopoietic cells and growth factors, stromal cells, endothelium, and extracellular matrix. These cell surface molecules influence induction, differentiation, and function of hematopoietic cells. They are also responsible for the retention and release of hematopoietic cells in the bone marrow (Verfaillie, 1998). Several major families of adhesion molecules exist, including the Ig supergene family, the integrins, and the selectins (Long, 1992).

Many extracellular matrix components interact with receptors on hematopoietic cells. These include fibronectin, thrombospondin, hyaluronic acid, hemonectin, laminin, and heparin sulfate. Receptors for some of these are known. CD44, receptor for hyaluronic acid, is an antigenically related group of inducible cell surface proteins variably expressed on all leukocytes. It is required for early granulopoiesis, as well as for trafficking of mature lymphocytes.

Another class of compounds, the chemokines, are important in regulating blood cell trafficking and homing. The chemokine SDF-1 is expressed by bone marrow stromal cells and microvascular endothelium. HSCs express CXCR4, the receptor for SDF-1. The interaction of SDF-1 and CXCR4 is involved in HSC engraftment. G-CSF–induced mobilization of HSCs is likely due to disruption of the interaction between SDF-1 and CXCR4 (Campbell, 2003; Papayannopoulou, 2008).

Laboratory assays are available for most hematopoietic growth factors and cytokines and are helpful in the diagnostic workup of a wide variety of diseases. Disease states caused by selective deficiency of a growth factor, such as anemia of renal failure due to low EPO levels, can be treated by administration of recombinant protein.

Hematopoietic Tissues

EMBRYONIC AND FETAL HEMATOPOIESIS

Beginning in the first month of prenatal life, primitive hematopoiesis starts outside the embryo in the mesenchyme of the yolk sac as **blood islands.** These contain predominantly **primitive erythroblasts,** which are large and megaloblastic, are formed intravascularly, and retain their nuclei. Definitive hematopoiesis in mammals takes place in the aorta-gonad-mesonephros (AGM) region of the embryo, from which hematopoietic cells migrate to the liver and spleen. At the sixth week, hematopoiesis begins in the liver, and this becomes the major hematopoietic organ of early and midfetal life. **Definitive erythroblasts,** which become non-nucleated red cells, are formed extravascularly in the liver, and granulopoiesis and megakaryocytes are present to a lesser degree. In the middle part of fetal life, the spleen and to a lesser extent lymph nodes have a minor role in hematopoiesis, but the liver continues to dominate. In the latter half of fetal life, the bone marrow becomes progressively more important as a site of blood cell production. As this occurs, the liver's role diminishes.

POSTNATAL HEMATOPOIESIS

Shortly after birth, hematopoiesis in the liver ceases, and the marrow is the only site for the production of erythrocytes, granulocytes, and platelets. Hematopoietic stem cells and committed progenitor cells are maintained in the marrow. Lymphocytes (of the B cell type) continue to be produced in the marrow, as well as in the secondary lymphoid organs, whereas T lymphocytes are produced in the thymus and also in the secondary lymphoid organs (see Lymphocytes).

At birth, the total marrow space is occupied by active hematopoietic (red) marrow. As body growth progresses and marrow space increases during infancy, only part of that space is needed for hematopoiesis; the remaining space is occupied by fat cells. Later in childhood, only the flat bones (the skull, vertebrae, thoracic cage, shoulder, and pelvis) and the proximal parts of the long bones of the upper and lower limbs are sites of blood cell formation. The remaining marrow space is fatty or yellow marrow that can be replaced by hematopoietic cells if continuous, intensive stimulation exists.

The marrow circulation is closed, that is, arterioles deriving from central longitudinal arteries (i.e., in long bones) connect directly with broad venous sinuses that anastomose and eventually empty into central longitudinal veins. The flattened endothelium of the sinuses is partially covered by adventitial reticular cells, a form of fibroblast that elaborates argentophilic reticulin fibers. These reticular cells and fibers form the supporting meshwork of the marrow stroma, where the hematopoietic cells reside. The reticular cells are but minimally phagocytic; they may swell and take up water, may become fat cells, and may induce hematopoietic stem cells to become committed progenitor cells. After proliferation and maturation have occurred in the marrow stroma, blood cells gain entrance to the blood through or between the endothelial cells of the sinus wall. This requires displacement of adventitial cells. Stromal mesenchymal cells and sinusoidal endothelial cells produce a variety of cytokines and chemokines involved in hematopoiesis.

Erythrocyte Production

The erythrocyte is a vehicle for the transport of hemoglobin, which is produced in precursor cells of the erythrocytes, the normoblasts. The function of hemoglobin is the transport of oxygen and carbon dioxide. The erythrocyte is also metabolically capable of keeping hemoglobin in a functional state.

NORMOBLASTIC MATURATION

The earliest recognizable erythroid precursor is the **pronormoblast** (Fig. 31-2). At about 20 μm diameter, it is the largest of the erythroid precursors. The nucleus has a fine, uniform chromatin pattern that is somewhat more distinct and more intensely stained than that of the myeloblast. The nuclear membrane is prominent. One or more prominent nucleoli are present. The cytoplasm has a heterogeneous quality and is moderate in amount and basophilia; no granules are present. The pronormoblast undergoes mitosis and forms two basophilic normoblasts.

The **basophilic normoblast** (Fig. 31-3) is somewhat smaller and has slightly coarser chromatin that stains intensely; the chromatin may be partially clumped, and the pattern may suggest a wheel with broad spokes. The parachromatin (the nonchromatin part of the nucleus) is distinct and stains pink. Nucleoli are present but are not often visible. The nuclear/cytoplasmic (N/C) ratio is moderate; about one fourth of the total cell area appears to be cytoplasm. The cytoplasm is deeply basophilic, owing to the abundance of RNA; much of this is evident as polyribosomes on electron micrographs. The cell borders of early normoblasts frequently appear irregular owing to the presence of pseudopodia.

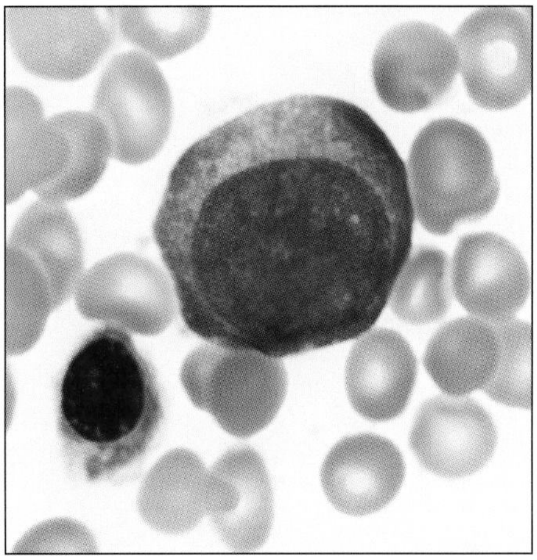

Figure 31-2 Pronormoblast with a large round nucleus, fine chromatin, and basophilic cytoplasm (Wright–Giemsa, 1000×).

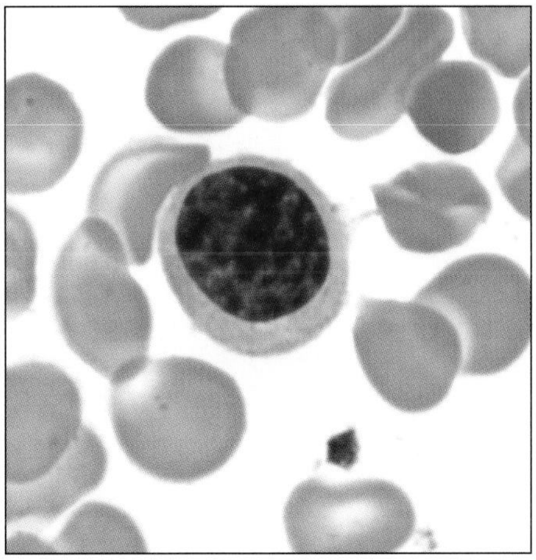

Figure 31-3 Basophilic normoblasts with chromatin condensation and deeply basophilic cytoplasm (Wright–Giemsa, 1000×).

After mitosis of the basophilic normoblast, evidence of continuing hemoglobin production becomes visible in the cytoplasm of the two daughter cells as polychromasia, that is, mixtures of the red-staining of hemoglobin with the blue of RNA in varying shades of gray. This cell is the **polychromatophilic normoblast** (Fig. 31-4), which is slightly smaller than the basophilic normoblast. The nucleus occupies about half of the area of the cell, stains intensely, and has moderately condensed chromatin that is sharply distinct from the pink parachromatin. The polychromatophilic normoblast undergoes one or two mitotic divisions.

After the last mitosis, the nucleus becomes small and dense (pyknotic), and the **orthochromatic normoblast** stage is reached (Fig. 31-5). Mitosis is no longer possible. The cell is smaller than the polychromatophilic normoblast and has a lower N/C ratio. The cytoplasm contains more abundant hemoglobin and fewer polyribosomes and remains slightly polychromatophilic.

Finally, accompanied by cytoplasmic contractions and undulations, the nucleus and a small rim of cytoplasm are ejected from the orthochromatic normoblast, forming the **reticulocyte** (Fig. 31-6). On air-dried films with Romanowsky-type stains, the reticulocyte is polychromatophilic as a result of the retention of RNA.

In the marrow, developing erythroid cells are usually in contact with macrophages in what are termed **erythroblastic islands** (Fig. 31-7). These erythroblastic islands are usually broken up when aspirated marrow is

PART 4

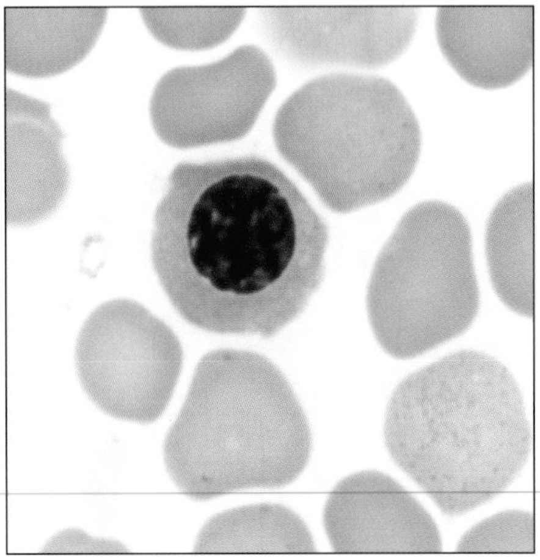

Figure 31-4 Polychromatophilic normoblast with light blue cytoplasm due to accumulation of hemoglobin (Wright–Giemsa, 1000×).

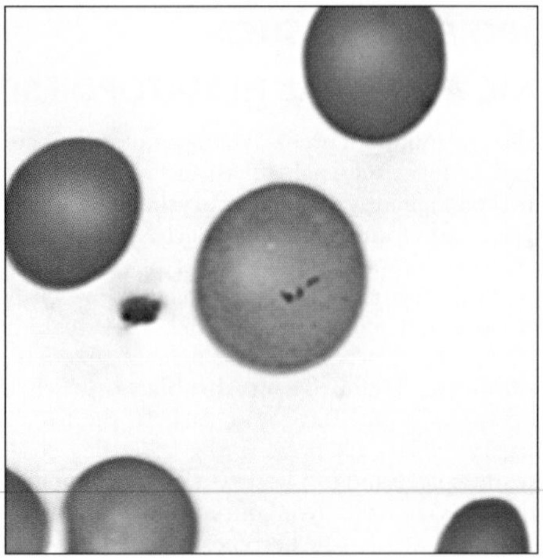

Figure 31-6 Reticulocyte (polychromatophilic erythrocyte) with pink-gray cytoplasm due to residual RNA (Wright–Giemsa, 1000×). *RNA,* Ribonucleic acid.

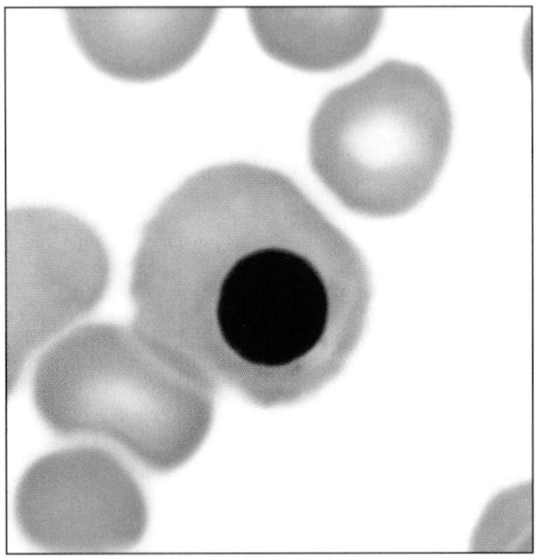

Figure 31-5 Orthochromatic normoblast with pyknotic nucleus and pink-gray cytoplasm (Wright–Giemsa, 1000×).

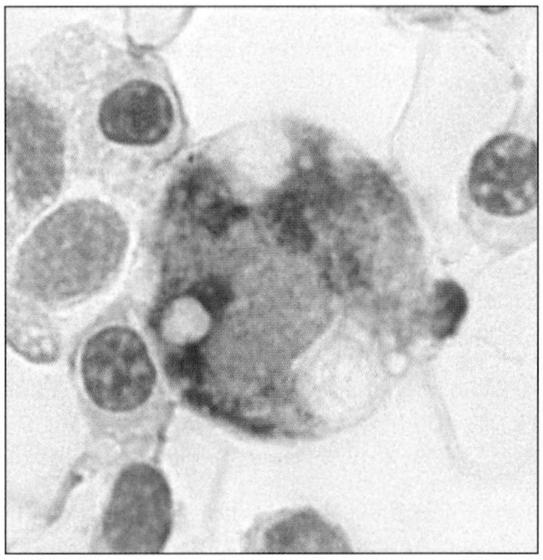

Figure 31-7 Siderophage with associated normoblasts (part of an erythroblastic island) in the bone marrow (Prussian blue, 1000×).

spread on slides, but fragments of macrophage cytoplasm may sometimes be seen attached to the separated normoblasts, especially on Prussian blue–stained films.

During proliferation and maturation, iron is transferred from plasma transferrin into the cells in the normoblastic series. The pronormoblast and the basophilic normoblast have the highest content of RNA, which begins to decline in the polychromatophilic normoblasts as hemoglobin increases in amount. Synthesis of RNA gradually decreases in each stage through the orthochromatic normoblasts. When the nucleus is no longer present (in the reticulocyte), RNA synthesis ceases, yet the RNA already present remains for a few days, and protein and heme synthesis continue in the reticulocyte until the cell loses its RNA and mitochondria.

During this maturation process, three or four mitotic divisions occur in a period of 3 days, resulting in the potential production of 16 reticulocytes from each pronormoblast. The reticulocytes are larger than mature red cells and remain in the marrow stroma for 1–2 days before being released into the blood.

In the marrow, the reticulocytes are about equal in number to the nucleated erythrocytes and slightly greater in number than the reticulocytes in the circulating blood. If sufficiently severe hypoxia is present, this marrow pool of reticulocytes can be released. This approximately doubles the number of circulating reticulocytes.

Normally, reticulocytes remain as such, slowly synthesizing hemoglobin, for 2–3 days in the marrow and for 1 day in the blood. Residual ribosomes, mitochondria, and other organelles are then removed, and the mature erythrocytes circulate for about 120 days. During this time, they gradually age, certain enzymatic activities diminish, and they are finally destroyed within phagocytic cells of the mononuclear phagocyte system (reticuloendothelial system).

MEGALOBLASTIC MATURATION

Abnormal maturation of erythroid precursors that occurs in vitamin B_{12} deficiency or folic acid deficiency is known as megaloblastic maturation, and the abnormal erythroid cells are called **megaloblasts.** Because of impaired ability of the cells to synthesize DNA, the intermitotic and mitotic phases are prolonged. This results in enlarged cells, with nuclear maturation lagging behind cytoplasmic maturation (nuclear–cytoplasmic dissociation). The nuclear chromatin pattern is more delicate and more "open," with prominent parachromatin. Karyorrhexis, or breaking up of the nucleus, and Howell-Jolly bodies are frequently noted. Megaloblastic development parallels normoblastic maturation; the stages of promegaloblast, basophilic megaloblast, polychromatophilic megaloblast, and orthochromatic megaloblast may be recognized.

REGULATION OF ERYTHROCYTE PRODUCTION

The number of erythrocytes in the blood may be regulated by changing the rate of production. The rate of erythrocyte destruction does not vary appreciably in normal individuals. Increased production of erythrocytes occurs when oxygen transport to the tissues is impaired, as in anemia, in cardiac or pulmonary disorders, and in the low oxygen tension of high altitudes. Erythrocyte production decreases when an individual is hypertransfused or exposed to high oxygen tension.

Oxygen affinity of hemoglobin is modulated by the concentration of phosphates, in particular 2,3-diphosphoglycerate (2,3-DPG) in the red cell. These phosphates combine with the β-chains of reduced hemoglobin

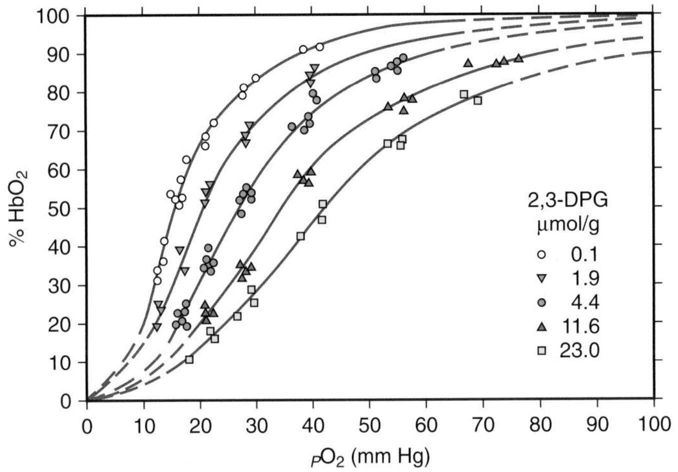

Figure 31-8 Oxygen dissociation curves of hemoglobin at different concentrations of 2,3-DPG. The curve is sigmoidal and shifts to the right with increasing concentrations of 2,3-DPG; this results in decreased affinity of hemoglobin for oxygen and increased delivery of oxygen to the tissues. *(Reprinted from Duhm J. Oxygen affinity of hemoglobin and red cell acid base status, p. 583, Copyright 1972, with permission from Elsevier.) DPG,* diphosphoglycerate.

and diminish its affinity for oxygen (Fig. 31-8). In areas of tissue hypoxia, as oxygen moves from hemoglobin into the tissues, the amount of reduced hemoglobin in the red cells increases, binding more 2,3-DPG, further reducing its oxygen affinity so that more oxygen can be delivered to the tissues. If hypoxia persists, depletion of free 2,3-DPG leads to increased glycolysis, production of more 2,3-DPG, and a persistently lower oxygen affinity of the hemoglobin.

Tissue hypoxia induces formation of EPO via production of the transcriptional factor, hypoxia-inducible factor-1 (HIF-1). HIF-1 is a heterodimer consisting of α- and β-subunits, of which the α-subunit is regulated by hypoxia. Under conditions of normal oxygen tension, HIF-1α undergoes proteosomal degradation, but it is stable under hypoxic conditions. EPO effects the production of more red cells in the bone marrow. It acts by inducing committed progenitor cells (CFU-E and BFU-E) in the marrow to proliferate and differentiate into pronormoblasts by shortening the generation time of normoblasts, and by promoting early release of reticulocytes into the blood. The result is increased numbers of marrow normoblasts in a normal ratio of cell types, a condition known as normoblastic hyperplasia. Increased cellular expression of HIF-1α can result from a 598C→T mutation in the von Hippel–Lindau gene (the von Hippel–Lindau protein is involved in HIF-1α degradation). This results in elevation of EPO levels and an autosomal recessive form of hereditary polycythemia known as Chuvash polycythemia (Gordeuk, 2004).

Measurement of EPO is accomplished by in vitro immunologic methods utilizing serum or plasma, with ethylenediamenetetraacetic acid (EDTA) plasma providing greater sensitivity (Lindstedt, 1998). Elevated levels are detected in patients with secondary polycythemia and in those with aplastic anemia. Decreased levels below the normal range are found in normal individuals after transfusion and in those with primary polycythemia (polycythemia vera). However, considerable overlap exists, and normal EPO levels may be found in both primary and secondary polycythemia (Spivak, 2002). Anti-EPO antibodies have been described in pure red cell aplasia and systemic lupus erythematosus (Casadevall, 1996; Schett, 2001); these may interfere with immunoassays for EPO and may contribute to anemia.

SYNTHESIS OF HEMOGLOBIN

Heme Synthesis

Heme synthesis occurs in most cells of the body, except the mature erythrocytes, but most abundantly in the erythroid precursors. Succinylcoenzyme A condenses with glycine to form the unstable intermediate α-amino β-ketoadipic acid, which is readily decarboxylated to δ-aminolevulinic acid (ALA) (Fig. 31-9). This condensation requires pyridoxal phosphate (vitamin B_6) and occurs in mitochondria.

ALA is excreted normally in small amounts in the urine, but in certain abnormalities of heme synthesis (e.g., lead poisoning), excretion is increased. Two molecules of ALA condense to form the monopyrrole porphobilinogen, catalyzed by the enzyme ALA-dehydrase. Porphobilinogen is also normally excreted in small amounts in the urine. Markedly elevated amounts appear in the urine in acute intermittent porphyria, and are easily detected by a color reaction with Ehrlich's aldehyde reagent.

Four molecules of porphobilinogen react to form uroporphyrinogen III or I (Fig. 31-10). The type III isomer is converted, by way of coproporphyrinogen III and protoporphyrinogen, to protoporphyrin. In certain diseases when this pathway is partially blocked, the type I isomers of uroporphyrinogen and coproporphyrinogen are formed, and their oxidized excretion products, uroporphyrin I and coproporphyrin I, are increased in amount.

Protoporphyrin is normally found in mature erythrocytes. In lead poisoning and in iron deficiency, levels of free erythrocyte protoporphyrin (FEP) are increased. Iron is inserted into protoporphyrin by the mitochondrial enzyme ferrochelatase to form the finished heme moiety.

Other abnormalities of heme synthesis (the porphyries) are discussed later in this chapter.

Globin Synthesis

Globin synthesis occurs in the cytoplasm of the normoblast and reticulocyte. The polypeptide chains are manufactured on the ribosomes. Specific small soluble RNA (sRNA) molecules determine the placement of each amino acid according to the code in the messenger RNA (mRNA). Progressive growth of the polypeptide chain begins at the amino end. This process of protein synthesis occurs on ribosomes clustered into polyribosomes, which are held together by the mRNA. Because the reticulocyte can synthesize hemoglobin for at least 2 days after loss of its nucleus, it appears that the mRNA for hemoglobin is quite stable. The polypeptide chains released from the ribosomes are folded into their three-dimensional configurations spontaneously.

Control of hemoglobin synthesis is exerted primarily through the action of heme. Increased heme inhibits further heme synthesis by inhibiting the activity and synthesis of ALA synthase. Heme also promotes globin synthesis, mainly at the site of chain initiation, and the interaction of ribosomes with mRNA.

STRUCTURE AND FUNCTION OF HEMOGLOBIN

In each hemoglobin (Hb) molecule, one heme group is inserted into a hydrophobic pocket of one folded polypeptide chain (Bunn, 1986). Normal adult HbA consists of four heme groups and four polypeptide chains (two α-chains and two β-chains), which form a roughly globular hemoglobin molecule (Fig. 31-11). The ferrous iron atoms have six coordination bonds: four to the pyrrole nitrogens of heme, one to the imidazole nitrogen of histidine of the globin chain (87-α or 92-β), and one that is reversibly bound to oxygen. As the oxygen partial pressure increases, each of the four heme groups sequentially binds one molecule of oxygen. In the process, a change in the overall configuration of the hemoglobin molecule occurs, which favors the additional binding of oxygen.

The sigmoid-shaped oxygen dissociation curve of hemoglobin reflects this increasing affinity for oxygen with increasing partial pressure of oxygen in the lungs (see Fig. 31-8). In the tissues, conversion of oxygenated Hb to Hb, decreasing pH, and increasing temperature produced by metabolic processes, as well as the binding of more 2,3-DPG to Hb, result in a shift of the Hb-oxygen dissociation curve to the right, favoring the release of oxygen from hemoglobin.

Carbon dioxide (CO_2) is transported in erythrocytes as well as in plasma. A small part of red cell CO_2 is dissolved and is bound to amino groups of hemoglobin as carbamino-CO_2, but most is in the bicarbonate form. The enzyme carbonic anhydrase catalyzes the transformation of carbon dioxide to bicarbonate in the red cell while in the tissue capillary bed and catalyzes the reverse reaction (the release of carbon dioxide from bicarbonate) in the erythrocyte when it is in the capillary bed of the lungs.

ERYTHROCYTE DESTRUCTION

The erythrocyte gradually undergoes metabolic changes over the course of its 120-day life span, at which time the less viable senescent cell is removed from the circulation. Certain glycolytic enzymes diminish in activity as the cell ages. Older red cells have a smaller surface area and an increased mean cell hemoglobin concentration (MCHC) compared with younger cells. Furthermore, aged red cells lose sialic acid from their

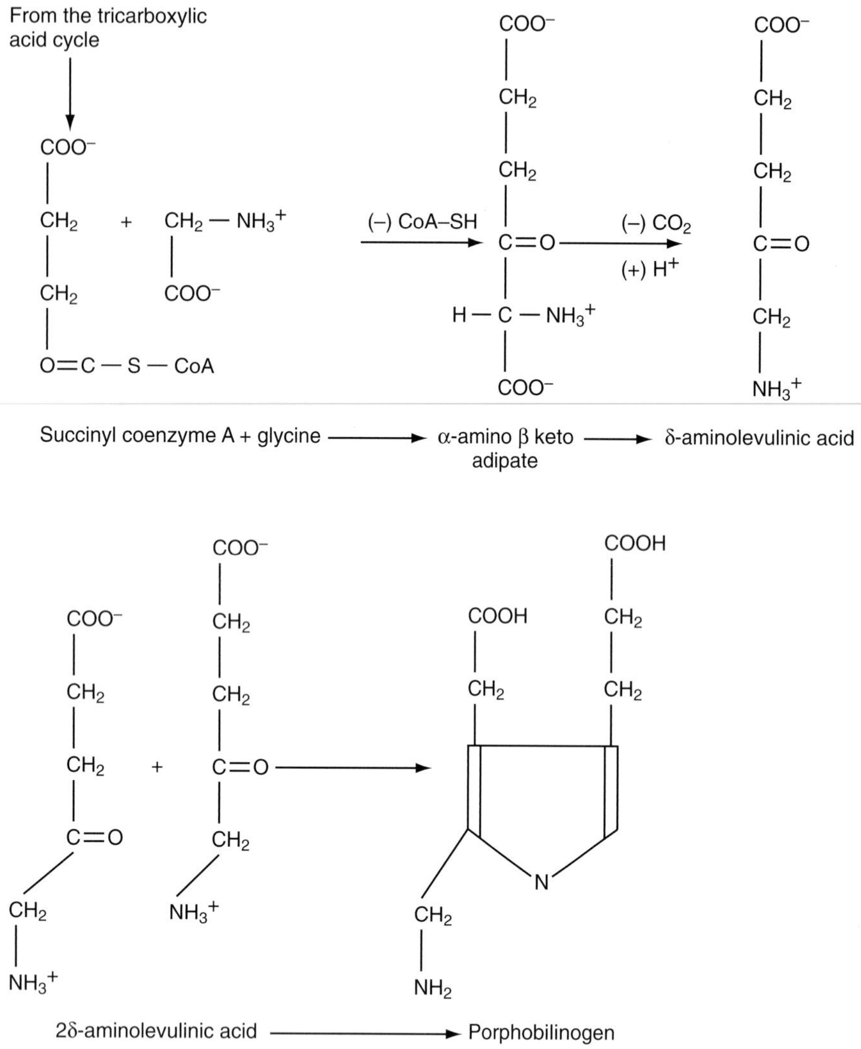

Figure 31-9 Formation of porphobilinogen from succinylcoenzyme A and glycine. *(From Leavell BS. Fundamentals of clinical hematology. 4th ed. Philadelphia: WB Saunders; 1976, with permission.)*

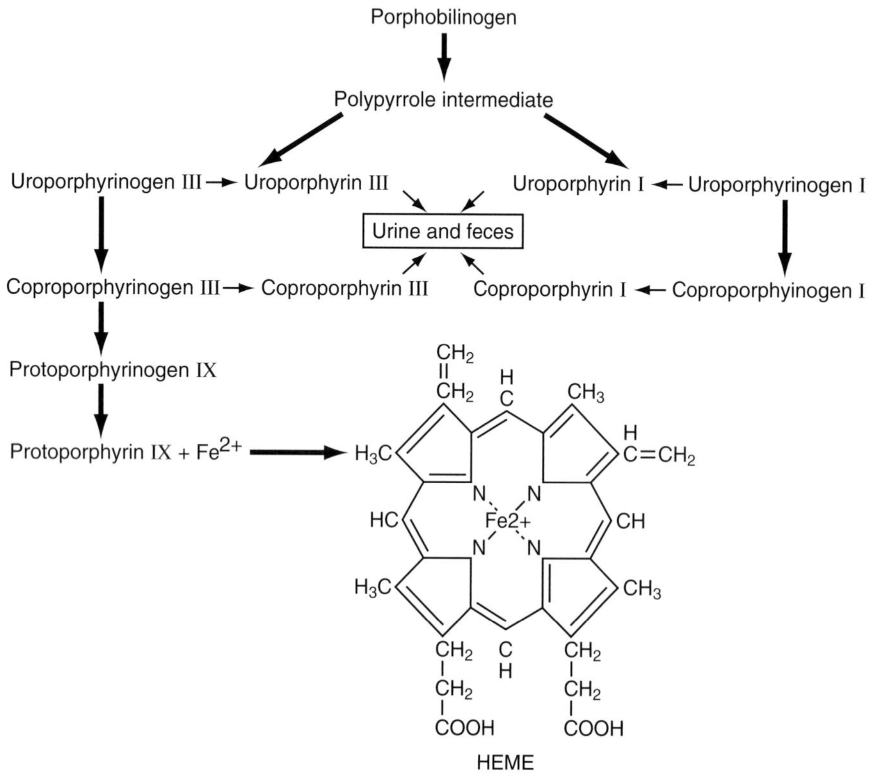

Figure 31-10 Formation of heme from porphobilinogen. *(From Leavell BS. Fundamentals of clinical hematology. 4th ed. Philadelphia: WB Saunders; 1976, with permission.)*

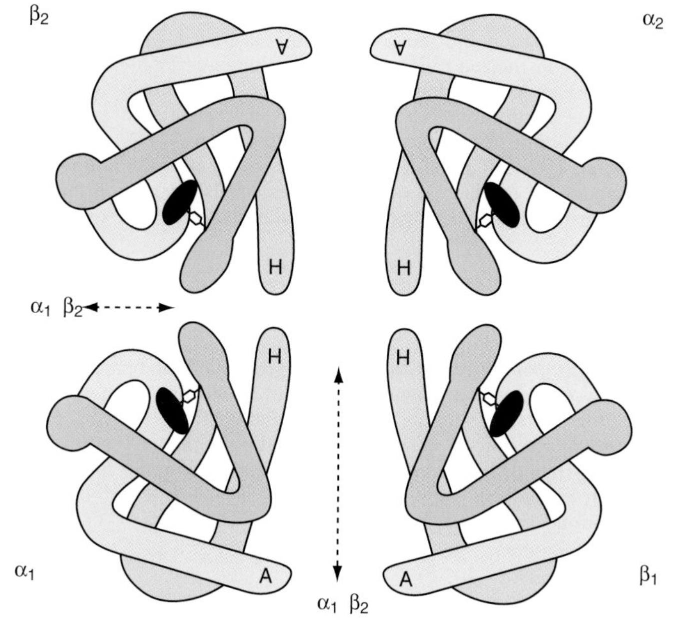

Figure 31-11 The hemoglobin molecule (tetramer, molecular weight 64,500 Da). The heme group for each monomeric polypeptide chain is depicted as a black disk, connected to an imidazole group of histidine and located near the surface of the molecule in a "pocket" formed by the polypeptide chain. The letters *A* and *H* designate α-helix segments of each polypeptide chain: A is the amino-terminal segment, and H is the carboxy-terminal segment. The four monomers are separated in this drawing but actually make contact along a relatively large area (α1β1), which is thought to be the relatively fixed or stabilizing contact area, and a smaller (α1β2) area thought to be the functional contact area, where movement occurs during oxygenation and deoxygenation, changing the molecular configuration. *(Redrawn from White JM, Dacie JV. Prog Hematol 1971;7:69, with permission.)*

membranes, exposing an asialoglycophorin. This senescent antigen is recognized and an autoantibody is synthesized by the host. After binding of the autoantibody, the senescent cell is removed from the circulation by the mononuclear phagocyte system, primarily within the spleen. About 3 million cells are normally removed from the blood per second with no demonstrable histologic evidence of erythrophagocytosis.

In some pathologic states, the mononuclear phagocyte system removes younger sensitized or abnormal red cells at a rapid rate. Subsequently, erythrophagocytosis is often evident. In autoimmune hemolytic anemia, the mononuclear phagocyte system removes red cells following the binding of autoantibodies or complement to reticulocytes and young red cells. In other pathologic states, red cells are removed because of structural defects that interfere with their normal passage through the microcirculation of the mononuclear phagocyte system.

DEGRADATION OF HEMOGLOBIN

After removal of the red cell from the circulation, hemoglobin is broken down within the macrophages of the mononuclear phagocyte system into its three constituents: iron, protoporphyrin, and globin. The iron goes into storage and may be completely reutilized. The globin may be degraded and returned to the amino acid pool of the body. In contrast, the protoporphyrin ring is split, converted to bilirubin, and excreted from the body.

In the macrophage, the protoporphyrin ring is cleaved by a heme oxidase enzyme at the α-methene bridge, yielding 1 mol of carbon monoxide (CO) and 1 mol of biliverdin. The CO appears in the blood as HbCO and is eventually exhaled. Biliverdin is reduced to bilirubin in the macrophage, and bilirubin is transported to the liver by plasma albumin. It is removed from the plasma by the liver cell, conjugated mainly with glucuronide, and excreted in the bile. In the intestine, reduction by bacteria occurs, and bilirubin is transformed into urobilinogen, mesobilirubinogen, and stercobilinogen, compounds that are collectively designated urobilinogens.

Estimation of exhaled CO, HbCO, or fecal urobilinogen can be used as a measure of hemoglobin breakdown. When production of red cells is diminished and the level of circulating hemoglobin is low, as in aplastic anemia, urobilinogen excretion is reduced. When destruction of erythrocytes is increased, as in hemolytic anemia, all three are increased in amount.

In normal humans, about 80%–90% of the excreted bile pigment measured as fecal urobilinogen is derived from breakdown of senescent erythrocytes that have lived 100–120 days. However, about 10%–20% of the pigment is excreted within the first few days. This early labeled bile pigment comes from nonhemoglobin heme formed in the liver, as well as from the breakdown of newly formed hemoglobin in the bone marrow. Much of the latter may represent hemoglobin from the pieces of cytoplasm of the orthochromatic normoblast that are lost during the process of nuclear extrusion.

In certain hematologic diseases, notably thalassemia, megaloblastic anemia, myelodysplasia, and erythropoietic porphyria, this early labeled bile pigment fraction may be markedly increased. This intramedullary destruction of hemoglobin, which never appears in circulating erythrocytes, is known as **ineffective erythropoiesis.**

ERYTHROKINETICS

The balance between delivery of erythrocytes to the blood and removal of erythrocytes from the blood results in a relatively constant hemoglobin mass in the circulation. Anemia occurs when removal of erythrocytes from the blood is increased and cannot be compensated for by increased production, or when delivery of erythrocytes to the blood is decreased, or when both processes exist together.

When anemia develops, tissue hypoxia leads to elevated levels of erythropoietin in the plasma. Resultant normoblastic hyperplasia produces more erythrocytes for delivery to the circulation. The marrow in a normal individual is capable of six to eight times the normal output of erythrocytes with extreme stimulation. This capacity must be compared with the output actually attained when one is evaluating the marrow response of a given patient.

Measurements that assess **effective erythropoiesis** (production and delivery of erythrocytes to the circulation), **ineffective erythropoiesis,** and destruction of erythrocytes may be necessary to determine the mechanism and the cause of anemia.

MEASUREMENTS OF TOTAL PRODUCTION OF ERYTHROCYTES OR HEMOGLOBIN

The **total mass of erythropoietic cells** in the body cannot be easily measured. An estimate is made by examining a sample of bone marrow from a normally active site and determining the cellularity and the percentage of total nucleated cells that are erythropoietic (see Bone Marrow Examination, Chapter 29). When marrow activity increases, usually the additional hematopoietic cells replace the fat in the red marrow sites before extension occurs into the yellow marrow of the long bones. One assumes that the sample is representative of the marrow as a whole—an assumption that usually is valid.

The **plasma iron turnover** is calculated from the serum iron level and the rate of removal of injected radioactive iron from the plasma. About 25%–30% of the iron is not used in erythropoiesis and is primarily taken up by the liver. The remaining 70%–75% is taken up by erythropoietic cells and is therefore a measure of total erythropoiesis, both effective and ineffective.

MEASUREMENTS OF TOTAL DESTRUCTION OF ERYTHROCYTES OR HEMOGLOBIN

Determination of **fecal urobilinogen** is an estimate of the total excretion of bile pigments—the breakdown products of heme. This measurement includes pigment derived from hemoglobin formed and destroyed in the marrow without ever reaching the circulating erythrocytes. Limitations include diminished conversion of bilirubin to urobilinogen caused by oral administration of broad-spectrum antibiotics, and failure of pigment to reach the intestine in obstructive jaundice.

A portion (up to 50%) of the excreted urobilinogen is reabsorbed into the portal circulation and is reexcreted into the bile, without conjugation, by the liver. Only a small amount is normally excreted in the urine. Increased urinary urobilinogen is seen with severe liver disease, as well as with conditions associated with increased heme catabolism that overwhelm the metabolic capacity of the liver. Thus, hepatocellular damage, cirrhosis, hepatic congestion due to congestive heart failure, obstructive liver disease, cholangitis, hemolytic anemia, and ineffective erythropoiesis are all associated with elevation of urinary urobilinogen.

MEASUREMENTS OF EFFECTIVE PRODUCTION OF ERYTHROCYTES

Reticulocyte Count

Because the RNA of the reticulocyte disappears about a day after its entry into the blood, enumeration of reticulocytes will be a measure of the number of cells being delivered by the marrow to the blood each day, that is, a measure of effective erythropoiesis. The absolute reticulocyte count is calculated by multiplying the reticulocyte percentage by the erythrocyte count. To give a meaningful expression of erythropoiesis, the absolute reticulocyte count, or some estimate of it, and not simply the percentage, must be used. The normal absolute reticulocyte count is approximately 50 $\times 10^9$/L, or 1% of circulating erythrocytes. Because the normal maturation time for reticulocytes in the blood is 1 day, production of reticulocytes is 50 $\times 10^9$/L/day.

A second consideration is an adjustment for increased maturation time of reticulocytes in the blood as a result of accelerated release from the marrow, an effect of erythropoietin. The need for this is recognized by the presence of large, polychromatic cells or nucleated red cells in the blood film, indicating a shift of excessively immature reticulocytes from the marrow into the blood. To avoid an overestimate of daily erythrocyte production, a correction factor is used that is based on estimated maturation time of reticulocytes in the blood. This varies inversely with hematocrit as follows (Hillman, 1996):

Hematocrit, %	Reticulocyte maturation time, days
45	1.0
35	1.5
25	2.0
15	2.5

If a patient has a Hct of 0.25, a red count of 2.89 $\times 10^{12}$/L, and a reticulocyte count of 7%, he will have an absolute reticulocyte count of 202 $\times 10^9$/L. Because the average normal absolute reticulocyte count is 50 $\times 10^9$/L, the patient has

$$(202\times10^9/\text{L})/(50\times10^9/\text{L})$$

or four times as many reticulocytes as normal. However, this must be corrected for the increased maturation time: $4 \times \frac{1}{2} = 2$. Therefore, two times as many reticulocytes are entering the blood per day as in a normal individual, that is, red cell production is two times normal.

If only the hematocrit is available, the same correction can be made as follows:

Correction for anemia:

$$\text{Patient's reticulocyte count (7\%)/Normal reticulocyte count (1\%)} \times \text{Patient's Hct (0.25)/Normal Hct (0.45)} = 4$$

Correction for shift:

$$\text{Corrected reticulocyte index (4)} \times 1/\text{Maturation time (2)} = 2$$

These corrections are necessary to assess the degree of red cell production in response to anemia.

A normal individual with a normal supply of iron can increase red cell production by two times normal within a week if the hematocrit drops to 0.35, or by three times normal if the hematocrit drops to 0.25. Only if there is a parenteral supply of iron (such as in hemolysis) can the maximal red cell production of six to eight times normal be achieved.

If an appropriate marrow response to anemia has not been reached in 1–2 weeks, some impairment of red cell production exists.

The **erythrocyte utilization of iron** is a measure of the amount of an injected dose of iron that appears in the hemoglobin of circulating erythrocytes. It is derived from the plasma iron turnover and the percentage of radioactive iron that has been injected and that appears in the circulating erythrocytes after 2 weeks, assuming that none of the newly formed cells have been destroyed in that time interval. This, too, is a measure of effective erythropoiesis.

MEASUREMENTS OF EFFECTIVE SURVIVAL OF ERYTHROCYTES IN BLOOD

The **erythrocyte survival** can be determined by removing a sample of blood, labeling the erythrocytes with chromium-51 (^{51}Cr), inactivating the excess ^{51}Cr remaining in the plasma, and reinjecting the labeled erythrocytes into the patient. The ^{51}Cr is bound to the β-chain of the hemoglobin molecule and for the most part is not released until the red cell is removed from the circulation and the hemoglobin is degraded. Measurements of radioactivity in the red cells are made at 2 hours or 24 hours (the zero time, or 100% level) and at 1- to 3-day intervals until over 50% of the activity has disappeared. The results are usually expressed as the ^{51}Cr half-survival time. The normal range is 28–38 days. (The reason it is not 60 days is that ^{51}Cr is eluted from the hemoglobin at the rate of about 1% per day.) If production of erythrocytes equals destruction (i.e., if a steady state exists), the erythrocyte survival is also a measure of effective production of erythrocytes.

SUMMARY

Total erythropoiesis refers to the total production of hemoglobin or red cells; effective erythropoiesis refers to production of hemoglobin or red cells that reach the circulation; and ineffective erythropoiesis refers to production of hemoglobin or red cells that never reach the circulating blood. These concepts of the **erythrokinetic** approach to the study of anemia are useful, especially in anemias that defy easy classification.

THE PORPHYRIAS

PHYSIOLOGY

Heme biosynthesis is an essential pathway that occurs in all metabolically active cells containing mitochondria and is most prominent in bone marrow and liver. The erythroid marrow is the major heme-forming tissue in the body, producing 85% of the daily heme requirement. Heme complexed with globin is preserved in circulating red blood cells for approximately 120 days, whereas heme produced in liver for cytochromes and enzymes is subject to much more rapid turnover, measurable in hours. A brief sequence of the heme biosynthesis pathway, with the disease states associated with specific enzyme deficiencies along the pathway, is shown in Figure 31-12.

Porphyrins are compounds composed of four pyrrole rings connected by methene bridges, differentiated by substituents found in the eight peripheral positions. The arrangement of four nitrogen atoms in the center of the porphyrin ring enables porphyrins to chelate various metal ions, such as iron, or in disease states, zinc. The biosynthetic intermediates between porphobilinogen (PBG) and protoporphyrin are not porphyrins, but rather their reduced, precursor forms: the porphyrinogens. Porphyrins that leak out of capillaries into the skin are the cause of photosensitivity, and the precursor substances have been linked to the neurovisceral manifestations. δ-Aminolevulinic acid seems to be the chief offender here (Sassa, 2006).

CLINICAL PORPHYRIAS AND THEIR BIOCHEMICAL BASIS

The porphyrias make up a group of inherited and acquired disorders of heme biosynthesis caused by a deficiency of a specific enzyme in the biosynthetic pathway, culminating in the excess production and increased excretion of precursors formed in the steps before the enzyme defect. The porphyrias can be classified by their clinical presentation, and this scheme may be a helpful starting point for the consulting pathologist, as clinicians will call with information about their patients' signs and symptoms, and then will ask for help with ordering laboratory studies (Tables 31-2 and 31-3).

Neurovisceral Symptoms in Isolation

Acute Intermittent Porphyria (AIP)

AIP is the most common acute and probably the most common inherited porphyria (Chemmanur, 2004). It is inherited in an autosomal dominant fashion with incomplete penetrance, making family studies more challenging. PBG deaminase deficiency has been demonstrated in all examined tissues, at levels of about 50% during attacks and quiescent periods. Diagnosis may be made most easily with demonstration of elevated levels of ALA and PBG in urine during acute attacks (with PBG greater in amount than ALA), but the PBG enzyme assay can be performed at any time on RBCs. Frequently, patients have urine metabolite levels at or near the

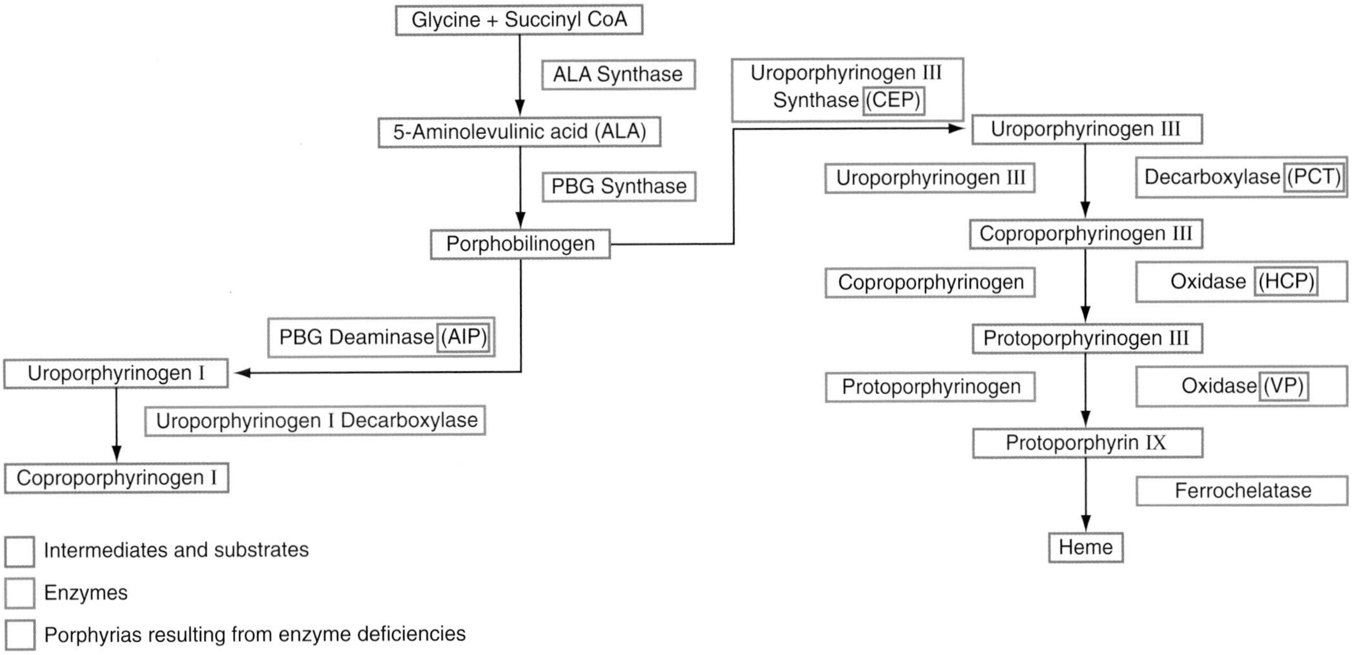

Figure 31-12 Biosynthetic pathway of heme and pathogenesis of the porphyrias.

TABLE 31-2
Key Features of the Major Porphyrias

Porphyria	Inheritance	Enzyme deficiency	Excess metabolites	Clinical features	Exacerbating factors
Acute intermittent porphyria	Autosomal dominant	PBG deaminase	PBG (U) ALA (U) Darkened urine on standing	Abdominal pain; psychiatric symptoms	Steroid hormones
Congenital erythropoietic porphyria	Autosomal recessive	Uroporphyrinogen I synthase and/or UPG III cosynthase	UP (U) CP (U) UP (E) Red, fluorescent pigment in urine	Photosensitivity; red urine, teeth; hemolysis	Sunlight
Hereditary coproporphyria	Autosomal dominant	Coproporphyrinogen oxidase	CP III (F, U) PBG (U) ALA (U) Red, fluorescent pigment in urine	Photosensitivity	Stress
Variegate porphyria	Autosomal dominant	Protoporphyrinogen oxidase	PBG (U) ALA (U) UP (U, F) CP (U, F) Red, fluorescent pigment in urine	Photosensitivity	Stress
Porphyria cutanea tarda	Autosomal dominant Acquired	Uroporphyrinogen decarboxylase	UP I (U) UP III (U) Acid induces pink fluorescence	Photosensitivity	Alcohol, hepatic injury, iron overload

ALA, Aminolevulinic acid; *CP,* coproporphyrin; *E,* erythrocyte; *F,* feces; *PBG,* porphobilinogen; *U,* urine; *UP,* uroporphyrin; *UPG,* uroporphyrinogen.

reference range during quiescent periods, although this is not always the case. Characteristically, the urine of AIP patients turns dark red upon exposure to air and light, as PBG is oxidized to a porphyrin spontaneously. It is interesting to note that the patient is often hyponatremic during acute attacks. The acute patient typically presents with colicky abdominal pain, nausea and vomiting, mental confusion, tachycardia, and, in half, a motor neuropathy (Chemmanur, 2004). Symptoms typically begin at the time of puberty, reflecting the influence of steroid hormones on the disease. Prevention is the mainstay of management, with avoidance of particular drugs (barbiturates and sulfonamides among many others), hormonal changes, and fasting. Specifically, a low-carbohydrate diet may trigger an attack. At a time when such diets are popular with the general public, clinicians may wish to caution all acute porphyria patients on the risks that these diets carry. A recent case series discussed the possible benefit of liver transplant in patients with severe AIP (Seth, 2007).

Aminolevulinic Acid Dehydratase Deficiency Porphyria (ADP)

ADP is the rarest of the porphyrias, with just six reported cases (Sassa, 2006). Clinically indistinguishable from AIP, it may be differentiated in the laboratory by the presence of excess ALA alone in the urine (Sassa suggests that it may indeed be ALA that is the chief offender causing neurovisceral symptoms) and decreased D-aminolevulinic acid dehydratase in the red blood cells of affected patients. Of note, this type of porphyria must be distinguished from tyrosinemia and heavy metal intoxication.

Neurovisceral Symptoms Plus Photosensitivity

Variegate Porphyria (VP)

Similar to AIP and HCP, VP is inherited as an autosomal dominant disorder with low penetrance. It is sometimes referred to as South African

TABLE 31-3
Test Results for the Porphyrias

Porphyria	Urine	RBC	Feces
Acute intermittent porphyria	↑ PBG, ALA	↓ PBGD activity	Noncontributory
ALA dehydratase deficiency porphyria	↑ porphyrins (ALA alone is increased) Note: Rule out organic acids and heavy metals in urine.	↓ D-aminolevulinic acid dehydratase activity	Noncontributory
Variegate porphyria	↑ porphyrins, PBG	Noncontributory	↑ coproporphyrin III/I ratio (<10)
Hereditary coproporphyria	↑ porphyrins, PBG	Noncontributory	↑ coproporphyrin III/I ratio (>10)
Porphyria cutanea tarda	↑ porphyrins	↓ UROD in Type II, UROD WNL in Types I, III	Noncontributory
Congenital erythropoietic porphyria	↑ porphyrins	↓ UPG III cosynthase	Noncontributory
Erythropoietic protoporphyria	Noncontributory	↑ free protoporphyrin	Noncontributory

ALA, Aminolevulinic acid; *PBG,* porphobilinogen; *PBGD,* porphobilinogen deaminase; *UPG,* uroporphyrinogen; *UROD,* uroporphyrinogen decarboxylase; *WNL,* within normal limits.

porphyria because of its prevalence in the Caucasian population in this region. It is called **variegate** because of the spectrum of patient presentations. Some have only the cutaneous manifestations, others just the neurovisceral, others both features. Thus, the clinician need not check both boxes to entertain this diagnosis, especially in patients of Afrikaner descent. Patients have approximately 50% activity of protoporphyrinogen oxidase. Thus, they excrete fecal protoporphyrins and coproporphyrins and urine ALA, PBG, and coproporphyrins. Induction of hepatic ALA synthase I by precipitating factors, such as barbiturates, oral contraceptives, or a low-carbohydrate diet, specifically results in increased ALA and PBG during acute attacks (Chemmanur, 2004). Cutaneous manifestations in the form of erosions or bullae following trauma to sun-exposed skin are seen at a younger age than is observed with porphyria cutanea tarda. Diagnosis is made by conventional measurements of metabolites, family history, and DNA analysis. Avoidance of triggering factors remains the major approach to patient care.

Hereditary Coproporphyria (HCP)

Also inherited in an autosomal dominant fashion with incomplete penetrance, HCP is less common than AIP. It is due to a deficiency of coproporphyrinogen oxidase. Clinically, HCP resembles a milder form of AIP with its neurovisceral attacks, but cutaneous manifestations are seen in roughly a third of patients (Chemmanur, 2004). Fecal coproporphyrinogen III is excreted both during and between attacks, and ALA and PBG are seen in urine during an acute crisis. ALA excretion usually exceeds that of PBG, and this, coupled with the cutaneous findings (if present) helps to differentiate HCP from AIP. Prevention, including sunscreen, is central to management.

Photosensitivity Plus Hemolytic Anemia

Porphyria Cutanea Tarda (PCT)

PCT is the most common of the porphyrias in the United States. Three types have been identified: I is sporadic; II and III are inherited in dominant fashion. The deficient enzyme is uroporphyrinogen decarboxylase (UROD), and researchers have postulated the presence of an inhibitor of UROD, possibly secondary to iron and metabolites of uroporphyrinogen. In Type I, only hepatic UROD is decreased; erythrocyte activity is within the reference range. In Type II, levels of both hepatic and erythrocyte UROD activity are decreased. In Type III, hepatic UROD activity is low, but family studies may aid in distinguishing this subgroup from Type I. It is interesting to note that patients with hemochromatosis are at increased risk for acquired PCT (Chemmanur, 2004). Patients present with cutaneous findings alone, and these are due to mild trauma to sun-exposed areas, not simple photosensitivity. Diagnostic laboratory findings include increased uroporphyrins with smaller increases in urine coproporphyrins. Exacerbating factors, such as alcohol, an inducer of hepatic ALA synthase I, and estrogens, should be avoided. Additional management strategies involve phlebotomy to reduce the hepatic iron load, chloroquine to complex porphyrins for urinary excretion, and the use of sunscreen (Chemmanur, 2004).

Congenital Erythropoietic Porphyria (CEP)

CEP is distinct from the other porphyrias discussed earlier in both its inheritance (it is a recessive disorder) and its severity. Patients present shortly after birth with red-pigmented urine, hemolytic anemia, and severe cutaneous photosensitivity. Erythrodontia is striking and may be a useful clue if the diagnosis has not already been made. The deficient enzyme is uroporphyrinogen III synthase, and ALA synthase activity is increased. Coproporphyrin I and uroporphyrin I are present in urine. The prognosis for CEP is significantly worse than for the other porphyrias, with death occurring at an early age in many cases.

Hepatoerythropoietic Porphyria (HEP)

HEP is a rare form of porphyria that causes hemolysis and photosensitivity. It is not discussed further in this text.

Photosensitivity in Isolation

Erythropoietic Protoporphyria (EPP)

EPP is due to a partial deficiency of the enzyme ferrochelatase, the final enzyme in the heme biosynthetic pathway. The molecular basis of this disorder is complex. Some cases are autosomal recessive, but others involve two different genetic aberrations. Clinical symptoms begin in childhood, earlier than in other porphyrias (which have their onset at puberty) and painful, itching erythema occurs within a short time (minutes) of sun exposure. Neuropsychiatric symptoms are absent, but a recent case series described a child who was sent for psychiatric care after screaming in pain when outside (Wahlin, 2006). This article makes a useful point regarding the emotional sequelae of painful skin lesions: Emotional distress follows many diseases and must be carefully distinguished from the specific, although myriad, neurovisceral symptoms that characterize other porphyrias. Uniquely among the porphyrias, EPP has a normal urine profile, and RBC testing must be performed to render a diagnosis.

ANALYTIC TECHNIQUES

Testing of urine, red blood cells, and feces for various porphyrins, which are typically increased in the porphyrias, and for specific enzymes of the heme biosynthetic pathway, which may be decreased, takes place in reference laboratories. The pathologist should select a laboratory that is well familiar with the porphyrias, and that follows a logical algorithm, so that disease, if present, can be properly classified. Neither the ordering clinician nor the general pathologist needs to attempt classification of the porphyria by selecting one or two specific assays. The algorithmic approach is the rational one and begins with a quantitative evaluation of porphyrins: PBG and ALA in the urine, and porphyrins and PBGD (porphobilinogen deaminase) measurement in the erythrocytes. Although the Watson-Schwartz test has provided an adequate screening tool for decades, it does not offer the expected sensitivity of today's medical practice and is not even available at some of the reference laboratories that conduct porphyria workups. High-performance liquid chromatography (HPLC) and fluorometry are the mainstays of analytic technique. HPLC can separate individual porphyrins; this, combined with measurement of total fecal porphyrins, reliably distinguishes between AIP and HCP (Deacon, 2001). VP may be diagnosed by measurement of fecal and urine metabolites, and also by the fluorescence emission peak of 624–627 nm, which is unique among the porphyrias (Poh-Fitzpatrick, 1980). DNA testing for specific mutations should be restricted to patients with an established diagnosis based on clinical signs and urine/RBC/feces analysis, and to kindreds. Recall that

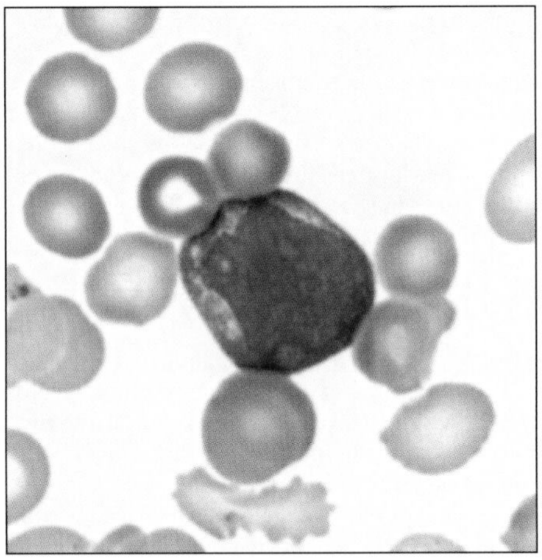

Figure 31-13 Myeloblast with high nuclear/cytoplasmic ratio, fine chromatin, visible nucleoli, and basophilic cytoplasm (Wright–Giemsa, 1000×).

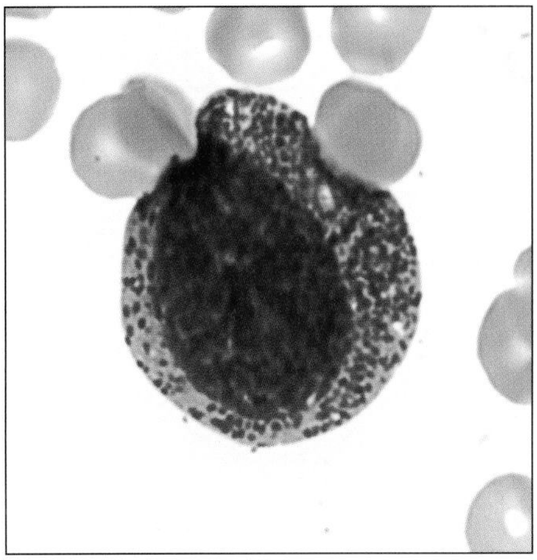

Figure 31-14 Promyelocyte *(center)* with azurophilic granules in the cytoplasm; the nuclear chromatin is still fine (Wright–Giemsa, 1000×).

the porphyrias are characterized by incomplete penetrance. Thus, a patient's signs and symptoms *may* be due to one of the porphyrias, or they may not. It is possible that the patient carries the genetic mutation but has another reason for his complaints. If the manifestations *are* due to porphyria, then urine and RBC tests will bear that out. Only then should one turn to DNA testing for the patient and his kindreds. The proper samples to submit for testing are urine (a 24-hour sample is strongly preferred, with the appropriate preservative dictated by the reference laboratory) and blood. A stool sample should be provided if VP or HCP is being considered but is less critical for the other porphyrias. Finally, testing is optimally performed during an attack to diagnose the acute porphyrias (AIP, ADP, VP, HCP). Thus, a negative test that was performed during quiescence may be repeated when the patient is again symptomatic.

NEUTROPHILS

The common progenitor cell for neutrophils and monocytes (CFU-GM) divides and gives rise to the progenitor cells for granulocytes (CFU-G) and for monocytes (CFU-M). CFU-G and CFU-M cells give rise to myeloblasts and monoblasts, respectively, under stimulation of colony-stimulating factors for granulocytes and monocytes (see Fig. 31-1).

MORPHOLOGY OF NEUTROPHIL PRECURSORS

The **myeloblast** (Fig. 31-13) is a cell about 15 μm in diameter with a moderately high N/C ratio; a large oval to quadrangular nucleus; a very fine, uniform chromatin pattern; a delicate nuclear membrane; and two to five nucleoli. The cytoplasm is pale, clear blue, and without granules. The appearance of azurophilic (primary) granules (≈0.5-μm diameter) heralds the earliest promyelocyte (Fig. 31-14) and indicates that the cell is to be a neutrophil. The **promyelocyte** stage encompasses the entire period of production of azurophilic granules. The promyelocyte is slightly larger than the myeloblast. The nuclear chromatin begins to condense, and the nucleoli are less obvious. The cytoplasm is basophilic and is filled by more and more azurophilic granules. The **neutrophil myelocyte** stage begins with the appearance of specific neutrophil (secondary) granules, at first only in the Golgi region; as more specific granules develop, they spread throughout the cytoplasm (Fig. 31-15). With successive mitoses, the number of azurophilic granules (whose production has ceased at the end of the promyelocyte stage) is diminished. The early neutrophil myelocyte, therefore, has a rather fine, dispersed nuclear chromatin pattern, many azurophilic granules, and few specific granules. The late neutrophil myelocyte has a somewhat more condensed chromatin pattern, a cytoplasm well filled with specific granules, and rather few azurophilic granules. The myelocyte is the latest stage capable of cell division. The next stage, the **neutrophil metamyelocyte,** is distinguished by an indented, kidney-shaped nucleus with more condensed chromatin (Fig. 31-16). From this stage on, changes in the cytoplasm are insignificant. In the **band neutrophil** (stab form), the nucleus has more condensed chromatin and a rather uniform elongated shape (Fig. 31-17). Partial constriction of the nucleus

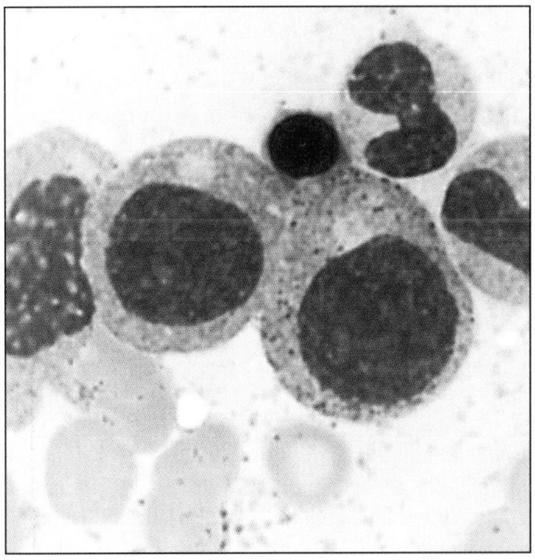

Figure 31-15 Myelocytes have secondary granules in the cytoplasm and show condensation of nuclear chromatin. Persistent primary granules are seen in early myelocytes *(center-right)* and are lost as myelocytes mature. A band neutrophil and an orthochromatic normoblast are also seen (Wright–Giemsa, 1000×).

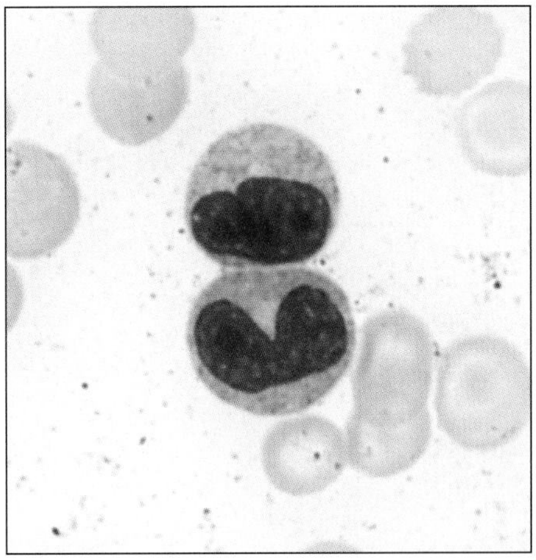

Figure 31-16 Metamyelocytes show nuclear indentation and increased chromatin clumping (Wright–Giemsa, 1000×).

occurs in the band stage, until a fine filament (length but no breadth) is formed between two of the lobes, at which point the cell is classified as a **segmented neutrophil** (Fig. 31-18).

During development and maturation, neutrophilic precursors express various cell surface markers that can be used for immunophenotypic recognition. Myeloblasts express the HSC marker CD34, as well as HLA-DR

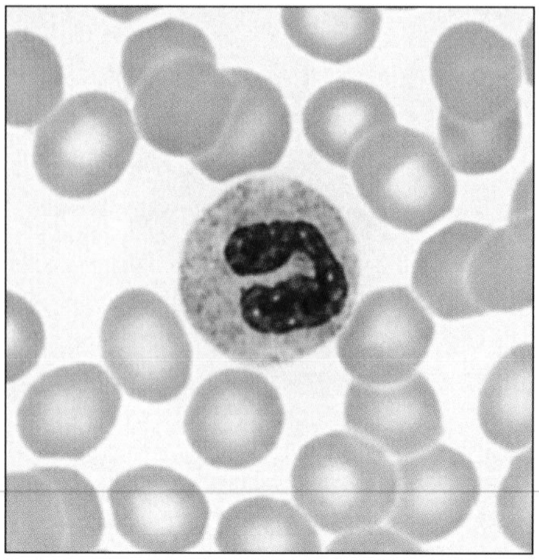

Figure 31-17 Band neutrophil with mature nucleus with clumped chromatin but without segmentation (Wright–Giemsa, 1000×).

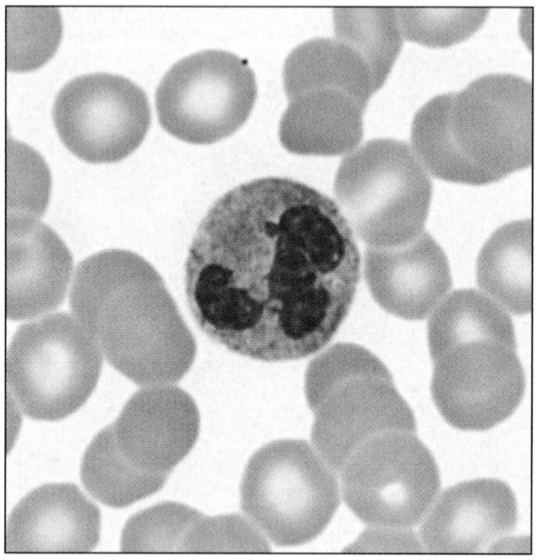

Figure 31-18 Segmented neutrophil with multiple nuclear lobes joined by fine chromatin filaments (Wright–Giemsa, 1000×).

TABLE 31-4
Neutrophil Constituents and Functions

Azurophilic granules (formed in promyelocyte stage)
Lysosomal enzymes: acid hydrolases, acid phosphatase, β-glucuronidase
Myeloperoxidase
Elastase
Arylsulfatase
Cationic antibacterial proteins
Specific granules (formed in myelocyte stage)
Lysozyme
Lactoferrin
Collagenase
Plasminogen activator
Aminopeptidase
Tertiary granules
Gelatinase
Cytoplasmic organelles
Alkaline phosphatase
Neutrophil functions
Phagocytosis
Bactericidal activity

and myeloid lineage specific markers CD13, CD33, CD15, and CD117. Mature neutrophils express CD13, CD15, CD16, and CD11b, but lose HLA-DR and CD33.

The mature human neutrophil has twice as many specific granules as azurophilic granules (Table 31-4). The azurophilic granules (formed in the promyelocyte stage) contain lysosomal enzymes (e.g., acid hydrolases: acid phosphatase, β-glucuronidase), myeloperoxidase, elastase, arylsulfatase, and cationic antibacterial proteins, along with other enzymes and proteins. The specific granules (formed in the myelocyte stage) contain lysozyme, lactoferrin, collagenase, plasminogen activator, aminopeptidase, and vitamin B_{12}–binding protein, as well as other enzymes and proteins. Tertiary granules, similar in size to the specific granules, contain gelatinase. Alkaline phosphatase is located in yet another type of cytoplasmic organelle lighter in density than specific granules. These organelles first appear during the late myelocyte stage.

DISTRIBUTION AND KINETICS

For each neutrophil in the blood vessels, about 16 precursors are present in the marrow. From the time of differentiation into a myeloblast, through about five mitotic divisions (three of which occur at the myelocyte stage), it takes about 14 days until the progeny of that cell reach the blood. The last 6–7 days are spent in the maturation and storage pool. When a neutrophil enters the blood, it moves readily between a circulating granulocyte pool, which is sampled in the leukocyte count, and a marginal granulocyte pool, which is not, but is either marginated along vessel walls or sequestered in capillary beds. In less than a day after it arrives, the neutrophil emigrates from the circulation in a random manner and enters the tissues. Migration into tissues is dependent on adhesion molecules of the selectin family (and their corresponding ligands) expressed on neutrophils and endothelial cells. From there, if not utilized in an inflammatory exudate, neutrophils leave the body within a few days via secretions in bronchi, saliva, gastrointestinal tract, and urine, or they are destroyed by the mononuclear phagocyte system.

FUNCTION

Neutrophils are able to move in a zigzag manner, but their motion changes to a straight line path if a chemotactic attractant or factor (e.g., a bacterium coated with certain components of complement) is within a certain distance. Neutrophils express chemokine receptors CXCR1 and CXCR2, which are responsible for neutrophil migration in response to chemokines. Neutrophils also have receptors for the Fc portion of IgG, as well as for complement (C3) and bind and phagocytose the coated particle. Phagocytosis occurs with the formation of a phagocytic vacuole that contains the ingested particle; accompanying this process is an increase in metabolic activity and energy production. Specific granules, followed shortly by azurophilic granules, empty their contents into the phagocytic vacuoles—a process known as degranulation. Bactericidal activity occurs within the vacuole, mediated by H_2O_2, superoxide anion (O_2^-), myeloperoxidase, and a halide ion generating free halogen, or by other enzymatic activity. Other substances can act as chemotactic factors too. The C5a fragment is a chemotactic factor and is also an anaphylatoxin that causes smooth muscle contraction. Substances liberated by bacteria and metabolic products of arachidonic acid may also act as chemotactic factors for neutrophils. Neutrophils are thus important in defense against infectious disease. If their enzymes are activated and released outside the cell, neutrophils can cause tissue necrosis, tissue injury, and inflammation.

EOSINOPHILS

Eosinophils are produced in the bone marrow. In vitro culture studies show that there is a separate eosinophilic committed progenitor cell (CFU-Eo) in the marrow that is distinct from CFU-GM, CFU-G, and CFU-M. Three growth factors (GM-CSF, IL-3, IL-5) produced by T lymphocytes influence eosinophil development. IL-5 promotes terminal maturation, functional activation, and prevention of apoptosis of eosinophils.

MORPHOLOGY OF EOSINOPHIL PRECURSORS

The cell that is the precursor for the earliest recognizable eosinophil, the eosinophil myelocyte, is presumably a distinctive myeloblast. However, it is morphologically indistinguishable from that which gives rise to neutrophils and monocytes or to basophils (see Figs. 31-1 and 31-13). In the early eosinophil myelocyte, the granules are large and take the basophilic stain. As the cell matures, the granules appear olive-green, and finally the characteristic red-orange color (Figs. 31-19 and 31-20). Nuclear maturation is similar to that of the neutrophil. Eosinophils are slightly larger than neutrophils and have fewer nuclear lobes. Mature eosinophils express CD16 and CD32.

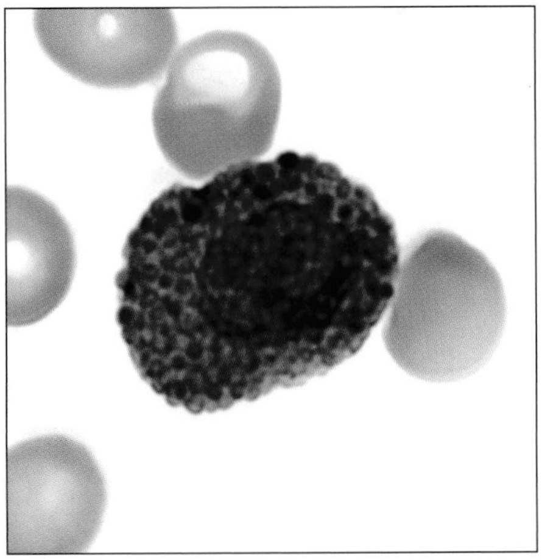

Figure 31-19 Eosinophil myelocyte with ovoid nucleus and eosinophilic secondary granules in the cytoplasm (Wright–Giemsa, 1000×).

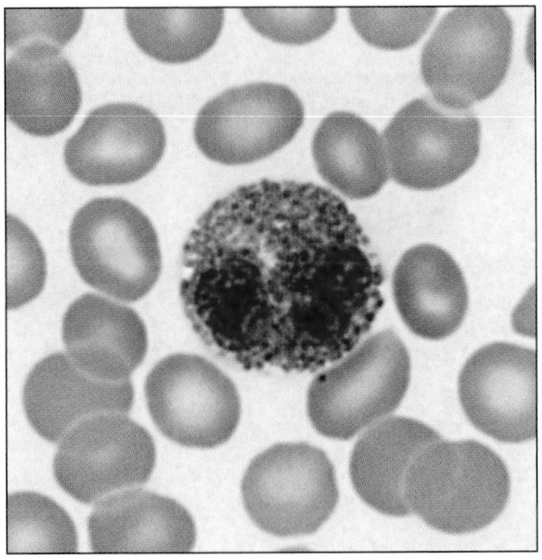

Figure 31-20 Mature eosinophil with bilobed nucleus and large eosinophilic cytoplasmic granules (Wright–Giemsa, 1000×).

Electron micrographs of eosinophils show characteristic granules that have a dense crystalloid core in a less dense matrix. Immature granules, appearing in the myelocyte, at first have no crystalloids but develop them as maturation proceeds. Mature granules are of two types: a larger granule (0.5–1.5 µm in largest diameter) with a dense crystalloid, and a smaller granule (0.1–0.5 µm diameter) without a crystalloid. The smaller granules appear later during maturation, after the myelocyte stage.

Eosinophil-specific granules (Table 31-5) contain major basic protein (MBP) in the crystalloid core; MBP is toxic to parasites and cells, neutralizes heparin, and induces histamine release from basophils. Granule constituents in the matrix include acid hydrolases, peroxidase, phospholipase, and cathepsin. The specific granules also contain eosinophil cationic protein (ECP), eosinophil-derived neurotoxin (EDN), and eosinophil peroxidase (EPO). ECP shortens coagulation time and alters fibrinolysis; it also inhibits lymphocyte proliferation and is a potent neurotoxin. EDN is a strong neurotoxin (Gleich, 1986). The smaller granules contain arylsulfatase; both granule types contain peroxidase and acid phosphatase. Eosinophil peroxidase is different from the type of peroxidase present in neutrophils and monocytes; also, eosinophils contain no alkaline phosphatase or muramidase. Eosinophils secrete IL-1, IL-3, IL-6, IL-8, TNF-α, and GM-CSF. TNF-α appears to be the cause of fibrosis in Hodgkin's disease (Roberts, 1999).

DISTRIBUTION AND KINETICS

The kinetics of eosinophils are similar to those of neutrophils. They are stored in the bone marrow for several days after going through various maturational stages. The half-life in the blood is approximately 18 hours before entering the tissues, where they survive for at least 6 days. Eosinophils in the tissues, however, are at least 100 times as numerous as the total number of eosinophils in the blood; they are located primarily in skin, lung, and gastrointestinal tract (i.e., the epithelial barriers to the outside world).

TABLE 31-5
Eosinophil Constituents and Functions

Eosinophil-specific granules
Larger granules
Major basic protein
Acid hydrolases
Peroxidase
Phospholipase
Cathepsin
Eosinophil cationic protein
Eosinophil-derived neurotoxin
Smaller granules
Arylsulfatase
Peroxidase
Acid phosphatase
Eosinophil functions
Anthelmintic activity—major basic protein, eosinophilic cationic protein, peroxidase
Phagocytosis
Allergic response
Dampen inflammatory reactions

FUNCTION

Eosinophils act as phagocytes and modulate inflammatory responses (see Table 31-5). Eosinophils leave the blood when adrenal corticosteroid hormones increase. They proliferate in response to immunologic stimuli, and this proliferative response is mediated, at least with some antigens, by T lymphocytes, monocytes, and mast cells. Eosinophils destroy helminths by generating potent oxidants and releasing cationic proteins. Eosinophils participate in some inflammatory conditions, particularly allergic reactions, asthma, and certain myocardial diseases (Gleich, 1986). Although eosinophils phagocytose foreign particles and antigen–antibody complexes, this is not their only activity. Another major function of eosinophils is to dampen hypersensitivity and inflammatory reactions. Evidence indicates that eosinophils modulate reactions that occur when tissue mast cells and basophils degranulate. Eosinophils express the chemokine receptor CCR3. Among the chemotactic factors that attract eosinophils, eosinophil chemotactic factor of anaphylaxis (ECF-A) is present in basophils and mast cells; also, eosinophils contain substances that inactivate factors released by mast cells and basophils, such as histamine, slow-reacting substances of anaphylaxis, and platelet-activating factor (PAF).

When an intense or prolonged eosinophilic inflammatory reaction occurs, there is often the formation of Charcot-Leyden crystals. These hexagonal bipyramidal crystals are composed of lysophospholipase localized in the cytoplasm of eosinophils (Jandl, 1996).

BASOPHILS AND MAST CELLS

Basophils and mast cells are derived from hematopoietic precursors and probably share a common precursor with other granulocytes and monocytes.

MORPHOLOGY

Basophils develop from a cell resembling a myeloblast. The first recognizable stage is a **basophil myelocyte,** with the appearance of specific basophil granules. These granules (about 0.2–1 µm in diameter) are larger than the azurophilic granules of the promyelocyte and often are irregular in shape. As the cell matures, the granules become more metachromatic (red-purple) because of increasing acid mucopolysaccharide (heparin) content. During maturation, cytoplasmic RNA decreases, and the nucleus partially segments. Because of incomplete nuclear segmentation, stages analogous to the neutrophil are not readily identified. In mature basophils, the nucleus has condensed but smudged chromatin, and the background cytoplasm lacks basophilia (residual RNA) (Fig. 31-21). Mature basophils express CD32.

In contrast, **tissue mast cells** are connective tissue cells of mesenchymal origin that contain metachromatic cytoplasmic granules. They are

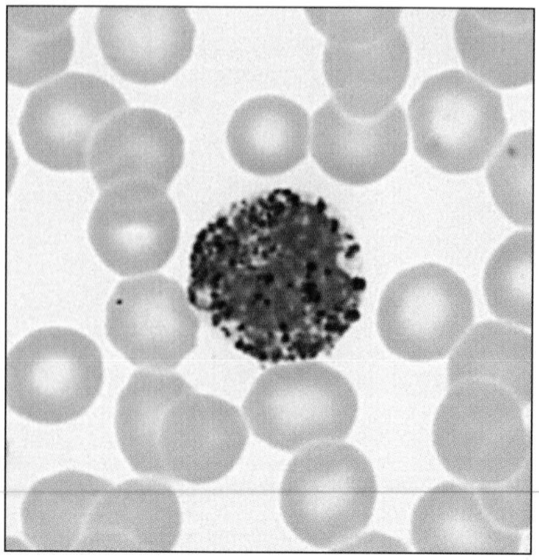

Figure 31-21 Mature basophil with large dark red-purple basophilic granules that partially obscure the nucleus (Wright–Giemsa, 1000×).

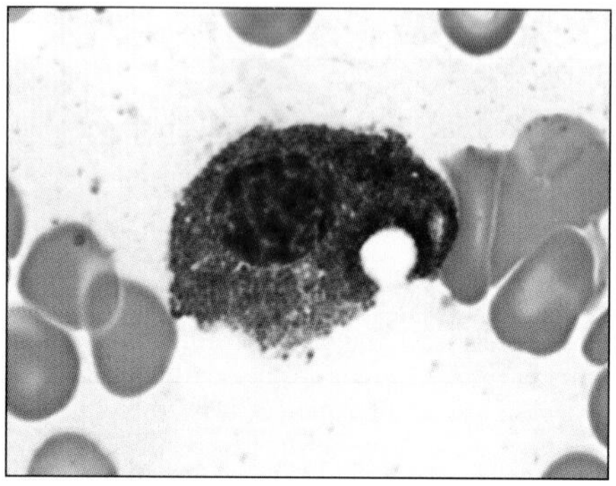

Figure 31-22 Bone marrow mast cell shows numerous uniform purple granules in the cytoplasm that partially obscure the nucleus (Wright–Giemsa, 1000×).

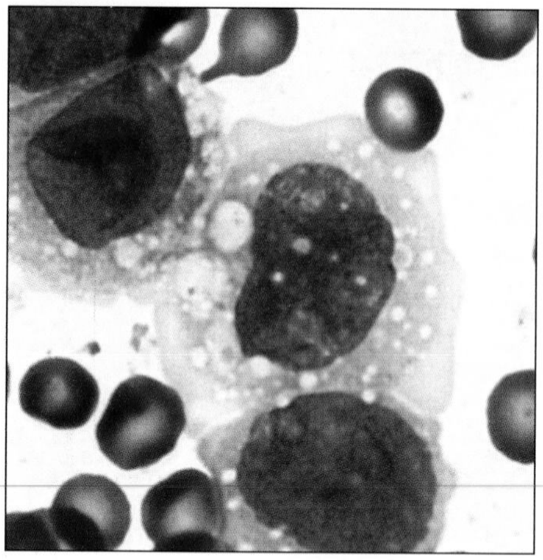

Figure 31-23 Promonocytes have fine nuclear chromatin, often with visible folds and basophilic cytoplasm that may contain vacuoles (Wright–Giemsa, 1000×).

TABLE 31-6
Basophil Constituents and Functions

Basophil-specific granules
Histamine
Heparin
Peroxidase
Eosinophilic chemotactic factor A
Other cellular constituents
Slow-reacting substance of anaphylaxis
Platelet-activating factor
Basophil functions
Immediate hypersensitivity reactions
Some delayed hypersensitivity reactions

widely distributed throughout the body, including bone marrow, thymus, and spleen, but they do not normally appear in blood. On Romanowsky-stained films (Fig. 31-22), they are usually larger than basophils and have a low N/C ratio and a round or oval reticular nucleus that is usually obscured by abundant red-purple granules. The granules are smaller, more round and regular, and less soluble than basophil granules. The cytoplasmic granules are often spindle-shaped rather than round.

DISTRIBUTION AND KINETICS

Basophils have a life span similar to eosinophils. The maturation time in the marrow is approximately 7 days. Basophils circulate in the blood and are not normally found in tissues, in contrast to mast cells, which can spend 9–18 months in connective tissue (Jandl, 1996). GM-CSF, IL-3, and IL-5 influence basophil production. However, IL-3 is the principal growth factor for basophilic growth, whereas *c-kit* ligand enhances the number and activation state of mast cells (Lyman, 1998).

FUNCTION

With regard to circulating numbers, basophils respond to adrenal corticosteroids in similar fashion to eosinophils. Basophil granules contain histamine, heparin, and peroxidase (Table 31-6). Basophils synthesize and store histamine and ECF-A. They synthesize and release slow-reacting substance of anaphylaxis (SRS-A) and probably PAF at the time of stimulation but do not store them. Basophils lack hydrolytic enzymes such as alkaline and acid phosphatase, at least in cytochemically demonstrable amounts. Glycogen is abundant outside the granules. Although ultrastructurally different, mast cells have similar cytochemical characteristics, except for the presence of proteolytic enzymes and serotonin, which basophils lack. In tissues, the two cell types appear to function in a similar manner.

Basophils (as well as mast cells) appear to be involved in immediate hypersensitivity reactions, such as allergic asthma. IgE binds readily to basophil and mast cell membranes. When a specific antigen reacts with the membrane-bound IgE, degranulation occurs with the release of mediators of immediate hypersensitivity (e.g., histamine, SRS-A, PAF, heparin, ECF-A). The latter leads to the accumulation of eosinophils, which contain substances that tend to counteract these mediators. Basophils are also involved in some delayed hypersensitivity reactions, or **cutaneous basophil hypersensitivity,** such as contact allergies, in which they appear to undergo a different type of degranulation response.

MONOCYTES AND MACROPHAGES

Monocytes share the same committed progenitor cell as neutrophils, the CFU-GM (see Fig. 31-1).

MORPHOLOGY

In normal marrow, it is not possible morphologically to distinguish the "monoblast" from the myeloblast. The earliest recognizable cell in this series is the **promonocyte,** which is 15–20 μm in diameter—somewhat larger than the myeloblast. The N/C ratio is moderate, and the nucleus may be oval or indented with a fine uniform or slightly streaked chromatin pattern and two to five nucleoli. The cytoplasm is basophilic with a ground-glass appearance and a variable number of fine azurophilic granules (Fig. 31-23). The **monocyte,** which is present in both blood and marrow, is only slightly smaller; it has a moderate to low N/C ratio and an indented or lobed nucleus with a finely-streaked, only slightly condensed, delicate chromatin pattern. Nucleoli are indistinct or obscured. The cytoplasm is opaque, more gray than blue, and contains an abundance of fine azurophilic granules (Fig. 31-24).

Macrophages, the tissue component of the monocyte system, arise from emigrated blood monocytes. Macrophages are larger than monocytes and measure 15–80 μm in diameter. They have irregular cell membranes, often with blebs and pseudopodia. The N/C ratio is high with an oblong and/or indented nucleus. Although macrophages are located in virtually all tissues of the body, the greatest numbers are found in the bowel, liver, bone marrow, and spleen.

In promonocytes, monocytes, and macrophages, the granules (Table 31-7) contain acid hydrolase, arylsulfatase, nonspecific esterase, and

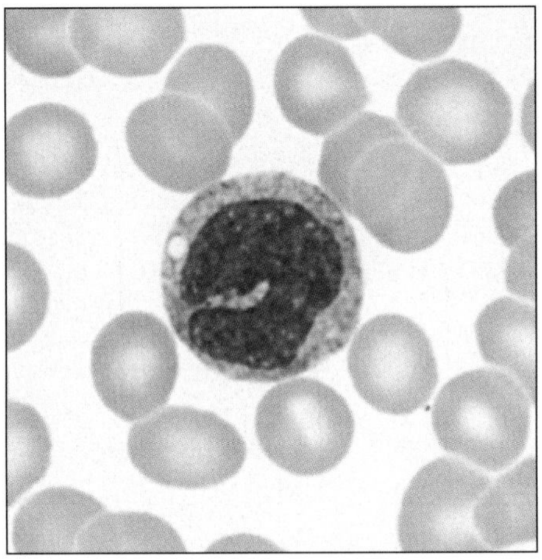

Figure 31-24 Mature monocyte with an indented nucleus, delicate chromatin, basophilic cytoplasm, and fine azurophilic granules (Wright–Giemsa, 1000×).

TABLE 31-7
Monocyte/Macrophage Constituents and Functions

Granules and other constituents
Acid hydrolase
Arylsulfatase
Nonspecific esterase
Peroxidase
Acid phosphatase
Monocyte/macrophage functions
Phagocytosis—bacteria, cellular debris, senescent cells
Antigen processing
Cell-mediated immunity—antibody-dependent cellular cytotoxicity
Synthesis of bioactive molecules

peroxidase. More than one type of granule may be present. As the cell matures, peroxidase activity diminishes, and acid phosphatase, arylsulfatase, and nonspecific esterase activity increases. The enzyme activity occurs in the rough endoplasmic reticulum, Golgi zone, coated vesicles, and digestive vacuoles, suggesting that in the macrophages the coated vesicles are a second form of primary lysosome that shuttles hydrolytic enzymes from the Golgi to the digestive vacuoles.

In addition to these enzymes, monocytes and macrophages possess numerous surface receptors and surface antigens. Monocytes and macrophages possess class I (HLA-A, B, C) antigens and class II (HLA-DR, DP, DQ) gene complex molecules. The CD4 T cell antigen (molecule) not only is present on T-helper cells but is also present on monocytes and macrophages. Because the CD4 molecule acts as a receptor for the human immunodeficiency virus type-1 (HIV-1), the virus infects monocytes and macrophages along with T-helper cells. Monocytes and macrophages express CD11 (CD11a, b, c) antigens, markers that define surface adhesion glycoproteins. CD14, CD64, and CD68 antigens are also present on monocytes and macrophages. These surface molecules are often used to identify the lineage of mononuclear cells in hematologic malignancies.

DISTRIBUTION AND KINETICS

After promonocytes are formed, they respond to M-CSF and undergo two or three mitotic divisions in a period of about 50–60 hours before being released into the blood. Under conditions of increased demand, the cycle time can shorten, with earlier release of more immature cells into the blood. Blood monocytes are distributed in a circulating monocyte pool and a marginal monocyte pool, in a ratio of 1:3.5. Once monocytes enter the blood, they leave randomly with a half-time of 8.4 hours; this time period is shortened in splenomegaly or acute infection and may be prolonged in monocytosis. After monocytes leave the blood, they spend several months, perhaps longer, as tissue macrophages.

FUNCTION

The monocyte is formed in the marrow and transported by the blood; it migrates into the tissues, where it transforms into a histiocyte or a macrophage to spend most of its life span. Blood monocytes and tissue macrophages make up a mononuclear phagocyte system (reticuloendothelial system).

The mononuclear phagocyte system has an important role in defense against microorganisms, including mycobacteria, fungi, bacteria, protozoa, and viruses (see Table 31-7). The cells are motile and respond to chemotactic factors (complement components, as well as lymphokines and γ-interferon from activated T lymphocytes); they become immobilized by migration-inhibition factor from activated lymphocytes. They engage in phagocytosis, a process that is enhanced if the particle is coated by IgG or complement for which the macrophages have membrane receptors. After phagocytosis, they kill ingested microorganisms.

These mononuclear phagocytes are an integral part of both humoral and cell-mediated immunity. They handle or process antigens, providing contact of the antigen (or antigenic information) with lymphocytes. They also respond to various lymphokines and monokines and act as effector (e.g., cytotoxic) cells in the cell-mediated immune response. Monocytes and macrophages function in antibody-dependent cellular cytotoxicity. They have the ability to kill a variety of malignant cells (Weinberg, 2004) by promoting both cytostasis and cytolysis. Some of the ability of macrophages to destroy malignant cells may be attributed to the production of hydrogen peroxide (H_2O_2), nitrous oxide (NO), and reactive oxygen intermediates.

Macrophages remove and process senescent cells and debris through phagocytosis and digestion, for example, erythrocytes, leukocytes, and megakaryocyte nuclei are removed by macrophages in the marrow; inhaled particulate material is removed by alveolar macrophages in the lungs.

Macrophages may be activated by specific factors (e.g., cytophilic antibody) or nonspecific factors (e.g., in response to phagocytosed material). Activation results in enlargement of the cell and enhanced metabolism, phagocytosis, microbicidal activity, cytotoxicity, secretion of cytolytic proteins (including TNF-α), and the like.

Macrophages synthesize and secrete a large number of biologically active molecules, including enzymes, complement components, binding proteins, coagulation factors, cytokines and growth factors, chemotactic factors, angiogenesis factors, and bioactive lipids. This system, therefore, has multiple functions that include host defense, control of hematopoiesis, and policing of the environment within the body (Johnston, 1988).

MEGAKARYOCYTES

Platelets originate from polyploid megakaryocytes, the largest of all hematopoietic cells, which account for less than 1% of the total nucleated marrow cells. Megakaryocytes arise from the multipotential hematopoietic stem cell, and then from a committed progenitor cell, the CFU-Meg (see Fig. 31-1). Megakaryocyte proliferation is largely regulated by thrombopoietin. Additional growth factors, including kit-ligand, IL-3, IL-6, and IL-11, support megakaryocytic development in the presence of thrombopoietin (Kaushansky, 1995). Serum thrombopoietin levels are generally inversely proportional to platelet count; however, levels are elevated in liver disease and inflammatory states, probably through hepatocyte or marrow stromal cell responses (Kaushansky, 2003).

MORPHOLOGY

Committed progenitor cells are not morphologically distinguishable from lymphocytes. Megakaryocyte development is characterized by **endomitosis,** nuclear division without cytoplasmic division, which results in ploidies varying from 2N to 64N. Most are 8N and 16N, with smaller numbers on either side. Nuclear lobes do not correlate precisely with ploidy. Nuclear chromatin is intensely staining, rather dispersed early, more compact and dense later. Nucleoli are small at all stages of megakaryocyte development.

The earliest recognizable **megakaryoblast** has overlapping nuclear lobes and a small amount of basophilic cytoplasm. During the course of maturation, nuclear lobes increase and spread out, and red-pink granules become visible, first in the center of the cell. In the **mature megakaryocyte,** the nucleus is more compact, basophilia has disappeared, and the granules are clustered into small aggregates (Fig. 31-25).

The formation of individual platelets is a complex process. Megakaryocytes develop invaginated surface membranes (demarcation membranes) that provide a membrane reserve for proplatelet formation (Italiano, 2003). Proplatelets are pseudopodial extensions of megakaryocytes that progressively branch and thin out. Microtubular action is important in the formation of proplatelets and in bringing granule and organelle constituents into

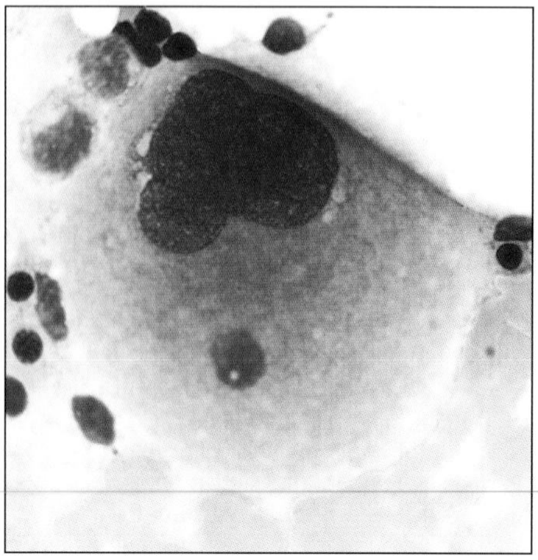

Figure 31-25 Megakaryocyte with a large, lobated nucleus and abundant granular cytoplasm (Wright–Giemsa, 1000×).

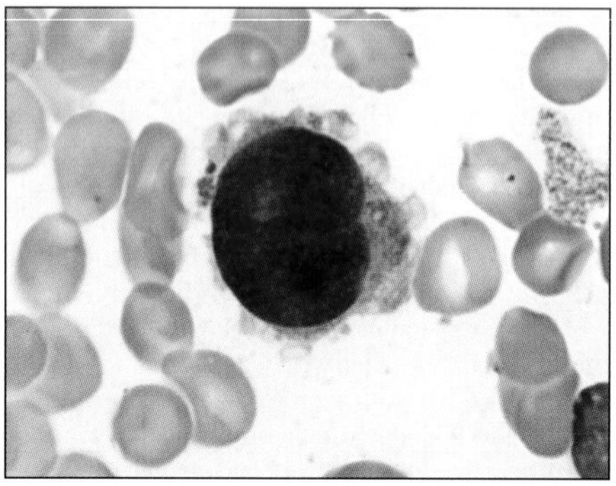

Figure 31-26 Dwarf megakaryocyte with bilobed nucleus and scant granular cytoplasm; a few giant platelets are also seen. These cells are most often associated with myeloproliferative neoplasms or myelodysplastic syndromes (Wright–Giemsa, 1000×).

the proplatelets. Platelets are formed at the ends of proplatelets and are released by microtubular action (Hartwig, 2003).

MEGAKARYOCYTES IN BLOOD

Whole megakaryocytes or fragments may occasionally be found in normal blood films. If buffy coat films are examined, they are consistently present. Megakaryocyte fragments in blood films may be as small as lymphocytes and are recognized by the deeply stained chromatin (with a sharper chromatin–parachromatin separation than in lymphocyte nuclei) and by fragments of attached megakaryocyte cytoplasm. They are found more frequently than normal in myelophthisic processes and myeloproliferative neoplasms, or after stress or injury to the marrow.

Dwarf or micromegakaryocytes (Fig. 31-26) show evidence of abnormal megakaryopoiesis: agranular cytoplasm with hyaloplasmic zones or pseudopods, and association with large atypical platelets having similar cytoplasmic characteristics. These abnormal dwarf megakaryocytes are rarely found in any condition except myeloproliferative neoplasms or myelodysplastic syndromes.

DISTRIBUTION AND KINETICS

The maturation time for megakaryocytes in the marrow is about 5 days in humans. Platelets are released into the marrow sinuses over a period of several hours (Hartwig, 2003), and the megakaryocyte nuclei are phagocytosed by macrophages. Newly released platelets appear larger, more active metabolically, and more effective hemostatically. Platelets circulate at a stable concentration that averages 275×10^9/L. At any one time, about two thirds of the total platelets are in the circulation, and the remaining third are present in the spleen. In asplenic individuals, all platelets are circulating. In diseases characterized by splenic enlargement, 80%–90% of platelets may be sequestered in the spleen, resulting in decreased concentrations of circulating platelets (thrombocytopenia).

Platelets survive for 8–11 days in the circulation. Some platelets are utilized in maintaining vascular integrity and in plugging small vascular injuries (random loss); others are removed by the mononuclear phagocytic system when they become senescent.

TABLE 31-8
Key Cell Surface Markers in Lymphocyte Development

Cell name	CD markers
Progenitor B cell	CD19, TdT, CD79a, HLA-DR
Pre-B cell	CD19, TdT, CD10, CD20, cytoplasmic μ
Naive mature B cell	CD19, CD20, Bcl-2, surface IgM
Centroblasts	CD19, CD20, CD10, Bcl-6
Mature B cells (peripheral blood)	CD19, CD20, CD21, CD22, CD24, CD38
Plasma cells	CD38, CD138, cytoplasmic Ig

FUNCTION

Platelets normally function in (1) maintaining the integrity of blood vessels, and (2) forming hemostatic plugs to stop blood loss from injured vessels and, in the process, promoting coagulation of plasma factors.

LYMPHOCYTES

PRIMARY LYMPHOID TISSUE

During fetal life, lymphocyte precursors originate in the bone marrow and undergo antigen-independent lineage commitment. Maturation and selection of T cells occur primarily in the thymus, and of B cells, in the marrow and peripheral lymphoid organs. The T cell population is largely self-renewable following thymic involution. B cells are capable of only limited self-renewal. They are dependent on recruitment from marrow stem cells to replenish programmed B cells and plasma cells that are incapable of self-renewal (Jandl, 1996). NK cells are derived from CD34+ HSCs, but details of development and maturation are not completely understood.

B Cell Development: Bone Marrow (Table 31-8)

A distinct organ, the bursa of Fabricius, is present in birds and serves as the primary site of B cell development. In the human, B cells develop in the bone marrow after the hematopoietic stem cells have populated that organ. During adult life, generation of B cells occurs in the bone marrow.

B cell differentiation can be divided conveniently into two stages. The initial stage of B cell differentiation involves the antigen-independent generation of diversity through rearrangement of the Ig heavy and light chain genes. The second stage is regulated by antigen triggering, T cell interaction, macrophages, and various growth factors (Fig. 31-27). This stage occurs predominantly in the secondary lymphoid organs (LeBien, 2008).

A progenitor cell gives rise to the first recognizable B cell in man and mammals. This cell in humans is the pro-B (progenitor) cell that is characterized by receptor CD19 and terminal deoxynucleotidyl transferase (TdT) but contains no cytoplasmic or surface bound Ig (Hagman, 1994). Differentiation of pro-B cells requires Ig gene rearrangement. The pre-B cell is characterized by the presence of intracytoplasmic μ heavy chains with no surface-bound immunoglobulin ($sIg^-c\mu^+$). It also contains HLA-DR antigens, CD19, CD79a, and other surface markers. Humoral proteins influence pre-B cell differentiation.

In becoming a pre-B cell, a lymphoid stem cell undergoes *DJ* and *VDJ* gene segment rearrangement to form a functional *V* gene for the μ heavy chain (Fig. 31-28). A productive heavy chain gene rearrangement is then followed by a rearrangement of the *VJ* gene segment of the light chain. Rearrangement of the κ light chain gene on chromosome 2 occurs first. If the κ rearrangements at both loci are nonproductive, rearrangement of the λ light chain gene on chromosome 22 follows. The controls exerted during pre-B cell development allow only one productive *VH* and *VL* gene to emerge, limiting each B cell to one unique antibody structure (Bertoli, 1988). The combination of the μ heavy chain and the κ or λ light chain allows the pre-B cell to generate an intact Ig molecule and express surface IgM. Isotype switching (changing from IgM/IgD to IgG1, etc.) and constant heavy gene deletions occur in pre-B cells and more differentiated B cells. The switching of μ cells to γ1 or α2 cells occurs by the formation of a DNA loop in which all intervening constant heavy genes are deleted (Fig. 31-29). IgD can be coexpressed with IgM through alternative RNA processing.

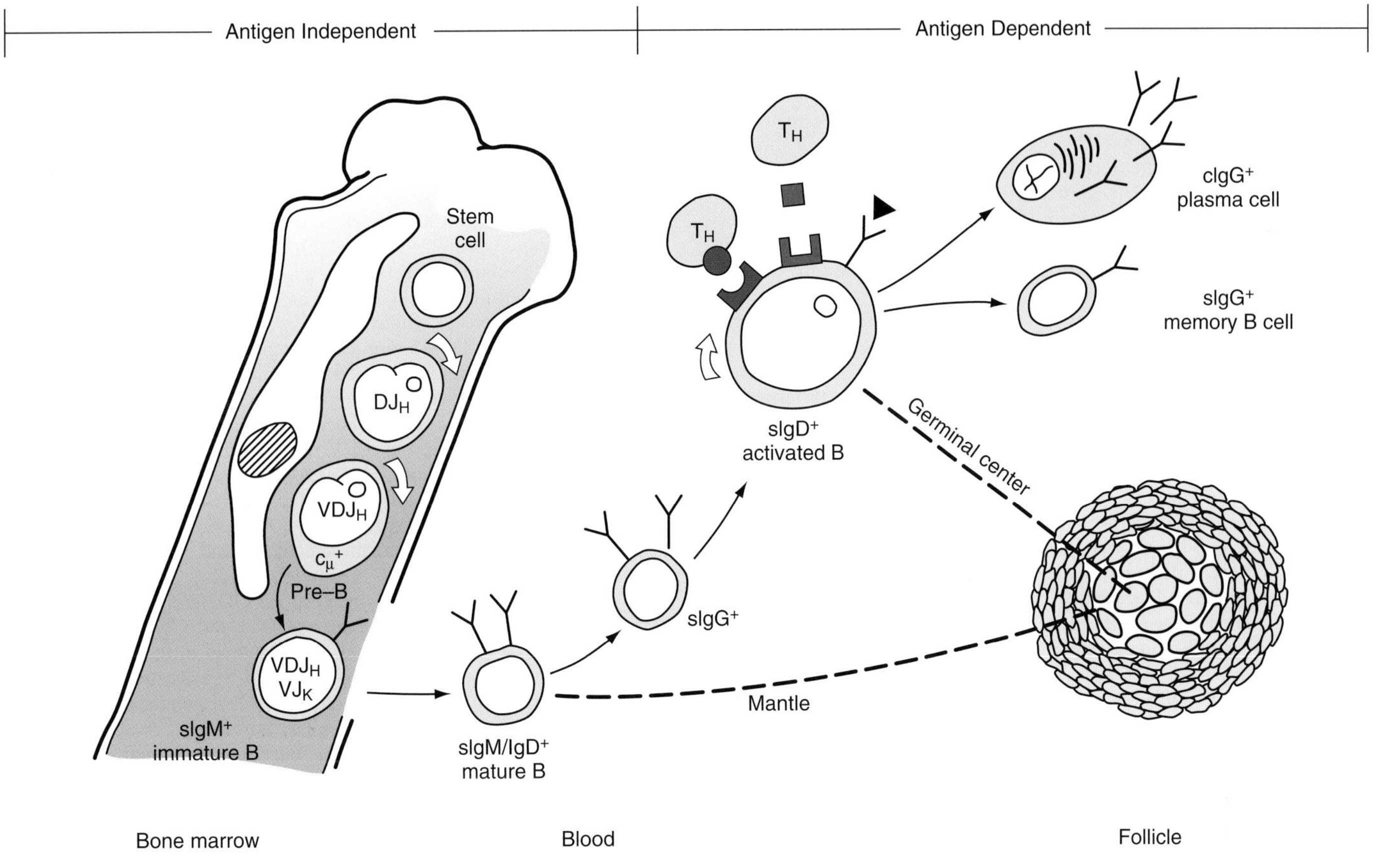

Figure 31-27 Differentiation of pre-B cells into B cells occurs independently of antigen, whereas proliferation and terminal differentiation of B cells are antigen driven. Hematopoietic stem cells with stromal cell help give rise to pre-B cells. These proliferate *(open arrow denotes cell cycling),* rearrange *DJ* and *VDJ* gene segments, then express μ chains in the cytoplasm ($c\mu^+$). A small, resting pre-B cell *(not shown)* with rearranged *VJk* gene assembles a complete IgMk molecule, becoming an immature B cell and leaving the bone marrow. Expression of sIgD marks entry of the cell into the mature, resting phase (or G_0) characteristic of most blood and mantle zone B cells. Switching to an alternative isotype (IgG in this case) may occur before an encounter with antigen or afterward. Antigen triggers the resting B cell to enlarge (in G_1 phase of the cell cycle) and present processed antigen and DR to the antigen-specific T cell receptor–CD3 complex. T-helper cells (T_H) secrete growth factors that bind to newly expressed receptor, further enhancing proliferation (S and M phases) in germinal centers. The activated B cell can be induced to differentiate into plasma cells, which secrete their abundant cytoplasmic IgG. Alternatively, it can become a memory B cell with refined specificity poised to deliver an anamnestic immune response on its next encounter with antigen. *(From Bertoli LF, Burrows PD. Normal B-lineage cells: their differentiation and identification. Clin Lab Med 1988;8:15, with permission.) IgG,* Immunoglobulin G.

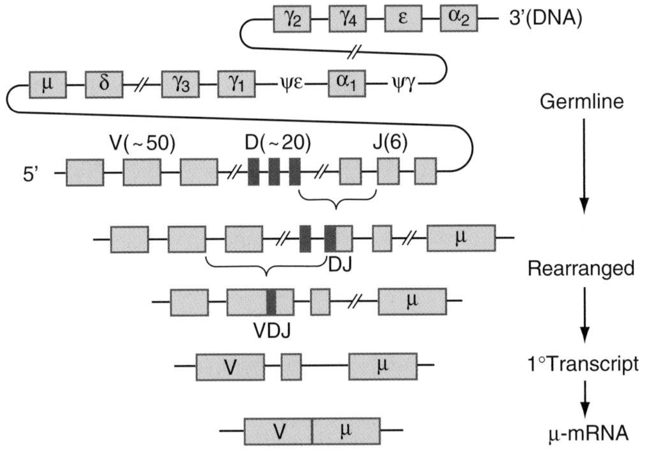

Figure 31-28 Generation of a functional *Ig* gene requires DNA rearrangement. In the germline and in somatic nonlymphoid cells, *V, D,* and *J* gene segments are widely separated in the DNA of chromosome 14. A cell committed to the B lineage first undergoes D to J rearrangement, juxtaposing the D and J segments and deleting intervening DNA sequences. This is followed by *V* to *DJ* rearrangement, generating a complete VDJ exon. The primary RNA transcript is processed to yield a contiguous V (VDJ) mRNA. *(From Bertoli LF, Burrows PD. Normal B-lineage cells: their differentiation and identification. Clin Lab Med, 1988;8:15, with permission.) DNA,* Deoxyribonucleic acid; *Ig,* immunoglobulin.

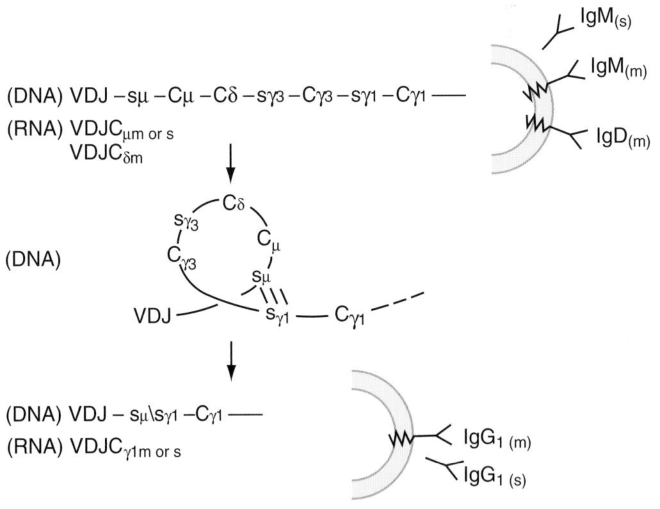

Figure 31-29 Alternative strategies for expression of non-IgM isotypes. IgD can be coexpressed with IgM, by alternative processing of a primary RNA transcript of VDJ-Cμ-Cδ, to yield μ membrane (m), μ secretory (s), and δm RNAs. The production of IgG, IgA, or IgE isotypes involves DNA rearrangement. During the switch from IgM to IgG, for example, intrachromosomal recombination between homologous switch (s) regions results in deletions of C_μ, C_δ, and $C_{\gamma 3}$, so that $C_{\gamma 1}$ is now the first *C* gene 3′ of the VDJ exon. Thus, the same variable region is expressed with a different constant region. *(From Bertoli LF, Burrows PD. Normal B-lineage cells: their differentiation and identification. Clin Lab Med 1988;8:15, with permission.) Ig,* Immunoglobulin; *RNA,* ribonucleic acid.

Pre-B cells give rise to naive mature B cells that characteristically express surface-bound Ig. These cells are present in primary lymphoid follicles, in follicular mantle zones, and in the circulation. In addition to IgD and IgM, these cells often express CD5 and are positive for Bcl-2.

In the second stage of differentiation, naive B cells interact with antigen and undergo transformation in the presence of T cells and macrophages. This process occurs in the germinal center. The B cells transform into blastic cells (centroblasts) that express Bcl-6 and CD10. Rapid division and expansion of B cell clones occur in an attempt to identify cells with Ig that provides the best fit for the stimulating antigen. Antigenic specificity is further refined through the process of somatic hypermutation in the variable region gene. Centroblasts give rise to centrocytes, which are cleaved follicle center cells. These cells express the modified Ig (following somatic hypermutation). Cells with lower affinity for the antigen are destroyed through apoptosis (cells in the germinal center do not express Bcl-2; therefore, they can undergo apoptosis). Surviving centrocytes differentiate into plasma cells that produce circulating Ig, or memory B cells that provide rapid humoral response the next time the same antigen is encountered. Memory B cells are present in the marginal zone of the follicle.

The state of Ig genes is, therefore, a good indicator of the developmental stage of B cells. The presence of Ig gene rearrangement identifies primitive B cells. Somatic hypermutation resulting in variable region sequences that are different from germline sequences identifies a B cell that has been stimulated by antigen. Germinal center B cells can be distinguished from post–germinal center B cells by the presence of intraclonal diversity in the former due to ongoing somatic hypermutation.

In the peripheral blood, approximately 6%–15% of B cells express surface-bound IgM (90% of these coexpress IgD), 1%–3% IgG, and 0.5%–2% IgA. Mature B cells express receptors for Fc portions of Ig isotypes, C3b and C3d fragments of complement, interferon, and IL-4. Mature B cells also express CD19, CD20, CD21, CD22, CD24, and CD38.

Plasma cells are characterized by abundant cytoplasmic Ig, reflecting the Ig commitment of the activated B cell. At this stage, Fc and C3 receptors, HLA-DR antigen, and surface-bound Ig are greatly reduced, but the cells express CD38 and CD138. Thus, the lymphocytes bearing sIg give rise to cells committed to the synthesis of IgM, IgG, and IgA.

T Cell Development: Thymus (Table 31-9)

The microenvironment of the thymus is necessary for the differentiation of T cells. The human thymus has two parts: the cortex and the medulla. The cortex is subdivided into two portions—the subcapsular cortex and the inner cortex—and is populated predominantly by small lymphocytes with a few scattered epithelial cells. Fibrous septa extend from the capsule to the medullary region. The medulla is composed mostly of epithelial cells with a small component of lymphocytes. In the medulla, Hassall's corpuscles, small islands of partially hyalinized epithelial cells, are present.

Pro-T cells from the bone marrow or fetal liver migrate to the thymus, where they undergo T cell receptor (TCR) gene rearrangement and are processed into functionally mature T cells for circulation in the blood and to the peripheral or secondary lymphoid tissues. TCR genes are organized in a similar manner to Ig genes. They possess V, D, J, and C regions and undergo rearrangement during early T cell maturation. In addition to the heterodimeric glycoproteins (α/β or γ/δ), the TCR/CD3 complex consists of the following subunits: CD3-ε, -ξ, and -η (Blumberg, 1990). The TCR recognizes foreign peptides held in an association with self-MHC molecules. In early T cell development, the γ- and β-chain genes rearrange simultaneously, with TCR commitment dependent on expression of surrogate α-chain and development of a pre-TCR (Haks, 1998; Kang, 2001). Successful passage of thymocytes with β-chain-containing pre-TCR through a developmental checkpoint is followed by rearrangement of the TCR α-chain and formation of α/β T cells. During this process, developing T cells first coexpress both CD4 and CD8 (double positive cells), with subsequent downregulation of one or the other. In the thymic medulla, pre-T cells lose the ability to make TdT as they convert to mature T cells (third stage) and then circulate in the blood and peripheral lymphoid tissues.

The earliest T cells in the thymus express CD2 and CD44 (Schattner, 2001). Subsequently, these cells express CD25 and CD3. The TCRs of CD4+ α/β T cells recognize nonself peptides held in the groove of class II MHC molecules, and TCRs of CD8+ α/β T cells recognize nonself polypeptides bound to the class I molecules (MacLennan, 1999).

The maturation of T cells is complex, however; at least three stages with multiple intermediate substages have been defined (Paraskevas, 2009b). In the first stage, pro-T cells migrate from the bone marrow or the fetal liver to the cortex of the thymus. In the second stage, pro-T cells migrate from the subcapsular cortex to the inner cortex and then to the thymic medulla (see Table 31-9). During this time, T cells with the ability to recognize foreign antigens are retained, and T cells with the ability to recognize self-antigens are eliminated.

Thymic function decreases with age, although it persists throughout life. Thymic function and T cell reconstitution can be assessed by measuring newly generated T cells utilizing a PCR assay for extrachromosomal DNA circles called **TCR rearrangement excision circles (TRECs)** (Kong, 1998).

A majority of postthymic (peripheral) T cells express α/β TCR; a small minority do not, but rather express γ/δ chains. NK cells express only ε chains with cytoplasmic CD3. Mature T cells are of at least three types. CD4 (helper) T cells possess α/β TCR chains and express CD2, CD3, CD4, CD5, and CD7 cell markers. CD8 (suppressor or cytolytic) T cells have α/β TCR chains and express CD2, CD3, CD5, CD7, and CD8 cell markers. Mature T cells with γ/δ TCR chains exhibit CD2, CD3, and CD7, lack CD4 and CD8, and seem to function as another population of cytotoxic cells (Paraskevas, 2009b).

CD4 T cells can develop into at least four subgroups with different functions (Zhu, 2008). Th1 cells produce interferon (IFN)-γ, TNF-β, and IL-2 and mediate immune response against intracellular pathogens. Th2 cells produce IL-4 and IL-5 and are important in defense against extracellular parasites. Th17 cells produce IL-17, IL-21, and IL-22 and mediate immune responses against extracellular bacteria and fungi. Induced regulatory T (iTreg) cells produce TGF-β, IL-10, and IL-35 and are involved in maintaining self-tolerance and regulating immune responses. Antigen-independent development of T cells is controlled by interaction with thymic epithelial cells and thymic fibroblasts, as well as by the influences of cytokines, growth factors, and thymic hormones. IL-1, IL-2, IL-3, IL-4, IL-7, and SCF are critical in the growth and differentiation of thymic lymphocytes. Thymic hormones produced by thymic epithelial cells also induce T cell function.

In the T-zone area of the peripheral lymphoid system, the T cell antigen–dependent pathway occurs through the binding of the TCRs to antigen peptides associated with appropriate MHC I and MHC II molecules on macrophages or interdigitating dendritic cells (IDCs). This results in the release of IL-1 by the activated macrophages, which, in turn, leads to the formation of IL-2 receptors on T cells and the subsequent synthesis and release of IL-2 by these activated T cells. In this activation process, many other cytokines (including IL-4, IL-6, IL-10, TNF, and interferon) are released, and appropriate cytokine receptors are upregulated. These events result in the activation and maturation of T-helper cells, T-suppressor

TABLE 31-9
Summary of T Cell Maturation

Stage	Maturation events	Cell surface markers
Pro-T cell	Migration from marrow to thymic cortex	CD2, CD44
α/β Pre-T cell	Migration from thymic cortex to medulla, elimination of self-recognizing T cells, α/β TCR rearrangement (for T cells destined for the helper or suppressor subset)	TdT, CD1, CD2, CD3, CD4, CD5, CD7, CD8
γ/δ Pre-T cell	Migration from thymic cortex to medulla, elimination of self-recognizing T cells, γ/δ TCR rearrangement (for T cells destined for the cytotoxic subset)	TdT, CD1, CD2, CD3, CD7
Mature T cell	Loss of ability to make TdT, circulation in peripheral blood as helper, suppressor, or cytotoxic subset	Helper T: CD2, CD3, CD4, CD5, CD7 Suppressor T: CD2, CD3, CD5, CD7, CD8 Cytotoxic T: CD2, CD3, CD7

TCR, T cell receptor; *TdT,* terminal deoxynucleotidyl transferase.

cells, T-cytotoxic cells, and other immunoregulatory cells. This activation process not only increases the number of antigen-specific T cells, it also alters the immunophenotype and changes the expression of certain adhesion molecules on T cells. For example, LFA-1 (a heterodimer formed from CD11a and CD18) and VLA-4 (a heterodimer of CD29 and CD49d, CD44, and CD2) are upregulated, and L-selectin (CD62L) is downregulated (MacLennan, 1999). Changes in the expression of adhesion markers allow for the proper circulation of T cells in the body.

Natural Killer Cells: Bone Marrow

Immunophenotypic and functional data suggest that NK cells and T cells have a close developmental relationship. Expression of CD3 proteins has been found in human fetal NK cells. Thus, it is likely that NK cells and T cells have a common precursor cell. Although NK cells can develop in the thymus, the thymic environment is not required for NK cell differentiation. NK cells can develop in secondary lymphoid tissues and bone marrow (Caligiuri, 2008). Fetal NK cells possess CD3γ, δ, ε, and CD28; adult NK cells express CD2, CD3ξ, CD7, CD8α, CD16, and CD56. SCF, IL-7, and IL-2 are critical in the development of NK cells (Spits, 1995). NK cells proliferate in the presence of IL-2, and their activity can be augmented by exposure to IFN-γ. NK cells appear to be targeted against virus-infected cells unable to signal cytotoxic T cells (usually as a result of low expression of class I MHC molecules). Because NK cells possess the Fc portion of IgG, they participate in antibody-dependent cell lysis (MacLennan, 1999).

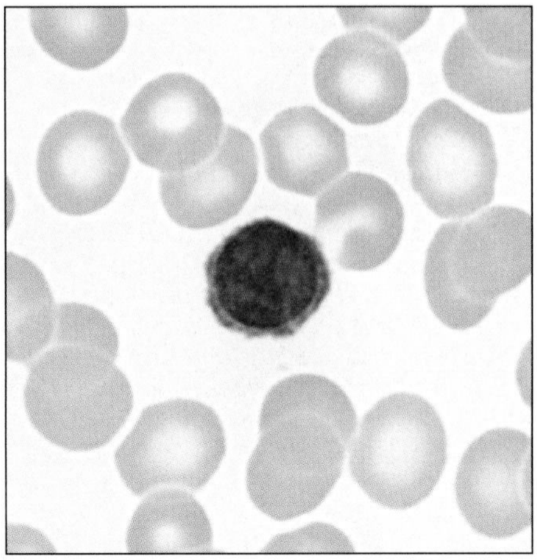

Figure 31-30 Small lymphocyte with high nuclear/cytoplasmic ratio, condensed chromatin, and scant basophilic cytoplasm (Wright–Giemsa, 1000×).

SECONDARY LYMPHOID TISSUE

In late fetal and postnatal life, lymphocytes are produced in the secondary lymphoid tissue: spleen, lymph nodes, and intestine. Lymphocytes of the secondary lymphoid organs are progeny from stem cells that have been influenced by primary lymphoid organs. The secondary lymphoid organs are thus composed of a mixture of B cells and T cells. Lymphopoiesis in secondary lymphoid organs depends solely on antigenic stimulation. B cells and T cells tend to localize in anatomically distinct parts of the lymphoid tissues, where proliferation can take place.

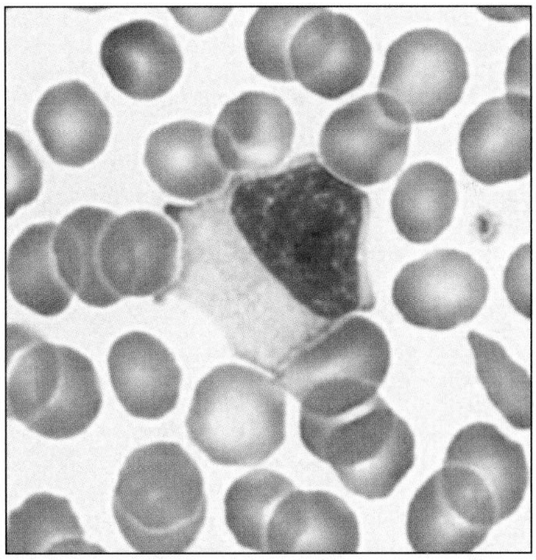

Figure 31-31 Atypical lymphocyte with large nucleus, finer chromatin, and abundant basophilic cytoplasm scalloping around adjacent red blood cells (Wright–Giemsa, 1000×).

LYMPHOCYTE FUNCTION AND PHYSIOLOGY

T cells and their progeny function in cell-mediated immunity, which includes delayed hypersensitivity, graft rejection, graft-versus-host reactions, defense against intracellular organisms (such as tubercle bacillus and *Brucella*), and defense against neoplasms. B cells and their progeny perform in humoral immunity, or in the production of antibodies, either as a lymphocyte or after transformation into a plasma cell.

A majority of circulating lymphocytes are T cells that have a life span of months to years. The B cells are a minor population (10%–20% of the lymphocytes), probably have a short life span measured in days (with the exception of memory B cells), and are distinguished by the presence of considerable Ig on their surface membranes.

Lymphocytes circulate in the blood and home to appropriate lymphoid organs. During fetal development, lymphocytes migrate from fetal liver to bone marrow or thymus. Later, pro-T cells migrate from the bone marrow to the thymus and immature B cells home to secondary lymphoid tissues. After thymic processing, virgin T cells also home to specific areas in the peripheral lymphoid tissues. The circulation of lymphocytes is regulated by multiple cell surface adhesion molecules and chemokines, including integrins, selectins, and leukocyte (L) selectin. The circulation and homing of lymphocytes is a very complex, multistep phenomenon, reviewed elsewhere (Springer, 1994; Paraskevas, 2009a). However, in the postcapillary venule of lymphoid tissue, the lymphocyte travels from the blood through the endothelium and into the lymphoid tissue, where it may stay or percolate through and return to the blood via the thoracic duct lymph. Small lymphocytes (Fig. 31-30) have little cytoplasm and, in electron micrographs, few organelles and relatively little RNA. After antigenic stimulation, small lymphocytes (B cells or T cells, depending on the nature of the antigen) become activated, increase their RNA synthesis, and undergo blast transformation. On Romanowsky-stained films, these blasts are large cells (15–25 μm) with abundant, rather deep blue cytoplasm, a large reticular nucleus with uniform chromatin, and prominent nucleoli. This cell is called the **reticular lymphocyte** (nonleukemic lymphoblast; **immunoblast**). If the blasts are derived from B cells, the new lymphocytes function

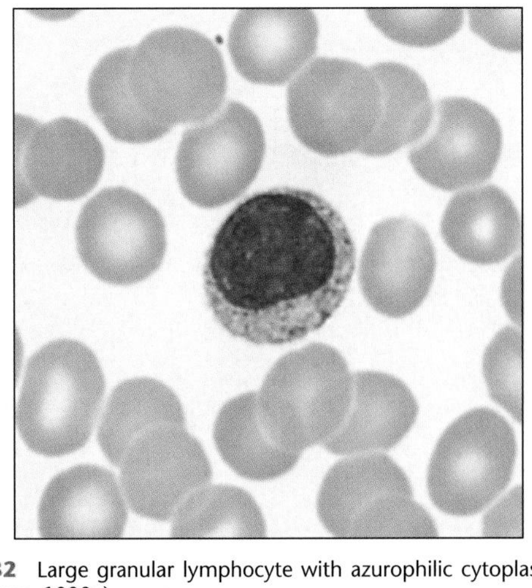

Figure 31-32 Large granular lymphocyte with azurophilic cytoplasmic granules (Wright–Giemsa, 1000×).

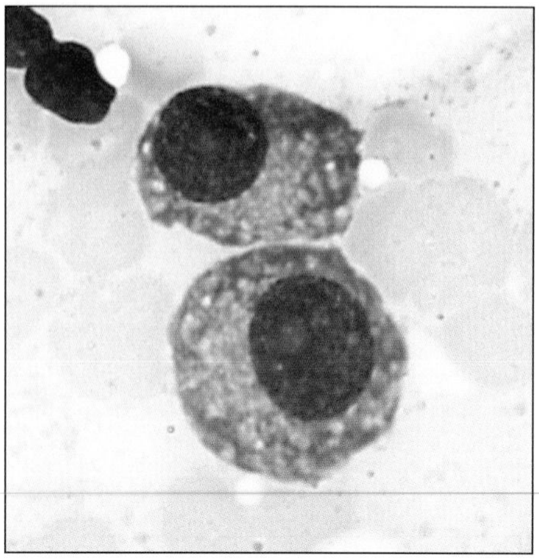

Figure 31-33 Plasma cells with abundant basophilic cytoplasm, eccentric nucleus, and perinuclear clear Golgi zone (Wright–Giemsa, 1000×).

in the production of antibodies (B cells, plasma cells); if the blasts are derived from T cells, the progeny act in the cellular immune response. The latter is mediated by several soluble factors produced by the activated T cell, including IL-2, which induces the proliferation of T cells; IL-3, which is a multipotential colony-stimulating factor; IL-4, which promotes the proliferation of B cells; IL-5, which enhances the proliferation of eosinophils as well as B cells; IL-6, which promotes differentiation of B cells; lymphotoxin, which is directly toxic to cells; and migratory inhibitory factor, which promotes adherence of macrophages and keeps them at the site. Atypical lymphocytes (Fig. 31-31) are seen in certain viral infections such as infectious mononucleosis. These cells have large nuclei with fine chromatin and more abundant cytoplasm that often scallops around adjacent red blood cells. Large granular lymphocytes (Fig. 31-32) contain azurophilic granules in their cytoplasm; these cells most often represent cytotoxic T cells or natural killer cells.

Plasma cells have abundant blue cytoplasm, often with light streaks or vacuoles, an eccentric round nucleus, and a well-defined clear (Golgi) zone adjacent to the nucleus. The nucleus of the plasma cell has heavily clumped chromatin, which is sharply defined from the parachromatin and is often arranged in a radial or wheel-like pattern (Fig. 31-33).

SELECTED REFERENCES

Abboud CN, Lichtman MA. Structure of the marrow and the hematopoietic microenvironment. In: Lichtman MA, Beutler E, Kipps TJ, et al, editors. Williams hematology. 7th ed. New York: McGraw-Hill; 2006, p. 35–72.

This reference put hematopoiesis into the essential context of the bone marrow microenvironment.

Deacon AC, Elder GH. Best Practice No. 165: front line tests for the investigation of suspected porphyria. J Clin Pathol 2001;54:500–7.

Reviews the laboratory diagnosis of porphyrias, including optimal specimens, techniques, quality control, and interpretation of results.

Dessypris EN, Sawyer ST. Erythropoiesis. In: Greer JP, Foerster J, Rogers GM, et al, editors. Wintrobe's clinical hematology. 12th ed. Baltimore: Williams & Wilkins; 2009, p. 106–25.

Essentials of erythroid commitment, colony formation and development, heme and globin, and control of erythropoiesis.

Hillman RS, Finch CA. Red cell manual. 7th ed. Philadelphia: FA Davis; 1996, p. 58.

Updated classic work illustrating the morphology of red blood cells, with descriptions of red cell disorders and pathophysiology, diagnosis, and treatment of anemias.

Kaushansky K. Thrombopoietin: a tool for understanding thrombopoiesis. J Thromb Haemost 2003;1:1587.

A review of the effects of the primary hormonal regulator of platelet production and the underlying mechanisms through which it works.

Koury MJ, Mahmud M, Rhodes MM. Origin and development of blood cells. In: Greer JP, Foerster J, Rogers GM, et al, editors. Wintrobe's clinical hematology. 12th ed. Baltimore: Williams & Wilkins; 2009, p. 79–105.

This reference provides a concise overview of blood cell development.

Paraskevas F. Lymphocytes and lymphatic organs. In: Greer JP, Foerster J, Rogers GM, et al, editors. Wintrobe's clinical hematology. 12th ed. Baltimore: Williams & Wilkins; 2009a, p. 300–25.

This provides an excellent basic discussion of post–bone marrow lymphopoiesis.

Paraskevas F. T lymphocytes and NK cells. In: Greer JP, Foerster J, Rogers GM, et al, editors. Wintrobe's clinical hematology. 12th ed. Baltimore: Williams & Wilkins; 2009b, p. 358–401.

This reference provides a thorough discussion of the bases of T and NK biology.

Sieff CA, Zon LI. Anatomy and physiology of hematopoiesis. In: Nathan and Oski's hematology of infancy and childhood. 7th ed. Philadelphia: WB Saunders; 2009, p. 195–273.

A thorough but readable reference on hematopoiesis from marrow anatomy through progenitor cells, molecular signaling, growth factors and receptors, differentiation, clinical disorders, and treatment considerations.

REFERENCES

Access the complete reference list online at http://www.expertconsult.com

CHAPTER 32

ERYTHROCYTIC DISORDERS

M. Tarek Elghetany, Katalin Banki

KEY POINTS

- Anemia may result from decreased marrow production or shortened red cell survival.
- Nonmarrow diseases, such as endocrine, renal, and inflammatory disorders, significantly influence bone marrow function.
- Stem cell disorders, such as inherited and acquired aplastic anemias, and paroxysmal nocturnal hemoglobinuria usually affect more than one cell line.
- Hemolytic anemia may be caused by extrinsic factors, usually acquired, such as chemical agents or antibodies, or intrinsic factors, usually inherited, such as disorders of the red cell membrane or enzymes, or hemoglobinopathy.
- Polycythemia is defined by laboratory parameters and may be absolute with an increase in total red cell mass as a result of increased erythropoietin production, or relative as a result of a decrease in plasma volume.

ANEMIAS

GENERAL MANIFESTATIONS

Anemia is considered to be present if the hemoglobin (Hb) concentration or the hematocrit (Hct) is below the lower limit of the 95% reference interval for the individual's age, sex, and geographic location (altitude) (Table 32-1). This means that 2.5% of normal individuals will be classified as anemic. Conversely, an individual whose Hb falls within the reference intervals for age and sex yet significantly below his or her own reference values should be considered anemic.

Anemia may be absolute, when red blood cell mass is decreased, or relative, when associated with a higher plasma volume. Causes of absolute anemia fall into two major pathophysiologic categories: impaired red cell production and increased erythrocyte destruction or loss in excess of the ability of the marrow to replace these losses. Several authors have included posthemorrhagic anemia in the latter category (Hillman, 1996; Erslev, 2001b). The presence of anemia may be a sign of an underlying disorder

PART 4

TABLE 32-1
Reference Values Below Which Anemia Is Considered to Exist at Sea Level

Age, years	Hb, g/dL
Both Sexes	
1–2	11
3–5	11.2
6–11	11.8
Females	
12–15	11.9
16–69	12
≥70	11.8
Males	
12–15	12.6
16–19	13.6
20–49	13.7
50–69	13.3
≥70	12.4

From Looker AC, Dallman PR, Carroll MD, et al. Prevalence of iron deficiency in the United States. JAMA 1997;277:973–6.
Hb, Hemoglobin.

whose cause should be identified because correction may be very important to the individual. Relative anemia may occur with pregnancy, with macroglobulinemia, and in postflight astronauts. However, recent studies suggest that prolonged exposure to weightlessness and return to sea level after a period of high altitude acclimatization are associated with selective loss of young red cells, also known as neocytes, as a result of erythropoietin (EPO) withdrawal (Risso, 2007).

Anemia may be classified by red cell morphology as macrocytic, normocytic, or microcytic—an approach that is useful in differential diagnosis (see later discussion). Both pathophysiologic and morphologic classifications should be understood. Some anemias (e.g., blood loss anemia) have more than one pathogenetic mechanism and go through more than one morphologic stage.

Clinical signs and symptoms result from diminished delivery of oxygen (O_2) to the tissues and, therefore, are related to the lowered Hb concentration and blood volume, and are dependent on the rate of these changes. Modifying factors include compensatory adjustments in cardiac output, respiratory rate, and O_2 affinity of Hb. When anemia develops slowly in a patient who is not otherwise severely ill, Hb concentrations as low as 6 g/dL may develop without producing any discomfort or physical signs, as long as the patient is at rest.

In general, the anemic patient complains of easy fatigability and dyspnea on exertion, and often of faintness, vertigo, palpitations, and headache. The more common physical findings are pallor, a rapid bounding pulse, low blood pressure, slight fever, some dependent edema, and systolic murmurs. In addition to these general signs and symptoms, certain clinical findings are characteristic of the specific type of anemia.

IMPAIRED PRODUCTION—IRON DEFICIENCY ANEMIA

Iron Metabolism

(Andrews, 2009).

Iron is an essential component of Hb, of myoglobin (in muscle cells), and of certain enzymes (in most body cells). The major "pools" of iron in the body are illustrated in Figure 32-1. Two thirds or more of the body's total iron is in the erythron (normoblasts and erythrocytes); each milliliter of red cells contains about 1 mg of iron. Storage iron is present in macrophages of the reticuloendothelial system in two forms: ferritin and hemosiderin. Ferritin is a water-soluble complex of ferric salt and a protein, apoferritin. Apoferritin has a molecular weight of approximately 450,000 Da and consists of 24 subunits with a variable ratio of H (heavy) and L (light) types. Apoferritin forms a shell around a crystalline core of predominately ferric oxyhydroxide (FeOOH). The genes for the H and L subunits have been located on chromosomes 11 and 19, respectively. Hemosiderin is water insoluble and consists mostly of aggregates of ferric oxyhydroxide core crystals with partially or completely degraded protein shells. Protein degradation usually occurs in lysosomes. The iron in hemosiderin is much more difficult to release than that of ferritin. Most of the iron utilized in Hb synthesis is that recently released from degraded Hb in macrophages and transported to the normoblasts by plasma transferrin

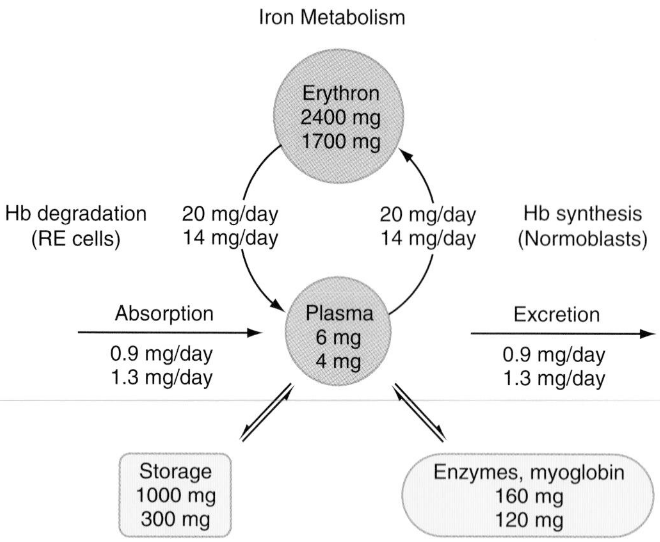

Figure 32-1 Scheme of iron metabolism. The upper figure in each position is average for an 80-kg man; the lower figure is for a 65-kg woman. (Data from Hillman and Finch, 1974.) The plasma iron, bound largely to transferrin, is central in this scheme. It completely turns over several times a day in supplying iron for heme synthesis. Each day, about 1/120 of total circulating red cells are destroyed, and the same number of new red cells is delivered to the blood. That proportion of the total erythron iron enters the plasma from the site of hemoglobin (Hb) degradation, the macrophages of the reticuloendothelial (RE) system, and travels (bound to transferrin) to the normoblasts in the marrow. Storage iron largely resides also in the macrophages of the RE system. Absorbed iron enters the plasma pool, bound to transferrin. Iron is largely excreted by loss of cells.

(a β-globulin, molecular weight 80,000 Da, gene located on chromosome 3). Each molecule of apotransferrin binds two atoms of ferric iron. Subsequently, transferrin binds to transferrin receptors (TfRs) (CD71) on the cell membrane of erythroid precursors, reticulocytes, and most body cells. The transferrin–transferrin receptor complex is rapidly internalized, iron is released, and apotransferrin returns to the circulation and binds more iron. In addition to transferrin receptors, hepatocytes express a related molecule designated as transferrin receptor 2. Although its physiologic function is not clearly understood, mutations in the transferrin receptor 2 gene have been associated with hemochromatosis.

Very little iron is lost from the body; this small iron loss occurs mainly as loss of cells from the gastrointestinal (GI) tract and to a lesser extent from the skin and through the urine. The iron excreted in women averages more than that excreted in men because of menstrual blood loss. About 1 mg is lost each day, except in menstruating females, whose iron loss averages about 2 mg/day. Iron balance is maintained by control of absorption. In the United States, dietary iron averages 15 mg/day with 7% absorption in men, and 11 mg/day with 13% absorption in women. Absorption can be increased in iron deficiency, but only to about 20% of ingested iron in meat-containing diets, and less in vegetarian diets (Hillman, 1996). Absorption takes place largely in the small intestine, most efficiently in the duodenum and upper jejunum, with heme iron absorbed more efficiently than inorganic iron. Iron absorption is facilitated by ascorbate and citrate and is inhibited by phytates and tannins. Acid production by the stomach lowers the pH in the duodenum, thus enhancing the solubility and uptake of nonheme ferric iron. Although the mechanism of iron entry into mucosal cells of the upper GI tract remains largely unknown, more than one pathway seems to be in place, including an independent mechanism for heme absorption.

Recent studies suggest the presence of an iron transport channel called the divalent metal transporter (DMT), which is regulated by iron regulatory proteins 1 and 2. DMT-1 regulates iron transport from intestinal surface to inside the cell. This process is aided by the recently discovered duodenal cytochrome *b*–like ferroreductase, which reduces iron to the ferrous form. The export of iron from enterocytes, macrophages, and hepatocytes to plasma involves another transport system, which includes ferroportin-1 and hephaestin (Fleming, 2008). Ferroportin-1 is located at the basolateral membrane of apical enterocytes and functions as a transport protein delivering iron to the plasma. Hephaestin, named after the Greek god **Hephaestus,** who forged iron, has a ferroxidase activity that contributes to iron transport by transforming iron to the ferric form to enable its uptake by circulating apotransferrin. Ceruloplasmin also has ferroxidase activity and is involved as well in the release of iron from the cells. Because both ceruloplasmin and hephaestin are copper-containing ferroxidases, copper deficiency affects iron release and can produce iron deficiency anemia. Another recently identified 25-amino-acid antimicrobial peptide, hepcidin, has been shown to play a major role in iron homeostasis, possibly through a hormonal effect. Hepcidin is produced by the liver, is filtered by the kidney, and accumulates in urine. Hepcidin negatively controls the release of iron from cells, such as intestinal epithelium and macrophages, to the plasma. Hepcidin combines with ferroportin-1, leading to internalization and lysosomal degradation of both proteins; thus it limits the release of intracellular iron into the plasma (Fleming, 2008). Several proteins play a role in the regulation of hepcidin expression, which proved to be an intricate process that is still under study. These include a glycosylphosphatidyl inositol (GPI)-membrane–linked protein called hemojuvelin, TfRs 1 and 2, and human hemochromatosis protein, in addition to other groups of mediator proteins (Anderson, 2009).

In the plasma, total iron averages 110 μg/dL (19.7 μmol/L). The great majority of this is bound to the transferrin, which has a capacity to bind 330 μg of iron per deciliter (or 59.1 μmol/L) and therefore is about one-third saturated. A very small amount of iron in plasma is in ferritin. Plasma (or serum) ferritin averages about 100 μg/L in men (less in women—about 50 μg/L).

Iron Deficiency Anemia

When iron loss exceeds iron intake for a time long enough to deplete the body's iron stores, insufficient iron is available for normal Hb production. When well developed, iron deficiency is characterized by a hypochromic microcytic anemia.

Iron deficiency typically results when the need for iron is increased (e.g., during rapid growth in infancy and childhood, during pregnancy) or when excessive loss of blood has reduced the body's reserves of iron (e.g., following repeated hemorrhages, excessive menstruation, or multiple pregnancies).

Iron deficiency is probably the most common cause of anemia on the planet, affecting at least one third of the world's population (Brittenham, 2009). Children between the ages of 6 and 24 months are particularly susceptible. It is caused by insufficient dietary iron to meet the needs of rapid growth. After the first 4–6 months of life, the iron stores present from birth have been exhausted, and the infant depends on dietary iron. An infant maintained on milk and carbohydrates without supplements of iron-containing foods is likely to develop iron deficiency anemia—one component of the "milk anemia" of infancy. This anemia is also frequently related to intestinal blood loss due to cow's milk protein intolerance in young children when cow's milk is introduced too early. In a study in the United States, iron deficiency anemia was reported in 3% of toddlers aged 1–2 years and in 2%–5% of adolescent girls and women of childbearing age, with iron deficiency (absent anemia) noted in higher (>9%) proportions (Looker, 1997). Defective absorption of iron and eventual iron deficiency anemia occur after total gastrectomy or even subtotal gastrectomy. Prolonged treatment of peptic ulcer and acid reflux by H_2 blockers and acid pump blockers may cause defective iron absorption. Except for the sprue syndrome, causes of malabsorption of iron are extremely rare. Because iron deficiency increases the rate of absorption of both iron and lead, lead intoxication may accompany iron deficiency.

If an adult male had absolutely no iron intake or absorption (which would be extremely unlikely), his body iron stores of 1000 mg would last for 3–4 years before he would even begin to become iron deficient. Therefore, almost all cases of iron deficiency anemia in adult males are due to chronic blood loss. Hemorrhagic lesions, such as benign and malignant tumors, chronic ingestion of some medications, and helminthic infections are common causes of iron deficiency in males and postmenopausal females.

The sequence of events in developing iron deficiency anemia is usually as follows (Hillman, 1996): When blood loss exceeds absorption, a negative iron balance exists. Iron is mobilized from stores, storage iron decreases, plasma ferritin decreases, iron absorption increases, and plasma iron-binding capacity (transferrin) increases. This stage is known as **iron depletion.** After iron stores are depleted, the plasma iron concentration falls, saturation of transferrin falls below 15%, and the percentage of sideroblasts decreases in the marrow. As a result of lack of iron for heme synthesis, red cell protoporphyrin increases. This second stage is **iron-deficient erythropoiesis;** anemia may not yet be present. The third stage is **iron deficiency anemia;** in addition to the abnormalities just discussed, anemia is detectable. The anemia at first is normochromic and normocytic, gradually becomes microcytic, and finally becomes microcytic and hypochromic.

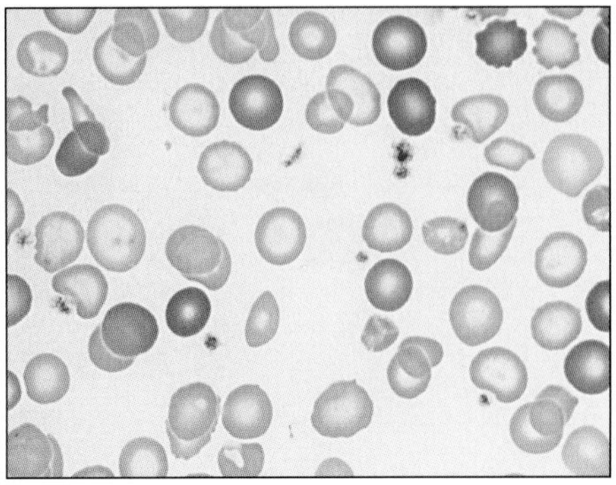

Figure 32-2 Iron deficiency anemia, post transfusion. The cells are pale with an enlarged central pallor, in sharp contrast to the transfused normochromic cells.

Clinical Features

Clinical findings may be due to the underlying cause of the blood loss itself, to the general manifestations of anemia (see previous discussion), or to iron deficiency. Those that are probably attributable to lack of tissue iron include paresthesias, such as numbness and tingling; atrophy of epithelium of the tongue with burning or soreness; fissures or ulcers at the corners of the mouth (angular stomatitis); chronic gastritis, which leads to decreased gastric secretions but few symptoms; "pica," which is the craving to eat unusual substances such as dirt or ice; concave or spoon-shaped nails (koilonychia); and difficulty swallowing due to "webs" of tissue or partial strictures at the junction of the esophagus and hypopharynx. The latter two findings are relatively uncommon. The combination of glossitis, sore mouth, dysphagia, and iron deficiency is called Plummer-Vinson syndrome. Splenomegaly may occur in iron deficiency but is uncommon. A high prevalence of iron deficiency with or without anemia has been reported in patients with restless legs syndrome (Brittenham 2009).

Laboratory Features

Blood. In early iron deficiency anemia, the stained blood film often shows normochromic normocytic erythrocytes (Hillman, 1996). In later stages, the picture is one of microcytosis, anisocytosis, poikilocytosis (including elliptical and elongated cells), and varying degrees of hypochromia. The plasma membranes of iron-deficient cells are abnormally stiff, and this abnormality contributes to the development of poikilocytes, particularly elongated hypochromic elliptocytes (pencil cells). Anisocytosis may be identified by automated blood counters as increased red cell distribution width (RDW). This finding, however, is not specific for iron deficiency anemia. Reticulocytes are usually decreased in absolute numbers, except following iron therapy. The mean corpuscular volume (MCV) is low, and Hb and Hct are relatively lower than the erythrocyte count. Osmotic fragility may be decreased because the red cells are thinner than normal (see Figs. 30-10 and 32-2).

The leukocyte count is normal or slightly lowered. Granulocytopenia and a small number of hypersegmented neutrophils may be present. Megaloblastic changes in severe iron deficiency may be related to decreased activity of the enzyme ribonucleotide reductase, which contains an essential nonheme iron atom (Beck, 1991). However, the detection of hypersegmented neutrophils should raise suspicion for a mild folate deficiency, which may become more overt after iron therapy (Dallman, 1993). Platelets may be increased, whether the lack of iron is due to blood loss or dietary deficiency, but tend to be decreased in severe anemia.

Marrow. Normoblastic hyperplasia occurs early, but in later stages the limiting effect of severe iron deficiency restricts erythropoiesis to the basal level. The normoblasts are smaller than normal, deficient in the amount of Hb in the cytoplasm, and irregular in shape with frayed margins (Fig. 32-3). Giant neutrophil bands or metamyelocytes, if present, are rarely due to iron deficiency **per se;** usually, they indicate an associated cobalamin or folate deficiency (see later under Megaloblastic Anemia). Iron stains should be performed routinely (Figs. 32-4 and 32-5). **Storage iron** is absent, unless iron has recently been administered in some form. The proportion of normoblasts that are **sideroblasts** is decreased (<20%); this proportion is usually about the same as the percent saturation of transferrin (or total iron-binding capacity [TIBC]) and is a measure of iron delivery to the normoblasts.

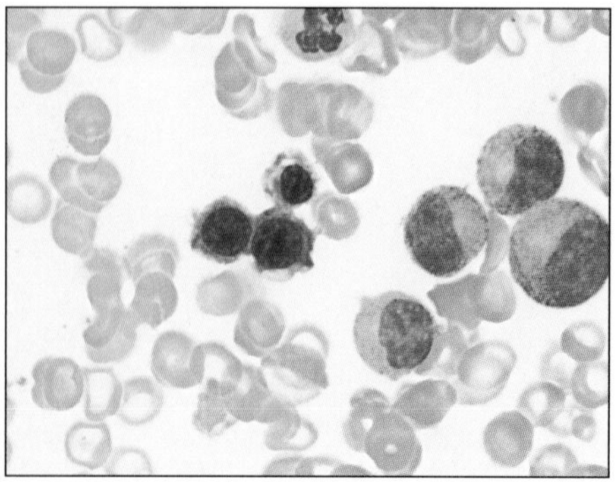

Figure 32-3 Marrow film, iron deficiency anemia. The three normoblasts have irregular margins and irregular clear spaces, reflecting lack of hemoglobin synthesis (i.e., defective cytoplasmic maturation).

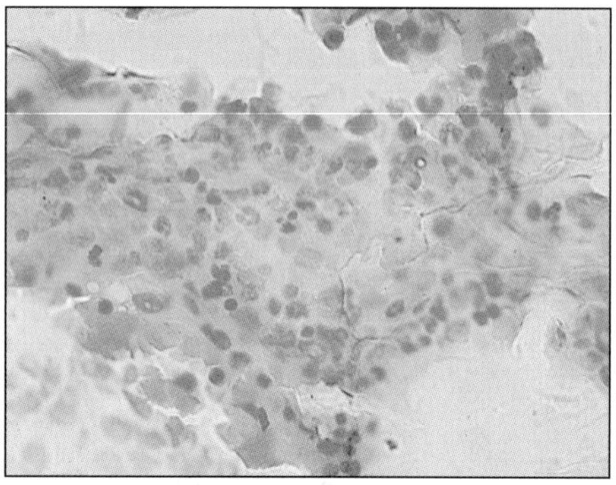

Figure 32-4 Marrow film, Prussian blue reaction. Depleted iron stores: No blue-green staining iron is visible. On a scale of 0–5+, the iron is normal from 1+ to 3+ for women and from 2+ to 3+ for men.

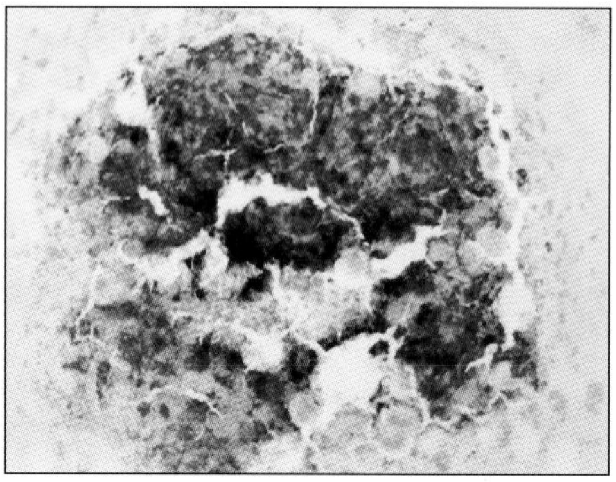

Figure 32-5 Marrow film, Prussian blue reaction. On a scale of 0–5+, the amount of storage iron is judged at 5+, which is markedly increased.

Serum Iron. The reference interval is 50–160 μg/dL (9–29 μmol/L) in adults. The level is lower in iron deficiency and in infection and anemia of chronic disease.

Serum (Total) Iron-Binding Capacity. The reference interval for adults is 250–400 μg/dL (45–72 μmol/L). In iron deficiency anemia, the serum TIBC is increased. It is normal or decreased in the anemia of chronic disease. If chronic infection coexists with chronic blood loss, the TIBC may not be increased, even though the patient is iron deficient.

Percent Saturation of TIBC. The ratio of serum iron to TIBC is the percent saturation of the TIBC. Normally, this is 20%–55%; values below 15% indicate iron-deficient erythropoiesis.

A marked diurnal variation in serum iron by as much as 30% normally occurs, with highest values in the morning and lowest values late in the day. Consequently, fasting morning blood specimens are preferred for the diagnosis of iron deficiency. The TIBC remains relatively constant in a normal individual. Pregnancy and oral contraceptives increase TIBC.

Serum iron is usually higher in the first 90 days of life; then it dips to somewhat lower reference intervals for the second month of life, and the value gradually increases with age, until it reaches the adult range approximately at the age of 15 years (Ritchie, 2002b; Soldin, 2004). On the other hand, the TIBC gradually rises with age until it reaches values that are comparable to those of adults at the age of 15 years (Soldin, 2004). Similarly, percent saturation in children is less than in adults; it reaches the adult value between the ages of 15 and 18 years (Ritchie, 2002b).

Serum Ferritin. In adults, the reference values are 12–300 μg/L, with higher values in men than in women. Serum ferritin appears to be in equilibrium with tissue ferritin and is a good reflection of storage iron in normal subjects and in most disorders. The equivalence of 1 μg/L of serum ferritin with 8–10 mg storage iron has been suggested. In patients with some hepatocellular diseases, malignancies, and inflammatory diseases, serum ferritin is a disproportionately high estimate of storage iron because serum ferritin is an acute phase reactant. In such disorders, iron deficiency anemia may exist with a normal serum ferritin concentration. In the presence of inflammation, persons with a serum ferritin level of less than 50–60 μg/L are likely to respond to iron therapy. On the other hand, hypothyroidism and ascorbate deficiency may lower plasma ferritin levels independent of iron stores (Brittenham, 2009).

In infancy and childhood, between the ages of 6 months and 15 years, the reference interval for serum ferritin is somewhat lower than in early infancy or adult life (Soldin, 2004). In men, serum ferritin gradually rises between the ages of 18 and 30 years, whereas in women, it does not. However, postmenopausal women have a much higher ferritin level than premenopausal women, and it is comparable with that of men (Van den Bosch, 2001). Serum ferritin levels do not display diurnal variation.

Erythrocyte Porphyrins. Because heme is formed by insertion of iron into protoporphyrin IX, the latter is increased in iron-deficient erythropoiesis, whether owing to iron deficiency or to anemia of chronic disease. It is also increased in lead poisoning and in some cases of sideroblastic anemia but is normal in thalassemia. Zinc usually becomes attached to protoporphyrin, forming zinc protoporphyrin (ZPP). A relatively simple micromethod measuring ZPP in whole blood has been shown to be useful in distinguishing microcytosis due to iron deficiency from that due to β-thalassemia minor (Labbé, 2004). The normal reference interval was 10–99 μg/dL of erythrocytes; in iron deficiency, erythrocyte porphyrins became elevated before the development of anemia, and this may be one of the earliest indicators of iron deficiency (Labbé, 2004).

Serum Transferrin Receptors. TfRs also exist in a soluble form in the circulation. Serum TfRs (STfRs) are produced by shedding of membrane TfRs during erythrocyte maturation. STfRs vary with the rate of erythropoiesis. Patients with aplastic anemia (AA) have lower than normal levels of STfRs, and patients with autoimmune hemolytic anemia have higher values. Iron deficiency anemia is associated with increased serum levels of TfRs, probably as a result of increased membrane TfR synthesis and expression secondary to iron starvation. Unlike serum ferritin, STfRs are usually not affected by inflammation (Clark 2009).

Serum Transferrin Receptor–to–Serum Ferritin Ratio. The serum transferrin receptor–to–serum ferritin (TfR/F) ratio has been suggested as a new approach to estimate total body iron stores. However, it appears to have limited value in identifying anemia of chronic disease (ACD). The TfR/F ratio may be better utilized in identifying iron deficiency anemia coexisting with ACD (Clark, 2009).

Reticulocyte Hemoglobin Content. Some automated hematology analyzers offer an assay of Hb content within reticulocytes (CHr; in pg/cell). By measuring CHr, the status of erythropoiesis in the previous 3–4 days may be assessed using reticulocytes as a guide (Clark, 2009).

Hepcidin Level. Measuring plasma hepcidin may serve as a valuable tool in the study of abnormalities of iron metabolism and iron deficiency. Hepcidin level measurement is currently undergoing numerous studies.

Differential Diagnosis

Anemia due to iron deficiency usually needs to be distinguished from other causes of microcytosis with or without anemia. These include the thalassemia traits, long-standing ACD, and the sideroblastic anemias (see later

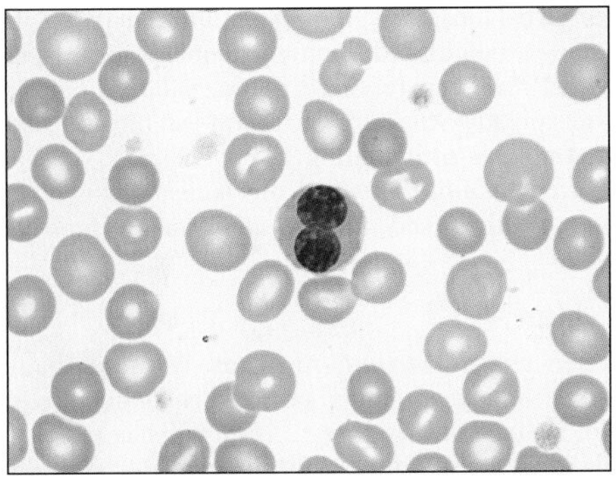

Figure 32-6 Blood film, megaloblastic anemia. Macrocytosis and a circulating megaloblast with abnormal, binucleated nucleus and open chromatin.

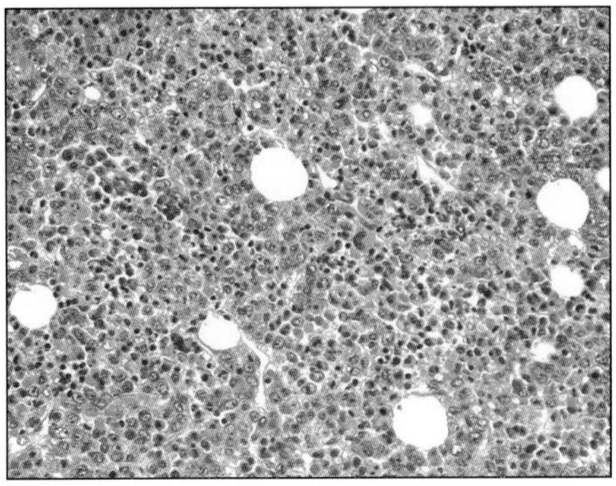

Figure 32-7 Hypercellular marrow in megaloblastic anemia. Cellularity is over 95%.

discussions of these entities). Bone marrow storage iron and serum ferritin will be decreased in iron deficiency and normal or elevated in all others. In **thalassemia trait,** the ZPP is normal, serum iron is normal, and the condition is present in family members. In β-thalassemia trait, Hb A_2 and sometimes fetal hemoglobin (Hb F) are increased. Yet, Hb A_2 is often decreased in iron deficiency. In **ACD** (chronic infection, rheumatoid arthritis, or neoplastic disease), although the serum iron is low, as in iron deficiency, the TIBC is low or normal. In the **sideroblastic anemias,** which include chronic lead poisoning, the serum iron and percent TIBC saturation are increased, and pathologic "ring" sideroblasts are present in the marrow.

Management

The first principle in therapy of iron deficiency anemia is that the underlying cause can be identified and corrected. Ferrous iron is given orally—at about 200 mg/day—in three doses between meals. This will provide 40–60 mg of absorbed iron per day, which, with the iron produced by turnover of senescent red cells, will be sufficient to increase production to two or three times normal (Hillman, 1996). The reticulocyte count will reach a maximum at 5–10 days, then will gradually decrease toward normal. Monitoring the Hb is best; Hb should increase by 0.1–0.2 g/dL/day after the fifth day, and by at least 2 g/dL for each of the subsequent 3 weeks. After the Hb has returned to normal, iron therapy should be continued for at least 2 months to replenish storage iron. Patients refractory to treatment need to be investigated for continued underlying diseases, particularly chronic gastritis and *Helicobacter pylori* gastritis (Clark, 2009).

IMPAIRED PRODUCTION—MEGALOBLASTIC ANEMIA

Macrocytosis With Normoblastic Marrow

Macrocytic anemias that are not megaloblastic may be due to early release of erythrocytes from the marrow, so-called shift reticulocytes. This may occur in response to acute blood loss, hemolysis, bone marrow infiltration, and high levels of EPO associated with bone marrow failure diseases such as aplastic anemia, refractory anemia, and Diamond-Blackfan anemia. Nonmegaloblastic macrocytosis is also found in hypothyroidism, in individuals with excessive alcohol intake, and in liver disease (Hillman, 1996).

Megaloblastic Anemia

Blood

Macrocytic anemias associated with megaloblastosis differ from nonmegaloblastic macrocytic anemia in that macroovalocytes and giant hypersegmented neutrophils are present in the blood (Figs. 30-11, 30-15, and 32-6). Pancytopenia is the rule. The anemia is macrocytic with an elevated MCV and is characterized by macroovalocytes and often extreme degrees of anisocytosis and poikilocytosis. Microcytes and dacrocytes are common. Basophilic stippling, multiple Howell-Jolly bodies, nucleated red cells with karyorrhexis, and even megaloblasts may be seen. Leukopenia is present. Granulocytes have increased numbers of lobes, presumably as a result of abnormal nuclear maturation. Five lobes in more than 5% of the neutrophils constitute hypersegmentation (Herbert, 1985), as do any neutrophils with six or more lobes. Thrombocytopenia is usually encountered and on rare occasions is sufficiently severe to be responsible for bleeding. It is worth noting that significant morphologic changes may occur in the blood in the absence of anemia, and that neurologic symptoms may be present in the absence of anemia.

Marrow. Megaloblastic anemia is characterized by enlargement of all rapidly proliferating cells of the body, including marrow cells. The major abnormality is the diminished capacity for deoxyribonucleic acid (DNA) synthesis. In cobalamin or folate deficiency, marked reduction in intracellular 5,10-methylene tetrahydrofolate occurs and is required to transform deoxyuridine monophosphate to deoxythymidine monophosphate. This reaction is mediated by thymidylate synthase and is essential to maintain the normal rate of DNA synthesis (Antony, 2009). With such deficiency, the cells have both a prolonged intermitotic resting phase and a block early in mitosis. The number of mitotic figures is increased. Ribonucleic acid (RNA) synthesis is less impeded than DNA synthesis; hence, cytoplasmic maturation and growth continue, accounting for enlargement of the cells. The delicate chromatin and the prominent parachromatin result in a distinctly more "open" chromatin pattern than is seen in the erythroid precursors (Figs. 30-28 and 32-6). The nuclei undergo karyorrhexis readily, and multiple Howell-Jolly bodies may be present. Usually more cells analogous to the pronormoblast and the basophilic normoblast are noted (i.e., promegaloblast and basophilic megaloblast) than are seen in normal erythropoiesis. This has sometimes been termed **maturation arrest,** or nuclear-cytoplasmic asynchrony. Giant polychromatic megaloblasts are especially distinctive. The same general features are seen in the other cell lines. In the granulocytic series, the cells are larger, with retarded nuclear maturation and large cytoplasmic mass; often the specific granules themselves are distinctly larger. The chromatin pattern is less condensed (more "open"), and as a result the nucleus appears to stain poorly. Abnormally contorted nuclear configurations are common. The giant metamyelocyte is the most characteristic of the abnormal granulocytes. Megakaryocytes, too, are large and have separated nuclear lobes or nuclear fragments.

The bone marrow is hyperplastic (Fig. 32-7). The fat is replaced, and red marrow extends into the long bones. The number of erythroid precursors (megaloblasts) is increased, and the myeloid/erythroid ratio is decreased. If the megaloblastic process is incompletely developed, or if the patient has been inadequately treated, the findings may be only partial. Because they persist longer, granulocytic alterations are especially helpful in assessing recently treated megaloblastic anemia. Marrow findings result from the effects of impaired nucleic acid synthesis, leading to megaloblastosis and hypoxic stress, giving rise to increased numbers of erythroid cells. If the patient is transfused with packed red cells, the number of erythroid precursors diminishes, but the cytologic abnormalities persist.

Erythrokinetics. In megaloblastic anemias, the mass of erythroid tissue is increased, plasma iron turnover is rapid, and urine and fecal urobilinogen are increased. These measures indicate an **increase in total erythropoiesis** that may be up to three times normal. The decreased rate of appearance of iron in the Hb of circulating erythrocytes and reticulocytopenia indicate **ineffective erythropoiesis.** In addition to increased destruction of defective erythroid precursors in the marrow, survival of circulating erythrocytes is short, indicating hemolysis. Indirect serum bilirubin is increased, serum iron is increased, endogenous carbon monoxide (CO) production is increased, and serum lactate dehydrogenase is usually greatly elevated. Serum muramidase may be elevated, implying ineffective granulocytopoiesis.

Megaloblastic anemia is nearly always due to cobalamin or folic acid deficiency. The aforementioned findings are similar for either.

Cobalamin (Vitamin B_{12}) Metabolism

Vitamin B_{12} (cyanocobalamin) has a molecular weight of 1355 Da. The molecule's two major parts are (1) a **planar group** (the corrin nucleus), a ring structure surrounding a cobalt atom; and (2) a **nucleotide group,** which consists of the base, 5,6-dimethylbenzimidazole, and a phosphorylated ribose esterified with 1-amino,2-propanol. A cyanide group is in coordinate linkage with the trivalent cobalt. Different forms of vitamin B_{12} result from replacement of the cyanide by hydroxy, adenosyl, or methyl groups; generically, these are termed **cobalamins.**

Cobalamin is the only vitamin exclusively synthesized by microorganisms. It is found in practically all animal tissues and is stored primarily in the liver in the form of adenosylcobalamin. The human liver contains approximately 1 μg/g of liver. Cobalamin is initially bound to R binders (cobalamin-binding proteins with *R*apid electrophoretic mobility) present in saliva or food, is released by peptic digestion, and is then bound by other R binders at the acid pH of the stomach. On entering the duodenum, cobalamin is released by pancreatic enzymes to finally bind to gastric intrinsic factor (IF), a 44-kDa glycoprotein produced in the parietal cells of the stomach. The gene for IF is located on chromosome 11. This cobalamin–IF complex, which is highly resistant to digestion, then adheres to specific receptor sites on the epithelial cells of the ileum, at which site the cobalamin is absorbed. A recent study indicates that the cobalamin–IF receptor is a combination of two proteins: a 460-kDa protein called cubilin, and a 45–50-kDa protein called amnionless. Both proteins are also present in renal tubules. Mutation of any of the two genes can produce megaloblastic anemia with proteinuria, also known as Imerslund-Gräsbeck syndrome (Fyfe, 2004). The concentration of the receptor in the ileum increases progressively until it reaches its maximum near the terminal ileum. The cobalamin–IF complex is taken into the cell, where cobalamin is released and the IF is destroyed. The receptor recycles to the surface of the cell (Babior, 2001).

Cobalamin is transported in the plasma as methylcobalamin, while bound to a group of proteins named transcobalamin II (TC II) and haptocorrins (variously called TC I, TC III, R binder, cobalophilin *[vide infra]*). Ninety percent of newly absorbed cobalamin is bound to TC II, which serves as the chief transport protein, rapidly delivering the vitamin to the liver, hematopoietic cells, and other dividing cells. Some cobalamin binds to haptocorrins—a step that prevents its loss from the plasma; this cobalamin is a passive reservoir in equilibrium with body stores in the liver but not taken up by other body cells. The reference values for plasma cobalamin depend on the method of assay, but they commonly are 200–900 ng/L (150–670 pmol/L). One third of the binding sites on transcobalamins are normally occupied: 70%–90% of plasma cobalamin is bound to haptocorrins, mostly TC I; this is very slowly cleared from the plasma. The remainder is bound to TC II, which remains only about 5% saturated; much of newly absorbed cobalamin bound to TC II is removed from the plasma during the first few hours, but a small fraction remains bound for several weeks.

The relative importance of the transcobalamins is illustrated by the clinical effects of congenital deficiency. Lack of TC II results in severe megaloblastic anemia in infancy; yet the serum cobalamin level is normal. Lack of TC I is not accompanied by anemia or megaloblastosis; yet the serum cobalamin level is decreased (Antony, 2009).

TC I and III are R-type proteins. TC III is probably an isoprotein of TC I, which is unsaturated with cobalamin and thus less charged. Much of the serum TC III is released from granulocytes during blood clotting in vitro; TC III does not appear to bind significant amounts of plasma cobalamin under normal conditions. Haptocorrins (TC I and III) may arise from granulocytes, salivary glands, and liver, as well as from other tissues. Elevation of TC I and III accounts for the elevation of total cobalamin-binding proteins in myeloproliferative neoplasms. TC II is also synthesized by a variety of cells, including renal cells, enterocytes, and hepatocytes. TC II acts as an acute phase reactant; its levels are increased in inflammatory and infectious conditions (Carmel, 1999).

The daily requirement for cobalamin is in the range of 2–5 μg/day. The body's stores of 2–5 mg will last for several years if intake is cut off, as is the case when total gastrectomy is performed (Beck, 1991).

Cobalamin Deficiency

Although the true prevalence of cobalamin deficiency in the general population is unknown, it increases with age. Approximately 15% of adults older than 65 years have laboratory findings of vitamin B_{12} deficiency. This prevalence may be attributed to the high frequency of hypochlorhydria of 25%–50%, which has been reported in the elderly population (Antony, 2009). The widespread use of proton pump inhibitors to control gastric secretion is becoming a contributing factor (Oh, 2003). Cobalamin deficiency is produced by any of several mechanisms which are not always exclusive of each other and involve inadequate intake and reduced absorption.

Inadequate Intake

A dietary deficiency is an *extremely rare* cause of megaloblastic anemia in the United States and is seen only in persons who completely abstain from animal food, including milk and eggs. Only strict vegetarians are known to develop this form of cobalamin deficiency.

Defective Production of Intrinsic Factor

This is the most common cause of cobalamin deficiency.

Pernicious Anemia

Pernicious anemia (PA) is a "conditioned" nutritional deficiency of cobalamin that is caused by failure of the gastric mucosa to secrete intrinsic factor. This abnormality is genetically determined but usually is not manifested until late in life; less than 10% of cases occur in persons younger than age 40. The annual incidence of PA is approximately 25 new cases per 100,000 individuals over the age of 40 years. Positive family history is obtained in approximately 30% of patients (Antony, 2009). Modern surveys indicate that PA is as common in blacks as in Caucasians (Carmel, 1999).

Clinical Features

The disorder is equally common in males and females. Symptoms of **anemia** and the combination of skin pallor and jaundice giving a lemon-yellow appearance to the skin are often present. The tongue may be sore, smooth, and pale (atrophic glossitis) or red and raw (acute glossitis). **GI symptoms** may be prominent and include episodic abdominal pain, constipation, and diarrhea. Diffuse and irregular degeneration of the white matter of the **central nervous system (CNS)** characteristically involves the posterior and lateral columns of the spinal cord (subacute combined degeneration) and sometimes other sites. Symmetrical sensations of "pins and needles" of the distal extremities, numbness and tingling, loss of position sensation (difficulty with balance and gait), and loss of vibratory sensation (perhaps the most constant sign) are indicative of peripheral neuropathy and posterior column lesions. Lateral column involvement gives rise to weakness, spasticity, and increased deep tendon reflexes. Sometimes, the brain may be affected, and the patient shows irritability, emotional instability, or a change in personality. Neuropsychiatric disorders may be associated with cobalamin deficiency even without accompanying hematologic manifestations (Lindenbaum, 1988). Recent studies suggest that cobalamin is essential for the maintenance of certain levels of cytokines and growth factors in the CNS. Cobalamin deficiency has been reported to cause an increase in CSF levels of myelinotoxic cytokines, such as tumor necrosis factor-α, while decreasing myelinotrophic cytokines, such as interleukin (IL)-6 (Scalabrino, 2009).

Gastric Findings

Atrophic gastritis of varying degrees is found in most adults with PA, and gastric atrophy involving all coats of the wall in the remainder. IF and hydrochloric acid (HCl) are secreted by gastric parietal cells in the human; in adult PA, IF secretion is absent, and almost always histamine-refractory achylia and achlorhydria—decreased volume of gastric juice and lack of HCl secretion—are present.

Immune Abnormalities

Autoantibodies have been found in the serum of patients with pernicious anemia (Antony, 2009). **Anti–parietal cell antibodies** react with gastric parietal cells and are present in more than 90% of patients. These anti–parietal cell antibodies are also present in patients with chronic gastritis, such as that associated with iron deficiency, and in some patients with thyroiditis and myxedema; they are seen in 4%–5% of age-matched healthy individuals. When these antibodies are chronically injected into rats, they decrease gastric HCl, IF, and pepsin secretion and produce gastric atrophy. The major antigen to which these antibodies are produced is the acid-producing enzyme H^+,K^+-ATPase, a 92-kDa protein present on the luminal membrane of parietal cells, which is the target of proton pump inhibitors. A recent study suggests that antibodies to *H. pylori* are common in PA, particularly in young patients. Infection may be the first step toward initiation of an autoimmune response (Hershko, 2007).

Another type of autoantibody is directed against intrinsic factor. **Anti-intrinsic factor antibodies** occur in the serum, saliva, and gastric juice of about 75% of patients with PA. Two types of anti-IF antibodies occur: "blocking" antibodies, which block the binding of cobalamin to IF; and "binding" antibodies, which bind to the cobalamin–IF complex and prevent the complex from binding to receptors in the ileum. Although these antibodies can cause some functional impairment in vivo, it is not clear whether the antibodies are the cause or an effect of the disease. IF antibodies in the absence of PA occur in a small percentage of individuals with hyperthyroidism (Graves' disease), and similarly in persons with insulin-dependent diabetes. Therefore, IF antibodies are considered highly specific and confirmatory for PA, although their absence does not exclude the diagnosis (Antony, 2009).

Family studies in patients with pernicious anemia have shown an increased incidence of the disease in relatives, and many relatives have achlorhydria and partial defects of cobalamin absorption. Relatives of patients with pernicious anemia also have a higher incidence of gastric parietal cell antibodies and of thyroid antibodies than normal individuals.

It is possible that adult pernicious anemia is a genetically determined autoimmune gastritis. However, the relationship of the gastric lesion to the antibodies remains unclear.

Pernicious Anemia in Children

Two forms of PA are known to occur in children. **Congenital pernicious anemia** usually appears early in the second year of life. IF secretion may be lacking, or the secreted IF may be functionally defective, but acid secretion and the appearance of the gastric mucosa are normal. Antibodies to parietal cells and to IF are absent. **Juvenile pernicious anemia** occurs usually in older children and is like that of adults, with gastric atrophy, achlorhydria, and serum antibody to IF and parietal cells, although the latter may be absent in a subset of patients (Rosenblatt, 1999).

Gastrectomy

Surgical removal of the stomach (total or even subtotal occasionally) will remove the source of intrinsic factor. This will lead to megaloblastic anemia after the body's stores of cobalamin have been exhausted—in 3 to 6 years—if cobalamin therapy has not been given. Frequently, the anemia is due in part to iron deficiency.

Defective Absorption of Cobalamin

Malabsorption Syndromes. Celiac disease, tropical sprue, resection of the small bowel, or inflammatory disease of the small bowel may be associated with multiple defects of absorption, including other vitamins. Folic acid deficiency (absorbed principally in the upper small bowel) is more commonly seen than cobalamin deficiency (absorbed principally in the lower small bowel) in diseases leading to malabsorption. The reason for this is probably the lesser time necessary for depletion of body stores of folic acid.

The Imerslund-Gräsbeck syndrome is an autosomally recessive inherited defect in the intestinal absorption of cobalamin that occurs in the presence of normal intrinsic factor. In many patients, proteinuria of the tubular type is also found. As mentioned earlier, the syndrome is caused by a defect in the cubilin/amnionless receptor (Fyfe, 2004).

Lack of Availability of Cobalamin. In certain countries, infestation with the fish tapeworm *Diphyllobothrium latum* is common enough that cobalamin deficiency may occur occasionally when it is present. The worm successfully competes with the host for the ingested cobalamin. Most common in Finland, it is rarely seen in the United States.

Bacteria in a blind loop of intestine may also preferentially utilize ingested cobalamin to the detriment of the host.

Vitamin B_{12} or folate deficiency may exert indirect cardiovascular effects. Both deficiencies are associated with hyperhomocystinemia, which is an independent factor for atherosclerosis and vascular thrombosis (Oh, 2003).

Diagnosis of Cobalamin Deficiency

Recognition of megaloblastic anemia indicates the likelihood of cobalamin deficiency or folic acid deficiency. In addition, evidence of neurologic involvement favors cobalamin deficiency. This diagnosis can be established by one of four methods.

Therapeutic Trial. With the patient on a diet low in cobalamin and folate, a parenteral physiologic dose of cobalamin (10 μg/day) is given. Optimal hematologic response indicates deficiency and consists of reticulocytosis beginning on the third or fourth day, reaching a peak on the seventh day. Erythropoiesis becomes normoblastic by 2 days, and leukopoiesis becomes normal by 12 to 14 days. Within a week, leukocyte and platelet counts have returned to normal, and the Hb concentration begins to rise.

Serum Cobalamin Assay. This is the usual method of detecting a cobalamin-deficient state. The original microbiological assay of serum cobalamin employed an organism (e.g., *Euglena gracilis*) that requires cobalamin for growth. Although the microbiological method is precise and reliable, it requires at least 48 hours of incubation and is subject to the inhibitory effects of antibiotics. Radioisotopic dilution and chemiluminescence assays are more rapid and widely used and give results comparable with those of the *Euglena* assay, provided that the binding protein is specific for biologically active cobalamin; a standardized intrinsic factor preparation is most satisfactory. However, these methods may produce false-normal values in approximately 10% of patients with cobalamin deficiency (Zittoun, 1999).

Reference values are 200–900 ng/L. In megaloblastic anemia due to cobalamin deficiency, serum cobalamin is usually less than 100 ng/L. Individuals with folate deficiency and mild cobalamin deficiency and who are pregnant have borderline values between 100 and 200 ng/L. Patients with human immunodeficiency virus (HIV) infection or multiple myeloma and those receiving megadose vitamin C therapy often have low serum cobalamin levels in the absence of clinical manifestations (Ward, 2002; Antony, 2009). Spuriously normal cobalamin levels have been recorded in patients with cobalamin deficiency associated with overgrowth of intestinal bacteria, which produce biochemically inert B_{12} analogs, and in patients with autoimmune disorders, myeloproliferative neoplasms, and active liver disease (Ward, 2002; Antony, 2009). Measurement of TC II–bound cobalamin (holotranscobalamin II) may provide additional information, in that its levels fall below the normal range long before total serum cobalamin does and probably represent a state of negative cobalamin balance (Zittoun, 1999). However, its clinical utility has been limited (Ward, 2002).

Methylmalonic Acid and Homocysteine Assays. Because a cobalamin coenzyme is essential for the isomerization of methylmalonate to succinate, urine excretion of increased amounts of methylmalonate is found in cobalamin deficiency. Provided that the rare inborn error of metabolism, methylmalonic aciduria, is not present, this is a sensitive test for cobalamin deficiency, but it is not usually necessary for the diagnosis. In addition, plasma levels of methylmalonic acid and homocysteine are increased. However, plasma levels of methylmalonate are normal in folate deficiency in the absence of cobalamin deficiency (Antony, 2009). Following several weeks of therapy, their plasma concentration returns to normal. Plasma levels of these metabolites should be interpreted with caution in patients with chronic renal failure because of the tendency of these metabolites to accumulate (Zittoun, 1999).

Deoxyuridine Suppression Test. This measures the ability of marrow cells in vitro to utilize deoxyuridine in DNA synthesis. Normally, in marrow cells, the major source of thymidine for DNA is de novo synthesis from deoxyuridine, which requires intact cobalamin and folate enzymes; therefore, less than 10% of added tritium-labeled thymidine (^{3}H-Tdr) is incorporated into DNA. In megaloblastic marrows due to cobalamin or folate deficiency, deoxyuridine cannot be efficiently converted to thymidine, and more ^{3}H-Tdr is taken up into DNA. An abnormal deoxyuridine suppression test indicates cobalamin or folate deficiency. This test is very sensitive and produces abnormal results before anemia or macrocytosis is observed (Zittoun, 1999). A lymphocyte microdeoxyuridine suppression test (Herbert, 1985) requires only 1 mL of blood, making this diagnostic modality available to infants and children.

Detecting the Cause of Cobalamin Deficiency

Clinical history is useful in suggesting whether cobalamin or folate deficiency is the cause of megaloblastic anemia. Clinical associations of pernicious anemia include a family history of PA in one third of patients, along with certain endocrine deficiencies (thyroid disease, diabetes mellitus, hypothyroidism, and Addison's disease) and immune disorders (immune thrombocytopenic purpura, autoimmune hemolytic anemia, and acquired hypogammaglobulinemia). Cobalamin deficiency is likely to occur in strict vegetarians and in patients with paresthesias, neuropathy, or a previous gastrectomy.

In cobalamin-deficient patients, it is important to determine whether IF is lacking. To do so, the ability of the patient to absorb an oral dose of radioactive cobalamin may be measured. The usual method is the Schilling test, which measures radioactivity in a 24-hour sample of urine. Two hours after oral administration of 0.5–2.0 μg of radioactive cobalamin, a large "flushing" dose of nonlabeled cobalamin is given parenterally. Normal individuals will excrete more than 7% of a 1-μg dose of ingested cobalamin in the urine in 24 hours, whereas patients lacking IF will excrete less. If excretion is low, the test must be repeated using the same procedure, except that hog IF is given orally, along with labeled cobalamin. If 24-hour excretion is normal, the low value in the first part was due to IF deficiency. If excretion remains abnormal in the second part of the procedure, an explanation for malabsorption of cobalamin on the basis of intestinal disease must be sought. The test may be repeated after 7–10 days of antibiotic administration if bacterial overgrowth is suspected, and pancreatic extracts may be added to investigate the possibility of pancreatic dysfunction (Antony, 2009). The validity of the results depends on good renal function and accurate urine collection. The Schilling test will be abnormal in PA even after the patient is treated with cobalamin and is in remission. Some patients may absorb vitamin B_{12} in water (as given in the original Schilling test) but fail to absorb vitamin B_{12} bound to protein in food. A modification of the Schilling test is being introduced to include protein-bound B_{12} using egg yolk or chicken serum (Zittoun, 1999).

Other tests that will establish the diagnosis of PA include direct assay of IF in gastric juice. The combination of megaloblastic anemia, decreased serum cobalamin, and serum antibodies to IF is essentially diagnostic of PA, obviating the need for the Schilling test (Lindenbaum, 1983).

Folic Acid Metabolism

Folic acid or pteroylmonoglutamic acid contains three parts: pteridine, *p*-aminobenzoate, and L-glutamic acid (Beck, 1991). In nature, folic acid occurs mainly as less soluble polyglutamates, with multiple glutamic acid residues attached to one another. Folic acid is present in a wide variety of foods, such as eggs, milk, leafy vegetables, yeast, liver, and fruits, and is formed by intestinal bacteria as well. Folates are extremely thermolabile, and prolonged cooking (>15 minutes) in large quantities of water in the absence of reducing agents destroys folate.

Polyglutamates are hydrolyzed to monoglutamate by folate hydrolase, which is present in the brush border of proximal jejunum and has maximal exopeptidase activity at pH 5.5 (Antony, 2009; Hamid, 2009). Folates are transported across the intestinal membrane by a variety of carriers, including reduced folate carrier and proton-coupled folate transporter (Hamid, 2009). Another transport system carries folate across the basolateral membrane of the cell. In the plasma, one third of the folate is free, and two thirds is nonspecifically and loosely bound to serum proteins. A small amount of folate is specifically bound to folate-binding proteins, the physiologic significance of which is unclear (Antony, 2009). Folate is rapidly removed from plasma to cells and tissues for utilization. The principal form of folate in serum, erythrocytes, and liver is 5-methyltetrahydrofolate (5-methyl-FH_4); the liver is the chief storage site. Intracellular folates exist primarily as polyglutamates. A significant enterohepatic circulation is present, and bile contains 2–10 times the folate concentration of normal serum. Moreover, folates that are filtered in the renal glomeruli are extensively reabsorbed back into the renal circulation (Hamid, 2009). The minimal daily requirement is about 50 μg of pteroylmonoglutamate or 400 μg of total folate; a typical reference interval for serum folate is 5–21 μg/L (11–48 nmol/L), and for red cell folate, 150–600 μg/L (340–1360 nmol/L) of red blood cells.

The Folate–Cobalamin Relationship

Anemia of cobalamin deficiency is partially corrected by folate even in the absence of cobalamin supplementation, but the reverse is not true. Therefore, some of the megaloblastic manifestations in cobalamin deficiency are actually caused by abnormalities in folate metabolism (Antony, 2009). The most accepted theory for their interrelationship is the methylfolate trap theory. This theory is based on the observation that the methyl form of tetrahydrofolate (FH_4) would leak out of cells unless conjugated to form polyglutamates. Methyl FH_4 is a poor substrate for the conjugating enzyme. Cobalamin is essential for the process of conversion of methyl FH_4 to FH_4. Accumulation of methyl FH_4 is followed by its leakage out of the cells (Babior, 2001).

Folic Acid Deficiency

(Antony, 2009).

Inadequate Intake of Folate

Evolution of Laboratory Abnormalities. Herbert delineated the sequence of events in the onset of folate-deficient megaloblastic anemia. After a folate-deficient diet was initiated, various abnormalities were established as follows: 3 weeks, low serum folate; 5 weeks, hypersegmented neutrophils in bone marrow; 7 weeks, hypersegmented neutrophils in peripheral blood, with bone marrow showing increased and abnormal mitoses and basophilic intermediate megaloblasts; 10 weeks, bone marrow showing some large metamyelocytes and polychromatophilic intermediate megaloblasts; 13 weeks, high excretion of formiminoglutamic acid (FIGLU) in urine; 17 weeks, low erythrocyte folate; 18 weeks, macroovalocytosis of erythrocytes with many large metamyelocytes in bone marrow; 19 weeks, overtly megaloblastic bone marrow; and 20 weeks, anemia (Herbert, 1985).

At this time, changes in the intestinal epithelium have not yet appeared. Therefore, in the human, with no dietary intake of folic acid, anemia will appear in 3 to 6 months. The peripheral blood and bone marrow features of megaloblastic anemia due to folic acid deficiency are similar to those of cobalamin deficiency; however, leukopenia and thrombocytopenia are less constant. Folic acid deficiency has usually been found in association with some complicating factor.

Nutritional Folate Deficiency. Megaloblastic anemia due to lack of folate is most commonly associated with insufficient dietary intake. The usual diet does not contain much above the minimal requirements, and body stores in the adult are sufficient for only about 3 months' needs. Dietary folate deficiency is especially common in the tropics and in India, and even in those locations, it is usually associated with increased demand for folate in pregnancy, rapid growth in infancy, infection, or hemolytic anemia. Elderly persons on inadequate diets in the United States may develop folate-deficient megaloblastic anemia.

Folate deficiency in infancy is uncommon in the United States. Human milk or fresh cow's milk contains sufficient folate, but heated milk, powdered milk, and goat's milk do not. If the infant's milk lacks folate, if the diet is low in ascorbic acid, or if infection or diarrhea is a problem, megaloblastic anemia may occur.

Megaloblastic anemia in pregnancy is not uncommon because of the fetal requirements for folate. The mother's plasma folate level gradually falls during pregnancy, and at birth the plasma level in the newborn averages five times that of the mother. Megaloblastic anemia is more frequent in multipara, may be precipitated by infection, and is usually due to folate deficiency rather than cobalamin deficiency. Pregnant women should receive, in addition to iron, folic acid supplements. Recent studies indicate that folate supplementation for pregnant women reduces the risk of giving birth to babies with neural tube defects, with anencephaly and spina bifida being the most common defects.

Liver Disease. Liver disease associated with alcoholism may lead to folate-deficient megaloblastic anemia because of the grossly inadequate diet of the alcoholic, and because the liver is the major site for folate storage and metabolism (Zittoun, 1999). With adequate dietary folic acid intake, however, the anemia that is found with liver disease is macrocytic and normoblastic—not megaloblastic.

Defective Absorption of Folate

Defective absorption of folic acid occurs in association with malabsorption syndromes discussed previously and in the blind loop syndrome, in which bacteria preferentially utilize folate.

Nontropical sprue, or adult celiac disease, is an important cause of malabsorption in adults or children that is related to dietary gluten (wheat protein). Included among the signs of malabsorption may be megaloblastic anemia due to folic acid deficiency (Beck, 1991). Jejunal biopsy shows villous atrophy. The folate deficiency, as well as the malabsorption, responds to a gluten-free diet. Folic acid therapy (parenteral) corrects the folate deficiency, but not the general malabsorption.

Tropical sprue is a poorly understood malabsorptive disorder that is common in the Caribbean, India, and Southeast Asia. Evidence of malabsorption includes megaloblastic anemia due to folate deficiency. Treatment with folic acid brings considerable improvement in general malabsorption, as well as in the anemia, but additional antimicrobial treatment is recommended.

Megaloblastic anemia or decreased serum and red cell folate without anemia has been associated with the long-term use of anticonvulsant drugs such as phenytoin, phenobarbital, and primidone. The problem appears to be a drug-induced malabsorption of pteroylpolyglutamate. Oral contraceptives cause malabsorption of folate in a small proportion of women, owing to impaired deconjugation of pteroylpolyglutamate (Beck, 1991).

Increased Requirement for Folate

The increased need in pregnancy and in infants has been mentioned. Increased cell turnover that occurs in neoplasia and in the markedly stimulated hematopoiesis of hemolytic anemias may result in megaloblastic erythropoiesis. The basis for this is the increase in need for a marginal supply of folate.

Inadequate Utilization of Folate

Inadequate utilization of folic acid is relatively rare. Folic acid antagonists such as methotrexate block folic acid metabolism and because of this are used in therapy of some malignant neoplasms. In addition to inhibiting growth of the tumor, they induce megaloblastic hematopoiesis.

In addition to the previously mentioned nutritional problem in alcoholics, **alcohol** may exert a direct effect in suppressing hematopoiesis by blocking the metabolism of folate. In addition, alcohol can interfere with folate absorption and folate enterohepatic circulation, usually resulting in increased loss of folate in urine (Hamid, 2009). Plasma homocysteine is usually elevated in alcoholics (Zittoun, 1999).

Diagnosis of Folate Deficiency

Folic acid deficiency or cobalamin deficiency is suspected when the blood and bone marrow show findings characteristic of megaloblastic anemia; usually, serum folate and cobalamin levels are then determined.

Serum and Red Cell Folate. A microbiological assay for folic acid activity employing *Lactobacillus casei* is a reliable method for definitive diagnosis (Beck, 1991). Radioisotopic and chemiluminescence methods employing different folate binders are widely used because of their rapidity and greater convenience. Although correlation with the microbiological assay is generally good, discrepancies seem to be frequent and, on the basis of other data, tend to be resolved in favor of the microbiological assay. False-normal red cell folate levels have been reported in 16%–40% of patients identified by microbiological assays (Zittoun, 1999). Unlike serum folate (which is entirely 5-methyltetrahydrofolate), red cell folates are a heterogeneous mixture of different forms with varying polyglutamate chain lengths, which pose challenges to nonmicrobiological assays.

The serum folate level is decreased (<3 μg/L) in megaloblastic anemia due to folate deficiency but is usually normal or increased in cobalamin deficiency. A low serum folate level precedes a decrease in red cell or tissue folate; it indicates a negative folate balance but does not by itself indicate tissue folate deficiency. Serum folate is highly sensitive to folate intake and may normalize after a single adequate meal, despite the presence of true underlying deficiency (Antony, 2009). In cobalamin deficiency, serum folate is decreased in 10% of cases, increased in 20%, and normal in the remainder (Tietz, 1990).

The red cell folate is a better test of body folate stores and is decreased in megaloblastic anemia due to folate deficiency. In cobalamin deficiency, however, red cell folate is low in almost two thirds of cases, so this needs to be excluded before a low red cell folate is taken as proof of severe folate deficiency. Therefore, three measurements are often useful in distinguishing between deficiencies of folic acid and cobalamin (Table 32-2).

Physiologic doses of folic acid (parenteral, 50–200 μg/day) will allow an adequate reticulocyte response in patients with folic acid deficiency, but not with cobalamin deficiency. On the other hand, the usual therapeutic doses of folic acid (5–15 mg/day) or larger doses of cobalamin (500–1000 μg) may induce a partial response in a patient with megaloblastic anemia due to the other deficiency. Treatment of cobalamin deficiency with folic acid is hazardous in that although a reticulocyte response may occur, neurologic damage will progress.

Urinary Formiminoglutamic Acid

Folic acid coenzymes are required for the conversion of FIGLU to glutamic acid in the catabolism of histidine. When oral histidine is given, FIGLU will appear in increased amounts in the urine if folate deficiency is present. The test is useful in patients with megaloblastic anemia due to antifolate drugs; these patients have normal serum folate levels but greatly decreased tissue coenzyme levels (Beck, 1991).

Deoxyuridine Suppression Test. See earlier discussion.

TABLE 32-2
Correlation of Vitamin B_{12} and Folate Levels With Clinical Status: Three Laboratory Tests Needed to Separate Four Clinical Situations

Clinical situation	Serum vitamin B_{12}, pg/mL	Serum folate, ng/mL	Red cell folate, ng/mL
Normal*	Normal (200–900)	Normal (5–16), indeterminate (3–5), or low (<3)	Normal (>150)
Vitamin B_{12} deficiency	Low (<100)	Normal (5–16) or high (>16)	Low (<150)
Folic acid deficiency	Normal	Low	Low
Deficiency of both	Low	Low	Low

From Herbert V. Megaloblastic anemias. Lab Invest 1985;52:3–19.
*Normal includes transient states of negative folate balance.

Plasma Homocysteine Assay. As with cobalamin deficiency, total plasma homocysteine is increased in approximately 75% of patients with folate deficiency. The level of methylmalonic acid is normal (Zittoun, 1999).

Acute Megaloblastic Anemia

Acute megaloblastic anemia may develop over the course of only a few days. The most common cause has been related to nitrous oxide (N_2O) anesthesia. N_2O rapidly destroys methylcobalamin, causing a rapidly progressive megaloblastic anemia. Acute folate deficiency may occur in some patients in intensive care units because of a combination of factors (decreased intake, total parenteral nutrition, dialysis, surgery, sepsis, medications). Serum folate may be normal (Antony, 2009).

Therapy for Megaloblastic Anemia

Although it may be necessary to treat severely anemic patients with both vitamins, it is usually possible to determine which deficiency is the cause, and treat only for it.

The maximal reticulocyte response occurs in 5 to 7 days. Within 4 to 6 hours after the initial therapy (if parenteral), the marrow shows decreased early megaloblasts and the appearance of pronormoblasts. Within 2–4 days, the marrow is predominantly normoblastic. Granulocytic abnormalities return to normal more slowly, and hypersegmented neutrophils disappear from the blood only after 12–14 days.

PA is treated parenterally with 1000 μg of cyanocobalamin daily for 1 week, twice weekly for the second week, once weekly for 4 weeks, then monthly for the lifetime of the patient (Antony, 2009). High concentrations of oral cobalamin (e.g., 1000 μg per day) force absorption of some cobalamin through an alternate system. Some reports recommend the use of oral cobalamin therapy instead of injections (Oh, 2003).

In folate deficiency, oral therapy is generally used at a dosage of 1–2 mg/day. Cobalamin deficiency must be excluded and corrected if present, to avoid the occurrence of neuropathies of cobalamin deficiency. Supplemental dietary folic acid during pregnancy is reported to reduce the incidence of neural tube defects in the baby.

Other Defects of Nucleoprotein Synthesis

Other defects of nucleoprotein synthesis may lead to megaloblastic anemias that do not respond to cobalamin or folic acid.

Congenital Defects

Orotic aciduria is a very rare autosomal recessive condition in which certain enzymes required for pyrimidine synthesis are absent. Findings include excessive urinary excretion of orotic acid, failure of normal growth and development, and megaloblastic anemia that is refractory to cobalamin and folate but that responds to uridine.

Inborn defects in enzymes involved in folate metabolism, including methyltetrahydrofolate reductase and glutamate formiminotransferase deficiencies, have also been described.

Synthetic Inhibitors

Synthetic inhibitors of purine synthesis (6-mercaptopurine, thioguanine, azathioprine), of pyrimidine synthesis (5-fluorouracil), or of deoxyribonucleotide synthesis (cytosine arabinoside or hydroxyurea) are used in chemotherapy for neoplasia and may concomitantly produce megaloblastosis.

Refractory Anemias

Anemias that are megaloblastic and that fail to respond to cobalamin or folic acid are considered with the myelodysplastic syndromes (see Chapter 33). The megaloblastic changes are usually atypical and do not include the characteristic granulocytic features, but other dysplastic changes are present.

IMPAIRED PRODUCTION—OTHER

Anemia of Chronic Disease

(Means, 2003).

ACD designates an anemia syndrome typically found in patients with chronic infections or inflammatory or neoplastic disorders; it is characterized by reduced reticulocyte response accompanied by low serum iron, despite adequate iron stores. It is also termed anemia of chronic disorder, inflammation, or cytokine response. ACD occurs in approximately 50% of hospitalized patients, as identified by laboratory studies. The frequency is higher in the elderly population. ACDs have also been observed in acute trauma and critical care patients.

Erythrocytes are usually normocytic and normochromic, although in 20%–50% of patients, the anemia is microcytic and hypochromic. Anisocytosis and poikilocytosis are slight. The reticulocyte count usually is not elevated. Leukocytes and platelets are not distinctively altered, except by the causative disease.

The marrow is normocellular or minimally hypocellular or hypercellular, and the cell distribution is not greatly disturbed. The normoblasts may have frayed hypochromic cytoplasm, and the appearance of Hb in the cells may be delayed (as in iron deficiency anemia). Sideroblasts are decreased, but storage of iron is normal or increased.

The serum iron concentration is characteristically decreased, the TIBC is decreased or normal (in contrast to iron deficiency anemia, in which the TIBC is elevated), and the percent saturation is decreased. Erythrocyte protoporphyrin and serum ferritin are elevated.

The most important pathogenetic mechanism of ACD is the presence of high levels of cytokines, which may result in decreased red cell survival, altered iron metabolism, direct inhibition of hematopoiesis, and decreased EPO secretion. Tumor necrosis factor-α (TNF-α) plays a significant role in inflammation and immune response. TNF-α levels are increased in patients with cancer, rheumatoid arthritis, infection, and the acquired immunodeficiency syndrome. In vitro inhibition of human erythroid colony formation, burst forming units-erythroid (BFU-E), and colony forming units-erythroid (CFU-E) by TNF-α has been reported. Similarly, an inhibitory action of IL-1 and interferon-γ (IFN-γ) on erythropoiesis has been implicated. Ceramide, a product of cytokine-induced enzymatic hydrolysis of cell membrane sphingomyelin, plays a role as a messenger in the inhibitory effects of IFN-γ (Means, 2003).

EPO levels, although above normal, have been disproportionate to the degree of anemia, indicating relative EPO deficiency in ACD. Inhibitory effects of cytokines on EPO synthesis sites such as renal and liver cells have been suggested. The relative deficiency of EPO induces neocytolysis (i.e., selective hemolysis of the youngest red blood cells). Thus, a mild hemolytic event usually accompanies ACD (Risso, 2007).

Recently, hepcidin has been shown to be elevated in ACD through induction by IL-6 and is considered an acute phase reactant. As mentioned earlier, hepcidin interferes with the release of intracellular iron. Recent evidence also suggests that hepcidin may exert an inhibitory effect on erythroid colony formation at certain levels of EPO, and thus may provide a bone marrow inhibitory effect (Dallalio, 2006).

The anemia usually fails to respond to iron therapy. However, patients treated with EPO have shown improvement.

Anemia of Renal Insufficiency

A normocytic normochromic anemia is commonly encountered in patients with chronic renal failure (CRF). The correlation between severity of anemia and degree of elevation of blood urea nitrogen (BUN) is positive but not strictly linear. When creatinine clearance falls below 20 mL/min, the Hct is usually below 0.30 (Caro, 2006).

Several factors are often involved in the anemia of chronic renal failure. Decreased production of EPO by the damaged kidney is probably the important factor in most cases in which the BUN exceeds 100 mg/dL. Both ineffective erythropoiesis and impaired ability of the marrow to respond to EPO appear to be present to some degree.

Inhibitors of erythropoiesis have been demonstrated in the plasma of patients with chronic renal failure. The nature of these inhibitory factors is not known; however, parathyroid hormone and spermine have been implicated as inhibitors of erythropoiesis. Recent studies indicate the presence of a high level of inflammatory cytokines, such as IL-1, IL-4, IL-6, and TNF-α, in patients with CRF. As discussed under Anemia of Chronic Disease, these cytokines exert a bone marrow suppressive effect and probably contribute to the development of anemia (Stenvinkel, 2003). The role of hepcidin in this type of anemia is also being investigated.

Hemolysis is a significant feature in many cases of CRF. There appears to be an extracorpuscular factor in uremic plasma that has a detrimental effect on red cell metabolism and results in morphologically deformed cells (echinocytes and spiculated red cells). Numerous irregularly contracted and fragmented cells are seen in the hemolytic-uremic syndrome and in malignant hypertension as a result of traumatic damage incurred by the red cells in traversing damaged small blood vessels. Changes in red cell membrane adenosine triphosphatase (ATPase) and transketolase may render the red cells more sensitive to oxidant drugs or chemicals.

In addition, bleeding is a common problem in chronic renal disease, probably owing to thrombocytopenia, in some patients, or to platelet functional defects, which are present in most patients. Anemia due to iron deficiency from blood loss should always be suspected. Folic acid deficiency may be a problem in patients in a dialysis program, in that folic acid is readily moved into the dialysis bath.

Anemia in Liver Disease

Chronic posthemorrhagic anemia; hypoplastic anemia secondary to viral-induced marrow suppression; folate-deficient megaloblastic anemia due to poor nutrition in alcoholic cirrhosis; and acquired hemolytic anemia associated with Coombs'-positive red cells, congestive splenomegaly, or lipid disturbances may occur in liver disease (Gallagher, 2009). Iron deficiency anemia is the most common in approximately 50% of patients, followed by hypersplenism in approximately 25% of patients (Ozatli, 2000). IFN-α and ribavarin (Rbv) are common therapies for hepatitis C infection. Rbv induces suppression of erythropoiesis, possibly through downregulation of EPO receptors. In addition, Rbv can cause a dose-dependent hemolytic anemia. IFN-α can produce anemia through suppression of hematopoietic progenitor cell proliferation and induction of apoptosis of erythroid progenitor cells (Dieterich, 2003).

In addition to these, an anemia associated with liver disease is characterized by shortened red cell survival and relatively inadequate red cell production. It is exaggerated by an increased blood volume that appears to correlate with the degree of portal hypertension. The red cells are normocytic or macrocytic (thin macrocytes). Frequently, target cells are present, especially in obstructive jaundice; these have increased surface membrane with increased cholesterol and lecithin content. However, the phospholipid/cholesterol ratio is normal. Reticulocytes may be slightly increased, and platelets may be normal or decreased. The bone marrow may be slightly hypercellular, and erythropoiesis is macronormoblastic rather than megaloblastic. Changes in leukocytes, such as those seen in megaloblastic anemias, are not seen, and this type of anemia does not respond to cobalamin (vitamin B_{12}) or folic acid. The anemia is of unknown origin.

A small proportion of patients with severe cirrhosis have a hemolytic anemia associated with "spur cells," which are red cells with thorny projections similar to acanthocytes. As with target cells, the spur cells occur secondary to lipid abnormalities in the plasma; they have increased surface membrane with increased cholesterol, but normal phospholipid content in the membrane. The increased membrane cholesterol tends to associate with the outer membrane leaflet, making it more rigid. The spleen attempts to remodel the membrane, resulting in characteristic membrane projections (Gallagher, 2001).

Anemia in Endocrine Disease

Uncomplicated anemia in hypothyroidism is mild to moderate, with Hb concentration rarely less than 8–9 g/dL; it is normochromic and normocytic without reticulocytosis and with normal red cell survival. It reflects decreased marrow production due to a smaller tissue O_2 requirement and subsequent reduced EPO secretion. Because plasma volume is decreased in hypothyroidism, the apparent degree of anemia may not be proportional to the decrease in red cell mass. Hypothyroidism may be complicated by iron deficiency anemia, producing a microcytic anemia, particularly in females, as a result of menorrhagia, although in males, it may be caused by achlorhydria and diminished iron absorption. Macrocytosis is frequently observed. Although the incidence of pernicious anemia in patients with hypothyroidism may be increased, most cases of macrocytosis are due to folate deficiency. Approximately 10%–25% of patients with hyperthyroidism have anemia, which is mainly due to increased plasma volume (Greg, 2006).

In adrenal cortical hormone deficiency, a mild normochromic normocytic anemia is present. The cause is unclear, but the condition is corrected by hormone replacement.

Deficient testosterone secretion in men results in a decrease in red cell production of 1–2 g Hb/dL (to a value comparable with that of women). This appears to be due to a stimulatory effect of androgens on EPO secretion and occurs through enhanced EPO action on the marrow, and possibly as a direct effect on a subset of marrow cells, such as stromal cells.

Pituitary deficiency also causes moderately severe normocytic anemia, which is associated with marrow hypoplasia. The mechanism is probably complex and related to loss of function of multiple endocrine glands and possibly loss of growth hormone effect.

A small number of patients with hyperparathyroidism have a normocytic, normochromic anemia. Earlier studies suggested that the parathyroid hormone may suppress normal erythropoiesis. More recent studies failed to support this theory. The cause of the anemia is unknown but is likely related to marrow fibrosis (Greg, 2006).

Anemia Associated With Bone Marrow Infiltration (Myelophthisic Anemia)

This anemia is associated with marrow replacement by (or involvement with) abnormal cells or tissue component, such as metastatic carcinoma, multiple myeloma, leukemia, lymphoma, lipidoses or storage diseases, and certain other conditions.

Normochromic and normocytic (occasionally macrocytic) anemia of varying severity is present. Reticulocytes are often increased, and the number of normoblasts is usually out of proportion to the severity of the anemia. The leukocyte count is normal or reduced (occasionally elevated), and immature neutrophils and even myeloblasts may be found. Platelets are normal or decreased, and bizarre, atypical platelets can sometimes be seen.

Examination of the marrow will usually reveal the condition responsible for this reaction. Mechanical crowding out of the hematopoietic tissue by the pathologic process has been assumed but not proved and probably is not the usual cause. Often the amount of erythropoietic tissue in the marrow as determined by morphologic and kinetic studies is normal or increased. The mechanism described earlier under Anemia of Chronic Disease may often play a role, but the reason for the outpouring of immature cells into the blood is not clear.

In addition to myelophthisic anemias, circulating normoblasts and immature neutrophils can be seen in hemolytic anemias, severe anemias due to other causes, severe infections, and congestive heart failure, but usually the normoblasts are not as numerous.

The **leukoerythroblastotic reaction** associated with myelophthisic anemias cannot always be distinguished from the blood picture of primary myelofibrosis, which is one of the myeloproliferative neoplasms. In primary myelofibrosis, enlargement of the spleen and liver is almost always found. In the blood film, more severe red cell abnormalities, leukocytosis, myeloblasts and immature granulocytes of all varieties (not just neutrophils), increased basophils, more atypical platelets, more numerous megakaryocyte fragments, and dwarf megakaryocytes are all findings more characteristic of primary myelofibrosis than of a leukoerythroblastotic reaction of some other cause. Examination of the bone marrow biopsy is necessary for the final diagnosis.

Aplastic Anemia

AA usually refers to pancytopenia associated with a severe reduction in the amount of hematopoietic tissue that results in deficient production of blood cells in the absence of a bone marrow infiltrative process or increased reticulin (Marsh, 2009). Usually two of the following three blood parameters are needed to diagnose AA: Hgb less than 100 g/L, granulocyte count less than 1.5×10^9/L, and platelet count less than 50×10^9/L. The marrow, although hypocellular, may have patchy areas of normocellularity, or even hypercellularity. The diagnosis of **severe AA** is made in pancytopenic patients when at least two of the following three peripheral blood values—granulocyte count less than 0.5×10^9/L, platelet count less than 20×10^9/L, or reticulocyte count less than 20×10^9/L, or 1% (corrected for Hct)—are present and the bone marrow is less than 30% cellular (Young, 2002; Marsh, 2009). The term **very severe AA** is used when granulocyte count is less than 0.2×10^9/L (Young, 2002). Otherwise, the AA would be classified as moderate or nonsevere. The incidence of AA is 2 per million per year based on retrospective studies in Europe and North America, and is about 2–3 times higher in East Asia (Marsh, 2009).

Clinical Features

The clinical course may be acute and fulminating, with profound pancytopenia and a rapid progression to death, or the disorder may have an insidious onset and a chronic course. The symptoms and signs depend on the degree of the deficiencies: bleeding from thrombocytopenia, infection from neutropenia, and signs and symptoms of anemia. As a rule, splenomegaly and lymphadenopathy are absent. Bleeding is the most common presentation of AA, occurring in approximately 40% of patients (Young, 2009). Bleeding usually manifests as easy bruisability, gum bleeds, and episodic nosebleeds. Less than 5% of patients present with infection.

Etiology

Aplastic anemias are of diverse origin. Since 1980, in approximately 70% of cases, no specific etiologic agent could be correlated with the disease; such cases are considered idiopathic. Drug- and chemical-related aplastic anemias account for 11%–20%, and those associated with infectious hepatitis account for 2%–9% of cases (Young, 2009).

Pathogenesis

Hematopoietic failure may occur at any level in the differentiation of bone marrow precursor cells. Insufficient stem cells may be assayed as long-term culture-initiating cells, or committed stem cells (progenitor cells) may be insufficient. The CD34+ cells in the bone marrow, which contain most of the stem cells and committed progenitor cells, are markedly decreased in patients with AA. Although in theory AA could result from a defective marrow microenvironment, these defects do not appear to be causative for most patients (Young, 2002).

The mechanism of AA is suggested to fall under two main categories: direct damage and immune-mediated destruction of marrow cells. Direct damage to the hematopoietic stem and progenitor cells could be caused by a known agent, such as cytotoxic drugs, irradiation and viruses, or an unknown agent, which in some way alters the ability of the cell to proliferate or differentiate. Immune-mediated destruction of stem and progenitor cell compartments results from cytotoxic lymphocyte activation, cytokine production, and specific cell elimination. Recent studies favor immune-mediated mechanisms for AA and suggest that chemical and viral antigens may initiate the destructive immune process (Young, 2009). In fact, acquired AA is being viewed now as an immune-mediated disease.

Prognosis

Complications are due to infection, bleeding, and problems of iron overload from repeated transfusions. The prognosis appears to depend on the severity of marrow damage. However, the initial blood count and response to therapy during the first few months of treatment are important prognostic factors (Young, 2009). In a series of 101 patients treated by conventional methods (Williams, 1978), 25% of patients died within 4 months of onset of symptoms, 50% died within 12 months, and 71% within 5 years. Those who died within 4 months had significantly lower reticulocyte, neutrophil, and platelet counts; a lower percentage of myeloid cells in the marrow; and a shorter interval between onset of symptoms and visit to the physician (Lynch, 1975). Other factors that correlated with a poor prognosis included male gender, but not age of the patient or cause of the aplasia (Williams, 1978). Yet, the age of the patient usually influences the decision regarding which therapy the patient should receive. In some survivors, partial recovery is common. With the introduction of modern treatment protocols by immunosuppressive therapy and bone marrow transplantation, long-term survival rates greater than 60% are reported. Survivors have a much higher risk of developing myelodysplastic syndrome, paroxysmal nocturnal hemoglobinuria, acute leukemia, and solid tumors (Young, 2002; Marsh, 2009).

Management

Treatment includes bone marrow transplantation for patients younger than 40 years of age with severe disease if there is an HLA-matched donor. Children and young adults have a much higher survival probability compared with older adults (Young, 2009). Immune suppression using antilymphocyte globulin and cyclosporin A may induce hematologic remission in some patients. Androgens appear to be least helpful in the stimulation of any residual marrow. Supportive care must be used with caution. Certainly, appropriate antibiotics should be used to combat infection; however, the risk for sensitization should be considered with the administration of blood products. Single-donor platelets or platelets from HLA-matched donors are preferred (Alter, 1998).

Idiopathic Aplastic Anemia

In patients with pancytopenia and a hypocellular marrow, a search should be made for evidence of significant exposure to radiation, drugs, and chemicals of known or possible propensity to injure the marrow, so that further exposure can be eliminated. Nevertheless, in approximately 70% of cases of aplastic anemia, no suspected causal relationship to toxic agents can be found, and it is these that are designated as idiopathic.

The symptoms and signs do not differ, but the onset is commonly more insidious than in toxic or hypersensitive aplastic anemias.

Blood

The red cells are usually normal to increased in size with a varying degree of anisocytosis and poikilocytosis, particularly oval macrocytes. Macrocytosis may be a prominent feature, particularly in response to high levels of EPO. The RDW may be increased, even without transfusion (Elghetany, 1997). Polychromasia, stippling, and normoblasts are most often conspicuously absent. Leukopenia with marked decrease in granulocytes and a relative lymphocytosis are observed. In severe leukopenia, there is often an absolute lymphocytopenia. Neutrophil granules may be larger than normal and may stain dark red (unlike the "toxic" granules found in infections), and the neutrophil alkaline phosphatase may be elevated. However, neutrophil left shift is not seen in the absence of infection (Elghetany, 1997). Thrombocytopenia is part of the picture. Monocytopenia may be present. The serum iron is usually increased, and serum cobalamin and folate levels are usually normal. Although an occasional patient is hypogammaglobulinemic, most patients have normal levels of serum immune globulins.

Bone Marrow. In most cases, the aspirate consists of red cells, lymphocytes, some plasma cells, mast cells, and fatty particles. Marrow sections will show fatty tissue with inconspicuous fibrosis and islands of lymphocytes and plasma cells (Fig. 32-8). Although focal areas of predominantly erythroid normocellularity or hypercellularity (hot spots) may sometimes be present, the overall cellularity is decreased. The hot spots usually show erythroid precursors with delayed nuclear maturation at a high proliferative rate. Storage iron is increased.

Erythrokinetics. The increased serum iron concentration is a valuable early sign of erythroid hypoplasia and reflects decreased plasma iron turnover. In addition, erythrocyte utilization of iron is decreased. Both effective and total erythropoiesis, therefore, are decreased in aplastic anemia.

Aplastic Anemia Associated With Chemical or Physical Agents

Toxic Aplastic Anemias. A number of physical and chemical agents produce marrow damage in all humans and animals exposed to a sufficient dose. Examples include ionizing radiation; mustard compounds; benzene; and antineoplastic agents such as busulfan, urethane, and antimetabolites. Benzene, although strongly linked to AA, is now considered less of a problem than in the past because of reduction in exposure.

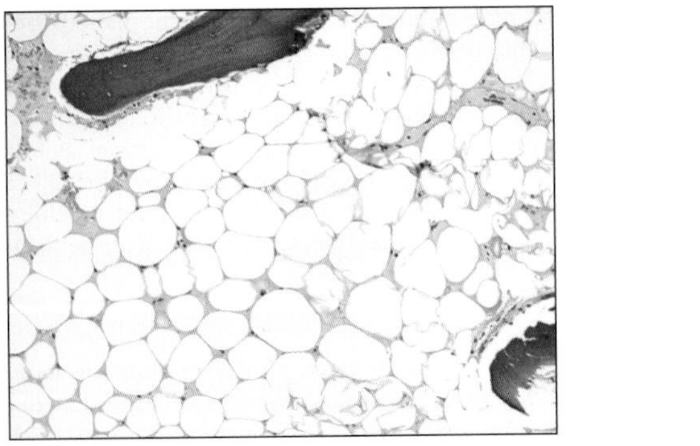

Figure 32-8 Section of hypocellular marrow, aplastic anemia. Cellularity is less than 5%.

Ionizing Radiation. Effects depend on the radiosensitivity of the cells and the capacity of the cells to regenerate, as well as the survival rate of cells in the blood. Erythroid cells are most sensitive, granulocytes have intermediate sensitivity, and megakaryocytes are the least sensitive of the three. Stromal cells are relatively insensitive.

After acute exposure to radiation, the reticulocyte count falls, but the red cells decline slowly because of their long survival. Within the first few hours, a neutrophilic leukocytosis occurs as the result of a shift from marginal and probably marrow storage pools. A fall in lymphocytes occurs after the first day and is responsible for the early leukopenia, because lymphocytes are sensitive to irradiation and are directly killed. After 5 days or so, granulocytes begin to fall. The platelets decrease later. Platelets are often the last to return to normal in the recovery phase. Quiescent marrow stem cells are remarkably resistant to a single dose of irradiation. However, chronic exposure to low-dose irradiation, including localized radiation for ankylosing spondylitis, is associated with delayed increased risk for AA because of its impact on the stem cell replicating pool (Young, 2009).

Hypersensitive Aplastic Anemias. A large number of drugs produce marrow damage in some individuals after single or repeated exposures. Effects are not dose related as they are in the previously discussed toxic aplasia. Agents include antimicrobial drugs (salvarsan, chloramphenicol, sulfonamides, chlortetracycline, streptomycin), anticonvulsants (mephenytoin, trimethadione), analgesics (phenylbutazone), antithyroid drugs (carbimazole), antihistaminics (tripelennamine), H_2-histamine receptor antagonists (cimetidine), insecticides (dichlorophenyltrichloroethane [DDT]), and other chemicals—some known (gold compounds, quinacrine, chlorpromazine, hair dyes, bismuth, mercury) and others unknown. The nonsteroidal antiinflammatory medications are becoming more linked to an increased risk for developing AA following marked reduction in the use of chloramphenicol.

Chloramphenicol is an important drug in this category. This antibiotic was considered to be the most common cause of AA at the peak of its use, which began in 1949. Reactions of the marrow to chloramphenicol are of two types, which are possibly unrelated (Alter, 1998).

In about half of patients who receive chloramphenicol, increased serum iron, reticulocytopenia with anemia, neutropenia, and thrombocytopenia are found. The marrow may show decreased erythroid cells and vacuolization of primitive erythroid and granulocyte precursors. These changes are dose related, time dependent, and reversible.

In a very small proportion of persons receiving chloramphenicol, an irreversible AA develops that may be fatal. Pancytopenia occurs 3 weeks to 5 months from the last dosage. No relationship has been established between the reversible erythropoietic lesion and the development of aplastic anemia; it may be that individual susceptibility is responsible for the latter. For this reason, it is essential that restraint be employed in using the drug; monitoring its administration with blood cell counts is not an effective preventive measure.

Aplastic Anemia Associated With Other Disease

Infection. Viral infections are frequently associated with limited marrow suppression, typically neutropenia and less commonly thrombocytopenia. Marrow aplasia has been described as a rare sequela to viral hepatitis, occurring a few months after onset when the hepatitis is resolving. It is estimated at less than 0.07% of hepatitis cases in children and 2% of patients with non-A, non-B hepatitis. Almost all cases are seronegative for hepatitis A, B, C, and G. These patients are usually males younger than age 20; the prognosis is usually grave, and bone marrow transplantation is considered early in the course of the disease (Young, 2002). Parvovirus has been associated with transient erythroid aplastic crisis in patients with chronic hemolytic disorders (Young, 2002). Human immunodeficiency virus and Epstein-Barr virus may also cause hematopoietic depression. The mechanism of virus-induced bone marrow failure may be related to direct cytotoxicity, or, more likely, to immune-mediated mechanisms secondary to molecular mimicry, antigen spread, and danger signals caused by the infection (Young, 2002).

Paroxysmal Nocturnal Hemoglobinuria. This rare hemolytic process (see later discussion) may be followed by aplastic anemia. Usually in paroxysmal nocturnal hemoglobinuria (PNH), a variable degree of marrow hypofunction coexists. Alternatively, in some patients who present with AA, the red cell defect of PNH may be present or may appear during the course of the disease. Recent studies using sensitive techniques, such as flow cytometry, to detect cells with PNH defect indicate that as many as 40%–50% of patients with AA may have some surface marker evidence of PNH. However, hemolytic disease occurs in approximately one third of these patients. The clonal expansion of PNH cells may have an immunologic background, as evidenced by the strong association of HLA-DR2 and PNH (Young, 2002).

Pregnancy. Pregnancy occurring in a patient with acquired AA may make the pancytopenia more severe. Occasionally, however, AA occurs during pregnancy and remits following delivery. In some such cases, aplasia recurs during a second pregnancy. Infants may be anemic, thrombocytopenic, or leukopenic. Survival rates for AA in pregnancy have been relatively high for the mother (83%) and the baby (75%). Hemorrhage is the most common cause of death in these patients (Young, 2009).

Thymoma. Although thymomas are usually associated with pure red cell aplasias, other bone marrow elements may also become depressed. Pancytopenia, often with hypoplastic bone marrow, occurs in rare cases with thymoma. AA may occur as a late complication after the treatment of thymoma (Ritchie, 2002a).

Immunologic Diseases. AA occurs in approximately 10% of cases of eosinophilic fasciitis. The prognosis of AA in this setting is usually poor. AA may be associated with systemic lupus erythematosus (SLE) and rheumatoid arthritis (RA), although the role of drug therapy in the pathogenesis of AA has been considered (Young, 2009). AA may also complicate multiple sclerosis, congenital immunodeficiency syndromes, and immune thyroid disease.

Inherited Aplastic Anemia

The term **inherited AA** designates individuals with a genetic predisposition to chronic bone marrow failure, which may be associated with other congenital anomalies. Between 30% and 35% of childhood AA cases are inherited. In a study of 134 children with AA, 40 patients were diagnosed with inherited aplastic anemia. Twenty-six had Fanconi's anemia (FA), 10 patients had familial AA without classic signs of FA, and 4 patients presented with amegakaryocytic thrombocytopenia that later developed into complete aplasia (Alter, 1998).

Fanconi's Anemia. FA is an autosomal recessive disorder with a carrier frequency of 1/300 in the United States and Europe (Alter, 2002). Often more than one member of a family is affected. The pancytopenia becomes obvious after infancy and is usually significant by the eighth year of life. The anemia is usually normochromic and may be macrocytic; increased levels of Hb F and i antigen may be observed; the marrow is generally hypocellular. Developmental anomalies are present and may include hyperpigmentation, short stature, hypogonadism, malformations of the extremities (e.g., aplasia of the radius, abnormalities of the thumbs), microcephaly, and malformation of other organs (e.g., heart, kidneys). Chromosomal defects consisting of random breaks and rearrangements characteristically are present in blood lymphocytes, as well as in marrow cells. Chromosomal breakage becomes more evident when the cultured cells are challenged with alkylating and DNA cross-linking agents such as mitomycin C and diepoxybutane. A breakthrough in investigating FA evolved from the observation that hybrid cells from FA and normal cells resulted in correction of the abnormal chromosome fragility, a process known as complementation. More than 13 complementation groups have been distinguished to date (Freedman, 2009). The most common is complementation group A (FANCA), which occurs in approximately 70% of FA patients. Several FA proteins form a nuclear complex that is involved in DNA repair (Alter, 2002). The predicted median survival in FA is 19 years. Patients with FA are at higher risk of developing leukemia and nonhematologic tumors, particularly in the head and neck, liver, lower esophagus, vulva, and anus, with an overall incidence of neoplasia of 15% (Alter, 1998). The median age for all cancers in patients with FA was 16 years (Freedman, 2009).

Other Inherited Aplastic Anemias. A few children present with bleeding manifestations secondary to amegakaryocytic thrombocytopenia. As their disease progresses, they develop a pancytopenia and a hypocellular marrow. Chromosome breakage studies are usually normal. The mode of inheritance is autosomal recessive. The molecular defect is related to a mutation in the gene for thrombopoietin receptor, *c-mpl*, which maps to 1p35 (Alter, 2002).

Pancytopenia and hypoplastic anemia may develop in a subset of patients with other familial disorders. Some patients with dyskeratosis congenita (reticulated hyperpigmentation of skin, dystrophic nails, and mucous membrane leukoplakia) and Shwachman-Diamond syndrome (exocrine pancreatic insufficiency and neutropenia) develop AA during the course of their disease (Alter, 2002).

Pure Red Cell Aplasia

Transitory Arrest of Erythropoiesis (Transient Aplastic Crises)

This may occur during the course of a hemolytic anemia (often preceded by an infection), and the combination of aplasia and hemolysis becomes a life-threatening situation. Red cell production may occasionally cease during or following rather minor infections in normal children or adults, at which time the marrow will show absence of all but a few of the most immature erythroid precursors. Aplastic episodes in chronic hemolytic anemias often appear to be due to parvovirus B19 infection. This virus inhibits erythropoiesis by infecting mature CFU-Es. The morphologic hallmark of the disease is the presence of scattered giant pronormoblasts in the bone marrow aspirate with marked reduction in the more mature erythroid precursors. Nuclear inclusion may be difficult to identify with Wright's stain. The aplastic crises resulting from parvovirus infection are transient, with erythroid marrow recovery in 1 to 2 weeks after onset (Erslev, 2001c).

Transient Erythroblastopenia of Childhood

Transient erythroblastopenia of childhood (TEC) occurs in previously healthy children, usually younger than 8 years of age, with most affected children between 1 and 3 years of age. It is characterized by a moderate to severe normocytic anemia, severe reticulocytopenia, transient neutropenia (20%), and increased platelet counts (60% of patients). Macrocytosis is usually observed during recovery because of the effects of reticulocytes. A history of a viral infection within the previous 3 months is frequently elicited. The bone marrow is generally normocellular and shows virtual absence of erythroid precursors, except for a few early forms. Granulocytic maturation arrest may occur in some neutropenic patients. Patients recover within 1–2 months without therapy. TEC can occur in siblings simultaneously and in seasonal clusters. Transient neurologic manifestations, such as hemiparesis and seizures, may accompany TEC (Freedman, 2009). In most cases, the pathogenesis involves humoral inhibition of erythropoiesis; cell-mediated immune suppression was identified in about 25% of cases, but parvovirus has not been proven to be the cause of TEC (Alter, 2002; Freedman, 2009).

Congenital Red Cell Aplasia (Diamond-Blackfan Anemia; Congenital Hypoplastic Anemia)

This is a rare, congenital red cell aplasia that usually becomes obvious during the first year of life but may occur as late as 6 years of age. Severe anemia is usually macrocytic, reticulocyte level is low, leukocytes are normal or slightly decreased, platelets are normal or increased, and the marrow usually shows a reduction in all developing erythroid cells, except normal granulocytic and megakaryocytic cell lines. In a small number of cases, residual erythroid precursors are detected. These precursors are mostly pronormoblasts. Hb F is elevated (5%–25%) to a degree not expected for the patient's age, and the antigen i is often present. Red cell adenosine deaminase (ADA) is usually increased. These findings contrast with TEC, in which the red cells are normocytic, the Hb F is normal, the antigen i is absent, and red cell enzymes are at a lower level (characteristic of an older cell population) (Alter, 1998).

Approximately half of cases have an autosomal dominant pattern of inheritance with variable penetrance. The defect appears to be in the erythroid-committed progenitor cells. CFU-Es and BFU-Es are decreased in the marrow, and BFU-Es, which normally circulate, are absent or decreased in the blood. In addition, these progenitor cells exhibit an acceleration in programmed cell death (apoptosis) and fail to respond in in vitro culture systems to normal T cells and to usual levels of EPO, suggesting a qualitative defect. A mutation in the *RPS19* gene was detected in 25% of patients. This gene encodes a ribosomal protein subunit of nucleolar localization (Alter, 2002).

About 75% of patients respond at least partially to corticosteroids, and the overall long-term survival is about 65%, although many patients require long-term steroid use (Alter, 1998).

Acquired Pure Red Cell Aplasia

Among middle-aged adults, selective failure of red cell production occurs rarely. Reticulocytopenia and a cellular marrow devoid of all but the most primitive erythroid precursors are characteristic. Leukocyte and platelet production is normal. About half of reported cases have been associated with thymoma, usually a noninvasive spindle cell type. However, only 5%–10% of patients with thymoma have the anemia. Remission of the anemia occurs in about one fourth of cases following surgical removal of the thymoma. Chronic acquired red cell aplasia has also been associated with other conditions, such as drugs, collagen vascular disorders, viral infections such as HIV, lymphoproliferative disorders of granular lymphocytes, or other disorders with immunologic aberrations. Most of these anemias appear to be part of a spectrum of autoimmune cytopenias in which the target cells are erythroid stem cells or normoblasts. In some patients, antibodies that react with these cells have been identified. Corticosteroids and immunosuppressive drugs have been used as therapy, but less than half of patients achieve satisfactory remission (Erslev, 2001c).

Sideroblastic Anemia

Sideroblastic anemia is characterized by hypochromic red cells, which are microcytic in the hereditary forms and often macrocytic in the acquired forms of the disease (Wiley, 2009). The red cells may be mixed with normochromic cells, so that the appearance is dimorphic (see Fig. 30-13). The serum iron concentration is increased, the TIBC is decreased, and the percent saturation of the iron-binding protein is greatly elevated. The marrow shows markedly increased storage iron (see Fig. 32-5), erythroid hyperplasia with evidence of defective hemoglobinization, and increased numbers of sideroblasts. In addition, increased numbers of siderotic granules per cell and granules surround the nucleus (with most authors requiring five or more iron granules encircling at least one third of the circumference), forming "ring sideroblasts" (Swerdlow, 2008) (see Fig. 32-17). In the latter case, iron loading of mitochondria is seen by electron microscopy. These findings are associated with defective synthesis of heme, which may be due to any of several possible enzyme defects. Occasionally, megaloblast-like changes are seen in the erythroid cells, but changes typical of cobalamin or folate deficiency are not seen in granulocytes unless folate deficiency coexists.

Hereditary Sideroblastic Anemias

Hereditary sideroblastic anemias include several modes of inheritance (i.e., X-linked, autosomal dominant, and autosomal recessive). The X-linked forms generally exhibit low levels of δ-aminolevulinic acid synthase (ALAS) enzyme. This occurs in males and may not appear until adolescence. It is rare, but a few family studies have been well documented. In contrast to acquired sideroblastic anemia, the ring sideroblast abnormality is usually found in late, nondividing erythroblasts (Bottomley, 1982). The gene for ALAS-2 isoenzyme (erythroid ALAS) has been localized to the X chromosome, and a point mutation of this gene *(Xp11.21)* seems to occur in most X-linked sideroblastic anemiaa (Wiley, 2009). Mutations of the *ALAS-2* gene may result in enzyme low affinity for pyridoxal phosphate, structural instability, abnormal catalytic site, or increased susceptibility to mitochondrial proteases. The degree of anemia improves with pyridoxine supplementation when the mutation disrupts the catalytic association between the enzyme and pyridoxal phosphate (Alcindor, 2002). Hereditary sideroblastic anemias may be due to a defect in the mitochondria (i.e., mitochondrial cytopathy). Most of these disorders are produced by deletions in the mitochondrial genome, which may account for as much as 30% of the entire mitochondrial genome (Alcindor, 2002). These rare diseases are usually associated with systemic manifestations such as Pearson's syndrome (pancreatic insufficiency, vacuolation of bone marrow cells, ring sideroblasts, and a variable degree of marrow failure).

Acquired Sideroblastic Anemias

Refractory Anemia With Ring Sideroblasts. Refractory anemia with ring sideroblasts (RARS) is a category of myelodysplastic syndromes (Swerdlow, 2008; see also Chapter 33). The dimorphic anemia has both hypochromic-microcytic and macrocytic red blood cells, and the MCV is usually high (see Fig. 30-15). At least 15% of erythroblasts (early and late forms) in bone marrow are ring sideroblasts. Other manifestation of dysplasia in the erythroid cell line may be seen. When dysplastic features involve myeloid and megakaryocytic cell lines as well, the designation **refractory cytopenia with multilineage dysplasia** is given. Growing evidence suggests that RARS may be caused by mutations of mitochondrial DNA (Swerdlow, 2008).

Secondary (Drug- or Toxin-Induced) Sideroblastic Anemia

This form of sideroblastic anemia is secondary to some agent that interferes with heme synthesis; recognition is important because hematologic improvement occurs if the agent is removed.

The **antituberculosis drugs** isoniazid, cycloserine, and pyrazinamide cause sideroblastic abnormalities in some patients on long-term therapy.

Lead poisoning is an important member of this group because environmental exposure to lead is usually unrecognized and needs to be detected. Lead interferes with heme synthesis by blocking the enzymes ALAS, ALA dehydratase, and heme synthase. These blocks are only partial and of different degrees; ALA and coproporphyrin are increased in the urine. **Chloramphenicol** also results in ring sideroblast formation, probably by inhibiting mitochondrial protein synthesis. **Copper deficiency** or **zinc overload** can produce sideroblastic anemia, vacuolated marrow cells, and neutropenia. Large quantities of ingested zinc interfere with copper absorption and produce manifestations of copper deficiency. Copper chelators in large doses, such as penicillamine, can produce sideroblastic anemia.

Ethanol-induced anemia is perhaps the most common of the reversible sideroblastic anemias. Folate deficiency, hypomagnesemia, and hypokalemia are concomitant findings. Alcohol may produce ring sideroblasts through decreased plasma levels of pyridoxal phosphate, along with decreased activity of ALA dehydratase and ferrochelatase (Wiley, 2009). After withdrawal of alcohol intake, abnormal sideroblasts usually disappear within a few days.

Primary pyridoxine deficiency, often associated with malnutrition, is occasionally associated with sideroblastic anemia. However, other manifestations, such as peripheral neuropathy and dermatitis, dominate the clinical presentation. Sideroblastic anemia as the sole manifestation of pyridoxine deficiency has not been reported in humans, although it occurs in animals (Alcindor, 2002).

Refractory Anemia

An ill-defined group of chronic anemias usually occurs in individuals over the age of 50. Normocytic or macrocytic anemia, reticulocytopenia, often pancytopenia, and a hypercellular marrow showing erythroid hyperplasia with a variable degree of dyserythropoiesis are present. Often the patient has been treated with cobalamin, folic acid, and iron without response. The process is usually unremitting, and in a small proportion of cases additional dysplastic changes in marrow cells and increased blast cells evolve into an acute leukemia. Refractory anemias, therefore, are considered one of the myelodysplastic syndromes (see Chapter 33).

Congenital Dyserythropoietic Anemias

Congenital dyserythropoietic anemias (CDAs) represent a family of inherited refractory anemias characterized by ineffective erythropoiesis and marrow erythroid multinuclearity.

At least three types have thus far been separated on the basis of marrow and serologic findings (Heimpel, 2004). CDA-I has megaloblastic changes with some binuclearity in approximately 5% of marrow erythroblasts, internuclear chromatin bridges, and a macrocytic anemia. Some cases have an abnormality in the *CDAN1* gene located on the long arm of chromosome 15 (Heimpel, 2004). CDA-II is more common than the others and shows binuclearity and multinuclearity of 10%–40% of erythroid precursors with pluripolar mitoses and karyorrhexis. The anemia is normocytic. CDA-II is distinguished from the others in that it has a positive acidified serum test (with some but not all normal sera) and a negative sucrose hemolysis test. It is known as hereditary erythroblastic multinuclearity with positive acidified serum test (HEM-PAS). The red cells have an antigen not present on normal or PNH cells, and about one third of normal sera contain the corresponding immunoglobulin (Ig)M antibody. In addition, red cells in CDA-II react strongly with anti-i and anti-I. Electron microscopy demonstrates an excess of endoplasmic reticulum parallel to the cell membrane, which gives the appearance of a double membrane in late erythroblasts and some erythrocytes. CDA-II is thought to be related to abnormal membrane glycosylation. The gene for CDA-II *(CDAN2)* has not been identified but maps to 20q11.2 (Freedman, 2009). CDA-III has giant erythroid precursors, with more pronounced multinuclearity (gigantoblasts) in 10%–40% of erythroid precursors, along with a macrocytic anemia. A putative gene for CDA-III *(CDAN3)* has been recently localized on chromosome 15 near the *CDAN1* gene (Heimpel, 2004). In contrast to CDA-I and CDA-II, which are autosomal recessive, CDA-III has autosomal dominant inheritance. Other variants have been described in a small number of families.

BLOOD LOSS ANEMIA

Acute Posthemorrhagic Anemia

Blood may be lost from the circulation externally or internally into a tissue space or body cavity. If blood is lost over a short time in amounts sufficient to cause anemia, **acute posthemorrhagic anemia** occurs. Normal healthy individuals are able to compensate for rapid blood loss of up to 20% of circulating blood volume with few symptoms (Hillman, 1996). After a single episode of excessive bleeding, the major manifestations are those due to depletion of blood volume (hypovolemia). After a day or so, blood volume is returned to previous levels by movement of fluid into the circulation, and anemia becomes evident.

The earliest hematologic change is a transient fall in the platelet count, which may rise to elevated levels within an hour. The next development is a moderate neutrophilic leukocytosis with a shift to the left; a maximum leukocyte count of 10–35 × 10^9/L may occur in 2–5 hours. Hb and Hct do not fall immediately but only slowly as tissue fluids move into the circulation to compensate for lost blood volume. The fall in Hb and Hct may not reveal the full extent of red cell loss until 2 or 3 days after the hemorrhage.

The anemia that develops at first is normochromic and normocytic, with a normal MCV and mean cell hemoglobin concentration (MCHC) and only minimal anisocytosis and poikilocytosis. Increased EPO secretion stimulates erythroid proliferation in the marrow, and reticulocytes begin to reach the circulation in 3–5 days, reaching a maximum by 10 days or so. During this period, transient macrocytosis (increased MCV), increased polychromasia, and normoblasts may appear in the blood. It takes about 2–4 days after blood loss for the leukocyte count to return to normal, and about 2 weeks for the morphologic changes to disappear. Return of red cell values is slower.

Chronic Posthemorrhagic Anemia

If blood is lost in small amounts over an extended period, both clinical and hematologic features that characterize acute posthemorrhagic anemia are lacking. Regeneration of red cells occurs at a slower rate.

The reticulocyte count may be normal or slightly increased. Significant anemia does not usually develop until after storage iron is depleted; the anemia, therefore, is one of iron deficiency. The anemia is at first normochromic and normocytic, and gradually the newly formed red cells become microcytic, then hypochromic. The leukocyte count is normal or slightly decreased, owing to neutropenia. Platelets are commonly increased, and only later, in severe iron deficiency, are they likely to be decreased.

The cause of blood loss must be identified because a hidden malignancy, particularly of the GI tract, may be the cause of the anemia.

HEMOLYSIS—GENERAL

Anemias that are due primarily to increased red cell destruction are **hemolytic anemias.** A shortened red cell survival, therefore, proves that hemolysis is present; this measurement is usually unnecessary in practice.

Hemolytic anemias may be due to a defect of the red cell itself, an **intrinsic hemolytic anemia:** These are usually hereditary and are commonly grouped as **membrane, metabolic,** and **hemoglobin** defects. Alternatively, hemolysis may be due to a factor outside the red cell and acting upon it, an **extrinsic hemolytic anemia:** These are almost always acquired. The terms **intravascular hemolysis** and **extravascular hemolysis** refer to the **site** of destruction of the red cell: within the circulating blood and outside it, respectively.

Erythrocyte Survival Studies

Shortened red cell survival defines hemolysis. If the hemolytic process is moderate or severe, evidence of increased red cell turnover will suffice to show that hemolysis is present. If the hemolytic process is mild or obscure, red cell survival studies may be necessary.

Radioactive chromium (^{51}Cr) is convenient and is widely used for red cell survival studies. Labeled chromate is added to a blood sample in vitro and binds to β-chains of Hb. The chromated red cells are injected intravenously, and their disappearance is measured by counting blood, which is sampled every 1–2 days for 10–14 days. Residual activity is an index of the intravascular life span of the labeled red cells. Because ^{51}Cr emits γ-rays, external scanning can detect sites of red cell destruction.

The erythrocyte life span is usually expressed as the period during which one half of the radioactivity remains in the blood (the T½ ^{51}Cr; Fig. 32-9). Chromium normally elutes from the red cells at a rate of 1% per day. Thus, the half-life of the ^{51}Cr-labeled erythrocytes in normal individuals is 25–32 days instead of 60 days. Blood loss, changes in Hct, and recent blood transfusions significantly complicate the interpretation of survival data; therefore, a steady state is necessary for usable results.

In autoimmune hemolytic anemias, the slope of red cell survival produces a straight line when plotted on semilogarithmic paper (see Fig. 32-9). In other hemolytic anemias, two cell populations may exist. In these situations, the survival curve may be composed of an initial steep slope followed by a flatter component (Fig. 32-10). This type of curve has been seen in hereditary enzyme-deficiency hemolytic anemias, sickle cell anemia, and PNH (Dacie, 1991).

CO production measures heme catabolism immediately before and during the time of the assay. This is the only available method to study short-term fluctuations in red cell destruction (Franco, 2009).

Flow cytometry has been applied in some centers to measure red cell survival. Most techniques use ex vivo labeling of red cells by biotin. The rate of cell disappearance is then measured using fluorochrome-conjugated avidin or streptavidin. With multicolor flow cytometry additional parameters, such as reticulocytes and Hgb F content, may be monitored simultaneously (Franco, 2009).

Hemoglobin Destruction

Laboratory findings differ, depending on the site of blood destruction, the amount of destroyed blood, and the rate of destruction. If the destruction is **intravascular** and the quantity of destroyed blood is large, free Hb and

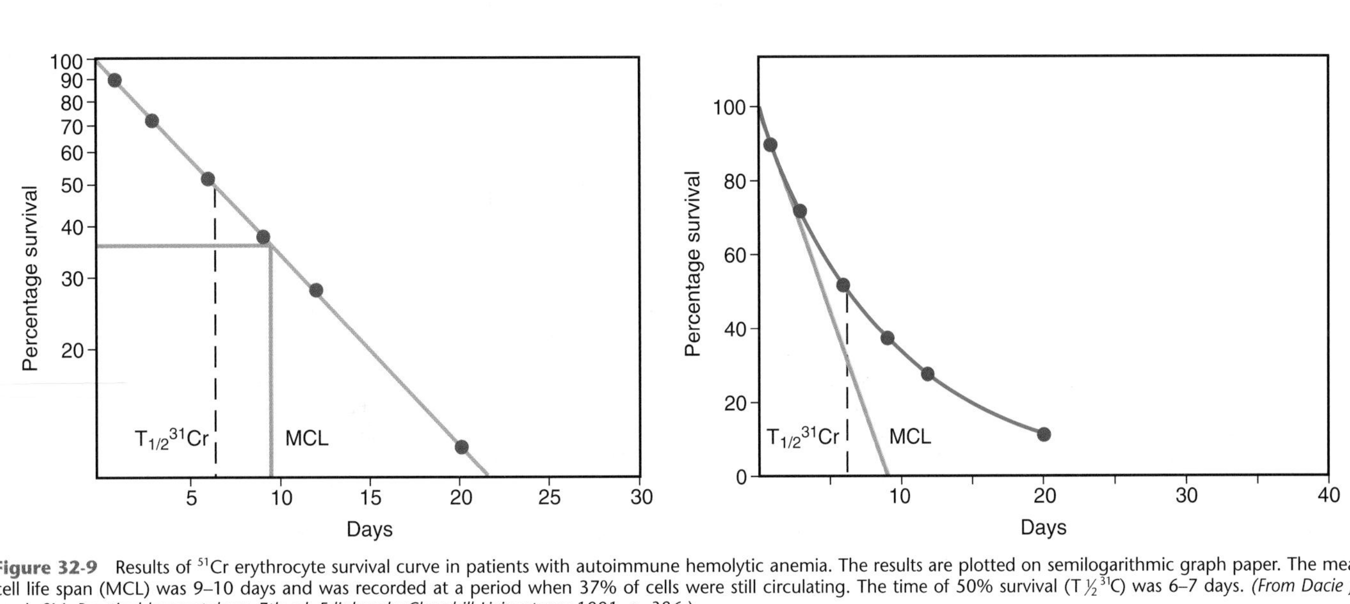

Figure 32-9 Results of ^{51}Cr erythrocyte survival curve in patients with autoimmune hemolytic anemia. The results are plotted on semilogarithmic graph paper. The mean cell life span (MCL) was 9–10 days and was recorded at a period when 37% of cells were still circulating. The time of 50% survival (T½ ^{31}C) was 6–7 days. *(From Dacie JV, Lewis SM. Practical haematology. 7th ed. Edinburgh: Churchill Livingstone; 1991, p. 386.)*

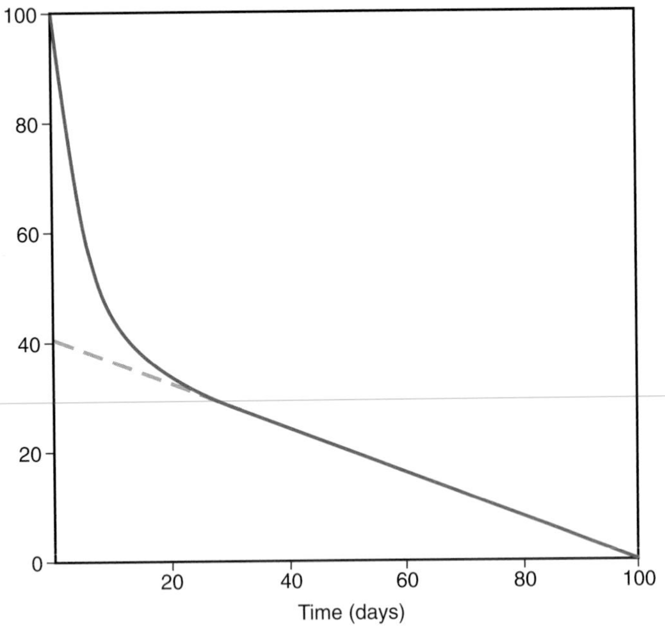

Figure 32-10 Results of radioactive chromium (^{51}Cr) erythrocyte survival curve in a patient with hemolytic anemia containing two cell populations. The percent survival is on the ordinate. By extrapolating the flatter curve to time 0, it can be estimated that 40% of the cells have a mean life span of 100 days. Sixty percent of cells have a mean life span of 5 days. *(From Bentley SA. Red cell survival studies reinterpreted. Clin Haematol 1977;6:601–23.)*

methemalbumin will be present in the plasma (hemoglobinemia and methemalbuminemia). The urine may contain free Hb and also hemosiderin.

Free Hb readily dissociates into αβ-dimers ($\alpha_2\beta_2 \rightarrow 2\alpha\beta$). These are bound to haptoglobin, an α_2-globulin, and the Hb–haptoglobin complex is rapidly removed from the circulation and catabolized by the liver parenchymal cells. This process prevents Hb from appearing in the urine. However, when the plasma Hb level exceeds 50–200 mg/dL (8–31 μmol/L), which is the capacity of haptoglobin to bind Hb, the free αβ-dimers of Hb readily pass through the glomerulus of the kidney. Part of the Hb is then absorbed by the proximal tubular cells, where the Hb iron is converted to hemosiderin. When these tubular cells are shed into the urine later, **hemosiderinuria** results. If the amount of Hb in the tubular lumen exceeds the capacity of the tubular cells to absorb it, it reaches the urine **(hemoglobinuria).** In the process, it may be oxidized to methemoglobin (hemiglobin). Plasma Hb not bound to haptoglobin or removed by the kidney is oxidized to hemiglobin. The oxidized heme groups (hemin) are bound to **hemopexin,** a β-globulin, and the complex is rapidly cleared by the hepatic parenchymal cells. If hemopexin is depleted, hemin groups bind to albumin, forming methemalbumin. Once hemopexin again becomes available, it removes the hemin groups from albumin for hepatic clearance (Hillman, 1996).

Lactate dehydrogenase (LD) is released from red cells and is increased in serum in hemolysis, especially in intravascular hemolysis; it is cleared more slowly than Hb. If the upper reference value is 207 IU/L, the LD in hemolytic anemia may be increased by as much as 800 IU/L. In megaloblastic anemia, associated with marked ineffective erythropoiesis, the LD is greatly increased to several thousand units. Serum LD is also increased in other forms of cellular injury. In hemolytic anemias, reversal of the LD isoenzyme pattern is seen, with LD_1 exceeding LD_2.

The normal plasma Hb level is 0.5–5 mg/dL (0.08–0.78 μmol/L). A rise to 10 mg/dL imparts to the plasma a yellow to orange color. With further increase, the color becomes pink. Levels up to 25–30 mg/dL are common in hemolytic anemia. Higher levels usually indicate intravascular hemolysis and are seen in hemolytic transfusion reactions and in paroxysmal cold and nocturnal hemoglobinurias.

If hemolysis is primarily **extravascular,** no hemoglobinemia, hemoglobinuria, or hemosiderinuria is present. Hemolysis is detected by measuring an increase in one of the products of heme catabolism (see Chapter 31):

1. An increase in CO expired, or in the blood carboxyhemoglobin level.
2. An increase in indirect-reacting serum bilirubin; because this is bound to albumin, it will not appear in the urine.
3. An increase in urine urobilinogen or, more consistently, in fecal urobilinogen.

The normal urobilinogen in a 24-hour specimen is 0.5–4 mg (0.8–6.75 μmol) in urine and 40–280 mg (0.068–0.470 mmol) in the stool. Following excessive hemolysis, it may increase to 5–200 mg in the urine and to 300–400 mg in the stool. Examination of feces is more dependable than examination of urine because feces may show an increase when the urine shows none. It may show an increase even when the serum bilirubin concentration is not raised because the normal liver can remove large amounts of (indirectly reacting) bilirubin and of reabsorbed urobilinogen from the blood.

Hemolytic anemia is characterized also by increased red cell production. Because of the availability of maximal amounts of iron for Hb formation, red cell production reaches the maximal degree possible (about eight times normal) in severe chronic hemolytic anemia, if complicating factors such as folate deficiency do not intervene. If red cell destruction exceeds the capacity of the marrow to replace red cells at the same rate, hemolytic anemia occurs. With less severe hemolysis, the marrow may be able to produce enough red cells that anemia does not occur; this is called compensated hemolysis.

Sudden worsening of the degree of anemia may occur in chronic hemolytic anemia and may be due to either of two basic mechanisms. Occasionally, episodes of bone marrow failure (transient arrest of erythropoiesis; see earlier discussion) characterized by erythroid hypoplasia and reticulocytopenia may upset the equilibrium between production and destruction of red cells. In most instances, these **aplastic crises** are probably due to parvoviral infection (Young, 1984). On the other hand, an increased rate of red cell destruction may occur, associated with infection or other illness that increases splenic size. This is not associated with erythroid aplasia and is called a **hemolytic crisis.**

Blood Film

The anemia is normocytic or macrocytic. Macrocytosis is due to the presence of immature red cells, which are larger than normocytes. Polychromasia is usually prominent; it may be excessively basophilic and normoblasts may be present, both of which indicate a "shift" of marrow reticulocytes into the blood. Other red cell abnormalities may give a clue to the nature of the hemolytic process. Spherocytes suggest hereditary spherocytosis (HS) or autoimmune hemolysis (see Fig. 30-12); schistocytes imply microangiopathic hemolytic anemia (see Fig. 30-19); sickle cells, target cells, or crystals suggest a hemoglobinopathy. When hemolytic anemia is acute, increased numbers and younger forms of leukocytes and platelets are often released from the marrow, together with erythrocytes. The result is leukocytosis with a "shift to the left" and thrombocytosis with both normal and giant platelets.

Bone Marrow

Normoblastic hyperplasia is present and may be striking in degree. Storage iron is usually increased and sideroblasts are normal or increased in number, reflecting the abundance of available iron for Hb synthesis.

HEMOLYSIS—MEMBRANE DISORDERS

Hereditary Spherocytosis

HS affects 1 in 5000 of the population, occurring predominantly in those of Northern European ancestry. Prevalence in other ethnic groups is unknown, although HS has been reported worldwide, particularly in Japanese and African populations. The reported prevalence may be an underestimation in that milder forms may be clinically asymptomatic (Gallagher, 2009). HS is characterized by spherocytic red cells that are intrinsically defective, splenomegaly, and familial occurrence (most often autosomal dominant). In about 15%–30% of cases, however, neither parent is affected. The hemolytic process is variable in severity and is corrected by splenectomy, although the spherocytosis remains.

The laboratory findings are those of a chronic extravascular hemolytic process: evidence of increased pigment catabolism, erythroid hyperplasia, and reticulocytosis. The direct antiglobulin test is negative. The red cells characteristically have increased osmotic fragility. On the blood film, spherocytes have a smaller diameter and are more intensely stained than normal cells. They have no central pallor, which if present may be eccentric (see Fig. 30-12). The MCV is low-normal and the MCHC is often increased, reflecting a decrease in cell surface. In compensated cases, reticulocytosis may be a sensitive indicator.

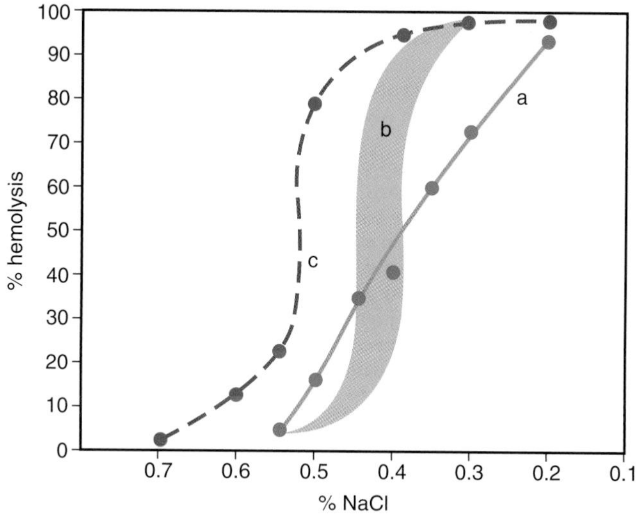

Figure 32-11 Erythrocyte osmotic fragility. **a,** Thalassemia, showing a small fraction of cells with increased fragility *(lower left)* and a larger fraction of cells with decreased fragility *(upper right)*. **b,** Normal curves fall in the shaded area. **c,** Hereditary spherocytosis, showing increased osmotic fragility.

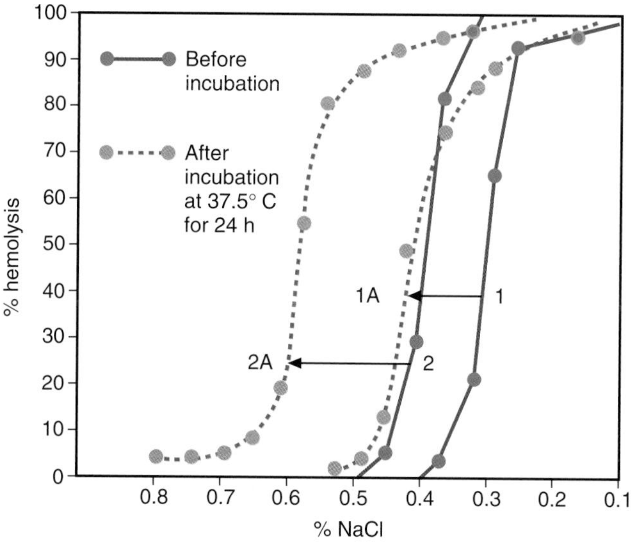

Figure 32-12 The effect of incubation on erythrocyte osmotic fragility. The change in the osmotic fragility curve from "before incubation" to "after incubation" is illustrated for normal blood (1→1A) and for blood from a patient with hereditary spherocytosis (HS) (2→2A). Blood in HS characteristically shows a greater increase in fragility with incubation than does normal blood or even blood of acquired spherocytosis (e.g., autoimmune hemolytic anemia).

Osmotic Fragility Test

Red cells are suspended in a series of tubes containing hypotonic solutions of NaCl, varying from 0.9%–0.0%, incubated at room temperature for 30 minutes, and centrifuged. The percent hemolysis in the supernatant solutions is measured and plotted for each NaCl concentration. Cells that are more spherical, with a decreased surface/volume ratio, have a limited capacity to expand in hypotonic solutions and lyse at a higher concentration of NaCl than do normal biconcave red cells. They are said to have increased osmotic fragility. Conversely, cells that are hypochromic and flatter have a greater capacity to expand in hypotonic solutions, lyse at a lower concentration than normal cells, and are said to have decreased osmotic fragility (Fig. 32-11).

The osmotic fragility of freshly drawn blood is usually increased in HS but may be normal in mildly affected patients. In blood that is incubated at 37° C for 24 hours before the test is performed, the osmotic fragility is almost always increased (Fig. 32-12).

The increased osmotic fragility of freshly drawn blood is characteristic but not specific; it may occur in acquired spherocytic anemias, such as immune-mediated hemolytic anemia. A greater difference in median fragility (after incubation from before incubation) occurs in HS cells than in control normal cells; this is an important diagnostic feature in HS. A tail of very fragile cells conditioned by the spleen is usually seen. The tail usually disappears after splenectomy. Cells with increased surface/volume ratio are osmotic resistant. These cells are seen in iron deficiency, thalassemia, liver disease, and reticulocytosis.

Autohemolysis Test

Sterile, defibrinated blood is incubated at 37° C for 48 hours (Dacie, 1991). During this time, red cells undergo a complex series of changes, lose membrane, and become more spherocytic. In normal blood, without added glucose, the amount of autohemolysis at 48 hours is 0.2%–2.0%. In normal blood, incubated with added glucose, the amount of autohemolysis is less—0%–0.9%.

In HS, autohemolysis is virtually always increased; with glucose, the lysis is diminished to a variable extent. This test is being used less frequently and is probably no more sensitive than the incubated osmotic fragility test (Gallagher, 2009).

Red blood cells in HS are characterized by an unstable lipid bilayer, which facilitates the release of lipids from the membrane, resulting in loss of surface area and formation of poorly deformable spherocytes that are selectively retained and damaged in the spleen. The erythrocytes are abnormally permeable to sodium, and there is no defect in energy metabolism, which is, in fact, increased. The increased metabolic activity has been explained as an attempt to compensate for a membrane defect that leaks cations, with degenerative changes and loss of cell membrane accelerated by the metabolic and physical stresses of passage through the spleen.

The genetic defects in HS are heterogeneous but affect the skeletal proteins of the red cell membrane. HS can be divided into the following pathogenetic categories: (1) isolated partial deficiency of spectrin, (2) combined partial deficiency of spectrin and ankyrin, (3) partial deficiency of band 3 protein, (4) deficiency of protein 4.2, and (5) other, less common defects. Most of these abnormalities are related to the synthesis of abnormal protein, mostly through point mutations or frameshift (Gallagher, 2009).

Hereditary Elliptocytosis

This autosomal dominant condition probably includes more than one genetic variant. In the U.S. population, the prevalence is approximately 3–5 per 10,000. It is more common in individuals of African and Mediterranean ancestry. All cases of hereditary elliptocytosis (HE) are associated with weakening of the membrane skeleton and defective association of proteins that hold the skeleton together (Gallagher, 2009). On the basis of red cell morphology, HE can be divided into three groups: (1) common HE (including hereditary pyropoikilocytosis [HPP]), with elliptocytes that may be rod shaped, (2) spherocytic HE, and (3) Southeast Asian ovalocytosis. The most commonly defined abnormality appears to be a defect in spectrin, resulting in impaired association of spectrin dimers into spectrin tetramers and spectrin oligomers. Other abnormalities include a defect in protein 4.1 and deficiency of glycophorin C. HPP is associated with two abnormalities: a mutation in spectrin that disrupts spectrin heterodimer self-association, and a partial deficiency of spectrin that results in a decreased spectrin/band 3 ratio.

Common HE

Most persons with the common form of HE (≈90% of cases) are nonanemic; a minority of this group (perhaps 10%–20%) have mild hemolysis. Nonhypochromic elliptocytes are abundant in the blood film, numbering approximately 15% (see Fig. 30-16), whereas in normal individuals less than 5% of the red cells are elliptical (Gallagher, 2009). The deformity is increased in sealed, moist preparations.

In a subgroup of common HE, especially in black families, affected neonates transiently have moderate poikilocytosis, red cell fragmentation, and budding, with hemolytic anemia; during the first year of life, hemolysis declines and typical HE emerges. Worsening of hemolysis in the neonatal period has been attributed to the presence of fetal hemoglobin, which binds poorly to 2,3-diphosphoglycerate (2,3-DPG). Higher levels of the latter exert a destabilizing effect on spectrin-protein 4.1-actin interaction (Gallagher, 2009).

Hereditary Pyropoikilocytosis

HPP is a severe congenital hemolytic anemia, which is characterized by microcytosis, striking micropoikilocytosis and fragmentation, and autosomal recessive inheritance. HPP represents a subtype of common HE. It occurs primarily in blacks. In contrast to normal red cells, which show budding and fragmentation when heated to 49° C, HPP red cells fragment at 45°–46° C.

Spherocytic HE

This subgroup accounts for 10% of cases. A mild to moderate hemolytic anemia and splenomegaly are present, with both elliptocytes and spherocytes, along with abnormal osmotic fragility and autohemolysis tests. Poikilocytes and fragments are usually absent. The molecular basis of this subtype is unknown.

Southeast Asian Ovalocytosis

This subgroup occurs with high frequencies (20%–30%) in certain populations of the Far East, particularly Malaysia. Hemolysis is usually absent or mild. The erythrocytes are less elongated, and some have the appearance of stomatocytic ovalocytes. Many cells contain one or two transverse ridges or a longitudinal slit. This condition is associated with increased resistance to malaria. The underlying defect is related to a deletion of 27 bases from the band 3 gene (Gallagher, 2009).

Hereditary Stomatocytosis (Hereditary Hydrocytosis)

This is a rare, autosomally transmitted disorder. Heterozygotic individuals have no anemia, and 1%–25% of stomatocytes are seen on the blood film. In presumed homozygotic individuals, about one third of the red cells are stomatocytes, and there is a mild to moderate hemolytic anemia. The membrane abnormality results in increased permeability of the membrane to Na^+ and K^+ (and therefore water), resulting in hydrated, macrocytic red cells. The MCV may be as high as 150 fL. Osmotic fragility and autohemolysis are increased. Although the exact membrane defect is not known, several reports indicate the absence of a membrane protein located in the band 7 region called stomatin. Although stomatin is decreased or absent from red cells of affected individuals, the loss may be maturational in the marrow or circulation rather than causing the disease by itself (Gallagher, 2009). Individuals with Rh deficiency syndrome, either absent (Rh_{null}) or markedly reduced (Rh_{mod}), usually have hemolytic anemia with stomatocytosis.

Paroxysmal Nocturnal Hemoglobinuria

PNH is an acquired clonal stem cell disorder characterized by the production of abnormal erythrocytes, granulocytes, and platelets (Brodsky, 2009). The red cell defect renders them more susceptible to complement-mediated intravascular lysis. Three types of erythrocytes have been described according to their in vitro sensitivity: type I with normal sensitivity, type II with medium sensitivity (three to five times normal), and type III with extreme sensitivity (15–25 times normal). Several complement defense proteins are decreased or absent in PNH. These proteins include: decay accelerating factor (DAF, CD55), membrane inhibitor of reactive lysis (MIRL, CD59), and C8-binding protein (a homologous restriction factor). DAF is a glycoprotein that antagonizes the convertase complexes of complement. MIRL is a protein that controls the membrane attack complex, C5b-9. Other proteins that are deficient in PNH include CD58 (leukocyte function antigen 3), CD14 (endotoxin-binding protein receptor), CD24, and CD16a (Fcγ receptor). Membrane-associated enzymes such as acetyl cholinesterase and leukocyte alkaline phosphatase may be deficient as well. Recent work indicates that deficient proteins and enzymes are attached to the cell membrane by a common glycolipid anchor called GPI. Deficiency of GPI results in secondary deficiency of the attached proteins. Therefore, PNH can be redefined as partial or complete lack of GPI-linked proteins on a population of cells of the hematopoietic system.

PNH is a rare disease with an estimated annual incidence of 4 per million (Brodsky, 2009). The disease is characterized by chronic intravascular hemolysis with or without obvious hemoglobinuria. However, hemosiderinuria is almost constantly present. Typical nocturnal or sleep-related hemoglobinuria is present in a minority of patients. Bouts of hemolysis could be initiated by infection, surgery, whole blood transfusion, injection of contrast dyes, or even severe exercise. The proposed relationship between mild drop in pH during sleep and nocturnal hemoglobinuria has not been confirmed (Brodsky, 2009).

The blood usually shows a normocytic anemia with a reticulocytosis that is often less than expected for the degree of anemia. Hypochromic microcytic anemia is not uncommon, however, and is due to loss of iron in the urine. Neutropenia occurs in three fifths and thrombocytopenia in two thirds of patients at some time during the course of disease, so that pancytopenia is common. The direct antiglobulin test is usually negative.

The marrow may be hypercellular with erythroid hyperplasia, but it may be hypocellular. In some patients, marrow failure may occur during the course of PNH; in others, AA is the initial diagnosis, with signs of PNH manifesting simultaneously or later. As mentioned earlier, approximately 40% of patients with AA have evidence of PNH clone at diagnosis (Young, 2002).

Thrombotic complications are common, occurring in approximately 40% of patients, and represent a major cause of mortality. Thrombosis commonly occurs in hepatic, cerebral, and abdominal veins. The absence of CD59 on platelets results in externalization of phosphatidylserine, a site for prothrombinase complexes, and thus increases the propensity for thrombosis. The disease may undergo partial remissions and exacerbations. In more than half of patients, both the proportion of abnormal cells and the clinical severity decrease with time. Abnormal cytogenetics can be found in up to 20% of PNH patients. In approximately 3%–5% of PNH patients, the disease progresses to acute leukemia.

Sucrose Hemolysis Test

This test should be performed whenever the diagnosis of PNH is considered, also in hypoplastic anemias and in any hemolytic anemia of obscure origin (Hartmann, 1970). The principle of the test is that sucrose provides a medium of low ionic strength that promotes the binding of complement to the red cells. In PNH, a proportion of red cells are abnormally sensitive to complement-mediated lysis. Suspicious results can be seen in some other hematologic diseases, especially megaloblastic anemia and autoimmune hemolytic anemia. False-negative results occur if the serum lacks complement activity. A simpler screening test, called the sugar water test, applies the same principle of mixing blood with sugar and observing for hemolysis.

Acidified Serum Test (Ham Test)

Definitive diagnosis of PNH used to depend on a positive acidified serum test (Ham, 1939; Dacie, 1991). In acidified serum, complement is activated by the alternate pathway, binds to red cells, and lyses abnormal PNH cells that are unusually susceptible to complement. The patient's washed red cells are mixed with ABO compatible normal serum (fresh or properly stored) and acid; after an hour's incubation at 37° C, the PNH cells are lysed, as indicated in Table 32-3. The patient's own serum may or may not result in lysis, depending on residual complement, and the other tubes provide controls.

In PNH, usually 10%–50% of the cells are lysed. If lysis also occurs with heat-inactivated serum, the test is not positive, as spherocytic or antibody-sensitized cells may be responsible. A positive acidified serum test occurs in congenital dyserythropoietic anemia, type II (CDA-II), or HEM-PAS (see earlier discussion). In this situation, however, lysis does not occur with the patient's own serum, and occurs with only about 30% of normal sera. Also, the sugar water screening test is negative in CDA-II.

Flow cytometry using immunofluorescent staining of red cells with a monoclonal antibody against deficient proteins such as CD55, CD58, and CD59 is gradually becoming the standard method of diagnosing PNH. Granulocytes provide excellent diagnostic targets for flow cytometry. A fluorescein-labeled proaerolysin variant (FLAER) is increasingly being used for the diagnosis of PNH. It binds selectively to the GPI anchor.

The gene responsible for the PNH phenotype has been identified on the X chromosome and designated phosphatidyl inositol glycan A or

TABLE 32-3
Acidified Serum Test

	1	2	3	4	5	6	7
Fresh normal serum		0.5	0.5			0.5	0.5
Patient's serum			0.5				
Heat-inactivated normal serum				0.5			0.5
0.2 N HCl		0.05	0.05	0.05		0.05	0.05
50% patient's red cells	0.05	0.05	0.05	0.05			
50% normal red cells					0.05	0.05	0.05
Pattern of lysis in positive test	Trace	+++	+	–	–	–	–

Modified from Dacie JV, Lewis SM. Practical haematology. 7th ed. Edinburgh: Churchill Livingstone; 1991, p. 261.
HCl, Hydrochloric acid.

PIG-A. More than 120 somatic mutations of the *PIG-A* gene have been described.

HEMOLYSIS—HEMOGLOBIN DISORDERS

There are two main groups of inherited disorders of Hb: (1) structural variants, with defects in the structure, and (2) thalassemias, with defects in the synthesis, of a globin chain. An overlap has been noted between these groups; 44 structural variants also have a thalassemic phenotype with decreased synthesis, and hence, level of the abnormal globin chain. Hereditary persistence of fetal hemoglobin (HPFH) is related to the thalassemias, although the phenotype is not clearly thalassemic. Most thalassemias involve α- or β-globin chains. δ-, γ-, and $\varepsilon\gamma\delta\beta$-thalassemias are known, but are clinically less significant.

Normal Hemoglobins

The heme group is identical in all Hbs. The protein part of the molecule is a tetramer, made up of two dimers; each dimer contains an α-like and a β-like globin. Postnatally, only one α-like globin is present, and this forms three distinct Hb tetramers with the three different β-like globins present. Three additional embryonic Hbs are present only in the first 3 months of gestation (Fig. 32-13).

Hb A ($\alpha2\beta2$)

Hemoglobin A is the major normal adult Hb, accounting for about 97% of the total. It consists of two identical α-chains, each with 141 amino acids; and two identical β-chains, with 146 amino acids each. Each chain is linked with one heme group. The molecule is ellipsoidal, with the four heme groups at the surface of the molecule, where they function by combining reversibly with O_2.

Hb F ($\alpha2\gamma2$)

Hemoglobin F is the major Hb of the fetus and the newborn infant. The increased O_2 affinity of fetal blood versus adult blood is due to its lower affinity for 2,3-DPG. The two α-chains are identical to those of Hb A, and the two γ-chains, with 146-amino-acid residues, differ from β-chains. In normal individuals, Hb F has two types of γ-chains, which differ by one amino acid, having either alanine (Aγ) or glycine (Gγ) at position 136. The ratio of Gγ to Aγ chains changes from 3 : 1 at birth to 2 : 3 by age 12 months (Weatherall, 2001). There is a common polymorphism of the Aγ gene, in which threonine replaces isoleucine at position 75. This Hb F variant is called Hb F Sardinia and is without functional abnormalities. Approximately 10% of total Hb F is a negatively charged variant, designated Hb F1, owing to posttranslational acetylation of the amino-terminal ends of the γ-chains.

During fetal life, Hb F predominates, as γ-chain production is high. β-Chain production begins before the 20th week of prenatal life, so that Hb A is 10% of the total between 20 and 35 weeks and between 15% and 40% at the time of birth. Around birth, production of Hb F is turned down; by 6 months, Hb F is usually less than 8%, and by 12 months, it is less than 5%, in about 90% of infants. Between 12 and 24 months of age, Hb F is usually less than 3% but varies from 3%–10% in about 20% of infants. After the age of 2 years, Hb F is normally less than 2%, and only traces of Hb F (<0.8%) are present in most adults. However, among healthy adults, 5%–10% have slightly raised Hb F level (up to 5%). During fetal life, all red cells produce and contain Hb F, whereas in adults only 3%–5% do so; these are termed F cells (Weatherall, 2001). Adult production of Hb F is regulated by multiple genetic loci, including the Xmn1-HBG2 site in the β-globin locus, the HMIP locus at 6q23, and the bcl11A locus on chromosome 2 (Thein, 2009). Polymorphic variants at these loci cause a modest increase in Hb F in otherwise healthy adults and probably underlie most cases of Swiss-type or heterocellular hereditary persistence of fetal Hb.

F cells may increase in number when reactivation of Hb F synthesis occurs in normal pregnancy and in some disorders of erythropoiesis, particularly chronic bone marrow failure syndromes. In certain acquired hematopoietic disorders, the Hb F level may also be elevated. These include megaloblastic anemia, myelofibrosis, aplastic anemia, paroxysmal nocturnal hemoglobinuria, refractory anemias, leukemias, and solid tumors (up to 5%–10%). In the second trimester of pregnancy, there could be a slight increase, and in hydatidiform moles, a more significant increase—up to 6%. The highest levels of Hb F are found in juvenile myelomonocytic leukemia, Fanconi's anemia, and erythroleukemia (30%–50%). Elevated Hb F is found in a few hemoglobinopathies, in β- and $\delta\beta$-thalassemias, and in HPFH. The switch from γ-globin to β-globin and the decrease in Hb F are delayed in sickle cell patients, who might not reach their stable Hb F level until adolescence (Huisman, 1980). A similar delay in decline in Hb F is also seen in thalassemia trait (Schroter, 1981).

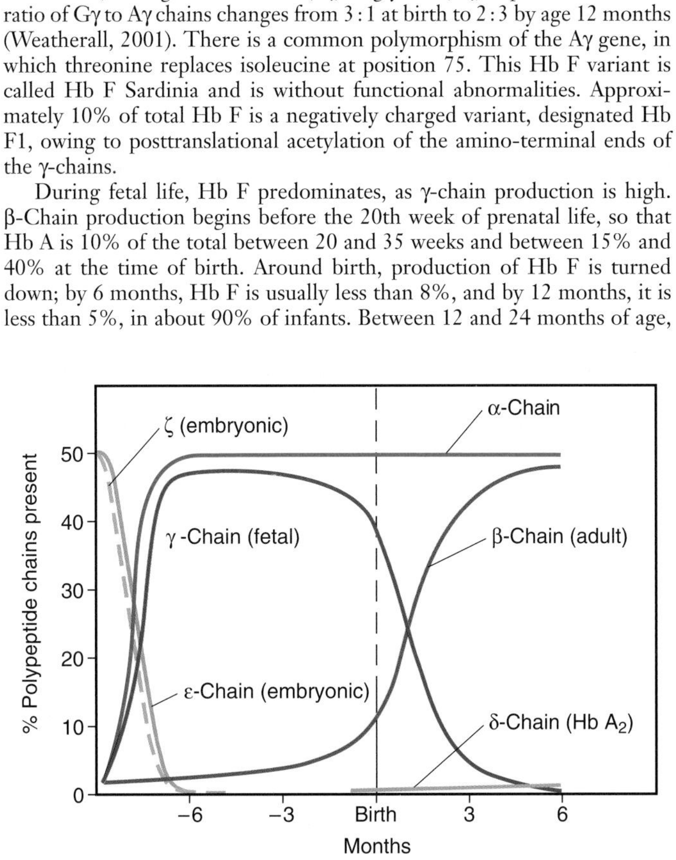

Figure 32-13 Relative proportions of polypeptide chains of hemoglobin present during fetal and neonatal life. *(From Bentley SA. Red cell survival studies reinterpreted. Clin Haematol 1977;16:601–23.)*

Hb A_2 ($\alpha_2\delta_2$)

Hemoglobin A_2 accounts for 1.5%–3.5% of normal adult Hb. Its two α-chains are the same as in Hb A; its two δ-chains differ from β-chains in only 10 of their 146 amino acids. Less efficient transcription of the δ-globin gene compared with the β-gene is the result of differences in the promoter area (Delvoye, 1993; Tang, 1997) and the second intron (Kosche, 1985). δ-Chain synthesis begins late in fetal life. The level of Hb A_2 gradually increases during the first year of life, at which time the adult level is reached.

Increased Hb A_2 is seen almost exclusively in β-thalassemias. It rarely reaches 6% and never more than 12%. Hb A_2 is occasionally increased in hyperthyroidism and megaloblastic anemia; it has been reported to be increased in sickle cell trait (Whitten, 1981) and sickle cell disease, but the increase is only modest and the level stays below 4.5%. It may be decreased in iron deficiency anemia and α-thalassemia. If the patient with β-thalassemia trait has concomitant severe iron deficiency, the increase in Hb A_2 might be dampened down and appear equivocal; in these instances, retesting should be performed after the iron deficiency is corrected. Because of its developmental delay, Hb A_2 might not be useful in diagnosing β-thalassemia trait in young infants.

Embryonic Hemoglobins. The zeta (ζ) chain is the embryonic analog of the α-chain and may combine with epsilon (ε) chains to form Hb Gower-1 ($\zeta2\varepsilon2$) or with γ-chains to form Hb Portland ($\zeta2\gamma2$). The ε-chain is the embryonic counterpart of the γ-, β-, and δ-chains and combines with α-chains to form Hb Gower-2 ($\alpha2\varepsilon2$). Hb Gower-1, Hb Portland, and Hb Gower-2 are the embryonic Hbs and are found in normal human embryos and fetuses with a gestational age of less than 3 months.

The Globin Gene Clusters. Globin synthesis is controlled by two separate gene clusters. The ζ-gene and two α-genes (α-like globins), together with nonfunctioning pseudogenes, are on chromosome 16. Genes for the ε-, δ-, β-chains, and the two γ-chains (β-like globins), and two pseudogenes are located on chromosome 11 (Fig. 32-14). Note that there are two functioning α-genes on a haploid chromosome (balanced by only one β-gene). The different globin genes evolved from a common ancestor by gene duplication. There is considerable polymorphism of regulatory sequences within these clusters, accounting for normal variations and wide phenotypic differences in hemoglobinopathy and thalassemia syndromes.

Glycosylated Hemoglobins. The term glycation or glycosylation implies the linkage of a sugar to a protein. Approximately 5% of Hb A undergoes posttranslational glycosylation, resulting in linkage of sugars to serine, asparagine, and hydroxylysine residues. The glycosylated Hbs have been designated Hb AIa (<1%), Hb AIb (<2%), and Hb AIc (3%). Glycosylation of Hb increases linearly over the 120-day life span of the red cell. Hb AIc contains a molecule of glucose attached nonenzymatically by a

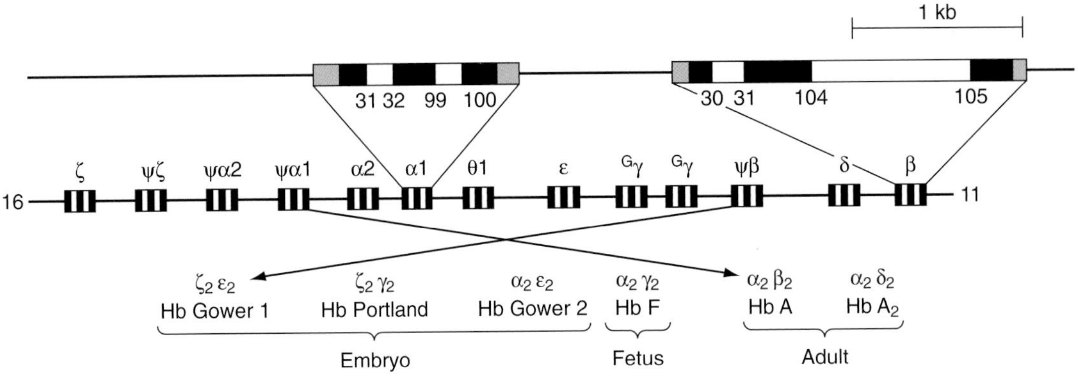

Figure 32-14 The α- and β-globin gene clusters on chromosomes 16 and 11, respectively. In the extended α- and β-globin genes, the introns are shaded dark, the 5′ and 3′ noncoding regions are hatched, and the exons are unshaded. *(From Weatherall DJ, Clegg JB. The thalassemia syndromes. 4th ed. Oxford: Blackwell Scientific Publications; 2001.)*

ketoamine linkage to the amino-terminal amino group of each β-chain. Hb AIc is elevated twofold to threefold in patients with diabetes mellitus. The measurement of Hb AIc has been used as an index of metabolic control of diabetes during the preceding 2–3 months (Bunn, 1994). Hb AIc may be falsely decreased in conditions associated with rapid red cell turnover, such as hemolytic anemia.

Laboratory Investigation of Hemoglobinopathies and Thalassemias

Current recommendations include automated complete blood count (CBC) with accurate MCV, RBC, MCH, and MCHC values; Hb H test; ferritin; and high-performance liquid chromatography (HPLC) for Hb A_2 and Hb F measurement and detection of Hb variants, followed by alkaline and acid electrophoresis when a variant is found and additional studies (Sickledex) as necessary (Clarke, 2000).

Cation-Exchange HPLC. Numerous automated systems have been developed in the last 20 years, and HPLC is now the method of choice for initial screening of Hb variants and for separation and determination of percentages of Hb A, Hb A_2, and Hb F (Wilson, 1983). A cation-exchange HPLC system, Bio-Rad Variant by Bio-Rad Laboratories (Philadelphia, Pa.), emerged as the leading commercial kit. Resolution of this system is claimed to be similar to that of isoelectric focusing, and data banks of retention times are available (Figs. 32-15 and 32-16) (Riou, 1997; Globin Gene Server). Variants detected by HPLC are confirmed by an alternative technique, such as electrophoresis.

Hemoglobin Electrophoresis and Isoelectric Focusing. Hb molecules in an alkaline solution have a net negative charge and move toward the anode in an electrophoretic system. A practical method for routine Hb electrophoresis is cellulose acetate at alkaline pH (Briere, 1965). It is rapid and reproducible and separates the major Hb variants S, D, G, C, and E from Hb A (Figs. 32-17 and 32-18). Quantification of the major bands is easily accomplished. Those with an electrophoretic mobility greater than that of Hb A at pH 8.6 are known as the "fast Hbs"; these include, in order of increasing mobility, Hbs K, J, Bart's, N, I, and H. Hbs A_2, C, E, and O Arab at the slow end are unresolved from each other, as are S, D, G, and Lepore. Citrate agar electrophoresis at an acidic pH (Milner, 1975) provides ready separation of Hbs that migrate together on cellulose acetate: S from D and G, and C from E and O (Fig. 32-19). Isoelectric focusing separates Hbs based on their isoelectric point along a pH gradient with a high resolution (Fig. 32-20). Capillary electrophoresis is a rapidly developing automated system with a performance similar to that of HPLC (Mario, 1997).

Alkali Denaturation Test for Hb F. Fetal hemoglobin resists alkali denaturation; adult Hb does not (Singer, 1951). A hemolysate is alkalinized and then neutralized, and the denatured adult Hb is precipitated by ammonium sulfate. A filtrate will then contain only alkali-resistant Hb, which is measured and expressed as a percentage of the total. The modification of Betke (1959) is reliable for Hb F less than 15% but underestimates Hb F at higher levels. The reference interval is 0.2%–1.0% for adults. This method has been largely replaced by HPLC or capillary electrophoresis estimation of Hb F.

Acid Elution Slide Test for F Cells. Modification of the original method of Kleihauer and Betke by Shepard (1962) is useful for analyzing the distribution of Hb F among red cells. Hemoglobins other than Hb F are eluted from the red cells on an air-dried blood film by a citric acid–phosphate buffer (pH 3.3). Only Hb F remains in the fixed red cells, and the distribution can be determined after staining. In normal adults, almost all red cells appear as ghosts; 1%–5% of red cells contain residual Hb (F cells). In most types of HPFH, Hb F is distributed evenly among red cells (pancellular distribution). In all other conditions, such as thalassemia or a hemoglobinopathy, and in Swiss-type HPFH, the distribution of Hb F is heterogeneous or uneven among red cells (heterocellular distribution). Flow cytometry is also used to detect F cells.

Hb A_2 Quantitation. Hb A_2 quantitation is challenging for two reasons: (1) Its level is low with a narrow range and only a modest increase in disease, requiring a high degree of precision, and (2) Hb variants with similar charge or retention time interfere with its estimation. Several laboratory methods of varying accuracy and precision are being used. Cation-exchange HPLC (Head, 2004), microcolumn chromatography (Steinberg, 1991), and cellulose acetate electrophoresis with elution are considered to be sufficiently precise. Densitometry of electrophoretic bands on cellulose acetate membrane is unreliable (Schmidt, 1975). Increasingly, cation-exchange HPLC is the method of choice; it provides accurate measurement of Hb F, along with separation of Hb variants. In the presence of Hb S, however, its level is falsely elevated because Hb S adducts have similar retention times (Suh, 1996). In the presence of Hb S, microcolumn chromatography gives an accurate measurement of Hb A_2 (Head, 2004).

Hb A_2 estimation is used principally in diagnosis of β-thalassemia trait, in which it is elevated up to 7%. Hb A_2 values from normal individuals do not overlap with those of individuals with β-thalassemia trait when performed by microchromatography or HPLC; however, there is some overlap with the cellulose acetate electrophoresis method (Huisman, 1986). Reference intervals for Hb A_2 are 1.5%–3.5% of total Hb.

Sickling Test—Metabisulfite Slide Test. Adding sodium metabisulfite, a reducing substance, to blood enhances deoxygenation of Hb and sickling of Hb S (Fig. 32-21). The test does not distinguish sickle cell anemia from sickle trait or other Hb S syndromes because all red cells sickle; however, sickling occurs more rapidly with greater amounts of Hb S in the cells. Positive tests may occur with other rare sickling hemoglobins (Hbs S Travis, C Harlem), Hb I, and high concentrations of Hb Bart's. Hb I, an α-chain variant, has normal functional properties. False-negative tests may occur if Hb S concentration is less than 10% (as in very young infants), or if deoxygenation is inadequate (e.g., deterioration of reagent).

Sickle Solubility Test. In this nonquantitative test, red cells are lysed with saponin, and Hb is reduced by dithionite (sodium hydrosulfite). Reduced Hb S is insoluble in concentrated inorganic buffer (2.3 M phosphate buffer), and the polymers of deoxy-Hb S obstruct light rays to produce opacity. The test is useful in screening large numbers of people for the presence of Hb S or other sickling Hbs. False-positive reactions (turbid solution) occur also in the presence of many Heinz bodies, as in unstable Hb disorders after splenectomy, and in blood protein disorders due to precipitation of plasma proteins. False-negative reactions (clear

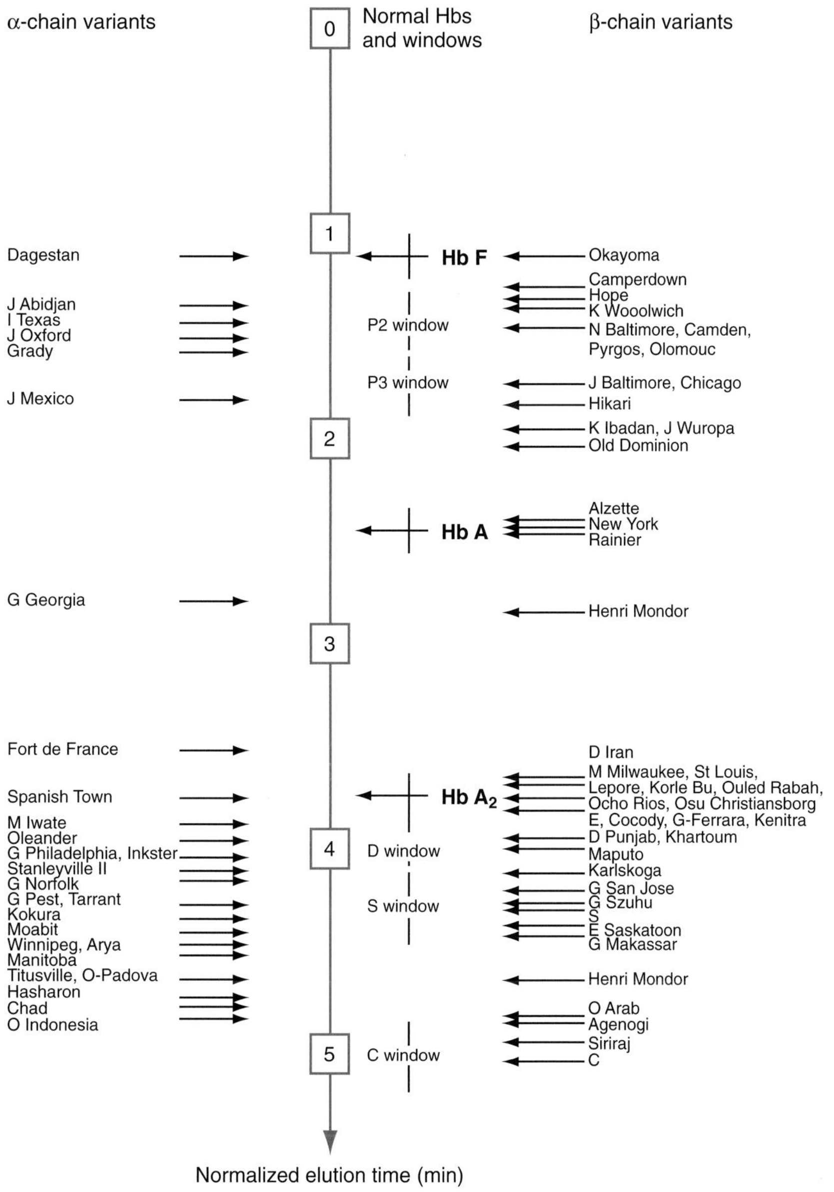

Figure 32-15 Elution times of 74 hemoglobins. Elution times were normalized to a reference value of 3.8 minutes for Hb A_2. Cation-exchange high-performance liquid chromatography (HPLC) separation by the Bio-Rad Variant system, using the β Thalassemia Short Program. *(From Riou J, Godart C, Hurtrel D, et al. Cation-exchange HPLC evaluated for presumptive identification of hemoglobin variants. Clin Chem 1997;43:34–9.)*

solution) occur if the amount of Hb S is too small, as in severe anemia, or if the reagent has deteriorated.

DNA Analysis (Old, 2001). Gap PCR is used for detection of common deletions in α- or, less often, in the other thalassemia syndromes. In gap PCR, primers bind to the region flanking the deletion. PCR product is obtained only from the affected alleles, as the primers are located far apart in the normal gene. Additional primers that amplify the normal allele are used to assess for heterozygosity/homozygosity. Southern blotting is still used and can assess all alleles and confirm PCR results. PCR-based techniques have been developed to screen for common point mutations in β-thalassemia and Hb variants. In reverse dot blotting or reverse hybridization, mutant oligonucleotides are fixed to a nylon membrane (ViennaLab) or microplate (Bio-Rad), and hybridized with the patient's amplified DNA. In ARMS (amplification refractory mutation system), amplification takes place only when the primer matches perfectly the genomic DNA sequence. ARMS primers are available for the detection of all common β-thalassemia mutations (Old, 1996). PCR-based sequencing is utilized for confirmation of single nucleotide mutations and small deletions.

Structural Hemoglobin Variants

As of 2005, 893 Hb variants had been identified (Huisman, 1998; Globin Gene Server). Ninety percent of these are due to single amino acid substitutions; in the remaining 10%, the polypeptide chain is abnormally long or short as a result of termination errors, frameshift mutations, insertions, deletions, or fused or hybrid chains.

A majority affect the α- or β-globin chains. Involvement of the γ-chain and the δ-chain occurs, but because of the small amount of Hb involved, their variants are less often detected and are rarely of clinical significance. A large number of Hb variants that do not cause disease have been discovered in surveys.

New Hbs were assigned letters of the alphabet, then geographic names—usually to distinguish different Hbs with similar electrophoretic mobilities. Several variants of Hb D, G, and J, for example, are known. Sometimes, a variant is known by multiple names, based on independent discoveries. Hb M indicates a variant that forms methemoglobin. Amino acid substitutions in some of the known Hb variants are listed and classified by functional characteristics in Table 32-4.

Hbs S, C, E, and D are, by far, the most important variants (Table 32-5). Together with the thalassemias, they reached polymorphic frequencies in regions where falciparum malaria was/is endemic, owing to partial protection against this parasite by mechanisms still not fully understood.

Abnormal Hemoglobin Syndromes

In homozygous β-chain structural variants, both allelic genes for the abnormal β-chains are present, so that no normal β-chains (hence, no Hb

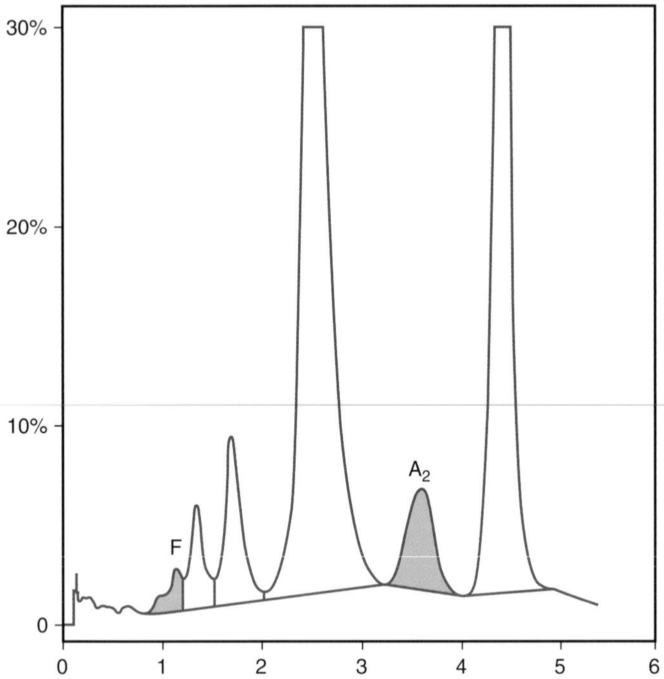

Figure 32-16 Ion-exchange high-performance liquid chromatography (HPLC) separation of hemoglobins (Hbs): patient with sickle cell trait: Hbs F, A, and A_2 and an abnormal Hb in the S window are detected. Hemoglobin A_2 cannot be quantified because of the presence of Hb S. *(Bio-Rad Variant Classic Hb Testing System, Bio-Rad Laboratories, Philadelphia.)*

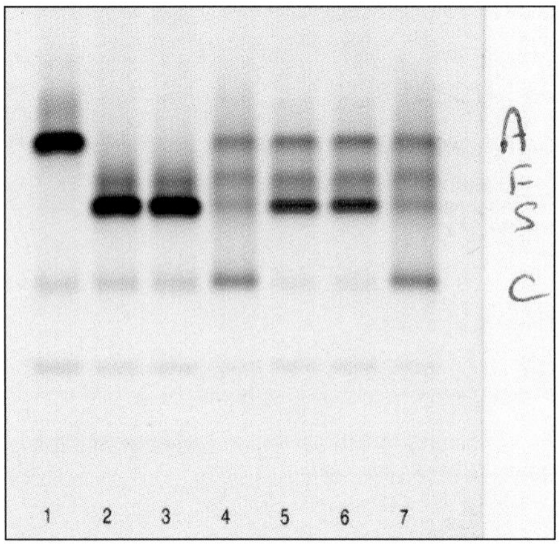

Figure 32-17 Electrophoretic separation of hemoglobins at alkaline pH. **1,** Normal adult; **2** and **3,** 17-year-old with sickle cell anemia; **5** and **6,** patient with sickle cell anemia, recently transfused; **4** and **7,** Hbs A/F/S/C standard (Hydragel 7 Hemoglobin/Hydrasys System, Sebia Electrophoresis, Norcross, Ga).

A) are produced. Because α-, γ-, and δ-genes are normal, the Hb F and Hb A_2 are structurally normal, although they may be increased in amount.

In heterozygous β-chain structural variants, the abnormal Hb is present, in addition to Hb A, F, and A_2. Its level depends on its rate of synthesis and stability, but also on its readiness to form dimers with α-chains. This latter process is driven by electrostatic forces between the positively charged α-globin and the negative β-globin. Because most β-globin variants acquire positive charge, their assembly with the positive α-chain is slower. As a result, the percentage of abnormal Hb is usually less than that of Hb A. In the presence of coexistent α-thalassemia, when β-chains compete for an insufficient number of α-globins, these effects are exaggerated and the level of structural variant decreases further. Similar forces influence the levels of Hb A_2. δ-Globin, the subunit of Hb A_2, has a significant positive charge, not favorable for dimer formation. Positively charged β-chain variants also have little affinity for α-chains, leaving excess α-chains for assembly with δ-globin and resulting in a slight increase in Hb A_2. This has been described in Hbs S and C trait, but the increase is so minimal that its existence was always questioned.

TABLE 32-4
Functional Classification of Hemoglobin Variants

I. Homozygous: hemoglobin (Hb) polymorphisms: the variants that are most common

Hb S	$\alpha_2\beta_2^{6Val}$	Severe hemolytic anemia: sickling
Hb C	$\alpha_2\beta_2^{6Lys}$	Mild hemolytic anemia
Hb D	Punjab $\alpha_2\beta_2^{121Gln}$	No anemia
Hb E	$\alpha_2\beta_2^{26Lys}$	Mild microcytic anemia

II. Heterozygous: hemoglobin variants causing functional aberrations or hemolytic anemia in the heterozygous state
- A. Hemoglobins associated with methemoglobinemia and cyanosis
  - Hb M Boston $\alpha_2^{58Tyr}\beta_2$
  - Hb M Iwate $\alpha_2^{87Tyr}\beta_2$
  - Hb M Saskatoon $\alpha_2\beta_2^{63Tyr}$
  - Hb M Milwaukee $\alpha_2\beta_2^{67Glu}$
  - Hb M Hyde Park $\alpha_2\beta_2^{92Tyr}$
  - Hb FM Osaka $\alpha_2\gamma_2^{63Tyr}$
  - Hb FM Fort Ripley $\alpha_2\gamma_2^{92Tyr}$
- B. Hemoglobins associated with altered oxygen affinity
  1. Increased affinity and polycythemia
     - Hb Chesapeake $\alpha_2^{92Leu}\beta_2$
     - Hb J Capetown $\alpha_2^{92Gln}\beta_2$
     - Hb Malmo $\alpha_2\beta_2^{97Gln}$
     - Hb Yakima $\alpha_2\beta_2^{99His}$
     - Hb Kempsey $\alpha_2\beta_2^{99Asn}$
     - Hb Y psi (Ypsilanti) $\alpha_2\beta_2^{99Tyr}$
     - Hb Hiroshima $\alpha_2\beta_2^{146Asp}$
     - Hb Rainier $\alpha_2\beta_2^{145Cys}$
     - Hb Bethesda $\alpha_2\beta_2^{145His}$
  2. Decreased affinity—may have mild anemia or cyanosis
     - Hb Kansas $\alpha_2\beta_2^{102Thr}$
     - Hb Titusville $\alpha_2^{94Asn}\beta_2$
     - Hb Providence $\alpha_2\beta_2^{82Asn}$
     - Hb Agenogi $\alpha_2\beta_2^{90Lys}$
     - Hb Beth Israel $\alpha_2\beta_2^{102Ser}$
     - Hb Yoshizuka $\alpha_2\beta_2^{108Asp}$
- C. Unstable hemoglobins
  1. Hb may precipitate as Heinz bodies after splenectomy: "congenital Heinz body anemia"
     - a. Severe hemolysis: no improvement after splenectomy
       - Hb Bibba $\alpha_2^{136Pro}\beta_2$
       - Hb Hammersmith $\alpha_2\beta_2^{42Ser}$
       - Hb Bristol $\alpha_2\beta_2^{67Asp}$
       - Hb Olmsted $\alpha_2\beta_2^{141Arg}$
     - b. Severe hemolysis: improvement after splenectomy
       - Hb Torino $\alpha_2^{43Val}\beta_2$
       - Hb Ann Arbor $\alpha_2^{80Arg}\beta_2$
       - Hb Genova $\alpha_2\beta_2^{28Pro}$
       - Hb Shepherd's Bush $\alpha_2\beta_2^{74Asp}$
       - Hb Koln $\alpha_2\beta_2^{98Met}$
       - Hb Wein $\alpha_2\beta_2^{130Asp}$
     - c. Mild hemolysis: intermittent exacerbations
       - Hb L-Ferrara $\alpha_2^{47Gly}\beta_2$
       - Hb Hasharon $\alpha_2^{47His}\beta_2$
       - Hb Leiden $\alpha_2\beta_2^{6\text{ or }7}$ (Glu deleted)
       - Hb Freiburg $\alpha_2\beta_2^{23}$ (Val deleted)
       - Hb Seattle $\alpha_2\beta_2^{70Asp}$
       - Hb Louisville $\alpha_2\beta_2^{42Leu}$
       - Hb Zürich $\alpha_2\beta_2^{63Arg}$
       - Hb Gun Hill $\alpha_2\beta_2^{91\text{-}}97$ (5 a. a. deleted)
     - d. No disease
       - Hb Etobicoke $\alpha_2^{84Arg}\beta_2$
       - Hb Dakar $\alpha_2^{112Gln}\beta_2$
       - Hb Sogn $\alpha_2\beta_2^{14Arg}$
       - Hb Tacoma $\alpha_2\beta_2^{30Ser}$
  2. Tetramers of normal chains: appear in thalassemias
     - Hb Bart's γ_4
     - HbH β_4
     - Hb α_4

Data from Winslow RM, Anderson WF. The hemoglobinopathies. In: Stanbury JB, Wyngaarden JB, Fredrickson DS, et al, editors. The metabolic basis of inherited disease. 5th ed. New York: McGraw-Hill; 1983, p. 2281–317.

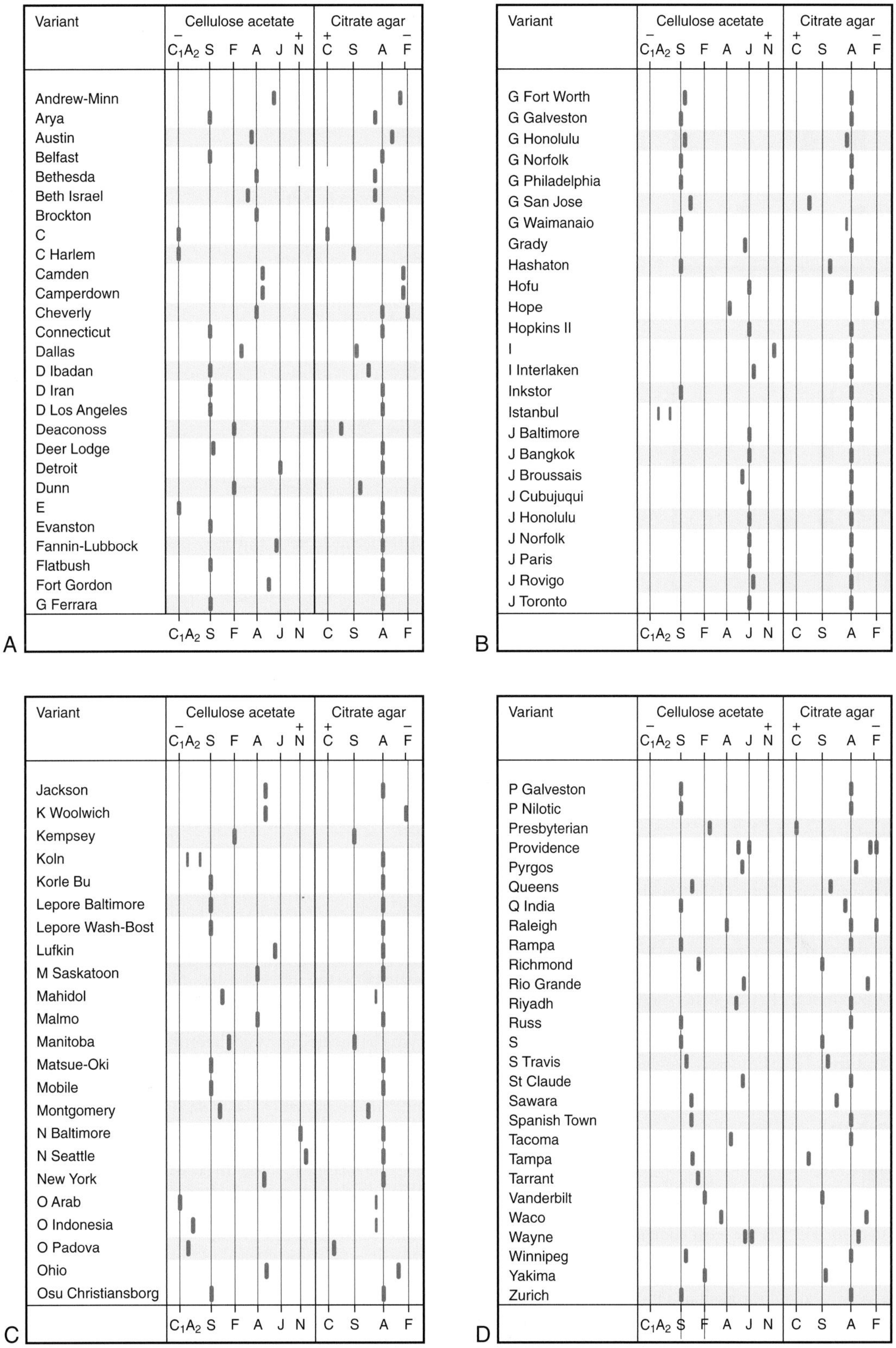

Figure 32-18 Electrophoretic mobility of 102 hemoglobin variants at alkaline (cellulose acetate) and acidic (citrate agar) pH. *(Courtesy of Winston Moo-Penn and Danny Jue.)*

PART 4

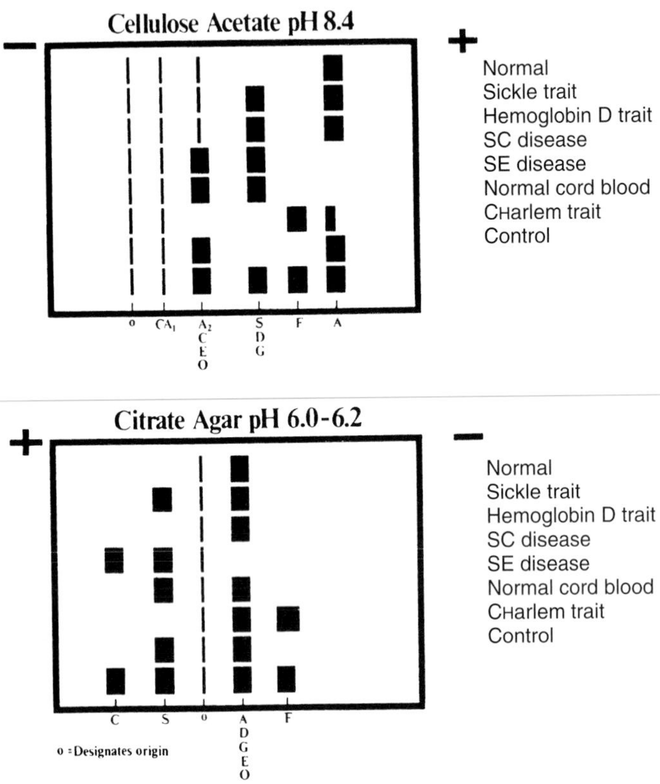

Figure 32-19 Hemoglobin (Hb) electrophoresis. Comparison of various Hb samples on cellulose acetate (at pH 8.4) and citrate agar (at pH 6), showing relative mobilities. The control is a composite sample. The relative amounts of Hb are not necessarily proportional to the size of the band. *(From Schmidt RM, Brosious EF. Basic laboratory methods of hemoglobinopathy detection. 6th ed. Atlanta: U.S. Department of Health, Education and Welfare, Centers of Disease Control; 1976. HEW Publ. No. CDC 77-8266.)*

Double heterozygotes for a β-chain structural variant and β^+-thalassemia are well known. Here, the quantity of abnormal Hb exceeds that of Hb A, in contrast to the heterozygous β-structural hemoglobinopathies, in which the reverse is true.

In heterozygous α-chain structural variants, the abnormality in the α-chain will affect all three Hb types. Therefore, six different hemoglobins are found—the three normal hemoglobins and the three abnormal forms. Examples are Hb D Baltimore, Hb Ann Arbor, and Hb M Boston.

Double heterozygotes for two β-chain abnormalities produce two different abnormal β-chains; therefore, there are two abnormal Hbs and no Hb A. An example of this is Hb SC disease. Double heterozygotes for β- and δ-chain abnormalities and for α- and β-chain abnormalities are rare but have provided important information. The latter will have four major Hb types on electrophoresis.

Sickling Disorders

Sickle Cell Trait (Hb AS)

The heterozygous state for Hb S is the most common hemoglobinopathy in the United States. It is present in about 8% of African Americans (Schneider, 1976) and in as many as 45% of the population in certain areas of West Africa. The gene is found throughout sub-Saharan Africa and, at a much lower frequency, in the Mediterranean, Middle East, and India. Hb S trait is a completely benign condition without clinical symptoms or hematologic abnormalities. Added risk associated with sickle cell trait is minimal, at the most, and is seen only in very rare circumstances. Extreme low O_2 tensions can trigger sickling, and a few people have sustained splenic infarction when flying at very high altitude in unpressurized airplanes. Slightly increased incidences of hematuria, impaired ability to concentrate urine, and bacteriuria in women have been reported. Sickle cell trait confers protection to children from the lethal effects of falciparum malaria, which accounts for the major distribution of Hb S in central Africa.

The stained blood film appears normal, except perhaps for a few target cells. Blood cell counts are normal. The sickle cell slide preparation is positive, and almost all red cells eventually sickle. The solubility test is positive.

TABLE 32-5
Prevalence of Common Hemoglobin Disorders Among African Americans

	%
Traits	
Silent α-thalassemia (αα/−α)	24
Hb AS	8.6
α-Thalassemia trait (−α/−α)	5.7
Hb AC	2.4
β-Thalassemia trait	1.5
HPFH	0.1
Hbs D and G	0.026
All others	0.3
Sickling Disorders	
Hb SS	0.16
Hb S/C	0.13
Hb S/thal	0.06
Hb S/HPFH	0.004
Other Disorders	
Hb CC	0.02
Hb C/β-thalassemia	0.02
Homozygous β-thalassemia	0.005

Data from Motulsky (1973), Schneider (1976), and Pierce (1977).
Hb, Hemoglobin; *HPFH,* hereditary persistence of fetal hemoglobin.

Hemoglobin separation shows 60% Hb A, 40% Hb S, normal Hb F, and normal to slightly increased Hb A_2, up to 4.5%.

The proportion of Hb S is decreased in the presence of α-thalassemia; Hb S is less than 35% when one α-gene is deleted, and less than 29% when two genes are lost (Head, 2004). In the latter, cells are hypochromic and microcytic. Because 27% of African Americans carry the α^+-thalassemia gene, it is not surprising that this diagnostic dilemma is quite common. Hb S level may also be diminished in iron and folate deficiency. Clinically, the combination of sickle cell trait and α-thalassemia trait is benign, with possible mild microcytic anemia due to the thalassemia trait.

Sickle Cell Disease (Hb SS)

Homozygous Hb S disease is a serious chronic hemolytic anemia, first manifested in early childhood and often fatal before the age of 30 years. With modern medical care, many patients live longer, but the median age of death in the United States is still only in the 40s. Hb S is found mostly in the black population; 1 of every 600 black persons in the United States has sickle cell anemia (Steinberg, 1999).

In Hb S (β6 glu→val), the glutamic acid in the sixth position on the β-chain is replaced by valine. Hb S is freely soluble when fully oxygenated; when O_2 is removed, Hb S polymerizes, with formation of tactoids (fluid crystals) that are rigid and deform the cell into the shape that gave the cell its name. A strong interaction between the side chain of β6 valine and the hydrophobic pocket of β85 phenylalanine and 88 leucine of another Hb S molecule is probably the basis of polymer formation. In homozygous Hb S disease, sickling occurs at physiologic O_2 tensions, and the rigidity of the red cells is responsible for the hemolysis, as well as for most of the complications. These irreversibly sickled cells result from membrane reorganization during repeated episodes of sickling and unsickling, in addition to cell dehydration that markedly reduces cellular deformability. Sickle cells contain high calcium levels, which stimulate potassium and water loss (Gardos effect) and exaggerate cell dehydration (Weatherall, 1999). The hemolytic component is mostly extracellular and is caused by clustering of band 3 of the cell membrane, with the consequence of increased IgG binding and recognition by macrophages. Integrins (α4β1) on the sickle cell surface attach to fibronectin and adhesion molecules expressed on endothelial cells; this is enhanced by inflammatory cytokines, von Willebrand factor, and platelet activation, and together these interactions cause vaso-occlusion.

Complications. In early childhood, bilateral painful swelling of the dorsa of the hands or feet occurs as a result of sickling and capillary stasis; this is known as the **hand-foot syndrome,** or sickle cell dactylitis. It lasts about 2 weeks, is accompanied by changes of periostitis as observed by X-ray, and does not occur after the age of 4.

The spleen is central to three complications: A **sequestration crisis** refers to sudden pooling of blood and rapid enlargement of the spleen, resulting in hypovolemic shock. This may occur in early childhood when

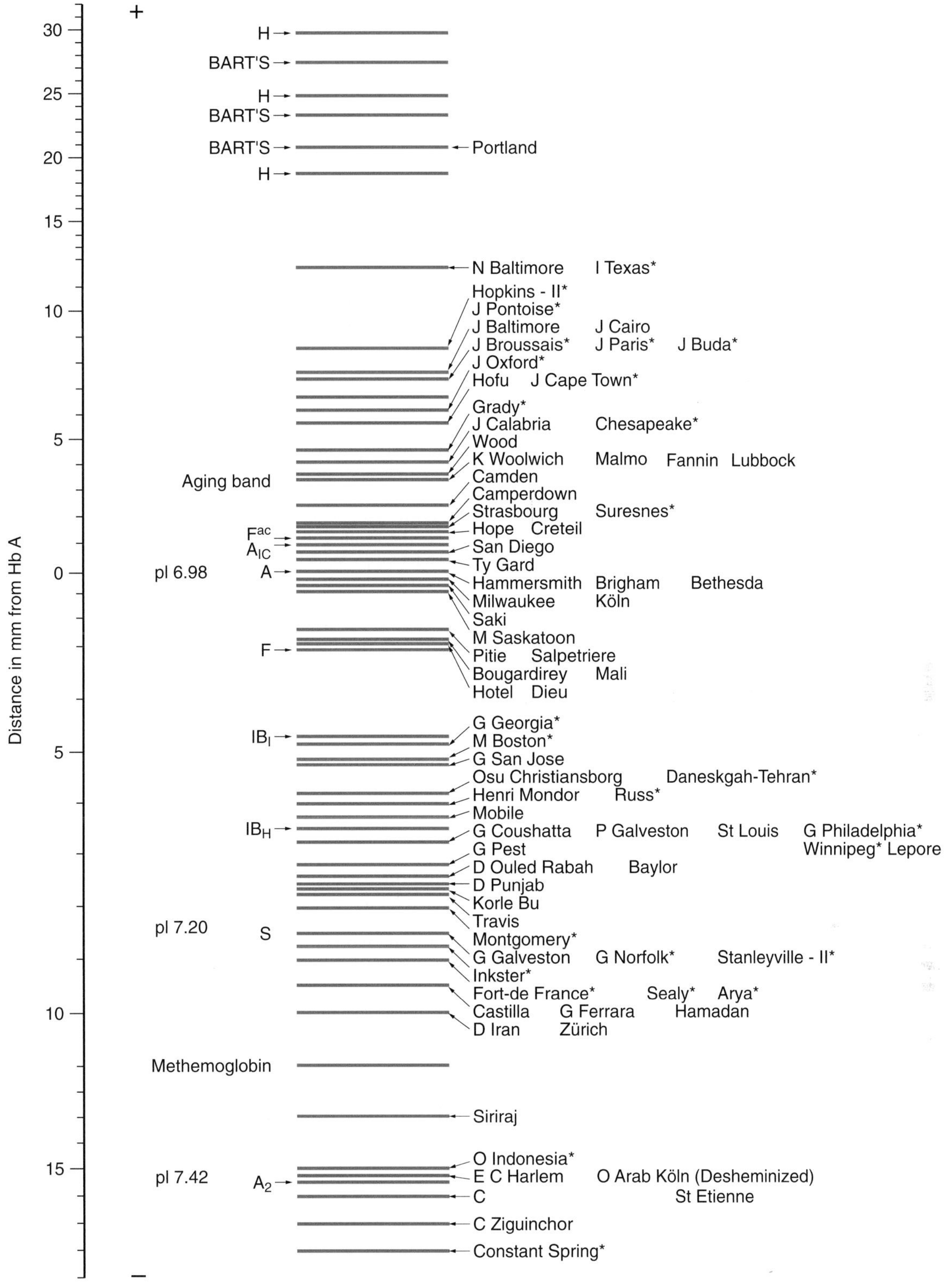

Figure 32-20 Comparison of 57 hemoglobin variants by isoelectric focusing. Asterisk denotes α-chain variants. *(From Basset P, Braconnier F, Rosa J. An update on electrophoretic and chromatographic methods in the diagnosis of hemoglobinopathies. J Chromatogr Biomed Appl 1982;227:267–304.)*

splenomegaly is present and is often preceded by infection. **Functional asplenia** (Pearson, 1969) consists of inadequate antibody responses under some conditions and an impaired ability of the reticuloendothelial system to clear bacteria and particulate material from the blood, probably owing to reticuloendothelial blockade. This may explain in part the increased risk of infection in children with the disease. Salmonellal and pneumococcal infections are unusually prevalent in children with sickle cell anemia. Vaso-occlusive episodes result in progressive infarction, fibrosis, and contraction of the spleen—so-called **autosplenectomy.** Although splenomegaly is present in childhood, a small fibrotic remnant is the rule in the adult.

From early childhood, patients cannot produce concentrated urine, apparently as a result of anoxic damage in the medullae of the kidneys. Hematuria as a result of papillary necrosis is common. Renal insufficiency occurs in 5%–20% of adults (Steinberg, 1999).

Vaso-occlusive crises are debilitating episodes of abdominal and bone or joint pain, accompanied by fever, which are probably due to plugging of small blood vessels by masses of sickled cells. Bone necrosis occurs in 10%–50% of patients and may be a focus for salmonellal osteomyelitis. Acute chest syndrome represents episodes of acute chest pain often associated with a new infiltrate in the chest film. Approximately 40% of patients

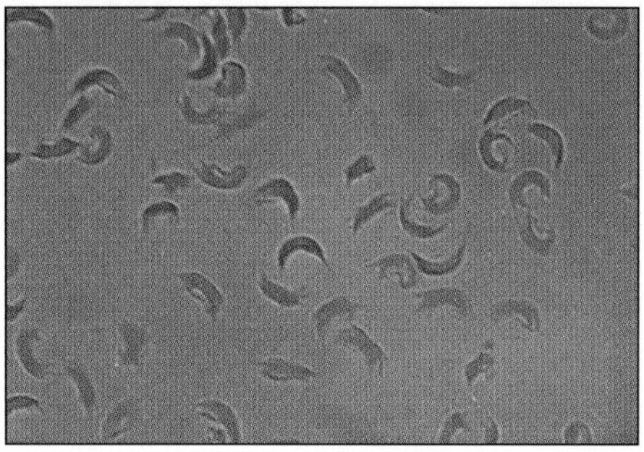

Figure 32-21 Sickle cell preparation, in sodium metabisulfate; sickle cell anemia. Even in sickle cell trait, all cells eventually sickle.

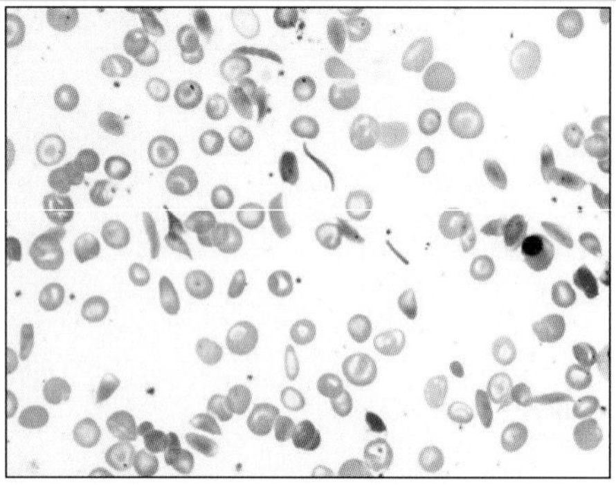

Figure 32-22 Blood film, sickle cell anemia. The erythrocytes are far from one another, suggesting a severe anemia. Numerous pointed sickle cells and target cells are present. Close to the nucleated red blood cell, elliptical cells are seen. These cells have a dense center, instead of the usual central pallor, suggesting that they are incipient sickle cells (500×).

experience at least one episode of acute chest syndrome. Although an infectious origin has been suspected in earlier studies, fat embolism is now considered to play a major role in this syndrome. The various complications that result from recurring vaso-occlusive crises involve many body organs (Steinberg, 1999).

Aplastic crises occasionally can afflict any patient with chronic hemolytic anemia. Temporary failure of red cell production that would not be noticed in a person with a normal red cell life span will cause a serious fall in Hb concentration in chronic hemolytic anemia. This may be the result of infection, particularly parvovirus B19, exposure to toxic drugs, or folic acid deficiency; sometimes no cause can be found. Hemolytic crises due to a further increase in hemolysis are rare.

Diagnosis. The anemia is normochromic and normocytic; polychromasia is increased, and nucleated red blood cells are present. Sickle cells are almost always found in the stained smear (Fig. 32-22). Target cells are numerous, and Howell-Jolly and Pappenheimer bodies are regularly seen in older children and adults as a result of asplenia. The microhematocrit as an estimate of degree of anemia is unreliable because of excessive plasma trapping. Neutrophilia and thrombocytosis are usual. The marrow shows normoblastic hyperplasia.

No Hb A is found if the patient has not been transfused recently; more than 80% of the hemoglobin is Hb S, 1%–20% Hb F, and 2%–4.5% Hb A_2 (Wrightstone, 1974). The fetal hemoglobin is distributed unevenly among the red cells. Hb S and several D and G hemoglobins have the same electrophoretic mobility at alkaline pH, but of these, only Hb S gives a positive sickling test.

Hemoglobin SC Disease

The frequency of Hb SC disease is almost the same as that of Hb SS disease in African Americans. It causes a mild hemolytic anemia. Crises are less frequent and less painful than in sickle cell anemia. Onset is usually in childhood, but the disease might be undetected until later in life. The life expectancy is only modestly shortened. The body habitus is normal or stocky in contrast to the asthenic features in sickle cell anemia. Splenomegaly might be the only finding on physical examination. Fatigue, dyspnea on effort, frequent upper respiratory infections, attacks of mild jaundice, and arthralgias are seen. Constant hip and low back pain may be present with aseptic necrosis of the head of the femur. Hematuria from renal medullary infarction and splenic infarcts has been described. In pregnancy, crises are more frequent and there is an increase in thrombotic tendency, which can cause massive thromboembolism and sudden death following childbirth. A higher incidence of retinopathy is seen in Hb SC disease than in SS disease.

Anemia varies from moderate to very mild and is normochromic-normocytic. Anisocytosis and poikilocytosis are mild to severe, and target cells are numerous—up to 85% of the erythrocytes. Plump and angulated sickled cells are often present on the film. The sickling test is positive. Hb S is 50% and Hb C is slightly less. Hb F is usually under 2%. The proportions of Hbs are the same in patients with coexistent α-thalassemia (Steinberg, 1983).

Hb S/β-Thalassemia

This is the third most common sickling disorder after Hb SS and Hb SC in African Americans, and the most common one in people from the Mediterranean. It usually runs a milder course in black people (usually S/β^+-thalassemia) but causes a severe sickling disorder with manifestations similar to those of sickle cell anemia in people of Italian, Turkish, or Greek descent.

In Hb S/β^0-thalassemia, Hb A is absent; Hb S is 75%–90%, Hb F is 5%–20%, and Hb A_2 is 4%–6%. This disorder clinically and hematologically resembles sickle cell disease, except for the spleen, which remains enlarged after childhood and into adult life. The main difference is that in Hb S/β^0-thalassemia, the MCV and MCH are decreased, and the Hb A_2 might be significantly increased. Family study is often necessary for a clear distinction (Wrightstone, 1974; Lehmann, 1977). On the blood smear, pronounced microcytosis, variable hypochromia, and many target cells are present. As a consequence of reduced cellular hemoglobin, Hb S polymers are formed more slowly, and fewer sickled cells are present on the smear.

In Hb S/β^+-thalassemia, Hb A is 15%–30%; Hb S is over 50%, Hb F is 1%–20%, and Hb A_2 is 4%–6%. Although these individuals clinically may resemble those with sickle trait (Hb AS), in S/β^+-thalassemia, the amount of Hb S always exceeds Hb A, and in Hb AS, Hb A always exceeds Hb S.

Hb SS/α-Thalassemia

Thirty to forty percent of patients with sickle cell anemia are heterozygous, and 2%–3% are homozygous for α^+-thalassemia (Higgs, 1982). MCV (83 fL in heterozygotes and 72 fL in homozygotes) and MCH are decreased. Hb level is higher and reticulocyte count is significantly lower, as compared with sickle cell anemia. On the smear, sickled cells are uncommon similarly to Hb S/β^0-thalassemia. Although anemia is less severe, the vaso-occlusive disease is not, and some studies even show increased morbidity and mortality. As described earlier, δ-chains successfully compete with positively charged S-chains for a limited number of α-chains, and Hb A_2 levels increase. Hematologically, this cannot be separated from Hb S/β^0-thalassemia (Table 32-6). Whenever microcytosis and increased Hb A_2 are present in sickle cell anemia, family or molecular studies are to be done to differentiate these entities.

Hemoglobin SD Disease

(Hb S/D–Los Angeles). SD disease simulates but is less severe than sickle cell anemia, and thus may also resemble SC disease. It is occasionally seen in the African American population. On routine (alkaline) electrophoresis, the pattern is indistinguishable from sickle cell anemia because Hb S and Hb D cannot be separated. Agar gel electrophoresis at pH 6.2 will separate Hb S and Hb D.

Hb S/O Arab. Compound heterozygotes of Hb S and Hb O Arab (β121 glu→lys) have a severe sickling disorder. Hb O Arab is found in black and Arabic people. Hb E and a few other, less frequent β-variants also cause sickling disorders with Hb S. Coexistence of an α-chain variant and a sickle cell trait does not cause a sickling disorder.

Other Common β-Chain Variants

Hb C Trait (β6 glu→lys). Hemoglobin C is prevalent in West Africans and in about 2%–3% of black people. The heterozygous state (Hb AC) is asymptomatic, without anemia, with normal or minimally reduced MCV and normal red cell life span. The MCHC might be slightly elevated. Target cells are present on blood film. Hb C makes up about 40% of the total hemoglobin. When significant microcytosis is present, it is usually caused by coexistent α-thalassemia, and Hb C is reduced to 38%, 32%, and 24% in patients with three, two, and one α-gene, respectively (Huisman, 1977).

TABLE 32-6
Differential Diagnosis of Sickle Cell/Thalassemia Syndromes

Genotype	Clinical expression	Hb	MCV	Hb F	Hb A_2	Hb A
SS	Severe	7–8	85–95	2–20	2–4	
S/β^0 thal	Moderate to severe	8–10	65–75	5–20	4–6	
SS/α thal	Moderate to severe	8–10	70–85	2–20	3–5	
S/HPFH	Asymptomatic to mild	13–14	75–85	20–30	1–3	
S/β^+ thal	Mild to moderate	11–12	70–80	1–13	3–6	10–30

Data from Bunn (1986) and Steinberg (2001).
Hb, Hemoglobin; *Hb A*, accounts for 97% of normal adult hemoglobin; *Hb A_2*, accounts for the remaining 3% of normal adult hemoglobin; *Hb F*, fetal hemoglobin; *HPFH*, hereditary persistence of fetal hemoglobin; *MCV*, mean corpuscular volume.

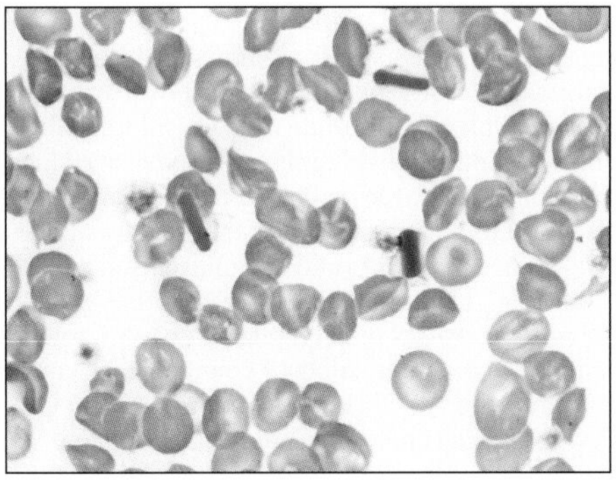

Figure 32-23 Hemoglobin (Hb) C disease, after splenectomy. Before splenectomy, the only morphologic abnormality was the presence of target cells. After splenectomy, Howell-Jolly bodies and Hb crystals, such as those in the center, were present. Note that almost all of the Hb in this particular cell is in the dark bar, and the membrane is still visible. Some such crystals are distinctly hexagonal (1000×).

Hb C Disease. Homozygous Hb C disease is a mild hemolytic anemia with splenomegaly that is often asymptomatic but occasionally results in jaundice and abdominal discomfort. Life expectancy is normal. In the United States, 0.02% of black people have Hb C disease (Schneider, 1976). Reticulocytosis is low for the degree of anemia. The anemia is largely a consequence of low O_2 affinity of Hb C (Bunn, 1986) and should not be treated. The MCV is normal or decreased, and the MCHC is normal or increased. Numerous target cells with an admixture of microspherocytes and minimal polychromasia are seen in the blood. Osmotic fragility is biphasic, with both increased and decreased fragility, but is not used in the diagnosis today. Hexagonal or rod-shaped crystals may be seen in erythrocytes in the stained smear, especially after splenectomy or after slow drying of the smear (Fig. 32-23). As opposed to Hb S, crystals of Hb C tend to melt at low partial pressure of oxygen (pO_2) and do not cause vaso-occlusive disease. The red cells are dehydrated (causing the increased MCHC), owing to loss of cations and water as a result of interaction of Hb C with the red cell membrane. As a consequence, the cells are more rigid and less deformable than normal, increasing their likelihood of being trapped and destroyed in the spleen. Hb F is elevated at 2%–4%, and Hb A_2, when measured by HPLC, might be slightly increased; the remainder of hemoglobin is Hb C.

Hb C/β^+-Thalassemia. This occurs mainly in black people, in whom it tends to result in little disability, except for anemia in pregnancy. Red cell indices are typical of β-thalassemia trait, but there is anisocytosis and 20%–50% target cells. Usual values are 65%–80% for Hb C, 16%–30% for Hb A, and 2%–5% for Hb F.

Hb C/β^0-thalassemia. People of Mediterranean extraction usually have a moderately severe hemolytic anemia with β^0 or a severe β^+ genotype. This combination is extremely rare in the African population. Hb C/β^0-thalassemia may be difficult to distinguish from Hb C disease in that Hb A is absent in both, and there is an overlap in Hbs A_2 and F levels. Hb A_2 is elevated to about twice normal, and Hb F is elevated at 3%–10%.

Hb E (β 26 glu→lys). This is probably the most prevalent hemoglobin variant worldwide and the third most common in the United States, behind S and C. It is found primarily in Southeast Asia, especially in people of Thai and Burmese extraction, but is also found in blacks and Caucasians. Hb E is associated with a β-thalassemia phenotype, as well as with a structurally abnormal globin chain. The mutation that causes amino acid substitution also activates a cryptic splice site that competes with the normal RNA splice donor site, and normally processed RNA is decreased. In the laboratory, Hb E can be demonstrated to be unstable. It precipitates abnormally in the heat denaturation test and with isopropanol, yet this has no in vivo significance; the red cell survival is normal (Fairbanks, 1980).

Hb E Trait (Hb AE). Hb AE is asymptomatic, with borderline microcytosis (MCV = 84 ± 5) and no anemia. Hb A is 65%–70% of the total hemoglobin, Hb E is 30%, and Hb F is normal. Coexistence of one α-thalassemia gene does not change any of the above parameters and can be proven only by DNA analysis. If two or three α-thalassemia genes are also present, the proportion of Hb E decreases to 21% and 14%, respectively. The proportion of Hb E is also significantly lower in iron deficiency.

Hemoglobin E Disease. This is also asymptomatic; it resembles a thalassemia trait, with microcytosis (average MCV = 70 fL), erythrocytosis, normal MCHC, and slight anemia. Thus, Hb E behaves as an extremely mild thalassemia. The reticulocyte count is normal, but 20%–80% target cells are evident on the blood film. Hb E accounts for more than 90% of the hemoglobin, with Hb F from 1%–10% and no Hb A.

Hb E/β-Thalassemia. In sharp contrast with Hb E disease, this is a severe condition. It is one of the most important thalassemia syndromes and is most common in Southeast Asia. Clinical variability is marked; rarely, there are very few symptoms, but the usual picture is that of thalassemia intermedia or thalassemia major. Most of the thalassemia alleles are of the β^0 or severe β^+ variety. Ineffective erythropoiesis, a consequence of excess α-globins, red cell indices, red cell morphology, and clinical manifestations are similar to those in homozygous β-thalassemia. Hbs E, F, and A_2 are present. Hb F shows extreme variation, from 5%–85%; the mean Hb F is 42%, and Hb E is 58% (Steinberg, 2001).

Hb D Los Angeles (Punjab) (β121 glu→gln). This constitutes the most common D variant in African Americans (<0.02%). In the Punjab region of India, heterozygosity reaches 3%. Homozygotes have normal red cell indices, no evidence of hemolysis, and 95% Hb D with normal Hbs F and A2 (Bunn, 1986). Double heterozygotes for Hb D Punjab/β^0-thalassemia have a mild hemolytic anemia with thalassemic red cell indices and increased Hbs F and A_2.

The significance of Hb D Punjab is that compound heterozygosity with Hb S produces a moderately severe sickling disorder (see Hb SD Disease earlier). Other, less frequent D hemoglobins (D Iran, D Ibadan) and G hemoglobins do not cause sickling—a major difference for genetic counseling. D and G hemoglobins migrate with Hb S on alkaline electrophoresis but are separated from S at acidic pH, migrating with Hb A. It is more difficult to separate them from each other. Careful analysis of isoelectric focusing and HPLC are helpful in most cases.

Common α-Chain Variants

Hb G Philadelphia (α 68asn→lys). This is the most common α-chain variant in black people (Schneider, 1976). Almost invariably, the linked α-gene is deleted ($-\alpha^G$). Simple heterozygotes ($-\alpha^G/\alpha\alpha$) have 30% Hb G and normal red cell indices, but double heterozygotes with α-gene deletion on the other chromosome as well ($-\alpha^G/-\alpha$) have 45% Hb G and a thalassemia trait phenotype. As with other α-chain variants, a minor hemoglobin, a combination of α^G with δ, is present close to Hb A_2 and helps to differentiate Hb G Philadelphia from β-chain variant G and D hemoglobins.

Disorders of Hemoglobin Function and Stability

A number of amino acid substitutions occur in the heme pocket, where they may increase the stability of the methemoglobin form (Hb M) or alter the affinity of the heme for O_2; the latter usually alters the stability of the molecule as well. Other substitutions affect the αβ contact sites; these also can change stability and O_2 affinity of the molecule (Bunn, 1994).

These functionally significant hemoglobinopathies are heterozygous; usually, the concentration of the abnormal Hb is less than 50%. Generally, Hbs with abnormal α-chains form a smaller proportion of the total (10%–25%) than those with abnormal β-chains (35%–50%).

Hemoglobins Associated With High Oxygen Affinity and Polycythemia

Eighty-six abnormal Hbs with high O_2 affinity that are associated with familial erythrocytosis are known today (Globin Gene Server). Some are listed in Table 32-4. The O_2 dissociation curve is shifted to the left. The p_{50}, the pO_2 at which Hb is 50% saturated, is decreased. Under physiologic conditions, the normal p_{50} of whole blood is 26 mm Hg; in this disorder, it has ranged from 5–23 mm Hg. Because the Hb has high affinity for O_2, the tissues are relatively hypoxic at any given p_{50}, resulting in increased EPO production and polycythemia. These disorders are autosomal dominant; only heterozygotes have been described. The Hb concentration has ranged from 15–23.8 g/dL. Measurement of O_2 affinity is required to establish the diagnosis (Bunn, 1986). Because the amino acid substitution is inside the molecule, often the abnormal hemoglobin is indistinguishable from Hb A on electrophoresis or HPLC.

Hemoglobins Associated With Low Oxygen Affinity

There are far fewer variants with decreased O_2 affinity (see Table 32-4; Bunn, 1986). The Hb–O_2 dissociation curve is shifted to the right (increased p_{50}). These individuals have mild "anemia," as they can unload more O_2 to the tissues and they simply do not need that much Hb. A handful of variants with markedly decreased affinity are associated with cyanosis. In these, O_2 uptake is impaired in the lung and the level of deoxyhemoglobin is more than 5 g/dL, causing cyanosis. These patients have a slate gray color to their skin and mucous membranes. They have no anemia. Many of the unstable Hbs also have decreased O_2 affinity; however, the hemolytic state dominates the clinical picture.

M Hemoglobins: Pseudocyanosis

Nine abnormal Hbs are associated with clinical methemoglobinemia and cyanosis that do not respond to methylthioninium chloride (methylene blue) (Globin Gene Server; Bunn, 1994). The color is similar to cyanosis—a brownish color, caused by methemoglobin. The common feature is that all have an amino acid substitution at or near the heme group, so that methemoglobin is unusually stable, and reduction to ferrous heme and hence reversible binding of O_2 are prevented. Methemoglobin constitutes no more than 3% of the total Hb in normal humans.

Cyanosis from birth is seen in Hb M disease with α-chain abnormalities, or in fetal Hb M (Hb FM Osaka). In the latter, cyanosis will disappear after the γ-chains have been replaced by β-chains by 6 months of age. Cyanosis does not appear until nearly 6 months of age in Hb M variants with β-chain abnormalities, for the same reason (Bunn, 1994). Of course, the cyanosis is not associated with enzyme abnormalities in the red cell, toxic drugs, or cyanotic heart disease—conditions that must be considered in the differential diagnosis. Patients usually have no other symptoms.

All Hb M disorders thus far discovered have been reported in heterozygotes, probably because homozygosity is lethal. Some types of Hb M will not separate from Hb A on alkaline electrophoresis. If the hemolysate is first converted to methemoglobin, the Hb M will migrate differently from normal methemoglobin at pH 7.1. The absorption spectra of the eluted Hb M, which may be distinctive, can be compared with those of normal methemoglobin (Bunn, 1994).

Unstable Hemoglobins (Bunn, 1998)

More than 100 Hb variants have been described in which the Hb precipitates within the red cell as Heinz bodies. Some are listed in Table 32-4. About 75% of the abnormalities are β-chain. Rare unstable hemoglobins such as Hb F Poole are related to unstable γ-chain variants. Amino acid substitution or deletion renders the Hb molecule unstable. Precipitated Hb attaches to the cell membrane and shortens its survival; the cells are inflexible. Heinz bodies are removed by the spleen, and further damaged cells have a shortened survival. The O_2 affinity is usually abnormal and may be increased or decreased. Some of these unstable Hbs cause "congenital Heinz body hemolytic anemias."

All patients have been heterozygous. Clinical features have shown considerable variation, from severe hemolytic anemia in the first year of life (e.g., Hb Hammersmith, Hb Bristol) to a very mild chronic hemolytic anemia (e.g., Hb Louisville, Hb Hasharon) that may be exacerbated by drugs (e.g., Hb Zurich). A few unstable Hbs have been discovered incidentally in clinically normal individuals (e.g., Hb Tacoma, Hb Sogn).

Jaundice and splenomegaly are common, as in other hemolytic anemias. More distinctive in some cases is the excretion of darkly pigmented urine (only during hemolytic crises in mild variants). The urine pigment appears to be dipyrrole, probably a breakdown product of heme molecules after separation from globin (Dacie, 1991). Cyanosis is present in some patients and is due to methemoglobinuria and sulfhemoglobinemia or to low O_2 affinity.

The anemia is normocytic and normochromic to hypochromic, the latter because of the removal of precipitated Hb from aging red cells by macrophages of the spleen and other reticuloendothelial organs. Prominent basophilic stippling, probably related to excessive clumping of ribosomes, is a common feature. Occasional "bite cells" may be seen. Patients with relatively high Hb concentrations in the steady state usually have Hb variants with a high O_2 affinity and an unexpectedly high reticulocyte count (e.g., Hb Köln, Hb Gun Hill). On the other hand, patients with rather low Hb concentrations may be relatively asymptomatic if their Hb has a low O_2 affinity; their reticulocyte counts are unexpectedly low for the Hb concentration (e.g., Hb Hammersmith). Heinz bodies are rarely seen in circulating red cells before splenectomy, although sometimes they may be generated by incubating the red cells with brilliant cresyl blue or new methylene blue. After splenectomy, Heinz bodies are readily demonstrable in a large proportion of cells; the blood film shows irregularly contracted cells and basophilic stippling that may be pronounced.

In splenectomized patients, the Heinz bodies may interfere with Hb determinations and with electronic platelet and white cell counts. Before the absorbance of the hemolysate is measured, it should be centrifuged to remove the Heinz bodies. Platelet and leukocyte counts should be performed by visual methods. Hb electrophoresis is normal in about one fourth of patients. Hb A_2 may be elevated in β-chain variants because of the loss of abnormal Hb from the cells; this phenotype may resemble thalassemia intermedia. Hb F may be increased to a level of 10%–15%. Key laboratory determinations include heat instability and isopropanol precipitation tests.

Heat Instability Test. Most unstable Hbs precipitate more rapidly than normal Hbs when incubated at 50° C (Dacie, 1991). Both normal and unstable Hbs precipitate more rapidly in Tris-buffer than in phosphate buffers. In a hemolysate in tris-buffer, an easily visible precipitate forms within an hour if unstable Hb is present; the control sample is clear or slightly cloudy. Slight precipitation is equivocal; the test should be repeated and the isopropanol precipitation test performed as well. Precipitates accounting for 10%–40% of the total Hb are found in unstable Hb disorders.

Isopropanol Precipitation Test. A relatively nonpolar solvent weakens the internal bonds of Hb and decreases its stability (Carrell, 1972). An unstable Hb precipitates within 20 minutes in the nonpolar solvent isopropanol, whereas a normal hemolysate remains clear for 30–40 minutes. False-positive results occur with high levels of Hb F.

THALASSEMIAS

In thalassemias, globin chains, usually of normal structure, are produced at a decreased rate. β-Thalassemia refers to decreased production of β-chains; α-thalassemia and δβ-, δ-, and γδβ-thalassemias refer to reduced synthesis of the respective polypeptide chains. As a result, there is an overall deficit of Hb tetramers in the red cells, and MCV and MCH are reduced. However, it is not the lack of the affected globin chain, but the accumulation of the unaffected one, that causes hemolysis and, primarily in β-thalassemia, ineffective hematopoiesis in severe forms of the disease.

Thalassemia occurs predominantly in persons of Mediterranean, African, and Asian ancestry as, similarly to Hb variants or glucose-6-phosphate dehydrogenase (G6PD) deficiency, thalassemia genes are under selective pressure by malaria. In Greece and Southern Italy, the prevalence of β-thalassemia is around 10%, and that of α-thalassemia is 5%.

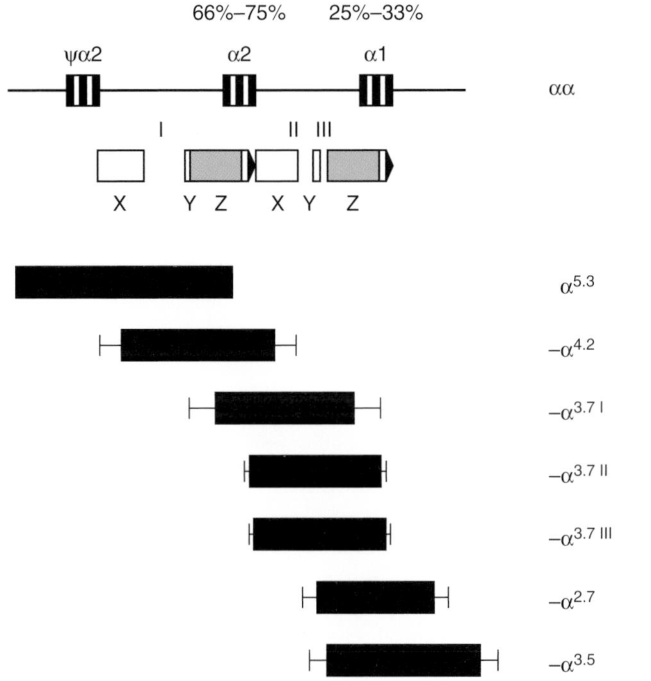

Figure 32-24 Deletions that cause α^+ thalassemia. The homologous boxes (X, Y, and Z) are interrupted by nonhomologous segments (I, II, and III). Black bars show the extent of each deletion and thin bars show the breakpoint areas. In each case, only one α-gene is deleted.

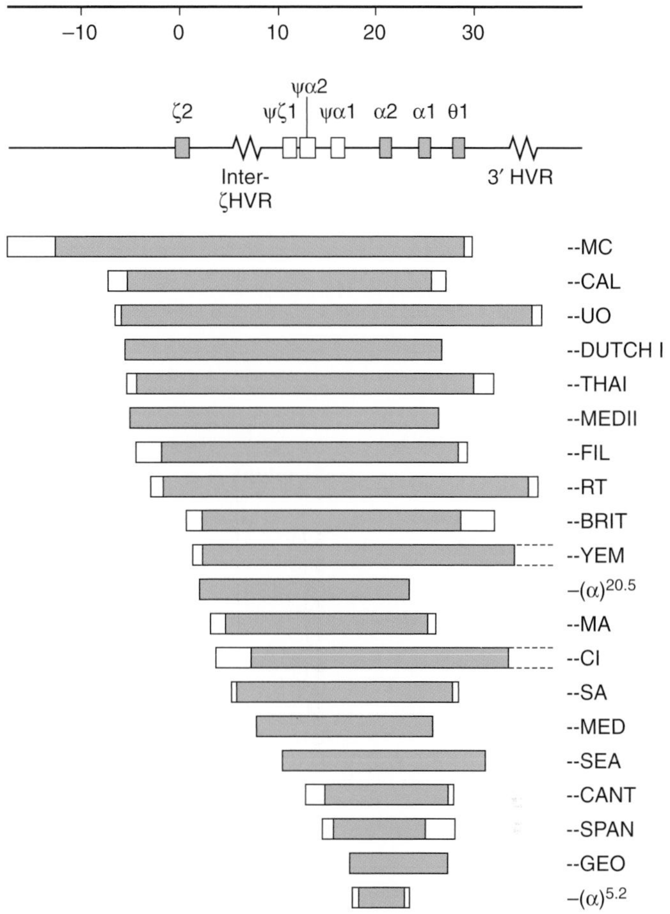

Figure 32-25 Large deletions of the α-gene complex cause α^0-thalassemia. No α-chain synthesis is directed from the chromosome. MED (Mediterranean) and SEA (South East Asian) deletions are the most frequent.

Twenty-five to 30% of black people and 20% of Thai people carry an α-thalassemia gene. Because structural variants and thalassemias occur in the same population, a wide variety of diseases emerge from their interactions.

Several classifications are used. The clinical classification defines thalassemia major, a severe and transfusion-dependent form; thalassemia intermedia, with less severe symptoms; and thalassemia minor (carrier state or trait), without clinical symptoms, but with hematologic abnormalities. The genetic classification is based on gene(s) affected by the mutation, heterozygous/homozygous state, absent/reduced rate of globin synthesis, and so forth. Finally, specific mutations cause well-defined syndromes and can be used for classification.

Molecular Defects

In β-thalassemia, considerable heterogeneity in molecular defects is noted. One hundred ninety-seven different mutations have been identified as the cause of β-thalassemia. Most are associated with single base substitutions that produce defects in promoter activity, RNA processing/splicing, or translation, resulting in decreased or unstable mRNA. Large deletions are uncommon. In rare structural variants, the production of highly unstable β-chains results in the phenotype of β-thalassemia (Bunn, 1998). Despite this diversity, 20 common mutations account for 80% of β-thalassemia alleles in the world population (Weatherall, 1999). In β^0-thalassemia, β-chain synthesis is absent on the affected chromosome. Messenger RNA (mRNA) is absent or may be present but nonfunctional. In β^+-thalassemia, β-globin chains are present but reduced in quantity because molecular defects have resulted in the production of unstable or decreased amounts of mRNA.

In $\delta\beta^0$-thalassemia, large deletions involve the δβ– or Aγδβ–gene complex. As a result, no Hb A or Hb A_2 synthesis is supported from the affected chromosome, but the γ-gene is upregulated and Hb F production is increased. Lepore Hbs have δβ-fusion globins that are the result of unequal crossover between δ- and β-globin genes during meiosis.

The α-thalassemias are generally due to gene deletion of various lengths. Two α-globin genes are present on each chromosome 16, surrounded by two highly homologous duplication units, each containing three homologous segments (Z, X, and Y). Unequal crossing over between the Z segments produces a chromosome with one α-gene ($-\alpha^{3.7}$) and another with three (ααα). Similar nonreciprocal crossing over between X boxes causes another common deletion ($-\alpha^{4.2}$) (Fig. 32-24). This recombination has a high probability, and chromosomes with missing or extra α-genes are found in every civilization; nonetheless, only the thalassemic alleles became frequent in certain populations, under pressure from malaria. These defects, affecting only one of the genes, are called α^+-thalassemia. The heterozygous genotype can be written (–α/αα). Nondeletion defects are less common ($\alpha^T\alpha$/αα). α^0-Thalassemia results from deletion of both α-globin genes on the chromosome (Fig. 32-25), which leads to no α-chain synthesis (—/αα).

Hb Constant Spring is due to an abnormal termination codon in an α-globin gene that results in an elongated α-chain with 31 extra amino acids. Because of marked reduction in mRNA stability, the clinical phenotype of α-thalassemia is seen (Orkin, 1998).

β-Thalassemias

Clinical and Hb findings in the β-thalassemias are summarized in Tables 32-7 and 32-8. The disorders are very heterogeneous phenotypically, as well as at the level of the molecular defects. The terms thalassemia major, thalassemia intermedia, and thalassemia minor refer to clinical severity and are not genetic designations.

Homozygous β-Thalassemia (Thalassemia Major; Cooley's Anemia)

With absence of (β^0) or a marked decrease in (β^+) β-chain production, there is an excess of α-chains. Aggregates of α-chains are unstable and precipitate in the normoblast or red cell and damage the cells. Excess α-chains and their degradation products—heme, hemin, and iron, which serve as foci for the generation of reactive O_2 species—result in the partial oxidation of band 4.1 and a reduced spectrin/band 3 ratio in red blood cell precursors. Precipitates and cells are removed, causing ineffective erythropoiesis and severe hemolytic anemia. Furthermore, clustering of band 3 in the membrane may be followed by opsonization with autologous IgG and complement and removal by macrophages (Weatherall, 1999).

Clinical findings include jaundice and splenomegaly, which become evident early in childhood. Prominent frontal bones, cheekbones, and jaws impart a mongoloid appearance. These changes and X-ray findings of a

TABLE 32-7

β-Thalassemias and Their Associated Biochemical and Molecular Defects

	Typical DNA defect	β-Chain	δ-Chain	γ-Chain	Hb F distribution	α: non–α-globin imbalance
β^+ thalassemia	Mutation	↓	+	+	Heterocellular	+++
β^0 thalassemia	Mutation	0	+	+	Heterocellular	++++
δβ thalassemia	Deletion	0	0	+++	Heterocellular	++
HPFH	Deletion	0 or ↓	0	++++	Pancellular	+

Data from Forget BG. Molecular studies of genetic disorders affecting the expression of the human β-globin gene: a model system for the analysis of inborn errors of metabolism. Recent Prog Horm Res 1982;38:257–77.
DNA, Deoxyribonucleic acid; *Hb,* hemoglobin; *Hb F,* fetal hemoglobin; *HPFH,* hereditary persistence of fetal hemoglobin.

TABLE 32-8

Major Categories of β-Thalassemia Syndromes

Syndrome	Genotype	Clinical features	Hemoglobin pattern
Homozygous States			
β^+-thalassemia	β^+/β^+	Thalassemia major or intermedia	↓↓Hb A, ↑↑Hb F, variable Hb A_2
β^0-thalassemia	β^0/β^0	Thalassemia major	>95% Hb F, rest Hb A_2
$\delta\beta^0$-thalassemia	$\delta\beta^0/\delta\beta^0$	Thalassemia intermedia	100% Hb F
Hb Lepore	Lepore/Lepore	Thalassemia major	85% Hb F, 15% Hb Lepore
Heterozygous States			
β^+-Thalassemia	β^+/β	Thalassemia minor	Hb A, ↑Hb A_2, ±↑ Hb F
β^0-Thalassemia	β^0/β	Thalassemia minor	Hb A, ↑Hb A_2, ±↑ Hb F
$\delta\beta^0$-Thalassemia	$\delta\beta^0/\delta\beta$	Thalassemia minor	Hb A, 5%–20% Hb F, ±↓Hb A_2
Hb Lepore	Lepore/β	Thalassemia minor	Hb A, ↑Hb F, ↓Hb A_2, 10% Hb Lepore

Modified from Orkin SH, Nathan DG. The thalassemias. N Engl J Med 1976;295:710–4.
Hb, Hemoglobin.

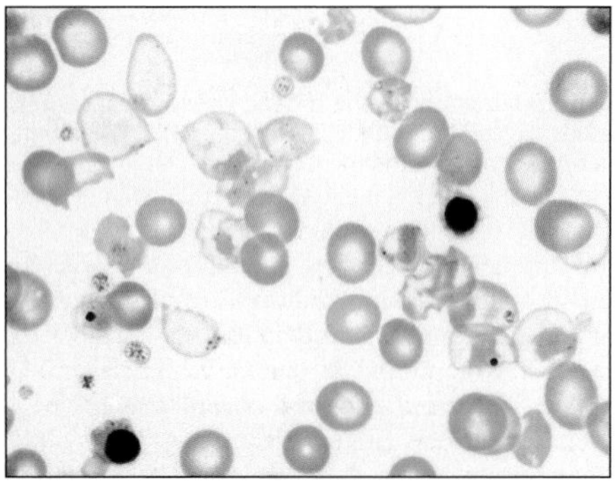

Figure 32-26 Homozygous β-thalassemia. A few cells contain hardly any hemoglobin (Hb), and the Hb is often precipitated at the membrane. Bizarre target cells, Howell-Jolly bodies, and poorly hemoglobinized nucleated red blood cells are seen.

thinned cortex of the long and flat bones and thickening of the skull with osteoporosis ("hair-on-end" appearance) reflect extreme bone marrow hyperplasia. Growth is stunted and puberty is delayed. Most patients require regular transfusions and develop problems caused by iron loading. Iron overload commonly develops, and the major cause of death is cardiac failure due to myocardial siderosis by the end of the third decade.

Unlike most hemolytic diseases, the anemia is hypochromic and microcytic. Extreme poikilocytosis with bizarre shapes, target cells, ovalocytosis, Cabot rings, Howell-Jolly bodies, nuclear fragments, siderocytes, anisochromia, anisocytosis, and often extreme normoblastosis are present (Fig. 32-26). Poikilocytosis is more striking in patients with an intact spleen; normoblastosis is more severe after splenectomy. Normoblasts have hypochromic cytoplasm and, especially after splenectomy, aggregates of densely staining Hb, which probably represent precipitated α-chains. Incubation of the blood with methyl violet stains these precipitates in both red cells and normoblasts. The reticulocyte count is less elevated than expected for the degree of anemia because of destruction of erythroid precursors in the marrow. Osmotic resistance of the red cells, serum iron, and indirect-reacting bilirubin are increased.

In the marrow, marked normoblastic hyperplasia is present. Many late normoblasts show inclusion bodies as in the blood. Gaucher-like cells are present. Storage iron and sideroblasts are increased.

In β^0-thalassemia, Hb A is absent, Hb F is as high as 98%, and Hb A_2 is about 2%. In β^+-thalassemias (Mediterranean), Hb F is 60%–95%, with Hb A present. Although Hb A_2 may or may not be increased, the ratio of A_2 to A is always increased. In black people with β^+-thalassemia, the clinical features are less severe (thalassemia intermedia), and transfusion is usually unnecessary; Hb F is 20%–40%, Hb A_2 is 2%–5%, and the rest is Hb A (Table 32-8).

Heterozygous β-Thalassemia (β-Thalassemia Trait; Thalassemia Minor; Cooley's Trait)

This is caused by the β^0-thalassemia gene with absent, or the β^+-thalassemia gene with reduced, β-globin chain synthesis. There are usually no symptoms or abnormal physical signs. The only clinical presentation might be a refractory anemia of pregnancy (Weatherall, 2001).

Most β-thalassemia heterozygotes have a mild anemia, but occasionally, Hct and Hb might be normal. Those of African origin have higher Hb levels than people from the Mediterranean region, reflecting their milder genotype. Characteristically, the RBC is elevated (5–7 M/μL), the MCH is low (usually less than 22 pg), and the MCV is low (between 55 and 70 fL). The MCHC is sometimes low but often normal. The reticulocyte count is twice the normal value. On stained films, the cells have a moderate degree of microcytosis, hypochromia, anisocytosis, and poikilocytosis; target cells and basophilic stippling are often, but not always, present (Fig. 32-27). Osmotic fragility is decreased. In the marrow, there is mild normoblastic hyperplasia with ragged cytoplasmic borders—a sign of defective hemoglobinization.

Hb A_2 is elevated in the 3.5%–7% range; Hb F is slightly elevated (1%–3%) in about half of cases. In the few cases where Hb F exceeds 4%, it is likely that a gene for HPFH is also present (Mazza, 1976). Relatively rare deletional forms tend to have higher levels of Hb F (up to 9%), and in a few families, in which the deletion included the promoter region, Hb F was found to be unusually high (up to 14%) (Weatherall, 2001). In infants, a slower than normal decline in Hb F level is observed, and the adult steady-state level is not reached until adolescence. This is a particularly important consideration in double heterozygosity for β-thalassemia and Hb S, when Hb F level is used to predict prognosis.

In a few cases, both Hb A_2 and F are normal. These are difficult to distinguish from the α-thalassemia trait, and only molecular studies might be definitive. Studies indicate that the bulk of these cases result from the coinheritance of β- and δ-thalassemia (Weatherall, 1994), either in *trans* or

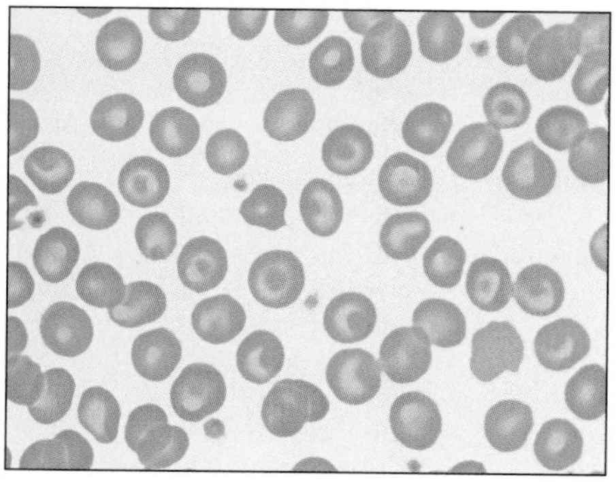

Figure 32-27 β-Thalassemia trait. Hypochromic, microcytic red blood cells with frequent targeting. Mild anemia.

in *cis*, to the β-thalassemia gene. In other patients with normal Hb pattern, only minimal hematologic changes are noted (the "silent" β-thalassemia gene), and only a more severe β-thalassemia syndrome in a family member suggests the presence of a very mild β-thalassemia mutation.

Iron studies are little different from normal (Weatherall, 2001), although iron deficiency often complicates thalassemia trait in childhood and during pregnancy. In severe iron deficiency, the level of Hb A_2 may fall into the normal range, thus obscuring the diagnosis of β-thalassemia trait, but this is unusual. Most often, although the level of A_2 falls, it remains elevated above the normal range (Weatherall, 2001). Nevertheless, when iron deficiency is present, repeat measurement of Hb A_2 is recommended after replenishment of iron.

The differential diagnosis between iron deficiency and β- or α-thalassemia trait can be difficult. Increased RBCs in the presence of decreased MCV is the hallmark of thalassemia trait. An MCV/RBC ratio <13 suggests thalassemia trait; a ratio >13 is more consistent with iron deficiency, but this and other formulas are not conclusive enough for diagnosis.

$\delta\beta^0$-Thalassemia

This is sometimes called F-thalassemia, a helpful name, as you have to think of it when there are thalassemic indices and significantly increased levels of Hb F. β- and δ-chains are not produced; this is nearly, although not completely, compensated for by increased output of γ-chains. The heterozygous state is similar to a mild β-thalassemia trait, except that Hb A_2 is not increased or is even slightly reduced (mean level is 2.4%), and Hb F is significantly increased (5.4%–20%). In the homozygous state, hemoglobin consists of only Hb F.

Clinically, $(\delta\beta)^0$-thalassemia behaves as a mild form of β-thalassemia. In the heterozygous state, the Hb is normal or slightly reduced, the MCH is between 21 and 26 pg, and the MCV is 65–79 fL. There are no clinical symptoms. Homozygotes have a mild form of thalassemia intermedia with a Hb level of 10–13 g/dL, mildly thalassemic red cell indices, and only minimal hepatosplenomegaly. It is most common in the Mediterranean population. The mild phenotype is the result of increased production of γ-chains, which compensate to some degree for the lack of β-chains.

The molecular defect is a long deletion involving the β- and δ- and often also the Aγ-gene. Twenty-one different deletions have been described (Globin Gene Server), but the hematologic findings are essentially the same. When the Aγ-gene is also deleted, the accurate nomenclature is $(A\gamma\delta\beta)^0$-thalassemia; homozygotes have a somewhat more severe phenotype.

$\delta\beta^+$-Thalassemia: Lepore Hemoglobins

In the Lepore hemoglobins, an abnormal δβ-fusion chain is produced, a result of chromosome crossing-over and fusion of genetic material at the δβ-genes. No δ- or β-chain synthesis is directed from the affected chromosome. Because Hb F production is only slightly increased and the composite δβ-chain is synthesized at a very slow rate, a severe thalassemic phenotype is produced. Hematologic abnormalities are similar to those seen in β^0-thalassemia. Hb Lepore migrates slightly faster than Hb S on alkaline electrophoresis and usually constitutes about 10% of total Hb in the heterozygotes; Hb A_2 averages 2%, and Hb F is 2%–3% (Efremov, 1978). In homozygotes, Hb Lepore is 10%–15%, and the rest is Hb F. Different Hb Lepores have been described, depending on the point of fusion, but they behave similarly. This is a much more severe thalassemia gene than the $(\delta\beta)^0$ form and causes transfusion-dependent thalassemia major in the homozygous state.

Hereditary Persistence of Fetal Hemoglobin

A group of conditions with persistence of fetal hemoglobin production beyond infancy, but without significant hematologic abnormalities, is known as HPFH. There are two major types: pancellular and heterocellular (or Swiss) HPFH.

The pancellular form of HPFH is closely related to β- and δβ-thalassemias, with which it forms a continuous spectrum. At one end of the spectrum is minimal γ-chain production with no compensation for deficiency of β-chains in β-thalassemia; at the other end, Hb F production is up and almost entirely compensates for the deficit in HPFH (Weatherall, 2001). As a result, at least in heterozygotes, there is no clear evidence of thalassemia (except maybe borderline microcytosis in a few cases), and this serves as a criterion in diagnosis. In clinical practice, a patient with significantly elevated Hb F and reduced Hb A_2 is suspected to have HPFH if red cell indices are normal but is diagnosed with $\delta\beta^0$-thalassemia if the indices are thalassemic. Nevertheless, there is a slight α/non–α-chain imbalance, and HPFH could be considered a mild form of $\delta\beta^0$-thalassemia. Hb F is homogeneously (evenly) distributed among the red cells (pancellular). This is in contrast to β- or δβ-thalassemia, in which the distribution is heterocellular. Pancellular HPFH is rare. It is found in about 0.1% of African Americans and even less frequently in other ethnic groups.

Deletional Pancellular HPFH. In the six deletional forms, the δβ-gene complex is deleted. The black and Ghanaian forms are the most common, but Indian, Italian, and Southeast Asian forms are also well documented. Homozygotes have slightly microcytic, hypochromic red cells, but no anemia. Hb F is 100%; no Hb A or Hb A_2 is present. The Hct can even be high—a result of high O_2 affinity of Hb F. In the heterozygote, no hematologic abnormalities are found. Hb F is 15%–30%, and Hb A_2 is decreased at 1%–2.1%.

Hb Kenya. This is a Hb analogous to the Lepore Hbs, which is associated with an HPFH phenotype. It contains an Aγβ-fusion gene. In the heterozygote, Hb Kenya is around 10%, F is 7%, and A_2 is reduced.

Nondeletional Pancellular HPFH. A mutation in the promoter region of one of the γ-genes results in increased synthesis of Hb F. Output from the δ- and β-genes in *cis* is reduced. Levels of Hb F range from 3%–31% in the different forms, Hb A_2 is invariably low, and the red cell indices are close to normal. There are two particulars to keep in mind. First, β-chain synthesis is decreased, but not absent from the affected chromosome, and compound heterozygotes of this form of HPFH and Hb S on the other chromosome do have Hb A (≈30%). The hemoglobin composition is similar to that seen in Hb S/β+-thalassemia, except that Hb A_2 is reduced. Second, it is not rare to find it together with an α-thalassemia gene, which is highly prevalent in African Americans.

Heterocellular or Swiss-type HPFH has less Hb F, ranging from 2%–5%. The distribution of Hb F is uneven (heterocellular): F cells and erythrocytes without Hb F are present. It was first described among healthy Swiss army recruits but is present in other populations and is quite common. It is caused by polymorphic variations at three well-known and other lesser known loci that regulate adult Hb F production (Thein, 2009). In normals or in carriers of β-thalassemia or Hb S, there is only a minimal increase in Hb F. When inherited with Hb SS or homozygous β-thalassemia, however, the result could be an unusually high level of Hb F and milder disease.

α-Thalassemias

α-Thalassemia is probably the most common single-gene disorder in humans. Its distribution is largely limited to tropical and subtropical regions of Asia and Africa and the Mediterranean (Higgs, 1989), where it reaches extremely high frequencies.

Two α-globin genes are present on each chromosome 16. α-Thalassemias are classified according to the total output of these two linked α-globin genes. In α^0-thalassemia, both genes are inactive (—/), but in α^+-thalassemia, only one gene is defective as the result of deletion (–α/) or, less frequently, of mutation ($\alpha^T\alpha$/). Nondeletional forms usually result in less globin output from the linked α-gene and more severe phenotypes. Rarely, the chromosome has a deletion and a separate mutation (α^T–/). Previously, α^0 and α^+ were called α-thalassemia 1 and 2. This was rather confusing, as the milder defect with one affected gene was called α-thalassemia 2, and the more severe genotype with two defective genes, α-thalassemia 1. Alternatively, these terms were also used to describe clinical phenotypes.

TABLE 32-9
α-Thalassemia Syndromes

Syndrome	Defective genes	Genotype	Clinical features	Newborn	After first year
Hydrops fetalis	4	—/—	Fetal or neonatal death with severe anemia	Hb Bart's >80% Hb H, Hb Portland	
Hb H disease	3	—/–α (—/αα^{CS})	Chronic hemolytic anemia	Hb Bart's 20%–40% (Hb CS)	Hb H 5%–30% (Hb CS 2%–3%)
Thalassemia minor	2	—/αα –α/–α $\alpha^T\alpha$/–α	Asymptomatic, mild anemia, thalassemic indices	Hb Bart's 5%–10%	None
Silent carrier	1	–α/αα (αα/αα^{CS})	No clinical or hematologic abnormality	Hb Bart's ±1%–2% (Hb CS)	None (Hb CS 1%)

Modified from Wintrobe MM, Lee GR, Boggs DR, et al. Clinical hematology. 8th ed. Philadelphia: Lea & Febiger; 1981.
Hb, Hemoglobin.

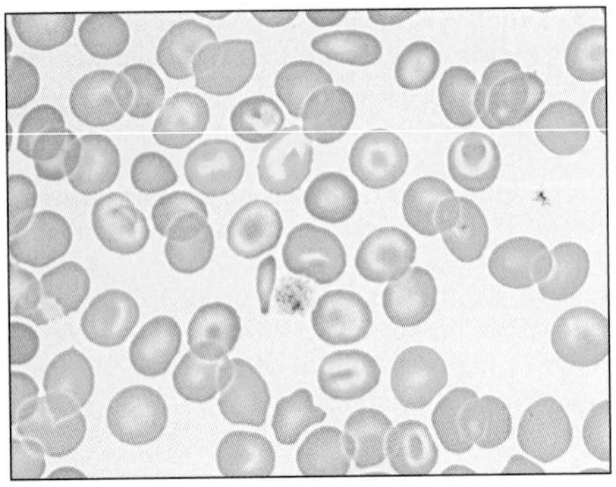

Figure 32-28 Hemoglobin H disease. Mild anemia and target cells.

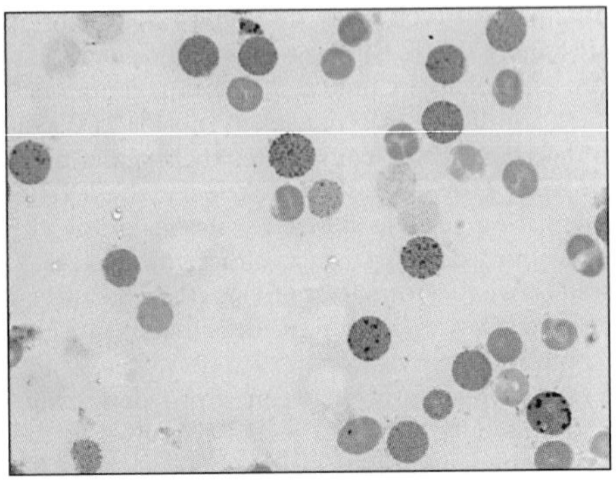

Figure 32-29 Hemoglobin H preparation. Film made after incubation of blood with brilliant cresyl blue. Several red cells contain multiple small pale blue inclusions.

Unlike the extremely unstable α-chains in β-thalassemia, excess β- and γ-chains can form stable tetramers, hemoglobin H (β_4), and Bart's (γ_4). These precipitate in aging red cells and, through interaction with the cell membrane, cause hemolysis. This is mostly a hemolytic anemia, whereas in β-thalassemia, ineffective erythropoiesis predominates.

α-Thalassemia Syndromes

Four α-thalassemia syndromes result from the combination of these genotypes (Bunn, 1986), which roughly correspond to a loss of 4, 3, 2, or 1 genes from the normal complement (αα/αα) (see Table 32-9). In the following discussion, nondeletion forms are not always depicted separately, for the sake of simplicity.

Hemoglobin Bart's Hydrops Fetalis (—/—). Complete absence of α-chains is incompatible with life. Infants are stillborn with severe edema, marked anemia, and marked hepatosplenomegaly. The blood shows marked anisocytosis, poikilocytosis, microcytosis, and erythroblastosis. ABO or Rh incompatibility is absent. Because of the absence of α-chains, no Hb A or Hb F is present. Large quantities of Hb Bart's (γ_4), a variable amount of Hb Portland, and traces of Hb H (β_4) are present; all of these migrate faster than Hb A on alkaline electrophoresis. Hb Bart's is functionally useless for O_2 transfer, causing extreme intrauterine hypoxia.

Hemoglobin H Disease (–α/—). Three of the four α-genes are absent. A chronic hemolytic anemia occurs with the clinical picture of thalassemia intermedia in a minority of cases, although the severity varies, and most patients do well. Hb H disease is very common in Southeast Asia but is also seen in the Mediterranean and the Middle East; it is very rare, however, in black people, as α°-thalassemia is uncommon in this group. Splenomegaly and sometimes hepatomegaly are present. Hb values average 3 g/dL less than in age- and sex-matched controls. Transfusion is rarely needed. Anemia may become more severe during pregnancy, but the Hb rarely falls below 7 g/dL. The MCV (60–70 fL) and MCH (17–21 pg) are decreased (Higgs, 1989), and RBC is increased (6–6.2 M/μL). The blood film shows hypochromia, basophilic stippling, and anisopoikilocytosis with target cells (Fig. 32-28). Reticulocytes range from 4%–5%.

Hemoglobin electrophoresis shows a rapidly migrating band of Hb H (β4), accounting for approximately 9% (from 1%–40%) of the hemoglobin, and the slightly less rapidly migrating Hb Bart's in half of cases. Hb H can be precipitated in vitro and lost from the hemolysate by careless handling or prolonged storage. In old hemolysates, a series of bands migrates as Hb H. Hb Bart's is alkali resistant and may be measured with Hb F (which is not increased in Hb H disease). The percentage of Hb Bart's is 2%–40% at birth; it gradually falls thereafter, averaging 4.8%, but the level in adults is variable. As in other α-thalassemia syndromes, more Hb Bart's is present at birth than Hb H in adult life. Hb A_2 is diminished.

Hemoglobin H Preparation. Vital staining of the blood with an oxidizing dye such as brilliant cresyl blue induces inclusion bodies (Hb H precipitates) in many of the red cells. During incubation of two parts of blood in one part of 1% brilliant cresyl blue stain, the unstable Hb H (β_4) gradually precipitates as multiple small pale blue inclusions uniformly distributed on the red cell membrane (Fig. 32-29) (Jones, 1981). Hb H inclusions must be distinguished from (1) the granules and reticular networks in reticulocytes, which are darker blue in color; and (2) pre-formed Heinz bodies, which are larger, also darker blue, and often are attached to the membrane. After 20 minutes of incubation at room temperature, Hb H inclusions are present in at least half of the red cells in Hb H disease, and in a very rare red cell in α-thalassemia trait. The larger, single Heinz bodies may be found after splenectomy in Hb H disease.

α-Thalassemia Trait: Heterozygous α°-Thalassemia (—/αα) or Homozygous α$^+$-Thalassemia (–α/–α). Absence of two α-genes results in clinical features similar to β-thalassemia minor with very mild anemia and thalassemic indices, with MCV ranging from 65–75 fL (Higgs, 1989). The α-chain/β-chain synthesis ratio is decreased (≈0.6). Diagnosis is best made by finding 5%–10% Hb Bart's in cord blood; normally, only trace amounts (<0.5%) are found. In adults, Hb Bart's is undetectable, and Hb studies are perfectly normal, except that Hb A_2 might be slightly reduced. Hb H inclusions are found in α°-thalassemia, but rarely in heterozygous or homozygous α$^+$-thalassemia, and only in a very small percentage of red cells, if exhaustively sought after (Wasi, 1974), and if the sample is enriched for Hb H-containing red cells (Jones, 1981). Otherwise, no evidence of Hb imbalance is detectable by standard techniques, and the diagnosis is one of excluding iron deficiency, anemia of chronic disease, and β-thalassemia trait. In contrast to β-thalassemia, Hb F is normal, and Hb A_2 is normal or decreased. This condition is absolutely benign, and most patients are diagnosed on routine screening. Hematologic findings are identical in the two distinct genotypes found in different populations: (—/αα), common in Southeast Asia and the Mediterranean and exceedingly rare in black people; and (–α–α), most common in those of African descent.

Silent Carrier α-Thalassemia (Heterozygous α^+-Thalassemia) (αα/–α). In this condition, one of four α-globin genes is absent. Hematologic findings are normal, except that the MCV might be slightly reduced, with a mean value of 81 fL and a range of 75–85 fL, and the MCH might be minimally decreased; many times, however, the red cell indices are perfectly normal. During the neonatal period, heterozygous α^+-thalassemia can be diagnosed by a raised level of Hb Bart's (1%–2%) in the cord blood. Hb Bart's disappears by the age of 6 months, and the diagnosis can be made only by molecular or globin chain synthesis studies. Because only 40% of newborns with the heterozygous α^+-thalassemia genotype have detectable Hb Bart's in their cord blood (Higgs, 1982), failure to detect Hb Bart's in the newborn does not rule out silent carrier α-thalassemia, and newborn screening should not be used to rule out this entity.

From large studies comparing hematologic findings of different genotypes, it became apparent that there is a continuum between normal, silent carrier, and α-thalassemia trait. Because there is no clear separation between one- and two-gene defects, some authors group these together as milder α-thalassemia phenotypes. None of the α-thalassemia genes or their combinations can be identified with certainty without molecular studies.

Hemoglobin Constant Spring (αCSα/). Hb Constant Spring is due to an abnormal termination codon in an α-gene that results in an elongated α-chain with 31 extra amino acids. It is by far the most common of the elongated α-chain variants. Because of marked reduction in mRNA stability, the clinical phenotype of α-thalassemia is seen (Orkin, 1998). Similar to other nondeletional α^+-thalassemia genes, it causes a more severe phenotype. The homozygous state appears as an asymptomatic, mild hemolytic anemia, with a Hb level of 9–11 g/dL. The red cell indices are unusual for thalassemia: The MCV is normal (88 fL) and the RBC is low (3.9 M/μL). Hemoglobin consists of 5%–8% Hb CS, normal Hb A_2, trace amounts of Hb Bart's, and the rest Hb A (Weatherall, 1994). Heterozygotes have a silent carrier phenotype with no hematologic abnormality and about 1% Hb CS. Abnormal Hb migrates more slowly than Hb A_2 at alkaline pH and is easily missed. Hb CS is common in Southeast Asia, where it is found in about 50% of cases of Hb H disease (αCSα/—).

Screening and Prenatal Diagnosis of Hemoglobin Disorders

In populations in which there is a significant incidence of severe forms of thalassemia or sickle cell anemia, women should be screened early in pregnancy for thalassemia and the sickle cell trait (Weatherall, 1985, 1994; Alter, 1988). If both parents are carriers, prevention of severe disease is possible through genetic counseling and offering prenatal diagnosis with the option of therapeutic abortion. In high-frequency regions, screening of school children or premarital counseling has been implemented. Initial tests include MCV (<80 fL), MCH (<27 pg), and HPLC to estimate Hb A_2 (>3.5%) and to detect common Hb variants (cutoff values are in parentheses). In prenatal diagnosis, fetal DNA analysis of chorionic villi replaced fetal blood analysis by the early 1990s.

HEMOLYSIS—METABOLIC DISORDERS

Deficient enzyme activity in the erythrocyte may result in abnormalities that lead to premature destruction and hemolytic anemia; these disorders are usually inherited. However, interference with, or oxidative stress on, erythrocyte metabolism can sometimes result in hemolysis in individuals who have normal erythrocytes.

Erythrocyte Metabolism

The mature red cell lacks mitochondria and, therefore, lacks oxidative phosphorylation and Krebs cycle activity. Energy production is mainly glycolytic, 90% of which occurs through the Embden-Meyerhof pathway, as glucose goes to lactic acid with the net production of 2 mol of adenosine triphosphate (ATP) (Fig. 32-30). ATP is needed for energy-requiring reactions in the cell: for active cation transport across the membrane, for maintaining membrane deformability, and for preserving the cell's biconcave shape. Glucose uptake by red cells is independent of insulin. Approximately 90% of glucose is consumed in the glycolytic pathway, while 10% is utilized in the pentose phosphate pathway (hexose monophosphate [HMP] shunt). One step of the glycolytic pathway replenishes NADH (reducing agent derived from nicotinamide adenine dinucleotide [NAD]), which plays a major role in protecting Hb from oxidative stress. Most of the hemiglobin (methemoglobin) produced in the normal cell (about 3% of the total per day) is reduced by NAD-linked methemoglobin (Met Hb) reductase. The HMP shunt generates nicotinamide adenine dinucleotide phosphate (NADPH) in the first two steps through the enzymes G6PD and 6-phosphogluconate. NADPH production is linked to glutathione reduction and, through this mechanism, to preservation of vital enzymes and Hb from oxidation. Small amounts of oxidized hemoglobin (methemoglobin) are reduced by glutathione (GSH). The activity of the HMP shunt increases when the cell is exposed to an oxidant drug, probably as a result of increased NADP production. If an enzyme in this pathway lacks activity, GSH cannot be produced, and Hb will be oxidized by the oxidant stress. Oxidation in the red cells is mediated by high-energy derivatives of O_2, referred to collectively as activated O_2 (Prchal, 2000). Oxidized globin chains denature and precipitate as Heinz bodies, which adhere to the membrane, inducing rigidity and a tendency to lyse. Moderate enzyme deficiencies in this pathway (e.g., in G6PD) may not be associated with anemia under normal conditions; however, an acute hemolytic episode occurs if the cells are challenged by oxidant stress (e.g., drugs, infection).

Deficiencies in the Embden-Meyerhof pathway result in impaired ATP generation and a chronic hemolytic anemia. The mechanism of red cell destruction here is less clear. Heinz bodies are not formed. Lack of cell deformability and impaired cation pumping are important in the hemolytic process. However, ATP deficiency is difficult to demonstrate in many patients, and other disorders associated with more severe ATP deficiency are not associated with significant hemolysis (Prchal, 2000).

The Rapoport-Luebering shunt provides for the conversion of 1,3-diphosphoglycerate (1,3-DPG) to 2,3-DPG instead of directly to 3-phosphoglycerate (3-PG) (see Fig. 32-30). If this shunt is operating, generation of 2 mol of ATP (per mole of glucose) is bypassed; the result is no net energy production in glycolysis. However, 2,3-DPG combines with the β-chain of Hb and decreases the affinity of Hb for O_2. At a given pO_2, therefore, increased 2,3-DPG allows more O_2 to leave Hb and go to the tissues; the O_2 dissociation curve is shifted to the right. Increased activity of this shunt is apparently stimulated by hypoxia.

Glucose-6-Phosphate Dehydrogenase Deficiency

About 10% of male American blacks who were given the antimalarial drug primaquine during the Korean War developed a self-limited, acute hemolytic anemia (Beutler, 1994; Prchal, 2000). The relationship between antimalarial drugs and hemolysis had been observed earlier in the 1920s (Beutler, 1999). Only the older red cells were destroyed, and it was eventually determined that the deficiency in susceptible red cells was in G6PD. Reticulocytes have five times higher enzyme activity than the oldest erythrocyte population (Prchal, 2000). It has since been found that G6PD deficiency is widespread throughout the world. Among whites, the highest incidence is in Kurdish Jews; the deficiency is common in the Middle East, in Mediterranean countries, and in Asia. G6PD deficiency is the most common human enzyme defect and is present in more than 400 million people worldwide (Cappellini, 2008).

G6PD is present in all cells; however, its concentration varies in different tissues. In healthy red cells, the enzyme operates at only 1%–2% of its maximal potential, allowing for a large reserve of reductive potential (Cappellini, 2008). Because G6PD is determined by a gene on the X chromosome, full expression of the deficiency is found in the male hemizygote. Partial expression may be found in the heterozygous female, who has two populations of red cells—one normal and one deficient. The deficiency of G6PD limits the regeneration of NADPH, which renders the cell vulnerable to oxidative denaturation of Hb. Because, normally, G6PD is highest in young cells and decreases as the cell ages, in persons with G6PD deficiency, the older cells are preferentially destroyed.

Hemolytic susceptibility in affected persons can increase greatly during intercurrent illness or upon exposure to various drugs that have oxidant properties (Table 32-10).

The genetic heterogeneity is great, and approximately 400 biochemical variants have been defined. This genetic heterogeneity is expressed as variations in stability and the electrophoretic and catalytic properties of the enzymes, in the degree of deficiency, in the types of cells in the body affected, in the types of drugs that will produce hemolysis, and in susceptibility to chronic hemolysis or to neonatal jaundice. The most common

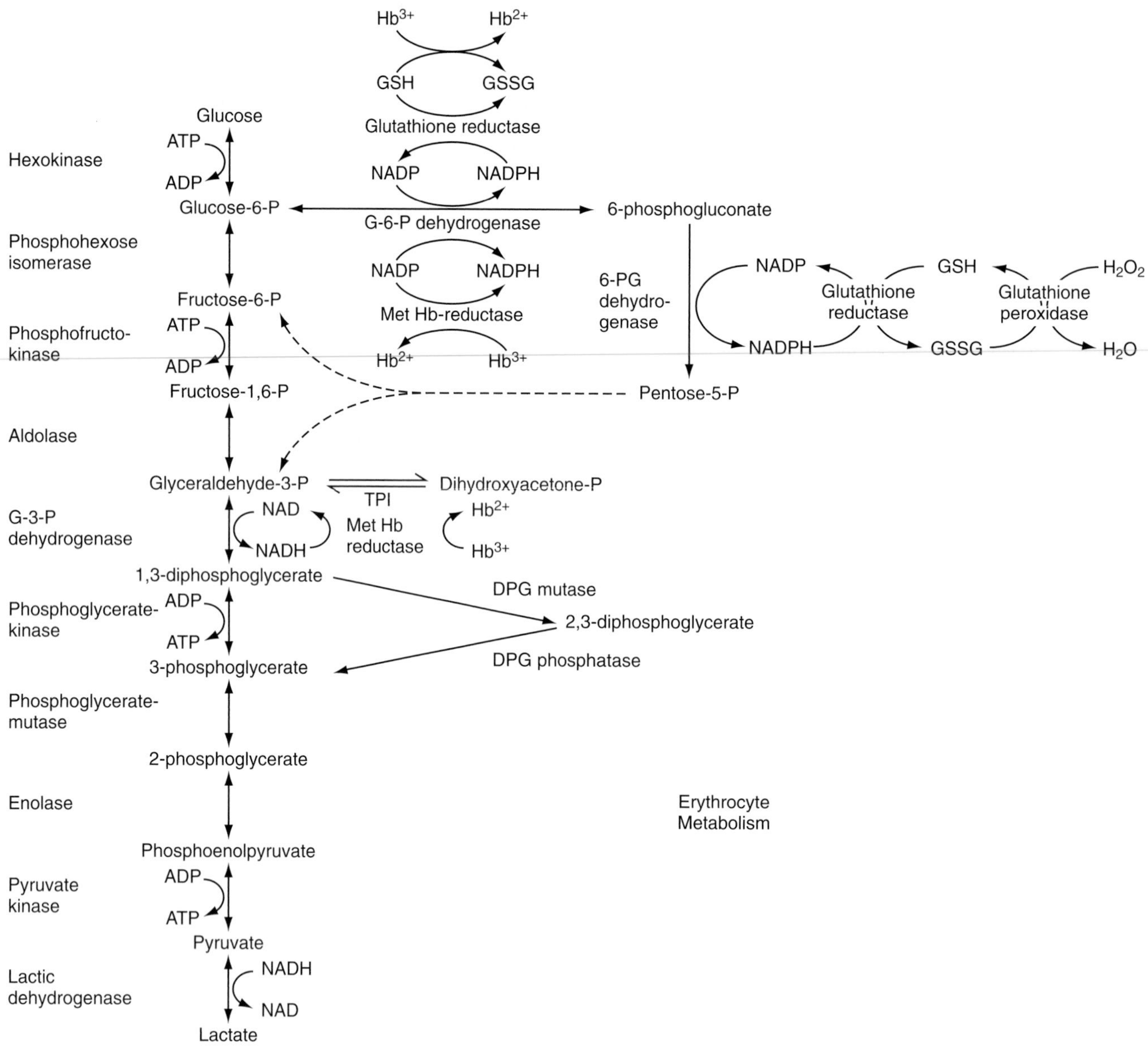

Figure 32-30 Erythrocyte metabolism is discussed in the text. Normally, most hemiglobin (methemoglobin, Hb^{+}++) is reduced to hemoglobin (Hb^{+}+) by nicotinamide adenine dinucleotide–linked methemoglobin reductase (NAD, Met Hb reductase). Nicotinamide adenine dinucleotide phosphate (NADP)-linked methemoglobin reductase requires methylene blue for activation and is more effective in drug-induced methemoglobinemia than the normal cell mechanism. *GSH,* Reduced glutathione; *GSSG,* oxidized glutathione.

("normal") G6PD isoenzyme in all population groups is designated as B. In blacks, an electrophoretically more rapid variant, A, is prevalent and has almost the same activity; 20% of black males have this variant. Eleven percent of black males have the A type of G6PD, which involves only 5%–15% of normal enzyme activity; it is these individuals who are susceptible to hemolysis after ingesting oxidant drugs or during infection. The most common variant in whites is G6PD-Mediterranean, found in Mediterranean populations; the level of enzyme activity in affected males is low—often less than 1%. These individuals usually are not anemic but may have somewhat more severe and non–self-limited hemolytic anemia with infection, and with a wider variety of drugs than the black variant. In a subgroup of G6PD-deficient subjects, severe hemolysis may occur within hours after eating fava beans ("favism"). Although the vast majority of G6PD-deficient subjects worldwide are not anemic, a small proportion of persons with G6PD-Mediterranean (and persons with some rarer variants) have a chronic nonspherocytic hemolytic anemia. G6PD deficiency is a common cause of neonatal jaundice, occurring in approximately one third of all male neonates with jaundice (Cappellini, 2008). Jaundice is usually evident by 1–4 days of age and is more severe in premature babies than in full-term infants.

Laboratory findings during active hemolysis are those of hemolytic anemia in general. In the blood film, one finds poikilocytes, some spherocytes, bite cells, and irregularly contracted cells that stain densely and have contraction of Hb from a part of the cell membrane. These probably are cells from which Heinz bodies have been removed by the spleen. After supravital staining with methyl violet, Heinz bodies may be present early in an acute hemolytic episode. G6PD deficiency may be detected by one of the screening tests: the dye reduction test, the ascorbate cyanide test, or a fluorescent spot test. Confirmation is made with a quantitative assay.

Heinz Bodies

When a globin chain denatures, it forms precipitates that are known as Heinz bodies (Dacie, 1991). These precipitates cannot be detected in Romanowsky's-stained, air-dried blood films, but after vital staining with methyl violet or crystal violet, Heinz bodies stain deep purple. They vary from 1 to 4 μm in diameter and often attach to the red cell membrane. They also stain, but less intensely, as pale blue inclusions in reticulocyte stains (e.g., new methylene blue) (Fig. 32-31).

The presence of Heinz bodies in freshly drawn blood indicates that (1) an oxidizing drug or chemical (e.g., phenylhydrazine, chlorate, naphthalene, dapsone) has been ingested in sufficient amount to overwhelm the normal protective mechanisms of the red cell and denature Hb; (2) a drug such as primaquine has been ingested by an individual with

TABLE 32-10
Drugs and Chemicals That Have Clearly Been Shown to Cause Clinically Significant Hemolytic Anemia in G6PD Deficiency

Acetanilid
Methylene blue
Nalidixic acid (NegGram)
Naphthalene
Niridazole (Ambilhar)
Nitrofurantoin (Furadantin)
Pamaquine
Pentaquine
Phenylhydrazine
Primaquine
Sulfacetamide
Sulfanilamide
Sulfamethoxazole (Gantanol)
Sulfapyridine
Thiazolesulfone
Toluidine blue
Trinitrotoluene (TNT)

From Beutler E. Hemolytic anemia in disorders of red cell metabolism. New York: Plenum Medical Book Company; 1978.
G6PD, Glucose-6-phosphate dehydrogenase.

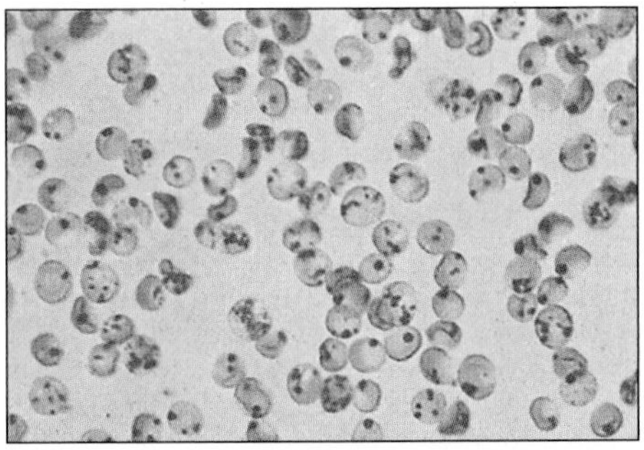

Figure 32-31 Heinz bodies. Normal red cells incubated with an oxidant drug and stained while in suspension with methyl violet; finally, an air-dried film was made and stained with Wright's stain. Purple-staining Heinz bodies are precipitates of denatured hemoglobin that tend to attach to the cell membrane.

G6PD deficiency (or another defect resulting in a deficiency of reduced glutathione), so that Hb is not protected from oxidative denaturation; or (3) the subject has an unstable Hb.

Ascorbate Cyanide Test

When blood is incubated with a solution of sodium cyanide and sodium ascorbate, hydrogen peroxide is generated from the coupled oxidation of ascorbate and oxyhemoglobin (Dacie, 1991). Cyanide inhibits catalase, hydrogen peroxide is available to oxidize Hb, and the brown color of methemoglobin is discernible. This occurs more rapidly in G6PD-deficient cells than in normal cells.

The ascorbate cyanide test is not specific, in that abnormalities in the glutathione synthesis or maintenance pathways can produce positive results.

Fluorescent Spot Test

Whole blood is added to a mixture of glucose-6-phosphate (G6P), NADP, saponin, and buffer, and a spot of this mixture is placed on filter paper and is observed for fluorescence with ultraviolet light. If G6PD is present, NADP is converted to NADPH. Because phosphogluconate dehydrogenase is present in most hemolysates, further NADP is converted to NADPH (see Fig. 32-30). NADPH fluoresces, but NADP does not. The normal control sample fluoresces brightly, and lack of fluorescence indicates G6PD deficiency. By reoxidizing any small amounts of NADPH formed, oxidized glutathione (GSSG) enhances the ability of the test to detect mild G6PD deficiency. This is the recommended screening test for G6PD deficiency (Beutler, 1979b).

Quantitative Assay of G6PD. For G6PD, most assays are based on the rate of reduction of NADP to NADPH, measured spectrometrically at 340 nm, when a hemolysate is incubated with G6P (Beutler, 1984). In heterozygotes or in acute hemolysis in black subjects with G6PD deficiency, the diagnosis may be obscured even with the assay, because of increased levels of G6PD in reticulocytes and younger erythrocytes. Usually, however, the ascorbate cyanide screening test will be positive in these instances.

Pyruvate Kinase (PK) Deficiency

The most common red cell enzyme deficiency involving the Embden-Meyerhof glycolytic pathway, PK deficiency results in mild to moderately severe nonspherocytic chronic hemolytic anemia with splenomegaly. The prevalence of PK deficiency is estimated to be 1:20,000 in the general white population (Zanella, 2005). The anemia may be detected in infancy, or not until adult life in milder cases. Neonatal jaundice occurs in more than half of cases, which may require exchange transfusion. Patients tend to tolerate the anemia rather well because of high levels of 2,3-DPG, which occur as a result of the block in glycolysis. The blood film may show no notable red cell abnormalities until after splenectomy, when echinocytes, irregularly contracted cells, and crenated red cells may be prominent. Reticulocyte counts are elevated and increase further after splenectomy.

PK isoenzymes are produced by two separate genes: one on chromosome 15, encoding the M (muscle) isoforms, and the other on chromosome 1, encoding the L (liver) and R (red cell) isoforms. The complexity of PK isoforms is further complicated by the fact that functional enzyme is a tetramer. Inheritance is autosomal recessive, but this is probably true only in consanguineous families. PK mutants are numerous and are not detected in phenotypically normal heterozygotes that have one half the normal PK activity. Most individuals with PK-deficient hemolytic anemias are therefore probably double heterozygotes for two mutant genes (Valentine, 1979). Acquired PK deficiency occurs occasionally in myelodysplastic disorders and leukemias (Valentine, 1979; Miwa, 1981).

The autohemolysis test gives variable results. Some patients show only a mild increase in autohemolysis that is partially prevented by glucose (type I), and others have a greater increase that is not prevented by glucose (type II). Heinz bodies are not found. The diagnosis is made by a specific screening test or enzyme assay.

The reticulocyte count in unsplenectomized patients is usually increased, although not proportional to the degree of anemia, because younger PK-deficient erythrocytes are selectively sequestered in the spleen (Zanella, 2005). Splenectomy is indicated in cases requiring transfusions. After splenectomy, the Hb concentration usually increases by 1–2 g/dL and the reticulocytes increase sharply, although hemolysis persists (Miwa, 1981).

Fluorescent Spot Test. Pyruvate kinase catalyzes the phosphorylation of adenosine diphosphate (ADP) to ATP by phosphoenolpyruvate (PEP) with the formation of pyruvate (Beutler, 1984). Pyruvate then reduces any NADH present to NAD with the formation of lactate (see Fig. 32-30). Loss of fluorescence of NADH under ultraviolet light is observed as evidence of the presence of PK.

Leukocytes must be removed from the sample because they normally contain about 300 times as much PK as red cells do, and in PK deficiency, the red cells but not the leukocytes are deficient.

Quantitative Assay of PK. The same principle is employed as in the screening test, but the rate of decrease of absorbance at 340 nm is measured. A negative screening test or a normal PK assay (using the standard high substrate [PEP] concentrations) does not rule out PK-deficient hemolytic anemia. Because mutant PK enzymes may have normal activity at high PEP concentrations and decreased activity at low PEP concentrations, it is necessary to perform the assay both ways (Beutler, 1984).

Other Glycolytic Enzyme Deficiencies

Other enzyme deficiencies in the **Embden-Meyerhof pathway** are rarer (Beutler, 1994; Prchal, 2000). When severe, they produce hemolytic anemia, with two exceptions: (1) LD deficiency has no clinical manifestations; and (2) deficiencies of 2,3-DPG mutase and 2,3-DPG phosphatase activities occur together and result in erythrocytosis as a result of lack of 2,3-DPG, shifting the O_2 dissociation curve of Hb to the left.

Other enzyme deficiencies in the **hexose monophosphate shunt** are rare. They include the two enzymes involved in glutathione synthesis: γ-glutamyl cysteine synthase and glutathione synthetase. As in G6PD deficiency, hemolysis increases with oxidant drug exposure or infection.

No good evidence is available, however, for the causation of chronic hemolytic anemia by 6-phosphogluconate deficiency, glutathione reductase (GR) deficiency, or glutathione peroxidase (GP_x) deficiency (Beutler, 1994). GR contains flavine-adenine dinucleotide and is often partially deficient because of dietary riboflavin deficiency. GP_x is one-half normal in about 30% of the Jewish population as a result of homozygosity for a gene with low GP_x activity; in addition, GP_x activity is dependent on selenium intake in the diet. In neither case is there an association with a hematologic disorder.

Pyrimidine-5′-Nucleotidase Deficiency

When RNA is degraded in the reticulocyte, pyrimidine nucleotides must be dephosphorylated by pyrimidine-5′-nucleotidase (PN) to cross the red cell membrane (Paglia, 1981). Autosomal recessive PN deficiency results in accumulation of pyrimidines, and the impaired degradation of RNA results in pronounced basophilic stippling in red cells on the blood film. This is probably one of the more common enzyme deficiencies responsible for nonspherocytic hereditary hemolytic anemia, once G6PD and PK deficiencies are excluded (Rees, 2003).

The disorder is characterized by mild to moderate chronic hemolysis, jaundice, reticulocytosis (≈10%), marked basophilic stippling (about 5% of the red cells), and splenomegaly without notable improvement after splenectomy. However, no cases of transfusion dependency associated with PN deficiency have been reported (Rees, 2003). A screening test compares the ultraviolet absorption of deproteinized extracts of red cells at 260 nm with that at 280 nm. In PN deficiency, the major absorption peak is shifted from the normal 260 nm to 280 nm, which is the maximum for the pyrimidines uridine diphosphate and cytidine diphosphate. Confirmation requires an assay showing decreased nucleotidase activity (Beutler, 1984).

Acquired PN deficiency occurs in lead poisoning and is probably responsible for the basophilic stippling in that condition. It has been also reported in β-thalassemia trait, acute leukemias, chronic myeloid leukemia, chronic lymphocytic leukemia, and lymphomas (Rees, 2003).

HEMOLYSIS—ACQUIRED; EXTRINSIC

Chemical Agents

Agents Hemolytic to Normal Cells

The action of chemical agents depends on the dose and on other factors, many of which are known only vaguely. They range from simple substances, such as water, to some that are highly complex. When used as irrigating fluid, distilled water may be found responsible for acute hemolytic anemia as a result of entry into venous channels during transurethral resection. Also, drowning in fresh water may be associated with red cell hemolysis, particularly in the lungs, although drowning in salt water could cause profound red cell hydration (Schrier, 2009).

In addition to anemia, some chemicals produce methemoglobinemia, which can manifest as cyanosis (toluene, trinitrotoluene, nitrobenzene, acetanilide, and phenacetin). Some may lead to AA (toluene and trinitrotoluene). Promin, a sulfone derivative, makes blood turn chocolate brown because of the formation of sulfhemoglobins. As mentioned earlier, ribavirin, a drug used in the treatment of hepatitic C virus infection, may produce a dose-dependent hemolytic anemia in about one third of patients.

Lead toxicity may produce progressive anemia, with basophilic stippling, reticulocytosis, normoblastemia, Cabot rings, Howell-Jolly bodies, and leukocytosis. Lead not only causes damage to the red cell and hemolysis, but also produces defects in the heme synthetic pathway. In cases of chronic exposure to lead, basophilic stippling, more in the marrow than in the peripheral blood, and coproporphyrinuria are the characteristic findings. These changes produce defective erythrocytes, which are removed by the spleen.

Agents Hemolytic to Abnormal Cells

Certain drugs and chemicals that have oxidizing activity may produce hemolytic anemia in individuals with G6PD deficiency or other defects resulting in glutathione deficiency. In addition, unstable hemoglobins, such as Hb Zürich, have a propensity for drug-induced hemolytic anemia. Premature infants, although they have high levels of G6PD, have glutathione instability and low levels of glutathione and may develop hemolytic anemia when given large doses of synthetic water-soluble analogs of vitamin K.

It must be remembered that, if exposure to these oxidant substances is great enough, acute hemolytic anemia may be produced in normal individuals.

During the acute hemolytic episode, Heinz bodies can be demonstrated frequently by direct staining of blood with methyl violet. Red cells with Heinz bodies are removed from the circulation by the spleen, or the Heinz bodies are extracted from the red cells by splenic action. Therefore, Heinz bodies may not be found in the blood if the spleen is effectively removing them, or after the acute hemolytic process has abated.

Tests for G6PD deficiency, the most common underlying cause of drug-sensitive hemolytic anemia, are described earlier in this chapter.

Physical Agents

Heat

Extensive burns produce hemolytic anemia, probably because of direct damage to red cells. Gross hemoglobinuria may occur in patients with severe burns. The blood film may show remarkable morphologic abnormalities of the red cells, including budding fragmentation of the membrane and microspherocytosis. The most severe abnormalities are often found immediately after extensive burns before a reticulocyte response has had time to develop. Badly damaged cells are rapidly removed from the circulation.

Traumatic Hemolysis

Hemolytic anemia characterized by striking morphologic abnormalities of the red cells, which include fragments (schistocytes) and irregularly contracted cells (triangular cells, helmet cells), has been attributed to physical trauma to the red cells. The basis of the hemolytic process is probably damage to the red cells in their contact with loose fibrin meshworks (intravascular coagulation) or with pathologic vascular lesions. Fragmentation of the cells results with or without intravascular lysis. Two general categories are recognized in this group of disorders, aptly termed the "red cell fragmentation syndrome": macroangiopathic and microangiopathic.

Macroangiopathic Hemolytic Anemia (Cardiac Valvular Disease and Prostheses). Chronic intravascular hemolysis associated with low serum haptoglobin, hemosiderinuria, reticulocytosis, and red cell abnormalities (e.g., schistocytes, irregularly contracted cells) may occur after surgical replacement of a diseased heart valve with a prosthesis or after surgical repair of a septal defect with a plastic patch (Erslev, 2001d). This has been attributed to mechanical damage of red cells in the turbulent environment of a leaky valve or of a roughened surface uncovered by endothelial cells. Repair of the valve or coverage of the patch by endothelium has improved the hemolytic process. Other studies have shown that some patients with cardiac valvular disease have a hemolytic process that may be altered by surgery.

External mechanical trauma has been reported in **march hemoglobinuria,** a condition that is seen in soldiers after a long march and in joggers and other athletes following long practices, particularly on hard surfaces. In this condition, anemia and reticulocytosis are uncommon. The chronic intravascular hemolysis may lead to iron deficiency as a result of loss of Hb in the urine.

Thrombotic Microangiopathy (Microangiopathic Hemolytic Anemia). Thrombotic microangiopathies (TMAs) are microvascular occlusive disorders characterized by systemic or intrarenal aggregation of platelets, thrombocytopenia, and mechanical injury to erythrocytes. Fragmented red cells (e.g., schistocytes, irregularly contracted cells) are probably produced when blood flows through turbulent areas in the microcirculation that are partially occluded by platelet aggregates (Moake, 2002). TMA may be idiopathic or precipitated by drugs such as mitomycin C, transplantation, malignancy, pregnancy, collagen vascular disease, or HIV (Ahmed, 2002).

The classification of TMA has been controversial for many years. In routine clinical practice, the term thrombotic thrombocytopenic purpura (TTP) is often used for adult cases with predominant neurologic symptoms, whereas the term hemolytic-uremic syndrome (HUS) has been used to describe childhood cases with thrombotic microangiopathy and predominant renal involvement (Moake, 2002). However, the distinction is not always possible, and overlapping symptoms may be observed. Authors suggested the inclusion of both entities under TTP/HUS, presuming a similar pathogenetic mechanism with variable organ tropism. Others group sporadic cases of HUS with TTP under idiopathic TMA and separate most cases of HUS under toxin-associated TMA (Ahmed, 2002).

Recent studies indicate a difference in pathogenetic mechanisms between HUS and TTP, as discussed later.

Hemolytic-Uremic Syndrome

HUS is classified into diarrhea-associated (D+) or typical form, and diarrhea-negative (D−) or atypical form. D+ HUS constitutes approximately 95% of cases in children and is less common in adults (Zheng, 2008). D+ HUS occurs most commonly in infants younger than 2 years of age, but it affects all ages. It is caused by one of several serotypes of *Escherichia coli* that produce a verotoxin (named for its toxicity against African green monkey kidney [vero] cells). The most common is *E. coli* O157:H7, which produces Shiga toxins 1 and 2. The annual incidence of infection with *E. coli* O157 is approximately 8 per 100,000 people in North America. The percentage of cases with bloody diarrhea that progress to HUS is 3%–7% for sporadic cases and 20%–30% for some outbreaks (Zheng, 2008). HUS usually occurs 4–6 days after the onset of diarrhea. Shiga toxins cause bloody diarrhea, then enter the circulation and travel in the plasma on the surface of platelets or monocytes (Moake, 2002). Recent studies suggest that these toxins become attached to glomerular capillary endothelium and other renal epithelial cells. Shiga toxins, together with locally secreted cytokines, cause the release of unusually large multimers of von Willebrand factor (vWF), which promote platelet aggregation in renal vasculature (Moake, 2002). Endothelial cell damage is the hallmark of D+ HUS in children, and endothelial swelling may be severe enough to occlude the capillary lumen. The thrombi of D+ HUS are composed predominantly of fibrin with few platelets and little vWF (Zheng, 2008). Hemolytic anemia with schistocytes (due to interaction of red cells with microvascular thrombotic lesions), variable thrombocytopenia, and uremia are the cardinal features. Death formerly occurred in almost half of cases; the renal pathology has included acute glomerulonephritis and thrombotic and necrotic vascular lesions associated with patchy, bilateral renal cortical necrosis. With supportive therapy, including transfusions and dialysis, some investigators have reported mortality reduced to 5%–15%. Nonetheless, minor to major renal impairment has been reported in approximately 50% of patients. Five to ten percent of patients with HUS have D− HUS, with no antecedent diarrhea of Shiga-toxin–producing organisms, and some of these patients have familial history of the disease (Zheng, 2008). Approximately 50% of patients with D− HUS have mutations in one of the complement regulatory proteins: factor H, factor I, membrane cofactor protein (MCP), or factor B. These patients have a much higher mortality rate (Moake, 2002). Approximately 5% of D− HUS patients have antibodies against factor H, raising the possibility of using plasma exchange or immunosuppressants for therapeutic strategy (Zheng, 2008).

Thrombotic Thrombocytopenic Purpura (TTP)

TTP may occur at any age but has a peak incidence in the third decade; it occurs more often in females than in males. The annual incidence is 3.7 cases per 100,000 (Ahmed, 2002). The triad of clinical manifestations present in most patients includes hemolytic anemia, thrombocytopenia, and neurologic symptoms; in addition, fever and renal diseases are often present. This constitutes the classic pentad. Pathologically, microvascular occlusive lesions with hyaline thrombi and endothelial proliferation are widespread throughout the body. Until 1997, the origin was unknown. Different theories included endothelial injury by oxidant stress, antiendothelial antibodies, anti-CD36 (glycoprotein IV located on microvasculature) antibodies, platelet aggregating factors, and release of large vWF multimers into the plasma. In 1996, a protease that cleaves vWF subunits was identified in normal plasma. In 1997 and the following years, several reports indicated deficient vWF-cleaving protease in patients with TTP due to low enzyme levels (in familial cases) or to the presence of IgG enzyme inhibitor (in nonfamilial cases). These observations were confirmed by additional studies, which showed normal levels of vWF-cleaving protease in HUS (Moake, 2004). The enzyme has been further characterized as number 13 in a family of 19 distinct ADAMTS-type enzymes identified to date (*a* *d*isintegrin *a*nd *m*etalloprotease with eight *t*hrombo*s*pondin-1-like domains). Therefore, the vWF-cleaving metalloprotease is now referred to as ADAMTS13 (Moake, 2004). In the absence of vWF-cleaving protease, ultra-large vWF multimers secreted by endothelial cells would not be processed normally. These highly adhesive multimers may induce platelet clumping in the microcirculation under shear stress, resulting in the clinical manifestation of TTP. The disease is acute and until the 1980s was fatal in well over half of cases. With the therapy of plasma exchange by plasmapheresis and plasma transfusions (in addition to platelet inhibitors), the remission rate has improved, and long-term survival now approaches 90% (Moake, 2004). TTP can now be classified into three main categories: familial, idiopathic, and secondary. The familial form (Upshaw-Schulman syndrome) results from a mutation in the *ADAMTS13* gene and is associated with a very low activity of the enzyme. More than 50 mutations have been described to date. Approximately 50% of patients with familial TTP experience their first episode during childhood, and exacerbations may occur in association with minor infections (Zheng, 2008). The idiopathic form is caused by antibodies to ADAMTS13. The secondary form may occur along the course of other conditions, such as malignancies, hematopoietic stem cell transplantation, chemotherapy, infection, and certain medications, such as cyclosporine, quinine, ticlopidine, and clopidogrel. The mechanism of TTP under these circumstances is unknown, although direct endothelial cytotoxicity and drug-induced autoimmunity are possible mechanisms (Zheng, 2008).

Preeclampsia/Eclampsia

Preeclampsia and eclampsia are microangiopathic disorders occurring with pregnancy and sharing some features of HUS or TTP. Approximately 4% to 39% of patients with severe preeclampsia develop HELLP syndrome: *h*emolysis, *e*levated *l*iver enzymes and *l*ow *p*latelet count. The syndrome becomes manifest usually during the third trimester, although some patients may develop it during the postpartum period. Most patients recover within a few days after delivery. In a small subset of patients, severe persistent multisystem disease requires plasma exchange (McMinn, 2001).

Infectious Agents

Destruction of erythrocytes by plasmodia is responsible for the anemia in malaria. This is supported by the observation that the osmotic and mechanical fragility of parasitized erythrocytes is increased. Inhibition of marrow activity may be an additional factor. Fulminant hemoglobinuria (blackwater fever) is a complication of *P. falciparum* malaria.

Oroya fever, a frequently fatal disease that occurs in Peru, is characterized by a hemolytic anemia and leukocytosis. *Bartonella bacilliformis* is the responsible agent.

Babesiosis, a protozoan infection transmitted by ticks from rodents or cattle, is associated with hemolysis; parasites may be seen in red cells in Romanowsky's-stained blood films.

Hemolytic anemia with cold agglutinins may complicate mycoplasmal pneumonia and infectious mononucleosis. This is due to the effect of antibody on the red cells.

Hemolytic anemia of varying severity is frequent in some bacterial infections. A notable example is *Clostridium perfringens* septicemia following septic abortion or biliary tract surgery, which may be accompanied by a dramatic and life-threatening hemolytic crisis.

Immune Hemolytic Anemias

Immune hemolytic anemias are disorders in which erythrocyte survival is reduced because of the deposition of immune globulin and/or complement on the red cell membrane. The immune hemolytic anemias can be grouped according to the presence of autoantibodies, alloantibodies, or drug-related antibodies (Table 32-11).

Autoimmune Hemolytic Anemia

The autoimmune hemolytic anemias (AIHAs) are due to an altered immune response, resulting in the production of antibody against the host's own erythrocytes, with subsequent hemolysis. The incidence of AIHA is estimated at 10–30 cases per 1 million population (Gehrs, 2002).

TABLE 32-11
Classification of Immune Hemolytic Anemias

Autoimmune hemolytic anemias
Associated with warm antibodies
Associated with cold antibodies
Combined warm and cold antibodies
Alloimmune hemolytic anemias
Transfusion-associated hemolytic anemia
Hemolytic disease of newborn
Rh incompatibility
ABO incompatibility
Drug-induced hemolytic anemia
Drug adsorption
Autoantibody induction
Neoantigen formation

TABLE 32-12
Autoimmune Hemolytic Anemia (AIHA)*

Condition	Warm AIHA	COLD AIHA CHAD	PCH	Mixed AIHA
Idiopathic	282 (23)	194 (16)	5 (<1)	47 (4)
Drug-induced disorders	184 (15)	0	0	2 (<1)
Neoplasia	165 (14)	81 (7)	0 (0)	26 (2)
Non-Hodgkin's lymphoma	27	25	0	8
Chronic lymphocytic leukemia	65	4	0	8
Hodgkin's lymphoma	11	7	0	5
Carcinomas	37	30	0	4
Miscellaneous	25	15	0	1
Infections	9 (<1)	76 (6)	14 (1)	2 (<1)
Pneumonia—*Mycoplasma*	0	21	0	0
Viral pneumonia	2	19	0	0
Infectious mononucleosis	0	11	1	0
Miscellaneous	7	25	13	2
Collagen diseases	30 (2)	15 (1)	0 (0)	20 (2)
Systemic lupus erythematosus	7	4	0	16
Rheumatoid arthritis	21	6	0	4
Others	2	5	0	0
Miscellaneous disorders	45 (4)	20 (2)	0	6 (<1)
Totals	715 (58)	386 (32)	19 (2)	103 (8)

Data from Sokol RJ, Hewitt S. Autoimmune hemolysis: a critical review. Crit Rev Oncol Hematol 1985;4:125–54.
CHAD, Cold hemagglutinin disease; *PCH,* paroxysmal cold hemoglobinuria.
*Numbers in parentheses are percentages.

The AIHAs can be classified according to serologic or clinical characteristics (Table 32-12). Some AIHAs are mediated by antibodies with maximum binding affinity at 37° C, and other AIHAs are mediated by antibodies with maximum binding affinity at 4° C. In addition, AIHAs could be viewed according to their association with other disorders. In a study of 1834 patients, approximately 40% of cases of AIHA have been associated with an underlying disease, while the remainder were idiopathic (Sokol, 1992). Lymphoproliferative disorders account for approximately half of cases of both warm and cold AIHA (Gehrs, 2002).

Etiology and Pathophysiology. The cause of the production of autoantibody in patients with AIHA is unknown. However, several mechanisms have been suggested. Autoimmune antibodies, particularly cold-reacting antibodies, are sometimes produced following an infection. This is typically seen with the elaboration of anti-I in patients with *Mycoplasma pneumoniae* infections and anti-i in patients with infectious mononucleosis. The cold agglutinins of anti-I and anti-i specificity are strikingly similar to one another in the structure of antigen binding sites. These antibodies react with antibodies that also identify the product of the *VH4-34* gene segment in B-cells. It has been hypothesized that infections can cause the production of antibodies of B cell, utilizing this gene segment. These antibodies will also have cold agglutinins activity against the I/i antigens (Rosse, 2004).

The amount of antibody, its avidity for the erythrocyte autoantigen, and its ability to fix complement are significant variables. Opsonization of red cells can destroy them in the circulation (intravascular hemolysis) or can cause their accelerated removal from the circulation by tissue macrophages (extravascular hemolysis). Major sites for these macrophages are the spleen and, to a lesser extent, the liver (Gehrs, 2002).

The development of AIHA in patients with lymphoproliferative disorders or with autoimmune disorders may relate to some abnormality with B cells, T cells, or macrophages, or the interaction among these cells. Perhaps loss of T cell suppressor function could result in unrestrained production of red cell antibody by B cells. This hypothesis is strengthened by the observation that methyldopa, a drug known to cause the development of anti–red cell antibodies, inhibits the activation of suppressor T lymphocytes (Gehrs, 2002).

In AIHA associated with warm-type antibody, there is IgG coating of erythrocytes with or without complement fixation. Clearance of red cells occurs mostly in the spleen. In the absence of complement fixation, it appears that the Fc portion of the red cell–bound IgG interacts with the Fc receptor present on the membrane of splenic macrophages located along the cords of Billroth. Thus, sensitized erythrocytes are retained, phagocytosed, or fragmented by splenic macrophages during their passage through the spleen.

In AIHA associated with the production of cold-type autoantibody, erythrocytes are usually coated with IgM. Under these circumstances, the fixation of complement frequently occurs. In paroxysmal cold hemoglobinuria, the offending antibody is an IgG that fixes complement. If the entire complement sequence is activated, there may be intravascular hemolysis. This phenomenon may occur in cases of cold hemagglutinin disease, as well as in paroxysmal cold hemoglobinuria. If complement activation fails to proceed to completion but is halted at an intermediate stage, intravascular lysis of the erythrocytes may not occur. However, extravascular hemolysis can still continue. In this situation, sensitized cells with C3b on the membrane are bound in the liver by the interaction of C3b and its receptors on Kupffer's cells. Erythrocytes may be phagocytosed entirely, or portions of the cells may be removed, resulting in fragmentation and spherocyte formation.

Approximately 7% of patients with AIHA satisfy diagnostic criteria for both warm and cold autoantibodies (Sokol, 1992). In these cases, IgG and C3d sensitize the erythrocytes. The serum contains IgM cold autohemagglutinins (optimally reactive at 4° C, but with a high thermal amplitude to 37° C) and IgG warm autoantibodies.

AIHA Associated With Warm Antibody. The warm antibody type of AIHA is slightly more frequent in females than in males and is most likely to occur in individuals 40 years or older; peak incidence occurs around the seventh decade. This age distribution may be related to the higher frequency of lymphoproliferative disorders with age (Packman, 2008). Idiopathic warm-antibody AIHA accounts for approximately 50% of cases. Chronic lymphocytic leukemia and lymphomas account for about half of secondary warm-antibody AIHA, and autoimmune disorders, such as SLE, account for most of the remaining cases (Packman, 2008). Clinical signs and symptoms frequently are those of an underlying disorder. However, the patient with idiopathic AIHA may have noted the presence of a mild upper respiratory tract infection just before the onset of hemolysis. As the disorder progresses, weakness, dizziness, and fever may be noted. Jaundice can be a presenting complaint. Pregnancy carries a fivefold risk of developing autoantibodies compared with the control population (Gehrs, 2002).

Laboratory findings include the presence of moderate to severe anemia. The neutrophil count may be increased. In a small proportion of cases, thrombocytopenia can exist. The peripheral film frequently shows spherocytosis, red cell fragmentation, polychromasia, and a few normoblasts. Reticulocyte percentage is high in approximately 50% of patients and is often associated with increased MCV. However, as many as one third of patients have transient reticulocytopenia, despite the presence of normal or hyperplastic erythroid precursors in the marrow (Packman, 2008). The lack of reticulocytosis should not keep one from making a diagnosis of AIHA. The bone marrow exhibits normoblastic erythroid hyperplasia, sometimes with mild megaloblastic changes.

There is usually a decrease in serum haptoglobin and an increase in unconjugated bilirubin and LD. The osmotic fragility and autohemolysis test can be normal or abnormal.

Direct and indirect antiglobulin tests indicate the presence of erythrocyte antibodies. The specificity of the autoantibodies is usually directed against antigens of the Rh system, membrane protein band 3 and band 4.1, and glycophorin A. However, activity against U, LW, Kell, jk^a, and Fy^a antigens may also occur. The warm antibody is most likely an IgG with subclass IgG1 and less frequently with IgG3. When IgG2 or IgG4 is present on the red cells alone, no hemolytic reaction is associated (Packman, 2001a). Occasionally, the antibody may be an IgA immune globulin, or rarely an IgM immune globulin. Complement may be detected on the erythrocyte membrane in slightly more than half of cases. Although many warm antibodies fix complement, intravascular complement–mediated hemolysis and hemoglobinuria are unusual, possibly because of the ability of complement regulatory proteins in plasma and on red cell surfaces to abort fixation of terminal complement components (Packman, 2008).

In some cases, sensitized red cells contain less immune globulin than can be detected using commercially prepared antiglobulins, which are normally sensitive to 250 to 500 molecules of IgG per red cell (Gilliland, 1976). Under these circumstances, the autoantibody at times can be detected with an antiglobulin consumption test.

The clinical course of AIHA associated with warm antibody is characterized by periods of remission and relapse. In secondary AIHA, the course and prognosis are related to the nature of the underlying disorder. In idiopathic AIHA, complications of the hemolytic disorder may be severe, leading to the demise of the patient. Pulmonary emoboli, infection, and cardiovascular collapse are causes of death, and deep vein thrombosis and splenic infarcts are common complications during active hemolysis (Packman, 2008).

AIHA Associated With Cold Antibody. AIHA associated with cold antibody can be mediated by an IgM and less frequently by an IgG. The IgM autoantibody is associated with a syndrome known as cold agglutinin disease, whereas the IgG autoantibody is seen with paroxysmal cold hemoglobinuria.

Cold Agglutinin Disease

Cold agglutinin disease occurs in individuals usually over the age of 50 years and in females more often than in males. In some cases, cold agglutinin disease is associated with a lymphoproliferative disorder or infection (especially with *M. pneumoniae* or infectious mononucleosis). Cases unassociated with an underlying disorder are listed as idiopathic. Virtually all sera from healthy individuals contain low-titer cold agglutinins, regarded as benign or harmless, and are polyclonal. Postinfectious cold agglutinins are usually polyclonal. By contrast, monoclonal cold agglutinins are generally pathogenetic and may arise from B cell lymphoma (Gehrs, 2002). Cold agglutinin disease represents approximately 20% of AIHA.

Symptoms and signs vary widely. Some individuals may complain of acrocyanosis or Raynaud's phenomenon. Others will have episodes of hemolysis, including hemoglobinuria, following exposure to cold. Temperatures of 30° C and lower are normally attained in the superficial skin vessels of those body parts exposed to cold. The thermal range of the antibody is clinically more important than the agglutination titer (Petz, 2008).

Laboratory findings usually indicate an anemia. Spherocytes and polychromatophilic erythrocytes are present to a variable degree in the blood film. There may be marked red cell agglutination, which should be differentiated from rouleaux formation (see Figs. 30-25 and 30-26). A mild leukocytosis can exist. Red cell agglutination may interfere with automated hematology counts, particularly MCHC, which tends to be high.

The cold antibody is usually an IgM with anti-I or, less frequently anti-i, specificity. Rarely do other specificities exist. In the chronic idiopathic form of cold agglutinin disease, the antibody tends to be monoclonal IgM, *k* with anti-I specificity (Gehrs, 2002). The autoantibody is also capable of fixing complement. When the titer of cold antibody is very high, the thermal range of antibody activity may extend up to 37° C. The direct antiglobulin test is positive only if the reagents contain anticomplement activity. Thus, one usually observes a positive antiglobulin reaction with broad-spectrum and non–γ-reagents, but no agglutination with only the γ-reagent. On cold exposure and antibody binding to red cells, the complement may be activated to the stage of C3b, which adheres to the red cells after entering the systemic circulation. In the hepatic circulation, macrophages carry specific receptors for C3b. However, cells usually escape hepatic destruction. Most patients experience chronic mild to moderate anemia, which they tolerate well, and patient outcome is significantly better than with warm-antibody AIHA (Petz, 2008). Some authors remain with the opinion that chronic cold agglutinin disease is a variant of Waldenström's macroglobulinemia in which the IgM M-component has cold agglutinin activity.

Paroxysmal Cold Hemoglobinuria

Paroxysmal cold hemoglobinuria is a very rare disorder that can occur in an individual of any age. However, more cases are now being reported in young children (Petz, 2008). Females are as frequently involved as males. Patients have symptoms of acute hemolysis following exposure to the cold. Chills, fever, pain in the back and legs, and hemoglobinuria are reported. The acute form may follow an acute upper respiratory illness or immunization by 1–2 weeks, but the chronic form is associated with congenital syphilis. Hemoglobinuria following exposure to cold is rare in the acute form.

Laboratory features consist of anemia, elevated reticulocyte count, increased concentration of indirect bilirubin, and the presence of Hb in the urine. Anemia is frequently severe and rapidly progressive.

The serum contains a cold hemolysin with biphasic activity. This antibody, first described by Donath and Landsteiner (1904), is an IgG that fixes the first components of complement (C1–C4) in the cold (4° C). As the temperature rises to 25°–37° C, the antibody dissociates, but the remainder of the complement proteins are activated, and erythrocyte lysis results; this biphasic hemolysis is the basis for the Donath-Landsteiner autohemolysis test for the diagnosis of this condition. The direct antiglobulin test is positive with anti-C3 but is generally negative with anti-IgG unless performed at colder temperature. The specificity of the antibody is directed against the P antigen. In general, the prognosis is good.

AIHA Associated With Warm and Cold Antibodies

AIHA associated with both warm and cold autoantibodies is mediated by IgG warm antibodies and complement, as well as IgM cold hemagglutinins. Females are more likely involved than males. There appears to be an association between the combined warm and cold antibody AIHA and SLE in that 15%–42% of patients have SLE (Shulman, 1985; Sokol, 1985). In one study (Shulman, 1985), 6 of 12 patients (50%) had idiopathic AIHA, and 4 of these (33%) had concomitant thrombocytopenia (Evans' syndrome); all 12 patients had severe hemolysis that responded dramatically to corticosteroid therapy.

Alloimmune Hemolytic Disease of the Newborn

Alloimmune hemolytic disease of the newborn (HDN) usually occurs following the transplacental passage of maternal antifetal red cell antibodies. HDN most frequently results from incompatibility in Rh and ABO erythrocyte antigens between mother and fetus. In rare cases, some other red cell antigen may be responsible for this disorder.

In HDN due to **Rh incompatibility,** prior sensitization is necessary to initiate the disease process. This sensitization usually occurs during pregnancy when Rh(D)-positive fetal red cells cross the placenta and enter the circulation of a mother with Rh-negative cells. Most women have less than 1 mL of fetal blood in their circulation following delivery. However, intrapartum fetomaternal hemorrhage of more than 30 mL occurs in approximately 1% of pregnancies (Ramasethu, 2001). Maternal sensitization can also occur by a previous incompatible transfusion. Under either of these circumstances, maternal IgG antibodies are produced against the fetal cells. If a subsequent pregnancy occurs in a sensitized mother, fetal erythrocytes again reach the maternal circulation and restimulate an antibody response, resulting in transfer of anti-Rh(D) antibody across the placenta and reduced fetal red cell survival.

In the **ABO system,** anti-A or anti-B antibodies of the IgG class may arise spontaneously in the mother; their presence does not require prior transfusion or pregnancy. As a result, first-born children may suffer from HDN when ABO incompatibility exists. Although ABO incompatibility occurs in 15% of group O pregnancies, ABO hemolytic disease is estimated to occur in only 3% of all births (Ramasethu, 2001).

The clinical features of HDN due to Rh incompatibility vary greatly. Some newborns experience only mild jaundice. Others initially appear markedly pale and then develop jaundice. They can have prominent hepatosplenomegaly. The disease may be complicated by a bleeding diathesis, marked acid-base abnormalities, and kernicterus. In very severe cases, patients can present with hydrops fetalis.

Early examination of the blood usually reveals an increase in nucleated erythrocytes, which may include forms as immature as pronormoblasts. Although this finding gave the disease its name, **erythroblastosis fetalis,** erythroblastosis is not always present, especially if the examination is not performed immediately after birth.

Up to 2.0×10^9 nucleated red cells per liter in term infants and up to 5.0×10^9/L in premature infants are commonly seen in this disorder. Normally, nucleated red cells average 0.5×10^9/L in term infants and $1.0–1.5 \times 10^9$/L in premature infants. Blood from the umbilical vein for early examination is more reliable than peripheral (capillary) blood because the erythrocyte count and the Hb may be significantly altered between birth and ligation of the cord.

Generally, there is macrocytic anemia of varying severity and an increase in reticulocytes. Occasionally, anemia may develop suddenly on the second or third day. The leukocyte count is frequently elevated, with immature leukocytes. Normoblastic hyperplasia of the marrow is pronounced.

In severely affected infants, thrombocytopenia, depression of prothrombin complex procoagulants, or diffuse intravascular coagulation may occur.

A direct antiglobulin test on fetal erythrocytes indicates the presence of an IgG antibody. When the maternal serum and an eluate from the fetal erythrocytes are incubated separately with a panel of O cells, one can usually demonstrate the presence of antibody with Rh(D) specificity. In

Rh-negative pregnant women known to be sensitized to Rh(D), the titer of anti-Rh(D) antibody is measured periodically during pregnancy to serve as a guide for performing amniocentesis.

HDN associated with **ABO incompatibility** is less severe than that observed with Rh incompatibility. Occasionally, the diagnosis is suggested by the presence of unexplained hyperbilirubinemia in a group A or B newborn infant from a group O mother.

Laboratory findings usually show a mild anemia and modest reticulocytosis. In contrast to Rh isoimmune disease, spherocytosis in ABO isoimmune disease may be prominent. However, there may be no anemia. Fetal cells are usually weakly positive with the antiglobulin reagents. Serum from the newborn and eluates from the cells should contain anti-A or anti-B antibody. In addition, maternal serum should contain high titers of anti-A or anti-B antibodies of the IgG subclass.

Drug-Induced Immune Hemolytic Anemia

Immune hemolytic anemia may occur following the administration of drugs. Most cases in the 1970s were associated with methyldopa or high-dose intravenous penicillin therapy. Recently, this picture has changed, with second- and third-generation cephalosporins being the most common causative agent and accounting for more than 80% of drug-induced immune hemolytic anemia (Garratty, 2007). Four mechanisms appear to mediate immune hemolysis (Packman, 2001b).

Formation of Ternary Complexes (Neoantigen Formation). Numerous drugs are known to weakly bind to red cell membrane, even when given in small doses (Table 32-13). Antibodies recognize the combined drug and red cell membrane components as antigen and bind to them, forming a ternary complex. The drug-induced antibody is usually IgM and tends to fix complement, resulting in lysis of cells. In addition, red cells may be sequestered in the liver and spleen because of their coating with C3b.

Patients present with acute intravascular hemolysis, hemoglobinemia, and hemoglobinuria. The direct antiglobulin reaction is positive if the reagents contain anticomplement activity. The reaction usually is negative with the γ-reagent because it contains little anti-IgM or complement specificity.

The diagnosis can be determined by incubating the patient's serum with the offending drug in the presence of target erythrocytes, while observing agglutination, lysis, or sensitization of the erythrocytes.

Adsorption of Drug to Red Cell Membrane. Penicillin and cephalosporin, particularly in high doses, bind firmly to proteins, including red cell membrane. These drugs induce an antibody response to them, but the antibody specificity is not directed against a red cell membrane. Both IgM and IgG antibodies are made, but only the IgG antibodies are associated with immune hemolysis. Complement is not involved. The erythrocytes, coated with IgG antibody, are presumably removed via the Fc receptors on macrophages in the spleen.

The direct antiglobulin test is strongly positive. Antibody eluted from patients' erythrocytes will react only with red cells previously treated with penicillin or cephalosporins.

TABLE 32-13
Examples of Drugs Implicated in Causing Immune Hemolytic Anemia and Their Mechanism of Action

Drug Adsorption Mechanism	
Penicillins	Cephalosporins
Tetracyclines	Tolbutamide
Ternary Complex Mechanism	
Stibophen	Quinidine
Quinine	Cephalosporins
Rifampicin	Diethylstilbestrol
Chlorpropamide	Amphotericin B
Autoantibody Mechanism	
α-Methyldopa	L-Dopa
Procainamide	Cephalosporins
Mefenamic acid	Fludarabine

Modified from Packman CH. Drug related immune hemolytic anemia. In: Beutler E, Lichtman MA, Coller BS, Kipps TJ, Seligsohn U, editors. Williams hematology. 6th ed. New York: McGraw-Hill; 2001b, p. 657.

Induction of Autoantibody by Drugs. In approximately 15% of patients using the antihypertensive drug methyldopa, a positive direct antiglobulin reaction is present. The antibody is of the IgG class and in some studies appears to have Rh specificity (Packman, 2001b). The actual mechanism of autoantibody production is not known. However, it has been hypothesized that methyldopa causes activation of T cells and increased secretion of γ-IFN, which upregulates MHC class I and class II molecules on antigen-presenting cells and induces antibody production by B cells (Baier, 1994).

Development of the positive antiglobulin reaction occurs after a lag period of 3–6 months and is dose dependent. Thirty-six percent of patients have a positive antiglobulin reaction when consuming 2 g or more of methyldopa per day, and 11% have a positive reaction when taking only 1 g daily. An immune hemolytic anemia occurs in less than 1% of patients and is not dose dependent. Methyldopa also decreases mononuclear phagocytic activity, which may explain the rarity of hemolytic anemia despite the common presence of autoantibodies (Sokol, 1992). Levodopa, procainamide, fludarabine, and mefenamic acid are additional drugs that have been reported to cause an AHA in a fashion similar to methyldopa.

Nonimmunologic Adsorption of Immunoglobulins to Red Cell Membrane. Drugs such as cephalosporins and cisplatin appear to alter the erythrocyte membrane, resulting in the nonspecific adsorption of plasma protein to its surface. As a result, IgG and IgM may be loosely bound to red cell membrane. This phenomenon can then cause a positive direct antiglobulin reaction. It is now believed that this mechanism can cause hemolytic anemia (Garratty, 2007).

LABORATORY DIAGNOSIS OF ANEMIA

The diagnosis and study of anemia require the proper use and interpretation of laboratory measurements. Prerequisites for the efficient use of the laboratory are a careful history and physical examination, both of which lead to initial laboratory measurements and provide important guidance in determining the nature of the anemia.

Whether the patient is anemic can be ascertained by determining whether the Hb, Hct, or erythrocyte count lies below (1) the reference intervals for age and sex, or (2) the patient's previous values, even though these are within the reference intervals. The task then is to define the underlying cause or mechanism for the anemia.

Usually, complete blood count (WBC, RBC, Hb, Hct, MCV, MCH, MCHC) and examination of a Wright's-stained film are parts of the routine examination of blood. It is possible that all these values could be normal in the presence of a mild macrocytic anemia, in which the RBC count does not fall below the normal range and the macrocytes present (and detectable on the blood film) do not elevate the MCV above the normal range.

Once anemia is discovered, the basic examination of the blood should include the following: (1) Hb, Hct, RBC count, and erythrocyte indices; (2) blood film examination; (3) leukocyte count; (4) platelet count; and (5) reticulocyte count.

With current multichannel instruments, all red cell values and their indices have comparable precision. Indices are **mean** values, however, and will not detect different populations of cells that balance each other. For example, combined deficiencies of folate and iron may give rise to populations of macrocytic and hypochromic microcytic cells, which could yield normal indices. Careful examination of the blood film is essential, and red cell volume RDW is very useful in defining this type of abnormality (see Chapter 30).

The size of the erythrocytes, determined by the MCV and by examination of the blood film, will determine the morphologic type of anemia. In addition, certain findings on the blood film will suggest mechanisms that are involved.

Increased numbers of **polychromatic** macrocytes, with or without normoblasts, suggest increased erythropoiesis, and in the untreated patient, this is usually due to hemorrhage or hemolysis. In this situation, the history (of blood loss) or physical examination (jaundice or splenomegaly) will help.

Findings suggestive of hemolysis are **poikilocytes** (abnormally shaped red cells), **sickle cells, irregularly contracted forms** (including red cell fragments or schistocytes), and **spherocytes.** Sometimes it is difficult to detect spherocytes in HS because of minimal anisocytosis. Morphologic findings in red cells that are helpful in this situation include the presence of a low MCD (mean cell diameter), between 6.0 and 6.5 μm (normal =

7.0–7.4 µm), red cells with small eccentric or no pallor, and red cells with slightly more intense staining due to Hb density.

Target cells may be found in hemoglobinopathies, especially in the presence of Hb C, Hb D, and Hb E, and in the thalassemias. They may be present in any **hypochromic** anemia, although usually in smaller numbers. Target cells without microcytosis are also found in liver disease and in the absence of the spleen or of splenic function.

Fine **basophilic stippling** (which is due to precipitation of RNA) may be found in polychromatic red cells associated with a significant increase in the generation of erythrocytes, as in response to hemorrhage or hemolysis. **Coarse basophilic stippling** suggests an abnormality in Hb synthesis. It is found in megaloblastic anemias, thalassemias, refractory anemias, some red cell enzyme deficiencies, unstable Hbs, and lead poisoning. In particular, hypochromasia or microcytosis with stippling is against the diagnosis of iron deficiency anemia and is more suggestive of thalassemia or lead poisoning. As mentioned earlier, some cases of iron deficiency may be associated with lead poisoning (see Iron Metabolism).

The combination of **oval macrocytes** (especially egg-shaped macrocytes) and **hypersegmented neutrophils** indicates the very likely existence of megaloblastic anemia.

Finally, examination of the blood film allows the evaluation of **qualitative abnormalities in leukocytes and platelets,** as well as an estimate of their numbers. Blood diseases that may be first suspected or detected in this manner are many and include compensated hemolytic anemia; early megaloblastic anemia; and anomalies of red cells, such as hereditary elliptocytosis, or of leukocytes, such as the Pelger-Hüet nuclear anomaly.

After the basic studies just mentioned, the choice of additional procedures depends on the morphologic type of the anemia, as determined by the indices and the blood film.

Macrocytic Anemia (Increased MCV)

The macrocytic anemias are normochromic, as determined by appearance on the film and by the MCHC. The first step is to ascertain whether the anemia is megaloblastic. Clues from the film have been mentioned. A **bone marrow aspiration** should be performed to confirm the presence of megaloblastosis.

Megaloblastic Marrow

If the marrow is **megaloblastic,** with characteristic changes in both red cell and white cell precursors, the anemia in all likelihood is due to folate or cobalamin deficiency.

See earlier sections on diagnosis of cobalamin deficiency and of folate deficiency. Once the **type** of deficiency is defined, the **cause** must be determined.

Nonmegaloblastic Marrow

If the marrow is **not megaloblastic,** conditions that can be associated with macrocytosis should be investigated. These include liver disease; hemolytic anemias; hypothyroidism; excessive alcohol intake; hypoplastic anemias; and refractory anemias with hyperplastic bone marrow, which include the myelodysplastic syndromes. Anemias associated with these disorders, although they *may* be macrocytic, are more usually normocytic, and thus are considered with the normocytic anemias as well.

Microcytic and Hypochromic Anemias (Decreased MCV and MCH)

If the counts are performed on a multichannel instrument, the MCHC is likely to be in the normal range, with slight to moderate degrees of hypochromia. Consequently, the MCV has assumed the leading role in the detection of microcytic hypochromic anemias. These anemias reflect a quantitative defect in Hb synthesis. Major causes of microcytic anemia include the following:

1. **Iron deficiency anemias** are due to increased requirement or blood loss not balanced by intake.
2. **ACD** is associated with infection, neoplasia, or collagen disease. This anemia may be normochromic and normocytic, but in long-standing disease is often hypochromic and microcytic.
3. **Thalassemia** is a genetically determined impairment in the rate of globin synthesis.
4. **Sideroblastic anemia** is that group of refractory anemias with erythroid hyperplasia of the marrow in which a defect in Hb synthesis creates a population of hypochromic microcytic cells. The blood film is dimorphic and macrocytes may prevail, making the MCV normal or high, particularly in acquired forms of sideroblastic anemia.

Because **iron deficiency** is the most common anemia, the first step is to determine whether the body lacks iron.

When blood loss cannot be documented, serum ferritin, serum iron and iron-binding capacity, or bone marrow study for iron should be performed. These will usually discriminate between the two most common anemias in this category: iron deficiency and simple chronic anemia associated with some other disease, frequently chronic infection or cancer. In both, the serum iron concentration is low, but in iron deficiency, the TIBC is elevated, whereas in simple ACD it is normal or decreased. Storage iron in the marrow is depleted in iron deficiency but is normal or elevated in anemia of chronic disease. Iron deficiency anemia in an adult male almost always means chronic blood loss; the source must be found and corrected, if necessary.

Hypochromic anemias (or erythrocytoses) with basophilic stippling and normal or increased serum iron are most likely **thalassemias,** and the next examinations to perform are Hb electrophoresis and determination of Hb A_2 and Hb F. Family studies are often necessary.

Sideroblastic anemias include refractory anemia with ring sideroblasts, which are part of myelodysplastic syndromes (see Chapter 33), as well as anemias that occur after therapy with certain drugs (e.g., isoniazid) or in chronic lead poisoning. Coarse basophilic stippling is common in this group of anemias.

Table 32-14 summarizes some laboratory distinctions within the microcytic anemias.

Normocytic and Normochromic Anemias (Normal MCV)

This large group of anemias has many causes. A useful approach is evaluation of the erythrokinetics in a given patient (see Chapter 31). Often, the reticulocyte production index (RPI) and examination of the bone marrow will suffice. The RPI is the simplest measure of effective erythropoiesis.

Optimal Marrow Response: Reticulocyte Production Index Greater Than Two

If the output of reticulocytes has exceeded two times normal, as determined by the absolute reticulocyte count, or RPI, it can be assumed that the marrow has reached an optimal response. The cause for the anemia is then **acute blood loss** or **hemolysis.** If blood loss cannot be proved, evidence that hemolysis is in fact present must be sought.

TABLE 32-14
Laboratory Features in Microcytic Hypochromic Anemias

				MARROW					
	Serum iron	**Serum TIBC**	**% saturation**	**% sideroblasts**	**Iron stores**	**Serum ferritin**	**ZPP**	**Hb A_2**	**Hb F**
Iron deficiency	↓	↑	↓	↓	↓	↓	↑	N-↓	N
β-Thalassemia trait	N (↑)	N	N	N	N-↑	N-↑	N	↑	N-↑
ACD	↓	N-↓	↓	↓	N-↑	N-↑	↑	N	N
Sideroblastic anemia	↑	↓	↑	↑	↑	↑	↑ (↓)	N	N-↑

ACD, Anemia of chronic disease; *N,* normal; *TIBC,* total iron-binding capacity; *ZPP,* zinc protoporphyrins; ↓, decreased; ↑, increased.

Erythroid hyperplasia of the marrow, serum bilirubin, and urine or fecal urobilinogen will indicate whether erythropoietic activity and destruction are increased. Red cell survival determination may be needed to prove hemolysis in some cases. Low serum haptoglobin and high LD point to hemolysis, but a normal level does not exclude it. None of these measurements will specify whether hemolysis is intravascular or extravascular, but elevated plasma Hb, hemoglobinuria, and hemosiderinuria indicate intravascular hemolysis.

Once it is determined that excessive hemolysis is occurring, the type of hemolytic mechanism must be ascertained.

Direct Antiglobulin (Coombs') Test. If the direct antiglobulin reaction is *positive* using broad-spectrum reagents, tests to determine the presence of IgG, IgM, or complement on the red cells should be undertaken. If immunoglobulin is present on the red cells, tests for antibody specificity, cold agglutinins, Donath-Landsteiner antibody, and serum protein electrophoresis may help to define the process.

If the direct antiglobulin reaction is *negative*, the examinations performed next will depend on the clinical findings and the results of measurements already made.

If HS is suspected, osmotic fragility before and after 24-hour incubation at 37° C and family studies will be necessary.

If a nonspherocytic congenital hemolytic anemia is suspected, screening for G6PD and PK deficiencies, Hb electrophoresis, and a sickle cell test will be helpful. If these are negative, the heat instability test, isopropanol solubility test, and autohemolysis test should be considered.

If thalassemia seems likely, determinations of Hb A_2 and Hb F and perhaps looking for Hb H inclusions are appropriate. Thalassemias are usually microcytic and hypochromic anemias; β-thalassemia major, β-thalassemia intermedia, and Hb H disease are hemolytic disorders and may have an increased RPI.

If drug-induced hemolysis is suspected, a test for Heinz bodies, a screening test for G6PD, and, if possible, tests for a drug-dependent autoantibody are indicated.

If the nature of the hemolytic anemia is obscure, a flow cytometry test for PNH should be performed.

Inadequate Marrow Response: Reticulocyte Production Index Less Than Two

The mechanism of the anemia may be ineffective erythropoiesis. Conditions with the greatest degree of ineffective erythropoiesis appear in other categories (e.g., megaloblastic anemia, thalassemia), but most of the myelodysplastic syndromes have a hyperplastic bone marrow and impaired delivery of cells to the blood. In some of these, morphologic changes in erythroid precursors may overlap with megaloblastic anemia, but granulocytic and megakaryocytic changes usually seen in megaloblastic anemia are lacking.

A low reticulocyte count may indicate decreased production caused by inadequate stimulation of the marrow. Chronic renal disease may result in impaired production of EPO. Certain endocrinopathies, such as hypopituitarism or hypothyroidism, may result in regulation of Hb production at a lower level as a result of decreased tissue need for O_2.

A large group of normochromic anemias associated with various chronic diseases form a heterogeneous group characterized by failure of the marrow to meet the need for slightly decreased red cell survival. Some of these are ACDs associated with infection, cancer, or rheumatoid arthritis; they have the defect in iron metabolism noted previously in the section on hypochromic microcytic anemias.

Inability of the marrow to respond to EPO may be due to damage to the marrow by drugs or toxic chemicals, to unknown causes, or to infiltration of the marrow by neoplastic cells or fibrous tissue.

In those conditions with low reticulocyte counts in which the marrow is not effectively producing erythrocytes, it is usually helpful to examine the bone marrow. Other studies conducted to determine the underlying disease process can then proceed according to the marrow picture, the assessment of erythrokinetics, and the clinical findings.

POLYCYTHEMIA

Polycythemia (erythrocytosis) is classically defined as an elevated Hct level above the normal range. In the clinical setting, polycythemia exists when Hb and red cell count are increased, reflecting an elevation of the total red cell volume (Maran, 2004). Yet, the recent World Health Organization (WHO) classification of hematologic malignancies has defined polycythemia as Hgb >18.5 g/dL for men, >16.5 g/dL for women, Hct >99th percentile of the method-specific range, or lower values but with a documented unexplained Hgb increase of at least 2 g/dL (Swerdlow, 2008).

Absolute polycythemia refers to an increase in the total red cell mass in the body; in **relative polycythemia,** the total red cell mass is normal, but the Hct is elevated because the plasma volume is decreased. Polycythemia may be classified as in Table 32-15. Some classifications are based on EPO response (Cazzola, 2004), and others are based on the underlying mechanism (i.e., primary or secondary, and congenital or acquired) (Gordeuk, 2005).

TABLE 32-15
Pathophysiologic Classification of Polycythemia

Relative Polycythemia
1. Diminished plasma volume: dehydration; shock
2. Spurious polycythemia (stress polycythemia; Gaisböck's syndrome)

Absolute Polycythemia
1. Secondary polycythemia with appropriately increased EPO production
   a. Decreased oxygen (O_2) loading: hypoxia; high altitude; pulmonary disease; cyanotic heart disease; carboxyhemoglobinemia; methemoglobinemia; Hb M
   b. Decreased O_2 unloading: high O_2 affinity hemoglobinopathy; biphosphoglycerate deficiency
2. Secondary polycythemia with inappropriately increased EPO production
   a. Neoplasms: Wilms' tumor; renal carcinoma; cerebellar hemangioma; hepatoma
   b. Localized tissue hypoxia: polycystic kidney; renal artery stenosis
   c. Postrenal transplant
   d. Acute hepatitis
3. Genetic polycythemia
   a. Primary familial congenital polycythemia (mutated EPO receptor)
   b. Chuvash polycythemia (mutated *VHL* gene)
4. Primary marrow disorders
   a. Polycythemia vera

Modified from Cazzola M. Serum erythropoietin concentration as a diagnostic tool for polycythemia vera. Haematologica 2004;89:1159–60.
EPO, Erythropoietin; *Hb M,* methemoglobin.

RELATIVE POLYCYTHEMIA

Relative polycythemia refers to an increase in Hct or red cell count as a result of decreased plasma volume; total red cell mass is not increased. This occurs in acute dehydration (e.g., severe diarrhea, burns) and in patients on diuretic therapy.

In **spurious polycythemia** (apparent polycythemia, Gaisböck's syndrome), the red cell mass is often high normal and the plasma volume is low normal; these patients have been regarded as an extreme of the normal physiologic state. Almost all are men; they have a high incidence of tobacco smoking and tend to be obese and to have hypertension. Sleep apnea and diuretics may be contributory factors. Serum EPO level is normal (Cazzola, 2004).

ABSOLUTE POLYCYTHEMIA

Appropriately Increased Erythropoietin Production Due to Hypoxia

Cellular response to hypoxia is controlled by a family of α-β heterodimeric transcription factors, known as hypoxia-inducible factors (HIFs), which regulate the transcription of EPO. There are three HIF isoforms—HIF1α, HIF2α, and HIF3α—with HIF2α being the major isoform regulating EPO expression. In the presence of normoxia, HIF1α is rapidly destroyed by the collaborative effect of O_2, prolyl hydroxylase domain–containing enzymes, and the von Hippel–Lindau tumor suppressor protein (VHL). Under hypoxic conditions, degradation of HIFα is slowed, resulting in increased transcription of its target genes, which include EPO. Binding of EPO to its receptor results in autophosphorlyation of the receptor-associated Janus kinase 2 (JAK 2), which has tyrosine kinase activity (Patnaik, 2009).

Arterial Oxygen Unsaturation

Lack of O_2 reaching the blood for whatever reason results in arterial unsaturation, impaired O_2 delivery to the tissues, increased production of EPO, erythroid hyperplasia in the marrow, and resultant erythrocytosis. The red cell mass is increased. As a response to the hypoxia, the red cell 2,3-DPG and the p_{50} are increased. In contrast to polycythemia vera, there is usually no leukocytosis or thrombocytosis, and the neutrophil alkaline phosphatase is normal. Arterial O_2 unsaturation may be the cause of polycythemia in persons living at high altitudes; in patients with chronic pulmonary disease and a block in diffusion of O_2 into the blood; in cyanotic heart disease in which there is right-to-left shunt; and in caroboxyhemoglobinemia mostly related to cigarette smoking. In case of CO poisoning, hypoxia is caused by two mechanisms: direct reduction of O_2 saturation and interference with O_2 release from Hb (Landaw, 1990).

High Oxygen Affinity Hemoglobinopathy

Another cause of tissue hypoxia is the presence of structurally abnormal Hb that has a high affinity for O_2 (Prchal, 2003) (see earlier under Hemoglobins Associated With Altered Oxygen Affinity). As in other functional hemoglobinopathies, the disorder occurs in the heterozygote. More than 100 Hb mutations associated with increased O_2 affinity have been identified (Prchal, 2003). Abnormal Hb releases less O_2 to the tissues than does normal Hb at the same pO_2; the O_2 dissociation curve is shifted to the left, and the p_{50} is decreased. The red cell 2,3-DPG is not increased. As in arterial O_2 unsaturation, EPO production and erythrocytosis are increased. It must be emphasized that routine Hb electrophoresis often does not detect these Hb variants because the amino acid substitution occurs at one of the αβ-contact sites, or near the heme pocket. A low p_{50} therefore is presumptive evidence for a hemoglobinopathy. Some high-affinity Hbs associated with polycythemia are unstable; in these instances, the heat instability test is positive.

Other causes of altered O_2 affinity include Hb M and deficiency of red cell enzyme 2,3-DPG mutase, which is involved in the generation of 2,2-DPG (Gordeuk, 2005).

Inappropriate Erythropoietin Production

Neoplasms

Neoplasms, benign or malignant, have been associated with polycythemia. Renal neoplasms account for the majority. In almost all cases, erythrocytosis has disappeared after resection of the tumor. These neoplasms have been shown to express high levels of EPO mRNA. These tumors include cerebellar hemangiomas, renal cell carcinomas, Wilms' tumors, some hepatomas, uterine leimyomas, pheochromocytoma, parathyroid adenomas, and meningiomas (Patnaik, 2009).

Renal Disorders

In other neoplasms or growths (e.g., renal cysts, hydronephrosis, ovarian carcinoma, some hepatomas), it appears that the mass impinging on the kidney induces increased renal production of EPO as a result of increased pressure or local hypoxia within the kidney. Renal artery stenosis is also associated with polycythemia. Posttransplant erythrocytosis occurs in 10%–20% of renal transplant recipients. The therapeutic effects of angiotensin-converting enzyme inhibitors in this condition suggest a role for angiotensin II in regulating erythropoiesis (Prchal, 2003).

Familial Polycythemia

The most common familial polycythemia is due to the presence of a **high oxygen affinity hemoglobin,** which is inherited as an autosomal dominant trait. Congenital polycythemia may be due to a defect in the hypoxia-sensing mechanism. Von Hippel–Lindau syndrome is an autosomal dominant disorder associated with mutations in the *VHL* gene. These mutations result in increased levels of HIF-1α and increased levels of EPO (Prchal, 2003; Gordeuk, 2005). Chuvash polycythemia is an autosomal recessive congenital polycythemia that is endemic in the Chuvash population of the Russian federation. It has been reported to be associated with a high mortality rate caused by thrombotic and hemorrhagic complications.

Congenital polycythemia may occur secondary to a defect in the EPO receptor in the presence of a normal hypoxia-sensing mechanism. Primary familial and congenital polycythemia (PFCP) is an autosomal dominant disorder that is present at birth. PFCP is associated with low serum EPO levels and in vitro hypersensitivity of erythroid progenitors to EPO. Sixteen germline mutations in the EPO receptor gene *(EPOR)* with resulting truncated receptors have been described in PFCP to date (Patnaik, 2009). As mentioned earlier, marked decrease in red cell 2,3-DPG associated with **deficiency of 2,3-DPG mutase** activity results in polycythemia and appears to be inherited as an autosomal recessive condition.

Polycythemia Vera

Polycythemia vera is a panmyelosis, that is, a condition in which excessive proliferation occurs in megakaryocytes and granulocytes, as well as in erythrocytes. It is manifested by erythrocytosis, leukocytosis, and thrombocytosis of varying degrees. Mutation in the *JAK2* gene is now described as a constant finding. Polycythemia vera is discussed with the myeloproliferative neoplasms.

MEASUREMENT OF ERYTHROCYTE AND PLASMA VOLUME

The diagnosis of absolute polycythemia depends on reliable measurements of erythrocyte and plasma volumes. Erythrocyte and plasma volumes are measured with the use of radioactive isotopic tracers and the dilution principle. The most commonly employed tracers are ^{51}Cr in the form of sodium chromate bound to erythrocytes for measurement of erythrocyte volume. ^{125}I or ^{131}iodine is bound to albumin and can be used to measure plasma volume.

For a detailed description of measurement of red cell and plasma volume, see the report of the International Committee for Standardization in Hematology (1980).

Erythrocyte Volume

In brief, blood is collected from the patient, and the erythrocytes are labeled with ^{51}Cr. The chromated erythrocytes are washed in saline. An aliquot of the ^{51}Cr erythrocytes diluted in saline is injected intravenously into the patient. After a period of equilibration, usually 10–20 minutes, a sample of blood is withdrawn from the opposite arm. In cases in which the equilibration time is likely to be prolonged (as in splenomegaly, heart failure, or shock), another sample should be withdrawn 60 minutes after injection.

Radioactivity of each sample is recorded by a scintillation counter. The erythrocyte volume (EV) is calculated using the following formula:

$$\text{EV (mL)} = I \text{ (cpm)}/C \text{ (cpm/mL)}$$

where I is the total injected radioactivity (counts/minute) and C is the radioactivity in erythrocytes after mixing is complete (counts/minute/mL of erythrocytes).

Plasma Volume

Approximately 20 mL of blood is withdrawn from a patient. After centrifugation, the plasma is removed, and radioiodine-labeled albumin is added. After mixing, the labeled plasma is injected intravenously into the patient. At 10, 20, and 30 minutes following injection, 5 mL of blood is removed and radioactivity is counted in a well-type scintillation counter. The radioactivity at zero time (P_0) is determined by plotting the three points on semilogarithmic graph paper and extrapolating to zero time. A standard is prepared by diluting an aliquot of the radioiodine-labeled albumin with saline containing a small amount of detergent.

The plasma volume (PV) is calculated using the following formula:

$$\text{PV (mL)} = S \text{ (cpm/mL)} \times D \times V \text{ (mL)}/P_0 \text{ (cpm/mL)}$$

where

S = counting rate of standard (counts/minute/mL)
D = dilution of diluted standard solution
V = volume of radioiodine-labeled albumin solution injected
P_0 = counting rate of plasma sample corrected to zero time (counts/minute/mL).

Interpretation

The normal erythrocyte volume for men is 20–36 mL/kg, and for women, it is 19–31 mL/kg. The plasma volume for men is 25–43 mL/kg; for women, 28–45 mL/kg. In newborns and premature infants, the red cell volume and plasma volume in milliliters per kilogram are higher than in adults.

Patients with polycythemia have red cell volumes exceeding 36 mL/kg for men and 32 mL/kg for women. Changes in erythrocyte volume and plasma volume in a variety of conditions are recorded in Table 32-16.

TABLE 32-16
Clinical Effect of Variable Relationship Between Red Cell Volume and Plasma Volume

Red cell volume	Plasma volume	Cause	Effect
Normal	High	Pregnancy Cirrhosis Nephritis Congestive cardiac failure	Pseudoanemia
Normal	Low	Stress Peripheral circulatory failure Dehydration Edema Prolonged bed rest	Pseudopolycythemia
Low	Normal	Anemia	Accurate reflection of degree of anemia
Low	High	Anemia	Anemia less severe than indicated by blood count
Low	Low	Hemorrhage Severe anemia (when hematocrit <0.2)	Anemia more severe than indicated by blood count
High	Normal to low	Polycythemia	Accurate reflection of polycythemia or polycythemia less severe than apparent
High	High	Polycythemia (when hematocrit >0.5)	Polycythemia more severe than apparent
Normal or even high	High	Marked splenomegaly	Pseudoanemia

From Dacie JV, Lewis SM. Practical haematology. 5th ed. Edinburgh: Churchill Livingstone; 1975.

SELECTED REFERENCES

Bunn HF, Forget BG. Hemoglobin: molecular, genetic and clinical aspects. Philadelphia: WB Saunders; 1986.

This classic book provides elegant descriptions of major hemoglobinopathies and includes essential clues to differential diagnosis in a concise manner.

Cappellini MD, Fiorelli G. Glucose-6-phosphate dehydrogenase deficiency. Lancet 2008;371:64–74.

A concise and informative review of glucose-6-phosphate dehydrogenase deficiency.

Fyfe JC, Madsen M, Hojrup P, et al. The functional cobalamin (vitamin B12)-intrinsic factor receptor is a novel complex of cubilin and amnionless. Blood 2004;103:1573–9.

The first article to investigate the mechanism of Imerslund-Gräsbeck syndrome.

Garratty G, Arndt PA. An update on drug-induced immune hemolytic anemia. Immunohematology 2007;23:105–19.

A detailed review about the prevalence and mechanism of cephalosporin-induced hemolytic anemia.

Globin Gene Server. Available from: http://globin.cse.psu.edu/

An up-to-date interactive database of Hb variants and thalassemias.

Moake JL. Thrombotic microangiopathies. N Engl J Med 2002;347:589–600.

An excellent review of pathophysiologic mechanisms, clinical presentation, and management of thrombotic microangiopathy. The accompanying figures are exceptionally well designed and simple.

Steinberg MH, Forget BG, Higgs DR, Nagel RL. Disorders of hemoglobins. 1st ed. Cambridge: Cambridge University Press; 2001.

Comprehensive reference book on disorders of hemoglobin; detailed account of hemoglobin variants.

Weatherall DJ, Clegg JB. The thalassaemia syndromes. 4th ed. Oxford: Blackwell Scientific Publications; 2001.

A complete study of thalassemias and their interaction with variant hemoglobins.

Young NS. Acquired aplastic anemia. Ann Intern Med 2002;136:534–46.

This article highlights the most recent thoughts on the immunologic mechanism of aplastic anemia and provides a short discussion of its relationship to myelodysplastic syndrome and paroxysmal nocturnal hemoglobinuria.

REFERENCES

Access the complete reference list online at http://www.expertconsult.com

CHAPTER 33

LEUKOCYTIC DISORDERS

Robert E. Hutchison, Katherine I. Schexneider*

Continued

*Acknowledgment: The authors wish to thank Drs. Douglas A. Nelson, Frederick R. Davey, and Naif Z. Abraham, who authored earlier versions of this work, and whose words continue to echo throughout.

KEY POINTS

- Leukocytes are regulated by complex homeostatic mechanisms which direct their responses to infection and inflammation.
- Leukocytosis often reflects an underlying abnormality; leukopenia, especially neutropenia, places a patient at risk for infection.
- Hematopoietic neoplasms have been categorized by a World Health Organization classification according to cell of origin, cytogenetic and molecular abnormalities, immunophenotype, and clinical features.
- Acute leukemias are rapidly progressing neoplasms of precursor myeloid or lymphoid cell origin. An understanding of biology is associated with improvements in therapy.
- Chronic myeloproliferative disorders and myelodysplastic syndromes are heterogeneous disorders of differentiated myeloid cells. They often are initially indolent but ultimately progress.
- Non-Hodgkin lymphomas most often arise from mature B cells. They are pathologically and clinically heterogeneous. T cell lymphomas are less common, also heterogeneous, and often difficult to treat successfully.
- Hodgkin lymphoma is now considered a neoplasm of defective B cells. Much of its pathology is due to an associated inflammatory milieu.

LEUKOCYTES

Leukocytes, or white blood cells, are found within the bone marrow (BM), the peripheral blood, and the tissues. Leukocytes are among the essential elements of the hematopoietic-lymphoreticular-immune system, which functions to protect the human body from nonself cells (infection) and altered-self cells (cancer). Normal leukocyte development is reviewed in Chapter 31.

Leukocyte function involves cell adhesion molecules (CAMs), proteases, and cytokines (Table 33-1). Molecular interactions with endothelial cells direct leukocytes to their ultimate destination. Tissue- or organ-specific molecules on endothelium, including selectins and integrins, influence specific leukocyte trafficking, as well as passage across the endothelium; chemokines also influence migration (Ruoslahti, 2000; Sallusto, 2000; Alon, 2002; Patel, 2002; Moser, 2004; Rot, 2004).

One very important leukocyte homeostatic mechanism is apoptosis, or programmed cell death. In B and T cell development, it eliminates those with nonfunctional or autoreactive antigen receptors and regulates activation of the inflammatory response (Marsden, 2003; Ivanovska, 2004). It also plays a critical role in granulocyte development by increasing their relatively short life span at sites of infection and downregulating inflammation at completion, and it prevents the release of enzymes and inflammatory mediators from senescent granulocytes into surrounding healthy tissue. Abnormalities of apoptosis are involved in numerous pathologic states (cancer, degenerative disease, persistent infection, autoimmune disease). Apoptosis occurs at the mitochondrial level through an intrinsic system that induces activation of a cascade of caspase enzymes, modulated by bcl-2 family proteins (Schultz, 2003; Martin, 2004; Petros, 2004; Saelens, 2004). An extrinsic pathway involves death receptors (DRs), including Fas/CD95 and tumor necrosis factor (TNF) receptor-1 (TNFR1). These transmit apoptotic signals via a transmembrane death domain to induce activation of caspases and other associated enzymes (Green, 2003; Ivanovska, 2004; Jiang, 2004). Fas can also activate nuclear factor (NF)-κB that regulates a number of immune and inflammatory processes (Aggarwal, 2004; McDonald, 2004). This factor functions as a tumor promoter in a variety of tumors, including inflammation-associated cancer, myeloma, and Hodgkin lymphoma (HL) and non-Hodgkin lymphoma (NHL) (Pikarsky, 2004; Baud, 2009; Schmitz, 2009).

Although the underlying biology of leukocytes is complex, the task of the general pathologist is to interpret complete blood counts, peripheral blood smears, and occasionally BM samples; integrate clinical data; and

TABLE 33-1
Characteristics of Key Cell Signaling Biomolecules

Biomolecule	Target	Function
G-CSF	Myeloid bone marrow precursors	Increase proliferation and development of neutrophils
L-Selectins	Endothelial cell integrin receptors	Bind leukocytes to endothelial cells to facilitate adhesion and diapedesis
Chemokines	Leukocytes via chemokine receptors	Direct migration and activation of leukocytes via cytokine chemoattractant properties
Fas/CD95 ligand (membrane protein)	Fas/CD95 (membrane receptor)	Apoptosis via death-inducing complex
Caspases	Protein substrates	Apoptosis via enzymatic cascades
Bcl-2 antiapoptotic protein family (Bcl-2, Bcl-xL)	Mitochondrial outer membrane (MOM), nuclear membrane, endoplasmic reticulum	Decreases cell sensitivity to apoptosis
Bcl-2 proapoptotic protein family (Bax, Bok, Bak)	MOM, nuclear membrane, endoplasmic reticulum	Increases cell sensitivity to apoptosis

G-CSF, Granulocyte-colony stimulating factor.

render a diagnosis. Hematopathologists, in addition, perform more detailed analyses of hematologic specimens.

Nonneoplastic Disorders

Currently, laboratory examination of leukocytes occurs as part of the automated complete blood count (CBC) for almost every patient. The total leukocyte or white blood cell (WBC) count, as well as the relative and absolute concentrations of neutrophils, lymphocytes, monocytes, eosinophils, and basophils, is determined and compared with normal values for the patient's age and sex. Absolute concentrations (i.e., the product of the WBC count and the percentage of the respective cell series, such as lymphocytes or neutrophils) are of greatest value in identifying abnormalities. Abnormal results from the automated count are "flagged" and are then reviewed by a skilled laboratory technologist.

These abnormalities include leukocytosis, which is an increase in the total WBC count, and leukopenia, which is a decrease in the total WBC count, each compared with normal values for age and sex. The differential count, usually first performed on an automated instrument, quantifies the relative and absolute concentrations of the various forms of white cells and the maturation state for neutrophils. Increases in the absolute concentration of cells in each series are termed neutrophilia (neutrophilic leukocytosis), lymphocytosis, monocytosis, eosinophilia (eosinophilic leukocytosis), and basophilia (basophilic leukocytosis). Decreases in the absolute concentration are termed neutropenia, lymphopenia (or lymphocytopenia), monocytopenia, eosinopenia, and basopenia. Increased numbers of band neutrophils and/or the presence of immature neutrophils (metamyelocytes and earlier) is noted and enumerated and often confirmed or modified by a manual differential count. Nucleated red blood cells (RBCs) are also enumerated, noted, and subtracted from the WBC count, by automated or manual methods. Abnormalities may occur in neoplastic conditions (e.g., leukemia, marrow infiltration by metastatic tumor) and in nonneoplastic conditions (e.g., infection, drug effect, nutritional deficiency). An increase in any cell type may be clinically important, but a decrease is usually significant only for neutrophils. Usually an isolated monocytopenia, eosinopenia, or basopenia identified in a CBC is not considered pathologic. Functional neutrophil abnormalities occasionally occur. One purpose of the examination of leukocytes is to help in establishing a diagnosis. Occasionally, this alone may furnish a specific diagnosis, for example, in leukemia. The leukocyte differential count and cytologic appearance are frequently helpful diagnostically when interpreted with other data, for example, in acute appendicitis, infectious mononucleosis, or another type of infection. Another purpose is to help in establishing a prognosis. For example, leukopenia in acute appendicitis or pneumonia is considered prognostically unfavorable.

Finally, study of the leukocytes is helpful in following the course of disease. For example, toxic effects of radiotherapy and chemotherapy may be recognized and recovery monitored by examination of leukocytes.

GRANULOCYTIC AND MONOCYTIC DISORDERS

The pathologist should grasp the mechanisms and deteminants or causes, both quantitative and qualitative, of the following disorders and should be able to consult with clinical colleagues as they consider their differential diagnosis.

TABLE 33-2
Key Causes of Neutrophilia

- Acute inflammatory—collagen vascular, vasculitis
- Acute infectious—bacterial, some viral, fungal, parasitic
- Drugs, toxins, metabolic—corticosteroids, growth factors, uremia, ketoacidosis
- Tissue necrosis—burns, trauma, MI, RBC hemolysis
- Physiologic—stress, exercise, smoking, pregnancy
- Neoplastic—carcinomas, sarcomas, myeloproliferative disorders

MI, Myocardial infarction; *RBC,* red blood cell.

Neutrophilia

Neutrophilic leukocytosis or neutrophilia refers to an absolute concentration of neutrophils in the blood above normal for age. The normal reference interval (established for each laboratory separately) is approximately 1.8–7.0 × 10^3/μL for adults, with a slightly wider range (1.0–8.5 × 10^3/μL) in young children. The neutrophilias are acquired disorders; none is inherited. Key causes of neutrophilia are listed in Table 33-2.

Mechanisms

The primary factors influencing the neutrophil count are (1) the rate of inflow of cells from the BM (mitosis/proliferation, maturation/storage, and release); (2) the proportion of neutrophils in the marginal (cells adhering to vessel walls) granulocyte pool (MGP) and the circulating (nonadhering cells) granulocyte pool (CGP) of the blood—MGP and CGP are approximately equal in size and in equilibrium in health; and (3) the rate of outflow of neutrophils from the blood (i.e., migration from and through vessels into tissue, both randomly and at sites of inflammation, infection, etc.).

Physiologic leukocytosis is produced by factors or situations that are not related to underlying tissue pathology. Severe exercise, hypoxia, stress, or injection of epinephrine will lead to a decrease in the MGP and a corresponding increase in the CGP, resulting in a **pseudoneutrophilia** (i.e., no change in total blood granulocyte pool, or TBGP). This simple redistribution of cells between the CGP and the MGP, also known as demargination, is the release and detachment of leukocytes from molecular receptors on vessel luminal walls. This may be due, in part, to epinephrine-induced activation of β-receptors on endothelial cells, releasing cyclic adenosine monophosphate (cAMP), which ultimately alters or modulates the properties and characteristics of cell surface adhesion molecules and increases the release of neutrophils (as well as other leukocytes) into the circulation (Gabriel, 1998; Heine, 2001; Shephard, 2003).

Stress of greater severity or injection of endotoxin or corticosteroids also results in increased inflow of cells to the blood from the marrow maturation/storage pool. Interleukin-6, an important regulator of the acute phase response, appears to play a significant role in both the demargination of circulating cells (initial wave of circulating neutrophils) and the release of neutrophils from the marrow (second wave of circulating neutrophilic granulocytes) (Suwa, 2000). As a result, the mitotic pool appears to be increased to replenish the maturation/storage pool from which more mature cells exit into the TBGP, and both the MGP and the CGP are enlarged. A "greater" neutrophilia is possible in this situation because of the additional egress of cells from the maturation/storage pool (in addition to demargination); immature cells, such as band neutrophils and metamyelocytes, are likely to be present (Suwa, 2000).

As mentioned earlier, neutrophilia may be produced by corticosteroids, which increase the release of neutrophils from the marrow, decrease the egress of neutrophils from the blood, and increase demargination.

Pathologic leukocytosis is an increased WBC count that occurs as a result of disease, usually as a response to tissue damage. This leukocytosis is most often a neutrophilia.

In addition to the random loss of neutrophils from the circulation in various body secretions, neutrophils leave the blood by ameboid movement when attracted to a focus of inflammation in tissues, presumably responding to a multitude of chemotactic molecules and gradients. It is from the MGP that the neutrophils leave the blood, pass between capillary endothelial cells, and reach the tissues.

In acute infection, increased margination of neutrophils and outflow from blood to tissues would lead to neutropenia were there not a flow of neutrophils from the marrow storage compartment into the blood. Because the latter overcompensates, the result is a neutrophilia. Usually, production and storage compartments then increase in the marrow and are able to sustain the increased CGP (neutrophilia) and MGP in the face of increased flow of neutrophils from the blood into the inflammatory site. In these instances, the marrow will show granulocytic hyperplasia (increased myeloid to erythroid [M:E] ratio and increased cellularity), with maturation intact. An increase in immature peripheral blood granulocytes is usually present, often termed "shift to the left."

If the demand for neutrophils is extremely great, as in severe infection, there may be depletion of the marrow storage pool and decreased CGP (neutropenia) and MGP, because the supply of cells is insufficient for the demand. In these instances, the marrow will show increased numbers of early neutrophil precursors, through the myelocyte stage, but decreased numbers of metamyelocytes, bands, and neutrophils.

Determinants

Certain host factors modify the degree of neutrophilic response. Children respond more intensely than adults. The degree of neutrophilia may be impaired by the same factors that impair erythrocyte production (iron, folate, or cobalamin deficiency) or by marrow failure due to other causes. Imperfectly defined factors that enable the body to localize an infection may play a role: the more localized the process, the more pronounced is the neutrophilia.

Other factors modifying the neutrophilic response are due more to the microorganism than to the host. Pyogenic bacteria, especially, induce neutrophilia. Within limits, a more virulent agent results in a higher neutrophil count. When the infection is overwhelming, however, there is apt to be a neutropenia and a greater shift to the left.

Treatment of infections with antibiotics may modify the leukocytic response to infection. Steroid therapy, although causing neutrophilia, tends to impair the host response to infection, probably because of diminished movement of neutrophils into the tissues and increased lysosomal stability.

Neutrophilia, sometimes pronounced, is occasionally seen in patients with nonhematologic neoplasms and may be secondary to several factors, including response to tissue necrosis and underlying infection, as well as to the production of hematologic growth factors (Peterson, 1993; Granger, 2009). Neutrophilia can also be seen with gastrointestinal and hepatic tumors, HL, renal cell carcinoma, and metastatic BM disease (Blay, 1997; Hernandez, 2002). It is thought that cytokine production by tumor cells is, at least in some situations, responsible for hematologic changes such as neutrophilia, monocytosis, thrombocytosis, and lymphocytopenia in patients with malignancy (Ruka, 2001).

Neutropenia

Neutropenia is a reduction in the absolute neutrophil count (ANC) below ≈1.5–2 × 10^9/L for white adults and below ≈1.2–1.3 × 10^9/L for black adults. Remember that the ANC is the product of the WBC count and the percentage of neutrophils and bands that have been enumerated in the WBC differential count. The term ***agranulocytosis*** has been used for severe neutropenia, usually <0.5 × 10^9/L; this can also be associated with depletion of eosinophils and basophils. The term severe chronic neutropenia (SCN) refers to patients with ANC <0.5 × 10^9/L for months or years, usually with diseases that primarily cause neutropenia in the absence of other cytopenias (Dale, 2002a). If the neutrophil count is less than 1 × 10^9/L, the risk of infection is considerably increased over normal, and if the neutrophil count is less than 0.5 × 10^9/L, the risk of infection is greater still.

TABLE 33-3
Key Causes of Neutropenia*

- Drugs—cancer chemotherapy, chloramphenicol, sulfas/other antibiotics, phenothiazines, benzodiazepine, antithyroids, anticonvulsants, quinine, quinidine, indomethacin, procainamide, thiazides
- Radiation
- Toxins—alcohol, benzene compounds
- Intrinsic defects—Fanconi's, Kostmann's, cyclic neutropenia, Chédiak-Higashi
- Immune-mediated—collagen vascular disorders, RA, AIDS
- Hematologic—megaloblastic anemia, myelodysplasia, marrow failure, marrow replacement
- Infectious—any overwhelming infection
- Others—starvation, hypersplenism

AIDS, Acquired immunodeficiency syndrome; *RA,* rheumatoid arthritis.
*Brief, partial list.

The mechanisms by which neutropenia occurs include (1) decreased flow of neutrophils from marrow into blood as a result of lack of production or ineffective production (i.e., a proliferation or maturation defect); (2) increased removal of neutrophils from the blood (survival defect); (3) altered distribution between CGP and MGP; and (4) combinations of these mechanisms. Further, neutropenias may be inherited, acquired as part of an autoimmune disorder, or acquired secondary to a toxic or drug-associated insult. Neutropenias are not as neatly classified as anemias. It should be noted that drugs induce neutropenia through several mechanisms and are a very important consideration in any differential diagnosis of leukopenia. Partial lists of causes and conditions associated with neutropenia are shown in Table 33-3.

Intrinsic defects or constitutional disorders associated with neutropenia usually present at birth or in early infancy and are rare. Those due to myeloid hypoplasia or a proliferation defect include Fanconi's anemia (FA), Kostmann's syndrome, Schwachman-Diamond syndrome, and cyclic neutropenia. Those that are due to maturation defects include myelokathexis and Chédiak-Higashi syndrome.

FA is an inherited BM failure syndrome that usually occurs in childhood and rarely presents in adulthood. This condition is heterogeneous in its clinical manifestations but was classically defined by the presence of aplastic anemia and congenital physical malformations. The aplastic anemia of FA patients appears to be indistinguishable from acquired aplasia. FA patients are also susceptible to hematopoietic and certain solid organ malignancies. Diagnosis is made by cytogenetic analysis while looking for chromosome breakage after exposure to diepoxybutane or mitomycin C.

In keeping with variation in clinical presentations and manifestations of this syndrome, the underlying molecular pathology is complex. Currently, at least 11 FA genetic subtypes exist and 7 FA genes have been cloned. One gene, *FANCD1*, is actually *BRCA2*, which, like *BRCA1*, is a DNA repair gene that appears to be a putative breast and ovarian cancer susceptibility gene identified in certain families with an inherited predisposition to breast and ovarian cancer. These genes probably function as tumor suppressor genes and appear to be involved in the molecular pathway(s) responsible for the disruption of DNA repair in FA (Levitus, 2004; Tischkowitz, 2004). The mechanism of pathogenesis appears varied, but identification of DNA repair abnormality is useful for diagnosis (Auerbach, 2009).

Kostmann's syndrome, originally termed **infantile genetic agranulocytosis,** is a rare severe (ANC usually <200/μL) congenital neutropenia appearing in early infancy. Initially identified as showing an autosomal recessive pattern of inheritance, autosomal dominant and sporadic cases also occur. The marrow usually shows the presence of early granulocytes (promyelocyte/myelocyte arrest), but few maturing forms are seen; neutrophil survival is normal. Although the underlying genetic defect in myeloid precursor cells is not entirely elucidated, mutations in the gene *(ELA2)* encoding neutrophil elastase appear to be present in most patients with autosomal dominant disease and with antiapoptotic gene *HAX-1* in recessive cases (Carlsson, 2007). These mutations may be responsible for the untimely initiation of apoptosis in myelocytes, producing their premature destruction and interrupting the normal cycle of maturation. In addition, other underlying molecular/genetic changes may produce DNA mutations and genome instability, which contribute to initiation and progression of this disease (Zeidler, 2002; Christensen, 2004).

Patients with cyclic neutropenia typically present with recurrent episodes of symptomatic infection (fatigue, mouth ulcers, cervical lymphadenopathy, fever) due to cyclic episodes of severe neutropenia. The latter is due to the periodicity or cycling of neutrophil production. The disease usually presents in childhood but may present in adulthood. Typically, oscillations of neutrophil and monocyte levels (between near normal levels and very low levels) occur over an approximately 21-day period. Mutations in *ELA2*, the gene for neutrophil elastase, have been identified in many patients (Dale, 2002b). This appears to be responsible for selective apoptotic death of neutrophil progenitors, a mechanism similar to that seen in Kostmann's syndrome, as discussed earlier.

Chronic familial neutropenia or benign familial neutropenia refers to a lower than "normal" neutrophil count, as found in some ethnic populations. It is an incidental and clinically stable finding with no predisposition to infection and is considered a genetic variation.

It is important to note that the two most common causes of congenital neutropenia are neutropenia of pregnancy-induced hypertension (PIH—most common) and overwhelming bacterial infection. Typical signs of infection, including a granulocytic left shift, toxic granulation, and Döhle bodies, accompany the latter, but these changes are not seen in PIH. Neither usually continues beyond the first week of life, and other causes should be searched for in infants with persistent neutropenia (Christensen, 2004).

Patients with congenital or primary immunodeficiency diseases may exhibit some degree of neutropenia. Males with X-linked agammaglobulinemia (XLA) are often neutropenic, and XLA should be considered in the differential diagnosis of chronic neutropenia in an infant. An abnormal nonreceptor tyrosine kinase, associated with signal transduction and differentiation of hematopoietic cells, appears to be involved. This is due to various mutations in the gene *Btk* (*B*ruton's or *B* lymphocyte *t*yrosine *k*inase) on the long arm of the X chromosome (q22). Other congenital syndromes having a prominent association with neutropenia include selective immunoglobulin (Ig)A deficiency, common variable immunodeficiency, and hyper IgM syndrome (Cham, 2002).

Certain autoimmune diseases can also be associated with chronic neutropenia. Both rheumatoid arthritis (RA) and systemic lupus erythematosus (SLE) show this association (Starkebaum, 2002). The combination of chronic neutropenia and RA is termed Felty's syndrome (FS), and patients develop symptoms owing to both RA (e.g., subcutaneous nodules, contractures, erythema, warmth, tenderness, symmetrical involvement of large and small joints, musculoskeletal pain) and chronic neutropenia (symptoms of recurrent bacterial and fungal infections). A portion of these cases are associated with large granular lymphocyte (LGL) leukemia (Shah, 2009). SLE may present with multisystem involvement, making presenting symptoms highly variable. Organ systems frequently affected include the skin, kidney, BM, and central nervous system (CNS); symmetrical involvement of the joints is also seen. Again, the pathophysiology is complex; alterations in neutrophil proliferation and survival with neutropenia due, at least in part, to immune-mediated destruction, occur in both SLE and FS, and increased neutrophil apoptosis may be noted in SLE (Starkebaum, 2002).

Primary autoimmune myelofibrosis (Bass, 2001; Pullarkat, 2003; Rizzi, 2004) is a relatively rare but recently described clinicopathologic entity in patients who do not have SLE or another well-defined autoimmune disease. Although this entity is still being defined, patients present with chronic peripheral blood cytopenias, BM fibrosis with variable marrow cellularity, and BM lymphoid aggregates in the absence of other disorders that typically cause myelofibrosis. These include primary marrow hematologic neoplasia, infection, metastatic cancer, or osteopathy such as Paget's disease or hyperparathyroidism. Prognosis for these patients appears to be very good with corticosteroid therapy.

Drugs (Andres, 2004; Bhatt, 2004) are an important cause of neutropenia, may act in different ways, and may affect progenitor or mature cell populations. Drugs are the most common cause of acute neutropenia **(agranulocytosis)** and typically show a lack of granulocytic cells in the marrow. In some patients, however, a pronounced progenitor hyperplasia may be present, sometimes termed **maturation arrest** or **promyelocytic hyperplasia.**

Drugs may initiate immune-mediated destruction via immune complex formation (quinidine) or complement-mediated cell lysis (propylthiouracil). Some drugs, including penicillin, aminopyrine, and gold, act as haptens. Inhibition of granulopoiesis or myeloid toxicity occurs with chemotherapeutic agents, chlorpromazine, and others. These effects tend to be dose dependent and reversible. Important and limiting side effects of cancer chemotherapy are severe neutropenia with its risk of infection, as well as severe thrombocytopenia with risk of bleeding; anemia is more readily controlled with transfusion.

Radiation damages, alters, and destroys BM progenitor cells, as well as marrow stromal elements. Radiation type, dose, and duration are all factors that determine the extent of BM damage, such as aplasia or hypoplasia. Radiation affects a number of molecules and processes, including DNA structure, gene translation and transcription, apoptosis, and other signaling pathways. Lymphocytes are most sensitive and are directly killed by exposure. The lymphocyte count correlates with, and has been used to assess, dose and severity of exposure (Dainiak, 2002). In addition, hematopoietic precursors undergoing mitosis are very sensitive to injury and death.

Isolated neutropenia or agranulocytosis is fairly uncommon in adults. When a myelophthisic process, such as metastatic carcinoma, disseminated tuberculosis, or Gaucher's disease, infiltrates the BM, the damage is not limited to granulopoiesis but affects normoblasts and megakaryocytes as well. Because of the short life span of granulocytes, however, neutropenia is the earliest recognizable effect in the blood. It may take weeks before damage to the erythropoietic tissue becomes manifest because of the usually long life span of erythrocytes. Platelets have a rather short life span; on the other hand, megakaryocytes are more resistant to damage.

Neutropenia due to increased ineffective granulocytopoiesis occurs in megaloblastic anemias and with drugs that have an antifolate effect. In these conditions, anemia and thrombocytopenia are usually associated. The marrow is usually hyperplastic. In megaloblastic anemia due to nutritional deficiency, drug-induced suppression of DNA synthesis, or an inborn error of metabolism, asynchronous nuclear/cytoplasmic maturation (megaloblastic change or megaloblastosis) is identified in marrow progenitor cells. Ineffective granulocytopoiesis may also occur in myelodysplasia, discussed in the section on neoplastic disorders.

In starvation, cellularity tends to be decreased, and a morphologic marrow change termed serous fat atrophy or gelatinous transformation of the BM is present. This change shows a loss of hematopoietic cells within the marrow stroma replaced by small or shrunken fat cells expanded by an intercellular, homogeneous, eosinophilic material. BM hypocellularity is typically seen with advanced disease. Neutropenia with BM hypoplasia can be associated with a decrease in plasma or serum lysozyme (muramidase).

Transient neutropenia may occur early in some infections, followed by leukocytosis once marrow production catches up with the demand. As previously noted, in severe, extensive bacterial infection, neutropenia with a shift to the left may be due to inability of marrow production to keep up with peripheral utilization. Some bacterial infections, notably brucellosis and *Salmonella* infections, are prone to be associated with neutropenia; they may have some depressing effect on the marrow as well. Patients with viral infections such as measles and rubella have neutropenia for several days after appearance of the rash; this is probably due in part to increased utilization. Other acute viral infections, such as hepatitis, infectious mononucleosis, and influenza, may also cause acute neutropenia. Lymphocytosis is present and persists after the neutropenia subsides.

The neutropenia of hypersplenism has been attributed to selective removal of neutrophils by the spleen. It is associated with neutrophilic hyperplasia of the marrow and is corrected by splenectomy. Splenomegaly due to many causes may result in shortened neutrophil survival and neutropenia; these include congestive splenomegaly, Felty's syndrome, Gaucher's disease, and lymphoma. In some cases of Felty's syndrome (neutropenia and splenomegaly in rheumatoid arthritis), a neutrophil-specific antibody may be involved. Ramirez (2004) recently showed enhanced apoptosis in patients with cirrhosis and ascites, which appeared to be dependent upon elevated activity levels of caspase-3 in these patients. Patients are prone to neutropenia and infection; in the past, this was largely attributed to hypersplenism with increased splenic clearance of neutrophils. However, these recent findings suggest that other mechanisms, at least in part, may also be contributory.

Pseudoneutropenia may be caused by increased margination of neutrophils in some individuals, without a decrease in total granulocyte count. Rather than showing an equal distribution between MGP and CGP, an increased proportion of neutrophils appear to be present in the MGP. Small doses of endotoxin will cause a shift of neutrophils into the MGP from the CGP, giving an apparent neutropenia, before causing leukocytosis. In animals, anesthetic agents such as ether will cause the same type of pseudoneutropenia.

TABLE 33-4
Morphologic Alterations in Neutrophils

Toxic granulation—azurophilic cytoplasmic granules seen in severe infections, other toxic conditions, and reactive conditions
Cytoplasmic vacuoles—seen in infection, indicating phagocytosis
Döhle bodies—pale blue, oval cytoplasmic remnants of ribosomes seen in infection and other toxic conditions
May-Hegglin anomaly—rare autosomal dominant condition with pale blue cytoplasmic ribosomal inclusions resembling Döhle bodies
Alder-Reilly anomaly—prominent azurophilic granulation not related to infection
Pelger-Huët anomaly—bilobed or rounded nuclei with pince-nez shape
Chédiak-Higashi syndrome—autosomal recessive disorder with giant granules, likely representing giant fused lysosomes, and abnormal leukocyte function

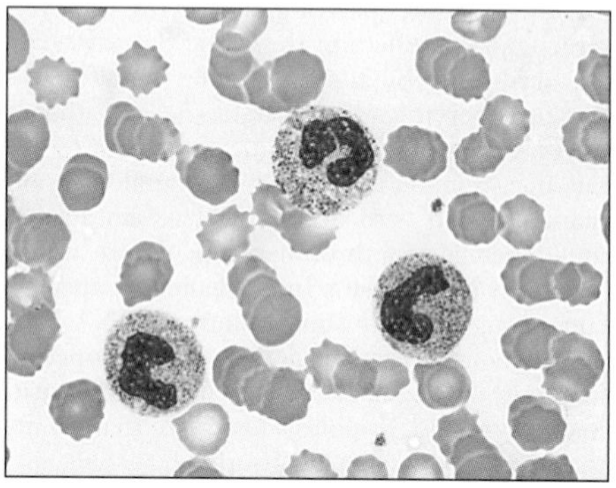

Figure 33-1 A neutrophil with toxic granulation is pictured, along with two bands. Basophilic inclusions (Döhle bodies) are present as well (×1000).

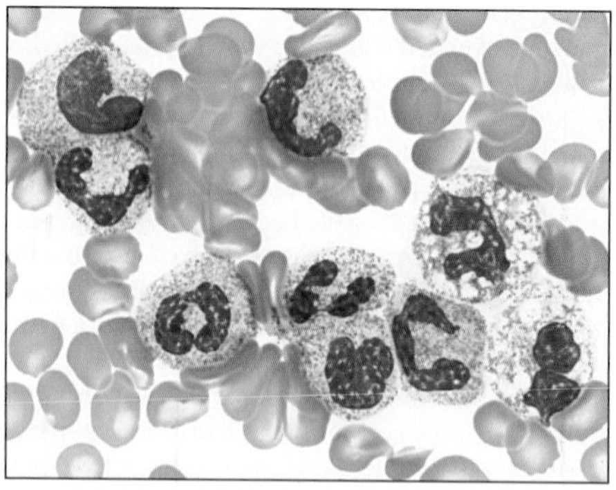

Figure 33-2 Leukemoid toxic neutrophilia with left shift and toxic vacuolization (×1000).

Morphologic Alterations in Neutrophils

In addition to quantitative changes, qualitative morphologic alterations occur in neutrophils, and these too may be inherited or acquired. Some of these, such as toxic granules or cytoplasmic vacuoles, are acquired and disappear after the stimulus that provoked them is gone. Others are hereditary and persist through life, with or without functional impairment (Table 33-4). These are well illustrated and reviewed by Brunning (1970), and more recently by Kroft (2002).

It should be noted that disorders of leukocyte function may exist with no structural abnormality detectable with the usual modes of morphologic examination.

Toxic Granulation

Toxic granules are dark blue to purple cytoplasmic granules in the metamyelocyte, band, or neutrophil stage. They are peroxidase positive and may be numerous or few in number; less peroxidase activity may be seen in toxic than in normal neutrophils. Toxic granulation is noted in infections or other toxic conditions but may also be seen in noninfectious reactive conditions (Figs. 33-1 and 33-2).

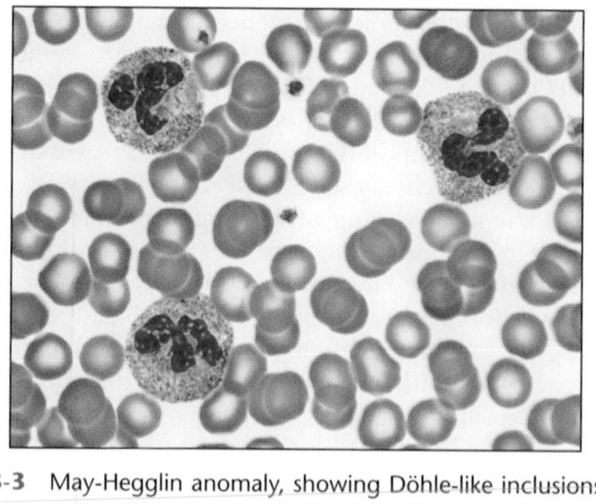

Figure 33-3 May-Hegglin anomaly, showing Döhle-like inclusions (×1000).

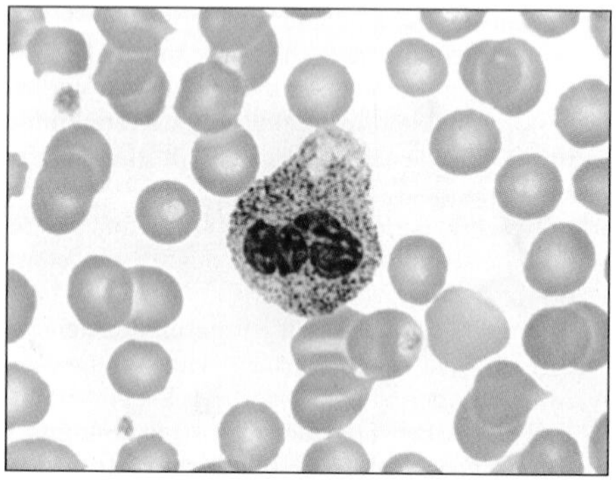

Figure 33-4 The Alder-Reilly anomaly may be found in healthy individuals or in those with mucopolysaccharidoses, in which granules are metachromatic (×1000).

Döhle Inclusion Bodies

These small, oval inclusions in the peripheral cytoplasm of polymorphonuclear neutrophils stain pale blue with Wright's stain (see Fig. 33-1). They are remnants of free ribosomes or rough-surfaced endoplasmic reticulum, persisting from an earlier stage of development.

May-Hegglin Anomaly

This rare autosomal dominant condition involves the nonmuscle myosin heavy chain 9 gene (*MYH9*) linked to chromosome 22q12-13 (Kelley, 2000; Martignetti, 2000; Seri, 2000). The mutations appear to alter the assembly and stability of myosin and may be responsible for the underlying pathophysiology and changes seen in leukocyte and platelet structure and function. It appears that at the molecular level, various mutations in *MYH9* are, at least partially, responsible for a phenotypic spectrum of illness. This spectrum appears to include May-Hegglin anomaly and Sebastian, Fechtner, and Epstein platelet syndromes (Heath, 2001; Seri, 2003). This spectrum may be phenotypically modified by aberrant fibulin-1 gene expression, which also may be responsible for the clinical variability of disease (Toren, 2003). Fibulin-1 is a gene encoding for a secreted glycoprotein present in the basal membrane of many organs.

Although clinically variable, this anomaly is characterized by the presence of pale blue inclusions resembling Döhle bodies in neutrophils, by giant platelets, and, in some persons, by thrombocytopenia (Fig. 33-3). The inclusions are larger and more prominent than the Döhle bodies found in infections. They have been described in eosinophils, basophils, and monocytes, as well as in neutrophils (Brunning, 1970). The blue staining of the inclusions can be abolished by prior treatment of the cells with ribonuclease. With electron microscopy, the appearance of the inclusions differs from that of Döhle bodies (composed of parallel strands of rough endoplasmic reticulum), suggesting structural alterations in RNA and ribosomes (So, 2003). Granulocyte function is normal.

Alder-Reilly Anomaly

Dense, prominent, larger than normal azurophilic granulation in all white blood cells was described by Alder in 1939 (Fig. 33-4). In neutrophils, it may resemble toxic granulation, but it is unrelated to infection and is not transient. In 1941, Reilly described similar granulocytes in some but not all patients with gargoylism, Hurler's syndrome, or, more generally, the genetic mucopolysaccharidoses (Reilly, 1941). Other observations have

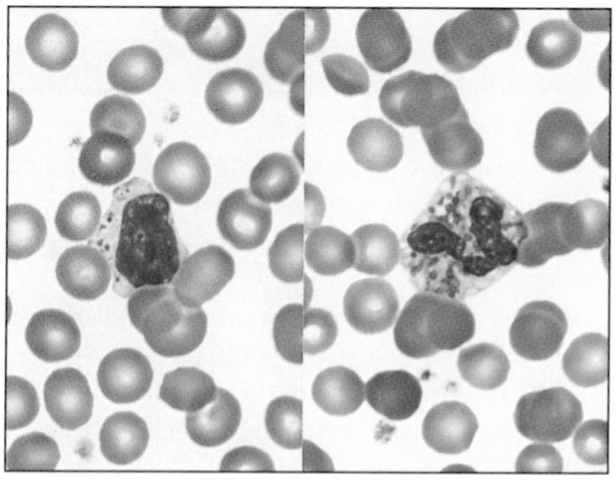

Figure 33-5 Genetic mucopolysaccharidoses often show abnormal lymphocyte granules with surrounding halos. In these cells from the same blood film, neutrophils showed similar changes (×1000).

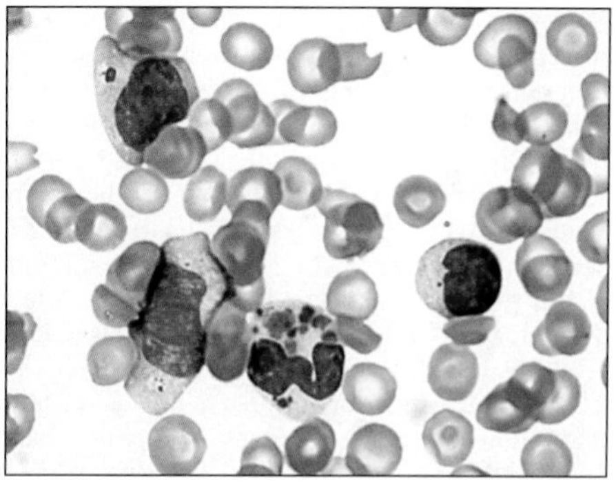

Figure 33-7 Chédiak-Higashi neutrophils and lymphocytes with large granules (×1000).

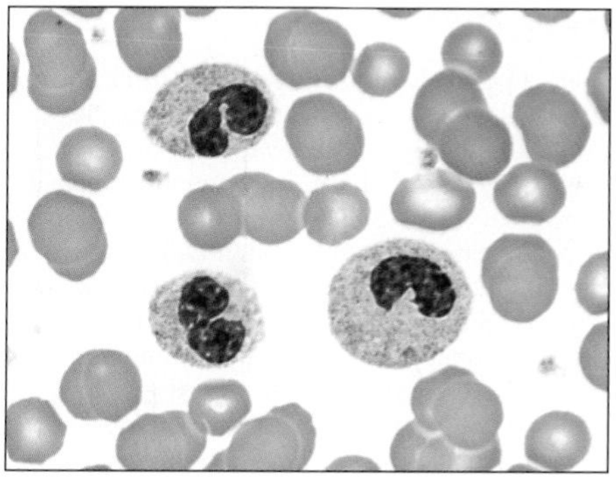

Figure 33-6 Inherited Pelger-Huët anomaly (×1000).

shown that the heavy granulation in neutrophils can occur as a feature of the genetic mucopolysaccharidoses or independently in otherwise healthy persons (Brunning, 1970).

Occurring more often than the Alder-Reilly anomaly in the genetic mucopolysaccharidoses is a metachromatic inclusion in the lymphocytes surrounded by a clear space (Fig. 33-5). Macrophages in the marrow frequently contain similar granulation. This group of disorders is inherited and is characterized by deficiencies or derangement in various lysosomal enzymes required for degrading mucopolysaccharides. The result is abnormal deposition and storage of mucopolysaccharides in multiple organs. Skeletal abnormalities are prominent.

Pelger-Huët Anomaly

This hereditary, autosomal dominant condition involves failure of normal segmentation of granulocytic nuclei. Most nuclei are bilobed and rounded, with a characteristic spectacle or pince-nez shape (Fig. 33-6). The chromatin is quite coarse, and these are not normal young band forms. When a large number of band-like neutrophils appear in the differential count in a patient without infection or other cause, careful analysis of the blood films of the patient and of family members will occasionally establish the presence of the Pelger-Huët anomaly. The cells are functionally normal, and the underlying abnormality is mutation of the lamin B receptor gene (Speeckaert, 2009).

A similar appearing, acquired disorder of nuclear segmentation in granulocytes may be found in cases of granulocytic leukemia, myelodysplastic and some myeloproliferative disorders, and some infections, and after exposure to certain drugs (Brunning, 1970); this is called the pseudo–Pelger-Huët anomaly. In addition to band forms and neutrophils with only two segments, mature cells with round, nonsegmented nuclei and coarse chromatin are common. In contrast to the congenital Pelger-Huët anomaly, ring-shaped and other abnormal nuclei may be seen, and the cytoplasm is usually hypogranular.

Chédiak-Higashi Syndrome

Partial oculocutaneous albinism, photophobia, immune deficiency, abnormally large granules in leukocytes and other granule-containing cells, neurologic defects, and frequent pyogenic infections characterize this rare, autosomal recessive disorder (Introne, 1999). An accelerated lymphoma-like phase occurs, with lymphadenopathy, hepatosplenomegaly, and pancytopenia; lymphoid infiltrates are widespread, and death ensues at an early age. Granulocytes, monocytes, and lymphocytes contain giant granules (Fig. 33-7), which appear to be abnormal lysosomes. The pathogenesis of this disorder is linked to an abnormality of granule maturation, causing enlargement and apparent fusion of granules and vesicles (such as lysosomes, melanosomes, and platelet dense granules) in all cell types. Leukocyte functional abnormalities exist. Although the mechanism is not fully elucidated, a mouse genetic model, ***beige***, has revealed a mutation in the gene *CHS/beige*, coding for the CHS1 or Lyst protein. The *LYST* (lysosomal trafficking regulator) gene appears to be involved in regulation of vesicular size, trafficking, and intracellular movement, such that vesicular migration and release are abnormal (Ward, 2002).

Myelokathexis applies to peripheral neutropenia with the presence of BM neutrophils. WHIM (*w*arts, *h*ypogammaglobulinemia, *i*nfection, and *m*yelokathexis) syndrome is a rare, autosomal dominant disease of leukocyte trafficking involving chromosome 2q21. The disease appears to be due to mutations in the chemokine receptor gene *CXCR4* and altered leukocyte response to its functional ligand CXCL12. Hematologic changes include severe peripheral neutropenia with lymphopenia also common, but with granulocytic hyperplasia of the BM (Gorlin, 2000; Hernandez, 2003; Gulino, 2003, 2004).

Functional Disorders of Neutrophils

Inherited and acquired disorders affecting neutrophils and other leukocytes may result in abnormal function and susceptibility to infections. Deficiencies of humoral factors (antibodies, components of complement) may result in defective chemotaxis or opsonization. As described previously, some inherited disorders, such as the May-Hegglin, Alder-Reilly, and Pelger-Huët anomalies, have altered morphologic appearances but apparently normal granulocytic function. Other inherited conditions, such as the Chédiak-Higashi syndrome and specific granule deficiency (SGD), display alterations in both morphology and function. Inherited conditions such as chronic granulomatous disease (CGD), myeloperoxidase deficiency (MYD), and leukocyte adhesion deficiency (LAD) exhibit functional disorders with essentially normal morphology on Wright's- and Giemsa-stained films.

Chronic granulomatous disease (Lakshman, 2001; Vignais, 2002; Heyworth, 2003; Jurkowska, 2004) is a rare, primary immunodeficiency affecting neutrophils, eosinophils, macrophages, and monocytes; it results from the inability of these phagocytic cells to kill intracellular microorganisms. Patients present with recurrent bacterial and fungal infections (skin, liver, mouth, lymph nodes). These lead to chronic granulomatous lesions (a hallmark of the disease) that may, in turn, obstruct vital organ systems and ultimately lead to death. Symptoms occur early in life, and both autosomal recessive (≈66%) and X-linked (≈33%) modes of inheritance are known.

The disease results from genetic defects in any of the membrane-bound or cytoplasmic components of nicotinamide adenine dinucleotide phosphate (NADPH) oxidase. This enzyme complex is not assembled and thus is inactive in the resting cell, but, with cell stimulation, the membrane and cytoplasmic components come together and are assembled into the active NADPH oxidase–protein complex, which can begin functioning. Once assembled, this enzyme is responsible for production of superoxide anion ($NADPH + 2O_2 \rightarrow 2O^{-}_2 + NADP^+ + H^+$), as well as hydrogen peroxide and hypochlorous acid—molecular mediators of microbial cell death. The production of these highly reactive oxygen free-radical species is often referred to as the **respiratory burst,** indicating the increased oxygen consumption that occurs with NADPH oxidase activation. Thus, any defect in this enzyme, which prohibits or significantly reduces its activity, will allow intracellular microorganisms to remain viable and ultimately spread (by cell mobility and seeding of adjacent tissue), producing recurrent infection and granulomatous disease. Global gene expression profiling studies (Kobayashi, 2004) suggest that both an increase in proinflammatory activity and defective neutrophil apoptosis may also be involved.

Myeloperoxidase (MPO) is present in neutrophils (in azurophil/primary granules) and monocytes (in lysosomes) but is not present in promonocytes and tissue macrophages. MPO catalyzes the cellular production of hypochlorite (ClO^-) or hypochlorous (HOCl) acid ($H_2O_2 + Cl^- \rightarrow H_2O + ClO^-$). HOCl is a strong oxidant normally involved in the destruction of intracellular microorganisms, as well as possibly tumor cells (Hoy, 2002). Although a single gene encodes MPO, the translation product undergoes a number of complex modification reactions, including insertion of heme, to produce the final active enzyme molecule (Nauseef, 2004).

Primary MYD is a congenital disorder that is not uncommon and that is easily identifiable with automated cell counters incorporating measurement of MPO activity in the differential count. Secondary MYD, which can be transient and corrected with treatment of the underlying disease, may occur secondary to conditions such as myeloid neoplasms, drugs, severe infectious diseases, diabetes mellitus, and pregnancy (Lanza, 1998). Primary MYD may be total or partial and does not show an increased frequency of infection in most individuals (Lanza, 1998; Lakshman, 2001; Suzuki, 2004), although an increase has been reported occasionally (Kutter, 2000).

Human eosinophil peroxidase is structurally related to MPO but is not identical and is encoded by a different gene. Deficiency is thought to be extremely rare, is unrelated to MYD, may show autosomal recessive inheritance, and appears to be without clinical symptoms (Nakagawa, 2001).

Patients with an extremely rare condition, SGD, present with multiple bacterial infections, atypical bilobed nuclei within neutrophils, and lack of secondary/specific cytoplasmic granules within neutrophils on Wright's-stained peripheral blood films. SGD also affects eosinophils. In addition to granule deficiencies and impaired bactericidal activity, neutrophils are defective in chemotaxis, receptor upregulation, and disaggregation. A mutation in a myeloid transcription factor gene (*C*CAAT/*e*nhancer *b*inding *p*rotein-*e*psilon or *C/EBPe*) appears to play a role in this disease (Rosenberg, 1993; Gombart, 2001; Khanna-Gupta, 2001).

Because proper neutrophil function is dependent upon cell–cell adhesion via the integrins, it is not surprising that LAD diseases exist. Integrins are essentially nonadhesive surface molecules in circulating leukocytes, which, upon proper stimulation, become adhesive or develop increased binding properties for their specific ligands. This appears to occur via conformational change in the integrin molecule structure and/or clustering of increased numbers of molecules on the cell surface. Ultimately, defective leukocyte adhesion and migration occur, resulting clinically in recurrent infection and leukocytosis.

Three types of leukocyte adhesion deficiencies have been described (Bunting, 2002; Gabius, 2002; McDowall, 2003; Etzioni, 2004). In LAD I, expression of integrin on the leukocyte cell surface is absent or abnormal because a mutation in the β_2-subunit (of CD18) produces a lack of normal expression of the integrin, causing its absence or dysfunction at the cell surface. Recurrent severe infections, neutrophilia with severe infection, and delayed separation of the umbilical cord are seen. LAD II is due to a mutation affecting fucose transport, leading to the impaired expression of selectin ligands on leukocytes (CD15a or sialyl Lewis X), as well as other cells. Neutrophilia (with and without infection) and developmental abnormalities occur. In LAD III, CD18 and CD15a are normally expressed on leukocytes. Instead, there seems to be a defect in integrin activation (via endothelial chemokines) caused by a mutation in leukocyte-expressed G protein–coupled receptors (GPCRs). If binding between leukocyte GPCRs and endothelially expressed chemokines does not occur, integrin activation and leukocyte adhesion cannot occur. Recurrent severe infections, neutrophilia with infection, and bleeding tendencies have been noted. The latter is seen because platelet GPIIbβ3 integrins are not activated. Some forms of LAD can be diagnosed by flow cytometry, by revealing the lack of expression of CD18 or CD15a on neutrophils (Roos, 2001).

Eosinophilia

Eosinophilia exists if blood eosinophils exceed $\approx 0.35 \times 10^9/L$ when large numbers of cells are counted, as with automated instruments or direct chamber counts; or $\approx 0.5 \times 10^9/L$ when the count is calculated from the 100- or 200-cell differential and the total leukocyte count. Increased eosinophils are chiefly acquired disorders and quantitative in nature, although Mathur has described impaired eosinophil function with aging, in the areas of degranulation, superoxide anion production, and adhesion (Mathurs, 2008). Eosinophilia is typically associated with allergic processes (the most common cause in ambulatory outpatients in North America) (Brigden, 1999) and parasitic infections; both are common secondary or reactive types of eosinophilia. Classically, the major function of eosinophils appeared to be the release of granule contents or reactive oxygen species generated by the cell membrane to damage the target organism or offending cell (Shurin, 1988). At present, eosinophil function appears more complex, in that additional functions with immunoregulatory and proinflammatory signaling roles also appear to exist. Thus, the eosinophil appears to be capable of acting as both an effector and/or a regulatory cell.

TABLE 33-5
Key Causes of Eosinophilia

- Allergic—urticaria, hay fever, asthma
- Inflammatory—eosinophilic fasciitis, Churg-Strauss syndrome
- Parasitic—trichinosis, filariasis, schistosomiasis
- Nonparasitic infections—systemic fungal, scarlet fever, chlamydial pneumonia of infancy
- Respiratory—pulmonary eosinophilic syndromes (Löffler's, tropical pulmonary eosinophilia), Churg-Strauss syndrome
- Neoplastic—CML, Hodgkin lymphoma, T cell lymphomas
- Idiopathic hypereosinophilic syndromes—affecting heart, liver, spleen, CNS, other organs
- Others—certain drugs, hematologic and visceral malignancies, GI inflammatory diseases, sarcoidosis, Wiskott-Aldrich syndrome

CML, Chronic myelogenous leukemia; *CNS,* central nervous system; *GI,* gastrointestinal.

Similar factors influence the eosinophil count as described previously for the neutrophil count. These factors include (1) mitosis/proliferation, maturation/storage, and release in, and from, the BM; (2) the rate of outflow of eosinophils from the blood (rolling, tethering, adhesion, and migration); (3) trafficking of eosinophils to specific sites of accumulation; and (4) the survival and rate of eosinophil destruction in the tissues. Eosinophil production is stimulated by interleukin (IL)-5, migration is influenced by the chemokine eotaxin, and the two factors interact in producing eosinophilia (Palframan, 1998). Causes and conditions associated with eosinophilia are shown in Table 33-5.

Identification of a cause of secondary eosinophilia is often difficult, and extensive overlap between conditions has been noted. It may be more important to distinguish reactive eosinophilia from eosinophilia due to clonal hematopoietic neoplasms and from idiopathic hypereosinophilic syndrome.

The presence of an abnormal karyotype or other evidence of a myeloproliferative disorder suggests eosinophilia arising from a leukemic clone, although eosinophilia arising in lymphoid leukemias is likely reactive (Bain, 1996). Eosinophilia is usually present in chronic myeloid leukemia (CML), and some cases present with marked eosinophilia as the primary feature (Gotlib, 2003). Chronic eosinophilic leukemia is distinct from CML and shows different but varied cytogenetic abnormalities (Swerdlow, 2008).

A number of hematologic neoplasias may be accompanied by eosinophilia, including acute leukemias, systemic mast cell disease, plasma cell dyscrasias, and myelodysplastic and myeloproliferative diseases. It may also occur with a primary neoplasm originating in another organ, such as lung, soft tissue, or colon. Rare case reports in the literature describe associations of an eosinophilic leukemoid reaction with metastatic melanoma (Oakley, 1998), malignant fibrous histiocytoma (MFH) (Melhem, 1993), and lung carcinoma (Varindani, 1982). It appears that abnormalities in cytokine expression and regulation are responsible, at least in part, for this reaction. A granulocytic leukemoid reaction was reported in one patient with MFH (Melhem, 1993).

Eosinophilia is often a prominent component in tissue affected by HL, and extensive involvement has been reported to impart an adverse prognosis (von Wasielewski, 2003). Tissue and blood eosinophilia is also seen in T cell lymphomas and may similarly be a negative prognostic feature (Tancrede-Bohin, 2004). Eosinophilia is sometimes prominent in acute lymphoblastic leukemia, particularly those with t(5,14)(q31;q32), in which the eosinophilia is considered to be reactive (Swerdlow, 2008).

Hypersensitivity and allergic reactions and atopic conditions such as bronchial asthma and seasonal rhinitis (hay fever) are characterized by eosinophilia. These immune reactions are mediated by IgE, which results in mast cell and basophil degranulation with the release of a chemotactic factor for eosinophils. Eosinophils are found in the blood, marrow, and sputum (in bronchial asthma), and in nasal and conjunctival discharges (in hay fever). Blood eosinophilia usually is only mild or moderate ($0.4–1.0 \times 10^9/L$).

In asthma, absolute eosinophil counts have been useful in management because the level of eosinophils positively correlates with pulmonary performance, indicates the adequacy of steroid therapy, and may indicate the presence of complicating infections.

A variety of skin disorders exhibit cutaneous eosinophilc infiltrates. Some are commonly associated with peripheral eosinophilia, and others are not (Christophers, 2000). Atopic dermatitis and eczema are often accompanied by blood eosinophilia, especially in children. In pemphigus, eosinophilia is characteristic. Eosinophilia is frequently associated with acute urticarial reactions but is uncommon in chronic urticaria. In any case, it is important to recognize that the recruitment of eosinophils is dependent upon the proper interaction of chemokines (IL-5) and their receptor molecules, as well as their interaction with specific subset lymphocyte populations (T-helper type 2 [Th2] lymphocytes) in these cutaneous responses and conditions.

Moderate to severe peripheral blood eosinophilia is most commonly associated with infection by helminths (parasitic worms, including nematodes, trematodes, and cestodes), constituting the most common cause of eosinophilia in the world (Brigden, 1999). Eosinophilia is more pronounced if tissues are invaded (e.g., trichinosis) than when parasites inhabit the lumen of a viscus (e.g., tapeworm). Some parasites, such as *Taenia solium* (cysticercosis), produce little inflammatory response while alive but trigger an inflammatory response upon degeneration of the organism. Other parasites, such as *Trichinella spiralis* (trichinosis), incite peripheral eosinophilia upon larval invasion of the muscles and encystment. Note that the absence of eosinophilia does not exclude a parasitic infection (Schulte, 2002).

In trichinosis, eosinophil levels begin to rise in the blood within days after infection. The peak of the eosinophilia is seen during the third or fourth week. Eosinophilia may be absent, however, in severe infestation with trichinae.

Leukocytosis and eosinophilia extending over months are seen in toxocariasis or visceral larva migrans. Migrating larvae of the dog *(Toxocara canis)* or the cat *(T. cati)* nematode cause this infestation. In this condition, pulmonary lesions (Löffler's syndrome or simple eosinophilic pneumonia) may be present; an immune hypersensitivity reaction to the nematode *Ascaris lumbricoides* has been classically associated with Löffler's syndrome.

Another parasitic infestation with eosinophilia is creeping eruption (cutaneous larva migrans) caused by larvae of the dog *(Ancylostoma braziliense)* or cat *(A. caninum)* hookworm. Eosinophilia in these infections is T cell dependent (Basten, 1970) and, as indicated earlier, is dependent upon multiple chemokine and chemotactic molecules and receptors and intercellular interactions.

Eosinophilia of various degrees is seen in some infectious diseases. In scarlet fever, eosinophilia is commonly associated with the cutaneous rash, which is probably allergic in nature. Chorea may be associated with eosinophilia, but other forms of rheumatic fever are not.

Eosinophilic pneumonias with acute presentations typically include simple pulmonary eosinophilia or **Löffler's syndrome,** parasitic infections, drug-induced eosinophilic pneumonias, and idiopathic acute eosinophilic pneumonia. A number of pulmonary eosinophilic syndromes with more chronic presentations also exist. Other classification schemes divide eosinophilic pneumonia into idiopathic (of unknown cause) and secondary (infection, drug, immunologic and/or systemic disease) pneumonia.

Löffler's syndrome (simple eosinophilic pneumonia) affects all age groups and is characterized by repeated, transient pulmonary exudates accompanied by fever and clinical symptoms of bronchitis, often producing sputum that contains eosinophils. The syndrome resolves in a few weeks. It may be caused by a variety of exposures, including certain drugs, inhaled antigens, or helminth (see earlier) infestation. The latter occurs during periods of dissemination or migration when parasites pass from the blood into the alveoli of the lung. Löffler's syndrome may also be idiopathic.

Many drugs are associated with blood or pulmonary eosinophilia and pulmonary infiltrates. Symptoms may be mild, or more severe, leading to fulminant respiratory failure. However, the prognosis is favorable in most cases, with resolution of the disease occurring with elimination of the offending drug. Thus, a careful drug history is critical for diagnosis in these patients. Implicated drugs include pilocarpine, physostigmine, digitalis, *p*-aminosalicylic acid, sulfonamides, chlorpromazine, phenytoin, some

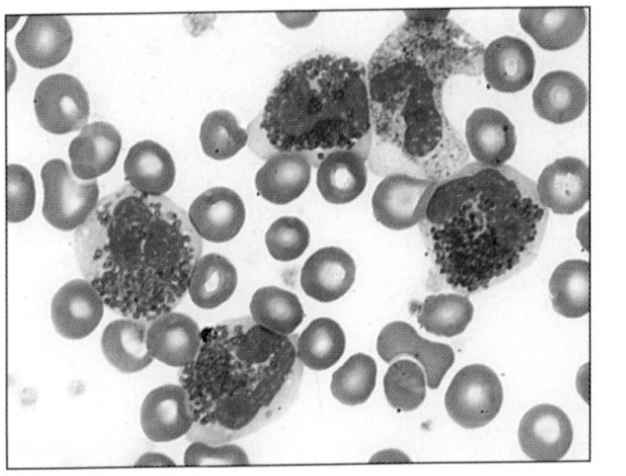

Figure 33-8 Marked eosinophilia of unknown cause, suggesting hypereosinophilic syndrome, peripheral blood (×1000).

antidiabetic drugs, some anticancer agents, and many others. A common mechanism for the production of eosinophilia has not been identified. Patients with kidney and/or liver disease have a higher incidence of drug reaction, including eosinophilia, than others.

Tropical pulmonary eosinophilia is a syndrome of paroxysmal cough and bronchospasm associated with marked eosinophilia. It is found mainly in India, Africa, Southeast Asia, and the South Pacific. However, it may be seen in any racial group living in an endemic area. *Wuchereria bancrofti* (a parasite of humans that inhabits the lymphatics) is the most common and widely distributed cause of this disease. Very high titers of serum IgG and IgE levels against microfilarial antigens are present. The disease is probably a hyperimmune reaction to microfilariae, which may be found occasionally in lung or lymph node biopsy specimens, but not usually in blood. Response to the antifilarial drug diethylcarbamazine is curative.

Persistent high levels of eosinophils for long periods of time, no evidence of known causes of eosinophilia, and signs and symptoms of organ damage and injury are criteria for inclusion of patients in idiopathic hypereosinophilic syndrome (HES) (Fig. 33-8). HES appears to be a heterogeneous syndrome composed of a number of different disorders of varying severity. Although the pathogenesis of HES is not entirely understood, dysregulation of intracellular or intercellular molecular communication(s) appears to be involved, at least in some forms of HES. This dysregulation leads to persistently activated eosinophils, which release eosinophil granule proteins and enzymes, lipid mediators, and cytokines, chemokines, and growth factors; this not only produces tissue damage and injury, but also sets up an **autocrine loop** that continually activates cells and continues to produce eosinophil degranulation, causing further cell and tissue damage. Some forms appear to be T cell mediated, involving a subset of Th2–type lymphocytes. At least two distinct forms or hematologic variants appear to exist: the myeloid variant and the lymphoid variant, differing in clinical presentation, long-term behavior, and risk for malignant transformation (Brito-Babapulle, 2003; Roufosse, 2003). Clonal populations of eosinophils have been found in some patients with HES (Chang, 1999). In other patients with HES, abnormal clonal populations of T cells have been identified; these clonal populations may be precursors of malignancy (Simon, 1999).

The organ most consistently affected in HES is the heart, with mural thrombi formation, myocarditis, endocardial and myocardial fibrosis, constrictive pericarditis, and fibroplastic endocarditis (Brito-Babapulle, 2003). Hepatosplenomegaly is common. Other organ systems may be involved and include the CNS, retina, lungs, skin, gastrointestinal (GI) tract, and kidney.

Occasional reports describe persistent eosinophilia occurring in families in the absence of any known cause. This condition is known as **familial** or **constitutional eosinophilia** and appears to be benign (Naiman, 1964). The exact prevalence of familial eosinophilia is unknown.

Basophilia

Basophilia is an increase in the absolute basophil count above $0.2 \times 10^9/L$. Causes of basophilia are listed in Table 33-6. Reactive basophilia is an uncommon finding overall. Basophilia is seen most frequently in hypersensitivity and allergic reactions, CML (Fig. 33-9), myeloid metaplasia (extramedullary myelopoiesis), and polycythemia vera. Relative basophilia may be transient following irradiation. Basophilia may be present in hypothyroidism and chronic hemolytic anemia and following splenectomy.

TABLE 33-6
Key Causes of Basophilia

- Myeloproliferative disease
- Allergic—food, drugs, foreign proteins
- Infectious—variola, varicella
- Chronic hemolytic anemia—especially post splenectomy
- Inflammatory—collagen vascular disease, ulcerative colitis

TABLE 33-7
Key Causes of Monocytosis

- Infectious—tuberculosis, subacute bacterial endocarditis, syphilis, protozoan, rickettsial
- Recovery from neutropenia
- Hematologic—leukemias, myeloproliferative disorders, lymphomas, multiple myeloma
- Inflammatory—collagen vascular disease, chronic ulcerative colitis, sprue, myositis, polyarteritis, temporal arteritis
- Others—solid tumor, immune thrombocytopenic purpura, sarcoidosis

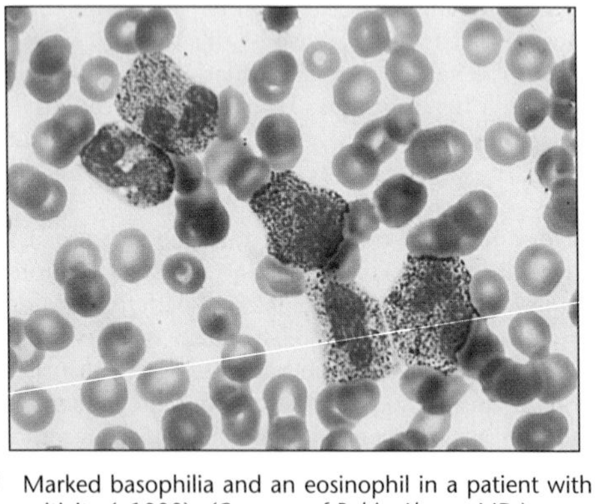

Figure 33-9 Marked basophilia and an eosinophil in a patient with Philadelphia chromosome positivity (×1000). *(Courtesy of Robin Abaya, MD.)*

Monocytosis

Monocytosis is an increase in monocytes above the upper reference value, especially when greater than $1.0 \times 10^9/L$. The most common causes are recovery from neutropenia and indolent infections. Causes and associations of monocytosis are shown in Table 33-7.

Monocytosis is present during the recovery stage from acute infection and from agranulocytosis, in which it is considered a favorable sign. Monocytosis may be present in subacute bacterial endocarditis. In this condition, monocytes may show phagocytosis of other blood cells, red blood cells, and leukocytes. It may be present in mycotic, rickettsial, protozoal, and viral infections.

Infectious disease, however, is an uncommon cause of monocytosis. In a classic study of 160 successive cases of absolute monocytosis (Maldonado, 1965), more than half (85) were associated with **hematologic disease.** These included acute monocytic and granulocytic leukemias, lymphoma (HL most frequently), multiple myeloma, and myeloproliferative disorders.

Monocytopenia

Monocytopenia is a decrease in circulating monocytes below the lower reference value of $0.2 \times 10^9/L$. Few studies have dealt with monocytopenia because of (1) the large number of cells that must be counted in a differential to obtain reliable counts; (2) the distributional bias of wedge blood film for monocytes compared with the spinner-made blood film; and (3) the unavailability, until fairly recently, of automation allowing large numbers of cells to be counted routinely.

During therapy with prednisone, monocytes fall during the first few hours after the first dose but return to above original levels by 12 hours. Monocytopenia has also been observed in hairy cell leukemia (HCL). Monocytopenia is uncommon as an isolated finding.

TABLE 33-8
Key Causes of Lymphocytosis

- Infectious—many viral, pertussis, tuberculosis, toxoplasmosis, rickettsial
- Chronic inflammatory—ulcerative colitis, Crohn's
- Immune mediated—drug sensitivity, vasculitis, graft rejection, Graves', Sjögren's
- Hematologic—ALL, CLL, lymphoma
- Stress—acute, transient

ALL, Acute lymphoblastic leukemia; *CLL,* chronic lymphocytic leukemia.

LYMPHOCYTIC AND PLASMACYTIC DISORDERS

In these disorders, the pathologist should consider neoplastic conditions, which are covered in the later sections of this chapter, as well as the benign causes, discussed in the following sections.

Lymphocytes in Normal Individuals

In normal individuals, the absolute numbers of lymphocytes and T cells are highest in young children. The percentage of lymphocytes in the blood is normally up to about 50% for the first 5 years. During the first decade of life, the absolute lymphocyte count and the absolute number of T cells decrease but remain higher than observed in the adult. By the time of adolescence, the absolute lymphocyte count and the absolute number of T cells have leveled off to values observed throughout adulthood. The absolute number of B lymphocytes remains stable during all stages of life (Davey, 1977; Perkins, 2004). In adolescence and adulthood, lymphocytes constitute about 20%–40% of all leukocytes, or $1.5–4.0 \times 10^9/L$ cells/L.

Some disagreement is ongoing regarding the absolute numbers of lymphocytes and of T cells in aged individuals. Although some studies (Diaz-Jouanen, 1975) indicate that there is a decrease in total lymphocyte count and T cell numbers, other investigators have reported no significant change in total lymphocytes or T cells in aged individuals (Weksler, 1974; Davey, 1977). The normal CD4/CD8 ratio is between 1.0 and 3.4, but we have seen values as high as 12 in reactive conditions. In the neonate, the numbers of total T cells and CD8+ T cells may be similar or decreased compared with adults, whereas CD4+ T cells may be similar or increased (De Waele, 1988).

Lymphocytosis

Lymphocytosis is an increase in the number of lymphocytes in the peripheral blood; reference intervals are $\approx 1.5–4.0 \times 10^9/L$ in the adult and $\approx 1.5–8.8 \times 10^9/L$ in the child. Relative lymphocytosis (an increase in the percentage of lymphocytes) is present in various conditions and is especially prominent in disorders with neutropenia. Lymphocytosis is unusual in acute bacterial infections but is commonly associated with viral infection (Epstein-Barr virus [EBV], hepatitis) (Table 33-8).

Acute Infectious Lymphocytosis

Acute infectious lymphocytosis (AIL) is a contagious condition characterized by lymphocytosis and occurring mainly in children. The incubation period is 12–21 days. Antibody and viral studies have indicated a relationship between infectious lymphocytosis and coxsackievirus A, coxsackievirus B6, echoviruses, and adenovirus type 12. No association has been noted with EBV, cytomegalovirus, or herpesvirus. The disease has variable systemic manifestations, from mild and nonspecific to more marked symptoms such as vomiting, fever, abdominal discomfort, signs suggesting involvement of the nervous system, cutaneous rashes, upper respiratory infection, and diarrhea. Leukocytosis ($20–5 \times 10^9/L$, occasionally $>10 \times 10^9/L$) precedes the clinical manifestations.

In AIL, from 60%–95% of blood leukocytes are small mature lymphocytes and are probably of T cell origin (Cassuto, 1977). In contrast to infectious mononucleosis, atypical lymphocytes are uncommon. Eosinophilia is usually present. The lymphocytosis usually lasts 3–5 weeks, sometimes longer. Other blood changes are unusual. The marrow has no characteristic changes; an increased percentage of lymphocytes has been observed but is probably an artifact of an admixture of peripheral blood. Lymph node enlargement is rare and minimal when present. The spleen and the liver are rarely, if ever, enlarged. Lymph node biopsy may show reactive follicular hyperplasia but no characteristic changes. In some cases, white cells in the cerebrospinal fluid (CSF) are increased, with about 40% lymphocytes.

A chronic form of infectious lymphocytosis also occurs in children. The leukocyte count is 10–25 × 10^9/L, with 60%–80% lymphocytes of normal appearance. Slight eosinophilia, monocytosis, and plasmacytosis are also present. As a rule, children have enlargement of tonsils, lymph nodes, and spleen and a history of recurrent upper respiratory infection. The marrow shows no abnormalities.

Pertussis

Whooping cough (pertussis), although reduced by routine immunization, still occurs in unimmunized children and is most severe in infants. It also occurs in adults with immunity reduced since childhood vaccination. The etiologic agent is *Bordetella pertussis*, a highly infectious agent that produces an inflammatory reaction of the entire respiratory tract. The incubation period is approximately 6–20 days, and the first symptoms are those of a head cold. Later, the patient develops paroxysms of coughing productive of thick sputum. The paroxysms typically end with a "whooping" sound, due to deep inspiration, giving the disease its descriptive name. There is frequently pain over the trachea and bronchi. The disease typically lasts 6–12 weeks.

Patients frequently develop significant lymphocytosis with counts higher than 30 × 10^9/L recorded. The lymphocytes are small, mature T cells with a normal CD4/CD8 ratio (Hudnall, 2000). The lymphocyte count is highest during the first 3 weeks of the illness, and then decreases during the fourth and subsequent weeks (Lagergren, 1963). The lymphocytosis is at least partially due to the release of lymphocytosis-promoting factor (LPF) or pertussis toxin from the organism. This factor may cause transient increased mobilization of lymphocytes from lymphoid organs, followed by inhibition of recirculation of lymphocytes from blood into the lymph flow. Thus, the lymphocytosis is due to redistribution of lymphocytes into the peripheral circulation without increased lymphopoiesis (Rai, 1971; Spangrude, 1985). At the molecular level, this absolute lymphocytosis appears to be due, at least in part, to the absence of L-selectin on many circulating lymphocytes (Hudnall, 2000). This seems reasonable in that L-selectin is an endothelial adhesion and lymph node homing receptor, and absence of this surface molecule would essentially prevent circulating lymphocytes from finding their "home" in most lymph nodes. They would remain in the circulation for longer time periods and cause an increase in number (lymphocytosis) in the blood. The exact mechanism of loss of L-selectin from the lymphocyte cell surface is not presently known.

Chronic Lymphocytosis/Persistent Polyclonal B Cell Lymphocytosis

Persistent reactive lymphocytosis is an uncommon event in adults, and significant lymphocytosis should raise suspicion of neoplastic disease, such as chronic lymphocyte leukemia. Coexistence of neutropenia or classic Felty's syndrome suggests LGL leukemia. Often tissue biopsy and/or immunophenotyping of peripheral blood will point toward a specific disease or diagnosis. Mononucleosis or lymphocytosis due to other viruses occasionally presents in later life, however.

A rare condition, persistent polyclonal lymphocytosis, has been reported in adults, predominantly in female smokers, and in the postsplenectomy state (Himmelmann, 2001). Persistent polyclonal B cell lymphocytosis appears to be a benign polyclonal B cell proliferation, showing binucleated atypical lymphocytes in the peripheral blood. Polyclonal serum IgM is usually increased. A majority (65%–85% vs. 15%–20% in normal individuals) of the peripheral B cells appear to be IgM+/IgD+/CD27+ memory B cells (Loembe, 2002). Occasional *bcl-2/Ig* gene rearrangements (t[14;18]), commonly associated with follicular lymphoma, have been found (Delage, 1997). Although the cause is unknown, dysregulation of Fas-mediated apoptosis and the CD40 survival pathways appear to be involved (Loembe, 2001; Roussel, 2003).

Retrovirus-Associated Diseases and Conditions

Human T lymphotropic virus type 1 (HTLV-1), discovered in 1980 by Poiesz and Gallo, is a retrovirus associated with adult T cell leukemia/lymphoma (ATL) (Poiesz, 1980). It is endemic in areas of Japan, the Caribbean basin, and the southeastern United States. HTLV-2, a second human retrovirus, was found in a patient with HCL (Kalyanaraman, 1982). A third human retrovirus, human immunodeficiency virus type 1 (HIV-1), was recognized and confirmed as the cause of acquired immunodeficiency syndrome (AIDS [discussed further later]) over the next 2 years. Later, in 1985, a second but distinct type of HIV—HIV-2—was identified.

HIV-1 infects both monocyte/macrophages and T cells (both essential cells for normal immune system function), using cell surface chemokine receptors (CCR5 on the former and CXCR4 on the latter); infection ultimately causes progressive loss of CD4+ lymphocytes, disrupts normal immune function, and produces immunodeficiency and disease. Disease encompasses not only many different types of infection, but also an increase in neoplastic disease, including lymphoma. At present, it appears that HIV-1 plays an indirect role (through immune dysregulation and not by direct induction) in the development of these lymphomas (Knowles, 2003). HTLV-1 and -2 also infect and transform T cells, primarily CD4+ cells with HTLV-1 and CD8+ cells with HTLV-2. HTLV-1 immortalizes CD4+ lymphoblasts in some patients, producing ATL. Although HTLV-2 was originally identified in a patient with HCL, a definitive link between HTLV-2 infection and human disease does not currently exist.

Several cases have now been reported of a transient T cell lymphocytosis in patients infected with HTLV-1 (Kinoshita, 1985; Ehrlich, 1988). In most patients, the disorder is characterized by few clinical symptoms consisting of fever, limited lymphadenopathy, and occasional skin rash. The peripheral blood lymphocyte count is usually less than 20 × 10^9/L; however, 10%–40% of these lymphocytes are immature forms. In most of these cases, the lymphocytosis is monoclonal and, therefore, leukemic. Although some patients with this infection progress to ATL, most (90%–95%) patients with antibodies against HTLV-1 are symptom free. Most individuals exhibit only a viral-like syndrome; however, others manifest a chronic progressive leukemia, and still others develop tropical spastic paraparesis (Davey, 1991). ATL typically develops decades after initial infection, and thus is usually seen in older patients.

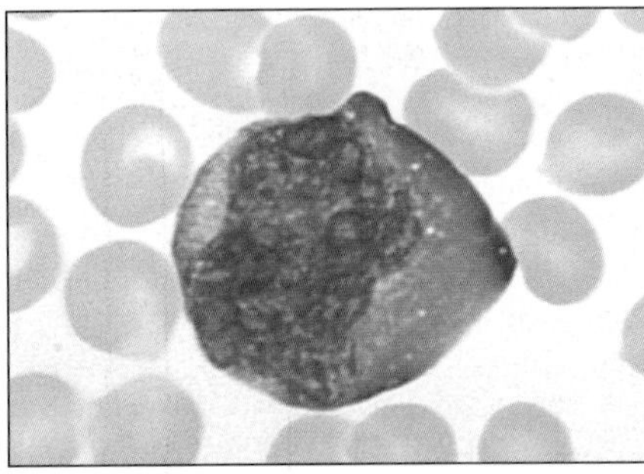

Figure 33-10 Infectious mononucleosis, showing a large activated lymphoid cell in the blood (×1000).

Infectious Mononucleosis and Epstein-Barr Virus Infection

Infectious mononucleosis (IM) is usually a self-limited infectious disease characterized by sore throat, prolonged malaise, atypical lymphocytosis with the presence of large transformed lymphocytes (Fig. 33-10), lymphadenopathy (most often posterior cervical), and often splenomegaly. In immunocompromised patients, EBV is associated with benign B cell hyperplasia, malignant lymphoma, and posttransplantation lymphoproliferative disease (Hess, 2004; Thompson, 2004).

Etiology and Pathophysiology. IM is a disorder that occurs secondary to infection with EBV (human herpesvirus 4). When the primary infection occurs in healthy individuals during early childhood, the disease often goes unnoticed. However, when the infection involves healthy adolescent individuals or adults, the resultant disorder is the IM syndrome. In most cases, the virus gains entry into the body through the oropharyngeal epithelial and lymphoid tissues, and the virus appears to infect both tissues. The virus attaches to C3d complement receptors (CD21) on B lymphoid cells and enters into the cells. The EBV then stimulates DNA synthesis in these B cells and induces the formation of several new antigens, including the viral capsid antigen (VCA), the membrane antigen (MA), early antigen (EA)—both diffuse (EA-D) and restricted (EA-R) subtypes—Epstein-Barr nuclear antigens (EBNA), and the lymphocyte-detected membrane antigen (LYDMA) (Harrington, 1988). Thus, the earliest phase of this disease is characterized by an infection of B cells that proliferate, develop neo-antigens, circulate, stimulate an immune response, and synthesize immunoglobulin (Sixbey, 1984). VCA, EA, and EBNA are the viral proteins most important for serodiagnosis in immunocompetent patients (Hess, 2004). Clinical and laboratory features are summarized in Table 33-9.

Typically, the humoral immune response is characterized by the rise in titer of IgG and IgM viral capsid antibodies during the incubation and

PART 4

TABLE 33-9

Summary of Features of Infectious Mononucleosis (IM) in Immunocompetent Patients

Epstein-Barr Virus (Human Herpesvirus-4)

Pathophysiology
- Virus enters through oropharyngeal epithelial and lymphoid cells
- Virus attaches to CD21 on B cells
- Viral antigens—viral capsid antigen (VCA), early antigen (EA), Epstein-Barr nuclear antigen (EBNA)—are produced and elicit antibody production

Humoral Immune Response
- Immunoglobulin (Ig)M against VCA rises during incubation and prodrome, falls over few weeks to months
- IgG against VCA rises during incubation, decreases during convalescence, remains detectable for life
- Antibodies to EA rise 2–3 weeks after onset of illness, then fall
- Antibodies to EBNA rise during convalescence, detectable for life

Cellular Immune Response
- T cells activated during second week of illness
- CD8-positive cytotoxic T cells kill infected B cells
- Natural killer cells kill infected B cells
- Some resting memory B cells remain latently infected

Clinical Features
- 2- to 5-week incubation period
- Vague onset of symptoms
- Fever, sore throat, lymphadenopathy
- Adolescents, young adults more often symptomatic than younger children

Laboratory Features
- Leukocytosis with absolute lymphocytosis and atypical lymphocytes
- Transient monocytosis
- Relative and absolute neutropenia early on
- Mild thrombocytopenia in half of cases
- Hemolytic anemia in 1%–3% of cases, often with anti-I specificity
- Elevated transaminases in 85%–100% of cases, but clinical jaundice rare
- Spot test is simple, rapid, specific, based on agglutination of horse red blood cells (RBCs)
- Heterophil antibody (HA) test is based on differential absorption of IM-specific HA by beef RBC stroma and guinea pig kidney

early prodrome periods. The titer of IgM capsid antibody starts to fall during the second and third weeks of illness, and then diminishes to undetectable levels within the following several months. The IgG viral capsid antibody decreases during convalescence but remains detectable for life. Approximately 2–3 weeks after the onset of illness, Epstein-Barr virus antibodies against the early antigens appear and then decline over the succeeding 2 months. The titer of the Epstein-Barr virus nuclear antigen antibodies rises during the latter portion of convalescence and is apparently detectable throughout life.

The cellular immune response in IM is characterized by proliferation and activation of T cells, usually during the second week of illness, in response to EBV-induced B cell infection and activation. Because these activated T cells are derived mostly from the cytotoxic/suppressor cell subpopulation, marked suppression and destruction of EBV-infected B cells occur. Indeed, most of the atypical lymphocytes observed in the peripheral blood of patients with IM during the second week of illness possess the CD8 antigen. These cytotoxic/suppressor T cells kill infected B cells and diminish polyclonal antibody production induced by the Epstein-Barr virus. In addition to T-cytotoxic cells, the activity of natural killer (NK) cells has a profound effect on limiting the proliferation of EBV-infected B cells in patients with IM (Purtilo, 1981). It is also likely that EBV-infected B cells are destroyed, at least in part, through the mechanism of antibody-dependent cellular cytotoxicity—a process requiring the presence of both cytotoxic cells and antibody. This process of B cell proliferation followed by the inhibitory and destructive effects of EBV-directed antibody production, as well as T cell and NK cell cytotoxic effects, occurs within the patient's peripheral blood, BM, lymphoid tissues, and, perhaps to a limited degree, all tissues of the body.

Most (over 90%) immunocompetent adults have serologic evidence of past EBV infection. EBV has the capacity not only to infect cells (many of which are destroyed by an intact immune system) but to produce a latent infection in resting memory B cells and, in some cases, produce transformation of lymphocytes to malignant lymphoma (Kuppers, 2003; Thorley-Lawson, 2004). However, a majority of latently infected individuals show no disease manifestations throughout their lifetimes.

The resting memory B cells can act as a reservoir of EBV, because viral antigens (easily recognized by an intact immune system) are not expressed on the lymphocyte surface. In this model of EBV infection, mechanisms of viral persistence and transformation appear to be dependent on the interaction between the stage of maturation of the infected lymphocyte and the genetic expression of different groups (or "programs") of viral proteins within the infected lymphocyte (Kuppers, 2003; Thorley-Lawson, 2004). In addition, different types of EBV-associated tumors (such as African Burkitt lymphoma [BL], nasopharyngeal carcinoma, B cell lymphoproliferative disease or posttransplant lymphoproliferative disease in immunocompromised individuals, and HL) appear to exhibit different groups of viral protein expression (Wong, 2002).

In IM, a spectrum of EBV expression patterns (programs) is found in different cells (Klein, 2007). In type III latency-growth program, cells express a full set of EBV-encoded proteins, including six nuclear proteins (EBNA1–6) and three latent membrane proteins (LMP1, -2 and -3).

LMP1 has strong immunogenic activity and is present only in acute infection, except in immunocompromised hosts. Type I latency program involves expression of only one nuclear protein, EBNA-1, and is found in some memory B cells. Type IIa latency involves expression of EBNA-1, LMP-1, and LMP-2. Type IIb latency expresses all EBNAs (EBNA1–6) but not LMP-1. Tumor cells in posttransplant lymphoproliferative disorders (PTLDs) correspond to latency type III, BL cells to latency type I, and cells in EBV+ HL and EBV+ nasopharyngeal carcinoma (NPC) to latency type IIa, with LMP-1 expression. T/NK cells are not normally infected by EBV and in extranodal nasal T/NK cell lymphoma; infection is complex, involving inflammatory tissues, is of latency type II with abundant LMP-1, and is dependent on IL-2.

Given the diversity of EBV-related protein expressions, assay for more uniformly expressed molecules is warranted for diagnostic identification of EBV. EBV-encoded RNAs EBER-1 and EBER-2 are reliably expressed at high levels in virtually all latent EBV infections, and are detected with high sensitivity by in situ hybridization assays that are currently the standard for EBV identification (Gulley, 2008).

Clinical Features. IM has been observed in patients from 3 months–70 years of age but is most common in adolescents and young adults. A 2- to 5-week incubation period prior to onset of symptoms usually occurs. Onset is vague, indefinite, and similar to the onset of other infectious diseases. Patients usually have fever, sore throat with ulcerative pharyngitis, and lymphadenopathy.

Complications. Of the rare anemias associated with IM, hemolytic anemia is the most common, occurring in 1%–3% of cases. The cause now appears to be related to the anti-I antibody produced frequently in this disease.

Mild thrombocytopenia occurs in about half of cases, but the platelet count is not often less than 100 × 10^9/L. Thrombocytopenic purpura with hemorrhagic complications is exceedingly rare. Splenic rupture may also occur. Neutropenia, pancytopenia, and hemophagocytic syndrome may rarely occur and be fatal (Mroczek, 1987). Two rare conditions resulting from EBV infection in healthy individuals are chronic active EBV infection (CAEBV) and EBV hemophagocytic syndrome (EBVHS). Both conditions show high morbidity and mortality and appear to be related to ectopic EBV infection in T cells and natural killer cells, in contrast to the usual B cell infection that commonly occurs in IM (Kasahara, 2002).

Abnormal liver function tests indicative of hepatitis occur in 85%–100% of patients with IM. Clinical jaundice is rare, but cases have been reported in which jaundice and acute pharyngitis were the only clinical manifestations of IM, with positive hematologic and serologic findings. Although uncommon, complications may also involve the nervous system, heart, kidney, and lungs.

Approximately one third of patients with IM carry β-hemolytic streptococci in the pharynx. Thus, one should give attention to strict clinical, hematologic, and serologic criteria in distinguishing IM from streptococcal pharyngitis.

Hematologic Features. Leukocytes are increased, usually ranging from 12–25 × 10^9/L. Rarely, counts as high as 80 × 10^9/L have been recorded. The leukocytosis is usually due to lymphocytosis (60%–90%) composed of a variety of atypical lymphocytes. The total leukocyte count, as a rule, returns to normal within 3 weeks. The atypical lymphocytes have nuclear alterations and an increase in the amount and basophilia of cytoplasm.

Lymphocytes include **monocytoid** lymphocytes, which likely correspond to immunoblasts in lymph nodes (see Fig. 33-10). Other atypical lymphocytes, which are more numerous, include plasmacytoid lymphocytes and those with small nuclei but abundant cytoplasm.

Often the number of monocytes rises transiently. The term **mononucleosis** refers to an increase in lymphocytes, not in monocytes.

Cytologic alterations are not pathognomonic of IM. Similar cells are found in a variety of disorders, including cytomegalovirus mononucleosis, toxoplasmosis, and infectious hepatitis, and usually to a lesser extent in viral pneumonia, varicella, mumps, and viral exanthemas of children.

Neutrophils are relatively and absolutely decreased in most cases during the first week of illness. During this time, a shift to the left may occur, with an increase in band cells and metamyelocytes. Toxic granules and Döhle bodies may be seen. The eosinophils are within normal limits.

The BM from patients with IM usually shows increased cellularity. Numbers of lymphocytes, macrophages, plasma cells, megakaryocytes, and erythroid cells are increased. The neutrophilic series appears decreased. About half of cases may have collections of mononuclear cells forming loose granulomas.

Serologic Findings in Immunocompetent Patients

Heterophil Antibody. Paul (1932) first described the presence of sheep cell agglutinins in the sera of patients with IM. Sheep cell agglutinins are not, however, specific for IM and can be present in other disorders.

Davidsohn (1937) demonstrated that the heterophil antibodies in patients with IM are absorbed by beef erythrocytes, in contrast to heterophil antibodies present in other disorders. The latter are absorbed by Forssman's antigen, such as that found in guinea pig kidney. The differential absorption test (Paul-Bunnell-Davidsohn test) is highly specific for IM (Davidsohn, 1969).

The spot test for IM (Lee, 1968) is based on the principle that horse erythrocytes are more sensitive than sheep erythrocytes in testing for IM. A positive test for IM shows agglutination of horse erythrocytes by serum absorbed with guinea pig kidney, but not by serum absorbed with beef erythrocyte stroma. The spot test has proved to be a simple, rapid, highly specific, and sensitive test for the heterophil antibodies of IM. False-positive tests occur but are very rare. The spot test is still in use, as are other similarly performing immunoassays and latex-based detection tests for heterophil antibody (Rogers, 1999). False-negative tests occur particularly in young children who produce heterophil antibodies (IgM) in limited amounts. In heterophil-negative IM, the diagnosis may be substantiated by assay for antibody to EBV.

As previously mentioned, several antibodies are produced by the host in response to a variety of Epstein-Barr virus antigens (see Table 33-9). Antibody to the viral capsid antigen arises within the first 2 weeks of onset. This antibody, measured by an immunofluorescent or other method, is used for determining exposure to EBV. Assaying for the presence of EBV antibody is usually limited to the few cases of heterophil-negative IM.

In addition to heterophil and EBV antibodies, patients with IM frequently produce antibodies to a wide variety of antigens. Antibodies against human erythrocytes, leukocytes, and platelets have been described. Patients with IM have an increased frequency of cold agglutinins. Positive tests for rheumatoid factor and antinuclear factor have been reported.

In immunocompromised patients, serologic tests are of limited value, and direct detection methods are considered more reliable. Determination of EBV viral load by polymerase chain reaction (PCR) appears to be one of the better tests for this patient population (Hess, 2004).

Differential Diagnosis. Clinical, hematologic, and serologic features of IM permit an accurate diagnosis to be made in more than 90% of cases. When the heterophil test is negative, one must consider several possibilities. The patient could still have EBV antibody–positive but heterophil-negative IM. Cytomegalovirus infection, however, is the most common cause of heterophil-negative mononucleosis. Other possibilities include toxoplasmosis, infectious hepatitis, human herpesvirus 6, human immunodeficiency virus types 1 and 2, and ingestion of drugs (*p*-aminosalicylic acid, phenytoin [Dilantin], and diaminodiphenylsulfone) (Tsaparas, 2000; Taylor, 2003).

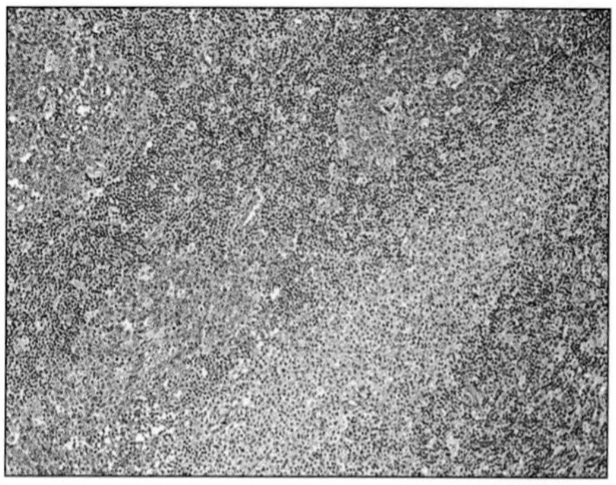

Figure 33-11 Toxoplasmosis lymphadenitis shows follicular hyperplasia with monocytoid B cell hyperplasia *(lower right-center)* and scattered individual and aggregates of histiocytes, often impinging on the germinal center/mantle zone border (×200).

Course. Classic IM is a benign disorder, and complications occur in less than 5% of patients. The disorder usually resolves in 3–4 weeks. Fatalities are extremely rare but tend to occur in members of the same family (Purtilo, 1979). Additional studies indicate that affected individuals frequently suffer from X-linked lymphoproliferative disease (XLP). This group of immunosuppressed individuals possess a rare, familial, fatal form of combined immunodeficiency, apparently involving both B and T cells. All untreated patients die by approximately 40 years of age. EBV infection can produce any one of three severe complications in XLP: fulminant IM, life-threatening lymphoproliferative disease and B cell lymphoma, and dysgammaglobulinemia. Although classically associated with EBV infection, XLP can occur in patients seronegative for EBV. XLP has been mapped to human chromosome Xq24-25, which codes for a cell surface receptor present on T and NK cells, but not B cells. An uncontrolled cytotoxic T cell response is thought to be responsible for liver necrosis and BM failure, ultimately causing death (Thompson, 2004). In addition to XLP, EBV-associated lymphoproliferative disorders can occur in individuals with congenital and acquired immunodeficiencies.

Cytomegalovirus Infection

Some individuals infected with cytomegalovirus develop a syndrome similar to infectious mononucleosis. This disorder can occur following massive blood transfusion (posttransfusion mononucleosis) or spontaneously in previously healthy individuals (cytomegalovirus mononucleosis). The patient has fever, chills, profound malaise, and myalgia. Sore throat (but not exudative pharyngitis) and lymphadenopathy may be noted. Occasionally, splenomegaly is found, but hepatomegaly does not occur. Commonly involved systems in immunocompromised patients are the CNS, GI, and pulmonary systems, although disease may be found in almost any organ system.

Leukocytosis is characteristic with absolute lymphocytosis. Usually 20% or more of the leukocytes are atypical lymphocytes. BM aspirates have shown increased numbers of normal lymphocytes and atypical lymphocytes. Abnormal liver function test results are the most frequent abnormal laboratory finding (Wreghitt, 2003). In a small percentage of patients, titers of cold agglutinins, rheumatoid factor, or antinuclear antibodies may be increased. No rise in heterophil, Epstein-Barr virus, or *Toxoplasma gondii* antibodies occurs. The diagnosis is usually made by isolating the cytomegalovirus from urine, saliva, blood, or tissue biopsy, or by serology.

Toxoplasmosis

Toxoplasma gondii, a protozoan parasite, can produce in both young and old a disease (toxoplasmosis) similar to infectious mononucleosis. Diagnosis is critical in congenitally infected fetuses and newborns, women infected during pregnancy, immunocompromised patients, and patients with chorioretinitis (Remington, 2004).

Only a small proportion (≈10%) of immunocompetent individuals are symptomatic. These patients typically present with lymphadenopathy, commonly cervical. Some patients may also show fever, headache, sore throat, hepatosplenomegaly, chorioretinitis, and an increased number of atypical lymphocytes in the peripheral blood. In immunocompromised patients, disease commonly involves the CNS and eyes but may also involve the lungs and heart.

The histopathology of lymph nodes is usually distinctive, with scattered epithelioid histiocytes which often blur the germinal center/mantle zone border, and with sinus monocytoid B cell hyperplasia (Fig. 33-11).

TABLE 33-10

Key Causes of Lymphopenia

- Destructive—radiation, chemotherapy, corticosteroids
- Debilitative—starvation, aplastic anemia, terminal cancer, collagen vascular disease, renal failure
- Infectious—viral hepatitis, influenza, typhoid fever, TB
- AIDS associated—HIV cytopathic effect, nutritional imbalance, drug effect
- Congenital immunodeficiency—Wiskott-Aldrich syndrome
- Abnormal lymphatic circulation—intestinal lymphangiectasia, obstruction, thoracic duct drainage/rupture, CHF

AIDS, Acquired immunodeficiency syndrome; *CHF,* congestive heart failure; *HIV,* human immunodeficiency virus; *TB,* tuberculosis.

Morphology correlates closely with elevated *Toxoplasma* antibody titers (Dorfman, 1973). BM biopsy specimens have no specific pathologic lesion.

The diagnosis is established by demonstrating an elevation of *Toxoplasma* antibodies in immunocompetent patients. In immunocompromised patients, serologic tests are not sensitive, and direct detection of the organism from blood, from body fluids, or in tissue is necessary for definitive diagnosis.

Autoimmune Lymphoproliferative Syndrome

Autoimmune lymphoproliferative syndrome (ALPS) is an uncommon cause of lymphadenopathy, splenomegaly, and autoimmune cytopenias with onset in childhood that is caused by an inheritable genetic defect, a mutation in one of the genes encoding Fas, or CD95, or occasionally a caspase gene. Fas is a key component of apoptosis. The disease has variable penetrance and is characterized by chronic lymphoid hyperplasia with presence of CD4/CD8 double negative T cells, and the above symptoms (Oliveira, 2010).

Other Nonneoplastic Causes of Lymphadenopathy

Other causes of benign or reactive lymphadenopathy include autoimmune disease and infection—in addition to the specific entities noted previously, Castleman's disease, Rosai-Dorfman disease (sinus histiocytosis with massive lymph node hyperplasia), Kikuchi histiocytic necrotizing lymphadenitis, Kawasaki disease, and others. Each has specific findings and is reviewed in detail elsewhere (Weiss, 2008).

Lymphocytopenia

Lymphocytopenia is present when the absolute lymphocyte count is below $\approx 1.0 \times 10^9$/L in adults and below $\approx 2.0 \times 10^9$/L in children. Normally, about 80% of circulating peripheral blood lymphocytes are CD3+ T cells, and a majority ($\approx$65%) of these cells are CD4+ helper T cells. A number of immunologic deficiency disorders that are genetically determined have lymphocytopenia, along with various other immunologic defects of humoral or cell-mediated immunity. Lymphocytopenia in these disorders is due to impaired lymphopoiesis. Increased levels of adrenocortical hormones, administration of chemotherapeutic drugs, or irradiation will result in lymphocytopenia. Impaired drainage of the intestinal lymphatics with loss of lymphocytes into the intestines due to a number of causes has been implicated as a mechanism for lymphocytopenia. In advanced cases of NHL and HL, as well as in terminal cases of carcinoma, lymphocytopenia is often observed. Causes and conditions associated with lymphocytopenia include those listed in Table 33-10.

Acquired Immunodeficiency Syndrome

Acquired immunodeficiency syndrome (AIDS), once a progressively fatal infectious disorder with characteristic clinical, hematologic, and serologic abnormalities, can now be controlled in most patients with highly active antiretroviral (HAART) therapy.

Etiology. AIDS is a disorder secondary to infection with HIV-1 and HIV-2—RNA retroviruses that are cytotropic for CD4+ T cells and for other cells, including macrophages, monocytes, megakaryocytes, and CNS microglial cells. Viral entry into a cell results from interaction with the CD4 receptor and with chemokine coreceptors that determine target cell tropism (Starr-Spires, 2002). HIV is responsible for both direct killing of infected cells and indirect killing of neighboring cells, utilizing both apoptotic-dependent and apoptotic-independent mechanisms of cell destruction (Badley, 2003).

HIV infection is spread by contamination with secretions, excretions, blood, and tissues that contain the virus. Because of the cytotropic effect of the AIDS viruses for CD4+ cells, there is a marked decrease in the number of T-helper cells and an imbalance in T-suppressor/cytotoxic cells in the blood and lymphoid tissues of the body. As a result, a profound cellular immune depression occurs, characterized by infection with a variety of opportunistic organisms. Initially, B cells are not involved and immunoglobulin levels are normal or increased. However, as the disease progresses, the frequency of malignancy in these patients is increased. AIDS-associated cancers include Kaposi's sarcoma, non-HL, and cervical cancer (all AIDS-defining cancers), as well as HL and anogenital cancers (Bellan, 2003; Mbulaiteye, 2003). Although the cause of these malignancies is undoubtedly multifactorial, recent studies suggest that HIV may possess oncogenic potential (Lazzi, 2002; De Falco, 2003). In addition, the functions of monocytes and NK cells are abnormal.

Hematologic Features. The most common hematologic abnormality in patients with AIDS is anemia of chronic disease and lymphopenia (80%–85% of cases), particularly of the T-helper/inducer (CD4) subset. Thrombocytopenia occurs in approximately 30% of cases and neutropenia in 40%, often with a left shift; the former is often immune mediated (Hoxie, 1995).

The peripheral blood film usually displays atypical lymphocytes that have a plasmacytoid appearance. Monocytes are often large with a fine nuclear chromatin and cytoplasmic vacuoles. Immune-mediated anemia, thrombocytopenia, and neutropenia in AIDS have also been described.

The BM is usually normocellular to hypercellular (Castella, 1985). Often increased numbers of immature myeloid precursor cells, macrophages laden with iron, and plasma cells occur. Defects occur in BM progenitor cells such as colony-forming unit-granulocyte, monocyte (CFU-GM); colony-forming unit-granulocyte, erythrocyte, monocyte, megakaryocyte, pluripotential stem cell (CFU-GEMM); colony-forming unit-megakaryocyte (CFU-MK); and burst-forming unit-erythrocyte (BFU-E). Many drugs used to treat AIDS and its infectious complications are also myelosuppressive. Suppression of the marrow is, in many patients, multifactorial, resulting from an interaction of direct HIV cytopathic effect, dysregulation of the immune system and of apoptosis, possible complicating infection and/or nutritional imbalance, and drug effect. The most clinically valuable information of BM biopsy is usually the identification of infection or malignancy in the marrow. The disease course has been converted to a relatively indolent chronic course in those who receive and adhere to HAART therapy, but remains a tragic illness in disadvantaged populations and in those not treated.

Functional Disorders of Lymphocytes

Functional disorders of lymphocytes can be inherited or acquired. The immune deficiency may be due to a disorder of maturation or function of monocytes and antigen-presenting cells, B cells, T cells, stem cells, suppressor cells, or a combination. These may cause antibody production defects or a combination of antibody production and T cell function defects. Acquired disorders may be due to malnutrition, infection, or malignancy, as well as any insult that may significantly perturb immune regulation and cellular communication. Acquired functional abnormalities of lymphocytes are frequently observed in lymphoid malignancies. For example, decreased B cell function is observed in chronic lymphocytic leukemia, in which two thirds of patients have hypogammaglobulinemia. In multiple myeloma, synthesis of normal immunoglobulin in the presence of high levels of paraprotein is diminished.

Diminished T cell activity has been described in patients with HL, sarcoidosis, and leprosy. In HL, diminished T cell activity may be the result of the suppressive effects of monocytes. In autoimmune disease, loss of suppressor T cells has been observed.

In severe malnutrition and in terminal malignancies, both humoral and cell-mediated immunity are diminished.

The diagnosis of functional disorders of lymphocytes requires the use of skin tests, enumeration of B and T cells and their subsets, measurement of serum immunoglobulin and antibodies, and a variety of in vitro lymphocyte assays that record their responses to mitogens and antigens. Molecular testing, including cytogenetic and fluorescent in situ hybridization (FISH) analysis, flow cytometry, and PCR, may be required for definitive diagnosis. A thorough history and physical examination should always precede any testing. It is probably best to begin a workup with less expensive and easily obtainable tests.

TABLE 33-11
Key Causes of Plasmacytosis

- Viral—infectious mononucleosis, measles, rubella, HIV
- Bacterial—tuberculosis, syphilis, streptococcus, staphylococcus
- Parasitic—malaria, trichinosis
- Inflammatory—SLE, RA, inflammatory bowel disease, alcoholic liver disease
- Neoplastic—plasma cell leukemia, myeloma
- Immune stimulation—immune complex disease (serum sickness), drug sensitivity, transfusion
- Trauma

HIV, Human immunodeficiency virus; *RA,* rheumatoid arthritis; *SLE,* systemic lupus erythematosus.

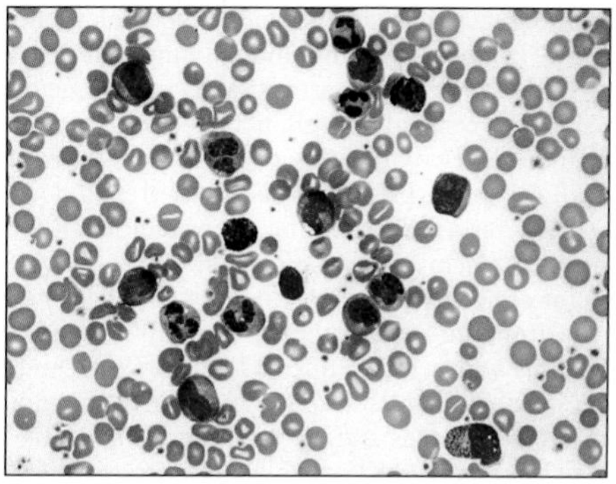

Figure 33-12 Chronic myeloid leukemia with increased segmented neutrophils, myelocytes, and basophils and an occasional blast (×500).

This topic is covered more fully in Part 6, Immunology and Immunopathology.

Plasmacytosis

Plasma cells are not normally present in circulating blood. They are increased in a variety of chronic infections, in allergic states, in the presence of neoplasms, and in other conditions in which the serum γ-globulin concentration is elevated. Plasma cells have also been recorded in the blood of patients with viral disorders, including rubella, measles, chickenpox, and mumps. They are moderately increased in cutaneous exanthemas, infectious mononucleosis, syphilis, subacute bacterial endocarditis, sarcoidosis, and collagen disease. Rarely, bacterial sepsis may show a peripheral plasmacytosis mimicking plasma cell leukemia (Shtalrid, 2003). Their increase is usually linked with increases in lymphocytes, monocytes, and eosinophils. Causes and conditions associated with plasmacytosis include those illustrated (Table 33-11).

In the marrow, an average of 1%–2% of plasma cells are present in adults. An increase beyond 4% is significant; lower values are found in children. Increases of up to 20% of plasma cells may be found in a variety of conditions other than multiple myeloma, including metastatic carcinoma, chronic granulomatous infection, conditions linked with hypersensitivity, and following administration of cytotoxic drugs. They are often increased in aplastic anemia, but this is probably just a relative increase. On the other hand, they are decreased or absent in agammaglobulinemia.

LEUKEMOID REACTIONS

A leukemoid reaction is an excessive leukocytic response in the peripheral blood. It includes leukocytosis of 50×10^9/L or higher with a shift to the left; lower counts, even below normal, with considerable numbers of immature granulocytes; and similar quantitative or qualitative changes in lymphocytes or monocytes. Depending on the predominant cell, leukemoid reactions may be neutrophilic, eosinophilic, lymphocytic, or monocytic. No clear explanation for these apparent temporary aberrations in normal regulatory control mechanisms is yet available, although in some instances they appear to be due to elevation of cytokines or granulocyte colony-stimulating factor by tumor (Melhem, 1993; Nara, 2003; Nimieri, 2003). The reactions are irregular in degree, even when associated with the same inciting agent.

Neutrophilic Leukemoid Reactions

Excessive neutrophilia may occur in many situations, including hemolysis, hemorrhage, malignancy with bone involvement, HL, myelofibrosis, infection (especially tuberculosis), severe burns, eclampsia, and certain intoxications.

Examination of the blood is usually more helpful than marrow examination. Leukemoid reactions lack the characteristic differential count that is seen in CML, including the myelocyte "peak," eosinophilia, and basophilia (Fig. 33-12).

Eosinophilic Leukemoid Reactions

Cells as immature as eosinophilic myelocytes rarely appear in the blood in reactive eosinophilia, in which the leukocyte count may exceed 50×10^9/L (see Fig. 33-8). Eosinophilic leukemoid reactions usually occur in children and usually are caused by parasitic infection. As with granulocytic leukemoid reactions, some eosinophilic leukemoid reactions have been associated with tumor (Melhem, 1993; Oakley, 1998).

Erythroblastosis and Leukoerythroblastosis

In patients with or without anemia, circulating normoblasts frequently are accompanied by a neutrophilic leukemoid reaction; this, then, is a **leukoerythroblastotic reaction.** A moderate anemia with normoblasts in the peripheral blood is fairly common in metastatic carcinoma involving BM. Leukoerythroblastosis may also be associated with marrow infection and/or fibrosis, and may be seen in benign conditions such as GI bleeding and hemolytic anemia (Weick, 1974).

Lymphocytic Leukemoid Reactions

Extremely high counts of normal-appearing lymphocytes may occur in infectious lymphocytosis and in pertussis (see earlier). When atypical lymphocytes are strikingly increased or immature (which may occur in conditions such as infectious mononucleosis), the distinction from leukemia may be difficult.

Examination of the marrow may be useful because lymphocytes are minimally increased, if at all, in most leukemoid reactions in contrast to leukemia. Flow cytometric studies of peripheral blood and/or BM would reveal a nonclonal population of lymphocytes with a normal combination of cell surface markers in benign proliferations.

NEOPLASTIC DISORDERS PRIMARILY INVOLVING LEUKOCYTES

OVERVIEW OF HEMATOPOIETIC NEOPLASMS

Hematopoietic neoplasms consist of a diversity of disorders which have in common their derivation from hematopoietic stem cells of the BM or lymphoid organs, and which are known or assumed to be clonal processes arising as the result of genetic errors. Given the diversity and regulatory complexity of hematopoietic cells, it is not surprising that neoplasms involving these tissues are quite diverse, differing in predominant cells within a neoplasm, degree of differentiation, rates of proliferation and apoptosis, clinical features, and response to therapy. Diagnosis and classification of hematopoietic tumors have changed with our understanding of disease. In the 19th century, "leukemia" referred to the white or pale color of blood, which contained increased leukocytes compared with red corpuscles, neither of which could be microscopically seen in detail without differential staining. **Chlorosis** and **chloroma** referred to the grossly greenish tinge of granulocytic cells. **Lymphoma,** first used by Virchow, referred to tumors of the lymph glands.

After the development of Romanowsky's stains (such as Wright-Giemsa), and later, hematoxylin and eosin (H&E), as well as improvements in microscopes, hematopoietic tumors could be classified by morphology, clinical features, and location of the abnormal proliferations. Hematopoietic tumors were referred to as leukemias when they primarily involved the blood and BM, and as lymphomas or sarcomas when they primarily involved the soft tissue. "Acute" referred to diseases with aggressive clinical courses, and "chronic" to those which progressed more slowly. Morphologic subtyping based on predominant cell types progressed into the 1950s and 1960s with the development of cytochemical stains to differentiate subtypes of myeloid cells and some lymphoid cells (such as HCL).

Since about 1970, an explosion of knowledge and new technology has occurred which provides many new tools for understanding these tumors. These include the discovery of B cells; T cells and other immunologic compartments; monoclonal antibodies and leukocyte differentiation antigens; cytogenetic karyotyping; immunoglobulin and T cell gene rearrangements; PCR; nucleic acid arrays; and, most recently, proteomic assays. Many, although certainly not all, hematopoietic tumors can now be characterized at the level of the genetic abnormality and the resultant intracellular pathway perturbations. This offers tremendous opportunity to develop therapies targeted to specific abnormalities. Examples include (1) chronic myeloid leukemia, with a t(9;22)(q34;q11) *BCR/ABL* translocation and resultant abnormal tyrosine kinase, which has been targeted by the drug Gleevec (imatinib mesylate) (Druker, 2004), and (2) acute promyelocytic leukemia with t(15;17)(q22;q12) *PML/RARα* and an abnormal receptor for retinoic acid, which responds to all-*trans* retinoic acid.

Classification of leukemias and, particularly, lymphomas became confusing in the 1970s and 1980s as knowledge progressed. The French-American-British (FAB) Cooperative Group developed consensus criteria for leukemias and myelodysplastic syndromes (Bennett, 1976, 1982), and lymphoma classification varied internationally. In North America, the standard lymphoma classification became the National Cancer Institute (NCI) Working Formulation for Clinical Usage (Non-Hodgkin Lymphoma Pathologic Classification Project, 1982), and in Europe, the updated Kiel Classification (Stansfeld, 1988). These were synthesized in the Revised European American Lymphoma Classification (Harris, 1995). Most recently, hematopathologists and oncologists began to recognize that uniform diagnostic criteria are essential for all hematopoietic neoplasms. The current global classification of hematopoietic tumors sponsored by the World Health Organization (WHO) (Swerdlow, 2008) recognizes the predominance of the abnormal biology of each tumor and utilizes a combination of diagnostic techniques, varying with each tumor, to arrive at the diagnosis. Morphology, immunophenotype, cytogenetics, and molecular genetics are all utilized, and cytochemical assays are used in some cases. Many tumors may present as leukemias or soft tissue tumors (lymphomas), and these terms remain descriptively useful. The WHO classification also utilizes a two-tiered approach for acute myeloid leukemias, which recognizes that in many areas of the world, molecular and cytogenetic testing is not available, and where it is available, it is not always productive. For such cases (acute myelogenous leukemia [AML], not otherwise specified), morphologic criteria are based on the earlier FAB classification.

CHRONIC MYELOPROLIFERATIVE DISORDERS

The chronic myeloproliferative disorders recognized by the WHO are chronic myeloid leukemia, BCR-ABL1–positive CML, chronic neutrophilic leukemia (CNL), polycythemia vera (PV), primary myelofibrosis (PMF), essential thrombocythemia (ET), chronic eosinophilic leukemia, not otherwise specified (NOS), mastocytosis, and myeloproliferative neoplasm, unclassifiable (Swerdlow, 2008). These are clonal proliferations of a pluripotential stem cell that can differentiate along granulocytic, erythroid, and megakaryocytic lines (Adamson, 1976; Fialkow, 1977). Each has a chronic course that may terminate as acute leukemia, myelofibrosis, or a coagulopathy. One, CML, has a characteristic genetic translocation (Nowell, 1960); another, PV, exhibits a mutation of *JAK2 V617F* that is shared with approximately 50% each of ET and PMF, while mastocytosis is characterized by *KIT* mutation. Key features of the major disorders and of myelodysplastic/myeloproliferative diseases are summarized in Table 33-12.

Chronic Myelogenous Leukemia

Clinical Features

CML occurs in young and middle-aged adults. The age-specific incidence, however, increases markedly after 50 years of age. Onset is insidious, and the disorder may be discovered accidentally on a routine blood test. The patient may have symptoms of anemia and weight loss or simply may complain of malaise. The spleen enlarges progressively, and the patient begins to lose weight and have fever and night sweats associated with increased metabolism as a result of granulocyte turnover. The discomfort associated with an enlarged spleen may bring the patient to the doctor. Infarcts in the spleen may produce left upper quadrant pain. Excessive bleeding or bruising may occur in the later stages of the disease. Lymphadenopathy, although often present, is rarely prominent (Cortes, 2004).

Laboratory Features

Blood. The leukocyte count is usually over 5×10^9/L and may exceed 30×10^9/L. The differential count is characteristic. There is a complete spectrum of granulocytic cells, from a few myeloblasts to mature neutrophils, with myelocytes and neutrophils exceeding the other cell types (Savage, 1997). This bimodal distribution helps to exclude other myeloproliferative disorders and reactive leukocytosis (see Fig. 33-12). Myeloblasts account for less than 10% of the cells. The relative percentage of neutrophil myelocytes increases as the total leukocyte count increases. Basophilia is consistently present and eosinophilia is almost always noted, along with the presence of eosinophil myelocytes. Monocytes are also absolutely increased in most patients.

Normocytic anemia is present in the majority of patients at diagnosis, and a few normoblasts can usually be found. Thrombocytosis is present in more than half, and less than 15% have thrombocytopenia.

Marrow. The marrow is markedly hypercellular, primarily as a result of granulocytic proliferation, with all stages represented. Eosinophil and basophil precursors are usually increased. Normoblasts tend to be relatively decreased. Frequently, the marrow cannot be aspirated because of the density of cellularity or (especially later in the disease) because of increased reticulin, which can be demonstrated on marrow biopsy. Macrophages laden with blue pigment (sea-blue histiocytes) or macrophages indistinguishable from Gaucher's cells are found in some patients.

It is good to remember that even a typical BM is not diagnostic of CML. On the other hand, the diagnosis can be made from the peripheral blood film in most cases.

Neutrophil Alkaline Phosphatase. The neutrophil alkaline phosphatase (NAP) is greatly reduced or absent in more than 90% of patients with CML. It is greatly elevated in polycythemia vera; elevated, normal, or low in idiopathic myelofibrosis; and normal or elevated in leukemoid reactions. During remission of CML with a normal-appearing blood picture, in most cases the NAP continues to be low; in about one third of patients, it returns to normal. The NAP increases in the accelerated and blastic phases of the disease. It may also increase in response to infection, as it does in normal individuals.

Cytogenetic Abnormalities. In more than 95% of patients with typical CML, cultured cells from the blood or bone marrow possess the cytogenetic abnormality t(9;22)(q34;q11), involving the *ABL1* gene on the long arm of chromosome 9 and the *BCR* gene on the long arm of chromosome 22. An abnormally small chromosome formed by this translocation is called the Philadelphia (Ph′) chromosome (Nowell, 1960). The *BCR-ABL1* gene fusion results in a novel RNA transcript and subsequently a protein growth factor with tyrosine kinase activity higher than that of the normal p145 protein coded for by *ABL1*. Variant translocations involving additional genes and cryptic translocations requiring molecular detection occur. Most translocations involve a *BCR* breakpoint at the major breakpoint region (M-BCR) with resultant p210 protein, and an occasional breakpoint at the μ region results in a p230 protein. Minor breakpoint region (m-BCR) translocations with resultant p190 protein are usually associated with acute lymphoblastic leukemia (ALL), but rare m-BCR translocations in CML are associated with increased monocytosis, and small amounts of p190 may be found in standard CML (Vardiman, 2008).

Other Findings. Serum cobalamin and transcobalamins are usually increased considerably as a result of increased transcobalamin I, and are thought to reflect the size of the total blood granulocyte pool. Serum muramidase (lysozyme) is also increased.

Course

Treatment with busulfan or hydroxycarbamide (hydroxyurea) in the past usually controlled the disease in the chronic phase, but without hematologic BM remission or clearing of the Ph′ chromosome. Improved results were obtained with recombinant interferon-α or allogeneic transplant (Silver, 1999). A synthetic protein kinase inhibitor, STI-571 (imatinib mesylate; Gleevec), specifically targets the BCR-ABL protein and, along with newer analogous inhibitors, provides remarkably improved results. This treatment usually results in clinical remission, although drug resistance and relapses occur (Kantarjian, 2010).

Except for those cases cured by transplantation, the disease changes after a variable period, depending in part on therapy, into a more aggressive or accelerated phase (Cortes, 2003). This is characterized by one or more features of progressive myeloproliferation: increased blood or marrow blasts of 10%–19%; peripheral blood basophilia >20%; persistent thrombocytopenia unrelated to therapy $<100 \times 10^9$/L; thrombocytosis $>1000 \times 10^9$/L; increasing leukocytosis and splenomegaly unresponsive to

TABLE 33-12

Key Features of Major Myeloproliferative and Myelodysplastic/Myeloproliferative Disease

Disorder	Demographics	Laboratory features, morphology	Cytogenetics	Prognosis
CML	Middle-aged	*BCR-ABL* present	t(9:22)(q34;q11) *BCR-ABL1*	Dependent on response to TKI
PV	Middle-aged, M > F	Major criteria: Hb >18.5 g/dL in M or >16.5 g/dL; *JAK2 V617F* Minor criteria: hypercellular marrow with panmyelosis; ↓EPO; endogenous erythroid colony formation in vitro; 2 major plus 1 minor, or first major plus 2 minor criteria	*JAK2 V617F,* negative t(9;22)	10–20 years
PMF	>50 years	Major criteria: megakaryocyte proliferation/atypia with marrow fibrosis; CML, PV, MDS ruled out; *JAK2 V617F* Minor criteria: leukoerythroblastosis, ↑LD, anemia, splenomegaly; all 3 major plus 2 minor criteria	+8, +9, del(20q), del(13q), del(1p), negative t(9;22)	Dependent on phase: ≈10 years in early prefibrotic phase; ≈5 years in fibrotic phase
ET	5th decade (M = F), second peak in 30s (F > M)	Platelet count >450 K; BM with proliferation of mature megakaryocytes; PV, PMF, CML, MDS ruled out; *JAK2 V617F* NOTE: All four criteria must be met.	*JAK2 V617F* in 50%; del(13q22), +8, +9 seen in 5%–10% of cases; negative t(9;22)	Stable for many years (most cases)
CMML	Median, 65–75 years, M > F	Monocytosis >1000, cytopenias, myeloid dysplasias, <20% blasts	+8, −7, 12p abn in 20%–40% of cases; negative t(9;22)	20–40 months with progression to AML in 15%–30%
JMML	Younger than 3 years, M > F	Monocytosis >1000, blasts <20%, plus 2 of ↑Hb F, immature grans, WBC >10K, clonal abn, GM-CSF hypersensitivity	Monosomy 7, negative t(9;22)	Poor; possible benefit from BMT
Myeloid/lymphoid neoplasms w/↑eos and *PDGFR/ FGFR1*	M 25–55 years	PB w/inc eos, BM eos with mast cells	*FIP1L1-PDGFRA, PDGFRB, FGFR*	Variable response to TKI
Mastocytosis	All ages	Mononuclear w/central nuclei, variable basophilic granules (often not seen in fixed tissue); dense aggregates of spindle cells	*KIT D816V*	Cutaneous, indolent; systemic, variable; leukemia, aggressive
CEL NOS, idiopathic HES	Usually adult M; any age or sex	PB ≥1.5 K eos/µL, <20% blasts	+8, i(17q) 8p11 w/various partners	Indolent, 80% 5-year survival

Abn, Abnormalities; *AML,* acute myelogenous leukemia; *BM,* bone marrow; *BMT,* bone marrow transplant; *CEL,* chronic eosinophilic leukemia; *CIM,* chronic idiopathic myelofibrosis; *CML,* chronic myeloid leukemia; *CMML,* chronic myelomonocytic leukemia; *eos,* eosinophils; *EPO,* erythropoietin; *ET,* essential thrombocythemia; *F,* female; *GM-CSF,* granulocyte-macrophage colony stimulating factor; *grans,* granulocytes; *Hb,* hemoglobin; *HES,* hypereosinophilic syndrome; *inc,* increased; *JMML,* juvenile myelomonocytic leukemia; *LD,* lactate dehydrogenase; *M,* male; *MDS,* myelodysplastic syndrome; *NAP,* neutrophil alkaline phosphatase; *NOS,* not otherwise specified; *PB,* peripheral blood; *PMF,* primary myelofibrosis; *PV,* polycythemia vera; *TKI,* tyrosine kinase inhibitor; *WBC,* white blood cell.

therapy; or cytogenetic clonal evolution. Granulocytic dysplasia, increased small dysplastic megakaryocytes, and reticulin fibrosis are also suggestive.

Blast phase is essentially a progression to acute leukemia and is defined by >20% blasts in the blood or BM and large aggregates of blasts in the marrow or in extramedullary locations. Blast lineage is myeloid in 70% of cases and may include any myeloid cell types (neutrophilic, eosinophilic, basophilic, monocytic, erythroid, or megakaryocytic), although Auer rods are rarely found. In approximately one third of cases, however, the appearance is that of ALL (Rosenthal, 1977). Usually, these are of precursor B-lineage, with expression of terminal deoxyribonucleotidyl transferase (TdT), CD34, CD19, and CD10 but negative surface Ig. Occasional cases are precursor T-lineage with TdT, CD3, cytoplasmic CD3 (cCD3), and CD7. Myeloid antigens are often coexpressed, and bilineal myeloid/lymphoid cases also occur. Blast transformation appears because of secondary genetic changes involving *p53*, retinoblastoma *(Rb)*, and other genes (Calabretta, 2004).

Chronic Neutrophilic Leukemia

Chronic neutrophilic leukemia is a rare myeloproliferative disorder characterized by persistent and unexplained neutrophilia of >25 × 10^9/L mature granulocytes resembling reactive neutrophilia (Elliott, 2001; Bain, 2008). It typically affects older adults and presents with splenomegaly and sometimes hepatomegaly, often with mucocutaneous bleeding, pruritus, or gout. There may be a left shift with bands present and toxic granulation. BM findings include hypercellularity with granulocytic hyperplasia showing a myeloid/erythroid ratio of up to 20 : 1 and a predominance of mature neutrophils to myelocytes. Erythroid cellularity and megakaryocytes may be increased, but dysplasia is not present. Cytogenetics are usually (90%) normal, with some cases showing abnormalities including +8, +9, del(20q), and del(11q). Cases with variant Ph′-positive chromosome and neutrophilia are considered CML.

Because there is not a genetic marker for this disease, it is likely that many of these are reactive processes due to occult malignancy or other causes of inflammation. Multiple myeloma has most often been implicated, but other neoplasms may induce marked neutrophilia with or without marrow involvement.

Polycythemia Vera

Polycythemia vera is a clonal stem cell proliferation affecting primarily the erythroid series, characterized by excessive proliferation of erythroid and also usually granulocytic and megakaryocytic elements in the marrow (panmyelosis). It is genetically characterized by mutation of Janus 2 kinase, *JAK2V617F,* or another functionally similar mutation such as *JAK2* exon 12 mutation (Levine, 2008). *JAK2* mutation occurs in essentially all patients with PV but is also present in approximately 50% of patients with thrombocythemia and primary myelofibrosis. The disease is manifested in the blood by an absolute increase in red cell mass, leukocytosis, and thrombocytosis. Serum and urine erythropoietin are decreased. The production of erythrocytes is autonomous with **endogenous erythroid colonies**

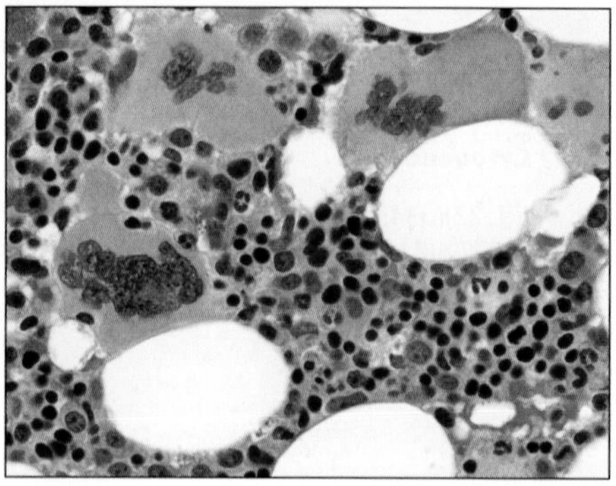

Figure 33-13 Bone marrow biopsy in polycythemia vera shows panmyelosis with normoblastic hyperplasia (×500).

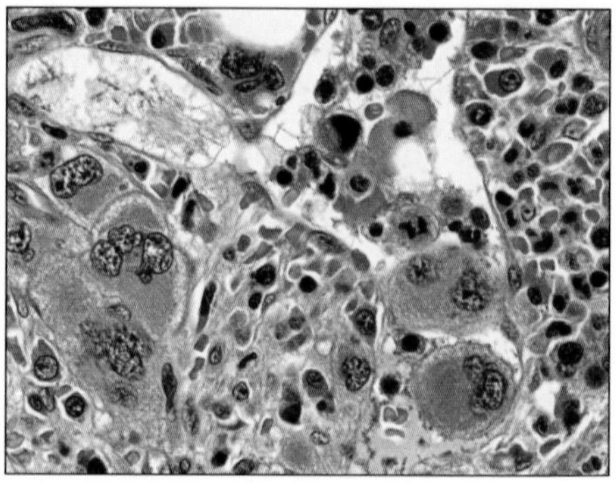

Figure 33-14 Bone marrow biopsy in chronic idiopathic myelofibrosis, with increased spacing between cells suggesting fibrosis and intrasinusoidal hematopoiesis (×500).

(EECs) growing in vitro without erythropoietin, but it does respond to erythropoietin when the patient has become anemic through blood loss (Pierre, 2001). Pathology may be related to decreased expression of the thrombopoietin receptor c-Mpl (Kaushansky, 2003), and overexpression of the polycythemia rubra vera-1 messenger RNA (Pahl, 2004). There is initially a proliferative phase and eventually a spent phase with anemia, marrow fibrosis, increased splenomegaly, and extramedullary hematopoiesis.

Clinical Features

The disease is slightly more frequent in men than in women. It usually begins in middle age. Affected patients exhibit ruddy cyanosis, and splenomegaly is present in two thirds. Thrombotic or hemorrhagic phenomena occur in about half of patients, and thrombosis is most common (Chomienne, 2004). Myocardial infarction, cerebral thrombosis, splenic or pulmonary infarcts, and thrombophlebitis account for the most frequent thrombotic episodes; upper gastrointestinal bleeding, often from peptic ulcer, is the most common bleeding problem. Pruritus, especially after bathing, is common.

Laboratory Features

Blood. Erythrocytes exceed $6–12 \times 10^{12}$/L, and the hemoglobin is >18.5 g/dL (males) or >16.5 g/dL (females). Mean cell volume (MCV), mean cell hemoglobin (MCH), and mean cell hemoglobin concentration (MCHC) are normal or low. The erythrocytes become hypochromic and microcytic if chronic blood loss has occurred. Macrocytes, polychromatic cells, and normoblasts may be found but are not a prominent feature of the disease. Red cell production is increased. Red cell destruction is normal during the period of erythrocytosis; later in the disease, as splenomegaly develops, red cell survival diminishes. The total blood volume is increased, primarily because of increased red cell mass, and the plasma volume may also be elevated to a lesser degree. Blood viscosity is high, and it may be difficult to prepare good blood films. The erythrocyte sedimentation rate (ESR) is reduced.

The platelet count is increased in about two thirds of patients, often to levels exceeding 1000×10^9/L. In 80% of untreated patients, functional platelet abnormalities are present (Gilbert, 1975) with decreased aggregation in response to adenosine diphosphate (ADP) and epinephrine. Functional defects may be related to decreased expression of c-Mpl on platelets (Moliterno, 1998), although megakaryocytes are increased (Bock, 2004). No consistent abnormality of secondary hemostasis is present.

Moderate neutrophilic leukocytosis in the range of $10–30 \times 10^9$/L is common. Immature granulocytes are seen in about one half of cases, and basophils are often absolutely increased. The NAP is markedly elevated in 80% of patients, and serum transcobalamins and serum muramidase are usually elevated.

The arterial oxygen saturation is normal. Hyperuricemia appears in many patients with PV as a result of increased nucleic acid metabolism; in some patients, secondary gout or renal uric acid stones occur.

Marrow. The marrow is moderately to markedly hypercellular, with prominent normoblastic erythroid hyperplasia in panmyelosis. Megakaryocytes show an increase in and clustering of variable small and large megakaryocytes associated with an increase in dilated sinuses (Michiels, 1997) and frequently cluster around sinusoids (Fig. 33-13). Increased reticulin is often present, and storage iron is decreased or absent in 95% of cases.

Diagnosis

Criteria of the WHO (Swerdlow, 2008) for the diagnosis of polycythemia vera are as follows:

1. Elevated Hb >18.5 (males) or 16.5 (females) g/dL, or other evidence of increased red cell volume.
2. Presence of *JAK2 B617F* or similar mutation such as *JAK2* exon 12 mutation.

Both of these major criteria must be present, along with any single minor criterion: BM biopsy showing panmyelosis with prominent erythroid and megakaryocytic proliferation, low serum erythropoietin, or endogenous colony formation in vitro. Alternatively, the diagnosis may be made by the first major and two minor criteria.

Polycythemia vera is a chronic disease; patients usually live 10–20 years under good control. Phlebotomy, chlorambucil, radioactive phosphorus (^{32}P), and hydroxycarbamide (hydroxyurea) have been used to control the manifestations of the disease.

In about 20%–40% of patients, the spent or postpolycythemic phase occurs with progressive anemia, gradual splenic enlargement, and further elevation of the leukocyte count, with more immature granulocytes and more circulating nucleated red cells. Many erythrocytes become oval, and teardrop cells (dacryocytes) become prominent. BM aspiration becomes impossible because of myelofibrosis, and splenomegaly increases, owing to extramedullary hematopoiesis. Manifestations at this stage of the disease are indistinguishable from those of myelofibrosis with myeloid metaplasia. Another late complication of polycythemia vera is acute leukemia or myelodysplastic syndrome (MDS) (Landaw, 1986). A slight increase, 2%–3%, is seen in patients treated with phlebotomy alone, and a greater increase (10%) is seen in those treated with cytotoxic agents.

Primary Myelofibrosis

This is a chronic, progressive clonal panmyelosis characterized by megakaryocytic and often granulocytic hyperplasia with varying degrees of reactive fibrosis of the marrow and extramedullary hematopoiesis (Swerdlow, 2008). Typically, leukoerythroblastic anemia occurs with marked red cell abnormalities, circulating normoblasts, immature granulocytes, and atypical platelets. Chronic idiopathic myelofibrosis (CIM) is an uncommon disease with an incidence one-third that of CML. It occurs typically in persons over the age of 50 and has an insidious onset, with weight loss, anemia, and abdominal discomfort due to the large spleen. Often the liver is enlarged as well, and the patient may be slightly jaundiced. Radiograph shows patchy osteosclerosis in up to half of patients, but osteoporosis may also be seen.

A prefibrotic stage in 20%–30% of cases is characterized by mild normocytic anemia with poikilocytosis, including dacryocytes, nucleated RBCs, thrombocytosis, and mild leukocytosis with some immature forms. The marrow is hypercellular and contains abnormal megakaryocytes, which cluster around sinuses and trabeculae. The histopathology of the BM is dominated by atypical, enlarged, and immature megakaryocytes with cloud-like immature nuclei (Michiels, 1999), and also small megakaryocytes. Fibrosis may be minimal initially. Intrasinusoidal hematopoiesis is often present (Fig. 33-14).

Characteristic findings of presentation in the fibrotic stage include moderate normochromic, normocytic anemia (often with some hypochromic cells and basophilic stippling), moderate anisocytosis, and marked poikilocytosis, including prominent teardrop forms (dacryocytes) and elliptocytes. Normoblasts are often increased out of proportion to the degree of anemia with slight reticulocytosis. The anemia may have a complicated origin, with components of marrow failure, ineffective erythropoiesis, and hemolysis. Splenomegaly due to extramedullary hematopoiesis is typical.

The leukocyte count is moderately increased; immature neutrophils and occasionally myeloblasts are present. Basophils are often increased. Platelets are normal or decreased in number (rarely increased) and often atypical with distinct clear "zones." Micromegakaryocytes the size of lymphocytes with both nucleus and cytoplasm or small megakaryoblasts may usually be found if searched for; on rare occasions, they are present in considerable numbers.

In vitro blood cell culture shows increased colonies (CFU-GM) similar to those in CML. Serum GM-CSF is high, serum uric acid is frequently increased, and cobalamin is normal or elevated.

It is usually impossible to aspirate marrow, and biopsy is necessary. The marrow is fibrotic, with residual islands of atypical megakaryocytes, erythroid, and granulocytic precursors. The fibrosis is of loose connective tissue with scanty collagen, but reticulin fibers are abundant. Foci of osteoid and/or new bone formation in endophytic plaques (Thiele, 2001b) may be found, and bony trabeculae may be irregularly thickened (myelosclerosis). The marrow may show a mixture of hyperplasia and fibrosis in one sample or may vary in different sites of the body. Megakaryocytes with abnormal nuclei cluster or form sheets which may be found in sinuses with other marrow precursors. Extramedullary hematopoiesis is found in the spleen and liver.

Biology

Although the proliferating megakaryocytes are neoplastic, the stromal proliferation is reactive because of inappropriate release of megakaryocyte/platelet-derived growth factors, including platelet-derived growth factor (PDGF), transforming growth factor (TGF)-β, basic fibroblast growth factor (bFGF) and calmodulin (Reilly, 1998).

Approximately 50% of patients show *JAK2 V617F* mutation. A small number, up to 5%, have an *MPL W515K/L* gene mutation. Chromosomal studies show absence of *BCR/ABL*, but variable cytogenetic changes: +8, +9, del(20q), del(13q)(q12-22), partial trisomy 1q, del(5q), and der(6)t(1;6)(q21-23;p21.3). Additional cytogenetic abnormalities may be associated with cytotoxic therapy and/or progression of disease.

Course

The natural course is increasing fibrosis with progressive anemia and enlargement of the spleen. Hemolysis frequently becomes an increasing element in the anemia, and infection may be a serious problem. Portal hypertension occurs in 10%–20% of cases and may result in bleeding esophageal varices. Hypertension may be due to portal vein thrombosis or intrahepatic obstruction as a result of myeloid metaplasia coupled with increased portal blood flow.

Androgen preparations, corticosteroids, and erythropoietin are helpful in control of anemia (Tefferi, 2003). Median survival has been about 5 years—considerably less than that of polycythemia vera; however, some patients live longer, and in those patients, the terminal event is frequently an acute leukemia. Recent therapeutic advances with durable remission of cytopenias have been reported with thalidomide and prednisone (Mesa, 2004). Hydroxyurea is used in patients who require control of excess myeloproliferation.

Occasionally, patients exhibit cytopenias and marrow fibrosis due to other causes, some of which may show favorable response to specific therapies. These include metastatic tumors, primary hematopoietic tumors such as HCL or plasma cell dyscrasia (Meerkin, 1994), damage from radiation, and rarely autoimmune myelofibrosis (Hasselbalch, 1987; Pullarkat, 2003). Malnourished children with vitamin D deficiency (rickets) sometimes show myelofibrosis. A role of solvents in myelofibrosis has been postulated (Brandt, 1987) but is not clear or well documented; neither is it known whether solvent-associated cases are neoplastic or secondary myelofibrosis. Benzene has been most often suspected and is a known inducer of AML at threshold levels of exposure. General environmental exposure appears much lower than that likely to be associated with hematologic malignancies (Duarte-Davidson, 2001). Peritrabecular marrow fibrosis occurs in primary hyperparathyroidism or secondary hyperparathyroidism of chronic renal failure.

Essential Thrombocythemia

Thrombocythemia is a clonal myeloproliferative disorder primarily affecting the megakaryocytic lineage with the principal manifestation of sustained thrombocytosis. Forty percent to 50% carry a *JAK2 V617F* mutation (Levine, 2008). It most often occurs in the fifth decade, with equal sex distribution and a second peak of incidence in females in their 30s (Thiele, 2008a).

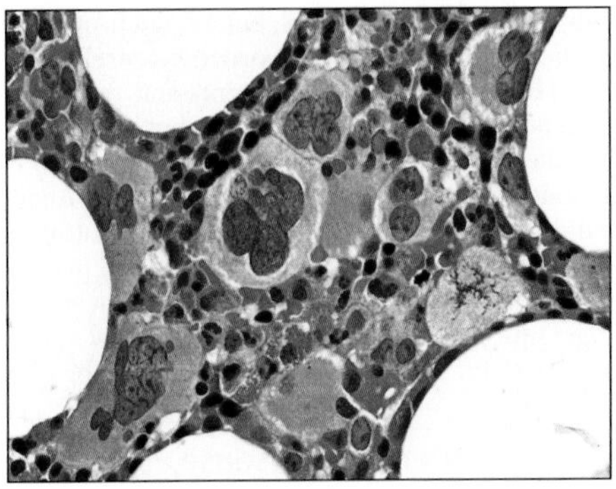

Figure 33-15 Bone marrow biopsy in essential thrombocythemia, with increased and clustered megakaryocytes (×500). Nuclei in this case are unusual, resembling primary myelofibrosis.

Clinical Features

Patients often (50%) present with asymptomatic thrombocytosis, but up to half of patients present with hemorrhage or thrombosis. The latter occurs as arterial or venous thrombosis or as microvascular occlusion resulting in transient ischemic attacks (TIAs) or digital ischemia. Characteristic recurrent, spontaneous mucosal hemorrhages are most common in the GI tract or the upper airway. Hemorrhages are occasionally preceded or accompanied by thrombosis. Mild splenomegaly occurs in 50% of cases.

Laboratory Features

Blood. The most striking feature is the marked increase in platelets (≥450 × 10^9/L; usually >1000 × 10^9/L), often with abnormal and giant forms, and usually accompanied by fragments of megakaryocytes. Neutrophilic leukocytosis is sometimes present. Hypochromic microcytic anemia due to chronic blood loss is present in many cases. Platelet function defects in thrombocythemia are frequently demonstrable. The most typical finding is decreased aggregation in response to epinephrine.

Marrow. The marrow shows increased and enlarged megakaryocytes with mature cytoplasm and multilobulated nuclei and a tendency to cluster in a normal or only slightly hypercellular BM (Michiels, 1999) (Fig. 33-15). Megakaryocyte nuclei are not described as atypical but often are distinctive and resemble other myeloproliferative disorders (MPDs). Erythroid proliferation may be present secondary to blood loss. Biopsy features may be indistinguishable from those of PV, but usually with less erythroid prominence. Splenic extramedullary hematopoiesis may be present.

Cultured marrow typically shows in vitro spontaneous colony formation of megakaryocytes and also erythroid colonies (Niittyvuopio, 2004). Abnormal (decreased) labeling of BM for the thrombopoietin (TPO) receptor c-Mpl may aid in separating ET from reactive thrombocytosis (Gale, 2003).

Diagnosis

Criteria of the WHO for the diagnosis of thrombocythemia are as follows (Swerdlow, 2008):

1. Sustained platelet count ≥450 × 10^9/L.
2. BM biopsy showing proliferation of mainly megakaryocytes with enlarged mature nuclei, no increase or left shift of granulopoiesis or erythropoiesis.
3. Not meeting WHO criteria for polycythemia vera, PMF, BCR-ABL1–positive CML, MDS, or other myeloid neoplasm.
4. Demonstration of *JAK2 V617F* mutation or, in its absence, no evidence of reactive thrombocytosis.

Genetics

Forty percent to 50% of cases carry a *JAK2 V617F* mutation. BCR/ABL translocations must be ruled out to exclude CML. Ph′-positive thrombocytosis is likely an early form of CML and differs morphologically by lack of the characteristic large clustered megakaryocytes (Michiels, 2004). Some cases show +8 abnormalities of 9q or del(20q) (Swerdlow, 2008). Other abnormalities such as del(5q) or abnormalities of 3q21q26.2 suggest MDS with thrombocytosis.

PART 4

Most cases are stable for many years, but a small proportion may merge into other chronic myeloproliferative disorders or, rarely, may develop into acute leukemia. Historically, alkylating agents and radiophosphorus have been used to treat essential thrombocythemia, but these were complicated by secondary leukemias. Hydroxycarbamide (hydroxyurea) has been used more recently, but it too has leukemogenic potential. Anagrelide is currently in use and is considered more safe and reliable (Silverstein, 1999). Development of erythrocytosis with increased red cell mass raises the possibility of polycythemia vera, and there is some crossover between the two entities. Endogenous erythroid colony formation may allow early identification of cases at risk for PV (Griesshammer, 2004). Fibrosis rarely occurs.

Chronic Myeloproliferative Disease, Unclassifiable

Chronic myeloproliferative disease, unclassifiable (CMPD, U) includes disorders with features of MPD but which do not meet criteria for a specific entity or have intermediate features (Swerdlow, 2008). Examples of CMPD, U include prefibrotic CIM, prepolycythemic PV, and postpolycythemic PV (without prior diagnosis), as well as cases with features of MPD but presenting with some dysplasia or increased blasts. BCR/ABL and other specific cytogenetic abnormalities are absent. This category overlaps with myelodysplastic/myeloproliferative disease, unclassifiable. Often, with follow-up, characteristic findings develop which allow definite diagnosis (Swerdlow, 2008).

Chronic Eosinophilic Leukemia, Not Otherwise Specified, and Idiopathic Hypereosinophilic Syndrome

Chronic eosinophilic leukemia (CEL) is a clonal proliferation of eosinophils with a chronic increase in the blood and often organ damage due to tissue infiltration. The blood contains $\geq 1.5 \times 10^9/L$ mostly mature eosinophils and often increased but less than 20% blasts in the blood or marrow. If blasts are not increased, if there is no evidence of underlying cause or monoclonality, or if organ involvement or dysfunction occurs and eosinophilia has persisted at least 6 months, the term idiopathic hypereosinophilic syndrome may be used. HES is, however, a diagnosis of exclusion (see Fig. 33-8), and causes of reactive eosinophilia must be ruled out. The differential diagnosis of reactive processes includes parasitic infection, Löffler's syndrome, cyclic eosinophilia, cutaneous angiolymphoid hyperplasia, Kimura's disease, autoimmune disease including vasculitides, and granulomatous disease. Neoplasms, including T cell lymphoma, HL, systemic mastocytosis, acute leukemias, and myeloproliferative diseases, are often causes of secondary eosinophilia due to cytokine production (IL-2, IL-3, IL-5, GM-CSF) or, in some cases, clonal involvement of the eosinophil series. When associated with a defined CMD, the eosinophilia is considered a component of that disease and is not termed CEL. Myeloproliferative diseases with eosinophilia and *PDGFRA*, *PDGFRB*, or *FGFR1* gene abnormalities are classified separately.

Some cases of CEL have clonal cytogenetic abnormalities, such as +8, i(17q), or 8p11 translocations, including t(8;13)(p11;q12), t(8;9)(p11;q32-34), and t(6;8)(q27;p11). The 8p11 translocation may also occur in AML, precursor acute lymphoblastic leukemia of B-lineage (B-ALL), or precursor ALL of T-lineage (T-ALL). Other abnormalities, including *JAK2 V617F* mutation and trisomy 10, may occur (Swerdlow, 2008). The clinical outcome of CEL and HES is usually indolent with 5-year survival of about 80%.

Mastocytosis

Mastocytosis is a clonal neoplastic proliferation of mast cells involving skin, BM, lymph nodes, and/or spleen (Swerdlow, 2008), with variable degrees of malignancy. Subtypes are described based on distribution of disease and clinical manifestations. Symptoms are complex and arise from secretion of vasoactive amines, including histamine and serotonin, as well as from mass effects.

Mastocytosis is associated with mutations of the *KIT* proto-oncogene that encodes the tyrosine kinase receptor for stem cell factor (SCF), most frequently, *KIT D816V* with CD117 expression. Morphologically, increased mast cells are found in involved organs, often with associated fibrosis. Mast cells normally are mononuclear cells with central nuclei, clumped chromatin, and dense basophilic granules. They are frequently difficult to identify, however, as mast cell granules are not well preserved in fixed tissue, and cells may appear like bland clear cells, histiocytes, fibroblasts, or others. Mast cells may be identified in tissue using Giemsa or toluidine blue stain and immunohistochemistry. Mast cell tryptase is the most specific marker, but cells also express CD117, as well as CD45, CD33, CD68, CD2, and CD25. Mast cells lack myeloperoxidase but often express chloroacetate esterase. Diagnostic testing should include immunologic assays (immunohistochemistry and/or flow cytometry) for CD117, CD2, CD25, and tryptase, as well as assays for *KIT D816V* mutation in marrow, blood, or other extracutaneous organs for systemic disease.

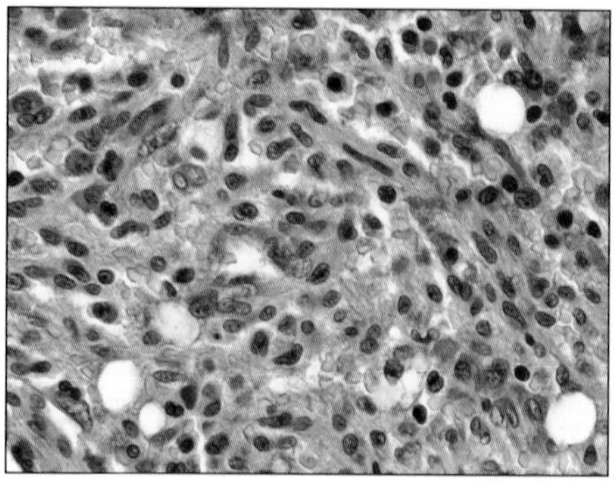

Figure 33-16 Mastocytosis in the bone marrow, presenting after treatment for acute myeloid leukemia (×500).

Urticaria with melanin pigmentation is common with skin involvement and is referred to as **urticaria pigmentosa (UP)** or **maculopapular cutaneous mastocytosis (MPCM).** This form occurs in both children and adults. In children, lesions are often large and papular, or are associated with blistering in children younger than 3 years old. It is often self-limited or may spontaneously regress. Histology shows aggregates of spindle-shaped mast cells filling the papillary dermis and extending into reticular dermis (Swerdlow, 2008). A diffuse cutaneous variant is referred to as **diffuse cutaneous mastocytosis,** and a localized variant as **mastocytoma of skin.**

Systemic mastocytosis is defined by involvement of at least one extracutaneous organ with or without skin involvement. It presents with variable cutaneous and constitutional symptoms, including urticaria, pruritus and dermatographism, symptoms of systemic histamine release, bone pain, arthralgia and fractures, splenomegaly, hepatomegaly, or lymphadenopathy.

BM involvement is sometimes difficult to identify, with paratrabecular and perivascular aggregates of increased lymphocytes, eosinophils, neutrophils, mast cells, and fibroblasts. Marrow biopsy of most cases shows multifocal, sharply demarcated compact aggregates of mast cells. These may be spindle shaped and lacking in apparent granules on H&E stain, or may consist of mixed infiltrates of mast cells, lymphocytes, eosinophils, histiocytes, and fibroblasts, with a peripheral rim or central core of lymphocytes. Compact infiltrates of hypergranular mast cells also occur and are referred to as **tryptase-positive round cell infiltrates,** or TROCI. The latter may also be seen in basophilic leukemia or acute myeloid leukemia. Mast cells are frequently increased in hematologic neoplasms such as HCL, lymphoplasmacytic lymphoma, and myeloid neoplasm and are most apparent around BM particles on aspirate smears. Reactive mast cells do not typically show compact aggregates.

In addition, systemic mastocytosis (SM) not infrequently presents simultaneously with or in close temporal relationship with other hematopoietic neoplasms, including acute leukemia, myeloproliferative and/or myelodysplastic neoplasms, and occasionally other hematopoietic neoplasia. SM is sometimes detected only after treatment for an acute process (Figs. 33-16 and 33-17). These cases are referred to as systemic mastocytosis with associated clonal non–mast cell lineage disease (SM-AHNMD). The non–mast cell (MC) disease is categorized by criteria for the same disorder without SM.

Mast cell leukemia also occurs and is defined by the presence of atypical mast cells constituting more than 20% of a marrow aspirate. More than 10% of the circulating cells are usually mast cells (Swerdlow, 2008).

Mast cell sarcoma refers to localized, destructive extramedullary tumors of highly atypical mast cells, occurring in larynx, bowel, meninges, bone, and skin. Extracutaneous mastocytoma of mature granulated mast cells occurs rarely in the lung.

The outcome is highly variable, with cutaneous disease usually indolent. In children, it usually regresses. Systemic disease without skin

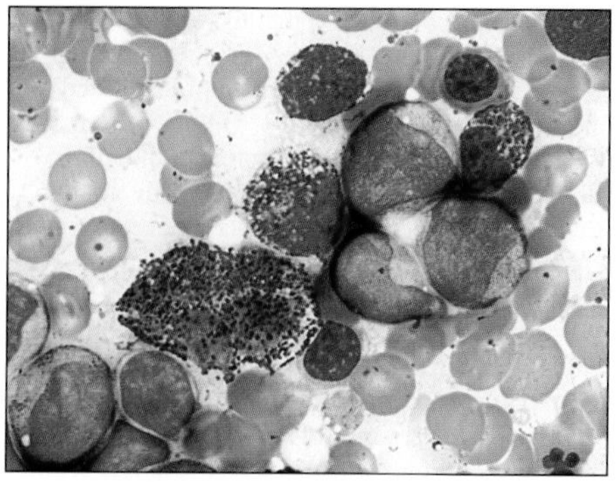

Figure 33-17 Acute leukemia with early mast cell disease before therapy (earlier specimen from case shown in Fig. 33-16) (×1000).

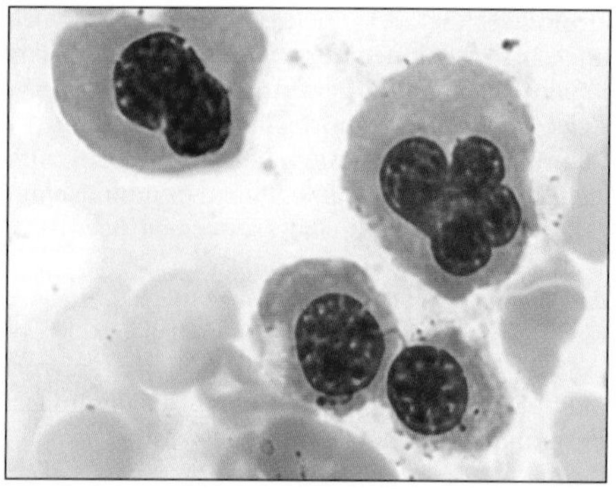

Figure 33-18 Drug-induced dyserythropoiesis, with irregular nuclear lobation in the cells above right, compared with two relatively normal normoblasts (×1000).

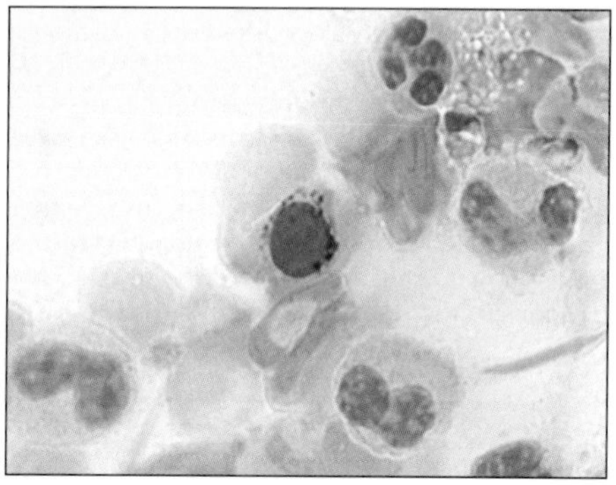

Figure 33-19 A ring sideroblast is present in the center of the field (×1000).

involvement is more aggressive than with skin disease, and mast cell leukemia and sarcoma are highly aggressive.

Myeloproliferative Neoplasm, Unclassifiable

These are disorders with features of myeloproliferative neoplasm (MPN) but which do not meet criteria for a specific entity or have intermediate features (Swerdlow, 2008). Examples of CMPD, U include prefibrotic CIM, prepolycythemic PV, and postpolycythemic PV (without prior diagnosis) cases with features of MPN but presenting with some dysplasia or increased blasts, and those with convincing evidence of MPN that is, however, obscured by a concurrent inflammatory or neoplastic condition. *BCR/ABL* and other specific cytogenetic abnormalities are absent. This category overlaps with myelodysplastic/myeloproliferative disease, unclassifiable. Often, with follow-up, characteristic findings develop which allow definitive diagnosis.

Myeloid and Lymphoid Neoplasms with Eosinophilia and Abnormalities of *PDGFRA, PDGFRB*, or *FGFR1*

This disease category was established in the 2008 WHO Classification for a group of myeloid neoplasms associated with eosinophilia that have genetic abnormalities resulting in abnormal tyrosine kinases that may be successfully treated with tyrosine kinase inhibitors, of which the prototype is imatinib. It and related drugs have been used successfully in the first two conditions listed in this group.

PDGFRA rearrangement is most often associated with a FIP1L1-PDGFRA fusion protein resulting from a cryptic deletion at 4q12. The disease usually presents as chronic eosinophilic leukemia with peripheral eosinophil counts >1.5 × 10^9/L, with multisystem involvement and organ damage. BM eosinophilia is often accompanied by increased mast cells that are considered part of the disease. It usually occurs in men between 25 and 55 years, but also may occur in others. Presentation also occurs as AML and as T-lymphoblastic lymphoma/leukemia (T-LBL). Diagnosis and appropriate therapy depend on identification of the genetic abnormality by reverse transcriptase polymerase chain reaction (RT-PCR) or by cytogenetic FISH assay for deletion of the *CHIC2* gene, or use of a break-apart probe encompassing *FIP1L1* and *PDGFRA*. Other genetic variants have been described and are generally imatinib sensitive (Swerdlow, 2008).

Rearrangement of *PDGFRB* at 5q31~33, usually due to t(5;12)(q31~33;p12) with production of *ETV6- PDGFRB*, resembles CMML with eosinophilia. Variant translocations involving *PDGFRB* may be associated with other morphologies, including CEL, MPN, and others. This disease occurs most often in middle age, but with a wide age range and a 2 : 1 M/F ratio. The morphology is similar to CMML with increased eosinophils and sometimes increased mast cells but is now classified by the genetic abnormality. The disease is sensitive to imatinib. Diagnostic testing is completed by cytogenetics to detect t(5;12) and/or by RT-PCR. Secondary trisomy 21 is frequent.

Hematologic neoplasms involving *FGFR1* at chromosome region 8p11 are heterogeneous and may present as MPN, AML, T or less often B lymphoblastic leukemia/lymphoma, or mixed phenotype acute leukemia. Eosinophilia is present in 90% of cases overall. Although an abnormal tyrosine kinase is produced, it is not imatinib sensitive, and no specific inhibitor is yet described. The genetic abnormalities are most often translocations and karyotyping may be diagnostic. Prognosis is poor.

Myelodysplastic and Myelodysplastic/Myeloproliferative Neoplasms

Myeloproliferative diseases, in general, are disorders in which proliferation of hematopoietic cells outpaces apoptosis, and cellular elements in the blood are increased while the morphology of hematopoiesis is near normal. Myelodysplastic diseases or syndromes are disorders in which apoptosis predominates, hematopoiesis is ineffective, and cytopenias occur. The myelodysplastic/myeloproliferative disorders show features of both, with variable increases in cells, as well as cytopenias and morphologic dysplasia. These include chronic myelomonocytic leukemia, atypical chronic myeloid leukemia, *BCR-ABL1*–negative, juvenile chronic myelomonocytic leukemia, and myelodysplastic/myeloproliferative neoplasm, unclassifiable.

MDS occurs primarily in persons over age 50 and usually present as an anemia refractory to hematinics, with or without neutropenia and thrombocytopenia. Liver, spleen, or lymph nodes are not usually enlarged. The marrow is hypercellular with abnormal maturation in one or more of the three hematopoietic cell lines, and blast cells are often increased. This group of disorders has also been called dysmyelopoietic syndromes or **preleukemias** because of the high proportion of cases that ultimately progress to overt acute leukemia. The FAB Cooperative Group (Bennett 1976, 1982) described and classified these disorders, and their nomenclature remains useful with certain modification, per the WHO classification (Swerdlow, 2008). A scoring system for predicting survival and risk of acute leukemic transformation has been developed based on percentage of blasts, cytogenetics, and extent of cytopenias. In general, blast count >5% elevates risk and >10% increases risk further; complex chromosomal abnormalities or chromosome 7 abnormalities are high risk; del(5q), isolated del(2q), -Y, and normal cytogenetics are low risk; other cytogenetic findings are intermediate risk; and more than one cytopenia increases risk.

Types of Abnormal Cellular Maturation

Dyserythropoiesis resembles megaloblastic change and includes nuclear fragmentation or karyorrhexis, multinuclearity, nuclear budding or bridging, basophilic stippling, and ring sideroblasts (Bennett, 1986). These features may also be seen in toxicity due to drugs, chemotherapy, heavy metals, alcohol, and other toxins (Swerdlow, 2008) (Figs. 33-18 and 33-19). Erythroid cells may be decreased or increased in number. Erythrocytic abnormalities in the blood film include presence of oval macrocytes, anisochromia, basophilic stippling, dacryocytes, and reticulocytopenia.

Dysgranulopoiesis includes nuclear/cytoplasmic asynchrony, hypogranulation, nuclear hyposegmentation with increased chromatin condensation, occasionally abnormal large azurophilic granules, inappropriately prominent nucleoli, or other abnormalities. Neutrophil precursors and monocytes often resemble one another. Neutrophils with mature chromatin but with decreased granulation and bilobed or unilobed nuclei resemble the cells of Pelger-Huët anomaly and are termed **pseudo Pelger-Huët** cells (Figs. 33-20 and 33-21).

Dysmegakaryocytopoiesis includes large megakaryocytes with unsegmented nuclei, micromegakaryocytes, and megakaryocytes with two or more small, unconnected nuclei (Fig. 33-22). Megakaryocytes may be decreased in number. In the blood film, giant hypogranular platelets are frequent, and micromegakaryocytes are seen rarely.

Myelodysplastic/Myeloproliferative Neoplasms

Chronic Myelomonocytic Leukemia

CMML is a clonal stem cell disorder in which the predominant feature is persistent monocytosis (>1 × 10^9/L for longer than 3 months) for which other causes have been excluded (Swerdlow, 2008). Typically, cytopenias are present in the blood (anemia, thrombocytopenia, and/or neutropenia), but neutrophilia with morphologic abnormalities also occurs. There is absence of a Philadelphia chromosome or *BCR/ABL*, dysplasia of one or more myeloid lineages, and less than 20% blasts plus promonocytes in the marrow (Fig. 33-23). The marrow also shows monocytosis and often has increased promonocytes, which may be distinguished from abnormal myelocytes by nonspecific esterase (α-napthyl acetate, or α-napthyl butyrate esterase) staining or strong labeling with antilysozyme or CD68. Eosinophilia or basophilia may be present, and plasmacytoid-appearing monocytes are seen frequently. When eosinophils exceed 1.5 × 10^9/L, the WHO recommends the subcategory of CMML with eosinophilia.

In CMML and also in the acute myeloid leukemias with monocytic differentiation, promonocytes are considered equivalent to blasts and are included with them for determining the blast percentage. Promonocytes are monocytic precursors which have recognizable monocyte morphology but immature chromatin and finely convoluted or cerebriform nuclei (Fig. 33-24). Blast percentages typically are <5% in the blood and <10% in the marrow, and such cases are referred to as CMML-1. The subcategory CMML-2 refers to cases with 5%–19% blasts in the blood, with 10%–19% in the marrow, or with the presence of Auer rods. This indicates aggressive disease with likely impending transformation to acute leukemia.

The immunophenotype is CD13/CD33+, with variable CD14/CD68/CD64/CD4-positive. Plasmacytoid monocytes may be seen and may express CD14, CD43, CD56, CD68, and CD4, with variable CD2/CD5. Cytogenetic abnormalities in 20%–40% of cases include +8, -7/del, and abnormalities of 12p.

CMML occurs most often at older age (median, 65–75 years) with a male predominance. Symptoms are usually those related to cytopenias (fatigue, infection, bleeding) or hypermetabolic state (fever, weight loss, night sweats). Hepatosplenomegaly may be present, particularly in patients with elevated WBCs. Lymphadenopathy may be associated with granulocytic sarcoma and evolution to acute leukemia. Median survival is 20–30 months, with progression to AML in 15%–30%.

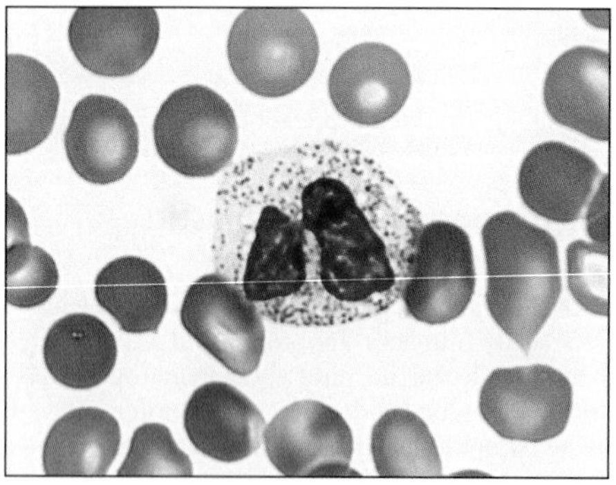

Figure 33-20 Pseudo–Pelger-Huët neutrophil (×1000).

Atypical Chronic Myeloid Leukemia, BCR-ABL1 Negative

This disease shows myelodysplastic and myeloproliferative features, a predominant component of increased neutrophils and precursors with dysplastic features, and dysplasia of other cell lines (Swerdlow, 2008). Ph′ chromosome or BCR/ABL is absent. These cases were previously considered along with CML or CMML, but they are Ph′ chromosome and BCR/ABL negative, and, although monocytosis is often present, it is less prominent than neutrophilia. Clinical features may include anemia, thrombocytopenia, or splenomegaly. The marrow is hypercellular with variable features of each lineage. A variant, "syndrome of abnormal chromatin clumping," shows exaggerated chromatin condensation, as well as other dysplastic features.

Cytogenetics show +8, +13, del(20q), i(17q), or del(12p) in up to 80% of cases. There is no *BCR-ABL1* fusion gene, and cases with *PDGFRA* or *PDGFRB* rearrangements are excluded. This disease usually occurs in later

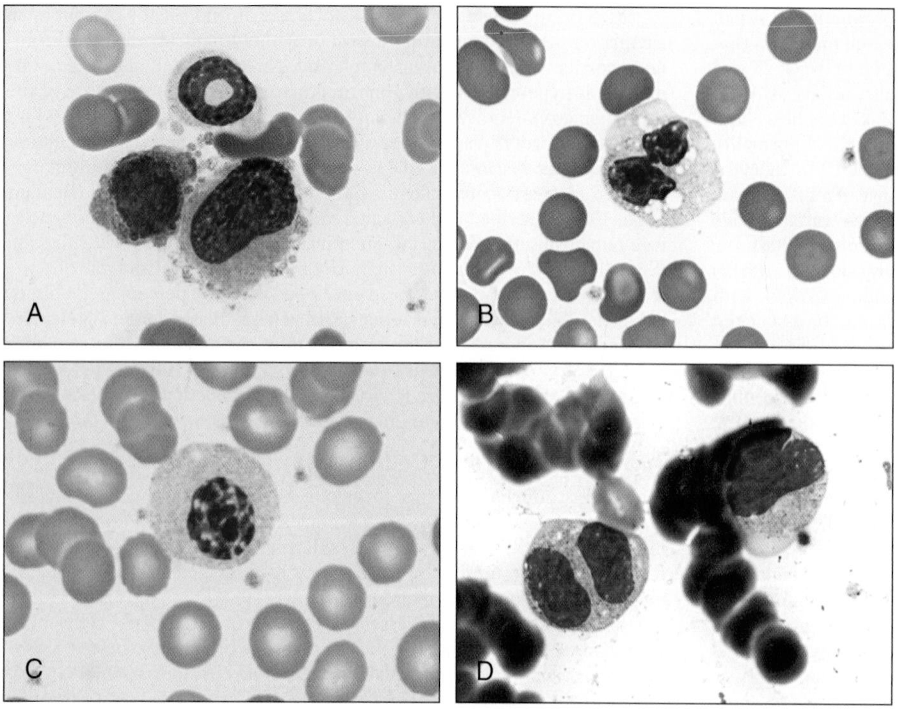

Figure 33-21 Other forms of neutrophil dysplasia. **A,** Ring neutrophil along with dysplastic erythroid and megakaryocytic cells in the marrow (×1000). **B,** Pelger-Huët neutrophil resembling a monocyte (×1000). **C,** Mononuclear Pelger-Huët cell (×1000). **D,** Large, irregularly lobulated and granulated neutrophil precursors (×1000).

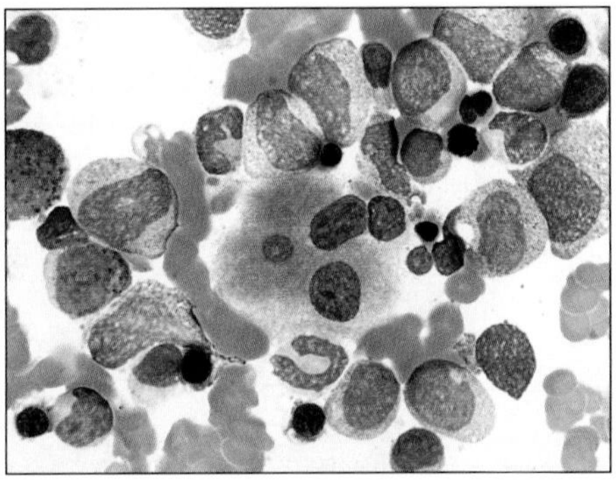

Figure 33-22 A dysplastic megakaryocyte showing unconnected nuclear lobes. Mononuclear forms are also frequent in myelodysplasia (×500).

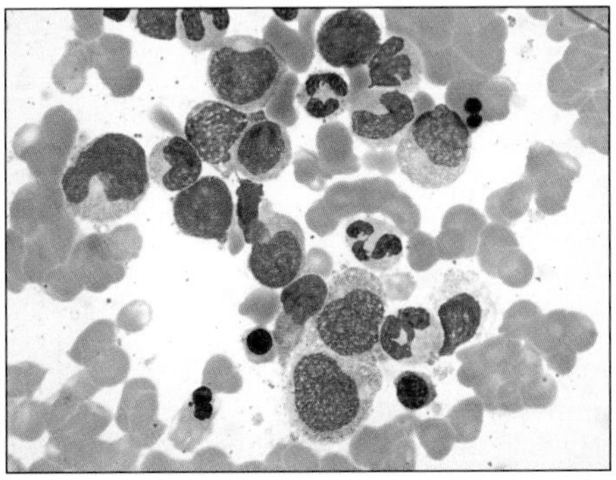

Figure 33-23 This case of chronic myelomonocytic leukemia shows moderate trilineage dysplasia and monocytosis (×500).

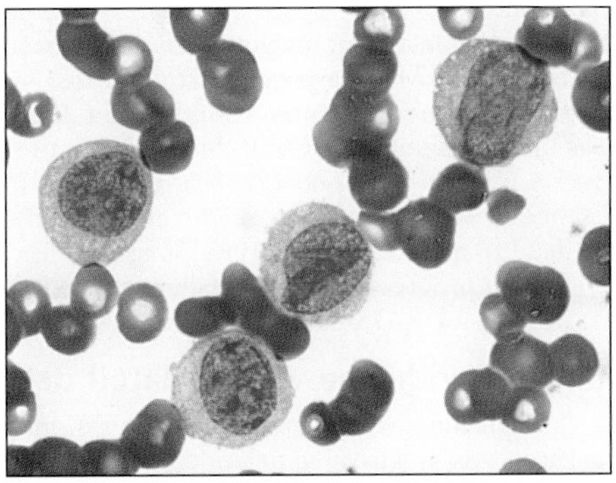

Figure 33-24 Promonocyte *(center)* shows immature chromatin and finely convoluted nuclear folds in comparison with monoblasts.

years, although with a wide reported age distribution down to the teen years. It has a generally poor outcome with median survival of 20 months, and a 25%–40% transformation to acute leukemia.

Criteria for diagnosis of aCML include the following (Swerdlow, 2008):

- Leukocytosis (WBC ≤13 × 10^9/L) due to increased neutrophils and precursors with prominent dysgranulopoiesis
- Prominent dysgranulopoiesis
- No Ph′ chromosome or *BCR/ABL-1* fusion gene
- No rearrangement of *PDGFRA* or *PDGFRB*
- Neutrophil precursors (promyelocytes, myelocytes, metamyelocytes) ≥10% of WBCs
- Minimal absolute basophilia; basophils usually <2% of leukocytes
- No or minimal absolute monocytosis; monocytes <10% of WBCs
- Hypercellular marrow with granulocytic proliferation and granulocytic dysplasia, with or without dysplasia of erythroid and megakaryocytic lineages
- Less than 20% blasts in blood or marrow

Juvenile Myelomonocytic Leukemia

Juvenile myelomonocytic leukemia (JMML) is a clonal disorder of predominantly granulocytic and monocytic lineages, with dysplasia in these and frequently other lineages, occurring in children or young adolescents (Luna-Fineman, 1999; Swerdlow, 2008). *BCR/ABL-1* is absent, and *RAS/MAPK* pathway mutations are characteristic. The occurrence is 1.3 cases per million children younger than 14 years, and most affected children are younger than 3 years of age, with a 2:1 male predominance. JMML is frequent in children with neurofibromatosis type 1.

In all, 25% of patients show monosomy 7, 35% exhibit mutations of *PTPN11* (encoding *SHP2*), and 20% each have mutations in *NRAS*, *KRAS2*, and *NF1*. Some infants with Noonan syndrome and *PTPN11* mutation may have spontaneous recovery or accelerated disease. Patients with normal karyotype often have markedly increased hemoglobin F. Immune phenomena of hypergammaglobulinemia and autoantibodies are frequent.

Blood shows leukocytosis, thrombocytopenia, and often anemia. The WBC is relatively high, usually 25–30 × 10^9/L, and mature neutrophils predominate, while monocytosis is also present. Circulating nucleated red blood cells (NRBCs) are frequent. The marrow is hyperplastic with granulocytic hyperplasia, variable erythroid cellularity, and often decreased megakaryocytes. Cutaneous leukemic infiltrates are common.

The prognosis is poor, and death is usually due to organ failure from leukemic infiltrates, although some patients benefit from BM transplant.

Criteria for diagnosis of JMML follow here (Swerdlow, 2008):

- Peripheral blood monocytosis >1 × 10^9/L
- Absence of Ph′ chromosome or *BCR/ABL-1*
- Blasts and promonocytes less than 20% of blood and marrow
- Plus two of the following:
  - Hemoglobin F increased for age
  - Immature granulocytes in the blood
  - WBCs >10 × 10^9/L
  - Clonal chromosomal abnormality (may be monosomy 7)
  - GM-CSF hypersensitivity of myeloid progenitors in vitro

Myelodysplastic/Myeloproliferative Disease, Unclassifiable

This category of the WHO classification is used for those cases with features of myelodysplastic disease, but with the addition of prominent myeloproliferative features, including thrombocytosis ≥450 × 10^9/L with megakaryocytic hyperplasia or WBC >13 × 10^9/L, with or without splenomegaly, no previous CMPD or MDS, and absence of a chromosomal abnormality specific to another disease (no *BCR/ABL* or rearrangement of *PDGFRA*, *PDGFRB*, or *FGFR1;* no del[5q], t[3;3][q21;q26] or inv[3][q21;q26]) (Swerdlow, 2008).

Refractory Anemia with Ring Sideroblasts Associated With Marked Thrombocytosis

This disorder is included in the WHO classification under the category of MDS/MPD, unclassified, because of not-yet-resolved questions regarding whether it is truly a distinct entity or an overlap syndrome of coexisting disorders. It is characterized by features of myelodysplastic neoplasm and refractory anemia with ring sideroblasts (RARS; see description later), along with features similar to essential thrombocythemia, with peripheral thrombocytosis ≥450 × 10^6/L, and increased, large atypical BM megakaryocytes. A majority of cases (60%) carry a *JAK2 V617F* mutation identical to that in MPN; occasional cases show a *MPL W515K/L* mutation.

Myelodysplastic Syndromes

These are clonal hematopoietic neoplasms characterized by cytopenias due to ineffective hematopoiesis and increased apoptosis. They show morphologic dysplasia of at least one and usually more lineages and have varied cytogenetic findings (but not typically those associated with myeloproliferative neoplasms), and many have a propensity to progress to acute leukemia (Table 33-13).

Refractory Cytopenia with Unilineage Dysplasia

This category consists of neoplasms, with dysplasia affecting >10% of one myeloid cell lineage, and cytopenia of the affected cell line, with <10% dysplasia of other lineages.

Refractory Anemia

This clonal disorder involves primarily the erythroid lineage with ineffective erythropoiesis but without increased blasts. Anemia (Hb <10 g/dL) with reticulocytopenia and abnormal erythrocytes are the presenting

TABLE 33-13

Key Features of the Major Myelodysplastic Syndromes

Disorder	Demographics	Laboratory features, morphology	Cytogenetics	Risk group
Refractory cytopenia with unilineage dysplasia, anemia (RA), thrombocytopenia, or neutropenia	Median age, 65–70 years	Peripheral blood (PB) with unicytopenia or bicytopenia, blasts <1%; bone marrow (BM) with >10% unilineage dysplasia and <5% blasts	Del (20q), +8, abnormalities of chromosome 5 or 7	Low
Refractory anemia with ringed sideroblasts	Median age, 60–73 years	Similar to RA with >15% ringed sideroblasts in BM	Rare abnormalities of single chromosome	Low
Refractory cytopenia with multilineage dysplasia	Median age, 70 years	PB with cytopenias of ≥2 cell lines, <1% blasts, <1 × 10^9/L monocytes; BM with dysplasia of ≥10% of precursors of ≥2 cell lines, <5% blasts	+8, –5, –7, del(7q), del(20q), complex in up to 50%	Intermediate
Refractory anemia with excess blasts (RAEB)	Over age 50	RAEB-1: PB with <5% blasts, <1 × 10^9/L monocytes; BM with hypercellularity, dyspoiesis, 5%–9% blasts without Auer rods; RAEB-2: PB with 5%–9% blasts, or 10%–19% BM blasts, or Auer rods	+8, –5, del(5q), –7, del(7q), del(20q)	RAEB-1, intermediate; RAEB-2, high
5q– syndrome	Middle-aged to older females	PB with thrombocytosis, <5% blasts; BM with increased, hypolobulated megakaryocytes, <5% blasts	5q– is sole abnormality	Low

findings. Abnormal granulocytes are rare, and blasts are less than 1% in the blood. The marrow is normocellular to hypercellular with erythroid hyperplasia and/or dyserythropoiesis and less than 5% blasts. Survival is relatively good (>5 years), and progression to acute leukemia (AL) low (6%).

Refractory Neutropenia

The absolute neutrophil count is <1.8 × 10^9/L. Dysplasia usually consists of nuclear hypolobation and hypogranulation. Toxic/secondary neutropenia is excluded.

Refractory Thrombocytopenia

Platelets are <100 × 10^9/L. More than 10% of at least 30 megakaryocytes evaluated in smears and sections show dysplastic features of hypolobation, binucleation or multinucleation, and/or micromegakaryocytes.

Refractory Anemia with Ring Sideroblasts

In RARS, in addition to the findings of RA, ring sideroblasts are present and constitute 15% or more of marrow erythroid precursors. These are nucleated RBC precursors in which stainable iron particles (iron-encrusted mitochondria) form a ring of 10 or more closely associated with and encircling at least one third of the nucleus (see Fig. 33-19). Defective cytoplasmic maturation and anisochromic erythrocytes are associated abnormalities. Survival is similar to RA, with a lower progression to AL (≤2%).

Refractory Cytopenia with Multilineage Dysplasia

Refractory cytopenia with multilineage dysplasia (RCMD) is a clonal disorder with bicytopenias or pancytopenia and dysplasia of 10% or more of the precursors of two or more lineages. Blasts are not increased, with <1% in the blood and <5% in the marrow. Ring sideroblasts may be present; when numerous (>15%), the case is still classified as RCMD and is not categorized separately, as in prior classifications.

This disease usually occurs in older individuals (median age, ≈70 years). In contrast to RA and RARS, which infrequently show cytogenetic abnormalities (<10%), RCMD and RCMD with ring sideroblasts (RCMD-RS) show them in up to 50%. These include trisomy 8, monosomy 7, del(7q), monosomy 5, del(5q), del(20q), and complex karyotypes. Survival is ≈33 months, and AL conversion is 11%.

Refractory Anemia with Excess Blasts

In refractory anemia with excess blasts (RAEB), the blood shows cytopenia in two or three of the cell lines, and less than 5% circulating blasts. The marrow is hypercellular, with variable erythroid or granulocytic hyperplasia. Dyspoietic changes are present in all three cell lines, and 5%–9% of marrow cells are blasts. Less than 5% blasts are present in the blood, and no Auer rods are found. Clusters of 5–8 blasts and promyelocytes in the marrow interstitium are frequently seen on sections and have been referred to as abnormal localization of immature precursors (ALIP). Hypocellular marrow is seen in a minority of cases (10%–15%). These may be difficult to interpret, as the patients are often older, with decreased cellularity to begin with, and because marrow stress in hypoplastic anemia often causes some dysplasia. A diagnosis of MDS should be made cautiously when the marrow is hypoplastic.

Cases of RAEB with concurrent myelofibrosis are referred to as **RAEB with fibrosis (RAEB-F).** Megakaryocytes are increased and dysplastic, and reticulin fibrosis is significant, often resulting in a dry tap.

RAEB-2 has findings similar to RAEB, but with any of the following: (1) greater than 5% blasts in the blood, (2) 10%–19% blasts in the marrow, or (3) the presence of Auer rods. Cytogenetic abnormalities include +8, -5, del(5q), -7, del(7q), and del(20q). Survival is usually less than 2 years in RAEB-1 or -2, with progressive marrow failure and cytopenias or progression to AL in 25% for RAEB and in 33% for RAEB-2.

Myelodysplastic Syndrome with Isolated del(5q)

This disorder is characterized by anemia and/or thrombocytosis with increased megakaryocytes and isolated deletion of chromosome region 5q. Some cases also exhibit a *JAK2 V617F* mutation. Blasts are less than 5% in the marrow and blood; lymphoid aggregates are often present. Megakaryocytes are usually small and hypolobulated. Anemia may be severe and macrocytic, and an otherwise normocellular to hypercellular marrow may have erythroid hypoplasia. Outcome is relatively favorable.

Myelodysplastic Syndrome, Unclassified

The myelodysplastic syndrome, unclassified category is used when clinical and hematologic findings of myelodysplasia exist, but without specific features to allow placement in one of the other categories. Patients usually have neutropenia or thrombocytopenia with a hypercellular BM and dysplasia of granulocytic or megakaryocytic lineage. Less than 5% blasts are found in the BM, and they are not increased in the blood.

Childhood Myelodysplastic Syndrome; Refractory Cytopenia of Childhood

In the WHO classification, it is recognized that MDS, although rare in children, does occur but tends to show different features than in adults. Refractory cytopenia of childhood (RCC) is defined as MDS with persistent cytopenia with <5% blasts in the BM and <2% in the blood and dysplasia, at least unilineage but usually multilineage, in the marrow. The marrow is also frequently hypocellular. Pancytopenia is frequent, with macrocytic anemia showing anisopoikilocytosis. The cytogenetic abnormality of monosomy 7 is the most common genetic abnormality and is associated with progressive disease. Cases with trisomy 8 may show a long stable period. This disorder may be morphologically indistinguishable from results of infection, vitamin deficiency (B_{12}, folate, vitamin E), metabolic or autoimmune disease, paroxysmal nocturnal hemoglobinuria (PNH), or acquired aplastic anemia.

ACUTE MYELOID LEUKEMIA

AML is the most common form of acute leukemia during the first few months of life, but during childhood and adolescence it accounts for approximately one third of AL. In the middle and later years of life, it becomes the most frequent AL, with a median age of 60, and an occurrence of 10/100,000 per year in those older than 60 years. Viruses, radiation, cytotoxic chemotherapy, benzene, and smoking have been linked to increased incidence, but most cases are not known to be associated with such factors.

The onset often resembles acute infection and includes signs of granulocytic insufficiency, with ulcerations of mucous membranes (especially of the mouth and throat) and fever. Enlargement of lymph nodes, spleen, and liver is not pronounced. Marked prostration and general malaise may be present. In untreated cases, the course is rapidly progressive (Table 33-14).

AML classification currently utilizes a multilayered approach which recognizes recurrent acquired cytogenetic abnormalities associated with specific types, history of predisposing factors (prior cytotoxic therapy), association with MDS or related abnormalities, and morphologic stratification for those for which none of these can be appreciated. This approach requires, or at least encourages, attempts to define the morphology, cytogenetics, and immunophenotype of each case. With advances in molecular cytogenetics and FISH, and with widespread adoption of these and other methods, it is likely that most cases will eventually be categorized by their genetic abnormalities. Knowledge of these changes is particularly important because therapies may be targeted to the biochemical pathways or even to the nucleic acid perturbations involved (Gilliland, 2004). See Tables 33-15 and 33-16.

The French-American-British Cooperative Group published proposals in 1976 for the classification of acute leukemias (Bennett, 1976) and subsequently revised criteria for the classification of ALL (Bennett, 1981) and AML (Bennett, 1985a, 1985b) based on morphology of cells in Romanowsky's-stained blood and marrow films and certain supplemental cytochemical reactions or serum lysozyme levels. These criteria have been superseded by the current WHO classification (Swerdlow, 2008), but basic morphologic tenets remain, and FAB criteria serve as the basis for subtyping AML, not otherwise specified.

The diagnosis of AML requires the presence of 20% blasts in the marrow or blood. Myeloblasts generally have central nuclei with fine, uncondensed chromatin and often prominent nucleoli (usually three to five) but have variable cytoplasm and may have some cytoplasmic granules. Primitive myeloblasts are identified by monoclonal antibodies against myeloid-associated antigens (MPO, CD13, CD33, CD117). More mature myeloblasts can also be identified by cytochemical reactions with granulocyte-associated enzymes using MPO, Sudan black B (SBB), and chloroacetate esterase (CAE) assays, although flow cytometric assays are utilized more often in current practice. Monoblasts are frequently large with abundant cytoplasm, diffuse chromatin, and often prominent nucleoli. Monoblasts are characterized by strong reaction with α-napthyl acetate esterase (ANA), which is inhibited in monocytes by sodium fluoride, or with α-napthyl butyrate esterase (ANB), or antibodies including anti-lysozyme, CD68, CD64, and CD36. For cases with monocytic differentiation, promonocytes are considered equivalent to blasts (Fig. 33-24). Promonocytes are immature recognizable monocytes with some chromatin condensation but with fine nuclear convolutions. Abnormal

TABLE 33-14
Clinical and Laboratory Features of Acute Myeloid Leukemia

- Affects all ages, but increases with older age (>60 years)
- May resemble acute infection at presentation
- Requires 20% blasts in blood or marrow for diagnosis
- Key myeloid antigens: myeloperoxidase, CD13, CD33, CD117, and CD14/CD64
- Recurrent cytogenetic abnormalities that characterize defined subtypes
- Classification made by morphology, cytogenetics, flow cytometry, cytochemistry

TABLE 33-15
Key Features of the Major Acute Myeloid Leukemias

Category	Cell morphology	Cell surface markers	Cytogenetics	Prognosis
AML with t(8;21)	≥20% blasts, ≥10% maturing granulocytes, Auer rods, dysplasia, abnormal granules	CD13, CD33, CD117, CD19, CD34	t(8;21)(q22;q22) AML1/ETO	More favorable
AML with inv(16)	Blasts with both monocytic and neutrophilic differentiation, increased eosinophils/immature eosinophils	CD13, CD33, CD14, CD4, 64	inv(16)(p13;q22) or t(16;16)(p13;q22)	More favorable
APL with t(15;17)	Promyelocytes with azurophilic granules, Auer rods	CD13, CD33 CD2, ± CD117	t(15;17)(q22;q12) PML/RARα; Variants all involve 17q12	More favorable if responsive to ATRA
AML with t(9;11)	Monoblasts and promonocytes predominate	CD33, CD65, CD4, HLA-DR	t(9;11)(p22;q23) MLLT3-MLL	Intermediate
AML, therapy related	Multilineage dysplasia, RS, increased basophils	CD13, CD33, CD34, ± CD56, CD57	11q23 abnormality seen with topoisomerase II inhibitor–associated AML	Less favorable
AML with t(6;9)	Any morphology may be seen but myelomonocytic is most common	CD13, CD33, CD38, HLA-DR, CD117	DEK-NUP214; t(6;9) (p23;q35)	Less favorable
AML with inv(3) or t(3;3)	Any morphology may be seen except APL	CD13, CD33, HLA-DR, CD34, CD38	Inv(3)(q21;q26.2) or t(3;3) (q21;q26.2) RPN1-EVI1	Less favorable
AML with t(1;22)	Megakaryoblastic morphology with small and large megakaryocytes	CD41, CD61, ± CD13, CD33	t(1;22)(p13;q13) RBM15-MKL1	Less favorable
AML with *FLT3* mutation/duplication	Any	Any	t(6;9)(p23;q34), t(15;17) (q22;q12) or normal	Less favorable
AML with *NPM1* mutation	Myelomonocytic and monocytic features	CD13, CD33, CD34 is negative	*NPM1* mutation, cytoplasmic expression	More favorable in absence of *FLT3*
AML with *CEBPA* mutation	Variable, generally similar to less differentiated AMLs in FAB scheme (M1, 2)	CD13, CD33, CD65, CD11b, CD15	*CEBPA* mutation	More favorable

AML, Acute myeloid leukemia; *APL,* acute promyelocytic leukemia; *ATRA,* all-*trans* retinoic acid; *PML,* promyelocytic leukemia; *PB,* peripheral blood; *RARα,* retinoid acid receptor gene-α.

TABLE 33-16
Key Features of the Acute Myeloid Leukemias, Not Otherwise Specified

Category	Cell morphology	Cell surface markers
All categories	≥20% blasts in BM and/or blood	Myeloid differentiation, any lineage
AML, minimally differentiated	Myeloblasts, <3% positive for SBB, MPO, or ANA	CD13, CD33, CD117
AML without maturation	Myeloblasts ≥90% of nonerythroids in BM, ≥3% positive for MPO	CD13, CD33, CD117
AML with maturation	Same as for AML with t(8;21)	CD13, CD33, CD117
Acute myelomonocytic leukemia	Monocytic and granulocytic cells, each 20%–80%,	Variable CD13, CD33, CD14, CD4, CD11b, CD11c, CD64, CD36, CD68
Acute monoblastic/ monocytic	≥80% of nonerythroid monoblasts (M5a) or differentiating monos (M5b)	CD13, CD33, CD117, CD14, CD4, CD11b, CD11c, CD64, CD68, CD36
Erythroleukemia	≥50% erythroid precursors and ≥20% of nonerythroids are myeloblasts; pure erythroleukemia without myeloid blasts is rare	Glycophorin A in erythroids; CD13, CD33, CD117 in myeloblasts
Acute megakaryoblastic leukemia	Blasts with cytoplasmic blebs, often clusters; PB may show megakaryocytic fragments; MPO negative	CD41, CD61, CD36, often CD13, CD33

AML, Acute myeloid leukemia; *ANA,* antinuclear antibody; *BM,* bone marrow; *MPO,* myeloperoxidase; *PB,* peripheral blood; *SBB,* Sudan black B.

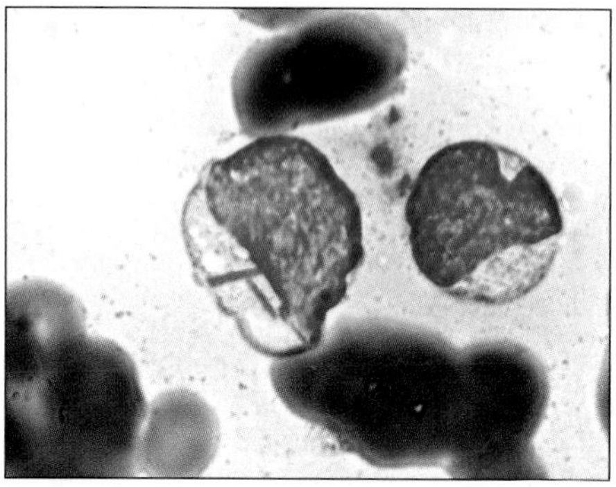

Figure 33-25 Auer rods vary from prominent, as in this cell, to thin and delicate.

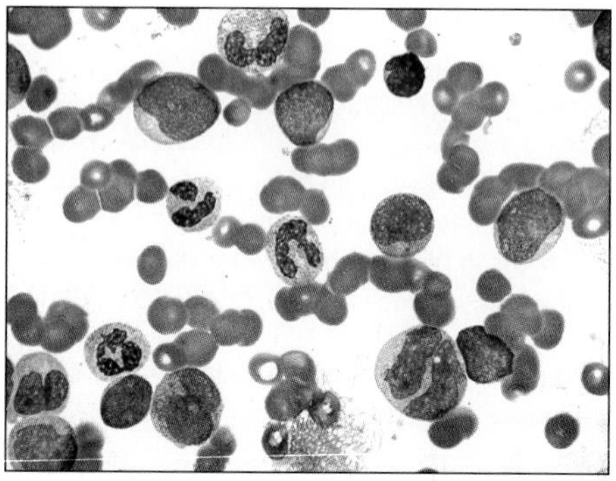

Figure 33-26 This case of acute myelogenous leukemia with t(8;21) shows granulocyte maturation with abnormal granulation and bilobed precursors (×500).

promyelocytes are also considered blast equivalents for the diagnosis of acute promyelocytic leukemia. Megakaryoblasts are identified by antibodies against platelet-associated antigens or electron microscopy for platelet peroxidase.

Initial assessment for suspected AML is based on a differential WBC count of the blood and a 500-cell count of the marrow aspirate. Acute leukemia is diagnosed when blasts exceed 20% of the marrow or blood. Otherwise, it is necessary to calculate the percentage of erythroid precursor cells. The diagnosis of AML-erythroleukemia is established when more than 50% of BM cells are erythroid precursors, and when myeloblasts represent more than 20% of the remaining nonerythroid (NE) cells (i.e., nucleated cells not including erythroid precursors, lymphocytes, or plasma cells). MDS is suggested when less than 20% of the nucleated marrow cells, or less than 20% of nonerythroid cells (when RBC precursors exceed 50%), are myeloblasts. Once the diagnosis of AML has been made, only nonerythroid cells should be considered in the differential count for the further assignment of morphologic subtypes.

A helpful finding in the diagnosis of AML is the presence of Auer rods, eosinophilic rod–like cytoplasmic inclusions derived from myeloperoxidase-positive primary granules. Phi bodies, which appear as strings of eosinophilic bead-like granules, are derived from catalase-positive microperoxisomes and are seen in larger numbers in AML and also in MDS (Cardullo, 1981). They are not, however, generally given the same diagnostic import as Auer rods. With Romanowsky's stains, Auer rods are linear or spindle-shaped, red-purple inclusions in myeloblasts or promyelocytes (Fig. 33-25). Less commonly, they may be seen in more mature neutrophils (in AML with t[8;21]). Auer rods, derivatives of azurophilic granules, stain positively for SBB, MPO, CAE, and acid phosphatase. Auer rods can be found in any of the subtypes of AML, but they are especially associated with those with granulocytic differentiation.

The main categories of AML in the WHO classification are (1) AML with recurrent cytogenetic abnormalities; (2) AML with multilineage dysplasia; (3) AML, therapy related; and (4) AML, not otherwise specified (subclassified by morphology and immunophenotype).

Acute Leukemia with Recurrent Genetic Abnormalities

(Swerdlow, 2008).

AML with Balanced Translocations/Inversions

AML with t(8;21)(q22;q22), RUNX1-RUNX1T1. The morphology usually corresponds to acute myeloid leukemia with neutrophilic maturation, and these represent 5%–12% of AML, with predominance in young patients. Blasts are 20% or greater in the marrow (or blood), and maturing neutrophilic precursors constitute more than 10% of marrow nucleated cells (not including NRBCs, lymphocytes, and plasma cells). Morphologic findings are characteristic but variable: large blasts with abundant basophilic cytoplasm; maturing neutrophil precursors with peripheral cytoplasmic basophilia; frequent Auer rods, often long, sharp, and tapered, and sometimes present in myelocytes and mature forms up to segmented neutrophils; abnormal granulation, including giant Chédiak-Higashi–like or secondary granules or homogenous waxy-appearing secondary granulation; and nuclear dysplasia with bilobed nuclei which may be widely separated (Fig. 33-26). Monocytosis is not prominent, and monocytes are less than 20% of the marrow. Eosinophilia is common, and basophils or mast cells may be increased. The immunophenotype is distinctive with high-intensity CD34 along with myeloid markers MPO and CD13, but relatively weak CD33 and sometimes CD56. One or more B cell markers—CD19, PAX5, and cytoplasmic CD79a—are often coexpressed.

The presence of t(8;21) is diagnostic of AML, even when blasts appear to be less than 20%. This disease is referred to as a **core binding factor leukemia** because RUNX1, also known as AML1 or core binding factor α (CBFA), encodes a transcription factor required for hematopoieses. The outcome of AML with t(8;21) is generally more favorable than AML without recurrent genetic abnormalities, or with MDS-associated abnormalities. Additional genetic abnormalities also occur, including *KIT* mutations associated with less favorable outcome.

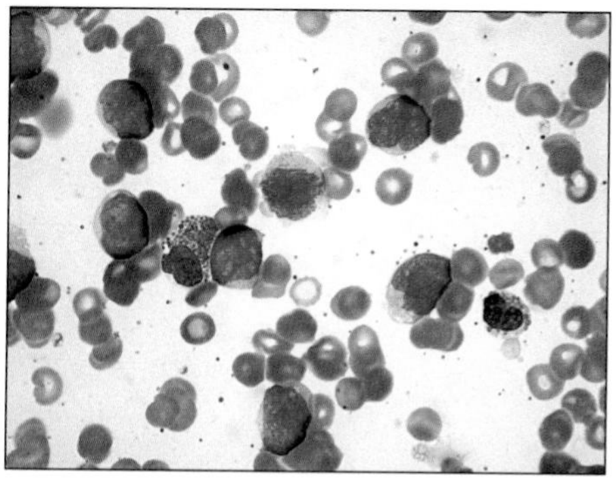

Figure 33-27 Acute myelogenous leukemia with inv16 shows myelomonocytic differentiation with eosinophilia. (Two eosinophils are present in this view.)

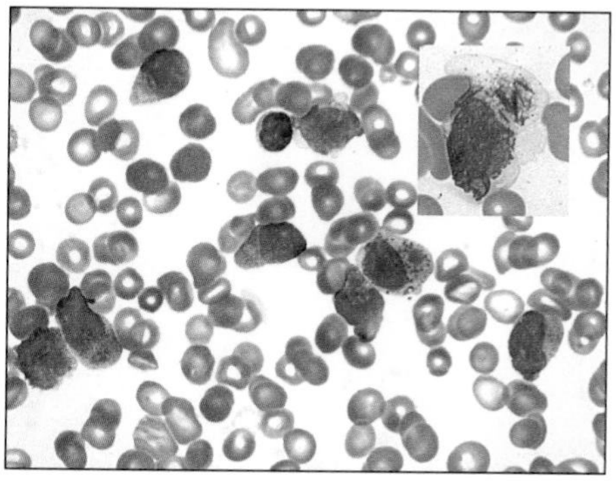

Figure 33-28 Acute promyelocytic leukemia with t(15;17) shows predominantly abnormal promyelocytes (×500). *Inset (top right):* Abnormal promyelocytes with bundles of Auer rods are known as **faggot cells** from their resemblance to bundles of firewood, or faggots (×1000).

AML with inv(16)(p13q22) or t(16;16)(p13.1;q22), CBFβ/MYH11. These correspond to acute myelomonocytic leukemia with abnormal eosinophils (Bitter, 1984). Occurrence and outcome are similar to AML with t(8;21). These cases show >20% blasts in marrow and/or blood with differentiation to monocytic and neutrophilic lineages (≥20% each). Eosinophils are characteristically increased (Fig. 33-27), including those with large basophilic granules (as in eosinophil promyelocytes), and cytoplasmic positivity is often weak for chloroacetate esterase. This type is associated with the chromosomal abnormality inv(16)(p13q22) or its variant t(16;16)(p13.1;q22) with fusion of the *CBFB* gene on 16q and *MYH11* on 16p and variable resultant chimeric mRNAs (due to differing breakpoints) and a BCGB-MYH11 fusion protein. This additional core binding factor leukemia generally has relatively favorable outcomes compared with other AMLs. In addition to karyotyping, RT-PCR or FISH is useful for timely diagnosis. Secondary genetic abnormalities are common, including trisomy 22, which is relatively specific for this disease, and *KIT* mutations.

The immunophenotype typically shows both granulocytic (CD13, CD15, CD33, CD65, MPO) and monocytic (CD4, CD14, CD64, CD36, CD11b, CD11c, and lysozyme) markers, sometimes with CD2 coexpression.

Acute Promyelocytic Leukemia with t(15;17)(q22;q12), PML/RARα, and Variants. Promyelocytes instead of myeloblasts predominate in the marrow in hypergranular promyelocytic leukemia (PML) (M3) (McKenna, 1982) (Fig. 33-28). Azurophilic granules are abundant and intensely stained. Auer rods are found in most cases and frequently are multiple (10 or more) in a given cell (see Fig. 33-28). Hemorrhagic complications are frequent as the result of disseminated intravascular coagulation (DIC), apparently initiated by procoagulant material from leukemic cell granules.

The characteristic chromosomal abnormality t(15;17)(q22;q21) shows fusion of the retinoid acid receptor gene-α *(RARA)* on chromosome 17 with the *PML* gene on chromosome 15. The *RARA-PML* fusion gene is transcribed as a chimeric mRNA. Leukemia usually responds to therapy with all-*trans* retinoic acid (ATRA), which is usually given in addition to chemotherapy, and the prognosis is relatively favorable. The molecular genetic abnormality may be detected in the laboratory by cytogenetics, RT-PCR, or FISH. Achievement of remission often occurs as a slow "maturation" process, rather than therapy-induced aplasia followed by remission as seen in treatment of other acute leukemias.

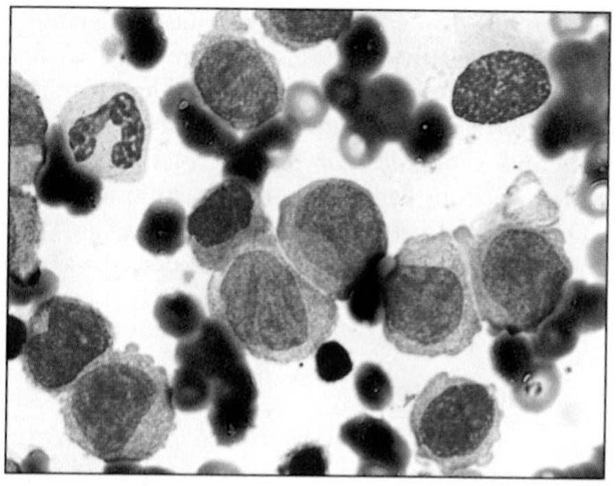

Figure 33-29 Acute myelogenous leukemia with monocytic differentiation and 11q23 abnormality (×1000).

Variant translocations include t(11;17)(q23;q21), t(5;17)(q32;q12), and t(11;17)(q13;q21). Some variants, such as t(11;17)(q23;q21), do not respond to ATRA. *FLT3* mutations are present in ≈40% and are associated with higher WBC count, microgranular morphology, and a bcr breakpoint of PML.

Hypogranular or microgranular variants of M3 (M3V) occur in which cytoplasmic granules appear sparse by light microscopy, and numerous but smaller by electron microscopy (Bennett, 1980; Golomb, 1980). Nuclei of most leukemic cells are bilobed or reniform, and confusion with an atypical monocytic leukemia is frequent. Cytochemical staining reactions are somewhat less positive than in the hypergranular M3. Auer rods, single or multiple, and typical hypergranular promyelocytes are found in variable numbers, and there appears to be a spectrum between typical and hypogranular types. The WBC may be high.

In acute promyelocytic leukemia, a majority of leukemic cells stain for MPO, SBB, and CAE, along with ANA in 25%. The immunophenotype is typically bright CD33; heterogeneous CD13, CD64, and CD117; and dim to absent HLA-DR, CD34, CD11a, CD11b, CD15, CD18, and CD64.

AML with t(9;11)(p22;q23); MLLT3-MLL. The 11q23 abnormalities are present in a more diverse group of leukemias than other recurrent genetic abnormalities. Chromosome band 11q23 abnormalities, which involve the *MLL* gene, are not specific for AML, but are also found in ALL, mixed lineage leukemias, and occasionally in lymphomas. The most common translocation in AML involving this region is t(9;11)(p22;q23). Others include t(6;11)(q27;q23), t(10;11)(p12;q23), t(11;17)(q23;q21), and t(11;19)(q23;p13) (Caligiuri, 1997). Most cases of t(9;11) show monocytic differentiation (monoblastic or myelomonocytic) (Fig. 33-29). In general, the prognosis of AML with 11q23 abnormalities is less favorable than that of other AML with standard chemotherapy, but evidence suggests that children with t(9;11) respond similarly to patients without 11q23 abnormalities (Martinez-Climent, 1999).

AML with t(6;9)(p23;q34); DEK-NUP214. This disease shows variable morphology and granulocytic and/or monocytic differentiation but is usually associated with multilineage dysplasia and basophilia of marrow and blood (>2%). Immunophenotype includes usual MPO, CD13, CD33, CD38, and HLA-DR, with variably positive CD117, CD34, CD64, and Tdt, but not lymphoid lineage-associated antigens. A DEK-NUP214 fusion protein acts as an abnormal transcription and nuclear transport factor. *FLT3-ITD* mutations are present in most cases. Prognosis is generally poor.

AML with inv(3)(q21q26.2) or t(3;3)(q21;q26.2); RPN1-EVI1. This disease show multilineage dysplasia, increased atypical megakaryocytes with monolobed or bilobed nuclei, and normal to increased platelet counts. Pseudo–Pelger-Huët cells are common, and differentiation may be granulocytic and/or monocytic. Marrow eosinophils, basophils, and/or mast cells are often increased. EVI1 is a transcription factor which, likely promoted by RPN1, induces proliferation and transformation while impairing differentiation. This is an aggressive disease with short survival.

AML (Megakaryoblastic) with t(1;22)(p13;q13); RBM15-MKL1. This is an acute leukemia of infants and young children, more often reported in girls, presenting as acute megakaryoblastic leukemia with hepatosplenomegaly. This form is not associated with Down syndrome. Blasts are usually medium-sized to large with fine reticular chromatin, one to three nucleoli, and basophilic cytoplasm with blebs or pseudopods. Cytochemistry/immunophenotype shows absence of MPO and SBB and expression of platelet markers CD41 and CD61 (best demonstrated by cytoplasmic labeling techniques), CD36, and variable CD13, CD33, and CD34. Micromegakaryocytes are often found, and biopsy sections show reticulin fibrosis. Patients may respond well to chemotherapy.

AML with Gene Mutations

Although many cases of AML have been associated with recurring translocations or inversions, many have shown normal karyotype. Most if not all of these carry genetic mutations not detectable by Giemsa banding morphology; mutations are also found in cases with karyotypic abnormalities. Several carry prognostic implications. As these continue to be investigated, new, specific categories of AML are certain to be described. Biological and clinical associations are available for some common AML-associated mutations, and two of these are recognized by provisional categories in the WHO classification.

Mutations of fms-related tyrosine kinase 3 *(FLT3)*, encoding a tyrosine kinase receptor involved in hematopoietic proliferation and differentiation, occur in about one third of cases of AML. Two types of *FLT3* mutations have been noted: one change of length type involving internal tandem duplications (*FLT3*-ITD), and another affecting the tyrosine kinase domain (*FLT3*-TK) at codon 835 or 836. *FLT3* mutations are seen in any AML, but primarily those with t(6;9), t(15;17), and normal karyotype. *FLT3*-ITD mutations are associated with less favorable prognosis, particularly in cases with normal karyotype.

AML with *NPM1* Mutation. This constitutes a provisional entity in the WHO classification. Most cases have monocytic or myelomonocytic differentiation, but cases with multilineage dysplasia and erythroid differentiation are also found. Mutations of *NPM1*, encoding the nuclear shuttle protein nucleophosmin, are found in similar frequency as *FLT3*, or one half of cases with normal karyotype, but are associated with better prognosis. This favorable association is especially noted in cases with normal karyotype and without *FLT3* mutation. *NPM1* mutation may be detected by immunohistochemical assay of sections, in which affected cells show abnormal cytoplasmic localization of NPM protein, or it may be detected by PCR assays.

AML with CEBPA. *CEBPA* encodes the CCAAT/enhancer binding protein-α, another hematopoietic proliferation- and differentiation-inducing transcription factor. Similar to *NPM1* mutation, it is associated with improved prognosis in AML with normal karyotype and without *FLT3* mutation. It is found in less than 20% of cases of AML. The morphology is most often AML without differentiation or AML with differentiation, although monocytic differentiation may also occur. Immunophenotype includes usually CD34, frequently CD7, with myeloid markers HLA-DR, CD11b, CD13, CD15, CD33, and CD65.

KIT mutations are also seen in cases of AML, as well as in GI stromal tumors and mast cell disease. In AML with t(8;21) and t(15;17), *KIT* mutation is associated with diminished prognosis. Other AML-associated mutations include those involving *WT1*, *MLL*, *NRAS*, and *KRAS*.

Acute Myeloid Leukemia with Myelodysplasia-Related Changes

(Swerdlow, 2008).

These leukemias show morphologic features of myelodysplasia or history of prior MDS or MDS/MPN, or they have MDS-related cytogenetic abnormalities. Patients with a history of cytotoxic chemotherapy or radiation for another malignancy are not included. These cases are characterized by 20% or more blasts in blood and/or marrow, as well as dysplasia in ≥50% of cells of at least two lineages. Dysplastic features are similar to those of MDS of various types (Fig. 33-30).

Cytogenetic abnormalities qualifying for this disorder include -5/del(5q), i(17q)/t(17p), -13/del(13q), del(11q), del(12p)/t(12p), del(9q), idic(X)(q13), t(11;16)(q23;p13.3.), t(3;21)(q26.2;q22.1), t(1;3)(p36.3;q21.1), t(2;11)(p21;q23), t(5;12)(q33;p12), t(5;7)(q33;q11.2), t(5;17)(q33;p13), t(5;10)(q33;q21), and t(3;5)(q25;q34). The immunophenotype often includes primitive blasts with myeloid phenotype and CD34 expression, CD56, and/or CD7. Prognosis is generally poor.

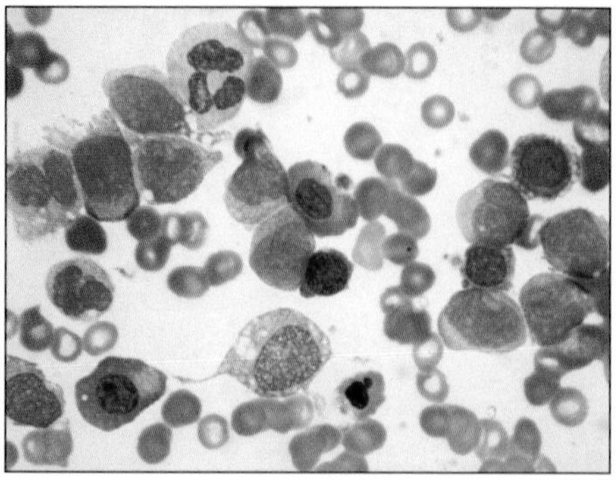

Figure 33-30 Acute myelogenous leukemia with multilineage dysplasia showing dysgranulopoiesis and dyserythropoiesis (×1000).

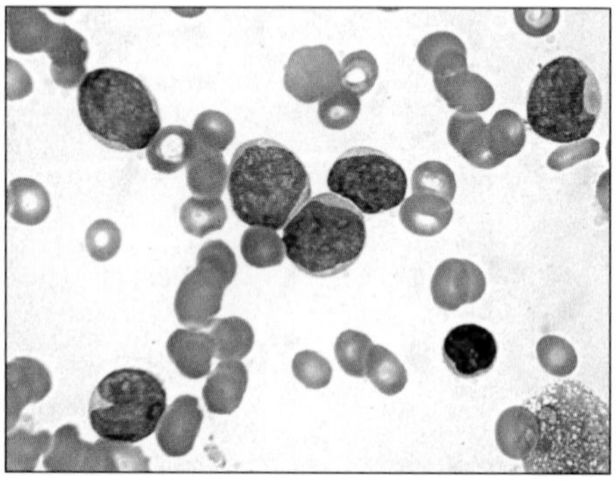

Figure 33-31 Acute myelogenous leukemia, minimally differentiated, resembles acute lymphoblastic leukemia and requires immunophenotyping for diagnosis (×500).

Therapy-Related Myeloid Neoplasms

These disorders are related to prior radiation or cytotoxic chemotherapy utilizing alkylating agents or topoisomerase inhibitors. They include cases of AML, MDS, and MDS/MPN. Most patients have been treated for prior malignancies, but some have been treated for nonneoplastic conditions.

Most commonly, disease is related to mutagenic effects of alkylating agents (including chlorambucil, cyclophosphamide, thiotepa, and busulfan) or radiation. These effects usually occur 5–10 years post exposure and most often present as MDS. Cytogenetic features are similar to those of MDS and AML with multilineage dysplasia. Loss of portions of chromosome 5 or 7 is common. Response to therapy and outcomes are poor.

Cases secondary to prior chemotherapy with topoisomerase II inhibitors (including epipodophyllotoxins etoposide and teniposide, and doxorubicin) occur after a shorter latency period of 1–5 years and most often are associated with overt AML with balanced chromosomal translocations involving 11q23 (*MLL*) or 21q22 (*RUNX1*). These most often show AML with maturation, monocytic or myelomonocytic morphology. Response to therapy is possibly similar to de novo AML.

Acute Myeloid Leukemia, Not Otherwise Specified

These cases do not fulfill criteria for the previous categories, or cytogenetic studies were unsuccessful or could not be performed. Categorization is similar to French-American-British Cooperative Group criteria.

Acute Myeloblastic Leukemia, Minimally Differentiated

In acute myeloblastic leukemia, minimally differentiated, myeloblasts display less than 3% positivity with SBB, MPO, or ANA (Bennett, 1991). When examined for myeloid and lymphoid markers using flow cytometry or immunocytochemistry, however, at least 20% of the blasts exhibit myeloid-associated antigens (CD13, CD33, CD117, and/or MPO). Stem cell antigens CD34, CD38, HLA-DR, and TdT are often expressed, while lineage-specific lymphoid markers cCD3, cCD20, and cCD79a are absent. Some primitive markers often associated with lymphoid lineage, including CD2, CD7, and CD19, are not lineage specific and are sometimes expressed (Fig. 33-31).

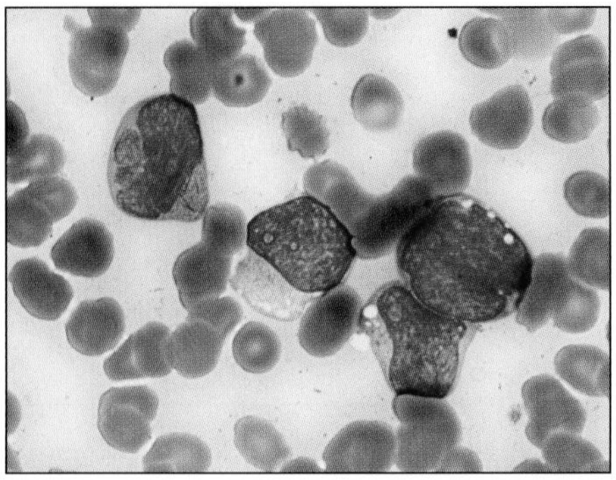

Figure 33-32 Acute myelogenous leukemia without maturation shows blasts with less than 10% maturing neutrophils. Auer rods are present in the cell at upper left.

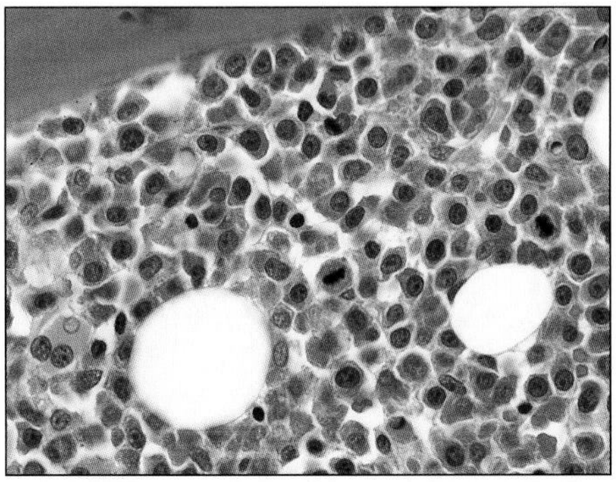

Figure 33-33 Acute myelogenous leukemia with maturation shows maturing granulocytic cells on this biopsy (×200).

Acute Myeloblastic Leukemia without Maturation (M1)

In this category, myeloblasts represent at least 90% of nonerythroid cells in the BM (Bennett, 1985a, 1985b) and at least 3% of blasts labeled with MPO or SBB. Positive staining for CAE is sometimes also present but is less sensitive. CD13, CD33, CD117, and/or MPO antigens are usually detectable, as are other, less specific markers. CD3, CD20, and CD79a are usually absent (Fig. 33-32).

Acute Myeloblastic Leukemia with Maturation

Myeloblasts represent 20% (per WHO) to 89% of total marrow cells, granulocytes from promyelocytes to neutrophils are greater than 10% of nonerythroid cells, and monocytes and their precursor cells are less than 20% (Fig. 33-33). Most blasts stain with MPO, SBB, and CAE.

Cases with t(8;21)(q22;q22) are categorized as AML with recurrent cytogenetic abnormality t(8;21).

Acute Myelomonocytic Leukemia

In acute myelomonocytic leukemia, myeloblasts constitute more than 20% of total marrow cells. The sum of the monoblasts, promonocytes, and monocytes is greater than 20% but is less than 80% of nonerythroid cells. Cells of the granulocytic series (myeloblasts, promyelocytes, myelocytes, and other more mature forms) also represent 20%–80% of nonerythroid cells (Fig. 33-34). Peripheral blood monocytosis ($\geq 5 \times 10^9$/L) is usually present.

In myelomonocytic leukemia, variable staining of leukemic cells with MPO, SBB, CAE, and periodic acid–Schiff (PAS) has been noted. In most cases, leukemic cells exhibit diffuse and intense staining with ANA and ANB. In some cases, these nonspecific esterases cannot be demonstrated, and the diagnosis may be made on the basis of Romanowsky's stains and/or immunophenotyping.

Immunologic markers are variable but usually show myeloid antigens CD13 and/or CD33, as well as variable expression of monocytic markers CD14, CD4, CD11b, CD11c, CD64, CD36, CD68, and lysozyme. Some pure myeloblasts may be present, including those with CD34 and CD117 expression, and a second population of variably mature monocytes. Cases with recurrent cytogenetic abnormalities are categorized separately.

Acute Monoblastic and Acute Monocytic Leukemia

In this disorder, 80% or more of marrow nonerythroid cells are monoblasts, promonocytes, or monocytes (see Figs. 33-24 and 33-35). Two subtypes are recognized. The monoblastic subtype is characterized by large blasts accounting for 80% or more of marrow monocytic cells. The monocytic subtype has fewer monoblasts (<80% of marrow monocytic cells) and greater numbers of promonocytes and monocytes (Bennett, 1985b). In both, ANA and ANB label the leukemic cells diffusely and intensely (80% or more of leukemic cells). Occasional cases fail to show nonspecific esterases, and the diagnosis is made from Romanowsky's stains and/or immunophenotypic techniques. Antilysozyme and CD68 are particularly useful on slides. Both myeloid and monocytic markers are frequently expressed, as in acute myelomonocytic leukemia. The translocation t(8;16)(p11;p13) has been associated with AML-M5 (or M4) with erythrophagocytosis.

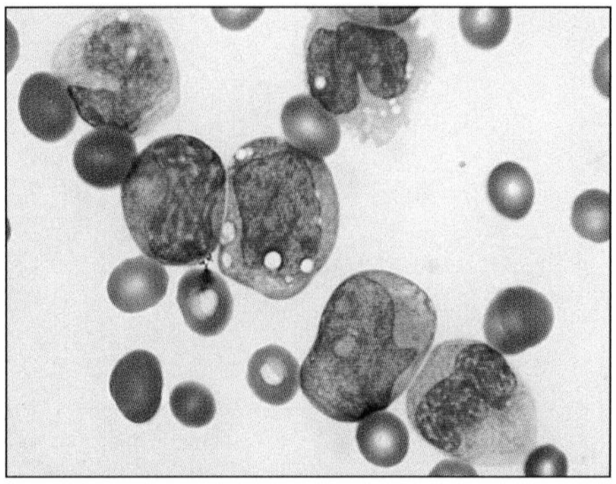

Figure 33-34 Acute myelomonocytic leukemia shows blasts and dual differentiation to granulocytes and monocytes (×1000). Acute monocytic leukemia shows monoblasts and maturing monocytes. Promonocytes are counted as blasts and show finely convoluted nuclei (×1000).

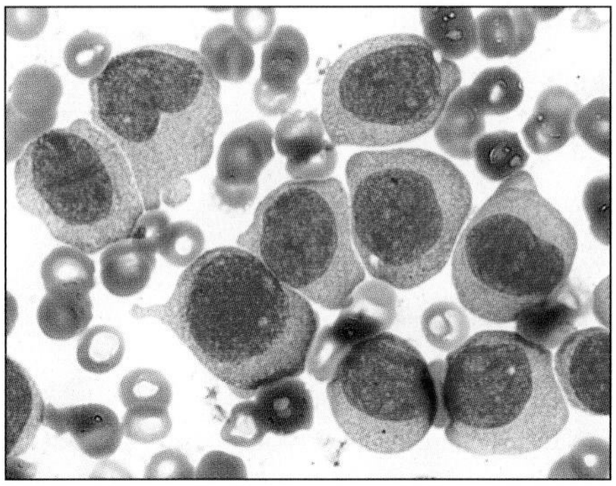

Figure 33-35 Acute monoblastic leukemia shows predominantly monoblasts (×1000).

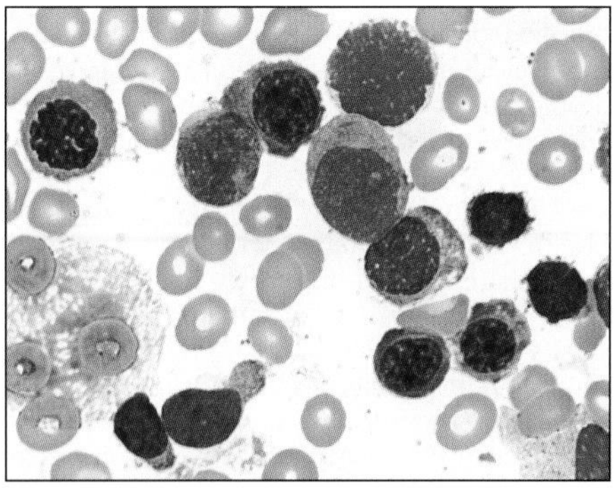

Figure 33-36 Erythroleukemia, erythroid/myeloid, shows predominance of erythroid precursors with myeloblasts constituting 20% or more of nonerythroid cells. An Auer rod is seen in the blast at upper center (×1000).

Erythroleukemia

The diagnosis of erythroleukemia is made when more than 50% of nucleated cells of the BM are erythroblasts, and 20% or more of nonerythroid cells are myeloblasts. In most cases, termed erythroleukemia (erythroid/myeloid), a mixture of variable proportions of erythroid precursors and myeloblasts (sometimes abnormal monocytic and megakaryocytic elements are present as well) is seen (Fig. 33-36).

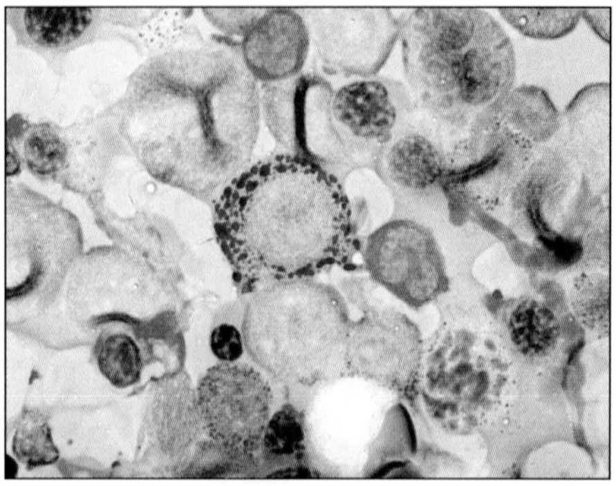

Figure 33-37 Coarse periodic acid–Schiff-positive granules are often seen in erythroid precursors in erythroleukemia (×1000).

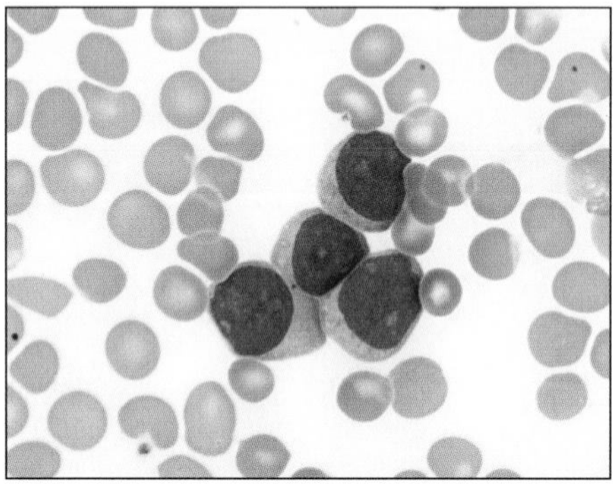

Figure 33-38 Blasts sometimes cluster in acute megakaryocytic leukemia (×1000).

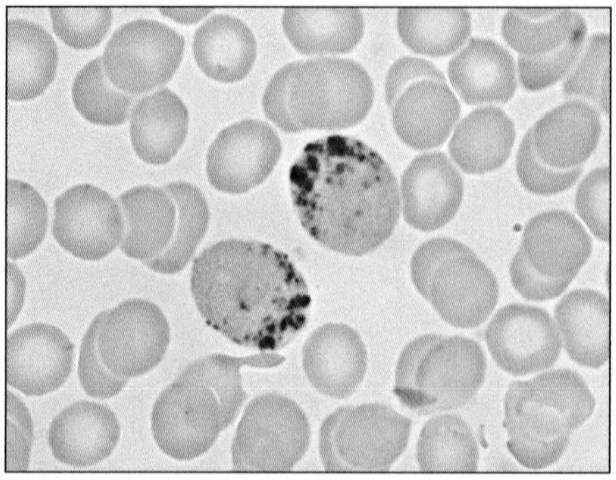

Figure 33-39 Alpha naphthyl acetate esterase-positive granules in megakaryoblasts.

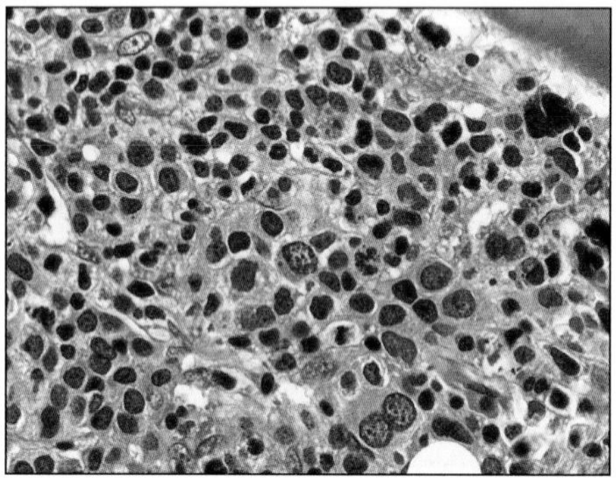

Figure 33-40 Acute panmyelosis with myelofibrosis shows involvement of all three myeloid lineages, with fibrosis (×200).

Very rarely, there is virtually no granulocytic involvement in the neoplastic process, and primitive erythroblasts predominate. This has been known as **erythremic myelosis** and is now known as **pure erythroid leukemia.** Morphologic abnormalities of erythroblasts are often pronounced, with atypical megaloblastic features, bizarre nuclear shapes, and multinucleated giant forms. The cytoplasm may contain pseudopods and/or vacuoles, particularly in the probasophilic and basophilic erythroblasts.

In some cases, erythroid cells may show strong cytoplasmic PAS positivity (Fig. 33-37). This is granular in early erythroid precursors and diffuse in later stages. Erythroid precursors are PAS negative in normal individuals and in most diseases, including nutritional megaloblastic anemia. They are sometimes positive, however, in iron deficiency anemia, thalassemia, and RARS. In erythroleukemia, myeloblasts usually stain with SBB, MPO, and CAE. A nonspecific esterase-positive monocytic component may also be present. Neoplastic erythroid precursors are sometimes positive for ANA and ANB (Hayhoe, 1984).

Acute Megakaryoblastic Leukemia

The diagnosis of acute megakaryoblastic leukemia, like other forms of acute myeloid leukemia, requires ≥20% blasts in the marrow. Megakaryoblasts are highly polymorphic; some blasts simulate lymphoblasts, while others are larger and have pseudopods or stringy cytoplasmic projections. The cytoplasm is usually light blue and may or may not possess granules (Fig. 33-38). The nuclei often have one to three nucleoli. Micromegakaryocytes may be present and are not counted as blasts.

The blasts are cytochemically undifferentiated. They do not stain with SBB, MPO, CAE, or ANB. However, ANA is usually positive in a focal cytoplasmic pattern (Fig. 33-39). The PAS reaction shows diffuse and peripheral granular (often in large blocks) staining.

Megakaryocytic lineage is most often (Bennett, 1985a) demonstrated by immunophenotyping using monoclonal antibodies against platelet glycoprotein Ib (CD41) or IIb/IIIa (CD61) (Erber, 1987). Blasts are often also positive for myeloid antigens CD13 and CD33, and characteristically for CD36. Care must be taken to differentiate this disease from AML with minimal differentiation by flow cytometry, which may show artifactual positivity for platelet markers due to adherence of platelets to blasts; this can be done by immunochemical examination of cytospins. Truly positive cells show membrane and/or cytoplasmic labeling rather than adherent platelets.

In the peripheral blood, there is usually pancytopenia with marked leukopenia and anemia. Megakaryocytic fragments are sometimes present in the blood. The BM shows variable and sometimes pronounced myelofibrosis, often resulting in futile attempts at obtaining marrow aspirate films.

Clumping of blasts may simulate metastatic tumor such as neuroblastoma or small cell carcinoma. Infants with t(1;22)(p13;q13) often show marrow infiltration mimicking neuroblastoma.

Young children (1–4 years of age) with Down syndrome (trisomy 21) have an increased incidence of megakaryoblastic leukemia, which may be transient and spontaneously remit in 1–3 months. Subsequent transient or persistent relapses may occur. Blasts also tend to show erythroid features, indicating derivation from a multipotential erythroid/megakaryocytic precursor (Zipursky, 1992). Patients often respond well to therapy but tolerate intensive therapy less well than others (Gamis, 2005).

Acute Basophilic Leukemia

Acute basophilic leukemia is a rare form of AML in which the blastic cells differentiate along the basophil lineage. The peripheral blood usually demonstrates anemia and thrombocytopenia with leukocytosis. The BM is infiltrated by blastic cells simulating lymphoblasts or myeloblasts. Blasts are generally negative for Sudan black B and myeloperoxidase. An increase in mature basophils or in blasts staining with toluidine blue may occur. Diagnosis historically rests on the identification of blasts with basophilic granules by ultrastructural methods (Brunning, 1994).

Acute Panmyelosis with Myelofibrosis

This is a rare form of acute leukemia with panmyeloid proliferation and marrow fibrosis. Pancytopenia is typically seen. Red blood cells show minimal poikilocytosis, but dysplastic features in myeloid cells are often seen, as are atypical platelets.

The BM sample frequently shows a dry tap; on biopsy, clusters of blasts, late erythroid precursors, and dysplastic megakaryocytes are seen in a variably fibrotic background (Fig. 33-40). This is differentiated from acute megakaryoblastic leukemia by involvement of all three myeloid lineages, rather than only the megakaryocytic.

Myeloid Sarcoma

This neoplasm has been called myeloblastic sarcoma, granulocytic sarcoma, extramedullary myeloid cell tumor, and chloroma. It represents a localized

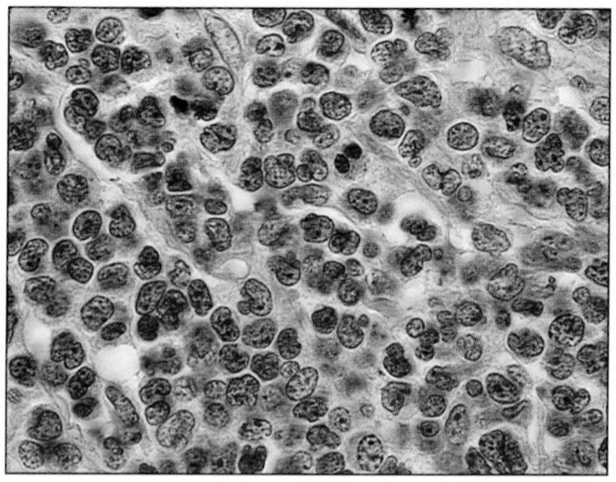

Figure 33-41 Granulocytic sarcoma, in this case presenting in the skin, resembles lymphoma but with large blastic or monocytoid cells. Eosinophils or precursors are frequently present (×500).

TABLE 33-17
Lineage Requirements in Mixed Phenotype Acute Leukemia

Myeloid lineage
Myeloperoxidase or monocyte differentiation markers (NSE, lysozyme, CD14, CD64, CD11c)
T lineage
Cytoplasmic or surface CD3
B lineage
Strong CD19 + strong CD79a, cytoplasmic CD22, or CD10
or
Weak CD19 + at least two: strong CD79a, cytoplasmic CD22, or CD10

From Swerdlow (2008).
NSE, Neuron-specific enolase.

tumor of myeloblasts or monoblasts infiltrating extramedullary sites (Fig. 33-41). These tumors have been reported to occur in the skin, lymph nodes, nasopharyngeal and upper respiratory tract tissues, breast, ovary, bone, perineural and epidural structures, and the eye and other orbital structures, as well as in a variety of soft tissues (Neiman, 1981). Myeloid sarcomas have been reported in 3%–8% of autopsied cases of chronic myelogenous leukemia and may precede the occurrence of acute myeloid leukemia in <1% of cases (Muss, 1973).

Myeloid sarcomas may occur at any age. Three clinical settings are found: (1) no known disease, (2) a known myeloproliferative disorder, and (3) acute myeloid leukemia (Neiman, 1981). The diagnosis depends on recognizing the nature of the primitive cells that can often be mistaken for solid tumors, including non-HLs, amelanotic melanomas, or undifferentiated carcinoma (Hutchison, 1990). The diagnosis is facilitated by making touch imprint preparations of cut sections of the tumor and staining them with Romanowsky's stains, by cytochemical reactions, and by immunophenotyping. Anti-MPO and CD68 are particularly useful for granulocytic or monocytic lineage in paraffin sections.

Myeloid Proliferations Related to Down Syndrome

Children and adults with Down syndrome have a much higher frequency of leukemia than those without the syndrome. This includes ALL and AML, and diagnostic considerations for most are similar to leukemia occurring outside the syndrome. In addition, two specific and likely related disorders are unique to this group of patients.

Transient Abnormal Myelopoiesis

Transient abnormal myelopoiesis (TAM) occurs in 10% of neonates with Down syndrome and in a small number who are phenotypically normal but have trisomy 21 mosaicism. It presents as acute megakaryoblastic leukemia, frequently with thrombocytopenia and leukocytosis, often with higher blast proportions in blood than in marrow, and hepatosplenomegaly. Blasts are of megakaryocytic/myeloid lineage and express CD41 and CD61, as well as CD34, CD117, CD13, CD33, CD7, CD4, CD36, and CD71. Genetics show trisomy 21 and *GATA1* mutations.

Uniquely, this disorder resolves spontaneously in the vast majority of cases. However, 20%–30% subsequently develop nonremitting AML, as described later.

Myeloid Leukemia Associated with Down Syndrome

AML of Down syndrome occurs most often in the first 3–5 years at an incidence greater than 50 times that of others. It is usually of megakaryocytic lineage and may be preceded by a preleukemic phase similar to RCC, or by TAM. Compared with TAM, blasts are similar but lack CD34 and often CD56 and/or CD41. Trisomy 8 is frequent, as is trisomy 21. *GATA1* mutations are usually absent.

Blastic Plasmacytoid Dendritic Cell Neoplasm

This tumor used to be included in the WHO classification with the lymphomas and was called blastic NK-cell lymphoma or CD4+ CD56+ hematodermic neoplasm. It is now known to be derived from plasmacytoid dendritic cell precursors and presents in skin with frequent involvement of blood and marrow, and often lymph nodes. Skin lesions may be nodules, plaques, or patches. Tumors resemble lymphoblastic lymphomas with monomorphic dermal infiltrates of blasts with fine chromatin and irregular nuclei, along with agranular cytoplasm. Cytochemical stains for myeloid precursors are absent, and immunohistochemistry shows characteristic findings of CD4, CD56, CD43, and CD45RA. Plasmacytoid dendritic cell markers CD123, TCL1, CLA, MxA, and BDCA-2/CD303 are positive. CD99 is reported positive (Shapiro, 2003). CD7, CD68, and CD33 are often expressed, and CD3, CD5, CD13, CD34, CD117, CD20, and CD79a are negative. Cytotoxic T cell markers are also negative in tissue sections. Immunoglobulin and usually T cell receptor genes are germline. The disease is aggressive, usually relapsing after initial therapy, but occasionally responding well to aggressive therapy.

Acute Leukemias of Ambiguous Lineage

(Swerdlow, 2008).

Some cases of acute leukemia have features that are indeterminate between lymphoid and myeloid lineage, or have features of more than one lineage. This is a controversial area of difficult-to-classify leukemia. Many leukemias that appear to be of defined lineage have one or more immunologic markers which are aberrant, or show lineage infidelity. A single such marker is usually insignificant. ALL with myeloid markers responds similarly to other types of ALL, and lymphoid markers in AML are clinically important, mostly if they help suggest a subtype, such as CD19 expression in AML with t(8;21). CD117 has been proposed as a good indicator of myeloid lineage (Bene, 1998), but CD117, CD13, and CD33 are not considered adequate to assign myeloid lineage in an otherwise lymphoid blast proliferation (Swerdlow, 2008).

Ambiguous acute leukemias fall into two main categories per the WHO classification: acute undifferentiated leukemia (AUL) and mixed phenotype acute leukemia (MPAL). MPAL is divided into several entities. In the past, the term **bilineal acute leukemia** has been applied to rare disorders in which there are distinct blast populations of more than one lineage. Biphenotypic leukemia has referred to those with one population of leukemic cells with multiple lineage expression (mixed lineage). These concepts remain, and criteria are established to assign more than one lineage to a blast population (Table 33-17). Subcategories of MPAL are listed in the following sections.

Undifferentiated Acute Leukemia

These are rare acute leukemias in which the predominant cells are blast forms that cannot be classified using morphologic, cytochemical, ultrastructural, immunologic, or DNA analytic methods (Raghavachar, 1986; Sobol, 1988). CD34, CD38, and HLA-DR are frequently expressed, and CD7 and TdT may be expressed as well.

Mixed Phenotype Acute Leukemia with t(9;22)(q34;q11.2); BCR-ABL1

These are cases of MPAL with t(9;22) translocation and associated *BCR-ABL1*. They are rare disorders, more common in adults than in children. Cases with prior CML are excluded.

Mixed Phenotype Acute Leukemia with t(v;11q23); MLL Rearranged

This disease is more common in children than in adults. Dimorphic blast populations are frequent and consist of monoblasts and lymphoblasts. Prognosis is generally poor.

Mixed Phenotype Acute Leukemia, B/Myeloid, NOS

Myeloperoxidase or monocytic differentiation and CD19 with CD79a, cCD22, and/or CD10; neither t(9;11) or 11q23 translocation occurs.

Mixed Phenotype Acute Leukemia, T/Myeloid, NOS

Myeloperoxidase or monocytic differentiation and cytoplasmic or surface CD3; neither t(9;11) or 11q23 translocation occurs.

Mixed Phenotype Acute Leukemia, NOS—Other Rare Types

This category includes T- and B-lineage disease and cases with trilineage differentiation.

Natural Killer Cell Lymphoblastic Leukemia/Lymphoma

This category considers the possibility of bilineage NK and T-lineage lymphoblastic leukemia/lymphoma, but such an entity remains ambiguous.

PRECURSOR LYMPOID NEOPLASMS

Historically, lymphoid leukemias and lymphomas have been classified separately. Leukemias are hematopoietic malignancies primarily involving BM and blood and have been most extensively categorized by the FAB group. Lymphomas are those primarily involving lymphoid organs or other soft tissues and have been subject to numerous classification schemes that evolved rapidly because of advances in immunology, oncology, and genetics. Since publication of the Revised European–American Lymphoma (REAL) classification (Harris, 1994), lymphoid leukemias and lymphomas have been classified by biological features of the disease, rather than by the anatomic distribution, and an international consensus in classification has generally been attained (Berard, 1997). The WHO classification focuses on cytogenetic and molecular findings whenever possible (Swerdlow, 2008).

B Lymphoblastic Leukemia/Lymphoma

Clinical Features

This category of malignancy most often presents as leukemia and is the prototype of ALL. The other major type of ALL is T lymphoblastic, which is less common and tends to present as lymphoma or concurrently as both leukemia and lymphoma. ALL is generally thought of as a clinical entity which is pathologically subtyped and warrants some general discussion.

Acute lymphoblastic leukemia is the most common malignancy of children and adolescents. In the United States, 3000–4000 new cases are reported per year, two thirds of which affect children. The evolution of treatment with combination chemotherapy, CNS treatment, and intensified therapy for high-risk categories has led to cure rates of nearly 80% in children. Favorable factors are age 5–10 years, hyperdiploidy (best, 54–62 with trisomy 4, 10, and/or 17), t(12;21), and normal or low WBC. Poor risk factors include age younger than 1 year, t(9;22), and t(4;11). Among adults, only 30%–40% are cured, in part because of the higher frequency of adverse genetic abnormalities (Pui, 2004). Adult ALL incidence increases in middle to older age, similarly to genetically high-risk AML. Individuals with this disorder often present with symptoms of fatigue, fever, and bleeding. Generalized lymphadenopathy, splenomegaly, and hepatomegaly are common findings. Because leukemic cells infiltrate many tissues of the body, other symptoms may occur. Leg pain can be associated with periosteal infiltrates, as well as headache, nausea, and vomiting with meningeal leukemia. Rapid onset of unconsciousness may indicate subarachnoid hemorrhage.

Presentation occurs occasionally in skin, bone, and/or lymph node without BM involvement (<25% blasts in the marrow). These cases are referred to as lymphoma. They most often occur in young people (<18 years) and show overlapping features with precursor B-ALL, TdT, and B-lineage markers, and frequently additional 21q chromosome material (Maitra, 2001). Morphology in tissue sections shows diffuse infiltrations of small cells (nuclei smaller than histiocyte nuclei) with diffuse chromatin, inconspicuous nucleoli, scant cytoplasm, high mitotic rate, and frequently a "starry-sky" pattern of admixed histiocytes (indicating high apoptotic rate).

Anemia is present in precursor B-ALL if clinical manifestations are fully developed. It is usually normocytic. Frequently, nucleated red cells are present. Thrombocytopenia of moderate to marked degree is the rule. The leukocyte count occasionally is very high ($>100 \times 10^9$/L) and often is slightly elevated, but it is perhaps most frequently normal or decreased. The predominant cell is the lymphoblast.

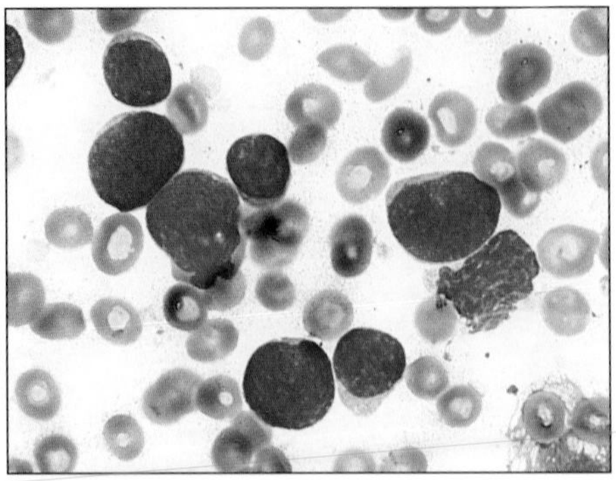

Figure 33-42 Precursor acute lymphoblastic leukemia of B-lineage, with small to medium-sized blasts and lack of conspicuous nucleoli (×1000).

Marrow

By the time the patient is symptomatic, hematopoietic cells and fat are usually replaced by a diffuse infiltration of lymphoblasts. Blast percentage is usually greater than 50%. Predominance of small blasts with high nuclear/cytoplasmic (N/C) ratios and inconspicuous nucleoli (L1 type in the FAB classification) is most common in childhood ALL (Fig. 33-42). Chromatin is diffuse in some cells but may show variable condensation, and blasts may be difficult to distinguish from the normal lymphocytes of young children. Larger blasts with more abundant cytoplasm, prominent nucleoli, and often irregular nuclei (FAB L2) also occur and tend to predominate in adult ALL.

The blasts are negative for SBB, peroxidase, and naphthol ASD CAE. Azurophilic granules may be present, but they are SBB and peroxidase negative. In other cases, ALL blasts may exhibit some SBB reactivity, but peroxidase is negative.

Blasts characteristically express TdT, cytoplasmic CD22 and CD79a, CD19, and HLA-DR. CD10 (common ALL antigen) is expressed in many, and expression of CD34 is variable. Cytoplasmic μ immunoglobulin heavy chain (cyt-μ) indicates a slightly more mature state, but surface immunoglobulin is negative. Myeloid-associated antigens CD13, CD33, and CD15 may be expressed.

Cytogenetics

Cytogenetic findings are increasingly important in diagnosis and prognostication in ALL and have been previously reviewed (Mrozek, 2004). The current WHO classification divides B-ALL into groups based on frequently found (recurrent) cytogenetic findings.

B Lymphoblastic Leukemia/Lymphoma with t(9;22)(q34;q11.2); BCR-ABL1

The Ph′ chromosome t(9;22) with production of a fusion BCR-ABL occurs in about 30% of cases of adult (20% detected at karyotyping) and 6% of cases of childhood ALL. The t(9;22) is the most frequent adult ALL translocation and is associated with poor prognosis. Two types are found: that identical to CML, involving the bcr region of BCR with resultant p210 kD fusion protein, occurring in half of adult cases of Ph′-positive ALL; and another with breakpoint upstream of bcr, producing a smaller chimeric message and p190 kD protein. The latter occurs in most childhood Ph′-positive cases. Ph′-positive ALL is most often of precursor B cell lineage but also may present with biphenotypic myeloid differentiation.

B Lymphoblastic Leukemia/Lymphoma with t(v;11q23); MLL Rearranged

Abnormalities of the *MLL* gene at chromosome region 11q23 are seen in 5%–7% of cases of ALL (Le Beau, 2000), as well as in AML, and are often associated with *FLT3* overexpression. ALL with t(4;11)(q21;q23) is associated with poor prognosis, high WBC count, and immature B-lineage phenotype with lack of CD10 or CD24 but with CD15 expression. It involves *MLL* and the partner gene *AF4*. It is most common in infants, and many cases of ALL with this abnormality are biphenotypic. Translocation t(11;19)(q23;p13.3) is the next most frequent MLL abnormality in ALL but also occurs in AML (monocytic). Overall, 11q23 (MLL) abnormalities, with the possible exception of t(9;11) in AML, confer poor prognosis.

B Lymphoblastic Leukemia/Lymphoma with t(12;21)(p12;q22); TEL-AML1 (ETV6-RUNX1)

This constitutes approximately 25% of B-ALL, correlates with high-density CD10 and HLA-DR expression with negative CD9 and CD20, and is associated with good prognosis. The *TEL* gene at 12p12 is fused with the *AML1* gene at 21q22 with a resultant fusion protein. *AML1 (RUNX1)* is a transcription factor involved in hematopoietic differentiation/proliferation. The abnormality is difficult to detect by karyotyping but can be detected by RT-PCR analysis for the chimeric mRNA or by FISH.

B Lymphoblastic Leukemia/Lymphoma with t(1;19)(q23;p13.3); E2A-PBX1 (TCF3-PBX1)

Another translocation, t(1;19)(q23;p13), and variants are associated with pre-B cell ALL (with cytoplasmic μ Ig). It involves the *E2A* gene at 19p13, which encodes transcription factors, and *PBX* at 1q23. This has also been associated with decreased response to therapy.

B Lymphoblastic Leukemia/Lymphoma with t(5;14)(q31;q32); IL3-IGH

This rare variant of B-ALL is associated with eosinophilia. The rearrangement results in constitutive expression of *IL3* and interleukin effects. Immunophenotype is CD19+, CD10+.

B Lymphoblastic Leukemia/Lymphoma with Hyperdiploidy

B-ALL with multiple trisomies and between 50 and 66 chromosomes (normal = 46) is referred to as hyperdiploid. This usually occurs in children and implies favorable prognosis. Trisomies of chromosome 4,10, and 17 are considered markers for low-risk disease in pediatric leukemia protocols. Blasts usually express CD19, CD10, and CD34 but often are CD45 negative.

B Lymphoblastic Leukemia/Lymphoma with Hypodiploidy

Hypodiploid B-ALL shows fewer than the normal 46 chromosomes. Prognosis is unfavorable, especially when chromosomes are fewer than 45, and even more so when fewer than 44.

B Lymphoblastic Leukemia/Lymphoma, Not Otherwise Specified (Refers to All Other B-ALL)

Precursor T Lymphoblastic Leukemia/Lymphoblastic Lymphoma

Precursor T lymphoblastic leukemia (T-LBL), which accounts for 10%–20% of cases of ALL, occurs predominantly in boys who tend to be slightly older than children with precursor B lymphoblastic ALL. Patients with T-lineage ALL often have a high leukocyte count and mediastinal involvement. Blast morphology is heterogeneous, similar to B-ALL, and immunophenotyping is required for diagnosis. The immunophenotype reflects thymic T cells which have a distinct maturation pattern (Reinherz, 1980), and the blasts show varying maturity. Most cases exhibit TdT, CD7, and cytoplasmic CD3 with variable CD1a, CD2, and CD5. Some cases, of early thymic phenotype, lack CD4 or CD8, but most (midcortical thymic phenotype, particularly in lymphoma presentation) coexpress CD4 and CD8. In late cortical thymic phenotype, CD4 or CD8 alone may be present, and in these, TdT and/or CD1a is particularly helpful for diagnosis. Myeloid markers such as CD13, CD33, and/or CD117 may be present, and CD79a may be present occasionally.

Presentation as lymphoma often shows a more mature thymic phenotype than leukemic presentation (Crist, 1988). These are relatively common lymphomas of adolescents and young adults (one third of pediatric NHLs) and also occur later in life. They typically present in the mediastinum and/or peripheral lymph nodes, and pleural effusions are common. Airway compromise or superior vena cava syndrome is frequently present, resulting in emergent need for therapy and limiting diagnostic procedures.

Morphology. T-LBL usually shows diffuse tissue involvement by blasts with nuclei smaller than those of histiocytes or reactive endothelial cells (Fig. 33-43), although some show nuclei similar in size to Burkitt lymphoma. Chromatin is usually finely dispersed to slightly clumped, but rarely as much as Burkitt lymphoma. Mitotic rates are high, and there is often a "starry sky" pattern similar to Burkitt. Neoplastic cells sometimes show selective T-zone involvement of lymph nodes and/or a leukemia-like infiltration pattern in soft tissue.

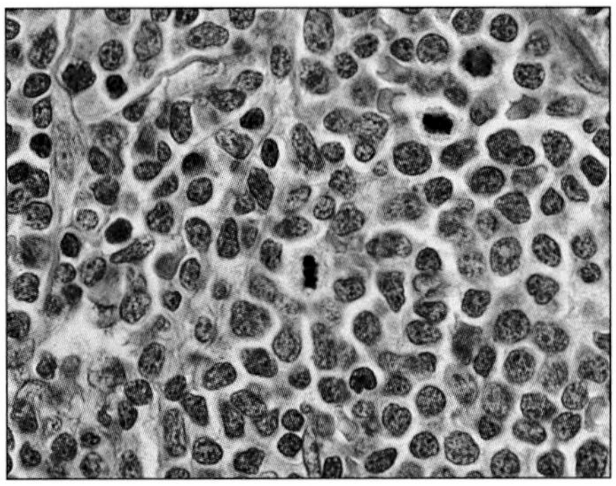

Figure 33-43 Precursor T lymphoblastic lymphoma (×500).

The differential diagnosis of T-LBL in young patients primarily involves it, BL, and occasionally large B cell lymphoma (LBCL). Mediastinal location favors T-LBL over BL, but not LBCL. In adults, the differential diagnosis includes blastoid and blastic variants of mantle cell lymphoma. Granulocytic sarcoma is also in the differential in any age group. Expression of TdT and lineage-specific T cell markers without B or myeloid markers is usually diagnostic.

Genetics. T cell receptor genes are frequently rearranged, but Ig heavy chain genes may also be rearranged (Racke, 2011). Patients with T cell ALL frequently show translocations of α and δ T cell receptor loci at 14q11.2, the β locus at 7q35, or the γ locus at 7p14-15, usually with genes encoding transcription factors. Partner genes include *MYC* (8q24.1), *TAL1* (1p32), *RBTN1* (11p15), *RBTN2* (11p13), *HOX11* (10q24), *HOX11L2* (5q35), and *LCK* (1p34.3-35). TAL1 regulatory gene deletions occur in 25% of cases, and del(9p) involving *CDKN2* is also frequent (Mrozek, 2004).

MATURE B CELL NEOPLASMS

These constitute the most numerous and possibly the most diverse group of hematopoietic neoplasms. Overall rates vary from 1.2/100,000 population/year in China to 15/100,000 in the United States. Geographic variation is seen in mature lymphoma/leukemia, with follicular and diffuse large B cells predominating in Western developed countries, constituting 50% of NHLs; myeloma is also common (Catovsky, 2008). The cells affected in mature B cell malignancies are those making up the humoral immune system, which itself is very complex and includes innumerable clones of B lymphocytes with genetically distinct immunoglobulin gene rearrangements. They exist at many states of maturation and are influenced by and affect many regulatory pathways. Normal cells and tumors are influenced by immune status and perturbations, viruses, other microorganisms, and antigenic stimuli. Tremendous variation in growth rates and in aggressiveness of tumors is seen in this large group, corresponding to high proliferative rates of some cells and quiescence of others. A correspondingly variable tendency toward apoptosis influences response to antineoplastic therapies. Clinical behaviors relate to clonal escape from regulation, the balance of proliferation and apoptosis, and modulation by therapy. Features of major categories are shown in Table 33-18.

Monoclonal B Cell Lymphocytosis

Diagnosis of chronic lymphocytic leukemia requires the presence of leukocytosis of ≥5 × 10^9/L monoclonal lymphocytes with **chronic lymphocytic leukemia** (CLL) phenotype (see later) for at least 3 months, or lower counts with the presence of cytopenias and/or disease-related symptoms. Otherwise, a diagnosis of **monoclonal B cell lymphocytosis** is made, analogous to the concept of monoclonal gammopathy of unknown significance (MGUS).

Chronic Lymphocytic Leukemia/Small Lymphocytic Lymphoma

This is a clonal proliferation of small B lymphocytes involving BM, blood, and lymph nodes. It is common, usually indolent, at least initially, but

TABLE 33-18
Key Features of Major Mature B Cell Neoplasms

Lymphoma	Demographics, clinical and laboratory presentations	Morphology	CELL SURFACE MARKERS Positive	Negative	Cytogenetics
CLL/SLL	M > F, over 60 years; insidious onset of fatigue, lymphadenopathy; WBC >5 K/μL, anemia, thrombocytopenia, occasionally AIHA	Small lymphocytes with condensed chromatin	CD19, CD20, CD5, CD22, CD23, CD79a, dim sIg	CD10, bcl-6, FMC-7	+12, del(13q14.3), del(11q22-23), del(17q)(TP53)
B cell PLL	M > F, mean age 65 years; massive splenomegaly, minimal lymphadenopathy, WBC >100 K	Prolymphocytes ≥55%	CD19, CD20, FMC-7, bright sIg	CD5, CD23, often negative	Occ del(17p), del(13q14)
Hairy cell leukemia	M > F, median age 50 years; insidious onset with splenomegaly, leukopenia with monocytopenia	Medium-sized cells with round to oval indented nuclei, reticular chromatin, frayed cytoplasmic borders	CD20, CD22, CD79a, CD103, CD25, CD11c	CD5, CD10, CD23	
Lymphoplasmacytic lymphoma	M > F, mean age 63 years; BM, nodal and splenic involvement, symptomatic IgM paraprotein	Plasmacytoid lymphocytes and plasma cells with PAS-positive inclusions (Dutcher bodies)	CD19, CD20, CD22, CD25, CD38, CD79a, bright sIgM, cIgM	CD5, CD10, CD23, CD103, bcl-6	del(6q), +3, +4, +18, none specific
Heavy chain disease (α-HCD, immunoproliferative small intestinal disease, prototype)	Younger adults in poorer Mediterranean communities with malabsorption, diarrhea	Lymphoplasmacytic infiltrate of intestinal mucosa, variant of MALT	NA	NA	
Marginal zone lymphomas: splenic, nodal, MALT	F > M, median age 61 years; indolent course involving stomach, other mucosal sites, spleen, or nodes	Lymphocytes with condensed chromatin and moderate cytoplasm; lymphoepithelial lesions in MALT type	CD20, CD79a, sIgM, bcl-2	CD5, CD10, CD23, bcl-6	+3, t(11;18)(q21;q21) in MALT type, 7q abnormalities
Follicular lymphoma	F > M, median age 59 years; lymphadenopathy, BM and splenic involvement frequent	Follicle-like structures with centrocytes and varying numbers of centroblasts	CD19, CD20, CD22, CD23, CD79a, CD10, bcl-2, bcl-6, sIgM	CD5, CD43	t(14;18)(q32;q21)
Mantle cell lymphoma	M > F, median age 60 years; lymphadenopathy, splenomegaly, BM involvement; typically refractory	Atrophic germinal centers, prominent mantle zones, small lymphs with irregular nuclei; blastoid/pleomorphic variants	CD5, CD43, FMC-7, bcl-2, cyclin D1, sIgM	CD10, CD23, bcl-6	t(11;14)(q13;q32)
Diffuse large B cell lymphoma	M > F, all ages, moderately aggressive but responds to chemo and anti-CD20	Diffuse infiltrate of large B cells, variable morphology	CD19, CD20, CD22, CD79a, sIg, bcl-2±, bcl-6±, CD30±, MUM1 in post-GC types	CD5 (usually)	t(14;18) in 20%, 3q27 (bcl-6) abnormalities in 30%, occ secondary *myc* translocations
Mediastinal large B cell lymphoma	F > M, young to middle-aged adults; airway compression, superior vena cava syndrome	Sclerotic lesions with clear, multilobulated, or RS-like cells	CD19, CD20, CD22, CD79a, CD30	CD5, CD10	Amplifications of 9p24, 2p15, others
Primary effusion lymphoma	Rare, associated with HHV-8 in immunosuppressed younger male homosexuals; pleural effusion	Immunoblastic or anaplastic cells	CD45, CD30, CD38, CD138	CD19, CD20, CD79a, sIg, bcl-6	
Plasmablastic lymphoma	Rare, associated with EBV in immunosuppressed	Plasmacytoid	CD45, CD38, CD138, CD79a	CD45, CD20, PAX-5 negative or weak	
EBV associated; chronic inflammation, of the elderly, lymphomatoid granulomatosis, post transplant	Immunosuppressed, elderly, others	Variable	CD20, EBV-EBER		

TABLE 33-18
Key Features of Major Mature B Cell Neoplasms—*Cont'd*

Lymphoma	Demographics, clinical and laboratory presentations	Morphology	CELL SURFACE MARKERS Positive	Negative	Cytogenetics
Burkitt lymphoma	1. Endemic: children in Africa, jaw mass M > F 2. Sporadic: children to young adults, worldwide, M > F 3. Immunodeficiency-associated: HIV patients	Uniform cells with round to oval nuclei, multiple nucleoli, high mitotic rate	CD19, CD20, CD10, bcl-6, sIg	TdT, bcl-2	t(8;14)(q24;q32), t(2;8)(p12;q24), t(8: 22)(q24;q11)
Intermediate BL/ DLBCL lymphoma	Children w/ rapidly growing mass, adults	Intermediate between BL and DLBCL	CD19, CD20, CD10, bcl-6, sIg		t(8;14)(q24;q32), 8q24/MYC, variable, others

AIHA, Autoimmune hemolytic anemia; *BL,* Burkitt lymphoma; *BM,* bone marrow; *cIg,* cytoplasmic immunoglobulin; *CLL,* chronic lymphocytic leukemia; *EBER,* EBV-encoded RNA; *DLBCL,* diffuse large B cell lymphoma; *EBV,* Epstein-Barr virus; *F,* female; *GC,* germinal center; *HHV,* human herpesvirus; *HIV,* human immunodeficiency virus; *Ig,* immunoglobulin; *M,* male; *MALT,* mucosa-associated lymphoid tissue; *MYC,* c-Myc gene; *NA,* not applicable; *PAS,* periodic acid–Schiff; *PLL,* prolymphocytic leukemia; *RS,* Reed-Sternberg; *sIg,* surface immunoglobulin; *SLL,* small lymphocytic lymphoma; *TdT,* deoxyribonucleotidyl transferase; *WBC,* white blood cell.

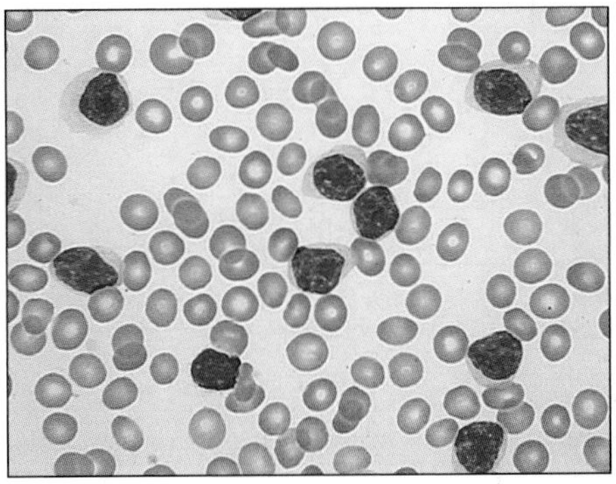

Figure 33-44 B cell chronic lymphocytic leukemia (×1000).

difficult if not impossible to cure (Muller-Hermelink, 2008). Cases with predominant involvement in the marrow and blood are traditionally called CLL, and lymphomas are called small lymphocytic lymphoma (SLL), but these are considered manifestations of a single entity. A majority of cases are leukemic and constitute 90% of chronic lymphoid leukemias in the United States and Europe. It is rare in those younger than age 40; most cases occur over the age of 60, and the condition is more than twice as common in men as in women. Onset is insidious, and the disease is commonly discovered by chance during the investigation of another problem. Most patients are >50 years of age.

The tumors show diffuse infiltrates of small mature lymphocytes with clumped chromatin and scant to moderate cytoplasm (Fig. 33-44). Admixed prolymphocytes and proliferation centers (containing increased prolymphocytes and lymphocytes with increased cytoplasm) are characteristic. Mitotic rates are very low.

CLL/SLL shows a characteristic phenotype of monoclonal B cells (CD19/CD20/CD79a) with dim surface Ig (single light chain with IgM or IgM and IgD), coexpression of usual T cell marker CD5, and expression of CD23. CD22, CD10, and cyclin D1 are negative. This pattern is very useful in distinguishing CLL/SLL from mantle cell, follicular, and marginal zone lymphomas. Bcl-6 is negative, and bcl-2 variable.

Ig heavy and (monotypic) light chain genes are rearranged, and Ig heavy chain (IGH) genes have undergone somatic hypermutation in 50%–60%. Mutation is associated with adverse prognosis and is associated with expression of the tyrosine kinase ZAP-70, normally expressed in T cells. ZAP-70 can be detected by flow cytometry, but the protein undergoes degradation in vitro and is imperfectly associated with gene expression.

Cytogenetic studies show del 13q14.3 in 50%, trisomy 12 in 20%, del(11q22-23) and/or mutations in this region in 20%, del(17p13) at the p53 locus in 10%, and del(6q21) in 5%. The first of these is associated with favorable outcome, and the latter three with adverse outcome. Cytogenetic abnormalities vary with mutation status. These abnormalities often cannot be detected by karyotype because CLL cells do not grow well in culture, but they are detectable by FISH probes. Other adverse features include expression of CD38, doubling of lymphocyte count in <12 months, and elevated β_2-microglobullin.

The leukocyte count is usually between 30 and 20 × 10^9/L. In the typical type of CLL, 90% or more of the cells are small lymphocytes that are monotonously similar in appearance and usually look normal. Nuclear chromatin may be coarsely condensed and more sharply separated by parachromatin than in normal lymphocytes, or, in some cases, the chromatin is less condensed than normal. Nucleoli are evident in many of the lymphocytes. Size variation is minimal, and the amount of cytoplasm is slight to moderate. Less than 10% of lymphocytes are prolymphocytes or reticular lymphocytes (transformed lymphocytes).

Often there is neither anemia nor thrombocytopenia at the time of diagnosis. Anemia due to impaired production does develop as the marrow is replaced by leukemic cells. In addition, erythrocyte life span in some patients with CLL may be reduced. This is especially true when there is marked splenomegaly. Autoimmune hemolytic anemia develops in about 10% of patients. Thrombocytopenia is often slight and occasionally becomes severe as the disease progresses, so that hemorrhagic manifestations appear. Thrombocytopenia is usually due to hypoproliferation but may also be secondary to an immune process or splenic sequestration. Patchy, nodular, or interstitial involvement of the BM by neoplastic lymphocytes is associated with a relatively good outcome. A diffuse infiltrate of the BM, however, usually correlates with a poor prognosis and/or advanced disease (Bartl, 1982b; Montserrat, 1987). An increased proportion of prolymphocytes (between 10% and 55%) has been referred to as mixed CLL/prolymphocytic leukemia (PLL) and may correlate with aggressive disease (Melo, 1987; Bennett, 1989). Expression of markers CD38 and ZAP-70 and *p53* abnormalities have been investigated for possible prognostic value, but results are inconclusive (Kim, 2004; Mainou-Fowler, 2004). Anemia, B symptoms, and International Prognostic Index (IPI) may provide the best prognostic information (Nola, 2004). The median survival for patients with CLL is about 7 years, but recent therapy such as fludarabine shows promise for better survival.

B Cell Prolymphocytic Leukemia

Prolymphocytic leukemia was originally described as a variant of CLL (Galton, 1974). The male/female ratio is 6.5 : 1, and mean age is 65 years. PLL is characterized by a very marked lymphocytosis (usually greater than 100 × 10^3/µL), massive splenomegaly, moderate hepatomegaly, and inconspicuous lymphadenopathy. The malignant lymphoid cells have a large vesicular nucleolus, condensed nuclear chromatin, and a moderate amount of cytoplasm (Fig. 33-45). More than 55% of blood leukemic cells are prolymphocytes. Immunophenotype varies from SLL/CLL by bright surface Ig (monoclonal IgM with or without IgD), lack of CD5 in two thirds of cases, and usually lack of CD23 and presence of FMC-7. Abnormalities of *p53* are frequent, and deletions at 11q23 and 13q14 occur. Prolymphocytic leukemia is usually less responsive to treatment than CLL in general, and it has a poorer prognosis.

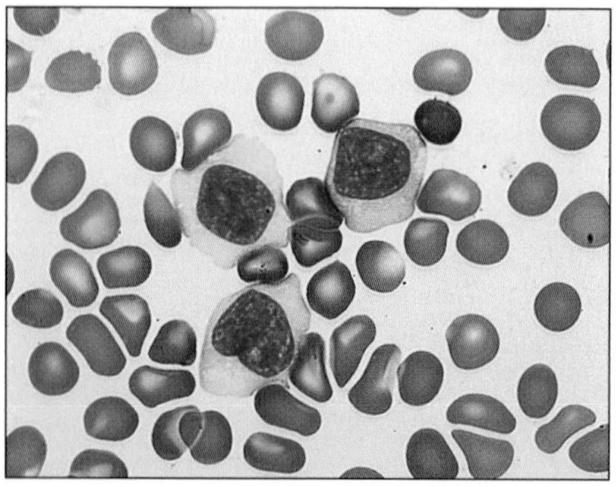

Figure 33-45 B cell prolymphocytic leukemia typically shows high white blood cell count, large lymphocytes with moderately abundant cytoplasm, and prominent nucleoli, although variability is noted (×1000).

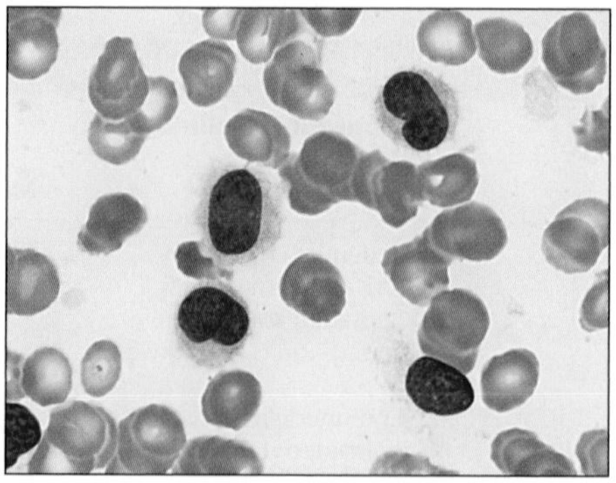

Figure 33-48 Hairy cell leukemia shows lymphoid cells with foamy cytoplasm and cytoplasmic projections, and oval or indented nuclei with reticular chromatin (×1000).

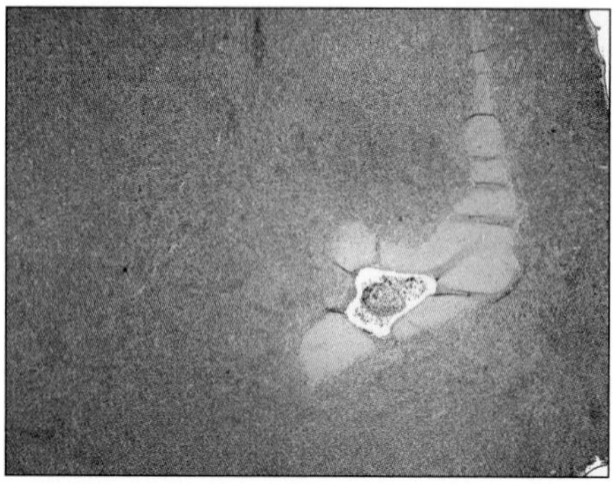

Figure 33-46 Splenic marginal zone lymphoma showing mild white pulp expansion and patchy red pulp involvement (×100).

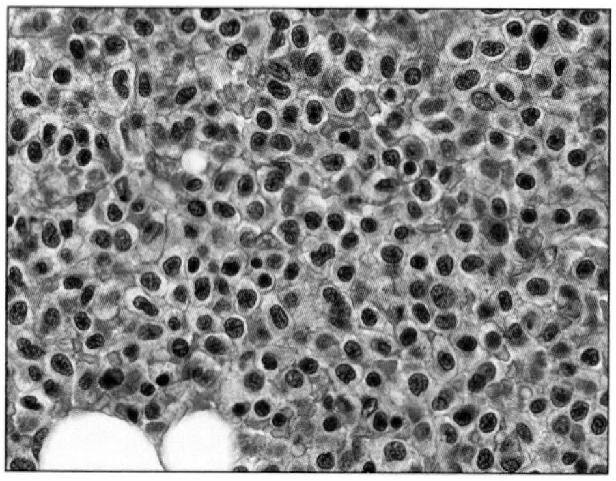

Figure 33-49 Hairy cell leukemia in a bone marrow biopsy shows small nuclei with moderate cytoplasm and distinct cytoplasmic boundaries (×500).

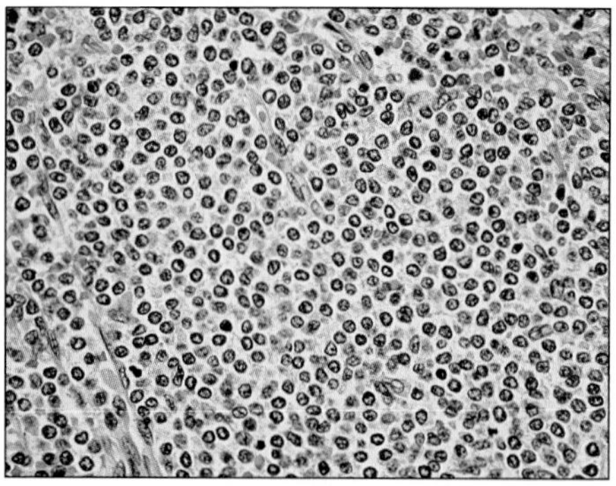

Figure 33-47 Higher-power view of splenic red pulp involvement by monocytoid splenic marginal zone cells in splenic marginal zone lymphoma (×200).

Splenic Marginal Zone Lymphoma

Splenic marginal zone lymphoma (SMZL) has many clinical, laboratory, and morphologic features similar to HCL and features similar to SLL/CLL (Swerdlow, 2008). The disease is more common in men than in women. Patients are often in their seventh decade of life when they present with splenomegaly.

In the spleen, the neoplastic infiltrate expands from the white pulp into the red pulp. Some patients (≈⅓) show a small monoclonal gammopathy, usually IgM. The BM may demonstrate patchy infiltrates or massive involvement. The tumor arises from splenic marginal zones, which in reactive processes are seen as an outer zone of pale lymphocytes with moderately abundant cytoplasm surrounding the white pulp and imparting a target-like appearance. In some cases, reactive follicles with germinal centers are present, and an expanded marginal zone surrounds the white pulp and involves the red pulp. Marginal zone hyperplasia may mimic this disorder. Other cases show predominantly red pulp involvement (Figs. 33-46 and 33-47). Red cell lakes are not present, and lymph nodes are not characteristically involved. The tartrate-resistant acid phosphatase (TRAP) stain is usually negative, although positive reactions have been recorded.

The immunophenotype is mature B cell with surface IgM/IgD (similar to SLL/CLL), positive CD20, CD79, and other pan–B cell markers. CD5, CD10, CD23, cyclin D1, CD103, annexin A1, and CD43 are characteristically negative.

Immunoglobulin genes are clonally rearranged, and half of cases show somatic mutations. Translocation/loss of 7q21-32 is noted in 40% of cases, and trisomy 3q in some (Dogan, 2003). Bcl-2 is variable and is typically expressed according to some studies (Pawade, 1995) but not others (Menendez, 2004). Hepatitis C may play a role in the pathogenesis in some cases (Weng, 2003; Iannitto, 2004; Kelaidi, 2004).

SMZL is indolent but has shown poor response to therapy. New approaches utilizing chemotherapy combined with anti-CD20 therapy appear promising (Arcaini, 2004).

Hairy Cell Leukemia

Bouroncle (1958) initially described this disorder, which is clinically variable in its manifestations. HCL occurs more frequently in males than in females. The mean age of afflicted patients is 50 years. It has an insidious onset and is characterized by proliferation of abnormal cells in the reticuloendothelial organs and blood. Splenomegaly is the predominant physical finding (Foucar, 2008). Pancytopenia or depression of only two cell lines is the usual finding, with variable numbers of hairy cells. Monocytopenia is characteristic and hairy cells are usually infrequent in the blood, although they may result in leukocytosis. In most cases, BM aspiration is difficult. Marrow biopsy shows a marrow that varies in cellularity, often having both hypocellular and hypercellular areas and reticulin fibrosis. Hypocellular cases of HCL occur and mimic aplastic anemia. Morphologically, the cells are medium sized (10–20 μm in diameter) with round to oval nuclei, although many are notched or dumbbell or bean shaped. The chromatin pattern is usually uniformly reticular, and nucleoli are small and inconspicuous. In some cells, chromatin is more condensed, resembling that of a lymphocyte. The cytoplasm is moderate in amount, is light blue-gray, and exhibits numerous hair-like projections and frayed borders, most prominent on electron micrographs (Fig. 33-48).

In marrow sections, cells with small central nuclei, abundant cytoplasm, and reticulin fibrosis produce a characteristic fried-egg appearance, which may resemble erythroid islands when involvement is not extensive (Fig. 33-49). Chromatin is usually more delicate and nuclei more irregular than

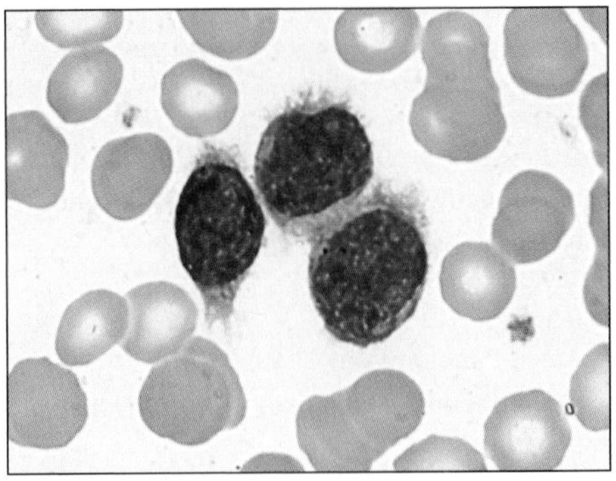

Figure 33-50 Villous lymphocytes (×1000).

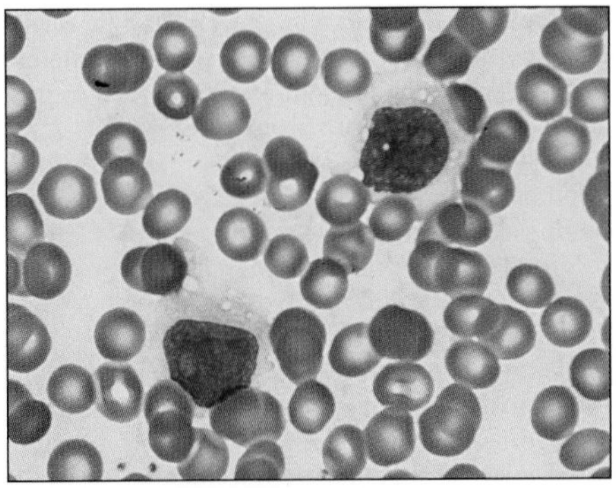

Figure 33-51 Hairy cell leukemia (HCL) variant shows morphology intermediate between usual HCL and prolymphocytic leukemia.

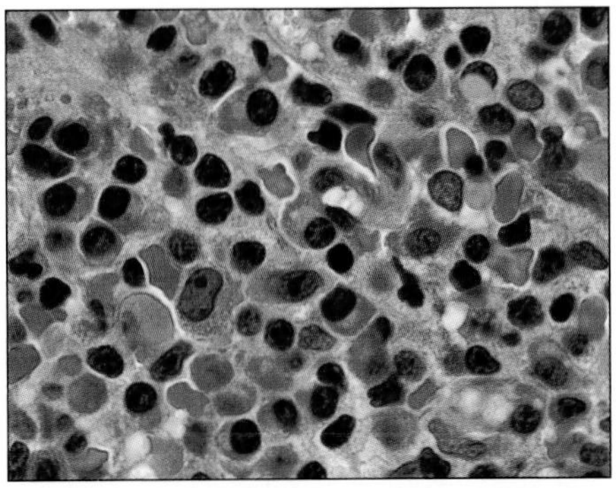

Figure 33-52 Lymphoplasmacytic lymphoma involving the marrow, with associated Waldenström's macroglobulinemia. Lymphocytes, plasma cells, plasmacytoid lymphocytes, and a rare Dutcher body *(upper right)* can be seen (×1000).

in erythroid precursors. In small or poorly preserved biopsies, HCL may be mistaken for large B cell lymphoma.

Splenectomy specimens are usually diagnostic, with red pulp infiltrates of cells similar to those in the marrow. In addition, the cells tend to line splenic sinuses, obliterating the endothelium and producing red cell "lakes," which lack visible endothelium. Lymph nodes may show paracortical infiltrates, and the liver may show sinus infiltration.

Cytochemically, these cells contain acid phosphatase, which is resistant to inhibition by tartrate-resistant acid phosphatase; this is in contrast to the isoenzymes of acid phosphatase present in other hemic cells (Yam, 1971).

Immunophenotype is mature B cell (CD19, CD20, CD22, CD79a, DBA.44, FMC-7, and surface membrane immunoglobulin [SMIg]) with expression of hairy cell–associated markers CD103, CD25, CD11c, annexin A1 (ANXA1), and (dim) cyclin D1 (Falini, 2004). Cells are negative for CD5, CD10, and CD23. Immunoglobulin heavy and light chain genes are rearranged, with somatic mutation of V gene regions. No specific genetic abnormalities are yet described.

The clinical course is usually chronic but may be acute or subacute. Median survival is between 5 and 6 years. Traditionally, splenectomy has offered significant benefit to many patients. Treatment with α-interferon provided the first chemotherapy remissions, but 2′-deoxycoformycin and 2-chlordeoxyadenosine now produce more durable remissions.

Splenic B Cell Lymphoma/Leukemia, Unclassifiable

Splenic Diffuse Red Pulp Small B Cell Lymphoma

This is a lymphoma of small B cells with diffuse splenic red pulp involvement and involvement of BM sinusoids and blood. At least some cases were previously referred to as splenic lymphoma with circulating villous lymphocytes due to circulating neoplastic cells with short cytoplasmic villi, often with a polar distribution (Fig. 33-50). Neoplastic lymphocytes show clumped chromatin and moderate basophilic cytoplasm. Patients have massive splenomegaly but often low levels of lymphocytosis. Neoplastic cells may circulate in the blood, even in the absence of marrow involvement. The phenotype is B cell with expression of DBA.44 and surface IgG, but usually absent CD103 and absent Annexin A1.

Hairy Cell Leukemia Variant

Most cases of **hairy cell variant** are described as lymphoproliferative disorders resembling HCL but with high WBCs and the presence of prominent nucleoli (Sainati, 1990), and not closely related biologically. These cases have morphology and clinical features intermediate between HCL and PLL (Fig. 33-51). Response to chemotherapy is poor, but the clinical course is chronic, and remission may be attained with splenectomy. TRAP and CD103 are variable, and CD25 and Annexin A1 are usually negative. A very rare form of variant HCL has been described, mostly in Japanese patients, and is referred to as **Japanese variant** (Machii, 1993). This disorder shows slightly more prominent nucleoli than typical HCL, but less so than prolymphocytoid variants, also variable CD103 and TRAP, negative CD25, and usually lack of surface Ig (Yamaguchi, 1996; Wu, 2000). It shows clonal rearrangement of Ig genes and must be distinguished from polyclonal B cell lymphocytosis with similar morphology (Machii, 1997).

Lymphoplasmacytic Lymphoma

Lymphoplasmacytic lymphomas (LPL), a term derived from the Kiel Classification (Stansfeld, 1988), refers to tumors of small lymphocytes with plasmacytoid differentiation and plasma cells, secretion of a monoclonal IgM paraprotein, and lack of CD5 expression. They usually involve BM, lymph nodes, and spleen (Fig. 33-52).

Lymph nodes show diffuse infiltrates of lymphocytes, plasmacytoid lymphocytes, and plasma cells. Proliferation centers are not present, and monocytoid B cells are not seen. The infiltrate may be paracortical with sparing of sinuses. PAS-positive inclusions are often seen in the cytoplasm, and Golgi-centered inclusions frequently invaginate into the nucleus of the lymphoid cells, forming **Dutcher bodies.** Tissue mast cells are frequently increased.

The BM usually shows nodular and/or diffuse interstitial infiltrates of similar cells. Blood involvement may be present, but with lower WBCs than CLL.

The immunophenotype shows B cell markers CD19, CD20, CD22, and CD79a with bright surface and cytoplasmic IgM (occasionally IgG or IgA) but not IgD, and a monoclonal κ or λ light chain. It differs from CLL by absence of CD5 and bright immunoglobulin expression. CD10 and CD23 are also negative; CD38 is positive, and CD43 is variable.

Ig heavy and light chain genes are clonally rearranged, and there is somatic mutation of variable regions, consistent with a postantigen selection (post germinal center) state of maturation and differing from CLL (Swerdlow, 2008).

Del6q21 and trisomy 4 are frequent in LPL, and trisomies 3 and 18 and other abnormalities are sporadically reported.

The term **Waldenström's macroglobulinemia** refers to LPL with BM involvement and a monoclonal IgM paraprotein. It has a peak incidence between the ages of 60 and 70. Symptoms of increased viscosity include visual disturbances, neurologic symptoms, impaired kidney function, and congestive heart failure. Hemorrhagic phenomena may occur as the result of interference of complexes with platelets and clotting factors. Cryoglobulinemia occurs somewhat more frequently than with myeloma and often results in Raynaud's phenomenon.

Normochromic, normocytic anemia is sometimes associated with thrombocytopenia or pancytopenia. Relative or slight absolute lymphocytosis is usually found. Marked rouleaux formation is evident on the blood film, and the sedimentation rate is usually extremely rapid, although it may be low if macrocryoglobulins are present and the test is carried out at a lower temperature. Anemia is occasionally hemolytic with a positive Coombs' test.

Serum globulin is usually markedly increased. The relative serum viscosity may be simply measured using an Ostwald viscometer. The average time for descent of the serum at room temperature is expressed as a ratio to that of distilled water. The normal range is 1.4–1.8. It is considerably elevated in most patients with macroglobulinemia. Symptoms of hyperviscosity appear in most patients when the relative serum viscosity is between 6 and 8, although the threshold varies among patients. The paraprotein is identified by immunoelectrophoresis. Light chain proteinuria occurs in about 10% of patients.

Many cases previously placed in this category are now believed to represent low-grade lymphoma of mucosa-associated lymphoid tissue (MALT) lymphoma with plasmacytoid expression. No definite biological marker can be used to separate the two, but MALT lymphomas typically involve epithelial organs, and macroglobulinemia is not the presenting feature. Many cases of cryoglobulinemia due to LPL and MALT lymphoma are associated with hepatitis C virus (Sansonno, 1996).

Heavy Chain Diseases

A small number of patients produce and excrete heavy chain fragments without associated light chains. Some of these proteins show structural mutations. The classification of associated lymphoproliferative disorders is somewhat ambiguous. Lymphoproliferative disorders associated with γ heavy chain disease often resemble LPL or plasmacytoma; μ heavy chain disease may resemble CLL, and α heavy chain disease is associated with MALT lymphoma.

γ Heavy Chain Disease

γ heavy chain disease (HCD) is a lymphoproliferative disorder characterized by secretion of a truncated γ-chain without light chain binding sites. It presents with lymphadenopathy, hepatosplenomegaly, fever, and propensity to infection. Anemia is constantly present, often with leukopenia and thrombocytopenia. Atypical lymphocytes or plasma cells are frequently present in the blood, and a few cases have terminated in plasma cell leukemia. The marrow is usually abnormal, with increased plasma cells, lymphocytes, and eosinophils. A rather broad serum protein "spike" has been found in the βγ-region in most patients, accompanied by hypogammaglobulinemia. The diagnosis is made by showing that the protein reacts on immunoelectrophoresis with antisera to γ-chains but not to light chains. The protein is also found in the urine in varying amounts, although concentration techniques may be necessary to demonstrate it.

α Heavy Chain Disease

α heavy chain disease appears to be more common than γ-HCD and involves a younger age group. The uniform clinical pattern in most patients is malabsorption and diarrhea accompanying a massive lymphoplasmacytic infiltration of intestinal mucosa, sometimes evolving to large B cell lymphoma. It has also been referred to as Mediterranean abdominal lymphoma and immunoproliferative small intestinal disease (IPSID). In a few patients, the respiratory tract has been involved instead. BM and other lymphoid organs have not been involved. Usually, routine protein electrophoresis is negative, but small amounts of α-chain may be detected in the serum and sometimes in the urine with immunoelectrophoresis. The abnormal protein does not contain light chains. It is most common in Mediterranean areas and is associated with poor living conditions in low socioeconomic groups. Similar to MALT lymphoma, many cases may initiate an infectious antigen-driven proliferation.

μ Heavy Chain Disease

The few patients who have been described with μ heavy chain disease have had chronic lymphocytic leukemia with vacuolated plasma cells in the marrow. Routine serum electrophoresis showed only hypogammaglobulinemia. The μ heavy chain was detected by serum immunoelectrophoresis; it was not found in the urine. In most patients, however, the urine contained κ light chain in large amounts (Franklin, 1975).

Plasma Cell Neoplasms

Clonal neoplasms of mature plasma cells are common neoplasms that have been difficult to treat and are greatly feared. They are now known, however, to consist of a spectrum of disease varying from indolent and nonprogressive to highly aggressive and refractory to therapy. The best measures of disease course are the clinical findings themselves, and treatments using new agents are rapidly evolving to increase efficacy and improve outcome. Major categories now are monoclonal gammopathy of undetermined significance, that is, usually indolent (but may be associated with amyloidosis), asymptomatic myeloma and symptomatic myeloma (Table 33-19).

TABLE 33-19

Diagnostic Criteria for Monoclonal Gammopathy of Undetermined Significance, Indolent and Smoldering Myeloma, and Plasma Cell Myeloma

Monoclonal Gammopathy of Undetermined Significance
M-protein in serum <30 g/L
Marrow plasmacytosis <10%
No lytic bone lesions
No myeloma-related symptoms (no CRAB)
Asymptomatic (Smoldering) Myeloma
Serum M-component >30 g/L
Marrow plasmacytosis >10%
No organ or tissue impairment (no CRAB)
Plasma Cell Myeloma
M-protein in serum or urine (no specific level need be met)
Bone marrow clonal plasma cells
Organ or tissue impairment (hypercalcemia, renal insufficiency, anemia, bone lesions; CRAB)

CRAB, Hypercalcemia, renal insufficiency, anemia, or bone lesions.

Monoclonal Gammopathy of Undetermined Significance

Monoclonal gammopathy of undetermined significance is the term utilized when a monoclonal serum immunoglobulin is present but no myeloma is detectable. Most cases (75%) are IgG, with smaller proportions of IgM (15%) and IgA (10%). It is a preneoplastic condition with progression to myeloma in about 1% of affected patients per year. The condition consists of a monoclonal Ig (M-component) of <30 g/L IgG, <10% clonal plasma cells in the marrow, absence of lytic bone lesions, no melanoma-related organ or tissue impairment (CRAB: hypercalcemia, renal insufficiency, anemia, or bone lesions), and no evidence of other B cell lymphoproliferative disorder. Cytogenetic and immunophenotypic abnormalities are similar to those in myeloma, and none is known to be predictive of progression.

Plasma Cell Myeloma

Plasma cell myeloma is a neoplastic proliferation of plasma cells, occurring primarily in the BM. Although plasma cells also proliferate in lymph nodes and spleen, these organs are rarely enlarged (Swerdlow, 2008). Symptomatic myeloma is defined by the WHO 2008 classification simply as the presence of M-protein in serum or urine, BM clonal plasma cells or plasmacytoma, and the presence of related organ or tissue impairment (CRAB, see previously).

Multiple myeloma is rare in those younger than 40 years of age. The mean age at the time of diagnosis is 62 years with an equal sex distribution. Bone pain is the most common symptom, and pathologic fractures are frequent. Neurologic symptoms may be prominent from encroachment of tumor that has broken through the bony cortex on spinal nerves or spinal cord. Bone destruction leads to calcium mobilization, with increased calcium in the serum and metastatic calcification. Growth of myeloma cells in the marrow produces multiple tumors, which appear on a radiograph as multiple punched-out osteoporotic lesions; occasionally, the growth is diffuse and appears as diffuse osteoporosis. A propensity to infection is common because of impaired production of antibodies. Plasma cell disorders may be associated with human herpesvirus type 8 (HHV-8).

A normochromic, normocytic anemia usually occurs, and normoblasts may be present in the blood. The leukocyte count is slightly decreased, normal, or slightly increased. Occasional myeloid left shift to the myeloblast may be noted. The platelet count is usually normal but may be decreased. The most striking feature of the blood film is the marked degree of rouleaux formation.

The BM shows the presence of plasma cells or myeloma cells, ranging from less than 1% to over 90%, depending on the degree of involvement at the site of the aspirated marrow. Diagnosis of myeloma and its variants is based on both pathology and clinical findings, including serum monoclonal immunoglobulin and radiologic evidence of lytic bone lesions (Durie, 2003; Swerdlow, 2008). Lytic bone lesions are associated with increased osteoclastic activity, hypercalcemia, and neurologic changes. This may be related to activity of the receptor activator for NF κB (RANK)

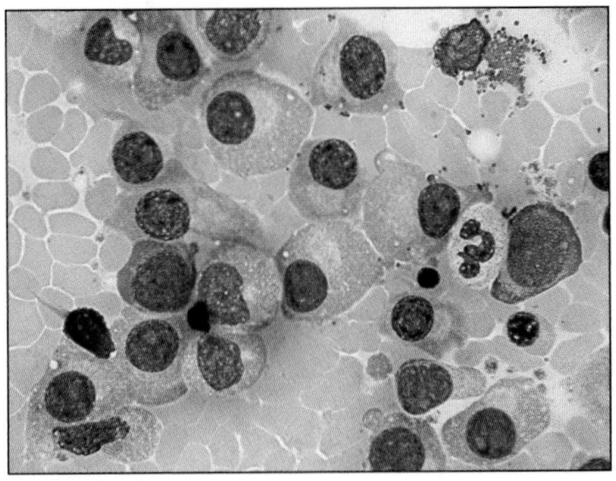

Figure 33-53 Myeloma in the bone marrow showing large plasma cells with nucleoli (×1000).

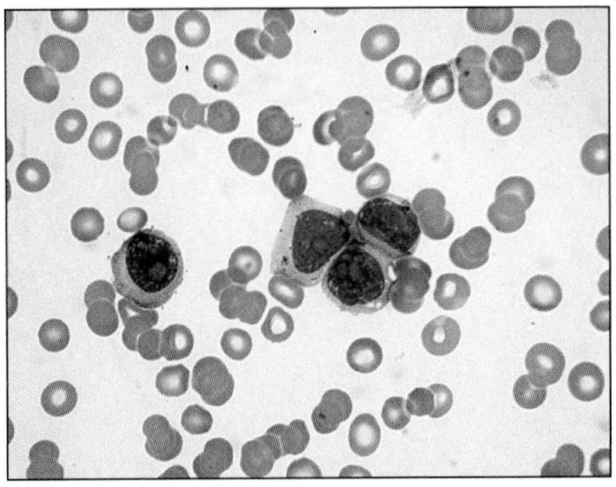

Figure 33-54 Plasma cell leukemia with cells resembling immunoblasts (×1000).

ligand (Sezer, 2003) and has stimulated interest in its receptor, osteoprotegerin (OPG).

Cytologically, the cells may be indistinguishable from normal plasma cells, but they usually show abnormal chromatin, such as less clumping of nuclear chromatin, large nucleoli, lack of perinuclear clear zone, lighter blue cytoplasm, or varying degrees of anaplasia (Fig. 33-53). Immature, plasmablastic, and anaplastic variants are described.

The immunophenotype is variable, most typically with expression of CD38 and CD138, loss of CD19 expression (normally present on plasma cells), and absence of CD20, but with abnormal acquisition of CD56 and often CD117. Immunohistochemical labeling or mRNA in situ hybridization of BM sections for κ and λ usually identifies monoclonal plasma cells. Cyclin D1 expression is associated with t(11;14).

Cytogenetic analysis divides myeloma into two main groups: hyperdiploid with multiple trisomies involving odd-numbered chromosomes and associated with good prognosis; and hypodiploid associated with adverse prognosis. Karyotype and FISH studies show frequent del13q14 (50% of cases), translocations t(4;14), t(14;16) or t(14;20), or deletion of TP53 (del 17p13) that, along with aneuploidy, are unfavorable when detected by karyotype, or t(11;14) or t(6;14) that is favorable when detected only by FISH. The translocation t(11;14)(q13;q32) involves the same gene as that in mantle cell lymphoma, but the breakpoints are different. Losses of 8, 13, 14, and X are common. Elevated serum β_2-microglobulin is also an adverse feature. A high-risk molecular signature has been described (Zhou, 2009).

Serum globulin is usually increased, often strikingly so. This increase is responsible for the tendency toward rouleaux formation and an elevated ESR. Serum protein electrophoresis usually shows an M-spot, a homogeneous band in the γ- or β-region; less commonly, there is hypogammaglobulinemia (when only light chains are produced by the neoplastic plasma cells). Immunoelectrophoresis indicates that the monoclonal protein is IgG in over 50% of cases, IgA in about 20%, IgD in less than 1%, and IgE very rarely. Roughly 5% of myeloma proteins are cryoglobulins, that is, proteins that precipitate from cooled serum and redissolve on warming. Some tumors secrete free monoclonal light chains (Bence Jones protein), in addition to the whole immunoglobulin molecule, and in about 25%, only light chains are produced. Hypogammaglobulinemia is found in the latter group because light chains are filtered through the renal glomerulus, leaving little or none in the serum, in addition to the fact that immunoglobulin production by nonmalignant plasma cells is greatly reduced. If renal damage has occurred, albumin and whole immunoglobulin molecules are also found in the urine. Excretion of light chains sometimes results in obstruction and loss of nephrons and so-called myeloma kidney. Renal insufficiency is common and is the presenting feature of multiple myeloma in some cases. Amyloidosis, which is present in about 10%–15% of cases of multiple myeloma, may be a factor in renal failure.

Median survival after diagnosis of multiple myeloma has been approximately 3–4 years, but new drugs are likely altering this.

Clinical Variants

Asymptomatic (Smoldering) Myeloma. Smoldering myeloma shows M-protein at myeloma levels (>30 g/L) and/or 10% or more clonal plasma cells in the marrow with no related organ/tissue impairment (CRAB). Patients with solitary plasmacytoma and bone lesions detected only by magnetic resonance imaging (MRI) are included. These asymptomatic patients differ from those with MGUS primarily by a higher rate of progression: 10% per year for the first 5 years, 3% for the next 5 years, and then 1% per year.

Nonsecretory Myeloma. These patients are similar to others with myeloma, except that tumor cells do not produce (15%) or secrete (85%) immunoglobulin. The incidences of renal insufficiency, hypercalcemia, and depression of normal Ig are less.

Plasma Cell Leukemia. Often in multiple myeloma, a few plasma cells are found in the peripheral blood. Only in the rare instances of myeloma in which large numbers of plasma cells circulate (either >20% of blood leukocytes, or $>2 \times 10^9$/L) is the term plasma cell leukemia used (Fig. 33-54). Patients with plasma cell leukemia tend to have tissue infiltration, advanced-stage disease, and poor survival (Woodruff, 1978).

The immunophenotype varies from usual myeloma in that CD56 is often absent.

Solitary Plasmacytoma of Bone. These patients show no clinical features of myeloma but may have a monoclonal immunoglobulin without suppression of normal immunoglobulin. Tumors are controlled by radiation, but two thirds of cases eventually progress to myeloma.

Extraosseous Plasmacytoma. Extramedullary solitary plasmacytomas occur in GI tract, bladder, CNS, breast, thyroid, testis, parotid gland, lymph nodes, or skin and are irradiated. They recur in one quarter of patients but progress to myeloma in only about 15%.

Monoclonal Immunoglobulin Deposition Diseases

Primary Amyloidosis

Primary amyloidosis, an uncommon presentation of plasma cell neoplasms of various types, results from abnormal polymerization of immunoglobulin into β-pleated sheets in connective tissue. A variety of amyloid types occur, including hereditary, secondary associated with chronic inflammation, the type associated with Alzheimer's disease, and others. All amyloid is biochemically composed of an A protein component and a P component. In plasma cell dyscrasia, the A component is derived from immunoglobulin light (L) chains and is referred to as AL amyloid. It may be detected by homogeneous pink staining of thickened blood vessels in abdominal fat, BM, rectum, or other tissues. Congo Red stain shows characteristic apple-green birefringence under polarized light. It may also be detected by thioflavin T, antibodies against amyloid P, and antibodies against immunoglobulin light chains. It may involve the heart with subsequent congestive failure, liver with hepatomegaly, kidney with nephrotic syndrome or renal failure, nerves with sensory/motor loss, and other organs. It may occur in overt myeloma (20%), but most often it is seen in patients with disease otherwise fulfilling criteria for MGUS.

Monoclonal Light and Heavy Chain Deposition Diseases

Nonamyloid immunoglobulin deposition may result in organ dysfunction in rare disorders known as light chain deposition disease (LCDD) or heavy chain deposition disease (HCDD) (Swerdlow, 2008).

Osteosclerotic Myeloma

This is a syndrome of polyneuropathy, organomegaly, endocrinopathy, monoclonal gammopathy, and skin changes (POEMS) associated with osteosclerotic multiple myeloma showing marrow fibrosis and sclerosis, and with lymph node changes resembling plasma cell Castleman's disease.

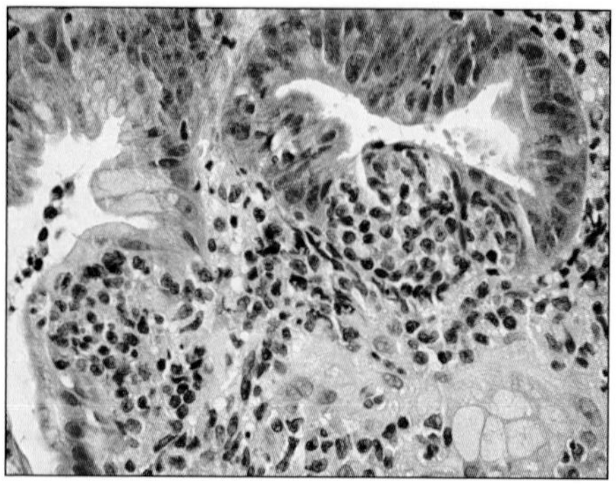

Figure 33-55 Mucosa-associated lymphoid tissue lymphoma with nests in lymphocytes in gastric epithelium (×500).

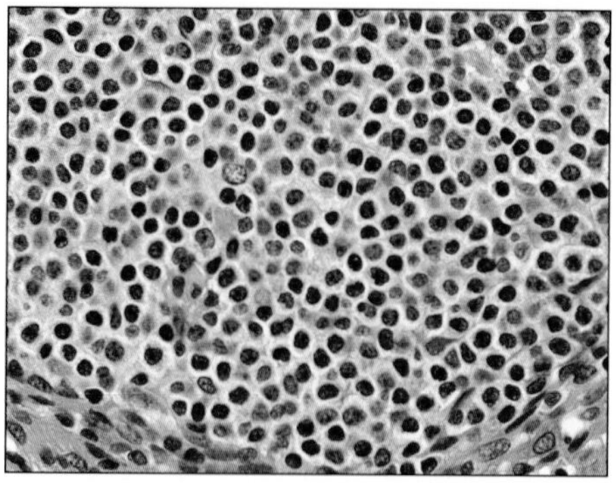

Figure 33-56 Nodal marginal zone lymphoma showing a nodule of monocytoid B cells (×200).

The plasma cells usually express λ light chain, and heavy chain is IgG or IgA.

Extranodal Marginal Zone B Cell Lymphoma of Mucosa-Associated Lymphoid Tissue

Extranodal marginal zone B cell lymphoma of mucosa-associated lymphoid tissue is an indolent lymphoma of mucosal tissue, including stomach, other GI tract, bronchi, salivary glands, thyroid, skin, and other areas. MALT lymphoma of the stomach is in many cases an antigen-driven clonal B cell proliferation related to infection by *Helicobacter pylori*, which is also associated with gastric ulcer; early cases may respond to antibacterial therapy. Other patients have autoimmune disorders such as Sjögren's syndrome or Hashimoto's thyroiditis. The terminology of MALT lymphomas refers only to those of predominantly small cells, although large cell and other aggressive lymphomas may arise in the same tissues. α heavy chain disease, or IPSID, is considered a special subtype of this disease (see earlier).

Gastric or other mucosa is infiltrated by small lymphocytes that form clusters within the epithelium, referred to as lymphoepithelial lesions (Fig. 33-55). Submucosa contains diffuse infiltrates of small lymphocytes, centrocytes, monocytoid lymphocytes, and plasma cells. Germinal centers, apparently reactive to the entire process, are usually present. Plasma cells often are abundant at the periphery of the lesions and generally are monoclonal.

The immunophenotype is B cell (CD19, CD20, CD22, CD79a) with surface Ig. CD5, CD10, bcl-6, and usually CD23 are negative. Bcl-2 is frequently positive, and CD43 is variable (Isaacson, 2008). Follicular dendritic cell–associated markers CD21 and CD35 often reveal expanded follicular meshworks and colonized germinal centers.

Immunoglobulin genes are clonally rearranged with somatic mutations of V regions. Trisomies 3 and 18 are frequent. t(11;18)(q21;q21), involving the apoptosis-inhibiting gene *API2* with *MLT* at 18q21, is common in pulmonary and gastric tumors. t(1;14)(p22;q32) is associated with ocular adnexae, orbit, and salivary gland lesions; t(14;18)(q32;q21), with activation of NF-κB–mediated antiapoptotic pathways, is common in thyroid, ocular adnexae, and skin lesions (Gascoyne, 2003). These tumors are typically indolent with good response to radiation therapy.

Nodal Marginal Zone Lymphoma

These tumors are derived from post–germinal center marginal zone B cells and show small lymphocytes surrounding reactive follicles and expanding in the interfollicular zones. They may resemble nodal involvement by MALT lymphoma or splenic marginal zone lymphoma (Fig. 33-56). Germinal center colonization is frequent, as are plasma cell differentiation and occasional eosinophilia. Increased large cells may be present and do not apparently affect prognosis, although transformation to diffuse large B cell lymphoma may occur.

The immunophenotype is similar to MALT or SMZL, with surface Ig (IgM/IgD, IgM, less often IgA or IgG), B cell markers (CD19, CD20, CD22, CD79a), expression of CD23, variable CD43, and absence of CD5 or CD10. Bcl-2 is expressed in a majority of cases, and survivin is overexpressed in about 50%, suggesting activation of antiapoptotic pathways. Nodal MZL is heterogeneous at the molecular and immunohistochemical levels (Camacho, 2003). Ig heavy and (monotypic) light chain genes are rearranged. Trisomies 3, 7, and 18 may occur, and 5-year survival is greater than 50%.

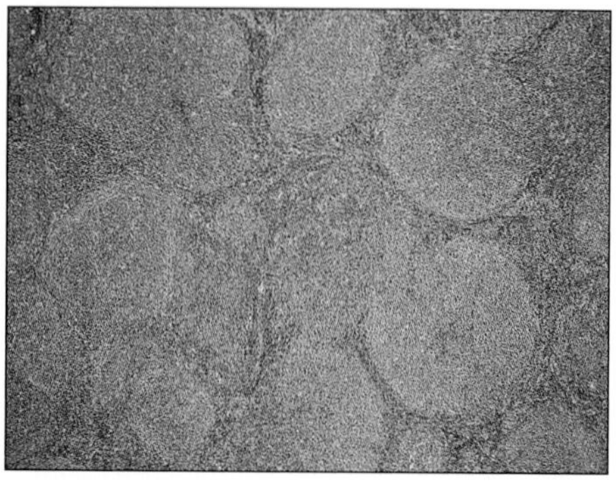

Figure 33-57 Low-power view of follicular lymphoma, recapitulating lymph node germinal centers (×200).

Pediatric Nodal Marginal Zone Lymphoma

A clinical subtype of nodal marginal zone lymphoma occurs in the pediatric age group, usually in boys, with localized lymphadenopathy of the head and neck. Tumors contain progressively transformed germinal center and resemble reactive lymphadenopathy, but show clonal immunoglobulin gene rearrangement. Children have excellent outcomes with conservative treatment.

Follicular Lymphoma

Follicular lymphoma (FL) is a group of related lymphomas of germinal center–derived B cells. Morphologic distinction between the subgroups is based on the numbers of centroblasts in the neoplastic follicles (Harris, 2011).

The overall morphologic pattern (Fig. 33-57) shows recapitulation of lymph node follicles, but with limited diversity of cell type and lack of proliferation of other lymph node structures. The tumors generally show crowded follicles of more than usual uniformity, lacking distinct mantles and with little intervening paracortex, and lacking normal germinal center **tingible body** macrophages and polarization. Most often, small irregular cells (small cleaved cells or centrocytes) predominate with variable numbers of admixed large cells (large cleaved and noncleaved cells or centroblasts). There may be diffuse infiltrates as well. The term **follicular** indicates a greater than 75% follicular pattern; **follicular and diffuse** refers to cases that are 25%–75% follicular; **focally follicular** refers to cases with less than 25% follicular pattern; and **diffuse** indicates that no follicular component is present (Table 33-20). BM involvement is frequent and usually first involves the paratrabecular regions, often in a spotty fashion.

Cytologic grading is based on the average number of centroblasts (CBs) per high-power field (hpf) within neoplastic follicles (Figs. 33-58 and 33-59). It is now recommended that grades 1 and 2 be combined into grade 1-2. An hpf is defined as that with a 40× lens and a 10× ocular with an 18-mm field of view. A 50× lens with a 22-mm 10× ocular, often used in wet hematology, provides a nearly equivalent field of view.

Marginal zone or monocytoid B cell differentiation occurs in up to 10% of cases. It usually appears around follicles and in interfollicular areas and resembles a composite lymphoma. FL shows an immunophenotype of mature B cells with bright monoclonal surface Ig, CD19, CD20, CD22, CD23, CD79a, and CD10 expression. Bcl-2 (cytoplasmic) and bcl-6 (nuclear) are both usually expressed, which helps to separate FL from

TABLE 33-20
Follicular Lymphoma: Grading and Variants

Grading	Definition
Grade 1	0–5 centroblasts per hpf*
Grade 2	6–15 centroblasts per hpf*
Grade 3	>15 centroblasts per hpf*
3a	Centrocytes present
3b	Solid sheets of centroblasts
Reporting of pattern	**Proportion follicular**
Follicular	>75%
Follicular and diffuse	25%–75%†
Focally follicular	<25%†
FOLLICULAR LYMPHOMA: VARIANTS	
Diffuse large B cell lymphoma with follicular lymphoma	Presence of diffuse areas with >15 centroblasts/hpf

From Swerdlow (2008).
*hpf = high-power field of 40× lens with 10× 18-mm eyepiece or 50× lens with 10× 22-mm eyepiece (average of 10 fields within follicles).
†Give approximate percentage in report.

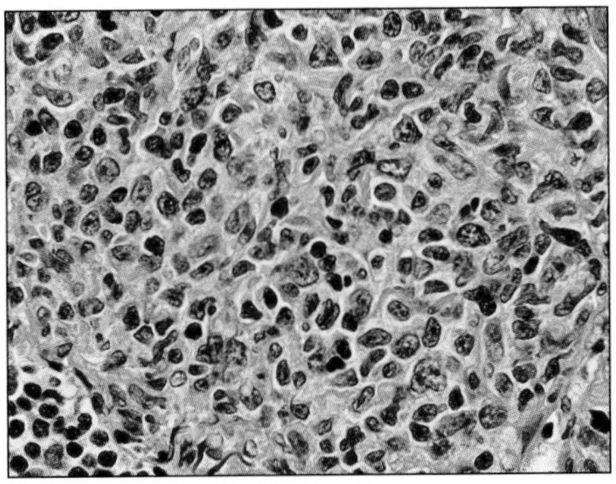

Figure 33-58 Follicular lymphoma, grade 2, showing centrocytes with 5–15 centroblasts per high-power field (hpf). Grade 1 shows <5 centroblasts per hpf.

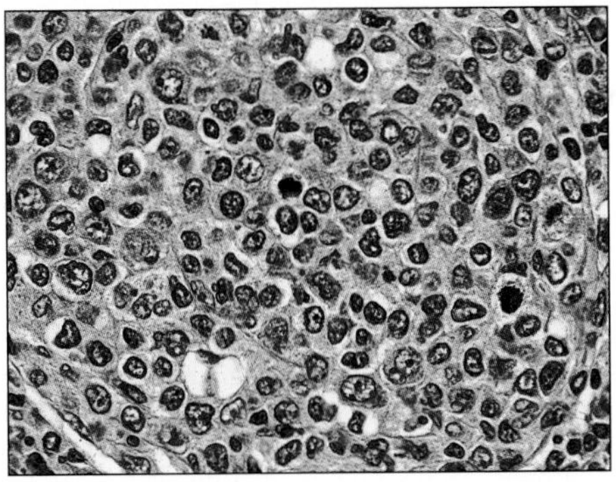

Figure 33-59 Follicular lymphoma, grade 3a, shows centrocytes with >15 centroblasts per high-power field (hpf) (×500).

reactive hyperplasia (bcl-2–negative/bcl-6–positive) and other lymphomas not of germinal center cell (GCC) derivation (bcl-6–negative). CD5 and CD43 are typically absent.

IgH is clonally rearranged along with a light chain Ig gene, and there is t(14;18)(q32;q21) with juxtaposition of IgH and *BCL-2*. Bcl-2 protein is inappropriately expressed, and subsequent inhibition of apoptosis is considered a primary pathogenic mechanism of FL. Standard PCR assays are relatively insensitive for IgH and t(14;18) because only 75% of IgH breakpoints are in the major breakpoint region (MBR) or minor cluster region (mcr) targeted by standard primers. Quantitative real-time PCR and FISH assays provide improved sensitivity (Jenner, 2002; Jiang, 2002). Other abnormalities may be seen, including a variant Bcl-2 rearrangement, t(2;18)(p12;q21), 6q23-36 abnormalities, and deletions/abnormalities of 9p or 17p13 involving TP53 (both associated with large cell transformation), rearrangements or mutations of BCL-6 at 3q27, and abnormalities of X, 1, 2, 4, 5, 7, 12, 13, and 18 (Nathwani, 2001).

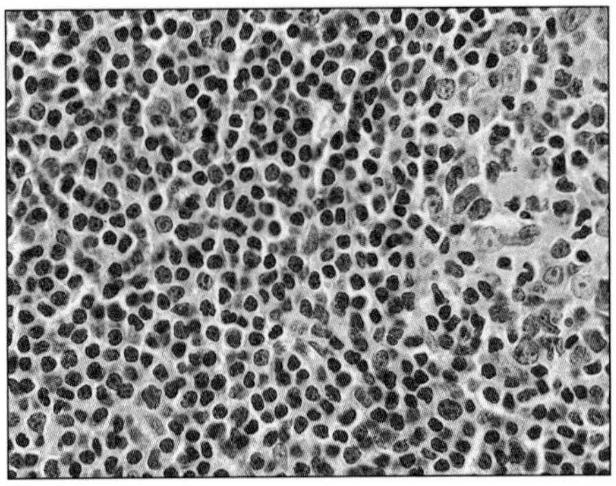

Figure 33-60 Mantle cell lymphoma, showing an expanded mantle around residual germinal center.

Prognosis is variable, with grade 1 and 2 disease generally showing an indolent course but lack of cure. Grade 3 is more aggressive but likely more curable. Attempts to identify patients requiring aggressive therapy have led to a follicular lymphoma international prognostic index (FLIPI) (Solal-Celigny, 2004) based on age, stage, hemoglobin, number of nodal areas involved, and lactate dehydrogenase, which appears to be valid at least for FL in first relapse (Montoto, 2004). Diffuse large B cell lymphoma (DLBCL) is considered by WHO authors to be a different entity even when it arises in FL (Swerdlow, 2008). In these situations, two diagnoses are recommended, such as "follicular lymphoma, grade 3/3 (75%), with diffuse large B cell lymphoma (25%)," when the DLBCL occupies 25% of the sampled tumor. Leukemic involvement by FL may also occur and is sometimes known as **lymphosarcoma cell leukemia.** Flow cytometry is helpful to distinguish between that, CLL, and leukemic mantle cell or marginal zone lymphomas.

Diffuse follicular lymphoma is essentially a diffuse transformation of grade 1 or 2 FL. Diagnosis requires phenotyping and/or cytogenetic studies to rule out mantle cell or marginal zone lymphoma, and includes previous categories of diffuse small cleaved cell, centrocytic diffuse, diffuse mixed small cleaved, and large cell and centrocytic/centroblastic diffuse.

Follicular lymphoma occurring in the pediatric age group (pediatric follicular lymphoma) is a distinct entity that usually lacks t(14;18) or bcl-2 expression and behaves in an indolent fashion. Most cases are grade 3. Primary intestinal follicular lymphoma may occur in duodenal polyps and is usually indolent, as are many other extranodal follicular lymphomas. Intrafollicular in situ follicular lymphoma of bcl-2–positive follicle cells has been described.

Primary Cutaneous Follicle Center Lymphoma

This is the most common primary cutaneous B cell lymphoma and consists of variably distinct follicular to diffuse lesions in the dermis composed of bcl-6/CD20/CD79a–positive centrocytes and admixed centroblasts, with a background of CD21/CD35 positive follicular dendritic cells. Bcl-2 is usually negative, and CD10 is associated with more distinct follicular patterns. A bcl-2–positive follicular lymphoma in the skin suggests extension of disease from another location. Prognosis is excellent with typical response to radiation.

Mantle Cell Lymphoma

Since the REAL classification was published, it has become recognized that mantle cell lymphoma (MCL) is a dangerous form of lymphoma that combines refractoriness to therapy with an aggressive clinical course and poor survival (ILSG, 1997). Refractoriness is likely due in part to strong expression of Bcl-2, also seen in normal mantle cells, follicular lymphomas, and some other leukemias, lymphomas, and solid tumors (Korsmeyer, 1999). Bcl-2 inhibits apoptotic pathways.

The tumor usually shows a diffuse or sometimes mantle zone pattern (Swerdlow, 2008). In the mantle zone pattern, atrophic germinal centers are often seen in the center of nodules, and these may be seen as occasional small naked follicles within a diffuse infiltrate. Nuclei are small to medium sized with clumped to moderately dispersed chromatin and a moderately increased mitotic rate. Nuclear membranes are typically slightly irregular with occasional small round and cleaved nuclei also present. Scattered histiocytes with lightly eosinophilic cytoplasm are often present. A blastic or "blastoid" variant shows slightly larger nuclei with blast-like chromatin and a higher mitotic rate, simulating lymphoblastic lymphoma (Fig. 33-60).

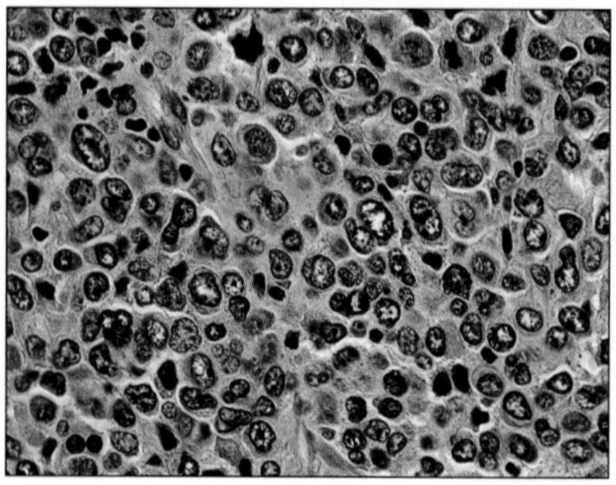

Figure 33-61 Diffuse large B cell lymphoma with centroblasts and admixed centrocytes (×500).

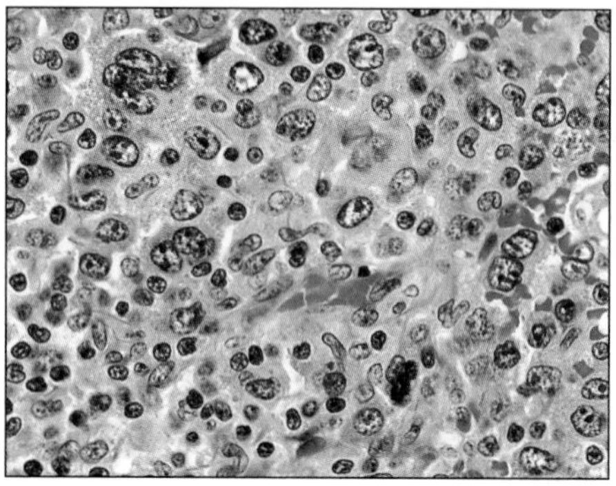

Figure 33-62 Diffuse large B cell lymphoma, with polymorphism and Reed-Sternberg–like cells (×1000).

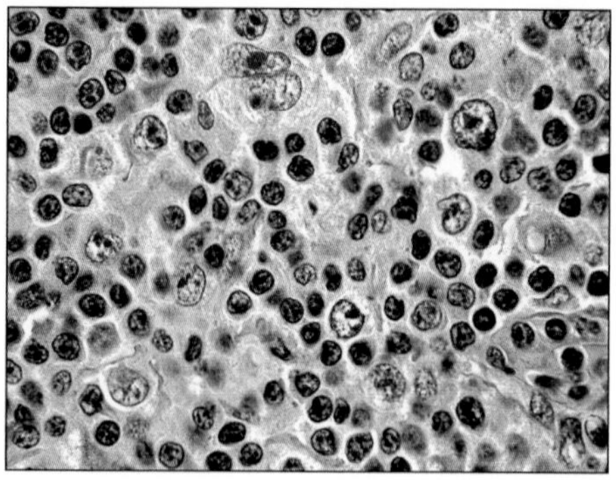

Figure 33-63 T cell and histiocyte-rich large B cell lymphoma resembles lymphocyte predominant Hodgkin lymphoma, but most small cells are T cells (×500).

These are monoclonal (monotypic surface IgM and IgD) B cells (CD19, CD20, CD22) with characteristic coexpression of CD5 (and CD43) and absence of CD23. Bcl-2 and cyclin-D1 are expressed while bcl-6 and CD10 are negative. Rare cases occur without CD5 expression (Liu, 2002).

Immunoglobulin heavy and (monotypic) light chain genes are rearranged. A majority of cases have t(11;14)(q13;q32) involving the Ig heavy chain gene and bcl-1 with overexpression of PRAD-1, which encodes cyclin-D1. In diagnostic laboratories, many cases do not show demonstrable bcl-1 translocation by PCR, and cyclin-D1 expression may not be detected for technical reasons. FISH assay, which may be performed from fresh cell suspensions, nuclei extracted from paraffin, or, in some cases, thin sections from paraffin blocks, is usually confirmatory. Complex karyotype is often seen in advanced, blastoid, or pleomorphic variants, and secondary 8q24 abnormalities are associated with blastic/blastoid morphology and leukemic presentation (Viswanatha, 2000; Au, 2002; Hao, 2002). BCL-2 rearrangements are absent.

Diffuse Large B Cell Lymphoma, NOS

DLBCL includes a variety of morphologies, all of which share a diffuse pattern, large cells, and mature B cell phenotype (Swerdlow, 2008). It occurs in both nodal and extranodal sites and at all ages. It is frequent in immunosuppressed patients (often in association with EBV in these) and is the most common lymphoma of the CNS. Various morphologies are mimicked by peripheral T cell lymphomas, and phenotyping is required for diagnosis.

DLBCL presents with diffuse infiltration by large B cells (nuclei larger than histiocytes or endothelial cell nuclei) with variable morphology. They may be centroblasts and/or centrocytes with scant cytoplasm and multiple nucleoli (centroblastic morphologic variant) (Fig. 33-61). Some cases show plasmacytoid immunoblasts with large nuclei, one or more prominent nucleoli, and abundant amphophilic cytoplasm that may be eccentric (immunoblastic variant). Other cases of DLBCL show polymorphic cell morphology with large and small cells and Reed-Sternberg–like giant cells (anaplastic variant) (Fig. 33-62). Still others occasionally show large cells with clear cytoplasm.

Neoplastic cells show surface Ig, sometimes cytoplasmic Ig, and B cell markers (CD19, CD20, CD22, CD79a). CD30 is occasionally present in variable numbers of cells. CD20 expression by immunohistochemistry (IHC) is usually very helpful in paraffin-section diagnosis. CD10 and/or BCL6 suggests germinal center differentiation, and IRF4/MUM1 suggests post–germinal center differentiation.

In DLBCL, Ig heavy and (monotypic) light chain genes are rearranged. Bcl-2 and/or bcl-6 abnormalities and protein expression are frequent (Skinnider, 1999; Capello, 2000).

Gene array studies have separated DLBCL into at least four major expression groups: GCC-like, activated B cell (ABC)-like, type 3, and mediastinal large B cell lymphoma (Rosenwald, 2002, 2003; Savage, 2003). Of the first three, GCC-like shows better response to therapy than ABC or type 3. BCL-2 and BCL-6 are in the gene cluster of GCC-like tumors and may be surrogates for this category. In the GCC category, cases with t(14;18) show lower proliferation but do not differ in outcome by treatment (Iqbal, 2004). Bcl-2 protein is associated with resistance to apoptosis and chemotherapy, but this may be overcome with humanized monoclonal anti-CD20 (Mounier, 2003).

Subgrouping by immunophenotyping roughly follows expression grouping. Cases with CD10 expression (>30% of cells) or CD10-, BCL-6+, and IRF4/MUM1 are considered germinal center types. All others are non–germinal center types. A variety of other specific types of DLBCL are also described by the WHO classification, as follows (Swerdlow, 2008).

T Cell/Histiocyte-Rich Large B Cell Lymphoma

T cell/histiocyte-rich large B cell lymphoma (TCHRLBCL) variant is very difficult to distinguish from nodular lymphocyte predominant HL (NLPHL), but the distinction is important, as this is a usually aggressive tumor which presents with advanced stage, while lymphocyte predominant HL (LPHL) is often localized and indolent and requires less therapy. TCHRLBCL exhibits a diffuse infiltrate of large B cells, which may appear as centroblasts or immunoblasts or resemble lymphocyte and histiocytic (L&H) cells of LPHL and include Reed-Sternberg–like cells (Fig. 33-63). Large B cells constitute 10% or less of total cells, and T cells constitute the majority. The phenotype is similar to LPHL, with CD20, CD79a, and epithelial membrane antigen (EMA) positivity. J-chain, Oct-2, and Bob-1 are also expressed. Surface/cytoplasmic Ig, if monoclonal, is somewhat helpful, but LPHL is also now considered a clonal B cell disease. Helpful distinctions are the diffuse infiltrate, T cell background, lack of CD3/CD57 rosettes around neoplastic cells in a nodular B cell background as seen in nodular LPHL, lack of residual IgD-positive mantle cells, and lack of a follicular dendritic meshwork by CD21/CD23/D35 staining. Advanced-stage presentation also suggests TCHRLBCL, but rare cases of NLPHL may present with disseminated disease.

Primary DLBCL of the CNS

CNS DLBCL usually presents in middle age as supratentorial tumors with various neurologic symptoms. Homogeneous to focally necrotic on MRI, they frequently show characteristic perivascular tumor cell accumulations on biopsy. These express pan-B cell markers with BCL-6 and strong IRF4/MUM1 positivity in most and variable BCL-2 expression, and they are typically EBV negative. Tumors typically respond to modern chemotherapy.

Primary Cutaneous DLBCL, Leg Type

These are aggressive B cell lymphomas that typically arise in older adults, women more often than men, and often on the lower legs, although they may occur anywhere in the skin. They are composed of monotonous sheets of large B cells with expression of pan-B cell markers, with monotypic Ig,

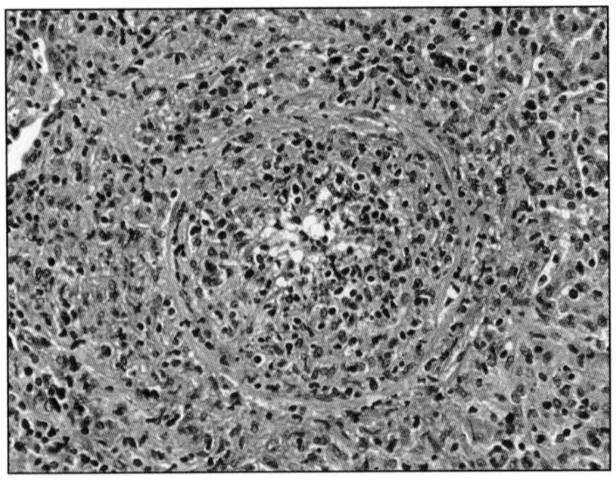

Figure 33-64 Lymphomatoid granulomatosis, showing a polymorphous angiodestructive pulmonary infiltrate (×200). *(Courtesy Dr. Anna-Luise Katzenstein.)*

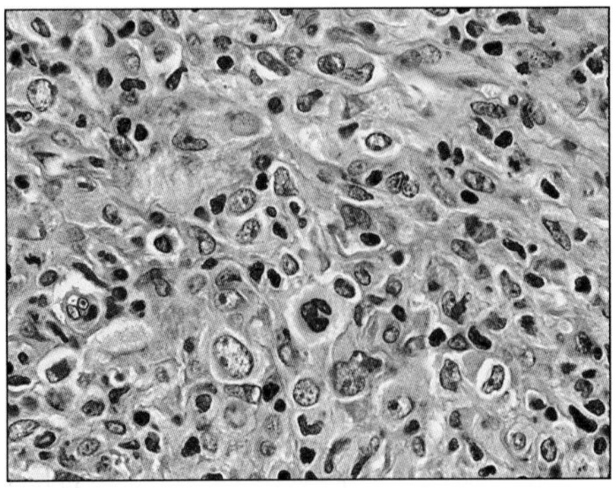

Figure 33-65 Mediastinal large B cell lymphoma with sclerosis (×500).

strong BCL2, IRF4/MUM1, and FOX-P1. BCL-6 is usually positive, and CD10 negative.

EBV-Positive DLBCL of the Elderly

These are DLBCLs arising in patients older than 50 years of age and associated with EBV. Histology varies from mostly large cells to a more polymorphic distribution of cell sizes, often geographic necrosis, with EBV demonstrable by antibody staining for EBV LMP-1 and by ISH for EBV-encoded ribonucleotides. CD10 and BCL6 are negative, IRF4/MUM1 is usually positive, and CD30 is frequently expressed. These aggressive tumors are similar to DLBCL arising in immunosuppressed patients, and a form of age-related immunosuppression is surmised.

DLBCL Associated with Inflammation

This is another EBV-associated tumor that arises in situations with protracted chronic inflammation, the prototype being pyothorax-associated lymphoma (PAL). Features are similar to EBV+ DLBCL of the elderly.

Lymphomatoid Granulomatosis

This is an angiocentric lymphoproliferative disorder involving the lung and/or other sites, including brain, kidney, liver, skin, upper respiratory tract, and GI tract (Katzenstein, 1979). It is considered to be an EBV-driven B cell neoplasm with a prominent reactive T cell component, sometimes in a setting of immunosuppression (Katzenstein, 1990; Wilson, 1996). It has histologic features similar to NK/T cell lymphoma of nasal type (Pittaluga, 2008).

Presentation is usually cough, dyspnea, and chest pain with constitutional symptoms, including fever, malaise, weight loss, GI symptoms, myalgias, and neurologic symptoms. Bilateral mid to lower lung nodules are most commonly seen, often with nodules in the brain, kidney, skin, and subcutaneous tissue.

Histology shows an angiocentric and angiodestructive infiltrate of polymorphic lymphocytes, plasma cells, immunoblasts, and histiocytes, with inconspicuous neutrophils and eosinophils and without well-formed granulomas. Fibrinoid necrosis of vessels is often seen (Fig. 33-64), as is tissue infarction.

Immunophenotyping shows variable numbers of CD79a, usually CD20-positive B cells with EBV LMP-1 expression, variable CD30 expression, and lack of CD15. EBER is generally positive in some studies (Myers, 1995). A majority of background cells are reactive T cells with CD4 predominance. Higher-grade lesions (with more B cells) show clonal rearrangement of the IgH receptor genes. T cell receptor genes are not clonally rearranged.

Grading is related to the number of clonal EBV-positive lymphocytes. Grade I lesions are polymorphic with only occasional large cells. Grade II is mixed with large pleomorphic cells in a mixed inflammatory background. Grade III is essentially diffuse large B cell lymphoma.

Outcome is variable, with waxing and waning, sometimes spontaneous remissions, and often progression to pulmonary failure in a median of 2 years. Appropriate therapy is related to determination of grade. Grade III lesions are treated with systemic chemotherapy, and grades I and II may be treated with α-interferon.

Primary Mediastinal (Thymic) Large B Cell Lymphoma

Primary mediastinal (thymic) large B cell lymphoma (PMBL) often appears in young adulthood to middle age and is more frequent in women. Histology is variable, but diffuse or compartmentalizing sclerosis is frequent, and clear cells, multilobulated cells, or Reed-Sternberg–like cells may be present (Fig. 33-65). Symptoms are often related to location, with airway compression or superior vena cava syndrome and often local invasion and local recurrence after therapy. CD45, CD19, and CD20 are expressed, but not CD5 or CD10 (Swerdlow, 2008). CD30 is expressed in some cases, but not with the phenotype of classical HL. Ig genes are clonally rearranged; *IgV* and *Bcl-6* gene hypermutations are consistent with GCC cell derivation but occur similarly to normal thymic B cells (Csernus, 2004). Gene expression array analysis shows MLBCL to be similar to classical HL (Savage, 2003). A majority of patients respond to standard CHOP (cyclophosphamide, hydroxydaunorubicin, Oncovin, and prednisone/prednisolone) chemotherapy, but long-term survival may be better with more aggressive approaches (Zinzani, 2001; Andreopoulou, 2004).

Intravascular Large B Cell Lymphoma

Intravascular large B cell lymphoma is a rare tumor which is largely restricted to the intravascular lumina of small vessels (Swerdlow, 2008). It is very aggressive, widely disseminated at diagnosis, and often undiagnosed until autopsy. Findings often include hemorrhage, thrombosis, and/or necrosis of tissues throughout the body, with tumor only inconspicuously present in the small vessels. B cell markers are expressed (CD19, CD20, CD22, D79a) and CD5 in some. Clonal Ig gene rearrangements are present with somatic hypermutation consistent with post-GCC derivation (Kanda, 2001). Rare T cell cases are described (Merchant, 2003). Vascular adhesion molecules CD29 (β 1 integrin) and CD54 (CAM-1) have been reported absent (Ponzoni, 2000).

ALK-Positive Large B Cell Lymphoma

Diffuse large B cell lymphomas with expression of full-length anaplastic lymphoma kinase (ALK) protein resemble T cell anaplastic large cell lymphoma (ALCL) in morphology and expression of ALK, but lack t(2;5) and NPM-ALK fusion protein. Most described cases show t(2;17)(p23;q23) with clathrin gene involvement (CLTL-ALK); other rare abnormalities include t(2;5)(p23;q23), as in typical ALCL. These are of B cell derivation with expression of CD79a but absent CD20 and frequently lack CD30 expression (Laurent, 2010).

Plasmablastic Lymphoma

Plasmablastic lymphoma expresses plasma cell antigens CD38 and CD138 and is associated with EBV. CD20, CD45, and PAX5 are weak to absent, but CD79a and IRF4/MUM1 are positive. There is cytoplasmic IgG. It has an aggressive behavior and has been reported primarily in the oral cavity of HIV patients, but is now known to occur in other patients and other locations as well.

Large B Cell Lymphoma Arising in HHV8-Associated Multicentric Castleman's Disease

This tumor, arising in multicentric Castleman's disease and frequently in patients with HIV, resembles an IgM-producing plasmablastic lymphoma. CD20 and CD38 are variably expressed, CD79a and CD138 are negative, and EBER is negative. HHV-8 is detectable by IHC. The disease is aggressive.

Primary Effusion Lymphoma

This is another rare tumor presenting in serous effusions but without tumors. Cytology is usually immunoblastic or anaplastic. It is associated

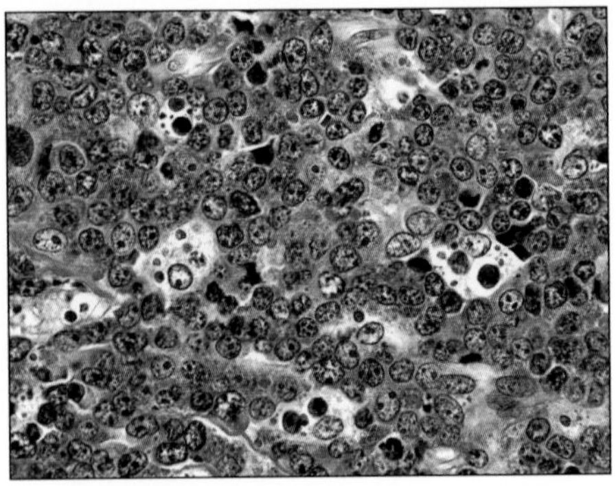

Figure 33-66 Burkitt lymphoma (×500).

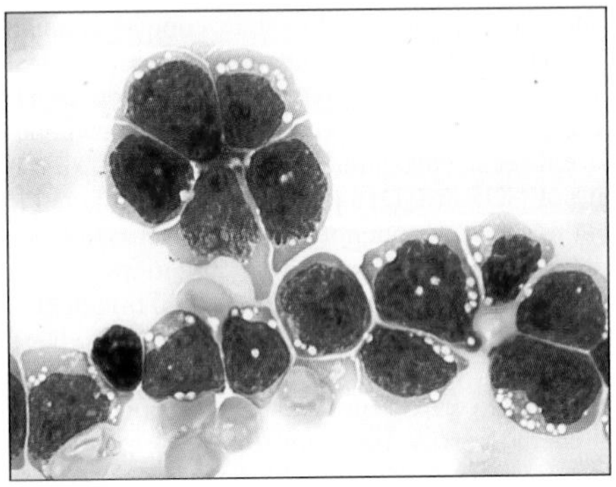

Figure 33-67 Burkitt lymphoma cytology (×1000).

with the Kaposi's sarcoma virus human herpesvirus-8 (HHV-8) in immunodeficient patients. Tumor cells label as B cells and have Ig rearrangements, although T cell varieties have been reported. EBV can usually be detected using in situ hybridization (ISH) for EBER, but EBV-latent membrane protein-1 is absent by immunohistochemistry (Said, 2011). The pathogenesis may be related to viral activation of the alternative NF-κB pathway (Matta, 2004).

Burkitt Lymphoma

BL was first described in the jaws of African children by Dennis Burkitt in 1958 (Burkitt, 1958). It was first defined as a distinct tumor entity by the WHO in 1968 (Berard, 1985) and remains so in the current WHO classification (Leoncini, 2008). It represents approximately one third of pediatric NHL, but also occurs in adults. Several epidemiologic types of BL exist. The prototype is **endemic** BL, which occurs predominantly in children in Africa and other equatorial regions and is associated with EBV. **Sporadic** BL occurs worldwide in children and adults and is not usually associated with EBV. Patients with HIV or other immune suppression often have EBV-related BL, which is, however, different from the endemic form at the molecular level. BL is a highly proliferative tumor that grows very rapidly.

The tumor shows a diffuse infiltrate with pushing borders of medium-sized relatively uniform cells with round to oval nuclei containing three to five moderately prominent nucleoli in relatively clear parachromatin (Fig. 33-66). Cytoplasm is moderate and basophilic, and tends to square off between adjacent cells. Lipid-laden cytoplasmic vacuoles are seen in imprints (Fig. 33-67). Both high mitotic and high apoptotic rates are noted, along with a prominent pattern of "starry sky" macrophages. In most cases, the histology is distinctive, but some overlap is seen with both DLBCL and occasionally lymphoblastic lymphoma.

Burkitt leukemia/lymphoma exhibits leukemic cells with moderately clumped chromatin and basophilic vacuolated cytoplasm (see Fig. 33-66) with surface immunoglobulin restricted to one light chain. Typically, they show lack of TdT, presence of B cell antigens CD19, CD22, CD20, CD79a, and often CD10, and expression of monoclonal surface Ig. Rare cases show lack of surface membrane immunoglobulin or expression of TdT, and these require cytogenetic confirmation. Burkitt leukemia/lymphoma shows very high proliferative rates and rapid disease progression. Although the condition is rapidly fatal if untreated, recent results of therapy in pediatric patients have shown long-term survival of better

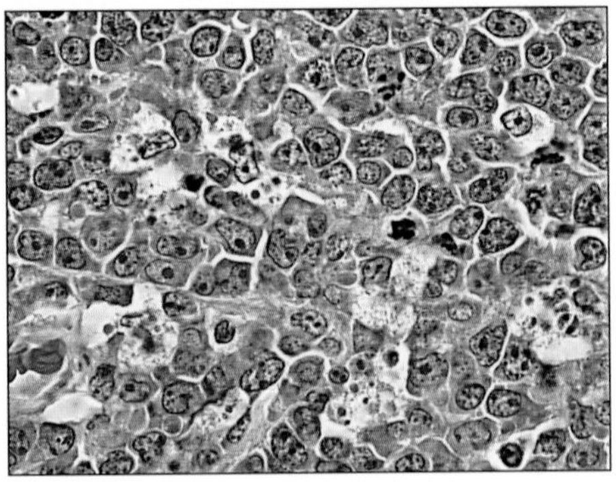

Figure 33-68 Atypical Burkitt or Burkitt-like lymphoma, with moderate pleomorphism and increased numbers of prominent nucleoli (×500).

than 90% (Patte, 2001). Outcome in adults has also improved, but long-term survival is less than in children (50%–70%) (Blum, 2004; Kasamon, 2004).

Burkitt leukemia/lymphoma shows characteristic cytogenetic abnormalities consisting of translocation of c-myc on chromosome region 8q24 to one of the immunoglobulin genes (heavy chain-14q32, κ-2q11, or λ-22q11) to give t(8;14), t(2;8), or t(8;22). Most cases show t(8;14)(q24;q32). C-myc promotes both proliferation and apoptosis (Le Beau, 2000) and presumably causes uncontrolled proliferation of immunoglobulin-bearing B cells. These cells are sensitive to chemotherapy, however.

B Cell Lymphoma, Unclassifiable, with Features Intermediate Between DLBCL and Burkitt Lymphoma

Cases of lymphoma occur with histologic and clinical features intermediate between Burkitt and large B cell lymphoma. The histology is similar to BL, except that generally more pleomorphism is seen with the presence of large cells (up to 25%) and medium-sized cells, and with greater irregularity of nuclei and more prominent nucleoli than in typical Burkitt (Fig. 33-68). Cytoplasm is usually less distinct than in BL.

Previously called Burkitt-like, non-Burkitt, or atypical Burkitt lymphoma, some cases were found to have bcl-2 and not c-myc abnormalities (Yano, 1992). The REAL classification placed most cases with this histology in the category of diffuse large B cell lymphoma.

In children, the clinical presentation is similar to Burkitt (Hutchison, 1989), although cytogenetic studies in one report did not show c-myc translocations (Lones, 2004). In other studies in adults, 8q24/MYC translocations have been reported in nearly half of patients (McClure, 2005) REF Bcl-2 along with c-myc translocations have been identified in some patients and are adverse features (MacPherson, 1999).

In a child with a rapidly growing tumor and presentation similar to Burkitt (such as ileocecal or other abdominal site, extranodal site with effusions, endocrine or gonadal sites, etc.), these are treated as BL (Cairo, 2003). Fixation and other technical artifacts blur the morphologic distinction, and classification shows greater interobserver variation than other pediatric lymphomas (Lones, 2000).

In adults, children with slower growing tumors, children with tumors with 90%–95% proliferation rates, and those with complex karyotypes, the classification becomes murky. The trend in treatment of large B cell lymphoma in young people is to use therapies designed for BL (Patte, 2001). In adults, the condition is often treated as DLBCL. There may be a role for more aggressive therapy, but this generally means increased morbidity, so it is controversial. However, aggressive pediatric regimens have been successfully tested in adults with BL (Nicola, 2004).

B Cell Lymphoma, Unclassifiable, with Features Intermediate Between DLBCL and Classical Hodgkin Lymphoma

These are essentially **gray zone tumors** with overlap features that prevent precise diagnosis. Mediastinum is often involved, and the differential diagnosis is usually between PMBL and classical HL. These disorders have shown overlap by gene expression studies, so it is not surprising that morphologic overlap occurs.

MATURE T CELL AND NATURAL KILLER CELL NEOPLASMS

T cell and NK cell lymphomas and leukemias are a diverse group of neoplasms which are uncommon to rare compared with B cell lymphomas. Although they account for only about 12% of lymphomas overall, an approximately equal number of categories is recognized by the WHO. Most of these are typified by clonal rearrangement of genes encoding CD3, the T cell receptor complex which is an antigen receptor of the immunoglobulin supergene family, although true NK cell neoplasms do not show clonal rearrangement by clinical tests (Cheuk, 2011). Features of major T/NK neoplasms are summarized in Table 33-21.

A majority of postthymic (peripheral) T cells express αβ-chains of the T cell receptor (TCR); a small minority do not, but rather express γδ-chains. NK cells express only ε-chains with cytoplasmic CD3. T cell clonality studies in the laboratory usually focus on γδ-receptor rearrangement, which is present in all or most T cells. This is because in early T cell development, the γ- and β-chain genes rearrange simultaneously, with TCR commitment dependent on expression of surrogate α-chain and development of a pre-TCR (Haks, 1998; Kang, 2001). The repertoire of significant γ-gene "families" is much smaller (four to six) than β-families, and TCR-γ PCR assay is far more efficient for routine use than is TCR-β PCR, which requires approximately 25 different primer sets (Shadrach, 2004). TCR-γ PCR is also effective with DNA extracted from formalin and has largely replaced Southern blot analysis of TCR-β. Flow cytometry assays using antibodies for each TCR V β-family is also useful and rapid but requires a large number of antibodies, and RT-PCR for V β-family transcripts may be utilized (Langerak, 2001; Morice, 2004).

Mature αβ T cells express CD2, CD3, CD5, CD7, and either CD4 or CD8. They are negative for TdT and CD1. Normal resting lymphoid tissue usually shows a CD4/CD8 ratio of 2 : 1. Differentiation to one or the other in the thymus involves activation or silencing of CD4 or CD8 from CD4+CD8+ cells, but is poorly understood (Yasutomo, 2000). Primarily mature CD4 cells proliferate in the postthymic environment (Foa, 1980). The CD4/CD8 ratio drops in acute inflammation and rises to often high levels in recovery and chronic inflammation, so that these are not good markers of clonality. Peripheral T cell neoplasms often lose expression of a normal pan-T cell antigen such as CD7 and show predominance of CD4 or CD8 (Knowles, 1989). Care must be taken to distinguish abnormal αβ T cells from normal NK cells.

γδ T cells typically are doubly negative for CD4 and CD8 and are also often CD5 negative with CD2 expression and show a maturation sequence of CD7. Because they usually account for only 1%–2% of normal T cells, an increase in these cells is a suspicious finding in itself. NK cells are highly variable in expression of pan-T cell antigens CD2 and CD7, are often CD5 negative, and typically express CD16 (a low-affinity Fc receptor also found on monocytes and granulocytes), with variable CD56 and CD57. CD3 is detectable in the cytoplasm with polyclonal antibodies but is also present on the surface in some NK neoplasms. Cytotoxic granule constituents TIA-1, granzyme-B, and perforin are usually present in NK cells and cytotoxic T cells.

T-Prolymphocytic Leukemia

T-prolymphocytic leukemia is an uncommon disorder with a median age of 69 years, and the disease is slightly more frequent in males than in females. Patients present with a marked lymphocytosis (>100 × 10^9/L), anemia, and thrombocytopenia. In most cases, the neoplastic cell is a prolymphocyte with a prominent **punched-out** nucleolus showing distinct perinucleolar chromatin and moderately abundant cytoplasm. In approximately 20% of patients, however, the lymphocytes lack distinctive features and do not possess a prominent nucleolus. Hepatosplenomegaly, lymphadenopathy, and skin involvement are common (Campo, 2008).

The immunophenotype is most often CD4+ peripheral T cell (60%), with CD4/CD8 coexpression in 25%, and CD8+ in 15%. CD7 is strong, and surface CD3 weak.

There is clonal TCR αβ (and γδ) rearrangement. In all, 80% show inv(14)(q11;q32) and 10% t(14;14)(q11;q32) involving TCR αβ locus and oncogenes TCL1 and TCL1b. Chromosome 8 abnormalities t(8;8)(p11-12;q12) or trisomy 8q is seen in 70%; other abnormalities include t(X;14)(q28;q11) and deletions at 11q23.

T-prolymphocytic leukemia is a rapidly progressive malignancy with survival usually less than 1 year. Recent progress has been made with new therapies, including alemtuzumab (Campath-1H) (Dearden, 2001; Cao, 2003).

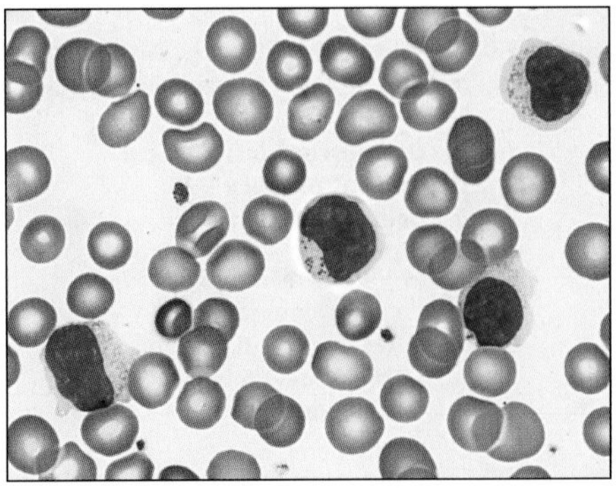

Figure 33-69 Large granular lymphocyte leukemia (×1000).

Large Granular Lymphocyte Leukemia

The median age of these patients is 63 years. Sixty percent to 70% of patients are symptomatic with recurrent infections due to neutropenia. Anemia or rheumatoid arthritis is also common (Lamy, 2003). Lymphocytosis is usually mild (up to 20 ×10^9/L), and lymphocyte number may be normal. Large granular lymphocyte (LGL) cells are usually at least 2 × 10^9/L (Chan WC, 2008). Chronic neutropenia is frequent, splenomegaly may be present, and there may be anemia and/or thrombocytopenia. LCLs are at least relatively increased and show moderate size with abundant light blue cytoplasm and condensed chromatin. Azurophilic cytoplasmic granules vary in number and size (Fig. 33-69). The BM exhibits a moderate interstitial infiltrate of granulated lymphocytes. Erythroid and myeloid elements may be normal or hypoplastic in occasional cases. The spleen typically shows red pulp infiltrates.

The common variant is CD3/CD8/CD57/TCR αβ+, CD4 negative. Uncommon variants express CD4 (Lima, 2003), dually express CD4 and CD8, show doubly negative CD4/CD8, and/or have variable expression of CD57 and CD56. Cases reactive with CD3 and CD56 tend to behave aggressively (Gentile, 1994). Cases of LGL leukemia following renal transplant have been seen (Gentile, 1998), along with those of donor origin following BM transplant (Au, 2003). Benign LGL lymphocytosis following BM transplant is likely related to the early emergence of LGL cells (Niederwieser, 1987).

TCR γ-gene rearrangement is usually clonal by PCR, and TCR-β is usually rearranged. Although a single clonal band usually confirms a suspicious diagnosis, PCR assays may show a dominant clone emerging from an oligoclonal population of autoimmune disorders. This, along with a typically indolent course, makes cases with low WBCs very difficult to diagnose. Low-dose methotrexate, cyclosporine, or cyclophosphamide often induces long-lasting remission (Lamy, 2003).

Chronic Lymphoproliferative Disorders of NK Cells

Chronic lymphocytosis of LCLs of NK phenotype occurs rarely. These are generally indolent asymptomatic processes that come to light as incidental findings or may be associated with neutropenia and/or anemia. They resemble LGL leukemia but are CD3 negative, with expression of CD16, dim CD56, cytotoxic granule markers TIA-1 and granzyme B and M, and variable CD2, CD7, and CD57. CD5 and CD8 are often expressed. KIR NK-receptors (NKRs) are abnormally expressed in restricted or negative fashion, but are not frequently assayed in clinical laboratories. T cell receptors are not clonally rearranged, and no characteristic cytogenetic abnormalities of EBV are associated.

Aggressive NK Cell Leukemia

This is a rare aggressive leukemia of NK cells associated with EBV and usually occurring in Asian teens and young adults. It usually presents with constitutional symptoms. The WBC is variable and hepatosplenomegaly is common; it sometimes shows lymphadenopathy, hepatosplenomegaly, coagulopathy, hemophagocytic syndrome, and/or multiorgan failure (Cheuk, 2011).

Morphology of leukemic cells is variable, sometimes resembling LGL leukemia, sometimes showing larger lymphoid cells with condensed chromatin and basophilic cytoplasm, and sometimes showing blastic or transformed cells.

TABLE 33-21
Key Features of the Major Mature T and NK Cell Neoplasms

Lymphoma	Demographics; clinical and laboratory presentations	Morphology	CELL SURFACE MARKERS (TYPICAL PROFILE) Positive	Negative	Gene rearranged, involved
T cell PLL	M > F; median age, 65 years; lymphocytosis >100 × $10^3/\mu L$, anemia, thrombocytopenia, HSM, skin lesions	Prolymphocyte	CD7; CD4 (60%), CD4/8 (25%), CD8 (15%)		TCR-γδ TCR-αβ inv(14) (q11;q32)
LGL leukemia	Median age, 63 years; neutropenia causing infection, anemia, mild lymphocytosis (>2 × $10^3/\mu L$)	Moderately sized cell with condensed chromatin, abundant pale blue cytoplasm, azurophilic granules	CD3, CD8, CD57, TCR-γδ; some variants are CD4+ or CD4/8+ or CD4/8−	CD4	TCR-γδ TCR-αβ
Aggressive NK cell leukemia	Asian teens to young adults; constitutional symptoms, HSM, variable WBC count	Variable, may resemble LGL cells or appear blastic	cCD3ε, CD2, CD56	sCD3, 57	TCR-γδ TCR-αβ Clonal EBV, del(6) (q21;q25)
Adult T cell leukemia/ lymphoma	Associated with HTLV-1, frequent in Japan, Caribbean, Central Africa; acute variant with skin, lymph node involvement, hypercalcemia	Moderately large blastic cells with convoluted nuclei (floret cells), agranular, basophilic cytoplasm	CD2, CD3, CD4, CD5, CD25, often CD30	CD 7, 8	TCR-γδ TCR-αβ
Extranodal NK/T cell lymphoma, nasal type	Most prevalent in Asia, Native Americans of Mexico and Central and South America	Angiocentric and destructive, involving upper aerodigestive tract	CD2, CD56, cytotoxic granules, cyto CD3ε	Surface CD3	Germline receptor genes
Enteropathy-associated T cell lymphoma	All ages and regions; increased in celiac disease (may present concurrently), jejunum and ileum	Large cells with inflammatory background, occasionally monomorphic (type II) medium-sized cells	CD3, CD7, CD103; CD3, CD8, CD56 (type II)	CD4, CD5	TCR-γδ TCR-αβ
Hepatosplenic T cell lymphoma	Rare, increased in adolescents and young adults and with chronic immunosuppressive therapy; involves liver/ spleen/marrow	Medium-sized cells involving splenic red pulp and sinuses of liver and marrow	CD3, CD8±, CD56±	CD4, CD5, often CD4/CD8 double negative	TCR-γδ
Subcutaneous panniculitis-like T cell lymphoma	Rare, F > M; subcutaneous panniculitis with neoplastic cells	Involves fat lobules, spares septa, variable-sized monomorphic cells, rimming of fat cells, histiocytes	CD3, βF1, CD8, cytotoxic granules	CD4, CD56	TCR-γδ TCR-αβ
PTCL, NOS	Peripheral nodes, disseminated disease, sometimes cutaneous	Varies in cell size and from polymorphic to monomorphous	Variable with CD3, CD4, other pan-T cell markers	CD7, CD5, others often lost	TCR-γδ TCR-αβ
Angioimmunoblastic T cell lymphoma	Middle-aged and elderly; generalized disease, systemic symptoms, hypergammaglobulinemia	Partial nodal effacement involving paracortex, increased venules, clear cell clusters, EBV+ B cells	CD3, CD2, CD5, CD4, (reactive CD8), CD10, CXCL13	CD8	TCR-γδ TCR-αβ+3, +5, +X
Mycosis fungoides/ Sézary syndrome (SS)	M > F, middle-aged to older; dermatitis progressing to ulcerated lesions; PB involvement in SS	Dermal band-like infiltrates of lymphocytes with cerebriform nuclei, microabscesses	CD2, CD3, CD4	CD7, CD8	TCR-γδ TCR-αβ
Primary cutaneous CD30-positive	M > F, adults to elderly; limited to skin lesions	Polymorphic lymphoid cells, some anaplastic	CD4, CD30	Often CD2, CD3, CD5, ALK	TCR-γδ TCR-αβ
Anaplastic large cell lymphoma	M > F, teens, young adults; peripheral, abdominal adenopathy, extranodal and BM involvement, frequent B symptoms	Pleomorphic large cells, wreath-like nuclei, multiple nucleoli, abundant cytoplasm	CD30 (cytoplasmic and Golgi), CD2, CD4, CD5	CD3, CD7, EBV	TCR-γδ TCR-αβ t(2;5)(p23;q35) Other variants involve 2p23

BM, Bone marrow; *EBV,* Epstein-Barr virus; *HSM,* hepatosplenomegaly; *HTLV,* human T lymphotropic virus type 1; *LGL,* large granular lymphocyte; *NK,* natural killer; *NOS,* not otherwise specified; *PB,* peripheral blood; *PLL,* prolymphocytic leukemia; *PTCL,* peripheral T cell lymphoma; *TCR,* T cell receptor; *WBC,* white blood cell.

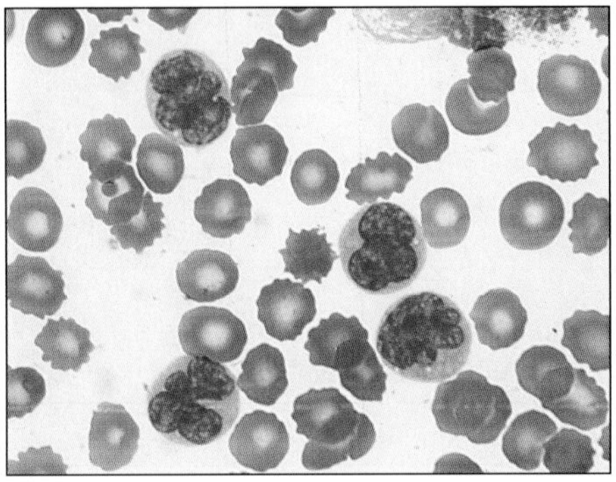

Figure 33-70 Natural killer cell leukemia in an adult, with floret cells resembling adult T cell leukemia.

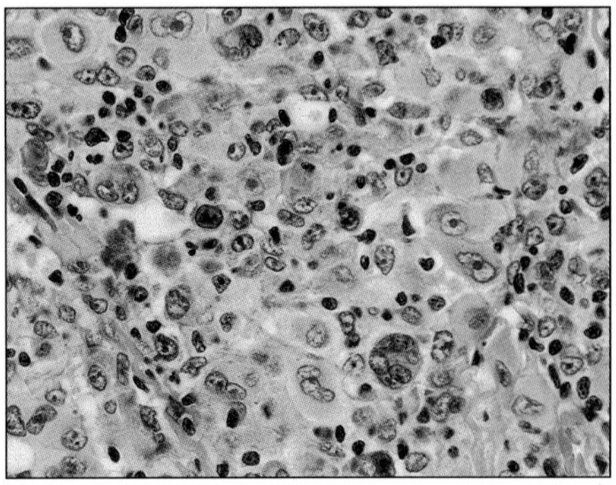

Figure 33-71 Adult T cell leukemia/lymphoma, with anaplastic features (×500).

The immunophenotype is surface CD3 negative and cytoplasmic CD3 ε/CD2/CD56 positive, and it expresses cytotoxic molecules (TIA-1, granzyme-B, and/or perforin). CD16 is variable, and CD57 negative.

TCR genes are not rearranged. Clonality may be established by detecting clonal episomal EBV (analyzing tandem repeats by Southern blot) or finding clonal cytogenetic abnormalities such as del(6)(q21;q25).

Indolent NK cell proliferation also occurs and is characterized by adult onset, lack of constitutional symptoms, lack of EBV, and a CD57+ phenotype (along with CD2, CD16, and CD56, with negative surface CD3) (Fig. 33-70).

EBV-Positive T Cell Lymlphoproliferative Disorders of Childhood

These are rare lymphomas occurring most often in Asian or Native Americans from Central or South America that are associated with EBV. **Systemic EBV-positive T cell lymphoproliferative disease of childhood** is an aggressive, often fulminant disease following acute or chronic EBV infection and characterized by indistinct monoclonal infiltrates of small T cells, occasionally with some pleomorphism, associated with hepatosplenomegaly and hemophagocytic syndrome involving these organs and BM. Cells are mature T cells with CD2, CD3, and TIA-1 expression, variable CD4 (chronic EBV) or CD8 (acute EBV), and negative CD56. **Hydroa vacciniforme-like lymphoma** is an EBV-positive cutaneous T cell lymphoma of sun-exposed skin. The infiltrate is that of CD56+ cytotoxic T or NK cells predominantly involving the dermis. The disease course is variable and tends to be initially indolent, but more aggressive following dissemination.

Adult T Cell Leukemia-Lymphoma

Adult T cell leukemia-lymphoma (ATLL) is a highly variable but often clinically aggressive T cell leukemia/lymphoma associated with HTLV-1 retrovirus infection (Poiesz, 1980). It is most endemic in southwestern Japan but also in the Caribbean basin, the southeastern United States, and central Africa. Transmission of HTLV-1 may occur vertically (from mother to child), or through sexual contact, intravenous drug abuse, or blood transfusion. Only a minority of individuals infected with HTLV-1 (2.5%) develop ATLL, typically after a latent period of many years. Acute infection results in a flu-like syndrome.

The acute variant typically shows leukemia, skin involvement, generalized lymphadenopathy, lytic bone lesions, and hypercalcemia. The blood film demonstrates anemia and thrombocytopenia with the presence in blood and marrow of moderately large blastic cells with convoluted or clover-leafed nuclei and condensed chromatin **(floret cells).** Nucleoli are small or absent, and the cytoplasm is agranular and basophilic. Admixed blast-like cells are present. Marrow involvement is often patchy with increased osteoclastic activity. Skin lesions resemble mycosis fungoides, including the presence of Pautrier's microabscesses, but often with more pleomorphic cells.

Lymph nodes in acute or lymphomatous variants show highly variable morphology, often with features and diversity reminiscent of anaplastic large cell lymphoma (Jaffe, 2011). Histology may resemble common ALCL, small cell variant, HL, or typical large cell lymphoma (Fig. 33-71).

The chronic variant often resembles mycosis fungoides, and the smoldering variant shows low-level leukemic involvement with <5% circulating neoplastic cells. Clonal integration of HTLV-1 is an invariable finding and

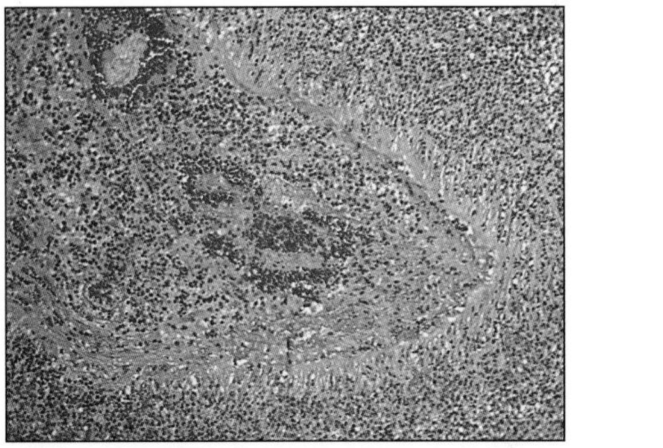

Figure 33-72 Nasal/nasal-like T/natural killer cell lymphoma, showing angioinvasion and destruction (×200).

is essentially diagnostic (Yamaguchi, 2002), but it should be noted that HTLV-1 infection is chronic, and these patients may have other hematologic diseases, just as other people do.

The immunophenotype of ATLL is CD2/CD3/CD5/CD25 positive, usually CD4+ and CD7 negative. CD30 is often positive, but ALK is negative. Cytotoxic markers are negative. TCR genes are clonally rearranged. Occasional patients with smoldering disease show a Hodgkin-like lymphoproliferative disorder of EBV-infected B cells with CD30 and CD15 expression, likely related to chronic immunosuppression. It may be noted that both HTLV-1 and EBV are potent inducers of CD30.

Extranodal NK/T Cell Lymphoma, Nasal Type

These lymphomas have been referred to as lethal midline granulomas, polymorphic reticulosis, and angiocentric T cell lymphoma. They are extranodal lymphomas usually of NK cell derivation which are associated with EBV and are most common in Asia and Latin America. They typically involve nasopharynx, palate, skin, GI tract, testes, or other sites. The hemophagocytic syndrome is sometimes associated (Cheuk, 2011).

The histology shows diffuse infiltrates of lymphoid cells of varying, often polymorphic, cytology, from small lymphocytes to large cells, immunoblasts, and/or anaplastic cells. Typically, mucosal ulcerations are present and some areas show an angiocentric and angioinvasive pattern (Fig. 33-72) with fibrinoid necrosis of vessels and associated infarction-like necrosis.

Immunophenotype is usually CD2/CD56 positive, with cCD3-ε and expression of cytotoxic molecules. CD43, CD45Ro, HLA-DR, CD25, CD95, and FAS ligand are also expressed, but CD4, CD8, CD5, CD16, and CD57 are negative.

TCR αβ and γδ and IgH genes are germline, but clonal episomal EBV is present. EBER ISH is positive. Del(6)(q21;q25) is occasionally described. Prognosis is variable.

Enteropathy-Associated T Cell Lymphoma

This is a clonal T cell malignancy of intraepithelial T cells. It is associated with celiac disease, but patients often present simultaneously with malabsorption and lymphoma (Swerdlow, 2008). It usually occurs in the jejunum or ileum, with other locations in or outside of the GI tract reported.

Morphology shows variable small, medium-sized to large neoplastic cells, often with pale to eosinophilic cytoplasm and eccentric angulated nuclei. In some cases, the cytology is similar to anaplastic large cell

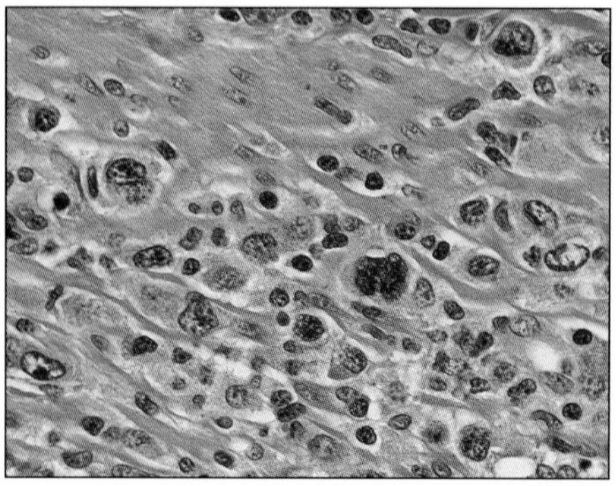

Figure 33-73 Enteropathy-associated T cell lymphoma infiltrating the muscularis of the small bowel (×500).

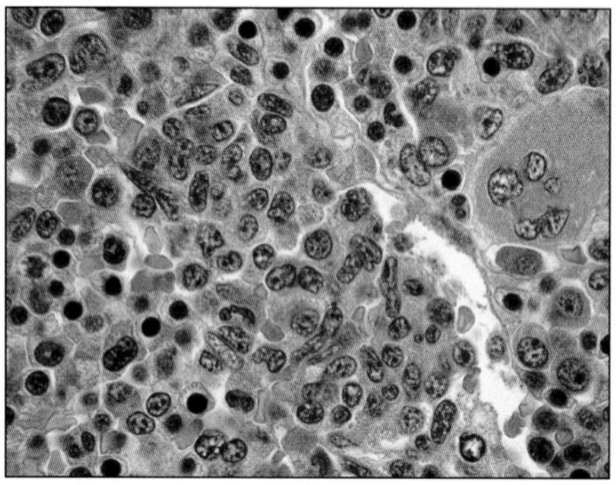

Figure 33-74 Hepatosplenic T cell lymphoma showing intrasinusoidal involvement of the bone marrow (×500).

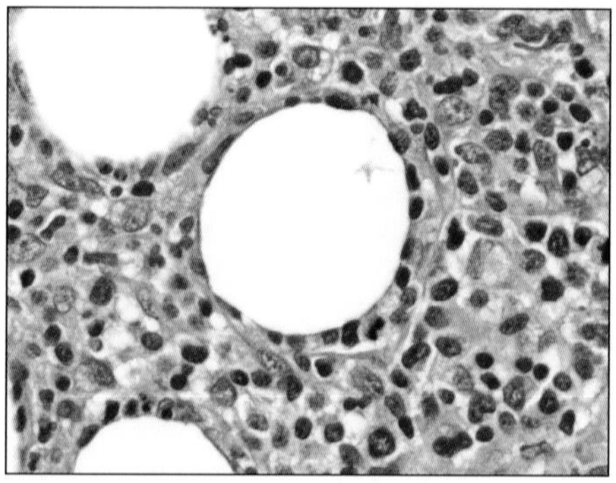

Figure 33-75 Subcutaneous panniculitis-like T cell lymphoma (×500).

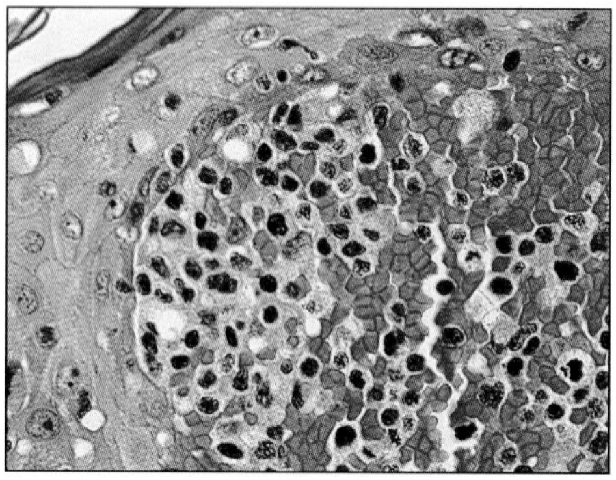

Figure 33-76 Cutaneous T cell lymphoma, showing a large Pautrier's microabscess (×20).

lymphoma with wreath-like multinucleation and horseshoe nuclei (Fig. 33-73). Other cases have bland-appearing small lymphocytes. Histiocytes and eosinophils are often abundant.

The phenotype is CD3, CD7, CD103 positive, CD8 variable, CD4 negative, often with double-negative CD4/CD8. Small cell variants are CD8/CD56 positive. Cytotoxic molecules are expressed. TCR genes are clonally rearranged, and patients with celiac disease typically have HLA DQA1*0501 and DQB1*0201. This is usually an aggressive disease.

Hepatosplenic T Cell Lymphoma

This is a rare neoplasm, usually of $\gamma\delta$ T cells, which shows sinusoidal infiltration of spleen, liver, and BM. It is most common in adolescent or young adult males. Patients present with massive splenomegaly, hepatomegaly, pronounced thrombocytopenia, and sometimes leukocytosis and anemia (Swerdlow, 2008).

Histology shows diffuse splenic red pulp involvement by small to medium-sized lymphoid cells with slightly dispersed chromatin and moderate cytoplasm. Liver shows similar cells in sinuses. Diagnosis is best made in the BM with presence of a characteristic infiltration of sinuses but otherwise intact architecture and hematopoiesis (Fig. 33-74). Immunophenotyping of sections is extremely helpful because of inconspicuous morphology on H&E.

The immunophenotype is CD3 and TIA-1 positive, with double-negative CD4 and CD8, negative CD5, granzyme B, and perforin (Belhadj, 2003). TCR $\delta 1$ antibodies are positive and TCR $\alpha\beta$ negative, although some cases of $\alpha\beta$ type occur.

TCR γ PCR is positive, and TCR β occasionally positive. Most cases are EBV negative, but EBV-positive cases may occur (Taguchi, 2004). Isochromosome 7q is usually described, with occasional trisomy 8. The disease is aggressive, with early responses to therapy but usual relapse and progression. No data have been obtained from clinical trials.

Subcutaneous Panniculitis-like T Cell Lymphoma

Subcutaneous panniculitis-like T cell lymphoma (SPLTCL) is a neoplasm of cytotoxic T cells that usually occurs as multiple nodules in the subcutaneous fat of the trunk or extremities and mimics benign panniculitis. The overlying epidermis and dermis are not involved, but the septa of subcutaneous adipose are infiltrated. The lymphoid infiltrate is polymorphic and may be deceptively bland, although some large cells are usually present (Fig. 33-75). There is rimming of fat cells by lymphocytes and usually vascular involvement with areas of necrosis and histiocytic infiltrates. Acute inflammatory cells are not typically present as they are in benign panniculitis, and multinucleated giant cells usually are not seen.

The immunophenotype is usually mature CD8+ T cell with expression of granzyme B, perforin, and TIA-1, with a genotype of clonal $\alpha\beta$ T cell type (Go, 2004). Twenty-five percent are $\gamma\delta$ T cell with double-negative CD4/CD8 and expression of CD56 (Swerdlow, 2008).

The disease is typically aggressive, and hemophagocytic syndrome is seen in about 37%. Median survival is approximately 27 months, but long-term remissions may be obtained with anthracycline-based therapy (Go, 2004).

Mycosis Fungoides and Sézary Syndrome

Mycosis fungoides (MF) occurs twice as frequently in men as in women. It usually affects individuals in their middle to late years.

The disorder first appears as an eczematoid, psoriasiform, or nonspecific exfoliative dermatitis. The lesions tend to form plaques and then tumors that often ulcerate. Some patients develop generalized erythroderma.

Biopsies of the skin reveal band-like lymphocytic infiltrates in the dermis (see Fig. 33-71), often with admixed histiocytes and occasional eosinophils (LeBoit, 2011). T cells with irregular nuclei (Fig. 33-76) show single-cell infiltration of the epidermis and often form clusters known as Pautrier's abscesses (Fig. 33-77). These are usually accompanied by parakeratosis and acanthosis, typically with minimal or no spongiosis, and elongation of rete pegs. The nuclei of at least a portion of neoplastic cells typically have a cerebriform appearance. The extent of the cutaneous infiltrate is not always directly correlated with severity of disease. Communication with the dermatologist or other treating physician is important, and even subtle changes in a clinically suspicious patient should be taken seriously.

Phenotype is usually mature T cell with CD8 expression and lack of CD7, but this is not usually conclusive. *TCR* genes are clonally rearranged, and PCR analysis of formalin-fixed biopsy tissue should be attempted in suspicious cases.

In advanced stages of the disease, neoplastic cells infiltrate the lymph nodes, liver, spleen, and other organs. Early nodal involvement (category I) shows dermatopathic changes with scattered atypical cerebriform

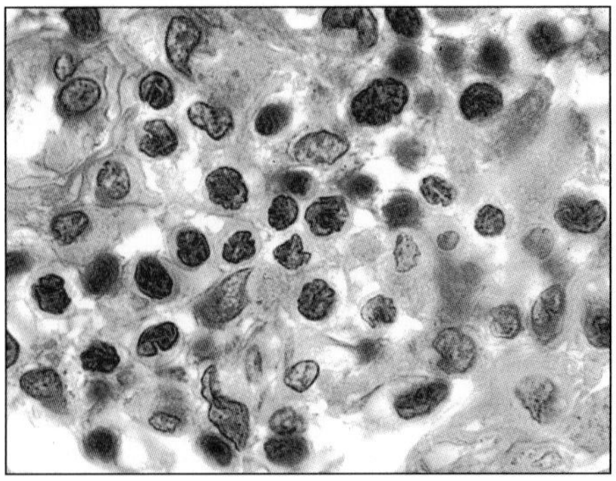

Figure 33-77 Neoplastic lymphocytes with convoluted nuclei in mycosis fungoides (×1000).

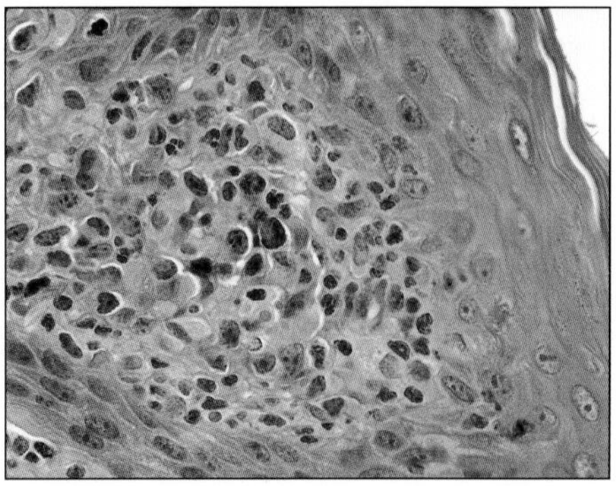

Figure 33-79 Cutaneous anaplastic large cell lymphoma (×1000).

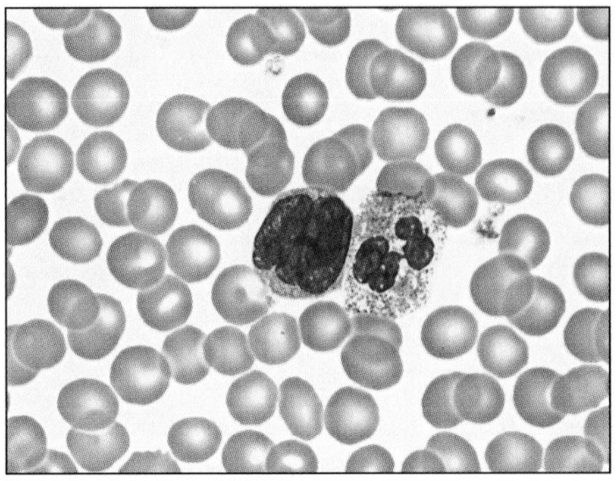

Figure 33-78 Sézary cell in the blood, along with a neutrophil (×1000).

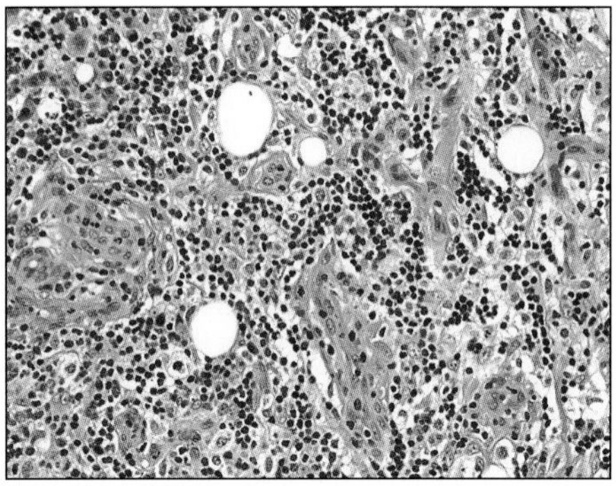

Figure 33-80 Angioimmunoblastic lymphoma showing arborizing vessels and lymphoid infiltrate infiltrating fat. In other areas of this case, plasma cells and immunoblasts are present. Clear cells are also frequently present (×200).

lymphocytes. Category II shows partial nodal effacement, and category III shows diffuse involvement.

Rare atypical mononuclear cells with cerebriform nuclei (Sézary cells) may be present in the peripheral blood (Fig. 33-78). Lymphocytosis with these cells (especially in the erythremic patient) is called Sézary syndrome.

The disorder may follow a prolonged chronic course. However, following lymph node infiltration, the disease becomes more progressive, and death, usually due to infection, occurs within 2 years.

Therapy is topical in early cases. More advanced disease has been treated with PUVA, retinoids, α-interferon, and, more recently, alemtuzumab (Campath) (Pichardo, 2004) or vorinostat (Duvic, 2009).

Primary Cutaneous CD30-Positive T Cell Lymphoproliferative Disorder

This category in the WHO classification includes primary cutaneous ALK negative, lymphomatoid papulosis, and borderline lesions (Kadin, 2011). These disorders share the features of dermal infiltrates of polymorphic lymphoid cells, including variable proportions of anaplastic or Reed-Sternberg–like cells with expression of CD30, and a typically relapsing/remitting clinical course.

Cutaneous ALCL resembles systemic ALCL (Fig. 33-79), except that it is indolent and does not exhibit detectable ALK expression or genetic translocations. Lymphomatoid papulosis has been considered a variant of pityriasis lichenoides et varioliformis acuta (PLEVA), with an inverted vase-like lymphoid infiltrate containing variable numbers of CD30-positive large cells. It has been associated with HL in a number of instances.

Both disorders share the phenotype of CD4-positive mature T cells with variable loss of pan-T cell antigens, expression of cytotoxic molecules, and strong CD30 expression. ALK is negative, and *TCR* genes are clonally rearranged. Atypical regressing histiocytosis is an older term used for both disorders.

Primary Cutaneous γδ T Cell Lymphoma

Primary cutaneous γδ T cell lymphoma is a rare lymphoma of adults consisting of a heterogeneous pattern of presentation (dermal, epidermal, and/or subcutaneous) in the skin of adults comprising γδ T cells. These express CD3, CD2, and CD56, often dually negative for CD4 and CD8 or CD8 positive, with lack of CD5 and βF1. They express TCR γ receptor, and TCR-γ is clonally rearranged. Histologically, they may mimic SPLTCL or MF.

Primary cutaneous CD8-positive aggressive epidermotropic cytotoxic T cell lymphoma is another rare cutaneous T cell lymphoma of cytotoxic T cells. Cells are small-medium or medium-large and often pleomorphic or blast-like. They express CD3, βF1, CD8, and granzymes B and TIA-1, with variable CD2 and CD7, but negative CD4 and CD5. These often resemble MF in their epidermotropism. The disease is aggressive.

Primary cutaneous CD4-positive small-medium T cell lymphoma is characterized by pleomorphic CD-positive T cells, without clinical patches or plaques (as seen in MF). They are CD3 and CD4 positive without CD30. Lesions are often localized. *TCR* genes are clonally rearranged, but the disease is indolent and is often treatable by excision.

Angioimmunoblastic T Cell Lymphoma

This disorder has been termed angioimmunoblastic lymphadenopathy with dysproteinemia (AILD) and abnormal immune response. It is a clonal T cell lymphoma that presents with constitutional symptoms and polyclonal hypergammaglobulinemia. Although once thought to be initially a reactive process with a spectrum of progression to lymphoma, it is now believed to be neoplastic from the onset.

Histology shows paracortical lymph node hyperplasia with depletion of lymphocytes, increased plasma cells, and prominent high endothelial postcapillary venules with PAS-positive hyalinization and "burned-out" residual follicles (Fig. 33-80). Clusters of lymphocytes with small nuclei but moderately abundant clear cytoplasm are usually present and increase in prominence with progression. The tumor is derived from follicular T-helper cells (THCs). The immunophenotype is mature T cell with CD4 predominance but often abundant reactive CD8 cells, coexpression of CD10, CXCL13, and PD-1, polyclonal plasma cells and B-immunoblasts, and prominent dendritic cells near vessels detected by CD21/CD23. CD20 is occasionally expressed, and secondary clonal B cell proliferations occur (Warnke, 2007).

TCR genes are usually rearranged and *IgH* genes are also rearranged in a minority of cases, at least some of which are associated with EBV and/or immunosuppression. Trisomy 3 or 5 or an additional X chromosome has been described. The disease is aggressive, and infectious complications are common (Swerdlow, 2008).

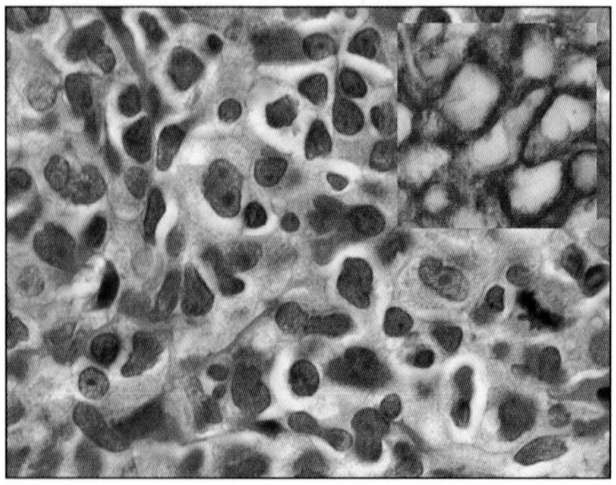

Figure 33-81 Peripheral T/natural killer cell lymphoma, unspecified; CD3 expression is seen in inset (×1000).

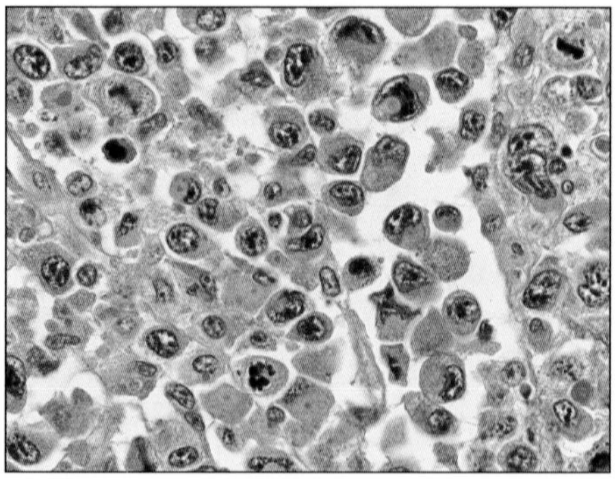

Figure 33-82 Anaplastic large cell lymphoma in an adolescent (×500).

Peripheral T/NK Cell Lymphoma, Unspecified

Peripheral T/NK cell lymphoma (PTCL), unspecified, are characteristically diverse and may consist of sheets of large cells (Fig. 33-81), paracortical lymph node expansion by mixed small and large cells, clear cells, predominantly small cells, and cases with striking pleomorphism resembling ALCL or HL. Abnormal patterns of T-antigen expression are helpful for diagnosis. Pan-T cell antigens (CD3, CD2, CD5, CD7) are usually present in some combination, but one or more are often aberrantly not expressed. CD4+ cases are more frequent than CD8+, but both double-positive and double-negative cases may occur (Swerdlow, 2008). In paraffin sections, CD3, CD45Ro, and CD43 are helpful if positive, but the latter two are also present in myeloid tumors and some B cell lymphomas. CD68 is rarely expressed.

T-zone variant of PTCL, unspecified, shows paracortical expansion with preserved GCC. The cytomorphology is variable with small and medium-sized cells, lymphocytes, plasma cells, endothelial hyperplasia, and sometimes clusters of clear cells and/or cells resembling those in HL.

The lymphoepithelioid variant, formerly known as Lennert's lymphoma, exhibits clusters of epithelioid histiocytes.

These tumors are typically aggressive and often belie their sometimes bland or reactive appearance. Clonal rearrangement of *TCR* genes is essential for confident diagnosis.

Anaplastic Large Cell Lymphoma

ALCL was first recognized relatively recently as NHL reactive with the Hodgkin-associated antibody Ki-1 (anti-CD30) (Stein, 1985). Primary ALCL is most common in adolescents and young adults and accounts for about 10%–15% of pediatric lymphomas. Cases in young people were likely overlooked previous to routine immunophenotyping, and retrospective review shows that about half of pediatric large cell lymphomas have been of T cell phenotype with **polymorphic immunoblastic** morphology, which is now associated with ALCL (Hutchison, 1991). In addition, the morphology is variable and is not of itself diagnostic, and a variety of secondary ALCLs (including progressions of other lymphomas, post-transplant tumors, and EBV- and HTLV-1–associated lymphomas) also express CD30.

Primary ALCL appears associated with chromosomal abnormalities involving chromosome region 2p23 such as t(2;5)(p23;q35), in which the gene for a tyrosine kinase anaplastic lymphoma kinase is fused to that of the nucleolar shuttle protein nucleophosmin, with a resultant NPM-ALK fusion protein that is highly expressed (Morris, 1994). The terms ALKoma and ALK lymphoma have been proposed (Benharroch, 1998). Variant genetic abnormalities involving ALK also occur, usually with ALK overexpression (Falini, 1999). Secondary ALCL and primary cutaneous ALCL are usually ALK negative. The clinical implications of primary or secondary ALCL have not yet been fully elucidated.

ALCL usually shows diffuse infiltrates or aggregates of large, sometimes pleomorphic cells with abundant cytoplasm and indented or horseshoe-shaped nuclei and sometimes wreath-like multilobulated nuclei (Fig. 33-82). Lymph node sinus and superficial paracortical involvement are common, cohesive sheets of tumor cells often simulate carcinoma, and some cases show a polymorphic Hodgkin-like pattern. True Reed-Sternberg cells are not seen. Histologic variants include small cell and lymphohistiocytic types, but these also express ALK and show similar phenotype otherwise.

Essentially all exhibit CD30. Most primary cases in young people express ALK, which is usually both nuclear and cytoplasmic, but is only cytoplasmic in some genetic variants. Slightly more than half show peripheral T cell phenotype by IHC, but with variable expression of CD3, CD43, and CD45Ro. Variable expression of CD45, CD25, and EMA has also been noted. CD68 or CD15 is only occasionally expressed. T cell surface marker–negative cases have been referred to as **null**, but recent evidence suggests that even though up to 90% show *TCR* rearrangements, expression of TCR is typically defective (Bonzheim, 2004).

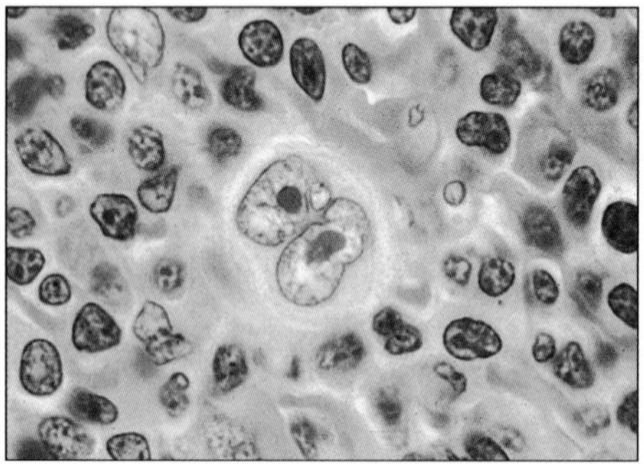

Figure 33-83 A Reed-Sternberg cell in a case of mixed cellularity Hodgkin lymphoma (×1000).

CD56 expression occurs and is related to adverse prognosis (Suzuki, 2000). Cytotoxic granules with labeling by marker TIA-1 are also described (Felgar, 1999). Signal transducer and activator of transcription 3 (STAT3) is often overexpressed, with activation of antiapoptotic pathways and increased expression of bcl-2, bcl-xl, surviving, and others, and decreased caspase-mediated apoptosis (Amin, 2004). Survivin expression in about half of cases is possibly associated with adverse outcome (Schlette, 2004). ALCL differs from HL in that ALK expression abrogates CD30 induction of NF-κB, whereas CD30 activates NF-κB in HL (Horie, 2004).

A majority exhibit t(2;5)(p23;q35), but variants are also seen, including t(1;2)(q25;p23) involving *TPM3*, which encodes a tropomyosin; inv(2)(p23;q35) involving *ATIC;* and t(2;3)(p23;q35) involving *TFG* (TRAK-fused gene). These all show cytoplasmic without nuclear ALK. Other partner genes include *TPM4*, *CLTC*, *MSN*, *ALO17*, and *MYH9* (Lamant, 2003). Those with translocations involving the clathrin gene (CLTC-ALK) have been identified as large B cell lymphoma (CD20-negative, CD79a+), each with *IgH* rearrangement and *TCR* rearrangement combined. They show granular cytoplasmic staining with ALK. Cytogenetics showed t(2;17)(p23;q23) (De Paepe, 2003). Rare cases of B cell ALCL, with or without ALK, are classified by the WHO with LBCL.

HODGKIN LYMPHOMA

The nomenclature of HL, formerly called Hodgkin's disease, is little changed from that of the Rye Conference (Lukes, 1966). The hallmark of HL is the Hodgkin Reed-Sternberg (HRS vs. RS) cell, which is a large binucleated, multinucleated, or mononuclear (Hodgkin) cell with each nucleus bearing a very large inclusion-like nucleolus (Fig. 33-83). These neoplastic cells appear in an immunoproliferative background containing variable numbers of lymphocytes, histiocytes, eosinophils, and plasma cells. Degenerating "mummified" neoplastic cells are also often present.

TABLE 33-22
Key Features of Hodgkin Lymphomas

Lymphoma	Demographics, clinical presentation	Morphology	Cell surface markers	Prognosis
Nodular, lymphocyte predominant (NLPHL)	M > F, 30–50 years, with peripheral lymphadenopathy	Mononuclear cells with convoluted nuclei (popcorn or L&H cells) loosely aggregated in nodules of small B cells	CD45, CD20, bcl-6, J-chain, Oct-2, BOB.1, EBV absent in LP cells	Excellent for stages I, II
Nodular sclerosis	M = F, <30 years with mediastinal mass, occasional spleen or lung involvement; 40% have B symptoms; most patients present with stage II disease	Broad bands of collagen, nodules of lymphoid tissue with aggregates of HRS cells and lacunar cells, multinucleated variants	CD15, CD30, CD45-EBV in 1%–40%	Good with systemic therapy
Mixed cellularity	M > F; median age, 38 years; peripheral lymphadenopathy common, spleen, BM; B symptoms common; patients often stage III or IV	Classic HRS cells in mixture of lymphocytes, plasma cells, eosinophils, histiocytes	CD15, CD30, CD45-EBV in 75%	Good with systemic therapy
Lymphocyte depletion	M > F; median age, 30–37 years; B symptoms, advanced stage common; associated with HIV	Classic HRS cells common with paucity of background lymphocytes; pleomorphic HRS cells mimic sarcoma	CD15, CD30, CD45-EBV pos in HIV-affected patients	Associated with advanced stage
Lymphocyte-rich classical	M > F, older age; peripheral lymphadenopathy; B symptoms rare; most patients with stage I or II disease	Scattered classic HRS cells among numerous small lymphocytes; nodular growth pattern	CD15, CD30; Oct2 and BOB.1 vary; J-chain absent; EBV in 40%–75%	Good, similar to NLPHL

BM, Bone marrow; *CHL,* classical Hodgkin lymphoma; *EBV,* Epstein-Barr virus; *F,* female; *HIV,* human immunodeficiency virus; *HRS,* Hodgkin Reed-Sternberg; *L&H,* lymphocytic and histiocytic; *LP,* lymphoplasmacytic; *M,* male.

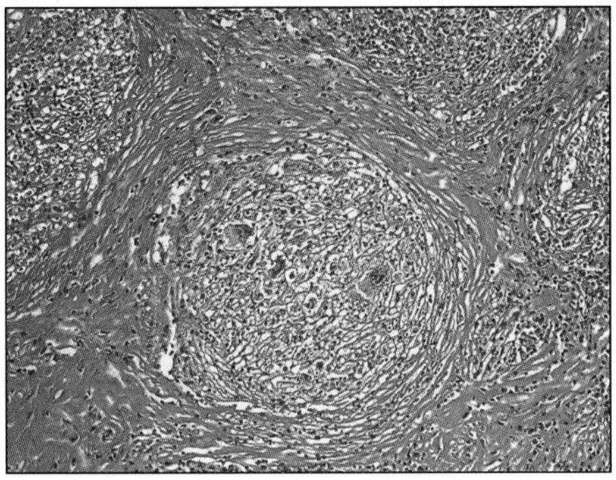

Figure 33-84 Dense fibrosis in a case of nodular sclerosis Hodgkin lymphoma (×200).

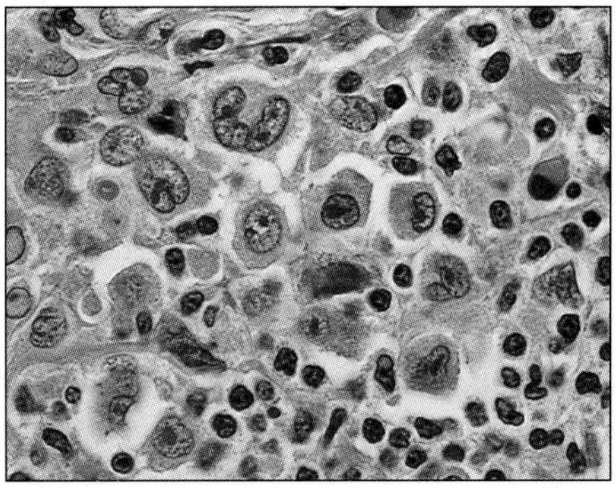

Figure 33-85 A cluster of Hodgkin Reed-Sternberg cells in a nodule of nodular sclerosis Hodgkin lymphoma (×500).

Classical Hodgkin Lymphoma

Mixed cellularity, nodular sclerosis, lymphocyte-depleted, and lymphocyte-rich classical subtypes have similar biology and are all referred to as "classical" HL (Stein, 2008). NLPHL appears to be a different entity (Fig. 33-84).

The most common phenotype of HRS cells in classical HL is expression of CD30, CD15, and fascin with absence of CD45 and T cell markers. B cell–associated markers CD20 and/or CD79 are expressed in a minority of cases (<30%) and are usually focal and weak. Occasional cases show strong CD20 expression. B cell transcription factors Oct2 and Bob.1 are absent, as is immunoglobulin J chain. Light chain immunoglobulin antibodies may show generalized cytoplasmic labeling. Standard Ig and *TCR* gene rearrangement studies are negative in classical HL, but sequencing of amplified single-cell *IgH* genes suggests that most cases of HL are derived from clonal B lymphocytes (Stein, 1999). EBV is associated with a substantial portion of cases of classical HL (Herbst, 1992).

HL may occur from early childhood to old age. Increased frequency is noted between 15 and 35 years and after age 50. Males predominate, especially in childhood; disease in females younger than age 30 is usually nodular sclerosis in type (Table 33-22).

Nodular Sclerosis

Nodular sclerosis (NS) is characterized by broad bands of collagen separating nodules of lymphoid tissue and the presence of **lacunar variants** of HRS cells with pale cytoplasm and variable nucleoli (Figs. 33-85 and 33-86). Classic HRS cells are variable in number. Fibrosis may be inconspicuous in early lesions, but neoplastic cell clustering is usually present.

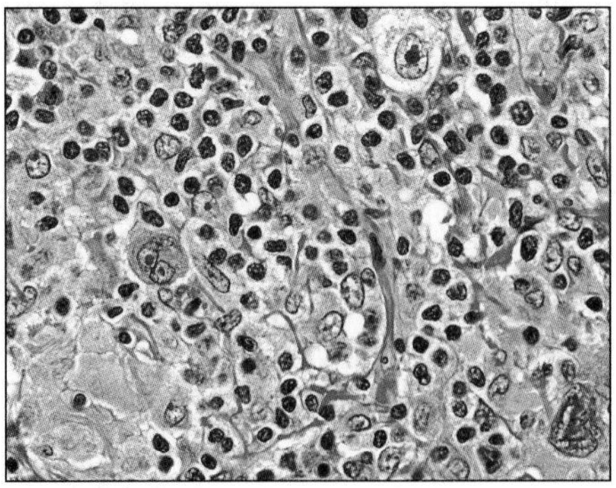

Figure 33-86 Scattered Hodgkin Reed-Sternberg cells in mixed cellularity Hodgkin lymphoma (×500).

NS HL is graded on the basis of the number of neoplastic cells. When sheets of neoplastic cells are present in 25% or more of nodules, the tumor is designated grade 2. This is frequently associated with necrosis and has

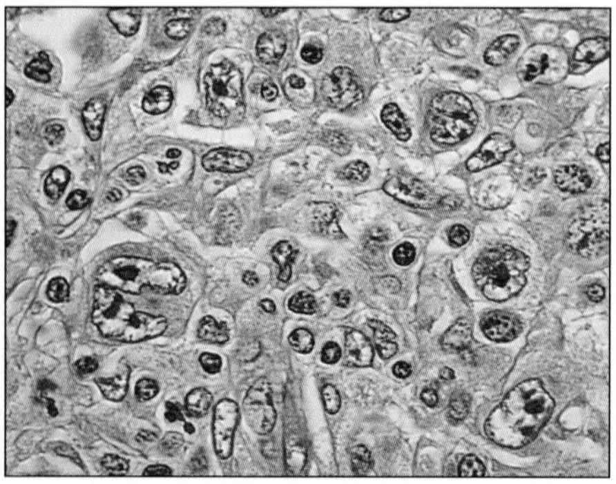

Figure 33-87 Lymphocyte-depleted Hodgkin lymphoma shows predominance of neoplastic cells with few lymphocytes (×500).

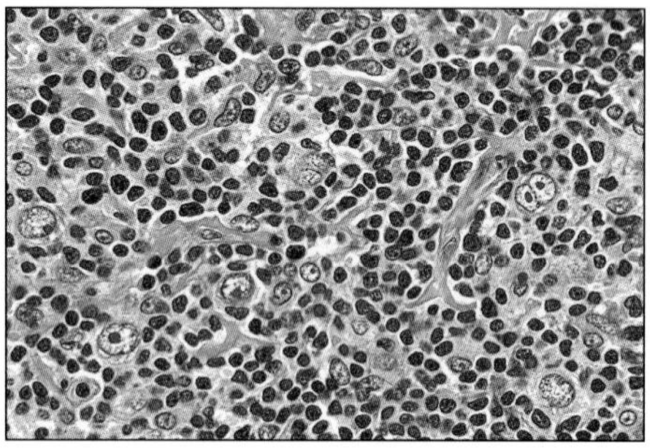

Figure 33-88 Lymphocyte predominant Hodgkin lymphoma, with lymphocyte and histiocytic cells showing round rather than popcorn nuclei (×500).

been termed syncytial variant. The NS variety of HL is common, often presenting as a mediastinal mass in a young woman.

Mixed Cellularity

Mixed cellularity shows a diffuse polymorphic infiltrate of lymphocytes, plasma cells, eosinophils, histiocytes, and Reed-Sternberg cells, which sometimes are numerous (Fig. 33-87). Necrosis and disorderly fibrosis may be present. This subtype is less common in young people than is NS, and it is the most frequent subtype with EBV involvement.

Lymphocyte Depletion

This type is uncommon, often presents at older age, and may be associated with diffuse fibrosis. Neoplastic cells predominate and lymphocytes are relatively diminished compared with other forms of HL (Fig. 33-88). It is sometimes associated with an acute febrile illness accompanied by pancytopenia and lymphocytopenia. BM involvement is common, but lymphocytosis and thrombocytosis, often seen in other types of HL, are usually absent (Neiman, 1973).

Normocytic anemia is seen in about 50% of HL cases. Leukocyte and platelet counts are variable, and eosinophilia may be present. Blood and marrow findings and many of the histologic features appear to be manifestations of host responses to the disease. Immunologic studies in HL have shown that cell-mediated immunity is defective when extensive disease is present.

Clinical staging defines Stage I disease as limited to lymph nodes in one anatomic region or two contiguous regions on one side of the diaphragm. Stage II disease involves more than two contiguous regions or two noncontiguous regions on one side of the diaphragm. Stage III disease is present on both sides of the diaphragm but is confined to lymphoid tissue. Stage IV disease involves BM or any other organ, in addition to lymphoid tissue. The incidence of BM involvement in untreated cases of HL is approximately 10% (Bartl, 1982a). All stages are additionally classified as "A" if systemic symptoms are absent and "B" if they are present. An aggressive approach to the management of HL has resulted in improved survival with many cures, especially in young patients.

Nodular Lymphocyte Predominant HL

The histology of NLPHL consists of effacement of lymph node architecture by a nodular infiltrate of small B cells with an associated follicular dendritic network and clustered or scattered large cells referred to as L&H cells, after the original Lukes and Butler terminology of lymphocytic and histiocytic HL. Nodularity may be vague. L&H cells are variable in cytology from case to case, although they are usually more uniform within a case. The appearance most often described exhibits large nuclei with vesicular chromatin, moderately prominent nucleoli, and convoluted nuclei resembling popcorn ("popcorn cells"). Cytoplasm is moderate in amount and clear, retracted, or slightly eosinophilic. Probably more often, the neoplastic cells show round to oval nuclei with distinct eosinophilic or basophilic nucleoli, but less prominent than in HRS cells (see Fig. 33-84). With experience, these cells become distinctive. Occasional HRS cells may be seen but are not always present and rarely predominate. Their phenotype, however, is different from that of classic HRS cells. L&H cells are usually loosely aggregated in the centers of nodules but are scattered elsewhere.

The phenotype of L&H cells is mature B cell, expressing CD45, CD20, CD22, CD79a, bcl-6, BOB.1, Oct-2, CD75, and usually J-chain. CD30 is absent or weak, and EMA is frequently expressed. The nodules are composed mostly of B cells but with abundant admixed CD3 and CD3/CD57-positive T cells, which tend to form rosettes around L&H cells. These are not always present, but are diagnostically helpful when they are. Nodules contain a follicular dendritic network which may be illuminated by CD21, CD35, or CD23 antibodies (Pileri, 2002). Cytoplasmic Ig is present but does not appear clonal, even though B cells have been proven to be monoclonal by single-cell PCR (Atayar, 2011).

IgH is clonally rearranged by sensitive assays in the research setting, but this usually is not detectable in routine clinical laboratory settings. L&H cells are of germinal center or post–germinal center derivation with somatic mutations of *Ig* genes which are ongoing in about half of studied cases (Braeuninger, 1997; Pileri, 2002).

Progressive transformation of lymph node germinal centers (PTGC) has been described as a precursor lesion to NLPHL, but no relationship has been proven. Most cases of PTGC do not lead to lymphoma.

Nodular Lymphocyte-Rich Classical HL

Nodular lymphocyte-rich classical Hodgkin lymphoma (NLRCHL) is a type of HL that morphologically and clinically resembles NLPHL but shows immunophenotypic characteristics of classical Hodgkin lymphoma (CHL). Typically, germinal centers are preserved and HRS cells are found in the mantle zones. It usually presents in peripheral lymph nodes with early-stage disease. The HRS cells in this type express CD30 and uniformly lack immunoglobulin J-chain that is present in NLPHL (Agnagnostopoulos, 2000). Recent studies show overlap between NLRCHL and NLPHL in expression of B cell factors bcl-6, Oct-2, and Bob.1, which are variable in NLRCHL but nearly constant in NLPHL, with less frequent CD20 and EBV. (However, EBV-EBER positivity is rarely seen in LPHL.) CD15 and MUM-1 are more frequent in NLRCHL, and Pax-5 is expressed in most cases of both types (Nam-Cha, 2009). A large clinical study has shown that patients with NLRCHL are older than those with other CHL, and that response and outcome are excellent, resembling NLPHL (Shimabukuro-Vornhagen, 2005).

IMMUNODEFICIENCY-ASSOCIATED LYMPHOPROLIFERATIVE DISORDERS

Lymphomas and uncontrolled polyclonal lymphoid proliferations occur with increased frequency in patients with immune dysfunction. These dysfunctional states fall into three main categories: primary (congenital) immune deficiency states, HIV infection, and iatrogenic immunodeficiency, particularly due to posttransplant immunosuppression but also due to prolonged immunosuppressive therapy for other reasons.

Most of these are B cell lymphoproliferative disorders associated with infection or reactivation of EBV or other virus and include large B cell lymphoma and variants, BL, and polymorphic B cell hyperplasia. Hodgkin and peripheral T cell lymphomas occur rarely. See Table 33-23 for a summary of lymphoid diseases associated with EBV.

Primary immune deficiencies are rare disorders and include Wiskott-Aldrich syndrome (WAS), ataxia-telangiectasia (AT), common variable immunodeficiency syndrome (CVID), severe combined immunodeficiency (SCID), X-linked immunoproliferative disorder (XLP), Nijmegan breakage syndrome (NBS), and hyper-IgM syndrome (Lim, 2011).

ALPS is an autoimmune disorder that also causes lymphadenopathy and involves inherited mutations of the *FAS* gene, which blocks apoptosis. This involves different mutations of varying effect; it may be more common than was previously thought and may show adult onset in some cases (Oren, 2002). Hyper-IgM syndrome results from mutations in CD40

TABLE 33-23
EBV Associations

Mononucleosis-type illness
Hodgkin lymphoma: MC > LR > NS; LD seen in HIV patients
Immunodeficiency-associated lymphoproliferative disorders
Posttransplant lymphoproliferative disorders
Some DLBCL cases (associated w/inflammations, in elderly)
Lymphomatoid granulosis
Primary effusion lymphoma
EBV+ lymphoproliferative disorders of childhood
Burkitt lymphoma (endemic and HIV associated)
Nasal NK-T cell lymphoma
Angioimmunoblastic lymphoma
Plasmablastic lymphoma

DLBCL, Diffuse large B cell lymphoma; *EBV*, Epstein-Barr virus; *HIV*, human immunodeficiency virus; *LD*, lymphocyte depletion; *LR*, lymphocyte rich classical; *MC*, mixed cellularity; *NS*, nodular sclerosis.

ligand with inhibition of T/B cell interaction and B cell maturation. AT and NBS are abnormalities of DNA repair. WAS is a syndrome of thrombocytopenia, skin rash, and recurrent infections which is fatal but curable by allogeneic BM transplantation.

Fatal EBV infectious mononucleosis is a common occurrence in XLP and SCID. Large B cell lymphomas are the most common tumors in most primary immunodeficiencies, and lymphomatoid granulomatosis is increased in WAS.

HIV-Associated Lymphomas

Inadequately treated HIV shows a markedly increased incidence of high-grade B cell lymphomas associated with EBV (Knowles, 1988; Said, 2011). These are primarily Burkitt, atypical Burkitt, and large B cell lymphoma. HIV-associated BL is similar to endemic Burkitt with EBV association and c-myc translocation but with different breakpoints (Haluska, 1989). BL with plasmacytoid differentiation is unique to HIV. MALT lymphomas occur even in children with HIV; HL and NK lymphomas occur rarely. Primary effusion lymphomas in HIV are due to KHSV/HHV-8 infection and are associated with Kaposi's sarcoma and multicentric Castleman's disease. The incidence of HIV-associated lymphoma has dropped substantially in developed nations since the introduction of HAART.

Posttransplant Lymphoproliferative Disorders

These are also EBV associated and result from chronic infection and/or reactivation (Collins, 2002). PTLDs are composed of a unique spectrum of lymphoproliferative disorders, which have been divided into morphologic categories (Swerdlow, 2011). In many cases, these tumors regress when immunosuppressive therapy is reduced, but this is unpredictable.

Plasmacytic hyperplasia (PH) is composed of numerous plasma cells and scattered immunoblasts. Infectious mononucleosis–like PTLD shows paracortical expansion of lymph nodes with increased immunoblasts. Both are early or low-grade lesions with a slow progression.

Polymorphic PTLD shows increased immunoblasts and plasma cells in a lymphoid background. Monomorphic PTLD is essentially diffuse lymphoma, usually large B cell. A Hodgkin-like PTLD is likely to be a large B cell lymphoma with Hodgkin-like features, previously called polymorphic immunoblastic in the Working Formulation (Fig. 33-89). Monomorphic T cell lymphomas also occur rarely.

A disorder similar to PTLD also may occur with chronic immunosuppression for other reasons, such as the use of methotrexate in the treatment of rheumatoid arthritis. (See also previous descriptions of large B cell lymphomas of the elderly and those occurring in chronic inflammation, which are also EBV related.)

HISTIOCYTIC AND DENDRITIC CELL NEOPLASMS

These are rare disorders that affect lymph nodes and soft tissues, and occasionally the BM (Jaffe, 2008a).

Histiocytic sarcoma, also known as true histiocytic lymphoma, is a malignant tumor of noncirculating cells of monocyte macrophage lineage (Chang, 2011). The differential diagnosis includes monocytic leukemia

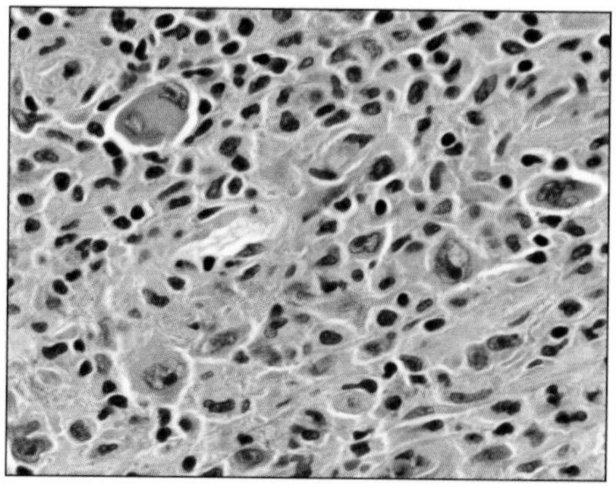

Figure 33-89 Large B cell lymphoma (anaplastic subtype) arising in polymorphic posttransplant lymphoproliferative disorder, in the gastrointestinal tract (×500).

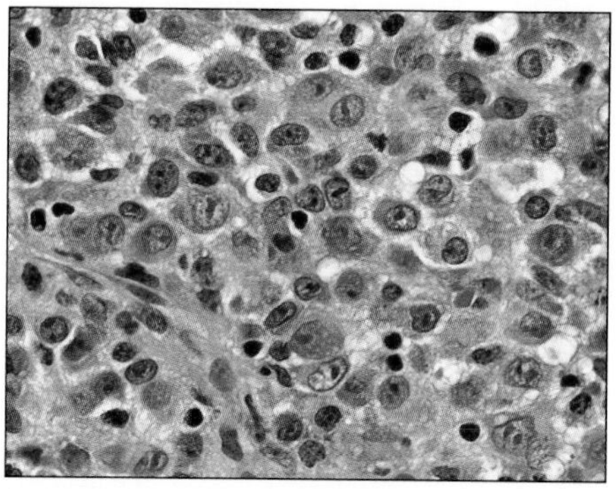

Figure 33-90 Histiocytic sarcoma in a child. This case showed expression of monocytic markers and enzymes, lack of lymphoid markers, and lack of lymphoid gene rearrangements (×500).

and large B or peripheral T cell lymphoma. It resembles a large cell lymphoma or histiocytic sarcoma of monocytic lineage (Fig. 33-90). Tumor cells show nuclear features of malignancy. These label with CD68, lysozyme, α_1-antitrypsin, and antichymotrypsin; others label with other monocyte macrophage markers (e.g., CD64, CD14). Some hemophagocytosis may be seen.

Hemophagocytic Syndromes

These are often mistaken for histiocytic malignancy. They present with hepatosplenomegaly, fever and other constitutional symptoms, cytopenias, and infiltrates of macrophages in involved organs, including BM with hemophagocytosis primarily of red blood cells (Fig. 33-91). Hemophagocytosis may be difficult to identify in occasional otherwise usual cases. These are usually associated with recent viral infection, EBV, or cytomegalovirus (CMV), but familial hemophagocytic syndromes may also occur.

The cause of the disorder is often cryptic, but frequently an aggressive course is followed. Approximately 60% of patients succumb within 2 months (Chen, 2004; Karras, 2004), but some patients respond to immune therapy.

Langerhans Histiocytosis

Langerhans cell histiocytosis (LCH) is a neoplastic proliferation of Langerhans cells, which are dendritic cells normally found primarily in the skin (Jaffe, 2008b). It presents in a variety of ways, including unifocal disease, usually in the bone, and occasionally in the lymph node, skin, or lung, of an adolescent or young adult. These have been termed eosinophilic granuloma. Multifocal unisystem disease usually involves bone of children with frequent spread to adjacent soft tissues, also known as Hand-Schüller-Christian disease. Skull involvement may lead to diabetes insipidus, tooth loss, or exophthalmos. Multiple lung lesions may be seen in adults. Multifocal multisystem disease, that is, Letterer-Siwe disease, occurs in infants. It is an aggressive disease with fever, skin rash, hepatosplenomegaly, lymphadenopathy, bone involvement, and pancytopenia.

Histologically, the disease consists of infiltrates of Langerhans cells. They resemble benign histiocytes but have a coffee bean–shaped nucleus with a linear central groove (Fig. 33-92). Variable numbers of eosinophils and lymphocytes are usually present. The infiltrates form nodules in bone, involve the upper dermis of the skin, and may involve lymph node sinuses and splenic red pulp. Giant cells are sometimes present but differ from

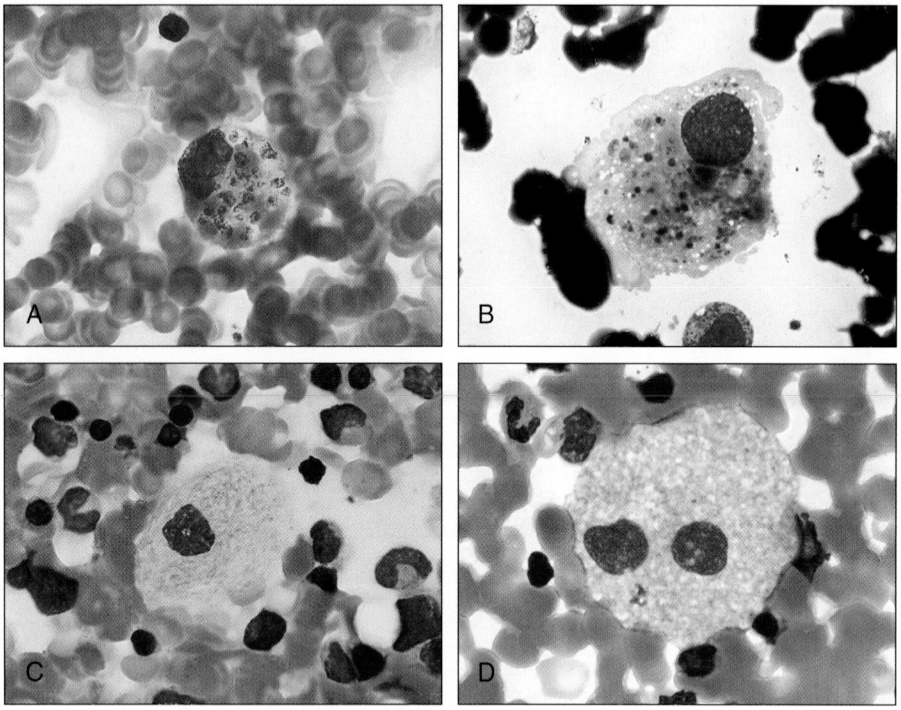

Figure 33-91 **A,** Histiocytic hyperplasia occurring in infection-associated hemophagocytic syndrome; this macrophage contains platelets as well as erythrocytes (×1000). Compare with **B,** a histiocyte containing cell debris in a patient with human immunodeficiency virus (×1000); **C,** an abnormal macrophage in Gaucher's disease (×1000); and **D,** one in Niemann-Pick disease (×1000).

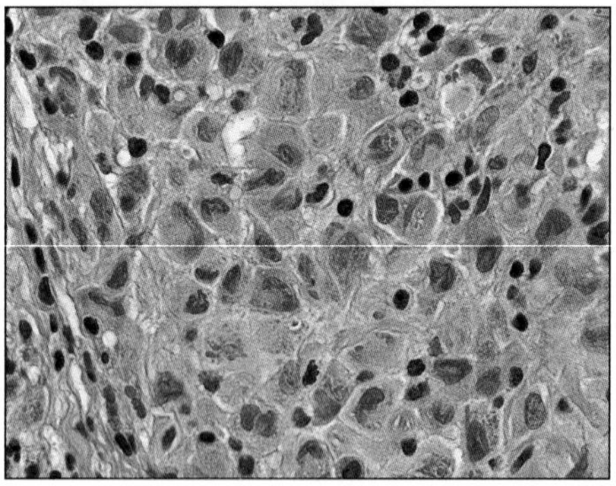

Figure 33-92 Langerhans cell histiocytosis, showing typical nuclear folding and grooves (×500).

multinucleated histiocytes (as in juvenile xanthogranuloma) by the presence of characteristic nuclei.

Immunophenotyping shows reactivity for CD1a and S-100 protein and may be weakly reactive with CD45 and CD68, but is negative for T and B cell–specific antibodies and follicular dendritic markers CD21 and CD35. Electron microscopy remains useful in some cases because of characteristic Birbeck granules, which are pentalaminar racket-shaped structures pathognomonic of Langerhans cells.

Outcome is largely dependent on extent of organ involvement, with localized disease showing a high rate of event-free survival and extensive disease showing only a variable response to chemotherapy. Pulmonary disease in adults may remit spontaneously on cessation of smoking.

A cytologically malignant form of LCH has been termed Langerhans cell sarcoma (Swerdlow, 2008). Patients usually present with multiorgan disease, a high mitotic rate, and aggressive behavior.

Interdigitating Dendritic Cell Sarcoma/Tumor

Interdigitating dendritic cell sarcoma/tumor (IDCS) is a rare tumor of lymph node paracortical interdigitating dendritic cells (Weiss, 2008b). It has the gross and microscopic appearance of a sarcoma and is tan in color, with a firm lobulated appearance, sometimes with hemorrhage or necrosis and microscopic fascicles, whorls, and/or a storiform pattern. Lymphocytes are scattered throughout, and plump epithelioid cells may be present. Atypia is variable.

Immunophenotyping is essential to diagnosis. The tumor cells are positive for S-100, with variable weak positivity for CD45 and monocyte markers CD68 and lysozyme. CD1a, CD21, and CD35 are negative. Other myeloid B and T cell markers, EMA, and CD30 are also negative. Background lymphocytes are reactive T cells. Prognosis is variable.

Follicular Dendritic Cell Sarcoma/Tumor

This is another rare dendritic cell tumor derived from follicular dendritic cells, which are phenotypically different from IDCS (Chan JKC, 2008). Involvement is usually with cervical lymph nodes, with axillary, mediastinal, mesenteric, and retroperitoneal node involvement also described. Microscopically, nodes show fascicles, a storiform pattern, and/or complete whorls.

The immunophenotype shows positivity for CD21, CD23, and CD35, with variable S-100 and CD68, negative CD1a, and occasional CD45 and CD20. Other myeloid T and B cell markers, cytokeratins, and HMB-45 are negative. CD117 is also negative (Hornick, 2002).

These tumors are indolent, with frequent good response to simple resection.

Dendritic Cell Sarcoma, Not Otherwise Specified

Dendritic cell sarcomas which do not fall into the previous specific categories may be termed DCS, not otherwise specified (Weiss, 2008a). They include indeterminate cell sarcomas that express CD1a and S-100 without Birbeck granules, and fibroblastic reticular cell tomor.

SELECTED REFERENCES

Bhatt V, Saleem A. Review: drug-induced neutropenia—pathophysiology, clinical features, and management. Ann Clin Lab Sci 2004;34:131–7.

This is a recent review of the mechanisms of action, clinical features, diagnosis, and management of drug-induced neutropenia, including the use of filgrastim and pegfilgrastim in patients undergoing chemotherapy.

Dainiak N. Hematologic consequences of exposure to ionizing radiation. Exp Hematol 2002;30:513–28.

This article reviews common forms of ionizing radiation, including measurement, as well as dose response for normal marrow elements, effects on cells at the cellular level, and clinical effects of exposure.

Gilliland DG, Jordan CT, Felix CA. The molecular basis of leukemia. Hematology (Am Soc Hematol Educ Program) 2004;80–97.

This paper describes the molecular genetics of adult and pediatric leukemias and relates recent findings to current and future therapies.

Hernandez AM. Peripheral blood manifestations of lymphoma and solid tumors. Clin Lab Med 2002;22:215–53.

This article describes the correlation of findings identified on peripheral blood films in patients with various types of lymphoid leukemia and lymphoma, including morphology of various lymphoma cells in the circulating blood during disease.

Jaffe ES, Harris NL, Vardiman JW, et al, editors. Hematopathology. Philadelphia: WB Saunders, 2011.

This is a comprehensive, authoritative, and up-to-date review of hematopathology, incorporating the 2008 WHO classification.

Kroft SH. Infectious diseases manifested in the peripheral blood. Clin Lab Med 2002;22:253–77.

A review of both nonspecific hematopoietic changes in the peripheral blood during infection as well as findings for the few diseases in which peripheral blood film review plays a primary diagnostic role.

List AF, Vardiman J, Issa JP, Dewitte TM. Myelodysplastic syndromes. Hematology (Am Soc Hematol Educ Program) 2004;297–317.

This overview of myelodysplastic syndromes covers the spectrum from microscopic diagnosis to laboratory science and the translation of recent findings into therapeutic strategies.

Pui CH, Relling MV, Downing JR. Acute lymphoblastic leukemia. N Engl J Med 2004;350:1535–48.

This review describes the molecular genetic alterations, prognostic factors, molecular epidemiology, and pharmacogenetics of pediatric and adult acute lymphoblastic leukemia.

Rot A, von Andrian UH. Chemokines in innate and adaptive host defense: basic chemokinese grammar for immune cells. Annu Rev Immunol 2004;22:891–928.

This recent article presents an overview of chemokine communication and signaling mechanisms in immunity.

Schultz DR, Harrington WJ Jr. Apoptosis: programmed cell death at a molecular level. Semin Arthritis Rheum 2003;32:345–69.

This article reviews mechanisms and regulatory and effector proteins of the extrinsic and intrinsic apoptotic pathways and includes a glossary of terms in the appendix.

Swerdlow SH, Campo E, Harris NL, et al, editors. WHO classification of tumours of haematopoietic and lymphoid tissues. 4th ed. Lyon, France: IARC; 2008.

This provides a comprehensive and uniform classification of hematopoietic neoplasms. It was commissioned by the WHO through the major organizations of hematopathology, with clinical input from cooperative groups and cancer centers, and is intended to provide standard diagnositic criteria for worldwide use. Updated in 2008.

REFERENCES

Access the complete reference list online at http://www.expertconsult.com

CHAPTER 34

THE FLOW CYTOMETRIC EVALUATION OF HEMATOPOIETIC NEOPLASIA

Brent L. Wood, Michael J. Borowitz

KEY POINTS

- Flow cytometry is a powerful, rapid, and cost-effective technique for the identification and monitoring of hematopoietic neoplasms.
- Successful implementation of flow cytometry requires careful attention to details of instrument and reagent performance.
- Normal hematopoietic cells are characterized by a reproducible gain and loss of antigen expression with maturation.
- Hematopoietic neoplasms show deviation from the normal patterns of antigen expression, allowing for their diagnosis and classification.
- The flow cytometric detection of residual disease following therapy allows for the monitoring of therapeutic response.

The diagnosis, classification, and post-therapeutic monitoring of hematopoietic neoplasms have greatly benefited from the widespread application of immunophenotypic studies over the past two decades. The subdivision of hematopoietic neoplasms by their correspondence to normal hematopoietic lineages and stages of differentiation is a basic tenet of current classification systems (e.g., the World Health Organization [WHO] classification) (Swerdlow, 2008). This information is largely provided by immunophenotyping and has resulted in the incorporation of immunophenotypic data into the definition of many hematopoietic neoplasms to the extent that certain diagnoses cannot be confidently made without immunophenotypic studies.

Flow cytometry is a rapid and convenient technique for generating immunophenotypic data. The ability to perform multiparametric analysis on an individual cellular basis is a unique feature of the technique and offers distinct advantages over competing immunophenotypic methods such as immunohistochemistry. Guidelines on the use of flow cytometry for the immunophenotyping of leukemic cells in the clinical laboratory have been published (Clinical and Laboratory Standards Institute, 2007), and National Institutes of Health-sponsored consensus conferences on the flow cytometric analysis of leukemia and lymphoma were convened in 1995 (U.S.-Canadian Conference, 1997) and 2006 (Davis, 2007; Wood 2007) to attempt standardization of clinical practice. Despite these efforts, considerable heterogeneity exists in the clinical application of this technique to the evaluation of leukemia and lymphoma, and this lack of standardization represents a significant challenge to the ability to consistently provide high-quality results.

Medical indications for performing flow cytometry in a clinical setting currently can be divided into four basic areas:

1. The diagnosis and classification of hematopoietic neoplasms. The ability to accurately identify abnormal subpopulations of cells, assign lineage, and determine maturational stage adds improved reproducibility to the diagnosis of hematopoietic neoplasms, particularly for chronic lymphoproliferative disorders and acute leukemias. Flow cytometry is widely used for this purpose.
2. Assessment of biological parameters associated with prognosis. The expression of specific molecules at the time of diagnosis has been associated with long-term clinical outcome and can be easily assessed by flow cytometry. An example is the expression of CD38 or Zap-70 in chronic lymphocytic leukemia (CLL), where increased expression of either has been associated with poor long-term survival (Damle, 1999; Crespo, 2003).
3. Detection of antigens used as therapeutic targets. A variety of immunologic reagents are now available for therapeutic use that specifically target antigens expressed by hematopoietic neoplasms (e.g., CD20, CD52, CD33). Confirmation of expression of the antigen of interest by the tumor is a necessary prerequisite for use of these expensive therapies.
4. Detection of residual neoplastic cells following therapy. The ability of flow cytometry to routinely identify and quantitate the presence of abnormal hematopoietic cells with a sensitivity of 0.01% is increasingly being used as a surrogate measure of response to therapy and impending relapse (Campana, 2003).

TECHNICAL CONSIDERATIONS

INSTRUMENTATION

The basic principle of flow cytometry relies on the injection of a monodisperse suspension of particles (cells) into the center of a flowing stream of fluid (sheath) that then passes through a small quartz capillary tube at a constant velocity (Shapiro, 2003). The sheath fluid serves to maintain the particles in the center of the flowing stream, where they may be illuminated by one or more focused light sources, typically lasers. The light scattered by the particles is collected by detectors positioned at a variety of angles around the capillary to obtain information about the cross-sectional area, and hence size (low angle or forward scatter) or complexity/granularity (high angle or side scatter), of each individual particle as it transits the capillary. In addition, if fluorescent molecules or fluorochromes are attached to the particles, they may be excited by the incident light, giving rise to fluorescent emission that can be collected with the use of additional detectors and optical filters (Fig. 34-1). The net result is a

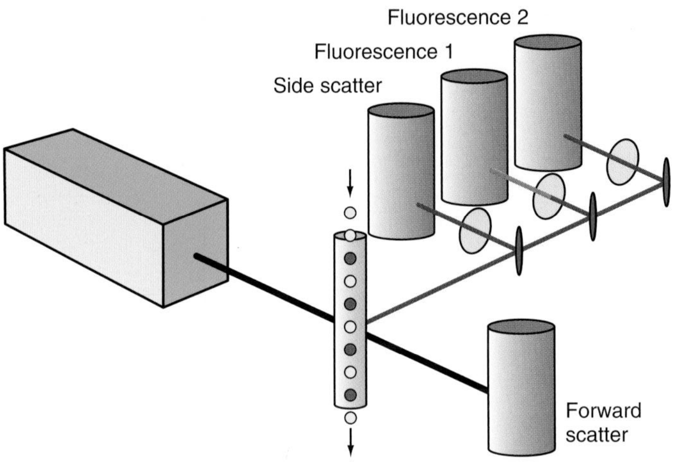

Figure 34-1 Schematic of a flow cytometer. A flowing stream of particles *(center)* is illuminated by a laser *(left)* and the resulting low angle (forward scatter) or right angle (side scatter) light scatter collected by appropriately positioned detectors. In addition, fluorescent molecules attached to the particles may be excited by the laser light and the resulting emission routed through a series of optical mirrors and filters to the appropriate detectors (fluorescence 1 and fluorescence 2).

multiparametric analysis of each individual particle with the number of parameters evaluated dependent on the number of fluorescent molecules used and the complexity of instrument design. Modern clinical instrumentation is capable of assessing up to 10 simultaneous fluorochromes (Wood, 2006).

Optimization and standardization of instrument performance are critical for the success of any flow cytometric study, but are of particular importance in the analysis of hematopoietic neoplasms because of the wide range of signal intensities that must be detected. The preferred approach is to define a set of instrument conditions that allow for optimal instrument performance and perform daily quality control of the instrument to consistently achieve that level of performance. Adherence to a consistent and fixed level of instrument performance greatly simplifies quality control and provides reproducible data for subsequent interpretation. Daily assessment of the fluorescence intensity and coefficient of variation, using particles that have stable, moderately bright fluorescence and assessment of instrument noise using nonfluorescent particles, is the cornerstone of instrument quality control.

The operator has control over relatively few instrument variables on a flow cytometer, principally detection threshold, detector gain, rate of sample flow and, for some multilaser instruments, laser delay time. The detection threshold or discriminator is associated with a single parameter and is the value that must be achieved for the system to recognize that a particle has passed through the capillary to initiate signal processing. Typically, forward scatter is used to identify particles that have a size greater than some desired value (e.g., cells equal to or larger than lymphocytes). Of particular importance is the gain or voltage supplied to each detector, commonly a photomultiplier tube, as this has a direct impact on the ability to separate signals of interest from background instrument noise (signal-to-noise ratio). The voltage applied to each detector should be adjusted to optimize the signal-to-noise ratio and allow detection of the weakest required signals for each detector. This often results in positioning of negative cellular populations in such a way that they completely occupy the lowest decade of a logarithmic scale. Finally, for instruments having multiple lasers that intersect the capillary stream at different points (spatially separated lasers), a parameter must be supplied to allow synchronization of signal processing to account for the different times at which a single particle encounters each laser as it transits through the capillary. This laser delay time should be adjusted to maximize signal intensity for each laser. It should be noted that the laser delay time is highly dependent on the transit time of the particle through the capillary, and so requires a stable fluidic system to remain constant—a problem historically on certain instruments.

The rate at which the sample is introduced or aspirated through the system can be controlled by the operator but is limited by two factors: the rate at which the instrument electronics can process signals that are generated, and sample concentration. If particles pass through the instrument more rapidly than they can be processed by the electronics, the data for a subset of the particles will be lost, and another subset will show unusual and undesirable artifacts, typically variable loss of signal intensity over a wide range. It is critically important to select a sample aspiration rate and concentration appropriate to the instrument to be used. One additional phenomenon related to sample concentration is termed **coincidence,** the simultaneous presence of more than one particle in the laser, resulting in a single recorded event that has composite characteristics of the particles involved. Coincidence can represent a significant problem for rare event detection and can be minimized using methods for doublet discrimination during analysis—techniques beyond the scope of this chapter (Wood, 2006).

REAGENTS

The identification of cellular characteristics beyond those provided by light scatter measurements commonly utilizes fluorochromes that directly interact with cellular structures such as DNA or that indirectly interact through conjugation to antibodies. Each fluorochrome has a unique excitation and emission spectrum that partly determines the performance characteristics of the reagent and dictates which fluorochromes may be used simultaneously (Fig. 34-2). In an effort to increase the number of usable simultaneous fluorochromes possible from a single excitation source, tandem fluorochromes have been devised (e.g., PE-Cy5) that rely on excitation of a primary fluorochrome that transfers its energy to a secondary fluorochrome (Cy5), providing the predominant fluorochrome emission at a longer wavelength. Tandem fluorochromes are required for high-level multicolor flow cytometry, but they have more complex emission spectra, as well as decreased fluorochrome stability under some circumstances. The other important fluorochrome characteristic, the intensity of emission, is related to the relative efficiency of excitation by the light sources utilized and the quantum efficiency of the fluorochrome itself (Fig. 34-3). Differences in emission intensity directly correlate with differences in detection sensitivity and are a key consideration in the design of reagent panels, as discussed later.

The use of multiple simultaneous fluorochromes (i.e., multicolor flow cytometry) is required for the analysis of leukemia and lymphoma, with three being the minimum number recommended under current consensus guidelines (U.S.-Canadian Consensus, 1997). Because most fluorochromes have overlapping emission spectra, determination of the fluorescence due to a specific fluorochrome in a single detector requires subtraction of the portion of the signals contributed by each of the other fluorochromes in the sample, a process termed **compensation.** The appropriate amount of each signal to subtract (i.e., compensation coefficient) may be represented by an n-by-n matrix, where n is the number of fluorochromes. Consequently, as the number of fluorochromes used increases, the number of compensation coefficients that must be determined increases geometrically, and software rapidly becomes required to do this process correctly. To determine the compensation coefficients, a series of samples singly labeled with each fluorochrome are evaluated, with the positive population as bright as the brightest signal one plans to evaluate. Because the spectral characteristics of the tandem fluorochromes can vary significantly between lots and manufacturers, separate compensation controls are often required for each lot and conjugate of these reagents. Software, either on the instrument or on offline computers, is used to analyze the resulting data and to calculate compensation coefficients.

Although the process of determining and correctly applying compensation is now made simple through software, the use of multiple fluorochromes can result in significant display artifacts that reflect compromised low-level detection sensitivity (Roederer, 2001). This is a particular problem when one attempts to detect low-level signals in the presence of brightly overlapping fluorochrome emissions. Understanding the impact of compensation-related effects is the single most difficult aspect of multicolor flow cytometry and the least understood by most users. The implications of overlapping fluorochrome emission have direct consequences for panel design and data interpretation (Fig. 34-4). When compensation settings are not appropriate for the reagents used, artifacts arise that can lead to both the misattribution of low-level positivity and an inability to recognize the presence of subpopulations (Fig. 34-5). The use of software compensation provides a nondestructive method for data collection and allows the adjustment of compensation settings following acquisition, thereby supplying a way to correct for inadvertent compensation errors.

Antibodies are an integral part of the immunophenotypic evaluation of leukemia and lymphoma. It is important to determine the correct amount of each antibody to use by evaluating a series of samples labeled with different concentrations of antibodies (i.e., titering) (Stewart, 2000). The object of titering is to maximize the signal-to-noise ratio by providing as bright a signal as possible on positive populations, while maintaining a low

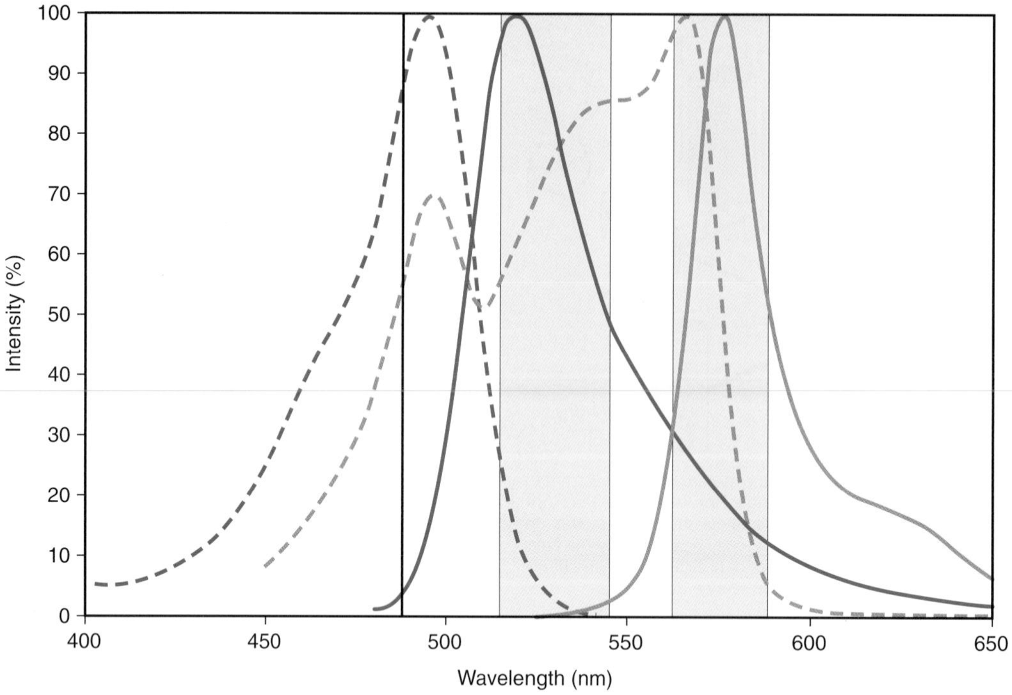

Figure 34-2 Fluorochrome emission spectra. Each fluorescent molecule possesses a characteristic absorption *(dotted line)* and emission spectrum *(solid line)* whose wavelength maxima are spectrally separated; the degree of separation is termed the **Stokes shift.** Although a small amount of fluorescein emission occurs at the same wavelength as phycoerythrin, the fluorescence emission of fluorescein *(green)* can be separated from that of phycoerythrin *(orange)* using appropriate optical filters *(shaded areas).* The 488-nm laser commonly used to excite each of these fluorochromes is indicated by a black, vertical line.

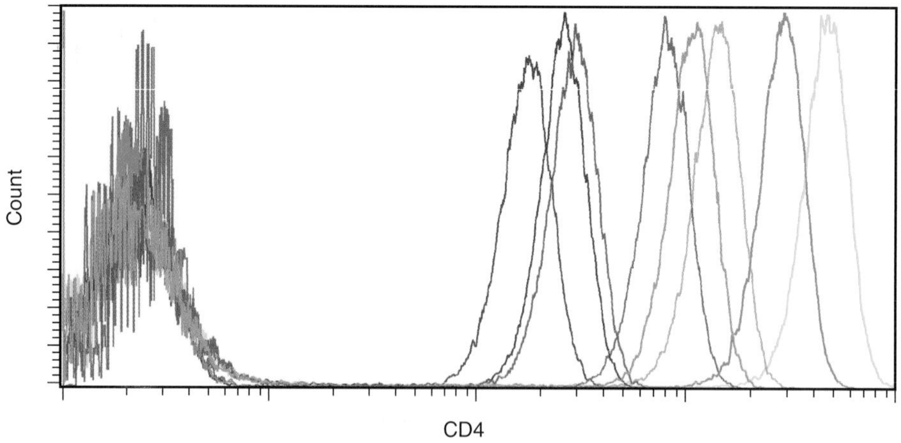

Figure 34-3 Comparison of fluorochrome emission intensity. Fluorochromes are characterized by differences in relative intensity of emission that are important to take into account to achieve optimal sensitivity. The relative fluorescence intensity for CD4 expression on lymphocytes is pictured for fluorescein (FITC) *(blue),* phycoerythrin (PE) *(green),* PE-Texas-Red *(orange),* PE-Cy5 *(yellow),* PerCP-Cy5.5 *(red),* PE-Cy7 *(light blue),* allophycocyanin (APC) *(magenta),* and APC-Cy7 *(purple).* The actual intensities observed are dependent on the clone of antibody used, the ratio of fluorochrome to protein in the antibody conjugate, the method of specimen preparation used, the instrument performance characteristics, and the method of instrument setup.

level of background nonspecific binding. For high-specificity antibodies used for cell surface labeling, one should be able to achieve saturation, a consistent intensity on positive populations at higher antibody concentrations, without significant increases in background on negative populations. The inability to do so indicates a poor-quality antibody. For intracellular labeling, saturation typically is not achieved because of relatively high levels of nonspecific antibody binding by intracellular constituents, generally a linear function of antibody concentration, and optimization of signal-to-noise by titering becomes critical for adequate reagent performance.

PANEL DESIGN

The pairing of reagents with appropriate fluorochromes is a key factor in ensuring appropriate signal intensity and detection sensitivity. The following four steps can aid in the construction of appropriate reagent panels:

1. Determine the purpose for each potential combination of reagents. Each reagent combination should have a clearly defined objective or should not be further pursued.
2. Select a group of cellular targets. The selected group of targets or antigens should be able to successfully address the purpose of the reagent combination and should be relatively independent of fluorochrome or availability of commercial conjugates. The reagent combination should be the minimum needed to answer the question being asked. Antibodies are commonly combined in a variety of ways for use in the identification of abnormal hematopoietic populations, but these generally fall into one of the categories outlined in Table 34-1.
3. Assign a fluorochrome to each target. The basic principle is that highly expressed antigens should be coupled with dim fluorochromes, and dimly expressed antigens should be coupled with bright fluorochromes. This principle provides reasonable signal intensities and avoids compensation problems due to excessively bright fluorescence. Commercial availability often limits the choice of fluorochromes, although most companies offer custom conjugation services that can provide reagents that might be better suited to a particular purpose than those more generally available.

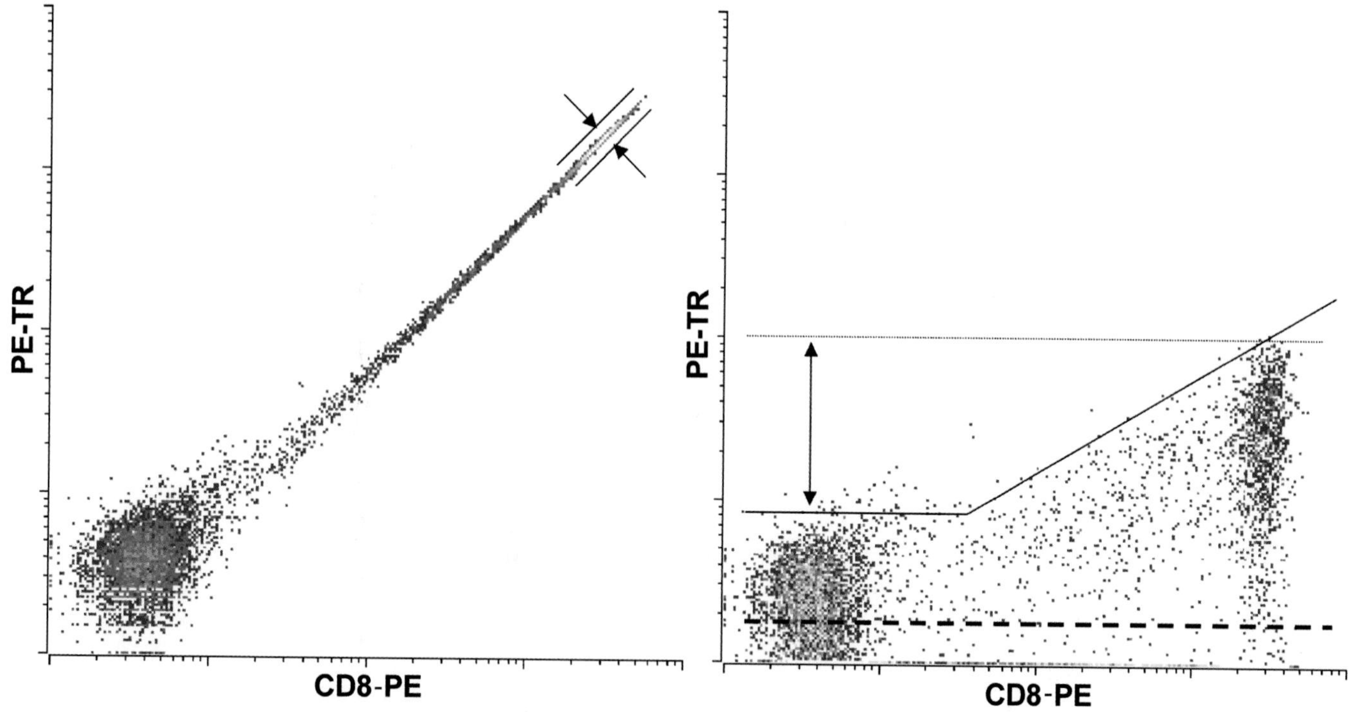

Figure 34-4 Compensation. The fluorescence emission of lymphocytes labeled with CD8-PE appears in both PE and PE-Texas Red detectors as the result of emission of PE in both regions of the spectrum examined by these detectors. Note that no PE-Texas Red conjugated antibody is used in this experiment. Without compensation applied *(left),* cells expressing abundant CD8 show bright signals for both PE and PE-Texas Red with a width to the population *(arrows)* due to measurement errors inherent in the method. Once compensation is correctly applied *(right),* the centers of the positive and negative populations have the same low level of PE-Texas Red emission *(dotted line),* with many events lying on the horizontal axis. However, the PE-positive population shows a much broader degree of apparent PE-Texas Red background fluorescence than the PE-negative population *(solid line and arrow).* If a PE-Texas Red conjugated antibody had been used, CD8-positive cells might have been erroneously interpreted as doubly positive, but this apparent "positivity" is a direct result of measurement errors and logarithmic data display. The practical result is that the sensitivity for the detection of low-level PE-Texas Red is compromised in the presence of bright PE fluorescence.

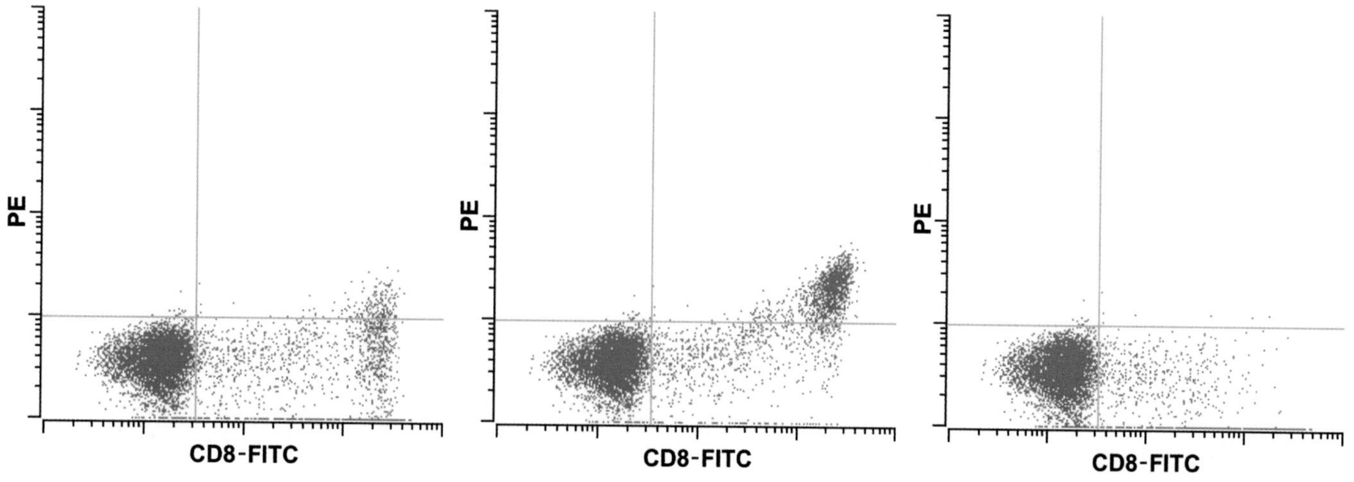

Figure 34-5 Inappropriate compensation. The fluorescence emission of lymphocytes singly labeled with CD8-FITC shows minimal apparent PE fluorescence when 8% of the FITC signal is subtracted from the PE signal (i.e., appropriate compensation) *(left).* If the degree of compensation is decreased to 7.2% *(center),* the CD8-positive population appears to express low PE and could be misinterpreted as immunophenotypic aberrancy, depending on the PE antibody included. Note the lack of symmetry and the pointed end of the positive population as a clue to the inaccurate compensation. If the compensation is increased to 8.8%, the positive population is compressed on the *x*-axis and appears not to exist.

4. Test reagent combinations. The reagent combination must be empirically tested to ensure that signal intensities are as expected, that low-level sensitivity is appropriate where important, and that unexpected interactions between reagents do not occur. A sample prepared with all reagents of interest should be compared with the same sample prepared with a series of preparations, each lacking one of the component reagents (fluorescence-minus-one controls), as well as with a second series containing each single reagent independently (single-stained controls). Unexpected changes in intensity of one or more reagents indicate potential problems with the reagent combination.

SPECIMEN HANDLING AND SAMPLE PREPARATION

Any specimen from which a single cell suspension can be generated is suitable for flow cytometric immunophenotyping, including peripheral blood, bone marrow, and lymph node, to name a few. Blood and bone marrow may be anticoagulated with ethylenediaminetetraacetic acid, heparin, or acid citrate dextrose, with heparin generally preferred because of improved stability with specimen age. Tissue specimens are best transported and stored in tissue culture media, such as RPMI 1640, and a single cell suspension is generated by mechanical dissociation using scalpel and

TABLE 34-1
Reagent Panel Design Strategies for the Detection of Hematopoietic Neoplasms

Principle	Example implementation
At least one reagent for population identification	CD45 for general cell type Lineage-associated antigen for specific cell lineage (e.g., CD19 for B cells)
Multiple antigens of same lineage and maturational stage to identify inappropriate expression levels	Use of CD2, CD3, CD4, CD5, CD7, or CD8 simultaneously to evaluate mature T cells
Multiple antigens of same lineage but different maturational stages to identify normal maturation and asynchronous expression	Use of CD13 and CD16 simultaneously to demonstrate neutrophilic maturation
Separation of different cell lineages	Use of CD11b and CD15 simultaneously to separate monocytic and neutrophilic maturation
Demonstration of clonality	Use of κ and λ in combination with a B cell lineage reagent (e.g., CD19)
Identification of frankly aberrant antigen expression	Use of T or NK cell–associated antigens such as CD7 or CD56 in combination with CD34

NK, Natural killer.

forceps, needle and syringe, or wire screen mesh (Braylan, 1989), followed by filtration through fine-gauge wire mesh to remove aggregates. Specimens of all types are commonly stored at room temperature before preparation, although refrigeration will retard degradation when preparation must be delayed.

Analysis of white blood cells in peripheral blood or bone marrow requires erythrocyte removal for efficient evaluation. Density-gradient centrifugation (e.g., ficoll-hypaque) was historically used for this purpose, but it leads to selective loss of cellular subpopulations and gives relatively poor recovery on bone marrow specimens. Erythrocyte lysis using ammonium chloride or a variety of commercial preparations has become the standard technique for sample preparation in clinical laboratories (Carter, 1992). Currently recommended methods involve the addition of antibodies to an aliquot of blood or marrow, followed by erythrocyte lysis and washing with a buffered salt solution such as phosphate buffered saline to remove cell debris, the lysing reagent, and unbound antibody. Inclusion of a small amount of formaldehyde (0.25%–0.5%) with the lysing reagent or following washing is a convenient way to stabilize both antibody binding and specimen stability. When analysis of light chain expression on B cells is required, plasma immunoglobulin (Ig) must be removed by repeated washing before antibody addition. Once prepared, samples should be acquired on the instrument as soon as reasonably possible to avoid sample and fluorochrome degradation, although fixation and refrigerated storage will delay degradation.

DATA ACQUISITION

As the prepared sample is evaluated on the flow cytometer, it is important to collect enough events to allow detection of the population of interest. For populations that represent a large percentage of the total, relatively few events need to be acquired, but infrequent populations require the acquisition of larger numbers of events. Because in the evaluation of hematopoietic neoplasms, one rarely knows what the likely population frequency will be for a given sample, it is most convenient to acquire a fixed number of total events that ensures the desired minimum level of sensitivity. For example, if a sensitivity of 0.1% is desired and 50 events are determined to be adequate for confident population identification, then 50,000 total white blood cell events will need to be acquired. The acquisition of fewer events will compromise the ability to detect low-frequency populations—an important consideration when evaluating for residual disease following therapy and in situations where the acquisition of a larger number of events is often desirable.

Instrument carryover between samples becomes a significant concern when evaluating for the presence of small abnormal populations. Most commercial instruments have a manufacturer's specification for carryover of roughly 1%—a relatively high level when one is looking for infrequent populations. To minimize carryover, a small amount of water should be run between each aliquot of sample acquired until background returns to an acceptably low level. Failure to do so will result in the sporadic appearance of populations having unexpected immunophenotypes that can be mistaken for neoplastic disease.

INTERPRETIVE CONSIDERATIONS

The identification of hematopoietic neoplasia by immunophenotyping relies on the principle that neoplastic cells express patterns of antigen expression that are distinctly different from those of their normal counterparts. Antigen expression in normal cells is a tightly regulated process, resulting in a characteristic pattern of antigen acquisition and loss with maturation that is cell lineage specific. Neoplastic cells commonly show nonrandom alterations in antigen expression that include the following:

1. Gain of antigens not normally expressed by cell type or lineage.
2. Abnormally increased or decreased levels of expression (intensities) of antigens normally expressed by cell type or lineage, including the complete loss of normal antigens in some instances.
3. Asynchronous antigen expression (i.e., expression of antigens normally expressed by cell type or lineage), but at an inappropriate time during maturation.
4. Abnormally homogeneous expression of one or more antigens by a population that normally exhibits more heterogeneous expression.

The consequence is that the immunophenotypic identification of hematopoietic neoplasia rests on a thorough knowledge of the normal patterns of antigens expressed by hematopoietic cells.

NORMAL PATTERNS OF ANTIGEN EXPRESSION

All hematopoietic cells arise from the hematopoietic stem cell, a quiescent cell population that possesses long-term regenerative potential and is present at a low frequency in the bone marrow. The stem cell population in humans can be identified if a sufficient number of cells are evaluated and show expression of bright CD34 and CD133, intermediate CD45, dim to absent CD38, variable CD90, and dim CD123, CD117, HLA-DR, CD13, and CD33. Maturation toward lineage-committed progenitors is accompanied by a slight decrease in CD34 and CD45, loss of CD133 and CD90, and an increase in CD38 and HLA-DR. Further maturation along each lineage occurs in the bone marrow until mature, functional, albeit naive progeny are released into the peripheral blood. The one exception is T cells, whose earliest precursors migrate to the thymus, where maturation to functional forms occurs. The patterns of antigenic change with maturation for B cell, T cell, neutrophilic, monocytic, and erythroid lineages have been elucidated by multiple investigators (Loken, 1987, 1988; Inghirami, 1990; Terstappen, 1990a; Terstappen, 1990b; Terstappen, 1990c; Terstappen, 1992b; Harada, 1993; Hoffkes, 1996; Ginaldi, 1996b; Almasri, 1998; Lucio, 1999; McClanahan, 1999; Wood, 2004), and a summary of each lineage is presented in Figures 34-6 through 34-10, respectively.

ABNORMAL PATTERNS OF ANTIGENIC EXPRESSION IN HEMATOPOIETIC NEOPLASIA

Most hematopoietic neoplasms have abnormal immunophenotypes that are characteristic enough to allow their detection, even at relatively low levels of involvement. In some cases, the immunophenotype is characteristic enough to allow classification using immunophenotypic data alone. However, each group has sufficient variability that correct diagnosis relies on recognition of the overall immunophenotypic pattern, and not on the expression of individual antigens or the rigid application of immunophenotypic profiles. The following discussion emphasizes general immunophenotypic principles useful for the diagnosis and classification of hematopoietic neoplasia, as a complete discussion of the antigenic abnormalities seen in each subtype of disease is beyond the scope of this chapter (Craig, 2008).

Acute Leukemia

Diagnosis and Classification

The diagnosis of acute leukemia relies on enumeration of the percentage of blasts in the peripheral blood or bone marrow; the current criterion in

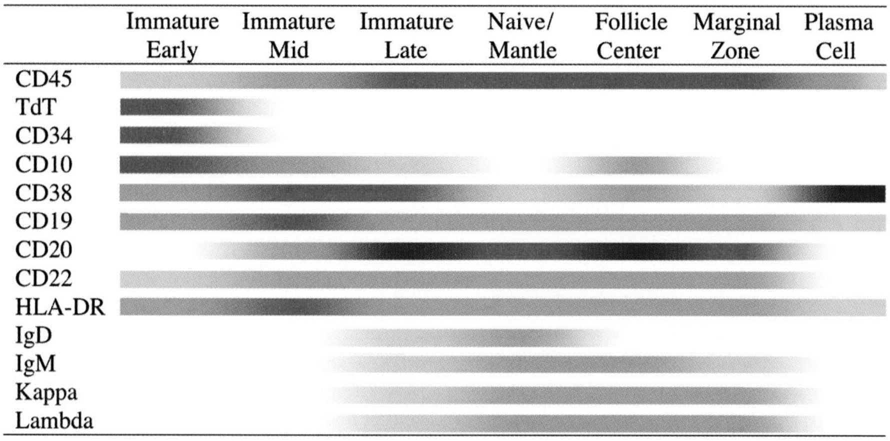

Figure 34-6 B cell differentiation. The intensity of antigen expression throughout B cell maturation is depicted for antigens commonly used in the clinical laboratory. Normal mature B cells express κ or λ light chains, never both. Darker colors represent higher levels of antigen expression.

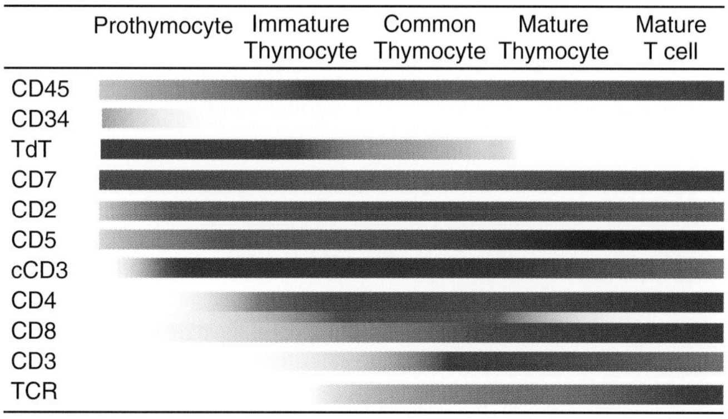

Figure 34-7 T cell differentiation. The intensity of antigen expression throughout T cell maturation is depicted for antigens commonly used in the clinical laboratory. T cell maturation occurs largely in the thymus, and most maturational stages will not be seen outside of that organ. At the common thymocyte stage, immature T cells express both CD4 and CD8, with subsequent stages showing expression of one or the other, but not both. Darker colors represent higher levels of antigen expression.

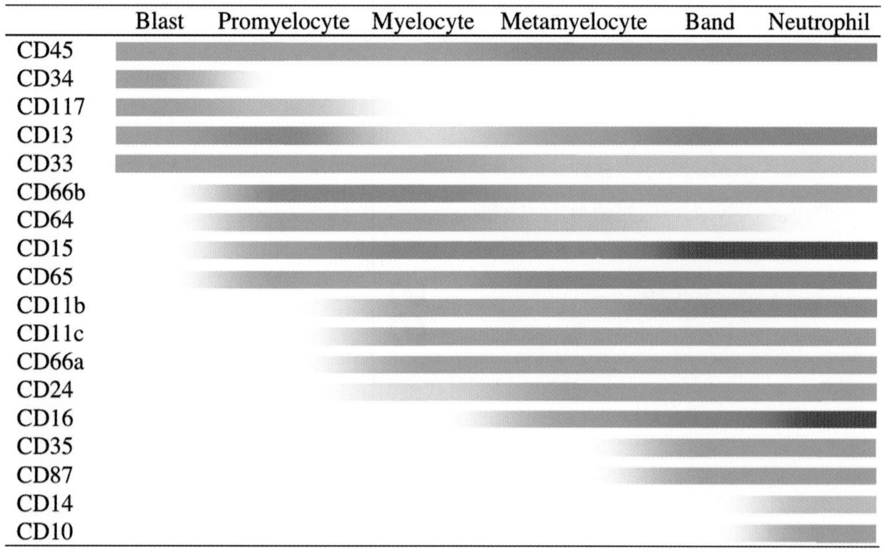

Figure 34-8 Neutrophil differentiation. The intensity of antigen expression throughout neutrophil maturation is depicted for antigens commonly used in the clinical laboratory. Darker colors represent higher levels of antigen expression.

the WHO classification for the diagnosis of acute leukemia is greater than 20% blasts (Swerdlow, 2008). In flow cytometry, identification of blasts relies on the demonstration of expression of immature antigens by a population having appropriate CD45 expression and light scatter characteristics. Although it is the overall immunophenotype that allows identification of blasts, antigens commonly used for blast identification include CD34, CD117, CD133, and terminal deoxynucleotidyl transferase (TdT). White blood cells express CD45 at distinct levels of intensity characteristic of both lineage and stage of differentiation that when used in conjunction with orthogonal light scatter (side scatter) allow delineation of the basic white blood cell populations (Borowitz, 1993; Stelzer, 1993) (Fig. 34-11). This technique is particularly useful for the identification of blasts, given their expression of intermediate CD45 and low side scatter; CD45 versus side scatter analysis has become standard practice in the clinical laboratory for this purpose.

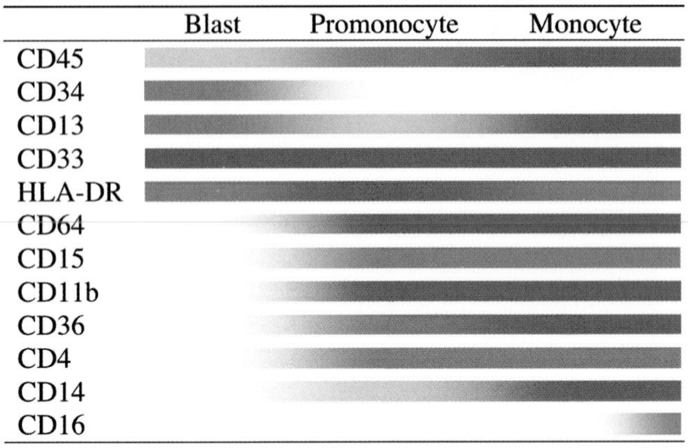

Figure 34-9 Monocyte differentiation. The intensity of antigen expression throughout monocyte maturation is depicted for antigens commonly used in the clinical laboratory. Darker colors represent higher levels of antigen expression.

Although flow cytometry is excellent at identifying and enumerating blasts, two issues suggest caution in utilizing flow cytometric blast percentages for making an initial diagnosis of acute leukemia. First, the blast percentage obtained from bone marrow specimens is often inaccurate because of a combination of peripheral blood dilution (artifactual decrease) and compromise of nucleated erythroid precursors during specimen processing using lysing reagents (artifactual increase). Second, blasts identified by immunophenotyping do not always directly correspond to blasts as identified by morphology. This is true because leukemic populations, similar to normal populations, consist of a maturational continuum, and there is not perfect concordance between specific antigenic changes and the arbitrary morphologic changes that distinguish blasts from more differentiated cells. Moreover, in some types of leukemia, early neutrophilic (promyelocytes) and monocytic (promonocytes) precursors are intentionally included in morphologic blast counts. Nevertheless, if one pays attention to these limitations, the diagnosis of acute leukemia can generally be correctly suggested.

Although in most cases of acute leukemia the diagnosis (i.e., recognition of the presence of 20% blasts) is made by morphology, flow cytometry can be extremely useful in excluding a diagnosis of acute leukemia when the marrow is populated by cells that may mimic acute leukemia. A common situation in which this can occur is the presence of increased normal B cell precursors that may resemble primitive lymphoblasts morphologically, especially in suboptimal specimens. Although these cells superficially resemble leukemic precursor-B lymphoblasts immunophenotypically, multiparameter flow cytometry can readily distinguish these normal immature precursors (hematogones) from acute leukemia (Lucio,

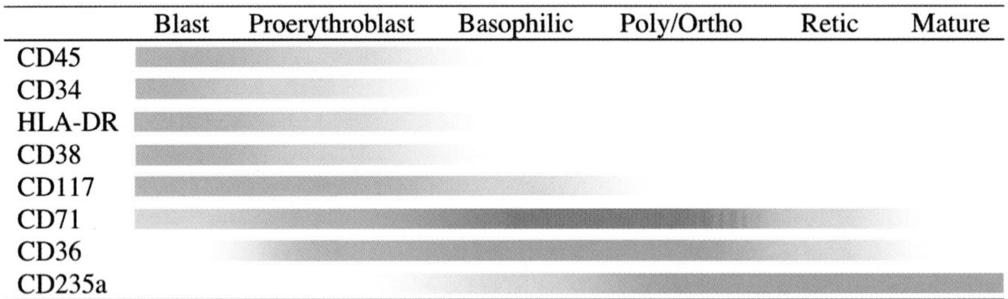

Figure 34-10 Erythroid differentiation. The intensity of antigen expression throughout erythrocyte maturation is depicted for antigens commonly used in the clinical laboratory. Darker colors represent higher levels of antigen expression.

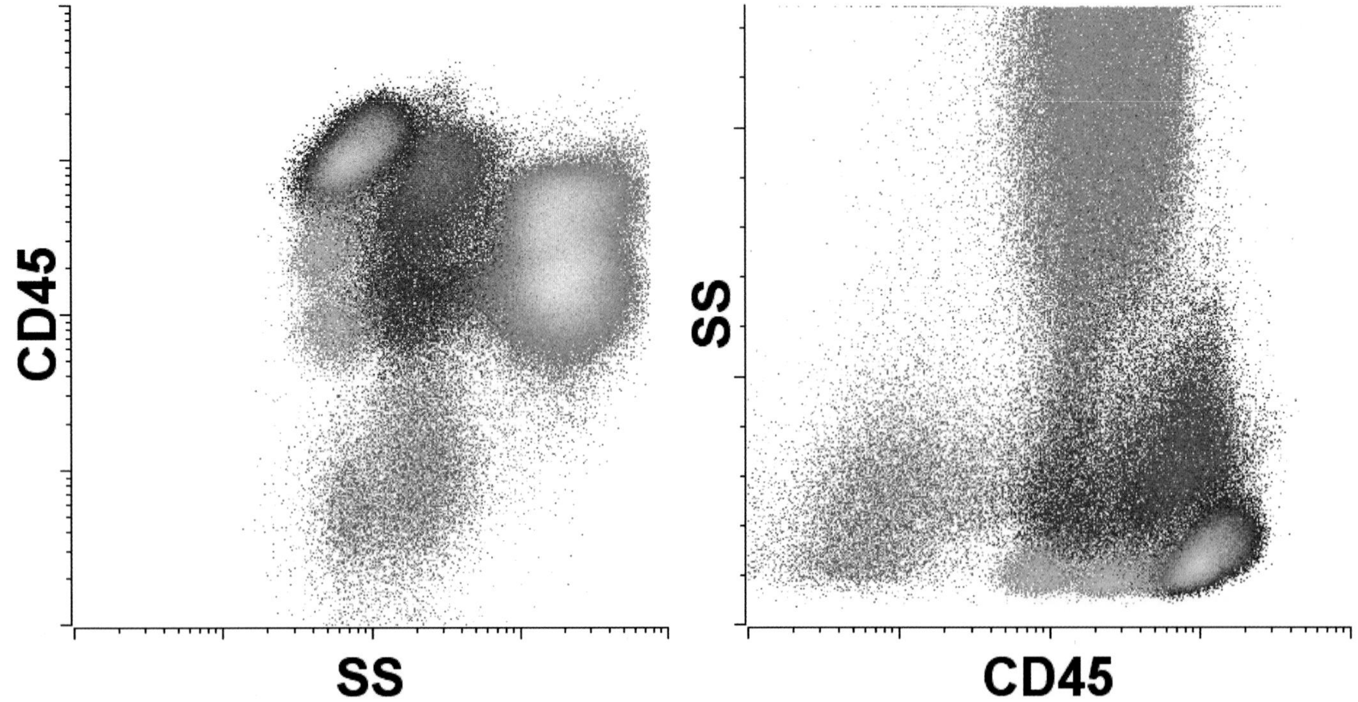

Figure 34-11 CD45 versus side scatter. The display of CD45 versus side scatter is increasingly used in the clinical laboratory as a starting point for the identification of white blood cell populations. Data are commonly displayed with side scatter on a logarithmic *(left)* or linear *(right)* scale. Major white cell populations colored are lymphocytes *(blue)*, B cells *(light blue)*, monocytes *(purple)*, maturing neutrophils *(green)*, blasts *(red)*, basophils *(dark purple)*, and maturing erythrocytes *(orange)*.

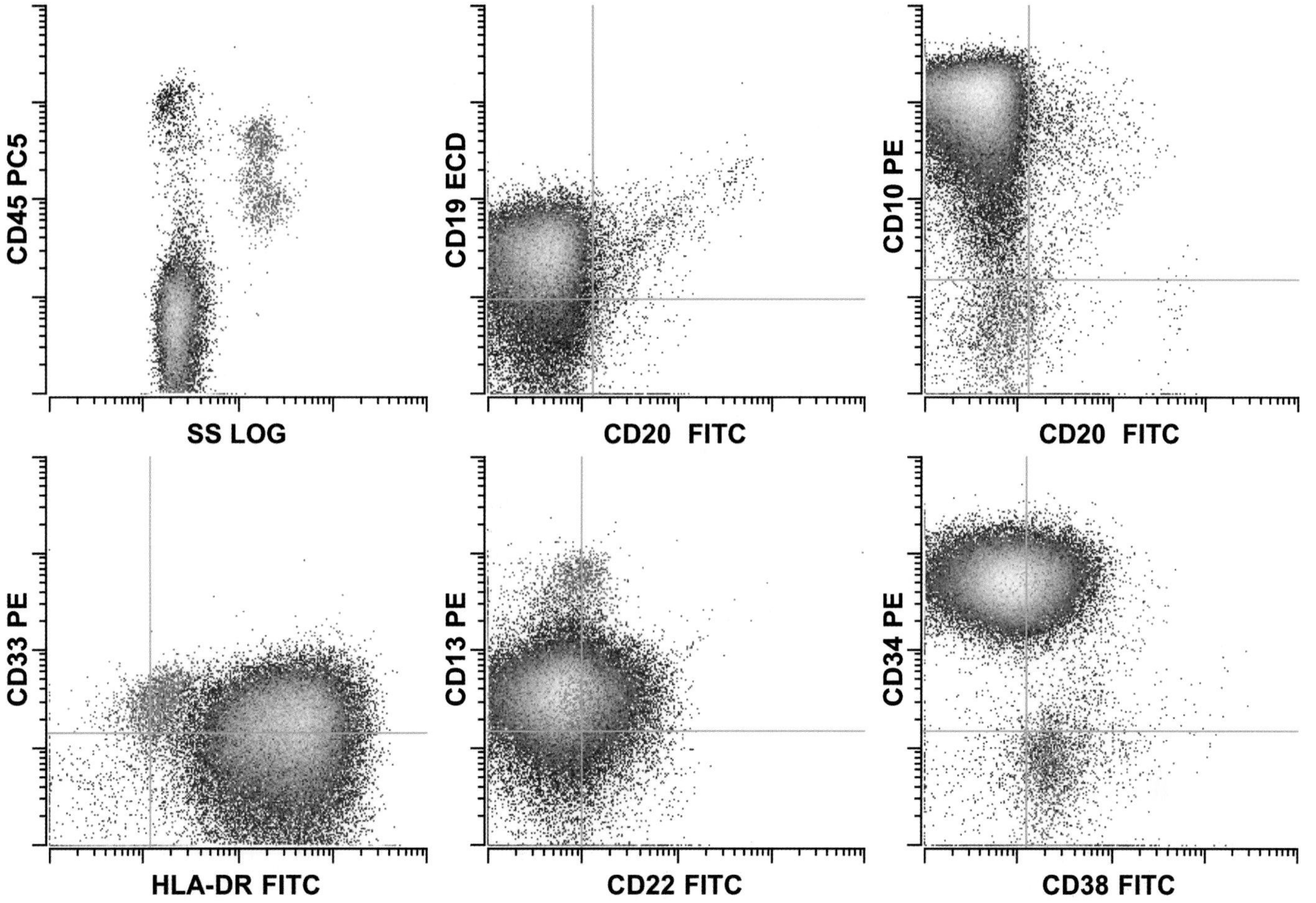

Figure 34-12 Precursor B cell lymphoblastic leukemia/lymphoma (acute lymphoblastic leukemia). The neoplastic cell population *(red)* in comparison with normal immature B cells shows abnormal expression of B cell–associated antigens CD19 (dim), CD22 (very dim), and CD10 (bright), along with aberrant expression of CD45 (absent), CD34 (bright), and CD38 (dim). In addition, the low-level expression of myeloid-associated antigens CD13 and CD33 is seen—a feature frequently seen in this disorder and not suggesting myeloid differentiation by itself. The cells have low side scatter, as is typical of lymphoid blasts.

1999; Weir, 1999; McKenna, 2001). Additionally, some nonhematolymphoid tumors such as small cell carcinoma or pediatric small round cell tumors can resemble leukemic blasts on smears but are readily distinguished from leukemic blasts by flow cytometry, where they appear as CD45-negative cells lacking specific markers of B cell, T cell, or myeloid lineage, often with higher side scatter than might be expected for a cell with so little cytoplasm (Chang, 2003).

The major role for flow cytometry in acute leukemia is classification. Classification is largely a matter of lineage assignment and correlation with normal maturational stage. The determination of lineage in particular is a decision of major therapeutic importance, with the primary distinction being whether the leukemia is of myeloid or lymphoid lineage. The immunophenotypic characteristics of acute myeloid leukemia (Terstappen, 1992a; Reading, 1993; Bradstock, 1994; Macedo, 1995a, 1995b; Weir, 2001; Orfao, 2004) and acute lymphoblastic leukemia (Farahat, 1995; Khalidi, 1998; Weir, 1999) and their similarities to normal populations have been well described in numerous publications. In general, it is the overall pattern of antigen expression rather than expression of any single antigen that allows determination of lineage. This is due in part to the lack of lineage specificity of many antigens commonly used for immunophenotyping. As a rule, the more closely an antigen is expressed at the level commonly seen in cells of that lineage, the more likely it accurately reflects lineage differentiation, for example, dim expression of the B cell antigen CD19 has relatively poor lineage specificity, as it may be seen in acute myeloid leukemia, but brighter and more uniform CD19 expression at the level seen on normal B cells is more typical of precursor B cell lymphoblastic leukemia. A subset of cytoplasmic antigens are the most lineage-restricted antigens currently known and are used to arbitrate lineage assignment in cases where the surface immunophenotype is unclear. Table 34-2 lists antigens commonly used for lineage assignment. In rare cases, the leukemic cells may show differentiation along more than one lineage (Hanson, 1993; Bene, 1995; Matutes, 1997), most commonly either myeloid and B cell or myeloid and T cell, as evidence of the stem cell nature of these forms of acute leukemia. If a single blast population shows such differentiation, it is commonly termed **biphenotypic acute leukemia;** if two abnormal blast populations are present, each having a distinct and different lineage, this is termed **bilineal acute leukemia.** Examples of immunophenotypic patterns seen in acute leukemia are provided in Figures 34-12 through 34-15.

TABLE 34-2
Antigens Used for Lineage Assignment in Acute Leukemia

	AML	ALL–B cell	ALL–T cell
Definitive	Cytoplasmic MPO	None	Cytoplasmic CD3 Surface CD3 T cell receptor
Strongly associated	CD117	Cytoplasmic CD79a Cytoplasmic CD22 CD19 CD10—bright	CD7—bright
Moderately associated	CD13 CD33	TdT—moderate to bright	CD5 CD2

ALL, Acute lymphoblastic leukemia; *AML,* acute myeloid leukemia. *MPO,* myeloperoxidase.

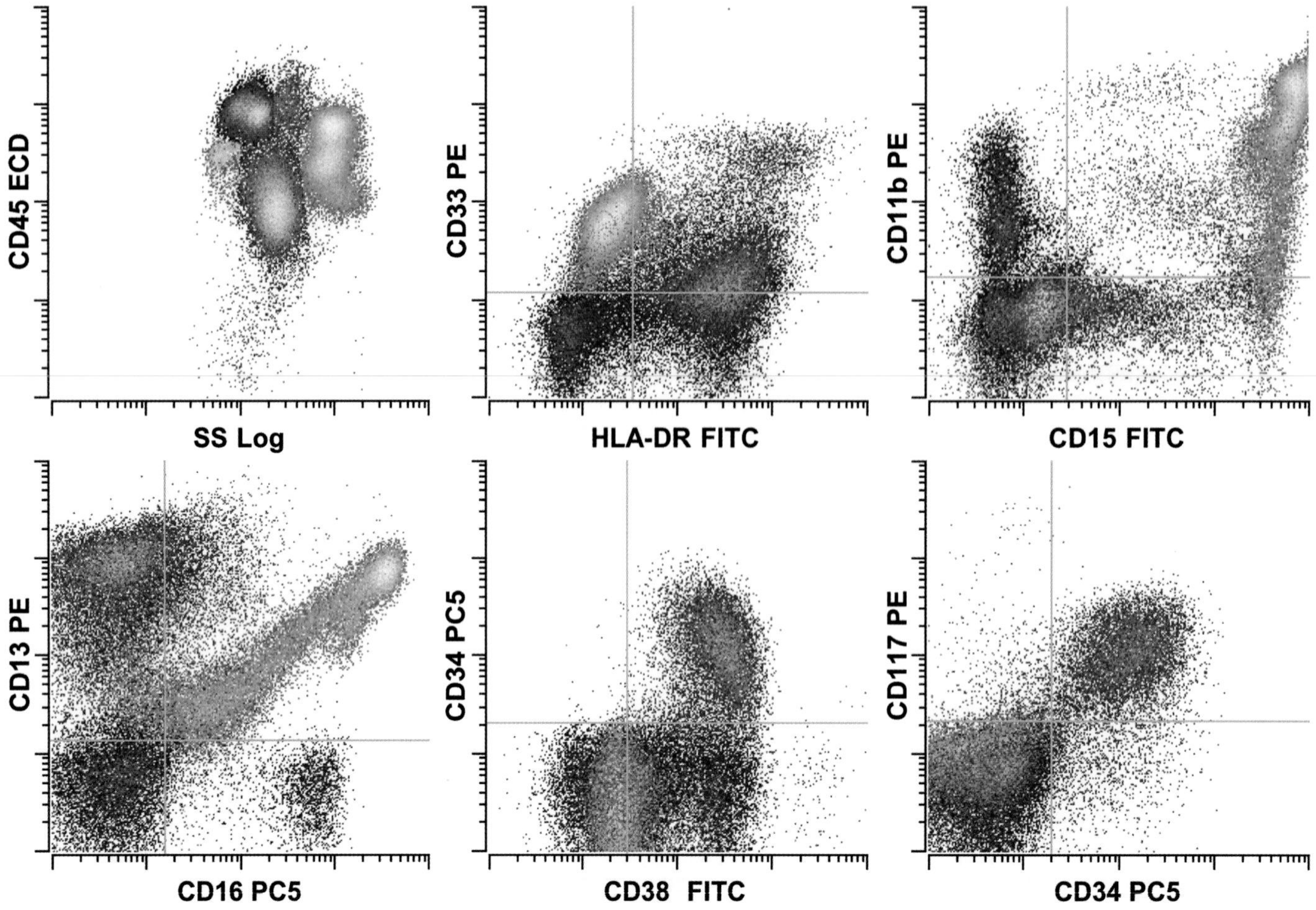

Figure 34-13 Acute myeloid leukemia with differentiation. The neoplastic cell population consists of blasts *(red)* showing abnormal expression of the myeloid-associated antigens CD33 (dim), CD13 (bright), and CD15 (dim partial) in association with immature antigens CD34 and CD117. The blasts do not express the more mature neutrophilic antigens CD11b and CD16, and are typical of the relatively immature forms seen in many cases of acute myeloid leukemia. Background maturing granulocytes are present *(green)* that are normal and are not part of the leukemic population.

Prognostic Factors

Although several reports have discussed the prognostic significance of particular surface markers in both acute lymphoid and myeloid leukemia (Schabath, 2003), for the most part, these have not stood the test of time, and they currently do not have a significant impact on therapy. One reason for this is that the presence of recurrent cytogenetic or molecular abnormalities in acute leukemia is now recognized as an important prognostic feature that has therapeutic implications; these are now an integral part of the WHO classification of acute leukemia. In many cases, the underlying cytogenetic abnormality is associated with characteristic immunophenotypic features that aid in suggesting an appropriate classification (Orfao, 1999; Hrusak, 2002); with few exceptions, once cytogenetic abnormalities are accounted for, immunophenotype is no longer prognostic. However, some markers, such as CD56 expression in acute myeloid leukemia (AML) with t(8;21) (Baer, 1997), have been associated with an adverse prognosis within that cytogenetically defined leukemia. A summary of phenotypic features associated with cytogenetic or molecular abnormalities is provided in Table 34-3.

Therapeutic Targets

In AML, the most commonly used therapeutic target is anti-CD33 (gemtuzumab ozogamicin). CD33 is expressed in the great majority of cases of AML, although its level of expression correlates with response to anti-CD33 therapy (Walter, 2007). Relatively little is known about the role of monitoring changes in CD33 expression. In acute lymphoblastic leukemia (ALL), to date few studies have used targeted monoclonal antibodies, although anti-CD22 (epratuzamab) and CD52 (alemtuzamab) are now used in some clinical trials (Raetz, 2008). The near ubiquitous expression of CD22 in B precursor ALL limits the role of flow cytometry in determining eligibility for such trials.

TABLE 34-3
Association of Immunophenotype with Cytogenetic Abnormalities in Acute Leukemia

	Immunophenotype
Acute Myeloid Leukemia	
t(15;17)	HLA-DR negative, CD15 low to absent, CD33 bright, CD34 low to absent
t(8;21)	CD34 bright, CD56 positive, CD19 dim, TdT positive, CD15 positive
Acute Lymphoblastic Leukemia	
t(12;21) (by FISH)	CD10 positive, CD20 low to negative, CD9 low to negative
MLL (e.g., t[4;11])	CD10 negative, CD15 positive

MLL, Mixed lineage leukemia.

Residual Disease Monitoring in Acute Leukemia

Many of the large number of antibodies that can be used to help classify acute leukemia are not, in and of themselves, essential for determination of lineage. However, a larger panel of antibodies, properly selected, can be very useful in identifying specific differences between the leukemic population and background normal elements, thereby enhancing the ability to use flow cytometry to detect small abnormal populations. Thus, the purpose of flow cytometric immunophenotyping in acute leukemia at diagnosis goes beyond simple assignment of lineage and extends to the description of a "leukemia-associated immunophenotype" characteristic of

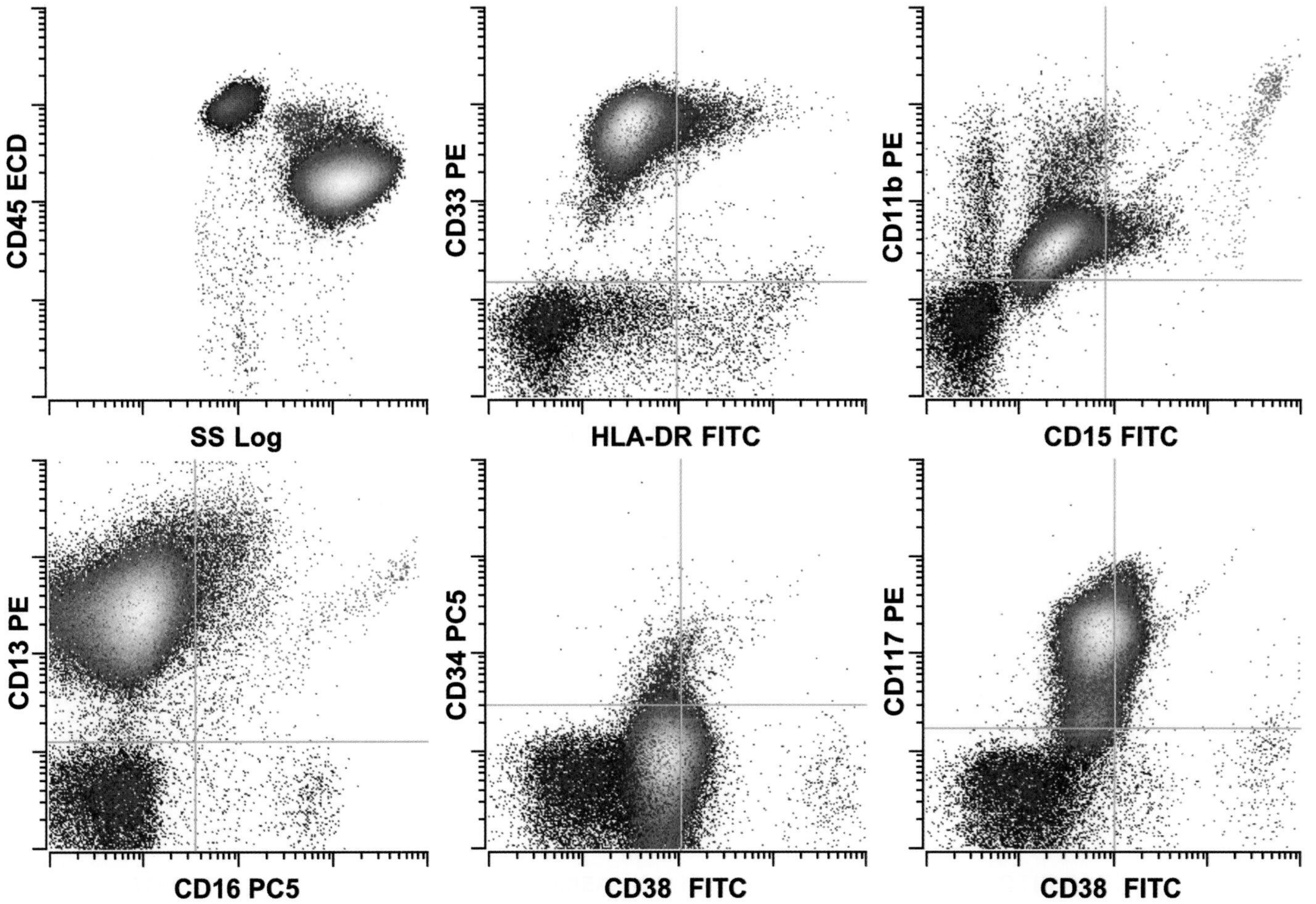

Figure 34-14 Acute promyelocytic leukemia. The neoplastic cell population consists of promyelocytes *(red)* showing abnormal expression of the myeloid-associated antigens CD33 (bright) and CD13 (intermediate), with high side scatter indicating abundant cytoplasmic granularity. The population lacks expression of CD34 and HLA-DR, antigens commonly present on true myeloid blasts, and retains expression of CD117, as is seen on a subset of normal promyelocytes. However, in contrast to normal promyelocytes, abnormal cells lack significant expression of CD15, a characteristic and common abnormality in this disorder.

that leukemia, knowledge of which is useful in assessing follow-up samples (Campana, 2003). An important caveat is that immunophenotypic changes between diagnostic samples and persistent or recurrent disease are frequently observed in both ALL (Borowitz, 2005; Galpa 2008) and AML (Baer, 2001; Voskova, 2004). Accordingly, it is necessary that one monitor more than one antigenic pattern and not expect exactly the same immunophenotype seen at diagnosis to persist after therapy. Examples of particularly informative combinations useful for detecting aberrant expression of antigens in minimal residual disease are shown in Table 34-4. The detection of minimal residual disease in acute leukemia has been demonstrated to be correlated with risk of relapse and overall survival for both AML (San Miguel, 2001; Feller, 2004; Maurillo, 2008) and ALL (Coustan-Smith, 2000; Dworzak, 2002; Borowitz, 2008), and is increasingly used to guide therapeutic decision-making. An example of minimal residual disease detection in ALL is shown in Figure 34-16.

TABLE 34-4

Four-Color Antibody Combinations Useful for Minimal Residual Disease Detection

Acute myeloid leukemia	Acute lymphoblastic leukemia–B cell
CD34/CD33/HLA-DR/CD45	CD20/CD10/CD19/CD45
CD34/CD117/CD33/CD45	CD9/CD34/CD19/CD45
CD115/CD117/CD33/CD34	CD58/CD10/CD38/CD19
CD15/CD13/CD33/CD34	CD38/CD10/CD34/CD19
HLA-DR/CD117/CD33/CD34	CD20/CD10/CD19/CD34
Chronic lymphocytic leukemia	**Acute lymphoblastic leukemia–T cell**
CD20/CD79a/CD19/CD5	TdT/CD5/CD3/CD7

Antibody combinations from Weir (1999), Rawstron (2001), and Vidriales (2003).

Lymphoma

Diagnosis and Classification

As with leukemia, flow cytometry can contribute both to the diagnosis and to the classification of lymphoma. The immunophenotypic diagnosis of lymphoma relies on the identification of an expanded population of abnormal mature lymphocytes. By far and away, the most common way in which such an expansion is assessed by flow cytometry is through the demonstration of light chain restriction in B cell proliferations. As with all neoplastic cells, neoplastic lymphocytes arise from a single precursor that undergoes clonal expansion. However, unlike most cells, each lymphocyte normally expresses one of a series of polymorphic molecules on its surface that provides a unique identity; in the case of B cells, this identifying molecule is Ig. Because individual Ig molecules contain one of two forms of light chain—κ or λ—reagents directed against light chains can be used as markers of clonality for B cells (Braylan, 1993; Geary, 1993; Fukushima, 1996).

In the case of T cell proliferations, the T cell receptor genetic locus is more complex, but a larger series of reagents directed against the β-chain families of the T cell receptor can be used to demonstrate clonality for T cells (Lima, 2001; Morice, 2004). The use of reagents directed against killer-inhibitory receptors (KIR antigens) has even been suggested to allow demonstration of natural killer cell clonality (Morice, 2003). The assumption behind all of these assays is that clonality equates with malignancy.

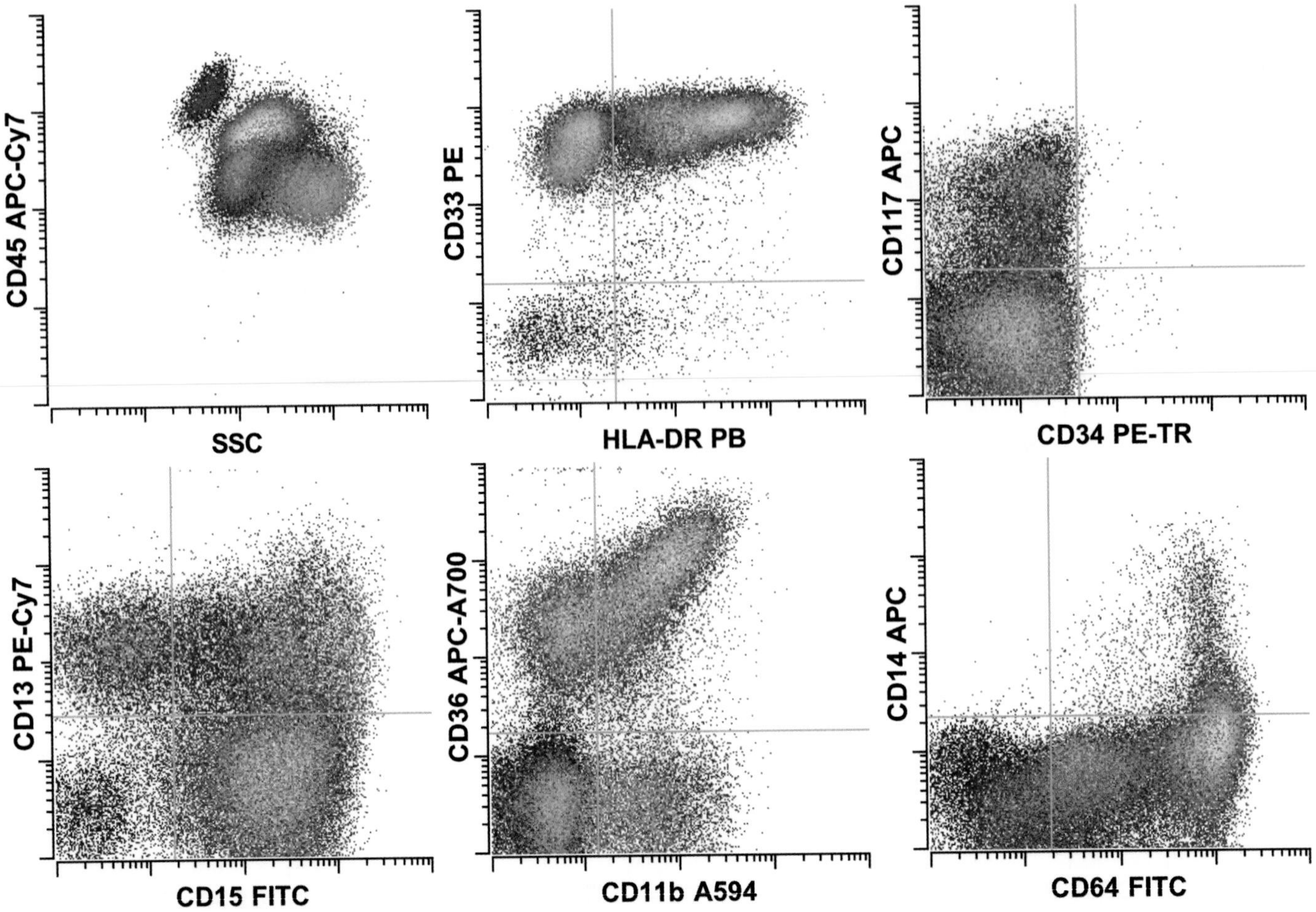

Figure 34-15 Acute myelomonocytic leukemia. The neoplastic cells consist of a relatively small population of blasts *(red)* with a larger population of cells showing monocytic differentiation *(violet)*. The blasts show abnormal expression of CD33 (bright), CD13 (intermediate), HLA-DR (intermediate), and CD117 (intermediate) without CD34. The monocytic differentiation is reflected in the acquisition of early monocyte antigens CD64 (bright) and CD36 (intermediate to bright), along with other more mature myelomonocytic antigens CD15 (intermediate) and CD11b (low to intermediate), without significant acquisition of the mature monocyte antigen CD14 (absent) or marked gain in the expression of CD45, as is seen in mature monocytes. This finding suggests differentiation to the promonocyte stage, a population usually included in morphologic blast counts. In addition, a lesser degree of neutrophilic differentiation *(green)* is present.

Although clonality is a necessary consequence of neoplasia, clonal expansion is also a normal and necessary component of the immune response following antigenic stimulation, so the demonstration of clonality by itself is not entirely sufficient for the diagnosis of lymphoma.

It is increasingly recognized that a subset of otherwise normal individuals may contain small clonal populations of lymphocytes, best documented in the case of B cells (Rawstron, 2002; Chen, 2004; Kussick, 2004). It is not clear whether these clonal populations represent an early subclinical stage of disease, a precursor population without the full complement of genetic abnormalities required for neoplasia, or an incidental finding of no clinical consequence. Nevertheless, the term **monoclonal B cell lymphocytosis** has been adopted to describe such small populations in the peripheral blood, and numeric criteria have been suggested to allow their distinction from true neoplasia (Shanafelt, 2009). Consequently, it is necessary that flow cytometric findings suggesting lymphoma be put in a morphologic and clinical context before a definitive diagnosis of lymphoma is made.

In addition to light chain restriction, or restricted T-cell receptor β-chain usage, lymphomas, like leukemias, show alterations in antigen expression that deviate from normal maturation. In many cases, these alterations also provide evidence of neoplasia. Moreover, specific alterations are seen in specific types of lymphoma, thereby permitting classification as well as diagnosis in many cases, for example, increased expression of the T cell–associated antigen CD5 in CLL or mantle cell lymphoma (Matutes, 1994b; Tworek, 1998). Alteration in the intensity of Ig expression is also a common abnormality in B cell lymphoma and can be useful even when Ig expression is entirely absent (Li, 2002). Similarly, T cell lymphoma often shows alterations in the expression of one or more T cell antigens (Picker, 1987; Ginaldi, 1996a). However, special care must be taken in interpreting small populations of phenotypically abnormal T cells, especially in unusual sites, because a large number of reactive conditions can be associated with expansions of populations that are not commonly seen in normal blood or lymph nodes (McClanahan, 1999).

An even more powerful method to diagnose lymphoma is to combine the detection of clonality with the ability to identify alterations in antigen intensity through multicolor flow cytometry. For instance, coupling the identification of follicle center B cells using CD19 and CD10 with the detection of κ and λ light chains in a four-color analysis allows one to identify the presence of light chain restriction specifically within the follicle center B cell population, greatly increasing both the specificity and the sensitivity of the analysis. Examples of immunophenotypic patterns seen in lymphoma are provided in Figures 34-17 through 34-21. One important limitation of this type of analysis is that neoplasms containing relatively rare, large abnormal cells (e.g., Hodgkin lymphoma) may be difficult to recognize unless an appropriate antibody combination is used and a sufficiently large number of events are acquired (Fromm, 2009). In this regard, the approach is essentially similar to minimal residual disease detection. An example of the flow cytometric detection of classical Hodgkin lymphoma is shown in Figure 34-22.

The classification of lymphoma relies on the recognition of specific patterns of antigenic expression that are similar to some normal maturational stage, yet deviate sufficiently to allow identification of the abnormal population. Among B cell lymphoma, there are two entities that can be both diagnosed and classified with a high degree of confidence based on immunophenotypic data alone: chronic lymphocytic leukemia/small lymphocytic lymphoma (CLL/SLL) and hairy cell leukemia. CLL/SLL is

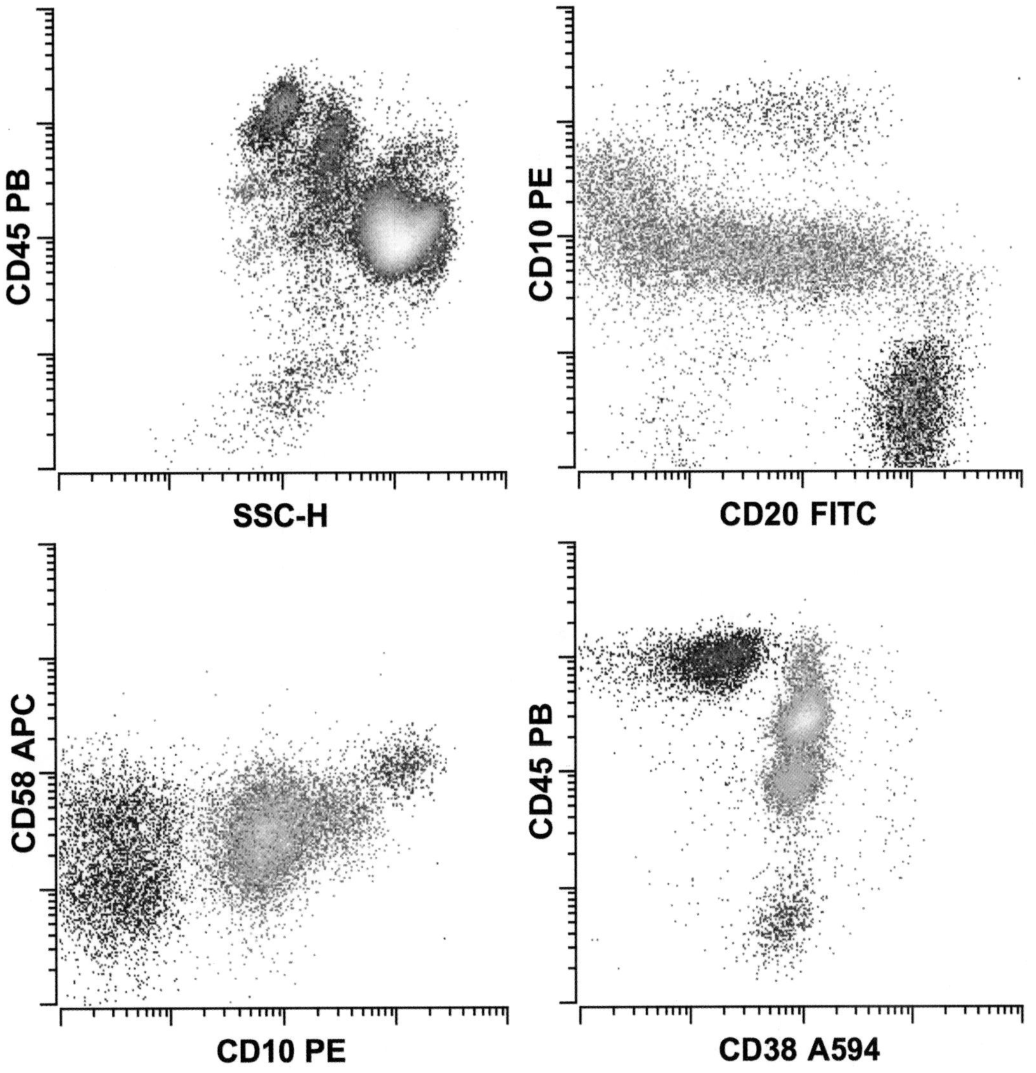

Figure 34-16 Minimal residual disease detection. An abnormal population of immature B cells is identified *(red)* that have abnormally increased expression of CD10 and CD58, abnormally decreased expression of CD45, and normal expression of CD20 and CD38. This composite immunophenotype is different from normal immature B cells *(cyan)* or mature B cells *(dark blue),* allowing its discrete identification at a level of 0.1% of white cells.

characterized by the coexpression of CD5 by abnormal B cells, decreased intensity of clonal light chain expression, decreased expression of a variety of mature B cell antigens, including CD20, CD22, and CD79b, and presence of the activation antigen CD23 without significant FMC7, an activation epitope of CD20 (Serke, 2001) (see Fig. 34-17). This constellation of immunophenotypic findings is diagnostic for CLL/SLL (Matutes, 1994b; Tworek, 1998). The only other B cell neoplasm that consistently expresses CD5 is mantle cell lymphoma, a more aggressive lymphoma that is important to distinguish from CLL/SLL. In contrast to CLL/SLL, mantle cell lymphoma shows relatively bright expression of mature B cell antigens such as CD20 and CD79b, expresses clonal Ig at a relatively normal to high level, and expresses FMC7 without significant CD23 (see Fig. 34-18). Although mantle cell lymphoma generally can be readily distinguished from CLL/SLL, because some other low-grade lymphoproliferative disorders can occasionally express CD5 and mimic the mantle cell phenotype, a definitive diagnosis requires either fluorescent in situ hybridization (FISH) demonstrating t(11;14) or overexpression of cyclin D1 by immunohistochemistry. These other rare CD5-positive B cell neoplasms cannot be distinguished by their immunophenotypic criteria, and a combination of clinical history, morphology, and cytogenetic abnormalities is often required to reach a correct classification.

Hairy cell leukemia is characterized by increased expression of a variety of B cell antigens, including CD19, CD20, and CD22, clonal surface light chain restriction, markedly increased expression of the cell adhesion molecules CD11c and CD103, and expression of the α-chain of the interleukin-2 receptor CD25 (see Fig. 34-19) (Robbins, 1994; Matutes, 1994a). In addition, the cells exhibit a variable degree of increased side scatter caused by the abundant cytoplasm they possess, often giving the cells light scatter characteristics similar to those of monocytes. This finding, in combination with the monocytopenia that is common in this disorder, is a frequent cause of false-negative results, particularly when one relies on relatively tight gates to identify the lymphocyte population by light scatter parameters alone or with CD45 versus side scatter.

Another immunophenotypic finding which aids in the classification of B cell lymphoma is expression of CD10, an antigen present on immature B cells and on normal mature B cells as they transit through the follicle center. Among B cell lymphomas, CD10 is expressed in most cases of follicular lymphoma (Almasri, 1998) (see Fig. 34-20), in a significant subset of large B cell lymphomas, and in Burkitt's lymphoma, in each of these cases indicating origin from the follicle center. In follicular lymphoma, the expression of CD10 is often coupled with decreases in CD19, CD20, and CD38 intensity (Yang, 2005; Mantei, 2009) that differ from the normal somewhat higher levels seen in normal germinal center B cells. Demonstration of bcl-2 overexpression by the CD10-positive B cell population can be useful in confirming neoplasia (Cook, 2003), particularly in cases lacking surface light chain expression, and reflects the presence of an underlying t(14;18) characteristic of follicular lymphoma. Although CD10 positivity alone does not allow definitive classification, its presence significantly reduces the possible entities that must be considered, with morphology generally being required to allow definitive classification.

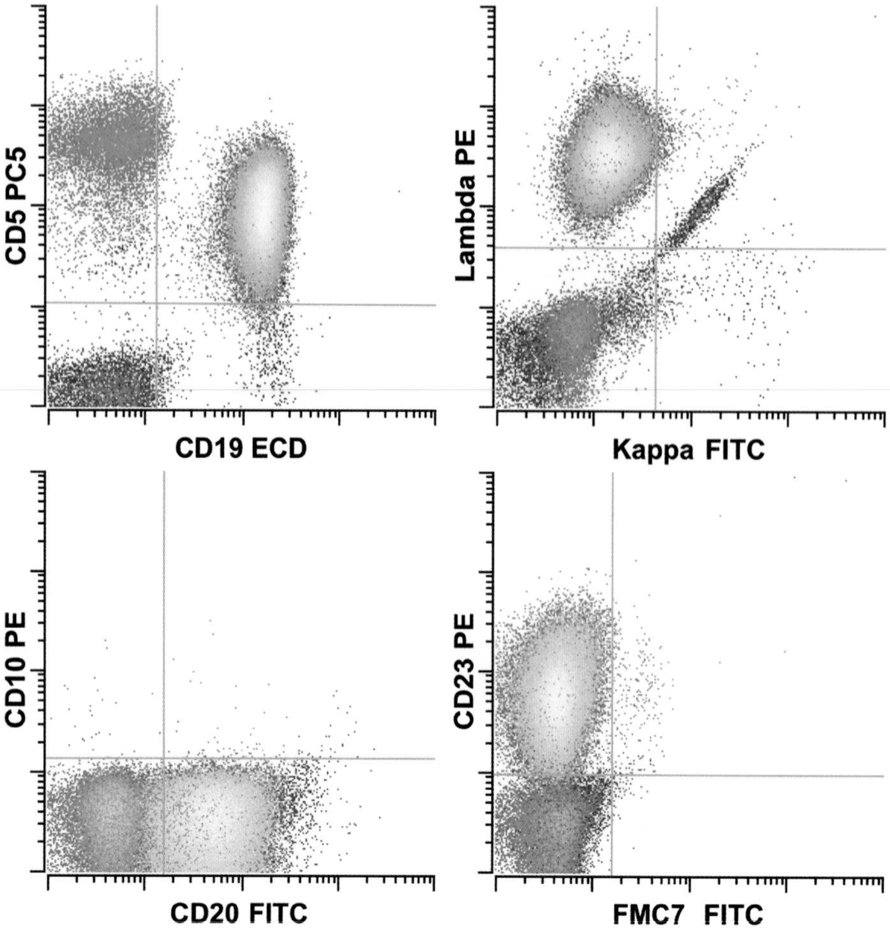

Figure 34-17 Chronic lymphocytic leukemia/small lymphocytic lymphoma. The neoplastic B cell population *(gold)* shows abnormal expression of the B cell antigens CD19 (intermediate) and CD20 (low) with surface λ light chain expression (low) and coexpression of CD5 and CD23 (intermediate). The combination of CD5 coexpression, low-level light chain restriction, and low-level CD20 and CD23 without FMC7 is diagnostic for this particular disorder. The important differential is seen with mantle cell lymphoma (see Fig. 34-18).

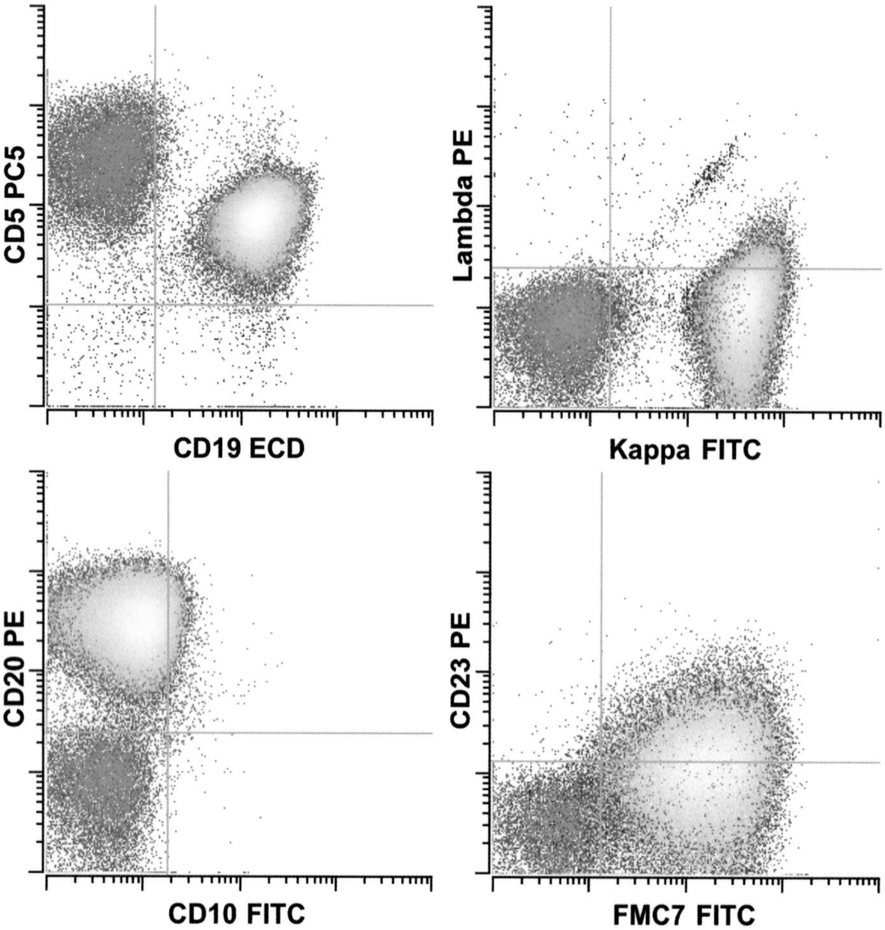

Figure 34-18 Mantle cell lymphoma. The neoplastic B cell population *(gold)* shows expression of B cell antigens CD19 (intermediate) and CD20 (intermediate) and κ light chain restriction (bright), along with coexpression of CD5 (intermediate) and FMC7 (intermediate) with only low CD23. The overall pattern of antigen expression differs from that seen in CLL/SLL (see Fig. 34-17) and suggests mantle cell lymphoma. Definitive diagnosis would require demonstration of t(11;14) by FISH or cyclin D1 overexpression by immunohistochemistry.

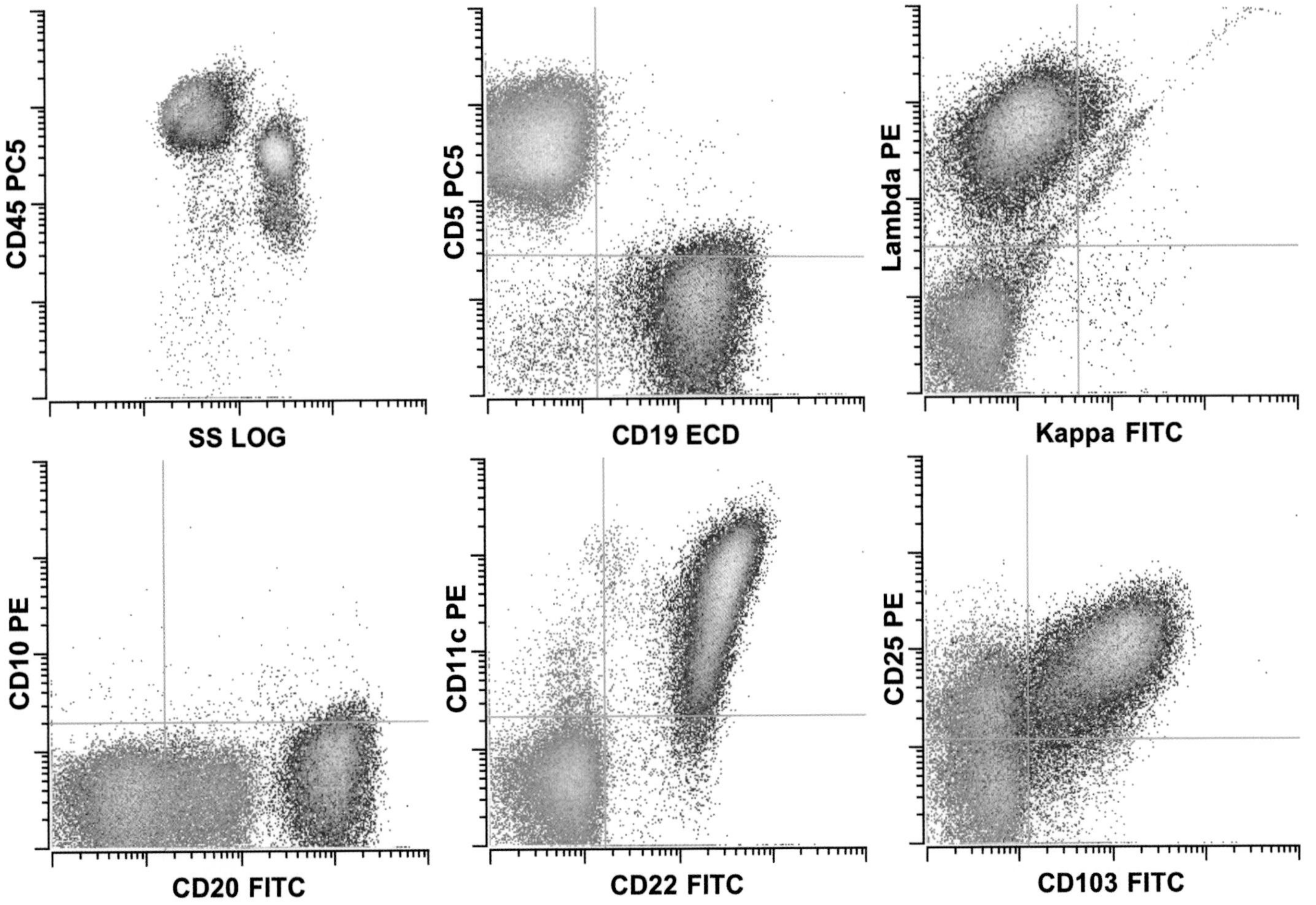

Figure 34-19 Hairy cell leukemia. The neoplastic B cell population *(red)* shows expression of B cell antigens CD19 (intermediate), CD20 (bright), CD22 (bright) and surface λ light chain restriction (intermediate) with aberrant expression of the adhesion molecules CD11c (variably bright), CD103 (intermediate), and CD25 (intermediate). This immunophenotype is diagnostic for hairy cell leukemia. Note the absence of monocytes by CD45 versus side scatter, a characteristic finding in hairy cell leukemia.

The role of immunophenotyping in the classification of T cell lymphoma is less well described, although certain associations have been noted that require larger studies for validation. As a general rule, a majority of T cell lymphomas are composed of CD4-positive T cells and exhibit abnormal patterns of antigenic expression. In angioimmunoblastic T cell lymphoma, abnormal T cells are CD4-positive and commonly show loss or decreased expression of surface CD3 (Serke, 2000) with abnormal coexpression of CD10 (Attygalle, 2002) (see Fig. 34-21). In mycosis fungoides/Sézary syndrome, abnormal T cells are also typically CD4-positive and can show a variety of immunophenotypic abnormalities, commonly including alterations in the intensity of CD3 and CD4 and decreased expression or loss of CD7 (Bogen, 1996; Lima, 2003). However, CD7 is normally variably expressed on CD4-positive T cells, decreased expression is associated with a normal memory immunophenotype, and expanded subpopulations with this immunophenotype may be seen in a variety of reactive conditions, including inflammatory skin lesions (Murphy, 2002). Consequently, demonstration of the loss of CD7 by itself does not allow definitive classification nor a definitive diagnosis of lymphoma and generally requires the presence of additional antigenic abnormalities to be informative. Expression of CD30 in combination with an aberrant pattern of T cell antigen expression can be useful in the identification of anaplastic large cell lymphoma (Juco, 2003). Finally, a large granular lymphoproliferative disorder (large granular lymphocytic leukemia) is generally characterized by clonal expansion of CD8-positive T cells having variably decreased expression of CD5 or CD7 and expression of NK cell–associated antigens such as CD57 or CD16 (Richards, 1995). However, similar clonal expansions may be seen in a wide variety of nonneoplastic conditions, and knowledge of the clinical context is required for an understanding of the clinical significance.

Prognostic Factors

As noted earlier, flow cytometry is widely used to assess markers of prognostic significance in CLL, including CD38 (Damle, 1999) and ZAP-70 (Crespo, 2003). Although these assays are widely available, problems with interpretation and standardization have been reported. The distribution of CD38 on CLL cells is often continuous, not discrete, and arbitrary criteria have been used to distinguish positive from negative cases. This problem is even greater in the case of ZAP-70 assessment, where expression is often very dim, and where questions have been raised about the best method to determine positivity. Nonetheless, most cases are either clearly positive or clearly negative for each of these markers, and many papers, using varying techniques, have demonstrated their prognostic significance (Rassenti, 2008). However, a certain number of cases with borderline positivity are best considered as indeterminate for expression. To date, there are no prognostic markers in other types of lymphoma that are as well established as those in CLL/SLL.

Therapeutic Targets

The most widely used therapeutic antibody is anti-CD20 (rituximab). Determination of CD20 expression is essential to establish the suitability of this therapy, although it is expressed by the great majority of B cell lymphomas. Following therapy, B cells may persist but show loss of CD20 expression. Assessment of samples with more than one B cell marker, such as the combination of CD19 and CD20, is helpful in demonstrating the presence of residual B cells lacking CD20. Anti-CD52 (alemtuzamab) is occasionally used to treat cases of refractory lymphoma; because of the profound immunosuppression associated with this therapy, documentation of expression is important, although the great majority of lymphomas will express CD52.

Minimal Residual Disease Detection

Detecting low levels of involvement can be important in accurately staging patients with lymphoma (Douglas, 1999). This is particularly applicable to studies of bone marrow, where detection of small populations of light chain–restricted B cells can be seen in cases in which morphology is either negative or equivocal (Duggan, 2000; Palacio, 2001; Sanchez, 2002;

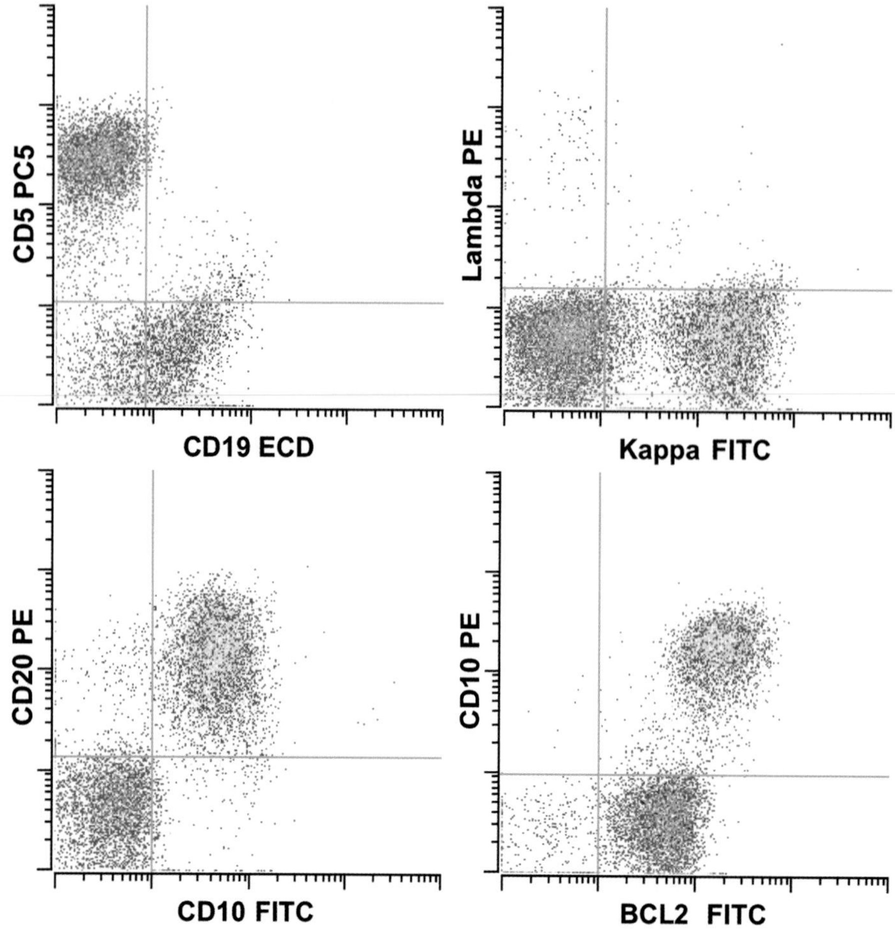

Figure 34-20 Follicular lymphoma. The neoplastic B cell population *(gold)* shows abnormal expression of the B cell antigens CD19 (dim), CD20 (intermediate), and surface κ light chain restriction (intermediate) with coexpression of the follicle center–associated antigen CD10 (intermediate). In addition, the neoplasm shows overexpression of cytoplasmic Bcl-2 due to the presence of the t(14;18) characteristic of follicular lymphoma. Overexpression of Bcl-2 by itself is not diagnostic of follicular lymphoma, but its combined expression with CD10 is much more specific, as normal CD10-positive follicular B cells would be expected to be negative.

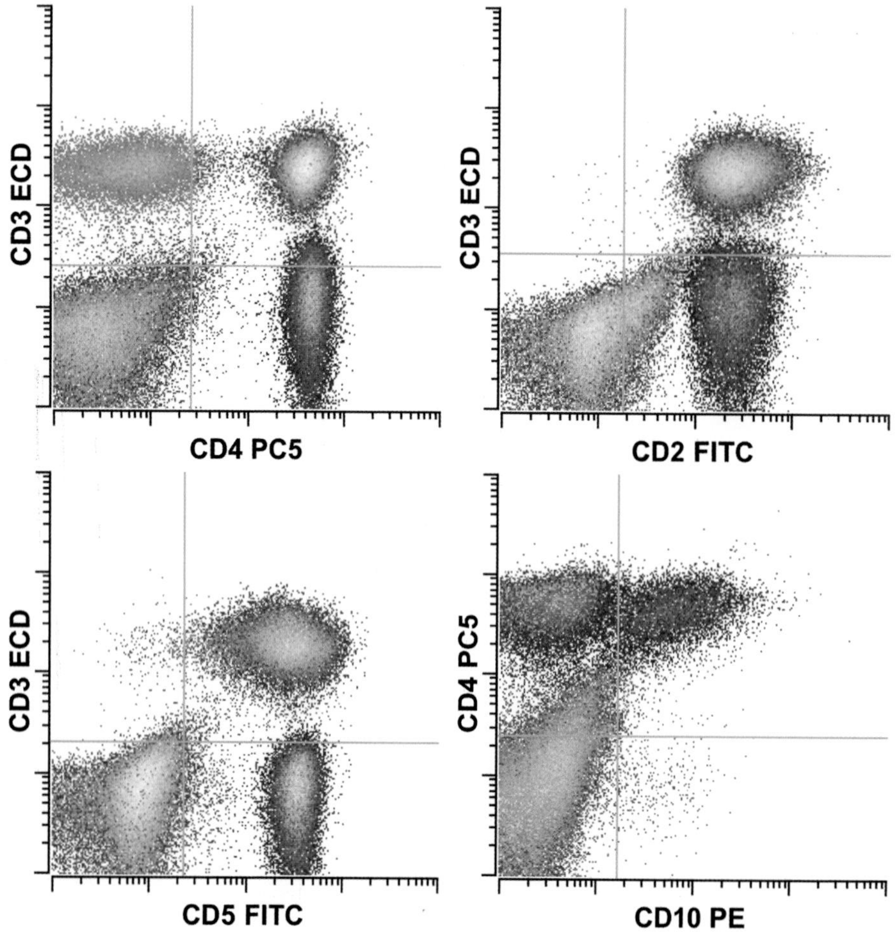

Figure 34-21 Angioimmunoblastic T cell lymphoma. The neoplastic T cell population *(blue)* shows expression of the T cell–associated antigens CD2 (intermediate) and CD5 (intermediate), along with the helper T cell antigen CD4, but without surface CD3. In addition, the neoplastic cells coexpress CD10. The composite immunophenotype is characteristic of that seen in angioimmunoblastic T cell lymphoma.

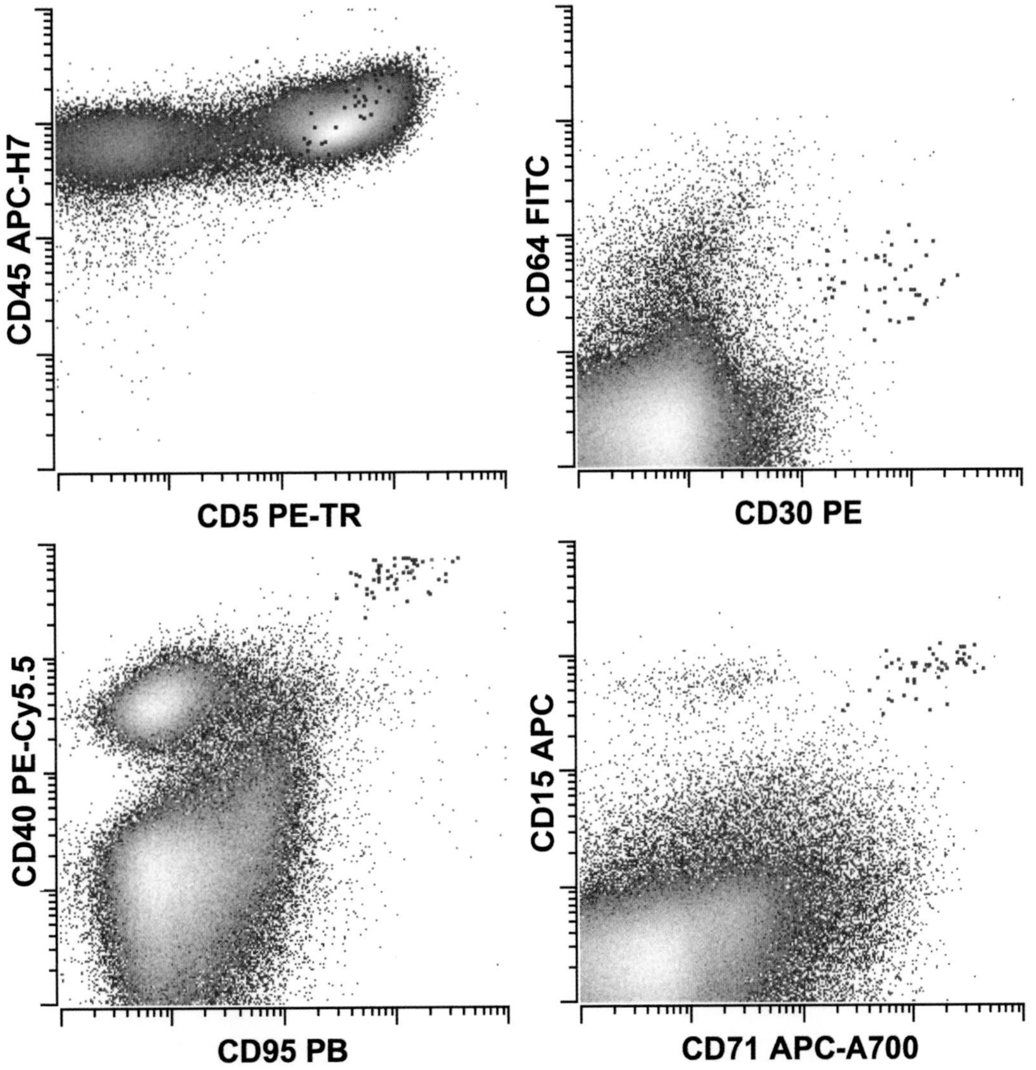

Figure 34-22 Classic Hodgkin lymphoma. A discrete population of cells is identified that differs from normal lymphocytes and macrophages, having expression of CD15, CD30, high CD40, high CD71, and high CD95. This immunophenotype is typical for classical Hodgkin lymphoma. Note that these cells commonly show increased autofluorescence that appears as apparent low positivity for FITC-labeled reagents (CD64 in the current example). Also note that Hodgkin cells commonly are rosetted by T cells, giving apparent positivity for CD5 and CD45 *(top left panel).*

Stacchini, 2003), although the cost-effectiveness of this approach has been questioned (Hanson, 1999). Similarly, the peripheral blood may be evaluated for lymphoma to aid in the timing or advisability of stem cell collection, and the resulting harvested stem cell product may be tested for the presence of residual lymphoma to minimize the amount of tumor reinfused in patients undergoing bone marrow transplantation. In addition, as in acute leukemia, minimal residual disease studies have been used in patients with CLL and have demonstrated an association between the presence of residual disease following therapy and both event-free and overall survival (Rawstron, 2001; Moreton, 2005). In these cases, methods to demonstrate clonal populations of light chain–restricted B cells are not as sensitive as methods that rely on the presence of small phenotypically aberrant populations using principles similar to those used in acute leukemia.

Plasma Cell Neoplasms

Plasma cell neoplasms generally are not difficult to identify by flow cytometry (Ruiz-Arguelles, 1994; Ocqueteau, 1998), and their immunophenotype at diagnosis (Paiva, 2009) and detection following therapy are associated with outcome (Paiva, 2008). The expression of bright CD38 and/or CD138 is used to identify the plasma cell population, with common abnormalities being decreased CD45, decreased CD19, and abnormal coexpression of CD56 or CD117 in combination with the identification of cytoplasmic light chain restriction. An example of immunophenotypic abnormalities seen in plasma cell neoplasms is presented in Figure 34-23. It is important to recognize that flow cytometric analysis typically underestimates the percentage of plasma cells present in a specimen, sometimes dramatically, possibly because of plasma cell aggregation, apoptosis, and peripheral blood dilution.

Myelodysplastic Syndromes and Myeloproliferative Disorders

The same principles used to identify other hematopoietic neoplasms can be used to identify myelodysplastic syndromes and myeloproliferative disorders (Elghetany, 1998; Wells, 2003, Kussick, 2003a, 2003b; Wood, 2007; Matarraz, 2008). Abnormalities in antigen expression can be identified on myeloid blasts, maturing neutrophils, and maturing monocytes; common abnormalities include (1) alterations in the intensity of expression of CD34, CD117, and HLA-DR, and aberrant expression of antigens such as CD7 or CD56 on myeloid blasts (Wells, 2003; Kussick, 2003b; Matarraz, 2008), (2) abnormal patterns of CD13 and CD16 expression and decreased side scatter on maturing neutrophils, and (3) aberrant CD56 expression on maturing monocytes (Wells, 2003; Kussick, 2003b). Abnormalities in erythroid maturation have also been described (Della Porta, 2006). Similar abnormalities in addition to basophilia may be identified in myeloproliferative disorders (Kussick, 2003a), although this has been less well studied. Although abnormalities can be demonstrated in essentially all cases having cytogenetic abnormalities, low-grade myelodysplasia

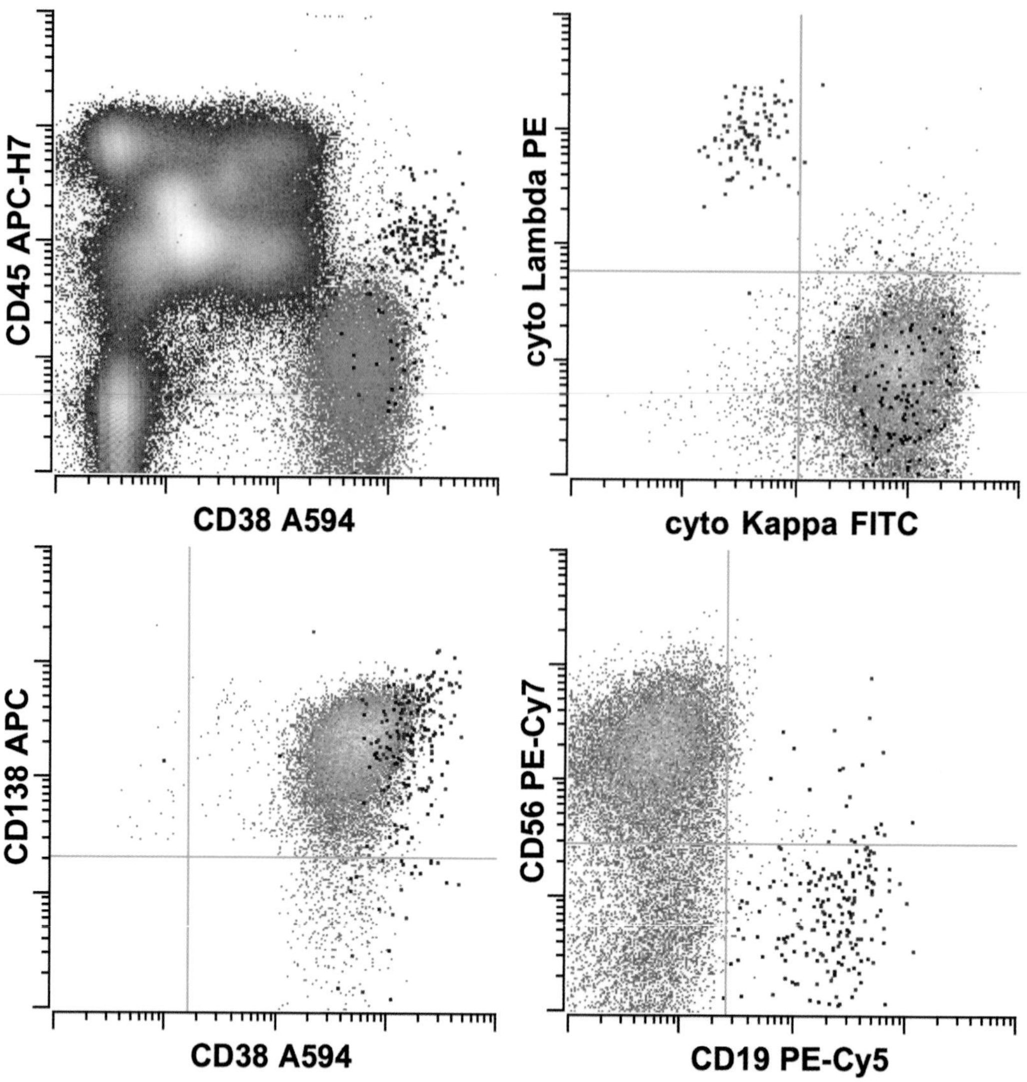

Figure 34-23 Plasma cell neoplasm. The neoplastic plasma cell population *(green)* is identified by the bright expression of CD38 and CD138, but both are slightly decreased in comparison with the few normal polyclonal plasma cells *(emphasized in blue and red)*. Abnormal plasma cells show abnormal expression of CD45 (low to absent) and CD19 (absent) and cytoplasmic κ light chain restriction, with aberrant expression of CD56. This immunophenotype is characteristic of that seen in a variety of plasma cell neoplasms, including multiple myeloma, plasmacytoma, and monoclonal gammopathy of uncertain significance (MGUS). Definitive classification requires clinical and laboratory correlation.

predominantly affecting the erythroid lineage, as well as polycythemia vera and essential thrombocythemia, is not consistently identified currently, and new methods are needed. An example of immunophenotypic abnormalities seen in myelodysplasia is presented in Figure 34-24.

Paroxysmal Nocturnal Hemoglobinuria

Certain nonneoplastic hematopoietic disorders can be diagnosed using the same principles used to identify hematopoietic neoplasms. Paroxysmal nocturnal hemoglobinuria (PNH) is an acquired clonal stem cell disorder characterized by the loss of a variety of cell surface proteins on all progeny of the hematopoietic stem cell, including erythrocytes, neutrophils, monocytes, lymphocytes, and platelets. The loss of these proteins is the result of mutation of a key enzyme required for synthesis of the glycosylphosphatidyl-inositol (GPI) linkage used to attach these proteins to the cell surface. Detection of the loss of GPI-linked proteins is readily accomplished by flow cytometry (Richards, 2000) and serves as the principal diagnostic method for this disorder. For clinical testing, it is recommended that at least two GPI-linked antigens be evaluated on at least two different cell lineages, with commonly evaluated antigens being CD55 and CD59 on both erythrocytes and white blood cells, CD14 on monocytes, and CD66b on granulocytes. Platelets and lymphocytes generally are not evaluated. Another reagent increasingly used for the diagnosis of PNH is the fluorescent derivative of a mutant form of the bacterial toxin aerolysin, which binds specifically to the GPI linkage and can identify GPI-deficient cells with a high degree of sensitivity and specificity (Brodsky, 2000). An example of PNH is shown in Figure 34-25.

SUMMARY

Flow cytometry is a powerful, rapid, and cost effective technique for the identification and monitoring of hematopoietic neoplasms. Successful implementation requires careful attention to instrument and reagent performance, as well as a strong working knowledge of normal patterns of antigenic expression on hematopoietic cells.

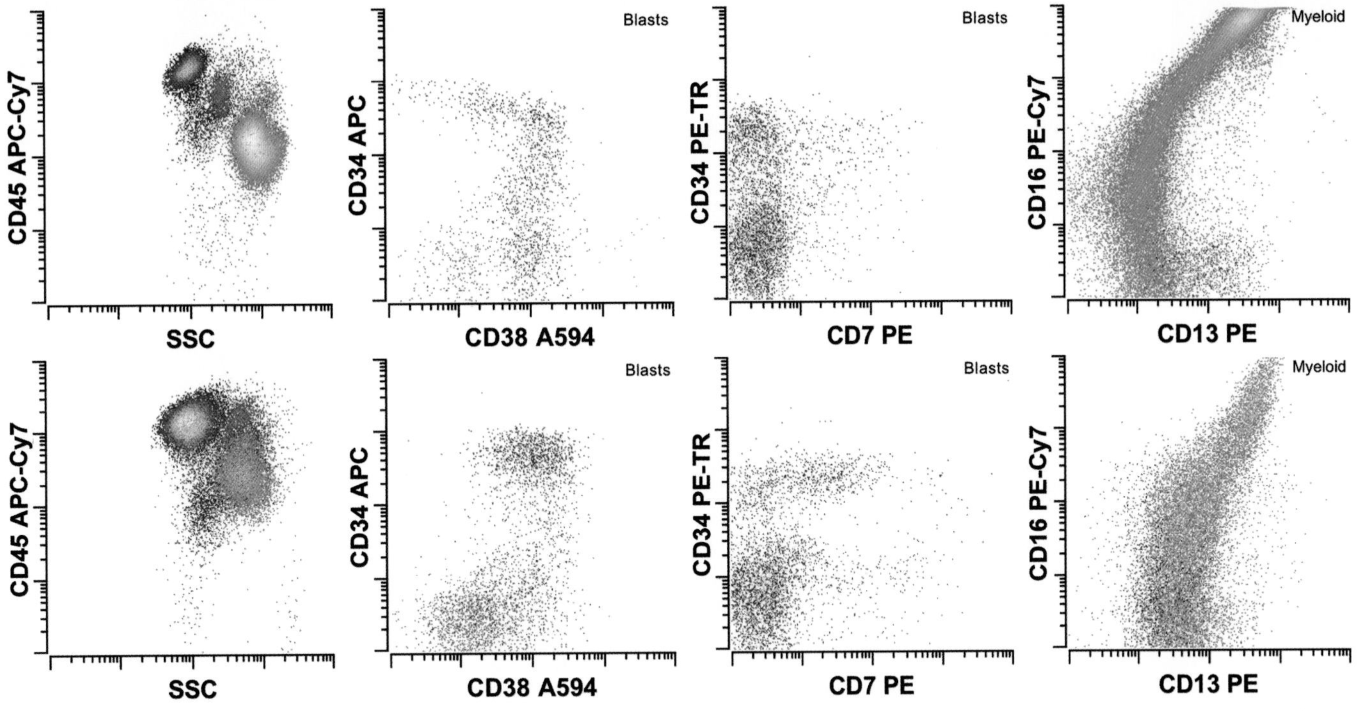

Figure 34-24 Myelodysplasia. A sample from a patient with low-grade myelodysplasia *(lower row)* is compared with normal bone marrow *(upper row)*. Abnormalities commonly seen in myelodysplasia include neutrophil hypogranularity as indicated by decreased side scatter *(left)*, decreased CD45 expression by the blasts *(red, left)*, homogeneity of the myeloid blasts *(red, left center)*, acquisition of lymphoid-associated antigens (CD2, CD5, CD7, and CD56) by myeloid blasts *(right center)*, and abnormal patterns of myelomonocytic maturation, such as abnormal CD13 and CD16 on maturing neutrophilic forms *(right)*. Decreased side scatter is best noted by comparing the relative positions of neutrophils *(green)* and monocytes *(magenta)*. It is the combined presence of these abnormalities that suggests the presence of a myeloid stem cell disorder, such as myelodysplasia.

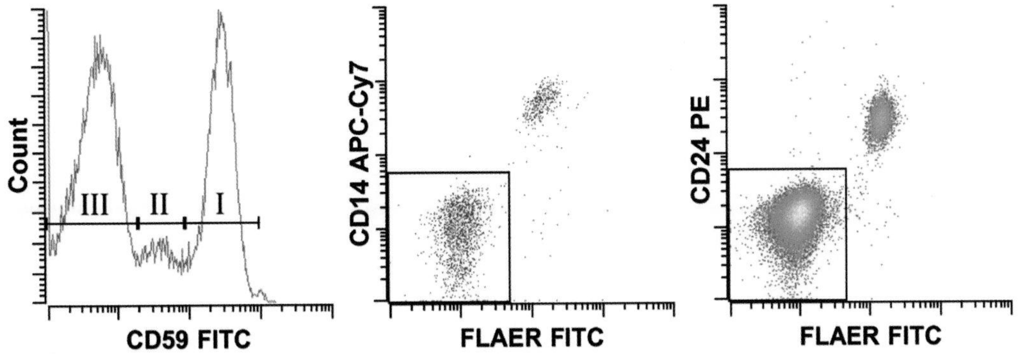

Figure 34-25 Paroxysmal nocturnal hemoglobinuria. Erythrocytes *(left panel)* identified by light scatter properties show differing levels of CD59 expression, corresponding to normal (Type I, 36%), partially deficient (Type II, 9%), and completely deficient (Type III, 54%) forms. Monocytes *(center panel)* identified by a combination of CD45, CD15 (low), CD33 (high), and side scatter (intermediate) show a mixture of normal (positive for CD14 and fluorescent aerolysin [FLAER]) and GPI-deficient forms (gated, 81%). Granulocytes *(right panel)* identified by a combination of CD45, CD15 (high), CD33 (low), and side scatter (high) show a mixture of normal (positive for CD24 and FLAER) and GPI-deficient forms (gated, 85%). Note the greater percentage of GPI-deficient monocytes and granulocytes compared with GPI-deficient erythrocytes, a common finding in PNH.

SELECTED REFERENCES

Clinical and Laboratory Standards Institute (CLSI). Clinical flow cytometric analysis of neoplastic hematolymphoid cells: approved guideline. 2nd ed. Wayne, Pa: Clinical and Laboratory Standards Institute; 2007. CLSI Document H43-A2.

Useful reference document on technical issues related to the clinical performance of flow cytometry for leukemia and lymphoma.

Shapiro HM. Practical flow cytometry. 4th ed. New York: Wiley Liss; 2003.

The definitive exposition of technical issues related to flow cytometry.

Swerdlow SH, Campo E, Harris NL, et al, editors. World Health Organization classification of tumours of haematopoietic and lymphoid tissues. Lyon, France: IARC Press; 2008.

A definitive and well-illustrated text expounding the first revision of the most modern and comprehensive classification of human hematopoietic disease achieved through international consensus.

Stewart CC, Mayers GL. Kinetics of antibody binding to cells. In: Stewart C, Nicholson JKA, editors. Immunophenotyping. 1st ed. New York: Wiley-Liss; 2000. p. 1–22.

The entire volume is an excellent, modern general reference on the use of immunophenotyping in a variety of settings.

U.S.-Canadian consensus recommendations on the immunophenotypic analysis of hematologic neoplasia by cytometry. Bethesda, Md., November 16-17, 1995. Cytometry 1997;30:213–74.

Comprehensive description of consensus guidelines for the practical performance of clinical flow cytometry for the diagnosis of leukemia and lymphoma.

REFERENCES

Access the complete reference list online at http://www.expertconsult.com

CHAPTER 35

IMMUNOHEMATOLOGY

Laura Cooling, Theresa Downs

Continued

KEY POINTS

- Blood group antigens play a variety of physiologic roles as membrane structures involved in maintaining erythrocyte cytoskeleton integrity, as well as in membrane transport, cell signaling, and immune complement regulation, and as receptors/modulators of disease.
- The ABO histo-blood group antigens are widely expressed throughout the body and are the single most important blood group for selection and transfusion of blood products, as well as a major consideration in solid organ and bone marrow transplantation.
- The recipient immune response to exposure to foreign red cell antigens through transfusion or pregnancy may include antibody production and complement activation resulting in hemolysis (e.g., transfusion reaction, hemolytic disease of the fetus and newborn).
- Pretransfusion and perinatal blood testing is performed to prevent transfusion reactions and hemolytic disease of the fetus and newborn, and must include the key serologic evaluations of ABO and Rh antigen typing, antibody detection/identification, and crossmatching.
- Antihuman globulin reagents as used in direct or indirect testing are integral to virtually all red cell antibody detection and identification techniques.
- Patients with complex serologic problems such as antibodies to high-frequency antigens and autoantibodies may require utilization of a variety of special immunohematologic studies (enzymes, adsorption, elution) to identify compatible blood for transfusion.

BASIC IMMUNOHEMATOLOGIC CONCEPTS

The term immunohematology refers to the serologic, genetic, biochemical, and molecular study of antigens associated with membrane structures on the cellular constituents of blood, as well as the immunologic properties and reactions of blood components and constituents. Fundamental discoveries in the area of immunohematology have played an integral role in the development of transfusion medicine, which includes the transfusion of blood, its components, and its derivatives (see Chapter 36). In this integrated relationship, immunohematologists perform and interpret a wide variety of serologic and molecular assays to aid in the diagnosis, prevention, and management of immunization associated with transfusion, pregnancy, and organ transplantation. Over the years, research in the field of immunohematology has contributed significantly to the fundamental understanding of human genetics and immunology, with broad applications to membrane physiology and function, epidemiology, anthropology, and forensic science.

BLOOD GROUP ANTIGENS

The term blood group refers not only to genetically encoded erythrocyte antigens but also to the immunologic diversity expressed by other blood constituents, including leukocytes, platelets, and plasma. Most blood group genes, with few exceptions, are located on the autosomal chromosomes and are inherited following Mendelian rules of inheritance. A majority of blood group alleles demonstrate codominance as well, meaning that genetic heterozygotes at a particular locus will express both gene products.

Many membrane-associated structures on blood cells may be defined as antigens because they have the capability of reacting with a complementary antibody or cell receptor. A majority of these antigens are also immunogens, in that they are able to elicit an antibody-mediated immunologic response in a responsive host. Each antigen may have a variety of different epitopes or specific antigenic determinants. Epitopes are discrete, immunologically active regions of the antigen, whose molecular configuration can interact with specific lymphocyte membrane receptors or secreted complementary antibody. Clinically, about a dozen antigen systems are significant and are commonly encountered on the transfusion service. In general, these antigens demonstrate polymorphic epitopes with varied distribution, often along racial or ethnic lines, in the population. Patients who lack certain antigens may form antibodies when exposed to them, and these antibodies may be detected on routine testing in the blood bank.

Immunogenicity

The ability of an antigen to elicit an immune response is known as its immunogenicity. The immunogenicity of an antigen is determined not only by certain innate characteristics of the antigen itself but also by the host's genetically determined immune responsiveness. Characteristics of antigens that determine their immunogenicity include degree of foreignness; molecular size and configuration, which may change with temperature, pH, and ionic environment; and antigenic complexity, as measured by the number of available epitopes or antigenic determinants.

Blood group antigens vary greatly in their ability to elicit an immune response. The A, B, and RhD antigens are certainly the most immunogenic; thus all blood transfused must be matched for these antigens between the blood donor and the recipient. Approximately 50%–75% of D-negative individuals would produce anti-D if transfused with only one unit of D-positive blood. After the D antigen, K is the next most immunogenic, followed by Fy^a and common Rh antigens, based on the frequency with which their corresponding antibodies are encountered. Using the same criteria, other common blood group antigens such as Fy^b, Jk^a, Jk^b, and s are much less immunogenic. The relative immunogenicities of some clinically important red cell antigens are listed in Table 35-1.

Chemical Characteristics

The chemical composition, complexity, and molecular size of an antigen determine most of its physical and biological properties, including immunogenicity. As a general rule, pure polysaccharides are not immunogenic except in certain species such as humans and mice (Virella, 2001). Pure lipid and nucleic acids are not immunogenic but can be antigenic because they can serve as haptens. Haptens are well-defined chemical groupings that are too small to be immunogenic by themselves but can induce an antibody response when attached to a carrier protein.

Although pure protein may be immunogenic, the most potent immunogens are usually complex macromolecular glycoproteins and lipoproteins. Thus, it is not surprising that red blood cell (RBC) antigens are glycoproteins, lipoproteins, and glycolipids. Experiments with peptide chain polymers have shown that aromatic amino acids, such as tyrosine and phenylalanine, can contribute significantly to overall immunogenicity (Virella, 2001). In glycoproteins, immunogenicity may also be influenced by the extent of branching in the polysaccharide side chains. Whereas the immunogenicity of an antigen relates to the total complex molecular structure, the areas where antigen combines with specific antibody (i.e., the epitopes) are usually limited to one or a few simple structures (terminal sugars, amino acids) exposed on the exterior, mobile surface of the molecule (Delves, 2006). These are often referred to as immunodominant structures because they determine the specificity and optimal binding energy of antigen–antibody interactions.

Antigen Density

The number of antigenic sites on a foreign substance, whether a complex molecule or a cell, will contribute to the strength of an immunologic response. Studies of blood group antigens have demonstrated that antigen density contributes to the efficiency of antibody binding and the extent of complement activation, thus determining the likelihood of RBC hemolysis.

Various techniques have been used over the years to determine the number of copies of specific blood group antigens on the RBC membrane. Historically, radioimmunoassay, enzyme-linked immunosorbent assay, electron microscopy using ferritin-labeled antiimmunoglobulin, and flow cytometry have been used to indirectly calculate the number of antigen sites on RBC membranes. Table 35-2 lists the estimated densities of common RBC antigens.

BLOOD GROUP ANTIBODIES

Immunoglobulins and Antigen Binding

Immunoglobulin (Ig)s are protein molecules that are produced in response to antigenic stimulation and that demonstrate specific antibody activity. To understand antibodies, one first must be familiar with Ig structure and function. Information on Igs that is relevant to blood banking is summarized in Tables 35-3 and 35-4.

The specificity of an antibody is determined by the hypervariable or complementarity-determining regions of an Ig molecule. Three hypervariable regions are included in each of the light and heavy chains that make up the Ig molecule (Delves, 2006). Amino acid sequence heterogeneity in the hypervariable regions, which allows for variation in the configuration of the peptide chains in the variable loops, determines the combining specificity for each antibody. The combining site of an antibody, where it is in physical contact with an antigenic determinant or epitope, is called the paratope. For simple, linear antigens (sequential epitopes), the combining site may be in contact with five or six amino acids or hexose units. In the case of a globular protein antigen, as many as 16 amino acids of what is generally a discontinuous or conformational epitope may be in contact with the antibody-combining site (Delves, 2006).

Binding involves formation of multiple noncovalent bonds between the antigen and amino acids of the paratope. The attractive forces between antigen and antibody, which include electrostatic and van der Waals forces, hydrogen bonds, and hydrophobic interactions, become significant when the distance between the interacting groups is small. As a result, the better the physical fit between epitope and paratope, the higher is the overall binding energy and the greater is the affinity of the resulting reaction between antibody and antigen (Delves, 2006).

TABLE 35-1
Relative Immunogenicity of Selected Clinically Important Blood Group Antigens*

Antigen	Relative potency	Antigen	Relative potency
D	0.70	K	0.10
C	0.041	E	0.0338
k	0.030	e	0.0112
Fy^a	0.0046	C	0.0022
Jk^a	0.0014	S	0.0008
Jk^b	0.0006	s	0.0006

*These figures represent the approximate percentage of persons negative for a specific antigen who, if transfused with one unit of corresponding antigen-positive blood, would develop antibodies to that specific antigen. When the relative potency of K antigen is 0.1, as estimated by Kornstad (1958), the relative potency of other blood groups can be estimated as shown by Klein (2006).

TABLE 35-2
Number of Membrane Sites for Selected Native Erythrocyte Antigens Estimated by Radioimmunoassay*

Antigen	Phenotype	Number of antigenic sites
A	A_1 adult	810–1170 × 10^3
	Newborn	250–370 × 10^3
	A_2 adult	240–290 × 10^3
	Newborn	140 × 10^3
	A_1B adult	460–850 × 10^3
	Newborn	220 × 10^3
	A_2B adult	140 × 10^3
B	B adult	750 × 10^3
	A_1B adult	430 × 10^3
I	I+	500 × 10^3
K	K+k–	6.1 × 10^3
	K+k+	3.5 × 10^3

Antigen	Phenotype	Number of antigenic sites
D	DCce	9.9–14.6 × 10^3
	Dce	12–20 × 10^3
	DcEe	14–16.6 × 10^3
	DCe	14.5–19.3 × 10^3
	DcE	15.5–33.3 × 10^3
	DCcEe	23–21 × 10^3
	D– –	110–202 × 10^3
	Weak D (D^u)	0.8–3 × 10^3
c	c+C–	70–85 × 10^3
	c+C+	37–53 × 10^3
e	e+E–	18.2–24.4 × 10^3
	e+E+	13.4–14.5 × 10^3
E	e–E+	0.45–25.6 × 10^3

*Figures taken from Klein (2006).

TABLE 35-3
Important Properties of Human Immunoglobulin (Ig) Classes

	IgG	IgM	IgA	IgD	IgE
Heavy chain isotype	γ	μ	α	δ	ε
Light chains	K or λ	K or λ	K or λ	K or λ	K or λ
No. of four-peptide units	1	5	1–2	1	1
Valency (Ag binding)	2	5(10)*	2–4	2	2
Development in immune response	Late primary, secondary	Early primary			
Half-life in vivo, days	21	10	6	3	2
Serum concentration, mg/mL	8–16	0.5–2	1.4–4	0–0.04	Trace
Percentage of total serum Ig	80	6	13	0–1	
Extravascular distribution	Tissue	Fluids	Secretions		Secretions
Inactivated by sulfhydryl reagents	–	++++	±		
Crosses placenta	Yes	No	No	No	No
Induces agglutination	+	++++	++		
Fixes complement	++ (classical)	+++ (classical)	+ (alternative)	–	–
Binding to Fcγ receptors	+++	–	+	–	+

Data from Delves P, Martin S, Burton D, Roitt I. Roitt's essential immunology. 11th ed. Somerset, N.J.: Wiley-Blackwell; 2006.
*Valency of 10 is observed only with very small haptens.

TABLE 35-4
Some Known Properties of the Four Immunoglobulin (Ig)G Subclasses

Subclasses of IgG	IgG1	IgG2	IgG3	IgG4
Heavy chain subclass	γ1	γ2	γ3	γ4
Allotypic markers	a, x, f, z	N	b0, b1, b3, g, s, t, etc.	4a, 4b (isoallotypes)
Half-life in vivo, days	21	21	7	21
Relative serum concentration, %	64–70	23–28	4–7	3–4
Placental transfer	++	±	++	++
Complement fixation	+++	++	++++	±
Macrophage binding	+++	+	+++	±
Binding to staph A protein	Yes	Yes	No	Yes
Antibodies showing subclass restriction	Anti-Rh	Anti-dextrans		Anti-AHF

Data from Delves P, Martin S, Burton D, Roitt I. Roitt's essential immunology. 11th ed. Somerset, N.J.: Wiley-Blackwell; 2006.

Blood Group Alloantibodies and Autoantibodies

A majority of clinically significant blood group antibodies are IgG or IgM, although occasionally an IgA antibody is encountered. Blood group antibodies are usually classified as (1) an **alloantibody**, which reacts with a foreign antigen not present on the patient's own erythrocytes, or (2) an **autoantibody**, which reacts with an antigen on the patient's own cells. RBC autoantibodies are discussed later in this chapter.

Some alloantibodies to erythrocyte antigens are called **naturally occurring,** that is, the antigenic stimulus is unknown. Naturally occurring antibodies may appear regularly in the serum of persons who lack the corresponding antigen, such as in the ABO blood group system. Other naturally occurring antibodies are produced only in a small subset of individuals.

Most blood group alloantibodies are produced as the result of immunization to foreign erythrocyte antigens by exposure through transfusion of blood components or through pregnancy. Alloantibodies to RBCs frequently require the selection of specific antigen-negative components for transfusion. Identification of alloantibodies and selection of compatible blood components remain the most important functions of a transfusion medicine service.

THE COMPLEMENT SYSTEM AND BLOOD BANKING

Complement plays a key role in the pathophysiology of hemolysis through its involvement in the sensitization and destruction of transfused RBCs by alloantibody, or the destruction of autologous RBCs by autoantibody. Complement is also important in immunohematologic testing.

Role of Complement in Erythrocyte Destruction

Antibody binding to RBC antigens is the most common reason for complement activation on the RBC membrane in vivo. Complement may also be activated on RBCs via a carrier–hapten antibody complex such as penicillin-coated RBCs and antipenicillin antibodies. Complement components may also be attached to the membrane via a nonspecific mechanism induced by certain drugs, or when erythrocytes are **innocent bystanders** in another immune reaction.

RBC–antibody complexes usually activate complement by the classical pathway. However, the mode of destruction and the extent of RBC hemolysis depend primarily on the class of Ig involved and the activity of an individual's reticuloendothelial (RE) system.

Intravascular Hemolysis

Intravascular RBC hemolysis is usually caused by antibodies directed against the ABO antigens. Rarely, other IgM blood group antibodies, as well as some complement-fixing IgG antibodies (e.g., anti-Kidd antibodies), can induce intravascular hemolysis. Intravascular lysis occurs when large amounts of complement are rapidly activated, resulting in complete activation of the complement cascade with assembly of the terminal membrane attack complex (C5b6789). This complex polymerizes to form pores in the RBC membrane, so that extracellular fluid enters the cell, causing it to swell and burst by osmotic lysis.

Extravascular Hemolysis

IgG antibodies cause the majority of extravascular hemolysis via the RE system, which removes complement-coated RBCs. When IgG antibodies bind RBCs and activate complement, complement regulatory proteins generally stop the activation process at the C3/C4 level. RBC-bound C3b

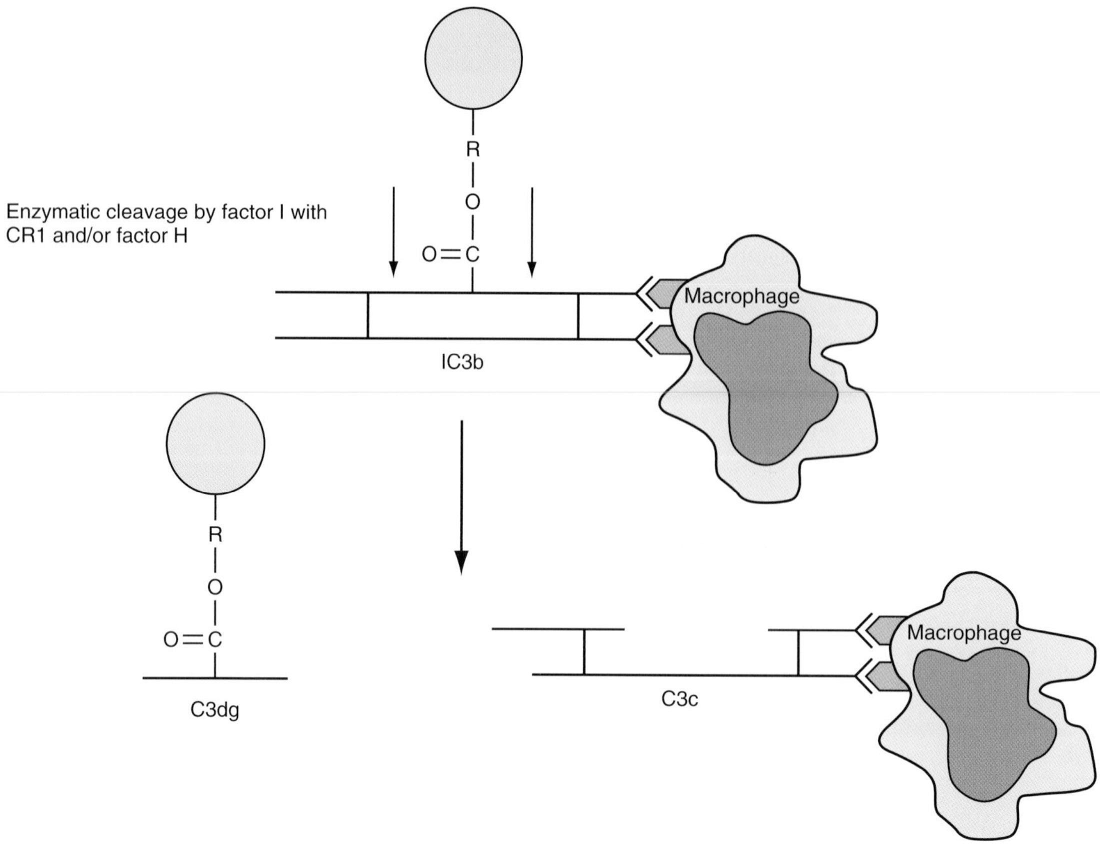

Figure 35-1 Action of factor I in the release of C3b-coated erythrocytes from reticuloendothelial system sequestration.

TABLE 35-5
Complement Receptors on Human Cells

Receptor	Ligand	Distribution
CR1 (CD35)	C3b, C4b	Erythrocytes, neutrophils, monocytes, macrophages, B lymphocytes, follicular dendritic cells
CR2 (CD21)	C3d, C3dg, iC3b	B cells
CR3 (CD11b/CD18)*	iC3b	Monocytes, macrophages, neutrophils, natural killer cells
CR4 (CD11c/CD18)*	iC3b	

*Members of the integrin receptor family.

is degraded to iC3b, which is enzymatically inactive, by factor I and factor H. iC3b is further degraded to C3c and C3dg by factor I and CR1, a cofactor and C3b/C4b receptor (Freedman, 1994) (Fig. 35-1). Decay accelerating factor (DAF) participates by inhibiting C3 convertase (C4b2b) formation and by promoting C3 convertase degradation. On RBCs, CR1 and DAF carry the Knops and Cromer blood group antigens, respectively.

Initially, C3b/iC3b-coated RBCs are rapidly sequestered in the liver by monocytes and macrophages, which have receptors for C3b (Table 35-5). Although phagocytic cells also have receptors for C4b, the role, if any, of C4b in immune hemolysis of erythrocytes is not defined (Freedman, 1994). A portion of the RBCs sequestered in the liver are immobilized and destroyed by phagocytosis with a half-life of about 2 minutes (Klein, 2006). Within 15–20 minutes, however, destruction slows, and many of the cells escape extravascular destruction through the action of the complement regulatory protein, factor I, as previously described. C3dg, the iC3b fragment produced by factor I cleavage, remains attached to RBCs but has no enzymatic or opsonic properties. As a result, sequestered C3dg-coated RBCs are released back into the circulation and survive normally (see Fig. 35-1). In the circulation, C3dg is cleaved, leaving C3d attached to the RBC membrane.

In the absence of complement activation, IgG-coated RBCs are removed by phagocytic cells via Fcγ receptors. Although phagocytosis is not complement dependent, Mollison (1989) demonstrated that RBCs coated with both IgG and complement tend to show accelerated removal by the liver, whereas RBCs coated only with IgG tend to be destroyed more slowly in the spleen, displaying a linear pattern of removal with a minimum half-life of 20 minutes. Theoretically, RBCs coated only with IgG antibody could also be the targets of antibody-dependent cellular cytotoxicity mechanisms (Klein, 2006), because natural killer cells possess Fcγ receptors.

ERYTHROCYTE ANTIGENS AND ANTIBODIES

More than 700 erythrocyte antigens have been reported in the literature and have been organized into 30 blood group systems by the International Society of Blood Transfusion (ISBT) (Table 35-6). Many described erythrocyte antigens are high-frequency or public antigens expressed by most donors (>90%–99%), whereas others are extremely rare (private antigens). In the following section, we review the more common RBC antigens and antibodies encountered on the transfusion service. Table 35-7 summarizes several commonly encountered RBC alloantibodies according to their Ig class, serologic phase of detection, clinical significance, and statistics on finding compatible blood.

ABO AND H BLOOD GROUP SYSTEMS (ISBT NO. 001 AND 018)

Originally discovered in 1900, the ABO blood group system is the single most important blood group for the selection and transfusion of blood. As histo-blood group antigens, ABO epitopes are found on many tissues and body fluids, including RBCs, platelets, and endothelial cells (Issitt, 1998). Because they are so widely expressed, ABO antigens are a major consideration in solid organ and bone marrow transplantation (Wu, 2003).

The ABO blood group system consists of two antigens—A and B—and four phenotypes—groups A, B, AB, and O. A and B are autosomal codominant antigens (ISTB No. 001) and are expressed on group A, B, and AB

TABLE 35-6
Terminology for Blood Group System Genes and Gene Products

TRADITIONAL NOMENCLATURE		ISBT NOMENCLATURE		ISGN NOMENCLATURE		
Name	**Symbol**	**Symbol**	**Number**	**Gene**	**Chromosome**	**Gene product name**
ABO	ABO	ABO	001	*ABO*	9q34.1	α1,3 *N*-acetyl-galactosaminyltranferase (A antigen) α1,3-galactosyltransferase (B antigen)
MNS	MNS	MNS	002	*GYPA* *GYPB* *GYPE*	4q28.2	Glycophorin A (CD235 A) Glycophorin B (CD235B) Glycophorin E (CD235E)
P1Pk	P1	P1	003	*A4GALT1*	22q13	P1 antigen
Rh	Rh	RHD RHCE	004	*RHD* *RHCE*	1p36.1	RhD protein (CD240) RhCE protein
Lutheran	Lu	LU	005	*LU*	19q13.3	Lutheran glycoprotein, B-CAM
Kell	K	KEL	006	*KEL*	7q34	Kell glycoprotein
Lewis	Le	LE	007	*FUT3*	19p13.3	α-3/4-fucosyltransferase
Duffy	Fy	FY	008	*DARC*	1q23	Duffy-associated receptor cytokine glycoprotein
Kidd	Jk	JK	009	*SLC14A1*	18q12	Urea transporter (HUT11)
Diego	Di	DI	010	*SLC4A1*	17q21.3	Anion exchanger 1 (AE1, Band 3)
Yt	Yt	YT	011	*ACHE*	7q22	Acetylcholinesterase
Xg	Xg	XG	012	*XG*	Xp22.3	Xg glycoprotein (CD99)
Scianna	Sc	SC	013	*ERMAP*	1p34	Human erythroid membrane–associated protein
Dombrock	Do	DO	014	*ART4*	12p13.2	ADP-ribosyltransferase (CD297)
Colton	Co	CO	015	*AQPI*	7p14	Aquaporin-1 (CHIP)
Landsteiner-Wiener	LW	LW	016	*LW*	19p13.3	ICAM (CD242)
Chido/Rodgers	Ch/Rg	CH/RG	017	*C4A,C4B*	6p21.3	C4A, C4B complement glycoproteins
Hh	Hh	H	018	*FUT1*	19q13.3	α1,2-fucosyltransferase
Kx	Kx	XK	019	*XK*	Xp21.1	Kx glycoprotein
Gerbich	Ge	GE	020	*GYPC*	2q14	Glycophorin C and glycophorin D (CD236)
Cromer	Cromer	CROM	021	*DAF*	1q32	Decay-accelerating factor (CD55)
Knops	Kn	KN	022	*CR1*	1q32	Complement receptor 1 (CD35)
Indian	In	IN	023	*CD44*	11p13	CD44
Ok	Ok	OK	024	*CD147*	19p13.3	CD147, extracellular matrix metalloproteinase inducer
Raph	Raph	RAPH	025	*CD151*	11p15.5	Tetraspanin (CD151)
John Milton Hagen	JMH	JMH	026	*SEMA7A*	15q24.3	Semaphorin (CD108)
I	I	I	027	*GCNT2*	6p24.2	β1,6 *N*-acetylglucosaminyltransferase
Globoside	P(Gb4)	GLOB	028	*B3GALNAcT1*	3q26	β1,3 *N*-acetylgalactosaminyltransferase
GIL	Gill	GIL	029	*AQP3*	9p13	Aquaglyceroporin
RHAG	RHAg	RHAG	030	*RhAG*	6p21-qter	Rh-associated glycoprotein (CD241)

From Daniels (2002, 2004) and Reid (2004).
ADP, Adenosine diphosphate; *CHIP,* channel-forming integral protein; *ICAM,* intercellular adhesion molecule; *ISBT,* International Society of Blood Transfusion; *ISGN,* International Society for Gene Nomeclature.

red cells, respectively. In contrast, the group O phenotype is an autosomal recessive phenotype, reflecting the absence of a functional ABO gene. Group O individuals express the H antigen (ISBT No. 018), the biosynthetic precursor of both A and B antigens (Fig. 35-2). Group O is the most frequent ABO phenotype in most populations tested, particularly among Native Americans. Expression of ABO antigens on RBCs is usually accompanied by the presence of naturally occurring antibodies against the missing antithetical antigen(s). Table 35-8 shows the serologic reactions and frequencies of the four major ABO phenotypes.

Null and Weak Phenotypes

The ABO system also contains several phenotypes associated with weakened, anomalous, or complete absence of ABO antigen expression. The most common ABO subtypes encountered in the blood bank are A_1 and A_2 (Table 35-9). A_1 red cells are distinguished from A_2 (and other weak A subtypes) by agglutination with the lectin *Dolichos biflorus*. Comparison of A_1, A_2, and other weak A subtypes indicates both quantitative and qualitative differences in A antigen expression (Issit, 1998; Swensson, 2005). The ABO system contains additional weak A and weak B phenotypes. The serologic characteristics of some weak group A, B, and O subtypes are shown in Table 35-10.

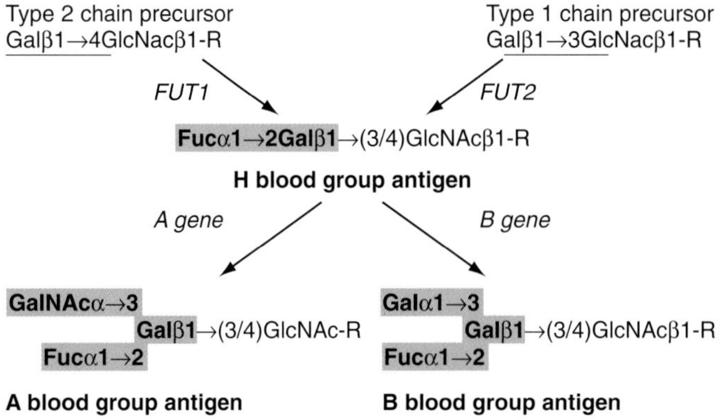

Figure 35-2 Synthesis of type 1 and type 2 chain H and AB antigens. Type 1 chain and type 2 chain precursors *(underlined)* are fucosylated by *FUT1* and *FUT2* fucosyltransferases to form H antigen. H antigen then serves as a substrate for *A* and *B* glycosyltransferases. The terminal carbohydrate epitopes denoting blood group H, A, and B antigens are highlighted in amber. *Fuc,* Fucose; *Gal,* galactose; *GalNAc, N*-acetylgalactosamine; *R,* other oligosaccharide.

TABLE 35-7
Serologic Characteristics and Clinical Significance of Red Cell Alloantibodies

Antibody	Usual Ig class	MOST COMMON PHASE OF REACTIVITY			CLINICAL SIGNIFICANCE		APPROXIMATE % OF COMPATIBLE DONORS	
		Sal	Alb	AGT	HTR	HDFN	Caucasian	Black
D	IgG	Few	X	X	Yes	Yes	15	8
C	IgG		X	X	Yes	Yes	30	68
E	IgG	Few	X	X	Yes	Yes	70	98
c	IgG		X	X	Yes	Yes	20	1
e	IgG		X	X	Yes	Yes	2	2
Cw	IgG/IgM	Some	X	X	Yes	Yes	98	100
K	IgG	Rare		X	Yes	Yes	91	97
k	IgG		X		Yes	Yes	0.2	0.1
Kp^a	IgG	Rare		X	Yes	Yes	98	99.9
Kp^b	IgG		X		Yes	Yes	<0.1	0.1
Js^a	IgG		X		Yes	Yes	>99.9	81
Js^b	IgG		X		Yes	Yes	<0.1	1
Fy^a	IgG		X		Yes	Yes	34	90
Fy^b	IgG		X		Yes	Yes	17	77
Jk^a	IgG		X		Yes	Yes	23	9
Jk^b	IgG		X		Yes	Yes	28	5
M*	IgM	X			Few	Yes	22	30
N	IgM	X			Rare	Rare	28	26
S	IgG/IgM		Some	X	Yes	Yes	45	69
s	IgG			X	Yes	Yes	11	3
U	IgG			X	Yes	Yes	0	1
Lu^a†	IgM	X			?	Yes	92	96
Lu^b†	IgG			X	Yes	Mild	<0.1	<0.1
P1‡	IgM	X	Some		Rare	No	21	6
P	IgM	X	Some	Some	Probable	Yes	<0.1	0.1
PP_1P^k†	IgG/IgM	X	Some	Some	Probable	Yes	<0.1	0.1
Le^a‡	IgM	X	Some		Yes	No	78	77
Le^b‡	IgM	X			Yes	No	28	45
I	IgM	X	Few		Rare	No	<0.1	<0.1
i	IgM	X	Few		?	No	<0.1	<0.1

AGT, Antihuman globulin test; *Alb,* albumin; *HDFN,* hemolytic disease of the fetus and newborn; *HTR,* hemolytic transfusion reaction; *Sal,* saline.
*Most examples of anti-M also have a small but significant IgG component.
†Exhibits characteristic mixed-field agglutination pattern.
‡May occasionally show in vitro hemolysis.

TABLE 35-8
Routine ABO Grouping Results and Phenotype Frequencies

CELLS AGAINST KNOWN ANTISERA		SERUM AGAINST RED CELLS OF KNOWN PHENOTYPE			FREQUENCIES IN U.S. POPULATION, %			
Anti-A	Anti-B	A	B	Interpretation	Caucasian	Black	Native American	Asian
–	–	+	+	O	45	49	79	40
+	–	–	+	A	40	27	16	28
–	+	+	–	B	11	20	4	27
+	+	–	–	AB	4	4	<1	5

Composite figures calculated from Mourant (1976).

Anomalous ABO expression can be inherited (*cis*-AB, B[A]) or acquired (acquired B). In the *cis*-AB phenotype, A and B antigens are synthesized by the same enzyme and are inherited as a single, autosomal dominant allele. Likewise, the B(A) phenotype, an autosomal dominant phenotype characterized by trace A antigen expression on group B RBCs, is due to synthesis of A antigen by the *B*-gene enzyme. The acquired B phenotype, on the other hand, is an acquired enzymatic modification of group A_1 red cells in vivo. The acquired B phenotype usually occurs in the setting of bacterial infection or cancer and reflects enzymatic deacetylation of group A antigen to form a B-like antigen on RBCs. The *cis*-AB, B(A), and acquired B phenotypes are usually detected because of discrepancies in ABO typing (Issitt, 1998; Roback, 2008).

Bombay and para-Bombay are two rare null phenotypes characterized by an absence of all ABH antigens on RBCs. In the classic Bombay phenotype (O_h), neither AB nor H antigens are present on RBCs or in secretions. Para-Bombay also shows few or no ABH antigens on RBCs, sometimes accompanied by normal expression of ABH antigens in secretions and body fluids.

Biochemistry

The ABO antigens are carbohydrate antigens and, therefore, represent a posttranslation modification of glycoproteins and glycolipids. On RBC glycoproteins and polylactosaminylceramides, ABO antigens are usually expressed on type 2 chain oligosaccharides, characterized by repeating

TABLE 35-9
Differentiating Characteristics of the A_1 and A_2 Subgroups

Group		A_1	A_2
Quantitative Differences			
Reaction with diluted anti-A		++++	++
No. of antigen sites	Adult Newborn	1,000,000 310,000	250,000 140,000
Quantitative Differences			
Reaction with *Dolichos biflorus* (anti-A_1) lectin		++++	0
Anti-A_1 in serum		No	1%–8%
Biochemistry/Molecular Differences			
Glycolipid erythrocyte variants containing antigens		A^a, A^b: linear A^c, A^d: branched Type 3A Type 4A	A^a, A^b (linear chains only) Type 4H
N-acetyl-galactosaminyltransferase activity		Normal activity Optimal at pH 6	Decreased activity Optimal at pH 7
Gene		Consensus *A101* allele	*1059-101delC* Frameshift + 21 extra amino acids

TABLE 35-10
Serologic Differentiation of the ABO Groups

	RED CELLS WITH ANTI-					SERUM WITH RED CELLS					
Phenotype	**A**	**A_1**	**B**	**A,B**	**H**	**A_1**	**B**	**O**	**Substances in saliva of secretors**	**Level of transferase in serum**	**Antigen sites per RBC3103**
A_1	++++	++++	0	++++	0/+	0	++++	0	A,H	Normal (optimal activity at pH 6.0)	810–1170
A_{int}	++++	++	0	++++	++	0	++++	0	A,H		
A_2	++++	0	0	++++	+++	*	++++	0	A,H	Decreased (optimal activity at pH 7.0)	240–1290
A_3	++mf	0	0	++mf	+++	*	++++	0	A,H	Low	30
A_x	0/±	0	0	++	++++	+†	++++	0	H	Very low	4
A_m	0‡	0	0	0	++++	0	++++	0	A,H	Low (A_1 or A_2 enzyme may be present)	0.2–1.9
B	0	0	++++	++++	++	++++	0	0	B,H	Normal	750
B_3	0	0	++mf	++mf	+++	++++	0	0	B,H	Low	
O	0	0	0	0	++++	++++	++++	0	H	Normal	1700
O_h	0	0	0	0	0	++++	++++	++++	None§ (classic Bombay)	Normal	

mf, Mixed field (minor population of agglutinates).
*May have anti-A_1 in serum.
†Ax subgroups usually have anti-A_1, but not always.
‡A antigen specificity demonstrated only after adsorption/elution procedures.
§Bombay secretors (para-Bombay) have been reported.

lactosaminyl (Galβ1–4GlcNAcβ1–3)$_n$ motifs (see Fig. 35-2). On glycosphingolipids, ABO antigens can be expressed on multiple (type 1, 2, 3, and 4 chain) oligosaccharide precursors. ABH antigens expressed on RBC glycoproteins and most glycosphingolipids (type 2, 3, and 4 chain) are of RBC origin. In contrast, type 1 chain ABO antigens are synthesized by gastrointestinal mucosa, secreted into plasma, and passively adsorbed onto red cell membranes. Synthesis of type 1 chain ABO antigens is linked to the Lewis blood group system.

The first step in the synthesis of ABH antigens is the synthesis of the H or group O antigen, the immediate biosynthetic precursor of both A and B antigens. The H antigen is formed by the addition of fucose (Fuc), in an α1–2 linkage, to a terminal galactose. This reaction is catalyzed by two different enzymes, depending on whether the fucose is being added to a type 1 or type 2 chain oligosaccharide acceptor. Fucosyltransferase type 1 (*FUT1*), the product of the H or *FUT1* gene, catalyzes the formation of type 2 chain H antigen. In contrast, fucosyltransferase type 2 *(FUT2)*, the product of the *Secretor* gene, catalyzes the transfer of fucose to type 1 chain precursors to form type 1 chain H or Le^d antigen (Lowe, 1994). Inactivating mutations in *FUT1* are responsible for the Bombay and para-Bombay phenotypes (Kelly, 1994). Bombay and para-Bombay nonsecretors also have inactivating mutations in *FUT2* (Lowe, 1994; Daniels, 2002).

Once H antigen is formed, it can serve as a substrate for *A* gene and *B* gene glycosyltransferases. The A antigen is formed by *A* gene glycosyltransferase, which adds an *N*-acetylgalactosamine (GalNAc), in an α1–3 linkage, to the subterminal galactose of H antigen. Likewise, the B antigen is formed by the addition of an α1–3 galactose (Gal) to the same galactose by the *B* gene glycosyltransferase. Biochemically, the A and B antigens are very similar, differing only by the presence of an *N*-acetyl group. It is fascinating that such a minor chemical modification should have such profound immunologic consequences. Removal of the *N*-acetyl group on A antigen by circulating deacetylase enzymes is responsible for the acquired B phenotype (Issitt, 1998).

Molecular Biology

FUT1 (*H* gene) and *FUT2* (*Se* gene) are located together on chromosome 19q13.3 and reflect a gene duplication (Lowe, 1994). FUT1 is a 365 amino acid, type II transmembrane glycoprotein, composed of a large, 240 amino acid, carboxy-terminal catalytic domain, which is anchored within the Golgi lumen by a short transmembrane and a cytosolic domain. More than 20 mutant *FUT1* alleles have been described (Issitt, 1998; Reid, 2004).

The *ABO* gene locus is located on chromosome 9q34 and encodes the A and B glycosyltransferases (Yamamoto, 1995). The gene is large,

TABLE 35-11
Key Amino Acids in Distinguishing A, B, and Hybrid Glycosyltransferases*

RBC phenotype	AMINO ACID NUMBER OF A/B GLYCOSYLTRANSFERASE 176	234	235	266	268	Gene type†
A	Arg	Pro	Gly	Leu	Gly	*AAAA*
B	Gly	Pro	Ser	Met	Ala	*BBBB*
Cis-AB	Arg	Pro	Gly	Leu	**Ala**	*AAAB*
Cis-ABTaipei	Arg	Pro	Gly	**Met**	Gly	*AABA*
Cis-AB	Gly	Pro	**Ser**	Leu	Ala	*BBAB*
B(A)	Gly	Pro	Gly	**Met**	**Ala**	*BABB*
B(A)	**Gly**	**Ala**	**Ser**	**Met**	**Ala**	*BBBB*
O03	Arg	Pro	Gly	Leu	**Arg**‡	*AAAX*

RBC, Red blood cell.
*Modified from Reid (2004) and Daniels (2002). Amino acids that differ from the A101 (A_1 type) consensus allele are highlighted in bold.
†Gene type refers to amino acid positions 176, 235, 266, and 268. These four positions differ between A (AAAA) and B alleles. Amino acids at 235, 266, and 268 strongly influence substrate specificity. Hybrid glycosyltransferases have amino acids matching both A and B consensus alleles at these positions.
‡*O03* allele (historically O^2), associated with a group O phenotype, possesses an inactivating missense mutation at amino acid 268.

spanning 18kb, and contains seven exons, although exons 6 and 7 encode the majority of the active enzyme. The product of the *ABO* gene is a 41-kD, 353 amino acid type II transmembrane glycoprotein. Comparison of A and B enzymes shows nearly 98% identity, differing by four key amino acids at residues 176, 235, 266, and 268 (Table 35-11). Amino acid 268 is absolutely critical in determining the activity and substrate specificity (UDP-GalNAc vs. UDP-Gal) of the enzyme. Substrate specificity is also influenced by amino acid residues 235 and 266. The polymorphism at residue 176 is not biologically significant. To date, more than 200 ABO alleles have been identified.

The cloning and sequencing of the *ABO* gene locus have also uncovered the molecular basis of group O and ABO subtypes. Two deletion mutants (O^1, O^{1var}) are the most common and the ancestral genes for most other group O alleles (Roubinet, 2004). It is interesting to note that the O^2 allele (*O03*), found in many Europeans, contains a single missense mutation at amino acid residue 268 (see Table 35-11) (Yamamoto, 1995). *O03* and a related allele (*Aw08*) have been linked to ABO typing discrepancies by an absence of anti-A and/or anti-B in these individuals (Wagner, 2005). It has been suggested that the absence of anti-A or -B is the result of weak residual enzyme activity (Seltsam, 2005); however, this has not been confirmed (Yazer, 2008).

Several ABO subtypes are also the result of mutations at the *ABO* gene locus, including single-nucleotide polymorphisms (SNPs) and nonsense, frameshift, and translation-initiator mutations (Yamamoto, 1995; Reid, 2004; Seltsam, 2006). For example, the A_2 and A_{el} phenotypes are associated with a single nucleotide deletion (nucleotide 1060) and frameshift, resulting in the loss of a stop codon and synthesis of a longer A enzyme with decreased enzyme activity. Single point mutations appear to be responsible for the decreased enzyme activity of A_3, A_x, A_{finn}, A_{end}, B_3, B_x, and B_v alleles (Yamamoto, 1995; Reid, 2004). In contrast, the *cis*-AB and B(A) alleles, which can synthesize both A and B antigens, are molecular chimeras with characteristics of both A_1 and *B* gene consensus alleles (see Table 35-11) (Yamamoto, 1995).

ABO Antibodies

Antibodies against ABO antigens are the most important antibodies in transfusion medicine. The practicing pathologist should note that the routine antibody screen does not test for ABO antibodies. All reagent cells in the antibody screen are group O. Patients demonstrate anti-A or anti-B on reverse typing (vide infra).

In general, ABO antibodies are naturally occurring. It is believed that the immune stimulus for the formation of ABO antibodies may be exposure to ABH-like substances found in nature, particularly on the bacterial polysaccharides. It is interesting that ABO titers have progressively decreased over the past two decades with increasing consumption of pasteurized, commercially packaged foods that are relatively sterile (Mazda, 2007). This trend may be reversed with increasing use of probiotic nutritional supplements that contain live bacteria. The latter have been shown to stimulate ABO antibodies, with marked increases in ABO titers within several months (Daniel-Johnson, 2009).

ABO antibodies are weak or absent in the sera of newborns until 3–6 months of age. Adult levels of ABO antibodies are reached by 5–10 years of age and decrease only slightly with advancing age (Auf der Maur, 1993). Anti-A,B is found exclusively in group O individuals and appears to recognize an epitope common to both A and B antigens. Before the development of anti-A and anti-B monoclonal antibody typing reagents, anti-A,B was useful in identifying Ax and weak B subgroups. Anti-A,B is still used for typing donor units and cord samples (see ABO Grouping section).

In general, ABO antibodies are detected as room temperature, saline agglutinins with optimal reactivity at 4° C (see Table 35-7). Most naturally occurring ABO antibodies are of IgM isotype, although IgA and IgG antibodies with ABO specificity are also present (Rieben, 1991). ABO IgG antibodies, reactive at 37° C, can also occur following immune stimulation by transfusion or pregnancy. These antibodies generally are of higher titer and are less readily neutralized by soluble blood group substances. ABO antibodies can fix complement and can cause hemolysis in vivo and in vitro.

Clinically, ABO antibodies are a cause of hemolytic transfusion reactions and hemolytic disease of the fetus and newborn (HDFN). ABO antibodies are also a cause of acute rejection in solid organ transplantation. As a result, solid organ transplants should be ABO compatible with the recipient's sera. Rare exceptions to the latter are heart transplantation in children younger than 6–8 months of age, who have not yet developed ABO antibodies (West, 2001), and transplantation of A_2 organs, which have very weak ABO expression on epithelium and vascular endothelium (Wu, 2003). In ABO-incompatible bone marrow transplantation, ABO antibodies can result in hemolysis and a delay in erythroid and megakaryocyte engraftment (Cooling, 2007). For additional information on ABO-incompatible marrow and organ transplants, see section on Antibody Titers.

Less Common ABO Antibodies

Anti-A_1. Anti-A_1 is a naturally occurring antibody found in the sera of some A_2, A_2B, and other weak A subtypes. Anti-A_1 hemagglutinates A_1 RBCs, but not A_2 and other weak A phenotypes. Although uncommon, anti-A_1 has been implicated in transfusion reactions and solid organ rejection.

Anti-H. Anti-H is usually a benign, naturally occurring antibody in the sera of A_1 and A_1B nonsecretors. Anti-H reacts most strongly with group O erythrocytes, followed by A_2, B, A_2B, A_1, and A_1B (refer to Table 35-48 later in this chapter). Because H antigen is present to some degree on all RBCs, anti-H is an autoantibody in most individuals. In contrast, alloanti-H is a clinically significant alloantibody in Bombay (O_h) and para-Bombay individuals. Because all RBCs express some H antigen, finding compatible RBCs can be extremely difficult in these patients.

Biological Role

The biological role of ABH antigens is still not known. Multiple studies have linked specific ABO types with a higher incidence of many diseases, including autoimmune, neoplastic, and infectious disorders. Depression of A and B antigen expression can occur in malignancy and is often associated with increased metastatic potential. Malaria has been shown to bind A and B antigens with rosette formation, a possible risk factor in cerebral malaria (Cserti, 2007). Genotyping studies suggest a "parent of origin effect" between severe malaria and inheritance of a functional maternal ABO allele (Fry, 2008). A and B antigen expression may also stabilize the clustering and spatial organization of sialoglycoproteins, which also serve as malaria receptors (Cohen, 2009). For a complete review of ABH and human disease, the reader is referred to Issitt (1998) and Garratty (1994).

MNS BLOOD GROUP SYSTEM (ISBT NO. 002)

Discovered in 1927, the MNSs blood group was the second blood group system identified after ABO. Today, the MNSs blood group system consists of more than 46 antigens, of which only four (M/N and S/s) are commonly encountered in the clinical setting (Reid, 2009). As shown in Table 35-12, the M and N antigens are fairly evenly distributed in both blacks and

TABLE 35-12
Phenotypes of the MNSs System

GLYCOPHORIN A ANTIGENS			GLYCOPHORIN B ANTIGENS					PHENOTYPE FREQUENCIES, %	
M	**N**	**En (a)**	**'N'**	**S**	**s**	**U**	**Phenotype**	**White**	**Black**
+	0	+					M+N–	28	26
+	+	+					M+N+	50	44
0	+	+					M–N+	22	30
			+	+	0	+	S+s–U+	11	3
			+	+	+	+	S+s+U+	44	28
			+	0	+	+	S–s+U+	45	69
Null Phenotypes									
0	0	0	+	+/0	+/0	+	En (a–)	Rare	Rare
0	0	0	0	0	0	0	M^kM^k	Rare	Rare
			0	0	0	0	S–s–U–	Rare	<1
			0	0	0	wk+	S–s–U^{var} (23% Henshaw+)	Rare	<1

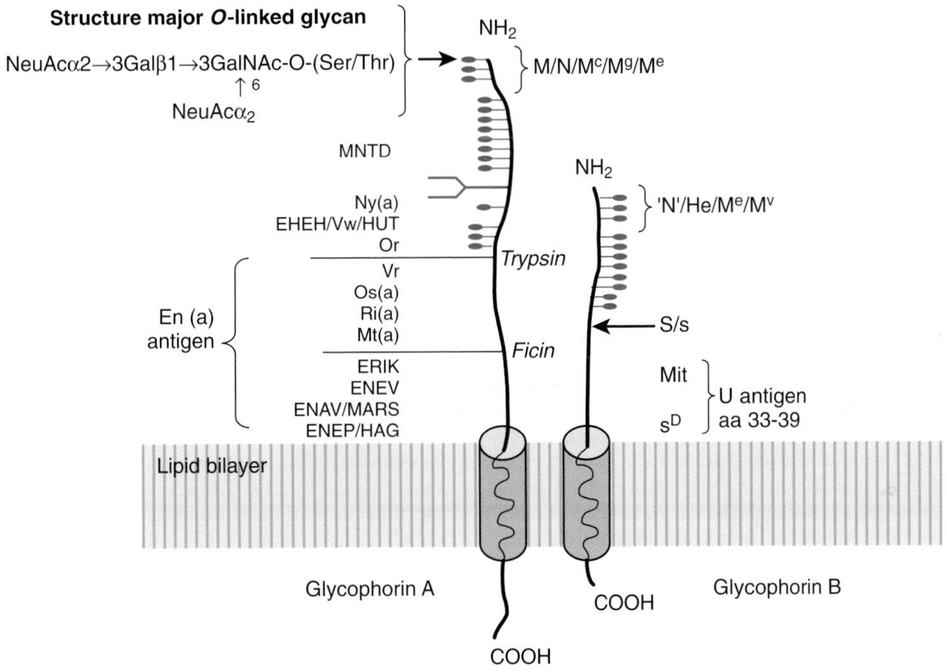

Figure 35-3 Glycophorin A (GYPA) and B (GYPB). GYPA and GYPB possess 11–15 O-linked glycans (—●), consisting predominantly of a disialotetrasaccharide (78%), along the amino-terminal half of the extracellular domain. GYPA also possesses a single, biattenary *N*-glycan, indicated by a branched structure. The single transmembrane domain for both molecules is indicated by a solid amber cylinder. The allelic antigens, M and N, reside at the extreme amino-terminus of GYPA and differ by only two amino acids at residues 1 and 5. The N antigen is also present at the amino-terminus of GYPB and is designated "N" antigen. The S/s antigens are located at amino acid 29 of GYPB. The locations of high- and low-incidence antigens are shown. The En (a) and U antigens involve large stretches of protein near the lipid bilayer and are missing in deletion and recombinant glycophorins.

Caucasians, with approximately 25% of donors homozygous for M or N antigen. In contrast, the S antigen is nearly twice as frequent in Caucasians (57%) as in black people (30%). In a minority (<1%) of blacks, an S–s– or null phenotype can be observed. As with Rh antigens, the MNSs blood group antigens are expressed only on RBCs. Approximately one million M/N and 170–250 thousand S/s epitopes are present per RBC.

Null Phenotypes

Three major null phenotypes are present in the MNSs system: U–, M^k, and En (a–). The U– phenotype is the most common and is observed exclusively in blacks. In S–s–U– individuals, complete loss or a recombination of glycophorin B occurs, leading to altered expression of S/s and U antigens. Recombinant glycophorin B, such as the Henshaw phenotype, can react weakly with some examples of human anti-U and are known as U variants (S–s–U^{var}). The En (a–) phenotype is the result of recombination between glycophorin *A* and *B* genes to form a Lepore-type A-B hybrid (exons A1-B2-B5) lacking most of glycophorin A (GYPA). The M^kM^k phenotype lacks all MNSs antigens, including En(a), as the result of recombination and deletion of glycophorins A and B (GYPA and GYPB). Loss of GYPA can coincide with loss of Wr^b expression, an antigen on Band 3. It is believed that Wr^b requires an electrostatic interaction between a glutamic acid (Glu658) on Band 3 and the ENEP antigen on glycophorin A (Poole, 1999).

Biochemistry

The M/N antigens reside on GYPA (CD235A), a major RBC membrane glycoprotein. In the membrane, GYPA is present as a dimer, usually in association with Band 3, the erythrocyte anion exchanger. Structurally, GYPA is a 31-kD, 131 amino acid, type 1 glycoprotein composed of a large, 72 amino acid extracellular domain, a transmembrane domain, and a short cytoplasmic tail (Fig. 35-3). The molecule is heavily glycosylated, possessing 15 *O*-linked and one *N*-linked carbohydrate side chain. The

O-linked glycans consist predominantly of a disialotetrasaccharide linked to a serine or threonine residue. Because of the large number of sialylated *O*-linked glycans on GYPA, nearly 60% and 50% of the total molecular weight is carbohydrate and sialic acid, respectively. Not surprisingly, GYPA is the major sialomucin on RBCs and contributes significantly to the overall negative charge or ζ potential (Huang, 1995). The M and N antigens reside on the extreme amino-terminus of GYPA.

The S/s and U antigens reside on GYPB, a related RBC glycoprotein (see Fig. 35-3). GYPB (CD235B) is a 20-kD, 72 amino acid glycoprotein composed of a large, extracellular *N*-terminal domain containing 11 *O*-linked glycans. Although GYPB shares considerable homology with GYPA at the amino-terminus, GYPB is smaller, lacking both an *N*-glycan and a cytoplasmic tail. In the membrane, GYPB appears to be closely associated with the Rh immune complex. The S/s epitope is located at amino acid 29 (Daniels, 2002).

Molecular Biology

The genes for GYPA and GYPB reside on chromosome 4q28-q31 as part of a 330-kb gene cluster encoding GYPA, GYPB, and glycophorin E (GYPE) (5′-A-B-E-3′). Studies indicate that GYPB and GYPE arose from GYPA by gene duplication and nonhomologous recombination. Similar to many erythroid-specific genes, the promoter region contains consensus sequences for Sp1 and GATA-1, an erythroid transcription regulatory binding factor (Rahuel, 1994). The greater stability of GYPA mRNA (>24 hours) over GYPB mRNA (<17 hours) may explain the greater numbers of GYPA on RBCs (Rahuel, 1994).

The biochemical nature of the MNSs antigens has long been known. The M and N antigens lie at the extreme amino-terminus of GYPA (amino acids 1–5) and include both protein and carbohydrate as part of the immune epitope. It is amino acid differences at positions 1 and 5, however, that define the M/N antigens (Table 35-13). It is not surprising that several low-incidence M and N antigen variants are the result of different amino acid substitutions (M^g, M^c) and/or altered expression of *O*-linked glycans (M_1, Tm, Can). In addition to GYPA, the N antigen is expressed on the extreme amino-terminus of GYPB. The latter is referred to as the 'N' antigen to distinguish it from N antigen on GYPA (Issitt, 1998). GYPA also possesses several high-incidence antigens (see Table 35-13).

Unlike the complexity of the M/N antigens, the S/s antigen is a single amino acid polymorphism on GYPB (Met29Thr). The U antigen is a high-incidence antigen involving amino acids 33–39 on GYPB. Loss of S–s–U antigens can be observed with M^k and other recombinant GYPB alleles such as Henshaw. It is estimated that 90% Henshaw+ RBCs are U– or U^{var} and account for 23% of all S–s–U– patients.

Recombination resulting in recombinant glycophorin proteins is associated with the loss of high-frequency antigens and the generation of new, low-frequency antigens (see Table 35-13). Historically, these were classified as the Miltenberger subsystem. Misalignments with single crossovers leading to A-B Lepore-type (e.g., Hil) and B-A anti-Lepore (Dantu) variants are known, as are gene conversion or double crossover events, in which segments of one glycophorin are inserted into the other to form B-A-B and A-B-A hybrids (Reid, 2004, 2009). Mutant GYP molecules can express MNSs antigens more strongly or weakly than normal and display unusual resistance or sensitivity to enzyme treatment (Reid, 2009). Some mutant GYPs are associated with increased Band 3 (Diego) expression (Hsu, 2009).

MNSs Antibodies

Anti-M and -N

Antibodies against M and N antigens are naturally occurring antibodies of IgM isotype, usually detected as room temperature saline agglutinins (see Table 35-7). Anti-M and anti-N may show dosage, reacting more weakly with heterozygous (M/N) cells than with homozygous (M/M or N/N) cells. Because the M and N antigens reside on GYPA, the reactivity of anti-M and anti-N is destroyed by pretreatment of RBCs with proteolytic enzymes or neuraminidase. Some examples of anti-M and anti-N can be enhanced by acidification of serum to pH 6.5, use of an albumin diluent, or preincubation of RBCs in a glucose-containing solution.

Clinically, anti-M is a commonly encountered antibody in the blood bank. In contrast, anti-N is distinctly uncommon, despite the fact that 25% of patients are negative for N antigen (M homozygous). The rarity of anti-N is due to the presence of 'N' antigen on GYPB. When observed, anti-N is usually an autoantibody, reacting with both N and 'N' antigens. An autoanti-N (anti-N_f) was reported in hemodialysis patients in the past, caused by the use of formaldehyde to sterilize membranes. Formaldehyde reacted with the terminal leucine on N and 'N' antigens, creating a neoantigen (Issitt, 1998). In general, anti-M and anti-N are clinically insignificant antibodies and only rarely cause hemolytic transfusion reactions or HDFN. In contrast, potent hemolytic alloanti-N is observed in patients lacking GYPB (M+N–S–s– phenotype). In these patients, severe hemolytic transfusion reactions and HDFN can occur after transfusion of N+ RBCs.

Anti-S, -s, and -U

Unlike anti-M and anti-N, antibodies against S, s, and U antigens are always clinically significant (see Table 35-7). All are antibodies of IgG isotype, reactive at 37° C, arising from immune stimulation. Some examples of anti-S and anti-s show dosage. Enzymatic modification of RBCs with proteases, but not neuraminidase, can decrease the reactivity of some anti-S and anti-s. The reactivity of anti-U is resistant to proteolytic digestion. Anti-S, -s, and -U are causes of hemolytic transfusion reactions and HDFN.

Biological Role

Despite the prevalence of GYPA and GYPB on RBCs, their biological role is still unknown: Their absence is not associated with any known hematologic or pathologic sequelae. Because they are rich in *O*-glycans and sialic acid, GYPA and GYPB contribute significantly to the ζ potential of red cells, decreasing homotypic and heterotypic red cell adhesion. GYPA also facilitates transport and expression of Band 3 (AE1/Diego), a critical protein in gas exchange. Increased Band 3 expression and osmotic resistance can be observed with Miltenberger type III red cells, a GYP B-A-B hybrid (Hsu, 2009). Finally, GYPA and GYPB may play a role in *Plasmodium falciparum* infections. *P. falciparum* can adhere to RBCs via sialic acid, which is highly expressed on glycophorins. Glycophorin-deficient phenotypes, such as En (a–), are relatively resistant to *P. falciparum* in vitro. Similar results can be obtained after neuraminidase treatment of RBCs (Garratty, 1994).

P BLOOD GROUP SYSTEM (ISBT NO. 003 AND 028)

The P blood group system historically consists of one antigen (P1, ISBT 003) and two members of the GLOB collection, P^k and P (ISBT 028). Similar to the Lewis system (see later), the P blood group antigens are glycosphingolipids, consisting of an antigenically active carbohydrate moiety covalently linked to a ceramide lipid tail. P^k and P antigens are high-frequency antigens on most donor RBCs (>99.9%). RBCs are particularly rich in P antigen, which makes up nearly 6% of the total RBC lipid (van Deenen, 1974). P^k and P antigens are also expressed on nonerythroid cells, including lymphocytes, platelets, plasma, kidney, lung, heart, endothelium, placenta, uroepithelium, fibroblasts, and synovium (Cooling, 1995, 1998; Spitalnik, 1995). In contrast, the P1 antigen is uniquely expressed on RBCs (Cooling, 1998). Approximately 79% of Caucasian and 94% of black donors express P1 on their RBCs (Table 35-14). P1 expression is variable between individuals and can be lost with in vitro storage.

Null/Weak Phenotypes

Several P blood group phenotypes have been described (see Table 35-14). The P_1 and P_2 phenotypes account for >99% of donors. Both possess P^k and P antigens and differ only in expression of the P1 antigen. Three autosomal recessive null phenotypes have been identified, as well as weak variants (Issitt, 1998; Kundu, 1978, 1980). The molecular basis for the null phenotypes has been elucidated (Steffensen, 2000; Hellberg, 2002). An association between the P^k variant and Luke (LKE)-negative phenotype has been noted in some donors (Cooling, 2001, 2003a). Because they lack P antigen, p and P^k individuals are resistant to parvovirus B19 (Brown, 1994).

Biochemistry

Synthesis of the P^k, P, and P_1 antigens proceeds from the stepwise addition of sugars to lactosylceramide, a ceramide dihexose (CDH) (Fig. 35-4). The first step is the synthesis of the P^k antigen, the ultimate precursor of all globo-type glycosphingolipids. To make P^k antigen, Gb_3 synthase (α4GalT1) adds a galactose, in an α1–4 linkage, to CDH. The P^k antigen can then serve as a substrate for Gb_4 synthase (β3GalNAcT1). In some cells, including RBCs, the P antigen is further elongated to form

TABLE 35-13
MNSs Blood Group Antigens

HIGH FREQUENCY						LOW FREQUENCY	
ISBT	**Name**	**Frequency**	**Glycophorin***	**Amino acid change (high→low)**	**Frequency**	**Name**	**ISBT**
MNS1	M	78%	GYPA	Ser^1-Ser-Thr-Thr-Gly^5			
MNS2	N	72%	GYPA	Leu^1-Ser-Thr-Thr-Glu^5			
MNS4	s	89%–93%	GYPB	Thr29>Met	31%–55%	S	MNS3
MNS5	U	≥99%	GYPB	Amino acids 33–39			
			B-AM-B	Trp^1-Ser-Thr-Thr-Gly^5	3%–7% blacks	He	MNS6
			B-A-B/A-B-A	Mutant GYP: exons A2- Bψ^3	Rare	Mi^a	MNS7
			GYPA	Ser^1-Ser-Thr-Thr-Glu^5	Rare	M^c	MNS8
MNS40	ENEH	100%	GYPA	Thr28>Met	Rare	V^w	MNS9
			GYPA	Thr28>Lys	Rare	HUT	MNS19
			B-A-B	Mutant GYPB: pseudoexon 3	6%–9% Asians	Mur	MNS10
			GYPA	Leu^1-Ser-Thr-Asn^4-Glu^5	Rare	M^g	MNS11
			GYPA	Ser47>Tyr	Rare	Vr	MNS12
MNS13	Me	78%	GYPA/GP:He	Gly^5 of GYPA and Henshaw+			
			GYPA	Thr58>Ile	1% Thai	Mt^a	MNS14
			B-A	Mutant GYP: exons B2–A2/A4	2% Asian	St^a	MNS15
			GYPA	Glu55>Lys	Rare	Ri^a	MNS16
			Unknown	Unknown	Rare	Cl^a	MNS17
			GYPA	Asp27>Glu	Rare	Ny^a	MNS18
			A-B/A-B-A	Mutant GYP: exons A3–B4	6% Chinese	Hil	MNS20
			GYPB	Leu^1-Ser-Ser-Thr-Glu^5	Rare	Mv	MNS21
				Unknown	Rare	Far	MNS22
			GYPB	Pro39>Arg	Rare	sD	MNS23
			GYPB	Arg35>His	Rare	Mit	MNS24
			B-A	Mutant GYP: exons B4–A5	0.5% blacks	Dantu	MNS25
			GYPA	Arg49>Thr	0.7% Thai	Hop	MNS26
MNS29	ENKT	100%	GYPA	Arg49>Thr; Tyr52>Ser	Rare	m	MNS27
MNS28	En (a–)	100%	GYPA	GPA molecule			
MNS30	"N"	>99%	GYPB	Leu^1-Ser-Thr-Thr-Glu^5			
			GYPA	Arg31>Trp	Rare	Or	MNS31
			A-B-A	Mutant GYP: Asn45	0.4% Danish	DANE	MNS32
			A-B	Mutant GYP: exons A3–B4, S+	Rare	TSEN	MNS33
			A-B/B-A-B	Mutant GYP: exons A3–B4	6% Chinese	MINY	MNS34
			B-A-B/A-ψB-A	Mutant GP: Anti Mur+HUT	6% Chinese	MUT	MNS35
			A-B	Mutant GYP: exons A4–B5	Rare	SAT	MNS36
			GYPA	Gly59>Arg	Rare	ERIK	MNS37
			GYPA	Pro54>Ser	Rare	Os^a	MNS38
MNS39	ENEP	100%	GYPA	Ala65>Pro	Rare	HAG	MNS41
MNS42	ENAV	100%	GYPA	Glu63>Lys	15% Native Americans	MARS	MNS43
MNS44	ENDA	100%	A-B-A	Mutant GYP: DANE+Mur+			
MNS45	ENEV	100%	GYPA	Val62>Gly			
			GYPA	Thr17>Arg	Rare	MNTD	MNS46

From Daniels (2002, 2007) and Reid (2004, 2009).
ISBT, International Society of Blood Transfusion.
*Glycophorin A (GYPA), glycophorin B (GYPB) or hybrid, recombinant glycophorins containing elements of GYPA and GYPB. ψB refers to GYPB pseudoexons.

additional, globo-family antigens such as Luke (LKE), Forssman, NOR, and type 4 chain ABH antigens (globo-ABH) (Roback, 2008).

Unlike P^k and P antigens, the P1 antigen is not a globo-glycosphingolipid but is a member of the neolacto-family (type 2 chain glycosphingolipids). In P_1 individuals, a terminal α1,4 galactose is added to paragloboside to form P1. The P1 antigen is not expressed on RBC glycoproteins despite the presence of multiple type 2 chain precursors (polylactosamine) on *N*-linked glycans (Yang, 1994).

Molecular Biology

The genes responsible for P^k, P1, and P have been cloned. It is believed that both P^k and P1 antigens are synthesized by α4GalT1, an α1,4 galactosyltransferase (Steffensen, 2000; Iwamura, 2003). The *α4GalT1* gene resides on chromosome 22q13 and is organized into two exons, of which only one (exon 2) encodes the enzyme. The α4GalT1 enzyme is a 353 amino acid type II glycoprotein containing two *N*-glycosylation sites and five cysteine residues. Similar to many galactosyltransferases, it possesses a DXD motif or a UDP-Gal binding site. Several missense and frameshift mutations (insertions and deletions) in the enzyme catalytic domain have been identified among p individuals (Steffensen, 2000; Koda, 2002). The absence of P1 antigen in P_2 individuals was originally reported as the result of decreased transcription arising from mutations in the *α4GalT1* promoter (-551C-500; Iwamura, 2003); however, subsequent studies questioned these findings (Tilley, 2006). A more recent study indicates that P1 synthesis arises from an alternate start codon and α4GalT1 transcript (Thursson, 2009). As a result, the P1 system has been renamed P1PK by the ISBT.

Globoside or P antigen, a β1,3 *N*-acetylgalactosaminyltransferase, is the product of β3GalNAcT1 (β3GalT3 in original literature; Okajima, 2000). The gene resides on chromosome 3q25 and contains six exons,

TABLE 35-14
P Blood Group System

			MOLECULAR BASIS		FREQUENCIES, %	
RBC phenotype	**RBC antigens**	**Possible antibodies**	**A4GalT1**	**B3GALNAcT1**	**Caucasian**	**Black**
P_1	P^k, P, P_1	None	Normal	Normal	79	94
P_2	P^k, P	Anti-P_1	Alternate start codon*	Normal	21	6
Null Phenotypes						
P_1^k	↑P^k, P_1	Anti-P	Normal	Null allele†	Rare	Rare
P_2^k	↑P^k	Anti-P, anti-P_1	Alternate start codon*	Null allele†	Rare	Rare
p	None	Anti-$P^k PP_1$ (Tj^a)	Null allele‡	Normal	Rare	Rare
Weak Phenotypes						
Variant P^k	↑P^k, ↓P	Anti-P	Unknown	Unknown	Rare	Rare
Weak P	↓P^k, ↓P	None	Unknown	Unknown	Rare	Rare

RBC, Red blood cell.
*Recent study suggests that P_1 is transcribed by an alternate α4GalT1 transcript (Thursson, 2009).
†Multiple inactivating mutations have been identified in β3GalNAcT1 open reading frame associated with the P^k phenotype (Hellberg, 2002).
‡Multiple inactivating mutations have been identified in α4GalT1 open reading frame associated with the p phenotype (Steffensen, 2000; Koda, 2002).

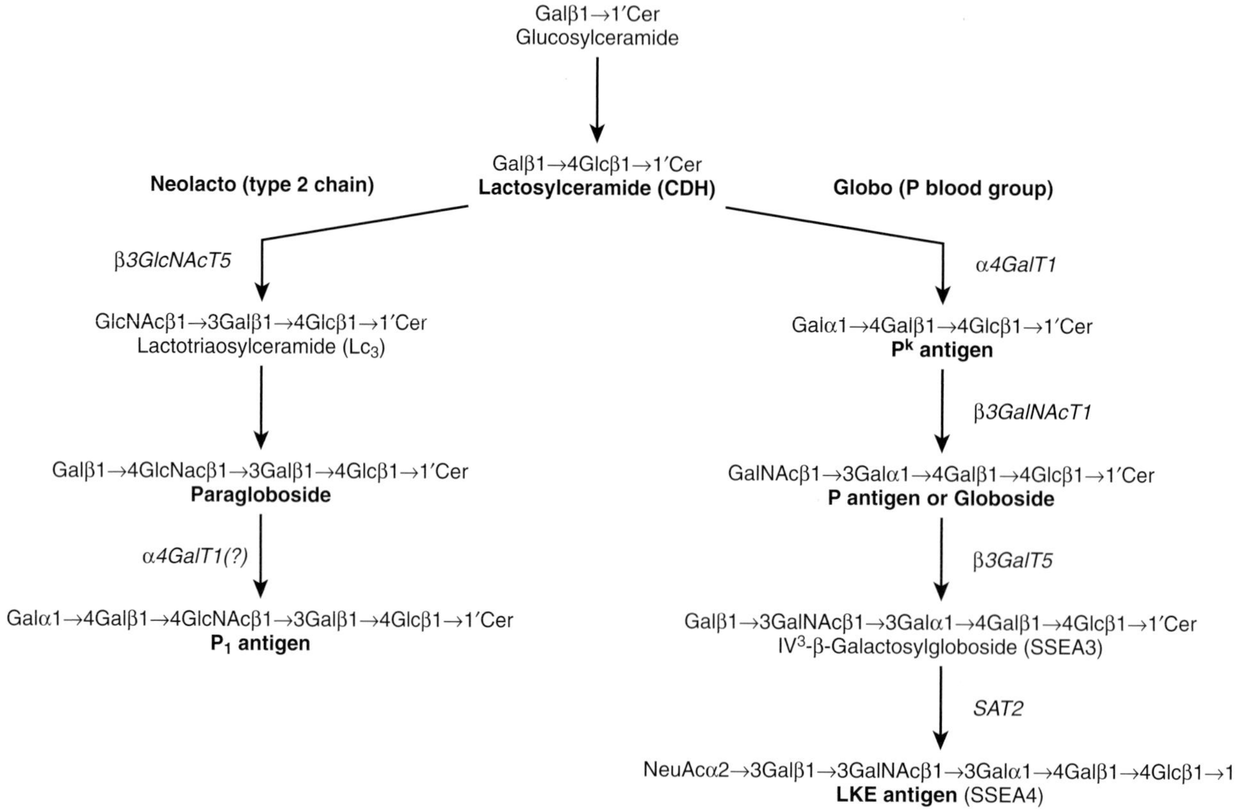

Figure 35-4 Synthesis of P blood group antigens. *Cer,* Ceramide; *Gal,* galactose; *GalNAc,* N-acetylgalactosamine; *Glc,* glucose; *GlcNAc,* N-acetylglucosamine; *SSEA,* stage-specific embryonic antigen; *NeuAc,* acetylneuraminic acid.

although only exon 6 encodes the enzyme. A member of the β1,3 galactosyltransferase family, β3GalNAcT1 possesses seven conserved domains common to most β1,3 galactosyltransferases, as well as a DXD motif. A variety of mutations have been identified in P^k individuals (Hellberg, 2002). In mice, the absence of β3GalNAcT1 is lethal (Vollrath, 2001).

P Blood Group Antibodies

Anti-P_1

Clinically, the most common antibody observed is anti-P_1, which is detected in one quarter to two thirds of P_2 donors (Issitt, 1998). Anti-P_1 is a naturally occurring antibody of IgM isotype and is often detected as a weak, room temperature agglutinin. Rare examples of anti-P_1 are reactive at 37° C or show in vitro hemolysis. Because P1 expression varies in strength between individuals, anti-P_1 may not react with all P1-positive cells tested. Anti-P_1 can bind complement and may be detected in the indirect antiglobulin test (IAT) if polyspecific antihuman globulin (AHG) is used. Antibody reactivity can be eliminated by prewarming sera or by adding soluble P1 substance from hydatid cyst fluid, earthworms, and bird eggs. Anti-P1 titers are often elevated in patients with hydatid cyst disease or fascioliasis (liver fluke), and in bird fanciers (Issitt, 1998). Some examples of anti-P_1 have I blood group specificity (anti-IP_1).

In general, anti-P_1 is not clinically significant, and its presence rarely requires transfusion of antigen-negative blood. The exception is seen in patients with an anti-P_1 showing in vitro hemolysis. Because of the risk of immediate and delayed hemolytic transfusion reactions, these patients should receive P1-negative (P_2), crossmatch compatible units. Anti-P_1 is not a cause of HDFN.

Alloanti-PP$_1$P^k

Anti-PP$_1$P^k (historically known as anti-Tj^a) is a separable mixture of anti-P, anti-P$_1$, and anti-P^k in the sera of p individuals. These antibodies are naturally occurring and may be IgM only or IgM plus IgG (IgG3). Because anti-PP$_1$P^k antibodies are potent hemolysins, patients can be transfused only with p RBCs. In women, alloanti-PP$_1$P^k and alloanti-P are associated with HDFN and spontaneous abortion. Early and frequent plasmapheresis has been used with therapeutic success in alloimmunized pregnant women of the p and P^k phenotypes (Spitalnik, 1995).

Alloanti-P

Anti-P is also a naturally occurring IgM alloantibody in the serum of P^k (and p) individuals. It is a potent hemolysin and can cause in vivo hemolysis following transfusion of P-positive (P$_1$ and P$_2$) RBCs. Alloanti-P is a cause of HDFN and is associated with spontaneous abortions.

Auto-Anti-P (Donath-Landsteiner)

An autoantibody with anti-P specificity is seen in patients with paroxysmal cold hemoglobinuria (PCH), a clinical syndrome that may occur in children following viral infection. In PCH, autoanti-P is an IgG, biphasic hemolysin capable of binding RBCs at colder temperatures, followed by intravascular hemolysis at body temperature. This characteristic can be demonstrated in vitro in the Donath-Landsteiner test. See full description in later sections on immunohematologic methods.

Biological Role

Unlike many antigens, the physiologic role of the P blood group antigens is not known. Evidence suggests that the P^k antigen may be associated with the α-interferon and major histocompatibility class II receptors (Ghislain, 1994; George, 2001) and may modulate cell signaling via lipid rafts (Kovbasnjuk, 2001). The P blood group antigens may also play a role in cellular differentiation and neoplasia. The P^k and P antigens are differentially expressed during embryogenesis, hematopoiesis, and intestinal mucosal differentiation (Jacewicz, 1995; Cooling, 2003b). The P^k antigen is a marker of apoptosis in germinal center B cells, Burkitt lymphoma, and lymphoblastic leukemia (Mangeney, 1991). LKE is a marker of embryonic and mesenchymal stem cells (Gang, 2007) and is implicated in adhesion, cell signaling, and metastasis in renal cell and breast carcinoma (Satoh, 1996; Steelant, 2002).

Several P blood group antigens are receptors for microbial pathogens. The P blood group antigen is the receptor for parvovirus B19, a single-stranded DNA virus associated with multiple clinical sequelae, including aplastic crises (Brown, 1994; Cooling, 1995). P^k can bind human immunodeficiency virus (HIV) and may confer resistance to HIV infection (Lund, 2009). The P1 and P^k antigens are receptors for shiga toxins, produced by *Shigella dysenteriae* and enterohemorrhagic *Escherichia coli* (EHEC) strains. In addition to gastroenteritis, EHEC infection is the most common cause of community-acquired hemolytic-uremic syndrome, probably reflecting toxin binding to P^k antigen on glomerular vascular endothelium and platelets (Boyce, 1995; Cooling, 1998; Karpman, 2001). P, P^k, and LKE blood group antigens on uroepithelium are cell receptors for P-fimbriae, a bacterial adhesin and colonization factor expressed on uropathogenic *E. coli* strains. The P^k antigen also serves as a receptor for *Streptococcus suis* and *Pseudomonas aeruginosa* (Spitalnik, 1995).

RH AND RHAG BLOOD GROUP SYSTEMS (ISBT NO. 004 AND 030)

The first and most clinically important characterization of the Rh system antigens came when Landsteiner and Wiener (1940) published studies of animal experiments involving the immunization of guinea pigs and rabbits with rhesus monkey RBCs. The resulting antiserum agglutinated 85% of human RBCs, and the antigen defined was called the Rh (rhesus) factor. This anti-Rh was later reported to have the same specificity as antibodies studied earlier by Levine and Stetson (1939) that were responsible for HDFN. It is interesting to note that the anti-Rh developed by Landsteiner and Wiener was later shown to recognize a different blood group antigen, named LW for its discoverers.

Today, the Rh system is probably the most complex red cell antigen system in humans, encompassing some 50 antigens, many phenotypic variants, and complex serologic relationships. Hence, the following review is basic and highlights the most current information. For a detailed, historical review of the Rh system, readers should consult Issitt (1998) and Daniels (2002).

TABLE 35-15
Comparison of Wiener, Fisher-Race, and Rosenfield Nomenclatures for Antigens of the Rh Blood Group System

Wiener	Fisher-Race	Rosenfield
Rho	D	RH1
rh′	C	RH2
rh″	E	RH3
hr′	c	RH4
hr″	e	RH5

TABLE 35-16
Wiener and Fisher-Race Nomenclatures for the Rh Haplotypes and Their Population Frequencies*

		FREQUENCIES IN U.S. POPULATION			
Wiener	Fisher-Race†	Caucasian	Black	Native American	Asian
R0	Dce	0.04	0.44	0.02	0.03
R_1	DCe	0.42	0.17	0.44	0.70
R_2	DcE	0.14	0.11	0.34	0.21
Rz	DCE	0.00	0.00	0.06	0.01
r	ce	0.37	0.26	0.11	0.03
r′	Ce	0.02	0.02	0.02	0.02
r″	cE	0.01	0.00	0.01	0.00
r^y	CE	0.00	0.00	0.00	0.00

*Composite figures calculated from Mourant (1976).

†In historical Fisher-Race nomenclature, RhD-negative was designated as "d." At this time, RhD-negative phenotypes using Fisher-Race denote only the RHCE antigens present on red cells.

Theories of Rh Inheritance and Classification System

Using five basic antisera—anti-D, anti-C, anti-E, anti-c, and anti-e—Wiener identified five different factors or antigens (Table 35-15) that, from population and family studies, appeared to be inherited as two complexes of up to three factors each. Eight possible combinations of three-factor complexes were identified if one included "d" as designating the lack of D, because no anti-d had ever been demonstrated. Wiener proposed a single-locus inheritance system with eight alternative common alleles coding for two Rh agglutinogens, capable of expressing up to three different antigenic determinants. Wiener's nomenclature for the eight different genes and allelic frequencies is provided in Tables 35-16 and 35-17.

Fisher and Race later proposed a different inheritance theory and nomenclature system based on genetic evidence of the antithetical or allelic nature of the C/c and E/e antigens (Race, 1948). These investigators proposed a system of three closely linked loci or subloci on each chromosome, which were inherited as a block of genes (haplotype). They also introduced the DCE nomenclature to name the alleles, including the use of "d" to designate the lack of D locus (see Table 35-15). Rosenfeld proposed a numeric system of naming the antigens in 1962, because the increasing number of Rh antigens rendered an alphabetic notation impractical (Table 35-18). It was also appreciated that this nomenclature contained no inferences as to the genetic inheritance of the antigens.

Biochemistry

Tremendous progress has been made in deciphering the biochemistry and molecular biology of the Rh blood group system. It is now clear that Rh complex consists of three integral membrane proteins: RhD, RhCE, and Rh-associated glycoprotein (RhAg). RhD and RhCE are highly homologous proteins, differing by approximately 30 amino acids. Both are 30-kD, 416 amino acid multipass proteins containing 12 transmembrane domains, six extracellular loops, and a cytoplasmic amino- and carboxy-terminus (Fig. 35-5). Both proteins possess two to three molecules of palmitate (C16 fatty acid) covalently linked to transmembrane cysteine residues. Palmitoylation of Rh proteins may help maintain the phospholipid asymmetry of the RBC membrane (Avent, 1999).

TABLE 35-17
Frequencies of Common Rh Phenotypes*

REACTION WITH ANTI-†					PHENOTYPE		GENOTYPE		FREQUENCIES, n (%)‡			
D	C	c	E	e	Rh	DCE	Rh	DCE	Caucasian	Black	Native American	Asian
+	+	+	+	+	Rh_1Rh_2	DCcEe	R^1R^2	DCe/DcE	0.1176 (89)	0.0374 (100)	0.2992 (89)	0.294 (97)
							R^1r''	DCe/cE	0.0084 (6)		0.0088 (3)	
							$r'R^2$	Ce/DcE	0.0056 (5)		0.0135 (4)	0.0084 (2.8)
							rR^z	ce/DCE		0.0132 (4)	0.0006 (0.2)	
+	+	+	−	+	Rh_1rh	DCce	R^1R^0	DCe/Dce	0.0168 (5)	0.1495 (63)	0.0176 (15)	0.042 (50)
							R^1r	DCe/ce	0.3108 (95)	0.0884 (37)	0.0968 (85)	0.042 (50)
+	−	+	+	+	Rh_2rh	DcEe	R^2R^0	DcE/Dce	0.0112 (10)	0.0968 (63)	0.0136 (15)	0.0126 (50)
							R^2r	DcE/ce	0.1035 (90)	0.0572 (37)	0.0748 (85)	0.0126 (50)
+	+	−	−	+	Rh_1Rh_1	DCe	R^1R^1	DCe/DCe	0.176 (91)	0.029 (81)	0.194 (92)	0.490 (93)
							R^1r'	DCe/Ce	0.017 (9)	0.007 (19)	0.017 (8)	0.028 (7)
+	+	−	+	+	Rh_1Rhz	DCEe	R^1R^z	DCe/DCE		0.053 (100)		
+	−	+	+	−	Rh_2Rh_2	DcE	R^2R^2	DcE/DcE	0.02 (88)	0.012 (100)	0.116 (94)	0.044 (100)
							R^2r''	DcE/cE	0.003 (12)		0.007 (6)	
+	+	+	+	−	Rh2Rhz	DCcE	R^2R^z	DcE/DCE			0.041 (100)	
+	−	+	−	+	Rh_0Rh_0	Dce	R^0R^0	Dce/Dce	0.0016 (5)	0.1936 (46)	0.0004 (8)	0.0009 (33)
							R^0r	Dce/ce	0.0296 (95)	0.2286 (54)	0.0044 (92)	0.0018 (67)
−	−	+	−	+	rhrh	ce	rr	ce/ce	0.1369 (100)	0.0676 (100)	0.0121 (100)	0.0009 (100)
−	+	+	−	+	rh′rh	Cce	rr′	ce/Ce	0.0055 (100)	0.0014 (100)	0.0044 (100)	0.0012 (100)
−	−	+	+	+	rh″rh	cEe	rr″	ce/cE	0.0028 (100)		0.0022 (100)	

*Estimated from haplotype frequencies (p, q from Table 35-16) using p2 for homozygotes and 2pq for heterozygotes.
†+, Positive; −, negative.
‡%, Percentage of genotypes within a given phenotype.

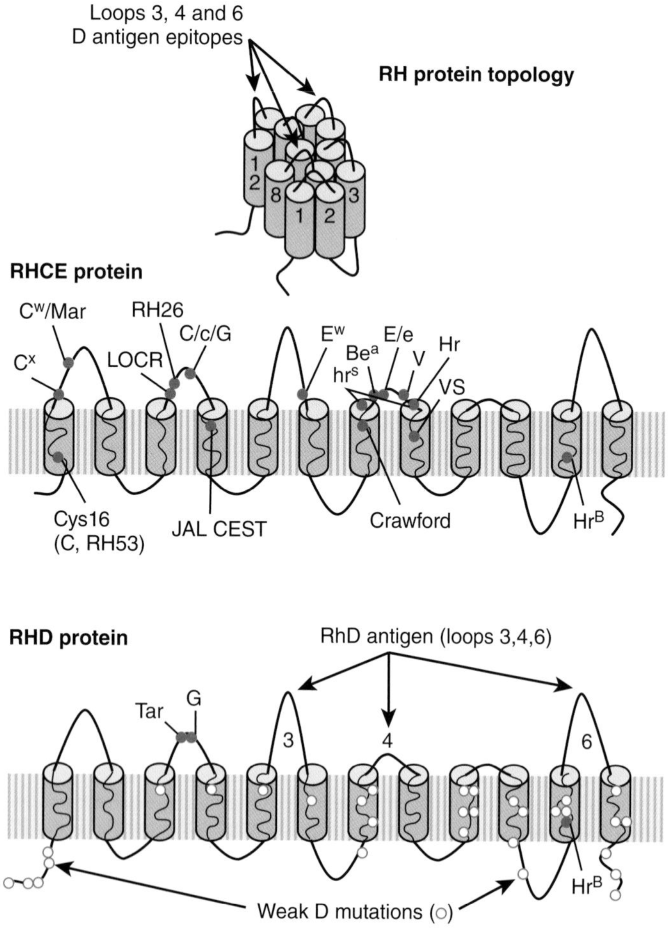

Figure 35-5 RH proteins. Both RHD and RHCE proteins are multipass proteins with 12 transmembrane domains, indicated by solid amber cylinders. The location of Rh antigens denoted by single–amino acid polymorphisms is denoted (•). The RhD epitope is a complex antigen involving structures on the third, fourth, and sixth extracellular loops. Missense mutations in RHD, leading to weak D expression, are indicated by open circles (o).

RhAg is a 45–70-kD multipass glycoprotein, evolutionarily related to RhD and RhCcEe glycoproteins. RhAg is a 409 amino acid glycoprotein with 12 transmembrane domains and a single, large *N*-linked carbohydrate side chain on the first extracellular loop. Overall, approximately 170,000 molecules each of Rh and RhAg proteins are present per RBC. RhD, RhCE, and RhAg are erythroid-specific proteins (Avent, 1999).

In the RBC membrane, RhD, RhCE, and RhAg proteins exist as part of an Rh immune complex, composed of two molecules of Rh (RhD and RhCE) and two molecules of RhAg (Eyers, 1994). The importance of RhAg for the expression and correct assembly of Rh proteins cannot be understated. In the absence of functional RhAg protein, neither RhD nor RhCE proteins will be expressed (Rh_{null} and Rh_{mod} phenotypes). In addition to RhAg, Rh proteins may be topologically associated with CD47 (Lutheran), ICAM4 (LW), DARC (Duffy), Band 3 (Diego), and GYPB. At least two non-Rh antigens, Fy5 and U, may require noncovalent interactions between Rh, DARC glycoprotein (Fy5), and GYPB (U), respectively (Ridgwell, 1994).

Molecular Biology

The genes for RhD (*RHD*) and RhCE (*RHCE*) proteins span 65kb on chromosome 1p34-36.1 and share nearly 92% sequence identity. The two genes are separated by only 30kb and have opposite orientations, facing each other at their 3′ ends (Fig. 35-6). The *RHD* gene is also flanked by two homologous sequences known as rhesus boxes. The *RHAG* gene (*RHAG*) resides on chromosome 6p11.1 and shares 36% homology with the *RHD* and *RHCE* genes. All three genes possess 10 exons and at least one GATA-1 consensus sequence in the promoter region (Cherif-Zahar, 1994; Iwamoto, 1998). It is believed that *RHAG* and *RH* genes arose by gene duplication 250–350 million years ago. A second gene duplication 8–11 million years ago resulted in the ce and D alleles (cDe or R_0 haplotype). The remaining RHCe alleles are believed to be the product of point mutations, recombination, and gene conversion of the *RHD* and *RHCE* genes (Avent, 1999).

D Antigen

The cloning of *RHD* and *RHCE* genes opened the door to understanding the complex immunology of many Rh antigens and phenotypes. The D antigen, the most immunogenic of all the Rh antigens, resides on the RHD protein. Current evidence suggests that D is a highly complex antigen, depending on both specific amino acids and the tertiary structure of the RHD protein itself. At least nine "D-specific" amino acids (Met169,

TABLE 35-18
Molecular Basis for RH and RHAG Antigens

ISBT	Name	Frequency, %	RH protein (D or CE)	Molecular basis (protein or gene exon)	Comments
RH (ISBT 004)					
RH1	D	85–92	D	RHD, loops 3,4,6	
RH2	C	68% Caucasian people 27% black people	CE	Ser103 + Cys16	Antithetical RH4
RH3	E	22–29	CE	Pro226	Antithetical RH5
RH4	c	80	CE	Pro103	Antithetical RH2
RH5	e	80	CE	Ala226 Dependence on Arg229	Antithetical RH3
RH6	f	65	CE	Pro103 + Ala226 Dependence on Arg229	Compound antigen
RH7	Ce	27–28	CE	Ser103 + Ala226	Compound antigen
RH8	C^w	1–2	CE	Gln41>Arg	Antithetical RH51
RH9	C^x	<0.01	CE	Ala36>Thr	Antithetical RH51
RH10	V	30% black people	CE	Leu235>Val, +Gly336	Often with RH20
RH11	E^w	<0.01	CE	Met167>Lys	E variant type I
RH12	G	84–92	D, CE	Ser103	Anti-C+D
RH17	Hr_0	100	CE	RHCE loops 3,4,6	
RH18	Hr	100	CE	Met238	
RH19	hr^S	98	CE	Ala226, Met238	
RH20	VS	40% black people	CE	Leu226>Val	Often with RH10
RH21	C^G	68	CE	Ser103	
RH22	CE	1	CE	Ser103 + Pro226	Compound antigen
RH23	D^w	<0.01	Partial D	Gln233, RHD loop 3,6	
RH26	c-like	80	CE	Gly96 + Pro103	
RH27	cE	22–28	CE	Pro103 + Pro226	Compound antigen
RH28	hr^H	<0.01	?	Unknown	
RH29	Total Rh	100	CE + D	RHD + RHCE	Made by Rh_{null}
RH30	Go^a	2% black people	Partial D	On DIV^a	
RH31	hr^B	98	CE	Unknown	Missing on R2R2
RH32	RN	<1% black people	Partial D	Exons D4–CE5	Antithetical RH46
RH33	Har	<0.01	Partial D	Exons CE4–D5	R_0^{Har}
RH34	Hr^B	100	D + CE	Cys336	
RH35	1114(CeMA)	<0.01	CE	Unclear; CeMA is JAL+	Weak C,e
RH36	Be^a	<0.1	CE	Pro221>Arg	Weak c,e,f
RH37	Evans	<0.01	D–CE hybrid	Exons D6–CE7	
RH39	C-like	100	?	Unknown	On C– and C+ RBCs
RH40	Tar	<0.01	D	Leu100>Pro	
RH41	Ce-like	70	CE	Exon 2, Ala226	
RH42	Ce^S	2% black people	Partial D	Leu245>Val	Associated $dCce^S$
RH43	Crawford	0.7% D- blacks	CE	Gln223>Glu, VS+	ce^S variant; VS+, V+
RH44	Nou	100	?	Unknown	
RH45	Riv	<0.01	Partial D	On DIVa	
RH46	Sec	100	CE	CE exon 4	Antithetical RH32
RH47	Dav	100	CE	Exon 7	
RH48	JAL	<0.01	CE	Arg114>Trp or Glu	Antithetical RH57
RH49	STEM	0.4% Indian people	?	Unknown	
RH50	FPTT	<0.01	Partial D	Exons CE4–D5	
RH51	MAR	>99	CE	Ala36, Gln41	Antithetical RH8,9
RH52	BARC	<0.01	Partial D	Exons CE6–D7	
RH53	JAHK	<0.01	CE	Exon D2 (Ser103), no Cys16	
RH54	DAK	<0.01	Partial D	Unknown	
RH55	LOCR	<0.01	CE	Gly95>Ser	Weak c,e,f ; Rh26±
RH56	CeNR	<0.01	CE–D hybrid	Complex epitope	D– –; RH32+
RH57	CEST	>99	CE	Arg114	Antithetical RH48 (Jal)
RHAG (ISBT 030)					
RHAG1	Duclos	>99	RhAg	Gln106>Glu	
RHAG2	Ol^a	<0.01	RhAg	Ser227>Leu	Weak Rh expression
RHAG3	DSLK	>99	RhAg	Lys164>Gln	

From Wagner and Flegel (2004), Reid (2004), Westhoff (2004), Coghlan (2006), Daniels (2009), Hue-Roye (2009), and Hustinx (2009).
ISBT, International Society of Blood Transfusion.

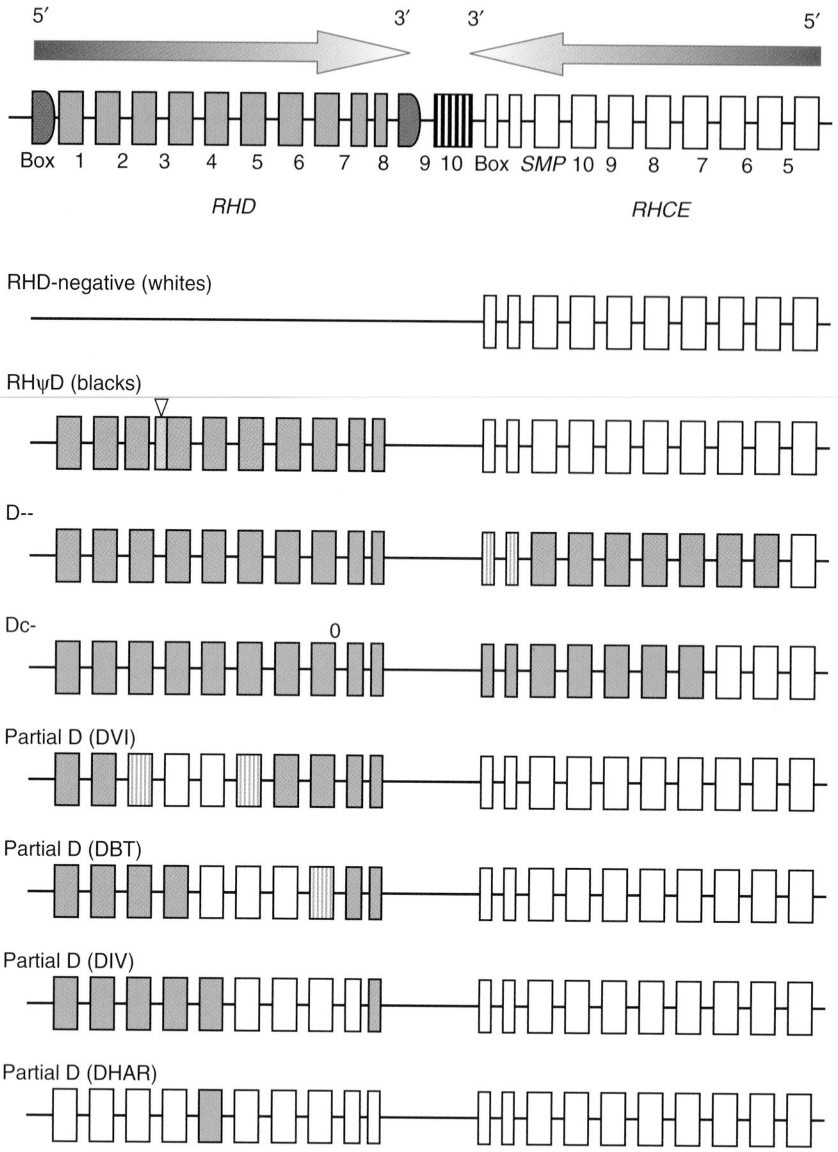

Figure 35-6 The *Rh* gene cluster. *RHD* and *RHCE* genes are closely situated and face each other at their 3′ ends. The *RHD* gene is also flanked by Rh boxes. *SMP* is an unrelated gene. RHD-negative phenotype can result from deletion of the *RHD* gene or, in black people, a 37–base pair (bp) insertion leading to a frameshift (pseudogene). Also shown are examples of partial D and CE phenotypes that are the result of recombination between *RHD* and *RHCE* genes.

Met170, Ile172, Phe223, Ala226, Glu233, Asp350, Ala353, and Gly354) have been identified as functional D epitopes. The nine amino acids lie along the third, fourth, and sixth external loops of the RHD protein, creating six distinct D-epitope clusters or footprints (see Fig. 35-5). How the immune system recognizes these clusters is a matter of intense investigation (Avent, 1999).

Weak D Antigen

Approximately 1% of D-positive individuals type as weak D (historically known as D^u), characterized by weak or absent RBC agglutination by anti-D during routine serologic testing. In weak D individuals, the D antigen usually requires enhancement with AHG owing to a quantitative decrease in RhD protein. In these individuals, the number of RhD molecules is decreased 40–100-fold, ranging from 66–5200 molecules per red cell (Reid, 2004).

A weak D phenotype can occur with many partial D phenotypes, Ce *in trans* with suppression of RHD, in the Rh_{mod} phenotype, and via autosomal recessive inheritance of two weak RHD alleles. The latter accounts for the majority of weak D phenotypes present in the general population. To date, more than 40 different weak RhD alleles have been identified. Nearly all possess missense mutations, leading to amino acid substitutions, along the transmembrane and cytoplasmic domains (see Fig. 35-5). Because of their location, it is hypothesized that these mutations may interfere with the assembly or efficient insertion of the RhD protein. Furthermore, because all the mutations are intramembranous or intracellular, it is assumed they do not significantly alter the presentation of D epitopes on the extracellular loops (Wagner, 1999). This may explain why most weak D individuals do not make alloanti-D when transfused with D-positive blood (see later).

Partial D Antigen

Partial D antigens are RHD proteins with missing D epitopes. Although they type as D-positive, persons with partial D antigens can make alloanti-D antibodies reactive with allogeneic, but not autologous, RBCs. The alloanti-D produced by these individuals recognizes D-specific epitopes missing on their own RBCs (see Fig. 35-6). Partial D can result from missense mutations or from genetic recombination of *RHD* and *RHCE* genes (Avent, 1999). Partial D phenotypes arising from genetic recombination are frequently associated with the generation of new, low-incidence antigens (see Table 35-18).

Rh-Negative Phenotype

Rh-negative (D–) occurs in approximately 15% of white donors, almost always in association with a ce/ce or rr phenotype. In most Caucasian people, D– reflects a deletion of the entire *RHD* gene (see Fig. 35-6). In blacks, D– can result from gene deletion or from inheritance of an *RHD* pseudogene. Nearly 60% of D-negative black people inherit a mutant RHD allele (RHψD) containing a 37–base pair (bp) internal duplication, frameshift, and premature stop codon (Avent, 1999). *RHD* genes containing nonsense mutations and nucleotide deletions have also been reported in some D-negative Japanese and Caucasian donors (Daniels, 2002; Reid, 2004).

C/c, E/e, and Compound Rh Antigens

In contrast to the complexity of the D antigen epitope, the C/c and E/e antigens are single–amino acid polymorphisms on the RhCE protein (see Fig. 35-5). Three additional amino acid polymorphisms (Cys16Trp, Ile-60Leu, and Ser68Asn) may help stabilize the C and c antigens. Arg229 appears critical to e and f expression (Chen, 2004). Because C/c and E/e epitopes are present on the same protein, alloantibodies dependent on the expression of both C/c and E/e antigens can occur. Four alloantibodies with "compound" Rh specificity have been described: anti-ce (f or RH6), anti-Ce (RH7), anti-cE (RH27), and anti-CE (RH22). These antibodies react only with RBCs carrying the appropriately paired antigens, in *cis*, on the same RhCE protein (see Table 35-18). The RHCE protein is home to several additional high- and low-incidence antigens.

G Antigen

The G antigen (RH12) is a high-frequency antigen present on virtually all D-positive and C-positive RBCs. G has been identified as Ser103, a C-type antigen, on RHD and RHCE proteins (see Fig. 35-5). It is not surprising that anti-G alloantibodies have both anti-C and anti-D specificity (anti-C + D) and are frequently accompanied by anti-C (anti-G + anti-C) (Shirey, 1997).

Weak and Deletion C/c and E/e Phenotypes

Similar to D, phenotypes with weakened or absent C/c and E/e are known. *RHCE* alleles with point mutations, deletions, and recombinations can lead to weakened CcEe expression. African ethnic groups, in particular, show significant molecular diversity in *RHCE* alleles. A recent study reported partial C [(C)ce^S] phenotype in nearly 25% of sickle cell patients (Noizat-Pirenne, 2009). Although these patients serologically type as C+c+, rare patients can produce an alloanti-c (Ong, 2009; Pham, 2009). Likewise, point mutations and rearrangements resulting in weakened e expression and alloantibody formation (anti-e, hr^S) are well known (Reid, 2004; Vege, 2009).

The deletion phenotypes D••, D— (↑D+, C–c–E–c–), DC– and Dc– are the result of genetic recombination between *RHCE* and *RHD* genes to yield RHCE-D-CE hybrids (see Fig. 35-6). As a consequence, total ablation of Ee and/or Cc epitopes occurs, with many recombinants expressing new low-frequency Rh antigens (see Table 35-18). Furthermore, many recombinants (e.g., D••, D—) demonstrate exalted D antigen expression on serologic testing owing to a double dose of some D epitopes on both RHD and mutant RHCE-D-CE proteins. For a detailed summary, the reader is referred to Reid (2004).

RHAG Alloantigens

RHAG is a new blood group system with three antigens; Ol^a, Duclos, and DSLK (Tilley, 2010). All three are the result of an amino acid polymorphism in the RhAg protein. Both Duclos and DSLK are associated with weak U expression, suggesting an interaction between RhAg and GYPB.

Rh_{null} Phenotype

Rh_{null} erythrocytes lack all Rh antigens as a result of an apparent absence of RhD and RhCE proteins. In addition, Rh_{null} erythrocytes lack the high-frequency antigens Fy5 and LW and may have markedly decreased expression of S/s and U antigens. The absence of these non-Rh antigens reflects the complex topologic association of Duffy, LW, and GYPB proteins with Rh proteins on RBC membranes.

Extremely rare (<1 in 6 million), Rh_{null} cells have abnormalities in RBC morphology (spherocytes, stomatocytes), water content, cell volume, cation fluxes, carbon dioxide (CO_2) permeability, and phospholipid asymmetry (Issitt, 1998; Endeward, 2006). Rh_{null} cells show increased osmotic fragility and a shortened circulating half-life, often accompanied by a mild hemolytic anemia (Rh deficiency syndrome). Because Rh_{null} individuals can become sensitized to multiple Rh antigens, including high-frequency antigens, transfusion support can be quite difficult. Some alloimmunized Rh_{null} individuals can produce anti-RH29, which reacts with all RBCs except Rh_{null}.

The Rh_{null} phenotype can arise from two distinct genetic backgrounds—regulator and amorph. The Rh_{null}-amorph type is the result of nonsense mutations in the *RHCE* gene in D-negative people. Because of the absence of RhD and RhCE proteins, Rh_{null}-amorph RBCs have reduced (but not absent) expression of RhAg protein (Daniels, 2002). The Rh_{null} regulator type arises from mutations in *RHAG* (Reid, 2004).

Rh_{mod} Phenotype

Mutations in *RHAG* are also observed in the Rh_{mod} phenotype. Rh_{mod} RBCs have markedly decreased Rh and RhAg expression, detectable only by careful adsorption and elution studies. Similar to Rh_{null} individuals, persons with Rh_{mod} may have laboratory evidence of Rh deficiency syndrome with a mild hemolytic anemia. Three Rh_{mod} samples have been studied, each containing a single, different missense mutation in the *RHAG* gene (Reid, 2004).

Rh Antibodies

Antibodies against Rh antigens are routinely encountered in the blood bank (see Table 35-7). D is the most immunogenic Rh antigen, followed by c, E, C, and e (Harmening, 2005). In general, antibodies against Rh antigens are the result of immune stimulation by transfusion or pregnancy. Exceptions include some examples of anti-C^w and anti-E, which can be naturally occurring. Most antibodies against Rh antigens are of IgG isotype (IgG_1 and IgG_3), although rare examples of IgM and IgA are known. Anti-Rh antibodies are reactive at 37° C and are usually detected in the AHG phase of testing. The reactivity of anti-Rh antibodies can be enhanced with enzyme-treated RBCs. The gel method is extremely sensitive for the detection of Rh antibodies (Weisbach, 2006).

Clinically, antibodies against Rh are associated with hemolytic transfusion reactions. However, because Rh antibodies do not fix complement, incompatible RBCs are almost always cleared through extravascular destruction. To prevent sensitization to the D antigen, Rh-negative patients should be transfused with Rh-negative RBCs. This is particularly true for young girls and women of childbearing age. For transfusion in alloimmunized patients, RBC units should be negative for the Rh antigen of interest and crossmatch compatible with the recipient's serum through the AHG phase of testing. One possible exception may be R_1R_1 (DCe/DCe) patients who have developed anti-E alloantibodies. Because these patients are at increased risk of delayed hemolytic transfusion reactions because of the subsequent development of anti-c, many blood bankers advocate transfusing only R_1R_1 units to R_1R_1 patients (Shirey, 1994).

Antibodies against Rh antigens are also a major cause of HDFN. All Rh-negative women should receive Rh immune globulin (IgG anti-D) prophylactically in midpregnancy, following an invasive procedure (i.e., amniocentesis), and immediately after delivery to prevent alloimmunization. Rh immune globulin prophylaxis is also recommended in women with partial D phenotypes because these women can be at risk for D alloimmunization (Ansart-Pirenne, 2004). Rh immune globulin may also be given following transfusion of RhD+ platelet concentrates or after accidental transfusion of RhD+ RBCs. In the latter, Rh immune globulin is given after two-volume RBC exchange with RhD-negative RBCs (Nester, 2004). Administration of one vial of Rh immune globulin is recommended for every 30 mL whole blood or 15 mL packed RBCs transfused (Roback, 2008). Rh immune globulin should be given within 72 hours of exposure to prevent active immunization. Rh immune globulin is not given to Rh-negative women who are already immunized to D antigen (i.e., have anti-D).

It is also recommended to give Rh immune globulin to Rh-negative women with anti-G alloantibodies. As stated earlier, anti-G behaves as an anti-C + anti-D because of recognition of a Ser103 or C-type antigen on both RhD and RhCE proteins. In general, HDFN secondary to anti-G or anti-C + anti-G is mild when compared with HDFN due to anti-D. However, because these women may still become immunized to D-specific epitopes on the RhD protein, many blood bankers advocate giving Rh immune globulin to Rh-negative women with anti-G antibodies (Shirey, 1997). Separation of anti-G from a true anti-C + anti-D is very laborious, requiring sequential adsorption and elution (Yesus, 1985). One clue suggesting the presence of anti-G is an anti-C titer at least fourfold higher than anti-D (Shirey, 1997). It is not necessary, however, to separate anti-G from anti-C + anti-D for routine transfusion. With very rare exceptions, RBCs negative for D and C antigens are also negative for G antigen.

Biological Role

The specific physiologic function of the Rh proteins is still unclear; however, there is a strong belief that Rh proteins may constitute a membrane transporter. The Rh proteins are homologous with ammonium transporters of the Mep/Amt family. In addition, Rh-like homologs have been discovered in invertebrate life forms such as the nematode worm *Caenorhabditis elegans* and a marine sponge, *Geodia cydonium* (Avent, 1999). Evidence suggests that RhAG is capable of facilitating NH_4 transport. It is speculated that the Band 3/Rh complex may serve as an O_2/CO_2 gas exchange metabolon (Daniels, 2007).

TABLE 35-19
Phenotypes of the Lutheran System

REACTIONS WITH ANTI-				FREQUENCY U.S. POPULATION, %		
Lu^a	**Lu^b**	**Lu-3**	**Phenotype**	**Caucasian**	**Black**	**Comments**
+	0	+	Lu (a+b–)	0.1	0.1	
+	+	+	Lu (a+b+)	7	5	
0	+	+	Lu (a-b+)	93	95	
Null Phenotypes (Lu$_{null}$)						
0	0	0	Lu (a–b–)	Very rare	Very rare	Autosomal recessive Normal CD44, i/I, CD75 Make an anti-Lu-3
0/W*	0/w*	w*	Lu (a–b–)	Very rare	Very rare	In (Lu), autosomal dominant ↓CD44, I/i; ↑CD75 *ELKF* mutation
0/W*	0/w*	w*	Lu (a–b–)	Very rare	Very rare	X-linked recessive, GATA1 mutation Absent CD75

*Weak Lu antigens detected only by adsorption and elution techniques.

LUTHERAN BLOOD GROUP SYSTEM (ISBT NO. 005)

The Lutheran (Lu) blood group system contains 19 antigens including four pairs of allelic antigens and 11 high-incidence antigens. Lutheran is a minor constituent of RBC membranes, averaging only 2000–5000 molecules per cell, and can vary in strength between donors (Issitt, 1998). Even within a single individual, considerable heterogeneity in Lutheran expression is seen, with only 40%–50% of red cells positive for Lutheran antigens by flow cytometry (El Nemer, 1998). Lutheran appears on red cells at the orthochromatic erythroblast stage, concurrent with binding of red cells to laminin (Daniels, 2009). Lutheran antigens are ubiquitously expressed on human tissues. In addition to RBCs, Lutheran glycoprotein is expressed by colon, small intestine, ovary, testis, prostate, thymus, spleen, pancreas, kidney, skeletal muscle, liver, lung, placenta, brain, heart, and bone marrow (Rahuel, 1996).

Null/Weak Phenotypes

A Lu(a–b–) phenotype can occur in three settings with distinct patterns of inheritance: autosomal recessive, autosomal dominant (*In[Lu]*), and X-linked recessive (Table 35-19). The autosomal recessive phenotype is a true null phenotype, characterized by complete absence of all Lutheran antigens on RBCs. As a consequence, these individuals can make an alloantibody to Lutheran glycoprotein (anti-Lu3) which reacts with all Lu-positive RBCs. The Lu$_{null}$ phenotype is extremely rare and is not associated with altered expression of other red cell antigens.

The autosomal dominant and X-linked recessive forms are characterized by very weak Lutheran expression, often detected only after adsorption and elution. *In(Lu)* is an autosomal dominant Lu$_{mod}$ phenotype with an incidence of 0.02%–0.12% (Daniels, 2009). In addition to Lutheran antigens, *In(Lu)* red cells can show weakened expression of P_1, i, Indian/CD44, and Knops/CD35 antigens and enhanced expression of CDw75 (Daniels, 2002, 2009). The X-linked Lu$_{mod}$ phenotype has weakened Lutheran, enhanced i and CDw75, and normal P_1, i, and CD44 expression. Because both *In(Lu)* and X-linked recessive Lu$_{mod}$ phenotypes express some Lutheran antigen on RBCs and other tissues, neither is associated with the development of anti-Lu3. *In(Lu)* RBCs can display subtle abnormalities, including increased poikilocytosis and increased hemolysis, during in vitro storage (Ballas, 1992).

Biochemistry

The Lutheran antigens reside on two isomeric, type 1 glycoproteins: Lu-glycoprotein (85kD) and epithelial cancer antigen (B-CAM, 78kD) (Daniels, 2009). The 85-kD glycoprotein is the predominant isoform found on RBCs and normal tissues. Members of the Ig superfamily, the 78- and 85-kD glycoproteins share a common, large (518 amino acid) extracellular domain with five Ig regions and five potential *N*-glycosylation sites (Fig. 35-7). Three Ig domains are of the constant-region-2 (C2) type, whereas the remaining two are variable-region (V) domains. A laminin binding site resides in a flexible hinge region between C2 and V domains.

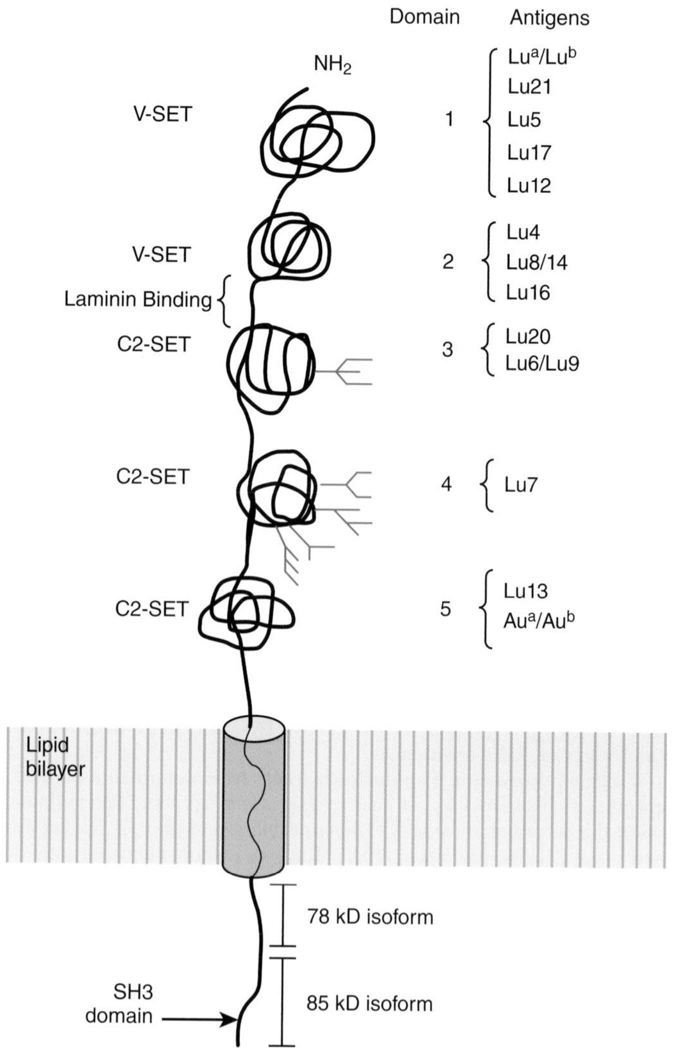

Figure 35-7 Lutheran glycoprotein. The Lutheran antigens reside on one of five immunoglobulin domains (V, C2-like). The transmembrane domain is indicated by a solid amber cylinder. The length of the cytoplasmic domain can vary from 19 amino acids (78-kD form) to 59 amino acids (85-kD isoform). The latter also possesses a consensus-binding motif for Src protein (SH3 domain).

TABLE 35-20
Lutheran Blood Group Antigens

HIGH-FREQUENCY ANTIGENS				LOW-FREQUENCY ANTIGENS		
ISBT	**Name**	**Frequency, %**	**Amino acid change (high→low)**	**Frequency, %**	**Name**	**ISBT**
LU2	Lu^b	99.8	Arg77>His	5–8	Lu^a	LU1
LU3	Lu^{ab}	>99	Unknown	Rare		
LU4	Barnes	>99	Arg175>Gln	Rare		
LU5	Beal	>99	Arg109>His	Rare		
LU6	Jan	>99	Ser275>Phe	1–2	Mull	LU9
LU7	Gary	>99	Unknown (4th IgSF)	Rare		
LU8	Taylor/MT	>99	Met204>Lys	1.8	Hof	LU14
LU11	Reynolds	>99	Unknown	Rare		
LU12	Much	>99	Heterogeneous Deletion Arg34 + Leu35 Arg140>Gln	Rare		
LU13	Hughes	>99	Ser447>Leu Gln581>Leu	Rare		
LU16		>99	Arg227>Cys	Rare		
LU17	Delcol	>99	Glu114>Lys	Rare		
LU18	Au^a	90	Ala539>Thr	51% Caucasians, 68% blacks	Au^b	LU19
LU20		>99	Thr302>Met	Rare		
LU21		>99	Asp94>Glu	Rare		

ISBT, International Society of Blood Transfusion.

The 7-kD difference between the 78-kD and 85-kD isoforms reflects the length of the COOH-terminal cytoplasmic tail. In addition to its longer length, the cytoplasmic domain of the 85-kD isoform possesses an SH3 motif, a potential binding site for Src protein. The cytoplasmic domain also interacts with spectrin, a cytoskeletal protein (Kroviarski, 2004). Because it is a highly folded protein, stabilized by disulfide bonds, Lutheran is destroyed by sulfhydryl-reducing agents and many proteases.

Molecular Biology

The gene for Lutheran (*LU*) resides on chromosome 19q13.2-13.3. It is a 12.5-kb gene containing 15 exons: Alternate splicing of exon 13 is responsible for the 78-kD minor isoform (Rahuel, 1996; El Nemer, 1997). Although no TATA or CAAT boxes are present in the 5′ flanking or promoter region of the gene, it does possess consensus sequences for several *cis*-regulatory elements, including the ubiquitous Sp1, AP2, EGR-1, EKLF, Ets, and GATA-1, an erythroid transcription binding protein (El Nemer, 1997; Singleton, 2008).

The molecular basis for most Lutheran antigens is now known (Table 35-20). Most are the result of SNPs (Daniels, 2002, 2009). The autosomal recessive, true Lu_{null} phenotype arises from inheritance of two silent amorph LU alleles due to nonsense mutations and deletions (Daniels, 2009). The molecular basis for the autosomal dominant *In(Lu)* phenotype was finally identified in 2008. Most *In(Lu)* individuals are heterozygous for a mutant *EKLF* gene, an erythroid transcription factor active in late erythroid differentiation (Singleton, 2008). The *In(Lu)* phenotype, therefore, is the result of reduced transcriptional activation and expression of LU glycoprotein. Reduced EKLF activity likely accounts for decreased expression of other blood group antigens. The basis for the X-linked recessive (XS2) has been identified as mutations in the transcription factor GATA1, which resides on the X chromosome.

Lutheran Antibodies

In general, Lutheran antibodies are not clinically significant and are only rarely associated with HDFN and hemolytic transfusion reactions. Anti-Lu^a is the most common Lutheran alloantibody encountered in the blood bank and is often an IgM, room temperature agglutinin. Because not all RBCs express detectable Lu antigens (El Nemer, 1998), anti-Lu^a can display mixed field agglutination. Antibodies against Lu^b and other Lutheran antigens are most often of IgG isotype, reacting best in the IAT. Reactivity of anti-Lu^a, Lu^b, and other Lutheran antibodies can be inhibited by pretreatment of RBCs with chymotrypsin, trypsin, 2-aminoethylisothiouronium bromide (AET), and dithiothreitol (DTT).

Biological Role

Biologically, Lutheran is a high-affinity receptor for laminin, a basement membrane protein involved in cell differentiation, adhesion, migration, and proliferation. Overexpression of LU glycoprotein in ovarian carcinoma and other cancers is hypothesized to facilitate tumor cell adhesion and metastasis (Rahuel, 1996). In sickle cell patients, increased Lutheran expression on reticulocytes and sickle cells may contribute to the pathophysiology of vaso-occlusive crises. Patients with sickle cell disease have indirect evidence of chronic vascular injury with shedding of microvascular endothelial cells and exposure of vascular basement membrane (Solovey, 1997). In these patients, increased exposure of laminin on the thrombotic subendothelium, coupled with increased expression of laminin receptor on reticulocytes and sickle cells, may promote red cell adhesion and circulatory stasis (El Nemer, 1998; Parsons, 2001). Likewise, LU glycoprotein may contribute to thrombosis in polycythemia vera. The *JAK2* mutation was shown to increase phosphorylation of LU glycoprotein and red cell adhesion (Daniels, 2009). In normal erythropoiesis, LU may play a role in migration of maturing erythroid cells out of the marrow (Daniels, 2009).

KELL AND KX BLOOD GROUP SYSTEMS (ISBT NO. 006 AND 019)

First identified in 1945, the Kell blood group system currently consists of 46 high- and low-frequency antigens (Table 35-21). Eleven Kell antigens belong to five sets of allelic antigens, whereas the remainder are predominantly high-incidence antigens (>99% of the population). Many low-incidence Kell antigens (K, Js^a, Ul^a, Kp^a, Kp^c) show distinct racial differences. The Kell antigen is found on RBCs, erythroid and megakaryocyte progenitors, skeletal muscle, and testis. RBCs express approximately 2000–6000 copies of Kell protein per cell (Issitt, 1998).

Null and Weak Phenotypes

K_0K_0 is an autosomal recessive, null phenotype that completely lacks all Kell antigens (Table 35-22). As a consequence, these individuals can make an alloantibody to the Kell glycoprotein (anti-Ku). Unlike McLeod RBCs (see later), K_0K_0 RBCs have enhanced expression of Kx antigen, present on the XK protein. Unlike Rh_{null} red cells, K_0K_0 red cells have no decrease in CO_2 permeability (Endeward, 2006). A K_0K_0 RBC can be produced in the laboratory by treating Kell-positive RBCs with sulfhydryl-reducing agents.

TABLE 35-21
Kell and XK Blood Group Antigens*

ANTIGEN (HIGH FREQUENCY)					ANTIGEN (LOW FREQUENCY)	
ISBT	**Name**	**Percent donors**	**Amino acid change (high→low frequency)**	**Percent donors**	**Name**	**ISBT**
KEL2	k	99.8	Thr193>Met	9	K	KEL1
			Thr193>Ser	Rare		
			Ala423>Val	Unknown		Weak KEL2
KEL4	Kp^b	99.9	Arg281>Trp	2	Kp^a	KEL3
			Arg281>Gln	<0.1	Kp^c	KEL21
KEL7	Js^b	>99.9	Leu597>Pro	<1% Caucasians 19.5% blacks	Js^a	KEL6
KEL11		>99.9	Val302>Ala	0.3	Wk^a	KEL17
KEL14		>99.9	Arg180>Pro	<2	cls	KEL24
KEL5	Ku	>99.9	Heterogeneous	0.8	K_0	K_{null}
			Heterogeneous	Rare	K_{mod}	
			Glu494>Val	2.6% Finnish <0.1% other	UL^a	KEL10
KEL12		>99.9	His548>Arg			
KEL13		>99.9	Unknown			
KEL16		>99.8	Unknown			
KEL18		>99.9	Arg130>Trp			
			Arg130>Gln			
KEL19		>99.9	Arg492>Gln			
KEL20	Km	>99.9	Unknown			
KEL22		>99.9	Ala322>Val			
			Gln382>Arg	>0.1		KEL23
			Arg248>Gln	Rare	VLAN	KEL25
			Arg248>Trp		VONG	KEL28
			Arg406>Gln	Rare	TOU	KEL26
KEL27	RAZ	>99	Glu249>Lys			
KEL29	KALT	>99	Arg623>Lys			
KEL30	KTIM	>99	Asp305>Asn			
			Arg292>Gln	Rare	KYO	KEL31
KEL32	KUCI	>99	Ala424>Val			
KEL33	KANT	>99	Arg428>Leu			
KEL34	KASH	>99	Try253>Cys			
XK1	Kx	>99.9	Mutation XK protein	Rare	McLeod	

ISBT, International Society of Blood Transfusion.
*As referenced in Daniels (2002, 2004, 2007, 2009) and Reid (2004).

TABLE 35-22
Phenotype Frequencies in the Kell System

REACTIONS WITH ANTI-										FREQUENCY IN U.S. POPULATION, %	
K	**k**	**Kp^a**	**Kp^b**	**Js^a**	**Js^b**	**Ku**	**Km**	**Kx**	**Phenotype**	**Caucasian**	**Black**
+	0					++*	++	w*	K+k–	0.2	Rare
+	+					++	++	w	K+k+	8.8	2
0	+					++	++	w	K–k+	91	98
		+	0			++	++	w	Kp(a+b–)	Rare	0
		+	+			++	++	w	Kp(a+b+)	2.3	Rare
		0	+			++	++	w	Kp(a–b+)	97.7	100
				+	0	++	++	w	Js(a+b–)	0	1
				+	+	++	++	w	Js(a+b+)	Rare	19
				0	+	++	++	w	Js(a–b+)	100	80
Null Phenotypes											
0	0	0	0	0	0	0	0	++	K_0	Exceedingly rare	
0/w	0/w	0/w	0/w	0/w	0/w	w	w	++	K_{mod}	Rare	
0/w	0/w	0/w	0/w	0/w	0/w	0/w	0	0	McLeod	Rare	

*++, Strong reactivity; *w,* weak reactivity.

Kell antigens are significantly depressed/absent on McLeod RBCs, an X-linked recessive phenotype characterized by the absence of XK protein on RBCs (Kx antigen, XK1; ISBT 019), acanthocytes, and neuromuscular disorders. Because McLeod individuals lack XK and Kell proteins, these individuals can make alloantibodies directed against both proteins. As a consequence, McLeod individuals are incompatible with both Kell-positive and K_0K_0 RBCs. Depressed Kell expression is also observed on K_{mod} and Gerbich-negative RBCs, two autosomal recessive phenotypes. As with the K_0K_0 phenotype, some $Kell_{mod}$ individuals have increased Kx (KEL15) expression and can develop an anti-KEL5 (anti-Ku) following RBC transfusion. Transient depression and masking of Kell antigens have been reported in septic patients and in autoimmune hemolytic anemia due to anti-Kell autoantibodies (Judd, 1981; Issitt, 1998; Bosco, 2009). Kell antigens are also depressed (up to 80%) in alleles bearing KEL3 in *cis* (e.g., KKp^a, KEL*1,3; kKp^a, KEL*2,3) (Poole, 2006; Kormoczi, 2009).

Biochemistry

The Kell antigens (ISBT No. 006) reside on a 93-kD, 732 amino acid glycoprotein (CD238), possessing a short 47 amino acid amino-terminal cytosolic domain; a single transmembrane domain; and a large, 665 amino acid extracellular domain that includes the carboxy-terminus and 4-5 *N*-linked glycans (Fig. 35-8). In the KEL1 phenotype, a Thr183>Met substitution voids a glycosylation site, resulting in only four *N*-linked glycans (Lee, 1997).

Overall, the molecule has a complex, folded tertiary structure due to the formation of multiple disulfide bonds by the 15 cysteine residues present in the extracellular domain of the molecule (Lee, 1997). Because of its highly folded nature, the Kell glycoprotein is fairly resistant to proteolytic digestion but is exquisitely sensitive to sulfhydryl-reducing agents such as DTT, AET, 2-mercaptoethanol (2-ME), and ZZAP, a combination of DTT and cysteine-activated papain.

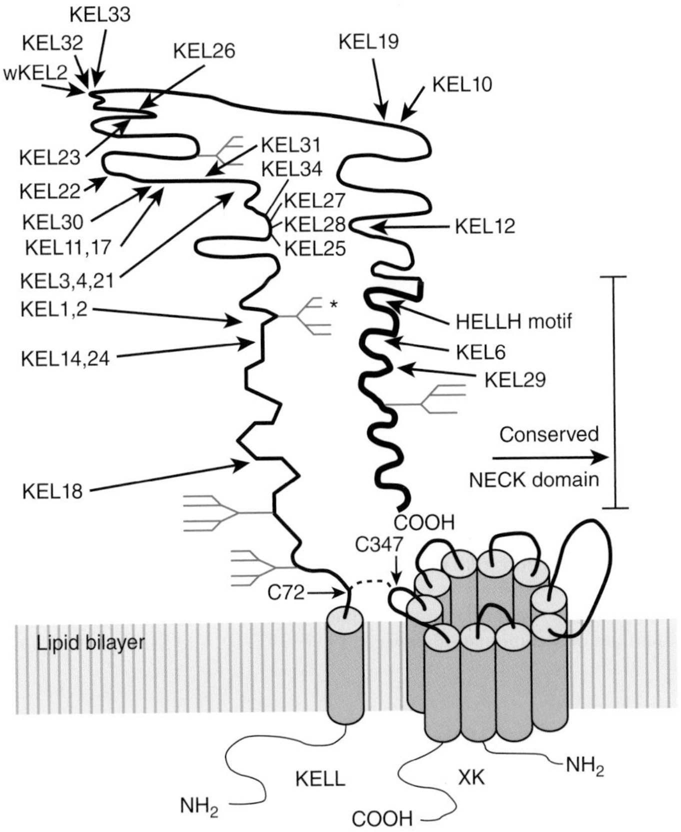

Figure 35-8 Diagram of KELL and XK protein. KELL is covalently linked to the XK protein by a disulfide bond (- - - -) through Cys72 of Kell and Cys347 of XK. The sites of different Kell antigens are indicated by solid lines. The highlighted area at the carboxy-terminus of KELL represents the domain sharing the most homology to other NECK family proteins (NEP-24.11, ECE-1, PEX). The zinc-binding motif (HELLH) is a consensus sequence shared by zinc-dependent metalloproteinases. The transmembrane domains of KELL and XK protein are indicated by solid amber cylinders. The *N*-glycosylation sites are indicated by branched structures. The *N*-glycosylation site marked by an asterisk is not present in individuals of the KEL1-positive phenotype.

In the RBC membrane, the Kell glycoprotein is covalently linked to the XK protein (ISBT No. 019), a 444 amino acid, nonglycosylated, multipass protein containing 10 transmembrane domains. Encoded by a gene on chromosome Xp21, the XK protein is hypothesized to be a membrane transport protein. On RBCs, the XK protein is covalently linked to the Kell protein through a disulfide bond at C347 on the fifth extracellular loop of XK protein and C72 of Kell. In the absence of XK protein (McLeod phenotype), Kell expression is decreased on RBCs, suggesting that XK protein may help transport Kell. Transfection studies in COS cells, however, show normal transport and folding of the Kell protein in the absence of XK protein (Russo, 1998). Nor is expression of XK dependent on Kell expression. The XK protein is expressed on several nonerythroid tissues, including liver, skeletal muscle, heart, brain, and pancreas (Ho, 1994).

Molecular Biology

Cloned in 1991, the Kell gene (*KEL*) contains 19 exons spanning 21.5kb on chromosome 7q34 near the cystic fibrosis gene. The promoter region and exon 1 contain several consensus-binding sequences for GATA-1, an erythroid transcription regulatory binding factor. Kell is a member of the M13 neprilysin family of zinc neutral endopeptidases and shares homology with common acute lymphocytic leukemia antigen (CALLA, CD10), endothelin-converting enzyme-1 (ECE-1), neutral endopeptidase 24.11 (NEP-24.11), and PEX. The region of greatest homology lies in the carboxy-terminal half of the molecule (amino acids 550–652) and is sometimes referred to as the NECK domain (N-24.11, EC-1, K family). This relatively conserved region shares 34%–36% homology with the carboxy-terminal catalytic domains of NEP-24.11 and ECE-1, as well as a pentameric zinc-binding motif (HELLH), a common feature of zinc-dependent metalloproteinases (Lee, 1997).

With cloning of the Kell gene, the molecular and biochemical basis of several Kell antigens became possible. As shown in Table 35-21, all the Kell alloantigens identified and sequenced are single–amino acid polymorphisms in the translated Kell protein. Furthermore, nearly every amino acid polymorphism occurs in the amino half of the molecule (Lee, 1997).

Several individuals with absent or depressed Kell expression have also been studied. K_0K_0 phenotype arises from homozygosity for a silent *KEL* amorph gene. Multiple inactivating mutations of the *KEL* gene have been identified, including splice-site mutations and premature stop codons (Reid, 2004). Missense mutations, sometimes leading to premature stop codons, are responsible for the K_{mod} phenotype (Reid, 2004). Several mutations have been identified in the XK protein on Xp21, responsible for the McLeod phenotype (Russo, 2002). The molecular basis for decreased Kell antigen expression with Gerbich-negative phenotypes is unknown. It is speculated that Kell and glycophorin C (Gerbich) may be near neighbors on the RBC membrane.

Kell Antibodies

Alloantibodies against antigens in the Kell blood group system are clinically significant (see Table 35-7). They can be associated with both immediate and delayed hemolytic transfusion reactions. Anti-Kell antibodies are also associated with HDFN. HDFN secondary to maternal anti-Kell antibodies is often characterized by reticulocytopenia, with little or no bilirubinemia. It is now known that maternal anti-Kell (anti-KEL1 or K1) directly suppresses erythroid progenitors, leading to a severe reticulocytopenic anemia in the fetus (Vaughan, 1998) with up to 30% of affected infants presenting with fetal hydrops (van den Akker, 2008). Anti-K1 is present in approximately 1% of pregnancies, with HDFN affecting 40% of K1-positive infants (Finning, 2007). Several centers now routinely screen and refer prenatal patients with Kell antibodies, with improved perinatal outcomes (Kamphuis, 2008). Reports have also described neonatal thrombocytopenia due to suppression of marrow megakaryocytes (Wagner, 2000). In general, thrombocytopenia is mild, with only 2% of infants having platelet counts of $<100 \times 10^9/L$ (van den Akker, 2008). Similar to RHD, fetal genotyping can be performed on maternal plasma (Finning, 2007).

The most commonly encountered antibody against the Kell blood group system is anti-K1, which is second only to Rh D in immunogenicity. Antibodies against Kell antigens are of IgG isotype, arising from immune stimulation via transfusion or pregnancy, although examples of naturally occurring anti-Kell alloantibodies are known (Judd, 1981). Because Kell antigens are sensitive to sulfhydryl-reducing agents, the activity of anti-Kell antibodies can be eliminated by pretreatment of RBCs with AET, DTT, 2-ME, or ZZAP.

Biological Role

Kell cleaves endothelin-3, a vasoactive peptide that functions in endothelial cell migration, neovascularization, axonal growth, and neural crest development. In a murine $Kell_{null}$ model, absence of Kell led to only subtle effects, including decreased blood pressure, blunting endothelin-3 activation of Ca^{++}-dependent K^{+} channels, decreased microvascular formation, and mild changes in motor function (Zhu, 2009). Because endothelin-3 is also cleaved by ECE-1, a related endothelin converting enzyme, Kell may have only a minor physiologic role in endothelin-3 homeostasis. The ability of anti-Kell to suppress fetal erythropoiesis also suggests a possible role for Kell during erythroid differentiation and maturation (Vaughan, 1998); however, only minor differences in mean corpuscular volume, mean corpuscular hemoglobin, hemoglobin (Hg), and reticulocyte counts were observed in $Kell_{null}$ mice (Zhu, 2009).

In contrast to Kell, the absence of XK protein is strongly associated with several abnormal clinical and laboratory findings. McLeod RBCs have shortened survival, decreased permeability to water, and abnormal morphology (acanthocytes). The McLeod syndrome, characterized by both hematologic and neuromuscular abnormalities, typically presents with areflexia, dystonia, and choreiform movements late in life. Late-onset muscular dystrophy and cardiomyopathy can also be seen. Both hematologic and neuromuscular defects in McLeod patients are believed to result from the absence of XK protein on red cells, brain, heart, and skeletal muscle (Ho, 1994). It is interesting that the Huntington's disease gene, another neurodegenerative disorder, is located near the *XK* gene on the X chromosome (Issitt, 1998).

The McLeod phenotype can also be associated with chronic granulomatous disease (CGD), a functional neutrophil defect resulting in severe, recurrent, life-threatening bacterial infections. In two thirds of patients, CGD results from a deletion or mutation of the cytochrome *b* gene *(CYBB)* on the X chromosome. Because of the proximity of the *CYBB* and *XK* genes on the X chromosome, approximately 7% of patients with X-linked CGD also express a McLeod phenotype (Curnutte, 1995).

LEWIS BLOOD GROUP SYSTEM (ISBT NO. 007)

The Lewis blood group system is unusual in that the Lewis antigens are not of erythroid origin. It primarily consists of two antigens: $Lewis^a$ (Le^a) and $Lewis^b$ (Le^b). Four additional antigens (Le^{ab}, Le^{bH}, ALe^b, BLe^b) reflect the influence of ABO on Lewis synthesis and antigenicity. On RBCs, the Lewis antigens reside on glycosphingolipids, composed of a Lewis-active carbohydrate head group linked to a ceramide (*N*-acyl sphingosine) lipid tail. Lewis antigens are synthesized in the gastrointestinal tract and passively adsorbed onto RBCs from a soluble pool of secreted Lewis substance in plasma (Hauser, 1995). Tissues and fluids expressing Lewis include plasma, saliva, RBCs, platelets, lymphocytes, endothelium, uroepithelium, and bowel mucosa. In some tissues, Lewis antigens are expressed on glycosphingolipids, glycoproteins, and mucins (Issitt, 1998).

Three Lewis phenotypes are observed in adults: Le (a+b–), Le (a–b+) and Le (a–b–). The Le (a+b+) is only rarely observed, usually on RBCs of very young children and some individuals of Polynesian, Japanese, or Taiwanese ancestry (Issitt, 1998). As shown in Table 35-23, the Le (a–b–) phenotype is five times more common in blacks than in Caucasians. The Le (a–b–) phenotype is also increased in neonates owing to developmentally delayed expression of the *Lewis* and *Secretor* genes. By 5 years of age, most children will express adult levels of Lewis antigens on their RBCs. The amount of Lewis antigen on RBCs is also influenced by ABO type. Le (a–b+) RBCs from group O donors appear to have more Le^b than A_1 and B cells. As will be discussed later, group A_1 and B donors can convert Le^b to ALe^b and BLe^b, respectively (Issitt, 1998).

Biochemistry

Although biosynthetically related to each other, the Le^a and Le^b antigens are not allelic antigens. They represent the complex interaction of two distinct glycosyltransferases: fucosyltransferase type II (FUT2) and fucosyltransferase type III (FUT3). FUT3 is the product of the Lewis gene *(Le/FUT3)* and is an α1–3/4 fucosyltransferase. FUT2, the product of the *Secretor* gene *(Se)*, is an α1–2 fucosyltransferase related to the *H* gene, FUT1. How *Le*, *Se*, and *ABO* genes interact to yield the different combinations of RBC and plasma phenotypes is shown in Table 35-23 and Figure 35-9.

The precursor molecule for Lewis and related antigens is a type 1 chain precursor, historically known as the Le^c antigen. In Le (a+b–) donors, FUT3 or Lewis adds an α1–4 linked fucose to Le^c to form the Le^a antigen. Because these donors lack the *Se/FUT2* gene *(se/se)*, no type 1 chain H (Le^d) is made. As a result, only Le^a antigen is present in plasma, saliva, and RBCs. The Le (a–b+) red cell phenotype results from the inheritance of both *Le* and *Se* genes. FUT3 still converts a small amount of type 1 chain precursor to Le^a antigen. However, most Le^c substance is converted to type 1 chain H or Le^d by FUT2 (see Fig. 35-9). FUT3 subsequently adds a second fucose to form Le^b antigen (Lowe, 1994). In group A and B persons, type 1 chain H is further modified by the A/B glycosyltransferase to form type 1 chain A and B antigens. Similar to type 1 chain H and Le^c antigens, these molecules can serve as substrates for FUT3 to form ALe^b and BLe^b (see Fig. 35-9). In group A_1 donors, ALe^b is the major Le^b antigen found in plasma (Lindstrom, 1992).

The Le (a–b–) red cell phenotype occurs in individuals who lack the *Le/FUT3* gene. Individuals who are negative for both *Le* and *Se* alleles *(le/le, se/se)* are unable to synthesize Le^a antigen or type 1 chain H antigens. As a result, only type 1 chain precursor or Le^c antigen is present in secretions and plasma. In contrast, individuals who inherit at least one Se allele can express type 1 chain glycolipids with ABH activity.

Molecular Biology

The *FUT3* or *Lewis* gene resides on chromosome 19p13.3 near two other α1–3 fucosyltransferase genes, *FUT5* and *FUT6*. All three α1–3 fucosyltransferases are highly homologous, consistent with gene duplication (Weston, 1992). The gene encodes a 361 amino acid type II glycoprotein with both α1→4 (Le^a) and α1→3 (LeX) fucosyltransferase activity. FUT3 is highly expressed in colon, stomach, small intestine, lung, and kidney, with weaker expression in salivary gland, bladder, uterus, and liver. FUT6 is coexpressed with FUT3 in most tissues (Cameron, 1995).

The Le (a–b–) or null phenotype arises from inactivating mutations in *FUT3*. More than 10 missense mutations in the *FUT3* gene have been identified, with most *FUT3* null alleles possessing at least two mutations (Daniels, 2002; Reid, 2004). The Lewis weak (Le^w) phenotype, characterized by a Le (a–b–) RBC phenotype and the presence of Lewis-active substance in saliva, is due to a single missense mutation in the transmembrane domain (T59>G). The latter has normal enzyme activity but decreased Golgi retention (Mollicone, 1994).

The *FUT2 (Se)* gene resides on chromosome 19q13.3 as part of a 100-kb gene cluster that includes the *H* gene *(FUT1)* and *Sec1*, an inactive *FUT2*-like pseudogene (Kelly, 1995). Multiple null alleles have been reported, with distinct geographic and ethnic distributions. Most null alleles are the result of nonsense mutations (Daniels, 2002). There are also examples of recombination between FUT1, FUT2, and Sec1 (Koda, 1996;

TABLE 35-23
The Lewis Blood Group System

	FREQUENCIES IN U.S. ADULTS, %		POSSIBLE GENOTYPE		ABH AND LEWIS SUBSTANCES IN SALIVA AND PLASMA		
Phenotype	**Caucasian**	**Black**	***Le* Gene**	***Se* Gene**	**Group O**	**Group A**	**Group B**
Le (a+b–)	22	23	*Le/Le* or *Le/le*	*se/se*	Le^a	Le^a	Le^a
Le (a–b+)	72	55	*Le/Le* or *Le/le*	*Se/Se* or *Se/se*	Type 1H Le^a, Le^b	Type 1H, A Le^a, Le^b, ALe^b	Type 1H, B Le^a, Le^b, BLe^b
Le (a–b–)	6	22	*le/le* *le/le*	*Se/se* *se/se*	Type 1H Type 1 chain precursor (Le^c)	Type 1H, A Type 1 chain precursor (Le^c)	Type 1H, B Type 1 chain precursor (Le^c)

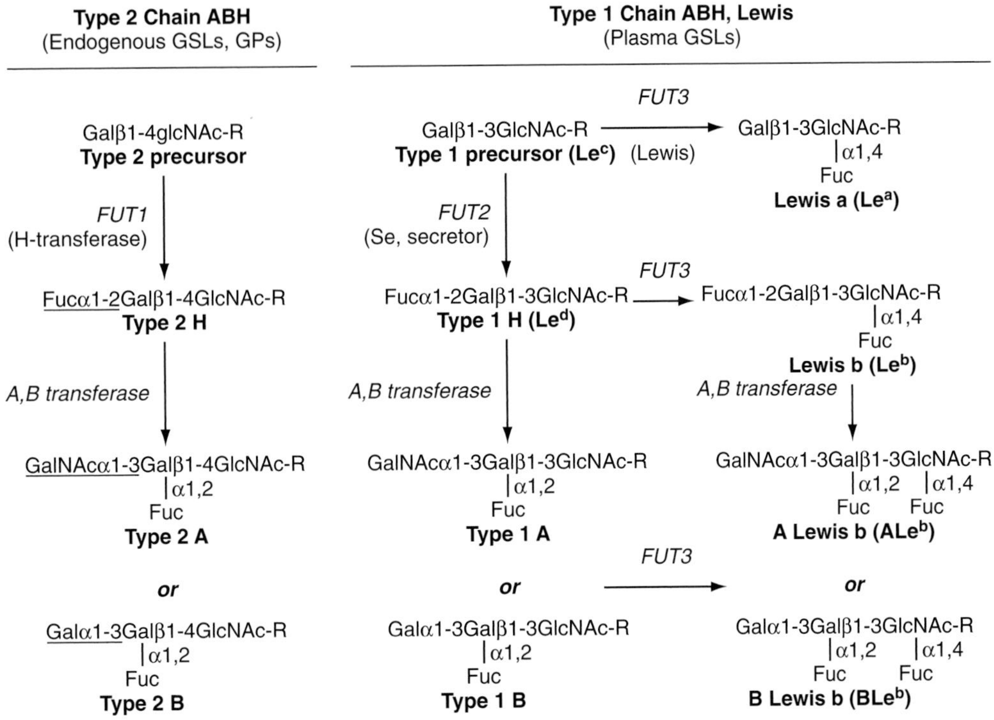

Figure 35-9 Synthesis of Lewis and type 1 chain ABH antigens. *Fuc,* Fucose; *Gal,* galactose; *GalNAc,* N-acetylgalactosamine; *Glc,* glucose; *GlcNAc,* N-acetylglucosamine; *Le,* Lewis; *R,* ceramide.

Soejima, 2008). The partial secretor phenotype has been linked to an Ile129>Phe mutation (Yu, 1995).

Lewis Antibodies

Similar to ABO, antibodies against Le^a and Le^b antigens are naturally occurring IgM antibodies (see Table 35-7), but unlike ABO antibodies, Anti-Lewis antibodies are seldom clinically significant. Most examples are detected as room temperature agglutinins; however, some examples are reactive in the IAT. Although uncommon, some examples demonstrate in vitro hemolysis. Because Le^a and Le^b are glycosphingolipids, antibody reactivity can be enhanced by pretreatment of RBCs with enzymes. Antibody reactivity is neutralized by the addition of commercially available soluble Lewis substance or plasma containing the soluble Lewis antigen of interest. Anti-Le^b can be observed in individuals of Le (a+b–) or Le (a–b–) phenotype, whereas anti-Le^a is observed only in Le (a–b–) individuals. Anti-Le^a is not observed in the Le (a–b+) phenotype because these individuals synthesize a small amount of Le^a. It is interesting to note that some Le (a–b+) women can transiently become phenotypically Le (b–), with the development of anti-Le^b, during pregnancy. Some examples of anti-Le^b can demonstrate ABH specificity (anti-LebH, anti-ALe^b, anti-BLe^b), reacting more strongly with Le^b-positive RBCs of specific ABO types.

They are not associated with HDFN and are only rarely associated with hemolytic transfusion reactions. It is speculated that they could play a role in renal graft rejection in black, Le (a–b–) individuals (Spitalnik, 1984). For transfusion, patients with anti-Lewis antibodies reactive only at room temperature may be safely transfused with crossmatch–compatible RBCs. In contrast, rare examples of anti-Le^a or anti-Le^b that are hemolytic in vitro should receive antigen-negative, crossmatch–compatible RBCs. If antigen-negative blood is not available, infusion of plasma containing the soluble Lewis antigen of interest may be helpful in neutralizing or inhibiting circulating antibody before RBC transfusion (Klein, 2006).

Biological Role

The Lewis blood group antigens play an important role in disease. *Helicobacter pylori*, a causative agent of gastritis and ulcers, binds H, Le^b, and Le^y antigens via BabA recognition of a terminal Fucα1–2Gal epitope (Boren, 1993). The latter appears to explain the increased incidence of ulcers and stomach cancer among blood group O secretors (Yamaoka, 2008). A Lewis null and/or nonsecretor phenotype has also been linked with a higher incidence of recurrent *Candida* vaginitis and urinary tract infection (Sheinfeld, 1989; Hilton, 1995). A Le (a–b–) phenotype is associated with an increased incidence of heart disease (Ellison, 1999). Conversely, a nonsecretor phenotype protects against Norovirus infection, a highly contagious RNA virus responsible for 23 million gastrointestinal infections a year (Lindesmith, 2003). Aberrant expression of sialyl-Le^a occurs in many gastrointestinal and uroepithelial cell cancers and may contribute to tumor metastasis. Sialyl-Le^a is a ligand for the endothelial adhesion molecule E-selectin and may mediate tumor cell–endothelium interactions (Takada, 1993). Sialyl-Le^a is also the epitope for the tumor marker CA 19-9, a useful serologic marker for monitoring patients with gastrointestinal and other malignancies.

DUFFY BLOOD GROUP SYSTEM (ISBT NO. 008)

The Duffy (FY) blood group system is best understood in terms of its interaction with *Plasmodium vivax* and its racial heterogeneity. Discovered in 1951, it contains five antigens: Fy^a, Fy^b, Fy3, Fy5, and Fy6. Fy^a and Fy^b are autosomal codominant antigens, whereas Fy3, Fy5, and Fy6 are high-incidence antigens present on all RBCs except the Duffy null phenotype. The Fy4 antigen, originally described on Fy (a–b–) RBCs, is now thought to be a distinct, unrelated antigen and is no longer included in the FY system. Fy^a and Fy^b antigens are common in Caucasians, whereas the Duffy null or Fy (a–b–) phenotype is the predominant phenotype in blacks (Table 35-24). Fy^x, characterized by extremely weak Fy^b expression, is somewhat rare. In addition to RBCs, the Duffy antigens are expressed on cerebellar Purkinje cells and postcapillary venule endothelial cells. Duffy antigens have also been reported on endothelial cells of renal glomeruli, vasa recta, thyroid, and pulmonary capillaries, as well as on alveolar type 1 squamous cells and epithelial cells of renal collecting tubules (Chaudhuri, 1997; Hadley, 1997). RBCs possess approximately 12,000–14,000 copies of DARC glycoprotein (DARC) per cell (Daniels, 2002).

Biochemistry

The Duffy antigens reside on DARC or Duffy antigen receptor for chemokines (Fig. 35-10). The latter is a 338 amino acid, integral membrane glycoprotein, containing a 62 amino acid extracellular amino-terminus, seven transmembrane domains, and an intracellular carboxy-terminus rich in serine and threonine residues. The amino-terminal domain possesses three *N*-glycans (Czerwinski, 2007) and is linked to the third extracellular loop by a disulfide bond to form a hepatohelical structure. A second disulfide bond exists between the first and second extracellular loops. DARC exists as a homodimer or as a hetero-oligomer with CCR5, a β-chemokine receptor that plays a role in HIV internalization (Chakera, 2008).

TABLE 35-24
Phenotype Frequencies in the Duffy System

REACTIONS WITH ANTI-				CAUCASIAN PEOPLE		BLACK PEOPLE	
Fy^a	**Fy^b**	**Fy3**	**RBC phenotype**	**Frequency***	**Genotypes†**	**Frequency***	**Genotypes†**
+	−	+	Fy (a+b−)	17	FY*A/FY*A	9	FY*A/FY*A FY*A/FY*Fy
+	+	+	Fy (a+b+)	49	FY*A/FY*B	1	FY*A/FY*B
−	+	+	Fy (a−b+)	34	FY*B/FY*B	22	FY*B/FY*B FY*B/FY*Fy
−	−	−	Fy (a−b−)	Very rare	FY*amorph	68	FY*Fy/FY*Fy
+/−	w	w	Fy (a+b^w) Fy (a−b^w)	<0.1%	FY*A/FY*X FY*X	Very rare	FY*A/FY*X FY*X FY*X/FY*Fy

*Frequency (%) U.S. population.
†Abbreviations: *FY*A,* Fy^a allele; *FY*B,* Fy^b allele; *FY*Fy,* FY*B allele carrying a GATA-1 promoter mutation; *FY*X, FY*B* gene containing missense or Sp1 promoter mutation with weak Fy^b expression; *FY*amorph,* silent *FY* gene containing disruptive mutations (deletion, frameshift, nonsense). See accompanying text.

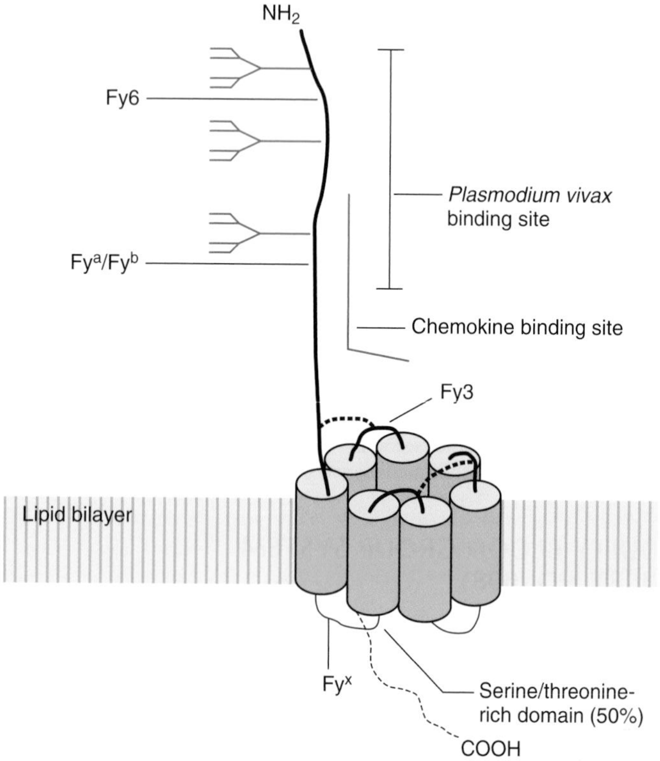

Figure 35-10 Duffy glycoprotein or Duffy antigen receptor for chemokine molecule (DARC). DARC contains a 62 amino acid, extracellular amino-terminal domain and seven transmembrane domains, indicated by solid amber cylinders. A disulfide bond exists between the amino-terminal domain and the third extracellular loop. A second disulfide bond exists between the first and second extracellular loops. Three *N*-glycosylation sites are indicated by branched structures. The sites of the Fy3, Fy6, and Fy^a/Fy^b antigens are indicated by arrows. The binding site for *Plasmodium vivax* exists between amino acids 8 and 44 and includes the Fy6 and Fy^a/Fy^b antigens. The chemokine-binding site lies in a cleft between the amino-terminal domain and the third extracellular loop. The mutation leading to the Fy^x phenotype, characterized by weak Fy^b expression, is present in the first cytoplasmic loop.

The Fy^a, Fy^b, and Fy6 antigens reside on the amino-terminal domain of DARC and are sensitive to proteolytic cleavage. The amino-terminal domain is also the binding site for *P. vivax* and plays a role in chemokine binding. Site-directed mutagenesis has confirmed that amino acids 19–26 are critical for *P. vivax* binding (Tournamille, 2005). The high-incidence antigen Fy3 is believed to reside on the third extracellular loop (Hadley, 1997; Wasniowska, 2004).

Molecular Biology

Located on chromosome 1q22-23, the Duffy gene *(FY)* is a 1014-bp gene containing two exons, a small upstream exon encoding the first seven amino acids, and a second exon encoding the rest of the molecule (Hadley, 1997). The promoter region contains consensus sequences for multiple *cis*-regulatory elements, including AP-1, Sp1, and GATA-1, an erythroid transcription activator binding protein that controls transcription of DARC in erythroid cells (Iwamoto, 1996). Phylogenetic studies indicate that *FY*B* is the ancestral gene of human and nonhuman primates (Li, 1997). Genetic studies have identified four Duffy alleles—*FY*A, FY*B, FY*Fy,* and *FY*X*—responsible for the Fy^a, Fy^b, Fy_{null}, and Fy^x phenotypes, respectively (see Table 35-24). The codominant alleles, *FY*A* and *FY*B,* differ by a single amino acid (Asp42Gly). The Fy^x phenotype *(FY*X),* characterized by extremely weak Fy^b expression, arises from an R89C substitution in the first cytoplasmic loop, leading to protein instability (Yazdandakhsh, 2000; Reid, 2004).

Three distinct mechanisms are responsible for the Fy_{null} or Fy (a−b−) serologic phenotype. In Caucasians, the *FY* gene is disrupted *(FY*amorph),* leading to complete absence of DARC on all tissues (Daniels, 2002; Reid, 2004). As a result, these individuals can make alloantibodies to all Duffy antigens, including high-incidence antigens (Fy3, Fy5). In contrast, black Fy (a−b−) individuals are homozygous for *FY*Fy* (FY^*B^{-33}), a *FY*B* variant allele that possess a point mutation in the *FY* gene promoter (−33T>C) that abrogates the consensus binding site for GATA-1. The latter is an erythroid transcription binding factor that regulates the expression of *FY* and other genes in RBCs (Iwamoto, 1996). As a result, FY transcription is absent in RBCs but is present in endothelial and epithelial cells, which utilize other promoter enhancer elements. Because Fy^b is expressed on nonerythroid cells, black Fy (a−b−) individuals do not make anti-Fy^b and only rarely make anti-Fy3. Finally, there is increasing recognition that some individuals, particularly donors, who historically typed as Fy (a−b−) by serology, are actually Fy (a−b^x) on genotyping.

Duffy Antibodies

Antibodies against Fy^a, Fy^b, and other Duffy antigens are clinically significant. They are associated with HDFN and both immediate and delayed hemolytic transfusion reactions. They are usually of IgG isotype, reactive at 37° C, and are detected only in the IAT. Antibodies against Fy^a, Fy^b, and Fy6 antigens, which reside on the long amino-terminal domain of DARC, can be inhibited by prior protease digestion of RBCs. In contrast, Fy5 and Fy3 antigens are relatively resistant to protease digestion. Antibodies against Duffy antigens can demonstrate dosage.

Clinically, anti-Fy^a is the most common alloantibody encountered and can be observed in Fy (a−) individuals of all races. Anti-Fy^b is relatively uncommon and is observed primarily in nonblacks. Alloantibodies against the high-incidence antigens Fy3 and Fy5 are relatively rare, occurring predominantly in white, Fy_{null} individuals. Anti-Fy3 behaves like an anti-Fy^{a+b}, reacting with all Duffy-positive RBCs. Occasionally, potent anti-Fy3 can be produced by sickle cell, Fy (a−b−) patients despite the expression of Fy^b on nonerythroid tissues (Castilho, 2009). Anti-Fy5 also reacts like an anti-Fy^{a+b} but requires the presence of Rh antigens for reactivity. Anti-Fy6 has not been observed clinically but is the epitope for an anti-Duffy monoclonal antibody that blocks *P. vivax* binding (Tournamille, 2005).

Biological Role

DARC is a chemokine-binding protein, capable of binding several inflammatory chemokines from the C-X-C and C-C families (Gardner, 2004), including interleukin-8, RANTES (regulated upon activation, normal T

TABLE 35-25
Phenotypes of the Kidd System

REACTIONS WITH ANTI-				FREQUENCY (%) U.S. POPULATION		
Jk^a	Jk^b	Jk3	Phenotype	Caucasian	Black	Comments
+	0	+	Jk (a+b–)	28	57	Autosomal codominant
+	+	+	Jk (a+b+)	49	34	Sensitive 2M urea
0	+	+	Jk (a–b+)	23	9	
Null Phenotypes (Jk$_{null}$)						
0	0	0	Jk (a–b–)	Very rare	Very rare	Autosomal recessive Resistant 2M urea
0/w*	0/w*	w*	Jk (a–b–)	–	–	*In (Jk),* autosomal dominant Rare, Japanese only Partially resistant 2M urea

*Weak Jk antigens detected only by adsorption and elution techniques.

cell expressed, and presumably secreted), and monocyte chemotactic protein-1 (see Fig. 35-10). Because DARC lacks a DRY motif, DARC does not transmit an intracellular signal upon binding chemokines. DARC can form heterodimers with the β-chemokine and HIV receptor CCR5, suppressing CCR5 signaling (Chakera, 2008). DARC may facilitate leukocyte recruitment to sites of inflammation by establishing a chemokine gradient and transporting chemokines across activated endothelium (Horne, 2009). In murine models, DARC functions in chemokine homeostasis and neutrophil recruitment, particularly during inflammatory insults. It is interesting to note that the absence of DARC in mice was protective against acute lung injury (Zarbock, 2010).

In humans, no distinct clinical syndrome is associated with a Fy$_{null}$ phenotype; however, the Fy$_{null}$ phenotype has been linked to lower neutrophil counts, susceptibility to infection, renal disease, and reduced graft survival following renal transplantation. A recent study linked low neutrophil counts in people of African ancestry to the *FY*Fy* (-33C) allele (Reich, 2009), leading to speculation regarding the impact of the Fy$_{null}$ phenotype and recovery from chemotherapy and other marrow insults. The role of DARC and Fy phenotype in renal transplantation is mixed, with some studies showing an increase in rejection and chronic lesions (Lerut, 2007; Horne, 2009). In patients with sickle cell disease, the Fy$_{null}$ phenotype is associated with increased chronic organ damage and proteinuria (Afenyi-Annan, 2008).

DARC is also the receptor for *P. vivax*, which binds DARC at the Fy6 epitope. Fy$_{null}$ individuals are resistant to most *P. vivax* strains, providing a selective advantage to populations living in malaria endemic areas (Storti-Melo, 2009). The latter likely explains the prevalence of the Fy$_{null}$ phenotype among blacks. Likewise, the Fy$_{null}$ phenotype (–33C/C) may provide a survival advantage in HIV infection, particularly in patients with baseline neutropenia (Kulkarni, 2009). Vigorous controversy is ongoing regarding reports linking Fy$_{null}$ with increased susceptibility to HIV infection (Winkler, 2009).

KIDD BLOOD GROUP SYSTEM (ISBT NO. 009)

The Kidd blood group system is strongly associated with delayed hemolytic transfusion reactions and with intravascular hemolysis (recall that most hemolysis with non-ABO antibodies is extravascular). It consists primarily of two allelic antigens: Jk^a and Jk^b. Inheritance is autosomal codominant with three predominant phenotypes (Table 35-25). A fourth phenotype, Jk$_{null}$ or Jk (a–b–), is very rare, except among Polynesians (≤1%) and Finns. Weak or altered Jk expression due to novel JK alleles is also known (Whorley, 2009). In addition to RBCs, Kidd antigens are expressed along descending vasa recta endothelial cells of the renal medulla. Evidence suggests low-level, constitutive expression of Kidd on heart, skeletal muscle, colon, small intestine, thymus, brain, pancreas, spleen, prostate, bladder, and liver (Olives, 1996). More than 14,000 Kidd epitopes are present per human RBC (Lucien, 2002).

Null Phenotypes

Jk$_{null}$ is autosomal recessive, reflecting homozygosity for a JK^{null} or amorph allele (see Table 35-25). *In(Jk)* is a second Jk (a–b–) phenotype that is characterized by very weak Kidd expression. Similar to *In(Lu)*, the *In(Jk)* phenotype is autosomal dominant owing to a suppressor gene at a distant, unrelated locus. It is interesting to note that Jk$_{null}$ RBCs are resistant to lysis by 2M urea, a lytic agent used by some automated hematology analyzers. *In(Jk)* RBCs have intermediate resistance to urea (Issitt, 1998). No change in gas permeability is seen with Jk$_{null}$ cells (Endeward, 2006).

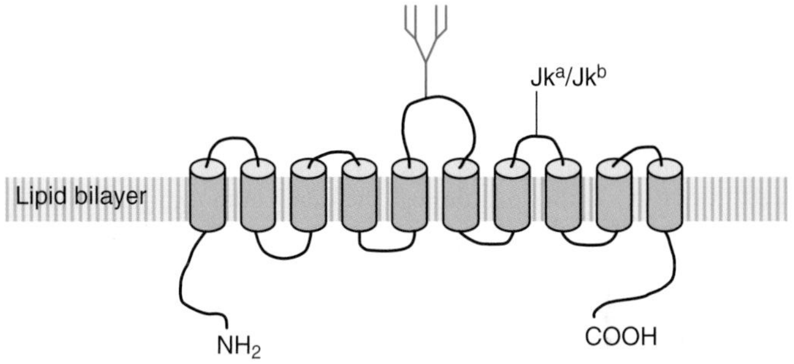

Figure 35-11 The Kidd/urea transporter glycoprotein. The site of Jk^a/Jk^b polymorphism at residue 280 is indicated by a solid line. The *N*-glycosylation site is indicated by a branched structure on the third extracellular loop. The 10 transmembrane domains are represented by amber cylinders.

Biochemistry

Apparent resistance to urea by Jk$_{null}$ RBCs became clear with cloning and isolation of the human erythroid urea transporter (UT-B). The latter is a 43–45-kD multipass glycoprotein, which shares 60% homology with the vasopressin-sensitive urea transporter of rabbits (UT2) and humans (HUT2, UT-A) (Lucien, 1998). The molecule is a 391 amino acid protein with 10 transmembrane domains and a cytosolic amino- and carboxy-terminus (Fig. 35-11). A single *N*-glycan is present on the third extracellular loop (Asn222) and expresses ABO antigens (Lucien, 2002). The Jk^a/Jk^b antigens reside on the fourth extracellular loop at amino acid 280. The third extracellular loop may play a key role in urea transport.

Molecular Biology

The Kidd glycoprotein is encoded by a 30-kb gene *(JK, SLC14A1, UT-B)* on chromosome 18q12-21. This is the same location as the human HUT2/UT-A urea transporter (61% homology), suggesting that the two genes arose by gene duplication. The *JK* gene is organized over 11 exons, although only exons 4–11 encode the mature protein (Lucien, 1998). Similar to many blood group genes, the promoter region contains a GATA-1 consensus sequence, as well as other *cis*-regulatory elements (AP-2, AP-3, NF-ATp, Sp1, Ets-1). A single-bp transition (G823A) is the molecular basis of the Jk^a/Jk^b polymorphism, resulting in an Asp280 (Jk^a) or Asn280 (Jk^b) (Lucien, 2002). Three novel missense mutations associated with JK*A (W171R, E44K) and JK*B (A183V) alleles have been reported, resulting in weak and/or discrepant phenotyping with different commercial typing reagents (Whorley, 2009). In the autosomal recessive Jk$_{null}$ phenotype, more than 10 distinct inactivating mutations have been identified, including splice-site, nonsense, and missense mutations (Reid, 2004; Wester, 2008; Liu, 2009). The etiology of the *In(Jk)* phenotype is unknown.

Kidd Antibodies

Clinically, anti-Jk or Kidd antibodies are a common cause of hemolytic transfusion reactions, accounting for nearly one quarter of all delayed hemolytic transfusion reactions and 75% of those with true hemolytic sequelae (Ness, 1990). They are usually of IgG1 or IgG3 isotype and are capable of activating complement (see Table 35-7). Antibody reactivity can be enhanced with enzyme-treated RBCs and by the presence of complement. Anti-Jk is not enhanced by polybrene (Liu, 2009). An anti-Jk3, which reacts with all RBCs except Jk_{null}, is observed in Jk_{null} individuals (see Table 35-25). Anti-Jk3 was also reported in one individual carrying the JK^*A^{44K} allele (Whorley, 2009).

Anti-Jk antibodies can be difficult to detect or identify in the blood bank. Anti-Jk antibodies are often of low titer with weak avidity and can display dosage in vitro. Furthermore, anti-Jk antibodies are frequently transient, disappearing rapidly after immune stimulation. As a consequence, patients previously sensitized to Kidd antigens may be negative for anti-Jk antibodies in later blood samples. Following transfusion of crossmatch–compatible, Jk-positive RBCs, sensitized patients can mount a brisk anamnestic antibody response with rapid and extensive in vivo hemolysis as RBCs are cleared by extravascular and intravascular hemolysis. Although uncommon, anti-Jk can cause a mild HDFN.

Biological Role

Biologically, JK/UT-B functions in the facilitated transport of urea. In kidney, transport of urea by JK/UT-B on vasa recta endothelial cells is thought to help stabilize osmotic gradients in the renal medulla during the concentration of urine. On RBCs, JK/UT-B may help preserve the osmotic stability of RBCs as they pass through the kidney. Although Jk_{null} individuals exhibit a slightly decreased capacity to concentrate urine, the absence of JK/UT-B is not associated with a clinical syndrome. It is likely that other mechanisms exist to compensate or reduplicate the function of JK/UT-B on tissues (Lucien, 1998).

DIEGO BLOOD GROUP SYSTEM (ISBT NO. 010)

The Diego blood group system consists of 21 antigens, including four sets of allelic antigens (Table 35-26). Nineteen antigens are rare, low-incidence antigens present on less than 1% of donors. In general, there are no apparent racial differences in the expression of most Diego antigens except Di^a. Initially described in 1955, Di^a antigen is rare in all populations except those of Mongolian ancestry, Asian people, and native South American Indians. In some South American Indian populations, the frequency of Di^a can reach 50% (Issitt, 1998). In addition to RBCs, Diego antigens are expressed by human kidney along the collecting ducts (Tanner, 1993). One million copies of Diego glycoprotein (AE1) are present per RBC.

Biochemistry

The Diego blood group system resides on Band 3, also known as AE1. AE1 is a 100-kD, 991 amino acid glycoprotein containing two functionally distinct domains: a large 40-kD amino-terminal cytoplasmic domain and a transmembrane domain comprising the carboxy-terminal half of the molecule (Fig. 35-12). On RBCs, AE1 is an oligomer, usually existing as a dimer or tetramer through the formation of intramolecular disulfide bonds. The amino-terminal cytoplasmic domain binds several key cytoskeletal proteins (band 4.1, band 4.2, and ankyrin) and three glycolytic enzymes: glutaraldehyde-3-phosphate dehydrogenase, aldolase, and phosphofructokinase. Binding of hemochromes or denatured Hg to the extreme amino-terminus of AE1 is believed to play a role in Heinz body formation. There is also an apparent, noncovalent association of AE1 with GYPA on RBC membranes (Low, 1986). Miltenberger type III cells (Gp.Mur), a glycophorin B-A-B hybrid, have increased AE1 on red cells (Hsu, 2009).

The remainder of AE1 is membrane associated, containing 12–14 transmembrane domains, which constitute the carboxy-terminal half of the molecule. Whereas the amino-terminal domain is involved in membrane stability, the carboxy-terminal domain functions as an anion transporter, facilitating transfusion of Cl^- and HCO_3^- anions across the cell membrane (Tanner, 1993). The carboxy-terminal, transmembrane domain is also the site of all the Diego antigens described to date. There is a single *N*-glycosylation site, which displays a massive, highly branched, polylactosaminoglycan with both ABO and I blood group activity (Fukuda, 1984). It is estimated that nearly half of all ABO epitopes on RBCs are associated with AE1.

Molecular Biology

AE1 is the product of a 20-exon, 17-kb gene *(SLC4A1)* on chromosome 17q21-q22. The cloning of the *AE1* gene was invaluable in assigning several orphan antigens to the Diego system. Like so many blood group antigens, every Diego antigen identified to date is the result of a point mutation, leading to an amino acid polymorphism in the translated protein (see Table 35-26 and Fig. 35-12). Most of these amino acid polymorphisms occur among nonconserved amino acid residues, based on a comparison of AE1 with the sequences of other anion transporters (Reid, 2004). The Diego system also contains two examples of allelic, low-incidence antigens: Mo^a/Hg^a and Jn^a/KREP. In each case, two distinct amino acid substitutions at the same amino acid residue lead to different

TABLE 35-26
Diego Blood Group Antigens

ANTIGEN (HIGH FREQUENCY)					ANTIGEN (LOW FREQUENCY)	
ISBT	**Name**	**Percent donors**	**Amino acid change* (high→low frequency)**	**Percent donors**	**Name**	**ISBT**
DI2	Di^b	>99.9	Pro854>Leu	Very rare†	Di^a	DI1
DI4	Wr^b	99	Glu658>Lys	1	Wr^a	DI3
			Val557>Met	<0.1	Wd^a	DI5
			Pro548>Leu	<0.1	Rb^a	DI6
			Thr552>Ile	<0.1	WARR	DI7
			Arg432>Trp	<0.1	ELO	DI8
			Gly565>Ala	<0.1	Wu	DI9
			Asn569>Lys	<0.1	Bp^a	DI10
			Arg656>His	<0.1	Mo^a	DI11
			Arg656>Cys	<0.1	Hg^a	DI12
			Tyr555>His	<0.1	Vg^a	DI13
			Lys551>Asn	<0.1	Tr^a	DI19
			Arg646>Gln	<0.1	Sw^a	DI14
			Glu429>Asp	<0.1	NFLD	DI16
			Pro566>Ser	<0.1	Jn^a	DI17
			Pro566>Ala	<0.1	KREP	DI18
			Pro561>Ser	<0.1	BOW	DI15
			Glu480>Lys	<0.1	Fr^a	DI20
			Arg646>Trp	<0.1	SWI	DI21

ISBT, International Society of Blood Transfusion.
*Referenced in Daniels (2004) and Reid (2004b).
†Di^a antigen has a much higher incidence among North and South American Indians, Asian people, and people of Mongolian ancestry (e.g., Eastern Poland).

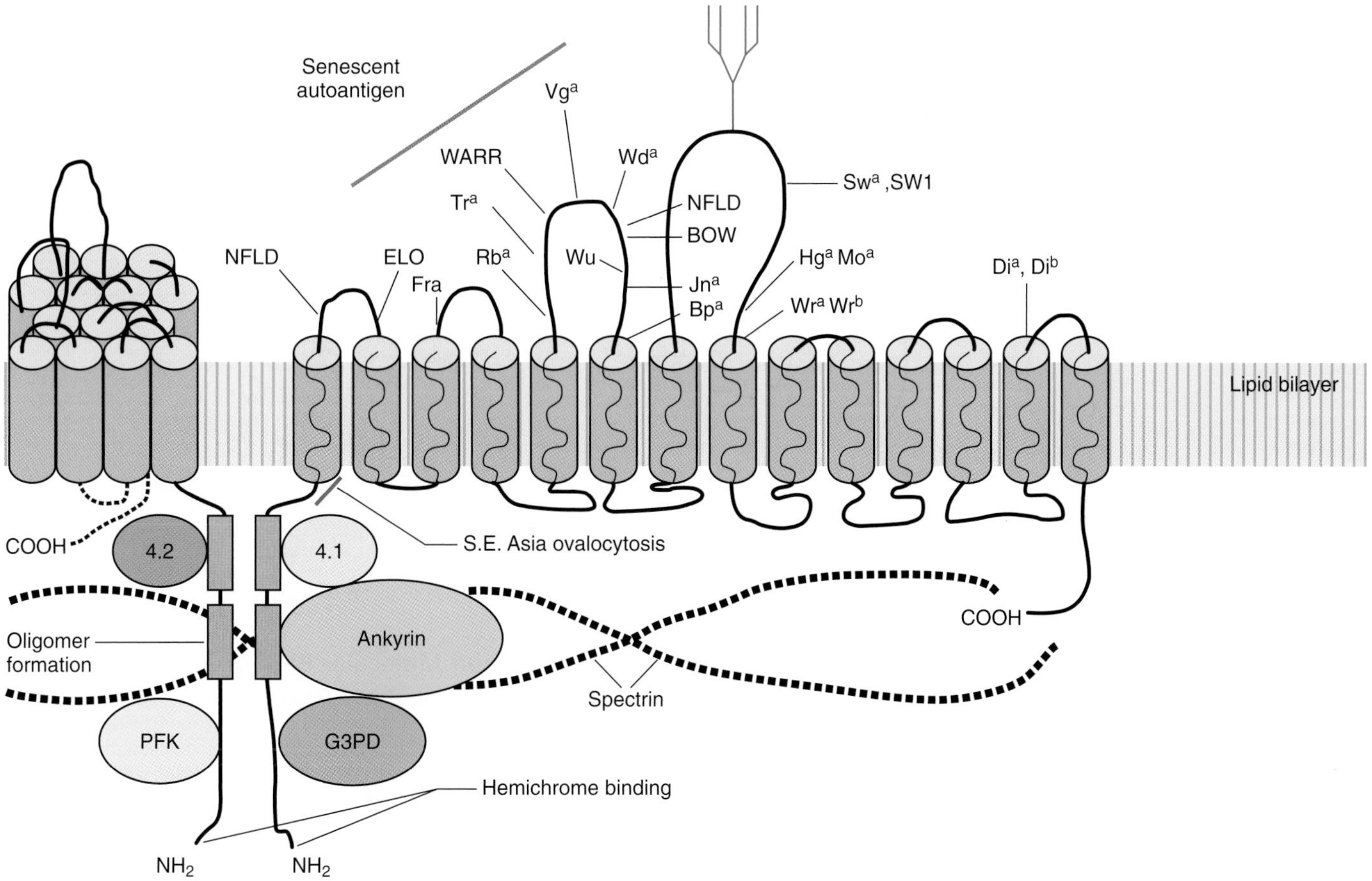

Figure 35-12 Structure of anion exchange protein AE1 (Band 3). AE1 is a multipass glycoprotein with 14 transmembrane domains, indicated by solid amber cylinders. The Diego blood group antigens reside along the extracellular loops and are indicated by solid lines. The AE1 senescent autoantigen is on the third extracellular loop between Rb^a^ and Vg^a^ antigens. The massive *N*-glycan is shown by a branched structure on the fourth extracellular loop. The large cytoplasmic domain has binding sites for cytoskeletal proteins 4.2, 4.1, and ankyrin, as well as the glycolytic enzymes phosphofructokinase (PFK) and glutaraldehyde-3-phosphate dehydrogenase (G3PD). In the red cell membrane, AE1 exists as oligomers (dimers, tetramers) linked by interchain disulfide bonds along the amino-terminal cytoplasmic domain *(solid rectangles)*. An 8 amino acid deletion at the boundary of the amino-terminal cytoplasmic domain and the first transmembrane domain is responsible for Southeast Asia ovalocytosis (SAO).

alloantigens. A similar example exists in the Kell system (Kp^a, Kp^b, and Kp^c).

The most interesting Diego antigen, however, is Wr^b. As stated earlier, AE1 is topically associated with GYPA in the RBC membrane. RBCs lacking GYPA (En [a–] phenotype) are phenotypically Wr (a–b–), implying that Wr^b is on GYPA. Available evidence now suggests that Wr^b is formed by an electrostatic interaction between GYPA and a glutamic acid (Glu658) on AE1 (Poole, 1999). Which specific amino acid on GYPA is critical to Wr^b formation is still a matter of debate, but clearly part of the Wr^b epitope involves amino acids on GYPA (see Fig. 34-3).

Diego Antibodies

Antibodies against Diego blood group antigens can be immune stimulated or naturally occurring. Antibodies against Di^a, Di^b, Wr^b, and ELO are usually immune stimulated. These antibodies are of IgG isotype and are detected in the AHG phase of testing. Anti-Di^a, Di^b, and Wr^b can be associated with decreased red cell survival, hemolytic transfusion reactions, and HDFN. Anti-Wr^b is also associated with autoimmune hemolytic anemia (Issitt, 1998).

In contrast, antibodies against the majority of other Diego antigens are usually naturally occurring, room temperature, saline agglutinins. Anti-Wr^a is particularly common, occurring in 1 in 100 donors. Antibodies against Wd^a and WARR are also fairly common, with anti-WARR reported in 13%–18% of donors (Issitt, 1998).

Biological Role

Functionally, AE1 plays a critical role in gas transport and acid-base equilibrium. To facilitate the removal of CO_2, RBCs hydrate CO_2 via carbonic anhydrous to form bicarbonate ion (HCO_3^-), which is readily soluble in plasma. As the level of intracellular HCO_3^- rises, RBCs exchange HCO_3^- ions for Cl^- in plasma (the Cl^- shift, or Hamburger shift). This process is mediated by AE1 as RBCs pass through capillaries and small capillary venules. Because of the high copy number of AE1 on the RBC membrane, anion exchange is 90% complete within 0.4–0.5 second. An increase in HCO_3^- capacity and osmotic resistance is observed with Miltenberger III red cells owing to significantly higher AE1 expression (Hsu, 2009). In the kidney, AE1 is expressed along the basolateral membrane of type A intercalated cells of renal collecting ducts, where it functions in acid secretion and bicarbonate readsorption (Tanner, 1993). Given the physiologic importance of AE1, it is not surprising that no Diego null phenotype has been described to date.

AE1 also plays a role in the RBC cytoskeleton (see Fig. 35-12). The long, amino-terminal half of the molecule binds several peripheral proteins involved in the stability of the RBC membrane. AE1 tetramers bind ankyrin, protein 4.2, and protein 4.1, which help to anchor and stabilize the RBC membrane to the underlying cytoskeleton (Tanner, 1993). AE1 protein may contribute to red cell senescence. Cold storage is rapidly associated with the formation and clustering of large, AE1 oligomers, which could promote red cell clearance (Karon, 2009). In addition, at least one senescent autoantigen on RBCs is located on AE1, between amino acids 538 and 554 (between Rb^a and Vg^a antigens; see Fig. 35-12) (Kay, 1994).

CARTWRIGHT BLOOD GROUP SYSTEM (ISBT NO. 011)

Discovered in 1956, the Cartwright (Yt) blood group system consists of two autosomal codominant antigens: Yt^a and Yt^b. Yt^a is a high-incidence antigen expressed by 99.8% of Caucasian donors. The incidence of Yt^b varies by race, ranging from 0% in Japanese to 24%–26% in the Mideast (Issitt, 1998). Yt antigens are missing on PNH III RBCs, which are devoid of all glycophosphoinositol (GPI)-linked glycoproteins. In addition to RBCs, Cartwright antigens are expressed on neural synapses and neuromuscular junctions (Masson, 1994). A total of 7000–10,000 molecules of Yt glycoprotein are present per RBC.

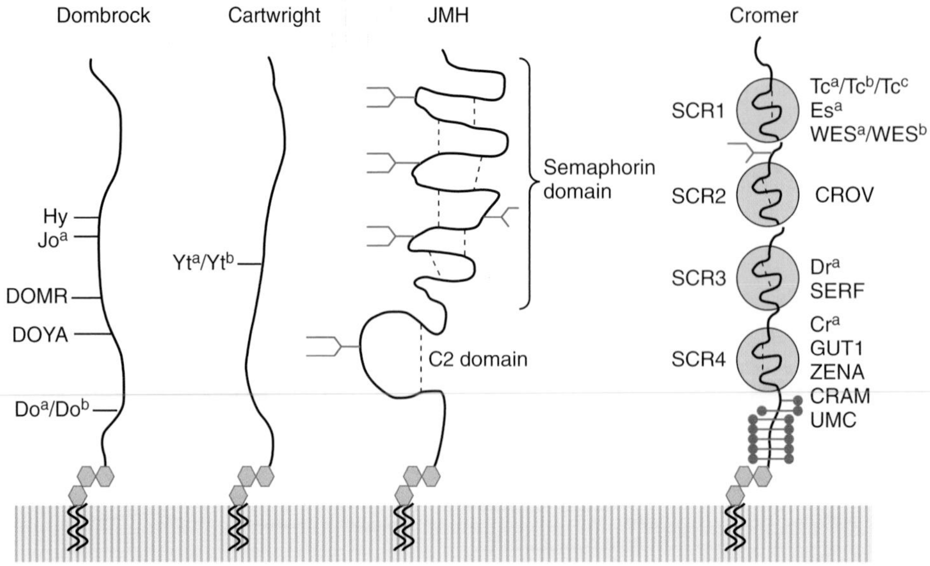

Figure 35-13 Blood group antigens on glycophosphoinositol-linked glycoproteins.

Biochemistry

The Cartwright antigens are located on acetylcholinesterase (AChE), a β-carboxyesterase responsible for degradation of the neurotransmitter acetylcholine. Several different molecular forms of AChE have been isolated, including large heteromeric forms composed of several catalytic subunits covalently linked to collagen. On RBCs, AChE is expressed as a palmitoylated, GPI-linked glycoprotein (Fig. 35-13) (Li, 1991). Human erythrocyte AChE is unique in the palmitoylation or covalent linkage of a palmitic fatty acid to the inositol ring, which renders the molecule resistant to phospholipase C. In RBC membranes, AChE usually exists as a 160-kD dimer and possesses both *N*- and *O*-linked glycans.

Molecular Biology

The gene for AChE possesses four exons, spanning 4.5–4.7kb, on chromosome 7q22. Alternate splicing of exon 3 is responsible for the GPI-linked form of AChE observed in RBCs (Li, 1991). The Yt^a and Yt^b antigens represent a single–amino acid polymorphism at residue 322, where His322 is Yt^a and Asn322 is Yt^b (Bartels, 1993). The Yt^a/Yt^b polymorphism is not located near the catalytic site of the enzyme and has no effect on enzyme activity (Masson, 1994).

Cartwright Antibodies

In general, anti-Yt^a and Yt^b are usually clinically benign, although shortened red cell survival and even delayed hemolytic transfusion reactions have been reported. Neither antibody is associated with HDFN (Issitt, 1998). Anti-Yt^a and anti-Yt^b are of IgG isotype, arising from immune stimulation, and are usually detected in the IAT. Despite the high incidence of Yt^a in the general population, anti-Yt^a is more common than anti-Yt^b, suggesting that Yt^a is the more immunogenic antigen. Anti-Yt^a is also more likely to cause a positive monocyte-monolayer assay with decreased red cell survival (Arndt, 2004).

Biological Role

AChE is a critical enzyme required for the rapid degradation of acetylcholine on postsynaptic membranes of nerves and muscles. The role of AChE in RBCs is unknown.

XG BLOOD GROUP SYSTEM (ISBT NO. 012)

The Xg blood group system contains a single antigen, Xg^a. As a result, only two phenotypes are known: Xg^a-positive and Xg^a-negative. Because the Xg^a antigen is encoded by a gene on the X chromosome, the incidence of the Xg^a-positive phenotype is higher among women. Among Caucasians, approximately 89% of women and 66% of men are Xg^a-positive. Similar results have been found in other ethnic populations (Byrne, 2004). Xg appears to be specific for RBCs. Approximately 9000 molecules of Xg^a are present per RBC (Reid, 2004).

Biochemistry and Molecular Biology

The Xg^a antigen is located on a 24–29-kD, 180 amino acid glycoprotein named XG protein. A type 1 glycoprotein, XG protein possesses a large, 117 amino acid, amino-terminal extracellular domain, a single transmembrane domain, and a short, carboxy-terminal cytoplasmic tail. Of 11 potential *O*-glycosylation sites, only three appear to be glycosylated. The protein is encoded by a 2.4-kb gene *(XG)* located on the X chromosome at the pseudoautosomal boundary/X-specific boundary (pAB1X).

In the RBC membrane, the XG protein may be topologically associated with a second protein, MIC2 or CD99. The latter is a 32.5-kD glycoprotein biochemically similar to XG protein. Evidence suggesting a near-neighbor relationship of the XG and MIC2 proteins includes MIC2 inhibition of anti-Xg^a antibodies and coimmunoprecipitation of MIC2 by anti-Xg^a. And finally, high MIC2 expression is observed on Xg^a-positive, but not Xg^a-negative, erythrocytes (Daniels, 2002).

Xg^a Antibodies

Anti-Xg^a is not associated with hemolytic transfusion reactions or HDFN (Byrne, 2004). Anti-Xg^a may be immune stimulated or naturally occurring. Most examples are of IgG isotype, including some capable of activating complement. Because of differences in Xg^a-positive phenotype between men and women, most examples (>85%) of anti-Xg^a are observed in men.

SCIANNA BLOOD GROUP SYSTEM (ISBT NO. 013)

The Scianna (Sc) blood group system contains seven antigens. Sc1 and Sc2 are antithetical antigens, with most individuals typing as Sc:1,-2. Sc2 and Sc4/Rd are low-incidence antigens, whereas Sc3, Sc5, Sc6, and Sc7 are high-incidence antigens (Table 35-27) (Wagner, 2003; Flegel, 2005; Hue-Roye, 2005). Sc3 is a high-incidence antigen present on all RBCs except Sc_{null} (Sc: −1, −2, −3). Scianna appears to be specific for RBCs and erythropoietic tissues.

Biochemistry

Scianna antigens reside on *e*rythrocyte *m*embrane-*a*ssociated *p*rotein (ERMAP), a 60–68-kD, 446 amino acid glycoprotein. Similar to Lutheran, Ok, and LW proteins, ERMAP is a member of the Ig superfamily. The molecule is a type 1 single-pass transmembrane protein possessing a single IgV domain and a large cytoplasmic domain that is likely involved in signal transduction. The latter possess both SH3 and B30.2 domains, as well as multiple phosphorylation sequences for protein kinase C, tyrosine kinase, and casein kinase II (Su, 2001). The molecule possesses 11 cysteine residues and is sensitive to sulfhydryl-reducing agents.

Molecular Biology

The *ERMAP* gene resides on chromosome 1p34 and consists of 11 exons spanning 19kb. Most Sc antigens are the result of an SNP and amino acid polymorphism (see Table 35-27). Of three Sc_{null} studied to date, one was the result of a deletion and frameshift mutation (307del2) and two were the result of an SNP leading to a stop codon (Wagner, 2003; Flegel, 2005). An additional amino acid polymorphism (His26>Tyr) has been identified in the leader sequence, which is not expressed on the mature red cell protein (Flegel, 2005; Fuchisawa, 2009). Approximately 25% of Caucasians are positive for the His26>Tyr polymorphism (Fuchisawa, 2009).

Scianna Antibodies

Anti-Scianna antibodies are rare and generally benign. They are usually of IgG isotype with some examples binding complement. Most examples are immune stimulated; however, naturally occurring anti-Sc2 antibodies are known. The antigens are relatively resistant to enzymes but can be weakened with DTT and AET. They are not a cause of transfusion reactions. Anti-Sc4 and anti-Sc2 have been associated with HDFN. Autoantibodies against Sc1 and Sc3 antigens have been associated with warm autoimmune hemolytic anemia (Issitt, 1998). Anti-Scianna antibodies can be neutralized with soluble recombinant ERMAP protein (Seltsam, 2009).

Biological Role

The biological role of ERMAP is unknown, although its structure suggests that it may play a role in RBC adhesion and signaling. The IgV domain possesses a C1q recognition sequence that may mediate adhesion between marrow macrophages and erythroblasts in erythroid islands. Because ERMAP shares homology with the B7 family of proteins (CD80, CD86) and neural autoantigens, it is speculated that ERMAP could be involved in immune recognition and autoimmune anemia (Su, 2001).

DOMBROCK BLOOD GROUP SYSTEM (ISBT NO. 014)

The Dombrock blood group system contains seven antigens. Do^a (DO1) and Do^b (DO2) are autosomal codominant antigens expressed by 67% and 82% of white donors, respectively (Table 35-28). Gy^a, Hy, Jo^a, DOYA, and DOMR are high-incidence antigens found on virtually all donors. In addition to RBCs, Dombrock mRNA has been identified in fetal liver and spleen (Gubin, 2000).

Null/Weak Phenotypes

The Do_{null} or Gy(a–) phenotype is a rare, autosomal recessive phenotype (see Table 35-28). An acquired Do_{null} phenotype can be observed in paroxysmal nocturnal hemoglobinuria type III (PNH-III). A hematopoietic stem cell disorder, PNH III is characterized by chronic hemolysis due to an absence of all GPI-linked glycoproteins, including Cromer, Dombrock and Cartwright antigens.

Loss of one high-incidence Dombrock antigen is often accompanied by weakened expression of other Dombrock antigens (see Table 35-28). This is due to the heterogeneity of Dombrock alleles, which carry different combinations of Dombrock antigens (Reid, 2005; Baleotti, 2006). Hy(–) and DOMR(–) individuals typically have weakened Do^b and Gy^a and weak/absent Jo^a expression, whereas Jo(a–) is often associated with weak Do^a, Hy, and Gy expression (Reid, 2005; Costa, 2009). The one example of DOYA(-) types as Co(a--b–) with weakened expression of Gy, Hy, and Jo^a (Daniels, 2009).

Biochemistry

Dombrock antigens reside on an adenosine diphosphate (ADP)-ribosyltransferase (CD297), which catalyzes the transfer of ADP-ribose from nicotinamide adenine dinucleotide (NAD) to a protein acceptor. The cloned molecule is a 47–58-kD, 314 amino acid glycoprotein that is anchored into the RBC membrane via a GPI glycolipid tail (GPI-linked; see Fig. 35-13). The molecule has five potential *N*-glycosylation sites, two myristoylation sites, and five cysteine residues (Gubin, 2000; Daniels, 2002). As a consequence, Dombrock can be destroyed by disulfide-reducing agents and phosphatidylinositol phospholipase C, which cleaves GPI-linked proteins (Gubin, 2000).

Molecular Biology

The gene for Dombrock *(ART4)* spans 14 kb on chromosome 12p13.2-12.1. The gene consists of three exons, although exon 2 encodes more than 70% of the translated protein and includes all seven Dombrock antigens. Do^a, Do^b, Jo^a, Hy, DOYA, and DOMR are the result of a single–amino acid polymorphism (see Table 35-28). The Do_{null} or Gy(a-) phenotype is the result of mutations that abolish exon 2 (Reid, 2005).

Dombrock Antibodies

Anti-Dombrock antibodies can be clinically significant, although many examples are benign. They are commonly found in mixtures of alloantibodies and can be difficult to identify. Anti-Dombrock antibodies are capable of causing shortened RBC survival and acute and delayed hemolytic transfusion reactions. Transfusion reactions and accelerated clearance due to anti-Dombrock antibodies can be missed in routine testing, with implicated units often testing as **crossmatch–compatible,** even in a full IAT crossmatch. Moreover, a posttransfusion direct antiglobulin test and eluate can be negative with no observable rise in antibody titer with

TABLE 35-27
Scianna Blood Group Antigens

Antigen (high frequency)	Percent donors	Amino acid change (high→low frequency)	Percent donors	Antigen (low frequency)
Sc1	99	Gly57>Arg	0.7	Sc2
Sc3	100	307delGA Arg332stop	Rare	SC_{null}
		Pro>Ala	Rare	(Rd) Sc4
Sc5 (STAR)	100	Glu>Lys		
Sc6 (SCER)	100	Arg81>Gln		
Sc7 (SCAN)	100	Gly35>Ser		

From Wagner (2003), Reid (2004), Flegel (2005), and Hue-Roye (2005).

TABLE 35-28
Phenotypes of the Dombrock System

REACTIONS WITH ANTI-DOMBROCK ANTIBODIES										FREQUENCY (%) U.S. POPULATION	
Do^a	Do^b	Gy^a	Jo^a	Hy	D06	DOMR	Phenotype	ISBT	Amino acid change	Caucasian	Black
+	0	+	+	+	+	+	Do (a+b–)	D01	Asn265	18	11
+	+	+	+	+	+	+	Do (a+b+)			49	44
0	+	+	+	+	+	+	Do (a–b+)	D02	Asp265	33	45
Null/Weak Phenotypes											
0	0	0	0	0	0	0	Gy(a–) or Do_{null}†	D03	Loss exon 2*	Rare	Rare
0	w	w	0/w	0	w	+	Hy(–)	D04	Gly108>Val	Rare	Rare
w	0/w	+	0	w	w	0/w	Jo(a–)	D05	Thr117>Ile	Rare	Rare
0	0	w	w	w	0	?	DOYA(–)	D06	Tyr183>Asp	Rare	Rare
0	+	0	w	w	?	0	DOMR(–)	D07	Ala144>Glu	Rare	Rare

ISBT, International Society of Blood Transfusion.
*Loss of exon 2 has been associated with splice-site, frameshift, and nonsense mutations (Reid, 2003a; 2004b).
†Also associated with PNH III red blood cells (RBCs), which lack all glycophosphoinositol (GPI)-linked glycoproteins, including Dombrock, Cartwright, and Cromer antigens.

time (Reid, 2005; Baumgarten, 2006). Anti-Dombrock is not associated with HDFN.

Antibodies against Dombrock antigens are usually of IgG isotype, arising from immune stimulation by transfusion or pregnancy. Antibody reactivity can be enhanced by the use of papain- or ficin-treated RBCs. Conversely, antibody reactivity is reduced or abolished by the treatment of red cells with sulfhydryl-reducing agents (DTT, AET), trypsin, chymotrypsin, and pronase. Anti-Dombrock can deteriorate with in vitro storage, complicating pretransfusion testing (Baumgartner, 2006). In addition, Dombrock titers may decrease over time in vivo, falling below the level of detection (Reid, 2005).

Biological Role

Although Dombrock is an ADP-ribosyltransferase, no enzyme activity has been reported on RBC membranes (Reid, 2005). No known clinical syndrome is associated with a Do_{null} phenotype. It has been hypothesized that Dombrock may play a role in clearing circulating NAD+ and/or post-translational modification of proteins (Reid, 2005). Dombrock may also contribute to integrin-mediated cell adhesion via an RGD motif at the Do^b antigen; the RGD motif is abolished in the Do^a phenotype.

COLTON BLOOD GROUP SYSTEM (ISBT NO. 015)

The Colton blood group system was initially identified in 1967 and consists of two autosomal codominant antigens, Co^a and Co^b, and a third high-incidence antigen ("TOR") (Arnaud, 2008). Co^a is a high-incidence antigen present on 99.7% of donors. Co^b is expressed by less than 11% of donors, with only 0.3% being Co (a–b+). Although very rare, a Co (a–b–) or null phenotype is reported. Colton antigens are expressed on RBCs, renal proximal tubules, thin descending limb of Henle, renal vasa recta endothelium, choroid plexus, ciliary body, microvessels, gallbladder, placenta, and some epithelial cells. More than 120,000–160,000 molecules of Colton glycoprotein are present per RBC.

Biochemistry

The Colton blood group antigens reside on aquaporin 1 (AQP-1) or channel-forming integral protein, a water-selective membrane channel (Fig. 35-14). Cloned in 1991, AQP-1 is a 269 amino acid multipass integral membrane protein containing six transmembrane domains. Crystallographic studies suggest that the first intracellular and third extracellular loops fold back into the plasma membrane, overlapping at two Asp-Pro-Ala (NPA) sequences to form a water channel. A single *N*-glycosylation site (Asn42), capable of expressing ABH antigens, is found in the first extracellular loop near the Co^a/Co^b and TOR epitopes (residues 45 and 47). The latter is variably glycosylated in vivo, leading to a spectrum of AQP-1 glycoforms, ranging from 40–60kD (Agre, 1994). In RBC membranes, AQP-1 exists as a homotetramer, a square array of AQP-1 monomers, which may help stabilize the structure and functional integrity of individual monomers (Knepper, 1994).

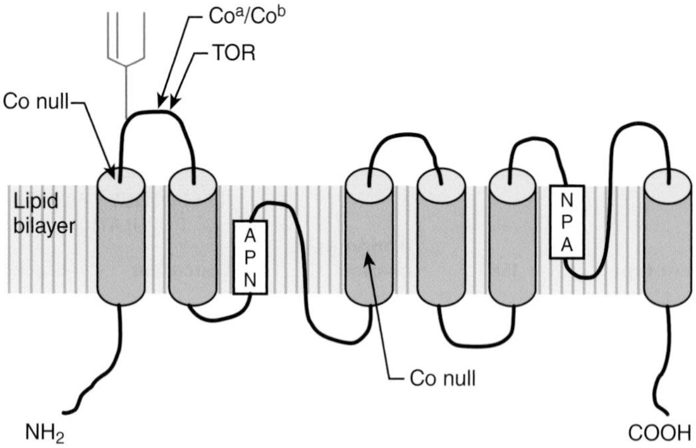

Figure 35-14 Structure of aquaporin-1 (AQP-1, channel-forming integral protein [CHIP]). AQP-1 is a multipass protein containing six transmembrane domains, indicated by solid amber cylinders. The first cytoplasmic and third extracellular loops fold back into the lipid bilayer, overlapping at two Asp-Pro-Ala (NPA) motifs, to form a water channel. The *N*-glycosylation site is indicated by a branched structure on the first extracellular loop. The Co^a/Co^b polymorphism at amino acid 45 is indicated by a solid line. TOR is a rare antigen adjacent to the Co^a/Co^b polymorphism at amino acid 47. The sites of two mutations leading to a Colton null phenotype are also shown.

Molecular Biology

AQP-1 is a 17-kb gene on chromosome 7p14. The gene has four exons and both TATA and Sp1 consensus sequences in the promoter region (Moon, 1993). The Co^a and Co^b antigens are the result of an A314T polymorphism, leading to Ala45 (Co^a) or Val45 (Co^b) (Smith, 1994). A third polymorphism (Gln47>Arg) just distal to the Co^a/Co^b polymorphism was recently identified in an alloimmunized Turkish patient (TOR) with an apparent anti-Co3 (Arnaud, 2008). Several different inactivating mutations of the AQP-1 gene are associated with the Co_{null} phenotype, including deletion of exon 1 and frameshift and missense mutations. An acquired Co_{null} phenotype is also reported in rare patients with monosomy 7 and congenital dyserythropoietic anemia (Agre, 1994).

Colton Antibodies

Anti-Colton antibodies can be clinically significant: They can be associated with shortened RBC survival, hemolytic transfusion reactions, and HDFN (see Table 35-7). Antibodies to Co^a and Co^b are usually of the IgG isotype, resulting from immune stimulation by transfusion or pregnancy. Some examples of anti-Co^a and anti-Co^b are reported to bind complement. Anti-Colton antibodies are detectable in the AHG phase of testing and are enhanced with protease-treated RBCs. Rare Co_{null} and "TOR-negative" individuals can make an anti-Co3 (anti-Co^{a+b}), an alloantibody that reacts with both Co (a+b–) and Co (a–b+) RBCs (Reid, 2004; Arnaud, 2008).

Biological Role

Biologically, AQP-1 is a major molecular water channel on RBCs that facilitates the concentration of urine in kidney (Verkman, 2009). Co_{null} red cells also have decreased CO_2 permeability (Endeward, 2006). Despite its importance in water regulation, Colton-null individuals show few or no adverse clinical effects. Co_{null} RBCs appear morphologically normal in appearance and number, although mild decreases in RBC life span are reported (Mathai, 1996). The absence of any clinically significant hematologic sequelae in Co_{null} individuals is most likely due to the presence of a second aquaporin, AQP-3. A glycerol and, perhaps, urea transporter, AQP-3 (GIL blood group) is moderately permeable to water and appears to account for the residual water permeability on Co_{null} RBCs (Roudier, 1998; Verkman, 2009).

LW BLOOD GROUP SYSTEM (ISBT NO. 016)

Named in honor of its discoverers, the LW, or Landsteiner-Wiener, blood group system is most important for its role in the history of the Rh blood group system. Landsteiner and Wiener originally developed antibodies against the LW antigens by immunizing rabbits with rhesus monkey red cells. The resulting "anti-Rh" antibodies were initially believed to recognize the RhD antigen; however, later investigators proved that the antibodies developed by Landsteiner and Wiener recognized a non-Rh (LW) antigen.

The LW blood group system consists of two allelic antigens: LW^a and LW^b. LW^a is a high-frequency antigen (99% of white donors). Expression of LW antigen is dependent on RhD protein expression, with the highest expression observed on RhD-positive red cells and weaker expression on RhD-negative cells. LW antigens are absent from Rh_{null} erythrocytes. An LW (a–b–) or null phenotype can also be seen in very rare individuals who are homozygous for a silent LW allele. The LW antigen is expressed on RBCs and placenta. Approximately 3600–5000 molecules of LW glycoprotein are present per RBC (Issitt, 1998).

Biochemistry

The LW antigens reside on intracellular adhesion molecule type 4 (ICAM-4, CD242), a 40–47-kD type 1 glycoprotein. A member of the Ig superfamily, ICAM consists of two extracellular C2-like domains: a single transmembrane domain and a short cytoplasmic tail. Four *N*-glycosylation sites are present, along with evidence of *O*-glycosylation, which may influence adhesion (Toivanen, 2008). Although several amino acids are critical for ICAM-4/integrin binding, the first C2 or Ig domain is most critical (Toivanen, 2008). The molecule has three disulfide bonds and is sensitive to reducing agents such as DTT (Reid, 2004).

TABLE 35-29
Chido/Rodgers Blood Group Antigens

Chido (Ch) antigens		Name	Frequency*	Amino acid	Frequency*	Name	Rodgers (Rg) antigens	
CH/RG3†	CH/RG1	Ch1	96%	Arg1191>Leu Ala1188>Val	98%	Rg1	CH/RG11	CH/RG12†
	CH/RG6	Ch3	93%	Conformational epitope	95%	Rg2		
		Ch6	96%	Ser1157>Asn	95%	Rg3	CH/RG13	
CH/RG7†		WH	Rare	Conformational epitope (Ch6+Rg1)				
CH/RG2†	CH/RG4	Ch4	96%	His1106>Asp Ile1105>Leu Ser1102>Lys Leu1101 Pro				
		Ch2	91%	Conformational epitope (Ch4+Ch5)				
	CH/RG5	Ch5	94%	Gly1054>Asp				

*Calculated from Giles (1987) and Issitt (1998).
†Conformational epitopes Irequire the presence of two Ch/Rg antigenic determinants.

Molecular Biology

The *ICAM4* gene resides on chromosome 19p13. The LW^a and LW^b antigens arise from an SNP (A308G), leading to Gln70 (LW^a) or Arg70 (LW^b). Of two LW_{null} individuals studied, one possessed a 10-bp deletion in the coding sequence (Hermand, 1995).

LW Antibodies

Clinically benign, anti-LW antibodies are rarely a cause of hemolytic transfusion reactions or HDFN. They usually are of IgG isotype and are detected in the IAT. Antibody activity can be reduced by ethylenediaminetetraacetic acid (EDTA) and pretreatment of RBCs with sulfhydryl-reducing agents (DTT, AET). In addition to anti-LW^a and -LW^b, LW_{null} individuals can make an anti-LW^{ab}, which reacts with both LW (a+b–) and LW (a–b+) erythrocytes.

Biological Role

LW glycoprotein is a potential counterreceptor for the β2-integrin protein Mac1 (CD11b/CD18), LFA-1 (CD11a/CD18), and platelet GPIIb/IIIa. It is hypothesized that the LW glycoprotein may participate in adhesive interactions during early erythroid development. Mice lacking ICAM-4 have a decrease in erythroblastic islands in their marrow, although peripheral red cell mass is normal (Toivanen, 2008). LW expression is elevated in sickle cell patients and may be involved in microvascular occlusion (Reid, 2004). LW glycoprotein may also be involved in red cell senescence by binding to CD11/CD18 integrin on splenic macrophages (Issitt, 1998; Toivanen, 2008).

CHIDO/RODGERS BLOOD GROUP SYSTEM (ISBT NO. 017)

The Chido/Rodgers (Ch/Rg) blood group system contains 10 antigens, including two pairs of antithetical antigens and three conformational antigens. The latter require coexpression of two spatially distinct Ch/Rg antigens that together generate a third, conformational antigen (Table 35-29). Most Ch/Rg antigens are high-incidence antigens (>90%). Similar to Lewis blood group antigens, Ch/Rg antigens are of plasma origin and are passively adsorbed onto RBC membranes. Ch/Rg antigens are weakly expressed on cord RBCs and some GYPA-deficient RBCs (Issitt, 1998).

Biochemistry/Molecular Biology

Ch/Rg antigens are antigenic determinants on the C4d fragment of the C4 complement molecule. C4 is the product of two highly homologous genes (99% identity), *C4A* and *C4B*, on chromosome 6p21.3 near the HLA locus. At present, more than 50 C4 alleles have been identified, including null alleles, making the genetics of this system difficult. Each gene spans approximately 22kb and is organized into 41 exons. Four amino acids in exon 26 are responsible for distinguishing C4A from C4B. Most Ch/Rg antigens are determined by amino acid polymorphisms encoded in exons 25 and 28 (Giles, 1988). In general, Chido antigens are on C4B and Rodgers antigens are on C4A, although examples of C4B-expressing Rodgers antigens (and vice versa) are known (Giles 1987, 1988). On protein electrophoresis, C4A migrates faster than C4B.

Chido/Rodgers Antibodies

Antibodies against Ch/Rg antigens do not cause hemolytic transfusion reactions or HDFN. Rare reports have described anaphylaxis following transfusion of plasma and platelets (Westhoff, 1992). Anti-Ch/Rg antibodies are of IgG isotype and are usually detected with AHG. Antibody reactivity can be enhanced by incubating RBCs in a low–ionic sucrose solution. Antibody reactivity can be inhibited by plasma or by treatment of RBCs with proteases (Reid, 2004).

Biological Role

C4 deficiency is associated with autoimmune disorders and susceptibility to bacterial meningitis. Specific C4 allotypes have been linked to several autoimmune disorders, including rheumatoid arthritis and Graves' disease.

GERBICH BLOOD GROUP SYSTEM (ISBT NO. 020)

The Gerbich (Ge) blood group system contains seven antigens: three high-frequency (>99%; Table 35-30) and four low-frequency antigens. The Gerbich glycoproteins (GPC/D; Fig. 35-15) are on fetal and adult RBCs, platelets, and kidney and fetal liver. Between 180,000 and 250,000 molecules of Gerbich are present per RBC (Reid, 2004).

Null/Weak Phenotypes

Three autosomal recessive phenotypes are associated with the loss of high-incidence Gerbich antigens: Yus (Ge-2,3,4), Gerbich (Ge-2,-3,4), and Leach (Ge-2,-3,-4). Gerbich antigens are decreased in patients with hereditary elliptocytosis due to protein 4.1 deficiency (Daniels, 2002).

Biochemistry

Gerbich antigens are expressed on two biosynthetically related type 1 glycoproteins: glycophorin C (GYPC; see Fig. 35-15) and glycophorin D (GYPD). GYPC is a 40-kD, 128 amino acid glycoprotein bearing one *N*-linked and 12 *O*-linked glycans. GYPD is a 107 amino acid variant, lacking 21 amino acids at the amino-terminus (Reid, 2004b). The cytoplasmic domain interacts with several cytoskeletal proteins, including spectrin, protein 4.1, and p55.

Molecular Biology

GYPC and GYPD are the products of a single gene, *GYPC*, on chromosome 2q14-121. The gene spans 13.5kb and is organized into four exons. Exons 1–3 encode the extracellular domain; exon 4 is responsible for the transmembrane domain and the cytoplasmic tail. The promoter region contains classical CCAC and TATA sequences, as well as transcription factor binding sites for Sp1, GATA-1, and NF-E6. GYPD is the product of leaky translation at a downstream, alternative AUG residue (Met22).

TABLE 35-30
Gerbich Blood Group Antigens

HIGH FREQUENCY						LOW FREQUENCY	
ISBT	Name	Frequency	GP*	Amino acid change (high→low)	Frequency	Name	ISBT
GE2	Ge2	>99%	GYPD	N′ terminus			
GE3	Ge3	>99%	GYPC	aa 43–50			
			GYPD	aa 22–29			
GE4	Ge4	>99%	GYPC	N-terminus			
GE5	Webb	>99%	GYPC	Ser8>Asn	Rare	(Webb–)	
			GYPC+D	Duplication of exon 3	2% blacks 1.5% Finnish	Lsa	GE6
GE7	An^a	>99%	GYPD	Ser2>Ala	0.01%	An(a–)	
GE8	Dh^a	>99%	GYPC	Leu14>Ala	<0.01%	Dh(a–)	
Gerbich Null Phenotypes†							
			GYPC	Deletion exon 2	Rare	Yus	(Ge–2,3,4)
			GYPC	Deletion exon 3	10%–50% Melanesians	Gerbich	(Ge–2,–3,4)
			GYPC	Deletion exons 3+4	Rare	Leach	(Ge–2,–3,–4)

ISBT, International Society of Blood Transfusion.
*Glycophorin C (GYPC) or glycophorin D (GYPD).
†Yus and Gerbich phenotypes are the result of mutant GPC alleles. No GPD is found in Yus, Gerbich, or Leach phenotypes.

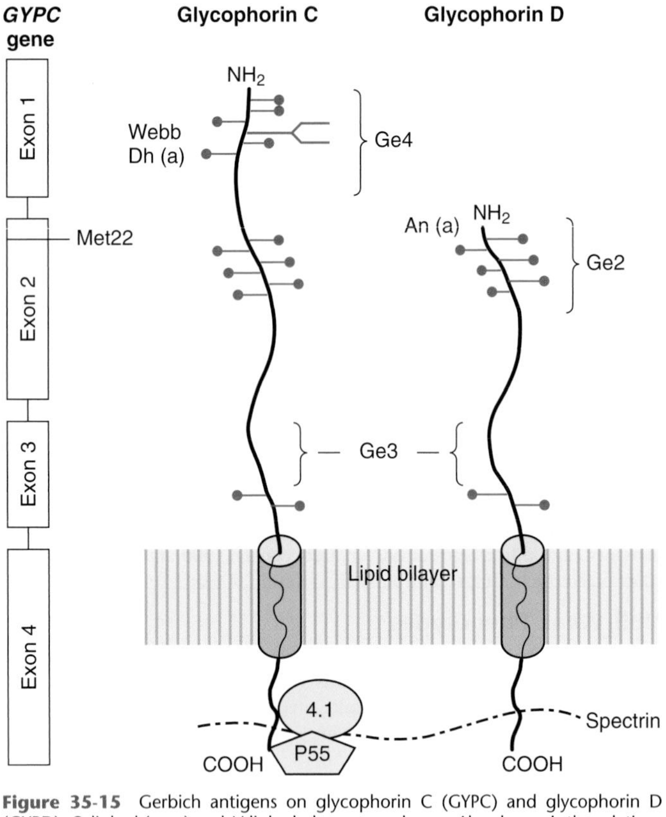

Figure 35-15 Gerbich antigens on glycophorin C (GYPC) and glycophorin D (GYPD). O-linked (—●) and *N*-linked glycans are shown. Also shown is the relationship of the *GYPC* gene to both proteins. GYPD is the result of alternative translation at Met22 in exon 2. Deletions of different exons are responsible for the three Gerbich null phenotypes. GYPC and GYPD may interact with spectrin, protein 4.1, and p55 of the cytoskeleton.

As shown in Table 35-30, the high-frequency antigens Ge2 and Ge4 are the NH_2-termini of GYPD and GYPC, respectively. Ge3 is encoded by exon 3 and is shared by both molecules. With the exception of Ls^a, low-frequency Ge antigens are the result of single–amino acid polymorphisms. The Leach phenotype results from deletion of exons 3 and 4. As a result, no GYPC nor GYPD protein is expressed (see Fig. 35-15). The Yus and Gerbich phenotypes are deletion mutants characterized by variant GYPC synthesis and complete loss of GYPD synthesis. As a result, Yus and Gerbich can express high-incidence antigens present on GYPC (Ge3, Ge4) but not on GYPD (Ge2).

Gerbich Antibodies

Anti-Gerbich antibodies are usually, but not always, clinically significant. Reports have described shortened RBC survival and delayed hemolysis following transfusion of Gerbich-incompatible RBCs. One report described severe HDFN. Autoantibodies against Gerbich antigens have been associated with severe autoimmune hemolytic anemia (Reid, 2004).

Anti-Gerbich antibodies can be of IgM or IgG isotype. Most are immune stimulated, although naturally occurring anti-Ge are known. They may be detected at room temperature and are enhanced by AHG. Gerbich antigens are resistant to chymotrypsin but are sensitive to other proteases (trypsin, pronase).

Biological Role

Similar to Diego/Band 3, GYPC and GYPD help anchor the membrane to the underlying cytoskeleton. In patients with protein 4.1 deficiency and hereditary elliptocytosis, GYPC and GYPD are decreased (75% normal). Likewise, the Ge null (Leach) phenotype is associated with marked elliptocytosis due to reduced membrane stability and deformability (Daniels, 2002). Because they are rich in sialic acid, GYPC and GYPD can bind influenza virus. GYPC may also bind specific *P. falciparum* strains owing, in part, to its *N*-glycan (Mayer, 2006). Evolutionary studies have presented the odd finding that GYPD is the ancestral protein and is shared among all primates. The formation of an upstream start codon with synthesis of GYPC is relatively new and is limited to humans (Wilder, 2009).

CROMER BLOOD GROUP SYSTEM (ISBT NO. 021)

The Cromer system (Cr/CROM) contains 15 antigens, including five antithetical antigens and 10 high-incidence antigens (Table 35-31). Cromer antigens are present on DAF (CD55), which is widely expressed on tissues and in secretions. DAF has been identified on all hematopoietic cells, vascular endothelium, gastrointestinal and genitourinary epithelium, brain, and body fluids (Storry, 2002). Cromer is expressed on cord RBCs and placental trophoblasts.

Null/Weak Phenotypes

Inab or Cromer null phenotype is a rare autosomal recessive phenotype, characterized by complete absence of all Cromer antigens but normal expression of CD59 and other GPI-linked glycoproteins. Many individuals with the Inab phenotype suffer from chronic gastrointestinal disorders, particularly a chronic protein-losing gastroenteropathy. CD55/Cromer is also missing on PNH III RBCs, which lack all GPI-linked glycoproteins. Weak Cromer expression (40% normal) is observed in the Dr(a–) phenotype.

TABLE 35-31
Cromer Blood Group Antigens

HIGH-FREQUENCY ANTIGENS			Amino acid change (high→low)	LOW-FREQUENCY ANTIGENS		
ISBT	Name	Frequency		Frequency	Name	ISBT
CROM1	Cr[a]	>99%	Ala227>Pro	Rare		
CROM2	Tc[a]	>99%	Arg52>Leu	6% blacks 0% Caucasians	Tc[b]	CROM3
			Arg52>Pro	Rare	Tc[c]	CROM4
CROM5	Dr[a]	>99%	Ser199>Leu	Rare	Dr(a–)	
CROM6	Es[a]	>99%	Ile80>Asn	Rare		
CROM7	IFC	>99%	Heterogeneous	Rare	Inab	
CROM9	Wes[b]	>99%	Leu82>Arg	2% blacks <0.5% Caucasians	Wes[a]*	CROM8
CROM10	UMC	>99%	Thr250>Met	Rare		
CROM11	GUT1	>99%	Arg240>His	15% Muapuche Indians	GUT1(–)	
CROM12	SERF	>99%	Pro216>Leu	1% Thai	SERF(–)	
CROM13	ZENA	>99%	His242>Gln			
CROM14	CROV	>99%	Glu156>Lys			
CROM15	CRAM	>99%	Gln247>Arg			

ISBT, International Society of Blood Transfusion.
*Because of their proximity, Wes[a] weakens Es[a] expression.

Biochemistry

CD55/DAF is a highly glycosylated, 381 amino acid, 70-kD GPI-linked glycoprotein (see Fig. 35-13). The extracellular domain consists of four short consensus repeat (SCR) domains, capable of binding complement components (C3b/C4b), followed by a 70 amino acid stretch rich in *O*-linked glycans (50% serine/threonine) that may protect the molecule from proteolysis. X-ray crystallography indicates that the molecule is rod-like, held by a rigid stalk composed of the serine/threonine-rich regions (Lublin, 2005). Each SCR domain contains four highly conserved cysteine residues, resulting in two intrachain disulfide bonds per SCR. As a consequence, DAF is sensitive to sulfhydryl-reducing agents. The molecule contains a single *N*-glycosylation site near SCR1 (Medof, 1987). SCR2 and SCR3 are the binding sites for the C3 convertase complexes C3bBb or C4b2a (Lublin, 2005).

Molecular Biology

The *DAF* gene spans 40kb on chromosome 1q32 and is organized into 11 exons. Most Cromer antigens reflect single–amino acid polymorphisms (see Table 35-31) (Hue-Roye, 2007). The Inab phenotype is the result of nonsense or splice-site mutations. The origin of the Dr(a–) phenotype is interesting. A single–amino acid polymorphism (596C>T) leads to both an Ser199>Leu polymorphism and an alternative splice site. In Dr(a–) individuals, two mRNA species are observed, encoding a truncated mutated protein arising from alternate splicing (major transcript) and the full DAF bearing the Leu165 polymorphism (minor transcript). Dr(a–) RBCs have weakened expression of DAF and all Cromer antigens (Storry, 2002).

Cromer Antibodies

The clinical significance of anti-Cromer antibodies is variable. In some individuals, anti-Cromer antibodies are associated with decreased RBC survival and hemolytic transfusion reactions. Cromer antibodies do not cause HDFN owing to adsorption of antibodies by DAF on trophoblast epithelium (Storry, 2002; Lublin, 2005). In several cases, a transient loss of anti-Cromer antibodies was noted in the second and third trimesters with reappearance of the antibody following delivery (Hue-Roye, 2007).

Anti-Cromer antibodies are usually of IgG isotype, arising from immune stimulation. They are detected in the IAT and can give weak, variable results (historically, high-titer, low-avidity [HTLA] antibodies). Anti-Cromer can be inhibited by plasma, urine, and platelet concentrates. Antibody reactivity is highly sensitive to pretreatment of RBCs with chymotrypsin and pronase, but not with other proteases. Cromer antigens are weakened, but not destroyed, by AET and DTT.

Biological Role

CD55/DAF protects cells from complement by promoting the decay of two C3 convertases: C4b2a and C3bBb. In murine models of induced autoimmune disease, CD55 knockout mice demonstrate increased disease severity (Lublin, 2005). CD55 is also a receptor for uropathogenic and intestinal *E. coli* strains bearing Afa/Dr and X adhesins, echovirus, and coxsackie B virus.

KNOPS BLOOD GROUP SYSTEM (ISBT NO. 022)

The Knops blood group contains 10–12 antigens, including six antithetical antigens (Table 35-32). Several Knops antigens (Kn[b], Mc[b], Sl[a], KCAM) are racially segregated. Knops antigens are present on adult and cord RBCs, neutrophils, B lymphocytes, and dendritic cells (Reid, 2004). Knops can vary in strength between individuals, with approximately 1% of donors showing extremely weak Knops expression (10% normal, Helgeson phenotype).

Biochemistry

Knops resides on complement receptor 1 (CR1, CD35), a 220-kD glycoprotein (Daniels, 2002; Reid 2004). The extracellular domain consists of 30 SCRs, arranged into four long homologous regions (LHRs) that are capable of binding C4b and C3b. The molecule also possesses six to eight *N*-glycosylation sites.

Molecular Biology

The *CR1* gene resides on chromosome 1q32. Four CR1 alleles (CR*1–4) are present, of which CR1*1 is the most common (Daniels, 2002). Variation in CR1 strength and copy number appears to be genetically determined. To date, all Knops antigens arise from amino acid polymorphisms (see Table 35-31; Moulds, 2002; Covas, 2007). KN4/7 (Sl/Vil) antigens may be expanded to include five antigens, reflecting the influence of a second amino acid polymorphism (Ser1610>Ser) and a conformational antigen (Sl3) that requires Sl1 and Sl4 coexpression (Moulds, 2002).

Knops Antibodies

Knops antibodies are clinically insignificant. Knops-incompatible RBCs have normal survival following transfusion. Knops antibodies are of IgG isotype, arising from immune stimulation, and are usually detected only with AHG. Historically classified as an HTLA antibody, Knops antibodies are notoriously difficult to work with because of their low avidity, biological variation in Knops expression, antigen degradation, and the common presence of additional alloantibody specificities. Knops antigens are resistant to proteases but are weakened by sulfhydryl-reducing agents (AET, DTT).

Biological Role

A complement regulatory protein, CR1 can bind C3b/C4b immune complexes, promoting their degradation by factor 1. CR1 also enhances

TABLE 35-32
Knops Blood Group Antigens

HIGH FREQUENCY					LOW FREQUENCY	
ISBT	Name	Frequency	Amino acid change (high→low)	Frequency	Name	ISBT
KN1	Kn[a]	99%	Val1561>Met	4% Caucasians	Kn[b]	KN2
KN3	Mc[a]	99%	Lys1590>Glu	45% blacks	Mc[b]	KN6
KN4	Sl1 (Sla)	98% Caucasians 52% blacks	Arg1601>Gly	Blacks only	Sl2 (Vil)	KN7
	Sl4*	100% blacks 96% Caucasians	Ser1610>Thr	4% Caucasian people	Sl5*	
KN8	Sl3†		Arg1601+Ser1610			
KN9	KCAM	80%–98% Caucasians	Ile1615>Val	70%–80% West Africans, Afro-Brazilians	KCAM(−)	
KN5	Yk[a]	92% Caucasians 98% blacks	Unknown			

ISBT, International Society of Blood Transfusion.
*Sl4 and Sl5 are theoretical antigens not formally added to the Knops family at this time.
†Sl3 is a conformational antigen that requires the presence of both Sl1 (Arg1601) and 'Sl4' (Ser1610).

phagocytosis of C3b/C4b-coated particles and could play a role in *Leishmania, Legionella,* and *Mycobacterium* infections (Daniels, 2002). CR1 also binds *P. falciparum* with rosette formation—a clinical finding associated with severe malaria. Because Sl(a−) RBCs show reduced *P. falciparum* binding and rosetting, it was hypothesized that the Sl 1/Sl 2 phenotype, which is present in 70% of African black people, may provide protection against severe malaria. A later study, however, found no correlation among Sl1/Sl2 phenotype, malaria infection, or disease severity (Zimmerman, 2003). Despite the latter, the extremely high incidence of the Sl(a−) or Sl 2 phenotype in Africa suggests a past selective advantage for the Sl(a−) phenotype in this population.

INDIAN BLOOD GROUP SYSTEM (ISBT NO. 023)

The Indian (IN) blood group contains two autosomal codominant antigens: In[a] (IN1) and In[b] (IN2). In[b] is a high-frequency allele (99% white people), whereas In[a] is relatively rare except among Indian (4%) and Arab populations (11%–12%). Three additional high-incidence antigens are known: IN3, IN4, and AnWj. Rare IN3- and IN4- have been identified only in Moroccans and Pakistanis, respectively (Poole, 2007). Indian antigens are carried by the CD44 glycoprotein and are widely expressed on all hematopoietic cells, epithelial cells, and neural tissue. Approximately 6000–10,000 CD44 molecules are present per RBC (Byrne, 2004; Reid, 2004).

Null/Weak Phenotypes

Indian antigens, including AnWj, are depressed on *In(Lu)* RBCs. They are transiently depressed on cord RBCs during pregnancy and autoimmune hemolytic anemia as a result of autoanti-AnWj (Daniels, 2002).

Biochemistry

Indian antigens are present on CD44, a ubiquitous glycoprotein on many cell membranes. CD44 is heterogeneous between tissues owing to tissue-specific differences in mRNA processing and glycosylation. In RBCs, CD44 is an 80–85-kD, 341 amino acid type 1 glycoprotein bearing a large, heavily glycosylated extracellular domain containing six cysteine residues, six *N*-glycans, three chondroitin sulfate glycans, and several *O*-linked glycans. Similar to Diego/Band 3, CD44 can bind the cytoskeletal proteins, protein 4.1, and ankyrin (Daniels, 2002).

Molecular Biology

CD44 resides on chromosome 11p13. The gene spans 50kb and contains 20 exons, which are able to generate an array of splice-form variants. In RBCs, CD44 is encoded by exons 1–5, 16, 17, 18, and 20. A single–amino acid polymorphism is responsible for the In[a] (IN1, Pro46) and In[b] (IN2, Arg46) antigens. Missense mutations are responsible for the loss of high-incidence antigens IN3 (H85Q) and IN4 (T163R) (Poole, 2007). The basis of the AnWj antigen is unknown.

Indian Antibodies

Antibodies against both Indian and AnWj antigens can be clinically significant, with shortened RBC survival and transfusion reactions. They are not associated with HDFN. Autoimmune anemia due to autoanti-AnWj has been reported. Anti-Indian antibodies are usually of IgG isotype, arising from immune stimulation. They can present as saline agglutinins and are enhanced by AHG. With the exception of AnWj, Indian antigens are destroyed by proteases and AET. Anti-Indian antibodies are also inhibited by plasma, which contains soluble CD44.

Biological Role

CD44 is a major adhesion molecule on leukocytes. CD44 binds a spectrum of extracellular matrix proteins, including collagen, fibronectin, laminin, and hyaluron. In bone marrow, CD44 may participate in the adhesion of erythroid progenitors to stromal fibroblasts. In leukocytes, CD44 may facilitate white blood cell (WBC)–endothelial adhesion, helping to localize WBC to sites of inflammation. CD44 has been implicated in tumor metastasis, wound remodeling, and embryonic differentiation. AnWj/CD44 is also a receptor for *Haemophilus influenzae*.

OK BLOOD GROUP SYSTEM (ISBT NO. 024)

The OK system contains a single high-frequency antigen, Ok[a] (>99% donors), residing on CD147. CD147 is present on RBCs, WBCs, hematopoietic progenitors, endothelial cells, brain, and many tumor cell lines.

Biochemistry and Molecular Biology

Ok[a] resides on CD147, a 35–68-kD, 251 amino acid *N*-linked glycoprotein. A member of the Ig superfamily, CD147 possesses IgC2 and IgV domains. The gene for CD147 resides on chromosome 19p13.2-pter. The Ok(a−) phenotype arises from a E92K polymorphism (Daniels, 2002).

CD147 Antibodies

Anti-Ok[a] is rare and has been described only in Japan. Anti-Ok[a] is of IgG isotype, arising from immune stimulation, and is associated with shortened RBC survival following transfusion of Ok[a]-incompatible RBCs. It is not associated with HDFN. The Ok[a] antigen is resistant to enzymes, sialidases, and sulfhydryl-reducing agents. Three monoclonal antibodies against Ok[a] were recently developed by the New York Blood Center (Tian, 2009).

Biological Role

On WBCs, CD147 is a leukocyte activation–associated protein and may participate in cell adhesion, tumorigenesis, and wound healing via stimulation of enzymes required for remodeling of the extracellular matrix (Daniels, 2002). CD147 may also play a role in the trafficking of red cells out of the spleen. In a murine model, CD147 blockade was associated with anemia, splenomegaly, and de novo erythropoiesis (Coste, 2001). It is interesting to note that red cell aging is accompanied by progressive loss of CD147, suggesting a possible role for CD147 in splenic removal of senescent red cells (Khandelwal, 2006).

RAPH BLOOD GROUP SYSTEM (ISBT NO. 025)

The RAPH blood group system contains a single antigen, RAPH or MER2, located on CD151 or tetraspanin (TM4). CD151 is widely expressed on epithelium, fibroblasts, endothelium, muscle, renal glomeruli and tubules, CD34 cells, early erythroid precursors, megakaryocytes, and platelets. CD151 is strongly expressed in early erythroblasts but is progressively lost with increasing maturation. As a result, MER2 expression is variable among adult donors, with 92% typing MER2-positive and 8% typing MER2-negative. MER2-negative donors strongly express CD151 on other cell lines such as platelets and lymphocytes.

Null Phenotypes

A MER2-negative, autosomal recessive phenotype was identified in three individuals of Indian ancestry (Crew, 2004). All three individuals had nephrotic syndrome with end-stage renal disease and neurosensory deafness. In addition, two individuals had severe pretibial epidermolysis bullosa, bilateral lacrimal duct stenosis, and nail dystrophy. Renal biopsies revealed splitting and fragmentation of the tubular and glomerular basement membranes, respectively. Likewise, skin biopsies showed classic separation of the epidermis with focal edema.

Biochemistry

CD151 or tetraspanin is a 253 amino acid, 28–32-kD multipass protein with four transmembrane domains, four cysteine residues, two extracellular loops, and a single *N*-glycosylation site. The second, large extracellular loop contains a QRD motif for integrin binding (aa 194) and is the site of polymorphisms associated with alloantibody formation (Crew, 2008). In the cell membrane, tetraspanins are associated with integrins ($\alpha3\beta1$, $\alpha6\beta1$, $\alpha7\beta1$) and are implicated in cell adhesion, tumor metastasis, and signaling.

Molecular Biology

CD151 (TSPAN24) is located on chromosome 11p15 and consists of eight exons: exons 2–8 encode the translated protein. The MER2 null phenotype with renal disease has been linked to a nucleotide insertion (exon 5, G383) and a frameshift mutation, leading to a 140 amino acid, nonfunctional protein (Crew, 2004). In addition, two SNPs (R171C, R178H) have been identified in three individuals with MER2 alloantibodies (Crew, 2004, 2008).

MER2 Antibodies

Six examples of anti-MER2 are known in patients of Indian, Turkish, and Pakistani origin (Crew 2004, 2008). All were of IgG isotype, arising from transfusion and pregnancy. Three examples fixed complement. Reactivity is sensitive to disulfide-reducing agents and most proteases except papain (Crew, 2004). No reports have described HDFN due to anti-MER2. MER2 can cause hemolytic transfusion reactions in some patients. A monocyte-monolayer assay may be helpful in determining the clinical significance of anti-MER2 antibodies (Crew, 2008).

Biological Role

The occurrence of renal disease and neurosensory deafness in all three patients with frameshift mutations suggests that CD151 is critical for basement membrane assembly in kidney and inner ear. The clustering of tetraspanin (CD151) and $\beta1$ integrins, which are important in laminin adhesin, also supports a role for CD151 in basement membrane function and assembly (Crew, 2004).

JMH BLOOD GROUP SYSTEM (ISBT NO. 026)

The JMH (John Milton Hagen) system contains six high-incidence antigens and can vary in strength between individuals. In addition to RBCs, JMH is found on lymphocytes, activated macrophages, thymus, brain, respiratory epithelium, placenta, testes, and spleen (Reid, 2004).

Variant and Null Phenotypes

JMH weak, JMH variant, and JMH negative have been described (Seltsam, 2007). An acquired, JMH weak to negative phenotype can occur in the elderly, accompanied by the occurrence of JMH autoantibodies. Five distinct, autosomal recessive JMH variants have been described as the result of single missense mutations. At least one example of an autosomal dominant, JMH-negative phenotype has been described.

Biochemistry

JMH is carried on CD108 (SEMA-L), a semaphorin family glycoprotein (see Fig. 35-13). The protein is a 666 amino acid protein composed of a large 500 amino acid SEMA domain, a C2-type Ig domain, and five *N*-glycosylation and six myristoylation sites. The molecule contains an RGD sequence essential for promoting axonal growth (Seltsam, 2007). The molecule is anchored into the cell membrane by a GPI tail (GPI-linked) and is absent on PNH III RBCs. The molecule contains 19 cysteine residues and is sensitive to sulfhydryl-reducing agents.

Molecular Biology

SEMA7A resides on chromosome 15q24.1 and consists of 14 exons ranging from 42–362 bp in size (Seltsam, 2007). JMH variants are the result of missense mutations at two mutational hotspots in propellar 3 (R207W, R207H) and propellar 7 domains (R460H, R461C). All four mutations may lead to conformational changes based on molecular modeling. An additional missense mutation has been identified among four Native Americans (R347L; St Louis, 2009).

No mutations were identified among JMH-weak and JMH-negative samples. It is interesting to note that SEMA7A mRNA can be identified in reticulocytes from JMH-negative individuals, suggesting that the absence of JMH on red cells is posttranscriptional. The absence of JMH on red cells was not due to PNH or related defects in GPI biosynthesis: CD55 and CD59 expression on JMH-negative red cells was normal (Seltsam, 2007).

JMH Antibodies

Anti-JMH antibodies do not cause hemolytic transfusion reactions or HDFN, although shortened RBC survival has been documented in some patients. The latter may reflect true alloantibodies in JMH-variant individuals. The antibodies are of IgG isotype and can be naturally occurring. The JMH antigen is sensitive to proteases and DTT. An assay for detection of anti-JMH antibodies was recently developed for gel using immobilized recombinant SEMA7A on polystyrene beads (Seltsam, 2008).

Biological Role

Semaphorin proteins are implicated in cell signaling. In hematopoietic cells, SEMA7A can modulate cellular immunity via effects on T cells, monocytes, and natural killer (NK) cells. SEMA7A inhibits NK cell proliferation (Figueiredo, 2009) and is a negative regulator of T cell activation. Conversely, SEMA7A stimulates chemotaxis, secretion of inflammatory cytokines, and dendritic cell maturation in monocytes (Ji, 2009).

I BLOOD GROUP SYSTEM (ISBT NO. 027)

The I blood group system contains two biosynthetically related antigens: I and i. The system was named I for "individuality" after an extensive search of 22,000 individuals identified only five I- adult donors (Cooling, 2010). The biosynthetic precursor to I antigen, the i antigen, is strongly expressed on cord cells because of developmental delays in the enzyme responsible for I antigen synthesis. By 3 months of age, there is a perceptible decrease in i antigen, accompanied by increased I antigen, with an adult I+i– phenotype by 18–24 months of age (Marsh, 1961). Increases in I antigen are accompanied by parallel increases in A and B antigens (Cooling, 2010). Both I and i antigens are ubiquitously expressed on glycolipids and glycoproteins on red cells and other tissues.

Null Phenotype

The i_{adult} phenotype is a rare, autosomal recessive phenotype found in <1/10,000 donors. In Asia, the i_{adult} phenotype can be associated with congenital cataracts (Inaba, 2003; Yu, 2003). Elevated i antigen is also observed on cord RBCs and reticulocytes and in megaloblastic anemia, leukemia, and chronic hemolytic states as a sign of stressed erythropoiesis (Cooling, 2010). Elevated i antigen is also observed in HEMPAS (hereditary erythroblastic multinuclearity with positive acidified-serum test), a congenital dyserythropoietic anemia associated with chronic hemolysis, binucleated erythroblasts, and altered red cell glycosylation (Deneke, 2009). The molecular basis of HEMPAS was recently identified as altered Golgi trafficking due to mutations in SEC23B, a COPII protein (Schwarz, 2009).

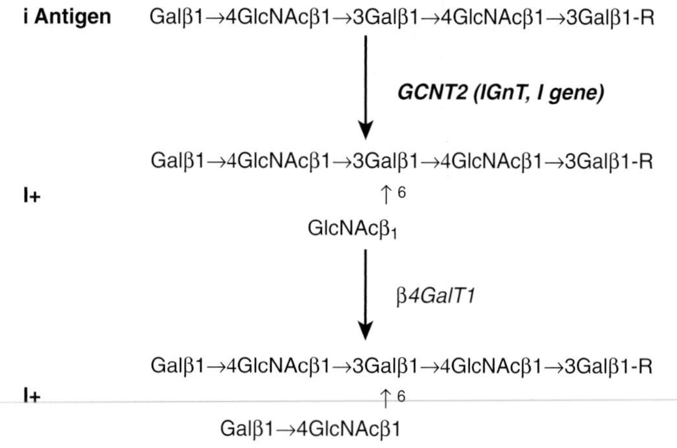

Figure 35-16 Structure of the I and i antigens. The I antigen is composed of two successive lactosaminyl subunits. I antigen requires the action of GCNT2, a 1-6-*N*-acetylglucosaminyltransferase. (*Gal,* Galactose; *GlcNAc, N*-acetylgalactosamine; *R,* other oligosaccharide.)

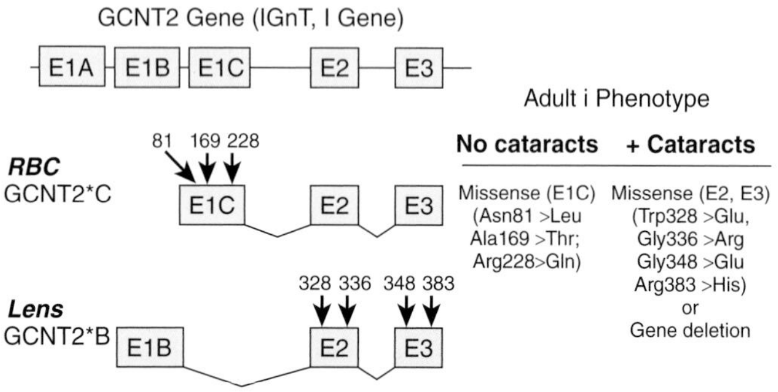

Figure 35-17 The *I* gene, showing three different exons 1. In human red blood cells (RBCs) and lens, a different GCNT2 mRNA is translated, based on which exon 1 is utilized. Mutations in *GCNT2* gene can result in an i_{adult} phenotype and cataracts. In Europeans, mutations usually are seen only in exon 1C and affect I antigen synthesis in RBCs. In Asia, i_{adult} phenotype involves gene deletion or mutations in exons 2 and 3. As a result, loss of GCNT2 activity is seen in all tissues.

Biochemistry

Type 2 chain oligosaccharides, both i and I antigens, terminate in a Galβ1→4GlcNAc or lactosaminyl epitope and differ only in complexity and multivalency. As shown in Figure 35-16, the i antigen is a linear oligosaccharide containing at least two successive lactosamine epitopes. The I antigen is derived from i antigen by the action of a β1–6 *N*-acetylglucosaminyltransferase, a first step in the synthesis of large, branched multivalent complex polylactosamines (see Fig. 35-16). Both i and I can be further modified by other glycosyltransferases to yield ABH, LeX, and related antigens (Cooling, 2010).

Molecular Biology

The I antigen, a β1–6 glucosaminyltransferase, is the product of the *GCNT2* or *IGnT* gene. The gene spans approximately 100 kb on chromosome 6p24. The gene contains five exons, including three tissue–specific exon 1 (Fig. 35-17). As a consequence, three different GCNT2 spliceforms are possible, depending on which exon 1 is utilized (Inaba, 2003). GCNT2*A is ubiquitously expressed, whereas GCNT2*B is primarily expressed in human lens epithelia, fetal brain, and cerebellum (Yu, 2003). GCNT2*C, composed of exons E1C, E2, and E3, is the predominant transcript in erythroblasts and reticulocytes. In hematopoietic stem cells, erythroid differentiation is accompanied by transcriptional upregulation of GCNT2*C (Twu, 2007). The promoter for GCNT2*C contains transcription factor binding sites for Sp1, Oct-2, and C/EBPα. C/EBPα phosphorylation and binding is critical for transcriptional activation (Twu, 2007).

The translated GCNT2 protein consists of 402 amino acids with five *N*-glycosylation sites and 9 conserved cysteine residues. Unlike most galactosyl- and glucosaminyltransferases, GCNT2 does not contain a DXD motif. The enzyme is likely highly folded, based on crystallography data from C2GnT, a closely related β1,6 glucosaminyltransferase (Pak, 2006; Cooling, 2010). Sequence differences in exon 1, which encodes 77% of the translated enzyme, may account for the enhanced enzyme activity observed with the GCNT2*C isoform (Yu, 2003). Oligosaccharide analysis and enzyme studies indicate that the minimum acceptor for enzyme activity is a tetrasaccharide composed of two lactosamine motifs (Cooling, 2010).

Both the i_{adult} phenotype and congenital cataracts have been linked to mutations in *GCNT2*. In i_{adult} individuals without cataracts, missense mutations have been found in exon E1C, leading to an isolated loss of GCNT2*C activity in RBCs (Inaba, 2003; Cooling, 2010). In contrast, i_{adult} with cataracts is the result of mutations in exon E2 or E3 or a major deletion of the *IGnT* gene. As a result, GCNT2 activity is lost in all tissues, including RBC and lens (Yu, 2003; Cooling, 2010). Loss of GCNT2*B activity in the lens is believed to underlie the formation of cataracts in humans; however, a direct causal link has yet to be established. No increase in cataracts was observed in a GCNT2 knockout mouse model (Chen, 2005).

Anti-I and -i Antibodies

Anti-I and anti-i are antibodies of IgM isotype, reactive at room temperature (see Table 35-7). Autoantibodies to I are relatively common and are usually low-titered cold agglutinins. Some anti-I can have IH specificity, reacting stronger with group O and A_2 RBC (refer to Table 35-48). Although generally benign, hemolysis secondary to high-titered anti-I is observed in cold autoimmune hemolytic anemia (CAIHA). CAIHA can occur in the setting of malignancy and occasionally infection (e.g., *Mycoplasma pneumoniae*). These antibodies display high thermal amplitude, often agglutinating RBCs at temperatures of 30°–34° C. In contrast, alloanti-I is relatively rare and is found as a naturally occurring antibody in i_{adult} individuals. Anti-i is also uncommon but has been reported in CAIHA, infectious mononucleosis, choriocarcinomatosis, and alcoholic cirrhosis.

Biological Role

Despite the common occurrence of major maternal-fetal ABO incompatibility, severe HDFN due to ABO incompatibility is rare (0.04%). It is hypothesized that the developmental delay in I antigen synthesis may play a protective role against HDFN-ABO by minimizing the number of ABH antigens expressed on fetal red cells (Cooling, 2010). This is supported by parallel increases in I and ABH during the first 2 years of life. Additional evidence comes from extended studies of the *N*-glycan on Band 3, which accounts for 50% of the ABH antigen on red cells. Adult red cells had a fourfold increase in ABH expression on Band 3 owing to chain extension and branching (Fukuda, 1984; Cooling, 2010).

GIL BLOOD GROUP SYSTEM (ISBT NO. 029)

The GIL blood group system contains one high-incidence antigen, GIL (100% donors). The GIL protein is highly expressed on RBCs, kidney, small intestine, stomach, colon, spleen, eye, and respiratory tract (Reid, 2004).

Biochemistry

GIL is carried by aquaglyceroporin (AQP-3), a member of the major intrinsic protein family of water channels. Similar to Colton (AQP1), AQP3 is a 46-kD, 292 amino acid multipass protein containing six transmembrane domains and a single *N*-glycosylation site. The molecule is present in the cell membrane as dimers, trimers, and tetramers (Daniels, 2002).

Molecular Biology

The *AQP3* gene spans 6kb on chromosome 9p13 and is organized into six exons. The one example of a GIL-negative phenotype is the result of splice site and frameshift mutations, resulting in a truncated 218 amino acid protein. In general, AQP3 is highly conserved; no missense mutations in the translated protein were identified in a recent study of European and African individuals. Two SNPs were identified in the promoter region (A-14G, C-46A); however, neither polymorphism had an impact on AQP3 mRNA levels (Bahamontes-Rosa, 2008).

GIL Antibodies

Anti-GIL is associated with hemolytic transfusion reactions. No reports have described clinical HDFN due to anti-GIL despite a positive DAT.

Anti-GIL is usually of IgG isotype, reactive at 37° C and enhanced with AHG. The antigen is resistant to proteases, sialidases, and DTT.

Biological Role

AQP3/Gil is a membrane channel capable of transporting urea and glycerol. On red cells, AQP3 may play a role in malaria infection. AQP3 was shown to be internalized during *P. falciparum* infection as part of the parasitophorous vacuole (Bietz, 2009). Because AQP3 protects against hydroxyl radicals and osmotic stress, internalization and loss of AQP3 from the red cell extracellular membrane may contribute to the pathology and severity of malarial infections (Bahamontes-Rosa, 2008).

AQP3 is highly expressed in epidermis, where it plays a significant role in skin differentiation and hydration through regulation of glycerol content and metabolism (Boury-Jamot, 2009). A decrease in AQP3 is associated with decreased skin elasticity, poor wound healing, and eczema. Conversely, increased AQP3 is observed in basal cell carcinoma. Dermal AQP3 expression can be modulated by inflammatory mediators, ultraviolet radiation, and topical glycerol (Boury-Jamot, 2009; Horie, 2009). It is not surprising that cosmetic and pharmacologic companies are actively pursuing topical agents capable of modulating AQP3 expression in the skin.

IMMUNOHEMATOLOGY TESTS AND PROCEDURES

BASIC PRINCIPLES—HEMAGGLUTINATION

Specific hemagglutination is the single most important in vitro immunologic reaction in blood banking because it is the endpoint of almost all test systems designed to detect RBC antigens and antibodies. The hemagglutination process actually occurs in two stages. The first stage, often referred to as RBC sensitization, is simply the combination of paratope and epitope in a reversible reaction that follows the law of mass action and has an associated equilibrium constant. Antigen and antibody are held together by noncovalent attractions. In stage two, multiple RBCs with bound antibody form a stable latticework through antigen-antibody bridges formed between adjacent cells. This latticework is the basis of all visible agglutination reactions.

Formation of the latticework during the second stage of hemagglutination is naturally impeded by the fact that RBCs in solution normally repel each other. This is due to the net negative charge of the RBC membrane created by sialic acid. If RBCs are suspended in an ionic medium such as normal saline, cations arrange themselves around each cell to form an ionic cloud. Cations closest to the cell membrane are firmly bound and move with the RBC, while the outer cations move freely. The difference in charge at the surface between the inner and outer cation layers, called the surface of shear, creates an electrical potential named the ζ potential (Fig. 35-18). The ζ potential keeps RBCs in solution about 25 nm apart (Harmening, 2005). Another factor that may be important in keeping RBCs apart is the water of hydration. Proponents of this theory suggest that the hydrophilic polar heads of lipid molecules making up the outer cell membrane bilayer attract water molecules. The water thus creates a surface tension that helps to keep the cells apart.

One situation whereby the natural influence of the ζ potential to keep RBCs apart is circumvented is the phenomenon of rouleaux formation or "pseudoagglutination." Patients with multiple myeloma, Waldenström's macroglobulinemia, and hyperviscosity syndromes have high concentrations of abnormal serum proteins that change the net surface charge on the RBC membrane. The cells thus cluster together in clumps that resemble macroscopic hemagglutination. Plasma expanders, such as dextran and hydroxyethyl starch, as well as some intravenous X-ray contrast materials can also cause rouleaux formation. Rouleaux can be differentiated from true agglutination by direct microscopy (1) by the classical "stacked-coin" formation in rouleaux, and (2) by the loss of rouleaux after washing and resuspension in saline. Nonspecific agglutination can also be seen in cord blood samples contaminated with Wharton's jelly. The presence of hyaluronic acid and albumin in cord blood is responsible for this problem.

Factors Affecting Specific Hemagglutination

The extent of RBC sensitization and the facilitation of second-stage latticework formation are influenced first by inherent characteristics of the specific antigens and antibodies involved. In most immunohematology procedures, IgM antibodies can facilitate the second stage of hemagglutination because of their large diameter (35 nm) and multivalency, which allows them to span the distance between two adjacent RBCs in solution

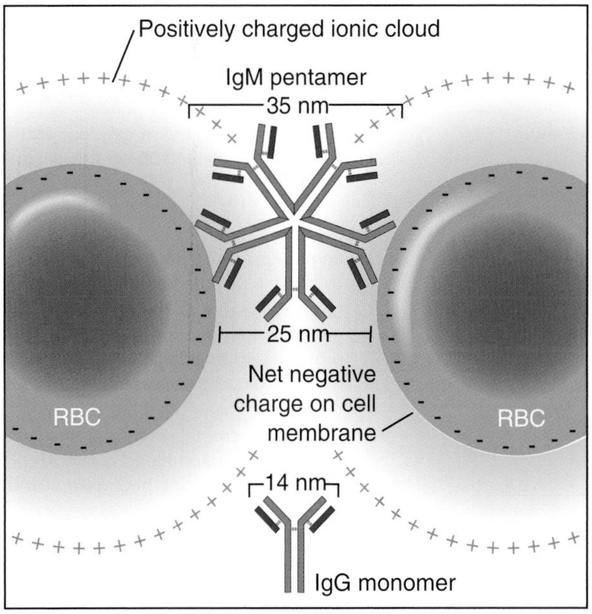

Figure 35-18 Erythrocytes are kept apart in an ionic medium by the ζ potential, which in turn influences the agglutinating capacity of immunoglobulin (Ig)G and IgM.

(see Fig. 35-18). Because of their innate agglutinating ability, IgM antibodies are frequently referred to as direct agglutinins. Most IgG antibodies, on the other hand, are considerably smaller (14 nm) and are unable to induce visible agglutination without the assistance of secondary enhancing reagents. Thus, IgG antibodies are commonly referred to as indirect agglutinins.

The density and accessibility of specific antigens on the RBC membrane are also critical in second-stage latticework formation. This can be illustrated by comparing the ABO and Rh antigens. Approximately 1 million ABO antigens are present per RBC, displayed on large *N*-glycans of extramembranous glycoproteins. Because of their high density and easy accessibility, ABO antibodies can readily bind exposed ABO antigens and agglutinate RBCs. In contrast, only 10,000–30,00 Rh antigens are readily accessible per RBC and, as multipass integral membrane proteins, are considered intramembranous. As a consequence, Rh antigens are less easily agglutinated by Rh antisera. In another example of the influence of antigen density, RBCs that are homozygous for a particular blood group gene will often give stronger reactions than heterozygous cells. This is because homozygotes express twice as many copies, or a double dose, of antigen per cell. In immunohematologic testing, this phenomenon is frequently referred to as dosage.

Secondarily to inherent antigen and antibody characteristics, the first and second stages of the hemagglutination reaction may also be influenced by manipulating various physical and/or chemical parameters of the reaction environment. An outline of how these various parameters may be controlled is shown in Table 35-33.

Grading of Hemagglutination Reactions

Hemagglutination in blood bank testing is observed and graded according to the strength of the reaction. Currently, three methods are available for evaluating visual hemagglutination reactions: Tube testing, column aggutination (gel technology), and solid-phase technology. In test tube reactions, reagents and patient sample are added to a test tube and centrifuged, creating a cell button at the bottom of the test tube. The cell button is gently dislodged while observing for macroscopic agglutination. Column agglutination or gel technology utilizes a dextran acrylamide gel microtube prepared by the manufacturer. The gel traps agglutinates at the top of the chamber if hemagglutination has occurred, while unagglutinated cells pass through the gel layer and form a pellet at the bottom of the microtube. In solid-phase technology, a microplate is the vessel for the reaction. Reagent or reagent cells (as a monolayer of cells or cell stroma) coat the well to which patient sample is added. Following incubation and washing, indicator cells are added. When hemagglutination occurs, there is a diffuse adherence of RBC to the well. If no reaction occurs, the RBCs settle to the bottom of the well.

TABLE 35-33
Factors Affecting the Hemagglutination Reaction

Reaction parameter	Effect	Manipulation
Temperature	Influences the equilibrium constant and/or reaction rate depending on the class of antibody involved	Decreasing the temperature to 24° C or even to 4° C enhances the reaction of IgM antibodies Prewarming or maintaining a reaction temperature of 37° C provides the optimum temperature for detection of IgG antibodies, while preventing most IgM antibodies from reacting
Incubation time	Different Ag/Ab reactions reach equilibrium over different time periods	Increasing the time of incubation in a given test system may enhance the detection of a weakly reactive antibody
pH	At a pH range of 6.5–7.5, chemical groups on Ag and Ab are oppositely charged, providing optimal ionic forces of attraction for most blood group antibodies	Changing the pH affects the equilibrium constant for selected antibodies that may react preferentially in a more acidic environment (e.g., anti-M, anti-Pr)
Ionic strength	In an isotonic saline medium, sodium cations and chloride anions cluster around erythrocyte Ag and blood group Ab, respectively, acting to neutralize Ag/Ab attractive forces	Addition of LISS reduces the shielding effect on oppositely charged Ab and Ag, thus increasing the rate of reaction and the equilibrium constant for red cell sensitization
Antibody concentration	Can affect first- and second-stage agglutination by influencing the number of antibody molecules attached to each erythrocyte	Increasing the serum-to-cell concentration increases the rate and/or affects the equilibrium constant of red cell sensitization by IgG antibodies May help to induce second-stage agglutination by IgM antibodies Addition of PEG, a large space-occupying molecule, effectively increases the relative concentrations of ag and ab respective to the volume of the reaction, greatly increasing the rate of reaction; is used only in AHG testing to detect IgG antibodies
ζ Potential	Causes red cells to repel each other in solution; if the ζ potential can be reduced or the red cells brought together by physical means, second-stage agglutination of sensitized red cells can be facilitated	Centrifugation—forcing cells closer together facilitates latticework formation Enzymes—cleave sialic acid residues to lower the ζ potential and improve accessibility of certain blood group antigens Albumin—reduces ζ potential and/or water of hydration to allow red cells to approach each other more closely Polybrene/protamine—provides an excess of cations that neutralize the repulsive force between red cells, producing both nonspecific aggregation and antibody-mediated latticework formation; the final addition of sodium citrate disperses nonspecific aggregates, while specific ag/ab agglutinates remain

ab, Antibody; *ag,* antigen; *AHG,* antihuman globulin; *LISS,* low–ionic strength saline; *PEG,* polyethylene glycol.

Tube Reactions

Hemolysis is considered the strongest positive reaction that can occur and indicates the presence of a potent, complement-fixing antibody. After recipient serum and reagent RBCs are incubated and centrifuged at 37° C, the serum should first be examined for hemolysis before the cell button is resuspended. When reading for agglutination, the tube should be shaken, using a gentle wrist action, until all cells are dislodged. This is most easily accomplished by gently holding the test tube at the top of the tube in a vertical fashion and using the wrist to gently dislodge the cell button, while watching closely for agglutinates. As the cell button begins to resuspend, tip the tube gently to observe for agglutinates. Proper illumination with a concave mirror is an invaluable aid for macroscopic reading. By placing the tube about 2.5 inches above a 3-inch concave mirror, aggregates can be differentiated easily from the free cells by looking at the mirror, not at the tube.

Table 35-34 lists two protocols for evaluating the strength of agglutination using numeric grading and/or scoring. Figure 35-19 shows the appearance of different agglutination grades. Although the agglutination grade gives an approximate idea regarding the potency or strength of a particular antibody, the scoring method is much more useful in semiquantitative procedures, particularly when used in conjunction with titration to compare the relative antibody strengths of two different sera.

Unlike tube testing, microcolumn gel technology and solid-phase red cell adherence reactions are fixed after the centrifugation phase. The card or well is ready to read without the need to dislodge the cell button. (See Figures 35-22 and 35-23 for examples of reactions in gel and solid phase).

TABLE 35-34
Grading and Scoring of Hemagglutination

Grade	Appearance	Score
H	Hemolysis—presence of free hemoglobin in the serum	10
4+	One solid aggregate	10
3+	Several medium to large aggregates	8
2+	Many small to medium aggregates with a clear background	5
1+	Many small aggregates with a turbid background	3
+ or w	Few small aggregates with many unagglutinated cells	2
$\pm^m$ or $+^m$	Aggregates visible only under microscopic magnification	1
0	Negative—absence of aggregates; all cells unagglutinated	0
mf	Mixed-field agglutination—presence of minor population of agglutinated cells superimposed on a negative background	NA
R	Rouleaux—nonspecific aggregation appearing like a stack of coins; disappears with addition of saline	NA

NA, Not applicable.

THE ANTIHUMAN GLOBULIN TEST

Many IgG antibodies are not able to directly produce detectable hemagglutination, even after centrifugation and the use of enhancement media and techniques such as polyethylene glycol, low–ionic strength saline (LISS), albumin, or enzymes. To visualize reactions by these antibodies, AHG reagents, which contain specific antibodies to human Igs or complement components, must be utilized. The antibodies in AHG sera act as bridges between RBCs already sensitized with antibody or complement to produce the characteristic latticework of second-stage hemagglutination (Fig. 35-20). This is the basis of the AHG test.

The AHG test is also called the Coombs' test, in honor of one of the investigators who first developed the test for laboratory use (Coombs, 1945), although the principle was actually described much earlier (in 1908) by Moreschi (Harmening, 2005). When the test is used to detect

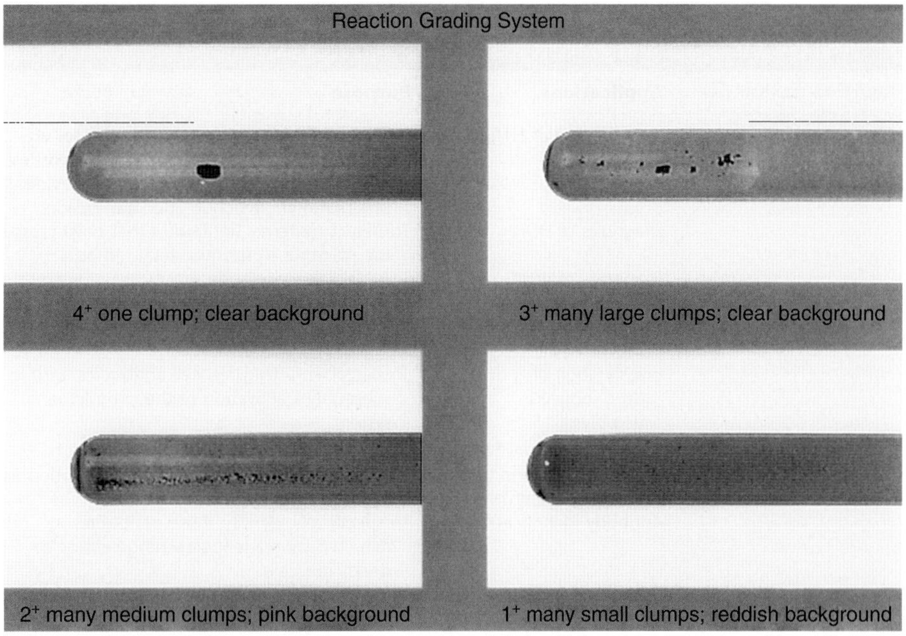

Figure 35-19 Agglutination grading system showing macroscopic hemagglutination reactions.

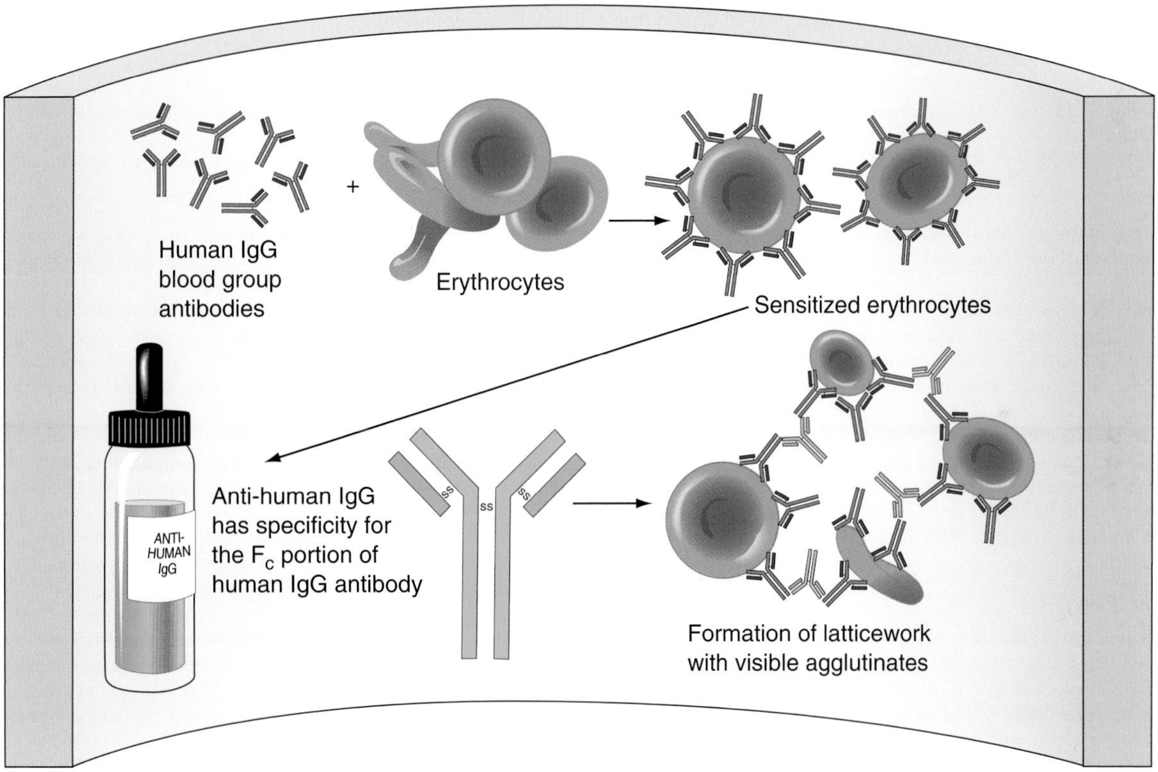

Figure 35-20 Antihuman globulin antibodies form a bridge between adjacent erythrocytes sensitized with human immunoglobulin (Ig)G or complement components.

antibodies or complement bound to RBCs in vivo, it is called the direct antiglobulin test (DAT). When the test is used to detect the reaction of antibody and RBCs in vitro after an appropriate incubation phase, it is called the indirect antiglobulin test (IAT). The red cell antibody screen is an example of an IAT.

Antihuman Globulin Reagents and Procedures

Various preparations of AHG sera are available for blood bank testing, depending on the application (direct or indirect) and whether one wishes to detect RBC sensitization by IgG, complement, or both.

Polyspecific Reagents

Polyclonal, polyspecific AHG reagents are produced by hyperimmunizing animals, usually rabbits, with purified Ig or complement to produce high-titered, high-avidity IgG antibodies. For a given batch of reagent, animal sera are harvested, pooled, adsorbed to remove heterophil agglutinins, and then titrated to ascertain the dilution necessary for optimal reactivity in routine use. Conventional polyspecific (also called broad-spectrum) AHG contains polyclonal IgG antibodies to the spectrum of human IgG subclasses and the C3 complement cleavage products C3b and C3d. Some anti-C4b and anti-C4d activity may also be present. However, most manufacturers adsorb out anti-C4 activity from their polyspecific AHG reagents because it has been shown that in vitro complement activation by clinically insignificant cold agglutinins results in much more C4d than C3d binding (Klein, 2006). Excluding anti-C4 activity thus reduces the number of false-positives in both DAT and IAT testing using polyspecific reagents. Because immunization against IgG will also produce anti–light chain antibodies in a polyclonal response, one should remember that

PART 4

TABLE 35-35
Applications for Direct and Indirect Antiglobulin Techniques

	Applications	Purpose	What is detected
Direct antiglobulin test (DAT)	Investigation of HTR	To detect circulating donor red cells that are sensitized with recipient antibody. A positive DAT is the first immunohematologic evidence of a hemolytic reaction after transfusion	DAT positive owing to IgG and/or C3d depending on the antibodies responsible
	Diagnosis of HDFN	To detect maternal antibodies that have crossed the placenta to sensitize fetal red cells	DAT almost always positive as a result of IgG; occasionally C3d if ABO antibodies involved
	Diagnosis of AIHA	To detect autoantibody sensitizing a patient's own red cells	Warm autoantibodies: DAT almost always positive owing to IgG Cold autoantibodies: DAT may be due to C3d only
	Investigation of drug-induced hemolysis	To detect anti-drug/red cell antibodies and/or subsequent activation of the complement system	DAT may be positive owing to IgG, C3d, or both, depending on the mechanism involved (see under Investigation of Autoimmune Hemolytic Anemia section)
Indirect antiglobulin test	Antibody detection (or antibody screen)	To detect clinically significant IgG alloantibodies in the recipient	Recipient IgG antibodies bound to reagent screening cells*
	Antibody identification	To specifically identify those antibodies detected by reagent screening cells or by donor red cells	Recipient IgG antibodies bound to reagent cells from a panel of 10–12 donors*
	Crossmatching	To detect antibodies that may have been missed by the antibody screen because of absence of the corresponding antigen or presence of a dosing antibody	Recipient IgG antibodies bound to donor red cells*
	Red cell antigen typing	To type patient or donor red cells for antigens that can be detected by IgG antisera reactive only by the AGT. A common example of this would be the weak D test	Specific binding of reagent IgG antibodies to red cells positive for the corresponding antigen

AGT, Antihuman globulin test; *AIHA,* autoimmune hemolytic anemia; *HDFN,* hemolytic disease of the fetus and newborn; *HTR,* hemolytic transfusion reaction; *Ig,* immunoglobulin.
*If complement is fixed in vitro, it may be detected if polyspecific antiglobulin is used.

polyclonal antiglobulin sera may cross-react with IgA or IgM light chains unless the manufacturer specifies that the anti-IgG component is heavy chain specific.

At present, the most commonly used polyspecific AHG reagents consist of rabbit polyclonal anti-IgG blended with murine monoclonal antibodies to C3b and C3d complement components. Also available is a polyspecific reagent derived exclusively from murine monoclonal antibodies to IgG, C3b, and C3d. The activity of anti-IgG and anti-complement in polyspecific antisera, whether polyclonal or monoclonal, will vary somewhat among different manufacturers and between lots produced by the same manufacturer. However, all AHG sera must contain levels of anti-IgG and anti-C3d activity that meet or exceed the reference standards of the FDA (21CFR660.52; Code of Federal Regulations, 2001b).

Monospecific Reagents

Commercially available FDA-licensed monospecific reagents include anti-IgG, anti-C3b+C3d, and anti-C3d. Monospecific anti-IgG or anticomplement may also be polyclonal or monoclonal in origin. For monoclonal anti-IgG, manufacturers must blend monoclonals against a variety of IgG epitopes or select a clone with specificity for an epitope common to all variants of IgG to ensure that the spectrum of human IgG subclasses will react with their reagent. With polyclonal monospecific anti-IgG, again one should keep in mind that it may contain anti–light chain activity unless the manufacturer labels it as heavy chain specific. Production of murine monoclonal blends of monospecific anticomplement has allowed manufacturers to develop reagents containing quantities of purified anti-C3b and -C3d of known potency that are less likely to give false-positive results by other anticomplement activities found in polyclonal reagents (Harmening, 2005).

Choosing Which AHG Reagent to Use

The DAT is an important diagnostic serologic technique used for the detection of antibody binding to RBC membranes in vivo. Polyspecific AHG reagents containing both anti-IgG and anticomplement activity are typically used for initial DAT evaluation. This is especially important when the DAT is being performed to aid in the diagnosis of CAIHA and some forms of drug-induced hemolytic anemia in which complement may be the only evidence of immune-mediated hemolysis. Circulating red cells that have been involved in complement activation will have mostly C3d on their surface as the result of complement regulatory protein degradation of C3b (see Fig. 35-1). Therefore, polyspecific AHG sera used in DAT testing must contain anti-C3d reactivity and usually contain some anti-C3b reactivity as well. One notable exception to the use of polyspecific AHG for DAT testing is cord blood. Because *only* IgG can cross the placenta, the DAT may be performed with an anti-IgG reagent only (see Prenatal and Postnatal Testing section).

A positive DAT with all reagents tested (polyspecific, IgG, C3) may indicate spontaneous agglutination or autoagglutination. Cells already heavily coated with IgG can agglutinate upon centrifugation in the absence of AHG reagent. IgM cold autoagglutinins that were not dissociated during the washing procedure can also cause autoagglutination. All positive DAT tests should be tested with an inert control such as saline or 6% albumin before positive test reactions are concluded.

The IAT is used for detection of in vitro antibody binding to RBCs, regardless of the antibody's ability to fix complement. It is unclear whether polyspecific AHG, which contains anticomplement reactivity, improves serum antibody detection by the IAT. Rare reports have described antibodies that were detected only by their ability to bind complement in vitro and would have been missed with the use of monospecific anti-IgG reagents (Roback, 2008). In addition, polyspecific AHG can yield stronger reactions in the IAT than monospecific anti-IgG alone (Wright, 1979). A major disadvantage of polyspecific AHG is unwanted detection of complement activation by clinically insignificant cold-reactive autoagglutinins or alloantibodies. As a result, many laboratories choose to use monospecific anti-IgG in antibody detection and identification tests and in crossmatch procedures.

Table 35-35 compares various applications for DAT and IAT techniques. Antiglobulin testing may be performed using test tubes, capillary tubes, microtiter plates, or gel microtube techniques (see later section on Compatibility Testing). These procedures may be semiautomated or fully automated, particularly in facilities that perform large-volume testing, such as blood collection centers. Unless otherwise specified, procedures referred to in this chapter employ tube testing. *The American Association of Blood Banks Technical Manual* (Roback, 2008), *Judd's Methods in Immunohematology* (Judd, 2008), and *Immunohematology Methods* (Mallory, 1993) are excellent general references for most common procedures, as well as more specialized techniques.

TABLE 35-36

Basic Procedures for Direct and Indirect Antiglobulin Testing by Tube Method

Procedure		REASONS FOR INVALID REACTIONS IN ANTIGLOBULIN TESTING	
		False-positive	**False-negative**
Direct antiglobulin test (DAT)	1. Prepare a 3%–5% suspension in normal saline of the red cells to be tested. 2. Add 1 drop of red cell suspension to a tube and wash three to four times with saline. 3. Blot the tube after the last wash. 4. Add 2 drops of polyspecific AHG (anti-IgG + anticomplement). 5. Centrifuge and examine for agglutination.* 6. Add check cells to all negative tubes (see Quality Control of the Antihuman Globulin Test section). Note: For DAT, blood samples should be collected in EDTA to prevent fixation of complement in vitro by clinically insignificant cold autoagglutinins.	• Overcentrifugation • Direct agglutination by strong cold agglutinins • Overincubation with enzyme-treated cells • Improper use of PEG or polycation enhancement reagents • Inadequate resuspension of cell button • Rouleaux formation‡ • Dirty glassware • Small fibrin clots may trap cells and mimic agglutination • Cells with a positive DAT will yield false-positive results in any indirect antiglobulin test	• AHG reagent failure† • Failure to add AHG reagents† • Improper or inadequate washing† • Delayed washing (elution of weakly attached antibody) • Serum/cell ratio too low • Failure to add test serum or enhancement reagents • Undercentrifugation • Resuspension of cell button too vigorous
Indirect antiglobulin test (IAT)	1. Add 2–3 drops of patient serum or the recommended number of drops of commercially prepared antisera to each tube. 2. Place 1 drop of the 3%–5% red cell suspension to be tested in a tube (e.g., donor cells, reagent screening cells). 3. Add recommended number of drops of enhancement media (e.g., LISS, PEG) if indicated. 4. Incubate at 37° C for the time period indicated for the assay being performed (from 15–60 minutes). 5. If indicated in the procedure, centrifuge and examine the serum for hemolysis and the cells for agglutination. 6. Whether step 5 is performed or not, continue by washing the tube(s) three to four times with normal saline. 7. Blot tubes dry after the last wash. 8. Add 2 drops of antiglobulin sera (polyspecific or monospecific anti-IgG) to all tubes. 9. Centrifuge and examine for agglutination.* 10. Add check cells to all negative tubes,		

AHG, Antihuman globulin; *EDTA,* ethylenediaminetetraacetic acid; *Ig,* immunoglobulin; *LISS,* low–ionic strength saline; *PEG,* polyethylene glycol.
*Protocol may include optional microscopic examination to confirm macroscopically negative tests.
†Will be detected by the use of Coombs' control cells.
‡Rouleaux will cause false-positive results in indirect tests read after 37° C incubation.

Quality Control of the Antihuman Globulin Test

To standardize antiglobulin sera and to confirm true-negative antiglobulin reactions, two types of quality control RBCs are normally used: those coated with IgG and those coated with C3b and/or C3d. To sensitize RBCs with IgG, Rh antibodies are usually used. RBCs coated with C3b are prepared by incubation of whole blood in low ionic strength saline (LISS) or with human anti-Le^a or anti-I. C3d-coated RBCs are prepared by incubating C3b-coated cells with fresh serum or trypsin to split C3b→C3d. IgG or complement-coated control cells should give a 1+ to 2+ reaction (see Fig. 35-19) when tested with anti-IgG or anti-C3b+C3d.

Quality control cells for the antiglobulin test are referred to as check cells, Coombs' control cells, and sensitized cells. In a true-negative test, free active antiglobulin reagent should remain. Control cells, sensitized with IgG and/or C3, are added to all negative tests and centrifuged. Hemagglutination of check cells confirms both the presence and the reactivity of the AHG reagent, thus validating a negative test result. If the control cells fail to agglutinate in any tube, the tests must be repeated because they are invalid and may have yielded false-negative results. False-negative tests can occur for a variety of reasons and are listed in Table 35-36.

Sensitivity of the Antihuman Globulin Test

Although the antiglobulin test is extremely sensitive, a negative test does not exclude the possible presence of antibodies on RBCs. It is estimated that 200–500 IgG or C3 molecules bound per cell are required for detection by antiglobulin antibodies (Issitt, 1998). A negative reaction can occur with small quantities of bound IgG and C3. In addition, AHG sera may possess greater activity against some subclasses of IgG than against others. Consequently, certain AHG sera may produce negative results with RBCs coated by a particular IgG subclass.

COMPATIBILITY TESTING

The term compatibility testing has historically been used synonymously with the serologic crossmatch test. In its broader context, however, compatibility testing is an entire quality process composed of many procedures designed to provide the safest blood product possible for the recipient of a transfusion. These procedures include proper record keeping, accurate donor and recipient identification, and actual serologic testing of the recipient specimen before transfusion. Outlined in the following sections and in Table 35-37 are the steps in compatibility testing required by the American Association of Blood Banks (AABB) Standards for Blood Banks and Transfusion Services (Price, 2009), referred to henceforth as the AABB Standards.

Specimen Requirements

Recipient Sample Identification

A physician order is required before blood is drawn for a type and screen. The order may be verbal (followed by a written order) or may be given on paper or electronically. Proper identification of patient blood samples and donor units is absolutely essential in blood banking. Recipient blood specimens must be labeled by the phlebotomist at the bedside directly from information on the patient's wristband. If the patient's wristband is not attached for any reason, signed confirmation of the patient's identity by nursing staff should be obtained before the blood is drawn. The recipient's blood specimen label should be legible and should include at least the patient's full name, hospital identification number, and specimen collection date, and it should be securely attached to the specimen tube when it is accepted by blood bank personnel. Unlabeled or improperly labeled blood

TABLE 35-37
Required Steps in Pretransfusion Compatibility Testing*

Physician (or other authorized health professional) order	Written (paper or electronic) order for type and screen test • Type and screen • Crossmatch red blood cells • Special requests such as irradiation, cytomegalovirus (CMV)-negative, etc. • Oral orders may be accepted if followed by the written request
Phlebotomy/recipient identification	Phlebotomist must positively identify the recipient and the recipient's blood sample • Transfusion request and labeled patient blood sample must contain at least two pieces of independent identifying information for that patient (e.g., name, hospital number, date of birth) • Mechanism to identify the date of sample and the phlebotomist (paper or electronic) • Transfusion service will ensure that identifying information on the requisition and sample label is in agreement
Recipient testing	Perform ABO and Rh typing on recipient's blood specimen—red cell and serum or plasma testing are required Review previous records for comparison with current typing results • Clinically significant antibodies • Significant adverse events to transfusion • Special transfusion requirements Test recipient's serum or plasma to detect clinically significant antibodies • Method must include 37° C incubation with conversion to antihuman globulin using reagent red cells that are not pooled
Donor testing	Confirm ABO and Rh types on donor red cell units as required • Confirmation testing for ABO group required on all units (serum testing not required) • Comfirmation of Rh type required only on those units labeled as Rh-negative (weak D testing is not required)
Crossmatch	Select ABO- and Rh-compatible red cell components for transfusion Perform serologic or electronic crossmatch of red cell components • Full antiglobulin crossmatch required if current antibody screen is positive or the patient has a known history of clinically significant antibodies
Labeling	Label all red cell products or other components with the recipient's identifying information • Label must contain at least two independent patient identifiers, donor unit number, and compatibility test results, if performed

*Requirements paraphrased from Roback (2008). See American Association of Blood Banks (AABB) Standards (Price, 2009) for specific wording.

specimens are unacceptable under any circumstances. During testing, all test tubes or other types of aliquot or reaction containers must be accurately identified directly from the label on the recipient sample.

Each pretransfusion blood sample should be accompanied by an appropriate order or requisition, containing at least the patient's full name and hospital identification number. The signature or initials of the phlebotomist should be on the requisition, as the test requisition is a permanent record of that particular specimen collection. With increasing use of electronic order entry, a computer-based system may record the physician order and capture the person performing the phlebotomy. The phlebotomist, however, should still sign the specimen for verification and matching against the electronic record. Upon specimen receipt, the label on the tube is compared with the information on the requisition for any discrepancies. If there is any doubt as to the proper identity of the sample, another sample must be obtained.

Type of Sample

Although serum has traditionally been the preferred specimen for compatibility testing, plasma is increasingly used owing to newer testing technologies (e.g., gel test). If serum is used, blood samples should be collected in siliconized plain tubes without serum separator gel. Other test methods, such as gel column agglutination, microtiter plates, and automated testing systems, may require a specific type of sample per manufacturer instructions.

Problems with plasma in conventional antiglobulin techniques are primarily technical. Plasma can be associated with small fibrin clots which can trap RBCs and resemble agglutination. Fibrin may also trap serum and cause neutralization of AHG reagent if not removed before washing. Finally, plasma can enhance rouleaux formation if fibrinogen levels are particularly high.

Appearance

Most blood bank laboratories have policies in place to reject grossly hemolyzed recipient blood samples as unacceptable for pretransfusion testing unless there is no other choice. Using serum that is already hemolyzed may mask antibody-induced hemolysis that would ordinarily be detectable in antibody screening tests. Lipemia may rarely cause difficulty in evaluating agglutination results, although lipemia is not usually a cause for rejection of a pretransfusion sample. Automated instruments may have additional specifications regarding sample appearance. For example, a grossly hemolyzed or lipemic sample can give false-positive readings with an automated gel technology instrument.

Age of Sample

According to AABB Standards, a pretransfusion specimen for testing and red cell transfusion is valid for 72 hours. After 72 hours, a new sample must be drawn. Requiring a new pretransfusion sample every 72 hours on previously transfused or pregnant individuals ensures that the sample being tested is fairly representative of the patient's current immune status.

In elective surgery patients, some facilities will extend the age of a preoperative sample up to 1 month provided that the patient (1) has a negative antibody screen, (2) has no history of clinically significant antibodies, (3) is not pregnant, and (4) has not been transfused within the preceding 3 months. Patients failing to meet these criteria are required to have a sample drawn within 72 hours of planned surgery (King, 2008).

Sample Storage

AABB Standards require that all pretransfusion samples be stored at 1°–6° C for at least 7 days after testing is completed, along with at least one representative segment from each of the donor units crossmatched on the recipient. The purpose of this is to ensure that repeat or additional testing of the donor or patient may be performed later if the patient experiences a delayed hemolytic reaction or other adverse effect of transfusion.

Documentation and Record Keeping

General Considerations

All blood banks must have a manual or computerized system of record keeping that contains the results or outcomes of all tests and activities carried out in the blood bank. Records must be complete and retrievable within a reasonable time frame. Transfer or dissemination of information from any patient records must conform to requirements of the institution's confidentiality policies in accordance with federal and state laws and

TABLE 35-38
Some Causes of ABO Grouping Discrepancies

	Problems with red cell testing	Problems with serum testing
Unexpected positive reactions	Acquired B antigen associated with colon and gastric cancers, intestinal obstructions Cord cells contaminated with Wharton's jelly Autoagglutination caused by cold autoantibodies Cells heavily coated with warm autoantibody Polyagglutination Acriflavine antibody (against dye used in anti-B) Genetic chimerism* Bone marrow transplants* Administration of red cells outside ABO group* B(A) phenomenon Fetomaternal hemorrhage*	Rouleaux-forming proteins present (e.g., plasma expanders, monoclonal gamma globulins) Room temperature alloantibody present (e.g., anti-M, N, P1) Room temperature alloantibody in immunoglobulin (Ig)M phase (e.g., anti-c) Cold autoagglutinin present (e.g., anti-I, IH) Passively acquired ABO antibodies, (e.g., incompatible plasma transfusion) Passenger lymphocyte-derived antibody associated with minor incompatible bone marrow or solid organ transplant Subgroup of A with anti-A1 in serum *Cis*-AB with weak anti-B in serum
Unexpected negative reactions	A or B subgroups Antigen depression due to leukemia or other disease state High levels of soluble blood group substances Massive transfusion with compatible red cells outside of ABO group Bone marrow transplants	Age of patient (elderly, newborn) Hypogammaglobulinemia Immunosuppression Bone marrow transplants ABO subgroups Long-term parenteral nutrition Snake venom

*Look for mixed-field appearance of reactions with reagent antisera.

regulations. Records must be preserved for different periods of time, depending on federal, state, and accrediting agency requirements.

Documentation of the entire compatibility testing process must include records of patient identification, order entry, individual special transfusion needs, date and time of testing, results of patient testing, identity of the technologist who performed the testing, and blood component issues. A computerized system is ideal for capturing this information and enables rapid and easy retrieval of these data for a given patient, including records of ABO and Rh type, antibody problems, transfusion history, and requirements for special types of blood products. From a more global perspective, computerized retrieval of data for groups of patients also greatly enhances the monitoring of blood product utilization within the facility, including blood ordering and transfusion practices of physicians.

Results and interpretations of all patient testing should be documented on appropriate manual worksheets or entered into the computer immediately upon observation of the results. In a manual record-keeping system, all forms should be filled out with ink, not pencil. If results must be changed on manual worksheets, original results must not be obliterated; a single line should be placed through them, and the new results dated and initialed by the technologist making the change. A continuously updated list of initials used by all personnel working in the blood bank on all shifts must be part of the permanent blood bank records. Changes to computerized results must also be completely documented as part of the computerized result record with ability to track both original and corrected data (Roback, 2008).

Check of Previous Records

Manual or computerized records must be checked for previous results on a given patient when a new sample is received. ABO and Rh tests on the current specimen should be checked against previous results, if available, to help verify that the specimen was collected from the correct individual. Information on any unexpected antibodies identified previously is also extremely important because the titer of an antibody may fall to levels that cannot be detected by antibody screening procedures. If a clinically significant antibody was previously identified, the patient must receive RBCs negative for the corresponding antigen (antigen-negative) even if current antibody screening tests are negative. Previous significant adverse events to transfusions and special requirements should also be reviewed before crossmatching is done.

ABO Grouping

Antisera and reagent RBCs for ABO grouping are standardized and readily available commercially. Most blood bank laboratories use monoclonal reagent antisera derived from antibodies produced by hybridoma cell lines. ABO grouping consists of two parts, commonly referred to as red cell grouping (forward type) and serum grouping (back type). In forward grouping, a 3%–5% RBC suspension is tested with commercially prepared anti-A and anti-B to test for antigens on the RBC membrane. In reverse grouping, patient or donor serum is tested against reagent cells of known A_1 and B phenotype to test for the expected ABO antibodies in the patient's serum (see Table 35-8). ABO grouping is carried out at room temperature, with only an immediate-spin centrifugation step required to promote a macroscopic agglutination reaction. The manufacturer's directions must be followed for all commercial reagents.

ABO Grouping of Donors

The collecting facility is required to perform a forward and reverse ABO type on all donors. The transfusion service or other laboratory responsible for compatibility testing must confirm the ABO group of all units of RBCs or whole blood received. RBC forward grouping is performed from an integral segment attached to each donor unit. For units labeled as group O, anti-A,B alone may be used for donor confirmatory testing because only group O RBCs will fail to hemagglutinate with anti-A,B.

ABO Grouping of Recipients

Every pretransfusion patient blood specimen must also be tested for ABO group. Both cell and serum groupings are required for initial ABO testing of all patient samples, and the results of RBC and serum testing should agree with each other (see Table 35-8) before any results are reported and blood is transfused.

Some blood banks routinely include the use of anti-A,B in the RBC grouping procedure, although this reagent does not usually yield any additional useful information except for the detection of A_x or B_x subgroups. Anti-A,B is used as a convenient reagent in repeat testing to confirm initial typing of a group O patient. Anti-A,B can also be used for confirmatory typing with neonate and infant samples, especially when the infant has been transfused with Group O RBCs. Infant red cells can give weaker reactions on forward typing owing to the decreased number of ABO antigens on infant red cells (see ABO and I Blood Group sections).

ABO Grouping Discrepancies

Interpretation of ABO blood grouping results is generally straightforward. In the event that the results of RBC and serum grouping do not agree, testing is repeated to rule out any clerical or technical error. If results still disagree, an ABO discrepancy is present owing to problems with the patient's serum or cells that must be resolved before an ABO type can be confirmed. Table 35-38 lists some of the many reasons for ABO discrepancies. Several references are available that provide a complete description of these problems and the protocols for resolution (Harmening, 2005; Roback, 2008).

If a blood transfusion is needed emergently and an ABO discrepancy occurs that cannot be resolved in a timely manner, group O packed RBCs, AB plasma components, or both may be given. However, it is important to be certain that a sufficient pretransfusion blood specimen is obtained from the patient so that the workup may be continued. In some cases, it may be necessary to send a pretransfusion specimen to a reference laboratory for further evaluation.

Rh Typing

Several types of antisera are available for detection of the RhD antigen. Today, the most commonly utilized anti-D typing reagents in tube testing are (1) a saline-reactive, low-protein, monoclonal/polyclonal blend containing murine monoclonal IgM anti-D for immediate direct agglutination of D-positive red cells, and (2) a human polyclonal IgG anti-D necessary for weak D (formerly called D^u) testing. Also available is a reagent blend of monoclonal IgM and monoclonal IgG anti-D from human/murine heterohybridoma lines suitable for both direct and subsequent weak D testing of RBCs.

Before monoclonal blended reagents became available, most routine D typing was performed using rapid tube anti-D made from pooled human sera and containing high molecular weight protein additives that enhanced the direct agglutinating capability of human IgG anti-D. However, because of the high protein concentration in these rapid tube reagents, spontaneous, false-positive aggregation can be observed in patients with abnormal serum proteins, or whose RBCs are heavily sensitized with autoantibody. As a control, manufacturers of high-protein Rh typing sera recommend running a parallel diluent control containing no antibody to detect false-positive reactions. For saline-reactive Rh typing reagents in use today, a concurrent negative reaction with anti-A or anti-B is a sufficient negative control. However, patients who appear to be AB, RhD-positive should be retyped for D with anti-D and an inert control reagent such as 6%–8% bovine albumin.

Direct typing for the D antigen is carried out at room temperature by the immediate spin technique, after mixing one drop of saline-suspended 3%–5% RBCs and one drop of commercial anti-D. If weak D testing is necessary, RBCs are tested by IAT with an IgG anti-D. A parallel test with a negative diluent control is always included for the weak D test.

Rh Typing of Donors

As required by the AABB Standards, all whole blood donor units are tested by the collecting facility for the D antigen by direct agglutination methods. All donor units testing as Rh-negative by direct agglutination are tested for a weak D phenotype by the IAT. If routine D testing or weak D testing is positive, the unit is labeled Rh-positive. The transfusion service must reconfirm the D type of all RBC units labeled Rh-negative by testing red cells from an integral attached segment by a direct anti-D agglutination method. Repeat testing of donor units by the transfusion service for weak D is not required by the AABB Standards.

Rh Typing of Recipients

Every pretransfusion recipient blood specimen must be tested for the D antigen by direct typing. Indirect testing for weak D in recipients is not necessary: Patients who fail to agglutinate after direct agglutination are typed as Rh-negative. Some blood banks do perform weak D testing for prenatal specimens; however, more recent data show that many individuals typing as weak D possess a partial D phenotype and are at risk for RhD alloimmunization. Erythrocyte typing for the C, c, E, and e antigens of the Rh system is not performed routinely but may be done to determine the most probable Rh genotype in the evaluation of antibody problems, in parentage studies, and in patients with long-term transfusion requirements.

ANTIBODY DETECTION

All specimens submitted for pretransfusion testing must be screened for clinically significant antibodies in the recipient serum (antibody screen). Because clinically significant antibodies typically react at body temperature, most laboratories omit room temperature incubation entirely. AABB Standards require that the method used incorporate incubation at physiologic or body temperature (37° C) followed by conversion to the IAT. If a method other than the IAT is used, it must have documented and validated equivalent sensitivity in its ability to detect clinically significant antibodies (Roback, 2008). A variety of different antibody screening protocols, utilizing different technologies, are in use today. Currently, none of the available technologies is capable of detecting all RBC antibodies.

Reagent Red Blood Cells

Reagent RBCs or screening cells used for the detection and identification of antibodies in a patient's serum are usually obtained from commercial manufacturers. AABB Standards require that antibody detection in recipients be performed using reagent cells that are not pooled. Typically, antibody screening cells consist of two to three group O reagent cells selected from different donors of known phenotype. Sets of cells are prepared so that all antigens to the most commonly encountered blood group antibodies are represented and must include C, c, D, E, e, Fy^a, Fy^b, Jk^a, Jk^b, K, k, Le^a, Le^b, P_1, M, N, S, and s antigens. An **antigram** that lists the blood group antigenic makeup of each cell (Fig. 35-21) accompanies each lot of screening RBCs. When possible, cells that are homozygous for selected antigens are used, which increases the likelihood of detecting weak or dose-dependent antibodies. A three-cell screening panel ensures homozygosity for more antigens such as Jk^a, Jk^b, Fy^a, Fy^b, S, and s, against which the corresponding antibodies are likely to exhibit dosage, but the additional cell adds expense to pretransfusion testing. Several studies (Cordle, 1990; Judd, 1997) have shown that use of three red blood samples for antibody detection rarely reveals a clinically significant antibody not detected by a two-cell screening procedure.

Antibody Detection Protocols

Tube Tests

In conventional test tube methods, one volume 3%–5% screening reagent cells and two volumes patient serum (giving an average volume/volume ratio of serum to cells of approximately 50 : 1) are incubated at 37° C with an enhancement medium for the time specified by the manufacturer, and are centrifuged and examined for hemolysis or agglutination. The screening cells are then washed three to four times with saline, and AHG reagent is added for final detection of IgG alloantibodies.

Because different blood group antibodies commonly show characteristic reaction patterns by IAT technique (see Table 35-7), close examination at different phases of testing in this conventional protocol may yield helpful information in evaluating cases in which the screen is positive:

- Direct agglutination of the cells in albumin or LISS after 37° C incubation frequently indicates the presence of an Rh antibody.
- IgM antibodies possessing a wide thermal range, such as anti-I, anti-P_1, and Lewis antibodies, may show reactions in albumin or LISS. However, these reactions generally become much weaker after conversion to the IAT.
- With rare exceptions, in vitro hemolysis of reagent cells after 37° C indicates the presence of Lewis, Kidd, Ii, P, PP_1P^k, or Vel antibodies.
- The vast majority of IgG antibodies, with the exception of Rh, will not be detected until after washing and conversion to the IAT.

Screening Cell Master List

		Rh								Kell				Duffy		Kidd		Sex linked	Lewis		MNSs				P	Lutheran	
Vial	Donor	D	C	E	c	e	f	C^w	V	K	k	Kp^a	Js^a	Fy^a	Fy^b	Jk^a	Jk^b	Xg^a	Le^a	Le^b	S	s	M	N	P1	Lu^a	Lu^b
I	R1R1	+	+	0	0	+	0	0	0	+	+	0	0	0	+	+	0	+	0	+	+	+	+	0	+	0	+
II	R2R2	+	0	+	+	0	0	0	0	0	+	0	0	+	0	0	+	+	+	0	0	+	0	+	+	0	+

Figure 35-21 The "antigram" accompanying each lot of reagent screening red blood cells.

- Reactions of different screening cells in multiple phases or with varying strengths usually indicate that more than one antibody is present.

Column Agglutination Technologies

Column agglutination is an alternative method for alloantibody detection used by many transfusion services. This technology utilizes the differential migration of RBC agglutinates through a small microtube containing a dextran acrylamide size exclusion gel column (Lapierre, 1990). The ID-Microtyping System gel agglutination test (ID-MTS, Ortho-Clinical Diagnostics, Raritan, NJ) commercially available in the United States is a 5 × 7-cm plastic card holding six microtubes containing gel matrix infused with anti-IgG. With six microtubes per card, a two-cell screen for three different patients can be performed with one gel card. In addition to antibody detection, anti-IgG gel cards can be used for antibody identification, red cell crossmatching, and DAT testing. Gel cards for ABO/Rh typing are also available.

For testing, precisely measured volumes of screening reagent RBCs (0.8% suspension in LISS) and plasma are incubated at 37° C in the reaction chamber above the column matrix. Following incubation, the plastic cards are centrifuged under carefully controlled conditions. IgG-coated RBCs agglutinate as they come into contact with the AHG reagent in the matrix and are trapped. Reaction strength and size determine the migration of the agglutinates, ranging from the largest (4+) agglutinates at the top to migration of weaker, smaller agglutinates farther into the gel column (Fig. 35-22). Unagglutinated RBCs pass easily through the column and are found as a pellet at the bottom. Because the plasma or serum remains in the reaction chamber above the matrix, repeated washing steps and addition of control cells to check the activity of the AHG reagent are unnecessary. The endpoint hemagglutination reactions are very stable, allowing the cards to be kept for supervisory review of questionable reactions. The cards can be photocopied or digitally photographed and downloaded as permanent laboratory data.

Column agglutination or gel technology has equivalent sensitivity to standard LISS tube testing for antibody detection and is particularly sensitive for detection of anti-Rh antibodies (Weisbach, 2006). Gel testing can offer several advantages over conventional tube procedures. It is more standardized than conventional tube testing with a reliable, stable agglutination endpoint, making it an attractive method for small facilities with cross-trained generalists. It is also less sensitive to clinically insignificant cold antibodies, eliminating unnecessary antibody workups. Additional time savings are achieved through the elimination of repetitive washing steps and manual macroscopic and/or microscopic readings. Finally, testing can be automated (ProVue, Ortho-Clinical Diagnostics, Rochester, NY), permitting high-throughput testing, electronic interpretation and validation, and digital documentation of results.

Solid-Phase Adherence Tests

Another alternative to tube tests for alloantibody detection is indirect solid-phase adherence test systems. In this application, reagent RBCs are bound to the bottom of microplate wells. Serum and an enhancement reagent are added and incubated at 37° C, allowing the alloantibody to bind to the solid phase. After washing to remove unbound serum globulins, indicator RBCs coated with antihuman IgG are added, and the plates are centrifuged. If a reaction has occurred between the reagent cells and the serum alloantibody, the antiglobulin-coated indicator cells will bind and cover the bottom surface of the well, whereas a discrete button in the bottom of the well indicates a negative reaction (Fig. 35-23). Wells may be read manually or with an automated reading device. As with column agglutination, positive reactions are very stable, so the plate may be covered, stored at 2°–8° C, and read up to 2 days later.

Direct solid-phase test systems are also available for applications such as ABO and Rh typing of red cells. For these tests, microplate wells are coated with the appropriate antibodies. Test cells are added and incubated, and the plates are then centrifuged. For positive reactions, the RBCs adhere to the entire bottom surface of the antibody-coated well; negative reactions result in a tightly packed cell button in the bottom of the well. Instrumentation is available for automated and semiautomated testing using solid-phase technology (Galileo, Immucor, Inc., Norcross, GA).

Antibody Identification

When red cell alloantibodies are detected in the serum of a prospective blood recipient, as indicated by a positive antibody screen, the antibody must be identified so that antigen-negative blood can be provided for transfusion, if required. Antibody identification is accomplished by first testing an extended panel of reagent RBCs of known phenotype against the recipient's serum by the IAT technique. An autocontrol is always included as part of the testing to help differentiate whether autoantibody, alloantibody, or both are present. The immunohematologist then compares the pattern of positive and negative serum reactions against the antigen phenotype pattern on the printed worksheet that accompanies each panel to find a match.

Interpreting the Results of Antibody Identification

Table 35-39 is a simple example of an antibody panel. Serum Y reacts with cells No. 1 through 3, which are positive for the D antigen, but does not react with cells No. 4 through 6, which are negative for the D antigen. The pattern of positive and negative serum reactions matches the phenotype pattern for the D antigen; therefore serum Y appears to contain anti-D. Similarly, the pattern of reactivity for serum Z matches the phenotype pattern for the E antigen; thus serum Z appears to contain anti-E.

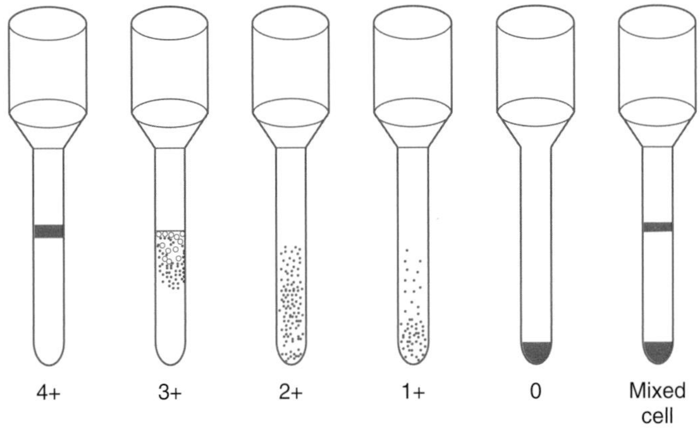

Figure 35-22 Appearance of reaction patterns and grading for gel or column agglutination technology.

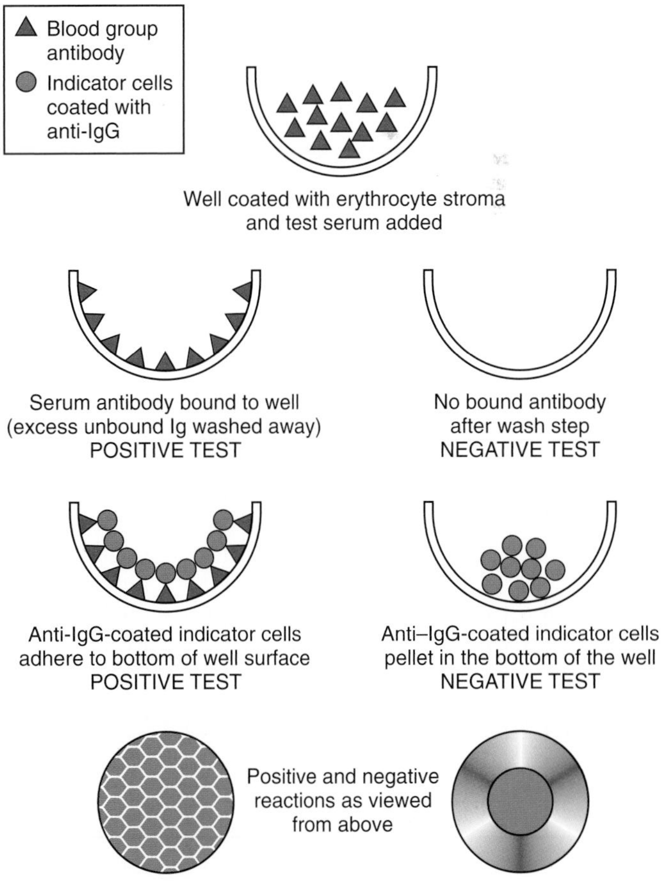

Figure 35-23 Principle of solid-phase adherence technology with appearance of positive and negative reactions.

Before such identification can be conclusively stated, one must be sure that enough cells of differing antigenic composition are tested to definitively identify a single antibody or combination of antibodies in a given serum.

Fisher's exact method has traditionally been used to statistically calculate the probability that a single antibody has been correctly identified within a confidence interval of 95% (i.e., the probability that the same results would be obtained by random chance because of a different antibody is 1 in 20). This method compares the numbers of positive and negative results against the number of cells tested that express or lack the corresponding antigen and against the total number of cells tested (Race, 1975).

Table 35-40 lists the probability values calculated by Fisher's exact method that are achieved with differing combinations of positive and negative cells in the total number tested. It can be seen that a p value of 0.05 can be achieved with a minimum of six cells, with three cells being positive for an antigen reacting with the antibody, and three cells negative for the antigen failing to react with the antibody. Most manufacturers supply reagent cell panels with 10–11 cells, with at least one of the combinations of positive and negative cells from Table 35-40, for most of the antigens to which unexpected antibodies are commonly encountered. Consequently, most simple antibody identifications are valid at a p value considerably less than 0.05, except in cases where there are antibodies to low- or high-frequency antigens, or where multiple antibodies are present in the same serum. In these situations, additional cells from other panels may have to be tested to achieve identification within the 95% confidence interval.

Figure 35-24 shows the results of a panel tested against patient serum with a conventional tube antiglobulin testing method and examined for agglutination after the 37° C incubation phase, and finally after the addition of AHG. In a quick overview of the panel results, an immunohematologist will at once notice that there is agglutination with different cells after centrifugation in both phases of the test, indicating the probable presence of multiple antibodies.

Following is an outline of the strategy used in evaluating antibody identification results:

1. The autocontrol is negative, indicating that the serum reactivity is most probably due to alloantibodies. However, if the autocontrol is positive, it is important that DAT testing be performed to confirm or rule out prior in vivo sensitization of the patient's cells. The DAT should be examined closely for the appearance of mixed field agglutination. In recently transfused patients, attachment of alloantibody to a minor population of transfused donor RBCs causes classic mixed field agglutination and is frequently the first sign of a developing immune response that may result in a delayed hemolytic transfusion reaction. In a massively transfused patient, only a small percentage of cells may be DAT-positive.
2. The first step that is performed by many immunohematologists in evaluating antibody identification results is to rule out those antibodies where the serum has failed to react with a cell known to carry

TABLE 35-39
Simple Panel Example

Cells in a panel	KNOWN ANTIGENIC COMPOSITION D	C	c	E	e	TEST SERUM Y	Z
No. 1	+	+	+	0	0	+	0
No. 2	+	+	0	+	+	+	+
No. 3	+	0	+	0	+	+	0
No. 4	0	0	+	0	+	0	0
No. 5	0	0	+	0	+	0	0
No. 6	0	+	0	+	+	0	+

TABLE 35-40
Probability Values Based on Fisher's Exact Method

Total number of cells tested	Antigen-positive cells that react with antibody	Antigen-negative cells that do not react with antibody	*p* value
5	3	2	0.100
6	4	2	0.067
6	3	3	0.050
7	5	2	0.048
7	4	3	0.029
8	6	2	0.036
8	5	3	0.018
8	4	4	0.014
9	7	2	0.028
9	6	3	0.012
10	8	2	0.022
10	7	3	0.008
10	6	4	0.005
10	5	5	0.004

Name *John Doe*

Hospital number *0001234.56*

		Rh								MNSs				P	Lewis		Lutheran		Kell*				Duffy		Kidd			Vial			
	Rh phenotype	D	C	E	c	e	f	C^w	V	M	N	S	s	P_I	Le^a	Le^b	Lu^a	Lu^b	K	k	Kp^a	Js^a	Fy^a	Fy^b	Jk^a	Jk^b	Xg^a		37C	AHG	CC
1	rr	0	0	0	+	+	+	0	0	+	0	+	0	+	+	0	0	+	0	+	0	0	+	+	+	0	+	1	0	1	
2	rr	0	0	0	+	+	+	0	0	+	+	0	+	+	0	+	0	+	+	+	0	0	0	+	0	+	+	2	0	3	
3	r′r	0	0	0	+	+	+	0	0	+	0	+	+	+	0	+	0	+	0	+	0	0	0	+	0	+	0	3	0	0	2
4	r″r	0	0	+	+	+	+	0	0	+	+	+	+	0	0	+	+	+	0	+	0	0	0	+	0	+	0	4	1	2	
5	rr	0	0	0	+	+	+	0	0	0	+	+	+	+	0	+	0	+	0	+	0	0	0	+	0	+	+	5	0	0	2
6	R_0r	+	0	0	+	+	+	0	+	+	+	0	+	+	0	0	0	+	0	+	0	0	0	0	+	0	0	6	0	0	2
7	R_1R_1	+	+	0	0	+	+	0	0	+	0	+	+	0	+	0	0	+	0	+	0	0	0	+	+	+	0	7	0	0	2
8	R_1R_1	+	+	0	0	+	+	0	0	+	+	+	+	+	0	+	0	+	+	+	0	0	+	0	0	+	+	8	0	3	
9	$R_1R_1^w$	+	+	0	0	+	+	+	0	+	+	0	+	+	0	+	0	+	0	+	0	0	+	+	+	+	+	9	0	1	
10	R_2R_2	+	0	+	+	0	+	0	0	+	+	0	+	+	+	0	0	+	0	+	0	+	0	0	+	+	+	10	1	2	
11	rr	0	0	0	+	+	+	0	0	0	+	0	+	+	0	+	+	+	0	+	+	0	+	+	+	0	0	11	0	1	
																												Auto	0	0	2

Figure 35-24 A typical panel worksheet showing an example of antibody identification results. *AHG,* Antihuman globulin; *CC,* Coombs' control cells. *Unless otherwise specified, it is understood that all cells are positive for the high frequency antigens Kp^b and Js^b.

the corresponding antigen. Although not required, whenever possible it is best to rule out antibodies based on lack of reactivity with cells demonstrating the homozygous form of an antigen, so as not to erroneously rule out weakly reactive antibodies that show dosage. Using the homozygous "rule of thumb" for ruling out antibodies, cells No. 3, 5, 6, and 7 are not reactive with the serum and may be used to rule out anti-D, anti-C, anti-c, anti-e, anti-M, anti-N, anti-s, anti-P_1, anti-Lu^b, anti-k, anti-Fy^b, anti-Jk^a, and anti-Jk^b. Expression of the antigens f, V, Le^a, Le^b, and Xg^a cannot be characterized as homozygous owing to the mechanisms of their inheritance, but because at least one of the four cells above is positive for these antigens and the serum did not react with them, the corresponding antibodies may be eliminated from consideration.

3. Because of reactions seen in different phases and demonstrating different agglutination strengths, at least two antibodies are likely present in the serum:
   - Cells No. 4 and 10 show direct agglutination in the 37° C phase, followed by stronger agglutination in the AHG phase, which is very typical of Rh system antibodies. These are the only two cells on the panel positive for the E antigen, which has not been ruled out. Thus, it is likely that anti-E is one of the antibodies involved.
   - Cells No. 2 and 8 show very strong agglutination in the AHG phase only. Upon examining the antigens across the top of the panel that have not been ruled out, one sees that the phenotype of the panel cells for the K antigen fits the serum reactivity of these two cells. Thus, it is likely that anti-K is a second antibody involved.
   - The remaining serum reactions with cells No. 1, 9, and 11 cannot be explained by anti-E or anti-K but may be explained by anti-Fy^a, because all three of these cells are positive for the Fy^a antigen, and Fy^a has not been ruled out.
4. Anti-S should be ruled out by testing another cell positive in the homozygous state for S antigen that at the same time is negative for Fy^a, K, and E antigens.
5. Antibodies to low-frequency antigens such as C^w, Lu^a, Kp^a, and Js^a may be ruled out by testing appropriate cells if available. When antibodies to low-frequency antigens are not ruled out, an antiglobulin crossmatch is used to detect any potential incompatibility between donor cells and the theoretical presence of one or more of these antibodies in the patient's serum.
6. Ruling out of additional antibodies may sometimes be accomplished by typing the patient's cells for selected antigens. This is particularly helpful when a patient's serum contains multiple antibodies and the reagent cell resources available to the blood bank are limited. If one of the antibodies that must be ruled out in a mixture of antibodies is anti-Jk^b, for example, the patient's cells may be typed for the Jk^b antigen with specific antisera. If the patient expresses the Jk^b antigen, then the presence of an alloantibody to Jk^b can be conclusively eliminated.
7. On the panel in Figure 35-24, there are at least three cells negative for all three antigens—Fy^a, K, and E—that do not react with the serum. However, to conclusively identify all three antibodies within the 95% confidence interval, three separate cells must be positive only for Fy^a antigen, three positive only for K antigen, and three positive only for E antigen that do react with the serum. Thus, anti-Fy^a can be identified with confidence; however, two more cells positive for K antigen and one more cell positive for E antigen must be tested with the serum to conclusively identify the presence of anti-K and anti-E.
8. If antibody identification is being performed for the first time on a particular patient, it is common practice to type patient RBCs for the antigens to which he or she has developed antibodies, as a confirmation of the antibody identification. The patient's RBCs should lack the antigens corresponding to the antibodies present.

Crossmatching

For many years, a major serologic crossmatch was required before the transfusion of whole blood or packed RBCs. This protocol required a 37° C incubation followed by conversion to the IAT. In 1984, this requirement was eliminated by the AABB Standards as long as (1) the current antibody screen on the patient is completely negative, and (2) there is no past history of clinically significant antibodies. For patients who meet these criteria, an abbreviated procedure designed to detect ABO incompatibility may be used. This may consist of an immediate spin crossmatch or an electronic crossmatch.

Immediate Spin Serologic Crossmatch

The serologic test to detect ABO incompatibility commonly consists of an immediate spin protocol employing a 3%–5% saline suspension of donor RBCs prepared from an integral segment taken from the selected donor unit. Cells usually are washed once to remove any anticoagulant or plasma protein that could interfere with the testing. A drop of donor cell suspension is mixed with recipient serum, centrifuged immediately, and examined for hemolysis and/or agglutination. This procedure has come to be known as the abbreviated or immediate-spin crossmatch.

Use of the immediate-spin crossmatch procedure in clinical settings has shown it to be a safe and cost-effective alternative to the antiglobulin crossmatch (Judd, 1988; Cordle, 1990; Shulman, 1990), although reports indicate that this technique may fail to detect ABO incompatibility when recipient ABO antibodies are of low titer, or when donor cells belong to a weak ABO subgroup (Berry-Dortch, 1985; Shulman, 1987). Rare false-negative results can occur as the result of a prozone effect in Group O/Group A major incompatibility, particularly if a delay in centrifugation occurs (Judd, 1988). The prozone/delay apparently allows for the fixation of C1 complement on RBC membranes, which sterically hinders hemagglutination. Suspension of donor cells in EDTA-saline eliminates this problem by chelating calcium necessary for formation of the C1 complement complex. In addition to false-negatives, the immediate-spin crossmatch can cause false-positive results due to rouleaux, cold-reactive antibodies, and fibrin—all of which may cause delays in issuing the blood for transfusion. In a recent College of American Pathologists (CAP) challenge, approximately 70% of participating hospitals reported using the immediate-spin crossmatch for patients with no clinically significant antibodies (Downes, 2009). In a multicenter study involving 1.3 million immediate-spin crossmatches, the observed risk of acute hemolytic reaction using the immediate-spin crossmatch technique was 0.0004% (Shulman, 1990).

Electronic Crossmatch

In 1994, Butch et al. first reported on a proposed standard operating procedure that would replace the immediate-spin serologic crossmatch with a computer **electronic crossmatch,** or EXM. Similar to the immediate-spin crossmatch, the electronic crossmatch may be used only for patients who have no currently detected clinically significant antibodies or any history of alloantibodies. The EXM reduces human error by assigning final verification of ABO compatibility between donor and recipient by the laboratory computer system (Judd, 1991). In addition, it eliminates time-consuming investigation of false-positive serologic reactions. In a recent CAP survey, nearly 20% of 3216 responding hospitals currently performed or were in the process of implementing the EXM (Downes, 2009).

The EXM is permissible provided that specific testing criteria are met and extensive validation of the blood bank information system has been performed to meet current AABB Standards and FDA requirements as outlined in a 1997 FDA internal document (Judd, 2002). Critical elements required in computer validation for the EXM (Judd, 1998) include updated hardware, instrumentation interfaces, historical records checks, reaction interpretation algorithms, prevention functions and warnings for ABO assignment/release, and personnel competency assessment. Because the safety of this procedure will be only as good as the electronic information that is entered and stored in the system, maximal use of bar codes to identify both donors and patients should be implemented. After extensive experience with electronic crossmatching at the University of Michigan, Judd (1998) recommends that bar-coded patient identification be mandatory, both at the time of sample collection and prior to transfusion, and that pretransfusion specimen labels be generated at the bedside from the bar code on the patient identification wristband. The FDA requirement that facilities wishing to implement the EXM must submit a request for variance to the Code of Federal Regulations for Compatibility Testing (21CFR606.151; 2001a) has been eliminated. Table 35-41 summarizes the AABB Standards requirements.

Antiglobulin Crossmatch

If the pretransfusion antibody screen detects a clinically significant antibody, or a check of patient records indicates that such antibodies have been detected previously, a major or long crossmatch must be performed. In the antiglobulin crossmatch, compatibility between recipient serum and donor red cells is tested by the antiglobulin method that is routinely used by the laboratory. Red cell units chosen for transfusion should lack the antigen of interest (antigen-negative) by phenotyping units with commercially available antisera. In the future, units may be chosen on the basis of donor genotyping by the blood center.

TABLE 35-41
Requirements for Implementation of the Electronic Crossmatch*

- Computer system has been validated onsite to ensure that only ABO-compatible red cell components are selected for transfusion.
- There have been at least two determinations of the recipient's ABO group, one of which is from the current sample.
- The donor unit blood type has been confirmed serologically from an integrally attached segment.
- The system contains the following data items:
  - Donation identification number
  - Component name
  - ABO/Rh type of component
  - Confirmed unit ABO group
  - Two unique identifiers for recipient
  - Recipient's ABO group/Rh type
  - Recipient's current antibody screen results[†]
  - Interpretation of compatibility
- A method exists to verify the correct entry of data prior to the release of components.
- The software contains logic to warn user of discrepancies between donor unit labeling and confirmatory test results, or of ABO incompatibilities between the recipient and the donor unit.

*Requirements paraphrased from Roback (2008). See Price (2009) for specific wording.
[†]The electronic crossmatch can be used only if current antibody detection tests on the recipient are negative and there is no known history of clinically significant blood group antibodies.

Some blood bank laboratories still choose to perform a full antiglobulin crossmatch for all transfusions, regardless of history and pretransfusion testing results. For patients with a negative antibody screen, the full crossmatch may *rarely* detect alloantibodies to low-frequency antigens not present on the screening cells (e.g., Kp^a, Wr^a). In addition, antibody detection tests could theoretically fail because of the presence of an antibody displaying dosage, deterioration of antigen from the reagent cells during storage, or technical error. Despite these concerns, the actual incidence of missing a clinically significant antibody with an abbreviated crossmatch is very low—less than 0.05% (Mintz, 1982; Cordle, 1990).

Compatibility Testing in Emergencies

In urgent situations, blood may have to be released for transfusion before the completion of compatibility tests, or even before a patient blood specimen is available. If the ABO and Rh types of the patient are not known, group O packed RBCs are released. Practice varies when selecting the Rh of emergency blood components. Some facilities use Rh-negative only for females <50 years of age, whereas others may start with Rh-negative and switch to Rh-positive after 4 (or more) units. If a blood specimen is available and there is time to perform ABO and Rh typing, type-specific blood may be released. All units must be conspicuously labeled to indicate that they are uncrossmatched, and that the patient's serum has not been screened for unexpected antibodies. In these situations, the patient's physician must sign a release form stating that the clinical situation warrants the release of uncrossmatched blood. In such cases, the antibody screen is promptly completed, and crossmatches are performed according to the laboratory's protocol. In the event of a positive screen or incompatible crossmatch, the physician should be notified immediately of any antibodies or incompatibility detected.

Massive transfusion occurs when the number of emergently transfused RBCs equals or exceeds the patient's blood volume in a relatively short time frame (<24 hours). Under these circumstances, many blood banks initiate a massive transfusion policy that permits switching to an immediate-spin or electronic crossmatch, even in a patient with known RBC alloantibodies. In these instances, serum antibody is typically diluted and undetectable in vitro owing to the large volume of donor blood and fluids transfused. Most protocols for massive transfusion return to use of the routine crossmatch procedure within 24 hours of the time the patient is stabilized. Transfusion of antigen-positive units could result in an increase in antibody titer and lead to a delayed hemolytic transfusion reaction in patients with alloantibodies. Communication with the patient's physician is critical in such cases to monitor the patient for hemolysis.

Preoperative Crossmatch Protocols

Most transfusion services have adopted a type and screen–only protocol for elective surgical procedures that do not routinely require transfusion. Blood orders for elective surgical procedures requiring transfusion are set at a level that reflects actual usage patterns for a given operative procedure at a particular institution. The type and screen–only protocol, when used in conjunction with preoperative blood ordering guidelines (maximum surgical blood order schedule; Friedman, 1976; Henry, 1977), allows for much more efficient blood inventory management and reduction in the crossmatch/transfusion (C/T) ratio. For blood ordering guidelines to be successful, they should come under periodic review and revision as new surgical procedures are adopted and techniques are refined.

The preoperative type and screen protocol requires no further serologic work as long as the patient's antibody screen is negative and there is no known history of clinically significant antibodies. If a patient unexpectedly requires transfusion during surgery, ABO- and Rh-compatible units are selected, and an immediate-spin crossmatch or EXM may be performed. If no ABO incompatibility is detected, the blood can be safely released to the operating room with a minimal turnaround time. If the preoperative antibody screen is positive, or if previous records indicate a known clinically significant antibody, standard operating procedures should specify a minimum number of antigen-negative units that would be held by the blood bank for use by the patient during surgery. These units must be crossmatched with the patient's serum using a full antiglobulin crossmatch procedure prior to transfusion.

Prenatal, Postnatal, and Infant Testing

All women should be screened as soon as possible for red cell alloantibodies and the potential for HDFN. The initial test is generally a blood type and antibody screen. If clinically significant antibodies are detected, the pregnancy is monitored with titration studies and other clinical diagnostic tests at specific intervals. Note that RhD-negative women who have received Rh immune globulin prophylaxis can have a weak anti-D on testing. In addition, Rh immune globulin can cross the placenta and cause a positive antibody screen in fetal and cord samples.

At birth, all cord samples are typed for ABO, RhD, and DAT, if indicated: A type and screen is not routinely performed because cord samples are frequently contaminated with maternal blood. Because only IgG antibodies cross the placenta, the DAT can be tested with anti-IgG only. A comparison should be made between mother and infant blood type to evaluate the potential for ABO HDFN. If the mother has clinically significant antibodies, the cord should have a DAT and be phenotyped for the corresponding antigens of interest. An antibody identification should be performed using maternal or cord sample, although maternal blood is often used owing to insufficient serum/plasma in cord samples. If the cord DAT is positive, and the mother does not have clinically significant antibodies, the laboratory should decide whether an eluate procedure should be routinely performed. The cord sample may be used for antibody identification and for eluates if needed.

In RhD-negative women, special precautions and testing are taken both prepartum and postpartum in an effort to prevent RhD alloimmunization (see Rh System). Prepartum, the father may be typed for RhD to determine the risk for HDFN. Alternatively, the fetus may be genotyped to determine RhD status (Finning, 2007). Unless the fetus or the father is confirmed as RhD-negative, the mother must receive prophylatic Rh immune globulin at 28 weeks and after invasive procedures. Once delivery has occurred, a fetal RhD type is performed on cord blood to determine the need for additional Rh immune prophylaxis. If the infant is RhD-negative or if the mother has become sensitized, Rh immune globulin is not given. However, if the infant is RhD-positive and the mother is not sensitized, the mother should receive additional Rh immune globulin. To determine how much Rh immune globulin should be administered postpartum, the mother should be screened for a possible maternal fetal bleed.

The most common screening test for a possible fetal bleed in an RhD-negative mother is the rosette test, which can detect approximately 10 mL of fetal cells in the mother's circulation (Bayliss, 1991). To perform the test, maternal blood is incubated with anti-D, which will bind circulating RhD-positive fetal red cells but not maternal RhD-negative red cells. After incubation and washing, indicator red cells are added and the sample is centrifuged and then examined under a microscope. If fetal red cells are present, indicator red cells will bind to anti-D on fetal red cells, forming a rosette. If no fetal red cells are present, the mixture will be smooth without rosettes.

If the fetal bleed screen is positive, additional studies are necessary to quantitate the extent of the bleed. The Kleihauer-Betke test and flow

TABLE 35-42
Special Techniques in Antibody Identification: Serum Procedures*

	Procedure	Application/effect
Hemagglutination inhibition	Inhibit antibody reactivity by mixing serum with a specific soluble antigen source in parallel with a dilution control; retest against known antigen-positive cells	Confirm specificity by neutralizing the following antibodies: anti-P1, anti-Le^a and Le^b, anti-Sd^a, anti-ABH, anti-I, anti-Ch/Rg. May also allow for easier identification of other antibodies in a mixture
Serum adsorption	Adsorb serum antibodies with autologous cells, selected allogeneic cells, or rabbit erythrocyte stroma (REST) at appropriate temperature for reactivity of antibody	Physically removes broadly reactive autoantibodies or alloantibodies from serum by reacting with absorbing cells to allow for detection of underlying IgG antibodies—particularly useful in cases of WAIHA. May be combined with elution in complicated cases involving identification of multiple antibodies
Sulfhydryl reagents	Pretreat serum with sulfhydryl reagents such as 2-mercaptoethanol (2-ME) or dithiothreitol (DTT)	Destroys pentameric structure of agglutinating IgM antibodies, effectively bypassing cold reactive autoantibodies and alloantibodies to allow for detection of underlying IgG alloantibodies
Titration	Prepare serial twofold dilutions of serum and test against antigen-positive indicator cell	Aids in identification of HTLA antibodies (titer of 1 : 64 or greater) Used to measure increase in production of IgG antibodies during pregnancy ABO-incompatible organ transplantation May rarely be useful in identifying alloantibodies of a higher titer present with a warm autoantibody
Prewarming	Keep all test components (test tubes, cells, serum, saline) at 37° C prior to testing; use monospecific anti-IgG AHG reagents	Bypasses reactivity of cold autoagglutinins or alloagglutinins of limited titer and thermal amplitude—prevents direct agglutination of test cells and/or in vitro complement activation in antibody detection and identification tests
Saline replacement	For tests in which patient or test red cells are suspended in serum and are suspected to have formed rouleaux, the serum is removed and replaced with equal volume of saline	Useful in obtaining valid results in ABO serum grouping or evaluating the presence of apparent agglutination when examining screening cells after 37° C incubation and centrifugation. Pseudoagglutination due to rouleaux will be dispersed by removal of the offending proteins and addition of a high–ionic strength medium.

AHG, Antihuman globulin; *HTLA*, high-titer, low-avidity; *Ig*, immunoglobulin; *WAIHA*, warm autoimmune hemolytic anemia.
*See also Table 35-33 for effects of antibody concentration, pH, incubation time, etc.

cytometry are two methods used to calculate the quantity of fetal red cells in maternal circulation. The Kleihauer-Betke test is based on the resistance of fetal Hg to acid, which looks bright pink in a sea of adult red cell ghosts on a peripheral blood smear. The percentage of fetal red cells present is manually determined and then multiplied by 50 to determine the volume (mL) of fetal blood present (Roback, 2008). Flow cytometric methods are less labor intensive and are used to calculate the percentage of RhD-positive fetal cells by immunofluorescence (Radel, 2008). Once the size of the bleed is determined, the mother should receive sufficient Rh immune globulin to neutralize all circulating fetal red cells. Calculations to determine the size of the fetal bleed and the number of Rh vials required are available in the *AABB Technical Manual* (Roback, 2008). In general, one vial of Rh immune globulin will suppress immunization of 15 mL of RhD-positive red cells.

SPECIAL ANTIBODY IDENTIFICATION TECHNIQUES

Patients who have undergone repeated transfusions may respond by forming multiple unexpected blood group antibodies. Autoantibodies and alloantibodies to high-frequency antigens will react with all cells tested, including all RBCs used for antibody identification, making it extremely difficult to detect other underlying alloantibodies. When complicated problems such as these are encountered, special techniques are required to resolve the problem and find compatible units for transfusion. Special techniques used in antibody identification frequently involve (1) an attempt to eliminate selected antibody reactivity that is interfering with identification of other specificities in the same serum, or (2) an effort to enhance or more clearly characterize the reactivity of an antibody that thus far has escaped definitive identification. Some of these techniques are outlined later in this chapter, as well as in Tables 35-42 and 35-43. The reader is also referred to the American Association of Blood Banks *Technical Manual* (Roback, 2008), *Applied Blood Group Serology* (Issitt, 1998), *Judd's Methods in Immunohematology* (Judd, 2008), and *Immunohematology Methods* (Mallory, 1993) as excellent references for most common procedures, in addition to more specialized techniques.

Serum Procedures to Eliminate Antibody Reactivity

Hemagglutination Inhibition

Hemagglutination inhibition is used to neutralize selected blood group antibodies with their corresponding antigen found in soluble form in human saliva, serum, or other body fluids, as well as in substances in nature (Table 35-44). Recently, reagents for antibody neutralization have been synthesized using modern molecular techniques (Seltsam, 2009). The identity of a suspected antibody is confirmed if it no longer agglutinates antigen-positive reagent cells after addition of soluble antigen. Hemagglutination inhibition may be particularly useful when working with a serum specimen containing multiple specificities. The principle of hemagglutination inhibition is also used to determine the secretor status of individuals with weak ABO subgroups (see Table 35-10). Care must be taken in interpreting results because weak reactions may be diluted by the inhibition substance. A control set of tubes containing an inert substance (typically saline) should be used in parallel to verify that a negative reaction was the result of inhibition and not of sample dilution.

Antibody Adsorption

Adsorption is a process used to physically remove antibodies from sera. The adsorption procedure may be performed using washed and/or enzyme-treated autologous RBCs, phenotypically matched allogeneic cells, cells selected to be positive for a specific combination of blood group antigens, or RBC stroma. The incubation temperature and times used in the adsorption process depend on the Ig class and the thermal range of the antibodies being adsorbed. In general, using a low antibody/cell ratio will increase adsorption efficiency.

Adsorption using allogeneic cells is helpful in separating multiple alloantibodies in a complex mixture (differential adsorption) or in eliminating the reactivity of an alloantibody to a high-frequency antigen. In patients with autoantibodies, adsorption with autologous RBCs, phenotypically matched cells, and rabbit erythrocyte stroma (REST) is often used to selectively remove warm and cold-reactive autoantibodies, respectively. Removal of autoantibodies is necessary to identify any potential underlying alloantibodies that the patient may have (see later in Investigation of Autoimmune Hemolytic Anemia section; Fig. 35-25).

TABLE 35-43
Special Antibody Identification Techniques: Red Cell Procedures

	Procedure	Application/effect
Enzyme treatment	Two-stage procedure (preferred): • Incubate test red cells with enzyme solution at 37° C. • Wash cells thoroughly to remove enzyme completely and retest cells with serum being investigated	• Eliminates some antibody reactivity by destroying corresponding antigen structures—MNS, Duffy, Ch/Rg; may be easier to pick out different specificities in a serum containing multiple antibodies • Enhances sensitization, agglutination, and/or hemolysis by other antibodies—Rh, Kidd, many IgM blood group antibodies; may allow for easier identification of weakly reactive antibodies
AET/DTT	Pretreat test red cells with AET or DTT; wash away reagent and retest cells with serum being investigated	Effectively creates Kell "null" cells for use in identifying alloantibodies in a mixture containing antibody to a high-frequency antigen in the Kell system
Elution	Remove and recover antibody from red cells by techniques such as glycine acid, organic solvents	Concentrates antibody that was coating red cells into a solution suitable for further identification procedures. Used in investigating positive DAT in cases of HDFN, HTR, autoimmune hemolytic anemia
Chloroquine diphosphate	• Washed packed red cells are incubated in a 1 : 4 ratio with chloroquine at room temperature. • Reagent is removed by multiple saline washes	Dissociates IgG from patient red cells with a positive DAT so that they may be typed with blood grouping reagents that require an indirect antiglobulin technique. Only anti-IgG should be used as the AHG reagent, as complement proteins are not dissociated with chloroquine
ZZAP	For adsorption purposes, aliquots of washed, packed red cells are incubated with ZZAP at 37° C. Cells are then washed with large volumes of saline to remove ZZAP. The combination of DTT and enzymes destroys coating of IgG autoantibodies	• Removal of autoantibodies from patient cells provides free antigen sites for adsorption of autoantibody from the serum • ZZAP also can be used to destroy Kell, Cartwright, Gerbich, and Dombrock system antigens
Dispersal of IgM-mediated autoagglutination	Incubate cell suspension with sulfhydryl reagents or wash cells multiple times with 37° C saline	Dissociation of cold autoagglutination permits valid ABO red cell typing and may aid in evaluating DAT results
Lectin typing	Reagents commonly derived from plant seeds are used to test for the presence or absence of a specific blood group antigen on the red cell membrane—used in place of an antibody reagent	Useful in typing for specific antigens such as A_1, H, and N and in classifying different polyagglutinable red cell conditions
Cell separation techniques	• Washed cells from the patient are centrifuged in microhematocrit tubes, and the top 5 mm containing the lightest cells is harvested • Differential agglutination may be performed based on known differences in antigen phenotype between donor and recipient	Useful in the following: • Phenotyping of autologous cells in recently transfused individuals • Evaluating whether a DHTR may be evolving in a patient with autoimmune hemolytic anemia • Estimating survival of transfused cells

AET, 2-Aminoethylisothiouronium bromide; *AHG*, antihuman globulin; *DAT*, direct antiglobulin test; *DHTR*, delayed hemolytic transfusion reaction; *DTT*, dithiothreitol; *HDFN*, hemolytic disease of the fetus and newborn; *HTR*, hemolytic transfusion reaction; *Ig*, immunoglobulin; *ZZAP*, combination of DTT and cysteine-activated papain.

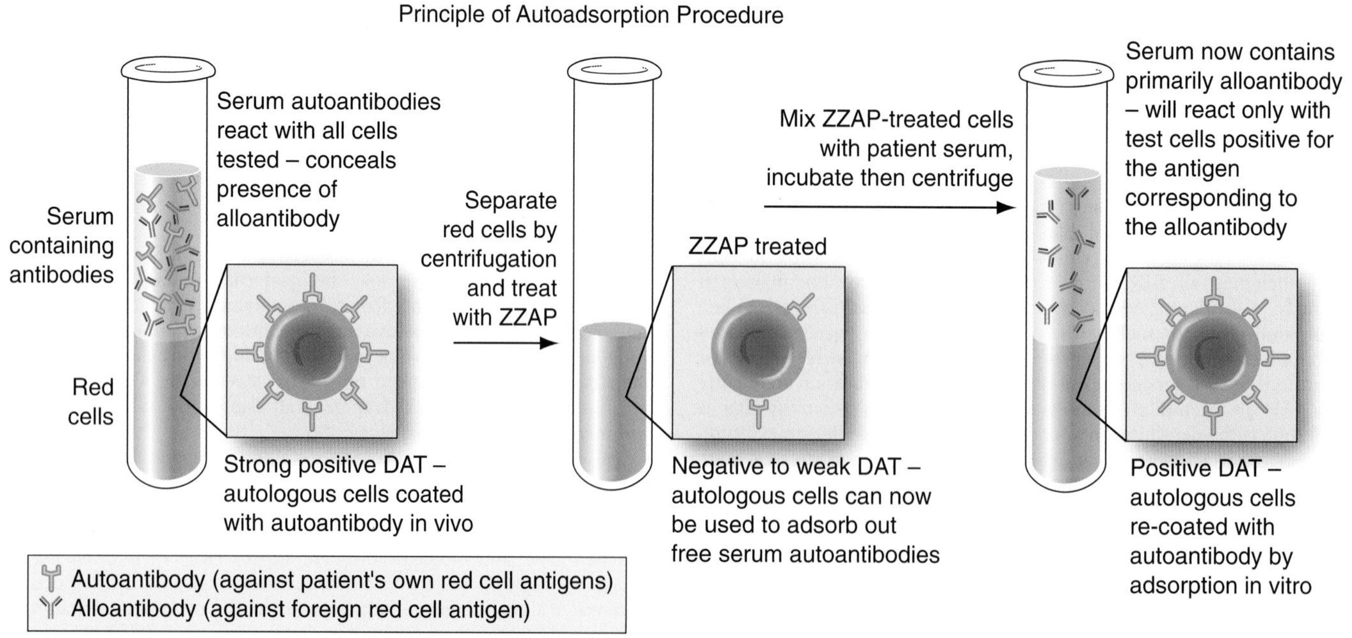

Figure 35-25 Autoadsorption procedure used to evaluate whether underlying alloantibodies are present in a patient with autoimmune hemolytic anemia.

TABLE 35-44
Sources of Soluble Antigens for Hemagglutination Inhibition

Soluble substance	Source
ABH	Secretor saliva
Le^a, Le^b	Secretor saliva
P1	Hydatid cyst fluid or pigeon eggs
Sd^a	Human or guinea pig urine
Ch, Rg	Plasma from Ch/Rg (+) individuals
I	Human milk

It is crucial to verify transfusion information before performing an adsorption because recently transfused individuals will have multiple red cell populations. In these patients, circulating donor cells could adsorb an alloantibody of interest. If the patient's phenotype is available, testing can be performed with allogeneic phenotype-matched red cells. If the phenotype is not known, three separate adsorptions with R_1R_1, R_2R_2, and rr cells can be performed and tested, and the results compared.

Thiol Reagents

Sulfhydryl compounds such as 2-ME or DTT cleave disulfide bonds and are frequently used to inactivate the agglutinating capacity of IgM antibodies by cleaving intersubunit disulfide bonds, as well as bonds linking IgM subunits to the J-chain (Klein, 2006), thus destroying the pentameric structure of the IgM molecule. These reagents are useful in investigating the presence of clinically significant IgG alloantibodies in a serum that contains broadly agglutinating IgM cold autoantibodies. They can also be used to dissociate autoagglutination caused by cold antibodies that may interfere with ABO/Rh typing and DAT testing. In prenatal studies, sulfhydryl reagents are frequently utilized to evaluate a serum containing an antibody such as anti-M that commonly has both IgM and IgG components. By destroying the agglutinating anti-M, the serum can be tested for IgG anti-M that is capable of crossing the placenta to cause a mild HDFN.

Serum Antibody Titration

Serum titration is a method used to semiquantitatively determine the amount of antibody present in a given serum/plasma. Serial twofold dilutions of serum are prepared and then tested with RBCs possessing the corresponding antigen. Each dilution is read for macroscopic agglutination, and the titer of the antibody is expressed as the reciprocal of the highest serum dilution that gives macroscopic agglutination. Titers are performed in obstetric patients, ABO-incompatible solid organ and bone marrow transplantation, and, occasionally, antibody identification studies.

In prenatal studies, clinically significant IgG alloantibodies capable of causing HDFN are titrated periodically in the maternal serum during pregnancy (Judd, 2005). An increasing titer usually indicates that fetal cells possess the corresponding antigen and are stimulating the mother to produce more antibody, thus providing valuable information to the physician regarding how the pregnancy should be managed. Because of the clinical importance of consistency in prenatal titer reporting, some laboratories require that the initial titer be performed by two technologists for agreement. If a discrepancy exists, a third technologist should perform the titration. The intial sample should be frozen for future studies. When the next titer request is submitted, the initial sample should be tested in parallel with the new sample.

Titers are also performed in the rare setting of major ABO-incompatible solid organ transplantation, which has risen in popularity with improvements in immunosuppressive therapy. ABO-incompatible heart transplants can be performed in children younger than 6–8 months owing to low-titer ABO antibodies in early infancy (West, 2001). ABO incompatible living donor kidney transplants, once unthinkable because of the risk of hyperacute rejection, have also been performed in adult patients. To prevent hyperacute rejection, intended recipients undergo an aggressive course of immunosuppression and therapeutic apheresis before and after transplant to reduce ABO titers below a critical threshold (Tobian, 2009). Similar to obstetric patients, these patients require a series of ABO titers to monitor treatment efficacy and screen against humoral rejection. Finally, ABO titers may be necessary in ABO-incompatible allogeneic bone marrow transplants. In contrast to peripheral blood stem cells, bone marrow contains significant quantities of red cells and can place the recipient at risk for a severe acute hemolytic transfusion reaction. ABO titers are performed before transplant to assess the risk of hemolysis and the need for pretransplant therapeutic apheresis (Cooling, 2007).

Antibody titration can also be used in the presumptive identification of HTLA antibodies. Most antibodies (excluding HTLA) that initially give weak (+/- or +/-[m]) reactions in IAT tests will seldom react at dilutions greater than 1 : 2. In contrast, HTLA antibodies characteristically give the same weak reactions at multiple serum dilutions, often reacting at dilutions equal to or greater than 1 : 64. If such an antibody is suspected, a titration is performed to demonstrate that the weakly reactive antibody is still reactive at a high dilution, thus allowing its classification as an HTLA. These antibodies are often directed against Ch/Rg, JMH, and Knops antigens.

It is important to note that both serologic technique and cell selection can affect titer results. For example, if the initial titer was tested against a cell with homozygous antigen expression, all subsequent titers should also be tested with a homozygous cell. Likewise, some laboratories use a tube technique without additives (saline), and others may use a LISS, tube, or gel method—all of which can yield significantly different end titers in parallel testing. Each laboratory should have a policy regarding appropriate cell selection and should perform titers using a technique approved by the laboratory director with proper validation. Titer results and their meaning should be communicated clearly to the physician. Any change in procedure or method *must* be communicated because this can affect titer results and have a direct impact on patient care.

TABLE 35-45
Effect on Antigen Expression/Antibody Reactivity by Enzyme* Treatment of Test Cells

Effect	Antigens
Destroyed	Fy^a, Fy^b M, N HTLA- Ch/Rg, JMH Pr Xg^a
Variable	Lu^a, Lu^b S, s Yt^a, Yt^b
Enhanced	ABH I/I Jk^a, Jk^b Le^a, Le^b P1 Rh U Di^a, Di^b
Usually unaffected	Kell

Data from Issitt (1998) and Roback (2008).
HTLA, High-titer, low-avidity; *JMH,* John Milton Hagen.
*Using ficin or papain.

Special Red Cell Procedures for Antibody Identification

Reagent or patient RBCs can be modified in various ways by the immunohematologist to abolish or enhance the reactivity of corresponding antibodies. Patient cells are also subjected to procedures designed to remove antibody that has bound in vivo, so that the antibody may be recovered and identified (eluate) and/or may provide RBCs for further testing.

Destruction of Red Cell Antigens

Available reagents for treating RBCs for the purpose of destroying certain blood group antigens include various proteolytic enzymes (e.g., papain, ficin), neuraminidase (removes sialic acid), ZZAP, AET, and DTT. In a serum containing multiple alloantibodies, selective pretreatment of RBCs with enzymes can destroy specific antigens, eliminating specific alloantibody reactivity. Enzymes are also thought to remove the water of hydration and decrease the ζ potential, allowing RBCs to more closely approach each other. As a result, they can enhance the reactivity of a weak, potentially significant antibody and facilitate its identification. Table 35-45 lists antibodies whose reactivity will be enhanced or eliminated by enzyme treatment of test RBCs. Note: AET and DTT can be used to create RBCs negative for all antigens of the Kell blood group system (except Kx); these reagents may also destroy certain antigens reacting with HTLA antibodies.

TABLE 35-46
Antibody Elution Techniques

Method	Principle*	Application
Heat	Addition of heat changes equilibrium constant of antigen–antibody reaction, and antibodies are released	• Recovery of ABO antibodies in cases of ABO HDFN • Gentle heat elution (at 45° C) may be useful for removing antibody from cells that is causing false-positive direct hemagglutination tests
Freeze-thaw	Damage to the red cell membrane by hemolysis alters complementary fit between antigen and antibody	Recovery of ABO antibodies in cases of ABO HDFN
Acid (e.g., digitonin acid, glycine acid/EDTA)	At an acid pH, antigen and antibody become negatively charged and repulse each other	• Good recovery of most IgG blood group antibodies (may be less sensitive for Kidd) • Glycine/EDTA also used to dissociate antibody but leaves red cells intact for phenotyping
Organic solvents (e.g., chloroform, xylene, ether)	Disrupts lipid bilayer of red cell membrane, altering complementary fit and/or reversing selected attractive forces between antigen and antibody	High-yield recovery of most IgG blood group antibodies

EDTA, Ethylenediaminetetraacetic acid; *HDFN,* hemolytic disease of the fetus and newborn; *Ig,* immunoglobulin.
*From Issitt (1998).

Antibody Elution

Elution is the process used to remove antibodies bound to RBCs, as indicated by a positive DAT. Elution is commonly used to concentrate and solubilize antibodies from RBCs for subsequent identification studies. The elution of an antibody with known blood group and/or drug specificity can be diagnostic in the evaluation of acute and delayed hemolytic transfusion reactions, HDFN, autoimmune hemolytic anemia, and immune hemolytic anemia induced by medication.

Elution may be accomplished by a variety of methods that alter or reverse the forces of attraction that hold the antigen and antibody together. Various methods involve adding heat, disrupting antigen structure by exposing the RBC membrane to freezing and thawing, using organic solvents, and altering the pH to dissociate RBC–antibody complexes. Freeze-thaw and heat elution techniques work well for removal of cold-reactive antibodies, whereas organic solvents and pH alteration are used to remove warm reactive IgG antibodies. Because organic solvents are carcinogenic, many laboratories have a commercially available acid elution kit.

All methods require numerous washes before elution to remove any serum containing unbound antibody. To ensure the complete removal of serum antibody, the saline from the last wash must be tested against appropriate cells to detect any residual unbound antibody. The last wash control should show an absence of antibody reactivity before the elution procedure is performed. Optimally, eluates should be tested on the same day they are prepared but may be stored at −20° C or lower if there is a delay in testing. Table 35-46 lists some of the common elution methods and their applications. For a more comprehensive listing and specific descriptions of elution procedures, see Mallory (1993) and Judd (2008).

Removal of Antibody From Red Cells to Facilitate Antigen Typing

Many antisera used for RBC antigen typing require the IAT technique. As a result, RBC samples with a positive DAT cannot be used for antigen typing because these cells are already coated with IgG antibody and will yield a false-positive result. Most elution methods that remove blood group antibodies from the surface of erythrocytes destroy the cells or the antigens. However, treatment of antibody-coated RBCs with chloroquine diphosphate dissociates antibody while leaving the antigens relatively intact (Edwards, 1982). Glycine/EDTA can also be used under carefully controlled conditions to dissociate IgG from RBCs, but overtreatment with this reagent can cause irreversible damage to the RBC membrane. After chloroquine or glycine treatment, RBCs can be antigen typed with AHG-reactive antisera. Note that glycine/EDTA-treatment destroys Kell protein. As a result, glycine/EDTA cells cannot be phenotyped for Kell system antigens.

Care should be exercised when interpreting antigen typing results with chloroquine-treated cells. Reports indicate that Rh antigens, and possibly other blood group antigens, can be weakened, resulting in false-negative reactions. Saline-reactive antisera, including monoclonal grouping reagents, should not be used with chloroquine-treated cells (Gamma Biologicals Inc., 2001). For chloroquine or glycine/EDTA, it is prudent to treat known antigen-positive cells in parallel as a control. Only monospecific anti-IgG should be used in the IAT because complement components are not dissociated by chloroquine from DAT-positive RBCs.

Red Blood Cell Typing With Lectin Reagents

Lectin typing reagents contain proteins that will recognize specific carbohydrates on the RBC membrane, causing direct hemagglutination. Lectin reagents are usually derived from plant seeds, but these receptor proteins are also found in some invertebrate animals and lower vertebrates. Because the potency of lectin reagents may vary with the preparation, each lot should be standardized before use. Although many lectins have been described, only a few have been found useful in blood banking (Bird, 1988). Sources for selected lectin reagents and their applications are listed in Table 35-47. Procedures for preparation of purified lectins may be found in *Judd's Methods in Hematology* (2008).

Separation of Autologous From Transfused Red Cells

In transfused patients, it may be necessary to separate autologous from transfused cells. Autologous RBCs for antigen typing may be necessary (1) in a transfused patient with multiple alloantibodies, (2) with a warm autoantibody and possible alloantibodies, or (3) with an antibody to a high-incidence antigen. Performing a DAT, and possibly even elution, on separated autologous and/or transfused cells can help determine whether a recently transfused individual with a warm autoimmune hemolytic anemia (WAIHA) is developing a delayed hemolytic transfusion reaction (DHTR) due to new alloantibodies. In rare cases, DAT testing on separated autologous RBCs may be required to differentiate a WAIHA from a DHTR involving a high-incidence antigen. In a final application, one could roughly estimate the proportion of surviving, transfused RBCs when a DHTR is suspected.

Two basic techniques for separating autologous from transfused RBCs are differential agglutination and density separation using centrifugation. In the first technique, antibodies are used to agglutinate only one population of cells, based on known antigenic differences between recipient and donor. Unagglutinated cells are physically removed from the agglutinates and are sequentially reacted with more antisera until no more agglutinates are formed. In the second technique, washed packed RBCs are centrifuged in multiple sealed microhematocrit tubes. Transfused cells are older, smaller, and denser than newly formed autologous cells (reticulocytes) and will spin toward the bottom of the tube. After centrifugation, the top 5 mm of each tube is cut away, and the cells are harvested from these small segments. These sections will contain the larger and lighter autologous cells. This method will be effective only if the patient is producing normal or high numbers of reticulocytes. When testing separated red cells, nonseparated cells should be tested in parallel as a control. The separated red cells should show clear positives and negatives, and the nonseparated cells should show mixed field agglutination.

TABLE 35-47

Lectins Useful in Immunohematologic Testing

Lectin	Activity inhibited by	Serologic specificity	Application
Ulex europaeus	α-L-fucose	Anti-H	Secretor status testing, classification of weak A subgroups, investigation of possible Bombay phenotype
Vicia graminea	O-linked *N* blood group tetrasaccharides (galactose [β1,3] *N*-acetyl-galactosamine)	Anti-N	Red cell antigen typing
Griffonia simplicifolia I*	α-D-galactose	Anti-B, Tn	• Red cell antigen typing • Investigation of acquired B/polyagglutination
Dolichos biflorus	Terminal α-*N*-acetyl-D-galactosamine	Anti-A, Tn, Cad	Classification of A subgroups, investigation of polyagglutination
Griffonia simplicifolia II*	α- or β-*N*-acetyl-D-glucosamine	Anti-Tk	Confirmation of Tk polyagglutination
Helix pomatia	α-*N*-acetyl-D-galactosamine	Anti-A, Tn, Cad	Gives distinctive mixed-field reaction with VA polyagglutination
Arachis hypogaea	β-D-galactose	Anti-T, Tk, Th, Tx	Investigation of polyagglutination
Glycine soja (max)	α-*N*-acetyl-D-galactosamine	Anti-T, Tn	
Leonurus cardiaca	α-*N*-acetyl-D-galactosamine	Anti-Cad specific at appropriate dilution	
Salvia sclerea	α-*N*-acetyl-D-galactosamine	Anti-Tn specific	
Salvia horminum	α-*N*-acetyl-D-galactosamine	Anti-Tn, Cad (separable)	
Vicia cretia	Galactose (β1,3) *N*-acetyl-galactosamine	Anti-T, Th	

*Formerly known as *Bandeiraea simplicifolia* I and II.

Hypotonic cell lysis is a third method that is available for harvesting autologous red cells in patients with sickle cell disease. The method is based on the resistance of Hg S red cells to hypotonic saline. The patient sample is repeatedly washed with 0.3% hypotonic saline to lyse normal donor red cells until gross hemolysis is no longer present. The cells are then washed and resuspended in 0.9% saline for antigen typing. Because sickle cell patients are regularly transfused, this technique is useful for facilities that provide antigen-matched red cells for their sickle cell patients.

Molecular Typing

Because most common blood group antigens are the consequence of SNPs, several commercial and home-brew assays have been developed to genotype donors and patients. The ability to genotype individuals for blood group antigens is extremely useful for multitransfused patients in whom standard serologic typing cannot be performed as a result of circulating donor red cells. Several transfusion services routinely genotype all hemoglobinopathy patients (e.g., sickle cell anemia, β-thalassemia) who have long-term transfusion needs and require antigen-negative units. Genotyping is also useful in patients with multiple alloantibodies or autoantibodies, in whom it can be difficult to exclude an antibody to a high-incidence antigen because of the lack of commercial reagents (e.g., Dombrock). Likewise, serologic phenotyping often cannot be performed in patients with a positive DAT because many reagents require the addition of anti-IgG for typing. Genotyping is commonly used in prenatal testing to identify a fetus at risk for HDFN. Fetal genotyping can often be performed with a maternal blood sample, offering a significant safety advantage over serologic testing, which requires fetal blood sampling (Finning, 2007). Finally, large-scale genotyping of donors has the potential to increase the availability of antigen-negative units for patients with clinically significant alloantibodies (Montpetit, 2006).

Several methods have been developed for red cell and platelet genotyping, including restriction fragment length polymorphism, allele-specific PCR, real-time PCR, direct sequencing, and microarray technology (see Chapters 65, 66, and 67). High-throughput screening methods, such as microarray, are amenable to semiautomated processes and permit extended typing for high- and low-incidence antigens. It is important to stress that genotype does not always reflect red cell phenotype because most genotyping methods focus on known common polymorphisms. Unknown polymorphisms may alter protein or gene expression not detected by the primers used. A well-known example is Fy(a–b–) phenotype in blacks, who genotype as FY*B but lack Fy expression on red cells because of a promoter mutation. Likewise, many partial RhD and RhCE phenotypes can lead to discrepancies between phenotype and genotype (see Rh section).

INVESTIGATION OF AUTOIMMUNE HEMOLYTIC ANEMIA

Autoantibodies, in general, are produced by an individual's own immune system against self or an antigen that is present in that same individual. Although produced against self-antigens, these antibodies typically react with the same antigen found in other normal individuals. If the antibodies produced are against blood cell constituents, the pathologic result could be hemolytic anemia, thrombocytopenia, or leukopenia. In many cases, these autoantibodies cause no demonstrable clinical symptoms.

The DAT is integral to the diagnosis of autoimmune hemolytic anemia (AIHA) because it can confirm the presence of antibody that has attached to the patient's own red cells in vivo. The DAT can help differentiate AIHA from congenital anemias caused by abnormalities in RBC cytoskeleton, enzymes, or Hg. The DAT may be positive owing to IgG and/or complement components, depending on the class or subclass of autoantibody involved. A positive DAT by itself, however, does not mean that an individual has AIHA. Approximately 8% of hospitalized patients have a positive DAT without any signs of hemolysis (Petz, 1993). In patients with suspected AIHA, the antibody screen may also be positive because of free autoantibody in the serum.

Autoantibodies are categorized as cold (usually IgM) or warm (usually IgG), based on the temperature of in vitro reactivity in the IAT. In some cases, patients may have mixed-type AIHA with both cold and warm reactive autoantibodies. The causative antibodies of these categories of anemias will be described here; additional information regarding the origin and pathophysiology of AIHA is provided in Chapter 32.

Warm Autoimmune Hemolytic Anemia

Individuals with warm reactive autoantibodies account for approximately 70%–80% of cases of AIHA, having an overall incidence of about 1 in 50,000 to 1 in 80,000 (Issitt, 1998). WAIHA may be classified as primary or idiopathic (of unknown origin), or as secondary. Secondary WAIHA is often observed in autoimmune diseases (frequently systemic lupus erythematosus), in lymphoproliferative disorders, and following viral infections. With the advent of improved diagnostic procedures, the percentage of WAIHA classified as idiopathic has dropped to about 30% of cases (Issitt, 1998). Patients with warm autoantibodies and a positive DAT will not all present with symptomatic anemia but may exist in a chronic compensated state for some time before progressing to overt clinical anemia.

Serologic Characteristics

Autoantibodies in WAIHA are usually IgG and polyclonal in nature, showing optimal in vitro reactivity at 37° C. A vast majority of warm autoantibodies present in serum and/or recovered in eluates from patients' RBCs can be demonstrated only by the IAT technique. The DAT will be positive in approximately 80% of cases. The DAT profiles in several large studies show that 40%–50% are due to IgG only, 45%–60% are caused by IgG and complement, and 0–15% are the result of complement only (Issitt, 1998). In those instances where the DAT is negative, the use of more sensitive techniques, such as radioisotope or enzyme-labeled DAT, can demonstrate low levels of IgG or, less frequently, IgM and IgA on red cells (Englefriet, 1992).

Ig subclass studies in WAIHA indicate that causative antibodies are predominantly IgG1 and/or IgG3. Despite the ability of these subclasses to activate complement, immune destruction of the patient's autologous cells occurs largely through the spleen and liver via extravascular pathways. Patients whose RBCs are coated with IgG3 antibodies are more likely to show overt anemia, apparently because of the greater capacity of IgG3 for binding to Fc receptors on macrophages (Englefriet, 1992). A more recent study shows that the presence of multiple IgG subclasses, rather than a single subclass, has a synergistic effect on the severity of hemolysis (Fabijanska-Mitek, 1997).

In general, warm autoantibodies display a broad specificity, reacting with all normal RBCs. Many broadly reactive antibodies can show Rh specificity, as evidenced by weak or absent reactivity to Rh_{null} red cells. On occasion, autoantibodies will demonstrate Rh pseudospecificity such as anti-e (most frequently), anti-c, and anti-E. Studies with recombinant cell lines show that in most instances, these antibodies are broadly reacting with the RhCE, RhD, and Band 3 proteins, regardless of Rh phenotype (Iwamoto, 2001). Notable exceptions to the latter are African Americans with partial RhCE proteins, who serologically type as c- and/or e-positive, but can produce true alloanti-c and alloanti-e after immune stimulation (see Rh section). Autoantibodies with apparent specificity for Kell, Kidd, MNSs, ABO, Vel, and LW antigens have also been reported. Relatively few individuals with WAIHA will show a single simple specificity (Issitt, 1998).

Serologic Testing Beyond the DAT

Transfusion is usually avoided for as long as possible in patients with WAIHA. If transfusion is necessary, it is important to characterize the autoantibody and exclude the presence of RBC alloantibodies (Eder, 2005). Typical investigation strategies should always include adsorption of the serum, followed by antibody detection and identification on the adsorbed serum. Subsequent testing can also be performed on eluted antibody, although it seldom yields further useful information *unless* the serum is nonreactive.

Autoadsorption. Because a strong, broadly reactive serum autoantibody can mask the presence of significant alloantibodies, adsorption studies should be performed in these patients. Autoadsorption using autologous cells can be performed on patients who have not been recently transfused (within the last 3 months). For patients who have a strong positive DAT, autologous cells should be treated with ZZAP (Branch, 1982) before adsorption. ZZAP contains DTT, which reduces disulfide bonds in the IgG autoantibodies coating the RBCs. This destabilizes the Ig structure, rendering the autoantibodies susceptible to digestion by cysteine-activated papain, the second component of ZZAP. By stripping bound autoantibody from cells, ZZAP treatment increases the adsorptive capacity of autologous RBCs (see Fig. 35-25). If the serum contains a high concentration of autoantibody, multiple, sequential autoadsorptions may be necessary to remove all autoantibody activity. If available in sufficient quantity, autoadsorbed serum may be used to perform crossmatching, particularly if antibody detection studies reveal the presence of underlying alloantibodies.

If the patient has had recent RBC transfusions, and the patient's red cell phenotype is known, adsorption may be performed using allogeneic cells of the same phenotype as the patient. Alternatively, if the patient's RBC phenotype is unknown, differential adsorptions may be performed on three separate aliquots of the patient's serum with different red cell samples of R_1, R_2, and rr phenotypes. One of the red cell samples should lack Jk^a and one should lack Jk^b (Roback, 2008). ZZAP treatment of the adsorbing cells will effectively destroy Fy^a, Fy^b, all Kell system antigens, and the M, N, S, and s antigens, thereby conferring on the adsorbing cell samples the capacity to remove autoantibody activity while preserving potential alloantibodies in the serum. The different aliquots of serum are then tested against cells of known phenotype to detect and/or identify alloantibody specificity.

Elution. In most cases of WAIHA, an eluate of the patient's cells will demonstrate the same broadly reactive antibody seen in serum. In the rare instances where the serum is only weakly reactive or negative, an eluate may concentrate the warm autoantibody to facilitate identification and evaluation of its spectrum of reactivity. If the eluate is nonreactive with normal reagent RBCs, the presence of drug-induced autoantibodies should be investigated (see later).

Cold Autoimmune Hemolytic Anemia

Cold autoantibodies may be detected in the serum of many normal individuals if tested under the right conditions. However, most of these antibodies are benign cold agglutinins that show optimal reactivity at 4° C and little or no reactivity at 37° C. Cold agglutinins are often a nuisance that can interfere with ABO/Rh typing, antibody detection, and crossmatching when polyspecific AHG is used. Although usually ignored as clinically insignificant, cold agglutinins may become pathologic by virtue of expanded thermal amplitude and a significant increase in titer, frequently in association with certain disease states. DAT, serum titration, and characterization of thermal amplitude are the most important serologic tests in evaluating a possible diagnosis of CAIHA. Table 35-48 outlines some of the serologic differentiating characteristics of various cold agglutinating autoantibodies, both pathologic and benign.

Cold Agglutinin Disease

Cold agglutinin disease (CAD) accounts for about 20% of total cases of AIHA (Issitt, 1998). As with WAIHA, CAD may be idiopathic or secondary following infection or malignancy. Anti-I is the most frequent autoantibody in idiopathic CAD and *M. pneumoniae* infections. In contrast to the anti-I cold agglutinins found in normal sera (usually less than 1:64 when tested at 4° C), anti-I in CAD is often of very high titer, with ranges of 1:10,000 to 1:1,000,000 (Cooling, 2010). The antibody also has expanded thermal amplitude, reacting with RBCs at temperatures in the range of 30°–34° C in vitro, especially in tests with albumin-suspended RBCs (Issitt, 1998). The DAT is typically positive with polyspecific and anti-C3 reagents.

In vivo hemolysis is the result of binding of antibody to a patient's RBCs in the peripheral vessels of the extremities, which are cooler (32° C and lower). As the cells recirculate to the body core and warm to 37° C, complement is activated and cells are destroyed. Hemolysis of cells may occur intravascularly but occurs more commonly via extravascular (C3b) pathways by macrophages in the reticuloendothelial system. Hemolysis may be chronic or episodic, depending on the thermal range of the antibody, and may be triggered by exposure to cold temperatures.

Because anti-I reacts broadly with virtually all adult RBCs, the antibody can cause great difficulty in compatibility testing. As with warm autoantibodies, one of the primary concerns is to detect and identify any potential underlying IgG alloantibodies. Techniques to circumvent the autoanti-I in serum testing may include prewarming, cold autoadsorption, adsorption with REST, or treatment of the serum with sulfhydryl reagents such as DTT or 2-ME (see Special Antibody Identification Techniques section).

Anti-i and anti-Pr are two additional specificities associated with CAD. Anti-i can be observed in patients with infectious mononucleosis and certain lymphoproliferative disorders. Up to 10%–20% of patients with infectious mononucleosis will have elevated cold agglutinin titers; however, few will actually develop clinical hemolysis (Eder, 2005; Cooling, 2010). Anti-i is usually an IgM, reacting more strongly with cord cells than with adult cells. Distinguishing anti-i from anti-I may require titrating patient sera with group O adult and cord red cells at 4° C, 24° C, and 37° C (Roback, 2008).

Anti-Pr specificities may initially react similarly to anti-I, but may be differentiated by equally strong reactions with cord and adult RBCs (see Table 35-48). In addition, anti-Pr is nonreactive with enzyme-treated red cells, whereas anti-I is enhanced by enzyme treatment. Anti-Pr in patients with CAD is usually monoclonal and may be IgG, IgM, or IgA (Issitt, 1998).

Paroxysmal Cold Hemoglobinuria

PCH is an autoimmune hemolytic syndrome most often seen in children following infection by mumps, chickenpox, measles, and other viruses. Historically, PCH was also seen in syphilitic patients. It can present suddenly with severe hemolysis with an initial Hg of 7 g/dL or lower. In addition to laboratory findings of intravascular hemolysis, PCH patients may have erythrophagocytosis on peripheral blood smear. The latter is highly unusual and should trigger an investigation for possible PCH (Eder, 2005).

TABLE 35-48
Differentiating Characteristics of Cold Red Cell Autoagglutinins

Antibody specificity	Clinical significance	IAT antibody screen*	Ig class	RELATIVE REACTION STRENGTHS WITH SELECTED RED CELLS AT ROOM TEMPERATURE†				
				O adult	O cord	A_1 adult	A_2 adult	Autologous
I	Acute CAD associated with *Mycoplasma pneumoniae* with antibody titers >1000 at 4° C	Pos	IgM	3+	w+	3+	3+	3+
i	Acute CAD associated with mononucleosis	Pos	IgM	w+	3+	w+	w+	Weaker than O cord
Pr	Rare cause of CAD‡	Pos	Reported cases of IgM, IgA, IgG	3+	3+	3+	3+	3+
P	PCH associated with certain viral infections in children	Neg	IgG§	Negative in routine agglutination tests; autoanti-P is a biphasic hemolysin (Donath-Landsteiner antibody)				
H	Benign except as alloantibody in Bombay phenotype	Weak to neg	IgM	3+	3+	1+	2+	0 to w+
IH	Benign	Weak to neg	IgM	3+	1+	1+	2+	0 to w+

CAD, Cold agglutinin disease; *Ig,* immunoglobulin; *Neg,* negative; *PCH,* paroxysmal cold hemoglobinuria; *Pos,* positive.
*Antigen expression: O adult (I+i– H+s); O cord (I–i+ H+s); A_1 (I+i– H+w); A_2 (I+i– H+).
†Reagent cells showing agglutination in 37° C phase may be much weaker after conversion to indirect antiglobulin test (IAT).
‡May be differentiated from anti-I by enzymes or increasing pH; anti-Pr reactivity is decreased by both techniques.
§Autoanti-P is the only pathologic cold autoantibody known to be routinely of the IgG class to IAT.

Autoanti-P, also known as the Donath-Landsteiner (DL) antibody, is the most common causative antibody in PCH. It is an IgG, biphasic autohemolysin capable of binding to RBCs at cold temperatures and causing intravascular hemolysis of those cells at body temperature (see Table 35-48). This characteristic can be demonstrated in vitro by the diagnostic DL procedure to aid in the confirmation of PCH. In this test, three sets of tubes containing patient serum and group O cells are incubated—one at 4° C followed by 37° C, one only at 4° C, and one only at 37° C. If the first set shows hemolysis, but the other two do not, this indicates the presence of the biphasic hemolysin characteristic of PCH. The DL test requires that a fresh blood sample be used to ensure that an adequate supply of complement is available, because complement is relatively unstable and deteriorates during storage. The sample should be drawn and immediately stored at 37° C until clot formation. It is also important not to draw the blood into an anticoagulant such as EDTA because chelation of calcium ions will prevent complement activation and thus in vitro hemolysis.

Because the autoantibody in PCH rarely reacts above 4° C in vitro, routine antibody detection tests are usually negative, and crossmatches are compatible. Patient RBCs sensitized by the DL antibody will most commonly give a positive DAT owing to C3 only. In addition, the DAT is positive only during or immediately after an episode of hemolysis (Eder, 2005). Because the antibody dissociates easily from RBCs during washing, the DAT is usually negative with anti-IgG. IgG may be detected, however, if the cells are washed with cold saline and tested with cold anti-IgG reagent (Roback, 2008).

Because the antibody is biphasic, many clinicians recommend keeping the patient warm and utilizing a blood warmer for transfusion. Although PCH is due to an autoanti-P, it is not necessary to transfuse the patient with rare, P-negative red cells. Most patients will have an acceptable transfusion response with routine allogeneic red cells (Eder, 2005).

Mixed-Type AIHA

A "mixed" AIHA occurs in <10% of patients and is characterized by the presence of warm and cold autoantibodies (Eder, 2005). The DAT is usually positive with both C3 and IgG, and the patient's serum will react in all phases of testing (at room temperature and at 37° C) in the IAT. The cold-reactive antibody is typically anti-I or anti-i, and the warm-reactive antibody is typically a 37° C reactive IgG autoantibody. To adsorb autoantibody in a mixed AIHA, the sample is sequentially adsorbed at 37° C to adsorb warm-reactive autoantibody, followed by incubation in an ice bath for 30 minutes to adsorb cold-reactive antibody. Clinically, mixed AIHA usually is similar to WAIHA, although some patients may have symptoms of both WAIHA and CAD.

Positive Direct Antiglobulin Tests and Hemolytic Anemia Induced by Medication

At this time, more than 130 drugs have been implicated in drug-induced hemolytic anemia, with an incidence of 1 in 1–2 million individuals (Salama, 2009). An even larger number of therapeutic drugs can be associated with a positive DAT (Table 35-49). It is also well documented that a positive DAT may be produced in patients receiving high-dose intravenous gammaglobulin therapy owing to passively acquired specific blood group antibodies, as well as nonspecific binding to RBCs by IgG dimers and aggregates in the gammaglobulin preparation (Knezevic-Maramica, 2003). Several theories regarding the immunologic process underlying drug-induced antibodies have been put forth, many of which remain unproven. Moreover, some drugs appear to work by more than one mechanism, further complicating the picture. An example of the latter is the group of cephalosporins, which now account for 93% of drug-induced hemolysis (Garratty, 2004).

Historically, drug-induced hemolytic anemia has been subclassified into four types, based on its serologic characteristics. Drug-independent antibodies do not require the addition of drug into the test system for detection, even though the drug is responsible for inducing hemolytic anemia. Drug-dependent antibodies, on the other hand, require the presence of the drug for serologic reactivity. Drug-dependent antibodies can be subclassified into two types, depending on whether antibody reactivity requires drug-coated red cells or simply the presence of drug in serum. Antibody reactivity against drug-coated red cells appears to be directed against the drug itself. Alternatively, reactivity observed after concurrent incubation of red cells, serum, and free drug is believed to reflect immune complex formation between drug and "anti-drug" antibody. Finally, nonimmunologic protein adsorption proposes that a change in the red cell membrane causes immune globulins and other plasma proteins to be adsorbed nonspecifically to the red cell membrane.

A unifying model has been suggested that may be applicable to many different drugs thought to be operating via the mechanisms mentioned previously (Garratty, 2004). The hypothesis suggests that the immune process is initiated by a primary interaction between RBCs and the drug or its metabolites, even though the drug may be only loosely bound to RBCs in vivo. This provides the composite determinants (or neoantigen) necessary for production of drug-dependent antibodies, as in the drug adsorption and immune complex mechanisms, or of drug-independent autoantibodies that recognize subtle alterations in the RBC membrane.

TABLE 35-49
Selected Drugs Associated With a Positive DAT and/or Hemolysis Due to Drug-Induced Autoantibodies

Reported mechanism	Drug
Drug-independent autoantibody induction	Cladribine, fludarabine, levodopa, mefenamic acid, methyldopa, procainamide
Drug dependent (reactivity with drug-coated cells)	Aminopyrine, amoxicillin, carbromal, cefamandole, cefazolin, cephalexin, erythromycin, insulin, nafcillin, penicillin, tetracycline, tolbutamide
Drug dependent (reactivity with uncoated cells)	Acetaminophen, amphotericin B, antazoline, butizide, ceftriaxone, chlorpropamide, diethylstilbestrol, etodolac, 9-hydroxy-methyl-ellipticinium, naproxen, phenacetin, probenecid, propyphenazone, quinine, sodium pentothal, stibophen, sulfamethoxazole, sulfasalazine, trimethoprim
Nonimmunologic protein adsorption	Clavulanate potassium, diglycoaldehyde, sulbactam sodium, suramin, tazobactam sodium
Combination mechanisms	Ampicillin, carbimazole, carboplatin, cefixime, cefotaxime, cefotetan, cefoxitin, ceftazidime, ceftizoxime, cephalothin, chlorinated hydrocarbons, chlorpromazine, cisplatin, cyanidanol, diclofenac, dipyrone, fenoprofen, fluorescein, hydrochlorothiazide, isoniazid, mefloquine, methotrexate, nomifensine, oxaliplatin, piperacillin, quinidine, ranitidine, rifampicin, streptomycin, sulindac, suprofen, teicoplanin, teniposide, ticarcillin, tolmetin, triamterene, zomepirac

Data from Roback J, editor. Technical manual. 16th ed. Bethesda, Md: American Association of Blood Banks; 2008.
DAT, Direct antiglobulin test.

Stimulation of Red Cell Autoantibody Production

Drug-Independent Autoantibodies. About 20% of hypertensive patients who receive methyldopa (Aldomet) for longer than 3–6 months will eventually develop a positive DAT, but only 0.8% will develop a hemolytic anemia (Petz, 1993). The DAT gradually becomes negative after stopping methyldopa treatment, although it may take months to longer than 2 years. Serologically, autoantibodies eluted from RBCs, or free in the serum, are indistinguishable from autoantibodies found in patients with WAIHA. The antibodies are usually of the IgG class, with both κ and λ light chains, and many show Rh specificity. The antibody reactivity is independent of the drug being added to the laboratory test system. Drug-independent antibodies may be found alone as warm autoantibodies (methyldopa, procainamide, and fludarabine) or in combination with drug-dependent antibodies (cefotetan). About 10% of patients with Parkinson's disease receiving L-dopa, a closely related drug, develop RBC autoantibodies, but these rarely result in overt hemolysis (Petz, 1993).

Drug-Dependent Autoantibodies (Two Types)

Reactivity With Drug-Coated Cells. About 3% of patients receiving large doses of penicillin intravenously (>10 × 10^6 IU/day) develop a positive DAT, although only a few of these patients will have hemolytic anemia (Salama, 2009). Breakdown products of benzyl penicillin exhibit a high binding affinity for the RBC membrane, which results in the formation of haptenic benzylpenicilloyl determinants. Certain patients can form high-titered antibodies against penicillin metabolites and, to a lesser extent, red cell membrane components. The resulting antibody–drug–RBC complex yields a positive DAT with IgG and sometimes with anti-C3. The DAT becomes negative again within days to several weeks after discontinuing penicillin. Both the patient's serum and eluates prepared from the patient's RBCs usually react only with penicillin-coated RBCs in in vitro testing.

Penicillin antibodies may consist of IgM or IgG. IgM antibodies are very common if a sensitive method is used for detection. Those antibodies associated with immune hemolytic anemia are usually of IgG isotype (Salama, 2009). Hemolysis occurs usually through extravascular destruction mediated by cells of the RE system, although rare cases of complement-mediated intravascular hemolysis have been reported. Several cases of acquired hemolytic anemia have also been reported in association with cephalosporins through a mechanism similar to that of penicillin (Garratty, 2004; Salama, 2009).

Reactivity With Uncoated Cells. A wide variety of drugs may cause hemolytic anemia via the so-called immune complex mechanism (see Table 35-49). In the unifying concept, these drugs loosely bind to the RBC membrane with subsequent formation of antibodies reacting with both drug and membrane components. The cell–drug–antibody complex then may stimulate activation of the complement cascade. Drugs acting by this mechanism most often are associated with episodes of acute intravascular hemolysis with hemoglobinemia and hemoglobinuria that may prove fatal (Petz, 1993). The DAT in these cases is usually positive with anti-C3d only. The antibodies implicated may be IgM or IgG (Roback, 2008). They can be detected only in test systems where serum/eluate, test cells, and free drug are all present simultaneously. Although the mechanism leading to antibody production may be similar to that of so-called drug adsorption, the drugs in this category are classified separately primarily by the DAT result (C3d+) and characteristic severe intravascular hemolysis.

Nonimmunologic Adsorption of Serum Proteins. Patients taking high-dose cephalothin (6–14g/day) for prolonged periods have been reported to develop a positive DAT, with a frequency ranging widely from 3%–81% (Garratty, 2004). Hemolysis is rarely, if ever, associated with the phenomenon (Roback, 2008). It was subsequently shown that RBCs exposed to cephalothin in vitro are able to nonspecifically adsorb plasma and serum proteins (albumin, Igs, complement). In the case of some cephalosporins, a decrease in CD55 and CD58 can be documented (Garratty, 2004). These proteins can be detected by polyspecific AHG sera in the DAT. It has been hypothesized that adsorption occurs because of a change in erythrocyte membrane properties induced by cephalothin and other drugs.

SELECTED REFERENCES

Daniels G. Human blood groups. 2nd ed. Oxford: Blackwell Science; 2002.
Summarizes each blood group system, including serology, biochemistry, and molecular basis for the major blood group antigen systems.

Friedman BA, Oberman HA, Chadwick AR, et al. The maximum surgical blood order schedule and surgical blood use in the United States. Transfusion 1976;16:380–7.
The historical standard for the design, use, and implementation of the MSBOS for blood ordering.

Issitt PD, Anstee DJ. Applied blood group serology. 4th ed. Durham, N.C.: Montgomery Scientific Publications; 1998.
A comprehensive text detailing the history, serology, disease associations, and possible biological roles of blood group antigens and antibodies.

Price T (Committee Chair). Standards for blood banks and transfusion services. 26th ed. Bethesda, Md.: American Association of Blood Banks; 2009.
Regulatory standards governing the collection, testing, processing, dispensing, transfusion, and tracking of blood components.

Reid RE, Lomas-Francis C. The blood group antigen facts book. 2nd ed. San Diego: Academic Press; 2004.
A succinct listing of the required serologic and molecular testing for each blood group antibody and antigen.

Roback J, editor. Technical manual. 16th ed. Bethesda, Md.: American Association of Blood Banks; 2008.
Techniques and policies for the collection, processing, testing, and dispensing of blood components.

REFERENCES

Access the complete reference list online at http://www.expertconsult.com

CHAPTER 36

TRANSFUSION MEDICINE

Robertson D. Davenport, Paul D. Mintz

PART 4

KEY POINTS

- Criteria for blood donor eligibility are established by the U.S. Food and Drug Administration to minimize risks to both the donor and the transfusion recipient.
- Blood components (red blood cells, platelet concentrates, fresh frozen plasma, cryoprecipitate) are manufactured and stored in a manner to minimize functional loss of desired constituents.
- Leukocyte reduction of blood components reduces alloimmunization to human leukocyte antigens, cytomegalovirus transmission, and febrile reactions. Irradiation of blood components can prevent graft-versus-host disease.
- Accurate identification of the pretransfusion blood sample and the intended recipient is the most important step in preventing acute hemolytic transfusion reactions.
- Restrictive red cell transfusion (hemoglobin target 7–9 g/dL) is associated with improved survival in critically ill patients younger than 55 years old or with lower Acute Physiology and Chronic Health Evaluation II scores.
- Platelet transfusion is generally indicated for microvascular bleeding, platelet count <10,000/µL, or platelet count <50,000/µL before an invasive procedure.
- Failure to respond to platelet transfusion may be due to immune causes (human leukocyte antigens or platelet-specific antibodies), nonimmune clinical causes (bleeding, splenomegaly, disseminated intravascular coagulation, medications), or product-specific causes (ABO incompatibility, age of component).
- Plasma transfusion is generally indicated for coagulation factor deficiency, disseminated intravascular coagulation, dilutional coagulopathy, urgent warfarin reversal, and thrombotic thrombocytopenic purpura.
- Potentially severe adverse effects of transfusion include hemolytic reactions, allergic reactions, transfusion-related acute lung injury, bacterial contamination, and graft-versus-host disease.
- Current risks of transfusion-transmitted human immunodeficiency virus or hepatitis are very low, but the risks of other transfusion-transmitted diseases (cytomegalovirus, parvovirus B-19) may be significant in some populations.

BACKGROUND

Transfusion medicine is a multidisciplinary specialty encompassing all aspects of blood donation, blood component preparation, blood cell serology, and blood transfusion therapy. The term **blood banking** has largely been superseded by transfusion medicine to emphasize the importance of patient care and clinical outcomes.

Operationally, transfusion medicine is divided between blood centers and transfusion services. Blood centers recruit and collect blood from donors and manufacture and distribute blood components. Transfusion services perform pretransfusion compatibility testing, select and issue blood components for patients, and provide medical support for blood transfusion. Most hospital transfusion services do not collect their own blood, but rather rely on regional blood centers.

Blood centers and transfusion services (collectively known as blood establishments) are regulated by the FDA. All blood establishments must be registered with the FDA, and blood centers that manufacture blood components must be licensed. Criteria for the acceptability of blood donors, performance of pretransfusion testing, manufacture of blood components, donor infectious disease testing, and evaluation and reporting of adverse events associated with transfusion are all defined by the FDA. Blood establishments are subject to periodic unannounced inspections by the FDA. Compliance with federal regulations is an essential aspect of

TABLE 36-1
Requirements of Allogeneic Donor Qualification

Category	Criteria
Age	At least 17 years
Whole blood volume collected	Maximum of 10.5 mL/kg
Donation interval	8 weeks after whole blood donation 16 weeks after two-unit red cell collection 4 weeks after infrequent apheresis At least 2 days after plasma, platelet, or leukocyte apheresis
Blood pressure	≤180 mm Hg systolic ≤100 mm Hg diastolic
Pulse	50–100 beats per minute, without pathologic irregularities <50 acceptable if an otherwise healthy athlete
Temperature	≤37.5° C orally
Hemoglobin/hematocrit	≥12.5 g/dL/0.38
Drug therapy	Finasteride, isotretinoin—defer 1 month after last dose Dutasteride—defer 6 months after last dose Acitretin—defer 3 years after last dose Etretinate—defer indefinitely Bovine insulin manufactured in the United Kingdom—defer indefinitely Ingestion of medications that irreversibly inhibit platelet function (aspirin) within 36 hours of donation precludes use of donor as sole source of platelets
General medical history	Free of major organ disease, cancer, abnormal bleeding tendency Family history of CJD or recipient of dura mater or human pituitary growth hormone—defer indefinitely
Pregnancy	Defer for 6 weeks
Recipient of blood transfusion or tissue transplant	Defer for 12 months
Vaccinations and immunizations	Recipient of toxoid, synthetic or killed viral, bacterial, or other vaccine—no deferral Recipient of life attenuated viral or bacterial vaccine—2- or 4-week deferral Smallpox vaccine—refer to current FDA guidance Other vaccines including unlicensed vaccines—12-month deferral
Infectious diseases—indefinite deferral	Viral hepatitis after 11th birthday Positive test for hepatitis B surface antigen Repeat reactive test for anti-HBc on more than one occasion Clinical or laboratory evidence of HCV, HTLV, or HIV infection by current FDA regulations Previous donation associated with hepatitis, HIV, or HTLV transmission Behavioral risk factors for HIV infection according to current FDA guidance History of babesiosis or Chagas' disease Stigma of parenteral drug use Injection of nonprescription drugs Risk of vCJD according to current FDA guidelines
Infectious diseases—12-month deferral	Mucous membrane exposure to blood Nonsterile skin or needle penetration Sexual contact with an individual with a confirmed positive test for hepatitis B surface antigen Sexual contact with an individual with viral hepatitis Sexual contact with an individual with HIV infection or at higher risk for HIV infection Incarceration in a correctional institution for longer than 72 consecutive hours History of syphilis or gonorrhea
West Nile virus	Defer according to current FDA guidance
Malaria	Confirmed diagnosis—defer for 3 years after becoming asymptomatic Travel to or residence in an endemic area as defined by the CDC—defer according to FDA guidance

CDC, Centers for Disease Control and Prevention; *CJD,* Creutzfeldt-Jakob disease; *FDA,* U.S. Food and Drug Administration; *HCV,* hepatitis C virus; *HIV,* human immunodeficiency virus; *HTLV,* human T cell lymphotropic virus; *vCJD,* variant of Creutzfeldt-Jakob disease.

transfusion medicine. In addition, professional organizations such as AABB (formerly known as the American Association of Blood Banks), the College of American Pathologists, and The Joint Commission have put forth accreditation standards for transfusion services and conduct voluntary peer inspections.

Blood Collection

Approximately 60% of the adult U.S. population is eligible to donate blood, although only about 5% actually do so annually. Approximately 16 million units of whole blood and red blood cells (RBCs) are collected annually in the United States (U.S. Department of Health and Human Services, 2009). Virtually all donors are voluntary and noncompensated. The average blood donor is a college-educated male between the ages of 30 and 50, who is married and has above average income. However, donations among women and minority groups are increasing. As the utilization of blood components increases and donor eligibility requirements are tightened, efforts to recruit additional donors will be critical to ensure an adequate blood supply.

Donor criteria are established for the protection of the blood donor and the transfusion recipient. Current (2010) donor qualification criteria are listed in Table 36-1. Criteria for donor protection include a minimum age of 17 years, a minimum weight of 110 pounds, normal vital signs, a minimum hemoglobin (Hb) concentration, and a specified donation interval. Criteria for the protection of the recipient include history or risk factors for infectious disease transmission (hepatitis, human immunodeficiency virus [HIV], malaria, and others), risk of bacteremia, ingestion of certain medications, and history of malignancy. Blood centers are required to maintain a registry of deferred donors, and each donor must be checked against this registry before any donation is made. Finally, every donation must be tested for infectious disease markers as defined by FDA regulations. Current (2010) donor testing requirements are indicated in Table 36-2.

Blood must be collected in a manner to minimize the risk of bacterial contamination. The skin at the venipuncture site must be prepared with

TABLE 36-2
Current U.S. Donor Infectious Disease Testing

Hepatitis B surface antigen (EIA)
Hepatitis B core antibody (EIA)
Hepatitis C virus antibody (EIA)
HIV-1 and HIV-2 antibodies (EIA)*
HTLV-I and HTLV-II antibodies (EIA)
Trypanosoma cruzi antibodies (EIA)
Serologic test for syphilis
Hepatitis C RNA (nucleic acid test)
HIV RNA (nucleic acid test)
West Nile virus DNA (nucleic acid test)

EIA, Enzyme immunoassay; *HIV*, human immunodeficiency virus; *HTLV*, human T cell lymphotropic virus.
*Combined HIV p24 antigen, HIV-1 antibodies, and HIV-2 antibodies acceptable.

an antibacterial scrub. Whole blood is collected into sterilized bag sets containing anticoagulant and attached satellite bags to facilitate component manufacture in a closed system. The rate of blood flow must be sufficient to prevent clot formation during phlebotomy. The volume of blood withdrawn is less than 10.5 mL/kg, including samples for testing. Typically, whole blood donations are 450 or 500 mL.

Blood components can also be collected by apheresis. The advantage of apheresis donation is that a greater volume of the desired components may be obtained from a single donation. The most common use of the apheresis donation is the collection of platelets (commonly called single donor platelets). Plasma may also be collected, typically concurrently with platelets. Apheresis donation allows for the collection of two units of RBCs from suitable donors. Leukocytes may also be collected by apheresis. This is most commonly utilized for the collection of hematopoietic progenitor cells for autologous or allogeneic transplantation. Granulocytes or mononuclear cells may be collected by apheresis for special applications.

Autologous donation is the collection of blood from a patient in advance of scheduled surgery for transfusion during or after the procedure to compensate for expected blood loss. Autologous transfusion prevents the transmission of blood-borne pathogens from allogeneic donors and is desired by some patients. It is not completely free of risk, however, particularly of bacterial contamination. Whether or not autologous transfusion actually decreases the need for allogeneic transfusion or improves patient outcome is controversial. Benefit in reducing allogeneic blood exposure or improving outcome has not been shown in controlled prospective randomized trials. Candidates for autologous donation must not have underlying disease that would put them at risk from this procedure. They must not be significantly anemic, although a lower Hb level than allowed for allogeneic donation may be acceptable. They must not be at risk for bacteremia because the most serious adverse consequence of autologous transfusion is bacterial contamination. Patients with heart disease, particularly aortic stenosis, may be unable to tolerate phlebotomy. Pregnancy does not itself constitute a contraindication to autologous donation; however, the value of autologous donation except in certain high-risk situations such as placenta previa is minimal. Autologous donations can occur more frequently than allogeneic donations. Typically, two or three units may be collected several weeks before surgery. Optimally, there should be sufficient time from donation to surgery to allow for recovery of a substantial portion of the collected red cell mass. This may require iron supplementation. Erythropoietin stimulation has been used as an adjunct to autologous donation.

Some patients desire to select donors for themselves (directed or designated donation) rather than receiving blood from the community blood supply. This provides some patients with the perception of greater safety, although no evidence suggests that directed donation reduces the risk of transfusion-transmitted disease. Directed donors must meet all criteria for allogeneic blood donation. In addition, directed donors must be compatible with the intended recipient. In certain situations, directed donation is contraindicated. Donation of any plasma-containing blood component from a mother to her child is particularly problematic because the formation of human leukocyte antigens (HLA) antibodies to fetal antigens is common in pregnancy, and transfusion of such antibodies can precipitate transfusion-related acute lung injury (see later). Transfusions from close relatives should be avoided in recipients of hematopoietic progenitor cell transplants because of the risk of immunization to HLA and other histocompatibility antigens, which may endanger graft survival. There are rare circumstances under which directed donation may be desirable. These include rare blood group compatibility requirements and limitations of donor exposure for patients with long-term expected transfusion requirements such as aplastic anemia. In cases of neonatal alloimmune thrombocytopenia, collection of maternal platelets may be the best way of providing compatible antigen-negative platelets. In the past, donor-specific transfusion was utilized in kidney transplantation. However, with current immunosuppressive regimens, the value of donor-specific transfusion in prolonging renal graft survival is questionable.

Adverse effects of donations may occur. Minor reactions, mostly presyncope, occur in 2.5% of whole blood donations (Eder, 2009). Major reactions, including loss of consciousness, nerve or arterial injury, allergic reaction, and citrate reaction, occur in about 0.07% of whole blood and 0.05% of apheresis platelet collections. Up to 36% of donors interviewed 3 weeks after donation report some adverse effect, mostly minor, such as arm bruise or soreness (Newman, 2003). More serious adverse effects such as vasovagal symptoms occur in about 5%, and nausea and vomiting in about 1%. Repeat donors are less likely to have reactions than first-time donors. Smaller donors are at greater risk of postdonation syncope. Most syncope reactions occur shortly after donation. However, delayed reactions can occur, and if the donor is at work or is driving, these can be very serious. Seizures following blood donation have been reported, although it is unlikely that there is a causal relationship (Krumholz, 1995). Some highly apprehensive donors hyperventilate, leading to respiratory alkalosis and tetany. This can usually be managed easily by having the donor breathe into a paper bag.

Personnel at a collection site should be prepared to treat donor reactions. Vasovagal syncope can usually be managed easily by placing the donor into a supine position and applying a cold compress to the forehead. It is rare that intravenous fluids are required. A physician should be available to donor site personnel for consultation, and emergency medical support should be available, if necessary. Vasovagal reactions can be minimized by prior hydration of the donor, or by the use of caffeine (Sauer, 1999; Newman, 2007).

Blood Component Manufacture

Whole blood donations are commonly manufactured into components. This facilitates the treatment of different patients with requirements for RBCs, plasma proteins, or platelets. The goals of component manufacture are to maintain viability and function, and to prevent detrimental changes or contamination of desired constituents.

RED BLOOD CELLS

RBCs are prepared from whole blood by centrifugation and removal of plasma. The most commonly used anticoagulant-preservative solution for RBC is CPDA-1. This is supplemented with dextrose and adenine to preserve red cell adenosine triphosphate levels. RBCs in CPDA-1 may be stored for up to 35 days at 1°–6° C. RBCs may also have an additive solution containing glucose and other substrates added during manufacture. Such additive solutions permit a longer storage period (42 days) and have a lower hematocrit (Hct). During storage, red cells undergo senescence changes similar to aging in vivo, such that a portion of transfused red cells are rapidly cleared by the spleen. The maximum allowable storage time for RBCs is defined by the requirement for recovery of 70% of transfused cells 24 hours after transfusion. Leakage of intracellular potassium occurs during red cell storage. The potassium concentration in the supernatant of RBCs can reach levels of 76 mmol/L, which may appear alarmingly high. However, the total amount of potassium in a unit of RBC at outdate is small compared with daily physiologic requirements, and hyperkalemia following transfusion is rare except in special circumstances (see later). Red cells lose intracellular 2,3-diphosphoglycerate (2,3-DPG) during storage, resulting in a shift of the Hb-oxygen dissociation curve to the left. Thus, shortly after transfusion, stored red cells have relatively high oxygen affinity. Normal levels of 2,3-DPG are restored within 24 hours of transfusion. The shift in oxygen association with storage is rarely clinically significant.

PLASMA

Plasma may be stored in the liquid state at 1°–6° C, or it may be frozen for extended preservation. In the liquid state at refrigerator temperatures, there is loss of labile clotting factors, particularly factor VIII and factor V.

Fresh frozen plasma (FFP) is separated from the RBCs and is placed at −18° C within 8 hours of collection. Plasma frozen within 24 hours after phlebotomy (FP24) is manufactured similarly to FFP but may not be frozen for up to 24 hours after collection. The coagulation factor content of FP24 is equivalent to FFP (Scott, 2009). Frozen plasma may be stored for up to 1 year at −18° C or lower. Before transfusion, both FFP and FP24 are thawed at 37° C and must be transfused within 24 hours. Thawed plasma not used within 24 hours may be relabeled as "Thawed Plasma." Thawed plasma can be kept at refrigerator temperatures for up to 5 days, while adequate levels of factors V and VIII are maintained (Downes, 2001; Scott, 2009).

CRYOPRECIPITATED ANTIHEMOPHILIC FACTOR

Cryoprecipitated antihemophilic factor (cryoprecipitate or cryo) is the cold insoluble portion of plasma remaining after FFP has been thawed at refrigerator temperatures. It contains approximately 50% of the factor VIII and 20%–40% of the fibrinogen present in the original plasma unit. Cryo also contains von Willebrand factor (vWF) and factor XIII. FDA regulations require that a unit of cryoprecipitate contain at least 80 IU of factor VIII, although most blood centers achieve higher levels routinely. A unit of cryoprecipitate contains approximately 250 mg of fibrinogen, but testing for the fibrinogen content is not required. Cryoprecipitated antihemophilic factor was a major advance in the treatment of hemophilia A before the development of safe purified clotting factor concentrates. Currently, cryo is used mainly as a source of fibrinogen.

PLATELET CONCENTRATES

Platelet concentrates (PCs) are prepared from whole blood by centrifugation of platelet-rich plasma and expression of platelet-poor plasma. Platelet concentrates must contain at least 5.5×10^{10} platelets per unit. They are stored at room temperature (20°–24° C) because platelets stored at refrigerator temperature (1°–6° C) have greatly diminished posttransfusion survival. Current FDA regulations allow PCs to be stored for up to 5 days with continuous gentle agitation. At the end of storage, the pH of the PCs must be 6.0 or higher. Platelet concentrates typically contain a small number of red cells, which are visibly apparent and can cause alloimmunization to red cell antigens. PCs contain 30–50 mL of plasma. It is typically necessary to pool five or more PCs to obtain a therapeutic dose for a typical adult patient.

PCs that are pooled using an open system must be transfused within 4 hours. PCs can be pooled and leukocyte reduced at the time of manufacture, using a system that maintains sterility, often referred to as prepooled platelets. Because the integrity of the container is not compromised in this process, prepooled platelets can be stored for up to 5 days.

PCs prepared by apheresis (platelets, pheresis, or single-donor platelets) are stored and handled in the same manner as platelet concentrates prepared from whole blood. Each apheresis platelet unit should contain a minimum of 3.0×10^{11} platelets. It is possible to collect two platelet units in a single apheresis session from some donors. One apheresis platelet unit will typically provide a therapeutic dose for an adult patient.

LEUKOCYTE COMPONENTS

Granulocytes can be prepared by apheresis. Granulocytes may be stored at room temperature for up to 24 hours. However, after even brief in vitro storage, granulocytes may have reduced ability to circulate and migrate to areas of inflammation (McCullough, 1983). It is desirable that they be transfused as soon as possible after collection. Donor stimulation with granulocyte colony-stimulating factor (G-CSF) is usually necessary to obtain a sufficient number of granulocytes to be a therapeutic dose for an adult patient (Heuft, 2002). Granulocyte units contain a substantial number of RBCs and must be ABO compatible with the recipient.

Mononuclear cells collected by apheresis can be a source of hematopoietic progenitor cells (HPCs) for autologous or allogeneic transplantation. The number of circulating HPCs can be increased by growth factor (G-CSF or granulocyte-macrophage colony-stimulating factor [GM-CSF]) stimulation, recovery from chemotherapy, or the chemokine receptor blocker plerixafor (Cashen, 2009; Nakasone, 2009). Autologous HPCs for transplantation in patients with lymphoma or other malignancies are typically collected when the bone marrow is recovering from chemotherapy because there are relatively high numbers of circulating stem cells at that time. HPCs may be stored frozen after addition of a cryoprotective agent, such as DMSO, for an extended period of time. After thawing at 37° C, HPCs should be transfused as soon as possible. Mononuclear cells can also be used as a source of lymphocytes for induction of graft-versus-tumor effect, known as donor lymphocyte infusion (Gilleece, 2003).

LEUKOCYTE-REDUCED BLOOD COMPONENTS

Leukocytes present in blood components, particularly RBCs and PCs, may cause adverse effects. Such untoward effects include febrile nonhemolytic transfusion reactions, immunization to leukocyte (particularly HLA) antigens with subsequent refractoriness to platelet transfusions, transmission of leukocyte-associated viruses, and graft-versus-host disease. To minimize most of these adverse impacts, many blood centers and transfusion services have instituted the use of leukocyte-reduced components for all transfusions (universal leukocyte reduction). It must be noted that leukocyte reduction has not been shown to prevent posttransfusion graft-versus-host disease and is not used for this purpose. To be considered leukocyte reduced, blood components must be prepared by a method known to reduce the total number of residual leukocytes to fewer than 5×10^6 per unit for RBC and fewer than 8.3×10^5 for whole blood–derived PC (Fridey, 2003).

Leukocyte reduction is typically accomplished by filtration at the time of component manufacture (prestorage leukocyte reduction) or at the time of transfusion (poststorage leukocyte reduction). Both methods are effective for removing leukocytes. However, prestorage leukocyte reduction has the advantage of preventing accumulation of leukocyte-derived biological response modifiers, particularly cytokines, which may cause adverse reactions (Heddle, 1999). In addition, filtration at the time of manufacture allows for better process control. Certain apheresis devices can reliably produce platelet concentrates containing fewer than 1×10^6 leukocytes. Subtle differences have been noted in the distribution of leukocyte subsets between such components and those produced by filtration (Pennington, 2001). These differences, however, are unlikely to be clinically significant.

Leukocyte reduction failures may occur during filtration of blood from donors with sickle trait. Such filtration failures are due to Hb S polymerization in an environment of low oxygen tension and high osmolality (Beard, 2004). Leukocyte reduction is not an effective means of preventing graft-versus-host disease (Hayashi, 1993). Clearly, granulocytes and hematopoietic progenitor cells cannot be leukocyte reduced.

SPECIAL COMPONENTS

Cryoprecipitate-reduced plasma (cryopoor plasma) is the supernatant remaining from the production of cryoprecipitate. It is relatively deficient in high molecular weight forms of vWF but retains normal levels of the vWF-cleaving metalloprotease ADAMTS 13 (Blackall, 2001). For these reasons, cryoprecipitate-reduced plasma is an attractive alternative to FFP for the treatment of patients with thrombotic thrombocytopenic purpura. However, at present, no definitive evidence indicates that plasma exchange with cryoprecipitate-reduced plasma results in improved patient outcome.

Red blood cells can be stored in the frozen state after addition of a cryoprotective agent, such as glycerol. Frozen RBCs can be stored in mechanical freezers or liquid nitrogen for up to 10 years. Frozen units are thawed rapidly at 37° C. The cryoprotective agent must be removed by progressive addition of washing solutions with decreasing osmolality. Failure to properly deglycerolize frozen RBCs can result in hemolysis. Cryopreservation and deglycerolization of sickle trait red cells by standard methods can result in the formation of a jelly-like mass. This can be overcome by using a modified process (Meryman, 1976). After deglycerolization, red cells can be stored for up to 1 day at 1°–6° C if processed by an open method, or up to 14 days if processed by a closed method. The main use of frozen RBCs is to maintain an inventory of rare antigen-negative units.

RBCs and PCs can be washed to remove plasma proteins and electrolytes. Washing can be accomplished by manual or automated methods. Loss of cells during the washing process can be substantial. In addition, washing of platelets can result in clumping and activation with reduced viability (Pineda, 1989). Because this is an open process, washed red cells may be stored for 24 hours at refrigerator temperatures, and washed platelets must be transfused within 4 hours of preparation. The main use of washed components is the prevention of severe allergic reactions. Washing is not an effective means of leukocyte reduction.

Transfusion-associated graft-versus-host disease (TA-GVHD) can be prevented by irradiation of components containing viable lymphocytes (RBCs, PCs, granulocytes, and nonfrozen plasma). This can be accomplished by exposure to γ-rays or X-rays. The minimum dose should be 25 Gy delivered to the center of the blood container and no less than 15 Gy to the periphery. Irradiation causes chromosomal damage, which prevents replication of transfused lymphocytes in the recipient. However, irradiated cells are immunogenic. Thus, irradiation is not equivalent to leukocyte reduction. Irradiation also causes damage to red cell membranes with increased potassium leakage and decreased posttransfusion survival (Moroff, 1999). Irradiated red cells must have the outdate shortened to no more than 28 days from the date of irradiation. Platelets appear to sustain minimal damage from irradiation, and so their expiration date need not be altered, although the increment in platelet count may be reduced (Sweeney, 1994; Slichter, 2005). Clearly, hematopoietic progenitor cells must not be irradiated. Irradiation is not sufficient to prevent transmission of viral infections, including cytomegalovirus, or bacterial contamination.

PATHOGEN REDUCTION

Although great progress has been made in reducing the risks of transfusion-transmitted diseases, some risk remains. In addition, it is possible that a new transmissible disease may emerge as a threat to blood safety. For these reasons, strategies to inactivate contaminating microorganisms (pathogen reduction) are presently under active development. Blood derivatives such as albumin, coagulation factor concentrates, and immunoglobulins are commonly treated by a variety of methods, including heat and solvent-detergent, which are highly effective against viruses, including HIV, hepatitis B virus (HBV), and hepatitis C virus (HCV). The solvent-detergent treatment process disrupts the lipid envelope of viruses such as HIV, HBV, and HCV. However, it is ineffective against nonlipid-enveloped viruses. In addition, it destroys cell membranes and so is not applicable to cellular blood components. Solvent-detergent–treated plasma is available in Europe and is approved by the FDA, although it is not presently available in the United States. Solvent-detergent–treated plasma contains predictable levels of all coagulation factors and is effective in the treatment of thrombotic thrombocytopenic purpura (TTP) (Horowitz, 1992; Moake, 1994). It may, however, contain reduced levels of protein S and has been associated with thrombotic complications (Doyle, 2003).

Presently, two pathogen reduction methods for platelets and plasma, not available in the United States but marketed elsewhere, are Intercept (Cerus Corporation, Concord, Calif.) and Mirasol PRT (Navigant Biotechnologies, Lakewood, Colo.) (McClaskey 2009). Psoralen compounds used in the Intercept system intercalate between bases of RNA and DNA and, when exposed to ultraviolet (UV) light, form covalent cross-links that prevent replication. Both treatments are effective against viruses, bacteria, and protozoans (Lin, 2004; Ruane, 2004). Intercept-treated platelet concentrate has been shown to be safe and effective in a randomized trial (McCullough, 2004). The treatment process does result in a statistically significant, and possibly clinically significant, reduction in posttransfusion platelet recovery. Riboflavin, used in the Mirasol PRT system, causes strand cleavage of nucleic acids when activated by UV light. Because these methods require exposure to light, their applicability to RBCs is limited. Both the Intercept and Mirasol processes have been shown to preclude the need for irradiation of blood components to prevent transfusion-associated graft versus host disease (Mintz, 2009). Although each of these techniques is promising, questions of efficacy, toxicity, and immunogenicity remain.

SELECTION OF BLOOD COMPONENTS

Blood components must be serologically compatible with the recipient. ABO compatibility is the primary consideration. Transfused red cells must be compatible with recipient antibodies, and transfused plasma must be compatible with recipient red cells. Therefore, whole blood must be of identical ABO type to the recipient. Red blood cells contain a limited amount of plasma and need to be compatible but not necessarily identical to the ABO type of the recipient. Similarly, plasma and platelet concentrates contain few, if any, red cells. ABO-compatible blood component selection is summarized in Table 36-3. Red blood cells must also be negative for clinically significant antigens when transfused to alloimmunized recipients. It is highly desirable to transfuse only Rh-negative red cells to Rh-negative recipients because there is approximately a 30% risk of immunization to Rh(D) (Frohn, 2003). This is particularly important for women of childbearing potential because of the risk of hemolytic disease of the newborn in subsequent pregnancies.

TABLE 36-3
ABO Compatibility

	RECIPIENT TYPE			
Donor type	**O**	**A**	**B**	**AB**
O	R P	R	R	R
A	P	R P		R
B	P		R P	R
AB	P	P	P	R P

P, Plasma-containing components (platelets, fresh frozen plasma) are compatible; *R*, red cells are compatible.

Special considerations apply to recipients of ABO-incompatible hematopoietic progenitor cell transplants. During the course of transplantation, such individuals will change their blood type. Transfused red cells should be compatible with both donor and recipient isohemagglutinins, and transfused plasma–containing components should be compatible with both donor and recipient red cells. Thus, the optimal choice for such a patient will depend on current and expected future typing results.

RED BLOOD CELLS

The primary consideration in selection of RBCs is serologic compatibility for the prevention of hemolytic transfusion reactions. Because the post-transfusion survival of red cells is inversely related to length of storage, it is desirable to select fresh (typically less than 10 days old) units in situations where it is particularly desirable to limit the number of transfusions, such as intrauterine and neonatal transfusion. For large-volume transfusions of pediatric patients (such as exchange transfusion or cardiac surgery), it may be desirable to select Hb S–negative (sickle-negative) units. It is also preferable to select sickle-negative red cells for transfusion to patients with sickle cell disease because the presence of Hb S in donor red cells may complicate monitoring of the effectiveness of transfusion therapy. However, it has never been shown that red cell transfusion from asymptomatic sickle trait donors is deleterious, and in some cases such as rare blood requirements, the use of a sickle trait donor may be the only option. Heavily transfused patients, particularly those with sickle cell disease, are at risk of alloimmunization and hemolytic transfusion reactions (Vichinsky, 1990). Such patients may benefit from prophylactic administration of antigen-matched red cells, particularly Rh and Kell (Ambruso, 1987; Castellino, 1999).

Exchange transfusion of the neonate with hemolytic disease of the newborn (HDN) is a special case. In this situation, antigen-negative red cells and plasma (for oncotic pressure and bilirubin-binding capacity) are needed. Red cells must be compatible with the maternal antibodies, including ABO antibodies. Reconstituted whole blood, prepared by combining RBC and compatible FFP to a desired Hct (typically 50%), is commonly used, although whole blood may be used if available.

PLATELETS

Major ABO compatibility is less of an issue in platelet transfusion than in red cell transfusion. ABO antigens are expressed weakly on platelets. ABO-incompatible platelet transfusions may result in lower posttransfusion survival, although this usually is not clinically significant. Transfusion of isohemagglutinins contained in the plasma of apheresis platelets from donors with high-titer anti-A or anti-B can cause an acute hemolytic reaction (Larsson, 2000). Therefore, if non–ABO-identical platelets must be transfused, overriding consideration is typically given to plasma compatibility with the recipient. Some centers will screen apheresis platelets to ensure that high-titer incompatible anti-A or anti-B (e.g., <1 : 200 reactivity at immediate spin) is not transfused.

Failure to achieve an expected platelet count increment after platelet transfusion on two or more occasions is commonly considered refractoriness. Failure to respond with an appropriate increase in platelet count after transfusion (platelet refractoriness) may be due to immune causes (HLA or platelet-specific antibodies), nonimmune clinical causes (bleeding, splenomegaly, disseminated intravascular coagulation [DIC], medications), product-specific causes (ABO incompatibility; older products give lower increments), or the fact that some donors' platelets store poorly. A poor increment following a single platelet transfusion must not be presumed to be due to alloimmunization. The refractoriness is often multifactorial and changes with the patient's underlying condition and therapy. HLA antibodies are the most common cause of immune-mediated platelet refractoriness. HLA class I antigens are expressed on platelets, and class I antibodies are common in patients who have been previously pregnant or transfused with non–leukocyte-reduced blood components. Leukocyte reduction has been shown to effectively prevent both alloimmunization and platelet refractoriness in previously unexposed patients with leukemia (Trial to Reduce Alloimmunization to Platelets Study Group, 1997). Antibodies to platelet-specific antigens are a relatively rare cause of platelet refractoriness. Several effective strategies are known for selection of platelets for the alloimmunized refractory recipient. The use of cross-match–compatible platelets is usually the first line (O'Connell, 1990). If the patient's HLA antibody specificities can be defined, it may be possible to select antigen-negative donors (Petz, 2000). Donors matched for HLA class I antigens may be selected. However, owing to constraints of donor availability, finding optimal matches may be very difficult. Even with a large donor base, many "HLA-matched" transfusions are mismatched for at least one antigen (Dahlke, 1984).

Pretransfusion Testing

The most critical step in pretransfusion testing is proper collection and identification of the recipient blood sample. The most common cause of an acute hemolytic transfusion reaction is misidentification of the sample or patient (Sazama, 1990; Linden, 2000). Each transfusion service must develop and implement policies and procedures for patient identification and specimen collection. The pretransfusion samples should be labeled at the time of phlebotomy by comparison with the patient's permanent identifier (typically a wristband). The label should contain at least two unique identifiers, such as patient name and hospital registration number. The date of sample collection and the identity of the phlebotomist must also be documented. In emergency situations when the patient's identity is unknown, a unique identifier must be assigned. This identifier must remain with the patient throughout the course of transfusion even if the patient is subsequently identified. Policies and procedures must be in place for management of patients with confidential or alias names.

Samples for pretransfusion testing should be collected no more than 3 days before transfusion, unless it is known that the patient has not been pregnant or transfused within the preceding 3 months. The common practice of patient admission on the same day as elective surgery presents special challenges. In this setting, pretransfusion samples may be collected during a preceding outpatient visit. One option is to require such patients to wear an identification wristband, although many patients find this undesirable. Another alternative is to assign a unique number to the pretransfusion specimen and affix this number to an identification form that the patient must provide on the day of surgery (Butch, 1994). Pretransfusion samples must be retained until at least 7 days after each transfusion. Typically, transfusion services retain pretransfusion samples for a fixed time.

Routine pretransfusion testing consists of ABO and Rh(D) typing and screening for unexpected red cell antibodies. If the antibody screen is positive, antibody identification tests should be performed. Results of current testing should be compared with records of the previous testing, if available. Clinically significant red cell antibodies may become undetectable over time but may cause delayed hemolytic reactions owing to an anamnestic response. Therefore, a history of a clinically significant red cell antibody should be honored by providing only antigen-negative red cells for transfusion. Any discrepancy in current testing or disagreement with previous records must be resolved before pretransfusion testing can be concluded.

Some patients present particular challenges in pretransfusion testing. Newborns typically have weak or absent isohemagglutinins. Expected ABO antibodies may not be present until 6 months of age. Recently transfused patients may show a mixture of circulating red cells, if they have not received ABO-identical units. Unexpected red cell antibodies can be acquired passively from transfusion of platelet concentrates or immunoglobulins. Some patients may lack expected isohemagglutinins because of disease or immunosuppressive therapy. Recipients of allogeneic HPC transplants may have complex and variable typing results, which necessitate conclusion of a "declared" blood type. In urgent situations when the blood type cannot be concluded, selection of group O red cells and group AB plasma is usually safe. If antibody identification tests cannot be completed, a medical judgment must be made regarding the urgency of transfusion and the risks of incompatibility. It may be desirable to issue red cells lacking antigen specificities that cannot be excluded, if available. The occurrence of a weakly expressed Rh(D) antigen may complicate pretransfusion testing.

The final step of pretransfusion compatibility testing is the cross-match. The purpose of the cross-match is a final check of ABO compatibility and, to a lesser extent, detection of unidentified antibodies. A major cross-match is performed between the recipient's serum or plasma and donor red cells. A minor cross-match, between recipient red cells and donor or plasma, is usually unnecessary. In the absence of unexpected red cell antibodies, a cross-match can be performed by direct agglutination ("immediate spin") for detection of ABO incompatibility. When unexpected red cell antibodies are present, the cross-match should be performed by antiglobulin technique. For antibodies judged to be clinically significant, antigen-negative cells are selected for cross-match. An alternative for ensurance of ABO compatibility is the so-called computer cross-match. This is applicable when at least two determinations of the recipient's ABO group have been made, at least one on a current sample, and there are no unexpected antibodies (Butch, 1997). A validated computer system can then ensure that issued blood complements are ABO compatible. The presence of red cell autoantibodies presents a special problem. In this setting, it is essential that alloantibodies be excluded. Typically, the cross-match will be positive. Many transfusion services have a policy of issuing "least reactive" units, although the value of this policy has been called into question (Petz, 2003).

In urgent situations, emergency release of blood complements before completion of compatibility testing may be indicated. The goals of emergency release are to provide red cells for oxygen-carrying capacity and plasma for coagulation factor content to a rapidly bleeding patient. ABO compatibility is the first priority (see earlier discussion of component selection). Antibodies to other blood group antigens typically do not cause acute hemolytic reactions and therefore are of lower priority. However, when there is a history of prior antibodies, or when antibody identification tests are partially complete, it may be preferable to select antigen-negative RBCs, if available. Finally, documentation of the medical order for emergency release of blood components should be obtained, usually after the fact.

Transfusion Administration

The transfusion service is responsible for developing and implementing policies and procedures for the administration of blood components. A physician's order is required to prepare, dispense, and administer blood components. Optimally, venous access should be established before a blood component is issued. The selection of location and type of access depends on the volume, timing, and expected duration of transfusion therapy. Peripheral access with an 18-gauge needle or catheter is typically sufficient. Smaller catheters may be used; however, high-pressure flow through a small lumen may cause hemolysis (de la Roche, 1993). Central venous access is desirable for high-volume administration or long-term therapy.

Before administration of a transfusion, accurate identification of the component and the intended recipient is essential. This process should include at least two unique identifiers, such as name and registration number, and comparison with a permanent identifier, such as a wristband. Additionally, the unit identifier on the blood container should be checked against the associated documentation (transfusion form or attached tag). The ABO and the Rh type on the unit label must agree with the associated documentation, and compatibility with the patient's recorded blood type should be verified. The expiration time and date of the blood component should be verified as acceptable. Many institutions require that two qualified individuals perform the identity check before transfusion. The physician's order and the patient's consent for transfusion should also be verified.

All blood components must be administered through a filter intended to retain clots and particles, typically 170–260 μm pore size. Administration sets should contain a drip chamber, attached compatible intravenous solution, and a means of controlling the flow rate. During surgery, it is routine practice to add a microaggregate filter through which the blood component flows first. This decreases the metabolic burden placed on the recipient to process aggregates of fibrin and cellular debris that accumulate during storage, and helps to preserve the patency of the intravascular line. Care should be taken to avoid admixture of the blood components with incompatible intravenous solutions. Normal saline is the preferred solution for all transfusions. Calcium-containing solutions should be avoided, as these may precipitate clotting. RBCs should not be administered with 5% dextrose, as this may cause hemolysis. Medications should not be added to blood components. Leukocyte reduction filters may be used for transfusion of RBCs or PCs to reduce the incidence of febrile transfusion reactions, HLA alloimmunization, or cytomegalovirus (CMV) transmission. The appropriate filter must be selected for the blood component because clogging or filter failure may occur if improperly used.

It may be desirable to administer refrigerated blood components (RBCs or plasma) through a blood-warming device. Transfusion of cold components faster than 100 mL per minute for 30 minutes may increase the risk of cardiac arrest (Boyan, 1963). Blood-warming devices should have a visible thermometer and an audible alarm to avoid exceeding temperature limits. Blood components should never be warmed by the use of tap water, conventional microwave ovens, or any other nonapproved warming device.

The desirable rate of administration depends on the patient's blood volume, cardiac status, and hemodynamic state. Except for urgent resuscitation, the transfusion should be started slowly (approximately 2 mL/minute for the first 15 minutes). The patient should be carefully observed for the first 15 minutes of infusion because severe reactions such as hemolysis, anaphylaxis, or sepsis may manifest after a small volume has entered the circulation. Subsequently, the administration rate may be increased. In general, it is desirable to complete a red cell transfusion within 2 hours and a platelet or plasma transfusion within 30–60 minutes. Any transfusion should be completed within 4 hours of initiation. Patients at risk of volume overload may require slower administration. If the total administration time exceeds 4 hours, smaller-volume blood components should be provided. When high flow rates are required, such as in some resuscitation or surgical situations, a pressure infusion device may be used. When such devices are used, care must be taken to avoid mechanical hemolysis or air embolism. During transfusion, the patient's vital signs should be checked at regular intervals, and any suspected reaction should prompt interruption of the transfusion and immediate investigation.

BLOOD COMPONENT THERAPY

All transfusion decisions are clinical judgments that should be made while taking into account clinical and laboratory data. There are no absolute indications, and few contraindications, to blood transfusion.

Red Cell Transfusion

Red blood cells provide oxygen-carrying capacity. Red cell transfusion may be used to treat acute or chronic anemia. A patient's ability to tolerate anemia depends on the degree of anemia, physiologic adaptive mechanisms, and cardiac or respiratory disease. Normal physiologic adaptations to anemia include increased cardiac output, redistribution of blood flow, increased oxygen extraction, and increased red cell 2,3-DPG, resulting in rightward shift of the oxygen-Hb dissociation curve. General guidelines for red cell transfusion are summarized in Table 36-4. Symptomatic anemia, regardless of Hb concentration, in a euvolemic patient is an indication for transfusion. Symptoms of anemia include fatigue, tachycardia, tachypnea, dyspnea on exertion, postural hypotension, and impaired mentation. Anemia may precipitate angina in patients with coronary artery disease. Generally, acute blood loss of greater than 15% of a patient's blood volume may be an indication for red cell transfusion. Studies of postsurgical morbidity in patients who refused blood transfusion have indicated that for patients with a preoperative Hb of at least 6 g/dL, without underlying coronary artery disease, and sustaining operative blood loss of less than 2 g/dL of Hb, there is little relationship between mortality and degree of preoperative anemia (Carson, 1996). Mortality increases with preoperative Hb levels below 6 g/dL (Spence, 1990). However, with a Hb loss of 2–4 g/dL, perioperative mortality increases with preoperative Hb levels below 10 g/dL. This risk is magnified by the presence of cardiovascular disease (angina, myocardial infarction, congestive heart failure, or peripheral vascular disease). One study of patients undergoing elective operations demonstrated no mortality despite Hb levels as low as 6 g/dL, provided that the blood loss was less than 500 mL (Carson, 1988).

The Transfusion Requirements in Critical Care (TRICC) study has been the largest randomized prospective trial to date comparing restrictive and liberal transfusion strategies (Hebert, 1999). The TRICC trial enrolled 838 critically ill patients with Hb levels <9.0 g/dL. Subjects were randomized to receive liberal or restrictive transfusion regimens. The liberal regimen was a transfusion trigger of 10 g/dL with a target of 10–12 g/dL. The restrictive regimen was a transfusion trigger of 7.0 g/dL with a target of 7.0–9.0 g/dL. The primary result was no statistically significant difference in 30-day mortality, although a trend favoring lower mortality was noted in the restrictive strategy group (18.7% vs. 23.3%; $p = 0.11$). Cardiac events, primarily pulmonary edema and myocardial infarction, occurred more frequently in the liberal than in the restrictive transfusion group (21.0% vs. 13.2%; $p < 0.001$). Subgroup analysis showed lower mortality in the restrictive strategy group among patients with lower disease severity measured by APACHE II scores (8.7% vs. 16.1%; $p = 0.03$) and among patients younger than 55 years of age (5.77% vs. 13.07%; $p = 0.02$). Thus, it appears that many critically ill adult patients can tolerate Hb levels less than 10 g/dL.

Whether the results of the TRICC trial are generalizable to patients with acute coronary syndromes is open to debate. A large retrospective cohort study of patients >65 years of age with acute myocardial infarction has examined the association between admission Hb and 30-day mortality (Wu, 2001). This showed a clear relationship between increasing mortality and lower initial Hb. Furthermore, among patients who received transfusion, lower adjusted odds of 30-day mortality were noted when the admission Hct was less than 33%, whereas the odds of death were higher for transfused patients with admission Hct >36% after adjustment for clinical factors, medication, and predictors of transfusion. These results suggested that red cell transfusion may result in lower short-term mortality among elderly patients with acute myocardial infarction who survived at least 2 days, if the Hct on admission is 30% or lower. However, inherent drawbacks of the retrospective study design, such as survivor bias, limit the conclusions that can be drawn from this study. An analysis of transfusion effects on 30-day mortality in patients with acute coronary syndromes presented somewhat different results (Rao, 2004). This was a reanalysis of three interventional drug trials with the primary outcome measure being 30-day mortality. Ten percent of subjects in the study were transfused. Transfused subjects were more likely to have comorbidities, including a higher Killip class, than nontransfused subjects. Cumulative mortality among transfused subjects was greater than in nontransfused subjects ($p < 0.001$). For subjects with a nadir Hct of 20%, no statistically significant difference in odds of death was observed between transfused and nontransfused individuals.

The recent Transfusion Trigger Trial for Functional Outcomes in Cardiovascular Patients Undergoing Surgical Hip Fracture Repair (FOCUS) addressed the red cell transfusion trigger in surgical patients with cardiac disease (Carson, 2006). The goal of this randomized clinical trial was to determine whether a more aggressive transfusion strategy in patients with cardiovascular disease or cardiovascular disease risk factors undergoing surgery for repair of hip fracture is associated with improved functional recovery and decreased risk of adverse postoperative outcomes. Subjects were randomly allocated to a 10 g/dL transfusion threshold or a symptomatic strategy. The study population consisted of patients 50 years of age or older who underwent surgical repair of a hip fracture, with Hb concentrations below 10 g/dL within 3 days after surgery, and who had clinical evidence of cardiovascular disease or cardiovascular risk factors. The primary outcome measure was ability to walk 10 feet (or across a room) without human assistance at 60 days after randomization, and the major secondary outcome measure was in-hospital acute coronary syndrome or death within 30 days. The FOCUS trial enrolled more than 2600 subjects, making it the largest and best powered clinical trial to date in transfusion medicine. The results of this trial will likely have a major impact on red cell transfusion in the surgical patient.

Transfusion of the patient with sickle cell disease (SCD) presents unique challenges. The indications for transfusion are to augment oxygen-carrying capacity in severe anemia and to improve microvascular circulation by decreasing the proportion of sickle red cells. Oxygen delivery in

TABLE 36-4
Red Cell Transfusion Guidelines

Symptomatic anemia in a euvolemic patient
Acute blood loss of >15% of estimated blood volume
Preoperative Hb <9.0 g/dL with expected blood loss >500 mL
Hb <7.0 g/dL in a critically ill patient
Hb <8.0 g/dL in a patient with an acute coronary syndrome
Hb <10.0 g/dL with uremic or thrombocytopenic bleeding
Sickle cell disease:
Acute sequestration: Hb <5.0 g/dL or decrease of 20% from baseline
Acute chest syndrome: Target Hb = 10 g/dL, HbS fraction <30%
Stroke prophylaxis: Target HbS fraction <30%
General anesthesia: Target Hb = 10.0 g/dL, HbS fraction <60%

Hb, Hemoglobin.

TABLE 36-5
Platelet Transfusion Guidelines

Thrombocytopenia due to decreased production
Stable patient: platelet count <10,000/μL
Fever: platelet count <20,000/μL
Bleeding, invasive procedure, or surgery: platelet count <40,000–50,000/μL
Retinal or central nervous system (CNS) bleeding: platelet count <100,000/μL
Microvascular bleeding due to platelet dysfunction

SCD represents a balance between oxygen-carrying capacity and blood viscosity. Optimal oxygen delivery is usually achieved when the posttransfusion Hct is about 30% (Schmalzer, 1987). No universally accepted laboratory parameters are available for transfusion in SCD. Hb values less than 5 g/dL and an acute drop of 20% from baseline during an acute illness are general indications for red cell transfusion. Acute splenic sequestration can produce sudden hypovolemia and cardiovascular collapse, necessitating prompt transfusion. In this setting, the rise in Hb following transfusion may be greater than expected because of release of sequestered red cells. Careful monitoring is essential to avoid overtransfusion (Powell, 1992). Acute chest syndrome may be life threatening. Prompt transfusion may prevent progression to respiratory failure (Mallouh, 1988). Exchange transfusion with a goal of achieving Hb S level of 30% or less and Hct of 30% is a typical approach. Long-term transfusion therapy can reduce the risk of stroke in SCD. In children, transfusion with the goal of maintaining Hb S levels below 30% can reduce the risk of stroke (Adams, 1998). How long a chronic transfusion regimen must be maintained is an open question. Termination, even after several years of therapy, can result in reversion to high risk of stroke (Adams, 2004). Before general anesthesia is administered, transfusion is indicated to achieve an Hb of 10 g/dL and an Hb S level of approximately 60% (Vichinsky, 1995). In uncomplicated pregnancy, prophylactic red cell transfusion is not beneficial. However, transfusion may be indicated in high-risk pregnancy or with a history of previous fetal loss (Seoud, 1994).

In autoimmune hemolytic anemia, transfusion may be indicated if cardiac or neurologic symptoms are present. Most patients with autoimmune hemolytic anemia tolerate transfusion of incompatible red cells, if alloantibodies have been excluded (Salama, 1992). Transfused red cells usually are not cleared any more rapidly than the patient's own red cells. It is important to note that a necessary red cell transfusion must never be withheld because of cross-match incompatibility. It is far more dangerous not to give such a transfusion to a patient with autoimmune hemolytic anemia than it is to provide it.

Red cell transfusion may be beneficial in bleeding associated with uremia. An inverse relationship between Hct and bleeding time has been noted in patients with chronic renal failure. Transfusion to an Hb of 10 g/dL may be beneficial in the bleeding uremic patient (Fernandez, 1985).

Transfusion of one unit of RBCs to an adult patient can usually be expected to raise the Hb by 1 g/dL and the Hct by 3%. However, the expected Hct increase may range from about 2%–9%, depending on the patient's vascular volume (Gorlin, 2000).

Platelet Transfusion

Platelet transfusion is indicated for prevention or treatment of hemorrhage due to thrombocytopenia or platelet dysfunction, as summarized in Table 36-5. Prophylactic transfusion is indicated when the platelet count is lower than 5000/μL. For stable patients undergoing chemotherapy, a prophylactic platelet transfusion threshold of 10,000/μL is often used (Rebulla, 1997). The goal of prophylactic therapy is to achieve platelet counts above 25,000/μL (Schlossberg, 2003). If the patient is febrile, a threshold for prophylactic transfusion of 20,000/μL is typically used. For bleeding patients, or for those undergoing an invasive procedure, including endoscopy or surgery, the goal of platelet transfusion therapy is to achieve sustained levels above 40,000–50,000/μL (British Committee for Standards in Haematology, Blood Transfusion Task Force, 2003). This usually ensures hemostasis, although it may take longer than normal to achieve. For this reason, for patients experiencing bleeding in critical spaces, such as the retina or central nervous system, a target of 100,000/μL is the standard of practice, as this level typically ensures no abnormal delay in hemostasis. In bleeding associated with platelet dysfunction, or thrombocytopenic bleeding associated with coagulopathy, there is no single transfusion threshold, and therapy must be guided by the patient's clinical condition. Cardiopulmonary bypass may result in a transient acquired platelet dysfunction that may manifest as microvascular bleeding. The platelet count is not usually a useful indicator in such situations. Prophylactic platelet transfusion in routine cardiopulmonary bypass is not indicated.

The recent Prophylactic Platelet Dose (PLADO) trial addressed the optimal prophylactic platelet dose in patients with hypoproliferative thrombocytopenia from stem cell transplantation or chemotherapy (Slichter, 2010). Subjects were randomized to one of three arms: a low platelet dose of 1.1×10^{11} platelets/m^2 (half the medium dose), a medium dose of 2.2×10^{11}/m^2, or a high dose of 4.4×10^{11}/m^2 (twice the medium dose). The primary outcome measure was the percentage of patients in each dose arm who had at least one episode of World Health Organization (WHO) grade 2 or higher bleeding. The incidence of grade 2 bleeding, higher grade bleeding, and other adverse events was similar among the three groups. The median number of platelets transfused in the low-dose group was significantly lower than in the other groups, but the number of platelet transfusions was higher. Bleeding events were more common on days when the platelet count was 5,000/μL or lower, regardless of treatment assignment. This trial demonstrated that low-dose prophylactic platelet transfusion is safe in hypoproliferative thrombocytopenia, but may not reduce total platelet transfusions.

The platelet transfusion is relatively contraindicated in immune thrombocytopenic purpura. In this setting, posttransfusion platelet survival is extremely brief, and platelet transfusion is indicated only if there is severe hemorrhage. Clearly, transfusion in the setting of intravascular platelet consumption should be undertaken with great caution. Platelet transfusion in heparin-induced thrombocytopenia or thrombotic thrombocytopenic purpura can be deleterious (Harkness, 1981; Gordon, 1987).

Transfusion of one apheresis platelet unit, or an equivalent pool of whole blood–derived platelet concentrates, can typically be expected to raise the platelet count of an adult by 20,000–40,000/μL. As a practical matter, it can be estimated that approximately 1 hour post transfusion, the blood platelet count should increase by 8000–10,000/μL for each 1×10^{11} platelets transfused for each square meter of body surface area (Strauss, 1995). However, there are many reasons why this increment may not be achieved. Consumption or bleeding, splenomegaly, platelet antibodies, and drugs are all causes of a poor response to platelet transfusion. Drugs that can cause an inadequate platelet increment include antibiotics, heparin, antiplatelet agents (clopidogrel, tirofiban), quinidine, and antithymocyte globulin, along with many others. In assessing platelet transfusion effectiveness, it is useful to take into account dose and body size by calculating the corrected count increment (CCI).

$$CCI = \frac{\textit{Platelet count increment} \times BSA}{\textit{Number of platelets transfused}\,(\times 10^{11})}$$

where *BSA* is the body surface area (m^2).

Example

Pretransfusion platelet count = 8000/μL
Posttransfusion platelet count = 36,000/μL
BSA = 1.5 m^2
Platelet dose = 3.0×10^{11}

$$CCI = \frac{24{,}000 \times 1.5}{3} = 12{,}000$$

A CCI >7500 at 1 hour or a CCI >4500 at 24 hours generally indicates a successful transfusion. Obtaining a platelet count within 1 hour of completing the transfusion may be helpful in distinguishing immune from nonimmune causes of platelet refractoriness. Typically, immune refractoriness will result in an inadequate platelet increment when measured at 1 hour. Typical nonimmune refractoriness will manifest as an adequate CCI at 1 hour but shortened survival time, so that the platelet count by 24 hours may be back to baseline. It must be appreciated that the CCI does not indicate that an adequate platelet count has been achieved. It indicates only the adequacy of a platelet count increment in relation to the number of platelets transfused.

Plasma Transfusion

Guidelines for plasma transfusion are summarized in Table 36-6. Plasma may be used to replace any plasma protein deficiency. Purified protein concentrates, such as factor VIII, albumin, or immunoglobulin, are preferable for replacement of specific deficiencies because these are highly

TABLE 36-6
Plasma Transfusion Guidelines

Coagulation factor deficiency, factor concentrate unavailable
Dilutional coagulopathy
Hemorrhage in liver disease
Disseminated intravascular coagulation (DIC)
Coumadin reversal
Thrombotic thrombocytopenic purpura (TTP)
Acute trauma resuscitation

TABLE 36-7
Cryoprecipitate Transfusion Guidelines

- Factor VIII deficiency, factor concentrate unavailable
- von Willebrand disease, factor concentrate unavailable
- Hypofibrinogenemia
- Factor XIII deficiency
- Uremic bleeding (DDAVP preferred)
- Topical fibrin sealant (commercial product preferred)

DDAVP, Desmopressin.

purified and standardized, and carry extremely low risk of infectious disease transmission. Plasma is most commonly used for replacement of coagulation factor deficiencies when no factor concentrate is available. Multifactorial deficiencies are common in liver disease, massive bleeding, multiorgan system failure, and warfarin therapy. The degree to which factor deficiency may contribute to bleeding in such cases is controversial. Standard coagulation tests such as prothrombin time (PT) and activated partial thromboplastin time (APTT) are commonly used to assess the need for plasma transfusion; however, these tests are poorly predictive of bleeding risk. In general, if the PT and APTT are less than 1.5 times the midpoint of the reference range, no benefit will be obtained from plasma transfusion. If the international normalized ratio (INR) is used, in general, no benefit will be derived from plasma transfusion if it is less than 1.5, although for nervous system and retinal hemorrhage, plasma may be reasonably used unless the INR is less than 1.3. For maximal hemostatic effect, plasma should be transfused immediately before an invasive procedure is performed. For the bleeding patient, plasma transfusion may have to be repeated every 3–4 hours to maintain adequate coagulation factor levels. In general, a dose of 10–20 mL per kilogram is necessary to achieve a hemostatic effect. Plasma is the preferred choice for rapid reversal of warfarin, although factor IX complex concentrate is also effective (Boulis, 1999). Plasma is a source of vWF protease activity, which may be deficient in thrombotic thrombocytopenic purpura.

Cryoprecipitate Transfusion

General guidelines for the transfusion of cryoprecipitate are summarized in Table 36-7. Cryo can be used for factor VIII or vWF replacement. High purity or recombinant factor concentrates, however, are better alternatives. Cryo is a good source of fibrinogen and factor XIII. Most patients with hypofibrinogenemia also have deficiencies of other coagulation factors and are better treated with FFP. Some evidence suggests that cryo may be effective in the treatment of uremic bleeding, possibly by providing high molecular weight forms of the vWF (Triulzi, 1990). Desmopressin (DDAVP) is a preferred therapy for this situation, however. DDAVP may become ineffective after repeated short-term use, at which point cryo transfusion could be initiated. Cryo, when mixed with calcium and thrombin, can be used to make a topical fibrin sealant for surgery, although more concentrated, virally inactivated commercial products are available. Each unit of cryoprecipitate can be assumed to contain at least 80 units of factor VIII activity and 250 mg of fibrinogen, although the actual content is variable.

MASSIVE TRANSFUSION

Massive transfusion, usually defined as replacement of one blood volume within 24 hours, necessitates a systematic approach. Large-volume blood loss is often due to trauma but also occurs in gastrointestinal hemorrhage (particularly with chronic liver disease), ruptured aortic aneurysms, and some surgical procedures such as liver transplantation. No single massive transfusion protocol will be optimal for all patients, although establishing an institutional policy is helpful because these cases can become chaotic. Special attention should be paid to patient and sample identification to avoid transfusion errors.

The priorities in transfusion management of massive bleeding are prevention or treatment of hypovolemic shock, maintenance of adequate oxygen-carrying capacity, maintenance of oncotic pressure, correction or prevention of coagulopathy, and avoidance of adverse effects of transfusion. Initial patient evaluation should include pertinent medical history (especially liver, kidney, cardiovascular, and hematologic diseases), history of previous transfusions or pretransfusion testing problems, examination for microvascular bleeding, complete blood count (CBC), and coagulation profile (PT, APTT, fibrinogen). Note that in hypovolemia, the CBC will underestimate blood loss. A sample for pretransfusion testing should be obtained and processed as soon as possible. Initial resuscitation is usually provided with crystalloid fluids. Red cell transfusion should be considered if greater than 15% loss of estimated blood volume (about 1000 mL in a typical adult) occurs with ongoing bleeding. RBC transfusions should be fully crossmatched if possible; however, the patient should not suffer adversely for want of serologically compatible RBCs. Transfusion can be started with group O uncrossmatched RBCs. If the patient's Rh type is unknown, Rh(D)-negative RBCs are preferable, especially for females with childbearing potential.

Coagulopathies may occur during massive transfusion as the result of dilution, consumption, or dysfunction. During resuscitation with RBCs and fluids, measured factor levels and platelet counts are often higher than would be expected on a purely dilutional basis (Counts, 1979; Murray, 1995), with considerable variation between patients. Consumptive coagulopathies occur with DIC, burns, brain injury, hyperthermia, and sepsis. These usually manifest by prolonged PT and APTT, lower than expected fibrinogen and platelet counts, and the presence of fibrin degradation products or D-dimers. Platelet or coagulation factor dysfunction can occur in hypothermia, acidosis, liver disease, or renal failure.

No single protocol has been established for plasma or platelet transfusion in massive bleeding. However, in retrospective studies, several protocols have been associated with improved outcomes (Cotton, 2009; Dente, 2009; Riskin, 2009). Such protocols call for transfusion of RBCs, plasma, and platelets in fixed ratios. Several retrospective studies in both military and civilian acute trauma resuscitation have suggested that more aggressive plasma transfusion is associated with lower mortality and improved outcomes (Holcomb, 2008; Cotton, 2009; Zehtabchi, 2009; Zink, 2009; Mitra, 2010). However, many confounding factors in these studies make causal inference problematic. Lacking randomized clinical trials, it is not possible to say definitively that a protocol-driven approach is superior to individualized clinical judgment. In a laboratory-driven approach, plasma is typically given if PT or APTT is greater than 1.5 times the reference range, and platelets are typically given for counts less than 50,000. It may be prudent to reserve platelet transfusion until after surgical control of major bleeding has been attained because it is likely to be ineffective during rapid blood loss. Cryoprecipitate may be given if the fibrinogen is less then 100 mg/dL, but hypofibrinogenemia is usually accompanied by deficiency of other factors, so plasma is often a better choice. Therapy is best guided by frequent assessment of coagulation parameters.

Complications of massive transfusion include hypothermia, hypocalcemia, and acid-base disorders. Hypothermia can be avoided with the use of high-flow warming devices. When the transfusion rate exceeds about 100 mL/minute, a clinically significant drop in ionized calcium may occur as the result of accumulation of citrate, and calcium supplementation may be indicated. Liver disease, hypotension, and hypothermia may exacerbate hypocalcemia. Monitoring the corrected QT interval is useful. Measurement of total calcium will not accurately indicate the level of ionized calcium. During rapid transfusion of RBCs, a modest decrease in arterial pH may be seen (Vretzakis, 2000); metabolic alkalosis is common after massive transfusion because of metabolism of citrate.

NEONATAL AND PEDIATRIC TRANSFUSION

Neonates particularly receive RBC transfusions because of anemia of prematurity, HDN, or iatrogenic blood loss. The unique physiology of the neonatal period and the relative fragility of the developing brain vasculature necessitate some differences from the approach to older children or adults. Guidelines for neonatal transfusion are summarized in Table 36-8. RBC transfusion of 15 mL/kg will typically increase the Hb by 2–3 g/dL, and platelet transfusion of 10 mL/kg will typically increase the platelet

TABLE 36-8
Guidelines for Neonatal Transfusion

RBC Transfusion	
Hct <20% with symptomatic anemia	
Hct <30% with supplemental O_2 <35% or mechanical ventilation with MAP <6 cm H_2O	
Hct <35% with supplemental O_2 >35% or mechanical ventilation with MAP >6 cm H_2O	
Hct <45% with cyanotic congenital heart disease or extracorporeal oxygenation	
Plasma Transfusion	
Coagulation factor deficiency, factor concentrate unavailable	
Disseminated intravascular coagulation (DIC)	
Platelet Transfusion	
Platelet count <30,000/μL in term infant with platelet production failure	
Platelet count <50,000/μL in stable premature infant	
Platelet count <100,000/μL in unstable premature infant	

Adapted from Roseff SD, Lugan NLC, Manno CS. Guidelines for assessing appropriateness of pediatric transfusion. Transfusion 2002;42:1398–413.
Hct, Hematocrit; *MAP,* mean arterial pressure.

count by 40,000–50,000/μL. For large-volume transfusion, as in exchange transfusion or cardiac surgery, selection of fresh RBCs (typically <10 days old) may be indicated. However, with transfusion of 15 mL/kg, most infants tolerate transfusion of RBCs stored until outdate, without adverse effects (Strauss, 1996). For a premature infant with an expected ongoing transfusion requirement, the use of aliquots of a single unit until outdate can significantly reduce donor exposures. Premature and low-birthweight infants are at greater risk of CMV infection and graft-versus-host disease (see later).

Exchange transfusion of the neonate for hyperbilirubinemia is usually indicated if the total bilirubin is greater than 25 mg/dL. Relating the total bilirubin to hours since birth is predictive of kernicterus risk (Bhutani, 1999). A two-blood volume exchange is typically used, which can be expected to reduce the total bilirubin by 25% and the fetal red cell mass by about 70%. Whole blood or RBCs reconstituted with compatible plasma to Hct of 45% can be used.

Transfusion Reactions

Transfusion reactions are a diverse group of adverse reactions to transfusion that usually present during or shortly after transfusion. The workup and treatment of a transfusion reaction must be predicated on the clinical picture, especially in atypical cases. If a transfusion reaction occurs while a transfusion is in progress, the transfusion should be stopped immediately, and the intravenous line should be kept open with saline. It is important to recognize that the unit a patient is reacting to is not necessarily the one that is being infused. All suspected transfusion reactions should be reported to the blood bank or transfusion service.

FEBRILE NONHEMOLYTIC REACTIONS

A febrile transfusion reaction is defined as a rise in temperature of 1° C or greater, possibly accompanied by chills or rigors. Symptoms usually occur during the transfusion but may be delayed for up to 1 hour after the procedure has been completed. A patient who is hypothermic at the start of a transfusion and then manifests an expected temperature rise to normal, without symptoms, is not having a febrile reaction. In some patients, it may be impossible to distinguish between a febrile transfusion reaction and disease-related fever.

It is important to rule out a hemolytic transfusion reaction or bacterial contamination of the unit. Antipyretics, such as acetaminophen (325–500 mg) can be administered. Antipyretics are not necessarily required, as the fever of nonhemolytic transfusion reactions is self-limited and usually resolves within 2–3 hours. Diphenhydramine (50–100 mg) is commonly administered in this setting but probably has no effect on the course of febrile reactions.

Controversy continues as to whether the transfusion can be restarted after a reaction has been diagnosed and the patient has been treated. The principal argument in favor of restarting the transfusion is the reduction in the number of donor exposures, especially if pooled platelet concentrates are involved (Oberman, 1994). Arguments against restarting the transfusion include the possibility that the patient may have a continued febrile reaction to the unit, and, if a hemolytic reaction or bacterial contamination has not been definitely excluded, a severe reaction may ensue (Widmann, 1994). The decision to restart the transfusion should be driven by the clinical condition of the patient and the results of transfusion reaction testing.

Premedication with antipyretics is often used to prevent febrile reactions, although the efficacy of premedication has not been established. A randomized, placebo-controlled trial failed to show prevention of febrile reactions by acetaminophen and diphenhydramine, but the number of subjects may have been insufficient to demonstrate a relatively small difference (Wang, 2002).

Some, but not all, studies have shown a reduction in the incidence of febrile reactions since the introduction of universal leukocyte reduction (Uhlmann, 2001; Dzik, 2002; Ibojie, 2002). It is clear though that leukocyte reduction does not prevent all febrile reactions. Febrile reactions also have been attributed to the accumulation of pyrogenic cytokines in units during storage (Muylle, 1993). These biological mediators are produced primarily by leukocytes. Febrile reactions to platelet transfusion can be reduced by using platelet concentrates less than 4 days old (Kelley, 2000). Filtration at the time of transfusion will not remove pyrogenic cytokines from blood units, although it may remove other cytokines and activated complement components (Snyder, 1996). The use of prestorage leukocyte reduction has been shown to reduce the generation of cytokines in stored platelets and red cells and may be more effective than poststorage leukocyte reduction in preventing febrile reactions (Federowicz, 1995). Accumulated cytokines can be removed by plasma reduction or the washing of cellular blood components (Heddle, 1994). Plasma removal appears to be equivalent to prestorage leukocyte reduction in prevention of febrile reactions (Heddle, 2002). Plasma removal will not prevent all febrile reactions.

ALLERGIC REACTIONS

Mild allergic reactions to transfusion are commonplace. They may occur with any type of blood component, including autologous RBCs (Domen, 2003). Presenting symptoms include pruritus, urticaria, erythema, and cutaneous flushing. About 10% of allergic reactions have pulmonary signs and symptoms but not cutaneous involvement. Gastrointestinal involvement may include nausea, vomiting, abdominal pain, and diarrhea.

Should an allergic reaction occur, the transfusion should be discontinued and intravenous access maintained. If there is upper airway involvement, prompt intubation may be necessary. Oxygen should be administered if there is dyspnea or evidence of desaturation. Mild allergic reactions usually will respond to intravenous antihistaminics such as diphenhydramine (50–100 mg). More severe reactions may require epinephrine. In mild cutaneous reactions, the transfusion usually can be restarted after treatment without recurrence or worsening of the symptoms. In more serious reactions, particularly if there is airway involvement, restarting the transfusion is not advisable.

With the exceptions of IgA and haptoglobin deficiencies, the specific antigen to which the patient is reacting cannot usually be identified. Premedication with an antihistaminic, such as diphenhydramine, 25–50 mg, administered orally or intravenously, may prevent mild allergic reactions. Steroids such as methylprednisolone (125 mg) may help patients who manifest repeated allergic reactions, although the efficacy of steroids has not been proven.

Patients who have had repeated or significant allergic reactions may benefit from the concentration of cellular blood components through the removal of most of the plasma or by the washing of red cells and platelets. However, the routine use of washed components for patients with cutaneous allergic reactions is unwarranted.

SEVERE ALLERGIC (ANAPHYLACTIC) REACTIONS

In addition to the signs of typical milder allergic reactions, anaphylactic or anaphylactoid reactions manifest cardiovascular instability, including hypotension, tachycardia, loss of consciousness, cardiac arrhythmia, shock, and cardiac arrest. Respiratory involvement with dyspnea or stridor may be more pronounced than is seen usually in typical allergic reactions.

If an anaphylactic reaction occurs, the transfusion should be discontinued and intravenous access maintained. Supportive care, including intubation, oxygen, intravenous fluids, and placement of the patient in the Trendelenburg position, should be instituted promptly. Epinephrine should be available immediately. For hypotension unresponsive to supportive measures or for significant bronchospasm, subcutaneous epinephrine 0.3–0.5 mg (0.3–0.5 mL of a 1 : 1000 solution) can be given. This dose can be repeated every 20–30 minutes for up to three doses. Alternatively, 0.5 mg of epinephrine may be given intravenously (5 mL of a 1 : 10,000 solution) and repeated every 5–10 minutes for refractory hypotension.

An antihistamine such as diphenhydramine, 50–100 mg, can be given intravenously, particularly when there are cutaneous manifestations such as urticaria. Aminophylline (6 mg/kg loading dose) may be useful when there is bronchospasm. Steroids are probably not effective in the acute situation, but if symptoms persist, a drug such as hydrocortisone (500 mg) may be given.

Patients with IgA deficiency who develop anti-IgA can have anaphylactic reactions (Vyas, 1969). Patients who have significant allergic reactions should be evaluated for their quantitative IgA levels. Recent transfusion may elevate serum IgA levels falsely. However, if IgA deficiency has been established, anti-IgA testing should be done, usually by a reference laboratory. IgA-deficient plasma can be obtained from rare donor registries, if necessary. Red cells and platelets can be washed to remove sufficient amounts of IgA to prevent reactions.

Patients with haptoglobin deficiency can have similar anaphylactic transfusion reactions due to IgG or IgE antihaptoglobin (Shimada, 2002). Haptoglobin deficiency is rare in North American populations but is more common than IgA deficiency among Japanese patients suffering anaphylactic reactions.

ACUTE HEMOLYTIC REACTIONS

Acute hemolytic transfusion reactions (AHTRs), by definition, present within 24 hours of transfusion. Intravascular hemolysis is much more common in acute hemolytic reactions than is extravascular hemolysis. Presenting signs include fever and chills, nausea, vomiting, pain, dyspnea, tachycardia, hypotension, bleeding, and hemoglobinuria. Fever may be the initial sign of an AHTR. Therefore, any increase in temperature of 1° C or greater should result in a red cell transfusion being stopped and a laboratory evaluation initiated. Renal failure is a later complication. Pain during an AHTR has been reported as localizing to the flanks, back, abdomen, chest, head, and infusion site. A subjective feeling of distress is reported sometimes. Unexpected bleeding may be due to DIC. During surgery, hypotension and excessive bleeding may be the only signs of an AHTR. Both may be attributed to other causes; therefore, physicians must be mindful of the possibility of a hemolytic reaction in this circumstance.

Laboratory findings in AHTRs include hemoglobinemia, hemoglobinuria, elevated lactate dehydrogenase, hyperbilirubinemia, and low haptoglobin. The blood urea nitrogen and creatinine will be elevated if renal injury has occurred. The direct antiglobulin test (DAT) may show positive results with a mixed-field pattern if transfused incompatible red cells are present in the circulation. Red cell antibody identification studies may or may not show positive results, depending on the specificity of the antibody involved and the amount of antibody in the serum. ABO incompatibility due to a clerical error is the most common cause of AHTRs.

In the event of an AHTR, the transfusion should be discontinued and intravenous access maintained. The identity of the patient and the unit or units of RBCs should be reconfirmed, and other units of RBCs that have been dispensed for the patient should be located and quarantined. The reaction must be reported to the blood bank promptly. If a misidentification is discovered, another patient (e.g., with a similar name) may also be at risk of receiving incompatible blood.

Treatment of an AHTR must be guided by the clinical response of the patient. Patients who have minimal symptoms may be managed best by careful observation. However, in severe reactions, early vigorous intervention may be lifesaving. It bears repeating that the severity of AHTRs is related directly to the volume of incompatible blood transfused. Thus, early recognition, discontinuation of the transfusion, and prevention of the transfusion of additional incompatible units are the essential first steps of treatment. Initial attention must be paid to cardiovascular support. If hypotension is present, fluid resuscitation and pressor support may be indicated. Care should be taken to avoid fluid overload, however, especially in patients with impaired cardiac or renal function.

Because the load of incompatible red cells in the circulation dictates the severity and course of AHTRs, an exchange transfusion with antigen-negative blood may be considered. Again, the decision to perform an exchange transfusion must be guided by the clinical response of the patient. It is not appropriate to expose a patient to the added risk of infectious disease if the hemolytic process is well tolerated. With ABO incompatibility, however, an exchange transfusion may greatly reduce the chance of morbidity or death.

Because renal failure is a significant problem in some patients, attention should be given to prevention. Early treatments of hypotension and DIC are the most important interventions to limit the extent of possible renal impairment. Maintenance of urine output with intravenous fluids and diuretics, mannitol or furosemide, early in the course of the reaction has been used successfully. Hydration with normal saline and 5% dextrose (1 : 1 ratio) at a rate of 3000 mL/m^2 per day and administration of sodium bicarbonate to maintain the urine pH above 7.0 have been recommended (Nussbaumer, 1995). Infusion of an initial dose of 20% mannitol 100 mL/m^2 given over 30–60 minutes followed by 30 mL/m^2 per hour for the next 12 hours has also been recommended (Slavc, 1992). However, if oliguria in the face of euvolemia is present, fluid loading may be contraindicated.

Further transfusion of red cells should be avoided until the cause of the reaction has been established. Foremost, however, no patient should be allowed to exsanguinate for lack of serologically compatible blood. Group O RBCs lacking other known clinically significant antigens to which the patient currently has an antibody should be obtained, if possible. The results of serologic tests performed up to this point must be considered, and clinical judgment exercised. Although the focus of attention in most AHTRs is on red cells, care should be taken to avoid the transfusion of plasma or platelets that may aggravate hemolysis, especially when ABO incompatibility is a possible cause. Undue haste in both serologic evaluation and decision-making must be avoided because human errors are committed most often under pressure.

DELAYED HEMOLYTIC REACTIONS

By definition, delayed hemolytic transfusion reactions (DHTRs) occur at least 24 hours after transfusion of the offending unit. The time from transfusion to diagnosis of a DHTR is variable. Most patients present within the first 2 weeks after receiving the transfusion. However, clinical DHTR may be recognized more than 6 weeks later. Almost all DHTRs are due to an anamnestic response to a red cell antigen to which the patient has previously made an antibody, the concentration of which was too low to detect in pretransfusion testing. Rarely, a DHTR may be due to primary alloimmunization to a red cell antigen. Typically, hemolysis is extravascular, but intravascular hemolysis may occur also. Fortunately, these reactions tend to be much less severe than AHTRs; accordingly, they may be overlooked. Some patients will present with only unexpected anemia. Other clinical signs include fever or chills, jaundice, pain, or dyspnea. Rarely renal failure may ensue. In patients with sickle cell disease, DHTRs may precipitate a sickle crisis (Mintz, 1986).

Laboratory findings in DHTRs include anemia, elevated lactate dehydrogenase, hyperbilirubinemia, low haptoglobin, leukocytosis, the presence of a new red cell antibody, and a positive reaction on a DAT. The degree of hyperbilirubinemia will depend on the rate and amount of hemolysis, as well as on liver function. Typically, unconjugated bilirubin levels are elevated during active hemolysis. Depressed haptoglobin levels do not necessarily indicate intravascular hemolysis, as they may be seen with extravascular hemolysis as well.

Many patients tolerate DHTRs well and may need only to be followed carefully. Generally, fluid loading and diuresis are not indicated unless there is active intravascular hemolysis. Complications, such as renal failure or sickle crisis, should be treated as such. If there is a large burden of antigen-positive red cells, an exchange transfusion should be considered. In general, transfusion should be avoided until the causative antibody can be identified and antigen-negative units obtained. However, as with AHTRs, a patient should not be allowed to have significant morbidity from anemia for lack of serologically compatible blood. The selection of red cells for transfusion needs to be based on the results of serologic testing and good communication between the medical director of the blood bank and the patient's physician.

Because extravascular hemolysis is similar to autoimmune hemolytic anemia, in which high-dose intravenous immunoglobulin (IVIG) infusion may be useful, IVIG may be considered in the treatment of DHTRs also. A single dose of IVIG, 400 mg/kg, infused within 24 hours of transfusion, has been used successfully to prevent transfusion reactions in alloimmunized patients for whom compatible blood could not be obtained (Kohan, 1994). Five patients so treated had sustained increases in Hct. No transfusion reaction developed in any of the cases.

BACTERIAL CONTAMINATION OF BLOOD COMPONENTS

The clinical presentation of a transfusion reaction caused by bacterially contaminated blood components is usually dramatic. Onset of symptoms in most cases occurs during the transfusion or shortly after it; delayed presentation of more than 1 day has rarely been reported with contaminated platelet transfusions. Fever, chills, hypotension, shock, nausea, and vomiting are the most commonly reported symptoms (Kuehnert, 2001; Perez, 2001). Dyspnea, pain, and diarrhea also may occur. High fever and hypotension during or shortly after transfusion are particular clues that a contaminated unit may have been transfused. The clinical complications due to bacterial contamination are significant, often resulting in shock, renal failure, DIC, and death. The mortality rate is high and depends on the type of component involved, the identity and amount of the causative organism, and the clinical condition of the patient. Patient factors associated with clinical reactions include thrombocytopenia and pancytopenia. Risk factors for fatality include contamination by gram-negative rods, greater patient age, smaller volume of component transfused, and younger age of stored platelet concentrate. The latter two factors most likely reflect greater numbers of organisms in the component. The organism involved depends on the type and storage of the blood component. RBCs have been found to contain *Acinetobacter*, *Escherichia*, *Staphylococcus*, *Yersinia*, and *Pseudomonas* species. Gram-positive cocci such as *Staphylococcus* and *Streptococcus*, gram-negative rods such as *Acinetobacter*, *Klebsiella*, *Salmonella*, *Escherichia*, and *Serratia*, and gram-positive rods such as *Propionibacterium* have been reported in platelet concentrates (Kuehnert, 2001; Andreu, 2002). Some transfusion services culture for bacteria all platelet concentrates that have caused a febrile transfusion reaction because, if a red cell concentrate from the same donation exists, it can be withdrawn.

Usually, treatment must be initiated before the causative organism has been identified. If a reaction occurs, the transfusion should be discontinued, the unit with its associated tubing should be removed, and any other blood bags that have been recently transfused should be recovered. Supportive care of circulation and respiration should be initiated as required. Antibiotic therapy initially should include broad-spectrum coverage such as a β-lactam and an aminoglycoside until microbiological stains or cultures indicate the causative organism.

AABB standards require that blood banks and transfusion services have methods to detect and limit bacterial contamination of platelets. FDA approved methods include culture, measurement of oxygen consumption, and rapid qualitative immunoassay (AuBuchon, 2002; Ortolano, 2003). Measurements of pH or glucose and inspection for "swirling" have been used as indicators of contamination but are not sufficiently sensitive to meet current AABB standards (Wagner, 1996). Some studies have found that apheresis platelets have a lower incidence of septic reactions than pooled whole blood–derived platelets (Ness, 2001). Because skin flora, if present, enter the collection at venipuncture, diversion of the first 8 mL decreases the risk by 50% (Eder, 2009). Most blood centers culture apheresis platelets and prepooled platelets at the time of manufacture. The components then are held for a brief time (typically 12 hours) and are released for distribution if the culture is negative. Although this approach is operationally efficient, it is not optimal in that the culture is taken at a time when the bacterial load is low. The residual risk of a septic reaction with culture-negative apheresis platelets is approximately 1:75,000 (Eder, 2007). A rapid immunoassay has recently been approved by the FDA for detection of bacterial contamination in platelets (Platelet PGD Test, Verax Biomedical Incorporated, Worcester, MA). Although this test holds promise for significantly reducing the risk of septic reactions, this has not yet been shown in peer-reviewed publications. Pathogen reduction technology in the future may significantly reduce, if not eliminate, bacterial contamination.

TRANSFUSION-RELATED ACUTE LUNG INJURY

Transfusion-related acute lung injury (TRALI) usually presents during or within hours of transfusion. Its symptoms include dyspnea, hypoxemia, tachycardia, fever, hypotension, and cyanosis (Kleinman, 2004). Fever and hypotension, when present, are usually moderate and respond quickly to antipyretics and fluids. Characteristically, there is a lack of abnormal breath sounds. A chest X-ray usually shows pulmonary edema. By definition, there are no signs of cardiac failure. Patients with hematologic malignancy or cardiac disease appear to be at higher risk for TRALI (Silliman, 2003). This may reflect the fact that these patient groups receive the majority of platelet transfusions. Reported mortality is approximately 20%, depending on the severity of the lung injury and the underlying clinical status of the patient. A wide range of severity is seen in this transfusion reaction; milder forms may not be readily recognized.

The differential diagnosis includes circulatory overload, bacterial contamination, allergic reactions, acute respiratory distress syndrome (ARDS), pulmonary embolism, and pulmonary hemorrhage. The diagnosis is established by findings of noncardiogenic pulmonary edema. Pulmonary artery wedge pressure is not elevated. Characteristically, TRALI resolves within 48–96 hours from outset (Popovsky, 1992). Failure of the patient to improve substantially after this time should call the diagnosis into question. Although chest X-ray findings may persist beyond 7 days, unlike with ARDS, no permanent pulmonary sequelae are evident. A decrease in leukocyte or platelet count may be a useful clue in TRALI caused by transfusion of HLA class I antibodies (Cooling, 2002).

The treatment of TRALI is supportive. If a transfusion is in progress, it should be discontinued, and blood bags from recently transfused units should be recovered. The blood bank should be consulted regarding the evaluation of TRALI. Usually, oxygen is indicated. Severely affected patients may require mechanical ventilation. Corticosteroids appear to be of little, if any, value. Diuresis is not indicated in the absence of signs of fluid overload.

TRALI has been attributed to the presence of antibodies in the plasma of the transfused unit that are directed against HLA or granulocyte antigens present on recipient leukocytes (Kopko, 2002). Plasma from multiparous female donors may carry a greater risk of TRALI (Palfi, 2001). It also has been attributed to the presence in the unit of lipid inflammatory mediators that activate already primed recipient neutrophils (from surgery, trauma, or inflammation) to cause capillary injury and leakage (Silliman, 2003).

GRAFT-VERSUS-HOST DISEASE

Transfusion-associated graft-versus-host disease can occur when viable donor T cells proliferate, are not recognized by the recipient's immune system as foreign, but recognize and reject the host as foreign. Patients with marked cellular immunodeficiencies are at risk of TA-GVHD (Table 36-9). These include congenital cellular immunodeficiencies (DiGeorge syndrome, severe combined immunodeficiency syndrome), immaturity of the immune system (intrauterine transfusions, very-low-birthweight infants), disease-associated immunodeficiencies (Hodgkin lymphoma), and therapy-associated cellular immunodeficiencies (hematopoietic progenitor cell transplantation, fludarabine treatment). Humoral immunodeficiencies, such as common variable immunodeficiency (CVID), are not a risk factor for GVHD. HIV infection, although it may cause marked T cell dysfunction, does not increase the risk of TA-GVHD. Common immunosuppressive regimens for solid organ transplantation and typical chemotherapy regimens for solid tumors do not increase the risk of TA-GVHD. However, TA-GVHD has been reported with highly aggressive chemotherapy for neuroblastoma and some other tumors. Patients with normal immunity may be at risk of TA-GVHD if the recipient is homozygous for an HLA haplotype and the donor is heterozygous but shares one haplotype. In this case, recipient lymphocytes are unable to recognize transfused lymphocytes as foreign, but transfused cells see recipient cells as foreign (Fig. 36-1). This is most likely to occur with donations from close (first- or second-degree) relatives but may also occur owing to chance, particularly in populations that are relatively homogeneous (Aoun, 2003).

TA-GVHD typically manifests 2–50 days after transfusion. Characteristic findings include rash, diarrhea, fever, liver dysfunction, and pancytopenia. Mortality is greater than 90%, with most patients dying of infection. In contrast to the expected GVHD of allogeneic HPC transplantation, the bone marrow in TA-GVHD is of recipient type and is a target organ. Aggressive immunosuppressive treatments have been tried but with rare exceptions have been unsuccessful. Thus, preventive measures are of paramount importance.

The minimum number of viable transfused T cells necessary to cause TA-GVHD has not been established, but it is clear that current leukocyte reduction methods are not sufficient (Hayashi, 1993). Exposure to ionizing radiation (γ-rays or X-rays) can cause chromosomal damage and prevent replication of transfused leukocytes. Current FDA guidance suggests a midplane dose of 25 Gy, with a minimum dose of 15 Gy to any point of the blood container (see earlier discussion of special components). It is possible that pathogen reduction technology based on nucleic acid modification may be effective in preventing TA-GVHD, but this remains to be established.

TABLE 36-9
Indications for Irradiation of Blood Components for Prevention of TA-GVHD

Absolute Indications
Congenital cellular immunodeficiency
Hematopoietic progenitor cell transplantation
Hodgkin lymphoma
Granulocyte transfusions
Intrauterine transfusions (IUTs)
Transfusion to neonates who have received IUT
Transfusions from biological relatives
Chemotherapy with purine analogs (fludarabine)
Probable Indications
Low-birthweight infants (<1200 g)
Hematologic malignancies other than Hodgkin lymphoma
HLA-matched platelet concentrates
High-dose chemotherapy, radiation therapy, and/or aggressive immunotherapy
Controversial Indications
Solid organ transplantation
Large-volume or exchange transfusion of infants who did not receive IUT
Aplastic anemia
Absolute lymphopenia (Absolute lymphocyte count <500/mL)
Irradiation NOT Indicated
HIV infection
Hemophilia
Small-volume transfusions of term infants who did not receive IUT
Elderly patients
Typical dose immunosuppressive therapy (other than purine analogs)
Immunocompetent surgical patients
Pregnancy
Red cell membrane, metabolic, or hemoglobin disorders (e.g., thalassemia, SCD)

Adapted from Gorlin JB, Mintz PD. Transfusion-associated graft-vs-host disease. In: Mintz PD, editor. Transfusion therapy: clinical principles and practice. 3rd ed. Bethesda, Md: AABB Press; 2011, p. 650.
HIV, Human immunodeficiency virus; *SCD,* sickle cell disease; *TA-GVHD,* transfusion-associated graft-versus-host disease.

HYPOTENSIVE REACTIONS

Transfusion-associated hypotension is defined as hypotension that occurs during transfusion in the absence of signs or symptoms of other transfusion reactions, such as fever, chills, dyspnea, urticaria, or flushing. The degree of hypotension required for the diagnosis is controversial but could be defined reasonably as a drop of at least 10 mm Hg in systolic or diastolic arterial blood pressure from the pretransfusion baseline. However, if the immediate pretransfusion blood pressure is elevated from the patient's typical blood pressure and the arterial pressure does not fall below the patient's usual blood pressure, this should not be considered a hypotensive reaction. Hypotension begins during the transfusion and resolves quickly when the transfusion is discontinued. If hypotension persists beyond 30 minutes after discontinuation of the transfusion, another diagnosis should be strongly considered. Hypotensive reactions have been associated with red cell and platelet transfusions. Some reactions have been associated with the use of leukocyte reduction filters (Fried, 1996; Abe, 1997).

If hypotension occurs, the transfusion should be discontinued and intravenous access maintained. The patient should be positioned with head down and feet elevated (Trendelenburg position), and isotonic fluids should be administered. Pressor support is indicated only if the hypotension is severe and refractory to intravenous fluids.

The cause of transfusion-associated hypotension has not been established definitively. However, the condition is most likely due to the release of bradykinin through activation of the contact pathway of coagulation. Some reactions have been associated with angiotensin-converting enzyme (ACE) inhibitor drugs in the recipient and/or the use of leukocyte reduction filters. ACE is the major enzyme that breaks down bradykinin in the circulation. Some filters, particularly those with a net-negative surface charge, appear to cause activation of kallikrein and cleavage of high

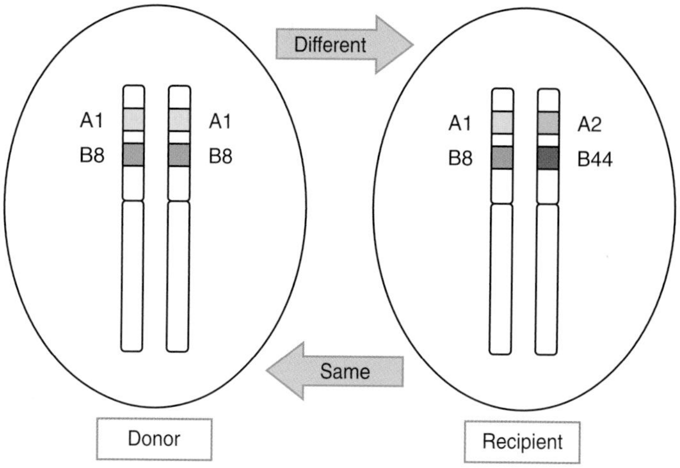

Figure 36-1 Mechanism of TA-GVHD in immunocompetent patients. The donor is homozygous at the HLA class I locus. The recipient is heterozygous and shares one haplotype with the donor. Engrafted donor T cells recognize the recipient as foreign, but the recipient's T cells do not identify donor T cells as foreign. (*HLA,* Human leukocyte antigens; *TA-GVHD,* transfusion-associated graft-versus-host disease.)

molecular weight kininogen, which results in the release of bradykinin (Davenport, 1997; Shiba, 1997; Mair, 1998). However, there is variability because not all such filtered units show activation.

NONIMMUNE HEMOLYSIS

Lysis of red cells can occur as a result of storage, handling, or transfusion conditions. Hyperosmotic or hypo-osmotic fluids mixed with red cells can result in significant lysis. Patients who receive lysed red cells may tolerate them remarkably well. However, transient hemodynamic, pulmonary, and renal impairment may occur, and death due to transfusion of lysed red cells has been reported (Sazama, 1990). The transfusion of autologous blood from a patient with sickle Hb can result in hemolysis and death (DeChristopher, 1990). The clinical signs are usually hemoglobinemia and hemoglobinuria. Hyperkalemia may occur, particularly in patients with renal failure. Fever also may occur. Finding lysis of RBCs in the transfused unit and excluding other causes, such as hemolytic transfusion reactions, establishes the diagnosis. All RBC units will show a slight degree in hemolysis with prolonged storage, but this will not result in clinical signs after transfusion. The principal reported complications of nonimmune hemolysis are renal failure and cardiac arrhythmia due to hyperkalemia. Hemolytic transfusion reactions can rarely occur when no red cell antibody is identifiable (Davey, 1980). Differentiation of this condition from nonimmune hemolysis may be impossible without careful investigation of the transfusion circumstances.

Should nonimmune hemolysis occur, the transfusion should be discontinued and intravenous access maintained. The blood bag, together with attached tubing and intravenous fluids, should be saved for further investigation. A hemolytic transfusion reaction needs to be ruled out. The serum potassium level should be checked and an electrocardiogram obtained to assess hyperkalemia. Care is supportive. Urine output should be maintained with hydration unless there is a contraindication such as renal failure.

TRANSFUSION-ASSOCIATED CIRCULATORY OVERLOAD

Circulatory overload is an all-too-common and preventable transfusion reaction. It presents as congestive heart failure during or shortly after transfusion. Signs and symptoms can include dyspnea, orthopnea, cyanosis, tachycardia, elevated blood pressure, pulmonary edema, jugular venous distention, pedal edema, and headache. The differential diagnosis includes TRALI, allergic reactions, and causes of congestive failure not related to transfusion, such as valvular heart disease. Clearly, patients with preexisting heart disease are at risk of circulatory overload with transfusion. The diagnosis of circulatory overload on clinical and radiologic examination may be difficult. Elevation of brain natriuretic peptide can be helpful in making the diagnosis (Zhou, 2005; Tobian, 2008).

TABLE 36-10
Approximate Current Per-Unit Risks of Infectious Disease Transmission

HIV	1:1,467,000
HBV	1:280,000–1:357,000
HCV	1:1,149,000
HTLV-I/II	1:641,000–1:1,900,000
West Nile virus	≈1:7,000,000

Data from Busch (2005), Zou (2009) and Zou (2010).
HBV, Hepatitis B virus; *HCV,* hepatitis C virus; *HIV,* human immunodeficiency virus; *HTLV,* human T cell lymphotropic virus.

Volume overload should be anticipated in at-risk patients and prevented readily. Blood should be transfused slowly. Although a transfusion usually should be completed within 4 hours, the duration may be extended if medically indicated. If longer than 6 hours is required, however, alternative strategies should be considered. Small volumes can be transfused with adequate time between transfusions to allow for diuresis. To avoid additional donor exposures, a unit can be split using sterile technique and a portion retained in the blood bank for later transfusion. Units can also be concentrated by plasma removal. A diuretic can be administered before or during the transfusion.

TRANSFUSION-TRANSMITTED DISEASE

Improvements in donor screening and testing have resulted in dramatic reductions in transfusion-transmitted disease risk over the past two decades. For example, the risk of transmitting HIV by blood transfusion in the United States has been reduced from approximately 1 in 100 in certain urban areas in the early 1980s to approximately 1 in 1,500,000 throughout the country at present. It is virtually impossible to accurately measure current risks of hepatitis and HIV transmission by epidemiologic methods. Risk estimates for HIV, HBV, and HCV are now based on mathematical models that take into account the probability of marker-negative window-phase donations, viral strains not reliably detected by current assays, persistent antibody-negative carriers, and testing errors (Dodd, 2002). Current (2010) risk estimates are summarized in Table 36-10.

Hepatitis

Historically, HCV has accounted for the majority of cases of posttransfusion hepatitis (PTH). Approximately 10% of chronic HCV is attributable to blood transfusion (Alter, 1999). PTH is asymptomatic in the majority of cases. Three patterns of transaminase elevation have been observed: monophasic, polyphasic, and plateau (Pastore, 1985). Approximately 75%–85% of individuals have persistent HCV infection, and about 50% of these have evidence of chronic hepatitis. As many as 10% of patients with HCV PTH eventually manifest clinical liver disease (Seeff, 1992). Acute PTH due to HBV is typically more severe, with 25%–30% of individuals having jaundice, and with an incubation time of 40–60 days (Walsh, 1970; Seeff, 1975). Less than 10% of infected individuals progress to chronic hepatitis. If acquired before the age of 5 years, acute HBV infection is usually less severe, but the risk of chronic hepatitis is much greater. Hepatitis D virus (HDV) requires coinfection with HBV for replication. If acquired simultaneously with HBV, HDV can cause severe hepatitis and liver failure. If acquired during chronic HBV infection (superinfection), HDV significantly increases the risk of severe chronic liver disease. Transfusion-transmitted HDV is rare, and screening methods for HBV are also effective against HDV. Hepatitis A virus and hepatitis E virus have relatively short periods of viremia and do not progress to a chronic carrier state. Transmission of these viruses by transfusion is rare but has occurred (Sherertz, 1984; Matsubayashi, 2004). Hepatitis G virus (GBV-C) has a prevalence rate of about 1% in asymptomatic blood donors (Roth, 1997). Although it is clearly transmissible by transfusion, no causal relationship between GBV-C infection and hepatitis or chronic liver disease has been established (Alter, 1997).

Human Immunodeficiency Virus

The clinical manifestations of transfusion-transmitted HIV are similar to those of HIV infection acquired through other routes. An acute viral syndrome occurs in about 60% of cases. Untreated, asymptomatic infection persists for about 10 years before acquired immunodeficiency syndrome (AIDS)-defining illness occurs, although progression tends to be more rapid in older individuals (Blaxhult, 1990). The time to AIDS progression for transfusion recipients may be shorter than that for the implicated donor, but this may reflect the effects of age and other cofactors (Busch, 1994). Until recently, Group O viral isolates were not reliably detected by enzyme immunoassay (EIA) tests. Currently, the prevalence of group O HIV in the United States is low, but it is endemic in some parts of western Africa, and transfusion-transmission by emigrants from such areas has occurred (Pau, 1996). Therefore, residence in or emigration from such areas has been a reason for permanent donor deferral. However, a combined immunoassay for simultaneous detection of HIV p24 antigen and HIV-1 and HIV-2 antibodies that detects group O HIV has been FDA approved for donor testing (Sickinger, 2008). Blood centers implementing this test can discontinue geographic deferral for HIV group O.

Human T Cell Lymphotropic Virus

Human T-cell lymphotropic virus type I (HTLV-I) is causally associated with adult T cell lymphoma/leukemia and HTLV-associated myelopathy (HAM) (Hall, 1996; Manns, 1999). Most carriers are asymptomatic. ATL or HAM develops in a small minority of cases after a latent period of many years. HTLV-I is rare in the United States. HTLV-II is prevalent in intravenous drug users in the United States and is also associated with HAM (Murphy, 1997). Blood donors who are HTLV-II positive have a higher incidence of acute bronchitis, pneumonia, bladder or kidney infection, and arthritis; HTLV-I–positive donors have a higher incidence of bladder or kidney infection and arthritis (Murphy, 2004).

Cytomegalovirus

CMV is common in the general population. In immunologically competent individuals, it causes minor symptoms but becomes latent in virtually all cases (Larsson, 1998). Approximately 50% of blood donors are CMV seropositive, although the estimated risk of transmission by a seropositive transfusion is about 1% (Preiksaitis, 1988). In patients with cellular immunodeficiency, CMV can cause pneumonitis, hepatitis, retinitis, and multisystem organ failure. CMV transmission can be minimized by the use of seronegative blood components, although many studies have shown a low rate of CMV infection in such patients. Whether this is due to failure to detect potentially infectious donors or whether viral transmission occurred by other routes is unclear. Several studies, including a prospective randomized trial, have shown that leukocyte-reduced blood components are as effective as seronegative components in reducing the risk of CMV transmission (Bowden, 1995).

Parvovirus B-19

Parvovirus B-19 is also common in the general population. The incidence of viremia among blood donors is variable, with episodic peaks, but it averages around 1:5000 (Hitzler, 2002). In most individuals, parvovirus B-19 causes a mild self-limited febrile illness. However, it is trophic for erythrocyte precursors in the bone marrow and can cause aplasia, particularly in the setting of accelerated erythropoiesis. Transfusion-transmitted parvovirus infection has been implicated in causing chronic anemia after bone marrow transplantation and in thalassemia (Zanella, 1995; Cohen, 1997).

West Nile Virus

West Nile virus (WNV) arrived in the United States in 1999. From its initial outbreak in New York, it has spread across the country. Birds are the natural reservoir, with mosquitoes serving as the vector of transmission. Humans are an accidental host, with infection occurring during times of mosquito activity. Most acute WNV infections are asymptomatic, with a febrile illness occurring in about 1 in 5 infections and neuroinvasive disease in about 1 in 150 infections (Petersen, 2002). In 2002, 23 confirmed cases of transfusion-transmitted WNV were reported by the Centers for Disease Control and Prevention (Pealer, 2003). In areas of peak WNV activity in 2002, the estimated rate of viremia among blood donors was 1.5 in 1000 (Biggerstaff, 2002). Donor screening for WNV by nucleic acid testing (NAT) was implemented in July of 2003 in North America. Subsequently, rare cases of WNV transmission by blood transfusion have been reported, most likely due to the low viral copy number that escaped detection (Macedo de Oliveira, 2004).

Malaria

About 1300 cases of malaria are reported annually in the United States. Transfusion-transmission of malaria still occurs rarely (1–2 cases annually). Implicated donors usually have a history of travel to an endemic area (Mungai, 2001).

Babesiosis

Babesia species are endemic in North American mammals and are transmitted by ticks of the genus *Ixodes*. Many cases of babesiosis are asymptomatic or mild. However, it may be more severe in the asplenic or immunosuppressed patient. The parasite is capable of survival in refrigerated red cells. About 40 cases of transfusion-transmitted babesiosis have been reported in the United States, although it is possible that transmission in endemic areas may be as high as 1 in 1800 red cell units (Cable, 2001; Lux, 2003).

Trypanosoma cruzi

T. cruzi is the cause of Chagas' disease and is endemic in parts of Central and South America. There may be 50,000–100,000 chronic carriers of *T. cruzi* in the United States, largely as the result of immigration (Kirchhoff, 1987). Rare cases of transfusion-transmitted Chagas' disease have been reported in the United States (Nickerson, 1989). The risk is dependent on the demographics of the donor population. Seropositivity rates among blood donors have been estimated to be 1 : 25,000 nationally and as high as 1 : 2000 in Los Angeles (Leiby, 2002; Centers for Disease Control and Prevention, 2006–2007). Since the FDA approval of a donor screening EIA test, more than 1000 confirmed positive donors have been detected in the United States (AABB Chagas Biovigilance Network, 2010). Estimates of the residual risk of transfusion-transmitted Chagas' disease since implementation of donor testing in the United States have not been published to date.

Transmissible Spongiform Encephalopathies

Transmissible spongiform encephalopathies are caused by a protein, called a prion, that is capable of assuming an abnormal configuration that is resistant to enzymatic degradation and serves as a template for further abnormal prion deposition. Variant Creutzfeldt-Jakob disease (vCJD) is a human TSE that emerged from an epidemic of bovine spongiform encephalopathy, probably as a result of entry of the pathogenic prion into the human food supply from affected cattle. The transmissibility of vCJD by blood in experimental models suggests a possible risk of transmission by transfusion. The magnitude of such a risk is presently unknown. However, four cases of prion acquisition have been reported in individuals who received transfusions from donors who were themselves diagnosed with vCJD (Chohan, 2010). However, it is notable that no cases of transfusion transmission of sporadic or familial CJD have been found to date, despite ongoing surveillance (Dorsey, 2009).

Conclusion

Discovery of the A, B, and O blood groups by Carl Landsteiner in 1900 led to the widespread use of blood transfusion therapy early in the 20th century. This treatment directly afforded a remarkable evolution in surgical, trauma, and medical care. Although remarkable progress has been made in identifying and reducing transfusion-transmitted infection, the incidence of the principal noninfectious risks—TRALI and mistransfusion due to clerical error—has remained stable for many years. Increasing attention has been focused recently on these latter hazards, and it is hoped that this will lead to a substantial reduction in their occurrence. Despite the continuing risks of transfusion, a much greater threat is posed by withholding a blood component that is clinically indicated than by transfusing it.

SELECTED REFERENCES

Adams RJ, McKie VC, Hsu L, et al. Prevention of a first stroke by transfusions in children with sickle cell anemia and abnormal results on transcranial Doppler ultrasonography. N Engl J Med 1998;339:5–11.

This prospective randomized trial showed that chronic transfusion to maintain Hb S <30% reduced the risk of stroke in children with sickle cell disease.

Bowden RA, Slichter SJ, Sayers M, et al. A comparison of filtered leukocyte-reduced and cytomegalovirus (CMV) seronegative blood products for the prevention of transfusion-associated CMV infection after marrow transplant. Blood 1995;86:3598–603.

This prospective randomized trial demonstrated that leukocyte reduction is equivalent to CMV seronegative blood components in preventing CMV transmission. However, CMV disease was more common in the group receiving leukocyte-reduced components, which is a point of controversy.

Dzik WH, Anderson JK, O'Neill EM, et al. A prospective, randomized clinical trial of universal WBC reduction. Transfusion 2002;42:1114–22.

This prospective randomized trial showed that universal leukocyte reduction was associated with fewer febrile transfusion reactions, but not with in-hospital mortality, length of stay, or hospital costs. These latter points are controversial.

Hebert PC, Wells G, Blajchman MA, et al. A multicenter, randomized, controlled clinical trial of transfusion requirements in critical care. N Engl J Med 1999;340:409–17.

This prospective randomized trial showed that a restrictive strategy of red-cell transfusion is at least as effective as, and possibly superior to, a liberal transfusion strategy in critically ill patients, with the possible exception of patients with acute myocardial infarction and unstable angina.

Heddle NM, Klama L, Singer J, et al. The role of the plasma from platelet concentrates in transfusion reactions. N Engl J Med 1994; 331:670–1.

This prospective randomized trial showed that most febrile reactions to platelet transfusion are due to a constituent in the plasma supernatant, most likely pyrogenic cytokines released during storage.

Kleinman S, Caulfield T, Chan P, et al. Towards an understanding of transfusion related acute lung injury: statement of a consensus panel. Transfusion 2004;44: 1774–89.

This consensus panel statement summarizes the current understanding of the causes, incidence, outcomes, and strategies for reducing transfusion-related acute lung injury.

Linden JV, Wagner K, Voytovich AE, Sheehan J. Transfusion errors in New York State: an analysis of 10 years' experience. Transfusion 2000;40:1207–13.

This analysis of transfusion errors reported to the New York State Department of Health showed that transfusion errors are a significant risk. Most errors result from human actions and thus may be preventable. A majority of events occur outside the blood bank.

McCullough J, Vesole DH, Benjamin RJ, et al. Therapeutic efficacy and safety of platelets treated with a photochemical process for pathogen inactivation: the SPRINT trial. Blood 2004;104:1534–41.

This prospective randomized trial showed that photochemically treated platelets are substantially equivalent to conventional platelets, although posttransfusion platelet count increments and days to next transfusion were decreased compared with conventional platelets.

Petz LD, Garratty G, Calhoun L, et al. Selecting donors of platelets for refractory patients on the basis of HLA antibody specificity. Transfusion 2000;40:1446–56.

This retrospective study showed that a strategy of selecting platelet donors based on the recipient's HLA antibody specificities was as effective as HLA matching or cross-matching and allowed for a much larger pool of potential donors.

Rebulla P, Finazzi G, Marangoni F, et al. The threshold for prophylactic platelet transfusions in adults with acute myeloid leukemia. N Engl J Med 1997;337: 1870–5.

This prospective randomized trial demonstrated that prophylactic platelet transfusion at <10,000/μL is as safe and effective as transfusion at <10,000/μL in acute leukemia and substantially reduces the number of transfusions.

Trial to Reduce Alloimmunization to Platelets Study Group. Leukocyte reduction and ultraviolet B irradiation of platelets to prevent alloimmunization and refractoriness to platelet transfusions. N Engl J Med 1997;337:1861–9.

This prospective randomized trial demonstrated that reduction of leukocytes by filtration and ultraviolet B irradiation of platelets are equally effective in preventing alloantibody-mediated refractoriness to platelets during chemotherapy for acute myeloid leukemia. Platelets obtained by apheresis from single random donors provided no additional benefit as compared with pooled platelet concentrates from random donors.

Vichinsky EP, Haberkern CM, Neumayr L, et al. A comparison of conservative and aggressive transfusion regimens in the perioperative management of sickle cell disease. N Engl J Med 1995;333:206–13.

This prospective randomized trial showed that a conservative transfusion strategy (increase hemoglobin level to 10 g/dL) is as effective as an aggressive transfusion regimen (decrease the hemoglobin S level to <30%) in preventing perioperative complications in patients with sickle cell anemia and results in substantially fewer transfusions.

REFERENCES

Access the complete reference list online at http://www.expertconsult.com

CHAPTER 37

HEMAPHERESIS

Jeffrey L. Winters

KEY POINTS

- Hemapheresis is the process of removing normal or abnormal components from circulating blood.
- Cytapheresis involves the removal of cellular components; plasmapheresis involves the removal of plasma, the liquid component.
- Separation of the blood components is based on size (filtration instruments), density (centrifugation instruments), or a combination of both.
- Donor apheresis maximizes the collection of a scarce resource by allowing donors to donate only what is needed, returning the remaining components back to the donor.
- Donor apheresis is highly regulated. Donor eligibility requirements, frequency of donation, and amount of product allowed to be collected vary according to the components being collected, the instruments being used for the collection, and the frequency of the apheresis donations.
- Hematopoietic progenitor cell–apheresis collection has advantages over hematopoietic progenitor cell–marrow harvest, including faster time to engraftment, avoidance of general anesthesia for the donor, quicker donor recovery, and decreased expense.
- There is a dearth of randomized placebo-controlled clinical trials involving apheresis. To address this, the American Society for Apheresis categorizes diseases treated with apheresis according to the strength of the evidence supporting its use.
- Therapeutic cytoreduction for leukocytosis or thrombocytosis is indicated for primary disorders where symptoms of hyperviscosity or risk factors for complications are present.
- A 1–1.5 plasma volume plasma exchange will remove 70% of a substance located within the plasma. The treatment of additional plasma volumes results in the removal of a fixed percentage of the remaining substance, leading to diminishing returns in treating greater than 1.5 plasma volumes.
- Plasma exchange is nonselective, removing pathologic substances as well as beneficial substances such as coagulation factors and protein-bound drugs.
- Complications of donor apheresis are less common than complications seen with whole blood donation, although the rate of reactions requiring hospitalization has been reported to be greater.

Continued

- The most common reactions to donor apheresis, in decreasing frequency, are hematoma/pain; hypocalcemia due to the citrate anticoagulant; vasovagal reactions with syncope; and vasovagal reactions without syncope.
- Complications have been reported to occur in approximately 5% of patients undergoing therapeutic apheresis treatments. If complications due to central venous access placement are included, the complication rate has been reported to be 17%.
- The most common reactions due to therapeutic apheresis procedures, in decreasing frequency, are transfusion reactions from replacement fluids; hypocalcemia due to citrate anticoagulant; hypotension; vasovagal reactions; tachycardia; respiratory distress; tetany/seizure; and rigors/chills.

OVERVIEW

DEFINITIONS

The word **apheresis** is derived from the Greek word "aphaeresis," which means "to separate," "to take away by force," or "to remove." Hemapheresis is the process of removing normal or abnormal blood constituents from circulating blood. It can be divided into cytapheresis, removal of the cellular component of blood, and plasmapheresis, removal of the plasma fraction. Cytapheresis can be selective with removal of red blood cells (erythrocytapheresis), platelets (plateletpheresis), or white blood cells (leukocytapheresis). If the red blood cells removed during an erythrocytapheresis are replaced with donor red blood cells in a therapeutic procedure, this is referred to as a red blood cell exchange. When a plateletpheresis procedure is performed as a therapeutic procedure, it is referred to as a thrombocytapheresis. If during a plasmapheresis procedure the removed plasma is replaced with a replacement fluid, the procedure is referred to as a plasma exchange. It is important to realize that the terms **plasmapheresis** and **plasma exchange** are not equivalent, even if they are commonly used in this way.

BASIC PRINCIPLES

All of the early apheresis instruments separated whole blood into its components by centrifugation. Centrifugal force is applied to whole blood such that the various components separate according to their specific gravity (density), with the most dense component layering the farthest from the axis of rotation and the least dense layering closest. Those components with intermediate densities would layer in between in order of increasing density. The order of density of blood components from least to most dense is shown in Figure 37-1 as follows: plasma, platelets, lymphocytes,

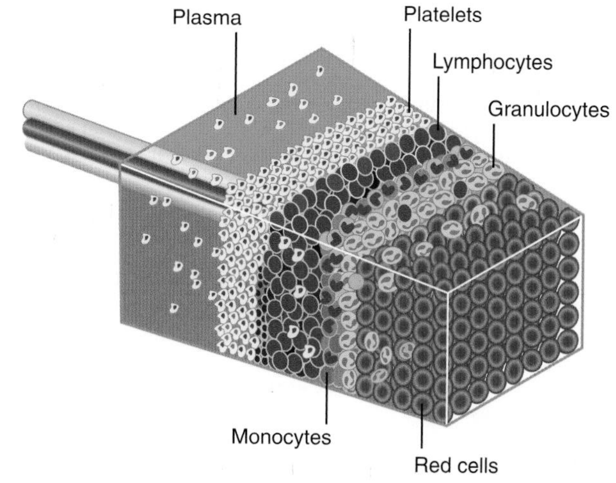

Figure 37-1 Separation of blood components within a centrifugal separation chamber. Blood components placed in a centrifuge are separated based on their density. The densest elements (red blood cells) are farthest from the axis of rotation, and the least dense element (plasma) is closest. *(Image courtesy of Sergio Torloni, MD, Director of Transfusion Medicine, Mayo Clinic, Scottsdale, Ariz.)*

granulocytes, and red blood cells (Burgstaler, 2010). Some mixing does occur at the interfaces of the various layers, resulting in some contamination with components of the adjacent layers. For example, red cells are present within the granulocyte layer and vice versa.

Centrifugation separators can be divided into two classes: intermittent flow and continuous flow centrifuges. In intermittent flow centrifuges, the bowl is filled with the whole blood to be separated and centrifugal force is applied. After the components are separated, the component of interest is removed. The centrifuge is then stopped and the bowl is emptied with contents returned to the patient/donor. The cycle is then repeated with whole blood being processed in discrete batches. In continuous flow centrifuges, each of the individual component layers is removed, with the layer of interest being retained, while the others are mixed together outside of the separation chamber and returned. This means that as volume is removed from the separation chamber, it can be continually replaced by whole blood, resulting in continuous separation. The chamber is not emptied until the entire procedure has been completed (Burgstaler, 2010).

In addition to centrifugation, apheresis can be accomplished by filtration. In this method, components of whole blood are separated based not on density but on size. The whole blood flows over a membrane containing pores that are of a size such that only the component of interest can pass through. The remaining elements are then returned. These separators may be hollow fiber or flat plate systems. The former consists of bundles of tubes containing pores within their walls. The blood enters into the tubes with the plasma exiting through the pores, where it is then collected, while the cellular elements exit from the opposite end of the tubes. The flat plate separators consist of two porous membranes. Whole blood flows between the membranes with the cellular elements being retained and collected at the opposite end of the plates, while the plasma passes through the membranes and is collected from the exterior surface of the plate (Burgstaler, 2010).

Centrifugation and filtration can be combined. In these instruments, blood enters a stationary chamber containing a central rotating filter. As the filter rotates, the blood begins to move and separate into layers. The result is that the more dense elements move away from the filter with the plasma being located directly adjacent to the filter. The plasma can then pass through the filter and can be drawn off while the cellular elements are collected from the periphery of the stationary chamber. The advantage of the combination of centrifugation and filtration in this arrangement is that the cellular elements cannot clog the pores of the filter. This means that filters with smaller surface areas, in comparison with filtration instruments, and lower *g* forces, in comparison with centrifugation instruments, can be used (Burgstaler, 2010).

Another basic aspect of apheresis involves determining the blood volume of the donor/patient. This is necessary because of the need to limit the amount of blood within the instrument and tubing connected to the donor/patient—the extracorporeal circuit—to avoid hypotension and complications. Previously, Standards for Blood Banks and Transfusion Services limited the extracorporeal blood volume for donors to 15% of total blood volume (Standards Committee of the American Association of Blood Banks, 1997). It was therefore necessary to determine the donor's blood volume. This is most often accomplished through nomograms or as a calculation performed by the instrument used for the procedure. This requires the input of donor/patient-specific data by the instrument operator, typically height, weight, gender, and hematocrit (Hct). A number of equations and rules are available for this determination (Nadler, 1962; Gilcher, 1996). For example, Equations 37-1 and 37-2 can be used to determine blood volume in males and females, respectively (Nadler, 1962):

$$\text{Males: } BV = (0.3669 \times H^3) + (0.03719 \times W) + 0.6041 \quad \textbf{(37-1)}$$

$$\text{Females: } BV = (0.3561 \times H^3) + (0.03308 \times W) + 0.1833 \quad \textbf{(37-2)}$$

where

BV is blood volume in liters.

H is height in meters.

W is weight in kilograms.

Because the blood volume of tissues varies according to the ratio of adipose tissue present, such calculations may overestimate the blood volume in obese patients and underestimate it in muscular patients. These biases are partially corrected by formulas that cube the height of the patient (Mollison, 1998). The regulatory necessity to calculate blood volume has been simplified, beginning with the 19th edition of Standards for Blood Banks and Transfusion Services. Instead of limiting the extracorporeal volume to 15%, the maximum amount allowed to be within the extracorporeal circuit is 10.5 mL/kg of the donor's weight (Standards Committee of the American Association of Blood Banks, 2009). Calculations of blood volume, however, are still necessary to "prescribe" appropriate processing volumes during therapeutic cytapheresis. Additionally, for plasma exchanges, the blood volume can be used to further calculate the plasma volume, as given by Equation 37-3 (Buffaloe, 1983):

$$PV = BV[1-(0.91)(0.96)VCH/100] \quad \textbf{(37-3)}$$

where PV is plasma volume in liters, and VCH is venous centrifuge Hct.

Finally, the plasma volume can be used to calculate the exchange volume, the volume processed in a plasma exchange procedure as given by Equation 37-4 (Buffaloe, 1983):

$$EV = PV \times PVE \quad \textbf{(37-4)}$$

where EV is exchange volume in liters, and PVE is desired number of plasma volumes to exchange.

These equations allow for the determination of appropriate volumes to be processed in the various therapeutic procedures described in this chapter.

The final basic aspect of hemapheresis that is applicable to all procedures, therapeutic and donor, is venous access. In donor hemapheresis, peripheral venous access is used, usually the veins of the antecubital fossa. The use of central venous access in this setting, with the potential for serious complications, would be too risky for the donor. If a donor's peripheral venous access is such that it cannot be used, then another donor should be located. The possible exception to this would be the setting of allogeneic peripheral hematopoietic progenitor cell harvest, where an alternative donor may not be available. Obviously, the risks to the donor and the benefits to the recipient must be carefully considered, and the donor must give informed consent before central venous access can be used.

In the setting of therapeutic hemapheresis procedures, it is often assumed that central access is essential because of damage to peripheral veins from previous medical treatment (e.g., chemotherapy), as well as the need for long-term therapy for some diseases. The Canadian Cooperative Multiple Sclerosis Study Group (Noseworthy, 1989) found that among 294 multiple sclerosis patients undergoing weekly plasma exchange procedures for 20 weeks, only 4.4% of patients could not be treated because of poor peripheral venous access. Of those who started the course of therapy, only 5.4% lost peripheral venous access such that the course could not be completed (Noseworthy, 1989). In a similar study, Grishaber (1992), looking at 46 patients with neurologic diseases requiring hemapheresis, found that 50% of patients could complete their course of therapy using peripheral access alone. Factors associated with the requirement of central venous access included Guillain-Barré syndrome or hospitalization within a medical intensive care unit (Grishaber, 1992). Contrary to popular belief, these authors also found no difference between peripheral venous access and central venous access with regard to the time required to perform the therapeutic procedures (Grishaber, 1992). These studies indicate that peripheral venous access, with its lower rate of complications, should be tried initially in therapeutic hemapheresis. Central venous access should be reserved for occasions in which peripheral access fails.

When peripheral venous access is not possible, then both the hemapheresis service and the physician placing the catheter must determine the type of central catheter to be placed. Many routinely used central venous catheters are inadequate for hemapheresis because their walls are too soft and collapse, their length is too long, or their diameter is too small. These characteristics result in pressure alarms from the instruments. The ideal catheters have relatively rigid walls to prevent collapse and large diameter with relatively short length to allow for maximum flow. Appropriate catheters include the Mahurkar dual-lumen catheter (Kendall, Mansfield, Mass.), PermCath (Kendall), Hickman Hemodialysis and Plasmapheresis Catheters (C.R. Bard, Inc., Cranston, R.I.), and the Neostar Pheres-Flow catheter (Horizon Medical Products, Inc., Manchester, Ga.). Other catheters may be used, such as the Hickman dual-lumen vascular access catheter (C.R. Bard, Inc.) or triple-lumen catheters, but often these can be used only as return lines and not as draw lines, requiring peripheral access as well. Grishaber (1992) found unacceptable failure rates with these catheters and could not recommend their insertion solely for apheresis procedures. A rule of thumb is that if a catheter can be used for dialysis where flow rates are greater than those seen in apheresis, it can be used for apheresis.

DONOR CYTAPHERESIS

DONOR PLATELETPHERESIS

Benefits of Apheresis Platelets

The use of apheresis platelets has increased from 25% of platelets transfused in 1987 (Wallace, 1993) to 83% in 2006 (Whitaker, 2008). In part, this is due to the inability to increase platelets derived from whole blood donations. In addition, there is a perception that apheresis platelets offer advantages over those produced from whole blood. The reported benefits of apheresis platelet products are given in Table 37-1.

An additional advantage of apheresis platelets over pooled nonapheresis products is simplification of inventory management. Pooled products, because they are prepared in an open system, have a 4-hour shelf life after pooling. Apheresis products do not need to be pooled and as a result retain their 5-day shelf life. In situations where platelet products are initially requested but then are not transfused, the use of apheresis products could avoid wastage. The disadvantages of apheresis platelets are the additional expense to obtain them and limited availability in some areas.

Platelet Product Requirements

Standards for Blood Banks and Transfusion Services require that the minimum number of platelets in an apheresis product be 3.0×10^{11} in 90% of units tested (Standards Committee of the American Association of Blood Banks, 2009); the Food and Drug Administration (FDA) requires a minimum of 3.0×10^{11} in 75% of units tested (CFR, 2009). The result of these requirements, however, is that an apheresis platelet product contains at least as many platelets as a pool of platelets from six whole blood donations.

Plateletpheresis Donor Selection

The donor requirements for plateletpheresis are the same as those for whole blood donation (Standards Committee of the American Association of Blood Banks, 2009). The FDA has issued additional requirements, as outlined in guidance issued in December of 2007, "Guidance for Industry and FDA Review Staff: Collection of Platelets by Automated Methods" (Division of Blood and Blood Products, Center for Biologics Evaluation and Research, 2007). FDA guidance includes a proscription on the collection of apheresis platelets from a donor who has ingested aspirin or piroxicam (Feldene) within 2 days of donation. Standards for Blood Banks and Transfusion Services (2009) also require that the use of platelets from a donor taking "medications known to irreversibly inhibit platelet function shall be evaluated." Finally, donors who have taken clopidogrel (Plavix) or ticlopidine (Ticlid) are deferred from apheresis platelet donation for 14 days after the last dose (Division of Blood and Blood Products, Center for Biologics Evaluation and Research, 2007).

Additional plateletpheresis-specific requirements include restrictions on the frequency and number of donations, as well as on the number of products donated. First, donors can donate as often as twice per week, but there must be a 2-day interval between hemapheresis procedures. A donor cannot donate more than 24 times in 12 months. This limit on the number of donations is based on the fact that early instruments produced platelet products containing significant numbers of lymphocytes (Strauss, 1994). This resulted in concerns that long-term platelet donation could result in lymphocyte depletion with subsequent disturbance in immune function. Finally, if a donor donates multiple plateletpheresis products, such as a double- or triple-platelet product, the donor is deferred from additional hemapheresis donation for 1 week. This restriction arises from concern

TABLE 37-1
Reported Benefits of Apheresis Platelet Products

Decreased donor exposure with decreased risk of transfusion-transmitted disease
Decreased donor exposure with delay in alloimmunization to HLA (Sintnicolaas, 1981)
Decreased risk of septic platelet transfusion reactions (Ness, 2001)
Prestorage leukocyte reduction with delay in alloimmunization to HLA (Trial to Reduce Alloimmunization to Platelets Study Group, 1997), decreased febrile transfusion reactions (Heddle, 1995), and decreased cytomegalovirus infection (Bowden, 1995)

HLA, Human leukocyte antigen.

about exhaustion of platelet production with frequent donation and high product yields. Both of these concerns will be discussed further in the section dealing with plateletpheresis donor concerns.

Donors must have a minimum platelet count of 150,000/μL to be eligible to donate. FDA guidance requires that a sample for a platelet count be drawn prior to collection. This count should be used for eligibility determination (current collection or future collections) and to program the hemapheresis instrument to determine the platelet yield of the collection. The count may be completed before the procedure starts or immediately following the start of the procedure. If the platelet count cannot be obtained before the collection starts or immediately afterward (e.g., collections on a mobile drive), an average of previous measurements from the donor or a default count can be used to program the instrument. If one of these surrogate counts is used, a triple-platelet collection cannot be performed. The sample collected, however, must be tested. Finally, the FDA also requires that the hemapheresis device be programmed such that the donor's platelet count will not fall below 100,000/μL (Division of Blood and Blood Products, Center for Biologics Evaluation and Research, 2007).

Individuals donating after whole blood donation, or after an instrument failure resulting in the inability to return the extracorporeal blood volume, must wait 8 weeks before donating by apheresis. Exceptions are if the extracorporeal volume of the instrument is less than 100 mL, or if the loss of red cells is less than 200 mL. In these cases, the donor is eligible to donate by apheresis after the normal deferral period (Standards Committee of the American Association of Blood Banks, 2009). The FDA has provided further guidance on donor eligibility after red blood cell loss, as outlined in Table 37-2. Finally, the FDA has also defined limits on the total amount of plasma that can be removed during an apheresis platelet collection. Donors weighing less than 175 lb can have no more than 500 mL removed; in those weighing greater than or equal to 175 lb, 600 mL can be collected. An exception to these limits exists in that the manufacturer of the plateletpheresis collection device can define a different volume in the labeling of the device (Division of Blood and Blood Products, Center for Biologics Evaluation and Research, 2007).

Donor selection for plateletpheresis may be influenced by a number of factors, in addition to regulatory considerations. The yield of a plateletpheresis procedure is determined, to a large extent, by the platelet count of the donor, with higher counts associated with a higher yield (Glowitz, 1980; Goodnough, 1999). Some collection centers will screen whole blood donors for high normal platelet counts and will recruit these individuals for plateletpheresis to maximize the yield of each collection procedure. Female donors, on average, have higher platelet counts than males (Glowitz, 1980; Goodnough, 1999). Some authors have found higher platelet yields in female donors compared with males (Glowitz, 1980). In addition, the presence of a higher plasma volume in females enhances the separation and collection of platelets by some instruments, and this could also contribute to the higher yield. The difficulty with female donors is that because of prior pregnancies, they are at increased risk of sensitization against human leukocyte antigen (HLA) and neutrophil antigens. Antibodies toward these antigens have been implicated in the development of transfusion-related acute lung injury (TRALI). The American Association of Blood Banks (AABB) issued association bulletin #06-07 in November 2006 to address the risk of TRALI. In this bulletin, the AABB requires collection centers to "implement interventions to minimize the preparation of high plasma-volume components from donors known to be leukocyte-alloimmunized or at increased risk of leukocyte alloimmunization" (Strong, 2007). Because of this, collection centers have adopted policies of deferring all females from plateletpheresis donation, deferring females who have been pregnant from plateletpheresis donation, or testing female donors for the presence of HLA and neutrophil antibodies (Powers, 2008).

Additional donor considerations arise in the selection of platelet products for alloimmunized patients. These patients, through transfusion or previous pregnancies, develop antibodies to antigens expressed on platelets, most frequently antibodies to HLA class I. The result is the development of an immune refractory state as defined by inadequate post-transfusion platelet increments as measured by platelet count collected between 10 minutes and 1 hour after the completion of a platelet transfusion. Antibodies toward platelet antigens are solely or partially responsible for a third of patients being refractory to platelet transfusion (Doughty, 1994). The presence of such a state requires the search for compatible platelet donors. Three general strategies have been employed to achieve this. First, if the specificities of the HLA alloantibodies and the HLA class I phenotype of the plateletpheresis donor are known, attempts can be made to obtain platelets from a donor lacking these antigens (Schiffer, 1987; Hussein, 1996). A second strategy that is used if the HLA class I type of the patient is known and the HLA antibody specificities are unknown or broad, is to attempt to match the HLA type of the patient and of the donor as closely as possible (Duquesnoy, 1978). Finally, if the HLA class I types of the recipient or potential donors are unknown, or if poor increments continue despite HLA matching, platelet cross-matching can be performed. Such testing involves combining donor platelets with recipient serum in a solid-phase red blood cell adherence assay (Schiffer, 1987; Bock, 1989; Murphy, 1991; O'Connell, 1992).

TABLE 37-2

Donor Eligibility Following Red Blood Cell Loss

Initial red blood cell loss	Second red blood cell loss within 8 weeks	Eligibility
<200 mL	<200 mL	No deferral
<200 mL	>200 mL but ≤300 mL	Defer for 8 weeks from second donation
>200 mL but ≤300 mL	NA	Defer for 8 weeks from first donation
<200 mL	Total loss from first and second loss >300 mL	Defer for 16 weeks from second loss
≥300 mL	NA	Defer for 16 weeks from loss

Division of Blood and Blood Products, Center for Biologics Evaluation and Research, 2007.
NA, Not available.

Plateletpheresis Donor Concerns

The typical platelet donor experiences a drop in platelet count following donation of 20%–29% (Szymanski, 1973; Katz, 1981; Heyns, 1985), with that among females typically being greater (Rogers, 1995; Dettke, 1998). The fall in platelet count does not correlate with the yield of the plateletpheresis procedure, that is, the fall is less than that predicted by the yield and represents mobilization of platelets from the spleen (Heyns, 1985). The time required for return to baseline following apheresis platelet donation is 4 days in males. A delay in increase of thrombopoietin levels causes delayed return to normal platelet counts in females (Dettke, 1998). In donors undergoing alternate day collections, platelet count and apheresis yields have been shown to return to baseline levels by day 10 of collection, with stable counts and yields obtained during subsequent collection procedures (Glowitz, 1980). A rebound elevation in platelet count with increased platelet yield following repeat procedures has also been seen (Szymanski, 1973). In donors with low platelet counts (150,000–180,000/mL), plateletpheresis using prolonged collection times to achieve the platelet yield required by regulations demonstrated no clinically significant problems in 291 procedures, despite postprocedure platelet counts as low as 69,000/mL (Rogers, 1995). The results of these studies indicate that even in donors undergoing repeated plateletpheresis, platelet counts return to normal levels promptly, and bleeding complications are uncommon.

Although studies have shown that platelet counts recover quickly following platelet donation, initial studies of the long-term effects of platelet donation suggested that donation could result in declines in baseline platelet counts (Lazarus, 2001). Lazarus retrospectively studied 939 donors who had donated 11,464 platelets over 4 years and found a significant and sustained decrease in platelet count that directly correlated with donation frequency (Lazarus, 2001). Although regular donation resulted in lower platelet counts, clinically significant thrombocytopenia was not seen (Lazarus, 2001). These findings raised concerns that frequent apheresis platelet donations could produce thrombocytopenia, and prompted the FDA to suggest restrictive policies on donation. Subsequent studies have failed to demonstrate declines in platelet count with long-term donation or with donation of high-yield products such as double- or triple-platelet products (Richa, 2008). As a result, less restrictive guidance was provided by the FDA in the form of the 2007 guidance document mentioned previously.

Plateletpheresis using early hemapheresis instruments was associated with losses of donor lymphocytes as great as 5–10 × 10^9 per procedure (Strauss, 1994). Based on studies involving therapeutic lymphocytapheresis and chronic thoracic duct drainage, it had been shown that abnormal cell-mediated immunity could be achieved by the loss of 1–1.5 × 10^{11} lymphocytes within a few weeks (Strauss, 1994). As a result of this and studies showing decreased total lymphocytes, T lymphocytes, and immunoglobulin (Ig)G levels 8 months after donation, concerns about inducing immune suppression arose. This resulted in regulations limiting the number of plateletpheresis donations to 24 per year (Standards Committee of the American Association of Blood Banks, 2009) and warning potential plateletpheresis donors about the possibility of lymphocyte depletion (Division of Blood and Blood Products, Center for Biologics Evaluation and Research, 1988), as well as some authors suggesting that donors should be deferred if their lymphocyte counts were below 1.2×10^9/L (Strauss, 1994). More recent studies of donors donating with newer hemapheresis instruments have shown no differences in lymphocyte counts, lymphocyte subsets, or IgG levels when nondonors, plateletpheresis donors, and whole blood donors were compared (Lewis, 1999). In fact, the loss of lymphocytes over the course of 24 donations using modern hemapheresis equipment is equivalent to the loss of lymphocytes in a single whole blood donation (Strauss, 1994).

DONOR LEUKOCYTAPHERESIS

Granulocyte Transfusions

Granulocytes are sometimes transfused to neutropenic patients with infections that are refractory to antibiotic therapy, but clinical trials testing their efficacy are few. Seven controlled trials comparing antibiotics versus antibiotics and granulocyte transfusions have appeared in the literature and were reviewed by Strauss (1993). In these studies, the granulocyte donors were stimulated with steroids, and granulocyte colony-stimulating factor (G-CSF) was not used. Five of seven trials reported at least partial success of granulocyte transfusion in treating infections in neutropenic patients whose infections were unresponsive to antibiotics. The data from these studies were subsequently analyzed by quantitative meta-analysis and demonstrated that the dose of neutrophils transfused, as well as the survival rate of the controls, was primarily responsible for the differing success rates reported in the studies (Vamvakas, 1996). The authors stated that granulocyte transfusions should be considered in neutropenic patients with infections carrying a high mortality rate, and that the highest possible granulocyte doses ($>4 \times 10^{10}$ neutrophils) should be used (Vamvakas, 1996). Since these early studies, only one randomized trial involving G-CSF–stimulated donors has been published. This study demonstrated no difference between study groups with regard to survival (Hubel, 2002). Most of the studies and reports describing granulocyte transfusions in adults have dealt with neutropenic patients with unresponsive bacterial infections. Studies have looked at the utility of granulocyte transfusions in patients with fungal infection, but the results of such trials have been mixed (van Burik, 2003).

Another group of patients frequently considered for granulocyte transfusions are septic neonates. Six controlled studies have been published evaluating granulocyte transfusions in this setting, four of which found benefit (Laurenti, 1981; Christensen, 1982; Baley, 1987; Cairo, 1987, 1984; Wheeler, 1987). Quantitative meta-analysis of these studies identified granulocyte dose as the primary reason for disagreement in study outcomes. Those studies using buffy coat–derived granulocytes demonstrated no advantage, and those using leukocytapheresis-derived granulocytes demonstrated benefit (Vamvakas, 1996). Again, all of these trials were conducted before G-CSF became available. No trials of transfusion of G-CSF–stimulated granulocytes have been reported.

Granulocyte transfusions may benefit neutropenic patients, especially if large doses can be collected. Recommendations regarding who should be considered for granulocyte transfusions include adult patients who are profoundly neutropenic and are anticipated to remain neutropenic for at least 1 week, and those whose infections have progressed despite appropriate antibiotic therapy (Schiffer, 1990). In addition, the patient should have a possibility of recovery of granulocyte production. In neonates, indications for granulocyte transfusion include evidence of bacterial sepsis with an absolute neutrophil count below 3000/µL and decreased marrow store of neutrophils with less than 7% (of nucleated cells) metamyelocytes or more mature forms (Blanchette, 1991; Strauss, 1991).

Granulocyte Product Requirements

One of the critical factors in the success of granulocyte transfusions is the dose of granulocytes provided. Standards for Blood Banks and Transfusion Services require that 75% of granulocyte components collected have a minimum of 1.0×10^{10} granulocytes (Standards Committee of the American Association of Blood Banks, 2009). It must be realized that this dose represents a minimum, and that higher doses are desirable.

Granulocytes are stored at room temperature (20°–24° C) without agitation and have an expiration date of 24 hours (Standards Committee of the American Association of Blood Banks, 2009). Neutrophils, however, undergo apoptosis throughout storage. Accumulation of transfused granulocytes at sites of inflammation decreases with increasing time of storage; they should therefore be transfused as soon as possible after collection (Price, 1979).

Granulocyte Donor Selection

As with plateletpheresis, leukocytapheresis donors must fulfill all of the requirements applicable to whole blood donation. In addition, platelets are removed during the collection, and application of the 150,000/µL platelet count requirement to granulocyte donors may be prudent. Another consideration in selecting donors is the ABO type of both recipient and donor. Significant numbers of red blood cells are present within granulocyte products. Because the red cell content is greater than 2 mL, Standards for Blood Banks and Transfusion Services require that the product be cross-match compatible (Standards Committee of the American Association of Blood Banks, 2009). If a granulocyte product could be generated with less than 2 mL of red cells, then ABO type could be ignored, as it does not influence transfused granulocyte survival or migration (McCullough, 1988).

Another consideration in donor selection is the cytomegalovirus status of the donor and recipient. Granulocyte transfusions have been linked to cases of cytomegalovirus (CMV) infection in CMV seronegative recipients (Winston, 1980; Buckner, 1983). Therefore, donors for CMV seronegative patients must also be CMV seronegative.

Finally, it is critical that HLA- or crossmatch-compatible donors be selected for alloimmunized patients. Studies of alloimmunized patients have demonstrated minimal to no recovery, survival, or localization to sites of infection using granulocytes from random donors (Dutcher, 1983; McCullough, 1986).

Granulocyte Donor Stimulation

Granulocyte dose is critical for the effectiveness of granulocyte therapy. The most commonly used method to increase granulocyte yield is to administer steroids to donors 10–12 hours before collection. Administration of oral prednisone (MacPherson, 1976; Jendiroba, 1998) or dexamethasone (Higby, 1977) increases granulocyte yield up to twice that of unstimulated donors. The effects of steroids appear to result from mobilization of granulocytes from marrow stores. Studies have shown no effect of steroid stimulation on the ability of neutrophils to phagocytose particles, phagocytose fungi, kill bacteria, or undergo chemotaxis when compared with granulocytes from nonstimulated donors (Glasser, 1977). In addition, steroid stimulation has been shown not to affect accumulation of transfused granulocytes at sites of injury (Price, 1979), and it inhibits apoptosis during storage (Liles, 1995).

The availability of G-CSF has resulted in the ability to generate even larger granulocyte doses and has led to a resurgence of interest in granulocyte transfusions. Administration of 5 µg/kg of G-CSF every other day resulted in granulocyte collections four to five times those seen in unstimulated donors and greater than those seen with prednisone stimulation (Jendiroba, 1998). The use of G-CSF–stimulated granulocyte transfusions has been shown to result in significant and sustained increments in neutrophil counts in patients (Adkins, 1997b). The optimum timing for granulocyte collection in G-CSF–stimulated donors is 12 hours after administration of the G-CSF (Price, 1998).

As with steroids, concerns have arisen over the function of G-CSF–stimulated granulocytes. Studies have demonstrated normal phagocytosis, chemotaxis, chemiluminescence, and superoxide anion production (Caspar, 1993) and normal accumulation at sites of injury (Adkins, 1997a). G-CSF has been shown to enhance microbicidal activity (Lieschke, 1992), as well as inhibit neutrophil apoptosis during storage (Adachi, 1994). Concern has also been raised as to whether repeated doses of G-CSF will adversely affect granulocyte function. Again, enhanced phagocytosis and oxidative burst were seen with multiple G-CSF administrations (Joos, 2002).

Studies have been performed to evaluate the effect of the combination of steroids and G-CSF (Dale, 1998; Liles, 1997). Eight milligrams of dexamethasone with 300 or 600 µg of G-CSF resulted in higher granulocyte yields than either agent alone, leading to a 10-fold increase in neutrophil count at 12 hours. The combination of dexamethasone and 600 µg resulted in a significantly greater yield than dexamethasone and 300 µg of G-CSF (Liles, 1997). Granulocyte function with this combined regimen demonstrated no defects (Dale, 1998). Subsequent studies comparing 450-µg versus 600-µg doses of G-CSF with 8 mg of dexamethasone found

TABLE 37-3
Short-Term Side Effects of Medications Used in Granulocyte Mobilization

Medication	Side effects
Corticosteroids	Headache Flushing Insomnia Euphoria Palpitations Epigastric acidity Hyperglycemia
G-CSF	Bone pain Myalgias Arthralgias Headache Fever Chills Gastrointestinal discomfort Paresthesias Chest pain Edema Fatigue

From Volk (1999).
G-CSF, Granulocyte-colony stimulating factor.

TABLE 37-4
Diseases/Conditions That Are Relative Contraindications to Medications Used for Granulocyte Mobilization

Medication	Condition
Corticosteroids	Hypertension Diabetes Peptic ulcer disease
G-CSF	Inflammatory conditions Gout Risk factors for thrombosis

From Korbling (1998) and Technical Manual Committee (2008).
G-CSF, Granulocyte-colony stimulating factor.

equivalency with regard to both the donor's absolute neutrophil count (ANC) at 12 hours and donor side effects (Liles, 2000).

Finally, the route of administration of G-CSF, when given with dexamethasone, also influences granulocyte kinetics. Subcutaneous administration gives a higher sustained ANC compared with IV administration (Stroncek, 2002).

Granulocyte Collection Procedure

Granulocyte yields can also be increased by enhancing the separation of red blood cells and granulocytes during the centrifugation process. Red blood cells and granulocytes have similar densities and sedimentation rates, resulting in poor separation during centrifugation. The addition of sedimenting agents such as hydroxyethyl starch (HES) can improve this separation and thereby enhance granulocyte collection (Iacone, 1981). The mechanism of action of HES is the induction of rouleaux formation among red blood cells. The resulting greater red cell sedimentation rate and a greater upward flow of plasma during centrifugation enhance separation (Lee, 1995b). Different types of HES include the high molecular weight hetastarch and the low molecular weight pentastarch. Both of these agents have been shown to have equivalent safety profiles (Strauss, 1986, 1987), although pentastarch has the benefit of being rapidly excreted. As a result, there is less danger of accumulation of the HES and possible complications (see discussion at end of chapter). Although the safety profile of pentastarch may be superior, a controlled study has shown greater granulocyte yields with hetastarch (Lee, 1995b).

Granulocyte Donor Concerns

In addition to granulocytes, platelets and significant numbers of red blood cells are present in the leukocytapheresis product. The donor's Hct typically drops by 7% following a granulocyte collection (Hester, 1995). This drop is due not only to loss of red blood cells but also to dilutional effects of volume expansion caused by the HES used during the procedure. Platelet count typically drops by 22% after each procedure—an equivalent drop to that seen with plateletpheresis (Hester, 1995). Again, a degree of dilutional effect is present. An additional cause for a fall in platelet count is seen in donors stimulated with G-CSF (Bensinger, 1993). Healthy donors receiving G-CSF for 10 days typically have a decline in platelet count starting at day 8, with significant differences from baseline at days 10 and 11. The mechanism behind this effect is uncertain and may represent changed platelet distribution, decreased platelet production, or increased intravascular volume (Korbling, 1998). In addition, recovery of platelet count appears to be prolonged, requiring 7–10 days among stem cell donors versus 4–6 days among platelet donors (Stroncek, 1996b).

G-CSF and corticosteroids can cause a number of other side effects (Table 37-3). These side effects are very common, occurring in 90% of allogeneic donors receiving G-CSF for apheresis collection of hematopoietic progenitor cell (HPC-A) (Stroncek, 1996a), are usually mild, and are treated symptomatically. For example, bone pain and headache, which tend to be dose related (Stroncek, 1996a; Murata, 1999), typically respond to mild analgesics. Nausea and vomiting are more common in women, and headache is more common in those younger than 35 years (Murata, 1999). More significant but rare side effects of G-CSF include splenic rupture, anaphylaxis, acute iritis, marginal keratitis, gouty arthritis, autoimmune thyroiditis, rheumatoid arthritis exacerbation, thrombosis, erythema multiforme, acute lung injury, and capillary leak syndrome (Korbling, 1998; Volk, 1999; Azevedo, 2001; Arimura, 2005; Tigue, 2007; Veerappan, 2007). These are believed to represent exacerbation of underlying donor/patient illnesses. Donors, whether for granulocyte or HPC-A collection, should be evaluated for these illnesses in determining suitability for donation (Table 37-4).

Although the short-term effects of G-CSF are predominantly mild, the long-term effects are uncertain. Concerns have been expressed over the possibility of recipients developing hematologic diseases such as myelodysplasia or chronic myelogenous leukemia (CML) (Korbling, 1998; Volk, 1999). This is due in part to the occurrence of leukemic transformation after G-CSF therapy in 10%–15% of patients with congenital neutropenia receiving long-term G-CSF therapy (Bonilla, 1994). In addition, studies of normal donors receiving G-CSF have demonstrated the induction of a small population of tetraploid myeloid cells (Kaplinsky, 2003); temporary asynchronous allele replication and persistent aneuploidy, up to 265 days following G-CSF administration (Nagler, 2004); abnormal DNA relaxation and de novo DNA synthesis (Shapira, 2003); and alterations in gene expression (Hernandez, 2005; Amariglio, 2007). These findings were similar to those that have been seen in hematologic malignancies. It has been estimated that to detect a 10-fold increase in the frequency of leukemia above the population background of 0.05%, a study following 2000 stimulated donors for a minimum of 10 years would be needed (Pamphilion, 2008). Two registries have published data that almost meet these requirements. The European Bone Marrow Transplant Registry examined unstimulated bone marrow donors and HPC-A donors collected between 1990 and 2003. Among bone marrow donors, 9 of 28,134 (0.032%) donors developed hematologic malignancies compared with 5 of 16,432 (0.030%) stimulated HPC-A donors (Grupp, 2006). The National Marrow Donor Program examined 4015 healthy unrelated allogeneic donors who had donated between 1997 and 2007. Twenty cases of malignancy were identified, and this incidence was consistent with the age-adjusted U.S. incidence of cancer in adults. No cases of hematologic malignancy were seen (Confer, 2007). Despite these reassuring findings, donors undergoing G-CSF stimulation should give informed consent before stimulation, and appropriate institutional review should be obtained for use of G-CSF in this non–FDA-approved role.

Long-term steroid treatment is associated with a number of well-known side effects, including the development of posterior subcapsular cataracts (PSCs). Because these complications appear with long-term use, it would seem that short-term steroid stimulation of granulocyte donors should not be associated with them. This may not be the case, however. A single-center double-blind study compared the presence of cataracts in 9 apheresis platelet donors and 11 granulocyte donors matched for age, gender, and number of respective donations (Ghodsi, 2001). The frequency of cataracts not associated with steroid administration was equivalent between the two groups, but those associated with steroid administration—PSCs—were statistically more frequent in the granulocyte donors when all eyes were considered (5 of 22 eyes vs. 0 of 18; $p = 0.040$) (Ghodsi, 2001). A subsequent multicenter study examined 89 granulocyte donors and 89 control donors (Burch, 2005). The granulocyte donors had donated a mean of 13 donations (range, 5–39). Six of the granulocyte donors and 4 of the control donors had evidence of PSC

TABLE 37-5
Advantages and Disadvantages of Double Red Blood Cell Collections

Advantages	
Decreased incidence of donor reactions compared with whole blood donation (Wiltbank, 2002)	
Decreased number of donors necessary to produce a given number of red blood cell units (Gilcher, 2003)	
Standardized red blood cell dose (Gilcher, 2003)	
Decreased amount of component processing (i.e., one set of laboratory tests for two units of red blood cells) (Beeler, 1997)	
Decreased donor exposure if a patient receives both parts of a double red cell collection (Gilcher, 2003)	
Disadvantages	
Greater complexity of collection (Gilcher, 2003)	
Greater time necessary for donation (Gilcher, 2003)	

on photographic examination. This was not a statistically significant difference (Burch, 2005). This better powered study suggests that cataract formation may not be a concern among granulocyte donors.

DONOR ERYTHROCYTAPHERESIS

Benefits of Erythrocytapheresis

A single unit of red blood cells or the equivalent of two units of red blood cells can be collected by apheresis. With the current shortages of red blood cells in the United States and the decreasing size of the donor pool, the collection of red blood cells, with the concurrent collection of other blood products or as double red blood cells, can maximize collection of this scarce resource. Advantages and disadvantages of double red blood cell collections are given in Table 37-5.

Erythrocytapheresis Product Requirements

The Standards for Blood Banks and Transfusion Services requires that apheresis red blood cells be collected and prepared by a method that is known to result in a mean hemoglobin (Hb) >60 g or a packed red cell volume of 180 mL. In addition, at least 95% of the units sampled must have >50 g of Hb or 150 mL packed red cell volume (Standards Committee of the American Association of Blood Banks, 2009). If the red blood cell units are leukocyte reduced, then the mean Hb must be >51 g or 153 mL packed red cell volume. Here, at least 95% of tested units must have >42.5 g of Hb or 128 mL packed red blood cell volume (Standards Committee of the American Association of Blood Banks, 2009).

The FDA does not define product requirements for red blood cells—single or double—collected by apheresis but instead states that 95% of the products collected must meet "expected or target RBC volume" and "any other target parameters specified in the device's operator manual" (Division of Blood and Blood Products, Center for Biologics Evaluation and Research, 2001). The FDA also defines how such validation and testing is to be performed, with the initial validation consisting of testing "100 consecutive RBC units," while subsequent testing must include at least 50 units per month, consisting of both single and double red blood cell products. If a center collects less than 50 units, all units must be tested (Division of Blood and Blood Products, Center for Biologics Evaluation and Research, 2001).

Erythrocytapheresis Donor Selection

Allogeneic apheresis red blood cell donors must meet the criteria defined by the FDA and the AABB for whole blood donation. In addition, they are required to meet any other selection criteria defined by the device's operator manual (Division of Blood and Blood Products, Center for Biologics Evaluation and Research, 2001).

The FDA and the AABB do not define a minimum Hb/Hct for double red cell donation. Instead, it is required that the collection center follow the instrument manufacturer's recommendations (Division of Blood and Blood Products, Center for Biologics Evaluation and Research, 2001; Standards Committee of the American Association of Blood Banks, 2009). The FDA does, however, require that the Hb/Hct be determined by a quantitative method (Division of Blood and Blood Products, Center for Biologics Evaluation and Research, 2001). As a result, the copper sulfate method cannot be used to qualify a donor for double red cell donation.

The AABB limits the total volume of red blood cells removed, such that the donor's Hct and Hb are not <30% and <10 g/dL, respectively, after volume replacement (Standards Committee of the American Association of Blood Banks, 2009). The FDA makes no specific limitations, requiring that the manufacturer's recommendations be followed (Division of Blood and Blood Products, Center for Biologics Evaluation and Research, 2001).

The type of product collected determines the donation interval following hemapheresis red blood cell donations. Donors donating a single unit of red blood cells are deferred for 8 weeks. The exception to this would be that, as described in the section on donor plateletpheresis, they could donate platelets or platelets with concurrent plasma, as long as the extracorporeal red blood cell volume of the collecting instrument is less than 100 mL (Division of Blood and Blood Products, Center for Biologics Evaluation and Research, 2001). Donors donating two units of red blood cells are deferred for 16 weeks, and no automated or manual collections are allowed during this time (Division of Blood and Blood Products, Center for Biologics Evaluation and Research, 2001).

If a donor experiences an incomplete procedure, that is, the targeted collection is not reached, the FDA defines the length of deferral based on the absolute loss of red blood cells during the initial collection and subsequent collections, as outlined in Table 37-2 (Division of Blood and Blood Products, Center for Biologics Evaluation and Research, 2007).

Erythrocytapheresis Donor Concerns

Owing to the removal of two units of red blood cells, one of the most frequent concerns is whether reactions are more frequent with double red blood cell collections when compared with whole blood collections. Studies have demonstrated no increase in reactions with automated double red cell collections when compared with whole blood donation (Wiltbank, 2002; Gorlin, 2003). Wiltbank reported lower rates of moderate and severe reactions with automated double red blood cell collection (6.8/10,000 and 1.2/10,000 collections, respectively) compared with whole blood donations (14.5/10,000 and 1.2/10,000 collections, respectively) (Wiltbank, 2002). The lower rate of reactions, despite the removal of a greater red blood cell mass, results from the fact that donors are isovolemic at the end of the collection as a result of the infusion of saline.

Donors undergoing double red cell donation experience a transient fall in Hct of 9% (Taylor, 2002). This is due to red cell loss, as well as volume expansion from saline administration. Despite this fall, studies have shown minimal effects on donors following double red blood cell donations. Meyer (1993) found in a study of 40 blood donors that double red blood cell donors took 1–2 days longer than whole blood donors to regain their baseline sense of well-being. Smith (1996) found no significant differences in ambulatory monitored blood pressure and pulse among one-unit red blood cell collections, two-unit red blood cell collections, and sham collections (Smith, 1996). Quintana (1995) found that double red blood cell donation did not have a significant effect on exercise capacity, as determined by examining maximal oxygen consumption decrease, anaerobic threshold, maximum heart rate, respiratory exchange ratio, and maximum power on days 0, 2, 7, and 14 following donation.

A final concern with double red blood cell donations is whether donors making such donations are at greater risk of developing iron deficiency than whole blood donors. Meyer (1993) followed double red blood cell donors and whole blood donors for 1 year, measuring serum ferritin, serum iron, total iron-binding capacity, transferrin saturation, and zinc protoporphyrin/heme ratios. Half of the donors in each group received iron supplementation. No significant differences were found in iron balance between double red cell donors and the whole blood donors (Meyer, 1993).

MULTICOMPONENT APHERESIS DONATION

With current instrumentation, different combinations of blood products can be collected from the same donor. This allows for the optimum utilization of each donor. For example, the maximum amount of plasma would be collected from an AB donor, while his or her red blood cells, which frequently outdate before they are transfused, would not be collected. An O Rh-negative or Rh-positive donor would provide a double red blood cell collection, but plasma, which is usually in adequate supply, would not be collected. The various combinations of collections currently available are given in Table 37-6. It should be mentioned that all of the various regulations that apply to individual apheresis collections with regard to donor criteria and donor frequency apply to multiple-component collections. For example, a donor undergoing a double red cell collection with

TABLE 37-6
Combinations of Blood Products Available for Multicomponent Collections

• Red blood cell and plasma	• Double or triple platelet
• Red blood cell and platelet	• Platelet and single or double plasma
• Red blood cell, plasma, and platelet	• Double platelet and single plasma
• Double red blood cell	• Double or triple plasma

a concurrent plasma collection would have to meet the requirements for a double red cell collection, as well as the requirements for frequent or infrequent plasma collection, as applicable. This would include tracking red blood cell loss (see Table 37-2) and total plasma volume loss (see discussion of plasma donation later).

HEMATOPOIETIC PROGENITOR CELL COLLECTION BY APHERESIS

Benefits of Hematopoietic Progenitor Cell Collection

HPC-A provides a number of advantages for both the donor and the recipient that have resulted in replacement of the collection of hematopoietic progenitor cells by bone marrow harvest (HPC-M) in many patients. Donors tolerate hemapheresis better than bone marrow harvest as it does not require an operative procedure with the need for general anesthesia. As a result, the procedure is less expensive, is more convenient as it can be undergone as an outpatient, and avoids the potential complications seen with general anesthesia and surgery. Also, the donor recovers more quickly from the procedure without the pain and temporary disability that often accompany bone marrow harvest (Lee, 1995a). The use of peripheral blood HPCs in transplantation restores hematopoietic and immune function more rapidly than bone marrow. This means fewer days of immune suppression and fewer exposures to allogeneic blood products in the recipient (Moog, 1998; Bensinger, 2001). Additionally, in autologous transplantation, collection of peripheral HPCs by hemapheresis can be performed when marrow involvement by malignancy or prior pelvic irradiation is present and would preclude bone marrow harvest (Lee, 1995a).

Although HPC-A collection provides a number of benefits over bone marrow harvest, it also has disadvantages when compared with bone marrow harvest. Disadvantages include possible adverse effects of mobilization regimens, a greater length of time required for collection, the possibility of a larger volume of component to be transfused at the time of transplantation, and the necessity for central venous access in many cases, along with the accompanying risks and complications (Lee, 1995a). In addition, conflicting evidence in allogeneic transplantation suggests a greater frequency of chronic graft-versus-host disease (GVHD) (Duhrsen, 1988; Brown, 1997) or GVHD more refractory to standard therapy (Flowers, 2002). This may result from the larger number of T cells within peripheral blood stem cell products compared with bone marrow.

Autologous versus Allogeneic Hematopoietic Progenitor Cell Harvest

At first, HPC-A collections were limited to autologous transplantation. This was due to the use of chemotherapy as the method for mobilizing HPCs. Transplantation of HPCs collected in this way was limited to diseases such as solid malignancies, Hodgkin disease and non-Hodgkin lymphomas, and multiple myeloma. The use of HPCs has subsequently expanded to include transplantation for leukemias, including CML (Lee, 1995a; Gillespie, 1996; Moog, 1998). As methods for mobilization that do not depend upon chemotherapy have become available, HPC-A collection has been used for allogeneic donations as well. Initial use of HPC-A collection in this setting was limited to retransplant in recipients with recurrent disease or failure to engraft (Lee, 1995a; Gillespie, 1996; Moog, 1998). Currently, the use of allogeneic HPC-A in initial transplants is widespread.

Hematopoietic Progenitor Cell Dose

An important factor in determining the success of HPC transplantation is the dose of HPCs infused. Unfortunately, a method for definitively enumerating HPCs is not available. It is known that HPCs are found within the mononuclear cell component of blood; as a result, the mononuclear cell count (MNC) has been used as an indicator of when to discontinue HPC collection. Studies have shown that a total dose of 6.0–6.5 $\times 10^8$ MNC/kg is sufficient to produce rapid engraftment (Kessinger, 1989, 1995). Although MNC does not correlate directly with HPC dose, it is convenient and easily measured.

A more exact way of measuring HPC dose is by assessing colony-forming unit granulocyte-macrophage (CFU-GM) colonies grown on soft agar. HPC collections that contain $0.5–2.0 \times 10^5$ CFU-GM/kg are associated with rapid engraftment (Bender, 1992). Unfortunately, CFU-GM assays are technically challenging and difficult to standardize. As a result, direct comparison of data between institutions and studies should be made with caution. In addition, the assay requires 2 weeks to complete.

A third method of determining HPC dose is the measurement of CD34+ cell count within the product. HPCs represent a subset of CD34+ cells. As a result, the measurement of CD34+ cells gives a better indication of HPC dose than MNC and also correlates with CFU-GM (Lee, 1995a). A minimum dose of CD34+ cells necessary for engraftment appears to be 2.5×10^6 CD34+ cells/kg (Bensinger, 1995; Korbling, 1995). This dose of CD34+ cells results in prompt engraftment of white blood cells. Bensinger (1995), however, found that the higher dose of 5.0×10^6 CD34+ cells/kg resulted in an equivalent engraftment of white blood cells, as well as more rapid engraftment of platelets. Although CD34+ cell content is easier to measure than CFU-GM, it has been plagued by difficulties in standardization due to variations in methods used (Lee, 1995a). Fortunately, the availability of kits and instruments from numerous manufacturers appears to have solved this problem. It should be mentioned that in the setting of allogeneic HPC transplantation, as with many things in life, too much of a good thing may be bad. Although minimal numbers of CD34+ cells/kg are needed for prompt engraftment, too many cells have been associated with an increased risk of chronic graft-versus-host disease in some studies (Zaucha, 2001; Heimfeld, 2003). Zaucha (2001) found a higher incidence of extensive chronic graft-versus-host disease in allogeneic transplant patients receiving greater than 8.0×10^6 CD34+ cells/kg.

Some authors have suggested that the dose of CD34+ cells needed for engraftment may vary with the number of HPC collection procedures performed (Smolowicz, 1999). It is thought that a higher total dose is necessary when CD34+ cells are collected over multiple procedures. This is believed to be due to changes in CD34+ cell subsets seen during the course of multiple collections (Smolowicz, 1999).

Hematopoietic Progenitor Cell Mobilization

Early attempts at harvesting hematopoietic progenitor cells from peripheral blood were successful but labor and resource intensive. Peripheral blood contains only 10% of the fraction of CD34+ cells found in bone marrow (Lee, 1995a). This means that when HPCs are collected during steady state (i.e., without mobilization), the number of procedures necessary to achieve a sufficient dose may be large, for example, 12 procedures in one study (Moog, 1998). This limits the utility of hemapheresis collection of HPCs during steady state. The discovery that peripheral hematopoietic progenitor cells could be mobilized from the bone marrow meant that therapeutic doses of HPCs could be collected by hemapheresis in fewer procedures, making the method more attractive. Chemotherapy, cytokines, or a combination of chemotherapy and cytokines can mobilize HPCs from bone marrow (Lee, 1995a; Gillespie, 1996; Moog, 1998). Table 37-7 gives a general comparison of the effectiveness of these three mobilization regimens.

The regimen initially used for mobilization was chemotherapy. During the period of rebound hematopoiesis following chemotherapeutic treatment, the number of HPCs present within the peripheral blood increases dramatically (see Table 37-7). This allows for the effective collection of HPC-A and serves to decrease the tumor burden within the donor/recipient. The limitation of such a method of mobilization, however, is that it can be applied only to autologous transplants.

Cytokines such as G-CSF and granulocyte-macrophage colony-stimulating factor (GM-CSF) dramatically increase the presence of HPCs within the peripheral blood and have the additional benefit of providing minimal short-term toxicity (see Table 37-3). This therefore allows for the mobilization of HPCs in normal donors and the use of hemapheresis in allogeneic transplantation. The mechanism of action of these cytokines is an indirect one with regard to their effects on HPCs. HPCs in the marrow are bound to stromal cells by adhesion molecules. These molecules include VLA-4 and CXCR4 on the HPCs and VCAM-1 and SDF-1 on the stromal

TABLE 37-7
Comparison of Mobilization Regimens

Regimen	Approximate day when peak HPC concentrations are reached	Increase in HPCs above steady state
Chemotherapy	Day 14 after completion of chemotherapy	5–15×
Cytokines (G-CSF and GM-CSF)	Day 5 after initiation of cytokine therapy	60×
Chemotherapy and cytokines	Day 5 after initiation of cytokine therapy	1000×

Data from Gillespie TW, Hillyer CD. Peripheral blood progenitor cells for marrow reconstitution: mobilization and collection strategies. Transfusion 1996;36:611–24.
G-CSF, Granulocyte-colony stimulating factor; *GM-CSF,* granulocyte-macrophage colony stimulating factor; *HPC,* hematopoietic progenitor cell.

TABLE 37-8
Factors That Negatively Influence Mobilization in Autologous Stem Cell Collections

- Age*
- Presence of marrow involvement
- Follicular NHL compared with diffuse NHL
- Prior radiation therapy
- Greater number of cycles of chemotherapy
- Low platelet count
- Low NK cell numbers
- Prior rituximab therapy

Data from Kessinger A, Sharp JG. The whys and hows of hematopoietic progenitor and stem cell mobilization. Bone Marrow Transplant 2003;31:319–29.
NHL, Non-Hodgkin lymphoma; *NK,* natural killer.
*Not important if mobilized by chemotherapy. When granulocyte-colony stimulating factor (G-CSF) is given alone, younger donors/patients mobilize better than older ones (Bensinger, 1995; Moog, 1998).

cells. G-CSF increases the number of neutrophils in the marrow. This results in increases in proteolytic enzymes such as elastase and MMP-9, which are released by the neutrophils. These enzymes cleave VCAM-1 and SDF-1, resulting in the release of HPCs from the stromal cells, allowing them to enter the peripheral circulation (Lapidot, 2002).

Overall, the magnitude of increase in CD34+ cells with G-CSF and GM-CSF is the same, but differences in recipient recovery of hematopoiesis and donor side effects exist between the two agents. Recipients of GM-CSF–mobilized HPCs experience a longer time until recovery of platelet production than do recipients of G-CSF–mobilized HPCs (13 days vs. 18 days) (Gillespie, 1996). Although donors receiving GM-CSF experience the same symptoms as those receiving G-CSF, they tend to have more severe side effects (Bolwell, 1994). The use of G-CSF or GM-CSF in normal donors is associated with a peak in CD34+ cells at approximately 5 days following initiation of cytokine therapy (Bensinger, 1996). The use of G-CSF in normal donors for periods longer than 5 days has been associated with a decrease in the number of CD34+ cells collected after day 10 of stimulation (Stroncek, 1996a).

In December of 2009, a new medication was approved by the Food and Drug Administration for the mobilization of HPC-A from patients with non-Hodgkin lymphoma and multiple myeloma. This medication, plerixafor, is a CXCR4 inhibitor that was initially investigated as an anti–human immunodeficiency virus (HIV) medication. As described earlier, CXCR4 on the HPCs binds to SDF-1 on marrow stromal cells. Plerixafor blocks this interaction, resulting in mobilization of HPCs from the marrow (Cashen, 2009). Currently, plerixafor has been approved for the mobilization of HPC-A from patients who have failed previous mobilization and is given in addition to G-CSF. Plerixafor cannot be used to mobilize stem cells in patients with leukemia, as it has been shown to mobilize leukemic cells (Cashen, 2009).

In addition to G-CSF and GM-CSF, a number of other cytokines and monoclonal antibodies against stem cell adhesion molecules are being evaluated for their effects on HPC mobilization. These include stem cell factor, Gro-β, and hrPTH (Pusic, 2008).

Finally, the effects of chemotherapy and cytokine mobilization are independent of one another. This means that by combining the two mobilization regimens, even greater numbers of HPCs can be collected than when either regimen is used alone. In healthy allogeneic donors, the optimum mobilization regimen appears to be 10–16 μg/kg of G-CSF split into two doses and administered subcutaneously (Kroger, 2002). Although G-CSF demonstrates a dose response, doses larger than 10–16 μg/kg result in more donor adverse effects without significant improvement in CD34+ cell yield. If a donor is a poor mobilizer, however, higher doses can be given (Kroger, 2002). Twice-daily dosing has been shown to be superior to single dosing in this setting. This is thought to be due to the relatively short half-life of G-CSF of 3–4 hours (Kroger, 2002).

In autologous donors, mobilization is complicated by the underlying disease, as well as by previous therapy. In autologous HPC collection, G-CSF doses >16 μg/kg are needed. If poor mobilization occurs, the patient/donor may need to be remobilized with chemotherapy followed by growth factor, higher doses of growth factor, sequential stimulation with G-CSF and GM-CSF, or the use of plerixafor (Kessinger, 2003; Pusic, 2008; Cashen, 2009).

In addition to these mobilization regimens, HPCs are mobilized by the collection procedure itself. Studies of the kinetics of HPCs during hemapheresis procedures have shown that larger numbers of HPCs are recovered than would be expected based solely on the number of cells present in the peripheral blood. This means that during the procedure, as HPCs are removed, additional HPCs are released from the marrow (Smolowicz, 1999).

Unfortunately, despite attempts to optimize mobilization regimens, not every patient collects a dose of peripheral blood HPCs sufficient for transplantation. Factors that have been found to adversely affect HPC harvest are given in Table 37-8. Some authors have found that the number of CD34+ cells within the bone marrow is a predictor of the ability of a patient to mobilize and could be used to assist in deciding whether a patient should undergo hemapheresis or bone marrow harvest (Passos-Coelho, 1995a).

Although mobilization increases the number of HPCs present in the peripheral blood, it can also have detrimental effects on the donor and on the HPC product. As discussed in the section on donor concerns in granulocyte collection, the use of G-CSF is associated with minimal short-term side effects, as well as unknown long-term side effects. In the setting of autologous harvest, these effects and concerns are unimportant relative to the risks that the patient faces from the disease. In addition, the use of such agents in this setting accelerates white cell recovery following chemotherapy—a beneficial effect. In the setting of allogeneic donation, the uncertainty of long-term risks of cytokine mobilization must be explained to the donor during the consent process. The delay in platelet recovery seen following G-CSF treatment and granulocyte collection is also seen with HPC harvest (Gillespie, 1996; Stroncek, 1996b). In autologous donors, this combined with marrow suppression from recent chemotherapy may result in the need for platelet transfusion. Mobilization is also associated with increased risk of catheter thrombosis (Lee, 1995a). Finally, in addition to mobilizing HPCs, the regimens described previously have been shown to mobilize tumor cells into the peripheral blood by some (Brugger, 1994; Gazitt, 1996) but not all authors (Passos-Coelho, 1995b). The study by Brugger (1994) demonstrated mobilization of tumor cells on days 1 through 7 following the start of chemotherapy in patients without bone marrow involvement, and on days 9 through 16 in those with marrow involvement. Mobilization of tumor cells in these latter patients occurred within the time frame of HPC collection. Similarly, Gazitt (1996) found that mobilization of plasma cells in multiple myeloma patients occurred later—days 5 and 6—than mobilization of stem cells—days 1 through 3. Differences in mobilization of tumor cells versus HPCs have led many to suggest that single collections early in the course of mobilization may be better than multiple collections. It should be realized that although tumor contamination does occur, the effect of this contamination on relapse is uncertain.

Hematopoietic Progenitor Cell Collection Procedure

One of the first things to consider in performing an HPC collection is when to initiate the collection. In allogeneic donors, initiating collection on the fifth day after the start of G-CSF administration appears to be the preferred practice. This is due to the relatively reproducible response of healthy allogeneic donors to G-CSF administration (Kroger, 2002). For autologous donors, a number of criteria can be used in determining whether to initiate therapy. Criteria that have been used include myelocytosis and rising monocyte levels (Lee, 1995a), a twofold increase in total white blood cell count in 24 hours (Lee, 1995a), time of first platelet count increase (Gillespie, 1996), day 14 after initiation of chemotherapy (Gillespie, 1996), and a white blood cell (WBC) count of 10,000/μL (Dreger, 1993). With regard to this last indicator, Dreger (1993) demonstrated a peak in CFU-GM 1–2 days after the WBC count reached 10,000/μL. Starting collection at this time avoided missing the subsequent peak in CFU-GM. Another widely used method is serial CD34+ cell counts by flow cytometry. This can be used to detect a rise in CD34+ cells and to trigger HPC harvest. Trigger levels described in the literature should be viewed with caution because of the current lack of standardization in CD34+ cell measurements (Lee, 1995a). Individual institutions must determine their own trigger criteria.

Once the decision to initiate collection has been made, a number of aspects of the procedure can be modified that will influence the quality of the product. First, the instrument used to collect the HPCs determines the characteristics of the product. A number of instruments are available, including the Amicus (Fenwal Inc., Lake Zurich, Ill.), the CS3000 Plus (Fenwal Inc.), and the COBE Spectra (CaridianBCT Inc., Lakewood, Colo.). Direct comparison of the CS3000 Plus and the COBE Spectra demonstrated no differences in their efficiency of collecting CD34+ cells (Stroncek, 1997). It was found that the product produced by the COBE Spectra contained more neutrophils (Stroncek, 1997). Studies comparing the Amicus and the COBE Spectra demonstrated similar CD34+ cell collection efficiency, but the COBE Spectra removed significantly more platelets from the donor (Ikeda, 2003; Adorno, 2004). The Amicus HPC-A product contains fewer neutrophils than the COBE Spectra (Snyder, 2000). The presence of fewer neutrophils could be a significant finding if the HPC product is to be modified, such as T cell depleted, as these additional cells can interfere with the depletion process. In addition, studies have found a correlation between HPC-A neutrophil content and adverse reactions at the time of stem cell transplant (Calmels, 2007).

Another variable to consider is the whole blood flow rate during the procedure. It would seem that higher flow rates would result in a higher volume processed and a concurrent larger number of HPCs collected. With the COBE Spectra, this does appear to be the case (Lin, 1995). With the CS3000, however, increased flow rates were associated with the detrimental effect of decreased mononuclear cell content of the product, as well as the beneficial effect of decreased platelet count (Lin, 1995). This may have resulted from insufficient dwell time within the centrifugal field to allow adequate centrifugation at the higher flow rate.

Although the whole blood flow rate can adversely affect collection efficiency, the concept of increasing the amount of blood processed to increase the HPC yield is a valid one. Standard HPC collection involves the processing of approximately 1.5–3 blood volumes per procedure (Lee, 1995a). Alternatively, large-volume leukocytapheresis (LVL) involves processing more than 5 blood volumes, or more than 15 L (Reik, 1997). The benefits of such procedures include the collection of large numbers of HPCs per procedure, with the resulting need for fewer collection procedures, as well as greater mobilization of HPCs during the procedure (Lee, 1995a; Moog, 1998). In addition to these, improved yield of HPCs in patients who mobilize poorly has been seen (Smolowicz, 1997). Disadvantages of LVL include longer time required to complete the procedure and an increased incidence of citrate reactions (see discussion at the end of the chapter) (Moog, 1998). In standard leukocytapheresis procedures, thrombosis of central catheters is the most common complication (Goldberg, 1995), but in LVL, citrate reactions predominate, occurring in 33% of donations (Lin, 1995). This is due to the greater amount of citrate anticoagulant that is infused. Some authors have attempted to minimize this by adding heparin to the anticoagulant before the procedure (Reik, 1997) and/or providing IV calcium supplementation during the procedure (Bolan, 2002; Buchta, 2003).

Hematopoietic Progenitor Cell Donor Concerns

In addition to the reactions associated with G-CSFs, as described in the section on granulocyte collections, and concerns seen with large-volume leukocytapheresis, thrombocytopenia is a matter of concern in both autologous and allogeneic HPC collections. Schlenke (2000) reported average platelet losses of 24.2 ± 12.5% during large-volume peripheral blood hematopoietic progenitor cell collections using the CS3000. Smaller platelet loss has been reported using the Amicus (Burgstaler, 2004). In addition, patients undergoing autologous peripheral blood stem cell collections may be thrombocytopenic from the chemotherapy routinely used as part of the mobilization regimen. Bleeding complications in these patients are uncommon (Goldberg, 1995). However, patients may require platelet transfusions before or after collections, depending on their platelet count, to avoid bleeding complications.

Donor Plasmapheresis

Plasma Products

Two types of plasma products are collected by donor plasmapheresis: fresh frozen plasma and source plasma. Source plasma is plasma that is subsequently used to manufacture derivative products. These derivative products include albumin, Igs, coagulation factor concentrates, and laboratory reagents. Fresh frozen plasma (FFP) is the liquid component of whole blood that has been frozen within 6–8 hours after collection. The benefit of collecting FFP by plasmapheresis is that 600–700 mL of plasma can be collected from a single donor. This can then be divided into multiple units of a volume equivalent to FFP derived from whole blood donations. Alternatively, the entire volume can be frozen as "jumbo plasma." These large units have the benefit of limiting donor exposure in patients requiring large volumes of FFP, such as in plasma exchange for thrombotic thrombocytopenic purpura (TTP). An additional benefit is that the large volume of collection can maximize the production of frequently used or rare products such as type AB FFP or IgA-deficient FFP.

Plasma Donor Selection

The donor criteria for plasmapheresis vary according to the frequency of donation. Donors donating plasma less frequently than every 4 weeks are classified as "infrequent" donors and must fulfill whole blood donor requirements. In addition, AABB Standards require that donors taking warfarin be deferred from plasma donation for 1 week following their last dose of medication (Standards Committee of the American Association of Blood Banks, 2009). This is due to the fact that the plasma of individuals taking this medication will have decreased vitamin K–dependent coagulation factor activity.

If the donor donates more frequently than every 4 weeks, he or she is classified as a "frequent" donor and must fulfill criteria outlined in the Code of Federal Regulations (CFR) (Standards Committee of the American Association of Blood Banks, 2009). These requirements are similar in many ways to those for whole blood donation, with differences in deferrals for malaria and transfusion-transmitted disease exposure (CFR, 2009). In addition, the CFR requires that frequent plasma donors have a total serum protein of at least 6.0 g/dL; this is determined before each donation. Donors must also have a serum protein electrophoresis or quantitative immunodiffusion performed every 4 months, as well as an annual physical examination by a physician (CFR, 2009). Frequent plasma donors are limited to two donations within a 7-day period with at least 2 days between donations (CFR, 2009).

Both frequent and infrequent plasma donors, as well as those donors donating multicomponent collections or plateletpheresis, are limited in the amount of plasma that they can donate within a 12-month period. Donors weighing 110 to 175 lb can donate up to 12 L; those weighing more than 175 lb can donate 14.4 L (Division of Blood and Blood Products, Center for Biologics Evaluation and Research, 1995).

Plasma Donor Concerns

The risks of donor plasmapheresis are those common to any hemapheresis procedure. In addition, concern arises over possible depletion of Igs or removal of coagulation factors faster than they can be replenished, especially in frequent donors. Studies of long-term donors (Wasi, 1991), as well as donors undergoing frequent donations (Ciszewski, 1993), have not supported these concerns.

Indications for Therapeutic Hemapheresis

Therapeutic apheresis procedures, both cytapheresis and plasma exchange, have been used to treat a wide variety of illnesses, often without a clear scientific basis for expecting any benefit. Limited numbers of randomized controlled trials have been conducted (Shehata, 2002). In this way, apheresis has been analogous to the bloodletting of the early 18th century, with which it has frequently been compared. As a result, it is difficult in some cases to determine for which diseases and disorders hemapheresis is truly indicated. To help determine when hemapheresis procedures are indicated, the American Society for Apheresis (ASFA) publishes regularly updated recommendations and guidance on the use of apheresis (Szczepiorkowski, 2010). Diseases are grouped into four indication categories, as given in

TABLE 37-9
ASFA Categorization of Apheresis Indications

Category	Description
I	Disorders for which apheresis is accepted as first-line therapy, either as a primary standalone treatment or in conjunction with other modes of treatment.
II	Disorders for which apheresis is accepted as second-line therapy, either as a standalone treatment or in conjunction with other modes of treatment.
III	Disorders for which published available evidence does not permit definitive determination of the role of apheresis. Treatment decisions should be highly individualized.
IV	Disorders for which published evidence demonstrates or suggests apheresis to be ineffective or harmful. Institutional review board (IRB) approval is desirable if apheresis is undertaken in these circumstances.

From Szczepiorkowski (2010).
ASFA, American Society for Apheresis.

TABLE 37-10
ASFA Recommendation Grades

Recommendation grade	Description
1A	Strong recommendation with high-quality evidence. Can apply to most patients in most circumstances without reservation.
1B	Strong recommendation with moderate-quality evidence. Can apply to most patients in most circumstances without reservation.
1C	Strong recommendation with low-quality or very-low-quality evidence. May change when higher-quality evidence becomes available.
2A	Weak recommendation with high-quality evidence. Best action may differ depending on circumstances or patient or societal values.
2B	Weak recommendation with moderate-quality evidence. Best action may differ depending on circumstances or patient or societal values.
2C	Weak recommendation with low-quality or very-low-quality evidence. Other alternatives may be equally reasonable.

From Szczepiorkowski (2010).
ASFA, American Society for Apheresis.

Table 37-9. In addition, each indication is assigned a recommendation grade that indicates the strength of the ASFA recommendation, as well as the quality of the evidence supporting the recommendation. These are defined in Table 37-10. Table 37-11 lists diseases that have been categorized by ASFA in the most recent publication of the categorization.

A discussion of all of the disorders listed in Table 37-11 is beyond the scope of this chapter. The interested reader is referred to three sources: the textbooks *Apheresis: Principles and Practice* (McLeod, 2010) and *Therapeutic Apheresis: A Physician's Handbook* (Winters, 2008), both published by the AABB, and the special issue of the *Journal of Clinical Apheresis* entitled "Guidelines on the Use of Therapeutic Apheresis in Clinical Practice—Evidence-Based Approach from the Apheresis Applications Committee of the American Society for Apheresis" published by the ASFA (Szczepiorkowski, 2010).

A final consideration is that not every possible disorder that has or could be treated by hemapheresis is included in the resources mentioned here. Similarly, not every potential disorder has been classified by the ASFA. In circumstances where requests are made to perform therapeutic hemapheresis procedures for category III indications, or for those indications that have not been categorized, a physician must evaluate the pathophysiology of the disease process and whether hemapheresis makes sense, the evidence that exists in the medical literature supporting the use of hemapheresis, and the risks of the hemapheresis procedure to the patient, including financial risks (Shaz, 2007). Hemapheresis procedures should not be attempted solely because, "We tried everything else," or because "When in doubt, pheresis it out." The interested reader is referred to the article "How We Approach an Apheresis Request for a Category III, Category IV, or Noncategorized Indication" (Shaz, 2007), for a discussion of clinical decision-making in such circumstances.

THERAPEUTIC CYTAPHERESIS

Therapeutic Plateletpheresis

Thrombocytosis

Thrombocytosis is defined as an increase in the number of platelets present in the blood. This can range from mild increases to increases resulting in platelet counts greater than 1,000,000/µL. It is in these latter patients that concern arises. Thrombocytosis can result from a number of disease processes (Table 37-12). These processes can be primary or secondary (reactive); the latter type accounted for the majority (82%) in one study of patients with platelet counts greater than 1,000,000/µL (Buss, 1994).

Both thrombotic and hemorrhagic events may complicate thrombocytosis. Hemorrhagic complications consist predominantly of mucocutaneous bleeding (Schafer, 1996). Thrombotic complications include both microvascular thrombosis, such as erythromelalgia, and macrovascular thrombosis, such as myocardial infarction. Of cases of macrovascular thrombosis, arterial thrombosis predominates, with the most frequent sites including the cerebrovascular, peripheral vascular, and coronary artery circulations (Schafer, 1996). These complications are rare in cases of secondary thrombocytosis (4%) but are relatively common in primary cases (56%) (Buss, 1994). Risk factors found to be associated with these complications in primary thrombocytosis are given in Table 37-13.

Because of concern over the occurrence of these complications, studies have focused on efforts to reduce elevated platelet counts. Treatments include chemotherapeutic agents such as alkylating agents, radiophosphorus (^{32}P), and hydroxycarbamide (hydroxyurea), as well as medications such as interferon-α and anagrelide (Schafer, 1996). All of these agents have been found to be effective in reducing platelet counts over a period of days to weeks; they also have significant side effects, including leukemogenesis with alkylating agents, ^{32}P, and hydroxycarbamide. As a result, and because of the low risk of complications in patients with secondary disorders, these interventions to reduce platelet count are not used in this setting, and the underlying disorder is treated (Buss, 1994). In primary disorders, however, the decision is more difficult and controversial. Still, unless the patient is symptomatic from the elevated platelet count, many authors recommend not treating. This is due in part to studies that have shown no convincing evidence that reducing the platelet count prevents complications (Schafer, 1984), as well as the fact that the platelet count does not correlate with the risk of thrombosis (Tefferi, 1994).

Therapeutic Thrombocytapheresis Indications

The role of hemapheresis in the treatment of thrombocytosis is to intervene when patients become symptomatic and to stabilize patients' condition until medical management reduces the platelet count. As stated previously, platelet count does not correlate with the risk of thrombosis, even when the count is >1,000,000/µL (Schafer, 1984, 1996; Buss, 1994; Tefferi, 1994). As a result, thrombocytapheresis should be used to treat those who are symptomatic from their elevated platelet counts. Additionally, thrombocytapheresis can be used in the preoperative setting to reduce the platelet count and possibly prevent bleeding, and in the treatment of pregnant women (Isbister, 1997). The benefit of thrombocytapheresis in this latter patient group is again uncertain, as there is a lack of correlation between platelet count and pregnancy outcome (Schafer, 1996). Although hemapheresis is an adjunct to therapy and not a primary treatment modality, Baron (1993) did note that apheresis appeared to increase the sensitivity of patients to busulfan therapy. This produced a greater platelet response but also a greater danger of pancytopenia (Baron, 1993). It must be stressed that the effects of thrombocytapheresis in thrombocytosis are temporary, lasting hours to days, and medical management must be instituted at the same time.

Thrombocytapheresis procedures in this setting can be performed on any instrument that can collect platelets from donors. Typically, the goal of the procedure is to process 1–1.5 blood volumes (Baron, 1993), or to process for a defined length of time such as 3 hours (Burgstaler, 1994). In a study comparing the ability of apheresis systems to reduce platelet counts, Burgstaler and Pineda (1994) found that processing for 3 hours resulted in a 43% reduction in platelet count using the COBE Spectra. Just as there is no defined level at which thrombosis occurs, no target for

TABLE 37-11

Diseases Treated by Hemapheresis*

Disorder	Hemapheresis procedure	ASFA category	ASFA recommendation grade
ABO-incompatible stem cell transplant			
Hematopoietic progenitor cell (HPC)-M (marrow)	Plasma exchange	II	1B
HPC-A (apheresis)	Plasma exchange	II	2B
ABO-incompatible solid organ transplant			
Kidney	Plasma exchange	II	1B
Heart (<40 months of age)	Plasma exchange	II	1C
Liver	Plasma exchange	III	2C
Acute disseminated encephalomyelitis (ADEM)	Plasma exchange	II	2C
Acute inflammatory demyelinating polyneuropathy (Guillain-Barré syndrome)	Plasma exchange	I	1A
Acute liver failure	Plasma exchange	III	2B
Age-related macular degeneration (AMD)			
Dry AMD	Double-filtration plasmapheresis	III	2B
Amyloidosis	Plasma exchange	IV	2C
Amyotrophic lateral sclerosis (ALS)	Plasma exchange	IV	1B
Antineutrophil cytoplasmic antibody (ANCA)-associated rapidly progressive glomerulonephritis (Wegner's granulomatosis)			
Dialysis independent	Plasma exchange	III	2C
Diffuse alveolar hemorrhage	Plasma exchange	I	1C
Dialysis dependent	Plasma exchange	I	1A
Anti–basement membrane antibody disease (Goodpasture's syndrome)			
Dialysis independent	Plasma exchange	I	1A
Diffuse alveolar hemorrhage	Plasma exchange	I	1B
Dialysis dependent	Plasma exchange	IV	1A
Aplastic anemia	Plasma exchange	III	2C
Autoimmune hemolytic anemia			
Warm autoimmune hemolytic anemia	Plasma exchange	III	2C
Cold agglutinin disease	Plasma exchange	II	2C
Babesiosis			
Severe	Red cell exchange	I	1B
High-risk patient	Red cell exchange	II	2C
Burn shock resuscitation	Plasma exchange	IV	2B
Catastrophic antiphospholipid antibody syndrome (CAPS)	Plasma exchange	II	2C
Chronic focal encephalitis (Rasmussen's encephalitis)	Plasma exchange	II	2C
	Immunoadsorption	II	2C
Chronic inflammatory demyelinating polyneuropathy (CIDP)	Plasma exchange	I	1B
Coagulation factor inhibitors	Plasma exchange	IV	2C
	Immunoadsorption	III	2B
Cryoglobulinemia			
Symptomatic/severe	Plasma exchange	I	1B
Secondary to hepatitis C	Plasma exchange	II	2B
Cutaneous T cell lymphoma			
Erythrodermic	Extracorporeal photopheresis (ECP)	I	1B
Nonerythrodermic	ECP	III	2C
Dilated cardiomyopathy (New York Heart Association functional Class II–IV)	Plasma exchange	III	2C
	Immunoadsorption	III	2B
Familial hypercholesterolemia			
Homozygotes	Low-density lipoprotein (LDL) apheresis	I	1A
Heterozygotes	LDL apheresis	II	1A
Heterozygotes with small blood volume	Plasma exchange	II	1C
Focal segmental glomerulonephritis	Plasma exchange	I	1C
Graft-versus-host-disease			
Chronic cutaneous	ECP	II	1B
Acute cutaneous	ECP	II	2C
Acute or chronic noncutaneous	ECP	III	2C
Heart transplant rejection			
Prophylaxis of acute cellular rejection (ACR)	ECP	I	1A
Treatment of ACR	ECP	II	1B
Treatment of antibody-mediated rejection (AMR)	Plasma exchange	III	2C

Continued

PART 4

TABLE 37-11
Diseases Treated by Hemapheresis—*Cont'd*

Disorder	Hemapheresis procedure	ASFA category	ASFA recommendation grade
Hemolytic-uremic syndrome (HUS)			
Atypical HUS due to complement factor gene mutations	Plasma exchange	II	2C
Atypical HUS due to autoantibody to factor H	Plasma exchange	I	2C
Diarrhea-associated HUS (typical HUS)	Plasma exchange	IV	2C
Hyperleukocytosis			
Leukostasis	Leukocytapheresis	I	1B
Prophylaxis	Leukocytapheresis	III	2C
Hypertriglyceridemic pancreatitis	Plasma exchange	III	2C
Hyperviscosity in monoclonal gammopathy			
Symptomatic	Plasma exchange	I	1B
Prophylaxis for rituximab	Plasma exchange	I	1C
Immune thrombocytopenic purpura (ITP)	Plasma exchange	IV	1B
Immune complex rapidly progressive glomerulonephritis	Plasma exchange	III	2B
Inclusion-body myositis	Plasma exchange	IV	2B
	Lymphocytapheresis	IV	2C
Inflammatory bowel disease	Adsorptive cytapheresis	II	2B
Lambert-Eaton myasthenic syndrome	Plasma exchange	II	2C
Lung allograft rejection	ECP	II	1C
Malaria	Red cell exchange	II	2B
Multiple sclerosis			
Acute central nervous system (CNS) demyelination	Plasma exchange	II	1B
Chronic progressive	Plasma exchange	III	2B
Myasthenia gravis			
Moderate to severe	Plasma exchange	I	1A
Prophylaxis prethymectomy	Plasma exchange	I	1C
Myeloma cast nephropathy	Plasma exchange	II	2B
Nephrogenic systemic fibrosis	Plasma exchange	III	2C
	ECP	III	2C
Neuromyelitis optica	Plasma exchange	II	1C
Overdose and poisoning			
Mushroom poisoning	Plasma exchange	II	2C
Snake bites	Plasma exchange	III	2C
Monoclonal antibody with progressive multifocal leukoencephalopathy (PML)	Plasma exchange	III	2C
Other compounds	Plasma exchange	III	2C
Paraneoplastic neurologic syndromes	Plasma exchange	III	2C
	Immunoadsorption	III	2C
Paraproteinemic polyneuropathies			
Immunoglobulin (Ig)G/IgA	Plasma exchange	I	1B
IgM	Plasma exchange	I	1B
Multiple myeloma	Plasma exchange	III	2C
Pediatric autoimmune neuropsychiatric disorders associated with streptococcal infections (PANDAS)	Plasma exchange	I	1B
Pemphigus vulgaris	Plasma exchange	IV	2B
	ECP	III	2C
Phytanic acid storage disease (Refsum's disease)	Plasma exchange	II	2C
Polycythemia vera and erythrocytosis			
Polycythemia vera	Erythrocytapheresis	III	2C
Secondary erythrocytosis	Erythrocytapheresis	III	2B
POEMS syndrome	Plasma exchange	IV	2B
Polymyositis/dermatomyositis	Plasma exchange	IV	1B
	Lymphocytapheresis	IV	1B
Posttransfusion purpura (PTP)	Plasma exchange	III	2C
Psoriasis	Plasma exchange	IV	1B
Pure red cell aplasia	Plasma exchange	II	2C
Red cell alloimmunization in pregnancy	Plasma exchange	II	2C
Renal transplant			
Antibody-mediated rejection	Plasma exchange	I	1B
Desensitization living donor with donor-specific human leukocyte antigen (HLA)	Plasma exchange	II	1B
High panel reactive alloantibody (PRA) cadaveric donor	Plasma exchange	III	2C
Rheumatoid arthritis	Plasma exchange	IV	1B
Scleroderma (progressive systemic sclerosis)	Plasma exchange	III	2C
	ECP	IV	1A
Schizophrenia	Plasma exchange	IV	1A

TABLE 37-11
Diseases Treated by Hemapheresis—*Cont'd*

Disorder	Hemapheresis procedure	ASFA category	ASFA recommendation grade
Sepsis and multiorgan failure	Plasma exchange	III	2B
Sickle cell disease			
Acute stroke	Red cell exchange	I	1C
Acute chest syndrome	Red cell exchange	II	1C
Prophylaxis for second stroke	Red cell exchange	II	1C
Prophylaxis for iron overload	Red cell exchange	II	1C
Multiorgan failure	Red cell exchange	III	2C
Sydenham's chorea	Plasma exchange	I	1B
Systemic lupus erythematosus (SLE)			
Severe (e.g., cerebritis, diffuse alveolar hemorrhage)	Plasma exchange	II	2C
Nephritis	Plasma exchange	IV	1B
Thrombocytosis			
Symptomatic	Thrombocytapheresis	II	2C
Prophylactic or secondary	Thrombocytapheresis	III	2C
Thrombotic microangiopathy, drug-associated			
Gemcitabine	Plasma exchange	IV	2C
Cyclosporine/Tacrolimus	Plasma exchange	III	2C
Quinine	Plasma exchange	IV	2B
Ticlopidine/Clopidogrel	Plasma exchange	I	2B
Thrombotic microangiopathy, hematopoietic progenitor cell transplant associated	Plasma exchange	III	1B
Thrombotic thrombocytopenic purpura (TTP)	Plasma exchange	I	1A
Thyrotoxicosis	Plasma exchange	III	2C
Wilson's disease with fulminant hepatic failure and hemolysis	Plasma exchange	I	1C

From Szczepiorkowski (2010).
ASFA, American Society for Apheresis.
*See Table 37-8 for explanation of ASFA categories and Table 37-9 for explanation of recommendation grades.

TABLE 37-12
Diseases Associated With Thrombocytosis

Primary	Essential thrombocythemia Agnogenic myeloid metaplasia Polycythemia vera Chronic myelogenous leukemia
Secondary (reactive)	Splenectomy Acute hemorrhage Iron deficiency Chronic inflammatory diseases Solid malignancies Rebound after myelosuppression

Reprinted from Buss DH, Cashell AW, O'Connor ML, et al. Occurrence, etiology, and clinical significance of extreme thrombocytosis: a study of 280 cases. Am J Med 1994;96:247–53, Copyright © 1994, with permission from Excerpta Medica, Inc.

TABLE 37-13
Factors Associated With Complications in Primary Thrombocytosis

Thrombosis	Increasing age Previous thrombotic event Longer duration of thrombocythemia
Hemorrhage	Platelet count >2,000,000/μL NSAID ingestion

From Cortelazzo (1990) and Tefferi (1994).
NSAID, Nonsteroidal anti-inflammatory drug.

platelet reduction has been defined. The patient's symptoms should be treated, with improvement/resolution being the desired endpoint.

Thrombocytapheresis for symptomatic thrombocytosis is a category II indication with a 2C recommendation grade, and prophylactic thrombocytapheresis for asymptomatic thrombocytosis is a category III indication with a 2C recommendation grade, according to the ASFA (Szczepiorkowski, 2010).

Therapeutic Leukocytapheresis

Hyperleukocytosis

Hyperleukocytosis is an extreme elevation in white blood cell count. The causes of such elevations include malignant and nonmalignant disease, with the former resulting in the highest counts. This can produce a number of syndromes, including central nervous system (CNS) leukostasis, characterized by neurologic deficits, and pulmonary leukostasis, characterized by poor oxygenation and chest pain (Isbister, 1997). Traditionally, extremely elevated white blood cell counts have been believed to result in increased viscosity with changes in blood flow within the microvasculature. White blood cells, especially granulocytes, are more rigid than red blood cells (Isbister, 1997). It has been believed that, at these very high white blood cell counts, occlusion of the microvasculature can occur, resulting in leukostasis and ischemia. However, this may not represent the entire picture. White blood cell count does not necessarily correlate with the onset of symptoms. More recent evidence suggests that the interactions of adhesion molecules expressed on the leukemic blasts and endothelial cells may also contribute to vascular occlusion and endothelial injury (Liesveld, 1997; Porcu, 2000; Stucki, 2001).

In addition to vascular occlusive symptoms of hyperleukocytosis, another potential problem resulting from markedly elevated white blood cell count is the tumor lysis syndrome (Isbister, 1997). This occurs during the patient's initial chemotherapy and results from the release of tumor cell breakdown products, producing damage to the kidneys and/or initiating disseminated intravascular coagulation.

Higher mortality rates occur during the first week of therapy among patients with white blood cell counts greater than 100,000/μL. These deaths were associated with a significantly greater number of CNS hemorrhages than in those with white cell counts <50,000/μL (Dutcher, 1987). Similarly, the presence of pulmonary leukostasis is also associated with early mortality (Lester, 1985). In one study, average survival of patients with pulmonary leukostasis was 0.2 months versus 15.4 months in those with CNS leukostasis and 10.8 months in patients lacking leukostasis (Lester, 1985). As in thrombocytosis, the definitive treatment of these elevated white blood cell counts is to treat the underlying disease, in this case leukemia.

Therapeutic Leukocytapheresis Indications

As in therapeutic thrombocytapheresis, the role of leukocytapheresis in hyperleukocytosis is to decrease the white cell count to relieve symptoms and/or prevent tumor lysis syndrome. As with thrombocytapheresis, the indication for treating a patient is the presence of symptoms indicating leukostasis. Additionally, leukocytapheresis can be used to treat pregnant women to prolong pregnancy until the child can be delivered and the mother started on chemotherapy. Again, hemapheresis represents an adjunct to therapy and not a primary treatment modality. The definitive therapy is chemotherapy that should be begun at the same time or shortly after hemapheresis is initiated, as the reduction in white blood cell counts with leukocytapheresis is temporary. With this said, two things should be stated. Although hemapheresis can reverse or lessen leukostasis symptoms in some patients, no correlation has been found between the degree of leukoreduction, as an absolute value or as a percentage, and overall survival (Porcu, 1997). In addition, although leukocytapheresis may improve 2- to 3-week mortality rates after diagnosis, it does not appear to affect the long-term or overall survival rates of these patients (Thiébaut, 2000; Giles, 2001).

Leukocytapheresis procedures share similarities with granulocyte collections, as previously described. HES can be used to enhance the separation of cellular components during centrifugation, resulting in more efficient white cell removal. This is especially important when the cells are more mature granulocytes, as seen in chronic phase CML. The total blood volume processed is usually 8–10 L or two blood volumes (McLeod, 1993). With this strategy, reductions in white blood cell count of 50%–85% have been reported (Steeper, 1985; Burgstaler, 1994). As in therapeutic thrombocytapheresis, no goal has been defined for the reduction in white blood cells, and improvement/resolution of the patient's symptoms is the endpoint. Hyperleukocytosis with leukostasis is a category I indication with a 1B recommendation grade for leukocytapheresis. Prophylactic leukocytapheresis for asymptomatic hyperleukocytosis is a category III indication with a 2C recommendation grade, according to the ASFA (Szczepiorkowski, 2010).

Red Cell Exchange

Red cell exchange (RCE), or therapeutic erythrocytapheresis, is a form of cytapheresis that removes the patient's red blood cells and replaces them with allogeneic red blood cells. This form of hemapheresis has been used occasionally to treat hyperparasitemia in malaria and other parasitic infections of red blood cells such as babesiosis (Powell, 2002). It is most commonly used in the treatment of sickle cell anemia.

Sickle Cell Anemia

Sickle cell anemia is an autosomal recessive disorder present in 1 in 200–500 African American newborns (Wayne, 1993); it is also seen in people from sub-Saharan and Western Africa, Arab countries, the Mediterranean basin, and India (Davies, 1997). Sickle cell anemia results from a mutation that substitutes a valine for a glutamic acid at position six of the β-globin chain of Hb, producing Hb S (Davies, 1997). This change decreases the solubility of Hb when deoxygenated, such that crystals form which alter the shape of the red blood cell and damage its membrane. Repeated episodes lead to irreversible sickling of the cell. Even in the absence of sickling, the red cells in sickle cell anemia are abnormally "sticky." The combination of this "stickiness" and sickling leads to occlusion of small vessels, endothelial damage, and thrombosis (Wayne, 1993; Davies, 1997).

Sickle cell anemia is characterized by chronic hemolytic anemia and crises—episodes of acute illness. Crises are most often due to vascular occlusion and infarction and include crises of pain, aplasia, splenic sequestration, hemolysis, cerebrovascular accidents, acute chest pain syndrome, and priapism. They are treated by correcting factors that enhance sickling, namely, dehydration, hypoxia, and acidosis. This is done through hydration, alkalinization, and the administration of supplemental oxygen (Wayne, 1993; Davies, 1997). In addition, painful crises are treated by the administration of analgesics. These crises can also be treated by red blood cell transfusion.

Red cell transfusion in sickle cell anemia can be divided into three categories: acute simple transfusion, chronic simple transfusion, and red cell exchange transfusion. Acute simple transfusion consists of the transfusion of red blood cells to increase oxygen-carrying capacity and is indicated for the treatment of symptomatic anemia, splenic sequestration crisis, aplastic crisis, blood loss, accelerated hemolysis, and preoperative preparation (Wayne, 1993). Chronic simple transfusion consists of regular transfusions of red blood cells in an attempt to suppress endogenous red cell production with the goal of keeping the percentage of red cells containing Hb S below 30%. This form of therapy is indicated for cerebrovascular disease and debilitating vaso-occlusive symptoms. It can also be used to treat sickle cell disease complicated by pulmonary disease, cardiac disease, high-risk pregnancy, and preoperative preparation (Wayne, 1993).

RCE in sickle cell anemia is used to remove Hb S–containing red blood cells, while replacing them with Hb A–containing red cells. The goal of RCE is to leave the patient with a Hct of approximately 30% and a "sicklecrit"—the percentage of cells containing Hb S—of less than 30% (Wayne, 1993; Davies, 1997). To do this, the fraction of red cells remaining (FCR) must be calculated based on the patient's current Hb S percentage and the desired Hb S percentage. This can be calculated by Equation 37-5. If the patient's Hct is to be increased by the procedure, then the adjusted FCR must be calculated according to Equation 37-6 (COBE BCT, 1997). It should be noted that increasing the Hct too much can result in decreased oxygen delivery as a result of increased viscosity. This results from the fact that the sickle cells, as well as the endothelium, of these patients are "stickier" than normal.

$$\text{Desired FCR\%} = (\text{Desired Hb S}/\text{Current Hb S}) \times 100 \qquad \textbf{(37-5)}$$

$$\text{Adjusted FCR\%} = \text{Desired FCR\%} \times (\text{Current Hct}/\text{Desired Hct}) \times 100 \qquad \textbf{(37-6)}$$

These are then entered into the hemapheresis instrument along with other values to determine the volume of red blood cells necessary to perform the procedure. The benefits of RCE over the other strategies of transfusion are given in Table 37-14.

TABLE 37-14 Benefits of Red Blood Cell Exchange by Apheresis Compared With Simple or Chronic Transfusion

Decreased amount of hemoglobin S without increasing hematocrit and, therefore, viscosity
Use of fewer units of red blood cells to achieve the same percentage of hemoglobin S
Decreased contribution to iron overload in chronically transfused patients

From American Society for Apheresis Clinical Applications Committee, McLeod BC. Clinical applications of therapeutic apheresis. J Clin Apheresis 2000;15:1–5. Copyright © 2000 J Clin Apheresis. Reprinted with permission of Wiley-Liss, Inc., a subsidiary of John Wiley & Sons, Inc.

Acute chest syndrome is a crisis characterized by respiratory symptoms, chest and abdominal pain, infiltrates on chest radiograph, and an abnormal chest examination. It is thought that pain from rib splinting or fat embolism results in hypoventilation leading to atelectasis. This, in turn, causes hypoxia leading to occlusion of small vessels in the lung and possible thrombosis of the pulmonary arteries (Davies, 1997). It occurs in 20%–50% of sickle cell patients and has a mortality rate of 2%–14%. Repeated episodes may progress to chronic pulmonary disease (Wayne, 1993). RCE is used to remove Hb S–containing cells and has been associated with marked improvement (Wayne, 1993).

Priapism is a painful, sustained erection that results from occlusion of vessels in the corpus cavernosum by sickled cells. It is associated with dehydration and acidosis and is treated with supplemental oxygen, hydration, and analgesics (Wayne, 1993). If prolonged (over 6 hours), priapism is referred to as fulminant priapism and may require surgical intervention or RCE. A significant percentage of patients will suffer from impotence if not treated (Davies, 1997). Although RCE has been reported as effective in treating priapism, it is not without risks. A syndrome of neurologic events called ASPEN syndrome (association of sickle cell disease, priapism, exchange transfusion, and neurologic events) has been reported to occur in some patients treated with RCE. It consists of neurologic events ranging from headache and seizure activity to obtundation requiring ventilator support. The syndrome is thought to be due to decreased cerebral blood flow from the abrupt elevation in Hct, as well as the release of vasoactive substances from the penile detumescence. Aggressive treatment has been associated with complete neurologic recovery (Siegel, 1993). Patients suffering from priapism undergoing RCE should be monitored for symptoms of ASPEN syndrome.

Additional crises and disorders in sickle cell patients for which RCE is indicated include cerebrovascular accident, retinal artery vaso-occlusion, hepatic failure, and septic shock. RCE has also been used to decrease the

TABLE 37-15

Characteristics Indicating Best Responders to Extracorporeal Photopheresis Among CTCL Patients

• Erythrodermic skin stage	• Immunocompetent patient
• WBC count <15,000/mm^3	• Absence of bulky lymph nodes or visceral disease
• Disease of short duration	• Presence of Sézary cells in the circulation
• Normal percentage of CD8 cells	

Data from Zic JA. The treatment of cutaneous T-cell lymphoma with photopheresis. Dermatol Ther 2003;16:337–46.
CTCL, Cutaneous T cell lymphoma; *WBC,* white blood cell.

TABLE 37-16

Factors Associated With the Development of Chronic Graft-Versus-Host Disease

• Increased donor age	• Unrelated donor
• Increased recipient age	• Prior acute graft-versus-host disease (GVHD)
• Human leukocyte antigen (HLA) disparity	• Alloimmunized female donor

Data from Foss FM, Gorgun G, Miller KB: Extracorporeal photopheresis in chronic graft-versus-host disease. Bone Marrow Transplant 2002;29:719–725.

percentage of Hb S at the initiation of chronic simple transfusion therapy, to prevent sickling due to contrast dye during cerebral angiograms, and in preparation for surgery (Wayne, 1993). It should be noted that a study has shown no benefit of RCE versus a conservative transfusion regimen designed to increase Hb to 10 g/dL in preventing complications of surgery (Vichinsky, 1995).

Stroke in sickle cell anemia is a category I indication with a 1C recommendation grade for RCE. Acute chest syndrome, stroke prophylaxis, and prophylaxis for iron overload in sickle cell anemia are all category II indications with 1C recommendation grades for RCE. Primary or secondary stroke prevention is a category II indication for RCE with a 1C recommendation grade. Finally, multiorgan failure in sickle cell anemia is a category III indication with a 2C recommendation grade for RCE according to the ASFA. Severe malaria is a category II indication with a 2B recommendation grade for RCE. Severe babesiosis is a category I indication with a 1B recommendation grade, and treatment of high-risk patients without severe symptoms is a category II indication with a 2C recommendation grade for RCE (Szczepiorkowski, 2010).

Extracorporeal Photopheresis

Extracorporeal photopheresis, also called extracorporeal photochemotherapy (ECP) or photopheresis, is a form of leukocytapheresis. In this procedure, a small percentage of a patient's white blood cells are collected by hemapheresis. These cells are then treated by incubation with a psoralen compound and are exposed to ultraviolet A (UVA) irradiation within the instrument. Following this, the cells are reinfused into the patient (Zic, 1999). This then appears to result in an immunomodulatory effect. Depending on the disease being treated, this may stimulate or suppress an immune response. Currently, this therapy is approved by the FDA only for the treatment of cutaneous T cell lymphoma (CTCL). In December of 2006, the Centers for Medicare Services approved coverage of the use of photopheresis for the treatment of chronic graft-versus-host disease and acute cardiac allograft rejection. Previously, Medicare had covered the use of photopheresis in the treatment of CTCL.

Extracorporeal Photopheresis Indications

Cutaneous T Cell Lymphoma. The first disease treated by photopheresis was CTCL—a skin-based T cell lymphoma characterized by a long premalignant phase (4–10 years) of eczematous skin lesions. Following this, the disease progresses through a series of phases characterized by increasing skin involvement until the development of the tumor phase, characterized by cutaneous masses. CTCL may then progress to a leukemic phase known as Sézary syndrome, in which malignant T cells are found circulating in the blood. Median survival depends on the stage of the disease at diagnosis; 10-year survivals range from 20% for the tumor stage to 85% for the initial plaque phase (Zic, 1999).

In 1987, Edelson reported responses in 64% of 37 CTCL patients treated with photopheresis. Subsequently, the use of photopheresis for the treatment of CTCL received FDA approval (Zic, 2003). Combined analysis of more than 400 patients reported in the literature has found an overall response rate of CTCL to photopheresis of 55.7%, with 17.6% of patients having a complete response. Response rates vary from 64% for stage IB patients (generalized patches and plaques) to 27.3% for stage IVB patients (visceral involvement) (Zic, 2003). Factors predictive of response to photopheresis are given in Table 37-15. The median time until clearing of skin lesions in such patients is 11 months; patients who show an early response (clearing in 6–8 months) maintain their response (Zic, 1999). Extracorporeal photopheresis has also been associated with longer survival from time of diagnosis (longer than 60 months among photopheresis-treated patients vs. 31 months for patients receiving chemotherapy) (Christensen, 1991).

The mechanism of action of photopheresis in CTCL has not been completely elucidated. Extracorporeal photopheresis is known to induce a CD8+ T cell response toward expanded pathologic T cell clones within the patient (Zic, 2003). It is thought that this is due to the fact that upon exposure to UVA, 8-methoxypsoralen (8-MOP) reacts with cellular constituents, irreversibly binding to DNA, proteins, and lipids. This induces an increase in the number of HLA class I molecules present on the exposed cell, as well as apoptosis. It is interesting to note that apoptosis occurs in exposed lymphocytes, including malignant T cells, but not monocytes. Monocytes, as a result of their exposure to subphysiologic temperatures and contact with walls of the tubing during collection and photoactivation, differentiate into immature dendritic cells (DCs). These DCs are then capable of phagocytosing the apoptotic malignant T cells and can present the tumor antigens from these cells within their HLA class I molecules. Upon reinfusion of the UVA-exposed photopheresis product, these antigen-presenting cells can then activate cytotoxic T cells, resulting in an immune response toward abnormal T cell clones (Zic, 2003). This is associated with a shift in the patient's cytokine profile from that of a Th2 response to a Th1 response (Zic, 2003). The beneficial effects of the procedure do not result from direct cytotoxicity of 8-MOP and UVA on abnormal T cells or tumor cells, as only 10%–15% of the lymphocyte pool is harvested, and less than 5% of cutaneous T cell lymphoma cells are treated (Christensen, 1991).

Erythrodermic CTCL is a category I indication with a 1B recommendation grade for extracorporeal photopheresis, according to the ASFA (Szczepiorkowski, 2010). Nonerythrodermic CTCL is a category III indication with a 2C recommendation grade for extracorporeal photopheresis (Szczepiorkowski, 2010).

Graft-Versus-Host Disease and Solid Organ Rejection. Chronic graft-versus-host disease (cGVHD) occurs in 27%–50% of matched related sibling donor transplants and in 42%–72% of unrelated bone marrow or peripheral blood stem cell transplants (Foss, 2002). Factors associated with cGVHD are given in Table 37-16.

A number of studies have reported the use of extracorporeal photopheresis in cGVHD (Foss, 2002). In these studies, patients with cGVHD unresponsive to other therapies have shown improvement in skin, oral, and visceral (hepatic) lesions. These have been associated with normalization of CD4/CD8 ratios and decreased numbers of NK cells. Treatment allowed for tapering of steroid doses and maintenance of the response for a median of 12 months. No increase in infection rates or CMV activation was noted in the patients studied (Foss, 2002). Those patients who were more likely to respond were those who started therapy within 10 months of transplant.

As with CTCL, the mechanism behind photopheresis in cGVHD is unclear. It is remarkable that therapy associated with immune activation in one disease is associated with immune suppression in another. In cGVHD patients, photopheresis is associated with a decrease in antigen recognition and processing by DC, as well as decreased numbers of DCs. This, in turn, decreases CD8 stimulation, with a shift in Th1 response to a Th2 response through inhibition of Th2 cytokine secretion (Foss, 2002). The result is decreased alloreactivity by T cells.

Similar to cGVHD, solid organ rejection is a disorder of alloreactive T cells. Extracorporeal photopheresis has similarly been used to treat rejection in heart, lung, kidney, and liver transplant. In cardiac transplantation, the use of extracorporeal photopheresis has been reported to histologically reverse 89% of treated rejection episodes without side effects. Similar rates have been reported with other transplant types (Dall'Amico, 2002).

Chronic cutaneous GVHD is a category II indication with a 1B recommendation grade. Acute cutaneous GVHD is a category II indication with a 2C recommendation grade. GVHD involving organs other than the skin, whether acute or chronic, is a category III indication with a 2C recommendation grade for extracorporeal photopheresis, according to ASFA (Szczepiorkowski, 2010). Treatment of cardiac allograft rejection is a category II indication with a 1B recommendation grade for extracorporeal photopheresis, and prophylaxis of rejection is a category I indication with a 1A recommendation grade (Szczepiorkowski, 2010).

Other Diseases. Additional diseases that have been treated with extracorporeal photopheresis are listed in Table 37-17. Many, but not all, of these diseases have a common thread of T cell alloreactivity or autoreactivity. Some of these diseases have been assigned categories and recommendation grades by ASFA; the reader is referred to Table 37-11.

Extracorporeal Photopheresis Procedure

The extracorporeal photopheresis procedure is performed using the UVAR XTS or CELLEX photopheresis system (Therakos, Inc., Exton, PA) with the UVAR XTS scheduled for discontinuation by 2016. For the UVAR XTS, following venipuncture, 125 mL or 225 mL of whole blood is collected in a Latham centrifuge bowl, where the components are separated. Heparin or acid-citrate-dextrose (ACD) can be used as the anticoagulant. The buffy coat is retained in a collection bag, and the remaining blood components are returned to the patient. Because this is an intermittent centrifuge, six cycles (125 mL bowl) or three cycles (225 mL bowl) of whole blood collection are performed to collect a 270-mL MNC suspension. This consists of 80 mL of plasma, 90 mL of saline, and 100 mL of MNC. After completion of the collection, 8-MOP is added to the bag. The MNC suspension is then pumped through a photoactivation chamber. This consists of transparent acrylic plates between which is sandwiched a tortuous channel. Adjacent to the plate is a UVA light source that irradiates the 8-MOP–containing buffy coat. The MNC suspension is photoactivated for 30 minutes. Following completion of photoactivation, the buffy coat is then reinfused. The general process for the CELLEX device is similar to that for the UVAR XTS, in that a buffy coat is harvested, exposed to 8-MOP, photoactivated, and reinfused to the patient. CELLEX differs from UVAR XTS, however, in that it is a continuous flow device, can be used to perform a double- or single-needle procedure, and has peristaltic pumps, as opposed to pneumatic pumps. This device also has only a single-size centrifugation bowl. Results of these changes are that the extracorporeal volume of the CELLEX is less that that of the UVAR XTS (216–266 mL for the CELLEX vs. 220–620 mL for the UVAR XTS), and the total procedure time is less (1.5 hours for the CELLEX vs. 3 hours for the UVAR XTS). In addition, the CELLEX provides greater flexibility in programming of the device (Burgstaler, 2010). This means that much smaller patients, including pediatric patients, who could not be treated previously can now receive photopheresis. A typical course of photopheresis for CTCL consists of two treatments on consecutive days every 4 weeks (Christensen, 1991). Following improvement in disease symptoms, the interval between procedures may be prolonged, and the patient weaned from extracorporeal photopheresis. For other indications, the frequency of treatment varies; the reader is referred to the ASFA guidelines for additional information (Szczepiorkowski, 2010).

An important aspect of this procedure is the clean separation of whole blood into plasma and buffy coat. The product must allow the transmission of UVA light to photoactivate the 8-MOP. The presence of significant numbers of red blood cells within the leukocytapheresis product will reflect or absorb the UVA irradiation, resulting in failure to photoactivate the product. As a result, it is critical that the Hct of the leukocytapheresis product be less than 7% (Zic, 1999). Similarly, it is important that excess plasma not be present. Excess plasma will dilute the white blood cells, resulting in fewer passages of each cell through the photoactivation chamber (Zic, 1999).

Two complications of this procedure are photosensitivity and possible leukemogenesis. Patients undergoing extracorporeal photopheresis are sensitive to sunlight (Knobler, 1993). They should avoid direct or indirect sunlight exposure for 24 hours following completion of the procedure by covering exposed skin, using sunscreen, and wearing wrap-around ultraviolet (UV) protective eyewear. Another possible complication of extracorporeal photopheresis could be mutagenesis from DNA damage caused by photoactivation of the 8-MOP. This theoretically could result in the reinfusion of cells with damaged DNA still capable of cell division. These cells could then give rise to hematologic malignancies. Although evidence has not been found to support this concern, it is still a theoretical risk of the procedure (van Iperen, 1997).

TABLE 37-17
Diseases in Which Extracorporeal Photopheresis Has Been Reported as Effective

Malignancy	Cutaneous T cell lymphoma (CTCL)
Graft-versus-host disease (GVHD)	Mucocutaneous GVHD Hepatic GVHD
Organ rejection	Heart Kidney Lung
Autoimmune diseases	Systemic lupus erythematosus Rheumatoid arthritis Juvenile dermatomyositis Pemphigus vulgaris Epidermolysis bullosa acquisita
Infectious diseases	Chronic Lyme arthritis AIDS-related complex (ARC)
Other diseases	Severe atopic dermatitis Psoriasis Nephrogenic systemic fibrosis

From van Iperen (1997), Zic (1999), and Mathur (2008).

THERAPEUTIC PLASMA EXCHANGE

Efficacy of Removal

The goal of therapeutic plasma exchange is to remove a pathologic substance present within the plasma by removing the patient's plasma and replacing it with a substitution fluid. The removal is nonspecific in that all of the substances present in the plasma, including normal substances, are removed. Removal of a substance can be predicted by Equation 37-7, as shown in Figure 37-2 (Derksen, 1984b):

$$Y/Y_0 = e^{-x} \qquad \textbf{(37-7)}$$

where

Y is the final concentration of the substance
Y_0 is the initial concentration of the substance
x is the total number of times the patient's volume is exchanged.

This model assumes that the intravascular compartment is closed, and that exchange between the intravascular and extravascular compartments does not occur. Based on this equation, 30% of the initial quantity of a substance will remain within the patient's plasma after one plasma volume exchange, and 10% will remain after the exchange of two plasma volumes.

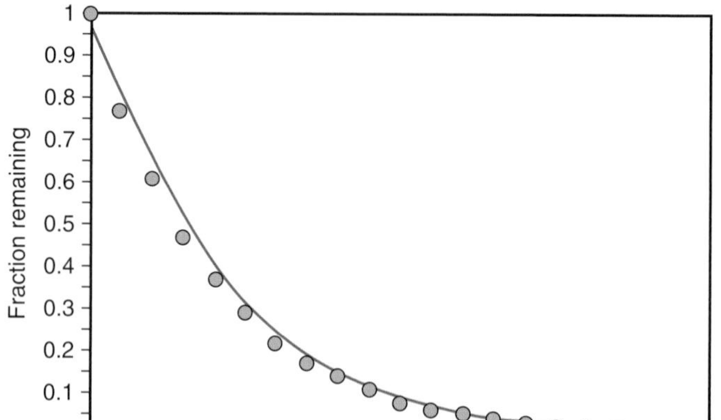

Figure 37-2 Removal of substances during plasma exchange. The removal of substances limited to the intravascular compartment, whether pathologic or normal, can be predicted by an exponential equation (see Equation 37-7). A fixed percentage of the remaining substance is removed with each blood volume. This means that as the number of blood volumes processed increases, a progressively smaller amount of the substance is removed, resulting in diminishing returns.

As more plasma volumes are exchanged, a fixed percentage of the remaining substance is removed (approximately 70%), such that a smaller and smaller total amount is removed. As can be seen in Figure 37-2, the marginal benefit of removing additional plasma volumes declines after 1.5–2 plasma volumes, so most therapeutic plasma exchange procedures are limited to 1–1.5 plasma volume exchanges.

The assumption that no exchange occurs between intravascular and extravascular compartments during the procedure is not valid for all substances. As a result, the amount removed as well as the concentration in the plasma at the end of the procedure may not match that predicted. For example, IgM is located predominantly within the intravascular space (76%), with negligible influx from the extravascular space (Derksen, 1984b). As a result, during a plasma exchange procedure, the equation will accurately predict the removal of IgM. IgA, however, is evenly distributed between the intravascular space and the extravascular space and can move between the two compartments. During plasma exchange, as the concentration of IgA within the intravascular space falls, IgA within the extravascular space follows its concentration gradient and moves into the intravascular space. The result of this is that after the procedure has been completed, the plasma concentration of IgA is not as low as predicted; this would lead one to believe that the procedure was not as efficient as expected (Derksen, 1984b). If one looks at the amount of substance removed by measuring the IgA within the collection bag, one would see that the total amount of IgA removed was greater than predicted, and that the procedure was more efficient than expected. Not only was IgA being removed from the intravascular compartment, it was also being removed from the extravascular compartment (Derksen, 1984b).

Four patterns of removal in plasma exchange using 5% albumin as the replacement fluid have been identified. In the first pattern, seen with fibrinogen and C3, the concentration decreases to a greater extent than expected. This is probably due to the combination of removal and consumption of these factors during the hemapheresis procedure. In the second pattern, such as with IgM, cholesterol, and alkaline phosphatase, the change in concentration is what is predicted. These substances are confined to the intravascular space or have little exchange between compartments. In the third pattern, as seen with lactate dehydrogenase (LD) and creatinine phosphokinase (CPK), the concentration is less than predicted owing to movement of these substances between compartments. Finally, in the fourth pattern, concentrations are much greater than predicted or do not change at all, which may be due to rapid equilibration. This pattern is seen with small inorganic and organic molecules such as potassium, bicarbonate, and glucose (Orlin, 1980).

The pattern of removal of Igs during plasma exchange depends on whether normal Ig or a paraprotein is involved. The removal of normal IgG has been reported to be predictable by Equation 37-7; it behaves as if it is entirely intravascular (Chopek, 1980; Orlin, 1980). Others, however, have reported behavior similar to that of a substance equilibrating between the two compartments (Derksen, 1984b). In the case of paraproteins, the removal of Igs may appear to be half of what is expected when looking at plasma concentrations (Chopek, 1980). This difference is attributed to expansion of the patient's plasma volume due to the presence of the paraprotein (Chopek, 1980). In other words, the plasma volume of the patient is greater than what is predicted by standard equations (e.g., Equation 37-3), such that if these are used to calculate a 1.5 plasma volume exchange, the real volume exchanged will be less.

In addition to the effect on removal of the substance from the plasma, the distribution between the intravascular and extravascular compartments and the ability to move between these compartments will influence the rise in plasma levels of the substance following plasma exchange. The concentrations of substances that diffuse rapidly and have a large extravascular component will rise rapidly. The increase in concentrations of those substances that are predominantly intravascular will depend on the rate of synthesis of the substance. Most substances return to normal levels within 48–72 hours. Exceptions to this include fibrinogen, complement, and Igs, for which mean recoveries at 48 hours were 65%, 65%, and 44% of initial values, respectively. Cholesterol also shows a slow recovery, with 67%–72% of preapheresis values achieved 1 week after hemapheresis (Orlin, 1980).

For the majority of substances removed by plasma exchange, the rate of synthesis does not increase following the procedure (Derksen, 1984a). For some substances, especially the Igs, rebound may occur. Rebound is an increase in concentration after completion of a procedure to a level greater than that seen initially (Derksen, 1984a; Dau, 1995). This may result from the removal of inhibitory substances by the procedure or the removal of negative feedback on the responsible cell. As a result of this, concurrent treatment with cytotoxic agents during the procedure is suggested to prevent rebound (Dau, 1995). In addition, plasma exchange may enhance the efficacy of cytotoxic agents by increasing the metabolic activity of autoreactive immune cells, making them more sensitive to such agents (Dau, 1995). Another point related to this is that plasma exchange will only temporarily decrease the level of a pathologic substance unless additional therapy is instituted to stop its production. This means that in most cases, plasma exchange should be viewed as an adjunct to other therapies.

Replacement Fluids

In therapeutic plasma exchange, 1–1.5 plasma volumes are removed; therefore, this volume must be replaced with another fluid. A number of replacement fluids are available, each of which has advantages and disadvantages. Replacement fluids used in plasma exchange include 5% albumin, FFP, plasma cryoprecipitate reduced (cryopoor plasma), saline, and HES.

Albumin in a concentration of 5% is the most widely used replacement fluid. It is a hyperoncotic fluid for most patients and therefore will result in the net flow of fluid from the extravascular space. This can result in a mild dilutional anemia (Chopek, 1980). The main advantage of 5% albumin is that it does not transmit viral diseases. Disadvantages, however, are that it is expensive and has at times been in short supply because of FDA-mandated recalls. Hypotensive reactions due to prekallikrein activation (Alving, 1978) and febrile reactions due to pyrogens have been reported (Pool, 1995). Both of these reactions are rare. In addition, the albumin may not function comparably to the albumin present in the plasma before exchange. Although exchange with 5% albumin provides physiologic concentrations of the protein, the drug- and metabolite-binding sites of this albumin are occupied by preservatives such as sodium caprylate and may not be available for normal physiologic functions (Koch-Weser, 1976). Standard practice is to use a 5% albumin solution for 60%–70% of the replacement volume. The remaining volume is replaced by crystalloid (normal saline).

FFP is used as the primary replacement fluid in treating TTP (see later discussion of this disease) and may also be used to prevent the dilutional coagulopathy seen with repeated plasma exchanges. FFP can be used in the treatment of severe factor XI deficiency in a patient known to bleed from this defect who is to undergo a surgical procedure. Because a concentrate for factor XI is not available and the quantity of FFP that would need to be infused to reach therapeutic levels would cause volume overload, exchange with FFP immediately before the surgical procedure can provide hemostasis. Advantages of FFP are that it is relatively inexpensive and provides physiologic concentrations of coagulation factors. Disadvantages include the danger of transmission of transfusion-transmitted viral diseases, transfusion reactions, the need to have an ABO-compatible product, and an increase in the frequency of citrate reactions (see discussion at the end of the chapter). This last disadvantage results from the fact that the patient is infused not only with citrate anticoagulant but also with the citrate within the FFP. When used to treat TTP, 60%–70% of the replaced volume will be FFP, and the remainder will be normal saline. When used to prevent coagulopathy, two units of FFP can be given at the end of the procedure, with most of the replacement volume being 5% albumin.

Plasma cryoprecipitate reduced is also used in the treatment of TTP, specifically in those unresponsive to plasma exchange with FFP. The advantages and disadvantages of plasma cryoprecipitate reduced are the same as those for FFP, with the exception that plasma cryoprecipitate reduced does not provide physiologic concentrations of all coagulation factors, thereby lacking fibrinogen and factor VIII.

Saline is used for a portion of most plasma exchange procedures (30%–40%); it is used to prime the instrument and to make the anticoagulant solution. The use of saline for greater volumes is problematic in that it is a crystalloid and not a colloid and can redistribute into the extravascular space, resulting in hypotension and edema following the procedure. The advantages of saline are that it is inexpensive and does not carry the risks of transmitting disease.

The final option is the use of synthetic colloidal fluid such as HES. HES is derived from plant starches and consists of large starch molecules that can be added to saline to generate a colloidal solution. Plasma exchanges using HES as the replacement fluid have been described (Burgstaler, 1990; Rock, 1997). The benefits of HES are that it is inexpensive and does not transmit disease. A disadvantage is that a small percentage of individuals will have an allergic reaction to HES (see discussion at end of chapter). Also, high molecular weight HES hetastarch has a half-life of 25.5 hours, so significant amounts can persist after frequent plasma

TABLE 37-18
Effects of Plasma Exchange on Medications as Reported in the Literature

Medications That Do Not Require Dose Supplementation Because of Insignificant Removal, Redistribution From Tissue Stores, or Drug Binding to Red Blood Cells	Medications That Are Removed and May Require Dose Supplementation
• Acyclovir	• Basiliximab
• Azathioprine	• Ceftazidime
• Carbamazepine	• Ceftriaxone
• Cyclophosphamide	• Chloramphenicol
• Cyclosporine	• Cisplatin
• Digitoxin	• Diltiazem
• Digoxin	• Interferon-α
• Oxcarbazepine	• Intravenous immune globulin (IVIG)
• Phenobarbital	• Palivizumab
• Phenytoin	• Propoxyphene
• Prednisolone	• Propranolol
• Prednisone	• Rituximab
• Propranolol	• Tobramycin
• Quinine	• Verapamil
• Tacrolimus	• Vincristine
• Valproic acid	
• Vancomycin	

From Kale-Pradhan (1997), Kintzel (2003), and Ibrahim (2007).

exchange procedures, resulting in volume expansion and alterations in partial thromboplastin time (PTT), total protein, albumin, Hct, and fibrinogen (Rock, 1997). These changes are less frequent with pentastarch, a low molecular weight HES, because of its shorter half-life. HES has been associated with changes in hemostasis (Rock, 1997) but is an alternative replacement solution for those who have reactions to albumin or FFP (Burgstaler, 1990). It can also be used in those who require plasma exchange, but whose religious beliefs preclude the use of replacement fluids derived from blood.

Patient Concerns

Plasma exchange is a nonselective method of removing substances from plasma; many of the concerns about patients undergoing plasma exchange involve the removal of unintended substances such as therapeutic drugs and coagulation factors. Despite the fact that plasma exchange has been a treatment modality for a variety of diseases for almost 30 years, little information is available regarding its effects on therapeutic drugs. Theoretically, drugs that are highly protein or lipid bound should be efficiently removed by plasma exchange. As in the previous discussion, the volume of distribution influences the removal of a drug. For example, a highly protein-bound drug that is limited predominantly to the intravascular compartment should be efficiently removed, and a highly protein-bound drug that is distributed throughout the body will not be efficiently removed. A poorly bound drug will also not be efficiently removed.

The effect of plasma exchange on drug concentrations can be determined by calculating the drug half-life during plasma exchange (Kintzel, 2003). These calculations could then be used to determine the additional dosing that might be needed following plasma exchange. This has not been done with the majority of medications. The effects of plasma exchange on a variety of medications are given in Table 37-18. From a practical standpoint, because plasma exchange may remove a portion of a drug dose, drugs that are given once daily should be withheld until after the procedure, if possible. Drugs that are administered more often should also be scheduled, so they are not given directly prior to plasma exchange.

Another possible way in which plasma exchange and therapeutic drugs may interact is through the removal of enzymes necessary for metabolism and proteins necessary for transport. Plasma pseudocholinesterase is removed during plasma exchange; as a result, neuromuscular blockade agents such as succinylcholine or mivacurium may have a prolonged effect in patients who have recently undergone plasma exchange (Wood, 1978; Naik, 2002). Such agents should be avoided immediately following plasma exchange.

Following plasma exchange using 5% albumin as a replacement fluid, decreases in the levels and activities of coagulation factors (Flaum, 1979; Orlin, 1980), as well as abnormal coagulation tests (Flaum, 1979), have been seen. Flaum (1979) demonstrated significant decreases in the levels of factors V, VII, VIII, IX, and X, and von Willebrand factor (vWF) activity following plasma exchange. These deficits returned to normal by 24 hours following plasma exchange, with the exception of factors VIII and IX and vWF activity, which had returned to normal at 4 hours (Flaum, 1979). Orlin (1980) noted reductions in fibrinogen levels to 25% of preapheresis levels. Fibrinogen levels had reached 66% of preapheresis levels at 72 hours (Orlin, 1980). These studies indicate that a risk of bleeding exists in hemostatically challenged patients following plasma exchange. This is especially true in patients undergoing serial procedures on consecutive days, when sufficient time for recovery of hemostatic levels may not be possible. At-risk patients, such as those who have undergone or will undergo surgical procedures or biopsies in proximity to their plasma exchange, may require FFP as a portion of their replacement fluid. This should be given at the end of the procedure to prevent its removal.

In addition to increased risk of bleeding, increased risk of thrombosis is possible. Because of the nonspecific nature of removal, inhibitors of coagulation, such as antithrombin, are also removed during plasma exchange (Chirnside, 1981; Volkin, 1982). This could theoretically lead to thrombosis.

Finally, platelets are also lost during therapeutic plasma exchange (Perdue, 2001). In a study of 71 patients undergoing therapeutic plasma exchange with the COBE Spectra, Fresenius AS104 (Fresenius HemoCare, Redmond, WA), or the Haemonetics LN9000 (Haemonetics, Braintree, MA), platelet losses ranged from 0–71% (Perdue, 2001). Factors found to influence platelet losses included the instrument used, with the Fresenius AS104 having the greatest losses (18.6% vs. 2.6% and 1.6% for the Haemonetics LN9000 and the COBE Spectra, respectively), and the disease for which patients are being treated. Of patients treated in the study, those with hyperviscosity syndrome due to dysproteinemia had the greatest losses (Perdue, 2001). In this study, however, no bleeding complications occurred (Perdue, 2001). Greater losses with the Fresenius AS104 in comparison with the COBE Spectra were felt to be due to differences in *g* force and dwell time between the two instruments (Burgstaler, 2001).

Procedures for Selective Removal of Plasma Components

As previously discussed, plasma exchange is nonselective. Each plasma exchange removes approximately 150 g of plasma proteins (110 g of albumin and 40 g of globulin) (Randerson, 1982; Lysaght, 1985) to eliminate 1–2 g of pathologic substance. Repeated plasma exchanges can result in bleeding due to loss of coagulation factors and immunodeficiency due to loss of Igs. If other replacement fluids are used, additional risks may be present, including disease transmission and allergic reactions. Because of these disadvantages, a number of procedures have been developed to selectively remove a plasma component, allowing return of the patient's "cleansed" plasma. The benefits of such procedures are that depletion of normal plasma components and the need for substitution fluids are avoided. The drawbacks to such procedures are that they are more expensive to perform than plasma exchange because of the costs of selective removal columns. In addition, although many devices are available worldwide to perform these types of procedures, only two are available in the United States and have been licensed by the Food and Drug Administration.

Selective removal procedures most often involve an initial separation step, in which the cellular elements of whole blood are separated from the plasma. The plasma is then perfused through the selective removal device, where the substance of interest is removed by chemical, physical, or immunologic means. The treated plasma is then recombined with the cellular components and reinfused. The selective removal device may then be regenerated, and the bound substance removed and diverted to a waste collection bag. Following this, the selective removal device is used to treat additional plasma. If the device cannot be regenerated, then it is discarded. Examples of selective removal procedures are discussed in the following sections.

Selective Removal of Low-Density Lipoproteins

Selective removal of low-density lipoproteins (LDLs), also called LDL-apheresis, is indicated for the treatment of familial hypercholesterolemia

TABLE 37-19

Criteria for Use of Low-Density Lipoprotein (LDL) Apheresis in Familial Hypercholesterolemia (FH)

U.S. Food and Drug Administration Criteria
• Functional FH homozygotes with an LDL cholesterol >500 mg/dL
• Functional FH heterozygotes with an LDL cholesterol ≥300 mg/dL who have failed a 6-month trial of maximal drug therapy and an American Heart Association Step II diet
• Functional FH heterozygotes with an LDL cholesterol ≥200 mg/dL and documented coronary artery disease who have failed a 6-month trial of maximal drug therapy and an American Heart Association Step II diet
German Committee of Physicians and Health Insurance Funds
• Homozygotes for FH
• Patients with severe hypercholesterolemia in whom maximal dietary and drug therapies for >1 year have failed to lower cholesterol sufficiently
International Panel on Management of FH
• Homozygotes for FH
• Heterozygotes for FH with symptomatic coronary artery disease in whom LDL cholesterol is >4.2 mmol/L or decreases by <40% despite maximal medical management
Heart—United Kingdom
• Homozygotes for FH in whom LDL cholesterol is reduced by <50% and/or >9 mmol/L with drug therapy
• Progressive coronary artery disease, severe hypercholesterolemia, and Lp(a) >60 mg/dL in whom LDL cholesterol remains elevated despite drug therapy.

Data from Thompson GR, HEART-UK LDL Apheresis Working Group. Recommendations for the use of LDL apheresis. Atherosclerosis 2008;198:247–55.

(FH) in homozygotes and in heterozygotes unresponsive to drug therapy (Thompson, 2008). This disorder results in accelerated atherosclerosis due to the inability of the liver to clear LDL cholesterol from the blood caused by mutations in the hepatic LDL receptor. Criteria for the treatment of patients with LDL apheresis vary worldwide and are given in Table 37-19. Comparisons of the life expectancy of patients treated with these techniques and their untreated siblings (Thompson, 1985), as well as series (Kamanabroo, 1988) and case reports (Leren, 1993) of treated patients, have been reported. Significant reductions in cholesterol, improvements in xanthomas, disappearance of electrocardiographic (ECG) abnormalities, regression of coronary artery lesions, improvement in exercise tolerance, and prolongation of life span have been seen (Thompson, 1985; Kamanabroo, 1988; Leren, 1993; Matsuzaki, 2002). A number of methods are available for the selective removal of LDL.

The first method used after plasma exchange was double-filtration plasmapheresis (DFPP). LDL is one of the largest plasma components; as such, filters can be constructed to allow its removal. In DFPP, plasma is separated from whole blood by filtration. The plasma is then passed through a second filter with a pore size too small to allow passage of the LDL. The resulting plasma filtrate contains 83% of the albumin, 68% of the IgG, and 47% of the HDL cholesterol present in the original plasma. The filter, however, retains 94% of the LDL cholesterol, 92% of the IgM, and 90% of the fibrinogen. In comparison with plasma exchange, secondary filtration produced a similar decrease in LDL cholesterol but resulted in a smaller loss of HDL cholesterol (Leitman, 1989). Because lipids in the plasma can clog the second filter, a heater is used in modern DFPP instruments to heat the plasma before it reaches the second filter. This keeps the lipids from gelling (Klingel, 2004).

A second method of LDL-apheresis is heparin-induced extracorporeal low-density lipoprotein precipitation (HELP) (B Braun Medical Inc., Bethlehem, PA). With this technique, plasma is separated from whole blood using a hollow fiber separator. A sodium acetate buffer of pH 4.84 containing heparin is added to the plasma to precipitate the LDL. This precipitate is then removed by filtration, with the heparin being adsorbed from the plasma by a diethylaminoethyl cellulose filter. The acetate and extra volume are then removed through bicarbonate dialysis/ultrafiltration. The treated plasma is combined with the cellular elements and returned to the patient (Bambauer, 2003). Results of treatment in one trial demonstrated reductions in LDL cholesterol of greater than 30%, with reductions in HDL and fibrinogen of 15% and 58%, respectively (Lane, 1993).

A third method of removal is dextran sulfate absorption (Liposorber, Kaneka, Osaka, Japan). In this method, two columns of dextran sulfate are used to continuously remove LDL cholesterol. Plasma is separated from whole blood using a hollow fiber separator and is pumped through the dextran sulfate column. Treated plasma is then mixed with the cellular elements and returned to the patient. In the column, the negatively charged dextran sulfate interacts with the positively charged apolipoprotein B-100 of the LDL cholesterol, resulting in its removal. When the first column becomes saturated, flow is switched to the second column and the first is rinsed with 4.1% NaCl to remove the LDL cholesterol. Following this, the column is flushed with lactated Ringer's solution, then is ready to be used again. A salinometer monitors the effluent of the column to make certain that the hyperosmolar saline is not infused into the patient (Bambauer, 2003). Studies using this system have demonstrated a 53% reduction in cholesterol with one plasma volume exchange (Thompson, 1995), as well as a 36% reduction in fibrinogen and a 5% loss of high-density lipoprotein (HDL) (Schulzeck, 1992).

The fourth method of LDL removal is immunoadsorption (Therasorb-LDL, Miltenyi Biotec, Cologne, Germany). In this system, two columns containing agarose beads covalently linked to sheep polyclonal antihuman apolipoprotein B-100 antibodies are used. Similar to other methods, one column is perfused with plasma as the second one is regenerated. In this case, a glycine/HCl buffer is used to remove the bound ApoB–containing LDL (Bambauer, 2003). A study of the use of this form of LDL-apheresis demonstrated its ability to maintain cholesterol at levels of 165 mg%, as well as to increase HDL (Richter, 1993).

The fifth available method is direct adsorption of lipoproteins from whole blood (DALI, Fresenius, St. Wendel, Germany). This system consists of columns that contain polyacrylate-coated polyacrylamide beads. Similar to dextran sulfate, these beads are negatively charged, resulting in binding of the positively charged ApoB-containing LDL. For this column, plasma separation need not occur, as anticoagulated whole blood can be passed through the column. Unlike the systems previously described, the column is not regenerated but is used only once. Different sizes of columns are available to treat different blood volumes (Bosch, 2001a; Bambauer, 2003).

The final system is the dextran sulfate whole blood perfusion system (Liposorber D, Kaneka, Osaka, Japan). As with the DALI column, plasma separation is not needed because whole blood is perfused through the column. Using different dextran sulfate beads than those used in the Liposorber system, LDL binds to the negatively charged dextran. As with the DALI columns, these cannot be regenerated and are discarded once saturated. Again, the columns come in different sizes for use in treating different blood volumes (Otto, 2003).

Of all the systems described previously, only the dextran sulfate system and the HELP system are currently FDA approved for use in the United States. Comparisons of these systems have shown similar reductions in LDL cholesterol, lipoprotein a (Lp[a]), HDL, and other plasma components (Matsuda, 1994; Parhofer, 2000; Bambauer, 2003; Otto, 2007); reductions in HDL, fibrinogen, and other plasma components are less than those seen with plasma exchange. These systems have also demonstrated similar reaction rates but differ in terms of cost and simplicity of the operation (Matsuda, 1994).

Some systems, such as the HELP system and secondary filtration, remove additional plasma components such as fibrinogen. Because of the removal of large macromolecules other than LDL, these systems have been used to alter blood flow characteristics in certain disease states. This form of apheresis has been referred to as Rheophoresis. These devices have been used to treat age-related macular degeneration (Klingel, 2003), sudden sensorineural hearing loss (Suckfull, 1999, 2002), stroke (Jaeger, 1999), and myocardial ischemia (Jaeger, 1999).

According to ASFA, homozygous FH is a category I indication for LDL apheresis with a grade 1A recommendation. Heterozygous FH is a category II indication for LDL apheresis with a grade 1A recommendation. Plasma exchange is a category II indication with a grade 1C recommendation for FH homozygotes whose blood volume is too small for them to be treated with a selective removal system (Szczepiorkowski, 2010).

Therapeutic Plasma Exchange Indications

Table 37-20 lists selected disorders for which plasma exchange is indicated and which will be briefly discussed.

TABLE 37-20
Conditions for Which Plasma Exchange Is Accepted

Neurologic disorders	Acute inflammatory demyelinating polyneuropathy (AIDP)
	Chronic inflammatory demyelinating polyneuropathy (CIDP)
	Myasthenia gravis
Hematologic disorders	Thrombotic thrombocytopenic purpura
	Hyperviscosity syndrome
Metabolic disorders	Familial hypercholesterolemia
Other disorders	Anti–basement membrane antibody disease (Goodpasture's syndrome)
	Cryoglobulinemia
	Glomerulonephritis
	Conditioning for renal transplant

Neurologic Disorders

Therapeutic plasma exchange (TPE) is well described for acute inflammatory and chronic demyelinating polyneuropathy and for myasthenia gravis; these diseases are common indications for TPE.

Acute Inflammatory Demyelinating Polyneuropathy. Guillain-Barré syndrome (GBS) is a neurologic disorder of immune origin and is the most frequently encountered paralytic disorder (Guillain-Barré Syndrome Study Group, 1985; Ropper, 1992). It affects males more frequently than females and is more common with increasing age (Hughes, 1993). The disorder is characterized initially by leg weakness, which progresses proximally to involve the arm, face, and oropharyngeal muscles (Ropper, 1992). Sensory loss is mild but may include paresthesias of fingers and toes. Disease progression stops by the third week of the illness and then improves after a variable period of stability (Ropper, 1992).

The pathophysiology of GBS is thought to be one of antibody-mediated damage to peripheral nerve myelin followed by inflammatory response. Complement-fixing antibodies to peripheral myelin have been identified in patients (Koski, 1985). The titers of these antibodies correlate with the clinical course of patients (Koski, 1986), as well as to the response to plasma exchange and relapse following plasma exchange (Vriesendorp, 1991). Treatment of GBS consists of supportive care to provide adequate nutrition, ventilatory support, and avoidance of infection and pulmonary embolism (Ropper, 1992). Intravenous immune globulin (IVIG) is also beneficial in the treatment of GBS (Plasma Exchange/Sandoglobulin Guillain-Barré Syndrome Trial Group, 1997), but corticosteroids are not (Hughes, 1978) and may interfere with the response to hemapheresis (Mendell, 1985).

Plasma exchange is associated with improvement in disability, greater likelihood of recovering function, and a shortened course (Guillain-Barré Syndrome Study Group, 1985). Unfortunately, patients requiring ventilation support for several days before initiation of plasma exchange are not likely to benefit immediately from the procedure. However, they have been found to have a shorter course of ventilator dependency (Guillain-Barré Syndrome Study Group, 1985). Plasma exchange should be initiated within 14 days of the onset of symptoms (Guillain-Barré Syndrome Study Group, 1985; Plasma Exchange/Sandoglobulin Guillain-Barré Syndrome Trial Group, 1997) and should consist of five to six procedures over 8–13 days (Guillain-Barré Syndrome Study Group, 1985; Plasma Exchange/Sandoglobulin Guillain-Barré Syndrome Trial Group, 1997). Replacement fluid should be albumin. Treatments should continue for at least 10–14 days, as cessation of plasma exchange during the active phase of the disorder is characterized by relapse (Ropper, 1988). Ten percent of patients may relapse 16–21 days after therapy (Ropper, 1988).

A review of the Cochrane Neuromuscular Disease Group Register summarized the results of randomized and quasirandomized trials of plasma exchange versus sham exchange or supportive therapy (Raphael, 2002). A total of six trials involving 649 patients were identified which fulfilled the criteria for evaluation. According to the authors of the review, results showed that TPE is the "first and only treatment that has been proven to be superior to supportive treatment alone" (Raphael, 2002). In addition, the authors found that TPE was most effective if started within 7 days of disease onset; two sessions of TPE are superior to none in mild acute inflammatory demyelinating polyradiculoneuropathy (AIDP), four sessions are superior to two in moderate AIDP, and six sessions are no better than four in severe AIDP (Raphael, 2002).

AIDP is a category I indication with a 1A recommendation grade for plasma exchange, according to the ASFA (Szczepiorkowski, 2010).

Chronic Inflammatory Demyelinating Polyneuropathy. Chronic inflammatory demyelinating polyneuropathy (CIDP) is a neurologic disorder, probably of autoimmune origin, characterized by progressive or relapsing motor and/or sensory peripheral nerve dysfunction involving more than one limb and developing over 2 months (Cornblath, 1991). Hyporeflexia or areflexia is also present, with nerve conduction studies indicating demyelination, and nerve biopsy showing demyelination and remyelination (Cornblath, 1991). Other causes of polyneuropathy, such as toxin exposure, must be excluded. Patients demonstrate a male predominance with peak age of onset in the fifth and sixth decades (Dyck, 1975). Patients typically present with burning dysesthesias, muscle pain, and shooting pain, as well as distal muscle weakness (Dyck, 1975). The pathophysiology is thought to be immune-mediated damage to peripheral nerve myelin, causing demyelination and subsequent nerve degeneration. Evidence in support of an immune mechanism includes the presence of demyelination in monkeys when given patient-derived immune globulin (Heininger, 1984), deposition of Ig in nerve biopsies (Dalakas, 1980a), and monoclonal IgG in the cerebrospinal fluid (CSF) of some patients (Dalakas, 1980b). Some CIDP patients respond to corticosteroids but are prone to the complications of these medications because of the need for long-term treatment (Dyck, 1975). IVIG has been found to be beneficial (van Doorn, 1990), especially in a select group of patients demonstrating specific findings (van Doorn, 1991).

The first double-blind, sham-controlled crossover study of plasma exchange in CIDP demonstrated an improvement in 5 of 15 patients undergoing two procedures per week for 3 weeks. The benefits of therapy gradually disappeared 10–14 days following discontinuation (Dyck, 1986). A more recent study involving more frequent procedures (four the first week, three the second week, two the third week, and one the fourth week) demonstrated improvement in 80% of patients, usually becoming apparent on the third to sixth days of treatment (Hahn, 1996). Unfortunately, 66% of responders relapsed after stopping therapy (Hahn, 1996). Comparison of plasma exchange and IVIG has demonstrated similar rapid response with both treatment modalities (Dyck, 1994). Therapy usually consists of an initial intensive course of four to six procedures over 2 weeks, followed by one to two treatments per week or at longer intervals as tolerated. Improvement is usually seen within a week (Hahn, 1996) but lasts only 2 weeks (Dyck, 1986). Five percent albumin is used as the replacement fluid.

CIDP is a category I indication with a 1B recommendation grade for plasma exchange, according to the ASFA (Szczepiorkowski, 2010).

Myasthenia Gravis. Myasthenia gravis (MG) is an autoimmune disorder characterized by weakness of voluntary muscle groups. It may involve only the extraocular muscles or may be generalized, involving appendicular and trunk muscles. The presence of bulbar muscle weakness can lead to aspiration in the setting of a weakened diaphragm. This can result in severe respiratory compromise and was the major cause of death in these patients in the past. MG is caused by autoantibodies directed against the acetylcholine receptor on the motor endplate. These autoantibodies prevent normal functioning of the receptor by increasing receptor turnover, blocking the binding of acetylcholine, and fixing complement with degradation of the receptor (Lindstrom, 1976; Maselli, 1994). The disorder can be associated with other autoimmune phenomena and is associated with thymic abnormalities, including thymoma (Sanders, 1994). Treatment of myasthenia gravis is directed toward increasing the amount of acetylcholine at the motor endplate through the use of acetylcholine esterase inhibitors such as pyridostigmine and neostigmine, as well as decreasing antibody production through immunosuppressive medications such as corticosteroids or azathioprine (Sanders, 1994). In addition, IVIG has been used to treat MG with beneficial effects and has been found to produce effects similar to plasma exchange (Gajdos, 1997).

Plasma exchange is performed to lower the level of anti–acetylcholine receptor antibody, although it has also been reported to be successful in 10%–15% patients with symptoms of MG who do not have detectable antibody. Intensive courses of plasma exchange are recommended for those patients with MG who have severe disease with impaired respiratory function, swallowing, and locomotion (Sanders, 1994), as well as to prepare patients for thymectomy or surgery (Iwasaki, 1993). This may consist of 1–1.5 plasma volume exchanges performed daily for 5–6 days (Dau, 1977). Patients with stable chronic disease who experience mild exacerbations can be treated with shorter courses of 2–3 plasma exchanges (Antozzi, 1991); some patients can be treated with as few as 1–4 exchanges per month (Dau,

1980). The course of therapy should be individualized to the needs of the patient. Five percent albumin is used as the replacement fluid. Concurrent immunosuppressive therapy is also performed to prevent rebound of the antibody (Dau, 1977).

Moderate to severe myasthenia gravis is a category I indication with a 1A recommendation grade for plasma exchange, according to the ASFA. Prophylactic treatment prior to thymectomy is a category I indication with a 1C recommendation grade (Szczepiorkowski, 2010).

Hematologic Disorders

Thrombotic Thrombocytopenic Purpura. TTP is a disorder characterized by thrombocytopenia, microangiopathic hemolytic anemia, neurologic dysfunction, fever, and some degree of renal dysfunction. Laboratory abnormalities, in addition to thrombocytopenia, include schistocytes and nucleated red blood cells on peripheral smear, as well as elevated LD. Although it has been assumed that the elevation in LD is due to hemolysis, a study of 10 patients has demonstrated that in the majority of patients, it is of hepatic origin (Cohen, 1998). TTP can also be divided into primary (idiopathic) and secondary TTP. Causes of secondary TTP include systemic lupus erythematosus (Nesher, 1994), bone marrow transplant (Pettitt, 1994), cyclosporine (Wiener, 1997), pregnancy (McCrae, 1997), ticlopidine (Bennett, 1998), HIV infection (Hymes, 1997), and a number of chemotherapeutic agents.

Primary TTP can be divided into several variants. Idiopathic initial episode TTP consists of a single episode not associated with any other cause. Intermittent TTP is characterized by relapses following the initial episode. Chronic relapsing TTP also consists of recurring episodes, but these begin during childhood and recur at predictable intervals (Moake, 1995).

Histologic study of tissue from patients with TTP has demonstrated the presence of platelet thrombi within the microvasculature. Immunohistochemistry has demonstrated these to consist of platelets and vWF with little fibrin (Asada, 1985). In addition, studies have shown that early in the course of TTP, unusually large multimers of vWF (UL vWF) circulate in the patient's plasma (Moake, 1989). These multimers have an increased affinity for glycoprotein Ib-IX on platelets and are thought to induce platelet aggregation under high shear stress conditions. Normally, these UL vWF multimers are located within the endothelium, and when released into the circulation are cleaved into smaller fragments by a metalloprotease called **a**d**i**sintegrin **a**nd **m**etalloprotease with **t**hrombo**s**pondin Type I motifs **13** (ADAMTS13) (Levy, 2001a). It has been demonstrated that in patients with idiopathic initial TTP, intermittent TTP, and ticlopidine-associated TTP, an autoantibody is present that decreases ADAMTS13 enzyme activity (Furlan, 1998a,b; Rice, 1998; Tsai, 1998). In idiopathic TTP, autoantibodies are present in 44%–83% of cases (Moake, 2002; Zheng, 2004), with severe deficiency of ADAMTS13 activity (<5%) specifically associated with idiopathic TTP (Moake, 2002; Vesely, 2003; Zheng, 2005). In chronic relapsing TTP, ADAMTS13 activity has been shown to be absent without the presence of an autoantibody representing a genetic deficiency in enzyme production (Furlan, 1997). This congenital syndrome of TTP is also known by the eponym of Schulman-Upshaw syndrome. Other than in patients with ticlopidine-induced TTP, and possibly HIV-induced TTP, neither autoantibodies nor a deficiency in ADAMTS13 enzyme activity appears to be involved in secondary TTP. A study of bone marrow transplant–associated TTP showed normal ADAMTS13 activity (van der Plas, 1999). It is postulated that endothelial damage in many secondary cases results in release of UL vWF that may overwhelm protease activity. Similarly, studies of patients with diarrhea-associated hemolytic-uremic syndrome also show normal ADAMTS13 activity (Tsai, 2001).

The primary treatment of TTP is plasma exchange. Prior to the use of plasma exchange, the mortality rate of TTP was 95%. Following the widespread use of plasma exchange, the mortality rate has decreased to 15% (Rock, 1991). The mechanism of plasma exchange is thought to be the combination of autoantibody removal, UL vWF removal, and ADAMTS13 infusion. An alternative therapy to plasma exchange is plasma infusion. In most cases, however, this is not as effective as plasma exchange (Rock, 1991). This is due to the fact that the volume of plasma that can be infused is limited by the ability of the patient's cardiovascular system to withstand the volume. Coppo (2003) studied large-volume plasma infusion compared with plasma exchange. In their trial, they sought to infuse as much plasma as was given during a plasma exchange. They demonstrated no significant difference with regard to outcome between patients randomized to plasma exchange and those assigned to plasma infusion. They did, however, see greater complications in the plasma infusion group due to volume overload, and 8 of the 19 patients in that arm had to be switched to plasma exchange because of this complication (Coppo, 2003). There are two settings in which plasma infusion is indicated in the treatment of TTP. First, patients with a genetic deficiency of ADAMTS13 expressed as chronic relapsing TTP can be given regular fresh frozen plasma infusion to prevent exacerbation. In addition, plasma infusion can be used to treat a patient while arrangements are being made to perform plasma exchange. Additional therapies for TTP include antiplatelet medications (Amorosi, 1977), vincristine (Gutterman, 1982), splenectomy (Crowther, 1996), IVIG (Centurioni, 1995), cyclosporine (Hand, 1998), corticosteroids (Bell, 1991), and rituximab (Elliott, 2009).

Treatment of TTP consists of daily plasma exchange of 1–1.5 volumes using FFP as a replacement fluid until the platelet count is greater than 150,000/μL, the LD is normalizing, and no evidence of neurologic dysfunction is present (Bell, 1991; Dawson, 1994). If the patient remains stable for 48 hours on plasma exchange, then tapering can be started by performing apheresis every other day (Dawson, 1994). It should be noted, however, that the benefits of tapering have not been proven (Bandarenko, 1998), and at some centers this is not done. Because patients may have an abrupt worsening of signs and symptoms with a longer course following early cessation of plasma exchange (Bell, 1991), many recommend tapering. Regardless, close monitoring of neurologic status, platelet count, and LD should be performed during and after plasma exchange. It is important to note that the presence or absence of schistocytes at the time that plasma exchange is discontinued does not affect relapse and is not a criterion for the discontinuation of treatment (Egan, 2004). In patients not responding to plasma exchange with FFP, switching to plasma cryoprecipitate reduced as the replacement fluid may be beneficial and has been shown to induce remission in some patients (Rock, 1996). This is thought to be possibly due to the lack of vWF in plasma cryoprecipitate reduced. Because of this finding, a frequent question is whether plasma cryoprecipitate reduced should be routinely used as the replacement fluid in plasma exchange for TTP. The North American TTP Group performed a multiinstitutional prospective randomized trial comparing FFP and plasma cryoprecipitate reduced as replacement fluids in primary TTP during initial presentation. This trial showed the two replacement fluids to be equivalent in this population (Zeigler, 2001). A second trial by the Canadian Apheresis Study group also found no benefit of plasma cryoprecipitate reduced compared with FFP in the treatment of idiopathic TTP (Rock, 2005). In addition, plasma cryoprecipitate reduced is not routinely available in many blood centers, as it is discarded as a byproduct of cryoprecipitate production.

Although plasma exchange is effective in treating idiopathic TTP, its role in secondary cases lacking deficiency of ADAMTS13 is uncertain. Studies of plasma exchange in the setting of bone marrow transplant–induced TTP have shown it to be ineffective (Ho, 2005).

TTP is a category I indication with a 1A recommendation grade for plasma exchange, according to the ASFA (Szczepiorkowski, 2010).

Hyperviscosity Syndrome. Hyperviscosity syndrome is characterized by mental status changes, a bleeding diathesis involving the mucosa and gastrointestinal tract, retinopathy with hemorrhage and papilledema, and hypervolemia with congestive heart failure (Foerster, 1993b). Hyperviscosity syndrome occurs in less than 5% of multiple myeloma patients but in as many as 70% of patients with Waldenström's macroglobulinemia (Foerster, 1993b). It may rarely be seen with polyclonal increases in Ig. Differences in frequencies in plasma cell disorders are due to differences in the monoclonal proteins produced in these two diseases. In multiple myeloma, the Ig produced is usually IgG or IgA, but in Waldenström's macroglobulinemia, the protein is IgM. In hyperviscosity syndrome, the presence of large concentrations of paraprotein increases blood viscosity by causing sludging of the red blood cells and results in occlusion of the microcirculation with organ ischemia (McGrath, 1976). Symptoms usually occur when the viscosity increases to 4–6 Ostwald units (normal blood viscosity is 1.5–1.8 Ostwald units), but patients may be asymptomatic at very high protein concentrations and viscosities (Bloch, 1973). Although the viscosity is dependent on the concentration, demonstrating an exponential relationship (Bloch, 1973), it is also dependent on the nature of the protein. The exponential nature of the relationship between concentration and viscosity means that after a critical concentration, small changes result in a large increase or decrease in viscosity.

The treatment of hyperviscosity syndrome is twofold. First, the long-term goal is to decrease paraprotein production with chemotherapy. The second goal is to decrease the protein concentration and improve blood flow. This second goal can be achieved with plasma exchange by exchanging 1–1.5 plasma volumes with 5% albumin or equal volumes of albumin and saline. In hyperviscosity syndrome due to an IgM monoclonal protein, one to two plasma exchanges may be sufficient to remove enough protein to improve viscosity, as IgM is located almost entirely within the intravascular space. With IgG or IgA paraproteins, the Ig is also present within the extravascular space, and more procedures may be necessary to decrease paraprotein levels. The goal of therapy should be relief of symptoms, with the subsequent frequency tailored to the needs of the patient. In instances of Waldenström's macroglobulinemia resistant to therapy, repeated plasma exchange alone has been used to control hyperviscosity for extended periods of time—as long as 17 years (Salmon, 1997). It should be noted that because of the presence of extravascular Ig in multiple myeloma, patients might experience hypovolemia following procedures, as oncotic pressure results in movement of fluid from the intravascular space.

Symptomatic hyperviscosity is a category I indication and a 1B recommendation grade for plasma exchange, according to the ASFA. Prophylactic plasma exchange to treat hyperviscosity prior to the administration of rituximab is a category I indication with a 1C recommendation grade (Szczepiorkowski, 2010).

Myeloma With Acute Renal Failure

Acute renal failure occurs in multiple myeloma patients who excrete free light chains—Bence Jones proteins—in their urine. It occurs in 3%–9% of multiple myeloma patients (Bear, 1980; Johnson, 1980; Solling, 1988) and is associated with a poor prognosis. Myeloma with acute renal failure may be caused by the filtration of monoclonal light chains with deposition in the renal tubules leading to cast nephropathy. This eventually leads to dilation of the tubules, as well as tubular atrophy and renal failure (DeFronzo, 1978; Bernstein, 1982; Cohen, 1984). Unlike in hyperviscosity syndrome, the amount or characteristics of the light chain do not correlate with the disease. The diagnosis of cast nephropathy is made by renal biopsy, as other causes of renal failure may be seen in patients with multiple myeloma (Leung, 2008). Development of this complication is prevented by treatment of the underlying disease. Additional treatment includes alkalization of the urine to enhance excretion of the protein.

Plasma exchange is used in the treatment of cast nephropathy in multiple myeloma to decrease the quantity of light chains present. Although this can also be accomplished with dialysis, plasma exchange has been found to be more effective (Bear, 1980; Johnson, 1980; Solling, 1988). Renal failure in multiple myeloma is associated with poor prognosis; however, two controlled trials (Zucchelli, 1984; Johnson, 1990) have demonstrated recovery of renal function in some patients on dialysis with cast nephropathy by using the combination of chemotherapy and plasma exchange. A larger multicenter randomized controlled trial, however, failed to demonstrate efficacy of plasma exchange in myeloma kidney (Clark, 2005). This trial was criticized for using composite endpoints, failing to biopsy patients to ensure that cast nephropathy was present, and obtaining lower rates of dialysis dependency compared with other trials (Leung, 2006). The role of plasma exchange in myeloma kidney remains controversial (Leung, 2008). In cast nephropathy, the plasma exchange is performed daily to three times per week for 1–4 weeks until renal function improves. Subsequent therapy is performed as needed to maintain renal function (McGrath, 1976).

Multiple myeloma cast nephropathy is a category II indication with a 2B recommendation grade for plasma exchange, according to the ASFA (Szczepiorkowski, 2010).

Nephrologic Disorders

Anti–Basement Membrane Antibody Disease. Anti–basement membrane antibody disease (Goodpasture's syndrome) is a rare disorder characterized by the combination of pulmonary and renal hemorrhage. It affects men more commonly then women and is most frequent between 18 and 35 years of age. The disorder is autoimmune with an antibody directed against type IV collagen within the glomerular and pulmonary basement membrane. The antibody is usually transient and may be triggered by damage to the respiratory system, as the syndrome is frequently preceded by an infectious or chemical insult. Patients usually present with pulmonary symptoms of cough, hemoptysis, and dyspnea. Laboratory values show evidence of renal failure and renal inflammation. Mortality rate may be as high as 50%. Treatment of Goodpasture's syndrome focuses on suppressing antibody production and inflammation and removing the antibody. The former goals are accomplished through the use of immunosuppressive agents such as cyclophosphamide and prednisone (Wiseman, 1993).

Plasma exchange is used to remove the anti–basement membrane antibody. Treatment consists of 1–1.5 plasma volume exchanges using 5% albumin for replacement. Therapy is usually performed daily for 7–14 days and, in the presence of concurrent immunosuppression, results in decreased antibody levels and clinical improvement (Erickson, 1979; Pusey, 1983; Johnson, 1985). Because the antibody is only transiently present, treatment longer than 6 months is uncommon (Pusey, 1983). It should be noted that plasma exchange should be started early, as recovery of renal function is unlikely once scarring and atrophy of glomeruli and tubules occur (Johnson, 1978). Patients who present needing dialysis, who have a creatinine >6.8 mg/dL, who are oliguric, and who have 100% crescentic glomeruli on renal biopsy are unlikely to benefit from plasma exchange (Levy, 2001b). In this setting, plasma exchange may be reserved for the onset of pulmonary hemorrhage (Levy, 2001b). Patients with a creatinine of <5.7 g/dL and who have less than 50% crescentic glomeruli on renal biopsy have overall and "renal" survivals at 1 year of 100% and 95%, respectively (Levy, 2001b).

Anti–basement membrane antibody disease in dialysis-independent patients is a category I indication with a 1A recommendation for plasma exchange, according to the ASFA. If patients are dialysis dependent and lack pulmonary hemorrhage, plasma exchange is a category IV indication with a 1A recommendation grade. In patients with pulmonary hemorrhage, irrespective of renal function, plasma exchange is a category I indication with a 1B recommendation grade (Szczepiorkowski, 2010).

Cryoglobulinemia. Cryoglobulins are Igs that reversibly precipitate at cold temperature. Three categories of cryoglobulins exist. Type I cryoglobulin consists of a single monoclonal protein and is usually seen in multiple myeloma, Waldenström's macroglobulinemia, or other lymphoproliferative disorders. Usually, the immunoglobulin is IgG or IgM (Foerster, 1993a). Type II cryoglobulin consists of a mixture of polyclonal immunoglobulins with a monoclonal protein, usually IgM, directed toward polyclonal IgG. Type II cryoglobulinemia is associated with chronic hepatitis C infection, autoimmune disorders, and IgM-producing malignancies (Foerster, 1993a). Finally, Type III cryoglobulin consists of polyclonal immunoglobulins, usually IgM, that have activity toward polyclonal IgG. They are associated with autoimmune conditions, as well as infections (Foerster, 1993a). Cryoglobulins produce symptoms by precipitating in areas of low temperature, such as the skin or extremities, resulting in vascular occlusion. This produces a wide variety of symptoms, including acrocyanosis, Raynaud's phenomenon, skin ulcers, skin purpura, and glomerulonephritis (Foerster, 1993a).

Cryoglobulin precipitation is dependent on the concentration of the Ig. As the concentration of the Ig increases, the temperature at which the protein precipitates rises (Hillyer, 1996). As a result, some patients may experience symptoms with only small decreases in temperature, such as those occurring in the distal extremities when patients are exposed to the outdoor environment.

Treatment of cryoglobulinemia is directed at the underlying disease (Berkman, 1980). In addition, plasma exchange can be used to reduce the protein concentration, thereby decreasing the temperature at which precipitation occurs (Berkman, 1980; McLeod, 1980). Treatment usually consists of 1–1.5 volume exchanges using 5% albumin. Again, the intensity, duration, and frequency of therapy are determined by patient symptoms. As these proteins precipitate at room temperature, blood warmers (on both the draw and return lines) may be necessary to prevent precipitation in the apheresis instrument. In some patients with high cryoglobulin concentrations and resulting precipitation at higher temperatures, it may be necessary to perform hemapheresis procedures at room temperature of 37° C or higher to prevent precipitation (Hillyer, 1996).

Severe symptomatic cryoglobulinemia is a category I indication with a 1B recommendation grade for plasma exchange, according to the ASFA. Cryoglobulinemia secondary to hepatitis C viral infection is a category II indication with a 2B recommendation grade for the use of immunoadsorption (Szczepiorkowski, 2010).

Glomerulonephritis. Many of the glomerulonephritides result from deposition of antigen–antibody complexes within the glomeruli, leading to glomerular damage. These complexes, as well as their constituent components, can be found circulating within the bloodstream. Because of this, it is theoretically possible for plasma exchange to be used to remove these substances, thereby halting and possibly reversing further glomerular injury. A number of glomerulonephritides have been treated with plasma exchange. As with many of the diseases treated by hemapheresis, investigations have been limited to case studies and small case series without randomized, controlled trials. Treatments for some selected glomerular kidney diseases are given in Table 37-21.

TABLE 37-21
Glomerulonephritides Treated With Plasma Exchange

Disease	Putative substance removed	Reported efficacy
Primary focal segmental glomerulosclerosis (Bosch, 2001b)	50 kD permeability factor	Partial or complete remission of proteinuria in 44% of patients
Recurrent focal segmental glomerulosclerosis following renal transplant (Bosch, 2001b)	50 kD permeability factor	Long-term remission in 44% of adults and 74% of children
Lupus nephritis (Mistry-Burchardi, 2001)	Antinuclear antibodies, anti-DNA antibodies	No benefit over immunosuppression alone or as adjunct therapy
Pauciimmune rapidly progressive glomerulonephritis (Gaskin, 2001)	Antineutrophil cytoplasmic antibodies (ANCAs)	Possible benefit when renal function is impaired to the point where dialysis is required
Immune complex rapidly progressive glomerulonephritis (Walters, 2008)	Variety of antibodies, including immunoglobulin (Ig)A	No conclusive evidence supporting use in rapidly progressive glomerulonephritis due to immune complex deposition

Conditioning Therapy for Renal Transplantation

Kidney transplantation represents the current optimal therapy for chronic renal failure, and plasma exchange plays an adjunctive role by reducing ABO isoagglutinins. Unfortunately, the supply of deceased donor kidneys is inadequate to meet the need for organs in the United States, with approximately 86,728 people listed on the deceased donor kidney waiting list as of November 5, 2010 (Organ Procurement and Transplantation Network, 2010). The waiting time for deceased donor kidney transplantation exceeds 4 years (United Network for Organ Sharing, 2008). If a patient is blood group O or blood group B, the average waiting time is even longer. In addition, in 2007, 5000 of the 50,000 listed on the waiting list have panel reactive alloantibodies (PRA) >80% (United Network for Organ Sharing, 2008). Fewer than 300 of these patients are transplanted each year, with many of the most highly sensitized patients requiring a perfect HLA-matched kidney. Because so few of these highly sensitized patients receive deceased donor kidneys, a waiting time cannot be calculated for this group (Stegall, 2002).

While these individuals await an ABO- or HLA-compatible deceased donor kidney, their medical condition deteriorates. This wait is associated with a 5%–8% mortality rate per year. Attempts to transplant ABO- or cross-match incompatible kidneys have, in the past, been associated with the development of hyperacute rejection. Pre-formed ABO isoagglutinins or anti-antibodies bind to target antigens present upon the vascular endothelium of the incompatible organ at the time of reperfusion of the graft. The result is fixation of complement followed by endothelial injury, thrombosis, and occlusion of the microvasculature of the organ, resulting in immediate loss of the organ. To circumvent hyperacute rejection and increase the availability of organs, a number of protocols have been developed that use plasma exchange or immunoabsorption in combination with immunosuppression to reduce ABO isoagglutinin or anti-HLA antibody titers. These protocols have been reported to allow successful transplantation of incompatible kidneys from living donors.

Tanabe (1998) used three to four immunoabsorption procedures and/or one to two double-filtration plasma exchange procedures in an attempt to reduce ABO isoagglutinin titers to fewer than 16 before transplantation of ABO-incompatible living donor kidneys. This treatment, in conjunction with intensive immunosuppression and splenectomy at the time of transplantation, resulted in no instances of hyperacute rejection among 67 patients. Patient survival among ABO-incompatible transplant recipients was equivalent to that of ABO-compatible recipients. Graft survival was significantly less up to 3 years after transplant (79%) but showed equivalence at 4 years after transplant and beyond (Tanabe, 1998). Our group reported on the use of four plasma exchanges before transplant to reduce isoagglutinin titers to fewer than 4. This, and an intensive immunosuppression regimen with splenectomy, allowed for successful transplantation without hyperacute rejection among 26 ABO-incompatible transplants (Winters, 2004). One-year graft and patient survivals were slightly lower than in ABO-compatible transplants performed during the same time period (89 vs. 96% and 94 vs. 99%, respectively) (Gloor, 2003b).

Plasma exchange is associated with reductions in isoagglutinin scores and titers at the time of transplantation (Aikawa, 2001; Winters, 2004). Following transplant, however, titers will rise to levels greater than those seen at transplant but less than those seen initially (Aikawa, 2001; Winters, 2004). In addition, ABO antigen levels are maintained on the graft (Aikawa, 2001). Despite these increases in antibody titers, rejection episodes are limited to the early transplant course and can be reversed with plasma exchange and increased immunosuppression (Winters, 2004). Studies have suggested that "accommodation" occurs in the setting of ABO-incompatible kidney transplantation (Delikouras, 2003). This appears to be due to active self-protection of the graft through the alteration of gene expression (Park, 2003).

ABO-incompatible renal transplantation is a category II indication with a 1B recommendation grade for plasma exchange, according to ASFA (Szczepiorkowski, 2010).

A number of groups have reported success in transplanting cross-match incompatible living donor kidneys using the combination of plasma exchange, IVIG, immunosuppression, and splenectomy (Montgomery, 2000; Schweitzer, 2000; Gloor, 2003a). Four to six plasma exchanges with concurrent immunosuppressive therapy and IVIG were successful in converting patients with low-titer anti-HLA antibodies (<16) to cross-match compatibility on the day of transplantation. None of the patients treated developed hyperacute rejection. Acute humoral rejection episodes were seen in 43% of patients treated by Gloor (2003a), but these episodes were reversed with additional plasmaphereses and steroids. Graft survivals of 100% (Schweitzer, 2000) and 79% (Gloor, 2003a) have been reported at 12 months following transplantation. Unlike ABO-incompatible transplants, reports have described durable, sustained loss of donor-specific HLA antibodies following conditioning for and transplantation of cross-match incompatible kidneys (Zachary, 2003). In addition, as in ABO-incompatible accommodated transplants, cross-match incompatible accommodated transplants demonstrate altered gene expression that results in downregulation of apoptosis of the graft's endothelial cells (Salama, 2001).

Plasma exchange for desensitization in cross-match incompatible renal transplantation with a living donor kidney is a category II indication with a 1B recommendation grade, according to ASFA. Plasma exchange for desensitization in high-PRA patients awaiting a cadaveric renal transplant is a category III indication with a 2C recommendation grade (Szczepiorkowski, 2010).

Donor/Patient Complications Common to All Hemapheresis Procedures

Hemapheresis procedures, both donor and therapeutic, are safe procedures with minimal risk of complications. Those which do occur are generally traumatic and associated with venous access or physiologic complications that include citrate-mediated, allergic-type, and volume-related problems. Because citrate-mediated reactions are common and may require the attention of the physician, they are discussed in some detail in the following paragraphs. The reaction rates among donors undergoing hemapheresis procedures have been found to be 2.18% (McLeod, 1998) and 0.81% (Despotis, 1999), respectively. This is less than the 11%–21% reaction rate reported for whole blood donation (Newman, 1997). However, the rate of serious reactions—those requiring hospitalization—has been found to be 0.01% (2 out of 19,736 donations) (Despotis, 1999), which is 20 times greater than that reported to occur with allogeneic whole blood donation (1 out of 198,119 donations; 0.0005%) (Popovsky, 1995). Therefore, although apheresis donation appears to have a lower reaction rate than whole blood donation, the risk of serious reactions is greater.

TABLE 37-22
Reaction Rates Among Apheresis (McLeod, 1998) and Whole Blood (Newman, 1997) Donors

Reaction	Apheresis donations (%)	Whole blood donations (%)
Hematoma or pain	1.15	9–16
Citrate toxicity	0.4	N/A
Mild vasovagal	0.05	2–5
Vasovagal with syncope	0.08	0.1–0.3

N/A, Not available.

The most common of reactions seen by McLeod among apheresis donors were injuries due to venipuncture (McLeod, 1998). Table 37-22 lists the adverse effects to apheresis donation reported by McLeod, their frequency, and comparable frequency among whole blood donors. As with whole blood donation, first-time donors had reactions more frequently than repeat donors. Reactions were found to be more frequent among platelet donors than among plasma or granulocyte donors (5.9% and 9.4%, respectively, vs. 12%), which may have been due to a greater number of first-time donors in this group (McLeod, 1998). Despotis (1999) found associations of citrate and hypotensive reactions with donor weight, gender, and type of collection instrument used. For venipuncture-related complications, only female gender was associated as a risk factor (Despotis, 1999). The instrument used for collection also influenced reaction rates. McLeod found that the Fenwal CS3000 had fewer reactions than other instruments. This could possibly be due to lower citrate infusion rates with this instrument, as well as the ability to perform single-needle procedures with the other instruments. Such single-needle procedures, which alternate between drawing and returning through the single intravenous line, result in larger extracorporeal volumes (McLeod, 1998). Despotis (1999) noted that the relationship between donor weight and citrate reactions was different when the COBE Spectra and the Fenwal CS3000 were compared. Donors with lower weights had a higher probability of citrate reactions on the Fenwal CS3000, and those with higher weights had a higher probability on the COBE Spectra. The authors of this study believed that this was due to the methods by which these instruments determine the anticoagulant infusion rate (Despotis, 1999).

Reactions among therapeutic hemapheresis procedures have been reported to occur in 4.75% of procedures (McLeod, 1999). The reactions identified and their overall frequencies are given in Table 37-23. The rate of reactions varied with regard to procedure, replacement fluid, and patient. For example, the reaction rate for plasma exchange using albumin was 3.35% as compared with 7.81% for plasma exchange using plasma as the replacement fluid. Leukocytapheresis demonstrated a reaction rate of 5.71%, HPC-A collection had a rate of 1.66%, and no reactions occurred in the 18 patients who underwent therapeutic thrombocytapheresis. Patients with neurologic disorders were more likely than other categories of patients to experience vasovagal reactions (McLeod, 1999).

Shemin (2007) in a more recent review examined the frequency of complications during the performance of plasma exchanges. Of 1727 plasma exchanges in 174 patients, 614 procedures (36%) were complicated by a reaction. Most complications were mild, and no deaths occurred. Of the reactions, 0.2% required discontinuation of the procedure, and 0.1% required additional medical management beyond that available in the apheresis unit. The most common reactions were fever (7.7%), urticaria (7.4%), and hypocalcemic symptoms (7.3%). Similar to what was reported by McLeod, differences were seen based on the replacement fluid used. Urticaria and pruritus were more common with the use of FFP as a replacement fluid; hypotension was more common with the use of albumin and saline (Shemin, 2007).

It should be noted that the study by McLeod did not include complications or reactions due to venous access, but that by Shemin did. Studies that included these data have noted higher reaction rates with therapeutic hemapheresis. For example, Couriel (1994) noted adverse effects in 17% of therapeutic apheresis procedures. These were predominantly mild, consisting of citrate reactions, but 6.15% of procedures were complicated by severe reactions, reactions that were life threatening, or reactions that resulted in termination of the procedure. All of these reactions were due to central venous access and consisted of a pneumothorax, a hemopneumothorax, catheter-related bacteremia, and a sternocleidomastoid hematoma. The patient with the hemopneumothorax exsanguinated because of the complication (Couriel, 1994). Of the two severe reactions requiring additional medical intervention reported by Shemin (2007), one was due to arterial puncture during central line placement. Although only one death due to therapy was reported by Couriel, and no deaths attributable to therapeutic hemapheresis were reported in the studies by McLeod and Shemin, additional deaths have been reported by other authors. A majority of such deaths have been ascribed to cardiopulmonary arrest during hemapheresis; additional causes have included anaphylaxis, pulmonary embolus, and vascular perforation due to central venous access. Huestis (1989) estimated a mortality rate for therapeutic hemapheresis of 3 per 10,000 procedures (0.03%), and Mokrzycki (1994) estimated the mortality rate, based on a review of the literature available to that time, to be 0.05% of procedures.

TABLE 37-23
Reaction Rates Among Patients Undergoing Therapeutic Apheresis Procedures

Reaction	Frequency (%)
Transfusion reactions	1.6
Citrate toxicity	1.2
Hypotension	1.0
Vasovagal reactions	0.5
Pallor and diaphoresis	0.5
Tachycardia	0.4
Respiratory distress	0.3
Tetany and seizure	0.2
Chills or rigors	0.2

Data from McLeod BC, Sniecinski I, Ciavarella D, et al. Frequency of immediate adverse effects associated with therapeutic apheresis. Transfusion 1999;39: 282–8.

As discussed under the description of each procedure, specific complications are associated with specific procedures, such as those due to G-CSF administration in granulocyte harvest. A discussion of complications and risks common to all hemapheresis procedures follows.

ELECTROLYTE AND ACID-BASE DISTURBANCES

Citrate is used as the primary anticoagulant in both donor and therapeutic apheresis procedures because it effectively prevents coagulation while being short acting and easily reversible, unlike heparin. Citrate ions chelate calcium ions, producing a soluble complex. As a result, the chelated calcium ions are unavailable for biological reactions such as the coagulation cascade. Within the apheresis instrument, plasma citrate concentrations reach 15–24 mmol/L, lowering the calcium ion concentration below 0.2–0.3 mmol/L, the level necessary for coagulation (Strauss, 1996). This ionized calcium level requires the infusion of approximately 500 mL of ACD-A solution and would be incompatible with life. Death does not occur, however, because of compensatory mechanisms in the donor/patient. Upon return of blood from the apheresis instrument to the donor/patient, the citrate is diluted throughout total extracellular fluid. In addition, the liver, kidneys, and muscles rapidly metabolize citrate, releasing the bound calcium (Strauss, 1996). The body responds to the decrease in ionized calcium by increasing parathyroid hormone levels, resulting in mobilization of calcium from skeletal stores and increased absorption by the kidneys (Silberstein, 1986). Finally, calcium bound to albumin is also mobilized and buffers the decline (Bolan, 2003a).

In therapeutic plasma exchange procedures, the volume of plasma removed must be replaced by a similar volume of replacement fluid. In plasma exchange using FFP or plasma cryoprecipitate reduced as replacement fluid, an additional source of citrate is infused in the form of the anticoagulant present in these solutions. It is therefore common for symptoms of citrate toxicity to be seen in these patients. In plasma exchange using albumin as a replacement fluid, it would be expected that citrate toxicity would be less of a problem. However, this is not always the case. Normally, 40%–55% of serum calcium is bound to albumin, with the unbound portion representing the physiologically active ionized calcium. Albumin preparations are depleted of this calcium and, as a result, bind calcium when infused during plasma exchange. This can lead to a drop in ionized calcium with the subsequent appearance of symptoms due to hypocalcemia. Goss (1999) demonstrated a higher incidence of citrate reactions and greater decreases in ionized calcium levels in neurology patients receiving plasma exchange with 5% albumin as the replacement fluid when compared with those receiving 10% pentastarch as the replacement fluid. A subsequent study demonstrated that the addition of calcium gluconate to the albumin preparation before administration more effectively reduced the incidence of citrate toxicity when compared with IV calcium gluconate or oral calcium carbonate (Weinstein, 1996). The effect was due to the saturation of calcium binding sites on the albumin, thereby maintaining ionized calcium levels in the patient.

Despite compensatory mechanisms, citrate infusion can result in a decrease in ionized calcium levels to the point where symptoms develop in the donor/patient. These result from a decrease in ionized calcium to levels at which the excitability of nerve membranes increases to the point where spontaneous depolarization can occur (Strauss, 1996). Resulting signs and symptoms can include perioral paresthesias, acral paresthesias, shivering, light-headedness, twitching, and tremors. In addition, some patients experience nausea and vomiting. As the ionized calcium levels fall farther, these symptoms may progress to carpopedal spasm, tetany, and seizure (Strauss, 1996). It is therefore important to elicit the presence of early symptoms from the donor/patient, so that interventions can occur before the more severe symptoms. In addition to the symptoms described previously, prolongation of the QT interval on electrocardiogram, depressed myocardial contraction, and fatal arrhythmias have been reported (Strauss, 1996). Hypotension may also be seen with citrate reactions (Goodnough, 1999) and may be due to the depressed myocardial function mentioned and to vascular smooth muscle relaxation (Bunker, 1962).

Factors that have been found to influence the rate of citrate reactions in donor and therapeutic apheresis include alkalosis due to hyperventilation (Strauss, 1996); the type of anticoagulant solution used, with ACD-A having more reactions than ACD-B (Szymanski, 1978); the rate of infusion of the anticoagulant solution (Strauss, 1996); the amount of citrate infused (Strauss, 1996); and the donor's serum albumin level before the start of the procedure (Bolan, 2003a). It should be noted that intermittent flow hemapheresis procedures tend to have a greater frequency of citrate reactions, as the rate of citrate infusion is higher when the separation chamber is emptied than during continuous apheresis procedures. Also, the method by which an instrument calculates the dose of anticoagulant may influence the rate of reactions among certain donor subgroups (Despotis, 1999).

The treatment of citrate reactions is relatively simple when reactions are identified early. Treatment includes slowing the reinfusion rate to allow for dilution and metabolism of the citrate, increasing the donor/patient blood/citrate ratio to decrease the amount of citrate infused, giving oral calcium in the form of calcium antacids, and giving intravenous calcium (Strauss, 1996).

Administration of oral calcium carbonate and its effects on citrate toxicity in apheresis platelet donors were studied by Bolan (2003a, 2003b). It was found that administration of 2g of calcium carbonate was associated with a statistically significant reduction in the severity of paresthesias (Bolan, 2003b). Physiologically, this dose was also associated with the greatest improvement in ionized and total calcium levels among the doses examined (Bolan, 2003a), but it was not associated with a reduction in overall symptom development, and it did not affect the occurrence of more severe symptoms (Bolan, 2003b).

Administration of intravenous calcium, in the form of calcium gluconate or calcium chloride, usually is not necessary in donor procedures but is common in the setting of therapeutic apheresis procedures. In HPC-A collections, the continuous infusion of calcium gluconate or calcium chloride has been found to prevent hypocalcemic symptom development (Bolan, 2002; Buchta, 2003), with calcium chloride maintaining higher ionized calcium levels (Buchta, 2003). In a comparison of infusion of calcium gluconate continuously, prophylactically at the start of HPC collection, or at the time of symptom development, continuous infusion maintained higher calcium levels, and changes in calcium levels were insignificant with the other two modes of administration (Kishimoto, 2002). When given to treat symptoms, the usual dose is 10 mL of calcium gluconate IV infused over 10–15 minutes (Hester, 1983). In patients with low ionized calcium levels before the start of the procedure, calcium gluconate can be given prophylactically.

Magnesium is another physiologically important divalent cation. Similarly to calcium, magnesium is bound by citrate. As a result, the infusion of citrate in the setting of plateletpheresis decreases ionized magnesium by 30% (Mercan, 1997). Mercan (1997) also found that magnesium levels fall more rapidly than calcium levels during citrate infusion, and they recover more slowly. Hypomagnesemia can induce signs and symptoms similar to hypocalcemia, including muscle spasms, muscle weakness, decreased vascular tone, and impaired cardiac contractility. In addition, hypomagnesemia can impair calcium and potassium homeostasis, including inhibition of the release of parathyroid hormone when markedly decreased (Mercan, 1997). As a result, patients with low magnesium levels before undergoing apheresis may exhibit signs and symptoms of citrate toxicity due to hypomagnesemia and not hypocalcemia. Patients who cannot rapidly metabolize citrate, thereby releasing the bound cations, may also be at risk (Kamochi, 2002). These symptoms may be unresponsive to the administration of calcium supplementation. To avoid hypomagnesemia, it is common at some institutions to measure magnesium levels before initiation and to supplement magnesium before performing procedures if indicated. Reports have described the use of prophylactic magnesium infusions similar to those done with calcium. Haddad (2005) investigated prophylactic administration of magnesium to allogeneic HPC-A donors. Supplementation was associated with normal ionized magnesium levels during the procedure, as well as greater parathyroid hormone response and higher blood glucose levels. However, no differences were seen with regard to the symptoms (mild paresthesias, coldness, and nausea) (Haddad, 2005).

As described, citrate is rapidly metabolized. This process consumes hydrogen ions; as a result, metabolic alkalosis due to citrate infusion may develop. The risk of this occurrence is greatest in patients with renal disease, who cannot adequately excrete bicarbonate (Kelleher, 1987), and in those receiving replacement fluids containing citrate (Kelleher, 1987; Dzik, 1988). A study comparing patients with TTP undergoing plasma exchange with FFP replacement versus patients with myasthenia gravis undergoing plasma exchange with albumin demonstrated increased frequency of metabolic alkalosis in the former group (Marques, 2001). Patients with TTP demonstrated a mean creatinine level of 1.3 mg/dL and a mean blood urea nitrogen of 24.8 mg/dL (Marques, 2001). Although the metabolic alkalosis seen in these patients did not reach critical levels (>35 mEq/L HCO_3^-) and resolved following cessation of plasma exchange, it was associated with critical drops in potassium (<3.0 mEq/L) during the procedures (Marques, 2001). The presence of alkalosis can worsen hypocalcemia (Edmondson, 1975) and slow citrate metabolism (Dzik, 1988). Unfortunately, the symptoms of metabolic alkalosis are nonspecific, usually presenting as worsening symptoms of hypocalcemia. Alkalosis resolves with time or dialysis and can be avoided by reducing the amount of citrate infused by adjusting the blood/citrate ratio and/or using replacement fluids that lack citrate (Pearl, 1985).

Metabolic alkalosis results in a shift in hydrogen ions from intracellular locations (in an attempt to compensate pH) with a concurrent flux of potassium into these cells to maintain electrical neutrality. The result is that significant drops in potassium can occur during large-volume hematopoietic progenitor cell collections, in addition to those seen in the TTP patients described previously. Schlenke (2000) found an average drop in potassium levels of 11.3 ± 7% in a study of 96 large-volume leukaphereses. Despite this decline, none of the patients in this study experienced symptoms attributable to hypokalemia. Symptoms of hypokalemia include weakness, hypotonia, and cardiac arrhythmia (Schlenke, 2000). Treatment of such complications would consist of replacement of the potassium, orally or intravenously. A prudent option would be to prevent the reaction by determining the potassium level before the start of the procedure and supplementing if indicated.

ALLERGIC, ANAPHYLACTOID, AND ANAPHYLACTIC REACTIONS

Allergic, anaphylactoid, and anaphylactic reactions result from the release of vasoactive substances such as histamine, leukotriene C4, leukotriene D4, prostaglandin D2, and platelet-activating factor from mast cells and basophils. The release of these substances is mediated by the presence of IgE antibodies on the surface of these cells. When the target antigen binds to the IgE molecule, the substances listed previously are released. This in turn results in a variety of symptoms by causing contraction of smooth muscle, increased vascular permeability, and vasodilation. Mast cells and basophils can also be activated by complement-derived factors such as C3a and C5a, which can be produced by antigen–IgG interactions and other mechanisms (Vamvakas, 2001). These types of reactions can range from mild urticarial reactions to life-threatening anaphylactic reactions. Signs and symptoms of these reactions include pruritus, urticaria, erythema, flushing, angioedema, upper airway obstruction, lower airway obstruction, hypotension, shock, nausea, vomiting, and diarrhea (Vamvakas, 2001).

Allergic reactions have been reported in both donors and patients undergoing hemapheresis procedures. Among donors, reactions have been reported among platelet, plasma, and granulocyte donors. In platelet and plasma donors, reactions to ethylene oxide gas used to sterilize the tubing sets used for the procedures have been described (Leitman, 1986; Muylle, 1986). These reactions have occurred predominantly in donors who had undergone numerous previous procedures. It is thought that during the procedures, ethylene oxide present within the plastic binds to proteins within the plasma. The proteins serve as carrier molecules and the ethylene oxide as a hapten, with the result being an immune response with the generation of IgE antibodies toward ethylene oxide. In most of the donors who experienced allergic phenomena, IgE antibodies to ethylene oxide were identified (Leitman, 1986). Reactions ranged from urticaria, flushing, and periorbital edema (Leitman, 1986) to an anaphylactic reaction consisting of wheezing, flushing, swelling of the lips, and hypotension (Muylle, 1986). The overall rate of reaction in one study was 1.0% of platelet donors. The reactions also showed an increased frequency with the Fenwal CS3000 than with the Haemonetics V-50 (Haemonetics, Braintree, Mass.). This was thought to be because, at the start of processing with the CS3000, a mixture of saline and anticoagulant that was used to prime the bag was infused into the patient. This was not the case with the V-50. It was postulated that this resulted in a bolus of ethylene oxide that produced the symptoms (Leitman, 1986).

Reactions have been reported among granulocyte donors as well. Besides ethylene oxide reactions, another mechanism is possible. Granulocyte donors are exposed to low molecular weight or high molecular weight HES to enhance red cell sedimentation. Although these substances are poor immunogens and have not been able to induce antibody formation, allergic reactions have occurred in the setting of HES use in hemapheresis (Dutcher, 1984) and as a volume expander (Ring, 1977). The mechanism behind the production of anaphylactoid reactions with HES is thought to be due to the ability of HES to activate the alternative complement cascade. This would result in the production of C3a and C5a, both of which can cause mast cell and basophil release (Dutcher, 1984). Reactions reported to occur with HES include mild urticarial reactions and severe reactions with respiratory and cardiac arrest. The rate of reaction in a study of patients receiving HES for volume expansion was 0.085%, with severe (anaphylactic) reactions occurring in 0.006% (Ring, 1977). Reactions have occurred with both high molecular weight (hetastarch) (Ring, 1977) and low molecular weight (pentastarch) (Kannan, 1999) HES. Because of this risk, Dutcher (1984) recommended excluding people with a history of allergies as granulocyte donors.

Among therapeutic hemapheresis patients, reactions to ethylene oxide or HES could occur. In addition, therapeutic plasma exchange procedures frequently use plasma products—FFP or plasma cryoprecipitate reduced—as replacement solutions. As a result, patients are also at risk for allergic and anaphylactic reactions due to transfusion reactions. The most common allergic reaction within the setting of plasma product infusion is the urticarial reaction. This reaction occurs in 1%–3% of plasma infusions and consists of hives scattered over the body. In 1 in 20,000–47,000 transfusions, anaphylaxis occurs (Vamvakas, 2001). The most common cause of this last reaction is the infusion of plasma containing IgA into an IgA-deficient individual who possesses anti-IgA antibodies (Vamvakas, 2001).

The treatment of allergic, anaphylactoid, and anaphylactic reactions depends on their severity. In donor reactions, the procedure should be stopped. Simple reactions such as urticaria can then be treated with oral antihistamines (e.g., diphenhydramine). The same treatment can be provided with therapeutic procedures, although in this case the procedure can be restarted following antihistamine administration. In addition, the patient can be premedicated with antihistamines before subsequent procedures are performed.

Anaphylactic reactions are life threatening. The procedure, whether donor or therapeutic, must be immediately discontinued. Vascular access should be kept open using saline. For less severe reactions, epinephrine 0.3–0.5 mg can be given subcutaneously, with the dose repeated every 20–30 minutes for up to three doses. In addition, aminophylline 6 mg/kg can be given for bronchospasm. This loading dose should be followed by an infusion of 0.5–1 mg/kg/hour. Volume expansion with normal saline or lactated Ringer's solution can be given for hypotension. Oxygen should be given for respiratory distress. For severe reactions, epinephrine 0.5 mg can be given intravenously, with repeated dosing every 5–10 minutes. Dopamine can also be given for hypotension unresponsive to volume. The airway must be protected, and endotracheal intubation may be indicated (Vamvakas, 2001).

Obviously, the best course of action is to avoid such reactions. Donors who have experienced such reactions should be deferred from future donation. Patients with mild reactions should be premedicated with antihistamines. Those with severe reactions due to IgA should receive IgA-deficient replacement fluids. For most procedures, this could be albumin or saline. For procedures requiring plasma as a replacement fluid, as in plasma exchange for TTP, IgA-deficient plasma products must be used.

ANGIOTENSIN-CONVERTING ENZYME INHIBITORS

The use of angiotensin-converting enzyme (ACE) inhibitors by patients undergoing hemapheresis procedures is associated with reactions similar in many respects to the allergic reactions described previously. These reactions consist of flushing, hypotension, bradycardia, and dyspnea (Strauss, 1996) and have been seen in patients undergoing therapeutic plasma exchange (Owen, 1994), LDL-apheresis using dextran sulfate columns (Agishi, 1994), and treatment with staphylococcal A protein columns (Owen, 1994). These reactions result from activation of the kinin system and generation of bradykinin when patient plasma comes in contact with the negatively charged plastic of the apheresis set. Normally, bradykinin is rapidly inactivated by kininase I and II. ACE inhibitors, however, block the actions of these enzymes such that high levels accumulate, producing the symptoms described previously (Strauss, 1996). During plasma exchange with albumin, prekallikrein-activating factor present in the albumin can trigger the formation of bradykinin (Owen, 1994). Again, the presence of ACE inhibitors prevents degradation of this substance. These reactions can be avoided by withholding ACE inhibitors for 24–48 hours before hemapheresis procedures (Owen, 1994). Some newer ACE inhibitors have longer half-lives; withholding these drugs for longer periods or switching to ACE inhibitors with shorter half-lives may be necessary.

HYPOVOLEMIA AND VASOVAGAL REACTIONS

Hypotension can be seen during both donor and therapeutic hemapheresis procedures. This can be the result of two different pathophysiologic mechanisms. In the first, hypotension results from intravascular volume depletion due to too much volume being present within the extracorporeal circuit. Such reactions are characterized by both increased vascular tone and increased cardiac output as the sympathetic nervous system attempts to compensate for the hypovolemia (Strauss, 1996). Increasing both heart rate and contractility produces the increase in cardiac output. These reactions are not common among hemapheresis donors, as Standards for Blood Banks and Transfusion Services limit the amount of volume that can be present within the extracorporeal circuit to 10.5 mL/kg (Standards Committee of the American Association of Blood Banks, 2009), and the donors fulfill health and weight requirements. In therapeutic procedures, the patient has an underlying disease that may make hypovolemia more likely. For example, the presence of hypotension has been found to be more common in patients with neurologic disease (McLeod, 1999). Standards for Blood Banks and Transfusion Services do not prescribe limits on extracorporeal volume during therapeutic hemapheresis procedures, although application of the limits used during donor hemapheresis procedures would seem prudent (Strauss, 1996).

The second mechanism causing hypotension during hemapheresis procedures is the vasovagal reaction. In this reaction, hypovolemia results in a decrease in blood pressure. As stated previously, the compensatory response is to increase cardiac output and vascular tone. During a vasovagal reaction, parasympathetic output, which normally counteracts sympathetic output, increases disproportionately, resulting in slowing of heart rate and decreased vascular tone, leading to hypotension (Strauss, 1996). Factors that have been associated with such reactions in whole blood donors include younger age, low weight, first-time donation, and inattentive staff (Newman, 1997). Tomita (2002) examined the incidence of vasovagal reactions among apheresis donors and whole blood donors at the same collection center. They noted that the incidence of these reactions among apheresis donors increased with age, unlike what has been reported with whole blood donors. The age-related increase in vasovagal reactions was even more common in women and was thought to result from a lower circulating blood volume in these populations (elderly and women), leading to a greater percentage of the donor's blood being within the extracorporeal circuit during collection. The resulting greater drop in blood pressure during collection leads to additional reactions. It was also noted that the incidence increased with increasing cycles during a collection, and it was theorized that hypocalcemia was involved in the onset of vasovagal reactions (Tomita, 2002).

Hypovolemic and vasovagal reactions are treated similarly. The procedure should be temporarily interrupted, and a fluid bolus should be infused. If the reaction is due to hypovolemia, blood pressure should increase and pulse rate should decrease in response to this intervention. If the reaction is due to a vasovagal reaction, this may not occur. Additional treatments for vasovagal reactions include placing the donor/patient in the Trendelenburg position (head down), applying cold compresses to the forehead and neck, and reassuring the donor/patient (Strauss, 1996).

HYDROXYETHYL STARCH AND COAGULOPATHY

As discussed under the section dealing with plasma exchange, removal of plasma from a patient during a therapeutic hemapheresis procedure and replacement of the volume with albumin or some other fluid that does not contain coagulation factors can result in mild, temporary abnormalities in coagulation. These changes are usually short lived, with return of most coagulation factors to normal levels within 24–48 hours. The use of HES as volume replacement or as a sedimenting agent is also associated with changes in coagulation factor levels. Both high molecular weight HES, such as hetastarch, and low molecular weight HES, such as pentastarch, result in prolongation of the PTT, as well as decreases in fibrinogen levels. This is thought to result from the dilutional effects produced when these substances are infused. High molecular weight, but not low molecular weight, HES is also associated with decreases in factor VIII activity, factor VIII antigen, and vWF antigen, as well as with prolongation of bleeding time (Strauss, 1988). It is thought that this last effect is a result of the decrease in vWF antigen levels and may represent an acquired von Willebrand disease–like state. Because of these changes, a risk of coagulopathy exists with the use of these agents. This risk appears to be dose dependent. In the setting of volume expansion in critical care, the maximum dose of HES needed to avoid such complications has been suggested to be 20 mL/kg/24-hour period. Doses up to 3600 mL have been given in this setting without difficulty (Nearman, 1991). The danger in hemapheresis procedures is that multiple collections or therapeutic procedures may be necessary in a given donor/patient over consecutive days. Because HES, especially high molecular weight HES, has a long half-life, this may result in an accumulation of HES over the course of the hemapheresis procedures and the potential danger of coagulopathy.

HYDROXYETHYL STARCH AND OTHER SIDE EFFECTS

As has been mentioned, HES has a long half-life. This is dependent upon the metabolism of HES by α-amylase and subsequent renal excretion of the breakdown products (Yacobi, 1982). Persistent pruritus due to deposition of HES in the skin has been reported as one of the most frequent complications of HES administration. Skin deposits have been detected for up to 4 years following administration (Sirtl, 1999; Stander, 2001).

In addition to skin deposition, a case report has described marrow and organ failure in a patient undergoing chronic plasma exchange (20 months) with HES used as the replacement fluid. In this patient, foamy macrophages containing HES were found replacing bone marrow, as well as infiltrating duodenal mucosa, liver, peritoneum, and dura mater. These cells were also present in ascitic fluid (Auwerda, 2002).

AIR EMBOLUS

Air embolus is a rare complication of hemapheresis procedures. It occurs when air enters the venous system through a leak in the hemapheresis instrument or the venous access. Air entering the right ventricle and pulmonary artery results in obstruction to right ventricular output and pulmonary artery vasoconstriction (Montacer-Kuhssari, 1994). Symptoms of air embolism include dyspnea, tachypnea, cyanosis, tachycardia, and hypotension. The reason for the rarity of this complication is that all modern hemapheresis instruments possess sensors that can detect air within the extravascular circuit and stop the procedure. Should air embolism occur, however, treatment consists of placing the donor/patient in the Trendelenburg position on the left side. This traps the air in the apex of the right ventricle, away from the pulmonary outflow tract, improving right ventricular outflow. Over time, the air will dissolve.

SUMMARY

In summary, hemapheresis represents a safe and effective technique for the production of needed blood components, as well as for the treatment of a variety of diseases. Although hemapheresis is often compared with the 18th century practice of bloodletting, it shares little with this practice. Hemapheresis is selective in what is removed from the donor/patient. In addition, hemapheresis is grounded in evidence-based medicine. Hemapheresis procedures are safe; however, they are not without risk and should be applied only to those diseases and disorders for which the possibility of benefit exists, and for which evidence in support of this benefit has been shown.

SELECTED REFERENCES

Ibrahim RB, Liu C, Cronin SM, et al. Drug removal by plasmapheresis: an evidence-based review. Pharmacotherapy 2007;27:1529–49.

An extensive review of the literature concerning the effects of plasma exchange on drug clearance and metabolism. The article provides suggestions for therapy modification, as well as for future research.

McLeod BC, Weinstein R, Winters JL, Szczepiorkowski ZM, editors. Apheresis: principles and practice. 3rd ed. Bethesda, Md.: AABB Press; 2010.

A comprehensive textbook that addresses both donor and therapeutic apheresis, including the history of apheresis, currently available instrumentation, and an in-depth discussion of the mechanism of action and the physiology of apheresis.

Shaz BH, Winters JL, Bandarenko N, Szczepiorkowski ZM. How we approach an apheresis request for category III, category IV, or non-categorized indication. Transfusion 2007;47:1963–71.

A discussion of the clinical decision-making process to be used when considering performing a therapeutic hemapheresis procedure, which is not an ASFA category I or II indication.

Shehata N, Kouroukis C, Kelton JG. A review of randomized controlled trials using therapeutic apheresis. Transfus Med Rev 2002;16:200–29.

A summary of all randomized controlled trials involving therapeutic apheresis. Includes numerous tables summarizing the trials, as well as recommendations concerning treatment protocols.

Szczepiorkowski ZM, Winters JL, Bandarenko N, et al. Guidelines on the use of therapeutic apheresis in clinical practice: evidence-based approach from the Apheresis Applications Committee of the American Society for Apheresis. J Clin Apheresis 2010;25:83–177.

Comprehensive review of the use of therapeutic apheresis. Includes one-page summaries describing treatment recommendations and technical considerations for more than 50 diseases. Also provides categorization and strength of evidence for the use of apheresis in the diseases discussed.

REFERENCES

Access the complete reference list online at http://www.expertconsult.com

CHAPTER 38

TISSUE BANKING AND PROGENITOR CELLS

Charlene A. Hubbell, Lazaro Rosales

KEY POINTS

- Appreciate the wide range of allogeneic tissues used for transplantation.
- Allograft tissue is screened, tested, and processed to improve its safety.
- Allograft tissue is stored by a variety of methods, including cryopreservation.
- Risks and complications are associated with the use of allograft tissue.
- A wide range of assisted reproductive techniques are available to infertile couples and individuals.
- Hematopoietic progenitor cells can be derived from multiple sources and transplanted in different ways, depending on the needs of the recipient.
- Appreciate the balance between the graft-versus-host reaction and the graft-versus-leukemia effect.

Throughout the United States, tissue banks routinely provide hundreds of products that not only extend life but also in many instances significantly improve the quality of life for the patients they serve. More than 400,000 bone allografts (American Association of Tissue Banks, 2008) and 50,000 corneas (Eye Bank Association of America, 2008) are transplanted annually in the United States—a number that far exceeds the approximately 25,000 solid organ transplants per year (United Network for Organ Sharing, 2008). Clinical applications of allogeneic and autologous tissue and the types of tissue available have grown exponentially in the last two decades. Yet, aside from the patients and physicians served by these tissue banks, many people are unaware of the vast scope of activities in today's health care environment that are under the umbrella of tissue banking. Over the past 20 years, tissue banking in the United State has evolved from a system of incidental hospital bone or sperm banks to a system of regulated, accredited facilities, much like blood banks, providing an expanding variety of high-quality, carefully screened and tested products for use by physicians (Table 38-1).

Many tissue banks provide a wide range of products and services in skin, bone, and heart valve procurement, processing, and storage. Other tissue banks focus their services in specialized areas such as reproductive tissue or hematopoietic progenitor cells (HPCs). One bank may recruit donors and procure and process tissue such as skin for burn patients or bone for orthopedic repairs; another may collect, process, and store HPCs for life-saving bone marrow transplants. Processing of musculoskeletal tissues and cardiac valves, which requires extensive equipment, personnel, and quality assurance, is performed primarily by a few large tissue banks that subcontract with other tissue banks, which, in turn, collect, store, and issue these products. In addition, an exponential growth has occurred over the past two decades in reproductive banks that provide assistance to infertile couples or individuals.

SOURCES OF TISSUE

Tissues used for transplantation come from two primary sources: living donors and deceased donors. Living donors may be individuals who donate for their own use (autologous HPCs or sperm), as directed donors for a given individual (allogeneic HPCs or sperm donation), or altruistically for unknown recipients (surgical discard bone, sperm donation, allogeneic HPCs through the National Marrow Donor Program). A large majority of bone, skin, and cardiac valves used for transplantation, as well as eye tissue, come from deceased donors. Unlike solid organ donation, where there is a need for the organs to be obtained while circulation is maintained, deceased donor tissue can be obtained for several hours after death and up to 24 hours later if the body is refrigerated. This substantially increases the number of available tissue donors. Because corneal tissue has relatively minimal contact with the circulatory system, some individuals who would otherwise be excluded as tissue donors may still be eye donors.

Deceased donor tissue is procured primarily from hospital operating rooms or morgues and medical examiners' offices. Harvesting of tissue is performed in a sterile or clean environment using aseptic techniques. Many tissues, such as bone, are then frozen for subsequent processing and refreezing or freeze-drying. Specialized tissues such as cornea are processed immediately and stored for only a short time (48 to 72 hours) before use. Tissue from living donors is procured in the operating room (surgically salvaged bone or bone marrow) or in specialized clean environments that hemapheresis centers and sperm banks are equipped to provide. These tissues are collected under sterile conditions, processed immediately, and used in less than 24 hours or frozen for subsequent use.

TISSUE BANK ACTIVITIES

The major activities of tissue banks are outlined in Table 38-2. A major impetus for the movement to formal, accredited tissue banks in our nation was the concern about transfusion-transmitted disease. As with blood banks and transfusion services (see Transfusion Medicine and Hemapheresis chapters), donor recruitment, screening, and testing are critical functions of the tissue bank. Since the early 1990s, cases involving disease transmission documented that careful screening by both medical record review and serologic testing, as well as maintenance of detailed records, was critical to safe tissue banking practices and thus acceptance of allograft tissue by both the public and health care providers. Concerns still remain

TABLE 38-1
Categories of Transplantable Tissue

Musculoskeletal
Bone
Cartilage
Meniscus
Tendon
Ligament
Fascia
Skin
Cardiovascular
Heart valves
Saphenous vein
Corneal (eye)
Reproductive
Sperm
Ova
Embryo
Hematopoietic
Bone marrow
Peripheral blood progenitor cells
Umbilical cord blood progenitor cells
Other
Ear ossicles
Dura mater
Parathyroids
Pancreatic islet cells

TABLE 38-2
Tissue Banking Activities

Donor recruitment
Acquisition of tissues
Processing and storage of tissues
Provision of tissues for transplantation
Public and professional education
Quality assurance and record keeping
Recipient records

that physicians who utilize these tissues recognize and report these adverse reactions, primarily infection, to the originating tissue bank. The Joint Commission (TJC) has standards for tissue banking practices that are targeted primarily at the transplantation facility. These standards focus on the necessity for implantation facilities to keep clear, precise records regarding tissue receipt, storage, and use, so that all allogeneic tissues can be traced from donor to recipient. TJC standards also require institutions to establish a mechanism for physicians to report adverse reactions and the originating tissue bank to be notified. Accredited full service tissue banks, in the same manner as blood banks, investigate suspected reactions or complications extensively. "Look-back" reviews should include reviews of the complications associated with other tissue from the same donor, the current health of the donor, if living, and quarantining of other tissue from the same donor. The American Association of Tissue Banks (AATB)* provides strict standards and accreditation for organizations involved in any area of tissue banking. Several states also require tissue banks to be licensed, and the U.S. Food and Drug Administration (FDA) regulates the screening of donor tissue used for transplantation purposes (FDA CFR, 2009).

DONOR SCREENING

Tissue donors are carefully screened to prevent the transmission of bacterial, viral, and/or genetic disease, as well as to ensure the quality of the tissue obtained (Table 38-3). With deceased tissue donors, unlike blood donors, information regarding medical and social history is obtained from the family or close friends, as well as from physicians' records.

*AATB, 1350 Beverly Rd., #220A, McLean, Va.

TABLE 38-3
Comprehensive Donor Testing

Donor Screening
Review of medical history and medical records
Infectious diseases (including history of foreign travel)
Malignant disease
Collagen and immune complex diseases
History of genetic diseases
Trauma
Exposure to drugs, toxic substances, or biological hazards
Physical examination of living donors
Review of autopsy records for deceased donors
Review of social history for risk behaviors
Donor Serologic Testing
Antibody to human immunodeficiency virus (by nucleic acid testing)
Antibody to human T cell lymphotropic virus
Antibody to hepatitis C virus (by nucleic acid testing)
Hepatitis B surface antigen
Antibody to hepatitis B core antigen
Serologic tests for syphilis
Antibody to West Nile virus
Antibody to *Trypanosoma cruzi* (Chagas' disease)
Bacteriologic testing of tissue product

Reports of tissue transplant complications in the early 1990s focused on the transmission of human immunodeficiency virus (HIV) (Simonds, 1992) and hepatitis C (Conrad, 1995). More recently, attention has been focused on testing of tissue donors for additional disease transmission vectors (*Trypanosoma cruzi*, West Nile virus, and H1N1), as well as for transmission of nonscreened viruses such as Creutzfeldt-Jakob disease (Centers for Disease Control, 2003) and others (Kainer, 2004) by serologically negative tissue. It is likely, however, that there will continue to be isolated case reports of transmission of uncommon pathogens by tissue and organ donors. The impracticality of screening for all transmissible diseases emphasizes the continued need for careful screening of tissue and organ donors by medical history and family interview, as well as laboratory testing. Asking the right questions in the correct manner is a critical function that needs to be performed by well-trained, experienced individuals who are able to identify possible risks in the donor medical history, in information about possible risk behaviors, or in available laboratory data.

Other parts of the review process are targeted at ensuring the quality of the donated tissue. Musculoskeletal donors need to be carefully screened for any history of trauma that might result in a weakened structural bone graft. Sperm donations are reviewed not only for genetic disease but also to ensure viable sperm that will have a reasonable chance of resulting in successful fertilization. The use of umbilical cord blood for unrelated allogeneic bone marrow and peripheral blood transplantation requires screening and testing of the mother and of the cord blood. When tissue is procured from living donors, with the exception of HPC, the tissue is frozen and quarantined for a minimum of 180 days, at the end of which the donor serologic testing is repeated. This prevents the use of tissue from any donor who was in the "window" period for HIV or hepatitis C, that is, those who had been exposed to the virus but did not demonstrate antibody at the time of donation. The addition of nucleic acid testing for hepatitis C and HIV1/2 has also increased the safety of donated allograft tissue by decreasing the time between donor exposure and a positive laboratory test (AABB). Because of concerns about the sensitivity of testing specimens from deceased donors, tissue banks that process these tissues must utilize test kits that have been approved by the FDA for the testing of deceased donors (CFR, 2009).

CRYOPRESERVATION

Tissues such as HPCs, sperm, and skin and some types of musculoskeletal tissue require the presence of viable cells and have a very short shelf life at refrigerator temperatures, thus requiring cryopreservation. The goal of all cryopreservation techniques is to extend the usable storage period of the material being frozen by reducing the metabolic demand of cells at lower temperatures with no loss of viability due to the freezing or thawing procedures. Cryopreservation of animal sperm has been an established agricultural practice for decades, and human researchers have been able to gain from their experiences. Generally, cryopreservation of human tissues makes use of cryoprotectant agents such as dimethyl sulfoxide (DMSO) or glycerol, balanced tissue culture media, and some form of protein supplementation such as autologous plasma, albumin, or other colloidal suspensions. The actual freezing is often performed using a controlled-rate freezer, a mechanical device that controls the rate at which freezing of the tissue takes place, usually −1° C/minute down to temperatures of −80° C. DMSO is the cryoprotective agent of choice for tissues such as skin, HPCs, and other nucleated cell suspensions or tissues; glycerol is generally used for the freezing of sperm. Cryoprotectant agents function by preventing the formation of intracellular ice crystals during freezing and balancing the osmotic pressure and concentration of intracellular versus extracellular water during the thawing process. The formation of extracellular ice crystals or too rapid an increase in extracellular osmotic pressure with resulting dehydration of the cell during thawing can result in damage to the cells and thus loss of viability. Cryoprotectant agents, such as DMSO, work by slowing the rate at which this change occurs (Gorin, 1986). Most tissue banks make use of liquid nitrogen and controlled-rate freezing processors that are programmed to compensate for the heat released, called the **heat of fusion,** at the change from the liquid state to the frozen state (Gorin, 1986). Uncompensated, the heat of fusion can result in decreased viability of the cells or frozen tissue.

Once frozen, cryopreserved tissues are stored at varied temperatures from −80° C in a mechanical freezer to vapor (−100° C) or liquid (−196° C) phase liquid nitrogen. Expiration dates for cryopreserved tissues are generally 5 years after collection, although these are arbitrary limits and the actual length of storage possible for many tissues has not been determined. Other tissues that do not require the presence of viable cells, such as structural bone, may be frozen or freeze-dried by a variety of other methods. Some freeze-dried tissues have expiration dates of 5 years, and others may be stored indefinitely.

Skin Banking

The most common use of allogeneic skin grafts is as a temporary cover for patients with extensive third-degree burns, until autologous or autogeneic skin can be recovered and grafted. Because of the concentrations of histocompatibility antigens and antigen-presenting cells (APCs), all allogeneic skin grafts are eventually rejected (Medawar, 1946). When used to cover burns, the grafts are generally replaced periodically until autografting can be performed. Most deceased donor skin provided as an allograft is a split-thickness graft with a thin layer of epidermis without dermis, and therefore ABO matching is not required (Eastlund, 1998). As a temporary graft, however, split-thickness skin grafts provide vital, immediate cover, as a barrier against infection plus fluid, electrolyte, and heat loss from extensive burns, allowing for patient stabilization and eventual autografting.

Generally, skin is harvested from deceased donors with uninfected, unblemished skin who have a body surface area less than 1.75 m^2. The skin is harvested with a dermatome from areas of the back, legs, and upper arms. The skin is generally disinfected before harvest and is soaked in antibiotic-containing tissue culture solution until it is used or until it is frozen.

Skin can be stored at 2°–8° C for several days (Kagan, 2005) or cryopreserved and stored for several years. Because of today's need for extensive review of the donor's history and laboratory records, skin grafts are more commonly frozen for subsequent use. The cryoprotectant of choice is 10%–15% glycerol (American Association of Tissue Banks, 2002), and the graft is generally incubated for a period of time (20–30 minutes) in the freezing solution to allow the solution to permeate the graft. The skin is then frozen in strips supported by gauze mesh and is frozen flat (Eastlund, 1998). Skin can be frozen with or without controlled-rate freezing and is easily stored at −50° to −80° C; however, lower temperatures are commonly used for longer storage by many tissue banks (Kearney, 1998). Frozen skin allografts are thawed rapidly at 37° C and are used immediately or washed with physiologic solutions to dilute the cryoprotectant.

The limited supply of human skin allografts has stimulated efforts targeted at xenogeneic substitutions, such as pigskin and artificial barriers. More recently, attempts have been made to culture epithelial cells to expand the available supply of autologous skin (Wang, 2007). Another homologous tissue product, which has gained widespread use, is Alloderm,* an acellular dermal matrix graft that is processed from human allograft skin. The tissue is enzymatically processed to remove the immunologically active cells, leaving behind an acellular collagen framework. It allows for fibroblast infiltration, collagen deposition, and neoepithelization. Because the immunologically active cells are removed, the graft is tolerated (not rejected) significantly longer than traditional human skin allografts. It not only has been employed as skin graft for burns, it also has applications in opthalmic; plastic; ear, nose, and throat; and dental surgeries (Shorr, 2000). It is a product made from allogeneic human tissue that must be used with the identical patient consents and tracking required for other human tissue products.

Musculoskeletal Tissues

Bone banking began several decades ago, when physicians first stored surgical discard bone, mostly femoral heads from joint replacement surgery, for future use in spinal fusions and other orthopedic procedures. Generally, this involved simple storage of the bone in an unmonitored freezer somewhere in the hospital. Often, no testing or processing of the surgical discard bone was performed, nor were monitoring of storage conditions and tracking of tissue sources or recipients conducted. In some situations, the original donor/patient was not even asked for consent. Today, these practices have been almost eliminated by the use of musculoskeletal tissue from registered, accredited tissue banks, so that patients can confidently elect to have a bone allograft as part of a surgical procedure (Tomford, 1993). In addition to autogeneic bone grafts, living donor bone donation is still used as a source of some types of bone. Living donors are now screened and tested and must provide informed consent. In addition, the bone tissue obtained is further processed to reduce the risk of infectious disease transmission, and detailed records of the source donor and recipient are kept for tracking and follow-up purposes.

Surgical discard bone and deceased donor bone are processed in a similar fashion. Extraneous tissue, blood, and marrow elements are removed by high-pressure pulse washing, and the tissue is soaked in antibiotic solutions. Bacteriologic culturing of the tissue is done at collection, during processing, and before freezing. Tissue that requires the presence of viable cells such as cartilage, femoral head, tibia, whole bone, or tendon is usually washed, soaked, and frozen at temperatures between −60° and −150° C. With other tissues, where viability is not an issue, ethanol soaks may used to remove lipid content, generally in the preparation of demineralized, lyophilized bone, which also decreases the infectivity of the tissue. Most bone tissue is further sterilized by the use of low-dose irradiation. In addition, lyophilization, which is possible with bone products such as cancellous and cortical bone chips, appears to reduce the immunogenicity and the infectivity of these products. The use of ethlyene oxide to endsterilize bone tissue has been generally eliminated, as adverse reactions were reported in multiple recipients (Jackson, 1990). The bone tissue is cut and shaped and then is preserved by freezing or freeze-drying.

Bone allografts serve mainly as a mechanical support and a framework for the host's bone-forming cells to replace lost tissue. The osteoinductive function of the allograft bone is dependent in part on the presence of certain growth factor glycoproteins (Mohan, 1991), but they do not appear to cause any significant allograft reaction on the part of the host. Because bone tissue is processed to remove blood, marrow, and other extraneous tissue, most studies have failed to demonstrate the presence of ABO antigens (Ezra-Cohn, 1961). The antigenicity of the resulting product is low, thus histocompatibility or blood type matching is not required. Because large osteoarticular grafts, such as whole bone-patellar-tendon grafts, are not extensively processed, they may contain residual red blood cells, and instances of immunization to Rh system antigens have been reported (Hill, 1974). Many surgeons using these larger grafts will attempt to provide Rh-compatible tissue to Rh-negative females of childbearing age.

In addition to autogeneic bone, allograft bone is used for spinal fusion surgery, replacement of failed prosthetic joints, packing of benign bone cysts, reconstruction of maxillofacial deficits, restoration of alveolar bone in periodontal pockets, and even replacement of resected bone for tumors such as osteosarcoma (Kagan, 2005). Tendon and cartilage allografts are used primarily for knee repair surgery. Some patients will be confronted with the option of having autologous tissue recovered from their iliac crest for many elective orthopedic procedures, or of receiving allograft tissue from a tissue bank. Advantages and disadvantages are associated with each

*Lifecell Corporation, The Woodlands, Tex.

(i.e., autograft vs. allograft). Autografts appear to incorporate quicker, are not immunogenetic, and do not transmit disease; however, they are associated with longer anesthesia time, increased blood loss, and prolonged recovery from the donor site. Because of the wide supply of allografts, an exact fit can usually be made. No donor site recovery is needed, and the surgical procedure is generally shorter. However, although the risk of transmitted disease is greatly reduced by today's procedures, it is still present. Allografts also have a poorer capacity for osteoconduction and osteoinduction (Torroni, 2009), which makes them unsatisfactory for larger grafts.

Recent investigation and clinical trials have focused on the use of synthetic scaffolds or cages infused with the patient's own bone marrow stromal cells and various bone morphogenetic proteins to create a graft which is almost identical to an autologous graft without the necessity of a donor site (Torroni, 2009). Bone morphogenetic proteins allow the marrow stromal cells to differentiate into osteoprogenitor cells, eventually resulting in the formation of new bone.

Cardiac Valves

Aortic valve replacement may utilize human heart valves or pig valves. With the use of human valve tissue, anticoagulants are not required, and the incidence of thromboembolism or infection is lower. Human valves are ideal for use in children, pregnant women, or patients with a history of bacterial endocarditis. They are, however, utilized less often overall because procedures to place them are more technically difficult. Aortic and pulmonic valves are commonly procured from deceased organ donors when the whole heart is rendered unsuitable for transplantation because of events such as cardiac arrest that do not affect the integrity or function of the aortic or pulmonic valves. Procurement is performed in the operating room. The valves are carefully dissected with a cuff of myocardium, inspected for valve integrity, and frozen by controlled-rate freezing in liquid nitrogen using DMSO as the cryoprotective agent (O'Brien, 1988). Although blood group antigens have been demonstrated on the endothelium of cryopreserved hearts, the major mechanical function of these is dependent only on the nonviable connective tissue. After transplantation, host cells eventually replace the donor endothelium. Several studies have documented that neither ABO compatibility (Weipert, 1995) nor human leukocyte antigen (HLA) compatibility (Yap, 2006) is necessary for long-term function of these allograft valves. However, the use of allograft valves does induce the formation of HLA antibodies, especially in children, and may create difficulty in identifying a compatible donor for those patients later requiring whole heart transplantation (Hooper, 2005).

Recently, some cardiothoracic surgeons have attempted the use of saphenous vein allografts for performing coronary artery bypass procedures or for bypassing obstructed lower limb arteries when autografts are not available. Because the role of ABO matching in the long-term function of these tissues has been controversial, ABO-compatible tissue is generally used (Laub, 1992). Because thawing of the allograft valves is generally performed by operating room personnel, and not by experienced tissue bank technologists, detailed instructions and protocols are necessary to prevent cracking of the valve. Although the use of allograft valves has been a successful practice for several years, the results of most vein allograft studies to date are disappointing (Fahner, 2006).

Cornea

Corneal transplantation has been regularly performed in the United States since 1961, although the first corneal transplant is recorded to have taken place in 1905. Presently, more than 55,000 corneal transplants are performed each year (Eye Bank Association of America, 2008). There are 86 accredited eye banks in the United States involved in recruitment, screening, procurement, and transplantation of corneal tissue, as well as public and professional education. Loss of vision due to corneal disease can result from infection, trauma, burns, or congenital disease. Long-term (>10 years) success rates for corneal allografts are well above 90%.

Corneal donation is possible from many donors when other tissues are not retrievable because of age, trauma, or disease. Corneal tissue is recovered from donors up to 80 years of age. Generally, eye enucleation is performed in the operating room or morgue from deceased donors within 6 hours of death. Subsequently, the cornea is then removed in a sterile environment in the eye bank and is placed in supplemented, sterile tissue culture media. The corneas are stored at 4° C and are transplanted within 48–72 hours. This allows for appropriate serologic screening of the donor but ensures maximum viability of the graft.

The corneal graft has long been considered an "immunologically privileged site" (Medawar, 1948). Because the cornea is almost entirely avascular, host APCs and effector lymphocytes do not circulate through the allograft cornea. Histocompatibility and blood group matching therefore are not required. In a small percentage of corneal grafts, vascularization occurs, and some grafts are rejected. The use of HLA-matched corneal transplants in an attempt to provide successful grafts for this group of patients has met with varying success rates (Volker-Dieben, 1987).

Reproductive Tissue

Because of the exponential growth in knowledge of fetal development and reproductive technologies, particularly in vitro fertilization (IVF), 1%–3% of births in most Western countries now occur with assisted reproductive technologies (Evers, 2002). Reproductive banks are currently able to assist more individuals and couples who wish to maintain or achieve fertility. Most reproductive banks in the United States today function as for-profit corporations. Despite this, and because of a number of factors including consumer demand, the need for consumer confidence, and government regulation, sperm banks in the 21st century function in keeping with the highest medical and ethical standards, and physicians and patients can make use of their services without concern. Guidelines and standards for anonymous-donation sperm banking have been established by the American Society for Reproductive Medicine and the American Association of Tissue Banks.

Reproductive banks serve two types of donors: client-directed donors and anonymous bank donors. These include men and women who are about to undergo chemotherapy, radiation therapy, or surgery for malignant diseases that will affect their reproductive ability. Client-directed sperm donations are generally targeted to intimate partners of men who, for a variety of reasons, are concerned about future fertility. Other men will predeposit their sperm before vasectomy as insurance against life changes when they may wish to father additional children. Individuals with low sperm counts may bank their sperm to allow collection of sufficient gametes for fertilization of the intimate partner. Less frequently, males who have occupational exposure (such as nuclear power plant employees) that may lead to infertility or the potential for genetic defects may elect to store their sperm. Sperm collected and stored for intimate partners is tested in the same manner in which anonymous donor collections are screened. Semen from infected donors, which still may be usable by the intimate partner, must be quarantined and stored separately from other client deposits. Directed donations are also made to sperm banks for specific individuals who are not intimate partners.

Attempts at ova banking (egg banking) have not been as successful as embryo cryopreservation. Unfertilized ova have a very low rate of fertilization when they are subsequently thawed and attempts at IVF are made. Recently, attempts have been made at cryopreserving ovarian tissue for future implantation with very limited success in humans. One major concern is an increase in chromosomal abnormalities in both ova and ovarian tissue banking. Continuing research is needed in this area to provide women with the opportunity for future fertility with a chosen partner (Porcu, 2008).

Female patients confronted with loss of fertility due to age, disease, or chemotherapy, who have an intimate partner, are still frequently guided to IVF with cryopreservation of the resulting embryos for later implantation. Donor sperm and IVF are often recommended for females without an intimate partner until oocyte cryopreservation demonstrates more promising results. Many reproductive banks also provide donor ova collection for infertile individuals. These donors are screened in the same manner in which anonymous sperm donors are tested.

Sperm banks also provide sperm from anonymous donors for infertile couples or individuals. Sperm banks maintain libraries of sperm donors, so that individuals can select donors with similar physical characteristics such as hair and eye color, race, and the like. Anonymous sperm donors are rigorously screened not only to ensure the safety of the recipient and potential offspring, but also to provide the highest probability of successful fertilization. Sperm collected from anonymous donors is quarantined for 180 days before issue. During these 180 days, the donor is tested monthly, not only by the standard serologic assays employed for all tissue donors, but also for infections such as cytomegalovirus, *Neisseria gonorrhoeae*, and *Chlamydia*. Sperm donors are tested for genetic diseases such as Tay-Sachs disease, cystic fibrosis, sickle cell disease, and thalassemia. Generally, complete genetic karyotyping is performed on anonymous sperm donors. Collections are also examined for sperm number, function, and viability.

Not until all of these criteria have been met and reviewed by the medical director of the sperm bank are tissues released for use.

In vitro fertilization and embryo banking are also offered by many reproductive banks, as well as hospital-based fertility centers. Since the original success attained with IVF as a treatment for tubal obstruction in 1983 (Steptoe, 1983), significant advances have been made in this area which improve the success rate of IVF. They include technical innovations in culture media, embryo cryopreservation, and morphologic criteria for selection of the best embryo to transfer (Houghton, 2002). In addition to its use for women with fallopian disease, the success of intracytoplasmic sperm injection of the oocyte (Palermo, 1992) has made IVF the preferred technique for many infertile couples, utilizing either partner's sperm or donor sperm, as it results in higher fertilization rates as compared with artificial insemination (Boyle, 2004). In addition, IVF offers couples with certain genetic diseases, such as hemophilia and cystic fibrosis, the opportunity for preimplantation genetic diagnosis with subsequent selection of embryos in an attempt to reduce the risk of disease transmission to their offspring.

Collected semen is mixed with a glycerol–egg yolk solution that acts as a cryoprotectant, the egg yolk providing supplemental protein that assists in preserving the sperm during the thawing process. The semen-preservative mixture is aliquoted into straws or vials, precooled to a temperature of 5° C, frozen by controlled-rate freezing with liquid nitrogen, and stored in the liquid phase of liquid nitrogen at −196° C. Cryopreserved sperm can be used for artificial insemination or in vitro fertilization. Client-directed donations are kept indefinitely, and anonymous sperm bank donor samples are usually stored for 5 years. For those individuals desiring artificial insemination, these attempts are not always successful, and individuals are counseled to deposit adequate sperm for several reproductive procedures.

The advent of all these technologies has raised many ethical and scientific issues related to disposition of unused embryos, preimplantation screening of embryos, multiple gestations, and the possibility of unknown genetic risks to the health of children conceived through IVF (Lucifero, 2004). Thus a multidisciplinary approach to this field is needed to include members of the public, as well as scientific and medical professionals (Cetin, 2003).

Hematopoietic Progenitor Cell Banking

Hematopoietic cell transplantation had its beginning about 50 years ago with bone marrow transplants performed between genetically identical individuals (identical twins) in the setting of high-dose, myeloablative chemotherapy and/or radiation therapy as an attempt to cure hematopoietic malignancies (Thomas, 1959). Earlier work had demonstrated the presence of colony-forming units (CFUs) or cells in the spleen or marrow of mice that were able to restore hematopoietic function to their lethally irradiated, genetically identical littermates (Lorenz, 1951). Restoration of hematopoiesis in the human recipient is dependent on the transplantation of sufficient numbers of pluripotential HPCs that make up about 1% of normal marrow cells and are capable of both replication and differentiation into all lineages of blood cells (see Chapter 31, Hematopoiesis). Identification of the HLA system as the major histocompatibility system in man and the ability of tissue-typing laboratories to identify individuals' HLA types at the allele level allowed bone marrow transplantation to be performed between HLA-matched individuals, generally first-degree relatives, who were not genetically identical. Today, progenitor cell banks exist as highly specialized tissue banks that collect, process, store, and reinfuse HPC products obtained from bone marrow, peripheral blood, or even umbilical cord blood for patients with a wide variety of diseases (Table 38-4). Today, HPC grafts are performed in the traditional manner with the use of otherwise lethal doses of chemotherapy and/or radiation therapy (myeloablative transplants) in patients with malignant disease, and to restore normal function in patients with defects of hematopoiesis (aplastic anemia, sickle cell anemia). Hematopoietic transplants are also performed following minimal induction therapy in some patients (nonmyeloablative transplants). The success of these transplants depends on the "graft-versus-disease" effect of donor T lymphocytes to eliminate residual disease in patients with malignant disease. In the year 2000, approximately 18,000 patients worldwide were treated with some form of a hematopoietic graft (Storb, 2003). Terminology in transition is shown in Table 38-5. Data from both autologous and allogeneic hematopoietic transplants are now maintained by the Center for International Blood and Marrow Transplant Research (CIBMTR), which is a joint effort of the National Marrow Donor Program in the United States and the International Bone Marrow Transplant Registry. CIBMTR has been funded since 2006 by a contract from Heath and Human Services to gather and maintain data on clinical and research activities in hematopoietic transplantation (www.CIBMTR.org).

SOURCES OF HEMATOPOIETIC GRAFTS

Hematopoietic tissue for transplanting may come from one or more sources (Table 38-6). Individuals who have autologous or autogeneic grafts

TABLE 38-4
Indications for Hematopoietic Transplantation

Acute myeloid leukemia	Neuroblastoma
Acute lymphoblastic leukemia	Ewing's sarcoma
Chronic myelogenous leukemia	Rhabdomyosarcoma
Multiple myeloma	Aplastic anemia
Non-Hodgkin lymphoma	Sickle cell anemia
Myelodysplastic syndromes	Thalassemia
Hodgkin disease	Severe combined immunodeficiency

TABLE 38-5
Terminology in Transition

HPC	Hematopoietic progenitor cells, formerly hematopoietic stem cells
HPC, apheresis	Hematopoietic progenitor cells, apheresis, formerly peripheral blood progenitor cells or hematopoietic stem cells
HPC, marrow	Bone marrow–derived hematopoietic progenitor cells
HPC, umbilical cord blood	Cord blood–derived hematopoietic progenitor cells

HPC, Hematopoietic progenitor cell.

TABLE 38-6
Comparison of Hematopoietic Progenitor Cell Sources and Products with Collection and Complications

	Cord blood (HPC, UCB)*	Autologous (HPC, apheresis + marrow)*	Allogeneic (HPC, apheresis + marrow)*
Type of donor	Umbilical cord blood	Patient	Related or unrelated matched donor
Product	Cord blood progenitor/stem cells	Bone marrow or peripheral blood progenitor cells	Bone marrow or peripheral blood progenitor cells
Collection	Placenta umbilical cord at birth	Intraoperative marrow or hemapheresis	Intraoperative marrow or hemapheresis
Major complication	Insufficient progenitor cells	Recurrence of original disease	Graft-versus-host disease

*HPC (hematopoietic progenitor cell), apheresis = PBPCs (peripheral blood hematopoietic progenitor cells); HPC, marrow = BMPCs (bone marrow hematopoietic progenitor cells); and HPC, UCB (umbilical cord blood) = UCBPCs (umbilical cord blood hematopoietic progenitor cells).

donate their own cells, which are frozen and thawed before high-dose chemotherapy and/or radiation therapy. Immediately following this myeloablative therapy, the patient's own cells are thawed and reinfused. The patient's own hematopoietic progenitor cells in the transplant will home and reengraft in the marrow stroma and differentiate into mature blood cell–forming elements. Other patients who are not candidates for autologous transplantation, because of the presence of circulating tumor cells as in acute leukemia, will be candidates for an allogeneic transplant, where the hematopoietic tissue comes from a closely HLA-matched individual. Hematopoietic tissue contains viable lymphocytes that are capable of recognizing the foreign HLA antigens of the host and creating a graft-versus-host (GVH) reaction. This immune response of the graft to the host can vary from mild (Grade 1) to severe (Grades 3 and 4). The GVH reaction, particularly grades 3 and 4, remains one of the most significant morbidity and mortality risks associated with allogeneic hematopoietic cell transplantation. For this reason, donors are selected who are the best HLA match available. Donors may be HLA-matched siblings or other family members, or the patient may receive a graft from an unrelated HLA-matched individual identified through one of several worldwide donor registries. These registries, the largest in the United States being the National Marrow Donor Program, recruit healthy individuals who are willing to altruistically donate their bone marrow or peripheral blood progenitor cells (PBPCs) for an individual needing a transplant who does not have an HLA-matched related donor. Marrow or PBPCs from registry donors are obtained at a hospital or blood center close to their own home, and the graft is then transported by courier to the transplant center. Anonymity is maintained for both donor and recipient. Because of the need for an almost perfect HLA match, registries must have millions of volunteers if they are to have a reasonable chance of finding a match for a given patient. Because pluripotential hematopoietic progenitor cells do not express ABO antigens, they will engraft in the marrow stroma of ABO-incompatible individuals, thus abrogating the need for donors to be ABO compatible, but requiring the removal of mature red cells from these grafts.

Bone Marrow

Bone marrow is harvested from the iliac crest of the donor in the operating room under sterile conditions. Donors will elect to have general or spinal anesthesia. The amount of marrow to be collected is dependent on the recipient size. Generally, sufficient marrow is collected to provide 2×10^8 nucleated cells per kilogram of recipient body weight. For a 70-kg adult, this will generally require the collection of about 700 mL of marrow. The technique involves the collection of approximately 3–5 mL per aspiration into a heparinized syringe. Aspirating too large a volume from one site will result in dilution of the marrow with peripheral blood. Usually, two individuals will harvest marrow at the same time from each side of the donor iliac crest. As it is collected, the aspirated marrow is filtered through large-pore filters to remove bone spicules or clots, and supplemental anticoagulant is added. Because the hematopoietic progenitor cells are contained within the nucleated cell fraction, the collected marrow is often further processed to reduce the volume by separating the buffy coat from a large proportion of the red cells and plasma volume. The buffy coat may be further processed to remove all red cells if the donor and the recipient are ABO incompatible or T cell depleted if desired. Generally, bone marrow from allogeneic marrow donations is collected immediately before transplant, but it can be successfully frozen and stored for later use.

Although bone marrow harvested from the iliac crest was the original and long-standing source of HPCs for transplantation, the last 20 years have seen the development of technologies that allow the collection of these cells from the peripheral blood of both patients and normal donors and even from placental or cord blood.

Peripheral Blood Progenitor Cells

The stimulation for the development of technologies that would allow the collection of HPCs from peripheral blood was the potential for use in the autologous transplant setting, where concerns about marrow contamination with tumor cells are high. Because of the relative ease of hemapheresis collection over marrow harvest and the increased rate of engraftment, progenitor cells obtained from the peripheral blood are increasingly being used in the allogeneic setting as well. Currently, about 70% of allogeneic hematopoietic transplants employ HPCs from peripheral blood, and approximately 20% are obtained from marrow. This has positively affected the recruitment of volunteer donors in that more individuals may volunteer for the national marrow donor programs when hemapheresis is offered as an option over traditional bone marrow harvest. The instrumentation and procedures used for peripheral blood progenitor cell harvest are described in Chapter 37, Hemapheresis.

Clearly, the greatest advantage of peripheral blood progenitor cells over marrow is the time to neutrophil and platelet engraftment, averaging 8–12 days for mobilized peripheral blood progenitor cells compared with 2–4 weeks for bone marrow (Gianni, 1989). This rapid recovery clearly reduces morbidity and mortality associated with profound neutropenia/thrombocytopenia and reduces the costs associated with hospital stay, transfusion support, treatment of complications, and so forth.

HPCs were known three decades ago to be present in the peripheral blood following chemotherapy recovery (Richman, 1976). It was later, however, when hemapheresis systems were developed that would allow the safe collection of adequate numbers of these cells to provide for engraftment of the recipient after chemotherapy (Kessinger, 1988). In most patients undergoing autologous transplantation, large-volume apheresis collection (14–20 L/procedure) is now well established as an efficient means of collecting adequate numbers of HPCs in a reasonable number of procedures to provide for adequate hematopoietic recovery.

HPCs are morphologically indistinguishable from other mononuclear cells seen in the marrow or peripheral blood, yet collection of adequate numbers of cells is essential to ensuring marrow engraftment in the recipient. Bone marrow collections have traditionally been targeted at collecting sufficient nucleated cells to ensure a minimum number of progenitor cells. Bone marrow grafts could be assayed for progenitor cell activity by the use of colony-forming assays (Iscove, 1971). With this technique, a sample of mononuclear cells from the graft is cultured in methylcellulose media supplemented with hematopoietic growth factors and essential amino acids for 10–14 days. At the end of this period, the plates are examined for the numbers and types of characteristic CFUs, including burst-forming unit-erythroid, granulocyte-macrophage (CFU-GM), and mixed colonies—granulocyte, erythrocyte, monocyte, megakaryocyte. Clusters containing more than 50 cells are scored as a colony. Collections containing greater than 1×10^5 CFUs per kilogram of recipient weight are considered adequate.

With increasing use of peripheral blood hemapheresis procedures to obtain progenitor cell grafts, it became necessary to develop an assay that could be completed on the same day and used to determine the number of hemapheresis collections required. Quantitation of the number of cells bearing the CD34 antigen by flow cytometry has become the widely accepted method for assessing the adequacy of peripheral blood progenitor cell collections. The CD34 antigen is restricted to primitive cells of all lineages (Civin, 1989). Collection of hemapheresis products using CD34+ cell enumeration as an index of graft efficacy has proved to result in enduring hematopoietic engraftment (Berenson, 1991). Standardization of the CD34 cell assay and availability of flow cytometric analysis have resulted in the use of CD34+ cell measurements by most programs to determine the number and adequacy of peripheral blood progenitor cell collections (Keeney, 2004). Generally, peripheral blood progenitor cell collections containing greater than 3×10^6 CD34+ cells per kilogram of recipient body weight are considered adequate to provide for neutrophil engraftment in 8–10 days.

Collection of HPCs in the nonmobilized patient or donor would require multiple apheresis procedures or collections, as the numbers of HPCs in the peripheral blood are about $\frac{1}{10}$ to $\frac{1}{100}$ of the number in the marrow. Thus, **mobilization** therapies are required to increase the numbers of circulating HPCs and thus improve the efficiency of hemapheresis collection. Richman (1976) recognized that although there was a drop in the number of circulating CD34+ cells following chemotherapy, this was followed by a fourfold to fivefold increase in the percentage of circulating CD34+ cells just as the absolute neutrophil count began to recover, usually around 14–21 days following therapy. This increase in circulating CD34+ cells is greatest with chemotherapeutic agents such as cyclophosphamide and etoposide. If hemapheresis collection is performed in this window, large numbers of HPCs can be recovered with a limited number of procedures, even though the total white count may be less than 10,000/μL. Because the period of increased numbers of circulating CD34+ cells is short (2–3 days), close monitoring of the patient's white count and peripheral blood CD34+ cell counts and timing of the hemapheresis collection are critical. In addition, some investigators have felt that collecting autologous HPCs in the recovery phase of chemotherapy decreases the likelihood of tumor cells contaminating the apheresis product. The use of hematopoietic growth factors such as granulocyte-macrophage colony-stimulating factor (GM-CSF) and granulocyte colony-stimulating factor (G-CSF) also results in a significant increase in the numbers of circulating CD34+ cells in peripheral blood (Siena, 1989). Doses of 5–10 µg/kg of body weight for 4–5 days will result in a fivefold to 10-fold increase in the number of HPCs in the peripheral blood. The use of G-CSF alone has proved to be more efficient than chemotherapy priming for the collection of CD34+ cells. The combination of chemotherapy priming and the use of growth factors (primarily G-CSF) results in the maximum mobilization of PBPCs and the need for the fewest number of hemapheresis procedures to collect a transplant dose of HPCs—a strategy employed by most autogeneic transplant programs.

The use of G-CSF in the healthy allogeneic donor to mobilize HPCs has been investigated and, aside from mild effects such as bone pain and headache, is well tolerated (Anderlini, 1997). Increasingly, transplant programs are using peripheral blood instead of marrow as a source of HPCs for their allogeneic and autogeneic transplants. The higher risk of GVHD in allogeneic recipients of peripheral blood HPCs versus marrow (Cutler, 2001) has stimulated trials of new technologies to modify these grafts (see T Cell Depletion).

Umbilical Cord Blood

The fact that higher numbers of CFU cells or progenitor cells were present in umbilical cord blood was known for many years, but it was not until 1989 that the first attempts were made to use cells recovered from placenta umbilical cords for hematopoietic transplantation (Gluckman, 1989). The apparent success of many of these early cord blood transplants led to the organization of several cord blood banks in this country and in Europe in an attempt to provide another source of progenitor cell tissue for patients requiring an allogeneic transplant from an unrelated donor. The Cord Blood Transplantation Study (COBLT), which collected data from 1997–2004, established standardized procedures for donor screening, HLA matching, cord blood processing, and storage and data collection. These data clearly established that cord blood transplants in children with a wide range of malignant and nonmalignant conditions could result in a high degree of engraftment and 2-year event-free survivals of 55% for children with high-risk malignancies and 78% for children with nonmalignant conditions (Martin, 2006; Kurtzberg, 2009). In addition, because the progenitor cells are obtained from cord blood, there appears to be a greater degree of tolerance for some degree of HLA incompatibility between donor and recipient without the appearance of a Grade 3 or 4 GVH reaction; thus, hematopoietic transplantation might become available for some patients who otherwise have no HLA-matched donor (Barker, 2005). An additional advantage of cord blood HPC over both bone marrow and apheresis products is that the cord blood is banked and is more immediately available for use, thus reducing the time to transplantation.

Umbilical cord progenitor cells are harvested by cannulation of the placental vessels while the placenta is still in utero or, more commonly, following delivery, or by direct expression, of the cord blood from the placenta following delivery. The number of HPCs recovered is directly proportional to the volume of cord blood collected, which varies with the size of the infant/placenta and with the experience of the individual performing the collection (Wagner, 1992). Volumes ranging from 40–150 mL are common for experienced centers. This will result in the harvesting of approximately $4–11 \times 10^8$ nucleated cells. Collections that are not adequate in volume (<40 mL) are usually discarded. Generally, umbilical cord blood collections are not further processed to reduce their volume, and they are frozen directly with DMSO and liquid nitrogen storage. Specially trained staff deployed to the delivery room are not distracted by the care of the mother and/or the infant, and they also reduce the risk of bacterial contamination of the cord blood.

Careful screening and testing of the mother are essential to ensure the safety of the cord blood product, as well as the absence of genetic disease. In addition to standard laboratory measurements for serologically transmissible disease, testing is performed for viral and bacteriologic diseases.

Although umbilical cord blood banking offers the exciting potential for a lesser degree of histocompatibility and thus availability for more patients, the remaining critical issue is the lack of sufficient hematopoietic progenitor cells in most cord bloods to successfully engraft adults. Research efforts to expand these cells in vitro have met with limited success and are not yet ready for clinical trials. More recently, investigative efforts have focused on the use of more than one cord blood to provide sufficient HPCs to transplant adults (Haspel, 2008).

REDUCED-INTENSITY CONDITIONING OF HEMATOPOIETIC GRAFTS

Ablative conditioning regimens using high-dose chemotherapy and/or radiation therapy are not always successful in eliminating neoplastic cells before HPC transplant. These high-dose regimens are associated with increased morbidity and mortality, and many patients are excluded as candidates for traditional HPC grafts because of comorbidities. These factors, along with data demonstrating greater benefit from allogeneic versus autologous HPC grafts, led to the investigation of nonmyeloablative transplant protocols, now more commonly referred to as reduced intensity allogeneic HPC grafts.

Early murine studies had shown that recipients of allogeneic grafts had better survival than recipients of syngeneic grafts (Barnes, 1957). Later studies in humans showed a "graft-versus-leukemia effect" in patients transplanted for acute leukemias that appeared to correlate with the development of chronic graft-versus-host disease in the recipient (Weiden, 1981). That this effect was dependent upon donor T lymphocytes was further demonstrated by the high relapse rate that occurred in patients receiving T cell–depleted HPC grafts (Marmont, 1989). Initial efforts focused on the infusion of donor T lymphocytes after HPC grafting in patients who had relapsed (Kolb, 1990). This technique became known as donor lymphocyte infusion (DLI). Because these patients received no additional chemotherapy, the next approach was to attempt HPC peripheral blood grafts with no conditioning (Porter, 1999). It quickly became clear that some conditioning therapy, primarily immunosuppressive, was necessary to allow donor cells to engraft. Conditioning regimens in reduced-intensity conditioning of HPC transplants are now focused on providing sufficient immunosuppression to allow engraftment of donor cells without complete elimination of the tumor burden. The larger number of T lymphocytes in peripheral blood HPC grafts versus marrow appears to decrease the risk of graft rejection by overwhelming host T lymphocytes and favoring the development of a graft-versus-leukemia effect. DLI may also be given at a later date if insufficient donor T cell engraftment or disease relapse is evident.

In the reduced-intensity conditioning of HPC grafts, disease control is mediated by recognition of host residual tumor cells by donor T cells and requires establishment of at least partial donor T lymphocyte chimerism, if not full replacement by donor T cells. The kinetics of T cell engraftment in nonmyeloablative HPC transplants is such that up to a year may be required for the patient to achieve complete disease remission (Childs, 1999). Therefore, this therapy is not appropriate for patients with acute leukemia who are not in remission or for those with other aggressive malignancies likely to relapse at an early date. Although the morbidity and mortality associated with the conditioning regimen in nonmyeloablative HPC grafts are lower, the risk of GVHD is the same as that seen following high-dose conditioning regimens. Because of the higher risk of GVHD and graft rejection in unrelated HPC grafts, particularly HLA-mismatched ones, it remains to be seen whether this group of patients will benefit from nonmyeloablative HPC grafts (Koreth, 2009).

Reduced toxicity of the preparative regimen allows its use in older patients and is associated with less transfusion burden and shorter hospital stays (Weissinger, 2001). Studies are currently under way to look at the efficacy of reduced-intensity conditioning in such diseases as multiple myeloma (Cook, 2009), in which the patient population tends to be older. Reduced toxicity and improved outcomes seen with this therapy have contributed to its rapid growth in the hematopoietic transplant community.

PURGING

Once hematopoietic progenitor cells are collected from the marrow or from peripheral blood, it is often advantageous to further process the collected HPC product in an attempt to reduce possible tumor cell contamination or, in the allogeneic setting, to reduce the number of T lymphocytes. Two approaches, not mutually exclusive, have been taken. The first employs techniques targeted at eliminating tumor cells, so-called purging or negative-selection techniques. The second approach utilizes methods to separate and collect only the CD34+ hematopoietic progenitor cells, discarding the remaining cell fraction, which presumably contains contaminating tumor cells. These methods are usually referred to as **positive-selection techniques** (Table 38-7).

Purging techniques originally employed a variety of specific and nonspecific methods to remove the unwanted cell population. Original

TABLE 38-7
Stem Cell Purging Methods

Positive Selection
CD34+ cell selection
Solid-phase columns
Magnetic beads
Negative Selection
Pharmacologic
4-Hydroperoxycyclophosphamide (4HC)
Etoposide (VP-16)
Immunologic
Tumor cell + MoAb + toxin
Toxin = complement/ricin/other chemo
Tumor cell + MoAb + solid phase
Solid phase = bead column

MoAb, Monoclonal antibody.

methods used cytotoxic drugs such as 4-hydroperoxycyclophosphamide (4-HC) and etoposide to remove contaminating tumor cells (Yeager, 1986). These methods are the in vitro equivalent of high-dose chemotherapy, and thus the major negative effect is damage to HPCs. Other technologies included the use of lectins and/or rosetting to remove unwanted cell populations, particularly T cells. More recently, monoclonal antibodies targeted at a specific cell receptor have been used with complement or coupled to immunotoxins such as ricin to actually lyse the contaminating tumor cell population. Also, with the advent of immunomagnetic bead technology, the monoclonal antibody can be coupled to an immunomagnetic bead. The antibody-bead-tumor cell complex is then removed by passing the cell suspension over a magnetic field, where the unwanted cell populations will be retained, while the HPCs are rinsed through and collected.

Positive-selection techniques focus on the presence of CD34 on hematopoietic progenitor cells and the availability of monoclonal antibodies targeted to this antigen. Although the original technology used a column to which the monoclonal antibody was bound, current methods utilize an immunomagnetic bead or sphere. The mononuclear cell fraction from the bone marrow harvest or the progenitor cell hemapheresis collection is incubated with the monoclonal anti-CD34 or another monoclonal antibody of interest. A suspension of immunomagnetic beads labeled with a secondary antibody is then added that binds to the monoclonal anti-CD34, creating a bead–target cell complex. When the cell suspension is subsequently passed over a magnetic field, the CD34+ cell–magnetic bead complex will be retained, and the remaining mononuclear cell suspension containing unwanted tumor cells, T cells, and others will be removed. The CD34+ progenitor cells are then freed from the magnetic beads with the use of a releasing agent, and the beads are removed by reapplication of the magnetic field, leaving a cell suspension that is approximately 90% CD34+ cells. The reduction in total number of CD3+ T cells is about 3.5 $\log_{10}$ depletion. The median recovery of CD34+ cells is approximately 50% of the starting numbers of CD34+ cells in the hemapheresis product. The benefits of positive- and negative-selection purging of HPC grafts to reduce tumor cell contamination and reduce disease relapse rates have been controversial (de Lima, 2004). These techniques, with the exception of T cell depletion, have been widely investigated but are still considered experimental.

T Cell Depletion

Techniques to reduce the numbers of T lymphocytes in allogeneic hematopoietic grafts, primarily marrow, have been targeted at reducing the incidence and severity of GVHD. Many of the techniques mentioned previously for purging of tumor cells, such as positive selection for CD34+ cells, have also been applied to the reduction of T cells in the graft (Table 38-8). Other techniques specifically targeting T cells have included soybean lectin agglutination, E-rosette formation, combinations of the two, counterflow elutriation, monoclonal antibodies, and the application of monoclonal antibodies in vivo in the recipient post transplant to reduce donor T cells.

Soybean lectin produces an agglutinin specific for the CD2 receptor on lymphocytes, thus agglutinating CD2+ T cells. The addition of a rosetting step with sheep erythrocytes removes the remaining T cells not agglutinated by the soybean lectin. This method results in a 2 to 3 $\log_{10}$ depletion of T cells (Reisner, 1982). Current trials with monoclonal antibodies have focused on the use of anti-CD52 antibodies for in vitro treatment of the HPC product and in vivo to reduce host T lymphocytes (Chakraverty, 2002).

TABLE 38-8
T Lymphocyte Depletion Methods

Lectins	Immunologic
Soybean lectin with E-rosetting	Antibody
Counterflow centrifugation	Antibody + Complement
	Antibody + Solid phase
	Positive selection

Counterflow elutriation is a method used for the depletion of T cells that utilizes the separation characteristic of cells in a centrifugal field, based on the size and density of various cell populations. One of the advantages of the system is that no chemotherapeutic agents or antibodies are added to the hematopoietic progenitor cell population; thus, there is no impairment of cell function. Buffy coat concentrates from harvested marrow are introduced into the centrifuge at different flow rates, allowing for the collection of cell fractions of different sizes and densities. The system is highly efficient at separating a CFU-GM–rich fraction from a CD3+ lymphocyte fraction. Because no changes are made to the cells, the CD3+ fraction can be enumerated and partially added back to the CFU-GM fraction to provide a controlled dose of CD3+ cells, if clinically desired (Noga, 1990). Cell recovery is high, and because elutriation media are biocompatible, the product(s) can be reinfused without additional wash steps. The major disadvantages of the procedure are the cost of the required equipment and the need for experienced operators.

The introduction of immunomagnetic bead techniques for the positive selection of CD34+ cells has also led to the use of these techniques in the allogeneic setting for the resultant depletion of CD3+ T cells, particularly from peripheral blood progenitor cell collections. Immunomagnetic bead technology is easily applied to hemapheresis progenitor cell products and to the larger-volume bone marrow harvest products. Many centers have reported success with these newer methods to reduce CD3+ T cells in allogeneic transplantation, particularly when reduced-intensity conditioning is desirable (Handgretinger, 2008). Other centers have focused on in vivo protocols employing anti–T cell agents such as alemtuzumab for reduction of the donor T cell population in the recipient (Malladi, 2009).

One additional advantage of purging or positive-selection techniques is that they result in a significantly reduced volume of progenitor cell product to be frozen, thawed, and reinfused in the patient. This greatly reduces toxicities associated with the reinfusion of DMSO-containing products, as well as decreasing freezing and storage costs for the progenitor cell laboratory. Presently, licensed technologies for purging and/or positive selection to reduce tumor cell contamination are costly, and additional data are needed to assess the clinical efficacy of these procedures for tumor cell reduction.

Both positive- and negative-selection techniques incur a concomitant loss of as much as 50% of the original number of CD34+ cells from agent toxicity (chemotherapeutics, complement), entrapment by magnetic bead complexes, or loss during required wash steps. The initial hemapheresis or bone marrow collection of CD34+ cells must be increased to allow for subsequent loss in processing. This may be difficult to accomplish in patients who are hard to mobilize.

The major disadvantage of T cell depletion is the resultant increase in the incidence of disease relapse. Patients who demonstrate mild GVHD appear to have a lower incidence of relapse of neoplastic disease than do those patients who have no GVHD. The presence of the donor T cell population is apparently critical to "graft-versus-leukemia effect," with recognition of host antigens by donor T cells generating an immune response that eliminates residual host tumor cells. More recent studies have demonstrated a role for natural killer (NK) cells in the graft-versus-leukemia effect. Others have used combinations of techniques such as CD34+ selection and counterflow elutriation to create a CD34+ cell-rich fraction and an NK cell–rich/T cell–depleted fraction, taking advantage of the fact that NK cells do appear to have antitumor effects but do not contribute to GVH effects (Handgretinger, 2008).

CRYOPRESERVATION OF HEMATOPOIETIC GRAFTS

HPC grafts from all autogeneic and many allogeneic collections are cryopreserved and stored before use. The most common protocol involves the use of 10% DMSO as a cryoprotective agent, controlled-rate freezing, and liquid nitrogen storage, either vapor or liquid phase. The use of DMSO provides significant improvement in postthaw viability over agents such as glycerol. Because toxicities are associated with the postthaw infusion of progenitor cell products containing DMSO, other investigators have looked to the use of lower concentrations or the addition of hetastarch or other additives, but DMSO currently remains in use by most programs. Attempts to wash products following thaw to reduce the amount of DMSO present resulted in significant loss of progenitor cells; strategies are now targeted at reducing the volume of the prefreezing product, thus lowering the amount of DMSO necessary.

REINFUSION OF PROGENITOR CELL PRODUCTS

Regardless of the source of the progenitor cell graft, HPCs are infused to the recipient in a manner very similar to that of any blood product transfusion. Pluripotential progenitor cells, with their unique membrane receptors, will home to the marrow space, engraft, and replicate. Products that have been cryopreserved with DMSO in most cases are thawed and immediately reinfused without washing. HPCs collected by hemapheresis that are not further processed may contain large numbers of red blood cells. Cryopreservation in DMSO does not maintain red blood cell membrane integrity, and these products will contain a large amount of free hemoglobin when thawed. Recipient reactions will vary from mild, characterized by nausea, chills, or headache, to more severe reactions that can include hypotension, sepsis, renal failure, or even cardiac arrest (Stroncek, 1991). Such adverse reactions are shown in Table 38-9. Recipients of cryopreserved progenitor cell products are generally premedicated with antihistamines and/or antiemetics. Adequate hydration and the use of diuretics are indicated to decrease renal toxicities associated with free hemoglobin and larger-volume infusions.

TABLE 38-9
Adverse Reactions Observed in Patients Transfused with Cryopreserved Progenitor Cell Products

Common	Contributing Factors
Chills	Volume of product reinfused
Nausea	Type and amount of cryoprotectant reinfused
Emesis	Volume of incompatible red cells (allogeneic products)
Fever	Bacterial contamination
Headache	
Dyspnea	
Uncommon	
Renal failure	
Cardiac arrest	
Hypotension	
Sepsis	

SELECTED REFERENCES

Boyle KE, Vlahos N, Jarow JP. Assisted reproductive technology in the new millennium: part II. Urology 2004;63:217–24.

This, with part I, is an excellent review of current approaches to infertility.

Cetin I, Pardi G. A multidisciplinary approach to the future of reproduction. Placenta 2003;24:s3–4.

This is a good review of reproductive options for cancer patients.

Chakraverty R, Peggs K, Chopra R, et al. Limiting transplantation-related mortality following unrelated donor stem cell transplantation by using a nonmyeloablative conditioning regimen. Blood 2002;99:1071–8.

Outlines the risks, benefits, and new methods in hematologic transplants for patients without a matched related donor.

De Lima M, Shpall EJ. Ex-vivo purging of hematopoietic progenitor cells. Curr Hematol Rep 2004;3:257–64.

Good review of the methods and trials of ex vivo purging.

Gorin NC. Collection, manipulation and freezing of haemopoietic stem cell. In: Gladstone AH, editor. Clinics in haematology. London: WB Saunders; 1986, p. 19–48.

A lengthy but comprehensive description of cell freezing physiology and practices.

Kessinger A, Armitage JO, Landmark JD, et al. Autologous peripheral hematopoietic stem cell transplantation restores hematopoietic function following marrow ablative therapy. Blood 1988;71:723.

Provides the earliest work and later refinements in autologous hematopoietic transplants by one of the first groups to describe this therapy.

Kurtzberg J. Update on umbilical cord blood transplantation. Curr Opin Pediatr 2009;21:22–9.

This is an excellent review of the state of the art of cord blood transplantation by one of the leading experts in this discipline.

Storb R. Allogenic hematopoietic stem cell transplantation—yesterday, today, and tomorrow. Exp Hem 2003;31:1–10.

Interesting, nontechnical review by one of the leaders in hematopoietic transplantation.

REFERENCES

Access the complete reference list online at http://www.expertconsult.com

PART 5

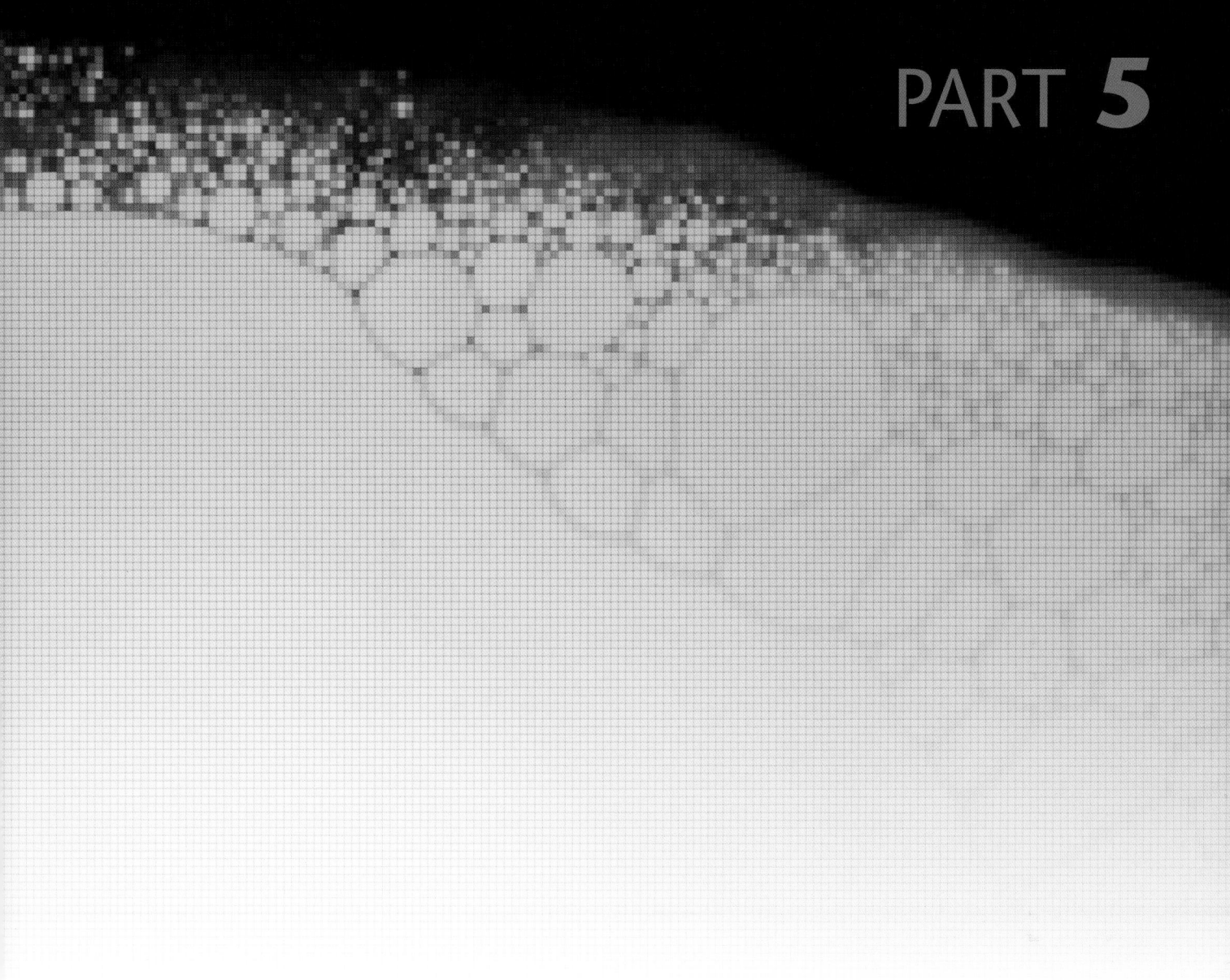

Hemostasis and Thrombosis

EDITED BY | Jonathan L. Miller

CHAPTER 39

COAGULATION AND FIBRINOLYSIS

Alvin H. Schmaier, Jonathan L. Miller

KEY POINTS

- Physiologic hemostasis consists of the plasma coagulation, fibrinolysis, and anticoagulation protein systems.
- Physiologic hemostasis is initiated by factor VIIa and tissue factor; thrombosis is also initiated by factor VIIa and tissue factor, but it is amplified by factor XII activation on injured tissue and platelet thrombus.
- The adequacy of physiologic hemostasis cannot be fully assessed by current assays to detect coagulation abnormalities such as the activated partial thromboplastin time and prothrombin time.
- Current assays to assess coagulation protein abnormalities have good diagnostic power to recognize specific defects in coagulation proteins.
- Acquired coagulation protein defects more commonly reflect general medical disorders than specific protein defects.

OVERVIEW OF COAGULATION AND FIBRINOLYSIS

Hemostasis, or cessation of bleeding, occurs within the intravascular compartment lined with endothelium. Normal hemostasis and thrombosis involve a number of factors. These factors include platelets, granulocytes, and monocytes, as well as the coagulation (clot forming), fibrinolytic (clot lysing), and anticoagulant (regulating) protein systems. The coagulation system serves to form thrombin that initiates the proteolysis of fibrinogen, leading to fibrin clot formation. The role of the fibrinolytic system is to lyse the clot formed by thrombin. The role of the anticoagulation system is to regulate all enzymes of the coagulation and fibrinolytic systems, so that no inappropriate excess of clotting or bleeding occurs. These three protein systems, together with the vessel wall endothelium, are in delicate balance to ensure adequate hemostasis with limitation on thrombosis formation.

Recent years have seen an evolution in our understanding of the physiologic hemostatic system (Fig. 39-1). For decades, the hemostatic system has been referred to as the **coagulation cascade,** based on the waterfall hypothesis of Ratnoff and Davies and MacFarland, who published, almost simultaneously, a sequence of proteolytic reactions starting with factor XII (Hageman factor) activation and ending with formed thrombin proteolyzing fibrinogen to form a clot (MacFarland, 1964; Ratnoff, 1964). However, at the onset, this hypothesis for physiologic hemostasis was untenable because it was known that factor XII (FXII) deficiency was not associated with bleeding (Ratnoff, 1955). Thus the physiologic basis of this pathway was questioned because FXII is not essential for hemostasis. Further, by the mid-1970s, the cofactors for FXII activation, that is, prekallikrein and high molecular weight kininogen, were identified, and deficiencies of these proteins were not associated with a bleeding state (Weuppers, 1972; Colman, 1975; Saito, 1975). Other mechanisms for physiologic hemostasis were sought. In 1977, Osterud and Rappaport recognized that FVIIa is able to activate FIX to FIXa (Osterud, 1977). Later, Broze and colleagues recognized that the kinetics of tissue factor pathway inhibitor (TFPI) was such that under physiologic circumstances the FVIIa–tissue factor complex cannot directly activate FX, but instead requires the involvement of FIX (Broze, 2003). These latter two studies indicate the important role of the FVIIa–tissue factor pathway in physiologic hemostasis. A key remaining question was how does FXI, whose deficiency is associated with bleeding,

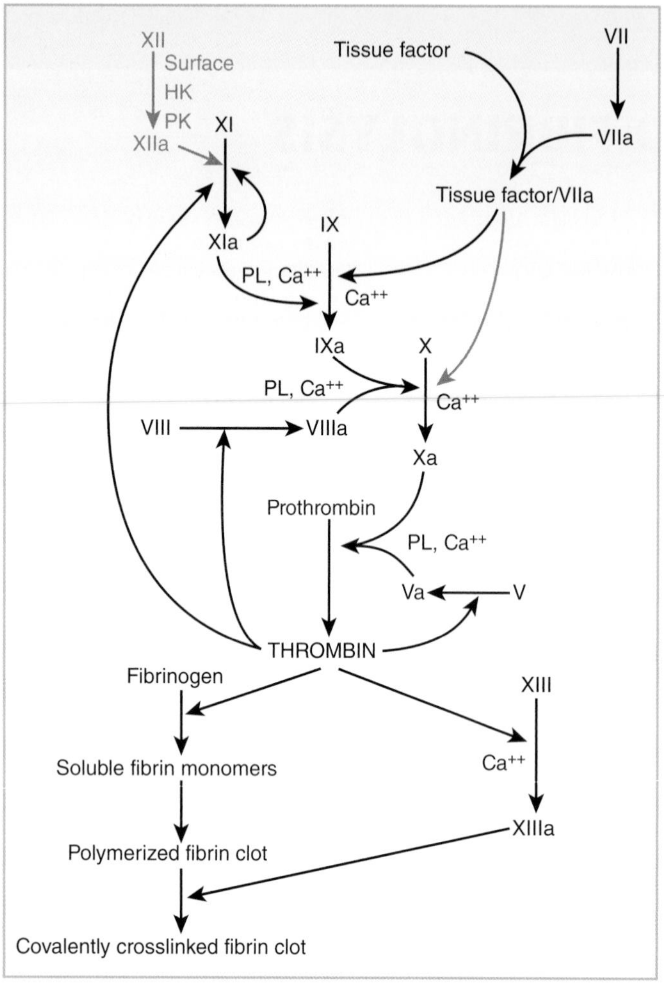

Figure 39-1 Schematic diagram of physiologic blood coagulation. Note that labels for the "contact phase" factors constituting factor XII (FXII), high molecular weight kininogen (HK), and prekallikrein (PK) are shown grayed. Although FXI is activated by FXIIa on a surface under artificial in vitro conditions, such as in the activated partial thromboplastin time (APTT), this pathway is not believed to contribute to normal physiologic hemostasis. Similarly, whereas tissue factor (TF)/FVIIa can directly activate X to Xa in the in vitro prothrombin time (PT) test under conditions in which supraphysiologic concentrations of TF are employed, this reaction is shown as grayed because it does not contribute significantly to clot formation under normal in vivo physiologic conditions. Normal clotting in vivo is initiated when sufficient TF/FVIIa becomes available to activate FIX to FIXa. Subsequently, FIXa in the presence of FVIIIa activates FX to FXa, which, in turn, activates prothrombin to thrombin in the presence of FVa. Thrombin not only then proceeds to clot fibrinogen and to activate platelets, but additionally exerts critically important positive feedback by activating both factor VIII and factor V. Physiologic amplification of thrombin formation is believed to result from thrombin activating FXI to FXIa, thereby providing an additional pathway for the activation of FIX. Phospholipid (PL) protein complexes present on the surface membranes of platelets in vivo; and Ca^{++}, calcium ions.

become activated under physiologic circumstances? In 1991, Gailiani and Broze found that formed thrombin activates FXI in the presence of dextran sulfate and high molecular weight kininogen, resulting in amplification of the coagulation system under stress (Gailiani, 1991). More recent evidence indicates that if FXI is poorly activated by thrombin, if FIX is poorly activated by FXIa, or if an antibody prevents FXIa activation of FIX, thrombin generation in plasma is reduced (Kravtsov, 2009). Under the same conditions, an antibody to FXIIa activation of FXI does not influence thrombin generation (Kravtsov, 2009). Furthermore, mice with total deficiency of FXII and low tissue factor (TF) are viable and phenotypically similar to low-TF mice with normal FXII expression. In contrast, superimposed FXI deficiency on the low-TF background results in death in utero (Spronk, 2009). Thus, FXII is not essential for hemostasis, but FXI is. Presently, physiologic hemostasis is understood to be an interacting system of activation and amplification of several zymogens that become serine proteases. The initiator of physiologic hemostasis is FVIIa when bound to its cofactor, tissue factor. Regulation of expression of tissue factor constitutes a major modulation of physiologic hemostasis. Thrombin in turn amplifies the process by activating FXI, leading to additional FIX activation.

It is important for the reader to understand the physiologic basis of hemostasis. However, clinical laboratory assays used to examine the coagulation system are based on the original coagulation cascade hypothesis. Although these tests do not represent physiologic hemostasis, they are still very useful for diagnosis of potential bleeding disorders. Thus one needs to understand the distinction between physiologic coagulation, fibrinolysis, and anticoagulation and the tests that we use to measure these systems. This chapter endeavors to clarify this distinction for the reader. In the first part of this chapter, the details of physiologic coagulation, fibrinolysis, and the regulation of coagulation will be presented. In the second part of this chapter, a description of the assays performed to measure bleeding disorders will be presented, together with a discussion of the limitations of these assays for characterizing physiologic hemostasis. In the third part of this chapter, an overview of congenital bleeding disorders will be presented. Last, this chapter will present the acquired bleeding disorders, the most common forms of bleeding states one actually encounters in clinical practice.

Physiologic Hemostasis

The physiologic hemostatic system, a tightly regulated balance between formation and dissolution of hemostatic plugs modulated by a series of enzymes and scaffolding proteins, has two major parts. The first part is its cellular component, which consists mostly of platelets and endothelial cells but also includes neutrophils and monocytes. The second part is a large group of plasma proteins, which participate in clot formation (coagulation), dissolution of clots (fibrinolysis), and the action of naturally occurring serine protease inhibitors (anticoagulation) that terminate activity of a number of enzymes of the coagulation and fibrinolytic systems.

ENDOTHELIUM AND PLATELETS

Normal hemostasis involves interplay among the cellular components and proteins involved in clot formation and lysis. Endothelium that lines the vascular compartment contributes to its constitutive anticoagulant nature. Endothelial cells have glycosaminoglycans that bind antithrombin (Marcum, 1984). Thrombomodulin on endothelial cell membranes is a locus at which protein C is activated by low levels of thrombin (Esmon, 1981). Intact endothelial cells secrete an ectonucleotidase, CD39, that degrades adenosine diphosphate (Pinsky, 2002). Endothelial cells also secrete prostacyclin and nitric oxide, which prevent platelet activation, thereby reducing the risk of arterial thrombosis (Hong, 1980; Palmer, 1987; Shariat-Madar, 2006). Endothelial cells additionally bind plasminogen, tissue plasminogen activator, and single-chain urokinase, all of which contribute to fibrinolysis and maintenance of an anticoagulant state (Barnathan, 1988; Cesarman, 1994). When a vessel wall is injured, collagen is exposed, and platelets adhere to the site of injury (van der Meijden, 2009). von Willebrand factor helps platelets adhere to the injured vessel wall by binding both to this exposed collagen and to the platelet receptor GP Ib/IX/V complex (He, 2003). This adhesion event activates platelets, initiating a signaling cascade within them (Zaffran, 2000). The stimulated platelets release the contents of their granules, recruit additional platelets to aggregate to those already adherent, and provide a surface favoring the activation of multiple coagulation factors. Furthermore, in flowing blood, factor XII autoactivates if exposed to collagen or in the milieu of activated platelets, leading to the cascade of proteolytic events producing thrombin (van der Meijden, 2009). Together, these events promote hemostatic plug formation as a physiologic event, and in pathophysiologic states may lead to thrombus formation.

Once prothrombin has been activated to thrombin in the intravascular compartment, the resulting thrombin stimulates endothelium to upregulate TF, and TF forms a complex with FVIIa. The complex of FVIIa–TF activates FIX to FIXa, which converts zymogen FX to enzymatically active FXa (see Fig. 39-1). In the presence of FVa from liver or injured endothelium, FXa activates prothrombin (FII) to thrombin (FIIa). Under normal circumstances, the rate-limiting component of prothrombinase complex formation and the ultimate generation of thrombin activity is the concentration of FXa (Rand, 1996). Thrombin then proteolyzes fibrinogen to form fibrin. In static, in vitro systems, as little as 5–10 pM TF is sufficient to induce clot formation, leading to a 1000–2000-fold amplification of the process that increases the concentration of thrombin to 10–20 nM, which is sufficient to initiate clot formation (Mann, 2003). In a static model of blood coagulation, the addition of 5 pM TF results in an average clot time

TABLE 39-1
Proteins of the Plasma Coagulation System

Surface-bound zymogens	Vitamin K–dependent zymogens	Cofactors/substrates
Factor XII	Factor VII	High molecular weight kininogen
Prekallikrein	Factor IX	Factor VIII
Factor XI	Factor X	Factor V
	Factor II	Fibrinogen
	Protein C	Protein S

of ≈5 minutes—a time sufficiently fast for physiologic hemostasis. Thrombin also is a major physiologic activator of platelets, together with other agonists such as collagen, ADP, platelet-activating factor, and epinephrine. Unactivated platelets probably circulate without promoting coagulation. When platelets are activated (see Chapter 40), their membranes become a site for additional thrombin formation. This pathway for thrombin formation conjoins with FXII autoactivation on exposed vessel collagen and downstream elaboration of thrombin as well (van der Meijden, 2009). Critical reactions to form FXa and thrombin are accelerated 300,000-fold on the platelet surface. Physiologically important coagulation and fibrinolytic reactions are likely to occur on the surface of cells in the intravascular compartment.

COAGULATION PROTEIN SYSTEM

Characterization of Coagulation Proteins

The proteins that constitute the coagulation system consist of zymogens and cofactors (Table 39-1). The zymogens (proenzymes) of the coagulation system can be grouped into the phospholipid-bound and the surface-bound. Phospholipid-bound zymogens make up the physiologically important hemostatic system. These proteins are vitamin K–dependent. Vitamin K is required for an essential γ-carboxylation reaction that takes place on the glutamic acid residue of each of these proteins located in their amino-terminal regions (see Chapter 42, Fig. 42-1). This carboxylation reaction allows these proteins to bind to phospholipid and cell membranes, where they are activated. Without this carboxylation reaction, these proteins do not function normally in the hemostatic system. Proenzymes include FX, FIX (Christmas factor), FVII, and FII (prothrombin). Protein C is a vitamin K–dependent phospholipid-bound zymogen, but when activated, it functions as an inhibitor (see later and Chapter 41). Protein S is a vitamin K–dependent cofactor for activated protein C.

The surface-bound proenzymes are proteins of the plasma kallikrein/kinin system (see Table 39-1). Surface-bound proenzymes include FXII (Hageman factor), prekallikrein (Fletcher factor), and FXI. These protein zymogens are also known as the **contact system** because FXII autoactivates when associated with a negatively charged surface such as a glass tube and several physiologic substances (see later) (Wiggins, 1979; Miller, 1980). The autoactivation phenomenon of FXII allows for a common laboratory test, the activated partial thromboplastin time (APTT), which is used to assess the integrity of the coagulation system (see later). This assay is an important diagnostic test that is performed more than 200 million times annually in the United States alone to assess many coagulation proteins. Thus, it is important to be aware that assays to assess coagulation proteins (e.g., APTT, activated clotting time) are based on the event of FXII autoactivation. Although absolutely essential for a normal APTT, the proteins of the plasma kallikrein/kinin system do not have a physiologic role in hemostasis. These proteins do participate in blood pressure regulation, fibrinolysis, inflammation, angiogenesis, and arterial thrombosis (Schmaier, 2002, 2003, 2004; Shariat-Madar, 2006; Maas, 2008; LaRusch, 2010). Under physiologic circumstances in vivo, prekallikrein when assembled on endothelial cells may be first activated by an endothelial enzyme, prolylcarboxypeptidase ($K_m = 9$ nM) with FXII activation secondary to the formed plasma kallikrein (Rojkjaer, 1998; Shariat-Madar, 2002). Finally, the role of the surface-activated proteins that participate in in vitro blood coagulation assays has been reevaluated. Although deficiencies of FXII, prekallikrein, and high molecular weight kininogen are not associated with bleeding, investigations suggest that they do have a role in arterial thrombosis. Mice deficient in FXII, kininogen, and the bradykinin B2 receptor are protected from arterial thrombosis (Renne, 2005; Shariat-Madar, 2006; Merkoulov, 2008). FXII participates in in vivo thrombus formation presumably by autoactivation on released polysomes from activated platelets, extracellular ribonucleic acid, aggregated proteins, or exposed collagen in the intravascular compartment in flowing blood (Smith, 2006; Kannemeier, 2007; Maas, 2008; van der Meijden, 2009). In the absence of the bradykinin B2 receptor, increased angiotensin II binds to the angiotensin receptor 2 to increase nitric oxide and prostacyclin to reduce arterial thrombosis risk (Shariat-Madar, 2006).

The hemostatic cofactors for the enzymatic reactions of the coagulation system may be considered to act as receptors for coagulation proteins. For example, high molecular weight kininogen serves as a receptor for prekallikrein binding to endothelial cells (Schmaier, 1988; Motta, 1998). Factors VIIIa and Va function as coreceptors of factors IXa and Xa, respectively (Miletich, 1978; Ahmad, 2000). All three of these proteins serve as cofactors that accelerate the reactions in which they participate. For example, high molecular weight kininogen accelerates the activation of prekallikrein and FXI by FXIIa. Factors VIIIa and Va accelerate FX and prothrombin activation, respectively, by factors IXa and Xa. Each cofactor also functions as a substrate of one or more enzymes that participate in their formation and inactivation. High molecular weight kininogen accordingly is a substrate of FXIIa, plasma kallikrein, and FXIa. Factors VIII and V are substrates of thrombin, and factors VIIIa and Va of activated protein C. Fibrinogen is a substrate of thrombin.

FVIII (antihemophilic factor) is a 330-kDa protein. When activated to FVIIIa, it is a cofactor for FIXa in the activation of FX. Its absence is associated with the most severe clinically recognized bleeding disorder, hemophilia A. FV is also a 330-kDa protein with homology to FVIII. When activated to FVa, it serves as a cofactor for FXa in the activation of FII (prothrombin) to thrombin. Fibrinogen is a 330-kDa protein that not only is the main substrate of thrombin (FIIa) but is also the principal adhesive molecule subserving platelet aggregation. When it is proteolyzed by thrombin, a fibrin monomer is formed. This monomer associates end-to-end and side-to-side to form a fibrin clot. The clot is stabilized by activated FXIII, a tissue transglutaminase that cross-links the strands of associating fibrin (Fig. 39-2). TF (47-kDa protein) is an essential cofactor for activated FVIIa. It is found in most tissues and cells. Upregulation of TF results in the formation of complexes with FVII that produce the initiation of hemostatic reactions. Last, high molecular weight kininogen (HK, also known as Fitzgerald factor or Williams factor) is a 120-kDa protein that acts as a cofactor for the activation of FXII, prekallikrein, and FXI.

Physiologic Protein Assemblies

Certain critical protein assemblies in hemostatic reactions accelerate these proteolytic events. The proteins of the coagulation system that are essential for hemostasis or control of bleeding were originally identified by observation of affected patients, and more recently through mouse knockout studies. Deficiencies in coagulation factors VIII and IX are the most prominent bleeding disorders that occur in patients who survive gestation and birth. The rare patients who have apparent congenital deficiencies of coagulation factors VII, X, V, and II usually do not have severe bleeding states. In contrast, murine models have demonstrated that mouse embryos containing complete genetic knockouts of factor VII, X, V, or II die of massive hemorrhage during gestation or at birth (Cui, 1996; Rosen, 1997; Sun, 1998; Dewerchen, 2000). This information suggests that the human patient who has a deficiency of factor VII, X, V, or II may have some factor, albeit less than 1%, to allow for a milder clinical phenotype than that seen in mouse models, or, alternatively, other compensatory mechanisms may be operative in the human patient. All of these proteins participate in two critically important assemblies that are essential for normal hemostasis: **tenase** and **prothrombinase.**

The tenase complex comprises the assembly of FIXa and thrombin-activated FVIIIa on phospholipid surfaces or cell membranes in an ordered structure, with FX to accelerate its activation to FXa. When all of these components are present, the rate of FX activation by FIXa is increased 1.4×10^8-fold over the rate of FX activation by FIXa alone. The prothrombinase complex in analogous fashion comprises the assembly of FXa and thrombin-activated FVa on phospholipid membranes or cell membranes in an ordered structure with FII (prothrombin) to accelerate its activation to FIIa (thrombin). When all of these components are present, the rate of FII activation by FXa is increased 1.7×10^8-fold over the rate of FII activation by FXa alone. Because these coagulation reactions occupy critical regulatory points within the physiologic hemostatic system, they are also the target of a number of anticoagulant agents for venous thrombosis that are currently in use or are being developed.

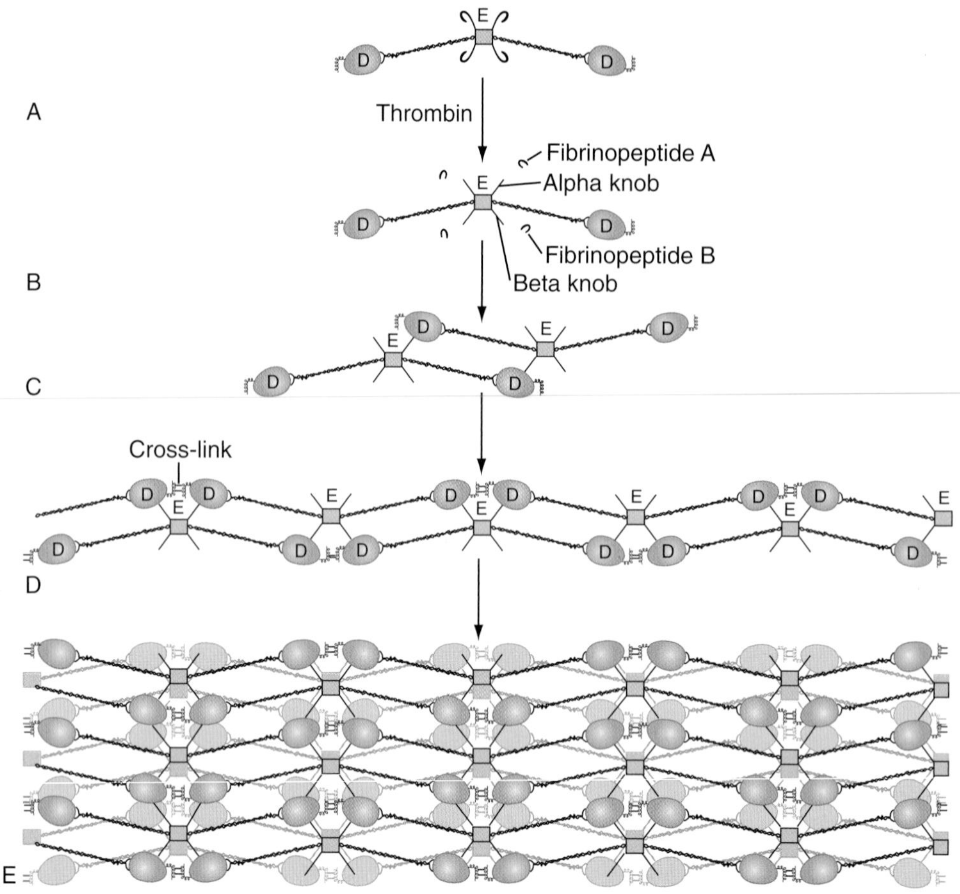

Figure 39-2 Formation of a fibrin clot. **A,** Schematic of fibrinogen. **B,** Thrombin proteolyzes fibrinopeptides A and B from fibrinogen to leave soluble fibrin monomer. Soluble fibrin monomer then associates side-to-side **(C)** and end-to-end (not shown, for clarity) to form fibrin polymers. **D,** Thrombin-activated factor XIII (factor XIIIa) covalently cross-links the fibrin polymers into an increasingly complex structure and an ultimately insoluble clot **(E).** Note that "E" corresponds to the central domain of the original fibrinogen molecule, and "D" to the peripheral domains. *(Modified with permission from Doolittle RF. Fibrinogen and fibrin. Sci Am 1981;245:126–35.)*

THE FORMATION OF FIBRIN AND THE FIBRINOLYTIC SYSTEM

The six peptide chains of the fibrinogen molecule are organized into a structure described as having a central E domain and two terminal D domains. When thrombin is formed, it cleaves fibrinopeptide A from the Aα chain and fibrinopeptide B from the Bβ chain of fibrinogen in the E domain region (Doolittle, 1981). The remainder of this thrombin-proteolyzed fibrinogen is called soluble fibrin monomer. Soluble fibrin monomers then assemble with end-to-end and side-to-side association to form a noncovalent fibrin polymer (see Fig. 39-2). Activated FXIII, a transglutaminase, cross-links fibrin monomeric subunits into an insoluble, cross-linked fibrin clot. When insoluble, cross-linked fibrin is made, a new linkage between the D domains of two adjacent fibrin monomers occurs, and in the process a neo-epitope of interaction is formed (see Fig. 39-2).

The fibrinolytic protein system consists of the zymogen plasminogen and its naturally occurring activators. Plasminogen is activated to the main clot-lysing enzyme, plasmin, by endogenous tissue plasminogen activator (tPA), single-chain urokinase plasminogen activator (ScuPA), and two-chain urokinase plasminogen activator (TcuPA). These activators are found in the endothelium as well as in granulocytes and monocytes. The natural plasminogen activators tPA, ScuPA, and TcuPA convert zymogen plasminogen to the active enzyme plasmin (Fig. 39-3). tPA is produced constitutively, and ScuPA is increased in inflammatory states. Plasminogen activator inhibitor-1 (PAI-1) is the major inhibitor of tPA and TcuPA. α_2-Antiplasmin, a serine protease inhibitor (serpin), is the major inhibitor of formed plasmin. However, the plasma concentration of α_2-antiplasmin is only about half the plasma concentration of plasminogen.

Following its activation from plasminogen, the active plasmin molecule recognizes multiple substrates. Plasmin will degrade soluble fibrinogen to produce fibrinogen degradation products (Fig. 39-4, *A*). Plasmin cleaves fibrinogen into an X fragment of similar molecular mass by eliminating portions of the α-chain (Marder, 1974). Plasmin then cleaves the X fragment asymmetrically between the D and E domains to produce fragment

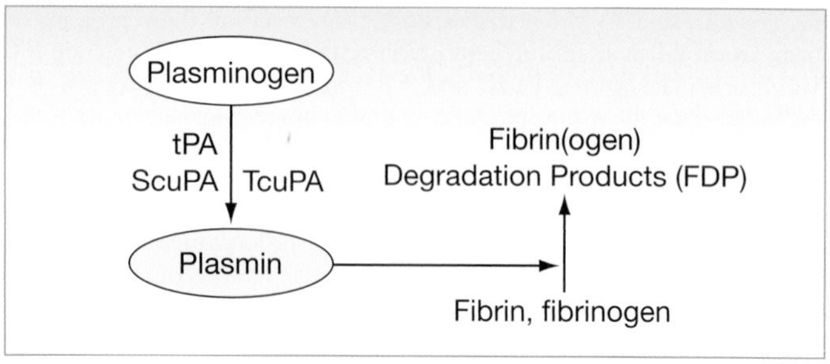

Figure 39-3 Fibrinolysis. Zymogen plasminogen is converted to plasmin by tissue plasminogen activator (tPA), single-chain urokinase plasminogen activator (ScuPA), and two-chain urokinase plasminogen activator (TcuPA). Formed plasmin degrades fibrinogen or fibrin to form fibrinogen or fibrin degradation products, respectively.

Y. Plasmin further degrades the Y fragment to produce soluble D and E domains that are called soluble fibrinogen degradation products or, in the case of fibrin digestion by plasmin, fibrin degradation products. Their presence indicates that plasmin has been formed. Plasmin will also degrade insoluble, crossed-linked fibrin (Fig. 39-4, *B*). When it does so, it liberates a D–D-dimer domain formed as result of the neo-epitope between these two domains (see Fig. 39-4, *B*) (Marder, 1976). The presence of soluble D-dimer indicates that first thrombin has been formed, then clotting has occurred, then the clot has been cross-linked by FXIIIa, and, finally, plasmin has been formed and has cleaved the insoluble, cross-linked fibrin clot.

THE ANTICOAGULATION PROTEIN SYSTEMS

(Fig. 39-5)

Three major anticoagulant systems regulate the enzymes of the coagulation protein system to help to inhibit clot formation. These systems are

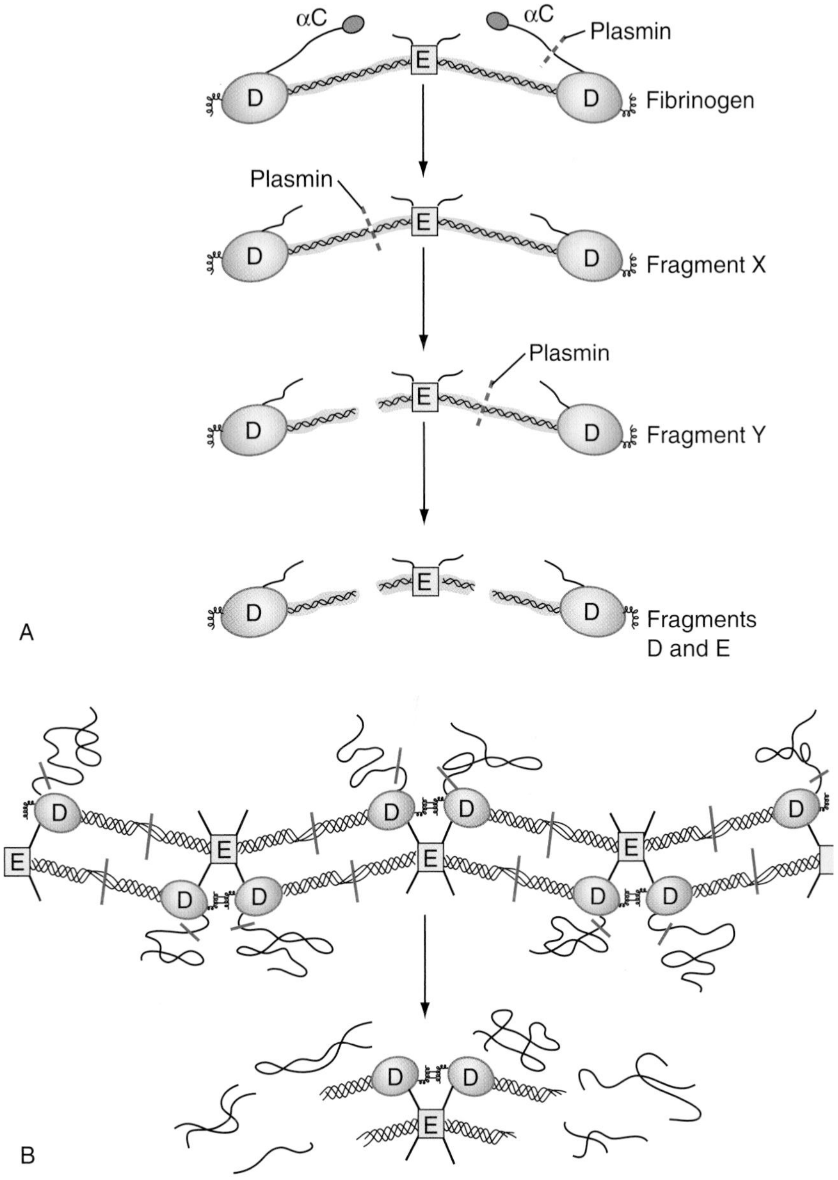

Figure 39-4 **Panel A,** Plasmin-cleaved soluble fibrinogen or fibrin. When plasmin cleaves fibrinogen, initially small portions from the α-chain (αC) are removed to make Fragment X. Fragment X is then asymmetrically cleaved into Fragment D and Fragment Y. Fragment 5Y is further cleaved by plasmin into Fragments D and E. *(Modified with permission from Greenberg CS, Lai T-S. Fibrin formation and stabilization. In: Loscalzo J, Schafer AI, editors. Thrombosis and hemorrhage. 3rd ed. Philadelphia: Lippincott, Williams & Wilkins; 2003, p. 83, Fig. 5-3, B.)* **Panel B,** Plasmin-cleaved insoluble, cross-linked fibrin. When insoluble, cross-linked fibrin is proteolyzed by plasmin, the neo-epitope between the D-domains is preserved, and the liberated fragment consists of the D-dimer together with an E domain. *(Modified with permission from Doolittle RF. Fibrinogen and fibrin. Sci Am 1981;245:126–35.)*

the protein C/protein S system, the plasma serine protease inhibitor system, and TFPI, a Kunitz-type serine protease inhibitor. Antithrombin (antithrombin III) is the main serine protease inhibitor of coagulation enzymes of the plasma serine protease inhibitor system. Each of these systems plays a critical role in proper regulation of the coagulation system. Moreover, in murine deletion models, complete deficiencies of protein C, protein S, antithrombin, and TFPI are incompatible with survival of mammalian gestation, delivery, or life ex utero (Huang, 1997; Jalbert, 1998; Hayashi, 2006; Burstyn-Cohen, 2009).

Protein C/Protein S System

When activated, protein C, a 62-kDa vitamin K–dependent protein, is an enzyme that functions as an inhibitor. Protein C is activated by thrombin when bound to an endothelial cell protein called thrombomodulin. Thrombomodulin forms a trimolecular complex with protein C and thrombin. Activated protein C inactivates factors Va and VIIIa to decrease the rate of thrombin formation. Protein S, a 69-kDa vitamin K–dependent protein, is not an enzyme. It is a cofactor, or receptor, for activated protein C on cell membranes. It allows activated protein C to bind to cell surfaces in such a manner as to orient itself to inactivate factors Va and VIIIa. The enzyme uses this cofactor as a receptor to localize its activity to perform its inhibitory function. Plasma protein S is in equilibrium between the free form and a bound form that is complexed to C4b-binding protein; only the free form functions as a cofactor for activated protein C. Activated protein C also binds to three receptors on endothelial cells: (1) endothelial cell protein C receptor to activate (2) protease-activated receptor (PAR)1 and (3) apolipoprotein E receptor 2 (ApoER2) (Esmon, 1999; Coughlin, 2000; Yang, 2009). Activation of PAR1 on endothelial cells may contribute to the anticoagulant function of activated protein C by liberating tPA. Activated protein C on endothelial cells also has an inflammatory effect via activation of sphingosine-1-phosphate receptor transactivation and activation of ApoER2 (Finigan, 2005; Yang, 2009). Thus activated protein C reduces thrombin formation, stimulates fibrinolysis, and initiates inflammation to reduce thrombosis risk.

Antithrombin

This serpin is a 58-kDa protein that inhibits each of the following hemostatic enzymes: IIa, Xa, VIIa, IXa, XIa, kallikrein, and XIIa. It exerts its anticoagulant effect primarily by inhibiting factors IIa and Xa (see Fig. 39-5). The ability of antithrombin to function as an inhibitor of coagulation protein enzymes is potentiated by heparin. In fact, it is the presence of antithrombin that gives heparin its anticoagulant properties. In the presence of heparin, antithrombin is 1000-fold more effective as an inhibitor of factor IIa. In addition to antithrombin, other serpins regulate the

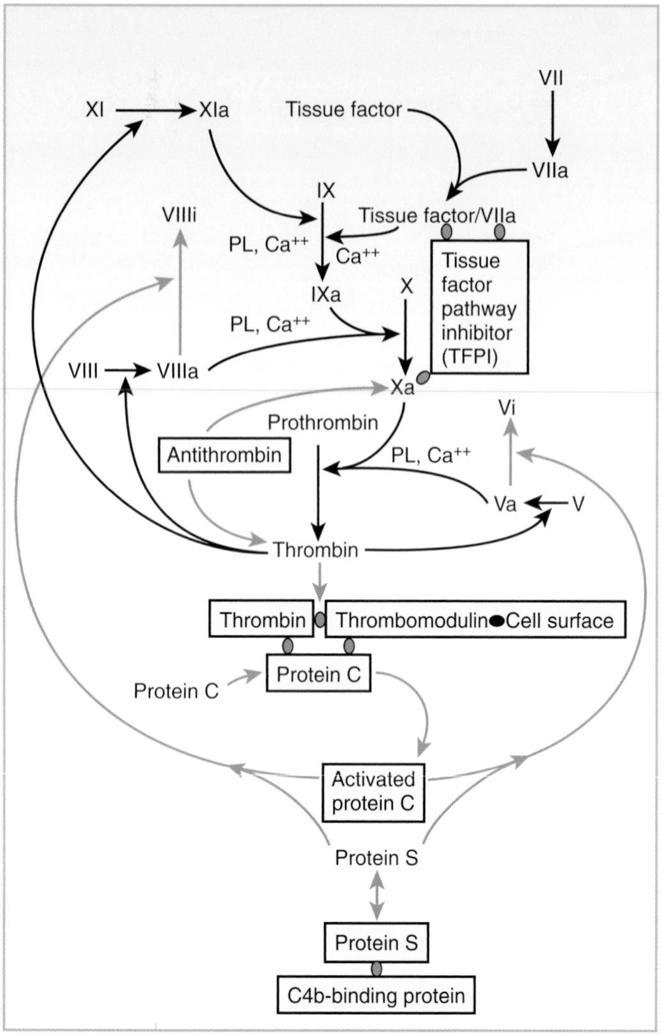

Figure 39-5 Natural inhibitors of coagulation: antithrombin (AT); components of the protein C pathway (thrombomodulin, protein C, protein S); and tissue factor pathway inhibitor (TFPI). Three major anticoagulant systems are recognized. Antithrombin inhibits factor Xa and thrombin to prevent thrombosis. It is important to note that antithrombin inhibits every enzymatic form of blood coagulation serine proteases (factor XIIa, plasma kallikrein, factor XIa, factor IXa, and factor VIIa), even though this is not indicated in the figure for readability purposes. The protein C system requires that this zymogen is activated to activated protein C by thrombin when bound to the endothelial cell membrane protein thrombomodulin. Protein S is a cofactor for activated protein C to inactivate factors Va and VIIIa. C4b binding protein regulates protein S activity. TFPI makes a quarternary complex with tissue factor/factor VIIa and factor Xa to inhibit both enzymes.

enzymes of the hemostatic and inflammatory systems. Heparin cofactor II is a serpin that specifically inhibits thrombin in the presence of dermatan sulfate. Protein Z inhibitor is a serpin that specifically inhibits factor Xa in the presence of its cofactor protein Z—a vitamin K–dependent protein. C1 inhibitor (C1 esterase inhibitor) is the most potent inhibitor of FXIIa, kallikrein, and FXIa in plasma. Its main function is to regulate the amount of free bradykinin in the intravascular compartment and reduce inflammatory events (Han, 2002; Schmaier, 2002; Maas, 2008).

Tissue Factor Pathway Inhibitor

In addition to the serpins, there is the Kunitz-type serine protease inhibitor, TFPI (Crawley, 2008). TFPI is the most potent inhibitor of the FVIIa–tissue factor complex. Under physiologic conditions, TFPI exerts its inhibitory effects by forming a quaternary complex with FVIIa, TF, and FXa (see Fig. 39-5). It is noteworthy that the murine TFPI knockout is embryonically lethal (Jalbert, 1998). Another family of Kunitz-type serine protease inhibitors, the amyloid β-protein precursor (AβPP) and related members, is present in platelets and brain and regulates factors XIa, IXa, Xa, VIIa/TF, and plasmin (Van Nostrand, 1990; Schmaier, 1993, 1995; Mahdi, 1995, 2000). This inhibitor does not inhibit thrombin. The exact function of this inhibitor is not completely known, but it is believed to be a cerebral anticoagulant (Del Zoppo, 2009). AβPP and amyloid precursor–like/protein 2 gene–deleted mice survive gestation but have an accelerated rate of thrombosis in a carotid artery thrombosis model (Xu, 2009).

CURRENT HYPOTHESIS FOR INITIATION OF THE HEMOSTATIC SYSTEM

More proteins participate in coagulation reactions in vitro than are critical for hemostatic reactions in vivo. The original coagulation cascade waterfall hypothesis initiated by FXII has been replaced by one whereby TF and FVIIa are initiators (Gailiani, 1991). TF is ubiquitous throughout the body, although it is rich in brain, lung, and placenta. Its expression is upregulated after injury. Regulation of the expression of TF is a major control mechanism for the initiation of hemostasis. Some investigators believe that a circulating form of TF is also present. The FVIIa–TF complex activates FIX, leading in turn to FX activation. It must be noted that at the concentrations of factors ordinarily present in the body, VIIa/TF does not directly activate appreciable amounts of FX because of the presence of TFPI—a point emphasized diagrammatically in Figure 39-1 by the graying of this reaction. Once FX has been activated to FXa, this Xa in turn contributes to the activation of thrombin from prothrombin. Thrombin then proteolyzes fibrinogen to form fibrin. Although TF-dependent coagulation reactions are rapidly inhibited by TFPI, if the stimulus for thrombin formation is sufficiently strong, coagulation is maintained through the activation of FXI by thrombin (Meijers, 2000). Activation of FXI to FXIa results in increased activation of FIX and eventually increased formation of thrombin. Further modulation of hemostatic balance in the direction of clot formation is exerted by TAFI, the thrombin-activatable fibrinolysis inhibitor (also known as carboxypeptidase U). Among its actions, TAFI cleaves C-terminal lysine residues from fibrin, thereby decreasing the binding of plasminogen to the clot and diminishing clot lysis (Leurs, 2005).

Clinical Laboratory Hemostasis

When faced with a bleeding patient, one must use an analytic diagnostic approach to determine the cause of the problem. The underlying cause in almost all cases will derive from a defect or deficiency in a plasma protein, a defect in platelet number or function, or a defect in adhesive interactions between platelets and the vessel wall.

Any coagulation protein defect can be a true protein deficiency, an inhibitor to the active site of the protein, an abnormal protein that cannot participate in its physiologic function(s), or an apparent deficiency that arises as the result of enhanced clearance of protein. In general, inhibitors to a coagulation protein are immunoglobulins, although hypergammaglobulinemic states or abnormal production of endogenous heparin, fibronectin, or cryoglobulins as acquired inhibitors to coagulation proteins have also been reported. Abnormal proteins that are present but do not function normally occur as a result of missense or deletion mutations, or translocations of DNA. Last, enhanced clearance of coagulation proteins usually occurs as a result of antigen–antibody complex formation. Resultant increased clearance of the protein gives the appearance of a deficiency, but the real mechanism is enhanced clearance.

Typical clinical presentations of bleeding disorders are shown in Table 39-2. In general, hemarthrosis and spontaneous soft tissue and intramuscular hemorrhage characterize plasma protein defects such as hemophilia A and B (factors VIII and IX deficiency). Soft tissue petechiae, purpura, or ecchymosis characterizes von Willebrand disease, or disorders of platelet number or function. However, at times, it is difficult to distinguish the potential mechanism for bleeding. Thus the clinical laboratory is essential for definitive diagnosis of a bleeding disorder in the patient.

PHYSIOLOGIC HEMOSTASIS VERSUS CLINICAL ASSAYS

In the practice of clinical hemostasis, a dichotomy is seen between physiologic hemostasis and assays used in the clinical laboratory to recognize coagulation protein defects. As indicated previously in Figure 39-1, physiologic hemostasis is initiated by an increase in the formation of TF–FVIIa complexes. At present, no good assays are available in the clinical laboratory to assess this early event specifically. Instead, the relatively late event of actual clot formation is monitored. The two assays most commonly used to examine the coagulation system are (1) the APTT induced by surface

TABLE 39-2
Patterns of Clinical Bleeding in Disorders of Hemostasis

Characteristics	Primary hemostasis (platelet/vascular problem)	Secondary hemostasis (coagulation factor problem)
Onset	Spontaneous, immediate after trauma	Delayed after trauma
Sites	Skin, mucous membranes	Deep tissues
Form	Petechiae, ecchymosis	Hematomas
Mucous membrane	Common (nasal, oral, gastrointestinal, genitourinary)	Less common
Other sites	Rare	Joint, muscle, central nervous system, retroperitoneal space
Clinical examples	Thrombocytopenia, platelet defects, von Willebrand disease, scurvy	Factor deficiency, liver disease, acquired inhibitors

(contact) activation of the system, and (2) the prothrombin time (PT) induced by the addition of excess tissue factor. Contact activation of the coagulation system occurs because FXII in the presence of artificial, negatively charged particles in the reagent autoactivates to FXIIa, which in turn initiates the cascade of proteolytic reactions of the coagulation system. As is discussed later, this test measures more proteins than those necessary for hemostasis. With the PT test, the addition of excess TF creates a very unphysiologic change in the normal stoichiometric relationships of factors, thereby allowing FVIIa to overcome the inhibitory effect of TFPI and favoring direct activation of FX to FXa. Both assays are extremely useful for assessing the integrity of the blood coagulation system and for recognizing potential bleeding problems in a patient (see later).

SCREENING TESTS FOR COAGULATION DISORDERS

When a patient with a bleeding problem is addressed in the clinical laboratory, several screening tests are used to classify and diagnose the basis of this disorder. The term **primary hemostasis** refers to platelet reactivity at the site of vessel injury; this topic is covered in Chapter 40. The platelet count is an example of a screening assay for primary hemostasis. This section describes assays for what has been called **secondary hemostasis,** that is, the coagulation of plasma. However, more recent studies employing animal model systems suggest the need for caution in accepting this distinction too literally, for example, in vivo visualization studies of arterial thrombus formation in at least some models suggest that platelet accumulation and fibrin generation may actually occur simultaneously (Falati, 2002; Furie, 2009). Regardless of the true order of events occurring in vivo, however, when performed simultaneously on a sample of plasma, these coagulation assays identify almost all of the diagnostic categories for a coagulopathy. The 50-year-old cascade hypothesis for hemostasis still has merit in explaining the mechanism(s) for clot formation seen in the screening tests for coagulation reactions. In this hypothesis, coagulation proteins are classified as members of the so-called **intrinsic system, extrinsic system,** or **common pathway** (Fig. 39-6). This approach allows for a practical differential diagnosis of which protein(s) may be affected, based on the results of a series of screening tests. The specific coagulation factors involved in each test are shown schematically in Figure 39-6. Methodologic aspects of these tests (Fig. 39-7) are discussed in the following paragraphs.

Activated Partial Thromboplastin Time (Fig. 39-7, *A*)

To perform this common coagulation assay, a mixture of a negatively charged surface, phospholipid, and anticoagulated patient plasma is incubated for several minutes. The recommended anticoagulant is 3.2 g% sodium citrate because less variation is seen in blood specimens from normal patients and those on anticoagulants collected in this concentration of anticoagulant (Adcock, 1997, 1998). Sodium citrate is a reversible chelator of calcium that prevents coagulation protein activation. When whole blood is collected, the ratio of anticoagulant to whole blood is 1 part

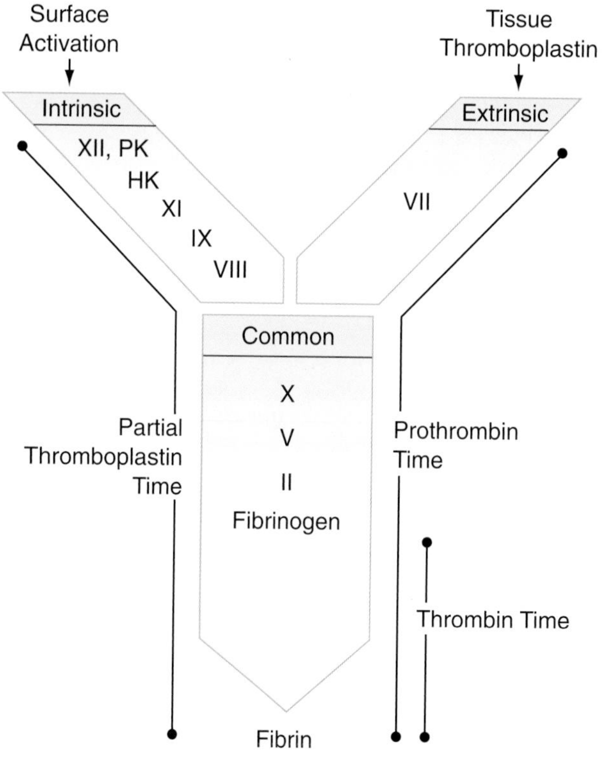

Figure 39-6 Organization of the coagulation system based on current assays. The **intrinsic** coagulation system consists of the proteins factors XII, XI, IX, and VIII and prekallikrein (PK) and high molecular weight kininogen (HK). The **extrinsic** coagulation system consists of tissue factor (tissue thromboplastin) and factor VII. The **common pathway** of the coagulation system consists of factors X, V, and II, and fibrinogen (I).

anticoagulant to 9 parts whole blood. After incubation of patient plasma with reagent for a prescribed time, depending on the assay, the sample is recalcified with excess calcium chloride, and the time required for clot formation is measured. The APTT assesses the coagulation proteins of the so-called intrinsic system and common pathways (see later). This assay is commonly referred to as the partial thromboplastin time (PTT), but it is really an "activated" PTT, in that its reagents contain a negatively charged surface that accelerates the rate of the reaction (Proctor, 1961).

Prothrombin Time (Fig. 39-7, *B*)

To perform this common coagulation assay, tissue thromboplastin (recombinant human or isolated animal tissue factor) and patient plasma are incubated for several minutes, after which the citrated plasma mixture is recalcified by the addition of excess $CaCl_2$, and the time required for clot formation is measured. The PT assesses the coagulation proteins of the so-called extrinsic system and common pathway (see later) (Quick, 1935). Tissue thromboplastin traditionally has been a crude preparation of animal brain TF. Presently, recombinant TF is used in the preparation of several commercial PT reagents. In general, the range of prolongation of time of an abnormal PT increases when recombinant TF is used. This fact makes for a more sensitive assay. The PT serves as the basis for the international normalized ratio (INR) value used to monitor patients on warfarin. As discussed in Chapter 42, the INR is the ratio of patient PT divided by geometric mean normal PT for the local laboratory (based on a population of normal individuals assessed with identical sample collection, reagents, and machines), raised to the power of the international sensitivity index. Although the INR is clearly the most appropriate measure to use in conjunction with oral anticoagulant monitoring, for hemostatic evaluation of the nonwarfarinized patient, actual PT values in seconds may be used, referencing the laboratory's locally established reference interval for the PT test.

Thrombin Time (Fig. 39-7, *C*)

To perform the thrombin time (also referred to as thrombin clotting time), purified exogenous thrombin is added to plasma to determine the time to clot formation. It is a direct measure of fibrinogen function and may be used to ascertain if there is a defect in fibrinogen function. The thrombin time will be prolonged in hypofibrinogenemic states, if an abnormal

PART 5

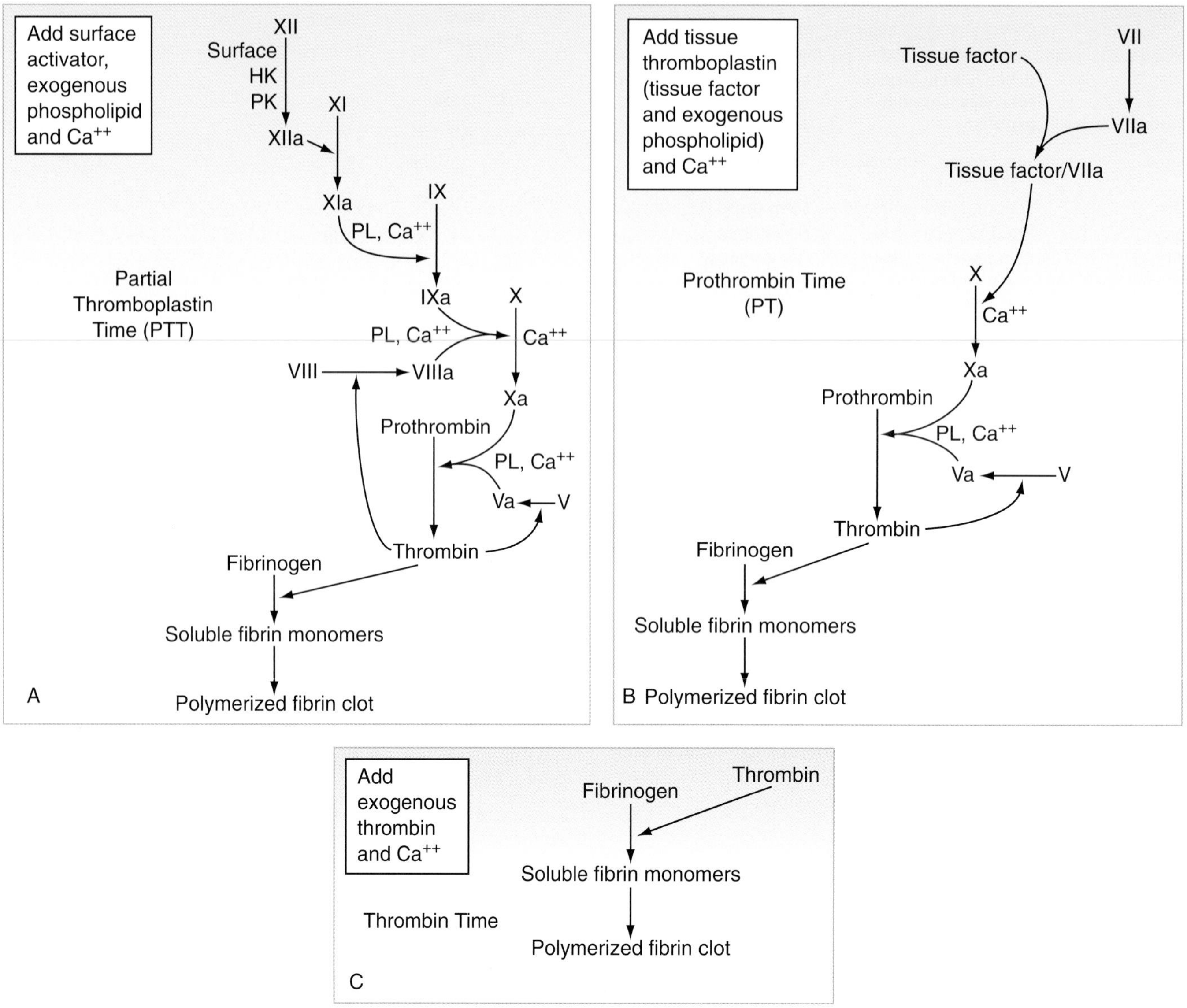

Figure 39-7 Coagulation screening tests. **Panel A,** Activated partial thromboplastin time (APTT, "PTT" on the figure) requires the presence of every protein except tissue factor and factor VII. **Panel B,** Prothrombin time (PT) requires tissue factor and factors VII, X, V, and II and fibrinogen. **Panel C,** In the thrombin time (or thrombin clotting time), exogenous thrombin is added to plasma to proteolyze (clot) fibrinogen. The endpoint in each of these tests is the number of seconds until detection of a clot, following addition of the indicated reagents to citrated platelet-free patient plasma. Because virtually all measuring systems employed detect the formation of a polymerized fibrin clot, whether or not any cross-linking of fibrin occurs, none of these tests will provide information with respect to factor XIIIa activity.

protein fibrinogen (dysfibrinogenemia) is present, or if a thrombin inhibitor is present.

ASSAYS USED IN CLINICAL COAGULATION TESTING

Clinical coagulation testing is based on functional assays that examine the rate of clot formation. In these assays, a sequence of proteolytic reactions takes place, leading to thrombin formation and its proteolysis of fibrinogen (Mann, 2003). Proteolysis of fibrinogen results in clot formation, precipitation of soluble proteins, which is detected by increased impedance or turbidity, or decreased optical clarity, based on the instrumentation used to measure the result. Any defect along the pathway to clot formation will give an abnormal final result. Furthermore, because a series of reactions need to take place for final clot formation to occur, any defect below a specific factor will lead to an abnormal result in measuring that factor. For example, a high-titer inhibitor of FVIII will produce an abnormal FXI assay. Similarly, deficient or abnormal fibrinogen will affect the results of all clotting tests.

All coagulation factors of the intrinsic system (XII, prekallikrein, high molecular weight kininogen, XI, IX, and VIII) are measured in assays using the APTT as its platform. These specific factor assays became readily available because of the recognition of patients and the commercial availability of specific factor-deficient plasmas that serve as substrate for them. For example, a FVIII assay is a mixture of APTT reagent, FVIII-deficient plasma, and test (unknown) plasma from the patient (Landell, 1953). After incubation for a few minutes, the time to clot is initiated by the addition of calcium chloride. FVII, together with coagulation factors of the common pathway (X, V, and II), is usually measured by assays using the PT as the platform. For example, an FX assay is a mixture of PT reagent that contains TF (thromboplastin), FX-deficient plasma, and test or patient (unknown) plasma. After incubation for a few minutes, time to clot is initiated by the addition of calcium chloride. The amount of factor present in a given patient sample is determined by comparing the patient sample against a standard curve made with plasma samples containing varying amounts of the specific factor to be assayed mixed with factor-deficient plasma, as well as the appropriate APTT or PT reagent for the assay.

Coagulation-based assays are sensitive and specific. They are much simpler to perform than antigen assays for each of the coagulation proteins. These assays provide information on the functional presence of the coagulation protein. Additional coagulant-based assays such as thrombin time (see earlier) and reptilase time (see later) specifically examine the integrity of fibrinogen to liberate its fibrinopeptides, resulting in fibrin clot formation. When establishing a clinically useful thrombin time, it is important to reduce the thrombin concentration to about 1–2 NIH U/mL (≈8–16 nM human α-thrombin at 3000 U/mg specific activity), so that the time of a normal assay is about 20 seconds. Such an assay will allow for reproducibility and sufficient sensitivity to detect subtle protein abnormalities. Coagulation-based assays examine the function of the protein; antigen assays establish the presence of the proteins; combined, the two assays characterize any protein with reduced function but with normal antigen. A dysfunctional protein has reduced protein function with normal levels of antigen. Such a situation arises commonly when fibrinogen is examined. The most useful means to determine whether fibrinogen is abnormal (i.e., dysfibrinogenemia) is to measure clottable fibrinogen and fibrinogen antigen. If fibrinogen clottability is less than 90% of the amount of fibrinogen antigen present, this finding would suggest that the protein produced is abnormal in some way.

Chromogenic assays are used to measure certain enzymes (plasmin, activated protein C) and various plasma protease inhibitors (antithrombin, C1 inhibitor, α_2-antiplasmin, PAI, tPA). Neutralizing the enzymatic activity of FXa or thrombin is a useful way to assay for the level of anticoagulants that inhibit FXa or thrombin (see Chapter 42). Presently, such assays are used to measure the therapeutic levels of unfractionated heparin, low molecular weight heparin, or fondaparinux. An assay for any future parenteral or oral FXa or thrombin inhibitor can be developed by using the agent's ability to neutralize its enzymatic activity. Last, a direct chromogenic assay for FXa has been useful in assessing the degree of anticoagulation for the occasional patient on warfarin who has a lupus anticoagulant (see Chapter 41) of sufficient potency to interfere not only with the APTT, but with the PT as well.

PRACTICAL APPROACH TO PATIENTS WITH COAGULATION DISORDERS

Using the coagulation cascade hypothesis and its grouping of proteins of the coagulation system, screening tests for coagulation proteins can identify various deficiencies or abnormalities among coagulation proteins (Table 39-3; see Fig. 39-6).

With the APTT, FXII autoactivation on an artificial, negatively charged surface initiates the sequence of reactions of the coagulation cascade. The APTT (labeled "PTT" in the figure) measures proteins of the intrinsic coagulation system (FXII, prekallikrein, high molecular weight kininogen, FXI, FIX, and FVIII) and proteins of the common pathway (factors X, V, II, and fibrinogen) (see Fig. 39-7, *A*). It is important to realize that a coagulation factor has to be decreased to different levels before screening assays are sensitive and show an abnormality. For example, most commercial APTT reagents will detect a decrease in FVIII when the level of the protein is down to 35%–45% of normal (i.e., 0.35–0.45 U/mL). In contrast, FXII and high molecular weight kininogen at a level of 10%–15% may not prolong an otherwise normal APTT. When evaluating new lots of coagulation reagents, it is important to determine their level of sensitivity to detect coagulation protein deficiencies. Additionally, very high levels of FVIII can mask a defect in other coagulation factors. High levels of FVIII can also mask a low protein C level in a clot-based activated protein C assay.

The PT measures the extrinsic coagulation pathway of coagulation, which consists of activated FVII (FVIIa) and TF and proteins of the common pathway (factors X, V, II, and fibrinogen) (see Fig. 39-7, *B*). FVII levels below 35%–40% will begin to be detected by prolongation of the PT. The thrombin time measures only the ability of exogenous thrombin to proteolyze (clot) fibrinogen (see Fig. 39-7, *C*). It is used to characterize fibrinogen function.

With knowledge of what each test measures, the following approach can be used to evaluate bleeding risk among patients who have one or more of these assays prolonged (see Table 39-3 and Fig. 39-6). For example, if a patient has an isolated prolonged APTT, determination of the patient's risk to bleed can begin with the addition of some historical information. If isolated prolongation of the APTT in a male patient is associated with bleeding, then the differential diagnosis in decreasing likelihood of frequency is FVIII, FIX, or FXI deficiency. These disorders will be discussed in the next section. If the APTT alone is prolonged and there is no history of bleeding, the most common cause is a lupus anticoagulant. The specific proteins of the so-called intrinsic coagulation system associated with a prolonged APTT but no bleeding history include, in decreasing frequency, FXII, prekallikrein, and high molecular weight kininogen. Knowing about these latter three proteins is essential in evaluating a prolonged APTT even though the patient is not at bleeding risk, so that patients neither get unnecessary plasma replacement therapy nor experience unnecessary delays in scheduled surgical procedures.

Alternatively, if the patient has an isolated PT prolongation that is associated with bleeding, this finding usually indicates partial FVII deficiency. Of note, FVII Padua (a substitution of glutamine for arginine at residue 304) renders the human FVII molecule less activatable in the presence of some nonhuman forms of TF (Girolami, 1979; Pollak, 2006). Individuals who may not even have a true bleeding disorder typically come to attention owing to a long PT performed with nonhuman TF. FVII assayed using this same source of TF may also appear to be decreased. Repeat assays employing recombinant human TF should provide more normal results for these tests. At times, defects in some common pathway proteins (fibrinogen, factors II, V, and X) may first produce an isolated PT prolongation, although, if severe, these latter protein defects will lead to prolongations of the PT and APTT. This arises because when a sensitive TF is used in the assay, a subtle abnormality in the common pathway proteins is first observed in PT-based assays. Usually, however, defects in the common pathway proteins (fibrinogen, factors II, V, X) result in prolonged PT and APTT. When confronted with patient laboratory results of prolonged PT and APTT, it is important not simply to consider the specific proteins mentioned earlier but also to address the differential diagnosis from general medical states such as anticoagulation therapy, disseminated intravascular coagulation, liver disease, vitamin K deficiency, and massive transfusion. Each of these entities will be described later in the section on acquired bleeding disorders.

A few rare bleeding disorders will not be recognized on routine blood coagulation and platelet screening tests. In order of frequency, these entities include FXIII defects, α_2-antiplasmin defects, PAI-1 defects, and α_1-antitrypsin$_{\text{PITTSBURGH}}$ (Aoki, 1980; Owen, 1983; Fay, 1992; Anwar, 1999; Hua, 2009). FXIII deficiency will be discussed below. α_2-Antiplasmin defects and PAI-1 defects, both congenital and acquired (see later), produce hyperfibrinolytic states as a result of reduced inhibition of plasmin, tPA, or urokinase. α_1-Antitrypsin$_{\text{PITTSBURGH}}$ is a rare entity and is a bleeding disorder that may result from a mutation in antitrypsin that leads to potent thrombin inhibition, thereby preventing any clot from forming.

When presented with a prolonged coagulation assay, the differential diagnosis is often between a true deficiency and inhibition of a specific coagulation protein. Two approaches can be used to obtain a specific diagnosis. In the first approach, the specific defect of a prolonged coagulation assay can be identified by performing all relevant coagulation factor assays. If any one test is decreased, then a specific coagulation factor inhibitor assay can be performed for that factor. One general approach to a specific inhibitor study can be employed by mixing various ratios of patient plasma to normal plasma (e.g., 1 : 1, 2 : 1, 4 : 1, 1 : 2, 1 : 4), incubating the samples for 2 hours at 37° C, and assaying the level of the specific factor in the mixture. Simultaneously, patient plasma and normal plasma used in the mixing study are also incubated under the same conditions. At the time of assay, the percentages of activity of the specific factor under study in normal plasma, patient plasma, and each of the mixtures are obtained. If the observed value at any given ratio of patient plasma to control plasma is less than the calculated expected value of mixing the two plasmas at various ratios (e.g., 1 : 1, 2 : 1, 1 : 2), then one can conclude that an inhibitor is present in patient plasma that transfers to the normal plasma sample. For example, if 100% activity (1 U/mL) of the factor being studied is observed in an undiluted sample, then a 1 : 1 dilution of normal plasma with factor-deficient plasma should yield a level of about 50% activity. If the same normal plasma was incubated with patient plasma at a 1 : 1 ratio, and the value came back as 32% activity, one should conclude that there is something in patient plasma that transfers and inhibits the factor's activity in normal plasma (i.e., the definition of an inhibitor). This approach serves as a general, nonquantitative method of assessing a coagulation factor inhibitor. In the section on hereditary coagulation protein defects

TABLE 39-3
Differential Diagnosis of Abnormal Coagulation Screening Tests

Abnormal Activated Partial Thromboplastin Time (APTT) Alone
Associated with bleeding: VIII, IX, and XI defects
Not associated with bleeding: XII, prekallikrein (PK), high molecular weight kininogen, lupus anticoagulants
Abnormal Prothrombin Time (PT) Alone
Factor VII defects
Combined Abnormal APTT and PT
Medical conditions: Anticoagulants, disseminated intravascular coagulation (DIC), liver disease, vitamin K deficiency, massive transfusion
Rarely dysfibrinogenemia; factor X, V, and II defects

PART 5

(later), a specifically quantitative method for determining inhibitors to FVIII will be presented; this approach is applicable to any factor that is measured by coagulant assay.

A second way to approach the problem of determining a specific coagulation factor defect is to begin with a mixing test of patient and normal plasma. Mixing studies based on the PT or APTT are interpreted with knowledge of the fact that a 50% level of any coagulation factor alone gives normal PT and APTT values. The reason that 50% of any coagulation factor will have normal PT and APTT values is that both of these screening assays have hyperbolic sensitivity curves (i.e., a decrease in any one factor does not lead to linear prolongation of either of these two assays). Only with values well below 50% will the PT and APTT start to be prolonged. As indicated earlier, the sensitivity of the PT and APTT to prolongation with lowering of clotting factors varies as to the factor and the reagent made by the manufacturer. Thus, if patient plasma is mixed 1 : 1 with normal plasma, the PT or APTT should be normal if no inhibitory factor was present in the patient plasma. If, however, the mixture does not correct to within normal values, one can consider that something in patient plasma interferes with function of the protein in normal plasma.

How one does screening assays for inhibitors has been somewhat subjective for individual laboratories; this is the main problem when a screening inhibitor assay is used as the first step in patient disease diagnosis. Almost no studies have provided evidence-based laboratory medicine on how to proceed with inhibitor screening studies. Some approaches to the use of mixing studies have been developed for testing for lupus anticoagulants, which has its own peculiar aspects (Brandt, 1995a, b). Critical issues in performing mixing studies include the ratio of patient plasma to normal plasma (1 : 1–4 : 1), the time of incubation from mixing to assay (immediate–2 hours), and the assays to be used to measure the result (PT, APTT). One investigation aimed to examine the sensitivity and specificity of mixing studies in assessing factor deficiencies and anticoagulants (Chang, 2002). In this study, patient plasma and normal plasma were incubated at 37° C for 1 hour before assay at a ratio of 1 : 1 or 4 : 1 (patient : normal). With an APTT mix of 1 : 1 and a percent correction of 70%–75% calculated by a specific formula (see reference for formula), the sensitivity/specificity for recognizing a factor deficiency or anticoagulant was 100%/33% or 33%/100%, respectively. When the percent correction was 50%, calculated from a ratio of 4 : 1 (patient : normal) in the plasma mix for APTT, the sensitivity/specificity in recognizing a factor deficiency or anticoagulant improved to 88%/100% or 100%/88%, respectively (Chang, 2002). Similarly, on a PT mix of 1 : 1 with a percentage correction of 70%–75% calculated by a specific formula (see reference for formula), the sensitivity/specificity in recognizing a factor deficiency or anticoagulant was 95%/50% or 50%/95%, respectively. When the percentage correction was greater than 40%, as calculated from a ratio of 4 : 1 (patient : normal) in the plasma mix for PT, the sensitivity/specificity for recognizing a factor deficiency or anticoagulant improved to 96%/100% or 100%/96%, respectively (Chang, 2002). Additional studies showed that the assay after an immediate mix versus 1-hour incubation at 37° C had lower sensitivity and specificity.

Multiple factor deficiencies, such as those seen when a patient is on warfarin, often do not correct, owing both to deficiencies in plasma levels of multiple proteins and to the production of abnormal coagulant molecules resulting from the carboxylation inhibition defect that proceed to function as inhibitors in coagulant-based assays. Once it is determined that an inhibitor is present, specific factor assays still need to be performed to isolate the specific protein toward which the inhibitor is directed. In general, most institutions start with a mixing study to diagnose a novel coagulation protein defect. Regardless of the diagnosis of a deficiency or inhibitor, all relevant factors that could be producing that defect need to be assessed. The alternative approach is to assay for all relevant factors initially to isolate the defect, and then to determine, if appropriate, whether an inhibitor is present. The latter approach usually speeds the time to patient diagnosis. If multiple factors are low, consideration should be given to the possibilities of factitious warfarin, heparin, myeloma proteins, hypodysfibrinogenemia, cryoglobulins, and so forth.

Hereditary Coagulation Protein Defects

As described earlier, protein or factor deficiencies can be quantitative or qualitative. In quantitative disorders, the factor level determined by routine clot-based methods (functional activity assays) is similar to that obtained by immunologic (antigen) assays. In qualitative disorders, the functional assay result is decreased, but the antigen level is significantly higher or normal, indicating the presence of a dysfunctional protein or an inhibitor to the function of that protein.

DEFICIENCY OF FACTOR VIII (HEMOPHILIA A) OR FACTOR IX (HEMOPHILIA B)

Hemophilia A (FVIII deficiency) is the most common severe congenital bleeding disorder that allows for normal gestation and delivery, affecting 1 in 5000–10,000 males. Hemophilia B (FIX deficiency, Christmas disease) is also a severe congenital bleeding disorder, affecting 1 in 25,000–30,000 males. The factor VIII and IX genes are both located on the X chromosome, with the result that hemophilia A and B are X-linked recessive disorders primarily affecting males. Females carrying a hemophilia mutation on one of their two X chromosomes are carriers. Hemophilia A can affect females when carriers have imbalanced Lyonization of the normal X chromosome or Turner's syndrome (XO), or when they are daughters of an affected male and a carrier female.

Bleeding manifestations of hemophilia A and B, which are coagulation factor problems, include hemarthrosis; soft tissue hematomas into muscles; easy bruising; excessive bleeding with surgery, trauma, dental extraction, and circumcision; bleeding in the gastrointestinal or genitourinary tract; epistaxis; poor wound healing; and, uncommonly, umbilical stump bleeding (see Table 39-2). Intracranial hemorrhage can occur, particularly following trauma. The severity of hemophilia is classified on the basis of plasma factor level (Table 39-4). Severe hemophilia presents with spontaneous bleeding two to four times per month and requires frequent treatment or prophylactic therapy with replacement factor products. At the other end of the spectrum, mild hemophilia presents with prolonged bleeding after trauma or major surgery, and patients rarely need intravenous factor replacement.

Hemophilia is suspected on the basis of bleeding symptoms or a family history of hemophilia. About one third of hemophilia A cases arise from spontaneous mutations. Laboratory evaluation of patients with such a bleeding history should include an APTT and PT. Diagnosis is confirmed by a FVIII or FIX assay. It is important to appreciate that two levels of the standard curve for FVIII coagulant activity assays need to be prepared to fully characterize patients with severe FVIII deficiency, because the curve is not linear at lower values. FVIII levels above 10% are evaluated with a standard curve that spans 10%–150% FVIII activity. Low FVIII levels are evaluated with a standard curve, e.g., that might range between 0.24% and 15% levels. The most common cause of severe hemophilia A is partial inversion of the FVIII gene up to and including intron 22, which accounts for up to 40%–45% of such patients (Naylor, 1992; Lakich, 1993). These inversions are due to homologous recombination between the region that includes the *F8A* gene in intron 22 and one of the two other homologous regions located more than 400kb 5′ (telomeric) to the FVIII gene (Lakich, 1993; Kaufman, 2001). Several types of these inversions have been described (Kaufman, 2001). If the intron 22 inversion is not detected, definition of the responsible mutation is difficult because of the large size of the FVIII gene (approximately 186,000 bp long). In contrast, the FIX gene is one-fifth the size of the FVIII gene, and the mutations responsible for hemophilia B are easier to define by genetic analysis.

More diagnostic testing may be required for patients with mild to moderate deficiency of FVIII for whom a diagnosis of hemophilia A may be less apparent (e.g., a female patient with low FVIII and apparent

TABLE 39-4
Classification of Hemophilia A and B

	CLASSIFICATION		
	Severe	**Moderate**	**Mild**
Percentage of patients	50–70	10	30–40
Factor VIII or factor IX activity, %	<1	1–5	6–30
Pattern of bleeding episodes	≈2–4 per month approximately	≈4–6 per year approximately	Uncommon
Cause of bleeding	Spontaneous	Minor trauma	Major trauma Surgery

autosomal inheritance). In patients with von Willebrand disease, a secondary deficiency of FVIII may occur (see Chapter 40) because FVIII is normally bound to von Willebrand factor in the plasma (Weiss, 1977). Further, a unique von Willebrand factor abnormality has been described in which a missense mutation in von Willebrand factor impairs the capacity of von Willebrand factor to bind to and promote FVIII secretion into plasma. This abnormality, first described in a French patient from Normandy, has been named von Willebrand disease "Normandy," or type 2N. It should be suspected in a patient with normal von Willebrand factor antigen and functional studies (see Chapter 40), but reduced FVIII levels, whose inheritance is autosomal recessive rather than sex-linked (Schneppenheim, 1996).

FIX activity levels during childhood remain at about 75% of adult levels. A 25% increment in FIX expression begins at puberty in both sexes (Andrew, 1992). It has been assumed that this is a result of steroid hormone action. It is interesting to note that a rare form of FIX deficiency, hemophilia B Leyden, undergoes postpubertal phenotypic resolution. Patients with this condition present with hemophilia B in early childhood, with FIX activity ranging from less than 1%–13% of normal. Plasma levels rise to as high as 70% of normal after the onset of puberty with resolution of bleeding complications (Reitsma, 2001). Mutations in hemophilia B Leyden have been identified in the promoter region of the FIX gene, within which a consensus sequence for steroid receptor binding is located (Crossley, 1992).

Evaluation of Carriers

Detection of carriers is useful for prediction of symptoms and prenatal counseling. Carriers may have low enough FVIII or FIX levels to be symptomatic with easy bruising, menorrhagia, and hemorrhagic complications of surgery and trauma (Arun, 2001). In hemophilia A, if the mutation is known, the potential carrier may be tested for that mutation. Otherwise, the woman should be tested for the common intron 22 inversion. Detailed genetic analysis of the woman, the affected male, and intervening family members may define the mutation. These techniques provide an extremely high likelihood of detection of carriers when all family members are available for study. Otherwise, the woman's ratio of FVIII activity to the level of von Willebrand factor antigen may be used to predict carrier status. Abnormally decreased ratios have been reported to identify 91%–99% of hemophilia A carriers (Fishman, 1982; Graham, 1986; Green, 1986). Prenatal diagnosis of the hemophilias can be performed at a number of high-risk obstetric centers by chorionic villous sampling at 12 weeks' gestation or by amniocentesis after the 16th week. If the genetic basis of the disease is known within a family, then mutational analysis or examination for the intron 22 inversion can be performed on the cell samples (Ljung, 1999; Arun, 2001). Fetoscopic blood sampling can be performed at 20 weeks' gestation for coagulation factor analysis, although it carries a higher risk and is less precise. In hemophilia B, 30%–40% of carriers will be missed by measurement of FIX activity, and mutation analysis is important for defining carrier status (Graham, 1979; Ljung, 1999). Similar to hemophilia A, hemophilia B arises spontaneously in one third of patients.

Treatment of Hemophilia

Recombinant factor products are now the standard of care for treatment of hemophilia A and B in developed countries. Clotting factors are dosed on the basis of weight and desired plasma activity. Plasma with 100% clotting factor activity has 1 U/mL of that clotting factor. By convention, one unit of a coagulation factor is the amount of that factor present in 1 mL of normal pooled human plasma. Each unit of recombinant FVIII/kg raises the plasma FVIII activity by about 2%, and each unit of recombinant FIX/kg raises the plasma FIX activity by about 1%. To raise the FVIII plasma activity of a 70-kg man by 100%, the calculated dose will be as follows:

$$\text{Body weight (kg)} \times 0.5 \text{ international units/kg}$$
$$\times \text{ FVIII activity increase desired (\%)} = \text{Dose required, or}$$
$$(70\text{ kg})\,(0.5)\,(100) = 3500 \text{ units to be infused.}$$

The plasma half-life of FVIII is about 12 hours. To raise the FIX plasma activity of a 70-kg man by 100%, the calculated dose will be as follows:

$$\text{Body weight (kg)} \times \text{desired FIX increase (\%)}$$
$$\times 1 \text{ international unit/kg} = \text{Dose required, or}$$
$$(70\text{ kg})\,(100) = 7000 \text{ units to be infused (Shapiro, 2005).}$$

About one third of FIX-deficient patients have a lower recovery after recombinant FIX infusion, requiring 20% higher dosing. The plasma half-life of FIX is about 24 hours.

Complications of Treatment

Inhibitor antibodies to FVIII or FIX represent significant complications of therapy. The incidence of inhibitors in patients with severe hemophilia A is approximately 15%–35%, and the incidence of inhibitors in patients with hemophilia B is approximately 1%–4%.

Studies to detect the emergence of an inhibitor may be undertaken periodically, and most particularly when doses of replacement factor therapy thought sufficient to control a bleeding challenge prove unsuccessful. It can be very helpful when trying to assess the emergence of an inhibitor to draw blood at multiple times following the infusion of the replacement factor. An acceleration in the fall-off rate of factor level plotted against time will typically occur with the development of an inhibitor against that factor.

Characterization of a specific inhibitor to FVIII or FIX or any other coagulation protein requires careful quantitation. This is important to perform because the degree of inhibitor titer has a major bearing on the choice of therapy for the patient. In general, lower-titer FVIII inhibitors (less than 5 Bethesda units [BU], see later) can be treated with replacement factor; in contrast, higher-titer inhibitors (above 10 BU, see later) typically can be treated effectively only with recombinant FVIIa or with a FVIII bypassing concentrate (activated prothrombin complex concentrates) (Hay, 2006). A simple mixing test as described previously for the APTT can underestimate the presence of an inhibitor. Further, as indicated earlier, there is no unanimity on how such mixing assays should be performed. In order to diagnose the presence of a FVIII or FIX inhibitor, a formal FVIII or FIX "Bethesda" inhibitor assay should be performed (Kasper, 1975). In general, this approach to assay for coagulation factor inhibitors is reliable for all coagulation protein inhibitors. This assay standardizes the amount of plasma in the mixture and the time of incubation and normalizes interpretation of the inhibitor, so that it is universally interpretable. In the classic Bethesda assay, 1 part patient plasma is mixed with 1 part normal plasma and is incubated for 2 hours at 37° C. The control is a 1:1 mix of normal plasma with buffer. In a variation of the original Bethesda assay, known as the Nijmegen modification, the control of pooled normal plasma is incubated with FVIII-deficient plasma, and the pooled normal plasma used in the assay is buffered to prevent pH shifts during the 2-hour incubation (Verbruggen, 1995). This modification is used less commonly in the United States (Peerschke, 2009). After incubation, the patient mixture and the control mixture are assayed for FVIII activity, and the percentage of residual FVIII activity is determined at each dilution by the ratio of patient mixture to control mixture. An arbitrary BU has been devised to quantify coagulation factor inhibitors determined by this method. Thus, in the case of FVIII, 1 BU is defined as the amount of patient plasma that destroys half the FVIII activity in the control plasma (Fig. 39-8). Therefore, patient plasma producing a residual FVIII activity of 50% is considered to contain 1 BU of inhibitor per milliliter. If this same plasma had been diluted tenfold before assaying for the inhibitor, then this result would indicate an inhibitor value of 10 BU/mL. This assay is sensitive, but at times is difficult to reproduce. A common observation is that varying dilutions of plasma may yield different estimates of the inhibitor titer. For assigning the level of BUs, the dilution that comes closest to the 50% residual factor is chosen for calculation of the FVIII inhibitor titer. Values on the standard curve should be read only at between 25% and 75% residual FVIII activity. If below 25%, higher dilutions of the sample are needed. If residual activity using the least diluted patient specimen is above 75%, a demonstrable inhibitor may not be present. It is in fact important for the laboratory to determine a lower limit of sensitivity for this assay, typically in the range of <0.4 to <0.6 BU, below which it reports lack of laboratory evidence for the presence of inhibitor. It is additionally of note that a plot made of residual FVIII activity versus increasing volume of original patient plasma in the Bethesda assay may distinguish between an inhibitor capable of reducing FVIII activity into the unmeasurable range (type I inhibitor) and an inhibitor that preserves some degree of residual FVIII activity, even at high inhibitor titer (type II inhibitor), presumably reflecting a target epitope at a less critical region of the FVIII molecule (Gawryl, 1982; Luna-Zaizar, 2009).

HEREDITARY DEFICIENCIES OF OTHER COAGULATION FACTORS

The other hereditary deficiencies of coagulation factors have autosomal inheritance (Table 39-5). With the exception of FXI deficiency, these disorders are very rare. However, they have a higher prevalence in areas where consanguineous marriage is practiced (Mannucci, 2004). In general,

TABLE 39-5
Characterization of Coagulation Factors and Their Deficiencies

Factor	Molecular weight, kDa	Gene location	Normal circulating half-life	Incidence	Inheritance	Bleeding severity
Fibrinogen	330	4q31.3–q32.1	2–4 days	1:1 million	Recessive	Mild–severe*
II	72	11p11.2	3–4 days	Very rare	Recessive	Mild–moderate
V	330	1q24.2	36 hours	1:1 million	Recessive	Moderate
V and VIII combined	–	LMAN1:18q21.32 MCFD2:2p21	36 hours for FV; 10–14 hours for FVIII	1:2 million	Recessive	Mild–moderate
VII	50	13q34	3–6 hours	1:500,000	Recessive	Mild–severe
VIII	330	Xq28	10–14 hours	1:10,000	Sex-linked	Mild–severe
IX	56	Xq27	18–24 hours	1:30,000	Sex-linked	Mild–severe
X	58	13q34	40–60 hours	1:500,000	Recessive	Mild–severe
XI	160	4q35.2	40–70 hours	Rare†	Recessive	Mild–moderate
XII	80	5q33-qter	50–70 days	Rare	Recessive	No bleeding
PK	88	4q33-q35	Not known	Very rare	Recessive	No bleeding
HK	120	3q27	9–10 hours	Extremely rare	Recessive	No bleeding
XIII	320	A:6p25.1 B:1q31.3	11–14 days	<1:1 million	Recessive	Moderate–severe

HK, High molecular weight kininogen; *PK,* prekallikrein.
*May be associated with thrombosis.
†Rare except in those of Ashkenazi Jewish descent.

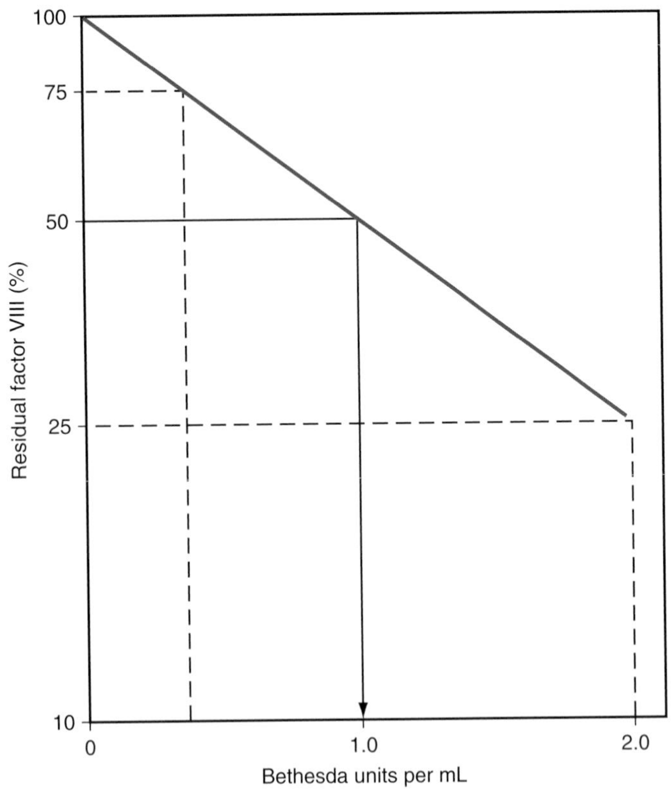

Figure 39-8 Expression of factor VIII inhibitor titer in Bethesda units. In this assay for an inhibitor to factor VIII, the percent residual factor VIII activity in normal plasma is determined after incubation with patient plasma. By convention, 1 international Bethesda unit of inhibitor is the amount of antibody that destroys 0.5 U factor VIII activity after 2 hours' incubation at 37° C. As shown in the figure, the percent residual factor VIII activity on a log scale is plotted against Bethesda units/mL in a linear scale. For a sample to be evaluable in this assay, the level of factor VIII activity should fall between 25% and 75%. Patient samples that produce residual factor VIII activity below 25% need to be diluted further so the 50% residual factor VIII activity point can be found. *(Redrawn with permission from Bockenstedt PL. Laboratory methods in hemostasis. In: Loscalzo J, Schafer AI, editors. Thrombosis and hemorrhage. 3rd ed. Philadelphia: Lippincott Williams & Wilkins; 2003, p. 370, Fig. 21-7.)*

most patients with coagulation protein deficiencies of factors VII, X, V, and II probably have partial defects because they have relatively mild bleeding disorders. Most coagulation-based assays have difficulty detecting these factors once their levels are below 5%–10%. In vivo, however, the presence of even this small level of coagulation factor can greatly influence bleeding risk. In contrast, findings with knockout mice indicate that a true null of each of these proteins is associated with virtually 100% mortality from hemorrhage before or at the time of birth. With hereditary factor deficiencies, heterozygous deficient individuals have approximately 50% (most commonly 30%–60%) of the normal level of the affected factor. The symptoms of these disorders are quite variable. Coagulation factor deficiencies may be suspected on the basis of symptoms, family history, or abnormal screening tests, and the laboratory confirms this diagnosis by specific factor assays. Once a specific protein deficiency is recognized, clinical history usually distinguishes a congenital from an acquired defect (see later).

Disorders With Prolonged APTT and Normal PT

Factor XI

Factor XI deficiency is common in Ashkenazi Jews, in whom heterozygote frequency is 8% (Asakai, 1991; Emsley, 2010). This ethnic population constitutes about 50% of the FXI-deficient patients seen in the United States. Most patients with FXI deficiency rarely have spontaneous hemorrhage. Bleeding typically occurs following injury or surgery, particularly involving areas of the body with high fibrinolytic activity (mouth, nose, genitourinary tract). Women can experience menorrhagia and postpartum hemorrhage. Bleeding can occur in heterozygotes and does not necessarily correlate with the residual FXI level (Leiba, 1965; Bolton-Maggs, 1988). However, the bleeding tendency may be modified by additional defects such as hemophilia, von Willebrand disease, and platelet function defects (Brenner, 1997). Diagnosis depends on determination of FXI activity below the reference range. Most widely used APTT reagents will have prolonged APTT results for patient samples with FXI activity below 20%–25% and mixed results when levels are 25%–60%. The lower limit of the normal range is probably between 60% and 70% (Bolton-Maggs, 1995). Therefore, a normal APTT does not rule out a mild FXI deficiency. In cases where marked elevation of FVIII may be present, the APTT can be normalized even when other factors are reduced (Lawrie, 1998). In all patients with FXI deficiency, preoperative management is critical to prevent bleeding complications. Patients with severe deficiency (FXI <10%–20%) should receive treatment with fresh frozen plasma to raise their FXI levels. Usually, replacement therapy of 20 mL/kg loading dose with a maintenance dose of 5–10 mL/kg every 24 hours is sufficient to cover patients with severe FXI deficiency through elective surgery (Kessler, 1996). Patients with levels from 20%–70% may bleed. A bleeding history and the nature of the proposed surgery will then guide management. The development of inhibitors to FXI in patients with FXI deficiency has been described, although these are rare (Salomon, 2003).

FXII, Prekallikrein, and High Molecular Weight Kininogen

As discussed previously, FXII, prekallikrein, and HK deficiencies are associated with prolonged PTT but are not associated with any bleeding risk. FXII deficiency is most common, occurring in all racial and ethnic backgrounds. It is associated with a very long PTT. Prekallikrein deficiency is less common but is seen in the United States in all ethnic groups. It is associated with a slightly prolonged APTT that corrects to normal when sitting on the bench for 1 hour at 37° C. HK deficiency is a rare disorder that also is associated with a very long APTT. These protein deficiencies are not associated with bleeding—a point emphasized diagrammatically in Figure 39-1 by graying of this portion of the coagulation "cascade." Because no replacement therapy for hemostasis is necessary for FXII, PK, or HK deficiency, it is important to recognize these defects to prevent unnecessary transfusion. Although deficiencies of FXII and HK have been associated with thrombosis risk, deletions of these proteins in mice are associated with delayed times to thrombosis in arterial thrombosis models (Renne, 2005; Merkoulov, 2008). When a deficiency in the proteins of the kallikrein/kinin system is suspected, a FXII assay should be performed first, because it is the most common.

Disorders With Prolonged APTT and PT

Observation of prolonged PT and APTT most commonly is due to general medical conditions described later under acquired disorders of blood coagulation. When hereditary disorders are considered, the following list, although much less common, should be considered.

Disorders of Fibrinogen

Fibrinogen deficiencies may prolong the PT and APTT if the plasma concentration of the protein is sufficiently low, usually less than 100 mg/dL. Afibrinogenemia is autosomal recessive and represents the total absence of fibrinogen. It results in a bleeding disorder of variable severity (Fried, 1980; Lak, 1999). Umbilical stump and mucosal bleeding are most common, as is an increased incidence of musculoskeletal and central nervous system bleeding. Patients also exhibit poor wound healing. Hypofibrinogenemia is a decreased level of normal fibrinogen and has a similar but milder pattern of bleeding. Both afibrinogenemia and hypofibrinogenemia are associated with recurrent miscarriage, as well as with antepartum and postpartum hemorrhage (Goodwin, 1989; Kobayashi, 2000). Paradoxically, reports have described thrombotic events in patients with afibrinogenemia (Chafa, 1995; Lak, 1999; Dupuy, 2001).

Dysfibrinogenemia is a qualitative fibrinogen deficiency characterized by the production of a dysfunctional fibrinogen (Miesbach, 2010). Most patients with congenital dysfibrinogenemia are heterozygous because of molecular defects in produced protein, although rare homozygous cases have been reported. Dysfibrinogenemias are most commonly acquired in association with liver disease. Acquired dysfibrinogenemias are most commonly due to posttranslational modifications of the fibrinogen protein as a result of synthesis in an abnormal liver. These defects are common in patients with hepatitis B and C. Patients with dysfibrinogenemia are usually asymptomatic or have mild bleeding, but in some cases, thrombosis has been reported, with or without a bleeding history (Hanss, 2001). The thrombin time and reptilase time, which measure clotting time during the conversion of fibrinogen into fibrin, are often prolonged in dysfibrinogenemia. When thrombin proteolyzes fibrinogen in the thrombin time, fibrinopeptides A and B are released from the Aα and Bβ chains of fibrinogen. Reptilase clots fibrinogen by liberating only fibrinopeptide A (Funk, 1971). Proteolysis of fibrinopeptide A from fibrinogen is sufficient to induce clot formation. Fibrinopeptide B liberation increases the rate of association of the fibrin monomers, but not the actual physiologic clot (Martinelli, 1980; Nawarawong, 1991). Bleeding risk is associated only with fibrinopeptide A release defects, not with fibrinopeptide B release defects. Therefore, a patient can have long PT and APTT from a fibrinopeptide B release defect and not have any bleeding risk, hence the reason for using both the thrombin time and reptilase time to assess dysfibrinogenemias. Assays that measure clottable fibrinogen will show lower levels than assays that measure fibrinogen antigen. A normal fibrinogen has a ratio of clottable fibrinogen activity to fibrinogen antigen greater than 95%. Ratios less than this raise the possibility of a dysfibrinogenemia. For many years, cryoprecipitate has served as a good source of fibrinogen when replacement is needed. A fibrinogen concentrate is now available for therapeutic administration both in Europe and in North America.

FII Deficiency

Prothrombin deficiency may be the rarest inherited coagulation factor deficiency (1 : 2,000,000) (Bolton-Maggs, 2004). A true prothrombin deficiency in the mouse is incompatible with life after birth (Sun, 1998). Hypoprothrombinemia (type I deficiency) manifests as a concomitant reduction in prothrombin activity and antigen levels. Bleeding symptoms include mucosal bleeding, hematomas, and hemarthrosis. Dysprothrombinemia (type II deficiency) presents with reduced activity and normal antigen levels. The clinical presentation of dysprothrombinemia is less predictable, and patients may be asymptomatic or may have only mild bleeding manifestations (Bolton-Maggs, 2004). Depending on the sensitivity of the reagents, both PT and APTT may be prolonged in prothrombin deficiency. However, a specific factor II assay is best if there is clinical suspicion or a positive family history in the presence of normal screening tests. A PT reagent-based prothrombin assay with factor-deficient plasma is most convenient. Prothrombin complex concentrates are the treatment of choice, although fresh frozen plasma can serve as an alternative source of prothrombin. Because the half-life of the protein is long, replacement every few days is typically sufficient.

FV Deficiency

Heterozygous FV deficiency is asymptomatic. Homozygous FV deficiency is rare (1 : 1,000,000), presenting in children with easy bruising and mucosal bleeding (Girolami, 1998; Lak, 1999). These individuals may well have some functional FV, considering that 50% of true null mice die at the time of development of the cardiovascular system (days 9–11), and the other half die at birth from hemorrhage (Cui, 1996). Hematomas and hemarthrosis may occur with injury but rarely spontaneously. It is associated with prolongation of both the APTT and PT (but a normal thrombin time) and is confirmed by a PT reagent-based, single-stage FV assay. Patients with FV deficiency should also have a FVIII assay performed to evaluate for combined deficiency of factors V and VIII (see later) (Nichols, 1998; Zhang, 2004). The only suitable replacement product available is fresh frozen plasma. It is interesting to note that human platelets contain 20% of total plasma FV and can also be a source of this protein for a bleeding state (Tracy, 1982). The replacement goal should be to elevate the FV level to at least 10%–15% (Peyvandi, 1999). Acquired inhibitors to FV are relatively common from the surgical use of topical bovine thrombin to aid incision hemostasis. Most cases are not severe, but the few encountered can be very serious and life-threatening owing to the lack of specific replacement therapy.

FX Deficiency

Heterozygous FX deficiency is asymptomatic. Homozygous FX deficiency is a severe bleeding disorder that presents in infancy. Symptoms include umbilical cord bleeding, mucosal bleeding, severe soft tissue hematomas, and hemarthroses (Peyvandi, 1998a). One-stage PT-based FX assays are sufficient for diagnosis, although additional assays are commercially available. As with all vitamin K–dependent clotting factors, it is important to exclude vitamin K deficiency or other acquired cause for the FX deficiency before the diagnosis of an inherited deficiency is made. For example, FX deficiency is the most common factor deficiency associated with primary amyloidosis, occurring in <10% of patients and probably due to adsorption of FX onto amyloid fibrils (Uprichard, 2002). Current therapy for factor X deficiency includes prothrombin complex concentrates, although recombinant FVIIa has been used successfully to treat FX deficiency associated with amyloidosis (Boggio, 2001).

Combined Deficiency of FV and FVIII

Combined FV and FVIII deficiency is a rare autosomal recessive disorder that results from a single gene defect rather than from coinheritance of defects in both FV and FVIII genes. Patients typically have FV and FVIII levels between 5% and 30%. In two thirds of patients, this results from null expression of LMAN1 (previously known as ERGIC-53) (Nichols, 1998). LMAN1 shuttles between the endoplasmic reticulum and the Golgi and is believed to facilitate protein trafficking through the secretion pathway (Zhang, 2003). Other patients have a mutation of *MCFD2*, which directly interacts with LMAN1 (Zhang, 2003). Bleeding manifestations include epistaxis, easy bruising, menorrhagia, and postpartum hemorrhage, as well as bleeding following surgery, dental extraction, and trauma (Seligsohn, 1982; Peyvandi, 1998b). Testing usually demonstrates disproportionate prolongation of the PTT compared with the PT. Replacement therapy includes both FVIII concentrates and fresh frozen plasma (as a source of FV).

Combined Deficiency of Vitamin K–Dependent Clotting Factors

Vitamin K–dependent clotting factor deficiency affecting multiple vitamin K–dependent coagulation factors (II, VII, IX, and X) occurs with vitamin K deficiency and hepatic dysfunction, but it also results from heritable dysfunction of hepatic enzyme γ-glutamyl carboxylase (type I) or the vitamin K epoxide reductase enzyme complex (type II) (Brenner, 1998; Zhang, 2004). Severely affected individuals may present as neonates with umbilical stump bleeding or spontaneous intracranial hemorrhage; in infancy or early childhood with hemarthroses, soft tissue hematomas, or gastrointestinal hemorrhages; or as adults with easy bruising, mucosal bleeding, and bleeding following surgery. Diagnosis is established by prolongation of both the APTT and PT and associated reductions in levels of vitamin K–dependent clotting factors. These patients may respond to vitamin K (oral or parenteral) with normalization of the APTT, PT, and factor levels, as well as resolution of bleeding symptoms. This fact makes the establishment of a diagnosis of an inherited abnormality difficult, in that other acquired causes of vitamin K deficiency (hemorrhagic disease of the newborn, liver disease, and prolonged use of broad-spectrum antibiotics) or factitious warfarin administration could present similarly. For patients who do not respond fully to vitamin K administration, fresh frozen plasma can be used for acute bleeding or surgery.

Disorders With Normal APTT and Prolonged PT

FVII Deficiency

FVII deficiency is common compared with the other rare hereditary coagulation factor deficiencies (Mariani, 2009). The bleeding manifestations are variable, with epistaxis, mucosal bleeding, and menorrhagia commonly reported (Peyvandi, 1997). Severe FVII deficiency is autosomal recessive, often presenting shortly after birth, and may have dramatic presentation with intracranial hemorrhage in 15%–60% of cases (Ragni, 1981). The diagnosis is suspected with the finding of isolated prolongation of the PT. However, FVII, a vitamin K–dependent clotting factor, is low in the newborn period and will also be low in the presence of vitamin K deficiency. Therefore, reevaluation of infants with mild deficiencies is required after they reach a few months of age, or after vitamin K replacement in older patients. Functional FVII activity is measured by a PT-based, FVII-deficient plasma clotting assay. The use of recombinant human thromboplastin will yield results that are more likely to reflect in vivo FVII levels. Samples for FVII testing should not be stored at 4° C, as this can lead to cold activation of FVII as result of C1 inhibitor inactivation and FXIIa formation in the tube with FVII activation (Kitchen, 1992). Cold activation of FVII results in an overestimation of the actual plasma FVII level. Therapeutic options include fresh frozen plasma, prothrombin complex concentrates, and recombinant FVIIa. For major surgery, plasma FVII levels of at least 20% are sufficient (Bolton-Maggs, 2004).

Disorders With Normal APTT and PT

FXIII Deficiency

FXIII stabilizes the clot after a fibrin clot has formed (Hsieh, 2008). Therefore, the PT and APTT will be normal even with a severe FXIII deficiency. Testing for FXIII deficiency is suggested for individuals with a positive bleeding history, particularly with features such as delayed bleeding, umbilical stump bleeding, or miscarriage, in which the PT and APTT are normal (Anwar, 1999). Thirty percent of severely FXIII-deficient patients die in middle age from spontaneous intracerebral hemorrhage unless they are receiving prophylactic therapy (Lorand, 1980). The diagnosis of severe FXIII deficiency (<5% activity) can be confirmed with the 5M urea clot solubility test or a chromogenic assay. Clots formed with normal FXIII activity remain stable in 5M urea, whereas clots from FXIII-deficient patients dissolve in urea. The reason for this is that FXIIIa initiates the formation of a new intermolecular γ-glutamyl–ε-lysine bridge between fibrin molecules (Lorand, 1980). This new interaction augments the mechanical rigidity of the clot structure and increases its resistance to lysis. The urea clot solubility assay is simple to perform but is sensitive only to very low levels of FXIII. More robust quantitative activity assays are based on cross-linking of glycine–ethyl ester into a specific peptide (Fickenscher, 1991), incorporation of an amine substrate into fibrinogen (Kohler, 1998), or incorporation of a biotinylated peptide to spermine attached to microtiter plates (Hitomi, 2009). Acquired deficiency of FXIII has been described in a variety of diseases, including Henoch-Schönlein purpura, isoniazid treatment for tuberculosis, various forms of colitis, erosive gastritis, and some forms of leukemia (Board, 1993), although FXIII level determination and therapeutic management are controversial. Because the half-life of FXIII is very long, replacement with fresh frozen plasma is usually sufficient for most patients. FXIII concentrates and recombinant FXIII are currently being evaluated in clinical trials (Lusher, 2010).

Hereditary Hemorrhagic Disorders of Fibrinolysis

Hereditary bleeding disorders resulting from excessive fibrinolysis are rare. Deficiency of α_2-antiplasmin has been reported in a few families with a bleeding tendency (Fay, 1992; Aoki, 1980). Although not recommended for routine use as a screening assay, the whole blood clot lysis time can be helpful as a first-order test to detect deficiencies of α_2-antiplasmin. In brief, whole blood is allowed to clot; following this, the time to clot lysis is recorded. In normal individuals, the presence of α_2-antiplasmin effectively prevents lysis from occurring in this in vitro setting, even 24 hours after initial clot formation. In contrast, in the presence of a severe deficiency of α_2-antiplasmin or in some fibrinolytic states, clot lysis can be observed after several hours. In such instances, follow-up testing specific for α_2-antiplasmin activity should be employed. Acquired α_2-antiplasmin deficiency commonly occurs in acute leukemia (Schwartz, 1986; Okajima, 1994). Also, plasma can be admixed with dilute acid to precipitate a fraction relatively rich in plasminogen activator, plasminogen, and fibrinogen but relatively poor in antiplasmins. This **euglobulin** fraction is then redissolved in buffer and clotted by recalcification, and the time for clot lysis is then measured. Euglobulin clot lysis is normally complete in 2–5 hours, but the time may be shortened with increased fibrinolysis associated with increased plasminogen activator activity. Plasminogen activator, plasminogen, and plasminogen activator inhibitor may be assayed directly.

Acquired Coagulation Disorders

Acquired bleeding disorders are due to anticoagulation, disseminated intravascular coagulation (DIC), liver disease, vitamin K deficiency, massive transfusion, and unique inhibitors to coagulation proteins. The topic of anticoagulation is addressed extensively in Chapter 42. In general, prolongations of the PT and APTT arising in a patient should raise the possibility, as discussed in the following sections, of anticoagulants, DIC, liver disease, vitamin K deficiency, and massive transfusion. Only after these clinical states have been excluded should attention be directed to specific protein defects influencing the PT and PTT.

THROMBOTIC DISORDERS AND DISSEMINATED INTRAVASCULAR COAGULATION

Risk factors underlying the development of thrombosis are discussed in detail in Chapter 41. Regardless of origin, however, the formation of a fibrin clot, cross-linking of that clot, and subsequent lysis of that clot by the fibrinolytic system are central features of the process.

DIC is a clinicopathologic condition in which activation of the coagulation and fibrinolysis systems results in the simultaneous formation of thrombin and plasmin with consumption of coagulation factors and inhibitors of the system, resulting in the clinical laboratory phenotype of prolonged PT, APTT, and thrombocytopenia. It arises in patients with sepsis, malignancy, obstetric complications, or massive tissue injury (Schmaier, 1991). DIC can arise during surgery as a result of the release of thromboplastic material within the tissue. In circulatory arrest operations on the arch of the aorta or the main pulmonary arteries, DIC is a frequent complication related to chilling of the patient and tissue destruction. Abruptio placentae and placenta previa are associated with acute hemorrhagic DIC, whereas retained dead fetus is associated with a DIC that is not hemorrhagic but prothrombotic. DIC due to sepsis can also occur in the postoperative period. DIC with sepsis is most commonly seen with gram-negative infection but can occur with gram-positive infection and in the immunosuppressed patient with fungemia. The balance between thrombin and plasmin formation in the individual patient clinically translates into a prothrombotic versus hemorrhagic state, respectively.

The diagnosis of DIC depends on appropriate clinical test results in the correct clinical setting. The finding of a prolonged PT and APTT with reduced fibrinogen and platelet count is highly suspicious for DIC in the hospitalized patient until proven otherwise (Colman, 1972). This clinical laboratory phenotype of DIC most probably results from a hyperfibrinolytic state and is the form of DIC most commonly recognized. A prothrombotic state as the result of DIC is usually associated with normal PT and APTT with mildly reduced platelet count and normal or elevated fibrinogen. The diagnosis of DIC is made by using a confirmatory test that shows the simultaneous presence of thrombin and plasmin formation. Currently, the D-dimer assay is the confirmatory test that, if positive, shows that both thrombin and plasmin have been formed. The D-dimer measures plasmin-cleaved, insoluble, cross-linked fibrin that originally arose from thrombin cleavage of fibrinogen (see Figs. 39-2 and 39-4, *B*). The D-dimer can be performed by immunonephelometric assay or by latex agglutination assay, and results can be obtained rapidly, facilitating the use of this test in clinical decision-making (Reber, 2009). As would be anticipated, the D-dimer is elevated in a wide variety of thrombotic conditions, including DIC (Koracevic, 2009). By careful establishment of a cutoff value, the D-dimer may be judiciously used in concert with clinical findings as a negative predictive test to exclude deep vein thrombosis or pulmonary embolism (Ceriani, 2010). The level of D-dimer may decrease in response to anticoagulation. In the past, fibrin degradation (split) products (FDPs) were used to recognize DIC (see Fig. 39-4, *A*). However, depending on the specificity of epitopes recognized by antibodies employed in the particular test systems, FDP may variably represent plasmin-cleaved fibrinogen, soluble fibrin, or insoluble fibrin. The finding of increased FDPs accordingly does not necessarily translate into a measure of plasmin-cleaved, insoluble, cross-linked fibrin equivalent to that obtained with the D-dimer assay. Fibrin monomer is the large molecular mass protein of fibrinogen that remains after fibrinopeptides A and B are liberated. It can be elevated in DIC, but if DIC is severe, it may be absent. Thus, it is an unreliable assay for use in recognizing DIC. A scoring system that combines in a quantitative fashion the results of four commonly employed laboratory tests that may be helpful, in the appropriate clinical setting, to evaluate the likelihood of DIC is presented in Table 39-6 (Levi, 2009).

LIVER DISEASE

It is important for liver disease to be recognized in patients because most coagulation factors are synthesized in the liver. Thus, patients with liver disease will have increased risk of bleeding. Patients with serious liver disease will have a prolonged PT and APTT. Not only is the synthesis of these proteins reduced, but the proteins made are at times abnormal, functioning as inhibitors of normal coagulation proteins. For example, abnormal fibrinogens (dysfibrinogenemias) are very common in patients with liver disease. As already mentioned, if these proteins have defects in fibrinopeptide A or B release, the thrombin time will be abnormal; the reptilase time is abnormal only in fibrinopeptide A release defects. Overall, abnormal fibrinogens can be appreciated by an abnormal ratio of clottable fibrinogen (an activity measure) to fibrinogen antigen (measured by radial immunodiffusion or another immunoassay). Finding less activity in relation to the mass of the protein is characteristic of an abnormal molecule. Similarly, all vitamin K–dependent proteins (factors II, VII, IX, and X and proteins C, S, and Z) are decreased in liver disease. These proteins may have abnormal γ-carboxylation reactions of the glutamic acid residues within their amino-terminal portion, thus producing reduced factor activity with relatively higher levels of that factor's antigen (see next section). In general, PK is one of the first proteins, and fibrinogen one of the last proteins, to be decreased in liver disease. Factors VIII and V become absent in the anhepatic stage of liver transplantation, but FVIII is elevated in patients with inflammatory hepatocellular disease. Moreover, antithrombin and other serpin plasma protein inhibitors are also decreased in liver disease.

TABLE 39-6
ISTH Diagnostic Scoring System for DIC

Risk assessment: Does the patient have an underlying disorder known to be associated with overt DIC?
- If yes, proceed.
- If not, do not use this algorithm.

Order global coagulation tests (PT, platelet count, fibrinogen, D-dimer)

Score the test results:
- Platelet count (>100 k/μL = 0, <100 k/μL = 1, <50 k/μL = 2)
- Elevated D-dimer (<0.4 μg/mL = 0, 0.4–4.0 μg/mL = 2, >4.0 μg/mL = 3)
- Prolonged PT (<3 sec = 0, >3 sec but <6 sec = 1, >6 sec = 2)
- Fibrinogen level (>100 mg/dL = 0, <100 mg/dL = 1)

Calculate score:
- If ≥5, compatible with overt DIC: Repeat score daily.
- If <5, suggestive (not affirmative) for nonovert DIC: Repeat next 1–2 days.

DIC, Disseminated intravascular coagulation; *ISTH,* International Society on Thrombosis and Haemostasis; *PT,* prothrombin time.
Note that in this example of score implementation, a D-dimer test having an upper normal limit of 0.4 μg/mL was employed. More generally, for the particular analyte employed as an "elevated fibrin marker," no increase = 0, moderate increase = 2, and strong increase = 3.

VITAMIN K DEFICIENCY

Vitamin K, a lipid-soluble vitamin, is provided by dietary intake of leafy green vegetables and by synthesis of intestinal flora. In clinical medicine, vitamin K deficiency is seen most often in the very ill patient on antibiotics who has subsisted on parenteral nutrition. Not infrequently, intravenous fluids are not supplemented with vitamin K. After 4–6 weeks of parenteral nutrition and antibiotic treatment, the patient becomes vitamin K–deficient. Vitamin K deficiency can also be seen in patients who have anatomic bypass of the small intestine, malabsorption, biliary tract obstruction, and, rarely, reduced dietary intake. For example, alcoholics are often vitamin K–deficient. Warfarin also inhibits the enzymatic pathway necessary for vitamin K utilization (see Fig. 42-1 in Chapter 42). Vitamin K has a critical role in the γ-carboxylation reaction of a number of glutamic acid residues within coagulation factors II, VII, IX, and X and proteins C, S, and Z. This γ-carboxylation is critical for the proteins to bind to cells and phospholipids, so that they can participate in physiologic coagulation reactions. Thus patients will have reduced clottable factor levels for the vitamin K–dependent factors II, VII, IX, and X. If antigen levels of these patients are measured, they will frequently be higher. In general, patients with a therapeutic level of warfarin (i.e., an INR between 2 and 3) have ≈5%–15% clottable factor activities, whereas their antigen factor levels are in the range of 25%–40%.

MASSIVE TRANSFUSION

Massive transfusion has been defined as the replacement of more than 1.5 blood volume in 24 hours. For example, in a 70-kg man, 7% of body weight, or 4.9 kg or L, is the blood volume (≈16–19 units, assuming that a unit of blood is 250–300 mL). Hemostatic failure can result from dilution of clotting factors, DIC, or acquired platelet dysfunction. Dilutional coagulopathy results from replacement with packed red blood cells and normal saline and lack of clotting factors or platelets. Tests of hemostasis typically show prolongation of the PT and APTT, reduced fibrinogen, and thrombocytopenia (Leslie, 1991). Additionally, in the massively transfused patient, an anticoagulant effect is seen as well, resulting from citrate in the transfused blood products.

ACQUIRED COAGULATION PROTEIN INHIBITORS AND LUPUS ANTICOAGULANT

Acquired inhibitors to coagulation proteins occur and, in some cases, increase the risk of bleeding. The clinical laboratory phenotype of these patients depends on the protein toward which the coagulation protein inhibitor is directed. The most common severe acquired coagulation protein inhibitor is that against FVIII. These patients present with bleeding and a long APTT. Characteristically, one sees this inhibitor in elderly patients, patients with B-cell malignancies, patients with connective tissue disorders such as systemic lupus erythematosus, and postpartum patients. These patients are managed acutely with high-dose FVIII, activated vitamin K–dependent coagulation factor concentrates, or rVIIa, but long term, management may require immunosuppression with Cytoxan, prednisone, or rituximab (Lian, 1989; Aggarwal, 2005). Management decisions in these patients are influenced by the severity of bleeding and by the titer of the inhibitor to FVIII, as determined by the Bethesda assay.

Acquired deficiencies or inhibitors are also seen in a number of medical conditions. Systemic amyloidosis is associated with decreases in plasma factor X or IX as a result of adsorption of the coagulation proteins onto the amyloid protein (McPherson, 1977; Furie, 1981; Mumford, 2000;

Thompson, 2010). In the case of factor X, the PT and APTT may be affected; in the case of factor IX, only the APTT. Hypergammaglobulinemic states seen with multiple myeloma or Waldenström's macroglobulinemia (IgM) can be associated with pan-inhibitors to coagulation protein function (Glaspy, 1992). Dysfibrinogenemias are also common in these patients.

The last type of inhibitor seen is the lupus anticoagulant or antiphospholipid antibody that influences coagulation protein reactions. Briefly, these inhibitors are antibodies directed to epitopes of proteins bound to phospholipids (Lafer, 1981; Levine, 2002). Lupus anticoagulants variably interfere with the APTT and, less commonly, with the PT. The degree of interference depends on the nature of the commercial reagent. Paradoxically, unless these patients have additionally developed an inhibitor against a specific coagulation factor, they are not at bleeding risk; rather, they may be at risk for thrombosis, which at times can be a vicious prothrombotic state (Mueh, 1980; Rand, 2003). Antiphospholipid antibodies may also interfere with several anticoagulation mechanisms such as annexin V, thus enhancing prothrombinase on endothelial cells and prostacyclin production from endothelial cells. For a more detailed discussion of lupus anticoagulants and the antiphosopholipid syndrome, see Chapter 41.

SELECTED REFERENCES

Adcock DM, Kressin DC, Marlar RA. Effect of 3.2% vs 3.8% sodium citrate concentration on routine coagulation testing. Am J Clin Pathol 1997;107:105–10.
Important paper that justifies the use of 3.2 g% sodium citrate as the anticoagulation standard for collection of samples for clinical coagulation testing.

Brandt JT, Triplett DA, Alving B, et al. Criteria for the diagnosis of lupus anticoagulant: an update. Thromb Haemost 1995a;74:1185–90.
Important paper that begins to define criteria for making the diagnosis of a lupus anticoagulant.

Chang SH, Tillema V, Scherr D. A percent correction formula for evaluation of mixing studies. Am J Clin Pathol 2002;117:62–73.
Helpful paper that begins to provide some evidence-based laboratory medicine on how screening mixing studies should be performed.

Colman RW, Robboy SJ, Minna JD. Disseminated intravascular coagulation (DIC): an approach. Am J Med 1972;52:679–89.
Classic paper on disseminated intravascular coagulation.

Gailiani D, Broze G. Factor XI activation in a revised model of blood coagulation. Science 1991;253: 909–12.
Classic paper that presents for the first time the modern view of assembly and interaction of proteins of the coagulation system.

Levine JS, Branch W, Rauch J. The antiphospholipid syndrome. N Engl J Med 2002;346:752–63.
Important paper that presents criteria for diagnosis of the antiphospholipid antibody syndrome.

Marder VJ, Budzynski AZ, Barlow GH. Comparison of the physio-chemical properties of fragment D derivatives of fibrinogen and fragment D-D of cross-linked fibrin. Biochim Biophys Acta 1976;427:1–14.
Classic paper describing the D-dimer.

Proctor RR, Rapaport SI. The partial thromboplastin time with kaolin: a simple screening test for first stage plasma clotting factor deficiencies. Am J Clin Pathol 1961;36:212–9.
Description of activated partial thromboplastin time.

Quick AJ, Stanley-Brown M, Bancroft FW. A study of the coagulation defect in hemophilia and in jaundice. Am J Med Sci 1935;190:501–11.
Description of prothrombin time.

Shariat-Madar Z, Mahdi F, Schmaier AH. Identification and characterization of prolylcarboxypeptidase as an endothelial cell prekallikrein activator. J Biol Chem 2002;277:17962–9.
Paper that identifies a physiologic activator of the plasma kallikrein/kinin system, the so-called contact activation system.

REFERENCES

Access the complete reference list online at http://www.expertconsult.com

CHAPTER 40

BLOOD PLATELETS AND VON WILLEBRAND DISEASE

Jonathan L. Miller, A. Koneti Rao

PART 5

KEY POINTS

- Platelets are highly complex cells that participate in critical steps central to hemostasis and thrombosis, including adhesion to subendothelium, secretion of granule contents, aggregation, and provision of membrane surface for activation of coagulation factors.
- Abnormalities of platelet number or of platelet function can play an important role in the balance of hemostasis and thrombosis.
- Almost unique to laboratory medicine and pathology, platelet pathology may be assessed in real time upon living cells obtained from the patient.
- von Willebrand factor is a multimeric protein synthesized by endothelial cells and megakaryocytes that plays a central role in platelet adhesive interactions.
- Platelet counts and platelet function are affected by a number of acquired disorders and autoimmune processes and by numerous drugs.

NORMAL PLATELET BIOLOGY

PLATELET STRUCTURE

Blood platelets are highly complex, anucleate cells that derive from bone marrow megakaryocytes. A well-prepared peripheral blood film offers the opportunity for evaluation of platelet number, size, distribution, and structure under the light microscope. Although subtle abnormalities of platelet structure usually require electron microscopy, gross absence or asymmetry of granules and grossly aberrant platelet surfaces may be evident. In films from nonanticoagulated fingerstick specimens, some platelet clumping is an expected feature. In instances of observed abnormalities, artifacts resulting from improper specimen collection or handling should always be considered, and a repeat specimen should be obtained if a satisfactory explanation for the abnormality is not apparent.

In cases of suspected platelet structural abnormalities, electron microscopy allows much more precise characterization of the defect (White, 2004) with the opportunity to examine in great detail each of the specific organelles within the platelet (Clauser, 2009). It is essential that established

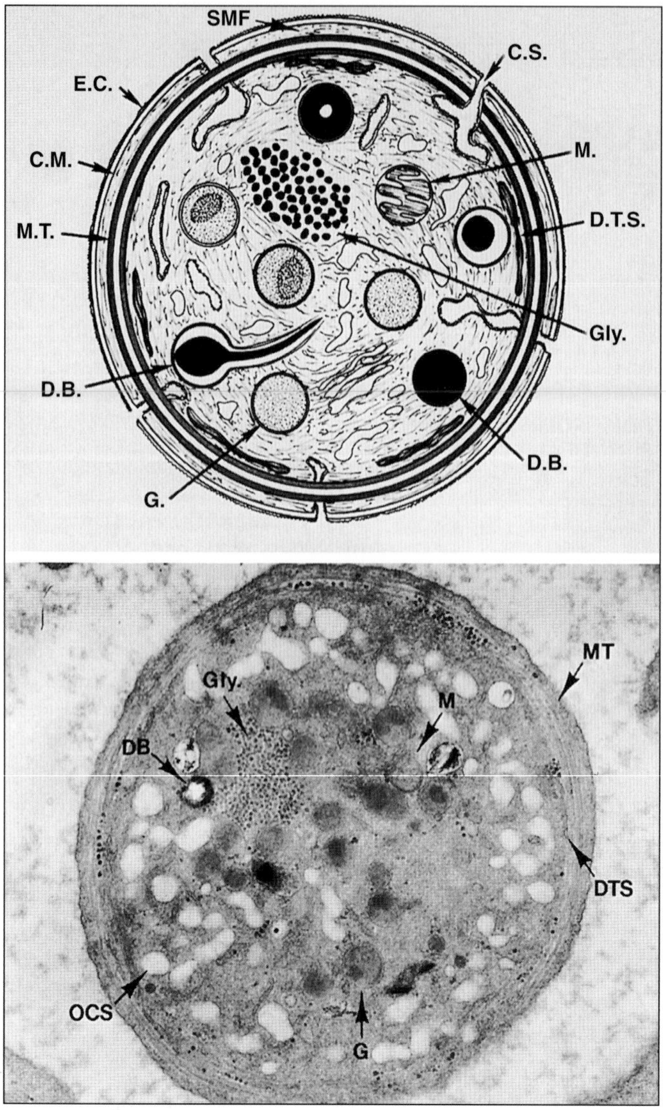

Figure 40-1 Discoid platelets. The diagram summarizes ultrastructural features observed in thin sections of discoid platelets cut in the equatorial plane. Components of the peripheral zone include the exterior coat (EC), the trilaminar unit membrane (CM), and the submembrane area containing specialized filaments (SMFs) that form the wall of the platelet and line channels of the surface-connected canalicular system (also referred to as the open canalicular system, or OCS). The matrix of the platelet interior is the sol-gel zone containing actin microfilaments, structural filaments, the circumferential band of microtubules (MTs), and glycogen (Gly). Formed elements embedded in the sol-gel zone include mitochondria (M), granules (G), and dense bodies (DBs). Collectively, they constitute the organelle zone. The membrane systems include the OCS and the dense tubular system (DTS), which serve as the platelet sarcoplasmic reticulum. The electron micrograph shows a platelet sectioned in the equatorial plane (×30,000) which reveals most of the structures indicated on the diagram. *(With permission from White JG, Bloom AL, Forbes CD, Thomas DP, Tuddenham EGD, editors. Hemostasis and thrombosis. New York: Churchill Livingstone; 1994.)*

protocols for the collection and processing of platelet specimens for ultrastructural study be followed meticulously to avoid attributing changes that occur because of inadvertent in vitro activation to abnormalities truly characteristic of platelets in vivo.

Normal features of the platelet that may be visualized ultrastructurally are shown in Figure 40-1. The outer surface of the platelet, the **glycocalyx,** is rich in glycoproteins. A submembranous band of **microtubules,** composed of the protein tubulin, provides structural support for the normally discoid cell. Contractile **microfilaments** may also be seen. These are composed principally of platelet actin and platelet myosin. An extensive **open canalicular system** within the platelet has been demonstrated by a variety of methods to be in direct communication with the extracellular environment. Often seen in close proximity to the open canalicular system is the **dense tubular system.** This system, apparently derived from the smooth endoplasmic reticulum, shows positive staining for platelet peroxidase activity (Breton-Gorius, 1972), in accord with its role as a site for arachidonic acid metabolism within the platelet. The dense tubular system also functions as a calcium-sequestering pump, providing low levels of cytoplasmic calcium within the resting platelet.

A variety of inclusions may be recognized within the platelet cytoplasm. Both **mitochondria** and **glycogen** may be identified. Lighter staining **α-granules,** less frequent **dense core** (or "bull's eye") **granules, lysosomes,** and **peroxisomes** may also be seen. The α-granules contain a number of different proteins, including platelet fibrinogen, platelet-derived growth factor (PDGF), von Willebrand factor (vWF), the factor V binding protein multimerin (Hayward, 1991, 1993), P-selectin (Stenberg, 1985; Berman, 1986), β-thromboglobulin (βTG), and the heparin-neutralizing platelet factor (PF)4. Dense core granules are known to be the locus of stored, nonmetabolic pools of adenosine diphosphate (ADP), adenosine triphosphate (ATP), 5-hydroxytryptamine, and calcium.

PLATELET MEMBRANE GLYCOPROTEINS AND PHOSPHOLIPIDS

Detailed study of the platelet membrane glycoproteins has led to an improved understanding of platelet function. Radioactive and biotin labeling (Fabris, 1992; Solum, 1995; Sachs, 2000) of surface glycoproteins and electrophoretic separation of solubilized proteins on polyacrylamide gels have permitted assessment of various platelet glycoproteins. In fact, application of this method to the platelets of patients with congenital bleeding disorders led to the discovery that some of these disorders were due to an absence of critical membrane glycoproteins, and that several major platelet glycoproteins existed as multichain complexes. A summary of platelet membrane glycoproteins that function as receptors for adhesive ligands is included in Table 40-1. Quantitatively, the glycoprotein (GP)IIb/IIIa receptor complex (also referred to as αIIbβ3) consists of two distinct proteins and dominates, with approximately 50,000 copies per platelet, followed by the GPIb/IX receptor complex at approximately 25,000 copies per platelet. (Note that this receptor complex may also be referred to as GPIb/IX/V or GPIb/V/IX, because GPV forms a tight, noncovalent association with GPIb and GPIX.) The copy number for other GP complexes is much lower.

Platelet membranes contain several phospholipids, including phosphatidylinositol, phosphatidylcholine, phosphatidylserine (PS), and phosphatidylethanolamine, that play a major role in platelet function. Phosphatidylinositides are the source of signaling molecules inositol trisphosphate and diacylglycerol that are produced following platelet activation. Negatively charged PS is expressed in the inner membrane leaflet of the resting platelet (Fig. 40-2) (Zwaal, 2005); on platelet activation, PS translocates to the outer leaflet—an essential step in the formation of a procoagulant platelet surface that is critical in several blood coagulation mechanisms (Solum, 1999). This activation-associated change in PS exposure can be assessed using flow cytometry as increased binding of annexin V to the platelet surface.

ROLE OF PLATELETS IN HEMOSTASIS AND PLATELET ACTIVATION MECHANISMS

Following injury to the blood vessel, platelets adhere to exposed subendothelium by a process (adhesion) which involves the interaction of a plasma protein, vWF, and a specific glycoprotein complex on the platelet surface, glycoprotein Ib-IX-V (GPIb-V-IX) (Fig. 40-3), which binds vWF, particularly under conditions of high shear stress. Adhesion is followed by recruitment of additional platelets, which interact with each other to form clumps in a process called aggregation. This involves binding of fibrinogen to specific platelet surface receptors—a complex comprising glycoproteins IIb/IIIa (GPIIb/IIIa, integrin αIIβ3). GPIIb/IIIa is platelet- and megakaryocyte-specific and has the ability to bind vWF as well. Resting platelets do not bind fibrinogen. Platelet activation induces a conformational change in the GPIIb/IIIa complex, which leads to fibrinogen binding, a prerequisite for aggregation. Activated platelets release contents of their granules (secretion or release reaction) such as ADP and serotonin from the dense granules, which cause recruitment of additional platelets. In addition, platelets play a major role in coagulation mechanisms; several key enzymatic reactions occur on the platelet membrane lipoprotein surface. During platelet activation, the negatively charged phospholipids, especially PS, become exposed on the platelet surface; this is essential for the role of platelets in accelerating specific coagulation reactions by

TABLE 40-1
Adhesive Platelet Membrane Glycoproteins

	Alternate designation	Molecular weight (reduced)* α-subunit, kDa	β-Subunit	Gene family	Ligand	Function	Glycoprotein expression†
GPIIb/IIIa	αIIbβ3, CD41/CD61	125, 23	110 kDa	Integrin	Fibr, vWF, FN, VN	Aggregation Adhesion	C, S
Vitronectin receptor	αvβ3, CD51/CD61	135, 25	110 kDa	Integrin	VN, vWF, fibr	Adhesion	C
GPIc/IIa	α5β1, VLA-5, CD49e/CD29	135, 27	130 Da	Integrin	FN, laminin	Adhesion	C
α6/IIa	α6β1, VLA-6, CD49/CD29	125	130 kDa	Integrin	Laminin	Adhesion	C
GPIa/IIa	α2β1, CD49b/CD29	167	130 kDa	Integrin	Collagen	Adhesion	C
GPIb/IX	CD42 A–C complex	145, 24	17 kDa	Leucine-rich glycoprotein	vWF, THR	Adhesion	C
P-Selectin	GMP 140, PADGEM, CD-62	140		Selectin	PSGL-1, O-linked carbohydrate	Platelet–leukocyte interactions	S
PECAM-1	CD31	130		Immunoglobulin		Platelet–endothelial cell interactions	C
GPIV	GPIIIb, CD36	88			TSP, Collagen	Adhesion	C
GPVI		61			Collagen	Signaling	C
PETA-3		27		Tetraspan		?Aggregation	C

Modified with permission and updated from Peerschke EIB, Lopez JA. Platelet membranes and receptors. In: Loscalzo J, Schafer AI, editors. Thrombosis and hemorrhage. 2nd ed. Baltimore: Williams & Wilkins; 1998, p. 253.
fibr, Fibrinogen; *FN,* fibronectin; *GMP,* guanosine monophosphate; *PADGEM,* platelet activation–dependent granule–external membrane protein; *PECAM,* platelet endothelial cell adhesion molecule; *PETA-3,* platelet–endothelial cell tetraspan antigen-3; *PSGL-1,* P-selectin–glycoprotein ligand-1; *THR,* thrombin; *TSP,* thrombospondin; *VN,* vitronectin; *vWF,* von Willebrand factor.
*Numbers separated by commas represent the molecular weight of disulfide-linked α- and β-chains of the respective receptor α- or β-subunit.
†C, Constitutive expression; S, membrane expression requires platelet stimulation.

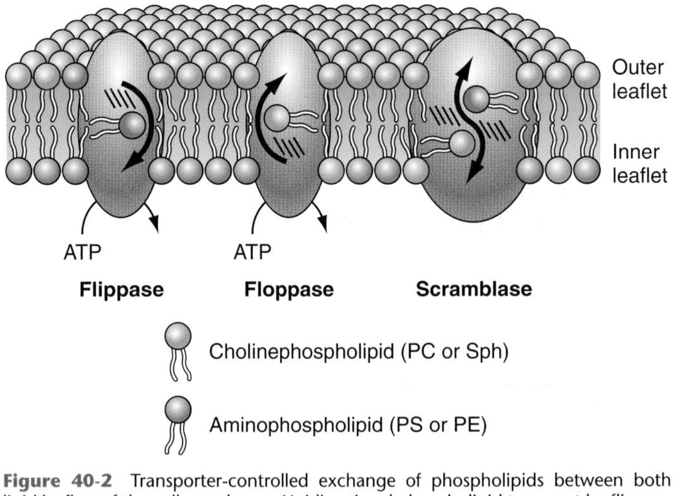

Figure 40-2 Transporter-controlled exchange of phospholipids between both lipid leaflets of the cell membrane. Unidirectional phospholipid transport by flippase is directed inward, whereas floppase promotes outward-directed transport. Both transporters are adenosine triphosphate (ATP) dependent and frequently move phospholipids against their respective concentration gradients. For example, aminophospholipid translocase (flippase) rapidly shuttles PS and PE from outer to inner leaflet, while ABCC1 (floppase) moves both cholinephospholipids and aminophospholipids more slowly toward the outer leaflet. The concerted action of both transporters is thought to create a dynamic asymmetrical steady state, in which the outer monolayer is rich in cholinephospholipids, whereas aminophospholipids predominantly occupy the inner leaflet. Bidirectional phospholipid transport is catalyzed by a scramblase, activation of which may occur following Ca^{++} influx or when cells go into apoptosis. Because scramblase activity moves all major phospholipid classes back and forth between the two leaflets, it promotes the collapse of membrane phospholipid asymmetry, with appearance of PS at the cells' outer surface. *(Modified with permission from Zwaal RF, Comfurius P, Bevers EM. Surface exposure of phosphatidylserine in pathological cells. Cell Mol Life Sci 2005;62:971–8.)* *PC,* Phosphatidyl choline; *PE,* phosphatidyl ethanolamine; *PS,* phosphatidyl serine; *Sph,* sphingosine.

promoting the binding of vitamin K–dependent factors (platelet coagulant activity). These events involving platelets are discussed in greater detail later.

Platelet Activation and Signaling Events

(see Fig. 40-3).

A number of physiologic agonists interact with specific receptors on the platelet surface to induce numerous events that culminate in well-recognized responses, including change in platelet shape from discoid to spherical (shape change), aggregation, secretion, and thromboxane A_2 (TxA_2) production (Shattil, 2004; Smyth, 2010). These agonists include ADP, collagen, thrombin, TxA_2, epinephrine, and platelet-activating factor, and they induce signaling events in platelets. Platelets possess at least three well-defined purinergic receptors that mediate responses to ADP: P2Y1, P2Y12, and P2X1. The P2Y1 receptor mediates the rise in cytoplasmic Ca^{++}. The P2Y12 receptor mediates inhibition of adenylyl cyclase to lower cyclic adenosine monophosphate levels in platelets and is the receptor targeted by the thienopyridine group of antiplatelet agents, including clopidogrel, ticlopidine, and prasugrel. A possible role in amplifying the initial phase of a platelet activation event is presently the subject of investigation of P2X1, which has attributes of an ion channel (Hu, 2010).

Thrombin induces platelet responses through interaction with protease-activated receptors (PARs); human platelets possess PAR1 and PAR4 receptors. GPVI is the principal collagen receptor in platelets and is a member of the immunoglobulin receptor superfamily. Ligation of platelet receptors by agonists such as thrombin, TxA_2, and ADP initiates the production and release of several intracellular messenger molecules, including products of hydrolysis of phosphoinositides by phospholipase C, diacylglycerol, and inositol 1,4,5-triphosphate (IP3) and conversion of arachidonic acid to TxA_2. These mediators induce or modulate the various platelet responses of Ca^{++} mobilization, protein phosphorylation, aggregation, secretion, and thromboxane production. The interaction between platelet surface receptors and key intracellular enzymes (e.g., phospholipases A_2 and C, adenylyl cyclase) is mediated by a group of distinct proteins (called G-proteins), which bind and are modulated by guanosine triphosphate. As in most secretory cells, platelet activation results in a rise in cytoplasmic ionized calcium concentration; inositol triphosphate functions as a messenger† to mobilize Ca^{++} from intracellular stores. This increase in cytoplasmic Ca^{++} levels regulates other events, such as activation of phospholipase A_2,

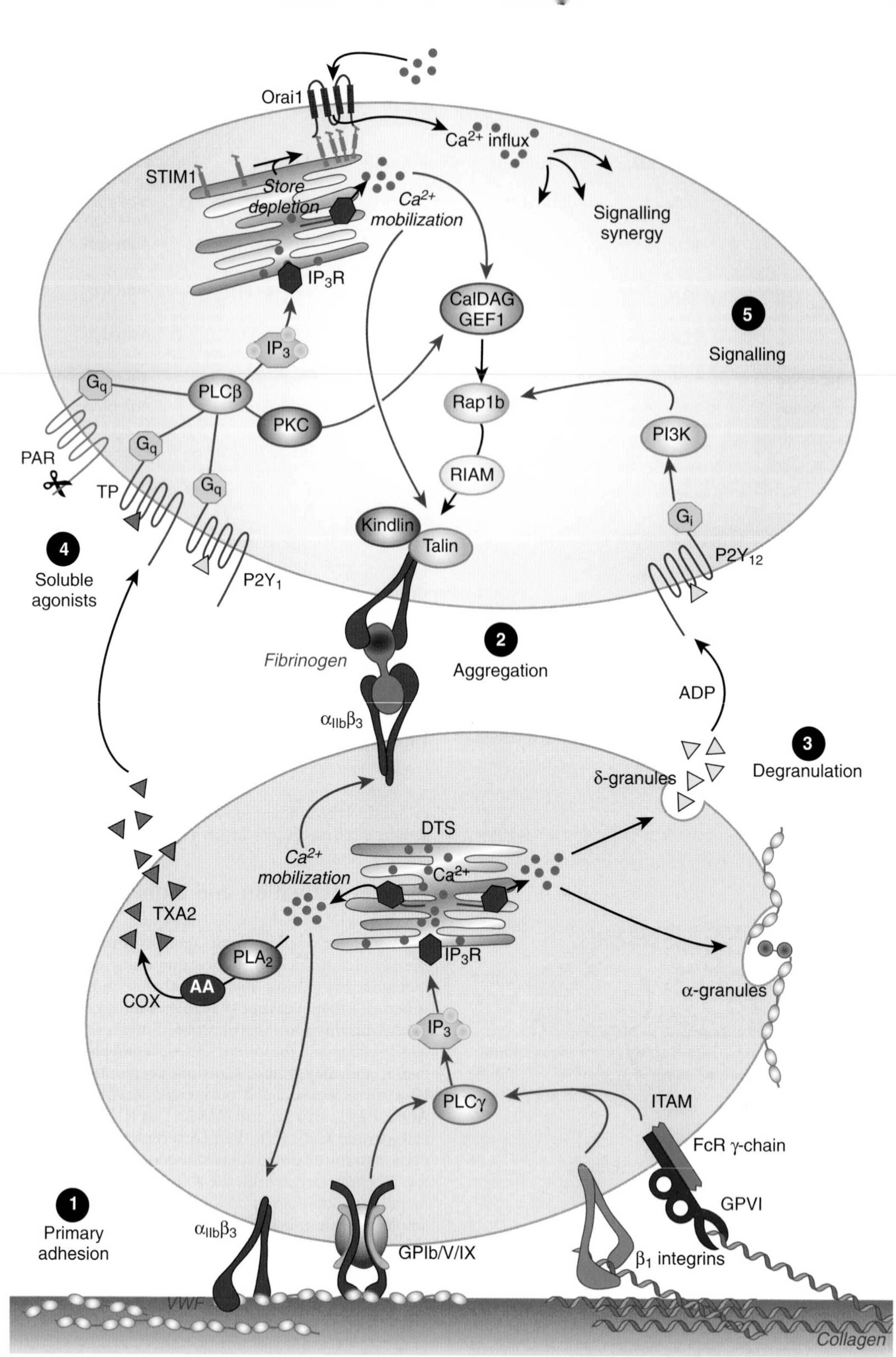

Figure 40-3 Platelet proteins and molecular pathways important for hemostasis. The stages of hemostatic plug formation are broadly divided into platelet adhesion and initial signaling events, platelet aggregation, degranulation, soluble agonist receptor activation, and subsequent signaling. *(For discussion in greater depth of these molecules and their roles in platelet activation, see Wei AH, Schoenwaelder SM, Andrews RK. New insights into the haemostatic function of platelets. Brit J Haematol 2009;147:415–30, from which this figure is reproduced with permission.)* *AA,* Arachidonic acid; *AC,* adenylyl cyclase; *Ca^{2+},* calcium; *CalDAG GEF1,* calcium and diacylglycerol-regulated guanine nucleotide exchange factor; *COX,* cyclooxygenase; *DTS,* dense tubular system; *IP3,* inositol (1,4,5)-trisphosphate; *IP3R,* IP3 receptor; *ITAM,* immunoreceptor tyrosine-based activation motif; *PAR,* protease-activated receptor; *PGH_2,* prostaglandin H_2; *PIP2,* phosphatidylinositol (4,5)-bisphosphate; *PI3K,* PI3-kinase; *PKC,* protein kinase C; *PLA_2,* phospholipase A_2; *PLC,* phospholipase C; *RIAM,* Rap1-GTP interacting adapter molecule; *Src,* Src family kinases; *STIM1,* stromal interaction molecule 1; *TP,* thromboxane receptor.

leading to TxA_2 production, and phosphorylation by myosin light chain kinase of the myosin light chain, which is involved in shape change and secretion.

Diacylglycerol activates the protein kinase C (PKC) family of enzymes, which phosphorylate several proteins, including pleckstrin. PKC activation is considered to play a major role in platelet responses, including secretion and activation of GPIIb/IIIa. Platelets possess several families of G-proteins that function as molecular switches in transmitting the signal from surface receptors to intracellular effectors. For example, phospholipase activation and calcium mobilization on activation by ADP (P2Y1), TxA_2, or thrombin are mediated by Gaq, and signaling through the P2Y12 ADP receptor and inhibition of adenylyl cyclase are mediated by Gai.

Another well-recognized response of platelets to activation is synthesis of TxA_2. The initial and rate-limiting step in TxA_2 production is the mobilization of arachidonic acid from phospholipids (predominantly phosphatidylcholine) by phospholipase A_2. Free arachidonic acid is converted by cyclooxygenase to prostaglandins G_2 and H_2, which are converted by thromboxane synthase to TxA_2. Binding of fibrinogen to the GPIIb/IIIa complex results in activation of tyrosine kinases and associated events, a process called **outside-in signaling** (Shattil, 2004). Numerous other mechanisms and events occur in platelets on activation, involving small GTPases, tyrosine kinases, and phosphatases; these are beyond the scope of the present review. Although the agonists mentioned previously activate platelets to function in hemostasis, other agonists, such as prostacyclin (PGI_2), produced by endothelial cells, inhibit platelet responses. PGI_2 does this by increasing platelet cAMP levels by activating adenylyl cyclase.

Through activation of the coagulation system, thrombin is produced and serves as a very potent stimulus for platelet activation. Upon stimulation by thrombin, collagen, or various other agents, platelets change in shape from discoid to spherical, extend pseudopods, undergo internal contraction resulting in centralization of their α-granules and dense core granules, and ultimately release from the cell the contents of these granules. Depending on the strength of the stimulus, the contents of the α-granules, dense core granules, or even lysosomal granules may be released. As a result of platelet activation, conformational changes in the glycoprotein IIb/IIIa complex occur (Frelinger, 1991; Phillips, 1991; Sims, 1991; Calvete, 1999), resulting in the formation of receptors capable of binding several plasma proteins, most notably fibrinogen (Bennett, 1979; Cox, 2004).

Following vascular injury, blood platelets rapidly adhere to the exposed subendothelium. Under lower shear conditions, such as those characteristic of the venous circulation, platelets may bind directly to exposed collagen by means of GPVI and GPIa/IIa (α2β1). Under higher shear conditions present in the arterial circulation, adhesion is believed to be initiated by binding of circulating vWF to exposed subendothelial collagen, followed by binding of surface-bound vWF to the platelet via the GPIb/IX receptor complex of the platelet (Auger, 2005).

Platelet Coagulant Activity

Platelets play a vital role in coagulation. The α-granules possess several coagulation factors, including factor V, fibrinogen, and several others. Most important, several of the key enzymatic reactions leading to activation of coagulation factors and thrombin generation require the platelet membrane surface to proceed at an optimum rate (Smyth, 2010). Following stimulation of platelets by agonists, progressive loss of platelet membrane phospholipid asymmetry results from increased bilayer movement, or "flip-flop," of PS and other phospholipids from the internal to the external surface of the membrane (see Fig. 40-2) (Hemker, 1983; Zwaal, 2005). A proline-rich, transmembrane protein termed **scramblase** (see Fig. 40-2) (Comfurius, 1996; Zhou, 1997) is believed to be involved in this process (Zwaal, 2005). The availability of highly ordered phospholipoprotein surfaces permits activation of factors IX and X and prothrombin to occur on the platelet surface. Platelet activation (e.g., by ADP or collagen) results in the generation of high-affinity binding sites for factor XI. High molecular weight kininogen and prothrombin may then serve as cofactors for activation of platelet-bound factor XI by thrombin (Baglia, 1998; Oliver, 1999). Platelets additionally contain endogenous factor V, which appears to play a key role in the formation of a receptor on the platelet surface for activated factor X (Miletich, 1978). Effector cell protease receptor-1, a platelet activation–dependent membrane protein (Bouchard, 1997), together with activated factor V, is required to mediate factor Xa binding to the surface of activated platelets to form a functional prothrombinase complex. Functional coagulation complexes are described further in the preceding chapter.

Laboratory Evaluation of Platelet Function Disorders

INITIAL LABORATORY EVALUATION

The initial laboratory evaluation of platelet disorders includes a platelet count. This measurement has become a routine component of the complete blood count in an era of electronic particle counting. The normal platelet count is 150–400 × 10^9/L. Many instruments additionally provide the mean platelet volume (MPV) and display a histogram of MPV. In healthy individuals the MPV varies inversely with platelet count, so that interpretation of MPV as low or high is best done with reference to the patient's platelet count (Bessman, 1981). Some automated instruments additionally assess platelet maturity, as reflected by the RNA content of **reticulated platelets**—analogous to reticulocyte measurements in the erythroid series. Such measurements offer the opportunity to detect a thrombopoietic response from the bone marrow 1 or more days earlier than it might be detected by more traditional approaches. Evaluation of the peripheral blood film provides a rough corroboration of the platelet count and size distribution.

Because platelets may undergo activation and spreading during preparation of the blood film, the apparent size distribution of platelets in the blood film in some cases may deviate significantly from actual volume distributions. In cases of severe thrombocytopenia below the established linearity of a given automated instrument, or whenever cellular fragments may be spuriously affecting the automated count, a manual phase contrast count with a hemocytometer chamber may be required. However, such manual counts performed on a relatively small number of platelets have a much higher coefficient of variation than is obtained when automated instruments are used within their linear ranges, and unless such counts are performed by an experienced individual, the counts may be unreliable.

SCREENING STUDIES OF PLATELET FUNCTION

No currently available laboratory test faithfully reflects the ability of platelets to accomplish their enormously complex series of functions in hemostasis. For many years, the template bleeding time test has been used by many laboratories as a global test for the adequacy of primary hemostasis. In this procedure, a disposable device is used that consists of a spring-loaded blade that descends vertically into the epidermis (described in detail by Hoyer [1982]) or a blade that cuts the epidermis as it makes a rotary arc (Buchanan, 1989). With these tests, a blood pressure cuff is placed around the upper arm and is inflated to maintain a pressure of 40 mm Hg. A standardized cut is then made on the volar surface of the forearm, a timer is started, and at 30-second intervals, the resulting drops of blood are blotted with filter paper (without directly touching the wound edge). When blood no longer stains the filter paper, the timer is stopped. At platelet counts above 100 × 10^9/L, bleeding times should fall within the laboratory's established reference interval. Prolonged bleeding times in such cases are associated with prior ingestion of drugs with an antiplatelet action (e.g., aspirin, clopidogrel), von Willebrand disease, and congenital and acquired disorders of platelet function (discussed later).

Whereas a carefully performed bleeding time test provides useful information during the evaluation of a patient with a history of bleeding manifestations, its usefulness is less clear in the context of preoperative hemostatic screening of asymptomatic patients. In an extensive review of publications reporting the extent of clinical bleeding in a wide variety of settings, Rodgers and Levin (Rodgers, 1990) concluded that the available data did not provide convincing evidence that the relationship between platelet count and bleeding time was predictively useful in the individual patient typically encountered in clinical practice. They additionally concluded that the degree of bleeding from a standardized template cut in the skin could not be relied upon in an individual patient to predict the risk of bleeding elsewhere in the body, such as at operative sites. A prospective study of 40 patients without a bleeding history and with no recent intake of nonsteroidal antiinflammatory drugs who underwent coronary artery bypass surgery found no predictive relationship between the preoperative bleeding time test and perioperative or postoperative bleeding (De Caterina, 1994). Although a dramatically prolonged bleeding time provides strong suspicion for an underlying disorder of primary hemostasis, the interpretation of mildly or moderately prolonged bleeding times is less clear. Because of the limitation in predictive value, the risk of scarring, and the considerable technical expertise and performance time associated with performance of bleeding times, use of this procedure has declined considerably in recent years. In parallel with this decline, the popularity of in vitro measures has increased, most notably the platelet function analyzer (PFA-100) instrument. With this instrument, anticoagulated whole blood is flowed under high shear force through a narrow hole punched out of a membrane coated with collagen and epinephrine or ADP. The combination of biophysical shear and chemical stimulation initially promotes platelet adhesion to the outer edges of the cut membrane; subsequently, platelet–platelet aggregation leads to full occlusion of the channel, which

TABLE 40-2

PFA-100 Closure Time (CT) Findings in Congenital and Acquired, Non–Drug-Induced Platelet Disorders

	Total number of subjects reported	CADP CT	CEPI CT
Disorders With Normal Platelet Counts			
Glanzmann thrombasthenia	23	P	P
Aspirin-like defect	6	N	P
$P2Y_{12}$ deficiency	4	N or P	N or P
Dense granule deficiency	30	N or P	N or P
Hermansky-Pudlak syndrome	44	N or P	N or P
Primary secretion defects	30	N	N or P
Platelet procoagulant defect	1	N	N
Disorders With Reduced or Normal Platelet Counts			
Bernard-Soulier syndrome	8	P	P
Platelet-type von Willebrand disease	3	P	P
Gray platelet syndrome	3	P	P
Wiskott-Aldrich syndrome	5	N or P	N or P
Hereditary macrothrombocytopenia associated with nonmuscle myosin heavy chain IIa syndromes	5	N	N or P
Macrothrombocytopenia of undefined cause	11	N or P	N or P
Undefined autosomal dominant thrombocytopenia	1	N	N
Primary Bone Marrow Disorders			
Myelodysplastic or myeloproliferative syndromes, with or without thrombocytosis	69	N or P	N or P

Modified with permission from Hayward CPM, Harrison P, Cattaneo M, et al. Platelet function analyzer (PFA)-100 closure time in the evaluation of platelet disorder and platelet function. J Thromb Haemost 2006;4:312–9.
Note: The data reported with CADP (collagen and ADP) and CEPI (collagen and epinephrine) cartridges, indicated as normal (N) or prolonged (P), are based on small numbers of reported cases.

is recorded as **closure time.** This process is dependent on plasma levels of vWF.

Whereas inhibition of the platelet cyclooxygenase by aspirin and other mild to moderate impairments of platelet function prolong closure times with the collagen/epinephrine membranes, only more profound impairment of platelet function or of vWF prolongs closure times with collagen/ADP cartridges. Thrombocytopenia or anemia also prolongs closure times. Although abnormal in some platelet disorders, the PFA-100 does not have sufficient sensitivity or specificity to be relied upon as a screening tool for platelet disorders (Table 40-2) (Hayward, 2006). Definitive identification of abnormalities of platelets or vWF requires more specialized studies.

Several additional ex vivo experimental systems have been developed in which shear forces play a major role. These include variations of cone-and-plate viscometers and parallel plate flow chambers (Michelson, 2002). These devices offer the potential to detect inherited and acquired disorders related to both platelets and vWF, but their role in clinical practice needs to be defined.

PLATELET AGGREGATION AND SECRETION STUDIES

Further evaluation of a suspected defect of platelet function can be performed through study of platelet aggregation and secretion in response to a battery of platelet-stimulating agents. These studies are performed using platelet-rich plasma (PRP) harvested from blood collected using sodium citrate as the anticoagulant. Sodium citrate lowers Ca^{++} in the blood to prevent clotting of blood, but not to the extent that it is lowered by ethylenediaminetetraacetic acid (EDTA), which is routinely used to collect samples for blood counts. EDTA dissociates the GPIIb/IIIa complexes on the platelet surface; thus, aggregation studies cannot be performed when such a sample is used. When citrated PRP is continuously stirred in a platelet aggregometer and a light beam is passed through the suspension, platelet aggregation in response to added agonists can be monitored by changes in light transmittance (Zucker, 1989). Discoid-to-spheroid shape change is seen as an initial decrease in transmittance, whereas subsequent formation of platelet clumps allows more light to pass through the suspension to the photodetector and is recorded as an increase in light transmittance. When instruments equipped with a second channel are used for monitoring secretion, the release of adenosine triphosphate (ATP) from platelet-dense granules is simultaneously measured (Fig. 40-4). This is accomplished by adding the firefly luminescence substrate and enzyme—luciferin and luciferase—to the PRP; released ATP then functions as a cofactor in the light-producing luciferin–luciferase reaction, and light emission is recorded with a second photodetector. Because of separation of wavelengths, the aggregation and release channels can be monitored independently (Miller, 1984). The release of ATP in most cases may be assumed to reflect the release of other constituents of dense granules, which are less easily measured (i.e., ADP, serotonin, calcium). Direct measurements of serotonin, ATP, and ADP can also be performed (Holmsen, 1989). As an alternative to lumiaggregometry studies, platelet secretion may be studied in parallel with aggregation by initially labeling platelets with radioactive serotonin and then measuring the release of radioactivity from platelets on activation (Lan, 2005).

Platelets have receptors for several agonists on their surface (see Figs. 40-3, 40-5, and 40-6). A number of these agonists may be used in the diagnostic laboratory to determine whether response to one or more of these agonists is impaired. Frequently employed agonists include collagen, epinephrine, ADP, U46619 (a TxA_2 analog), arachidonic acid, ristocetin, and the calcium ionophore A23187. Platelet responses to these agonists with the exception of ristocetin are dependent on active metabolic processes in platelets. In contrast, ristocetin-induced clumping of platelets occurs to a large degree even in the presence of metabolic inhibitors and in formalin-fixed platelets; therefore, it is often referred as **agglutination.**

Although of paramount importance as a platelet stimulus in vivo, thrombin is difficult to employ with PRP because of interference from the formation of fibrin. The partially trypsinized γ-thrombin, however, retains platelet-stimulating activity but largely lacks clotting activity and can be useful (Charo, 1977). Platelet responses to thrombin are mediated by a G-protein–coupled seven-transmembrane receptor that is cleaved by thrombin. Thus, thrombin receptor activating peptide, consisting of amino acid sequence SFLLRN, derived from the extracellular **tethered ligand** region of the thrombin receptor (Furman, 1998), is useful in platelet function testing. Agonists such as collagen, thrombin, and TxA_2 are capable of directly inducing secretion and further TxA_2 synthesis, in addition to inducing aggregation. In contrast, secretion and TxA_2 synthesis following platelet stimulation with the agonists ADP or epinephrine may be considered secondary responses after a threshold level of aggregation has first been achieved (Cattaneo, 2009). Mezzano and coworkers have recently reviewed the potential diagnostic yields and the limitations of aggregation and secretion studies (Mezzano, 2009).

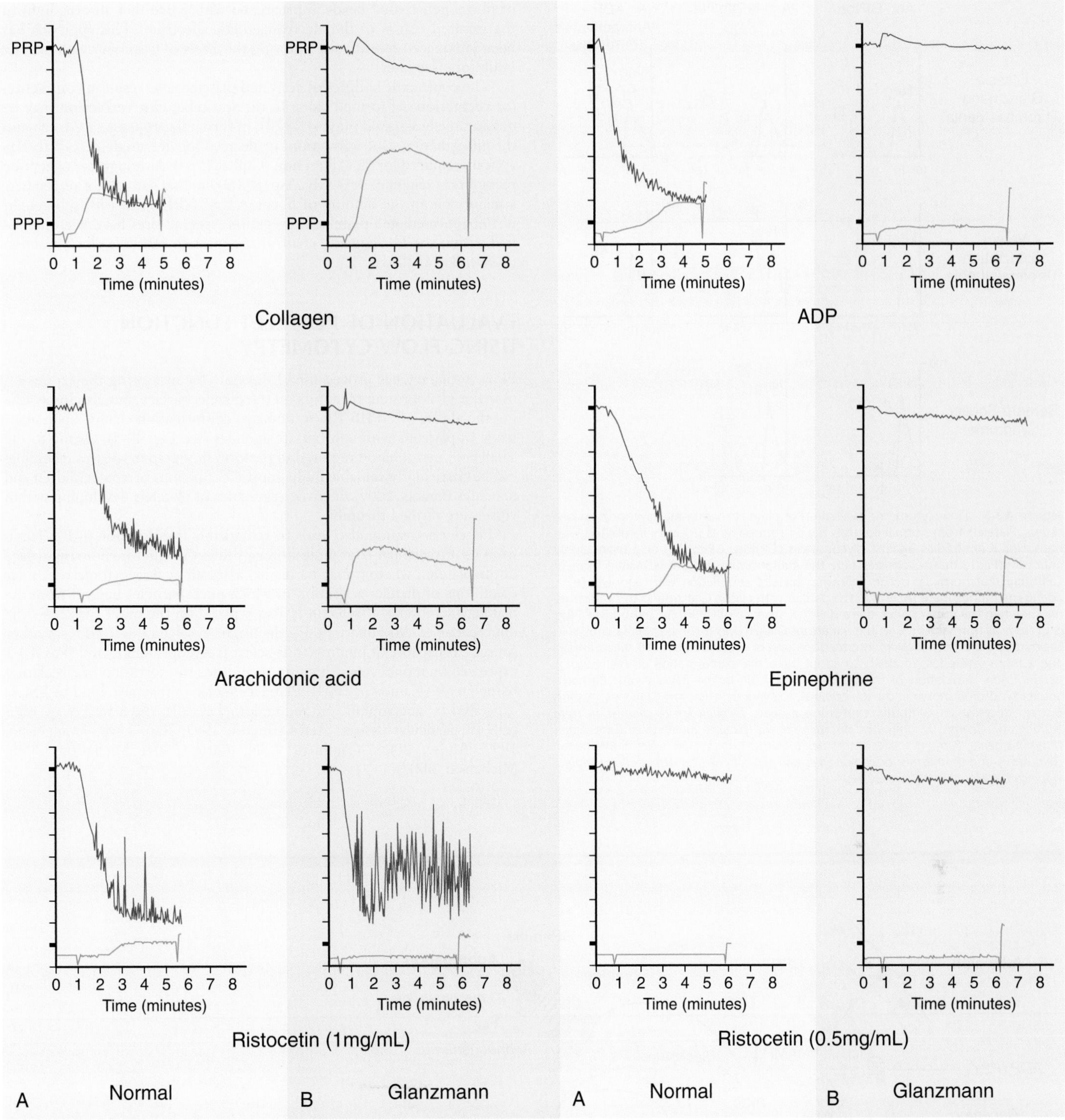

Figure 40-4 Platelet studies with lumiaggregometry in Glanzmann thrombasthenia. **A,** Normal pattern. Simultaneously measured platelet aggregation and secretion of adenosine triphosphate (ATP) (lumiaggregometry) in Glanzmann thrombasthenia. In each panel, the upper tracing displays platelet aggregation, with increasing light transmittance and aggregation shown as downward deflection. With platelet-rich plasma (PRP) initially set at 90% full vertical scale, and platelet-poor plasma (PPP) at 10%, the maximum possible downward deflection would be to the level of the PPP line. The lower tracing in each panel displays platelet secretion of ATP (monitored as luminescence when secreted ATP reacts with luciferin–luciferase reagent present in the cuvet) as an upward deflection. **B,** Patient with Glanzmann thrombasthenia. Simultaneous measurement of aggregation and a marker of dense granule secretion provide information on two responses of platelets to activation: aggregation and secretion. Note that the Glanzmann patient's platelets do aggregate in response to ristocetin: Even in the absence of glycoprotein (GP)IIb/IIIa, which functions as a receptor for platelet bridging by fibrinogen, ristocetin can facilitate the bridging together of platelets through the binding of plasma von Willebrand factor to the GPIbα chains present in normal numbers in Glanzmann platelets (see Fig. 40-6). *(Modified with permission from Miller JL, Schumackher H, Rock W, Stass S, editors. Handbook of hematologic pathology. New York: Marcel Dekker; 2000.)*

Other methods have also been developed to test platelet function. Impedance measurements, as opposed to monitoring of light transmission, have been used to study platelet aggregation, not only in PRP but also in whole blood (Cardinal, 1980). Following the addition of a platelet agonist to the stirred sample, conductance between two electrodes falls as platelets aggregate upon electrode surfaces. The resulting curves of electrical impedance over time share many similarities to those of light transmittance recordings, although characteristic differences between these two approaches have been noted (Ingerman-Wojenski, 1984; Joseph, 1987). When impedance aggregometry is combined with ATP secretion measurement on whole blood samples (Ingerman-Wojenski, 1984), relatively rapid evaluation of platelet function, requiring only a small volume of blood, may be performed (McGlasson, 2009). Additionally, platelet aggregation in whole blood may be monitored optically by means of the coaggregation

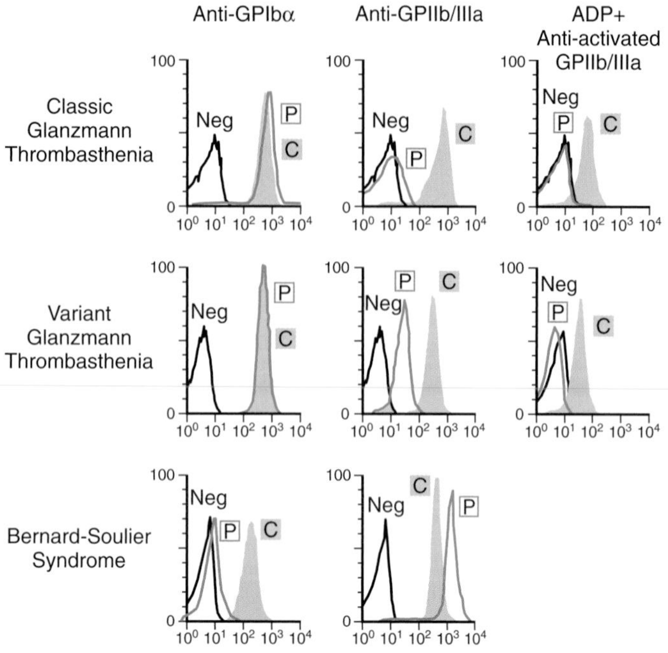

Figure 40-5 Flow cytometric evaluation of platelet membrane glycoprotein disorders. Platelets from normal controls (C) or from patients (P) were incubated with monoclonal antibodies against glycoprotein (GP)Ibα, GPIIb/IIIa, or a monoclonal antibody (Pac1) that recognizes only the conformationally altered active form of GPIIb/IIIa that normally occurs following platelet stimulation with agonists (e.g., adenosine diphosphate [ADP]). In the patient with classic Glanzmann thrombasthenia shown in the upper panel, there is virtual absence of GPIIb/IIIa, although GPIbα is present at normal levels. In the variant of Glanzmann thrombasthenia shown in the middle panel, although an intermediate level of expression of GPIIb/IIIa is apparent, a more severe loss of ability to adopt the active conformation of this receptor occurs upon stimulation of the platelets with ADP. In the patient with Bernard-Soulier syndrome shown in the lower panel, a severe deficiency of GPIbα expression but no decrease in GPIIb/IIIa expression is seen. *(Modified with permission from Nurden AT, George JN. Inherited disorders of the platelet membrane: Glanzmann thrombasthenia, Bernard-Soulier syndrome, and other disorders. In: Colman RW, editor. Hemostasis and thrombosis: basic principles and clinical practice. 4th ed. Philadelphia: Lippincott Williams & Wilkins; 2001.)*

of fibrinogen-coated beads impregnated with a dye that absorbs light in the infrared region of the electromagnetic spectrum. This approach has been introduced recently for assessing the effect of treatment with platelet inhibitors (see later).

The contractile abilities of activated platelets also result in contraction (or **retraction**) of formed clots. In the test tube, **clot retraction** may be quantitatively assessed (Taylor, 1970). In thrombocytopenia or Glanzmann thrombasthenia, clot retraction is delayed or incomplete. GPIIb/IIIa appears required for clot retraction (Coller, 1983). Although the tripeptide recognition sequence Arg–Gly–Asp (RGD) binding sites of fibrinogen play a major role in the binding of fibrinogen to GPIIb/IIIa with subsequent fibrinogen-mediated platelet aggregation, specific sites have been identified within the fibrinogen γ-chain that appear to subserve clot retraction (Podolnikova, 2003).

EVALUATION OF PLATELET FUNCTION USING FLOW CYTOMETRY

Flow cytometry has proved useful not only for measuring the expression of major glycoprotein receptors on the platelet surface, but also for assessing the ability of GPIIb/IIIa to undergo conformation change upon challenge of platelets with appropriate agonists (see Fig. 40-5). Owing to the small volumes of blood required to perform flow cytometry, this technique can be particularly valuable in diagnostic evaluations of small children and neonates (Israels, 2009). In vivo, aggregates of platelets developing within vessels are termed thrombi.

Platelet activation also leads to remarkable translocation of P-selectin from its intracellular α-granule storage site to the outer membrane surface of the platelet, where it may be readily assessed by flow cytometry. Under conditions of platelet activation in which microparticles bud off from the platelet membrane, P-selectin is also exposed on the outer surface of the microparticles. Microparticle P-selectin, or P-selectin derived from other sources, is capable of binding to P-selectin glycoprotein ligand (PSGL)-1 expressed by monocytes, which, in turn, leads to expression of circulating tissue factor (Cambien, 2004). Platelet P-selectin may also bind to PSGL expressed by neutrophils, injured endothelial cells, and a variety of other cells in particular disease states (Shattil, 1987; Rao, 1998; Evangelista, 1999; Andre, 2004; Cambien, 2004; Furie, 2004; Michelson, 2006; Michelson, 2007).

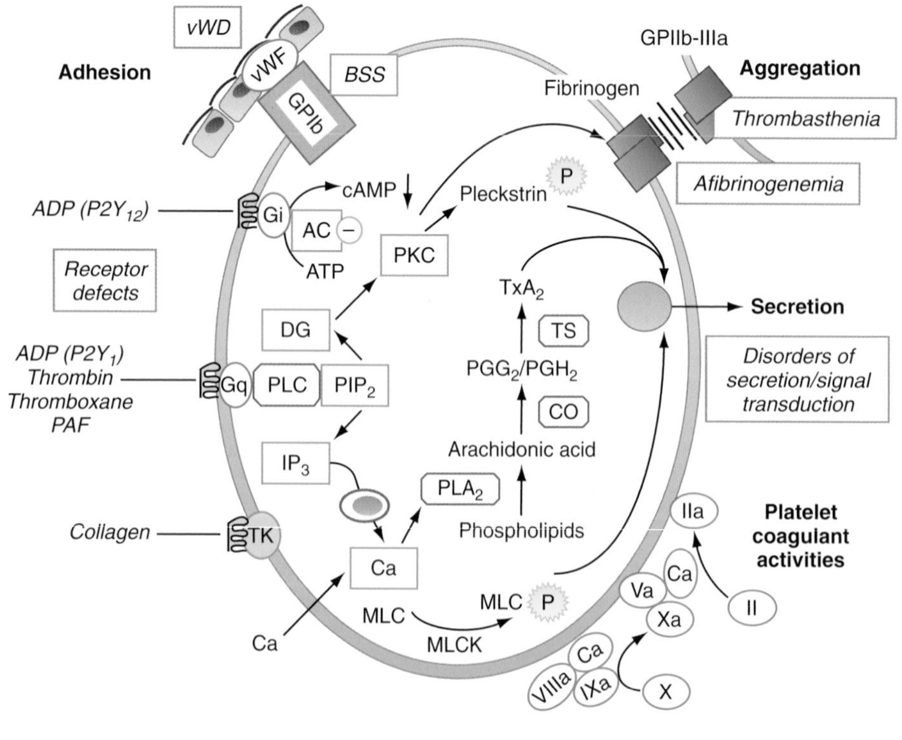

Figure 40-6 A schematic representation of selected platelet responses to activation and congenital disorders of platelet function. The Roman numerals in the circles represent coagulation factors. *(Modified with permission from Rao AK. Congenital disorders of platelet function: disorders of signal transduction and secretion. Am J Med Sci 1998;316:69–76.)* *AC*, Adenylyl cyclase; *BSS*, Bernard-Soulier syndrome; *CO*, cyclooxygenase; *DAG*, diacylglycerol; *G*, GTP-binding protein; *IP3*, inositol trisphosphate; *MLC*, myosin light chain; *MLCK*, myosin light chain kinase; *P2Y1, P2Y12*, G-protein–coupled adenosine diphosphate (ADP) receptors; *PAF*, platelet-activating factor; *PGG_2/PGH_2*, prostaglandin arachidonic pathway intermediates; *PIP2*, phosphatidylinositol bisphosphate; *PKC*, protein kinase C; *PLA_2*, phospholipase A_2; *PLC*, phospholipase C; *TK*, tyrosine kinase; *TS*, thromboxane synthase; *vWD*, von Willebrand disease; *vWF*, von Willebrand factor.

TABLE 40-3
Mechanisms of Platelet Destruction

Type of thrombocytopenia	Specific example(s)
Immune Mediated	
Autoantibody-mediated platelet destruction by reticuloendothelial system (RES)	Primary immune thrombocytopenic purpura; secondary immune thrombocytopenia associated with lymphoproliferative disease; collagen vascular disease; infections such as infectious mononucleosis; human immunodeficiency virus syndrome
Alloantibody-mediated platelet destruction by RES	Neonatal alloimmune thrombocytopenia; posttransfusion purpura; passive alloimmune thrombocytopenia; alloimmune platelet transfusion refractoriness
Drug-dependent, antibody-mediated platelet destruction by RES	Drug-induced immune thrombocytopenic purpura (e.g., quinine)
Platelet activation by binding of immunoglobulin G (IgG) Fc of drug-dependent IgG to platelet FcγIIa receptors	Heparin-induced thrombocytopenia
Non–Immune Mediated	
Platelet activation by thrombin or proinflammatory cytokines	Disseminated intravascular coagulation; septicemia/systemic inflammatory response syndromes
Platelet destruction via ingestion by macrophages (hemophagocytosis)	Infections; certain malignant lymphoproliferative disorders
Platelet destruction through platelet interactions with altered von Willebrand factor	Thrombotic thrombocytopenic purpura; hemolytic-uremic syndrome
Platelet losses on artificial surfaces	Cardiopulmonary bypass surgery; use of intravascular catheters
Decreased platelet survival associated with cardiovascular disease	Congenital and acquired heart disease; cardiomyopathy; pulmonary embolism

Modified with permission from Warkentin TE, Kelton JG. Thrombocytopenia due to platelet destruction and hypersplenism. In: Hoffman R, Benz EJ Jr, Shattil SJ, et al, editors. Hematology: basic principles and practice. Philadelphia: Elsevier Churchill Livingstone; 2005, p. 2305–25.

Quantitative Platelet Disorders

THROMBOCYTOPENIA

Decreased platelet production and increased platelet destruction (Table 40-3) constitute two of the major causes of thrombocytopenia. Additionally, decreased numbers of circulating platelets may be seen with splenomegaly of any cause, because of the resulting increase in sequestration of platelets by the spleen.

Congenital Thrombocytopenia

Congenital thrombocytopenias are being recognized with increasing frequency, and several distinct genetic abnormalities have been documented in such patients (Drachman, 2004; Althaus, 2009). Patients with these entities may present with isolated thrombocytopenia or with this disorder in conjunction with characteristic syndromes. From a practical point of view, they may be characterized based on inheritance patterns or on the size of the platelets. A diverse group of autosomal dominant syndromes, referred to as ***MYH9*-related macrothrombocytopenias,** include the May-Hegglin anomaly, Fechtner syndrome, Epstein syndrome, and Sebastian syndrome and share features of increased platelet size, cytoplasmic inclusions in leukocytes (Döhle bodies), and premature release of platelets. These entities arise from mutations in the *MYH9* gene encoding non-muscle myosin heavy chain IIA, a contractile cytoskeletal protein. All of the *MYH9* syndromes have macrothrombocytopenia; other features such as nephritis, sensorineural deafness, and cataracts serve to distinguish them (Althaus, 2009).

Other congenital thrombocytopenias inherited in an autosomal dominant manner include the velocardiofacial syndrome (VCF) and the DiGeorge syndrome, which arise owing to deletions within chromosome 22q11 and are associated with cardiac abnormalities, parathyroid and thymus insufficiencies, cognitive impairment, and facial dysmorphology (VCF only); and the Paris-Trousseau/Jacobsen syndrome, which is characterized by psychomotor retardation and facial and cardiac abnormalities, and arises as the result of deletion of a portion of chromosome 11,11q23-24, which encompasses the transcription factor *FLI-1* gene. Platelets in the latter disorder are increased in size and have giant α-granules. In patients who have the familial platelet disorder with predisposition to acute myeloid leukemia, autosomal dominant thrombocytopenia occurs secondary to mutations in the *RUNX1/CBFA2/AML1* gene. In these patients, platelet function is also abnormal (Song, 1999), and the platelets are of normal size. Patients with the Bernard-Soulier syndrome (BSS) have macrothrombocytopenia, which is inherited in an autosomal recessive manner, and the primary abnormality is a deficiency of the GPIb/IX/V complex on platelets (discussed later).

It is interesting to note that a dominant form of macrothrombocytopenia (Mediterranean macrothrombocytopenia) has been described in southern Europe; this has been associated with mutations in GPIbα and is considered a heterozygous form of the BSS (Savoia, 2001). Congenital amegakaryocytic thrombocytopenia is an autosomal recessive disorder associated with mutations in the thrombopoietin receptor *Mpl* and is characterized by severe thrombocytopenia and absence of megakaryocytes in the bone marrow. Patients with the Wiskott-Aldrich syndrome (WAS) and related X-linked thrombocytopenia have mutations in the *WAS* gene and characteristically have small platelets. Other causes of congenital thrombocytopenia include the gray platelet syndrome (GPS) (see later) and thrombocytopenia with absent radii syndrome, which is associated with skeletal abnormalities and is inherited in an autosomal recessive manner. In general, patients with congenital thrombocytopenia may have associated defects in platelet responses, in addition to decreased counts. Establishing the diagnosis of congenital thrombocytopenia is important because many patients with these entities often get labeled as having **chronic immune thrombocytopenia** and are subjected to inappropriate therapy.

Acquired aplastic anemias involving the erythroid and granulocytic lines, as well as the megakaryocytic line, are seen more commonly than are pure megakaryocytic aplasias. Toxic chemical exposures, viral illnesses, and, frequently, unexplained causes may underlie the aplasia.

Study of the bone marrow may be required to assess whether the thrombocytopenia is due to failure of platelet production. Bone marrow aspirates are often less reliable than bone marrow biopsies for enumerating the megakaryocytes present. In some instances, abnormalities in megakaryocyte structure may be found. In contrast to estimations of megakaryocyte numbers, it is usually difficult to assess abnormalities in megakaryocyte size or lobulation pattern from biopsy or clot sections. This is because one section may sample only a small portion of the relatively large megakaryocyte cell. For such purposes, a well-prepared Wright-Giemsa stain on an aspirate smear or on a biopsy touch preparation is typically most helpful.

Immune Thrombocytopenic Purpura

One of the most important and frequently encountered forms of enhanced consumption of platelets is the acquired disorder, immune thrombocytopenic purpura (ITP). As recently defined by an international consensus conference (Rodeghiero, 2009), **primary** ITP is a diagnosis of exclusion, made in the absence of other causes or disorders associated with thrombocytopenia—which, by contrast, would favor a diagnosis of **secondary** ITP (Table 40-4, *upper panel*). The clinical history is usually helpful in arriving at a tentative diagnosis, and in particular in distinguishing between the newly diagnosed, persistent, chronic, and severe forms of secondary ITP, as defined in Table 40-4. This group also recommended that a platelet count of <100,000 platelets/μL should be employed as a threshold for diagnosis. This threshold seeks to avoid overdiagnosis of disease in apparently healthy people with platelet counts of 100,000–150,000/μL and also to avoid inclusion of most women with pregnancy-related thrombocytopenia. A companion consensus conference report

TABLE 40-4
Immunologic Thrombocytopenic Purpura (ITP)

PROPOSED DEFINITIONS OF DISEASE

Primary ITP:

- Primary ITP is an autoimmune disorder characterized by isolated thrombocytopenia (peripheral platelet count $<100 \times 10^9$/L) in the absence of other causes and disorders that may be associated with thrombocytopenia.
- The diagnosis of primary ITP remains one of exclusion; no robust clinical or laboratory parameters are currently available to establish this diagnosis with accuracy.
- The main clinical problem with primary ITP is an increased risk of bleeding, although bleeding symptoms may not always be present.

Secondary ITP:

- All forms of immune-mediated thrombocytopenia except primary ITP*

Phases of the disease:

- Newly diagnosed ITP: within 3 months from diagnosis
- Persistent ITP: between 3 and 12 months from diagnosis; includes patients not reaching spontaneous remission and not maintaining complete response off therapy
- Chronic ITP: lasting for longer than 12 months
- Severe ITP: presence of bleeding symptoms at presentation sufficient to mandate treatment, or occurrence of new bleeding symptoms requiring additional therapeutic intervention with a different platelet-enhancing agent or an increased dose

RECOMMENDATIONS FOR THE DIAGNOSIS OF ITP IN CHILDREN AND ADULTS

Basic evaluation

- Patient history
- Family history
- Physical examination
- Complete blood count and reticulocyte count
- Peripheral blood film
- Quantitative immunoglobulin measurement*
- Bone marrow examination (in selected patients)
- Blood group (Rh)
- Direct antiglobulin test
- *Helicobacter pylori*†
- HIV†
- HCV†

Tests of potential utility in the management of an ITP patient

- Glycoprotein-specific antibody
- Antiphospholipid antibodies (including anticardiolipin and lupus anticoagulant)
- Antithyroid antibodies and thyroid function
- Pregnancy test in women of childbearing potential
- Antinuclear antibodies
- Viral PCR for parvovirus and CMV

Tests of unproven or uncertain benefit

- TPO
- Reticulated platelets
- PaIgG
- Platelet survival study
- Bleeding time
- Serum complement

Upper panel: ITP: Proposed definitions of disease.
Modified with permission from Rodeghiero F, Stasi R, Gernsheimer T. Standardization of terminology, definitions and outcome criteria in immune thrombocytopenic purpura of adults and children: report from an international working group. Blood 2009;113:2386–93.
*The acronym ITP should be followed by the name of the associated disease (for thrombocytopenia after exposure to drugs, the term "drug-induced" should be used) in parentheses, for example, "secondary ITP (lupus-associated)," secondary ITP (HIV-associated)," and "secondary ITP (drug-induced)."
Lower panel: Recommendations for the diagnosis of ITP in children and adults.
Modified with permission from Provan D, Stasi R, Newland AC. International consensus report on the investigation and management of primary immune thrombocytopenia. Blood 2010;115:168–86.
CMV, Cytomegalovirus; *HCV,* hepatitis C virus; *HIV,* human immunodeficiency virus; *PaIgG,* platelet-associated immunoglobulin G; *PCR,* polymerase chain reaction; *Rh,* rhesus; *TPO,* thrombopoietin.
*Quantitative immunoglobulin level measurement should be considered in children with ITP and is recommended in those children with persistent or chronic ITP as part of the reassessment evaluation.
†Recommended by the majority of international consensus panel members for adult patients regardless of geographic locale.

(Provan, 2010) proceeded to address a number of critical issues concerning the diagnosis and management of ITP. No single laboratory test for the diagnosis of ITP was awarded "gold standard" status by this group.

A variety of laboratory approaches were deemed to be of "potential utility" or of "unproven or uncertain benefit," as shown in Table 40-4 *(lower panel).* Of particular interest, antecedent infectious diseases appear to be present in approximately 60% of pediatric patients with ITP. Molecular mimicry, in which immune responses initially directed against an infectious organism cross-react with platelet antigens in both children and adults, appears likely in a number of instances, including infection with human immunodeficiency virus (Karpatkin, 1992, 1995) and hepatitis C virus (HCV) (Stasi, 2009; Zhang, 2009). In recent years, increasing attention has also been paid to the association between *Helicobacter pylori* infection and ITP (Semple, 2009; Stasi, 2009). A possible mechanistic explanation for the thrombocytopenia is that *H. pylori* organisms may trigger P-selectin–dependent platelet aggregation and increased PS expression (Yeh, 2010).

In addition to accelerated destruction of platelets in ITP, evidence suggests impairment in the production of new platelets by megakaryocytes (McMillan, 2007; Cines, 2009). This may be due to detrimental effects on megakaryocytes by infectious agents, as well as to immunologic mechanisms affecting platelet precursors. The observation that a number of patients with chronic forms of ITP do respond to new thrombopoietin mimetic agents would appear to add further support for suppression of platelet production as an important mechanism in some patients with ITP (McMillan, 2007).

The study of platelet-associated immunoglobulins in patients suspected of having ITP has been widely employed in an effort to identify immune-mediated processes. However, the predictive value of positive findings in such cases remains in serious question because immunoglobulins that do not influence platelet survival or function may be associated with platelets in various clinical settings (Kelton, 1982), and platelet-associated IgG may be nonspecifically elevated in disorders associated with elevated plasma IgG. Alternatively, a number of enzyme-linked immunosorbent assays (ELISAs) are available, whereby antibodies eluted from patient platelets or serum are reacted against purified glycoprotein complexes typically immobilized in wells by murine monoclonal antibodies. Many pathologic antibodies may fail to recognize their epitopes within the glycoprotein targets provided in this artificial manner (especially in the case of GPIb). Additionally, false-positive results may occur when patient serum is used if human antimouse antibodies are present in sufficient titer. Some laboratories have also used the monoclonal antibody immobilization of platelet antigen (MAIPA) approach to detect autoantibody obtained directly from patient serum or eluted from patient platelets, which is directed at specific platelet glycoprotein complexes (Kiefel, 1987; Hewitt 1994; Clofent-Sanchez, 1996; Cordiano, 1996). MAIPA assays preserve platelet target antigens in a more native form than most preceding techniques. Results closely matching those of the MAIPA assay have been reported by using a multicolor flow cytometric technique (Nguyen, 2004). However, a true "gold standard" assay for ITP still appears to be a goal for the future, rather than a present reality.

Drug-Induced Thrombocytopenia

Drug-induced thrombocytopenia must always be considered as a cause of acute thrombocytopenia. This disorder can be particularly difficult to identify in patients who are on multiple drugs. Certain drugs such as heparin, quinidine, gold, and sulfa antibiotics, however, have had a relatively higher frequency of causing thrombocytopenia than most other drugs. In this context, the laboratory may play a helpful role if a drug-dependent antibody interacting with the platelets can be demonstrated. It is interesting that whereas normal platelets possess a binding site for antiplatelet antibodies implicated in thrombocytopenia associated with quinidine or quinine, platelets from patients with BSS do not appear to have this receptor (Kunicki, 1978b). Berndt (1985) has provided evidence that such antibodies may be binding to GPIX, to the β-subunit of GPIb, or to a region defined by the association of GPIb and GPIX. It has been suggested by Pfueller (1988), however, that quinine- and quinidine-induced thrombocytopenia may result from antibodies that are heterogeneous among patients, with recognition of neoantigens composed of various epitopes on the platelet surface and the drug, or of new conformations of platelet glycoproteins induced by the drug. Additionally, in some patients, quinidine-dependent antibodies may be directed against epitopes present within the GPIIb/IIIa complex (Pfueller, 1988; Chong, 1991; Visentin, 1991; Nieminen, 1992).

Immune thrombocytopenia has been well described with administration of the platelet GP IIb/IIIa antagonist drugs abciximab, eptifibatide, and tirofiban. All three agents can cause acute severe thrombocytopenia, even following first exposure to the drug (Aster, 2007). Acute thrombocytopenia results from drug-dependent, preexisting antibodies that bind to the GPIIb/IIIa complex; additionally, drug-dependent antibodies may subsequently arise as an immune response to the drug administration (Aster, 2004).

Heparin-Induced Thrombocytopenia

See Chapter 42 for an extensive discussion of this entity.

Thrombotic Thrombocytopenic Purpura

The microangiopathic disorders referred to as thrombotic thrombocytopenic purpura (TTP) and the hemolytic-uremic syndrome (HUS) have long been considered to be close relatives better distinguished on the basis of clinical presentation than upon laboratory findings. This situation changed dramatically in 1998, with two independent groups (Furlan, 1998; Tsai, 1998) demonstrating that the pathogenesis of TTP was related to deficient activity of a plasma metalloproteinase, known as ADAMTS-13, which normally cleaves unusually large vWF molecules (so called UlvWF) released by endothelial cells. This enzyme deficiency results in the persistence of unusually large vWF molecules that are capable of binding both to endothelial cells and to platelets, leading to a meshwork of platelet-rich thrombi in the microcirculation (Moake, 1986; Tsai, 1998). Although an earlier study (Padilla, 2004) had suggested that P-selectin might function as the endothelial anchor for ULvWF, a more recent study using P-selectin–deficient mice concludes that P-selectin appears unnecessary for anchoring to occur, and raises an alternative hypothesis that electrostatic charges presented by endothelial glycosaminoglycans may serve as anchoring sites for UlvWF (Chauhan, 2007).

In HUS, plasma vWF–cleaving protease activity is not severely decreased as observed in TTP (Furlan, 1998). Nevertheless, in typical forms of *Escherichia coli*– or *Shigella* toxin–associated diarrheal HUS, long vWF strings have been observed to bind both to endothelial cells and to platelets, and the possibility has been raised that the toxin may interfere with ADAMTS-13 binding to vWF strings (Moake, 2009).

Application of ADAMTS-13 testing results has increasingly been found to be helpful both for the purpose of prognostication and for guidance in treatment, such as the decision to institute anti–B lymphocyte immunotherapy (Coppo, 2010; Hovinga, 2010; Zheng, 2010). However, both the sensitivity and the specificity of plasma ADAMTS-13 levels for the diagnosis of TTP have been called into question in a number of studies. Thus, neither the presence of a normal level of ADAMTS-13 (implying normal gene product) nor the absence of demonstrable neutralizing antibodies in the plasma of patients otherwise meeting clinical criteria for TTP is sufficient to exclude this diagnosis (George, 2004; Peyvandi, 2004). Patients with systemic connective tissue disorders (Mannucci, 2003), as well as those with ITP, disseminated intravascular coagulation (DIC), and a variety of other disorders, have also been found to have decreased levels of ADAMTS-13 (Moore, 2001). The extent to which these findings reflect idiosyncrasies of the particular testing approaches employed, as opposed to reflecting shared or distinct pathophysiologic mechanisms among these diverse disorders, is presently unresolved. The assays originally developed involved a number of steps in the testing process, including reacting the patient's plasma with a protease-free vWF substrate previously denatured with guanidine or urea, performing gel electrophoresis on degraded vWF, immunoblotting, and demonstrating an abnormal persistence of higher molecular weight vWF multimers. Continual efforts have been made to simplify the ADAMTS-13 assays. Early modification of this method was applied to the final step, where a technically less demanding ELISA of the residual ability of vWF to bind to a collagen-coated surface was substituted for vWF multimeric analysis (Gerritsen, 1999). Subsequently, efforts were directed toward the development of one-step, simplified assays of plasma proteolytic activity against molecules recapitulating the critical residues of vWF required for proteolysis by ADAMTS-13 (Kokame, 2004; Whitelock, 2004). Such assays offer the advantage of rapid turnaround times; their potential role in such diagnostic decision-making is not yet clear.

TABLE 40-5

Reactive Conditions in Which Elevated Platelet Counts May Be Found

Transient processes • Acute blood loss • Recovery (rebound) from thrombocytopenia • Acute infection or inflammation • Response to exercise Sustained processes • Iron deficiency • Hemolytic anemia • Asplenia (e.g., after splenectomy) • Cancer • Chronic inflammatory or infectious diseases	• Connective tissue disorders • Temporal arteritis • Inflammatory bowel disease • Tuberculosis • Chronic pneumonitis • Drug reactions • Vincristine • All-*trans*-retinoic acid • Cytokines • Growth factors

Reprinted with permission from Schafer AI. Thrombocytosis. N Engl J Med 2004;350:1211–9.

THROMBOCYTOSIS

Increased platelet count, or thrombocytosis, may arise as a result of a benign, reactive process (Table 40-5) or alternatively be a manifestation of a neoplastic disorder (Griesshammer, 1999; Schafer, 2004) (see later). The blood film should be reviewed to confirm the increase in platelets. Clues as to whether one is dealing with an autonomous clonal process or a reactive secondary process may be provided by a number of clinical and laboratory findings (Table 40-6).

It has been stated that reactive processes typically do not produce platelet counts over $1000 \times 10^9/L$; this criterion is not reliable for diagnosis. Patients with myeloproliferative syndromes may develop bleeding or thrombotic events. In a meta-analysis reviewing patients with essential thrombocythemia, platelet counts repeatedly failed to achieve significance as a risk factor for thrombosis (Finazzi, 2008). Unless additional risk factors are present, thrombotic events are less likely to occur in secondary than in primary thrombocytosis (Griesshammer, 1999). Patients with myeloproliferative syndromes may have abnormalities in platelet and megakaryocyte structure and platelet function (reviewed later). The abnormalities in aggregation studies do not have the ability to predict bleeding or thrombotic events. Despite statistically significant abnormalities when populations of patients with myeloproliferative disorders or with reactive thrombocytosis are compared, in the individual patient platelet sizing parameters and platelet function studies are unlikely to be capable of differentiating these disorders (Sehayek, 1988).

Inherited Disorders of Platelet Function

OVERVIEW

Table 40-7 provides a classification based on platelet functions or responses that are abnormal (see Fig. 40-6). Although several of these disorders are

TABLE 40-6
Clinical Findings That May Distinguish Between Clonal and Secondary (Reactive) Thrombocytosis

Finding	Clonal thrombocytosis*	Secondary (reactive) thrombocytosis
Underlying systemic disease	No	Often clinically apparent
Digital or cerebrovascular ischemia	Characteristic	No
Large-vessel arterial or venous thrombosis	Increased risk	No
Bleeding complications	Increased risk	No
Splenomegaly	Yes, in about 40% of patients	No
Peripheral blood smear	Giant platelets	Normal platelets
Platelet function	May be abnormal	Normal
Bone marrow megakaryocytes:		
• Number	Increased	Increased
• Morphologic features	Giant, dysplastic forms with increased ploidy; associated with large masses of platelet debris	Normal

Reprinted with permission from Schafer AI. Thrombocytosis. N Engl J Med 2004;350:1211–9.
*Clonal thrombocytosis includes essential thrombocythemia and other myeloproliferative disorders.

TABLE 40-7
Classification of Inherited Disorders of Platelet Function

1. Defects in platelet–vessel wall interaction (disorders of adhesion)
   a. von Willebrand disease (deficiency or defect in plasma von Willebrand factor)
   b. Bernard-Soulier syndrome (deficiency or defect in glycoprotein [GP] Ib/IX)
2. Defects in platelet–platelet interaction (disorders of aggregation)
   a. Congenital afibrinogenemia (deficiency of plasma fibrinogen)
   b. Glanzmann thrombasthenia (deficiency or defect in GPIIb/IIIa)
3. Disorders of platelet secretion and abnormalities of granules
   a. Storage pool deficiency
   b. Quebec platelet disorder
4. Disorders of platelet secretion and signal transduction defects (primary secretion defects)
   a. Defects in platelet–agonist interaction (receptor defects)
   b. Receptor defects: thromboxane A_2, collagen, adenosine diphosphate (ADP), epinephrine
   c. Defects in G-protein activation
      - $G\alpha_q$ deficiency
      - $G\alpha_s$ abnormalities
      - $G\alpha_{i1}$ deficiency
   d. Defects in phosphatidylinositol metabolism
   e. Phospholipase C–β_2 deficiency
   f. Defects in calcium mobilization
   g. Defects in protein phosphorylation (pleckstrin)
      - PKC-θ deficiency
   h. Abnormalities in arachidonic acid pathways and thromboxane A_2 synthesis
      - Impaired liberation of arachidonic acid
      - Cyclooxygenase deficiency
      - Thromboxane synthase deficiency
5. Defects in cytoskeletal regulation
   a. Wiskott-Aldrich syndrome
6. Disorders of platelet coagulant–protein interaction (membrane phospholipid defects)
   a. Scott syndrome
7. Miscellaneous

Modified with permission from Rao AK. Congenital disorders of platelet function: disorders of signal transduction and secretion. Am J Med Sci 1998;316:69–76.

rare, they shed enormous light on platelet physiology. Of note, not all of these disorders are due to a defect in the platelets per se. Some, such as vWD and afibrinogenemia, result from deficiencies of plasma proteins essential for normal platelet function. Moreover, in most patients with inherited abnormalities in platelet aggregation responses, the underlying molecular mechanisms remain unknown. In patients with defects in platelet–vessel wall interactions (adhesion disorders), adhesion of platelets to subendothelium is abnormal. The two disorders in this group are von Willebrand disease (vWD), due to a deficiency or abnormality in plasma vWF, and the BSS, in which platelets are deficient in GPIb (and GPV and GPIX); in both disorders, platelet–vWF interaction is compromised. Binding of fibrinogen to the GPIIb/IIIa complex is a prerequisite for platelet aggregation. Disorders characterized by abnormal platelet–platelet interactions (aggregation disorders) arise because of a severe deficiency of plasma fibrinogen (congenital afibrinogenemia) or because of a quantitative or qualitative abnormality of the platelet membrane GPIIb/IIIa complex, which binds fibrinogen (Glanzmann thrombasthenia). Patients with defects in platelet secretion and signal transduction constitute a heterogeneous group lumped together for convenience of classification, rather than on the basis of an understanding of the specific underlying abnormality. The major common characteristics in these patients, as currently perceived, are abnormal aggregation responses and an inability to release dense granule contents upon activation of PRP with agonists such as ADP, epinephrine, and collagen. In aggregation studies, the second wave of aggregation is blunted or absent. Platelet dysfunction in such patients may arise from diverse mechanisms. A small proportion of these patients have a deficiency of dense granule stores (storage pool deficiency). In some of the other patients, impaired secretion results from aberrations in signal transduction events that lead to secretion and aggregation. Another group consists of patients who have an abnormality in interactions of platelets with proteins of the coagulation system; the best described is the Scott syndrome, characterized by impaired transmembrane migration of procoagulant phospholipid PS. Defects related to platelet cytoskeleton or structural proteins may also be associated with platelet dysfunction, as, for example, in WAS. Recent studies document impaired platelet function associated with mutations in transcription factors (RUNX1, GATA1) that regulate expression of important platelet proteins. In addition to the groups discussed previously, some patients have abnormal platelet function associated with systemic disorders, such as Down syndrome and the May-Hegglin anomaly, where specific aberrant platelet mechanisms are unclear.

DISORDERS OF PLATELET ADHESION

Bernard-Soulier Syndrome

BSS is a rare autosomal recessive platelet function disorder resulting from an abnormality in the platelet GPIb/V/IX complex, which consists of four polypeptides and distinct gene products (GPIbα, GPIbβ, GPV, and GPIX). This complex mediates the binding of vWF to platelets and thus plays a major role in platelet adhesion to the subendothelium, especially at higher shear rates. GPIb exists in platelets as a complex consisting of GPIb, GPIX, and GPV. Approximately 25,000 copies of GPIb/V/IX complex are present on platelets, and these are reduced or abnormal in the BSS. Although GPV is also decreased in BSS platelets, it is not required for platelet surface GPIb/IX expression. Bleeding time is markedly prolonged, platelet counts are moderately decreased, and, on the peripheral smear, platelets are increased in size. In platelet aggregation studies, responses to the commonly used agonists ADP, epinephrine, thrombin, and collagen are normal. Characteristically, the aggregation in PRP in response to ristocetin is decreased or absent—a feature shared with patients with vWD. However, plasma vWF and factor VIII are normal in BSS. Secretion (dense granules) on activation with thrombin may be decreased.

The blood film from a patient with BSS may resemble that from ITP patients in terms of thrombocytopenia and enlarged platelet size. Findings in the aggregometer are almost the reciprocal of those in Glanzmann thrombasthenia: Aggregation and secretion are normal with all agents *except* ristocetin. In addition, the release reaction induced by thrombin may be decreased. Unlike vWD, in which platelet agglutination is diminished in response to ristocetin, in BSS the addition of exogenous vWF (present in plasma cryoprecipitate fractions) does not restore ristocetin-induced agglutination of platelets. This important difference is attributable to the finding that, whereas vWD is characterized by a deficiency in plasma vWF, in BSS the deficiency is seen in the platelet membrane receptor for vWF.

When platelet surface membrane glycoproteins from patients with BSS are analyzed, a striking decrease in GPIb is noted (Nurden, 1975; Whitelock, 2004). Molecular studies have identified a variety of specific point mutations or deletions in GPIbα, GPIbβ, and GPIX that, when present in homozygous or doubly heterozygous fashion, result in a classic BSS phenotype. Mutations in the gene encoding GPIbα are most common. A point mutation in the leucine-rich region of the GPIbα chain may also produce a Bernard-Soulier phenotype, even when expressed only by a single allele (Miller, 1992; Ware, 1993).

von Willebrand Disease

See later section on von Willebrand factor and von Willebrand disease.

DISORDERS OF PLATELET AGGREGATION

Glanzmann Thrombasthenia

Glanzmann thrombasthenia is a rare autosomal recessive disorder characterized by markedly impaired platelet aggregation, prolonged bleeding time, and relatively more severe mucocutaneous bleeding manifestations than most platelet function disorders (Nurden, 2001). It has been reported in clusters in populations where consanguinity is common. Normal resting platelets possess approximately 50,000–80,000 GPIIb/IIIa complexes on the surface. The primary abnormality in thrombasthenia is a quantitative or qualitative defect in the GPIIb/IIIa complex, a heterodimer consisting of GPIIb and GPIIIa whose synthesis is governed by distinct genes located on chromosome 17. Thus, thrombasthenia may arise owing to a mutation in either gene, with decreased platelet expression of the complex. Because of this, fibrinogen binding to platelets on activation and aggregation is impaired. A variety of distinct mutations involving GPIIb and GPIIIa have been described in patients with thrombasthenia (Franchini, 2010). Clot retraction, a function of the interaction of GPIIb/IIIa with the platelet cytoskeleton, is also impaired. The history of investigation of Glanzmann thrombasthenia has set the paradigm for the application of emerging technologies to platelet pathophysiology, as recently chronicled in a historical review of this topic (Coller, 2008).

In non–anticoagulated blood films prepared from patients with Glanzmann thrombasthenia, platelets are present in normal number and appearance but show a characteristic tendency to remain isolated, without the platelet–platelet clumping seen in normal blood films. The diagnostic hallmark of thrombasthenia is absence or marked decrease of platelet aggregation (see Fig. 40-4) in response to virtually all platelet agonists (except ristocetin), with absence of both primary and secondary waves of aggregation; the shape change response is preserved. Platelet-dense granule secretion may be decreased with some agonists (e.g., ADP) but normal on activation with thrombin. Heterozygotes have approximately half the number of platelet GPIIb/IIIa complexes, but platelet aggregation responses are completely normal.

Because the platelet antigen Pl^{A1} is associated with glycoprotein IIIa, this antigen is typically decreased in patients with Glanzmann thrombasthenia (Kunicki, 1978a; Von dem Borne, 1981). Relative estimation of platelet GPIIb/IIIa molecules through binding of specific monoclonal antibodies permits diagnosis of Glanzmann thrombasthenia by flow cytometry requiring only small volumes of blood (Kunicki, 1978a; Montgomery, 1983; Kempfer, 1991). Flow cytometry has become a very useful tool for the diagnosis of both inherited and acquired Glanzmann thrombasthenia (Giannini, 2008; Miller, 2009), as illustrated in Figure 40-5. Definitive characterization of true homozygosity or compound heterozygosity for mutations in GPIIb or GPIIIa may be undertaken by molecular techniques (Bray, 1994; French, 1998; Rosenberg, 1998; Ruan, 1998; Gonzalez-Manchon, 1999; Franchini, 2010). As recently emphasized by Nurden and coworkers, identification of mutations or deletions in the specific genes that produce abnormalities in a multichain receptor complex such as GPIIb/IIIa will become essential in gene therapy for such disorders (Nurden, 2009). Although congenital afibrinogenemia is characterized by a similar absence of platelet aggregation, in this disorder, prothrombin time, activated partial thromboplastin time, and thrombin time are markedly prolonged, although they are normal in thrombasthenia.

DISORDERS OF PLATELET GRANULES, SECRETION, AND SIGNAL TRANSDUCTION

As a unifying theme, patients lumped into this heterogeneous group generally manifest impaired secretion of granule contents and absence of the second wave of aggregation upon stimulation of PRP with ADP or epinephrine; responses to collagen, thromboxane analog (U46619), arachidonic acid, and platelet-activating factor (PAF) may also be impaired. Conceptually, platelet function is abnormal in these patients when granule contents are diminished (storage pool deficiency [SPD]), or when an aberration occurs in the activation mechanisms governing aggregation and secretion (see Table 40-7).

Deficiency of Granule Stores

The term SPD refers to patients with deficiencies in platelet content of dense granules (δ-SPD), α-granules (α-SPD), or both types of granules (αδSPD) (Hayward, 1997; Rao, 2005; Nurden, 2009).

δ-Storage Pool Deficiency

Patients with δ-storage pool deficiency (δ-SPD) have a mild to moderate bleeding diathesis associated with prolonged bleeding time. In platelet studies, the second wave of aggregation in response to ADP and epinephrine is absent or blunted, and the collagen response is markedly impaired. However, both impaired (Weiss, 1981) and normal (Ingerman, 1978) aggregation responses to arachidonic acid have been noted. Responses to epinephrine may also be variable; a second wave of aggregation is noted in some patients (Weiss, 1988). It is interesting to note that δ-SPD has been documented (Nieuwenhuis, 1987; Israels, 1990) in a number of patients with prolonged bleeding times and normal aggregation responses. Thrombin-induced secretion of acid hydrolases is also impaired in SPD platelets; this is corrected by addition of exogenous ADP.

Normal platelets possess three to eight dense granules/platelet (each 200–300 nm in diameter) (Nieuwenhuis, 1987; Israels, 1990). Under the electron microscope, dense granules are decreased in SPD platelets (White, 1971; Israels, 1990). Other methods to demonstrate a decrease in dense granules include (1) fluorescence microscopy after staining of platelets with mepacrine (quinacrine), which localizes in dense granules because of high affinity for ATP; and (2) specific staining by uranyl ions (uranaffin reaction) of both the membrane and the core of dense granules. Flow cytometry can also be applied to assess fluorescent staining of dense granules (Linden, 2004). By direct biochemical measurement, total platelet and granule ATP and ADP contents are decreased (Holmsen, 1979) along with other dense granule constituents such as calcium, pyrophosphate, and serotonin. Two thirds of platelet ATP and ADP resides in the dense granules and a smaller amount in the metabolic pool; proportionately more ADP than ATP is present in dense granules (Holmsen, 1979). Thus, in δ-SPD platelets, the ratio of total ATP to ADP is increased (>2.5) compared with that in normal platelets. Incubation of normal platelets with carbon-14–serotonin results in its incorporation into dense granules and subsequent secretion upon activation. In SPD platelets, the initial rate of uptake of carbon-14–serotonin is normal, but saturation levels and retention over 4–6 hours are decreased.

Other abnormalities reported in δ-SPD include decreased synthesis of prostaglandins, TxA_2, and malondialdehyde in platelets activated with collagen and epinephrine, but not arachidonic acid (Weiss, 1988); impaired liberation of arachidonic acid from membrane phospholipids (Rendu, 1978); and an enhanced ADP- but not thrombin-induced rise in cytoplasmic Ca^{++} levels (Lages, 1997). Platelet procoagulant activity

PART 5

(prothrombinase activity) induced upon activation has been reported to be impaired in association with an inability to maintain elevated intracellular Ca^{++} levels (Weiss, 1997).

δ-SPD has been reported in association with other inherited disorders such as the Hermansky-Pudlak syndrome (HPS) (oculocutaneous albinism and increased reticuloendothelial ceroid), the Chédiak-Higashi syndrome, WAS, thrombocytopenia with absent radii syndrome, and the Griscelli syndrome (Menasche, 2000; Gunay-Aygun, 2004). The simultaneous occurrence of δ-SPD and defects in skin pigment granules, as in HPS, points to the interrelatedness of the two types of granules with respect to genetic control—a concept further advanced by animal models (Novak, 1984; Menasche, 2000; Huizing, 2001; Gunay-Aygun, 2004).

Dense granule membranes possess the lysosomal proteins, lysosome-associated membrane protein 2 and CD63 (granulophysin or LAMP3) (Nishibori, 1993; Israels, 1996), as well as P-selectin and GPIIb/IIIa. Granulophysin is deficient in HPS platelets (Gerrard, 1991). Studies with antigranulophysin antibody demonstrated the presence of a normal number of granules in platelets of two nonalbino patients with SPD (McNicol, 1994); therefore, these patients have the granules but with reduced contents.

A substantial amount of information on SPD has been obtained from patients with HPS, which is characterized by oculocutaneous albinism, platelet SPD, and lipofuscinosis (Gunay-Aygun, 2004; Huizing, 2008). A large group of HPS patients reside in Northwest Puerto Rico, where HPS occurs in 1 in every 1800 individuals (gene frequency, 1 in 21) (Witkop, 1990). At least eight HPS-causing genes are known, leading to various subtypes of human HPS, with most patients being in HPS-1 and coming from Puerto Rico (Gunay-Aygun, 2004; Huizing, 2008). At least 14 mouse models of HPS have been reported to date; seven of these constitute models for the human subtypes (Gunay-Aygun, 2004). Together, human and mouse models have served as an invaluable source of information about vesicle formation and trafficking. Human HPS subtypes are autosomal recessive, and heterozygotes have no clinical findings. In addition to albinism, which is variable between HPS subtypes, most patients have congenital nystagmus and decreased visual acuity. Two additional manifestations have been noted in patients with HPS: granulomatous colitis and pulmonary fibrosis (Gunay-Aygun, 2004).

Chédiak-Higashi syndrome is a rare autosomal recessive disorder characterized by SPD, oculocutaneous albinism, immune deficiency, neurologic dysfunction, and the presence of giant cytoplasmic inclusions in different cells (Huizing, 2001). Chédiak-Higashi syndrome patients have defective cytotoxic T and natural killer cell function. It arises from mutations in the lysosomal trafficking regulator *(LYST)* gene on chromosome 1. The protein coded by this gene interacts with several proteins, including the SNARE complex protein HRS and signaling proteins, and participates in intracellular membrane fusion reactions and vesicle trafficking (Huizing, 2001; Tchernev, 2002).

Gray Platelet Syndrome

The term **gray platelet syndrome (GPS)** has been derived from the initial observation by Raccuglia (1971) of a gray appearance of platelets, with a paucity of granules in peripheral blood smears from a patient with a lifelong bleeding disorder. Characterized by an isolated deficiency of α-granule contents, GPS patients have a lifelong bleeding diathesis of autosomal recessive inheritance, mild thrombocytopenia, and prolonged bleeding time (Weiss, 1979; Gerrard, 1980; Nurden, 2008). Under the electron microscope, platelets and megakaryocytes reveal absent or markedly decreased α-granules (Levy-Toledano, 1981). Platelets are severely and selectively deficient in α-granule proteins such as platelet factor four (PF4), β-thromboglobulin, vWF, thrombospondin, fibronectin, factor V, high molecular weight kininogen, and PDGF (Gerrard, 1980; Nurden, 1982). Platelet aggregation responses have been variable. Responses to ADP and epinephrine were normal in most patients; however, in some patients, aggregation responses to thrombin, collagen, and ADP have been impaired. Impaired thrombin-induced Ca^{++} mobilization and an increase in Ca^{++} transport have been reported in some patients. GPS is a heterogeneous disorder associated with abnormalities in α-granule formation and maturation (Nurden, 2008).

Plasma levels of PF4 and βTG have been found to be raised in some patients (Gerrard, 1980), suggesting that the defect is not in their synthesis by megakaryocytes but in their packaging into granules. Studies on megakaryocytes cultured from peripheral blood of three GPS patients show that vWF is synthesized but is secreted into extracellular space instead of normal α-granule packaging (Drouin, 2001). The neutrophils from these patients also had decreased granules. Reticulin is increased in the bone marrow from GPS patients (Breton-Gorius, 1981; Levy-Toledano, 1981), which can be attributed to elevated plasma PDGF levels. Using complementary DNA (cDNA) microarrays, Hyman (2003) found upregulation of cytoskeletal proteins, including fibronectin 1, thrombospondins 1 and 2, and collagen VIα, in fibroblasts from a patient with GPS.

Quebec Platelet Disorder

The Quebec platelet disorder (QPD) is an autosomal dominant disorder associated with delayed bleeding and abnormal proteolysis of α-granule proteins caused by increased amounts of platelet urokinase-type plasminogen activator (Kahr, 2001; McKay, 2004). Patients are characterized by normal to reduced platelet counts, proteolytic degradation of soluble and membrane proteins of α-granules, deficiency of an α-granule factor V–binding protein called multimerin, and selective defective aggregation with epinephrine. Platelet factor V but not plasma factor V is degraded along with other α-granule proteins, fibrinogen, vWF, thrombospondin, osteonectin, fibronectin, and P-selectin. QPD appears to derive from pathologically increased expression of the urokinase plasminogen activator (uPA) in megakaryocytes caused by a *cis* regulatory defect linked to the *uPA* gene (Diamandis, 2009). This leads to an increase in platelet uPA stores, which are only partially inhibited, and in turn increased intraplatelet generation of plasmin, which degrades several platelet α-granule proteins. Additionally, the uPA released by activated QPD platelets leads to increased platelet-dependent fibrinolysis, which may contribute in a major way to the bleeding observed in QPD. Patients with QPD suffer from mucocutaneous bleeding, which often is delayed by 12–24 hours following injury and is unresponsive to platelet transfusions but responsive to fibrinolytic inhibitors (McKay, 2004).

Defects in Receptors, G-Proteins, and Platelet Signal Transduction

Signal transduction mechanisms encompass processes that are initiated by the interaction of agonists with specific platelet receptors and include responses such as G-protein activation and activation of effector enzymes such as phospholipase C and phospholipase A_2 (see Figs. 40-3 and 40-6, and also section on platelet activation and signaling events). If the key components in signal transduction are the surface receptors, the G-proteins, and the effectors, evidence now exists for specific platelet abnormalities at each of these levels.

Patients with defects in platelet–agonist interaction have impaired responses caused by an abnormality in the platelet surface receptor for a specific agonist. Such receptor defects have been documented for epinephrine, collagen, ADP, and TxA_2 (Rao, 2004; Coller, 2010). Hirata (1994) described an Arg 60-to-Leu mutation of the human TxA_2 receptor in a dominantly inherited bleeding disorder. Several patients with a defect in the P2Y12 ADP receptor, which is coupled to inhibition of adenylyl cyclase, have been described (Cattaneo, 1992; Nurden, 1995; Cattaneo, 1997; Daly, 2009). Because ADP and TxA_2 play a synergistic role in platelet responses to several agonists, patients with receptor defects manifest abnormal responses to multiple agonists. Specific deficiencies in the P2Y1 (Oury, 1999) and P2X (Oury, 2000) ADP receptors have been documented but are less well characterized.

A few patients with isolated blunting of platelet responses to collagen associated with deficiencies in platelet GPIa and GPVI have been described (Nieuwenhuis, 1985, 1986; Kehrel, 1988; Khan, 2004). Reduced surface expression by flow cytometry of GPIa on the platelets of 18 individuals from two unrelated families with an autosomally dominant bleeding disorder has been reported; Western blot analysis also showed mildly reduced GPIa. However, no mutations in GPIa or GPIIa could be demonstrated (Noris, 2006). Abnormalities of GPVI have been associated with increased bleeding tendency (Khan, 2004). Deficiency of platelet GPVI in some patients has been attributed to anti-GPVI antibody–mediated loss of this GP (Boylan, 2004). A familial defect in GPVI signaling has been described, the characterization of which involved flow cytometry, studies of aggregation and secretion, tyrosine immunoblotting, and GPVI shedding (Arthur, 2007; Dunkley, 2007). It has been proposed that metalloproteinase-mediated ectodomain shedding of GPVI may constitute a regulatory control on the reactivity of this receptor (Berndt, 2007). Last, polymorphisms of GPVI are being studied as possible risk factors for thrombosis (Moroi, 1989; Arai, 1995; Nieswandt, 2001; Cabeza, 2004; Nurden, 2004; Yee, 2004).

G-proteins make up a heterogeneous group of proteins that link surface receptors and intracellular effector enzymes; defects in G-protein activation can impair signal transduction (see Chapter 74). Patients with deficiencies at the level of Gαq (Gabbeta, 1997) and Gαi1 (Patel, 2003) have been described. A patient with the Gαq deficiency had a mild bleeding disorder, abnormal aggregation and secretion responses to a number of agonists, and diminished GTPase activity (a reflection of G-protein α-subunit function) on activation. Essentially identical abnormal platelet findings have been reported in Gαq-deficient knockout mice (Offermanns, 1997). Additionally, impaired platelet responses have been reported in association with Gαs hyperfunction (which leads to increased cAMP levels) and alterations in the Gαs gene (*GNAS1*) (Freson, 2001b).

Platelet signal transduction is also impaired by defects in phospholipase C activation, calcium mobilization, and protein phosphorylation. Several patients have been identified who have a relatively mild bleeding diathesis and impaired dense granule secretion, although their platelets have normal granule stores and, in general, synthesize substantial amounts of TxA_2. On laboratory testing, these patients have abnormal aggregation and secretion, particularly in response to some agonists (ADP, epinephrine, PAF); the response to other agonists such as arachidonate and high concentrations of collagen may be normal. Such patients appear to be more common than those with SPD or defects in TxA_2 synthesis. Defects in early platelet activation events, including Ca^{++} mobilization, phosphatidylinositol hydrolysis, and phosphorylation of pleckstrin (a protein phosphorylated by protein kinase C), have been described (Rao, 2004; Coller, 2010). Specific deficiencies at the level of phospholipase C-β2 (Lee, 1996; Yang, 1996) and protein kinase C-θ (Sun, 2004) have been documented. Activation of GPIIb/IIIa and platelet fibrinogen binding is a prerequisite for aggregation and is a signal transduction–dependent process. Defects in GPIIb/IIIa activation due to upstream signal transduction defects have been noted in some patients (Gabbeta, 1996). A major platelet response to activation consists of liberation of arachidonic acid from phospholipids and its subsequent oxygenation to TxA_2, which plays a synergistic role in the response to several agonists. Patients have been described with impaired liberation of arachidonic acid from membrane phospholipids related to an abnormality in phospholipase A_2 (Adler, 2008), as well as with congenital deficiencies of cyclooxygenase and thromboxane synthase (Rao, 2004; Coller, 2010); these lead to diminished TxA_2 production on platelet stimulation.

DEFECTS IN CYTOSKELETAL ASSEMBLY

WAS is an X-linked inherited disorder affecting T lymphocytes and platelets and characterized by thrombocytopenia, immunodeficiency, and eczema (Remold-O'Donnell, 1996). Bleeding manifestations are variable. Several platelet abnormalities, including dense granule deficiency and deficiencies of platelet GPIb, GPIIb/IIIa, and GPIa have been reported. WAS arises from mutations in the gene coding for the WAS protein of 502 amino acids that binds to several other signaling proteins, including Cdc42 (a GTPase) and p47nck (a SH3-containing adapter protein) (Remold-O'Donnell, 1996; Zigmond, 2000). This protein constitutes a link between the cytoskeleton and signaling pathways and is a key regulator of cytoskeletal assembly.

DISORDERS OF PLATELET PROCOAGULANT ACTIVITIES

Platelets play a major role in blood coagulation by providing the surface on which several specific key enzymatic reactions occur. As discussed previously, in resting platelets, asymmetry is seen in the distribution of some of the phospholipids, such that PS and phosphatidylethanolamine are located predominantly on the inner leaflet, and phosphatidylcholine has the opposite distribution. Platelet activation results in redistribution with expression of PS on the outer surface, mediated by phospholipid scramblase (see Fig. 40-2). Exposure of PS on the outer surface is an important event in the expression of platelet procoagulant activities. A few patients have been described in whom the platelet contribution to blood coagulation is impaired, but aggregation and secretion responses are normal; this is referred to as Scott syndrome (Weiss, 1994; Solum, 1999; Weiss 2009). In these patients, who have a bleeding disorder, bleeding time and platelet aggregation responses have been normal, as have PT and partial thromboplastin time. In a patient described by Weiss (1994), platelet factor Xa–binding sites and binding of factors IXa and VIIIa were diminished; this was associated with decreased surface expression of PS following platelet activation. A review of additional patients presenting with forms of Scott syndrome has recently been presented (Weiss, 2009).

TRANSCRIPTION FACTOR MUTATIONS AND ASSOCIATED PLATELET DYSFUNCTION

Transcription factors regulate the expression of proteins in platelets and megakaryocytes, megakaryopoiesis, and platelet production. Several reports have demonstrated impaired platelet function and congenital thrombocytopenia in patients with mutations in specific transcription factors.

RUNX1/CBFA2 (Familial Platelet Disorder With Predisposition to Acute Myelogenous Leukemia)

An association between inherited platelet function abnormalities, thrombocytopenia, and a predisposition to acute myeloid leukemia (AML) has been reported in several families and has been linked to mutations in the gene *RUNX1* (*AML1*, *CBFA2*) (Song, 1999; Sun, 2004; Coller, 2010) (see Chapter 77 for a discussion of *RUNX1* in AML). This disorder is inherited as an autosomal dominant trait. Platelet abnormalities include impaired aggregation and secretion, granule deficiency, abnormal αIIbβ3 activation, decreased platelet myosin light chain and pleckstrin phosphorylation, decrease in platelet protein kinase C-θ and 12-lipoxygenase, and decreased platelet thrombopoietin receptors (Mpl) (Song, 1999; Sun, 2004; Coller, 2010; Kaur, 2010). *RUNX1* regulates expression of several genes including *MYL9* (myosin light chain) (Jalagadugula, 2010), *PF4* (Aneja, 2011), 12-lipoxygenase (*ALOX12*) (Kaur, 2010), and protein kinase C-θ.

GATA-1

GATA-1 is a major transcription factor regulating both megakaryopoiesis and thrombopoiesis. *GATA-1* mutations have been associated with an X-linked syndrome consisting of dyserythropoiesis, anemia, thrombocytopenia, and large platelets (Drachman, 2004); selectively impaired responses to collagen and ristocetin related to abnormalities in GPIbβ; diminished levels of platelet GαS protein and messenger RNA (mRNA); and a form of GPS (Freson, 2001a; Drachman, 2004; Hughan, 2005; Tubman, 2007).

RELATIVE FREQUENCIES OF VARIOUS INHERITED PLATELET DEFECTS

The relative frequency of various disorders remains unknown. The entities commonly thought about—Glanzmann thrombasthenia, BSS, and SPD—are distinctly uncommon, with the exception of some local pockets on a worldwide basis. Thrombasthenia and BSS are rare disorders. Although no data have been published, patients currently lumped into the heterogeneous category of defects in platelet secretion and signal transduction probably exhibit the more frequently encountered inherited platelet function abnormalities, excluding vWD. In our experience, in most of them, the underlying mechanisms are unknown. SPD is present in less than 10%–15% of patients with congenital platelet defects. Abnormalities in thromboxane production occur in about 20% of these patients. A large proportion of remaining patients with abnormal aggregation and secretion demonstrate adequate dense granule stores and produce substantial amounts of TxA_2. In some of these patients, evidence suggests defects in the signaling mechanisms (Rao, 2004).

EVALUATION OF PATIENTS WITH SUSPECTED PLATELET DISORDERS

The evaluation of patients with a clinical history or symptoms suggesting a bleeding tendency involves consideration of the coagulation and fibrinolytic systems, as well as of the blood platelets. A carefully conducted history and physical examination can be the single most important factor leading to a diagnosis in many patients. Determination of whether the disorder is likely to be congenital or acquired is important, and a family history is critically important. A platelet count may help determine whether the bleeding tendency is explicable by decreased platelet numbers alone. Prolonged PFA-100 or bleeding time may help determine whether a platelet defect is present. However, both may be normal in patients with platelet function defects. Because vWD may be more common than congenital platelet defects in patients with mucocutaneous bleeding manifestations, simultaneous evaluation of plasma factor VIII and vWF would be indicated.

Bleeding manifestations in patients with inherited platelet function defects are highly variable. The usual reasons for referral for evaluation include mucocutaneous bleeding manifestations, excessive bleeding following a procedure or surgery, and prolonged bleeding time or PFA-100 with a reasonable platelet count. In patients suspected of having a platelet function defect, possible studies include platelet count, bleeding time, PFA-100, and studies to assess platelet aggregation and secretion responses in vitro. Platelet studies are usually performed using PRP harvested from anticoagulated blood, and responses to various agonists, including ADP, epinephrine, collagen, arachidonic acid, a TxA_2 analog (U46619), thrombin receptor peptides, and ristocetin, are monitored. The patterns of response observed may often provide clues to the nature of the underlying platelet defect, although specific techniques, largely available in research laboratories, are required to delineate the precise platelet mechanisms that are altered. Patients with classical thrombasthenia are characterized by the absence of both primary and secondary waves of aggregation in response to all commonly used agonists (except ristocetin) with a normal shape change response. Impaired or absent response to ristocetin with normal aggregation response to other agonists suggests vWD or BSS. In the latter disorder, platelet counts are decreased and platelet size is increased. Although these findings may occur in some variants of vWD (e.g., type 2B), plasma levels of vWF and factor VIII, as well as the multimeric pattern of vWF, are normal in BSS but abnormal in vWD. Patients with impaired granule secretion or diminished dense granule contents generally show a decreased or absent second wave of aggregation in response to ADP, epinephrine, and PAF, along with blunted responses to other agonists (collagen, U46619) associated with markedly decreased release of granule contents.

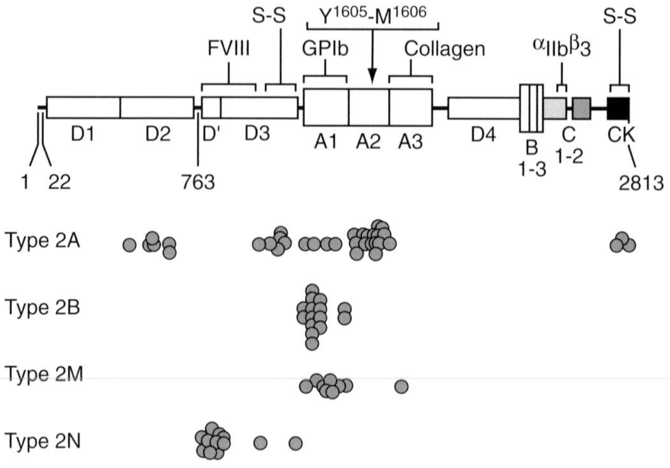

Figure 40-7 Structure of von Willebrand factor (vWF) and mutations in von Willebrand disease (vWD) type 2. The vWF precursor consists of a signal peptide (residues 1–22), a propeptide (residues 23–763), and the mature subunit (residues 764–2813). The locations are indicated for repeated domains (A, B, C, D, CK); binding sites for factor VIII (FVIII), platelet glycoprotein Ib (GPIb), collagen, and integrin αIIβ3; intersubunit disulfide bonds (S–S); and the Tyr–Met bond cleaved by ADAMTS13 (Y1605–M1606). Below, the schematic structure of vWF is shown, along with the locations of mutations that cause specific subtypes of vWD type 2. *(Sadler JE. New concepts in von Willebrand disease. Annu Rev Med 2005;56:175, Figure 1. Reprinted, with permission, from the Annual Review of Medicine, Volume 56, © 2005 by Annual Reviews at www. annualreviews.org.)*

THERAPY FOR CONGENITAL PLATELET FUNCTION DEFECTS

Platelet transfusions and 1-desamino-8D-arginine vasopressin (DDAVP) administration have been the mainstays of therapy for patients with inherited platelet defects. Because of wide disparity in bleeding manifestations, therapeutic approaches need to be individualized. Platelet transfusions are effective in controlling bleeding manifestations but are associated with potential risks involving blood products, including alloimmunization. Patients with thrombasthenia may develop antibodies against GPIIb/IIIa that compromise the efficacy of subsequent platelet transfusions. A viable alternative to platelet transfusions is intravenous administration of DDAVP, which was shown to shorten bleeding time in a substantial number of patients with platelet function defects (Rao, 1995; Mannucci, 1998). The effect on bleeding time lasted about 4–5 hours. This response appears to be dependent on the abnormalities leading to platelet dysfunction. Most patients with Glanzmann thrombasthenia have not responded to DDAVP infusion with shortening of the bleeding time. Responses in patients with disorders of platelet secretion, signal transduction, or storage pool deficiency have been variable, with shortening of bleeding time reported in some patients.

DDAVP administration induces a rise in plasma vWF, factor VIII, and tissue plasminogen activator. Abnormal in vitro platelet aggregation or secretion responses in patients with platelet defects are not corrected by DDAVP (Rao, 1995). Recently, recombinant factor VIIa has developed into an important drug for the management of bleeding events in patients with Glanzmann thrombasthenia and some other inherited defects (Poon, 2000; Almeida, 2003). Additional approaches that have been utilized to improve hemostasis in patients with inherited platelet defects include a short (3–4 day) course of prednisone (20–50 mg) (Mielke, 1981) and administration of antifibrinolytic agents such as ε-aminocaproic acid or tranexamic acid. Allogeneic bone marrow transplantation has now been successfully performed with complete correction in patients with thrombasthenia, although the development of antibodies directed against the GPIIb/IIIa complex remains a potential problem (Flood, 2005; Fujimoto, 2005).

VON WILLEBRAND FACTOR AND VON WILLEBRAND DISEASE

VON WILLEBRAND FACTOR BIOLOGY

von Willebrand factor is a pivotal protein in hemostasis, playing key roles both in primary hemostasis and in secondary hemostasis. In the latter role, vWF serves as a carrier protein for factor VIII; in the absence of vWF, factor VIII is rapidly cleared from the plasma (see Chapter 39). With respect to primary hemostasis, vWF serves as an adhesive platelet ligand that tethers the platelet to exposed collagen at sites of vascular injury. vWF circulating in the blood plasma is derived from secretion by endothelial cells. This secretion has a major constitutive component, but a releasable pool of vWF is also stored in the endothelial Weibel-Palade bodies. Megakaryocytes also synthesize vWF, which is stored in the platelet α-granules. This pool of vWF is released only upon platelet activation, as part of the more general platelet release reaction. Although such released vWF generally would not be capable of appreciably raising the overall level of vWF in the plasma, local increases in vWF at sites of injury may be significant.

The vWF gene is located on chromosome 12 and is 178 kB long, extending over 52 exons. The presence of a partial, but nonfunctional, duplication of the vWF gene on chromosome 22 (vWF pseudogene) is an important consideration in the design of primers for amplification of the vWF gene. Following cleavage of an N-terminal propolypeptide fragment, the mature 2050 amino acid vWF protein is composed of a series of functional domains, as shown in Figure 40-7. Individual vWF monomeric units are bound together by a series of disulfide bonds, which occur near both N-termini and C-termini (Tsai, 2003). The resulting multimers may achieve molecular weights exceeding 20 MDa. Soon after their secretion into the blood, however, vWF multimers undergo proteolytic trimming by the metalloproteinase ADAMTS13. Although a potential cleavage site exists between Tyr842 and Met843 within the A2 domain of each vWF multimer, following a certain degree of proteolysis, the ADAMTS13 proteolysis of potential sites within vWF comes to a halt—presumably as the result of steric hindrance of the ADAMTS13 penetrating deeper into the vWF multimeric structure. Deficiency of ADAMTS13, due to a congenital abnormality or to the formation of autoantibodies against the enzyme, results in the circulation of unusually large vWF multimers in the plasma. These forms are capable of spontaneously aggregating platelets, as well as forming large strands anchored to the endothelial surface that can result in RBC fragmentation—two characteristic attributes of the associated disorder, TTP.

At sites of vessel injury, vWF binds to exposed subendothelial collagen. Particularly under conditions of high shear, where relatively high blood flow occurs through smaller-diameter vessels, bound vWF and GPIbα on the surface of circulating blood platelets are able to bind together, effectively tethering the platelet to the injury site. This ligand–receptor interaction further produces outside-to-inside signaling across the platelet membrane, leading to platelet activation. One component of this platelet activation consists of a subsequent inside-to-outside signaling event within GPIIb/IIIa that makes this receptor complex competent to bind the aggregatory ligand fibrinogen. In the clinical laboratory, vWF may be assayed antigenically, functionally, and even structurally. Although vWF antigen was formerly quantified by a variety of gel electrophoretic approaches, it may now be measured with high precision by rapid methods such as ELISA or immunoturbidometric procedures.

TABLE 40-8
vWD Classification and Laboratory Values

Condition	Description	vWF:Rco (IU/dL)	vWF:Ag (IU/dL)	FVIII	vWF:Rco/vWF:Ag Ratio
Type 1	Partial quantitative vWF deficiency	<30*	<30*	↓ or Normal	>0.5–0.7
Type 2A	↓vWF-dependent platelet adhesion with selective deficiency of high molecular weight vWF multimers	<30*	<30–200‡	↓ or Normal	<0.5–0.7†
Type 2B	Increased vWF affinity for platelet GPIb; ± ↓platelet numbers	<30*	<30–200‡	↓ or Normal	Usually <0.5–0.7†
Type 2M	↓vWF-dependent platelet adhesion without selective deficiency of high molecular weight vWF multimers	<30*	<30–200‡	↓ or Normal	<0.5–0.7†
Type 2N	Markedly decreased vWF binding affinity for FVIII	30–200	30–200	↓↓	>0.5–0.7
Type 3	Virtually complete deficiency of vWF	<3	<3	↓↓↓ (<10 IU/dL)	Not applicable
"Low vWF"*		30–50	30–50	Normal	>0.5–0.7
Normal		50–200	50–200	Normal	>0.5–0.7

Modified with permission from Nichols WL. Am J Hematol 2009;84:366–70. Note that these values represent prototypical cases. Exceptions occur, and repeat testing may be necessary.

FVIII, Coagulation factor VIII activity; *GP,* glycoprotein; *vWD,* von Willebrand disease; *vWF,* von Willebrand factor; *vWF:Ag,* vWF antigen; *vWF:RCo,* vWF ristocetin cofactor activity; ↓, decrease in function or in the test result compared with the laboratory reference range.

*<30 IU/dL (or 30%) is recommended as the "cutoff" level for a definitive diagnosis of vWD, although some patients with type 1 or type 2 vWD will have levels of vWF:RCo and/or vWF:Ag of 30–50 IU/dL. This "cutoff" is recommended because (1) There is a high frequency of blood type O in the United States, which is associated with "low" vWF levels; (2) bleeding symptoms are reported by a significant proportion of normal individuals; (3) no abnormality in the vWF gene has been identified in many individuals who have mildly to moderately low vWF:RCo levels. This does not preclude the diagnosis of vWD in patients with vWF:RCo of 30–50 IU/dL if supporting clinical and/or family evidence of vWD is present, nor does this preclude the use of agents to increase vWF levels in those who have vWF:RCo of 30–50 IU/dL, and who may be at risk for bleeding.

†Until more laboratories clearly define a reference range, the vWF:RCo/vWF:Ag ratio of <0.5–0.7 is recommended to distinguish type 1 vs. type 2 vWD variants (A, B, or M).

‡Note that despite the higher value occasionally observed, the vWF:Ag in the majority of individuals with type 2A, 2B, or 2M vWD is <50 IU/dL.

VON WILLEBRAND DISEASE AND ITS SUBTYPES

As shown in Table 40-8, a variety of clinical conditions may be associated with vWF abnormalities. In type 1 vWD, qualitatively normal vWF molecules are present in the plasma but are quantitatively decreased. Accordingly, a normal distribution of vWF multimers is seen across the entire size spectrum, albeit lower than normal amounts of each multimer (Fig. 40-8). In one sense, type 3 vWD represents an extreme extent of the quantitative abnormality in that total absence of vWF gene product is evident. However, whereas inherited type 1 vWD is typically expressed in an autosomal dominant fashion, type 3 is autosomal recessive, with neither parent of an affected patient typically showing symptomatic disease. Because one of the key functions of vWF is to serve as a carrier molecule for factor VIII, type 3 patients not only suffer with respect to platelet function but are at further hemostatic risk because of vanishingly low amounts of circulating factor VIII.

Patients with type 2 vWD have one or another of the many described qualitative abnormalities of this complex protein. For practical purposes, these abnormalities have been grouped into a small number of subtypes. In type 2A vWD, lack of higher molecular weight multimers is seen (see Fig. 40-8), with corresponding loss of vWF functionality due to mutations that prevent proper multimerization or to mutations that increase the susceptibility of fully formed vWF to proteolysis by ADAMTS13 or other proteolytic enzymes. In some instances, vWF synthesized by megakaryocytes and stored in platelet α-granules appears to have a fuller complement of vWF multimers than does plasma vWF derived from secretion by endothelial cells; this may reflect the protective effects resulting from proteolysis due to sequestration within the α-granules. In type 2B vWD, point mutations within the vWF molecule actually confer an increase-of-function capability with respect to its ability to bind the platelet GPIb receptor. Binding of abnormal type 2B vWF molecules to circulating platelets in the absence of appropriate hemostatic insult leads to uncompensated depletion of the higher molecular weight multimers of plasma vWF (see Fig. 40-8) and typically also to mild to moderate thrombocytopenia. In the clinical laboratory, this increase-of-function can be demonstrated by the ability of abnormally low concentrations (typically 0.3–0.5 mg/mL) of the modulator ristocetin (a glycopeptide antibiotic produced by *Amycolatopsis lurida*) to aggregate the PRP of such patients.

In contrast, in the case of type 2A vWD or type 1 vWD, the extent and rate of aggregation are decreased to below normal at standard ristocetin concentrations of 1.0–1.5 mg/mL. Patients with type 2M vWD share a similar decrease-of-function phenotype with type 2A vWD, but the mutations responsible for this vWD subtype do not result in loss of normal vWF multimeric structure. If, in contrast to testing the patient's own PRP, the patient's platelet-free plasma is tested for ristocetin cofactor activity, the observed level is decreased not only in type 1, type 2A, and type 2M, but also in type 2B, because of acquired deficiency of high molecular weight multimers actually remaining in the patient's plasma. In type 1 vWD, the levels of vWF antigen and ristocetin cofactor activity generally

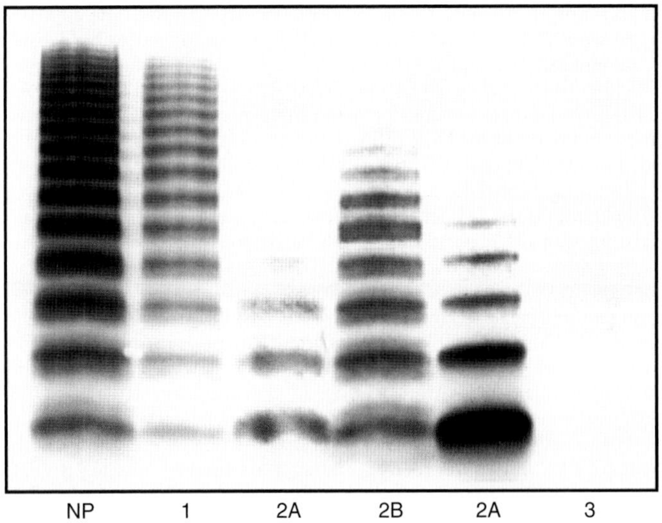

Figure 40-8 Multimer patterns in selected variants of von Willebrand disease (vWD). Plasma samples were analyzed for von Willebrand factor (vWF) by sodium dodecyl sulfate (SDS)-agarose gel electrophoresis and Western blotting. Patterns are shown for pooled normal plasma (NP) and patients with the indicated types of vWD. Note that in the 2A and 2B examples, there is relative loss of higher molecular weight multimers, although to varying extents. Of note, the extent of multimer loss is highly variable in each subtype, and the differences in extent of multimer loss between the 2A and 2B subtypes illustrated in these particular examples do not distinguish between these subtypes in diagnostic studies. Instead, functional studies are required to distinguish between the decrease-of-function 2A subtype and the increase-of-function 2B subtype (see text). *(Adapted with permission from Sadler JE. New concepts in von Willebrand disease. Annu Rev Med 2005;56:173–91; and Sadler JE. von Willebrand disease. In: Bloom AL, Forbes CD, Thomas DP, Tuddenham EGD, editors. Hemostasis and thrombosis. New York: Churchill Livingstone; 1994, p. 843–57.)*

decline in parallel. In contrast, in type 2 patients, a more dramatic decrease in ristocetin cofactor activity than in vWF antigen level is typically seen, because it is precisely the missing higher molecular weight multimers that are critical to the vWF–platelet interaction measured by this functional assay. A similar discrepancy may be observed between vWF collagen-binding activity and vWF antigen. Finally, patients with type 2N (Normandy) vWD have point mutations within the vWF molecule that specifically impair the ability of this molecule to bind factor VIII. Type 2N patients accordingly may show normal levels of vWF antigen and even of ristocetin cofactor activity, but will have abnormally low levels of circulating factor VIII. Because the vWF gene is transmitted autosomally, type 2N vWD should be suspected in cases where an autosomal inheritance pattern of factor VIII deficiency is noted. Definitive diagnosis is made by demonstrating impaired binding of normal factor VIII to the patient vWF, such as by ELISA assay and by molecular diagnostic methods.

Whereas, at least conceptually, the basis for diagnosing type 2 and type 3 vWD seems clear, the same cannot be said for type 1 vWD (Sadler, 2003, 2005). The level of circulating vWF is a result of multigenic influences. Not only genes encoding vWF, but also genes encoding intracellular transporter proteins, ABO genes affecting posttranslational modifications of the vWF molecule, genes affecting vWF proteolysis, and doubtless still other genetic factors may influence the quantity and functionality of vWF. For example, individuals inheriting the same vWF genes may be anticipated to have 20% or lower circulating levels of vWF if they are of type O rather than type AB blood group type. In some instances, this could mean the difference between being considered normal or deficient in vWF level. Additionally, Sadler (2003) has argued that, because of the relatively high prevalence of mild bleeding symptoms and of mild deficiencies of vWF, it may be erroneous to conclude that simple demonstration of a mild to moderate decrease in plasma vWF level is actually the *cause* of an individual patient's increased bleeding tendency. Thus, in such instances, it may be important to investigate additional possible causes for an apparent disorder of primary hemostasis, specifically, an abnormality of platelet aggregation or secretion in response to one or more platelet agonists. The approach to patients with mild deficiencies of vWF has continued to be debated (Gudmundsdottir, 2007; Onundarson, 2008). It has been proposed (Nichols, 2009; Sadler, 2009) that unless more diagnostic family or personal information is available for an individual presenting with a vWF level in the range of 30–50 U/dL, this condition may be better considered to be "low vWF" rather than "type 1 vWD" (see Table 40-8).

In the autosomal dominant bleeding disorder termed platelet-type von Willebrand disease (Miller, 1982; Weiss, 1982), patients characteristically have low-normal platelet counts, normal factor VIII coagulant activity, normal or decreased vWF antigen, and decreased plasma ristocetin cofactor activity. On agarose gel electrophoresis of plasma, a selective decrease in higher molecular weight multimers is seen, similar to that noted in type 2B vWD. However, unlike platelets from patients with type 2B vWD, platelets from patients with platelet-type vWD show an increased ability to bind normal vWF (Miller, 1983). In the diagnostic laboratory, this increased binding is reflected by the ability of unusually low concentrations of ristocetin (0.3–0.5 mg/mL) to produce strong aggregation of the patient's PRP in this disorder—a finding also observed in type 2B vWD (Ruggeri, 1980). Cryoprecipitate (which contains vWF), however, when added to platelet-type vWD platelets without additional aggregating agents, is capable of inducing aggregation; cryoprecipitate added to normal or type 2B vWD platelets, in contrast, does not produce aggregation. Platelets from patients with platelet-type von Willebrand disease also show unique agglutination reactions with desialylated vWF (asialo vWF) (Miller, 1987).

The molecular basis of platelet-type vWD has been shown to be due to a single base mutation resulting in the replacement of glycine by valine at amino acid residue 233 of the GPIb α-chain (Miller, 1991). Substitution of valine for methionine just 6 amino acids away at residue 239 has subsequently been reported in two additional kindreds (Russell, 1993; Takahashi, 1995). Each of these mutations is believed to produce conformational changes in the receptor, leading to abnormally heightened vWF binding (Pincus, 1991; Miller, 1996). Additionally, heightened binding in vivo between the mutant platelet protein and circulating vWF may induce a conformational change in the vWF that permits enhanced access for ADAMTS13 proteolysis (Nishio, 2004). Recently, a similar phenotype has been reported to result from a 9 amino acid deletion in an unexpectedly distant region of the GPIb α-chain (Othman, 2005). The incidence of platelet-type vWD is difficult to determine but appears to be far lower than even that of the relatively uncommon type 2B vWD disorder (Othman, 2010).

LABORATORY TESTS OF VON WILLEBRAND FACTOR

As is apparent from consideration of the domain structure of vWF (see Fig. 40-7), vWF is potentially capable of binding to a number of different molecules. Assessment of such binding comprises a group of functional tests of the vWF molecule. The principal functional tests of vWF currently employed in the evaluation of patients center around the binding of vWF to platelets, to collagen, and to factor VIII.

Although, as with a number of other plasma proteins, vWF does contain an RGD tripeptide sequence through which it can potentially bind to the platelet integrin GPIIb/IIIa, the major platelet receptor for vWF that is evaluated in the clinical laboratory is the GPIb/IX/V complex. Specifically, vWF binds to the α-chain of the GPIb molecule (GPIbα). Because platelets themselves contain a releasable store of vWF in their α-granules, and because the binding of exogenous vWF to normal, healthy platelets may lead to the release of that stored vWF (see earlier), assays of plasma vWF need to be designed to avoid the contribution of such released vWF. Fortunately, fixation of normal platelets with formalin preserves the reactivity of GPIbα to vWF, while effectively destroying the metabolic responses of the cell required to support secretion. Moreover, such fixed platelets may even be lyophilized and then reconstituted at the time of testing. When such platelets are incubated under stirring conditions with ristocetin, the rate and extent of their aggregation becomes a function of the amount of vWF contained in plasma samples used in the assay. This test of vWF reactivity with platelets is termed **vWF ristocetin cofactor activity** and may be performed manually in a standard platelet aggregometer or through a variety of more automated approaches.

Because measurements of ristocetin cofactor activity have traditionally suffered a relatively high coefficient of variation (i.e., low precision) compared with other tests performed in the coagulation laboratory (Kitchen, 2006), alternative measures of the interaction between vWF and platelet-associated GPIbα have been pursued, including assays based on ELISA, immunoturbidometric agglutination, flow cytometry, and other technologies (Vanhoorelbeke, 2000, 2002; Lattuada, 2004; Popov, 2006; Strandberg, 2006; Sucker, 2006; Pinol, 2007; Chen, 2008; Truss, 2009). As discussed earlier, it is characteristically the higher rather than the lower molecular weight multimers that are most active in binding to platelets, so that ristocetin cofactor activity will be expected to be diminished in instances where deficiency of the higher molecular weight multimers occurs, even if the total amount of vWF is normal (i.e., in instances where there is a relative abundance of only lower molecular weight multimers). Efforts to use recombinant GPIbα in functional ELISA assays to evaluate vWF functional activity (Federici, 2004; Hui, 2007; Flood, 2009) have also shown promise. Such assays may not always provide concordant results with traditional ristocetin cofactor assays, for example, not reporting out a comparably decreased value for some patient samples lacking the higher molecular weight multimers. On the other hand, an assay employing increase-of-function mutations in GPIbα corresponding to those seen in platelet-type vWD and that does not require the addition of ristocetin for vWF binding may be useful in demonstrating phenotypically normal variations in vWF that otherwise would be classified as a type 2M vWD by virtue of their failure to bind to the commonly employed reagent, ristocetin (Flood, 2009).

Measurement of the collagen-binding activity of vWF is more straightforward than ristocetin cofactor activity, usually assayed as the binding of vWF to collagen-coated wells by immunoassays such as ELISA. This activity is also greater in higher rather than lower molecular weight vWF multimers, so that frequently, vWF collagen-binding activity and vWF ristocetin cofactor activity will be similar. vWF collagen-binding activity, however, is generally considered a supplementary test rather than a replacement for tests assessing the interaction of vWF with platelets (Favaloro, 2007).

vWF multimeric analysis contributed significantly to the original foundation for defining the various phenotypes of vWD discussed previously. This technique traditionally has been sufficiently labor intensive to preclude its performance by all but a small number of reference laboratories, although the emergence of more automated approaches could potentially allow the performance of such analysis to become more widespread. At low resolution, multimeric analysis determines the relative distribution of vWF by molecular weight range. At higher resolution, abnormal patterns of multimers within a narrow size range may also be resolved. For example, vWF isolated from platelets will reveal higher multimers (also seen within endothelial cells) that are typically lost when vWF released into the circulating plasma comes in contact with ADAMTS13. Also apparent in these images is the production of additional bands reflecting proteolytic activity by ADAMTS13 that has not yet occurred on circulating vWF, along with vWF that had been protected within the platelet α-granules. Typical patterns of vWF multimers seen in the major vWD variants were discussed previously.

ACQUIRED VON WILLEBRAND DISEASE

Most patients with acquired vWD (AvWD) have been older than 40 years of age without previous manifestations or family history of a bleeding diathesis. Diverse associated disorders in these patients include both benign and malignant hematologic disorders (Federici, 2000; Kumar, 2002). About half of patients have had an underlying lymphoproliferative disorder or plasma cell proliferative disorder (Federici, 2000). In patients with myeloproliferative disease (chronic myelogenous leukemia, essential thrombocythemia, polycythemia vera) and with reactive thrombocytosis, an impressive correlation has been noted between abnormalities in plasma vWF and elevated platelet counts (Budde, 1997). AvWD has been reported in patients with autoimmune disorders, including systemic lupus erythematosus, scleroderma, mixed connective tissue disease, hypothyroidism, and antiphospholipid antibody syndrome (Federici, 2000; Kumar, 2002). Several therapeutic agents have been associated with AvWD: ciprofloxacin (Castaman, 1995), valproic acid, griseofulvin, and a plasma expander, hydroxyethyl starch. AvWD has been reported in patients with solid tumors, most notably Wilms' tumor, but case reports have associated AvWD with others as well (adrenocortical carcinoma, lung carcinoma, gastric carcinoma). Patients with aortic stenosis and congenital valvular heart disease may have excessive bleeding (particularly gastrointestinal), and several reports have documented AvWD in such patients (Gill, 1986; Vincentelli, 2003); of note, plasma abnormalities are corrected after surgery.

AvWD arises by diverse mechanisms. These include antibodies directed against functional domains of vWF (Kumar, 2002) with inhibition by patient plasma of ristocetin cofactor activity in normal plasma; enhanced clearance of vWF mediated by antibodies that are not targeted to a functional vWF region; increased proteolysis of vWF, induced by exposure of vWF to high stress, as, for example, in severe aortic stenosis (Sadler, 2005); and cellular adsorption and removal of vWF by malignant cells or by other cells (including platelets in myeloproliferative disease). Last, decreased vWF synthesis has been invoked in patients with hypothyroidism (Levesque, 1993) and in those receiving valproate (Kreuz, 1990).

ACQUIRED DISORDERS AFFECTING PLATELET FUNCTION

Alterations in platelet function occur in many acquired disorders of diverse origins (Rao, 2006). The specific biochemical and pathophysiologic aberrations leading to platelet dysfunction are poorly understood in most. In some, such as the myeloproliferative disorders (MPDs), intrinsically abnormal platelets are produced by the bone marrow. In others, dysfunction results from the interaction of platelets with exogenous factors, such as pharmacologic agents, artificial surfaces (cardiopulmonary bypass), compounds that accumulate in plasma owing to impaired renal function, and antibodies. In these disorders of platelet dysfunction, bleeding is usually mucocutaneous with a wide and often unpredictable spectrum of severity. The usual laboratory tests that identify platelet dysfunction include abnormal bleeding time, prolonged PFA-100 closure time, and abnormal in vitro platelet aggregation studies. Neither the PFA-100 nor the bleeding time is a reliable indicator of risk of clinical bleeding. For example, aspirin ingestion impairs platelet aggregation and secretion responses to usually used agonists (such as ADP, epinephrine, arachidonic acid, and low doses of collagen) in almost all individuals but prolongs bleeding time in only about half of subjects (Mielke, 1969; Mielke, 1983). Similarly, PFA-100 results may be normal in some patients with platelet defects (Hayward, 2006). In general, the correlation between abnormalities observed in bleeding time, PFA-100, or platelet aggregation studies and clinical bleeding remains weak.

MYELOPROLIFERATIVE DISORDERS

Bleeding tendency, thromboembolic complications, and qualitative platelet defects are all recognized in MPDs, which include essential thrombocythemia, polycythemia vera, chronic idiopathic myelofibrosis, and chronic myelogenous leukemia (Schafer, 1984; Landolfi, 1997) (see Chapter 33). Platelet abnormalities reflect their development from an abnormal clone of stem cells, but some of the alterations may be secondary to enhanced platelet activation in vivo. The clinical impact of in vitro qualitative platelet defects, which occur even in asymptomatic patients, is often unclear.

Numerous studies have examined platelet function and morphology in patients with MPD (Schafer, 1984; Landolfi, 1997). Under the electron microscope, platelet findings include reduction in dense and α-granules, alterations in open canalicular and dense tubular systems, and reduction of mitochondria (Maldonado, 1974). Bleeding time is prolonged in a minority (≈17%) of MPD patients and does not correlate with increased risk of bleeding (Schafer, 1984). Platelet aggregation responses are highly variable in MPD patients and often vary in the same patient over time. Decreased platelet responses are more common, although some patients demonstrate enhanced responses to agonists. In one analysis (Schafer, 1984), responses to ADP, collagen, and epinephrine were decreased in 39%, 37%, and 57% of patients, respectively. In patients with abnormally high circulating platelet counts, it has been a common laboratory practice to dilute patients' PRP with their own platelet-poor plasma to allow standardization of platelet aggregometry. However, recent studies have cautioned that decreases in aggregation observed in these patients may be at least partially artifactual, owing to inhibitory factors that appear to be present in the platelet-poor plasma employed as diluent (Cattaneo, 2007; Grignani, 2009). Impaired aggregation in response to epinephrine is more commonly encountered than with other agonists; however, a diminished response to epinephrine is not pathognomonic of an MPD. Impaired responsiveness to epinephrine in MPD has been attributed to a decrease in the number of platelet α_2-adrenergic receptors. Diminished epinephrine-induced TxA_2 production, dense granule secretion, and Ca^{++} mobilization have also been reported in patients with impaired epinephrine-induced aggregation response. On the platelet surface, decreases in GPIIb/IIIa complexes, GPIb, and GPIa/IIa have been documented in MPD. Evidence also reveals impaired signal transduction–dependent activation of GPIIb/IIIa (Kaplan, 2000). Platelet GPIV (CD36), another membrane GP related to platelet–collagen and platelet–thrombospondin interactions, has been noted to be increased in essential thrombocythemia (Legrand, 1991). Platelet receptors for the Fc portion of IgG have been reported to be increased in MPD platelets (Moore, 1981).

Platelet activation results in the release of free arachidonic acid, which is metabolized by two well-recognized pathways: the cyclooxygenase pathway, leading to TxA_2 production, and the 12-lipoxygenase pathway, leading to formation of 12-hydroperoxyeicosatetraenoic acid and 12-hydroxyeicosatetraenoic acid. Reduced platelet formation of lipoxygenase products has been reported in MPD patients (Schafer, 1982); this was associated with enhanced TxA_2 production (Schafer, 1982).

MPD patients have been reported to have defects in platelet signaling mechanisms, including calcium mobilization (Fujimoto, 1989), signaling through the TxA_2 receptor (Ushikubi, 1992), and protein phosphorylation due to deficiency of cyclic guanosine monophosphate-dependent protein kinase (Eigenthaler, 1993). Cooper (1978) reported a decrease in PGD_2-induced activation of adenylyl cyclase associated with a 50% reduction in platelet PGD_2 receptors, indicating impairment in platelet inhibitory mechanisms. Platelets from patients with polycythemia vera and idiopathic myelofibrosis, but not essential thrombocythemia or chronic myelogenous leukemia, have been shown to have reduced expression of the thrombopoietin receptor (Mpl) and reduced thrombopoietin-induced tyrosine phosphorylation of proteins (Moliterno, 1998).

Abnormalities in plasma vWF have been documented in MPD patients (and probably contribute to the hemostatic defect). Plasma vWF, particularly with large vWF multimers, is decreased, which is inversely related to platelet count, and has improved following cytoreduction (Budde, 1997). Changes in plasma vWF occur in patients with reactive thrombocytosis as well. Observed increases in the 140-kDa and 167-kDa proteolytic fragments of vWF raise the suspicion that enhanced vWF proteolysis by ADAMTS13 may be occurring, possibly because of platelet-induced conformational effects on the plasma vWF (Elliott, 2005).

ACUTE LEUKEMIAS AND MYELODYSPLASTIC SYNDROMES

The major cause of bleeding in these conditions is thrombocytopenia. However, in patients with normal or elevated platelet counts, bleeding complications may be associated with platelet dysfunction (Rao, 2005). Acquired platelet defects associated with clinical bleeding are more common in AML but have been reported in acute lymphoblastic and myelomonoblastic leukemias, hairy cell leukemia, and myelodysplastic syndromes. Reduced aggregation responses to ADP, epinephrine, and collagen have been reported, along with diminished nucleotide secretion, TxA_2 production, and platelet PDGF and βTG. Acquired forms of vWD and a Bernard-Soulier–like platelet defect have been described in hairy cell leukemia and myelodysplastic syndromes. In acute leukemias and myelodysplastic syndromes, platelets may be morphologically abnormal, and ultrastructural studies have shown decreased microtubules, reduced number and abnormal size of dense granules, and excessive membranous systems. The megakaryocytes exhibit dysplasia.

DYSPROTEINEMIAS

Excessive clinical bleeding may occur in patients with dysproteinemias; this appears to be related to multiple mechanisms, including platelet dysfunction, specific coagulation abnormalities, hyperviscosity, and alterations in blood vessels due to amyloid deposition. Qualitative platelet defects occur in some of these patients and have been attributed to coating of platelets by the paraprotein.

UREMIA

The pathogenesis of the hemostatic defect in uremia remains unclear, but platelet dysfunction and impaired platelet–vessel wall interaction are considered the major causes. Patients on dialysis have increased numbers of circulating reticulated platelets, indicating accelerated platelet turnover (Himmelfarb, 1997). Bleeding time was demonstrated many years ago to be prolonged in uremia. One major reason for this is the anemia frequently seen in uremia, and in fact, prolonged bleeding times are typically shortened following red cell transfusions or treatment with erythropoietin (Livio, 1982; Moia, 1987). Multiple platelet abnormalities are recognized in uremia (Boccardo, 2004). Adhesion of platelets to the subendothelium, an initial step in hemostasis, involves the interaction of vWF, platelets, and the subendothelium. Adhesion of platelets from uremic whole blood perfused over deendothelialized rabbit aorta has been reported to be impaired (Castillo, 1986). Most studies have found normal or increased plasma vWF antigen levels and activity (ristocetin cofactor), although in some vWF activity was consistently lower than the antigen level. The multimeric structure of vWF has been shown to be normal. The numbers of GPIb and GPIIb/GPIIIa sites per platelet have been reported to be normal in uremia (Gralnick, 1988). However, decreased platelet GPIb levels and a functional defect in vWF interaction with GPIIb/IIIa have been noted.

Many studies have shown impaired platelet aggregation responses to several agonists in uremia, sometimes with conflicting results. Plasma levels of PF4 and βTG are elevated in uremia and increase further with hemodialysis, reflecting reduced renal clearance, as well as platelet activation by membrane dialyzers. Several studies have shown reductions in products of arachidonic acid metabolism (PGG_2/PGH_2, TxA_2) in uremic platelets and have implicated these in observed defective aggregation and secretion. Reduced TXA_2 may arise as the result of a dysfunctional cyclooxygenase or through the liberation of arachidonic acid from phospholipids by phospholipase A_2 activation. Other platelet defects described in uremia include increased platelet cAMP levels and adenylyl cyclase (which can inhibit platelet responses), along with decreased agonist-induced Ca^{++} mobilization, clot retraction, and platelet procoagulant activity.

Convincing evidence suggests that pathogenesis of the hemostatic defect in uremia is linked to accumulation of dialyzable and nondialyzable molecules in the uremic plasma. One such compound, guanidinosuccinic acid, accumulates in uremic plasma, inhibits platelets in vitro, and stimulates generation of nitric oxide, which inhibits platelet adhesion and platelet responses by increasing levels of cellular cGMP (Boccardo, 2004). Exposure of human endothelial cells to uremic plasma leads to enhanced nitric oxide production. Enhanced prostacyclin-like activity has been observed in uremic plasma (Remuzzi, 1978). Aggressive dialysis is an important component of overall management and corrects the bleeding diathesis in some patients, but it is only partially effective in others. Elevation of the hematocrit with packed red blood cells or recombinant erythropoietin shortens bleeding time, improves platelet adhesion, and corrects mild bleeding in uremic patients.

ACQUIRED STORAGE POOL DISEASE

Several patients have been reported in whom the dense-granule SPD appears to be acquired (Rao, 2006). In general, this defect probably reflects in vivo release of platelet dense-granule contents due to activation or production of abnormal platelets by the marrow. Acquired SPD has been

TABLE 40-9
Drugs That Affect Platelet Function

Cyclooxygenase inhibitors
- Aspirin
- Nonsteroidal antiinflammatory agents
  - Indomethacin, phenylbutazone, ibuprofen, sulfinpyrazone, sulindac, meclofenamic acid

Adenosine diphosphate (ADP) receptor antagonists
- Ticlopidine, clopidogrel, prasugrel

Glycoprotein (GP)IIb/IIIa receptor antagonists
- c7E3 (abciximab), tirofiban, eptifibatride

Drugs that increase platelet cyclic adenosine monophosphate (cAMP) or cyclic guanosine monophosphate (cGMP)

Adenylate cyclase activators
- Prostaglandins I_2, D_2, E_1, and analogs

Phosphodiesterase inhibitors
- Dipyridamole
- Cilostazol
- Anagrelide
- Milrinone
- Methylxanthines
  - Caffeine, theophylline, aminophylline

Nitric oxide and nitric oxide donors

Antimicrobials
- Penicillins
- Cephalosporins
- Nitrofurantoin
- Hydroxychloroquine
- Miconazole

Cardiovascular drugs
- β-Adrenergic blockers (propranolol)
- Vasodilators (nitroprusside, nitroglycerin)
- Diuretics (furosemide)
- Calcium channel blockers
- Quinidine
- Angiotensin converting enzyme inhibitors

Anticoagulants
- Heparin

Thrombolytic agents
- Streptokinase, tissue plasminogen activator, urokinase

Psychotropics and anesthetics
- Tricyclic antidepressants
  - Imipramine, amitriptyline, nortriptyline
- Phenothiazines
  - Chlorpromazine, promethazine, trifluoperazine
- Selective serotinin reuptake inhibitors
  - Fluoxetine, sertraline, paroxetine
- Local anesthetics
- General anesthesia (halothane)

Chemotherapeutic agents
- Mithramycin
- Carmustine
- Daunorubicin

Miscellaneous agents
- Dextrans and hydroxyethyl starch
- Lipid-lowering agents (clofibrate, halofenate)
- ε-Aminocaproic acid
- Antihistaminics
- Ethanol
- Vitamin E
- Radiographic contrast agents
- Food items (omega-3 fatty acids, vitamin E, onions, garlic, ginger, cumin, turmeric, cloves, black tree fungus, gingko)

Modified with permission from Rao AK. Acquired disorders of platelet function. In: Colman RW, editor. Hemostasis and thrombosis: basic principles and clinical practice. Philadelphia: Lippincott Williams & Wilkins; 2006.

observed in patients with antiplatelet antibodies, systemic lupus erythematosus, chronic ITP, DIC, HUS, renal transplant rejection, multiple congenital cavernous hemangiomas, MPD, acute and chronic leukemias, and severe valvular disease, as well as in patients undergoing cardiopulmonary bypass and in platelet concentrates stored for transfusion.

ANTIPLATELET ANTIBODIES AND PLATELET FUNCTION

Binding of an antibody to platelets may induce several effects, including accelerated destruction, platelet activation, cell lysis, aggregation, secretion of granule contents, and outward exposure of PS. Platelet–antibody interaction may lead to impaired function, both as a consequence of activation and as a result of antibody binding to specific glycoproteins. Patients with ITP have decreased platelet survival and may have impaired platelet function and abnormally prolonged bleeding times, even at adequate counts. Antibodies can induce platelet dysfunction through multiple mechanisms. In many patients, antibodies are directed against specific platelet surface membrane glycoproteins GPIb (Woods, 1984), GPIIb/IIIa (Woods, 1984), GPIa/IIa (Deckmyn, 1994), and GPVI (Sugiyama, 1987; Boylan, 2004) and glycosphingolipids (van Vliet, 1987; Koerner, 1989). In one report, the anti-GPVI antibody induced clearance of the GPVI/FcR gamma complex from the platelet surface (Boylan, 2004). Some of these antibodies, in effect, induce acquired forms of BSS and thrombasthenia.

DRUGS THAT INHIBIT PLATELET FUNCTION

Many drugs may affect platelet function (Table 40-9). For several, the effects on platelets have been studied in vitro, and the relevance of such findings to drug levels achieved in clinical practice is not well established. Even among those shown to alter platelet responses ex vivo, the impact on hemostasis often remains unclear. Moreover, the impact of concomitant administration of multiple drugs, each with a mild effect on platelet function, is unknown, although it is clinically relevant. Because of their widespread use, aspirin and nonsteroidal antiinflammatory agents are an important cause of platelet inhibition in clinical practice. Aspirin ingestion results in inhibition of platelet aggregation and secretion upon stimulation with ADP, epinephrine, and low concentrations of collagen. Aspirin irreversibly acetylates and inactivates the platelet cyclooxygenase, leading to inhibition of synthesis of endoperoxides (PGG_2 and PGH_2) and TxA_2. Typically, 5–7 days is recommended after cessation of aspirin ingestion for studies intended to assess baseline platelet function. Several other nonsteroidal antiinflammatory drugs also impair platelet function by inhibiting the cyclooxygenase enzyme and may prolong bleeding time. Compared with aspirin, inhibition of cyclooxygenase by these agents is generally short-lived and reversible. In the case of ibuprofen, for example, 24 hours from cessation of this medication is a sufficient interval for testing of baseline platelet function.

Ticlopidine, clopidogrel, and prasugel are orally administered thienopyridine derivatives that inhibit platelet function by inhibiting the binding of ADP to the platelet P2Y12 receptor. These drugs prolong bleeding time and inhibit platelet aggregation responses to several agonists, including ADP, collagen, epinephrine, and thrombin, to various extents depending on agonist concentrations. GPIIb/IIIa receptor antagonists constitute a class of compounds that inhibit fibrinogen binding and platelet aggregation. These include a monoclonal antibody against the GPIIb/IIIa receptor (abciximab), as well as a synthetic peptide (eptifibatide) and a peptidomimetic (tirofiban) whose mechanism of action is based upon mimicking arginine-glycine-aspartic acid (RGD) sequences within fibrinogen,. These are potent inhibitors of aggregation (both primary and secondary) in response to all the usual agonists except ristocetin; they prolong bleeding time and are far more potent than aspirin as platelet inhibitors. Immune-mediated thrombocytopenia (secondary to drug-dependent antibodies) is a potential complication of the GPIIb/III antagonists (Aster, 2007) (see Chapter 42).

Growing evidence indicates that selective serotonin reuptake inhibitors (SSRIs) inhibit platelet function, and that this has clinical relevance. These include fluoxetine, setraline, paroxetine, fluvoxamine, citalopram, and escitalopram. Serotonin in plasma is taken up by platelets, incorporated into dense granules, and secreted on platelet activation. SSRIs inhibit uptake of serotonin and platelet aggregation and secretion responses to activation. In epidemiologic studies, patients on SSRIs have had increased gastrointestinal bleeding and increased bleeding with surgery (Movig, 2003; McCloskey, 2008).

β-Lactam antibiotics, including penicillins and cephalosporins, inhibit platelet aggregation responses and may contribute to a bleeding diathesis at high doses (Rao, 2006). These include carbenicillin, penicillin G, ticarcillin, ampicillin, nafcillin, azlocillin, cloxacillin, mezlocillin, oxacillin, piperacillin, and apalcillin. The platelet inhibition appears to be dose dependent, taking about 2–3 days to manifest and 3–10 days to abate after drug discontinuation. Cephalosporins may also impair platelet function. Moxalactam has been reported to induce platelet dysfunction associated with prolonged bleeding times and clinical hemorrhage; it inhibits synthesis of vitamin-dependent coagulation factors as well. Other third-generation cephalosporins appear to show little effect on normal platelet function. In general, the clinical significance of the effect of antibiotics on platelet function remains unclear. Because of the presence of concomitant factors (thrombocytopenia, DIC, infection, vitamin K deficiency), the general context in which bleeding events are encountered in patients on antibiotics prevents identification of the precise role played by the antimicrobials. Discontinuation of a specifically indicated antibiotic is usually not an option and is not necessary.

A host of other medications and agents, including food substances, inhibit platelet responses, but the clinical significance of many is unclear. They have been reviewed elsewhere (Rao, 2005). Given the increasing use of herbal medicines and food supplements, their role and interaction with pharmaceutical drugs need to be considered in the evaluation of patients with unexplained bleeding.

PART 5

SELECTED REFERENCES

Bennett JS, Vilaire G. Exposure of platelet fibrinogen receptors by ADP and epinephrine. J Clin Invest 1979;64:1393–401.

Classic paper demonstrating that fibrinogen serves as the critical adhesive ligand for platelet aggregation.

Charo IF, Feinman RD, Detwiler TC. Interrelations of platelet aggregation and secretion. J Clin Invest 1977;60:866–73.

Classic paper describing the relationships between aggregation and dense granule secretion.

Coller BS, Peerschke EI, Scudder LE. A murine monoclonal antibody that completely blocks the binding of fibrinogen to platelets produces a thrombasthenic-like state in normal platelets and binds to glycoproteins IIb and/or IIIa. J Clin Invest 1983;72:325–38.

Classic paper laying the foundation for antithrombotic therapy targeting platelet receptors.

Coller BS, Shattil SJ. The GPIIb/IIIa (integrin alpha IIb beta 3) odyssey: a technology-driven saga of a receptor with twists, turns, and even a bend. Blood 2008;112:3011–25.

Historical review of Glanzmann thrombasthenia providing both considerable breadth and depth.

Furlan M, Robles R, Galbusera M. von Willebrand factor-cleaving protease in thrombotic thrombocytopenic purpura and the hemolytic-uremic syndrome. N Engl J Med 1998;339:1578–84.

Landmark paper leading to the recognition of ADAMTS13.

Miller JL, Castella A. Platelet-type von Willebrand disease: characterization of a new bleeding disorder. Blood 1982;60:790–4.

Discovery of an increase-of-function mutation in the platelet receptor for vWF that mimics type 2B vWD.

Montgomery RR, Kunicki TJ, Taves C. Diagnosis of Bernard-Soulier syndrome and Glanzmann's thrombasthenia with a monoclonal assay on whole blood. J Clin Invest 1983;71:385–9.

Development of immunologic techniques for the diagnosis of inherited platelet disorders.

Nurden AT, Caen JP. Specific roles for platelet surface glycoproteins in platelet function. Nature 1975;255: 720–2.

Classic paper beginning the field of platelet glycoprotein biology and pathophysiology.

Provan D, Stasi R, Newland AC. International consensus report on the investigation and management of primary immune thrombocytopenia. Blood 2010;115: 168–86.

Recent consensus report on ITP.

Rodeghiero F, Stasi R, Gernsheimer T. Standardization of terminology, definitions and outcome criteria in immune thrombocytopenic purpura of adults and children: report from an international working group. Blood 2009;113:2386–93.

Recent consensus report on ITP.

Rodgers RPC, Levin J. A critical reappraisal of the bleeding time. Semin Thromb Hemost 1990;16: 1–20.

Landmark article (and entire journal issue) demonstrating the poor predictive value of bleeding time in a wide variety of clinical settings.

Ruggeri ZM, Pareti FI, Mannucci PM. Heightened interaction between platelets and factor VIII/von Willebrand factor in a new subtype of von Willebrand disease. N Engl J Med 1980;302:1047–51.

Classic article reporting discovery of the increase-of-function vWF mutation responsible for type 2B vWD.

Sadler JE. Von Willebrand disease type 1: a diagnosis in search of a disease. Blood 2003;101:2089–93.

Intriguing article questioning whether decreased levels of plasma vWF should be considered simply a risk factor for increased bleeding rather than an actual disease.

Tsai HM, Lian EC. Antibodies to von Willebrand factor-cleaving protease in acute thrombotic thrombocytopenic purpura. N Engl J Med 1998;339: 1585–94.

Landmark paper leading to the recognition of ADAMTS13.

Weiss HJ, Meyer D, Rabinowitz R. Pseudo von Willebrand disease: an intrinsic platelet defect with aggregation by unmodified human factor VIII/von Willebrand factor and enhanced adsorption of its high-molecular-weight multimers. N Engl J Med 1982;306:326–62.
Discovery of an increase-of-function mutation in the platelet receptor for vWF that mimics type 2B vWD.

White JG. Electron microscopy methods for studying platelet structure and function. Methods Mol Biol 2004;272:47–63.
Definitive methods of platelet electron microscopy.

REFERENCES

Access the complete reference list online at http://www.expertconsult.com

CHAPTER 41

LABORATORY APPROACH TO THROMBOTIC RISK

Richard A. Marlar, Louis M. Fink, Jonathan L. Miller

PART 5

KEY POINTS

- The amount of clot formed is regulated by several important regulatory mechanisms. Under normal conditions, these mechanisms control excess clot formation and halt venous thrombosis. Major systems are the antithrombin mechanism, the protein C–protein S system, and the tissue factor pathway inhibitor mechanism.
- Deficiencies, genetic or acquired, of the main regulatory proteins (antithrombin, protein C, and protein S) increase the risk for venous thrombosis.
- Increased levels of procoagulant factors or polymorphisms (causing functional change) increase the risk for venous thrombosis. A very common polymorphism in factor V (factor V_{Leiden}) reduces the ability of factor V to be downregulated by activated protein C. Relatively high levels of prothrombin (due to a specific polymorphism at base pair 20210) and elevated levels of factor VIII also increase the risk for development of thrombosis.
- Other inherited or acquired defects in hemostasis (dysfibrinogenemia and fibrinolysis) and in nonhemostatic systems (homocysteine) also increase the risk of venous thrombosis.
- Antiphospholipid syndrome and lupus anticoagulant (LA) are autoimmune disorders that affect the coagulation system and increase the risk of venous and arterial thrombosis. The LA antibodies are heterogeneous and present with a variety of laboratory abnormalities which can be detected only with a battery of tests. An approach for the identification of antiphospholipid syndrome and LA is presented.
- When evaluating a patient for thrombotic risk, it is important to plan the timing of testing so as to avoid misinterpreting decreased natural anticoagulants secondary to consumption by thrombosis or to anticoagulation from inherited deficiencies.

Hemostatic regulatory mechanisms limit the amount, location, and duration of clot formation. Dysfunction in the major regulatory systems of blood coagulation may lead to the pathologic condition of excessive clot formation (thrombosis). Both genetic and acquired deficiencies or abnormalities of such regulatory factors are capable of increasing the risk for thromboembolism. This chapter will discuss a number of factors that influence the balance toward bleeding or toward thrombosis, as well as the role of the laboratory in identifying abnormalities associated with these factors.

PHYSIOLOGIC ANTICOAGULANT PATHWAYS

(For a schematic overview of physiologic anticoagulant pathways, see also Fig. 39-5 in Chapter 39.)

Antithrombin (formally termed antithrombin III) is a circulating plasma serine protease inhibitor which regulates thrombin and factor Xa, and to a lesser extent factors IXa, XIa, XIIa, and VIIa (Stassen, 2004). The function of antithrombin is greatly enhanced on the endothelial cell surface by cell-bound glycosaminoglycans (heparan sulfate, dermatan sulfate, and small amounts of heparin) (Fig. 41-1) and pharmacologically by heparin (discussed extensively in Chapter 42).

A second major antithrombotic regulatory system is the protein C pathway, with an apparent multiprong mechanism consisting of a major anticoagulant component (Fig. 41-2) and an indirect profibrinolytic component (Esmon, 2009). The pathway is complex, with multiple factors which interact to generate a multitiered mechanism (Esmon, 2003a, 2003b, 2009). The central protein, protein C, is a vitamin K–dependent plasma proenzyme. The system is initiated with the generation of excessive non–clot-bound thrombin, which rapidly and tightly binds to an endothelial cell transmembrane glycoprotein, thrombomodulin (TM in Fig. 41-2). Thrombin bound in this complex undergoes a dramatic change in substrate specificity. Whereas it formerly was the sine qua non procoagulant enzyme of the coagulation system and a potent activator of platelets, its new ability to activate protein C effectively renders thrombin a potent anticoagulant enzyme. Thrombomodulin-bound thrombin, together with the endothelial cell protein C receptor, rapidly cleaves a small activation peptide from the protein C molecule (Stearns-Kurosawa, 1996; Esmon, 2004; Esmon, 2009). This process generates an active serine protease enzyme, activated protein C (APC). A second vitamin K–dependent inhibitory plasma protein, protein S (see Fig. 41-2), serves as a critical cofactor for APC. Protein S is a nonenzymatic cofactor molecule that binds in equilibrium to a large complement protein, C4b-binding protein (Rigby, 2004). Only the unbound (or "free") form of protein S possesses APC cofactor activity. The complex of APC and protein S on the phospholipid surface of platelets or other cells rapidly inactivates factor Va and factor VIIIa, thereby greatly diminishing thrombin generation in the procoagulant pathways (Esmon, 2003a, b). The protein C system also appears to exert significant, although indirect, profibrinolytic activity. This is believed to involve the thrombin-activated fibrinolytic inhibitor (TAFI) (van de Wouwer, 2004) and the plasminogen activator inhibitor-1 (PAI-1) (Madden, 1991; Meltzer, 2010). TAFI is a plasma carboxypeptidase which is rapidly activated by the thrombin–thrombomodulin complex (van de Wouwer, 2004). The active form of the carboxypeptidase cleaves C-terminal lysine residues from fibrin that has already undergone proteolytic cleavage by plasmin. Loss of these residues impairs the efficient binding of plasminogen-activating proteins to fibrin, thereby downregulating the fibrinolytic process. APC, via inactivation of factor Va, causes a decrease in thrombin generation, thus slowing TAFI activation. PAI-1 is inhibited by APC, thereby increasing overall fibrinolytic activity (Madden, 1991). Based on in vitro and animal experiments, the protein C system may also have other important defense properties, including anti-inflammatory activity and regulation of complement activity (Esmon, 2003a; Castellino, 2009).

As shown in Figure 41-3, tissue factor pathway inhibitor (TFPI) is another regulatory system that controls initiation of the tissue factor pathway (also referred to as the **extrinsic pathway**) of coagulation (Smithies, 2004; Crawley, 2008). This inhibitor has two reactive binding sites: one for factor Xa that has previously been activated by tissue factor–factor VIIa, and a second for the tissue factor–factor VIIa complex itself (Esmon, 2003b). After some factor Xa is generated, then and only then can TFPI inhibit the tissue factor–factor VIIa complex. Binding of these proteins by TFPI removes their ability to contribute further to clot formation. TFPI accordingly provides a negative feedback mechanism for downregulating the coagulation process (Esmon, 2003b). The protein C-protein S pathway and TFPI regulatory systems are interdependent, with some proteins playing multiple roles in several mechanisms (Marlar, 2007; Hackeng, 2009).

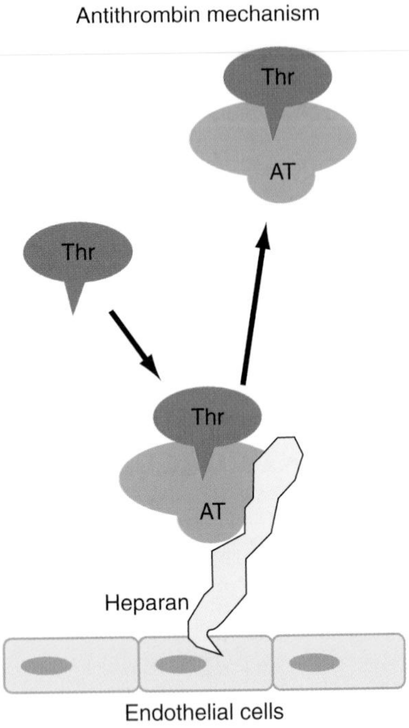

Figure 41-1 Antithrombin inhibitor mechanisms. *AT,* Antithrombin (formally termed antithrombin III); *Heparan,* heparan sulfate (a glycosaminoglycan); *Thr,* thrombin (or another coagulation enzyme such as factor X).

THROMBOPHILIC PROTEINS OR FACTORS

An imbalance between the procoagulant systems and the regulatory mechanisms can lead to bleeding or thrombosis. An increase in procoagulant factors or a decrease in regulatory factors will tip the balance to excessive fibrin production, resulting in thrombus formation. These imbalances can be caused by genetic or acquired factors, or by a combination of the two (Tables 41-1 and 41-2). However, the process leading to excessive fibrin formation is not as simple as a single factor being disproportionate to the other factors. Rather, it consists of a combination of moderately imbalanced factors, which leads to excessive fibrin formation at the initial site of injury (Marlar, 2007). This, in turn, leads to vessel occlusion and fibrin clot growth (Franco, 2001). This multifactorial model, in which these factors interact in a cooperative manner, will lead to significant risk for the development of thrombosis (Marlar, 2007). Therefore, a complete assessment of the recognized and established risk factors must be made to determine the overall risk potential for an individual (see Table 41-2). The following factors are the major known components involved in increased risk for thrombus development (see Table 41-1 for a summary of prevalence and relative risk).

ANTITHROMBIN

Both hereditary and acquired deficiencies of antithrombin have been identified (Egeber, 1965; Bloemenkamp, 2003; Patnaik, 2008). Genetic deficiency of antithrombin is a rare disorder (~1 in 10,000 individuals) in the general population, and about 1% of patients are diagnosed as having familial venous thrombosis (Adcock, 1997). Antithrombin is autosomal, having an apparent dominant expression and high penetrance, with a large

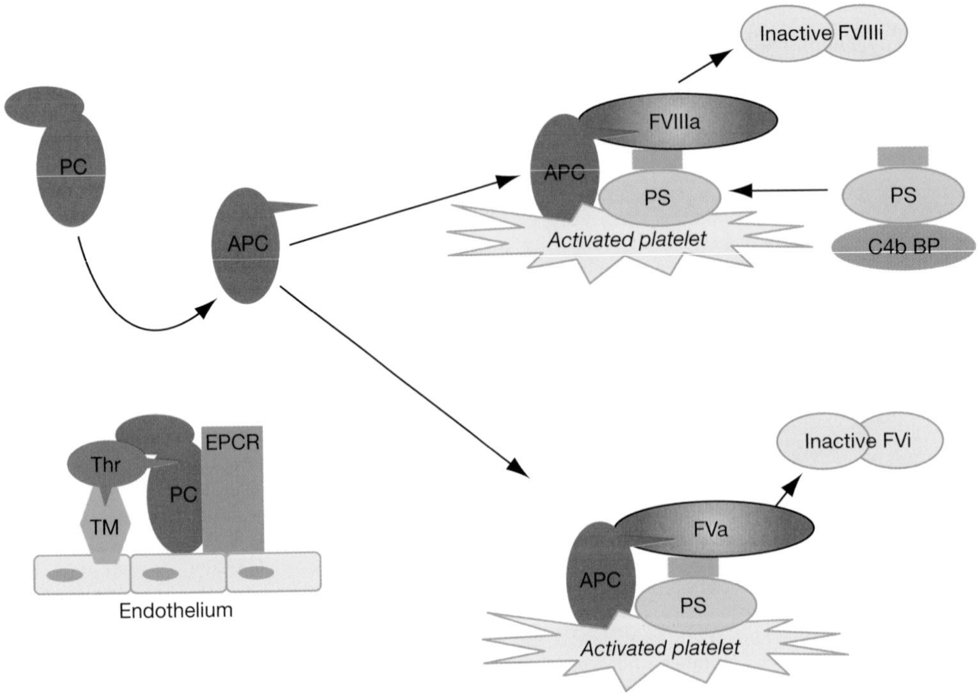

Figure 41-2 Protein C pathway. *APC,* Activated protein C; *C4b BP,* complement factor 4b-binding protein; *EPCR,* endothelial cell protein C receptor; *FVa,* factor Va; *FVIIIa,* factor VIIIa; *PC,* protein C; *PS,* protein S; *Thr,* thrombin; *TM,* thrombomodulin.

TABLE 41-1
Prevalence and Estimated Increased Thrombotic Risk of Thrombophilic Factors

Risk factors for thrombosis	Prevalence in general population, %	Prevalence in thrombophilic population, %	Estimated thrombotic risk, fold
Decreased antithrombin	<0.01	<1	12–20
Decreased protein C	0.3	4–8	8–10
Decreased protein S	0.2	7–12	10–15
Factor V_{Leiden} (heterozygous)	3–4*	10–40	1.8–2.6
Factor V_{Leiden} (homozygous)	<0.01%	2–4	10–15
Prothrombin G20210A	2–3*	10–15	1.5–2.2
Elevated factor VIII	10–15	20–35	2–4.5
Elevated fibrinogen	5–12	20–30	2–3
Dysfibrinogenemia	<0.01	0.3–0.8	1.5–3
Thrombomodulin mutations	<0.01	0.2–0.8	2–4
Elevated homocysteine	3–5	8–15	2–4.5
Lupus anticoagulant	1–5	10–30	2–10
Oral contraceptives	N/A	N/A	2–3
Pregnancy	N/A	N/A	4–8

N/A, Not applicable.
*Factor V_{Leiden} and Prothrombin 20210 prevalence for heterozygosity in Caucasian general population; however, both very low (<0.1%) in African and Asian populations.

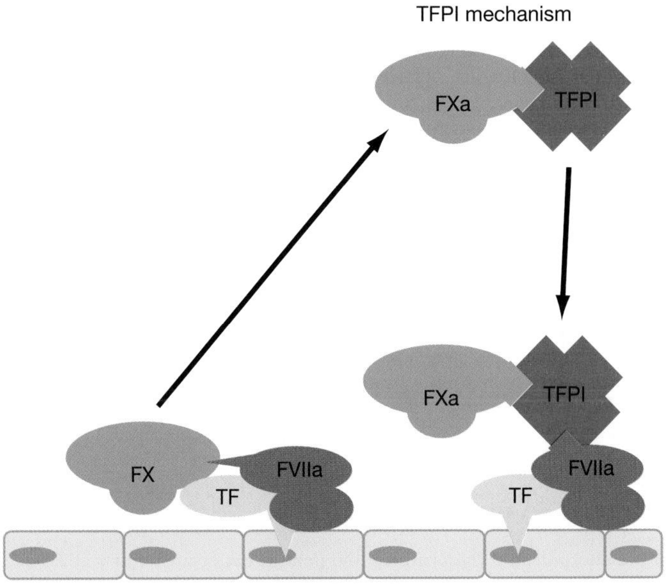

Figure 41-3 Tissue factor pathway inhibitor mechanisms. *FVIIa,* Factor VIIa; *FXa,* factor Xa; *TF,* tissue factor; *TFPI,* tissue factor pathway inhibitor.

number of known mutants throughout the gene (Adcock, 1997; Lane, 1997). Heterozygous individuals have plasma antithrombin levels around 50% of normal and are usually symptomatic (compared with heterozygotes of coagulation factor deficiencies, who usually are asymptomatic). Both type I (decreased activity with concomitant decreased antigen) and type II (decreased activity with normal levels of antigen) mutations have been described in antithrombin-deficient individuals (Lane, 1997). Homozygous antithrombin deficiency is incompatible with life, except for unique type II mutations in the heparin-binding region, where patients typically manifest venous thrombosis (Kuhle, 2001). The most common clinical presentation is deep venous thrombosis in the lower extremities and pulmonary embolus. It is noteworthy that thrombi may also occur in the retinal, mesenteric, and splenic veins (Bloemenkamp, 2003). Acquired deficiencies of antithrombin occur in disseminated intravascular coagulation (DIC) (Asakura, 2001), liver disease, the nephrotic syndrome, the acute period following venous thrombosis, and during heparin therapy (Marlar, 1990b). In some cases, acquired defects can cause plasma levels to drop to 30%–50% of normal and may be mistaken for genetic deficiencies. In the

TABLE 41-2
Estimated Thrombotic Risk for Cooperativeness of Multiple Factors

Risk factor 1	Risk factor 2	Combined risk (fold greater)
Protein C	Factor V_{Leiden} (heterozygous)	25–45
Protein S	Factor V_{Leiden} (heterozygous)	25–50
Factor V_{Leiden} (heterozygous)	Elevated factor VIII	12–20
Factor V_{Leiden} (heterozygous)	Oral contraceptives	8–20
Factor V_{Leiden} (heterozygous)	Pregnancy	25–40

newborn period, antithrombin is also characteristically low, reaching adult levels by the age of 6 months (Streif, 1999).

Both antithrombin activity and antigen in plasma can be determined using commercial kits. Antithrombin activity is determined by a chromogenic method utilizing factor Xa or thrombin as the inhibited enzyme. Antithrombin antigen is typically determined by enzyme-linked immunosorbent assay or by nephelometry. The normal ranges for both antithrombin activity and antigen are fairly narrow, usually around 80%–120% of normal (Adcock, 1997; Kuhle, 2001).

PROTEIN C

Protein C, the central protein in the protein C pathway, is a vitamin K–dependent protein. Both genetic and acquired deficiencies of protein C increase the risk for thrombosis. Protein C is autosomal, with variable penetrance phenotype expression. More than 100 mutations have been described with both type I (decreased activity with concomitant decreased antigen) and type II (decreased activity with normal levels of antigen) proteins (Marlar, 1990a, b; Lane, 1996). As shown in Table 41-1, surveys of the general population have found significant numbers of individuals with decreased levels of protein C. When plasma protein C levels, types of mutations, and lifestyles are compared, no differences are noted between symptomatic and asymptomatic individuals. The difference between asymptomatic and symptomatic protein C deficiencies is likely due to the further influence of additional thrombotic risk factors present within the symptomatic population. In homozygous protein C deficiency, severely deficient (<1% protein C activity) individuals manifest neurologic and ophthalmic complications during intrauterine development and subsequently develop purpura fulminans and DIC during the newborn period (Peters, 1988; Marlar, 1990c). This disorder is incompatible with life unless the patient is treated with protein C replacement (fresh frozen plasma [FFP] or protein C concentrate) and anticoagulant therapy. The plasma half-life of protein C is relatively short at 6–8 hours. The initiation of warfarin oral anticoagulant therapy (especially large loading doses) without overlap of prior heparin anticoagulation in individuals heterozygous for protein C deficiency can lead to an infrequent but devastating condition of thrombotic skin lesions known as warfarin-induced skin necrosis (Moll, 2004; Tai, 2004; Goldenberg, 2008).

Testing for protein C in plasma is performed using clotting activity or chromogenic activity assays, or one of several types of antigen assays. The activity assays measure the function of the molecule in plasma; however, chromogenic assays may erroneously report protein C molecules as functional that actually do not possess functionality with respect to their natural coagulant substrates (Marlar, 1990a). For this reason, a clotting-based assay is recommended to assess protein C functional activity (Rezende, 2004). In type I protein C deficiency, functional activity and antigen level are decreased to about 50% of normal, whereas in type II deficiency, the functional level is decreased on average to 50% of normal, but the antigen level is 100% of normal (Marlar, 1990a, b).

PROTEIN S

Both genetic and acquired deficiencies of protein S are associated with increased risk of thrombosis (Esmon, 2003a, 2009). As discussed previously, protein S together with APC binds to the phospholipid surface of a platelet or other cell, enhancing the enzymatic inactivation of factors Va and VIIIa (Hackeng, 1994; van Wijnen, 1996). About 40% of the protein S is free in plasma, whereas the remaining 60% is bound to the complement protein, C4b-binding protein (C4b BP) (Nelson, 1992). Many pathologic and physiologic conditions can change the ratio of free and bound protein S, thereby effectively modulating the protein C inhibitory pathway (Mackie, 2001). The level of protein S characteristically decreases during pregnancy, with values averaging only 60% of those of controls from the 10th week of pregnancy onward (Cerneca, 1997; ten Kate, 2008).

The autosomal gene encoding protein S is expressed with variable penetrance (Rezende, 2004). More than 50 mutations have been described with associated increased thrombotic risk (Simmonds, 1998). The traditional quantitative type I deficiency (decreased protein S activity with concomitant decreased total antigen) and a qualitative type II deficiency (decreased protein S activity with normal levels of free and total antigen) have been reported. Because of the equilibrium between protein S and C4b BP, a third type of mutation has been identified (Simmonds, 1998): Type III deficiency is similar to type I, but the decreased protein S activity is associated with normal free protein S, yet decreased total protein S. Several studies have shown, however, that these rare type III individuals actually may not have increased risk for thrombosis (Brouwer, 2005; Libourel, 2005). Homozygous protein S deficiency with severely decreased protein S activity (<1%) has been reported with the same presentation and similar treatment regimens as homozygous protein C deficiency (Brouwer, 2005). Symptoms include purpura fulminans and DIC during the newborn period, with ophthalmic and neurologic complications having developed in utero. This disorder is incompatible with life unless the patient is treated with replacement therapy (i.e., FFP) and anticoagulant therapy.

Plasma protein S levels are determined by protein S clotting activity assays, as well as by antigenic assays for free protein S and total protein S antigen. Definitive diagnosis of protein S deficiency can be very difficult owing to the complexity of protein S interaction with C4b BP (Nelson, 1992; Goodwin, 2002; Persson, 2003; ten Kate, 2008). The activity assay measures the functional fraction of protein S in the plasma sample, but falsely low protein S activity has been reported (Goodwin, 2002). Two types of antigen assays are available: Assays whose measurement includes both free protein S and the bound fraction are considered to be measuring the *total* amount of protein S in a plasma sample **(total protein S antigen).** Assays for free protein S measure only the unbound portion of protein S by employing a monoclonal antibody specific for unbound protein S or by including a precipitation step with polyethylene glycol in which the bound portion of the protein S molecules is removed (Comp, 1986; Goodwin 2002; Persson, 2003; ten Kate, 2008). Because clot-based functional assays have been reported to produce artifactually low values, it is recommended that free protein S antigen assays be used for the initial assessment of protein S. If the level is found to be decreased, reflex testing of both protein S activity and total protein S antigen should then be performed. Reaching a definitive diagnosis of congenital deficiency of protein S is challenging, given the complexity of the interaction of protein S with C4b BP, the acquired conditions which can change the equilibrium of free and bound forms, and the presence of vitamin K antagonists (Simmonds, 1998; Mackie, 2001; Goodwin, 2002; Rezende, 2004; ten Kate, 2008).

ACTIVATED PROTEIN C RESISTANCE AND FACTOR V_{LEIDEN}

Activated protein C resistance (APC-R) is said to be present when the addition of exogenous APC to plasma does not result in the anticipated prolongation of clotting time tests such as the activated partial thromboplastin time (APTT) (Dahlbäck, 1999; Castoldi, 2010). APC-R is considered one of the most common genetic risk factors for venous thrombosis; however, although the prevalence of this abnormality in the Caucasian population is on average 4%, prevalence is lower among African and Asian populations (Ridker, 1995; Heijmans, 1998). APC normally enzymatically inactivates factors Va and VIIIa, prolonging the clotting time of plasma. In APC-R, the ability of APC to enzymatically degrade factor Va is significantly reduced. The polymorphism at one of the cleavage sites in factor Va is an arginine residue substituted by a glutamine residue (R506Q) that renders the site resistant to APC cleavage (Aparicio, 1996). The amino acid substitution is due to a single nucleotide change in the gene, termed factor V_{Leiden} (Bertina, 1994). Factor V_{Leiden} increases the relative risk of thrombosis onefold to twofold in the heterozygous condition and tenfold to fifteenfold in the homozygous individual (Svensson, 1997; De Stefano, 1999; Castoldi, 2010). The presence of factor V_{Leiden} will typically produce a characteristic abnormality in functional APC-R assays. There are numerous variations of such assays, with an exogenous source of factor V–deficient plasma frequently employed to increase specificity for abnormalities attributable to a genetic abnormality of the patient's own factor V. Two clotting tests are performed: the first in the presence of added APC, and the second without the addition of APC. If the ratio of clotting time with added APC divided by clotting time in the absence of added APC is sufficiently high (usually >2.0), then APC-R or factor V_{Leiden} is excluded. Lower ratios, in contrast, suggest that the sample is APC resistant, and that the patient may have factor V_{Leiden} (or one of several other rare factor V mutations), which should be confirmed by genetic testing (Aparicio, 1996; Tripodi, 1997; Castoldi, 2010). Also of potential clinical importance, however, are those cases of acquired APC-R not associated with a genetic abnormality of the patient's factor V molecule. As shown in Figure 41-4, several abnormalities may affect regulation of the coagulation pathways and may additionally exert a prothrombotic influence by virtue of increasing APC-R (Cumming, 1995; Graf, 2003; Castoldi, 2010). Detection of such forms of APC-R will be more frequent when assays are employed that do not include the addition of exogenous factor V–deficient plasma.

PROTHROMBIN 20210

A polymorphism in the prothrombin gene at base pair number 20210 is a guanine-to-adenine substitution in the 3′-untranslated region of the gene (Colucci, 2004). Heterozygosity for this polymorphism imparts approximately a twofold greater risk for venous thrombosis (Eikelboom, 1999). Heterozygous individuals characteristically have levels of plasma prothrombin higher than those in individuals lacking this polymorphism, although even these higher levels usually fall within the established reference interval for prothrombin activity of most laboratories. Accordingly, molecular diagnostic procedures are required for the diagnosis of prothrombin 20210 (Poort, 1996; Grunwald, 2000). There is believed to be increased transcription of the gene into the gene product, probably as the result of an increase in time during which mRNA molecules are translated (De Stefano, 1999). Prothrombin 20210 is a common genetic risk factor for venous thrombosis in populations of European descent (about 3%), with lower prevalence in other, non-European populations (De Stefano, 1999).

ELEVATED COAGULATION FACTOR LEVELS

In addition to an elevated level of prothrombin acting as a risk factor for thrombosis, elevation of several other coagulation factors has been reported to impart an increased risk of thrombosis. As levels of factors VII, VIII, IX, XI, or fibrinogen are elevated, the relative risks for developing thrombosis are proportionately increased (one-and-one-half–fold to sixfold) (Kannel, 1987; O'Donnell, 1997; Kyrle, 2000; Meijers, 2000). The most

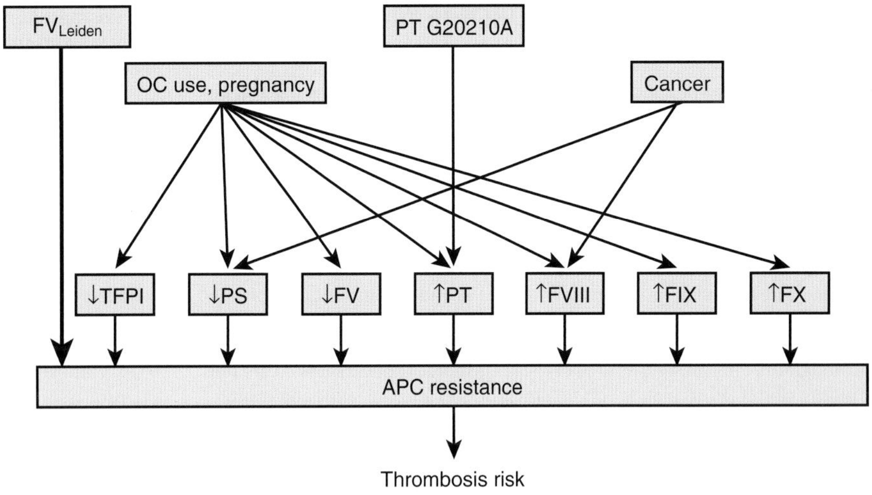

Figure 41-4 Activated protein C (APC) resistance as a complex phenotype. *(Redrawn with permission from Castoldi E, Rosing J. APC resistance: biological basis and acquired influences. J Thromb Haemost 2010;8:445–53.)*

studied and most complex of these reported risk factors is factor VIII. Factor VIII is regulated by genetic mechanisms and additionally by physiologic mechanisms that increase the release of stored factor VIII in times of stress and exercise. Some familial elevation of factor VIII has been reported, but transiently high levels can be seen in patients with a concomitant increase in plasma von Willebrand factor level and in patients with stress due to a variety of clinical conditions (Vormittag, 2009). Factor VIII levels of 120%–150% have a one-and-one-half–fold to twofold greater risk of thrombosis; levels of 300%–400% have an increased relative risk of threefold to sixfold (O'Donnell, 1997).

DYSFIBRINOGENEMIA

Fibrinogen is the final protein in the formation of a clot and the major component in a venous thrombus. Published reports of abnormalities associated with increased risk of thrombosis due to dysfunctional fibrinogen molecules are rare (Haverkate, 1995; de Moerloose, 2010). The incidence of recognized cases of dysfibrinogenemia in familial thrombosis is about 0.8%. Presently, the only assays commonly employed to assess fibrinogen are functional assays of clottability and antigenic assays. As discussed in Chapter 39, an imbalance in the ratio of such assays provides an indication of a decrease-of-function dysfibrinogenemia. Unfortunately, subtleties in the ability of fibrinogen—and perhaps more important, of the resulting fibrin—to bind proteins having an influence on the balance of hemostasis and thrombosis (e.g., tissue plasminogen activator) are not picked up by such assays. It is accordingly possible that the frequency by which dysfibrinogenemias underlie thrombotic events may be even higher than is presently recognized.

HYPOFIBRINOLYTIC MECHANISMS

Impaired function of the fibrinolytic system increases the risk of thrombosis, but there remains a lack of global clinical assays sufficiently robust to allow estimation of the degree of that risk (Collen, 1999; Meltzer, 2009). The euglobulin clot lysis time provides a measure of some aspects of the fibrinolytic system (Sartori, 2003). In brief, citrated plasma is diluted and acidified, resulting in the selective precipitation of many proteins that include fibrinogen, plasminogen activator, and plasminogen, whereas other molecules, including α_2-antiplasmin, remain in solution. This precipitated **euglobulin fraction** is then redissolved in appropriate buffer and clotted by thrombin, and the time to clot lysis measured. An abnormal rate of euglobulin clot lysis helps direct the subsequent laboratory evaluation to an underlying abnormality of a critical component of the fibrinolytic system. Such a result adds support to the decision to proceed to more detailed testing of the fibrinolytic system, such as specific assays for plasminogen activator, plasminogen, and other proteins upregulating or downregulating fibrinolysis (Meltzer, 2009).

Although a variety of defects in the fibrinolytic system may well be contributing to the increased risk of thrombosis, consensus has been difficult to achieve with respect to assessment through system-based assays, specific component functional assays, or molecular analysis studies with respect to the individual patient. Deficiencies of plasminogen, the zymogen precursor of plasmin—the major enzyme responsible for fibrin clot breakdown (see Chapter 39)—have been reported, but the association with increased thrombotic risk is not well founded (Schulman, 1996). Assessment of the mechanical properties of clots throughout the period of their formation and subsequent lysis with the Sonoclot, TEG thromboelastograph, or similar devices represents a quite different approach, which, with sufficient standardization, may permit the detection of abnormal fibrinolysis (Kamada, 2001; Salooja, 2001; Vig, 2001; Meltzer, 2009). These types of instruments work by detecting clot **rigidity** or **strength** during the clot formation and breakdown process (Kamada, 2001; Salooja, 2001; Vig, 2001; Meltzer, 2009; Kupesiz, 2010), and accordingly may offer the potential for real-time assessment of fibrinolytic state, which could be of particular benefit in conjunction with the monitoring of active antifibrinolytic therapy (Kupesiz, 2010).

OTHER POSSIBLE DEFECTS

Abnormalities in several other coagulation regulatory proteins and platelet proteins have been reported. However, difficulty in assessment of these proteins and lack of conclusive correlation with increased thrombotic risk have not yet established them as important risk factors for venous thrombosis.

Thrombomodulin (labeled as "TM" in Fig. 41-2) defects have been reported by several groups to have good association with thrombosis (2–6×). Numerous defects appear to span a large portion of the TM gene (Ohlin, 1995; Ohlin, 1997), with the result that it is still a challenge for clinical laboratories to detect such abnormalities.

Heparin cofactor II, a homologous inhibitor of antithrombin, has not been demonstrated to be associated with increased risk of thrombosis (Tollefsen, 2002). The PLA1/PLA2 polymorphism, as well as other platelet glycoprotein polymorphisms, has been of interest with respect to potential prothrombotic contributory roles (Lindoff, 1997; Heit, 2000; Robert, 2000; Paganin, 2003), with ongoing efforts to assess whether or not such variations actually achieve clinical significance (Ivanov, 2008; Zuern, 2010). Additionally, the non-O types of the ABO blood groups have been reported as increased thrombotic risk factors compared with type O, possibly owing to increased levels of von Willebrand factor and factor VIII (Wu, 2008).

ACQUIRED HYPERCOAGULABLE STATES

Numerous acquired conditions have been associated with increased risk of venous thrombosis. The relative risk for many of these has been determined and appears to combine with genetic causes to increase the overall risk for thrombosis. Common conditions that have a strong association with venous thrombosis include trauma, surgery and the postoperative state, pregnancy, immobility, obesity and diet, smoking, and previous thrombosis. Additionally, malignancy, chronic DIC, oral contraceptive use and hormone replacement use, heparin-induced thrombocytopenia, nephrotic syndrome, essential thrombocythemia, polycythemia vera, and inflammatory conditions have all been associated with increased risk of venous thrombosis. Finally, as discussed in Chapter 40, abnormalities of the enzyme ADAMTS13 have been associated with the thrombotic disorder thrombotic thrombocytopenic purpura.

ANTIPHOSPHOLIPID SYNDROME AND LUPUS ANTICOAGULANT

The antiphospholipid antibody syndrome (APS), a clinical disorder characterized by recurrent arterial and venous thrombotic events, is one of the most common risk factors for thrombosis, pregnancy complications, and fetal loss (Bizzaro, 2005; Palomo, 2009; Pengo, 2009). Venous or arterial thrombosis may occur, with venous manifestations being more common (Eby, 2009). The syndrome is an autoimmune disorder with antibodies directed against protein–phospholipid (PL) complexes. A strong association has been noted between immunoglobulin (Ig)G antibodies directed against domain I of β_2-glycoprotein I (β2GPI) and thrombotic and obstetric complications in APS. Autoantibodies directed against additional PL-binding proteins such as prothrombin or annexin A2 may also be seen, although the clinical significance of these antibodies appears less clear. The binding of β2GPI to platelet plasma membranes and the subsequent interaction of anti-β2GPI involving both platelet GPIbα and a truncated splice variant of LRP-8 (a member of the low density lipoprotein-receptor family present on platelets, also known as ApoER2) may trigger platelet activation (de Groot, 2005; Giannakopoulos, 2007; de Groot, 2010). A potentially significant interaction between anti-β2GPI and β2GPI complexes with platelet factor 4 has recently been suggested (Sikara, 2010).

When PL-specific binding antibody interactions occur in vivo, there is a prothrombotic action. However, it is ironic that when these interactions occur in vitro, there is inhibition of procoagulant reactions. The term **lupus anticoagulant** (LA) is misleading since the presence of an LA raises concern for clinical thrombosis rather than for clinical bleeding, and most patients with LA in fact do not have systemic lupus erythematosus. The original studies identifying the antiphospholipid antibodies (APAs) used cardiolipin in the binding assays (anticardiolipin antibodies [ACAs]). In occasional cases, testing may include antiphospholipid–protein complexes specifically with phosphatidylethanolamine, phosphatidylserine, or phosphatidylinositol. Many of the ACAs are responsible for the false-positive results observed in Venereal Disease Research Laboratory testing for syphilis. In turn, many infections and autoimmune diseases and a variety of medications are associated with a positive ACA (McCrae, 2001; Galli, 2003; Riboldi, 2003).

In a number of studies, abnormal LA or ACA have been reported to occur in 1%–5% of an asymptomatic general population, with many of these being transitory (Biggioggero, 2010). Patients who maintain a persistent LA together with high titers of anti-β2GPI show the highest correlation with thrombosis (de Laat, 2009). The combination of anti-β2GPI, ACA, and LA test positivity has the highest association with recurrent venous thromboembolism (Pengo, 2006).

The mechanisms by which APA affect coagulation and hemostasis are multifactorial owing to the diversity of PL-associated proteins. Reports on the in vivo mechanism for hypercoagulability include downregulation of TM, interference with protein S, platelet activation, and endothelial perturbation. In particular, platelet-associated binding of antibodies against β2GPI may cause platelet activation (see earlier). Although there is no uniform approach for in vitro diagnosis of LA, it is clear that because of the heterogeneity of these antibodies, the presence of an LA cannot be excluded by simply failing to detect it in any single assay. Most commonly, the APTT and the dilute Russell viper venom time (dRVVT) are employed. Because these assays recognize different aspects of PL-dependent coagulation reactions, the combination is best for detecting LA. In the dRVVT test, the coagulation cascade is initiated later than in the APTT, with direct factor X activation by the venom in a PL-dependent fashion.

Several reagents for the APTT are designed to be more sensitive to LAs. The clotting time of plasma from LA patients is prolonged in these assays. When mixed with equal parts of normal pooled plasma, the plasma from LA patients will prolong the clotting time of the mixture beyond the clotting time of the normal control plasma itself. Whereas specific factor inhibitors, such as those directed against factor VIII, are typically time- and temperature-dependent (see Chapter 39), LAs more commonly are immediate-acting even at room temperature. Of particular note, LAs are notorious for interfering with quantitative measurement of coagulation factors assayed in an APTT-based system. A tell-tale pattern that should itself arouse suspicion of an LA is a persisting increase in apparent factor activity with increasing dilutions of patient plasma used in the assay: Such apparent increases in factor activity result from corresponding dilutions of LA.

Preincubation of LA plasma with an appropriate source of PL can neutralize the LA and result in significant shortening of a subsequently performed clotting time. Sources of neutralizing PL that have been used for this purpose include purified hexagonal phase PLs and complex PLs derived from frozen and thawed washed platelets (platelet neutralization procedure [PNP]) (Favaloro, 2008, 2009).

Recent international consensus statements (Miyakis, 2006; Favaloro, 2009) combine the clinical criteria of vascular thrombosis and pregnancy complications with laboratory criteria. These laboratory criteria include a positive LA, an ACA of IgG or IgM of >40 IU and medium- or high-titer IgG or IgM anti–β_2-glycoprotein I antibodies. The tests should be abnormal when repeated at least 12 weeks apart before a diagnosis of APA is made. The clinical course of high-risk patients diagnosed with APS reveals an extensive increase in recurrence of thrombosis, which can be markedly reduced by adequate anticoagulation (Pengo, 2010). Current approaches deriving from recommendations by the International Society on Thrombosis and Haemostasis related to the diagnosis of APS are shown in Table 41-3. Important considerations in implementing such an approach include (1) processing to ensure that the specimen is platelet-poor, (2) choosing two tests, such as the dRVVT or a silica-activated APTT with low PL content, (3) eliminating the influence of anticoagulants in mixing studies, (4) correcting prolonged clotting time in the presence of excess PL, and (5) ensuring that specific comments on the laboratory's reference ranges and interpretations accompany the LA profile and the ACA and β2GPI antibody assays (Ledford-Kraemer, 2008; Pengo, 2009, 2010).

HYPERHOMOCYSTEINEMIA

Homocysteine is an amino acid that is an intermediate molecule for the production and regulation of the sulfur-containing amino acid methionine (Guba, 1996; Refsum, 1998; Cattaneo, 2001). Perturbations, genetic or acquired, in the regulatory mechanism of this pathway can lead to elevated levels of homocysteine and to an associated increased risk of thrombosis. The most devastating of these is the cystathione-β-synthetase gene, which, in the homozygous state, leads to severe thrombosis and atherosclerosis (Mudd, 1985). Acquired causes mostly associated with diet and vitamin intake also are significant factors raising homocysteine levels in plasma. The associated risk for thrombosis with elevated homocysteine levels is a graded response, in which the higher the plasma level, the greater is the risk. Of note, two common polymorphisms associated with the homocysteine-metabolizing enzyme, methylenetetrahydrofolate reductase (MTHFR), were initially thought to be associated with increased risk of thrombosis. More recent studies have failed to establish MTHFR as an independent risk factor for thrombosis in adults (Tosetto, 1997; Franco, 1999), although a possible relationship with childhood stroke remains less clear (Prengler, 2001). Accordingly, it is not presently recommended to evaluate MTHFR polymorphisms as a cause of venous thrombosis (Legnani, 1997; Franco, 1999) in adults; however, plasma levels of homocysteine often are determined as part of such an investigation.

General Aspects of the Laboratory Evaluation for Thrombotic Risk

Laboratory evaluation of thrombophilia is complex and rapidly changing, including the appropriate tests to order, when to order them, and on whom to perform the testing (Foy, 2009). There is no global test to grade the thrombotic risk status of an individual, so a series of individual tests must be ordered to obtain a good assessment of risk. Molecular diagnostic tests, in contrast, are not affected by such influences. From the laboratory perspective, appropriate assays to measure true functionality and concentration must be utilized. Whenever possible, activity assays should be performed to determine the functionality of the molecule; simply determining the antigen level may miss the type II molecule and misidentify the patient as normal (Rezende, 2004). A number of questions must be asked of every patient who is being considered for evaluation: Does the patient (and family) history justify an evaluation? Are the tests to be ordered appropriate for addressing major accepted risk factors? Is the timing appropriate to provide proper evaluation? Are there underlying therapeutic, pathologic, or physiologic conditions that interfere with interpretation of results?

Ideally, evaluations are performed when the patient is asymptomatic and is not on anticoagulation therapy. Unfortunately, during the immediate postthrombotic period before anticoagulation, plasma factors are consumed, thus inviting the potential for erroneous diagnoses. Heparin significantly decreases antithrombin levels, increases protein S levels, and

TABLE 41-3
Laboratory Detection of Lupus Anticoagulants (LAs)

A. Blood collection
  1. Blood should be collected before the start of any anticoagulant drug regimen or a sufficient period after its discontinuation.
  2. Fresh venous blood in 0.109 M sodium citrate (ratio 9 : 1)
  3. Double centrifugation removes residual platelets.
  4. Quickly frozen plasma required if LA assays are postponed.
  5. Frozen plasma must be thawed at 37° C.

B. Initial testing
  1. Use two separate screening tests based on different principles, each with a *low level of phospholipid (PL):*
     a. Dilute Russell viper venom time (dRVVT)
     b. LA-sensitive activated partial thromboplastin time (APTT) (preferably with silica activator)
  2. Exclude the presence of heparin, LMW heparin, direct thrombin inhibitors, or factor Xa inhibitors.
     a. Indirect (heparin) and direct thrombin inhibitors should be suspected from prolongation of the thrombin time.
  3. Results of screening tests are potentially suggestive of LA when their clotting times are longer than the local cut-off value.*

C. Mixing studies for prolonged LA-sensitive APTT or dRVVT
  1. Pooled normal plasma (PNP) for mixing studies should ideally be prepared in-house. Alternatively, adequate commercial frozen or lyophilized PNP can be used.
  2. Plasma with prolonged screening values should be mixed as 1 part patient plasma with 1 part PNP and reassayed without incubation (i.e., <30 minutes after mixing).
  3. Results of mixing tests are suggestive of LA when their clotting times are longer than the local cut-off value.†

D. Confirmatory tests for prolonged APTT or dRVVT
  1. Confirmatory tests are performed by increasing the PL concentration beyond that used in the screening tests.
  2. Bilayer or hexagonal (II) phase PL should be used to increase the concentration of PL.
  3. Results are confirmatory of LA if the % correction is above the local cut-off value.‡

E. A report with an explanation of the results should be given.§

Adapted from Pengo V, Tripodi A, Reber G, et al. Subcommittee on Lupus Anticoagulant/Antiphospholipid Antibody of the Scientific and Standardisation Committee of the International Society on Thrombosis and Haemostasis. Update of the guidelines for lupus anticoagulant detection. J Thromb Haemost 2009;7:1737–40.

APTT, Activated partial thromboplastin time; *LMW,* low molecular weight.

*The cut-off value is the 99th percentile of the distribution of clotting times performed on plasmas from healthy donors. Testing described should be performed with the *local* reagent/instrument combination on plasmas from at least 40 adult healthy donors younger than 50 years of age. Cut-off values established elsewhere should not be substituted, even if they refer to the same method and instrument.

†In the case of mixing studies, the cut-off value would be the 99th percentile of the distribution of clotting times when plasmas from healthy donors are mixed in equal parts with PNP; alternatively, the distribution may be of a derived "index of circulating anticoagulant" = [(b-c)/a] X 100, where a, b, and c are the clotting times of the patient plasma, mixture, and PNP, respectively.

‡In the case of confirmatory testing, a distribution of values for "% correction" = [(screen − confirm)/screen] × 100, based upon testing of plasmas from healthy donors at low (screen) and high (confirm) PL concentrations is first obtained. A patient result above the cut-off value assigned to this distribution (e.g., above the 99th percentile) would then be considered as a positive confirmatory test. Note that the clotting time of the confirmatory test in LA-positive samples is not always shortened to within the normal range of controls. Accordingly, to avoid false-negative results, confirmatory tests are recommended to be performed in all normal controls, and these results used to establish the cut-off value.

§International Society on Thrombosis and Haemostasis (ISTH) guidelines further state, "Results should be expressed as ratio of patient-to-PNP for all procedures (screening, mixing and confirm)." Additional ISTH subcommittee explanations and qualifications are reported in detail in the original source of this table.

may mask LAs (unless a heparin-neutralizing molecule such as protamine or polybrene, or the enzyme heparinase, is included in the assay). Warfarin decreases protein C and protein S levels. Only genetic risk markers can be evaluated at any time by molecular diagnostic techniques. Attempts have been made to circumvent the test abnormalities produced by oral anticoagulation by using ratios of protein C or protein S to one or another of the vitamin K–dependent coagulation factors. However, the variability of such ratios is considerable, inviting the opportunity for misdiagnosis. Thus, this approach is not recommended. An erroneous diagnosis can be made when plasma factor levels decrease during a variety of acquired conditions such as pregnancy, hormone therapy, and post surgery.

Perhaps even more than in many other areas of clinical medicine, it is of critical importance to communicate the implications of these laboratory results to the patient in a manner that neither underestimates nor overestimates the role that thrombotic risk factors play in that patient's life. Decisions such as whether or not to take oral contraceptives, how to manage pregnancies, and whether or not to undergo chronic anticoagulant therapy can be difficult for both patient and provider. In the case of inherited disorders, genetic counselors may play a critical role as well. In all such instances, knowledge not only of available testing, but also of limits in interpretation of these tests, can contribute greatly toward reaching the most appropriate clinical decisions.

SELECTED REFERENCES

Bertina RM, Koeleman BP, Koster T, et al. Mutation in blood coagulation factor V associated with resistance to activated protein C. Nature 1994;369:64–7.
Classic paper describing Factor V_{Leiden}.

de Laat B, Pengo V, Pabinger I, et al. The association between circulating antibodies against domain I of beta2-glycoprotein I and thrombosis: an international multicenter study. J Thromb Haemost 2009;7:1767–73.
Identification of critical epitope specificity for lupus anticoagulants.

Giannakopoulos B, Passam F, Ioannou Y, Krilis SA. How we diagnose the antiphospholipid syndrome. Blood 2009;113:985–94.
Recent review of the antiphospholipid syndrome.

Levine JS, Branch DW, Rauch J. The antiphospholipid syndrome. N Engl J Med 2002;346:752–63.
Comprehensive review of antiphospholipid syndrome and lupus anticoagulants.

Miyakis S, Lockshin MD, Atsumi T, et al. International consensus statement on an update of the classification criteria for definite antiphospholipid syndrome (APS). J Thromb Haemost 2006;4:295–306.
Consensus conference report on antiphospholipid syndrome.

Pengo V, Tripodi A, Reber G, et al. Subcommittee on Lupus Anticoagulant/Antiphospholipid Antibody of the Scientific and Standardisation Committee of the International Society on Thrombosis and Haemostasis. Update of the guidelines for lupus anticoagulant detection. J Thromb Haemost 2009;7:1737–40.
Consensus group report on standardization of lupus anticoagulant testing.

Poort SR, Rosendaal FR, Reitsma PH, Bertina RM. A common genetic variation in the 3′-untranslated region of the prothrombin gene is associated with elevated plasma prothrombin levels and an increase in venous thrombosis. Blood 1996;88:3698–703.
Classic paper describing prothrombin gene variant associated with elevated thrombotic risk.

REFERENCES

Access the complete reference list online at http://www.expertconsult.com

CHAPTER

42

ANTITHROMBOTIC THERAPY

Louis M. Fink, Richard A. Marlar, Jonathan L. Miller

PART 5

KEY POINTS

- Warfarin is the most commonly used oral anticoagulant. It acts as a vitamin K antagonist and blocks γ-carboxylation of a series of glutamic acid residues during the synthesis of factors II, VII, IX, and X, and proteins C and S. The resulting decreased functionality of the coagulation factors leads to prolongations of the prothrombin time, monitored by the international normalized ratio.
- Heparin binds to antithrombin and increases its ability to inhibit thrombin, factor Xa, and, to a lesser extent, other serine protease coagulation factors. Heparin is thus considered to be an "indirect" thrombin inhibitor. Heparin anticoagulant intensity is commonly monitored by prolongations of the partial thromboplastin time, with actual quantitation of heparin anticoagulant activity being assayed as anti–factor Xa activity. In instances where it is necessary to monitor low-molecular-weight heparin therapy, this must be done by measuring its anti–factor Xa activity.
- Heparin-induced thrombocytopenia (HIT) is a complication of heparin therapy in which antibodies develop against complexes of heparin and platelet factor 4. In the most severe cases, the resulting antibodies bind to platelets in such a manner as to cause activation, leading to arterial and/or venous thrombosis. Both immunologic and functional assays are employed in the evaluation of possible HIT.
- More recent anticoagulants function as direct thrombin inhibitors, or directly inhibit factor Xa. Effectively monitoring the activity of these inhibitors, as well as identifying possible interference by these inhibitors upon testing for other hemostatic abnormalities, presents new challenges to the diagnostic laboratory.
- Therapy directed toward inhibition of platelet reactivity is being used increasingly in both acute and chronic settings. The laboratory can monitor the resulting reactivity of platelets from treated patients, and in some instances can detect apparent resistance to aspirin or other therapeutic agents.

A wide array of agents may alter the synthesis or action of coagulation factors, affect platelet function, or modify blood vessel responses. Prescribed and over-the-counter medicines with anticoagulant or antiplatelet activity are among the drugs most commonly used. Such agents may behave as a "double-edged" sword in that they may prevent formation or extension of a thrombus, but they can also produce or exacerbate bleeding. The clinical laboratory has a major role in the monitoring of some antithrombotic therapy.

PREANALYTIC VARIABLES AND CONTROLS

All standards for accuracy and precision in monitoring anticoagulant therapy are of little use if the blood sample is not obtained and processed in a defined manner (Adcock, 2009). The Clinical and Laboratory Standards Institute (CLSI) has provided useful guidelines for the collection, storage, and preparation of blood or plasma before coagulation testing is undertaken (summarized in an Appendix at the end of this chapter [CLSI, 2008]).

For optimal reporting, the time and date of the sampling, as well as the time of the last dose of the anticoagulant, should be recorded. Laboratory results for monitoring antithrombotic therapy need to be interpreted in conjunction with the clinical history for optimal regulation. Whenever there is a computed manipulation of the analytic data, such as the conversion of prothrombin time (PT) from seconds to the international normalized ratio (INR), a periodic check must ensure that the appropriate constants and data manipulations are being used, as defined by the standard operating procedures for the laboratory.

VITAMIN K ANTAGONISTS

Warfarin is the most commonly prescribed oral vitamin K antagonist. It is a racemic mixture of the stereoisomers S-warfarin and R-warfarin. S-warfarin is more potent in producing an anticoagulant effect. Warfarin inhibits vitamin K reductase (vitamin K 2,3-epoxide reductase) and blocks regeneration of the active form of vitamin K, which is necessary for the formation of γ-carboxy-glutamic acid in a sequence of amino acid residues (termed the **Gla domain**) within factors II, VII, IX, and X and proteins C and S (Fig. 42-1). With the decreasing extent of γ-carboxylation of glutamic acid within the Gla domains, there is in turn a decreased ability of the affected proteins to be bound into the highly ordered protein–Ca^{++}–phospholipid complexes that are critical components of the coagulation cascade (Ansell, 2004). Tests dependent on proper functioning of these factors will become more abnormal with increasing intensity of oral anticoagulant therapy (Ansell, 2008).

The degree of warfarin anticoagulation is typically measured in the PT testing system, although prolongations of the activated partial thromboplastin time (APTT) also are typically observed. Because fibrinogen synthesis is not vitamin K–dependent, the thrombin time (TT) remains normal. It must be stressed that *initial* prolongation of the PT upon institution of warfarin therapy does *not* faithfully reflect the overall intensity of anticoagulation. The reason for this unintuitive observation is that although the relatively short half-life of factor VII (4–6 hours) underlies the contemporaneous prolongation of the PT, the half-lives of other vitamin K–dependent factors actually extend to several days. Only when all of these factors have reached a steady-state level of decreased γ-carboxylation should one anticipate that overall diminution of the

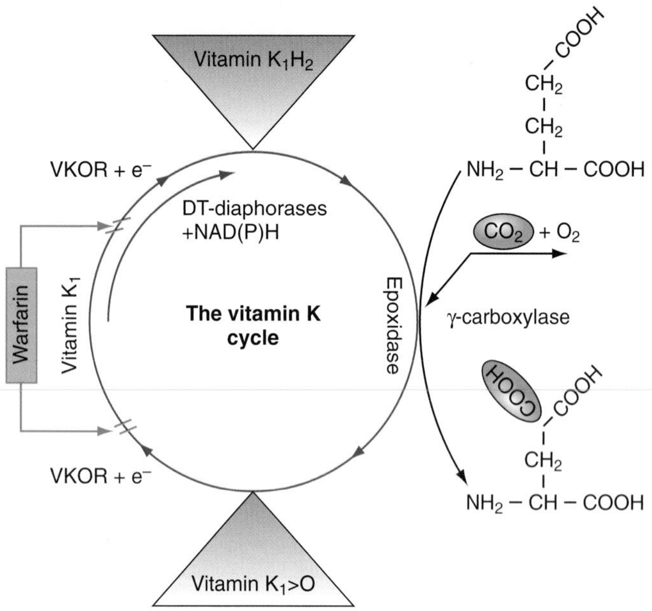

Figure 42-1 The vitamin K–dependent γ-carboxylation system. The γ-carboxylase converts vitamin K–dependent proteins to γ-carboxyglutamic acid (Gla) containing proteins by adding carbon dioxide (CO_2) to glutamic acid (Glu) residues in newly synthesized proteins. The γ-carboxylase requires reduced vitamin K_1 (vitamin K_1H_2) as a cofactor for this posttranslational modification reaction. Concomitant with γ-carboxylation, vitamin K_1H_2 is converted to vitamin K_1 2,3-epoxide (vitamin K_1>O). The epoxide is reduced by the warfarin-sensitive enzyme vitamin K_1 2,3-epoxide reductase (VKOR) to the vitamin K_1H_2 cofactor. This cyclic interconversion of vitamin K metabolites constitutes the vitamin K cycle. At high tissue concentrations, vitamin K_1 quinone (vitamin K_1) can be reduced to vitamin K_1H_2 by the alternative pathway of the cycle. This pathway is catalyzed by NAD(P)H dehydrogenases (DT-diaphorases), which are not inhibited by warfarin *(From Wallin R, Hutson SM. Warfarin and the vitamin K-dependent gamma-carboxylation system. Trends Mol Med 2004;10: 299–302.)*

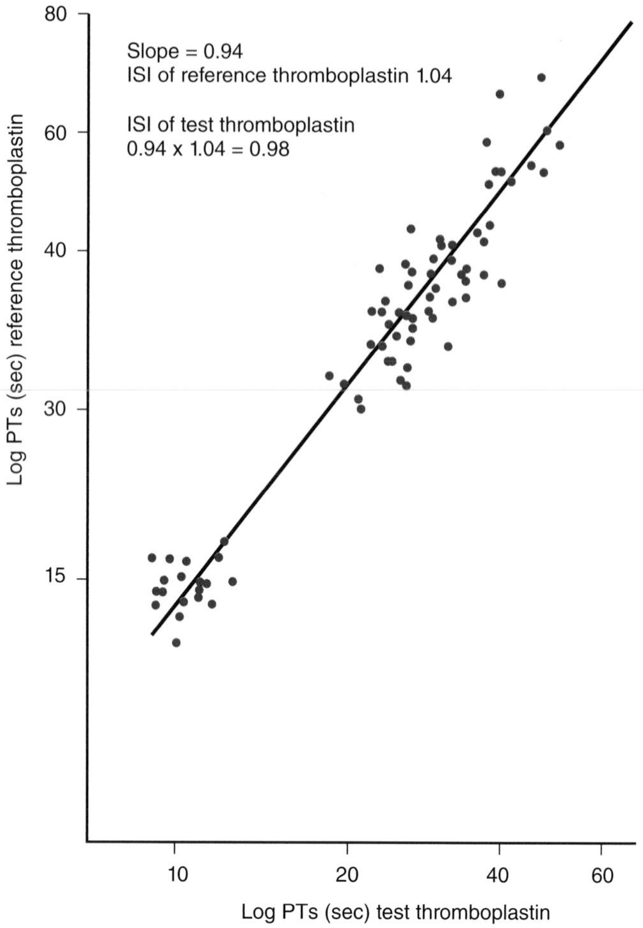

Figure 42-2 An example of a thromboplastin calibration using the World Health Organization (WHO) international sensitivity index (ISI) model. Prothrombin times were performed on a series of normal subjects and anticoagulated patients with a reference thromboplastin and a test thromboplastin under calibration. *(From Kitchen S, Preston FE. Standardization of prothrombin time for laboratory control of oral anticoagulant therapy. Semin Thromb Hemost 1999;25:17–25.)*

coagulation system (as reflected by actual thrombin generation) has been obtained. For this reason, a minimum of 4–6 days of oral anticoagulant therapy is generally recommended before assuming that laboratory monitoring actually reflects the steady-state level of anticoagulation. When more rapid onset of effective anticoagulation is necessary, heparin is given before or along with warfarin. After at least 4 days of combined therapy, heparin can be discontinued, and the warfarin dose can be adjusted to the prescribed target INR. Although warfarin therapy ordinarily produces a net anticoagulant effect, in certain settings (e.g., active HIT), the resulting decrease in carboxylation and hence activity of protein C and/or protein S may dominate the hemostatic imbalance, resulting in purpura fulminans or other manifestations of venous thrombosis (Martin, 1998).

As discussed in Chapter 39, the PT is performed by adding a source of phospholipid and tissue factor (thromboplastin), as well as excess calcium, to the citrated platelet-free plasma. The time in seconds to subsequent clot formation then is determined by mechanical or optical measurements. However, the actual degree of PT prolongation in response to warfarin therapy is highly dependent on the particular thromboplastin reagent and instrument system employed. Cooperation among a number of laboratories in different countries resulted in the development of the INR and the international sensitivity index (ISI), both of which are now universally used to improve standardization of PT reporting worldwide. In brief, the logarithms of PTs obtained on prescribed series of normal and warfarinized patients, using the primary international reference thromboplastin, are plotted against the logarithms of PTs obtained using an individual thromboplastin reagent (Fig. 42-2). The resulting slope of this plot is the ISI for that thromboplastin reagent and instrument combination (Kitchen, 1999; Poller, 2004; Adcock, 2002; van den Besselaar, 2004; Favaloro, 2008). The ratio of patient PT divided by geometric mean normal PT for the local laboratory (based on a population of normal individuals in which identical sample collections, reagents, and analyzers are used), raised to the power of the ISI, defines the INR as follows:

$$INR = \left(\frac{Patient\ PT\ in\ Seconds}{Mean\ of\ the\ Normal\ PT\ in\ Seconds} \right)^{ISI} \qquad \textbf{(42-1)}$$

Put in another way, the INR seeks to represent the PT ratio that would have been obtained if the international reference thromboplastin had actually been used in patient testing. However, attainment of a fully assay-independent INR may be very difficult in practice (Ng, 1993; Cunningham, 1994; Favaloro, 2010).

Because of the importance of proper monitoring of oral anticoagulant therapy, several additional points regarding ISI and INR must be emphasized: The ISI must be correctly specified not only for each type of PT reagent, but also for each new *lot* of thromboplastin, in conjunction with the specific instrument model being used in a given laboratory. Less responsive thromboplastins (typically derived from nonhuman tissues) have ISI values in the range of 1.7–2.2, whereas more responsive human-derived tissue-derived reagents have ISI values in the range of 1.0–1.7. Recombinant tissue factor is the most responsive thromboplastin, with ISI values approaching 1.0. Most laboratories report results simply as INR, but some also give the results as PT in seconds. During initiation of anticoagulation, more frequent measurements of PT may be required until the INR has stabilized. In plasma from patients treated with both heparin and warfarin, the anticoagulant contribution of warfarin can be assessed if heparin is first removed or neutralized before PT testing is performed (see later). Unless a method becomes available for removal or neutralization of direct thrombin inhibitors (DTIs), the therapeutic intensities of such inhibitors can be sufficient to prolong PT, and accordingly influence the INR value (Tobu, 2004; Walenga, 2004). This should be assessed when warfarin is to be started after DTI therapy (Bartholomew, 2005). Although most lupus anticoagulants exert a more pronounced effect upon the APTT than the PT, the presence of a lupus anticoagulant in some patients may render the PT inaccurate as a means of monitoring warfarin therapy. This may depend on the reagents used (Moll, 1997). In such instances, a direct chromogenic assay for factor X (rather than a clotting assay) may aid in monitoring of anticoagulant intensity (Rosborough, 2004). An additional consideration is that use of nonhuman tissue factor in some patients may lead to prolongation of the PT (and hence increased INR) that would not

TABLE 42-1

Phenotype Characteristics of Warfarin Metabolism Genotype Combinations

	GENOTYPE COMBINATION			
Warfarin sensitivity	***VKORC1***	***CYP2C9***	**Prevalence**	**Clinical considerations**
Very high	A/A G/A	*1/*3, *2/*2, *2/*3, *3/*3 *3/*3	23 (2.6%)	Dose decrease and frequent INR monitoring
High	A/A G/A G/G	*1/*2 *2/*3 *3/*3	36 (4.0%)	Dose decrease and frequent INR monitoring
Moderate	A/A G/A G/G	*1/*1 *1/*2, *1/*3, *2/*2 *2/*3	238 (26.6%)	Dose decrease and frequent INR monitoring
Mild	G/G	*1/*2, *1/*3, *2/*2	109 (12.2%)	Frequent INR monitoring
Normal	G/A	*1/*1	262 (29.2%)	Likely to experience normal response to warfarin
Less than normal	G/G	*1/*1	228 (25.4%)	Dose increase may be required to maintain optimal INR
Total			896 (100%)	

From Epstein RS, Moyer TP, Aubert RE, et al. Warfarin genotyping reduces hospitalization rates results from the MM-WES (Medco-Mayo Warfarin Effectiveness Study). J Am Coll Cardiol 2010;55:2804–12.
INR, International normalized ratio.
Prevalence values are N (%). Genotype is defined by the combination of measured allelic variations in CYP2C9 and VKORC1. Phenotype is the expected warfarin sensitivity based on genotype.

TABLE 42-2

Allele Frequencies in Derivation Cohort (N = 1015) and Relationship to Race and Therapeutic Warfarin Dose

SNP alleles	**Gene location**	**White (N = 838), %**	**African American (N = 153), %**	**Other or mixed race (N = 24), %**	**Univariate association with dose in total population, per allele (95% CI), %**
CYP2C9*2 (C>T)	3608C>T	13.1	5.2	10.4	−17 (−22 to −12)
CYP2C9*3 (A>C)	42614A>C	6.0	1.0	4.2	−30 (−36 to −24)
CYP2C9*5 (C>G)	42619C>G	0	1.3	2.1	NS
VKORC1 861 C>A	−4451C>A	36.0	8.8	26.1	14 (9 to 18)
VKORC1 3673 G>A	−1639G>A	36.6	9.5	41.7	−29 (−31 to 26)
VKORC1 5808 T>G	IVS1+324T>G	25.1	4.6	8.3	25 (29 to 22)
VKORC1 6853 G>C	IVS2+124G>C	37.2	24.3	41.7	−37 (−42 to −32)
VKORC1 9041 G>A	626G>A	39.4	51.3	41.7	18 (14 to 23)
F2 Thr165Met	494C>T	13.3	1.3	30.0	−5.8 (−11.4 to 0.0)

From Gage BF, Eby C, Johnson JA, et al. Use of pharmacogenetic and clinical factors to predict the therapeutic dose of warfarin. Clin Pharmacol Ther 2008;84:326–31.
CI, Confidence interval; *NS,* not significant; *SNP,* single-nucleotide polymorphism.
Frequency values are reported for the variant allele at each SNP. CYP2C9 gene locations taken from http://www.cypalleles.ki.se/cyp2c9.htm

have been obtained had human tissue factor been employed. This phenomenon has been reported in patients with **factor VII Padua,** who have a nonpathogenic polymorphism in their factor VII molecule that supports normal interaction with human tissue factor, but diminished interaction with tissue factor of various animal origins, notably including rabbit (Pollak, 2006; Kirkel, 2010).

The half-life of warfarin is between 20 and 60 hours, with a mean plasma half-life of 40 hours. The maximum effect of a dose lasts for up to 48 hours after administration. S-warfarin is metabolized by CYP2C9, and R-warfarin is metabolized by the CYP1AZ and CYP3A4 enzymes. VKOR controls the levels of reduced vitamin K reductase. There are polymorphisms of CYP2C9 and VKOR, and knowledge of the patient's specific gene alleles may have predictive value in determining which patients need higher or lower doses of warfarin (Higashi, 2002; Linder, 2002; Adcock, 2004). Warfarin dosing incorporating genotyping results has been reported to reduce patient hospitalization rates (Moore, 2008; Epstein, 2010). Specific allelic combinations of CYP2C9 and VKORC1 are associated with a wide range of warfarin sensitivities (Table 42-1). Allelic frequencies and their relationships to race and therapeutic warfarin dose are shown in Table 42-2. Pharmacologic algorithms have been developed to help guide warfarin dosing (Gage, 2008; Lubitz, 2010). They have become increasingly successful in predicting variabilities in response to warfarin dosing (Klein, 2009), and even in reducing hospitalization (Epstein, 2010).

Genetic resistance to warfarin therapy is uncommon. In instances where inappropriate responses to warfarin are marked and persistent, the metabolites can be measured using high-performance liquid chromatography (Lombardi, 2003). These measurements can also be used to check compliance. Drugs that affect S-warfarin metabolism may markedly alter the potency of warfarin treatment. Some drugs or herbal medications induce CYP2C9 and cause warfarin to be metabolized faster, thus decreasing the anticoagulant effect. Other drugs inhibit the metabolism of warfarin and thus enhance the effect of warfarin. Several hundred compounds are known to alter the metabolism of warfarin (Poller, 1996; Ansell, 2008). Antibiotics may interfere with the metabolism of warfarin, or they may suppress the gut flora, which supplies a significant amount of vitamin K in humans. Rifampin, e.g., may dramatically increase the metabolism of warfarin, thereby necessitating very high doses of warfarin to achieve anticoagulation (Krajewski, 2010). Foods, particularly green leafy vegetables rich in vitamin K, may make anticoagulation with warfarin more difficult. Warfarin products may have different potencies, so that switching between related medications may require more frequent monitoring and dosage adjustments (Bongiorno, 2004).

Warfarin is used most commonly for prevention of thromboembolic stroke in patients with atrial fibrillation. Additionally, warfarin is used both prophylactically and therapeutically in a wide range of clinical settings and may even be used on a lifelong basis in patients who are at particularly high risk for recurrent thrombotic events. The American Association of Chest Physicians periodically reviews the guidelines for anticoagulant therapy and publishes its consensus report in the journal *Chest* (Hirsh, 2008). The current recommendation for treatment targets an INR between 2 and 3 for most patients with venous thromboembolic disease and atrial fibrillation (Ansell, 2008).

Because warfarin is influenced by liver function, diet, absorption from the gut, and cotreatment with other drugs or herbal medications, it is not uncommon for patients to present with INRs that are elevated or decreased. Mild elevations of INR can be treated by changing the dosage schedule. More significant elevations can be treated with 2 mg of vitamin K given orally. If there is a high risk of bleeding, higher doses of vitamin K can be administered. However, the patient then may become resistant to further warfarin therapy, and another anticoagulant may have to be substituted. If the patient is bleeding, fresh frozen plasma, activated prothrombin complexes, or recombinant FVIIa may be transfused to achieve hemostasis (Ansell, 2008).

Extreme care should be used in treating patients with warfarin. Warfarin should not be used in patients with evidence of hemorrhage. If there is a suspicion of hemorrhage, a periodic assessment for blood loss and anemia should be made. Warfarin is teratogenic and should not be used in pregnant females (Bates, 2004). If a deficiency state of protein C is suspected, heparin or another anticoagulant should be started before or concomitantly with warfarin therapy. In patients with HIT, administration of warfarin is of particular concern, in that lowering the activity of protein C may potentially promote venous limb gangrene (Warkentin, 2008).

The INR is monitored to keep patients on warfarin therapy within a range that will prevent further thrombosis but will not lead to bleeding. Although an anticoagulant intensity goal INR of 2–3 defines the usual reference interval, still higher INRs may be sought in certain clinical settings. Patients, families, and caregivers should be educated about the therapy and should be informed about the importance of having the INR checked on a routine basis. In some instances, patients may be taught how to use point-of-care (POC) coagulometers to obtain an INR measurement (see following).

Many new developments have occurred in the technology of POC monitors for oral anticoagulant therapy. Mechanical technologies using the magnetic motion of iron filings, motion flow detectors, thrombin-cleavable fluorescent substrates, electrochemical detectors of impedance changes, and laser light dispersion technologies have been used to detect clot formation and to transform data into a reportable PT-INR. Each type of POC-PT measurement must be characterized for use with specific patients (NCCLS, 2004). Results obtained with different POC-PT instruments and laboratory-based instruments often are not comparable (Nutescu, 2004). Indeed, even the patient specimen itself will vary in terms of being whole blood directly sampled by a POC instrument, as opposed to the citrated plasma routinely used in the clinical laboratory setting. Quality assurance and quality control plans should be in place for POC coagulation testing (Gardiner, 2009; van Cott, 2009). Out-of-range POC INR should be retested by analyzing a sample of citrated blood in the clinical laboratory (Sunderji, 2005).

HEPARIN

Heparin is a natural polymer of sulfated glycosaminoglycans with a wide range of molecular weights. Unfractionated heparin (UFH) may be used prophylactically or therapeutically for venous and arterial thrombosis. The molecular weight of UFH ranges from 20,000–50,000 Da. UFH for systemic use is prepared from porcine intestine. Heparin is an **indirect** thrombin inhibitor that exerts its effects by binding to antithrombin in such a manner as to significantly increase the potency of the inhibitory action of antithrombin on the serine esterase activity of thrombin (Fig. 42-3). The anticoagulant effect is derived from inhibition of serine protease coagulation factors, with the most critical inhibition being that of factor IIa (thrombin) and factor Xa. However, additional effects of heparin include the release of tissue factor pathway inhibitor, an increase in tissue plasminogen activator and fibrinolysis, and impairment of platelet function (Salzman, 1980). Unfractionated heparin can be given subcutaneously or intravenously with a rapid onset of action (Bussey, 2004; Hirsh, 2004b). It is important to rapidly achieve effective anticoagulation in patients with veno-occlusive disease (e.g., venous thromboembolism [VTE]) because sequestered thrombin may allow subsequent propagation of the thrombus (Hull, 1997).

A variety of methods can be used to measure unfractionated heparin. These include the APTT, TT, protamine reversal, factor Xa inhibition, and activated clotting time (ACT). The APTT is the most commonly used assay. In contrast to the case of warfarin monitoring, for which the international community has established the INR to minimize performance variations in reagent/instrument combinations used by different laboratories, comparable standardization is presently lacking with respect to use of the APTT for monitoring heparin. This raises a particular problem for

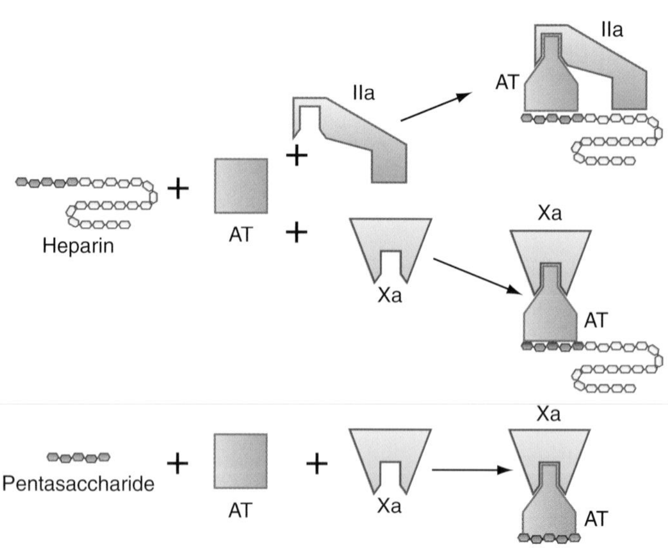

Figure 42-3 Hypothetical mechanisms for heparin/heparan sulfate regulation of protein–protein interactions. Binding of a specific pentasaccharide sequence of heparin present in unfractionated heparin (UFH) and low-molecular-weight heparin (LMWH) or in isolated form (fondaparinux) to antithrombin (AT) produces a conformational change in AT sufficient for inhibition of the serine protease factor Xa. Effective inhibition of thrombin (factor IIa) additionally requires direct interaction with a region of the heparin molecule distinct from the pentasaccharide. Such thrombin binding regions are characteristically more available in UFH than in the LMWH products. *(Modified from Nugent MA. Heparin sequencing brings structure to the function of complex oligosaccharides. Proc Natl Acad Sci U S A 2000;97:10301–3.)*

the laboratory with respect to serving those clinicians whose professional societies quote a heparin goal range in terms of actual seconds measured by APTT testing. Although there does appear to be a degree of convergence toward an increasingly standardized range for the normal APTT adult reference interval when products from a number of manufacturers are used, APTT testing systems with significantly different performance attributes are also available. Accordingly, it is important for the individual laboratory to consider the potentially considerable implications with respect to use of the APTT in therapeutic drug monitoring of heparin when deciding upon which reagent/instrument combination to adopt. A classic approach used by many clinicians for monitoring heparin therapy is to aim for a 1.5- to 2.5-fold increase in APTT over the patient's baseline APTT, or, alternatively, over the midpoint of the laboratory's normal reference interval for the APTT. However, the approach currently in general usage by clinical laboratories, and in fact mandated for many laboratories by their accreditation process, comprises performing a linear regression analysis of the APTT plotted against anti–factor Xa heparin levels for patients undergoing therapeutic heparin anticoagulation. An example of such an analysis is shown in Figure 42-4. Because recommendations from a number of professional societies as to goals for intensity of heparin therapy are expressed in anti-Xa units, the laboratory then translates the range of anti-Xa units (e.g., 0.3–0.7 anti-Xa units is commonly recommended in conjunction with treatment of deep venous thrombosis) into the corresponding range of APTT values that has been obtained with current lots of reagents for both the anti-Xa assay and the APTT. This relationship must be reevaluated each time a change in reagent lot (or instrument) occurs for either of these tests. Additionally, it should be noted that, owing to the complex pharmacokinetics of heparin, plasma samples must be obtained from patients actually undergoing heparin therapy; it is not acceptable simply to add exogenous heparin to normal plasma samples and then perform regression analysis on the resulting APTT and anti-Xa values (Olson, 1998; Hirsch, 2004b). As is apparent from the wide degree of scatter seen in Figure 42-4 (and an even greater range of scatter apparent in examples presented by Cuker [2009]), the relationship between APTT and anti-Xa values obtained from real patients is far from tight. When one considers the many contributors to variation in the APTT (see Chapter 39) such as factor VIII level and levels of contact factors and lupus anticoagulants, it is not at all surprising that the APTT will have considerable variation between patients, even though heparin levels may be identical. Less intuitive, however, may be the variability observed among anti-Xa heparin assays performed with the various available reagent/instrument combinations. One contributor to such variability is whether or not the particular assay system includes the addition of exogenous antithrombin

TABLE 42-3
Comparison of the Properties of LMWH, Fondaparinux, and Idraparinux

Feature	LMWH	Fondaparinux	Idraparinux
Mode of administration	Subcutaneous	Subcutaneous	Subcutaneous
Bioavailability, %	80–90	100	100
Half-life, hours	4	17	80
Target	Factor Xa > thrombin (2–4 fold)	Factor Xa	Factor Xa
Renal clearance	Yes	Yes	Yes
Neutralized by protamine sulfate	Partial	No	No

Modified from Bates SM, Weitz JI. New anticoagulants: beyond heparin, low-molecular-weight heparin and warfarin. Brit J Pharmacol 2005;144:1017–28.
LMWH, Low-molecular-weight heparin.

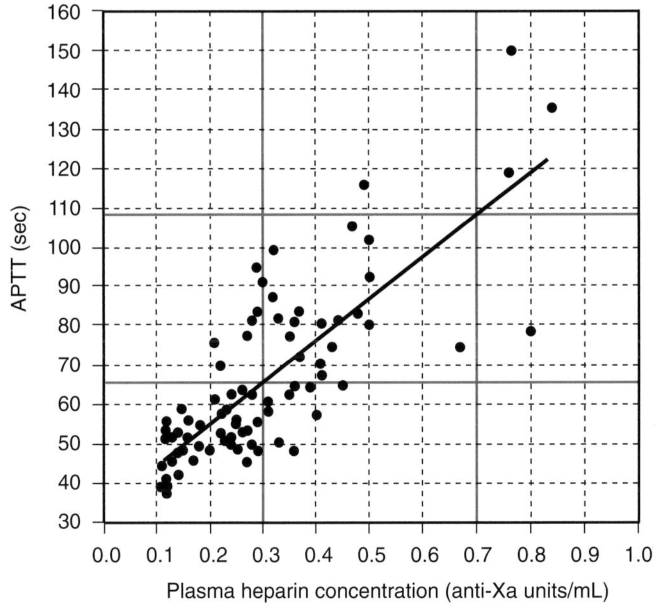

Figure 42-4 Linear regression analysis of relationship between activated partial thromboplastin time (APTT) and anti–factor Xa (Xa) heparin level performed on plasma samples from patients undergoing heparin therapy. With this particular reagent/instrument combination, the regression analysis yields an APTT range of 66–108 seconds that would correspond to an anti-Xa range of 0.3–0.7 U/mL.

(Lehman, 2006). Providing an excess of antithrombin may produce a higher heparin level for the patient who is deficient in endogenous antithrombin. In a sense, this yields the more accurate measurement. Viewed from a different perspective, however, the more appropriate measurement to guide dosing may be the one that reflects the actual inhibitory ability of infused heparin, that is, the method that remains dependent on the patient's own antithrombin level. It is interesting to note that in a recent interinstitutional study, when heparin dose adjustments were guided by APTT target ranges defined by their relationship to anti-Xa assays, concurrence in dose adjustment proved more difficult to achieve than when these adjustments were guided by simple fold-increase in the APTT, as described previously (Cuker, 2009). Regardless of how the continuing debate regarding optimal monitoring of heparin therapy is resolved, however, all would agree that for patients who have a quite prolonged baseline the APTT before initiation of heparin therapy, a more specific method such as the anti-Xa assay must be employed.

Heparin contamination is a frequent cause of prolongation of the APTT and TT, and in fact can interfere with the performance of clot-based tests. This is particularly true when samples are drawn from intravenous catheters. Some commercial test kits contain polybrene or other agents to neutralize heparin. The presence of heparin can be determined if a prolonged APTT shortens following treatment with heparinase (obtained from *Flavobacterium heparinum*). In specimens with a very prolonged APTT value, a second treatment with heparinase may be necessary to remove all heparin and produce a true APTT value. A similar approach can be used in which heparin-binding cellulose absorbs heparin from patient plasma. This absorption procedure has only minimal effects on the other coagulation factors, except for a slight reduction in factor IX (Hutt, 1972; Thompson, 1976; Cowan, 1981; Newman, 1995).

Patients may appear to be resistant to heparin, although the definition of such resistance may be dependent on the specific clinical setting:

> *"In the context of venous thromboembolism, heparin resistance is defined as the need for more than 35,000 U 24 h^{-1} to prolong the activated partial thromboplastin time into the therapeutic range. In contrast, during cardiac bypass procedures, the definition of heparin resistance is based on the ACT, with at least one ACT less than 400 s after heparinization and/or the need for exogenous antithrombin administration"*
>
> **(Anderson, 2002).**

Causes of heparin resistance include massive thrombosis with release of heparin-binding proteins; elevated factor VIII levels (often evidenced by short baseline APTT); treatment with nitroglycerin; severe obesity; antithrombin deficiency (<30%); HIT; and cancer (Edson, 1967; Bharadwaj, 2003; Francis, 2004a). In some instances of apparent heparin resistance as measured by the APTT, such as in the case of elevated factor VIII levels, simply changing to anti–factor Xa assays will provide a more accurate measure of the heparin level (Hirsh, 2004b). Additionally, a recent study has suggested that race may play a role in sensitivity to heparin (Shimada, 2010).

LOW-MOLECULAR-WEIGHT HEPARIN

Low-molecular-weight heparin (LMWH) (see Table 42-3) is derived from unfractionated heparin. LMWH does not as effectively inactivate thrombin as it does factor Xa. This has been explained by the observation that since distribution of the pentasaccharide with heparin chains is random, there will more frequently be insufficient room in adjacent regions for effective binding to thrombin in the shorter LMWH chains (Gray, 2008). Anti-Xa assays, rather than APTT, must be used when measurement of LMWH is needed (Boneu, 2001). The general therapeutic range for LMWH in patients being treated for venous thromboembolic disorders is different for each LMWH product. As a result of decreased binding to plasma proteins, a predictable response to LMWH can be expected in most cases, allowing LMWH to be given subcutaneously once or twice a day (Bounameaux, 2004; Harenberg, 2004). Plasma levels of LMWH usually are not monitored, except during treatment of children and newborns, pregnant women, markedly obese patients, and patients with renal failure. When monitoring is performed, blood is ordinarily drawn approximately 4 hours after the last dose because this is when the peak level is anticipated to occur (Bounameaux, 2004; Harenberg, 2004; Hirsh, 2008).

Complications of osteopenia and HIT (see later) occur less frequently when LMWH rather than UFH is used (Pettila, 2002; Schulman, 2002). However, patients with established HIT should not be anticoagulated with LMWH. Although LMWHs initially are less immunogenic, once antibodies have actually been produced following UFH administration, pathologic antigen–antibody interaction may occur upon subsequent administration of LMWH (Warkentin, 2007; Lobo, 2008).

FONDAPARINUX

Fondaparinux is a small synthetic pentasaccharide that targets factor Xa. This drug binds to antithrombin (AT) in an irreversible fashion, enhancing the reactive site of AT to complex with factor Xa. It has a longer half-life than heparin or LMWH and can be given subcutaneously once daily; dose is based on weight and does not ordinarily require measurement of blood levels. Fondaparinux is cleared by the kidneys, and its dose must be reduced in patients with compromised renal function (Weitz, 2010a). Only very rarely has fondaparinux been associated with HIT (Warkentin, 2007; Lobo, 2008).

HEPARIN-INDUCED THROMBOCYTOPENIA

Thrombocytopenias arising in the setting of heparin therapy occur in two forms. Nonimmune HIT is believed to result from platelet activation following the direct binding of heparin to platelets (Horne, 2001). The degree of thrombocytopenia is generally mild and transient. Of far greater concern are immune-mediated processes, sometimes referred to as **type II HIT,** but more commonly simply as **HIT.** Additionally, when venous and/or arterial thrombosis arises in the context of HIT, the entity may be referred to as **heparin-induced thrombocytopenia and thrombosis (HITT).** Studies have shown that UFH structures bind tetramers of PF4 into ultralarge complexes (ULCs) that are particularly antigenic (Rauova, 2005). If multiple IgG molecules bind to the ULC, the Fc regions of these antibodies may then be oriented in a manner favoring their binding to the Fc γRIIA receptors of the platelet, thereby causing signal transduction and subsequent platelet activation. Manifestations of such platelet activation include secretion of granular material and release of platelet microparticles whose outwardly facing phosphatidylserine may potentially promote thrombin generation and hence increased clotting. Antibodies to other chemokines which have shared sequence structures with PF4 (the CXC family of chemokines), including interleukin-8 (IL-8), interferon-gamma-inducible protein (IL-10), platelet basic protein and its proteolytic product β-thromboglobulin, and neutrophil-activating protein-2, may also cause HIT (Greinacher, 1994; Amiral, 1996). HIT-associated antibodies may also cause endothelial cells and monocytes to activate and express tissue factor on their surface (Fig. 42-5). HIT is more likely to arise in patients experiencing major trauma (Lubenow, 2010; Warkentin, 2010).

HIT occurs more frequently with exposure to bovine heparin than to porcine heparin, and with lower frequency following LMWH (Fig. 42-6). In the usual presentation, the platelet count drops at 5–10 days after exposure to heparin, with platelets falling to below 150,000/μL or decreasing to levels of less than 50% of peak platelet count before initiation of heparin. When this occurs, all heparin treatment should be discontinued (including heparin flushes of catheters). In most cases, the platelet decrease is seen at 4–5 days from initiation of therapy, but in some cases thrombocytopenia may occur as early as 2–3 days, and may even arise within a week or 2 following discontinuation of heparin administration. Although a fall in platelet count can certainly be a matter of concern in various clinical contexts, by far the most serious concern arises in that minority of patients with HIT who actually progress to thrombotic events (see Fig. 42-6). Venous thromboses are more common than arterial thromboses, and the lower limbs are more frequently involved. Formation of platelet microparticles with phosphatidylserine exposed on their outer surfaces, together with activation of monocytes that produce tissue factor, contributes to thrombin generation and subsequent venous thromboses (Kelton, 2008). Patients may have areas of skin necrosis at the site of heparin injections or acute systemic inflammatory reactions after a heparin bolus, and may show evidence of heparin resistance. Other causes of thrombocytopenia must be ruled out. If heparin is discontinued, thrombocytopenia frequently abates in 9–10 days. However, the patient can be at risk for thrombosis for several weeks after discontinuing heparin.

A presumptive diagnosis of HIT is often made on clinical grounds, particularly in cases where the time course and the extent of the drop in platelet count fit together convincingly with the patient's history of heparin therapy. In such cases, treatment decisions may be made independently of whether or not the results of laboratory testing also point in this direction (Warkentin, 2008). Several algorithmic approaches have been developed that attempt to assess the pretest likelihood of true HIT in the individual patient, most notably the **4T** system (Table 42-4). Establishing the correct diagnosis in a timely manner through laboratory testing has continued to represent a substantial challenge. As illustrated in Figure 42-6, a great many patients test positively on one or more immunologically based tests, and even a substantial number test positively on tests employing platelet functional responses, yet they may not actually have clinical HIT or HITT. Greinacher (2010) has postulated that a background level of antibody directed against PF4 bound to glycosaminoglycans may routinely arise as part of the body's antibacterial response to infectious organisms whose glycosaminoglycans also bind PF4. This hypothesis not only would account for a number of apparent biological false-positive results observed in HIT testing, but also would provide an explanation for what otherwise would appear to be an unusually short minimal time (≈5 days) to the appearance of antibodies following exposure to heparin.

Additionally, recent contributions by Rauova (2009), Kelton (2008), and others suggest that platelet content of PF4, in conjunction with the level of PF4 actually bound to the surface of both platelets and monocytes, may be a key determinant as to which patients will or will not manifest clinically significant HIT and HITT. Viewed from these perspectives, it may well be that present analytic approaches are not yet assessing critical pathophysiologic determinants. Until the time that such improved testing may become available, efforts will continue to establish algorithmic approaches intended to guide diagnosis using present technologies. Clearly, such algorithms must be expected to vary among themselves, based on the specific tests employed in a given laboratory. One example of such an algorithmic approach, as used in this instance by the Greinacher group in Greifswald, Germany, is illustrated in Figure 42-7.

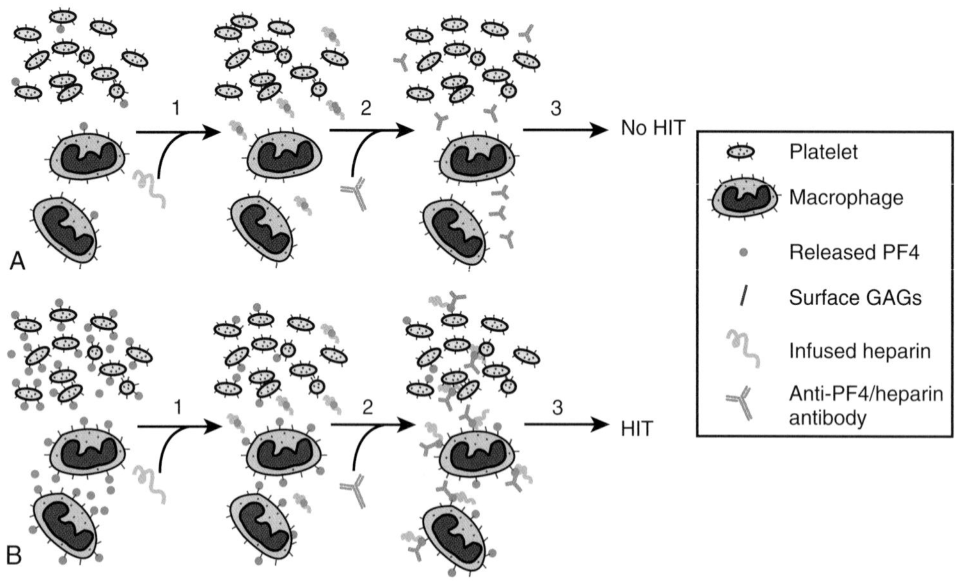

Figure 42-5 Mechanistic basis of heparin-induced thrombocytopenia (HIT). **(A)** shows the platelets and monocytes from a patient with little released platelet factor 4 (PF4) on the left. Following heparinization *(1)*, the small amount of surface-bound PF4 becomes complexed to the higher-affinity circulating heparin and induces anti-PF4/heparin antibody production *(2)*. Because there are not many surface PF4/GAG complexes for the antibodies to bind, they largely remain unattached to cells and do not activate the platelets or the monocytes *(3)*. The patient does not develop HIT. **(B)** is as **(A)**, but with a great deal of released PF4 bound to the GAGs on the surface of both platelets and monocytes. After heparinization *(1)*, some PF4/surface GAG complexes remain. Circulating free PF4/heparin induces antibody production *(2)*, and because there remain antigenic targets on platelets and monocytes, the antibodies bind to these cells and activate them *(3)*, resulting in both thrombocytopenia and the prothrombotic state seen in HIT. *(Modified from Kowalska MA, Rauova L, Poncz M. Role of the platelet chemokine platelet factor 4 [PF4] in hemostasis and thrombosis. Thromb Res 2010;125:292–6.)*

Considerations in the selection and interpretation of several of the more commonly used testing methods are discussed in the following paragraphs.

A test for HIT that had perfect sensitivity and specificity and that could be performed rapidly in a cost-effective fashion of course would be the ideal. Many laboratories, however, presently use a testing strategy in which the initial (or only) test is a readily performed PF4–enzyme-linked immunosorbent assay (ELISA) that has high sensitivity but lower specificity. Such assays accordingly may provide results that can be helpful in the effort to exclude the likelihood of HIT, with the degree of test positivity increasingly being associated with thrombotic risk (Fig. 42-8). However, if the value is higher than the established cutoff value (and particularly if

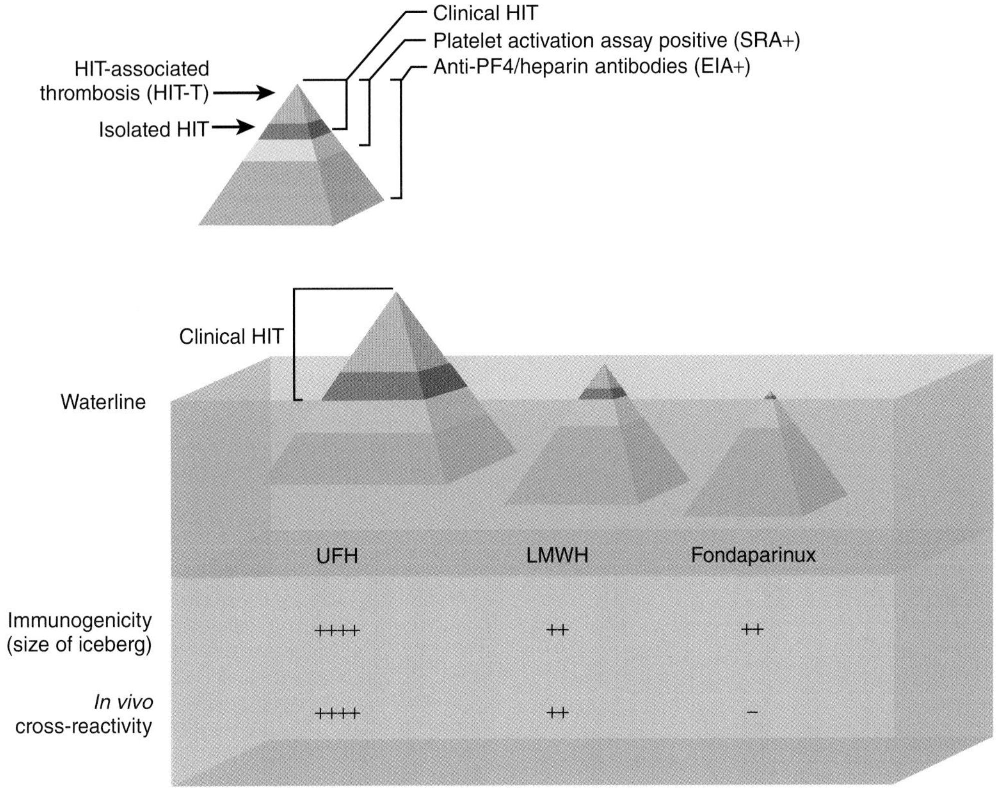

Figure 42-6 The relationship among the clinical expression of heparin-induced thrombocytopenia (HIT) (thrombocytopenia with or without thrombosis), the type of heparin used, and the antibodies that cause HIT. This can be conceptualized as an "iceberg." The visible component of the iceberg (the portion above the waterline) represents clinically evident features of HIT, such as thrombocytopenia and/or thrombosis. The mass of the iceberg corresponds to the entire spectrum of anti–platelet factor 4 (PF4)/heparin antibodies generated. Some of these antibodies will be biologically active (platelet activating), and others will be non–platelet activating, which may make them unlikely to cause clinical consequences. The type of heparin given to the patient determines the overall size of the iceberg, with unfractionated heparin (UFH) being the largest (most immunogenic), and low-molecular-weight heparin (LMWH) and fondaparinux having lesser immunogenicity. Also illustrated in this figure is in vivo cross-reactivity. UFH forms antigens that are readily recognized by HIT antibodies. In contrast, fondaparinux forms poorly recognized antigens. LMWH is intermediate. *(Illustration by AY Chen, from Kelton JG, Warkentin TE. Heparin-induced thrombocytopenia: a historical perspective. Blood 2008;112:2607–16.)*

TABLE 42-4
Pretest Scoring System for Heparin-Induced Thrombocytopenia: The 4 Ts

4 Ts	2 points	1 point	0 points
Thrombocytopenia	Platelet count fall >50% and platelet nadir ≥20 k/μL*	Platelet count fall 30%–50%, or platelet nadir 10–19 k/μL	Platelet count fall <30% or platelet nadir <10 k/μL
Timing of platelet count fall	Clear onset between days 5 and 10 or platelet fall ≤1 day (prior heparin exposure within 30 days)[†]	Consistent with day 5–10 fall, but not clear (e.g., missing platelet counts); onset after day 10[‡]; or fall ≤1 day (prior heparin exposure 30–100 days ago)	Platelet count fall <4 days without recent exposure
Thrombosis or other sequelae	New thrombosis (confirmed); skin necrosis[§]; acute systemic reaction post intravenous unfractionated heparin (UFH) bolus	Progressive or recurrent thrombosis[¶]; nonnecrotizing (erythematous) skin lesions[§]; suspected thrombosis (not proven)[¶]	None
o**T**her causes for thrombocytopenia	None apparent	Possible**	Definite**

From Lo GK, Juhl D, Warkentin TE, et al. Evaluation of pretest clinical score (4 Ts) for the diagnosis of heparin-induced thrombocytopenia in two clinical settings. J Thromb Haemost 2006;4:759–65.

*Greifswald, Germany (GW): platelet count fall >50% or nadir 20–100 k/μL; Hamilton, Canada (but not GW): Platelet count fall >50% directly resulting from surgery counts as 1 point, rather than 2 points.

[†]GW: onset from days 5–14 (rather than days 5–10); platelet fall within 1 day (heparin exposure within 100 days).

[‡]GW: onset after day 14.

[§]Skin lesions at heparin injection sites.

[¶]Progression refers to objectively documented increase in thrombus size (usually, extension of deep vein thrombosis by ultrasonography); recurrence refers to newly formed thromboembolus in previously affected region (usually, new perfusion defects in a patient with previous pulmonary embolism).

[¶]In GW, "suspected thrombosis (not proven)" was not included as a criterion.

**Determination of whether the presence of another apparent cause of thrombocytopenia was "possible" or "definite" was at the discretion of the investigator.

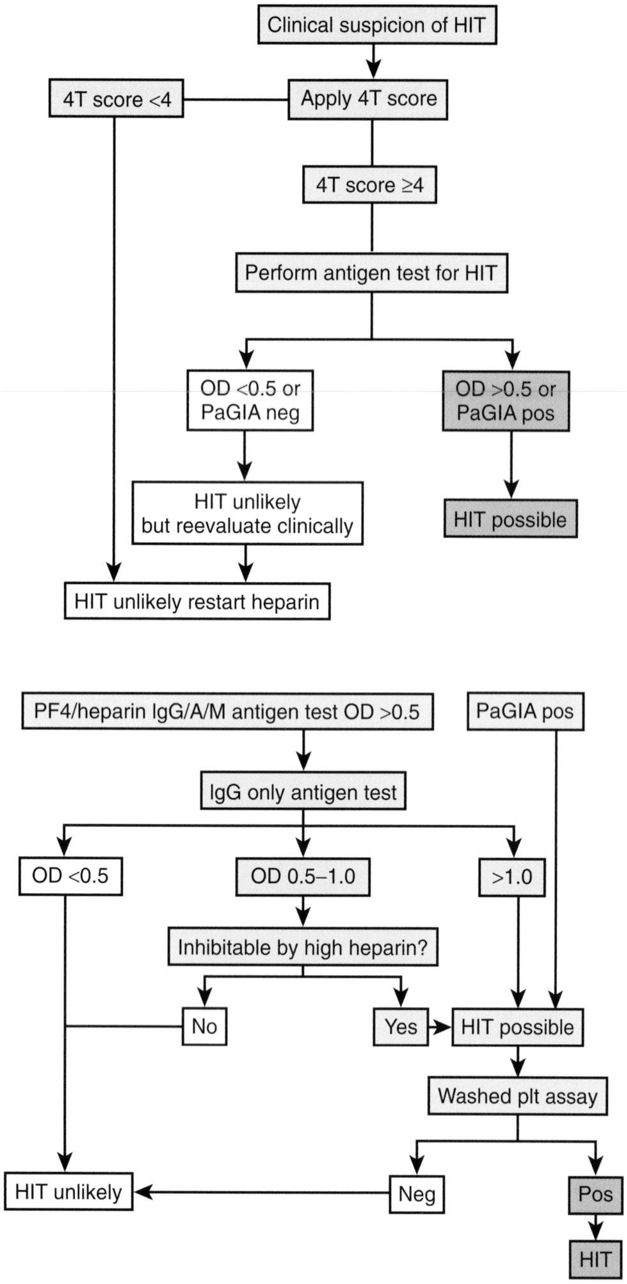

Figure 42-7 One example (among a variety of such efforts) of a diagnostic algorithm for heparin-induced thrombocytopenia (HIT):

1. Assess pretest probability for HIT (e.g., using the 4Ts). Patients with a low pretest probability (score ≤4) need no further testing, and heparin can be maintained.
2. If the enzyme immunoassay (EIA) or particle gel immunoassay (PaGIA) is negative, HIT is very unlikely, and heparin can be maintained. A positive result on a screening EIA or PaGIA indicates the presence of anti–platelet factor 4 (PF4)/heparin antibodies. If an immunoglobulin (Ig)G EIA is weakly positive (optical density [OD] <1.0), the antibodies are most likely non–platelet activating. A confirmatory step using high heparin should be performed; if reactivity is not inhibited, HIT is very unlikely, and heparin can be maintained.
3. An IgG EIA with OD >1.0 or positive PaGIA indicates increased risk for platelet-activating antibodies. These sera ideally should be assessed by a washed platelet activation assay. Demonstration of platelet-activating antibodies makes HIT very likely. A negative functional assay makes HIT unlikely, and heparin can be maintained/restarted.
4. Clinical reassessment should support final confirmation or exclusion of the diagnosis. However, it is a misconception to automatically retest patients whose EIA is negative (because EIA is positive even during the earliest phase of HIT). *(From Greinacher A, Althaus K, Krauel K, Selleng S. Heparin-induced thrombocytopenia. Hamostaseologie 2010;30:17–8, 20–8.)*

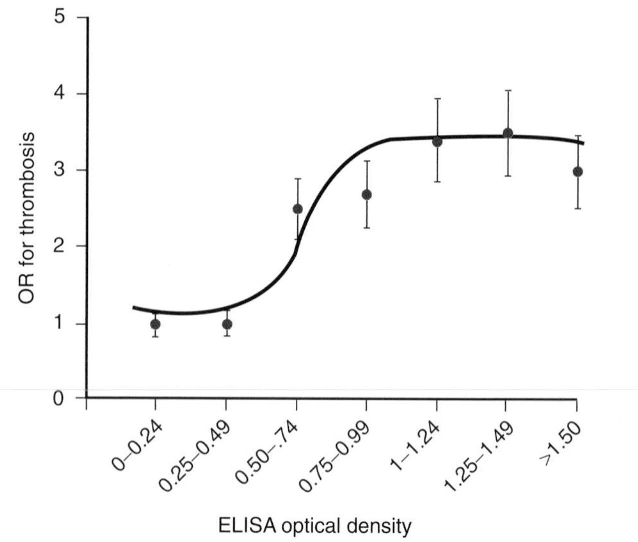

Figure 42-8 Relative risk of developing thrombosis related to quantitative results (mean ± SD) from an anti–platelet factor (PF4)/heparin enzyme-linked immunosorbent assay (ELISA) performed on 500 patients 6 days after coronary artery bypass graft surgery. *(From Mattioli AV, Bonetti L, Zennaro M, Ambrosio G, Mattioli G. Heparin/PF4 antibodies formation after heparin treatment: temporal aspects and long-term follow-up. Am Heart J 2009;157:589–95.)*

it is very high), then a functional test becomes pivotal to providing further laboratory support for the presence of HIT. Functional tests typically are much more demanding to perform but enjoy higher specificity, in addition to high sensitivity. A critical issue in the design of functional HIT tests is the choice of target upon which antibodies present in the patient's blood will act. Early tests employed platelet-rich plasma (PRP) of normal donors. However, as has been analyzed in considerable detail (Warkentin, 2001), washing of these target platelets so as to remove the accompanying plasma can greatly improve test performance. In North America, the gold standard of functional testing for HIT has been the serotonin release assay, in which washed platelets that have taken up exogenous serotonin are challenged with patient plasma in the presence of optimal heparin concentrations, and the amount of released serotonin is taken as the endpoint. Interestingly, in a number of European laboratories quite comparable results are obtained when aggregation in microtiter wells is employed as the functional endpoint using similarly washed platelets (Warkentin, 2001). An additional endpoint that has been explored is the formation of platelet microparticles, detectable by flow cytometric methods (Mullier, 2010).

A host of technical issues must be addressed in setting up any of these assays, including selection of platelet donors and whether or not to test these donors with respect to polymorphisms in Fc γRIIA. A number of studies have suggested that the use of serologic reagents in selectively detecting patient antibodies of the IgG (but not IgA or IgM) class may increase specificity for the diagnosis of HIT. However, concern that excluding IgA and IgM antibody detection may serve to decrease the sensitivity of HIT diagnostic testing still exists among a number of workers in the field. Because there appears to be a stoichiometric optimum for heparin interaction with PF4–glycosaminoglycan complexes, elimination of a proportion of false-positive reactions in some testing systems may be achieved by verifying that a (true positive) reaction is inhibited when the analysis is repeated in the presence of very strong heparin excess. Finally, it should be noted that in those instances where the target epitope is atypical (i.e., not the anticipated epitopes within platelet PF4), although the highly specific immunoassays may then fail to detect HIT-associated antibodies, this atypicality would not be expected to influence the functional assays. Correlation between ELISA heparin-platelet factor 4 (H-PF4) titers and the functional tests for HIT and heparin-induced platelet aggregation is greatest when H-PF4 antibodies are high (Javela, 2010). Given all of the complexities inherent in laboratory testing for HIT, it bears repeating that appropriateness of the clinical setting (most typically, falling platelet counts in a reasonable temporal relationship to heparin administration) remains of paramount importance with respect to evaluation of this disorder.

The laboratory sometimes will be called upon to perform HIT testing on presently asymptomatic individuals who have been positive for HIT at some time in the past. Given variability among patients in the rate of disappearance of detectable antibodies (Fig. 42-9), together with variability in their manifesting an anamnestic response upon reexposure to heparin, testing may be required before reexposure to heparin is considered, and of course subsequent to the initiation of such therapy if instituted.

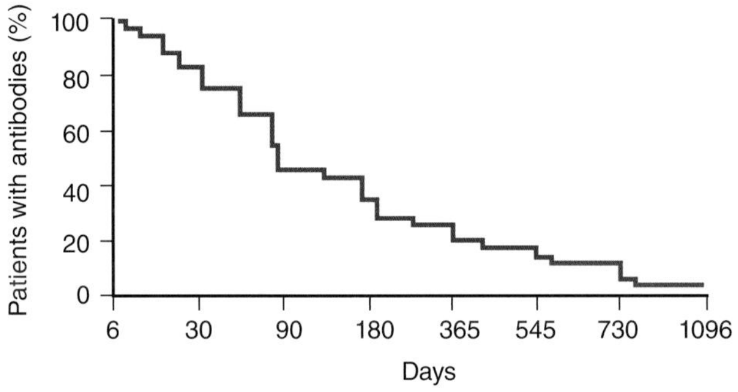

Figure 42-9 Rate of loss of demonstrable anti–platelet factor 4 (PF4)/heparin antibodies in a population of 131 serologically positive coronary artery bypass graft patients. The median time for persistence of measurable antibody was 90 days. *(From Mattioli AV, Bonetti L, Zennaro M, Ambrosio G, Mattioli G. Heparin/PF4 antibodies formation after heparin treatment: temporal aspects and long-term follow-up. Am Heart J 2009;157:589–95.)*

Guidelines to assist in monitoring of such patients have recently been endorsed by the American Society of Hematology, as presented in Figure 42-10. Although it has been demonstrated that most HIT-associated antibodies do not show an anamnestic reappearance if the patient is rechallenged with heparin more than 6 months following loss of detectable antibody, close laboratory monitoring of such rechallenged patients is critical. In the event that an anamnestic response does develop, the reemergence of antibody can be dramatic, requiring at least rapid detection of falling platelet counts, if not in fact more specific tests for HIT.

MONITORING OF HEPARIN THERAPY DURING PROCEDURES

Heparin is used extensively to prevent thrombi from forming during cardiac bypass surgery, as well as during a number of interventional vascular procedures. The ACT is frequently used to guide heparin therapy during the course of such procedures. In the ACT, glass beads, kaolin, or diatomaceous earth may be used to activate whole blood obtained from the patient. The ACT is used most frequently to monitor high levels of heparin (2–4 U/mL)—a range of heparin concentration beyond which the APTT does not perform optimally, and it is frequently used to monitor heparin reversal following injection of protamine. The importance of establishing local reference intervals using normal controls for ACT testing cannot be stressed too much. Only by this means can a testing

A. Cardiac and vascular surgery

Clinical picture	Laboratory profile		Recommended intraoperative anticoagulation*†
	Immunologic assay	Functional assay	
Remote HIT	Negative	Negative	1. Use UFH (Grade 1B)
Subacute HIT	Positive	Negative	1. Delay surgery, if possible, until immunologic assay becomes negative (Grade 1B) 2. If surgery cannot be delayed, use UFH (Grade 2C)
Acute HIT	Positive	Positive	1. Delay surgery, if possible, until functional and immunologic assays become negative (Grade 1B) 2. If surgery cannot be delayed, use bivalirudin (Grade 1B)

B. Cardiac catheterization/percutaneous coronary intervention

Clinical picture	Laboratory profile		Recommended intraprocedural anticoagulation†
	Immunologic assay	Functional assay	
Remote HIT	Negative	Negative	1. Use a non-heparin anticoagulant [bivalirudin (Grade 1B), argatroban (Grade 1C), lepirudin (Grade 1C), or danaparoid (Grade 1C)] 2. If a non-heparin anticoagulant is not available, use UFH
Subacute HIT	Positive	Negative	1. Use a non-heparin anticoagulant [bivalirudin (Grade 1B), argatroban (Grade 1C), lepirudin (Grade 1C), or danaparoid (Grade 1C)]
Acute HIT	Positive	Positive	

Figure 42-10 American Society of Hematology (ASH) practice guidelines for heparin reexposure in patients with a history of heparin-induced thrombocytopenia (HIT). HIT laboratory testing should be used to determine the safety of exposing a patient with a history of HIT to intraoperative heparin. *(From Cuker A, Crowther M. Quick reference: 2009 clinical practice guideline on the evaluation and management of heparin-induced thrombocytopenia. American Society of Hematology, 2009. Available from:* http://www.hematology.org/Practice/Guidelines/4678.aspx*)* *UFH,* Unfractionated heparin.
*If preoperative and postoperative anticoagulation is indicated, a non-heparin anticoagulant should be used. †American College of Chest Physicians Grading System: 1 = strong recommendation; 2 = weak recommendation; A = based on high quality evidence; B = based on moderate quality evidence; C = based on low quality evidence.

facility gain the experience necessary to monitor patients undergoing heparin therapy during procedures. For example, it is vital to obtain a baseline ACT value before heparinization is instituted and to realize that for occasional patients with a markedly prolonged baseline ACT (such as one who may have a lupus anticoagulant, or another who may have a severe contact factor deficiency), an alternative approach to monitoring should be considered—typically, an anti-Xa heparin assay. LMWHs have little effect on the ACT. However, the ACT may be considered in conjunction with monitoring of DTIs, as discussed in the following section (Rössig, 2010).

Direct Thrombin Inhibitors

Hirudin originally isolated from the salivary glands of leeches is available as a recombinant protein (Refludan, lepirudin). It forms an essentially irreversible complex with thrombin. Lepirudin has been used in patients with HIT. The half-life of lepirudin is between 90 and 120 minutes, and it is cleared by the kidneys. Anticoagulant activity has been monitored using the APTT, with a target range of 1.5–2.5 times baseline APTT (Call, 2004; Hirsch, 2008). However, in instances where a patient's baseline APTT is abnormal (e.g., in the presence of a lupus anticoagulant), monitoring by means of the APTT may be unreliable. One alternative to the APTT for monitoring DTIs is the ecarin clotting time (ECT), which uses the venom from *Echis carinatus*. The active enzyme of this venom is a metalloproteinase that converts prothrombin to meizothrombin—a reaction that is blocked by DTIs. A calibration curve for the ECT can be generated by directly spiking normal plasma with DTIs in vitro (Nowak, 2001; Kolde, 2004). The dilute thrombin time may also be used to monitor DTI therapy (Love, 2007). DTI may inhibit the PT/INR, and anticoagulant monitoring during the bridging transition between DTI and vitamin K antagonist therapy is accomplished by using a chromogenic assay for Factor X, or by discontinuing the DTI for several hours and then measuring the INR in patients after several days of vitamin K antagonist therapy (Hoppensteadt, 1997; Tobu, 2004; Walenga, 2004; Castellone, 2010).

A related DTI, bivalirudin, is a reversible, relatively short-acting molecule that has been approved for use in patients undergoing coronary angioplasty who have or are at risk for developing HIT (Merry, 2004; De Luca, 2009). It binds to the anion-binding exosite of thrombin.

Argatroban, a semisynthetic derivative of hirudin, is a short-acting reversible DTI that has also been approved for use in HIT. A rather wide window of 1.5–2.0 times baseline APTT has been suggested for the target therapeutic range of argatroban (Call, 2004). Alternative monitoring methods may help to narrow this range (Love, 2007). Argatroban is metabolized in the liver and can be used in patients with impaired renal function.

Dabigatran etexilate (see below) is the first oral anticoagulant in the direct thrombin inhibitor class to have received FDA approval in the U.S.

Clearly, DTIs are enjoying an increasing role in anticoagulation. At the present time, they are used primarily in patients with HIT. However, in the future, they may be anticipated to be used in a wider variety of clinical settings, particularly in patients for whom it has proven difficult to stabilize their anticoagulant intensity with more traditional agents (Weitz, 2010a).

New Oral Anticoagulants

Several newly developed oral anticoagulants have shown potential promise for their efficacy in preventing VTE and in treating VTE, for their role in stroke prevention with atrial fibrillation, and for their potential role in treating acute coronary syndrome (Weitz, 2010a, 2010b). The oral coagulation inhibitors include the DTI dabigatran etexilate and the Xa inhibitors rivaroxaban and apixaban (Turpie, 2009; Weitz, 2010b; Wittkowsky, 2010). These agents have relatively short half-lives of less than 15 hours, are significantly excreted by the kidney, and are irreversible; laboratory monitoring, although available, may not be required on a routine basis (Ng, 2009; Bounameaux, 2010; Mismetti, 2010). Dabigatran etexilate is actually a prodrug that requires activation to dabigatran. Rivaroxaban and apixaban are metabolized by CYP3A4, and drugs that inhibit or induce CYP3A4 may increase or decrease exposure to these drugs (Eikelboom, 2010; Wittkowsky, 2010).

Antiplatelet Therapy

Several classes of compounds are currently employed to diminish platelet functionality. These include aspirin, other cyclooxygenase inhibitors, adenosine diphosphate (ADP) receptor antagonists, and glycoprotein (GP) IIb/IIIa receptor antagonists. In contrast to treatment with oral anticoagulants or with heparin, antiplatelet therapy traditionally has not been as closely monitored in the laboratory. Increasingly, however, the laboratory is coming to play a greater role. Questions that can potentially be answered by laboratory testing include the following: (1) whether or not a patient's platelets are resistant to inhibition by a particular agent; (2) what dose of agent is required to achieve a desired intensity of inhibition; (3) when, following termination of therapy, platelet function has returned to an adequate level to subserve significant hemostatic challenges such as surgery; and (4) whether thrombocytopenia observed following antiplatelet therapy may reasonably be attributed to that therapy itself.

Certainly an agent that has enjoyed a long tenure in therapeutics is aspirin. As is widely known, aspirin irreversibly acetylates cyclooxygenase. In the case of the anucleate platelet, this effectively means that recovery from aspirin inhibition occurs only as platelets newly released from megakaryocytes enter the circulation. Although human platelets circulate in the blood for an average of 10 days, substantial normalization of platelet functional responsiveness occurs within 5–7 days following termination of aspirin therapy. This phenomenon may be due to the ability of thromboxane A_2, the active product from the platelet cyclooxygenase pathway of nonaspirinated platelets, to stimulate nearby platelets whose cyclooxygenase has been acetylated by aspirin. However, individual patient responses to therapeutic aspirin administration may vary (Mason, 2004; Sanderson, 2005). Because relative resistance to the platelet inhibitory effects of aspirin may imply the need for additional or alternative antiplatelet treatment in some clinical settings, the laboratory can play a useful role in measuring such resistance. Presently, two main approaches have been employed to assess platelet resistance to aspirin. Because platelets are the principal cell type to produce thromboxane, assay of this substance provides a measure of the activity of platelet cyclooxygenase. Because thromboxane A_2 undergoes conversion to thromboxane B_2 and thence to the more stable 11-dehydro-thromboxane B_2, plasma assay of this metabolite has been used as an indirect measure of platelet cyclooxygenase activity (Catella, 1986); subsequently, assay of urinary 11-dehydro-thromboxane B_2 was employed for this purpose (Eikelboom, 2002).

An alternative approach that more directly assesses actual platelet functionality is the measurement of platelet aggregation following stimulation of platelets in vitro by an agonist strongly dependent upon an intact cyclooxygenase pathway. Arachidonic acid and related compounds are frequently employed as agonists in such studies. Of great importance for the validation of such functional assays, if they are to be capable of identifying aspirin resistance, is very tight standardization of the testing procedure. Although this certainly may be accomplished by carefully performed platelet aggregometry on PRP (see Chapter 40), alternative methods have been developed to provide comparable information directly on anticoagulated whole blood. For example, the VerifyNow (Accumetrics, San Diego, Calif.) instrument permits optical platelet aggregation studies to be performed on a patient's whole blood. In this approach, fibrinogen-coated plastic beads impregnated with an infrared (IR) dye (i.e., a dye that absorbs light in the IR region of the electromagnetic spectrum) are added to citrated whole blood. Following addition of arachidonic acid, the fibrinogen-coated beads coaggregate with the platelets, presumably by virtue of the fibrinogen binding to the conformationally active forms of GPIIb/IIIa on stimulated platelets. Whereas absorbance by erythrocytes of light in the visible wavelength had previously precluded optical whole blood aggregometry, the introduction of IR techniques has permitted rapid quantitation of platelet aggregation (as increasing IR light transmittance) and of its inhibition by aspirin or other antiplatelet agents (Smith, 1999; Wang, 2003).

Whole blood or PRP aggregation studies have also proven helpful in defined clinical settings such as percutaneous transluminal coronary angioplasty (PTCA) for assessing the degree of residual platelet reactivity following inhibition of platelets by abciximab, eptifibatide, and other antagonists of the platelet GPIIb/IIIa complex (Hezard, 2000; Matzdorff, 2001). Detection of residual ADP purinergic receptors on the platelet surface following treatment by clopidogrel or other P2Y12 antagonists may be assessed in a similar manner (see later).

In addition to aggregometry, other methods may be employed to detect activation of the platelet by agonists, and consequently inhibition of that activation by antiplatelet therapies. Flow cytometry may be used for this purpose through the detection of markers of platelet activation. Translocation of P-selectin from the intracellular α-granule of the resting platelet to the extracellular membrane following sufficient platelet stimulation provides one such marker, although the relatively small number of P-selectin molecules detectable even on the fully activated platelet limits the dynamic range of this marker. Antibodies sensitive to conformational change in the GPIIb/IIIa molecule associated with platelet activation potentially offer a greater dynamic range of signal extending between fully nonactivated and fully activated platelets. Flow cytometric approaches have also been used to monitor residual functionality of the GPIIb/IIIa complex following treatment of patients with GPIIb/IIIa inhibitors (Hezard, 2000; Matzdorff, 2001), as well as to quantify platelet microparticles as an indicator of platelet activation (Craft, 2004).

Following the introduction of GPIIb/IIIa antagonists in PTCA and other invasive procedures, recognition that thrombocytopenia can complicate administration of this drug has been increasing (Abrams, 2004; Aster, 2009). In some instances, this fall in the platelet count appears to be due to an immediate interaction between drug and platelet, possibly caused by pre-formed drug-dependent antibodies (Aster, 2004). In other instances, the time course of the thrombocytopenia suggests the development of antibodies to the drug itself or to a neo-epitope formed by binding of the drug to its platelet target (Curtis, 2002, 2004; Nurden, 2004). Although definitively establishing such a drug-dependent cause by laboratory methods is difficult and at times may simply prove elusive, available methods currently employed for evaluation of such acquired thrombocytopenia include flow cytometry, monoclonal antibody-specific immobilization of platelet antigens, and related techniques.

Efforts to detect residual ADP purinergic P2Y12 receptors on the platelet surface following treatment by clopidogrel, prasugrel, or other P2Y12 receptor antagonists have arguably been more difficult still. The reasons for this difficulty are severalfold. First, the presence on the platelet surface of the additional P2Y1 class of ADP receptors that remain responsive to ADP following P2Y12 receptor antagonism complicates interpretation of residual responsiveness to ADP challenge in treated patients. Second, analysis of P2Y12 receptor antagonist therapy is almost universally undertaken in the setting of patient platelets that are being inhibited additionally by aspirin therapy. Third, it has become increasingly common for patients to be started on combined P2Y12 receptor antagonist and aspirin therapy very early in the course of their evaluation for possible acute coronary syndrome or other potentially catastrophic thrombotic disorders. Accordingly, there is no opportunity in such instances to establish a baseline platelet function study that might be used to assess reduction in responsiveness following initiation of P2Y12 receptor antagonist therapy. Rather than identifying a true reduction in responsiveness that can reliably be attributed to antiplatelet therapy, the laboratory will be able to provide only a snapshot of platelet responsiveness for the patient already under treatment.

Through comparison of response to ADP by the patient's platelets versus their responsiveness to other platelet agonists, derived estimates of the inhibition attributable to P2Y12 receptor antagonism have been proposed. As recently demonstrated, for levels of derived percent inhibition greater than ≈20%, the correspondence of these values to true percent reduction of posttreatment responses compared with pretreatment responses using the VerifyNow whole blood device (see earlier) (Fig. 42-11) appears reasonably good (Varenhorst, 2009). In addition to whole blood aggregation, assessments of responsiveness to ADP receptor antagonists may be made by traditional light transmittance aggregometry of patient PRP, arguably a gold standard for assessment of platelet function. Flow cytometric approaches have also been introduced that assess the phosphorylation of intracellular vasodilator-stimulated phosphoprotein—the degree of which reflects with some measure of specificity the downstream signaling following the binding of ADP to platelet P2Y12 receptors.

Efforts to sort out the relative merits of these different methods have been described in a number of recent publications (Alstrom, 2009; Gremmel, 2009; Varenhorst, 2009; Bidet, 2010; Bouman, 2010; Cuisset, 2010). Nevertheless, caution is still in order with respect to how much reliance can be placed upon current assays of platelet function to guide therapy. Lordkipanidze (2008) remarked at the conclusion of a double-blind study assessing four different methodologic approaches in 116 patients with coronary artery disease, "The assessment of platelet function inhibition by clopidogrel is highly test-specific. Decision to increase clopidogrel dosage may vary on the basis of the assay used, thus highlighting the need for unambiguous guidelines with respect to assay selection, as platelet function assays are not interchangeable. At present, platelet function testing evaluating clopidogrel efficacy cannot be recommended in routine clinical practice." Based on a study of 1069 patients on clopidogrel undergoing elective coronary stent implantation, caution was also expressed by Breet (2010), who concluded, "None of the tests provided accurate prognostic information to identify low-risk patients at higher risk of bleeding following stent implantation." Accordingly, it appears fair to say that the clinical usefulness of platelet function testing related to P2Y12 receptor inhibition to date has been only modest at best. It is important to note that limitations of available approaches must not be forgotten despite the understandably intense pressure from clinicians facing dosage decisions that carry the risk of increased thrombosis on the one hand, and increased bleeding on the other hand.

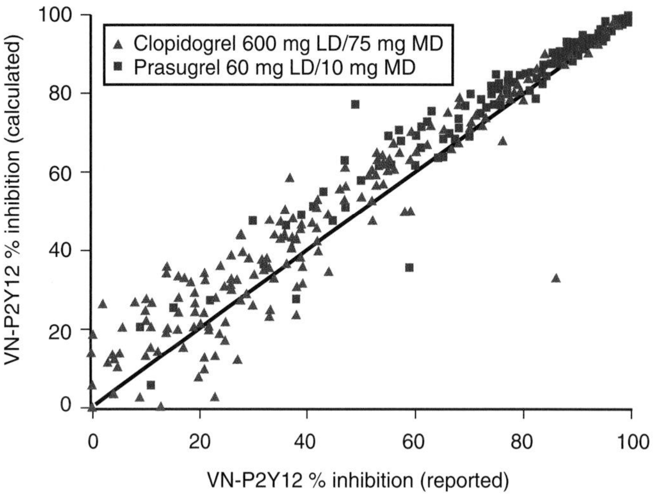

Figure 42-11 Association of "percent inhibition" reported by VerifyNow P2Y12 (x-axis) based solely on posttreatment measurement and calculated percent inhibition (y-axis) based on decrease in PRU (P2Y12 reaction units) posttreatment compared with pretreatment baseline PRU. Correlation coefficient (r) was calculated using Lin's concordance method. ■ represents prasugrel; ▲, clopidogrel; *filled line*, unity line. *(From Varenhorst C, James S, Erlinge D, et al. Assessment of P2Y(12) inhibition with the point-of-care device VerifyNow P2Y12 in patients treated with prasugrel or clopidogrel coadministered with aspirin. Am Heart J 2009;157:562.e1–9.)*

Analogous to the use of pharmacogenetics to guide oral anticoagulant therapy (see earlier), significant effort is being devoted to developing a role for assessing genotypic variations affecting the metabolism of P2Y12 inhibitors. Of particular note, clopidogrel is a prodrug that acquires its ability to antagonize P2Y12 receptors only after it has been transformed in vivo to active metabolite. The potential significance of this was spotlighted by a new warning label mandated for Plavix (clopidogrel) by the U.S. Food and Drug Administration (FDA) in March of 2010, accompanied by the following announcement on the FDA website, http://www.fda.gov/Drugs/DrugSafety/PostmarketDrugSafetyInformationforPatientsandProviders/ucm203888.htm.

> *"The liver enzyme CYP2C19 is primarily responsible for the formation of the active metabolite of Plavix. Pharmacokinetic and antiplatelet tests of the active metabolite of Plavix show that the drug levels and antiplatelet effects differ depending on the genotype of the CYP2C19 enzyme. The following represent the different alleles of CYP2C19 that make up a patient's genotype:*
> - *The CYP2C19*1 allele has fully functional metabolism of Plavix.*
> - *The CYP2C19*2 and *3 alleles have no functional metabolism of Plavix. These two alleles account for most of the reduced function alleles in patients of Caucasian (85%) and Asian (99%) descent classified as poor metabolizers.*
> - *The CYP2C19*4, *5, *6, *7, and *8 and other alleles may be associated with absent or reduced metabolism of Plavix but are less frequent than the CYP2C19*2 and *3 alleles.*
>
> *A patient with two loss-of-function alleles (as defined above) will have poor metabolizer status."*

Efforts to provide genotyping as referenced by the FDA announcement accordingly have intensified in the clinical laboratory arena, in an effort to keep pace with these rapidly moving developments. Additionally, as newer P2Y12 antagonists become available, attention must be paid increasingly to the pharmacogenomics of these compounds as well. Within the class of thienopyridines, for example, significant differences may be seen in the effectiveness of clopidogrel and of prasrugel, depending on CYP2C19 alleles. The extent to which genotyping of individual patients actually contributes to their clinical outcome continues to be a subject of intense investigation (Mega, 2009; Shuldiner, 2009; Momary, 2010; Sibbing, 2010). Study of such genotypes may prove of increasing use for managing drug–drug interactions, such as the effect of proton pump inhibitors on clopidogrel efficacy in inhibiting platelet reactivity (Laine, 2010).

APPENDIX: CLINICAL AND LABORATORY STANDARDS INSTITUTE PREANALYTIC GUIDELINES (CLSI, 2008)

1. Blood should be collected directly into the tube containing anticoagulant. Small syringes may be used and blood may be drawn through a vascular access device if it is flushed with saline and six dead space volumes of the vascular access device are discarded.
2. In a direct draw, the PT and APTT are not affected if the first tube drawn is tested. Collection of blood through lines that have been flushed with heparin is to be avoided.
3. The blood should be placed into an anticoagulated tube within 1 minute and mixed well, inverting at least 4 times. The tube should not be vigorously shaken.
4. The anticoagulant should be 3.2% sodium trisodium citrate. The ratio should be 9 parts blood and 1 part citrate.
5. Inadequately filled or clotted specimens should be discarded.
6. The specimen should be centrifuged and should be platelet-poor, which is defined as less than 20×10^9/L.
7. Hemolyzed specimens are discarded.
8. Grossly icteric, lipemic or slightly hemolyzed specimens should be analyzed using a mechanical method to detect clotting or with an instrument with a wavelength outside of the interfering substances absorption wavelength.

STORAGE OF SPECIMENS

- Specimens for PT determinations can be kept at 18°–24° C either on separated plasma or spun cells and testing should be performed within 24 hours. Cold activation of factor VII may occur at 2°–4° C.
- Routine unheparinized specimens can be kept centrifuged or uncentrifuged in an unopened tube on the cells at 18°–24° C and tested within 4 hours. Specimens with UFH should be centrifuged within 1 hour of collection, and plasma should be tested within 4 hours.
- If testing is not done within 24 hours for the PT or within 4 hours for the APTT, the plasma should be removed and frozen at −20° C and tested within 2 weeks, or stored at −70° C and tested within 4 weeks. These frozen samples should be rapidly thawed at 37° C with gentle mixing and assayed immediately. They may be kept at 4° C and assayed within 4 hours.

QUALITY CONTROL

- The quality control program should have a peer group for comparison. The laboratory should participate in a proficiency survey. Samples for this survey should be analyzed in the same manner as patient plasma samples.

SELECTED REFERENCES

Ansell J, Hirsh J, Poller L, et al. The pharmacology and management of the vitamin K antagonists: the Seventh ACCP Conference on Antithrombotic and Thrombolytic Therapy. Chest 2004;126(3 suppl): 204S–33S.

Excellent comprehensive review of oral anticoagulant therapy.

Aster RH, Curtis BR, Bougie DW. Thrombocytopenia resulting from sensitivity to GPIIb-IIIa inhibitors. Semin Thromb Hemost 2004;30:569–77.

Important review of thrombocytopenia secondary to antiplatelet therapy.

Cuisset T, Frere C, Poyet R, et al. Clopidogrel response: head-to-head comparison of different platelet assays to identify clopidogrel nonresponder patients after coronary stenting. Arch Cardiovasc Dis 2010;103: 39–45.

Assessment of methods for monitoring clopidogrel.

Cuker A, Ptashkin B, Konkle BA, et al. Interlaboratory agreement in the monitoring of unfractionated heparin using the anti-factor Xa-correlated activated partial thromboplastin time. J Thromb Haemost 2009;7:80–6.

Critical assessment of methods for monitoring heparin.

Gage BF, Eby C, Johnson JA, et al. Use of pharmacogenetic and clinical factors to predict the therapeutic dose of warfarin. Clin Pharmacol Ther 2008;84: 326–31.

Pharmacogenomics of warfarin.

Kelton JG, Warkentin TE. Heparin-induced thrombocytopenia: a historical perspective. Blood 2008;112: 2607–16.

Review of heparin-induced thrombocytopenia.

Mega JL, Close SL, Wiviott SD, et al. Cytochrome p-450 polymorphisms and response to clopidogrel. N Engl J Med 2009;360:354–62.

Pharmacogenomics of clopidogrel.

Varenhorst C, James S, Erlinge D, et al. Assessment of P2Y(12) inhibition with the point-of-care device VerifyNow P2Y12 in patients treated with prasugrel or clopidogrel coadministered with aspirin. Am Heart J 2009;157:562.e1–562.e9.

Assessment of methods for monitoring P2Y12 antagonist therapies.

REFERENCES

Access the complete reference list online at http://www.expertconsult.com

PART 6

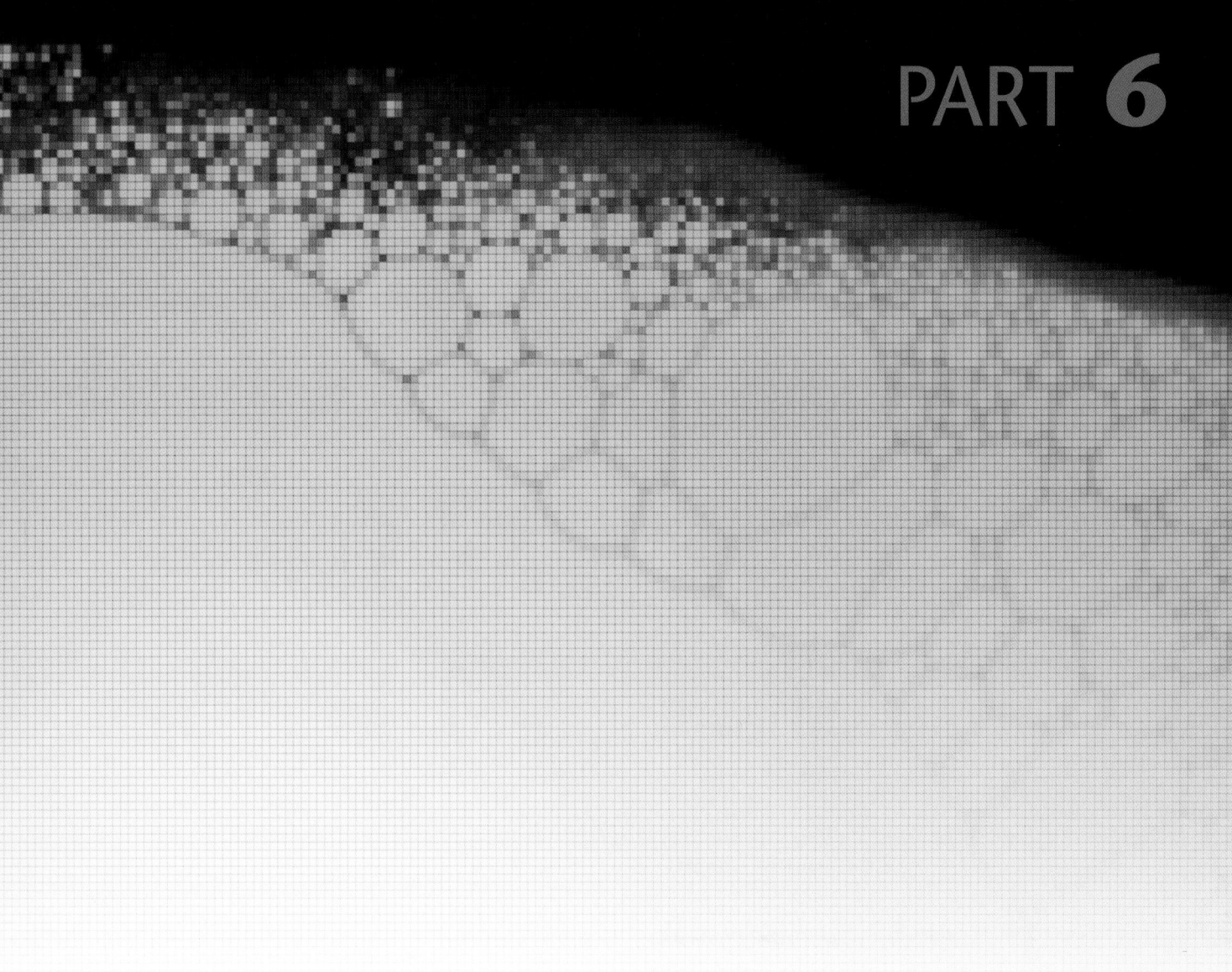

Immunology and Immunopathology

EDITED BY H. Davis Massey
Richard A. McPherson

CHAPTER 43

OVERVIEW OF THE IMMUNE SYSTEM AND IMMUNOLOGIC DISORDERS

Richard A. McPherson, H. Davis Massey

PART 6

KEY POINTS

- The immune system consists of cellular and humoral components that defend the body against invading microorganisms. Deficiency of individual factors of the immune system can leave an individual susceptible to different infections.
- The lymphoid cells of the immune system are composed of T cells, which act directly against foreign antigens, and B cells, which synthesize immunoglobulins that combine with foreign antigens. Antigen-presenting cells are crucial for cell-to-cell communication during the direction of an immune response.
- The mechanisms by which lymphocytes differentiate into T cells and B cells involve rearrangement of genes for the T cell antigen receptor and of genes for immunoglobulins, respectively.
- Lymphocytes from patient specimens are characterized by detection of surface proteins, termed cluster of differentiation markers, which designate their subset and function.
- Additional cellular elements are natural killer lymphocytes plus neutrophils, eosinophils, and the effectors of immunoglobulin (Ig) E-mediated hypersensitivity—basophils and mast cells.
- In addition to immunoglobulins or antibodies, humoral elements include a cascading series of proteins in the complement system that result in enzymatic destruction of foreign cells and recruitment of cellular infiltrates by cytokine actions.
- Histocompatibility antigens play a major role in antigen presentation to T cells and form the immunologic identity of an individual, which is important in rejection of organ transplants.
- Immunologic injury can occur as the result of excessive response to specific antigenic exposures, such as from allergies or from circulating immune complexes.
- Autoimmune disease results when the mechanisms for maintaining immunologic tolerance to self-(auto)antigens fail, resulting in the formation of various autoantibodies plus activation of the cellular immune system against the patient's own tissues.
- Laboratory measurements of the immune system involve relatively simple techniques for counting lymphocytes and their subsets, as well as for quantifying overall concentrations of immunoglobulins and complement proteins. More complex methods such as detection of gene rearrangements, autoantibody characterization, and allergen reactivity with IgE are useful for diagnosing various disorders of the immune system.
- Therapeutic approaches to disorders of the immune system include stimulation or replacement of deficient components and reduction or removal of other factors that are abnormal or are present in excess.

The immune system is structured to recognize, respond to, and destroy a wide variety of invading organisms such as bacteria, viruses, fungi, and parasites that otherwise would be capable of promoting infection that is harmful to the body. Discovery of components of the immune system has very often followed investigation of serious infections and the specific reactions that the body uses to combat pathogenic organisms. In general, this immunologic function can be summarized as searching for foreign (or nonself) antigens that do not belong in the body and then destroying them. In this process, the immune system also maintains surveillance over the appearance of new or foreign antigens on tumor cells and attempts to destroy them while leaving unharmed the normal (or self) antigens on healthy cells. Disease states may arise as a result of various aspects of immunologic function going awry, as in hypersensitivity reactions, autoimmune disease, and various immunodeficiency disorders. When functioning properly, the immune system is responsible for rejection of allogeneic organ/tissue transplants and graft-versus-host disease; the quest for tolerance in transplantation continues. This overview highlights components of the immune system and their functions, along with some of the significant clinical disorders of immunity.

LYMPHOID CELLS

The lymphoid cells of the body reside in the lymph nodes, the spleen, the mucosal surfaces, and the circulation. They derive from multipotential hematopoietic stem cells, with their production moving progressively from the yolk sac in the embryo to the liver in the fetus, and finally to the bone marrow in the infant through adult ages (Weissman, 1994). The various lymphoid cells are conveniently identified by the presence of unique protein markers on their surfaces that endow those cells with particular functions.

T LYMPHOCYTES

T lymphocytes undergo differentiation in the thymus. After originating in the bone marrow, prothymocytes pass from the cortex to the medulla of the thymus, during which time they undergo maturation. This process involves a selection process such that self-reactive thymocytes are eliminated, while thymocytes that can recognize antigens through interactions with molecules of the major histocompatibility complex (MHC) are retained (Nossal, 1994; von Boehmer, 1994). During maturation, they undergo genetic programming in which the gene for the T cell antigen receptor (TCR) is rearranged to produce protein receptors that are invariant in their antigen specificity for the life span of that T lymphocyte, as well as for all its descendent cells. T lymphocytes account for about 60%–70% of all lymphocytes in the blood; they are also found in paracortical areas of lymph nodes and within periarteriolar lymphoid sheaths in the spleen.

A majority (>95%) of T lymphocytes have antigen receptors made of α- and β-subunits linked with disulfide bonds to form a molecular heterodimer that resides on the outer membrane of the cell in association with the CD3 molecular complex (CD3 is a pan–T cell marker). The α- and β-subunit TCR proteins have variable, joining, and constant regions (α also contains a diversity region), with corresponding encoding regions in the *TCR* gene that undergo rearrangement, resulting in high specificity binding for a particular antigen. The CD3 proteins assist transduction of the signal to the interior of the cell when an antigen binds to the TCR on the lymphocyte surface (Janeway, 1994; Weiss, 1994). A small percentage of T lymphocytes have a TCR composed of γ- and δ-subunits that similarly interact with CD3; these cells are generally found at mucosal surfaces of the gastrointestinal and respiratory tracts. T cell proliferations may be characterized as neoplastic (clonal) or benign (polyclonal), according to whether their DNA shows predominantly a single form of *TCR* gene rearrangement or a complete spectrum of such rearrangements, as normally occurs in a heterogeneous lymphocyte population.

Examination of T lymphocytes by flow cytometry focuses on a variety of surface markers. CD4 is found on about 60% of $CD3^+$ cells; these are helper/inducer T cells that direct the functions of other cells of the immune system by secreting cytokines that stimulate various functions. Two distinct subpopulations of $CD4^+$ helper cells have been identified: Th1, which secrete interleukin (IL)-2 and interferon (IFN)-γ; and Th2, which secrete IL-4 and IL-5. Th1 cells facilitate macrophage activation delayed-type hypersensitivity and the production of antibodies with opsonizing action; Th2 cells direct synthesis of other antibodies such as IgE and activate eosinophils. The marker CD8 is found on about 30% of T cells (thus the normal ratio of $CD4^+$ to $CD8^+$ cells in the blood is typically 2 : 1). These $CD8^+$ T cells exhibit cytotoxicity and suppressor activity in the immune response.

The mechanism of antigen recognition is different between $CD4^+$ and $CD8^+$ subsets of T lymphocytes. CD4 molecules bind to the MHC class II molecules on antigen-presenting cells, whereas CD8 molecules interact with MHC class I molecules. Accordingly, $CD4^+$ T cells recognize antigens only in the context of MHC class II antigens, and $CD8^+$ T cells recognize them only through MHC class I antigens.

B LYMPHOCYTES

B lymphocytes make up roughly 10%–20% of peripheral lymphocytes in the blood; they also are found in the bone marrow, lymph nodes, spleen, and other lymphoid tissues. In the spleen and lymph nodes, they aggregate into lymphoid follicles. Differentiation of B lymphocytes occurs in the bone marrow, where both positive selection and negative selection take place, as well as at peripheral locations. Antigenic stimulation of B cells leads to the formation of plasma cells that secrete immunoglobulins—the basis of specificity in humoral immunity. The B cell antigen receptor complex uses surface IgM as the antigen-binding component. The antigen specificity of immunoglobulins derives from a rearrangement process in which both heavy and light chain genes are realigned. The heavy chain has variable, diversity, joining, and constant regions, whereas the light chain gene has variable, joining, and constant regions. Maturation of an antibody response entails switching from IgM to another heavy chain type (usually IgG) as the result of further gene rearrangement, although the light chain type remains fixed (Corcoran, 2005).

B cells have on their surfaces receptors for complement (CD21, which is also the receptor for Epstein-Barr virus [EBV] and thus makes these cells susceptible to EBV infection) and for the Fc region of immunoglobulins; they have CD19 and CD20, which are frequently used for immunologic identification of B cells.

ANTIGEN-PRESENTING CELLS

Macrophages function as mononuclear phagocytes in inflammation; they also process ingested antigens and present them to immune effector cells in association with MHC molecules on their membranes (Fig. 43-1). T cells are not activated by soluble antigens, and so presentation of antigens in this manner is necessary for T cell stimulation and induction of cell-mediated immunity (Germain, 1994; Trombetta, 2005). Macrophages also secrete cytokines such as IL-1 for modulation of inflammatory processes; they can directly lyse tumor cells in their role of immunosurveillance, and they are effector cells for some types of cell-mediated immunity (e.g., delayed hypersensitivity).

Dendritic cells (found in lymphoid tissues and in interstitial regions of other organs) and Langerhans cells (found in the epidermis) have extensive dendritic cytoplasmic processes that are rich in MHC class II molecules. Consequently, they are very efficient at presenting antigens (although they probably are not phagocytic) and are considered to be extremely important in that task within the entire immune system (Park, 2005).

NATURAL KILLER CELLS

Natural killer (NK) cells constitute 10%–15% of lymphocytes in the peripheral blood. They are neither T cells nor B cells and were formerly called **null cells.** NK cells have the function of lysing other cells without prior sensitization. They can attack tumor cells, cells infected with viruses, and others as well; consequently, they form the initial defense against aberrant cells. NK cells are characterized by the surface markers CD16 and CD56, which are commonly used for their identification. CD16 is the Fc receptor for IgG; hence NK cells are able to lyse selectively those cells that are coated with antibodies (antibody-dependent cell-mediated cytotoxicity, which is important in some hypersensitivity reactions). NK cells also secrete cytokines such as IFN-γ. It is interesting to note that NK cells are recognizable on examination of standard stained blood smears as large granular lymphocytes (Kronenberg, 2005).

NONLYMPHOID CELLS

These cells are not genetically programmed to recognize specific antigens or to interact with lymphoid cells in the induction of an immune response. Instead, they are effectors of immune reactions that are triggered by various factors.

NEUTROPHILS AND EOSINOPHILS

Neutrophils are drawn to regions of inflammation by chemoattractants such as IL-8; they then release from their granules toxic substances and enzymes that digest cellular structures indiscriminately; neutrophils also ingest cellular debris, as do eosinophils, and remove it from tissue sites.

BASOPHILS AND MAST CELLS

Basophils (and their counterparts in tissues, the mast cells) have on their surfaces high-affinity Fc receptors that bind circulating IgE. Uptake of IgE onto the membranes of basophils apparently is not antigen dependent; instead, it is driven by mass action between the amount of total IgE and the available basophils. When the antigen (or allergen) comes into contact with basophil surface-bound IgE that recognizes it, those basophils become activated and release substances such as histamine, which mediate some hypersensitivity reactions. Thus, basophil specificity is directed by the particular IgE that is bound to its surface from the blood; theoretically, a basophil could have multiple different IgE molecules on its surface and so could react with many different allergens.

HUMORAL FACTORS

IMMUNOGLOBULINS

Antibody molecules can be bound to B cell surfaces for stimulation of further immunoglobulin secretion; they also circulate in the blood and appear at mucosal surfaces of the respiratory and gastrointestinal tracts, where they are likely to come into contact with potentially pathogenic microorganisms. The major immunoglobulins in the blood are IgM, IgG, and IgA; these antibodies presumably arise following exposure to a multitude of foreign antigens and may remain for years with continued secretion to replace molecules that are lost through normal clearance of proteins from the circulation. At mucosal surfaces, the primary type of antibody is dimeric IgA, which is secreted at that site (Fagarasan, 2004) (see Chapter 46). The other immunoglobulins are IgD (which resides on B cell surfaces, where it may be involved in immune signal transduction but does not achieve substantial concentrations as free molecules in the blood) and IgE

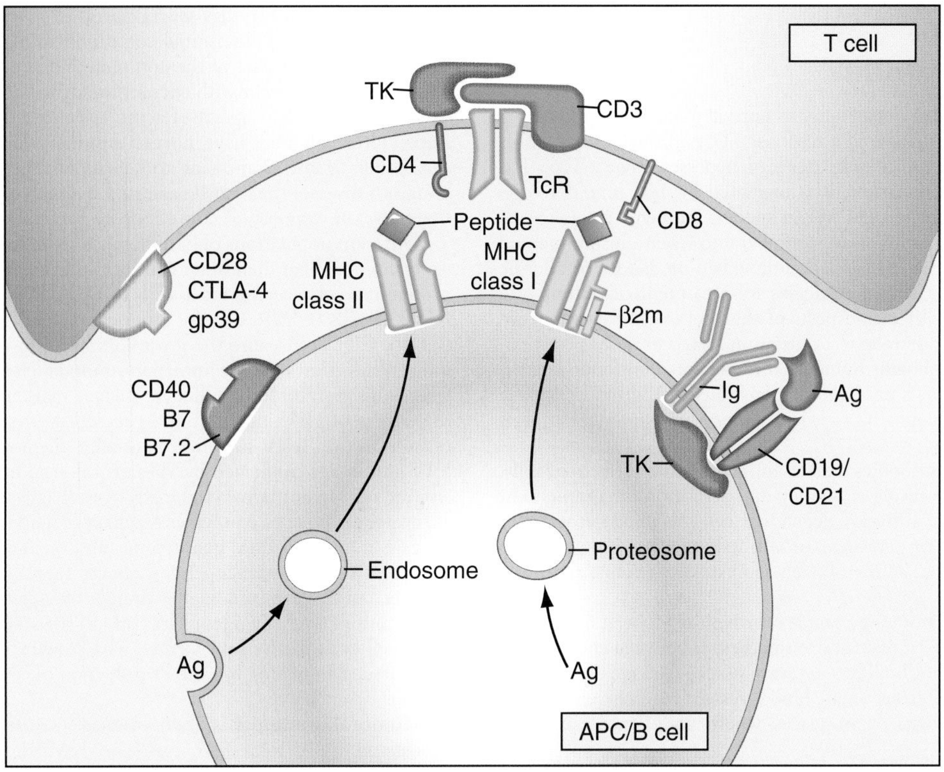

Figure 43-1 Cellular interactions in the immune system. Antigen-presenting cells (APCs) process external or internal antigens (Ag) and present antigen peptide fragments, in association with a major histocompatibility complex (MHC) molecule, to T cells. On the T cell, a specific antigen receptor (TcR), along with the co-receptor CD4 or CD8 molecule, recognizes the antigen–MHC complex. Cellular activation proceeds through the CD3 complex and activation of tyrosine kinases (TKs). The B cell receptor is composed of membrane-bound immunoglobulin (Ig) complexed to associated membrane proteins, and the CD19/21 coreceptor. On antigen recognition, cellular TKs are also activated. Co-stimulatory activation of T cells or B cells is provided by cellular receptors binding their ligands (the ligand B7 or B7.2 for T cell co-stimulation through CD28 and CTLA-4 molecules, and the gp39 ligand for the B cell CD40 molecule). *(Redrawn with permission from Paul W, Seder R. Lymphocytic responses and cytokines. Cell 1994;76:229; and Weiss A, Littman D. Signal transduction by lymphocyte antigen receptors. Cell 1994;76:263.)*

(which functions by binding to surfaces of basophils and stimulates the release of vasoactive substances from those cells in the presence of specific allergens).

Immunoglobulins in the blood function by attaching to antigens on the surfaces of foreign cells, bacteria, viruses, and the like, and by facilitating their destruction through nonspecific effectors such as complement and NK cell activation. Disease monitoring by immunoglobulin testing includes qualitative analysis for clonal versus polyclonal detection (e.g., for diagnosis of multiple myeloma) and quantitative analyses both for overall concentrations of IgM, IgG, and IgA (to detect possible selective or combined deficiencies or overproduction of immunoglobulin classes) and for titers of specific antibodies against individual antigens (e.g., isohemagglutinins, *Pneumococcus*, *Haemophilus*, tetanus, diphtheria).

COMPLEMENT

This set of interacting proteins has the role of enzymatically destroying targets (e.g., cells, bacteria) to which they have been directed by antibodies or through other means (see Chapter 47). Measurements of complement components have two major uses in clinical diagnosis: to detect congenital deficiencies (which are relatively rare) that may predispose to certain disorders such as infection or progression to autoimmune disease, and to detect acquired complement level reductions that reflect current activity of systemic autoimmune diseases such as systemic lupus erythematosus (Wen, 2004).

CYTOKINES

These soluble substances are the means by which cellular immune responses are regulated; they are short-acting mediators that are elaborated by some cells and diffuse to other cells, where they act (Leonard, 2003). Many cytokines are pleiotropic in that they can act on different cell types. They can act in an endocrine manner by stimulating cells at a distance, they can act on cells in their immediate vicinity (paracrine), and they can stimulate the same cells that secreted them (autocrine). The specific actions of cytokines include hematopoiesis through colony-stimulating factors that induce granulocyte and macrophage production, natural immune responses (through IL-1, tumor necrosis factor [TNF]-α, interferons, and IL-8), stimulation of lymphocyte growth and activation (through IL-2 and others), and activation of nonspecific inflammatory cells (see Chapter 47). Cytokines are still being discovered as more details emerge regarding cell-to-cell communication.

Clinical use of cytokines includes both suppression of the immune response in allogeneic organ transplantation by drugs such as cyclosporine, which blocks production of IL-2, and enhancement of the immune response in therapies against cancer or infection. These latter treatments are largely experimental, although it has been shown that pretreatment with antibodies against TNF-α can prevent deleterious Jarisch-Herxheimer reactions resulting from antibiotic treatment of *Borrelia recurrentis* infection in sheep (Fekade, 1996). This model very probably presages a host of new therapies by which immune responses will be selectively enhanced or suppressed according to particular clinical needs.

HISTOCOMPATIBILITY ANTIGENS

The MHC (also called the human leukocyte antigen [HLA] complex) is encoded on human chromosome 6 and includes class I molecules (HLA A, B, and C), class II molecules (HLA DP, DQ, and DR), and the intervening class III molecules of some complement components and TNF-α and -β (see Chapter 48). The functions of class I and class II antigens have already been discussed briefly in terms of how they participate in antigen presentation to T cells. These antigens were discovered and their highly polymorphic natures were described in studies of immune tolerance and rejection of transplanted allogeneic organs. Consequently, one of the most important clinical uses of HLA typing involves matching potential organ or tissue donors with recipients who are in need of a transplant. Another significant clinical application is seen in the typing of affected patients and their family members to establish their risk of developing some diseases that are associated with particular HLA types (e.g., ankylosing spondylitis with HLA B27) (see Chapter 49). Still another use of HLA typing involves providing matched platelets for patients who have become refractory to platelet transfusions as the result of HLA antibody formation after exposure to multiple donors (e.g., following transfusion support for chemotherapy or hematopoietic progenitor cell transplantation) (see Chapter 38).

PART 6

Mechanisms of Immunologic Injury

Immunologic responses can cause injury to normal tissues and to invading organisms that may have triggered a response. These injurious responses are conveniently classified into four types of hypersensitivity. Type I is anaphylactic or allergic in nature; it is mediated by IgE bound to the surface of basophils and mast cells. When specific antigens (or allergens) bind to surface IgE, the basophils are stimulated to release histamine and other vasoactive substances that are the immediate mediators of allergic reactions (Kemp, 2002). Clinical strategies for treatment of asthma and allergies have addressed different aspects of this sequence of events from counteracting the effects or release of histamine back to desensitization. Successful use of a recombinant humanized monoclonal antibody against IgE to treat such individuals has been demonstrated (Milgrom, 1999); in the future, this therapy could be based in part on measurement of IgE concentrations in serum.

Type II occurs when antibodies bind to antigens on the surfaces of cells; damage may occur as the result of binding and activation of complement (e.g., immune hemolysis), antibody-dependent cell-mediated cytotoxicity (e.g., lysis of tumor cells or parasites), or antibody-mediated interference with cellular functions (e.g., autoantibodies against acetylcholine receptors in myasthenia gravis).

Type III results from immune complex formation between exogenous antigens such as bacteria or viruses and antibodies, or between endogenous autoantigens and autoantibodies. Typical tissue damage occurs in organs that contain numerous small blood vessels wherein circulating immune complexes deposit, or in places where endogenous antigens naturally occur.

Type IV is cell-mediated or delayed hypersensitivity, which depends on functioning $CD4^+$ T cells or other cytotoxicity from $CD8^+$ T cells. Type IV is the basis of the immune reaction to viruses, fungi, protozoa, and parasites, and also to intracellular microbes such as mycobacteria. Patients with acquired immunodeficiency syndrome are susceptible to infection with these and other opportunistic agents when they lose $CD4^+$ T cells.

Laboratory Applications of Immunologic Assessment

Examinations of the immune system for evaluation of potential deficiencies or disorders are listed in Table 43-1.

Cellular immunity has several levels of investigation, beginning with leukocyte count and differential commonly available on automated hematology analyzers as part of the complete blood cell count. Deficiencies of neutrophils often occur with chemotherapy for malignancy, whereas elevation of neutrophils is a sign of acute infection, particularly with bacteria. Rare individuals may have normal numbers of neutrophils but may be susceptible to infection owing to defects of function (e.g., chronic granulomatous disease) that can be assessed by neutrophil activation (by oxidative burst) in response to stimuli, or by bacterial killing assays.

Different populations of lymphocytes are enumerated by flow cytometric techniques that quantitate cells according to the expression of surface protein markers specific for T cells (CD2, CD3), subsets of T cells (CD4, CD8), B cells (CD19, CD20), monocytes (CD14), and natural killer cells (CD16, CD56). Because the most common cause of lymphocyte disorder today is infection with the human immunodeficiency virus (HIV), the most frequently monitored lymphocyte surface markers are CD4 and CD8, for the effects of HIV infection and prediction of susceptibility to opportunistic infection. HIV infection is usually diagnosed by detection of anti-HIV antibodies confirmed by Western blot; monitoring of HIV infection also includes quantitative viral loads by molecular diagnostic methods such as reverse transcriptase polymerase chain reaction, and use of antiretroviral drugs is guided by HIV genotyping (and on rare occasion by phenotype testing of drug resistance). Lymphocyte function is not often measured directly, but this can be done by stimulation assays that look at lymphocyte proliferation (e.g., by incorporation of tritiated thymidine into DNA) or by cell cycle analysis performed with flow cytometry after stimulation. Of course, skin testing is a direct reflection of T cell response to antigens in vivo.

Humoral immunity is often assessed by quantitative immunoglobulin measurements of total IgG, IgA, and IgM; deficiency of one or more immunoglobulin classes can lead to increased susceptibility to infection. Measurement of IgG subclasses can also be useful in this type of evaluation. Serum protein electrophoresis and immunofixation electrophoresis provide additional information regarding the clonality of immunoglobulins. A monoclonal band of immunoglobulins indicates a clonal population of B cells or plasma cells that have escaped regulation and might result in a plasma cell dyscrasia such as multiple myeloma. In contrast, a polyclonal distribution of immunoglobulins is generally taken to indicate a reactive process of an otherwise normal immune system.

Direct measurement of immunoglobulin function is done by evaluating the titers of antibodies against specific antigens. The presence of isohemagglutinins against ABO blood group antigens is conveniently examined to detect anti-A and anti-B antibodies in persons who lack those blood

TABLE 43-1
Domains of Immunology Testing

Cellular Immunity • Complete blood count and differential • Lymphocyte enumeration (CD2, CD3, CD4, CD8, CD19, CD20, CD56) for T cells, B cells, NK cells • HIV antibodies/viral load/genotype • Skin testing for anergy • Lymphocyte function/activation • Neutrophil activation (oxidative burst) • Lymphocyte adhesion defect (CD11a, CD11b, CD11c, CD18) Humoral Immunity • Quantitative immunoglobulins (IgG, IgA, IgM) • IgG subclasses • Immunoglobulin function/stimulation (protein antigens: tetanus, diphtheria; carbohydrate antigens: *Pneumococcus, Haemophilus*); ABO blood group isohemagglutinins Complement • C3, C4 for consumption • Screening for deficiency: CH50 • Confirming deficiency: C1-C9 • C4d deposition • Circulating immune complexes	Cytokines • Interleukins • Interferons • Tumor necrosis factors Human Leukocyte Antigens (HLAs) • HLA antibodies for matching organs and bone marrow in allogeneic transplants • Identity testing • HLA genotyping (high resolution) • HLA typing for disease association (HLA-B27) Autoimmune Diseases • Systemic rheumatic diseases: Antinuclear antibodies; anti-dsDNA, anti-Sm, anti-RNP, anti-SSA, anti-SSB, anti-Scl70, anticardiolipin, anti-CCP • Organ-specific diseases: Antithyroid, anti–parietal cell, antiendomysial, antiadrenal, antiskin, antimitochondria, anti–smooth muscle • Vasculitis: Cryoglobulins (RF), c-ANCA, p-ANCA Allergy/Hypersensitivity/Asthma • Total IgE • Allergen-specific IgE: Foods, pollens, animals, insects, mold • Skin tests for allergy

c-ANCA, Classical antineutrophil cytoplasmic antibodies; *HIV,* human immunodeficiency virus; *NK,* natural killer; *p-ANCA,* protoplasmic-staining antineutrophil cytoplasmic antibodies; *RF,* rheumatoid factor.

groups. Common immunizations result in the presence of detectable antibodies against the protein antigens of diphtheria and the tetanus toxoid, and against the carbohydrate antigens of *Pneumococcus* and *Haemophilus*. Measurements of antibodies against these antigens are standard procedures for evaluation of immunodeficiencies; if they are lacking, reimmunization can be done to elicit evidence of an immune response.

The **complement system** is most frequently examined by measurement of C3 and C4 components to look for depressions that suggest consumption through activation. Although circulating immune complexes (CICs) are the presumptive cause of decreased C3 and C4 concentrations, CICs are rarely measured directly; however, deposition of CICs in tissues can be detected by immunofluorescent staining for immunoglobulin and C3 or C4d. Hereditary deficiencies of individual complement components are screened for by the CH50 test, which traditionally has used antibody-coated horse erythrocytes in a hemolysis assay (now often replaced by an equivalent assay using liposomes in place of erythrocytes), and then are confirmed with specific immunoasssays for deficiencies of individual complement proteins.

Determinations of **cytokine** concentrations are usually considered investigational procedures without definitive application, despite the understanding we have of the roles they play in pathophysiology. Some of the potential candidates for future monitoring are the interleukins IL-1β, IL-2, IL-2 receptor, IL-4, IL-5, IL-6, IL-8, IL-10, IL-12, and IL-13. These factors can be elaborated as locally acting messengers in many different inflammatory processes, and so lack specificity for distinguishing different etiologies such as infection versus autoimmune. They act at sites of tissue injury or inflammation and so do not reach easily measured concentrations in blood. Perhaps by looking at concentrations of multiple factors simultaneously both in blood and at the tissue level, interpretation will be feasible using patterns related to specific stimuli and physiologic insults. Other substances that fall into this category of immunomodulating agents include TNF-α and IFN-α, -β, and -γ. A recent clinical application utilizes the quantitation of IFN-γ released by lymphocytes in a peripheral blood specimen after in vitro stimulation with mycobacterial antigens to determine previous exposure status of a patient to that organism.

HLA testing and crossmatching between donors and recipients form the basis of solid organ and bone marrow transplantation. Traditional serologic testing for antigens and antibodies has now been expanded with high resolution HLA genotyping. HLA typing has also been used for matching platelet transfusions in select refractory patients. HLA typing has been used for identity testing, and some antigenic types (e.g., HLA-B27) are recognized to be associated with specific autoimmune disorders.

Applications of testing to **autoimmune diseases** are multiple. Systemic rheumatic diseases such as lupus erythematosus, rheumatoid arthritis, and scleroderma are commonly diagnosed with a battery of autoantibody assays, including the antinuclear antibody plus individual antibodies such as anti-DNA, anti-Sm, anti-RNP, anti-SS-A, anti-SS-B, Scl-70, anticardiolipin, rheumatoid factor, and anti–cyclic citrullinated peptide. Organ-specific autoimmune diseases are characterized by tissue or organelle reactive autoantibodies such as antithyroid, anti–parietal cell, antiskin, antiendomysial (antitissue transglutaminase), antimitochondrial, anti–smooth muscle, antiadrenal, and so forth. Antibodies important in vasculitis include cryoglobulins and classical antineutrophil cytoplasmic antibodies/protoplasmic-staining antineutrophil cytoplasmic antibodies. Although some autoantibodies are etiologic and serial measurements of their titers are important for monitoring disease progress, other antibodies are nonetiologic and so are most useful for diagnosis alone.

Allergies, hypersensitivities, and asthma have common pathways in which allergens are recognized by specific IgE that is bound to the surfaces of basophils and mast cells, thereby liberating histamine and creating allergic symptoms. Diagnostic evaluation of allergies includes measurements of total IgE plus allergen-specific IgE to determine which allergens are significant for particular patients. Typical allergens for this testing include foods, pollens, molds, animal dander, and insects. Skin testing in vivo with these allergens is complementary because a positive response depends on the presence of reactive IgE plus competent T cells with CD4.

Therapeutics in Immunology

Therapeutic targets in the immune system are important to consider because of the need to measure the effects of such treatments to make adjustments and guide clinical management (Table 43-2). Of course, one of the most common abnormalities of cellular immunity today is HIV infection, for which antiretroviral drugs are essential with monitoring that includes viral load measurements as well as genotyping to predict response to specific drugs.

Cellular immunity is the target of several different drugs that act against T cells and so are often used to suppress immune responses against allogeneic solid organ transplants, as well as graft-versus-host disease (GVHD) from allogeneic bone marrow transplants. These drugs include the cyclophilin binding drugs cyclosporine and tacrolimus, which inhibit calcineurin, and the immunosuppressants sirolimus and mycophenolate, both of which block activation of T cells and B cells. Therapeutic drug monitoring of blood concentrations of these immunosuppressants is useful to achieve therapeutic effect (usually as a synergistic action of agents from different drug classes) while avoiding drug toxicities. Polyclonal antilymphocyte globulin is used to reduce the circulating numbers of T cells in an effort to block transplant rejection. Also used is monoclonal anti-CD3 antibody, which binds to that molecule on T cells to reduce their numbers. Experimental anti–IL-2 receptor (CD25) antibody has also been used to block organ transplant rejection. Extracorporeal photopheresis has been successfully applied in the treatment of GVHD, and even for cellular rejection of transplanted solid organs, beyond its well-established role in controlling cutaneous T cell lymphoma.

TABLE 43-2
Therapeutic Targets in the Immune System

Cellular Immunity
- Glucocorticoids
- Anti–T cell drugs (e.g., calcineurin inhibitors)
- Anti-CD20 (e.g., rituximab)
- Antilymphocyte globulin
- Photopheresis
- Interleukin-2
- Antiretroviral drugs

Humoral Immunity
- Intravenous immunoglobulins (pooled)
- Plasma exchange (remove harmful antibodies, cryoglobulins)
- Humanized monoclonal/chimeric antibodies for target antigen neutralization (e.g., anti-CD20)

Complement
- Plasmapheresis to remove complement-activating immune complexes

Cytokines
- Interferons
- Anti–tumor necrosis factor-α
- Granulocyte-colony stimulating factor (G-CSF)

Human Leukocyte Antigens
- Organ transplant rejection: plasmapheresis
- Graft-versus-host disease: photopheresis

Autoimmune Diseases

Suppression of cellular or humoral immunity by
- Glucocorticoids
- Alkylating agents (e.g., cyclophosphamide)
- Antimetabolites (e.g., methotrexate, azathioprine)
- Nonsteroidal antiinflammatory drugs
- Anti–T cell drugs

Allergy/Hypersensitivity/Asthma
- Antihistamines
- Glucocorticoids
- Allergen desensitization injections
- Leukotriene antagonists
- β-Adrenergic agonists

Humoral immunity can be enhanced by passive intravenous infusion of immunoglobulin (IVIG) fractions pooled from multiple individuals who can be expected to contain antibodies against a multitude of infectious agents; high titer immunoglobulins against specific microorganisms are also available (e.g., against hepatitis B virus). IVIG is also used to modulate some autoimmune disorders such as myasthenia gravis, possibly by interfering with the attachment of harmful autoantibodies to tissue sites. Alternatively, harmful antibodies can be removed by plasma exchange using apheresis, in which plasma proteins are replaced by another protein solution such as 5% albumin.

Monoclonal antibodies designed to interact with very specific antigens on cell surfaces or in the blood are now in use for several clinical applications (Griggs, 2009). Because of the potential side effects of stimulating immune or even allergic responses, these large molecule drugs have been reconfigured to appear as naturally occurring proteins by humanizing them with constant regions derived from human immunoglobulin genes. An example of such a chimeric antibody is anti-CD20, which has application in treating B cell lymphomas, as well as in modulating the synthesis of some autoantibodies.

Complement consumption through CICs can be addressed therapeutically by plasmapheresis to remove those CICs (usually in the form of cryoglobulins) and thus lower the burden of harmful deposition in tissues such as the glomeruli or other vasculitides.

Cytokines in regular clinical use include IFN-α for combating infection with hepatitis B virus or hepatitis C virus, and IFN-γ for stimulating immune responsiveness. TNF-α can be neutralized in the circulation by specific therapeutic antibodies or a modified receptor molecule to decrease undesired inflammatory responses in conditions such as rheumatoid arthritis and Crohn's disease. Granulocyte-colony stimulating factor is used regularly in clinical practice to rescue patients who have developed leukopenia after chemotherapy, and to mobilize hematopoietic stem cells for collection from the peripheral blood to prepare for transplantation. Administration of IL-2 does succeed in raising CD4 counts, but this approach has not yet been found to improve outcome in HIV infection (INSIGHT-ESPRIT, 2009). It is likely that other stimulators or inhibitors of cytokines will come into clinical practice in the future.

HLA mismatches in allogeneic transplanted organs are typically dealt with by administration of immunosuppressant drugs but can also be treated with extracorporeal photopheresis to diminish cellular immune rejection, as well as with plasmapheresis to remove HLA antibodies that the host might have previously formed or later formed in response to the transplanted organ.

Autoimmune diseases have been treated with different groups of drugs to reduce the inflammatory response, such as corticosteroids, alkylating agents (e.g., cyclophosphamide), antimetabolites (e.g., methotrexate, azathioprine), nonsteroidal antiinflammatory drugs, and even some of the immunosuppressants normally used to reduce T cell activity in preventing organ transplant rejection. A new medication under trial for systemic lupus erythematosus is a monoclonal antibody against B lymphocyte stimulator, which is a member of the TNF family that acts to stimulate B cell proliferation and immunoglobulin secretion (Cancro, 2009). Other future therapies of autoimmune disorders will likely involve stimulation or suppression of specific sites in the immune response by specific monoclonal antibodies; bone marrow transplantation has also been successful in some cases.

Allergies and hypersensitivities are often treated long term by desensitization methods in which allergens are used to stimulate IgG that competes with IgE to neutralize those allergens that are known to cause problems in individual patients. Medications that are commonly used to control symptoms acutely and chronically are antihistamines, corticosteroids, leukotriene antagonists, and adrenergic agonists.

SELECTED REFERENCES

Kemp SF, Lockey RF. Anaphylaxis: a review of causes and mechanisms. J Allergy Clin Immunol 2002;110:341–8.

An excellent review article covering the immunopathology, the pathophysiology, and many causative agents of anaphylaxis, as well as its clinical management.

Kronenberg M. Toward an understanding of NKT cell biology: progress and paradoxes. Annu Rev Immunol 2005;26:877–900.

This comprehensive review discusses the present state of knowledge of natural killer T cells.

Park C, Chio YS. How do follicular dendritic cells interact intimately with B cells in the germinal center? Immunology 2005;114:2–10.

In this review, the function and interaction of follicular dendritic cells with B cells are nicely presented, along with good illustrations.

Trombetta ES, Mellman I. Cell biology of antigen processing in vitro and in vivo. Annu Rev Immunol 2005;23:975–1028.

This extensive review covers in detail the properties of antigen-presenting cells, as well as regulation, processing, and transport of antigen.

Wen L, Atkinson JP, Giclas PC. Clinical and laboratory evaluation of complement deficiency. J Allergy Clin Immunol 2004;113:585–93.

This article presents a brief description of the three complement pathways, an organ system review of the effect of complement deficiencies, and a diagnostic screening approach for complement deficient states.

REFERENCES

Access the complete reference list online at http://www.expertconsult.com

CHAPTER 44

IMMUNOASSAYS AND IMMUNOCHEMISTRY

Yoshihiro Ashihara, Yasushi Kasahara, Robert M. Nakamura†

Immunoassays and Immunochemistry

GENERAL CHARACTERISTICS OF ANTIGEN–ANTIBODY REACTION

Biological ligands based on the affinity between molecules, such as enzyme and substrate, hormone and receptor, antigen and antibody, play an important role in living organisms. Specific recognition characteristics of immunoassays (antigen–antibody [Ag–Ab] reactions) have become widely used as analytic tools, adding to the wide range of methods available in clinical laboratory testing.

Immunoassays can be used for the detection of antigens or antibodies. For antigen detection, the corresponding specific antibody should be prepared as one of the reagents. The reverse is true for antibody detection. The sensitivity of immunoassays has been enhanced through the development of new types of signal detection systems and solid-phase technology. Immunoassays have been optimized to detect less than 0.1 pg/mL of

†Deceased

antigen present in blood. They can be applied to the detection of haptens as small molecules; proteins and protein complexes as macromolecules; and any antibody to allergens, infectious agents, and autologous antigens.

CHARACTERISTICS OF ANTIGENS

An antigen can be defined as any substance that can represent antigenic sites (epitopes) to produce corresponding antibodies, from small molecules such as haptens and hormones to macromolecules such as proteins, glycoproteins, glycolipids, and other natural products. Artificial chemical compounds can also be antigens acting as haptens. Antigens should have at least one epitope. Epitopes that can be recognized by antibodies include amino acid sequences of peptides in proteins and high-dimensional protein structures such as neoantigenic sites.

CHARACTERISTICS OF ANTIBODIES

Immunoglobulin, an important plasma protein, refers to antibodies in the context of the biological functions of immunoglobulin specific to antigens. Antibodies, therefore, are produced in response to antigenic stimulation. Antibodies are formed of both functional and heterogeneous molecules that bind antigens via the antigen-combining site. Five classes (isotypes) of immunoglobulin have been identified: IgG, IgM, IgA, IgD, and IgE. IgG is further divided into four subclasses, and both IgA and IgM have two subgroups. All known antibody molecules have a heavy chain with a κ or a λ light chain. The molecular structure of antibodies is composed of variable regions and constant regions. The hypervariable domain (epitope-binding spot) can be assembled to interact with a wide variety of epitopes (antigen determinants). In laboratory medicine, two categories of antibodies can be distinguished: antibodies as reactants and antibodies as analytes. Antibodies as analytes are often classified by IgG, IgM, and IgA subtypes. Antibodies as reactants are prepared from antiserum obtained through animal immunization with purified antigen.

Polyclonal Antibodies

A polyclonal antibody can be obtained through immunization with an antigen, which presents various epitopes. In other words, the antibody generated is specific against each epitope. The avidity of a polyclonal antibody to a complex antigen is usually stronger than a single monoclonal antibody. Carrier proteins may be needed for the immunization of smaller molecules, such as haptens or hormones.

Monoclonal Antibodies

Monoclonal antibodies (Koehler and Milstein, 1975) have been developed using the following biotechnologies: somatic cell fusion, selection of the resulting hybridoma, and limiting dilution to ensure the clone is derived from a single cell. They are defined as uniform homogeneous antibodies directed to specific epitopes. An established cell line allows the secretion of all reactive immunoglobulin specific to single epitopes. Monoclonal antibodies have made it possible to analyze molecules on an epitope-to-epitope basis because of their narrow specificity. Yet monoclonal antibodies, in contrast to polyclonal antibodies, do not have the ability to recognize the entire molecule. For monoclonal antibodies, different antigens with a common epitope appear to be the same antigen. CA 19-9 antibody (Magnani, 1983) as a tumor marker can detect different sizes and shapes of molecules that have common carbohydrate epitopes. Monoclonal antibodies enable identification of isoenzymes, subtypes, and isotypes of protein, and conformational changes in molecules because they can discern the slightest differences in molecules.

Monoclonal antibodies may be cross-reactive with different antigens. This cross-reactivity can be explained by the probable existence of the same amino acid sequences, carbohydrates, or lipids on different molecules. Monoclonal antibody technology has allowed the development of extremely useful and nearly ideal immunoassay systems for clinical laboratory testing.

The production methods and applications of monoclonal antibodies have been extensively reviewed (Nakamura, 1983; Zola, 1987). Advantages of monoclonal antibodies are as follows:

- Monoclonal antibodies provide a well-defined reagent.
- Monoclonal antibody production can yield an unlimited quantity of homogeneous reagent with highly consistent affinity and specificity.
- Monoclonal antibodies can be prepared through immunization with a nonpurified antigen.
- Monoclonal antibodies have certain limitations in their use, as follows:
  - Insufficient reactivity is seen in precipitation or agglutination because network formation in the immunocomplex is weak or does not occur when single monoclonal antibodies are used.
  - Antigens with multiple heterogeneous epitopes are more difficult to characterize immunochemically with a single monoclonal antibody.

Antibody Production by Recombinant Technology

Skerra and Pluckthun (1988) have developed an expression system for the Fv fragment of variable domains of an antibody specific to phosphoryl choline using recombinant technology in *Escherichia coli*. This technology makes it possible to produce chimeric antibody fused to an enzyme.

A new technology called phage display has emerged for the production of antibodies (Winter, 1994). In this method, antibody fragments of predetermined binding specificity are constructed from a repertoire of antibody variable *(V)* genes, thereby eliminating the need for immunization and hybridoma technology. The *V* genes can be assembled in vitro. The phage selected from the repertoire by binding to antigen and antibody fragments is expressed in infected bacteria. Furthermore, the binding affinity of the antibodies is improved through mutation. In the near future, this technology will allow the use of specific antibodies with high avidity.

KINETICS OF ANTIGEN–ANTIBODY REACTION

Certain aspects of equilibrium or the law of mass action in chemistry can be applied to the Ag–Ab reaction. The kinetics of the reversible Ag–Ab reaction is as follows (Steward, 1986):

$$\mathrm{Ag} + \mathrm{Ab} \underset{K_2}{\overset{K_1}{\rightleftarrows}} \mathrm{AgAb}, \qquad \textbf{(44-1)}$$

where
Ag represents free antigen
Ab represents free antibody sites
AgAb represents the antigen–antibody complex concentration
K_1 and K_2 are the association and disassociation rate constants, respectively.

The rate of formation of the antigen–antibody complex is represented as follows:

$$d[\mathrm{AgAb}]/dt = K_1[\mathrm{Ag}][\mathrm{Ab}] - K_2[\mathrm{AgAb}] \qquad \textbf{(44-2)}$$

and at equilibrium, the net rate is zero. Therefore,

$$K_1/K_2 = [\mathrm{AgAb}]/[\mathrm{Ag}][\mathrm{Ab}] = K_a$$
$$\text{(association equilibrium constant or affinity constant).} \qquad \textbf{(44-3)}$$

K_a is the parameter limited to site-to-site reactions, although antigens and antibodies often have multiple binding sites on the molecule. The apparent association constant for multiple antigen and antibody reactions may be referred to as **avidity** instead of affinity. The K_a value may be obtained from the following equations and experimental data:

$$[\mathrm{Ab}] = [\mathrm{Ab}]_t - [\mathrm{AgAb}] \qquad \textbf{(44-4)}$$

where *[Ab]* is the antibody concentration at equilibrium, and $[Ab]_t$ represents the total original antibody concentration.

$$K_a = \mathrm{B}/([\mathrm{Ab}]_t - \mathrm{B})\mathrm{F} \qquad \textbf{(44-5)}$$

where *F* is free antigen or analyte, and *B* is bound antigen or analyte.

A Scatchard plot is produced when the amount of antigen bound (B) is plotted on the *x*-axis and the bound over free (B/F) ratio of analytes is plotted on the *y*-axis. The two parameters that can be determined from the Scatchard plot are the dissociation or affinity constant from the slope of the line and the concentration of antibody-binding sites from the X-intercept (Scatchard, 1949).

TABLE 44-1
Classification of Various Immunoassays and Their Characteristics

	Labels (reporter groups)	B/F separation*	Signal detection	Sensitivity
Precipitation immunoassays	Not required	Not required	Naked eye, turbidity, nephrometry	≈10 μg/mL[1]
Particle immunoassays	Blood cells, artificial particles (gelatin, particles, latex, etc.)	Not required	Naked eye, pattern analyzer, spectrophotometry, particle counting	≈5 ng/mL[2]
Radioimmunoassays	Radioisotopes (^{125}I, ^{3}H)	Required	Photon counting	≈5 pg/mL
Enzyme immunoassays	Enzymes	Required	Spectrophotometry, fluorometry photon counting (CL-EIA)	≈5 pg/mL ≈0.1 pg/mL[3]
Fluorescence immunoassays	Fluorophores	Required	Photon counting	≈5 pg/mL[4]
Chemiluminescence immunoassays	Chemiluminescent compounds	Required	Photon counting	≈5 pg/mL[4]

Data from (1) Ritchie R. Automated immunoanalysis, Part I and Part II. New York: Marcel Dekker; 1978; (2) Haux P, Dybois H, McGovern M, et al. Evaluation of the Tlna-quant ferritin assay on the Boehringer Mannheim/Hitachi 704 System. Clin Chem 1988;34:1174. Abstract; (3) Isomura M, Ueno M, Shimada K, et al. Highly sensitive chemiluminescent enzyme immunoassay with gelatin-coated ferrite solid phase. Clin Chem 1994;40:1830; and (4) Sgoutas DS, Barton EG, Hammarstrom M, et al. Four sensitive thyrotropin assays critically evaluated and compared. Clin Chem 1989;25:1785–9.
B/F, Bound over free.
*Washing step for separation of bound labels in immunocomplex from free labels. Homogeneous assays included are not required for B/F separation.

Overview of General Principles of Immunoassays

CLASSES OF IMMUNOASSAYS

A brief classification and a list of features of various immunoassays appear in Table 44-1. Precipitation immunoassays provide the simplest method for antigens and antibodies to react with each other without involving the detection of any labels. The resulting Ag–Ab complex in gel or liquid phase may be observed qualitatively as a precipitant by the naked eye and quantitatively with a detector.

The particle agglutination immunoassay (Kasahara, 1992b) uses inert particles as labels, as opposed to direct precipitation of the Ag–Ab complexes. Antigens or antibodies attached to particles such as erythrocytes, latex, or metal sol react with the analyte in the specimen. As a result of this immune reaction, large particles show significant agglutination patterns that may be seen by the naked eye. Yalow (1959) reported on the development of a radioimmunoassay (RIA) using radioisotopes as labels. This breakthrough allowed for the quantitative detection of a trace level of analytes and contributed to the advancement of basic research and clinical medicine. Insulin, for example, was quantified by RIA, which subsequently replaced the insulin bioassay. RIA may be formatted in a solid-phase procedure for easy separation of bound and free labels. Since the development of RIAs, the search for alternative labels to hazardous radioisotopes has intensified, with the aim of developing nonisotopic immunoassays using enzymes, fluorescent labels, and other reporter groups.

The enzyme immunoassay (EIA), using enzymes as labels, was developed in the early 1970s (Engvall, 1971; Van Weeman, 1971) and rapidly gained wide popularity. Enzymes can amplify signals depending upon the turnover of enzyme catalytic activity. Efforts to improve substrates and to increase sensitivity have led to the introduction of chromophore, fluorophore, and later chemiluminescent compounds. Depending on the substrate chosen, the assay method can be defined as a fluorescent enzyme immunoassay or as a chemiluminescent enzyme immunoassay (Thorpe, 1984).

Fluorescent immunoassays (FIAs) use fluorophores as labels. Fluorophores require optimal wavelength light energy for their excitation to produce detectable emission light. FIA sensitivity is likely to decrease because of the nonspecific background fluorescence present in biological specimens. Fluorophores that have a delayed fluorescence emission time of 100 ns (nanoseconds) are suitable for application on time-resolved FIA. The introduction of a new class of fluorescent compounds has resulted in improvements in FIA such as the elimination of background noise. Sophisticated instrumentation has been introduced that can detect low concentrations (10^{-15} M) of analytes using FIAs.

Chemiluminescent immunoassays use chemiluminescent compounds as labels. Chemiluminescent compounds include chemically synthesized molecules as well as natural products such as aequorin. Unlike fluorophores, most chemiluminescent compounds require chemical rather than light energy to generate emission light. The reduction–oxidation reaction is a process common to all chemiluminescent assays. Signal amplification is not expected of chemiluminescent labels because chemiluminescent molecules generate just one photon through molecular decomposition. A series of new and innovative compounds for electrochemiluminescence have proved suitable for application on immunoassays. Metal chelate with tribiphenyls emits light through a continuous reduction–oxidation reaction on the surface of electrodes (Blackburn, 1991).

In the various types of assays mentioned earlier, the main factors affecting assay sensitivity are the association constant (affinity or avidity) of the reactant, the signal intensity of the labels, and the signal/noise ratio of the detection signal reduced by background from the signals themselves or by a nonspecific reaction.

Iodine-125 (^{125}I) requires about 7 million molecules to generate 1 photon/second, based on half-life calculations of radioisotopes (Bounaud, 1987). Chemiluminescent substrates to enzymes can increase events by an order of magnitude six times greater than that of iodine-125. This is attributable to the catalytic amplification capacity of enzymes.

CONJUGATION CHEMISTRY

Depending on the assay chosen, the method of conjugation that couples one molecule to others, enzymes (or cofactors) to antigens (or antibodies), or antigens (or antibodies) to solid phase may vary. The coupling reaction applied should be performed under conditions that avoid the reduction of any of the biological activities of the protein. In the glutaraldehyde method (Avrameas, 1978), glutaraldehyde, along with two (or possibly more) aldehyde groups as coupling reagents, has been used for conjugation of protein amino groups. This method is based on mixed reactions, including aldol condensation at high pH (the pKa of the NH residue is 8.6–10.8). With this method, shown in Figure 44-1, the resulting conjugate has different forms because of the existence of multiple active sites for coupling. The periodate oxidation method (Nakane, 1966) for the conjugation of antibodies uses horseradish peroxidase, which contains carbohydrates in its molecules. The methods mentioned earlier are not suitable for regulation of site-specific reactions, such as when configurational stereospecificity of conjugates is required.

As shown in Figure 44-2, new coupling methods (Kato, 1975; Kitagawa, 1978) have been developed using a sophisticated coupling reagent, M-maleimidobenzyl-*N*-hydroxysuccinimide ester (MBS). The MBS is a bivalent reagent consisting of an activated ester and maleimide, and can react with an NH_2 group and an SH group, respectively. The carboxy group can also be used as a specific site for conjugating with α- or ε-NH_2 residues of proteins using *N*-hydroxysuccinimide (NHS) as the coupling reagent. The NHS coupling reagent extends to conjugate protein or the carboxyl group introduced on the solid phase.

CHARACTERISTICS OF THE SOLID PHASE

All heterogeneous immunoassays using conjugate with labels, including radioisotopes, require at least one separation step to distinguish the reacted immunocomplex (bound) from unreacted materials (free). Immobilization of antigens or antibodies for solid phase is performed by covalent binding or physical adsorption through noncovalent interactions. Gel particles made of agarose, polyacrylamide, and plastic beads, or titer plates composed of polystyrene, have been used as the solid phase, as well as particles coated with iron oxide that can be separated by a magnetic field.

The inner wall of a tube or a microtiter well is commonly used as a solid phase. With these relatively large solid phases, shaking of the reaction mixture may be needed to shorten the time required for the immune reaction to take place. The prozone phenomenon or hook effect caused by high concentrations of the analyte is likely to be observed in one-step immunoassay when limited quantities of solid-phase antibody or labeled antibody are employed. Microtiter or strip-type plates may cause an "edge effect." This effect can be explained by the different kinetics of the immune reaction or enzyme activity with variations in temperature. A difference in temperature may be present between the wells located at the edge of the microtiter plate and the center of the plate. A difference of about 2° C may be observed with an infrared thermometer between the edge and the center of wells at ambient temperature. The size and shape of the solid phase are critical factors affecting the immunoreaction kinetics and the capturing capacity of solid-phase antibody or antigen. Small spherical magnetic particles or latex particles with 3000 Å diameters provide a larger total surface area for immunoabsorbency than is usually obtained with other solid phases. The larger total surface area helps shorten the immunologic reaction time (Nishizono, 1991).

The particles used for the particle agglutination assay are listed in Table 44-2. The phenomenon of particle agglutination (direct agglutination) caused by an immunoreaction was first observed in tests after incubation with infected patient serum. Agglutination of erythrocytes after incubation with serum led to the discovery of ABO blood types. Particle immunoassays are based on the agglutination principle and use the reactant of an antibody or an antigen attached to the inert particle as a label, as opposed to direct precipitation of an Ag–Ab immunocomplex. As a label, the particle can significantly increase the immunoassay sensitivity, regardless of whether the resulting agglutination is detected by the naked eye or with spectrophotometric instruments for quantification.

Erythrocytes, gelatin particles, liposomes, metal sols, and various kinds of latex particles, including latex modified with iron oxide or dyes, are all suitable solid phases. The diameter of these particles used for agglutination reactions varies from 0.01–7 μm. No single theory can explain the kinetics of agglutination (Kasahara, 1992a) because of the wide variety of particle sizes used as labels. Brownian motion is not significant at room temperature for dispersed particles larger than 3–5 μm. However, the theory of potential energy of interaction between particles, or the theory of colloidal coagulation reaction, can apply to small particles such as latex microparticles. The IgM antibody, being multivalent, is estimated to be 750 times more efficient than the bivalent IgG antibody in an agglutination reaction. The distance between particles in flocculation should be less than or equal to 120 Å because of the molecular length of the antibody. In summary, important factors to consider in an immunoreaction are the surface properties of particles, such as charge and hydrophobicity, and the stability of dispersion.

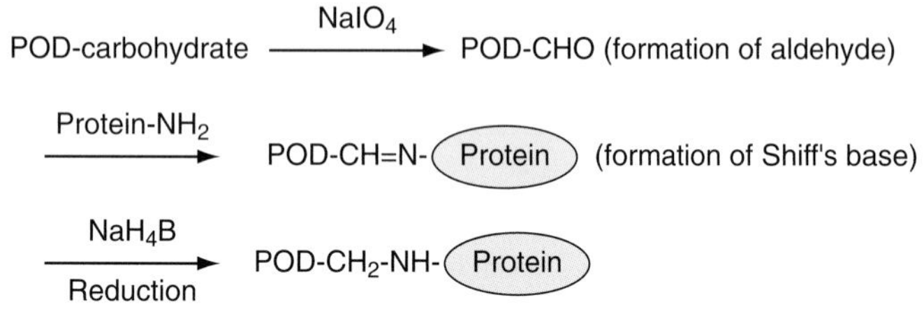

Figure 44-1 Coupling scheme for conjugation of protein with horseradish peroxidase (POD) based on the Nakane method.

PRECIPITIN AND NEPHELOMETRIC IMMUNOASSAYS

BACKGROUND AND PRINCIPLES OF PRECIPITIN REACTION

The precipitate that forms when large complexes of antigen and antibody combine to form an insoluble lattice has been widely used to identify and quantify immunoprecipitin reactions. The modes of application of

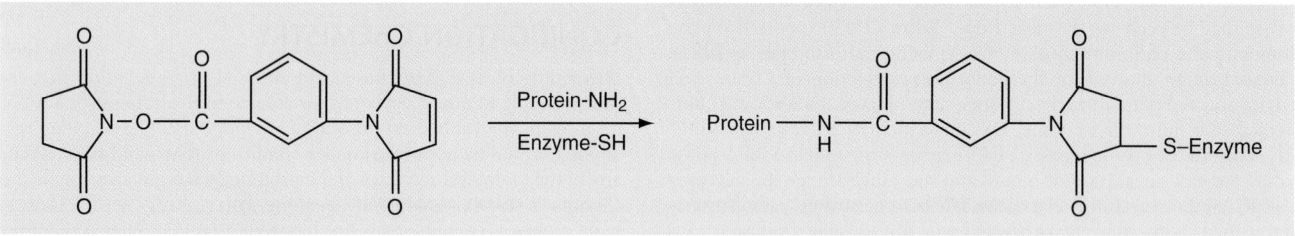

Figure 44-2 Preparation of enzyme–protein conjugate using hetero-bifunctional coupling reagent.

TABLE 44-2
Particles Used as Labels for Particle Agglutination Immunoassay

	Assay method	Supply
Human erythrocyte	Direct hemagglutination (Landsteiner) Erythrocyte antibody hemagglutination: titer plate/slide	ABO blood type Human immunodeficiency virus antibody
Avian erythrocyte	Direct hemagglutination	Human influenza virus antibody
Fixed animal erythrocyte	Passive hemagglutination: titer plate Reverse passive hemagglutination: titer plate	*Treponema pallidum* antibody Hepatitis B surface antigen (HBsAg)
Latex	Reverse passive agglutination: slide Reverse passive agglutination: turbidimetry Reverse passive agglutination	Chorionic gonadotropin Immunoglobulin (Ig)E Ferritin
Latex (color)	Immunochromatography	Human chorionic gonadotropin (hCG)
Microcapsule	Passive agglutination: titer plate	*T. pallidum* antibody
Gelatin particle	Passive agglutination: titer plate Reverse passive agglutination: charge-coupled device (CCD) camera	HIV, *T. pallidum* antibody Human hemoglobin (hHb)
Polypeptide particle	Passive and reverse agglutination	*T. pallidum* antibody, HBs antibody
Silicate particle	Passive agglutination: titer plate/CCD camera	*T. pallidum* antibody
Gold particle	Reverse agglutination enhancement photometry	Total estrogen
Metal sols	Reverse agglutination	hCG, hHb

From Nakamura RM, Kasahara Y. Heterogeneous enzyme immunoassays. In: Nakamura RM, Kasahara Y, Rechnitz GA, editors. Immunochemical assays and biosensor technology for the 1990s. Washington, DC: American Society for Microbiology; 1992. Reproduced with permission.

precipitin techniques have the advantages of sensitivity, specificity, and simplicity. The sensitivity limitation of these assays is a major consideration. Even under the best conditions of enhanced sensitivity afforded by newer light-scattering techniques, the lower limit of sensitivity of immunoprecipitin assays remains in the range of 0.1–0.5 mg/dL. This lower limit of sensitivity appears to be sufficient for the quantification of many major serum proteins. The precipitin reaction forms the basis for many quantitative and qualitative immunochemical techniques now used in the clinical laboratory (Kabat, 1961).

Factors affecting the precipitin reaction were extensively investigated by Heidelberg in 1935, who found that the relative proportions of reactants; conditions of temperature, pH, and ionic strength of the medium; and antibody characteristics of avidity and affinity were all important in the formation of the immune precipitate. On the pattern of precipitin formation, it can be noted that there is a point at which precipitation is maximum or optimal, which is designated as **the point of equivalence.** Continued addition of antigen once the point of equivalence has been reached produces a solubilizing effect on the precipitate. The dynamic range suitable for the determination of analytes should be up to the zone of equivalence. Optimization of the antibody concentration as a reactant is necessary, in addition to optimization of buffer solutions. Typical precipitant reaction methods are as follows:

1. Qualitative Precipitant Assay Methods
   - Single immunodiffusion (Williams, 1970)
   - Double immunodiffusion (Garvey, 1977)
   - Double immunodiffusion in two dimensions (Williams, 1970)
   - Electroimmunodiffusion reaction (Ritzmann, 1975)
   - Immunoelectrophoresis (Rose, 1973)
2. Semiquantitative Precipitant Assay Methods
   - Single radial immunodiffusion (Mancini, 1965, Fahey 1965)
   - Single-dimension electroimmunodiffusion ("rocket" electrophoresis) (Axelsen, 1975)

NEPHELOMETRIC IMMUNOASSAYS

A number of techniques for immunoprecipitin analysis have been developed that use light-scattering devices (Ritchie, 1978). The occurrence of immune complex formation has been related to the amount of such light scattering and has been used as a basis for antigen quantitation. Sophisticated instruments have been designed to rapidly measure light scattering. Measurements of scattered light are generally referred to as **turbidimetry** or **nephelometry.**

PARTICLE IMMUNOASSAY

PRINCIPLE OF PARTICLE AGGLUTINATION

The agglutination reaction may be used to detect antibodies in specimens with specific antigens sensitized to a particle (passive or direct agglutination; Fig. 44-3, *B*). Reverse agglutination using a corresponding antibody sensitized to particles can be employed to detect soluble antigens in the specimen (Fig. 44-3, *A*). A hapten unit single-binding site (for drugs, hormones, or small particles) does not form a cross-linking structure and hence cannot become agglutinated unless it is immobilized on the solid phase. As shown in Figure 44-4, *A* and *B*, when a particle or carrier immobilized with a hapten is used as a reactant, an agglutination inhibition reaction occurs that allows detection of the hapten. This assay is based on a competitive-type principle in which agglutination of hapten particles with a limited amount of antibody, whether free or sensitized on particles, is inhibited by the hapten present in the specimen. Also, labeled particles can react with reactants fixed on the solid phase of the membrane. After immunoreaction, particles within the immunocomplex can be developed to show color on part of the membrane. This type of assay has been popular as a simple device for the qualitative detection of human chorionic gonadotropin (hCG) and other analytes.

Hemagglutination

Hemagglutination tests (Boyden, 1951) are simple to perform and do not require special equipment. For this reason, both advanced and developing countries have adopted a variety of hemagglutination tests. A popular worldwide hemagglutination test is used for the detection of antibody to *Treponema pallidum*, marketed as Serodia-TP, by Fujirebio, Inc. (Tokyo, Japan). In the United States, the hemagglutination test for *T. pallidum* was approved in 1981 by the Centers for Disease Control and Prevention. It was also recommended by the World Health Organization because of its superiority over other tests in terms of specificity and sensitivity (Kasahara, 1992b).

In the *T. pallidum* agglutination test, the reagent consists of sensitized and unsensitized sheep red cells, as well as a serum diluent solution for the reconstitution of lyophilized sensitized cells as a positive control. Both qualitative and semiquantitative tests can be carried out using the following serum dilution protocol and a titer plate as a reaction container as follows: Using a 25 μL pipette dropper, place 4 drops 100 μL of serum diluent in well 1 (Fig. 44-5) and one drop in wells 2–4 for the qualitative assay (wells

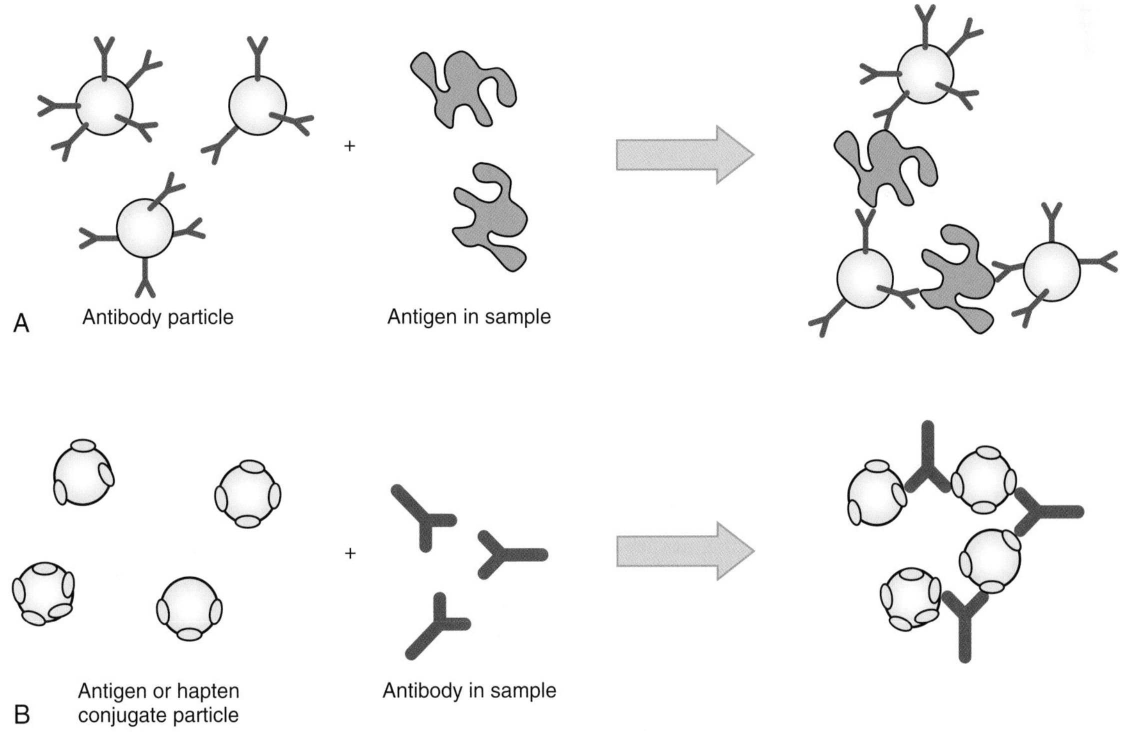

Figure 44-3 Principles of passive particle agglutination immunoassay for detection of antigen with multiple **A,** epitopes or **B,** antibodies. *(From Nakamura RM, Kasahara Y, Rechnitz GA, editors. Immunochemical assays and biosensor technology for the 1990s. Washington, DC: American Society for Microbiology, ASM Press; 1992.)*

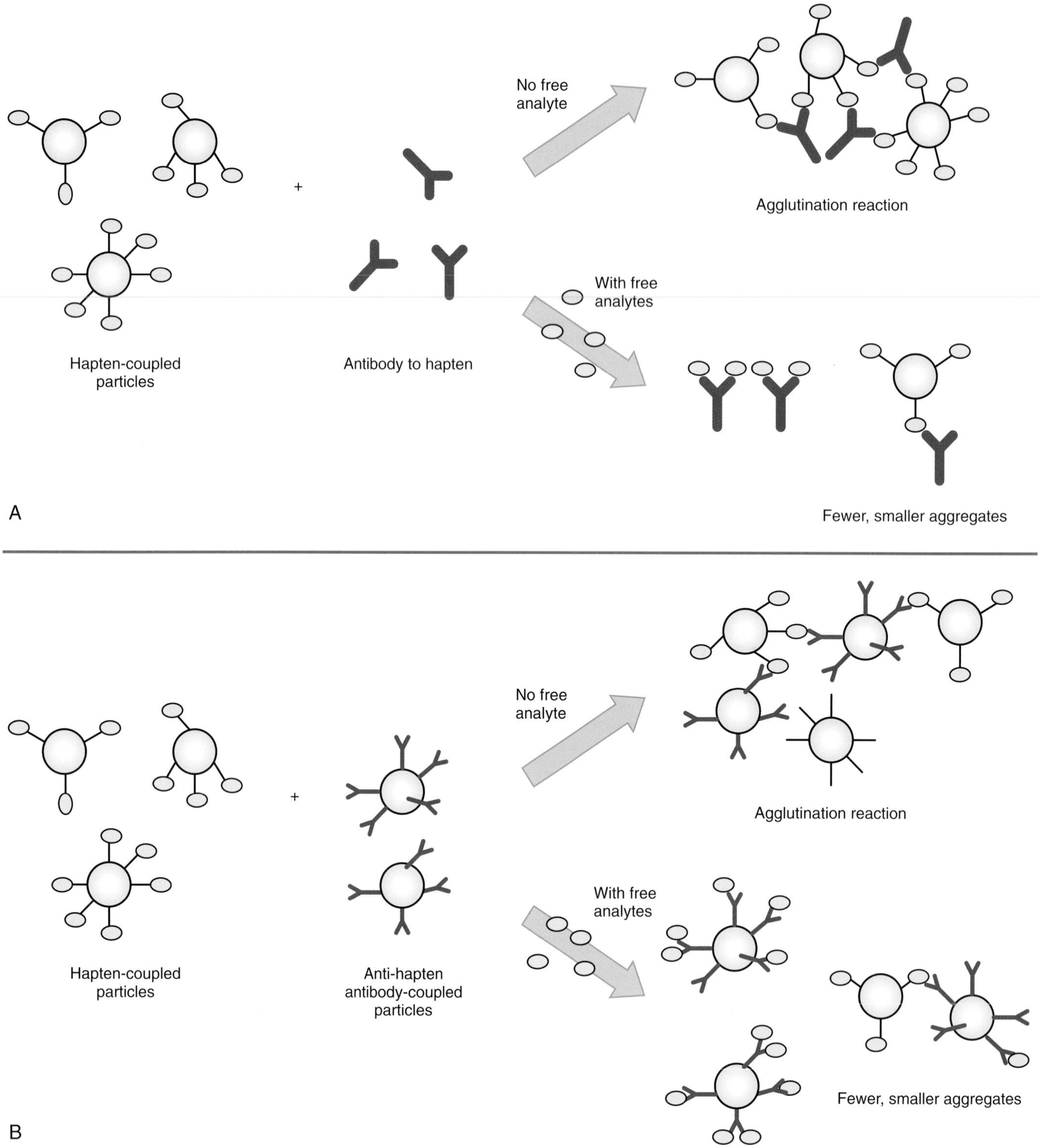

Figure 44-4 Principles of particle inhibition immunoassay for detection of antigen with single epitope (hapten), using antigen particle with **A,** free or **B,** fixed antibody. *(With permission from Nakamura RM, Kasahara Y, Rechnitz GA, editors. Immunochemical assays and biosensor technology for the 1990s. Washington, DC: American Society for Microbiology; 1992.)*

2–8 are used for the quantitative assay). The resulting agglutination patterns are shown in Figure 44-6. Negative patterns, indicating that immunoreaction has not taken place, show condensed flocculation particles with a cross-packing structure at the bottom of the microtiter well. On the other hand, positive patterns, indicating that immunoreaction has occurred, show an expanded agglutination pattern of particles. Agglutinated particles cannot be sedimented any further to obtain condensation as negative patterns, because their global shape is lost on account of the agglutination of particles. In the first and second rows, serum and unsensitized cells (negative control) were used, respectively. Specimens 1 and 2 show negative results. Specimens 3–8 show negative or positive results, depending on the specimen dilution. A positive result is observed for both specimens 7 and 8 up to 1:2560 (rows 3–8).

Hemagglutination kits are now available for the detection of antibodies to hepatitis type B virus (HBV), hepatitis type C (HCV), human immunodeficiency virus (HIV1/2), thyroglobulin, thyroid microsome, and other substances. Reverse hemagglutination tests are used for the detection of HBV surface antigen, α-fetoprotein (AFP), human hemoglobin in stool specimens, and so forth. The sensitivity of hemagglutination tests is approximately 50 ng/mL for antigen (analyte) detection. Kemp (1988) developed a hemagglutination assay that uses a mouse monoclonal antibody specific to the surface antigen of human erythrocytes. The antibody

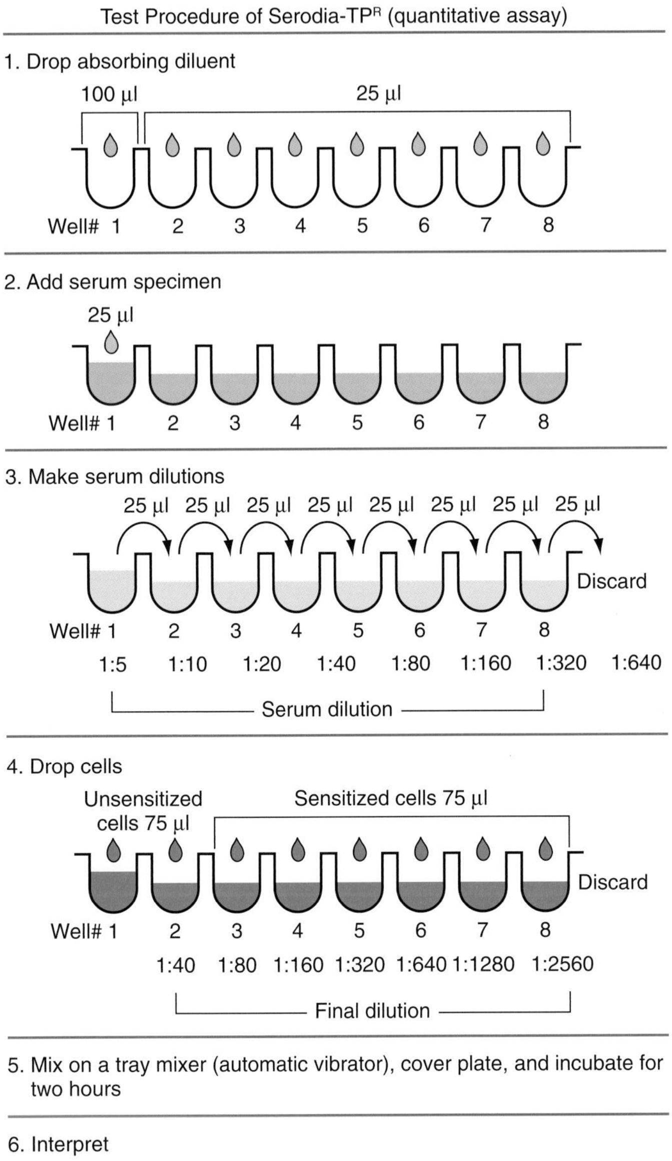

Figure 44-5 Hemagglutination assay for detection of *Treponema pallidum* antigen (Serodia-TP, Fujirebio, Inc., Tokyo, Japan) based on semiquantitative test protocols. *(With permission from Nakamura RM, Kasahara Y, Rechnitz GA, editors. Immunochemical assays and biosensor technology for the 1990s. Washington, DC: American Society for Microbiology; 1992.)*

can recognize an epitope common to different types of red cells or to abnormal cells, such as those found in sickle cell anemia. As shown schematically in Figure 44-7, blood cells in the specimens are used as solid-phase particles, and the resulting agglutination can be observed by the naked eye. Bivalent antibodies are conjugated chemically, so that one antibody specifically reacts with the surface epitopes of the blood cell, and the other is specific to the target antigen or analyte. The assay is applied for the detection of antibody to HIV, as well as for the detection of various antigens. Unlike conventional agglutination formats, the separation of plasma or serum is not required. This assay is simple, saves time, and offers safety advantages because it eliminates the need for serum separation for hazardous HIV- or HBV-positive specimens.

Gelatin Particle Agglutination

The development of a special gelatin particle with a highly hydrophilic surface that is able to prevent nonspecific binding of materials present in a specimen has provided an alternative to erythrocytes (Ikeda, 1984). This particle is made by phase separation and three-dimensional cross-linkage at 40° C and optimum pH. The resulting particle is fixed with formaldehyde or glutaraldehyde, and its diameter is about 3 μm. The physical properties of gelatin particles in comparison with those of erythrocytes are shown in Figure 44-8. A gelatin particle has no antigenicity and is therefore free from problems associated with heterophilic antibodies when erythrocytes are used as particles. This type of artificial particle requires much less serum dilution to avoid nonspecific binding and guarantees a more sensitive detection than with blood cells. Other synthetic particles (Hirayama, 1991) made from block copolymer composed of L-glutamic acid and derivatives have been developed by Hirayama (1991) as alternatives to gel particles. These synthetic particles can be stained with dye of any color because the particles themselves are colorless, as are gelatin particles. The gelatin particle agglutination test was initially applied to the detection of antibodies to human T cell lymphotropic virus, which was first discovered as a retrovirus in humans. This agglutination test (Ikeda, 1984) soon became very popular for blood screening for HIV, HBV, and HCV because of its high sensitivity and specificity and its simplicity, and the fact that strict temperature control is not required to perform the tests. Gelatin particle agglutination can replace any assay based on hemagglutination, with the exception of assays that use red blood cells in specimens as particles.

Latex Agglutination

Latex agglutination (Galvin, 1984), using latex as particles, has been employed for the detection of various analytes, such as hCG for qualitative pregnancy tests, and for the quantitative detection of other plasma proteins with or without instrumentation. The format of this qualitative assay is simple. For example, one might have to mix only a couple of drops of latex sensitized with reactant and specimen using a stick on a black slide. Two to three minutes later, phase inversion agglutination resulting from the immunoreaction can be observed by the naked eye. Latex agglutination was adapted for quantitative assays using light detection methods based on turbidimetry (light absorption) or nephelometry (light scattering). With these techniques, latex agglutination achieves an enhanced sensitivity of subnanograms per milliliter, while the sensitivity of the assay measuring intact precipitation of the Ag–Ab complex remains below 0.5 μg/mL.

Latex Turbidimetric Assay

Light adsorption (light loss by scattering on the surface of a particle) is proportional to the diameter of the particle and depends on the wavelength of light used. Most latex reagents commercially available use latex with a diameter of less than 1 μm and are applied in automated chemistry analyzers using photometric measuring principles. To further improve sensitivity, efforts were made to upgrade reagents and instrumentation, and to optimize particle size, selection of appropriate wavelength, and improvements in computer software for integration of data. Automated systems now use latex particles that can perform about 200 tests per hour at a subnanogram-per-milliliter sensitivity.

Particle-Counting Immunoassay

The particle-counting immunoassay (PACIA) (Masson, 1986) uses optical cell counting to assess the decrease in the number of unagglutinated particles after an immunoreaction. In the PACIA format, the rate assay, that is, the rate of decrease in the number of unagglutinated particles, or the endpoint of the assay reaction can be measured. The endpoint assay can be used to obtain a sensitivity at the nanogram-per-milliliter level; however, a longer incubation time is required for an endpoint immunologic reaction.

Other Particle Immunoassays

Quasielastic scattering immunoassays were developed using a measurement of the change in response to particle size distribution (Yarmush, 1987). This technique uses a laser light beam to measure the reduction in the mean diffusion coefficient of particles as a result of immunoreaction. Other methods measure the change in angular anisotropy of scattered light with the increasing average size of the particle. Particles with diameters about equal to the size of a wavelength achieve a size-dependent angular variation of scattered light.

SUMMARY

Indirect hemagglutination and gelatin particle agglutination tests using microtiter plates are popular procedures for qualitative and semiquantitative determination of various analytes. These tests do not require additional instrumentation or strict temperature control. Most important, they guarantee a sensitivity equal to or greater than conventional enzyme immunoassays when applied to antibody detection of infectious agents. Latex as a solid phase provides great kinetic advantages, such as a shorter immunoreaction time. For this reason, it was possible to adapt latex

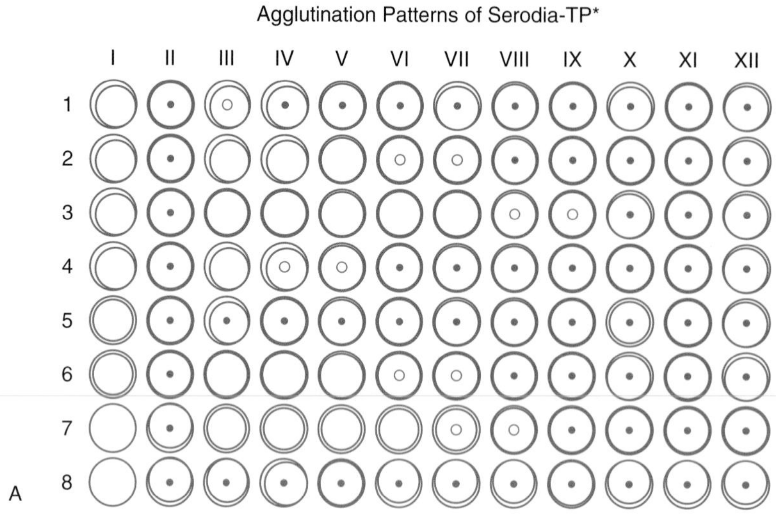

Row no.	I	II	III	IV	V	VI	VII	VIII	IX	X	XI	XII	
Type of cells added		Unsensitized cells	Sensitized cells										Result
Final dilution of serum specimen		1:40	1:80	1:160	1:320	1:640	1:1280	1:2560	1:5120	1:10240	1:20480	Medium control	Titer
Serum specimen													
No. 1	–	–		–	–	–	–	–	–	–	–	–	Inconclusive
No. 2	–	–	++	++	+	+	–	–	–	–	–	–	1:640
No. 3	–	–	++	++	++	++	++	+	–	–	–	–	1:2560
No. 4	–	–	+	+	–	–	–	–	–	–	–	–	1:160
No. 5	–	–	–	–	–	–	–	–	–	–	–	–	Negative
No. 6	–	–	++	++	++	+	–	–	–	–	–	–	1:640
No. 7	–	–	++	++	++	++	+	–	–	–	–	–	1:1280
No. 8	–	–	–	–	–	–	–	–	–	–	–	–	Negative

*Trademark for agglutination test for *T. pallidum* antibody, Fujirebio, Inc., Tokyo, Japan

B

Figure 44-6 Hemagglutination patterns for detection of **A,** anti-*Treponema pallidum* antibody and **B,** interpretation as positive or negative at final serum dilution. *(From Nakamura RM, Kasahara Y, Rechnitz GA, editors. Immunochemical assays and biosensor technology for the 1990s. Washington, DC: American Society for Microbiology, ASM Press; 1992.)*

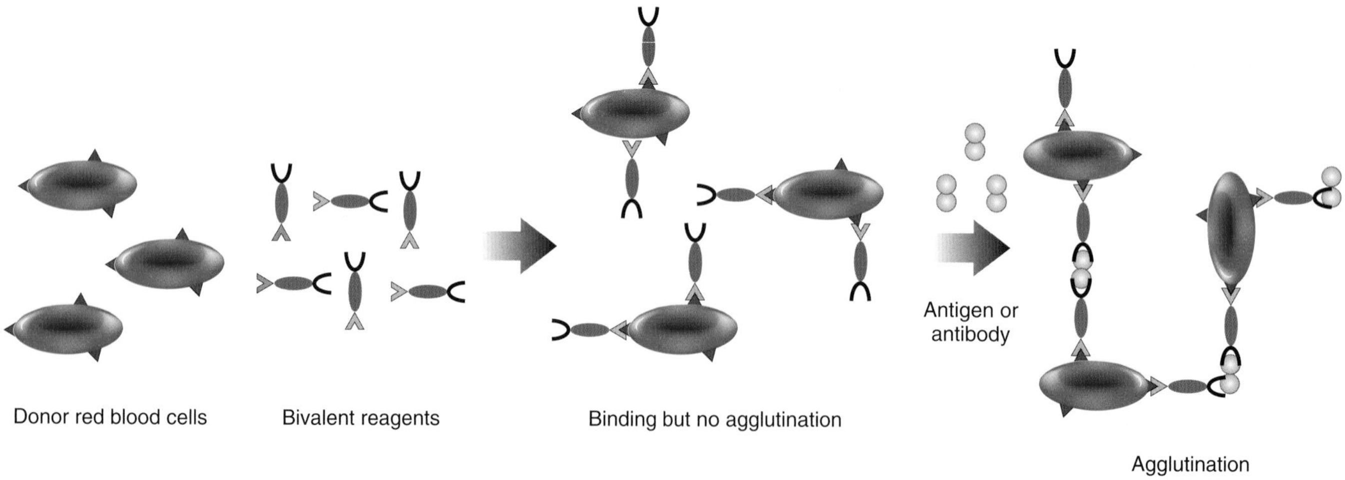

Figure 44-7 Schematic presentation of an assay based on autologous erythrocyte agglutination, using erythrocytes in the specimen as particles. *(With permission from Nakamura RM, Kasahara Y, Rechnitz GA, editors. Immunochemical assays and biosensor technology for the 1990s. Washington, DC: American Society for Microbiology; 1992.)*

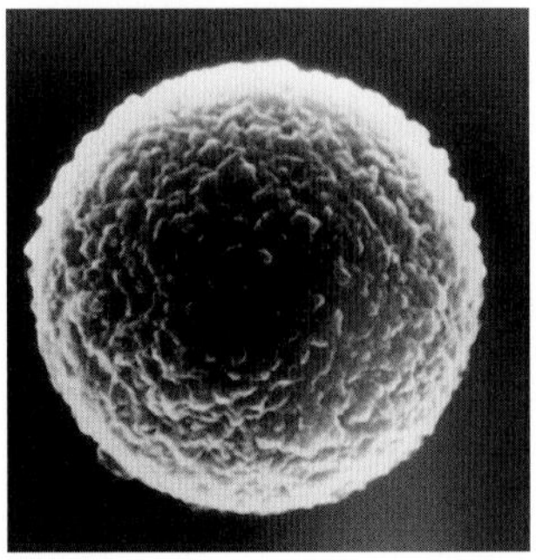

Physical properties	Carrier	
	Gelatin particles	Sheep erythrocytes
Diameter, μm	2 to 6	6
Specific gravity	1.05 to 1.10	1.10
Electrophoretic mobility; μm/s/V/cm	–0.75 to –1.85	–1.15

Figure 44-8 Electron micrograph (×25,000) and physical properties of gelatin particles in comparison with sheep erythrocytes. *(With permission from Nakamura RM, Kasahara Y, Rechnitz GA, editors. Immunochemical assays and biosensor technology for the 1990s. Washington, DC: American Society for Microbiology; 1992, p. 139.)*

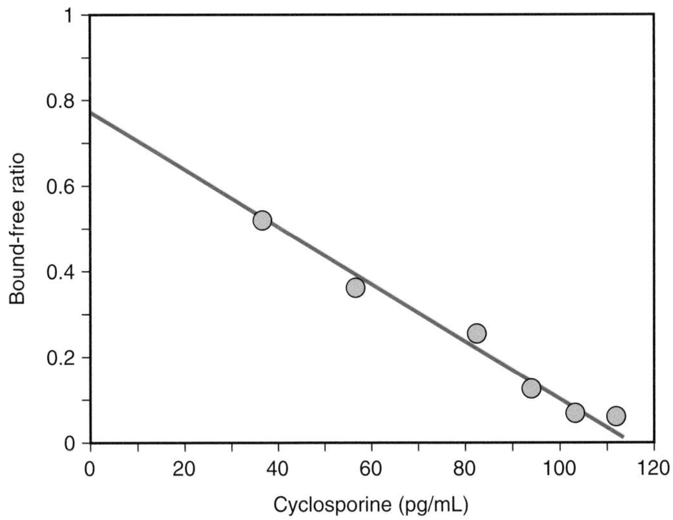

Figure 44-9 Scatchard plot of cyclosporine antibody binding characteristics (K_a = 8.1×10^9 L/M).

for use in existing or sophisticated instruments by applying different principles, resulting in an assay sensitivity of about three orders of magnitude greater than standard immunoprecipitation assays. Latex is susceptible to interferences from unknown factors present in specimens. To eliminate this problem, various absorbents have to be used in both the reagent and the incubation medium. The great advantage of particle immunoassay is its simplicity, because it does not require separation of bound and free reactants.

RADIOIMMUNOASSAY

BACKGROUND

Since RIA technology using radioisotopes as labels was first developed by Yallow and Berson (1959), it has been improved dramatically in sensitivity and precision. Numerous variations in the method have been introduced into the clinical laboratory. Two main RIA techniques, competitive and noncompetitive heterogeneous formats, require washing steps to separate bound and free labels (conjugates). The competitive assay follows the law of mass action, which specifies the reaction between analytes and binding proteins, receptors, and antibody. The key factor in assay optimization is the binding affinity of the antibody. The Scatchard plot of the ratio of bound to free antibody to analyte concentration is commonly used to evaluate antibody performance. Figure 44-9 shows the Scatchard plot for

TABLE 44-3
Properties of Radioisotopes Used as Labels for Radioimmunoassays

Isotope	Half-life	Type of decay	Specific activity (mCi/mmol)
^{125}I	60 days	γ	2,200
^{131}I	8.1 days	β^-, γ	16,100
^{3}H	12.3 years	β^-	29
^{14}C	5760 years	β^-	6,062
^{32}P	14.3 days	β^-	9,120

cyclosporine determination. As described earlier in Kinetics of Antigen-Antibody Reaction, from the following equation:

$$B/F = K_a([Ab]_t - B) \qquad \textbf{(44-6)}$$

the *y*-axis is the B/F ratio that is proportional to free [Ab] from $[Ab]_t$ – B, equal to free [Ag]. Therefore, K_a represents the slope of the plot. In Figure 44-9, the affinity constant K_a is 8.1×10^9 L/M for the antibody specific to cyclosporine. Radioactive emissions, such as γ-rays of iodine-125 labels, can be measured in terms of counts per minute (CPM) using a γ-scintillation counter. Typical radioisotopes used as labels and their properties are shown in Table 44-3. The choice of label affects the assay protocol considerably. For example, the most popular label, iodine-125, requires a rather short time for signal counting but has a limited shelf life because of its short half-life. On the other hand, the tritium (^3H) label requires a longer time for counting, thereby increasing the total assay time. Most RIAs now use iodine-125 as labels to expedite the conjugation process and to retain the biological activity of the reactants. A commonly used method for conjugation of iodine-125 with proteins is the chloramine-T method (Hunter, 1962). Tyrosine, in particular, has greater reactivity with iodate because of its hydroxy group at the para-position on the aromatic ring. The signal can be measured in terms of CPM as γ-ray emissions. Unlike enzymes, isotopes as labels with a small Stokes radius are not likely to disrupt antigenic activity because of the lack of steric hindrance when isotopes are conjugated with small antigens (haptens).

ASSAY PRINCIPLES AND METHODS

Various methods (antigen excess) based on the competitive binding reaction (Ekins, 1960) to antibodies between labeled antigens and nonlabeled antigens (analytes present in the specimen) have been developed for a wide variety of analytes. A conventional competitive method is shown in Figure 44-10. At first, known amounts of labeled antigen and antigen in the specimen are mixed and reacted competitively with a constant amount of antibody coated on a solid phase, such as sepharose beads or the inner wall of plastic tubes. After the immune reaction reaches its equilibrium, the mixture is washed to remove unreacted conjugates and antigens, and the immune complex trapped on the solid phase is separated. The washing step is referred to as B/F separation. Applying the competitive principle, the plot of antigen-bound percentage against logarithmic concentration of analyte provides the standard curve shown in Figure 44-10. The CPM plot on the standard curve gives the concentration of analytes.

A second antibody method is shown in Figure 44-11. The first antibody specific to a particular antigen (analyte) reacts competitively with both the conjugate and the antigen. Then, the immune complex is captured by the second antibody specific to the first antibody, on the solid phase. When the second antibody is coated on a fine solid phase, the immune complex on the second reaction can be separated as a precipitant from the unreacted molecules. For antibody determination, labeled antibody and antibody in the specimen react competitively with the antigen (analyte) fixed on the solid phase. The steeper slope of the standard curve provides more precise data. Competitive methods require lesser amounts of antibody or antigen (analyte) than the sandwich-type assays described later. Noncompetitive assays, originally demonstrated by Miles (1968), have recently gained greater popularity.

Immunoradiometric assays and sandwich assays (Fig. 44-12) have alternative relationships between analyte and antibody. The classical competitive assay achieves an immunologic response with a minimum amount of antibody; the sandwich assay uses a large amount of antibody on the solid phase. Monoclonal antibody technology has made it possible to manufacture large quantities of specific antibodies at moderate costs, thereby

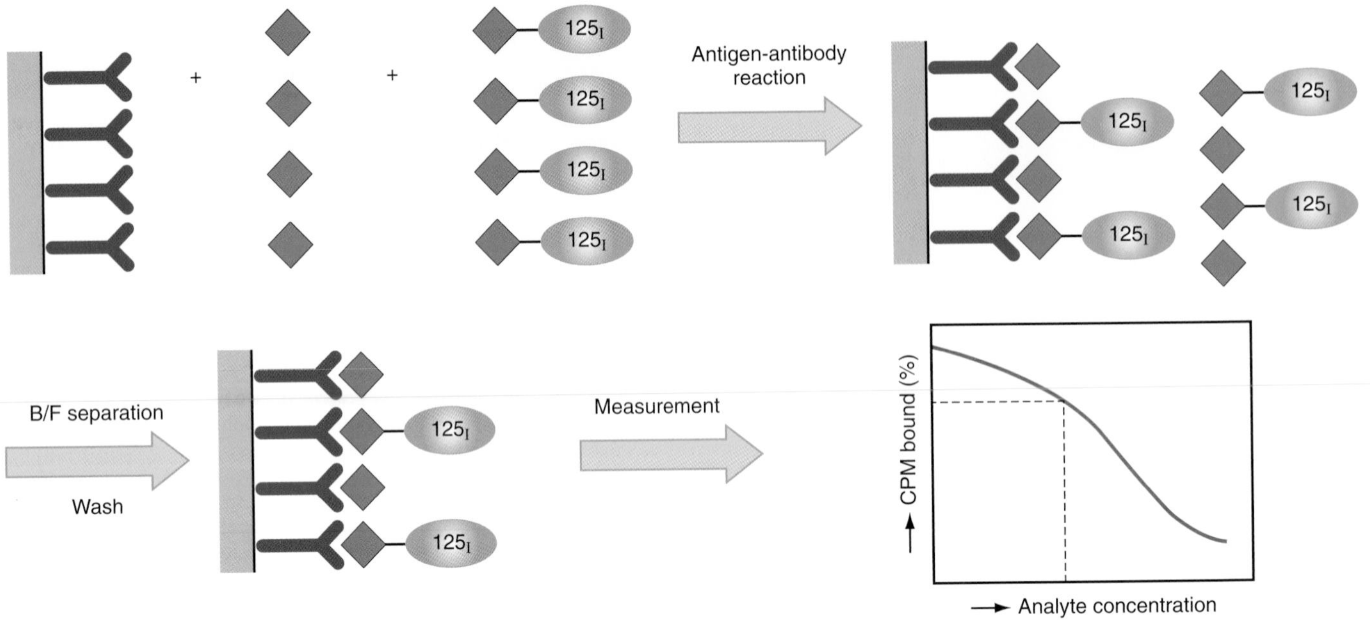

Figure 44-10 Assay principle of competitive radioimmunoassay (RIA) using first antibody as solid phase.

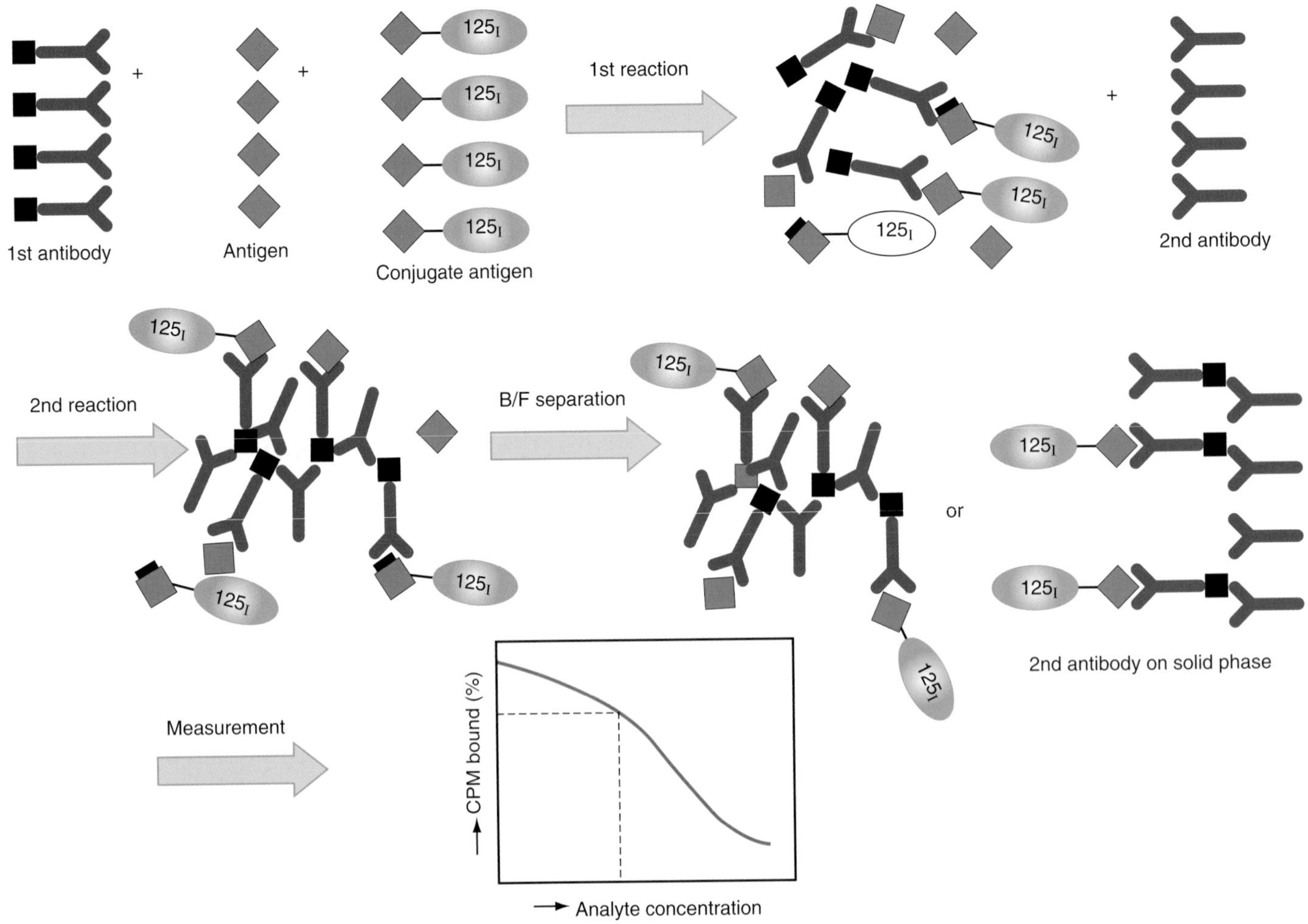

Figure 44-11 Assay principle of competitive radioimmunoassay (RIA) method using second antibody for B/F (bound/free) separation.

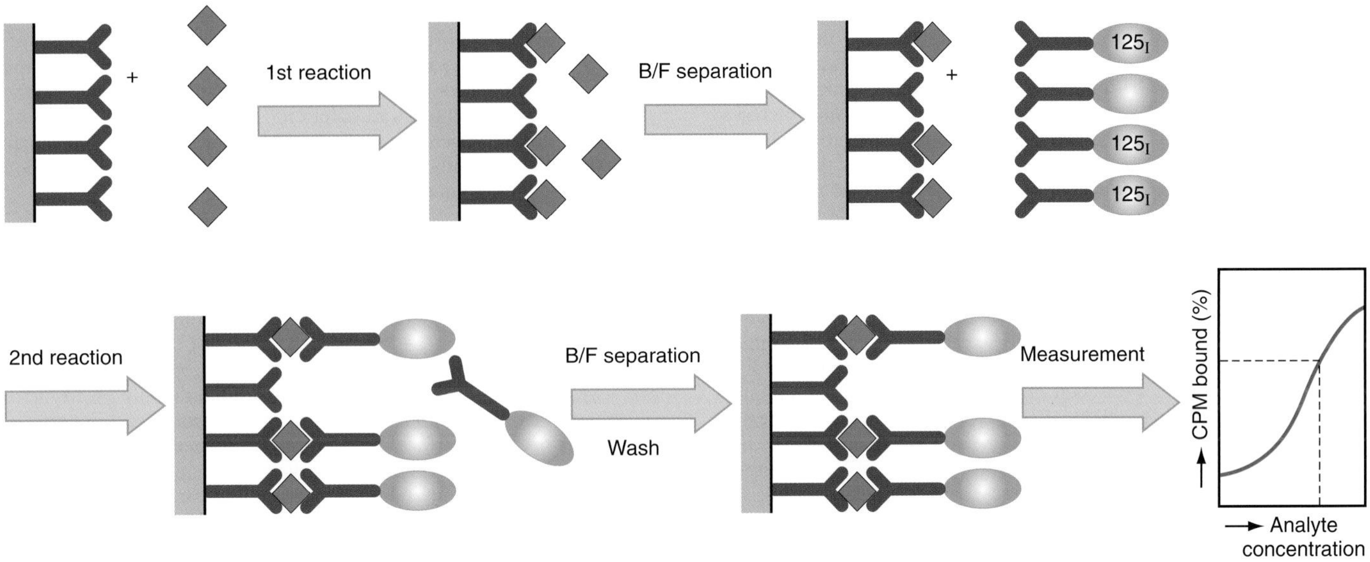

Figure 44-12 Assay principle of sandwich radioimmunoassay (RIA) method using solid phase, also referred to as immunoradiometric assay. *B/F,* Bound/free.

TABLE 44-4
Comparison of Radioimmunoassay, Heterogeneous Enzyme Immunoassay, and Homogeneous Enzyme Immunoassay

Assay	Immunologic reaction steps	Enzyme reaction steps	Signal detection steps
Radioimmunoassay Sample + (labeled analyte or Ab) – ^{125}I	Immunoreaction with washing steps for separation	Not required	Radioactive decay (γ-ray)
Heterogeneous enzyme immunoassay Sample + (labeled analyte or Ab) – enzyme	Immunoreaction with washing steps for separation	Enzyme reaction with additional reagent	Optical density Fluorescence Luminescence
Homogeneous enzyme immunoassay Sample + (labeled analyte or Ab) – enzyme or cofactors	Immunoreaction and/or systemic reaction is carried out in one solution, which includes reagent for signal development of enzyme.	Immunoreaction and/or systemic reaction is carried out in one solution, which includes reagent for signal development of enzyme.	Optical density Fluorescence Luminescence

Ab, Antibody.

allowing the sandwich assay to be exploited. The sandwich assay, which uses excess antibody, is more sensitive than the competitive assay. When background noise is completely omitted, the ultimate theoretical sensitivity of the sandwich assay is one molecule of analyte, which is possible when the amount of antibody used in the assay system approaches infinity. As shown in Figure 44-12, the antibody on the solid phase first captures the antigen (analyte) in the specimen. Following B/F separation, the conjugate reacts with the antigen (analyte) fixed on the solid phase; the signal can then be counted after the elimination of free conjugates through a washing step. This assay requires antigens with more than two antigenic sites. When two different antibodies (i.e., a solid-phase antibody specific to one antigenic site and a conjugate antibody specific to another antigenic site) are used, the assay protocol can be simplified by performing a one-step sandwich. Thus, the solid phase can mix together with the antigen in the specimen and the conjugate simultaneously. Interference does not occur because the antibodies on both the solid phase and the conjugate are capable of recognizing different antigenic sites. In this assay, the signal generated is proportional to the analyte concentration present in the specimen, as in the two-step sandwich assay. This assay method can be applied to antibody detection with an assay format using antigen as the solid phase or labeled antigen. For a two-step format, antigen as the solid phase or labeled antibody specific to the target antibody can be used. Using the sandwich format, assay sensitivity (Rodriguez-Espinosa, 1987) is high. An example is seen when an immunoradiometric assay is used for determination of the peptide hormone thyroid-stimulating hormone (TSH); the level of assay sensitivity is below 0.07 μU/mL of TSH, as compared with about 0.7 μU/mL with conventional competitive antigen-labeled assay.

SUMMARY

Compared with other immunoassays, RIAs are advantageous for a number of reasons: (1) precision and high sensitivity, (2) ease of isotope conjugation, (3) signal detection without optimization, and (4) stability against interference from the assay environment, among others. Disadvantages of RIAs are the short shelf-life of the reagents and the need to protect against hazardous radioactivity. Furthermore, as discussed later, RIAs may not be applied to homogeneous immunoassays because signals from isotopes cannot modulate Ag–Ab reactions.

ENZYME IMMUNOASSAY

BACKGROUND AND CLASSIFICATION

Quantitative immunoassays using enzymes as labels were developed as alternatives to radioisotopes (Avrameas, 1971; Engvall, 1971; Van Weeman, 1971). The most widely used are the enzyme-linked immunosorbent assay (ELISA), the EIA, and the enzyme-multiplied immunoassay technique (EMIT), which is a registered trade name of SYVA Co. (Dade Behring Inc., Cupertino, Calif.) (Rubenstein, 1972). Essentially, heterogeneous EIAs are similar to RIAs, except that they use enzymes as labels. Enzymes make it possible to develop homogeneous EIAs, eliminating the otherwise necessary washing steps for B/F separation. Table 44-4 compares the features of heterogeneous and homogeneous EIAs versus RIAs. Improvements in EIAs have provided many innovative formats with different degrees of speed, sensitivity, simplicity, and precision. Advantages and disadvantages of EIAs are listed in Table 44-5 (Nakamura, 1992a).

HETEROGENEOUS ENZYME IMMUNOASSAYS

The assay principle of heterogeneous EIAs is similar to that of RIAs, except that enzyme activity, not radioactivity, is measured. EIAs require a secondary process to obtain signals through the catalytic reaction of enzymes. Microtiter plate wells, plastic beads, plastic tubes, magnetic particles, and latex with filters, among others, can be used as the solid phase for the separation of bound and free conjugates. The use of small magnetic particles and latex allows shortening of the immunoreaction time, thereby reducing the total assay time. The development of substrates to be cleaved by enzymes was marked by the introduction of colorimetric and fluorometric substrates, and later chemiluminescent substrates, which increased the signal sensitivity. The enzymes commonly used in various heterogeneous EIAs are horseradish peroxidase, alkaline phosphatase, β-galactosidase, glucose oxidase, urease, and catalase. The most widely used enzymes and their characteristics are listed in Table 44-6. Assay sensitivity using enzymes may be determined by the turnover rate of each enzyme and by selection of signal measurement in which chemiluminometry is the most sensitive method.

The assay format of heterogeneous EIAs, similar to RIAs, can be divided into competitive and noncompetitive assays (Fig. 44-13). Competitive assays (analyte excess) use antigen–enzyme conjugates (Fig. 44-13, *A*), and noncompetitive assays (reactant excess) include two-site immunometric sandwich assays (Fig. 44-13, *B1*) and indirect assays to measure antibodies (Fig. 44-13, *B2*). Immunometric sandwich assays have gained much popularity for the determination of antigens such as tumor markers, plasma proteins, and infectious agents. Indirect assays for antibody measurement (Figs. 44-13, *B2*) have been adopted for the detection of antibodies to infectious agents (e.g., HIV, HBV, HCV) and to autoantibodies.

Heterogeneous EIA (see Fig. 44-13) consists of the following steps:

1. The solid phase with the attached reactants is mixed with analyte, regardless of whether the assay is based on the competitive or the noncompetitive format.
2. Following the addition of conjugate and incubation, washing steps are performed with a buffer solution containing a detergent, one or two steps after the immunoreaction. The immunoreaction should reach certain yields to obtain a stable and precise assay.
3. The solid phase, with the immunocomplex containing enzyme-labeled antigen or antibody, is incubated at constant temperature with the enzyme–substrate solution.
4. The enzyme reaction is stopped (stopping is not needed in rate assay), and the substrate reaction product is measured with various detectors, depending on the substrate used.

TABLE 44-5
Advantages and Disadvantages of Enzyme Immunoassay

A. Advantages
   1. Sensitive assays can be developed by the amplification effect of enzymes.
   2. Reagents are relatively cheap and can have a long shelf life.
   3. Multiple simultaneous assays can be developed.
   4. A wide variety of assay configurations can be developed.
   5. Equipment can be inexpensive and is widely available.
   6. No radiation hazards occur during labeling or disposal of wastes.

B. Disadvantages
   1. Measurement of enzyme activity can be more complex than measurement of the activity of some types of radioisotopes.
   2. Enzyme activity may be affected by plasma constituents.
   3. Homogeneous assays at the present time have the sensitivity of 10^{-9} M and are not as sensitive as radioimmunoassays.
   4. Homogeneous EIAs for large protein molecules have been developed but require complex immunochemical reagents.

EIA, Enzyme immunoassay.
From Nakamura RM, Kasahara Y. Heterogeneous enzyme immunoassays. In: Nakamura RM, Kasahara Y, Rechnitz GA, editors. Immunochemical assays and biosensor technology for the 1990s. Washington, DC: American Society for Microbiology; 1992. Reproduced with permission.

Colorimetric Enzyme Immunoassay

In this assay, enzyme reaction is performed by using chromogenic substrates to develop a color by prime catalytic reaction, for example, horseradish peroxidase, catalyzing ABTS (diammonium salt of 2,2′-azino-di[{3-ethyl-benzothiazoline-6-sulfonate}]) with H_2O_2 to form a green color, and alkaline phosphatase specific to the *p*-nitrophenylphosphate, to form a yellow color. Both enzymes are the most commonly used types of colorimetric enzyme immunoassays. A spectrophotometer is used to measure the optical density of the resulting chromogen. Many instruments are available for the measurement of optical density in tubes or microtiter plates, ranging from a fully automated system that performs sample pipetting and data printout to simpler manual devices. When the EIA reaction is performed on nitrocellulose membrane (Western blotting method) or other membranes, substrates that generate insoluble dyes are utilized. An hCG pregnancy test with an immunoassay format that is sold as an over-the-counter test commonly uses benzidine derivatives to react with peroxidase, or indoxyl phosphate derivatives to react with alkaline phosphatase, to generate insoluble dyes. The dye accumulating on the solid phase through enzyme reaction can be read by the naked eye. Theoretically, the measurement of optical density is limited to a range of 0–2.0. Therefore, the determination of optical density for analytes that require determination of a wide dynamic range can be problematic, even when an excess amount of conjugate and a solid phase with sufficient capturing capacity are used with a sandwich-type assay.

Efforts to improve EIAs, the milestone of nonisotopic immunoassays, have brought to light several disadvantages of RIAs, such as hazardous isotopic waste, radiolysis of labeled analytes, and the short half-life of iodine-125. Ishikawa (1989) developed an ultrasensitive EIA capable of detecting 3 fmol of specific IgG antibody. But to achieve this level of sensitivity, several tedious steps are required, such as immunocomplex transfer from a first solid phase to another solid phase to reduce background signals.

Fluorescent Enzyme Immunoassay

Fluorescent EIAs are identical to other EIAs, except that they use fluorescent substrates. In the fluorescent EIA, a fluorophore is generated by an enzyme reaction. Following excitation of the fluorophore at its optimal light excitation wavelength, light at a characteristic wavelength is emitted. Instruments such as a fluorometer require both a supplier of the excitation light source and a photomultiplier tube as a detector of the emission fluorescence. Substances that emit fluorescent light may be present in the specimen. These substances may increase the background signal, which may interfere with the assay's sensitivity. Thus, close attention should be paid to the selection of substrates for EIAs to avoid interfering factors. Compared with colorimetric EIAs, fluorescent assays generate a signal intensity that is at least one order of magnitude greater.

TABLE 44-6
Characteristics of Typical Enzymes Used as Labels for Enzyme Immunoassay

Enzyme characteristics	Peroxidase (EC1.11.1.7)	β-Galactosidase (EC3.2.1.23)	Alkaline phosphatase (EC3.1.3.1)
Source	Horseradish	*Escherichia coli*	Bovine intestine
Molecular weight, daltons	40,000	530,000	100,000
Specific activity	250 U/mg	600 U/mg	2500–5000 U/mg
Turnover rate*	10,000	318,000	250,000
Measurement of enzyme	Colorimetry, fluorometry, luminometry	Colorimetry, fluorometry, luminometry	Colorimetry, fluorometry, luminometry
Highly sensitive measurement	Luminometry	Fluorometry	Luminometry
Method for enzyme labeling	Periodate oxidation (Nakane method)	Dimaleimide method, cross-linking reagent†	Glutaraldehyde method, cross-linking reagent†

*Number of substrate molecules produced by a molecule of enzyme for 1-minute reaction; molecule number/minute.
†The reagent contains chemically reactive groups such as maleimide and succinimide.

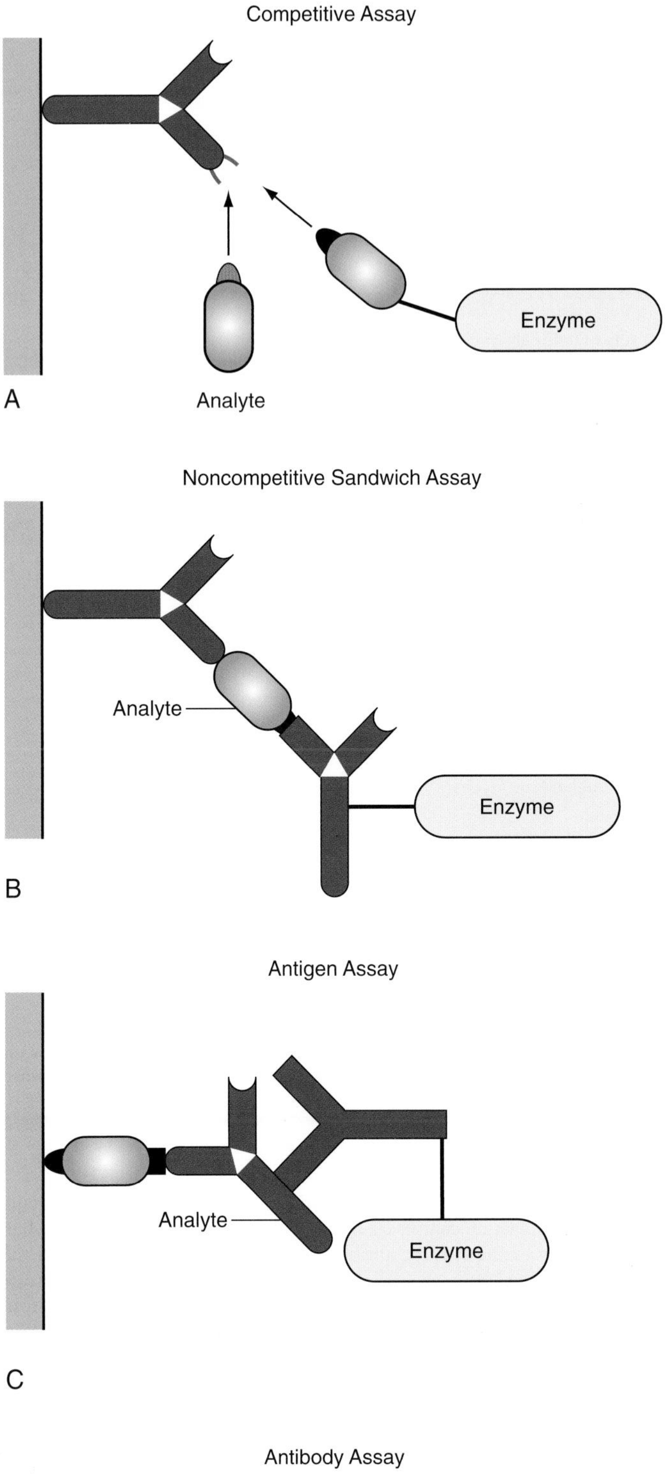

Figure 44-13 Assay principles of heterogeneous enzyme immunoassay (EIA) using solid phase. **A,** Competitive assay. **B** and **C,** Noncompetitive sandwich assay.

Chemiluminescent Enzyme Immunoassay

Chemiluminescent enzyme immunoassays (CL-EIAs) use chemiluminescent substrates that react with various enzymes employed as labels. The chemiluminescent enzymatic reaction generates light, similar to bioluminescence, which involves the use of natural substrates such as luciferin–adenosine triphosphate. Over the past 20 years, much attention has been paid to the application of chemiluminescence in immunoassays, and a variety of systems consisting of substrates and enzymes have been developed. Current systems using luminol derivatives to peroxidase with an enhancer or dioxetane derivatives to alkaline phosphatase achieve highly sensitive immunoassays. These assays are effective tools in practical diagnosis. The enzymatic oxidation reaction of luminol analogs has long been used for CL-EIA. Use of peroxidase with H_2O_2 is a common method that is interchangeable with an alternative coupling enzyme producing H_2O_2, such as glucose oxidase or uricase. The discovery of enhancers by Thorpe (1985) for luminol-based chemiluminescence remarkably improved the assay's sensitivity. Enhancers include phenol derivatives and aromatic compounds. For example, luminol-peroxidase with *p*-iodophenol as an enhancer achieves a light emission increase of up to 2800-fold in the optimized reaction mixture. This assay is able to detect TSH at 0.04 μU/mL when serum is used as the specimen. However, oxidative reactions, such as those for luminol, are likely to be interfered with by multiple factors that cause increased nonspecific background signals (noise).

Bronstein (1989a) developed a chemiluminescent substrate for alkaline phosphatase that differs considerably from other compounds. This new substrate is known as AMPPD (disodium 3-(4-methylspiro [1,2-dioxetane-3,2′-tricyclo-[3.3.1.1]decan]-4-yl) phenyl phosphate), an adamantyl dioxetane derivative. It requires no additional molecules for the emission of chemiluminescent light, unlike luminol, which needs oxidative compounds from outside the luminol molecules. AMPPD is a novel molecule that is a complete substrate because it is composed of the adamantyl group as a stabilizer of the entire molecule, the dioxetane bond as an energy source, and phosphoryl ester as a cleavage site of the enzyme, along with a phenyl group for chemiluminescence—all assembled within one molecule. The structure of the molecule and the reaction process for light generation are shown in Figure 44-14. Cleavage of the phosphoester bond of AMPPD by alkaline phosphatase triggers chemically initiated electron exchange luminescence by releasing electron-rich dioxetane. A chemiluminescent signal with maximum wavelength of 477 nm can be detected within a couple of minutes to a few hours, depending on substrate concentration. The alkaline phosphatase with AMPPD assay system has a sensitivity of less than 10^{-20} mol (Bronstein 1989b, 1991; Kricka, 1991).

CL-EIA uses AMPPD as a substrate to react with alkaline phosphatase, which is used as the enzyme label. CL-EIA can be performed on a fully automated instrument. This novel substrate made it possible to develop an extremely sensitive chemiluminescent enzyme immunoassay system. Ferrite particles 0.3 μm in diameter as the solid phase shorten immunoreaction time to within 30 minutes and provide a larger surface area for the immunoabsorbent. The relationship between the chemiluminescent signal and the concentration of analytes is linear up to about seven orders of dynamic range. The sensitivity of CL-EIA (Nishizono, 1991) was 10-fold greater than that of conventional RIAs when AFP was assayed; AFP was detected at a level of 30 pg/mL with an assay time of 30 minutes. Thus, the new chemiluminescent EIA systems are a definite improvement over RIAs in terms of sensitivity, time efficiency, and procedural simplicity, and they are increasing in popularity.

HOMOGENEOUS ENZYME IMMUNOASSAYS

Background

Two options are available to eliminate tedious assay procedures. One is to design fully automated instruments to access heterogeneous types of reagents, and the other is to develop innovative reagents that do not require complicated washing steps, such as those needed for heterogeneous EIAs. Enzymes and their cofactors are advantageous labels in homogeneous EIAs because enzyme activity can be modulated easily by changing factors in the microenvironment of the Ag–Ab reaction. This is not the case when radioisotope decay is used as the signal. At present, homogeneous EIAs are generally less sensitive than their heterogeneous counterparts. Conventional heterogeneous EIAs have equal sensitivity to RIAs in many applications, whereas homogeneous EIAs (Nakamura, 1988) remain one or two orders of magnitude less sensitive than RIAs. Homogeneous EIAs may require complex immunochemical reagents, but the assay systems are rapid and simple and are adaptable to conventional instruments. Various types of homogeneous EIAs are available. In each of these assays, the Ag–Ab interaction modulates the activity of the enzyme or enzyme label in the presence of the substrate. Modulation of the enzyme activity reflects the degree of the immunochemical reaction. Table 44-7 lists the characteristics of typical homogeneous EIAs. Homogeneous EIAs can be classified as competitive and noncompetitive binding assays. Competitive assays usually consist of enzyme-labeled antigens. However, the antigen (analyte) may be conjugated to the substrate or to a prosthetic group of the enzyme in other assay formats. In contrast, noncompetitive binding assays use a conjugate of antibody labeled with enzyme. Among the various methods reported, five homogeneous EIAs deserve our attention.

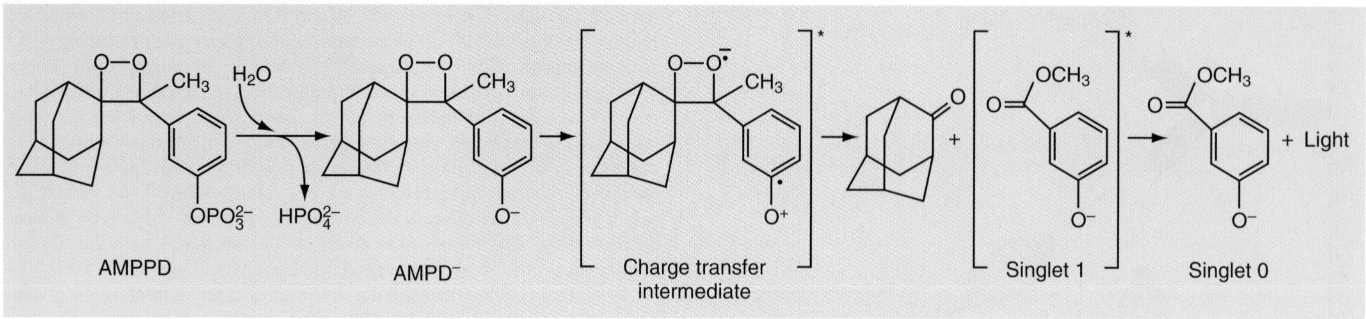

Figure 44-14 Adamantyl 1,2-dioxetane phenyl phosphate (AMPPD): a chemiluminescent substrate for alkaline phosphatase (ALP) detection. Hydrolytic phosphate cleavage by ALP triggers chemically initiated electron exchange luminescence (CIEEL) decomposition of AMPPD by releasing the electron-rich dioxetane phenolate ($AMPD^-$). Charge transfer from the phenolate to the dioxetane ring takes place, forming the charge transfer (CT) intermediate and subsequent breakdown of the cyclic peroxide. Release of energy occurs with light emission.

TABLE 44-7
Classification and Characteristics of Typical Homogeneous Enzyme Immunoassays*

Name and assay type	Conjugate	Manner of modulation
Competitive		
EMIT	Antigen with lysozyme, G6PD*	Steric hindrance
SLFIA	Antigen with substrate	Steric hindrance
ARIS	Antigen with prosthetic group	Steric hindrance
Enzyme-channeling immunoassay	Antigen with G6PDH* and hexokinase*	Enhancement by proximity
Biotin-enzyme avidin immunoassay	Antigen with avidin	Steric hindrance
CEDIA	Antigen with fragments of subunit	Steric hindrance
Noncompetitive		
Hybrid antibody immunoassay	Hybrid antibodies specific to antigen and to inhibitor	Steric hindrance
Proximal linkage immunoassay	Antibody with G6PDH* and hexokinase	Substrate cascade by proximity
EIHIA	Antibody with amylase*	Steric hindrance
Enzyme enhancement immunoassay	Antibody with β-galactosidase* and succinyl antibody	Charge effect
AEST	Antibody with peroxidase	Stabilization

From Kasahara Y. Principles and applications of particle immunoassay. In: Nakamura RM, Kasahara Y, Rechnitz GA, editors. Immunochemical assays and biosensor technology for the 1990s. Washington, DC: American Society for Microbiology; 1992. Reproduced with permission. *ARIS,* Apoenzyme reactivation immunoassay; *CEDIA,* cloned enzyme donor immunoassay; *EIHIA,* enzyme inhibitory homogeneous immunoassay; *EMIT,* enzyme-multiplied immunoassay technique; *G6PD,* glucose-6-phosphate dehydrogenase; *SLFIA,* substrate-labeled fluorescent immunoassay.
*Enzyme discussed in detail in the text.

Enzyme-Multiplied Immunoassay Technique

EMIT, the first homogeneous EIA, was developed by Rubenstein (1972). The EMIT system is illustrated in Figure 44-15. In EMIT, the conjugation of enzymes to haptens does not disrupt enzyme activity; however, the binding of hapten-specific antibodies to haptens results in inhibition of enzyme activity. Free haptens in the standard or sample relieve this inhibition by competing for antibodies. Thus, in the presence of antibodies, enzyme activity is proportional to the concentration of free haptens. As a general rule, the antibody inhibits the enzyme by inducing or preventing conformational changes necessary for enzyme activity (Rowley, 1975). The exception to this inhibition mechanism is the EMIT thyroxine assay, which uses malate dehydrogenase. In this assay, the thyroxine-malate dehydrogenase conjugate is enzymatically inactive, but it becomes activated when it is bound by thyroxine antibody (Ullman, 1979). It is believed that conjugated thyroxine inhibits the enzyme by binding to the active site, thus increasing the "apparent" K_m of the substrate. The antibody reactivates the enzyme by "pulling" the thyroxine out of the active site. In the EMIT assay system, malate dehydrogenase and glucose-6-phosphate dehydrogenase have been found to be most useful because they are less likely to be affected by serum constituents. These assays generally measure drugs at a concentration of milligrams per liter. However, the digoxin assay has a much lower limit of sensitivity in the range of 0.8–2 µg/L.

Substrate-Labeled Fluorescent Immunoassay

The substrate-labeled fluorescent immunoassay (SLFIA) (Burd, 1977) uses a characteristic fluorogenic substrate, umbelliferyl β-galactoside, attached to the antigen (analyte) as a conjugate. Umbelliferone is the fluorescent product produced when the substrate is cleaved with the enzyme β-galactosidase, which cannot cleave the substrate–antigen complex when it is reacted with the specific antibody. The free antigen (analyte) in the specimen solution competes with the antigen conjugated with the substrate to form the immunocomplex (Fig. 44-16). The antigen concentration in the sample is proportional to the fluorescent intensity of the cleaved fluorescent product. SLFIA can be used to assay drugs and haptens, as well as protein ligands such as IgG and IgM. A disadvantage of this method is that the amplification properties of the enzyme are not utilized, and thus the assay system has limited sensitivity in the range of 10^{-9}–10^{-10} molar concentration of the analyte.

Apoenzyme Reactivation Immunoassay

The apoenzyme reactivation immunoassay (ARIS) is a homogeneous assay developed by Morris (1981) using the prosthetic group consisting of flavin adenine dinucleotide (FAD)-conjugated antigen (analyte) and glucose oxidase apoenzyme. As shown in Figure 44-17, the antigen (analyte) and a constant amount of analyte–FAD conjugate compete for a limited amount of specific antibody. At equilibrium, the level of free conjugate is proportional to the amount of antigen (analyte) in the specimen. The apoenzyme combines with the free but not with the antibody-bound form of conjugate to reactivate glucose oxidase activity in proportion to the amount of free conjugate in the mixture. Active enzyme is generated in the procedure, and an amplification mechanism is built into this assay. ARIS has been used to assay for theophylline and IgG (Morris, 1981, 1985). This FAD-labeled conjugate assay is readily adapted to the measurement of high molecular weight proteins (e.g., thyroid binding globulin) (Schroeder, 1985), as well as other haptens such as phenytoin and hormones.

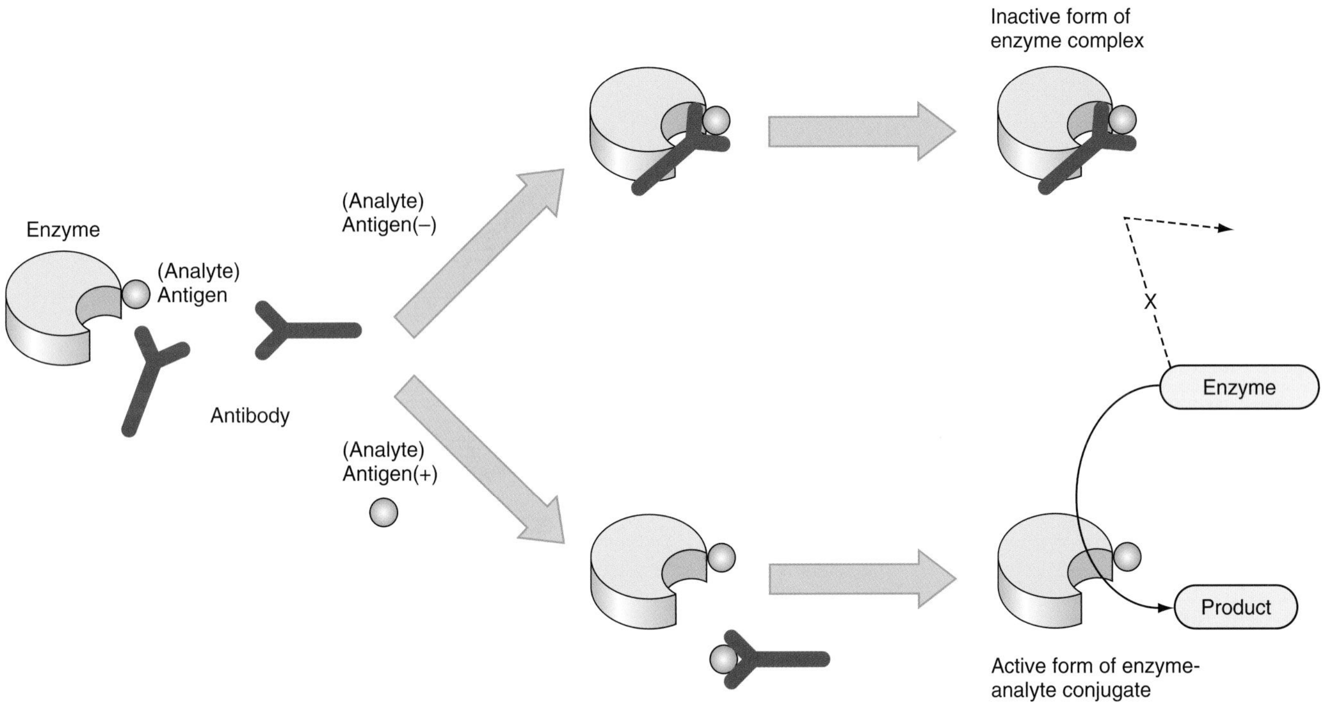

Figure 44-15 Enzyme-multiplied immunoassay technique (EMIT) system diagram: The activity of an enzyme as a label is inhibited by the binding of antibody to antigen (analyte) conjugated with enzyme. The analyte is usually a hapten. Glucose-6-phosphate dehydrogenase (G6PD) and lysozyme are usually used as enzymes. In the assay, enzyme activity is proportional to the concentration of the analyte. *(With permission from Nakamura RM, Kasahara Y, Rechnitz GA, editors. Immunochemical assays and biosensor technology for the 1990s. Washington, DC: American Society for Microbiology; 1992.)*

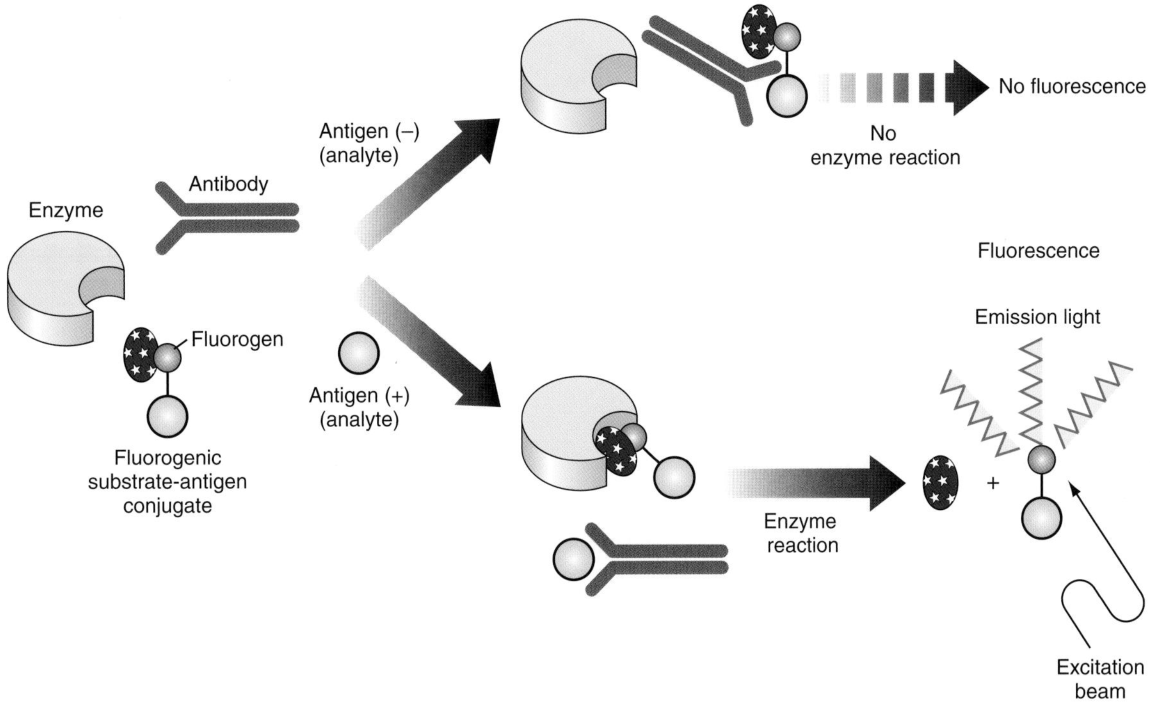

Figure 44-16 Substrate-labeled fluorescent immunoassay (SLFIA). The substrate β-galactosylumbeliferone is conjugated with the antigen (analyte) and forms a nonfluorescent substrate. The substrate can be cleaved by the enzyme β-galactosidase to form a fluorescent product. However, when the substrate–antigen conjugate is allowed to react with specific antibody to the antigen, no cleavage of the substrate complex with the β-galactosidase enzyme occurs. In this assay, the concentration of the antigen (analyte) is directly proportional to the fluorescent intensity measured. *(With permission from Nakamura RM, Kasahara Y, Rechnitz GA, editors. Immunochemical assays and biosensor technology for the 1990s. Washington, DC: American Society for Microbiology, ASM Press; 1992.)*

Enzyme Inhibitory Homogeneous Immunoassay

The enzyme inhibitory homogeneous immunoassay (EIHIA), developed by Ashihara (1988), consists of antibody conjugated with enzyme and insoluble substrate. This assay is most suitable for the determination of large antigens (analytes). The EIHIA can be made to be homogeneous because the immunocomplex of conjugate with large antigen blocks the enzyme reaction with the solid substrate (Fig. 44-18). α-Amylase has been used as a labeled enzyme for the determination of ferritin and AFP. The immunoreaction of analyte with enzyme-labeled antibody can reach a plateau within 10 minutes; thus, EIHIA based on a noncompetitive binding assay requires less incubation time to achieve a sensitive detection level. Using this method, the measuring range of ferritin in serum is 10–800 ng/mL,

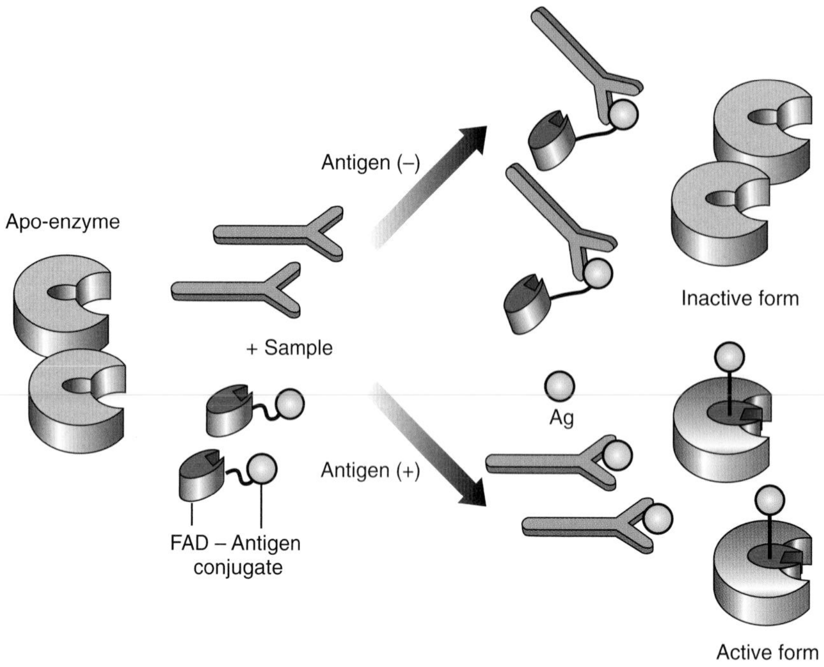

Figure 44-17 Apoenzyme reactivation immunoassay (ARIS). Flavin adenine dinucleotide (FAD) attached to the antigen is used. The apoenzyme is apoglucose oxidase, which requires FAD cofactor for activity. In the assay, the concentration of antigen (analyte) is proportional to the enzyme activity generated. *(With permission from Nakamura RM, Kasahara Y, Rechnitz GA, editors. Immunochemical assays and biosensor technology for the 1990s. Washington, DC: American Society for Microbiology; 1992.)*

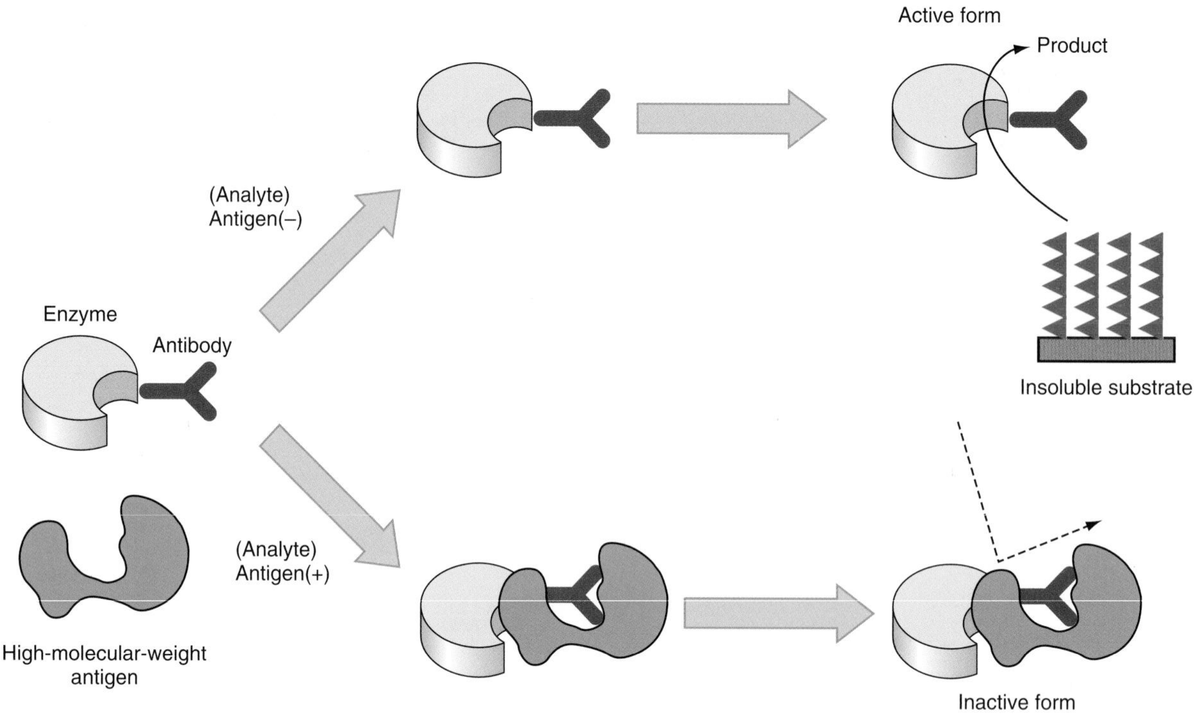

Figure 44-18 Enzyme inhibitory homogeneous immunoassay (EIHIA). The enzyme α-amylase from *Bacillus subtilis* or dextranase from *Chaetomium gracile* is conjugated to the specific antibody to the high-molecular-weight antigen. The high-molecular-weight antigen can be ferritin or α-fetoprotein. The α-amylase enzyme is inactive when the enzyme antibody conjugate reacts with specific antibody. The active enzyme form can react with the starch-insoluble substrate. The antigen concentration is directly proportional to the enzyme activity of the assay reaction. *(With permission from Nakamura RM, Kasahara Y, Rechnitz GA, editors. Immunochemical assays and biosensor technology for the 1990s. Washington, DC: American Society for Microbiology; 1992.)*

and for AFP it is 5–200 ng/mL. Dextranase has been used as an alternative enzyme (Nishizono, 1988). EIHIA has also been applied to a simple dry-film format (Ashihara, 1991). The dry film consists of three major layers, each containing a developing zone for immunologic and enzymatic reaction, a barrier zone, and a color-developing zone. An inhibitor specific to human amylase present in serum is used to prevent serum background. The assay for serum C-reactive protein is completed in only 6 minutes by simply placing the specimen on the slide using dry chemistry instrumentation. Nevertheless, the sensitivity of the system remains inadequate for application to analytes such as tumor markers.

Cloned Enzyme Donor Immunoassay

The cloned enzyme donor immunoassay was first achieved through the application of recombinant DNA technology to homogeneous

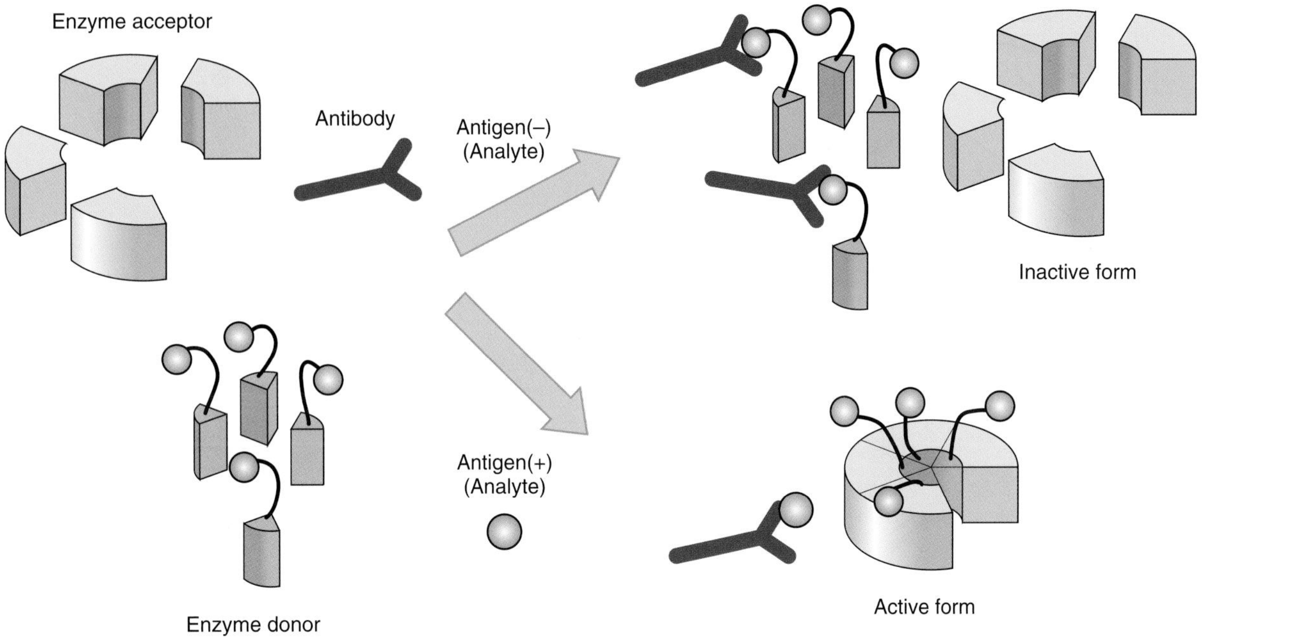

Figure 44-19 Cloned enzyme donor immunoassay (CEDIA). Enzyme acceptors associate with enzyme donors to form an active β-galactosidase tetramer. The antibody inhibits the association of enzyme acceptor with enzyme donor–antigen conjugate. *(With permission from Nakamura RM, Kasahara Y, Rechnitz GA, editors. Immunochemical assay and biosensor technology for the 1990s. Washington, DC: American Society for Microbiology; 1992.)*

PART 6

immunoassays by Henderson (1986). Microgenics Corp. (Concord, Calif.) was able to engineer β-galactosidase protein into a large polypeptide (an enzyme acceptor [EA]) and a small polypeptide (an enzyme donor [ED]). EAs and EDs assemble to form enzymatically active tetramers. In the assay (Fig. 44-19), a hapten antigen (analyte) is attached to an ED, and an analyte-specific antibody is used to inhibit spontaneous assembly of the active enzyme. The antigens (analytes) in patient serum compete with the analytes in the analyte–ED conjugate for antibody, modulating the amount of active β-galactosidase formed. The signal generated by enzyme substrates is directly proportional to the analyte concentration in the patient serum. The test for digoxin is a colorimetric assay that requires no serum pretreatment or predilution. The assay system is suitable for use with automated chemistry analyzers.

SUMMARY

EIAs can be applied to all Ag–Ab systems, including those involving serum protein, hormones, drugs, and other antigens and the antibodies directed against pathogens. Heterogeneous EIAs using chromogenic substrates can have a sensitivity comparable with that of RIAs, and they have gained wide acceptance for application in various immunoassays. Heterogeneous EIAs using sophisticated substrates that generate chemiluminescent light and small particles as the solid phase are sensitive enough to detect less than 1 pg/mL of analytes. Their sensitivity is thus much higher than that of RIAs. In addition, the assay manipulation is greatly simplified by fully automated instruments. Compared with heterogeneous EIAs, homogeneous EIAs have certain limitations in sensitivity, dynamic range, and large analyte application. Also, high background signals (noise) and relatively low assay signals are inevitable because of elimination of the washing steps for the separation of bound and free conjugates. Homogeneous EIAs are advantageous because they are based on a simple assay format and can be adapted to existing automatic instrumentation. At this time, heterogeneous EIAs with fully automated instruments remain the best choice in terms of sensitivity and simplicity, as well as for safety reasons, because they do not require the use of radioisotopes.

FLUORESCENT IMMUNOASSAY

BACKGROUND AND CLASSIFICATION

Coons (1941) first introduced the use of fluorescent compounds as immunochemical labels to detect antigens in tissue sections. Immunofluorescence assays on tissue sections are currently very well established in the pathology laboratory. Over the past several years, many FIA procedures have been developed to detect the concentrations of drugs, hormones, and a wide variety of proteins and polypeptides (Nakamura, 1992). In the initial stages of development, analytic FIAs were hindered by a decrease in sensitivity caused by background fluorescence of biological samples. Gradually, the sensitivity of fluorometric methods improved, and detection of analytes at concentrations of 10^{-15} M became possible. Further advancements were achieved through improvements in instrumentation and the introduction of unique substrates with various immunochemical and enzymatic reactions.

Selection of the fluorochrome label is important. The label should be stable and should demonstrate high molar extinction coefficiency and quantum yield. It should also emit at appropriate wavelengths without interference with ligand–antibody reactions. When most fluorophores or fluorescent molecules are irradiated with light at appropriate wavelengths, an electron in the ground state is transited into the excited state of the molecule. As the electron returns to the ground state, physical energy is released in the form of a photon of lower energy (longer wavelength) than the exciting light. The fluorescence spectrum reveals a wavelength of maximal emission, characteristic of a particular fluorescent compound. One of the typical labels, fluorescein isothiocyanate (FITC), has a less than 1 nanosecond time interval between excitation and emission, whereas other compounds (e.g., europium) exhibit delayed fluorescence with an interval of several hundred nanoseconds. The various FIAs may be classified as follows: (1) heterogeneous and homogeneous, (2) ligand or antibody labeled, (3) competitive or noncompetitive, and (4) solid or nonsolid phase. The most common methods are discussed here.

HETEROGENEOUS FLUORESCENT IMMUNOASSAY

Heterogeneous FIA procedures include a washing step to separate bound from free fluorescent labels. The assay procedure is similar to that of heterogeneous enzyme immunoassays and RIAs. Most commercially available assays use a solid-phase antigen or antibody system. The assay can be competitive or noncompetitive—a property shared by RIAs and EIAs.

FLUOROIMMUNOMETRIC METHOD

With the fluoroimmunometric method, the analyte reacts with excess labeled antibodies in the solution. Residual labeled antibodies bind to excess solid-phase bound antigens. The solid-phase matrix is washed, and

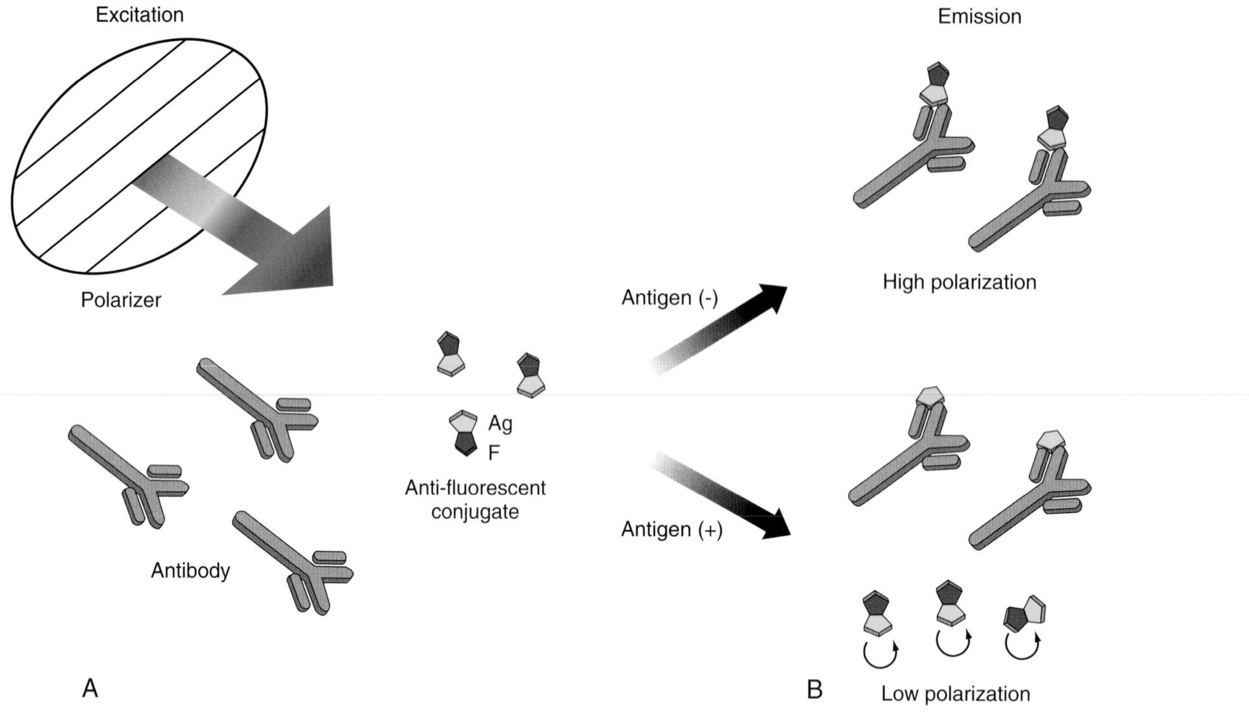

Figure 44-20 Assay principle of fluorescence polarization immunoassay (FPIA). **A,** A polarized beam can excite both an unbound conjugate and the conjugate bound to antibody (Ab) existing at the same angle as the irradiating beam. The conjugate consists of hapten (H) with a fluorescent molecule (F). **B,** Orientation of the molecules at the time of fluorescence emission. Small hapten conjugates free of antibody can quickly change their orientation and emit fluorescence at different angles that is not detected. However, the conjugate bound to the antibody still remains at the same angle because of its very slow movement, and it emits fluorescence that is detected.

fluorescence intensity is inversely related to the analyte concentration. This method can be adapted to the assay of haptens and complex proteins. Solid-phase FIA procedures were developed for the serologic assay of antibodies to rubella, toxoplasmosis, viral antigens, and antinuclear antibodies. Heterogeneous FIA methods for antigen determination were developed for serum proteins and hormones, including immunoglobulins, cortisol, progesterone, and thyroxine. The major advantage of heterogeneous FIAs is the significant reduction in interference by naturally fluorescent substances in patient samples, caused by the physical removal of interference factors during the separation step.

RADIAL PARTITION IMMUNOFLUOROMETRIC ASSAY

In radial partition immunoassays, radial chromatography is used and the assay is carried out on glass-fiber filter papers (Giegel, 1982). This procedure has been automated for the assay of hCG and several other analytes in serum (Rogers, 1986).

TIME-RESOLVED FLUOROIMMUNOASSAY

This method makes use of special instrumentation and fluorescent labels to increase assay sensitivity. It involves the use of fluorescent labels exhibiting delayed fluorescence with a time period of 100 ns or longer between excitation and emission. Because most substances responsible for background fluorescence have a short decay period, measurement of the delayed fluorescence signal will significantly reduce the effects of background fluorescence. This is accomplished with the time-resolved fluorometer, a special instrument that produces a fast light pulse that excites the fluorophore. Fluorescence is measured a little while after excitation. Thus, the effect of nonspecific background, which generally decays in less than 10 nanoseconds, can be removed (Halonen, 1973; Soini, 1983). Fluorophores exhibiting delayed fluorescence that have been used in these assays include (Soini, 1979) the following:

- Pyrene derivatives with a decay time of almost 100 ns
- Rare earth metal chelate labels with a very long decay time of almost 50–100 μs. These include europium (Eu^{3+}), samarium (Sm^{3+}), and terbium (Tb^{3+}).
- Time-resolved fluoroimmunoassays have been developed to measure many analytes, including hCG, IgG, cortisol, insulin, and others.

HOMOGENEOUS FLUORESCENT IMMUNOASSAY

By definition, these immunoassays are performed on homogeneous specimen samples. They do not require the separation of bound from free conjugates and usually are not sensitive to background interference in the samples. Homogeneous FIAs also have the advantage of being quick to perform. However, when compared with heterogeneous assays, they show certain disadvantages. Homogeneous FIAs have a limited sensitivity near 10^{-10} m/L with standard instrumentation. Labeled impurities in the sample may increase background interference. The assays require relatively pure labeled antigen or specific antibody, as well as special instrumentation, to achieve higher sensitivity.

FLUORESCENCE POLARIZATION ASSAY

A polarizing lens or prism can resolve light into rays in a single plane. When viewed at the right angle of an excitation beam of vertically polarized light, fluorescent compounds in solutions emit partially polarized fluorescence. The fluorescence polarization principle was first applied to immunoassay procedures by Dandliker (1970, 1973). Polarized light transmitted through the sample can excite the fluorescent label, regardless of binding to antibody. However, as shown in Figure 44-20, random thermal motion causes small molecules labeled with a hapten to tumble freely in solution, losing their polarized orientation. When the labeled antigen is bound to antibody with a molecular mass greater than 160 kDa, the molecular motion is slowed enough to increase the polarized signal.

Studies using labeled antibody or antibody fragments showed no change in polarization upon mixing antigen and labeled antibody, even though immunoreaction had occurred. This method is most useful for the measurement of small antigens and haptens (Jolley, 1981). Abbott Laboratories has adapted this approach for the assay of many therapeutic and abused drugs on the TDx (Abbott Diagnostics, Abbott Park, IL). They developed a next generation analyzer, the IMx, to measure molecules with large masses such as tumor markers, hormones, and infection-related antigens or antibodies (Fiore, 1988). They combined two assay principles—fluorescence polarization and microparticle enzyme immunoassay. The demand for random access capabilities led Abbott to develop a fully automated, high-throughput random access analyzer named the AXSYM. This system is being used in clinical laboratories (Smith, 1993).

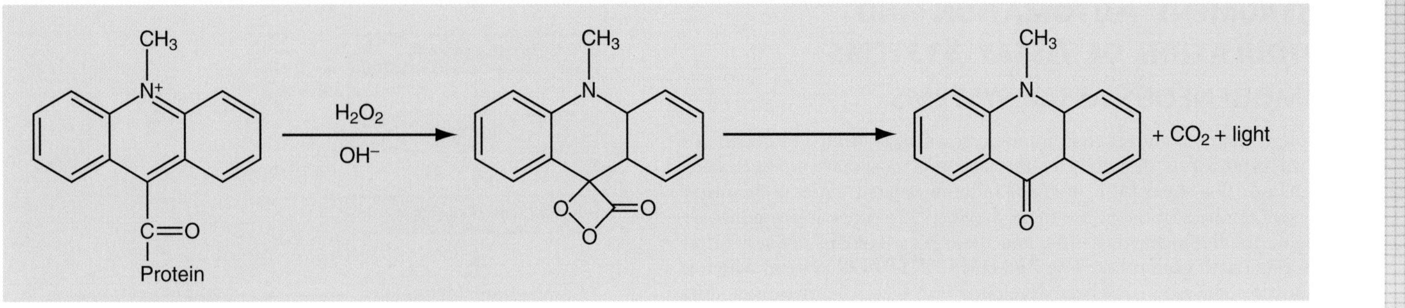

Figure 44-21 Chemiluminescent immunoassay mechanism with acridinium ester based on oxidative decomposition.

FLUORESCENCE EXCITATION TRANSFER IMMUNOASSAY

The fluorescence excitation transfer (FETI) method (Ullman, 1976) uses two labels: fluorescein as the donor fluorescent label and rhodamine as the acceptor or quencher. FITC has a maximum emission of 525 nm, and tetraethylrhodamine has a strong absorption peak at 525 nm. Therefore, when FITC-labeled antigen and rhodamine-labeled antibody bind, quenching of FITC fluorescence occurs. This phenomenon involves an energy transfer from an electronically excited fluorescent dye to an acceptor dye. The rate of energy transfer is inversely proportional to the sixth power of the distance between donor and acceptor molecules. For adequate reduction of fluorescence with quenching, the donor–acceptor distance between labels should be about 50–70 Å. This method is useful for the assay of antigen with multivalent antigenic determinants. Separate portions of specific antibody are labeled with fluorescein and rhodamine. The mixture of differently labeled fluorescein-tagged antibody and rhodamine-labeled antibody reduces the intensity of the fluorescein label by adjusting the ratio and amount of donor and acceptor molecules, so that they can react in close proximity to permit energy transfer. These problems have been overcome using new fluorescent compounds. The FETI method has been improved with the use of a fluorescence marker such as europium (III) (Eu[III]) trisbipyridine cryptate as a donor, and a fluorophore such as allopycocyanin as an acceptor (Alpha, 1987; Mathis, 1995). These transient compounds reveal a large Stokes shift in which the excited europium at 337 nm transfers energy through an acceptor molecule at an excitation of 620 nm and eventually emits fluorescent light at 665 nm, as in the time-resolved mode. Mathis (1993) has developed the fluorescence resonance energy transfer using cryptate-chelating rare metal and has applied it to the detection of AFP and carcinoembryonic antigen (CEA) in serum. CIS Bio International (Ceze, France) developed an automated homogeneous immunoassay system, KRYPTOR, for the detection of cancer markers such as CEA, CA 19-9, CA 125, and AFP, using the time-resolved amplified cryptate emission. The sensitivity for AFP was 0.25 ng/mL for 9 minutes' incubation.

FLUORESCENT PROTECTION IMMUNOASSAY

In this assay (Nargessi, 1979), the protein antigen is labeled with fluorescein and then is reacted with specific antibody to the antigen. The antigen-specific antibody will sterically inhibit the reaction of a second antibody specific to fluorescein, which functions to quench the fluorescence of fluorescein when it binds to the fluorophore. The ability of the specific anti-fluorescein antibody to interact with fluorescein coupled to the surface of the antigen will decrease. The procedure may be used to assay for antibody concentration or for antigen (analyte) concentration in a homogeneous system.

Chemiluminescent Immunoassay

BACKGROUND

Chemiluminescent immunoassays (CLIAs) use chemiluminescence-generating molecules as labels, such as luminol derivatives, acridinium esters, or nitrophenyl oxalate derivatives and ruthenium tri-bipridyl [$Ru(bpy)_3^{2+}$] with tripropylamine for electrochemiluminescence. Basically, the assay method does not differ from that of heterogeneous immunoassays, RIAs, and FIAs. Light generation of luminol derivatives requires OH^-/H_2O_2 as a chemical trigger or H_2O_2 with peroxidase as an enhanced chemiluminescent trigger. Acridinium esters chemically triggered with OH^-/H_2O_2 display a relatively high chemiluminescent quantum yield for light emission compared with luminol. Other chemiluminescent molecules include aequorin, a natural compound (Actor, 1998). Labels of chemiluminescent compounds produce light electrochemically on the surface of electrodes and can be applied to homogeneous assay formats. Both CLIAs using acridinium esters and electro-CLIAs are applicable for practical diagnostic testing. Their characteristics are described in the following section.

CHEMILUMINESCENT IMMUNOASSAY USING ACRIDINIUM ESTERS AS LABELS

In this method (Weeks, 1983), acridinium esters (Fig. 44-21) are directly conjugated with protein molecules. Acridinium esters can oxidatively react with H_2O_2 under alkaline conditions to produce high-energy intermediates that decompose to the excited fragment, generating light. The light emission of acridinium esters is extremely fast, within 5–10 seconds after initiation of the oxidation reaction. Flash-type chemiluminescence, as this process is called, has a much steeper spectrum of light emission to reactive time than glow-type chemiluminescence triggered by enzymes. The sensitivity of this assay is higher than that of RIA, and testing is less time consuming. The solubility of acridinium esters and the stability of conjugates with proteins in storage have been improved through modification of the molecule and conjugation chemistry. This technology is likely to bring improvements in the assay of haptens, such as hormones.

ELECTROCHEMILUMINESCENT IMMUNOASSAY

Electrochemiluminescent immunoassay (ECLIA) uses electrochemical compounds that generate light electrochemically, linked with the cycle reaction of the oxidative reduction. With optimization of reaction solutions, selection of appropriate conjugation method, and development of suitable compounds such as $Ru(bpy)_3^{2+}$ and TPA, it became possible to apply electrochemiluminescent technology to immunoassays (Blackburn, 1991). $Ru(bpy)_3^{2+}$ has a reaction site for the conjugation of analytes using activation reagent such as NHS. $Ru(bpy)_3^{2+}$, thus conjugated with antibodies, can be applied to sandwich-type assays for large molecules. The conjugate generates light on the surface of gold electrodes. $Ru(bpy)_3^{2+}$ on solid phase and TPA are oxidized on the surface of electrodes to form $Ru(bpy)_3^{2+}$ and TPA^+, respectively. TPA^+ spontaneously loses electrons. $Ru(bpy)_3^{3+}$ can generate emission light at 620 nm when it returns to $Ru(bpy)_3^{2+}$ as a ground state through reduction with TPA. The efficiency of light generation (quantum yield) depends on the proximity between the electrode and the conjugate, and thereby on the diffusion mobility of the conjugate. Free conjugates can generate more light than conjugates fixed on the solid phase as a result of immunoreaction. This allows easy access to the homogeneous assay format, but relatively high background noise interferes with assay sensitivity, as it does in other homogeneous assays. The assay protocol for the determination of analytes is as follows: Magnetic microparticles coated with antibody as the solid phase and sample mix together for immunoreaction. After washing for bound and free conjugates by magnetic separation according to the assay format, the solid-phase suspension is introduced into the detector with the electrode to measure chemiluminescence. The detection limit of ECLIAs has been reported as 0.2–0.4 ng/mL for CEA and 0.4 ng/mL for AFP. This assay does not require complicated instruments. A further advantage is that ECLIAs requires less time for signal detection, similar to FIAs and other CLIAs.

PART 6

Instrument Automation and Modulation of Assay Systems

HOMOGENEOUS ASSAY SYSTEMS

Although many homogeneous immunoassays have been developed for manual protocol as described in this chapter, most have not yet been automated. For the EMIT method, fully automated generic chemistry analyzers can be adapted to use these (Boyd, 1985). A few instruments are available for homogeneous FIAs, and these assay systems are not interchangeable with each other. The BRAHMS KRYPTOR system, which is the most recent system, has been developed with special features, including the use of a time-resolved fluorescence detector. It uses a two-wavelength method for internal standard correction of fluorescence intensity at 620 nm and 665 nm, making it possible to increase the sensitivity of the detection limit.

HETEROGENEOUS IMMUNOASSAY SYSTEMS

Until the early 1980s, most heterogeneous labeled immunoassays were manually performed. Then Boehringer Mannheim (which merged with Roche Diagnostics in 1998) developed a fully automated random access analyzer, the ES-600, based on colorimetric enzyme immunoassays, using horseradish peroxidase as the enzyme (Wu, 1987). From the late 1980s onward, many companies endeavored to develop fully automated EIA systems, which were high-throughput, sensitive, randomly accessible systems. Antigens associated with early onset of infectious disease, cytokines, growth factors, and hormones such as calcitonin exist at extremely low concentrations in serum, thus requiring a highly sensitive detection method for measuring these analytes (Nishizono, 1991; Isomura, 1994, 1999). Among the various methods, chemiluminescent immunoassays and their enzymes are the most sensitive assay systems capable of detecting analytes present at very low concentrations.

The fully automated instruments currently available are also capable of using fluorescent enzyme immunoassays. These assay systems are classified into several groups based on the generation and detection of signals and the type of solid phase. With respect to the detection signal, the AIA1200, 600 (Toso, Tokyo, Japan) and the AxSYM (Abbott, Abbott Park, Ind.) employ a fluorescent method of the EIA that uses alkaline phosphatase and a specific substrate, 4-methylumbelliferylphosphate. Three types of systems are available for chemiluminescent enzyme immunoassays. Lumipulse (Fujirebio, Tokyo, Japan), Access (Sanofi, Caska, Minn.), and Immulite (Diagnostic Products Corporation, Los Angeles) have used a stable chemiluminescent substrate, phenyl phosphoryl adamantyl dioxetane, for alkaline phosphatase (Babson, 1991; Nishizono, 1991; Patterson, 1994). Acridinium ester as a chemiluminescent label was applied to the ACS 180 (Bayer Diagnostics, Tarrytown, N.Y.) and later to the Centaur (Siemens, Tarrytown, N.Y.) In the ELECSYS 2010 (Roche Diagnostics, Indianapolis), $Ru(bpy)_3^{2+}$ is used as an electrochemiluminescent label (Erler, 1998).

PRACTICAL FLOW OF THE IMMUNOASSAY IN THE ANALYTIC SYSTEM

The market demands that instrumentation be able to perform a large number of tests with random access capability. To meet these criteria, it is necessary to improve reagents and avoid tediousness in performing heterogeneous immunoassays. To simplify the system for application in a fully automated assay system, individual cartridges of prepackaged reagents or predispensed reaction cuvette reagents were designed. A generic system for heterogeneous labeled immunoassays is depicted schematically in Figure 44-22. The operator selects the desired test items by means of a computer program and loads reagent cartridges or bottles for each test. For a particular analyte, the cartridges and the reaction cuvette are fed automatically into the instrument. Samples are transported to the appropriate position for dispensing. The assay is designed to use reaction trays or carousels that automate mixing and separation steps that depend on performance through first and second immunoreactions and the signal generation reaction. All steps of the assay are carried out sequentially on the reaction line, and the signals generated are measured by a detector. Test results are printed out within 20–40 minutes and are sent automatically online to the host computer. The system can treat about 60–200 tests per hour, processing 10–20 analytes in each sample specimen by the random access manner.

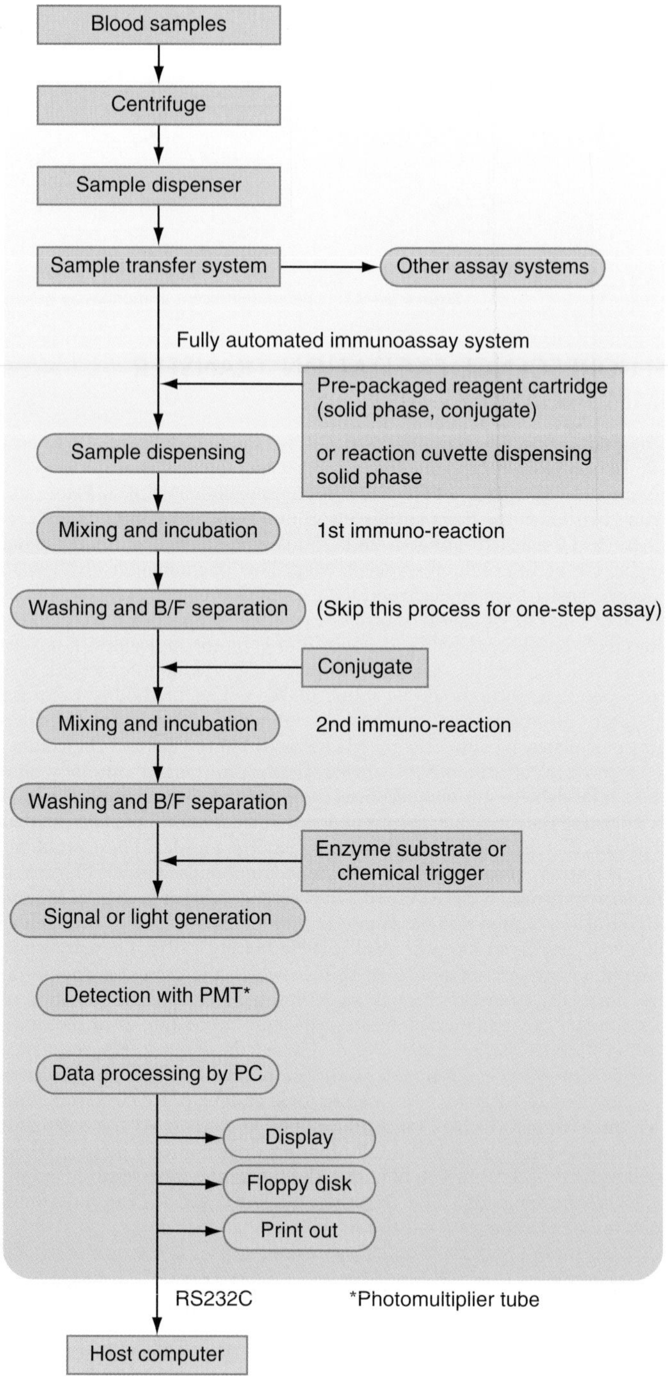

Figure 44-22 Brief diagram of fully automated immunoassay system in clinical laboratory automation.

INSTRUMENTATION AND KEY POINTS FOR THE HETEROGENEOUS IMMUNOASSAY

Although the assay principle is similar in many instruments, big differences among instruments may be noted with respect to sampling format, heating control, B/F separation, carryover, waste flow, and so forth. Thus we should pay attention to how well the instrument performs after implementation.

Reaction Cuvette

In an immunoassay system, the design of cuvette features is very important to obtain reproducible data. Manufacturers use certain types of cuvettes to

TABLE 44-8
New Generation of Heterogeneous Immunoassay Systems

	AIA-21, Tosoh	ACS: Centaur, Bayer Diagnostics	ARCHITECT i2000, Abbott	Lumipulse Presto II, Fujirebio	Cobas e411 Roche
Package of reagent	Freeze-drying in portion package	Reagent pack (solution)	Solution in bottle	Solution in bottle	Reagent pack (solution)
Reaction cuvette	Reagent cup	Disposable cuvette	Disposable cuvette	Disposable cuvette	Disposable cuvette
Reaction principle	Fluorescent enzyme immunoassay	Chemiluminescent immunoassay	Chemiluminescent immunoassay	Chemiluminescent enzyme immunoassay	Electro-chemiluminescent immunoassay
Labeled substance	Alkaline phosphatase	Acridinium ester	Acridinium ester	Alkaline phosphatase	Ruthenium
Enzyme substrate	4-Methylumbelliferyl phosphate	None	None	Adamantyl 1.2-dioxetane phenyl phosphate	—
Detector signal	Fluorescence	Chemiluminescence	Chemiluminescence	Chemiluminescence	Chemiluminescence
Assay format	S-1, S-2, competitive	S-1, S-2, competitive	S-1, S-2, competitive	S-1, S-2, competitive; delayed S-1	S-1, S-2, competitive; delayed backtitration
Pretreatment	Yes	Yes	Yes	Yes	Yes
Reaction flow	Turn table	Turn table	Turn table	Turn table	Turn table
Cycle time, seconds	30	15	18	15	42
Reaction time, minutes	10 or 40	7.5–36	29	20	9, 18, 27
Reaction temperature	37° C	37° C	37° C	37° C	37° C
Maximum analyte number	20	30	25	36	18
Throughput, tests/hour	120	240	200	240	86
Solid phase	Magnetic bead	Magnetic particle	Magnetic particle	Magnetic particle	Magnetic particle
First result time, minutes	50	8–40	15/29	32	9
B/F separation	Magnetic field	Magnetic field	Magnetic field	Magnetic field	Magnetic field
Sampling method	Pipetting probe	Disposable chip	Fixed probe	Disposable chip	Disposable chip
Sample auto dilution	Yes	Yes	Yes	Yes	Yes

B/F, Bound over free.

achieve easy access and rapid handling of reagents. An all-in-one–type cuvette containing the reagents and the reaction cell has been introduced in the Lumipulse system. The Immulite system utilizes a unique reaction cell for B/F separation. The AxSYM (Abbott) uses another unique reaction vessel consisting of a reagent, an incubation well, and a sample well within a cuvette for B/F separation. The system combines the content of this assay cuvette into a matrix cell. The latter can be used to capture the solid latex phase followed by B/F separation and the second immunoreaction of the labeled antibody and the solid phase.

Sampling and Fluid Delivery Type

In general, fluid delivery is selected from two different types: a disposable chip or a fixed probe nozzle. Cross-contamination of samples should be avoided in all assay systems. The disposable chip can completely prevent cross-contamination. In the case of the fixed probe system, even though the original sample is divided into several small aliquots, cross-contamination still occurs. Therefore, the disposable chip system is the best way to avoid cross-contamination and to minimize biohazardous waste. On the other hand, the running cost of using chips for the assay is higher than that of the probe assay. Environmental effects of the disposable chips must be considered.

Carryover

Carryover from an extremely high concentration of analyte in one sample to the next sample sometimes causes misjudgment in clinical diagnosis. A disposable plastic tube is the simplest way to prevent this problem. On the other hand, the fixed probe nozzle has several cost advantages, as mentioned earlier. Thus, most of the technologies concerned with sample engineering have focused on minimizing sample carryover through washing and tip maintenance steps. Now, several fixed probe tips have made it possible to limit carryover to less than the order of 10^{-7}. Even with such low carryover, some samples still create problems (e.g., a hepatitis B surface antigen [HBsAg] strong positive sample followed by a negative). In this case, a software system can be used to check the subsequent result by automatically retesting weakly positive values following strong positive results.

Bound/Fixed Separation and Washing Systems

In a heterogeneous immunoassay, the bound conjugate has to be separated from the free label. This B/F separation depends on the characteristics of the solid phase. The IMx and AxSYM systems use latex microparticles as the solid phase and employ a porous membrane to entrap the latex for separation of particles of the solid phase from particles of the liquid phase. The Diagnostics Product Corporation has developed a unique cell for B/F separation systems, in which the reaction solution spins out from an inner cell to an outer waste cell, while the bound phase stays in a solid-phase bead (¼-inch bead). Advantages of this format are the avoidance of cross-contamination or carryover from one reaction mixture to the next and the fact that no excess washing process is required. All other systems use magnetic particles and magnetic beads, for which easy and rapid separation can be achieved by applying a magnetic field.

NEW SYSTEMS FOR THE NEXT GENERATION (MODULAR SYSTEMS)

Table 44-8 compares several of the commercial high-throughput immunoassay systems that have been introduced in the past few years. It shows the instrument specifications of each analyzer. By reducing the incubation and reaction times, a rapid result can be obtained in 10–25 minutes. Thus a high-throughput machine performing 120–200 tests/hour is possible. Furthermore, several manufacturers have demonstrated a new system concept that aligns the different analytic systems needed in a clinical laboratory. Many clinical laboratories have introduced an automated sample transporting line, which is connected to different analytic instruments controlled independently. However, several analyzers are not amenable to this approach because the speed of the instrument throughput or cycle time cannot be harmonized easily. To solve these problems, ARCHITECT (Abbott Laboratories) is an example of a new machine concept in which one system computer can control several immunoassay analyzers connected to one chemistry analyzer. Several other combinations still under development are based on this concept, which will make it possible to simplify the clinical laboratory and to lower total assay cost.

Rapid and Simple Test Devices for Point-of-Care Testing

BACKGROUND

A strong demand for a home test (e.g., hCG for pregnancy diagnosis) has simplified the immunoassay format: The test must be simple, rapid, and reproducible. With these goals in mind, many hCG tests have been developed and have resulted in the first-generation test format with a flow-through enzyme immunoassay.

FLOW-THROUGH ASSAY DEVICES (IMMUNOFILTRATION ASSAY DEVICES)

Figure 44-23 illustrates schematically a typical flow-through–type device, the ICON hCG (Hybritech Incorporated, San Diego), which consists of a porous membrane with immobilized anti-hCG antibody and an absorbent pad below the membrane (Valkirs, 1985). The assay principle and the procedure are as follows. Several drops of urine sample are applied to the membrane. Urine is absorbed into the absorbent pad, and washing buffer is applied dropwise, followed by a solution of alkaline phosphatase–labeled anti-hCG antibody.

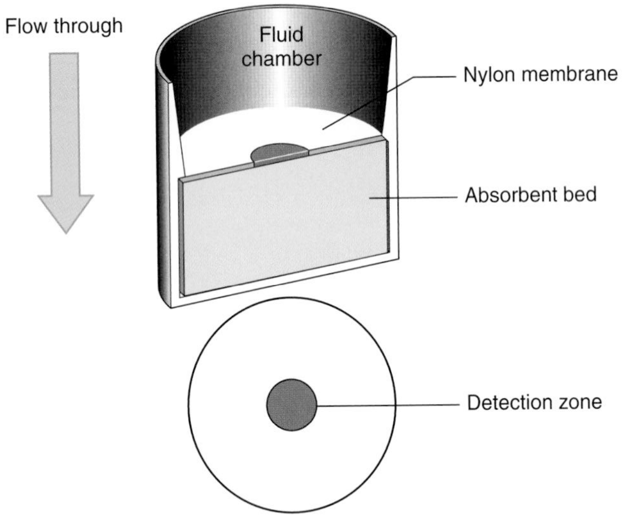

Figure 44-23 Flow-through immunoassay. Cross-section of Hybritech ICON and top view of the device. Capturing antibodies are immobilized at the center of a nylon membrane on which an absorbent bed is set to absorb unreacted sample fluid, labeled conjugate, and washing buffer. The assay can be performed sequentially, similar to a two-step enzyme immunoassay.

DIPPING STRIP

A dipping strip format has also been developed to reduce the cost of materials as compared with the flow-through format. In this format, the test strip contains a spotting area with antibody at one end of the strip. The assay is performed as follows:

- The strip is dipped in a sample cup containing the sample.
- The strip is then dipped in a washing cup.
- The strip is dipped in labeling solution.
- Finally, the strip is dipped in color developer, if needed.

IMMUNOCHROMATOGRAPHIC DEVICES

To eliminate stepwise reagent additions in these two formats, further improvement has been accomplished with the use of immunochromatographic techniques that ensure a simpler and quicker immunoassay. Immunochromatography consists of simultaneous B/F separation and signal generation followed by lateral flow on porous materials such as a nitrocellulose membrane or a glass-fiber sheet. Through the capillary action of the membrane, the analyte in the sample can migrate from the proximal end to the distal end, where an absorbent pad is set to maintain constant capillary flow rate. The sample loading zone, labeling zone, and detection zone are set between the two ends. The immunochromatographic method is classified into several formats. Figure 44-24 shows the typical immunochromatographic formats. The proximal end is employed as the sample loading port connected to a pad containing labeled antigen or antibody, under which a nitrocellulose membrane is in contact with the pad, which serves as a fixed detection zone. The distal end of the membrane is attached to the absorbent pad as a source of capillary force. The sample, loaded by means of a dropper, reconstitutes the conjugate antibody or antigen labeled with colloidal gold or colored latex, which forms an immunocomplex with the analyte being detected, and the complex migrates to the detection zone. The antibody or antigen immobilized in the detection zone can capture the complex and form a positive red or blue line. Excess labeling substance migrates to the absorbent pad. The mobile phase for sample migration is the sample itself. Therefore, samples strongly colored owing to the presence of a high concentration of bilirubin or hemoglobin may

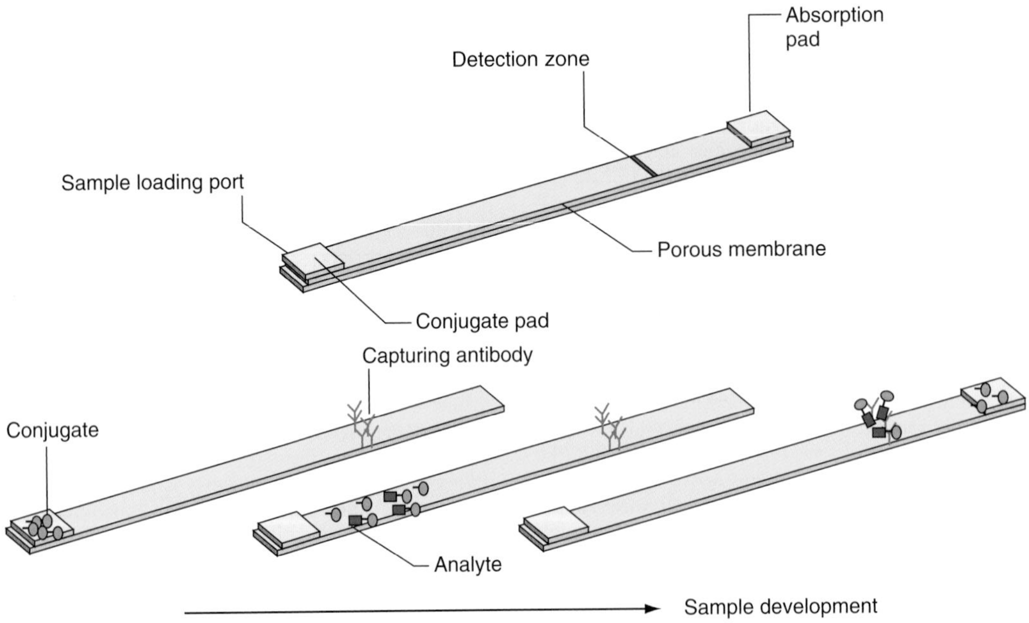

Figure 44-24 Typical immunochromatographic test strip by sample loading. Assay flows are illustrated in the lower part of the figure. In general, the proximal end of the lateral flow serves as the sample loading portion consisting of a pad containing antibody or antigen labeled with colored latex or colloidal gold. Analyte in the sample forms a complex with the conjugate and migrates to the detection zone, thereby immobilizing the capturing antibody to form a positive colored line. Excess amounts of conjugate and sample migrate to the distal end of the strip.

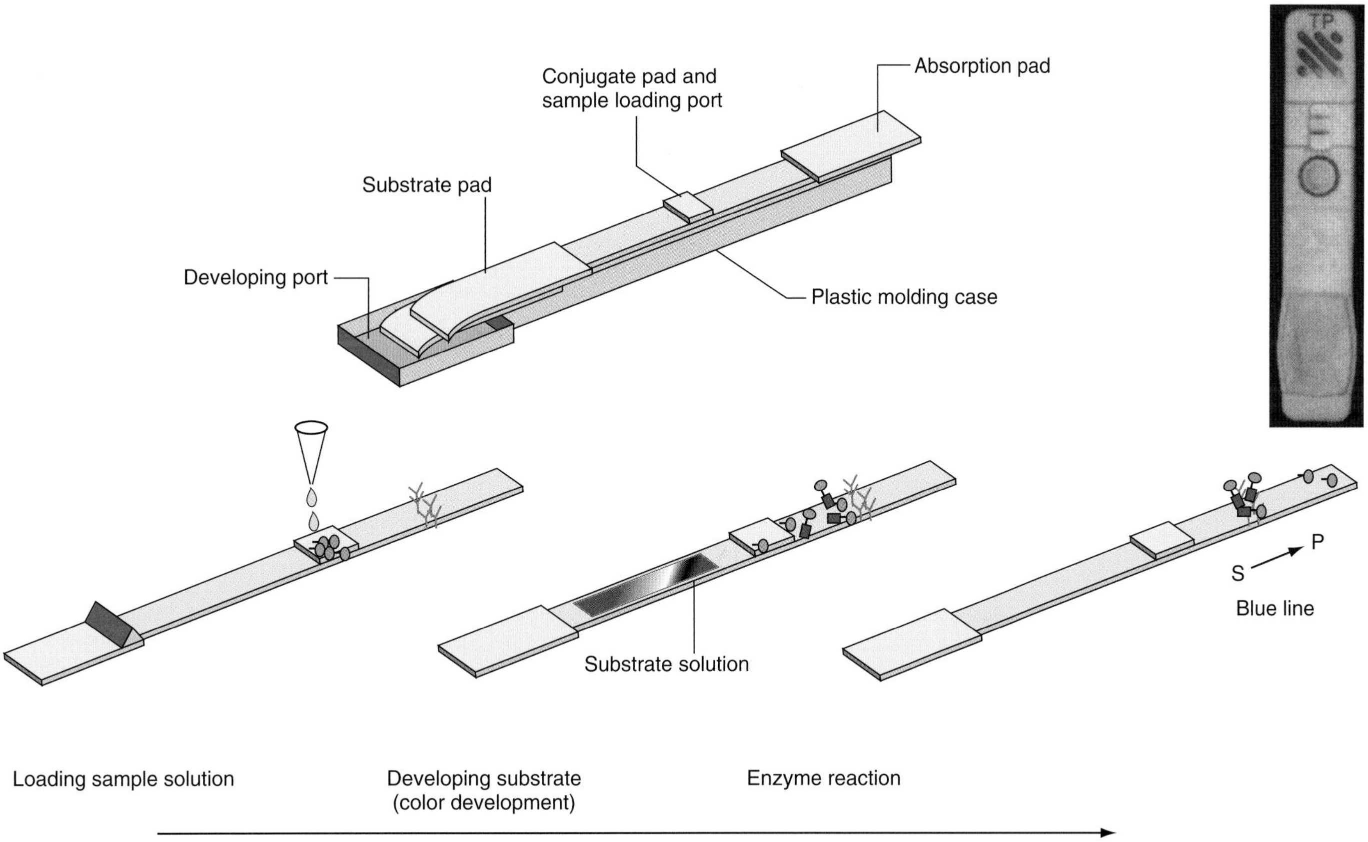

Figure 44-25 Immunochromatographic device using enzyme immunoassay (EIA). A sensitive amplification method is applied for immunochromatography using an enzyme. The sample is applied to the sample loading portion at the center of the strip. With this method, a developing solution is employed as the mobile phase and can serve as a washing buffer. The picture on the right part of the figure shows the plastic molded housing and assay results for *Treponema pallidum* (TP) antibody.

interfere with judgment in reading the results with the naked eye. In this format, the signal to be read is produced directly in the detection zone as a concentrated zone of colored particles.

Yamauchi (1997) established a novel platform format in which EIA can be performed automatically, including a washing procedure. The device is depicted schematically in Figure 44-25. In this format, the positioning of each of the zones is completely different from that of other immunochromatography formats mentioned previously. The proximal end has a developer solution, which makes it possible to carry out the washing process to take place spontaneously with capillary force. The sample is applied to a pad that is set in the center portion of the device and that contains the labeled conjugate in dry form. The distal end connects to an absorbent pad. Two drops of sample are dropped on the sample pad to react with the conjugate following reconstitution of the dried conjugate. The reaction mixture containing the immunocomplex formed between the analyte and the labeled antibody can spread to both ends. Once the reservoir of developing solution is ruptured, the dried substrate is reconstituted to become the soluble enzyme substrate in the detection zone. At this time, fluidic flow is directed toward the distal end. Serum components and excess nonreacted conjugate can be washed away to the absorbent. If the sample contains analyte, then the immobilized antibody captures the complex in the detection zone to form a colored line. This method has a number of advantages over other immunochromatographic devices developed by the sample. With such devices, hemolytic serum or lipemic serum may interfere with assay judgment by the naked eye owing to high background color. However, with this new device, which is equipped with a connected reservoir, interference by colored components does not occur. This device has been useful in detecting HBsAg, anti-HBs antibody (Yamauchi, 1997), and antibody to *T. pallidum* (Hasegawa, 1995). Most of its components, such as the membrane, the absorbent pad, and the sample compartment, have built-in molded plastic housing.

SUMMARY

Rapid and simple immunoassay devices are summarized in Table 44-9. These devices can be classified into three major types: flow-through, dipping, and immunochromatography, along with combination formats of these three types. Most immunochromatographic devices employ direct-labeled conjugate, colloidal metal, or colored latex. These types of formats are actually well suited for direct migration of the immunocomplex, along with migration of the sample solution. However, many of these devices require a large volume of sample, in the range of 100–200 µL. On the other hand, the EIA-type device allows the assay to be carried out using a smaller amount of sample—25 µL—but a developer is required. The current stream of rapid tests for point-of-care testing (POCT) is strongly oriented toward devices using immunochromatography because, unlike other immunoassay devices, special skills are not required to perform the test correctly; one simply needs to follow the manufacturer's directions (Kasahara, 1997). By further improving the time performance and simplifying the procedure of genetic testing, a certain number of protein assays could be shifted to nucleic acid assays, even in the field of POCT, particularly for the diagnosis of infectious diseases.

SIMULTANEOUS MULTIPLE IMMUNOASSAYS

BACKGROUND

Recent immunoassay advancements have led to the development of novel technology concepts that allow simultaneous multiple detection as a way to reduce the reagent cost. This means that anywhere from 5 to 100 analytes can be detected simultaneously in an individual sample. These technologies are classified into two broad categories in terms of the type of solid phase used. The first, microsectioning technology, is adapted to immunoassays using a microchip as the solid phase, and the second uses microparticles as the solid phase. In the second, two technologies have been applied to the recognition of individual assay analyte parameters. One is direct recognition of the solid phase using fluorolabeled latex, and the other involves the use of particles of different sizes. In the latter case, limited recognition is possible because the resolution is dependent on particle size. Miniaturized technologies such as these are considered highly

TABLE 44-9
Simple and Rapid Immunoassay Device Specifications

Assay principle	Kit name (analyte)	Sample specimens	Sample volume, μL	Mobile phase	Reaction time, min	Sensitivity	Housing	Manufacturer
Immunochromatographic Format								
One step (all in one)	Helisal One Step *(Helicobacter pylori)*	Blood	50	Plasma	5	Equal to ELISA	MP*	Cortics Diagnostics Ltd
	Biocard Troponin I test	Serum	150–200	Serum	15	0.1 ng/mL	MP	ANIBIOTECH OY
	Clear View hCG II	Urine	100	Urine	5	25 mIU/mL	MP	Unipath Limited
	QuickVue One Step hCG	Urine	3 drops (75)	Urine	3	25 mIU/mL	MP	QUIDEL
	CARD-I-KIT Troponin I	Serum	4 drops (100)	Serum	5–10	0.1 ng/mL	MP	AboaTech Ltd.
	TROPT Troponin T	Blood	150	Plasma	5–15	0.1 ng/mL	MP	Roche Diagnostics‖
	Determine HBsAg	Blood/serum	50	Plasma/serum	15	2.0–3.5 IU/mL	TS†	Inverness Medical Innovations
	BioSign Tumor	Blood/serum	50	Developer	5–10	—	MP	Princeton BioMeditech Corp.
	HBs Insta test	Blood/serum	200	Plasma/serum	15–20	0.5 ng/mL	MP	Morningstar Diagnostics
	EASY-SURE HBsAg Test	Serum	100–150	Serum	5–20	1 ng/mL	TC‡	West Wind Plus, Inc.
	PSA RapidScreen Test	Blood	1 hanging drop	Developer	≈15	>4 ng/mL	MP	Craig Medical Distribution, Inc.
	Triage Cardiac (Myoglobin CK-MB Troponin-I)	Blood	250	Plasma	15	—	MP	Biosite Diagnostics¶
	AMRAD ICT Hepatitis B	Blood/serum	—	Blood/serum	5–15	2 ng/mL	CC§	Amrad Corporation Ltd.
	Espline HBsAg	Plasma/serum	25	Developer	15	0.5 ng/mL	MP	Fujirebio Inc.
	TestPack PLUS hCG	Serum/urine	25	Serum/urine	5	50 mIU/mL	MP	Abbott
Two steps	EASY-SURE HIV1/2 Test	Plasma/serum	40	Developer	10	—	CC	West Wind Plus, Inc.
Dip Strip Immunochromatographic Method								
	AimStickPBD	Urine	Dipping volume	Urine	3	20 mIU/mL		Orgenics
	Dainascreen HBsAg	Plasma/serum	25	Plasma/serum + conjugate solution	15	3.1 ng/mL	TS	Dainabot
Flow-Through Format								
	ICON-II hCG	Serum						
	NycoCard CRP	Whole blood/plasma	50	Buffer, etc.	2	10 μg/mL	TC	Nyco Diagnostics
	Chagas Double Spot Test	Serum/plasma	1 drop	Buffer, etc.	10		MP	Morningstar Diagnostics
Immunochromatography and Flow-Through Combination								
	DoubleCheckGold HIV1/2	Serum/plasma	10	Buffer, etc.	15	—	MP	Orgenics

CRP, C-reactive protein; *ELISA,* enzyme-linked immunoabsorbent assay; *HBsAg,* hepatitis B surface antigen; *hCG,* human chorionic gonadotropin; *HIV,* human immunodeficiency virus; *PSA,* prostate specific antigen.
*MP represents molding plastic housing.
†TS represents test strip.
‡TC represents test card.
§CC represents card case.
‖From Towt J, Tsai SC, Hernandez MR, et al. ONTRAK TESTCUP: a novel, on-site, multi-analyte screen for the detection of abused drugs. J Anal Toxicol 1995;19:504–10.
¶From Bruni J, McPherson P, Buechler K. A STAT cardiac marker system for detecting acute heart attacks. Am Clin Lab 1999;18:14–6.

advantageous for minimizing the cost of reagents, saving energy, and protecting the environment, because of the small mass of reagent and sample volumes required.

MICROSPOT ASSAY

The microchip solid surface is fractionated into small areas using microdotting technology. A total of 100–200 reaction sites are produced in a 3 mm diameter area of a polystyrene flat plate (Ekins, 1998). In each site, a spotting area 80 μm in diameter receives a volume of less than 1 nL of solution ink-jetted automatically. With this method, the ambient assay theory established by Ekins has been applied, and the sensitivity and the detection limit depend on the antibody occupancy, but not on the surface area on the solid phase. The detection limit for TSH was found to be 0.01 mIU/L in an 18-hour assay, using this ambient analyte assay method. Therefore, it is evident that a highly sensitive assay can be achieved even on the microspot area. Boehringer Mannheim, which later merged with Roche Diagnostics, applied an avidin-coated solid phase uniformly to the surface area and then ink-jetted biotin-binding antibody or antigen on the spot. Multiple parameters, including HIV antibody, HBsAg, anti–hepatitis C antigens, and rubella, can be detected simultaneously on the microchip made of polystyrene. The assay format is a three-step fluorescent immunoassay. Finally, a confocal laser scanner detects the fluorescent signal on the chip. This chip assay is also available for the application of DNA detection.

MULTIANALYTE MICROARRAY IMMUNOASSAY

Silzel has developed an analyte mass assay that measures total analyte mass within a sample (1998). Therefore, the basic concept of this method is different from that of the ambient assay, which measures analyte concentration. A polystyrene film was used as the solid phase. An 80 pL droplet was ink-jetted onto the film, and DBCY5 was adopted as the labeling marker because of the long Stokes shift from the excitation wavelength at 670 nm to the emission wavelength at 710 nm, with near-infrared fluorescence emission. The detection apparatus used in this method consists of a microscope attached to a Pelitier-cooled charge-coupled device camera and a GaAlAs diode laser. In this format, 10^5 molecules of DBCY5 per 80 pL area could be detected in calibration solutions. The IgG subclass was applied to the present system for multiparameter detection. Four parameters—IgG1, 2, 3, and 4—were detected, and the sensitivity was shown to be comparable with that of ELISA, although a much smaller amount of antibody (100 times less) sufficed to cover the surface area as compared with an ELISA plate.

Protein chips microfabricated with highly dense spotting sites having 1250 reaction sites per 1×2 cm have been developed by Zyomyx (Hayward, Calif.) The protein chip is composed of silicon-based substrate as a solid phase and six lanes with a 5×50 array/lane (Peluso, 2003). Isomura has employed the chip and applied a simultaneous fluorescent sandwich immunoassay for some target proteins (e.g., AFP, interleukin [IL]-6, Erk-2, c-Jun, Grb2, c-Src, H-Ras) (Isomura, 2003). As shown in Figure 44-26, reaction sites are microfabricated to a pillar structure and then are coated with titanium oxide. The surface is coated with poly L-lysine polymer linking with polyethylene glycol-biotin. After binding of streptoavidin to biotin, the solid streptavidin can bind to biotinylated antibodies. The assay can be performed in a flow device. The detection limit for IL-6 was found to be 5–50,000 ng/L in a 3-hour assay with the use of this protein biochip assay method.

Efforts to find better diagnostic markers are ongoing. The proteomics assay based on matrix-assisted laser desorption/ionization is expected to serve as a tool for the discovery of new markers. Advancements in glycomics (Finkelstein, 2007), the systematic study of the structure and physiologic function of carbohydrates, should lead to the development of new markers as well. The combination of these with existing markers will be evaluated for the enhancement of multiple marker assays.

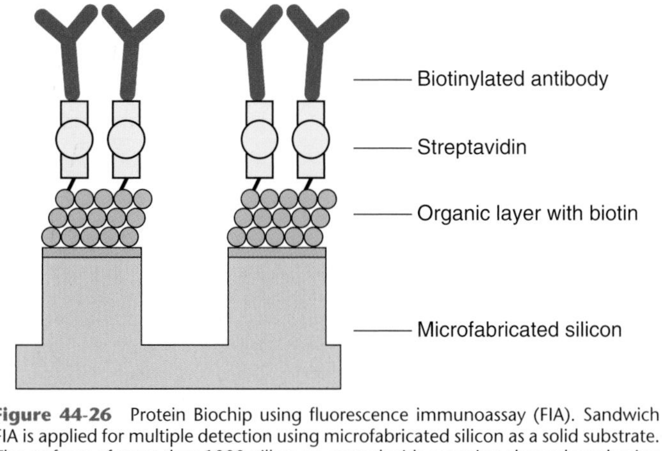

Figure 44-26 Protein Biochip using fluorescence immunoassay (FIA). Sandwich FIA is applied for multiple detection using microfabricated silicon as a solid substrate. The surfaces of more than 1000 pillars are coated with organic polymer layer having biotin. Streptavidin bound to biotin binds to biotinylated antibody specific to analyte and reacts with antigen in the sample. The silicon device arraying different antibodies specific to different antigens is set in a molded plastic device.

FLOW CYTOMETRIC IMMUNOASSAY

Luminex (Austin, Tex.) has developed a simultaneous multiparameter fluorescent immunoassay using flow cytometric technology in which two types of fluorophores for recognition of the analyte serve to mark the latex particles used as solid phase (Fulton, 1997; Oliver, 1998). Two different types of fluorophores and fluorescence intensities mark the analyte mapping of each particle. More than 60 analytes can be detected simultaneously in principle. The assay procedure is as follows. The sample is mixed with antibody labeled with R-phycoerythrin and a second antibody immobilized on latex as the solid phase. The mixture is incubated for 10–30 minutes and then is injected into the flow system. A total of 1000 particles are separated as in flow cytometry, and both an enhanced fluorescence signal from the excited R-phycoerythrin as a result of the labeling and two fluorescence signals on the particle are detected simultaneously by laser scanner. Carson and colleagues have applied this approach to the simultaneous detection of 15 cytokines such as IL-1, IL-2, IL-4, and IL-6 (Carson, 1999). Simultaneous detection was less sensitive than the assay of individual cytokines. However, it is still a sensitive assay compared with conventional ELISA, and sensitivity was 100 pg/mL for IL-2, 10 pg/mL for IL-4, 100 pg/mL for granulocyte-macrophage colony stimulating factor, and 200 pg/mL for interferon-γ.

MICROCHANNEL ASSAY USING COMPACT DISK

Gyros AB (Uppsala, Sweden) has developed a simultaneous microfluidic fluorescent immunoassay using a compact disk (CD) as microlaboratory technology in which the microfluidic flow can be obtained by centrifugal force (Poulsen, 2004). On the CD, 104 assays can be performed simultaneously by fluorescent column immunoassay. The solid phase consists of plastic microparticles bound to streptavidin. Specific antibody binding with biotin is applied to the column. A total of 100 nL of sample can be automatically metered by separation of the hydrophobic breaking valve in which the wall has been coated with hydrophobic polymer. The valve can open by centrifugal force, and several types of break settings in the channel of the CD make it possible to perform a rapid and simple assay by changing the rpm to control reactions. This assay has been applied to the detection of human IgG, with a sensitivity of 1 ng/mL.

SUMMARY

Remarkable technological advancements in simultaneous assays have been achieved in the current decade. However, one of the tasks that remain to be achieved is miniaturization of the assay in all of its aspects. For instance, mechanical or physicochemical difficulties in handling microvolumes of fluid and sample evaporation during handling remain inevitable. Before the assay can be introduced successfully in routine clinical laboratories, both device technology and assay environment layout in the laboratory need to be improved.

From the point of view of clinical application, simultaneous multiple assays may not appear as attractive as might have been expected. In some cases, the sensitivity and specificity of this technique need to be assessed more carefully. However, simultaneous multiple assays based on miniaturization technology should be the ultimate goal for laboratory diagnostics, given the advantages they offer in terms of cost containment, reduction of burden on patients from phlebotomy, and clinical utility.

The logistic regression model, using multiple markers, has improved the sensitivity and accuracy of diagnostic immunology but has met with only limited success. Recent advancements in laboratory pharmacogenomic testing for selection of the appropriate therapeutic drug in the right dosage for the right patient require further statistical calculation to obtain additional valuable test results. Pharmacogenomic testing is useful for protein assay as well. The Multivariate Index Assay by Vermillion Inc. (Fremont, Calif.), which was approved by the FDA in 2009, is a multiple-protein assay that comprises five conventional biomarker assays developed with certain types of algorithms. Several genetic testing methods based on algorithms have been approved by the FDA for laboratory testing, but not as kits. Genetic testing for multiple markers, as well as protein or carbohydrate testing, is likely to provide reliable options for diagnostics and for selection of therapeutic drugs.

PART 6

SELECTED REFERENCES

Ekins R. Ligand assays: from electrophoresis to miniaturized microarrays. Clin Chem 1998;44:2015–30.

A new sensitive immunoassay in a miniaturized microarray format is described in this report. This method can be applied to immunoassays and to DNA/RNA analysis and may well revolutionize the diagnostic and pharmaceutical fields as the DNA chip and the protein chip have done.

Kasahara Y. Homogeneous enzyme immunoassays. In: Nakamura RM, Kasahara Y, Rechnitz GA, editors. Immunochemical assays and biosensor technology for the 1990s. Washington, DC: American Society for Microbiology; 1992a, p. 169–82.

In this review, Kasahara describes the historical progression of immunoassay development, and reviews homogeneous enzyme immunoassays; it also addresses test sensitivity and procedure simplification and their applicability to small haptens and large proteins.

Kasahara Y, Ashihara Y. Simple devices and their possible application in clinical laboratory downsizing. Clin Chim Acta 1997;267:87–102.

Immunochromatographic assays are powerful tools for point-of-care testing and near patient testing. This report describes immunochromatographic assays in a simplified immunoassay format for point-of-care testing and near patient testing and discusses laboratory downsizing and laboratory automation, with specific reference to the situation in Japan.

Kricka LJ. Chemiluminescent and bioluminescent techniques. Clin Chem 1991;37:1472–81.

In this review, Kricka describes the characteristics and mechanisms of light emission from most of the chemiluminescent and bioluminescent molecules employed as detection signals in immunoassays and nucleic acid detection. This is an excellent review.

Nakamura RM, Kasahara Y. Heterogeneous enzyme immunoassays. In: Nakamura RM, Kasahara Y, Rechnitz GA, editors. Immunochemical assays and biosensor technology for the 1990s. Washington, DC: American Society for Microbiology; 1992b, p. 149–67.

In this reference, assay principles and assay performance are discussed, and practical application of heterogeneous enzyme immunoassays is described. This review will help the general reader gain an understanding of nonisotopic immunoassays and will assist the researcher in developing enzyme immunoassays.

REFERENCES

Access the complete reference list online at http://www.expertconsult.com

CHAPTER 45

LABORATORY EVALUATION OF THE CELLULAR IMMUNE SYSTEM

Roger S. Riley, Ronald Mageau, Jonathan Ben-Ezra

KEY POINTS

- Humoral immune tests assess production of specific antibody responses to past or recent infections, and cellular immune assays measure current immune responses.
- The immune system changes with age and nutritional status. Differences in immune responses of test subjects associated with immaturity, immunosenescence, or malnutrition should be taken into account when evaluating the results of specific tests.
- Primary immunodeficiency may be associated with an increased incidence of malignancy; malignancy, chemotherapy, and radiotherapy can significantly suppress the immune response and alter cellular immune assay results.
- Evaluation of the cellular immune response is undertaken in a graduated sequence of stages that may include both in vitro and in vivo testing to identify areas of immune deficiency.
- Measurement of lymphocyte activation may be accomplished in vitro by flow cytometry using activation-specific fluorescent-labeled monoclonal antibodies and vital dyes. The usefulness of this approach has increased significantly with the development of fluorochromes with different excitation spectra.

The understanding of the immune system is greatly enhanced by the detection of specific abnormalities in patients with suspected immune deficiency. These advances have come from studies of immune cell differentiation and function, experimental gene deletion, and detailed analysis of human immunodeficiency syndromes. New experimental approaches have helped to elucidate the mechanisms and functional basis of immune dysregulation in patients with primary (congenital) genetic mutations of the immune system or secondary (acquired) infections. Because some immune deficiencies cannot be accurately diagnosed by the combination of clinical symptoms and appropriate immune function assays, genetic information is becoming an increasingly important component of diagnostic testing and interpretation. The mission of the clinical immunology laboratory is to translate new research leads into highly standardized and clinically relevant tests for the individual patient.

Studies of the human cellular immune system have principally focused on three areas: (1) primary immune deficiency, which reveals the impact of congenital immune defects on host defense; (2) acquired immune deficiency, such as human immunodeficiency virus (HIV) infection, in which infection damages the immune system directly; and (3) autoimmune diseases, in which the effect of excessive or inappropriate immune activity is evident. In addition, cellular immune defects in patients with diseases with immune dysfunctional features, such as chronic infection, cancer, malnutrition, or traumatic injury, provide crucial insight into immune-mediated host defense.

The general concept of **immunity** is often equated with humoral immunity, because antibodies to infectious agents introduced by natural infection or by immunization have been studied for more than a century. Cellular immunology, as currently practiced in the clinical and research laboratory, is a relatively new science (Silverstein, 1979; Moulin, 1989; Good, 2002). The modern science of cellular immunology developed during the 1980s through a series of independent events and major research discoveries, including the use of monoclonal antibodies to identify immune cells, the development of analytic and sorting capabilities of the flow cytometer, the discovery of cytokine regulation of immune response, the birth of molecular immunology, and, above all, the tremendous need to understand and control the emerging HIV epidemic (Herzenberg, 2004). The appearance of HIV occurred virtually in parallel with the potential to identify $CD4^+$ T cells. The first analyses of cellular immune functional deficiency in the acquired immunodeficiency syndrome (AIDS) were based on analysis of lymphocyte proliferative response (Masur, 1981; Siegal, 1981) and have since evolved into a range of functional approaches (Perfetto, 1997; Rosenberg, 1997; Zhou, 1998).

In contrast to humoral immunity, cellular immune function is both fundamentally complex and difficult to measure. Basic humoral immune tests measure the specific antibody product of a past response to a specific virus or microbe; by contrast, most cellular immune assays measure current responses. Because a majority of peripheral blood lymphocytes are resting cells, the cellular immune reaction must be re-created or generated freshly within the test system. The system must be capable of triggering the response, supporting the reaction by providing all needed elements available in vivo, and having a measurable endpoint.

This chapter presents current cellular immunologic tests in light of future trends. Cellular immune assessment is moving away from single assays and single-number fixed endpoints toward an integrated analysis of cell function at several levels that reflect cellular interactions as a dynamic process.

General Principles of Cellular Immunology

Two main immune cell types are known: (1) T lymphocytes (T cells), and (2) B lymphocytes (B cells) (Silverstein, 2003; Janeway, 2004; Chaplin, 2010). T lymphocytes are defined by expression of the T lymphocyte receptor, which binds to antigen and CD3, a surface determinant associated with the T cell receptor that is essential for activation. T lymphocytes have different, clonally variable receptors for a large range of antigens, require thymic maturation for normal function, and mediate cellular immunity. B lymphocytes are identified by surface immunoglobulin (detected by monoclonal antibodies such as CD19 or CD20) and upon appropriate activation develop into plasma cells secreting specific antibody and thus mediating humoral immunity. Loss of the normal thymus will compromise T lymphocyte function and affect T-dependent B lymphocyte activation. Failure at the bone marrow level can affect both T lymphocyte and B lymphocyte immune responses, although specific linkages may be involved.

The distinction between a specific and a nonspecific immune response is a fundamental necessity because the system must be able to distinguish between self and nonself (LeGuern, 2003; Smith, 2004). In general, self-recognition is accomplished by incorporating the molecular major histocompatibility complex (MHC) self-antigen system into the antigen recognition phase. Antigen must be processed and presented in the context of self-MHC to be recognized and to lead to response and development of immune memory. The antigen-processing function is carried out by antigen-presenting cells (APCs); the best studied is the monocyte. This response triggers lymphocyte activation and proliferation, and may include production of effector cells and triggering of B lymphocytes to produce antibody. This type of immunity, often termed adaptive immunity, is retained as "memory" and typically is elicited following immunization or natural infection (Owen, 1993; Sprent, 2002). Lack of expression of MHC class II antigen can be detected on lymphocytes by flow cytometry using monoclonal antibodies against human leukocyte antigen (HLA)-DR or HLA-DQ and is a hallmark of MHC class II deficiency.

A second fundamental type of immunity can be described as innate immunity. This type of immunity is an ancient host response to infectious agents or self cells with absent or altered self-recognition molecules; it is encoded within the genome, does not have memory, and is not improved by repeated contact (Janeway, 2002; Turvey, 2010). The innate immune system consists of (1) external barriers (i.e, skin, mucosal surfaces) to prevent microorganisms from entering the body, and (2) a programmed, coordinated series of events to destroy microorganisms that penetrate the external barriers. These events include both chemically mediated (cytokines, complement, interferon) and cellular components (phagocytes, natural killer [NK] cells). The modern era of discovery about innate immunity began in 1989, when the late Charles Janeway, an immunologist at Yale University, predicted that sentinel cells (i.e., macrophages, dendritic cells) have nonclonal, germline "pattern recognition" receptors that directly recognize some invariant molecular signatures of microbes (pathogen-associated molecular patterns) not found in the host. In 1997, studies of *Drosophila melanogaster* (fruit fly) identified the toll-like receptor (TLR) as the major effector of the innate immune response in the fly, which has no adaptive immune system. Since that time, multiple TLRs have been found in humans, largely on macrophage and neutrophil membrane, as well as on epithelial cells lining the respiratory and gastrointestinal systems. TLRs can be thought of as a primitive, highly conserved alarm system that recognizes bacterial pathogens and stimulates the expression of molecules that initiate the local inflammatory response and phagocytosis (Beutler, 2009; Kumar, 2009). TLRs are highly conserved molecules characterized by an extracellular domain of leucine-rich repeats and an intracellular signaling domain with homology to that of the interleukin (IL)-1 and IL-18 receptor family. TLR signaling initiates the transcriptional expression of genes that constitute a core inflammatory response, including proinflammatory cytokines, such as IL-1α, IL-β, tumor necrosis factor (TNF)-α, and IL-6, as well as numerous chemokines and cell surface receptors that regulate T and B cell immune responses (Iwasaki, 2010; Kawai, 2010).

Other pattern recognition receptors are believed to play a less important role in the binding of bacteria and fungi by phagocytes in preparation for phagocytosis. These include a large family of lectin receptors (including the mannose receptor), some integrins, CD14, and scavenger receptors. Lectin receptors are carbohydrate receptors that specifically bind sugar residues found in the cell walls of certain bacteria. Scavenger receptors bind many anionic bacterial ligands.

Unlike phagocytic cells, NK cells are not functionally developed at birth, probably because the key cytokine, interferon (IFN)-γ, which is needed for development and maturation of this system, is also downregulated at birth. The NK cell, once called the "K" cell, "null" cell, or "third population," has neither surface immunoglobulin nor a rearranged T cell receptor (Cooper, 2009). The NK system is constitutively active and does not have to be primed by antigen to kill (Yokoyama, 2004; Hamerman, 2005). NK cells make up a diverse population that has eluded conventional classification by cell lineage analysis. However, CD56 is currently considered the most definitive immunophenotypic marker for the NK cell (Trinchieri, 1995). NK cells have been best known as cells that can kill nonspecifically (naturally) virus-infected cells and bacteria, and can prevent tumor cell metastasis. However, NK cells also regulate T and B cell functions, as well as hematopoiesis. These functions of NK cells are probably dependent on their ability to produce lymphokines, particularly IFN-γ. NK cells are important for antigen-independent activation of phagocytic cells early in infection and for favoring the development of antigen-specific T-helper type 1 (Th1) cells. When armed with specific antibody, however, these cells can kill specifically.

LYMPHOCYTE ACTIVATION AND PROLIFERATION

Although the immune system is classically divided into humoral and cellular components, this separation is in no way absolute, in that considerable interdependence is seen between B and T cells. The most commonly measured functional cellular immune parameter is lymphocyte proliferation (Perfetto, 2002). Measurement of lymphocyte activation/proliferation has evolved substantially since the late 1950s and early 1960s, when cell division was determined by counting the number of lymphocytes that had transformed into blasts. The latter method was later replaced by the quantitation of incorporated radiolabeled nucleic acid precursors (tritiated thymidine) into newly synthesized deoxyribonucleic acid (DNA). Although this "bulk assay" remains the most commonly used laboratory procedure for measuring cellular proliferation, new reagents and new procedures have recently become available to assess lymphocyte activation and proliferation. These include commercially available cell surface proliferation markers, the ability to measure the percentages of cells in specific phases of the cell cycle, the quantitation of cell-associated and secreted cytokines/

cytokine receptors, and the ability to assess the number of cell divisions in lymphocytes labeled with "tracking dyes." In this section, we review the molecular events involved in T lymphocyte activation and proliferation, and review some of the new methods that have been developed to assess the functions of the cellular immune system.

Unraveling the Biochemical Pathways of Lymphocyte Activation

Specific interaction of mitogen or antigen/MHC with the appropriate lymphocyte receptors leads to a cascade of cellular processes that include changes in membrane transport, rearrangement of the cytoskeletal system (polarizing the lymphocyte toward APC), and activation of several signaling pathways (Harding, 2005). These changes ultimately lead to a number of outcomes, including T cell differentiation, cytokine secretion, proliferation, anergy, or apoptosis. Ongoing investigations are unraveling the complex molecular and biochemical pathways that drive the activated T cell down these pathways. Specific abnormalities in these pathways are constantly being discovered and underlie many of the primary immunodeficiency diseases. Unfortunately, abnormalities in a bulk proliferation assay indicate only that there is limited or no cell division and provide no information regarding the underlying abnormality in lymphocyte activation. Therefore, more sophisticated assays are required to investigate underlying T cell abnormalities.

Antigen-Induced Activation of T Lymphocytes

Antigen/MHC-induced activation of T lymphocytes involves a series of complex and defined events that differ slightly between the activation of a naive T cell versus the activation of a memory T cell. Antigen is processed by B cells or monocytes, leading to the assembly of immunogenic peptides into class I or class II products of MHC genes (van der Merwe, 2003). The peptide–MHC complex is presented to T cells bearing the appropriate T cell receptor. In addition, the APC expresses a series of adhesion and costimulatory molecules that interact with appropriate ligand/counterreceptors on the T cell surface. Ligation of the T cell receptor alone is not sufficient for activation of the T cell, which has led to the development of the "two-signal model" for T cell activation (Bretscher, 1992, 2004). The first signal delivered via the T cell antigen receptor (TCR)/CD4/CD8 modulates transition of the T cell from the early stages of activation (i.e., G_0 to G_1). Signal two is delivered via the costimulatory pathways, most notably CD28, and to lesser extents, LFA-3, CD2, CD5, and CD7, and leads to the induction of IL-2 and other cytokine genes required for T cell proliferation and differentiation to effector cells.

T CELL RECOGNITION, ACTIVATION, AND SIGNAL TRANSDUCTION

Lymphocytes are unique in that they express surface receptors able to identify virtually any molecule or foreign substance (antigen). Structural diversity within these receptors is created by the differential rearrangement of T cell receptor genes. In general, only a limited number of circulating lymphocytes are able to recognize any single antigen. When a lymphocyte recognizes a foreign antigen in vivo, cells proliferate rapidly in a clonal manner to generate a large number of both effector and memory cells.

The TCR complex is composed of a both a heterodimeric antigen recognition structure (i.e., the TCR) and a noncovalently bound transducing complex referred to as CD3 (Malissen, 2003). The TCR cannot be expressed on the cell surface without CD3 (Weiss, 1991) and has no inherent signaling capabilities of its own. The antigen recognition structure is composed of structurally divergent α and β chains (or, less frequently, γ and δ chains), and the CD3-transducing complex is composed of five invariant polypeptide chains: α, β, ε, η, and a ζ chain dimer. Each of the CD3 proteins contains a motif called the immune tyrosine activation motif (ITAM), which binds the SH2 domains of protein tyrosine kinases. The ζ chain (which exists as a ζ homodimer, a ζ with an η, or a ζ with an Fc ε RI γ chain) contains three ITAMs and is the most significant component of the TCR complex involved in signal transduction from the TCR (Weiss, 1994; Alarcon, 2003). Originally described by Reth, these motifs play an essential role in early events following T cell activation (Reth, 1989; Irving, 1991). CD4 and CD8 molecules on the surfaces of T cells are also noncovalently attached to the TCR complex. They bind to HLA class II and class I molecules, respectively, on the APC and are also involved in transduction of activation signals (Fig. 45-1). Processed antigen is presented to T cells in the context of the MHC antigens. In general, $CD4^+$ T cells respond to exogenously processed antigens presented in the context of MHC class II, and $CD8^+$ T cells respond to endogenously processed antigens presented in the context of MHC class I. CD4 and CD8 are also associated with tyrosine kinases involved in the early events following T cell activation. In addition to these interactions and the costimulatory molecular interactions, another group of molecules present (adhesion molecules) on both the APC and the responding T cell bind to each other and serve to increase the avidity of the binding.

Costimulatory molecules identified on APCs include B7 (CD80) (Linsley, 1991), B7.2 (Azuma, 1993), and heat-stable antigen (HSA) (Liu, 1992), among others (Wingren, 1995; Foletta, 1998). On T cells, CD28 is the primary costimulatory molecule and binds B7; CTLA-4, on the other hand, binds both B7 and B7.2 and is involved in downmodulating T cell activation (Linsley, 1991). The receptor on T cells for HSA has not been identified. Antigen presentation in the presence of reagents that block the costimulatory molecules leads to anergic response (tolerance) on subsequent exposure to that specific antigen but does not affect the responses to other antigens (Tan, 1993). The ability to make nonimmunogenic transplantable tumors immunogenic by transfecting them with the *B7* gene (Chen, 1992; Baskar, 1993; Townsend, 1993; Janeway, 1994) suggests that costimulatory molecules play an important role in T cell activation in vivo.

SIGNAL TRANSDUCTION FOLLOWING ANTIGEN-SPECIFIC STIMULATION

The presentation of antigen to T cells leads to aggregation of the TCR–CD3 complexes and activation of protein tyrosine kinases (PTKs). The TCR itself has a small cytoplasmic tail with no known transducing activity. It is the associated ζ chains of the CD3 complex that contain the ITAM motifs and that have been shown to coprecipitate PTK activity. Two well-known classes of cytoplasmic PTK families are involved in the very early events following T cell receptor aggregation: Src and Syk/ZAP-70. Signaling cascades downstream from the TCR–CD3 complex and the CD28 costimulatory pathway are fairly well understood (Foletta, 1998; Samelson, 2002). Activation of TCR-associated tyrosine kinases ZAP70, $p59^{fyn}$, and $p56^{lck}$ leads to activation of three pathways: $p21^{ras}$, calcium/calcineurin, and protein kinase C (PKC). Activation of $p21^{ras}$ activates mitogen-activated protein kinases, which, in turn, phosphorylate several transcription factors, thereby regulating gene expression. Activation of the PTKs also activates phospholipase C, which hydrolyzes phosphatidyl inositol and leads to generation of the second messengers diacyl glycerol (DAG) and inositol triphosphate (IP_3). DAG activates PKC, and IP_3 leads to rapid and sustained increases in cytoplasmic calcium. The increase in free calcium activates the calmodulin-dependent phosphatase calcineurin. These events also lead to the induction of DNA-binding proteins and the transcription of numerous genes, including IL-2 and the IL-2 receptor required for T cell proliferation.

Understanding the pathways leading to T cell activation has led to the discovery of molecular defects in several acquired immunodeficiency diseases and may ultimately help provide therapeutic strategies to correct these deficiencies (Rosen, 2000). For example, mutations in the protein tyrosine kinase ZAP-70 have been reported and are associated with the autosomal form of severe combined immunodeficiency (SCID) syndrome in humans (Elder, 1998). Mutations in the common γ chain of the interleukin receptors IL-2, IL-4, IL-7, IL-9, and IL-15 lead to transduction abnormalities and are associated with the X-linked form of SCID (Noguchi, 1993). It is interesting to note that another form of autosomally inherited SCID is associated with mutations in the downstream Janus family protein tyrosine Jak3, the only signaling molecule associated with the common γ chain (Pesu, 2005). As more and more of the underlying abnormalities leading to T cell immunodeficiency are discovered, including at least 10 different molecular defects for SCID alone (Fischer, 2005), it has been proposed that these disorders be classified using a comprehensive system that would identify the disorders according to abnormalities in differentiation, maturation, and function (Gelfand, 1993). These designations would begin to focus on the actual physiologic or biochemical defect and may ultimately provide new options for therapy, including gene therapy (Buckley, 2004; Conley, 2005).

T CELL RESPONSES

Recently, the designation of T cell type I versus type II cytokine responses has been preferred for those T cell responses that lead to cytokine secretion patterns known to be involved in cellular immunity versus cytokine

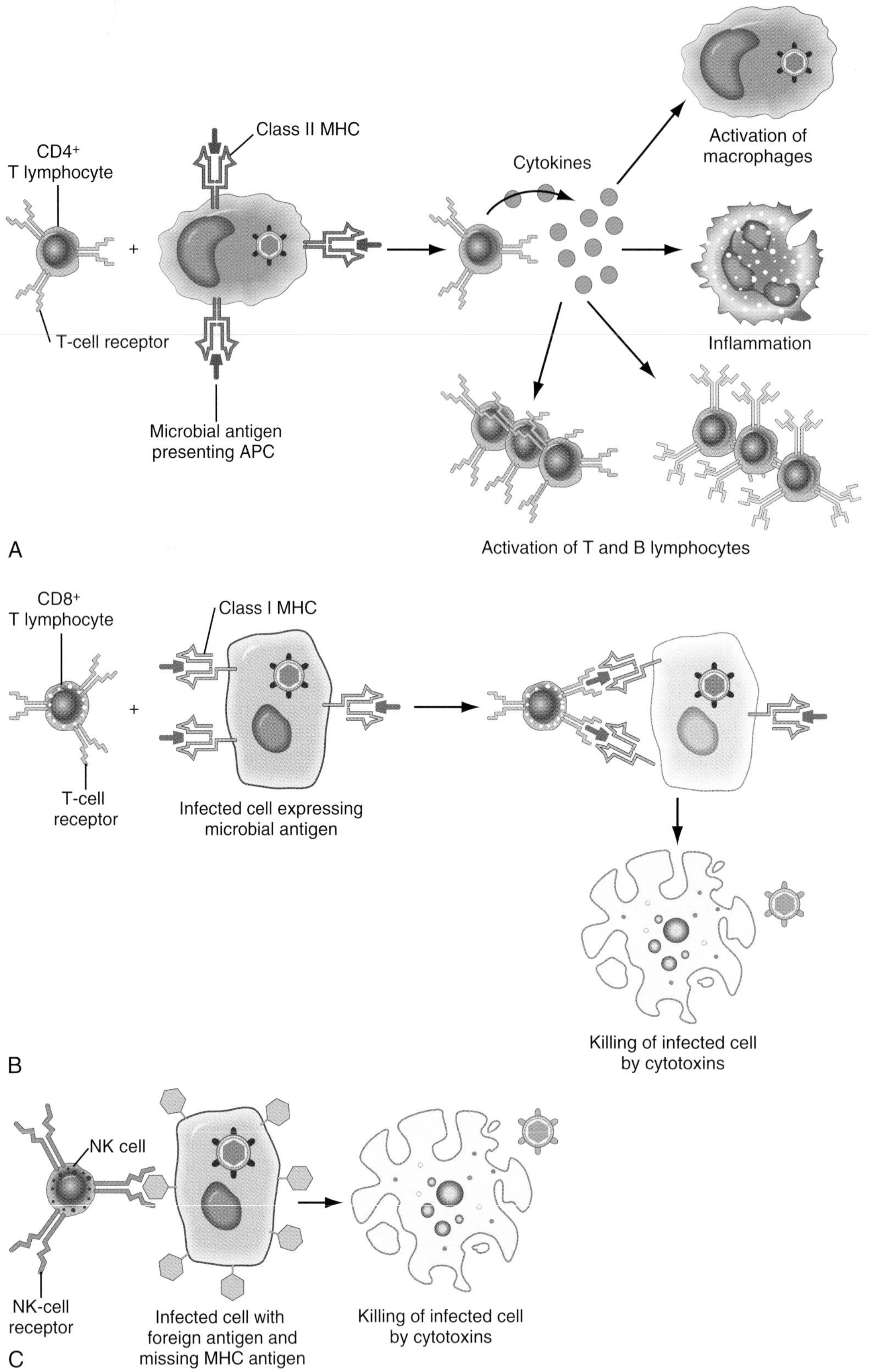

Figure 45-1 A schematic illustration of immune cell function. **A,** Function of helper T lymphocytes. Helper T cells are activated by contact with an antigen-processing cell (APC) that has ingested and processed a foreign or altered self substance and displays processed antigen fragments bound to a class II self–major histocompatibility complex (MHC) receptor. Simultaneous binding of the T cell receptor complex (TCR) in conjunction with a CD4 coreceptor activates the T cell primarily through a complex signaling mechanism involving the SRC kinase family. Activated T cell coordinates the immune response by secreting cytokines that have a multitude of effects, including recruitment and activation of macrophages, activation of the inflammatory system, and activation of cytotoxic T lymphocytes and other helper T lymphocytes. **B,** Function of cytotoxic T lymphocytes. Cytotoxic, CD8-positive cells are activated primarily by contact with infected, damaged, dysplastic, or neoplastic self-cells expressing processed microbial or abnormal self-antigens bound to the class I MHC. Activation of the cell occurs via the TCR in conjunction with the CD8 coreceptor that is specific for the class I MHC. The target cell is killed by the release of cytotoxic chemicals, including perforin, granzymes, and granulysin. **C,** Function of natural killer (NK) cells. NK cells are activated by cytokines or interferons and directly recognize "missing-self" virally infected or tumor cells that have only low levels of MHC I self-antigen. Unlike cytotoxic T cells, prior sensitization is not required. Killing of the target cell occurs via the release of cytotoxic chemicals, similar to cytotoxic T lymphocytes. *(Diagrams courtesy Dr. Peter Ping, Motifolio, Inc., Ellicott City, Md.)*

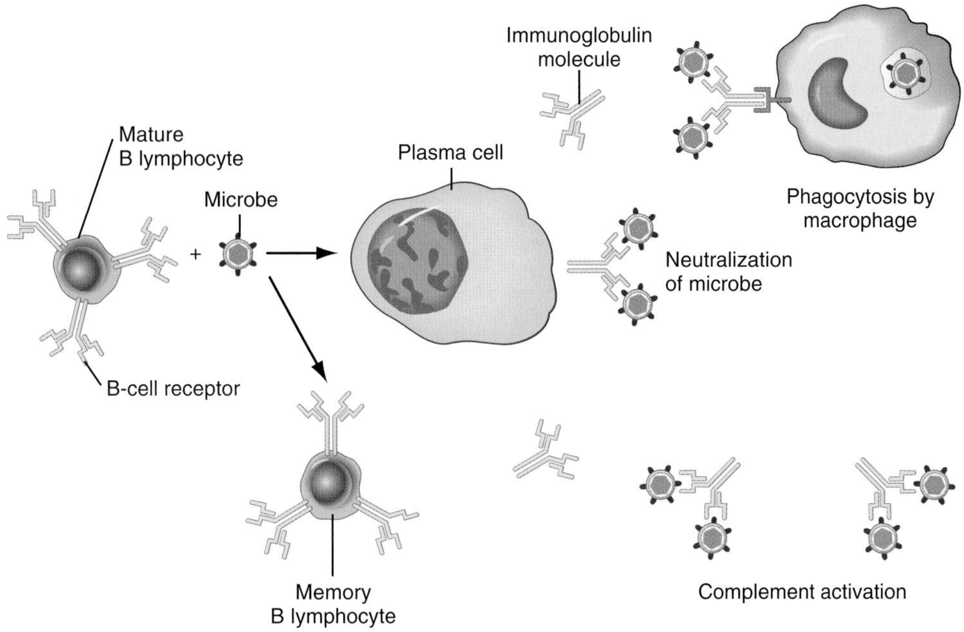

Figure 45-2 Function of B lymphocytes. Each B lymphocyte has a unique variable domain in its surface immunoglobulin molecules (B cell receptor) that permits it to recognize a specific antigen. An encounter with this specific antigen, in conjunction with a cytokine signal from a T helper cell, results in activation of the B cell. An activated B cell can differentiate into an antibody-producing plasma cell or a memory T cell. In the lymph node, the activated B cell may also undergo a germinal center reaction, resulting in hypermutation of the variable region of the immunoglobulin gene. *(Diagram courtesy Dr. Peter Ping, Motifolio, Ellicott City, Md.)*

secretion patterns observed in humoral immunity, respectively. Type I responses are characterized by the secretion of cytokines known to enhance inflammation (proinflammatory) and induce activation and proliferation of T cells and monocytes, namely, IL-2, IFN-γ, and IL-12. Type II responses are characterized by the secretion of cytokines that suppress inflammation (anti-inflammatory) and stimulate B cells to divide and differentiate into immunoglobulin-secreting cells (i.e., IL-4, IL-5, IL-10, and IL-13). Evidence suggests that secretion of type I cytokines regulates the secretion of type II cytokines and vice versa (Paul, 1993). For example, in the presence of IL-4 both in vivo (Chatelain, 1992) and in vitro (Seder, 1992, 1993), T cells will not develop into IFN-γ–secreting cells (i.e., this environment favors the development of a humoral immune response). It has been suggested that the relative amounts of IL-4 and IL-12 that are present during stimulation of naive T cells will shift the response one way or the other (Paul, 1994).

Several factors are involved in regulating the type of T cell response that ensues following antigenic stimulation. In addition to the cytokine environment, evidence suggests that the dose of antigen influences the type of response (Bretscher, 1992; Madrenas, 1995). The predominant response that develops following T cell activation has significant clinical implications. It has been postulated that the development of a type I response to HIV infection may lead to protective immunity (Clerici, 1994). Clearly, a type II response is not protective, as most infected persons seroconvert and eventually succumb to profound immunosuppression. Clerici and Shearer (1993, 1994) argue that repeated exposure to low-dose HIV-1 may lead to protective type I cellular immunity. Results reported by this group indicate that between 39% and 75% of peripheral blood mononuclear cells of HIV-1–seronegative and polymerase chain reaction-negative high-risk individuals (i.e., homosexual men, intravenous drug users, and infants born to HIV-1–positive mothers) secreted IL-2 in response to the env protein in vitro. These scientists propose that seronegative high-risk individuals develop protective cell-mediated immunity as a result of low-dose immunization or infection.

B CELL RESPONSES IN CELLULAR IMMUNITY

Antibody-producing B cells govern the humoral immune response to contain and eliminate primarily extracellular pathogens and, to a lesser extent, intracellular threats. Initiation of B cell activation involves initial antigen binding and requires costimulatory signals. These signals, in some cases, as in nonpeptide antigens for example, may be delivered by the antigen itself, by TLRs, by surface immunoglobulin cross-linking, or by other mechanisms (Mond, 1995). Alternatively, the Th2 subset of $CD4^+$ helper T cells provides important costimulatory triggers to activate B cells in response to peptide antigens (Fig. 45-2).

Surface immunoglobulin on naive B cells binds antigen and transmits intracellular signals. It also delivers antigen into the cell, where it is processed into peptide fragments and then distributed and bound to MHC class II surface receptors. Epitopes of these fragments are recognized by specific Th2 class helper T cells primed by related antigen exposure, and costimulatory signals are transmitted between CD40-ligand (CD154) on T cells and CD40 receptor molecules on B cells (Jones, 1981). These interactions generate T cell cytoskeletal changes and subsequent release of cytokines, including IL-4, which binds to B cells to favor cell cycle progression and hence clonal expansion, and also promotes isotype switching to immunoglobulin (Ig)G1 and IgE. These engaged T cells also release transforming growth factor (TGF)-β, which has been shown to induce isotype switching to IgG2B and IgA, along with IL-5 and IL-6, which promote B cell differentiation into plasma cells (Isakson, 1982). These cellular interactions occur in the T cell/B cell zone borders of primary lymphoid organs. Differentiation into effectors/plasma cells with antibody secretion appears to be sentinel for the primary/early focus of humoral immune response. Some activated B cells migrate into germinal centers and undergo further enhancement, including affinity maturation, IgH variable gene alteration, and isotype switching, to provide what is thought of as a more durable, prolonged response. A subset of memory cells is also produced that provide low-level surveillance with an associated rapid amnestic response upon antigen reexposure.

FLOW AND IMAGE CYTOMETRY IN EVALUATION OF CELLULAR IMMUNITY

Since its development three decades ago, laser-based single-cell analysis (flow and image cytometry) has become an essential tool for the medical research laboratory and the standard of laboratory clinical practice in the study of the cellular immune response (Goetzman, 1993; Lamb, 2002; Herzenberg, 2004; Shapiro, 2004). Measures of immune competence and immune modulation of specific surface markers and receptors, characterization of lineage by the immunophenotyping of lymphomas and leukemias, the definition of malignancy using specific chromosome probes, and the study of tumor heterogeneity by multiparameter DNA measures are analyses that are commonly performed in many laboratories, as detailed by many authors (Good, 2002; Goolsby, 2004; Herzenberg, 2004). Classification of cell types by these means enables the definition of biological and effector functions on a molecular basis, and allows these measures to be related to disease process and definition. These are but a few of the applications that are possible when laser-based technologies are applied.

Two major technologies are used. The first is flow-through, in which the particles that are being counted and their physical and chemical characteristics are measured by particles passing in a fluid stream in a single-cell suspension (Keren, 1989; Givan, 2004; Stewart, 2004). In the second, known as static analysis, the particles are stationary and the stage or the laser moves as in image analysis (Martin-Reay, 1994). Image analysis technology is slowly making its mark in the laboratory in the evaluation of touch preparations or cytospins, chromosome preparations, and tissue sections for certain applications, such as DNA and fluorescent in situ hybridization (FISH). Advances in recent years in the availability of fluorescent probes for use in FISH and chromosome painting will make these analyses more relevant and useful tools in the clinical laboratory (Weinberg, 1993; Stewart, 2002). As with many techniques, including cell cycle analysis in DNA, each of the new markers and new techniques must be defined and evaluated and correlated with patient outcomes before absolute clinical utility is imparted, or not. Development of instrumentation that combines the strengths of flow cytometry and the static advantages of image analysis has begun. These instruments, known as scanning laser cytometers, use the traditional flow cytometry measures of forward scatter, side scatter, and fluorescence on cells in suspension or fixed onto a glass slide. Experience with these systems will reveal whether this approach offers measurement advantages not available with the current flow cytometric and image system configurations (Martin-Reay, 1994). Scanning image cytometers and image analysis are not discussed further in this chapter.

Combined advances in electronic pulse processing, optics, and data storage, along with advances in computer technology and software, have allowed flow cytometry technology to become routine in the laboratory. Furthermore, the wide availability of workshop-clustered monoclonal antibodies now numbering 339 (Zola, 2002), labeled in multicolor, directly conjugated, and in premixed formats, has allowed the simultaneous detection of multiple surface antigens, as well as cytoplasmic and nuclear constituents. The ability to perform multiparameter analysis is the greatest strength of flow cytometry. Measurement of both phenotypic and intracellular markers is now done routinely in many laboratories. The major manufacturers have turned the art of flow cytometry into a routine laboratory measurement—a "black box" science—much to the dismay of many (Chapman, 2000). As described, this black box approach phenomenon is largely the result of the use of flow cytometry in the phenotyping of T cell subsets in monitoring patients with HIV (Mandy, 2004; H.M. Shapiro, 1993). Before the onset of the HIV epidemic, flow cytometry was used in the laboratory primarily for the characterization of leukemias and other hematologic malignancies, and for DNA analysis of tumors for synthesis phase (S phase) and DNA index (DI). Although flow cytometry technology may be more toward black box, the HIV epidemic has brought the power of the flow cytometer to a much larger number of institutions and laboratories. This has allowed the technology to become an integral part of many diagnoses, and to be used as an important adjunct in the treatment of patients. Despite its simplification, many issues with regard to U.S. Food and Drug Administration (FDA) regulation, proficiency testing, data management, and reproducibility of data remain. This is particularly true in the area of DNA analysis. It is not the purview of this chapter to describe all the nuances of a flow cytometer or an image cytometer. Current flow cytometers all can adequately perform routine immunophenotyping and other assays. Most laboratory problems are related to the nonavailability of standard quality control reagents and calibrators, and the lack of reliable, rapid methods for data transfer and storage that are compatible with laboratory information systems. More important for clinicians is an understanding of the technology, along with its strengths and pitfalls, and how it can be used for quality control and quality assurance, specimen preparation, and data interpretation.

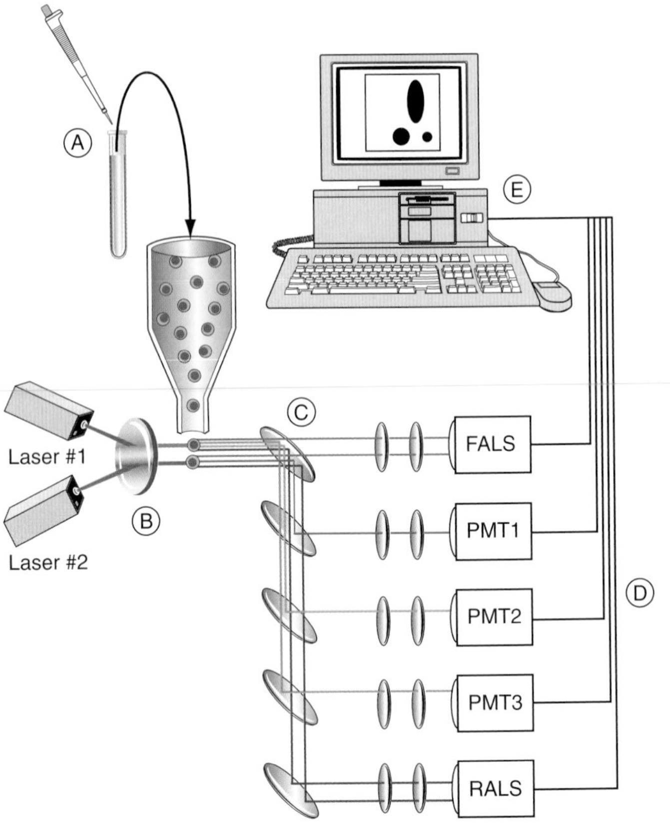

Figure 45-3 Structural components and function of the flow cytometer. **A,** Fluorochrome-labeled monoclonal antibody solutions are added to a cell suspension from peripheral blood, bone marrow aspirate, or a lymph node. The tubes are incubated at room temperature for a short time. **B,** Labeled cell suspensions are passed through the flow cell of a flow cytometer. Many flow cytometers are automated, but some models require the operator to process the tubes individually. More than 10,000 cells from each tube are typically analyzed to produce statistically valid information. **C,** Each cell passes individually through the highly focused laser beam of the flow cytometer, a process termed single cell analysis. The fluorochrome of each labeled monoclonal antibody attached to the cell is excited by the laser light and emits light of a certain wavelength. The cells also scatter light at multiple angles. Photodetectors placed at forward and right angles to the axis of the laser beam collect the emitted or scattered light. Forward and right angle scatter signals, and as many as five fluorochrome signals, can be detected from each cell (multiparametric analysis). **D,** The signals from each photodiode are digitized and passed to a computer for storage, display, and analysis. Typically, all data recorded from each cell are stored for possible later recall for further analysis (list mode data storage). **E,** A variety of histograms for visual display can be generated automatically or at the discretion of the operator. List mode data can also be transferred to a separate computer for analysis. Presently, most commercial flow cytometers utilize a standardized file format for list mode storage, and a variety of computer programs are commercially available for data analysis and display.

THE FLOW CYTOMETER AND OTHER TOOLS

The Light Source and Signal Processing

Today's clinical flow cytometer is rarely used for cell separation (i.e., cell sorting); this property continues to be associated with research instruments in the highly specialized laboratory. Most multifaceted clinical flow cytometers use a single argon ion–air cooled laser with a minimum of four photomultiplier tubes to perform three- or five-color immunophenotypic analysis (Fig. 45-3) (Shapiro, 1993; Chapman, 2000; Snow, 2004). Research laboratories interested in performing more than five colors of analyses with Hoescht's ultraviolet-stimulated probes use larger water-cooled 5W lasers in combination with air-cooled lasers, although new instrument systems with new lasers are eliminating the need for water-cooled lasers. At present, commercial manufacturers of flow cytometers include Becton Dickinson (San Jose, Calif.), Beckman Coulter (Fullerton, Calif.), and Partec GmbH (Munster, Germany). Analytic software is provided by the instrument manufacturers, as well as by several independent software companies, including Tree Star, Inc. (Ashland, Ore.), Verity Software House (Topsham, Maine), De Novo Software (Los Angeles), CyFlo Ltd. (Turku, Finland), Walter and Eliza Hall Institute of Medical Research (Melbourne, Australia), and Applied Cytometry (Sheffield, United Kingdom).

The Flow Cell

Two common flow cells are used in the clinical laboratory, but because most clinical instruments are used in the measurement of CD4 cells in the monitoring of HIV disease, a closed system is used as a biohazard precaution (Bogh, 1993; Chapman, 2000; McCoy, 2002). The first, known as a stream-in-air or flow-in-air flow cell, allows the optical measurement point to be directly on the sample stream. This type of flow cell minimizes the distance between the flow chamber and the sample injector tip and thus minimizes carryover between specimens and the sample wash time necessary between samples. This chamber allows greater sample flow rate

TABLE 45-1
Representative Fluorochromes Used in Flow Cytometric Analysis

Fluorochrome	Ex, nm	Em, nm	Excitation laser lines, nm	Comment
Hoechst 33342	343	461	355	Nucleic acid probe, AT-selective
DAPI	359	461	355	Nucleic acid probe, AT-selective
Pacific Blue	410	455	360, 405, 407	
Pacific Orange	400	551	360, 405, 407	
CFSE		517	488	
Fluorescein isothiocyanate (FITC)	493	525	488	pH sensitive
Alexa Fluor 488	495	519	488	Good photostability
Acridine Orange (AO)	510	530	488	Nucleic acid probe
R-Phycoerythrin (PE)	496, 565	575	488, 532, 561	High quantum yield, poor photostability
PE/Texas Red (Red 613)	496, 565	613	488, 532, 561	
Propidium iodide (PI)	305, 540	620	325, 360, 488	Nucleic acid probe, DNA intercalating, used as viability dye
Thiazole orange (TO)	510	530	488	Nucleic acid probe
7-Amino actinomycin D (7-ADD)	546	647	488	Nucleic acid probe, GC-selective, used as viability dye
PE/Cy5 conjugates	496, 565	670	488	Tandem dyes, Cychrome, R670, Tri-Color, Quantum Red
Peridinin chlorophyll protein (PerCP)	482	675	488	
PerCP/Cy 5.5	482	690	488	Tandem dye
PE/Cy 5.5	496, 565	695	488	Tandem dye
PE/Cy 7	496, 565	774	488	Tandem dye
Texas Red	589	615	595, 633	Sulfonyl chloride
Allophycocyanin (APC)	645	660	595, 633, 635, 647	
Alexa Fluor 647	650	668	595, 633, 635, 647	
APC/Cy7 (PharRed)	650, 755	785	595, 633, 635, 647	

Em (nm), Emission wavelength in nanometers; *Ex (nm),* excitation wavelength in nanometers.

variability than a closed system. Other advantages of the stream-in-air tips are important in cell sorting and are not considered here. With the closed system, often referred to as a quartz tip flow cell, the focal point is within the chamber. Disadvantages of these quartz systems include the thickness of the quartz and thus the diffraction of the laser beam or the scattering of the signal. Additionally, the relatively large cross-section (200 μm^2) makes the flow rate more difficult to control. The success of these quartz flow cells in the clinical system depends on illumination and collection optics. The major manufacturers have made many advances in these systems to provide both safety and maximum sensitivity with the use of low-power, laser-based systems (Bogh, 1993).

Many terms are used in the definition of flow cytometry systems, which include flow rate, sheath pressure, core size, resulting particle velocity, resulting coefficients of variation (CVs), and so forth. However, the most important factor for a laboratory worker to understand is that in DNA analysis, the cells are analyzed at a slow flow rate to increase the time a particle spends in the beam, allowing greater sensitivity and better CVs. In immunophenotyping, sensitivity typically is not an issue, and the particle flow rate can be increased. Most clinical systems were developed with compromises, to accommodate the most common application of immunophenotypic analysis (Baumgarth, 2000). Research flow cytometers offer much greater flexibility and operator control over sample flow rate, differential pressure, and time.

Colors and More Colors: Applications of Fluorochromes

Most laboratories are still using the most common fluorochromes, fluorescein isothiocyanate (FITC; 530-nm emission) and phycoerythrin (PE; 575-nm emission) for immunophenotyping, and propidium iodide (PI) (625-nm emission) in the measurement of DNA (McCoy, 2002). FITC and PE are directly conjugated by the antibody of interest and are simultaneously added to a patient's sample. Use of a secondary antibody such as a goat antimouse (GAM) IgG labeled with fluorescein is no longer necessary for extra sensitivity; therefore, the background fluorescence is minimized. Most clinically used antibodies in the study of HIV are premixed and prediluted for use in whole blood technologies. PI can be used simultaneously with cell surfaces made in multiparameter DNA analysis, although this requires preservation of the cell membrane (Clevenger, 1993).

New dyes that have become available to the clinical laboratory allow the simultaneous measurement of five or more colors with directly labeled monoclonal antibodies excited with a single 488-nm laser. This availability is revolutionizing the current performance of flow cytometry in laboratory practice. These dyes with a red and far red emission include PE Texas Red tandems (625-nm emission), PE-Cy-5 tandems (675-nm emission), and allophycocyanin (675-nm emission), to name a few (Table 45-1). The early tandems were problematic because of excess free PE in solution, leading to excess background fluorescence. New technologies for the synthesis of these dyes are exploding, solving most of the technical issues, and new dyes are constantly being added for use in the clinical laboratory (Clevenger, 1993). With the availability of the red and far red dyes, an HIV subset analysis can be performed in a single tube with greater surety (Nicholson, 1993). A single tube with 100 μL of whole blood is simultaneously stained with CD45 PE-Cy-5, CD3 PE-Texas Red, CD8 FITC, and CD4 PE. With the new digitized signal processing, compensation (vide infra) is easily performed, and the analysis is completed using CD45 as a gating agent with side scatter (SSC) and the simultaneous analysis of CD3, CD4, and CD8 (Fig. 45-4). Another interesting phenomenon is that these new dyes have allowed the use of fluorescence as a trigger in place of the usual forward light scatter parameter. This is possible because the far red dye spectra are not found in components of most cells, or they do not have autofluorescence competition in nature, as was found with FITC. Furthermore, they can be excited at wavelengths that minimize the autofluorescence from cell constituents such as riboflavin. Therefore, when performing a rare event (cells present at <0.1% of total population) analysis using a fluorescent trigger, many cells can be analyzed very rapidly. This method is also used to label leukocytes in unlysed blood using fluorescence as a trigger. A dye that marks the nuclei or cytoplasm of the leukocytes, and not the erythrocytes, is used.

The use of multicolor fluorescence has allowed the concept of multiparameter analysis to become a reality in most laboratories. The parameters can evaluate (1) different functional subsets of a particular cell population using an intracellular fluorescent probe; (2) use of several colors to identify small clusters of otherwise unidentifiable events (as in detection of minimal residual disease, MRD) ; (3) the activation status of cells at a

PART 6

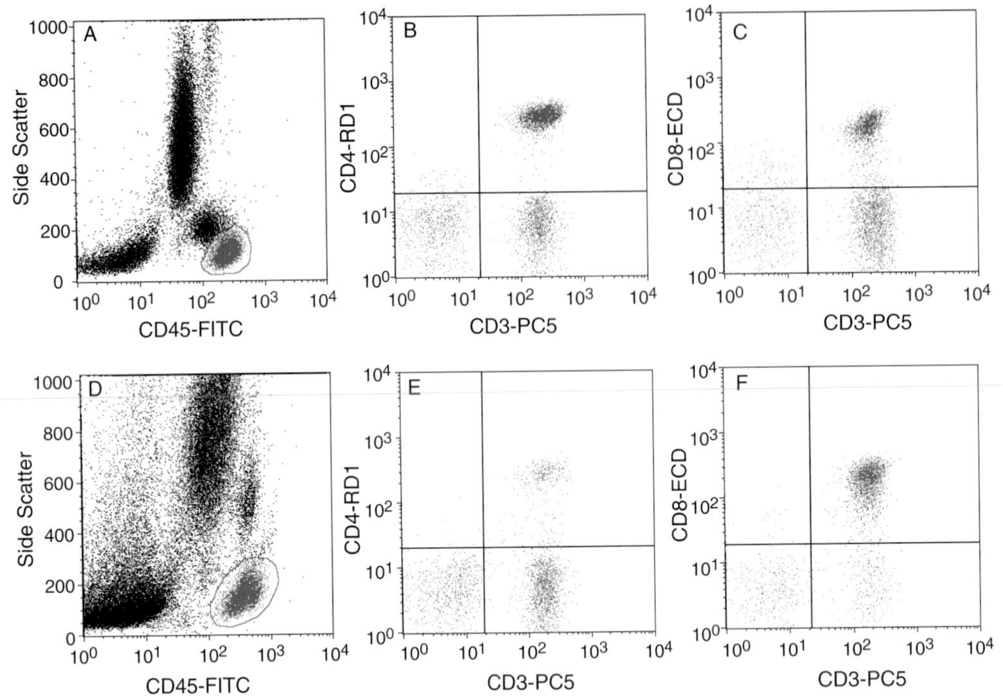

Figure 45-4 Flow cytometric immunophenotypic lymphocyte subset analysis. Use of four-color flow cytometry for the performance of peripheral blood lymphocyte subset enumeration. **A,** A dot-plot histogram of CD45 fluorescence intensity (CD45-FITC) versus side scatter (SS) as a gating strategy to discriminate lymphocytes (gated area) from other peripheral blood cells in a normal control individual. **B** and **C,** Dot-plot histograms of $CD3^+CD4^+$ and $CD3^+CD8^+$ cell populations. **D** through **F,** Corresponding histograms from a human immunodeficiency virus (HIV)-infected individual, demonstrating a marked decrease in $CD4^+$ lymphocytes and the corresponding relative increase in $CD8^+$ lymphocytes. Directly conjugated monoclonal antibodies were conjugated with fluorescein isothiocyanate (FITC), phycoerythrin (PE), energy-coupled dye (ECD), or a PE-Cy5 tandem (PC5).

particular disease stage (e.g., use of HLA-DR and CD38 on CD4 and CD8s in HIV staging using an anchor gate approach); and (4) cell surface expression and the DI or S phase of a particular cell population, as in defining the CD19 S phase in acute leukemia. Obviously, the possible combinations are nearly infinite and their sophistication is enhanced by the specific dyes and DNA/ribonucleic acid (RNA) probes that are now available. A discussion of some of these approaches and techniques follows.

Gating and Data Analysis

IMMUNOPHENOTYPIC ANALYSIS

Analysis of cell populations with the flow cytometer uses a combination of parameters that, when applied, define a specific cell population. Flow cytometry uses parameters similar to those that have been used for many years in hematology, including size (forward light scatter), cytoplasmic granularity (side scatter), and affinities for specific dyes, and combines them with the immunologic tools already mentioned. These include multiple fluorescent dyes bound to antibodies or probes, DNA measurements as obtained using PI or 4′6-diamidino-2-phenylindole, and other nuclear markers. The key is the simultaneous detection of these parameters with today's analytic systems. For many years, the clinical laboratory flow cytometer could use only three simultaneous measurements. Staining of cell populations was limited by the unavailability of directly conjugated monoclonal antibodies, necessitating the use of a secondary GAM reagent or the use of biotin-labeled antibodies. Definitions of positive and negative populations in high-background cases made it necessary to use a subtraction channel-by-channel algorithm to differentiate positive from negative (Bagwell, 1993). In cases in which the cell population had a defined boundary between negative and positive, a cursor was set so that no more than 2% of the events considered negative fell to the right of the cursor, thereby defining the positive events when a matched isotypic control was used. Although this approach seemed reasonable at the time (Lewis, 1993) and worked well with bright cell clusters, it has become cumbersome when identifying leukemic cells or performing analyses of cell activation markers. Leukemic cells are particularly problematic because each leukemia has its own "relative" fluorescent intensity, and isotype controls may have little relevance. Applying hard and fast rules to cursor settings led to the underestimation of positive clusters. The failure of this approach is especially dramatic in the analysis of monoclonality by κ and λ light chain expression where small, but significant differences were often lost.

Use of isotype controls in certain situations has been challenged on many fronts, both from technical aberrations associated with their use and from added costs to the laboratory. New software algorithms have the capability of making intensity measurements and defining clusters based on population means intensities, including relative fluorescent intensities, as well as actual molecules of equivalent soluble fluorochrome quantitation (vide infra). Clearly, the need to remember what we are measuring and an understanding of the biology of the population of interest need to be considered in designing an analysis protocol. Fortunately, some sophisticated software approaches and better reagents have allowed us to use multiparameter gating to define populations, rather than trying to make estimates of fluorescence expression using cursor values. Many investigators have used the multiparameter approach in defining cluster and other populations of interest (Loken, 1990; Baumgarth, 2000; Kraan, 2003; Stewart, 2004). These approaches take many forms, a few of which are reviewed here.

With the arrival of multicolor fluorescence came the need to analyze the numbers of cells expressing one or more colors at the same time in a particular cell population defined by forward angle light scatter (FALS) and SSC regions (Loken, 1976, 1977). When this method was first developed, scientists were thinking basically about the mathematics and the accounting of all cells and the numbers of these cells expressing one or more colors. A binary approach to this analysis was developed, known as Prism (Coulter, Hialeah, Fla). These analysis regions were hard-gated and were set into the instrument by the operator. They could not be redefined at a later time using list mode analysis, which caused a lot of frustration. This approach was later modified to allow some regating, and other manufacturers, as well as third-party software, made this Prism binary approach work on a postanalysis basis. Loken then defined bone marrow populations using CD45 versus SSC gating—a unique approach to defining the heterogeneous populations found in bone marrow (Loken, 1990; Stelzer, 1993). They and others (Borowitz, 1992) developed the concept of patterns defining specific leukemic states. Loken further promoted the use of CD45 and CD14 dual-parameter analysis gated on the lymphocyte region of FALS versus SSC for peripheral blood. Many agencies embraced and promoted this approach for most of the HIV flow cytometry panels to minimize the effects of contaminating monocytes in the lymphocyte population, because they might interfere with a true CD4 lymphocyte count, as monocytes have CD4 receptors on their surface (Passlick, 1989). Agencies that promoted this type of analysis included the Centers for Disease Control and Prevention (CDC, 1992), the National Institute of Allergy and Infectious Disease, Division of AIDS (DAIDS) (Calvelli, 1993), the National Committee for Clinical Laboratory Standards (NCCLS) (Standards, 1992), and the College of American Pathologists (CAP).

Unfortunately, even though this approach solved a lot of problems, it did not ensure that each tube in the panel had the same contents as the tubes containing CD45 and CD14, and the required purity correction might be overestimated, leading to incorrect values for CD4. These issues were reviewed during a conference held by the CDC a year after the HIV guidelines for the performance of CD4 counts were published (Stelzer, 1993). Other analyses of this approach have been performed by the AIDS Clinical Trial Group (ACTG) Flow Advisory Committee in the DAIDS Proficiency CD4/CD8 program (Kagan, 1993) and by CAP in its proficiency testing program (Homburger, 1993).

A new approach to gating was evaluated in HIV panels that followed from Loken's original approach to a bone marrow definition of clusters (Loken, 1990). The use of CD45 as a gating parameter has simplified the analysis of bone marrow, leukemias, and HIV panels. In bone marrow and leukemia workups, CD45 is usually set as the third or fourth color and is paired with forward light scatter or side scatter; this allows the definition of a blast (potentially malignant) population. The blast population is then defined using a panel of monoclonals and the three available color parameters. In the HIV, one-tube, four-color method, CD45 allows the definition of a large lymphocyte-gated region, which is secondarily gated for CD45. This can also be done without the use of light scatter parameters, as was previously described, or with the use of a two-tube, three-color panel. Newer analytic reagent products from some manufacturers include precounted beads in the monoclonal antibody–containing tube, thus permitting an absolute lymphocyte count, known as a flow differential, to be performed at the same time as the lymphocyte subset enumeration. This removes the requirement of needing a hematology counter when performing T cell enumerations and avoids the problems of white cell deterioration with shipping and the performance of an accurate differential to get accurate T cell numbers. These methods are just becoming incorporated into ACTG HIV trial work and that of other laboratories.

Another gating strategy is the use of two- or three-color definition of a particular subset of interest. This approach, commonly referred to now as an anchor gate, uses the particular properties of some cells to investigate another set of parameters. When applied specifically to T lymphocytes, it is referred to as a T gate (Mandy, 1992). An anchor gate (Paxton, 1995) is especially useful when looking at activation markers, as in the HIV subsets of CD3/CD8 expressing CD38 and HLA-DR, or when looking at the expression of CD45Ra and CD45Ro against CD3/CD4 or CD3/CD8. The advantage of this method is that it is intuitive, and each color acts as a quality control check for the other subset. Furthermore, one has the choice to define the expression of biologically relevant markers in relation to functional or biologically relevant populations. This approach lends itself well to quantitative fluorescence. Although the concept of quantitative fluorescence is not new, the techniques used to measure fluorescence equivalents or fluorescence thresholds or other similar designations are new. Quantitative fluorescence measurements will be described after DNA gating and analysis.

Another approach to anchor gating involves CD34 harvesting, which uses CD34 and CD45 staining with or without 7-amino-actinomycin D (7-AAD) as a viability assessment in the identification and enumeration of CD34 progenitor cells. With these methods, beads can also be used to obtain the number of cells recovered. These methods have great utility in bone marrow transplantation protocols in which progenitor cells are harvested from cord blood, bone marrow, or peripheral blood (e.g., the International Society for Hematotherapy and Graft Engineering) and reinfused. This approach has become the standard for most laboratories performing transplants. A commercial system called ProCount (Becton Dickinson) uses a similar approach and reagents to automate the process. Complex immunophenotypic analysis with five or more monoclonal antibodies is becoming more common in clinical and research laboratories for the detection of (1) minor lymphocyte subpopulations of clinical relevance in patients with autoimmune and immunodeficiency diseases, (2) small, immunologically aberrant subpopulations, and (3) minimal residual disease in patients with hematologic malignancy. In this regard, multiparametric flow cytometric analysis using 17 fluorescent colors was recently reported (Perfetto, 2004).

DNA ANALYSIS

General Aspects

Conceptually, DNA analysis should be less complex than immunophenotyping analysis, but a review of the literature and its prognostic capabilities, as well as performance by laboratories on proficiency tests, indicates otherwise (Nicholson, 1993; Coon, 1994; Tirindelli Danesi, 1997). Because publication of several thousand reports in the 1980s and the early 1990s yielded conflicting findings regarding the diagnostic and prognostic significance of ploidy and S phase activity in various human tumors, a DNA consensus conference was held and the proceedings published in *Cytometry* (Shankey, 1993). This report was a historical review of major tumor types (in fresh, frozen, and paraffin samples) and the clinical value of the performance of ploidy by DI and the value of the S phase. These parameters were analyzed in terms of their effectiveness as prognostic markers. The 1994 CAP Conference looked at the previous markers and some additional potential tumor surrogates. In each case, the DI and the S phase were less predictable as prognostic markers than was hoped. This was largely attributed to the variability in technical performance and analysis of these assays (both instrument and samples preparation) and the inherent risk of tumor heterogeneity and therefore of appropriate sampling of the tumor. Specific recommendations were made with each tumor type for appropriate quality control measures that should be taken and for proper deconvolution of the histograms. Since that time, the routine utilization of DNA analysis in the clinical laboratory has considerably declined. Because of the high degree of variability and the lack of prognostic significance, it was suggested by some that clinical DNA measurements be performed only by expert laboratories or be completely eliminated (ASCO, 1996). The FDA to date has not cleared any methods and still considers this a research test. However, several groups have made significant inroads into solving some of the issues associated with DNA analysis (Fig. 45-5) (Shankey, 2002). The future of this technique in clinical medicine is further discussed later in the chapter.

Sample Preparation

DNA preparative methods are reasonably simple and inexpensive to perform. Many references for the original methods exist, as do many modifications. The most common methods are those used on fresh and frozen tissues and developed by Krishan, Vindelov, Crissman, Steinkamp, and others (Rabinovitch, 1993; Vindelov, 1994), and those used on paraffin blocks (Hedley, 1983). In each case, whether the cells are enucleated or the cell membrane is preserved, the DNA dye PI is used most commonly in the majority of clinical laboratories and has already been described. PI staining is straightforward as long as timing, saturation, and removal of RNA parameters are followed. Measures of gross karyotypic abnormalities are made by comparing the peak (fluorescence intensity, PI uptake) of the tumor versus a diploid calibrator. Factors affecting this measurement include the CVs of the peaks for both the calibrator and the suspected tumor, the G_2/G_1 ratio, the linearity of the instrument, and linearity as measured by the deconvolution software package and the percent of tumor present (sampling) in the sample (Shankey, 2002). It is common to find laboratories reporting out a diploid tumor result on a sample containing "no" tumor. Tumors with near diploid values need stringent rules of interpretation, as does the definition of tetraploidy. Additional problems are associated with the definitions of aggregates, doublets, and debris; the treatment of sliced and cut nuclei; and the S phase population. The descriptive and semiquantitative acronym BAD is used by software analysis packages to model the effects of background, aggregates, and doublets (Rabinovitch, 1993, 1994). The impact of this parameter on the analysis is controversial.

The resulting S phase and DI measurements based on a single-parameter mode of analysis (PI only) are subject to these deconvolution algorithms, leading to great interlaboratory variability (Coon, 1994). These deconvolution algorithms for DNA have been studied extensively (Wheeless, 1991; Rabinovitch, 1993, 1994; Shankey, 1993; Coon, 1994), but many models used for analysis need further study. The DNA consensus document makes specific recommendations applicable to certain tumor types and suggests that laboratories perform their analyses accordingly, but even with these guidelines, a level of ambiguity remains in the interpretation and performance of the clinical laboratory that contributes to the discordance of results in comparative studies and in proficiency tests (Coon, 1988; Wheeless, 1991; Coon, 1994). Difficulty in achieving consensus makes interpretation of results more difficult for the novice laboratory, as well as for clinicians who are trying to compare their laboratory results with recent literature on the treatment of their patients. This is

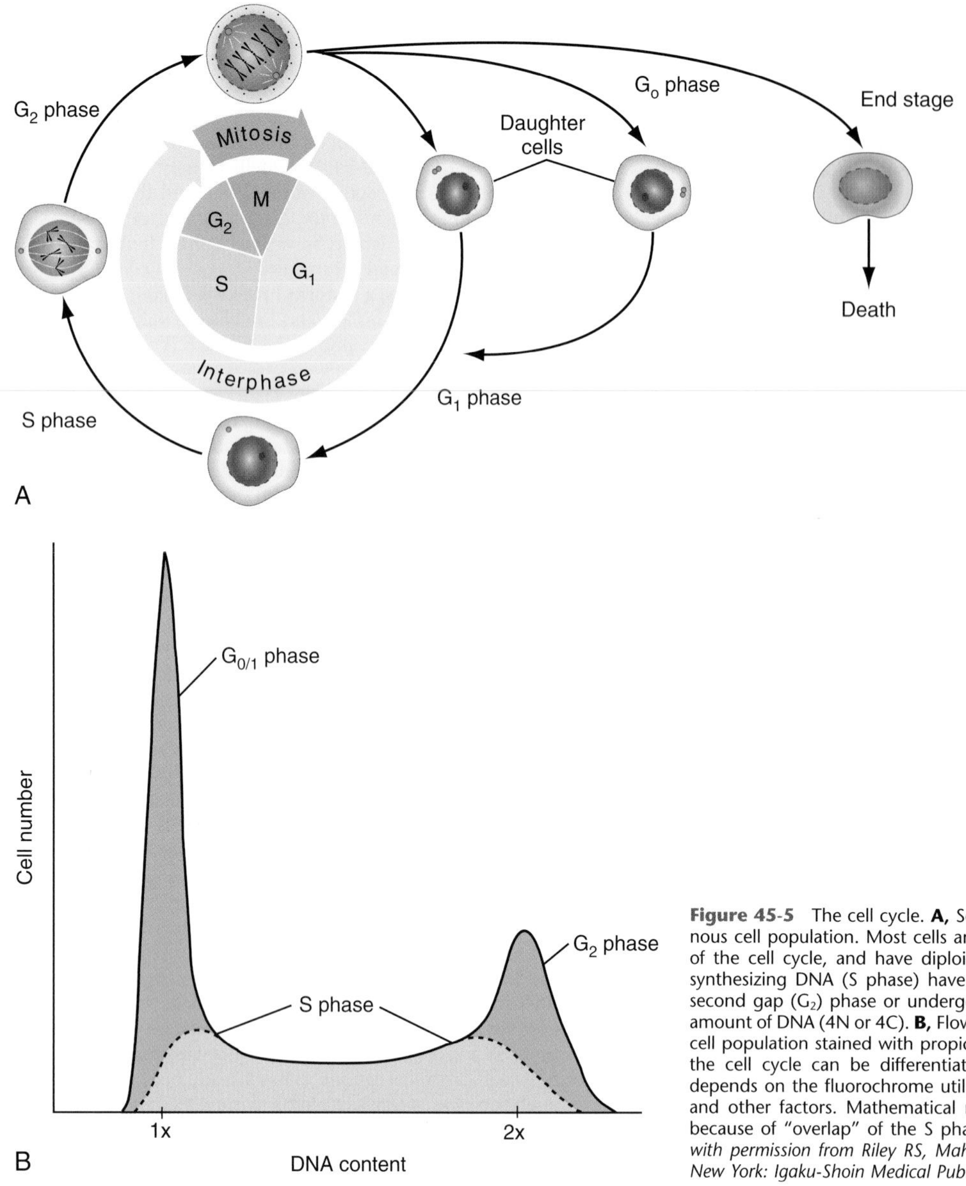

Figure 45-5 The cell cycle. **A,** Schematic illustration of the cell cycle of an asynchronous cell population. Most cells are in the resting (G_0) or early proliferative (G_1) stage of the cell cycle, and have diploid (2N or 2C) DNA content. Cells that are actively synthesizing DNA (S phase) have increased DNA content (2N–4N), and cells in the second gap (G_2) phase or undergoing mitosis (M) contain precisely twice the diploid amount of DNA (4N or 4C). **B,** Flow cytometric DNA histogram of a normal proliferating cell population stained with propidium iodide. Cells in the $G_0/_1$, S, and G_2M phases of the cell cycle can be differentiated by this technique. Resolution of DNA analysis depends on the fluorochrome utilized for staining DNA, resolution of the instrument, and other factors. Mathematical modeling is required for analysis of cell cycle data because of "overlap" of the S phase curve into the $G_0/_1$ and G_2M regions. *(Reprinted with permission from Riley RS, Mahin EJ, Ross W. Clinical applications of flow cytometry. New York: Igaku-Shoin Medical Publishers, 1993.)*

especially true in the classification of S phase values. S phase measures are subject to the effects of debris and aggregate modeling as described by Rabinovitch and others (Coon, 1988; Bagwell, 1993; Rabinovitch, 1993, 1994; Shankey, 1993). Furthermore, it is critical that decisions made with regard to which mathematical model is used for a particular tumor be kept constant, and that the list mode data be retained without modeling in case further analysis is necessary.

Other approaches using DNA and RNA probes, such as thymidine derivatives, bromodeoxyuridine and acridine orange (RNA), are used to improve the quality of the models in the estimation of proliferative and kinetic properties of a specific tumor. It is important to remember that proliferation measures are not the same as measures of S phase quantitation, which provide a static model or a picture in time of all cells being analyzed. Integration of the area for the number of cells between 2C and 4C in a DNA histogram is not capable of giving any information with regard to cells "stuck" in S_0 (cells actually stop DNA synthesis) nor of measuring the number of infiltrating normal cells that also might be proliferating. The S phase value may often be higher than the actual proliferative capacity owing to artifacts of tumor heterogeneity. The single-parameter histogram yields reasonable results when dealing with an asynchronous, relatively homogeneous cell population. Pulse labeling is most commonly used in larger academic settings and to measure the effectiveness of radiation and chemotherapy by obtaining true measures of G_0/G_1 cells and G_2 + M compartments, which are not possible to attain using single-parameter measures of S phase.

Other approaches using nuclear and cytoplasmic probes as well as surface markers can be used to separate a population of interest from a mixture of cell types. This type of multiparameter analysis is especially useful in the measure of S phase in hematologic malignancy. Specific blast populations can be identified by FITC fluorescence and FALS, and those events analyzed for DNA content and S phase using PI. Staining methods are altered to preserve cell surface properties or nuclear properties (Clevenger, 1993; Ramaekers, 1993; Bauer, 1994; Carothers, 1994). These methods usually involve staining the surface marker of interest (e.g., KI-67, cyclin B1, cytokeratin, CD10) with the monoclonal antibody, fixing it in an alcohol (or commercial fixation and permeabilization reagent), then treating it with a detergent to allow penetration of PI or another nuclear dye. Staining methods are selectively modified to preserve specific membrane and nuclear properties specific to the probe of interest (Bauer, 1994).

DNA Studies of Interest in Cellular Immunology

There has been an explosion of literature on the subject of apoptosis (i.e., programmed cell death) and its relevance to traditional DNA parameters and other phenotypic considerations. It is not within the scope of this chapter to handle this topic. Although many studies are ongoing, apoptotic measurements are still not part of the routine clinical laboratory.

As mentioned earlier, laboratory DNA analysis has recently come under much scrutiny, and in some regions, these studies are no longer being reimbursed. Several investigators in the field had challenged the wholesale expulsion of this test from the laboratory, as it is useful in certain tumors. The reexamination of a set of retrospective breast cases is being studied by Bagwell and others (2004) to attempt to develop a unified prognostic model for node-negative breast cancer patients. It is hoped that these studies and others will resurrect what could be a useful prognostic and diagnostic tool that perhaps was previously underestimated in its complexity.

QUANTITATIVE FLOW CYTOMETRY

The definition of cell types in immunologic terms such as effector cells implies the property of these cells to regulate, whether up or down, specific molecular functions through surface receptors. Known as immunologic phenotypes (Poncelet, 1993), these cells need other measurable properties to define their biological roles in maturation and in disease processes. One of the observed phenomena is the differential expression of cell surface antigens (CDs) in relative terms and in absolute quantitative terms. Before the availability of absolute measures, descriptive terms such as bright or dim, bimodal, and so forth, were used in the literature to describe a visual phenomenon of antigen density differences. Although descriptive, these terms are difficult to define and to standardize between laboratories and between patients. They also lack precision in defining an event and cannot be objectively used to monitor patients' treatment or cell definition (cell type) by measures of CD expression and overlapping expression. Evidence suggests that quantitative differences in antigen expression in chronic lymphocytic leukemia and other leukemias may be important in determining the prognosis (Poncelet, 1985). These measures are also used in the definition of MRD and in the investigation of a viral effect or activation in HIV disease (Poncelet, 1991). The percent of a specific cell present often does not give the true clinical picture. This is particularly true in leukopenic cases and when the blast population represents a relatively small percentage of total cells present.

Quantitative flow cytometry is defined as the quantitation of fluorescence intensity (FI) as determined by the antibody-binding capacity of a given fluorochrome antibody conjugate; it is an indirect measure of the amount of cell surface antigen present per individual cell (Stelzer, 1997; Marti, 2003). Investigators (Poncelet, 1985, 1986; Vogt, 1991, 1994) have described the use of polystyrene beads or cell lines coated with saturating amounts of antibody to determine the absolute numbers of receptors or antigenic sites per cell, also referred to as antigen density (Poncelet, 1993). ABC units are defined as a measure of relative antibody-binding capacity. This method does not need to match the fluorescein/protein ratio, as both the cells and the standards are being stained with the same antibody. Use of FI measurements should give the user a means to avoid this situation. More information can be obtained by referring to the 1997 U.S./Canadian consensus document that reviews the necessary parameters for standardization (Stelzer, 1997).

Although early in its development, quantitative phenotypes will help us define cluster analysis software programs for cell quantification and identification by establishing mean channel FI as a means of separating cells of different functional phenotypes.

Clinical Significance of Cellular Immune Testing

The decision to test the immune response is usually made in the context of the patient's clinical presentation, as described in Table 45-2. The most common reasons for the initiation of a clinical laboratory request include increased or unexplained susceptibility to infection, increased severity of common infections, or an unusual reaction to immunization. Unusual infections, especially those caused by opportunistic agents or severe infections that are unresponsive to treatment, and certain allergic or atopic states may also prompt immune testing. In recent years, potential HIV infection has replaced possible primary immune deficiency as the leading presumptive diagnosis. Because few, if any, cellular immune tests are totally and specifically diagnostic, and because they may be expensive and time consuming, the request for laboratory evaluation should be approached with caution and a clear understanding of how the result will lead to improved management of the patient. Under these circumstances, the responsibility of the clinical immunology laboratory is to establish a sufficient range of tests to enable judicious testing for determination of the nature and extent of the immune alteration, as well as interpretation of the results in the context of the current clinical presentation and past medical history.

TABLE 45-2
Presentation of Possible Immunodeficiency

- Frequent bacterial infection
- Unusually severe systemic reaction to a virus
- Development of infection with an unusual organism such as fungus or protozoa
- Systemic reaction following live virus vaccination
- Family history of recurrent infections
- Exposure to the human immunodeficiency virus

The principal task of the clinical immunologist, aided by the laboratory, is often to distinguish the features of primary immune deficiency, or suspected acquired immune deficiency due to HIV infection, from immune changes associated with other clinical conditions that may produce immune changes that could appear phenotypically identical to primary immunodeficiency. In this regard, immune changes may accompany many clinical entities such as malignancy, traumatic injury such as burns or accidents resulting in major blood loss or organ damage, hematologic disease such as Fanconi's anemia, hemophilia, immune thrombocytopenia, lymphoproliferative disorders such as histiocytosis, the hemoglobinopathies such as sickle cell anemia, thalassemia, and a fairly wide range of chromosomal abnormalities such as DiGeorge syndrome, Down syndrome, Bloom syndrome, William congenital dyskeratosis, epidermolysis bullosa, and Duncan syndrome (X-linked lymphoproliferative disorder). Autoimmune diseases such as rheumatic disease, mixed connective tissue disease, type 1 diabetes mellitus, systemic lupus erythematosus, amyotrophic lateral sclerosis, multiple sclerosis, and myasthenia gravis may be associated with cellular immune changes and are discussed further elsewhere in this textbook.

Primary immune deficiency disorders nearly always present in the context of infection or hematologic change. Laboratory evaluation of these disorders requires a stepwise approach to minimize blood drawing and to logically choose among available tests for the purpose of differential diagnosis. Some presumptive diagnoses may appear to be too frequently suspected, for example, Wiskott-Aldrich syndrome, although this does need to be ruled out in cases of unexplained thrombocytopenia. However, Wiskott-Aldrich syndrome may be missed if response to mitogens alone rather than to antigens as well is not tested, and the immune defect may become more marked with time, so that follow-up testing may be needed.

HIV infection can be readily diagnosed by direct testing, but the clinical immunology laboratory is sometimes used as a proving ground before the patient or guardian is approached for informed consent for HIV testing. This is based on the observation that an inverted CD4/CD8 ratio is virtually always found among HIV-positive adults. Thus, as a result of the current AIDS epidemic, the inverted CD4/CD8 ratio has become identified as a marker of HIV infection. However, a number of diseases other than HIV involve the immune system and can produce an inverted CD4/CD8 ratio, or extremely low CD4 cell numbers. These include, but are not limited to, DiGeorge syndrome, benign thymoma, the early phase of hepatitis C virus infection, Kawasaki disease, protein-calorie malnutrition, and malignancy.

Clinical Interpretation of Cellular Immune Testing

The clinician or laboratorian interpreting cellular immune function assays is often confronted by the issue of how to evaluate the potential clinical significance of an impaired in vitro immune response. Studies of even relatively well-defined disorders have shown that very significant differences in clinical symptoms may occur. However, newer testing strategies can be helpful in subclassifying patients by the level and extent of the defect.

For example, the DiGeorge syndrome (DiGeorge, 1974) is classically a triad of thymic and parathyroid aplasia and conotruncal defects. Patients with the DiGeorge syndrome show marked differences in severity of infection in spite of relatively similar findings of reduced numbers of mature T lymphocytes and a poor response to mitogens. Initially, a very high degree of fatality was associated with this syndrome. Improved surgical and anesthesia methods have led to a significant decrease in the incidence of severe infection, although some infants still develop intractable and ultimately fatal infection (Bastian, 1989). Recently, it has been possible to use more exact lymphocyte phenotype analysis to determine the severity of the immune defect and to more accurately predict clinical outcome. Using longitudinal testing over several months and a multiple parametric approach, it now seems that severity may be predictable from consistently low $CD4^+$ T cell numbers, an inverted CD4/CD8 ratio, and reduced lymphokine IL-2 production (Cunningham-Rundles, 1994). Investigation into the significance of monosomic deletions of chromosome 22q11.2, which are the leading causes of DiGeorge syndrome, velocardiofacial syndrome, and conotruncal anomaly face syndrome, illustrates the importance of new genetic information. Although only DiGeorge syndrome was originally described as an immunodeficiency disorder, new studies looking at the frequency of immunodeficiency in the other clinical syndromes associated with the chromosome 22q11.2 microdeletion have shown that more than 75% of patients have evidence of immunocompromise, the severity of which does not correlate with any particular phenotypic feature (Sullivan, 1998).

T cell function may be as important, or more important, in HIV infection than the loss of $CD4^+$ T cells or the rate of loss. In some viral-associated illnesses, considerable uncertainty exists as to how close the association is between an immune deficit detected ex vivo and the patient's in vivo immune function (Landay, 1991; Lloyd, 1992). In other diseases, immune abnormalities have been identified as disease markers, but there is no clear understanding of cause and effect. An example is seen in some forms of chronic fatigue syndrome associated with altered orthostatic response (Rowe, 1999) and increased plasma levels of TNF-α (Moss, 1999).

AGE AND THE IMMUNE RESPONSE

Current studies demonstrate that the immune system changes as part of the aging process (Weiskopf, 2009). Although considerable variation in this is seen, and much is a consequence of altered nutritional status (Mazari, 1998; Lesourd, 2004; Gorczynski, 2008), it is essential that the clinical laboratory provide relevant laboratory values for age-matched controls.

The study of pediatric patients presents particular issues for the laboratory diagnosis of immune deficiency. Development of the immune system in the child is not complete at birth; in addition, children have not been exposed to a wide variety of abnormal environmental agents and may have vulnerability to infection (Zola, 1996). Congenital viral exposure or prematurity alone may be associated with immune abnormalities. Key differences in the pediatric immune response include marked lymphocytosis at birth, elevated B cells, increased $CD4^+/CD8^+$ T cell ratio, few NK cells, and oligoclonal T cell expansions (Yabuhara, 1990; Fletcher, 1992; Cunningham-Rundles, 1993; Wedderburn, 2001). These differences are reflected in marked differences in the normal range of lymphocyte subsets and must be taken into account during evaluation of results (Denny, 1992; Bonilla, 1997). Also, marked differences in response to various activators have been noted as compared with adults. The neonatal response of premature infants to certain microbial activators may be stronger than that of adults or full-term infants because of rapid changes in immune regulation (Cunningham-Rundles, 1991, 2000), or because of fundamental differences in perinatal programming (Prescott, 1998). The immune system of elderly individuals also shows changes in comparison with that of younger adults. In particular, cumulative alterations in critical B and T cell subpopulations, altered cell signaling and cytokine production, and other changes may contribute to the increased incidence of autoimmune disease and cancer in this group (Ginaldi, 2000; Fulop, 2003; Hakim, 2004). The deterioration of immune responses with increasing age has been designated **immunosenescence** (Malaguarnera, 2001).

MALNUTRITION AND THE IMMUNE RESPONSE

Although it is generally believed that malnutrition is relatively rare in developed countries, growing evidence suggests that malnutrition is fairly common, especially in certain age groups (Pennington, 1996). Malnutrition is associated with immune deficiency and causes significant vulnerability to infection (Cunningham-Rundles, 1996; Keusch, 2003). For example, zinc deficiency can present as a profound immune deficiency that may be related to the primary lack of zinc uptake at the gastrointestinal tract, to acrodermatitis enteropathica, or to lack of adequate zinc in the diet (Moynahan, 1974; Prasad, 2009; Tuerk, 2009). Persons with hypogammaglobulinemia and associated malabsorption affecting zinc levels may show poor proliferative response in vitro and infections that resolve with zinc repletion (Cunningham-Rundles, 1981). This is associated with the fact that zinc is required for the biological activity of thymic hormone, is needed for the production of functionally mature T cells and for activation of T cells, and may play a role in intercellular signaling within the immune system (Cunningham-Rundles, 1998; Prasad, 1998; Haase, 2008; Hirano, 2008). Increasing evidence suggests that micronutrient imbalance will alter immune response through specific effects on the immune response (Amati, 2003). In many clinical settings, malnutrition may be a complicating factor. The interaction of infection with altered metabolism secondary to the acute phase response can cause temporal shifts in trace elements, leading to transient suppression of the immune response. Physical stress may have a similar effect and may lead to enhanced vulnerability to infection in the context of immune suppression (Cunningham-Rundles, 1999). This is a two-way process. Growth failure may be the first sign of HIV infection in an HIV-positive child (Peters, 1998). For this and other reasons, immune evaluation should be an ongoing process in the context of continuing treatment or other testing.

CANCER AND THE IMMUNE RESPONSE

Primary immunodeficiency is associated with an increased incidence of cancer (Cunningham-Rundles, 1987), and it is increasingly clear that tumors develop in association with HIV infection (Krown, 1996; Aoki, 2004; Engels, 2008). In the patient with cancer, generalized immune deficiency or reduction in response to antigenic challenge may appear in association with the development of primary malignancy, may occur during metastasis, or may be caused by the side effects of therapeutic intervention. Reduced immune response to nonspecific activators studied ex vivo in proliferation assays does correlate with stage of disease and has prognostic significance for survival (Heimdal, 1999). An inverted CD4/CD8 ratio and increased suppressor cell activity are often observed in untreated cancer patients, and changes in cytokine production have been observed (Livingston, 1987; Smyth, 2004). Experimental studies have shown that tumors may be surprisingly immunogenic but may drive the immune response toward a nonprotective response (Loose, 2009).

The development of new immunotherapeutic approaches is increasing, suggesting that response to tumor-specific antigens will be used more in the future (Schultes, 2004; Steinman, 2004; Waller, 2004). Immune response assays may also be used to track and evaluate response to treatments such as IL-2 (Lissoni, 1999) and cancer vaccines (Yannelli, 2004). In many patients, chemotherapy will produce transient suppression of immune response that resolves within a short time, and radiation may have longer-term effects (Katz, 1993). Assessment of immune response in the cancer patient requires highly selective and discriminating use of tests and activators, which reflect relevant processes, as well as specificity of response.

METHODOLOGIC APPROACH TO CELLULAR IMMUNE TESTING

Human studies have been based on observation of peripheral blood immune cells because the peripheral compartment is most accessible and readily measured, but this approach may not reflect regional events. Knowledge of the differences between systemic and mucosal immune response may ultimately explain many current paradoxes that arise when immune response measured in vitro or ex vivo is compared with host defense in vivo (Xu-Amano, 1993). Systemic cellular immune function appears to be regulated through functionally distinct T-helper–type cytokine patterns ("the cytokine network"), such that when Th1 cytokines, IL-2, and IFN-γ are produced, cellular immune host defense is favored. When Th2 cytokines, IL-4, IL-5, IL-6, and IL-10 are produced, B lymphocyte response is induced (Balkwill, 1989; Yamamura, 1991).

In contrast to systemic immunity, the primary activity of the mucosal immune response is to protect the mucosa by blocking microbial, toxin, and antigen entry through secretion and transport of IgA to the lumen of the gut—a process mediated by the innate immune system and a special type of memory T lymphocyte with reduced proliferative capacity capable of providing B cell help (Tlaskalova-Hogenova, 2002; Cheroutre, 2004; Nochi, 2006). Both lamina propria T lymphocytes and intraepithelial T lymphocytes develop in relative independence of the thymus and function differently from peripheral blood T cells in using the CD2 signal transduction pathway rather than the T cell receptor/CD3 pathway.

At present, tests of mucosal immunity usually are not performed in the clinical immunology laboratory, and, with rare exceptions, the immune cells under study are from the peripheral blood compartment. For this reason, use of in vivo skin testing and examination of humoral immune response to previously encountered vaccines are useful to the cellular immunologist, as these provide other means of assessment. In all cases, the use of a stepwise approach and repeated testing is highly informative.

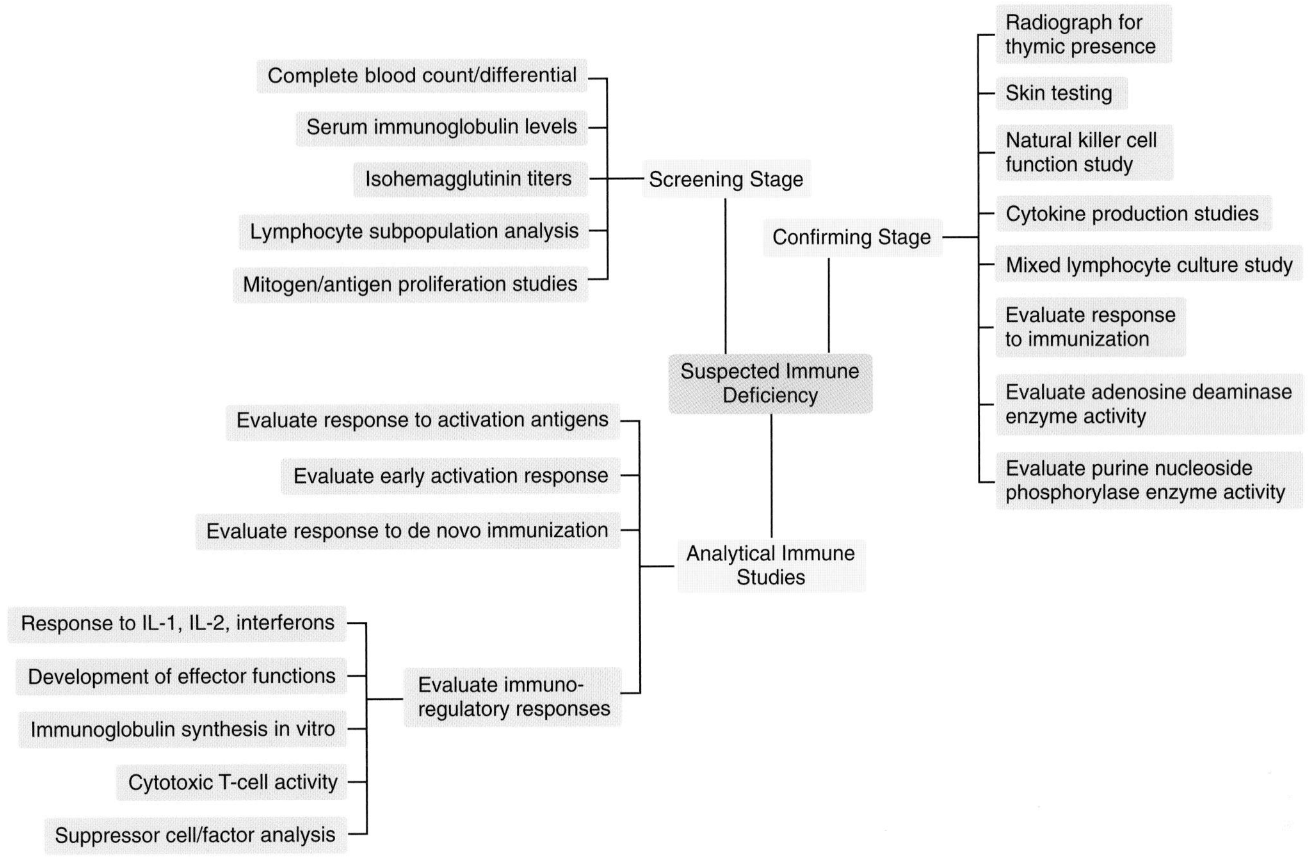

Figure 45-6 The three phases of the clinical evaluation of a suspected deficiency of cellular immunity.

TABLE 45-3
Basic Screening Immunology Studies

- Complete blood count with leukocyte differential count
- Isohemagglutinin titers
- Lymphocyte subpopulation analysis (numbers and percentages of T and B cells) by flow cytometry
- Lymphocyte activation in vitro to mitogens and microbial activators
- Serum immunoglobulins, including immunoglobulin subclasses if evidence of clinical infection with encapsulated bacteria. In some cases, immunoglobulin levels are normal but heterogeneous nonbinding antibodies are produced; thus, additional studies are needed.

STAGES OF STUDY: THE SCREENING STAGE

Evaluation of immune function in a patient with a possible immune deficiency is normally achieved in stages (Fig. 45-6). The first stage is a screening analysis of possible areas of deficiency in correlation with the medical history, the family history, and physical examination findings (Table 45-3). A complete blood count and leukocyte differential count must be obtained in all patients, and the peripheral blood film reviewed. Other critical assays include serum immunoglobulin levels (IgG, IgA, IgM, IgD, IgE), complement levels, and isohemagglutinin titers (Cassimos, 2009). These screening studies should be accompanied by appropriate flow cytometric analysis of lymphocyte subpopulations, and in children must include the use of a B cell marker to assess possible B cell shifts, which may occur transiently in the neonate and may be reflected in low T cell populations. The use of an NK cell marker is also strongly recommended in young children older than 3 months of age, because NK cell levels in this population may be reduced or absent at birth (Zola, 1983).

Although there is frequently a limitation on the quantity of blood to be drawn for such studies, it is essential that the first evaluation be performed on blood specimens obtained at the same time. Functional studies need to be performed on fresh anticoagulated blood whenever possible (or blood stored at room temperature in the dark for less than 24 hours) before mononuclear cells are isolated. When blood is being sent by air or transport to a distant laboratory, it is extremely important to include a control specimen drawn in parallel from a healthy person to serve as an internal standard for the shipping process. The type of tube chosen to draw the blood is important. The use of lithium heparin– or ethylenediaminetetraacetic acid–containing tubes is not recommended for any lymphocyte functional studies. Sodium heparin (preservative free) or acid citrate dextrose tubes must be used. Blood collected in heparinized tubes can also be used for flow cytometric analysis, although the timing of specimen preparation and analysis is critical (Standards, 1992; Nicholson, 1993).

The question of when the blood should be drawn is important. In general, most data have been obtained from blood drawn in the morning, and circadian effects may influence results. When this cannot be done, it is helpful to continue to maintain uniformity of drawing time for an individual patient. This is most critical when measuring absolute numbers of T lymphocyte subsets in the monitoring of HIV disease, or as part of a clinical trial (Malone, 1990).

The screening stage also includes a panel approach to assess mitogenic and antigenic proliferative response. The proliferative response of lymphocytes to a range of activators continues to be one of the most sensitive tools to assess normal function, and, when this includes an appropriate T cell and B cell activator, it can be useful in defining the areas of defect. Although this is not always done, the use of multiple concentrations of each activator is strongly recommended.

STAGES OF STUDY: THE CONFIRMING STAGE

General Aspects

Once the screening of the individual has been achieved and evidence of a potential immune deficiency has been observed, initial findings should be confirmed by repeated tests. Minimally, a positive and a negative (normal range and abnormal range) test should be carried out. Additional tests sometimes may be added to the panel; this may provide the beginning phase of analytic studies.

It is important to make appropriate arrangements to draw blood when the patient is in the most clinically stable state. Double baseline studies are

TABLE 45-4
Confirming and First-Stage Analytic Studies

Radiograph for thymic shadow	Response to immunization
Skin test	• Test for presence of age-appropriate specific antibodies
Natural killer cell activity (if child is 6 months or older)	• Naturally occurring antibody response to isohemagglutinins (anti-A and -B blood group substances) if patient has A, B, or O blood type
Cytokine production in response to activation T-helper 1, T-helper 2 (interleukin [IL]-2, interferon [IFN]-γ, IL-4, and so on)	Test for adenosine deaminase and purine nucleoside phosphorylase enzyme deficiency
Mixed lymphocyte culture reaction with patient as stimulator and patient as responder	

TABLE 45-5
Causes of Skin Test Anergy

• Lack of appropriate antigenic history when panel does not include ubiquitous activators	• Viral infection
• Primary immunodeficiency	• Malnutrition
	• Granulomatous disease
	• Neoplasia

recommended before intervention is undertaken, and these can encompass the confirming phase. In some cases of apparent immune deficiency, sequestration of immune cells is reflected in low percentages of T lymphocytes in the peripheral compartment. The confirmation stage should also include a careful reevaluation of the patient's medical history and family history. Studies that may be used at this confirming stage are shown in Table 45-4.

Thymic Presence

The roentgenogram for thymic shadow may be inadequate because the thymus is highly prone to stress depletion (Haynes, 1998; Chen, 2000). Although it is difficult to determine with accuracy, the actual size of the thymus assessed by magnetic resonance imaging has been found to correlate with $CD4^+$ T lymphocyte number in HIV infection (Vigano, 1999). Recent studies suggest that the human thymus can be thought of as a chimeric organ that comprises both central and peripheral lymphoid tissues. Haynes (1998, 2000) has postulated that thymic epithelial atrophy may derive in part from cytokines or other factors produced by peripheral immune cells within the thymic perivascular space. As described in the subsequent specific section on flow cytometric evaluation of T lymphocyte subsets, expression of normal maturation antigens acquired during thymic development will suffice to identify the presence of a working thymus.

Skin Testing

The use of a skin test panel can be important at this point. This approach to cellular immune assessment originally served as the departure point for the development of the cellular immune functional tests because it measures delayed-type hypersensitivity directly in vivo (McCormick, 2006). Experience with the delayed-type hypersensitivity skin test has shown good overall correlation between lack of reactivity, termed anergy, and immune deficiency (Deodhar, 1983; Maas, 1998), but it has not been useful as an analytic tool to dissect out the reason for lack of response. In addition, the skin test is not very quantifiable. Use of the purified protein derivative skin test to assess the possible presence of *Mycobacterium tuberculosis* is an exception, although anergic individuals do not respond; in addition, false-positives are seen in persons who have been vaccinated with bacille Calmette-Guérin (Huebner, 1993). The relative effectiveness of a standardized *Candida albicans* skin test product in children has been reported (Ohri, 2004).

Reasons for lack of skin test response are shown in Table 45-5. Some studies have been based on a de novo immunization skin test using dinitrofluorobenzene. Although this once was used rather extensively, the approach is no longer considered useful because of ambiguities in the underlying mechanism of reaction. The introduction of the "skin window" test may ultimately provide a more quantitative and informative measure of in vivo immune response because the reaction can be used to test autologous tumor response (Black, 1988). However, despite some reservations, the importance of the skin test as a convincing demonstration that immune defects noted in vitro may have prognostic significance in vivo should not be underestimated.

TABLE 45-6
Analytic and Immunoregulatory Studies

Development of activation antigens during response to stimulation, such as Tac antigen, transferrin receptor, upregulation for MHC class II on T cells, soluble receptors, and so on

Early activation response (e.g., calcium channels)

Immunoregulation
- Response to IL-1, IL-2, interferons
- Development of effector functions
- Immunoglobulin synthesis in vitro
- Cytotoxic T cell activity
- Suppressor cell/factor analysis

Gene activation, cell cycle analysis

Response to immunization: de novo immunization

IL, Interleukin; *MHC,* major histocompatibility complex.

TABLE 45-7
Immunophenotyping Lymphocyte Subpopulations

Basic peripheral blood panel (whole blood, lysed red blood cells*)
- CD45/CD14
- Isotype mouse immunoglobulin controls
- CD3/CD19
- CD3/CD4
- CD3/CD8
- CD3/CD56 and 16

Isolated mononuclear cells, activation panel†
- CD45/CD14
- Isotype mouse immunoglobulin controls
- CD3/CD25 (IL-2R)
- CD3/HLA-DR

HLA, Human leukocyte antigen; *IL,* interleukin.
*If low CD3, then repeat and add CD2. Further, monoclonals against T cell receptor paired with CD3 may be added. Monocyte markers also may be evaluated. These may be performed using three- or four-color reagents using CD45 gating.
†After 2 days of culture, remove cells and wash before staining with monoclonal antibodies listed; analyze control cells containing no activator, then analyze activated cells. Activators may include mitogen, IL-2, and/or interferon-γ.

STAGES OF STUDY: ANALYTIC IMMUNE STUDIES

Analytic studies are outlined generally in Table 45-6. Although a complete description of these approaches is beyond the scope of this discussion, in general these studies attempt to identify the underlying mechanism of immune defect by proceeding through a series of steps. Although there are different possible ways of doing this, one good way is to assess the general level of defect by following the general plan of assessing the presence of cell types and the relative proportions of all in light of areas of diminished general function, and then to perform studies of effector function.

If cell populations have been determined to be essentially intact in the absence of activation, the issue of intrinsic failure may be studied by many different approaches, including the use of expanded lymphocyte surface marker analysis, framework determinants to the TCR, and activation antigens such as CD25, CD38, and HLA-DR (Table 45-7). Absence of MHC class II upregulation in response to IFN-γ is one example. Although cell populations may express a reference normal differentiation antigen, they may also coexpress others inappropriately, and this may be a key to functional abnormality. For example, $CD8^+$ T cells coexpressing CD38 are not functionally the same as CD8 cells that do not express this marker and are expanded in HIV disease (Giorgi, 1989). Absence of expression of certain molecules, such as CD28, is another important indicator. In some primary immune deficiency syndromes, upregulation of the IL-2 receptor in response to IL-2 may be abnormal. Receptors may not be translocated normally, or receptors may be shed prematurely (Cunningham-Rundles, 1990).

Development of the immune response may be kinetically abnormal because of delayed secondary recruitment during the amplification phase. This should be tested by doing time course studies. In some cases, cytokines may not be made, or they may be functionally altered. Effector functions may be missing or impaired. Evaluation of this may require a detailed approach. Attempts to restore response by addition of cytokine may be useful, although this may circumvent the lesion through compensation rather than fill in the actual deficiency. New testing strategies may utilize whole blood rather than isolated mononuclear cells (Bocchieri, 1995). This system provides an excellent ex vivo mirror of immune response, because the actual relationships among cells are not altered. Furthermore, this system can be used to measure cytokine production (Petrovsky, 1995; Suni, 1998).

The cellular immunology laboratory is advised to choose basic analytic studies that are normally done on a routine basis, so a basis for comparison is available. Establishment of laboratory normal ranges and maintenance of reagent quality control, especially for certain variable elements, are essential for the accuracy and sensitivity of these tests.

LABORATORY EVALUATION OF LYMPHOCYTE FUNCTION

Developmental defects, inherited genetic abnormalities, and acquired infections cause profound immunodeficiency states. Additionally, severe burns, trauma, and therapeutic intervention may lead to immunodeficiency. Bulk assays can be used to ascertain whether or not an individual has a decreased T cell proliferative response and have been available for some time, but they are limited both by poor reproducibility and by the limited information garnered from bulk assays. Recent technological developments have allowed for the production of a variety of reagents that can be used to assess multiple activities along the pathway of T cell activation. These reagents include monoclonal antibodies specific for T cell activation markers, reagents and systems for the detection of intracellular cytokines, and tracking dyes and nonradioactive DNA precursors developed to assess lymphocyte proliferation.

LYMPHOCYTE TRANSFORMATION ASSAYS

Principles of Lymphocyte Transformation

The most common in vivo procedure used to assess cellular immunity is a simple skin test. A positive skin test for the detection of a delayed-type hypersensitivity response implies intact cellular immunity, as well as intact monocyte chemotaxis (Borut, 1980; Ananworanich, 2002). Although skin testing is easily performed, negative results are difficult to interpret, especially in young children, and skin testing is not as sensitive as in vitro lymphocyte stimulation assays (Borut, 1980). Other in vivo correlates of cell-mediated immunity include contact sensitivity, granuloma formation, and allograft rejection.

Mitogen-Induced Blastogenesis

Most laboratories assess the proliferative capacity of lymphocytes by measuring the rate of incorporation of radiolabeled DNA nucleosides (tritiated thymidine) following prolonged incubation of peripheral blood mononuclear cell cultures with mitogens (3–4 days) or antigens (5–10 days) (Maluish, 1986). In general, only a limited number of T cells respond to any one antigen in vitro; therefore, cells must be cultured from 5–10 days to detect a response. In vitro lymphocyte transformation in response to a mitogen was first reported by Nowell (1960). Mitogens and IL-2 in general are the most potent stimuli, as they induce the rapid proliferation of the largest proportion of lymphocytes. For this reason, proliferation can be detected in 3–4 days and thus provides an effective screening tool. Of the mitogens, phytohemagglutinin and concanavalin A (Con A) induce T cell blastogenesis, and pokeweed mitogen and staphylococcal protein A trigger B cell activation.

In the standard mitogen-induced blastogenesis procedure, lymphocytes are isolated with Ficoll-Hypaque density gradient centrifugation and cultured for several days with a mitogen or a specific soluble antigen in media enriched with human AB serum. Tritiated thymidine is added to the culture media, and the plates are incubated for an additional 4–24 hours. The cells are isolated (harvested) from the plates using a special device (cell harvester) and are transferred to disks of filter paper (Fig. 45-7). These

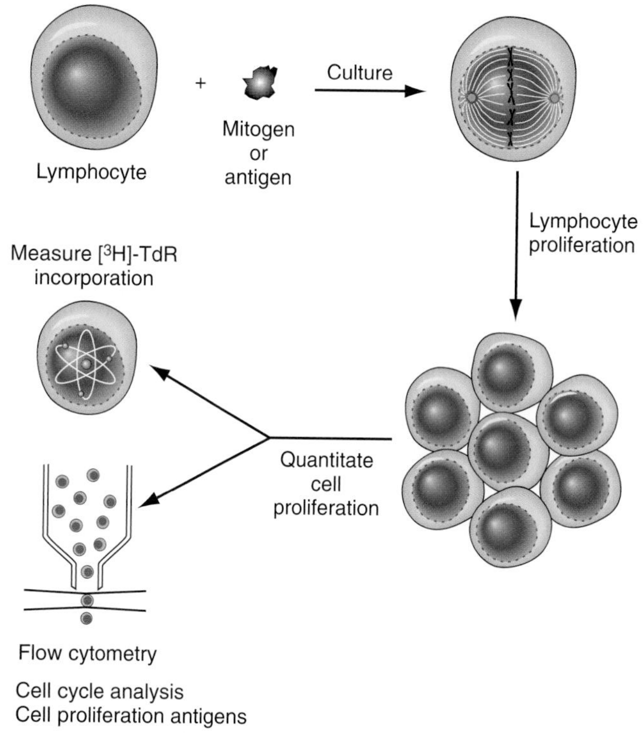

Figure 45-7 Principle of lymphocyte stimulation assay. Lymphocytes are cultured with antigen or mitogen. If stimulation occurs, a proliferative reaction takes place, with the formation of daughter cells. The amount of proliferation can be determined from tritiated thymidine (^{3}H-TdR) incorporation, by flow cytometric cell cycle kinetic analysis, or by measuring a cell proliferation antigen such as Ki-67. *(Reprinted with permission from Riley RS, Mahin EJ, Ross W. Clinical applications of flow cytometry. New York: Igaku-Shoin Medical Publishers; 1993.)*

disks are placed in scintillation fluid, and radioactive emissions are measured in a liquid scintillation counter. This technique is classified as a **bulk assay method** because the response of the entire cell population is measured.

Several controls are necessary in bulk assays of lymphocyte proliferation because the assays may be influenced by the number of cultured cells, incubation time and temperature, mitogen concentration, and various inhibitory factors that may be present. The results are expressed as a stimulation index, which is the ratio of radioisotope incorporation into the test versus control cells. The relative proliferation index is the ratio of the Δcounts per minute (cpm) of the test subject (cpm of stimulated cells minus unstimulated control cells) to the Δcpm of a panel of normal individuals tested simultaneously.

Bulk assays, in addition to their inherent technical problems, provide no information on the specific cell subsets that are responding. Cram and collaborators (1976) were among the first to resolve this problem through analysis of blastogenesis at the single cell level by flow cytometry. Since that time, flow cytometry with its inherent multiparameter potential has become the instrument of choice for analysis of lymphocyte transformation and other aspects of the cellular immune response. Comprehensive reviews of flow cytometry and methods used to assess lymphocyte activation and proliferation have been published by Maluish and Perfetto (Maluish, 1986; Perfetto, 2002).

Precise measurement of the proportion of lymphocytes in the various phases of the cell cycle (i.e., cell cycle analysis) is critical for flow cytometric studies of blastogenesis and lymphocyte proliferation. In general, two distinct approaches are used in cell cycle analysis. In the past, the preferred approach was to measure the level of fluorescence intensity emitted by DNA staining dyes. The most commonly used dye was propidium iodide, a phenanthridinium-based compound that intercalates stoichiometrically into DNA (i.e., the amount or intensity of fluorescence is proportional to the amount of DNA in a cell). Using complex mathematical modeling, the percentages of cells in the G_0/G_1, S, and G_2 phases can be determined from the distribution of FI. Most peripheral blood lymphocytes are in the resting phase of the cell cycle, with fewer than 5% of cells in the S phase. Many fluorescent dyes with different DNA binding affinities and spectral properties have also been used, including ethidium bromide, DAPI, Hoechst 33258, and Hoechst 33342. Bromodeoxyuridine

(5-bromo-2-deoxyuridine, BrdU) is another substance used to measure the proliferation of lymphocytes and other cells. BrdU is a synthetic analog of thymidine that is incorporated into the DNA of replicating cells, while substituting for thymidine. Fluorochrome-labeled antibodies specific for BrdU are used to measure BrdU incorporation and cell proliferation. The quantitation of cell cycle–related nuclear proliferation antigens is another approach for the measurement of cell cycling and proliferation in lymphocyte and other cell populations. Ki-67 antigen is a nuclear protein expressed by proliferating cells in all phases of the cell cycle, but not by resting cells (Sawhney, 1992). Labeled monoclonal antibodies specific for Ki-67 can be measured by flow cytometric or immunohistochemical techniques to obtain the **Ki-67 proliferation index.**

The use of dyes that stably integrate into the membranes of live lymphocytes or other cells is the most recently described means of measuring lymphocyte proliferation. After washing away excess dye, the lymphocytes are stimulated to divide. With each successive division, the amount of dye per cell is halved. The fluorescence emitted from the cells after culture can be modeled, and the number of cell divisions can be estimated. This method has been standardized into a kit that includes both the software required for analyses and the tracking dye (Sigma Immunochemicals, St Louis). An evaluation of 14 of the most commonly utilized tracking dyes reported that two of the dyes, PKH26 and carboxyfluorescein diacetate succinimidyl ester (CFSE), were most suitable for their ability to quantify lymphocyte proliferation (Hasbold, 1999; Parish, 1999, 2002; Hawkins, 2007; Quah, 2007; Gil, 2009). This assay may provide the most accurate assessment of cell proliferative response in in vitro culture systems with the substantial advantage over standard bulk assays of allowing the measurement of specific lymphocyte subsets. CFSE indices appear to correlate more closely with TdR assays than measurement of $CD69^+$ cells (Angulo, 1998). Measurements of lymphocyte proliferation using the tracking dyes PKH26 and CSFE have been developed, optimized, and tested for their utility in clinical applications (Allsopp, 1998; Angulo, 1998).

Some laboratories have replaced the tritiated thymidine incorporation assays with a combination of cell surface marker induction assays and measurement of the percentage of cells at various phases of the cell cycle following activation (Cost, 1993).

The recently developed ability to measure the production of cell-associated cytokines at the single-cell level also has significant potential as a clinical tool for evaluation of the cellular immune response. Cytokine flow cytometry (intracellular cytokine staining) is performed by stimulating target cells for 4 to 6 hours in the presence of membrane transport blocking reagents (brefeldin A or monensin) to prevent the secretion of cytokines (Ghanekar, 2006). Cells are then labeled with subset-specific monoclonal antibodies, fixed, permeabilized, and labeled with fluorescently tagged monoclonal antibodies specific for the cytokine of interest (Jung, 1993; Prussin, 1995; Maino, 2004; Maecker, 2005; Nomura, 2008). The assay has been developed with the presence of costimulatory antibodies for the sensitive detection of antigen responses in whole blood cultures after relatively short incubation periods (Suni, 1998). Special attention is being focused on the development of antibodies that recognize the nascent forms of the cytokines (within the Golgi) and optimization of the timing of culture to detect maximal cytokine response (Mascher, 1999). Clinical studies have begun to demonstrate the potential utility of this technique. For example, patients suffering very severe burns who show a shift to a Th2 cytokine response may be at increased risk for the development of multiple organ dysfunction syndrome (Zedler, 1999), and clinically active multiple sclerosis patients may show increased production of IL-10 (Inoges, 1999). Expansion of this technique to incorporate the ability to simultaneously measure proliferation and specific cytokine synthesis at the single-cell level has been reported but has not yet been evaluated in a clinical setting (Mehta, 1997).

Clearly, new assays are being developed that measure different events involved in T cell activation. Methods and reagents are available to measure the earliest phosphorylation/dephosphorylation events through signal transduction, gene transcription, and cell division. As these methods are adapted for routine clinical use, we will have a veritable armamentarium of methods to assess many of the processes involved in lymphocyte activation and proliferation. Although many of these new technologies are still within the domain of research laboratories, the methods are constantly being simplified and adapted for use and evaluation in clinical laboratories.

Mixed Lymphocyte Culture

The mixed lymphocyte culture assay (MLC) is a special type of lymphocyte stimulation assay based on the ability of histoincompatible lymphocytes from one individual to stimulate the lymphocytes of another individual (mixed lymphocyte reaction) (Bach, 1974; Dupont, 1976; Mickelson, 1990). Although complex in origin, the D locus of the HLA system is the major determinant of the MLC phenomenon. When two cells share common D loci, they are not able to stimulate each other, but when the D loci are different, the cells are stimulated. The MLC is unilateral (one way) when one group of cells are made incapable of responding (by treatment with radiation or mithromycin); it is bidirectional (two way) when no radiation or mithromycin is utilized. In the one-way MLC, untreated cells are termed the responder population, and treated cells are the stimulator population (Fig. 45-8).

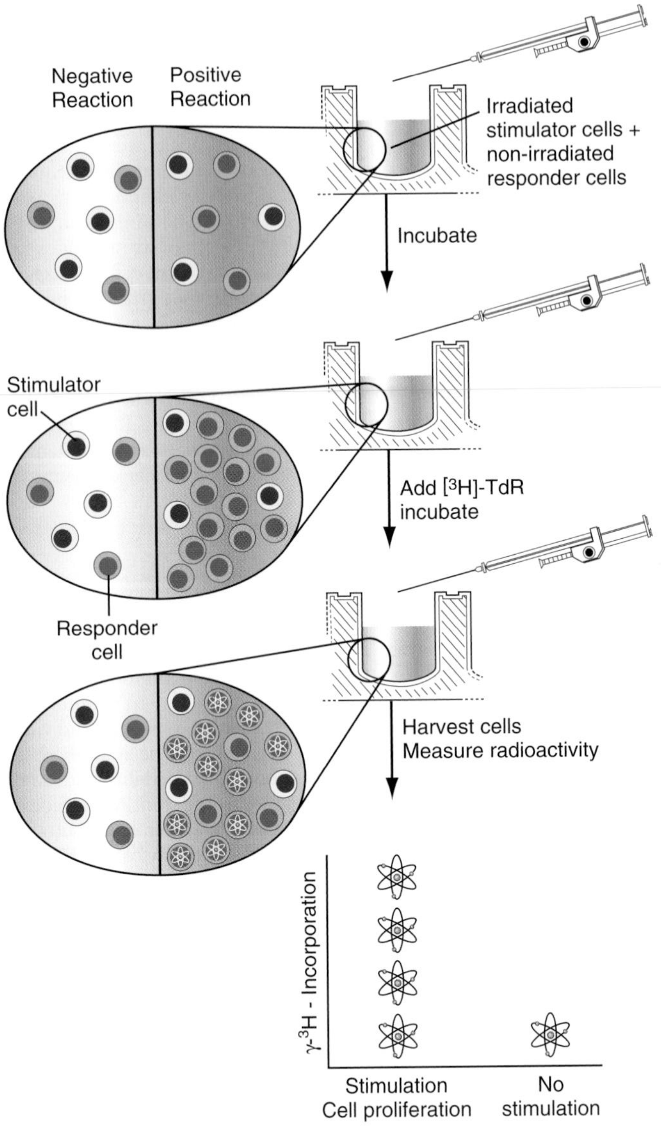

Figure 45-8 The one-way mixed lymphocyte culture assay (MLC). Irradiated stimulator cells, which are incapable of cell division, are mixed with nonirradiated responder cells, which can proliferate and divide. After incubation under cell culture conditions for approximately 1 week, responder cells proliferate in the presence of a disparity in the human leukocyte antigen (HLA)-D locus *(right side of diagram)*, but no proliferation occurs if the responder and stimulator cells are HLA-D compatible *(left side of diagram)*. Tritiated thymidine is added to the reaction mixture, and the degree of proliferation is determined by liquid scintillation counting. *(Reprinted with permission from Riley RS. Basic principles of immunodiagnosis. In: McClatchey KD, editor. Clinical laboratory medicine. Baltimore: Williams and Wilkins, 1994.)*

Numerous factors must be considered in performance and interpretation of the MLC. Because the reaction is complex, lack of stimulation between two cell types cannot be considered as conclusive evidence of histocompatibility at the HLA-D locus. Other minor histocompatibility loci may also be involved, as well as some non-HLA loci. In addition, specific and nonspecific serum factors can inhibit the assay, and lymphocytes from diseased individuals may not perform well. Numerous controls (including autologous controls) must be included, and the assay must be performed as expected for the results to be accepted as valid. The principal clinical use of the MLC assay is to assist in the selection of a compatible donor for a bone marrow transplant, because the MLC is a predictor of host response to a transplanted organ. To prevent graft rejection or graft-versus-host disease, donor and recipient cells must be mutually nonstimulatory (El-Agroudy, 2004).

Flow cytometric quantitation of the mixed lymphocyte reaction has been reported. In the method reported by Cram and by Kanda, nuclear DNA content during lymphocyte blastogenesis was determined with a DNA-specific fluorochrome (PI) (Cram, 1976; Kanda, 1985). With this technique, the proliferative index (percentages of cells in the S phase and G_2M phase of the cell cycle) is a direct measurement of de novo DNA synthesis. A good correlation ($r = 0.9493$) was observed between the flow cytometric measurement of the mixed lymphocyte reaction and the results using a traditional MLC with ^{3}H-thymidine incorporation. Other investigators have utilized BrdU, Ki-67, or CFSE for the flow cytometric quantitation of T cell proliferation in the MLR (Palutke, 1987, 1989; Bontadini, 1990; Marin, 2003; Onoe, 2003; Tanaka, 2005). Multiparametric analysis has also been used to measure nuclear DNA content in conjunction with T cell subsets, activation antigens, apoptosis, cytokine secretion, and other parameters during the MLR (Williams, 1984; Uchida, 1987, 1988; Lavergne, 1990; Nguyen, 2003).

CYTOTOXICITY ASSAYS

Cell death (cytotoxicity) is the endpoint commonly used in functional assays of the cellular immune system. In these assays, cell cytotoxicity may occur as the result of complement activity (complement-mediated cytotoxicity) or may be due to the direct effect of one cell on another (cell-mediated cytotoxicity). Conventionally, target cell lysis is determined by the release of a substance such as ^{51}chromium (^{51}Cr) from the target cell upon death, or by the incorporation of a vital dye such as eosin or tryptan blue. A variation of these assays, the microlymphocytotoxicity assay, is widely used in the clinical histocompatibility laboratory for human organ transplantation. However, the accuracy and reproducibility of these assays are often compromised by the length and technical complexity of the assays, technical problems such as poor uptake or nonspecific release of the marker, or the need for subjective interpretation of the results. The advent of new markers, in combination with the quantitative and multiparametric abilities of the flow cytometer, has made cytotoxicity assays much more practical for biomedical research studies. Other than in histocompatibility testing, these assays have not achieved widespread utilization in patient care.

Cytotoxic T Cell (CTL) Assays

Cytotoxic T cells (CTLs, T killer cells, cytolytic T cells, CD8$^+$ T cells, killer T cells) constitute a subset of T cells important in the host defense against altered class I MHC-positive self cells, especially cells infected with a virus or other pathogen. CTLs recognize altered target cells by the presence of peptide fragments produced by processing of the foreign antigen and presented by the class I MHC receptor to the T cell antigen receptor. Recognition of an MHC complex on a target cell by a CTL induces cell death by apoptosis by the granule-exocytosis pathway (granule endocytosis) or the FAS-FAS ligand pathway (Barry, 2002; Lieberman, 2003).

Transfused ^{51}Cr-labeled cells, especially red blood cells, have been used since the early 1950s to study cellular in vivo distribution and kinetics. In the mid-1960s, Goodman (1961), Sanderson (1964), and Wigzell (1965) independently described the use of ^{51}Cr-labeled mouse tumor of lymph node cells to study antibody-dependent complement-mediated cytotoxicity. Since that time, the **chromium release assay** has become the standard technique for the measurement of complement- or cell-mediated cytotoxicity. In the chromium release assay for cytotoxic T cell activity, the binding of CTLs to infected ^{51}Cr-labeled target cells with virus peptide on syngeneic class I MHC induces apoptosis with the proportional release of ^{51}Cr into the supernatant (Fig. 45-9) (Levin, 1978). Alternatives for the chromium release assay were developed because of the disadvantages of the assay, including its relatively limited sensitivity and use of a radioisotope. The most widely employed alternative techniques include flow cytometry and variations of the enzyme-linked immunosorbent assay (ELISA).

Measurement of antibody- or cell-mediated cytotoxicity by flow cytometry is based on the discrimination of viable and nonviable cells with fluorescent dyes. In addition to relatively high sensitivity, flow cytometry permits multiparametric analysis, with simultaneous detection of up to 12 markers at the single-cell level. The permeability of the cell membrane is

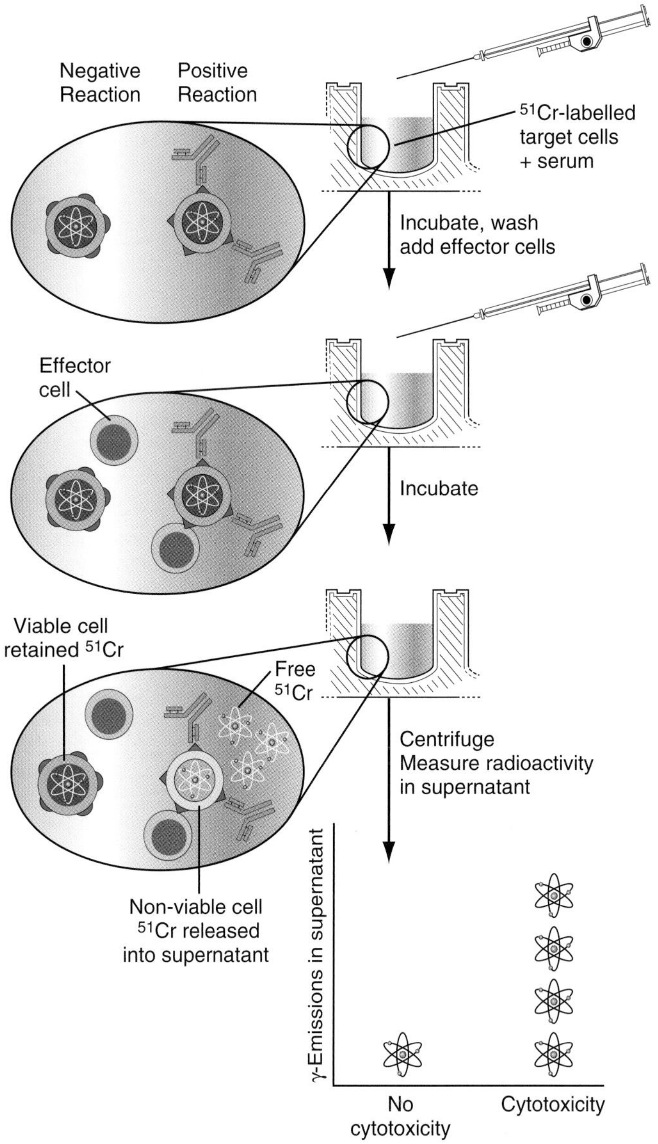

Figure 45-9 Principle of the antibody-dependent cell-mediated cytotoxicity (ADCC) assay. This assay is performed with mononuclear cells from a kidney organ donor or from several unrelated individuals (panel cells), which are stimulated with phytohemagglutinin (PHA) and labeled with ^{51}Cr. Following incubation with eluate from another nephrectomy specimen or from normal human serum, labeled cells are washed and incubated with effector cells from a normal unrelated individual. Radioactivity (γ-emissions) in the cells at the end of the experiment represents unlysed cells. The results are expressed as % cytotoxicity. *(Reprinted with permission from Riley RS. Basic principles of immunodiagnosis. In: McClatchey KD, editor. Clinical laboratory medicine. Baltimore: Williams and Wilkins, 1994.)*

the most widely used parameter of cell viability measured by flow cytometry. Damaged or nonviable cells have altered membrane permeability, and many leak some intracellular substances into the supernatant, while losing the ability to prevent other dyes from penetrating the cell membrane. PI and 7-AAD were the first fluorescent dyes to be used for flow cytometric measurements of cell viability because they are excluded by live cells but rapidly penetrate cells with damaged membranes. Fluorescein diacetate, carboxyfluorescein diacetate (CFDA), and calcein are lipid-soluble, nonfluorescent probes that are metabolized by cytoplasmic esterases to produce a charged, fluorescent product that is retained within the cell if the cell membrane is intact (Zarcone, 1986; Talbot, 1987). Other dyes used for viability determination include PKH-1 (Slezak, 1989), hydroxystilbamidine methanesulfonate (Fluoro-Gold [FG]) (Barber, 1999), SYTO13 (Shenkin, 2007), Cell Tracker Orange (Kim, 2007), and calcofluor white M2R (Berglund, 1987). In many cases, the simultaneous use of two or more markers permits the most accurate measurement of cytotoxicity. One example is the use of PKH-1 in conjunction with PI. PKH-1 is a fluorochrome that emits light in the green region of the spectrum, binds avidly to the cytoplasmic membrane, and is not transferred to other cells. In one

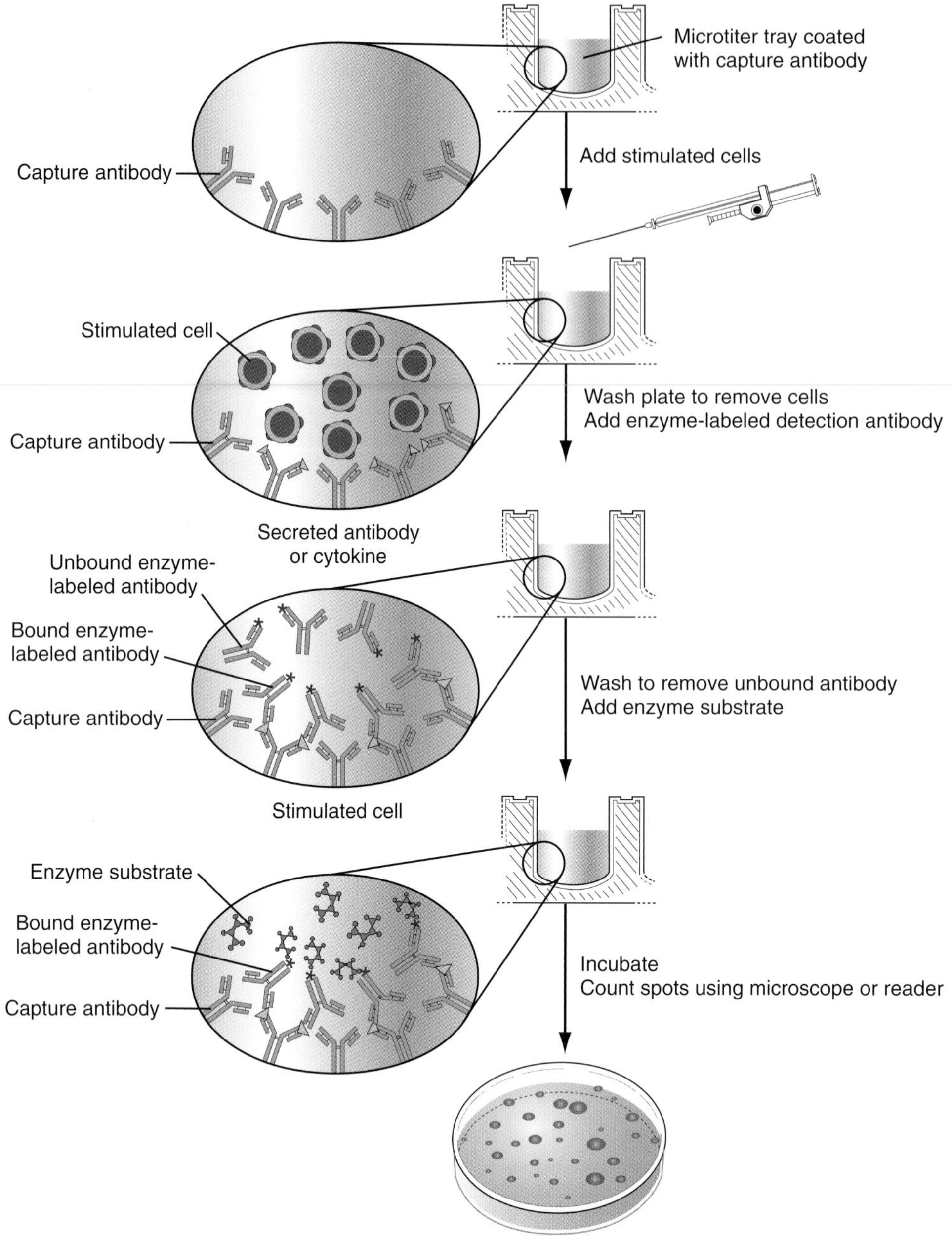

Figure 45-10 Principle of the enzyme-linked immunosorbent spot (ELISPOT) assay. ELISPOT assays bear many similarities to conventional sandwich enzyme-linked immunosorbent assays. A polyvinylidene difluoride (PVDF)-backed microplate is immobilized with an antibody specific for the analyte under evaluation. Immune cells are stimulated with an appropriate antigen or mitogen and then are pipetted into the wells of the microplate. The microplate is incubated in a humidified carbon dioxide (CO_2) chamber at 37° C for a specified period of time, during which stimulated immune products, such as cytokines and antibodies, are secreted. The secreted analyte binds to the immobilized antibody on the microplate. The microplate is washed to remove cells and unbound substances, and a biotinylated polyclonal antibody specific for the chosen analyte is added. Unbound biotinylated antibody is removed by washing, and streptavidin conjugated with alkaline-phosphatase conjugate is added. Following another wash to remove unbound enzyme, the reaction is completed by the addition of the enzyme substrate solution (BCIP/NBT). Dark, blue-black precipitate spots mark the original locations of analyte-secreting cells. The spots can be counted manually under a stereomicroscope, or automatically with a commercial automated ELISPOT reader system.

application, PKH-1 is used to label the target cells, while a second fluorochrome with a red emission signal (PI) is used to detect nonviable cells (Slezak, 1989). This combination of markers allows statistically valid quantitation of both dead and live effectors and targets, permitting the simultaneous determination of percent target lysis, effector-to-target ratio, viability of the effector cells at the termination of the assay, and viable effector-to-target cell ratios.

The enzyme-linked immunosorbent spot (ELISPOT) assay is a very sensitive, extremely versatile adaptation of sandwich ELISA (Shacklett, 2006). Originally described by Czerkinsky and coworkers in 1983 to detect individual B cells secreting antigen-specific antibodies, the ELISPOT was rapidly adapted to detect T cell cytokine excretion (Czerkinsky, 1983; Stott, 2000; Sedgwick, 2005; Kalyuzhny, 2009). Because the ELISPOT assay can reproducibility detect the proportion of antigen-specific or cytokine-secreting cells at a sensitivity of 1/100,000 to 1/1,000,000, it has achieved widespread use in research involving cancer, infectious disease, and immune disease. Clinically, the ELISPOT is used in immune monitoring and the detection of latent tuberculosis infection. The ELISPOT utilizes polyvinylidene fluoride (PVDF)-backed microplates coated with a monoclonal or polyclonal capture antibody specific for the desired analyte, usually IFN-γ (Kalyuzhny, 2005). A cell suspension and appropriate antigens or mitogens are added to the microplates, and they are incubated in a humidified carbon dioxide (CO_2) incubator at 37° C for a specified time. The plates are washed to remove cells and debris, a biotinylated polyclonal antibody specific for the analyte is added, the plates are washed a second time to remove unbound antibody, and avidin-horseradish peroxidase and a precipitating substrate is added to develop the assay. Colored spots on the plate represent individual analyte-producing cells (Fig. 45-10). The spots can be manually or automatically detected and counted. A variation of this assay using fluorochrome-labeled antibodies (Fluorospot assay) permits the simultaneous detection of two or three cytokines. A variation of the ELISPOT for the detection of granzyme B, rather than IFN-γ, has shown better correlation with the chromium release assay for the measurement of cytotoxic T cell activity (Shafer-Weaver, 2003; Malyguine, 2007).

Natural Killer Cell–Mediated Cytotoxicity

NK cells are critical members of the innate immune system characterized by their capability to lyse target cells without prior sensitization, termed **spontaneous cell-mediated cytotoxicity** (Sinkovics, 2005). NK cells can be subdivided into two functional and immunophenotypically distinct groups defined by the surface density of CD56 (i.e., CD56bright, CD56dim) (Cooper, 2001; Batoni, 2005; Whiteside, 2006; Morice, 2007; Milush, 2009; Poli, 2009; Bryceson, 2010). Release of ^{51}Cr from labeled target cells is the standard method for the characterization of NK cells. The chronic myeloid leukemia cell line K562 has been used as the standard target in these assays. A variety of other techniques are under evaluation because the ^{51}Cr-release technique has many disadvantages, including the use of radioisotopes, low sensitivity, and the spontaneous release of ^{51}Cr. These methods include the incorporation of radioactive nucleotides during cell proliferation, dye exclusion, target cell enzyme release, and flow cytometry (Bryceson, 2010). Flow cytometric analysis has been performed using a wide variety of markers to differentiate live and dead target cells, including CFDA, PI, Hoechst 33342, fluorochrome octadecylamine-fluorescein isothiocyanate (F-18), usually in combination with multiparametric analysis of cell surface makers, degranulation, cytokine production, and other parameters (McGinnes, 1986; Zarcone, 1986; Vitale, 1989; Kim, 2007; Chung, 2009; Bryceson, 2010).

Microlymphocytotoxicity Assay

The dye exclusion lymphocytotoxicity assay is the standard technique for the detection of an antibody–antigen interaction on a cell surface. The lymphocytotoxicity assay was introduced by Terasaki and McClelland in 1964, and was later accepted as the National Institutes of Health standard procedure for histocompatibility testing (Terasaki, 1964). In the histocompatibility laboratory, variations of the lymphocytotoxicity assay are used for HLA typing, detection of anti-HLA antibodies, and crossmatch testing.

In the lymphocytotoxicity procedure, viable cells (usually lymphocytes) are incubated with serum-containing antisera. If a cell surface antigen is present that is recognized by antibodies in the sera, an antigen–antibody complex will form on the surface. These complexes are detected by the sequential addition of rabbit complement and a vital dye, such as eosin, to the reaction mixture. The occurrence of complement fixation on the cell membrane leads to activation of the terminal complement components, and eventually to cell lysis and death. Dead cells are detected and counted by phase microscopy after differential uptake of the eosin dye and fixation with formalin. Antibody-bound lymphocytes will die, take up the eosin dye, and give a positive reaction; unbound lymphocytes will remain viable, exclude the eosin dye, and give a negative reaction (dye exclusion) (Fig. 45-11).

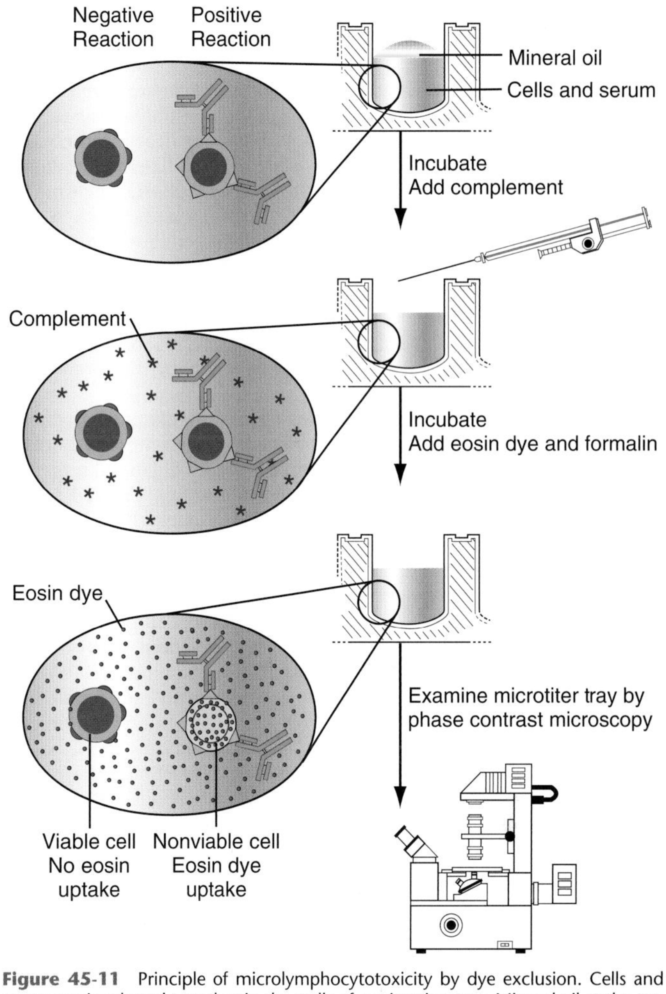

Figure 45-11 Principle of microlymphocytotoxicity by dye exclusion. Cells and serum are incubated together in the wells of a microtiter tray. Mineral oil at the top of the wells prevents fluid evaporation. Complement is added, and a second incubation is performed. The cells are washed, eosin is added, and the cells are fixed with formalin. Cells that fixed antibody and were killed through the action of complement take up eosin and appear dark and nonrefractive under a phase-contrast microscope. In contrast, living cells are refractive and are easily identified by phase-contrast microscopy. Variations of the microlymphocytotoxicity assay are used for human leukocyte antigen (HLA) typing, HLA crossmatch, and detection of anti-HLA antibodies. *(Reprinted with permission from Riley RS, Mahin EJ, Ross W. Clinical applications of flow cytometry. New York: Igaku-Shoin Medical Publishers; 1993.)*

Laboratory Evaluation of Granulocyte and Monocyte Function

Monocytes and granulocytes are extremely important in the early inflammatory response, and abnormalities in their functions lead to profound deficiencies in cellular immunity. The activity of neutrophils and macrophages is complex and involves activation of the cell, margination and passage through the vessel wall (diapedesis), movement toward an inflammatory stimulus (chemotaxis, chemokinesis), opsonization, engulfment of the offending agent (phagocytosis), and intracellular killing via the generation of toxic oxygen radicals (Seely, 2003; Zarbock, 2009). Until the modern era of flow cytometry, laboratory analysis of these nonspecific immune parameters was difficult to measure, with available assays being subjective and lacking standardized methods and quality control. In contrast to the subjective assays, many flow cytometric studies are rapid, reproducible, and statistically valid. In addition, the multiparametric capabilities of the flow cytometer permit the simultaneous determination of several cell functions, as well as an assessment of the interrelationship between cell function and other parameters. Flow cytometric assays have been described for the measurement of phagocytosis of microorganisms, degranulation and enzymatic activity, intracellular killing and degradation of microorganisms, exocytosis, osponization, oxidative metabolism, membrane potential, phagosomal pH, calcium mobilization, F-actin assembly, cell volume, apoptosis, receptor expression, adhesion and aggregation, and other parameters (Duque, 1987; Stelzer, 1988; Bjerknes, 1989; van Eeden, 1999; Elbim, 2009; Zarbock, 2009).

ASSAYS OF NEUTROPHILIC ACTIVATION

Neutrophil activation results when stimulatory substances (e.g., chemotactic factors, immune complexes, opsonized particles) bind to surface receptors to initiate metabolic and structural changes in the cell that result in locomotion, degranulation, phagocytosis, the oxidative burst, and other processes. Early studies of neutrophil activation utilized 7-nitrobenz-2-oxa-1,3-diazole-phallacidin, a fluorescent derivative of an acidic phallotoxin isolated from mushrooms of the *Amanita* genus, to measure changes in the equilibrium of F-actin that occur during cell activation (Belloc, 1990; Packman, 1990). However, the flow cytometric detection of neutrophil activation antigens, especially CD11b, CD13, and CD64, has become the standard technique for studies of neutrophil activation, usually performed in conjunction with other measurements of intercellular neutrophil function, such as the oxidative burst and measurement of the production and release of neutrophil secretion products such as myeloperoxidase, neutrophil elastase, and lactoferrin (Alvarez-Larran, 2005).

ASSAYS OF PHAGOCYTOSIS AND ENDOCYTOSIS

Conventional analysis of phagocytosis uses particles that are visible within the cell and can be counted after ingestion, or an ingestible substance that can be extracted from the cell and measured. Live or heat-killed *Candida albicans* or staphylococci fulfill the first criterion and permit a simple, convenient means of measuring phagocytosis. Target cells (i.e., neutrophils and monocytes) are incubated with yeast particles in the fresh serum, Giemsa-stained cell preparations are made, and 200 cells are examined and counted for the presence of ingested microorganisms (Lehrer, 1969, 1970). The results are expressed as the percentage of target cells showing phagocytosis and the number of particles per phagocytic neutrophil. Oil droplets containing dissolved oil red O stain and coated with *Escherichia coli* liposaccharide and C3 complement have also been used for the measurement of phagocytosis.

Flow cytometric assays of phagocytosis are quantitative and more accurate than subjective studies using visual counting of phagocytosed microorganisms. Different investigators have used a variety of labeled targets to study phagocytosis by both neutrophils and monocytes. Labeled targets have included fluorescent beads coated with opsonins (Bassøe, 1983a, 1983b, 1984a, 1984b, 1985; Bjerknes, 1983, 1984a, 1984b; Dunn, 1981; Steinkamp, 1982; Ogle, 1988), fluorescein-labeled *C. albicans* (Busetto, 2004), FITC-labeled zymosan particles (Nuutila, 2005), fluorescein-labeled *Staphylococcus aureus* (Carvalho, 2009), fluorescein-labeled *E. coli* (Hirt, 1994; Cacciapuoti, 2007; Danikas, 2008), enhanced green fluorescent protein (EGFP)-expressing *E. coli* (Gille, 2006; Bicker, 2008), and bis-carboxyethyl-carboxyfluorescein pentaacetoxymethylester-labeled *C. albicans* (Pattanapanyasat, 2007). For example, green fluorescent microspheres coated with C3b, iC3b, IgG, mixtures of these substances, bovine serum albumin, or human F(ab′)2 are utilized in the technique developed by Ogle and collaborators (1988). In this assay, neutrophils are incubated with coated microspheres alone or in the presence of cytochalasin D to inhibit phagocytosis. Externally bound microspheres are then stained with a red-labeled antibody against the immobilized ligand(s), and flow cytometric analysis is performed. The ratio of red-to-green fluorescence in the cytochalasin D–inhibited mixtures is used to correct the uninhibited mixtures for externally bound, nonphagocytosed particles. Net phagocytosis is thus represented by the corrected green fluorescence. The specificity of this technique was confirmed with the use of fluid phase C3b and iC3b and monoclonal antibodies to the receptors.

Receptor-mediated endocytosis is a common method for the cellular uptake of viruses, hormones, proteins, toxins, and other ligands. Endocytosis is a complex process that involves capping, internalization of the ligand, intracellular movement, and entry of the ligand into a subcellular compartment. Fluorescent dyes were first used to study endocytosis by Ohkuma and Poole (1978), who studied intralysosomal pH in living cells using a fluorometer and FITC-dextran. Subsequent investigators have used flow cytometry and fluorescent-labeled ligands or liposomes to follow the internalization of various ligands, while others have utilized changes in pH sensitivity to study internalization and/or intracellular movement (Metezeau, 1982; Murphy, 1982a, 1982b; Finney, 1983; Truneh, 1983; Murphy, 1984a, 1984b, 1984c, 1984d; van Deurs, 1984; Elguindi, 1985; Murphy, 1986; Ruud, 1986; Becker, 1997; Ruud, 1989). A different technique was utilized by Wang Yang (1988), who utilized flow cytometric pulse profiles to study capping and endocytosis by mouse B lymphocytes and BCL_1 cells. In this assay, the cells were stained with FITC-labeled anti-immunoglobulin, and were permitted to undergo changes in a temperature-controlled flow cytometer sample compartment. Cap formation resulted in decreases in area values from pH-dependent quenching as the internalized antibody entered the acidic subcellular compartments. Fattorossi (1989) described a related procedure utilizing FITC-conjugated, heat-killed *C. albicans* (F-Ca) opsonized with purified antibodies, or normal human serum. Neutrophils were first incubated with the labeled, opsonized *Candida* particles, and subsequently with ethidium bromide. Although ethidium bromide does not penetrate intact cell membranes, it binds to membrane-bound particles and causes a shift from green to red fluorescence through resonance energy transfer. Because internalized particles retain green fluorescence, the number of internalized or surface-bound particles can be ascertained by contour plot analysis. Fluoresceinated derivatives of α-fetoprotein and transferrin were used by Torres (1990) to study the endocytosis of these substances, and Fibach (1988) studied the uptake of a fluorescent fatty acid derivative [12-(1-pyrene) dodecanoic acid] by a variety of peripheral blood cells. Flow cytometry and electron microscopy were used by Kershaw (2009) to study the endocytosis and intracellular trafficking of chemokine CCR5.

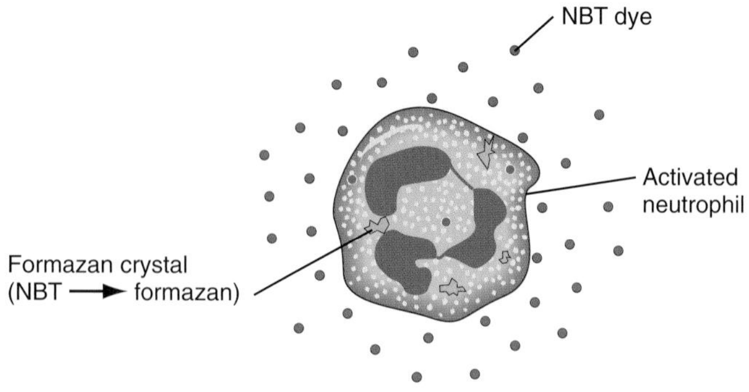

Figure 45-12 Principle of the nitroblue tetrazolium (NBT) reduction assay. Neutrophils are incubated with NBT. Enzymatic activity in the activated neutrophil converts NBT into an insoluble brownish-black precipitate (formazan), which is visible under the microscope. The proportion of neutrophils with intracytoplasmic precipitated material is determined. *(Reprinted with permission from Riley RS. Basic principles of immunodiagnosis. In: McClatchey KD, editor. Clinical laboratory medicine. Baltimore: Williams and Wilkins, 1994.)*

ASSAYS OF ENZYMATIC ACTIVITY AND INTRACELLULAR KILLING

Intracellular killing of microorganisms is mediated by complex enzymatic mechanisms. Oxygen-dependent mechanisms of cell killing are the most important, although oxygen-independent mechanisms have also been described. The increase in oxidative metabolism during phagocytosis is referred to as the **oxidative burst**. During this process, the key event is the activation of a membrane-bound pyridine nucleotide-dependent oxidase (NADPH oxidase), which reduces oxygen to O_2– (superoxide anion) and oxidizes NAD(P)H to $NAD(P)^+$. Subsequently, hydrogen peroxide (H_2O_2), hydroxyl radical (OH), and singlet oxygen are generated. All of these compounds are directly toxic to the cell, with the H_2O_2– halide-myeloperoxidase system being the most important mechanism of bacterial killing. In the presence of H_2O_2 and halide ions (I^-, Cl^-), myeloperoxidase catalyzes direct halogenation of the bacterial cell wall and causes damage to the cell wall by converting amino acids into aldehydes.

In the clinical laboratory, the nitroblue tetrazolium (NBT) reduction assay is the conventional method for determination of the oxidative capacity of the neutrophil. NBT is a yellow dye in its oxidized state, but when reduced, it forms formazan, a crystalline substance that has a deep blue color (Fig. 45-12) (Urban, 1979). NBT can be attached to latex particles or microorganisms to permit phagocytosis, or it can be ingested in soluble form by neutrophils that have been stimulated by endotoxin or other means. If the normal oxidizing environment in the phagolysosome is present, the resultant blue particles can be detected microscopically, or the formazan can be extracted and measured spectrophotometrically. Approximately 10% of normal unstimulated neutrophils ingest and reduce NBT, but this is increased to 80% with stimulated neutrophils.

A flow cytometric variation of the NBT assay has been described. With this technique, neutrophils are incubated for a short time with FITC-labeled Con A, rendering the cell membrane fluorescent (Fattorossi, 1990). The cells are then incubated with NBT and an agent to trigger respiratory activity, such as phorbol myristate acetate. The formazan that is subsequently produced has a distinct fluorescent peak at 520 nm that corresponds with the peak emission of fluorescein, and fluorescence quenching of surface fluorescence by formazan is proportional to the intensity of the respiratory burst. In addition, simultaneous changes in cell size and forward light scatter occur.

Bass (1983) described one of the first non–NBT-based flow cytometric–based assays to measure neutrophil oxidative metabolism and oxidative burst at the single-cell level. This technique uses the fluorogenic substrate dichlorofluorescein-diacetate (DCFH-DA) to quantitate H_2O_2 production during the oxidative burst (Bass, 1983). DCFH-DA is a small, nonpolar substance that is actively taken up by the cell and deacetylated by intracellular esterases into a nonfluorescent compound (2′,7′-dichlorofluorescein [DCFH]), which is trapped within the cell. In the presence of H_2O_2 and peroxidase, DCFH is oxidized into dichlorofluorescein, which is highly fluorescent in the green region of the spectrum (Fig. 45-13) (Bass, 1983). Other fluorochromes that have been used to directly measure the oxidative burst include dihydrorhodamine 123, dihydrotetramethylrosamine,

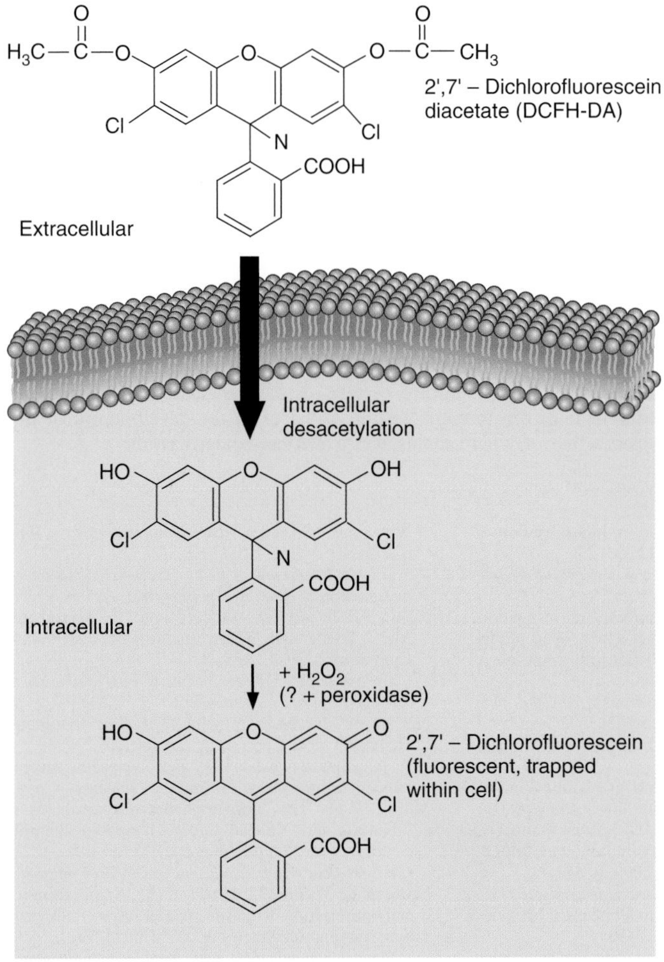

Figure 45-13 Flow cytometric analysis of the oxidative burst of polymorphonuclear leukocytes. In this assay, dichlorofluorescein-diacetate (DCFH-DA) is taken up by the cell and is trapped by deacetylation, with the formation of 2′,7′-dichlorofluorescein. During the oxidative burst, nonfluorescent 2′,7′-dichlorofluorescein is converted into the fluorescent product dichlorofluorescein. The fluorescent intensity in the green region of the spectrum is proportional to the oxidative capacity of the cell. *(Reprinted with permission from Bass DA, Parce JW, Dechatelet LR, et al. Flow cytometric studies of oxidative product formation by neutrophils: a graded response to membrane stimulation. J Immunol 1983;130:1910–17.)*

4-carboxydihydrotetramethylrosamine succinimidyl ester, and hydroethidine (Smith, 1993; Model, 1997; Walrand, 2003; Elbim, 2009).

Flow cytometric measurements of the oxidative burst have been combined with the quantitation of other metabolic or antigenic changes in the phagocytic cell to fully utilize the multiparametric power of the flow cytometer. In particular, several investigators have described flow cytometric techniques for the simultaneous measurement of phagocytosis and intracellular killing. In one of the earliest studies, phagocytic activity was determined by the internalization of viable, FITC-labeled *C. albicans* (Bjerknes, 1984). At selected intervals, fungi were extracted from the cells, and the fraction of killed fungi was measured by the uptake of PI. Later variations of this technique were developed to simultaneously measure phagocytosis and the oxidative burst (Trinkle, 1987; Prodan, 1995; Lehmann, 1998; McCloskey, 2000; Carvalho, 2009).

A technique for the assessment of surface antigen expression, phagocytosis, and cell proliferation in human bone marrow cells was described by Lund-Johansen (1990). With this technique, incubation of leukocytes with ethidium monoazide-labeled *C. albicans*, followed by staining with an FITC-labeled monoclonal antibody, permitted correlation of surface antigen expression with phagocytic capacity. After incubation with the labeled *C. albicans*, aliquots of the cells were fixed and stained with PI for cell cycle analysis. Haynes (1990) reported a novel method to measure protein digestion within the phagocytic vacuole based on the fluorescent quenching that occurs when rhodamine is attached to albumin at a high molar ratio. In the phagocytic vacuole, digestion of albumin releases free rhodamine and restores fluorescence. This method was affected less by vacuole pH than fluorescein-based methods and measured digestion even in the presence of abnormal phagocytosis.

ASSAYS OF OPSONIZATION

Phagocytosis of microorganisms and other foreign bodies is greatly enhanced by the presence of certain chemical substances (opsonins) on the surface of the foreign body. In patients with certain immunoglobulin and complement deficiencies, increased susceptibility to infection results in part from decreased opsonization. Opsonins in the serum can be detected by incubating the serum with normal neutrophils and yeast particles, and by visually quantitating phagocytosis of yeast particles by normal neutrophils. In addition, flow cytometric methods have been used for the measurement of serum opsonin function (Bassøe, 1984; Sjursen, 1987a, 1987b, 1989). In this assay, live FITC-labeled *Neisseria meningitidis* organisms were preopsonized by incubation with serum for 7.5 minutes, and then were incubated with human polymorphonuclear neutrophilic leukocytes (PMNLs) for 5 minutes at a bacteria-to-PMNL ratio of 20 : 1. Results were expressed in the number of bacteria incubated per phagocyte.

ASSAYS OF MEMBRANE PERMEABILITY

Fluorescein diacetate has been extensively utilized to monitor changes in membrane permeability. In this regard, fluorescein diacetate is enzymatically hydrolyzed within the cell, with the production of fluorescein. Free fluorescein is released into the extracellular environment across the cell membrane through a process that follows energy-dependent, first-order kinetics, and that is dependent on membrane integrity and permeability. The efflux of fluorescein is inhibited by metabolic poisons and glucose depletion, and has been used to study the effects of a variety of agents on the cell membrane (Prosperi, 1985, 1986). Prosperi (1990) showed that the fluorescein efflux is also related to the ionic gradient (membrane potential) of the cell.

Quality Control and Quality Assurance in the Cellular Laboratory

Throughout this chapter, we have tried to point out areas where the clinician and laboratory staff must pay particular attention to the methods used and the interpretations made in evaluation of the cellular response. Quality assurance and quality control parameters are not well defined in this area of the laboratory, and few absolute standards exist as compared with chemistry analytes or humoral antibody measures. The success of the cellular laboratory rests in its approach to the problem and the longitudinal assessment of the condition being diagnosed. It was clearly pointed out that baseline studies need to be repeated if the original evaluation is performed at a time of immunologic stress.

Basic parameters of diurnal variations in lymphocyte subsets are obvious but are often forgotten or overlooked. Malone (1990) pointed out that variability in CD4 measures of absolute counts is 50% owing to biology, with the other 50% related to other technical issues. Factors affecting the longitudinal evaluation of CD4 absolute counts in a clinical trial setting have been reviewed by Fei (1993). Furthermore, Fahey (1990) reviewed the prognostic value of both humoral and cellular assays in HIV. With other clinical cellular assays, variability is inherent in the assay owing to lack of standard formats and methods, as well as reagents. Furthermore, instrument calibration and sensitivity are not well monitored. Cytotoxic T lymphocyte assays are particularly difficult to standardize. Historic assays such as mitogen proliferation are also fraught with variability between laboratories. Therefore, laboratories that offer these immunologic tests must have an extensive database by which they can interpret an individual patient's result. Cellular laboratories must establish normal ranges for their assays and must be aware that adult normal ranges are not applicable to pediatric assays. This is particularly problematic because pediatric normal ranges are difficult to determine owing to lack of available subjects in the first year of life, and correct interpretation of laboratory results depends on these normal values. Data between laboratories should be compared carefully.

When available, a cellular immunology laboratory must use available standards in the performance of flow cytometry and DNA analysis, and should be aware of state and federal regulations with regard to the laboratory, including the Human Health and Services Clinical Laboratory

Improvement Act of 1988. Furthermore, laboratory staff should participate in proficiency testing, when available, and should be involved in continuing education seminars, including competency evaluations for all personnel involved in testing. All assays performed in the laboratory must include a normal control and, when possible, in-process controls to establish the validity of the assay. Shipped samples must be carefully monitored for exposure to heat and cold and time since patient procurement. A clinical history should accompany the samples for particular studies being ordered, so that the laboratory director can take the correct approach to testing.

A consensus document with recommendations on the immunophenotypic analysis of hematologic neoplasia by flow cytometry has been published (Braylan, 1997). This document was painstakingly developed by concerned providers in the medical community to cover laboratory procedures, selection of antibodies for identification of neoplasms, data analysis and interpretation, medical reporting, and indications in the absence of standardized kits and other devices. The FDA has put into effect the Analyte Specific Regulation (Analyte Specific Regulation, 1997), which moves reagents such as monoclonals from research use status to ASRs. This rule does not allow manufacturers to tell laboratory users how to use their reagents. They cannot specify intended use. The ASR rule does provide for stable, well-defined reagents manufactured under good manufacturing practices. All laboratories using these reagents as a "home brew test" must perform their own clinical trial and validation studies and must use a disclaimer in the final report. The consensus document allows a laboratory to perform its assays in a consistent manner and in keeping with the definition of clinical significance used across a large number of laboratories and institutions. The document is not a standard but is consistent with other published standards from NCCLS that are already in use.

The cellular laboratory is faced with a more difficult job of interpretation because the data are not easily standardized. Furthermore, quality assurance of the sample and the evaluation being performed depends on careful documentation of biological and logical parameters that may influence the results. The future of tests used in evaluation of the cellular component of the immune response resides in the development of new methods that may lend themselves to better standardization.

SELECTED REFERENCES

Allsopp CE, Nicholls SJ, Langhorne J. A flow cytometric method to assess antigen-specific proliferative responses of different subpopulations of fresh and cryopreserved human peripheral blood mononuclear cells. J Immunol Methods 1998;214:175–86.

The authors of this paper describe a useful approach to analyzing lymphocyte proliferative responses to antigen that makes use of a stable membrane-bound dye in combination with surface monoclonal antibody labels to identify subpopulations without the need for presorting.

Ananworanich J, Shearer WT. Delayed-type hypersensitivity skin testing. In: Rose NR, Hamilton RG, Detrick B, editors. Manual of clinical laboratory immunology. 6th ed. Washington, DC: ASM Press; 2002, p. 212–19.

This paper provides a practical and comprehensive review of skin testing for evaluation of the cellular immune response.

Balkwill FR, Burke F. The cytokine network. Immunol Today 1989;10:299–304.

A concise review of cytokines and cytokine function.

Barry M, Bleackley RC. Cytotoxic T lymphocytes: all roads lead to death. Nat Rev Immunol 2002;2:401–9.

This paper provides a thorough review of cytotoxic T cell function.

Baumgarth N, Roederer M. A practical approach to multicolor flow cytometry for immunophenotyping. J Immunol Methods 2000;243:77–97.

This article describes basic multicolor flow cytometry, technical problems that may be expected, and artifacts frequently encountered, and offers suggestions for handling them.

Beutler BA. TLRs and innate immunity. Blood 2009;113:1399–407.

This article is a succinct, up-to-date review of innate immunity and the role of toll-like receptors.

Bjerknes R, Bassøe C-F, Sjursen H, Laerum OD, Solberg CO. Flow cytometry for the study of phagocyte functions. Rev Infect Dis 1989;11:16–33.

The authors present a comprehensive review of the evaluation of phagocytic cell function by flow cytometry.

Bryceson YT, Fauriat C, Nunes JM, et al. Functional analysis of human NK cells by flow cytometry. Methods Mol Biol 2010;612:335–52.

This article is a current, thorough review of NK cell function analysis by flow cytometry.

Chaplin DD. Overview of the immune response. J Allergy Clin Immunol 2010;125:S3–23.

This article provides a concise, well-written, up-to-date summary of the immune system.

Elbim C, Lizard G. Flow cytometric investigation of neutrophil oxidative burst and apoptosis in physiological and pathological situations. Cytometry A 2009;75:475–81.

An excellent review of fluorescent probes and flow cytometric techniques for evaluation of neutrophil function, with an emphasis on primary immunodeficiency disease.

Ghanekar SA, Maecker HT, Maino VC. Monitoring of immune response using cytokine flow cytometry. In: Detrick B, Hamilton RJ, Folds JD, editors. Manual of molecular and clinical laboratory immunology. 7th ed. Washington, DC: ASM Press; 2006, p. 353–60.

A practical, useful review on cytokine flow cytometry.

Good RA. Cellular immunology in a historical perspective. Immunol Rev 2002;185:136–58.

A classic review of historical developments in cellular immunology, written by a pioneer in the field.

Herzenberg LA, Herzenberg LA. Genetics, FACS, immunology, and redox: a tale of two lives intertwined. Annu Rev Immunol 2004;22:1–31.

An historical account of the development of the flow cytometer from the inventors.

Janeway CA Jr, Medzhitov R. Innate immune recognition. Annu Rev Immunol 2002;20:197–216.

A classic review of the innate immune system from the immunologists who discovered the system.

Kalyuzhny AE. ELISPOT assay on membrane microplates. Methods Mol Biol 2009;536:355–65.

A recent, detailed review of the ELISPOT assay.

Keren DF. Surface marker assays in immunodeficiency diseases. In: Keren DF, editor. Flow cytometry in clinical diagnosis. Chicago: ASCP Press; 1989, p. 213–47.

A comprehensive review of the flow cytometric diagnosis of immunodeficiency diseases by a major leader in the field.

Malaguarnera L, Ferlito L, Imbesi RM, et al. Immunosenescence: a review. Arch Gerontol Geriatr 2001;32:1–14.

This review provides a good summary of age-related changes that occur in both arms of the immune system.

Maluish AE, Strong DM. Lymphocyte proliferation. In: Rose NR, Friedman H, Fahey JL, editors. Manual of clinical laboratory immunology. Washington, DC: American Society for Microbiology; 1986, p. 274–81.

An excellent summary of laboratory techniques for the measurement of lymphocyte proliferation.

Mandy FF. Twenty-five years of clinical flow cytometry: AIDS accelerated global instrument distribution. Cytometry A 2004;58:55–6.

An article highlighting the role of HIV evaluation in development of the flow cytometer.

McCoy JP Jr. Basic principles of flow cytometry. Hematol Oncol Clin North Am 2002;16:229–43.

An excellent summary of flow cytometric analysis, emphasizing instrument operation and function.

Morice WG. The immunophenotypic attributes of NK cells and NK-cell lineage lymphoproliferative disorders. Am J Clin Pathol 2007;127:881–6.

An excellent review of NK cells and NK cell function.

Nomura L, Maino VC, Maecker HT. Standardization and optimization of multiparameter intracellular cytokine staining. Cytometry A 2008;73:984–91.

A recent and important article on the standardization of flow cytometric analysis for cytokine analysis.

Perfetto SP, Chattopadhyay PK, Roederer M. Seventeen-colour flow cytometry: unravelling the immune system. Nat Rev Immunol 2004;4:648–55.

This paper describes a powerful form of flow cytometry capable of simultaneously examining several physical parameters and 17 fluorescent colors.

Perfetto SP, Currier J, Birx DL. T-lymphocyte activation and cell signaling. In Rose NR, Hamilton RG, Detrick B, editors. Manual of clinical laboratory immunology. 6th ed. Washington, DC: ASM Press; 2002, p. 224–37.

This paper provides a comprehensive review of the theoretical and practical aspects of T cell function and evaluation.

Sedgwick JD. ELISPOT assay: a personal retrospective. Methods Mol Biol 2005;302:3–14.

An historical account of the development of the ELISPOT assay.

Sinkovics JG, Horvath JC. Human natural killer cells: a comprehensive review. Int J Oncol 2005;27:5–47.

A thorough, comprehensive review of the NK cell.

Stewart CC, Goolsby C, Shackney SE. Emerging technology and future developments in flow cytometry. Hematol Oncol Clin North Am 2002;16:477–95.

A review of emerging applications and the future role of the flow cytometer in the medical sciences, from a leader in the field.

REFERENCES

Access the complete reference list online at http://www.expertconsult.com

CHAPTER 46

LABORATORY EVALUATION OF IMMUNOGLOBULIN FUNCTION AND HUMORAL IMMUNITY

Richard A. McPherson, H. Davis Massey

KEY POINTS

- Five different classes of antibody are known—immunoglobulin (Ig)M, IgG, IgA, IgD, and IgE—each with a distinct heavy chain.
- Two different light chain types have been identified: κ and λ.
- Antigens react with antibodies at the Fab region, which contains variable regions of both heavy and light chains.
- The Fc region on the heavy chains determines what other proteins will bind to the antibody (e.g., complement).
- IgG is prevalent in blood and tissue fluids; IgM is found mainly in the blood; secretory IgA is found primarily on epithelial surfaces; IgD is bound mostly to B cells; and IgE is bound largely to basophils and mast cells.
- Polyclonal increases in immunoglobulins occur as part of the immune response and may be found in chronic disease.
- Monoclonal increases in immunoglobulins suggest a plasma cell dyscrasia.
- Diagnosis of disorders of immunoglobulins is aided by their quantitative measurement, in addition to qualitative measures of their clonality by immunofixation electrophoresis and by determination of free light chain concentrations.
- Cryoglobulins can arise as excess monoclonal immunoglobulin (type I), which causes hyperviscosity, or as an IgM autoantibody against IgG (types II and III), which forms circulating immune complexes and causes vasculitis.
- Oligoclonal bands of immunoglobulin in cerebrospinal fluid suggest autoimmune disorders such as demyelinating disease or infection.

Antibodies are the effector molecules of humoral (B cell–mediated) immunity. They are immunoglobulins that react specifically and bind with the antigens that stimulated their production. By mass, immunoglobulins make up about 20% of plasma proteins in healthy individuals. Antibody activity is associated with the slowest migrating proteins on electrophoresis—the γ-globulins. The focus of this chapter is to discuss the general structural and functional properties of immunoglobulins, their laboratory evaluation, and their clinical significance.

STRUCTURAL PROPERTIES OF ANTIBODIES

ANTIBODY MOLECULES

The molecular structure of antibodies has been well elucidated (Padlan, 1991; Poljak, 1991; Tedford, 1991). An immunoglobulin molecule is a Y-shaped glycoprotein. It has two identical antigen-binding sites at the tips of the Y (Fab region) and binding sites for complement components and/or various cell surface receptors on the tail of the Y (Fc region). Each immunoglobulin molecule is composed of two identical heavy (H) chains and two identical light (L) chains. These polypeptide chains are held together by noncovalent interactions that are stabilized by disulfide bonds. Parts of both the H and L chains form the antigen-binding sites. Each immunoglobulin L and H chain consists of a variable region of about 110 amino acid residues at its amino-terminal end (the tips of the Y), which forms the antigen-binding site, linked to a constant region. The H constant region is three or four times larger than that of the L chain. Each chain is composed of repeating, similarly folded domains: An L chain has one variable region (VL) and one constant region (CL) domain, whereas an H chain has one variable region (VH) and three or four constant region (CH) domains (Fig. 46-1). The amino acid sequence variation in the variable regions of both L and H chains is for the most part confined to three small hypervariable regions that come together at the amino-terminal end of the molecule to form the antigen-binding site. Each antigen-binding site is only large enough to bind an antigenic determinant the size of five or six sugar residues.

Five different heavy chain isotypes (γ, α, μ, δ, ε) and two light chain isotypes (κ and λ) have been identified, with some of the isotypes having further subtypes. For example, γ has subtypes γ1, γ2, γ3, and γ4. The isotypes are formed as a result of variations in the constant regions of the heavy and light chains. These isotypic designations are the basis for the nomenclature of antibodies. Because the heavy chain alone determines effector functions, immunoglobulins are conveniently referred to by their heavy chain isotype (class) using an English letter terminology (IgG, IgA, IgM, IgD, and IgE).

Antibodies have two identical antigen-binding sites. An antigen-binding site is made up of amino acids from one H chain class and one L chain class. Thus, the four-chain Y monomer molecules (see Fig. 46-1) possess two identical antigen-combining sites and are said to be **bivalent.**

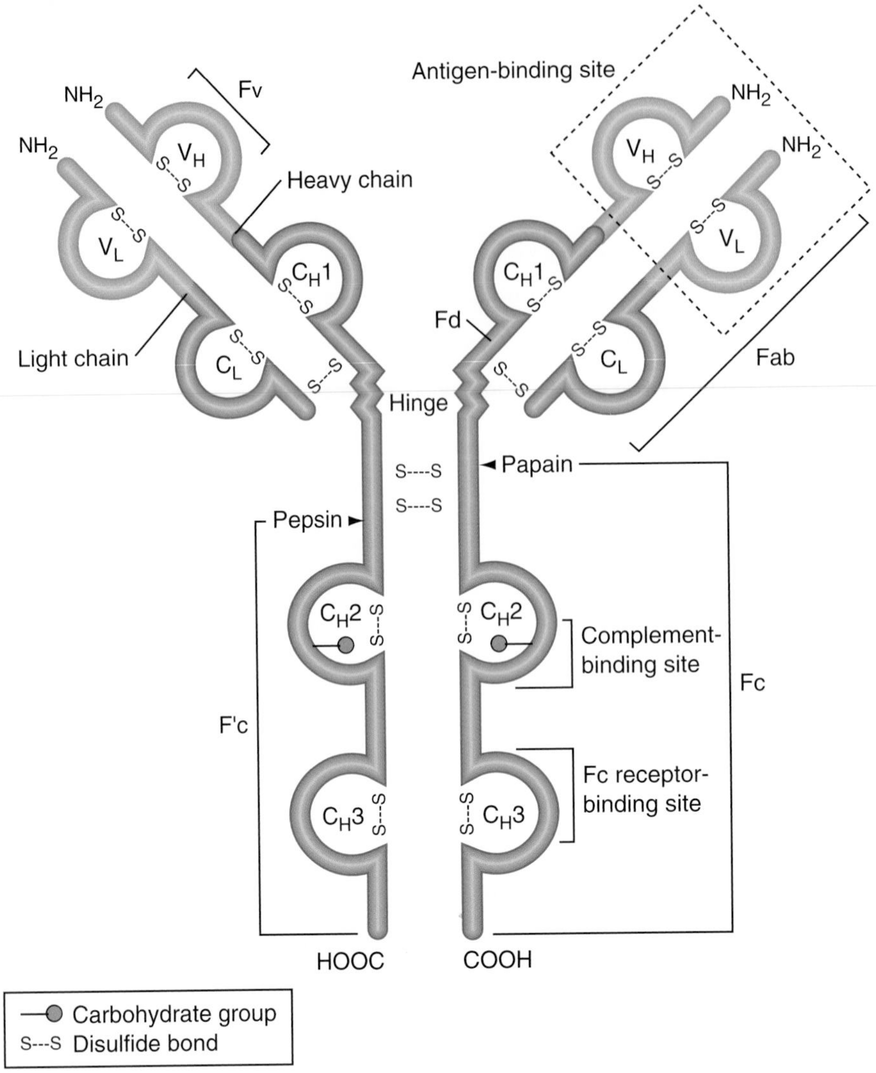

Figure 46-1 Schematic representation of immunoglobulin G molecule. The relative positions of the interchain disulfide bonds and the intrachain disulfide bonds that form the loop regions are shown. Each of the loops delineates the domain of the light and heavy chain labeled accordingly. Probable sites of enzymatic cleavage in the "hinge" region by papain or pepsin are indicated. The papain fragments are designated Fab and Fc. The pepsin fragments are Fc′ and Fab′2 (2 Fab fragments disulfide-linked). Digestion of Fab with pepsin under proper conditions yields the fragment Fv (VH and VL noncovalently associated). The part of the heavy chain that contributes to the Fab fragment is designated Fd.

Such antibody molecules can cross-link antigen molecules into a large lattice if the antigen molecules each have three or more antigenic determinants. Once the lattice reaches a certain size, it precipitates out of solution (Davies, 1983). This cross-linking is physiologically important because it enhances the engulfment of antigen, such as that expressed by bacteria and by phagocytic leukocytes. It is also involved in activation of the complement system. In addition, cross-linking may be required for the triggering of antibody-producing cells (B lymphocytes) by antigen. The efficiency of antigen-binding and cross-linking reactions by antibodies is greatly increased by a flexible hinge region, where the arms of the Y join the tail, allowing the distance between the two antigen-binding sites to vary.

Multivalence affects the avidity with which an antibody can bind certain types of antigens. A particulate antigen (such as a bacterium or virus) has repeating antigenic determinants on its surface. An antibody molecule may interact with a single particle in such a manner that both of its antigen-combining sites are bound to antigenic determinants on that particle rather than to antigenic determinants on two adjacent particles. When this type of binding occurs, the effective energy of interaction or avidity is greatly increased compared with that associated with monovalent attachments to two particles. This mechanism has been shown to be physiologically important in the neutralization of viruses by antibodies of relatively low binding affinity.

The protective effect of immunoglobulins is not due simply to their ability to bind antigen. They engage in a variety of biological activities mediated by the tail of the Y, the Fc region of the molecule. This part of the antibody molecule determines what will happen to the antigen once it is bound. Immunoglobulins with the same antigen-binding capacity can have a variety of different Fc regions and therefore different functional properties, such as activating the complement system and attaching to Fc receptors on macrophages, thereby aiding phagocytosis of antigens.

Because of its exposed location and loosely folded structure, the **hinge region** is readily attacked by various proteolytic enzymes. As the name suggests, the hinge region confers a certain amount of flexibility on the molecule, allowing it to assume the Y-shaped structure. This permits an antibody to become attached to a single particle (e.g., a bacterium) through both of its antigen-combining sites or, alternatively, to stretch out to its full length to join two particles. The unique properties conferred by the hinge region on Ig molecules are related to its rich content of proline and hydrophilic amino acid residues. The inter–H chain disulfide bonds of IgG, IgA, and IgD molecules are located in the hinge region (see Fig. 46-1).

The proteolytic enzymes papain and pepsin cleave antibody molecules into different characteristic fragments that lead to an understanding of the structure–function relationship of the protein. Papain cleavage produces two separate and identical Fab (fragment antigen-binding) fragments, each with one antigen-binding site, and one Fc fragment (so-called because in nonhuman primates, it readily crystallizes). On the other hand, pepsin cleavage produces one F(ab′)2 fragment, so-called because it consists of two covalently linked F(ab′) fragments (each slightly larger than a Fab fragment); the rest of the molecule is broken down into smaller fragments of various sizes (see Fig. 46-1). Because F(ab′)2 fragments are bivalent, they can still cross-link antigens and form precipitates. This is not true of the univalent Fab fragments. Neither of these fragments (subunits of

TABLE 46-1
Biological Properties of Immunoglobulin Domains

Domain	Known or probable function
CH3	1. Cytotrophic reactions involving: (a) Macrophages and monocytes (b) Heterologous mast cells (c) Cytotoxic killer (K) cells (d) B cells 2. Noncovalent assembly of heavy and light chains
CH2	1. Binding of complement (C1q) 2. Control of catabolic rate
CH1/CL	1. Noncovalent assembly of heavy and light chains 2. Covalent assembly of heavy and light chains 3. Spacers between interdomain interactions involving antigen binding and effector functions
VH/VL	1. Antigen binding 2. Noncovalent bonding of heavy and light chains

Used with permission from Dorrington KJ, Painter RH. Biological activities of the constant region of immunoglobulin G. In: Mandel TE, et al, editors. Progress in immunology III. Canberra: Australian Academy of Science; 1977.

antibodies) has the other biological properties of intact antibody molecules because they lack the tail (the Fc region) that mediates these properties. However, monovalent Fab is the form of postimmunization monospecific, affinity-purified ovine antibody that is used therapeutically in patients for such applications as removing toxic levels of digoxin (Digibind) or neutralizing crotalid snake venoms (CroFab).

Each B cell clone makes antibody molecules with a unique antigen-binding site. Initially, the molecules are inserted into the plasma membrane, where they serve as cell surface receptors for antigen. When antigen binds to the membrane-bound antibodies, B cells are activated to multiply, differentiate to a plasma cell, and synthesize a large amount of soluble antibody with the same antigen-binding site, which is secreted into the blood. Humoral antibodies defend humans and animals against infection by inactivating viruses and bacterial toxins via VH/VL domains and by recruiting complement and various cells to kill and ingest invading microorganisms via CL domains in the Fc region of the molecule. The biological properties of the various immunoglobulin domains are summarized in Table 46-1.

ANTIBODY–ANTIGEN INTERACTION

The binding of an antigen to antibody is reversible. The affinity and the number of binding sites contribute to the strength of an antibody–antigen interaction. This reversible binding is a result of many relatively weak noncovalent forces, including hydrophobic and hydrogen bonds, van der Waals forces, and ionic interactions. These weak forces are effective only when the antigen molecule is close enough to allow some of its atoms to fit into complementary recesses (regions) on the antibody surface. The complementary regions of a four-chain antibody unit are its two identical antigen-binding sites, whereas the corresponding region on the antigen is an antigenic determinant. Most antigenic macromolecules have many different antigenic determinants; if two or more of them are identical, the antigen is said to be multivalent.

The **affinity** of an antibody molecule reflects the tightness of fit of an antigenic determinant to a single antigen-binding site, and it is independent of the number of antigenic sites. However, the total **avidity** of an antibody for a multivalent antigen, such as a polymer with repeating subunits, is defined as the total binding strength of all of its binding sites together. A typical IgG molecule binds at least 10,000 times more strongly to a multivalent antigen if both antigen-binding sites are engaged than if only one site is involved.

For the same reason, if the affinity of the antigen-binding sites in an IgG and an IgM molecule is the same, the IgM molecule (because it is a pentamer and thus has 10 binding sites) will have much greater avidity for a multivalent antigen than an IgG molecule (which has two binding sites). This difference in avidity is important in view of the fact that antibodies produced early in an immune response usually have much lower affinities than those produced later. The increase in the average affinity of antibodies produced as time passes after immunization is called **affinity maturation.** This occurs because the antibody response to an antigen is heterogeneous, that is, antibodies with different antigen-combining sites are elicited against the antigen by the responding clones of B lymphocytes. Because

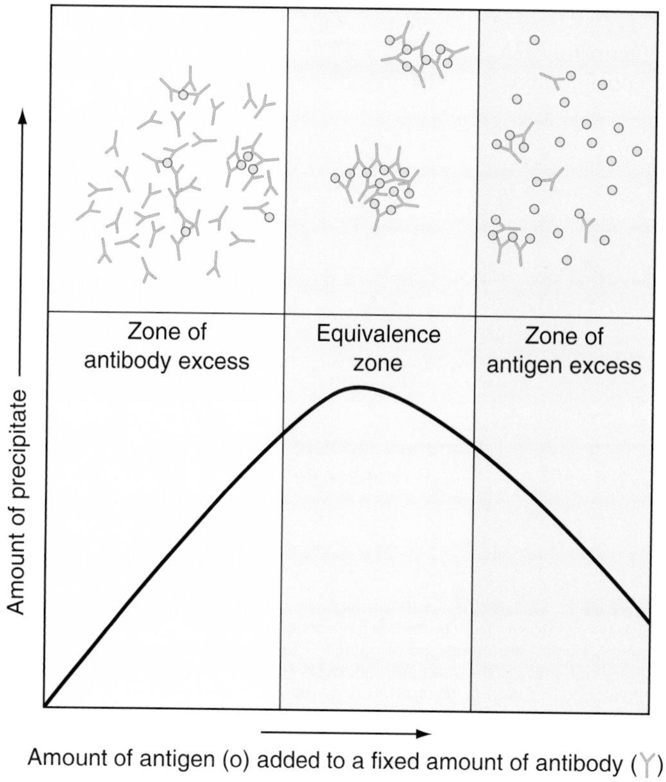

Figure 46-2 Antibody and antigen concentrations influence the size of antigen–antibody complexes formed. The largest complexes are formed when both molecules are present at approximately the same molar concentration (zone of equivalence), whereas the smallest complexes are formed when the antigen is present in great excess. Note that the small complexes formed in antigen excess have only a few antibody molecules per complex; for this reason, they are inefficiently cleared from the extracellular fluids by macrophages.

of its high total avidity, IgM (the major Ig class produced early in immune responses) can function even when each of its binding sites has only low affinity.

The size of the antigen–antibody complex is determined by the valence of the antigen and the relative concentrations of the antigen and the antibody. The antigen–antibody precipitation reaction is based on cross-linking of multivalent antigens by bivalent antibodies. If only one species of antibody (a monoclonal response) is present, molecules with only one antigenic determinant cannot be cross-linked. If an antigen is bivalent, it can form small cyclic complexes or linear chains with antibody, whereas an antigen with three or more antigenic determinants can form large three-dimensional lattices that readily precipitate. However, most antisera elicited against an antigen contain a variety of different antibodies (a polyclonal response) that react with different determinants on the antigen and can cooperate in cross-linking the antigen. By contrast, homogeneous (monoclonal) antibodies can precipitate molecules only if they contain repeating identical antigenic determinants.

Given valence conditions that allow the formation of large aggregates, the size of the antigen–antibody complexes that form depends critically on the relative molar concentrations of the two reactants. If an excess of antigen or antibody is present, large complexes are unlikely to form (Fig. 46-2). This property is crucial to understanding seemingly paradoxical reactions in some immunoassays that depend on antigen–antibody complex formation. For example, a vast excess of antigen can completely saturate all antibody-binding sites, leading to a negative signal (i.e., no agglutination). This phenomenon is sometimes referred to as the **prozone effect.** The prozone effect remains a potential problem for modern assay systems, including syphilis testing, in which extremely high titer antibodies can be missed unless the specimen is tested at dilutions (Smith, 2004) and even in immunofixation electrophoresis (see later, Fig. 46-6, *E*).

The size and composition of antibody–antigen complexes are not only important in influencing precipitation reactions in vitro, they are crucial in determining the fate of the complexes in the body. Complexes formed at equivalence or in antibody excess have multiple protruding Fc regions and therefore bind strongly to Fc receptors in macrophages, which ingest and degrade them. Small complexes, formed in antigen excess, have only one Fc region per complex. Therefore, they bind poorly to Fc receptors

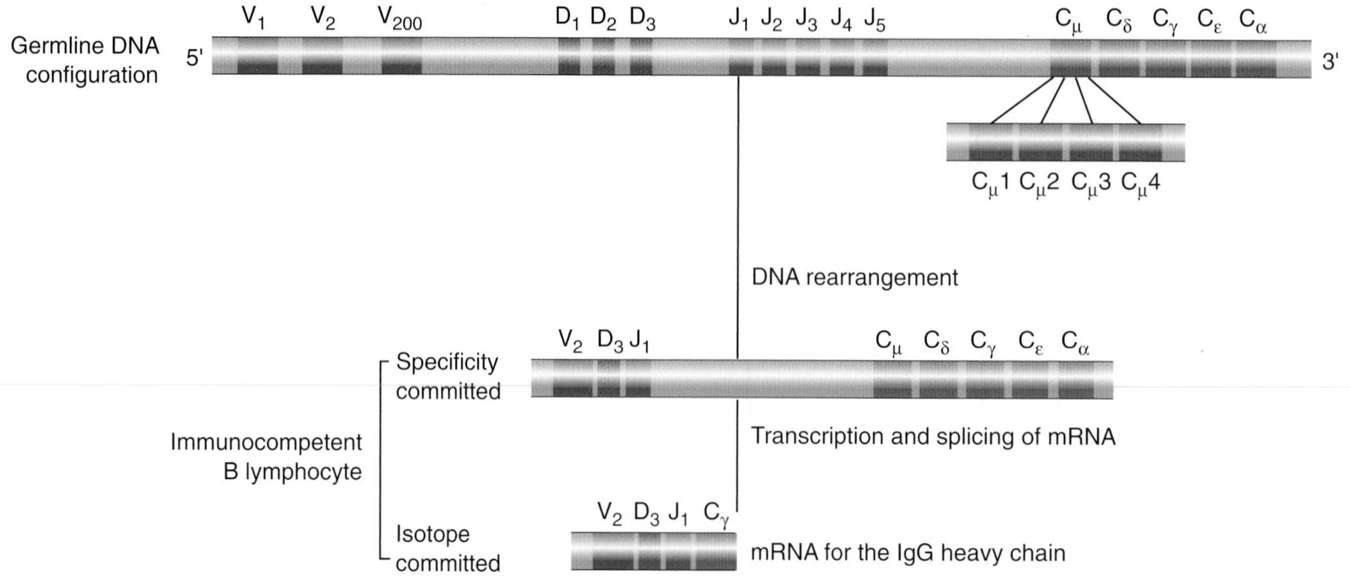

Figure 46-3 Organization and rearrangement of heavy chain immunoglobulin (Ig) genes (exons) on the mouse 12 chromosome. Each VH gene also has a leader sequence, which is not shown. The constant region genes are identified by the heavy chain isotype, and more than one gene exists for the Cγ and Cα isotypes. Unlike Cγ and Cα genes, CH genes are composed of multiple exons, as illustrated for the Cμ gene (Cμ1–Cμ4 domains). The switch sites are located at the 5′ end of each of the CH genes and are not shown. The solid line represents the intervening sequences (introns) between genes or gene segments. Each heavy chain is encoded by four distinct gene segments: V, D, J, and C. *(Redrawn with permission from Marcu KB. Immunoglobulin heavy-chain constant region genes. Cell 1982;29:719. Copyright © by Cell Press.)*

on macrophages and are less efficiently destroyed. Instead, they may be deposited in small blood vessels in the skin, kidneys, joints, and brain, where they may activate the complement system, causing inflammation and the destruction of tissue.

Although it appears that antigen–antibody complexes have a rigid "lock-and-key" appearance, antibodies are dynamic entities that undergo structural fluctuations (Karplus, 1983; Wilson, 1991). Conformational changes may even be required for binding. These adjustments include side chain shifts of up to 20–30 nm, aromatic ring rotations, conformational changes, and even small rotations between VH and VL domains (Bhat, 1990; Standfield, 1990; Herron, 1991).

The Genetic Basis of Antibody Diversity

It is estimated that a human is able to make at least 10^6–10^9 different antibody molecules. Special genetic mechanisms have evolved to produce the very large number of immunoglobulin molecules that develop in response to antigen stimulation without the need for an excessive number of genes (Max, 2003).

Immunoglobulin molecules are produced by three separate gene pools encoding the κ, λ, and H chains, respectively. The gene pools for light and heavy chains reside on different chromosomes. In each pool, separate gene segments that encode for different parts of the variable regions of light and heavy chains can be brought together by site-specific recombination events during B cell differentiation. The light chain gene pools contain one or more constant (C) genes and sets of variable (V) and joining (J) gene segments. The H chain gene pool contains a set of C genes and sets of V, diversity (D), and J gene segments. To make an antibody molecule, a VL gene segment is recombined with a JL gene segment to produce a V gene for the light chain; and a VH gene segment is recombined with D and JH segments to produce a V gene for the heavy chain (Fig. 46-3). Each of the assembled gene segments is then cotranscribed with the appropriate constant region sequence to produce a messenger RNA molecule that encodes for the complete polypeptide chain. By variously combining inherited gene segments encoding for VL and VH regions, vertebrates can make thousands of different light chains and thousands of different H chains that can associate to form millions of different antibody molecules.

The baseline repertoire of antibody molecules can be expanded still farther by somatic hypermutation, which seems to be activated by exposure to antigen. Thus, the selective role of antigen in the presence of somatic mutation appears to lead to fine tuning of the immune response and to a virtually unlimited diversity of antibody molecules. Somatic point mutations in immunoglobulin genes occur in B cells (not germ cells) during the lifetime of the animal or of humans (Tonegawa, 1983). The somatic hypermutations are largely confined to the H chain and L chain variable region genes and the introns immediately surrounding them. It is estimated that close to one mutation will occur in the H or L chain V region of an individual cell with each cell division. This not only increases antibody diversity but may cause a change in the affinity with which the antibody binds its ligand. Those emerging B cells that can bind the antigen more avidly have an advantage over other B cells that do not bind the antigen as avidly. As the concentration of antigen falls, those B cells that have more avid receptors dominate the population of responding cells. This results in greater affinity of the antibodies being produced on rechallenge than in the initial response. Thus, this process of somatic hypermutation can result in the presence in immunized individuals of high affinity antibodies that are much more effective on a weight basis.

All B cells initially make IgM antibodies. Some later switch to make antibodies of other classes (isotypes: IgG, IgA, etc.) that have the same antigen-binding site (idiotype) as the original IgM antibodies **(allelic exclusion)** (Table 46-2). Such class switching in combination with allelic exclusion allows the same antigen-binding sites (same VH and light chain) to be distributed among antibodies with many different biological properties (secondary effector functions) (Corcoran, 2005).

Thus, the gene organization mechanism permits the assembly of immunoglobulin molecules with a variety of specificities. Antibody diversity depends on the presence of multiple gene segments, their rearrangement into different sequences, the combination of different light and heavy chains in the assembly of immunoglobulin molecules, and somatic mutations.

General Properties of Immunoglobulins

The various classes of human immunoglobulins and their properties (Spiegelberg, 1974; Kolar, 2003) are summarized in Tables 46-3 and 46-4.

IMMUNOGLOBULIN M

This glycoprotein is the major class of antibody secreted into the blood in the early stages of a **primary** antibody response. Normally, the secreted form of IgM is a pentamer composed of five four-chain units, a macroglobulin with a 19S sedimentation rate, and a molecular weight of 900 kDa. However, in human autoimmune disorders, such as systemic lupus erythematosus (SLE), the monomeric 7S form may be detected in appreciable amounts in serum. Selective IgM deficiency is a rare disorder associated

TABLE 46-2
Summary of Immunoglobulin Variants

Type of variation	Distribution	Variant	Location	Examples
Isotypic	All variants present in serum of a normal individual	Classes	C_H	IgM, IgE
		Subclasses	C_H	IgA1, IgA2
		Types	C_L	κ, λ
		Subtypes	C_L	λOz+, λOz–
		Subgroups	V_L, V_H	$V_{\kappa I}$, $V_{\kappa II}$, V_{HI}, V_{HII}
Allotypic	Allelic forms not present in all individuals	Allotypes	Mainly C_H/C_L Occasionally V_H/V_L	Gm group (human γ chain; e.g., IgG1, G1m3, G1m17) b_4, b_5, b_6, b_9 (rabbit light chain)
Idiotypic	Antigenic individuality specific to each Ig molecule	Idiotypes	V_H/V_L	Determinant identified by antibody specific to an individual immunoglobulin

Modified with permission from Sell S. Immunology, immunopathology, and immunity. 4th ed. New York: Elsevier Science; 1987.

TABLE 46-3
Physical Properties of Human Immunoglobulins

WHO designation	IgM	IgG	IgA	IgD	IgE
Heavy chains	μ	γ	α	δ	ε
Heavy chain subclasses	μ_1, μ_2	γ_1, γ_2, γ_3, γ_4	α_1, α_2	–	–
Light chains	κ or λ	κ or λ	κ or λ	κ or λ	κ or λ
Molecular formula	IgM(κ) $(2\mu 2\kappa)_5$ IgM(λ) $(2\mu 2\lambda)_5$	IgG(κ) 2γ2κ IgG(λ) 2γ2λ	IgA(κ) $(2\alpha 2\kappa)_{1-3}$ IgA(λ) $(1\alpha 2\lambda)_{1-3}$ IgA(κ) $(2\alpha 2\kappa)_2$S† IgA(λ) $(2\alpha 2\lambda)_2$S	IgD(κ) 2δ2κ IgD(λ) 2δ2λ	IgE(κ) 2ε3κ IgE(λ) 2ε2λ
Number of four-chain units per molecule	5	1	1–3	1	1
Heavy chain molecular weight, kDa	70	50–60	55	62	70
Light chain molecular weight, kDa	23	23	23	23	23
Sedimentation coefficient, S20W	18.0–19.0	6.7–7.0	6.6–14.0	6.9–7.0	7.9–8.0
Molecular weight, kDa	900	143–160	159–447	177–185	187–200
Electrophoretic mobility	γ1–β1	γ2–α1	γ2–β2	γ1	γ1
Carbohydrate content, %	7–14	2.2–3	7.5–9.0	12–13	11–12
Heavy chain allotypes	–	Gm	Am	–	–
Light chain allotypes	Km(κ)*	Km(κ)*	Km(κ)*	Km(κ)*	Km(κ)
Valency for antigen binding	5 (10)	2	2.4 (? polymeric forms)	2	2
Number of domains on the heavy chains	5	4	4	4	5

*Formerly designated Inv marker.
†Dimer in external secretions carries secretory component -S.

with the absence of IgM and normal levels of other immunoglobulin classes. The cause of this disorder is unknown.

Because pentameric IgM has a total of 10 antigen-binding sites, it is more efficient than 7S monomeric IgM or IgG molecules in cross-linking antigen and in activating the complement system when bound to antigen. Thus, this high efficiency in binding and activating complement, coupled with its early appearance during the course of infection, makes IgM a particularly potent agent in combating microbial invasions.

Each IgM pentamer contains one copy of another polypeptide chain, called a **J (joining) chain,** which has a molecular weight of 15kDa. This accessory polypeptide is produced by IgM-secreting cells. It is an acidic glycoprotein with a high content of cysteine residues and thus is disulfide linked between two adjacent IgM monomeric Fc regions at the carboxy-terminal end. Presumably, oligomerization is initiated at this site.

IgM is also the first class of antibody to be produced by developing B cells. The immediate precursors of B cells, called pre-B cells, make μ chains but not light chains, which accumulate in the cells. Pre-B cells then begin to synthesize light chains, which combine with μ chains to form four-chain monomer IgM molecules. The two μ-chain and two light-chain component is inserted into the plasma membrane, where it functions as a receptor for antigen. At this point, the cells have become B lymphocytes and can respond to antigen.

Perhaps because of its large size, secreted pentamer IgM is not found to any significant extent in tissue spaces; it is confined to the blood circulation and does not cross the placenta. IgM is a minor component of secretory immunoglobulins at mucosal surfaces and in breast milk.

IgM is phylogenetically the most primitive of the immunoglobulins, and most variants of the genes from the μ chain appear to have evolved into heavy chain genes for the other immunoglobulin classes. Additional physical and biological properties of IgM, as well as the other classes of immunoglobulin, are given in Tables 46-3 and 46-4.

IMMUNOGLOBULIN G

IgG is the best studied isotype at both structural and functional levels (Burton, 1985). Antibodies of this class constitute the major immunoglobulin in the blood. They are copiously produced during the **secondary** immune response. The Fc region of IgG molecules binds to specific receptors on phagocytic cells, such as macrophages and polymorphonuclear leukocytes, thereby increasing the efficiency with which the phagocytic cells can ingest and destroy infecting microorganisms that have become coated with IgG antibodies in response to infection. These receptors on antibodies attached to target cells also guide natural killer (NK) lymphocytes to destroy them through the process of antibody-dependent cell-mediated cytotoxicity (ADCC). The best known function of IgG is complement activation via the classical cascade. The Fc region of IgG can bind to and thereby activate the first component of the complement system, which unleashes a biochemical attack that kills the microorganisms. At least two molecules of IgG are required for complement activation compared with one molecule of IgM, which has five Fc regions.

IgG molecules are the only antibodies that can pass from mother to fetus. Cells of the placenta that are in contact with maternal blood have receptors that bind the Fc region of IgG molecules and mediate their passage to the fetus. The antibodies first are ingested by receptor-mediated endocytosis and then are transported across the cell and released by exocytosis into the fetal blood. Other classes of antibodies do not bind to these receptors and therefore cannot pass across the placenta. The ability of IgG to cross the placenta provides a major line of defense against infection for

TABLE 46-4
Properties of Human Immunoglobulins

	IgM	IgG	IgA	IgD	IgE
Physiologic					
Normal adult serum concentration, mg/mL	1.2–4.0	8.0–16.0	0.4–2.2	0.03	17–450ng/mL
International units/mL	69–322	92–207	54–268	–	<100
Percentage total immunoglobulin	13	80	6	1	0.002
Intravascular distribution, %	41	48	76	75	51
Synthetic rate, mg/kg/day	2.2	35	24	0.4	0.003
Catabolic rate in serum, % per day (or half-life, days)	10.6 (5–6)	6 (18–23)	24 (5–6.5)	37 (2.8)	90
Biological					
Agglutinating capacity	+4	±	+2	–	–
Complement-fixing capacity via classical pathway	+4	+	–	–	–
Homologous anaphylactic hypersensitivity	–	–	–	–	+4
Heterologous guinea pig anaphylaxis	–	+	–	–	–
Fixation to homologous mast cells and basophils	–	±	–	–	+4
Cytophilic binding to macrophages	–	+	±	–	–
Placental transport to fetus	–	+	–	–	–
Rheumatoid factor–binding activity	–	+	–	–	–
Present in external secretions	±	+	+4	–	+2
Other Characteristic Properties					
IgM—Produced early in immune response, first effective defense against bacteremia					
IgG—Combats microorganisms and their toxins in extravascular fluids					
IgA—Defends external body surfaces					
IgD—Present on lymphocyte surface of immunocompetent cells, important for B cell activation and/or immunoregulation					

the first weeks of an infant's life. Normally, the human fetus begins to receive significant quantities of maternal IgG transplacentally at around 12 weeks' gestation. The quantity increases steadily until, at birth, cord serum contains a concentration of IgG comparable with that of maternal serum. Barring any immunologic disorders, adult levels of IgG are reached by the seventh year of life and remain relatively constant thereafter.

IgG antibodies have a high diffusion coefficient, which enables them to diffuse into the extravascular body spaces more readily than other Ig classes. IgG, being the predominant immunoglobulin in these spaces, carries the major burden of neutralizing bacterial toxins and of binding microorganisms to enhance their phagocytosis. Furthermore, only IgG antibodies coating target cells, such as tumor cells, can sensitize them for extracellular killing by ADCC; the NK cells responsible for ADCC also possess Fc receptors for IgG.

There are four subclasses of human IgG. These four subclasses reflect the existence of four antigenetically distinct H chains ($\gamma1$–$\gamma4$), which are similar but not identical in amino acid sequence and general properties. For example, IgG1 is the dominant subclass in adult humans. IgG3 is the most effective binder of complement, followed by IgG1 and IgG2. IgG4 in most cases fails completely to bind complement by the classical pathway. All the subclasses except IgG2 have been demonstrated to cross the placenta. A summary of the physical and biological properties of IgG is given in Tables 46-3 and 46-4, and for the subclasses in Table 46-5.

IMMUNOGLOBULIN A

Antibodies of this class constitute the major class of antibody in secretions (milk, saliva, tears, and respiratory and intestinal secretions). It exists as a four-chain monomer (like IgG) or as a dimer of two such monomer units. IgA molecules in secretions are dimers that carry a single J chain, similar to the one associated with pentameric IgM, and an additional glycopolypeptide chain of 70kDa called **secretory component** (SC). IgA dimers pick up SC from the surface of the epithelial cells lining the intestine, the bronchi, or the milk, salivary, or tear ducts. Secretory component is synthesized by the epithelial cells and is initially exposed on the nonluminal (external) surface of these cells, where it serves as a receptor for binding dimer IgA. The resulting dimer IgA–receptor complexes are ingested by receptor-mediated endocytosis and are transferred across the epithelial cell cytoplasm in the form of a membrane vesicle, which fuses with the plasma membrane on the luminal side of the epithelial cell. The extramembrane portion of the IgA receptor is then enzymatically cleaved and released as part of the secretory IgA molecule ($[\alpha_2,L_2,]_2 - J\alpha$) into the lumen. The amino-terminus of the dimer IgA receptor remaining attached to dimer IgA is the SC (Fig. 46-4). Thus, the fully assembled dimeric secretory IgA molecule is the synthetic product of two distinct types of cells: plasma cells and epithelial cells. In addition to this transport role, SC may protect the dimer IgA molecules from being digested by proteolytic enzymes in secretions.

In humans it has been possible to classify IgA antibodies into two subclasses—IgA1 and IgA2—based on differences in antigenic structure and variation in the arrangement of interchain disulfide bridges. Whereas IgA2 is a minor component of serum IgA, this subclass is the dominant form in secretions. Furthermore, secretory IgA reaches adult levels sooner than serum IgA. The IgA system in the intestinal tract of humans, for example, may be fully developed by 2 years of age, whereas serum IgA levels do not normally reach adult concentrations until 12 years of age.

Because of its presence near external membranes, secretory IgA constitutes a first line of defense against microorganisms in the external environment. It has been postulated that IgA inhibits the adherence of microorganisms to the surface of mucosal cells, thereby preventing their entry into body tissues. One property of secretory IgA that is important in this respect is its multivalence, which is associated with high avidity of binding to antigens; this may be especially relevant in the neutralization of viruses. Antiviral activity by IgA antibodies has been demonstrated in individuals given either of the polio vaccines. Secretory IgA may also combine with certain antigens in food, preventing their absorption into the bloodstream and thus reducing the incidence of allergic reactions. For example, IgA immunodeficiencies can lead to increased levels and incidence of humoral antibodies directed against antigens derived from food and intestinal organisms.

IgA possesses the following effective properties: It fixes complement through the alternative pathway; through a specific Fc receptor on macrophages it can serve as an opsonin for phagocytosis; and it can induce eosinophil degranulation through a specific receptor, which has implicated IgA in antiparasitic responses. The physical and biological properties of IgA are listed in Tables 46-3 and 46-4.

TABLE 46-5

Properties of Human Immunoglobulin G Subclasses

	IgG1	IgG2	IgG3	IgG4
Physiologic				
Percentage distribution of total normal serum IgG	66 ± 8	23 ± 8	7.3 ± 3.8	4.2 ± 2.6
Synthetic rate, mg/kg/day in serum	25	?	3.4	?
Fraction catabolic rate, % per day (half-life, day)	8 (23)	6.9 (23)	16.8 (7)	6.9 (23)
Ratio of κ/λ	1.4–2.4	1.0–1.1	1.1–1.3	5.0–7.0
Allotypic markers (Gm types)	a, z, f, x	n	bo, bi, bz, g, st, etc.	?
Biological				
Complement-fixing capacity via classical pathway	+2	±	+3	–
Heterologous skin-binding capacity	+	–	+	+
Placental transport to fetus	+	±	+	+
Macrophage receptor	+	–	+	–
Reaction with protein A	+	+	–	+
Dominant Antibody Activities				
Antitetanus toxoid	+2	+	+	±
Antidiphtheria toxoid	+2	+	+	±
Antithyroglobulin	+2	+	+	±
Anti-DNA	+2	+2	±	±
Anti-Rh	+2	–	–	±
Anti-factor VIII	–	–	–	+
Antidextran	–	+	–	–
Antilevan	–	+	–	–
Antiteichoic acid	–	+	–	–
Number of interheavy chain disulfide bonds in hinge region	2	4	5	2
Position of light–heavy chain disulfide bond on the heavy chain	N214	N131	N131	N131

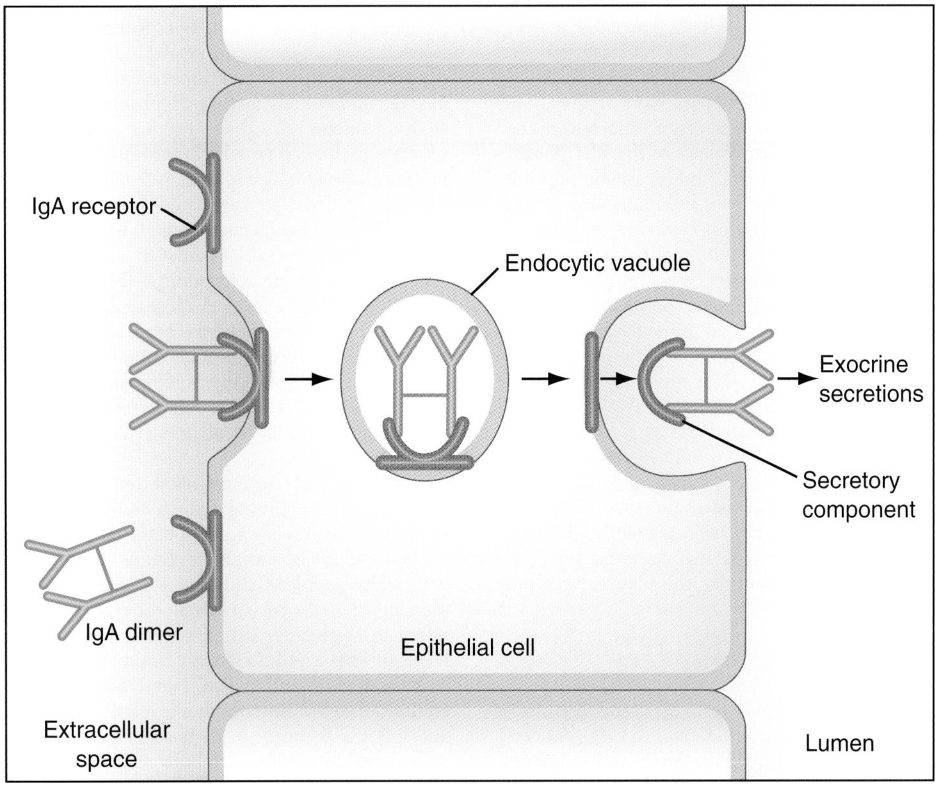

Figure 46-4 The mechanism by which the secretory component mediates the transport of a dimeric immunoglobulin (Ig)A molecule across an epithelial cell. The entire complex is transported from the extracellular fluid into the lumen of the epithelial tube. The secretory component is synthesized by the epithelial cell as a transmembrane glycoprotein and serves as a receptor on its basolateral surface for binding the IgA dimer. The receptor–IgA complex enters the cell in an endocytotic vesicle, which crosses the cell and is exocytosed at the apical surface. Cleavage of the receptor frees the dimer IgA for discharge at the exterior surface (lumen side). The portion of the receptor that remains attached to the IgA dimer is called the secretory component. This transport mechanism is responsible for depositing IgA in various exocrine secretions (e.g., saliva, milk, bile, tears, sweat), as well as in the mucous layer that protects the inner lining of the nasopharyngeal passages, intestine, and genitourinary tract.

IMMUNOGLOBULIN D

Although only a minor component of the serum, IgD is a major membrane immunoglobulin found on the surface of a high proportion of B lymphocytes, especially in newborns. During the course of B cell differentiation, these cells synthesize and display IgD molecules, as well as IgM molecules. Whereas this appears to contradict the "one-cell-one-immunoglobulin" rule, the antigen-binding sites (idiotype) of the two types of molecules and their light chains are identical. Only their CH regions differ. The membrane-bound IgD may serve as one of the receptors with which B cells bind antigen and are stimulated to undergo clonal proliferation. Some evidence suggests that IgM-bearing B cells can respond to certain T-independent antigens, and that the acquisition of IgD is needed for B cells (IgM- and IgD-bearing) to respond to the T cell help required for T-dependent antigen responsiveness.

Furthermore, if IgD molecules are selectively removed from IgM- and IgD-bearing B cells by taking advantage of the much greater sensitivity of the δ chain to papain, these cells are rendered susceptible to becoming tolerant. The precise role played by surface IgD in an immune response remains unknown, but the generally held view is that it turns on, turns off, or modulates (controls) B cell division or differentiation.

IgD usually is detected in serum at about 6 months of age, and its concentration throughout life is always very low. In disease states, however, IgD concentration can vary greatly. In chronic infection, IgD serum levels increase, as do those of the other immunoglobulins. To date, no specific increase in IgD has been associated with a particular disease. Patients with allergies and autoimmune diseases do not show an abnormal IgD concentration. IgD is usually absent in hypogammaglobulinemic individuals.

To date, IgD has not been assigned a specific biological role as a humoral antibody. IgD activity against a number of antigens has been reported on occasion. Surface IgD, which has proteins similar to those of surface IgM, is a marker for mature B cells, and its role as a receptor is generally accepted even though the nature and purpose of the signal it transmits remains controversial (Carsetti, 1993; Roes, 1993). IgD does not bind complement, does not cross the placenta, and does not bind to cells through its Fc region. The secreted form of IgD as well as that of the other immunoglobulins lacks the carboxy-terminal transmembrane peptide that anchors it to the surface of B cells. Tables 46-3 and 46-4 list additional properties of IgD.

IMMUNOGLOBULIN E

Of the various classes of immunoglobulin, IgE is present at the lowest serum concentration (see Table 46-4). It has the ability to attach to human skin (homocytotropic antibody) and to initiate aspects of the allergic reaction (reaginic antibody). The biological activity of IgE is accounted for by its property of binding through the Fc region to basophils and to their tissue equivalent—mast cells. IgE may also be important in the humoral immune response to parasitic disease because it is often found at high levels in the serum of patients with helminthic infection. IgE may play a part in allowing white blood cells (WBCs), antibodies, and complement components to enter sites of inflammation, leading to an immediate hypersensitivity reaction. IgE antibodies provide a striking example of the **bifunctional** nature of antibody molecules. The Fc portion of the molecule binds to the target cells, whereas the Fab portion binds the allergen (see Chapter 54 for the role of IgE in allergic diseases and related assays).

As with IgA, IgE is produced mainly in the linings of the respiratory and intestinal tracts and is part of the external secretory system of antibody. A deficiency of IgE has been inconsistently associated with deficiency of IgA in individuals with impaired immunity, who present with undue susceptibility to infection. IgE does not cross the placenta, and IgE–antigen complexes do not bind complement by the classical pathway (see Table 46-4).

SUMMARY

Five different classes of antibody (IgM, IgG, IgA, IgD, and IgE), four subclasses of IgG antibody (IgG1, IgG2, IgG3, and IgG4), and two subclasses of IgA antibody (IgA1 and IgA2) are present in humans. Each of these antibody isotypes possesses a distinct H chain (μ, γ, α, δ, ε, γ1, γ2, γ3, γ4; and α1, α2, respectively). The H chains contain the Fc region of the antibody, which determines what other proteins will bind to the antibody and therefore the biological properties of the class and subclass. Either type of L chain (κ or λ) can be associated with any class of H chain.

Structural differences among the five classes of immunoglobulins correspond to functional differences in their sites of production and action, their relative levels of production in primary and secondary immune responses, and their roles as physiologic effectors. For example, IgG is prevalent in both blood and tissue fluids, whereas IgM is chiefly confined to the blood, and secretory IgA is found primarily on epithelial surfaces. IgD and IgE are principally bound to cells, IgD to B cells, and IgE to basophils and mast cells.

CLINICAL SIGNIFICANCE OF IMMUNOGLOBULINS

Immunoglobulins play important roles in disease pathogenesis, diagnosis, prevention, and therapy.

DISEASE PATHOGENESIS

Monoclonal hyperimmunoglobulinemia is a prominent feature of multiple myeloma and Waldenström's macroglobulinemia. Antibodies against native antigens may result in autoimmune disease, as discussed in Chapters 51 and 53. Hypoglobulinemia or agammaglobulinemia is often the prime characteristic of some immunodeficiency disorders (see Chapter 50). Polyclonal hypergammaglobulinemia can result from chronic inflammation or other disorders such as cirrhosis of the liver due to excess pan–B cell stimulation.

Hyperimmunoglobulinemia

Serum Immunoglobulin Levels

Valid interpretation of serum immunoglobulin levels requires recognition of biological variations that exist throughout the life span of individuals. The most important of these variables are age, sex, and race. In neonates, levels of circulating immunoglobulins are much lower than at all other ages, as essentially all immunoglobulins at that stage were passively transferred from mother to fetus in utero. Immunoglobulin levels rise through childhood to more stable concentrations in mature adults. Normal IgG, IgA, and IgM concentrations at any particular age can vary as much as tenfold from lower to upper limits of the reference ranges. A very large study of immunoglobulin concentrations in a northern New England (99% Caucasian) population of 115,017 serum samples demonstrated the expected rise from infancy, more stable values after adolescence, and then in older individuals further slight increase in IgA, nearly stable IgG, and slight reduction in IgM (Ritchie, 1998). Little difference was noted between males and females in terms of IgA and IgG median levels, whereas males exhibited lower IgM than females at all ages except the very young. That study might be considered definitive for age and gender through the sheer number of subjects, although the population was not racially diverse.

A smaller but still reasonably large group of healthy white subjects (3213) from a single community (Tecumseh, MI) showed that mean concentrations of IgG and IgA increased with age, with slight but significant differences between the sexes. Females had higher serum levels of IgG and lower levels of IgA. Although these sex differences for IgG and IgA are statistically significant, their biological meaning is not apparent. IgM levels in these subjects remained relatively constant with age. However, females had higher mean levels of IgM (1.06 mg/mL) than males (0.77 mg/mL) (Cassidy, 1974).

Several studies have reported that immunoglobulin levels are higher in persons with pigmented skin. A study of a healthy biracial population in Evans County, Georgia, demonstrated that black people had higher levels of the three major immunoglobulins (IgM, IgG, and IgA) when compared with white people (Lichtman, 1967). The most prominent difference was seen in IgG. No urban–rural difference in immunoglobulin levels was noted in this study. White subjects in Rochester, New York, had serum levels of IgM and IgG similar to those of white subjects in rural Georgia. A triracial study in Durban, Natal, South Africa, showed that Bantu male adults had significantly higher levels of IgM (32% more), IgG (40% more), and IgA (32% more) in their sera than comparable white male adults in this community who were born in the same year and had the same ABO blood group. Healthy Asiatic male adults had about 20% more IgG, 23% more IgA, and 7% more IgM than comparable white male adults. A study of subjects in the Washington, DC, metropolitan area revealed that black people had significantly higher IgG levels than white people but similar IgA and IgM levels (Tollerud, 1995). Control groups used in these studies were matched for age, sex, and race, as well as for several environmental

TABLE 46-6

Polyclonal Hyperimmunoglobulinemias: Some Associated Disease States

Condition	Immunoglobulin (Ig) classes
Immunodeficiency Diseases	
Hyperimmunoglobulin E and recurrent infections	IgE
Wiskott-Aldrich syndrome	IgA, IgE
"Dysgammaglobulinemia type I"	IgM
Hyperimmunoglobulin A and recurrent infections	IgA
Acquired immune deficiency syndrome (AIDS)	All classes
Infections	
Congenital infections (syphilis, toxoplasmosis, rubella, cytomegalovirus)	IgM
Infectious mononucleosis	IgM or all
Trypanosomiasis	IgM or all
Intestinal parasitism	All classes
Several helminthic infections	IgE
Visceral larva migrans	All classes
Chronic granulomatous disease of childhood	All classes
Leprosy	All classes
Chronic infection in general	All classes, with a preference for IgG
Liver Diseases	
Chronic active hepatitis	IgG predominates
Acute hepatitis	IgG predominates
Biliary cirrhosis	IgM predominates
Lupoid hepatitis	All classes
Pulmonary Disorders	
Pulmonary hypersensitivity syndrome	All classes
Sarcoidosis	All classes
Berylliosis	All classes
"Autoimmune" Disorders	
Systemic lupus erythematosus	All classes
Rheumatoid arthritis	IgA or all
Many "autoimmune" states such as thyroiditis	All classes
Scleroderma	All classes
Cold agglutinin disease	IgM
Anaphylactoid purpura	IgA
Miscellaneous	
Down syndrome	All classes
Amyloidosis	All classes
Narcotic addiction	IgM
Renal tubular disease	All classes

factors. Increases in gammaglobulin often are first noted after serum protein electrophoresis, measurement of total protein, or measurements of albumin and γ-globulin fractions.

Increases in immunoglobulins are referred to as monoclonal or polyclonal. Monoclonal immunoglobulins from any one individual are structurally identical and are believed to result from the clonal expansion of a single immunoglobulin-producing lymphoid cell, and hence are specific for a particular antigen. Polyclonal immunoglobulins in the same individual are structurally different from each other in one or more important ways—by class, as polyclonal IgG, IgA, or IgM; by light chain; or by antigen specificity. Polyclonal immunoglobulins arise from the expansion of several to many different immunoglobulin-producing lymphoid cells.

Polyclonal Immunoglobulins

Polyclonal increases in immunoglobulins have been associated with many disease states (Table 46-6) (Cushman, 1973; Buckley, 1977). Serum protein electrophoresis is often sufficient to establish this condition. Immunoelectrophoresis, immunofixation, and determination of individual immunoglobulins or immunoglobulin light chains may be helpful at times to confirm a polyclonal distribution or an increased concentration in one or more immunoglobulin classes. Increases in serum immunoglobulins may result from decreased catabolism and increased synthesis. The control mechanisms for these events are not well understood. The implications of elevated immunoglobulins are unknown. Most immunoglobulins appear not to be directed toward a definable specific antigenic determinant, or set of specific antigenic determinants. It should also be noted that most autoantibodies are not monoclonal but polyclonal. In general, persistent polyclonal increases in gammaglobulin are thought to be related to antigenic stimulation of a chronic nature or loss of immunoglobulin regulation.

TABLE 46-7

Selected Conditions Associated With Monoclonal Immunoglobulins

- Multiple myeloma
- Macroglobulinemia of Waldenström
- Chronic lymphocytic leukemia
- Other leukemias
- Lymphomas
- "Benign" monoclonal gammopathy
- Systemic capillary leak syndrome
- Amyloidosis
- Chronic liver disease such as chronic active hepatitis, primary biliary cirrhosis
- Autoimmune disorders, including rheumatoid arthritis, systemic lupus erythematosus, thyroiditis, pernicious anemia, polyarteritis nodosa, Sjögren's syndrome
- Gaucher's disease
- Malignancies of various types
- Hereditary spherocytosis
- HIV infection, including AIDS

AIDS, Acquired immune deficiency syndrome; *HIV*, human immunodeficiency virus.

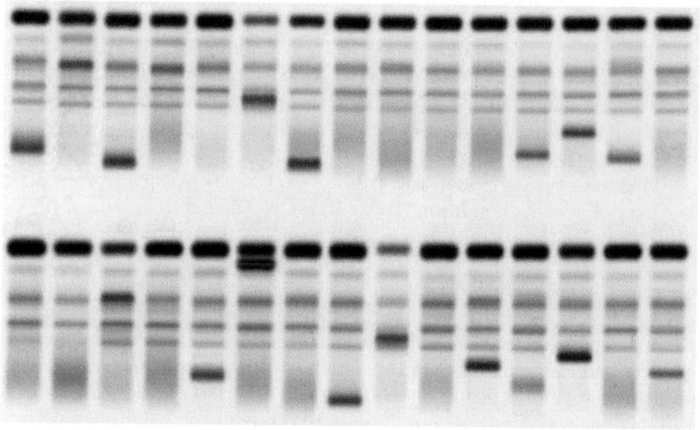

Figure 46-5 Serum protein electrophoresis performed in agarose gel. This gel demonstrates the variation in electrophoretic migration of monoclonal bands as typically encountered in diagnosing and monitoring patients with plasma cell disorders such as multiple myeloma. This routine analysis of serum specimens from 2 controls and 28 patients included 14 individuals with monoclonal bands.

Monoclonal Immunoglobulins

Monoclonal immunoglobulins or fragments of immunoglobulins have been associated with a number of disease conditions (Table 46-7) (Wells, 1974; Benbassat, 1976; Atkinson, 1977; Schaefer, 1978; Kelly, 1985). These immunoglobulins have also been referred to as immunoglobulins with restricted heterogeneity. Protein electrophoresis of serum and urine (Fig. 46-5) is commonly used to screen for monoclonal gammopathy.

The incidence of monoclonal immunoglobulins (M components) in unselected population studies is estimated to be 0.9% (Bachman, 1965; Axelsson, 1968; Cohen, 1985). Of course, a much higher percentage of positive results is found in clinical laboratories where the sera to be tested are preselected. Multiple myeloma, Waldenström's macroglobulinemia, and B cell neoplasms are some of the diseases that are associated with elevated levels of monoclonal immunoglobulins. It was earlier believed that monoclonal gammopathies were rare in cases of chronic lymphocytic leukemia or well-differentiated lymphocytic lymphoma. It has now been shown that when high-resolution electrophoresis and immunofixation are combined to study samples from these patients, most are found to have a monoclonal gammopathy (Keren, 1988). Monoclonal gammopathies have also been demonstrated in patients with Burkitt lymphoma and B cell acute lymphocytic leukemia.

Although the antigen-combining specificities of monoclonal gammopathies generally are not known, some result in paraproteinemic neuropathies. This clinical syndrome is generally due to the interaction of an IgM paraprotein with myelin-associated glycoprotein (MAG), gangliosides (e.g., GM1 in motor neuropathy, GD1b in sensory neuropathy), or other glycosphingolipids (Ropper, 1998).

The term *monoclonal gammopathy of undetermined significance* (MGUS) was coined by Kyle to categorize individuals in whom a monoclonal component is demonstrated in the serum but who lack other key features for diagnosing a malignant condition (Kyle, 1982). As many as 3% of individuals over the age of 70 have an MGUS (Kyle, 2003). Subjects with MGUS may have as many as 10% plasma cells in the bone marrow. This is considerably less than the bone marrow plasmacytosis associated with multiple myeloma. About 20% of individuals with MGUS will develop a malignant B cell lymphoproliferative disorder, most commonly multiple myeloma, over a 10-year period. Some of the other cases develop into chronic lymphocytic leukemia, amyloidosis, well-differentiated lymphocytic lymphoma, and other B cell proliferative diseases. Subjects with MGUS have quantities of M component ranging from 300 mg/dL to greater than 3000 mg/dL and usually do not have Bence Jones protein in the urine. It is recommended that such patients be followed with serum protein electrophoresis every 6–12 months to determine whether the process is progressing or regressing.

The risk of progression with MGUS is about 1% per year even after 25 years of a stable condition (Kyle, 2003). A 31-year follow-up study of MGUS in New Zealand showed progression to hematologic malignancy in 64% of 11 patients originally detected by screening 2192 subjects in a town in 1967 (Colls, 1999).

A special consideration is MGUS that is observed in organ transplant patients who have received immunosuppressive drugs that alter T lymphocyte functions, including the modulation of B cell responsiveness. These monoclonal gammopathies may be transient in up to 75% of cases (Radl, 1985). They may occur in both monoclonal and oligoclonal forms (Stanko, 1989), and they may coincide with infections of cytomegalovirus or Epstein-Barr virus (Drouet, 1999). Their progression is likely stimulated by high circulating levels of interleukin-6 (Nickerson, 1994).

Cryoglobulins

Cryoglobulins are immunoglobulins that precipitate upon storage at refrigerated temperatures (4° C), and as a group, are associated with hematologic, autoimmune, and chronic infections such as hepatitis C. Type I cryoglobulins consist of a single monoclonal immunoglobulin that precipitates in the cold without binding other proteins. This type of molecule is typically IgM encountered in Waldenström's macroglobulinemia, where it can produce a hyperviscosity syndrome due to very thick consistency of the circulating blood that can be exacerbated by cold ambient temperatures encountered by the patient.

Type II cryoglobulins are distinctly different from type I. The abnormality in type II is a monoclonal IgM autoantibody that is directed at the Fc region of normal polyclonal IgG (Cacoub, 2002). This autoantibody is the same as rheumatoid factor. It is also referred to as mixed cryoglobulin containing both IgM and IgG. It is commonly encountered in rheumatoid arthritis and in chronic hepatitis C virus infection for unknown reasons. The presence of IgM anti-IgG leads to formation of circulating immune complexes (CICs), with IgG normally occurring in the blood. These CICs then deposit in small blood vessels, causing vasculitis, glomerulonephritis, arthritis, and so forth.

Type III cryoglobulins have been described as a variant of type II in which the IgM autoantibody against IgG is polyclonal. Type III can be found in chronic infections and inflammatory states. Many such cases in the past could have been confused with type II because of methods that would not permit sensitive typing of the light chains in a minor band of IgM in the presence of large amounts of IgG, because both light chain types would appear in the cryoprecipitate.

DISEASE DIAGNOSIS

Laboratory evaluation of immunoglobulin levels and functions may be helpful in the diagnosis and management of disease. Complement fixation tests, hemagglutination assays, and other immunoassays can detect an increased or changing titer of antibodies against specific antigens such as those present on microorganisms.

Requests to examine sera for the presence of a monoclonal protein usually are generated by a physician who recognizes that a patient has clinical symptoms and signs of such a disorder, or by laboratory examination of a serum protein electrophoresis that suggests a monoclonal protein. Many times, the physician's suspicion of a plasma cell dyscrasia is triggered by findings of anemia (with one or more cytopenias), elevated total serum protein with elevated globulins, and proteinuria; other findings may include hyperuricemia, hypercalcemia, elevated alkaline phosphatase, bone pain, or lytic lesions of bone on x-ray. If indeed an M component is present in a serum protein electrophoresis, quantitative measurement of immunoglobulins by radial immunodiffusion, nephelometry, or another suitable technique can identify the specific immunoglobulin if only one of the major three classes is increased. Of course, this neither determines the light chain of a monoclonal immunoglobulin nor detects light chain myelomas. Biclonal gammopathies may be confusing.

Quantitative immunoglobulins are useful in monitoring the course of the disease and its treatment and may be helpful in separating a benign from a malignant condition. Monoclonal IgG levels of 2 g/100 mL or IgA levels of 1 g/100 mL (Isobe, 1971) or greater suggest a malignant condition. In many malignant immunocytopathies, the concentration of nonmonoclonal immunoglobulins is reduced. Thus, a deficiency of polyclonal immunoglobulins is suggestive of malignancy. Paradoxically, the patient with a malignant immunocytopathy is immunodeficient even though he possesses large quantities of a "nonsense" immunoglobulin produced by a poorly controlled clone of lymphoid cells.

Immunofixation

Confirmation of heavy chain and light chain types of a monoclonal band today is done almost exclusively by immunofixation electrophoresis (IFE). Immunoelectrophoresis (IEP) was an older procedure in which patient and normal serum specimens were electrophoresed in adjacent lanes, followed by diffusion of individual antisera against light and heavy chains from a trough cut into the agarose support medium. After overnight incubation, the pattern of precipitin arcs formed by the antisera with their target immunoglobulins was interpreted as monoclonal or polyclonal distribution. Readers are referred to earlier editions of this textbook for more information about IEP and pictures of the gels, which are no longer commonly used in modern clinical laboratories. IFE has virtually replaced IEP in the clinical laboratory because of its speed, sensitivity, and ease of interpretation. IFE has greater sensitivity for detecting small monoclonal bands in the presence of polyclonal immunoglobulins. IFE also has the advantage of a more rapid readout because diffusion through gel is not required. Replicate samples of patient serum are subjected to electrophoresis through high-resolution gel before monospecific antisera are applied directly to the separated serum proteins. The gel is washed, and the protein–antibody conjugates are stained and read directly (Fig. 46-6). One lane is treated with a precipitating reagent that fixes all proteins in the same pattern as the serum protein electrophoresis. Maintaining all serum proteins in register with the immunofixed immunoglobulins adds to the ease of confirming and identifying monoclonal paraproteins.

Occasionally, the concentration of the monoclonal protein in a patient's serum is so high that it exceeds the capacity of the reagent antibodies to form precipitating complexes by IFE. This phenomenon corresponds to the zone of antigen excess depicted in Figure 46-2. The result is a halo of precipitated complexes (where the concentrations are nearer to equivalence) with a clear central zone of antigen excess (see Fig. 46-6, *E*). Although this result appears atypical, it is straightforward to interpret and to confirm by repeating the IFE with a greater dilution of patient serum (Keren, 1999).

Either technique may be applied to other body fluids, most commonly urine. Monoclonal light chains in the urine (Bence Jones protein) may be detected in more than half of patients with multiple myeloma (Isobe, 1971; Wells, 1974). Polyclonal light chains may be detected in patients with other disorders, usually as part of complete immunoglobulin molecules. The original method to detect Bence Jones protein was based on precipitation in urine heated to 40°–60° C and then redissolution when further heated to 100° C. IFE of urine is more specific and more sensitive than the older Bence Jones assay. IFE may be performed on urine samples with sufficient protein or subsequent to concentration by lyophilization or by selective membranes (Minicon, Millipore Corporation, Billerica, Mass.).

Immunoglobulins at very high concentrations can significantly increase the viscosity of blood, leading to problems with organ perfusion. Measurements of the viscosity of serum have been done to assess this effect, but they are rarely used today because other methods for quantifying

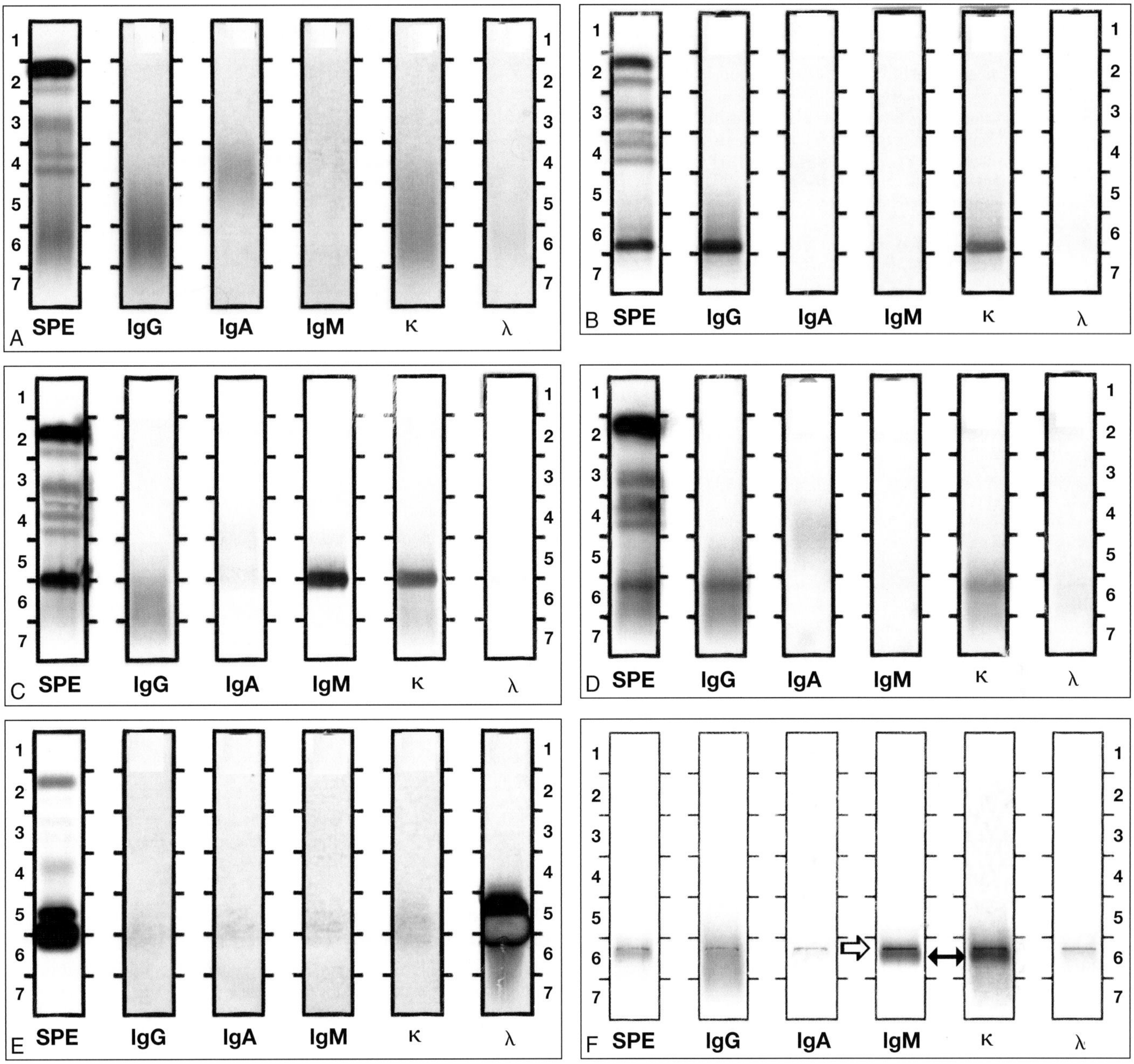

Figure 46-6 Monoclonal immunoglobulins (Ig) demonstrated by serum immunofixation. Replicate samples of patient serum were subjected to electrophoresis through agarose at pH 8.6. The separated proteins were allowed to react with monospecific antisera, and the gels were washed, fixed, and stained. **A,** Normal polyclonal pattern of immunoglobulins. **B,** Monoclonal IgG-κ immunoglobulin (M protein) in serum with loss of most normal polyclonal immunoglobulins. **C,** Monoclonal IgM-κ immunoglobulin in serum. **D,** Minor band of IgG-κ immunoglobulin in serum, along with normal appearing immunoglobulins—possible monoclonal gammopathy of undetermined significance (MGUS). **E,** Two bands of λ light chains in urine. The lower band demonstrates antigen excess with artifactual clearing in its central region surrounded by a ring of immunofixed protein. The upper smaller band sometimes results from dimerization of free light chains through disulfide bonds. **F,** Type II mixed cryoglobulin precipitated from serum containing monoclonal IgMκ *(solid arrow)* and polyclonal IgG. Some undissolved cryoglobulin *(open arrow)* remained at the application point of each lane. *IgA,* Sample reacted with anti-IgA (α-heavy chain specific); *G* or *IgG,* sample reacted with anti-IgG (γ-heavy chain specific); *κ,* sample reacted with anti-κ; *λ,* sample reacted with anti-λ; *IgM,* sample reacted with anti-IgM (μ-heavy chain specific); *SPE,* all proteins in sample precipitated with acid reagent (serum protein electrophoresis).

immunoglobulin concentrations such as nephelometry are widely practiced. Furthermore, serum viscosity by itself is a poor indicator of whole blood viscosity with cellular elements present, which is really the crucial factor clinically in the patient.

Immunoglobulin Free Light Chain Analysis

The synthesis of immunoglobulin heavy chains and light chains is regulated differently by virtue of their genes being on different chromosomes (heavy chain genes on chromosome 14; κ light chain genes on chromosome 2; λ light chain genes on chromosome 22). Light chains are normally synthesized in slight excess and are cleared from the circulation in a few hours so they do not accumulate in the blood; however, in some monoclonal plasma cell disorders, light chain synthesis can greatly exceed heavy chain production with the resultant release of variable quantities of free light chains. Because of the relatively rapid renal clearance of small light chains compared with that of an intact immunoglobulin, measurement of free light chains in serum or urine has been used to assess plasma cell mass and growth in monoclonal disorders. Although the concentration of the intact immunoglobulin of an M-spike has long been used in monitoring myelomas, this new and more rapidly responsive marker of light chain release has recently been introduced for clinical use.

Reagent anti–light chain antibodies used for IFE react with κ or λ light chains both as part of intact immunoglobulins and as free light chains. The principle of specifically measuring free light chains is to use reagent antibodies that react with epitopes on the light chains that are normally hidden by association with heavy chains. Consequently, the free light chain assay gives quantitative information that is complementary to results of quantitative immunoglobulin measurement, as well as protein electrophoresis (PEL) and IFE. One operational advantage of free light chain (FLC) analysis is its automation (Jaskowski, 2006).

Analysis of FLCs entails measurement of both κ and λ light chains in serum and/or urine. Results are abnormal if the κ or λ value is very high and the other is low. To accentuate differences, the ratio of κ to λ measurements is calculated (rFLC). If rFLC is abnormally high, the interpretation is that of plasma cell proliferation with a κ light chain type (i.e., a high κ value in the numerator). If rFLC is below the normal cutoff value, the interpretation is that of proliferation with a λ light chain type (i.e., high λ value in the denominator). Use of rFLC also allows application to patients who have renal disease and do not clear light chains from plasma normally, and so might have elevations of both κ and λ light chains.

Consensus guidelines for use of serum free light chain analysis have recently been developed by the International Myeloma Working Group (Dispenzieri, 2009). They include the following:

1. Serum screening for plasma cell disorders. The serum FLC assay combined with serum PEL and IFE is sufficient to screen for pathologic monoclonal plasmaproliferative disorders except for AL amyloidosis (light chain amyloidosis), for which the additional test of 24-hour urine IFE is essential. This recommendation allows FLC to replace the 24-hour urine IFE for all plasma cell disorders but AL. Avoiding 24-hour collections of urine is considered positively by many physicians and patients.
2. Serum FLC for prognosis. This assay should be performed at the time of diagnosis for MGUS, smoldering or active multiple myeloma, solitary plasmacytoma, and AL amyloidosis. The baseline values of FLC predict progression of these disorders and so can help to frame therapy or at least to make recommendations for frequency of monitoring and helping patients to understand the risks of their disease.
3. FLC for quantitative monitoring of response. The only recommended indications for routine serial use of FLC are seen in oligosecretory multiple myeloma and in AL amyloidosis. Other potential uses for which data were not sufficient to recommend use include light chain myeloma and measurable intact immunoglobulin disease. Also recommended is use in patients who have achieved a complete response to determine whether it is a stringent complete response.

The availability of FLC assays is an issue because the reagents have been provided by only one manufacturer, and they are not adaptable to a wide range of immunoassay instruments commonly found in clinical laboratories. Accordingly, these assays typically are sent out to reference laboratories. The commercial promotion of FLC assays has resulted in their use in far more situations than are covered by the recent consensus guidelines. Much more clinical outcome information needs to be accrued before it can be recommended that FLC assays should be used routinely for both diagnosis and monitoring of virtually any plasma cell disorder.

Cryoglobulin Testing

Accurate laboratory test results for cryoglobulins are especially sensitive to improper preanalytic handling, and clinicians must be aware of specimen temperature requirements when ordering these studies to avoid false-negative results (Shihabi, 2006; Chan, 2008). Testing for cryoglobulins in serum begins with a period of incubation in the cold (4° C) to detect turbidity or precipitate after 24 or 72 hours compared with an aliquot of the patient's serum kept at 37° C as a control for other precipitating substances not related to cold phenomena. Any cryoprecipitate is sedimented by centrifugation, washed briefly with cold saline to remove other serum proteins, and then redissolved (and dissociated) in warm saline for electrophoresis and immunofixation to identify immunoglobulin components (i.e., heavy and light chains).

Type I cryoglobulins typically form a relatively large volume of cryoprecipitate (e.g., up to 10% or even 20% of the serum volume—sometimes referred to as the "cryocrit") (Fig. 46-7). Upon immunofixation electrophoresis, type I cryoglobulins exhibit a single heavy chain and a single light chain type, often monoclonal IgM. The whole serum usually not treated with cryoprecipitation usually demonstrates a large amount of the same monoclonal band. The concentration of the band should fall after successful plasma exchange.

Type II cryoglobulins typically show only a small amount of cryoprecipitate that is less than 1% of the serum volume, and so quantitating the percentage of cryocrit is not analytically valid for serial measurements to monitor a patient's progress. IFE shows a monoclonal band of IgM plus polyclonal IgG (see Fig. 46-6, *F*). This pattern is observed frequently because of its association with chronic hepatitis C.

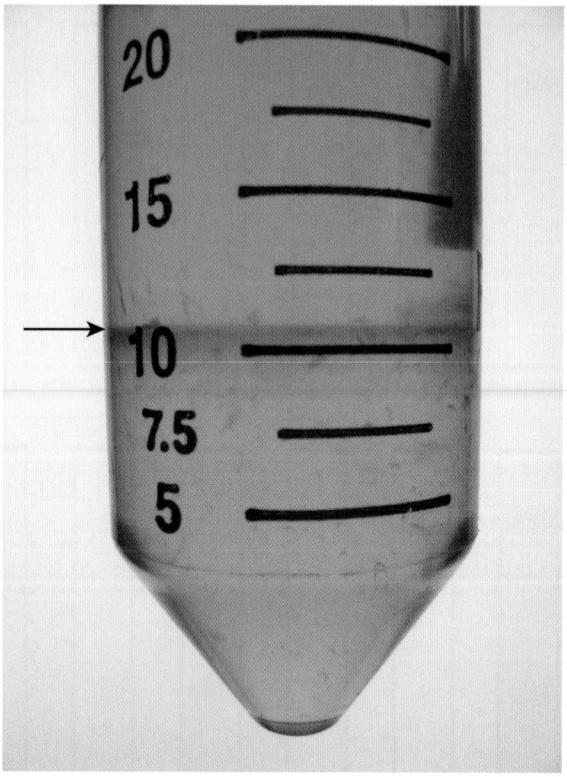

Figure 46-7 Type I cryoglobulin in the plasma of a patient undergoing plasmapheresis for hyperviscosity syndrome due to monoclonal immunoglobulin (Ig)M-κ. Plasma removed during plasma exchange was stored at 4° C in a 50-mL tube. The cryoglobulins that precipitated in the cold occupied approximately 20% of this patient's plasma volume. The *arrow* indicates the top of the cryoglobulin that settled in the tube.

IFE findings in type III cryoglobulin would be similar to those in type II with a relatively small amount of cryoprecipitate that demonstrates both polyclonal IgM and polyclonal IgG.

Oligoclonal Immunoglobulin Bands in Cerebrospinal Fluid

Evaluation of intrathecal synthesis of immunoglobulin is aided by high-resolution electrophoresis of cerebrospinal fluid protein that spreads out the γ region to display individual bands of different immunoglobulin clones. The interpretation of cerebrospinal fluid (CSF) protein electrophoresis requires simultaneous electrophoresis of the patient's serum to ensure that findings in the CSF are unique and do not just reflect the passive transfer of clonal immunoglobulins from the blood. Oligoclonal bands as a marker of synthesis of immunoglobulins in the central nervous system suggest the possibility of an autoimmune process such as a demyelinating disease. Another possibility is an immunologic response to central nervous system infection, so the interpretation of oligoclonal bands in CSF must be made in the context of other diagnostic findings such as cell counts, viral serologies, bacterial cultures, syphilis testing, nucleic acid amplification tests for viruses, and so forth.

The protein electrophoretic pattern of CSF and serum from a patient with multiple sclerosis is shown in Figure 46-8, *A*. The CSF was concentrated and the serum was diluted to achieve comparable amounts of stainable protein in each application. CSF has a relatively higher concentration of prealbumin than does serum. Albumin is the predominant band in both fluids. The other significant band in CSF is transferrin, because of its small molecular size that permits ultrafiltration from blood into CSF. The higher molecular weight proteins in serum (α2 plus β-lipoprotein) are absent from CSF. C3 is also identifiable in CSF, along with a band of asialotransferrin in the β2 region. After all these landmark proteins of CSF are recognized, oligoclonal bands should be evaluated in the γ region, which normally has only a small quantity of polyclonal immunoglobulins. The oligoclonal bands in Figure 46-8, *A*, are discrete and clearly separate from one another.

Examination of serum and CSF sometimes shows a clonal band of immunoglobulin present in both (Fig. 46-8, *B*); however, this finding is

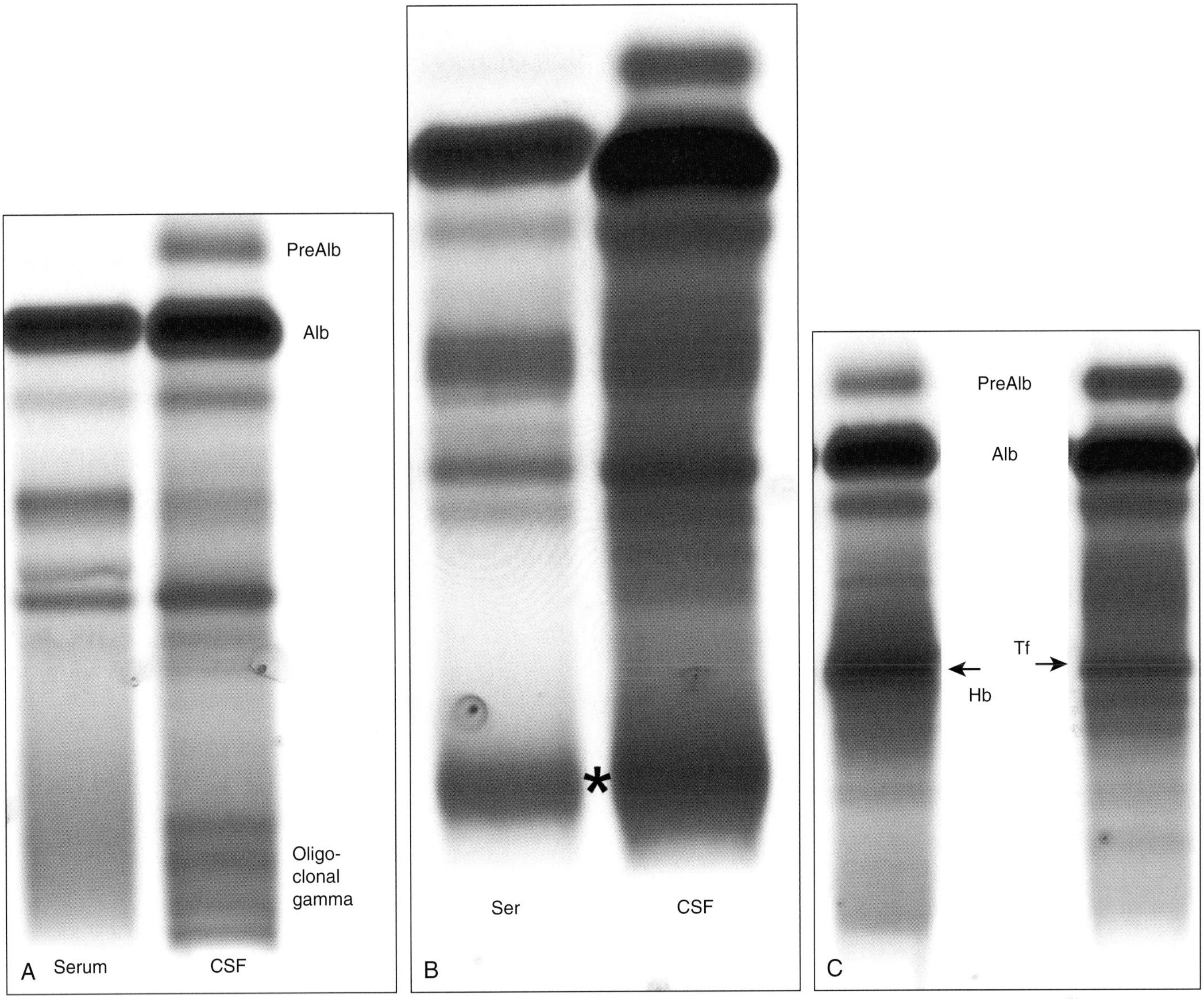

Figure 46-8 Protein electrophoretic patterns in serum and cerebrospinal fluid (CSF). **A,** Serum and CSF from the same patient showing positive oligoclonal bands in the γ region of the CSF but not in the patient's serum. **B,** Monoclonal band of immunoglobulin in both serum and CSF interpreted as negative for oligoclonal bands in CSF. **C,** Artifact of hemoglobin (Hb) in CSF *(left lane)* adjacent to the position of transferrin (Tf) *(right lane).*

not indicative of intrathecal synthesis and so is not a positive result for oligoclonal bands. Presumably, it represents clonal proliferation of plasma cells in the body with passive movement of the monoclonal antibody from blood into CSF.

Another distortion of the electrophoretic pattern occurs with release of hemoglobin (Hb) into the CSF, resulting in a major band in the β region close to transferrin (Fig. 46-8, *C*). This band of Hb should not be confused with clonal immunoglobulin in CSF. Confirmation that this band is Hb depends on visual examination of the CSF for blood or hemolysis (red color). A band of red Hb can also be seen in the β region before staining of the electrophoretic gel.

A consensus statement on analysis of CSF was commissioned from experts in multiple sclerosis by the Consortium of Multiple Sclerosis Clinics (Freedman, 2005). That group recommended qualitative assessment of CSF for IgG using IEF on unconcentrated CSF compared directly with a serum specimen from the same patient. Interpretation of the pattern should consist of one of the following:

Type 1: No bands in CSF and serum

Type 2: Oligoclonal bands in CSF, not in serum; indicates intrathecal IgG synthesis

Type 3: Oligoclonal bands in CSF plus other oligoclonal bands in CSF and serum; indicates intrathecal IgG synthesis

Type 4: Identical oligoclonal bands in CSF and serum; indicates systemic immune reaction with passive transfer to CSF; no intrathecal IgG synthesis

Type 5: Monoclonal band in CSF and serum; paraprotein; no intrathecal IgG synthesis

Problems in Detecting Monoclonal Bands

Clearly demarcated monoclonal bands are straightforward to identify when they are at high concentration and migrate separately from other serum proteins, particularly when the γ fraction is clear of normal polyclonal immunoglobulins owing to replacement of normal plasma cells with the malignant clone. Several examples of clear-cut monoclonal bands are presented in Figure 46-5. The area under the tracing for such bands can be readily integrated to calculate concentration of a monoclonal protein for monitoring in serial specimens.

Sometimes the monoclonal bands are much less pronounced and may be difficult to distinguish within a background of normal proteins. Figure 46-6, *D*, shows such a minor band of IgM-κ that can still be readily identified by IFE. However, when small monoclonal proteins migrate in the β or even α2 region, they can escape detection because of overlap with normal proteins such as transferrin or C3 (Fig. 46-9, *B*). A monoclonal band migrating between normal serum proteins may also be mistakenly disregarded (Fig. 46-9, *D*), so it is very important to interpret such electrophoreses with a firm expectation of where normal bands migrate and what their intensities should be.

False-positive interpretations of monoclonal bands can occur owing to the presence of fibrinogen from an unclotted specimen (Fig. 46-9, *C*), or when hemolysis occurs as the result of improper specimen collection

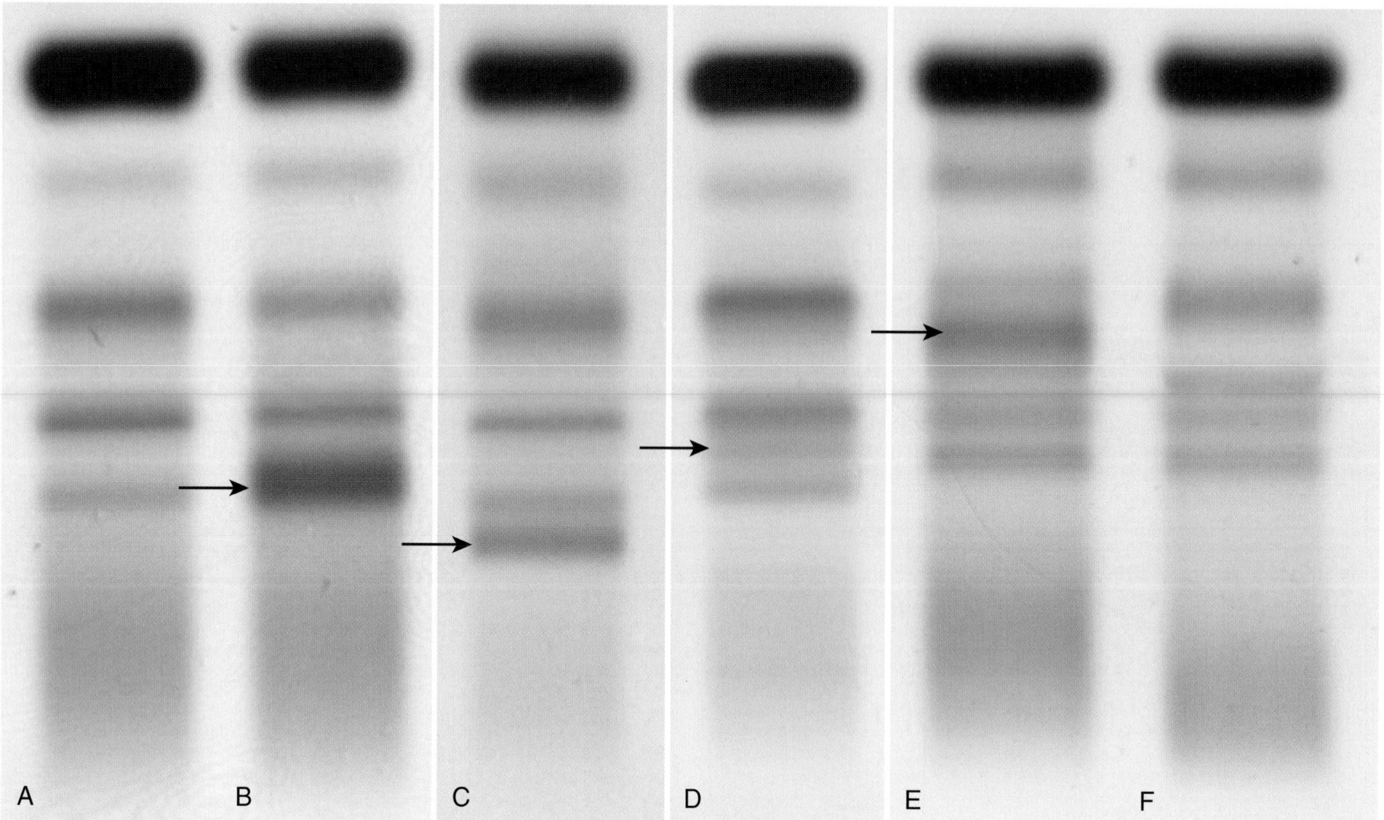

Figure 46-9 Low-intensity bands of monoclonal and other proteins migrating about the β region. **A,** Normal serum protein electrophoresis pattern. **B,** Minor band of immunoglobulin (Ig)A-κ *(arrow)* overlapping C3. **C,** Fibrinogen *(arrow),* not to be confused with a monoclonal band. **D,** Minor band of IgA-κ *(arrow)* migrating between transferrin and C3. **E,** Hemolysed specimen with a minor band of hemoglobin-haptoglobin *(arrow).* **F,** Redraw of serum without hemolysis from same patient as in **E. E** and **F** were electrophoresed on a different gel system from **A** through **D**; relative mobilities of normal serum proteins can vary in different systems.

(Fig. 46-9, *E* and *F*). Confirmation that a small band is a monoclonal paraprotein is typically done with IFE.

DISEASE PREVENTION AND THERAPY

Passive immunization is the administration of pre-formed antibodies obtained from another individual of the same species (homologous γ-globulins) or a different species (heterologous γ-globulins); it results in immediate protection against infection. The immunity is short-lived and decays as the antibodies are used and catabolized. Passive protection in neonatal life is based on transfer of maternal antibodies across the placenta or through colostrum (Pennington, 1991).

Pooled human γ-globulin is useful for temporary protection against several viral and bacterial infections (Berkman, 1990; Hammarström, 1990; Desai, 1991). Depending on the dose used and the time of administration, the disease may be modified to a mild form or entirely prevented. The effect is more complete and more predictable if one uses hyperimmune preparations made from the plasma of individuals who are convalescing from the disease in question, or who have recently been immunized against it. Such preparations contain a higher concentration of specific antibodies. Antibodies may also be produced in animals, such as horses, and in the past these antibodies found widespread use. However, prior sensitization to foreign proteins may lead to clinical reactions such as anaphylaxis, serum sickness, pyrexia, and local Arthus reactions.

Monoclonal antibodies have revolutionized many areas of medicine, including research, diagnostics, and therapy. Murine, human, and humanized monoclonal antibodies have been developed (Lefrano, 1990; Morrison, 1992; Mountain, 1992; Ward, 1992; Shin, 1993). Many monoclonal antibodies, often replacing polyclonal antisera, are used for diagnostic purposes (see Chapter 43). Perhaps the most important therapeutic applications of monoclonal antibodies are seen in the fields of transplantation and oncology (Stevenson, 1990; Vitetta, 1993; Neame, 1994). OKT3, a murine monoclonal antibody against the CD3 receptor on lymphocytes, is often used as an antirejection therapy to block the activity of cytotoxic T lymphocytes in renal transplant recipients (Ortho Multicenter Transplant Study Group, 1985). Many potential clinical applications of monoclonal antibodies are being evaluated. A recent example is the use of a monoclonal antibody against tumor necrosis factor-α to prevent Jarisch-Herxheimer reactions resulting from antibiotic treatment of *Borrelia* infection in sheep (Fekade, 1996). Anticytokine and antineutrophil adhesion molecule monoclonal antibodies may be effective in conditions associated with acute inflammation and cytokine release such as acid aspiration, ischemia, or reperfusion injury (myocardial infarction, hemorrhagic shock, aortic aneurysm repair); antibodies inhibiting neutrophil adhesion may be effective in asthma, pulmonary fibrosis, meningitis, and cerebral malaria; and recently, a monoclonal antibody directed against a component of the complement cascade suggests the possibility of eventual therapeutic regulation of specific arms of the inflammatory response (DiLillo, 2006). It seems reasonable to expect that a multitude of therapeutic applications will become available in the future, in which monoclonal antibodies will be designed to modulate the actions of one or more naturally occurring mediators of inflammation, infection, or malignant proliferation.

SELECTED REFERENCES

Cacoub P, Costedoat-Chalumeau N, Lidove O, Alric L. Cryoglobulinemia vasculitis. Curr Opin Rheumatol 2002;14:29.

This review presents an update on clinical findings in cryoglobulins with emphasis on patients with hepatitis C.

Chan AO, Lau JS, Chan CH, Shek CC. Cryoglobulinemia: clinical and laboratory perspectives. Hong Kong Med J 2008;14:55.

A good review of cryoglobulin testing with case studies.

Colls BM. Monoclonal gammopathy of undetermined significance (MGUS)—31 year follow up of a community study. Aust N Z J Med 1999;29:500.

This clinical series demonstrates the long-term significance of MGUS.

Dispenzieri A, Kyle R, Merlini G, et al. International Myeloma Working Group guidelines for serum-free light chain analysis in multiple myeloma and related disorders. Leukemia 2009;23:215.

This article provides official recommendations from the International Myeloma Working Group for clinical use of serum-free light chain testing based on a comprehensive review of the literature.

Fekade D, Knox K, Hussein K, et al. Prevention of Jarisch-Herxheimer reactions by treatment with antibodies against tumor necrosis factor α. N Engl J Med 1996;335:311.

This is an early clinical trial that showed how inflammatory reactions can be modulated by therapeutic antibodies.

Freedman MS, Thompson EJ, Deisenhammer F, et al. Recommended standard of cerebrospinal fluid analysis in the diagnosis of multiple sclerosis. Arch Neurol 2005;62:865.

This article is a consensus statement commissioned by the Consortium of Multiple Sclerosis Clinics that establishes the "minimum standard" for evaluation of CSF in patients suspected of having multiple sclerosis.

Keren DF. Procedures for the evaluation of monoclonal immunoglobulins. Arch Pathol Lab Med 1999;123:126.

This review of laboratory procedures provides insight into modern measurements of monoclonal gammopathies.

Kyle RA, Rajkumar SV. Monoclonal gammopathies of undetermined significance: a review. Immunol Rev 2003;194:112.

This is an updated and comprehensive assessment of patients with MGUS.

Ritchie RF, Palomaki GE, Neveux LM, et al. Reference distributions for immunoglobulins A, G, and M: a practical, simple, and clinically relevant approach in a large cohort. J Clin Lab Anal 1998;12:363.

This manuscript presents reference ranges for immunoglobulins in a very large population by age and gender.

Smith GS, Holman RP. The prozone phenomenon with syphilis and HIV-1 coinfection. South Med J 2004;97:379.

This recent case report reinforces the continuing need for vigilance in antigen–antibody–based testing, so as to avoid missing extremely high values of immune antibody caused by the prozone effect.

REFERENCES

Access the complete reference list online at http://www.expertconsult.com

CHAPTER 47

MEDIATORS OF INFLAMMATION: COMPLEMENT, CYTOKINES, AND ADHESION MOLECULES

H. Davis Massey, Richard A. McPherson

KEY POINTS

- The complement system is a group of circulating proteins that promote inflammation and host defense.
- Unregulated tissue damage is a possible complication of complement activation, and a large variety of circulating and membrane-bound proteins exist to regulate complement activity.
- Complement component C3 is the central convergence point for all complement activation pathways.
- It is frequently necessary to measure serum complement levels to track disease activity, but it is important to recognize that serum complement measurements are snapshots of a dynamic process involving variable rates of complement consumption and production.
- Methods are available that allow accurate determination of serum levels of complement components.
- Functional complement assays are sensitive and precise tools for providing information about the activity and integrity of a complement component or pathway.
- The simplest functional assay of the classical pathway (CH50) measures total hemolytic complement activity.
- Cytokines are soluble proteins released by cells over short distances to facilitate communication between cells, to assist in upregulation or downregulation of the immune response, to direct cell differentiation, and to orchestrate associated inflammatory and reparative activities.
- Adhesion molecules are complex glycoproteins that bind living tissues together and mediate cell migration during embryogenesis, wound healing, and the inflammation response.

Structure and Function of the Complement System

The term **complement** refers to a group of more than 30 circulating and membrane-bound regulatory and constitutive component glycoproteins that function to promote host defense against infectious agents, to promote the clearance of apoptotic cell debris and immune complexes, and to regulate the immune response. Unregulated tissue damage is a possible complication of complement activation, and a large variety of circulating glycoproteins, as well as tissue membrane-bound proteins, function to regulate complement activity and downregulate complement attack. The existence of this system of proteins was inferred late in the 19th century, when it became clear that fresh serum had the ability to lyse gram-negative bacteria and cholera vibrios in the presence of specific antibody. As techniques for protein purification and identification became more sophisticated over the years, it was recognized that complement is a very complex system with many interacting proteins.

In general, the system functions to identify foreign cells and microorganisms and destroy them. This may occur by direct lysis, by opsonization (the process of coating them with specific complement peptides recognized by specific receptors on phagocytes to aid ingestion), or by inflammation produced by the attraction of phagocytic cells. It also has become clear that complement plays a role in facilitating the immune response.

The complement system of proteins is phylogenetically older than the proteins associated with acquired immunity (immunoglobulin) and is present in primitive organisms that lack immunoglobulin. Complement is presumed to provide a level of innate or natural immunity and host defense, even in the absence of an antibody response. It accomplishes this via the mannan-binding lectin (MBL) pathway and the alternative

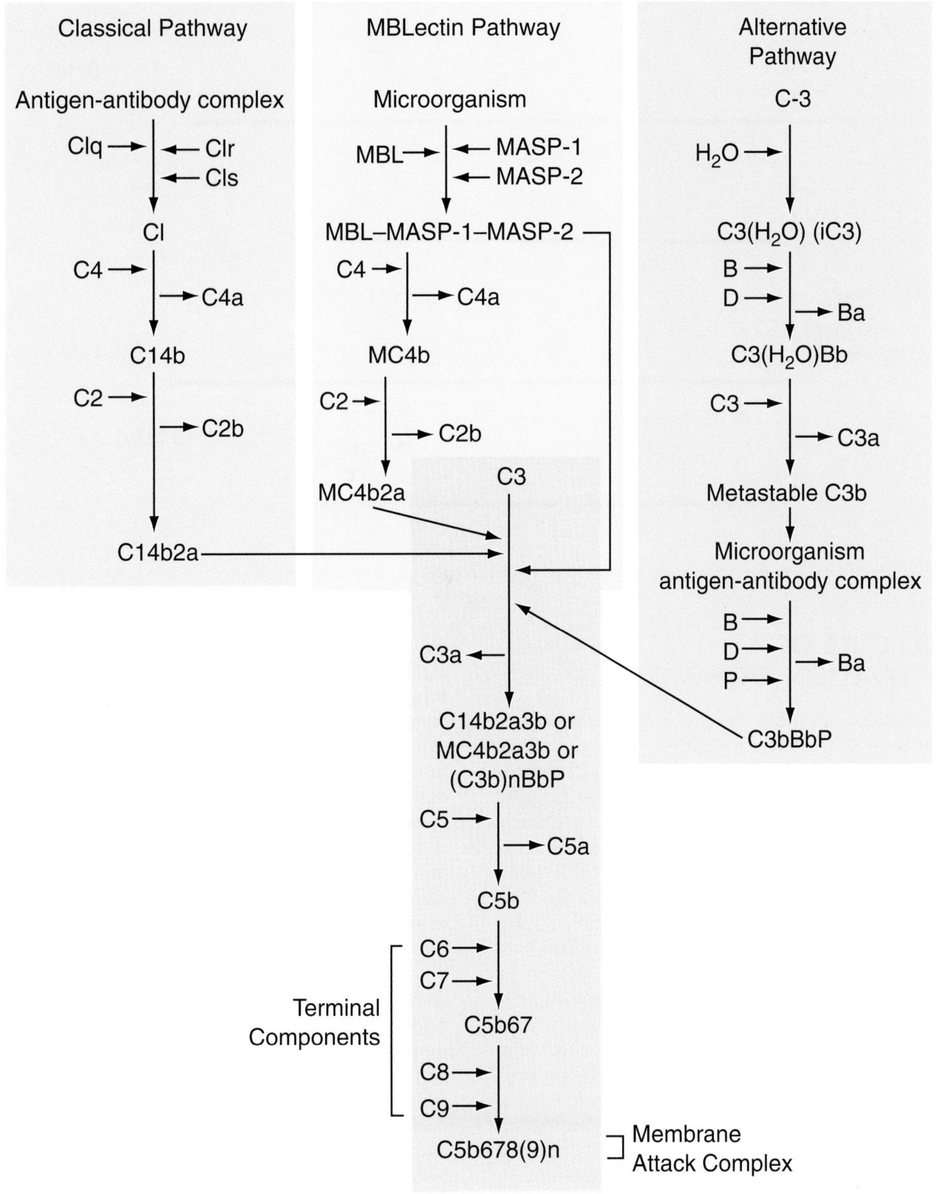

Figure 47-1 Components of the classical, MBLectin, and alternative pathways converge to form a convertase that cleaves C3. In the classical pathway, antigen–antibody complexes sequentially bind and activate C1, C4, and C2. In the MBLectin pathway, interaction of MBL with a carbohydrate on the surface of a microorganism leads to the formation of an enzymatic complex (MBL–MASP-1–MASP-2, termed M in the figure) that binds and activates C4 and C2. In the alternative pathway, C3 undergoes hydrolysis of its thioester bond, which induces a change in conformation. It then binds factor B (B), which is cleaved by factor D (D) to form a convertase that is stabilized by properdin (P). C3b, the cleavage product of C3, also has a cleaved thiolester bond and is capable of activating the alternative pathway. The C3b-containing convertase of all pathways continues sequentially by binding the late-acting component until the sequence of activation is complete.

complement pathway, both discussed later. Antibody provides a level of increased specificity and increased efficiency in mediating host defense. A detailed history of the discovery of complement and of the various complement pathways is provided elsewhere (Frank, 1998).

NOMENCLATURE

Three major complement activation pathways are present in human serum: the classical pathway, the alternative pathway, and the MBL pathway (or MBLectin pathway). Figure 47-1 illustrates the reaction sequence of each pathway. The nomenclature for proteins of the complement system generally follows two conventions (World Health Organization, 1968; IUIS-WHO, 1981). For historical reasons, the nine proteins of the classical pathway are designated by the upper case letter C, which is then followed by the number that relates to their order of appearance in the reaction sequence. A notable exception is C4, which acts before C2. Molecules that are part of the C1 complex are termed C1q, C1r, and C1s. Proteins reacting solely in the alternative pathway are called factors and are referred to by an upper case letter (e.g., factor B, factor D). Fragments of complement proteins resulting from proteolytic cleavage are designated by an appended lowercase letter (e.g., C4a, C4b), where "a" represents the smaller fragment, and "b" represents the larger fragment. The exception to this rule is C2, where C2a is the larger fragment and C2b is the smaller fragment. Further degradation fragments of the large complement fragment of one component are designated by lowercase letters (e.g., C3c, C3d). Components that have lost activity (i.e., are inactive) are usually designated by a prefixed lowercase "i" (e.g., iC3b, iC4b). Polypeptide chains of a native complement protein are designated by Greek lowercase letters (α, β, γ); with the exception of C1q, these chains are termed A, B, and C. Single components or multicomponent complexes that have enzymatic activity are designated by a bar over the component(s). Proteins of the MBLectin pathway are designated by abbreviations of the names of the proteins (e.g., MBL for mannan-binding lectin, MASP for MBL-associated serine protease). Regulatory proteins are designated by a descriptive title or letter (e.g., C4-binding protein, factor H). Membrane-bound regulatory proteins have been assigned CD numbers and descriptive titles (e.g., CD46 for membrane cofactor protein), and complement receptors are designated by numbers following the prefix CR (for complement receptors 1 to 4). The other complement receptors are designated by the component's symbol followed by the uppercase letter R.

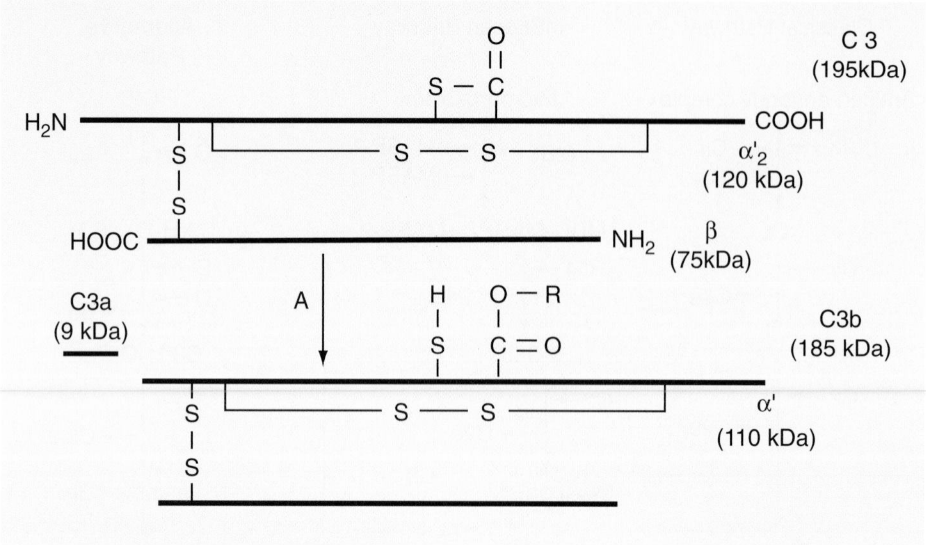

Figure 47-2 C3 cleavage by C3 convertase: The approximate molecular weight of each chain or fragment is given in kilodaltons (C3 convertase is represented by A).

C3: CENTRAL MOLECULE OF COMPLEMENT ACTIVATION PATHWAYS

The protein known as C3 is the central convergence point for the three complement activation pathways (the MBLectin pathway, the alternative pathway, and the classical pathway), which all proceed to lysis, phagocytosis, or regulation of the inflammatory response farther down the cascade.

C3 is a two-chain molecule synthesized in many cells, particularly hepatocytes, formed from a single-chain molecule, pro-C3, and released into the circulation, where it binds to foreign target surfaces. The α and β chains are stabilized by intrachain disulfide bonds; an interchain disulfide bond stabilizes α and β chain interaction (Fig. 47-2). The α chain contains a thiolester that imparts an unstable structure to the molecule. Although it is in the hydrophobic center of C3, the thiolester can be cleaved by gradual hydrolysis as water penetrates the molecule, activating the alternative complement pathway. C3 may also be cleaved rapidly by the action of C3 convertase in releasing the 9-kDa C3a fragment from the α chain amino-terminus, from the larger C3b. C3b will go on to coat target proteins, thereby marking them for destruction, and C3a in the role of anaphylatoxin activates nearby cells to release mediators of inflammation (Wen, 2004). Either avenue results in marked conformational alteration of C3 (now termed C3b) that permits it to interact with cells expressing C3b receptors, in particular CR1 (C3b/C4b receptor, CD35). (Native C3 will not interact with C3b receptors.)

C3 activation and conversion to C3b (with thiolester cleavage) lead to covalent binding of C3b to the surface of a target such as a microorganism. The target becomes coated with C3b capable of interacting with cells expressing C3b receptors, including all phagocytes, all B lymphocytes, and a subset of T lymphocytes. It is C3b that continues the complement cascade leading to lysis.

THE CLASSICAL PATHWAY

The classical pathway of complement activation, described around the year 1900, was the first to be studied, and for this reason is called "classical." It is evolutionarily the most recent of the three pathways described. The classical pathway is responsible for complement activation on most antibody-sensitized cells. Details of this pathway are published elsewhere (Fries, 1987; Volanakis, 1998). Nine numbered proteins make up the classical pathway. Activation of the classical pathway usually requires interaction between an antigen and a C1-binding **complementing** antibody. In humans, only immunoglobulin (Ig)M and IgG are effective at activating the classical pathway, except IgG4, which is unable to activate complement. A number of molecules other than immunoglobulins have the ability to activate the classical pathway via direct interaction with C1q. These include C-reactive protein, serum amyloid P component, β-amyloid, some gram-negative bacteria, certain viruses, mycoplasmas, protozoa, and intracellular components such as DNA, mitochondrial membranes, cytoskeletal filaments (Gewurz, 1993), and apoptotic cells (Korb, 1997). The latter might be of critical importance in the elimination of apoptotic cells and debris from the circulation. In some instances, infectious agents may exploit complement to their advantage, as with prion diseases such as transmissible spongiform encephalopathy, which may use complement components such as C3 and C1q to facilitate its localization within target cells (Mabbott, 2004).

Upon binding of immunoglobulin to a target, C1 binds to that immunoglobulin and becomes activated. C1 is a macromolecule of 740kDa that comprises a single molecule of C1q complexed with two C1r and two C1s chains held together in the presence of calcium ions. Once bound to immunoglobulin, C1q adopts a conformational change that leads to autoactivation of the two C1r chains. Activated $C1s_2$ cleaves the next component in the cascade, C4. The larger fragment, C4b, becomes attached to the activator surface, whereas the smaller fragment, C4a, is released in the fluid phase. C4a is an anaphylatoxin and is described in a subsequent section of this chapter. Most of the generated C4b is hydrolyzed and remains in the fluid phase. Nevertheless, some of the generated C4b molecules bind to the activator surface as a cluster around the antigen–antibody–C1 site. A single antibody–antigen–C1 site thus can lead to the deposition of many C4b molecules.

In the presence of magnesium ions, C4b acts as a site for the binding and subsequent cleavage of C2. $C1s_2$, in association with C4b, cleaves C2 into two fragments. The larger fragment, C2a, remains bound to C4b, whereas the smaller one, C2b, is released in the fluid phase. This molecular complex, C4b2a, is unstable and has a relatively short half-life because of decay that results from the tendency of C2a to break away from the complex in an inactive form. The C4b2a complex is the classical pathway C3 convertase required for C3 binding and cleavage (see Fig. 47-2). It is C2a as part of the C4b2a complex that enzymatically cleaves C3 in the next step of the activation cascade, and cleaves C5 in a later step. C2a cleaves C3 into a large fragment, C3b, which binds to the activator surface, and a smaller fragment, C3a, which is released into the fluid phase, where it serves as an anaphylatoxin. The newly generated C4b2a3b complex is the C5 convertase of the classical pathway that triggers deposition of terminal complement components on the target surface.

IgM and IgG differ in their ability to activate the classical pathway of complement. It appears that a single molecule of most IgM antibodies bound by multiple antibody sites to an antigen can bind one molecule of C1 and trigger a complete complement activation sequence. IgM, with its five antigen-binding sites, adopts a functionally active conformation on an antigenic surface that allows multiple interactions with antigens.

In contrast, C1 binding to IgG requires two molecules of IgG side by side in most experimental studies (Borsos, 1965). Because IgG antibodies bind to a target surface in a random fashion, and because antigens may not be evenly distributed on a target organism, the attachment of hundreds or thousands of IgG antibodies may be required to generate a C1-binding site. Classical pathway activation by IgG–antigen complexes is also shown to facilitate the alternative pathway (see next section) on the activator surface (Moore, 1981).

The ability of aggregated immunoglobulin to bind C1q has provided the basis for a number of tests designed to detect the presence of soluble immune complexes in patient blood samples. Radiolabeled C1q is added to the serum or plasma sample, and one of a number of techniques (e.g., polyethylene glycol precipitation) is used to separate free C1q from that bound to protein components of serum. The binding of C1q suggests the presence of immunoglobulin complexes in the serum or plasma sample (Zubler, 1976). Soluble immune complexes may also be measured by identification of C1q- or C3-bound immune complexes using enzyme-linked immunosorbent assay (ELISA) techniques (Stanilova, 2001). Detection of the presence of C1q in tissue specimens by direct visualization with immunofluorescently labeled anti-C1q antibodies may be used to identify immune complexes in biopsy specimens.

THE ALTERNATIVE PATHWAY

The presence of a second pathway of complement activation was first proposed by Pillemer in 1954 and was accepted by the scientific community almost two decades later. This complement activation pathway appears to be important in early defense against pathogenic microorganisms (Pangburn, 1984). Although antibodies can also activate this system, neither antibody nor lectin is required for activation. Initiation of the alternative pathway on an acceptor surface begins with deposition of active C3 on a surface that has no regulators of complement present on it, leading to the generation of C3b fragments and allowing the process to continue as an unimpeded amplification loop (Wen, 2004). This event depends on the ability of the carbonyl group of the exposed thiolester group of C3b to interact with an amide or a hydroxyl group of a protein or a carbohydrate present on the surface of a target (Law, 1979). In serum, C3 is hydrolyzed at a rate of 0.2%–0.4% of plasma pool per hour (Pangburn, 1981). C3 with a hydrolyzed thiolester undergoes a conformational change that allows it to interact with proteins that do not interact with native C3, and is termed C3(H_2O) (also termed iC3). C3(H_2O) then has the ability to interact with factor B in the presence of magnesium ions. Factor B, upon binding to C3(H_2O), can interact with factor D and is cleaved to generate the so-called initiation C3 convertase C3(H_2O)Bb and liberate a small fragment, Ba. This cleavage is mediated by factor D, a serine protease that adopts an active conformation upon recognition of its substrate and returns to an inactive conformation once proteolytic cleavage is accomplished (Volanakis, 1996).

The initiation C3 convertase cleaves C3 to generate metastable C3b at a continuously slow rate in the circulation. Metastable C3b can bind covalently to the activator surface and then, like C3(H_2O), can bind factor B. As in the initiation C3 convertase, factor D then cleaves factor B to generate the cell-bound C3 convertase C3bBb. This complex decays rapidly but is stabilized upon binding of properdin, which prolongs the half-life of the C3 convertase from 1 to 18 minutes (Fearon, 1975). This stabilized C3 convertase rapidly cleaves yet more C3, which can bind to the activator surface and therefore is referred to as the amplification C3 convertase of the alternative pathway. Amplification of C3b deposition to the activator surface leads to the formation of a C5 convertase (C3b2BbP) (Kinoshita, 1988), which has the ability to trigger activation of the terminal components of the complement system.

THE MANNAN-BINDING LECTIN PATHWAY

A third pathway of complement activation has been described recently that utilizes the serum protein MBL (also called mannose-binding lectin, or mannose-binding protein), which is present in serum at about 1.5 μg/mL. Formed in the liver, MBL is found in all mammals and birds and belongs to a family of molecules termed collectins (Epstein, 1996; Turner, 1996). The collectin family includes, in addition to MBL, lung surfactant proteins A and D (SP-A, SP-D), bovine conglutinin, bovine CL-43, and the ficolins (Epstein, 1996; Thiel, 2007). MBL and the ficolins are complement-activating soluble pattern recognition molecules, that is, they recognize pathogen-associated molecular patterns (PAMPs) on the surfaces of microbes. Once they bind their specific PAMP, these proteins undergo a conformational change that permits them to associate with the three MBL-associated serine proteases, MASP-1, MASP-2, and MASP-3, to activate the complement cascade (Thiel, 2007). MBL is structurally related to C1q and recognizes certain **pathogenic** carbohydrates expressed on the surface of microorganisms, but does not recognize carbohydrates such as galactose and sialic acid, which are the terminal sugars expressed on mammalian glycoproteins (Epstein, 1996). This allows MBL to discriminate between self and nonself, and it is reported that MBL may react with a wide range of acapsular gram-positive and gram-negative bacteria, viruses, yeasts, mycobacteria, parasites, and protozoa (Epstein, 1996).

The MASPs share structural homology with C1r and C1s, suggesting similarity with the C1 complex (C1qr_2s_2). After activation, MASP-2 cleaves C4 to generate the classical pathway C3 convertase C4b2a (Vorup-Jensen, 1998). MASP-1 has the ability to cleave C3 (Matsushita, 1998), suggesting that it might trigger alternative pathway activation directly (Schweinle, 1989). Following generation of the classical pathway C3 convertase C4b2a by the MBL–MASP-1–MASP-2–MASP-3 complex, complement activation proceeds as in the classical pathway, with possible recruitment of the alternative pathway as well (Suankratay, 1998). Specific antibody–antigen complexes can also trigger the MBLectin pathway. It was demonstrated that a fraction of IgG molecules that lack terminal galactose residues (termed IgG-G0), as found in the plasma of patients with pathologic conditions such as rheumatoid arthritis, have the ability to interact with MBL and activate the classical pathway (Malhotra, 1995). MBL may also play a role in the elimination of target organisms by phagocytes through interaction with a specific receptor present on those phagocytes (Tenner, 1995; Hansen, 1998). It may modulate inflammatory and allergic responses, affect apoptotic cell clearance, and modulate the adaptive immune system (van de Wetering, 2004; Thiel, 2007). Regulation of the MBLectin pathway appears to be mediated by C1 inhibitor (Matsushita, 1996) and α_2-macroglobulin (Terai, 1995).

TERMINAL COMPLEMENT COMPONENTS

The three complement activation pathways converge on the activation of C3 and the assembly of the membrane attack complex (MAC), formed by components C5 to C9. Upon formation of the classical, MBLectin (C4b2a3b), and alternative (C3b2Bb) pathway C5 convertases, C5 is cleaved. The larger fragment (C5b) can associate with the cell membrane and interact with C6. The next step involves the interaction of the C5b–6 complex with fluid-phase C7, forming a trimeric complex with amphiphilic properties (high affinity for the lipid constituents of the cell membrane) (Podack, 1979). C5b–7 inserts in the lipid bilayer of the cell membrane but is not sufficient for cell lysis to occur. C8 associates with this trimolecular complex via an interaction with exposed C5b. The C5b–8 complex penetrates the lipid bilayer further to form a small transmembrane pore that causes slow lysis of erythrocytes (Ramm, 1982). However, insertion of multiple copies of C9 through the lipid bilayer via an initial interaction with the α chain of C8 is needed to produce the full cytolytic activity of the MAC (Plumb, 1998). It is believed that the C5b–8 complex serves as an initiator of C9 polymerization within the cell membrane.

The MAC, by electron microscopy, has a hollow, cylinder-like structure formed by the assembly of its components in the presence of excess C9 (Podack, 1984). The mechanism by which the MAC disrupts the cell membrane is still controversial and may include distortion of the lipid bilayer to form **leaky patches** (Esser, 1991) or, more likely, formation of a transmembrane pore with a hydrophilic center through which ions can pass freely (Bhakdi, 1991). Formation of the MAC induces lysis of certain bacteria and viruses, and of heterologous erythrocytes. Most nucleated cells resist MAC-induced cytotoxicity. This protection, especially from attack by one's own complement proteins, is mediated by membrane-associated regulatory molecules that prevent MAC formation (see later, under "Regulation of Complement Activation"), as well as by shedding of the activated complement proteins by blebbing of the cell surface. Lysis of nucleated cells mediated by the MAC may occur but requires multiple MAC lesions to take effect (Koski, 1983).

It has been proposed that the deposition of sublytic amounts of the MAC might protect the cell from subsequent complement attack (Reiter, 1992). Nucleated cells are protected from the effects of the MAC in part because of its active elimination from the cell surface by membrane repair linked to lipid turnover (Mold, 1998). MAC formation has a stimulating effect on several nucleated cell types. Among others, these effects include production of reactive oxygen radicals from neutrophils and macrophages, release of eicosanoids from phagocytic cells, induction of procoagulant activity in platelets and endothelial cells, proinflammatory activity in endothelial cells and smooth muscle cells, proliferation of smooth muscle cells and endothelial cells, and triggering of signal transduction pathways (Niculescu, 1993, 1999; Benzaquen, 1994; Sims, 1995; Kilgore, 1996; Tedesco, 1997; Mold, 1998).

ANAPHYLATOXINS

Activation of complement via the classical, alternative, or MBLectin pathway leads to the generation of complement protein fragments that have important roles in various biological functions, including

TABLE 47-1
Complement Regulatory Proteins

Protein	Molecular weight, kDa	Target	Mechanism of action
Fluid Phases			
C1 inhibitor	105	C1	Dissociates the C1 complex by binding to C1r and C1s
Factor H	150	C3b	Cofactor for C3b inactivation by factor I
C4-binding protein	550	C4	Cofactor for C4b inactivation by factor I
S protein (vitronectin)	84	C5b–7	Inhibits insertion of the MAC into cell membranes
Clusterin	70	C5b–7	Inhibits insertion of the MAC into cell membranes
Factor J	20	C1, C3, B	Inhibits C1 complex formation, inhibits cleavage of C3 by Bb
Cell Associated			
CR1	190*	C3b, C4b	Dissociation of C3/C5 convertases, cofactor for C3b and C4b inactivation by factor I
DAF (CD55)	70	C3bBb, C4b2a	Dissociation of C3/C5 convertases
MCP (CD46)	45–70	C3b (C4b)	Cofactor for C3b inactivation by factor I
CD59 (protectin)	18–20	C8, C9	Inhibition of formation of the MAC
HRF	65	C8, C9	Inhibition of formation of the MAC

CR1, Complement receptor type 1; *DAF,* decay-accelerating factor; *HRF,* homologous restriction factor; *MAC,* membrane attack complex; *MCP,* membrane cofactor protein.
*Most common isoform of CR1.

opsonization, phagocytosis, immunomodulation, and generation of inflammatory reactions.

Complement activation leads to proteolytic cleavage of many complement proteins with the subsequent release of small biologically active fragments into the fluid phase. Three of these released fragments—C4a, C3a, and C5a—are called anaphylatoxins. The structural and functional characteristics of these molecules are described in an excellent review on the subject (Ember, 1998). C3a is a 9-kDa peptide fragment released during selective proteolytic cleavage of the C3α chain by C2a (as a component of C3 convertase) in the classical and MBLectin activation pathways. It is also released by proteolytic cleavage of C3 by the enzymatically active peptide Bb, a component of the alternative pathway C3 convertase. C4a is an 8.7-kDa peptide released from C4 upon cleavage by C1s2. C5a is an 11-kDa peptide released from the α chain of C5 by cleavage induced by C2a in the classical and MBLectin pathway C5 convertase, or by Bb in the alternative (and perhaps MBLectin) pathway C5 convertase. In general, anaphylatoxins are defined by their biological effects on smooth muscle cells, mast cells, small blood vessels, and peripheral blood leukocytes. Specific effects mediated by these peptides include degranulation of mast cells and basophils, with subsequent release of various mediators such as histamine and serotonin. They also induce human neutrophil aggregation and smooth muscle contraction, enhance vascular permeability, induce thromboxane release from guinea pig macrophages, and stimulate release of mucus from goblet cells (Marom, 1985). An especially important effect of the anaphylatoxins on basophils is vasodilation caused by histamine release, leading to increased blood flow to sites of inflammation.

The function of C4a is generally similar to that of C3a, but C4a is far less effective in its biological effects on a molar basis. C5a is by far the most potent of the human anaphylatoxins, having an effect 200-fold greater than C3a and 3000-fold greater than C4a in causing smooth muscle contraction of guinea pig ileum. It should be noted, however, that the relative effectiveness of these peptides is both tissue- and species-specific. For instance, C3a may be selectively effective in eosinophil localization to allergic sites, whereas C5a has an effect on many other cell types (DiScipio, 1999).

In addition to its role as an anaphylatoxin, C5a has many important biological properties. The binding of C5a to neutrophils produces an increase in adhesion and aggregation, induction of an oxidative response, and release of lysosomal enzymes. C5a is strongly chemotactic for monocytes and neutrophils, inducing the migration of these cells toward the source of complement activation in the tissues. Thus, a local complement-activating inflammatory reaction can induce increased blood flow to the affected tissue, adherence of neutrophils to a locally activated endothelium, and directed migration of phagocytes to inflamed sites along a chemotactic gradient. Neutrophils aggregated by C5a can embolize to the lung, causing changes in pulmonary gas exchange and even death. It is thought that C5a mediates much of the pulmonary inflammation caused by immune complex formation (Ward, 1997). In a rat experimental sepsis model, it has been demonstrated that C5a may block the bactericidal functions of neutrophils if produced in excessive amounts, suggesting a role for complement activation in the high mortality rates observed in sepsis (Czermak, 1999). The biological effects of anaphylatoxins are mediated via specific cell surface receptors described in the section on complement receptors.

REGULATION OF COMPLEMENT ACTIVATION

Complement activation, although important to host defense, may produce profound tissue damage. Organisms have evolved with internal control mechanisms to (1) limit overly widespread inflammation, (2) avoid excessive activation, and (3) protect host cells from inadvertent injury. A potent regulatory system consisting of fluid-phase and membrane-associated proteins controls complement activation at almost every step of the activation cascade (Table 47-1).

Fluid-Phase Regulators

Control of the first component of the classical pathway (C1) is mediated by C1 inhibitor (C1-Inh). C1-Inh blocks C1 autoactivation, C1 activation in the fluid phase, and C1 activation on weak activators of the classical pathway; it does not block activation on most immune complexes (Doekes, 1983). It is thought that C1-Inh has the ability to dislodge the entire $C1qr_2s_2$ complex from immunoglobulin with low binding affinity for C1q (Chen, 1998), and from targets sensitized with low doses of human IgG (Chen, 1998). In vitro, C1-Inh inactivates MASP (mannan-binding lectin-associated serine proteases) (Matsushita, 1996). C4b activity is regulated by factor I (formerly referred to as the C3b/C4b inactivator) (Fries, 1987), which cleaves the C4b α chain to generate two fragments, C4c and C4d; the latter fragment remains cell-bound. For proteolysis, a cofactor, C4-binding protein (C4BP), is required. C4BP is a 570-kDa protein that can also bind particle-bound and fluid-phase C4b and can displace C2a from the classical pathway C3 convertase C4b2a (Gigli, 1979). Because of its pivotal role in the three complement activation pathways, C3 is under rigid control. Fluid-phase C3b and $C3(H_2O)$ are rapidly inactivated by factor I, which cleaves three peptide bonds on the α chain of C3b (Davis, 1982), thus generating an inactive form of the molecule, iC3b, which is incapable of engaging C5 or factor B. This factor I–mediated cleavage requires factor H as a cofactor. Factor H is a 150-kDa protein that binds C3b and has decay-accelerating activity toward the alternative pathway C3 convertase, in addition to its cofactor activity for factor I–mediated cleavage of C3b. In addition to regulating C3b in the fluid phase, factor H binds to cell-bound C3b and triggers cleavage by factor I, thus limiting classical pathway activation (Ollert, 1995). Once C3b is cleaved into iC3b, which then remains bound to the target surface, it is free to interact with complement receptor type 3 (CR3) present on phagocytic cells, thereby promoting phagocytosis.

A number of fluid-phase inhibitors of the terminal complement components can prevent insertion of the MAC into cell membranes. S protein

TABLE 47-2
Cell Receptors for Complement Protein Fragments

Receptor	Molecular weight, kDa	Ligand	Physiologic role
CR1	190 (most common isoform)	C3b, C4b, iC3b	Phagocytosis, immune complex clearance
CR2	140	C3d, C3dg, iC3b	B cell activation
CR3	165 (α chain) 95 (β chain)	iC3b, C3d, C3b	Phagocytosis, cellular adhesion
CR4	150 (α chain) 95 (β chain)	iC3b, C3b	Cellular adhesion
C1qRp*	126	C1q, MBL, SP-A	Phagocytosis
C3aR	48	C3a	Chemotaxis, degranulation of serosal-type mast cells, increase in vascular permeability
C5aR	43	C5a, C5a desArg	Chemotaxis, degranulation of serosal-type mast cells, cellular adhesion, increase in vascular permeability

CR1, Complement receptor type 1; *C1qRp,* receptor for the collagenous region of C1q; *CR2,* complement receptor type 2; *CR3,* complement receptor type 3; *C3aR,* C3a receptor; *CR4,* complement receptor type 4; *C5a desArg,* C5a lacking the terminal arginine residue following inactivation by carboxypeptidase-N; *C5aR,* C5a receptor; *MBL,* mannan-binding lectin; *SP-A,* surfactant protein A.
*Other C1q receptors have also been described.

(not identical to protein S), also called vitronectin, binds the C5b–7 complex, thereby preventing its insertion in the cell membrane (Podack, 1977) and inhibiting C9 polymerization (Johnson, 1994). S protein binds C5b and C8 within the sC5b–9 complex (Su, 1996) and binds to the receptor C1q (Lim, 1996). Although the full role of S protein in regulating complement activation in vivo is uncertain, Peake (1996) showed that S protein forms a complex with sC5b–9 when complement is activated in rabbits, and that this complex still has the ability to block C9-mediated lysis of sensitized sheep erythrocytes bearing complement components 1–7. Clusterin (also called Sp-40, or apolipoprotein J) is another fluid-phase inhibitor of the terminal complement components. Similar to vitronectin, clusterin prevents insertion of the C5b–7 complex into the cell membrane (Choi, 1989) and regulates the MAC at both C5b–7 and C9 levels (Berge, 1997).

Cell-Associated Regulatory Proteins

Regulation of complement activation must occur on host cell surfaces to limit inadvertent injury to those cells. Many of these regulatory proteins also act as complement receptors. One such protein is complement receptor type 1 (CR1), which binds activated C4b and C3b and serves as a cofactor for their factor I–mediated cleavages (see next section for more). Control of cell membrane–deposited C4b and C3b is also achieved by membrane cofactor protein (MCP, CD46). This protein is expressed by almost every cell, with the notable exception of erythrocytes, and serves as a cofactor for factor I–mediated cleavage of C4b and C3b into C4c and C4d, and iC3b, respectively (Seya, 1986, 1989).

Another cell membrane–associated protein that controls complement activation at the level of the C3 and C5 convertases is decay-accelerating factor (DAF, CD55). DAF is expressed by all circulating cells, all endothelial cells, and a number of epithelial cells (Morgan, 1994b), and accelerates the decay of C3 and C5 convertases of both the classical and alternative pathways.

Regulatory control of terminal complement components of the MAC is achieved by homologous restriction factor (HRF), or C8-binding protein, and CD59 (also referred to as protectin, HRF-20, membrane inhibitor of reactive lysis, and P-18). HRF is expressed on erythrocytes, platelets, T lymphocytes, B lymphocytes, neutrophils, and monocytes (Morgan, 1994b), where it binds C8 and inhibits C9 polymerization (Morgan, 1994b). The second regulatory protein, CD59, is found on all circulating cells, endothelial cells, epithelial cells, spermatozoa, and glomerular podocytes (Morgan, 1994b), and on some cells of the central nervous system (Morgan, 1996). CD59 binds both the β chain of C8 and the b domain of C9 (Chang, 1994), inhibiting MAC formation on host cells. Because of their glycosyl phosphatidylinositol linkage to cell membranes, DAF, HRF, and CD59 are absent from the cells of patients with paroxysmal nocturnal hemoglobinuria (PNH) (Volanakis, 1988).

COMPLEMENT RECEPTORS

Receptors that bind activated complement components have been described in various cell types. These receptors control the biological effects of complement activation peptides and are linked to several other cellular functions as well (Table 47-2). The complement receptors that have been best studied are those that bind the degradation fragments of C3.

Complement receptor type 1 (CR1, CD35, C3b/C4b receptor) is a single-chain glycoprotein expressed on erythrocytes, mononuclear phagocytes, eosinophils, B lymphocytes, a subset of T lymphocytes, glomerular podocytes, follicular dendritic cells (Ahearn, 1998), and astrocytes (Morgan, 1996). It binds both C3b and C4b, to a lesser extent iC3b, and C1q as well (Klickstein, 1997). CR1 serves as a cofactor for factor I–mediated cleavage of C3b, iC3b, and C4b and has decay-accelerating activity for the classical and alternative pathway C3 and C5 convertases. A major physiologic role of CR1 is related to phagocytosis of complement-coated particles (opsonized particles). It is believed that erythrocyte CR1 has a major role in sequestering C3b- and iC3b-bearing immune complexes, removing them from the plasma and facilitating their transfer to degradation sites in the liver and the spleen (Birmingham, 1995). Decreased expression of erythrocyte CR1 may be associated with increased susceptibility to chronic forms of infection (Teixeira, 2001).

A receptor for the C3d fragment of C3 is found on human B cells, B cell lines, follicular dendritic cells, some peripheral T cells, some T cell lines, thymocytes (Ahearn, 1998), and astrocytes (Morgan, 1996), and is termed CR2 (CD21). CR2 has the ability to serve as a cofactor for factor I–mediated cleavage of iC3b bound to targets (Mitomo, 1987), and is the receptor for Epstein-Barr virus on B cells causing infectious mononucleosis (Fingeroth, 1984). The major function of CR2 is thought to be the regulation of B cell immune responses to antigen (Carroll, 1998).

A third complement receptor, CR3 (also referred to as Mac-1, CD11b/CD18) is a member of the β2 leukocyte integrin family of adhesion molecules. CR3 is expressed on mononuclear phagocytes, granulocytes, natural killer (NK) cells (Ahearn, 1998), and microglial cells (Morgan, 1996), and binds iC3b, C3b, and C3d (Brown, 1991). On phagocytes, CR3 triggers the phagocytic process in a fashion that parallels that of CR1. Another important role for CR3 is seen in the adhesion of monocytes and neutrophils to endothelial cells via interaction with its ligand, intercellular adhesion molecule type 1 (ICAM-1). This allows accumulation of phagocytes at sites of tissue injury where endothelial cells become activated. CR3 may serve as a receptor for both human immunodeficiency virus (HIV)-1 and *Neisseria gonorrhoeae* infection of follicular dendritic cells and cervical epithelial cells, respectively (Edwards, 2001; Batjay, 2004).

Complement receptor type 4 (CR4, CD11c/CD18) is a glycoprotein that shares characteristics with CR3. It is also a member of the integrin family of adhesion molecules and is expressed on myeloid cells, dendritic cells, NK cells, activated B cells, some activated T cells, platelets (Ahearn, 1998), and microglial cells (Morgan, 1996). CR4 binds iC3b, and C3b to a lesser extent (Brown, 1991). The exact role of CR4 in terms of complement activation is unknown, but because this glycoprotein is an adhesion molecule, it may serve to "assist" neutrophil adhesion to the endothelium during inflammatory processes (Sengeløv, 1995).

A receptor for the anaphylatoxin C5a (C5aR) is expressed on neutrophils, monocytes, basophils, eosinophils, platelets, mast cells, liver parenchymal cells, lung vascular smooth muscle cells, lung and umbilical vascular endothelial cells, bronchial and alveolar epithelial cells, astrocytes, microglial cells (Ember, 1998), and human T cells (Nataf, 1999). C5a binding to C5aR induces a wide variety of events, including chemotaxis of inflammatory cells; degranulation of mast cells; production of oxygen radicals; promotion of cell adhesion; production of leukotrienes and prostaglandins in neutrophils and eosinophils; and induction of acute phase proteins, cytokines, and antibodies (Ember, 1998).

COMPLEMENT BIOSYNTHESIS

It is estimated that about 90% of plasma complement components are synthesized in the liver and are acute phase proteins (i.e., their synthesis by the liver increases during inflammatory reactions to increase plasma levels). The hepatocyte produces the vast majority of complement components, with the exception of C1q, factor D, properdin, and C7 (Morgan, 1997a). C1q appears to be synthesized by epithelial cells, monocytes/macrophages, and fibroblasts. The main source of factor D is the adipocyte. Properdin is synthesized mainly by monocytes and macrophages, with some synthesis occurring in lymphocytes and granulocytes. Most plasma C7 also appears to originate from monocytes and macrophages, although neutrophils were shown to store C7. Monocytes, macrophages, cells of the synovial tissues, and astrocytes have the ability to synthesize all components of the classical and alternative pathways. This may have important implications in tissue-specific inflammation, where a localized mechanism of host defense must be present to eliminate foreign particles efficiently. Production of complement components usually synthesized by hepatocytes or by extrahepatic cells often requires stimuli generated in inflammatory reactions such as interleukin-1α, interleukin-6, or interferon-γ. A good description of the regulation of complement protein synthesis by various cells is provided elsewhere (Colten, 1998).

COMPLEMENT GENETICS

Most of the complement components are inherited in an autosomal codominant fashion. Genes that encode complement proteins, receptors, and regulatory molecules have been cloned and assigned a chromosome location (Table 47-3). Linkage exists for many of the genes that code for complement-related molecules. These linkage groups include major histocompatibility complex (MHC) class III genes (C2, factor B, and C4), genes for the regulators of complement activation (C4-binding protein, CR1, CR2, DAF, MCP, and factor H), and genes for proteins of the MACx (C6, C7, and C9) (Schneider, 1999). Molecules within each of these three groups share structural homology, suggesting that complement proteins may have arisen from gene duplication of a limited number of ancestral genes. Almost all complement-related proteins show polymorphism. The most polymorphic complement component is C4, with more than 35 identified alleles. Point mutations, insertions, or deletions of nucleic acids are usually linked to deficiencies in complement proteins (Schneider, 1997). Complement protein polymorphism is assessed by both phenotypic and genotypic analysis. Details of these methods will not be discussed in this chapter, and the reader is referred to Chapter 49 in this book, "The Major Histocompatibility Complex and Disease," as well as to other authors (Mauff, 1996; Schneider, 1997) for further reading.

COMPLEMENT AND ACQUIRED IMMUNITY

The complement system plays an important role in the establishment of acquired immune responses (Carroll, 2004). Evidence of this role came to light when depressed antibody responses to antigen stimulation were noted in animals transiently depleted in C3 (Pepys, 1974); in animals with genetic deficiencies in C2, C4, or C3 (Ochs, 1983; Böttger, 1985; O'Neil, 1988); and in patients who were genetically deficient in C2, C4, C3, or CR3 (Ochs, 1986). Studies of knockout mice lacking C4, C3, or CR1, and CR2, have furthered our understanding of the role that complement plays in the acquired immune response.

Complement may influence the antibody response to antigen in several ways. CR2 is present on the surface of B cells in association with CD19 and TAPA-1. When the B cell antigen receptor and CR2 are coligated (as would occur when antigen is complexed with C3d), the threshold for B cell activation and ultimately antibody production is dramatically lowered. Complement may also assist in the trapping of immune complexes by follicular dendritic cells, thereby facilitating the formation of lymphoid germinal centers, where B cells acquire the memory phenotype. Lack of one of the early components of the classical pathway of complement activation, or lack of CR1 and/or CR2, leads to an impaired immune response to antigen, and in some cases, to an inability to mount a secondary antibody response. Complement appears to play a role in the generation of CD5-positive B cells, which give rise to so-called **natural** antibodies (Carroll, 1998). Along with complement activation, these natural antibodies are important in proper B cell activation in response to antigenic challenge (Boes, 1998; Lutz, 1999).

Complement components C4, CR1, and CR2 play an important role in the maintenance of B cell tolerance to self-antigens (Prodeus, 1998). Complement, especially C3, is important in the generation of the acquired immune response to antigen via antigen-presenting cells (APCs). The presence of C3 cleavage products on antigen enhances uptake of that antigen by APCs (B cells and other professional APCs expressing CR1 and/or CR2), thereby increasing the efficiency of antigen presentation to T cells with enhancement of subsequent T cell–mediated responses (Boackle, 1998; Kerekes, 1998). Evidence suggests direct complement modulation of T cell immune response through interaction with complement receptors variably expressed on some T cell populations (Kemper, 2007). The role of complement in negatively regulating host immunity is also becoming apparent. For instance, cross-linking of C5a, C3b, and C1q receptors on macrophages and dendritic cells induces suppression of toll-like receptor mediated proinflammatory signaling, thereby contributing to induction of tolerance (Cummings, 2007). It thus appears that complement plays both inductive and inhibitory roles in acquired immunity.

TABLE 47-3
Complement Proteins in Human Plasma

Protein	Molecular weight, kDa	Chromosomal location	Concentration, mg/mL
Common to All Pathways			
C3	185	19p13.3–p13.2	1200–1300
Classical Pathway			
C1q	460	1p34.1–36.3	150
C1r	85	12p13	50
C1s	85	12p13	50
C4	205	6p21.3	300–600
C2	102	6p21.3	20
Alternative Pathway			
Factor B	93	6p21.3	200
Factor D	24	Unknown	2
Properdin	55 (monomer)	Xp11.4–p11.2	25
MBLectin Pathway			
MBL	200–400	10q11.2–q21	0.002–10
MASP-1	93	3q27–28	1.5–13
MASP-2	76	1p36.3–36.2	Unknown
Membrane Attack Complex			
C5	190	9q33	80
C6	110	5p13	45
C7	100	5p13	90
C8	150	1p32 (α, β chains), 9q22.3–q32 (γ chain)	55
C9	70	5p13	60
Control Proteins			
C1-Inh	105	11q11–q13.1	240
C4bp	550	1q32	250
Factor I	88	4q25	35
Factor H	150	1q32	300–450
S protein	84	17q11	500
Clusterin	70	Unknown	50
Factor J	20	Unknown	~5.4

MASP, MBL-associated serine proteases; *MBL,* mannan-binding lectin.

GENETIC COMPLEMENT DEFICIENCIES

Identification of individuals with complement deficiencies has contributed much to our understanding of the role that complement plays in host defense, especially against infectious agents, and in the development of autoimmune disease. Genetically controlled complement deficiencies are very rare but are estimated to account for as many as 6% of primary immunodeficiencies (Notarangelo, 2004). These deficiencies are

TABLE 47-4

Inherited Deficiencies in Complement and Complement-Related Proteins

Protein	Pattern of inheritance	Major clinical correlates*
Common to All Pathways		
C3	Autosomal recessive	Recurrent pyogenic infections, glomerulonephritis
Classical Pathway		
C1q	Autosomal recessive	Glomerulonephritis, SLE
C1r	Autosomal recessive	Glomerulonephritis, SLE
C1s	Autosomal recessive	Glomerulonephritis, SLE
C4†	Autosomal recessive	SLE, scleroderma, IgA nephropathy, membranous glomerulonephritis
C2†	Autosomal recessive	SLE, DLE, juvenile rheumatoid arthritis, glomerulonephritis
Alternative Pathway		
Factor B	Autosomal recessive	*Neisseria meningitidis* infection
Factor D	Autosomal recessive	Recurrent pyogenic infections
Properdin	X-linked	Recurrent pyogenic infections, fulminant meningococcemia
MBLectin Pathway		
MBL	Autosomal dominant	Recurrent infections
Membrane Attack Complex		
C5	Autosomal recessive	Recurrent disseminated neisserial infections, SLE
C6	Autosomal recessive	Recurrent disseminated neisserial infections
C7	Autosomal recessive	Recurrent disseminated neisserial infections, Raynaud disease
C8 (β or α–γ chains)	Autosomal recessive	Recurrent disseminated neisserial infections
C9	Autosomal recessive	None
Fluid-Phase Control Proteins		
C1-Inh	Autosomal dominant or acquired	Hereditary angioedema, autoimmune diseases‡
C4bp	Autosomal recessive	Angioedema, Behçet's-like syndrome
Factor I	Autosomal recessive	Recurrent pyogenic infections
Factor H	Autosomal recessive	Recurrent pyogenic infections, glomerulonephritis, age-related macular degeneration
Cell-Bound Proteins		
CR1	Autosomal recessive§	Association between low erythrocyte expression and SLE
CR3	Autosomal recessive	Leukocyte adhesion deficiency-1 (LAD-1), recurrent pyogenic infections, leukocytosis
DAF/CD59/HRF	Acquired	Paroxysmal nocturnal hemoglobinuria

dAF, Decay-accelerating factor; *DLE,* disseminated lupus erythematosus; *MBL,* mannan-binding lectin; *SLE,* systemic lupus erythematosus.

*Note that some people with complement deficiencies, especially C2 and components of the membrane attack complex, are clinically well. A substantial number of patients with defects in C5–C9 have had autoimmune disease. Deficiencies of C1–C9 are associated with a CH50 of 0. Deficiencies of C1, C4, and C2 are associated with SLE, and patients often have negative LE preps. Deficiencies of C3–C9 are associated with absent or low bactericidal activity in serum. Deficiency of C3 or C5 is associated with absent or diminished chemotactic activity of serum and may be associated with absent leukocyte response to infection.

†Deficiency in C4 genes (C4A andC4B) is referred to as "q0," for quantity zero. Such deficiency is designated C4Aq0 or C4Bq0. Patients with such deficiencies have a higher than normal incidence of autoimmune disease. Heterozygous C2-deficient individuals also have an increased incidence of autoimmune disease.

‡Approximately 85% of cases involve silent alleles, and 15% involve alleles encoding for acquired dysfunctional variant C1 inhibitor protein. In hereditary angioedema, the C1 level is normal or depressed, the C3 level is always normal, and the C4 level is depressed. In the acquired disease, C1 and C4 levels are depressed, the antigenic C1 inhibitor level usually is normal or high, and the functional C1 inhibitor level is very low.

§Homozygosity for low (not absent) numeric expression of CR1 on erythrocytes is detectable in vitro and may be associated with SLE. An acquired defect in the number of CR1 may also be operative. Low, but not absent, levels of leukocyte CR3 are detectable in both parents of most CR3-deficient children.

of interest because they allow us to determine the role of complement components in various biological phenomena and in various disease states. Knowledge of a specific genetic mutation associated with a deficiency would permit confirmation of the heritable nature of the complement deficiency and enable screening for carriers of the mutation within the family. Even so, because genetic analyses are difficult to undertake routinely and are generally more expensive to use for screening purposes, they are rarely used during the primary workup of complement component deficiencies (Mollnes, 2007). The absence of a complement component usually follows simple mendelian genetic principles and is most often inherited as an autosomal recessive trait, with some exceptions noted here. Heterozygous patients tend to have half the expected normal complement level or less, and homozygous (deficient) patients have little or no detectable complement component activity. Deficiencies are known for every protein linked to complement activation (Table 47-4). The incidence of complete complement deficiency is estimated to be 0.03% of the general population (Wen, 2004), but with the discovery of the MBL pathway came the surprising finding that deficiency in serum MBL is fairly common. In fact it is estimated that as much as 5% of the population has one of the three recognized gene mutations that lead to MBL deficiency (Sumiya, 1997).

A correlation between MBL deficiency (autosomal codominant) and upper respiratory tract infection, especially between the ages of 6 and 18 months, has been reported, demonstrating the importance of the MBL pathway in early childhood (Turner, 1996). One study suggested that variant MBL genes might be associated with as many as one third of all meningococcal infections in children (Hibberd, 1999). Purified MBL infusions are reported to correct the defect and susceptibility to infection in children with MBL deficiencies (Valdimarsson, 1998). Not surprisingly, the same tendency to acquire clinically significant infections is associated with MBL deficiency in those immunocompromised by chemotherapy. Furthermore, it has been suggested that MBL deficiency leads to autoimmune diseases such as systemic lupus erythematosus (SLE) (Turner, 1996) and is a risk factor for recurrent miscarriage (Christiansen, 1999). In contrast, deficiencies of early components of the classical pathway are rare, but are strongly associated with lupus-like disease with rash and glomerulonephritis (Botto, 2009).

Because complement is important in the clearance of immune complexes from the circulation, it may be true that early complement component deficiency leads to improper handling of immune complexes, along with their accumulation in tissues such as the kidney. Deficiencies of terminal complement components and alternate pathway components such

TABLE 47-5
Major Complement Deficiency Assays Performed on Peripheral Blood

Functional	Immunochemical single-protein quantification	Activation product	Autoantibodyanalysis	Surface proteins	Genetic mapping
Total Complement Activity	*Immunoprecipitation*	*ELISA Based on Antibody to Neo-epitopes Found on Activation Products*	*ELISA-Based Assays*	*Flow Cytometric Quantification*	*Detection of Disease-Associated Genetic Variants (Mutations, Polymorphisms)*
a. CH50 and AH50 hemolytic assays	a. RID	a. Split products: C3a, C4a, C5a	Anti-C1q in SLE, anti-C1-Inh in AE, anti-factor H in aHUS, others	CD55/DAF and CD59 in PNH	aHUS (factor H, factor I, factor B, C3)
b. ELISA for CP, AP, MBL (WIELISA)	b. Electroimmunoassay	b. Activated component complexes: C1rs-C1-Inh, others	Functional assays		MPGN (C3)
	c. Nephelometry and turbidimetry	c. Macromolecular complexes	a. C3 nephritic factor in MPGN, type 2		
Single-Component Activity	*Other Methods*				
a. Hemolytic assays using component deficient sera (e.g., C3, factor H)	a. ELISA				
b. ELISA (e.g., MBL and MASP functional activity with C4 as target)	b. TRIFMA				
c. Chromogenic substrate (C1-Inh)	c. WB				

Adapted from Botto M, et al. Complement in human diseases: lessons from complement deficiencies. Mol Immunol 2009;46:2774–83, Table 1.
AE, Angioedema; *aHUS,* atypical hemolytic-uremic syndrome; *AP,* alternate pathway; *CP,* classical pathway; *ELISA,* enzyme-linked immunosorbent assay; *MASP,* MBL-associated serine proteases; *MBL,* mannan-binding lectin pathway; *MPGN,* membranoproliferative glomerulonephritis; *PNH,* paroxysmal nocturnal hemoglobinuria; *RID,* radio-immunodiffusion; *TRIFMA,* time-resolved immunofluorometric assay; *WB,* Western blot; *WIESLA,* three-pathway ELISA (Wieslab, Lund, Sweden).

as factor B, factor D, and properdin (X-linked) are well described and are associated with elevated risk of recurrent infection with gram-negative cocci such as *Neisseria meningitidis* and septic shock. Deficiency in C1 inhibitor (autosomal dominant) leads to hereditary angioedema, a disease characterized by recurrent episodes of subcutaneous and submucosal edema. This deficiency can be inherited or acquired following the development of autoantibodies to C1 inhibitor. Deficiency of factor H due to a novel homozygous factor H gene mutation has been described in an 8-month-old child and was associated with thrombotic microangiopathy and ultimately renal failure (atypical hemolytic-uremic syndrome [aHUS]) (Licht, 2005). Table 47-5 lists complement deficiency assays in common use.

Assessment of Complement Activity in Disease

Complement promotes inflammation or tissue damage during the immune response, and plays an important role in the pathogenesis of some diseases. In the latter situation, complement is often activated by an abnormal antibody (autoantibody), by an immune complex, or by foreign material. To track disease activity in these cases, it is frequently necessary to measure serum complement levels (Table 47-6), as with SLE, in which depressed serum C3 or C4 correlates with disease activity. In such instances, nephelometric techniques are frequently employed (see "Assays of Complement," later).

It is important to recognize that serum complement measurements are only snapshots of a dynamic process involving variable rates of complement consumption and production. Many of the complement proteins behave as acute phase reactants, with their serum levels rising dramatically in some inflammatory states, while they may fall dramatically through catabolism in other inflammatory conditions such as autoimmune states. Depending on the rate of complement production and consumption, a normal serum complement level may be associated with tissue damage, just as a decreased serum complement level may be. For example, patients with biliary cirrhosis have an increased catabolic rate of C3, and it has been suggested that C3 may play a role in the development of this disease. Nevertheless, the level of C3 in the serum of patients with biliary cirrhosis is almost always elevated. In this case, increased synthesis obscures the increased catabolism. Along these lines, it is useful to bear in mind that complement levels in different anatomic compartments may differ. For instance, serum complement levels in patients with seropositive rheumatoid arthritis may be normal or elevated, while joint fluid complement levels may be severely depressed (where tissue damage is greatest).

TABLE 47-6
Complement Deficiency–Related Disease State and Recommended Analysis on Peripheral Blood

Disease	Complement analysis
Recurrent bacterial infections	CH50, AH50, WIELISA, C3, C3a/C3d, C5–C9 *(Neisseria),* properdin *(Neisseria),* MBL *(Neisseria)*
Systemic lupus erythematosus	CH50, C4 (C4A/B), C3a/C3d, anti-C1q autoantibodies
Angioedema	C1 inhibitor antigenic assay, C4, C1q, acquired anti-C1q autoantibody
aHUS	CH50, AH50, C3, C3a/C3d, C3 nephritic factor, factor H, factor B, factor I, anti–factor H antibodies
MPGN	CH50, AH50, C3, C3a/C3d, C3 nephritic factor, factor H, factor I, anti–factor H antibodies
PNH	CD55, CD59 (flow cytometry)

Adapted from Botto M, et al. Complement in human diseases: lessons from complement deficiencies. Mol Immunol 2009;46:2774–83, Table 2.
aHUS, Atypical hemolytic-uremic syndrome; *C3a/C3d,* to exclude excessive complement consumption; *MBL,* mannan-binding lectin pathway; *MPGN,* membranoproliferative glomerulonephritis; *PNH,* paroxysmal nocturnal hemoglobinuria; *WIESLA,* three-pathway enzyme-linked immunosorbent assay (ELISA) (Wieslab, Lund, Sweden).

Several investigators have attempted to identify which complement activation pathway predominates in mediating tissue damage in one illness or another by establishing a **complement profile.** The simplest approach to this problem examines the levels of various complement components and assumes that decreased levels of a given component of one of the pathways of complement activation are more likely to occur when that

TABLE 47-7

Complement Activation ELISA Results Using Peripheral Blood in Screening Suspected Complement Deficiencies

IMPAIRED FUNCTION OR DEFICIENCY	ELISA ACTIVITY		
Complement component	**Classical pathway**	**Alternative pathway**	**Lectin pathway**
C1q, C1r, C1s	Low	Normal	Normal
C4, C2	Low	Normal	Low
MBL, MASP	Normal	Normal	Low
B, D, P	Normal	Low	Normal
C3, C5, C6, C7, C8, C9	Low	Low	Low

Adapted from Mollnes TE, et al. Complement analysis in the 21st century. Mol Immunol 2007;44:3838–49, Table 1.

ELISA, Enzyme-linked immunosorbent assay; *MASP,* MBL-associated serine proteases; *MBL,* mannan-binding lectin pathway.

pathway is activated. So, if a patient has depressed levels of C3 and C4 and normal levels of factor B, the classical pathway is likely to be involved. If a patient has decreased levels of C3, factor B, and properdin, and normal levels of C4, alternative pathway activation is most likely. In this way, determining the levels of a limited number of components can provide a great deal of clinically useful information.

An important advance in this area is the use of ELISA to detect stable complexes formed in serum during complement activation. These assays are highly sensitive and can readily demonstrate which pathway of complement is activated in various disease states (Morgan, 1994a) (Table 47-7).

On activation, many complement proteins express new antigens (neo-antigens) that are not revealed on the native plasma protein. The neo-antigen present on the MAC, but not present on native terminal components, is perhaps the most interesting. Antibody to this neo-antigen exists and has been used to study serum neo-antigen levels by immunofluorescence and by ELISA (Falk, 1983; Sanders, 1985). The neo-antigen level is elevated in blood and spinal fluid in many patients with ongoing complement activation (Sanders, 1986), and the neo-antigen is present in tissues at sites of terminal complex deposition. For example, it is present in the glomeruli of patients with some forms of glomerulonephritis (Falk, 1983) and in lesional skin at sites of active SLE (Biesecker, 1982). Unlike C3 deposited in normal skin of patients with SLE and a positive lupus band test, the MAC neo-antigen is found only in lesions.

Complement in Disease States

RHEUMATOLOGIC DISEASES

Complement analysis in patients with autoimmune disease is useful for establishing the differential diagnosis and for following disease activity. A variety of autoimmune conditions are now linked to disorders of the complement systems, including the antiphospholipid syndrome, leukocytoclastic vasculitis, cryoglobulinemia (types I–III), and systemic forms of rheumatoid arthritis. Deficiency of an early complement component (C1, C4, or C2) is frequently associated with autoimmune disease (Wen, 2004), and the rheumatologic disease that has been evaluated most extensively in terms of the contribution of complement to disease activity is SLE (Agnello, 1986; Atkinson, 1986; Liu, 2004). The incidence of deficiency of complement components C1q, C4, and C2 is 90%, 75%, and 15%, respectively, in those with SLE (Pickering, 2000), and the incidence of SLE is increased in those with MBL deficiency (Kilpatrick, 2002). Large quantities of immune complexes, both circulating and tissue-bound, are formed in SLE. These immune complexes activate complement, and complement activation products contribute to the ongoing inflammation typical of SLE. It is postulated that removal of immune complexes from the circulation with the assistance of complement may reduce the formation of antibodies (autoantibodies) to these complexes. Extended exposure to circulating immune complexes, as well as to necrotic and apoptotic cell debris, due to impaired complement-related clearance mechanisms, especially in those with complement deficiencies, may be a factor in the loss of self-tolerance and the development of autoimmunity (reviewed in Markiewski, 2007). C3 and C4 levels are often reduced in SLE, and, in general, low levels are found in patients with active disease.

Some suggest that a low C4 level is the best indicator of ongoing active disease. However, some patients with active disease show normal C4 levels. Some believe that the level of circulating sC5b–9 or neo-antigen of the MAC might serve as a better indicator of active disease (Gawryl, 1988). As mentioned earlier, complement appears to play an essential role in the clearance of immune complexes from the circulation, particularly those that contain IgM or IgG complement-activating isotypes. C3b deposition on the immune complex resulting from complement activation allows interaction with cells that possess a C3b receptor (CR1). Upon binding to erythrocytes via CR1, immune complexes are prevented from diffusing from the plasma to tissues, where they could cause damage. Erythrocytes bearing immune complexes circulate to the liver, where immune complexes are removed by a process that does not shorten the life span of the red cell (Cornacoff, 1983; Birmingham, 1995). In diseases in which complement is activated and immunologically active products are formed in the circulation, the number of CR1s per red cell is decreased, possibly as the result of removal of CR1 from erythrocytes in the liver (Ross, 1985). In addition to those seen in SLE, erythrocytes from patients with chronic cold agglutinin disease, paroxysmal nocturnal hemoglobinuria (PNH), autoimmune hemolytic anemia, Sjögren's syndrome, and *Mycoplasma* pneumonia are reported to have reduced erythrocyte CR1, suggesting that immune deposits have been removed from erythrocytes in these diseases as well (Ross, 1985; Atkinson, 1986).

Complement proteins also act as acute phase reactants, so that complement levels may not be depressed even in situations in which complement activation occurs. For instance, normal or elevated serum complement levels may be found in juvenile rheumatoid arthritis (JRA), palindromic arthritis, pseudogout, gout, Reiter syndrome, and gonococcal arthritis. On the other hand, depressed complement levels may be found in the joint fluid in other rheumatologic conditions such as rheumatoid arthritis (RA). Depressed total hemolytic complement activity (CH50; see later under Assays of Complement) and the presence of cleavage products of C3 and factor B are thought to represent intra-articular complement activation (in the synovial fluid) in patients with seronegative rheumatoid arthritis, SLE, pseudogout, gout, Reiter syndrome, and gonococcal arthritis. This is not true of fluids obtained from patients with degenerative arthritis.

HEREDITARY ANGIOEDEMA

Hereditary angioedema (HAE) is a potentially life-threatening condition marked by submucosal, subcutaneous, nonpruritic, and nonerythematous swelling. It usually resolves within 48–72 hours but may instead be fatal when it involves the laryngeal mucosa. The cause of HAE is a heterozygous deficiency of C1-Inh. Because C1-Inh is the regulator of various components of the clotting, complement, and kinin-generating pathways, the actual pathway involved in the genesis of episodes of HAE is difficult to pinpoint. Several forms of HAE have been identified, including type I, in which patients have a reduced (30% or less) level of functional or antigenic C1-Inh, and type II, in which C1-Inh has reduced or absent activity, although it is present at normal levels (Wen, 2004).

INFECTIOUS DISEASES

As mentioned earlier and as evidenced by clinical findings in patients with genetically controlled complement deficiencies, the complement system plays a crucial role in defense against microorganisms. Patients with gram-negative septicemia and pyogenic infection often have deficiency of C3, or components of the alternative pathway. It is known that patients with hepatitis B surface antigen (HBsAg)-positive infectious hepatitis have an early fall in serum C3, which later returns to normal. This may be associated with signs of immune complex disease such as arthralgia. In a similar fashion, complement appears to play an important role in many parasitic infections, including leishmaniasis, trypanosomiasis, giardiasis, and malaria. In those with recurrent infections by *N. gonorrhoeae* or *Neisseria meningitidis*, a deficiency of MAC or properdin may be suspected. A thorough discussion of the interactions between the complement system and parasites, bacteria, and viruses may be found in several excellent reviews (Frank, 1988; Fishelson, 1994; Moffitt, 1994; Kozel, 1996; Cooper 1998). However, it is important to recognize that serum complement levels in general are not a reliable index of disease activity in these infectious conditions.

The role of complement in the adult respiratory distress syndrome (ARDS), a common occurrence in patients with severe trauma or overwhelming sepsis, has been studied. Evidence of massive activation of complement has been found in these patients, suggesting that bacteria and bacterial products activate complement (Hammerschmidt, 1980), with activation of the classical and alternative pathways (Langlois, 1988) and the formation of proinflammatory factors such as neutrophil-activating factor and C5a. Much of the pulmonary damage that occurs in ARDS may be due to neutrophil infiltration of the lung. Recent evidence suggests a role for complement receptors in the human immunodeficiency virus (HIV) infection of follicular dendritic cells (Doepper, 2002; Stoiber, 2005); a similar role for MAC has been suggested in prion disease (see "Neurologic Diseases," later).

RENAL DISEASES

Complement appears to play a key role in the glomerular damage found in many of the glomerulonephritides (West, 1998). This is usually demonstrated by the deposition of C3 or other complement components within or near damaged glomerular basement membranes. Also, the MAC has been identified in damaged glomeruli in patients with SLE-related glomerulonephritis. Patients with serum sickness and glomerular damage due to circulating immune complexes show evidence of activation of the classical or alternative pathway, or both. Traditionally, it has been believed that immune complexes are deposited in glomeruli during their passage through the kidney. Once deposited, these complexes activate complement, typically leading to depressed serum complement levels. Evidence of complement activation and deposition is routinely identified by immunofluorescence microscopy in the glomeruli of those with IgA nephropathy, membranous glomerulonephritis, and poststreptococcal glomerulonephritis, among other glomerulonephritides. An alternative view is that antibodies to glomerular structures form immune complexes in situ on the glomerular basement membrane (GBM), which then activate complement, causing local damage (Daha, 1979).

Although antibodies to GBM structures are clearly of importance in Goodpasture syndrome, their overall role in glomerulonephritis is questionable. In some patients with a rare form of glomerulonephritis, membranoproliferative glomerulonephritis, type II, with very low C3 levels, the protein known as C3 nephritic factor (C3NeF or NFa) stabilizes the alternative pathway C3 convertase. C3NeF is an autoantibody directed against Bb that extends the half-life of the alternative pathway C3 convertase by more than 10 times (Daha, 1976, 1979), and may protect it from decay dissociation by factor H (Fearon, 1980). Although C3NeF is thought to be responsible for the very low C3 levels present in these patients, it is not thought to play a central role in the development of nephritis. This is supported by experimental evidence using factor H–deficient and factor I–deficient mouse models (Thurman, 2006; Holers, 2008).

Dysregulation of the alternative complement pathway plays a role in aHUS, an atypical form of hemolytic-uremic syndrome that occurs without the usual bloody diarrhea prodrome. Most patients with aHUS have mutations of the genes encoding alternative pathway proteins such as factor H, factor I, and C3. The ability to identify mutations of complement-associated genes has useful clinical management applications. For instance, those with factor H gene mutations are recognized to have especially early and frequent recurrence of aHUS after renal transplant, leading to the practice of simultaneously transplanting both the liver, where factor H is manufactured, and the kidney, to improve allograft longevity (Thurman, 2006; Holers, 2008).

OPHTHALMOLOGIC DISEASES

Age-related macular degeneration (AMD) is the major cause of irreversible vision loss in developed countries. The risk of developing AMD is now known to be closely associated with a polymorphism of factor H, and possibly associated with genes encoding factor B and C3. This condition usually affects older patients and is characterized by progressive loss of retinal cells, retinal atrophy, subretinal bleeding and neovascularization, and retinal lesions known as drusen. The linkage of AMD to complement dysregulation was first suggested by the finding of components of complement, specifically C3 and C5a, in drusen typical of the condition (Markiewski, 2007; Holers, 2008).

DERMATOLOGIC DISEASES

Complement is thought to play a part in ongoing tissue damage in a variety of dermatologic illnesses. These include bullous pemphigoid, pemphigoid gestationis, cicatricial pemphigoid, epidermolysis bullosa acquisita, dermatitis herpetiformis, and pemphigus vulgaris (Yancey, 1998). Serum complement levels are usually normal or elevated in these inflammatory states, and the importance of complement in these conditions is suggested by immunofluorescence analysis of tissue biopsies and by studies of blister fluid. Gammon (1984) developed an in vitro model useful for the study of anti–basement membrane zone antibody-mediated skin disorders. These authors have shown conclusively that C5a is a key element in the pathogenesis of bullous pemphigoid and epidermolysis bullosa acquisita. C5a acts as the chemoattractant necessary for the influx of neutrophils into sites of subsequent tissue damage in these diseases.

HEMATOLOGIC DISEASES

In many types of autoimmune hemolytic anemia, complement plays an important role in the opsonization of erythrocytes, leading to their clearance by cells of the reticuloendothelial system. However, even in those cases in which complement is clearly involved, serum complement levels are usually normal. Complement is particularly important in the clearance of cells coated with IgM cold-reactive autoantibodies with anti-I specificity. These autoantibodies (cold agglutinins) are associated with lymphoproliferative disorders following infection, or they may occur as isolated findings, especially in the elderly. Cold agglutinins generally bind erythrocytes optimally at the subphysiologic temperatures found in some areas of the body such as the tip of the nose, fingers, and ears. They usually mediate cell lysis when circulating erythrocytes return to core body temperatures. Not all cold agglutinins are IgM antibodies. The syndrome of paroxysmal cold hemoglobinuria (PCH), for example, results from cold-reactive Donath-Landsteiner IgG antibodies, which bind to cells at temperatures below 37° C but mediate lysis upon warming. Although the antibody is different, the pathophysiologic effects are similar.

Other autoantibodies that activate complement bind more efficiently at warm temperatures. In general, these warm-reactive antibodies are of the IgG isotype. In some cases, these antibodies may be associated with lymphoproliferative malignancy and viral infection. Most IgG warm-reactive antibodies found in autoimmune hemolytic anemia have Rh specificity and are poor complement activators, as opposed to cold agglutinins and anti-A and anti-B blood group antibodies. However, some antibodies, such as Tja, activate complement well and cause lysis.

In PNH, patients experience recurrent episodes of intravascular hemolysis. Lysis of erythrocytes in these patients is believed to proceed via the alternative pathway (Rosse, 1998; Jarva, 1999), although serum complement levels are always normal, and the direct antiglobulin test is always negative. The defect in PNH is lack of glycosyl phosphatidylinositol-linked proteins on the surface of a patient's cells, resulting from mutations in the X-linked phosphatidylinositol glycan A *(PIGA)* gene. Among other proteins linked via this cell membrane anchor are DAF/CD55 and CD59, two molecules that control complement activation at the level of the C3 convertase, and C8 and C9, respectively (see earlier, under "Regulation of Complement Activation"). Alteration of these proteins caused by mutations of *PIGA* indicates that all cell lineages produced in the marrow, including erythrocytes, lack the ability to protect themselves from complement activation on their surfaces (Holers, 2008). Recently, the therapeutic mAb eculizumab (binds to C5 blocking C5 convertase) was approved for the treatment of this disease.

NEUROLOGIC DISEASES

The role of the complement system in diseases of the nervous system has become evident in recent years. This is somewhat surprising, in that the blood-brain barrier effectively blocks complement penetration into spinal fluid. Complement activation was demonstrated in diseases such as myasthenia gravis, multiple sclerosis, cerebral lupus, Guillain-Barré syndrome, and Alzheimer's disease (Morgan, 1994a, 1997b; Shin, 1998). Deposition of complement proteins was demonstrated in diseased tissue, and complement activation was shown in the cerebrospinal fluid of patients with most of these diseases. Presumably, inflammation causes a breakdown in the blood-brain barrier with local penetration of complement proteins. Moreover, some cells synthesize complement proteins. Evidence suggests that complement activation might be involved in myelin damage, thus leading to both central and peripheral nervous system illnesses. Complement was also shown to be involved in Alzheimer's disease and Pick disease. In Alzheimer's disease, a peptide derived from amyloid termed β-A4 binds C1q and activates complement in senile plaques of the diseased brain. The most abundant glial cell type, the astrocyte, was shown in vitro to synthesize all of the complement proteins under inflammatory conditions (Morgan, 1996). Furthermore, astrocytes and microglial cells express complement receptors in vitro (Morgan, 1997a). Therefore, despite the blood-brain barrier, the brain has the ability to mount a potent complement-dependent inflammatory reaction as a defense mechanism. Complement components may play a facilitating role in the neuropathology of prion diseases. The neuronal loss associated with transmissible spongiform encephalitis may be related to MAC formation on neuronal surfaces and the presence of extracellular C3b and C1q in disease-associated prion protein deposits (Kovacs, 2004).

CARDIOVASCULAR DISEASES

Involvement of the complement system in myocardial ischemia/reperfusion (I/R) injury is well accepted (Lucchesi, 1997). The mechanism by which complement contributes to acute myocardial infarction in patients is still unclear. Nevertheless, deposition of components of the classical and alternative pathways has been demonstrated in the affected myocardium, along with C5b–9. Production of anaphylatoxins that accompany complement activation appears to be responsible for the local inflammatory reaction. The most dramatic demonstration of an effect of complement, especially the terminal complement components (C5b–9), comes from an animal model of coronary artery occlusion (Kilgore, 1998). Rabbits with genetically controlled C6 deficiency showed significantly reduced infarct size as compared with normal rabbits. In addition, neutrophil infiltration was significantly reduced in C6-deficient rabbits, suggesting the crucial role of terminal complement components in the generation of local inflammation.

The role of complement in I/R-related injury following restoration of blood flow after cardiac (or other organ) infarction is becoming better appreciated. Reestablishment of blood flow to ischemically damaged tissue leads to increased vascular permeability with attraction and activation of inflammatory cells to the injured site. Newly arrived inflammatory cells release mediators of inflammation (cytokines) that further damage ischemically injured tissue and contribute to activation of the complement system. The actual means of complement activation in I/R is not yet elucidated, but binding of surface proteins found on damaged endothelial cells to pre-formed circulating antibodies may play an important role (Markiewski, 2007). Complement also appears to play a role in the development of atherosclerotic lesions (Torzewski, 1997) through mechanisms that are not yet clear. However, deposition of the terminal complement components (C5b–9) has been demonstrated in intimal plaque lesions of atherosclerosis, and activation of the complement system is associated with prelesional stages and progression of atherosclerotic lesions (Niculescu, 1987; Seifert, 1989). In keeping with this observation, C6-deficient rabbits were shown to be less susceptible than control rabbits to cholesterol-induced atherosclerotic lesions (Schmiedt, 1998).

A mouse model of autoimmune myocarditis suggests a role for complement in the human form of that condition, because protection from cardiac tissue injury is noted in animals lacking the C3 ligand CR2 (Kallwellis-Opara, 2007).

BIOCOMPATIBILITY

Many of the biomaterials implanted in the body activate complement, particularly the alternative complement pathway (Mollnes, 1997). On contact with blood or tissue fluids, these materials may activate complement and produce local inflammation or tissue damage. Materials must be tested for their complement-activating activity before they are widely used.

ORGAN TRANSPLANTATION

The success of organ transplantation has created a major problem—a shortage of human organs to meet the demands of an ever-growing number of patients awaiting such a surgical procedure. Therefore, use of animal donors such as the pig is proposed by many in the field as a logical alternative to human organs. However, vascularized porcine organs are susceptible to an intense rejection reaction, termed hyperacute rejection, when implanted in nonhuman primates or humans (Dalmasso, 1992; Platt, 1998). This reaction is mediated by antibody binding to vascular endothelial cells and complement activation. Complement activation was shown to be crucial in tissue damage in hyperacute rejection of xenografts. Complement activation on xenogeneic endothelial cells leads to their activation (i.e., endothelial cells adopt a procoagulant phenotype), which results in intravascular and interstitial thrombosis and hemorrhage. Such an intense reaction is due to the inability of porcine cell–associated complement-regulatory molecules such as DAF, MCP, and CD59 to control human complement activation. Therefore, the success of this promising therapeutic intervention relies on proper control of complement activation. The role of complement in the rejection of human organs (allografts) is becoming better appreciated, and it is likely that complement activation contributes to some extent to acute and chronic rejection episodes (Baldwin, 1995). Identification of C4d in the peritubular capillaries of renal transplant biopsies by immunofluorescence microscopy is a useful adjunctive study in the recognition of humoral rejection (Fig. 47-3) (Onitsuka, 1999).

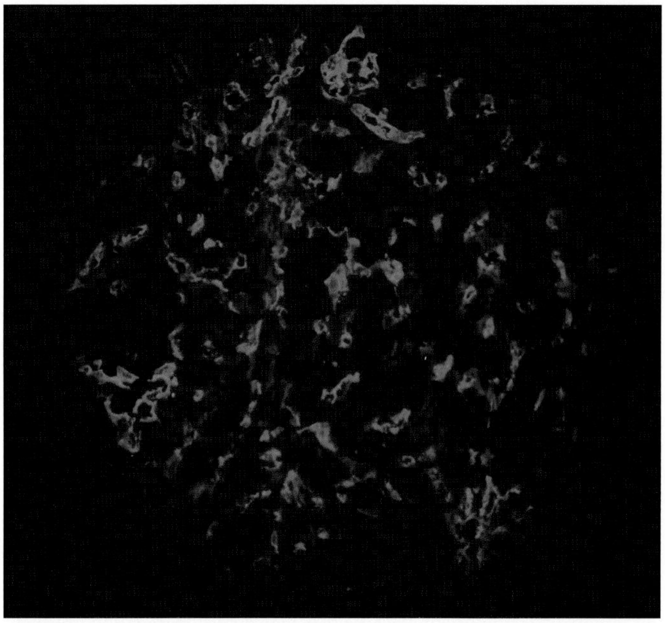

Figure 47-3 Fluorescence-labeled antibody to complement fragment C4d stains peritubular capillaries in a transplant kidney biopsy. In the early posttransplant setting, this staining pattern is a marker of humoral rejection. (40×, fluorescein isothiocyanate.)

CLINICALLY USEFUL COMPLEMENT INHIBITORS

Many complement inhibitors have been produced, and still more are in development. To be clinically useful, a complement inhibitor should avoid production of the proinflammatory byproducts of complement activation, such as the anaphylatoxins C3a and C5a. Inappropriate activation or inadequate regulation of complement activation is involved in a variety of human diseases. Therefore, the development of agents that selectively block complement activation would be useful in limiting tissue damage. Development of clinically useful complement inhibitors has been slow, but progress is being made, as evidenced by the recently approved mAb preparation eculizumab, a humanized long-acting mAb directed against C5 and marketed for the treatment of patients with PNH; other mAbs are in clinical testing phases and in preclinical development. As recently reviewed by Ricklin (2007), current strategies used to therapeutically regulate complement may be classed into five major categories: (1) purified plasma protease inhibitors, primarily C1-Inh (currently approved for treatment of hereditary angioedema); (2) soluble complement regulators, such as sCR1, which act to prevent complement attack on host cells; (3) therapeutic antibodies such as eculizumab, intended to selectively block various stages of complement activation; (4) small peptides, nucleotides, and synthetic molecules such as compstatin, which are used to sterically hinder or induce conformational changes in the elements of the complement cascade; and (5) anaphylatoxin receptor inhibitors, intended to reduce the proinflammatory signaling initiated by complement components such as C5a. Because of the critical role of complement in host defense, especially in infection, potential complement inhibitors will have to avoid interfering with intact and properly regulated elements of the system. As mentioned earlier, C1-Inh is absent or reduced in the serum of those with hereditary angioedema and has been administered as a therapeutic concentrate during acute attacks. Because C1 inhibitor is often reduced in severe inflammatory states as well, concentrates of C1-Inh have been shown to have promising clinical utility in conditions such as septic shock, reperfusion injury, hyperacute transplant rejection, and PNH (Kirschfink, 2001; Davis, 2004).

ASSAYS OF COMPLEMENT

GENERAL PRINCIPLES

Methods that allow accurate determination of levels of each of the components of the classical, alternative, and MBL pathways, as well as several enzymes and regulators of the complement system, are available. However, many of these assays are not available in routine clinical laboratories and are restricted to research laboratories. We focus our attention here on techniques that do not require a laboratory skilled in complement research for their performance. The reader is referred to other publications for details relative to methods that require more specialized techniques (Whaley, 1985; Harrison, 1986; Dodds, 1997; Giclas, 1997; Würzner, 1997; Mollnes, 2007). Complement assays can be divided into two types: those that measure complement proteins as antigens in biological fluids, and those that measure the functional activity of a given component. Both types of techniques have advantages and disadvantages. Methods used for antigenic (immunochemical) analysis are generally simpler to perform. These antigenic assays are highly specific, require fewer specialized reagents, are cheaper, and are considerably less time-consuming. In these assays, serum or plasma can be used, and commonly available methods of freezer storage (–20° C) are sufficient. For these reasons, antigenic assays are easily adaptable to a clinical laboratory.

On the other hand, antigenic assays do not provide information about the activity of a component, because they may detect degradation products, as well as functionally active components. The presence in serum of small fragments of a protein with antigenic activity may confuse the results. Some antigenic assays use radial immunodiffusion. In these assays, a protein fragment may diffuse more rapidly than the parent molecule, which may result in falsely high levels. As an example, the most commonly employed antigenic assays for C3 measure its major degradation product, C3c, by radial immunodiffusion. For accurate measurements of C3c, the specimen should be thawed at 37° C for a number of days to allow complete conversion of C3 to C3c. In fact, this is not usually done, which can represent a source of error, although the error is small and is not usually of clinical consequence. In general, antigenic assays are not as sensitive as functional assays and may not detect low levels of a component present in certain body fluids. The sensitivity of antigenic assays depends to some degree on the strength of the antibody employed; with the usual assays, as little as 10 μg/mL of protein antigen can be measured.

Kits are available that use inhibition of binding of radiolabeled substrate to detect various complement peptides. Such kits are available for measurement of C3a, C4a, and C5a. The usefulness of these measurements is still debated. Assays designed to measure the functional activity of the control proteins, factors H and I, in human serum have also been reported but require specialized reagents that may not be commercially available (Gaither, 1979). ELISA assays have been developed for the measurement of split products of complement proteins or complexes formed following complement activation. These kits measure breakdown products of complement proteins as they are generated after complement activation using specific monoclonal antibodies. Complement activation via the classical pathway can be measured by following the levels of C4d in serum versus those of C4. Also, ELISA of C1r–C1s–C1Inh complexes provides a measure of complement activation via the classical pathway. Activation of the alternative pathway can be measured by ELISA by assessing levels of Bb, or C3bBbP, or C3bP complexes in the circulation (Mayes, 1984). Measurement of as little as 10–20 ng/mL of C3bP in serum has been reported. This assay may also be used to measure surface-bound activation complexes. Activation via either pathway can be monitored by measuring levels of iC3b, or sC5b-9, the soluble form of the membrane attack complex.

Recently, an ELISA test for the measurement of serum or plasma MBL complex activity was developed that eliminates interference by components of the classical pathway (Petersen, 2001; Kuipers, 2002). In addition, ELISA kits are available that measure the generation of anaphylatoxins in serum/plasma. Because C3a and C5a are rapidly converted to their inactive desArg fragments by carboxypeptidase-N in serum, these assays utilize monoclonal antibodies specific for C3a-desArg and C5a-desArg. Because of their high sensitivity, ELISA assays serve as an excellent tool by which to assess complement activation in biological fluids via the classical pathway or the alternative pathway. Seelen (2005) describes a simple approach using three ELISAs that is suitable for screening deficiencies of all three pathways and is commercially available (WIELISA, Wieslab, Lund, Sweden). Advantages of this approach include the coverage of all three pathways simultaneously, the ability to detect properdin deficiency in the alternative pathway, and freedom from consideration of the availability of erythrocytes (Mollnes, 2007).

TABLE 47-8
CH50 and AH50 Interpretation

Test result	Interpretation
CH50 very low or 0 (AH50 normal)	Missing C1q, C1r, C1s, C2, or C4
AH50 very low or 0 (CH50 normal)	Missing properdin, or (very rarely) factor B or factor D
CH50 and AH50 very low or 0	Missing C3, C5, C6, C7, C8, or C9
Late components low (especially C3) CH50 and AH50 low	Missing factor H or factor I

Adapted from Wen BS, Atkinson J, Giclas PC. Clinical and laboratory evaluation of complement deficiency. J Allergy Clin Immunol 2004;113:585–93.

FUNCTIONAL EVALUATION OF THE CLASSICAL PATHWAY

Functional complement assays are sensitive and precise tools for providing information about the activity of a complement component. Some of these methods may be used to quantify activity at the molecular level, and others to express complement function in arbitrary units. Commercial reagents are available for titrating each component of classical or alternative pathways. Assays that measure the total hemolytic activity in a specimen (CH50) or the functional activity of isolated complement components in general use sheep erythrocytes as targets of complement-mediated lysis. Sheep erythrocytes are more sensitive to antibody- and complement-mediated lysis than erythrocytes from other species. The alternative pathway of complement activation (AH50) is easily measured using rabbit erythrocytes. These cells are particularly sensitive to antibody-independent lysis mediated by human serum. In addition, a functional hemolytic assay using chicken erythrocytes to assess functional MBL levels in serum has been developed, which the authors claim is useful for large-scale testing of patient samples (Petersen, 2001; Kuipers, 2002). A useful summary of the clinical significance of CH50 and AH50 testing is provided in Table 47-8.

The simplest functional assay of the classical pathway measures total hemolytic complement. Absence of any of the nine components, as occurs in homozygous genetically deficient patients, generally results in a total hemolytic complement titer (CH50) of zero. However, a normal value does not exclude the possibility of reduced levels of individual components in test subjects. When a patient's history and symptoms suggest a possible deficiency, hemolytic or antigenic titrations of individual components may be required. Often, a CH50 titer will be an adequate functional measure of complement activity. In the CH50 assay, commercially available antibodies added to sheep red blood cells react with antigen on red cell surfaces, forming immune complexes. Patient test serum is then added to the mixture as the source of classic pathway complement. Complement in the test serum will bind the immune complex previously formed on the sheep red cells, leading to activation of the classical complement pathway and to red cell lysis. By titrating the addition of patient test serum, it is possible to calculate the complement activity present in the patient sample, and to express that activity as the reciprocal of the dilution that causes lysis of 50% of red cells in the assay (the CH50). The complement titer is expressed in CH50 units (the reciprocal of the dilution of the complement source that lyses 50% of sensitized sheep erythrocytes).

Serial dilutions of the specimen are prepared and added to antibody-sensitized sheep erythrocytes. In this case, the 50% endpoint is determined by Von Krogh transformation of the data. This empirically derived formula converts the S-shaped dose-response curve into a linear function. Values of $Y/1\text{-}Y$ are calculated, in which Y is the fraction of red cells lysed in a test dilution. A graph is constructed in which the log of the relative volume of complement is plotted against the log of $Y/1\text{-}Y$ values. Usually, a straight line is obtained, and the titer is calculated by determining the relative volume of complement at which $Y/1\text{-}Y = 1.0$ (or 50% lysis). This value is divided into the reciprocal of original serum dilution (1:60 for human serum) to calculate the concentration of serum complement that lyses 50% of the cells. The complement titer represents the number of 50% hemolytic units present in 1.0 mL of undiluted serum (Mayer, 1961; Rapp, 1970). Clinical laboratories may use one of two commercially available variations of this classic test to perform the CH50 assay. One is based on the lysis of liposomes, releasing a marker enzyme, and the other is an ELISA that detects the final C9 neo-antigen formed with complete activation of the classical pathway.

FUNCTIONAL EVALUATION OF THE ALTERNATIVE PATHWAY

In this assay, human serum (usually first diluted 1 : 5) is serially diluted and is added to rabbit erythrocytes that are not sensitized with specific antibody, in a buffer that contains magnesium ions and ethylene glycol tetraacetic acid, to chelate calcium ions (calcium ions are required for classical pathway activation, not for alternative pathway activation) (Pangburn, 1988). The alternative pathway titer is designated AH50 and represents the final dilution of human serum in the assay that lyses 50% of the rabbit erythrocytes. A graph similar to that described for total hemolytic complement titration is produced to determine the AH50. Human serum may at times possess "natural" antibody to a carbohydrate widely expressed on cells of species other than humans and nonhuman primates. A high concentration of serum mixed with rabbit erythrocytes may induce agglutination, which can be misleading in interpreting an AH50 titer (Tomlinson, 1997). Therefore, it may be useful to absorb the serum with washed, packed rabbit erythrocytes on ice for 15–30 minutes to remove a certain proportion of natural antibodies, hence reducing cell agglutination in the assay.

FUNCTIONAL ASSAY OF C1-INHIBITOR AND FACTOR H

Assays for the assessment of C1-Inh function have been developed that are useful in the diagnosis of HAE. One that is in common use is an ELISA-based assay that measures formation of a complex between biotinylated C1s and C1-Inh on an avidin-coated solid phase. A second test makes use of steric hindrance created by the binding of inhibitor to C1r, preventing the subsequent binding of antibody to C1r. During radial immunodiffusion of C1r, unbound and therefore active C1r quantities will increase as the amount of C1-Inh present decreases. Factor H functional assays are important for the diagnosis of aHUS, membranoproliferative glomerulonephritis, type II (dense deposit disease), and AMD. A method described by Sánchez-Corral (2004) uses unsensitized sheep red blood cells incubated in serum. With this method, normal serum will provide factor H–conferred protection from hemolysis, whereas factor H–deficient serum will not prevent complement-mediated red cell lysis.

COMPLEMENT LEVELS BY ANTIGENIC ASSAYS

For use in antigenic assays, the specimen (serum or plasma) is stored frozen (−20° C or lower). Bacterial contamination may cause protein denaturation or fragmentation, whereas freezing and thawing do not usually have a major adverse effect on antigenic levels. For certain complement assays, the specimen is diluted in saline to achieve the correct concentration range for accurate measurement.

Antigenic analyses of complement proteins make use of one of several immune precipitin techniques. Single radial immunodiffusion using the method of Fahey or Mancini is commonly used to calculate specific protein quantities. With both methods, antigen is added to wells in a gel that contains antibody, and rings of precipitation are formed. The Fahey method employs antibody that is not in excess. The diffusion time at which results are read is thus critical. Diffusion endpoints are not reached, and this can lead to inaccurate measurement of antigenic complement levels. The Mancini method uses excess antibody in the gel and is more sensitive and accurate. Most commercial firms preparing immunodiffusion plates use the Mancini method. Radial immunodiffusion kits are available for all components of the classical and alternative pathways. These kits consist of plates coated with a thin layer of 2% agarose-containing monospecific antibody. Protein standard serum (a stabilized pool of normal human serum) is supplied, usually in prediluted solutions. Each standard solution contains a specific amount of the particular protein being measured for use in construction of the reference curve.

Nephelometric methods are also used to measure complement component levels, which in some instances may be comparable with those obtained with radial immunodiffusion (Bossuyt, 2002); they are commonly used in hospital laboratories to measure serum C3 and C4.

Ingvarrson (2007) recently described a proteomic approach that uses an antibody-based microarray platform employing recombinant human scFv antibodies, thus permitting protein expression profiling of serum complement-related proteomes. The microarray data correlated well with conventional clinical laboratory methods when plasma samples from both healthy and complement-deficient individuals were tested. Similarly, Janzi (2005) described a reverse array format in which serum samples are themselves spotted to a microarray slide in large sample numbers and are screened for the presence of a single serum protein, as proof of the principle that large numbers of serum samples may be simultaneously screened for clinically relevant proteins.

KININS AND THE KININ-GENERATING SYSTEM

The kinin-generating system is another inflammatory response pathway present in plasma that controls the generation of peptides important in the inflammatory response. Briefly, the most important biologically active peptide generated by the system appears to be bradykinin, a nonapeptide with potent activity in many biological systems. It is active in increasing vascular permeability, vasodilation, hypotension, induction of pain, contraction of many types of smooth muscle cells, and activation of the phospholipase A2 system, with activation of cellular arachidonic acid metabolism. Although in many respects it is similar to the complement system, the plasma kinin-generating system is simpler, because it is composed of only four plasma proteins. The major proteins of the kinin-generating system as currently understood are Hageman factor, clotting factor XI, prekallikrein, and high molecular weight kininogen.

On interacting with negatively charged surfaces, such as those supplied experimentally by glass or naturally by many biologically active materials such as lipid A of gram-negative bacterial endotoxin, Hageman factor is cleaved and activated. Proteolytic enzymes including kallikrein can cleave and activate Hageman factor as well. The cleaved Hageman factor (αHFa) has proteolytic activity and further activates and cleaves additional Hageman factor molecules to generate additional αHFa.

αHFa activates factor XI to factor XIa, resulting in activation of the intrinsic coagulation cascade. αHFa also cleaves the single-chain prekallikrein into a two-chain molecule, kallikrein, with the chains linked by disulfide bonds. Cleaved prekallikrein has proteolytic enzymatic activity located on the lower molecular weight chain. Activated kallikrein cleaves high molecular weight kininogen at several sites, thereby releasing bradykinin.

Bradykinin has a short half-life mainly caused by the activities of four membrane-bound and/or soluble zinc metallopeptidases: angiotensin 1–converting enzyme, aminopeptidase P, neutral endopeptidase 24.11 (neprilysin), and carboxypeptidases M and N (Moreau, 2005). These four act to convert bradykinin to inactive low molecular weight peptides lacking known biological activity.

Bradykinin has been postulated to play a role in a variety of diseases. Free bradykinin and lysyl-bradykinin have been found in the nasal fluid of patients with rhinitis. A pathogenic role for bradykinin has also been suggested in diseases ranging from asthma to hereditary or acquired angioedema. Bradykinin is an important mediator of the inflammatory response, and when administered locally, it produces the four cardinal signs of inflammation. Development of pharmacologic agents to block or ameliorate the effects of the kinin system has met with limited success but is ongoing (Dietrich, 2009).

CYTOKINES

Cytokines are soluble proteins acting at the picomolar to femtomolar range and released by many cell types to permit usually short-distance (autocrine and paracrine) communication between cells. The term cytokine encompasses lymphokines, interleukins, colony-stimulating factors (CSFs), interferons (IFNs), tumor necrosis factor (TNF), and chemokines. Although cytokines are produced by many cell populations (endothelial cells, fibroblasts, epithelial cells, and others), they are mainly the products of helper T cells (Th) and macrophages. These mediators are released to assist in upregulation or downregulation of the immune response and to orchestrate associated inflammatory and reparative activities, hematopoiesis, and immune cell proliferation and differentiation.

TABLE 47-9
Cytokines by Type and Function

Cytokine type	Cytokines	Actions
Adipokine (cytokine released from adipocytes)	IL-1α, TNF-α, IL-6, leptin, adiponectin, others	Proinflammatory, proatherogenic, antiinflammatory
Angiogenic	VEGF, IL-1, IL-6, IL-8	Neovascularization, prometastatic
Anti-inflammatory	IL-10, IL-13, TGF-β, IL-22, IL-1Ra, IFN-α/β	Upregulate inflammatory genes, depress cytokine-mediated lethality, downregulate autoimmune disease
Chemokine	IL-8, MCP-1, MIP-1α	Increase cell migration and activation
Colony stimulating	IL-3, IL-7, G-CSF, GM-CSF, M-CSF, erythropoietin	Hematopoiesis, proinflammatory, anti-inflammatory
gp130 signaling pathway	IL-6, IL-11, others	Growth factors, B cell activation, acute phase response
Lymphocyte growth	IL-2, IL-4, IL-7, IL-15	Clonal expansion, Th1/Th2/Th17 regulation
Mesenchymal tissue growth	FGF, TGF-β, others	Fibrosis, prometastatic
Nerve growth	NGFa, BNDF	Nerve and Schwann cell growth, B cell activation
Osteoclast-activating	RANKL	Bone resorption, immune stimulation
Proinflammatory	IL-1α, IL-1β, TNF-α, IL-12, IL-18, IL-23, MIF, IL-32, IL-33, CD40L	Upregulate inflammatory mediators and innate immune responses
Th1	IFN-γ, IL-12, IL-18	Upregulate Th1 response, clonal expansion of CTL
Th2	IL-4, IL-5, IL-18, IL-25, IL-33	Upregulate Th2 response, increase antibody production
Th17	IL-17, IL-23, IFN-γ	Upregulate Th17 response, autoimmune response
Type I IFN	IFN-α, IFN-β	Antiviral, upregulate MHC class I, antiangiogenic, antiinflammatory
Type II IFN	IFN-γ	Macrophage activation, upregulate MHC class II

BNDF, Brain-derived neurotrophic factor; *CSF,* colony-stimulating factor; *IFN,* interferon; *IL,* interleukin; *MCP-1,* monocyte chemotactic protein-1; *MHC,* major histocompatibility complex; *MIF,* macrophage migration inhibitory factor; *MIP-1α,* macrophage inhibiting protein-1α; *NGF,* nerve growth factor; *RANKL,* receptor activator of NFκB.

Secretion and binding of cytokines is the cellular equivalent of connecting to the Internet. The prevailing milieu of cytokines within the region of an organism creates a web of communication between cells. Cytokine signals are received at the cell surface not only as single messages but also in complex, subtle synergistic and antagonistic combinations that coordinate processes, including stimulation of hematopoiesis, orchestration of directed leukocyte migration (chemokinesis), activation of various inflammatory cells, stimulation of lymphocyte development and maturation, and processes related to the immune response. To respond to specific cytokine messages, cells display surface cytokine receptors, arrayed as so many antennae. Using these receptors, cells sample, process, and respond to combinations of soluble and substrate-bound cytokines in a manner dependent on surface receptor density and state of activation.

As mentioned, many cell types are capable of producing cytokines, but for the most part it is the T cell and the macrophage that are virtual cytokine factories; for this reason, many familiar cytokines are known as interleukins (ILs). The biological actions of a given cytokine, for instance, IL-1, may overlap with those of another cytokine such as TNF-α, as a form of built-in redundancy, and are often dependent on the circumstance in which the cytokine is secreted and the responding cell type. The same cytokine may have more than one effect or may function in regulating the immune response.

It is becoming more and more apparent that the family of cytokine proteins is extensive (now more than 100 known proteins), and classifying them conveniently requires examining them in more than one way. For instance, it might be convenient to think of the various cytokines as members of discrete functional classes, rather than solely as members of classes based on structural homology (Table 47-9). In this approach, there are two major classes of cytokine: the class that promotes cell-mediated immunity, and the class that promotes antibody-mediated immunity. The cytokines may be subdivided further according to their major activities, for example, proinflammatory, lymphocyte growth factor, anti-inflammatory, and CSF activities, among others.

Another means of classifying cytokines that may have clinical utility is to group them according to the structural homology of their receptors. To some degree, it is this receptor homology that accounts for cytokine functional pleiotropy and the redundancy mentioned earlier. Cytokine receptors may be divided into five major receptor types with subfamilies (Table 47-10): (1) the immunoglobulin superfamily receptor class shares structural homology with immunoglobulins and certain cell adhesion molecules; (2) the TNF receptor class members conserve a cysteine-rich common extracellular binding domain; (3) the G-protein–coupled seven transmembrane receptor class members contain seven transmembrane α-helices; and (4 and 5) the type I and type II receptor class members lack intrinsic tyrosine kinase activity. Receptors of this last type communicate with the nucleus through the STAT (signal transducers and activation of transcription) family of cytoplasmic transcription proteins via binding and activating of members of the JAK (Janus kinase) family of proteins. These receptors also make use of the RAS-RAF-MAP kinase and PI3 pathways to initiate gene transcription.

As mentioned, cytokines may be produced and released by several different cell types, including lymphoid cells, stromal cells (such as fibroblasts, osteocytes, and endothelial cells), and epithelial cells. The extent of influence of these soluble proteins may possibly extend over the long range (systemically) when released into the circulation (endocrine effect), as with the pyrogen IL-1, or their action may be local only, producing an effect on the cell releasing them (autocrine effect) or its neighboring cells (paracrine). For instance, IL-2 released by T cells has an autocrine proliferative effect through the IL-2 receptor (CD25). In the thymus, cytokines such as IL-7 released from thymic epithelial cells affect thymocyte maturation in a paracrine fashion. A majority of cytokines bind to high-affinity receptors that transduce signals to the cell nucleus through systems such as JAK/STAT signaling pathways, mitogen-activated protein kinase, cyclic adenosine monophosphate, and PI3-kinase, among others. Because of the profound biological effects of these powerful proteins, attempts at mass-producing and therapeutically administering them are ongoing. Clinical laboratory detection and measurement of them therefore is becoming more common. Bioassays are sometimes the "gold standard" for detecting cytokine activity, but they are usually time-consuming and unmanageable in the hospital laboratory. ELISA kits are widely available for many of the cytokines described in the text. Molecular techniques (polymerase chain reaction, in situ hybridization) are employed almost routinely now in hospital laboratories to identify the presence of cytokines with great sensitivity, and to localize a cytokine more precisely to a particular cell type.

Ever increasing interest in manipulating cytokine activity to treat disease has led to exploitation of several approaches (Table 47-11), including cloning and producing recombinant forms of cytokines or their receptor antagonists; delivering cytokines by gene and antisense nucleotide insertion through viral and nonviral vectors (commonly adenovirus or retrovirus vectors, or nonviral DNA plasmid vectors); vaccinating patients against their own (autologous) cytokines (Cutler, 2005); raising cytokine-blocking monoclonal antibodies; and genetically fusing molecules of interest, such as an enzyme, ligand, peptide, or extracellular domain of a surface receptor, to the Fc portion of human IgG1or albumin. This "fusion" approach has the advantage of conferring increased half-life and stability

TABLE 47-10
Selected Cytokines Grouped by Receptor Class

Receptor class	Structure and signaling pathway	Example receptors
Immunoglobulin superfamily	These receptors contain paired antiparallel β sheets forming the sandwich-like structure known as the Ig-fold seen in antibodies.	IL-1, IL-18, SCF (*c-kit*), M-CSF
Tumor necrosis factor	These receptors share a cysteine-rich common extracellular domain and activate the NFκB pathway.	TNF-α, TNF-β, NGF, CD40, CD27, CD30, CD120
G-protein–coupled receptor (serpentine receptors)	These receptors have a 7-transmembrane helix that couples to G-protein, ultimately activating MAP kinase via the cAMP and phosphatidylinositol signaling pathways.	IL-8, CCR1, CXCR4, MCAF, NAP-2
Type I (hemopoietin receptors)	These are transmembrane protein receptors with paired high-affinity α and β chains; these receptors share a common extracellular motif (WSXWS); they signal the nucleus through the JAK/STAT, RAS-RAF-MAP kinase, and PI3 pathways.	IL-2, IL-3, IL-4, IL-5, IL-6, IL-7, IL-9, IL-11, IL-12, IL-15, IL-21, GM-CSF, EPO, PRL, GH, G-CSF, LIF
Type II	These transmembrane protein receptors are similar to type I, but lack the WSXWS motif, while having conserved cysteine pairs in their extracellular domain; they signal the nucleus through the JAK/STAT, RAS-RAF-MAP kinase, and PI3 pathways.	IFN-α, IFN-γ, IFN-β, IL-10

cAMP, Cyclic adenosine monophosphate; *CSF,* colony-stimulating factor; *IFN,* interferon; *IL,* interleukin; *JAK,* Janus kinase; *NF,* nephritic factor; *STAT,* signal transducers and activation of transcription; *TNF,* tumor necrosis factor.

on the fusion product. In some instances, multiple ligands may be sequentially fused to a single gene to create a "trap" for the target by "trapping" or binding two target molecules on a single fusion protein, possibly as a result of the trap's high binding affinities (Huang, 2009).

Unfortunately, many disease states are complex conditions driven by an intricate interplay of numerous cytokines, so that a single "magic cytokine bullet" for those conditions is unlikely to arise in the very near future. For conditions in which dysregulation of a single cytokine is largely at fault, the challenge is less daunting. Several cytokine-related therapeutic agents have entered routine medical practice in recent years (see Table 47-11).

Cell Adhesion Molecules

The glue that binds living tissues into complex multicellular organisms comprises in part the cell adhesion molecules (CAMS) described subsequently. These complex glycoproteins permit cell migration during embryogenesis and wound healing, and govern the leukocyte trafficking and homing critical to lymphopoiesis and the immune response. Adhesion molecules are conventionally divided into five groups based on structural homology: cadherins, mucins, integrins, selectins, and immunoglobulin superfamily molecules. Cadherins are expressed most often on epithelial cells and interact with each other in a calcium-dependent manner. Mucins are heavily glycosylated proteins that interact mainly with selectins. Immunoglobulin superfamily members have immunoglobulin-like domains and interact with integrins, selectins, and each other. Integrins and selectins are discussed. Because of their ubiquitous presence and their critical importance in intercellular activity, significant investigation of CAMs and their role in disease activity is under way. The goal is to identify and target CAM interaction sites for therapeutic modulation with specific monoclonal antibodies, as well as sense/antisense oligonucleotides or other small molecules designed to block gene transcription (Mousa, 2008).

INTEGRINS

The integrin family (Gonzalez-Amaro, 1999) of adhesion molecules provides a critical physical link between those things external to the cell (other cells and the extracellular matrix [ECM]) and those things within the cell (cytoskeleton, intracytosolic molecules, and nucleus). Each integrin family member is composed of a heterodimer of noncovalently linked α and β subunits (Table 47-12). The major integrins are divided into four subfamilies, differing in patterns of expression and ligand specificity. The α1 integrins, also known as the very late activation antigens (VLAs), are created from the association of a β2 chain subunit (CD29) with any of the α chain subunits (CD49a–CD49h). They are expressed on all cells requiring firm anchoring to the ECM, and on circulating leukocytes, platelets, and some tumor cells. The β2 integrins, which tend to be expressed mainly by leukocytes and myeloid cells, result from association of the β2 chain subunit (CD18) with any of several α subunits. When combined with the αL (CD11a) subunit, the β2 integrin LFA-1 (lymphocyte function-associated antigen, CD11a/CD18) is formed. LFA-1 plays a crucial role in leukocyte adhesion to vascular endothelium during transendothelial migration. The β2 chain subunit, in association with the αM subunit (CD11b), forms Mac-1 (CD11b/CD18), an integrin expressed on myeloid cells and mononuclear phagocytes. The α integrin subunits are 120- to 180-kDa membrane proteins with short intracytoplasmic domains, a long extracellular fragment with seven homologous domains, and several metal ion–binding motifs (metal ion–dependent adhesion sites [MIDAS]) thought to function in converting an integrin from an inactive to an active conformation. Both α and β subunits bind to ligand, but the α subunit generally is thought to provide ligand specificity.

The intracytoplasmic tails of α and β integrin subunits associate with cytoskeletal components to transduce intracytoplasmic signals. In the process of signal transduction, integrins associate and interact with other cell membrane–associated proteins, cytoskeletal components, and noncytoskeletal cytoplasmic components. The integrin-associated protein (IAP or IAP 50) designated CD47, a member of the immunoglobulin superfamily, is one such membrane-associated protein that, mainly through association with β3 integrins, may function as a signal transducer. Other membrane-associated proteins involved in integrin signaling include caveolin-1 and CD9, which are involved in cell membrane caveola formation and platelet aggregation, respectively. Cytosolic molecules, including integrin cytoplasmic domain–associated protein (ICAP-1), help orchestrate the complex activity of β1-integrin–mediated cell migration.

Perhaps the best studied intracytoplasmic associations of integrin molecules are those with the cytoskeleton-associated proteins α-actinin, talin, filamin, vinculin, tensin, and paxillin. These cytoskeleton proteins, through their association with β1, β2, and β3 integrin subunits, bridge integrin and cytoskeleton and direct cell migration, phagocytosis, stress fiber formation at focal contact sites, and intracellular signal transduction, and link separate cytoskeletal proteins.

The pattern of integrin distribution is wide, especially among those integrins (mostly β1) involved in anchoring cells to components of the general ECM such as collagen and laminin. For those integrins mediating attachment to less widely distributed components, tissue distribution likewise is more restricted.

Monoclonal antibodies raised against specific integrin components (anti-integrins) are in clinical trials. β1 integrin is the target of the recently approved humanized monoclonal antibody natalizumab, which is used in the treatment of Crohn's disease and multiple sclerosis. Abciximab is an antithrombotic chimeric monoclonal antibody that is useful in preventing thrombosis and restenosis during some coronary artery procedures by blocking glycoprotein (GP)IIb/IIIa-dependent platelet aggregation. These novel therapies are not without serious risk, however, as several cases of therapy-related opportunistic infection and progressive multifocal leukoencephalopathy have been reported specifically with natalizumab (Stuve, 2007).

TABLE 47-11
Selected Engineered Therapeutic Agents

Class	Generic name	Agent/Action	Therapeutic indication
Cytokine			
	Aldesleukin (Proleukin)	Recombinant IL-2, binds and activates IL-2R	HIV
	IFN-β-1a (Avonex)	Recombinant IFN-β-1a, anti-inflammatory cytokine	Relapsing MS
	Sargramostim (Leukine)	Recombinant GM-CSF, modulates hematopoiesis	Leukemia, bone marrow stem cell transplant
Anticytokine Antibody			
	Adalimumab (Humira)	Recombinant humanized anti–TNF-α IgG1 mAb, binds and inhibits TNF-α	RA, CD, PA, AS
	Infliximab (Remicade)	Chimeric (75% human/25% mouse) IgG1 mAb binds TNF-α	RA, CD, AS
	Mepolizumab (Bosatria)	Recombinant humanized anti–IL-5 mAb	Allergic asthma
	Bevacizumab (Avastin)	Recombinant humanized anti–VEGF-A mAb, inhibits angiogenesis	Colorectal and non–small cell carcinoma
Small Molecule Antagonist			
	Thalidomide	VEGF and TNF mRNA inhibitor	ENL, MM, RCC
	AP12009	TGF-β2–blocking antisense oligonucleotide	High-grade glioma
Cytokine Receptor Antagonist			
	Anakinra	Recombinant IL-1Rα antagonist, competitively inhibits binding of IL-1α to its receptor	RA
	Tocilizumab (Actemra)	Recombinant humanized IL-6R mAb, acts as an immunosuppressant	RA
	Daclizumab (Zenapax)	Recombinant humanized IL-2Rα chain mAb, binds IL-2Rα (CD25) on T cells to prevent allograft rejection	Renal transplant
	Oprelvekin (Neumega)	Recombinant IL-11, stimulates stem cell and megakaryocyte progenitor growth	Chemotherapy-related thrombocytopenia
	Trastuzumab (Herceptin)	Recombinant humanized mAb, binds Her2/neu receptor overexpressed on some carcinomas; inhibits angiogenesis	Breast carcinoma
Fusion Protein			
	Etanercept (Enbrel)	Soluble TNF-αRII fused to human IgG1 Fc fragment; neutralizes membrane-bound and soluble forms of TNF-α	RA, AS, JRA, PA
	NBI-3001	Recombinant IL-4–*Pseudomonas aeruginosa* exotoxin fusion protein	Malignant high-grade gliomas
	Alefacept (Amevive)	LFA-3 fused to Fc domain IgG1, binds CD2 to inhibit T cell activation	Plaque psoriasis
Anti–Cell Adhesion Molecule			
	Natalizumab	Recombinant humanized leukocyte α_4/β_1 integrin mAb, blocks attachment of leukocytes to CNS endothelial cells	MS
	Abciximab	Anti-α_{II3}/β_3, α_v/β_3 chimeric mAb Fab fragment, antithrombotic	Angioplasty procedures
	Efalizumab (Raptiva)	Recombinant humanized anti-α_L/β_2 mAb, binds CD11a to act as an immunosuppressant	Psoriasis

AS, Ankylosing spondylitis; *CD,* Crohn's disease; *CSF,* colony-stimulating factor; *ENL,* erythema nodosum leprosum; *HIV,* human immunodeficiency virus; *IFN,* interferon; *IL,* interleukin; *JRA,* juvenile rheumatoid arthritis; *LFA,* lymphocyte functional antigen; *MM,* multiple myeloma; *MS,* multiple sclerosis; *PA,* psoriatic arthritis; *RA,* rheumatoid arthritis; *RCC,* renal cell carcinoma, *TNF,* tumor necrosis factor.

SELECTINS

The selectin family (Gonzalez-Amaro, 1999) contains three homologous proteins. L-selectin (CD62L) is expressed by most leukocytes, especially lymphocytes, and is thought to play an important role in naive and memory lymphocyte homing or trafficking to lymph nodes through high endothelial venules (HEVs). L-selectin also tethers neutrophils to activated endothelial cells in regions of inflammation. Its ligands include Glycam (glycan-bearing cell adhesion molecule)-1, MadCAM (mucosal addressin cell adhesion molecule)-1, and CD34. P-selectin (CD62P) is stored in the α granules and Weibel-Palade bodies of platelets and endothelial cells, respectively, and is expressed on the cell surface after cell activation. Once on the cell surface, P-selectin binds neutrophils, lymphocytes, and monocytes via its ligands, Lewis-X-, and Lewis-A-family–type complex carbohydrate groups. E-selectin (CD62E) is found on the surface of activated endothelial cells only and recognizes ligands similar to those recognized by P-selectin. It plays a recognition role for homing effector and memory T cells as they localize to sites of inflammation. Selectins interact with carbohydrate moieties such as sialyl-Lewis X and sialyl-Lewis A, and possibly other ligands, including integrins and glycolipids. The full extent of physiologic selectin ligands has not been determined, but it is expected that the list will include molecules expressed on leukocytes and endothelium because selectins are important for leukocyte–leukocyte and leukocyte–endothelium interactions.

The role of selectins is twofold: to mediate cell–cell interaction, and to contribute to cell activation by intracytoplasmic signaling. As with integrins, selectins are critical to the initial tethering and rolling of leukocytes along activated endothelium prior to extravasation. After binding a soluble form of the mucin-like glycoprotein GlyCAM-1 (a high endothelial venule product), L-selectin is able to mediate the activation of β1 integrins and their adhesion to fibronectin. P- and E-selectin may also serve as signal-transducing receptor molecules because a rise in intracellular free Ca^{2+} within leukocytes adhering to endothelial cells is linked to these selectin molecules (Huang, 1993). The most frequently used quantitative assays for soluble plasma or serum selectins are sandwich immunoassays (Mousa, 2008).

LEUKOCYTE EXTRAVASATION

Expression of integrin molecules is dependent on cell activation and may be upregulated or downregulated in response to specific cues from the external environment, including local cytokine stimulation or immune interaction. Leukocyte integrin interaction with endothelial cells is critical to the evolution of inflammatory and immune responses. In addition,

TABLE 47-12
Major Integrins and Their Ligands

Integrin	Name	Ligands
α1β1	VLA-1, CD49a/CD29	Collagen, LMN
α2β1	VLA-2, CD49b/CD29	Collagen, LMN
α3β1	VLA-3, CD49b/CD29	Collagen, LMN, FBN
α4β1	VLA-4, CD49d/CD29	VCAM-1, FBN
α5β1	VLA-5, CD49e/CD29	FBN
α6β1	VLA-6, CD49f/CD29	LMN
α7β1	CD49g/CD29	LMN
α8β1	CD49h/CD29	FBN
αLβ2	LFA-1, CD11a/CD18	ICAM-1, -2, -3
αMβ2	Mac-1, CD11b/CD18	ICAM-1, iC3b
αXβ2	p150, 95, CD11cCD18	FBGN, iC3b
αDβ2	—	ICAM-3, VCAM-1
αIIbβ3	GP IIb/IIIa, CD41/CD61	FBGN, vWF, FBN, VN
αVβ3	CD51/CD61	VN, FBGN
α4β3	CD49d/–	MadCAM-1, FBN, ICAM-1
αEβ7	—	E-cadherin

FBGN, Fibrinogen; *FBN,* fibronectin; *ICAM,* intercellular adhesion molecule; *LFA,* lymphocyte functional antigen; *LMN,* laminin; *VCAM,* vascular cell adhesion molecule; *VN,* vitronectin; *vWF,* von Willebrand factor.

homing of lymphoid cells to their sites of residence and intravascular spread of metastases involve similar endothelial interactions mediated through surface integrins and another set of cell adhesion molecules, the selectins and their ligands.

Extravasation of leukocytes occurs during cell homing, as with trafficking of γ/δ T cells to Peyer's patches, and as part of the inflammatory response. Both processes involve similar steps and the use of different adhesion molecules. In inflammation, the process begins with local release of proinflammatory cytokines such as TNF, IL-1, and IFN-γ, which activate the local endothelium to increase surface expression of adhesion molecules, including members of the immunoglobulin superfamily, vascular cell adhesion molecule (VCAM)-1 and ICAM-1. In addition, endothelial cells release chemotactic agents, including IL-8, forming a surface-bound and soluble chemotactic gradient recognizable by transmigrating inflammatory cells, which localize them to the inflammatory focus.

This process for white cells (Fig. 47-4) involves (1) tethering of the passing leukocyte to the endothelial surface mainly by endothelial selectins (E- and P-selectin) and their leukocyte ligand sialyl-Lewis X-modified glycoprotein; and (2) leukocyte rolling, in which, through rapid sequential surface expression of mainly leukocyte VLA-4 and α4β7 integrin, the shear force provided by the bloodstream rolls leukocytes along the endothelial surface, thereby bringing these integrins into contact with their endothelial ligands, VCAM-1 and MAdCAM-1, respectively. In the case of neutrophils, rolling is mediated by selectins alone. As they roll, leukocyte cell adhesion molecules trigger biochemical events, leading to (3) leukocyte

PART 6

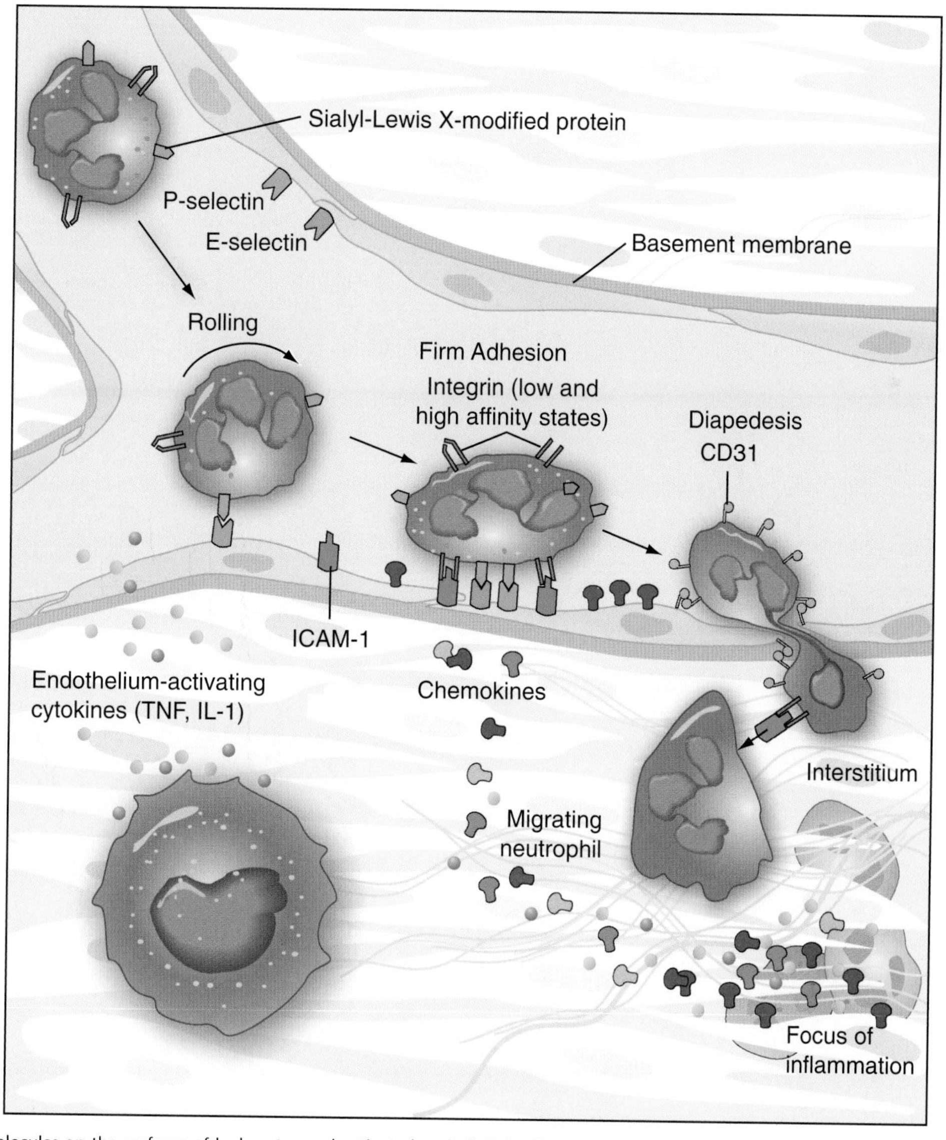

Figure 47-4 Adhesion molecules on the surfaces of leukocytes and activated endothelial cells guide the movement of white blood cells from the bloodstream to foci of tissue inflammation. Direction is provided by a chemotactic gradient. *ICAM,* Intracellular adhesion molecule; *IL,* interleukin; *TNF,* tumor necrosis factor.

activation and conversion of its integrins to an activated state of increased avidity. This leads to increased leukocyte–endothelial cell adhesion, and eventually to (4) arrest of leukocyte rolling, and (5) leukocyte transmigration of the endothelium with the assistance of the homotypic adhesion molecule CD31 expressed on both white cells and the endothelium, while following a chemotactic gradient. It is still a matter of debate whether leukocytes pass directly through individual endothelial cells or merely pass between adjacent endothelial cells. Endothelial cell retraction early in the inflammatory response would seem to make movement between endothelial cells easier. Once through the endothelium, integrin-mediated cell migration through the extracellular matrix along a chemotactic gradient completes the leukocyte journey to a focus of inflammation.

Deficiency states for β2 integrins (leukocyte adhesion deficiency type I) and congenital defects in the expression of selectins and their ligands demonstrate the indispensable role that these receptors play in producing the inflammatory response and in lymphocyte trafficking. In these patients, neutrophils are unable to exit the bloodstream and migrate to sites of inflammation or infection, creating in effect a state of immune suppression with increased susceptibility to bacterial infection and a paradoxical peripheral neutrophilia (Bullard, 1996). The events surrounding septic shock, thrombosis, reperfusion injury, and metastases also require integrin and selectin activity. This knowledge has led to the therapeutic use of monoclonal antibodies, soluble adhesion molecule ligands, and other interventions, including antisense oligonucleotides, to overcome adhesion molecule–mediated disease (Buckley, 1996; Gonzalez-Amaro, 1998).

PERSPECTIVES

Complement, cytokines, and adhesion molecules all play a role in disease states. In recognition of this, therapies have been designed to directly trigger or block various cytokine, cell adhesion molecules, and complement components as part of the treatment of disease. Clinical laboratory detection and measurement of native proteins and the clinically administered therapeutic agent continues to become more commonplace.

SELECTED REFERENCES

Carroll MC. The complement system in regulation of adaptive immunity. Nat Immunol 2004;5:981–6.

This article describes the intricate interaction that exists between complement activation products and T and B cell responses, and the nature of the link that exists between innate and adaptive immune responses.

Gonzalez-Amaro R, Diaz-Gonzalez F, Sanchez-Madrid F. Adhesion molecules in inflammatory diseases. Drugs 1998;56:977–88.

This article provides an excellent and in-depth review of the process of leukocyte diapedesis. Pharmacologic therapeutic blocking of this process is discussed.

Wen L, Atkinson JP, Giclas PC. Clinical and laboratory evaluation of complement deficiency. J Allergy Clin Immunol 2004;113:585–93.

This article provides a practical clinical approach to complement deficiency testing, as well as an overview of the complement system.

REFERENCES

Access the complete reference list online at http://www.expertconsult.com

CHAPTER 48

HUMAN LEUKOCYTE ANTIGEN: THE MAJOR HISTOCOMPATIBILITY COMPLEX OF MAN

Omar R. Fagoaga

KEY POINTS

- Major histocompatibility complex (MHC) class I molecules include HLA-A, HLA-B, and HLA-C; MHC class II molecules include HLA-DR, HLA-DQ, and HLA-DP; these are the classic “transplantation” antigens.
- MHC genes are closely linked and segregate en bloc to offspring.
- Characterization of human leukocyte antigen (HLA) alleles and molecules has been combined with clinical protocols to maximize donor and recipient compatibility, and to minimize the impact of the immune response on the transplanted organ. Advances in this area have contributed to the development of transplantation as a successful treatment modality for the replacement of diseased tissue.
- HLA matching usually includes evaluation of at least three loci: HLA-A, HLA-B, and HLA-DR. Individuals matched, at whatever resolution, for all three loci are termed 6/6 matches or 0 mismatches.
- Patients can be sensitized to specific foreign HLA molecules through transfusion, pregnancy, or prior transplantation. Assessment of compatibility between the recipient and the possible donor includes testing for this sensitization.
- Several methods are available for HLA typing, including serologic and cellular typing approaches and DNA-based typing. DNA-based typing has significant advantages over the other methods.

Survival depends on the ability of the immune system to recognize and respond to a multitude of foreign substances (antigens). Although this defense mechanism is basic to survival in a hostile world of microorganisms, this same defense system has a negative impact when tissue is transplanted from one individual to another, or when malfunctioning triggers autoaggressive reactions. The MHC genes encode proteins that are essential to immune recognition: the class I and class II molecules (Fig. 48-1).

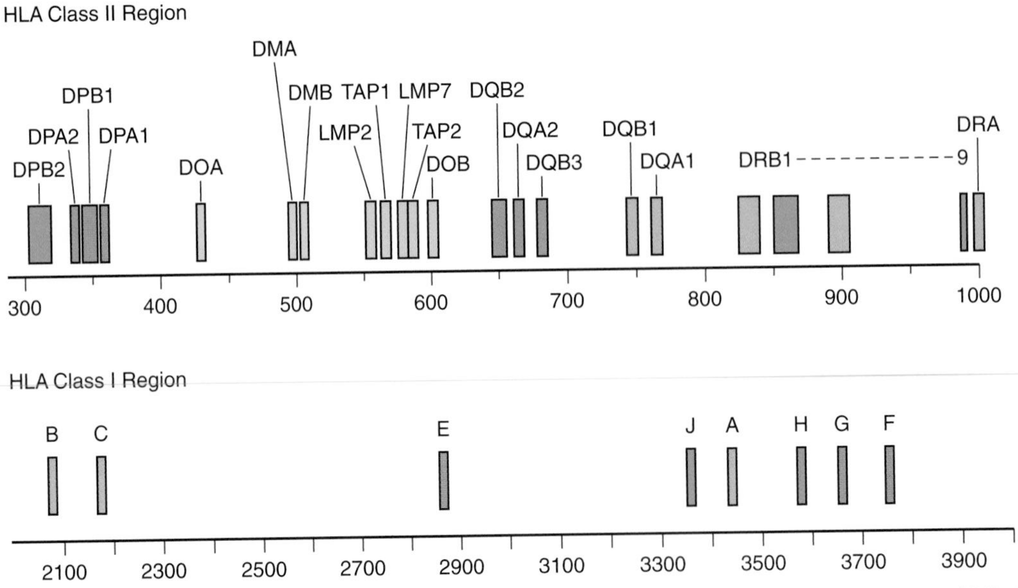

Figure 48-1 Map of the major histocompatibility complex (MHC) gene on chromosome 6. HLA-DPB2 in the human leukocyte antigen (HLA) class II region is located closest to the centromere. HLA-F is the most telomeric. The region between HLA-DRA and HLA-B is not shown. *(With permission from the Anthony Nolan Bone Marrow Trust, Available at: www.anthonynolan.org.uk/HIG.)*

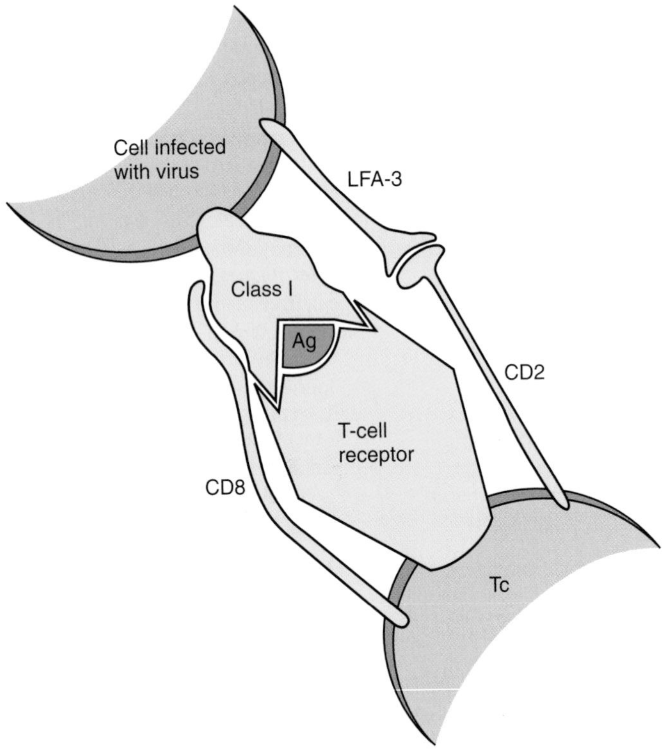

Figure 48-2 Model of the molecular interactions involved in antigen recognition.

In the human, class I molecules include HLA-A, HLA-B, and HLA-C, and class II molecules include HLA-DR, HLA-DQ, and HLA-DP. These molecules are the classical transplantation antigens. Other molecules encoded within the MHC are the class III molecules (see Chapter 49). These include the MHC-linked complement components (C2, C4, and Bf), 21-hydroxylase (CYP21), heat-shock protein (HSP)70, and tumor necrosis factor (TNF).

During an infection, the invading microorganism may infect or be engulfed by cells, and then may be degraded into peptide fragments. Inside the cell, MHC class I or class II molecules bind antigenic fragments derived from the microorganism. Once antigenic fragments have bound to the MHC molecules and have translocated to the cell surface, receptors on T lymphocytes interact with the complex of antigen fragment–MHC molecule, triggering humoral and cellular immune responses (Fig. 48-2). T cell specific cell surface molecules, CD4 and CD8, act to strengthen this cellular interaction and to transmit activation signals. Other cell surface molecules act to increase the affinity of cellular interactions (e.g., CD2 and its ligand, CD58 [LFA-3], or CD11a/CD18 [LFA-1] and its ligand, CD54 [ICAM-1]) and to transmit costimulatory signals (e.g., CD28 and its ligands, CD80/CD86 [B7], or CD40 and its ligand, CD154). Polymorphism in genes that specify MHC class I and class II molecules affects the antigen-binding specificity of the molecules, resulting in differences in immune responses among members of the species. The same pattern of interactions between a cell bearing an MHC class I or class II antigen fragment complex and a T lymphocyte occurs not only in recognition of invading pathogens but also in recognition of foreign class I and class II molecules (alloantigens) and in recognition of self-antigens (autoantigens) (see Chapter 49).

Because donor MHC class I and class II molecules are recognized by the recipient's immune system as foreign antigens, it is beneficial to ensure that donor and recipient are histo- (i.e., tissue) compatible (i.e., HLA-matched). Class I and class II molecules have great allelic diversity within a population, so ensuring compatibility between donor and recipient is often a difficult task that requires collaboration among medical staff, clinical HLA-typing personnel, and donor tissue coordinators (e.g., large organ-sharing networks, registries or banks of hematopoietic progenitor cell donors).

The genetics, structure, function, nomenclature, and techniques of detection of human MHC gene products—HLA-A, -B, and -C (class I) and HLA-DR, -DQ, and -DP (class II)—are discussed in this chapter. Also discussed is the importance of HLA matching for transplantation. In addition to references listed at the end of the chapter, Table 48-1 presents helpful websites that provide both reference material and updates of clinical outcomes.

GENETICS OF THE MAJOR HISTOCOMPATIBILITY COMPLEX

BASIC GENETICS

Mendel's first law, the law of segregation, is based on the principle that hereditary traits are determined by factors that are distributed to progeny. In any one individual, these factors, or genes as they are now called, are present on chromosomes (see Chapter 68). Each gene may have multiple forms (i.e., alleles). Because humans are diploid, two genes are included per pair of homologous chromosomes. In meiosis, the chromosomes segregate randomly during formation of the gametes (ova or sperm) so that only one of each pair of chromosomes (i.e., a haploid number) is transmitted by any given gamete. The double, or diploid, number of chromosomes is restored when the male and female gamete fuse to form the zygote.

TABLE 48-1

Websites on HLA Transplantation

Address	Information
www.ashi-hla.org	American Society for Histocompatibility and Immunogenetics, HLA typing standards
www.ebi.ac.uk/imgt/hla	HLA sequence database, tools for allele submission and sequence manipulation
www.anthonynolan.org.uk/hig	World Health Organization nomenclature information
www.ihwc.org or www.ihwg.org	International Histocompatibility Workshop
www.marrow.org	National Marrow Donor Program
www.bmdw.org	Bone Marrow Donors Worldwide
www.worldmarrow.org	World Marrow Donor Association
www.ibmtr.org	International Bone Marrow Transplant Registry
www.ctstransplant.org	Collaborative Transplant Study
www.unos.org	United Network for Organ Sharing
www.nhgri.nih.gov	National Human Genome Research Institute

Thus, for a trait determined by one gene, there will always be four possible genetic combinations in the offspring, each with equal probability of occurrence. These laws of segregation and random assortment apply to genes of the MHC system. Following are definitions for genetic terms that will be used in this chapter (Crow, 1976; www.nhgri.nih.gov):

Gene: Unit factor of inheritance

Chromosome: Carrier of the unit factors of inheritance

Locus: Position of a gene on a chromosome

Allele: An alternative form of a gene at a single locus

Homozygous: Having identical alleles at a locus, one on each chromosome

Heterozygous: Having different alleles at a locus, one on each chromosome

Codominance: The state in which the allele at each locus expresses its characteristic effect equally in the heterozygote

Genotype: Genetic composition of an organism or individual

Phenotype: Observable characteristics produced by the genes

Polymorphic: Having two or more common distinct genotypes maintained in a population

Homologous chromosomes: The two members of a chromosome pair that have corresponding gene loci, one derived from each parent

Crossing over: Exchange of segments between homologous chromosomes; also termed recombination.

Allo-(antigen, graft): Refers to antigenic differences between individuals of a single species

Auto-(antigen, graft): Refers to tissue or antigens of the same individual (i.e., self)

COMPOSITION OF THE MHC

The major histocompatibility gene complex in humans is located on the short arm of chromosome 6 (i.e., 6p21). It spans 3600 kb (kilobases) and includes 224 identified gene loci, of which 128 are predicted to be expressed. Approximately 40% of the expressed genes are estimated to have an immune system function (Aguado, 1999). HLA genes of the MHC are located in six subregions: HLA-A, HLA-C, HLA-B, HLA-DR, HLA-DQ, and HLA-DP (see Fig. 48-1). Each subregion encodes a minimum of one cell surface glycoprotein. With only one exception, the HLA genes are highly polymorphic, that is, each HLA gene has multiple alleles in the human population. Indeed, the HLA genes are the most polymorphic loci known in man (Parham, 1995; Table 48-2; www.anthonynolan.org/uk/hig). Because HLA genes specify molecules that play an important role in the immune response, polymorphism is believed to be essential to survival of the species and to be maintained in the population by selection; the introduction of molecular typing techniques in the 1980s allowed determination of the variability of the MHC region. As of December 2010 (http://hla.alleles.org/nomenclature/stats.html), more than 4383 class I and more than 1291 class II alleles had been identified (Fig. 48-3; http://hla.alleles.org/nomenclature/nomenclature_2009.html). In this newly found genetic variation, the HLA-B locus presents the greatest variability with 1927 alleles, and the HLA-C locus has the least with 960 alleles. In contrast, for class II alleles, the most variable locus is the DRB1 with 924 alleles.

TABLE 48-2

Examples of WHO-Recognized HLA Antigens (Specificities) Defined by Serologic Typing and HLA Alleles Defined by DNA Sequencing†

HLA-A antigens	HLA-DQ antigens	HLA-A alleles‡	HLA-DQA1 alleles§	HLA-DBQ1 alleles§
A1	DQ1	A*0101-0104N	DQA1*0101-*0105	DQB1*0501-*0504
A2	DQ2	A*02011-*0230	DQA1*0201	DQB1*06011-*0615
A203	DQ3	A*03011-*0304	DQA1*03011-0303	DQB1*0201-*0203
A210	DQ4	A*1101-*1105	DQA1*0401	DQB1*03011-*0309
A3	DQ5(1)	A*2301	DQA1*05011-*0505	DQB1*0401-*0402
A9	DQ6(1)	A*2402101-*2420	DQA1*06011-*06012	
A10	DQ7(3)	A*2501-*2502		
A11	DQ8(3)	A*2601-*2612		
A19	DQ9(3)	A*2901-*2904		
A23(9)		A*3001-*3007		
A24(9)		A*31012-*3104		
A2403		A*3201-*3203		
A25(10)		A*3301-*3304		
A26(10)		A*3401-*3402		
A28		A*3601		
A29(19)		A*4301		
A30(19)		A*6601-*6603		
A31(19)		A*68011-*6809		
A32(19)		A*6901		
A33(19)		A*7401-*7403		
A34(10)		A*8001		
A36				
A43				
A66(10)				
A68(28)				
A69(28)				
A74(19)				
A80				

Adapted from www.anthonynolan.org.uk/hig, with permission of SGE Marsh.

HLA, Human leukocyte antigen; *WHO,* World Health Organization.

†Each column of the table is independent. Numbers in parentheses indicate the broad serologic specificity. The serologic type may be listed without the broad specificity. For example, both A23(9) and A23 are correct designations.

‡HLA-A alleles specify HLA-A antigens. The antigen A1 is specified by either A*0101 orA*0102 or A*0103 alleles. A*0104N is a null or nonexpressed allele.

§HLA-DQA1 and HLA-DQB1 alleles specify HLA-DQ antigens. The antigen DQ5 (1) is specified by several different DQA1 and DQB1 combinations, including (1) DQA1*0101 and DQB1*0501 and (2) DQA1*0101 and DQB1*0502 alleles. In the past, serologic split designations were given to specificities that appeared to identify the antigen specified by a single HLA allele (e.g., A2 splits A203, A210; B7 split B703; B39 splits B3901 and B3902). It is now recognized that other alleles may also encode antigens that carry these serologic specificities, and the WHO Nomenclature Committee has recommended that these splits be discontinued.

LOCALIZATION OF MHC GENES

The genes of the MHC were assigned to the short arm of chromosome 6 (6p) on the basis of cytogenetic studies of aberrant chromosomes (i.e., chromosomes that have undergone a translocation). The map order and

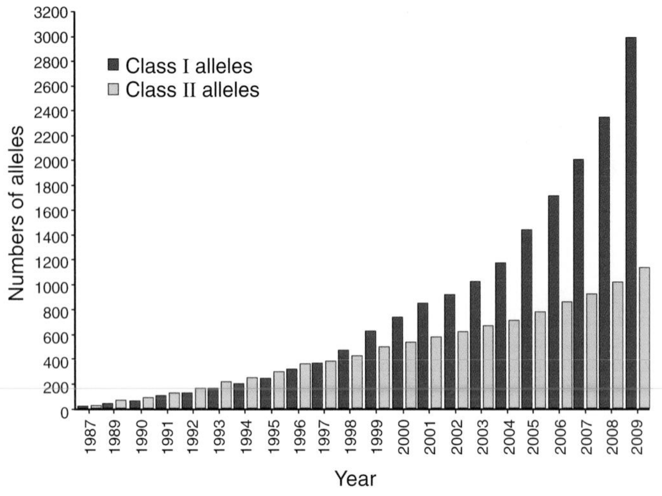

Figure 48-3 Numbers of class I and II alleles discovered from 1987–2009. The increase in the number of discovered alleles during this period has been made possible by the introduction of DNA typing methods; class I alleles include HLA-A, -B, and -Cw, and class II alleles include HLA-DRB1, -DQB1, -DQA1 and -DPB1. *(Data from Anthony Nolan Research Institute. Available at: http://hla.alleles.org/nomenclature/nomenclature_2009.html.)*

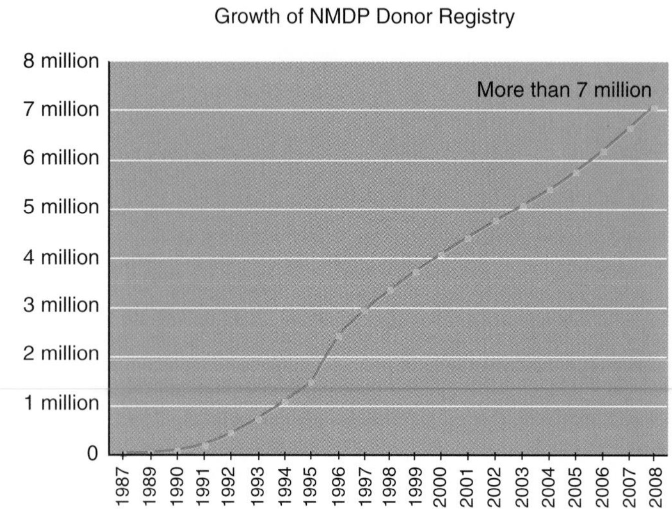

Figure 48-4 More than 7 million donors for hematopoietic stem cell and bone marrow transplantation were registered by the National Marrow Donor Program in 2008. *(Data from the National Marrow Donor Program. Available at: http://www.marrow.org/PHYSICIAN/images/NMDP_donor_growth_a.gif.)*

positioning of the MHC genes were determined by meiotic linkage analyses (i.e., studies of crossing over in families) and molecular biology techniques, including gene cloning, DNA sequencing, and pulsed field gel electrophoresis. The latter technique detects the presence of genes on single long fragments of DNA. The map order of genes within the MHC is HLA-A, -C, -B, -DR, -DQ, -DP, with HLA-A being distal to the centromere (see Fig. 48-1).

INHERITANCE

The MHC genes are closely linked, that is, they segregate en bloc to the offspring. The complex of linked genes that resides on one of the pair of homologous chromosomes and that segregates en bloc to the offspring is termed a haplotype. Each individual inherits two MHC haplotypes—one from each parent—and thus has two alleles for each of the genes. These alleles are codominantly expressed. The inheritance of the MHC genes follows the rules of segregation set down by Mendel. Within a family, each child inherits one MHC haplotype from the mother and one from the father. By convention, the paternal haplotypes are designated a and b, and the maternal haplotypes c and d. Thus, there are four possible MHC genotypes in the offspring: ac, ad, bc, and bd. Because the chance of inheriting a given haplotype is random, the probability of occurrence of any one of the four genotypes is one in four for each mating. In a family with five children, at least two of the children will be HLA-identical (assuming no crossing over). Although the MHC genes are closely linked, families have been reported in which a crossover has occurred. The frequency of crossing over between two linked genes was thought to be a measure of the distance separating the genes; however, molecular data have suggested the existence of recombination "hot" spots in the intervening DNA that can increase or decrease the likelihood of recombination during meiosis (Uematsu, 1988).

LINKAGE DISEQUILIBRIUM

The observation that alleles at different genetic loci occur in the population on the same haplotype significantly more frequently than would be expected on the basis of chance alone is called linkage disequilibrium. The expected frequency of two alleles (f_1, f_2) is the product of the gene frequency of each allele in that population ($f_{expected} = f_1 \times f_2$). The observed frequency is determined from family studies within the same population. Linkage disequilibrium is a hallmark of the human MHC and extends from HLA-A through HLA-DQ. The best known example of linkage disequilibrium is the A1,Cw7,B8,DR17(3),DR52,DQ2 haplotype in Caucasians, which is observed approximately four times more frequently than expected. The significance of linkage disequilibrium as it applies to immune competence and disease is discussed in Chapter 49 under Extended Haplotypes.

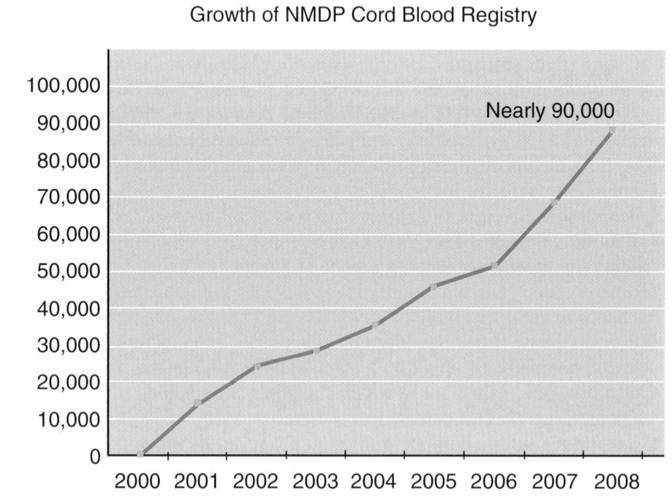

Figure 48-5 The number of umbilical cord units has increased in the last decade, primarily for the treatment of blood malignancies in pediatric patients; more than one HLA mismatch and more than one cord unit can be used in umbilical cord transplantation. *(Data from the National Marrow Donor Program. Available at: http://www.marrow.org/PHYSICIAN/images/NMDP_donor_growth_a.gif.)*

ETHNIC VARIATION

Accumulated data from the study of the world population groups (Dausset, 1973; Imanishi, 1992; Cadavid, 1997; Bugawan, 1999) demonstrate that the frequencies of HLA alleles differ significantly among ethnic population groups. MHC haplotypes and linkage disequilibrium of alleles also differ. These observations must be taken into account when unrelated allograft hematopoietic progenitor cell donor registries and banks such as the U.S. National Marrow Donor Program (NMDP) are established (Perkins, 1994). Both allele and haplotype frequencies dictate the number of volunteers required to find an HLA-matched unrelated donor for any patient. Some patients (e.g., those with rare or unusual types) cannot find closely matched unrelated donors from among the more than 7 million volunteers listed in all donor registries worldwide (Fig. 48-4). Currently, patients are more likely to find a match because the number of donors has increased, as has the use of umbilical cord blood units for transplantation (Fig. 48-5). It appears that cord blood transplantation may be more tolerant of HLA mismatches; this may be a result of reexposure to noninherited maternal antigens (NIMAs) found in the graft (Van Rood, 2009). Improvement in methods used for engraftment of progenitor cells from partially HLA-mismatched donors may allow transplantation in patients for whom close matches cannot be found (see Chapter 38).

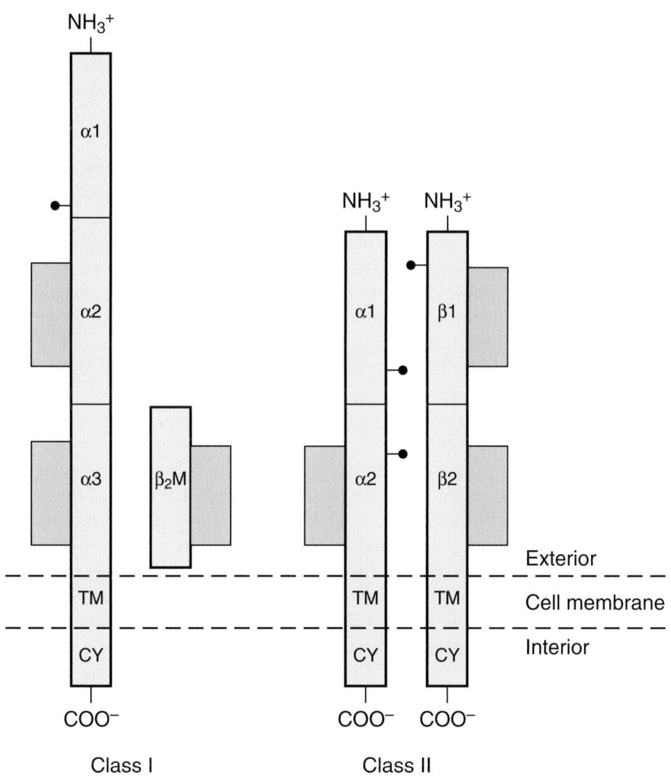

Figure 48-6 A schematic model of the structure of class I and class II molecules.

Class I Molecules—HLA-A, HLA-B, HLA-C Subregions

The HLA-A and -B molecules were the first MHC molecules to be described in humans (Dausset, 1981; van Rood, 1993). Because these molecules were defined by antibody responses to white blood cells (WBCs), they were called human leukocyte **antigens.** Leukocyte antibodies were observed in humans as early as the 1920s, but it was not until the 1950s that a systematic study began. In 1952, Dausset convincingly demonstrated the existence of leukocyte antibodies (leukoagglutinins). Because these leukoagglutinins did not react with leukocytes from the antibody producer but did react with a percentage of leukocytes from red cell group O unrelated individuals, he suggested that leukoagglutinins were alloantibodies. Shortly thereafter, Payne (1964) reported that sera from patients who had febrile nonhemolytic blood transfusion reactions frequently contained leukoagglutinins that demonstrated allospecificity. In 1958, Dausset described the first HLA alloantigen MAC (now HLA-A2 + HLA-28) and showed it to be genetically determined.

Originally, leukocyte specificities were thought to be the products of a single locus. A two-locus model, each locus with multiple alleles, was established through HLA studies in families by the identification of recombinational events that separated the two allelic series. These two allelic series were called the first, or LA (now HLA-A), and the second, or four, series (now HLA-B). These names were derived from descriptions of the LA 1, 2, 3 allelic series by Payne in 1967, and of the 4a, 4b allelic series by van Rood in 1969. A third locus was first proposed in 1970; however, it was not confirmed until 1975, when a family with a recombination between HLA-B and the new locus was identified. This third locus was designated HLA-C following the 1975 International Histocompatibility Workshop. Dausset (1981) was awarded the Nobel Prize for Medicine in 1980 for his original work on the human HLA system.

STRUCTURE OF CLASS I MOLECULES

The classical class I molecules, termed HLA-A, HLA-B, and HLA-C in the human, are heterodimers consisting of a transmembrane glycosylated polypeptide (heavy chain, 44 kDa) noncovalently associated with β2-microglobulin (12 kDa) (Fig. 48-6) (Bjorkman, 1990). The heavy chain of the class I molecule spans the cell membrane and is oriented with its amino-terminus on the outside of the cell. β2-Microglobulin is associated with the extracellular region of the heavy chain and is necessary for cell surface expression. The extracellular region of the class I heavy chain is divided into three domains designated α1, α2, and α3, each consisting of about 90 amino acid residues. The amino-terminal α1 domain contains a glycosylation site at the asparagine residue in position 86. The transmembrane segment of approximately 24 amino acids is mostly hydrophobic, whereas the intracellular carboxy-terminal segment of the molecule consists mainly of hydrophilic residues with a cluster of basic residues adjacent to the cytoplasmic surface of the cell membrane.

Polymorphism of class I molecules (see Table 48-2 and Figure 48-3) (Bodmer, 1997, 1999) is defined by the use of (1) class I specific antibodies (alloantisera and monoclonal antibodies) that bind to the HLA molecules; (2) cytotoxic T lymphocytes (CTLs) that recognize and kill in response to stimulation by foreign or allogeneic class I molecules in vitro; (3) isoelectric focusing of isolated class I molecules; (4) polymerase chain reaction (PCR)-based DNA typing of class I alleles; and (5) nucleotide sequencing of class I alleles. Most of the class I polymorphism arises from amino acid sequence differences clustered in the α1 and α2 domains of the heavy chain. The α3 domain is highly conserved among HLA class I molecules.

Fresh insights into the structure of the HLA molecule came when the three-dimensional structure of the class I molecule was defined using X-ray crystallography (Bjorkman, 1987). The structure of the extracellular portion is shown in Figure 48-7. The molecule consists of two pairs of structurally similar domains: α1 has the same tertiary conformation as α2, and α3- and β2-microglobulin have similar tertiary conformations. The α3- and β2-microglobulin domains are each composed of two antiparallel β-pleated sheets—one with four strands and one with three strands, connected by a disulfide bond. The α3 and α2 domains interact with one another through these β-pleated sheets, and their structure closely resembles that described for an immunoglobulin constant region domain. The α1 and α2 domains are paired to form an eight-strand β-pleated sheet. This sheet is topped by two α-helices forming a groove at the top of the molecule. This groove is the site for binding of antigenic peptide fragments by the class I molecule (Fig. 48-7). The sides and bottom of the groove are formed by side chains of the amino acids that constitute the helices and β-pleated sheets. Many of the amino acids that line this groove are polymorphic, creating allele-specific differences in antigen binding specificity among the different class I allelic products (Stern, 1994). Other residues in the helical regions of the groove interact with the T cell receptor during recognition of the class I antigenic fragment complex by a T lymphocyte (see Fig. 48-2).

ORGANIZATION OF CLASS I GENES

The HLA heavy chains are encoded within the MHC on chromosome 6 (see Fig. 48-1) (Shiina, 1999) and are highly polymorphic, whereas β2-microglobulin is encoded on chromosome 15 and is not known to be polymorphic in humans. The typical class I gene is encoded by eight exons. The first exon encodes the 5′ untranslated region and a hydrophobic leader peptide. Exons 2–4 encode the three extracellular domains; exon 5 encodes the transmembrane region. The sixth and seventh exons encode the cytoplasmic region, and the eighth exon encodes the 3′ untranslated region, including the poly(A) addition site. Intervening sequences (termed introns) between the exons are transcribed into RNA but are removed during messenger RNA (mRNA) splicing.

REGULATION OF CLASS I GENE EXPRESSION

HLA class I molecules are expressed as transmembrane glycoproteins on the surface of many cell types. However, the level of surface expression can vary extensively (Singer, 1990). The resting level of class I molecules is highest on β2-microglobulin lymphoid cells, and HLA-C expression is 10 times less than that of HLA-A or HLA-B (Le Bouteiller, 1994); this is a result of inefficient association and a mutated cis-regulatory element of transcriptional control found in region I of the HLA-C promoter (enhancer A) that reduces its expression (Neefjes, 1988). Differential expression of HLA molecules appears to reflect the level and antigenic specificity of the allogeneic sensitization seen in patients awaiting kidney transplantation, because these patients are subjected to multiple random blood transfusions while on dialysis; more kidneys are rejected because of the presence of HLA-A or -B or both A and B specific antibody, and far fewer are rejected by only HLA-Cw specific antibodies; class I molecules are undetectable on the membranes of certain other cell types such as brain cells, muscle

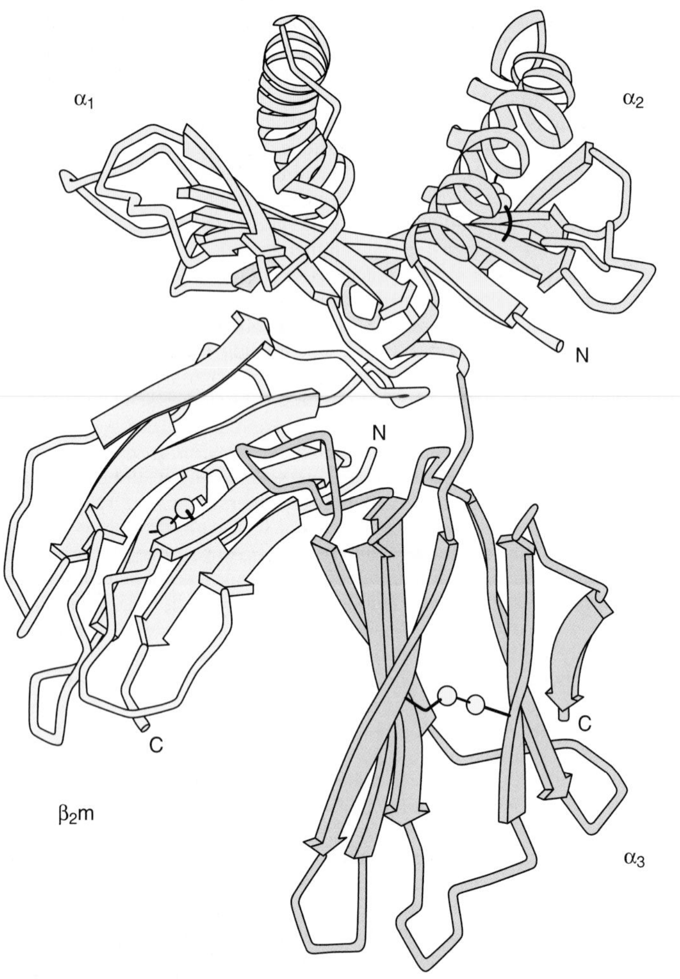

Figure 48-7 Three-dimensional model of the extracellular portion of a class I molecule. *(With permission from Bjorkman PJ, Saper MA, Samraoui B, et al. Structure of the human class I histocompatibility antigen, HLA-A2. Nature 1987;329:506.)*

cells, and sperm cells. Sequence elements located upstream of class I genes bind regulatory factors that control the cell surface expression of class I molecules. During an immune response, the cell surface expression of class I genes can be upregulated by binding of cytokine (e.g., interferon-γ, and TNF) to upstream regulatory elements. Tumors and certain viruses (e.g., human immunodeficiency virus) can suppress class I expression (Brodsky, 1999).

FUNCTION OF CLASS I MOLECULES

The HLA-A, -B, and -C molecules play key roles in an immune response. First, in the adaptive immune response, class I molecules bind peptides derived from proteins degraded or synthesized in the cytosol and display them on the cell surface for perusal by the antigen receptors on T lymphocytes (see Chapter 45). Presentation of antigen by class I molecules allows T cells to detect and mount a cytotoxic response to foreign material (e.g., a virus, abnormal proteins from a malignant cell). In the cytosol, intracellular antigens (including self-proteins and viral or abnormal proteins) are broken down into peptide fragments (Rock, 1999). These peptide fragments are transported to the endoplasmic reticulum, where they bind to the groove at the top of newly synthesized class I molecules and then are carried to the cell surface (Hansen, 1997b; Pamer, 1998) (see Fig. 48-2). Four genes, located in the class II region of the MHC (see Figs. 48-1 and 48-8), are involved in this process. Two of these genes (*LMP2* and *LMP7*) encode components of the proteosome complex, a macromolecular structure that degrades proteins within the cytosol (Tanaka, 1997). The other two genes (*TAP1* and *TAP2*) encode components of peptide transporters that move peptides from the cytosol into the endoplasmic reticulum (Momburg, 1998). $CD8^+$ CTLs recognize the processed peptide in conjunction with the class I molecule (Jorgensen, 1992). In the experimental system used to dissect this mechanism, CTLs were generated by in vitro stimulation with virally infected autologous cells. Recognition and lysis of the target cell were specific for the priming virus strain. Recognition also was affected by allelic polymorphism of class I molecules because only virally infected target cells sharing the appropriate class I allelic product(s) with the responder were lysed (Zinkernagel, 1997a, 1997b). The latter requirement is termed **MHC restriction.** Zinkernagel and his collaborator Doherty were awarded the Nobel Prize for Medicine in 1996 in recognition of the importance of the concept of MHC restriction to immunology.

Second, surface expression of class I molecules has a protective function in the innate immune response by preventing target cell lysis effected by natural killer (NK) cells. Unlike CTLs, NK cells do not require activation through the recognition of peptide bound to the class I molecule but can lyse and destroy target cells lacking classical HLA class I molecule expression on the cell surface. Through this innate mechanism, NK cells play an important role in surveillance against viruses and tumor cells that down-regulate expression of the class I molecule to avoid recognition by CTLs (Lanier, 1998; Long, 1999).

There are two groups of NK receptors: (1) the C-type lectin receptor CD94/NKG2, whose genes reside on chromosome 12, and (2) the killer cell immunoglobulin-like receptors (KIRs) encoded by genes on chromosome 19. NK cell function appears to be regulated by a balance between positive signaling receptors that initiate and inhibitory receptors that suppress cell activation. Both groups of receptors recognize HLA class I ligands. For example, the KIR2D receptors differentiate between HLA-C ligands based on the presence of specific amino acid residues at codons 77 and 80 (i.e., asn77lys80 vs. ser77asn80). Another NK receptor, KIR3D, recognizes the HLA-Bw4/Bw6 polymorphism. A third NK receptor, CD94/NKG2, recognizes the HLA-E molecule complexed with the HLA leader peptide from some of the allelic products of HLA-A, -B, -C, and -G molecules (Brooks, 1999).

NK cells can specifically recognize and lyse allogeneic cells that do not express the specific class I molecules expressed by the effector cell (i.e., "missing self") (Valiante, 1997). This could occur even in apparently HLA-matched transplant pairs where one member of the pair is homozygous and the other is heterozygous (e.g., donor: Bw4,Bw6; recipient: Bw6). Thus Bw4 specific NK cells from the donor might lyse cells without Bw4 from the recipient in a hematopoietic progenitor cell graft. This response may be unidirectional in some settings. In the example, the donor does not lack any HLA molecule present in the recipient; thus, the recipient NK cells will not detect any missing self. Because NK cells are relatively radioresistant and make up a subpopulation of about 10%–15% of peripheral blood lymphocytes, the NK response could be substantial; however, the extent of the role of NK activity in affecting transplant outcome is not known at present (Ruggeri, 1999).

OTHER CLASS I GENES

As many as 20 additional nonclassical or class Ib genes have been identified within the class I region of chromosome 6p by gene cloning (Aguado, 1999). Many of these are pseudogenes; however, several encode and express class I–like mRNA and/or molecules HLA-E, HLA-F, and HLA-G. These molecules may be key mediators of both adaptive and innate immune responses (O'Callaghan, 1998). Their genes are homologous to classical class I genes in structure, and the polypeptides encoded by these loci also associate with β2-microglobulin. However, just as a high level of allelic polymorphism is a hallmark of the HLA-A, HLA-B, and HLA-C loci, a low level of polymorphism of the HLA-E, HLA-F, and HLA-G loci is a defining feature of these genes. In addition, by comparison with classical class I molecules, the cell surface expression of nonclassical class I molecules is low, and the distribution of these class Ib molecules on specific cell types varies.

HLA-G

HLA-G is expressed principally on extravillous cytotrophoblast cells at the fetal/maternal interface, where it is thought to play a role in maternofetal tolerance (Le Bouteiller, 1999). HLA-G, as a ligand for at least three NK and other cell inhibitory receptors, protects the invading placental tissue from the cytolytic action of NK cells. Although HLA-G has the capability to bind and present processed antigen (i.e., peptides) to T cells, the diversity of peptides bound by HLA-G appears to be less than the diversity of peptides bound by classical class I molecules. Regulation of expression of HLA-G also differs from that of classical class I genes, as the gene contains no interferon response signal; thus, it is not interferon-inducible. It has been hypothesized that the soluble forms may act as specific immunosuppressors during pregnancy (Le Bouteiller, 1999). Recent evidence supports this hypothesis. HLA-G transcripts are present in great numbers in placental extravillous membranes in the first trimester, but at term, transcript numbers decline sharply, in keeping with the theory that HLA-G provides protection for the allogeneic embryo from maternal NK cell surveillance (Agrawal, 2003). This putative role raises the possibility that HLA-G may play a role in tolerance for transplanted tissues. Along these lines, it is interesting to note that liver–kidney transplant recipients with high concentrations of HLA-G in their sera had low numbers of acute rejection episodes and therefore may require less immunosuppressive therapy (Creput, 2003).

HLA-E

HLA-E may play a role in protecting a target cell from NK cell–mediated lysis. HLA-E molecules bind a set of almost identical hydrophobic peptides derived from the leader sequences of the classical class I and HLA-G heavy chains. HLA-E displays these bound peptides at the cell surface for recognition by NK cells, providing a check for the integrity of the antigen-presenting pathway (Lee, 1998a, 1998b; O'Callaghan, 1998). Skin grafting in a transgenic mouse model suggests that HLA-E may be recognized as a transplantation antigen (Pacasova, 1999). Recent studies suggest that host NK cells may be able to recognize HLA-E on allogeneic cells and possibly tolerate it, even when it is bound to donor peptides. With this finding comes the potential for exploiting this tolerance in pursuit of preventing NK cell–mediated graft rejection and graft-versus-host disease (GVHD) (Matsunami, 2002).

HLA-F

The role of HLA-F is unknown. Computer modeling predicts that certain amino acid residues of HLA-F could contribute to a putative peptide-binding groove, consistent with a role in antigen presentation by HLA-F (O'Callaghan, 1998). To date, HLA-F appears to be normally expressed only on the surfaces of extravillous trophoblasts that have invaded the maternal decidua, and has also been found on the surfaces of lymphoblastoid cell lines infected with Epstein-Barr virus (Ishitani, 2003).

Class II Molecules—HLA-DR, HLA-DQ, HLA-DP Subregions

The class II molecules in humans were first recognized by their ability to stimulate allogeneic T cells in the mixed leukocyte culture (MLC). During the 1975 International Histocompatibility Workshop, the MLC was used to define the HLA-D allelic series (Thorsby, 1975). Because MLCs required 7 days before results could be obtained, rapid serologic detection of HLA-D was sought. In 1975, it was determined that alloantisera contained antibodies reactive with molecules closely associated with the specificities previously identified as HLA-D by cellular techniques (Dausset, 1981). Following the 1977 International Histocompatibility Workshop, these serologic specificities were termed DR, for D-related specificities, because HLA-D and HLA-DR were observed to be associated but not identical to each other. Serologic testing coupled with genetic and immunochemical studies identified additional class II molecules: DR52, DR53, DR51, and DQ. Cellular techniques identified still another class II molecule in the late 1970s (Shaw, 1981). This molecule (now termed HLA-DP) was initially described as a secondary B cell antigen (SB) because it was usually weak or undetectable in a primary MLC and required secondary phase stimulation in culture for detection. Subsequently, the DNA coding sequences and locations of these genes within the MHC were further characterized using molecular biology techniques (Beck, 1999).

STRUCTURE OF CLASS II MOLECULES

The class II HLA-DR, -DQ, and -DP molecules are heterodimers consisting of two noncovalently associated transmembrane glycoproteins: an α chain (33–35 kDa) and a β chain (26–28 kDa) (see Fig. 47-3) (Gorga, 1992). Both polypeptide chains span the cell membrane and are oriented with their amino-termini on the outside of the cell. The extracellular regions of the α and β polypeptides are each divided into two domains, designated α1 and α2 and β1 and β2, and each domain consists of approximately 90 amino acid residues. The α chain has two carbohydrate moieties, one high-mannose and one complex-type glycan, at amino acids 78 and 118, respectively. β chains have one complex-type oligosaccharide at amino acid 19. The amino-terminal α1 and β1 domains of α and β chains contain the polymorphic residues, while the membrane proximal α2 and β2 domains are highly conserved and are homologous to immunoglobulin constant region domains. A region of approximately 12 amino acids in length connects the second extracellular domain to the hydrophobic transmembrane region (23 amino acids) and a small intracytoplasmic domain (8–15 amino acids).

Based on crystallography, the class II molecule is similar in structure to the class I molecule (Brown, 1993) (Fig. 48-7). In the class II molecule, the α1 and β1 domains of the α and β chains form an eight-stranded β-pleated sheet topped by two α helices to form the antigen-binding groove at the top of the molecule. The α2 and β2 domains each form two antiparallel β-pleated sheets that support the groove at the top. As with class I, many of the amino acids that line the antigenic peptide-binding groove are polymorphic, creating differences in peptide-binding specificities for the different class II allelic products.

Similar to the class I molecules, the class II molecules are highly polymorphic (see Table 48-2 and Figure 48-3) (Bodmer, 1997, 1999; Marsh, 2002). Class II polymorphism is defined by (1) class II specific antibodies (alloantisera and monoclonal antibodies), which bind to class II molecules; (2) alloproliferative T cells that recognize and proliferate in response to foreign class II molecules in vitro; (3) two-dimensional gel electrophoresis of isolated class II molecules; (4) hybridization of restriction endonuclease digests of DNA-encoding class II genes using locus-specific probes (a technique that detects restriction fragment length polymorphism); (5) PCR-based DNA typing of class II alleles; and (6) nucleotide sequencing of class II genes. Most of the class II polymorphism arises from amino acid sequence differences localized in the α1 and β1 domains of the two polypeptide chains.

ORGANIZATION OF CLASS II GENES

In contrast to the class I molecules, both the α and β chains of class II molecules are encoded within a 1100-kb section of the MHC region (see Figs. 48-1 and 48-8) (Beck, 1999). The class II region includes three subregions—DR, DQ, and DP—each of which encodes at least one expressed A (encoding an α chain) and B (encoding a β chain) gene. Sequence comparisons suggest that both class I and class II genes arose through a successive series of gene duplications during the evolution of this gene complex. The original duplication in the class II region most likely gave rise to primordial A and B genes. More recent gene duplications generated the DR, DQ, and DP subregions containing multiple genes.

A typical A gene contains five exons encoding (1) the 5′ untranslated region and leader sequence; (2) α1 domain; (3) α2 domain; (4) connecting peptide, transmembrane region, cytoplasmic tail, and a portion of the 3′ untranslated region; and (5) the remainder of the 3′ untranslated region, including the poly(A) addition signal. A typical β-chain gene is similar to the α-chain gene but has an extra exon for the cytoplasmic tail.

DR Subregion

The DR subregion encodes one or two DR molecules, depending on the haplotype (Bodmer, 1997, 1999). The subregion contains a single expressed DRA gene that is similar in different haplotypes, differing only in a single conservative amino acid substitution found in the cytoplasmic domain.

The most centromeric DRB gene, *DRB1* (Fig. 48-8), encodes a highly polymorphic β chain that, when associated with the α chain, exhibits serologic specificities DR1–DR18. This molecule is the predominant class II molecule on the cell surface, accounting for well over half of total cell surface class II molecules. There are multiple nucleic acids, hence amino acid sequence differences among DRB1 alleles.

The second expressed DRB gene, present only in some class II haplotypes, is located between the DRB1 locus and the DRA locus (see Fig. 48-8). In cells expressing DR alleles, DRB1*03, *11, *12, *13, and *14, the second DRB gene is termed *DRB3.* (HLA nomenclature is described subsequently.) The *DRB3* gene is polymorphic, although at present the number of identified alleles is approximately 10 times less than the number of DRB1 alleles. The DRB3 product combined with the DRA product forms the DR molecule, which carries DR52 serologic specificity. In cells expressing DRB1*04, *07, and *09 alleles, the second DRB gene is termed *DRB4.* The DRB4 product combined with the DRA product forms the molecule that carries the serologic specificity DR53. Last, in cells expressing DRB1*15 and *16 alleles, the second DRB gene is termed *DRB5.* This DRB5 product combined with the DRA product carries DR51 serologic specificity. Haplotypes expressing DRB1*01, *08, or *10 alleles do not usually carry a second expressed DRB locus. There are exceptions to these associations. For example, a haplotype carrying DRB1*15 without a DRB5 locus has been described (Wade, 1993).

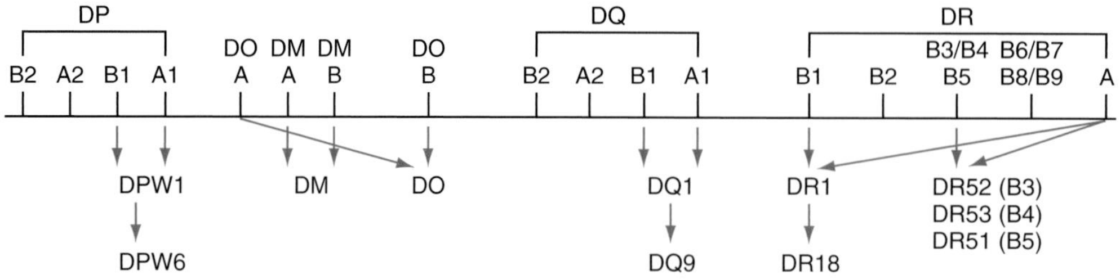

Figure 48-8 Map of the class II region of the human major histocompatibility complex (MHC). Gene products encoded by each subregion are listed. Not all genes are included.

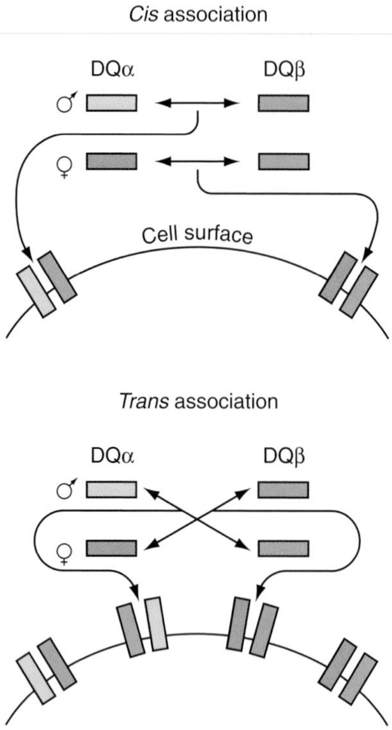

Figure 48-9 Model of the cis and trans associations of DQα and DGβ chains.

DQ Subregion

One set of A and B genes, *DQA1* and *DQB1*, encode the DQ heterodimer that carries DQ1–9 serologic specificities (see Table 48-2 and Fig. 48-8) (Bodmer, 1997, 1999). DQ molecules represent approximately 15%–20% of the total class II molecules expressed on the cell surface. Because both *DQA1* and *DQB1* loci are polymorphic, and because the protein products can associate in trans as well as in cis, heterozygotes may potentially express four different DQ molecules on their cell surfaces (Fig. 48-9). Other DQ-like A and B genes in the DQ subregion such as *DQA2* and *DQB2* are very similar to the *DQA1* and *DQB1* genes; however, no functional protein products are expressed.

DP Subregion

The DP subregion contains two sets of A and B genes (see Fig. 48-8). One set, *DPA1* and *DPB1*, encodes the DP protein product; the other set is made up of pseudogenes. Both *DPA1* and *DPB1* genes are highly polymorphic (Bodmer, 1997, 1999). The level of DP expression on the cell surface is very low.

LINKAGE DISEQUILIBRIUM OF GENES IN THE CLASS II REGION

Specific combinations of DRB1/DRB3, DRB1/DRB4, DRB1/DRB5, and DQA1/DQB1 alleles are common. The DQA1/DQB1 combinations found may be controlled in part by the ability of α and β chains to pair (Kwok, 1993). In addition, certain DR and DQ alleles are inherited together more frequently than expected, resulting in linkage disequilibrium in a population. The frequency of these combinations differs strikingly among different ethnic population groups. For example, both the DRB1*1101, DQB1*0501 (DR11[5]), DQ5[1] and the DRB1*0901, DQB1*0303(DR9, DQ9[3]) haplotypes frequently are found in populations of direct African heritage, whereas these DR–DQ combinations are rarely found in populations of Caucasoid heritage. Crossing over between the DP loci and the DR/DQ loci is common. Thus, minimal linkage disequilibrium is noted between the DR/DQ and DP alleles. Lists of common DRB1/DQA1/DQB1 haplotypes have been published (Begovich, 1992; Imanishi, 1992).

REGULATION OF CLASS II GENE EXPRESSION

Class II molecules, HLA-DR, -DQ and -DP, are constitutively expressed on antigen-presenting cells (APCs) of the immune system, including monocytes, macrophages, dendritic cells, B lymphocytes, and neoplastic cells. HLA class II expression is highest for HLA-DR, intermediate for HLA-DQ, and lowest for HLA-DP (Glimcher, 1992; Guardiola, 1993); as with class I, differential expression of HLA class II molecules is reflected in the antigenic specificity of allosensitization seen in patients awaiting kidney transplantation; more kidneys are rejected because of the presence of an HLA-DR or -DQ specific antibody, and fewer are rejected because of an HLA-DP specific antibody. DNA sequences found upstream of the coding sequences in class II genes are critical to expression. Binding of proteins to these regions regulates the expression of class II genes. Alterations in the ability of DNA-binding proteins to interact with the 5′ regulatory DNA sequences eliminating the expression of class II genes lead to an immunodeficiency called the **bare lymphocyte syndrome** (Kovats, 1994; Mach, 1996). Class II genes are inducible by interferon (IFN)-γ in many cell types (Glimcher, 1992; Mach, 1996), and expression may be affected by other cytokines (Guardiola, 1993). Expression of class II molecules in APCs may be modulated, particularly in dendritic cells, following antigen deposition and inflammation. The level of antigenic peptide class II complex expression and the presence of a costimulatory signal on the mature APC may play an important role in transplantation and in autoimmune disease (Nepom, 1991; Banchereau, 1998) (see Chapter 49).

FUNCTION OF CLASS II MOLECULES

Class II molecules act as antigen receptors in the immune response (see Fig. 48-2), binding antigenic peptide fragments processed from exogenous antigens such as bacteria. The exogenous antigens enter the cell through the endocytic pathway and are degraded into peptide fragments in late endosomes, where they encounter and bind to the newly assembled class II molecules (Watts, 1997). Binding of processed protein peptide fragments to the class II molecule is facilitated by two proteins encoded within the class II region of the MHC: DM and DO (see Fig. 48-8). Peptide binding is affected by polymorphic residues located in the groove of the class II molecule. The complex of antigenic fragment bound to the class II molecule is transported to the cell surface for display to and recognition by circulating T cells.

Antigen receptors on CD4⁺ T lymphocytes interact with the class II-antigenic fragment complex, triggering activation of the cell (Jorgensen, 1992). In the experimental system used to dissect this mechanism, effector T lymphocytes were stimulated in vitro with autologous APCs previously incubated with antigen. As observed for class I, recognition of the antigenic fragment by the effector T cell is influenced by MHC allelic polymorphism. The effector T cell is specific for the priming antigenic peptide in conjunction with the particular class II allelic product that originally presented the antigen (MHC restriction) (Rosenthal, 1973).

Each T cell activated by recognition of the complex of antigen fragment bound to class II molecule can perform one or several functions (Paul, 1994). The CD4+ T cell can help B lymphocytes differentiate to antibody-producing plasma cells, or it can help other T lymphocytes differentiate to either cytotoxic cells or cells with suppressor function. In addition, the T cell itself can function either as a cytotoxic cell, directly killing cells with the appropriate target (i.e., cells expressing class II MHC molecules complexed with the specific antigen), or as a cell with suppressor function, causing a dampening of the immune response. T cells also produce a number of biologically important molecules (such as IFN-γ) that augment the immune response and increase the expression of MHC molecules on target cells. In addition, T cells produce growth factors such as interleukin (IL)-2. These growth factors affect a wide range of cells from hematopoietic progenitor cells to mature lymphocytes.

OTHER CLASS II GENES

At least four other class II genes—*DOA*, *DOB*, *DMA*, and *DMB*—have been described that express protein products (see Fig. 48-8). The proteins encoded by the *DMA* and *DMB* genes form the DM heterodimer. The proteins encoded by the *DOA* and *DOB* genes form the DO heterodimer. These gene products are not detected on the cell surface, but rather are expressed inside the cell, localized to specialized intracellular compartments where newly synthesized class II (DR, DQ, DP) molecules bind their antigenic peptides. The DM molecule regulates peptide binding to HLA-DR, -DQ, and -DP, serving both chaperone-like and editor-like functions (Morris, 1994) that favor the presentation of stably bound peptides. The DO molecule negatively regulates the function of DM (van Ham, 1997).

CHARACTERISTICS OF ANTIGENIC FRAGMENTS BOUND BY MHC CLASS I AND CLASS II MOLECULES

The function of class I and class II molecules as antigen-binding receptors is similar; however, the peptides they bind have different characteristics (Cresswell, 1994; Engelhard, 1994). Peptides derived from proteins synthesized de novo in the cell (endogenous antigens such as viral antigens) associate with class I molecules in the endoplasmic reticulum. In contrast, peptides from soluble and particulate antigens taken up by the cell into the endocytic pathway (exogenous antigens) bind with class II molecules in an endosomal compartment. Both class I and class II molecules can alternatively bind self-peptides found in these compartments. Self-peptides result from the normal degradation of cellular proteins. Some of these self-peptides are fragments of histocompatibility molecules themselves. Usually, the self-peptides bound to MHC molecules do not trigger T lymphocytes, as they are molecules to which the immune system of the individual is tolerant. However, these self-peptides may trigger immune responses, initiating a self-destructive process leading to autoimmunity (Nepom, 1991) (see Chapters 51, 52, and 53).

Peptide binding to MHC molecules occurs only when the peptide fragment is of a suitable length and contains a particular amino acid sequence or motif that allows it to bind to one or more of the MHC molecules expressed in that individual. Examples of motifs for a peptide that binds to the HLA molecule encoded by A*0201 is leucine (or methionine or isoleucine) at residue 2 of the peptide, a hydrophilic amino acid at residue 3, and a valine (or leucine or isoleucine or alanine) at residue 9. The amino acids that make up the motif are referred to as **anchor** residues of the peptide. Different HLA molecules, either molecules encoded by different alleles at the same locus (HLA-A*0203, *0211, or *0301) or molecules encoded by different loci (B*4001 or DRB1*0406), bind peptides with different motifs. The amino acids forming the peptide motif bind to the MHC molecule in pockets found within the antigen-binding groove (Stern, 1994). The polymorphic amino acids of the MHC molecules line this groove and thus create differences in peptide-binding specificities for the different MHC molecules.

The peptides bound to class I molecules are 9–10 amino acids in length. Both the carboxy- and amino-terminal ends of the peptide are buried in the class I–binding groove, forming a **closed** peptide–MHC complex. The peptides bound to class II molecules vary in length from 12 to 30 amino acids. While maintaining the requirement for specific motif residues nested in the central portion of the peptide, both the carboxy- and amino-terminal ends of the peptide extend outside the class II–binding groove, forming an **open** peptide–MHC complex (Stern, 1994).

RECOGNITION OF FOREIGN MHC MOLECULES

Allorecognition involves the recognition by a T lymphocyte of a foreign MHC molecule on a cell from a second (allogeneic) individual. Upon recognition, the interaction triggers a series of events, resulting in activation of the T cell and initiation of an immune response not unlike the recognition of pathogens. Based on data from models of vascularized organ transplantation, two pathways of allorecognition have been hypothesized (Sayegh, 1996). The direct pathway for allorecognition involves the stimulation of recipient T cells by the donor MHC–peptide complex (i.e., direct recognition of intact foreign MHC molecules). The second route of allorecognition, the indirect pathway, involves stimulation of recipient T cells by self-MHC molecules presenting peptide fragments from donor cells. Indirect presentation occurs when antigen-processing cells of the recipient ingest cellular material from the grafted tissue, degrade the material intracellularly, and display the allogenic peptide(s) complexed with self-MHC molecules. Peptides derived from polymorphic regions of donor MHC molecules are the major candidates for stimulation of the indirect immune response (Suciu-Foca, 1998; Gould, 1999; Harris, 1999).

TANDEM REPEATS AND SINGLE NUCLEOTIDE POLYMORPHISMS IN THE MHC

More than 300 short tandem repeats (STRs) have been identified within the human MHC region (Foissac, 1997). Multiple single nucleotide polymorphisms (SNPs) are also present. A study by Abbal (1997) examined six STR loci within the MHC in a population of unrelated individuals and found strong linkage disequilibrium between specific HLA haplotypes and the STR markers. Because these markers cover a larger region of the MHC than the classical HLA markers now used, they may provide a more comprehensive approach to identifying MHC-identical individuals. These markers might, for example, be used to identify a recombinant MHC haplotype within a family (Carrington, 1996) or to enhance the probability that any unidentified histocompatibility genes in the MHC are matched. Molecular methods have been developed to identify both STRs and SNPs that are accurate and reproducible (Carrington, 1998).

MINOR HISTOCOMPATIBILITY MOLECULES

Minor histocompatibility antigens (mHags) are immunogenetic peptides that bind to MHC molecules and can be recognized by T cells to cause undesirable GVHD, but in the setting of leukemic recipients can produce the beneficial condition graft-versus-leukemia. Achieving the proper balance of acceptable GVHD and sufficient graft-versus-leukemia is problematic. In MHC-identical progenitor cell grafts, GVHD may be induced by mHag differences between the recipient and donor (Mutis, 1999). The mHags can be any polymorphic gene product encoded outside the MHC that differs between donor and recipient and that stimulates a T cell response (Goulmy, 1997; Simpson, 1998). Similar to other protein antigens, the polymorphic protein must be processed into antigenic fragments, and the polymorphic peptide fragment(s) must bind within the groove of MHC molecules. Because of the requirement for antigen presentation by MHC molecules, any polymorphic peptide must carry a motif suitable for MHC-specific binding. Thus, not all individuals can present and respond to all mHags even if there is a difference between donor and recipient. Most mHags are presented to CD8+ T cells by MHC class I molecules. T cell responses are initiated when the T cell receptor recognizes complexes formed by the polymorphic peptides of the mHags bound to the MHC molecules expressed on APCs.

The mHags were originally defined by skin graft rejection and by cytotoxic assays with T cell clones. These polymorphic peptides have restricted binding to class I MHC molecules, so biochemical definition of the minor histocompatibility antigenic peptide components was accomplished by elution, purification, and sequencing of the mHag peptide bound to a specific MHC molecule (den Haan, 1995). Recent studies have demonstrated the potential significance of mHags in clinical transplantation (Goulmy, 1997, 1996; Martin, 1997; Dupont, 1998). mHag-specific cytotoxic T lymphocytes have been demonstrated in patients with GVHD (Mutis, 1999). Recipient disparity for one mHag (HA-1) was associated with increased risk of acute GVHD after marrow transplantation using genotypically HLA-identical sibling donors, although this may not always be the case. Recently, HA-1 disparity has been shown to be associated with ongoing graft-versus-leukemia and suppression of progenitor leukemia cells in some patients (Kircher, 2004; Kloosterboer, 2004). The importance of matching for other mHags (HA-2, HA-3, HA-4, HA-5, H-Y) is less clear. DNA-based techniques to detect differences in mHags have been developed (Tseng, 1998; Wilke, 1998) and are being used in studies to measure the impact of these disparities on the outcome of transplantation.

HLA Nomenclature

SEROLOGIC AND CELLULAR SPECIFICITIES

HLA terminology is designated by a World Health Organization (WHO) Committee for HLA Nomenclature (see Table 48-2) (Bodmer, 1997, 1999). Historically, serologic and cellular defined specificities localized on the HLA protein molecules were assigned according to the results of international workshops during which typing reagents were exchanged among participating laboratories (13th International Histocompatibility Workshop website; see Table 48-1). (The 14th HLA and Immunogenetics Workshop convened during November 2005 in Melbourne, Australia). Assignments included the name of the HLA molecule and a numeric designation based on the order in which the serologically defined specificity was defined. For example, HLA-A1 (or just A1) was the first HLA-A specificity to be assigned, and HLA-A80 was the most recent. Over time, older serologically defined specificities were "split," as the definition became more discriminating. The narrowest definition of the specificity is called the subtypic or private specificity. The broader, shared specificities are called supertypic specificities. For example, B44 and B45 are subtypic specificities of the supertypic specificity B12. Thus, a cell that is either $B44^+$ or $B45^+$ must also be positive for B12.

In serologic testing, some alloantisera bind to more than one HLA allelic product—a phenomenon termed cross-reactivity. This serologic cross-reactivity among allelic products of HLA-A and HLA-B loci has been extensively studied and has been used to cluster molecules within cross-reactive antigen groups (CREGs) (Rodey, 1987). Class I molecules within a CREG share one or more determinants that are not shared by molecules in another CREG. An antigenic determinant (epitope) shared among members of a CREG is called a public specificity. Some of the CREG reactivity can be explained by the sharing of amino acid sequences among the HLA molecules in a CREG (Terasaki, 1992). Inclusion of HLA specificities within a CREG is not standard, as different sets of antibodies produce unique reaction patterns, and two different investigators with different sets of reagents may identify slightly different CREG groups. However, the various CREG groupings overlap considerably (Ellison, 1994). To be able to appropriately name newly discovered HLA alleles, a more logical format for HLA nomenclature assignment was implemented in 2010. This change was defined by the Update to HLA Nomenclature, 2009. The WHO Nomenclature Committee for Factors of the HLA System met during the 15th International Histocompatibility and Immunogenetics Workshop in Buzios, Brazil, in September 2008, and introduced colons into the naming scheme. These colons will allow for the discovery of more than 100 alleles in a given group; the following examples of these changes were listed in the WHO 2008 workshop report, http://hla.alleles.org/pdf/nomenclature_2009.pdf:

A*01010101 becomes A*01:01:01:01.
A*02010102L becomes A*02:01:01:02L.
A*260101 becomes A*26:01:01.
A*3301 becomes A*33:01.
B*0808N becomes B*08:08N.
DRB1*01010101 becomes DRB1*01:01:01:01.

For *antigen groups* that have more than 100 alleles such as the A*02 and B*15 groups, it will be possible to encode these in a single series. Thus the A*92 and B*95 alleles will now be renamed into the A*02 and B*15 allele series. For example,

A*9201 becomes A*02:101.
A*9202 becomes A*02:102.
A*9203 becomes A*02:103.

The HLA-Bw4 and -Bw6 specificities are broad, public epitopes that reside on the same molecule as the HLA-B locus subtypic specificities, but at a different site. Thus Bw4 and Bw6 are a diallelic system, and all B locus (and some A locus) molecules carry either Bw4 or Bw6 specificities. The region of the HLA molecule carrying the Bw4/Bw6 specificities has been identified in the $\alpha 1$ helix between amino acid residues 77 and 83 (Parham, 1991).

The WHO-designated serologic specificities localized to the class II molecules, HLA-DR and -DQ, have been assigned as described for the class I molecules (Bodmer, 1997, 1999) (see Table 48-2). Six HLA-DP types were originally defined by cellular techniques. Class II HLA-DP molecules are not adequately defined serologically.

Twenty-six HLA-D specificities were identified by MLC. All HLA-D specificities retain the "w" designation because these specificities are defined functionally by the measurement of stimulation of a responder cell. This stimulation is generated by differences in the DR molecules expressed on a stimulator cell and, to a lesser extent, by additional stimulation by the DQ and DP molecules.

DNA-BASED ALLELE DESIGNATIONS

Nucleotide sequencing has been used to identify the many different alleles encoding the HLA molecules. Currently, a single, serologically defined specificity may reside on two to more than 25 different allelic products (see Table 48-2). Each HLA allele is designated by the name of the gene locus followed by an asterisk and a four- to seven-digit number indicating the allele. For example, A*0201 is an allele of the HLA-A gene; B*1510 is an allele of the HLA-B gene; DPB1*0101 is an allele of the HLA-DPB1 gene; and DQA1*0601 is an allele of the HLA-DQA1 gene.

The first two numbers in the numeric designation of each allele are frequently based on the serologic type of the resultant molecule and/or the nucleotide sequence similarity to other alleles in the group. For example, the HLA-A molecule expressed by the A*0201 allele bears the A2 serologic specificity defining the HLA-A2 antigen. However, the HLA-B molecule expressed by the B*1510 allele does not bear the B15-associated serologic specificity, but rather the B71 serologic specificity defining the B71 antigen. It was designated B*1510 because of its predicted amino acid sequence similarity to B15 antigens. Cells expressing DRB1*0103 were serologically typed as DR-blank, DR1, or even DR13. Nucleotide sequencing identified an allele with a similar DNA structure to alleles bearing the DR1 serologic specificity (e.g., DRB1*0101 and *0102), and the name of this allele was based on that structural similarity. When a unique serologic specificity was later identified, the DR antigen determined by DRB1*0103 was given the DR103 serologic designation. The third and fourth numbers in the allele designation refer to the order in which the allele was described. For example, A*0201 was the first A2 allele to be sequenced, and A*0203 was the third.

Some alleles may differ in the DNA sequence of their coding regions, but their predicted amino acid sequence does not differ (often termed a silent or synonymous substitution). These combinations of alleles are identified by a five-digit designation. The first four numbers are shared, and the fifth digit is used to distinguish the unique nucleic acid sequences of the alleles (e.g., B*27051 and B*27052). In addition, two or more alleles may have a seven-digit name in which the first four digits are shared (e.g., DRB4*0103101 and DRB4*0103102). Digits five through seven indicate that the two alleles differ only outside the protein coding region. In the example listed here, the difference affects the RNA splice site of DRB4*0103102, resulting in loss of expression of the allele (Sutton, 1989). Finally, alleles that are not expressed as proteins at the cell surface may have an N added to their names (e.g., A*0215N, DRB4*0103102N) to indicate "null." Because each allele has a unique numeric designation, the N designation is not always written (i.e., A*0215 and A*0215N are the same allele).

New alleles are described in regular reports of the WHO HLA Nomenclature Committee (see Table 48-1; www.anthonynolan.com/hig/nomenc.html; Bodmer, 1999), and the nucleotide sequences of all alleles are deposited in a computerized databank (GenBank, EMBL, IMGT/HLA databases). Currently, for example, more than 349 HLA-A alleles have been assigned. New alleles are continually being identified and can be accessed through the website.

Techniques for Identifying HLA Polymorphism

Histocompatibility testing or HLA typing or tissue typing is performed in a limited number of laboratories because it uses specialized procedures and reagents. Commercially available kits can be obtained for both DNA-based and serologic testing; however, interpretation of the test results requires considerable experience and knowledge. Histocompatibility laboratories usually are found in medical centers that have organ and/or hematopoietic progenitor cell transplantation programs. HLA testing techniques are discussed in general in this section. For detailed procedures, the reader should refer to the American Society for Histocompatibility and Immunogenetics (ASHI) Laboratory Manual, 4th edition (2001) (see Table 48-1 for the ASHI website). HLA testing laboratories are accredited through ASHI, the European Foundation for Immunogenetics, and other organizations.

DNA-BASED TYPING OF CLASS I AND CLASS II ALLELES

Although serologic and cellular typing of HLA antigens has been extremely useful, there are a number of technical drawbacks to these techniques. With the advent of rapid and reliable methods for the isolation and characterization of class I and II genes and the determination of nucleotide sequences of class I and II alleles, it has become possible to use DNA-based methods for HLA typing. DNA-based typing of HLA alleles is now a commonly used technique in HLA typing laboratories (Hurley, 1997a; Middleton, 1999).

In contrast to other forms of testing, DNA-based typing has five significant advantages as follows:

1. It is specific. The specificity of each DNA typing reagent (i.e., synthetic oligonucleotide primers and probes) is clearly defined and is based on a specific, known nucleotide sequence. Because the oligonucleotides used as DNA typing reagents are synthetic, reagents are not limited and there should be no lot-to-lot variation in specificity.
2. It is flexible. New reagents can be designed as new alleles are discovered and unique nucleotide sequences identified. Testing can be carried out at several levels of resolution, depending on the typing requirements and the time available for testing.
3. It is more robust than other techniques. DNA typing does not require viable lymphocytes and is not influenced by the health of the patient. Furthermore, DNA-based testing is highly reproducible when standard methods such as sequence specific oligonucleotide probe (SSOP) testing are used in conjunction with a standard test protocol (Ng, 1996; Hurley, 2000a).
4. It can be used for large-scale typing. The batching of samples facilitated by automated and computerized methods reduces cost and errors. DNA-based methods are particularly applicable for the HLA typing of large numbers of volunteers for donor registries.
5. It can discriminate by detecting the full extent of HLA diversity. HLA alleles can specify HLA proteins that are indistinguishable using serologic typing. For example, an individual carrying the DRB1*0401 allele would have the same serologic type (DR4) as an individual carrying the DRB1*0412 allele (DR4). Thus, DRB1*0401 and DRB1*0412 are splits of the broad specificity DR4. These splits are identified by DNA typing. Serologic reagents specific enough to define this split are not available. Currently, more than 30 subdivisions of DR4 have been defined. There are many other examples of splits defined using DNA typing that cannot be identified using serologic typing; some are listed in Table 48-2.

The problems with serologic typing are particularly acute when typing some population groups. For example, populations of direct African origin can express class I and class II antigens that are difficult to identify with currently available serologic reagents (Bozon, 1997; Yu, 1997; Mytilineos, 1998). DNA-based HLA typing has greatly improved the ability to define HLA types in these populations.

Preparation and Amplification of DNA

Any cell with a nucleus can be used as a source of DNA. Although red blood cells do not contain nuclei, other cells in the blood, such as lymphocytes, are a good source of DNA. Cell lines such as Epstein-Barr virus–transformed B lymphocytes are also a good source of DNA. Because transformed cells can be grown in culture in the laboratory, they provide a replenishable supply of DNA and are used to provide reference DNA for quality control of typing procedures.

DNA is usually prepared from a small quantity (0.2–1 mL) of whole blood. Many different protocols can be used to isolate DNA from cells, and commercial kits are available for the preparation of DNA. The sensitivity of detection of HLA types is enhanced greatly by the amplification of DNA-encoding HLA genes using the PCR technique (Saiki, 1988). A pair of synthetic oligonucleotides (primers) should be complementary to sequences flanking a specific HLA gene and are utilized to generate millions of copies of that gene for use in the HLA typing reaction. Some typing reactions utilize primer sequences that are shared by all alleles at an HLA locus; other typing procedures utilize primer sets that are shared by only a subset of alleles at a locus. Annealing of the primers to sample DNA during the PCR reaction uses reaction conditions that guarantee that the primers will bind to perfectly matched sequences (target sequences) and not to sequences of other loci or other alleles that are not matched. By adjusting the temperature of the annealing component of the PCR reaction, the typing laboratory can control the specificity of the amplification.

Sequence-Specific Priming

One method of identification of HLA alleles uses sequence-specific primers (SSPs) in the PCR reaction (Olerup, 1992; Bunce, 1995). These primers anneal to denatured DNA containing the HLA alleles from which the primer sequences were derived. In the subsequent PCR reaction, only these selected alleles are amplified. DNA amplified by the primers is identified by gel electrophoresis or, if the DNA is labeled with a dye during amplification, by fluorescence. This procedure is useful in typing a small number of samples within a short time period. Commercial kits are available.

Sequence-Specific Oligonucleotide Hybridization

It has been possible to use hybridization of SSOPs to amplified DNA to identify alleles (Gao, 1991; Williams, 1997; Cao, 1999). The use of several different oligonucleotide probes to define a specific HLA allele or the use of sequence-specific priming coupled with hybridization with panels of probes is usually required. A set of oligonucleotides capable of identifying each allele is hybridized to denatured PCR-amplified DNA attached to a solid support. Hybridization conditions are adjusted so that the probes will anneal to denatured DNA containing the HLA alleles from which the oligonucleotide sequence was derived. The oligonucleotides are labeled with a tag for detection of hybridization. For example, the oligonucleotide might be coupled to an enzyme such as alkaline phosphatase. Following addition of a substrate, alkaline phosphatase cleaves the substrate to yield a colored compound or to produce light (chemiluminescence). After visualization, the pattern of hybridization can be read to determine the alleles present. Figure 48-10 illustrates the approach using an oligonucleotide probe for the DQB1 allele, DQB1*0302, to identify patients with insulin-dependent diabetes who carry this allele (Todd, 1987). The SSOP method is highly accurate, specific, and reliable (Ng, 1996; Hurley, 2000a). It is often used in situations where many samples are typed in large batches. Commercial kits using this method are available.

In a related procedure, called the reverse format, the oligonucleotide probes are bound to a solid support (Bugawan, 1994). DNA from the samples to be tested is amplified using primers labeled with, for example, biotin. The amplified DNA is then hybridized to the immobilized probes, which contain sequences found in the alleles present in the DNA. After visualization (using an avidin-linked detection system), the pattern of hybridization can be read to determine the alleles present. This procedure is useful for typing both small and large numbers of samples. Commercial kits utilizing this method are available.

Sequence-Specific Conformational Polymorphism or Heteroduplex Analysis

Another, although little used, method of identification of HLA alleles analyzes the mobility of amplified DNA, either denatured (sequence-specific conformational polymorphism [SSCP]) or as a renatured DNA duplex (heteroduplex analysis), following electrophoresis (Arguello, 1996). The mobility of the DNA is compared with the mobility of amplified DNA from known HLA alleles to define an HLA allele. This procedure is useful in typing a small number of samples, particularly in comparisons between individuals, for example, within a family.

```
            50                                               60
DQB1*0501  GTG ACG CCG CAG GGG CGG CCT GTT GCC GAG TAC
DQB1*0601  --- --C --- --- --- --- --- -AC --- --- ---
DQB1*0201  --- --- -T- -T- --- -T- --- -CC --- --- ---
DQB1*0301  --- --- --- -T- --- -C- --- -AC --- --- ---

DQB1*0302  --- --- --- -T- [--- -C- --- -CC ---] --- ---

DQB1*0303  --- --- --- -T- --- -C- --- -AC --- --- ---
DQB1*0401  --- --- --- -T- --- --- -T- -AC --- --- ---
```

A

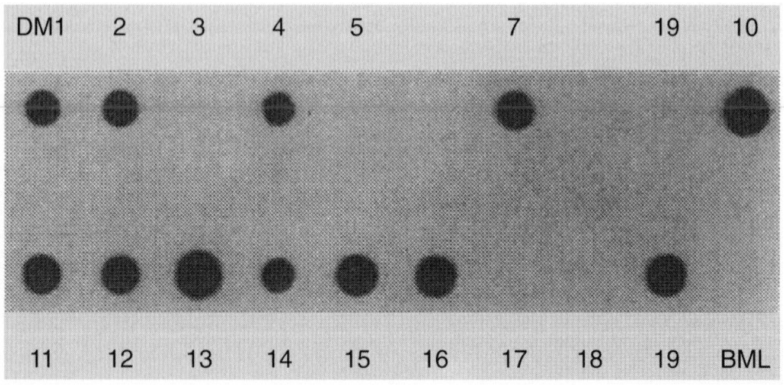

B

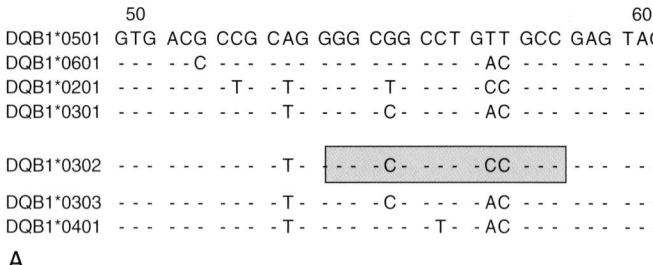

Figure 48-10 **A,** Nucleotide sequences of several DQB1 alleles. The sequences presented cover the codons for amino acids 50–60. A dash indicates that the nucleotide is identical to the top sequence. An oligonucleotide that is specific for the DQB1*0302 sequence is boxed. **B,** Oligonucleotide dot blot analysis of 17 insulin-dependent diabetes mellitus patients (DM1–19) and one control, BML. Amplified DNA containing class II DQB1 sequences for the patients was attached to a membrane and hybridized to the labeled oligonucleotide specific for the DQB1*0302 sequence (described previously). Positive hybridization signals indicate the patients who carry this DBQ1 gene sequence (patients DM1, 2, 4, 7, 10–16, 19). *(With permission from Todd JA, Bell J, McDevitt HO. HLA-DQ β gene contributes to susceptibility and resistance to insulin-dependent diabetes mellitus. Nature 1987;329:599.)*

Nucleic Acid Sequencing

A final method of identification of HLA alleles involves direct determination of the DNA sequences of the HLA alleles carried by an individual (sequence-based typing [SBT]). Alleles may be identified following PCR amplification to separate the alleles based on SSPs, or as a mixture of two alleles. Sequencing is labor-intensive and highly complex but will be used frequently to determine the HLA match at an allele level between hematopoietic progenitor cell transplant patients and their prospective donors (Petersdorf, 1995a; Rozemuller, 1996; Scheltinga, 1997). Efforts to develop automated SBT methods have yielded several potentially promising high-throughput approaches. These include the use of denaturing high-performance liquid chromatography (HPLC), which is reported to provide greater typing resolution than can be achieved by PCR-based sequencing approaches (Etokebe, 2003), and the so-called pyrosequencing technique. Pyrosequencing is a real-time, nonelectrophoretic DNA sequencing method that uses luciferase–luciferin light emission as a detection signal as nucleotides are incorporated into target DNA. A unique signal is created for each allelic variant, which is distinguished by recognition software (Nordstrom, 2000). Pyrosequencing by means of high-throughput systems permits processing of hundreds of individual specimens daily. In addition, reference-strand-mediated conformational analysis (RSCA) has been employed in high-throughput systems to achieve discrimination between HLA alleles differing by as little as one nucleotide. The technology detects differences between alleles by measuring their conformation-dependent mobility in polyacrylamide gels after they have been labeled with locus-specific fluorescent tags (Arguello, 1998).

Resolution of DNA-Based Typing

The level of resolution (i.e., the ability to discriminate among alleles) obtained by DNA typing methods is controlled by the choice and number of primers and/or probes used in the assay and the typing method. This choice may depend on the time available for performing the typing, the cost of the typing, the expertise of the laboratory personnel, and the purpose of the typing. Large-scale donor registry typing is usually carried out at low to intermediate resolution, while typing of a potential hematopoietic progenitor cell donor for a specific patient is carried out at allele-level resolution.

A multistep approach is often used to identify HLA alleles by DNA-based typing. For this reason, HLA types defined by DNA-based typing may be reported at different levels of resolution. Low-resolution (or generic or serologic)-level DNA-based typing produces a result that is similar in appearance and detail to a serologic type. For example, a DNA-defined type, DRB1*11 or DRB1*11XX, is the approximate equivalent of the serologic type DR11. The "XX" indicates that the allele was not further defined. At this level of resolution, it is not possible to determine which of the more than 30 DRB1*11 alleles is carried by the individual being tested. Although serologic typing can be as informative as low-resolution typing, results are more reliable with DNA-based testing. Intermediate resolution–level DNA-based typing may narrow the choices by listing several different possibilities for the type of an individual (e.g., DRB1*1101 or DRB1*1104). Finally, high resolution–level (or allele-level) DNA-based typing identifies the specific allele carried by an individual (e.g., DRB1*1104). Because identification of HLA alleles may be based on partial sequence information, it is possible that interpretation of the results will miss alleles that were unknown at the time of the typing (Hurley, 1997b). For this reason, laboratories are cautioned to maintain their raw typing data (i.e., which primers and probes were positive and negative and the nucleotide sequences of the reagents) so that the results can be reinterpreted as new alleles are described.

SEROLOGIC DETECTION OF CLASS I AND CLASS II MOLECULES

Lymphocyte microcytotoxicity testing, which originally was used in the mouse system by Gorer and Amos and later was modified by Terasaki and McClelland for use in the human system, has been used for HLA typing since the 1960s. Serologic testing for HLA-A, -B can be reproducible under controlled, standardized conditions; however, in large-scale testing (e.g., for registries), error rates may increase (Bozon, 1997; Yu, 1997). The reproducibility for serologically determined HLA-C and class II specificities is much lower. HLA-DP is not usually defined by serology. The microcytotoxicity serologic assay still is used fairly widely for class I specificities (HLA-A, -B) but has been supplanted by DNA-based testing for HLA-C and for class II specificities (HLA-DR, -DQ, -DP) in most typing laboratories. DNA-based testing with its greater resolution is used to determine the HLA type of unrelated individuals and of family members, especially if the segregation of HLA cannot be accurately discriminated by serology (e.g., families where parents are not available, families where parents share an HLA antigen). For example, an offspring inherits DR4 from each parent and so is DR4 antigen homozygous (DR4,DR4). However, high-resolution DNA typing might identify two distinct alleles of the DR4 antigen, DRB1*0401 and DRB1*0403 (DRB1*04 allele heterozygote), providing informative data for haplotype segregation analysis.

Lymphocyte Preparation

Lymphocytes used routinely in HLA serologic typing assays are readily obtained from peripheral whole blood by layering onto a Ficoll-Hypaque gradient to separate the blood cells by density centrifugation. The separated peripheral blood lymphocytes (PBLs) can be used for HLA-A, -B, -C typing. To test for HLA-DR, -DQ serologic specificities, it is necessary to enrich for B lymphocytes, or to use a special two-color fluorescent technique to simultaneously differentiate between unseparated B cells and T cells.

Lymphocyte Microcytotoxicity Assay

The HLA phenotype is determined by testing the unseparated lymphocyte preparation (PBL) or T lymphocytes (for HLA-A, -B, -C) or the enriched B lymphocytes (for HLA-DR, -DQ) against a panel of well-characterized HLA alloantisera. The assay is a two-stage test. During the sensitization stage, the lymphocytes are incubated with the antisera. Prescreened and standardized rabbit serum as a source of complement is added in excess, and the mixture is incubated for an additional period. If the lymphocytes carry a cell surface molecule recognized by complement-fixing antibodies in the alloantiserum, the antibodies bind to the cells and the cells are subsequently lysed following the addition of complement. The assay is terminated with the addition of fluorescein diacetate and ethidium bromide for fluorescent detection procedures, or of eosin and formalin or trypan blue and ethylenediaminetetraacetic acid for dye visualization methods. Reactions are read for percentage lysis and are numerically graded.

TABLE 48-3

Therapeutic Drugs, Mechanisms of Action, and Monitoring Methods

Drug	Mechanisms of action	Monitoring methods*
Azathioprine	Purine antagonist; blocks cell proliferation	Routine labs, pharmacokinetic studies, pharmacodynamic studies
Glucocorticoids	Blocks cytokine gene transcription; inhibits T cell proliferation and T cell–dependent immunity	Routine labs, pharmacokinetic studies
Cyclosporine	Inhibits expression of nuclear regulatory proteins and T cell activation genes	Routine labs, pharmacokinetic studies, pharmacodynamic studies
FK506	Inhibits expression of nuclear regulatory proteins and T cell activation genes	Routine labs, pharmacokinetic studies
Mycophenolate mofetil	Inhibits purine biosynthesis, thereby suppressing T and B cell proliferation	Routine labs, pharmacokinetic studies, pharmacodynamic studies
Rapamycin	Inhibits DNA and protein synthesis, blocking T cell proliferation; inhibits antigen-driven B cell proliferation	Routine labs, pharmacokinetic studies, pharmacodynamic studies

Adapted from Massey D, King A, Riley R. Renal allograft dysfunction in kidney transplant. American Society for Clinical Pathology, Clinical Chemistry Check Sample 2003;43:19–38.

*Routine labs include serum creatinine, blood urea nitrogen (BUN), complete blood count (CBC), liver enzymes, etc. Pharmacokinetic studies include measurement of trough levels and calculation of area under the curve (AUC). Pharmacodynamic study refers to measuring the biological effects of the drug at its target site.

HLA Typing Sera Trays

HLA typing reagents are derived from the sera of alloimmunized individuals (multiparous women, transplant recipients, multitransfused patients, and planned immunization of humans). Multiwell plates of human alloantisera (i.e., HLA typing trays) are commercially available. Because of the antigenic complexity of HLA antigens, several antisera should be used to define each specificity. Most laboratories use trays from at least two different vendors or may use locally derived alloantisera. Because many alloantisera are not truly monospecific and many exhibit some cross-reactivity, the reactivity of each antiserum must be thoroughly tested and known to the individual interpreting the results. This requires stringent quality control of each new lot of typing trays with well-characterized reference cells. The titer and the specificity of antibody formed by a sensitized individual may not remain constant over time; therefore, supplies of antisera are limited. In an attempt to create a consistent and unlimited supply of reagents, some companies have produced monoclonal antibodies. These monoclonal reagents are not available for all HLA specificities.

Cross-Reactivity

HLA alloantisera may react with more than one HLA allelic product. This phenomenon can result from polyspecificity of the antisera and/or from cross-reactivity and is responsible for the complex reactivity patterns of some alloantisera. Polyspecific sera contain two or more HLA-specific antibodies that can be adsorbed to remove one antibody with little effect on the reactivity of the other(s). Cross-reactive antisera contain, most frequently, a single antibody that reacts with an antigenic determinant shared among several different HLA allelic products (i.e., CREG or broad determinants, as previously discussed) (Rodey, 1994). Cross-reactions occur most frequently among allelic products encoded by the same locus but can occur between allelic products encoded by different loci (e.g., A2 + B17).

CELLULAR DETECTION OF CLASS II MOLECULES

The response of one cell in tissue culture to the alloantigens on the surface of a second cell is called the mixed leukocyte culture or mixed lymphocyte reaction (Hartzman, 1971). The MLC is considered an in vitro measure of class II disparity between individuals that recognizes determinants found on class II molecules, which are known collectively as HLA-D. The T cell response is made unidirectional by preventing cells from one of the two individuals from replicating by treating those cells with radiation or mitomycin C prior to addition to the culture. The MLC represents a summation response of a responder cell to differences in the multiple determinants on HLA class II molecules (DR, DQ, and DP) encoded by the irradiated stimulator cell haplotypes. The response to DR molecules appears to predominate.

Use of the MLC in clinical laboratories to determine histocompatibility has declined because of limitations inherent in the technique. The MLC can be influenced by the health of the patient, the type of disease, and the history of prior transfusion (Mickelson, 1996). For these reasons, the MLC assay has been replaced by more precise DNA-based typing methods. Currently, in some transplantation centers, the MLC is used to identify renal allograft recipients with specific hyporeactivity to donor HLA molecules following transplantation as a guideline for tapering of immunosuppression (Reinsmoen, 1993).

Limiting dilution analysis to define the frequency of donor cytotoxic or helper T lymphocytes has been used to predict the extent of allorecognition in hematopoietic progenitor cell transplantation (Madrigal, 1997). The correlations of these frequencies with subsequent events such as the extent of GVHD is still controversial.

TISSUE/ORGAN TRANSPLANTATION

Long-term survival of solid organ and hematopoietic progenitor cell grafts represents one of the most challenging goals in medical science. Renal transplantation is the therapy of choice for most patients with end-stage renal disease. Hematopoietic progenitor cell, heart, lung, liver, and pancreas transplantation is gaining wide acceptance as a therapeutic procedure with successful outcomes. The primary obstacle to solid organ and to hematopoietic progenitor cell transplantation is immunologically mediated rejection of the foreign tissue. Therefore, the success of allografting is dependent on the ability to deter the immune reaction, which may be accomplished by (1) histocompatibility matching between the donor and the recipient; (2) immunosuppressive therapy of the recipient (see Table 48-3 for a list of common immunosuppression drugs and laboratory approaches used to monitor them) (Suthanthiran, 1996); and (3) ultimately achieving specific unresponsiveness to donor alloantigen(s) (i.e., tolerance) (Remuzzi, 1995).

GENETIC BASIS OF TRANSPLANTATION

The genetic basis of transplantation was first determined in 1916 as a result of tumor transplantation experiments in mice and was subsequently extended to transplants of normal tissue (Snell, 1981). It was demonstrated that skin grafts within inbred strains that were homozygous at histocompatibility loci (i.e., syngeneic grafts) were successful, but grafts between two different inbred strains (allografts) were rejected. Furthermore, allografts from either parent inbred strain (two copies of the same MHC genes; homozygous) to first-generation (F1) hybrids (one copy of each of the two different sets of MHC genes from two homozygous parents) survived in all animals, whereas grafts from F1 hybrid offspring to either parent (one haplotype mismatch) did not survive. These observations established the laws of transplantation. In 1948, the factors or genes determining the fate of allografts were named histocompatibility or H genes. Also in 1948, the major histocompatibility locus in the mouse, H-2, was defined by Gorer (Snell, 1981). There are other histocompatibility or H antigens, which are termed mHags. Although called minor, mismatching for these antigens can have major effects (Goulmy, 1997; Dupont, 1998).

Because convincing evidence already existed in experimental animal models that molecules encoded by the MHC represent the major genetic barrier to successful allografting, HLA typing was used in humans to determine and to optimize compatibility between graft donor and recipient. Initially, the influence of HLA antigens on graft survival was investigated by grafting of nonvascularized skin between family members. As in studies with inbred mice, skin grafts between HLA-identical siblings survived significantly longer than grafts between one-haplotype–matched siblings, parents, or unrelated donors. These observations were extended to renal transplantation during the late 1960s and early 1970s. The most recent data from the international Collaborative Transplant Study (CTS) in Heidelberg and from the United Network for Organ Sharing (UNOS) Registry in the United States (analyzed at University of California, Los Angeles) confirm the MHC as the major genetic barrier to transplantation for renal grafts (Cecka, 1999; Opelz, 1999) (Fig. 48-11); for current updates, see the websites listed in Table 48-1. The data for hematopoietic progenitor cell transplantation also reaffirm the role of the MHC in transplant outcome as measured by both patient survival and GVHD (Hansen, 1999) (Fig. 48-12).

HISTOCOMPATIBILITY MATCHING

HLA Matching

Although the level of HLA match is an important element in transplant outcome, histocompatibility matching means different things in different settings, and strategies for matching vary. Criteria differ with variables that include the type of graft (e.g., solid vascularized organ vs. hematopoietic progenitor cell), the disease (e.g., chronic myelogenous leukemia vs. aplastic anemia), the age of the patient, and the clinical protocol (e.g., marrow vs. umbilical cord blood; T cell depletion of marrow vs. non–T cell depletion) (see Chapter 38).

Matching usually includes evaluation of at least three loci: HLA-A, HLA-B, and HLA-DR. Individuals matched, at whatever resolution, for all three loci are termed 6/6 matches or 0 mismatches. Zero mismatches (a term used in solid organ transplantation) may also refer to donor/recipient pairs where the donor has no detectable HLA differences from the recipient, that is, where the donor is homozygous for the alleles at one or more of the loci (e.g., homozygous donor: A*0101; B*0801; DRB1*0301; heterozygous recipient: A*0101, A*0301; B*0801, B*0702; DRB1*0301, DRB1*1501). Individuals matched for four of six alleles or antigens are termed 4/6 matches. Apparent differences in the level of match can arise because of the typing method used to assign HLA types (e.g., serologic vs. DNA-based typing). The serologic and DNA nomenclatures, although they are related, can differ. The definition of a match can also vary depending on the typing resolution. A patient and a donor may appear to be matched at the serologic level (e.g., recipient: A2, A26; donor: A2, A26); however, the pair may be mismatched at the level of HLA alleles (e.g., recipient: A*0201, A*2601; donor: A*0205, A*6601).

Matching for classical HLA molecules at the allele level could optimize outcome for all grafts (both vascular organs and hematopoietic progenitor cells) (Petersdorf, 1998; Opelz, 1999). However, because of the extremely large number of HLA alleles, allelic-level matching is difficult. Therefore, the level of matching that ensures a good outcome for the largest number of patients of all ethnic populations must be considered.

Following hematopoietic progenitor cell transplantation, subtypic determinants or allelic differences initiate important cytotoxic T cell responses leading to graft rejection and GVHD. Indeed, studies have shown that high-resolution matching for class I and class II alleles of the donor and recipient can improve outcome after unrelated marrow

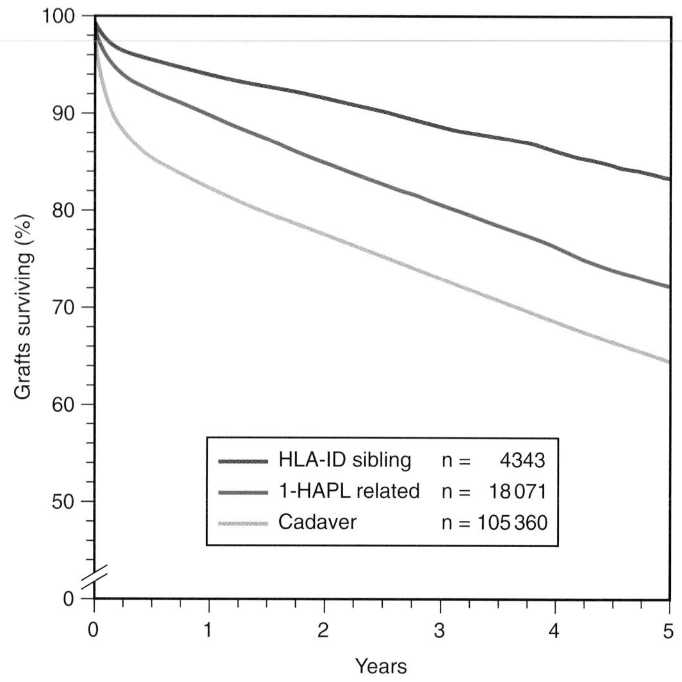

Figure 48-11 Five-year renal allograft (first transplant) survival of three categories of histocompatibility: human leukocyte antigen (HLA)-identical siblings; one-haplotype living-related; cadaver donor. Grafts from HLA-identical sibling donors (both HLA chromosomes matched) have the best outcomes. Numbers of transplants studied are indicated (regression, $p < 0.0001$). *(With permission from Opelz G, Wujcak T, Dohler B, et al. HLA compatibility and organ transplant survival. Rev Immunogenet 1999;1:334.)*

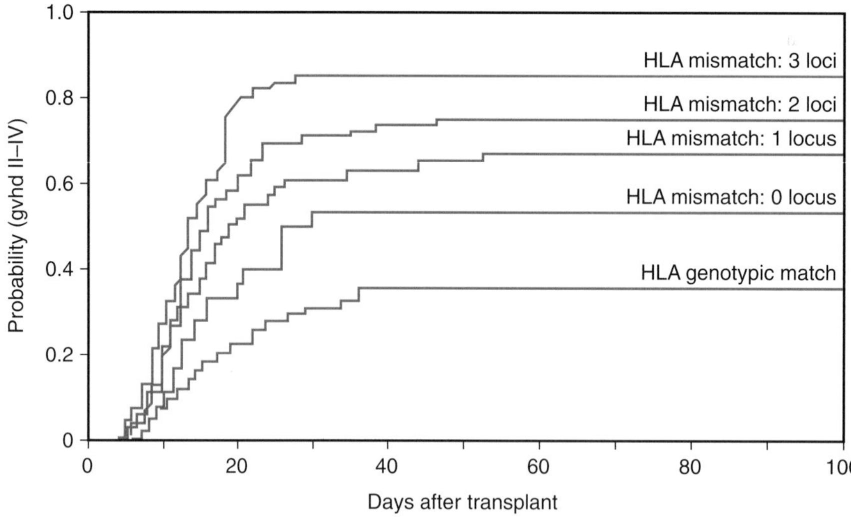

Figure 48-12 Probability of grades II–IV acute graft-versus-host disease (GVHD) in human leukocyte antigen (HLA)-identical sibling (HLA genotypic match) and haploidentical related marrow donor transplants variably matched for HLA-A, -B, or DR/Dw (HLA mismatch: 3 loci, 2 loci, 1 locus, or 0 loci). Matching for HLA-A, -B, and -DR was defined by serology, and matching for HLA-Dw was defined by mixed leukocyte culture (MLC) or by typing for HLA-DRB1 alleles with sequence specific oligonucleotide probe (SSOP). All patients received unmodified marrow (without T cell depletion) following a conditioning regimen that included total body irradiation. Cyclosporine and methotrexate were given for GVHD prophylaxis. *(With permission from Hansen JA, Yamamoto K, Petersdorf E, et al. The role of HLA matching in hematopoietic cell transplantation. Rev Immunogenet 1999;1:359. Copyright © 1999 Munksgaard International Publishers, Copenhagen, Denmark.)*

transplantation. Recent data suggest that multiple mismatches are detrimental to outcome; however, the impact of neither single mismatches nor specific loci has yet been well defined (Petersdorf, 1998; Sasazuki, 1998; Hansen, 1999). With respect to single allele mismatches and their impact on transplantation, a report by Flomenberg (2004) describes a differential impact of HLA mismatches at specific loci between donor and recipients; this multivariate analysis of more than 1800 donor–recipient pairs showed that single allele mismatches at HLA-C adversely affected engraftment; mismatches at HLA-A, -B, -C, and -DR were significant in terms of grade III–IV acute GVHD incidence, and in that the highest effect on this disease was given by mismatches at HLA-A, whether this was acute or chronic GVHD; mismatches at HLA-A, -B, -C, and -DR showed significant effects on mortality, and again HLA-A mismatches demonstrated the largest impact on survival, perhaps because single allele mismatches at this locus appeared to induce resistant GVHD. Only a minority of patients awaiting transplantation will receive grafts from fully allele-matched donors (Hurley, 2000b). To enable all patients to benefit from life-saving transplantation, identifying allele mismatches that are well tolerated would allow the selection of mismatched donors to be prioritized according to the biological risk of specific HLA mismatches.

Optimal matching for solid organ grafts may differ from matching requirements for hematopoietic progenitor cell transplantation. Recent data suggest that both the HLA loci matched and the level of resolution of HLA testing contribute to renal graft outcome (Opelz, 1999). Currently, UNOS facilitates sharing of cadaveric kidneys based on subtypic specificities. Because subtypic matches are infrequently identified, it has been proposed that the HLA class I molecules should be matched for the broader CREG determinants. CREG may define immunodominant determinants recognized in the humoral immune response. Rodey (1994) showed that 80%–90% of the HLA alloantibodies formed by kidney recipients following transplantation are directed to CREG determinants. CREG determinants are shared among different class I HLA molecules and, in contrast to subtypic specificities, have a similar distribution among ethnic population groups. Rare subtypic specificities are included within the CREG. Because the number of CREGs is less than the number of subtypic specificities, the probability of a CREG-level match is greater than for a subtypic or allele-level HLA class I match. Therefore, allocation of organs based on CREG matching should result in a higher probability of matched grafts being distributed equitably to recipients of all ethnic populations. CREG matching for the allocation of kidneys has been characterized as immunologically flawed, and its observed positive effect in prolonging graft survival and reducing immunosuppressant requirements has been attributed entirely to the effect of HLA matching (Egfjord, 2003). Others cite a positive role for CREG matching in reducing HLA sensitization among minority recipients of renal transplants (Crowe, 2003).

Other strategies focus on matching for biologically relevant fragments of MHC molecules (e.g., epitope matching) (Suciu-Foca, 1998; Harris, 1999). Until recently, direct recognition of alloantigens was thought to be the main pathway for graft rejection responses. However, studies suggest that the indirect response plays a significant role in graft rejection, at least of solid organ grafts (Sayegh, 1996). If the indirect pathway is activated, then the peptide epitopes generated by proteolytic breakdown of the HLA molecule and not the HLA molecule itself would be the immunogenic stimulus. Therefore, new innovative strategies can be designed for defining allowable mismatches based on recognition of the peptide fragments. For example, a strategy could consider whether the mismatched donor HLA molecules would be perceived as immunogenic in the recipient (i.e., whether the recipient HLA molecules would bind and present these epitopes). Theoretically, one could identify foreign HLA peptide sequences not presented by specific recipient HLA molecules and thus define allowable mismatches for given HLA molecules. The introduction of solid-based methods (Luminex, enzyme-linked immunosorbent assay [ELISA], and flow cytometry methods) for detecting antibodies to HLA molecules, in which eluted HLA molecules from cells are bound to polystyrene beads (or polystyrene microtiter plates), has allowed the more accurate identification of antibodies generated by patients awaiting transplantation. It is now possible to group HLA molecules based on the immunogenic epitope that is shared among them, thus allowing for better selection of donors for transplantation. The level of sensitization is more accurately interrogated by beads carrying a single HLA molecule, and absorption of alloantisera with these beads elucidates the epitope that the antibody is directed to and can be inferred by testing the unabsorbed and the absorbed serum with a panel of single-antigen beads; reduced panel reactivity in the absorbed serum defines the epitope specificity, and the HLA molecules that carry the epitope can be determined by evaluating Tables 48-4 and 48-5. Marrari (2009) and El-Awar (2007) have reported several epitopes or Eplets shared by multiple HLA class I and II molecules; some laboratories are currently using these epitope tables to determine unacceptable antigens in donors based on the patient's immune reactivity assessed using single-antigen Luminex bead methods and the HLAMatchmaker algorithm (Valentini et al., 2007), which predicts some of these epitopes.

The inherent complexity in interpretation of HLA typing results and in selection of a donor makes it critical to include an expert in histocompatibility testing. Experts in HLA typing will know the strengths and weaknesses of each method of typing, as well as the frequency of alleles and haplotypes in the population; this information is important in both the search for and the selection of a suitable donor.

HLA-Specific Antibody Detection in Recipient Serum

Patients can be sensitized to specific foreign HLA molecules through transfusion, pregnancy, or prior transplantations. Assessment of compatibility between the recipient and the possible donor includes testing for this sensitization. Recipient serum is tested prior to transplantation on a panel (lymphocytes or immobilized soluble HLA molecules) of known HLA profile to measure panel reactive antibody (PRA). At the time of transplantation, the recipient serum is tested with the prospective donor lymphocytes to identify specific reactivity to the potential donor in the donor-specific crossmatch. Although the techniques used to detect antibody binding may differ among laboratories, the purpose remains to obtain a profile of the immunologic risk factors of a recipient on the waiting list, which will aid the medical team in both pretransplantation and posttransplantation decisions. Binding of antibody in the current serum of the recipient to the T lymphocytes of the donor is a contraindication to renal transplantation.

Serum Screening (PRA)

Thorough characterization of the antibody profile in patients awaiting transplantation aids in interpretation of the pretransplantation donor-specific crossmatch. The goals of a PRA screen are as follows:

1. To identify the level of presensitization of the patient to HLA antigens. A patient with PRA in excess of 60% (i.e., serum from the patient reacts to specificities found in at least 60% of the panel) has a decreased likelihood of a negative donor-specific crossmatch and thus of receiving a transplant from an unrelated transplant.
2. To identify the HLA specificity of the antibodies to predict the HLA antigen(s) to be avoided when donors are selected.
3. To identify patients with irrelevant antibodies (e.g., immunoglobulin [Ig]M autoantibodies) so that appropriate techniques may be selected to avoid false-positive readings at the time of the donor-specific crossmatch.

Characterization of HLA-specific antibody present in the recipient serum requires testing on a selected panel of well-defined HLA specificities. Lymphocytes or soluble antigen from a sufficient number of individuals must be included in the screening panel to ensure that all but the rarest HLA-directed antibody will be detected. As far as possible, the screening panel should remain the same so that results are comparable over time. Renal transplantation recipients frequently form antibodies to CREGs rather than to subtypic specificities (Rodey, 1994, 1997), so the analyses of panel reactivity should consider identification of CREG, as well as of subtypic specificities. Identification of antibody specificities in patients awaiting transplantation aids in preselecting a potential donor for whom the recipient will have a negative final crossmatch. Computer programs assist in this selection (Claas, 1999; Duquesnoy, 1999).

The frequency of screening and the selection of assays used for the screening procedure are decisions based on the immunologic profile of the individual recipient. Decreased use of blood transfusions has negated the requirement for screening monthly serum samples on all patients (ASHI website; see Table 48-1). The presence of both HLA class I– and class II–specific antibodies is detected by serum testing on a panel of lymphocytes (e.g., by direct complement-dependent cytotoxicity or antiglobulin-augmented cytotoxicity assays) or on a panel of soluble HLA molecules immobilized on plates (i.e., ELISA) or on beads (i.e., flow cytometry). (The assays are described in detail in the ASHI manual [2001].) An advantage of the solid-phase soluble antigen assay is that it can be designed to detect only IgG, HLA class I–specific antibodies.

TABLE 48-4
Cross-Reactive Class I HLA Molecules Based on Epitope Sharing as Defined by Single-Antigen Bead Testing and HLAMatchmaker Algorithm

El-Awar, Terasaki, TerEp	Class I antibody reactive antigens	Marrari and Duquesnoy eplets
13	A01,02,03,11,24,36,68,69,80	143TK [145H/R] like 144TKR or 144TKH
238	A01,02,03,11,25,26,29,32,33,34,36,43,66,68,69,74; B57,58,63	65RA+56G [66K/N; 67M/V]
242	A01,02,03,1101,26,29,30,31,33,34,36,43,66,68,69,74,80	79GT+19E
208	A01,03,11,24,36,80	144KR
241	A01,11,25,26,34,36,43,6601,80	90D+m138M
16	A01,11,25,26,34,36,43,6601,80; B73; Cw04,06,07,18	90D
12	A01,11,25,26,43,6601	163R [166D/E; 167G/W]
14	A01,23,2402,80; B76	167DG (old166DG)
15	A01,26,29,36,43,80	76ANT
1	A01,36	44KM/152HA(151HA)/158V
201	A02	66RKH
210	A02,03,11,68,69	143TK+76VD [145H/R]
19	A02,23,24,68,69	127K
38	A02,25,26,29,31,32,33,34,43,66,68,69,74; B73; Cw07,17	253Q
18	A02,68,69	142MT/145H
2	A02,69	107W
17	A02; B57,58	62GE
6	A03	161D
404	A11	151AHA (149AAH)
209	A11,25,26,43,6601	163RW
30	A1102	19K
27	A203,25,26,34,43,66	150TAH (149TAH)
211	A203,25,26,34,43,66; B46,62,76	158WA
202	A23	65GKA+152RV/152RV+163TG
3	A23,24	65GKA
24	A23,24,25,32; B13,2705,37,38,44,47,49,51,52,53,57,58, 59,63,77	82LR (Aw,Bw)
23	A23,24,25,32; B38,49,51,52,53,57,58,59,63,77	79RI
212	A23,24,32; B38,49,51,52,53,57,58,59,63,77	79RI+90A
28	A23,24,80	62EE
213	A23,25,26,29,30,31,32,33,34,43,66,74	144QR+m138M
407	A24	65GKA+152HV/152HV+79RI/145KRA+79RI/142MI+151AHV
203	A2402	152HV+166DG
214	A25,26,33,34,66,68,69	62RN+m43Q
243	A25,26,33,34,66,68,69; B63	62RR [63E/N; 66K/N]
4	A25,26,34,43,66	145QRT
5	A29,43	62LQ
36	A30	17RS
31	A30,31	56R
204	A32,74; B08,18,37,38,39,41,42,54,55,59,64,65,67; Cw01,04,05,06,08,12,14,16,18	109L+163TW
215	A33,34,68,69; B08,18,37,38,39,41,42,54,55,59,64,65,67	62RN+193TW
220	A3301; B18,51,52,64,65,78	166EWH+103V
206	A36	44KM+163TW/152HA+163TW
222	A6602; B07,13,27,47,48,60,61,73,81; Cw02,17	163EW (163E)
29	A80	56E/163EG
408	B07	177DK
25	B07,08,18,2708,35,39,4005,41,42,45,46,48,50,54,55,56, 60,61,62,64,65,67,71,72,73,75,76,78,81,82; Cw01,03,07,08,12,14,16	79RN
216	B07,08,18,2708,35,39,4005,41,42,45,48,50,54,55,56,60, 61,62,64,65,67,71,72,75,76,78,81,82	80ERN (Bw6)
20	B07,08,41,42,48,60,81	180E
235	B07,13,27,47,48,60,61,73,81	65QI+163EW [62N/R; 67C/S/V; 70K/N/Q]
223	B07,13,27,47,48,60,61,81	76ER+163EW [77E/N/S; 80N/T]
224	B07,27,42,54,55,56,57,58,63,67,73,81,82	69AT [65Q/R; 70K/Q/S]
401	B07,27,42,54,55,56,57,58,63,67,81,82	69AT+76ER [7D/N/S; 80N/T]
229	B07,27,42,54,55,56,67,73,81,82	65QIA
11	B08	66QIF+71NT

TABLE 48-4

Cross-Reactive Class I HLA Molecules Based on Epitope Sharing as Defined by Single-Antigen Bead Testing and HLAMatchmaker Algorithm—*Cont'd*

El-Awar, Terasaki, TerEp	Class I antibody reactive antigens	Marrari and Duquesnoy eplets
22	B08,13,18,35,37,38,39,3905,4005,41,44,45,47,48,49,50, 51,52,53,59,60,61,62,64,65,71,72,75,76,77,78	71NT
227	B08,18,35,39,4005,41,45,48,50,60,61,62,64,65,71,72,75, 76,78	65QIT+73TS/65QIT+79RN/71NT+79RN
226	B08,18,37,38,39,41,42,54,55,59,64,65,67	62RQI+163TW [67C/F/S/Y; 70N/Q]
225	B08,59	66QIF+163TW
420	B08,64,65	71NT+163TW+158A
8	B13	144QL (144TQL)
217	B13,2705,37,44,47	79RT
21	B13,4005,41,44,45,47,49,50,60,61	41T
218	B13,57,62,63,75,76,77	76E+45RMA [77N/S; 80N/T]
35	B18,35,37,51,52,53,58,78	44RT
219	B18,35,37,51,52,53,78	44RT+71NT
228	B18,37,38,39,54,55,56,64,65,67	131S+163T
406	B2705	71KA+79RT/65QIA+79RT/44RE+73TD
411	B2708	71KA+80ERN/66QIK+73TS
221	B35,4005,46,49,50,51,52,53,56,57,58,62,63,71,72,75, 77,78	131S+163LW
245	B35,4005,46,49,50,51,52,53,56,57,58,62,63,71,72,75, 77,78; Cw09,10	163LW , 163L
9	B38,39,67	158T
230	B38,49,51,52,53,59,77	65QIT+79RI/71NT+79RI
10	B46	44RM+71QA
415	B46,57,58,63; Cw09,10	71AT+163LW
403	B46,62,75,76,77	45RMA+79RN
239	B46,73	80VM+M43p
246	B46,73; Cw01,07,08,09,10,12,14,16	80VRN
421	B46; Cw01,08,09,10,14,16	77TVS
419	B49,51,52,63,77	79RI+152RE
414	B49,52,63	62RE+76ENI
232	B54,55,59; Cw01,04,05,06,07,08,12,14,15,16,18	103L+163TW
236	B57,58	62GR+m43P/62GE+71SA/62GE+163LW/71SA+152RV
207	B57,58,63	71SA (70ASA)
237	B57,63,weak B58	44RM+71SA
409	B63	62RR+m43P [63E/N; 66K/N]
402/410	B07,42,54,55,56,67,81,82	70IAQ
41	B73; Cw07,17	267QE
240	B76	163LG
244	Cw02,04,05,06,15,17,18	79RK
40	Cw05,08	46GE/177KT
37	Cw07	193PL/267MQ/273SE
39	Cw02,09,10,15	21H

These antigen groups were generated from reports by Marrari M, Duquesnoy RJ. Correlations between Terasaki's HLA class II epitopes and HLAMatchmaker-defined eplets on HLA-DR and -DQ antigens. Tissue Antigens 2009;74:134–46; Marrari M, Duquesnoy, RJ. Correlations between Terasaki's HLA class I epitopes and HLAMatchmaker-defined eplets on HLA-A, -B and -C antigens. Tissue Antigens 2009;74:117–33; and El-Awar NR, Akaza T, Terasaki PI, Nguyen A. Human leukocyte antigen I epitopes: update to 103 total epitopes, including C locus. Transplantation 2007;84:532–40.

Serum samples from potential recipients should be stored at −70° C and protected from carbon dioxide and from evaporation. The stored characterized serum samples will be used in the donor-specific crossmatch to assess compatibility with a prospective donor.

Donor-Specific Crossmatch

The lymphocyte crossmatch tests for the presence of antibodies, if any, in the serum of the potential recipient that react with lymphocytes of the specific donor. In the crossmatch test, the lymphocyte is the target cell of choice because it expresses high levels of HLA molecules and is easy to isolate. This test is probably the most important contribution of the HLA tissue typing laboratory to clinical renal transplantation. The purpose of the crossmatch is to prevent hyperacute rejection and to detect antibodies that identify immunologic risk factors in patients awaiting transplantation. The occurrence of hyperacute rejection is significantly correlated with a positive direct complement-dependent cytotoxicity (CDC) crossmatch between donor T lymphocytes and recipient serum at the time of transplantation. Reactivity of current valid serum of the recipient to the T lymphocytes of the donor is a contraindication to renal graft transplantation. Detection of donor-reactive antibodies in noncurrent recipient serum samples is not a contraindication but may represent risk for graft loss other than immediate hyperacute rejection (Cardella, 1982; Geddes, 1999). A donor-specific crossmatch also is used in some centers to predict hematopoietic progenitor cell graft failure (Hansen, 1997a).

Requirements and methods for the donor-specific crossmatch are stated in the standards of the American Society for Histocompatibility and

TABLE 48-5
Cross-Reactive Class II HLA Molecules Based on Epitope Sharing as Defined by Single-Antigen Bead Testing and HLAMatchmaker Algorithm

Terasaki and El-Awar TerEplet	Class II antibody reactive antigens	Marrari and Duquesnoy eplets
1031	DR01; DR51	96EV
1032	DR07,08,09,10,11,12,13,14,17,18; DR52	96HV
1033	DR10,15,16; DR53	96QK
1034/1042/1605/1406	DR04	32FYH/96YL/98EN/180LT
1036	DR52	98QS
1027	DR17,18; DR52	77GNY
1026	DR17,18; (DR3*0101)	71QKGR+60Y
1040	DR04,08,10,12,13,14,17,18; (DR3*0301)	140TV
1041	DR08,11,12,13,14,17,18 (DR3*0301)	149H
1603	DR15,16	133L/140AM
1020	DR15 (DR5*0202)	71QAA
1402	DR51	108T
1017	DR11	57DE
1008/1405/1602	DR07	26QKF/71DRG
1001	DR07,09; DR53	4Q
1019	DR09,10,14; DR53	71RRA
1029	DR07,09	77TV/98ES
1043	DR07,09,10; DR53	180VM
1410	DR07,09,12 (DR3*0101,*0301)	60S+71R
1606	DR14	57AA/60H/112Y
1409	DR13	71DKA
1030	DR01,12 (DR5*0202)	85AV
1407	DR08,12	14GEY/71DRA
1024	DR08	25YRF/73ALDT
1023	DR09,14; DR53	71RAE
1014/1408	DR10; DR53	40Y+71RRA
1028	DR01,04,07,09,10,11,12,13,14,15,16; DR51; DR53	77T [73A/G & 78V/Y]
1025	DR07; DR52	74GQ [78V/Y]
1018	DR07,08,11,12,13,16,103; DR51	70D [67H/I/L, 71E/K/R, & 73A/G]
1022	DR07,17,18; DR52	73G [74Q/R & 77N/T]
1021	DR04,13,17,18; DR52	71K [70D/Q]
1035/1411	DR04,07,09	98E [120N/S]
1038	DR04,10; DR51; DR53	120N [98E/K]
1037	DR04,07,09; DR51; DR52	104A [105K/R]
1039	DR01,07,09,15,16; DR51; DR52; DR53	140A [105K/R]
2004	DQ05,06	52PQ/84EV/89GI
2015	DQ05	70GA/116I
2011	DQ05,0601	52PQ
2001	DQ02	45GE/52LL/71RKA
2006	DQ07,08,09	55PPP
2005	DQ07	45EV
2002	DQ04	57LD/70ED
2014	DQ04,07,08,09	52PL/140T/182N
2013	DQ02,04,07,08,09	84QL
2010	DQ04,05,06,08,09	45GV
2012	DQ08,09	45GV+55PPP
2009	DQ02,04,05,06,08,09	45G
2007	DQ04,05,06	55PR
2003	DQ04,05,06,07,08,09	46VY/52P
2008	DQ02,05,07,08,09 ?	Eplet not identified
2017	DQA02	47KL/53HRL
2019	DQA03	47QL/52FRR/187T
2018	DQA04,05,06	41GR/51VLQ
	Epitopes w/hidden residues that Duquesnoy considers uncommon	
1005	DR01,09,10	14FEH
1006/1604	DR11,13,14,17,18; DRw52	14SEH(11S, 12T)
1007	DR07; DRw51	48YR
1010	DR01,09; DRW51; DRw53	32IYN
1015	DR11,12,13,15,17	48FR
1016	DR04,08,13	57SA

TABLE 48-5

Cross-Reactive Class II HLA Molecules Based on Epitope Sharing as Defined by Single-Antigen Bead Testing and HLAMatchmaker Algorithm—*Cont'd*

Terasaki and El-Awar TerEplet	Class II antibody reactive antigens	Marrari and Duquesnoy eplets
1012	DR12	48FR/25YRL/71DRA+85AV
1401	DR09	32IYN/26KYH/74RAE+77TV
1404	DR09; DRw51	32IYN
1002/1403	DR01,07,15,16	32YN
1601/1041diff Eplet	DR08,11,12,13,14,17,18 same group as 1041, but different Eplet	96HK (or 149H)
1011	DR07,14	48YR
1004	DR04,10	140TV
1003	DR01,04,07,09,15,16; DRw51; DRw53	32Y
1009	DR04,08,11,13,14,15,16,17	Eplet not identified
1013	DR01,103,14,15	Eplet not identified

These antigen groups were generated from reports by Marrari M, Duquesnoy RJ. Correlations between Terasaki's HLA class II epitopes and HLAMatchmaker-defined eplets on HLA-DR and -DQ antigens. Tissue Antigens 2009;74:134–46; Marrari M, Duquesnoy RJ. Correlations between Terasaki's HLA class I epitopes and HLAMatchmaker-defined eplets on HLA-A, -B and -C antigens. Tissue Antigens 2009;74:117–33; and El-Awar NR, Akaza T, Terasaki PI, Nguyen A. Human leukocyte antigen I epitopes: update to 103 total epitopes, including C locus. Transplantation 2007;84:532–40.

Immunogenetics (see Table 48-1) and in the ASHI procedure manual (2001). Acceptable techniques at present include the Amos-modified CDC, the extended incubation time CDC, the antiglobulin-augmented CDC, and flow cytometry.

Antibody Detection Techniques

Different laboratories may use different combinations of assays to detect antibody. The level of sensitization detected will vary with the assay. The antibody specificity detected will vary with the target cell.

Direct Complement-Dependent Cytotoxicity

Direct CDC includes all assays that use the addition of complement to detect the direct binding of antibody to lymphocytes. Fixation of complement by the antibody–antigen complexes on the cell surface results in cell death or cytotoxicity. CDC methods include the basic technique (no wash step before addition of complement), the Amos-modified technique (wash step added before addition of complement), and extended-time incubation techniques. The wash step removes serum, which may contain substances that hinder complement activation. The advantages of direct CDC techniques are that they are reproducible, and that correlation with the incidence of hyperacute rejection is excellent.

Indirect Crossmatch Techniques

Indirect techniques include the anti-globulin augmented lymphocytotoxicity assay technique also known as anti-human globulin cytotoxicity assay, and flow cytometry. Both use a reagent specific for human immunoglobulin to augment detection of HLA-directed antibody. Indirect techniques detect the presence of antibodies specific for CREGs that frequently go undetected in direct CDC assays. Advantages of the flow cytometry assay include discrimination of the subclass of the cell-bound immunoglobulin (IgG vs. IgM) and characterization of the target cell binding the alloantibody (T lymphocyte vs. B lymphocyte vs. monocyte).

Autoantibodies

The presence of circulating autoantibodies in the recipient is not known to be deleterious. Thus, an autocrossmatch should be performed, preferably when the patient is put on the transplantation waiting list. If autoantibodies are present, the sera used for donor crossmatching should have the autoreactivity removed. Autoantibodies are primarily IgM, and HLA-specific antibodies are primarily IgG (Barger, 1989). Either heat inactivation at 63 ± 1° C or reduction with the chemical agent dithioerythritol or dithiothreitol (DTT) of any potential IgM antibodies is used to differentiate between IgM and IgG antibodies in the serum samples. If the heat-inactivated or DTT-treated serum sample is negative even though the untreated sample is positive, most centers will proceed with transplantation. However, DTT or heat inactivation should be used with caution because not all HLA-specific antibodies are IgG, and because if they are not properly controlled, both procedures can remove IgG activity, as well as IgM.

B Cell Antibodies

A crossmatch using donor B lymphocytes (B cell crossmatch) may be performed in sensitized patients in some centers. A positive donor-specific B cell crossmatch is not a contraindication to transplantation. The clinical significance has not been resolved, but a positive test may be a risk factor, particularly in patients who have previously been transplanted. Antibodies detected in a B cell crossmatch can be (1) class II, HLA-DR, -DQ specific, (2) weak HLA-A, -B, -C specific antibodies (B cells have a higher density of class I molecules and are more sensitive to complement-dependent assays than are T cells), and/or (3) non–HLA-specific antibodies (e.g., autoantibodies). To interpret a positive B cell crossmatch, it may be necessary to adsorb recipient sera with platelets before performing the donor crossmatch. (Platelets express class I but not class II molecules.) The two most commonly used B cell crossmatch techniques are the CDC and flow cytometry assays.

Selection of Recipient Serum Samples for Donor Crossmatch

For patients with no detectable sensitization (i.e., 0% PRA), the most recent serum sample available can be used for the donor-specific crossmatch. If the patient has preexisting antibodies or has had a recent sensitizing event, a current serum sample (i.e., within 48 hours of transplantation) should be collected. For sensitized recipients, representative samples, including the most reactive or "peak" serum sample, are tested in most centers; a donor-positive noncurrent sample may be considered to be a risk factor, particularly in the patient who rejected a primary graft early in the posttransplantation period (Mahoney, 1996).

RENAL TRANSPLANTATION

Current practice is to select donors for recipients who are ABO compatible, T cell, donor specific, crossmatch negative with appropriate recipient sera and the best available HLA match. The original finding that kidney grafts transplanted between HLA-identical siblings survive significantly longer than grafts transplanted between HLA-mismatched siblings or parent–sibling combinations has been consistently confirmed. Figure 48-11 shows a recent analysis of 5-year survival of renal allografts from the international CTS registry among three categories of donors: (1) HLA-identical sibling, 84% survival; (2) one-haplotype living-related, 73% survival; (3) all cadaver, 66% survival. The impact of matching for MHC in living-related transplantation is clearly observed by comparing categories 1 and 2. Similar results are observed in the UNOS database (Cecka, 1999).

Although outcome analyses of living-related grafts confirm the role of the MHC as the major genetic barrier to successful graft outcome, demonstration and acceptance of a positive influence of HLA matching in graft outcome for unrelated cadaveric transplantation have been more controversial. However, long-term survival data from collaborative, multicenter studies are consistent in showing a highly significant effect of HLA matching on graft survival in cadaveric renal transplantation (Cecka, 1999; Opelz, 1999). Moreover, two recent single-center studies—one from Europe (Oslo) and one from North America (Toronto)—have reported significant improvement in graft survival as a function of HLA match (Geddes, 1999; Leivestad, 1999). A single center may require prioritization based on HLA match to transplant sufficient recipients with well-matched grafts to achieve statistical significance in outcome analysis. Although the numbers are smaller, a highly significant influence of HLA matching has been observed on the outcome of kidney grafts from living-unrelated donors (Opelz, 1999).

Zero mismatched (0 MM) grafts from cadaver donors survive significantly better than and approximately as well as grafts from HLA-identical siblings (see Fig. 48-11); thus, UNOS mandates the sharing of 0 MM kidneys. Graft survival in patients following first kidney transplantations decreases stepwise as the number of mismatches increases from 0 MM to 6 MM (Cecka, 1999; Opelz, 1999). However, to ensure equitable sharing of organs for all recipients, including those with rare HLA haplotypes, new algorithms for prioritizing recipients on the waiting list have been adopted by organ-sharing programs (Opelz, 1999). The most recent outcome data for both graft and patient survival can be accessed through the CTS website (www.ctstransplant.org).

Matching of the initial graft not only increases survival time for that graft, but it decreases the probability of recipient sensitization and facilitates retransplantation. Accumulation of highly sensitized patients on the waiting list is a significant problem in many centers, as patients wait for long periods of time and may present difficult clinical management problems (Sanfilippo, 1992).

NONRENAL ORGAN TRANSPLANTATION

Survival of heart, liver, lung, and pancreas grafts is good, with between 58% and 67% of first grafts surviving at 5 years. Donors usually are not matched for HLA type, and a pretransplant donor crossmatch is not routinely performed. Serum antibody screens are recommended to identify the state of sensitization as an immunologic risk factor for the recipient. If feasible, the graft recipients and cadaveric donors of nonrenal vascularized grafts should be typed for HLA to allow for retrospective analyses. Recent international CTS data show no effect of HLA matching on outcomes of liver transplantation; however, the CTS data do show a significant impact of matching for HLA-A, -B, and -DR on outcomes of first heart transplants (Opelz, 1999). The acceptable period for cold ischemia preservation may limit the extent of HLA matching possible for heart transplantation.

ALLOGENEIC HEMATOPOIETIC PROGENITOR CELL TRANSPLANTATION

Allogeneic hematopoietic progenitor cell transplantation is performed for hematologic malignancies and disorders, bone marrow failure, certain inherited metabolic disorders such as lipid storage diseases, and congenital immunodeficiency syndrome. From a histocompatibility standpoint, the best donor is either self (autogeneic transplant), if the malignancy is not one that involves the bone marrow or the disease is not genetic, or an identical twin (syngeneic transplant). Progenitor cells from an HLA-identical sibling donor are a frequent source. These donor cells usually will be genetically identical to cells of the patient across the entire MHC region. Use of a sibling donor also increases the probability that non-HLA genes that might affect transplantation success and that are not well defined (i.e., minor histocompatibility genes) will be matched (Goulmy, 1997). Haploidentical family members may also be chosen as donors (Aversa, 1998), although a greater risk of severe GVHD is associated with mismatched HLA donors. Based on data from the International Bone Marrow Transplant Registry (IBMTR) (see Table 48-1; www.ibmtr.org), more than 16,000 allogeneic bone marrow transplants were performed from 1996 to 1997; 75% used related donors.

Most patients (≈70%) do not have an HLA-matched sibling and may be considered for transplantation with cells from an HLA-matched, unrelated donor. To facilitate the search for a matched donor, national registries of unrelated donors have been developed around the world (Hansen, 1996). The NMDP in the United States is such a registry and contains more than 3.9 million HLA-typed donors, making it the largest unrelated donor registry in the world (Perkins, 1994; see Table 48-1; www.marrow.org).

Hematopoietic progenitor cell grafts are among the most difficult of all clinical procedures for several reasons (Hansen, 1997a; Madrigal, 1997). First, at the time of transplantation, the recipients are nearly totally immunodeficient, either because of inherited deficiency (severe combined immunodeficiency) or because of pretransplantation conditioning (cytotoxic chemotherapy and irradiation). Conditioning is required to eliminate malignant cells and to prevent the immune system of the recipient from rejecting the donor progenitor cells, which are infused several days after conditioning. The amount of cytotoxic pretreatment is great enough to eliminate circulating leukocytes, nearly eliminate platelets, and abrogate production of new erythrocytes. Thus, the recipient is profoundly susceptible to all types of infection and would certainly die if not rescued by extraordinary medical care and transfused progenitor cells.

The second risk is the potential for immunologic attack of the recipient by the transplanted allogeneic progenitor cells, resulting in GVHD. GVHD has several forms and can be fatal. In spite of associated difficulties, a number of transplant centers have achieved exceptional success. Recent reports from single institutions and the IBMTR suggest leukemia-free survival of 40%–60% at 5 years after unrelated hematopoietic progenitor cell transplantation of patients with chronic myelogenous leukemia in chronic phase (see Table 48-1; www.ibmtr.org) (Hansen, 1998). Survival for patients with severe aplastic anemia transplanted with cells from unrelated donors varies from 30%–50% at 5 years, depending on patient age (see Table 48-1, NMDP, at www.marrow.org and www.ibmtr.org); survival rates of nearly 90% have been reported at some centers (Deeg, 1998).

In addition to marrow as a source of hematopoietic progenitor cells, collection of hematopoietic progenitor cells from growth factor–mobilized peripheral blood (Anderlini, 1997) or umbilical cord blood progenitor cells (Cairo, 1997) increases the availability of unrelated donors. New approaches to immunosuppression, including less aggressive conditioning protocols (e.g., “minitransplants”) (Storb, 1999), may extend the availability of progenitor cell transplantation as a therapeutic procedure to patients presently excluded by age or by organ dysfunction. Hematopoietic progenitor cell transplantation can also be used to generate immune responses directed at malignant cells. Relapse of disease following transplantation is greater for patients receiving an HLA-matched graft, suggesting that some degree of mismatching may be beneficial in stimulating an immune response against tumor cells (Beatty, 1993). As problems surrounding this most difficult procedure are overcome, hematopoietic progenitor cell transplantation may become one of the most widely used methods for the treatment of a variety of diseases (see Chapter 38).

HLA Typing for Progenitor Cell Transplantation

Many factors, including histocompatibility, influence the outcome of hematopoietic progenitor cell transplantation (Madrigal, 1997). The pretransplantation workup includes HLA-A, -B, and -DR typing of all available members of the immediate family to identify a matched related donor and to establish inheritance of haplotypes. DNA-based typing for class II genes has become standard, and DNA-based typing for class I genes has been implemented in many centers. Typing of the extended family, allele-level (i.e., high-resolution) typing of specific HLA class I and class II loci, typing of other loci within the MHC (i.e., short tandem repeats or complement loci), or use of other tests (e.g., crossmatching, cytotoxic T cell precursor measurements) to measure compatibility may also be appropriate (Hurley, 1999).

The level of HLA typing resolution required differs for hematopoietic progenitor cells and renal transplantation. It is likely that higher-resolution HLA typing is required to match donor and recipient for progenitor cell transplantation than is required for renal transplantation because progenitor cell transplantation involves the transfer of an entire immune system to the patient. Current research is focused on defining the loci that must be considered in donor selection, the level of resolution that must be used for matching, and the additive effect of multiple mismatches. The level of matching required may vary for each disease or protocol. Evidence suggests that matching unrelated donor and recipient for HLA-A, -B, -DRB1 alleles is related to improved outcomes. The impact of matching at other HLA loci (e.g., HLA-C, HLA-DQ) is under evaluation. Single mismatches may be tolerated; however, multiple mismatches appear to have a negative impact on outcome (Petersdorf, 1995b, 1998; Hansen, 1997a; Madrigal, 1997; Sasazuki, 1998). Furthermore, the positive effect of histocompatibility matching on outcome must be balanced by the positive impact of transplantation early in the course of the disease. Data from the IBMTR and the NMDP show that survival following transplantation is reduced as the disease phase advances (data on websites listed in Table 48-1).

Summary

The HLA class I and class II molecules encoded within the major histocompatibility complex have a significant role in the specificity and character of immune responses. Extensive polymorphism of these molecules provides the diversity needed to ensure survival in an environment of hostile and adaptive pathogens. Unfortunately, this ability of the immune system to distinguish self from nonself extends to the recognition of foreign HLA molecules following tissue transplantation. Definition and characterization of HLA alleles and molecules have been combined with clinical protocols to maximize compatibility and to minimize the impact of the immune response on foreign tissue. These advances have contributed to the development of transplantation as a successful treatment modality for the replacement of diseased tissue.

SELECTED REFERENCES

Aguado B, Bahram S, Beck S, et al. Complete sequence and gene map of a human major histocompatibility complex. Nature 1999;401:921.

Contains the first complete sequence and gene map of an MHC region and represents the collaborative effort of an international group of researchers.

Arguello JR, Little AM, Bohan E, et al. High resolution HLA class I typing by reference strand mediated conformation analysis (RSCA). Tissue Antigens 1998;52:57–66.

Describes the use of RSCA in separating polymorphic HLA alleles using an automated technology that may provide rapid high-throughput HLA analysis with the additional advantages of time and cost savings.

Etokebe GE, Opsahl M, Tveter AK, et al. Physical separation of HLA-A alleles by denaturing high-performance liquid chromatography. Tissue Antigens 2003;61:443–50.

Describes the application of HPLC to the task of identifying polymorphic HLA-A alleles in an automated high-throughput setting.

Nordstrom T, Ronaghi M, Forsberg L, et al. Direct analysis of single-nucleotide polymorphism on double-stranded DNA by pyrosequencing. Biotechnol Appl Biochem 2000;31:107–12.

Describes the technology behind pyrosequencing and its specific application to the tasks of sequencing and verifying the presence of single nucleotide polymorphisms in double-stranded DNA.

REFERENCES

Access the complete reference list online at http://www.expertconsult.com

CHAPTER 49

THE MAJOR HISTOCOMPATIBILITY COMPLEX AND DISEASE

Julio C. Delgado

KEY POINTS

- The major histocompatibility complex (MHC) genomic region contains several genes with immune-related functions.
- Recent identification of several genes within the MHC has increased the possibility of defining the genetic basis of immunity.
- The clustering of immune-related genes in the MHC region may not be coincidental and may be the result of evolutionary forces joining genes with similar functions.
- The MHC is associated with more diseases than any other region on the human genome.
- Nonrandom associations of fixed stretches of MHC DNA complicate the study of susceptibility genes but also provide the means for their identification.
- Methods are available for detecting associations or linkage between polymorphisms found with the MHC and disease.
- Although class I and class II encoded proteins are distinguished by structural and functional similarities shared by the members of each class, class III molecules can be defined only as non-I and non-II, because their genes and their products have no common features and are not recognized by T cells.
- Despite convincing genetic association studies showing the importance of the class III region in health and disease, neither the genes responsible for disease nor the underlying mechanism of pathology is known for many of the associated conditions.
- Almost half the genes within the MHC class III region play roles in the innate immune system, including members of the complement fixation cascade (*C4, C2, BF*) and tumor necrosis factor family.
- Deficiency of the second component of the complement system has been reported only in Caucasians, and it is the most common complement protein deficiency state in that population.
- Complete C4 deficiency is extremely rare. The level of C4 in the serum of patients with *C4 null* alleles is extremely variable and cannot be used reliably to detect heterozygotes for complete deficiency because there is no correlation between the level of C4 and the number of expressed *C4* genes.
- Extended haplotypes are highly characteristic of an ethnic subgroup and have lower frequencies or do not occur at all in other ethnic groups.
- It is critical to know the ethnic distribution of a disease-associated MHC allele to evaluate whether the allele in patients is increased compared with ethnically matched control populations and is in fact truly a marker for the ethnic distribution of the disease.
- A major problem with MHC gene associations is their incomplete penetrance, making ordinary formal segregation and linkage studies very difficult, if not impossible, to carry out.

Understanding the role of the MHC in immune responses and in the pathogenesis of disease requires defining polymorphisms in the class I and class II regions, as well as genes in the central region of the MHC, sometimes called the MHC class III region. The strong interest in the MHC genomic sequence originates from its established role in regulating inflammation and the innate and adaptive immune responses. Several genes in the MHC play important roles in cellular discrimination of self and nonself that require an essential knowledge of the effects of the MHC system in transplantation medicine and in susceptibility to autoimmunity. Variants of class I and class II genes were described in detail in the previous chapter. In this chapter, we discuss the non–human leukocyte antigen (HLA) region genes, disease associations, and methods for detecting the association of diseases with genetic markers.

Overview of the Human Major Histocompatibility Complex DNA Sequence

Completion of the MHC deoxyribonucleic acid (DNA) sequence preceded completion of the total human genome sequence by almost 4 years (The MHC Sequencing Consortium, 1999). The rush to complete the entire MHC sequence followed the need to understand the biology and genetics of the mouse MHC (H-2) and HLA regions, which were initially provided by murine inbred experiments and serologic typing (reviewed in Klein, 1986). Although the MHC was discovered more than 50 years ago, its nature has been resolved only in the last two decades, with the advent of DNA cloning and discovery of the structure of class I and class II molecules (Bjorkman, 1987; Brown, 1993).

The MHC located in the short arm of chromosome 6 spans approximately 4Mb and contains more than 250 identified loci, by far the most gene-dense region of the human genome sequenced to date (reviewed in Shiina, 2009). It encodes the most polymorphic human proteins—the HLA class I and class II molecules, some of which have more than 1000 allelic variants identified so far (Marsh, 2009). More than 40% of the total expressed loci in the MHC are associated with immune-related functions. This clustering of immune-related genes in the MHC region may not be coincidental and may be the result of evolutionary forces joining genes with similar functions.

Traditionally, the MHC region has been classified into three regions from telomere to centromere: HLA class I, non-HLA class (MHC class III), and HLA class II. HLA class I and class II gene functions were reviewed in detail in the preceding chapter. We will concentrate on the MHC class III region and will later return to HLA class I and class II genes to discuss disease associations.

Genes in the Central or Class III Region

The human MHC class III, or central MHC region, located between the HLA class I and class II regions, is the most gene-dense region of the human genome. Specifically, the MHC class III region contains 55 protein-coding genes in ≈900 kb sequence, with an average gene size of ≈8.5 kb (Xie, 2003), compared with the entire human genome, which contains, on average, fewer than 11 genes per megabase and has an average gene size between 27 and 45 Mb (Lander, 2001; Heilig, 2003). Although HLA class I and class II encoded proteins are distinguished by structural and functional similarities shared by the members of each class, MHC class III molecules can be defined only as non-I and non-II, because their genes and their products have no common features and are not recognized by T cells. Figure 49-1 shows a genetic map of the MHC class III region.

Despite convincing genetic association studies showing the importance of the MHC class III region in health and disease, neither the genes responsible for disease nor the underlying mechanism of pathology is known for many of the associated conditions. One reason for this is the fact that the functions of nearly half the genes in the MHC class III region are not completely known. Recently, a high-throughput yeast two-hybrid system was used to look into the function of several intracellular proteins encoded within the MHC class III region (Lehner, 2004). This study revealed that approximately one third of the analyzed proteins encoded within the MHC class III region may have a role in mRNA processing, which again suggests clustering of functionally related genes within this region of the human genome. Specifically, four of the proteins in the MHC class III region (LSM2, BAT1, DOM3Z, and SKIV2L) are orthologs of yeast proteins involved in mRNA processing, and another five proteins (BAT2, STK19, CLIC1, PBX2, and BAT5) interact with proteins previously implicated in RNA processing. Three proteins (STK19, PBX2, and RDBP) interact with proteins implicated in transcriptional regulation.

The region closer to HLA class II genes contains several genes of known function, including *TNXB* (Morel, 1989), which encodes tenascin X, a large extracellular matrix protein expressed in connective tissues, and *NEU1*, encoding neuraminidase 1, a lysosomal sialidase. Mutations of *TNXB* are a cause of the Ehlers-Danlos syndrome (Burch, 1997), and mutations of the *NEU1* gene are responsible for congenital sialidosis (Bonten, 1996).

Almost one half of genes within the MHC class III region play roles in the innate immune system, including members of the complement fixation cascade (*C4, C2, CFB*) and the tumor necrosis factor family (*TNF, LTα, LTβ*), which will be discussed in greater detail later in this chapter. Other members of the immunoglobulin superfamily are also located within the MHC class III regions: *NCR3* (natural cytotoxicity triggering receptor 3) and the less characterized *LY6G* genes. The *NCR3* gene encodes the NKp30 protein responsible for triggering natural killer (NK) cells (Pende, 1999), and it is involved in the killing of cells infected with *Plasmodium falciparum* (Mavoungou, 2007) and cytomegalovirus (Arnon, 2005). Increased expression of *NCR3* and the adjacent *LST1* (leukocyte-specific transcript 1) gene has been found in the blood of rheumatoid arthritis patients (Mulcahy, 2006). Both genes are also significantly upregulated in response to lipopolysaccharide, interferon-γ, and bacterial infection, suggesting a role for these gene products in autoimmune-related inflammation and dendritic cell/NK cell–associated functions.

The *NFKBIL1* (NF-κB-inhibitor-like) and *BTNL2* (Butyrophilin-like protein 2) genes are also located in the MHC class III region (Albertella, 1994; Stammers, 2000). Much interest has recently been focused on the NFKBIL1 and BTNL2 proteins after single mutations in their promoter regions were linked to rheumatoid arthritis (Okamoto, 2003) and sarcoidosis (Valentonyte, 2005), respectively. Other immune-related genes (e.g., *LY6* family members and *AIF1*) are likely to function as part of immune/inflammatory control (Utans, 1995; Autieri, 1996; Ribas, 1999; Mallya, 2002). Finally, the genes for the microsomal enzyme steroid P450 21-hydroxylase and three members of the major heat-shock protein 70 family are also contained in the MHC class III region and will be discussed later.

Tumor Necrosis Factor and Lymphotoxin α and β Genes

Tumor necrosis factor (TNF) and lymphotoxin α (LTα) are potent immunomodulatory cytokines produced in response to inflammatory stimuli. The biological functions of these cytokines and the laboratory methods used to measure them in body fluids were reviewed in great detail in Chapter 47. TNF and LTα proteins are each encoded by separate genes (*TNF* and *LTA*) and share approximately 34% amino acid identity (Carroll, 1987). TNF and LTα are either maintained as cell surface molecules nor

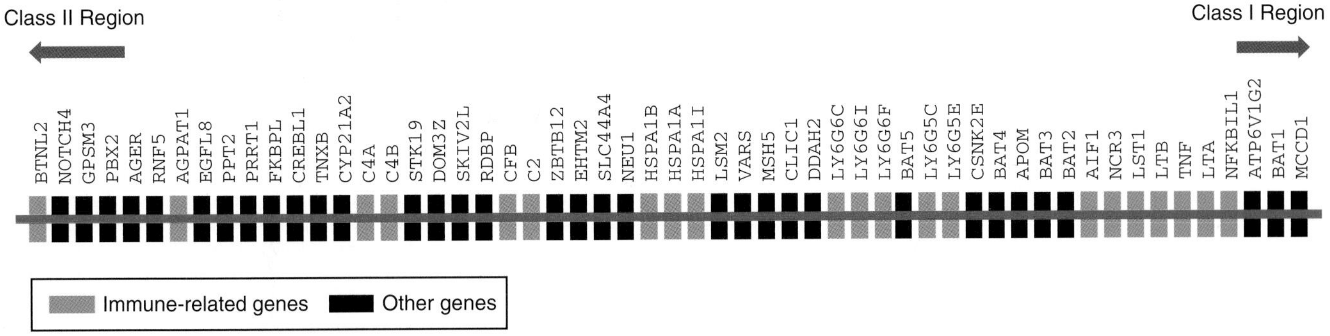

Figure 49-1 Gene map of the class III region of the major histocompatibility complex. Shown in order but not to scale are 55 genes from centromere to telomere. Genes presenting "immune loci" are marked by green boxes.

PART 6

released from cells. LTα is retained on the cell surface via a transmembrane region. Surface TNF results not from the presence of a transmembrane region, but rather from an association with lymphotoxin β (LTβ) (Browning, 1993). LTβ encoded by *LTB* has 21% and 24% amino acid identity with *TNF* and *LTα*, respectively.

To date, several *TNF* promoter polymorphisms, located at −1030, −862, −857, −851, −574, −376, −308, −244, −238, and +70 nucleotides relative to the transcription start site, have been identified (Wilson, 1992; Brinkman, 1994; Higuchi, 1998; Uglialoro, 1998). Throughout the past decade, the *TNF* loci have been the center of intense attention concerning the relevance of its promoter polymorphisms to susceptibility to various autoimmune and infectious diseases. This work remains controversial both at the genetic level and, more importantly, with regard to functional relevance. As recently demonstrated for some of the *TNF* promoter polymorphisms, these gene variations may be ethnic-specific markers for other linked and unidentified factors that may have an impact on host immune response in the development of autoimmune diseases and susceptibility or resistance to infectious diseases in a given population (Delgado, 2002). Polymorphisms in the *TNF* promoter region have been correlated in large-scale population studies with cerebral malaria (McGuire, 1994; Knight, 1999), rheumatoid arthritis (Criswell, 2004), coronary heart disease (Nicaud, 2002), type 2 diabetes (Kubaszek, 2003), Alzheimer's disease (McCusker, 2001), ankylosing spondylitis (McGarry, 1999), mortality to septic shock (Mira, 1999), and mucocutaneous leishmaniasis (Cabrera, 1995). In relation to *LTA* polymorphisms, large-scale analysis has linked both promoter and coding polymorphisms within the *LTA* gene to myocardial infarction (Ozaki, 2002).

HEAT-SHOCK PROTEIN 70 GENES

Stress proteins, or heat-shock proteins, are expressed by cells in response to a variety of stress stimuli. This response has been observed in all species examined to date. The family of stress proteins, 70 kDa in size, has a highly conserved amino acid sequence identity as found from primitive eukaryotes to humans. Several studies have identified loci for heat-shock protein 70 (HSP70) on chromosomes 6, 14, and 21 (Hunt, 1985; Sargent, 1989). Three genes encoding members of the HSP70 family are located telomeric to the *C2* locus (*HSPA1L*, *HSPA1A*, and *HSPA1B*, formerly known as *HSP70-Hom*, *HSP70-1*, and *HSP70-2*, respectively).

Sequence analysis of *HSPA1A* and *HSPA1B* genes has shown that they are intronless genes that encode an identical protein product of 641 amino acids. *HSPA1L* is also an intronless gene that encodes a protein of 641 amino acids and has 90% sequence identity with *HSPA1A* (Milner, 1990). Because of the high degree of sequence similarity between coding regions of the various *HSP70* genes, DNA probes corresponding to coding regions tend to cross-hybridize. However, sufficient sequence differences have been observed between the 5′ and 3′ untranslated regions to design oligonucleotide primers and probes to allow specific amplification and hybridization of the three genes (Milner, 1992).

The *HSP70* gene cluster lately has drawn attention because of a recent study that linked both *HSPA1L* and *HLA-B*5701* loci to hypersensitivity to the antiretroviral drug abacavir (Martin, 2004). Other polymorphisms in the *HSP70* genes have been correlated to cytokine response in trauma (Schroder, 2003; Wu, 2004), uveitis in patients with sarcoidosis (Spagnolo, 2007), and risk of clozapine-induced agranulocytosis in Ashkenazi Jews (Corzo, 1995).

C2, C4, AND *CFB* GENES AND TYPING

The C2, C4, and factor B proteins encoded within the MHC class III demonstrate inherited structural variants that can be studied by using techniques that detect differences in net surface charge due to amino acid differences. Two methods are used to separate these proteins: (1) high-voltage agarose gel electrophoresis, which detects variations in mobility due to charge differences between proteins at a given pH, and (2) isoelectric focusing in thin-layer polyacrylamide gels, which shows differences in isoelectric points. Proteins can be visualized by immunofixation electrophoresis using insolubility of antigen–antibody complexes, or by detection of functional hemolytic activity with overlay gels, in which antibody-sensitized sheep erythrocytes are combined with complement-deficient serum (Alper, 1983).

At the protein level, C2 shows minor polymorphism by isoelectric focusing. The alleles for C2 are *C* (common), a less common *B* (basic) allele with three rare basic variants, and four rare *A* (acidic) variants (Jahn, 1990). The polymorphic site for the *C2*B* allele is carried by the C2a complement fragment. The C2 protein is genetically polymorphic in a wide variety of ethnic groups, although *C2*C* accounts for more than 90% of *C2* genes in most populations (Alper, 1976; Meo, 1977). In Caucasian and Asian populations, *C2*B* accounts for 5%–10% of *C2* genes. A nonexpressed allele (*C2*QO*) is found in 2% of the Caucasian European population (Truedsson, 1993a). For C2 typing, proteins are separated by isoelectric focusing in polyacrylamide gels and are visualized by C2-induced hemolysis in overlay gels. Diluted normal human serum can replace C2-deficient serum as a reagent, because C2 is the limiting factor in the classical complement pathway.

Two distinct but closely related loci for the C4 protein (*C4A* and *C4B*), presumably the result of tandem gene duplication, encode for two forms of C4. The genetics of *C4* is extraordinarily complex, not only at the genetic level, but also at the protein level. It has been shown that the number of *C4* genes in humans varies from two to four, and in exceptional cases, six (Chung, 2002; Wu, 2007). Three quarters of *C4* genes carry endogenous retrovirus sequences that might confer intrinsic protection against exogenous retroviral infection (Schneider, 2001). Recent data suggest a negative correlation between the presence of endogenous retrovirus sequences and the level of C4 proteins, as well as a direct relationship between the number of genes and C4 protein levels (Yang, 2003).

At the protein level, C4A and C4B differ only by four amino acid residues in the α chain between positions 1101 and 1106. C4B is several times more hemolytically active than C4A, but C4A is more active at inhibiting the formation and dissolution of immune complexes than C4B. C4A variants usually carry Rodgers antigenic determinants (a Val–Asp–Leu–Leu epitope of the C4A chain), and C4B variants carry Chido determinants (an Ala–Asp–Leu–Arg epitope of the α chain of C4B). Extensive genetic polymorphism is detectable in C4A and C4B proteins among populations; more than 35 variants have been observed by agarose gel electrophoresis and DNA-based typing methods (Awdeh, 1980; Sim, 1986; Schneider, 1996; Hui, 2004). Among the C4A and C4B allotypes, the most common alleles are *C4A*3* and *C4B*1*. *C4A*4*, *C4A*2*, *C4B*2*, and *C4B*5* show a worldwide general distribution. *C4A*6* is also observed in many populations, with the exception of some Mongoloid groups. *C4B*3* is identified mainly in African and Caucasian groups.

C4 typing requires a combination of several techniques (Awdeh, 1980): (1) Immunofixation electrophoresis after treatment with neuraminidase. The patterns produced show three bands for each variant with some overlap occurring between certain variants. Additional treatment of the sample with carboxypeptidase reduces each variant to a single band. (2) Detection of C4A versus C4B by functional hemolytic assay. This method distinguishes C4A and C4B overlapping patterns because C4B variants have 5–10 times the hemolytic activity of C4A variants. (3) Rodgers (C4A) or Chido (C4B) serologic reactivity. The serum is incubated with human anti-Rodgers or human anti-Chido to test for inhibition of agglutination with appropriate positive erythrocytes. Alternatively, C4 variants can be typed for Chido or Rodgers reactivity by immunoblotting. Null alleles of *C4* heterozygotes can be detected in two ways. Electrophoresis of C4 null (*C4A QO* and *C4B QO*) samples demonstrates an absence of bands in homozygotes, but in heterozygotes requires quantification by visual inspection, crossed immunoelectrophoresis, or densitometric scanning of immunofixation patterns. An alternative method is to determine the presence and ratios of the C4A and C4B α chains after sodium dodecyl sulfate polyacrylamide gel electrophoresis of immunoprecipitates. More recently, DNA-based typing methods, including sequence-specific primer (SSP) amplification, restriction fragment length polymorphisms analysis, and direct DNA sequencing, have been used to complement inconclusive C4A and C4B protein allotyping (Schneider, 2003).

Factor B is synthesized by the *CFB* gene. Human factor B is highly polymorphic, with more than 20 variants identified to date, including several dysfunctional proteins, those present in low concentration, and null alleles. Factor B typing is normally performed by combining agarose electrophoresis and/or isoelectric focusing at the protein level with polymerase chain reaction (PCR) analysis at the DNA level (Geserick, 1998). By using these methods, it is possible to identify two very common alleles, *CFB*F* and *CFB*S*, two less common alleles, *CFB*F1* and *CFB*S1*, and a host of rare alleles. Variants are named for their decimal fraction migration in gel electrophoresis: CFB F to CFB F1 for fast variants, and CFB S to CFB S1 for slow variants. In European Caucasian populations, *CFB*F* has a frequency of 0.2, *CFB*S* of 0.77, *CFB*F1* of 0.01, and *CFB*S1* of 0.01; rare alleles account for only 0.002. *CFB*S* is most common in Caucasian, Mongoloid, and Australoid populations, and *CFB*F* is most common in Negroid populations. *CFB*F1* is observed in African groups, as well as in some Caucasian populations.

DISEASE ASSOCIATIONS WITH *C2, C4,* AND *CFB* GENES

Deficiency of the second component of the complement system has been reported in about 1 in 10,000 Caucasians, and is the most common complement protein deficiency state in that population (Silverstein, 1960; Klemperer, 1966). People with complete C2 deficiency are homozygous for null C2 alleles (*C2*Q0* for quantity zero). *C2*Q0* results from a 28-bp gene deletion that generates a frameshift and a stop codon 14 bp distal to the end of exon 6 (Johnson, 1992). Remarkably, *C2*QO* has a gene frequency of approximately 0.01 among Caucasians. Rarely, C2 deficiency is the result of missense mutations resulting in impaired C2 secretions that have been termed C2 deficiency type II (Wetsel, 1996). Although C2 deficiency can lead to disease, most patients remain asymptomatic. Up to 25% of homozygotes for C2 deficiency have increased susceptibility to bacterial infection due to immunoglobulin deficiency (Densen, 1991; Alper, 2003). Between 20% and 40% of reported patients with C2 deficiency have a systemic lupus–like disease (Truedsson, 1993b; Sullivan, 1994). A polymorphism in the *C2* gene has been correlated with reduced risk of age-related macular degeneration (Gold, 2006; Maller, 2006).

A high incidence of *C4 null* alleles is seen in the general population. *C4A*Q0* and *C4B*Q0* result from gene deletions, premature stop codons, and other mutations that cause transcription failure (Braun, 1990; Barba, 1993; Lokki, 1999). Thirty-five percent of individuals of all races do not express one *C4A* or *C4B* gene (i.e., carry *C4A*Q0* or *C4B*Q0*), 8%–10% carry two null alleles, and less than 1% do not express three alleles. Complete C4 deficiency (trans *C4A*Q0, C4B*Q0*) haplotypes are extremely rare (Hauptmann, 1986). The *C4A*Q0* allele, particularly in homozygous individuals or those with complete C4 deficiency, has been associated with systemic lupus erythematosus (Wilson, 1988; Huang, 1995). This susceptibility is probably related to defective handling of immune complexes (Fielder, 1983). Children homozygous for *C4B*Q0* have a 3.5-fold greater incidence of bacterial meningitis (Colten, 1992).

Increased frequency of the *C4B*Q0* allele has been found in patients with severe coronary artery disease who underwent bypass compared with healthy controls (Szalai, 2002).

Absence of homozygous factor B deficiency in humans has led to the notion that the condition might be lethal during embryonic development. Based on inheritance patterns and serum levels, some heterozygotes from *CFB*Q0* have been identified as having reduced protein products (Siemens, 1992). The *CFB F* variant has been associated with higher protein concentration but lower hemolytic activity than *CFB S* (Lokki, 1991). Mutations in the *CFB* gene have been associated with age-related macular degeneration (Gold, 2006; Maller, 2006) and hemolytic-uremic syndrome (Goicoechea de Jorge, 2007).

COMPLOTYPES

The four genes of the complement region occupy approximately 120 kb of genomic DNA (Carroll, 1984). The *C2* and *CFB* genes are located in very close proximity, separated by less than 2 kb, but *CFB* and *C4A* are separated by about 30 kb. *C4A* and *C4B* are about 10 kb apart. Alleles of the complement genes occur as a unit at the population level and show striking linkage disequilibrium in haplotypes determined by family studies. That is to say, they occur together as sets on the same chromosome more frequently than expected from the frequencies of their individual alleles and with no well-documented recombinations. For these reasons, haplotypes of the four complement loci have been called *complotypes*, as an abbreviation for "complement haplotypes" (Alper, 1983). Although their order from telomere to centromere is *C2, CFB, C4A, C4B* (see Fig. 49-1), for clarity in using variant alleles to designate complotypes, the positions of *CFB* and *C2* are transposed. Thus, *CFB*S, C2*C, C4A*QO, C4B*1* is a complotype that in abbreviated form is *SC01*. More than a dozen complotypes in Caucasians have frequencies of about 0.01 or higher (Table 49-1). In most populations, the *SC31* complotype is most common. In people of African descent, *FC31* is common, as is *SC42* in East and Southeast Asians.

TABLE 49-1
Common Complotypes in Normal Chromosomes of Caucasoid Populations*

Complotype	Frequency, %
SC31	0.430
SC01	0.127
FC31	0.096
SC30	0.053
SC42	0.040
SC61	0.034
FC30	0.031
FC01	0.029
SC02	0.029
SC21	0.022
SB42	0.019
SC33	0.014
SC2(1,2)†	0.013
SC32	0.011

*Complotypes are given as abbreviated letters and numbers, with four alleles in arbitrary order: *CFB, C2, C4A,* and *C4B.*
†*C4B* locus is heteroduplicated.

EXTENDED HAPLOTYPES

Based on the study of the distribution of complotypes in relation to *HLA-B* and *HLA-DR* specificities on normal Caucasian haplotypes determined in family studies, striking linkage disequilibrium involving the whole region became evident. One could easily recognize *HLA-B*, complotype, *DR* allele sets that showed statistically significant three-point linkage disequilibrium (Fig. 49-2) and that define what are regarded as extended haplotypes (Awdeh, 1983). A shorthand nomenclature for extended haplotypes has been designed by enclosing *HLA-B*, complotype, and *HLA-DR* variants in brackets. Thus, the most common extended haplotype in Caucasians is *[HLA-B8, SC01, DR3]*. Extended haplotypes are highly characteristic of an ethnic subgroup and have lower frequencies or do not occur at all in other ethnic groups (Alper, 1982; Fraser, 1990).

Initial studies defined extended haplotypes as the genomic interval between *HLA-B* and *DR*. It then became evident that other uncharacterized MHC alleles in the interval were likely to be included. Despite the fact that *HLA-A* alleles have shown limited variation for extended haplotypes, only half such haplotypes show unique and significant *HLA-A* allele associations (Alper, 1982). The *HLA-Cw* locus was by far the last to be characterized. Based on genetic distance and previously incomplete typing data of *HLA-B/Cw* pairs, it was evident that conserved haplotypes would also include the HLA-Cw genetic region. Thus, different *HLA-Cw* alleles have been recently associated with different extended haplotypes (Table 49-2) (Clavijo, 1998). Furthermore, several *TNF* and *HSP* allele systems and microsatellites have been studied in relation to extended haplotypes (Table 49-3). More recently, models have been created to describe the variable sizes of stretches of conserved DNA in the MHC, using the known frequencies of four different types of small blocks (<0.2 Mb) of relatively conserved DNA sequence: *HLA-Cw/B; TNF;* complotype*;* and *HLA-DR/DQ* (Yunis, 2003). Using HLA allele identification and TNF microsatellites, Yunis and colleagues have shown that some extended haplotypes extend to the *HLA-A* and *HLA-DPB1* loci, which form fixed genetic units of at least 3.2 Mb of DNA. Intermediate fragments of extended haplotypes also exist, which are, nevertheless, larger than any of the four small blocks. This complexity of genetic fixity at various levels should be taken into account in studies of genetic disease association, immune response control, and human diversity.

Extended haplotypes, which account for at least 30% of normal Caucasian haplotypes, have relatively fixed gross structure and DNA sequence and carry very similar, if not identical alleles, even when they are found in apparently unrelated individuals. The frequency of extended haplotypes is more likely to be underestimated than overestimated because haplotypes must be determined from family studies involving thousands of unrelated index cases. Recently, the MHC reference sequence (The MHC Sequencing Consortium, 1999) has been used as the starting point for numerous studies undertaken to ascertain multiple common and rarer extended haplotypes (Walsh, 2003; Stewart, 2004; Smith, 2006; Traherne, 2006). These studies will facilitate the identification of precise disease loci and may help us to better understand events such as recombination and polymorphism.

MHC DISEASE ASSOCIATIONS

The MHC is associated with more diseases than any other region on the human genome. We have reviewed concepts about complotypes and

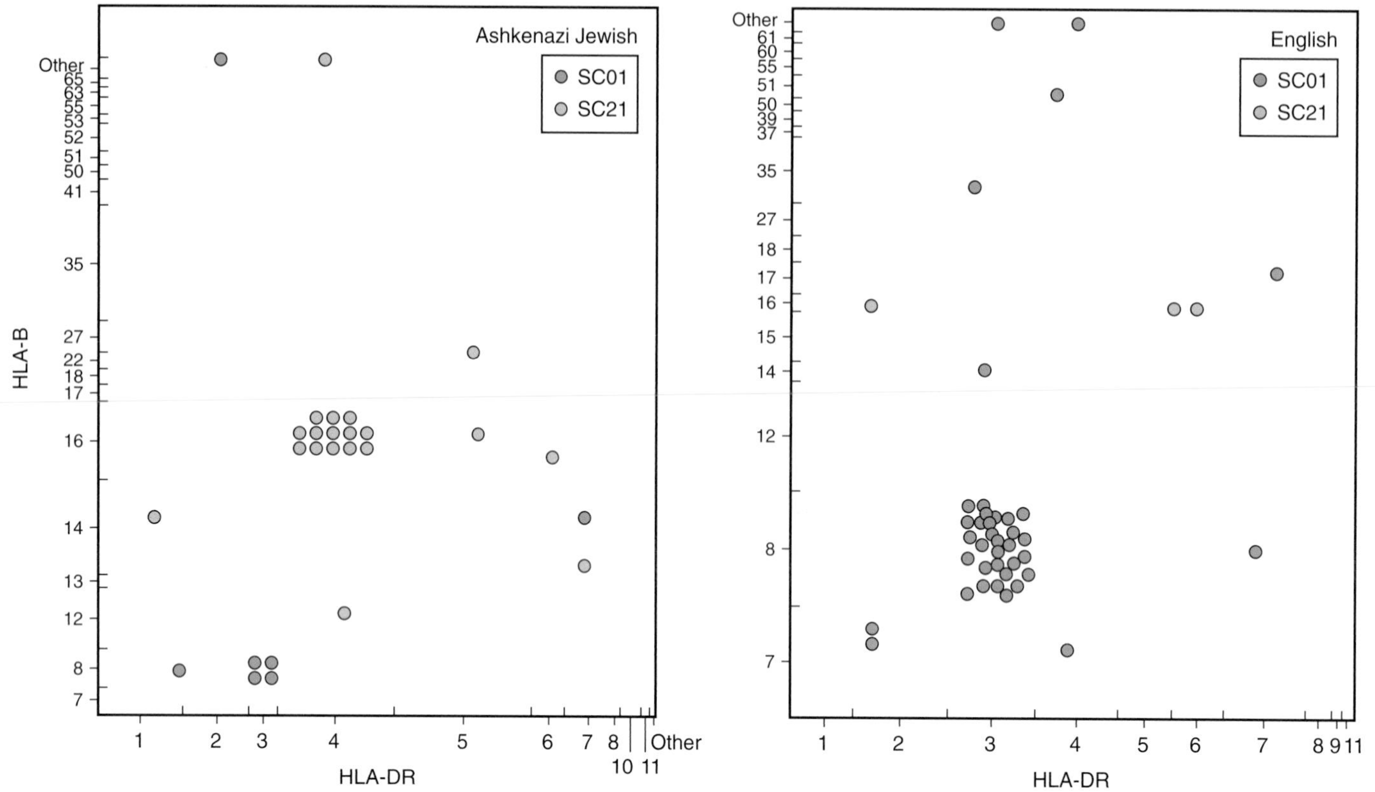

Figure 49-2 The haplotype distribution of the complotypes (haplotypes of complement alleles) *SC01 (CFB*S, C2*C, C4A*QO, C4B*1)* and *SC21 (CFB*S, C2*C, C4A*A, C4B*1)* in relation to *HLA-B* alleles on the ordinate and *HLA-DR* alleles on the abscissa. Heights and widths representing HLA specificity are proportional to allele frequencies for the respective populations. Clustering represents linkage disequilibrium and flags the extended haplotypes *[HLA-B16(38), SC21, DR4]* in Ashkenazi Jews *[HLA-B8, SC01, DR3]* and in the English and, to a much lesser extent, among Jews. *(From Alper CA, Awdeh ZL, Yunis EJ. Conserved, extended MHC haplotypes. Exp Clin Immunogenet 1992;9:58, Figure 4. Copyright © S. Karger AG, Basel.) HLA,* Human leukocyte antigen.

TABLE 49-2
Common Extended MHC Haplotypes*

Extended haplotype	HLA-Cw allele	Ethnicity
[HLA-B8, SC01, DR3, DQ2]	*0701*	Northern Europe
[HLA-B7, SC31, DR2, DQ6]	*0702*	Northern Europe
[HLA-B44, FC31, DR7, DQ2]	*1601*	Europe
[HLA-B44, SC30, DR4, DQ7/8]	*0501*	Europe
[HLA-B57, SC61, DR7, DQ2/3]	*0602*	Northern Europe
[HLA-B14, SC22, DR1, DQ1]	*0802*	Northern Europe
[HLA-B35, SC31, DR5, DQ3]	*0401*	Southern Europe
[HLA-B38, SC21, DR4, DQ8]	*1203*	Ashkenazi Jews
[HLA-B15, SC33, DR4, DQ8]	*0304*	Northern Europe
[HLA-B18, F1C30, DR3, DQ2]	*0501*	Basques, Sardinia, Spain
[HLA-B18, S042, DR2]†	*1203*	Northern Europe
[HLA-B42, FC(1,90)0, DR3]‡	*1701*	African

HLA, Human leukocyte antigen; *MHC,* major histocompatibility complex.
*Data from normal Caucasoid population chromosomes from Boston.
†Data from patients with C2 deficiency (Clavijo, 1998).
‡Data from chromosomes of normal black population living in Boston (Clavijo, 1999).

extended haplotypes to enhance our understanding of the relevance of a rather extensive literature on MHC disease associations. Most of the MHC disease associations reported to date are contained within extended haplotypes. It is probably because of this simple fact that so many MHC-allele–associated diseases have been reported, because it is not a single base pair but more than 3 million base pairs of conserved DNA that constitute the marker. For example, complement alleles such as *CFB*F1* and *C4B*3* have been linked to type 1 diabetes, because the extended haplotypes that carry them, *[HLA-B18]*, *F1C30*, *DR3]* and *[HLA-B62*, *SC01*, *DR3]*, are more common in these patients than in the general population. This association means that haplotypes comprising 3 million bases or more in length of conserved genomic DNA carry susceptibility alleles for type 1 diabetes. It is also critical to know the ethnic distribution of an associated MHC allele to evaluate whether the allele in patients is increased compared with that in ethnically matched control populations, or is in fact truly a marker for the ethnic distribution of the disease. Furthermore, it is more difficult to map the genes responsible for disease in Caucasian Americans than in African Americans or Asian Americans because the level of genetic diversity is lower in Caucasians.

A remarkable number of diseases show an association with MHC genes. Most diseases associated with MHC are autoimmune and do not show clear-cut mendelian inheritance. Many problems confound attempts to understand the inheritance mechanisms by which these diseases occur, and analysis of MHC markers in patients and their families has clarified the picture only marginally. A major problem with MHC gene associations is their incomplete penetrance, making ordinary formal segregation and linkage studies very difficult, if not impossible, to carry out. This is seen most clearly in monozygotic twins, who presumably have identical genes. If one such twin has one of these diseases (e.g., type 1 diabetes), the other twin does not necessarily have the same disease. For type 1 diabetes, the concordance rate appears to be no higher than 50% (Rubinstein, 1977; Barnett, 1981). This suggests that penetrance of a disease in a completely susceptible host is incomplete. Although there is excellent reason to consider genes in the MHC as determinants of type 1 diabetes susceptibility, only 15% of MHC-identical siblings of diabetic patients have insulin-dependent diabetes. This difference between 50% and 15% provides evidence for the influence of genes at a second, non–MHC-linked locus (or loci), and suggests the influence of other factors, such as environmental factors, in determining susceptibility.

Incomplete penetrance makes assignment of a specific mode of inheritance difficult and makes the likelihood of finding families with more than one affected member within one or more generations low. Families are frequently used to determine modes of inheritance. Another complicating factor is the inability to determine whether we are studying a group of patients that are homogeneous in terms of genetic determination. About 5%–6% of random families with a type 1 diabetic proband will have a second affected child. Of these sibling pairs, approximately 60% will be MHC-identical, 35% will be haploidentical, and a few percent will share

TABLE 49-3

TNF and *HSP* Gene Polymorphisms in Relation to Common Extended Haplotypes*

	COMPLOTYPE				*HSP*		*TNF* MARKERS								
HLA-DR	***C4B***	***C4A***	***CFB***	***C2***	***1B***	***1A***	***e***	***d***	***−308***	***−857***	***−863***	***a***	***b***	***HLA-B***	***HLA-Cw***
3	1	0	S	C	8.5	C	3	1	2	1	1	2	3	8	0701
2	1	3	S	C	9	A	3	3	1	1	1	11	4	7	0702
7	1	3	F	C	9	A	3	3	1	1	1	7, 8	4	44	1601
4	0	3	S	C	9	A	3	3	1	1	1	6, 7	5	44	0501
7	1	6	S	C	9	A	3	4	1	1	1	2	5	57	0602
5	1	3	S	C	9	A	3	3	1	1	1	5	5	35	0401
1	1,2	2	S	C	9	A	1	4	1	1	2	2	1	14	0802
4	1	2	S	C	9	A	3	3	1	2	1	10	4	38	1203
4	3	3	S	C	9	A	1	4	1	1	2	2	1	62	0304
2	2	4	S	0	9	A	3	3	1	2	1	10	4	18	1203
3	0	3	F1	C	8.5	C	3	4	1	1	1	1	5	18	0501

Data from Clavijo O, Delgado J, Awdeh ZL, et al. HLA-Cw alleles associated with HLA extended haplotypes and C2 deficiency. Tissue Antigens 1998;52:282–5.

*The numbers or letters under each column refer to a particular allele variant of the complement, heat-shock protein *(HSP)*, tumor necrosis factor *(TNF)* microsatellite, or *TNF* promoter polymorphisms that are associated with the human leukocyte antigen *(HLA)* specificities as noted. See text for explanation. In the case of *TNF-308*, 1 and 2 represent the *−308/G* and *−308/A* variants, respectively. The *TNF-857/C* allele is noted as 1, and the *TNF-857/T* allele as 2. The *TNF-863/C* TNF allele is noted as 1, and the *−863/A* as 2.

TABLE 49-4

MHC Monogenic Disease Associations

Disease	MHC gene	OMIM no.*
Bare lymphocyte syndrome type 1	*TAP1, TAP2, TAPBP*	604571
C2 deficiency	*C2*	217000
C4 deficiency	*C4A, C4B*	120810
Congenital adrenal hyperplasia	*CYP21A2*	201910
Ehler-Danlos syndrome	*TNXB*	606408
Hypotrichosis simplex of the scalp	*CDSN*	146520
Sialidosis	*NEU1*	256550

MHC, Major histocompatibility complex.

*OMIM number provides disease and gene association information at http://www.ncbi.nlm.nih.gov/omim.

no MHC haplotypes. This pattern suggests recessive inheritance of an MHC-linked susceptibility gene for the disease. At the very least, however, family studies provide highly useful haplotype data and usually allow the assignment of homozygosity for an HLA marker in probands. They have also established that MHC association in most diseases of interest is based on linkage between a susceptibility gene and the MHC.

Yet another unknown is the number of different susceptibility alleles for a disease in any specific population. In this regard, extended haplotypes can be helpful because, if increased in patients, they probably represent a single susceptibility allele that could be anywhere in the region of fixity. However, some patients have only portions of these haplotypes, and this provides little information about the location of specific allele involvement. Furthermore, it appears likely that many MHC-associated diseases are polygenic. Because of this, we will first discuss diseases associated with mutations of a single MHC gene; this will be followed by a discussion of polygenic diseases.

MHC MONOGENIC DISEASE ASSOCIATIONS

Table 49-4 lists MHC monogenic disease associations and their genes. We will discuss the most common diseases. We have already reviewed two of these disorders earlier in the chapter: C2 and C4 protein deficiencies.

Hereditary Hemochromatosis and the *HFE* Gene

Hemochromatosis is an autosomal recessive disease and is the most common hereditary metabolic disease in Caucasians. Hemochromatosis consists of an inherited metabolic defect in iron metabolism, resulting in failure to control iron absorption in the setting of increasing iron stores, leading to tissue iron overload and eventually to organ damage (reviewed in Adams, 2000). The most common manifestations of hemochromatosis are cirrhosis of the liver, hepatocellular carcinoma, diabetes mellitus, and cardiomyopathy. Discovery of the hereditary hemochromatosis (HH) gene in the MHC was based on the early finding of increased frequency of the *HLA-A3* allele in HH patients (Simon, 1976). After years of effort in the vicinity of the *HLA-A* locus, the *HFE* gene was found several megabase pairs away (Feder, 1996). *HFE* encodes a 343 amino acid protein that belongs to a group named MHC class I–related molecules because of their similarities to HLA class I molecules. The HFE protein interacts with the transferrin receptor and modulates enteric absorption of dietary iron (Waheed, 1999).

The *HFE* gene has two common missense mutations: the C282Y mutation, resulting in the substitution of a tyrosine for a cysteine, and the H63D mutation, resulting in the substitution of an aspartate for a histidine. Methods for diagnosis of hemochromatosis are discussed in detail in Chapter 70. The C282Y mutation, unlike the H63D mutation, interferes with protein interaction with β_2-microglobulin, abolishing the cell surface expression of HFE (Feder, 1997; Waheed, 1997). A homozygous C282Y mutation is present in the majority of HH Caucasian patients. The C282Y mutation has a remarkably high allelic frequency in northern European populations (0.05%–0.1%) and is rare in non-Caucasian populations. Penetrance of the C282Y homozygous state is as low as 10% or even 1% (Beutler, 2002). For this reason, population screening for this mutation is not recommended. The H63D mutation is present at high frequency in control Caucasians (>0.1%) and was also found in non-Caucasian populations; however, its role in HH remains unclear.

Congenital Adrenal Hyperplasia Due to 21-Hydroxylase Deficiency

Immediately 3′ to each *C4* locus are two loci for the adrenal steroid enzyme 21 hydroxylase (*CYP21A* and *CYP21B*) (Carroll, 1985; Higashi, 1986; White, 1986). The two genes are highly homologous, but three mutations cause premature termination of transcription of the *CYP21A* gene, rendering it a pseudogene (White, 1988). Congenital adrenal hyperplasia is clinically heterogeneous, with a severe salt-wasting form, a milder late-onset form manifested largely by masculinization in girls, and a mild cryptic form. The MHC linkage of this disorder was discovered before any MHC associations were detected, and before it was known that the *CYP21* loci were located within the MHC. Subsequently, studies found that 20% or more of European Caucasian patients with the salt-wasting form carried the rare extended haplotype *[HLA-A1, Cw6, B47, FC(91)0, DRB1*07, DRB4*0101, DQA1*0201, DQB1*0201]* (Fleischnick, 1983). It has been shown that this haplotype has a deletion of both *C4B* and *CYP21B*, thus explaining the severity of symptoms and the complete deficiency of the enzyme in homozygotes for this haplotype. Among patients with milder and cryptic disease, a different extended haplotype is common: *[HLA-B65, SC2(1,2), DR1]* (Sinnott, 1991). This haplotype is particularly common in southern Europe, and has a frequency of over 0.01% among Caucasians living in Boston. In all forms of 21-hydroxylase deficiency, the bulk of MHC haplotypes are not extended, and there is a great variety of

TABLE 49-5
Polygenic Diseases With MHC Associations

Disease	MHC gene	OMIM no.*
Abacavir hypersensitivity	*HLA-B57*	142830
Ankylosing spondylitis	*HLA-B27*	106300
Autoimmune thyroid disease	*HLA-DR3*	608173
Behçet disease	*HLA-B51*	109650
Celiac disease	*HLA-DQ2, DQ8*	212750
Multiple sclerosis	*HLA-DR, DQ*	126200
Narcolepsy	*HLA-DQ6*	161400
Rheumatoid arthritis	*HLA-DR4*	180300
Type 1 diabetes	*HLA-DR, DQ*	222100

MHC, Major histocompatibility complex.
*OMIM number provides disease and gene association information at http://www.ncbi.nlm.nih.gov/omim.

complotypes, suggesting that many independent mutations have led to deletion or derangement of the *CYP21B* gene.

POLYGENIC DISEASES WITH MHC ASSOCIATIONS

Table 49-5 lists some polygenic diseases and their MHC gene associations. This list is not exhaustive, and we will discuss only a few of the diseases in greater detail.

Abacavir Hypersensitivity

Abacavir is a reverse transcriptase inhibitor used in combination with other antivirals in the treatment of human immunodeficiency virus (HIV) infection. A severe hypersensitivity reaction occurs in 5% of abacavir patients; is characterized by symptoms such as fever, rash, and acute respiratory symptoms; and can lead to potentially life-threatening hypotension if drug therapy is not discontinued (reviewed in Clay, 2002). Patients with the *HLA-B*5701* allele are at risk for an abacavir hypersensitivity reaction (Hetherington, 2002; Mallal, 2002). Recent studies have demonstrated the cost-effectiveness of *HLA-B*5701* screening to reduce the risk of hypersensitivity reaction to abacavir in the treatment of HIV infection (Hughes, 2004; Mallal, 2008). *HLA-B*5701* genotyping can be performed by a variety of PCR or sequencing methods, as discussed in Chapter 48.

Ankylosing Spondylitis

A strong association has been noted between *HLA-B27* and ankylosing spondylitis (AS) in several populations (reviewed in Khan, 1992). About 90% of Caucasian patients with AS have *HLA-B27*, as compared with 5% to 10% of healthy controls (Rubin, 1994). *HLA-B27* shares sequence with proteins from enteric bacteria and peptides that both mimic and bind B27 and may constitute the molecular components of a mechanism for AS (Scofield, 1995). Another hypothesis suggests that "auto-display" occurring within or between B27 molecules provokes an autoimmune attack in AS (Luthra-Guptasarma, 2004). *HLA-B*27* genotyping is frequently performed by flow cytometry. However, *HLA-B27* screening is of limited usefulness given its poor positive predictive value, because among *HLA-B27*–positive individuals in the population at large, only 2% will develop AS (Gran, 1995).

Celiac Disease

Celiac disease (CD), also known as celiac sprue and gluten-sensitive enteropathy, is a disorder characterized by malabsorption resulting from inflammatory injury to the mucosa of the small intestine after ingestion of wheat gluten (reviewed in Green, 2007). Among Caucasians, two HLA-DQ alleles (*HLA-DQ2* and *DQ8*) are found in more than 99% of individuals with CD (Marsh, 1992; Goggins, 1994). Gliadin peptides, which were previously shown to exacerbate CD lesions in vitro and in vivo, have been found to bind to DQ2, lending further credence to the role of this *HLA-DQ* allele in the pathogenesis of CD (Kim, 2004). This finding suggests that HLA-DQ2 could present the gliadin peptide to T cells for autoimmune recognition. Another possible explanation for susceptibility to CD in HLA comes from recent studies showing the binding of atypical invariant chain fragments to HLA-DQ2 (Fallang, 2008; Wiesner, 2008). These studies suggest that HLA-DM–mediated exchange of invariant chain variants and other HLA-DQ2 peptides might be reduced compared with other HLA-DQ molecules, which may provide a basis for the association of CD and *HLA-DQ2*. HLA genetic testing before serologic screening in patients with suspected CD eliminates up to 60% of the population to be screened, and increases the cost-effectiveness of serologic workups (Chang, 2009).

Narcolepsy

Narcolepsy, also known as cataplexy, is a sleep disorder characterized by attacks of disabling daytime drowsiness and low alertness. Most patients with narcolepsy carry the specific *HLA-DQB1*0602* allele (Matsuki, 1992; Mignot, 1997). Patients with narcolepsy have a marked reduction of hypocretin-producing neurons in the hypothalamus compared with normal controls (Matsuki, 1992; Blouin, 2005). Findings of recent studies are consistent with immunologically mediated destruction of hypocretin-containing cells in patients with narcolepsy (Mignot, 2001). HLA testing in patients with narcolepsy has an excellent negative predictive value and is useful in ruling out the disease in patients with unexplained sleepiness (Hong, 2006).

Rheumatoid Arthritis

Rheumatoid arthritis (RA) is an inflammatory disease, primarily of the joints, with autoimmune features and a complex genetic component. The association between MHC markers and RA is well documented (Nepom, 1992; Ollier, 1992; Auger, 1998). For most of the populations studied, the primary associated marker is *HLA-DR4* (MacGregor, 1995). In Caucasians, for example, the most common RA-associated *DR4* alleles are *DRB1*0401* and *DRB1*0404*, and in Japanese, Israeli, and Chinese patients, it is *DRB1*0405*. Other *HLA-DR* specificities are also associated with RA: *DR1* has been reported in association with RA in Caucasian, Japanese, Spanish, Greek, and Israeli patients; *DR3* in Kuwaitis; *DR6* in Yakima American Indians; *DR9* in Chileans; and *DR10* in Spanish, Greek, and Israeli patients (reviewed in Zanelli, 2000).

To explain this broad spectrum of different *HLA-DR* associations with RA, it has been proposed that a shared DRB1 peptide epitope is involved in conferring RA susceptibility (Penzotti, 1996). The alleles associated with RA share a highly conserved sequence of amino acids in their third hypervariable region (amino acids 67–74). Individuals with RA frequently have autoantibodies to citrullinated peptides. Citrullination of self-antigens increases the affinity between these peptides and HLA-DR molecules carrying the shared peptide epitope (Hill, 2003; Lundberg, 2005). Thus, if a citrullinated arthritogenic peptide exists, it may bind preferentially to molecules with the RA DRB1 sequence. As yet, no such arthritogenic peptide has been identified. An alternative explanation may involve molecular mimicry between the shared RA DRB1 and antigenic sequences of a pathogen that can induce RA (Albani, 1992). Sequence homology has been found between the shared RA sequence and an HSP from *Escherichia coli* (Auger, 1998).

RA differs clinically from juvenile rheumatoid arthritis (JRA), and HLA associations with JRA are different as well. Furthermore, other *HLA-DR* associations vary among JRA clinical subsets (Stastny, 1993). For example, it has been reported that the frequency of haplotype *HLA-DRB1*0801, DQA1*0401, DQB1*0402* is increased in the whole pauciarticular group and in patients with the persistent pauciarticular form. The haplotype *HLA-DRB1*1301, DRB3*0101, DQA1*0103, DQB1*0603* was also associated with patients with persistent pauciarticular JRA (Fernandez-Vina, 1994). In keeping with the view that the polyarticular form of JRA is RA occurrence in the young, *DRB1*0401* shows a strong association.

Type 1 Diabetes

The most studied of all MHC-linked diseases is type 1 diabetes mellitus (Nepom, 1991; Thorsby, 1992; Winter, 1993; Lernmark, 1999). Type 1 diabetes is a disorder of glucose homeostasis that is characterized by susceptibility to ketoacidosis in the absence of insulin therapy. It is a genetically heterogeneous autoimmune disease affecting about 0.3% of Caucasian populations (Todd, 1990). Alleles of the HLA class II genes *DQ* and *DR* in the MHC region are major determinants of genetic predisposition to type 1 diabetes. Several alleles of these loci are associated with susceptibility to or protection from disease. Striking increases have been noted in the frequency of *HLA-DR3* and *HLA-DR4* among Caucasian patients (Thomson, 1984; Jenkins, 1991). Using molecular-based HLA typing analysis, the increase in *DR4* is found primarily in the subset of *DR4* in linkage disequilibrium with *DQB1*0302* (Kockum, 1993). Although the latter gene is now considered a major marker and perhaps a primary determinant of type 1 diabetes susceptibility, it is present in only 70% of Caucasian patients. Even among those who carry it, variability in the relative risk for diabetes is observed: *DRB1*0401*, *DQB1*0302* and *DRB1*0402*, and *DQB1*0302* are highly associated with the disease, but *DRB1*0404*, *DQB1*0302* is less so.

In many Caucasian patient populations with type 1 diabetes, there is an excess of *DR3/DR4* heterozygotes over the number of *DR3* or *DR4* homozygotes predicted by the Hardy-Weinberg equilibrium (Kockum, 1999). In addition, the relative risks for some *DR-DQ* genotypes are not simply the sum or product of relative risks for the single haplotype. For example, risk for the *DRB1*03–DQB1*02/DRB1*0401–DQB1*0302* genotype is often found to be higher than for the individual *DRB1*03–DQB1*02* and *DRB1*0401–DQB1*0302* homozygous genotypes. It has been hypothesized that this synergy occurs through the formation of highly susceptible *trans*-encoded HLA-DQB1 and HLA-DQA1 heterodimers (Nepom, 1987; Khalil, 1992). The DR-α molecules are not polymorphic, and mixed DR α-β dimers would not result in novel HLA molecules. On the other hand, both the α and β chains of *DQ* are polymorphic, and a DQ α-β dimer composed of transcomplementing chains would be unique to a heterozygous individual and would not be expressed in either parent. In the mouse, such transcomplementation has been demonstrated structurally, and epitopes newly formed in the resulting hybrid molecules allow for an altered functional immune response different from that of either parent (Charron, 1984; Long, 1984).

The *DRB1*1501*, *DQB1*0602* haplotype is negatively associated with type 1 diabetes. Individuals heterozygous for *DRB1*1501*, *DQB1*0602* who also carry a susceptibility gene for type 1 diabetes on the other haplotype are nonetheless not at risk for the disease (dominant protection), as would be expected with a recessive disorder (Noble, 1996). A recently proposed model for type 1 diabetes, which assumes that *DQB1* is a direct determinant of susceptibility, suggests a hierarchy of affinities among different class II molecules that compete for binding to the same type 1 diabetes peptide (Nepom, 1990). Susceptibility occurs if a gene product (e.g., DQB1*0302) binds and presents the type 1 diabetes peptide. In the presence of a high-affinity competitor (DRB1*1501), this event does not occur. Another model proposes that codon 57 of the *DQB*-encoded chain plays a critical role in the pathogenesis of type 1 diabetes. The presence of a nonaspartic acid at position 57 of *DQB1* has been suggested as an important determinant of susceptibility to type 1 diabetes mediated by the *DQB1* genes (Lee, 2001; Siebold, 2004). The excess presence of valine or serine at this position in diabetic patients carrying the *HLA-DR3* or *DR4* haplotype supports this concept.

Methods of Detecting Association or Linkage of Disease with Genetic Markers

GENETIC POLYMORPHISM

Genetic polymorphism is defined as the occurrence of two or more alleles at one gene, each with appreciable frequency in the same population. The frequency has been arbitrarily defined to be higher than 1%. Two groups of genetic polymorphisms are known: balanced or stable, and transient. A balanced or stable polymorphism occurs when two or more alleles are maintained in a population by selection. The heterozygous advantage is the classic example of a balanced polymorphism. A transient polymorphism represents a phase of allelic changes driven by genetic drift or by selection. Polymorphism of a gene can be stable in one population and transient in another, depending on the effect of selection.

GENE AND PHENOTYPE FREQUENCIES

To determine genetic polymorphism, it is necessary to find a representative sample of the population, assess the individuals, count the genes, and estimate the number of genes contained in the entire population. For example, assuming that a population of 100 individuals has been studied for a particular genetic trait or allele at a given gene, we can define the phenotype frequency as the number of individuals carrying the trait or the genetic variant. To calculate the frequency (f) of a given allele, divide the number of times that allele occurs (x) by the total occurrences of all alleles of that gene in the population ($x+y+z+...$):

$$f(x) = x/(x + y + z + \ldots) \qquad \textbf{(49-1)}$$

It is possible to calculate the gene frequency (g) without knowing the mode of inheritance by using the formula:

$$g = 1 - \sqrt{f} \qquad \textbf{(49-2)}$$

STRENGTH OF ASSOCIATION

Several methods have been devised for detecting the degree of association of genetic markers with hypothesized genes for disease susceptibility. One method is to compute the risk of disease among individuals carrying a specific allele of a polymorphic system. In this computation, the relative risk (RR), or odds ratio, calculates the risk of carrying a marker in a population of diseased individuals compared with a control population. This strength of association is the delta of Bergston and Thomson (Svejgaard, 1983), which is the same as the etiologic fraction (EF) (Miettinen, 1976). If, in a patient population, "a" individuals carry the specific character but "b" individuals do not, and in the control (normal) population, "c" individuals carry the character, we may write the information conveniently in the 2 × 2 table as follows:

	Character-Positive	Character-Negative
Patient	a	b
Control	c	d

The frequency of the character in this patient population (h_p) is:

$$h_p = \frac{a}{a+b} \qquad \textbf{(49-3)}$$

The RR, or odds ratio, is defined as follows:

$$\text{RR} = \frac{a \times d}{b \times c} \qquad \textbf{(49-4)}$$

Etiologic fraction is defined as follows:

$$\text{EF} = \frac{\text{RR} - 1}{\text{RR}} \times \frac{a}{a + b} = \frac{\text{RR} - 1}{\text{RR}} \times h_p \qquad \textbf{(49-5)}$$

Similarly, in decreased risk, for which the RR is less than 1, the preventive factor (PF) can be used:

$$\text{PF} = \frac{(1 - \text{RR})\, h_p}{\text{RR}\,(1 - h_p) + h_p} \qquad \textbf{(49-6)}$$

EF and PF fraction can vary between 0 (no association) and 1.0 (maximal association). Apart from providing estimates of having a marker if one already has a disease, these calculations ignore the mode of genetic determination of the disease in question. This is particularly problematic for recessive or more complicated modes, in which both haplotypes are important for determining disease, but heterozygotes and homozygotes for a given marker are given the same weight, that is, both are positive for the marker.

ANALYSIS OF MODE OF INHERITANCE BASED ON SIBLING PAIRS

Analysis of mode of inheritance based on sibling pairs was introduced to help overcome the problems of incomplete penetrance of disease genes and variations in the age of onset (Penrose, 1935). This analysis is based on the assumption that if HLA and/or genes closely linked to HLA have no influence on the development of a disease, then the affected sibling pairs will share HLA haplotypes with a normal frequency: 25% will share both haplotypes, 50% will share one, and 25% will share no haplotypes. Thus, observed and expected distributions of haplotype sharing are compared. If susceptibility genes or their closely linked markers are rare and fully penetrant in a purely recessively determined disease, the distributions of two-, one-, and no-haplotype–sharing sibs would be 100, 0, and 0. For dominant determination, the ratios would be 33, 66, and 0. What is observed in diabetes, for example (Rubinstein, 1977), is 60, 35, and 5—closer to recessive than dominant predictions. Once the mode of inheritance has been established, disease gene frequency and penetrance can be determined (Thomson, 1977).

ANALYSIS OF MODE OF INHERITANCE BASED ON POPULATION STUDIES

Investigators (Thomson, 1977) have devised a method for analyzing population data for markers closely linked to susceptibility loci for diseases with incomplete penetrance. In essence, this method predicts the proportions of homozygotes, heterozygotes, and noncarriers for the linked marker that are expected in cases of dominant or recessive inheritance. The greatest difference between the two modes of inheritance is observed in the proportions of individuals who are homozygous for the marker. Application of this method to *HLA-B27* and AS led, on statistical grounds, to rejection of a recessive mechanism. Thus, it was concluded that susceptibility to AS is inherited as a dominant trait.

The same method of analysis was applied to the distribution of *CFB*F1* among 1107 patients with type 1 diabetes mellitus (Raum, 1981). For dominant inheritance, 1.89 homozygotes were predicted, and for recessive inheritance, 6.2 homozygotes were predicted. Seven *CFB*F1* homozygotes were found—a result that is consistent only with recessive inheritance. Other modes of inheritance that could be rejected by these observations include simple dominant, epistatic (disease resulting from the presence of nonallelic genes), and overdominant (disease with greater penetrance when two specific alleles are present than when other combinations, including homozygosity for each specific allele, occur). Although a mixed model with different penetrance for homozygotes and heterozygotes could not be completely ruled out, other considerations make such a model unsatisfactory.

LOD SCORE METHOD

The logarithm of the odds (LOD) score is a statistical measure of linkage between a marker locus, such as in the MHC, and a disease susceptibility gene (Sutton, 1980). In the equation for calculating the LOD score, (1) the Z value is the ratio of the maximum likelihood of finding linkage ($P(F_1/\theta)$) to that of no linkage at a particular recombination value of θ, and (2) the $\theta(q)$ value, or recombination frequency, is a measure of the distance from a given locus corresponding to maximum Z value. The LOD score expresses the probability that alleles at two loci will segregate together, in terms of the ratio between the observed and the predicted recombination frequency if they assort independently. Various values of (q) from 0 to 0.5 are substituted into the following equation:

$$P(F_1/\theta) = 1/2\left[\theta^r(1-\theta)^{n-r} + \theta^{n-r}(1-\theta)^r\right] \quad \textbf{(49-7)}$$

where n = the number of children in a given family and r = the number of recombinants. The probability of obtaining a pedigree for a given value of θ (recombination frequency from 0 to 0.5), which is expressed as the ratio of $P(F_1/\theta)$ in a family at a given recombination fraction θ (from 0 to 0.5) to $P(F_1/0.5)$ in the same family assuming no recombination, can be expressed as the LOD score (Z). The LOD score is the sum of all z values where Z is

$$z = \log_{10}\frac{P(F_1/\theta)}{P(F_1/0.5)} \quad \textbf{(49-8)}$$

Values of Z greater than zero favor linkage, and those less than or equal to zero are against linkage. In general, a Z value greater than 3 (for some values of $\theta < 0.5$) means that the odds in favor of linkage are 1000 to 1 (p value = 0.05), as opposed to no linkage or independence. It is easier to calculate linkage for codominant traits (e.g., HLA) than for recessive traits. In studies that examine the linkage of HLA and disease, the parents may have recessive or dominant impenetrant susceptibility genes. Basic problems have been noted in using the LOD score method to detect linkage of partially penetrant genes, apart from impenetrant susceptible siblings. If susceptibility genes are common, as appears to be the case in type 1 diabetes, for example, apparent crossovers or nonidentical siblings could suggest additional susceptibility genes in a parent.

SUMMARY

The MHC comprises many alleles at many loci. The high resolution typing of class I and class II MHC genes and the identification of genes between and near them have increased the possibility of defining the genetic basis for immune responses and diseases of unknown origin, such as autoimmune diseases in man. The nonrandom association of markers with immune responses or associations with autoimmune diseases due to the presence of fixed stretches of MHC DNA and extended haplotypes and their fragments in the population complicate the study of susceptibility genes but also provide the means for their identification. Even though the human MHC is the most intensively investigated region of the genome, not all of the expressed genes within the MHC have been identified. It is probable that some unidentified MHC genes, rather than the one already identified, are susceptibility genes for some human MHC-associated diseases.

SELECTED REFERENCES

Brown JH, Jardetzky TS, Gorga JC, et al. Three-dimensional structure of the human class II histocompatibility antigen HLA-DR1 [see comments]. Nature 1993;364:33–9.

This landmark paper shows the first crystal structure of an HLA class II molecule associated with peptide.

Stewart CA, Horton R, Allcock RJN, et al. Complete MHC haplotype sequencing for common disease gene mapping. Genome Res 2004;14:1176–87.

This landmark report is the first of what will undoubtedly be many reports of the fine structure of MHC haplotypes to map the genetic variants that confer disease susceptibility.

Yunis EJ, Larsen CE, Fernandez-Vina M, et al. Inheritable variable sizes of DNA stretches in the human MHC: conserved extended haplotypes and their fragments or blocks. Tissue Antigens 2003;62:1–20.

A recent review of MHC haplotypes and smaller haplotype blocks, and an update of their allele compositions in the world's populations.

REFERENCES

Access the complete reference list online at http://www.expertconsult.com

CHAPTER 50

IMMUNODEFICIENCY DISORDERS

Kimberly W. Sanford, Susan D. Roseff

KEY POINTS

- Primary immunodeficiencies are a group of single gene disorders.
- Because of the complexity of diagnosing a primary immunodeficiency, the cooperation of the clinician, the research scientist, and the clinical pathologist is required.
- A logical approach to the diagnosis of primary immunodeficiency disorders based on staged diagnostic testing is necessary because of the complex nature of the immune system.
- Preparation for specimen collection, handling, and delivery to a specialty laboratory is required for performing complex immunologic assays.
- As a result of technological advances, molecular genetic testing is increasingly employed in diagnosing primary immunodeficiency disorders and will be paramount in guiding future treatment.

Primary immunodeficiencies are a group of single-gene disorders that result in defects in the immune system. The manifestations can vary in terms of degree of severity, types of symptoms exhibited, or both. These conditions, when unrecognized and left untreated, can result in death from infection. A genetic defect may result in loss of a critical enzyme, may cause developmental arrest in one aspect of the immune system, may cause loss of a structural component, or may create a nonfunctional protein. Most of these disorders are X-linked, resulting in a disproportionate number of affected males—approximately 70% of patients with primary immunodeficiency disorders (Puck, 1997a). A majority of primary immunodeficiencies are detected before 20 years of age, but diagnosis can be delayed because recognition requires a high degree of clinical suspicion. More than 100 primary immunodeficiency disorders have been described; however, more than 90% of such patients are affected by fewer than 20 primary immunodeficiency disorders (Puck, 1997a). Whereas primary immunodeficiency disorders are due to single gene mutations, secondary immunodeficiencies may be due to malnutrition, viral infection, hematologic and other types of malignancy, chemotherapeutic treatment for malignancy, and immunosuppressive medication for treatment of a variety of disorders.

The natural physical barriers of the body are the first line of defense against invading microbes and include skin, mucus at exposed mucosal surfaces, and ciliated cells of the respiratory, intestinal, and genital tracts. In addition to physical barriers, immunologic functions of the body exert continual surveillance through acquired and innate modes of action. The acquired immunologic response is specific, requiring previous antigen exposure for sensitization, and improves with each subsequent challenge from a given antigen. These responses are the result of a proliferation of antigen-specific B and T cells, which are stimulated after cellular receptors bind to antigens. B cells produce antigen-specific antibodies to eliminate extracellular antigens. T cells assist B cells to produce antigen-specific antibodies and also kill cells that are virally infected. Innate responses do not require prior antigen exposure and comprise phagocytic cells (macrophages, neutrophils, and monocytes), complement, cytokines, and acute phase reactants (Delves, 2000).

The immune system is an interlocking group of immune cells and immune functions, in which any defect may result in an immunodeficiency. The incidence of primary immunodeficiency diseases in the United States is estimated at about 1 in 200,000 liveborn infants, excluding selective immunoglobulin (Ig)A deficiency (Winkelstein, 2000). The most common immunodeficiency, selective IgA deficiency, has an incidence of 1 in every 1200 healthy blood donors, with IgA levels less than 0.05 mg/dL (Sandler, 1994). As a whole, the estimated incidence of diagnosed primary immunodeficiency disease is 1 in 10,000 (Immune Deficiency Foundation, 1992; Shearer, 1994; Smith, 1999). Data from Australia and Norway estimate the incidence of primary immunodeficiency at 2.1 per 100,000 (Baumgart, 1997) and 6.8 per 100,000, respectively (Ryser, 1988; Stray-Pedersen, 1997; Matamoros, 2000).

For unknown reasons, approximately half of reported immune defects involve defective antibody production due to low numbers of B cells or B cells with decreased production of antigen-specific antibody. Decreased antigen-specific antibody production most frequently manifests as recurrent pulmonary or sinus infection, as well as bacterial septicemia (Noroski, 1998). These infections are typically caused by encapsulated bacteria such as *Streptococcus pneumoniae* or *Haemophilus influenzae.* Defective T cell immunity is characteristically associated with opportunistic, viral, and fungal infections, such as *Candida albicans, Mycobacterium avium-intracellulare* (MAI), and *Pneumocystis (carinii) jiroveci* (Buckley, 2000). The type of infection a patient acquires may point toward the type of cellular immune defect that is present (Fig. 50-1). Primary immunodeficiency disorders are also associated with autoimmune diseases, as well as malignant neoplasms and especially lymphomas (Smith, 1999).

Clinical Signs and Symptoms of Immunodeficiency

Most frequently, increased susceptibility to recurrent infection is the first clinical indication of an immune defect. The type of recurrent infection provides insight into the immune defect and helps guide the clinician in evaluating the patient. Therefore, the most critical part of the medical evaluation is obtaining a complete medical history. Identifying children with immunodeficiency presents a significant challenge to pediatricians, because infections are a common occurrence in normal childhood but can be the principal manifestation of a primary immunodeficiency. Therefore, frequent and prolonged infections, coupled with failure to thrive, or opportunistic infections require a thorough immunologic workup (Puck, 1999). A confirmed report of an immunodeficiency disease occurring in a sibling or first-degree relative should also prompt careful clinical assessment and laboratory investigation, even without a history of severe or unusual infections. In one study of 70 patients with primary immunodeficiency disorders, approximately 18.6% had a family history of an immunodeficiency (Kobrynski, 2002).

Awareness of common clinical presentations can aid physicians in identifying individuals who are more likely to have a primary immune defect. Clinical signs and symptoms of primary immunodeficiency are presented in Figure 50-2. In addition to these warning signs, the physician should be alerted by elements in the history that are unusual, such as a history of autoimmune disease, significant lymphadenopathy, the need for an adult to have a myringotomy, severe herpes zoster or herpes zoster appearing in a young child, or intractable diarrhea or ulcerative colitis diagnosed in a child younger than 1 year old. These additional signs and symptoms should prompt evaluation for a possible immune defect.

It is not practical to investigate all immunologic systems in all patients, so the clinical picture and age of the patient will point the investigator to the portion of the immune system that is most likely to be affected. Taking a careful history and performing a thorough physical examination can narrow the possibilities to defects involving T cells, B cells, granulocytes, or the complement system. The roles of these host defenses and their correlation with different immunodeficiency disorders are presented in Figure 50-3.

It is also important to pay attention to the clinical circumstances and not to dwell exclusively on the number or severity of infectious episodes (Atkinson, 2000). For example, when an infectious process involves the same anatomic site repeatedly, the cause is more likely to be structural, not failure of one of the host defenses. Examples include chronic osteomyelitis in one location, recurrent episodes of pneumonia that affect only one lobe of the lung, and recurrent infection of a surgical wound. Additionally, some primary immunodeficiency disorders, such as chronic granulomatous disease, may present later in life than expected; however, it is still important to keep these disorders in the differential diagnosis (Lukela, 2005).

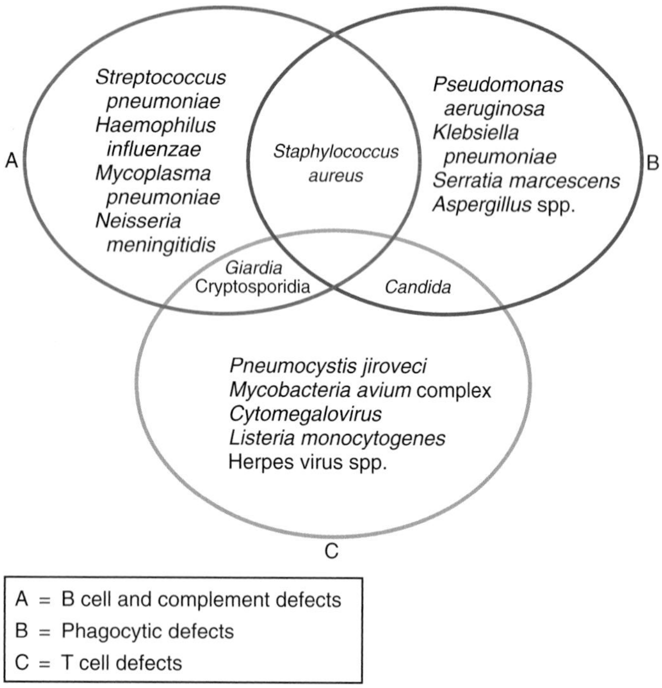

Figure 50-1 Infections associated with cellular immune defects.

Evaluation of the Immune System

Based on the previous considerations, when an immune defect is suspected, evaluation of the immune system is best approached in stages, with basic screening tests performed first and more complex testing conducted as indicated. For example, if a patient presents with strong clinical symptoms suggestive of a B or T cell disorder but a normal lymphocyte count, further investigation by a lymphocyte enumeration panel is warranted. An overview of this staged approach is given in Figure 50-4, and a basic testing algorithm for immunodeficiencies is provided in Figure 50-5.

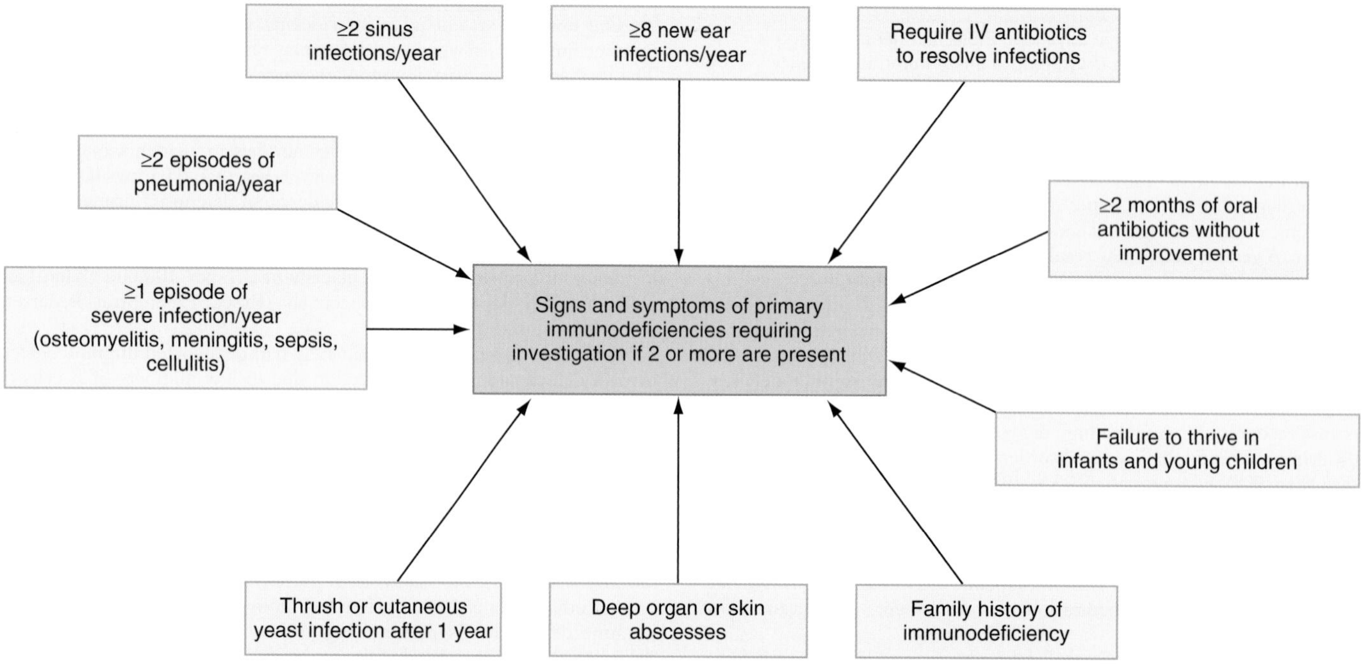

Figure 50-2 Clinical signs and symptoms of primary immunodeficiencies.

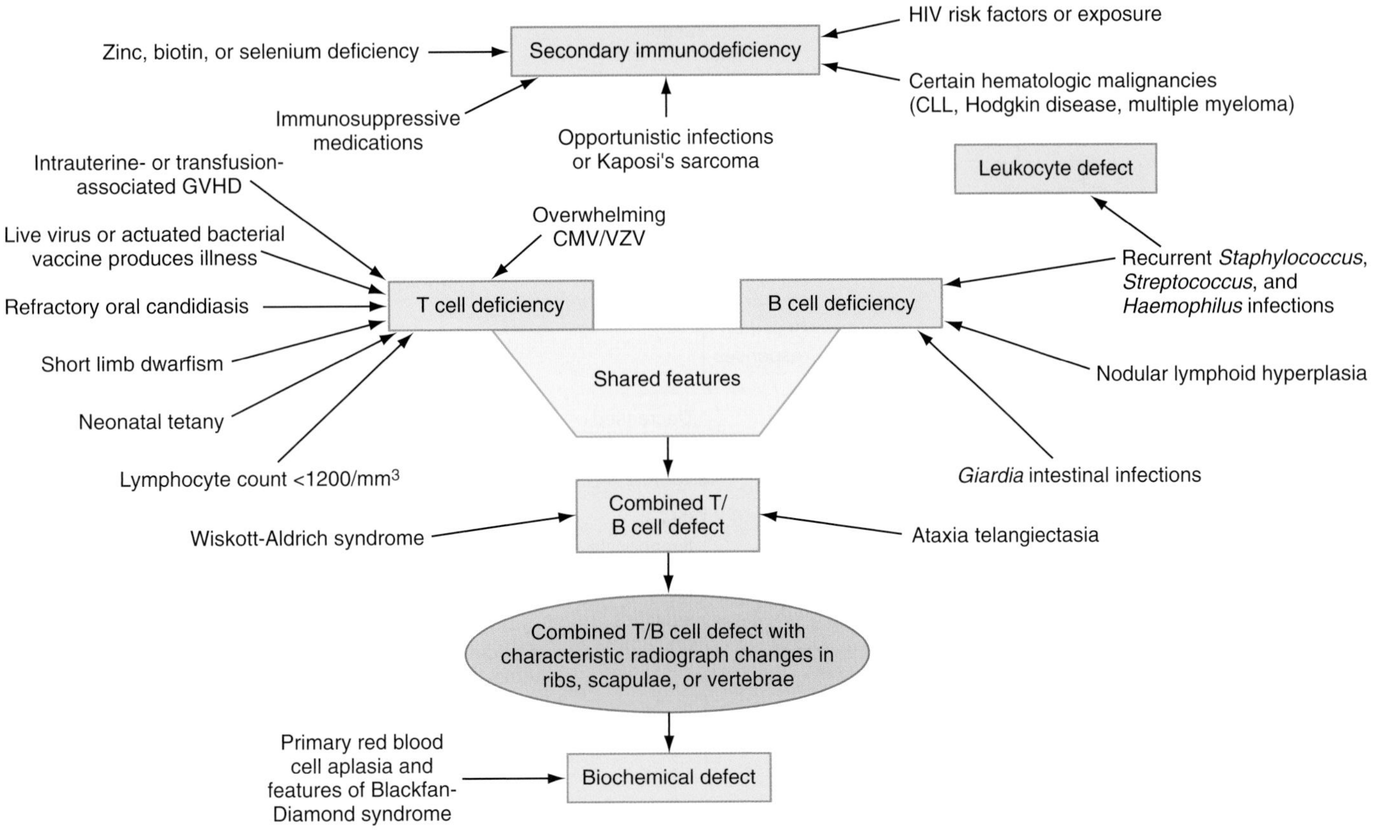

Figure 50-3 Patterns of immunodeficiency disorders. *CLL,* Chronic lymphoid leukemia; *CMV,* cytomegalovirus; *GVHD,* graft-versus-host disease; *HIV,* human immunodeficiency virus; *VZV,* varicella zoster virus.

Primary Investigation

- History and physical examination
- CBC/differential
- Radiographs
- Quantitative immunoglobulins (IgG, IgM, IgA)
- Review of previous culture results
- Pulmonary function testing

Secondary Investigation

- Titers for vaccines administered (tetanus, diphtheria, pneumococcus)
- IgG subclass analysis
- Lymphocyte enumeration panel (CD3, CD4, CD8, CD19, CD16, CD56)
- Complement levels (CH50, C3, C4)
- Skin testing
- Mononuclear cell proliferation studies
- NBT

Tertiary Investigation

- Enzyme studies (adenosine deaminase, purine nucleotide phosphorylase)
- NK cell cytotoxic studies
- Phagocyte studies
- Histology and immunohistochemistry analysis (or flow cytometry) of lymph nodes or lymphoid organs
- Cytokine production
- Advanced complement studies
- Molecular biology

Figure 50-4 Staged approach for laboratory investigation of primary immunodeficiency. *CBC,* Complete blood count; *NBT,* nitroblue tetrazolium slide test; *NK cell,* natural killer cell.

FIRST-LEVEL INVESTIGATIONS

Clinical History, Physical Examination, and Initial Blood Count

A thorough clinical history provides the primary clues in diagnosing a primary immunodeficiency disorder. The typical history includes recurrent, persistent infections or infections caused by unusual microbes. The clinician will be guided by the types of infection the patient has acquired. Patients with immunoglobulin deficiencies typically report an increased number of bacterial infections. Repeated viral, fungal, or other opportunistic infections are associated with T cell immunodeficiencies. Patients with phagocytic defects usually report a history of infections with catalase-positive bacteria, such as *Staphylococcus* spp. Complement deficiencies are most frequently associated with *Streptococcus pneumoniae* or *Neisseria* spp. infections (see Fig. 50-1) (Lindegren, 2004).

The physical examination may reveal findings that are characteristic for particular primary immunodeficiency disorders. Patients with primary immunodeficiency diseases are pale and lethargic, and appear chronically ill. Infants and young children affected with primary immunodeficiency disorders may present with failure to thrive, so monitoring height and weight is important. Small or absent peripheral lymph nodes, tonsils, or adenoids are indicative of X-linked agammaglobulinemia (Lindegren, 2004). In addition to respiratory infection, the infant may experience rhinitis, conjunctivitis, or hematologic, gastrointestinal, and autoimmune disorders (Fleisher, 2003). In contrast, patients with chronic granulomatous disease (CGD) and common variable immunodeficiency present with normal or enlarged peripheral lymph nodes (Buckley, 2000). The genetic defect in Wiskott-Aldrich syndrome causes immunodeficiency and thrombocytopenia, resulting in the combination of increased bruisability, petechiae, and eczematous skin rashes (Zhu, 1997).

The first test performed to examine the immune system is the complete blood count. A white blood count and differential will provide information on the morphology and number of small lymphocytes (diameter <10 μm). Normal parameters vary, based on the age of the patient, and therefore must be interpreted using age-appropriate normal ranges. At a minimum, regardless of age, one expects more than 1200 small lymphocytes per cubic millimeter. Because few (≈10%) of the lymphocytes are B lymphocytes, an

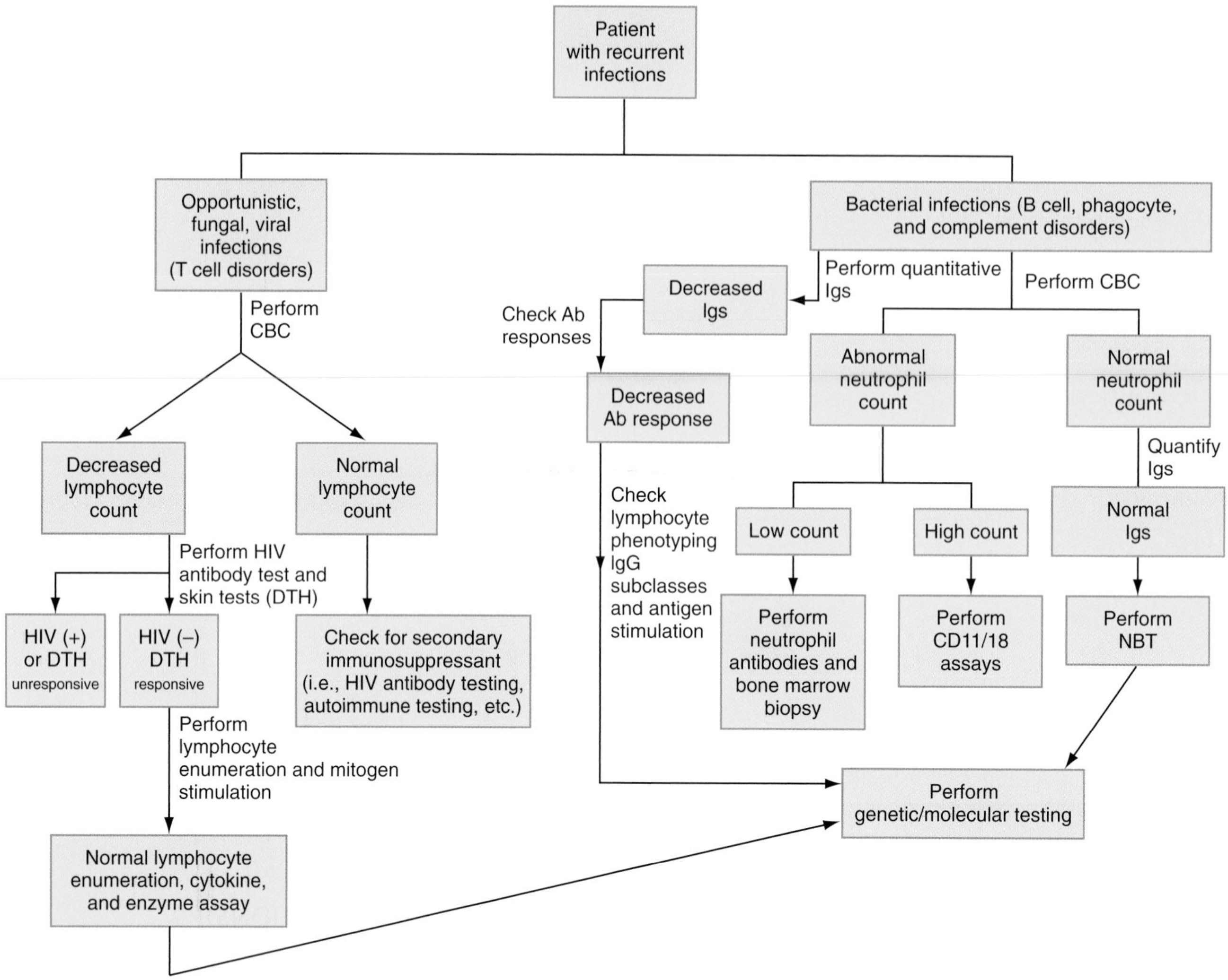

Figure 50-5 Testing algorithm for immunodeficiency. *Ab,* Antibody; *CBC,* complete blood count; *DTH,* delayed-type hypersensitivity skin test; *HIV,* human immunodeficiency virus; *Ig,* immunoglobulin; *NBT,* nitroblue tetrazolium slide test; *PPD,* purified protein derivative.

absolute lymphocyte deficiency primarily reflects T cell deficiency. Part of the first visit should include obtaining all previous medical records, including pathology reports or slides, and results of previous cultures and radiographs.

Immunoglobulins

Because antibody deficiency diseases are more common than other immune defects, first emphasis should be placed on investigation of immunoglobulins and their production (Stiehm, 1996). Approximately half of primary immunodeficiency disorders are related to inadequate antibody production or nonfunctional antibodies (Noroski, 1998). Quantitative immunoglobulin assays are readily available in all commercial and larger hospital laboratories and require only small volumes of serum to perform (see Chapters 19 and 46). Because immunoglobulin values increase with age, comparison with age-matched normal ranges is necessary for correct interpretation.

For the first few months of life, IgG is the major immunoglobulin found in infant serum and is maternal in origin. At approximately 3 months of age, dissipation of maternal IgG concentration, combined with a lag in production by the infant, creates a nadir in IgG levels. However, primarily IgM and secondarily IgA are synthesized by the infant; thus, the presence of these two immunoglobulins provides convincing evidence that X-linked agammaglobulinemia, characterized by pan-hypogammaglobulinemia, is not present. Therefore, IgA, IgM, and IgG should be quantified simultaneously.

Often, IgA is not present in significant amounts until 6 months of age; however, after 1 year of age, IgA levels that remain decreased indicate that this is a permanent defect (Plebani, 1986). IgA-deficient patients may be asymptomatic or may have mild symptoms such as increased respiratory or gastrointestinal infection; however, patients may experience severe or fatal anaphylactic reactions to plasma in blood products that contain IgA (Lindegren, 2004).

Hyper-IgM syndrome, an X-linked T cell inherited disorder, is characterized by normal to elevated levels of IgM with markedly low levels of IgA, IgG, and IgE (Levy 1997; Ramesh, 1998; Buckley, 2000). However, marked elevations of IgE are almost always part of the hyper-IgE syndrome (Buckley, 1978) and are common in immunodysregulation, polyendocrinopathy, enteropathy, immunodysregulation polyendocrinopathy enteropathy X-linked syndrome (IPEX), atypical complete DiGeorge syndrome, Wiskott-Aldrich syndrome (WAS), and Omenn syndrome (Ozcan, 2008). WAS characteristically shows marked elevation of serum IgA combined with low IgM concentrations (Ochs, 1998).

A simple way to assess functional antibody levels in children is to check for isohemagglutinins directed against ABO antigens that the patient lacks, because their presence will indicate active functional antibody production (Fleisher, 2003). Isohemagglutinins are naturally occurring antibodies that form at some point after 2–3 months of age; however, testing for these antibodies is not valid for children 4–6 months of age because of the persistence of maternal immunoglobulin. Additionally, because of relative immaturity, or perhaps inadequate exposure, children with normal immunity may have low concentrations of isohemagglutinins until 5–10 years of age (Cooling, 2008).

Radiologic Imaging

Radiographs, computed tomography (CT), and magnetic resonance imaging (MRI) studies can be helpful in assessing immunodeficiencies. Chronic interstitial pneumonia is common in infants, children, and adults with T cell deficiencies, and should be confirmed on chest radiograph. With time, many patients with primary B cell deficiency (agammaglobulinemia, common variable immunodeficiency) may develop chronic pulmonary fibrosis or bronchiectasis (Sweinberg, 1991; Cunningham-Rundles, 1999). Chest CT in a patient who has recurrent respiratory tract infection is the best means of investigating for bronchiectasis; if these changes have developed, further investigation is clearly warranted.

In the past, lateral views of the neck were used to assess pharyngeal lymphoid tissue in children. However, radiographs are not recommended for evaluation of cervical lymphoid tissue because the information they provide is more easily obtained by alternative methods. Frontal views of the chest may reveal an absence of the thymic shadow in infants, but because the thymus can shrink easily because of stress, evaluation of thymic size by this method is not reliable. Bony abnormalities, however, can alert the radiologist to an immunologic problem presenting in childhood. A subset of patients with immunodeficiencies involving abnormalities of T cells, or both T and B cells, have short-limbed dwarfism. These patients show characteristic lesions, usually in the metaphyseal regions of the long bones. Patients with infant-onset adenosine deaminase deficiency show readily identifiable skeletal abnormalities of ribs and hips (Lindegren, 2004). Bony abnormalities may be present in patients with the hyper-IgE syndrome; these abnormalities include diffuse osteoporosis, fractures that occur with little trauma, craniosynostosis, and midline bony defects (Grimbacher, 1999).

Pulmonary Functions

Immunodeficiency, especially if it has persisted for some time, will often affect the pulmonary system and its function, as previously mentioned. Therefore complete lung volumes, with forced expiratory volumes, should be tested, even if the chest radiograph is normal. Patients with both T and B cell defects are subject to pulmonary infection, often resulting in bronchospasm, restrictive or obstructive disease, or combinations of these abnormalities. Those patients who are both IgA and IgG2 deficient have significantly abnormal pulmonary function tests, and a causal relationship may be seen between these deficiencies and deterioration of lung function (Bjorkander, 1985).

SECOND-LEVEL INVESTIGATIONS

Antibody Production

Investigation of specific antibody production may require only monitoring of immune response to vaccine antigens and is the most direct method by which to assess B cell function. This is a useful approach for patients with a history of recurrent bacterial infection and low-normal quantitative immunoglobulin concentrations. The definitive method used to assess decreased quantitative immunoglobulins consists of measurement of antigen-specific preimmunization levels and postimmunization antibody levels approximately 4 weeks later. If the child or adult has received the usual immunizations in the past, antibody titers for these vaccine antigens can be measured. The most useful vaccine responses to assess are those associated with tetanus, diphtheria, *Haemophilus*, and *Pneumococcus;* many commercial laboratories have developed sensitive tests such as enzyme-linked immunosorbent assays (ELISAs) that can be used to assess antibody production. Evaluation of immune responses to vaccine must include pre-immunization serum antibody concentrations and the patient's age, because these factors affect antibody response. The testing laboratory provides guidelines for appropriate antibody responses. In general, a fourfold increase in protein antigens and a twofold increase in polysaccharide antigens are expected.

Antibody responses to tetanus toxoid and diphtheria toxoid are useful in evaluating responses to T cell–dependent protein antigens. Assessment of B cell function requires evaluation of responses to carbohydrate antigens, which activate B cells directly. It is important to use carbohydrate antigens that are not conjugated to proteins, such as meningococcal and pneumococcal polysaccharide antigens (Balmer, 2003). Children younger than 2 years old will not respond to unconjugated carbohydrate antigens (Barrett, 1984), and no live virus vaccines should be administered to the child, or any family member, until immunodeficiency is ruled out (Go, 1996).

IgG Subclasses

IgG consists of four subclasses, IgG1 through IgG4, which are distinguished by both structural and biological differences (Normansell, 1987; Schur, 1987). Although individual roles for each of the IgG subclasses have not been established, antibodies to carbohydrate antigens are concentrated in the IgG2 subclass, and many bacterial cell wall antigens are composed of carbohydrates (Scott, 1988). Thus, absence of an IgG2 response could result in failure to develop protection against bacterial infection. This relationship is most convincing in the occasional patient with IgA deficiency who also has a deficiency of IgG2 subclass and lacks an antibody response to vaccines for *Pneumococcus*. IgG subclass deficiency has also been implicated as the cause of recurrent infection in patients with normal or near normal IgG levels (Oxelius, 1979; Wedgwood, 1986; Shackelford, 1990; Gross, 1992; Popa, 1994).

The biological significance of IgG subclass deficiency is not always clear, and some individuals who completely lack genes for IgG2, IgA, and IgE are healthy (Lefranc, 1982; Migone, 1984). IgG1 is the first type of subclass response to carbohydrate antigens, and conversion to an IgG2 response occurs as the individual matures (Scott, 1988). No evidence indicates that those who are restricted to only IgG1 responses are at any disadvantage. To determine the biological significance of IgG subclass deficiency, testing of specific antibody production, usually by administering vaccines such as tetanus, diphtheria, *Haemophilus*, or a pneumococcal vaccine, is mandatory. Only patients with a clear antibody deficiency for multiple antigens would be considered to have a significant immune defect.

T Cell Immunity

Migration of stem cells from the bone marrow to the thymus results in development of T cells (Kruisbeek, 1999). During development of T cells in the thymus, many surface molecules are turned on and off in a regulated manner. These surface molecules are identified by their cluster of differentiation (CD). CD markers help distinguish the stage of maturation and the function of lymphocytes (Buckley, 2000). Despite regression of the thymus over time, T cell development persists throughout life (Jamieson, 1999). Unlike antibodies produced by B cells, which recognize antigens in their natural state, T cells recognize peptides along with MHC molecules after processing by antigen-presenting cells through CD3, the T cell receptor (Buckley, 2000).

Monoclonal antibodies are useful for detection of CD markers on lymphocytes and enable rapid enumeration of T cells and T cell subsets. This can be done by using small volumes of whole blood. The CD designation subdivides T cells (as a group, $CD3^+$) into two major subsets: $CD4^+$ and $CD8^+$ T cells. $CD4^+$ T cells are referred to as "helper" cells and are involved in initiation of immune reactions, cytokine secretion, and augmentation of B cell responses. $CD8^+$ T cells also release cytokines and are associated with cytolytic (killer) functions. $CD4^+$ and $CD8^+$ markers on T cells serve as signaling molecules and work in conjunction with major histocompatibility complex (MHC) class I and II antigens to amplify and stabilize engagement of T cell receptors (TCRs) with antigens. $CD4^+$ cells recognize antigens that are presented in the context of MHC class II antigens, and $CD8^+$ cells recognize antigens presented in context with MHC class I antigens (Buckley, 2000). Immunodeficiency diseases resulting from defective generation of T cells may result in total loss or low numbers of $CD3^+$ T cells, thereby creating similar effects on T cell subsets, $CD4^+$ and $CD8^+$ cells. For example, DiGeorge syndrome results in low numbers of $CD3^+$ cells (Hong, 1998). MHC class II deficiency results in a low number of $CD4^+$ cells (Klein, 1993), and an abnormality of Zap-70, a signaling molecule integral to the activity of the T cell receptor, leads to reduced numbers of $CD8^+$ T cells (Elder, 1998). If an immune defect is suspected, a panel of T cell markers is examined by flow cytometry, and the percentage and absolute count of cells in each set are compared with age-appropriate normal ranges (Illoh, 2004).

T Cell Functional Assessment

A clinical history of opportunistic infections and a decreased absolute lymphocyte count in a complete blood count should prompt further investigation of a patient's T cell function (Fleisher, 2003). Mucocutaneous candidiasis, another indication of defective T cell function, is characterized by extension of infection from the mucous membranes onto contiguous skin and may involve the fingernails with granulomatous inflammation (Atkinson, 2000; Lilic, 2001). Delayed-type hypersensitivity (DTH) skin tests are commonly used as measures of T cell function because they measure the ability to recall, recognize and present antigen, mobilize T cells, and generate a specific inflammatory response. Despite a normal absolute lymphocyte count, DTH skin tests should be performed when a T cell defect is suspected. However, these tests are difficult to interpret in infants because they may not have had sufficient exposure to respond to antigens to mount an immunogenic response, and a reduced or absent response may be normal. Hypersensitivity skin testing should incorporate more than one antigen (Kniker, 1985). To ensure proper administration and appropriate interpretation of test results, personnel must be well trained (Fleisher, 2003).

Insight into the capability of T cells can be gained by performing functional assessments of in vitro proliferative responses to different stimuli. Mitogens, antigens, and alloantigens are stimuli that cause proliferation of T cells. Mitogens are usually plant extracts that lack specificity and stimulate both $CD4^+$ and $CD8^+$ T lymphocytes. Alloantigens on unrelated donor cells also stimulate $CD4^+$ and $CD8^+$ cells in a relatively nonspecific way. Patients with significant T cell deficiency may still show proliferative responses to these stimulators, indicating the presence of T cells but not their ability to clear infectious agents from the host. Nonetheless, a proliferative response to specific antigens is a good indicator of the host's ability to resist infection (Lane, 1985). In the case of specific antigens, tetanus, diphtheria, and *Candida* are commonly used, although sufficient exposure to these antigens is required. Therefore, these are not reliable antigens for testing infants during the first year of life. A measure of specific T cell responses that is useful in infants consists of culturing peripheral blood mononuclear cells with mitogenic concentrations of anti-CD3 monoclonal antibody. This stimulator normally causes proliferation of all $CD3^+$ T cells, and absence of proliferation demonstrates a severe T cell defect (Hong, 1996).

Polymorphonuclear Killing Assays

Testing neutrophil function requires careful planning because specimens may be transported over long distances to large reference laboratories for testing. Blood collected from a patient should be submitted to the investigating laboratory as soon as possible because neutrophils undergo apoptosis rapidly after collection. If the blood must be stored or transported, it should be collected in a preservative such as ethylenediaminetetraacetic acid (EDTA) or citrate in a polypropylene tube and maintained at room temperature (20°–25° C). This decreases metabolic activity and minimizes adhesion of cells to the wall of the tube. Even under optimal conditions, cells can be maintained only for approximately 24–36 hours (Kuijpers, 1999).

Neutropenia or neutrophil dysfunction results in recurrent bacterial or fungal infection in the skin, lymph nodes, liver, lungs, or bones. This most commonly occurs with myelosuppressive therapies used to treat malignant neoplasms. These disorders must be distinguished from CGD, in which phagocytosis is normal, but intracellular killing of infectious organisms is defective, resulting in abscess or granuloma formation in the liver, bones, and lungs (Lekstrom-Himes, 2000). CGD inheritance is most commonly X-linked or autosomal recessive owing to mutations involving chromosome locations 16p24, 7q11.23, and 1q25. These changes result in defects in one of the four subunits of nicotinamide adenine dinucleotide phosphate (NADPH) oxidase, the enzyme that catalyzes the formation of hydrogen peroxide. This error causes failure of the metabolic burst in granulocytes following phagocytic ingestion of bacteria (Meischl, 1998). As a result, molecular oxygen is not reduced to superoxide and other free radicals, such as hydroxyl radical and hydrogen peroxide, which are important components of the intracellular mechanism of bacterial death (Babior, 1978). Therefore, CGD is characterized by recurrent infection with catalase-producing organisms, such as *Staphylococcus aureus*, which are capable of destroying the hydrogen peroxide produced by granulocytes. Therefore, catalase-positive organisms survive intracellular ingestion, multiply, and cause a granulomatous tissue response that, when excessive, can obstruct the gastrointestinal and genitourinary tracts. Chronic infection with *Serratia* spp., *Klebsiella* spp., *Burkholderia cepacia*, and *Aspergillus* spp. is particularly problematic (Gallin, 1983, 1990). However, patients with CGD do not experience this problem with catalase-negative organisms.

The fundamental biological characteristic of CGD leukocytes is that they will phagocytose bacteria normally but will not kill them. This provides the basis for a bacterial killing assay for CGD. Historically, the nitroblue tetrazolium (NBT) slide test has been the laboratory assay used to screen for CGD and is performed by reference laboratories (Park, 1968). In this assay, the patient's neutrophils are incubated with NBT, a pale yellow dye that is then activated by phorbol-myristate acetate (PMA), a strong, receptor-independent activation stimulus. Functional neutrophils phagocytose, reduce, and precipitate the NBT dye, forming intracellular deposits of black formazan. These deposits are indicative of rapid activation of NADPH-oxidase enzyme, causing reduction of oxygen by NADPH to superoxide that is subsequently catalyzed to hydrogen peroxide by superoxide dismutase (SOD). A technician then microscopically scores neutrophils that contain intracellular black formazan deposits (Kuijpers, 1999). However, the NBT slide test has been replaced in many laboratories by a flow cytometry test that detects intracellular oxidation of dichlorofluorescein diacetate or dihydrorhodamine 123 (O'Gorman, 1995). These nonfluorescent dyes, once oxidized, will produce intracellular fluorescent products that are detected by flow cytometry. Flow cytometry is a more objective and reliable method of identifying intracellular products.

The hyper-IgE syndrome (HIES) is phenotypically similar to CGD, with a classic triad of pneumonia, recurrent cutaneous and pulmonary abscesses, and elevated IgE levels; however, defective polymorphonuclear leukocyte function is not a predominant finding (Buckley, 1978; Ozcan, 2008). In addition, this syndrome includes bone abnormalities, unusual facies, and cutaneous candidiasis. Demonstration of IgE levels greater than 2000 IU/mL and (even as high as 20,000–60,000 IU/mL) with the appropriate clinical manifestations points toward the diagnosis. HIES is actually two distinct entities—autosomal dominant and autosomal recessive—based on inheritance patterns and nonimmunologic features. Each entity is characterized by different genetic mutations. Autosomal dominant HIES (AD-HIES) has been related to dominant-negative mutations of the signal transducer and transcription activator 3 (STAT3), causing impaired signaling of cytokines interleukin (IL)-6 and IL-10. However, signaling for IL-12 and interferon (IFN)-α remains intact. Patients with STAT3 mutations fail to generate helper T cells that secrete IL-17, which is important in providing epithelial and mucosal immunity against fungal and bacterial organisms. It also plays an important role in producing neutrophil chemoattractants. Autosomal recessive HIES (AR-HIES) is a distinct disease entity separated from AD-HIES by four major criteria: (1) The inheritance pattern is distinctly different; (2) patients lack connective tissue abnormalities; (3) the incidence of central nervous system complications is higher, and these patients have a higher frequency of varicella-zoster; and (4) herpes simplex virus occurs at a younger age with more complications (Renner, 2004). Of note is a case report of a patient with AR-HIES and a homozygous tyrosine kinase 2 (TYK2) mutation that resulted in a premature termination codon and absence of TYK2 protein. TYK2 belongs to the Janus kinase family, which is important in multiple cytokine signaling pathways, including type 1 IFN, IL-6, IL-10, IL-12, and IL-23. The patient exhibited severe defects in response to these cytokines and had impaired Type 1 helper T cells (T_H1) and accelerated Type 2 helper T cells (T_H2) differentiation. To date, this mutation has not been identified in any other patients with AR-HIES, which suggests that other, as yet undiscovered genetic mutations can result in this syndrome (Fischer, 2007; Ozcan, 2008).

Complement Evaluation

A number of congenital defects of the complement system have been described, although this is not a frequent cause of primary immunodeficiency disorder. The defects are typically associated with absence of one of the complement molecules or a nonfunctional complement protein, thereby reducing the ability of complement to bind to the surface of invading microorganisms. Individual defects lead to distinct clinical syndromes such as hereditary angioedema or paroxysmal nocturnal hemoglobinuria, a propensity for recurrent bacterial infection, or autoimmune disease (Schneider, 1999). Many of the genetically based deficiencies of the classical activating pathway (C1, C2, C3, C4) and of the terminal components (C5, C6, C7, C8, and C9) can be detected by using antibody-sensitized sheep erythrocytes in a total hemolytic complement assay (CH50). This assay tests for the functional integrity of C1–C9. Many commercial laboratories perform this assay, but to get accurate results, freshly drawn serum or plasma that is then frozen must be used. Therefore, logistics must be carefully coordinated if specimens must be sent to a distant location. Deficiencies of alternative pathway component factors D, H, and I and properdin are uncommon but can be detected by a hemolytic assay using unsensitized rabbit erythrocytes as potent activators of the alternative pathway. If one of these assays is abnormal, identification of individual deficient components rests on specialized functional and immunochemical tests that are specific for each component (see Chapter 47).

THIRD-LEVEL INVESTIGATIONS

Enzyme Measurements for Metabolic Defects

Deficiencies of the enzymes adenosine deaminase and purine nucleoside phosphorylase are related to purine metabolism and result in immunodeficiency. Patients with adenosine deaminase deficiency have findings similar to those of severe combined immunodeficiency (SCID) syndrome, a collection of genetic disorders characterized by a severe defect in the function or development of B and T cells. In contrast to SCID, patients deficient in adenosine deaminase have chondro-osseous dysplasia, resulting in skeletal abnormalities, and more severe lymphopenia. Deficient adenosine deaminase is caused by mutation of the gene located on chromosome 20q13.2–q13.11, resulting in toxic accumulation of metabolites that inhibit cell replication and cause apoptosis of lymphocytic cell lines

(Buckley, 2000). Lack of adenosine deaminase initially causes loss of T cells ($CD4^+$ T cells in particular) and subsequently B cells, leading to the common form of severe combined T and B cell deficiency (SCID) (Hirschhorn, 1995). As with many primary immune defects first recognized in the severe homozygous form, adenosine deaminase deficiency has been diagnosed as a heterozygous partial deficiency in adults with CD4 lymphopenia and significant T cell defects (Shovlin, 1994).

Purine nucleoside phosphorylase deficiency is characterized by recurrent infection, lymphopenia, neurologic abnormalities, and autoimmune disorders (Myers, 2004). This enzyme deficiency causes a decrease in T cells with minimal or no effect on B cells. Purine nucleoside phosphorylase enzymes are usually measured in erythrocyte lysates (Kizaki, 1977), but if blood products have been administered within the previous 3 months, the assay may be unreliable. More recently, capillary electrophoresis has been proposed as an alternative inexpensive assay that offers high separation flexibility in diagnosis of errors of metabolism and is capable of determining purine nucleoside phosphorylase or adenosine deaminase enzyme activity and the presence of toxic metabolites (Carlucci, 2003).

Natural Killer Cell Assays

Natural killer (NK) cells are a subset of lymphocytes that often function with T cells to eradicate intracellular organisms. Complete deficiency of NK cells is rare and is characterized by recurrent herpes infection (Fleisher, 2003). NK cells have the morphology of a large granular lymphocyte and express a unique group of cellular surface markers: CD16, CD56, and CD57 (Trinchieri, 1989). NK cells can be quantified easily by detecting these surface markers using flow cytometry. However, to assess the functional activity of NK cells, chromium release assays, which use chromium-51–loaded K-562 cell lines, have traditionally been performed (Biron, 1989). This older assay has limitations, in that it is more labor-intensive, incorporates radioactive materials, and cannot identify the cellular mechanisms for cell death of the target cells. These disadvantages have driven the development of newer, non–radioactivity-based methods, including fluorescent labeling techniques in combination with flow cytometry, to assess NK cell function. Another technique uses a colorimetric substrate to detect granzyme B, the serine protease found in the granules of cytotoxic T lymphocytes and NK cells, and plays a key role in granule-mediated apoptosis by cleaving cellular substrates (Hoppner, 2002; Ewen, 2003).

Additional Phagocyte Analyses

Genetic defects of the innate immune system are related to the formation or function of granules within neutrophils. Myeloperoxidase is the predominant enzyme detected in the primary granules of granulocytes and catalyzes the formation of hypochlorous acid (HOCL), which is capable of killing microorganisms (Kuijpers, 1999). However, its absence usually is not associated with clinical symptoms, with the notable exception of patients with diabetes mellitus, who experience increased susceptibility to disseminated candidiasis (Lanza, 1998). Myeloperoxidase deficiency, inherited as an autosomal recessive defect, is one of the most commonly inherited disorders of neutrophils, but its clinical significance is unknown (Lehrer, 1969; Klebanoff, 1999). Approximately half of affected patients have a deficiency of myeloperoxidase, and the remainder have normal concentrations, along with a structural defect in the enzyme (Nauseef, 1998).

Chédiak-Higashi syndrome and specific granule deficiency are congenital defects resulting in phagocyte granular disorders. Chédiak-Higashi syndrome is an autosomal recessive disorder in which all lysosome-containing cells have giant abnormal granules. In neutrophils, fusion of primary and secondary granules occurs, resulting in delay of fusion with phagosomes and recurrent bacterial infection. Patients with Chédiak-Higashi syndrome have a mild neutropenia, normal immunoglobulin levels, peripheral nerve defects, mild cutaneous and ocular albinism, mild platelet dysfunction, and periodontal disease (Introne, 1999).

Neutrophil-specific granule deficiency is a rare disorder characterized by recurrent bacterial infection of the skin and lungs. Patients lack secondary or specific granules of the neutrophils, which play an important role in acute inflammation and do not allow for proper migration of neutrophils. Morphologic examination of stained neutrophils shows characteristic abnormalities in specific granule deficiency (Ganz, 1988).

Patients with leukocyte adhesion deficiency (LAD) type 1 (a defect in the integrin CD18, the common β chain of LFA-1, Mac-1, and p150,95 molecules) (Anderson, 1987) are susceptible to all infections seen in CGD patients, along with otitis media and poor wound healing. Normally, because pathogens cause tissue damage and inflammation, adhesion molecules on vascular endothelium are upregulated and recognized by passing neutrophils bearing the appropriate counterligands, ultimately leading to accumulation of neutrophils at sites of inflammation (see Chapter 47). Patients with LAD lack the adhesion molecules necessary for diapedesis, resulting in tissue neutropenia and therefore more infection (Arnaout, 1993). This abnormality starts after birth and is marked by delayed cord separation, chronic skin ulcers, periodontitis, impaired wound healing, and leukocytosis. Deficient leukocytes demonstrate defects of adherence and adhesion-dependent functions such as spreading, phagocytosis, and chemotactic orientation (Anderson, 1987).

LAD type 2 predominantly affects neutrophils and macrophages, with faulty expression of the selectin ligand sialyl-LewisX and failure to convert GDP mannose to fucose, resulting in a clinical syndrome similar to type 1. It is also responsible for expression of the rare Bombay blood group (LAD-2) on red blood cells (Etzioni, 1993).

Leukocyte mobility is usually evaluated by directed migration through membrane filters or under agarose (Nelson, 1975; Cates, 1981). Counting the number of cells at a particular endpoint or "stop filter" microscopically, or radioactive labeling, has the disadvantage of measuring only the fastest cells. This may give an inaccurate assessment of most of the patient's neutrophils. It is actually better to count the number of cells at different points along the filter (Kuijpers, 1999). Injections of epinephrine and steroids, which cause polymorphonuclear leukocytes to demarginate and leave the marrow reserves, are used to further assess polymorphonuclear leukocyte mobility. A disorder of actin important in polymorphonuclear leukocyte migration has been described (Southwick, 1988).

Adhesion proteins on the surface of neutrophils can be functionally tested with different immobilized ligands bound to a monolayer of endothelial cells attached to a glass slide, and can be measured after pretreatment with chemoattractants. Rolling, attachment, and migration of neutrophils can be monitored over time by a video camera. Phagocytosis can now be assessed by flow cytometry, in which the neutrophils are incubated with fluorescence-labeled microorganisms, the sample is washed to remove labeled undigested microorganisms, and the cells with ingested labeled microorganism are counted (Kuijpers, 1999). Much in the same fashion, flow cytometry may be used to assess killing of microbes by employing vital dyes that distinguish live from dead organisms after incubation with neutrophils (Martin, 1992). Degranulation may be assessed by measuring expression of granule membrane proteins on the neutrophil cell surface by means of flow cytometry (Kuijpers, 1999).

Cytokines and Cytokine Receptors

Immune responses are regulated by soluble mediators called cytokines that produce a multiplicity of immune events through interactions with appropriate cytokine receptors on tissue and inflammatory cells. Cytokines play an important role as messengers within the immune system and in conjunction with the rest of the body to regulate immune responses (Mire-Sluis, 1998). By studying immunodeficient patients and gene knockout mice, our understanding of the role cytokines play in our host defenses has expanded. Deficiencies in IL-12 and IFN-γ increase susceptibility to *Salmonella* and mycobacterial infections (de Jong, 1998). Impaired secretions or responses to IL-12 impair granuloma formation and therefore allow unregulated growth of mycobacterial organisms (Jouanguy, 1999). Recent studies show that the pathophysiology of many of these disorders may be the result of defective cytokine signaling, which causes dysfunction or arrested development of B, T, and NK cells (Kelly, 2003). Most notably, human X-linked SCID is associated with defects in the interleukin receptor gene (IL2RG), which codes for a common γ chain (γc), a shared component of several cytokine receptors such as IL-4F, IL-7R, IL-9R, and IL-15R. Impaired production of γc leads to cytokine dysfunction and lack of development of affected lymphoid cells (Malek, 1999). Additionally, the *JAK3* gene encodes for a tyrosine kinase used in signal transduction through γc-containing cytokine receptors. Defects in this gene have been identified in patients with autosomal recessive SCID. IL-7 is a cytokine with a key role in T cell development, and a genetic defect in the α subunit of the IL-7 receptor has been identified in patients with a rare disorder of B^+ SCID (Notarangelo, 2000).

Additional Cell Surface Markers

MHC Class I and II Molecules

Congenital mutations affecting MHC class I and class II expression have been described. Class II molecules are found primarily on the antigen-presenting cells, which initiate the acquired immune response. As one might predict, genetic defects of MHC class II (from mutations involving MHC class II gene transcriptional activation) result in a profound immunodeficiency state (Klein, 1993) known as MHC class II deficiency, according to World Health Organization nomenclature. This is referred to as bare lymphocyte syndrome type II and is characterized by lack of expression of MHC II molecules on cellular surfaces. Thymic education and selection of immature T cells are compromised because of loss of antigen processing by MHC class II molecules. Quantities of B and T cells are normal in patients with bare lymphocyte syndrome; however, $CD4^+$ counts are decreased as a result of loss of proper antigen processing. Patients thus are unable to respond to foreign antigens and present with recurrent bacterial, fungal, viral, and protozoal infections. They do not respond to skin testing (type IV DTH), have a decreased ability to respond to mixed lymphocyte reactions, and have pan-hypogammaglobulinemia (Nekrep, 2003). An interesting facet of this syndrome is that there is no genetic defect of the MHC class II genes. Instead, a defect occurs in one of the four genes that encode the four regulatory factors essential for surface expression of MHC class II antigens (Reith, 2001).

Elimination of foreign antigen can be accomplished by $CD8^+$ T cell binding to MHC class I antigens expressed on nearly all nucleated cells. It is strange to note that immune defects resulting from MHC class I deficiency, a mutation involving either of the MHC class I cytoplasmic peptide transporters TAP-1 or TAP-2, produce an immune defect characterized by severe lung disease that becomes apparent in later childhood (Donato, 1995; de la Salle, 1999). This immunodeficiency was previously named type I bare lymphocyte syndrome, or human leukocyte antigen (HLA) class I deficiency, and is characterized by a decrease in $CD8^+$ cells and NK cell activity (Yabe, 2002). Diagnosis of both defects involves examining expression of these MHC antigens on peripheral blood lymphoid cells by flow cytometry (Illoh, 2004).

Treatment by Targeting Cell Surface Receptors

Recent case reports describe therapies that target cell surface receptors to treat complications associated with primary immunodeficiency disorders. An example is anti-CD20 (rituximab), a monoclonal antibody directed against the CD20 antigen found on B lymphocytes and used to deplete peripheral benign and malignant B lymphocytes. Successful treatment using these monoclonal antibodies has been reported for IgM autoantibody (reactive at 37° C)–mediated autoimmune hemolytic anemia in a child with common variable immunodeficiency, and for lymphoproliferative disorder in a child with WAS caused by depleting peripheral B cells in patients (Sebire, 2003; Wakim, 2004).

Using Novel Immunogens to Assess Antibody Production

Another valuable tool to evaluate specific antibody responses is vaccination with neo-antigens such as the bacteriophage ΦX174 and keyhole limpet hemocyanin. These neo-antigens may also be used to evaluate patients receiving immunoglobulin replacement therapy, because monitoring antibody responses to standard vaccines while receiving passive infusion of pooled immunoglobulins is not possible. Primary and secondary responses may be monitored because the neo-antigens provoke a primary IgM response, and then, upon reexposure, cause a secondary IgG response (Curtis, 1970; Ochs, 1971). Using ΦX174 clearance patterns and isotypes, a patient's response can be measured, thereby further defining various degrees and subsets of B cell deficiency (Ochs, 1971). Currently, this evaluation is available only in some academic institutions using research protocols (Fleisher, 2004).

Molecular Genetics and Prenatal Diagnosis

A number of the genes involved in the primary immunodeficiency syndromes have now been identified, cloned, and sequenced (Conley, 1992; Puck, 1993; Derry, 1994; Ramesh, 1998; Vihinen, 1999; Fischer, 2007; Zhang, 2009). In many cases, mouse knockout models have been produced to further study the effects of genes on immune function. In the past, more traditional methods of screening for genetic mutations responsible for immunodeficiencies were used, such as dideoxy fingerprinting and single-strand conformational polymorphism (Sarkar, 1992; Sheffield, 1993; Puck, 1997b). More recent advances using fluorescence-based sequencing, which uses fluorescently labeled dideoxynucleotide terminators, allow for simple and sensitive identification of deoxyribonucleic acid (DNA) sequence variations in individuals. Automated multichannel capillary sequences serve as an automated method of rapidly detecting fluorescence-based sequences for multiple patients within hours, and make direct sequencing for genetic mutations responsible for immune deficiencies practical (Niemela, 2000). Identification of mutated genes facilitates genetic counseling for prenatal diagnosis and aids in the detection of carrier status for defective genes. It also assists in the evaluation of previously undefined immune disorders. An excellent example of how these advanced techniques are enhancing our understanding of primary immunodeficiency disorders is exhibited by hyper-IgM syndrome. Previously, this was categorized as a single disorder, but genetic sequencing has revealed five distinct genetic defects affecting B or T cells with variable phenotypes (Durandy, 2004).

Analysis of immunodeficiencies with known genetic defects involves testing specific sites on DNA to detect specific mutations. Different methods such as polymerase chain reaction (PCR) may be used to detect the presence or absence of a particular gene, and immunoblotting or flow cytometry can be used to detect protein products and to confirm a diagnosis of primary immunodeficiency when the gene product is absent. High-resolution comparative genomic hybridization arrays detect microdeletions associated with complex immunodeficiency syndromes. For example, genomic hybridization arrays and targeted gene sequencing were performed on eight families with variant features of combined immunodeficiency characterized by recurrent sinopulmonary infection, cutaneous viral infection, and elevated serum IgE levels. The analysis revealed novel point mutations in the gene responsible for encoding the dedicator of cytokinesis 8 protein (DOCK8). Homozygous or compound heterozygous deletions in this gene lead to absence of DOCK8 protein in lymphocytes that regulate cytoskeletal rearrangements responsible for cell structure, adhesion, and migration, as well as other functions, resulting in this combined immunodeficiency (Zhang, 2009). An example of when it is important to determine the cause of an immunodeficiency is seen in SCID, a heterogeneous group of immunodeficiencies characterized by a number of different molecular defects. Distinguishing between various molecular defects in SCID has implications for treatment, antenatal diagnosis, and carrier testing. It is important to determine whether a patient has X-linked SCID because this may be treated using gene therapy. JAK3-deficient SCID is clinically indistinguishable from X-linked SCID, but gene therapy is not effective (Cavazzana-Calvo, 2000). Previously, testing to distinguish between these molecular defects took several weeks to complete because JAK3-deficient SCID is encoded by 23 exons. DNA analysis using single-stranded conformational polymorphism analysis and sequencing of all affected exons was required. More rapid screening methods can now be used to arrive at an expeditious diagnosis, with time-consuming genetic analysis being performed for subsequent confirmation. These protein-based assays employ flow cytometric analysis of γc, immunoblotting for JAK3 and γc, and detection of IL-2–induced tyrosine phosphorylation of JAK3 (Gilmour, 2001). However, with defects characterized by nonfunctional protein products, these assays are not useful. Table 50-1 lists the currently identified mutated genes and affected proteins associated with primary immunodeficiencies. Table 50-2 provides a summary of gene mutations with associated susceptibilities to pathogens.

With advances in technology, the ability to detect prenatally a wider range of immune defects is possible. If the specific mutation is known, or if the inheritance pattern is known to be X-linked, analysis of linked polymorphic markers or detection of specific mutations can be performed. Chorionic villous samples, amniocyte DNA prepared directly from fetal cells, or cultured and expanded cell lines can be analyzed (Durandy, 1985). In addition to prenatal testing, newborn blood screening (NBS), traditionally used to screen for genetically inherited metabolic disorders, is now used to screen for inherited immunodeficiencies. Several states have added TCR excision circles (TRECs) to the NBS by extracting DNA from the NBS cards to analyze episomal fragments of DNA formed during rearrangement of T cell receptors in the thymus. The δRec-ψJα TREC is produced by 70% of all T cells that produce α/β T cell receptors. Therefore, PCR quantitation of this TREC provides a marker for naive T cells and identifies infants with profound T cell lymphopenia associated with primary immunodeficiencies such as SCID or DiGeorge syndrome (Routes, 2009).

Many of the primary immunodeficiencies are rare disorders that can be difficult to diagnose; in these cases, genetic mutation detection is the most reliable method. These specialized tests are not readily available, and physicians may have difficulty locating laboratories to perform the necessary genetic analyses. Mutation registries and databases are available to provide information about tests for clinical data, immune status, antibody response, cellular function, and enzyme assays. Additionally, some online registries contain information about laboratories that perform these assays that increases awareness of testing availability and the ability to obtain an exact and prompt diagnosis (Samarghitean, 2004).

TABLE 50-1
Gene Mutations, Affected Proteins, and Primary Immunodeficiencies

Disease	Natural mutant	Protein	Function
Agammaglobulinemia		Btk	Cell activation
APECED		AIRE	Negative selection of T cells
AT		ATM	DNA lesion sensing
Atypical complete DiGeorge syndrome		Base pair deletion on 22a11.2	Oligoclonal T cells
CGD		gp91phox, p22phox, p47phox, p67phox	NADPH oxidase
DC		Dyskerin	Telomere maintenance
FHLH		Munc 13-4	Exocytosis of lytic granules
FHLH		Syntaxin11	Cytotoxicity
Griscelli	Ashen	Rab27a	Exocytosis of lytic granules
HIES AD/AR		STAT3/TYK2	Defective cytokine signaling
HIGM		CD40L	Activation of Ig CSR
HIGM		AID	Ig CSR and SHM
IPEX	Scurfy	FOXP3	Treg function
LAD		β2 integrin	Adhesion
NBS		Nibrin (NBS1)	DNA repair
Omenn syndrome		RAG, ARTEMIS, IL-7R, RMPR, IL-2Rγ, ZAP70, ADA, DNA ligase IV mutations	Oligoclonal T cells and absence of B cells
	SCID	DNA-PKcs	VDJ (NHEJ)
SCID		Artemis	VDJ (NHEJ)
SCID		Cernunnos, XLF	VDJ (NHEJ)
SCID		γc, JAK3	T (NK) cell development
SCN		HAX-1	Prevention of apoptosis
T cell deficiency		Orai-1, CRACMI	Ca channel
T cell deficiency (HLA II expression)		RFXAP, ANK, RFX5, CIITA	HLA class II transcription
Variant combined immunodeficiency		DOCK8	Cytoskeletal arrangements in lymphocytes
WAS		WASP	Cell cytoskeleton, migration
XLP		SAP	Coactivation (SLAM family), NKT
XLP2		XIAP	Control of apoptosis (NKT)
	lpr, gld	fas, fasL	Apoptosis
	Moth eaten	SHP-1	Phosphatase regulation

Data from Fisher A. Human primary immunodeficiency diseases. Immunity 2007;27:835–45.

AD, Autosomal dominant; *ADA,* adenosine deaminase deficiency; *AID,* activation-induced deaminase; *APECED,* autoimmune polyendocrinopathy candidiasis ectodermal dysplasia; *AR,* autosomal recessive; *AT,* ataxia telangiectasia; *Btk,* Bruton tyrosine kinase; *CGD,* chronic granulomatous disease; *DC,* dyskeratosis congenita; *DNA,* deoxyribonucleic acid; *DNA PKcs,* DNA-dependent protein kinase, catalytic subunit; *DOCK8,* dedicator of cytokinesis 8 protein; *FHLH,* familial hemophagocytic lymphohistiocytosis; *gld,* generalized lymphadenopathy disease; *HIES,* hyper-IgE syndrome; *HIGM,* hyper-IgM syndrome (Ig class switch recombination deficiency [CSR]); *HLA,* human leukocyte antigen; *IPEX,* immunoproliferative enteropathy X-linked syndrome; *LAD,* leukocyte adhesion deficiency; *lpr,* lymphoproliferation; *NADPH,* nicotinamide adenine dinucleotide phosphate; *NBS,* Nijmegen breakage syndrome; *NHEJ,* nonhomologous end-joining; *NK,* natural killer; *SAP,* SLAM-associated protein; *SCID,* severe combined immunodeficiency; *SCN,* severe congenital neutropenia; *SHM,* somatic hypermutations; *Treg,* regulatory T cells; *VDJ,* V(D)J recombination; *WAS,* Wiskott-Aldrich syndrome; *WASP,* Wiskott-Aldrich syndrome protein; *XIAP,* X-linked inhibitor of apoptosis; *XLF,* XRCC4-like factor; *XLP,* X-linked proliferative syndrome; *XLP2,* X-linked proliferative syndrome type 2.

Novel Approaches to Treating Immunodeficiency Disorders

Genetic analysis of primary immunodeficiencies is important not only for diagnosis of the disorder but as a guide for therapy. Understanding the pathophysiology of each immunodeficiency disorder will aid clinicians in providing the missing component and ameliorating symptoms. For example, enzyme replacement therapy has been used in the past to treat enzyme-deficient forms of SCID, such as adenosine deaminase and purine nucleoside phophorylase SCID; however, this requires prolonged treatment and results are variable, including decreased thymic output, lymphopenia, and increased viral infection (Gaspar, 2006). Direct genetic intervention may become a more suitable treatment as increasing numbers of successful case reports describe using autologous $CD34^+$ hematopoietic stem cells transduced with a retroviral vector containing the normal gene. In children affected with Adenosine deaminase deficiency-deficient SCID and SCID-X1, direct genetic intervention is a safe and effective treatment, resulting in reinitiation of thymopoiesis, restoration of cellular immunity, and correction of the metabolic disorder, without enzyme replacement therapy (Gaspar, 2006; Aiuti, 2009).

TABLE 50-2
Gene Mutations and Susceptibility to Pathogens

CD40L, CD40	*Pneumocystis jiroveci, Toxoplasma, Cryptosporidium*
IL12p40, IL12Rβ, IFNγR, STAT1	Mycobacteria
IRAK4	Encapsulated pathogens
SAP, XIAP	EBV
UNC93B, TLR-3	HSV encephalitis
Complement C5-C9	*Neisseria*
EVER 1,2, γc, JAK-3	HPV-epidermodysplasia verruciformis

Data from Fisher A. Human primary immunodeficiency diseases. Immunity 2007;27:835–45.

EVER 1,2, Epidermodysplasia verruciformis 1, 2 genes; *γc,* common cytokine γ chain; *IFNγR,* receptor of the interferon γ receptor; *IL12p40,* p40 subunit of interleukin-12; *IL12Rβ,* β chain of the IL-12 receptor; *IRAK4,* interleukin-1 receptor–associated kinase 4; *JAK-3,* Janus-associated kinase; *SAP,* SLAM-associated protein; *STAT1,* signal transducer and activator of transcription 1; *TLR-3,* Toll-like receptor 3; *UNC93B,* polytopic endoplasmic reticulum CERI-resident membrane protein; *XIAP,* X-linked inhibitor of apoptosis.

Other future strategies may include using chemicals to modify protein glycosylation to prevent protein unfolding and degradation resulting in primary immunodeficiency disorders (Vogt, 2007). Although these strategies have been demonstrated only in in vitro models, if the medications can be introduced at nontoxic levels with appropriate bioavailability in humans, clinical application may be practical in the future. Other medications such as gentamicin and Ataluren (formerly known as PTC 124) prevent premature translation termination at a premature stop codon and may be employed to treat disorders such as muscular dystrophy and cystic fibrosis, characterized by nonsense mutations resulting in absence of a critical protein causing the disorder. Although these treatments are still experimental, the hope of treating primary immunodeficiencies effectively lies in defining the genetic mutation and utilizing mutation-related strategies for treatment (Fischer, 2007).

SUMMARY

Assessment of host defenses is an extraordinarily complex process entailing the cooperation of the clinician, the research scientist, and the clinical pathologist. A logical approach, based on appreciation of the multiple systems involved in host defense and various diagnostic options, can lead to identification of the underlying disorder. The impressive success of modern therapy, incorporating new antimicrobials, recombinant DNA technology, bone marrow transplantation, and gene therapy, allows more precise delineation and characterization of the immunologic deficiency state. This in turn improves recognition, and ultimately treatment, of these patients.

SELECTED REFERENCES

Delves PJ, Roitt IM. The immune system, first of two parts. N Engl J Med 2000;343:37–49.

A general overview of the immune system and the function of innate and acquired responses, as well as the role of B and T cells. This article also provides a glossary of commonly used immunologic terms that clinicians may find useful.

Fleisher TA. Evaluation of suspected immunodeficiency. Medical Laboratory Observer 2003;February:10–21.

An overview of the application of laboratory methods to evaluate immune defects; includes a continuing education test.

Kuijpers TW, Weening RS, Roos D. Clinical and laboratory work-up of patients with neutrophil shortage or dysfunction. J Immunol Methods 1999;232:211–29.

This article provides a succinct overview of clinical signs and symptoms exhibited by patients, the physiology of the antimicrobial system of neutrophils, the mechanisms of assay to diagnose these aberrations, and potential treatments for affected patients.

Lekstrom-Himes JA, Gallin JI. Primary immunodeficiency diseases due to defects in phagocytes. N Engl J Med 2000;343:1703–14.

This review article provides an overview of immunodeficiencies due to phagocytic defects. Also features tables summarizing the syndromes with their corresponding genetic defects, as well as clinical and microscopic photographs to demonstrate the manifestations of the immunodeficiencies.

Lindegren ML, Kobrynski L, Rasmussen SA. Applying public health strategies to primary immunodeficiency diseases: a potential approach to genetic disorders. MMWR 2004;53:1–29.

Summary of a workshop convened by the CDC to discuss strategies to improve clinical outcomes of patients with primary immunodeficiencies. This summary discusses incidence and birth prevalence of primary immunodeficiency, newborn screening methods, morbidity and mortality data, and information for primary immunodeficiency registries.

REFERENCES

Access the complete reference list online at http://www.expertconsult.com

CHAPTER 51

CLINICAL AND LABORATORY EVALUATION OF SYSTEMIC RHEUMATIC DISEASES

Carlos Alberto von Mühlen, Robert M. Nakamura†

KEY POINTS

- Many types of autoantibodies to intracellular and nuclear antigens are present in the various systemic rheumatic diseases. Currently, it is considered important not only to detect the presence and quantity of intracellular and nuclear autoantibodies in the patient, but also to identify its immunologic specificity.
- Past studies have shown that distinct diagnostic profiles of autoantibodies are observed in many of the rheumatic diseases. Some diseases are characterized by the presence or absence of a specific antibody, or by differences in the quantitative level or titer of the autoantibody.
- Much progress has been made in improvement of sensitivity, specificity, and quality control of the many laboratory tests used for the detection of autoantibodies to intracellular and nuclear antigens.
- Immunofluorescence microscopy using human cellular extracts, such as HEp-2 cells, allows the sensitive detection of serum antibodies that react very specifically with various cellular proteins and nucleic acids.
- Widely used tests for screening of intracellular autoantibodies are immunofluorescence microscopy and the immunoenzyme tests. The secondary definitive tests for specific identification of autoantibodies to nuclear antigen are immunodiffusion, immunoprecipitation, particle agglutination, enzyme-linked immunosorbent assay, immunoblotting, and radioimmunoassay methods.
- Molecular biologists have used many of the autoantibodies as biological probes and have elucidated the biological functions of several of the autoantigens.

OVERVIEW AND CLASSIFICATION OF SYSTEMIC RHEUMATIC DISEASES

The rheumatic diseases are characterized by the presence of one or more autoantibodies that may be directed against components of the surface, cytoplasm, nuclear envelope, or nucleus of the cell. The last group, autoantibodies to nuclear antigens (ANAs), is a hallmark of the systemic rheumatic diseases (Tan, 1982a, 1989; Nakamura, 1985, 1986, 1992; von Mühlen, 1994). Many of the rheumatic diseases have a distinctive profile

†Deceased

TABLE 51-1
Systemic Rheumatic Diseases and Related Disorders

1. Systemic lupus erythematosus (SLE)
2. Discoid lupus erythematosus (DLE)
3. Lupus-like syndromes
4. Drug-induced lupus erythematosus
5. Sjögren's syndrome
6. Scleroderma/CREST syndrome (calcinosis cutis, Raynaud's phenomenon, esophageal dysmotility, sclerodactyly, and telangiectasia)
7. Rheumatoid arthritis (RA)
8. Dermatomyositis and polymyositis
9. Overlap syndromes
   a. Mixed connective tissue disease (MCTD)
   b. RA and SLE (Rupus)
   c. SLE and scleroderma (Lupoderma)
   d. Scleroderma and dermatomyositis (sclerodermatomyositis)
   e. Other
10. Systemic vasculitis
   a. Takayasu's arteritis
   b. Giant cell arteritis and polymyalgia rheumatica
   c. Wegener's granulomatosis
   d. Polyarteritis nodosa and Churg-Strauss syndrome
   e. Leukocytoclastic vasculitis
   f. Other
11. Poorly defined connective tissue disease syndromes

of autoantibodies with diagnostic and prognostic implications. Moreover, the biochemical and biological functions of many of the antigens involved in deoxyribonucleic acid (DNA) replication, splicing of ribonucleic acid (RNA) precursor, and RNA processing have been elucidated (Tan, 1989). Classification of the various rheumatic diseases has been difficult because of the lack of firm etiologic bases for most of them. A comprehensive classification developed by Decker and the Glossary Subcommittee of the American College of Rheumatology (Decker, 1983) is still in use. Our abridged classification of the systemic rheumatic diseases and related disorders is shown in Table 51-1.

Systemic Lupus Erythematosus and Related Lupus-like Disorders

Systemic lupus erythematosus (SLE) is the prototype systemic rheumatic disease and has the following significant features (Nakamura, 1994a):

1. SLE is a non–organ-specific autoimmune disease in which tissue injury is mediated primarily by DNA–anti-DNA immune complexes.
2. It is a multisystem disease that affects persons of all ages and both sexes, although it is most prevalent in women during childbearing years.
3. The disease demonstrates a hyperactive immune system with multiple abnormalities.
4. Patients with SLE demonstrate a heterogeneous and polyclonal antibody response, with autoantibody formation reaction involving similar mechanisms to those seen in a typical immune response to foreign immunogens (Fatenejad, 1998).
5. The typical case of SLE has an average of three different circulating antibodies present simultaneously. The prevalence of antibodies varies over a wide range, and more than 110 different types of autoantibodies have been identified in SLE (Sherer, 2004).

ETIOLOGIC FACTORS IN SYSTEMIC LUPUS ERYTHEMATOSUS

The origin is still not known. Some of the important causative factors in SLE include (1) endocrine–metabolic, (2) environmental, and (3) genetic (Chan, 1989). The strongest risk factor for the development of SLE is female gender (Hochberg, 1990). The presence of antinuclear antibodies was detected in female laboratory workers with varying degrees of exposure to blood from patients with SLE. The presence of antinative DNA antibodies was higher in laboratory workers than in an unexposed nonlaboratory group of women ($p < 0.001$) (Zarmbinski, 1992). These results help support the hypothesis that a transmissible agent that can cause autoantibody formation may exist in the blood of patients with SLE.

Certain chemicals have been implicated in SLE (Hochberg, 1990). The syndrome of drug-induced lupus with hydralazine, procainamide, and isoniazid has been studied for clues to the pathogenesis of SLE. Various reports show the acetylation mechanism as a risk factor in SLE. Studies have demonstrated a greater concordance rate of SLE among monozygotic and dizygotic twins (Block, 1975). Concordance of SLE was present in 11 (58%) of 19 monozygotic twins. The end result of the interaction of multiple etiologic factors is polyclonal activation of B cells in SLE patients with production of a wide spectrum of antibodies (Nakamura, 1994a; Sherer, 2004).

WHAT ARE THE DIAGNOSTIC CRITERIA FOR SYSTEMIC LUPUS ERYTHEMATOSUS?

In 1971, the American College of Rheumatology (ACR; previously the American Rheumatism Association [ARA]) published preliminary criteria for the classification of SLE (Cohen, 1971). Patients were considered to have SLE if four of the criteria were met sequentially or simultaneously during any interval of observation. In 1982, the Subcommittee for SLE Criteria of the ARA published revised criteria that incorporated new immunologic knowledge and improved the disease classification of SLE (Tan, 1982b). The 1982 revised criteria for classification of SLE included 11 categories, adding (1) abnormal titer of antinuclear antibody by immunofluorescence or an equivalent assay, and (2) antibody to native DNA and/or Sm antigen. In contrast to the 1971 criteria, the 1982 criteria removed Raynaud's phenomenon and alopecia because of their lack of sensitivity and specificity.

When the 1982 ARA criteria for classification of SLE were compared with the 1971 criteria, definite improvement in sensitivity and specificity was evident. The 1982 criteria showed 96.7% sensitivity and 96% specificity when evaluated with known SLE and control patients (Tan, 1982). In 1997, an update of the criteria were published, in which the lupus erythematosus (LE) cell test was dropped and anticardiolipin antibodies were added (Table 51-2)—changes emphasized in the "Guidelines for Referral and Management of SLE in Adults" put forth by the ACR Ad Hoc Committee on SLE Guidelines (Gladman, 1999).

WHAT ARE "LUPUS-LIKE" SYNDROMES AND DISEASES?

Many diseases and syndromes may share certain clinical features with SLE but are not SLE and have differing etiologies and pathogeneses. Diseases that have been listed in this category include vasculitis, cryoglobulinemia, relapsing polychondritis, lymphoproliferative disease, rheumatic fever, glomerulonephritis, syphilis, lupoid hepatitis, drug-induced lupus, and occult malignancy (Panush, 1993). There is a very broad category of patients who demonstrate fewer than four of the 1982 ARA classification criteria for SLE (Lazaro, 1989; Lom-Orta, 1980; Schurr, 1993) but are considered to have "lupus-like" illnesses. These patients have been classified as follows: (1) undifferentiated rheumatic disease, (2) nonrheumatic disease, (3) overlap syndrome, and (4) incomplete, latent, or incipient lupus. If these patients are followed, some stay with mild symptoms and as such remain labeled as having **undifferentiated connective tissue disease (UCTD)**, a few may develop definite SLE, but many evolve into other diseases with a better prognosis. Actually, up to 75% of patients with UCTD never fulfill diagnostic criteria for specific systemic rheumatic diseases (Mosca, 2004). In our hands, 99 patients with anti-U1nRNP antibodies followed for 10 years, many diagnosed as having UCTD when entering the cohort, developed characteristic signs and symptoms of rheumatoid arthritis, Sjögren's syndrome, systemic lupus, or scleroderma (Fig. 51-1), according to their human leukocyte antigen (HLA) profile and antibody titers (unpublished results).

AUTOANTIBODY PROFILE IN SYSTEMIC LUPUS ERYTHEMATOSUS

Characteristic of SLE is the presence of a broad spectrum of autoantibodies, including antibody to native DNA (ds-DNA), chromatin, Sm antigen,

TABLE 51-2

1997: Update of the 1982 Revised Criteria for Classification of Systemic Lupus Erythematosus*

1. Malar rash
2. Discoid rash
3. Photosensitivity
4. Oral ulcers
5. Nonerosive arthritis
6. Serositis (pleuritis or pericarditis)
7. Renal disorder (persistent proteinuria, cellular casts)
8. Neurologic disorder
9. Hematologic disorder
   a. Hemolytic anemia with reticulocytosis, OR
   b. Leukopenia $<4000/mm^3$ on ≥ 2 occasions, OR
   c. Lymphopenia $<1500/mm^3$ on ≥ 2 occasions, OR
   d. Thrombocytopenia $<100{,}000/mm^3$ in the absence of offending drug
10. Immunologic disorder
   a. Anti-DNA: antibody to native DNA in abnormal titer, OR
   b. Anti-Sm: presence of antibody to Sm nuclear antigen, OR
   c. Positive finding of antiphospholipid antibodies based on (1) an abnormal serum level of IgG or IgM anticardiolipin antibodies, (2) a positive test result for lupus anticoagulant using a standard method, or (3) a false-positive test result for syphilis known to be positive for at least 6 months and confirmed by *Treponema pallidum* immobilization or fluorescent treponemal antibody absorption test
11. Positive antinuclear antibody
   a. An abnormal titer of antinuclear antibody by immunofluorescence or an equivalent assay at any point in time and in the absence of drugs known to be associated with "drug-induced lupus" syndrome

From Hochberg MC. Updating the American College of Rheumatology revised criteria for the classification of systemic lupus erythematosus [letter]. Arthritis Rheum 1997;40:1725.

*The proposed classification is based on 11 criteria. For the purpose of identifying patients in clinical studies, a person shall be said to have SLE if any four or more of the 11 criteria are present, serially or simultaneously, during any interval of observation.

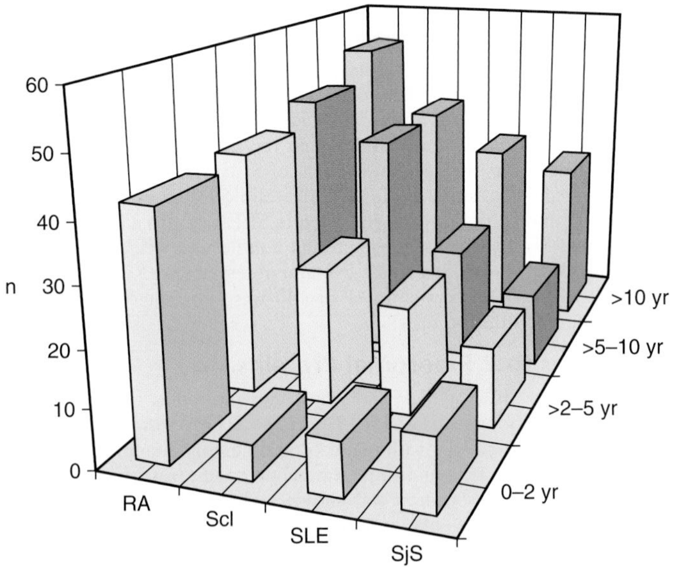

Figure 51-1 Classification criteria fulfilled by 99 patients with anti-U1nRNP antibodies over more than 10 years of observation. Many patients in this cohort were classified as having undifferentiated connective tissue disease (UCTD) in the first 2 years of clinical symptoms, and 43 individuals could be classified as having rheumatoid arthritis (RA). The number of RA-classified patients did not grow significantly toward the end of the study, but diagnoses of systemic lupus erythematosus (SLE) and scleroderma (Scl) were fulfilled ever more often ($p = 0.02$ and 0.0008, respectively, chi-square for trend). Patients developing SLE had low titers of anti-U1nRNP antibodies and were HLA-DR2/3. Those developing Scl had high anti-U1nRNP titers and were HLA-DR4. *SjS*, Sjögren's syndrome. *(From von Mühlen CA, Genth E, Mierau R, unpublished data.)*

U1nRNP, SS-A/Ro, SS-B/La, C1q, and several other nonhistone protein or nonhistone protein–RNA complexes (Nakamura, 1994a; Sherer, 2004). Polyclonality of antibodies is seen in SLE and scleroderma, and is rarely seen in the other systemic rheumatic diseases. Anti-native DNA, anti-Sm, anti-C1q, anti-ribosomal RNP, and anti–proliferating cell nuclear antigen (PCNA) are generally specific for SLE. The prevalence of autoantibodies varies over a wide range. Antibodies to native DNA and chromatin are detectable in up to 90% of patients, and antibodies to PCNA and cyclin or Alu-RNA protein are seen in 3% or less (von Mühlen, 1995) (Table 51-3).

Antibodies to Native DNA or Double-Stranded DNA

Anti–double-stranded DNA (ds-DNA) antibodies are rather specific for SLE and are observed at a frequency of 75%–90% in SLE patients with active disease (Buskila, 1992; Rekvig, 2003). Many earlier reports described antibodies to ds-DNA in diseases other than SLE. However, current thinking is that the reactive antibodies to DNA in the other diseases were actually anti–single-stranded DNA antibodies. The ds-DNA antibody tests often used ds-DNA preparations contaminated with denatured or single-stranded DNA. One possible exception could appear in primary Sjögren's syndrome, a disease sometimes difficult to differentiate from SLE in older people. Antibody to DNA plays a definite role in the pathogenesis of SLE. In studies of SLE patients, antibody to DNA is followed by the appearance of circulating DNA antigen—a sequence of events that results in the formation of immune complexes. Such DNA–anti-DNA immune complexes, mostly containing complement-activating IgG3, have a special tropism for basement membranes and are readily deposited in the kidney glomeruli. This initiates kidney damage through inflammatory mechanisms that end with complement activation and cell lysis (Okamura, 1993). Earlier methods for detection of DNA antibodies included the insensitive precipitation method, complement fixation, and passive hemagglutination. Current methods used are radioimmunoassay, indirect immunofluorescence on *Crithidia luciliae*, and enzyme-linked immunosorbent assay (ELISA) (Buskila, 1992; Kavanaugh, 2002). These can detect anti-DNA in 75%–90% of active untreated SLE patients. Transient increases in anti-DNA antibodies were described in rheumatoid arthritis (RA) patients treated with anti-TNF therapy (Allanore, 2004; Bobbio-Pallavicini, 2004). Occasional clinical lupus-like cases may occur in this situation (Swale, 2003; Eriksson, 2005).

Antibodies to Sm and Nuclear Ribonucleoprotein

Precipitating antibodies to Sm antigen have been considered highly specific markers for SLE (Tan, 1989). Antibodies to both Sm and nuclear ribonucleoproteins (nRNPs) are found in patients with SLE. The Sm and nRNP antigens were clearly associated because the nRNP could not be biochemically isolated from the Sm antigen. Lerner and Steitz (1979) used the tools of molecular biology to show that Sm and nRNP antigens were subcellular particles comprising small nuclear RNAs complexed with proteins. The particle bound by anti-nRNP is composed of an RNA component designated U1 (U for uridine-rich), complexed to at least seven proteins varying in molecular mass from 12–68 kDa (Tan, 1989), found at a frequency of 30%–40% in active SLE (Ter Borg, 1990).

The antigens of Sm consist of several proteins, conventionally called B1 (29 kDa), D (16 kDa), and E (13 kDa) (Tan, 1989). Purified anti-B1/B antibodies cross-react with the D protein and vice versa, but no cross-reaction is observed in smaller percentages of SLE sera. Thus, at least two epitopes on the B1/B protein are recognized by anti-Sm sera. Antigens reactive with anti-Sm and antinuclear RNA therefore are present in assemblies of interactive proteins and RNAs engaged in precursor nRNA splicing (Tan, 1989). No characteristic clinical features are apparent in SLE patients with anti-Sm antibodies (Barada, 1981), although some authors claim these autoantibodies to be associated with renal disease or with disorders of the central nervous system. Patients who have antibodies to only nRNP have a low frequency of antibodies to DNA and a low frequency of clinically apparent renal disease (Ter Borg, 1990). Anti-Sm and anti-nRNP antibodies may be detected by immunodiffusion, passive hemagglutination, or counterimmunoelectrophoresis. However, the previously mentioned methods do not accurately distinguish between antibodies against different small nuclear RNA-associated polypeptides. Reactivities with individual RNAs and polypeptides can be best demonstrated by RNA immunoprecipitation and immunoblotting techniques, respectively. Immunoblotting has been found to be more sensitive than conventional

PART 6

TABLE 51-3
Antigens and Autoantibodies in Systemic Lupus Erythematosus

Antigen	Molecular structure	Autoantibody frequency*
Native DNA	Double-strand DNA	40%–90%
Denatured DNA	Single-strand DNA	70%
Histones	H1, H2A, H2B, H3, H4	50%–70%
Chromatin (nucleosome)	DNA–histones complex	50%–90%
Sm	Proteins 29 (B′), 28 (B), 16 (D), and 13(E) kDa, complexed with U1,U2, and U4-U6 snRNA's; spliceosome component	15%–30%
Nuclear RNP (U1nRNP)	Proteins 70, 33(A), and 22 (C) kDa, complexed with U1 snRNA; spliceosome component	30%–40%
SS-A/Ro	Proteins 60 and 52 kDa, complexed with Y1–Y5 RNA's	24%–60%
SS-B/La	Phosphoproteins 48 kDa, complexed with Y1 nascent RNA Pol transcripts	9%–35%
Ku	Proteins 86 and 66 kDa, DNA-binding proteins	1%–19%
hnRNP protein A1	Nuclear protein 34 kDa	31%–37%
PCNA	Protein 36 kDa; auxiliary protein of DNA polymerase	3%
Ribosomal RNP	Phosphoproteins 38, 16, and 15 kDa associated with ribosomes	10%–20%
Hsp-90	Heat-shock protein 90 kDa	5%–50%
Golgi complex	Golgins, giantin	Unknown
HMG-17	DNA-associated proteins, 9–17 kDa	34%–70%
β2-glycoprotein I	Anionic phospholipids, cardiolipin	25%

Data from Nakamura and Bylund (1994); Krapf and von Mühlen (1996); and Sherer (2004).
DNA, deoxyribonucleic acid; *PCNA,* proliferating cell nuclear antigen; *RNA,* ribonucleic acid; *RNP,* ribonucleoprotein.
*Frequencies are mostly related to patients with active disease.

methods for the detection of anti-Sm and anti-nRNP (Nakamura, 1994b). Currently, the most widely used laboratory tests for the detection of anti-Sm and anti-nRNP antibodies are immunodiffusion and ELISA. These tests can differentiate between Sm and nRNP antibodies but cannot define the specific antibody epitopes present in patients' sera. Antibody specificity and epitopes are best determined by Western and Northern blotting methods.

Antibodies to SS-A/Ro and SS-B/La

Patients with SLE can have antibodies to SS-A/Ro alone, or they may have both anti-SS-A/Ro and anti-SS-B/La. Having anti-SS-A/Ro alone is strongly associated with HLA-DR2 and with being young (<22 years of age at onset). The presence of both anti-SS-A/Ro and anti-SS-B/La in SLE is associated with HLA-DR3 and is seen in older patients (>50 years of age at disease onset) (Hochberg, 1985). A study of 55 patients with SLE showed that patients with anti-SS-A/Ro alone had much more serious renal disease (Hochberg, 1985). SLE patients with only anti-SS-A/Ro also had a higher incidence of concomitant anti-DNA antibodies than SLE patients who had both anti-SS-A/Ro and anti- SS-B/La antibodies (Chan, 1989). Anti-SS-A/Ro autoantibodies have been closely associated with the appearance of nephritis, vasculitis, lymphadenopathy, photosensitivity, and leukopenia in SLE patients. Anti-SS-B/La antibodies, similar to anti-SS-A/Ro antibodies, are noteworthy for their strong association with Sjögren's syndrome, occurring in more than two thirds of patients with this disorder. The SS-B/La antigen is a cellular protein bound to a small RNA species, forming a small RNP that may function in processing of RNA polymerase III transcripts (Chan, 1989).

Recently, attention has been called to the differentiation between antibodies to SSA (SSA-60 kDa) in opposition to anti-SSB (SSA-52 kDa) (Schulte-Pelkum, 2009). Different clinical associations have been noted for each system, with anti-SSA 60 associated with primary Sjögren's syndrome and SLE, and anti-SSA 52 with scleroderma and myositis. Masked reactivities in up to 20% of tested sera were reported when both antigens were present in commercial ELISAs, pointing to the fact that each autoantibody should be tested separately.

Clinical Subsets of Systemic Lupus Erythematosus Associated With Antibodies to SS-A/Ro

Elevated levels of SS-A/Ro antibodies are related to several clinical autoimmune disorders, including (1) subacute cutaneous lupus erythematosus, (2) neonatal lupus erythematosus syndrome with congenital heart block and cutaneous lesions, (3) homozygous C2 and C4 deficiency with SLE-like disease, (4) primary Sjögren's syndrome vasculitis, rheumatoid factor positivity, and severe systemic symptoms, (5) ANA-negative SLE, and (6) SLE with interstitial pneumonitis (Bylund,1991). Precipitating antibodies to SS-A/Ro are seen in 65%–95% of patients with anti-SS-A/Ro associated subsets, and more than 90% of patients have anti-SS-A/Ro levels when detected by ELISA methods (Bylund,1991).

Anti-Ku and Anti-Ki Antibodies

The Ku antigen system consists of a pair of proteins called p70/p80 (Francoeur, 1986; Reeves, 1992). These proteins have a high affinity for DNA and are known to be DNA-binding proteins, interacting covalently with the ends of native DNA. With the use of both immunoprecipation and immunoblot assays, the Ku autoantibody was found in 10% of SLE sera and was not detected in 100 scleroderma sera examined. In studies with an enzyme immunoassay, Reeves showed that 39% of patients with SLE, 55% of those with mixed connective tissue disease (MCTD), and 40% of scleroderma patients had low levels of antibody to Ku protein (Reeves, 1992). Anti-Ki antibody was first reported in Japan (Tojo, 1981) and was observed in approximately 10% of SLE patients. A relationship was observed between anti-Ki and the clinical features of arthritis, pericarditis, and pulmonary hypertension in SLE patients. The Ki antigen was purified from rabbit thymus and had a molecular weight of 32 kDa. Sakamoto (1989) developed an ELISA and observed anti-Ki antibodies in 21% (30/140) of SLE patients; 11 of 140 were positive for anti-Ki by double-immunodiffusion tests.

Antibodies to P Ribosomal Proteins

Ten percent to 20% of SLE sera show autoantibodies targeting three ribosomal phosphoproteins of 15, 18, and 38 kDa in Western blot assays. Association of anti-rRNPs with major central nervous system disorders in SLE, mainly psychotic symptoms, was reported in a retrospective study (Bonfa, 1987). No association was shown with cognitive impairment or depression in lupus patients. Significant differences in the prevalence of anti-rRNP are found among races. These antibodies occur at a higher frequency together with anti-Sm and anti-U1nRNP antibodies in SLE (Yalaoui, 2002). An etiopathogenic role for anti-rRNP in the central nervous symptoms of lupus patients is not conclusively established (Nakamura, 1997; Isshi, 1998). Observations in larger multicentric samples of SLE patients showed association of anti-rRNP antibodies with hemolytic anemia, leukopenia, alopecia, malar rash, proteinuria, and neurologic complications (Hoffman, 2004; Mahler, 2006). One recent study found correlation with disease activity (Haddouk, 2009). Anti-P ribosomal autoantibodies, because of their high specificity, are proposed to join other criteria for SLE diagnosis and classification.

Proliferating Cell Nuclear Antigen Multiprotein Complex

Antibodies to PCNA proteins are detected in 3% of patients with active SLE with no distinctive clinical associations (Miyachi,1978; Kaneda, 2004). A possible association with central nervous system features, such as transverse myelitis, has been seen in our own patients (von Mühlen, unpublished results). The PCNA complex has been characterized as cell cycle related, and PCNA antibodies have served as useful probes in the study of agents regulating DNA replication, cell proliferation, and blast transformation.

Antiphospholipid Antibodies in Systemic Lupus Erythematosus

The lupus anticoagulant/antiphospholipid antibody syndrome is characterized by the presence of circulating antibodies to phospholipids and clinical features of arterial and venous thrombosis, thrombocytopenia, hemolytic anemia, miscarriage, and several systemic symptoms. Antiphospholipid antibodies have been found frequently in patients with SLE and other disorders such as infectious diseases (McNeil, 1991; Alarcon-Segovia, 1992). Antiphospholipid antibodies are found in up to 60% of patients with SLE. This is a very heterogeneous family of antibodies, functionally and immunochemically (McNeil, 1991). Cardiolipin (anionic phospholipid) has been widely used for the detection of antiphospholipid antibodies. A majority of anticardiolipin antibodies cross-react with zwitterionic phospholipids (McNeil, 1991). Antibodies to anionic phospholipids may be immunoglobulin (Ig)G or IgM, whereas antibodies to zwitterionic phospholipids are more frequently IgM.

Antibodies to phospholipids are identified in SLE patients in three ways (Alarcon-Segovia, 1992): (1) serologically false-positive test for syphilis (a positive Venereal Disease Research Laboratory test); (2) the lupus anticoagulant assay, which is a prolongation of the kaolin partial thromboplastin time that is not corrected by normal plasma; and (3) cardiolipin immunoassay with the use of cardiolipin or other negatively charged phospholipids as antigens and β2-glycoprotein I as cofactor. Patients with SLE will usually react with a negatively charged phosphate group present in cardiolipin, phosphatidic acid, phosphatidylserine, or phosphatidylinositol.

Harris (1987, 1990) convened international workshops to improve the precision and accuracy of antiphospholipid antibody immunoassays. Reference sera were prepared and standard IgG phospholipid units (GPL) and IgM phospholipid units (MPL) were defined. One GPL (MPL) unit is equivalent to 1 mg/mL of an affinity-purified standard IgG (IgM) sample. However, Lopez (1992) suggested that an IgA-specific assay for antiphospholipid antibody is important in assessing the antiphospholipid syndrome in patients with SLE. A higher prevalence of the IgA isotype seems to be found in black persons.

Newly developed assays for β2-glycoprotein I autoantibodies seem to bring specificity to the findings; it was described that β2-glycoprotein is the specific epitope for antiphospholipid autoantibodies (Obermoser, 2004). Furthermore, IgA antibodies targeting β2-glycoprotein I, or antibodies recognizing a complex of β2-GP I/oxLDL (oxidized low-density lipoprotein), seem to be pathogenic in atherosclerotic vascular disease (Staub, 2003; Matsuura, 2004; Ranzolin, 2004). Domain 4 of the molecule seems to be the target for proatherosclerotic anti-β2-GP I autoantibodies, and domain 1 seems to be involved in the antiphospholipid syndrome, as demonstrated by our group in deletion mutant studies (Iverson, 2006).

CHRONIC DISCOID LUPUS AND OTHER CUTANEOUS VARIANTS

A benign form of lupus may present as "discoid" (coin- or disk-shaped) cutaneous lesions without symptoms of systemic disease. This disorder is called chronic discoid lupus erythematosus (CDLE) (Sontheimer, 1992; Wallace,1992). The skin lesions of CDLE are as follows: (1) persistent localized erythema, (2) adherent scales, (3) follicular plugging, (4) telangiectasis, and (5) atrophy (Wallace, 1992). Subacute cutaneous lupus erythematosus (SCLE), a similar skin condition, consists of papulosquamous or nonscarring lesions with a major association with SS-A/Ro autoantibodies. Additional variants of CDLE, such as lupus panniculitis (also called lupus profundus) and urticarial lupus, have been described (Sontheimer, 1992).

Wallace (1992) has defined CDLE as the fulfillment of the description of CDLE or SCLE, or one of the variants of SLE, in which the 1982 ACR criteria for SLE are not met. Unfortunately, CDLE is a cutaneous autoimmune disorder that lacks any unifying diagnostic serologic abnormality. It is a mild form of lupus erythematosus that uncommonly disseminates to SLE. Otherwise, considerable overlap is seen between CDLE and SLE, in that up to 15% of patients with SLE have cutaneous discoid lesions. About 6%–12% of patients with SLE had discoid lupus for a varying number of years before the onset of systemic disease (Wallace, 1992). Antinuclear antibodies are commonly found, with estimates of prevalence in discoid lupus ranging from 6%–50%. The sex ratio of discoid lupus (2 females/1 male) is much less biased toward females than that of the systemic form. Figure 51-2 depicts some clinical aspects of cutaneous disease in SLE.

DRUG-INDUCED LUPUS ERYTHEMATOSUS, ANTIHISTONE AND ANTICHROMATIN ANTIBODIES

Characteristic of drug-induced lupus is the presence of histone autoantibodies. Histones are basic molecular proteins containing high molar ratios of positively charged amino acids, lysine, and arginine. Histones are found in eukaryotic cells closely associated with genomic DNA. The subunit of this histone–DNA complex is called a nucleosome, which has two molecules of each of the "core" histones (H2A, H2B, H3, and H4) and one molecule of H1, along with DNA about 200 base pairs in length (Rubin, 1985, 1987).

In studies of drug-induced lupus, the liver enzyme acetyltransferase appears to play an important role (Woosley, 1987). Acetyltransferase is an enzyme that can acetylate drugs such as hydralazine and procainamide, promoting detoxification and excretion of the drug. Patients with low levels of acetyltranferase were more prone to develop ANA and clinical symptoms than those who were treated with hydralazine, and had phenotypically high levels of acetyltransferase. Patients with high levels of enzyme who were rapid acetylators were not immune to the development of ANA. These patients, however, took a longer and larger cumulative dose of hydralazine before developing clinical disease. These findings related to acetyltransferase phenotypes have been confirmed in patients treated with procainamide (Rubin, 1988). Procainamide is the most common drug involved in drug-induced autoimmunity. Hydralazine, quinidine, and other drugs have also been implicated as causing drug-induced autoimmunity.

In drug-induced lupus, antibodies to single-stranded DNA and histones are present. In SLE, on the other hand, antibodies to double-stranded native DNA, Sm, and U1nRNP antigens are often present, in addition to antibodies to histones. Procainamide is used to treat patients with cardiac arrhythmias, and most patients eventually develop antihistone antibodies. However, only 10%–20% of procainamide-treated patients develop symptomatic autoimmune disease (Rubin, 1988). Patients with symptomatic disease develop a unique type of IgG antihistone antibody, which, rather than reacting with individual histones, shows specific reactivity with the histone H2A–H2B dimer complex (Rubin,1988). Thus, the IgG anti–(H2A-H2B) is a useful diagnostic marker, with high sensitivity and specificity for symptomatic disease, in contrast to the benign form of procainamide-induced autoimmunity, with IgM antibodies to the individual histone. Fifty percent of all patients treated with procainamide developed ANAs after 1 year of treatment (Tan, 1989). Slow acetylators developed ANAs more rapidly than rapid acetylators (Woosley, 1987). All patients on prolonged procainamide treatment developed a positive ANA response, irrespective of acetylator phenotype.

Because antihistone antibodies are found in many other conditions, more specific antibodies such as antichromatin are replacing assays for antihistones. Synonym names for antichromatin antibodies are LE cell factor, antinucleosome, antideoxyribonucleoprotein, and anti-(H2A-H2B-DNA). They are found in 75% of all patients with SLE, in up to 100% of drug-induced lupus patients, and in 20%–50% of patients with autoimmune hepatitis type I (lupoid hepatitis). In SLE patients, antichromatin antibodies correlate better with kidney disease than anti-dsDNA (Burlingame, 2002; Cervera, 2003; Burlingame, 2004), although recent emphasis on strong association with active lupus nephritis is being pushed toward the presence of antibodies to the first component of the classical complement cascade: anti-C1q autoantibodies (Tsirogianni, 2009).

SJÖGREN'S SYNDROME

Sjögren's syndrome is a chronic inflammatory exocrinopathy, that is, an autoimmune disease marked by dryness of the eyes, mouth, and other

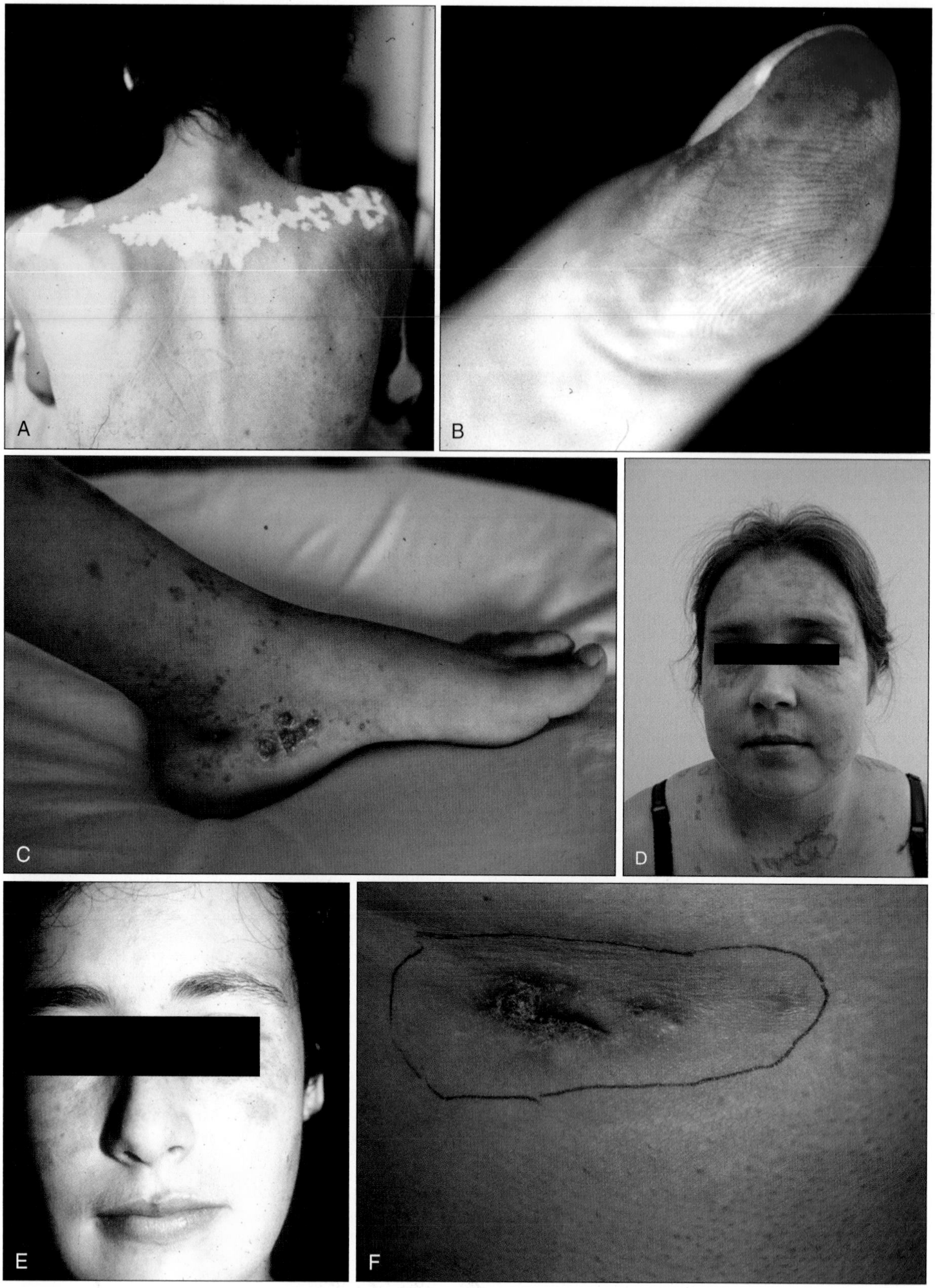

Figure 51-2 Typical cutaneous lesions in systemic lupus erythematosus (SLE). **A,** Scarring discoid lesions. **B,** Finger vasculitis. **C,** Vasculitis with ulcers. **D,** Subacute cutaneous geographic lesions. **E,** Typical malar rash. **F,** Lupus panniculitis.

mucous membranes (Schumacher, 1993; Ramos-Casals, 2005). The disease may evolve from exocrine glands to a systemic disorder, as well as to B cell lymphoproliferative transformation. It is much more frequently found in women than men, with an increasing prevalence throughout adult life. Often associated with Sjögren's syndrome is another rheumatic disease, such as RA, SLE, primary biliary cirrhosis, or systemic sclerosis (Table 51-4). Affected salivary or lacrimal glands are infiltrated with aggregates of lymphocytes. Extraglandular manifestations include lymphadenopathy, cutaneous vasculitis, and interstitial pneumonitis, among others.

The disease has been classified into (1) primary Sjögren's syndrome, which is not associated with another connective tissue disease, and (2) secondary Sjögren's syndrome, in which RA or some other autoimmune disorder is present. Sjögren's syndrome is known to occur in a primary form, with the sicca complex (keratoconjunctivitis sicca and xerostomia) as

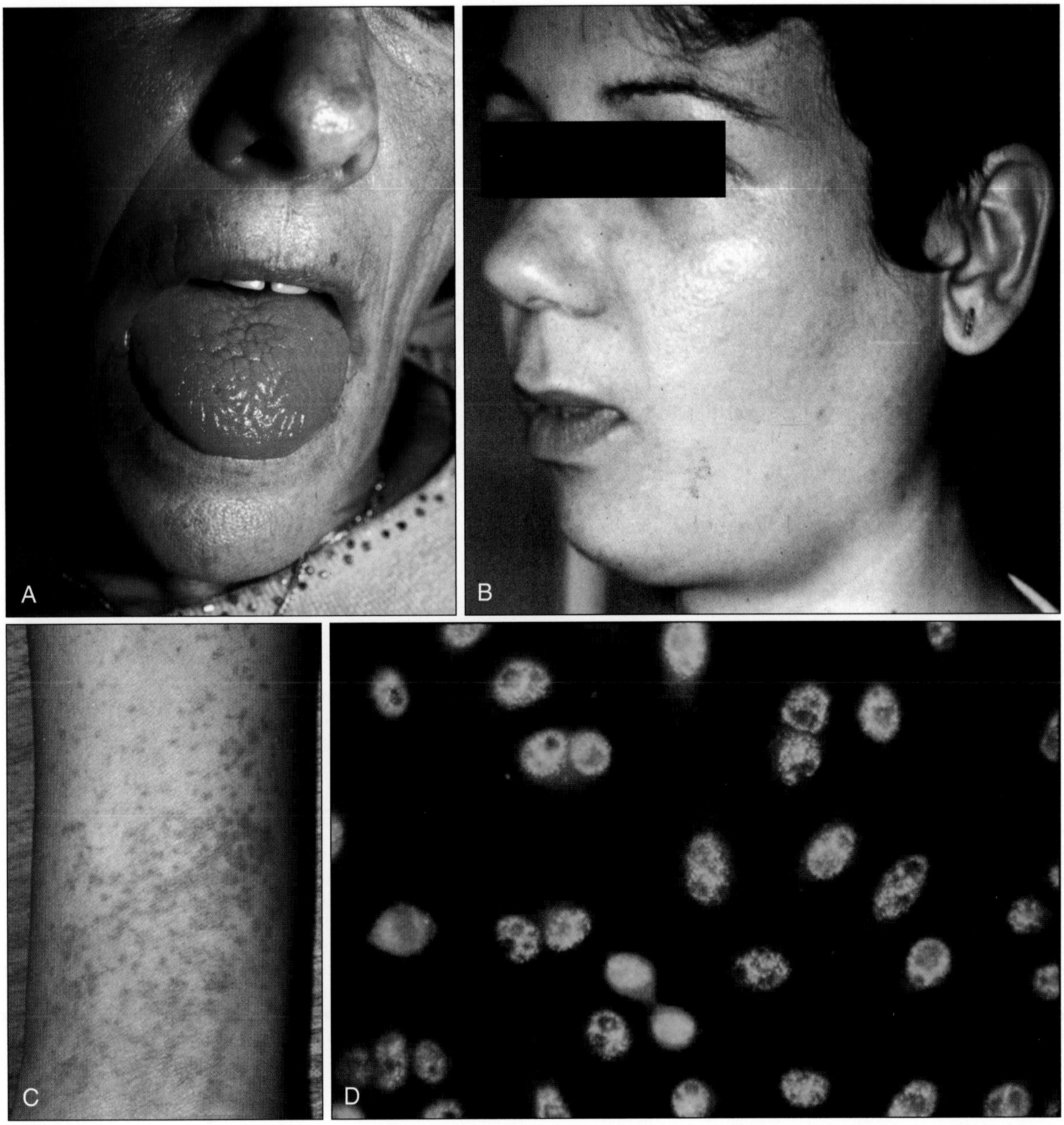

Figure 51-3 Clinical and laboratory characteristics of Sjögren's syndrome. **A,** Dry mouth and tongue. **B,** Parotid enlargement. **C,** Hypergammaglobulinemic purpura with photosensitivity (this patient with primary Sjögren's syndrome had a total immunoglobulin (Ig)G of 12 g/dL at the time this picture was taken). **D,** Fine speckled nuclear pattern in indirect immunofluorescence assay on HEp-2 cells, characteristic for the presence of anti-SSA/Ro autoantibodies.

its hallmark feature. Autoantibodies in Sjögren's syndrome are normally restricted to SS-A/Ro and SS-B/La antigens (Tan, 1989), but we have seen patients with other specificities alone, such as anti-Golgi complex or anti-NuMA. Anti-SS-A/Ro and anti-SS-B/La are present in SLE, but in lower prevalences than in Sjögren's syndrome. Anti-SS-B/La is seen in 60% of Sjögren's syndrome patients and in 35% of SLE patients; anti-SS-A/Ro is seen in 40% and 15%, respectively (von Mühlen, 1995). The presence of anti-SS-A/Ro, when associated with anti-SS-B/La, is indicative of primary Sjögren's syndrome, at times coexisting with SLE. The presence of anti-SS-B antibodies is less than 1% in RA (Tan, 1988). A striking association has been seen between anti-SS-A/Ro and the presence of both systemic and cutaneous vasculitis (Bylund, 1991). The association of SS-A/Ro antibody with vasculitis has been observed in patients with UCTD. Determination of anti-α-fodrin autoantibodies, which are also found in RA sera, does not add much to the diagnosis of Sjögren's syndrome (Ruffatti, 2004; Zandbelt, 2004). Clinical and laboratory characteristics of the disease are shown in Figure 51-3.

TABLE 51-4
Frequent Clinical Associations With Sjögren's Syndrome

1. Rheumatoid arthritis
2. Systemic lupus erythematosus
3. Polydermatomyositis
4. Mixed connective tissue disease
5. Primary biliary cirrhosis
6. Necrotizing systemic vasculitis
7. Autoimmune thyroiditis
8. Chronic active hepatitis
9. Mixed cryoglobulinemia
10. Hypergammaglobulinemic purpura

TABLE 51-5
Autoantigens and Autoantibodies in Scleroderma

Autoantigen	Molecular structure	Autoantibody frequency
Scl-70	100-kDa native and 70-kDa degradation product; DNA topoisomerase I	70% in diffuse scleroderma; 20%–59% in all patients; 13% in CREST
Centromere	Proteins 17, 80, and 140 kDa, localized at inner and outer kinetochore plates	57%–82% in CREST; 8% in diffuse form
RNA Pol I	RNA Pol I complex of subunit proteins, 210–211 kDa	4%–20% in scleroderma; 13% in diffuse form
RNA Pol II	Transcripts mRNA	4%
RNA Pol III	Transcripts 5S rRNA, tRNA	23% in scleroderma; 45% in diffuse form; 6% in CREST
Fibrillarin	Protein 34 kDa, component of U3 RNP particle	6%–8%; 5% in diffuse form; 10% in CREST
U1nRNP	Spliceosome complex	2%–5% in all patients; 24% in PM/scleroderma overlap
PM-Scl	Complex of 11 proteins,110–120 kDa	2%–5%; 24% in PM/scleroderma overlap
Ku	DNA-binding protein	1%–14% in scleroderma; 26%–55% in PM/scleroderma overlap
Th/To	Protein 40 kDa, complexes with 7S and 8S RNAs	4%–10% in scleroderma; 1%–11% in diffuse form; 8%–19% in CREST; up to 3% in PM/scleroderma overlap
NOR-90	Protein 90 kDa, human upstream binding factor, localized in nucleolus organizer region	Rare

CREST, **C**alcinosis cutis, **R**aynaud's phenomenon, **E**sophageal dysmotility, **S**clerodactyly, and **T**elangiectasia; *DNA,* deoxyribonucleic acid; *PM,* polymyositis; *RNA,* ribonucleic acid; tRNA, transfer ribonucleic acid.

Scleroderma

Systemic sclerosis (scleroderma) is a multisystem connective tissue disorder of unknown etiology in which vascular lesions and tissue fibrosis are prominent features. The cause of systemic sclerosis remains obscure. Patients with systemic sclerosis spontaneously produce autoantibodies against nuclear, nucleolar, and mitochondrial antigens (Reimer, 1990; Rothfield, 1992; Ho, 2003; Cepeda, 2004), which are of diagnostic and prognostic significance (Harris, 2003). A scleroderma patient usually has a restricted heterogeneity of autoantibody types. Table 51-5 lists the various types of autoantibodies described in scleroderma.

Patients with rapidly progressive and diffuse cutaneous involvement affecting the distal and often proximal extremities and trunk are at greater risk for early visceral involvement. Included in the classification of scleroderma is a large subset of patients who have a form of the CREST (**C**alcinosis cutis, **R**aynaud's phenomenon, **E**sophageal dysmotility, **S**clerodactyly, and **T**elangiectasia) syndrome. This subset of CREST patients may account for 20%–30% of all scleroderma patients (Fritzler, 1980). Patients with the CREST variant have limited cutaneous involvement confined to the distal extremities of fingers and face, and usually have a better prognosis and clinical course than those with diffuse cutaneous involvement (Fig. 51-4).

ANTIBODIES TO CENTROMERE ANTIGENS

The autoantibodies to centromere antigens were detected initially by immunofluorescence microscopy. The centromere antigen was localized to the region of the condensing metaphase chromosomes. In immunoblotting studies, the centromere antigens consist of three proteins: 16 kDa, 80 kDa, and 120 kDa. Autoantibodies to centromere proteins are present in 50%–80% of patients with the CREST subset. Twenty-five percent of those with idiopathic Raynaud's phenomenon with other signs or symptoms of CREST have anticentromere antibodies (Rothfield, 1992). Anticentromere antibodies are most often associated with lower frequency of pulmonary fibrosis and mortality, although an increased risk for pulmonary hypertension has been described (Cepeda, 2004).

ANTIBODIES TO SCL-70 (DNA TOPOISOMERASE I)

A major autoantigen is Scl-70, which was initially detected as a 70-kDa protein. This was later recognized as a degradation product of a 95-kDa protein, DNA topoisomerase I (Tan, 1989). The antigen was localized in punctate distribution in the nucleoplasm and nucleolus. In early studies, autoantibodies to Scl-70 were detected in 20% of unselected scleroderma patients by immunodiffusion studies (Bernstein, 1982). In later studies, Scl-70 autoantibodies were found in 75% of patients with the diffuse, severe form of scleroderma by immunodiffusion tests (Jarzabek-Chorzelska, 1986). This latter finding was probably caused by better preservation of topoisomerase I antigen in the tests, as well as by demonstration of higher prevalence of Scl-70 autoantibody in patients with the diffuse severe form of scleroderma (Nakamura, 1992). In summary, in many literature series, anti–Scl-70 autoantibodies are associated with diffuse and rapidly progressive cutaneous involvement, increased frequency of pulmonary fibrosis, and higher mortality.

ANTIBODIES TO RNA POLYMERASES

Three RNA polymerases catalyze the transcription of genes into RNA (von Mühlen, 1994). Autoantibodies targeting RNA polymerases tend to occur together in the same patients, appear to be specific for scleroderma, and are most often detected in individuals with diffuse scleroderma. Association with diffuse cutaneous disease, interstitial lung fibrosis, renal crisis, and higher mortality has been noted (Harris, 2003; Cepeda, 2004; Ioannidis, 2005). In one longitudinal cohort in the recent literature, investigators showed correlation of antibody titers with the scleroderma skin score (Nihtyanova, 2009).

AUTOANTIBODIES TO THE NUCLEOLAR ANTIGEN FIBRILLARIN (U3-snRNP)

The name fibrillarin comes from antigen localization in the dense fibrillar component of nucleoli. Antifibrillarin antibodies are seen most often in young men with scleroderma, minimal joint involvement, or pulmonary hypertension (von Mühlen, 1994; Harris, 2003).

ANTIBODIES TARGETING THE NUCLEOLAR ORGANIZING REGION

Nucleolar organizing region (NOR)-90 antibodies recognize the RNA polymerase I transcription factor hUBF (human upstream binding factor) in the fibrillar center of the nucleolus. NORs are regions where the nucleolus re-forms after mitosis, along with clusters of ribosomal RNA genes, and sites where Scl-70, U3-RNA/fibrillarin, NOR-90, and RNA polymerase I antigens can be detected (von Mühlen, 1994; Fritzler, 1995; Dagher, 2002).

Rheumatoid Arthritis

RA is a systemic autoimmune disorder characterized by chronic, symmetrical, and erosive arthritis of the peripheral joints. A large percentage of patients have elevated titers of serum rheumatoid factors. Nonarticular manifestations, such as subcutaneous nodules, vasculitis, interstitial

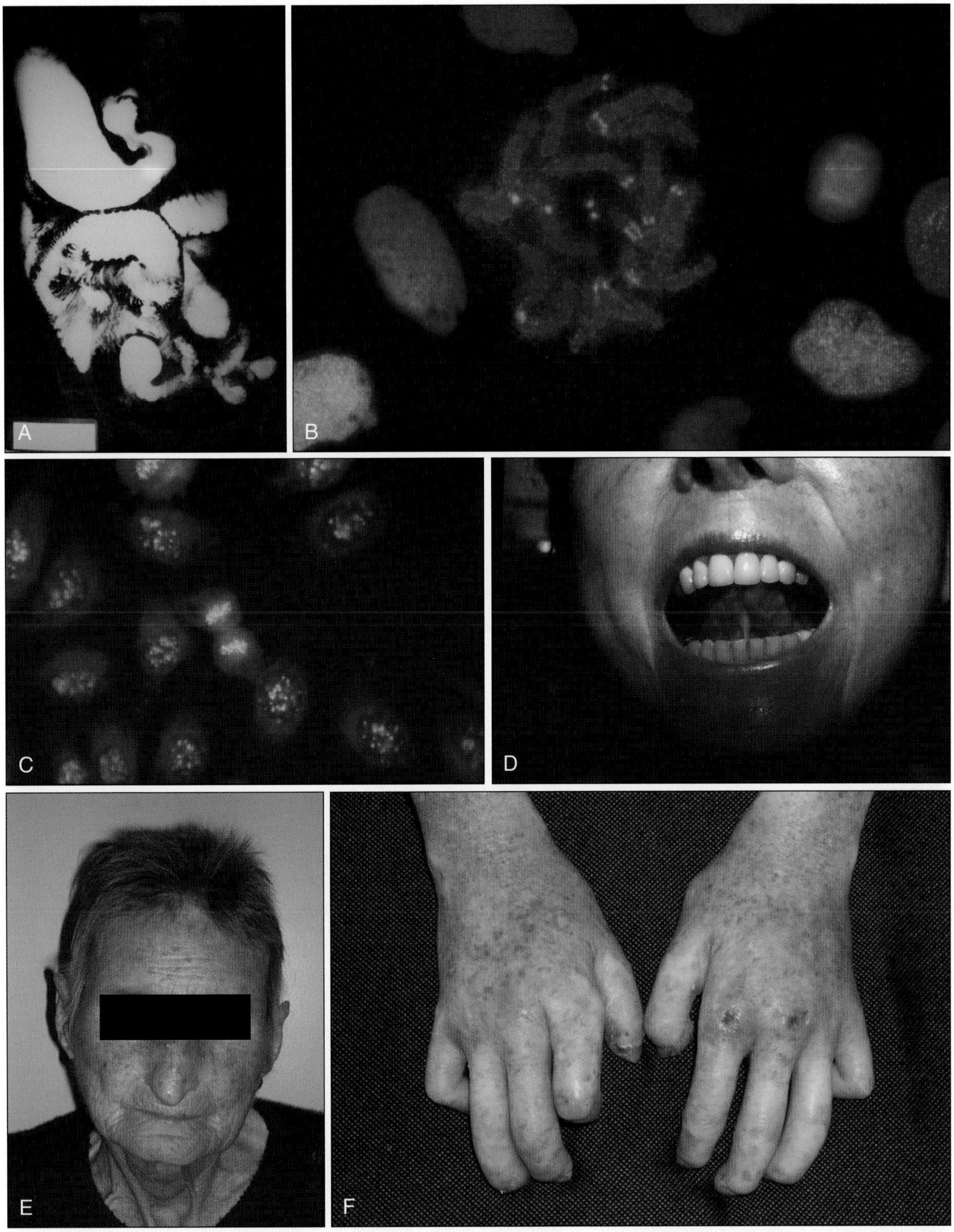

Figure 51-4 Systemic sclerosis (scleroderma): clinical and laboratory aspects. **A,** Intestinal malabsorption radiologic study showing diffuse dilation and hypoperistaltic waves. **B,** Centromere decoration in rat Indian Muntjac preparation. **C,** Centromeric pattern in indirect immunfluorescence assay on HEp-2 cells. **D,** Collagen deposition brings thickness to the lingual frenulum. **E,** Typical facial appearance in scleroderma: telangiectasias, lack of expression, thin lips and nose. **F,** Advanced sclerodactyly.

fibrosis, and anemia, may be associated. Sjögren's and Felty's syndromes commonly occur in RA. The primary cause of the disease is unknown. RA is associated with several autoantibodies, which can serve as diagnostic and prognostic markers (Aho, 1994; Viander, 1997; Firestein, 2003). These include the following:

1. Rheumatoid factor (RF)
2. Antifillagrin antibodies (also known as anticitrullinated protein antibodies; Table 51-6):
   - Antikeratin antibodies (AKAs)
   - Antiperinuclear factor (APF)
   - Antibodies to citrullinated peptides (often referred to as anti-cyclic citrullinated peptide [anti-CCP])
   - Anti-Sa antibodies, targeting citrullinated vimentin
3. Anti-RA33

All of these may precede the onset of clinical RA (Klareskog, 2004) (Fig. 51-5).

TABLE 51-6
Autoantibodies in Common Use in Rheumatoid Arthritis

	IgM RF (1940)	APF IIF (1964)	Anti-CCP 1st gen. ELISA (1998)	Anti-CCP 2nd gen. ELISA (2002)
Sensitivity (%)	66–85	60 (30–97)	68	73
Specificity (%)	72	95 (73–99)	90–98	95–98

APF, Anti-perinuclear factor; *CCP,* cyclic citrullinated peptide; *ELISA,* enzyme-linked immunosorbent assay; *RF,* rheumatoid factor. See text for references.

RHEUMATOID FACTOR

This antibody is directed against the Fc portion of the IgG molecule. Studies of monoclonal and polyclonal RF have shown polyreactive RF with binding specificity for substances other than IgG, such as nuclear components (Schumacher, 1993). Polyreactive RF is usually of the IgM class with low affinity. RF is not specific for RA and often is seen in cases of chronic infection and other systemic inflammatory conditions. RF in rheumatic disease has considerable immunochemical heterogeneity. In addition to the common IgM RF, both IgA RF and IgG RF have been detected. IgA RF has been related to more severe disease with erosions. The group of RFs consists of some of the only autoantibodies clearly shown to be involved in disease pathogenesis (Smolen, 1998).

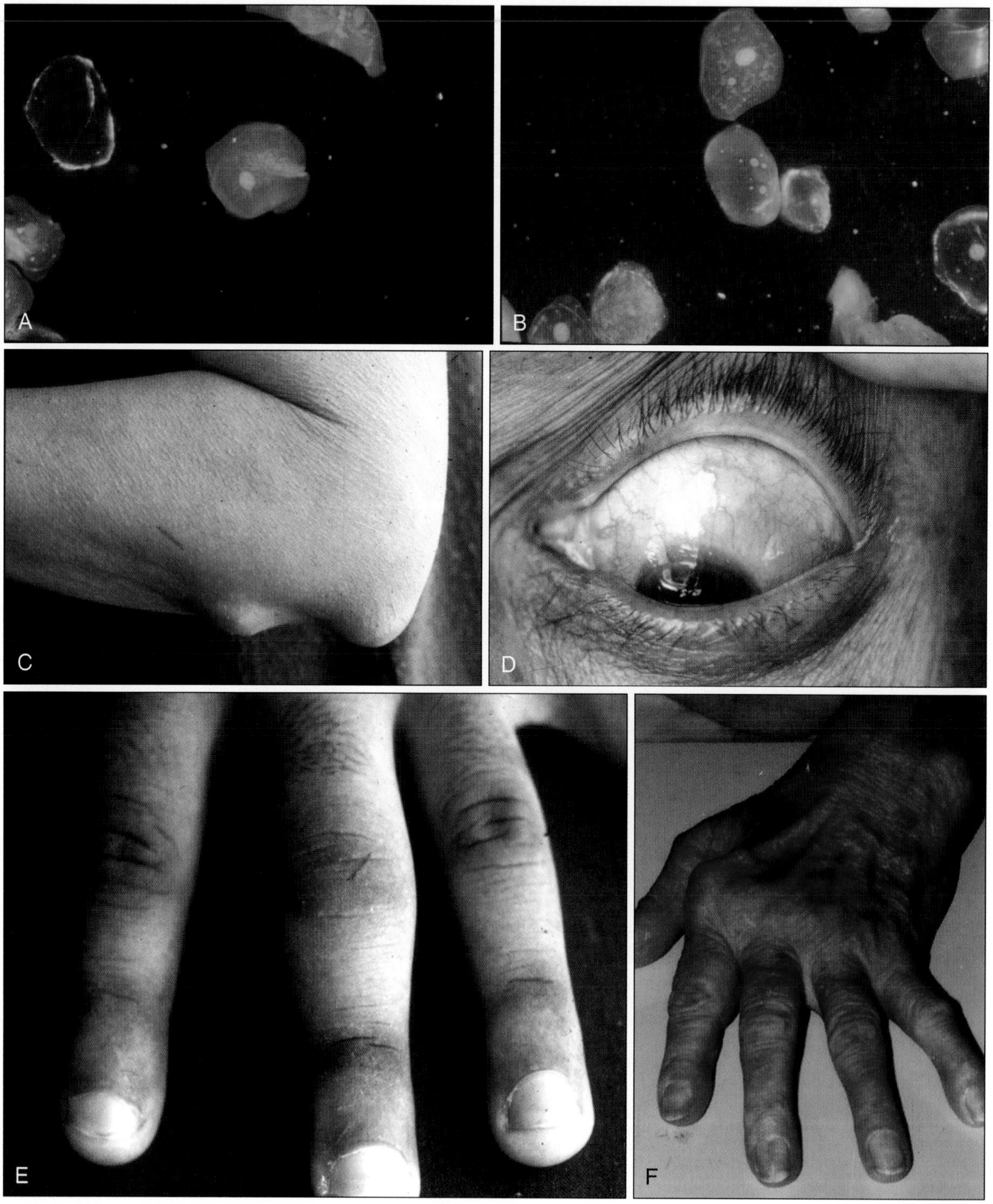

Figure 51-5 Rheumatoid arthritis (RA) with anti–perinuclear factor. **A,** Negative preparation for anti–perinuclear factor (APF) using oral mucosa cells as substrate in indirect immunofluorescence. **B,** Positive preparation for APF. Note the dense homogeneous granules around nuclei counterstained with ethidium bromide (orange color). **C,** Subcutaneous nodules in elbow region, common in seropositive RA. **D,** Episcleritis in RA. **E,** Proximal interphalangeal joint synovitis of the third finger in juvenile RA. **F,** Typical hand appearance in adult RA, with intrinsic muscle atrophy and cubital deviation of fingers.

TABLE 51-7
Autoantigens and Autoantibodies in Polymyositis and Dermatomyositis

Autoantigen	Molecular structure	Antibody frequency
Jo-1	Histidyl tRNA synthetase protein, 52 kDa	23%–36% in PM
PL-7	Threonyl tRNA synthetase protein, 80 kDa	4% in PM
PL-12	Alanyl tRNA synthetase protein, 110 kDa	3% in PM
Zo	Phenylalanyl-tRNA synthetase	<3% in PM
YRS	Tyrosyl-tRNA synthetase	<3% in PM
KS	Asparaginyl-tRNA synthetase	<3% in PM
Mi-2	Nuclear protein complex, proteins 53 and 61 kDa	15%–35% in PM; 5%–9% in DM
SRP	Protein 54 kDa complexed with 7 SL RNA	4%–5% in PM; does not occur in DM
PM-Scl	Complex of 11 proteins, 110–120 kDa	8%–12% in PM; 25% in PM/scleroderma overlap
U1nRNP	Spliceosome complex	4%–17% in PM/DM
SAE	Small ubiquitin-like modifier activating enzyme	4% in myositis patients, 8% in DM
p155(/p140)	p155-TIF1-γ (involved in nuclear transcription and cellular differentiation)	21% of myositis patients, 75% in adult DM associated with cancer
56 kDa	56 kDa, RNP component	80% of myositis patients
EJ	Glycyl-tRNA synthetase	<3% in PM
OJ	Isoleucyl-tRNA synthetase	<3% in PM

Data from Tan (1988), Nakamura (1992), von Mühlen and Tan (1994), Targoff (2006), Betteridge (2009), and Gunawardena (2008).
DM, Dermatomyositis; *PM,* polymyositis; *RNP,* ribonucleoprotein; *SRP,* signal recognition particle; *tRNA,* transfer RNA.

ANTIKERATIN ANTIBODY

This antibody reacts against the stratum corneum of rat esophagus (Young, 1979). AKA is a fairly specific but not very sensitive marker for RA. The occurrence of positive reactions in RA sera is 36%–59% and 0%–3% in normal healthy individuals (Aho, 1994). Most antikeratin-positive sera are also reactive with antiperinuclear factor, suggesting that these antigens share some similarities. Actually, it was demonstrated that AKA reacts with water-soluble acidic-neutral isoforms of fillagrin in the epidermis and with molecular forms of (pro)fillagrin in the rat esophagus epithelium, instead of cytokeratin (Simon, 1993; Sebbag, 2004).

ANTIPERINUCLEAR FACTOR

This antibody is reactive with perinuclear keratohyalin granules of buccal mucosa cells (Nienhuis, 1964). The amino acid citrulline seems to be an essential component of epitopes recognized by these autoantibodies (Schellekens, 1998). This immunofluorescence test is sensitive but less specific than AKA in RA patients. APF-positive tests in RA patients have been reported to range from 49%–87% (Janssens, 1988; Aho, 1994) and account for up to 5% in other connective tissue diseases or in normal controls. Both AKA and APF have been described in early seronegative RA, bringing a clear improvement to diagnosis of the disease.

ANTI-CYCLIC CITRULLINATED PEPTIDE

Antibodies to citrullinated peptides detected by ELISA constitute early, specific markers for RA (Sebbag, 2004; van Venrooij, 2004; Vossenaar, 2004; Hoffman, 2005). The antigen used in most assays is citrullinated fillagrin. The unusual amino acid citrulline is generated by action of the enzyme peptidyl arginine deiminase, which generates a posttranslational modification on peptides containing arginine. A second-generation ELISA is claimed to reach 98% specificity for the diagnosis of RA, with 70% sensitivity, representing major improvements over the RF test (Lee, 2003; Sebbag, 2004). Furthermore, anti-CCP antibodies can be detected in 50% of patients with early RA, at a time when RF is negative, allowing for improved diagnosis and early specific treatment. Many series in the literature point to associations with erosive, more severe and progressive disease (Forslind, 2004; Kastbom, 2004; Sebbag, 2004; Alexiou, 2008).

Anti-CCP antibodies are rarely found in other clinical conditions, such as viral infections (mainly hepatitis C), Lyme disease, Graves' disease, SLE, and Sjögren's syndrome (both with associated erosive articular disease). Children with juvenile RA generally do not benefit from this laboratory test, as its sensitivity is only 0.2%–3%. Positive results are seen in the polyarticular, RF-positive subset among children who commonly evolve to the erosive, adult form of RA (Low, 2004).

On the other hand, anti-CCP autoantibodies may better discriminate between patients with RA and those with polyarticular manifestations associated with hepatitis C virus infection (Bombardieri, 2004). Many authors now suggest that the anti-CCP test should greatly improve accuracy for RA disease classification, when added to the modified 1987 criteria of the American College of Rheumatology (Silveira, 2007).

ANTI-RA33

Hassfeld (1989) has reported an antinuclear antibody (anti-RA33) that may be specific for RA. From extracts of HeLa cells, an antigen of approximately 33 kDa was found to react with 36% of 95 sera from RA patients and with only 1 of 170 control patients. The antigen was termed RA33, and the autoantibody has no discernible relationship to other nuclear antibodies. Anti-RA33 was not related to antihistone. Immunoblot analyses with soluble extracts from HeLa cells showed an autoantibody targeting a 33-kDa antigen (anti-RA33) in 30% of Austrian RA patients and none in patients with ankylosing spondylitis or psoriatic arthritis (Aho, 1994). However, the prevalence of anti-RA33 in Finnish RA was found to be a low 6% (Aho, 1994). Anti-RA33 autoantibodies may also be found in MCTD, and in SLE (Steiner, 1996).

POLYMYOSITIS AND DERMATOMYOSITIS

Polymyositis (PM) is an inflammatory disease of striated muscle of unknown etiology. It is characterized by the presence of inflammatory infiltrates in the skeletal muscle, with associated muscle fiber necrosis and degeneration (Targoff, 1992). When the disease is accompanied by typical skin changes, it is called dermatomyositis (DM). PM is characterized serologically by the presence of a number of autoantibodies of various specifications directed against different transfer RNA (tRNA) synthetases (Targoff, 2002; von Mühlen, 1994) (Table 51-7). These autoantibodies define a subgroup of patients with PM, arthralgia, interstitial lung disease, and poorer prognosis than patients without the autoantibodies.

Antibodies to Jo-1 (histidyl tRNA synthetase) occur in 23%–36% of PM patients, most with interstitial lung disease (Targoff, 1992). Autoantibodies to threonyl and alanyl tRNA-synthetase occur at a lower prevalence in autoimmune myositis. In patients with a clinical syndrome showing overlapping features of PM and scleroderma, an antibody called anti-PM-Scl has been reported (Tan, 1988). The anti-PM-Scl antibody reacts with a complex of 11 polypeptides ranging from 110–120 kDa. Anti-PM-Scl shows staining of nucleolus and nucleoplasm in substrate cells by indirect immunofluorescence microscopy. Antibodies directed to Mi-2, a DNA-dependent, nucleosome-stimulated adenosine triphosphatase (ATPase) remodeling factor (Wang, 2001), are considered specific for dermatomyositis (von Mühlen, 1995). Attention is being called to the presence of antibodies to the 52-kDa component of SSA/Ro in a certain proportion of patients with PM/DM (Peene, 2002).

Concept of Overlap Syndromes

Overlap syndrome is a term used when patients exhibit symptoms of more than one disease (Pope, 2002). For example, patients who meet the diagnostic criteria for SLE and have typical manifestations suggestive of a second diagnosis, such as RA, have been described (Lazaro, 1989). It is uncertain whether overlap syndromes may represent the coexistence of two or more different diseases, or whether the syndrome is a distinct entity.

MIXED CONNECTIVE TISSUE DISEASE

The concept of MCTD was initially proposed by Sharp in 1972. The 20 patients described in the initial report had a combination of features usually associated with SLE, systemic sclerosis, and polymyositis. Characteristically, a high titer of autoantibody to a nRNP was found in all of the patients by hemagglutination (Sharp, 1972). The lack of renal and neurologic abnormalities and the excellent response of these patients to small doses of oral corticosteroids initially justified the classification as a separate group from SLE and systemic sclerosis. However, the concept of MCTD as a separate group has changed with time. Many think that MCTD represents an overlap of systemic sclerosis, SLE, and polymyositis (Nimelstein, 1980). A group of patients originally diagnosed as having MCTD was restudied 8 years later and showed a general evolution out of the overlap pattern to one of single disease; scleroderma was the most prevalent diagnosis (Nimelstein, 1980). There appears to be a large overlap that becomes apparent when the previously mentioned criteria are applied to a certain population of patients, and studies do not completely support the existence of MCTD as an individual clinical entity. Recently, it was shown that antibodies to a subunit of nRNP appearing in apoptotic blebs, named U1-70K, are a superior marker for early MCTD compared with autoantibodies to U1nRNP (Hof, 2005).

Molecular Biology and Functions of Certain Nuclear and Intracellular Autoantigens

Many of the intracellular autoantibodies, including ANAs, have been identified as diagnostic markers for rheumatic diseases such as SLE, scleroderma, Sjögren's syndrome, MCTD, drug-induced lupus, and polymyositis/dermatomyositis (Tan, 1989). Autoantibodies in human diseases have been used as tools to study various molecular biological functions and mechanisms. ANAs have been used to screen complementary expression libraries, with later identification of autoantigens. Biological functions that the autoantibodies have been demonstrated to inhibit are pre-mRNA splicing, DNA replication, DNA repair, transcription, transcription of rRNA, microtubule-based chromosome movement during mitosis, and aminoacetylation of tRNAs (Tan, 1988, 1989; Casiano, 1996; Tan 1997).

Profiles of Autoantibodies in Various Systemic Rheumatic Diseases

It has been observed that distinct profiles of ANA are seen in different systemic rheumatic diseases, characteristics of which include the presence or absence of certain antibodies and differences in the mean titers of these antibodies (Nakamura, 1986; Tan, 1988; Bizzaro, 2004). Nonetheless, one should be aware of the low positive predictive value of the ANA test in settings with low prevalence of systemic rheumatic disease and in aging populations (Slater, 1996). The following features are noteworthy:

1. Multiple ANAs frequently seen in SLE, often with high levels of anti-dsDNA antibodies in active disease.
2. Distinctiveness of anti-Sm, anti-rRNP, anti-C1q, and anti-PCNA for SLE.
3. Restriction of ANA in drug-induced lupus to antihistone and/or antichromatin (antinucleosome) antibodies.
4. Antibodies to U1nRNP or nuclear antibodies to RNP present in several rheumatic diseases with different frequencies.
5. Restriction of ANA in MCTD to U1nRNP (by disease definition), or nuclear RNP antibodies.
6. Sjögren's syndrome sera characterized primarily by the presence of antibodies to SS-A/Ro and SS-B/La.
7. Patients with scleroderma showing a profile consisting of antibodies to Scl-70, the centromere/kinetochore antigens, anti-RNA polymerases, and other nucleolar antigens such as fibrillarin and Th/To.
8. The frequent presence of RF and anticitrullinated proteins (AKA, APF, anti-CCP) in RA.
9. The presence of Jo-1, Mi-2, and PM-Scl autoantibodies in PM/DM.
10. Autoantibodies such as anticentromere, anti-CCP, and anti-ds-DNA may antedate overt clinical disease by many years.

TABLE 51-8

Decision Chart for the Identification of Some Autoantibodies Using HEp-2 Cells and Their Disease Association

1. Nuclear pattern
   Envelope (rim)
   - Punctate, mitotic figure negative → PBC
   - Continuous, mitotic figure negative → Chronic liver disease
   - Homogeneous, mitotic figure positive → SLE, drug-induced SLE

   Speckled
   - Large → hnRNP in SLE
   - Coarse → Sm, RNP in SLE, MCTD
   - Fine → SS-A/Ro, SS-B/La in SLE, SS
   - Pleomorphic → PCNA in SLE

   Discrete
   - Mitotic figure positive → Centromere in SCL
   - Mitotic figure negative → p95 (Sp100) in PBC
2. Nucleolar pattern
   - Homogeneous → PM-Scl in SCL
   - Clumpy → Fibrillarin in SCL
   - Speckled
     Mitotic figure punctate → RNA pol I, NOR-90 in SCL
     Mitotic figure homogeneous → Scl-70 in SCL
3. Cytoplasmic pattern
   - Dense fine speckles → Jo-1, PL-7, PL-12 in PM/DM
   - Homogeneous → rRNP in SLE and juvenile SLE
   - Fibrillar → Actin, myosin in MCTD, PBC, CAH
   - Segmental → α-Actinin, vinculin in MG, CD, UC
   - Reticular → Mitochondria in PBC
   - Polar → Golgi in SS, SLE, viral infections
   - Spindle apparatus → NuMA in SS, SLE; midbody, p330[d] in cancer
   - Discrete speckles → GWB bodies, EEA1, CLIP 170

Modified from Krapf AR, von Mühlen CA, Krapf FE, Nakamura RM, Tan EM. Atlas of immunofluorescent autoantibodies. Munich: Urban & Schwarzenberg; 1996.
CAH, Chronic autoimmune hepatitis; *CD,* Crohn's disease; *DM,* dermatomyositis; *MCTD,* mixed connective tissue disease; *NuMA,* nuclear mitotic-associated antigen; *PBC,* primary biliary cirrhosis; *PCNA,* proliferating cell nuclear antigen; *PM,* polymyositis; *RNP,* ribonucleoprotein; *SCL,* scleroderma; *SLE,* systemic lupus erythematosus; *SS,* Sjögren's syndrome; *UC,* ulcerative colitis.

Decision Chart for the Diagnostic Workup of Autoimmune Diseases

Immunofluorescence microscopy using human cellular extracts, such as HEp-2 cells, allows for the sensitive detection of serum antibodies that react very specifically with various cellular proteins and nucleic acids. This technique is essential nowadays in immunology laboratories committed to the routine diagnosis of human autoimmune disease. With a positive immunofluorescence, one is able to associate the specific pattern with the presence of a distinct autoantibody in that particular patient's serum. Because distinct autoantibody patterns occur in distinct diseases, as discussed earlier, the laboratorian offers the clinician the real possibility of narrowing down the diagnostic chase. A decision chart developed with those issues in mind is presented in Table 51-8, as is the cytoplasmic pattern classification for use in the routine laboratory (Table 51-9). Figures 51-6 through 51-8 depict some examples of immunofluorescence patterns as seen in our laboratories.

TABLE 51-9

Classification of Cytoplasmic Patterns in Indirect Immunofluorescence

Cytoplasmic patterns in IIF (cell substrate)	Representative antigens	Disease and clinical associations
1. Fibrous		
Stress fibers: linear cytoskeletal fibers, sometimes with small, discontinuous granular deposits (HEp-2, fibroblasts)	Actin Nonmuscle myosin	Both in chronic active hepatitis, liver cirrhosis, and myasthenia gravis; actin in autoimmune hepatitis, Crohn's disease, PBC, long-term hemodialysis, NHS, but rare in DCTD
Filamentous: filaments and fibrils spreading out from the nuclear rim (HEp-2, PtK2 epithelial cells)	Vimentin Keratin	Antivimentin often caused by cross-reaction with anti-α helix antibodies, detected in many types of infectious or inflammatory conditions, and in long-term hemodialysis; rare in DCTD; both seen in NHS; keratin is major system in ALD (69%), also common in DCTD and psoriasis
Segmental: just small segments of fibers (periodic dense bodies) are decorated (HEp-2, fibroblasts)	α-Actinin, vinculin tropomyosin	Myasthenia gravis, Crohn's disease, ulcerative colitis
2. Speckled		
Fine speckled: scattered small speckles, mostly with homogeneous or dense fine speckled background (HEp-2)	Many of the aminoacyl-tRNA-synthetases, mainly Jo-1	PM; "Jo-1 syndrome" (myositis and interstitial lung disease)
Dense fine speckled: cloudy, almost homogeneous throughout the cytoplasm (HEp-2)	rRNP, ribosomal phosphoproteins	Neuropsychiatric SLE
Granular pole: perinuclear, arrow-shaped, coarse granular, corresponding to the lamellar stacks of the Golgi complex (HEp-2)	Golgi apparatus	Rare in SLE, SjS, RA, MCTD, Wegener's granulomatosis, and other systemic rheumatic diseases; reported in idiopathic cerebellar ataxia, paraneoplastic cerebellar degeneration, and viral infections, including EBV and HIV
Coarse reticular: coarse diffuse reticular and granular (HEp-2)	Proteins in the inner mitochondrial membrane (mainly M2)	PBC; systemic sclerosis (43%); rare in other DCTD; centromere antibodies are frequently associated
Scattered small speckled: countable cytoplasmic speckles irregularly distributed (HEp-2)	Lysosomes/endosomes/peroxisomes/proteasomes	Limited scleroderma, glioblastoma and other neurologic diseases, idiopathic pleural effusion
Fine reticular: fine diffuse reticular and granular (HEp-2)	Endoplasmic reticulum (?); other unknown proteins	CLD; detected in all types of (chronic) inflammatory conditions
ANCA, pANCA: irregular perinuclear staining; cANCA: dense, fine, or coarse speckles (peripheral blood granulocytes, HL-60 leukemia cell line)	pANCA targets myeloperoxidase, other enzymes; cANCA targets PR3 (proteinase 3)	First reported in systemic vasculitis with necrotizing glomerulonephritis and inflammatory pulmonary disease; Wegener's granulomatosis (cANCA) and other necrotizing vasculitis (pANCA); cathepsin-G is the main antigen in ulcerative colitis, Crohn's disease, and primary sclerosing cholangitis; autoimmune hepatitis; vasculitis in PTU therapy; recently reported in RA (32%); IgM ANCA in tuberculosis and malaria

Data from Humbel (1993), von Mühlen and Tan (1994), and Stinton (2004).

ALD, Alcoholic liver disease; *ANCA*, antineutrophil cytoplasmic antibody; *cANCA*, cytoplasmic antineutrophil cytoplasmic antibody; *CLD*, chronic liver disease; *DCTD*, diffuse connective tissue disease; *EBV*, Epstein-Barr virus; *HIV*, human immunodeficiency virus; *Ig*, immunoglobulin; *IIF*, indirect immunofluorescence test; *MCTD*, mixed connective tissue disease; *NHS*, normal human serum; *pANCA*, perinuclear antineutrophil cytoplasmic antibody; *PBC*, primary biliary cirrhosis; *PM*, polymyositis; *PTU*, propylthiouracil; *RA*, rheumatoid arthritis; *RNP*, ribonucleoprotein; *SjS*, Sjögren's syndrome; *SLE*, systemic lupus erythematosus; *tRNA*, transfer ribonucleic acid.

Diagnostic Methods in Autoantibody Detection

Commonly used methods for autoantibody detection are listed in Table 51-10. Widely used tests for screening of intracellular autoantibodies are immunofluorescence microscopy and the immunoenzyme tests with many distinct antigens altogether (Nakamura, 1994b; Sahto, 2009), sometimes called **anti-ENA.** Secondary definitive tests for specific identification of ANA include immunodiffusion, immunoprecipitation, particle agglutination, immunoenzyme, immunoblotting, and radioimmunoassay methods (Teodorescu, 1992). Research for the presence of ANAs by immunofluorescence in HEp-2 cells will be positive 98% of the time when SLE patients with active disease are screened. In other words, a negative test most often will rule out an SLE diagnosis.

Standardization of the indirect immunofluorescence (IF)-ANA has been difficult (Nakamura, 1992; Feltkamp, 1996; Smolen, 1997). Many factors are involved in the performance of IF-ANA tests, including (1) substrate and fixative variations, (2) microscopic optics, (3) method and quantitation of results, (4) establishment of reference range, (5) interpretation of results, (6) reference sera, and (7) specificity and avidity of the ANA. The ANA Standardization Committee of the World Health Organization (WHO) recommends (1) that laboratories should report IF-ANA results at both 1:40 and 1:160 dilutions, and (2) that they should supply information on percentages of normal individuals who are positive at these dilutions in their own experience (Tan, 1997).

Bylund and Nakamura (1991) have shown the importance of SS-A/Ro autoantibody determination in screening tests for autoantibodies to nuclear antigens. Detection of anti-SS-A/Ro requires implementation and adherence to several technical and quality assurance recommendations. With use of appropriate substrate cells containing the SS-A/Ro antigen, many of the so-called ANA-negative lupus erythematosus patients will have a positive result on the indirect immunofluorescence test. Immunoprecipitation and double-immunodiffusion analysis have been used to determine the specificity of several ANAs. Assay specificity in double immunodiffusion is generally dependent on the quality of other control sera used in the procedure, as well as on the nature of the antigen preparation. Immunodiffusion tests are not very sensitive, but positive tests have a high degree of specificity. Immunodiffusion commercial kits are available for the detection of antibodies to RNP, Sm, SS-A/Ro, SS-B/La, and Scl-70, as well as other less prevalent markers (Nakamura, 1994b).

An increasing number of enzyme immunoassays have been developed with the use of standard purified and recombinant antigens (Saitta, 1992). Many of these enzyme immunoassays have proved to be more sensitive than comparable immunodiffusion methods. Thus, because of the high sensitivity of enzyme immunoassays, one needs to determine carefully the reference range of normal patients and the proper cutoff values. Compared with immunodiffusion tests, ELISA tests showed much greater sensitivity

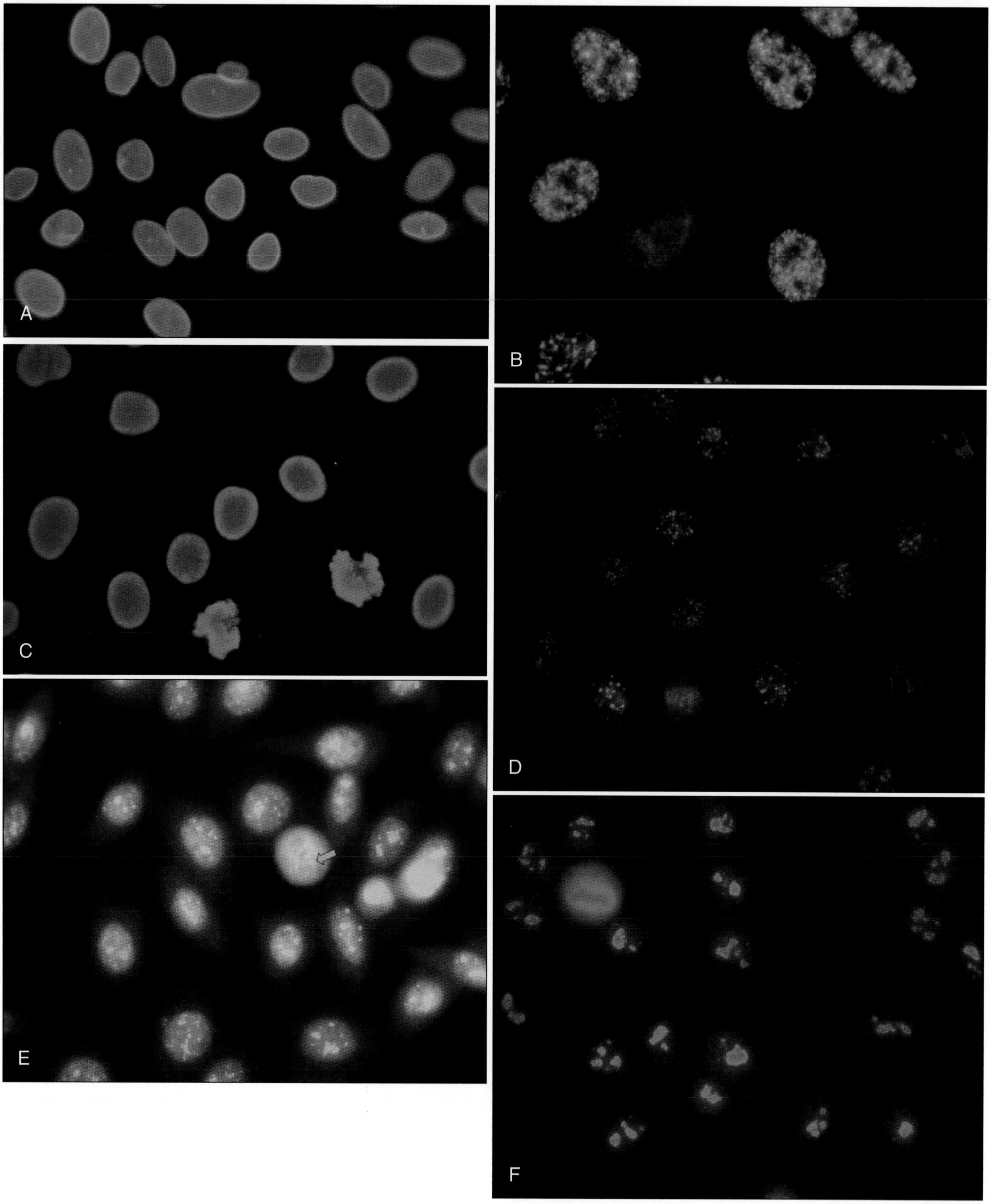

Figure 51-6 Indirect immunofluorescence with autoantibodies to nuclear and nucleolar antigens in HEp-2 cells (400×, fluorescein isothiocyanate [FITC] stain). In part **A,** autoantibodies to lamin proteins A, B, and C of the nuclear envelope give a homogeneous nuclear pattern in HEp-2 cells, associated with a continuous nucleoplasmic rim. No rim is seen when the antibodies are specifically directed to histones or double-stranded DNA (ds-DNA). Previous reports of a peripheral pattern elicited by anti-ds-DNA antibodies were probably due to fixation artifacts. The speckled nucleoplasmic pattern seen in part **B** is characteristic of autoantibodies directed to the so-called extractable nuclear antigens, like the anti-U1nRNP shown here. The nucleoli and metaphase cells are negative. Part **C** shows anti-ds-DNA autoantibodies, with homogeneous pattern in interphase as well as in metaphase cells. Part **D** is from a preparation with anticentromere autoantibodies, typically found in patients with the limited form of scleroderma (CREST syndrome), but also in primary biliary cirrhosis. Distinct speckles are seen in the interphase nuclei, one for each chromosome pair, which aggregate in the metaphase plates during cell division. Autoantibodies to NOR-90 and RNA-polymerase I elicit the same pattern in HEp-2 cells (**E**), with nucleolar speckles and dots along some spindles of metaphase cells. They can be differentiated by other assays, such as immunoblot or immunoprecipitation. Autoantibodies targeting fibrillarin (U3-nRNP) give clumpy staining of all nucleoli (**F**).

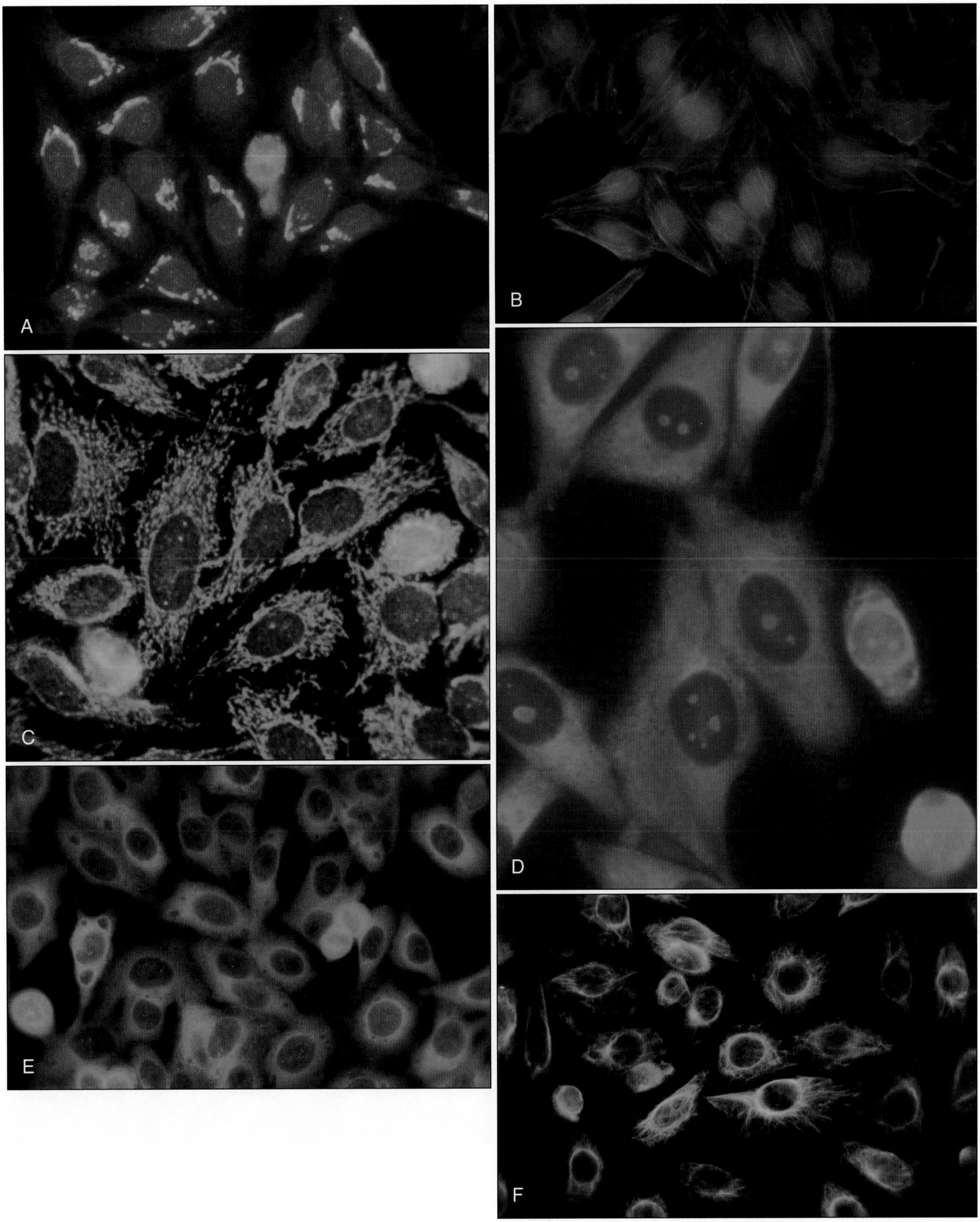

Figure 51-7 Indirect immunofluorescence of HEp-2 cells with autoantibodies to distinct cytoplasmic antigens (400×, fluorescein isothiocyanate [FITC] stain). In part **A,** the characteristic pattern of autoantibodies to the Golgi organelle is seen, with granules arranged in clusters at one pole of the cell and sparing the nuclei. Autoantibodies to nonmuscle myosin (**B**) decorate the stress fibers of the cytoskeleton (nuclei staining in blue with DAPI). These antibodies are found in patients with myasthenia gravis and chronic liver disease. Antimitochondrial autoantibodies display a coarse granular pattern involving the whole cytoplasm (**C**), mostly seen in primary biliary cirrhosis. Part **D** shows the dense granular, almost homogeneous, cytoplasmic pattern obtained with anti-rRNP antibodies. They target ribosomal phosphoproteins and are clinically associated with central nervous system manifestations in patients with systemic lupus erythematosus. As can be noticed in the picture, not uncommonly such antibodies also stain the nucleoli in a homogeneous pattern, although weakly. In part **E,** a homogeneous decoration of the cytoplasm was conferred by autoantibodies to PL-7 in polymyositis. Antikeratin antibodies (**F**) are seen as filamentar staining of cytoskeletal stress fibers and constitute the major specificity found in alcoholic liver disease (69%), also common in rheumatoid arthritis (36%–59%), psoriasis, and healthy individuals.

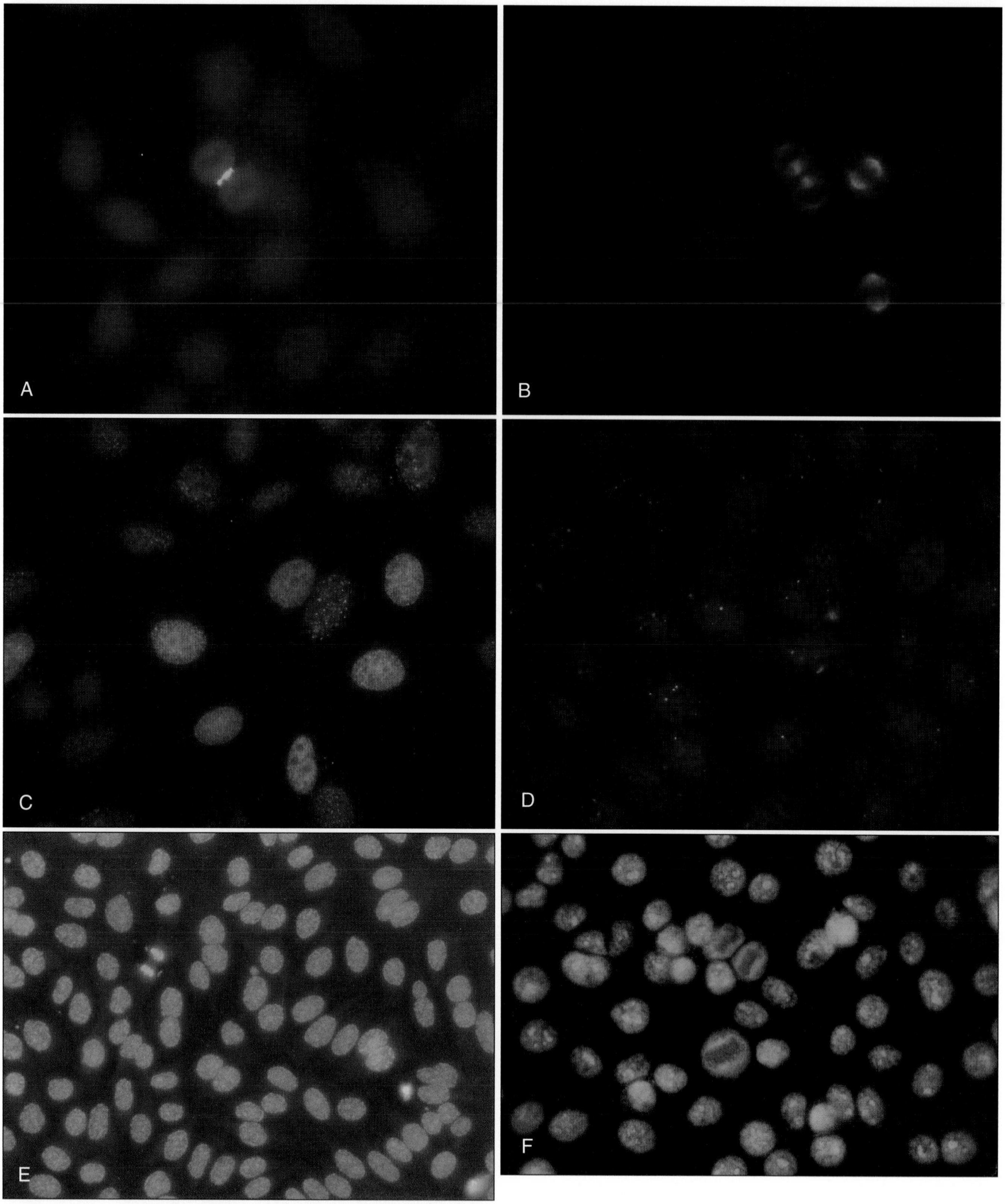

Figure 51-8 Some other distinct patterns in indirect immunofluorescence of HEp-2 cells (400×, fluorescein isothiocyanate [FITC] stain). In part **A,** cells at the end of metaphase show antigens condensing in the midbody, also called the intercellular bridge region. The spindle poles of dividing cells can be decorated, as in part **B,** with antibodies targeting the mitotic apparatus, such as NuMA (nuclear mitotic-associated protein). Proliferating cell nuclear antigen (PCNA) autoantibodies give a mosaic of nucleoplasmic patterns (**C**), ranging from homogeneous to distinct speckled, according to the phases of cellular division (details in the text). Part **D** shows the pattern obtained with anti-p80-coilin autoantibodies, where one can see from 1 to 8 nucleoplasmic dots. Part **E** shows one of the most common patterns seen in the routine laboratory—dense, fine, speckled nuclear in interphase as well as in mitotic cells. This is a nonspecific autoantibody found in systemic connective tissue disease, but also in interstitial cystitis, breast cancer, and allergic reactions. Nuclear and nucleolar stainings are seen with anti-Ku autoantibodies (**F**). Chromosomes in mitotic cells are negative (see clinical associations in text).

TABLE 51-10

Methods for Detection of Autoantibodies to Nuclear and Intracellular Antigens

Method	Antigen source	Sensitivity and use
Immunofluorescence microscopy	Tissue sections; cell lines	Sensitive assay; often used for screening
Double immunodiffusion (Ouchterlony)	Tissue and cell extracts	Requires precipitin reaction; high specificity but not very sensitive
Counterimmunoelectrophoresis	Tissue and cell extracts	Increased sensitivity and speed as compared with immunodiffusion procedure
Immunoblotting, Western blot	Cell extracts	Very sensitive; permits detection of antibodies against soluble and insoluble antigens
Dot blot, linear blot (line immunoassays)	Purified native or recombinant antigens	Qualitative assay; average sensitivity
ELISA	Purified native or recombinant antigens	Very sensitive, quantitative; high throughput; can determine antibody class; low cost
Microsphere multiplexed assay	Purified native or recombinant antigens	Very sensitive (compares with ELISA), semiquantitative, rapid, expensive proprietary technology

ELISA, Enzyme-linked immunosorbent assay.

but had lower specificity (Nakamura, 1992). Further, ELISA tests were frequently positive in low titers in sera of patients with rheumatic diseases other than SLE. For example, the presence of antibodies to Sm as assayed by immunodiffusion is considered to be highly specific for SLE. However, in ELISA tests, the Sm antibody was positive in 23% of 54 RA patients, 25% of 24 systemic sclerosis patients, 9% of 11 polymyositis patients, and 2% of 59 normal patients (Maddison, 1985). Increasing sensitivity and decreasing specificity might result in false-positive test results. Furthermore, clinical associations with distinct autoantibodies were determined mainly with the use of ID techniques.

New commercial ELISA kits developed for screening purposes claim to detect a variety of autoantibodies in a single assay, but having "total" fractions of cellular antigens in one ELISA well is not technically feasible nowadays. Those assays are not 100% sensitive for the screening of antinuclear antibodies, as they cannot detect certain autoantibodies such as antinucleolar specificities, PCNA or distinct NuMA types. Reported results using those kits, for the moment, should correctly specify to physicians which types of autoantibodies were tested, so as not to imply that a particular sample is "negative for all nuclear antibodies." Each ELISA test kit in such a situation should be validated for which antibody specificities it can actually detect (von Mühlen, 2002).

More recently, multiplexed assays are being incorporated into the routine work of bigger laboratories. The so-called multiplexed fluorescent microsphere immunoassay uses spectral addresses, allowing for the simultaneous determination of several autoantibodies—all in just one incubation and with no wash steps. We recently demonstrated that results for a proprietary multiplexed assay compared favorably with results from established ELISAs (Martins, 2004): agreement, sensitivity, and specificity, respectively, for five nuclear antigens evaluated were as follows: SSA, 99.1%, 100.0%, and 98.8%; SSB, 98.6%, 88.9%, and 99.5%; Sm, 97.6%, 95.8%, and 97.9%; RNP, 97.2%, 92.7%, and 98.8%; and Scl-70, 93.6%, 50.0%, and 99.0%. The multiplexed microsphere-based immunoassay seems to be a sensitive and specific method for the detection and semiquantitation of common antibodies in human sera. Clusters of clinically important autoantibodies, such as those in lupus or in systemic vasculitis, may be rapidly tested in a single batch. This is not to imply that the flow cytometry–based assay may be an alternative to screening autoantibodies with HEp-2 immunofluorescence, because there are clear limitations in identifying important autoantibodies in clinical samples by using current microsphere technology (Kroshinsky, 2009). One recent position paper of the American College of Rheumatology clarifies the state of the art in detecting autoantibodies and may be accessed at www.rheumatology.org/publications/position/ana_position_stmt.pdf.

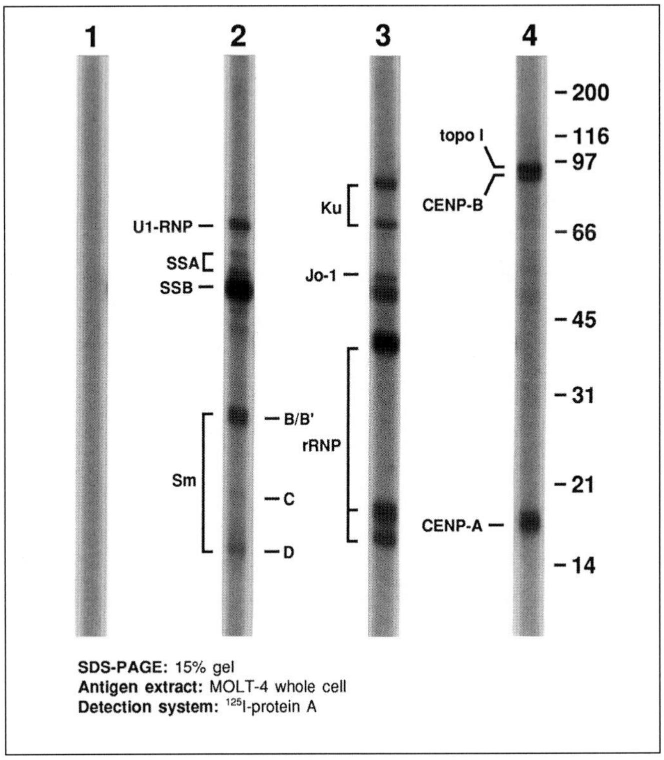

Figure 51-9 Immunoblotting analysis of common autoantibodies seen in rheumatic disease. In lane 1, the nitrocellulose strip was probed with a normal human serum (negative control), and no reactivity is seen as expected. The next three lanes show distinct bands obtained by mixing positive control sera containing known specificities. Lane 2 depicts reactivities to the ribonucleoproteins (RNPs) SSA (52 and 60 kDa), SSB (48 kDa), Sm (B/B', 28 kDa, and D, 14 kDa), and U1nRNP (the 70 kDa) and a faint band around 19 kDa, the C antigen. (The A protein, with 32 kDa and also characteristically recognized by U1nRNP antibodies, is not seen in this experiment.) Lane 3 shows the bands obtained by using the human prototype antisera to Jo-1 (52 kDa), Ku (two bands around the 70- and 80-kDa regions), and ribosomal RNP (15, 18, and 37 kDa). The small band above the 52-kDa antigen is not identified. Lane 4 displays the bands most commonly seen using sera from scleroderma patients (e.g., anti-DNA topoisomerase I [Scl-70, 95 kDa] and anticentromere antibodies [16 kDa, CENP-A, and 80 kDa, CENP-B]). On the left, positions in kilodaltons of the broad-range molecular weight standards can be seen. *(Used with permission from von Mühlen CA, Tan EM. Autoantibody specificities in autoimmune rheumatic diseases. Rev Bras Rheumatol 1994;34:173.)*

Variations in Methods Used for Detection of Autoantibodies to Nuclear and Intracellular Antigens

Most probably, the best studies regarding different methods for detection of autoantibodies to intracellular antigens were reported by a European Consensus Study Group. The European Consensus Study Group for the Detection of Autoantibodies to Intracellular Antigens in Rheumatic Diseases was formed in 1988 and conducted four annual workshops from 1989 to 1992 (van Venrooij, 1991; Charles, 1992). In 1988 and 1989, consensus workshops were conducted to define interlaboratory concordance in the detection of autoantibody specificities in rheumatic disease. Twenty-eight laboratories participated in the study and used various methods. The objectives of the consensus study initiated in 1989 were (1) to define the interlaboratory consensus in detecting autoantibodies and specificities, (2) to test whether discrepancies were due to the method used, and (3) to make recommendations for improved quality of results with improved sensitivity and specificity.

ENZYME-LINKED IMMUNOSORBENT ASSAYS

In the 1988 and 1989 studies, many false-positive reactions were noted. False-positive reactions were caused by poor blocking reagents in the procedure; also, impure antigen preparations were used. In the 1990 and 1991 cooperative study, the laboratory using ELISAs performed very well, with few false-positive or extraneous negative results. ELISA assays also performed well in sorting out sera with multiple specificities.

The percentage of clinical laboratories using ELISA increased from 25%–47% over a 4-year period, from 1989–1992. Homburger (1998) reported a comparison between a commercial ELISA and IF-ANA on HEp-2 cells, concluding that both methods were substantially equivalent for detecting clinically relevant ANA in patients with systemic rheumatic disease. Reaching an opposite conclusion, Emlen and O'Neill (1997) tested six commercial ELISA kits and concluded for the existence of significant differences in the detection of ANA by immunofluorescence and ELISA. A group of international scientists joined by the WHO reported on the performance of many commercial ELISAs, showing that (1) no single manufacturer was clearly superior to others in terms of overall sensitivity, specificity, and precision of products, and (2) areas that needed improvement were noted in kits used for the detection of antibodies to dsDNA and to Sm antigens (Tan, 1999). Great care should be exercised when selecting ELISA reagents and commercial kits. A good source of quality control data for the best commercial reagents is the periodic review of the College of American Pathologists in Immunology.

IMMUNOBLOTTING

This technique is very sensitive and is an important method for characterization of the specific nature of many autoantibodies. One important advantage is that a specific antibody can be identified with the use of crude cell extract antigen preparations (Fig. 51-9). The European Consensus Study observed the following with the immunoblotting test (Nakamura, 1994b):

1. The antigen preparation is very important in the immunoblotting procedure.
2. Detection of antibodies to nRNP, Sm, and Scl-70 was acceptable. This sensitive method is helpful in the detection of multiple specificities of antibodies in the same specimen.
3. The method requires careful controls to monitor molecular weight bands. For example, histone bands can be confused with a centromeric antigen (CENP-A, 19 kDa), and Scl-70 (topoisomerase I) can be confused with other 100-kDa bands.
4. Protein degradation can occur in the antigen cell extract used for immunoblotting, especially Scl-70 and centromere antigens.
5. The anti-Sm is distinguished by the presence of anti-D (the D antigen is a 16-kDa protein contained in all major nRNP particles).
6. Anti-SS-B/La is readily detected by immunoblotting. Anti-SS-A/Ro is poorly detected by immunoblotting and is insensitive because SS-A/Ro may not demonstrate the proper structure for recognition.

SELECTED REFERENCES

Burlingame RW. Recent advances in understanding the clinical utility and underlying cause of antinucleosome (antichromatin) autoantibodies. Clin Appl Immunol Rev 2004;4:351.

Antichromatin antibodies are a hallmark of lupus disease; this review brings all important data that justify the assertion.

Sebbag M, Chapuy-Regaud S, Auger I, et al. Clinical and pathophysiological significance of the autoimmune response to citrullinated proteins in rheumatoid arthritis. Joint Bone Spine 2004;71:493.

Very informative account, with historic highlights, of this important group of autoantibodies specifically seen in rheumatoid arthritis.

Sherer Y, Gorstein A, Fritzler MJ, Shoenfeld Y. Autoantibody explosion in systemic lupus erythematosus: more than 100 different antibodies found in SLE patients. Semin Arthritis Rheum 2004;34:501.

Most complete account of the prevalence and specificities of autoantibodies in systemic lupus erythematosus, comprising antibodies that target nuclear, cytoplasmic, phospholipid, and cell membranes, and other antigens.

Tan EM. Antinuclear antibodies: diagnostic markers for autoimmune diseases and probes for cell biology. Adv Immunol 1989;44:93.

This is a classic review paper in the field of autoantibodies that describes their clinical associations and the molecular nature of autoantigens; it was written by a scientist who discovered many of the most important autoantibody markers in rheumatology.

Tan EM, Smolen JS, McDougal JS, et al. A critical evaluation of enzyme immunoassays for detection of antinuclear antibodies of defined specificities. I. Precision, sensitivity, and specificity. Arthritis Rheum 1999;42:455.

This paper is the first to try to shed light on the difficult task of standardization of laboratory practices. Many useful recommendations from researchers, technicians, and clinicians enhance understanding of ELISA results.

von Mühlen CA, Tan EM. Autoantibodies in the diagnosis of systemic rheumatic diseases. Semin Arthritis Rheum 1995;24:323.

Very thorough description of major autoantibodies in systemic rheumatic disease, with clinical associations and molecular data for autoantigens.

Vossenaar ER, van Venrooij WJ. Anti-CCP antibodies, a highly specific marker for (early) rheumatoid arthritis. Clin Appl Immunol Rev 2004;4:239.

Historic and clinical discussion of anti-CCP autoantibodies, presenting some evidence for a possible etiologic role of these autoantibodies in rheumatoid arthritis.

REFERENCES

Access the complete reference list online at http://www.expertconsult.com

CHAPTER 52

VASCULITIS

Ankoor Shah, David J. Bylund, Rex M. McCallum

KEY POINTS

- The etiology and pathogenesis of vasculitides remain obscure and poorly understood, and may vary between different forms of vasculitis.
- There is no widely accepted standard classification system for idiopathic vasculitides, although the American College of Rheumatology and the Chapel Hill Consensus are the most widely used systems.
- The diagnosis of idiopathic systemic necrotizing vasculitides requires a high degree of suspicion.
- There are no pathognomonic clinical laboratory tests for patients with systemic necrotizing vasculitides.
- Antineutrophil cytoplasmic antibody (ANCA) tests are most valuable when selectively ordered in clinical situations where some form of ANCA-associated vasculitis is a serious consideration; they should not be used as screening tests.
- Detection of ANCA, particularly the association of cytoplasmic antineutrophil cytoplasmic antibody (c-ANCA) with Wegener's granulomatosis, has become an important adjunct in the diagnosis of systemic necrotizing vasculitis.
- c-ANCA immunofluorescence pattern should be confirmed using proteinase 3 enzyme-linked immunosorbent assay (ELISA).
- The pattern of perinuclear antineutrophil cytoplasmic antibodies (p-ANCAs) on indirect immunofluorescence is diagnostically nonspecific, so p-ANCA–positive sera should be tested in ELISA for myeloperoxidase-specific ANCA.
- Tissue biopsy with histologic confirmation of vasculitis remains the most important laboratory test for diagnosis of systemic necrotizing vasculitis.

The clinical, laboratory, and pathologic expressions of systemic necrotizing vasculitis are protean. Clinicians face a patient who presents with a wide array of confusing and conflicting symptoms and/or signs. Diagnosis of a systemic necrotizing vasculitic syndrome requires thorough evaluation that correlates an individual patient's history and physical examination with laboratory, imaging, and pathologic data. Although vasculitis can occur anywhere in the body, distinctive patterns of disease have been defined, and their identification points to particular disorders with specific treatment and prognosis (Langford, 1995, 2003).

Systemic necrotizing vasculitis is characterized pathologically by inflammation causing vascular lesions. These lesions may include the proliferation of intimal cells inside vessel lumina and narrowing or even closing of that space, causing ischemia and possible infarction to anatomic structures distal to the site of vascular injury. Also, the vessel wall may thin and weaken until an aneurysm forms or the vessel ruptures.

Idiopathic (primary) vasculitis occurs when vascular inflammatory damage is the principal clinicopathologic finding and no other underlying illness is present. Secondary vasculitis occurs when vasculitic lesions accompany underlying disorders such as infectious disease, connective tissue disease, and hypersensitivity reaction (Table 52-1). This chapter focuses on idiopathic vasculitis and those clinical laboratory tests useful for its diagnosis and management. Because methods of diagnosis and management in secondary vasculitides concentrate on the underlying disorders, they are discussed in appropriate chapters of this book. However, comments related to laboratory evaluation of end-organ damage in idiopathic vasculitis are relevant to secondary vasculitis.

CLASSIFICATION

No standard classification system for idiopathic vasculitides has been widely accepted. Historically, their classification has been based on various combinations of clinical and pathologic findings in an effort to provide standardization with regard to presentation, prognosis, and treatment (Jennette, 1997; 1998b). Working classifications have improved in recent years owing to efforts at standard nomenclature (Hunder, 1990; Jennette, 1994; Hoffman, 1998a; Langford, 2003). In the 1980s, the American College of Rheumatology began an effort to improve sensitivity and specificity in distinguishing individual types of primary vasculitis from others (Table 52-2). The classification scheme was not intended to provide diagnostic criteria for primary vasculitis, as diagnosis is defined primarily by clinical judgment. In 1993, this was further expanded upon by the Chapel Hill Consensus Conference (CHCC), which provided additional nomenclature (Jennette, 1994; Falk, 2004). Table 52-3 contains the names and definitions of vasculitides adopted by the CHCC. Both schemes rely largely on dividing different vasculitides by the caliber of the vessel involved, with the CHCC criteria including the ANCA as a biomarker that can be used to distinguish certain forms of small-vessel vasculitis.

PATHOGENESIS OF VASCULITIS

The etiology and pathogenesis of vasculitides remain obscure and poorly understood, and may vary between different forms of vasculitis (Langford, 2003). Most idiopathic vasculitides are attributed to immune-mediated vascular injury induced by any of several mechanisms, including (1) immune-complex deposits; (2) direct autoantibody binding to vessel wall structures (e.g., endothelium, basement membrane antigens) or to neutrophils when vasculitis is associated with ANCAs; and (3) cell-mediated inflammation (Jennette, 1994a) (Table 52-4). The pathogenic effects of these different mechanisms all unite in a final common pathway of vascular injury that activates humoral and cellular mediators of inflammation.

TABLE 52-1
Secondary Systemic Necrotizing Vasculitides

- Drug-related vasculitis
- Foreign protein–related vasculitis
- Vasculitis associated with infection
- Vasculitis in malignancy
- Lymphomatoid granulomatosis
- Hypocomplementemic urticarial vasculitis
- Hypergammaglobulinemic purpura
- Cryoglobulinemic vasculitis
- Radiation vasculitis
- Transplant vasculitis (vascular rejection)
- Connective tissue disease–associated vasculitis
- Rheumatoid arthritis
- Systemic lupus erythematosus
- Sjögren's syndrome
- Scleroderma
- Dermatomyositis/polymyositis
- Sarcoidosis
- Relapsing polychondritis
- Antiphospholipid antibody syndrome
- Behçet's disease

Adapted from Langford CA, McCallum RM. Idiopathic vasculitis. In Belch JJF, Zurier RB, editors. Connective tissue diseases. London: Chapman & Hall; 1995, p. 179, with permission.

TABLE 52-2
Idiopathic (Primary) Systemic Necrotizing Vasculitides

Small-Vessel Vasculitis
Wegener's granulomatosis
Henoch-Schönlein purpura
Primary angiitis of the central nervous system
Medium-Vessel Vasculitis
Churg-Strauss syndrome
Polyarteritis nodosa
Kawasaki disease
Large-Vessel Vasculitis
Giant cell (temporal) arteritis
Takayasu's arteritis

TABLE 52-3
Names and Definitions of Vasculitides from the Chapel Hill Consensus

	Definition
Large-Vessel Vasculitis	
Giant cell (temporal) arteritis	Granulomatous arteritis of the aorta and its major branches, with a predilection for the extracranial branches of the carotid artery. Often involves the temporal artery. Usually occurs in patients older than 50 and is often associated with polymyalgia rheumatica.
Takayasu's arteritis	Granulomatous inflammation of the aorta and its major branches. Usually occurs in patients younger than 50.
Medium-Sized Vessel Vasculitis	
Polyarteritis nodosa (classic)	Necrotizing inflammation of medium-sized or small arteries without glomerulonephritis or vasculitis of the arterioles, capillaries, or venules.
Kawasaki disease	Arteritis involving the large, medium-sized, and small arteries, and associated with mucocutaneous lymph node syndrome. Coronary arteries are often involved. Aorta and veins may be involved. Usually occurs in children.
Small-Vessel Vasculitis	
Wegener's granulomatosis	Granulomatous inflammation involving the respiratory tract, and necrotizing vasculitis affecting small to medium-sized vessels (capillaries, venules, arterioles, and arteries). Necrotizing glomerulonephritis is common.
Churg-Strauss	Eosinophil-rich and granulomatous inflammation involving the respiratory tract, and necrotizing vasculitis affecting small to medium-sized vessels and associated with asthma and eosinophilia.
Microscopic polyangiitis	Necrotizing vasculitis, with few or no immune deposits, affecting small vessels (capillaries, venules, or arterioles).
Henoch-Schönlein purpura	Vasculitis with immunoglobulin (Ig)A-dominant immune deposits, affecting small vessels (capillaries, venules, or arterioles).
Essential cryoglobulinemic vasculitis	Vasculitis with cryoglobulin immune deposits, affecting small vessels (capillaries, venules, or arterioles). Typically involves skin, gut, and glomeruli, and is associated with arthralgias and arthritis.
Cutaneous leukocytoclastic vasculitis	Isolated cutaneous leukocytoclastic angiitis without systemic vasculitis or glomerulonephritis.

T cells release interferon-γ and can also recruit monocytes and macrophages to vessel walls. These cells express increased levels of interleukin (IL)-1, IL-2, IL-6, tumor necrosis factor (TNF)-α, and TNF-β (Grau, 1989; Arimura, 1993). These mediators initiate the infiltration of inflammatory cells, activation of complement and coagulation cascades, and upregulation of other inflammatory molecules and growth factors such as platelet-derived growth factor and vascular endothelial growth factor. Sustained inflammation ultimately leads to extensive intimal thickening and vessel occlusion (Conn, 1993; Niles, 1995; Sneller, 1997; Langford, 2003; Guillevin, 2007). Substantial evidence of direct ANCA involvement in vasculitis tissue damage exists. In Wegener's granulomatosis (WG), ANCAs primarily target proteinase 3 (PR3), and in other vasculitides such as microscopic polyangiitis (MPA) and Churg-Strauss syndrome (CSS), myeloperoxidase (MPO) is a major target. Both of these antigens are enzymes contained in the granules of neutrophils and monocytes (Guillevin, 2007). Neutrophils that have been primed with low-dose TNF will have increased expression of MPO and PR3 and can release lytic enzymes when incubated with sera containing ANCA antibodies to these antigens (Kallenberg, 2006). In vitro studies also demonstrate that ANCA can increase attachment of rolling neutrophils to the endothelial layer (Radford, 2001). Finally, an association between the Birmingham Vasculitis Activity Score and the extent of disease and the number of activated B cells has been described (Seo, 2004b).

Perspective on Use of Clinical Laboratory Tests

When evaluating patients with complicated multisystem disease, the clinician's goal is accurate diagnosis to the level that defines proper treatment. Because no pathognomonic clinical or laboratory features of vasculitis have been identified, the physician must use combinations of clinical, laboratory, imaging, and pathologic findings to recognize patterns of disease. This may allow specific diagnosis or classification of the patient's disease as one in a group of vasculitic disorders requiring similar treatment, even when no specific entity is identifiable.

Deciding that a patient has vasculitis strictly on the basis of clinical symptoms is fraught with risks because of the large number of differential diagnostic possibilities and the lack of pathognomonic findings. Consequently, histologic or angiographic confirmation of vasculitis should be obtained from tissue biopsy or angiography for definitive diagnosis prior to therapy (Mandell, 1994; Langford, 2003).

Clinical laboratory tests are of limited value in establishing a specific diagnosis of vasculitis (Mandell, 1994; Langford, 2003), although clinicians use these tests to assist in identifying patterns of organ involvement characteristic of vasculitis, evaluating the extent and severity of end-organ damage, distinguishing idiopathic vasculitis from alternative secondary forms, and establishing baseline values for management. The association of ANCA with certain idiopathic vasculitides is an important aid in diagnosis and management. ANCAs are discussed in detail subsequently.

When evaluating a patient whose differential diagnoses includes vasculitis, utilize the following principles regarding the use and interpretation of clinical laboratory tests.

TABLE 52-4
Potential Mechanisms of Vessel Damage in Selected Primary Vasculitis Syndromes

Immune Complex Formation
Hepatitis B–associated polyarteritis nodosa
Henoch-Schönlein purpura
Essential mixed cryoglobulinemia
Production of Antineutrophil Cytoplasmic Antibodies
Wegener's granulomatosis
Microscopic polyangiitis
Churg-Strauss syndrome
Pathogenic T Lymphocyte Responses and Granuloma Formation
Giant cell (temporal) arteritis
Takayasu's arteritis
Wegener's granulomatosis
Churg-Strauss syndrome

ROUTINE TESTS

Patients whose history and physical examination findings suggest idiopathic vasculitis often have a confusing array of multisystem complaints that have been occurring for some time. First-order tests include the following: cultures for infectious agents (particularly if the patient has fever), complete blood cell count (CBC) with differential, markers of inflammation such as the erythrocyte sedimentation rate (ESR) or C-reactive protein (CRP), urinalysis, blood chemistry panel, and tests for specific organ function, such as the liver.

SPECIAL TESTS

Special tests help to differentiate idiopathic vasculitis from alternatives in the working differential diagnosis. Relevant laboratory tests would include those used to identify the circulating autoantibodies listed in Table 52-5 along with immune complexes. Directed tissue biopsy for histologic confirmation of vasculitis and/or angiography are considered the definitive tests for idiopathic vasculitis.

TEST PATTERNS IN VASCULITIS

Certain patterns of clinical laboratory test results are useful.

CBC

- Finding leukopenia and/or thrombocytopenia in idiopathic vasculitides is rare and suggests alternative diagnoses such as systemic lupus erythematosus (SLE), neoplasm, bone marrow disorders, lymphomatoid granulomatosis, or hypersplenism (Mandell, 1994).

TABLE 52-5
Antibodies Associated With Vasculitis

Antibody	Disease association	Principal test method(s)
ANCA, usually c-ANCA	Wegener's granulomatosis	IIF, ELISA
ANCA, c-ANCA, or p-ANCA	Microscopic polyangiitis	IIF, ELISA
Anti-C1q antibodies	Hypocomplementemic urticarial vasculitis	C1q binding
Hepatitis B antibodies	Hepatitis B–associated PAN	ELISA
ANA	Systemic lupus erythematosus	IIF, ELISA
Mixed cryoglobulins	Cryoglobulinemic vasculitis	Cryoprecipitation, IEP, IF
SSA (Ro), SSB (La)	Sjögren's syndrome	IIF, ELISA, ID
Rheumatoid factor	Rheumatoid arthritis	LA, ELISA
Hepatitis C antibodies	Hepatitis C–associated PAN	EIA
Anti-DNA	Systemic lupus erythematosus	IIF, ELISA

ANA, Antinuclear antibody; *ANCA,* antineutrophil cytoplasmic autoantibodies; *c-ANCA,* cytoplasmic ANCA; *DNA,* deoxyribonucleic acid; *EIA,* enzyme immunoassay; *ELISA,* enzyme-linked immunosorbent assay; *GBM,* glomerular basement membrane; *ID,* immunodiffusion; *IEP,* immunoelectrophoresis; *IF,* immunofixation; *IIF,* indirect immunofluorescence; *LA,* latex agglutination; *PAN,* polyarteritis nodosa; *p-ANCA,* perinuclear ANCA.

- Anemia with hemoglobin less than 9 g/dL results from conditions other than anemia of chronic disease, such as hemolysis, occult bleeding, or renal disease (Mandell, 1994).
- Peripheral blood eosinophilia occurs in a wide variety of inflammatory disorders. About 15%–20% of patients with polyarteritis nodosa (PAN) or WG may have eosinophilia, but not at the high levels seen in CSS.
- Vasculitis with histologic features of PAN associated with pancytopenia can be seen in patients with hairy cell leukemia (Mandell, 1994). Classic hairy cells may be observed on a peripheral blood smear.

ESR/CRP

- Markers of inflammation such as ESR or CRP, although nonspecific, are typically elevated in idiopathic vasculitides. If the ESR (before antiinflammatory therapy initiation) is not elevated, the diagnosis is probably not giant cell arteritis or WG.

Urinalysis

- First morning urine, both before and after centrifugation, should be carefully examined for protein, hematuria, cells, and casts that accompany glomerulonephritis, which may occur in vasculitides. If renal amyloidosis is in the differential diagnosis, proteinuria is typically seen without cells.

Viral Disease

- When PAN is suspected, serologic tests for liver function, hepatitis B virus (HBV), hepatitis C virus (HCV), and cytomegalovirus should be obtained (Langford, 2003; Golden, 1994; Mandell, 1994). Similarly, serologic tests for HBV and HCV are appropriate when a patient has cryoglobulins, leukocytoclastic vasculitis on cutaneous biopsy, and/or renal disease.
- Numerous vasculitides, including large vessel vasculitis, hypersensitivity vasculitis, a PAN-like syndrome, and primary angiitis of the central nervous system (CNS), have been described in association with human immunodeficiency virus (HIV) (Chetty, 2001).

Connective Tissue Disease

- Testing for antinuclear antibodies (ANAs) and rheumatoid factor (RF) is useful only when connective tissue disease or arthritis is suspected.
- Patients with rheumatoid vasculitis have high-titer RF.

ANTINEUTROPHIL CYTOPLASMIC ANTIBODY

ANCA reacts with neutrophil cytoplasmic antigens (Tervaert, 1991; Jennette, 1993a), which were previously shielded (Seo, 2004b). Identification of ANCA has become an important adjunct in the diagnosis of systemic necrotizing vasculitis (Niles, 1993; Seo, 2004b), although it must be stressed that because ANCA-associated vasculitides are relatively rare, the likelihood of false-positive results is increased if not used in the appropriate clinical context. Use of ANCA and autoantigen titers in monitoring disease activity is controversial.

DETECTION METHODS

Several laboratory methods, including indirect immunofluorescence (IIF), ELISA, radioimmunoassay, Western blotting, dot blotting, flow cytometry, immunoprecipitation, and capture enzyme immunoassay techniques, have been used to detect ANCA (Wieslander, 1991; Roberts, 1992; Seo 2004b). IIF and ELISA are the most common test methods used for this purpose. IIF is the most sensitive widely used method for ANCA detection.

IIF is done using isolated normal human neutrophils as substrate. These neutrophils are cytocentrifuged against multiwell glass slides, fixed with 99% ethanol, and then incubated with dilutions of patients' sera. Neutrophils may also be attached to slides by adherence, smear, or drop techniques (Roberts, 1990, 1992). Slides are stained with a fluorescein-labeled polyspecific antihuman immunoglobulin (Ig) conjugate; polyspecific conjugate is recommended because IgM and IgA c-ANCAs occur (Roberts, 1992). Slides are read on a fluorescence microscope by an experienced laboratory technician. With the use of IIF, three patterns of neutrophil staining are observed: c-ANCA, p-ANCA, and atypical patterns (Seo, 2004b).

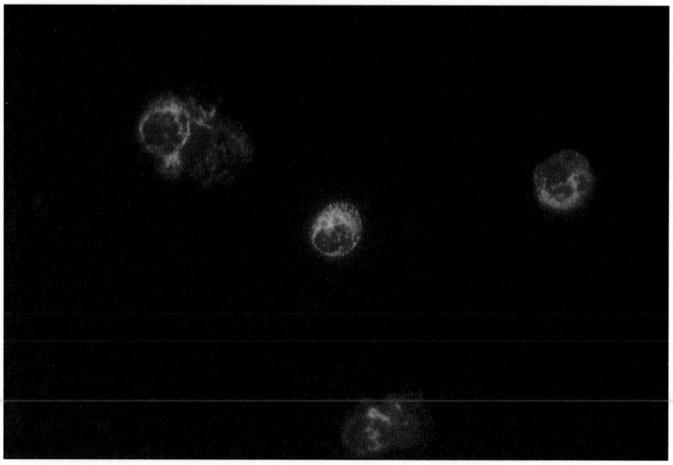

Figure 52-1 Antineutrophil cytoplasmic antibody cytoplasmic pattern (c-ANCA). Most ethanol-fixed neutrophils show finely granular, cytoplasmic fluorescence with central accentuation. There is no nuclear staining (×400).

c-ANCAs are characterized by finely granular staining of neutrophil cytoplasm with central accentuation between nuclear lobes; the nucleus itself does not stain (Fig. 52-1). Criteria useful for differentiating c-ANCA from nonspecific cytoplasmic staining due to other autoantibodies include the following: (1) lack of central accentuation; (2) less than 95% of neutrophils demonstrate cytoplasmic staining; (3) nonneutrophil specificity (e.g., lymphocytes on the slide should not stain when true ANCA is present); and (4) heterogeneous cytoplasmic granularity (Roberts, 1992; Savige, 1998).

p-ANCAs are characterized by staining of the perinuclear area (Fig. 52-2). The staining pattern that defines p-ANCA is caused by redistribution of target antigens from the neutrophil cytoplasm to the positively charged nuclear membrane when ethanol is used to prepare human neutrophils as substrate (Jennette, 1993a; Fig. 52-3). When formalin rather than alcohol is used to fix neutrophils, target antigen is immobilized and the immunofluorescent staining pattern is cytoplasmic (Jennette, 1993a). The use of formalin-fixed neutrophils to detect ANCA in routine diagnostic work remains controversial (Chowdhury, 1999). Nuclear staining mimicking ANAs may occur when this autoantibody is present in high titers (Niles, 1993). Distinguishing p-ANCA from atypical patterns is difficult (Seo, 2004b).

Atypical ANCA, which sometimes is referred to as X-ANCA, combines features of both c-ANCA and p-ANCA. Faint diffuse cytoplasmic staining typically occurs with strong linear perinuclear staining. This pattern is similar on methanol- or ethanol-fixed slides but can appear cytoplasmic or abolished altogether on formalin-fixed neutrophils (Beauvillain, 2008).

ANTIGENIC SPECIFICITY

The antigenic specificity of c-ANCA has been identified as a 29-kDa neutral serine protease, PR3, located within azurophilic granules of neutrophils and peroxidase-positive lysosomes of monocytes (Roberts, 1992; Niles, 1993; Seo 2004b). It has been implicated in the destruction of bacteria within phagosomes. PR3 is also found on the plasma membrane of resting neutrophils and monocytes in many patients (Seo, 2004b). It has been described as myeloblastin and is involved in differentiation of the HL60 promyelocytic cell line (Beauvillain, 2008). In the primary vasculitides, p-ANCA is usually produced by autoantibodies against MPO (Falk, 1988). MPO is also located within the primary granules of the neutrophil and acts to catalyze the formation of hypochlorite, a potent bactericidal agent (Beauvillain, 2008). Many p-ANCAs and atypical ANCAs are not directed at MPO or PR3, but rather are directed at other neutrophil cytoplasmic enzymes, including bactericidal agents, thereby increasing permeability protein, elastase, lactoferrin, lactoperoxidase, lysozyme, azurocidin, or cathepsin G (Jennette, 1993a; Niles, 1993; Hoffman, 1998b). ANCA patterns should be confirmed with more specific tests for PR3 and MPO, the antibodies most often associated with vasculitis (Savige, 2000; Langford, 2003; Seo, 2004b).

ELISAs for detecting autoantibodies to PR3 (PR3-ANCA) show good correlation with the presence of c-ANCA when experienced observers perform IIF (Roberts, 1992; Niles, 1993). An ELISA for detecting

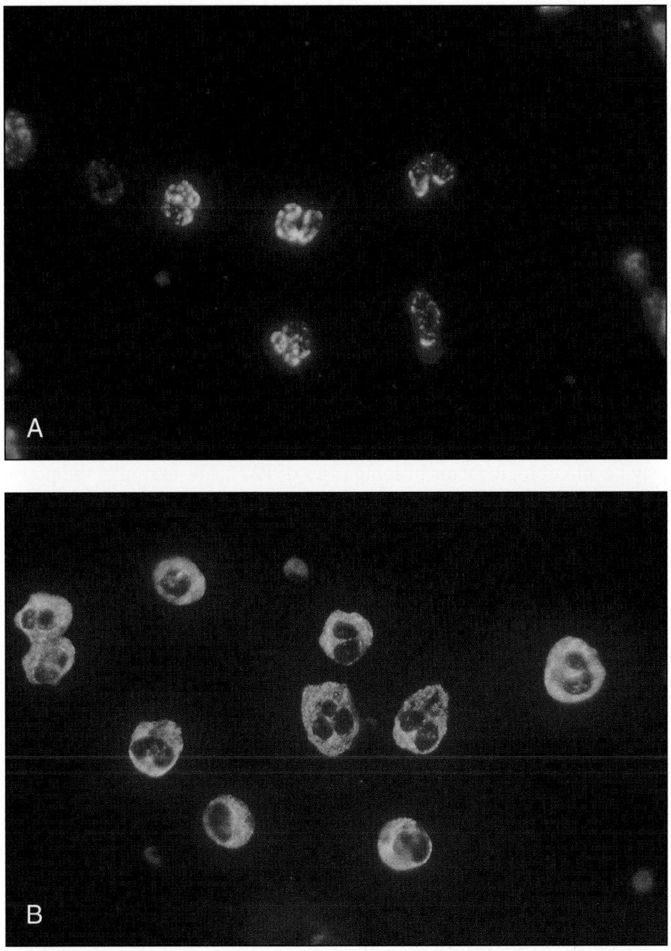

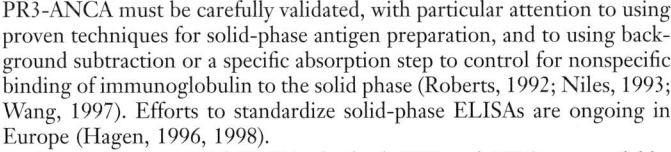

Figure 52-2 Antineutrophil cytoplasmic antibody perinuclear pattern (p-ANCA). Most ethanol-fixed neutrophils show perinuclear and nuclear fluorescence without cytoplasmic staining (**A,** ×400) that is cytoplasmic when formalin rather than alcohol is used to fix neutrophils (**B,** ×400).

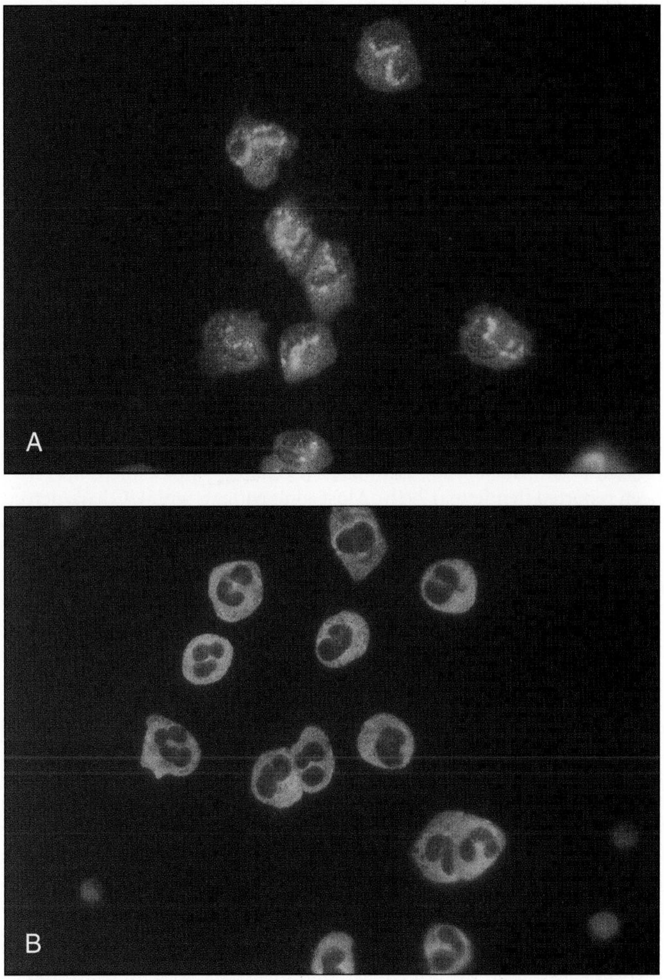

Figure 52-3 Atypical perinuclear antineutrophil cytoplasmic antibody pattern on ethanol-fixed neutrophils shows perinuclear fluorescence (**A,** ×500) but no fluorescence when formalin rather than alcohol is used to fix neutrophils (**B,** ×500).

PR3-ANCA must be carefully validated, with particular attention to using proven techniques for solid-phase antigen preparation, and to using background subtraction or a specific absorption step to control for nonspecific binding of immunoglobulin to the solid phase (Roberts, 1992; Niles, 1993; Wang, 1997). Efforts to standardize solid-phase ELISAs are ongoing in Europe (Hagen, 1996, 1998).

Licensed commercial ELISAs for both PR3 and MPO are available. Most use standard direct antigen coating of polystyrene microwell plates, so that antigen purity is of critical importance in defining analytic sensitivity and specificity (Roberts, 1992; Niles, 1993). Attempts to preserve native antigen conformation are important, in that ANCAs to PR3 are directed against conformational epitopes (Hoffman, 1998b). Loss of these epitopes through denaturation during antigen purification or coating onto the solid phase may partially explain detection of c-ANCA via IIF without a correlative PR3 titer. Capture ELISA utilizes monoclonal antibodies to capture the antigen on the ELISA plate, without obscuring the relevant epitopes. One study has suggested that this method has improved sensitivity for detecting PR3 compared with direct ELISA in WG (Csernok, 2004).

The correlation between p-ANCA and detection of myeloperoxidase on ELISA, however, is not good (Roberts, 1992). Several autoantibodies, including ANA, antineutrophil elastase, and granulocyte-specific ANA (GS-ANA), can produce a p-ANCA pattern on IIF. Therefore, sera that produce nuclear fluorescence on IIF require additional testing to confirm MPO. MPO-ELISA is recommended to confirm anti-MPO specificity because true ANA or GS-ANA and myeloperoxidase-specific ANCA (MPO-ANCA) are known to occur concurrently. IIF using HEp-2 cells (which are typically used for the detection of ANA) does not adequately make this distinction because ANA and MPO-ANCA can occur together, and GS-ANA may be negative on HEp-2 cells (Roberts, 1992; Specks, 1994).

ELISA has limitations; ultimately each laboratory must carefully verify a manufacturer's claims, so the clinician can receive information on performance characteristics. This proves especially important in confusing clinical situations in which there may be discrepancies between clinical presentation and laboratory results, and/or discordant results between IIF and ELISA tests.

In summary, it is recommended that a combination of IIF and ELISA be used to detect ANCA specific for PR3 MPO. By utilizing a combination of the two studies in the workup of suspected vasculitis, the specificity of both PR3 and MPO ELISA is near 99%. The sensitivity for newly diagnosed WG was 73%, and 67% for microscopic polyangiitis (Hagen, 1998). Disease-specific rates of ANCA positivity in the ANCA-associated vasculitides are described in the following sections.

DISEASE ASSOCIATIONS

Vasculitis

Both PR3-ANCA (c-ANCA) and MPO-ANCA (p-ANCA) are associated with WG, PAN, MPA, CSS, idiopathic pauci-immune necrotizing vasculitis and crescentic glomerulonephritis, and polyangiitis overlap syndromes (Niles, 1993; Langford, 2003; Seo, 2004b). PR3-ANCA is identified in about 70%–80% of patients with active WG, whereas MPO-ANCA is identified in less than 10% of such patients (Wiik, 2002; Seo, 2004b). Eighty to ninety percent of patients with active microscopic polyarteritis have PR3-ANCA (30%) or MPO-ANCA (60%) (Wiik, 2002). ANCA is found in about 30% of CSS patients, with an equal distribution of PR3 and MPO antibodies reported. In pauci-immune glomerulonephritis, ANCA is detected in 50%–80% of patients with active disease, typically MPO-ANCA (Langford, 2003; Seo, 2004b). Coexistence of ANCA and anti–glomerular basement membrane (anti-GBM) antibodies has been reported (Bonsib, 1993; Niles, 1993), and this may represent a crossover syndrome between WG and Goodpasture's syndrome, an autoimmune pulmonary-renal syndrome.

Inflammatory Disease of Gastrointestinal and Hepatobiliary Tracts

A variety of serologic tests, including p-ANCA, are emerging that are relevant to the diagnosis and treatment of ulcerative colitis, Crohn's disease (Sandborn, 2004), and disorders of the hepatobiliary system (Jennette, 1993b). p-ANCAs have been reported in about 75%–80% of patients with active ulcerative colitis (UC) or primary sclerosing cholangitis (Klein, 1991; Lo, 1993; Ellerbroek, 1994), about 75% of patients with chronic autoimmune hepatitis, about 30% of patients with primary biliary cirrhosis (Kallenberg, 1992; Mulder, 1993), and about 20% of patients with Crohn's disease (Roberts, 1992; Jennette, 1993b). Target antigen specificities in inflammatory bowel disease have not been fully defined, although autoantibodies against lactoperoxidase, bactericidal permeability-increasing protein (Hoffman, 1998b), lactoferrin (Peen, 1993), or cathepsin G have been reported (Jennette, 1993b). Most adult patients with UC have detectable p-ANCA that is sensitive to deoxyribonuclease, which helps differentiate p-ANCA in inflammatory bowel disease from p-ANCA in other disorders such as autoimmune hepatitis and primary sclerosing cholangitis (Nakamura, 2003). A subgroup of patients with Crohn's disease with p-ANCA may have colon involvement that mimics the clinical presentation of ulcerative colitis.

Other Diseases

ANCAs have been reported in other diseases, including drug-induced lupus erythematosus, SLE, Felty's syndrome and rheumatoid arthritis, Sjögren's syndrome, polymyositis and dermatomyositis, juvenile rheumatoid arthritis, reactive arthritis, relapsing polychondritis, antiphospholipid antibody syndrome, myelodysplastic syndromes, HIV infection, chromomycosis, invasive amebiasis, subacute bacterial endocarditis, cystic fibrosis, and certain neoplasms (Peter, 1993; Jennette, 1993b; Hoffman, 1998b; Choi, 2000). In the connective tissue disorders, ANAs that mimic p-ANCA must be excluded. Many patients treated with hydralazine appear to develop MPO-ANCA (Roberts, 1992). Propylthiouracil-associated vasculitis has been associated with positive ANCA (Hoffman, 1998b; Langford, 2003).

TEST INTERPRETATION

Interpretation of ANCA tests must consider several factors (Hagen, 1998; Hoffman, 1998a; Vassilopoulos, 1999; Seo, 2004a):

- ANCA tests should not be used as screening tests in nonselected patient groups in which the prevalence of vasculitis is low (Langford, 1998a).
- ANCA tests are most valuable when selectively ordered in clinical situations in which some form of ANCA-associated vasculitis is a serious consideration.
- c-ANCA immunofluorescence pattern should be confirmed using PR3 ELISA (Savige, 1999; Langford, 2003; Seo, 2004b).
- Anti-PR3 reactivity is most often seen in active WG or PAN but may be seen in idiopathic crescentic glomerulonephritis or CSS.
- c-ANCA in WG is considered highly sensitive in signaling active systemic disease (Vassilopoulos, 1999).
- Predictive value of an increased c-ANCA titer as a harbinger of WG relapse is controversial, in that not all increases in c-ANCA titer are followed by worsening WG (Specks, 1994; Langford, 2003).
- Rise in ANCA titer is a risk factor for a flare but is insufficient to adjust immunosuppressant medications on this basis alone (Langford, 2003; Seo, 2004).
- p-ANCA pattern on IIF is diagnostically nonspecific.
- p-ANCA–positive sera should be tested in ELISA for MPO-ANCA (Savige, 1999; Seo, 2004b), although several other antigens may be target antigens for p-ANCA.
- MPO-ANCA is most often seen in PAN, idiopathic crescentic glomerulonephritis, or CSS; however, it may be seen in WG.
- Neither a diagnosis of systemic necrotizing vasculitis nor a decision to treat should be based solely on a positive ANCA test result.
- A negative ANCA should not be used to exclude disease.

Ultimately, interpretation of a test for ANCA depends on the experience of individual clinicians who treat vasculitis and the pattern of disease manifested by the patient at hand (Jennette, 1998a, Langford, 2003; Seo, 2004b).

SYNOPSES OF MAJOR IDIOPATHIC VASCULITIC SYNDROMES

POLYARTERITIS NODOSA

Epidemiology

PAN, similar to all idiopathic vasculitides, is an uncommon disease. Estimates of the prevalence of PAN have varied from 4.6 per 1,000,000 in England, to 9.0 per 1,000,000 in Olmstead County, Minnesota (Conn, 1993; Langford, 1995). PAN may occur in either gender and at any age but is more common in men (male/female ratio = 2 : 1) between 40 and 60 years old (Langford, 1995). No racial predilection has been observed (Conn, 1993). Older series of patients with PAN include patients who now would be thought to have microscopic polyangiitis (Langford, 2003). HBV may be an etiologic factor in some cases of PAN. For example, the prevalence of HBV infection in an Alaskan Eskimo population hyperendemic for HBV was 77 per 100,000 (Langford, 1995). With increased knowledge regarding the transmission of HBV, in addition to the development of a preventive vaccine, the frequency of PAN due to HBV has decreased from 30% in the 1970s to 7% (Trepo, 2001).

Clinical Features

The clinical manifestations of classic PAN are highly variable. Patients often present with such nonspecific symptoms as fever, weight loss, and malaise. Hypertension is common and can be an important diagnostic clue. Although PAN can occur in virtually any organ system, symptomatic involvement of skin, joints, peripheral nerves, gastrointestinal (GI) tract, and nonglomerular renal vessels dominates the clinical picture (Conn, 1993; Savage, 2000; Langford, 2001, 2003). Tests indicating abnormal liver function suggest the possibility of concurrent hepatitis B infection (Langford, 1995, 2003; Savage, 2000). Pulmonary involvement in classic PAN is rare and even controversial. Although some investigators think that pulmonary PAN occurs (Lie, 1989), others think that such patients had CSS or WG, in which pulmonary disease is common (Langford, 1995; Fauci, 1998). The course of PAN is characterized by remissions, relapses, and, if untreated, high mortality (Fauci, 1998). Five-year survival with treatment is estimated to be 80%, and less than 10% of patients relapse (Langford, 2003).

Clinical Laboratory Findings

Results of clinical laboratory tests, although diagnostically nonspecific, reflect the systemic inflammatory nature of PAN. Typically, one finds normochromic anemia, neutrophilic leukocytosis, hypoalbuminemia, hypergammaglobulinemia, and a markedly elevated ESR. Measurement of serum creatinine and blood urea nitrogen (BUN) together with urinalysis to check for proteinuria, hematuria, and abnormal sediment is important for evaluating renal function. The positive ANA or RF found in 10%–40% of these patients may be associated with decreased levels of complement components C3 and C4. Serologic tests for HBV, HCV, and HIV should be obtained in all patients with PAN (Conn, 1993; Langford, 1995, 2003); eosinophilia is seen only rarely, and when present in high levels, should lead to consideration of CSS (Fauci, 1998).

Diagnosis

PAN can be difficult to diagnose given its nonspecific presentation, potential for diverse and diffuse organ involvement, and low prevalence. However, once suspected, a diagnosis of PAN is based on angiography and/or the histologic demonstration of PAN on biopsy of tissue from symptomatic site(s), such as muscle, nerve, kidney, and testes. Pathologically, PAN is a focal but pan-mural necrotizing arteritis of small- and medium-sized muscular arteries, preferentially occurring at vessel branch points (Fig. 52-4). Necrotizing mixed cell inflammation with fibrinoid necrosis, either circumferential or segmental in the vessel wall, is the hallmark lesion of active PAN. Microaneurysm or aneurysmal dilatation is also characteristic of acute phase PAN. The inflammatory process heals with fibrosis that may lead to proliferative endarteritis. An admixture of active and/or healing lesions adjacent to normal segments of blood vessel is a characteristic feature of PAN (Langford, 1995).

Angiography may be especially valuable in identifying GI abnormalities, or when a potential biopsy site is unavailable. In particular, angiography should be considered before attempting a closed needle biopsy of

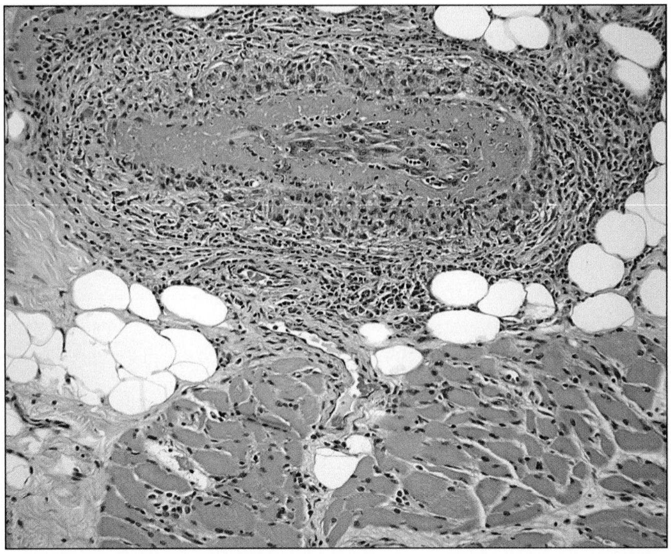

Figure 52-4 Polyarteritis nodosa. Skeletal muscle biopsy reveals circumferential pan-mural necrotizing arteritis of a small muscular artery with mixed cell inflammation, fibrinoid necrosis, and proliferative endarteritis. Eosinophils are a prominent component of the inflammation in this case, but there are no granulomas (hematoxylin and eosin [H&E], ×200).

the liver or kidney in patients suspected to have PAN, because the predilection for aneurysms at these sites increases the risk of severe bleeding (Langford, 1995).

Treatment and Prognosis

Patients with PAN are treated with glucocorticoids. The goal of glucocorticoid therapy is control of the disease without significant complications from the drug itself. Cyclophosphamide may be used for patients with severe PAN (GI, cardiac, and CNS involvement), for those failing corticosteroids alone, and to spare steroid in patients having significant corticosteroid adverse effects (Langford, 1995; Jayne, 2000; Watts, 2000; Langford, 2003). The prognosis for PAN patients has greatly improved with the use of glucocorticoids, extending the 5-year survival rate from 13% to 50%–60%. A majority of deaths occur within the first year, but whether before or after 1 year of disease, mortality most often results from infection as a complication of treatment, or from sequelae of vessel obliteration such as myocardial infarction or stroke (Langford, 1995). PAN associated with hepatitis infection or HIV should be accompanied by antiviral or antiretroviral therapy, respectively (Langford, 2003).

CHURG-STRAUSS SYNDROME

Epidemiology

CSS is thought to be a rare clinical condition, and a prevalence of 3 per one million people has been estimated (Conn, 1993; Langford, 2003). CSS typically begins between ages 15 and 69 years, with 38 years as the median age for onset of vasculitis (Langford, 1995).

Clinical Features

CSS, also called allergic angiitis and granulomatosis, is a systemic necrotizing vasculitis characterized by vascular and extravascular granulomatous inflammation, multiple organ involvement, and associations with allergic rhinitis, severe asthma, fever, and hypereosinophilia (Langford, 1995, 2003; Fauci, 1998). Clinical manifestations of CSS may resemble those of PAN in many respects but differ in that lung disease is typical and renal disease is uncommon, usually less severe in CSS than in PAN (Fauci, 1998).

The clinical course of CSS is often divided into three distinct phases, although in reality, these three phases are not always identifiable, or they may overlap (Langford, 1995, 2003): (1) a prodromal phase characterized by allergic respiratory disease; (2) an eosinophilic phase characterized by peripheral blood and tissue hypereosinophilia; and (3) a vasculitic phase. Cardiac involvement—either transmural eosinophilic carditis or coronary vasculitis—occurs in 25%–62% of CSS patients and is the major cause of death (Langford, 1995, 2003). Involvement with sites such as the heart, CNS, GI tract, and kidney is associated with a poor prognosis (Langford, 2003).

Clinical Laboratory Findings

A hallmark of CSS is striking peripheral blood eosinophilia, which may be seen at any phase of the disease. The peripheral blood eosinophil count reaches 1000 eosinophils per microliter in 80% or more of CSS patients (Conn, 1993); however, eosinophilia may not be found in all patients because of prior steroid treatments for asthma, or the wide and rapid fluctuation in the eosinophil count that can occur in this disorder. Normalization of the eosinophil count in response to steroid treatment is a feature of CSS, distinguishing it from the hypereosinophilic syndrome, in which eosinophilia may be steroid resistant. The degree of eosinophilia may correlate with the activity of vasculitic disease in some patients.

Other laboratory findings in CSS are nonspecific. Anemia, leukocytosis, and increased ESR frequently accompany the vasculitic phase. Serum IgE levels may be elevated. Serum RF may be identified, but the titer is usually low. Serum complement is reported as normal (Conn, 1993). Unlike PAN, no association between CSS and hepatitis B has been described (Langford, 1995).

Diagnosis

Historically, the diagnosis of CSS has been made solely on the basis of histologic demonstration of necrotizing eosinophilic vasculitis, eosinophilic tissue infiltration, and extravascular granuloma. In practice, however, few biopsy specimens contain all these findings. To increase the likelihood of identifying and diagnosing CSS, the emphasis can be shifted from these diagnostic indicators to include clinical features. One study has recommended the following criteria:

1. Asthma (Katzenstein, 2000).
2. Peripheral blood eosinophilia in excess of 1.5×10^3 cells/μL.
3. Systemic vasculitis involving two or more extrapulmonary organs (Conn, 1993).

Definitive diagnosis still requires demonstration of biopsy-proven vasculitis. Open-lung biopsy frequently does not confirm all histologic features of CSS and must be considered before the institution of therapy, if there is concern over possible infection. When clinical symptoms so indicate, useful biopsy specimens are most often obtained from muscle, sural nerve, prostate, and kidney. The differential diagnosis of CSS includes PAN, WG, and the hypereosinophilic syndrome (Langford, 1995, 2003).

Treatment and Prognosis

Corticosteroids are the basis for treatment of CSS. The utility of immunosuppressive therapy with azathioprine or cyclophosphamide is not well studied (Langford, 1995). Early diagnosis of CSS and corticosteroid treatment has led to a 5-year survival rate of 62%. Congestive heart failure and myocardial infarction cause 48% of all deaths in CSS. Cerebral hemorrhage, renal failure, GI perforation or hemorrhage, status asthmaticus, and respiratory failure also cause the demise of CSS patients. All of these features should lead to strong consideration of cytotoxic agent (cyclophosphamide) therapy in conjunction with corticosteroid (Langford, 1997). A short interval between the onset of asthma and the onset of vasculitis is considered an unfavorable prognostic sign.

MICROSCOPIC POLYANGIITIS

Epidemiology

MPA was recently distinguished from PAN, and little is known about its epidemiology.

Clinical Features

MPA occurs in a heterogeneous group of patients who, by definition, have a systemic necrotizing vasculitis of small vessels with few or no immune deposits (Langford, 2003). The sentinel features of MPA are glomerulonephritis, pulmonary hemorrhage, mononeuritis multiplex, and fever, similar to WG (Langford, 2003; Seo, 2004b). Presentation is often acute and severe. Neurologic disease (peripheral or central) manifests in 60%–70%, arthralgia/arthritis in 40%–60%, and cutaneous disease in 50%–65% of patients with MPA (Langford, 2003).

Clinical Laboratory Findings

Chest radiographs reveal a nodule, infiltrates, or alveolar hemorrhage in up to 70% of patients. Proteinuria and hematuria compatible with glomerulonephritis occur in 75%–90% of patients. Electromyography/nerve conduction velocity tests reveal evidence of peripheral neurologic disease in up two thirds of patients. CNS imaging may show evidence of central neurologic disease in 10% of people with MPA (Langford, 2003).

Diagnosis

MPA is diagnosed when tissue biopsy reveals small to medium-sized vessel nongranulomatous necrotizing vasculitis. In the lung, capillaritis is seen in the face of alveolar hemorrhage and the absence of linear immunofluorescence that would be seen in Goodpasture's syndrome. Renal biopsy reveals focal segmental necrotizing glomerulonephritis with few to no immune complexes (Langford, 2003).

Treatment and Prognosis

Patients with life-threatening disease in the lungs, kidneys, or nerves should be treated with cyclophosphamide (2 mg/kg/day) and prednisone (1 mg/kg/day) in a manner similar to the treatment of WG (see later) (Langford, 2003). Less severe disease may be treated with corticosteroids alone. Five-year survival is estimated to be 74%, and relapses occur in one third of patients (Langford, 2003).

WEGENER'S GRANULOMATOSIS

Epidemiology

Detailed annual incidence and prevalence data for WG are not available, but WG is estimated to be less common than PAN. WG occurs in persons of any age, race, or sex, although it affects predominantly Caucasians and has a slight male predominance (Conn, 1993). The mean age at onset is 41 years (Langford, 1995). Males and females are equally affected (Langford, 2003).

Clinical Features

WG is a clinicopathologic syndrome of unknown etiology characterized pathologically by necrotizing granulomatous inflammation of upper and lower respiratory tracts, focal segmental glomerulonephritis, and necrotizing vasculitis predominantly involving medium-sized and small arteries. WG presents in the ear/nose/throat regions with sinusitis, nasal obstruction or ulceration, otitis media, or hearing loss (Fauci, 1998; Lie, 1989). Forty-five percent of WG patients have lung involvement at presentation, and 85% manifest lung disease at some time during the course of their disease. Common lung manifestations include pulmonary infiltrates, pulmonary nodules, hemoptysis, or pleuritis (Fauci, 1998). Although renal disease initially afflicts only about 18% of these patients, 80% demonstrate glomerulonephritis at some time in the course of WG (Fauci, 1998). Other common signs of systemic illness include skin rash, arthralgias, fever, eye manifestations, and weight loss (Fauci, 1998; Lie, 1989). Although patients with WG limited to the respiratory tract without renal involvement have been described (**limited WG**), more than 50% of patients with such limited disease at presentation eventually develop more generalized disease (Langford, 1995).

Clinical Laboratory Findings

Clinical laboratory findings typical of WG include moderate leukocytosis without striking eosinophilia, mild normochromic anemia, and thrombocytosis (Conn, 1993; Langford, 1995). Leukopenia is not seen in the untreated patient and, thus, helps distinguish WG from other disorders. The presence of c-ANCA supports the diagnosis. Circulating immune complexes, measurable by C1q binding, may be found together with normal complement levels and hypergammaglobulinemia; quantities of the IgA subclass are often elevated (Conn, 1993; Langford, 1995). Indicators of glomerular involvement include microscopic or gross hematuria, proteinuria, red blood cell casts, and/or elevated serum creatinine and BUN. More than 50% of these patients are RF-positive, but ANAs are usually absent (Langford, 1995; Fauci, 1998). Serologic tests for anti-GBM autoantibody are negative. Prior to treatment, 80% of these patients have an elevated ESR.

Diagnosis

Although clinical and laboratory findings may be suggestive, a diagnosis of WG should be made only when there is biopsy-proven, histologic confirmation, or when c-ANCA is established in the patient with sinusitis, pulmonary infiltrate or nodule, and glomerulonephritis (Langford, 1998b, 2003). Pulmonary tissue obtained via open-lung biopsy offers the best opportunity to make an accurate diagnosis (Langford, 1995). Transbronchial biopsy does not yield adequate tissue for diagnosis more than 90% of the time. Although head and neck tissue is more directly accessible, characteristic pathologic features are found in fewer than 23% of such biopsy specimens. Diagnostically useful tissue from the head and neck region is best obtained from, in decreasing order of frequency, paranasal sinuses, nasal tissue, and the subglottic region. Glomerular changes in renal biopsy tissue, although suggestive of WG, are rarely diagnostic (Langford, 1995).

Although the morphologic spectrum of WG is broad, the hallmark pathologic lesion in WG is necrotizing granulomatous vasculitis. Affected vessels undergo fibrinoid necrosis with early infiltration by polymorphonuclear leukocytes followed by mononuclear cells. Pulmonary tissue may reveal any combination of necrosis, vasculitis, and granulomatous inflammation; microabscesses and scattered multinucleated giant cells in a highly inflammatory background may also occur (Yi, 2001) (Fig. 52-5). However, biopsy specimens often do not include all of these characteristic features.

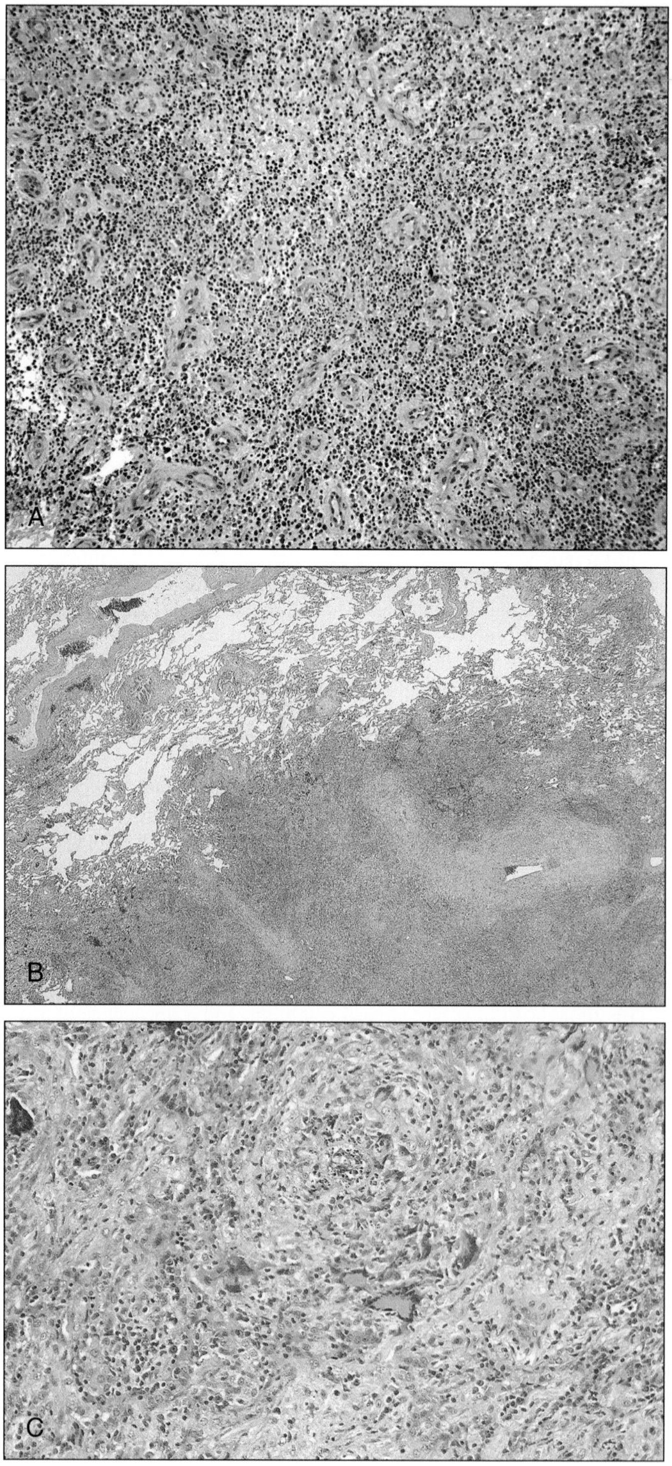

Figure 52-5 Wegener's granulomatosis. Paranasal sinus tissue reveals a florid mixed inflammatory cell infiltrate in a granulation tissue-type background. Inflammatory cells include multinucleated giant cells and neutrophil microabscesses (**A,** hematoxylin and eosin [H&E], ×200). Lung biopsy reveals nodular inflammation with necrosis (**B,** H&E, ×20) and granulomatous vasculitis (**C,** H&E, ×200).

The most common finding found on renal biopsy is segmental necrotizing glomerulonephritis, which is present to varying degrees in 80% of specimens. Renal vasculitis not related to glomeruli is unusual and is present in only 8% of biopsies.

Many disorders can mimic WG, including infectious or noninfectious granulomatous disease, CSS, Goodpasture's syndrome, idiopathic midline granuloma, lymphomatoid granulomatosis, and neoplasms of the upper airway or lungs (Fauci, 1998). Of these, infection is an important consideration because misdiagnosis can have fatal consequences when mistakenly treated with immunosuppressive therapy (Langford, 1995).

Treatment and Prognosis

A regimen of daily oral cyclophosphamide and corticosteroids is the therapy of choice for WG. Using this regimen, the National Institutes of Health reported that marked improvement or partial remission was achieved in 91% of patients, and complete remission in 75%. An overall mortality rate of 20% was noted, 13% of which could be completely or partially attributed to WG. Despite this marked improvement in survival and remission compared with 100% mortality in untreated patients, relapse and morbidity from both disease and treatment were noted. One half of the complete remissions were followed by one or more relapses, which occurred 3 months to 16 years after achieving remission (Langford, 1995; de Groot, 2001). Methotrexate is an alternative to cyclophosphamide in patients who do not have immediately life-threatening diseases (Langford, 1997). Also, methotrexate (20–25 mg/week) or azathioprine (2 mg/kg/day) can be given to maintain remission after 3–6 months of cyclophosphamide to induce remission. This therapy is given for an additional 1–2 years (Langford, 2003). Recently, rituximab, an anti-CD20 monoclonal antibody, has been utilized successfully in small case series of patients with disease limited to the eyes and ears, as well as in systemic disease affecting the lungs and kidneys (Sailler, 2008). Typically, rituximab is reserved for disease that is refractory to conventional treatments, and randomized controlled prospective trials of its use are under way.

During the first year of WG, the extent of renal disease is the factor most closely related to prognosis (Koldingsnes, 2002). Thereafter, lung involvement becomes the most important prognostic indicator, and glomerulonephritis does not appear to significantly affect prognosis.

LYMPHOMATOID GRANULOMATOSIS

Lymphomatoid granulomatosis (LG) is considered to be an unusual lymphoproliferative disorder that may evolve into malignant lymphoma in approximately 50% of patients. LG mainly affects the lungs, where it clinically mimics WG. Characteristic histologic findings include prominent blood vessel infiltration ("angiocentric") and destruction mimicking vasculitis (Fig. 52-6), but cellular morphology is more suggestive of lymphoma or lymphoproliferative disorder (Langford, 1995). No specific clinical laboratory tests are recommended.

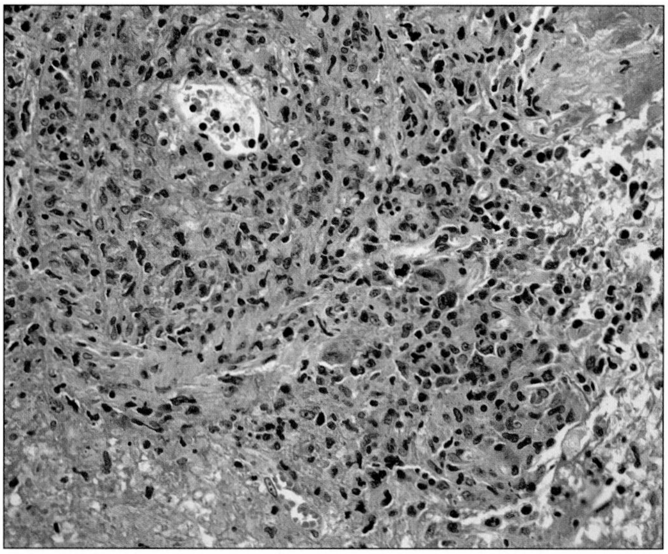

Figure 52-6 Lymphomatoid granulomatosis. Lung biopsy reveals admixtures of large atypical lymphoid cells and histiocytes with prominent blood vessel infiltration (**angiocentric**) and destruction mimicking vasculitis. The atypical lymphoid cells are malignant B cells. (Hematoxylin and eosin [H&E], ×400.) *(Case courtesy Dr. Robert W. Sharpe.)*

HENOCH-SCHÖNLEIN PURPURA

Epidemiology

Henoch-Schönlein purpura (HSP) occurs primarily in children between the ages of 4 and 11 years (Conn, 1993) but also afflicts some adults. HSP presents most commonly in the spring and classically follows an upper respiratory infection (Conn, 1993; Langford, 2003). HSP has a 3 : 2 male predominance (Langford, 1995).

Clinical Features

HSP, sometimes referred to as anaphylactoid purpura, is a systemic small vessel vasculitis classified as a subgroup of hypersensitivity vasculitis. The etiology of HSP is not known. Typical clinical findings in HSP include nonthrombocytopenic palpable purpura, arthralgias, renal disease, and GI tract abnormalities (Langford, 1995; Langford, 2003). Seventy percent of HSP patients manifest GI signs and symptoms that include colicky abdominal pain associated with nausea and vomiting, blood or mucus in the stool, life-threatening GI hemorrhage, and intussusception (Langford, 1995). Associated renal disease is characterized by focal proliferative glomerulonephritis that has variable clinical expression from isolated hematuria with red blood cell casts, to acute renal failure, to rare chronic renal failure (Lie, 1989; Langford, 1995; Fauci, 1998).

Clinical Laboratory Findings

Clinical laboratory studies in HSP are nonspecific and are primarily useful in excluding other disorders and seeking evidence of renal involvement. Leukocytosis and elevated ESR may be seen. Tests of CBC with platelet count and of coagulation are important in the evaluation of cutaneous purpura; in HSP, purpura is not the result of thrombocytopenia. Stool guaiacs should be performed intermittently to look for evidence of occult blood loss. Serum complement levels are usually normal, although an association between HSP and congenital absence of complement component C2 has been reported (Conn, 1993). Urinalysis and serum creatinine measurements should be performed at the onset of illness and twice weekly until systemic signs have ceased (Langford, 1995). Skin biopsy of the purpura reveals leukocytoclastic vasculitis with IgA deposition (Langford, 2003) (Fig. 52-7).

Diagnosis

Difficulty in diagnosing HSP is rare, except when the involvement of other major sites precedes the appearance of palpable purpura. Unlike other systemic necrotizing vasculitides, diagnosis is clinical, with laboratory studies used to rule out other disorders. Renal biopsy, which demonstrates proliferative glomerulonephritis, typically is not necessary for diagnosis, although it is used to assess disease severity and to estimate prognosis. Disorders to be considered in the differential diagnosis of HSP include any that cause acute abdomen, nephritis, or purpura (Langford, 1995).

Treatment and Prognosis

Treatment of HSP is supportive, and no specific treatment of proven benefit is available for HSP nephritis. Although glucocorticoids may be useful for decreasing edema, joint pain, and abdominal discomfort, sustained glucocorticoid therapy is not helpful because it does not decrease the risk of recurrent disease or improve renal prognosis (Langford, 1995). Nonsalicylate pain relievers for analgesia may soothe joint and soft tissue discomfort. Therapy for adults is similar to that for children, although hypertension in adults must be carefully controlled (Langford, 1995).

Prognosis for this generally self-limited disease, lasting from 6 to 16 weeks, is good (Conn, 1993). The mortality rate is about 1%–3% (Langford, 1995), and renal disease is the major cause of death (Langford, 1995). Those who have an acute nephritic presentation, particularly with nephrotic syndrome, have the worst outcome, with less than 50% returning to normal renal function and urinalyses in 2 years. The percentage of glomeruli with crescents may also be a useful prognostic indicator; however, it is important to realize that the course of HSP can be extremely variable. Patients who have severe clinical or histologic abnormalities may recover fully, and those with mild changes can progress to renal insufficiency. The disease recurs in 25%–40% of patients and largely consists of skin manifestations. Deterioration or improvement may be most notable during the first 2–3 years after resolution of the acute episode, although

PART 6

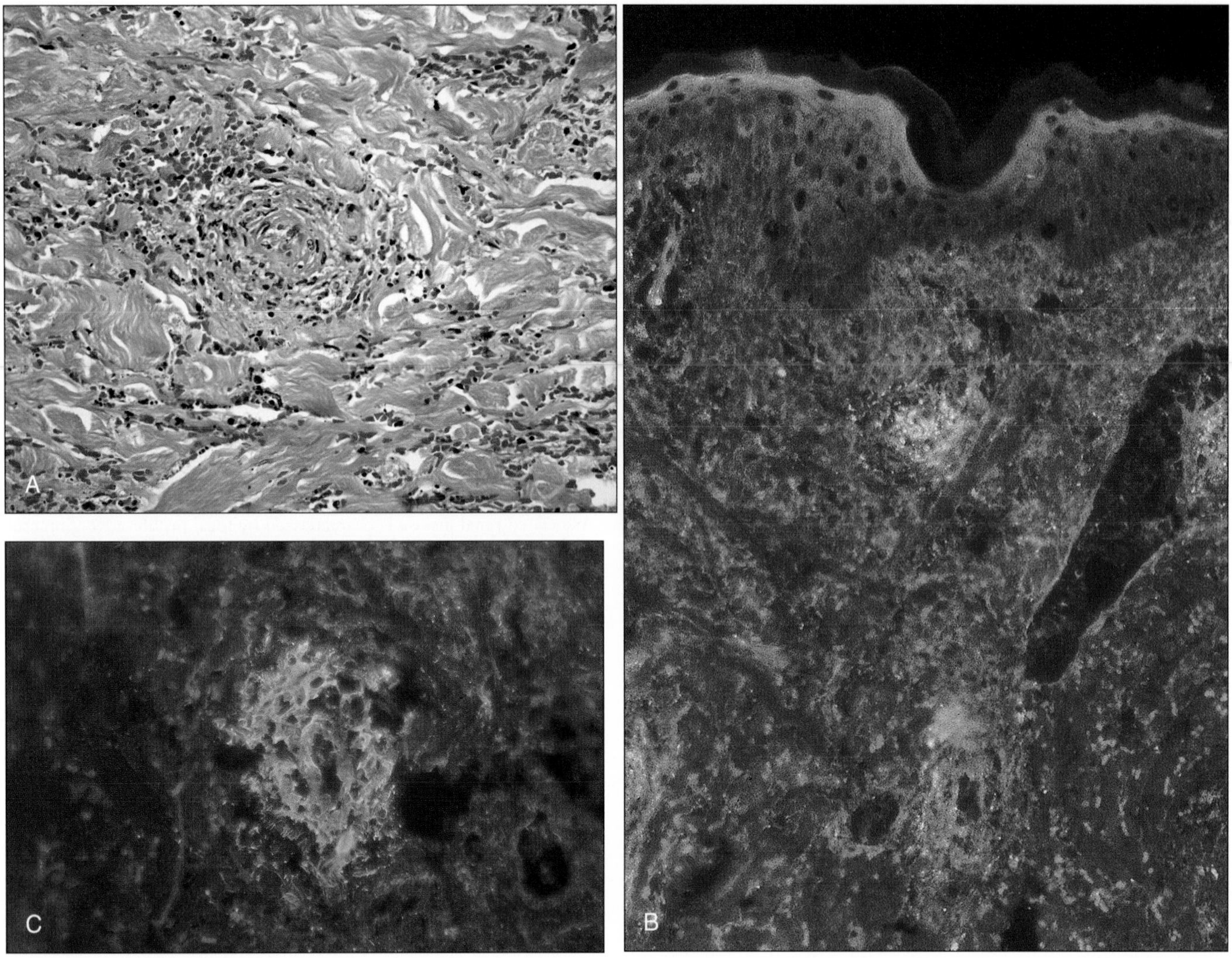

Figure 52-7 Henoch-Schönlein purpura. Skin biopsy reveals leukocytoclastic vasculitis with fibrinoid necrosis of small blood vessels in the superficial dermis associated with abundant perivascular nuclear leukocytoclastic debris (**A,** Hematoxylin and eosin [H&E], ×400). Direct immunofluorescence of the skin biopsy reveals granular vascular immunoglobulin (Ig)A immunofluorescence (**B,** ×200) and corresponding vascular and perivascular fibrinogen immunofluorescence (**C,** ×500).

significant changes in outcome have been seen later than that. Regular follow-up with measurements of blood pressure and urinalysis is extremely important for at least the first 5 years following an episode of HSP (Langford, 1995, 2003).

GIANT CELL (TEMPORAL) ARTERITIS

Epidemiology

Giant cell (GC) arteritis is a relatively common vasculitic disorder. Epidemiologic studies have shown increased incidence with age; one study that included biopsy-proven GC arteritis demonstrated an annual incidence rate of 23.3 per 100,000 persons older than 50 years (Conn, 1993). Nearly all cases of GC arteritis begin after age 50; women are involved twice as often as men (Langford, 2003).

Clinical Features

GC arteritis is a systemic disease characterized by granulomatous vascular inflammation involving medium-sized to large arteries. Although arteries in multiple sites can be affected, GC arteritis classically involves the temporal artery and/or other branches of the carotid artery (Fauci, 1998). Clinical manifestations include fever, headache, diplopia, and jaw claudication in patients older than 50 years of age. Ischemic optic neuritis can lead to sudden blindness, particularly in untreated patients (Fauci, 1998). GC arteritis is closely associated with polymyalgia rheumatica, which is characterized by stiffness and pain in the neck, shoulders, lower back, hips, and thighs that is worse in the morning and better with activity of the day (Fauci, 1998; Langford, 2003). Findings on physician examination can include temporal artery tenderness, nodularity, and absent pulsations (Langford, 2003).

Clinical Laboratory Findings

Characteristic laboratory findings include an elevated ESR and a normochromic anemia. Serum alkaline phosphatase is commonly elevated. Hypergammaglobulinemia and increased levels of complement and immune complexes have been reported (Fauci, 1998).

Diagnosis

Diagnosis is based on identifying typical clinical manifestations and a high ESR in an elderly patient who may or may not also have symptoms of polymyalgia rheumatica (Fauci, 1998). Diagnosis is confirmed by biopsy of the temporal artery showing pan-mural mononuclear cell infiltration, which can be granulomatous with giant cells and typically reveals disruption of the internal elastic lamina (Langford, 2003) (Fig. 52-8).

Treatment and Prognosis

GC arteritis is treated with glucocorticoids, and the clinical response to this therapy is usually dramatic. Prognosis is good, in that most patients achieve and maintain complete remission after glucocorticoid therapy (Fauci, 1998). Unfortunately, recovery of eyesight following blindness secondary to GC arteritis is rare, even with rapid and high-dose corticosteroid therapy (Hayreh, 2002). Treatment is begun with 60 mg of prednisone daily, with taper starting in 2–4 weeks and patients often requiring 2 years of corticosteroid therapy (Langford, 2003).

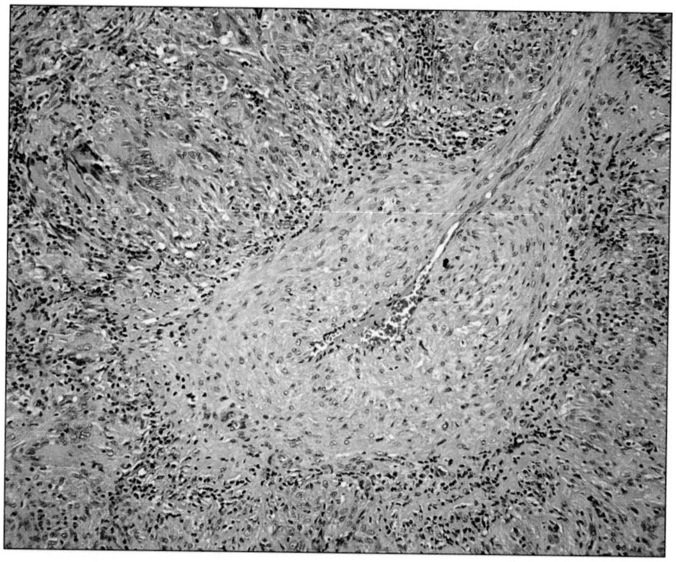

Figure 52-8 Giant cell (temporal) arteritis. Temporal artery biopsy reveals panmural mononuclear cell infiltration with prominent giant cells associated with disruption of the internal elastic lamina (hematoxylin and eosin [H&E], ×200).

TAKAYASU'S ARTERITIS

Epidemiology

Similar to many of the idiopathic vasculitides, Takayasu's arteritis is uncommon, and the epidemiology of the disease is not accurately known. This disorder is most prevalent in adolescent and young females between the ages of 10 and 30 years; in fact, 80%–90% of cases occur in females. Although more common in Japan, this disease has no proven racial or geographic restrictions (Conn, 1993; Fauci, 1998).

Clinical Features

Takayasu's arteritis is a granulomatous vasculitis of medium-sized to large elastic arteries that causes vascular stenosis or occlusion or aneurysm; there is a strong predilection for the aortic arch and its large branches, including pulmonary arteries (Langford, 1995; Fauci, 1998; Johnston, 2002; Langford, 2003; Seo 2004a). This disorder is sometimes called the aortic arch syndrome or pulseless disease. Patients present with acute systemic symptoms, including fever, malaise, night sweats, and weight loss. Ischemia in organs receiving their blood supply through the affected vessel(s) causes organ-specific symptoms and signs (Smetana, 2002). In the chronic obliterative phase, arterial pulses are decreased or absent in involved arteries (Langford, 1995), most commonly in the subclavian artery (Fauci, 1998). Vascular bruits and hypertension are common (Langford, 1995). Other findings include aortic regurgitation, cardiomegaly secondary to aortic or pulmonary hypertension, and stroke (Fauci, 1998). Takayasu's arteritis may progress slowly, may stabilize, or may rapidly cause death (Fauci, 1998).

Clinical Laboratory Findings

Laboratory studies of Takayasu's arteritis define a systemic inflammatory disorder (Langford, 1995). The ESR is elevated in 75%–100% of patients with active disease and tends to return to normal over time. ESR is thought to be a reliable index of inflammatory activity and has been used as a tool to monitor the effectiveness of therapy. Resolution of the disease, both symptomatically and angiographically, has been found to correlate with decline of the ESR, although one surgical series observed that 44% of patients thought to be quiet clinically were not upon arterial biopsy (Langford, 2003).

Hematologic studies often show mild to moderate normochromic anemia and/or mild leukocytosis. RF and ANA are usually negative. Hypergammaglobulinemia, hyperfibrinogenemia, and hypoalbuminemia may occur (Conn, 1993). Circulating immune complexes may be present in up to 50% of these patients but do not appear to correlate with disease activity.

Diagnosis

Takayasu's arteritis is diagnosed by correlating data from history, physical examination, and angiography. The disease should be considered as a diagnostic possibility in any young female who lacks or has a markedly decreased peripheral pulse rate, or who has blood pressure discrepancies and/or arterial bruits (Fauci, 1998). Characteristic angiographic findings help confirm the clinical diagnosis. Biopsy for tissue confirmation of diagnosis is seldom required or done (Fauci, 1998; Langford, 2003). The predilection of this syndrome for young females is an important feature that often separates it from other diagnostic considerations, particularly GC arteritis (Langford, 1995).

Treatment and Prognosis

In patients with active disease, corticosteroid therapy is the initial treatment of choice. If active disease persists despite corticosteroids, cyclophosphamide or methotrexate may be administered. Vasodilators, anticoagulants, and nonsteroidal antiinflammatory agents are used for symptomatic relief. Surgical intervention may be necessary for symptomatic vascular stenosis or occlusion (Langford, 1995; Hoffman, 2003).

The clinical course of Takayasu's arteritis is variable. Although spontaneous remissions occur, most patients require treatment. Prognosis appears to be related to the presence and severity of complications. Major complications include Takayasu's retinopathy, secondary hypertension, aortic valve insufficiency, and aortic/arterial aneurysm (Langford, 1995). Overall survival declines from 72%–97% at 5 years to 59% at 10 years, as the number and/or severity of these complications increases (Langford, 1995; Nordborg, 2003). Disease-related deaths usually occur from vascular complications, such as congestive heart failure, stroke, myocardial infarction, and aneurysm rupture (Langford, 1995).

PRIMARY ANGIITIS OF THE CENTRAL NERVOUS SYSTEM

Epidemiology

Primary angiitis of the central nervous system (PACNS) is a rare condition in which difficulty in making a definitive diagnosis hinders epidemiologic studies. PACNS is slightly more common in males than in females (4:3) and begins at a mean age of 43 years (Langford, 1995).

Clinical Features

Patients with PACNS present with headaches, focal neurologic deficits, altered mental status, paraparesis, quadriparesis, cranial neuropathies, seizures, and ataxia (Calabrese, 1997; Fauci, 1998). Initial symptoms are more generalized, and focal symptoms and signs generally develop later in the course of the disease (Langford, 1995). Fifteen percent of cases have spinal cord involvement (Calabrese, 1997). The course may be rapidly progressive or may wax and wane over a long time. Systemic symptoms are rare.

Clinical Laboratory Findings

Laboratory studies are not useful in making a diagnosis of PACNS, but they do play an important role in excluding other disease processes. The ESR is elevated in most, but not all, of these patients. Anemia has been seen in only 17% of them, and other hematologic parameters are usually normal. RF, ANA, and ANCA are typically absent. However, the cerebrospinal fluid (CSF) is usually abnormal with findings that include increased opening pressure, elevated protein, and lymphocytic pleocytosis. Because the CSF can also be completely normal, such testing does not always rule out the possibility of vasculitis (Langford, 1995).

Diagnosis

The diagnosis of PACNS remains one of exclusion. Proposed diagnostic criteria have included CNS dysfunction that is not explained by clinical, laboratory, or neurologic investigation; documentation by angiogram and/or biopsy of an arteritis within the CNS; and no evidence of a systemic vasculitis or other condition to which the angiographic or pathologic features could be secondary.

Given the difficulty with certainty regarding the last criterion and the poor discriminatory power of angiography regarding inflammatory versus noninflammatory vascular disease (Calabrese, 1997), CNS biopsies are underutilized. The role of brain biopsy in the diagnosis of PACNS remains controversial, although some advocate that such biopsy is essential to make a definitive diagnosis (Calabrese, 1997). Precluding the widespread application of brain biopsy has been not only its invasive nature but also the inconsistency of demonstrating histologic vasculitis, given the patchy nature of the process. Biopsy yield may be increased by obtaining samples of both parenchyma and leptomeningeal vessels. Given the difficulty in obtaining diagnostic certainty for this disease, biopsy is equally as important to rule out other possible etiologies. Histologically, segmental mixed inflammation with necrosis involves predominantly small and medium-sized cranial arteries. Granulomatous inflammation may be present. Thrombosis is often noted, and extracranial arteries are rarely involved (Langford, 1995; Rhodes, 1995). Therefore, differential diagnoses must be carefully considered in all cases and used in deciding appropriate tests to support a diagnosis of PACNS and to exclude other processes. The combination of normal magnetic resonance imaging and CSF has strong negative predictive value and excludes consideration of PACNS in most clinical situations (Calabrese, 1997).

Treatment and Prognosis

Aggressive treatment is indicated for patients in whom other disorders are ruled out, the diagnosis of PACNS is supported, and progressive neurologic difficulties are evident (Calabrese, 1997). Combination therapy using corticosteroids and daily cyclophosphamide is advocated; however, the prognosis of PACNS is poor, with 60%–70% of patients dying from their disease within 1 year of diagnosis (Langford, 1995).

KAWASAKI DISEASE

Kawasaki disease, or mucocutaneous lymph node syndrome, is a form of vasculitis involving small and medium-sized arteries (Fig. 52-9). This disease typically occurs in children who present with cervical lymphadenitis and alterations in skin and mucous membranes. Kawasaki disease is usually self-limited, but arteritis causes coronary aneurysms in 25% of patients. Death occurs in up to 3% of patients, usually from coronary vasculitis. Anti–endothelial cell autoantibodies have been demonstrated in patients with Kawasaki disease (Fauci, 1998).

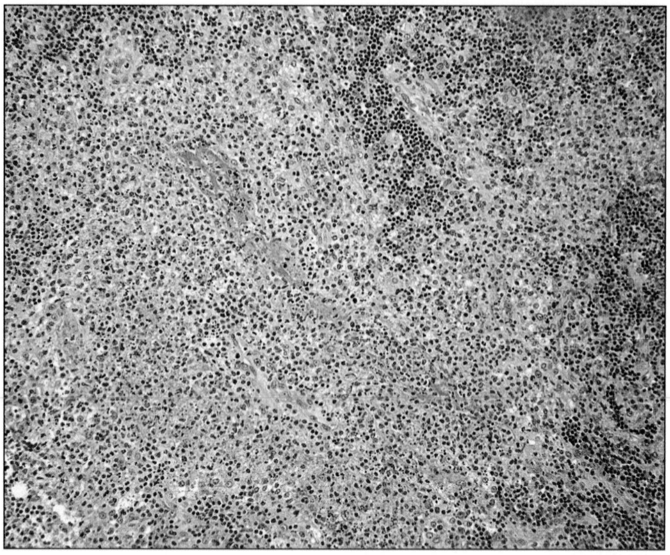

Figure 52-9 Kawasaki disease. Lymph node biopsy reveals necrotizing vasculitis with fibrin thrombi and mixed inflammation including neutrophils (hematoxylin and eosin [H&E], ×200). *(Case courtesy Dr. Robert W. Sharpe.)*

SUMMARY

The diagnosis of idiopathic systemic necrotizing vasculitides requires a high degree of suspicion and can be difficult because of the large number of differential diagnostic considerations. No pathognomonic clinical laboratory tests are available for patients with systemic necrotizing vasculitides, but such tests are useful for defining the extent and patterns of organ involvement. ANCA and their associations with systemic necrotizing vasculitis, particularly the association of c-ANCA with WG, have become an important serologic test used in the evaluation of these patients. However, clinicians and laboratorians using this test must thoroughly understand the operating characteristics, including limitations, of the test as performed in their laboratory. Tissue biopsy of symptomatic site(s) with histologic confirmation of necrotizing vasculitis remains the most important laboratory procedure for diagnosis of systemic necrotizing vasculitides.

SELECTED REFERENCES

Jennette JC, Falk RJ, Andrassy K, et al. Nomenclature of systemic vasculitides: proposal of an international consensus conference. Arthritis Rheum 1994;37: 187–92.

Outlines important conclusions and proposals made at the Chapel Hill Consensus Conference on the Nomenclature of Systemic Vasculitis.

Johnston SL, Lock RJ, Gompels MM. Takayasu arteritis: a review. J Clin Pathol 2002;55:481–6.

Excellent review of the history, clinical features, differential diagnoses, classification, immunology, and treatments of this rare but well-known disorder.

Langford CA. Vasculitis. J Allergy Clin Immunol 2003;111:S602–12.

Excellent current review of vasculitis.

Sandborn WJ. Serologic markers in inflammatory bowel disease: state of the art. Rev Gastroenterol Disord 2004;4:167–74.

State of the art review of emerging serologic tests relevant to ulcerative colitis and Crohn's disease.

Savige J, Davies D, Falk RJ, Jennette JC, Wiik A. Antineutrophil cytoplasmic antibodies and associated diseases: a review of the clinical and laboratory features. Kidney Int 2000;57:846–62.

Discusses a number of advances related to ANCA testing, diagnostic criteria for the ANCA-associated vasculitides, and the complications associated with treatment.

Seo P, Stone JH. The antineutrophil cytoplasmic antibody-associated vasculitides. Am J Med 2004b; 117:39–50.

Current review of the ANCA-associated vasculitides that discusses the role of ANCA assays in diagnosis and treatment, and outlines an approach to the evaluation and management of these diseases.

REFERENCES

Access the complete reference list online at http://www.expertconsult.com

CHAPTER 53

ORGAN-SPECIFIC AUTOIMMUNE DISEASES

David J. Bylund, Robert M. Nakamura[†]

PART 6

KEY POINTS

- The dominant clinical feature of organ-specific autoimmune disease is chronic inflammation, generally localized in a single organ specific for each individual disease.
- The etiology of virtually all organ-specific autoimmune diseases remains elusive.
- Direct immunofluorescence is essential for resolving the microscopic differential diagnosis of acantholytic and subepidermal bullous disorders.
- The presence of circulating autoantibodies at significant titers is often useful in establishing the etiology of autoimmune liver disorders.
- Antimitochondrial antibodies (AMAs) are the most specific and sensitive diagnostic markers for primary biliary cirrhosis (PBC). As a general guideline, an AMA titer greater than or equal to 1:160 is highly predictive of PBC.
- The prevalence of gluten-sensitive enteropathy/celiac sprue in the U.S. population is considered much greater than previous estimates.

Continued

[†]Deceased

- In gluten-sensitive enteropathy/celiac sprue, immunoglobulin A antiendomysial autoantibodies detect tissue transglutaminase (tTG), the primary autoantigen in gluten-sensitive enteropathy (GSE). Enzyme-linked immunosorbent assays are now available for the detection of anti-tTG. Their identification is considered diagnostically sensitive and specific for GSE alone or GSE associated with dermatitis herpetiformis.
- For specificity reasons, the use of assays to detect deoxyribonuclease-sensitive perinuclear antineutrophil cytoplasmic antibodies and antibodies to *Saccharomyces cerevisiae* should be limited to patients with colitis and should not be applied to the general population.
- Technical advances in enzyme-linked immunosorbent assays have made this technology available in most clinical laboratories, so that many assays for organ-specific autoantibodies (e.g., thyroid, kidney, pancreatic islet cells, peripheral and central nervous system) are more widely available when indirect immunofluorescence microscopy is not feasible.

Definition of Autoimmunity vs. Autoimmune Disease

Normally, each individual can distinguish **self** from **nonself** and can respond to invading foreign molecules without producing adverse reactions against self or host antigens (Nakamura, 2002). However, there are many pathways and alterations of self-recognition control mechanisms that can initiate an autoimmune response. **Autoimmunity** has been broadly defined as the failure of an organism to recognize its own healthy tissue as self. This autoimmune response includes any immune response to the host's own tissue, whether humoral (e.g., circulating autoantibodies) or cellular (e.g., delayed hypersensitivity). Autoimmunity can also be defined by the presence of autoantibodies and/or T cells that react against self antigens. Autoimmunity thus can explain "normal" regulatory physiologic mechanisms such as aging, physiologic clearance of dead cells and their components, and response to microbial infections. However, autoimmunity can also induce immunologic injury to the host and is the primary cause of diseases such as autoimmune thyroiditis and systemic lupus erythematosus (SLE). The term **autoimmune disease** is usually assigned to those conditions in which an autoimmune mechanism or injury has contributed to the pathogenesis of the disease.

Classification of Autoimmune Diseases

Human autoimmune diseases can be classified in several ways. They can be divided into the following categories:

1. Organ-specific autoimmune diseases, which include thyroid, adrenals, stomach and pancreas, etc.
2. Non–organ specific or systemic autoimmune diseases, such as SLE and rheumatoid arthritis.

This chapter will discuss various organ-specific autoimmune diseases in which the immune response is primarily against antigens localized to particular organs. Examples of organ-specific autoimmune diseases include insulin-dependent diabetes mellitus (IDDM), Hashimoto's thyroiditis, pernicious anemia with chronic atrophic gastritis, primary adrenal gland atrophy (Addison's disease), pemphigoid skin disorders, Grave's disease, and so forth.

Laboratory Tests for Evaluating Autoimmune Diseases

The patient history and the results of common clinical laboratory tests will help the physician select additional tests. Test selection is critical in determining the positive predictive value of autoantibody tests.

A direct approach in the diagnosis and evaluation of autoimmune disease is tissue biopsy of the affected organ for histologic and immunohistochemical and immunofluoresecent study examinations. This is most often used in autoimmune diseases that involve the kidney or skin. One can evaluate the tissue injury and determine the immunopathologic mechanism of injury, for example, by immunofluorescent localization of immunoglobulin and complement components in the basement membrane of the skin, glomerular basement membrane, or blood vessels.

TABLE 53-1
Methods for Autoantibody Detection

Methods	Use
Immunofluorescence	Sensitive assay for screening
Enzyme immunoassay	Sensitive assay for screening
Chemiluminescence	Sensitive assay for screening
Double immunodiffusion	Requires precipitin reaction, high specificity but low sensitivity
Counterimmunoelectrophoresis	Increased sensitivity and speed compared with immunodiffusion
Particle agglutination	More sensitive than immunodiffusion
Immunoblotting	Very sensitive, allows detection of antibodies to soluble and insoluble antigens

Antibody reactions may be (1) primary—the antigen and the antibody react by combining with each other (i.e., immunoenzymatic or immunofluorescence assays); (2) secondary—the antigen and the antibody initiate a secondary reaction, such as precipitation, agglutination, or complement fixation; and (3) tertiary—the antigen–antibody reaction initiates a biochemical reaction, such as IgE- and antigen-mediated histamine release from mast cells seen with skin lesions.

Primary, secondary, and tertiary antibody reactions vary in their relative sensitivities. The agar gel diffusion test may be considered a precipitin test with a sensitivity of 1. The electroimmunodiffusion (ED) method may increase the sensitivity 10 times, and an enzyme immunoassay or radioimmunoassay (RIA) may increase the sensitivity 10,000 times compared with the immunodiffusion assay. With the new, rapid, ultrasensitive nonisotopic immunoassays, analytes can be detected in pico(10^{-12})mole and subatto(10^{-18})mole concentrations.

The words zepto(10^{-21})mole and yocto(10^{-24})mole have been introduced into the vocabulary of clinical laboratorians for describing small numbers of molecules. Beginning with a mole consisting of roughly 6.022×10^{23} molecules, a zeptomole would correspond to about 600 molecules, and a yoctomole to only 0.6 or roughly 1 molecule.

The most commonly ordered clinical laboratory tests for autoimmune diseases involve detection of circulating antibodies. Immunofluorescent, enzyme-labeled, chemiluminescence antibody tests and RIA methods use primary antigen–antibody binding reactions. These primary direct antibody–antigen binding tests have high sensitivity and are preferred for use in the detection of circulating and tissue-bound antibodies and antigens (Table 53-1).

Tests that involve secondary antigen–antibody preparations such as complement fixation, agglutination, and precipitation in agar gel are not as sensitive as immunofluorescent enzyme tests, RIA, or chemiluminescence tests, but such secondary tests have higher specificity and may be more suitable for the identification of certain autoantibodies.

Cell-mediated studies may be useful laboratory tests in special circumstances. In summary, each clinical laboratory should also state on the report the immunologic method used as a screening tool to rule out the presence of a specific autoantibody.

Interpretation of Serum Autoantibody Levels in Autoimmune Diseases

Test results must be interpreted in the context of the patient's medical history and clinical disease state and with a clear understanding of the technical limitations of the test systems employed.

In general, the level of autoantibody is high in patients with autoimmune disorders and low in apparently healthy patients. A very high titer of autoantibody is significant, although a low or absent titer of autoantibody does not rule out the possibility of an autoimmune disorder. For example, at the height of severe thyroiditis, the gland may act as an immunoabsorbent and may remove circulating antibody. In addition, thyroglobulin may be released into the circulation during the acute stage and may neutralize circulating autoantibody. Therefore, the level or titer of a given antibody must be interpreted in relation to the stage or treatment of a particular disease. In contrast, serum antibody levels in pemphigus correlate with the severity and course of the disease. Also, in idiopathic inflammatory bowel disease, the higher titers of antibodies to common microbial antigens correlate with the severity of the disease, such as Crohn's disease (Dubinsky, 2008).

The incidence of certain autoantibodies increases with age. In patients older than 60 years, 50% demonstrated low titers of one or more autoantibodies. Antinuclear, anti-parietal cell, and antithyroid antibodies are age or sex dependent, with an increasing incidence in women and older people (Hooper, 1972; Whittingham, 1972; Hawkins, 1979). On the other hand, the incidence of smooth muscle antibody and rheumatoid factor does not correlate with age or sex and was similar in men and women. A study in Australia tested a normal population for the presence of 13 autoantibodies. Of 1830 individuals tested, 22% displayed one or more autoantibodies. Several of these antibodies appeared to be persistent, lasting 6 years or longer. The parietal cell antibody persisted in 75.3% of individuals. Antinuclear, thyroid microsomal, and smooth muscle antibodies also were persistent.

Recent Advances in Diagnostic Technologies for the Evaluation of Autoimmune Diseases

Within the last several years, advances in proteomic, microarray technology have allowed the simultaneous measurement of a number of autoantibodies within the same biological sample, called **multiplexing.** These multiplexing technologies, which use different addressable microbeads or non–bar-coded particles, have opened up new horizons in the diagnosis of autoimmune diseases. The new methods of multiplexing with arrays will allow testing of individual autoantibody profiles. The various autoantibody profiles will (1) improve understanding of the pathophysiology of specific diseases; (2) allow early diagnosis and prognostic information with predictive values of autoantibodies; and (3) allow more efficient implementation of specific therapies for treatment and prevention of autoimmune diseases (Tozzoli, 2008).

Several proteomic platforms have emerged that are capable of analyzing a large panel of known analytes (Balboni, 2006). At present, the main analytes that can be systematically studied in autoimmunity and autoimmune diseases include autoantibodies, cytokines, chemokines, components of signaling pathways, and cell surface receptors.

Much progress has been made on the multiplex antinuclear antibody (ANA) test profiles. Strong concordance has been noted between the multiplex ANA and conventional methods of assay for ANA (Xu, 2007).

One problem is that multiplex assays with limited numbers of autoantigens can miss some clinically important autoantibodies, which has led to a loss of confidence in them as screening tests for ANA by many physicians. This deficiency was addressed by the American College of Rheumatology (2009) with the position statement Methodology of Testing for Antinuclear Antibodies in which they recommend:

- IFA should remain the gold standard for ANA testing.
- Laboratories using bead-based multiplex or other solid phase assays for ANAs must provide data on that assay compared with IFA.
- In-house assays for ANA and other autoantibodies should be standardized according to national/international standards.
- When reporting results of ANA testing, the method of detection should be specified.

Simultaneously, considerable advances have been made in **biomedical informatics,** which will help in analysis of various multiarrays and autoantibody profiles (Baboni, 2006).

Autoantibodies as Predictors of Diseases

Several studies in the past have shown that autoimmune diseases are preceded by a long preclinical phase, and that many autoantibodies can be detected in the serum of asymptomatic patients years before the clinical manifestation becomes evident. Examples are IDDM and autoimmune thyroiditis. Therefore, tests for specific autoantibodies could be used for screening of high-risk populations to identify individuals predisposed to the development of diseases at an early stage. Identification may allow implementation of early treatment and preventive measures (Bizzaro, 2007; Rose, 2007).

Autoimmune diseases have a gender bias and represent the fifth leading cause of death by disease among females of reproductive age (Zandman-Goddard, 2007). Clinical studies indicate that the gender bias in autoimmunity may be influenced by sex hormones, as found in SLE.

Autoimmune disorders can be categorized broadly into systemic and organ-directed diseases (Nakamura, 2002). In this chapter, we discuss most of the organ-directed autoimmune diseases listed in Table 53-2.

The dominant clinical feature of these autoimmune disorders is chronic inflammation, generally localized in a single organ specific for each individual disease. Within this group of autoimmune disorders, familial clustering of diseases occurs with remarkable frequency. The relevant autoantibodies may or may not be species-specific, but they do exhibit specificity for an antigen present in the diseased organ or tissue.

Included in this chapter are some diseases with autoantibodies and inflammatory lesions restricted to one or a few organ(s) that combine clinicopathologic features of both organ-specific and systemic autoimmune diseases. Autoimmune liver disorders, such as PBC or autoimmune hepatitis, are examples of diseases in this group. Except for autoantibodies to thyroid receptors, the pathogenesis of autoantibodies in organ-specific diseases remains largely unproven.

DETECTION METHODS

Direct immunofluorescence microscopy (DIFM) is the laboratory method used to detect immune deposits in a patient's tissue. Indirect immunofluorescence microscopy (IIFM), briefly described in the following section, is the method most commonly used to detect circulating autoantibodies to specific target organs or tissues. Clinical laboratories are using enzyme-linked immunosorbent assays (ELISAs) more frequently because technical aspects of this method have improved.

Indirect Immunofluorescence Microscopy

This test procedure for IIFM is essentially the same as DIFM, except for the substrate used to bind target autoantibodies. The general procedure follows:

1. Prepare screening dilution of patient sera, or serial dilutions, and appropriate controls in phosphate-buffered saline (PBS).
2. Use a moisture chamber to incubate for 20–30 minutes diluted sera and controls layered over cryostat tissue sections of the substrate on multiwell glass slides. Do not allow the slides to dry.
3. Remove slides from the moisture chamber. Briefly but carefully wash each entire slide two to three times using PBS at room temperature. Then wash slides in PBS for 15 minutes, changing the wash once during this period.
4. Remove one slide at a time from the PBS wash, blot each slide dry, and place each in a moisture chamber. Dispense diluted fluorescein-labeled conjugate over each well. Incubate slides at room temperature for 20 minutes. Do not allow slides to dry.
5. Wash slides for 10 minutes in PBS that contains Evan's blue counterstain.
6. Mount coverslips.
7. View slides under a fluorescence microscope.
8. Store slides in the dark at 4° C.

Skin

Detection of autoantibodies is highly useful in the workup for cutaneous bullous disease. In patients with autoimmune skin diseases, autoantibodies include those to basement membrane zone (BMZ), epidermal intercellular spaces (ICSs), or dermal blood vessels, as summarized in Table 53-3. Several excellent technical reviews detail the use of immunofluorescence for examination of skin (Crosby, 1993; Flotte, 1995).

PEMPHIGUS

Pemphigus refers to a group of disorders that are characterized clinically by blisters and histologically by acantholysis. Three major subtypes of pemphigus are known: Pemphigus vulgaris, pemphigus foliaceus, and paraneoplastic pemphigus (Beutner, 1973; Ding, 1999; Nousari, 1999a). Each of these subtypes is characterized by autoantibodies to desmosomal adhesion molecules. Both IIFM to detect circulating autoantibodies and the more informative DIFM to identify tissue-bound autoantibodies are used for initial evaluations to maximize diagnostic sensitivity.

Antidesmoglein reactivity was detected in all patients with pemphigus and in none of the controls. Patients with a more benign form of

TABLE 53-2
Organ-Specific Autoimmune Diseases

Organ disease	Autoantibody	Detection method(s)
Thyroid Gland		
Autoimmune thyroiditis	Thyroid peroxidase	ELISA; IIFM using unfixed monkey thyroid
	Thyroglobulin	IIFM using methanol-fixed monkey thyroid; passive hemagglutination; latex agglutination
Graves' disease	TSH receptor	Radioreceptor binding assay; cAMP bioassay
Adrenal Gland		
Addison's disease	Adrenocortical	IIFM on unfixed monkey or human adrenal cortex
Parathyroid Gland		
Hypoparathyroidism	Parathyroid endothelial proteins	IIFM on unfixed bovine parathyroid gland
Pancreas		
Type 1A diabetes mellitus	Islet cells	IIFM on unfixed human pancreas, blood group O
	Insulin-associated	Radioimmunoprecipitation
	Antiglutamic acid decarboxylase	ELISA, RIA, immunoblotting
Muscle		
Dermatomyositis/polymyositis	PM-1, Jo-1	ELISA, immunodiffusion
Gastrointestinal Tract		
Atrophic gastritis	Gastric parietal cell	IIFM—mouse stomach/kidney
Pernicious anemia	Intrinsic factor	Radioactive vitamin B_{12} binding assay
	Salivary duct cells	IIFM—unfixed human salivary gland
	Gastric parietal cell	IIFM—human, monkey, mouse, or rat gastric mucosa substrate
Ulcerative colitis	Colon; lipopolysaccharide	IIFM—human or rat colon; hemagglutination
	DNase sensitive, p-ANCA associated	IIFM—ethanol-fixed neutrophils
Crohn's disease	ASCA IgA, ASCA IgG, OmpC, CB1r1	ELISA
Celiac disease	Tissue transglutaminase	ELISA
	IgA endomysial	IIFM—monkey esophagus
	Deaminated gliadin peptides	ELISA
Liver		
Autoimmune hepatitis	Smooth muscle	IIFM—mouse stomach/kidney
	Liver–kidney microsomal	IIFM—mouse stomach/kidney; ELISA
	ANA	HEp-2 cells
Primary biliary cirrhosis	Mitochondrial (M2)	IIFM—mouse stomach/kidney; ELISA
Primary sclerosing cholangitis	p-ANCA	IIFM—ethanol-fixed neutrophils
Neurologic		
Myasthenia gravis	AChR	Immunoprecipitation of iodine-125 α-bungarotoxin–conjugated AChR (human skeletal muscle); ELISA
Demyelinating diseases (e.g., multiple sclerosis)	Myelin; tubulin; myelin basic protein; myelin-associated glycoprotein	IIFM—mammalian spinal cord; ELISA; immunoblotting
Kidneys		
Anti-GBM disease	Glomerular and lung basement membrane	ELISA
Skin		
Pemphigus vulgaris	Intracellular space (ICS)	DIFM on skin biopsy
	Desmogleins	IIFM on monkey or guinea pig esophagus
	Dsg 1, Dsg 3, BP 180	ELISA
Pemphigus foliaceus	Dsg 1	
Paraneoplastic pemphigus	ICS and BMZ envoplakin, periplakin	DIFM on skin biopsy
		Immunoblotting
IgA pemphigus	IgA ICS	DIFM on human skin biopsy; IIFM on monkey esophagus
Bullous pemphigoid	BMZ (hemidesmosomal) proteins	
Mucous membrane pemphigoid		DIFM on skin biopsy
		IIFM on monkey esophagus
		DIFM—oral or ocular mucosa
Dermatitis herpetiformis	Tissue transglutaminase	
	Antigliadin	ELISA
	Anti–deaminated gliadin peptide	
	IgA endomysial	IIFM on monkey esophagus
Linear IgA dermatosis	IgA BMZ	DIFM on human skin biopsy; IIFM on monkey esophagus

AChR, Acetylcholine receptor; *ANA,* antinuclear antibody; *ASCA,* antibodies to *Saccharomyces cerevisiae; BMZ,* basement membrane zone; *cAMP,* cyclic adenosine monophosphate; *DIFM,* direct immunofluorescence microscopy; *DNase,* deoxyribonuclease; *ELISA,* enzyme-linked immunosorbent assay; *GBM,* glomerular basement membrane; *Ig,* immunoglobulin; *IIFM,* indirect immunofluorescence microscopy; *p-ANCA,* perinuclear antineutrophil cytoplasmic antibody; *RIA,* radioimmunoassay; *TSH,* thyroid-stimulating hormone.

TABLE 53-3
Autoimmune Skin Diseases

Immunologic Findings Essential for Diagnosis
Epidermal Intercellular Spaces
Pemphigus
Paraneoplastic pemphigus
Basement Membrane Zone
Pemphigoid
Gestational pemphigoid
Epidermolysis bullosa acquisita
Linear immunoglobulin A dermatosis
Chronic bullous dermatosis of childhood
Dermal Papillae ± Basement Membrane Zone
Dermatitis herpetiformis
Immunologic Findings Useful for Diagnosis
Cutaneous Manifestations in Systemic Rheumatic Diseases
Dermatomyositis/polymyositis
Lupus erythematosus
Mixed connective tissue disease
Relapsing polychondritis
Sjögren's syndrome
Systemic sclerosis
Vasculitis

pemphigus had anti-Dsy 1 antibodies, while patients with more severe deeper cutaneous lesions or mucosal involvement had both Dsy 1 and Dsy 3 reactivity, or Dsy 3 exclusively.

The BP 180–based assay was positive for 66.6% of patients with bullous pemphigoid and for none of those with mucous membrane pemphigoid (D'Agosto, 2004).

Pemphigus Vulgaris

Pemphigus vulgaris is a rare disorder that occurs in all racial and ethnic groups, although the incidence is slightly increased in the Jewish population. The disease affects both sexes and most commonly occurs in individuals between 40 and 60 years old (Becker, 1993). Desmoglein 3 is the major antigen in pemphigus vulgaris (Naparstek, 1993; Lin, 1998). ELISAs to detect anti-desmoglein-3 are available.

Direct Immunofluorescence Microscopy

DIFM of perilesional skin shows linear/granular IgG and C3 ICS immunofluorescence without BMZ staining (Fig. 53-1). This pattern is often described as "chicken wire" and preferentially stains the lower one half of the epidermis. IgG, especially IgG4, is present in nearly 100% of patients, whereas C3 is present in 50%–100% of patients, usually in acantholytic areas (Becker, 1993; Flotte, 1995; Lin, 1998). In 30%–50% of patients, IgA or IgM immunoreactants are seen (Izuno, 1986). C3 immunofluorescence only, without IgG, is described in drug-induced pemphigus and in impetigo (Nousari, 1997).

Indirect Immunofluorescence Microscopy

IIFM should detect circulating IgG autoantibodies to the surfaces of squamous epithelial cells in 100% of patients with active disease (Nousari, 1997). Monkey esophagus is considered the best tissue substrate (Fig. 53-2).

The presence of pemphigus vulgaris autoantibodies is abnormal at any titer. The titer generally correlates with disease activity, and increasing titers may be predictive of relapse (Becker, 1993; Crosby, 1993). Exceptions to this correlation do occur, however, so serial testing of IgG titers to monitor these patients must be carefully correlated with clinical findings. Patients who have only oral mucosal lesions may not have detectable circulating pemphigus vulgaris autoantibodies. In these patients, diagnosis is made using DIFM (Izuno, 1986).

Low titers of ICS-like autoantibodies may be infrequently detected in diverse conditions such as skin burns, penicillin or other drug allergy, toxic epidermal necrolysis, SLE, myasthenia gravis, pemphigoid, and lichen planus. Rarely, they are seen in healthy individuals (<1%) (Becker, 1993; Mutasim, 1993b; Nousari, 1997).

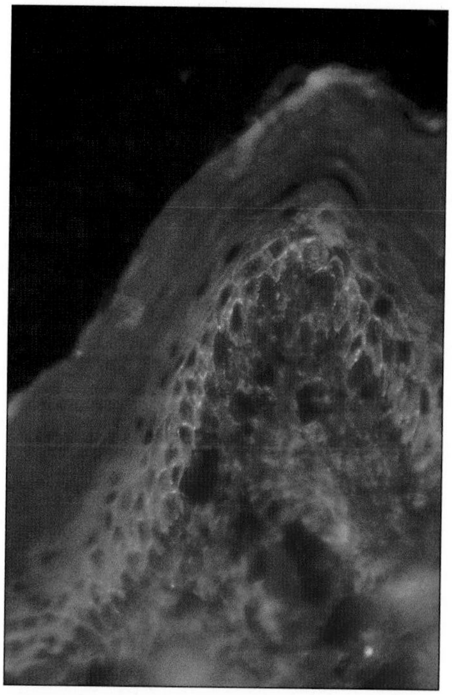

Figure 53-1 Direct immunofluorescence microscopy of skin lesions in pemphigus shows linear/granular C3 deposition on the cell surfaces (intercellular spaces) of mainly basal keratinocytes without basement membrane zone immunofluorescence (×400).

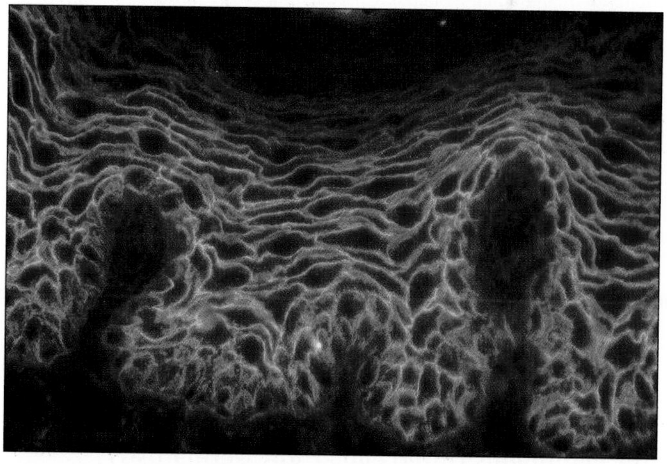

Figure 53-2 Indirect immunofluorescence microscopy in pemphigus shows linear immunoglobulin (Ig)G immunofluorescence on the cell surfaces of epithelial cells (intercellular spaces) using mouse esophagus as tissue substrate (×250).

Pemphigus Foliaceus

Subsets of pemphigus foliaceus include idiopathic pemphigus foliaceus, endemic pemphigus foliaceus (fogo selvagem), drug-induced pemphigus foliaceus, and pemphigus erythematosus. Desmoglein 1 is the major antigen in pemphigus foliaceus (Naparstek, 1993; Lin, 1998). ELISAs to detect anti-desmoglein-1 are available.

Direct Immunofluorescence Microscopy

For all forms of pemphigus foliaceus except pemphigus erythematosus, the DIFM pattern is similar to pemphigus vulgaris. In some cases, staining predominates in the superficial epidermis at the level of the stratum granulosum. In pemphigus erythematosus, linear IgG staining of epidermal ICS is combined with granular immunoreactants along the BMZ.

Indirect Immunofluorescence Microscopy

IIFM should detect circulating IgG ICS autoantibodies in virtually 100% of pemphigus foliaceus patients with active disease (Nousari, 1997). About 90% of these pemphigus foliaceus patients have detectable autoantibodies when monkey esophagus is used for indirect studies. Guinea pig esophagus is somewhat more sensitive in that it detects the remaining 10% of patients and the indirect titers tend to run higher than those obtained when monkey esophagus is used (Jiao, 1997).

Paraneoplastic Pemphigus

Paraneoplastic pemphigus, an uncommon disorder characterized by painful blisters or erosions of mucous membranes and skin, is a condition of patients with neoplasms. These blisters or erosions usually erupt in the mouth, but other mucosal sites have been reported. Malignant neoplasms that have been associated with paraneoplastic pemphigus include malignant lymphoma, chronic lymphocytic leukemia, thymoma, bronchogenic squamous cell carcinoma, and sarcoma. Rarely, paraneoplastic pemphigus is associated with benign neoplasms (Camisa, 1993; Mutasim, 1993c; Flotte, 1995; Kiyokawa, 1999).

The following criteria to define paraneoplastic pemphigus have been proposed by Mutasim (1993c), Flotte (1995), and Kiyokawa (1999).

- Painful mucosal erosions and a polymorphous skin eruption, with papular lesions progressing to blisters and erosive lesions affecting trunk, extremities, and palms and soles, associated with an occult or clinically known neoplasm.
- Suprabasilar acantholysis, keratinocyte necrosis, and vacuolar interface changes on light microscopic tissue sections
- IgG ICS combined with linear/granular complement and IgG along the BMZ
- Circulating ICS autoantibodies that bind to rodent bladder urothelium and monkey/guinea pig esophagus
- Immunoprecipitation of a complex of four keratinocytic proteins bound by the autoantibodies; this is mainly a research tool but may provide helpful clinical information in difficult cases

Paraneoplastic pemphigus associated with malignant neoplasms signals an extremely poor prognosis. Although clinical improvement or remission of mucocutaneous lesions after tumor resection has been reported, treatment for malignancy-associated paraneoplastic pemphigus is supportive. Paraneoplastic pemphigus associated with a benign neoplasm remitted after tumor resection (Mutasim, 1993c).

Direct Immunofluorescence Microscopy

DIFM of perilesional skin and/or mucosa from patients with paraneoplastic pemphigus detects IgG ICS immunoreactant with or without complement components. Granular or, less commonly, linear BMZ deposits of complement components (C3, C1q) are present, in addition to IgG ICS immunofluorescence (Mutasim, 1993c).

Indirect Immunofluorescence Microscopy

IIFM using monkey esophagus and rodent bladder urothelium demonstrates IgG immunoreactant both in ICS and along the BMZ. Binding to rodent (rat or mouse) bladder epithelium is an important differential finding that distinguishes paraneoplastic pemphigus from other types of pemphigus (Liu, 1993; Mutasim, 1993c).

IgA Pemphigus (Intercellular IgA Dermatosis)

Direct Immunofluorescence Microscopy

Intercellular IgA dermatosis is a rare intraepidermal vesiculobullous disorder. Direct studies show linear ICS immunofluorescence for IgA that is suprabasilar and particularly accentuated in the upper epidermis.

Indirect Immunofluorescence Microscopy

IIFM detects circulating IgA anti-ICS autoantibodies (Teraki, 1991; Flotte, 1995).

PEMPHIGOID

Bullous Pemphigoid

Bullous pemphigoid is a subepidermal bullous disease of unknown cause that can occur in patients of any age but mainly affects adults older than 60 years (Fig. 53-3, *A*). This disorder typically involves flexor surfaces of the arms, legs, groin, axilla, and lower abdomen. The oral mucous membranes may be affected, but such lesions are rarely the presenting or predominant sign—a point that differentiates pemphigoid from pemphigus vulgaris.

The major antigens in bullous pemphigoid are two keratinocytic hemidesmosomal proteins, an intracellular 230-kDa protein (bullous pemphigoid antigen 1), and a transmembrane 180-kDa protein (bullous pemphigoid antigen 2) (Nousari, 1997; Lin, 1998).

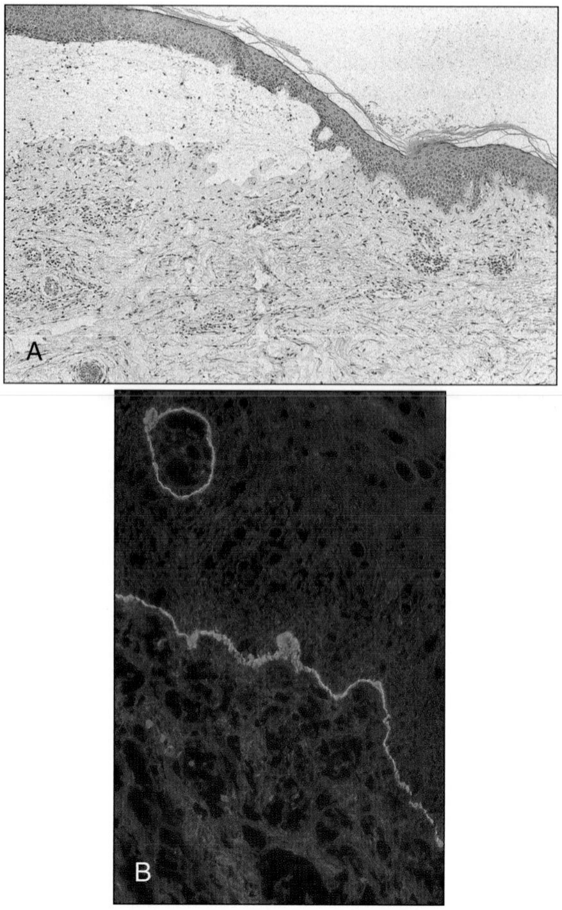

Figure 53-3 Skin biopsy of pemphigoid reveals a subepidermal split, nonnecrotic epidermis and variable inflammation, often with prominent eosinophils (**A,** Hematoxylin and eosin [H&E], ×100). Direct immunofluorescence microscopy reveals intense linear C3 deposition along the basement membrane zone (**B,** ×400).

Direct Immunofluorescence Microscopy

DIFM of unblistered, perilesional skin from the edge of a fresh blister is diagnostically sensitive and typically demonstrates linear BMZ immunofluorescence in nearly 100% of patients (Fig. 53-3, *B*). C3 and IgG or C3 alone is the predominant immunoreactant. Also, IgA and/or IgM may be present in up to 25% of patients, usually in weaker intensity and in combination with IgG (Izuno, 1986; Crosby, 1993; Korman, 1993).

A linear epidermal BMZ pattern can be identified in several disparate clinical disorders, including benign mucous membrane pemphigoid, epidermolysis bullosa acquisita, gestational pemphigoid (herpes gestationis), and bullous lupus erythematosus.

To help separate these disorders, salt-split direct skin biopsies are useful (Domloge-Hultsch, 1991). In bullous pemphigoid and gestational pemphigoid, linear IgG is localized to the epidermal side, or roof, of the split. Linear C3 immunofluorescence, however, may be seen along epidermal and dermal locations. In epidermolysis bullosa acquisita and bullous lupus erythematosus, immunoreactants are seen along the dermal side of the split (Nousari, 1997). Clinical correlation then becomes important in resolving diagnostic alternatives.

Indirect Immunofluorescence Microscopy

Bullous pemphigoid is serologically characterized by the presence of circulating autoantibodies to the BMZ, in the skin or the oral mucosa. IIFM detects circulating IgG anti-BMZ autoantibodies in about 50% of patients with pemphigoid, but sensitivity increases to 70%–80% if normal human salt-split skin is used as substrate (Izuno, 1986; Domloge-Hultsch, 1991; Nousari, 1997). In bullous pemphigoid, autoantibodies bind only to the roof of salt-split skin in 80% of patients. In epidermolysis bullosa acquisita and bullous lupus erythematosus, autoantibodies bind to the dermal base, or floor, of the split in 50% of patients (Domloge-Hultsch, 1991; Crosby, 1993; Korman, 1993).

Benign Mucous Membrane Pemphigoid

Benign mucous membrane pemphigoid, or cicatricial pemphigoid, consistently affects oral and ocular mucosa. Other mucosal sites of these lesions can be the nasopharynx, larynx, genitalia, rectum, and esophagus (Mutasim, 1993a). Scarring follows the healing of lesions, and blindness is the most feared complication.

Direct Immunofluorescence Microscopy

The DIFM pattern is similar to that seen in bullous pemphigoid. Sensitivity is 90% but increases if additional biopsies are taken. Chronic localized scarring pemphigoid, also known as cicatricial pemphigoid of Brunsting-Perry, is a variant of benign mucous membrane pemphigoid that is localized to the head and neck region (Sarret, 1991). In this variant, DIFM demonstrates IgG only along the BMZ without IgA or IgM; circulating anti-BMZ autoantibodies are also rare (Izuno, 1986).

Indirect Immunofluorescence Microscopy

IIFM detects circulating IgG autoantibodies in less than 33% of benign mucous membrane pemphigoid patients when oral mucosal substrate is used, but in only 5%–15% of patients using standard substrates (Sarret, 1991; Crosby, 1993; Nousari, 1997). Salt-split human skin studies may reveal deposits of IgA, IgG, or both in about 80% of these patients (Sarret, 1991).

No correlation has been noted between the presence and titer of autoantibodies and disease activity.

Gestational Pemphigoid

Infrequently, the subepidermal bullous disease gestational pemphigoid (herpes gestationis) develops during or soon after pregnancy (Izuno, 1986). Lesions typically are pruritic and are located predominantly on the abdomen and/or extremities.

Direct Immunofluorescence Microscopy

With DIFM, one typically finds linear C3 BMZ deposits. Associated IgG deposits are detected in 30%–40% of cases, but IgA and IgM are rare (Izuno, 1986).

Indirect Immunofluorescence Microscopy

Linear C3 deposits only may be visualized along the BMZ, but often autoantibody titers are too low to be seen using standard IIFM substrates. Complement may be detected, however, if complement immunofixation using normal human salt-split skin is used as substrate (Izuno, 1986; Nousari, 1997).

EPIDERMOLYSIS BULLOSA ACQUISITA AND BULLOUS LUPUS ERYTHEMATOSUS

Epidermolysis bullosa acquisita and bullous lupus erythematosus are acquired subepidermal blistering diseases characterized by the presence of autoantibodies to type VII collagen in BMZ protein (Gammon, 1993). Epidermolysis bullosa acquisita can occur at any age but most commonly presents in adults who are 40–50 years old. Neither an ethnic nor a sex predilection has been noted. All such patients are afflicted with a combination of blisters, erosions, scars, milia, and dyspigmentation of skin, most often located on trauma-susceptible extensor skin surfaces such as knees, elbows, and dorsa of hands and feet (Gammon, 1993). Bullous lupus erythematosus occurs in patients with lupus erythematosus.

Direct Immunofluorescence Microscopy

When DIFM is used, patients with epidermolysis bullosa acquisita and bullous lupus erythematosus have linear BMZ immunoreactants that most commonly consist of IgG and C3. When direct salt-split skin biopsy tissue is used, linear immunoreactants are localized at the dermal, or floor, aspect of the induced blister.

Indirect Immunofluorescence Microscopy

Only about 40% of epidermolysis bullosa acquisita patients have demonstrable autoantibodies when human skin without salt treatment is used as substrate. When indirect salt-split skin technique is used, circulating autoantibodies can be identified in about 50%–85% of patients (Fine, 1994; Nousari, 1997).

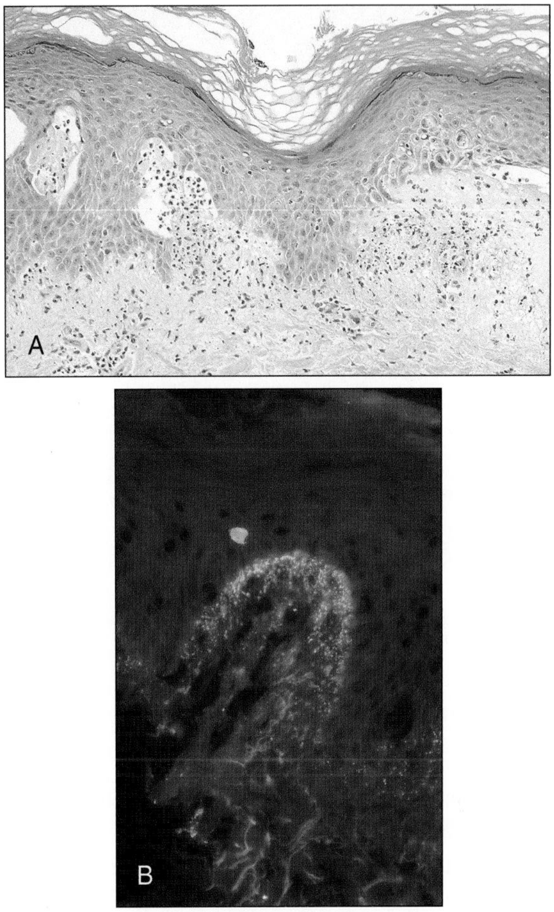

Figure 53-4 Skin biopsy of dermatitis herpetiformis reveals a subepidermal split, nonnecrotic epidermis and neutrophilic microabscesses in the tips of dermal papillae (**A,** Hematoxylin and eosin [H&E], ×200). Direct immunofluorescence microscopy reveals granular immunoglobulin (Ig)A immunofluorescence in the tips of dermal papillae and, to a lesser extent, along the basement membrane region (**B,** ×400).

DERMATITIS HERPETIFORMIS

Dermatitis herpetiformis is a severely pruritic subepidermal bullous disease associated with gluten-sensitive enteropathy (Fig. 53-4, *A*). Dermatitis herpetiformis is also associated with human leukocyte antigen (HLA)-B8, DR3 histocompatibility types (Crosby, 1993).

Direct Immunofluorescence Microscopy

The direct biopsy should focus on perilesional skin because a lesional skin biopsy may be negative. DIFM detects granular IgA in the tips of dermal papillae in approximately 80%–100% of dermatitis herpetiformis patients (Flotte, 1995) (Fig. 53-4, *B*). Concomitant IgA deposits may be seen along the BMZ. C3 deposits are often found with IgA, but IgG and/or IgM are detected infrequently (Izuno, 1986).

Indirect Immunofluorescence Microscopy

Patients with dermatitis herpetiformis do not have detectable anti-BMZ autoantibodies. However, antiendomysial IgA autoantibodies are detected in 80% of dermatitis herpetiformis patients. These autoantibodies are identified by their characteristic immunofluorescence pattern in the subepithelial muscularis mucosa of monkey esophagus (Peters, 1989).

LINEAR IgA DERMATOSIS

Linear IgA dermatosis is an uncommon acquired subepidermal blistering disorder that is now considered a distinct clinical entity, rather than a variant of dermatitis herpetiformis, as was once thought (Izuno, 1986; Crosby, 1993). Many cases are thought to be idiopathic but drug-induced, and systemic disorder–related forms are described (Kuechle, 1994; Nousari, 1995, 1999; Bouldin, 2000). Chronic bullous dermatosis of childhood is similar to linear IgA dermatosis, both clinically and immunopathologically (Elenitsas, 1995).

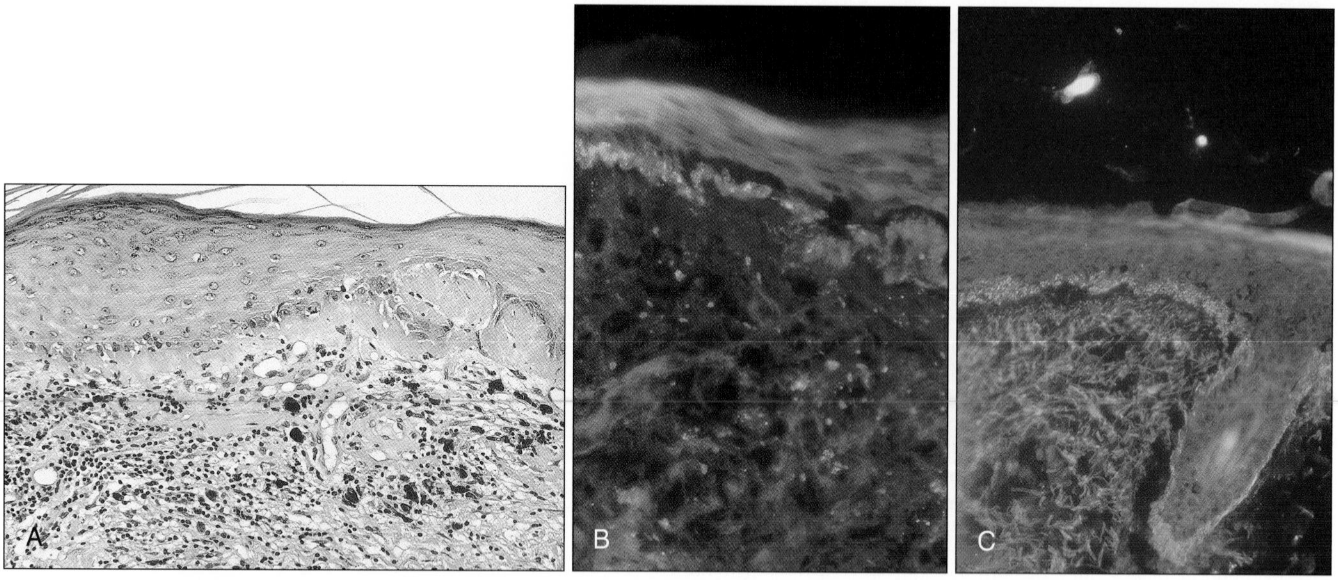

Figure 53-5 Skin biopsy of lupus erythematosus reveals epidermal atrophy, vacuolar alteration of basal keratinocytes, marked thickening of the basement membrane zone, perivascular and interstitial mainly lymphocytic inflammation, and melanin incontinence (**A**, Hematoxylin and eosin [H&E], ×500). Direct immunofluorescence microscopy reveals continuous granular C3 (**B**, ×500) and C1q (**C**, ×200) immunofluorescence along the basement membrane zone.

Direct Immunofluorescence Microscopy

In nearly 100% of cases, DIFM demonstrates intense linear IgA deposits along the BMZ but none in dermal papillae (Izuno, 1986). Although occasional cases may show concomitant weak C3 BMZ staining, immunoreactants other than IgA are not usually present.

Indirect Immunofluorescence Microscopy

Circulating IgA anti-BMZ autoantibodies can be detected with IIFM in about 10%–30% of cases (Crosby, 1993; Flotte, 1995).

LUPUS ERYTHEMATOSUS

Lupus erythematosus (Fig. 53-5, *A*) is a disorder characterized serologically by the presence of multiple autoantibodies, including antinuclear antibodies, anti-native DNA, antihistones, and anti-Sm.

Direct Immunofluorescence Microscopy

With DIFM, one sees characteristic coarse, granular, continuous deposits of immunoglobulins and complement along the epidermal BMZ in 50%–95% of SLE patients (Izuno, 1986). BMZ deposits of the complement membrane attack complex C5b–9 in lesional skin may be a marker for SLE (Helm, 1993).

Whereas these patients commonly have deposits of IgG, IgM, and complement component (C3 and/or C1q) (Fig. 53-5, *B* and *C*), immunoglobulins of all classes may be identified (Izuno, 1986). When nonlesional skin concurrently contains immunoglobulins IgG, IgA, and/or IgM in the typical pattern, the diagnosis is more likely than not SLE (Izuno, 1986).

Although characteristic, this reaction pattern can be seen in other disorders, such as mixed connective tissue disease, dermatomyositis, graft-versus-host reaction, drug eruptions, and vasculitis (Izuno, 1986). Therefore, it is mandatory to correlate direct results with both the clinical presentation and the results of light microscopic study of a skin biopsy. This information is then interpreted in the context of an individual's direct findings to categorize the clinical type of lupus erythematosus. Many publications cite the utility of DIFM for the purpose of diagnosing SLE from biopsied skin, with or without lesions, and from sun-exposed or sun-protected sites. In patients diagnosed with SLE, normal sun-exposed skin proves positive about 70% of the time, whereas normal sun-protected skin is positive in about 40% of patients (Izuno, 1986). However, the potential for predicting disease activity or renal involvement in this way remains controversial (Izuno, 1986). Perhaps the most practical clinical application of laboratory testing comes in the differential diagnosis of SLE from discoid lupus erythematosus. Up to 95% of individuals with discoid lupus erythematosus have coarse, granular, continuous BMZ deposits similar to those of SLE (Izuno, 1986). However, positive DIFM findings in discoid lupus erythematosus are confined to lesional skin, whereas skin with or without lesions can give positive DIFM findings in SLE (Izuno, 1986).

Subacute cutaneous lupus erythematosus is characterized clinically by arthritis, mild systemic manifestations, and anti-SS-A/Ro autoantibodies. DIFM of skin biopsies from these patients detects BMZ immunoglobulin and/or complement deposits in only 50% of lesional skin biopsies and 30% of uninvolved skin biopsies (Izuno, 1986). IIFM is positive in 50%–70% of patients with subacute cutaneous lupus erythematosus.

Other major systemic autoimmune diseases do not offer diagnostically specific findings by DIFM or IIFM. Although some patients have granular IgM deposits along the BMZ, this immunopathologic finding is considered to be a completely nonspecific marker that may be detected not only in autoimmune disease but also in a large number of inflammatory dermatitides, or in sun-exposed skin of clinically normal individuals (Izuno, 1986).

VASCULITIS

Vasculitis (see Chapter 52) in the skin has a number of synonyms, including leukocytoclastic vasculitis, allergic vasculitis, and hypersensitivity angiitis/vasculitis. Histologically, small blood vessels of the dermis show endothelial cell swelling, neutrophilic exocytosis, nuclear debris (**leukocytoclasis**), and necrosis in conjunction with extravasated red blood cells.

Direct Immunofluorescence Microscopy

Biopsy of such a lesion within 24 hours of onset may display vascular deposits of IgM, C3, fibrinogen, and sometimes IgG. A negative result does not exclude vasculitis. Biopsy of a lesion older than 24 hours may not be helpful, in that nonspecific fibrinogen staining may be the only finding. Histologic confirmation of the diagnosis is therefore essential. Henoch-Schönlein purpura is diagnosed when granular IgA, with or without C3, vascular immunofluorescence is seen in the appropriate clinical setting.

LIVER

AUTOANTIBODIES

Antinuclear Autoantibodies

ANAs are most commonly detected by IIFM, although ELISAs for identification of specific autoantibodies are becoming popular in clinical laboratories. ANAs are a very heterogeneous group, and almost all subtypes that occur in rheumatologic disorders are found in persons with autoimmune hepatitis. Homogeneous or speckled ANA patterns on HEp-2 cells are more commonly identified in patients with autoimmune hepatitis. Also reported in liver disease are specific autoantibodies to double-stranded DNA (Manns, 1992). ANAs in titers greater than 1:80 are detected in about 80% of patients with autoimmune hepatitis (Nakamura, 1991). However, ANAs may also be found in about 60% of patients with PBC, 50% of patients with alcohol-related liver disease, 40% of patients with

TABLE 53-4
Autoimmune Liver Diseases

	ANA	LKM	SLA	SMA	AMA	Anti-HCV	p-ANCA	ACA	Therapy
Autoimmune Hepatitis									
Type 1	+	–	–	+	–	–	±	–	Immunosuppression
Type 2a	–	+	–	–	–	–	–	–	Immunosuppression
Type 2b	–	+	–	–	–	+	–	–	
Type 3	–	–	+	±	±	–	–	–	Immunosuppression
Type 4	–	–	–	+	–	–	–	–	Immunosuppression
PBC	–	–	–	–	+	–	–	–	Supportive; transplant
PSC	–	–	–	–	–	–	+	–	Supportive; transplant
AiC	+	–	–	–	–	–	–	+	Immunosuppression

Modified from Manns MP. Autoimmune diseases of the liver. Clin Lab Med 1992;12:25–40.
ACA, Anti–carbonic anhydrase; *AiC,* autoimmune cholangitis; *AMA,* antimitochondrial antibodies; *ANA,* antinuclear antibodies; *HCV,* hepatitis C virus; *LKM,* liver–kidney microsomal antibodies; *p-ANCA,* perinuclear antineutrophil cytoplasmic antibodies; *PBC,* primary biliary cirrhosis; *PSC,* primary sclerosing cholangitis; *SLA,* antibodies against soluble liver antigens; *SMA,* smooth muscle antibodies.

viral hepatitis type B, and 25% of patients with autoimmune hepatitis who also have anti-liver–kidney microsomal autoantibodies (LKMs) (Nakamura, 1991). Anticentromere autoantibodies can be identified in 10%–15% of PBC patients.

Antimitochondrial Autoantibodies

Nine separate mitochondrial antigens have been identified that react with AMAs. AMAs directed at M2 and M9 antigens are considered the most important diagnostic markers of PBC (Bylund, 1992).

AMAs detected using IIFM on a substrate of rodent stomach/kidney tissue block show a typical pattern of fluorescence that reflects homogeneous cytoplasmic staining of kidney tubules and stomach parietal cell regions; distal tubules are also positive. This distal tubular staining is an important point in differentiating the reactivity of AMAs from that of LKMs, which do not stain distal renal tubules.

The M2 autoantigen is a heterogeneous mix containing several components of the mitochondrial 2-oxo-acid dehydrogenase complex. The dominant M2 autoantigen in patients with PBC is the 70-kDa E2 subunit of pyruvate dehydrogenase (Manns, 1992). The second most common mitochondrial autoantigen is the 50-kDa E2 subunit of branched-chain oxo-keto-acid-dehydrogenase (Manns, 1992). A group of serum autoantibodies called naturally occurring mitochondrial autoantibodies (NOMAs) have been found in persons having close contact with PBC patients and even in laboratory technicians processing PBC sera (Bylund, 1992). NOMAs are rarely produced in PBC patients but are observed in sera from patients with Epstein-Barr virus infection, cytomegalovirus infection, and other infectious disorders. NOMAs are directed at epitopes on the M2 and M9 antigens in PBC, but not to the same antigens as AMAs (Bylund, 1992). Although the significance of NOMAs is uncertain, their presence in persons associated with PBC patients has raised questions about possible contagious agents in the serum of these patients (Bylund, 1992).

Smooth Muscle Autoantibodies

Smooth muscle autoantibodies (SMAs) are found in approximately 50% of patients with classic autoimmune hepatitis and often occur with ANAs (Nakamura, 1991). When accompanying liver disease, SMAs are directed against F-actin, which is part of the liver cell cytoskeleton in close association with the liver cell plasma membrane (Nakamura, 1991). The SMA titer is typically greater than or equal to 1 : 80 in serum from a patient with autoimmune hepatitis. However, low titers of SMA can be detected in patients with other diseases, and in apparently healthy individuals (Nakamura, 1991).

IIFM on a tissue substrate of rodent stomach is commonly used to detect SMA, which stains the muscularis propria of stomach in a uniform and consistent pattern. Specific staining of muscularis mucosae and walls of blood vessels is characteristic. If a rodent stomach/kidney tissue block is used as substrate, faint staining may be noted in glomerular mesangial zones owing to the presence of F-actin in this region. If HEp-2 cells are used instead of other substrates, IIFM reveals "cable-like" cytoplasmic staining when SMA is present.

Liver–Kidney Microsomal Autoantibodies

LKMs stain the microsomes of hepatocytes and proximal renal tubules when detected using a rodent stomach/kidney tissue block as the substrate for IIFM. The distal renal tubules are characteristically negative for immunofluorescence. The simultaneous occurrence of AMA and LKM, although possible, is extremely unlikely.

ELISAs that detect LKM are becoming available for use in clinical laboratories. The presence of LKM can also be confirmed by using Western blotting, although this assay is not generally available outside of research laboratories.

Using the Western blotting procedure, LKMs have been grouped into three subtypes on the basis of their target antigens (Manns, 1992). A 50-kDa component of cytochrome P450 IID6 has been identified as the major antigen for LKM-1 (Manns, 1992). LKM-2, directed at cytochrome P450 IIC9, was found in patients taking ticrynafen (Manns, 1992), a drug that is no longer on the American market. LKM-3 has been identified in sera from patients with chronic viral hepatitis type D (Manns, 1992).

Other Liver Autoantibodies

The remaining groups of hepatic autoantibodies include anticytoskeleton, anticytosol, antiliver membrane, antinuclear lamins, liver-specific, and asialoglycoprotein receptor autoantibodies. All of these have been identified in patients with autoimmune liver disease, but their use as diagnostic markers is not currently widespread (Nakamura, 1991).

LIVER DISEASES

Table 53-4 lists typical serologic profiles in autoimmune hepatitis, PBC, and primary sclerosing cholangitis. These are typically chronic disorders defined by elevated concentrations of serum transaminases for at least 6 months.

Common clinical differential diagnoses include alcohol-related liver disease, drug-induced liver injury, viral hepatitides, and fatty liver of diabetes mellitus or obesity. Less common differential diagnoses include idiopathic hemochromatosis, Wilson's disease, α1-antitrypsin deficiency, and hepatic involvement in systemic diseases.

Autoimmune Hepatitis

Autoimmune hepatitis classically occurs in females around 35 years of age, who present with high concentrations of serum aminotransferases, hypergammaglobulinemia, amenorrhea, arthralgias, and circulating autoantibodies such as ANA, SMA, and LKM. By definition, these patients have no serologic evidence of viral hepatitis, Wilson's disease, or other diseases in the differential diagnosis. Histologically, liver biopsy typically shows chronic hepatitis with interface activity (Fig. 53-6, *A*). The patient's response to corticosteroids is dramatic, and failure to respond sheds doubt on the diagnosis of autoimmune hepatitis.

Autoimmune hepatitis is a heterogeneous group of disorders of uncertain etiology. There are no pathognomonic features. The International Autoimmune Hepatitis Group (IAHG) has integrated clinical and laboratory features at patient presentation into a scoring system for definite or probable diagnosis of autoimmune hepatitis. Table 53-5 lists clinical laboratory parameters used as criteria to diagnose autoimmune hepatitis; other criteria and scoring interpretations can be found in the reference section (Johnson, 1993; Manns, 1998). The absence of ANA, SMA, or LKM does not exclude this diagnosis.

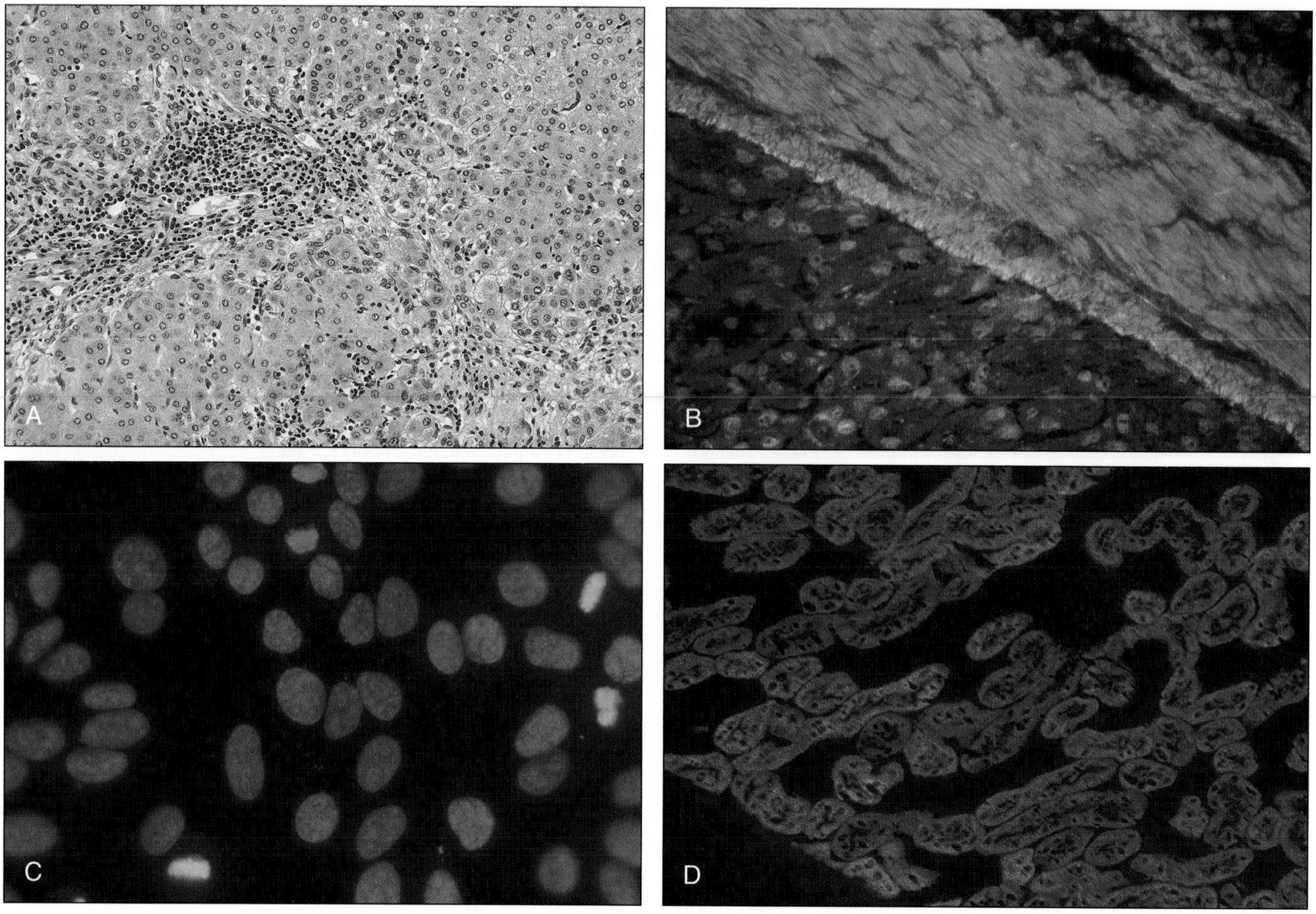

Figure 53-6 Liver biopsy in untreated autoimmune hepatitis shows prominent portal and lobular inflammation with interface activity and often numerous plasma cells at the leading edge of inflammation (**A,** Hematoxylin and eosin [H&E], ×500). Indirect immunofluorescence microscopy (IIFM) in this instance reveals combined smooth muscle antibodies and antinuclear antibodies using mouse stomach/kidney as substrate (**B,** ×200). The antinuclear antibody (ANA) pattern in liver disease is often homogeneous (**C,** ×400). IIFM of liver–kidney microsomal autoantibodies using mouse stomach/kidney as substrate. There is finely granular cytoplasmic immunofluorescence of proximal renal tubules, not distal tubules (**D,** ×200).

Although autoimmune hepatitis subtypes based on autoantibody patterns are presented in the medical literature, the clinical utility of such subtyping is uncertain, and the IAHG did not recommend subdivision of autoimmune hepatitis on the basis of autoantibody profiles. From a clinical perspective, autoimmune hepatitis can be viewed as a chronic liver disease characterized by the presence of a variety of autoantibodies. Most experts seem to agree that autoimmune hepatitis types 1 and 2 are the major forms of this disease, whereas additional subtypes are still at issue. Because the various subtypes are widely quoted, subclassification of autoimmune hepatitis according to its serologic profile is briefly discussed here.

ANAs characterize classical, type 1, autoimmune-type hepatitis. SMAs also are frequently detected (Fig. 53-6, *B* and *C*). Although AMAs are specific and sensitive diagnostic markers for PBC, as described later, AMAs can also be detected in about 15% of patients with both clinical and histologic features of autoimmune hepatitis, including clinical improvement in response to immunosuppressive therapy. Such patients are regarded as having a syndrome with features that "overlap" both autoimmune hepatitis and PBC. The AMA titer in this autoimmune hepatitis subgroup is rarely greater than 1:40 (Bylund, 1992). Additionally, the antigen specificity of these AMAs is similar to that seen in classical PBC (Manns, 1992). Liver disease in which LKMs are detected (Fig. 53-6, *D*), so-called type 2 autoimmune hepatitis, has been subdivided into two subgroups: types 2a and 2b. Usually, patients with this variant are negative for ANA and SMA. However, thyroid microsomal, thyroglobulin, and parietal cell autoantibodies are frequently detected. Type 2 autoimmune hepatitis is characterized by low IgA levels, and hypergammaglobulinemia is less prominent than in type 1 (Manns, 1992). Type 2a occurs in young females, who have high titers of LKM-1, negative serology for hepatitis C virus, and active but steroid-responsive disease.

The type 2b variant occurs in older patients, and less of a female preponderance has been seen. These patients have low titers of LKM-1, manifest milder liver disease, and often are serologically positive for hepatitis C virus. Their disease tends to be less responsive to immunosuppression than the 2a type.

A third subgroup of autoimmune hepatitis, separated from other subgroups on the basis of identifying serum anti-soluble-liver autoantibody (SLA), has been proposed by some investigators (Manns, 1992). Although this may become an important autoantibody to identify because it has been reported as the only serologic marker in about 25% of patients with autoimmune hepatitis, reliable tests to detect SLA are technically difficult and, as yet, are not routinely available in clinical laboratories (Manns, 1992).

It may be that high titers of SMA directed against F-actin characterize a fourth subgroup of autoimmune hepatitis that is frequently observed in young children (Manns, 1992).

Primary Biliary Cirrhosis

PBC is a chronic, progressive, cholestatic disorder typically occurring in young or middle-aged females. Patients may be asymptomatic or may have symptoms of cholestasis (itch). Laboratory studies demonstrate an elevation in alkaline phosphatase with or without hyperbilirubinemia, as well as increased IgM and AMA. Associated extrahepatic immunologic phenomena such as Raynaud's phenomenon, sicca complex, rheumatoid arthritis, thyroiditis, scleroderma, or celiac disease may occur (Bylund, 1992; Manns, 1992). Histologically, the liver shows various stages of nonsuppurative destructive cholangitis (Fig. 53-7, *A*).

AMAs are the most specific and sensitive diagnostic markers for PBC (Fig. 53-7, *B* and *C*). As a general guideline, an AMA titer greater than or equal to 1:160 is highly predictive of PBC, although about 10% of PBC patients have AMA titers of 1:16 or less (Bylund, 1992). About 95% of patients with typical features of PBC have been shown to have anti-M2 and/or anti-M9 AMA, whereas the remaining 5% of patients are AMA negative.

The cause of PBC is unknown, and several pathogenetic mechanisms are proposed regarding the immune-related bile duct injury characteristic

TABLE 53-5
Laboratory Parameters and Score for Autoimmune Hepatitis Diagnosis

Clinical laboratory parameters	Score
Biochemistry	
Ratio of increased alkaline phosphatase to aminotransferase	
>3.0	−2
<3.0	+2
Total serum globulin, γ-globulin, or IgG (× upper normal limit)	
>2.0	+3
1.5–2.0	+2
1.0–1.5	+1
<1.0	0
Autoantibodies (IIFM)	
Adults	
ANA, SMA, LKM	
>1:80	+3
1:80	+2
1:40	+1
<1:40	0
Children	
ANA, LKM	
>1:20	+3
1:10 or 1:20	+2
<1:10	0
SMA	
>1:20	+3
1:20	+2
<1:20	0
AMA	
Detected	−2
Not detected	0
Adults and Children (if ANA, SMA, LKM not detected)	
Other Liver Autoantibodies (SLA, ASGP-R, LC-1)	
Detected	+2
Not detected	0
Viral Markers	
Acute HAV or HBV	−3
HCV by ELISA and/or RIBA	−2
HCV RNA by PCR	−3
Other active viral infection	−3
Seronegative for known viruses	+3
Genetic Factors	
HLA B8-DR3 or DR4 allotype	+1

Adapted from Johnson PJ, McFarlane IG. Convenors on behalf of the panel. Meeting report: international autoimmune hepatitis group. Hepatology 1993;18:998–1008.

AMA, Antimitochondrial antibody; *ANA,* antinuclear antibody; *ASGP-R,* asialoglycoprotein receptor, *ELISA,* enzyme-linked immunosorbent assay; *HAV,* hepatitis A virus; *HBV,* hepatitis B virus; *HCV,* hepatitis C virus; *HLA,* human leukocyte antigen; *IIFM,* indirect immunofluorescence microscopy; *LC-1,* liver cytosolic-type 1; *LKM,* liver–kidney microsomal autoantibodies; *PCR,* polymerase chain reaction; *RIBA,* recombinant immunoblot assay; *SLA,* soluble-liver autoantibody; *SMA,* smooth muscle autoantibody.

of this disorder (Gershwin, 2000). Although this disease is classically associated with serum AMA, T cell–mediated immune injury to intrahepatic interlobular bile ducts dominates tissue lesions (Batts, 1991; Manns, 1991, 1988; Poupon, 1996). The discovery of retroviral antibody in PBC patients has been ascribed to either an autoimmune response or immune reactivity to viral proteins that share antigenic determinants with retroviruses (Mason, 1998).

The diagnosis of AMA-negative PBC derives from the clinical presentation, liver biopsy findings, and cholangiogram to exclude primary sclerosing cholangitis.

Primary Sclerosing Cholangitis

Primary sclerosing cholangitis typically occurs in males with a history of inflammatory bowel disease and/or diarrhea. In 50% of these patients, ulcerative colitis is the inflammatory bowel disease linked with primary sclerosing cholangitis. A diagnosis of primary sclerosing cholangitis is typically based on cholangiography, which reveals a characteristic beading pattern of bile ducts due to multifocal strictures at those sites (Fig. 53-8, *A*). The hallmark histologic lesion is fibrous cholangitis of large and/or small bile ducts, although in practice, a wide spectrum of chronic inflammatory lesions is seen on liver biopsy (Fig. 53-8, *B*).

Routine biochemical studies demonstrate an elevation in alkaline phosphatase and an increase in aminotransferases with or without hyperbilirubinemia. Although ANAs may be present, AMAs are not.

Furthermore, a high prevalence of atypical perinuclear antineutrophil cytoplasmic antibodies (p-ANCAs) detected with IIFM on ethanol- and formalin-fixed neutrophil displays has been reported (Manns, 1992; Lo, 1994; Gur, 1995; Bansi, 1996).

Autoimmune Cholangitis/Cholangiopathy

Autoimmune cholangitis/cholangiopathy is a chronic cholestatic liver disease that does not appear to be a variant of primary sclerosing cholangitis (Goodman, 1995; Tsui, 1997). The clinical presentation and histologic appearance of the liver resemble PBC, but serologic findings mimic autoimmune hepatitis type 1. AMAs are not detected. Additionally, an autoantibody to carbonic anhydrase has been detected in some autoimmune cholangitis patients (Gordon, 1995).

Although the connection between autoimmune cholangitis and PBC is not resolved, autoimmune cholangitis may be the same as AMA-negative PBC. Generally, autoimmune cholangitis patients respond to immunosuppression.

THYROID GLAND

THYROID DISEASES

Autoimmune thyroid diseases include Graves' disease and Hashimoto's thyroiditis (Burek, 1995).

Graves' Disease

The patient who has Graves' disease presents with symptoms of hyperthyroidism and diffuse goiter. The peak incidence is in the third to fourth decades of life, and the female/male ratio is 4–8:1; 60%–70% of these patients additionally manifest ocular disturbances (Patrick, 1993). Laboratory data show an increase in levels of triiodothyronine (T_3) and thyroxine (T_4) and in the uptake of T_3. Therapy is directed at reducing the thyroid's ability to respond to stimulation by autoantibodies. This can be achieved by subtotal thyroidectomy, by administration of radioactive iodine, or by use of antithyroid drugs such as propylthiouracil or methimazole (Patrick, 1993).

Hashimoto's Thyroiditis

Hashimoto's thyroiditis, the most common form of thyroiditis, is functionally characterized by a slow progression to hypothyroidism. In patients with hypothyroidism, T_3 and T_4 levels and T_3 uptake are low, and amounts of thyroid-stimulating hormone (TSH) increase abnormally (Patrick, 1993). The incidence of Hashimoto's thyroiditis peaks during the third to fifth decades, with a female/male ratio of 10:1. Autoantibodies directed against thyroglobulin (anti-Tg) and thyroid peroxidase (anti-TPO) antigens are clinically the most important for diagnosis (Patrick, 1993), but up to 20% of the adult female population with no clinical disease has detectable anti-Tg and/or anti-TPO, raising questions about their pathogenic significance (Patrick, 1993). Thyroid hormone replacement is reserved for patients with proven hypothyroidism.

Similarities between Graves' disease and Hashimoto's thyroiditis have been noted (Utiger, 1991). Both are associated with HLA-B8 and have a fundamentally similar pathogenesis, and it is believed that Graves' disease may progress to Hashimoto's thyroiditis (Utiger, 1991; Patrick, 1993).

AUTOANTIBODIES

Three major autoantibodies, including anti-TPO, anti-Tg, and autoantibody to thyroid stimulating hormone receptor (anti-TSHR), are important in autoimmune thyroid disease (Naparstek, 1993). Although anti-TPO and anti-Tg are considered markers of autoimmune thyroid disease, their

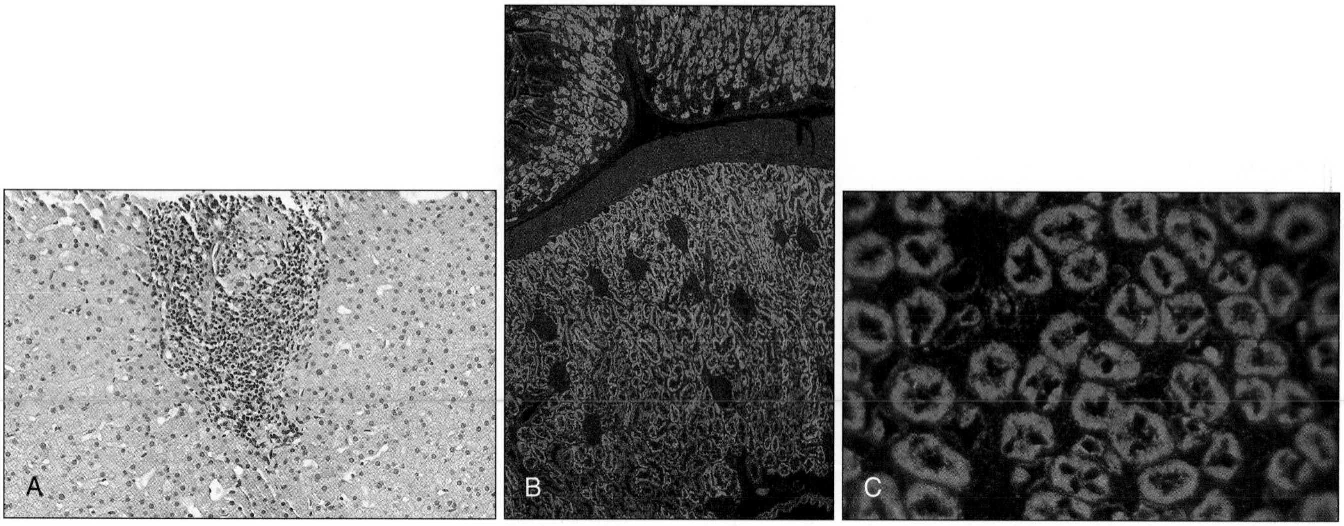

Figure 53-7 Liver biopsy in primary biliary cirrhosis shows variable portal inflammation with nonsuppurative lymphocytic cholangitis and, in this example, a florid duct lesion with granulomatous inflammation centered on an interlobular bile duct (**A,** Hematoxylin and eosin [H&E], ×200). Indirect immunofluorescence microscopy (IIFM) reveals diffuse immunofluorescence of renal tubules, including distal tubules (**B,** ×200), that has a homogeneous cytoplasmic appearance at higher power (**C,** ×500).

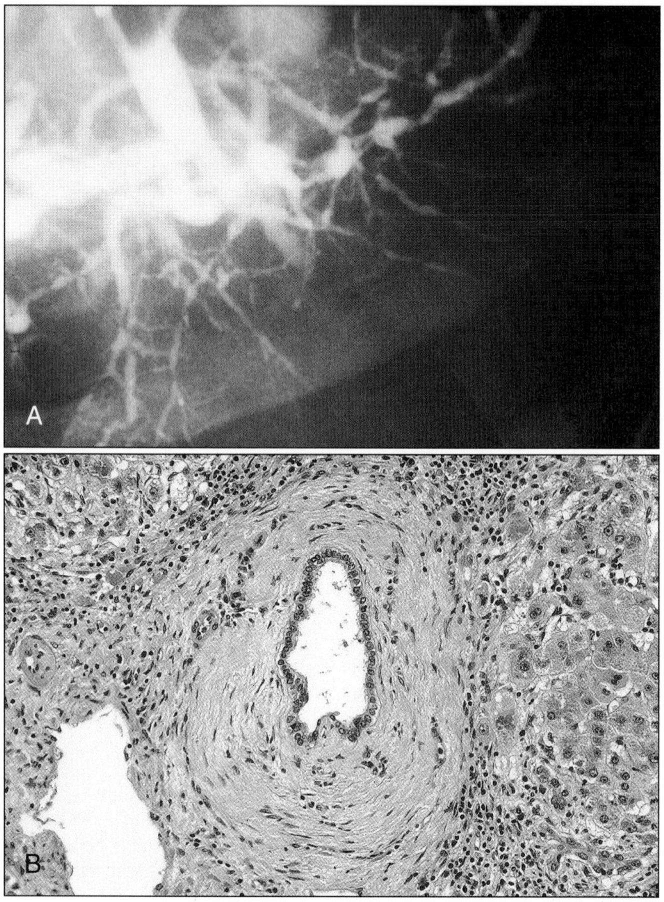

Figure 53-8 Cholangiogram in primary sclerosing cholangitis reveals the characteristic beading pattern of bile ducts due to multifocal strictures at those sites (**A**). Liver biopsy reveals prominent periduct fibrosis in the characteristic "onion-skin" pattern (**B,** Hematoxylin and eosin [H&E], ×500).

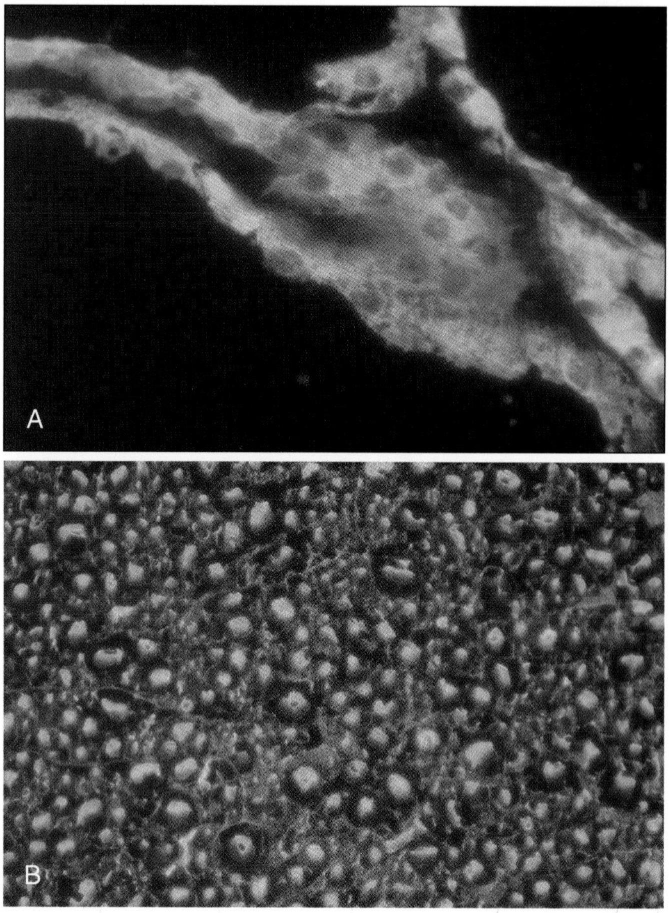

Figure 53-9 Indirect immunofluorescence microscopy of thyroid microsomal autoantibodies using unfixed monkey thyroid tissue as substrate (**A,** ×400) and of thyroglobulin autoantibodies using methanol-fixed cryostat tissue sections of monkey thyroid gland (**B,** ×200).

etiologic role has not been proved. They may occur as well in other organ-directed autoimmune diseases. Anti-TSHR, however, clearly plays a causal role in autoimmune thyroid disease (Naparstek, 1993).

Antithyroid Peroxidase Autoantibodies

Anti-TPO is directed to a 105-kDa antigen that is contained within the microsomal fraction of thyroid epithelial cell cytoplasm (Burek, 1995). ELISA is becoming a common and available method for detecting anti-TPO.

Historically, IIFM has been a popular and sensitive method for detecting anti-TPO (**antimicrosomal antibodies**). The IIFM test uses unfixed and air-dried human or monkey cryostat tissue sections as substrate. Positive sera stain the cytoplasm of thyroid follicular epithelial cells but do not stain their nuclei (Fig. 53-9, *A*). Anti-TPO must be differentiated from AMA when coarse granular cytoplasmic staining is noted; testing sera on mouse stomach/kidney tissue block can do this.

Anti-TPO can be detected in sera from patients with Graves' disease or Hashimoto's thyroiditis; its presence and titer correlate strongly with active clinical disease (Burek, 1995). Some controversy has arisen among investigators about whether determination of anti-TPO alone is sufficient to reliably detect autoimmune thyroid disease (Nordyke, 1993; Kaplan, 1999). The pathogenic role of anti-TPO remains unclear (Naparstek, 1993).

Antithyroglobulin Autoantibodies

Anti-Tg is targeted against thyroglobulin, which is the storage form of thyroid hormones within thyroid gland follicles (Burek, 1995). Several methods are available for measuring anti-Tg, including quantitative passive hemagglutination, IIFM, and ELISA.

Quantitative passive hemagglutination with chromic chloride hemagglutination or tanned red blood cells is the most widely used and sensitive method for detecting anti-Tg (Burek, 1995). Anti-Tg detected by hemagglutination is identified in titers greater than 1 : 1000 in about 80% of patients with Hashimoto's thyroiditis (Burek, 1995). Patients with Graves' disease (60%) or thyroid carcinoma (30%) or other autoimmune disorders such as pernicious anemia or Sjögren's syndrome, and 3%–18% of apparently normal individuals may also have anti-Tg, but their hemagglutination titers are usually (>90%) less than 1 : 1000 (Burek, 1995).

To locate anti-Tg, IIFM is done using methanol-fixed cryostat tissue sections of monkey thyroid gland (Fig. 53-9, *B*). Fixation is required to prevent loss of thyroglobulin during washing steps. Three patterns of immunofluorescence are described when anti-Tg is present (Burek, 1995): (1) floccular pattern, (2) dull colloid spaces but bright peripheral fluorescence, and (3) diffuse, bright, uniformly staining colloid in a "ground-glass" pattern attributed to the anti-Tg reaction with CA2 (Burek, 1995). CA2, or so-called second colloid antigen, is detected as the only serologic marker of autoimmune thyroiditis in the 5%–8% of patients who are positive by IIFM but negative for anti-Tg and anti-TPO using other methods (Bigazzi, 1992).

Anti–Thyroid-Stimulating Hormone Receptor Autoantibodies

Anti-TSHR autoantibodies consist of two groups of autoantibodies that can stimulate or block TSHRs, causing, respectively, hyperthyroidism or hypothyroidism. Anti-TSHR autoantibodies that bind to these receptors and stimulate thyroid hormone production are referred to as thyroid-stimulating immunoglobulins (TSIs), whereas anti-TSHR autoantibodies that bind to receptors and block the binding and function of TSH are referred to as thyroid-binding inhibitory immunoglobulins (TBIIs) (Mooij, 1993; Brunt, 1995). TSIs probably cause the hyperthyroidism in Graves' disease (Wilkin, 1990; Bigazzi, 1992; Brunt, 1995). Their prevalence varies from 55%–95%, depending on the method of detection (Bigazzi, 1992; Brunt, 1995). TSIs, which are usually of the IgG class, stimulate production of thyroid hormones by activating the adenylate cyclase system after binding to TSHRs (Patrick, 1993).

Detection of anti-TSHR is complex and is not part of routine clinical testing. The test may be useful for confirming Graves' disease in hyperthyroid patients with equivocal results in routine laboratory studies (Bigazzi, 1992). Additionally, one of the anti-TSHR assays may be used to monitor patients' hormone replacement therapy or to diagnose neonatal thyrotoxicosis (Bigazzi, 1992).

Two main classes of assays for anti-TSHRs are available, namely, bioassays and binding assays; their methodologic aspects are reviewed elsewhere (Gupta, 1988; Bigazzi, 1992; Patrick, 1993). Newer assays of a patient's serum based on stimulation of cyclic adenosine monophosphate (cAMP) in rat thyroid cells, maintained in tissue culture, may prove to be an improvement over the technically difficult bioassays (Burek, 1995).

TSIs are measured in bioassays that determine increased TSHR-mediated activity by measuring the release of cAMP or by measuring the uptake of iodide by thyroid cells maintained in culture (Brunt, 1995). TBIIs are measured by determining binding inhibition of radiolabeled TSH to its receptor, or by using cAMP bioassays (Brunt, 1995).

Kidney

GLOMERULONEPHRITIS

Glomerulonephritis is a major cause of primary renal disease. Immune-mediated mechanisms are thought to have an important role in the pathogenesis of glomerulonephritis, although experimental confirmation of such putative autoimmune mechanisms is still lacking.

DIFM has an important role in the study and diagnosis of glomerulonephritis (Fig. 53-10). The patterns of immune reactants can be divided broadly into those that cause granular or linear deposits within glomeruli or other kidney structures examined with DIFM. Granular deposits have been attributed to immune complexes that settle out of circulating blood or form in situ (McCluskey, 1995). DIFM patterns of immune deposits associated with major glomerular diseases are summarized in Table 53-6. Thorough reviews of these disorders are available in several texts (Heptinstall, 1992; McCluskey, 1995). However, for this discussion,

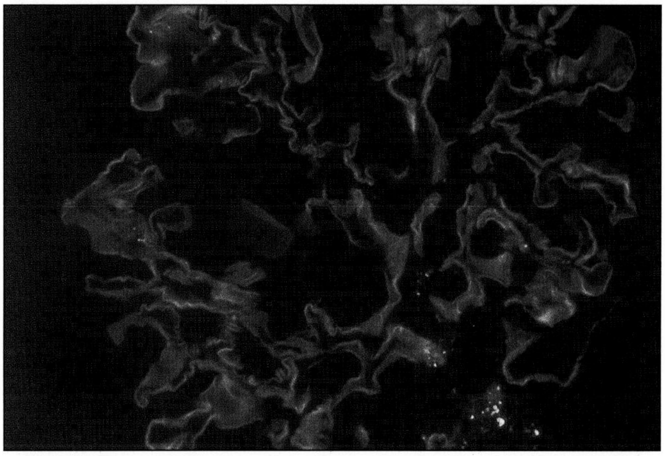

Figure 53-10 Direct immunofluorescence microscopy reveals global and linear glomerular basement membrane immunofluorescence in anti–glomerular basement membrane disease (×400).

TABLE 53-6
Major Glomerular Diseases With Direct Immunofluorescent Findings

Immunofluorescent pattern and disease	Immune reactant(s)
Granular, Mesangial, and GBM Deposits	
Acute poststreptococcal glomerulonephritis	Scattered C3 ± IgG, IgM
Diffuse proliferative lupus nephritis	IgG, IgA, IgM, C3
Membranoproliferative glomerulonephritis (MPGN, type I)	C3, IgG, IgM
Idiopathic immune complex crescentic glomerulonephritis	IgG, C3 ± IgM
Dense deposit disease (MPGN, type II)	C3 (globular) ± IgM
Chronic infections (e.g., bacterial endocarditis)	IgG, IgM, C3
Granular, Mesangial Predominant	
Lupus nephritis	
Mesangial	IgG, C3; usually IgM and IgA
Focal proliferative	IgG, C3, IgA; focal capillary loop deposits
Henoch-Schönlein purpura	IgA predominant; IgG, IgM, C3
IgA nephropathy	IgA predominant; often IgG, IgM, C3
Granular, GBM Predominant	
Membranous lupus nephritis	IgG, C3, IgA, IgM
Mixed cryoglobulinemia	IgM, IgG, C3; intravascular masses
Linear GBM	
Anti-GBM nephritis	IgG, C3; IgA and IgM infrequent
Light chain nephropathy	Usually κ light chain, may be in TBM, blood vessels, interstitium

Modified from McCluskey RT, Collins AB, Niles JL. Kidney. In: Colvin RB, Bhan AK, McCluskey RT, editors. Diagnostic immunopathology. 2nd ed. New York: Raven Press; 1995, p. 109.

GBM, Glomerular basement membrane; *Ig,* immunoglobulin; *MPGN,* membranoproliferative glomerulonephritis; *TBM,* tubular basement membrane.

only anti–glomerular basement membrane (anti-GBM) autoantibodies are presented in some additional detail.

ANTI–GLOMERULAR BASEMENT MEMBRANE DISEASE

Patients with anti-GBM disease vary in clinical presentation in that about 50% have renal-limited disease, and the other 50% have both renal and pulmonary symptoms. This latter presentation is often called Goodpasture's syndrome. Rarely, patients with anti-GBM disease may have pulmonary limited disease (Wilson, 1987).

Diagnosis of anti-GBM disease requires detection of anti-GBM autoantibodies to the NC1 domain of type IV collagen (McCluskey, 1995), the so-called Goodpasture's antigen. Methods for detecting circulating anti-GBM have included IIFM, ELISA, and RIA (Wilson, 1987; McCluskey, 1995); some investigators have additionally developed a sensitive Western blot test (McCluskey, 1995). Because IIFM is difficult to standardize and requires experience to perform, methods for detection have focused instead on validation of quantitative RIA or ELISA. Currently, a licensed commercial ELISA kit is available for the measurement of anti-GBM. This assay determines patient values from a standard curve and reports negative, borderline, or positive ranges. Most patients with active anti-GBM disease appear to have values greater than 100 units. Although borderline values can be seen in both active and quiescent anti-GBM disease, we have also seen such values in patients with renal disorders that are not anti-GBM disease.

The coexistence of antineutrophil cytoplasmic antibodies (ANCAs) has been documented in some patients with rapidly progressive glomerulonephritis (McCluskey, 1995). The coexistence of these two autoantibodies has varied from 0–40% of patients with rapidly progressive glomerulonephritis, accompanied by some evidence that the presence of ANCA in patients with anti-GBM disease affords a better renal prognosis (McCluskey, 1995).

ADRENAL GLAND

ADDISON'S DISEASE

Nontuberculous chronic adrenocortical insufficiency, or Addison's disease, has an estimated prevalence of 3–6 cases per 100,000 people (Muir, 1993). Among such patients, 65%–70% have circulating autoantibodies to adrenal cortex cells, demonstrable using IIFM on frozen sections of human adrenal cortex (Muir, 1993; Patrick, 1993; Burek, 1995). 21-Hydroxylase and 17α-hydroxylase are two autoantigens that have been identified as reactive with adrenocortical autoantibodies (Song, 1994; Devendra, 2004). Adrenocortical autoantibodies are not found in Addison's disease caused by tuberculosis or other exogenous agents (Patrick, 1993). About 45% of asymptomatic individuals with serum adrenocortical autoantibodies develop impaired adrenocortical function within 2.5 years after the autoantibody is identified (Muir, 1991).

Addison's disease associated with autoantibodies is most commonly diagnosed in persons between the ages of 20 and 50 years and is two to three times more frequent in females when diagnosed after the age of 30 (Muir, 1993; Patrick, 1993).

Laboratory tests show metabolic acidosis, hyperkalemia, hyponatremia, and low levels of serum chloride and bicarbonate. Plasma cortisol levels are also low and adrenocorticotropic hormone levels are elevated (Van Arsdel, 1993). Consequently, therapy consists of replacing glucocorticoids and mineralocorticoids (Patrick, 1993).

Addison's disease associated with autoantibodies can occur by itself but is more commonly accompanied by other autoimmune disorders as part of an autoimmune polyglandular syndrome (Muir, 1993). These companion diseases may include autoimmune thyroiditis, pernicious anemia, or insulin-dependent diabetes mellitus (Patrick, 1993).

In addition to adrenocortical autoantibodies, other adrenal autoantibodies have been detected in patients with Addison's disease, including steroid cell autoantibodies and autoantibodies that bind adrenocorticotropic hormone receptors (Muir, 1993).

PANCREAS

DIABETES MELLITUS

Diabetes mellitus (see Chapter 16) is the diagnostic term applied to a group of metabolic disorders that share hyperglycemia as their common link (Eisenbarth, 1995). That it is a serious diagnosis is documented by the fact that acute and chronic multiorgan diabetic complications account for about 15% of total U.S. health care expenditures. However, significant progress has been made in the care of diabetic patients, with the knowledge that aggressive blood glucose control reduces the risk for development of and progression to vascular complications.

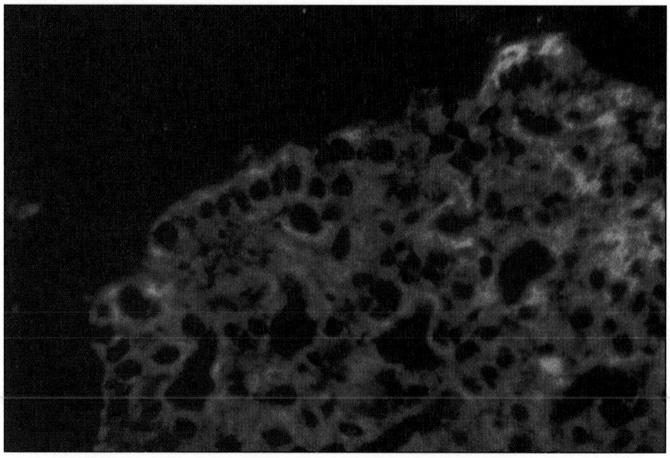

Figure 53-11 Indirect immunofluorescence microscopy of islet cell autoantibodies using human blood group O pancreas as substrate (×400).

Clinical Subtypes

The major clinical subgroups of diabetes mellitus are type 1A for immune-mediated diabetes, type 1B for non–immune-mediated diabetes with severe insulin deficiency, and a subgroup of adult type 2 diabetes with anti-islet autoantibodies that is termed latent autoimmune diabetes mellitus (American Diabetes Association, 1997; Devendra, 2004). Type 2 diabetes mellitus was formerly termed non–insulin-dependent diabetes and most commonly occurs in obese individuals older than 30 years.

Major types of circulating autoantibody in type 1A diabetes mellitus include the following: islet cell autoantibodies (ICAs); glutamic acid decarboxylase autoantibodies (anti-GAD); insulin autoantibodies (IAAs); and insulinoma-associated-2 and -2β autoantibodies (Lan, 1996; Schmidli, 1998; Devendra, 2004).

Islet Cell Autoantibodies

IIFM is the classical method used for detection of ICAs (Atkinson, 1993b). Frozen sections of human pancreas are used as the tissue substrate to detect specific, finely granular, cytoplasmic fluorescence in all cells of pancreatic islets (Fig. 53-11). Human blood group O is recommended as substrate to reduce nonspecific background interference due to ABO isohemagglutinins. Using IIFM, ICAs are detectable in about 80% of patients with newly diagnosed type 1A diabetes, 3%–4% of nondiabetic relatives of patients with type 1A diabetes, and only 0.5% of clinically normal subjects (Atkinson, 1994). ICAs include autoantibodies specifically reactive with anti-GAD, as well as non–GAD-reactive ICAs (Kaufman, 1992; Atkinson, 1993b).

ICA should be titered in Juvenile Diabetes Foundation (JDF) units in reference to an 80-unit standard serum from the Immunology of Diabetes Workshop; titers greater than 20 JDF units seem to have prognostic significance (Maclaren, 1992). Commercial ICA assays using primate substrate are available.

Insulin Autoantibodies

IAAs are identified in about 50% of patients with type 1A diabetes at the time of diagnosis and before insulin therapy begins (Atkinson, 1994). IAAs are usually measured using a technically demanding competitive radioimmunoprecipitation assay. This assay cannot distinguish between IAAs occurring spontaneously and those that occur as a result of insulin therapy. Therefore, IAAs need to be measured before insulin is administered.

Glutamic Acid Decarboxylase Autoantibodies

Anti-GADs are detected in most newly diagnosed type 1A diabetes patients and in about 80% of prediabetic, first-degree relatives of patients (Hagopian, 1993; Schatz, 1995). The two GAD autoantigens, classified by molecular mass, are designated GAD65 and GAD67 (Atkinson, 1993a). Anti-GADs are directed primarily at the GAD65 isoform, which is found

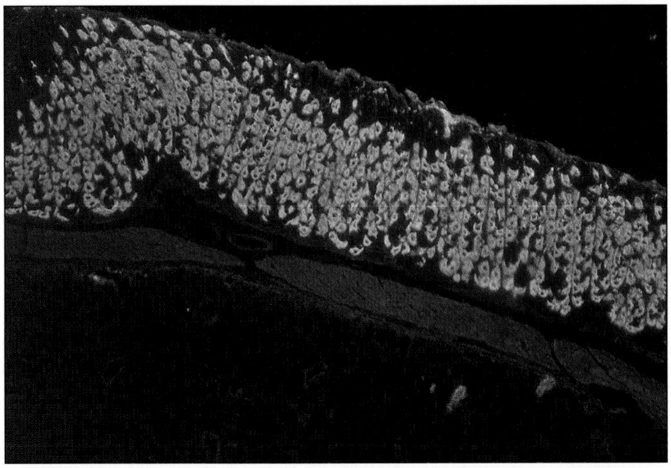

Figure 53-12 Indirect immunofluorescence microscopy of gastric antiparietal cell autoantibodies using mouse stomach/kidney as substrate (×400).

mainly in pancreatic islets and in the central nervous system (CNS), where it functions as an enzyme responsible for formation of the inhibiting neurotransmitter γ-aminobutyric acid (Maclaren, 1988; Barmeier, 1992; Kaufman, 1992; Luhder, 1994). The GAD67 form predominates in peripheral nerves (Atkinson, 1993; Falorni, 1994).

GAD autoantibodies are also associated with the rare stiff-man syndrome (Eisenbarth, 1995). A high percentage of these patients have type 1A diabetes.

Interpretation and Clinical Utility of Autoantibodies in Type 1A Diabetes

ICA, anti-GAD, IAA, and IA-2 autoantibodies are used currently as predictive markers for diabetes. ICA is a specific marker associated with an elevated risk of developing type 1A diabetes, but ICAs do not persist. Anti-GAD is usually detected before the diagnosis of diabetes and usually declines in titer after the onset of clinical diabetes (Schatz, 1994). Initial screening for autoantibodies associated with type 1A diabetes has been limited to ICA and IAA (Devendra, 2004).

Identification of islet autoantibodies can be used to confirm autoimmunity in patients with acute diabetes, which differentiates type 1A from type 1B diabetes. The use of these markers to identify individuals at risk for type 1A is being evaluated to determine the need for metabolic studies that would assess subclinical glucose intolerance and call for immunotherapy in the preclinical phase of diabetes (Maclaren, 1992). Measurement of anti-GAD using ELISA may eventually improve the feasibility of widespread screening for this autoantibody.

In addition to the autoantibodies discussed previously, patients with diabetes may have anti-TPO, antiparietal cell, and antiadrenocortical autoantibodies, so diabetes patients should be screened for these autoantibodies at least once (Maclaren, 1992).

Gastrointestinal Tract

PERNICIOUS ANEMIA

Pernicious anemia is an organ-specific autoimmune disease accompanied by cobalamin deficiency, megaloblastic anemia, neuropathy, and autoimmune gastritis with anti-intrinsic factor (anti-IF) (Gueant, 1997).

Pernicious anemia is characterized by histamine-fast achlorhydria, hypergastrinemia, and vitamin B_{12} deficiency (Brown, 1995). The insidious onset of neurologic symptoms and the development of megaloblastic anemia are typical features of the clinical course (Patrick, 1993). Morphologically, biopsy of the stomach body mucosa contains evidence of chronic atrophic gastritis.

Pernicious anemia is associated with circulating antiparietal cell (APC) autoantibodies in 90% of patients and with anti-IF in 60%–75% of patients, although anti-IF may be more specific for pernicious anemia (Brown, 1995; Burek, 1995). APCs are detected by IIFM performed on mouse stomach/kidney tissue blocks. This combined tissue block allows identification of specific parietal cell staining when there is no concomitant staining of renal tubules as would be seen in the presence of AMAs (Fig. 53-12).

The epitope domain of type I antibodies was found to be an amino acid sequence of 251–256 in the human IF (Gueant, 1997).

Anti-IF is most commonly detected by RIA. Of the two known types of anti-IF, type 1 anti-IF, or blocking autoantibody, prevents the binding of IF to vitamin B_{12}, and type 2, or binding autoantibody, reacts with free or complexed vitamin B_{12} to inhibit the action of IF (Patrick, 1993; Karen, 1994). Type 1 anti-IF is considered more diagnostically sensitive and specific for pernicious anemia (Karen, 1994). However, identification of APCs or anti-IF is not required for diagnosis of pernicious anemia. Pernicious anemia can occur in association with other autoimmune diseases, such as autoimmune thyroiditis or Addison's disease, and may be a part of autoimmune polyglandular syndrome 1 or autoimmune polyglandular syndrome 2 (Patrick, 1993).

CELIAC DISEASE (GLUTEN-SENSITIVE ENTEROPATHY)

Celiac disease is a lifelong inflammatory autoimmune disease of the gastrointestinal tract that affects genetically susceptible persons. Several other autoimmune diseases may be associated with celiac disease, such as type 1 diabetes mellitus and autoimmune thyroiditis (Shaoul, 2007). The common immunogenetic basis for this association is the fact that the diseases share common HLA and non-HLA genes.

More recently, deaminated gliadin peptides have been employed as targets for celiac disease–specific antibodies. Assay with the use of deaminated gliadin peptides measures a new species of antibodies, which differs from conventional gliadin antibodies (Mothes, 2007). The deaminated gliadin peptide antibody test showed a sensitivity of 90% and a specificity of 98% in celiac disease (Kaukinen, 2007). The deaminated gliadin peptide antibody test showed six of the nine cases with small-bowel mucosal damage persisting on a gluten-free diet, whereas tTG detected only two cases and the endomysial antibody test detected none (Kaukinen, 2007). The deaminated gliadin peptide antibody test has been recommended for workup of celiac cases, along with the tTG test. In a prospective study, almost all of the tTG-positive sera drawn from children who later developed celiac disease were also positive for gliadin peptide antibodies (Ankelo, 2007).

Susceptibility to celiac disease is genetically determined by possession of specific HLA-DQ alleles acting in concert with one or more non–HLA-linked genes (Bevan, 1999). Determination of HLA-DqZ and HLA-DQ8 is useful in the exclusion of celiac disease. Also, individual genetic testing will help to assess the risk of celiac disease among families in a high-risk population compared with the normal population (Karell, 2003; Liu, 2006).

Gluten-sensitive enteropathy (GSE), or celiac disease sprue, is a small-bowel disease characterized by malabsorption of gastrointestinal fat. Until recently, GSE was considered a rare disease in the United States, but now the prevalence is considered much greater than was previously estimated—about 1% of the U.S. population (Ferguson, 1997; NIH Consensus, 2004; Rostom, 2004). Patients may have nongastrointestinal manifestations that dominate the clinical presentation, such as anemia, neurologic symptoms, and autoimmune disease (Green, 2003). Hypersensitivity to gluten, or gluten derivatives, is the cause of GSE (Brown, 1995). Small-bowel biopsy from a patient with GSE is variably abnormal, but characteristic changes include villous atrophy, crypt elongation, intraepithelial lymphocytes, and crypt mitoses.

Patients with GSE manifest several humoral immune alterations. Serum IgA levels are usually elevated in GSE patients, except in those with an IgA deficiency, which does occur in GSE patients more commonly than in normal individuals (Brown, 1995). Patients with GSE may have circulating IgA antiendomysial, antireticulin, and/or antigliadin autoantibodies. IgA antiendomysial autoantibodies are detectable by IIFM using monkey esophagus as tissue substrate (Fig. 53-13). IgA antiendomysial autoantibodies detect tTG, the primary autoantigen in GSE (Dieterich, 1997). ELISA is now available for the detection of anti–tissue transglutaminase (anti-tTG). Their identification is considered diagnostically sensitive and specific for GSE alone or GSE associated with dermatitis herpetiformis (GSE-DH) (Talal, 1997). The titer of IgA antiendomysial autoantibody may be measured to monitor a patient's compliance with a gluten-free diet (Karen, 1994).

Antireticulin autoantibodies are detected by IIFM on a mouse stomach/kidney combined tissue block. These autoantibodies are detectable in adults (40%), in children with GSE (60%) and in adults with GSE-DH (20%). However, antireticulin autoantibodies are diagnostically nonspecific and generally are no longer considered useful in the diagnosis of GSE, being present also in patients with Crohn's disease, myasthenia gravis, Sjögren's syndrome, and other connective tissue disorders.

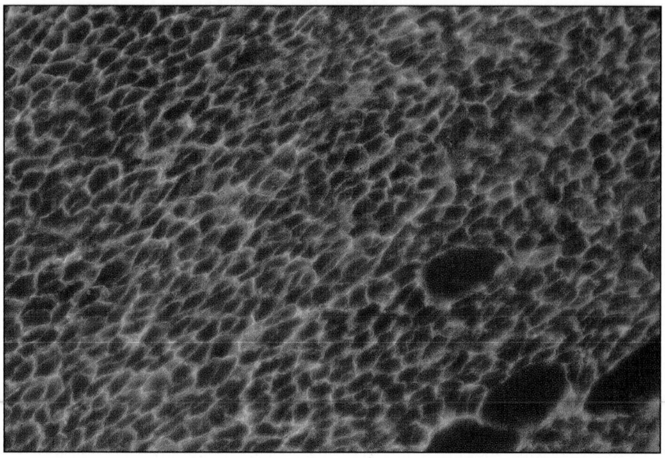

Figure 53-13 Indirect immunofluorescence microscopy of immunoglobulin (Ig) A endomysial autoantibodies using monkey esophagus as substrate (×400).

Antigliadin autoantibodies are detected by ELISA in almost all patients with GSE or GSE-DH (Brown, 1995). The target antigen, gliadin, is purified from gluten and is used in a solid-phase ELISA to detect these autoantibodies. Similar to IgA endomysial autoantibodies, antigliadin autoantibodies can be used to monitor a patient's adherence to a gluten-free diet. Antigliadin antibodies are less specific than anti-tTG and anti-endomysial antibodies.

A patient suspected of having GSE should be tested while on a normal, gluten-containing diet. In suspected patients without chronic liver disease, the presence of anti-tTG and/or IgA antiendomysial antibodies in the appropriate clinical setting is supportive of GSE. However, most clinicians consider histologic confirmation on small-bowel biopsy to be necessary to establish the diagnosis. Negative serology does not exclude a diagnosis of GSE, and IgA deficiency should be considered in patients with a suggestive clinical presentation. If IgA deficiency is identified, an IgG-tTg or IgG antiendomysial antibody test should be performed (NIH Consensus, 2004).

Compliance with a gluten-restricted diet can be monitored by anti-tTG, IgA antiendomysial, or deaminated gliadin peptide assay.

IDIOPATHIC INFLAMMATORY BOWEL DISEASE

Inflammatory bowel disease (IBD) is the term used to describe diseases that cause inflammation of the intestine. Crohn's disease (CD) and ulcerative colitis (UC) are the two major IBDs.

In CD, inflammation often occurs in the distal ileum but may affect any part of the digestive tract. In CD, inflammation is typically transmural with lymphoid aggregates and often forms granulomas. In UC, inflammation is mucosally based, with chronic active inflammation with ulcers involving the colon, especially the rectum.

Sensitive p-ANCA Associated With Ulcerative Colitis

p-ANCA, antineutrophilic cytoplasmic antibody, and a number of other (auto)antibodies have been described in patients with CD or UC (Nakamura, 2003; Vermeire, 2008). The antibody markers reflect a loss of tolerance toward bacterial and fungal antigens. These markers include p-ANCA, antibodies to *Saccharomyces cerevisiae* (ASCA), antipancreatic antibody, Omp C antibody, CBirl antibody, I-2 antibody, and others (Nakamura, 2003; Bossugt, 2006; Vermeire, 2008).

Most adult patients with UC (60%–80%) exhibit a positive test for p-ANCA. p-ANCA has been observed in 83% of children with UC. Billing (1995) provided evidence that the p-ANCA associated with UC is nuclear in location and differs from other types of p-ANCA.

It appears that the p-ANCA–associated antigen seen with IBD is located in the nuclei and most likely is a complex conformational epitope associated with histone (H-1), HMG-1, HMG-2 (high mobility group nuclear protein), and a nuclear envelope protein that is a 50-kDa nuclear envelope protein (Nakamura, 2003).

This p-ANCA pattern seen in IBD is the result of nuclear antigens that are sensitive to DNase digestion of substrate cells. In approximately 70% of cases of UC, convergence of the patterns and antigen occurs, and in 30% of cases, convergence to a homogenous cytoplasmic staining pattern is seen. The p-ANCA pattern is noted in 60%–80% of UC patients and in 10%–30% of CD patients.

IBD-associated ANCA was first reported by Faber and Elling (1967), who described "leukocyte specific anti-nuclear antibodies" in patients with CD and UC. It is now clear that the granulocyte-specific antibodies in IBD are in fact p-ANCA. The p-ANCA antibodies in IBD differ from antibodies observed in vascular diseases that are reactive with myeloperoxidase (see Chapter 52). Studies have shown that p-ANCA production takes place in the colonic mucosa.

p-ANCA is detected in 10%–30% of patients with CD. In CD, the expression of p-ANCA identifies a subgroup of CD characterized as "ulcerative colitis (UC)-like" phenotype, in which patients have clinical features of UC.

CD patients who are p-ANCA positive do not respond as well as the majority of CD patients to anti–tumor necrosis factor (TNF) monoclonal antibody therapy. On the other hand, 65% of CD patients respond well to anti-TNF monoclonal antibody therapy.

High levels of p-ANCA in CD patients were associated with later age of onset and UC-like inflammatory response, as well as a relatively decreased incidence of fibrostenosis and penetrating disease.

The p-ANCA pattern has been reported in 92% of patients with well-defined type 1 autoimmune hepatitis and in up to 70% of primary sclerosing cholangitis patients. The p-ANCA associated with UC-reactive antigen was associated with epitopes within the nuclei. Also, UC p-ANCA demonstrated as a dominant feature loss of antigen recognition after DNase-1 enzyme digestion of neutrophils.

In contrast, a majority of type 1 autoimmune hepatitis and primary sclerosing cholangitis patients showed a p-ANCA pattern–recognizing cytoplasmic constituent. Thus, UC-associated p-ANCA with nuclear epitopes is highly specific for IBD (Vidrich, 1995).

Anti-ASCAs have been found to be significantly more prevalent in patients with CD as compared with UC patients or healthy controls. These antibodies include both IgA and IgG classes directed against mannose sequences in the cell wall mannan of *Saccharomyces cerevisiae.* The presence of IgG or IgA ASCA has been shown to have a high specificity for CD. However, a subgroup of CD patients do not have ASCA antibodies. IgG and IgA ASCAs have been demonstrated in 60%–70% of patients with CD, 10%–15% of patients with UC, and 0–5% of control patients (Vasiliauskas, 2000; Bossugt, 2006).

Antibodies against exocrine pancreas have been described in CD patients with a prevalence of 30% (Joossens, 2006). The antigen has not been elucidated, and the antibodies are detected by IIFM.

NERVOUS SYSTEM

MYASTHENIA GRAVIS

Myasthenia gravis (MG) is a neuromuscular disorder characterized by use-associated muscular weakness, fatigue, and the presence of antiacetylcholine receptor (anti-AChR) autoantibodies. AChRs, located in postsynaptic membranes of skeletal muscle fibers, bind acetylcholine (ACh) from nerve endings, which causes a muscle contraction when enough ACh has been released (Naparstek, 1993; Rose, 1995). Anti-AChR autoantibodies interfere with this neuromuscular function, resulting in muscle weakness and fatigue.

Anti-AChR autoantibodies are detected in about 90% of MG patients (Rose, 1995). Radiolabeled α-bungarotoxin (α-BTx) is used in competitive RIAs to measure different forms of anti-AchR (Barna, 1995). α-BTx is a protein from snake venom that essentially irreversibly binds AChR, but it binds to ACh receptors at a site different from binding sites for anti-AchR (Rose, 1995). AChRs are obtained from extracts of denervated human skeletal muscle, such as from diabetic amputations, or from tissue cell culture. For testing, AChRs are labeled with α-BTx, then are incubated with patients' serum to allow any anti-AChR autoantibodies present to bind to AChRs at sites near the α-BTx binding site. After incubation, the radiolabeled complexes are precipitated by polyvalent antihuman immunoglobulin, and after correction for nonspecific binding, the washed precipitate is counted for radioactivity. The degree of radioactivity in the precipitate is directly proportional to the amount of anti-AChR in the patient's serum.

Modifications of this binding assay can be used to identify anti-AChR blocking and modulating autoantibodies. In a blocking assay, patients' sera containing anti-AChR are allowed to incubate with AChRs before α-BTx is added. The basis for this technique is the premise that anti-AChR capable of blocking α-BTx binding also blocks ACh binding to AChRs (Rose, 1995). The amount of radioactivity in the precipitate therefore is inversely proportional to the amount of anti-AChR in patients' sera.

Modulating anti-AChR autoantibodies are thought to accelerate AChR degradation, but their measurement in the clinical laboratory is technically difficult and is not widely performed.

Some MG cases have antibodies against skeletal muscle antigens, in addition to antibodies to AChR. A major epitope is the CA^{++} release channel of the sacroplasmic reticulum, called the ryandine receptor (RyR) (Skeie, 2008). These RyR antibodies are found mainly in MG patients with thymoma and correlate with severe MG symptoms. Also, antititin antibodies are a sensitive marker of thymoma-associated MG (Yamamoto, 2001). Titin is the major autoantigen recognized by antistriated muscle antibodies. Non-AChR muscle autoantibodies are present in many MG serum samples, mainly from patients with thymoma or late-onset MG (Mygland, 2000; Romi, 2000).

MULTIPLE SCLEROSIS

Multiple sclerosis (MS) is a relatively common demyelinating disease involving the white matter of the brain and spinal cord. It occurs more frequently in females than in males (2 : 1 ratio) and is usually evident during young adulthood, with a wide variety of possible clinical manifestations. About 50% of patients undergo alternating periods of active disease and remission, whereas the remainder follow a chronic progressive course (Steinman, 1993; McFarland, 1995). The diagnosis of multiple sclerosis derives from clinical findings and exclusion of all other disorders.

MS is a T cell–mediated autoimmune demyelinating disease that may be initiated by a virus infection (Kurtzke, 1993; Miller, 1997). However, the exact cause of MS is unknown, and autoimmune mechanisms are important in the pathogenesis of this disease (McFarland, 1995). No characteristic circulating autoantibodies have been noted in MS.

Laboratory examination of cerebrospinal fluid (CSF) provides important information that supports a diagnosis of MS in an appropriate clinical setting (Barna, 1995). Synthesis of IgG increases abnormally within the CNS of MS patients, so that measurement of the IgG index and the IgG synthetic rate provides useful, but not specific, test results (Valenzuela, 1995; Zweiman, 1991; Karen, 1994; McFarland, 1995). Evaluation of CSF for oligoclonal bands is also useful in the appropriate clinical setting, because they are identified in more than 90% of MS patients; however, their presence is not diagnostically specific, in that they can be detected in patients with such diverse disorders as neurosyphilis, CNS vasculitis, Lyme disease, subacute sclerosing panencephalitis, Creutzfeldt-Jakob disease, stroke, Guillain-Barré syndrome, and neoplasms (Karen, 1994). Serum protein electrophoresis must also be performed to ensure that CSF oligoclonal bands are not the result of serum leakage into the CSF. CSF oligoclonal bands are usually measured by high-resolution agarose electrophoresis of concentrated CSF (Karen, 1994).

NEUROPATHIES

Autoimmune disorders of the peripheral nervous system consist of a heterogeneous group of diseases that result from an aberrant immune response (Quattrini, 2003). Serum antibodies against ganglioside (GMI) and/or GDIb are frequently detected in autoimmune neuropathies, such as multifocal motor neuropathy, IgM paraproteinemic neuropathy, and Guillan-Barré syndrome. Some of them bind to GMI or EDIb monospecifically, but others can cross-react with both antigens (Kusunoki, 1993). These autoantibodies may interact with endothelial cell–bound antigens, which can affect the permeability of the blood-brain or nerve barrier to permit entry of autoantibodies into the nervous system (Yu, 1990).

The autoantibodies that bind to or block ganglionic AChRs identify a group of patients with autoimmune neuropathy (Vernino, 2000).

Considerable evidence indicates that many of the neuropathies of the peripheral nervous system have an immune-mediated pathogenic mechanism with development of various autoantibodies (Ho, 1998; Naparstek, 1993).

Autoantibodies to neural antigens have been demonstrated in both motor and sensory neuropathies. Patients with motor neuropathies show evidence of high IgM anti-GMI antibody levels (Carney, 2002).

TABLE 53-7
Antibodies in Common Paraneoplastic Neurologic Syndromes and Associated Tumors

Antibody	Clinical syndrome	Associated tumors and conditions
Anti-Yo	Cerebellar degeneration	Ovary, breast
Anti-Hu (ANNA-1)	Brain and cerebellar dysfunction	SCLC, neuroblastoma
Anti-Ri (ANNA-2)	Opsoclonus-myoclonus	Breast, ovary, SCLC
Antiamphiphysin	Stiff-man syndrome Encephalitis-neuropathy	Breast, ovary, SCLC Diabetes mellitus
Anti-VGCC	Lambert-Eaton myasthenia syndrome	SCLC

SCLC, Small cell lung cancer; *VGCC,* voltage-gated calcium channels (anti-body).

High titers of antisulfatide antibodies are also present in motor and sensory neuropathies, but are more frequently associated with demyelinating neuropathies. Neuropathies with evidence of demyelination often demonstrate antibodies to myelin-associated glycoprotein and sulfoglucuronyl paragloboside.

These autoantibodies may be detected by ELISA, IIFM, or immunohistochemistry. The importance of identifying such autoantibodies will undoubtedly increase as/if clinical studies correlate their presence with a particular disease or a therapeutic benefit. However, to date, these autoantibodies are not disease-specific and can occur even after trauma to the nervous system. Autoantibodies to primary neural components include those to neuronal proteins or to neuronal gangliosides (Zeballos, 1992; Darnell, 2003).

PARANEOPLASTIC NEUROLOGIC SYNDROMES

Paraneoplastic neurologic syndromes (PNSs) are diseases that occur as remote effects of tumors.

The most common types of tumors involved in PNS are small cell lung cancer (SCLC), thymoma, neuroblastoma, ovarian, breast, testicular, and Hodgkin lymphoma.

One of the reasons for PNS is that the tumor and the nervous system share antigens, so that the autoimmune response generated against the tumor initiates the neurologic problem (Anderson, 2008).

In Table 53-7 are listed various autoantibodies in the PNS.

Neurologic paraneoplastic syndromes may be the presenting feature of an occult tumor (Dalmau-Posner, 1999; Posner, 2000). For example, Lambert-Eaton syndrome is strongly associated with SCLC and P/Q-type voltage-gated calcium channel antibodies. Paraneoplastic sensory neuropathy is associated with SCLC or gynecologic tumors and with ANNA-1 anti-Hu antibodies.

The diagnostic value of a positive antineuronal antibody in patients with PNS is high, because the existence of an underlying malignancy can be seen in more than 90% of seropositive patients (Nakamura, 2002).

STIFF-MAN SYNDROME

Stiff-man syndrome is a rare disorder of the CNS of progressive fluctuating muscle rigidity with painful spasms. It is associated with IDDM and with epilepsy. (Solimena, 1998) reported evidence that impairment of neuronal pathways that operate through γ-aminobutyric acid is involved in the pathogenesis of stiff-man syndrome. Patients have antibodies to anti-GAD, which is the enzyme responsible for the synthesis of γ-aminobutyric acid.

In 1956, Moersch and Woltman, who coined the term **stiff-man syndrome,** described the syndrome as a neurologic clinical entity at the Mayo Clinic. Symptoms begin from age 30–50 and show evidence of anti-GAD in 60% of patients.

OTHER ORGANS

HEART

In idiopathic dilated cardiomyopathy (IDCM), evidence suggests that autoimmune reactions against certain myocyte antigens may play a pivotal role in the initiation and/or progression of IDCM (Jahns, 2008). These autoantibodies are probably "pathogenic" and can contribute in causing cardiac dysfunction and heart failure. Warraich (2006) presented evidence that human cardiac myosin autoantibodies can impair cardiac myocyte contractility. Other publications show evidence that autoantibodies could promote myocardial damage by inducing inflammation or interference with surface receptors on cardiomyocytes (Shmilovich, 2007). Also, organ-specific cardiac antibodies were seen more frequently in patients with dilated cardiomyopathy than in those with other cardiac diseases (Caforio, 1990).

Myocardial Autoantibodies

Autoantibodies to the myocardium have been reported as a part of several conditions that damage cardiac striated muscle, including myocardial infarction, post cardiac surgery, and cardiomyopathy; their identification may help differentiate immune-mediated cardiomyopathy from other causes of myocarditis (Naparstek, 1993; Burek, 1995). IIFM on frozen sections of monkey heart is used to detect myocardial autoantibodies. Specific myocardial staining can also be determined by excluding reactivity on noncardiac skeletal muscle. Unfortunately, AMA and/or heterophile autoantibodies can cause fluorescent staining that may be confused with that caused by myocardial autoantibodies.

MUSCLE

Skeletal Muscle Autoantibodies

Skeletal muscle autoantibodies have limited clinical applicability. Low titers (<1:30) may be seen in apparently healthy individuals, whereas some patients with myopathic disorders may have titers up to 1:60. Although high titers (>1:60) of skeletal muscle autoantibodies have been found in patients with MG, anti-AChR assays have greater clinical utility in diagnosing or monitoring MG.

About 50% of patients with thymoma have paraneoplastic MG. These patients with thymoma-associated MG produce autoantibodies to a variety of neuromuscular antigens, such as AChR, titin, skeletal muscle calcium release channel (RyR) and voltage-gated potassium channels (Mygland, 2000).

Skeletal muscle autoantibodies are detected by IIFM on frozen sections of monkey thigh skeletal muscle (Fig. 53-14).

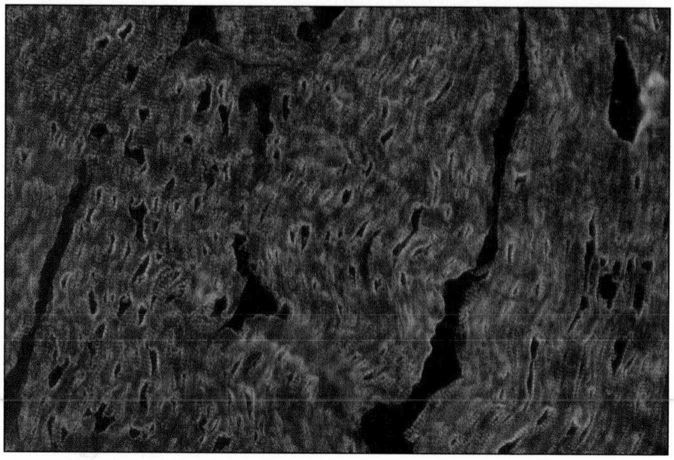

Figure 53-14 Indirect immunofluorescence microscopy of skeletal muscle autoantibodies on frozen sections of monkey thigh skeletal muscle (×400).

SUMMARY

Autoantibodies have an important role in the study of patients with organ-specific autoimmune disease. Detection of these autoantibodies may be important in the diagnosis of some organ-specific autoimmune diseases, such as Graves' disease, but more often they are supportive rather than essential for diagnosis. Similarly, although some of these autoantibodies are directly involved in pathogenesis of a disease (e.g., pemphigus), their presence is often a marker of underlying immunologic injury attributable to another disease mechanism, as is the case in type 1A diabetes mellitus. Newer techniques in molecular biology have disclosed, and will continue to disclose, the specific nature of many antigens targeted by these autoantibodies. It is hoped that this work will elucidate underlying disease mechanisms, allowing improved diagnostic tests and perhaps new directions in therapy. Technical advances in ELISA have made this technology available in most clinical laboratories, so that many assays for organ-specific autoantibodies are more widely available when IIFM is not feasible.

SELECTED REFERENCES

Darnell RB, Posner JB. Paraneoplastic syndromes involving the nervous system. N Engl J Med 2003;349;1543–54.

An up-to-date and comprehensive review of paraneoplastic antibodies.

Devendra D, Yu L, Eisenbarth GS. Endocrine autoantibodies. Clin Lab Med 2004;24:275–303.

State-of-the-art review of endocrine organ autoimmunity.

Green PHR, Jabri B. Coeliac disease. Lancet 2003;362:383–91.

Excellent review of celiac disease.

Johnson PJ, McFarlane IG. Convenors on behalf of the panel. Meeting report: international autoimmune hepatitis group. Hepatology 1993;18:998–1008.

Excellent summary of clinical laboratory parameters, including serology useful in the diagnosis and classification of autoimmune hepatitis.

Nakamura RM. Concepts of autoimmunity and autoimmune diseases. In: Nakamura RM, Bylund DJ, Keren DF, editors. Clinical and laboratory evaluation of human autoimmune diseases. Chicago: ASCP Press; 2002, p. 13–35.

Succinct overview of the immune system, tolerance, principal factors associated with development of autoimmune disease, and classification of autoimmune disease.

NIH Consensus. National Institutes of Health Consensus Development Conference Statement Celiac Disease, June 28–30, 2004. Available from: http://consensus.nih.gov/cibs/118/118celiacPDF.pdf

Consensus and state-of-the-science statements on celiac disease with summary statements of key elements for management and future research.

Nousari HC, Anhalt GJ. Skin diseases. In: Rose NR, Conway de Macario E, Folds JD, et al, editors. Manual of clinical laboratory immunology. 5th ed. Washington, DC: ASM Press; 1997, p. 997–1004.

Possibly the best synopsis of autoimmune skin diseases.

REFERENCES

Access the complete reference list online at http://www.expertconsult.com

CHAPTER 54

ALLERGIC DISEASES

Henry A. Homburger

KEY POINTS

- The prevalence of allergic disease has increased markedly in recent years throughout the world, especially in developed countries.
- IgE is the most important trigger molecule for allergic inflammation.
- Laboratory tests that establish a high likelihood of allergic disease have assumed increased importance. Test results support referrals to allergy specialists and enable primary care physicians to decide whether or not to manage patients within their own practices.
- New drug treatments for allergic diseases such as therapeutic monoclonal anti-IgE antibodies require demonstration of an elevated IgE level or the presence of IgE antibodies in serum prior to use.
- Clinical investigations of the natural history of allergic diseases in children have shown a reproducible sequence of sensitization to allergens that makes it increasingly important to establish the diagnosis of allergy at an early age to minimize exposure to allergen triggers and possibly ameliorate progression to serious diseases such as asthma.
- Tests for IgE and IgE antibodies are ordered principally for diagnosis.
- Measurement of serum total IgE in children and adults is of limited value in the diagnosis of allergic disease. The highest serum IgE levels typically occur in patients with hypersensitivity to several allergens and combinations of asthma, atopic dermatitis, and rhinitis. An elevated level carries a high predictive value for allergic disease, but a normal level does not exclude allergic disease.
- Measurement of IgE antibodies is useful and can be recommended in the following clinical situations:
  - Evaluation of children with early clinical signs of allergy, including eczema, gastrointestinal signs, or wheezing
  - Evaluation of children and adults suspected of having allergic respiratory disease to establish the diagnosis and to define the specificity of allergen sensitization to pollens, dust mites, fungal antigens, and foods
  - Confirmation of sensitization to food allergens and help in determining the presence of food allergy in children and adults with signs of immediate hypersensitivity on food ingestion
  - Evaluation of sensitivity to insect venom allergens, particularly as an aid in defining venom specificity in those cases in which skin tests are equivocal
  - Confirmation of the diagnosis of drug hypersensitivity in patients with anaphylactic sensitivity
  - Confirmation of the presence of IgE antibodies to occupational allergens, for example, natural rubber latex
- Testing for IgE antibodies is not routinely recommended for evaluating the effects of immunotherapy, or for excluding the diagnosis of anaphylactic sensitivity to insect venoms in treated patients. Tests for IgE antibodies are indicated only in patients who have had a thorough medical history and physical examination.

OVERVIEW

The prevalence of allergic disease has increased markedly in the United States and throughout the developed world (Bach, 2002). Estimates of the cumulative prevalence of allergic diseases in the United States range as high as 30% (Sly, 1999; Downs, 2001). According to recent data, up to 50 million persons in the United States are affected by allergies each year, including more than 31 million who suffer from asthma, of whom more than 9 million are children (Weiss, 2001). Seasonal allergies are estimated to have increased by more than 30% since 1985, childhood peanut allergies doubled in prevalence between 1997 and 2002, and asthma has increased from 35 cases per 1000 in 1982 to 56 cases per 1000 in 1994. Similar to many large categories of disease, estimates of the total yearly cost of allergic diseases run to the tens of billions of dollars. Simply stated, allergic diseases are a major public health concern.

Recent attempts to explain the increased prevalence of allergic diseases have focused on both genetic and environmental causes. Although it is clear that a host of genetic polymorphisms contribute to the development of allergic diseases (see later), genetic influences fail to account for the rapid changes in disease prevalence noted previously. Current theories emphasize the role of environmental influences in the changing prevalence of allergic disease. Several investigators have suggested that diminished exposure to microorganisms during early childhood in developed countries leads to aberrant development of the adaptive immune system and predisposes to both allergic disease and certain autoimmune diseases (Smits, 2005). This theory, called the Hygiene Hypothesis, postulates that early exposure to certain bacteria and parasites promotes development of mature dendritic cells and regulatory T cells, whereas diminished exposure leads to high levels of Th1 and Th2 effector T cells that participate in the pathogenesis of immune-mediated disease (see later). The proposed mechanism for the beneficial effect of exposure to bacteria, parasites, and even pets includes enhanced release of antiinflammatory cytokines interleukin (IL)-10 and transforming growth factor-β by dendritic cells, which induce antigen-specific regulatory T cells. This effect is postulated to be mediated by interactions between bacterial products (e.g., bacterial endotoxin, Toll-like receptors [TLR2 and TLR4]) and cells of the innate immune system, including dendritic cells, monocytes, and macrophages. Large-scale longitudinal studies are under way at several centers to investigate the epidemiology of allergic disease development and to validate aspects of the hygiene hypothesis.

At the clinical level, it has been well documented that the signs and symptoms of allergic diseases can be difficult to distinguish from those of other disorders (Host, 2003). Clinical manifestations may be relatively mild and self-limited, as in seasonal allergic rhinitis, or severe with marked morbidity, as in asthma. Laboratory tests are useful in the evaluation of patients with allergic disease, but knowledge of the basic mechanisms of immediate hypersensitivity and awareness of the empirical relationships between test results and their diagnostic predictive values are needed to optimize testing. This chapter addresses these subjects, beginning with a review of the biological mechanisms of immediate hypersensitivity and the "allergic phenotype," and proceeding to a detailed discussion of laboratory tests applied to the diagnostic evaluation of children and adults with allergic disease. Consideration is given to the chemical nature of common allergens. The distinction between sensitization and allergy is emphasized. Emphasis is also placed on identifying the minimum numbers of tests needed to achieve high positive and negative predictive values for allergic disease in different clinical situations. Clinical applications are identified in which laboratory testing is not cost-effective or may lead to erroneous clinical conclusions. Finally, new directions in the laboratory evaluation of allergic diseases are discussed, including testing for antibodies by microarray methods and testing for antibodies to purified native proteins and recombinant allergen components.

Pathogenesis of Allergic Disease

MECHANISMS OF IMMEDIATE HYPERSENSITIVITY

Immunoglobulin E is the most important trigger molecule for allergic inflammation. In the late 1960s, investigators working independently in two laboratories described a new class of human immunoglobulin that was responsible for the skin-sensitizing activity of serum from patients with allergic diseases (Ishizaka, 1966; Bennich, 1969). This immunoglobulin, originally called IgND, was later named IgE (Ishizaka, 1967). In the years that followed, investigators have focused on discovering the basic biological mechanisms of immediate hypersensitivity, including mechanisms that control IgE production by immunocompetent B lymphocytes, and that promote the recruitment of inflammatory cells and the release of vasoactive mediators from IgE-sensitized effector cells at sites of allergic inflammation. Recent studies have focused on investigating genetic determinants of the allergic (atopic) phenotype and on identifying the genes responsible for regulating IgE production.

THE ALLERGIC (ATOPIC) PHENOTYPE: GENETIC INFLUENCES AND CANDIDATE GENES

It is well known that the likelihood of developing allergic disease is strongly influenced by family history (Sibbald, 1980; Taylor, 1981). Genetically predisposed individuals are often called atopic, a synonym for the clinical allergic phenotype. The results of genetic epidemiologic studies suggest that serum levels of IgE are influenced by several genes, and clinical studies have shown that the levels of IgE protein in serum are several times greater for high IgE phenotypes (Martinez, 1994). At the structural level, a number of candidate genes have been identified that may act to determine the allergic phenotype, but the results are controversial and vary according to the populations studied (Ono, 2000; Sadeghnejad, 2009). Population-wide linkage analysis studies have identified the chromosomal locations of several candidate genes, and positional cloning studies support the relationship of putative allergy genes to known genes for molecules involved in regulating the immune response, including the human leukocyte antigens HLA-DRB1 and DQB1 (chromosome 6p21), the α-chain of the high affinity IgE Fc receptor (chromosome 11q), several cytokines including IL-4 and IL-13 and cytokine receptors (chromosome 5q31), the IL-4 receptor α-gene, and tyrosine kinases and nuclear transcription factors (Table 54-1) (Ono, 2000; Pykalainen, 2005).

TABLE 54-1
Genes and the Allergic Phenotype

Chromosome	Genetic locus	Phenotype
6p21-23	HLA D region (HLA-DRB1 and DQB1)	Responder or nonresponder to common allergens
11q13	Fc ε receptor β-chain	Enhanced responsiveness to aeroallergens; high total serum immunoglobulin (Ig)E
5q31	Cytokines interleukin (IL)-3, IL-4, IL-5, IL-9, and IL-13; β-adrenergic receptor	High total serum IgE; enhanced airway responsiveness
16	IL-4 receptor	High total serum IgE
20p13	*ADAM33* gene	Enhanced airway responsiveness, airway remodeling

HLA, Human leukocyte antigen.
Note: More than 120 candidate genes have been described to be associated with allergic disease. This table lists a selected sample of genes found in multiple studies.

Among the various candidate genes, some of the strongest evidence for a role in allergic disease is seen for genes of the major histocompatibility complex. Class II HLA alleles on chromosome 6p determine responsiveness to the common aeroallergens Derp p and Derp f peptides from dust mites (*Dermatophagoides pterynissinus* and *Dermatophagoides farinae*) and are found in linkage with other loci associated with bronchial hyperresponsiveness in asthmatic individuals (Hizawa, 1998; Lara-Marquez, 1999). A similar linkage has been proposed for an atopy gene that is closely linked to the IgE Fc receptor α-chain locus on chromosome 11q. This putative atopy gene has been described in several studies, including a study of African American families with asthma and enhanced responsiveness to *D. farinae* and grass pollen allergens (Sandford, 1995). Studies of the regulation of IgE synthesis have shown that the cytokines IL-4 and IL-13 induce IgE synthesis by B lymphocytes and promote the differentiation of helper/inducer T cells of the Th2 phenotype (see later). The cytokine gene cluster that includes IL-4 is found on chromosome 5q in linkage with a locus that influences IgE responses to several aeroallergens (Ober, 1998). Other loci that may play a role in the allergic phenotype include the gene encoding the IL-4 receptor α-chain (chromosome 16). This gene has been found to contain mutations that influence signal transduction by the transcription factor signal transducer and activator of transcription 6 (STAT6) (see later), which in turn promotes transcription of ε-immunoglobulin heavy chains (Hershey, 1997; Pykalainen, 2005).

A host of other genes have been implicated in genome-wide linkage studies of asthma, including genes associated with transmembrane proteins involved in cell migration, cell adhesion, and transmembrane signaling (Sadeghnejad, 2009). These genes influence asthma susceptibility and severity, and may play a role in airway remodeling.

REGULATION OF IgE SYNTHESIS: MOLECULAR AND CELLULAR INTERACTIONS

As noted previously, class II genes of the HLA D region strongly influence individual responses to exogenous antigens (Pieters, 2000; Wang, 2002). Gene products of the highly polymorphic HLA D region; DR, DQ, and DP molecules expressed on the plasma membranes of antigen-presenting dendritic cells: and B cells bind antigen for processing and presentation to immunocompetent T cells, thus initiating the immune response (Wang, 2002). The cellular and humoral immune responses that follow are determined by a complex interplay of cellular interactions involving both cell-to-cell contacts and secretion of stimulatory (and inhibitory) cytokines. Production of mature IgE antibodies by B lymphocytes exemplifies these mechanisms (Fig. 54-1). Initially, all B lymphocytes produce IgM

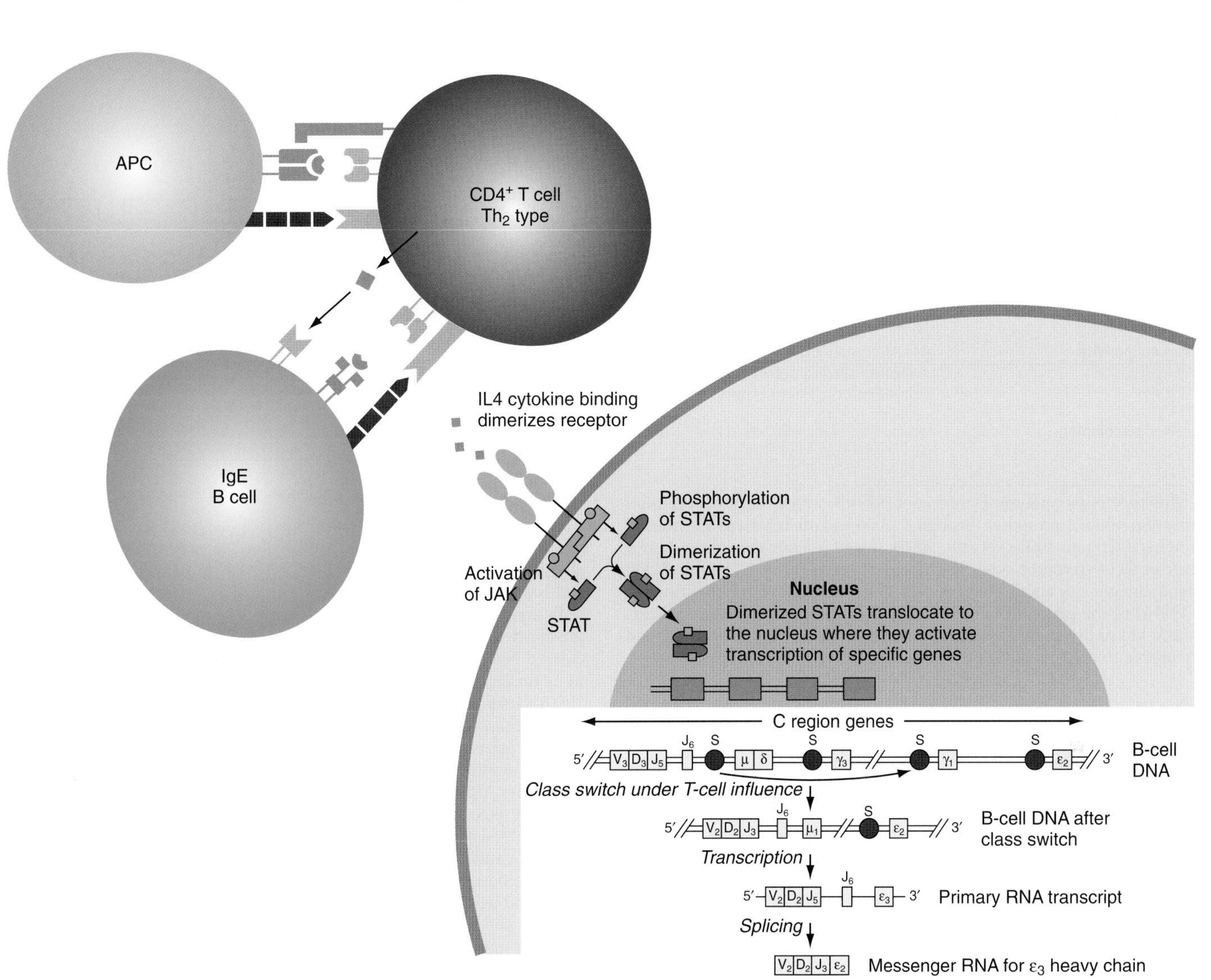

Figure 54-1 Cellular and molecular interactions regulating immunoglobulin (Ig)E synthesis.

antibodies. Antigen specificity is determined by rearrangement of V, D, and J exons that encode portions of the Ig variable region to create a variable region motif (VDJ) that encodes the antigen binding (Fab) portion of a mature Ig heavy chain. The rearranged VDJ motif is upstream from exons that encode the constant regions of the various Ig heavy chains, including the α-, γ-, and ε-exons. Production of mature transcripts for complete Ig molecules that bear these heavy chains requires additional rearrangements at the heavy chain (IgH) locus. These rearrangements result in a change in expression of heavy chain constant region domains from μ to another isotype (e.g., γ). This process is referred to as deletional switch recombination, because exons encoding domains of the μ-chain are excised by endonucleases in an irreversible process (Coico, 2003; Vercelli, 2009).

Synthesis of mature IgE molecules occurs in a series of steps that begin with expression of germline (sterile) transcripts of the ε heavy chain. Germline transcription must occur before deletional switch recombination can be completed. At the molecular level, this process involves interaction with a promoter exon upstream from the four exons that encode domains of the ε heavy chain (see later) (see Fig. 54-1). The ε-promoter contains binding sites for several transcription factors, including STAT6 and nuclear factor kappa B (NF-κB), which drive transcription by activating the promoter. Mutations at binding sites for these transcription factors block isotype switching to IgE. Because germline transcripts are "sterile" and do not encode a functional heavy chain, further metabolism of the germline transcript by endonucleases is required to create a functional heavy chain molecule. Endonucleases excise Cμ and ligate the now adjacent VDJ and Cε sequences. The process of deletional switch recombination involves rearrangement of double-stranded DNA at specific sites called S regions by enzymatically catalyzed breakage, cleavage, and recombination of DNA to create the functional heavy chain.

At the cellular level, IgE synthesis is initiated by cell-to-cell interactions and is driven by soluble cytokine mediators (Oettgen, 2001; Vercelli, 2009). Cytokines produced by T helper/inducer cells of the Th2 phenotype are required for the production of IgE heavy chain transcripts (Vercelli, 2009). This process is described by a two-signal model. The first signal for synthesis of IgE is provided by the cytokines IL-4 and IL-13. Th2 cells produce several cytokines that act as growth factors for B lymphocytes, including IL-4 and IL-13, which have been shown to induce production of germline ε-transcripts in human B lymphocytes (Vercelli, 1989; Defrance, 1994). These cytokines exert their effects by interacting with multimeric cell surface receptors. The receptors for IL-4 and IL-13 share a common, ligand-binding α-chain and a common transmembrane β-chain that participates in signal transduction (Palmer-Crocker, 1996). Binding of IL-4 and IL-13 to their receptors induces a series of phosphorylation reactions, which result in DNA transcription driven by phosphorylated transcription factors. Tyrosine kinases of the Janus family (JAK1, 2, and 3) are associated with intracellular domains of the IL-4 and IL-13 receptors and catalyze phosphorylation of the receptors, thus enabling them to bind intracellular transcription factors. The transcription factors, including STAT6 and NF-κB, in turn are phosphorylated, dimerize, and translocate to the nucleus, where they bind to the ε-promoter and induce expression of germline ε-transcripts (Oettgen, 2001; Vercelli, 2009).

Coincident with the interaction of antigen-presenting cells and T lymphocytes described earlier, which takes place through the T cell antigen receptor (TCR) and leads to production of IL-4 and IL-13, a second signal provided by cell-to-cell interaction is required to promote switch recombination from μ to ε heavy chain expression by B lymphocytes (Vercelli, 2009). This signal is provided by the interaction of CD40 and CD40 ligand (CD154). Engagement of the TCR results in upregulation of CD40 ligand on the T cell surface. CD40 ligand interacts with CD40 on the surface of

TABLE 54-2
Physicochemical Properties of Immunoglobulin E (IgE)

H chain class	ε
Molecular formula	ε_2L_2
Sedimentation coefficient(s)	8
Molecular weight, Da	190,000; H chain molecular weight is 70,000
Carbohydrate, %	18
Complement fixation (classic)	None
Serum half-life, days	1–5
Placental transfer	None
Reaginic activity	4+; Fc-containing fragments inhibit skin-sensitizing activity of native IgE, but Fab-containing fragments do not

Fab, Antigen binding.

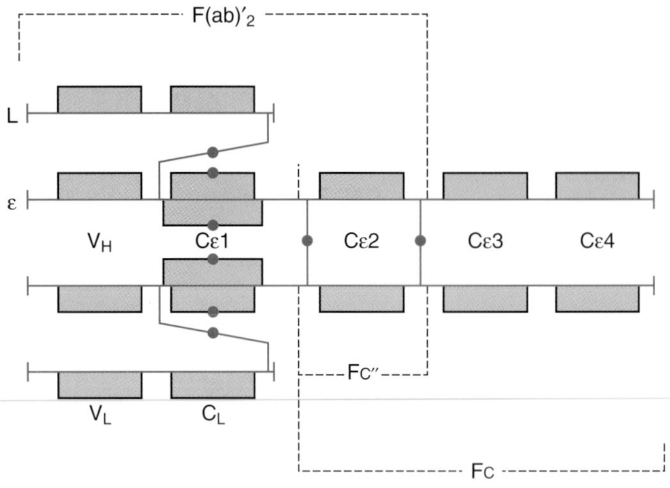

Figure 54-2 Immunoglobulin (Ig)E structure.

B lymphocytes to catalyze activation of NF-κB, which, in turn, facilitates activation of the ε-promoter through STAT6 and other activation-induced proteins (Oettgen, 2001; Vercelli, 2009). CD40 is a member of the tumor necrosis factor receptor superfamily, and engagement of CD40 by CD40 ligand antagonizes apoptosis of B cells. The importance of CD40 ligand (CD154) to the process of class switching is illustrated by some patients with X-linked hyper-IgM syndrome who are deficient in CD40 ligand and are unable to produce IgG, IgA, or IgE antibodies (Korthauer, 1993).

IMMUNOGLOBULIN E: STRUCTURAL AND FUNCTIONAL CHARACTERISTICS

The first demonstration that human IgE antibodies possess reaginic (skin sensitizing) activity and are different structurally from other immunoglobulins was put forth by the Ishizakas (Ishizaka, 1966). These investigators raised rabbit antisera to a reagin-rich immunoglobulin fraction isolated from the serum of an atopic patient. After absorption with purified immunoglobulins of all known isotypes (IgG, IgA, IgM, and IgD), the antiserum still reacted with γ_1-globulin present in the serum of allergic patients. After immunoprecipitation with this antiserum, the skin-sensitizing activity of serum from different atopic patients was abolished. Conclusive evidence of the immunochemical uniqueness and reaginic activity of IgE was obtained somewhat later, when it was discovered that human myeloma proteins reacted with the previously mentioned antiserum (Bennich, 1969). Experiments performed with isolated immunoglobulin fragments (Fab and Fab′2 fragments) prepared by enzymatic digestion of IgE myeloma proteins demonstrated conclusively that skin-sensitizing activity required an intact Fc ε-region, and that the antigenic determinants unique to IgE molecules were contained on the Fc ε-fragment (Bennich, 1969). The physicochemical properties and immunologic functions of different regions of the IgE molecule, as determined by experiments performed with purified human IgE myeloma proteins and immunoglobulin fragments prepared by enzymatic digestion, are summarized in Table 54-2 (reviewed in CLSI, 2009). Human IgE protein makes up only approximately 0.0005% of serum immunoglobulin and is catabolized at a rate of greater than 70% per day (the half-life of IgE in blood is 1 to 5 days). Individual IgE molecules have a functional valency of 2, as shown schematically in Figure 54-2.

Human IgE antibodies sensitize effector cells in the skin to release histamine—a phenomenon referred to as passive cutaneous anaphylaxis. The skin-sensitizing activity of IgE is heat-labile and requires an intact Fc fragment. Heating at 56° C for 2 hours irreversibly modifies the C ε 3 and C ε 4 domains of the IgE molecule and abolishes skin-sensitizing activity (Ishizaka, 1967). Binding to effector cells is also abolished by reduction and alkylation of inter-ε-chain disulfide bonds. Aggregated human IgE does not fix complement by the classical pathway, and no significant placental transfer of human IgE occurs.

CELLS AND MEDIATORS OF IMMEDIATE HYPERSENSITIVITY REACTIONS

Mast cells are the principal effector cells of immediate hypersensitivity reactions, although other cell types, including eosinophils, basophils, neutrophils, and lymphocytes, are involved in promoting and sustaining allergic inflammation (Church, 2003, reviewed in Barnes, 2009). Mast cells and basophils were once thought to be closely related cell types because both stain metachromatically with basic dyes and contain histamine in pre-formed granules. More recent evidence suggests that basophils are derived from granulocyte precursors, whereas mast cells are derived from mononuclear cell precursors and bear receptors for stem cell factor (Galli, 1990). Basophils develop in the bone marrow and enter the circulation as mature cells. Mast cells originate in the bone marrow as CD34+, protein tyrosine kinase Kit (CD117)+ progenitors and home to the tissues by binding to integrin and vascular cell adhesion molecule 1. Once located in the tissues, mast cell progenitors under the influence of the Kit ligand, stem cell factor, develop into mature cells. Two types of mast cells can be identified: Mast cells that predominate at mucosal surfaces require stem cell factor and T cell cytokines for development (IL-3, -4, -5, and -9); mast cells that develop in submucosal connective tissues require only stem cell factor and develop without cytokines from T cells.

Mast cells and basophils both contain histamine in pre-formed granules, but mast cells typically contain up to 10 times more histamine per cell than basophils. Two phenotypically distinct populations of mast cells have been identified and are termed MCt and MCtc, based on their content of tryptase (MCt) and tryptase and chymase (MCtc), respectively. MCt cells are found at mucosal surfaces at sites of allergic inflammation, often in proximity to T lymphocytes, whereas MCtc cells are more numerous in submucosal sites and in connective tissues and are not associated with allergic inflammation or T lymphocytic infiltration (Irani, 1986; Barnes, 2009). Mast cells are most numerous in the following tissues: lung (alveolar walls and bronchial epithelium and subepithelium), small intestine (epithelium and subepithelium), nasal mucosa, and skin. In all these locations, MCt cells predominate over MCtc cells.

Mast cells are the source of several important inflammatory mediators contained in pre-formed granules and are synthesized and released in response to signals associated with allergic inflammation (see later). The principal pre-formed mediators in mast cell granules are histamine, tryptase, chondroitin sulfates (proteoglycans), and tumor necrosis factor (TNF)-α. Newly generated inflammatory mediators include cyclooxygenase (prostaglandin) and lipoxygenase (leukotriene) products of arachidonic acid metabolism. In addition to these newly formed eicosanoid mediators, which are released within minutes of an allergic trigger, other cytokines and chemokine mediators are synthesized and released within hours of initiation of inflammation.

The primary mechanism of release of pre-formed mediators from mast cells involves transmembrane signaling mediated by cell surface (homocytotropic) IgE antibodies bound to high-affinity receptors for IgE (Fc ε RI) located diffusely on the plasma membranes of effector cells. Binding of IgE antibodies to Fc ε RI is reversible but of very high affinity (Ka = 10^{10} M^{-1}) (Wank, 1983). Although IgE antibodies in blood have a half-life of less than 5 days, the half-life of IgE antibodies bound to Fc ε RI on mast cells is estimated to be more than 10 days. The number of receptors per cell ranges from 40,000 to 500,000. Higher numbers of receptors are found on cells cultured in the presence of IgE, possibly reflecting upregulation of Fc ε RI expression by IgE. Fc ε RI is a multimetric receptor, composed of α-, β-, and γ-subunits as follows: α1, β1, and γ2. IgE

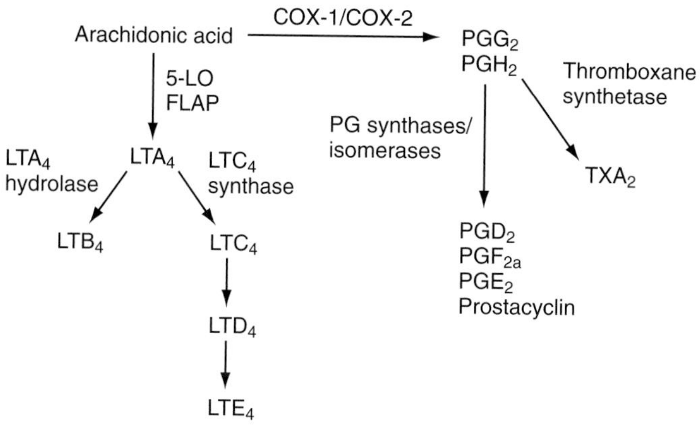

Figure 54-3 Metabolism of arachidonic acid. *COX,* Cyclooxygenase; *FLAP,* 5-lipoxygenase–activating protein; *5-LO,* 5-lipoxygenase; *LT,* leukotriene; *PG,* prostaglandin; *TX,* thromboxane.

antibodies are bound by the α-subunit; the β- and γ-subunits contain intracytoplasmic regions that function in transmembrane signaling (Ravetech, 1991; Metcalfe, 2009). Fc ε RI molecules are mobile within the plasma membranes of sensitized cells, as indicated by capping studies performed with fluorescein-conjugated anti-IgE antibodies. This mobility over short distances is believed to be important for the release of mediators from mast cells. Extensive studies with mast cells sensitized in vitro with IgE myeloma proteins or with intact allergen-specific IgE antibodies have shown that cross-linking (or bridging) of occupied IgE receptors by multivalent antigens or by intact anti-IgE antibodies or their F(ab′)2 fragments triggers release of histamine and other pre-formed mediators and initiates the synthesis and release of prostaglandin and leukotriene mediators. Univalent allergens, including haptens and Fab fragments of anti-IgE antibodies, do not promote mediator release.

The process of mediator release from sensitized mast cells is exquisitely sensitive and is dependent upon release of Ca^{++} from intracellular stores in the endoplasmic reticulum and influx of extracellular Ca^{++}. Aggregation of as few as 1000 molecules of IgE per cell can result in release of histamine and other mediators. Transmembrane signaling mediated by Fc ε RI aggregation is a complex process that is dependent upon phosphorylation of receptor subunit proteins by enzymes of the Src family. These phosphorylation steps in turn lead to phosphorylation of membrane phospholipids, including inositol triphosphate, which binds to receptors on membranes of the endoplasmic reticulum, resulting in release of stored Ca^{++}. Degranulation with release of pre-formed mediators is accomplished by a process of exocytosis. Receptor aggregation by allergen also leads to methylation of membrane phospholipids, followed by activation of adenylate cyclase, a transient increase in intracellular cyclic adenosine monophosphate (cAMP), and influx of extracellular Ca^{++} ions, which promotes fusion of granule and cell membranes during exocytosis. Increased intracellular Ca^{++} also activates cytosolic phospholipase A2, which promotes synthesis of arachidonic acid derived from membrane lipids. Free arachidonic acid is metabolized in mast cells to prostaglandin (PG)D_2 by enzymes of the cyclooxygenase (COX) pathway (COX-2, PG synthase, and isomerase), and to the cysteinyl leukotrienes LTB4, LTC4, LTD4, and LTE4 by enzymes of the 5-lipoxygenase pathway (Church, 2003; Metcalfe, 2009) (Fig. 54-3).

Histamine is the best known mediator of allergic inflammation. Injected intradermally, histamine produces a characteristic wheal and flare reaction that results from simultaneous vasoconstriction of postcapillary venules and neurogenic erythema (Petersen, 1997). Histamine in mast cells is contained in pre-formed granules with approximately 3–8 pg of histamine per cell. After release from mast cells, histamine interacts with specific G-protein–coupled receptors termed H1–H4 (Wess, 1997; Gether, 2000; Church, 2003). Engagement of the H1 histamine receptor leads to activation of phospholipase C with subsequent protein kinase C activation and Ca^{++} mobilization that causes the cellular responses associated with allergic inflammation. The effects of histamine are mediated by different receptors in different tissues. H1 receptors in the airway promote contraction of bronchial smooth muscle and mucous production, and H2 receptors in the stomach promote acid secretion. H3 and H4 receptors are found on histaminergic nerves and bone marrow cells, respectively. Histamine is degraded by two enzymatic pathways, with the major metabolite, *N*-methyl imidazole acetic acid (MIAA) resulting from sequential methylation and deamination of histamine by the enzymes histamine *N*-methyl transferase and monoamine oxidase. Most secreted histamine is excreted in the urine as MIAA, with small amounts appearing un-degraded.

The most abundant proteins in mast cell granules are neutral proteases, including tryptase and chymase. As noted previously, mast cells are characterized by their content of these two proteases. MCt cells predominate at epithelial surfaces in mucosa of the gut and airway, and MCtc cells are found in submucosal connective tissues of the skin and gut. Human mast cell tryptase is a tetramer comprising 29–40 kDa subunits with a molecular mass of approximately 134kDa (Schwartz, 1981). Two cDNA subunits of tryptase termed α and β have been cloned from human mast cells and bear approximately 90% sequence homology with one another (Miller, 1990). Most tryptase in human serum occurs in the form of α- and β-monomers and is believed to be released constitutively from mast cells. β-Tryptase is stored in secretory granules as a noncovalent complex with the proteoglycan heparin and is released upon cellular activation associated with allergic inflammation. Consequently, tryptase in serum provides an estimate of mast cell mass, and β-tryptase is a marker of mast cell activation and release of mediators resulting from allergic inflammation, including anaphylaxis (Schwartz, 1987). The half-life of tryptase in circulation is approximately 90 minutes (Schwartz, 1989). In addition to exhibiting enzymatic activity, tryptase promotes growth of fibroblasts and smooth muscle cells, activates mast cells, and promotes release of the chemoattractant IL-8 from epithelial cells (Cairns, 1996).

Newly synthesized prostaglandins and leukotrienes are important proinflammatory allergic mediators. The principal prostaglandin mediator of mast cells is PGD_2 (see Fig. 54-3), which is much more potent than histamine on a molar basis but is released in smaller quantities than histamine by activated mast cells (Church, 2003). PGD_2 and its metabolite, 9α,11β PGF_2, promote constriction of airway smooth muscle, peripheral vasodilatation, and inhibition of platelet aggregation. IgE-mediated mast cell activation also results in synthesis and release of the cysteinyl leukotrienes LTC4, LTD4, and LTE4 (see Fig. 54-3). These molecules are extremely potent bronchoconstrictors, up to 1000 times more potent than histamine, and they promote increased vascular permeability and mucous production. In the early allergy literature, the leukotrienes were referred to as slow-reacting substance of anaphylaxis (SRS-A). Their role in the asthmatic response is demonstrated by clinical trials that show effective elimination of much of the early asthmatic response to allergen by administration of leukotriene antagonists (Findlay, 1992).

Allergic inflammation often proceeds in two stages: an immediate response to allergen contact that occurs within minutes, followed by a late reaction that occurs up to 24 hours following allergen exposure. This biphasic response occurs commonly in asthma. Both stages of the allergic response depend on the presence and engagement of cell-bound IgE antibodies. The initial response reflects the effects of histamine, prostaglandin, and leukotriene mediators. The late response is caused by the recruitment of inflammatory cells, including eosinophils and neutrophils, at sites of allergic inflammation, followed by release of mediators from these activated cells. This late response is facilitated by the release of cytokines and chemoattractants from activated mast cells that promote the infiltration and degranulation of inflammatory leukocytes.

Laboratory Testing in the Evaluation of Allergic Diseases

THE RATIONALE FOR TESTING

Laboratory tests for allergic diseases have been available for longer than 30 years (Wide, 1967). Immunoassays for total IgE protein (IgE) and allergen-specific IgE antibodies (IgE antibodies) in serum have been the mainstays. During most of this time, there has been only modest interest in performing a full repertoire of IgE antibody tests onsite in hospital clinical laboratories, and many institutions have elected to send specimens to referral laboratories for testing. More recently, the use of laboratory tests in the evaluation of patients with allergic diseases has been driven by changes in the logistics of health care delivery, including the nearly universal adoption of managed care health plans. Other important developments favoring the use of laboratory tests in patients with allergic disease include the introduction of new therapeutic drugs for the treatment of allergic diseases, significant improvements in the analytic methods used for measuring IgE antibodies, better characterization of several classes of allergens, and improved knowledge of the natural history of development of allergic diseases, especially in children. Before the era of managed care, it was often possible for patients with symptoms and signs of allergy to be

TABLE 54-3
Protein Allergen Families

Protein family	Sensitivity to heat and proteases	Examples of plant food allergen sources	Clinical expression
PR-10 proteins (Bet v 1 homologues)	Sensitive*	Betulaceae: hazelnut* Rosaceae: e.g., apple, cherry, peach Apiaceae: e.g., carrot, celery,* fennel, parsley Fabaceae: e.g., peanut,* soybean,* mungbean	Oral allergy syndrome (OAS)
nsLTPs (nonspecific lipid transfer proteins)	Stable	Betulaceae: hazelnut Rosaceae: e.g., apple, cherry , peach Other: maize, peanut, barley, grape, cabbage	Systemic reactions common
Profilins (Bet v 2 homologues)	Sensitive	Profilins are widely distributed in plants. Typically: citrus fruits, melon, banana, tomato	Mainly OAS
Storage proteins (2S albumins, 7S/11S globulins)	Stable	Kennels/nuts/seeds: e.g., peanut/soybean, tree nuts, seeds, cereals	Systemic reactions common
CCDs (cross-reactive carbohydrate determinants)	Stable	CCDs are widely distributed in plant food. CCD allergenicity has been proposed for celery, tomato, and zucchini.	†

PR-120 proteins, Pathogenesis-related family 10 proteins from plants.
*Bet v 1 homologues in hazelnut, celery, peanut, and soybean have been found to be partially heat stable, and systemic reactions may occur.
†Immunoglobulin (Ig)E antibodies to profilins and CCDs in general are considered to have less clinical relevance than those to other allergen components.

seen by an allergy specialist without prior medical evaluation. This is no longer the case for most patients, who are evaluated initially by primary care physicians. In this paradigm, laboratory tests that establish a high likelihood of allergic disease assume increased importance, in that the results may justify referrals to allergy specialists and may enable primary care physicians to decide whether or not to manage patients within their own practices. New treatments for allergic diseases such as therapeutic monoclonal anti-IgE antibodies require demonstration of an elevated IgE level or the presence of allergen-specific IgE antibodies in serum as justification for their use (Soler, 2001; Lanier, 2003). Significant improvements have also been made to the analytic methods used for measuring IgE antibodies. As detailed later, the current generation of test methods bears little resemblance to the original tests introduced shortly after the discovery of IgE. Finally, and perhaps most important, clinical investigations of the natural history of allergic diseases in children have shown a reproducible sequence of sensitization to allergens that makes it increasingly important to establish the diagnosis of allergy at an early age to ameliorate progression to serious diseases such as asthma (Wahn, 2000).

In the field of clinical allergy, tests for IgE and IgE antibodies are ordered principally for diagnosis. In addition, test results may have prognostic significance for persistent allergy and may serve as a guide to specific therapies such as allergen avoidance or immunotherapy. The results of clinical studies are less clear about the role of laboratory data in evaluating the response to immunotherapy and in monitoring the course of disease. Ultimately, the medical usefulness of diagnostic test results is determined empirically by whether or not it is difficult to establish an accurate diagnosis on clinical grounds, and by studies of clinical outcomes that may justify trials of drug therapy without a specific etiologic diagnosis (so-called empirical therapy) (Gendo, 2004). Nevertheless, in many clinical situations, definitive management of allergic diseases requires that the offending allergens be identified unequivocally. For example, it is necessary to define allergen specificity in cases of anaphylactic sensitivity to foods, drugs, and insect venom allergens, in patients in whom allergen immunotherapy is indicated as treatment, and in patients who must practice rigorous allergen avoidance, as in occupational allergies or sensitivity to natural rubber latex.

ALLERGEN MOLECULES: STRUCTURE AND CROSS-REACTIVITY

Recent studies of common allergens have focused attention on the molecular basis of allergenicity and on the chemical properties of many important allergens (Kazemi-Shirazi, 2000; Shakib, 2008). Allergen proteins often have structural features that facilitate their recognition and binding by cells of the innate immune system and, in some cases, directly promote the synthesis of IgE antibodies by the adaptive immune system (Shakib, 2008). An example is Der p 1 antigen of the dust mite, *Dermatophagoides pteronyssinus. D. pteronyssinus* sensitivity is important in the pathogenesis of allergic asthma (see later), and Der p 1 has several properties that enhance its allergenicity. Der p 1 is a cysteine protease that acts in the airway to degrade protective surfactant molecules and α_1-antitrypsin, which normally offer a barrier to inhaled allergens. In addition, Der p 1 directly promotes mast cell degranulation and increased secretion of IL-4, and may act to inhibit the development of Treg cells that dampen the Th2-driven response to Der p 1 antigen exposure. Many other allergens also have intrinsic enzymatic activity or structural features that promote their allergenicity. Such intrinsic molecular features include patterns of glycosylation. An example is the storage glycoprotein Ara h 1 from peanut, which binds to cell surface receptors on dendritic cells and may promote synthesis of IL-4 and IL-13 by Th2 cells.

Knowledge of the chemical structure of allergens has been greatly facilitated in recent years by the study of recombinant allergen molecules (Kazemi-Shirazi, 2000). Recombinant protein technology has also fostered the development of a new generation of diagnostic reagents for measurement of IgE antibodies (see later) and has enhanced understanding of cross-reactivity between different classes of allergens. Studies of pollen and food allergens have focused on several classes of protein molecules, including pathogenesis-related family 10 proteins from plants (PR-10 proteins); nonspecific lipid transfer proteins from foods (LTPs); profilin proteins from foods; 2S albumin, 7S globulin, and 11S globulin storage proteins from foods; and cross-reactive carbohydrate determinants (CCDs) from glycoproteins in pollens and plants. The properties of these protein families are summarized in Table 54-3. Cross-reactive proteins from the PR-10 and profilin families are referred to as panallergens, reflecting the fact that these proteins are widely conserved in different plant species. Sensitization to panallergen proteins accounts for the presence in some allergic sera of IgE antibodies that are widely cross-reactive between seemingly unrelated allergens of common pollens and foods.

IN VIVO TEST TECHNIQUES: SKIN TESTS AND END-ORGAN CHALLENGE TESTS

It is not possible to discuss the use of laboratory tests in the diagnosis and management of allergic diseases without mentioning in vivo tests of immediate hypersensitivity, particularly the skin test and end-organ challenge tests. In vivo tests are regarded by many allergy specialists in the United States as the standards of diagnostic accuracy and reliability. The ability to reproduce a specific allergic reaction by in vivo challenge is considered the most sensitive technique for demonstrating the presence of immediate hypersensitivity and for defining its allergen specificity.

Skins tests are performed by skin prick and intradermal injection methods (Demoly, 1998). The response to intradermal injection of an allergen extract is graded by measuring the diameter of the wheal and erythema reaction immediately following the injection. A 1+ reaction corresponds to a 5–10-mm wheal. A response of this magnitude is usually considered as evidence of specific sensitivity to an allergen. Highly sensitive individuals may develop wheal diameters greater than 15mm with pseudopods. Skin tests performed by the prick method are used by most practicing allergists and make use of more concentrated allergen extracts—up to 1000-fold greater concentrations than are used for intradermal testing. Mean wheal diameters in millimeters are recorded as an indication of the degree of sensitivity. A more quantitative estimate of sensitivity to a given allergen can be obtained by the technique of end-point titration. Serial, tenfold dilutions of a standardized allergen extract are used, beginning with the most dilute solution. The endpoint of sensitivity is defined as the greatest dilution that produces a 1+ reaction.

End-organ challenge tests are useful in clinical management and for investigative purposes. Adaptations of challenge techniques include the bronchial provocation test in the diagnosis of asthma; the rhinoconjunctival challenge test in the diagnosis of allergic rhinitis; the double-blind, placebo-controlled food elimination and challenge test in the diagnosis of food allergy; and the sting challenge in the diagnosis of anaphylactic sensitivity to insect venom. The application of challenge tests in routine clinical situations is limited by the requirement for well-standardized allergen extracts of defined potency, and by the limited number of allergens that can be tested in an individual on a single occasion. As an example, food elimination and challenge procedures often require periods of abstinence of several days between introductions of suspected foods. Although generally regarded as the most reliable test for food allergy, the double-blind, placebo-controlled food challenge test is performed by relatively few practicing allergists at a limited number of tertiary care centers.

TABLE 54-4
Serum Immunoglobulin E (IgE) Reference Ranges in Children and Adults

Age	Mean (kU/L)	+1 SD (kU/L)
6 weeks	0.6	2.3
3 months	1.0	4.1
6 months	1.8	7.3
9 months	2.6	10
12 months	3.2	13
2 years	5.7	23
3 years	8.0	32
4 years	10	40
5 years	12	48
6 years	14	56
7 years	16	63
8 years	18	71
9 years	20	78
10 years	22	85
*Adults	13.2	41

SD, Standard deviation.
*In adults, the mean +2 SD cutoff is 127 kU/L. See text for explanation.

MEASUREMENT OF IgE: ANALYTIC METHODS AND REFERENCE RANGES

A variety of immunochemical methods have been used to measure IgE, including competitive displacement immunoassays, immunometric (sandwich) assays with radiolabeled and enzyme-labeled second-stage antibodies, and enhanced sensitivity nephelometry (Homburger, 1998; Hamilton, 2009). Nonisotopic immunometric assays are the most widely used methods. A popular commercial immunometric method uses monoclonal anti-IgE antibody bound to a high-capacity cellulose solid phase to capture IgE in a test sample, after which bound IgE is detected with a seccond enzyme-labeled, monoclonal antibody that generates a fluorescent product. The amount of product is proportional to the amount of IgE captured in the first stage of the assay. Currently available commercial immunoassays for IgE are capable of detecting less than 1 kU/L of IgE and are routinely calibrated to measure concentrations in the range of 2–5000 kU/L (1 kU equals approximately 2.4 micrograms of IgE). Assay calibrators used in commercial products are well standardized between manufacturers and are traceable to an international standard (World Health Organization [WHO] preparation 75/502 for human IgE). Results of interlaboratory proficiency surveys indicate that measurement of IgE is highly reproducible, with interlaboratory coefficients of variation <10% for survey samples with IgE concentrations in the normal range.

A number of studies have examined the serum concentrations of IgE in healthy, nonallergic children and adults. Synthesis of IgE occurs in the human fetus as early as the 11th week of gestation, but cord serum typically contains less than 1 kU/L of IgE (Homburger, 1998). Serum concentrations of IgE in children increase slowly with age and reach adult levels at approximately 10 years of age (Table 54-4). In both children and adults, studies of healthy subjects have yielded frequency histograms of IgE measurements that are strongly positively skewed, with upper 95th percentile confidence intervals that are seemingly very high compared with mean levels of IgE. The distribution of IgE concentrations in allergic subjects overlaps the skewed distribution of results in healthy controls. Many laboratories report reference ranges that are based on logarithmic transformations of skewed distributions, and the upper limits of "normal" are often portrayed as +1 standard deviation (SD) of an age-related, geometric distribution (see Table 54-4). This convention is confusing to many clinicians who are not aware of the skewed histogram of serum IgE concentrations in healthy nonallergic subjects.

MEASUREMENT OF IgE: CLINICAL APPLICATIONS

The measurement of IgE protein in serum has been thoroughly evaluated for its clinical usefulness as a screening test in the diagnosis of various allergic diseases, for its predictive value as an indicator of the likelihood of development of allergic disease in asymptomatic infants and children, and as a prognostic indicator in adults with certain types of chronic allergic disease. Measurement of IgE may also be useful in the evaluation of patients suspected of having immunodeficiency diseases, parasitic diseases, or the rare hyper-IgE syndrome.

The hyper-IgE syndrome was first described in 1972 by Buckley and colleagues, who reported two patients with greatly elevated serum IgE levels, diffuse dermatitis, recurrent furunculosis, and pneumonia with pneumatoceles secondary to *Staphylococcus aureus* infection. Subsequent reports of patients with this disorder have defined the clinical syndrome: elevations of serum IgE concentration are extreme (2000–50,000 kU/L), and patients have blood and tissue eosinophilia and strongly positive immediate wheal and flare reactions to inhalant allergens, pollens, foods, and bacterial and fungal antigens. Despite these findings, asthma is not common in patients with the hyper-IgE syndrome (Buckley, 1978).

The synthesis of IgE, as reflected by serum levels, has been studied in patients with a variety of primary immunodeficiency diseases. Increased IgE levels have been described in some patients with partial deficiencies of cellular immunity. Immunodeficiency diseases in which there is complete absence of synthesis of immunoglobulins G, A, and M, such as severe combined immunodeficiency disease, characteristically show diminished IgE synthesis and markedly decreased serum IgE levels. Serum IgE levels are variable in patients with IgA deficiency; ataxia telangiectasia patients typically have diminished levels, but patients with isolated IgA deficiency may have normal or modestly increased levels. Allergic disease is not common in patients with immunodeficiency diseases, with the exception of those individuals with selective IgA deficiency, who have elevated levels of serum IgE.

Parasitic infiltration of the gastrointestinal tract or parenchymatous organs stimulates IgE synthesis markedly, and studies in laboratory animals suggest that specific IgE antibodies are important in the host defense against parasites such as *Nippostrongylus brasiliensis* and *Schistosoma mansoni.* Serum IgE concentrations greater than 1000kU/L are regularly found in children in areas of endemic infestation with parasites. Other parasitic diseases known to be associated with increased serum IgE levels include visceral larva migrans *(Toxocara canis)*, intestinal capillariasis *(Capillaria phillippinensis)*, schistosomiasis, ancylostomiasis, and echinococcosis. In patients with intestinal parasitic disease, serum levels of IgE have been noted to decrease considerably following successful treatment with antiparasitic drugs.

In reviewing the usefulness of the serum IgE level as a diagnostic test for allergic disease, it is appropriate to discuss its use in children and adults separately. Elevated IgE levels in serum at birth or during infancy often antedate the development of clinical allergy (Kjellman, 1984). Serum IgE levels above the 95th percentile limit for age were described in 75% of children with a biparental family history of allergic disease; among healthy children with IgE levels more than 1SD above the mean for a given age, the incidence of development of allergic disease during the following 18 months was increased more than tenfold compared with a group with lower IgE levels. Although predictive of future development of allergic disease, these data provide relatively little information upon which to base specific clinical decisions.

Measurement of IgE in children is of limited value in the diagnosis of allergic disease. The principal value of IgE measurements in infants appears to be in alerting the physician to the likely possibility of an allergic disease. Serum IgE levels greater than +1 SD in such cases support the diagnosis of an allergic disease, but a normal IgE level does not exclude the diagnosis of allergic disease during infancy or later in life. The results of other diagnostic tests, including tests for IgE antibodies, are more specific (see later). In those clinical situations in which the presenting signs of allergic disease are unequivocal, for example, eczema and rhinitis in a child with an atopic family history, the serum IgE level provides little additional information. The situation is similar in older children and adults. Measurement of IgE in serum has limited diagnostic sensitivity for allergic disease. In general, children with hypersensitivity to several different allergens and multiple allergic diseases have elevated serum IgE levels, and those with hypersensitivity to fewer allergens and limited end-organ involvement often have normal levels. Diagnostic sensitivity is greatest in patients with clinical sensitivity to a number of different allergens. In atopic children, the presence of cutaneous disease and gastrointestinal manifestations increase the likelihood that the serum IgE level will be elevated. Children with allergic diseases that involve several organs tend to have elevations in serum IgE of greater magnitude than those with more limited disease. The diagnostic specificity of an elevated IgE level for allergic disease is excellent.

Measurement of serum IgE is also of modest diagnostic usefulness in most adults suspected of having an allergic disease. Results of clinical studies of adult respiratory allergy indicate that approximately 50% of adults with allergic asthma and fewer than 5% of adults with so-called intrinsic (nonallergic) asthma have elevated serum IgE levels. Asthmatic adults with hypersensitivity to a limited number of allergens usually have normal levels. The highest IgE levels in adults typically occur in those patients with hypersensitivity to several allergens and combinations of asthma, atopic dermatitis, and rhinitis. Just as in children, the limited diagnostic sensitivity of the serum IgE level limits the clinical usefulness of IgE measurements in those situations in which the diagnosis of allergic disease is most uncertain (Klink, 1990). This is not to say, however, that serum IgE should not be measured in such cases, as an elevated concentration carries a high positive predictive value for allergic disease.

Allergic bronchopulmonary aspergillosis is associated with a marked elevation in the serum level of IgE. This disease typically occurs in patients with allergic asthma, generally of long duration. Levels of IgE in serum are elevated during times of acute pulmonary infiltration, but IgE levels may fluctuate considerably during the course of the disease. A normal IgE level in a patient with active lung disease virtually excludes this diagnosis.

MEASUREMENT OF IgE ANTIBODIES: ANALYTIC METHODS AND REPORTING OF RESULTS

Two methods are commonly used to test for IgE antibodies: allergen skin testing by prick or intradermal methods (see previous discussion) and in vitro testing by immunometric assay. A third method involves measuring the release of inflammatory mediators or the expression of activation antigens on the surface of blood basophils exposed to allergens in vitro. Methods that involve blood cells are based on quantitation of histamine or LTC4 released from basophil leukocytes (leukocyte histamine release methods) or on flow cytometric detection of activation antigens (CD63 or CD203c) on the surface of basophils following exposure to allergen (de Weck, 1993; Nolte, 1993). These methods are commercially available but have not been widely adopted by clinical laboratories in the United States. Cellular assays require that blood samples be tested within 24 hours, and cells from up to 15% of individuals do not release histamine in vitro. Assays that rely on detection of activation markers do not require release of a mediator, but may be subject to false-positive results from IL-3 priming required before exposure to allergen. The results of early clinical studies of commercial cell-based assays indicate relatively poor sensitivity compared with skin tests for several allergens, including foods and insect venoms (Maly, 1997).

Immunometric assays for IgE antibodies were introduced in the late 1960s (Wide, 1967). Original (first-generation) methods utilized immunosorbents prepared by coupling allergens covalently to cyanogen bromide–activated Sephadex, paper disks, or microcrystalline cellulose particles as capture reagents for IgE antibodies. After incubating with serum, the solid phase was washed with buffer, and radiolabeled, affinity-purified, polyclonal anti-IgE antibody was added as a detection protein. These methods were semiquantitative, with results determined by comparison to an arbitrary dose-response reference curve that measured binding of IgE antibodies in calibrator solutions to a birch pollen immunosorbent. Results were reported in classes from 0 (negative) to 5+ (strongly positive). The original commercial method was referred to by the term radioallergosorbent test (RAST). First-generation tests for IgE antibodies had a number of limitations: The immunosorbents had limited capacity to bind IgE antibodies, which resulted in relatively poor analytic sensitivity; long incubation periods were required; and immunosorbents were susceptible to interference from competing IgG antibodies. In addition, the allergens used to prepare these early immunosorbents were poorly characterized and varied considerably from lot to lot and from manufacturer to manufacturer. These methods are no longer available commercially, and the term RAST should not be used to refer to current methods.

The development of improved (second- and third-generation) commercial methods for IgE antibodies in the1990s was marked by the ability to measure IgE antibodies quantitatively. This notable advancement was achieved by creating high-capacity allergen immunosorbents that had greatly increased antibody-binding capacity compared with earlier solid-phase reagents (Ewan, 1990). Calibration was based on WHO Reference Preparation 75/502. A different approach to quantification involved binding allergens to biotin, which enabled the use of a common avidin-coupled bead to capture fluid-phase allergen–IgE complexes (Iwamoto, 1990). Food and Drug Administration (FDA)-approved commercial assays based on both types of reagent are currently available. Second-generation and third-generation (automated) methods offer a number of improvements, including enhanced analytic sensitivity with detection of IgE antibodies at concentrations as low as 0.10 kUA/L, improved calibration with the ability to measure allergen-specific IgE quantitatively, resistance to interference by IgG antibodies, improved consistency of allergen immunosorbents from lot to lot, and rapid incubation times with results available within 6 hours.

Significant improvements have also been reported in the reagent allergens used to measure IgE antibodies, with better characterization of native allergens and preparation of a number of recombinant proteins from clinically important complex allergens. Recombinant proteins have been described for major allergens of dust mite, cat, and dog; *Alternaria tenuis;* pollen aeroallergens from trees, grasses, and weeds; numerous foods including peanut, tree nuts, wheat, milk, egg, and stone fruits; and natural rubber latex. Some recombinant proteins (e.g., Hev b 5 from *Hevea brasiliensis* 5 [natural rubber latex]) are now used in commercial allergen test reagents and contribute to increased diagnostic sensitivity (Bernstein, 2003). Although much improved over earlier assays, and despite having been approved by the FDA as quantitative methods, the previously mentioned new-generation assays from different manufacturers cannot be assumed to yield equivalent test results in all cases. Assays from different commercial manufacturers may differ in their allergen immunosorbents, and some differences in quantitation of IgE antibodies have been reported (Diagnostic allergy [SE-C] survey, College of American Pathologists, 2006). Clinicians and laboratorians must use caution in comparing test results obtained through different commercial test methods (Hamilton, 2004).

Tests for IgE antibodies have also been adapted to detect several different IgE antibodies simultaneously (so-called multiallergen tests), and a new commercial test of moderate Clinical Laboratory Improvement Act complexity has recently been introduced for point-of-care testing. By coupling several allergens to the same immunosorbent, it is possible to test a single aliquot of serum for the presence of several different antibodies without loss of analytic sensitivity (Ownby, 1984). Multiallergen tests yield qualitative results and enable simultaneous testing for IgE antibodies that occur commonly in atopic children and adults. The diagnostic sensitivity of multiallergen tests exceeds that of other single screening tests for allergy, including measurement of IgE (Ownby, 1984). In addition, multiallergen reagents can be used effectively to test sera for antibodies to several allergens of a common class (e.g. grass pollens or foods), with the use of algorithms in which testing for individual specificities is indicated only if the screening test is positive. The point-of-care test already mentioned uses a disposable cassette and whole blood to measure individual IgE antibodies simultaneously with a panel of common inhalant allergens. Although less sensitive analytically than complex immunometric methods, this test shows promise for use in primary care situations for rapid detection of IgE antibodies to common aeroallergens.

MEASUREMENT OF IgE ANTIBODIES: CLINICAL APPLICATIONS

Current recommendations for clinical use of the IgE antibody test are based on the results of clinical studies in which the sensitivity and predictive values of results of IgE antibody testing were compared with those of other diagnostic tests, including skin tests and challenge tests. Testing for IgE antibodies has certain advantages compared with skin testing. It poses no risk to the patient, and the results are not influenced by concomitant treatment with antihistamines or adrenergic bronchodilators. In addition, IgE antibody testing may be preferable to skin testing in certain groups of patients, such as infants, patients with dermographism, and patients with widespread dermatitis. Disadvantages have also been noted. Serologic testing is expensive if large numbers of individual tests are ordered indiscriminately, and the results are not available immediately. Recently, the multiallergen IgE antibody test performed with immunosorbents that have more than one allergen coupled to their surface has been shown to be a sensitive and cost-effective screening test for inhalant allergy.

It is difficult to define the absolute diagnostic sensitivity and specificity of IgE antibody results, because there is no universally accepted reference method (gold standard) for defining sensitivity to a given allergen. However, in most clinical studies, the results of IgE antibody tests have been compared with the results of in vivo diagnostic tests and allergic disease histories. It is clear from such studies that diagnostic sensitivity varies considerably, depending on the elapsed time between exposure to an allergen and testing, the class of allergen tested, the age of the patient, and the affected target organs. For the purposes of this chapter, it is useful to consider the following clinical applications separately: childhood allergic diseases including food allergy, adult allergic diseases, insect venom sensitivity, and drug and occupational allergies.

Children who are genetically predisposed to develop allergic diseases (atopic children) often develop symptoms and signs of disease in a predictable sequence as they progress throughout childhood. This concept has been called the **allergy march.** In genetically predisposed infants, eczema (atopic dermatitis) is often the first manifestation of allergic disease. Atopic infants and children younger than 3 years of age may also have gastrointestinal symptoms (colic, diarrhea, vomiting, and abdominal pain) or may suffer from chronic otitis. Children younger than 3 years may already suffer from recurrent wheezing. As the atopic child matures, cutaneous and gastrointestinal symptoms often give way to worsening respiratory symptoms with development of allergic rhinitis and asthma. The entire sequence of the allergy march is shown schematically in Figure 54-4.

Regardless of age, the presenting symptoms of allergic disease in children are not specific for immediate hypersensitivity and are easily mistaken for other etiologies. Increasingly, physicians have recognized that empirical therapy for suspected allergic diseases in children is not acceptable because it often results in unnecessary or inappropriate treatment with antihistamines, inhaled or systemic corticosteroids and leukotriene antagonists, and antibiotics. Empirical therapy allows the allergy march to proceed unchecked by missing the opportunity to lessen exposure to offending allergens. Although the results of clinical investigations are not yet conclusive, evidence suggests that avoidance of offending allergens and optimum pharmacotherapy may lessen the risk of sensitization to additional allergens and may interrupt the progression to serious allergic respiratory diseases later in childhood (Wahn, 1998; Platts-Mills, 2003).

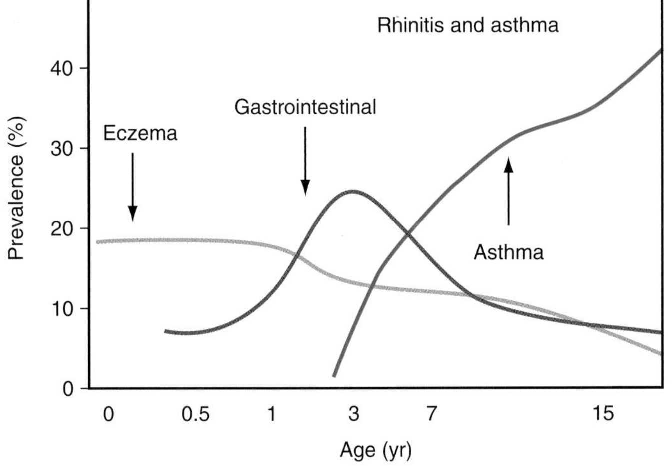

Figure 54-4 Relationship of age and clinical manifestations of allergic disease in children.

In a recent consensus document, the European Academy of Allergy and Clinical Immunology made the following recommendation (Host, 2003): Generally, all individuals with severe, persisting, or recurrent possible "allergic symptoms" and individuals with need for continuous prophylactic treatment should be tested for specific allergy, irrespective of the age of the child. Included in this description are children with cutaneous disease, gastrointestinal symptoms (colic, diarrhea, vomiting, or failure to thrive), recurrent wheezing, otitis, rhinitis, or asthma. Laboratory tests for IgE antibodies and skin tests were considered essentially interchangeable for the purpose of evaluating such children (Host, 2003).

The selection of appropriate allergens for testing is determined by clinical signs and symptoms and by the age of the child. The most frequent offending allergens in infants and children younger than 3 years of age are foods, notably protein allergens in cow's milk, egg white, wheat and soy, and dust mites (Nickel, 1997; Sampson, 2001). Immediate hypersensitivity to food allergens in infancy is commonly associated with eczema, gastrointestinal symptoms, chronic otitis, and wheezing. Less commonly, severely atopic children younger than 3 years may already have demonstrable IgE antibodies to house dust mites (*D. farinae* and *D. pteronyssinus*). These inhalant allergens are a common cause of asthma in older children. Except for the rare occurrence of a child with anaphylaxis whose symptoms are strongly associated with the ingestion of a particular food (e.g., peanut), it is seldom necessary to test for additional IgE antibodies to foods if the results of tests for common food allergens are negative. In addition, allergic respiratory disease caused by common seasonal inhalant allergens such as pollens is uncommon before age 3, and routine testing for IgE antibodies to these allergens is not recommended. In the age group younger than 3 years, the presumptive diagnosis of an allergic disease can be established with tests for IgE antibodies to common foods and dust mite allergens.

Positive test results for IgE antibodies to these allergens have dual significance: They establish a strong likelihood of immediate hypersensitivity disease, and they indicate an increased risk of sensitization to additional allergens later in childhood (Nickel, 1997; Wahn, 2009). For these reasons, the identification of IgE antibodies to common food allergens in symptomatic infants and children younger than 3 years is important for making proper treatment choices, and for deciding whether to seek referral to an allergy specialist. In children younger than 3 years, it is often more convenient to test sera for the presence of IgE antibodies than to perform skin prick tests. Levels of IgE antibodies that predict clinically significant, immediate hypersensitivity with high positive predictive values differ somewhat for different foods, and the clinical significance of low levels of IgE antibodies to common foods is limited (Sampson, 1997, 2001). Nevertheless, it is clear from the relationships shown in Figure 54-5 that the higher the level of IgE antibodies, the greater is the likelihood of clinically significant sensitivity to each food allergen. The receiver operating characteristic curves depicted in Figure 54-5 indicate cutoff concentrations for several common food allergens that have high predictive value for positive responses on subsequent food challenge testing. As illustrated by the graphs, a distinct advantage is associated with reporting results in quantitative units compared with the previous convention of class scores.

Allergic diseases in children older than 3 years typically manifest with respiratory signs and symptoms such as rhinitis, wheezing, and persistent cough (see Fig. 54-4). It is useful to think of the entire respiratory tract as a single allergic target organ. Allergic rhinitis and asthma often accompany one another. Most asthmatic children also suffer from rhinitis, and children with rhinitis often have asthma that may be clinically apparent or subclinical (Sly, 1999). With the development of disease affecting the respiratory tract, tests for IgE antibodies to inhalant allergens become much more important for clinical decision making (Host, 2003). Because a vast number of different inhalant allergens are available for testing, it is important to be selective in the initial testing of children with respiratory signs and symptoms, to avoid unnecessary testing. Data from clinical investigations support complementary approaches, such as the simultaneous use of small panels of individual inhalant allergens and of the multiallergen IgE antibody test for several antibodies.

The allergens chosen for testing in children with respiratory diseases depend on the age of the child and the scope of clinical manifestations (Table 54-5). After age 3 or 4, it is common for atopic children to develop IgE antibodies to indoor aeroallergens, including house dust mites, animal epithelia (cat and dog), cockroach, and moulds. The last antibody specificities to develop in children involve common outdoor aeroallergens,

PART 6

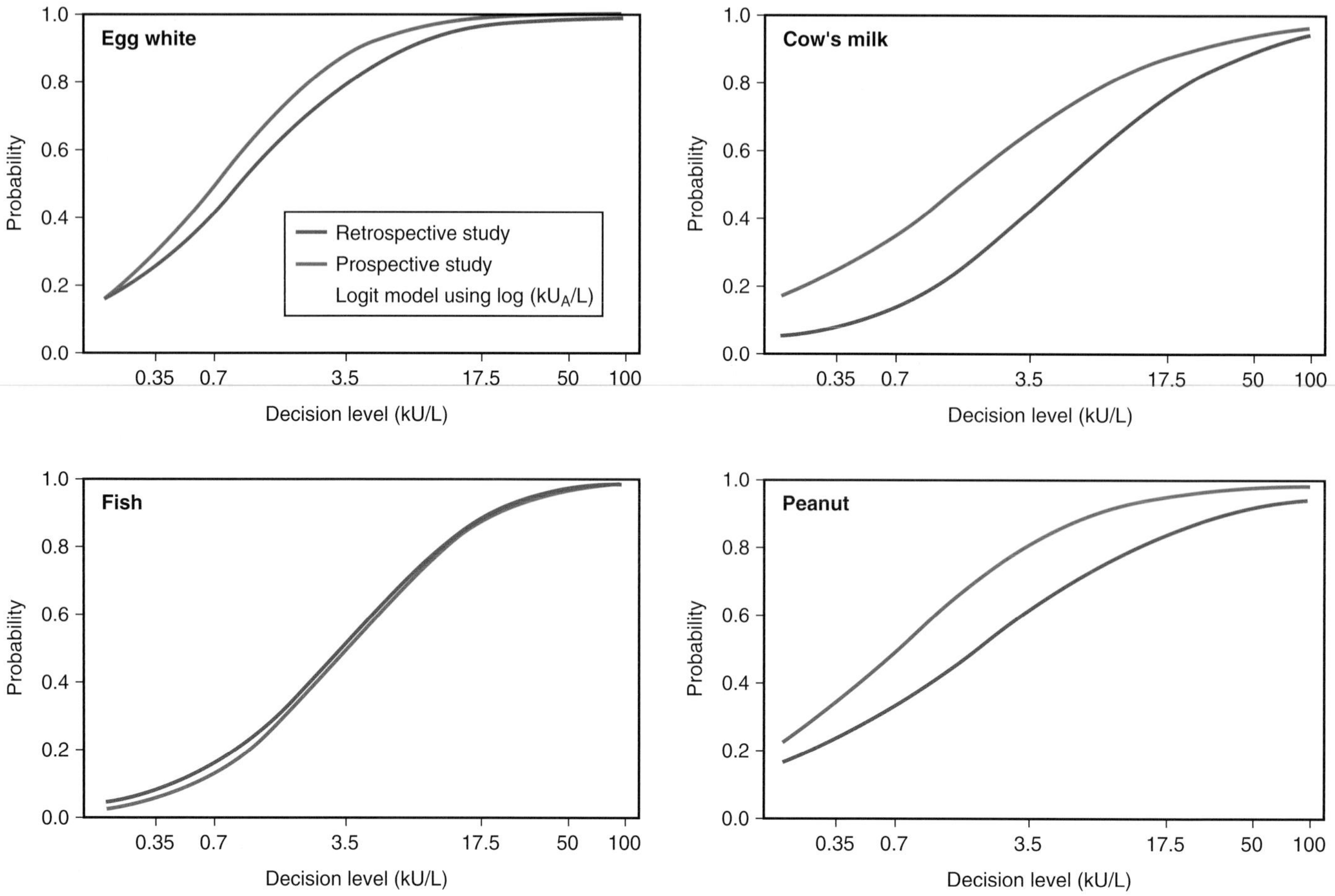

Figure 54-5 Probability of reacting to food allergens at increasing levels of immunoglobulin (Ig)E antibodies. *(With permission from Sampson HA. Utility of food-specific IgE concentrations in predicting symptomatic food allergy. J Allergy Clin Immunol 2001;107:891–6.)*

TABLE 54-5
Selected Immunoglobulin (Ig)E Antibody Tests for Evaluating Children With Clinical Signs of Allergy

Age, years	Signs of disease	Allergens
Younger than 3	Eczema with or without wheezing and otitis	Common foods: Egg white, milk, wheat, soy; house dust mites (*Dermatophagoides farinae* and *Dermatophagoides pteronyssinus*)
Older than 3 or 4	Rhinitis, wheezing, asthma	Common perennial inhalants: house dust mites, cat or dog, cockroach, *Alternaria tenuis*
Older than 3 or 4	Rhinitis, wheezing, asthma with seasonal exacerbations	Common perennial inhalants, as above, plus pollen inhalants (tree, grass, or weed pollens)

including pollen inhalants of trees, grasses, and weeds. No agreement has been reached on the minimum number of inhalant allergens that should be tested when evaluating children with respiratory symptoms, but consensus does indicate that testing should include house dust mites, cat or dog epithelium, a ubiquitous mould species (e.g., *A. tenuis*), and appropriate pollen allergens (Host, 2003). Testing for IgE antibodies to pollen allergens is indicated in older children, especially when symptoms are seasonal and tests can be performed at the time that symptoms are manifest. It is well known that levels of IgE antibodies to seasonal inhalants vary with the seasons, and there is little utility in performing tests for IgE antibodies to pollen inhalants when the allergens are not present in the environment, because false-negative results may be obtained. The multiallergen IgE antibody test is an efficient way to screen for the presence of IgE antibodies to pollen allergens. A positive result indicates the presence of IgE antibodies to at least one of the allergens on the immunosorbent but is not specific for a particular allergen. As such, a positive result is useful in identifying patients who might benefit from further testing with individual allergen reagents.

Longitudinal cohort studies of children with allergic respiratory disease point to the importance of IgE antibodies and exposure to allergens in predicting the severity of disease in children with wheezing. The likelihood of wheezing increases directly with the summed concentrations of IgE antibodies to dust mite and cat allergens. In addition, high concentrations of IgE antibodies to dust mite and animal epithelia in children with wheezing predispose to greater morbidity and increase the likelihood of hospital treatment in children with concomitant acute respiratory infection (Custovic, 2005).

In adults with allergic rhinitis or allergic asthma, tests for IgE antibodies are reliable for identifying sensitivity to all classes of allergen. The most common sensitivities are to common aeroallergens, including house dust mites, cockroach, animal epithelia, mould spores, pollen allergens, and organic dust allergens (Hamilton, 2004). Testing is indicated in cases in which the results are likely to influence the choice of treatment modality (Gendo, 2004). In adults suspected of having allergic rhinitis, IgE antibody tests are most useful in making the diagnosis when the pretest probability of disease is relatively low (less than 30%). Such patients typically do not have clinical findings that strongly suggest an allergic etiology. In this situation, positive test results greatly increase the posttest probability of disease for most common aeroallergens, including animal epithelia, moulds, and pollens. Among patients with a strong clinical history (prominent nasal symptoms and allergen triggers), testing is less likely to be useful and empirical treatment is often indicated. The results of several studies indicate that skin tests and second- and third-generation IgE antibody tests have essentially equivalent diagnostic utility in adults with allergic rhinitis, and either test modality can be used to identify allergens for inclusion in immunotherapy regimens (Gendo, 2004). The use of allergen immunotherapy in adults with asthma is more controversial, with only some studies showing clear efficacy. The decision to test for IgE antibodies in adults with asthma must be made on a case-by-case basis, with testing more likely to be useful in patients with clear-cut allergen triggers or occupational exposure to unique allergens.

New drug treatments for allergic diseases have become available in recent years. In particular, the treatment of severe persistent allergic asthma has been influenced by the introduction of anti-IgE pharmacotherapy (Busse, 2001; Soler, 2001; Lanier, 2003). Therapeutic anti-IgE is a recombinant humanized mouse monoclonal antibody to IgE that binds to the ε heavy chain of IgE, inhibits binding of IgE antibodies to Fc ε receptors on mast cells, and decreases antigen-induced mediator release from mast cells and basophils. Treatment with anti-IgE pharmacotherapy also decreases expression of Fc ε receptors on mast cells and decreases circulating IL-13. By interfering with binding of IgE antibodies to effector cells, anti-IgE antibody effectively blocks the release of inflammatory mediators that results from exposure to allergen. Results of clinical studies of anti-IgE pharmacotherapy for asthma have shown reduced rates of disease exacerbation and reduced requirements for corticosteroid drugs in treated patients (Soler, 2001; Lanier, 2003). Anti-IgE pharmacotherapy has also shown some efficacy in patients with food allergy, atopic dermatitis, or severe allergic rhinitis. For a physician to treat an asthma patient with anti-IgE, it must be documented that the patient has IgE antibodies to perennial aeroallergens and an elevated baseline level of serum IgE (30–700 kU/L). The dose of anti-IgE is determined by the serum IgE concentration and by body weight.

As noted earlier, the availability of quantitative assays for IgE antibodies has extended the usefulness of testing for several clinical applications (Yunginger, 2000). One such area is the evaluation of hypersensitivity to food allergens. Measurement of IgE antibodies is indicated to evaluate patients with food-induced symptoms that affect several end organs, including the skin, gastrointestinal tract, and airways, and even systemic reactivity. The gold standard for determining hypersensitivity to a food allergen is the double-blind, placebo-controlled food challenge. Recent data indicate that levels of IgE antibodies can be used to predict responses to food challenge for several common foods (see Fig. 54-5). These results define the levels of IgE antibodies above which a challenge is likely to be positive and therefore is not indicated. Similar attempts to define cutoffs for IgE antibody levels that predict reactivity to inhalant aeroallergens have failed to define levels that can be used across different practice situations (Soderstrom, 2003).

IgE antibody testing is also useful in the diagnosis of suspected sensitivity to Hymenoptera venom(s). Individuals sensitive to the venoms of honey bees, yellow jackets, hornets, or wasps may manifest signs of anaphylaxis following a sting; urticaria, angioedema, bronchospasm, or cardiovascular collapse may ensue. The reported death rate from sting-induced systemic reactions is at least 40 cases annually, but this figure probably underestimates the true incidence. The natural history of untreated venom sensitivity is not completely known. In many patients with documented venom sensitivity, it is possible to elicit a clinical history of progressively more severe reactions to successive sting episodes. On the other hand, venom sensitivity with anaphylaxis can occur in individuals with no prior history of allergic reactions, and venom sensitivity apparently ameliorates spontaneously in many individuals. The decision to treat a patient with venom immunotherapy is based on clinical assessment of the risk of anaphylaxis to possible future stings. The most reliable indicator of venom sensitivity is the response to a deliberate sting challenge, but this test is not widely performed and is rarely required in previously untreated patients to establish the diagnosis of venom sensitivity. Venom skin tests and IgE antibody tests are useful to confirm the clinical impression of venom sensitivity and to define its specificity. Comparative studies indicate that skin testing is a more sensitive diagnostic modality, with only approximately 80% of skin test–positive patients having elevated venom-specific IgE antibodies (Golden, 2003). Venom IgE antibody tests are useful primarily to confirm the results of skin tests, to define the allergen specificity of venom hypersensitivity, and in selected patients to identify venom sensitivity when a positive clinical history is not confirmed by venom skin testing (Golden, 2003).

With the exception of the sting challenge, no in vitro or in vivo test reliably predicts the clinical response to an insect sting in a treated patient following venom immunotherapy. Although levels of IgG antibodies in serum increase markedly with venom immunotherapy, no cutoff level has been defined that can be used to identify those patients who are no longer at risk. Semiquantitative estimates of IgG antibodies are not useful clinically, and levels of IgE antibodies following treatment bear no consistent relationship to clinical status. The decision to discontinue venom immunotherapy is based on clinical studies that show high protection rates after approximately 3 years of treatment (Yunginger, 1998).

Measurements of IgE antibodies have also been applied to the diagnosis of drug allergy. Although many drugs and their metabolites are capable of eliciting synthesis of antibodies, clinical data and the results of IgE antibody measurements are available for relatively few drugs, including penicillins and their metabolites and insulin. Penicillin and its isomer, penicillenic acid, combine with serum proteins through amide linkages to create allergenic moieties: penicilloyl-protein and penicillenic acid-protein are so-called major and minor antigenic determinants, respectively (Fig. 54-6). Measurable levels of IgM and IgG antibodies specific for the penicilloyl determinant occur commonly in penicillin-treated patients; although high titers of these antibodies persist in plasma for relatively short periods, lower titers can often be detected years after treatment (Shepherd, 1991). The diagnosis of hypersensitivity to penicillin has relied on skin testing with penicillin, penicilloyl-polylysine, and a minor antigen mixture. Positive skin test results occur infrequently, especially when testing is done remotely following treatment with penicillin. Less than 30% of patients with probable history of immediate hypersensitivity to penicillin have positive skin tests, and immediate hypersensitivity reactions to penicillin therapy are rare in patients with negative skin tests.

Using the results of skin tests as a diagnostic reference, clinical studies have reported finding measurable IgE antibodies to the penicilloyl determinant in 65% to 85% of patients with positive skin tests (Fontaine, 2007). Anti-penicilloyl antibodies are undetectable in control subjects. On the basis of these data, it is reasonable to recommend in vitro testing for penicilloyl-IgE antibodies only in patients with a history of recent hypersensitivity reactions. The absence of specific antibodies to penicilloyl-polylysine does not exclude the possibility of clinically significant IgE antibodies to other penicillin metabolites (Weiss, 1988; Fontaine, 2007). Genetically engineered recombinant drugs such as therapeutic monoclonal antibodies may also cause allergic reactions, including anaphylaxis (Chung, 2008). An example is the chimeric mouse-human monoclonal antibody against epidermal growth factor receptor used to treat patients with colon carcinoma and squamous cell carcinoma of the head and neck. Approximately one third of patients treated with the therapeutic antibody Cetuximab have signs of immediate hypersensitivity mediated by IgE antibodies to the oligosaccharide galactose-a-1,3-galactose present on the Fab portion of the antibody molecule. Diagnostic tests for this antibody can be anticipated for future clinical use.

Allergic diseases, particularly asthma, may be caused by a wide variety of allergens encountered in the workplace. Asthma may result from both allergic and nonallergic mechanisms. The list of causative agents associated with allergic occupational asthma is long and includes the following: animal proteins, enzymes, plant proteins, legumes, anhydrides, metallic salts, dyes, isocyanates, and wood dusts. Testing for IgE antibodies is available for several of these allergens. Recently, attention has been focused on natural rubber latex as an allergen in the health care workplace and in certain patients, for example, patients with spina bifida who have undergone several surgical procedures. Natural rubber latex is a complex allergen that contains several protein allergens. Testing for IgE antibodies to latex is useful for identifying sensitized individuals. Approximately 90% of skin test–positive patients have measurable IgE antibodies to latex allergens (Hamilton, 2003).

In concluding this section on testing for IgE antibodies with currently available tests, it is appropriate to summarize some of the major points made earlier. Measurement of IgE antibodies is useful and can be recommended in the following clinical situations: (1) to evaluate children with early clinical signs of allergic disease, including children with eczema, gastrointestinal symptoms, wheezing, and rhinitis; (2) to evaluate children and adults suspected of having allergic respiratory disease to establish the diagnosis of an allergic origin and to define the specificity of allergen sensitivity to pollens, dusts, fungal antigens, and foods; (3) to confirm sensitization to food allergens in patients with signs of clinical food allergy; (4) to identify allergens for use in immunotherapy regimens in patients with severe allergic rhinitis; (5) to evaluate the specificity of sensitization to insect venom allergens, particularly as an aid in defining venom specificity in those cases in which skin tests are equivocal; (6) to confirm the diagnosis of penicillin hypersensitivity in patients with recent clinical exposure; and (7) to confirm the presence of IgE antibodies to certain occupational allergens, for example, natural rubber latex. Testing for IgE antibodies is not routinely recommended for evaluating the effects of immunotherapy in treated patients, or for excluding the diagnosis of anaphylactic sensitivity to insect venoms in treated patients. Tests for IgE antibodies are indicated only in patients who have had a thorough medical history and physical examination.

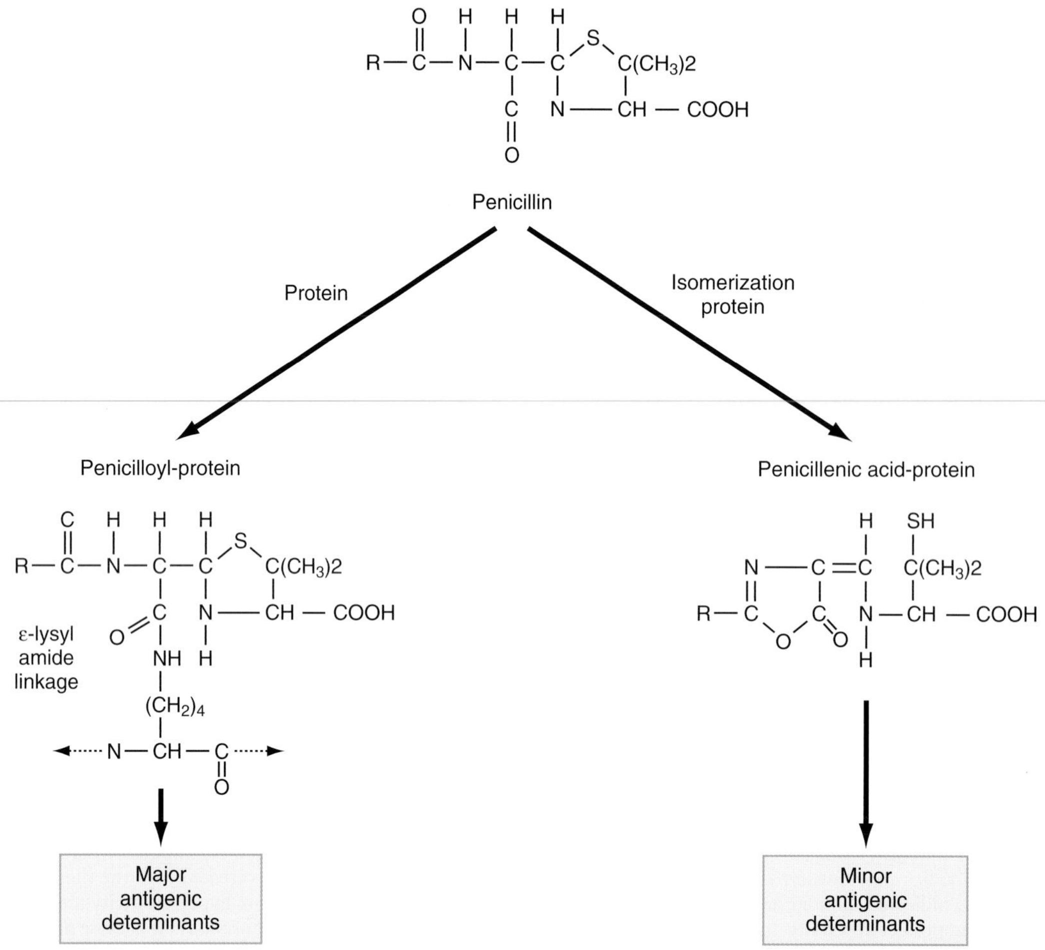

Figure 54-6 Allergens derived from penicillin.

FUTURE DIRECTIONS: COMPONENT-RESOLVED DIAGNOSTICS AND TESTING BY MICROARRAY METHODS

It is important in clinical allergy practice for clinicians to identify sensitization to an allergen and to differentiate novel sensitization from cross-reactivity. As noted in Table 54-3, many allergens from seemingly unrelated sources (e.g., tree pollens, weed pollens, foods) share components from protein and glycoprotein families (e.g., profilins, PR-10 panallergens, CCDs) with high degrees of structural similarity. Other allergenic proteins are unique to a particular source (e.g. storage proteins from many food sources). Recombinant technology has made it possible to synthesize large quantities of individual allergen proteins; these proteins are now being used in clinical investigations and (some are available) as diagnostic reagents for the detection of IgE antibodies (Valenta, 1999). A panel of recombinant protein components from a single source can be used to determine the serologic phenotype of response to a complex allergen (e.g., peanut, natural rubber latex) and will reveal whether reactivity to the complex allergen is caused by sensitization to one or more unique allergen components, or is attributable to cross-reactivity arising from sensitization to a panallergen. This distinction can be important, as the likelihood of severe or persistent allergy often increases with sensitization to unique allergen components (e.g., Ara h 2 in peanut, ovomucoid in egg white), and knowledge of cross-reactivity may help to determine the optimum allergens for use in an immunotherapy regimen.

Testing with component allergens may prove to be very helpful in distinguishing between sensitization and clinical allergy. Recent data from epidemiologic studies indicate that rates of sensitization to some allergens may greatly exceed incidences of clinical allergy. For example, approximately 10% of U.S. children have demonstrable IgE antibodies to peanut, but less than 2% display immediate hypersensitivity to peanut ingestion (Visness, 2009). The evolving clinical science of testing for IgE antibodies to component allergen proteins is referred to as component-resolved diagnostics. As more data become available from clinical studies of IgE antibodies to components, it is likely that additional recombinant reagents will be approved by the FDA for use in clinical practice.

Recombinant protein allergens have been used in combination with microarray technology to test for the presence of multiple IgE antibodies simultaneously. Up to 103 recombinant and purified allergen components from 47 allergens have been used in a single microarray panel. Results of microarray tests are consistent with established immunometric methods for IgE antibodies to aeroallergen and food component allergens (Jahn-Schmid, 2003). The results of a microarray analysis can be used to construct a serologic phenotype that displays reactivity to unique and cross-reactive allergen components. It is anticipated that microarray testing will be most cost-effective in the initial evaluation of suspected allergy to identify patterns of sensitization.

TESTS FOR MEDIATORS OF IMMEDIATE HYPERSENSITIVITY REACTIONS

As noted earlier, a number of mediators of immediate hypersensitivity reactions, including histamine, tryptase, the cysteinyl leukotrienes, and prostaglandin D_2, have been identified. Each of these mediators promotes inflammation in human allergic disease or in animal models of allergy and anaphylaxis. These mediators induce many of the characteristic biological effects of allergic reactions. Despite these findings, measurements of mediators in body fluids are of limited usefulness clinically in the differential diagnosis of allergic diseases. Measurements of histamine in plasma or urine can be of value in patients with anaphylaxis when tests are performed immediately following an anaphylactic episode (Friedman, 1989), but care is needed to obtain a suitable specimen. Hemolysis can lead to falsely elevated histamine levels in the blood and in histamine-rich foods, and bacterial colonization can lead to falsely elevated levels in urine. A more useful test in this clinical setting is measurement of tryptase in blood (Schwartz, 1987, 1989). Tryptase in serum consists primarily of α- and β-monomers of tryptase released constitutively from mast cells. Following anaphylaxis, mature β-tryptase (tetramers) is released from sensitized mast cells, and the level of tryptase increases rapidly (30 minutes to 1 hour) and remains elevated for up to 12 hours. By comparison, histamine is cleared rapidly from blood with a half-life of minutes. The leukotrienes are active locally and are present in minute concentrations in body fluids. Leukotrienes in blood are rarely measured for the diagnosis of allergic disease.

SELECTED REFERENCES

Busse W, Corren J, Lanier BQ, et al. Omalizumab, anti-IgE recombinant humanized monoclonal antibody, for the treatment of severe allergic asthma. J Allergy Clin Immunol 2001;108:184–90.

This article reviews the clinical indications for use of anti-IgE therapy and presents the results of early clinical studies of this new treatment modality.

Church MK, Shute JK, Sampson HA. Mast cell-derived mediators. In: Adkinson NF, Yunginger JW, Busse W, et al, editors. Middleton's allergy principles & practice. St Louis: Mosby; 2003. p. 189–212.

This chapter reviews mast cell inflammatory mediators and their roles in allergic inflammation.

CLSI. Analytical performance characteristics and clinical utility of immunological assays for human immunoglobulin E (IgE) antibodies and defined allergen specificities: approved guideline. 2nd ed. Wayne, Pa.: Clinical and Laboratory Standards Institute; 2009. CLSI document I/LA20-A2.

This guideline presents an overview of laboratory tests for IgE and IgE antibodies with emphasis on analytic concepts and quality control of clinical assays.

Gendo K, Larson EB. Evidence-based diagnostic strategies for evaluating suspected allergic rhinitis. Ann Intern Med 2004;140:278–89.

This article is a meta-analysis of studies that compare in vitro and in vivo diagnostic methods in the evaluation of patients with respiratory allergies.

Hamilton RG, Franklin Adkinson N Jr. In vitro assays for the diagnosis of IgE-mediated disorders. J Allergy Clin Immunol 2004;114:213–25; quiz 226.

This article is a comprehensive review of the evolution and performance of in vitro assays for IgE antibodies.

Host A, Andrae S, Charkin S, et al. Allergy testing in children: why, who, when and how? Eur J Allergy Clin Immunol 2003;58:1–11.

An excellent review of allergic diseases in children, this article presents the consensus recommendations of European allergy societies for evaluating children with suspected allergic diseases.

Oettgen HC, Geha RS. IgE regulation and roles in asthma pathogenesis. J Allergy Clin Immunol 2001;107:429–40.

This article presents a comprehensive review of the immunobiology of IgE synthesis.

Ono SJ. Molecular genetics of allergic diseases. Annu Rev Immunol 2000;18:347–66.

This article reviews basic and clinical studies of genes associated with allergic diseases.

Sadeghnejad A, Bleecker E, Meyers DA. Principles of genetics in allergic diseases and asthma. In: Adkinson NF, Bochner BS, Busse WW, et al, editors. Middleton's allergy principles & practice. St Louis: Mosby; 2009. p. 59–72.

This chapter summarizes studies of the genetic predisposition to allergic disease.

Sampson HA. Utility of food-specific IgE concentrations in predicting symptomatic food allergy. J Allergy Clin Immunol 2001;107:891–6.

This is a clinical article that discusses the use of IgE antibody levels to predict responses to double-blind placebo-controlled food challenges. Decision levels for several common food allergens are presented.

Shakib F, Ghaemmaghami AM, Sewell HF. The molecular basis of allergenicity. Trends Immunol 2008;29:633–42.

This review article presents a comprehensive discussion of the chemical properties of common allergens.

Vercelli D. Immunobiology of IgE. In: Adkinson NF, Bochner BS, Busse WW, et al, editors. Middleton's allergy principles & practice. St Louis: Mosby; 2009. p. 115–28.

This chapter reviews the subject of IgE synthesis and control by immunologic mechanisms.

Wahn U. Allergic factors associated with the development of asthma and the influence of cetirizine in a double-blind, randomised, placebo-controlled trial: first results of ETAC. Early Treatment of the Atopic Child. Pediatr Allergy Immunol 1998;9:116–24.

This article reviews the development of allergic diseases with age in children with a hereditary predisposition to atopy. The efficacy of early treatment of allergic children is discussed.

Wahn U. What drives the allergic march? Allergy 2000;55:591–9.

This article discusses the so-called allergy march. This concept is important for understanding the development of allergic diseases in children with age and sequential sensitization to allergens of different classes, including foods, perennial inhalants, and seasonal inhalants.

Yunginger JW, Ahlstedt S, Eggleston PA, et al. Quantitative IgE antibody assays in allergic diseases. J Allergy Clin Immunol 2000;105:1077–84.

This article reviews quantitative techniques for measuring IgE antibodies, including both in vivo and in vitro methods. The use of quantitative measurements in diagnosis and management of patients with allergic diseases is reviewed.

PART 6

REFERENCES

Access the complete reference list online at http://www.expertconsult.com

PART 7

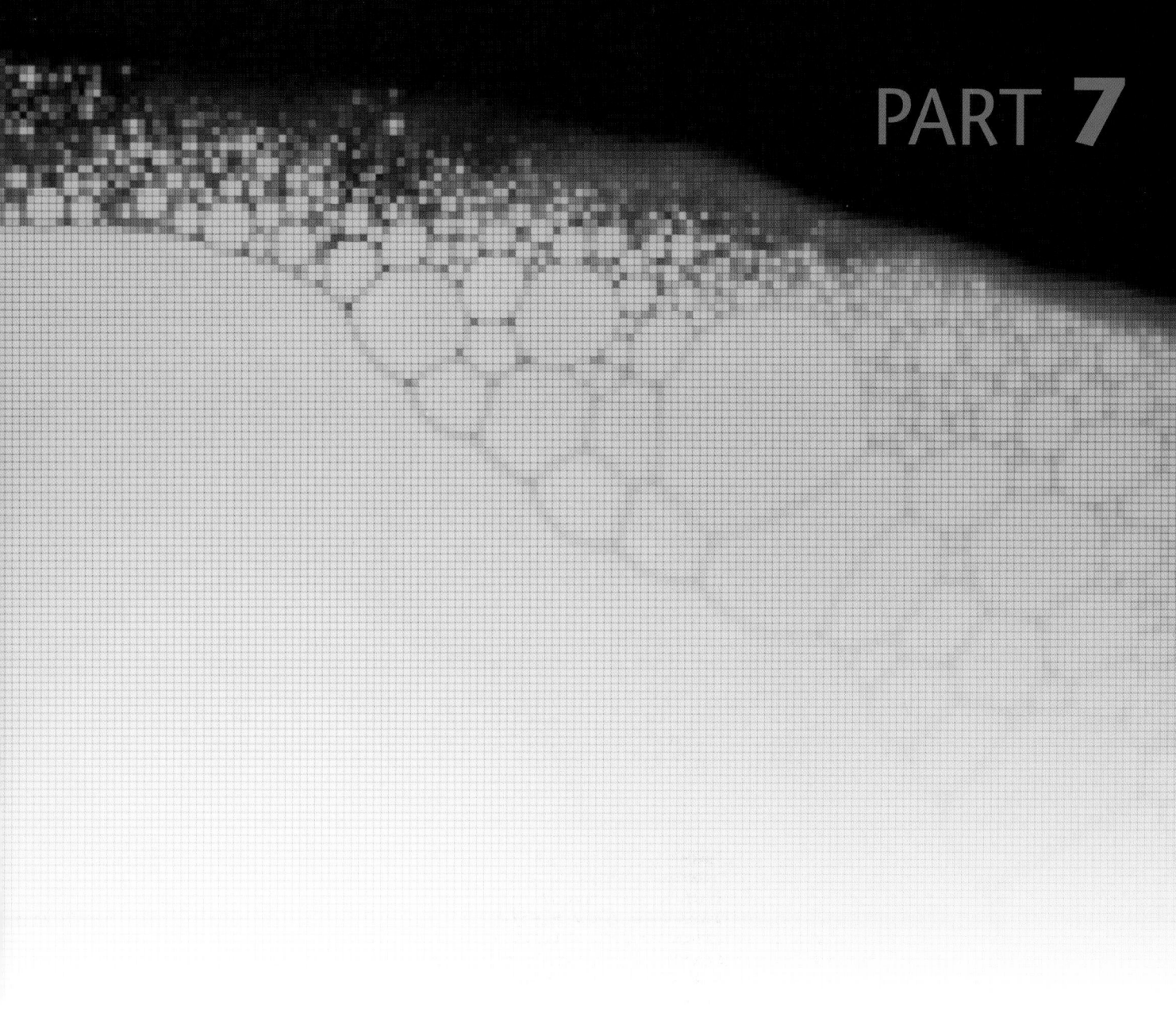

Medical Microbiology

EDITED BY
Gail L. Woods
Richard A. McPherson

CHAPTER 55

VIRAL INFECTIONS

Michael Costello, Linda M. Sabatini, Margaret Yungbluth

KEY POINTS

- Viruses cause more human infections than any other group of microorganisms and produce diseases that range from trivial upper respiratory infections to universally lethal rabies.
- Virus isolation in cell culture and viral antigen identification have been the traditional tests available in community hospital laboratories to diagnose genital and mucocutaneous, respiratory, gastrointestinal, central nervous system, and disseminated viral infections. However, several sensitive and specific molecular methods for detection of viral DNA and RNA are now available for routine diagnosis.
- Accurate and prompt viral diagnosis is fundamental for optimal patient management, for reasonable use of antiviral drugs, for reduction of unnecessary laboratory testing and inappropriate antimicrobial therapy, for application of infection control procedures, and for public health control of community outbreaks.
- Many common viruses grow in vitro in cell culture using primary, diploid, or heteroploid cell lines; viral growth produces distinct cytopathic changes in the cell culture monolayer or can be detected by staining the cell monolayer for viral antigen using fluorescein-labeled specific antibodies. Some fastidious viruses propagate only in newborn mice or embryonated egg tissue; some viruses have never been successfully grown in any culture system.
- The shell vial culture method uses a cell monolayer in a dram vial filled with culture medium; the specimen is inoculated by centrifugation onto the cell surface. After a shortened incubation (1–3 days), the monolayer is stained with fluorescein-labeled viral-specific antibodies. This method can be used for early identification of herpes simplex virus (HSV), cytomegalovirus (CMV), varicella zoster virus (VZV), respiratory viruses, and enteroviruses.
- Hybrid culture systems grow two cell lines together on the same shell vial coverslip. The cell mixture supports the growth of an expanded number of viruses and simplifies culture recovery of the common respiratory viruses (influenza, parainfluenza, respiratory syncytial virus [RSV], and adenovirus), enteroviruses, and HSV, CMV, or VZV from a single shell vial.
- Direct visualization of viral particles by electron microscopy (EM) can reveal unique morphologic features of several agents of viral gastroenteritis such as rotavirus, enteric adenovirus, norovirus, astrovirus, and calicivirus, none of which replicates in standard cell culture lines. EM has been largely supplanted by other methods in the clinical laboratory.
- Viral serology has two major applications: diagnosis of recent infection and determination of immunity. Demonstration of immunoglobulin (Ig)M-specific antibody during acute illness or a significant rise in IgG antibody between acute and convalescent sera defines acute infection. Serology may be helpful if culture, antigen assays, or nucleic acid–based testing is not available or feasible. Persistent specific IgG is a marker of immune status for measles, mumps, VZV, and hepatitis A and B viruses. Enzyme immunoassay methods are sensitive and are widely used for defining immunity.
- Nucleic acid hybridization and nucleic acid amplification tests detect virus by recognizing specific segments of the DNA or RNA viral genome; neither virus viability nor propagation is involved. In situ hybridization is a direct probe technique for detection of human papillomavirus (HPV), CMV, HSV, and parvovirus B19 in tissue; specificity is high, but sensitivity is suboptimal.

Continued

- Nucleic acid–based testing such as polymerase chain reaction (PCR), strand displacement amplification, and nucleic acid sequence–based amplification have raised the sensitivity of molecular diagnosis beyond culture or antigen detection methods. In addition to improved sensitivity, specimen transport is simpler because viable infectious virions are not needed. Combining several viral nucleic acid tests in a single multiplex or array assay has greatly expanded the clinical utility of molecular testing for viral infections. These assays generate a reliable answer within 24 hours.
- Real-time PCR transcription allows for the accurate quantization of viral load in a variety of specimen types. Quantitative analysis permits prognosis and monitoring of response to therapy for viral pathogens such as human immunodeficiency virus (HIV), hepatitis C virus, hepatitis B virus, CMV, Epstein-Barr virus, and BK virus.
- Detection of mutations associated with antiviral resistance is now available for HIV; resistance mutations may also have clinical significance for herpes viruses (CMV, HSV, and VZV) and influenza.

OVERVIEW

Viruses are responsible for an amazing spectrum of human illnesses that ranges from the annoying common cold to fatal immunoimpairment caused by HIV and some cancers. Virology has evolved rapidly from early characterization of viral morphology by EM to the development of techniques for virus replication in cell culture to sequencing of entire viral genomes and production of sophisticated nucleic acid–based diagnostic tests.

Established cell culture procedures for virus isolation are now being augmented or supplanted in clinical diagnostic laboratories by new, highly sensitive, and specific molecular techniques that can consistently detect as few as 10 virions per milliliter of specimen. Molecular tests have been developed to identify many common viruses and can also be used to quantitate viral load to gauge response to therapy. Both community hospitals and large medical centers now offer a broad range of molecular tests for common respiratory, skin, central nervous system, gastrointestinal, and disseminated viral infections.

Accurate and timely viral diagnosis is fundamental to optimize patient management, to appropriately use antiviral drugs, to reduce unnecessary tests and superfluous antibiotics, and to implement hospital precautions to limit nosocomial spread (Aitken, 2001; Dellit, 2007). Early and precise identification and sequencing of viral pathogens clearly benefit the general population through focused public health initiatives, as was recently demonstrated by identification of the coronavirus associated with severe acute respiratory syndrome (SARS) and the 2009 H1N1 influenza A virus pandemic. Prompt antigenic and genomic characterization of this novel influenza A strain permitted the rapid development of accurate diagnostic tests and an effective vaccine (Shinde, 2009; Trifonov, 2009).

Several excellent references provide detailed information about taxonomy and pathogenicity of human viruses (Knipe, 2007; Murray, 2008). This chapter reviews common viral syndromes that generate the majority of testing conducted in a typical hospital laboratory. Organization and staffing, equipment and supplies, and specimen collection and test selection are discussed, along with isolation and identification methods. Most hospitals have a case mix of common viral infections in healthy and immunocompromised children and adults to support a virology service. Table 55-1 summarizes test volumes and recovery rates for a Chicago-based hospital system, with adult and pediatric primary care and high-risk obstetrics, neonatology, hematology-oncology, transplantation, and HIV services. Viruses were detected by culture and antigenic detection methods in 2004. By 2008, these methods had been largely replaced by nucleic acid–based assays. Recovery rates reflect the increased sensitivity of nucleic acid–based assays. Increased volumes seen for 2009 reflect a large influx of inpatient and outpatient samples from the 2009 H1N1 influenza outbreak. Hospitals with different medical specialty profiles recover the same viruses, but with variations in relative isolation percentages.

Average detection time for most viruses is between 1 and 2 days (the same time scale as routine bacterial cultures); this reflects the combined use of rapid antigen assays, shell vial cultures with short incubation schedules, and nucleic acid amplification-based tests. Overall recovery rates for viruses in clinical samples are surprisingly high (16%–23%)—several times greater than for routine bacterial blood or stool culture, mycobacterial culture, or ova and parasite examination (Epsy, 2006; Leland, 2007). Many

TABLE 55-1
Viruses Detected by Conventional Virology (2004) vs. Molecular Methods (2008–2009)

	% POSITIVE SPECIMENS*†		
	2004	**2008**	**2009**
Viruses			
Herpes simplex	22	27	27.5
Cytomegalovirus	4	14.5	14.5
Enterovirus	10	9.2	11.4
Varicella zoster	<1	44.0	35.5
Respiratory Viruses			
Adenovirus	8	3.3	0.8
Influenza A	9	2.4	0.4
2009 H1N1	NA	NA	21.1
Influenza B	4	1.9	0.5
Parainfluenza 1–3	10	2.4	3
Respiratory syncytial virus	31	7.8	2.2
Human metapneumovirus (hMPV)	NA	2.7	1.1
Parainfluenza 4	NA	2.0	0.3
Coronavirus	NA	0.7	1
Enterovirus or rhinovirus	NA	24.2	16.1

Personal data, M. Costello and L. Sabatini, Multiple hospitals, Chicago area and southeast Wisconsin.
NA, Not available.
*2004: conventional virology testing methods; 2008: molecular testing methods; 2009: molecular testing methods; includes 2009 H1N1influenza epidemic.
†Average recovery of respiratory viruses from respiratory specimens was 47%.

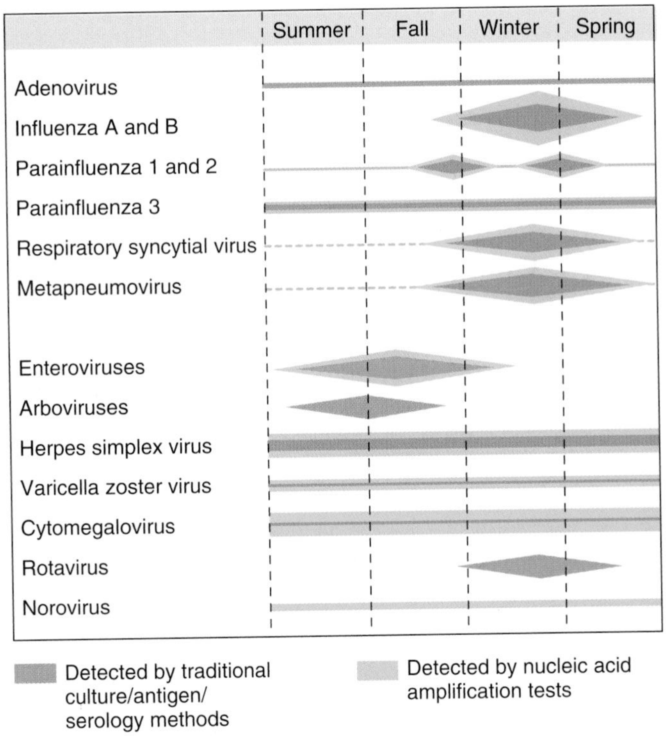

Figure 55-1 Seasonal variations in viral detection.

common viruses exhibit seasonal variations (Fig. 55-1). Influenza, RSV, and parainfluenza viruses 1 and 2 circulate every winter. Adenovirus, parainfluenza virus 3, CMV, and HSV infections occur year-round. Enterovirus disease clusters in late summer and early autumn. These temporal patterns have a direct impact on laboratory staffing needs and put the greatest demand on pediatric hospitals.

Four principal viral diagnostic laboratory methods are used: culture, antigen detection, nucleic acid detection, and serology. Each method has clear advantages and limitations (Fig. 55-2). Culture and antigen detection

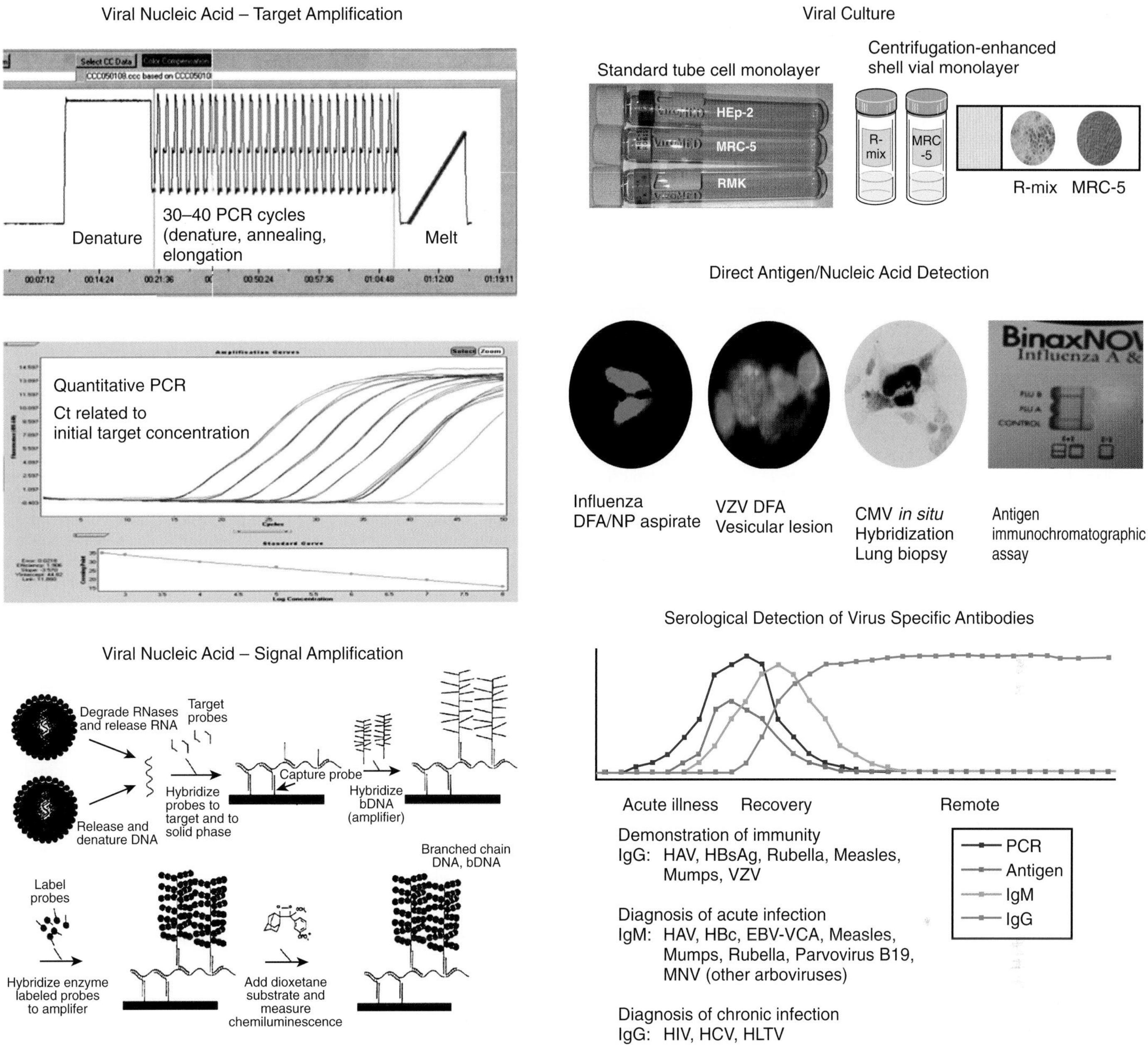

Figure 55-2 Laboratory methods for diagnosis of viral infection. *CMV,* Cytomegalovirus; *DFA,* direct fluorescent antibody; *EBV-VCA,* Epstein Barr virus-viral capsid antigen; *HAV,* hepatitis A virus; *HBc,* hepatitis B core antigen; *HBsAg,* hepatitis B surface antigen; *HCV,* hepatitis C virus; *HEp-2,* heteroploid cell line derived from laryngeal carcinoma; *HIV,* human immunodeficiency virus; *Ig,* immunoglobulin; *PCR,* polymerase chain reaction; *RMK,* Rhesus monkey kidney; *VZV,* varicella zoster virus.

requires viable virus or relatively intact viral fragments; specimens must be collected during active viral replication. Nucleic acid–based methods have the highest sensitivity and allow greater latitude in specimen collection and transport. The throughput time for most nucleic acid–based testing is 1 day or less and definitely outpaces timelines for standard culture. Nucleic acid–based tests are invaluable for identifying viruses that propagate slowly or not at all in cell culture. Viral nucleic acid fragments may persist into the recovery phase of illness, long after viable virions have been eliminated by the immune response; this limits their use as test of cure. Quantitative real-time PCR has become the standard of care in assessing viral loads and monitoring response to therapy for viruses such as HIV, CMV, HCV, HBV, and BKV. As the mechanisms of antiviral drug resistance are being defined, mutation detection is becoming the method of choice for appropriately targeting antiviral therapy.

Traditional serologic diagnosis requires paired sera from the acute and convalescent stages of infection to demonstrate a significant rise in specific viral antibody titer. Detection of virus-specific IgM antibody can diagnose acute illness from a single serum obtained during the acute or early convalescent period for some viral infections. Virus-specific IgG antibody tests are typically helpful to document immune status for selected viruses.

All necessary materials and reagents for virus isolation, antigen assays, and serologic procedures are available from commercial suppliers. The number of viruses that can be detected or quantified by nucleic acid–based tests continues to grow, and several assays are already commercially available. Laboratory-developed procedures require considerable technical expertise, and all molecular methods demand stringent quality control to guarantee accuracy and to minimize contamination. Despite these additional responsibilities, molecular approaches have enhanced overall sensitivity and quantitative accuracy, relative to conventional procedures. One should expect to see more molecular assays become standard of practice in clinical virology laboratories as available technologies continue to improve.

VIRAL CULTURE

Virus propagation in tissue culture was developed more than 60 years ago and remains a versatile, cost-effective, and comprehensive diagnostic approach. Many clinically significant viruses replicate in vitro, and virus recovery correlates well with acute disease. However, culture is labor-intensive, involves technical proficiency, requires at least 1-day turnaround for positive results, and frequently is less sensitive than nucleic acid–based detection methods (Leland, 2007).

Tissue culture cells are divided into three categories: primary cell cultures, diploid cell lines, and heteroploid cell lines, including genetically manipulated heteroploid cell lines that have been engineered for enhanced growth and detection of certain clinically significant viruses. Primary cell cultures are prepared directly from the parent organ (e.g., monkey or rabbit kidney) by mincing and trypsinization, and the mixture is transferred to tubes or shell vials, where the cells attach and form a confluent monolayer on the glass surface. Overlay medium with buffered isotonic inorganic salts, glucose, amino acids, vitamins, and cofactors at a physiologic pH sustains cell viability. Eagle minimum essential medium in Earl or Hanks balanced salt solution is a versatile nutrient system and is usually supplemented with a low concentration of protein-rich/immunoglobulin-poor fetal bovine serum to maintain a healthy monolayer but not promote ongoing cell proliferation. The most popular and versatile cell lines with a normal diploid karyotype are human diploid fibroblasts (HDFs) derived from lung or newborn foreskin. Cells are propagated in serum-rich growth medium and can be serially subcultured 20–50 times; examples include MRC-5, WI-38, and foreskin fibroblasts. Heteroploid cell lines are derived from malignant tumors and can be passaged indefinitely; they are aneuploid and divide rapidly. Heteroploid lines include HEp-2 (laryngeal carcinoma), HeLa (cervical carcinoma), and A549 (human alveolar adenocarcinoma). Heteroploid cell lines include genetically manipulated cells that have been engineered for enhanced detection of clinically significant viruses. Examples of genetically manipulated cells are ELVIS cells, which are stably transformed baby hamster cells containing an HSV-specific promoter sequence and the *Escherichia coli lacZ* gene (Stabell, 1993), and a buffalo green monkey kidney cell line (BGMK-hDAF) engineered to overexpress CD55, a receptor that some enteroviruses require for infection. Detailed additional information about cell lines, media formulations, propagation, and maintenance techniques is provided in other sources (Clarke, 2010).

Diploid and heteroploid cell lines should be tested periodically for *Mycoplasma* contamination and continued sensitivity to viral infection. Suppliers of purchased cells should perform these quality control measures and provide documentation. Cocultured cells are a mixture of two cell types that together support growth of a wide range of viruses. R-Mix contains A549 and mink lung cells with added trypsin and will recover the respiratory agents: influenzas, parainfluenzas, RSV, and adenovirus. Super E-Mix contains genetically engineered BGMK-hDAF and A549 cells to maximize recovery of enteroviruses. Viruses differ somewhat in their ability to replicate in culture, so critical specimens should be inoculated to a variety of cell lines to maximize recovery. A more extensive discussion of cell culture can be found elsewhere (Landry, 2000; Hodinka, 2010).

Each laboratory should select sufficient lines to cover the usual viral pathogens in its patient population and can vary the number and type to meet seasonal demands (Chapin, 2007; Leland, 2007). Primary cultures must be checked for contamination with endogenous virus. Viral replication in tube monolayers can be detected by inspecting the cell sheet with an inverted phase-contrast microscope for cytopathic changes associated with virus proliferation. Tube monolayers are versatile: A single cell line may support growth of several viruses, each producing distinctive cytopathic effect (CPE) or other measurable identifying features (hemagglutination, hemadsorption, interference). CPE may develop in 1–3 days (HSV) or may not be recognized for 5–20 days (RSV, VZV, CMV); therefore, cultures may need extended incubation for 2 weeks or longer (Clarke, 2010).

With the shell vial technique, the cell sheet rests on a round coverslip, monolayer side up, in a shell vial. The specimen is inoculated into the vial, which then is centrifuged to enhance viral attachment to the cell surface. After 1–3 days of incubation, the monolayer is tested for specific viral antigen, usually with a fluorescent antibody stain (Clarke, 2010). Shell vials are ideal for identification of a single virus (HSV) or a limited number of viruses (RSV and influenza), and for faster detection of slow-growing agents such as CMV and VZV. HSV vesicular genital lesions are excellent candidates for shell vial culture; sensitivity is almost 100% compared with traditional tube culture, and turnaround for negative specimens is decreased from 1 week to 1–2 days. Shell vials are comparable or superior to tube methods for recovery of CMV from urine, but backup tube culture is recommended to maximize CMV recovery from peripheral blood, body fluids, and tissue biopsies. Molecular methods will eventually replace cell culture as the "gold standard" for detection of most clinically significant viruses in clinical virology laboratories. This transformation is well under way, but the versatility of cell culture is still a valuable asset of this established technology.

SPECIMEN COLLECTION

Success with any diagnostic test begins with proper specimen collection and transportation. The laboratory must have realistic guidelines for optimal specimen handling and a specimen rejection policy, and then must communicate this information to the clinical staff and patient care sites (Table 55-2). Specimens for culture and antigen assays should be obtained early in acute illness, when virus shedding is highest; these testing methods are, at best, unreliable during convalescence. Nucleic acid amplification is more sensitive and has optimal value early in the course of disease.

Viral transport medium (VTM) contains a buffered salt solution, protein and saccharide nutrients, pH indicator, and antibiotics to inhibit bacterial and fungal contaminants, and is designed to stabilize virions and the patient's infected cells. Swab specimens, nasopharyngeal aspirates, and tissue biopsies should be placed in VTM for culture and antigen detection. Tissue should be frozen for molecular assays. Body fluids, lavages, blood, and bone marrow samples do not need VTM (Forman, 2007). Multipurpose transport media such as M4, Flextrans, Universal Transport, and others have been made for viral, chlamydial, and mycoplasmal culture. Most VTM formulations can stabilize viruses for 48 hours or less (Johnson, 1990). All specimens except blood samples should be transported and stored until setup at 4° C. Room temperature transport of specimens may be unavoidable in some circumstances, but physicians should appreciate the negative impact on recovery. Blood samples for virus isolation should be held at room temperature at all times and processed for culture on the day of collection. Viral cultures are best set up on the day specimens arrive in the laboratory, preferably within 36 hours of collection; at least one culture inoculation session should be scheduled during weekend shifts.

Equipment and Supplies

Most virology equipment is relatively inexpensive and is already in use in the microbiology and immunology laboratory sections. A class II biosafety laminar flow cabinet must be used for culture setup and whenever cultures are manipulated, to protect the technologist from infectious aerosol and to reduce tissue culture contamination. A centrifuge with covered carriers to accommodate shell vials should be available. Incubators to maintain uninoculated cells and to incubate inoculated cultures are needed, preferably with an internal outlet for hook-up of a roller drum. Also needed are an inverted phase-contrast microscope to identify CPE in cell culture monolayers, and an epifluorescence microscope for direct and indirect immunofluorescence assay (IFA) procedures; freezer space at −20° C (−70° C, if available) is also desirable for specimen and reagent storage. Liquid nitrogen for cell storage is expensive and is not essential for laboratories that purchase cell lines.

All essential supplies and reagents used to identify the common viruses are commercially available. Cell cultures are nourished by a balanced salt solution (Hanks or Earle) with added buffers, serum, and a nutrient mixture such as Eagle minimum essential medium (MEM). Eagle MEM is a precisely defined formulation of amino acids, sugars, vitamins, cofactors, and other metabolic requirements for the cell monolayer. Fetal bovine or calf serum (FBS) is a popular nutritional and hormonal supplement added to MEM; 5%–10% FBS is used for cell culture growth medium, and 2% for maintenance medium. Trypsin (0.25% solution), phosphate-buffered saline (PBS), glutamine and sodium bicarbonate solutions, VTM, and antibiotic mixtures for specimen decontamination should be stocked in the laboratory as needed.

Laboratories undertaking viral diagnostic services for the first time should consider beginning with straightforward testing such as HSV culture. Influenza, RSV, and rotavirus assays and cultures for other respiratory viruses can be added during the winter months. CMV identification is a priority for a hospital with immunocompromised patients. Enterovirus isolation could be offered initially for the summer and autumn. VZV, adenovirus, and parainfluenza virus cultures and antigen assays would be reasonable year-round additions as staff time and expertise increase. The laboratory should be familiar with specimen collection and transport requirements of public health laboratories and reference laboratories that provide supplementary culture, serology, antigen assay, and nucleic acid assays, so that send-out specimens are processed efficiently.

VIRAL ANTIGEN DETECTION

Rapid identification by direct methods is especially useful when specific antiviral therapy is available (for HSV, VZV, CMV, and influenza), and when nosocomial control is a factor (influenza, RSV, rotavirus, norovirus, and VZV). Viral antigen is detected with comparable sensitivity

TABLE 55-2
Specimen Collection for Common Viral Syndromes

Syndrome	Common viruses	Preferred specimen and transport conditions	Specimen quality validation	Most useful tests
Bronchiolitis/bronchitis Influenza Pneumonia	RSV, PIV, hMPV adenovirus, influenza A and B Influenza A and B RSV, hMPV, PIV, influenza A, adenovirus	NP swab, NP aspirate/wash; BAL; transport on ice for culture	Ciliated columnar cells or alveolar macrophages for NP aspirates and BAL	Nucleic acid amplification; EIA or DFA (in season); culture
Conjunctivitis	HSV, adenoviruses, enteroviruses, VZV	Conjunctival scrapings/swab in VTM; transport on ice for culture	Conjunctival Epithelial cells	Nucleic acid amplification; DFA; culture
Vesicular rash	HSV, VZV	Vesicular fluid/cells in VTM or slide smear for DFA; transport on ice for culture	Squamous Epithelial cells	Nucleic acid amplification; DFA; culture
Meningitis	Enteroviruses, HSV, VZV, EBV, West Nile virus and other arboviruses	CSF; transport on ice for culture	Abnormal CSF protein and cell counts	Nucleic acid amplification; culture (enteroviruses); IgM serology
Encephalitis	HSV, VZV, West Nile virus and other arboviruses, rabies	CSF, fresh brain tissue; transport on ice for culture	Abnormal CSF, protein and cell counts	Nucleic acid amplification; IgM serology
Enteritis	Rotavirus, norovirus, enteric adenoviruses	Fresh stool; transport promptly	Swab must be covered with stool	Rotavirus and adenovirus: EIA Norovirus: RNA amplification
Disseminated viral infection	CMV, EBV, HSV, VZV, adenovirus	Blood, tissue biopsy, BAL, CSF; transport immediately		Nucleic acid amplification; viral load for CMV, EBV; culture for CMV, HSV, VZV, adenovirus
	HIV	Blood		Serology; viral load; ARV resistance testing
Prenatal/neonatal viral infection	HSV1 and -2, CMV, enterovirus, parvovirus B19, rubella	CSF, vesicular fluid, tissue biopsy, amniotic fluid, urine; transport immediately		Nucleic acid amplification; culture; IgM serology

ARV, Antiretroviral therapy; *BAL,* bronchoalveolar lavage; *CMV,* cytomegalovirus; *CSF,* cerebrospinal fluid; *DFA,* direct fluorescent antibody; *EBV,* Epstein-Barr virus; *EIA,* enzyme immunoassay; *HIV,* human immunodeficiency virus; *HSV,* herpes simplex virus; *hMPV,* human metapneumovirus; *IgM,* immunoglobulin M; *NP,* nasopharyngeal; *PCR,* polymerase chain reaction; *PIV,* parainfluenza virus; *RSV,* respiratory syncytial virus; *VTM,* viral transport medium; *VZV,* varicella zoster virus.

and specificity by both direct fluorescent antibody (DFA) and enzyme immunoassay (EIA) methods. DFA has the advantage of microscopic visualization of the specimen's cell content so sample adequacy can be easily verified (Clarke, 2010), but DFA procedures are labor-intensive and may be unfeasible during seasonal respiratory viral outbreaks with high specimen demand. EIA methods require less subjective interpretive judgment than DFA, but assessment of sample quality is lost. DFA is best performed with an epifluorescence microscope, and positive and negative controls must be run routinely. Many EIA procedures are engineered for individual specimen testing with positive and negative control verification incorporated into a single-use cassette. Automated EIA procedures for batch testing combine washing, spectrophotometry, and data processing into a self-contained system; positive and negative controls are standard with each run, and the reading for the patient sample is interpreted using an established cutoff value. Sensitivity is highly dependent on adequate specimen collection, as illustrated by the variable sensitivity seen with these assays in the recent outbreak of 2009 influenza A (H1N1) (Ginocchio, 2009).

MOLECULAR DETECTION

Nucleic acid hybridization and amplification-based tests detect virus by targeting specific regions of the viral RNA or DNA genome. In situ hybridization (ISH) is a direct probe technique that can be used in anatomic pathology to detect a variety of viral pathogens. ISH is a useful method for the localization of specific viral nucleic acids inside individual cells with preservation of cellular morphology. ISH is particularly useful for diagnosis of EBV-related neoplasms (Fanaian, 2009). PCR can also be used for the diagnosis of viral infection in formalin-fixed, paraffin-embedded (FFPE) tissue biopsies, and is particularly useful for confirming the diagnosis of herpes viruses when histologic features are "nondiagnostic" (Böer, 2006).

Nucleic acid amplification technologies have raised the sensitivity of viral diagnosis beyond that of antigen assays or culture. Commonly employed target amplification technologies include PCR, real-time PCR, strand displacement amplification (SDA), nucleic acid sequence–based amplification (NASBA), and transcription-mediated amplification (TMA). Signal amplification technologies include hybrid capture, branched DNA (bDNA), invader chemistry, and gold nanoparticle probe technology. The clinical utility of PCR was greatly expanded with the introduction of real-time PCR, in which amplification and detection take place simultaneously in a closed tube or plate; crossing threshold (cycle number in which amplicon is detectable) is proportionate to viral copy, permitting accurate quantitation. Quantitative real-time PCR is now standard for monitoring HIV, HCV, HBV, CMV, and BKV viral loads. It is recommended to base clinical management on viral load assessment from a single laboratory to reduce the variability that is still inherent between laboratories and technologies (Hayden, 2008). Automation of nucleic acid–based testing, including extraction methods and incorporation of internal controls, has increased the precision of quantitative methods, reduced the risk of amplicon contamination, reduced the rate of false-positive or false-negative errors, and accelerated throughput.

Food and Drug Administration (FDA)-cleared commercial kits are still limited and include assays for HIV, HCV, HBV, HPV, CMV, enterovirus, and a variety of respiratory viruses. The Association for Molecular Pathology (AMP) website maintains a table of FDA-cleared assays, as well as available controls and proficiency panels (www.amp.org). The College of American Pathologists also provides proficiency testing (www.cap.org). Most nucleic acid–based viral assays are currently laboratory developed and utilize in-house designed primers and probes or commercially available analyte-specific reagents (ASRs). Strict adherence to specimen collection, storage, and processing requirements, proper handling and storage of extracted nucleic acid, particularly RNA, and routine monitoring for amplicon contamination are all essential for maximizing detection and reducing error. Analytic and clinical validation and verification are the responsibilities of the individual laboratories.

Equipment required to perform nucleic acid–based testing is becoming more accessible for community hospital laboratories. Most molecular virology methods currently require specialized facilities (separation of areas for reagents, specimen processing and amplification steps, and appropriate air handling) and highly skilled technologists. Many viruses contain RNA genomes, and sample processing requires a certain level of paranoia for accurate and sensitive diagnosis. However, this paradigm is rapidly changing; platforms have recently become available or are in development to support near point-of-care (POC) sample-to-report testing processes (e.g., enterovirus and influenza testing). Increasing availability of automation has greatly influenced the precision and ease of use of nucleic acid–based testing, particularly for quantitative analyses (e.g., HIV, HCV, HBV viral loads, HPV detection systems). Still many nucleic acid–based virology assays remain highly complex laboratory-developed methods requiring an appropriate level of oversight and monitoring. Extraction methods range from column-based manual methods to fully automated extraction and PCR setup. Automated extractors are available for small-volume to high-throughput laboratories. Additional equipment might include PCR workstations, temperature blocks, thermal cyclers (real-time and conventional), sequencers, centrifuges, micropipettors, gel electrophoresis systems, hybridization platforms, spectrophotometers, and storage areas of adequate capacity (4° C, –20° C, –70° C).

VIRAL SEROLOGY

Serologic diagnosis of viral infection has its attractions because serum specimens are easy to obtain, transport, and store. Viral serology has two major clinical applications: diagnosis of recent infection and determination of immunity (Hodinka, 1999). Evidence of current/recent infection requires demonstration of virus-specific IgM during the acute stage of illness, or demonstration of a significant rise in virus-specific IgG titer between acute and convalescent sera. Specific IgM is usually found in blood within the first week of primary infection and typically becomes undetectable within 1–3 months; in general, EIA methods are more sensitive, so detectable IgM may persist for approximately twice as long as immunofluorescent assays. The specificity and sensitivity of IgM assays are improved by removal of rheumatoid factor, by removal of IgG to eliminate competition with IgM for viral antigen, and by selective IgM or IgG capture methods. Virus-specific IgG is normally produced 1–2 weeks after primary infection, peaks at 4–8 weeks, and then declines but usually remains detectable indefinitely at low titer. The secondary immune response following viral reinfection or reactivation produces a different serologic profile: IgM may reappear transiently and in low titer, and IgG rapidly increases in titer. These are only general response patterns; intensity, specificity, timing, and class of antibody are influenced by the infecting virus, site of infection, and immune status of the host. In congenital infection, maternal IgG antibodies passively transfer across the placenta into the fetal circulation, but any IgM, IgA, or IgE detected in fetal, cord, or newborn blood represents antibody produced by the fetus or neonate following primary perinatal infection.

Serology is particularly helpful when specimen quality or transportation conditions are suboptimal for culture or direct antigen testing. If viral disease was not suspected at initial evaluation, then serology may be the only diagnostic tool available once the opportunity for culture, antigen assay, or nucleic acid amplification has passed. Serology is a logical diagnostic choice for viruses that require complex isolation procedures (EBV, human herpesvirus 6) or animal inoculation (arboviruses, some coxsackie A viruses), are a biohazardous risk (HIV, arboviruses, hemorrhagic fever viruses), or have no readily available nucleic acid amplification protocols. For some infections, serology is fast and relatively inexpensive; measles, mumps, and rubella infections can be diagnosed by culture, but IgM-specific antibody is detectable within 3 days of onset of illness and is more reliable. Virus may no longer be present when clinical symptoms develop; West Nile virus (WNV) and other arboviruses are often cleared from spinal fluid at the onset of clinical encephalitis, making serology a more useful diagnostic approach. Infections with a prolonged prodrome often have detectable antibody when the patient first develops symptoms (e.g., EBV and CMV mononucleosis). Specific situations for serologic diagnosis are listed in Figure 55-2.

CLINICAL VIRAL INFECTIOUS SYNDROMES

Our approach to laboratory diagnosis separates viral infections into specific clinical syndromes; this encourages the physician to associate a reasonable but limited group of viruses with the patient's presenting illness. The requisition form or order screen should be designed to require specific patient demographic data and a working clinical diagnosis, so that the laboratory can streamline testing and focus on rapid, high-yield, efficient testing. In this chapter, the following viral diseases and syndromes are discussed:

- Herpetic mucocutaneous infections
- Pediatric and adult respiratory syndromes
- Infectious mononucleosis
- Congenital and neonatal infections
- Viral central nervous system infections
- Viral exanthems and cutaneous infections
- Viral enteric infections
- Viral hepatitis
- Viral infections in the immunocompromised host
- Acquired immunodeficiency syndrome
- Virus-associated neoplasia

HERPETIC MUCOCUTANEOUS INFECTIONS

HSV and varicella zoster virus (VZV) are alpha herpesviruses, are commonplace worldwide, and characteristically produce infections in the skin and squamous mucous membrane surfaces of the body. Neither is usually life threatening; however, the effectiveness of acyclovir therapy has produced demand for prompt laboratory diagnosis, particularly for HSV (Schiffer, 2010).

HSV is ubiquitous and infects all racial groups worldwide. The two strains of HSV (serotype 1 and serotype 2) share many genomic and biological features, and both preferentially infect squamous epithelium; however, each has a unique antigenic profile and a somewhat distinctive epidemiology. HSV1 is transmitted via saliva to infect oropharyngeal and labiofacial surfaces. Lesions may develop on the exposed skin of athletes (herpes gladiatorum) or the hands of medical personnel (herpetic whitlow) after direct salivary contact. Initial HSV1 infection usually occurs in early childhood; primary infection is typically mild or asymptomatic, although a substantial minority of patients develops fever with painful gingivostomatitis. HSV1 is also responsible for an increasing number of genital herpetic ulcers (Ribes, 2001); melt curve analysis of genital herpes infections detected at a large metropolitan health care system in 2010 showed that approximately one third were serotype 1.

HSV1 directly infects ectodermal cells; viral replication depletes the host cells, so squamous cells lose their cytoplasmic integrity, leak fluid, and separate from one another to create a vesicle. Surface bacteria convert the vesicle to a pustule, which then ulcerates. Cutaneous herpes lesions heal without scarring as the epidermal cells regenerate. The immediate immune response involves natural killer cells, cytotoxic T lymphocytes, and production of neutralizing antibody. Despite cellular and humoral factors, HSV1 is able to migrate through sensory nerve fibers to the trigeminal ganglion and persists indefinitely in a dormant state in the neuronal nucleus (Schiffer, 2010). HSV episodically reactivates and travels back down neurosensory axons to the mouth and lips, where it again initiates replication in squamous cells. Most recurrent herpes infections are asymptomatic or produce transient vesicles with only cosmetic significance. With severe impairment of cell-mediated immunity (in acquired immunodeficiency syndrome [AIDS] and transplant patients), reactivation infection may be severe or even fatal. Encephalitis is another rare but devastating HSV1 infection. These complications are discussed in later sections of this chapter.

HSV2 infection is found principally in genital squamous surfaces and is transmitted through intimate sexual contact. At least 40 million Americans have been infected, with estimates of 1 million new cases annually. HSV2 recovery in children is most unusual and raises concerns about sexual abuse; however, beginning with adolescence, seroprevalence rises steadily through middle age and is proportional to the number of sexual partners (Fleming, 1997). In the United States, HSV2 seroprevalence in persons 13 years or older had progressively increased to a rate of 22%; however, a recent survey has shown a modest decrease to 17% (Xu, 2006). HSV2 produces the same pattern of primary and recurrent mucocutaneous lesions seen with oral HSV1. Latency is established in sacral neural ganglia, but reactivation rates are at least twice as high as with HSV1, and transient meningitis may occur. Primary and recurrent HSV2 lesions also heal completely in people with normal cellular immune function. The principal concern is exposure of infants during vaginal delivery; neonatal herpes is discussed later in this chapter.

Specimen Collection and Handling Guidelines

HSV is probably the easiest and fastest human virus to propagate in cell culture. Antigen assays are also relatively straightforward procedures. Nucleic acid amplification tests are now widely available and have superior sensitivity. Specimen collection is simple, and HSV is sufficiently durable and present in sufficient numbers that stat transport and laboratory handling are not essential. Swab specimens in VTM with antibiotics can tolerate a room temperature (22° C) transportation delay of 12 hours with only

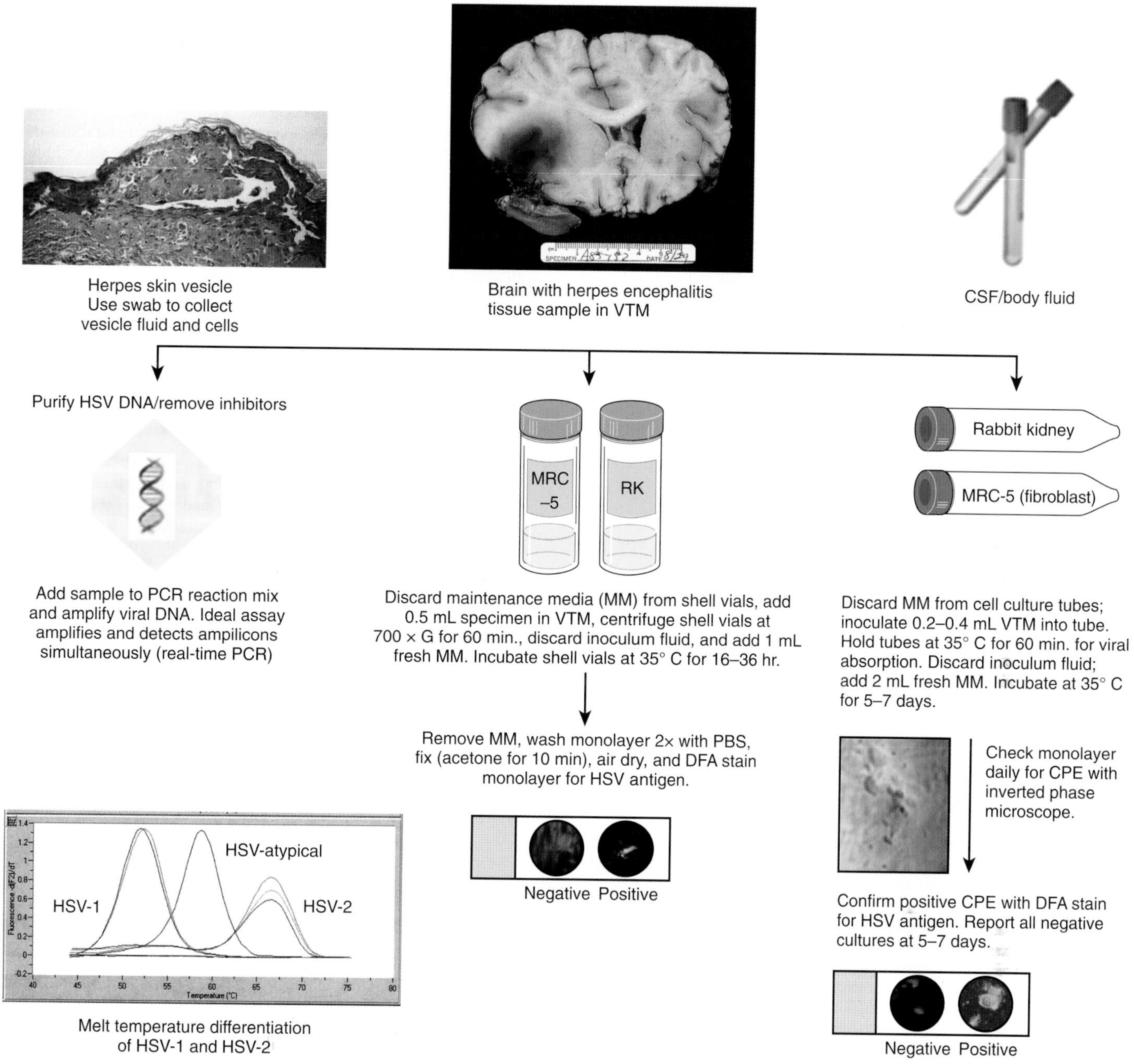
Herpes skin vesicle
Use swab to collect
vesicle fluid and cells
Brain with herpes encephalitis
tissue sample in VTM
CSF/body fluid
Purify HSV DNA/remove inhibitors
MRC
-5
RK
Rabbit kidney
MRC-5 (fibroblast)
Add sample to PCR reaction mix
and amplify viral DNA. Ideal assay
amplifies and detects ampilicons
simultaneously (real-time PCR)
Discard maintenance media (MM) from shell vials, add
0.5 mL specimen in VTM, centrifuge shell vials at
700 × G for 60 min., discard inoculum fluid, and add 1 mL
fresh MM. Incubate shell vials at 35° C for 16–36 hr.
Discard MM from cell culture tubes;
inoculate 0.2–0.4 mL VTM into tube.
Hold tubes at 35° C for 60 min. for viral
absorption. Discard inoculum fluid;
add 2 mL fresh MM. Incubate at 35° C
for 5–7 days.
Remove MM, wash monolayer 2x with PBS,
fix (acetone for 10 min), air dry, and DFA stain
monolayer for HSV antigen.
Check monolayer
daily for CPE with
inverted phase
microscope.
HSV-atypical
HSV-1
HSV-2
Negative Positive
Confirm positive CPE with DFA stain
for HSV antigen. Report all negative
cultures at 5–7 days.
Melt temperature differentiation
of HSV-1 and HSV-2
Negative Positive

Figure 55-3 Traditional tube and shell vial cultures for herpes simplex virus (HSV) and HSV DNA amplification.

modest viral loss. Specimens should be inoculated to cell culture on the day of receipt, but overnight refrigeration is acceptable.

Cell Culture Isolation of Herpes Simplex Virus

HSV grows exceptionally well in a variety of cell lines; human fibroblasts (WI-38, MRC-5, foreskin), rabbit kidney (RK), mink lung, HeLa, rhabdomyosarcoma (RD), Vero, and HEp-2 cell lines work well; however, primary monkey kidney (PMK) is not reliable. Two tissue culture tubes (e.g., one RK and one MRC-5) are usually inoculated; the procedure is summarized in Figure 55-3. HSV replicates rapidly with CPE usually apparent after 1 or 2 days of incubation. Genital cultures that fail to show HSV CPE after 5 days of incubation can be reported as negative. Incubation of cultures from central nervous system (CNS), corneal, oral, and other nongenital sites should be extended for 2 weeks, so other viruses (VZV, CMV, adenoviruses, enteroviruses, etc.) may be recovered. Individual HSV-infected cells become swollen and rounded, and this damage spreads rapidly across the monolayer. This CPE is characteristic of but not unique for HSV; changes caused by other viruses, toxins, or trichomonads may be confused with HSV, so confirmation with a DFA stain is needed. Reaction of infected cells with monoclonal HSV antibodies can distinguish HSV1 from HSV2 (Lipson, 1991). With the use of shell vial centrifugation-enhanced culture, HSV can be identified in the monolayer by DFA staining after only 1 day of incubation (Clarke, 2010).

The ELVIS HSV shell vial culture system uses genetically altered cells that develop blue nuclear color after 1 day or less of HSV replication; it is a simple and very sensitive method for HSV culture (Patel, 1999).

Nucleic Acid–Based Detection of Herpes Simplex Virus

Real-time PCR followed by melt curve analysis is commonly used for the detection and typing of HSV. A wide variety of specimen types can be accommodated with molecular methods, including swab specimens in VTM or universal transport media, cerebrospinal fluid (CSF), bronchoalveolar lavage (BAL), frozen tissue specimens, and FFPE tissue. PCR-quality DNA can be extracted by a variety of commercially available methods (manual or automated). Specimen DNA is combined with PCR reagents, which minimally include an appropriate buffer system containing Mg^{++} and K^{+} salts, deoxynucleotide triphosphates, target-specific primers, fluorescently labeled probes, and a DNA polymerase. The samples are placed in a real-time thermal cycler for temperature cycling and fluorescence monitoring, resulting in multiple rounds of DNA replication of specific regions of the viral genome with increasing levels of fluorescence. Costs are comparable with culture-based detection and typing methods; because of increases in sensitivity and rapid turnaround, nucleic acid amplification is quickly replacing conventional methods as standard of care.

Direct Detection of Herpes Simplex Virus

A direct smear from a herpetic skin vesicle can be stained with Giemsa reagent (Tzanck smear) to demonstrate viral multinucleated syncytial epithelial giant cells and intranuclear inclusions; however, these findings are not specific for HSV infection; identical changes are seen in VZV (chickenpox and shingles). Only 67% of herpetic lesions at the vesicle stage have a positive Giemsa Tzanck smear; sensitivity drops to only 30% for ulcerated skin lesions. Immunostaining of direct smears with fluorescein- or immunoperoxidase-labeled HSV antibodies eliminates confusion with VZV, and viral antigen can be identified in cells that do not yet have nuclear inclusions. However, when compared with culture, DFA staining has at best a 20%–30% false-negative error (Moseley, 1981; Lafferty, 1987). All negative direct specimen test results must be considered as possible false-negatives that should be validated by parallel culture. On the other hand, PCR diagnosis of mucocutaneous genital herpes infection is 20%–30% more sensitive than culture and has a more rapid turnaround time than culture (Espy, 2000). PCR is superior for identification of asymptomatic mucocutaneous viral shedding—eight times more sensitive than culture (Cone, 1994).

Serologic Diagnosis

Broad antigenic homology has been noted between HSV1 and HSV2, so accurate serologic testing requires antigens that are serotype-specific. EIA and Western blot methods that use unique HSV1 and HSV2 glycoprotein G (gG) envelope antigens do not detect cross-reacting antibodies (Ashley, 1988; Morrow, 2003). HSV2-specific antibody testing of pregnant women and their husbands helps predict neonatal transmission risk (Ashley, 1999; Cherpes, 2003). Positive HSV2 antibody in a patient with genital vesicles or ulcers is highly likely to represent true genital herpes (Jerome, 2007). IgM serology for HSV1 or HSV2, including gG IgM antibody, is not specific or sensitive and should not be used for diagnosis of primary infection.

VIRAL RESPIRATORY TRACT INFECTIONS

Every year, several million combined outpatient visits and hospitalizations in the United States are related to respiratory tract infections, most of which are viral in origin. All age groups are affected, and infections range from minor colds to serious laryngotracheobronchitis (croup), bronchiolitis, and pneumonia. Colds and pharyngitis have usually been managed with clinical judgment and no laboratory testing. Hospital laboratories have traditionally used a combination of antigen assay and culture to identify influenza viruses, parainfluenza viruses, RSV, and adenovirus among pediatric and adult patients. However, commercial multiplex nucleic acid panels in a single vial simultaneously test for influenza A and B, several influenza A hemagglutinin (H) antigens, parainfluenzas, RSV, adenoviruses, coronaviruses, metapneumoviruses, rhinoviruses, and enteroviruses. Most current assays are designed for batch testing with a throughput time of 4 to 8 hours (Li, 2007; Mahoney, 2007; Pabbaraju, 2008). Overall sensitivity compared with antigen assay and culture is excellent, with as many as 40% more viral infections identified, particularly when multiplex assay includes metapneumovirus, coronaviruses, and rhinovirus/enterovirus (Mahoney, 2007). The cost of an expanded amplified nucleic acid respiratory virus panel is competitive with the combined labor and reagent expenses charged for antigen testing, followed by virus culture of specimens with negative antigen results. During high-prevalence respiratory outbreaks, multiplex viral nucleic acid tests are the least costly diagnostic strategy for hospitalized children (Mahoney, 2009).

The obvious immediate advantage of these expanded test profiles for the individual patient is the far greater likelihood of prompt recovery of the viral pathogen for evidence-based use of antiviral drugs and for rapid implementation of appropriate infection control measures (Arnold, 2008). These assays should also help delineate the clinical effects of coinfection with multiple viral pathogens (Brunstein, 2008). With the addition of picornavirus/rhinovirus, coronavirus, and metapneumovirus pathogens, public health laboratories have used multiplex amplified molecular tests to successfully characterize additional viral respiratory infection outbreaks (Marshall, 2007; Wong, 2009).

Molecular techniques have been successfully applied in the rapid evaluation of recent novel viral respiratory disease outbreaks. An example is the initial emergence of worldwide SARS in 2003; the causative agent was sequenced and was promptly characterized as a novel coronavirus, and accurate diagnostic testing quickly became available (Ksiazek, 2003). In the spring of 2009, a novel H1N1 influenza A virus, first detected in Mexico, rapidly evolved into a global pandemic. Within a matter of weeks, the strain had been sequenced and accurate diagnostic reagents had been developed; within 6 months, a vaccine was mass-produced and distributed (Greenberg, 2009; Perez-Padilla, 2009; Sullivan, 2010). The wider implementation of molecular methods has also demonstrated that clinical respiratory tract symptoms can be caused by a more diverse range of viral agents than was previously presumed. Metapneumovirus has been defined as having epidemiologic and clinical properties similar to those of RSV (Kahn, 2006). Acute upper respiratory tract colds are caused by rhinoviruses and coronaviruses; more than 100 of these agents circulate almost continuously in the pediatric and adult communities. Healthy hosts get many colds over a lifetime, with up to 25% of total sick days severe enough to miss work or school. Rhinoviruses have been the only viral pathogen recovered by multiplex amplified nucleic acid testing in babies with typical bronchiolitis and acute exacerbations of asthma. Both coronaviruses and rhinoviruses have caused clinically severe lower respiratory illness in compromised hosts (Piotrowska, 2009; Talbot, 2009; Kuypers, 2010).

Influenza

Influenza A and B viruses cause predictable annual cold weather outbreaks of acute febrile upper and lower respiratory tract illness with characteristic accompanying systemic features (Fig. 55-4). Influenza A is usually more common than B and produces more serious disease. Influenza antigens change through point mutations in the genome (antigenic drift, influenza A and B) and through recombination of human and animal viral RNA segments (antigenic shift, influenza A), so antibodies from prior infections may not be protective in subsequent outbreaks (Sullivan, 2010; Treanor, 2010). Influenza is easily spread from person to person in aerosol droplets; the virus attaches to and replicates rapidly in the ciliated columnar epithelial cells of the pharynx and tracheobronchial tree. After incubation of 1 to 2 days, disease usually begins abruptly with the onset of fever and chills; viral respiratory epithelial necrosis causes sore throat and cough, but associated systemic myalgias, headache, and generalized weakness are typically more severe than respiratory symptoms. Uncomplicated influenza usually resolves after 4–5 days. However, during every influenza outbreak, a small number of patients develop severe acute primary pneumonia with viral necrosis extending into the alveolar lining cells. These patients are at risk for developing bacterial lower respiratory infection following acute influenza, because the bronchi are temporarily covered by metaplastic epithelium and have not yet reacquired normal ciliated mucosa; individuals with chronic lung and cardiac disease are most vulnerable and account for a majority of the deaths recorded each year for influenza epidemics (Yeldandi, 1994; Soto-Abraham, 2009).

Influenza outbreaks in a local community have a characteristic epidemiologic curve (Treanor, 2010); numbers of infected individuals rise rapidly, peak, and then decline rapidly over about a 6–8 week period. A second peak of influenza-related bacterial pneumonia then follows. Every year, approximately 100,000 hospitalizations and 20,000 deaths in the United States are linked to influenza, and most fatalities are caused by bacterial bronchopneumonia, usually affecting patients with preexisting chronic obstructive lung disease or congestive heart failure. Myocarditis, meningoencephalitis, Reye syndrome, and Guillain-Barré syndrome are relatively rare complications.

Influenza is diagnosed best during the first 2–3 days of illness, when viral shedding is maximal. Infected cells from the upper respiratory tract are the easiest to collect for testing. Nasopharyngeal aspirate (NPA) and pharyngeal swab specimens provide sufficient material for simultaneous testing for several viral agents, including influenza viruses. Proper specimen collection is critical. A video demonstrating collection of both specimen types is available at http://www.thepathologycenter.org/Education.asp. Nucleic acid testing by RT-PCR has been shown as the most sensitive method for diagnosis, and has surpassed culture methods in both accuracy and turnaround time (Erdman, 2003; Templeton, 2004). Culture is the next most sensitive diagnostic test; nasopharyngeal secretions/NPA samples are ideal; nasopharyngeal swabs and throat swabs may be satisfactory but often provide suboptimal samples. Shell vial culture with 1–2 days' incubation has excellent sensitivity (Dunn, 2004) and may still provide a diagnosis within a time frame to affect management of the index patient or prophylaxis of contacts. Hybrid mink lung and A549 shell vial monolayers are versatile and can recover influenza A and B, parainfluenzas, adenovirus, and RSV (Figs. 55-5 and 55-6). Culture with traditional cell

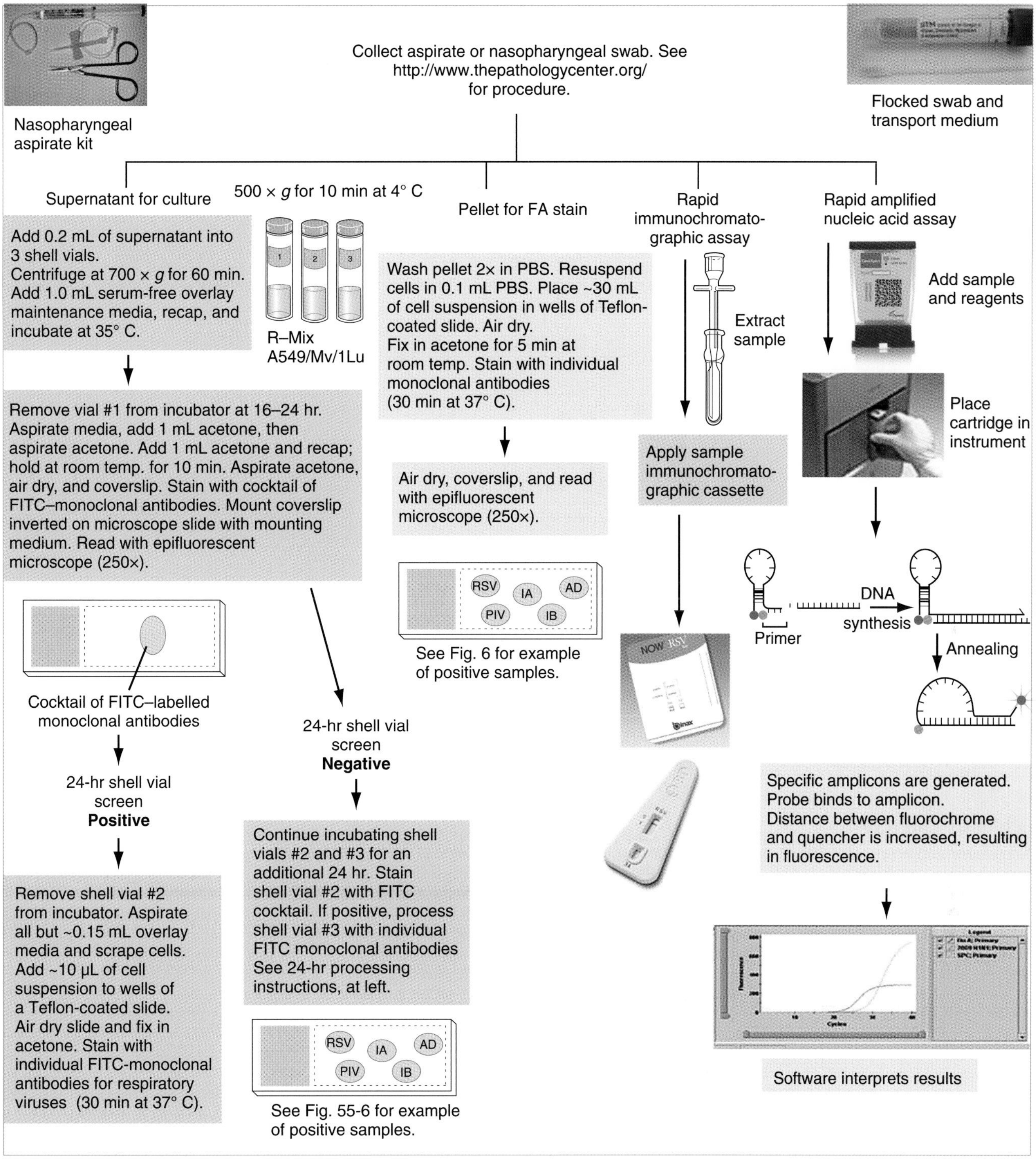

Figure 55-4 Laboratory diagnoses of respiratory viral infections with direct antigen assays (enzyme immunoassay [EIA] and direct fluorescent antibody [DFA]), shell vial culture, and nucleic acid assays.

monolayers and red cell hemadsorption attachment to influenza-infected cells expressing surface hemagglutinin antigen may not yield a positive result for 2–7 days, and currently is rarely used in hospital laboratories.

DFA stain can demonstrate virus-infected columnar epithelial cells in NPA samples, which provide the preferred specimen (see Fig. 55-6). Compared with cell culture, DFA sensitivity ranges from 77%–93% for detection of influenza A, and from 70%–80% for influenza B (higher in pediatric patients). Specificity is greater than 95%; however, good results are heavily influenced by the experience of the microscopist and by specimen quality. Throat and nasopharyngeal swabs generally lack sufficient columnar cells for DFA staining. Commercial immunochromatographic EIA methods are rapid and easy to perform but have only fair sensitivity for influenza antigen detection in NPA specimens during outbreaks. Specificity of any antigen testing during nonseasonal times of the year is poor, so laboratories should restrict ordering to high-prevalence months. Sensitivity with nasopharyngeal swabs is considerably lower, particularly for antigen assays and culture. Nasopharyngeal swab specimens collected during the 2009 H1N1 influenza outbreak were tested by DFA and two rapid EIA methods, along with a commercial RT-PCR multiplex test and an R-mix shell vial culture. DFA sensitivity was poor (46%), and EIA methods showed only 10%–40% sensitivity; all antigen assays had 6% false-positive results (Ginocchio, 2009). It is not surprising that RT-PCR was clearly superior to all other methods; however, antigen assays performed more poorly than anticipated. Comparison of an antigen assay with RT-PCR in a similar H1N1 influenza outbreak in the Chicago area also showed low sensitivity (50.5%) and a 39% false-positive rate (Sabatini, unpublished data).

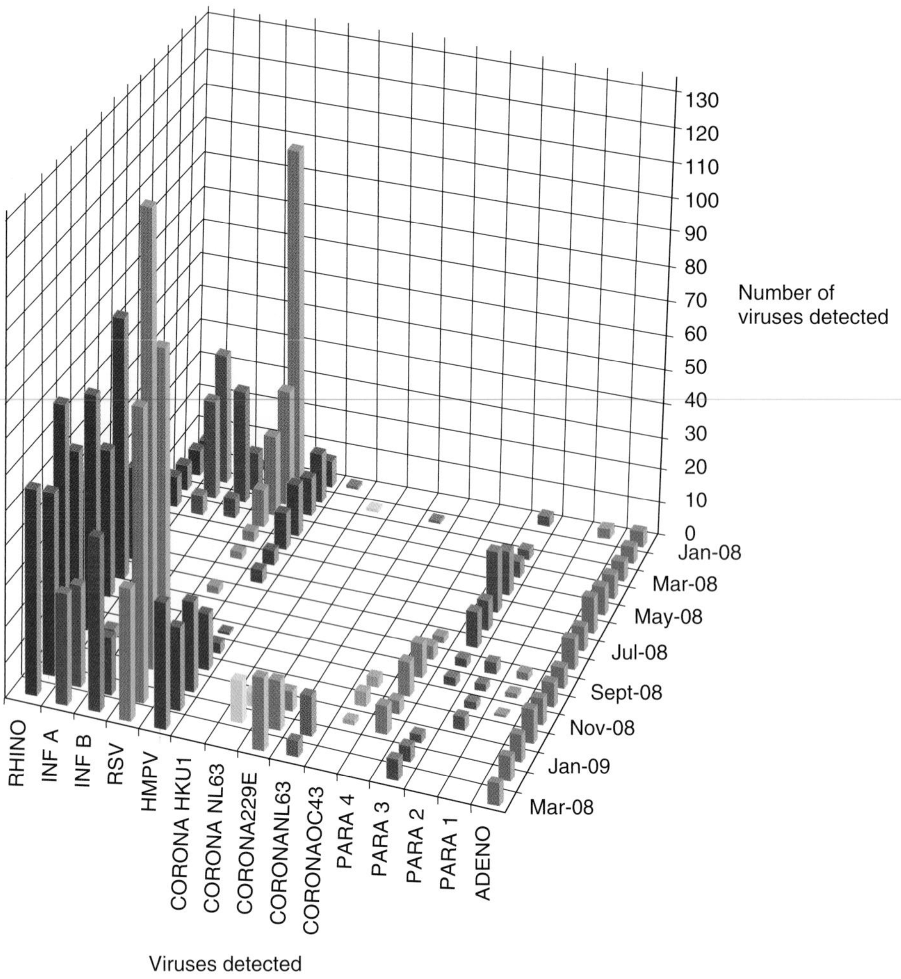

Figure 55-5 Seasonal variation in respiratory viral infections. Chicago area and southeast Wisconsin—January 2008 to April 2009.

Bronchiolitis and RSV

RSV is the most important cause of serious lower respiratory viral disease in infants and young children (Hall, 2001, 2010). Like influenza, RSV is transmitted by droplet aerosol, and outbreaks recur every winter. Currently, no vaccine for RSV is available; natural immunity to RSV is incomplete and of short duration, so multiple infections occur throughout life. RSV, similar to influenza, infects ciliated columnar epithelial cells from the nasopharynx to the distal bronchioles. Small babies experience the most serious infections because their narrow terminal airways become occluded by necrotic epithelial cells; bronchiolar obstruction leads to air trapping and hypoxia, which may be severe enough to require hospitalization. Acute symptoms usually resolve in a few days; administration of oxygen and other supportive measures are often the only medical interventions needed. Most critical RSV infections occur in premature infants, in children with underlying cardiopulmonary disease or immunodeficiencies, and in transplant recipients. Adults who are immunocompromised and the elderly may also have severe lower airway RSV disease (Falsey, 2005). Treatment with ribavirin or with the monoclonal antibody palivizumab is available but generally is prescribed only for severe cases (Empey, 2010).

RSV is a particularly fragile and labile virus that may not remain viable if specimen transport is delayed. It replicates slowly in cell culture, and recovery times range from 3–10 days (Tristram, 2003; Tang, 2008). Hep-2 and A549 cell lines are ideal for RSV replication; characteristic cytopathic changes are seen with fusion of adjacent infected cells into a large multinucleate syncytium (see Fig. 55-6). Shell vial culture improves RSV recovery somewhat and shortens isolation time to 1–2 days (Dunn, 2004). Use of shell vial monolayers with a hybrid mix of A549 and mink lung cells detects RSV, as well as influenza A and B, parainfluenzas, and adenoviruses (see Figs. 55-4 and 55-6). Detection of RSV antigen in respiratory secretions by DFA staining (see Fig. 55-6) or by EIA is as sensitive as or superior to culture, and availability of results is clinically relevant; therefore, rapid tests have remained popular and practical methods for RSV diagnosis in children (Ohm-Smith, 2004; Tang, 2008). EIA is easy and rapid to perform; DFA requires more time and interpretive expertise, but it can be expanded to assay multiple viruses, and confirmation of specimen quality is simple. Similar to rapid antigen assays for influenza, RSV antigen tests should be performed only during wintertime outbreaks; off-season testing has poor specificity, with false-positive results outnumbering true-positive results. RT-PCR has been shown to have superior sensitivity over all other methods, and transport conditions are not as restricted because viability is not required (Falsey, 2002; Perkins, 2005); RSV nucleic amplification is the ideal method for off-season specimens. With the advent of multiplex testing, other viruses, such as metapneumovirus, coronaviruses, bocavirus, parainfluenzas, and even rhinoviruses, have been shown to produce respiratory disease that clinically mimics RSV (Kahn, 2006; Falsey, 2010).

Croup

Croup is most commonly caused by parainfluenza viruses (PIVs) (Henrickson, 2003). PIV1, PIV2, and PIV4 are more common during cold weather; PIV3 causes disease year-round (see Fig. 55-5). PIVs (particularly PIV3) are the second most frequent cause of viral lower respiratory tract infection in young children. Viral epithelial necrosis and mucosal edema in the larynx, trachea, and large bronchi narrow the airway, producing hoarseness, barking cough, and the stridorous obstructed breathing pattern characteristic of croup. Immunity is transient, and repeat infections are common; however, in older children and adults, symptoms are less severe and are centered in the upper respiratory tract, possibly resembling rhinovirus colds. Antigen assay methods are limited to DFA staining of virus-infected nasopharyngeal cells (see Fig. 55-6), which shows 70%–85% compared with culture; all DFA-negative specimens should be cultured to maximize recovery (Costello, 1993). Multiplex viral nucleic acid tests, which include the parainfluenzas, are superior to both antigen assays and culture for clinical diagnosis (Mahoney, 2008, 2009).

Metapneumovirus

Human metapneumovirus (hMPV) is a recently recognized RNA myxovirus, genus Metapneumovirus (Falsey, 2010). Similar to RSV, hMPV causes a range of cold weather respiratory infections, including upper

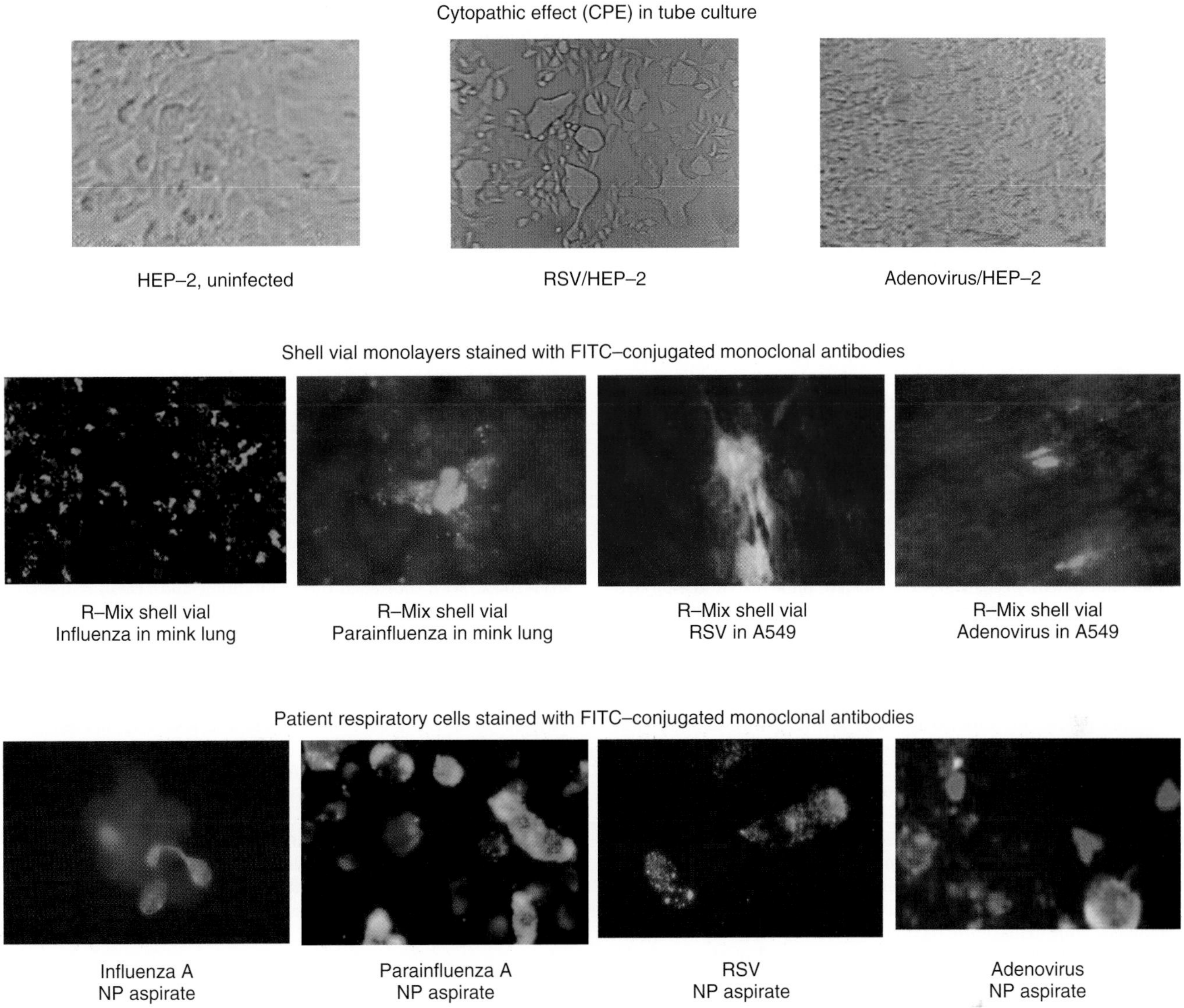

Figure 55-6 Viral growth in cell culture line and viral detection in patient samples.

airway disease, lower airway bronchitis and bronchiolitis, influenza-like syndrome, and pneumonia. hMPV bronchiolitis tends to be less harsh than RSV, but coinfection with RSV and hMPV can be more severe than infection with either one alone (Konig, 2004). hMPV ranks as the second or third most common cause of serious lower airway pediatric disease; the elderly and the immunocompromised also can experience severe respiratory tract infection (Bouscambert, 2005; Kahn, 2006; Dare, 2007; Lüsebrink, 2010).

Recovery in LLC-MK2 cells or Vero cells may take up to 7 days (Deffrasnes, 2005). Culture of NPA and bronchial lavage specimens using a shell vial culture format and anti-hMPV monoclonal antibody DFA staining can shorten recovery (Ebihara, 2005; Landry, 2005). However, nucleic acid testing is considered the "gold standard," and inclusion of hMPV in commercial multiplex RT-PCR assays has demonstrated that hMPV is a consistently recovered pathogen in a community hospital practice (see Fig. 55-5). During the early spring of 2010, as 2009 H1N1 abated, hMPV supplanted influenza in the Chicago area, accounting for up to 42% of viral respiratory infections. Wider availability of nucleic acid assays will better define the spectrum of hMPV disease and the true incidence of infection.

Other Viral Respiratory Tract Infections

Adenovirus has a consistent year-round epidemiology profile, and most clinical isolates are seen in patients with respiratory tract and conjunctival infections (see Fig. 55-5); most adenovirus respiratory disease is mild and self-limiting. However, outbreaks of severe respiratory infection have been reported in military personnel and in other populations living in crowded conditions. Outbreaks of a virulent adenovirus serotype 14 and a recombinant adenovirus with properties of serotypes 11 and 14 have recently been reported in otherwise healthy adults and children (Lewis, 2009; Tate, 2009; Yang, 2009). Serious adenoviral pneumonia can also develop in the immunocompromised; stem cell and solid organ transplant recipients are the most common patient groups involved, and disease is identified by standard culture and molecular methods (Rhee, 2010). Adenovirus can be demonstrated by DFA staining of nasopharyngeal aspirate cells (see Fig. 55-6). Adenovirus also grows well in R-Mix hybrid mink lung/A549 shell vial monolayers (see Fig. 55-6).

In 2003, an outbreak of highly contagious acute hemorrhagic pneumonia originated in China and was spread by international travelers within Asia and beyond; the responsible organism was identified as a coronavirus variant (CoV), the clinical disease was named severe acute respiratory syndrome, and the outbreak had a mortality rate of almost 10% (Peiris, 2003). With detailed molecular characterization of CoV, accurate diagnostic testing was developed within a matter of months. Strict infection control measures were implemented for all recognized cases to limit transmission. Nucleic acid amplification for CoV-SARS is available through public health laboratories. However, even though these diagnostic methods are available, only very rare cases of SARS have been reported since the 2003 epidemic, and these were connected to research facilities. The explanation for the dramatic disappearance of CoV-SARS is not clear, but public health facilities continue surveillance for a possible recurrence.

With the advent of multiplex nucleic acid tests, the significant impact of rhinoviruses, human coronaviruses, and human bocaviruses and the possibility of WU and KI polyomaviruses in both upper and lower respiratory tracts are better appreciated. Expanded availability of broad testing panels has highlighted the importance of these respiratory viral agents, with small children having the most frequent and most serious lower respiratory tract infections (Choi, 2006; Louie, 2009; Tregoning, 2010; Zorc, 2010).

Specimen Collection

The respiratory myxoviruses and adenovirus can infect ciliated columnar epithelial cells from the nasopharynx to the alveoli, so when lower airway disease (croup, bronchiolitis, pneumonia, or influenza) is suspected, the upper respiratory mucosa is still the easier and more accessible site to sample for culture, antigen assay, or nucleic acid assays. The upper respiratory tract is the most common site of infection for rhinovirus and coronavirus. Specimens should be collected during the first few days of illness, when viral replication is greatest. A throat swab placed in VTM with antibiotics may be accepted for influenza culture, but yield is 10%–20% less; expectorated sputum is also adequate for culture, particularly in adults who are coughing productively. Nasopharyngeal swab specimens vary considerably in quality but are adequate for nucleic acid assays; culture and a limited panel of viruses for direct antigen detection can also be performed on NP swabs. Collect swab specimens using sterile Dacron, rayon, or flocked swabs with plastic shafts; do not use cotton or calcium alginate. Nasopharyngeal specimens obtained with flocked swabs collect a larger volume of sample with more numerous epithelial cells, and consistently provide better samples than are provided by fiber swabs (Daley, 2006; Walsh, 2008).

NPA is straightforward and simple: a catheter attached to a syringe is inserted through the nares to the nasopharynx; 1–3 mL of saline is instilled, then saline and mucosal cells and secretions are immediately reaspirated directly back into the syringe. A video demonstrating collection of swab and aspirate samples can be reviewed at http://www.thepathologycenter.org/Education.asp. All specimens should be transported on ice promptly to minimize RSV loss. Specimen quality can be verified before performing culture or antigen assay. NPA with at least two ciliated columnar epithelial cells per 250× field yields a fourfold greater recovery of respiratory viral pathogens (Costello, 1993). Nasal swabs are never acceptable for testing by any method.

Virus Antigen Assays

Figure 55-4 outlines a strategy for specimen collection and testing by culture, antigen assay, and nucleic acid methods for respiratory virus diagnosis. Reproducible and accurate viral antigen detection by DFA requires interpretive expertise; therefore, if possible, both viral culture and antigen assay should be done to maximize recovery. Hospitals with a large pediatric service routinely test respiratory specimens for a panel of viruses (RSV, hMPV, influenza A and B, PIVs, and adenovirus) during winter months if budgets permit. Adults should be tested for influenza virus; RSV and possibly hMPV should also be considered for elderly patients. The NPA sample is used for EIA testing, and then is washed in PBS and centrifuged with the supernatant used for virus culture. If DFA stains for viral antigens are ordered, the cell button is resuspended in PBS, and drops of fluid/cells are spread on Teflon and poly-L-lysine–coated slides. Air-dried smears are fixed with 100% acetone and are stained for viral antigen(s) using specific fluorescein conjugated antibodies with Evans blue counterstain. NPA cytospin preparations increase cell recovery (Landry, 2000). Cell recovery is superior from flocked swab collections. Note the number of ciliated columnar epithelial cells and the degree of nonspecific staining caused by residual background mucus or neutrophils. Figure 55-6 shows that NPA DFA stains positive for influenza A, parainfluenza 3, RSV, and adenovirus. Fluorescein-conjugated antisera are tested for specificity with a panel of known positive tissue culture control cells; reagent lots should show consistent cellular stain distribution and intensity. Overall, DFA methods have excellent specificity and sensitivity.

Several EIAs are commercially available for RSV and influenza A and B. The specificity and sensitivity of these products are comparable with those of DFA staining (Ohm-Smith, 2004; Weinberg, 2005). NPA can easily be checked for the presence of ciliated columnar epithelial cells by scanning a wet mount slide prepared by mixing one drop of specimen with one drop of saline at 250× to verify that sufficient nasopharyngeal columnar cells are present. Swab specimens from the throat or nasopharynx contain too little cellular material for cytologic prescreening.

Virus Isolation

The same specimen requirements and restrictions used for antigen assays also apply to virus culture. Respiratory cultures in nonimmunocompromised adults and children can be modified throughout the calendar year to accommodate predictable seasonal epidemics of influenza, RSV, metapneumovirus, and PIV (see Fig. 55-5). At a minimum, virology laboratories should attempt to isolate RSV and influenza during the winter; if staffing permits, PIV, metapneumovirus, and adenovirus can be included for pediatric patients (Hodinka, 2010). Culture improves overall diagnostic yield beyond antigen assays by approximately 10%–20% for all agents except RSV, which is fastidious and may not remain viable in transport. Culture setup can be expanded to recover viruses that are not included in the antigen assay panel.

Nasopharyngeal swabs for influenza culture only should be placed in VTM with antibiotics at collection and transported promptly, preferably on ice. Sputum that contains lower respiratory tract cells and/or acute inflammation is also acceptable for influenza culture and should be placed in VTM with antibiotics. VTM vial specimens should be vortexed vigorously; culture inoculation should not be delayed past 24 hours; inoculation on the day of collection is obviously preferable. For prompt recovery, the supernatant is inoculated into duplicate shell vials (i.e., two trypsinized Madin-Darby canine kidney [MDCK], two Rhesus monkey kidney [RMK], or two hybrid R-Mix), which are refed after centrifugation with FBS-free MEM (bovine serum may contain antibodies to influenza virus). After 1–2 days' incubation at 35° C, shell vial monolayers are DFA-stained for influenza antigen.

Figure 55-4 outlines a shell vial culture procedure for NPA, using a "hybrid" cell monolayer (R-Mix) that contains both A549 and mink lung (MvL) cells, which together support growth of RSV, influenza A and B, adenovirus, metapneumovirus, and the parainfluenzas. Compared with traditional cell lines, this hybrid cell mix has overall recovery rates of 96%–100%, with shortened turnaround time and overall reduced cost of materials and labor (Schindler, 1999).

Laboratories that culture for only RSV should consider using shell vials in place of traditional tubes to reduce recovery time. HEp-2 or A549 cells in Eagle MEM supplemented with 2%–5% fetal bovine serum support RSV replication. Cell culture tube monolayers should be checked daily for CPE for 10 days. Figure 55-6 shows typical RSV multinucleated cellular syncytium CPE, a pattern that is influenced by cation content and freshness of the maintenance medium (Shahrabadi, 1988; Tristram, 2003). Adenovirus also replicates in HEp-2 and A549 cell lines and produces a grapelike rounding and swelling of monolayer cells, usually by 5–7 days; shell vial cultures shorten adenovirus detection to 3 days (see Fig. 55-6).

A number of serologic methods may be used to detect specific antiviral antibodies, but none is practical for rapid diagnosis and clinical management. Serologic diagnosis is most useful for public health epidemiology studies.

Molecular Detection Methods

Multiplexed nucleic acid and array based assays are consistently more sensitive than culture and, as this technology matures, will become the testing of choice for detection of common respiratory viral pathogens (Nolte, 2007; Mahony, 2008). Several commercial assays are available; some detect single agents, and some contain a minimum of influenza A and B and RSV; others detect a broad panel of respiratory viruses. Technology is rapidly evolving for POC rapid testing. A respiratory virus panel has recently been approved for moderate complexity laboratories and incorporates viral RNA extraction, RT-PCR amplification, and multiplexed detection in a fully automated system that requires only a single pipetting step. The clinical importance of subtyping influenza A virus varies seasonally, depending on the dominant circulating strains and their responses to antiviral therapies (http://www.cdc.gov/h1n1flu/diagnosis/). Simultaneous amplification of a panel of viral agents can provide sensitive and accurate results, typically within 24 hours. The currently available assays have all been approved for use with nasopharyngeal swabs in viral transport media. Clinical laboratories should consider incorporating these versatile molecular assays when possible into their service menu (see Fig. 55-4).

INFECTIOUS MONONUCLEOSIS AND RELATED INFECTIONS

Infectious mononucleosis is a common systemic lymphoproliferative disease usually caused by primary EBV infection. EBV is part of the Herpesviridae family and, similar to HSV, eventually infects the vast majority of the population worldwide. EBV is spread by saliva; primary infection in early childhood is usually asymptomatic, but if delayed until the teen or young adult years, it often leads to classic infectious mononucleosis. Approximately 150,000 mononucleosis cases are reported annually in the United States (Cohen, 2000; Johannsen, 2010).

TABLE 55-3
Serologic Profiles in Epstein-Barr Virus Infection*

Interpretation	Heterophile antibodies	VCA (IgM)	VCA (IgG)	EA (IgG)	EBNA-1 (IgG)
Never infected (susceptible)	–	–	–	–	–
Current primary infection	+/– (50%–85%)†	+ (70%–100%)	+ (>98%)	+ (60%–80%)	–
Infectious mononucleosis	++	++	++	++	–
Recent primary infection	–/+	–/+	++	+	–
Remote past infection	–	–	++	+	+
Immunodeficient patient with persistent activation	–/+	–/+	++	++	+/–

Adapted from Hess RD. Minireview: routine Epstein-Barr virus diagnostics from the laboratory perspective: still challenging after 35 years. J Clin Microbiol 2004;42: 3381–7.
EA, Early antigen; *EBNA,* Epstein-Barr nuclear antigen; *IgM,* immunoglobulin M; *VCA,* viral capsid antigen.
*Atypical serologic profiles may require further testing (VCA-IgG avidity testing, Western blot, or polymerase chain reaction) for evaluation.
†Positive results are lower in younger patients.

EBV first infects the pharynx; sore throat, fever, and tonsillitis typically mark the onset of infectious mononucleosis. EBV is strikingly lymphotrophic; it attaches to the C3d receptor (CD21) on the surface of B lymphocytes in the oropharynx and initiates a polyclonal proliferation of immortalized B lymphoblasts, which generates a polyclonal array of nonspecific IgM antibodies (detected in heterophile antibody assays for infectious mononucleosis). The cell-mediated immune system responds with natural killer cells and $CD8^+$ cytotoxic T lymphocytes to eradicate infected B cells. EBV-infected B lymphocytes accumulate in lymph nodes throughout the body, and defensive cytotoxic T lymphocytes infiltrate nodal interfollicular areas, spleen, and liver and circulate as atypical lymphocytes in the peripheral blood (Strickler, 1993; Luzuriaga, 2010). As the patient's cell-mediated factors bring EBV replication under control, infectious mononucleosis symptoms diminish, and lymphadenopathy, splenomegaly, and hepatitis subside.

Similar to other herpesviruses, EBV infection persists in a dormant asymptomatic state. A small percentage of the immortalized B lymphocytes evade eradication and remain latently infected, serving as a lifelong reservoir for reactivation. The EBV genome circularizes and persists as an episome in the lymphocyte nucleus; Epstein-Barr–encoded RNA (EBER) and the Epstein-Barr nuclear antigen (EBNA) and latent membrane protein antigens maintain the EBV genome in a dormant state, working in concert with $CD8^+$ cells. Asymptomatic EBV reactivation is common, and up to 20% of healthy adults sporadically shed infectious virus in the saliva. With impaired cell-mediated immunity (AIDS, organ transplantation, X-linked lymphoproliferative disease), EBV cannot be held in check; overt diseases such as oral hairy leukoplakia and B cell lymphoproliferative disease and lymphoma may develop. EBV DNA and EBER are identified by nucleic acid tests in the spinal fluid of patients with primary CNS lymphoma, and by nucleic acid amplification assay and in situ hybridization in transplant recipients who develop B cell lymphoproliferative disease during immunosuppressive therapy. EBV is also linked to nasopharyngeal carcinoma in Asians and to African Burkitt's lymphoma; EBV apparently functions as an initiator; then proliferative factors such as coinfection or immune dysregulation lead to malignancy (Johannsen, 2010).

Diagnosis of Infectious Mononucleosis

Cytotoxic T lymphocytes and apoptotic lymphocytes circulate in the bloodstream during infectious mononucleosis (Fisher, 1996); lymphocytosis (>50%) along with atypical lymphocytosis (>10% total lymphocytes) is relatively insensitive for diagnosing EBV mononucleosis, but the combined findings have a specificity of at least 95%. EBV can be cultivated in lymphoblastoid cell lines, but positivity does not differentiate primary infection from reactivation. Serologic testing is the principal laboratory method for infectious mononucleosis diagnosis (Johannsen, 2010). The polyclonal B lymphocyte proliferation of acute EBV infection generates a variety of transitory but generally harmless autoantibodies such as IgM anti-i (cold agglutinin), rheumatoid factor, and antinuclear antibody. Perhaps the most unusual immunoglobulins produced in infectious mononucleosis are the Paul-Bunnell heterophile antibodies. These IgM class antibodies have affinity for sheep, horse, and bovine erythrocytes, and are not directed against any EBV antigens. They are apparently random antibodies produced during EBV-induced B lymphocyte polyclonal proliferation; they emerge during the first week of infectious mononucleosis, decline during convalescence, and are usually undetectable by 3–6 months. Various heterophile antibodies can also develop during serum sickness and occasionally in other viral infections; however, heterophile antibody with strong affinity for beef erythrocyte antigens unchanged by adsorption with guinea pig kidney antigen (the differential absorption test) is specific for acute EBV infectious mononucleosis.

Several commercial rapid assays directly mix patient serum on a slide with a suspension of guinea pig kidney antigen; this is followed by addition of preserved equine or bovine erythrocyte antigen bound to latex particles; agglutination occurs almost immediately if the serum contains infectious mononucleosis heterophile antibody. Rapid agglutination tests and solid-phase modifications are approximately 80%–90% sensitive, have a false-positive rate of less than 2% and a positive predictive value of 95% or greater, and are excellent POC assays (Rogers, 1999; Hess, 2004). Their chief limitation is sensitivity: Heterophile antibody is present in more than 90% of teens and adults but in only 40% or less of young children with EBV infectious mononucleosis.

As EBV evolves from primary infection into latency, various EBV antigens are sequentially expressed, and the specific antibodies generated can be used as markers of the stage of infection. The structural nucleocapsid protein viral capsid antigen (VCA) is produced during acute lytic infection; VCA IgM is a specific and sensitive indicator of acute primary EBV infection and subsides with recovery; VCA IgG can usually be detected with onset of symptoms and then persists for life. The early antigens (EAs) (DNA polymerase and thymidine kinase) are produced during acute infection and active EBV replication; antibody to EA-D is present in recent infection, but EA-R antibody is a persistent late marker. As acute mononucleosis subsides, a small percentage of Epstein-Barr–immortalized B lymphocytes escape immune destruction and latently retain episomal EBV DNA; EBNA is responsible for duplication and survival of this episome. Therefore, EBNA IgG typically develops after acute EBV infection has resolved.

The serologic patterns encountered in the various stages of EBV infection are summarized in Table 55-3. IFA serologic assays use lymphoblastoid cell lines, and EBV production is arrested at specific stages for expression of specific antigens; IFA methods are sensitive and specific but have some interpretive subjectivity and require technical expertise. EIA methods using purified or recombinant VCA show better than 95% sensitivity and almost 100% specificity, and have the advantage of objective interpretation and automated processing (Chan, 1998; Tranchard-Bunel, 1999; Hess, 2004). Most primary care physicians rely upon demonstration of atypical lymphocytes in peripheral blood, rapid heterophile screens, and IgM and IgG VCA for diagnosis of infectious mononucleosis. Quantitative tube heterophile reference methods, IgG-EBNA, and IgG-EA are procedurally more complex and have less practical applicability in outpatient practice.

Heterophile-Negative Infectious Mononucleosis

Of the many patients who present with typical clinical features of infectious mononucleosis in the United States, 70% or more have a positive heterophile test, identifying EBV as the cause. Of the 30% who lack heterophile antibody, up to half are IgM-VCA positive, which also verifies acute EBV infection. In approximately 15% of patients with a febrile lymphoproliferative mononucleosis syndrome, primary infection with *Toxoplasma gondii,* CMV, human herpesvirus 6 (HHV6), or HIV is demonstrated; in the remaining 5%–10%, no etiology is established.

Toxoplasmosis is discussed in Chapter 62; accurate diagnosis is most critical in pregnancy, in immunocompromised hosts, and in chorioretinitis

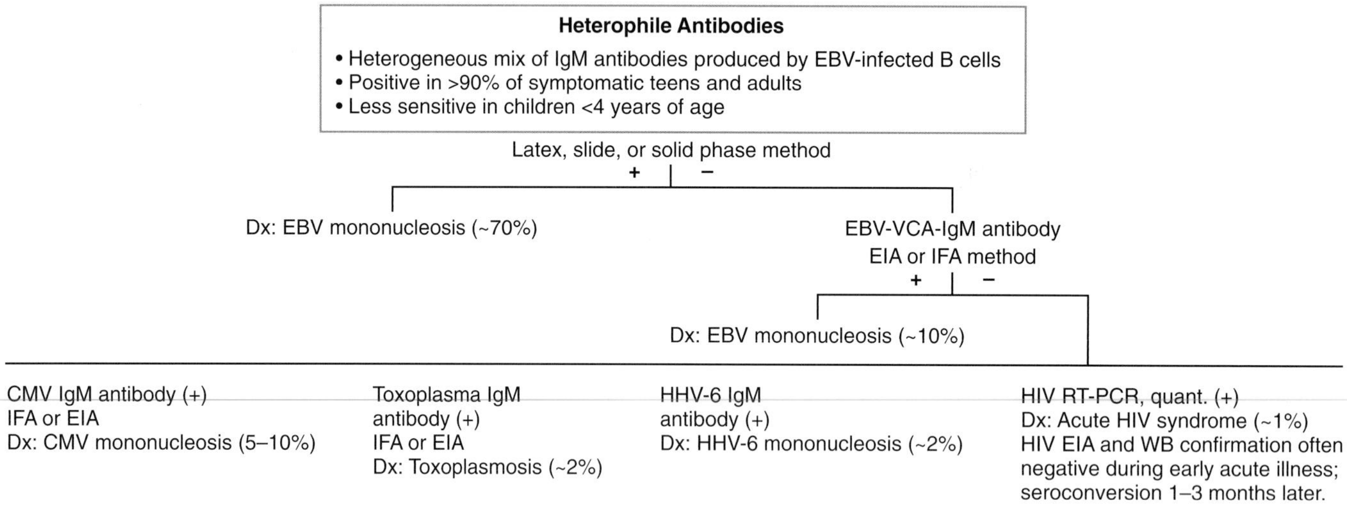

Figure 55-7 Serologic evaluation of patients with clinical symptoms of acute infectious mononucleosis and atypical lymphocytosis. No diagnosis is established in 5%–10% of cases. *CMV,* Cytomegalovirus; *Dx,* diagnosis; *EBV,* Epstein-Barr virus; *EIA,* enzyme immunoassay; *IFA,* immunofluorescent assay.

(Remington, 2004). Primary CMV infection acquired in childhood is usually asymptomatic, whereas teens and adults may have a systemic febrile lymphoproliferative illness that clinically overlaps with EBV infectious mononucleosis (Wreghitt, 2003; Crough, 2009). Isolation of CMV from saliva or urine is not helpful because asymptomatic reactivation and shedding is such a common event. Recovery of CMV from circulating leukocytes is valid and sensitive but is expensive and time-consuming compared with serodiagnosis. CMV IgM IFA serology is complicated by the fact that CMV-infected substrate cells express receptors for immunoglobulin Fc; the anticomplement IFA method (ACIF) is procedurally more complex but reduces this false-positive error. IgM-specific EIAs and enzyme-linked fluorescence assays have overall accuracy that is comparable with the ACIF-IFA IgM assay and have less interpretive subjective variation; pretreatment of serum to remove IgG and rheumatoid factor improves sensitivity (Hodinka, 2007).

HHV6 is another ubiquitous lymphotrophic virus with affinity for T cells. HHV6 causes roseola infantum (exanthem subitum), a common febrile exanthem in young children (Braun, 1997; Prober, 2005; Zerr, 2005). Most primary infections occur in young children; when first exposure is delayed until adulthood, infection is often symptomatic and clinically similar to mononucleosis (Braun, 1997). Both IFA- and EIA-specific IgM assays can diagnose acute infection; virus can also be identified in saliva and plasma with PCR. However, confirmatory testing is not practical for routine primary care practice (Steeper, 1990; Chiu, 1998; Zerr, 2005).

Infection with HIV1 can also produce an acute illness that clinically mimics EBV mononucleosis (Kassutto, 2004). One third or more of patients develop fever, lymphadenopathy, atypical lymphocytosis, and occasionally mild hepatocellular damage or meningoencephalitis. As many as 2% of EBV-negative mononucleosis cases may be caused by HIV acute retroviral syndrome. Standard anti-HIV EIA may fail to detect specific antibody if blood is collected during this early phase of infection, but quantification of plasma HIV by RT-PCR is typically high (10^5 copies/mL). EIA, Western blot, and IFA serologic tests all become positive for HIV antibodies within 1–3 months, as features of acute infection resolve (Schupbach, 2003). Figure 55-7 shows an algorithmic approach to the serologic evaluation of a patient with symptoms of acute mononucleosis. Despite extensive laboratory testing for these acknowledged causes of mononucleosis, no etiologic agent is identified in at least 10% of cases.

CHRONIC FATIGUE SYNDROME

Both the medical press and the lay press have discussed at length a clinical entity characterized by persistent disabling fatigue accompanied by fever, pharyngitis, tender lymphadenopathy, arthralgias, and myalgias (Holmes, 1988; Natleson, 2001). Although the clinical features of this syndrome suggest an infectious cause, none has yet been clearly identified. Initial reports implied that EBV, as chronically persistent primary or reactivated infection, was responsible because many patients had high titers to EBV VCA and EA. However, serologic tests were neither standardized nor reproducible, and EBV culture and ISH performed on saliva and circulating leukocytes showed no difference between chronic fatigue patients and normal controls. Some studies have suggested a role for CMV, enteroviruses, *T. gondii*, HHV6 and HHV7, and human T cell leukemia virus, but other reports have failed to verify a causative role (Reeves, 2000; Colby, 2006). Immunologic and serologic testing is not helpful for diagnosis or prognosis. Chronic fatigue syndrome remains defined by clinical signs and symptoms, rather than by laboratory test results (Lloyd, 1998; Gantz, 2001). A recent study has suggested a link between the retrovirus xenotropic murine leukemia virus and chronic fatigue syndrome (Lombardi, 2009); although this remains unproven, the preliminary association has prompted several blood banks to exclude donors with a clinical history of chronic fatigue syndrome.

CONGENITAL AND PERINATAL VIRAL INFECTIONS

The pregnant uterus is a sterile secluded environment that shelters the fetus from external microbial injury. Maternal vaginal bacteria that ascend through a flawed cervical barrier cause many infections in pregnancy, but maternal infection also can spread hematogenously to the fetus across the placenta, or can directly involve the baby at the time of vaginal delivery. These perinatal infections are collectively named TORCH infections, for toxoplasma (see Chapter 62), rubella, cytomegalovirus, HSV, and other organisms such as HIV, parvovirus B19, enterovirus, and *Treponema pallidum* (see Chapter 59). Infection with these agents may be silent or may cause only minor symptoms in the mother; however, the immature fetal immune system does not generate an effective cellular or humoral response, so fetal tissue necrosis may be severe or even fatal.

Diagnosis of perinatal infection centers on two issues: identification of acute maternal infection (particularly primary infection) and verification of involvement of the fetus or newborn. Maternal infection is best established by recovery of the suspected organism, but for many infectious agents this is impractical, and serologic demonstration of specific IgM antibody, although imperfect, is the first-line diagnostic test. Maternal infection crosses the placenta in 30%–60% of cases. Ultrasound may detect fetal organ damage (microcalcifications, microcephaly, hydrocephalus, organomegaly, hydrops, etc.), but recovery of the organism by culture, demonstration of its antigen or genome in fetal blood or tissues, or detection of specific antibody is required to prove specific fetal infection. Test selection for diagnosis of common perinatal and congenital infection is summarized in Table 55-4. Routine screening of all pregnant women for syphilis, for immunity to rubella, and also for HIV serostatus is standard of care; however, routine prenatal testing for toxoplasma, HSV, and CMV antibodies is not advised. IgM serologic methods in particular may show interlaboratory and intralaboratory variation, with false-negative and false-positive errors; IgG assays do not differentiate primary from recurrent or latent maternal infection and cannot predict fetal involvement. Testing should be reserved for mothers with suspected infection.

Cytomegalovirus

CMV, the most common intrauterine infection, affects 1% of liveborn babies in the United States. About 90% of these infants are asymptomatic

TABLE 55-4
Laboratory Testing for Congenital and Perinatal Infections

Pathogen	Maternal serology	Culture, antigen assays, nucleic acid amplification	Fetal or newborn serology
Cytomegalovirus 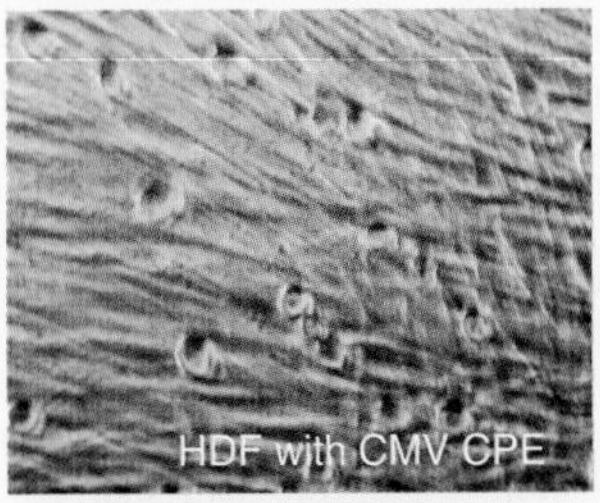 HDF cell monolayer with CMV cytopathic changes	IgM EIA IgG avidity	CMV culture, mother: blood CMV culture, newborn: urine, saliva, blood, tissues (first 2 weeks of life) CMV nuclear inclusions: tissues CMV PCR, in utero: amniotic fluid, umbilical cord blood CMV PCR, newborn: blood, urine (first 2 weeks), tissues	IgM EIA
Herpes simplex virus 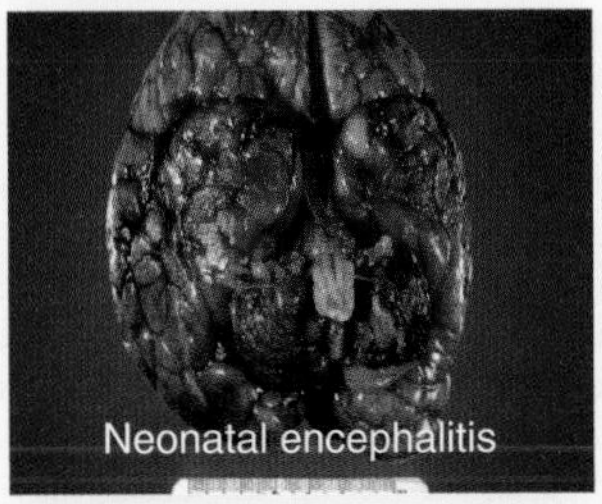	IgM EIA for HSV1 and HSV2 (gG)	HSV PCR or culture: newborn conjunctiva, oral mucosa, skin, CSF HSV nuclear inclusions: newborn tissues, skin lesions	IgM EIA or IFA
Enterovirus 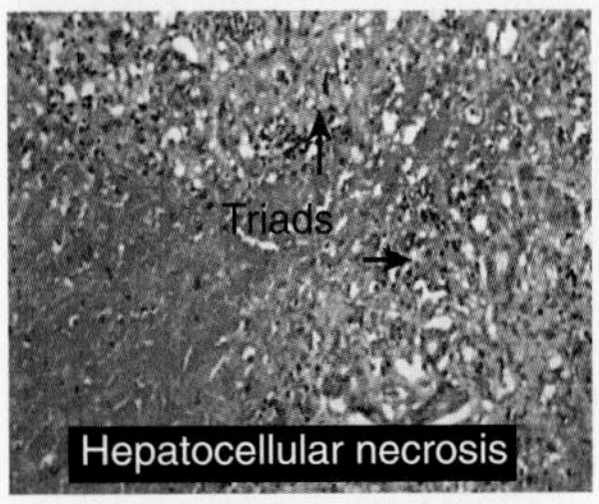		Enterovirus RT-PCR, newborn: CSF, blood, tissues, throat Enterovirus culture, newborn: blood, CSF, tissues, stool, throat Request enterovirus typing from Public Health Laboratory	
Parvovirus B19 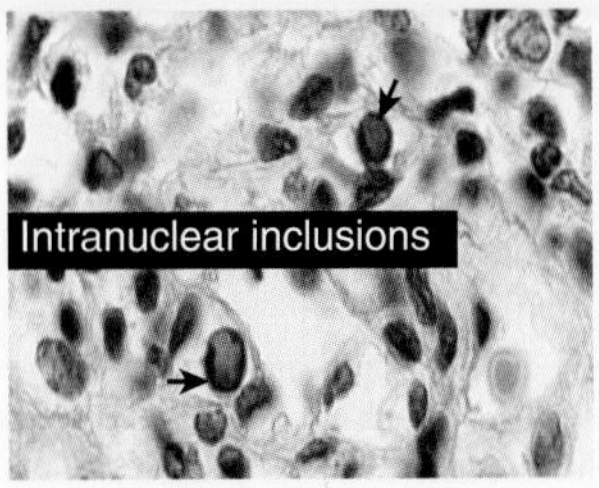	IgM EIA or IFA	PB19 PCR: maternal blood Ground glass viral nuclear inclusions: newborn erythroblasts PB19 ISH, newborn: erythroblasts PB19 PCR: placenta, fetal tissues, blood	IgM EIA
Hepatitis B virus	HBsAg, HBc-IgM, anti-HBsAg	HBV PCR quantitative viral load: newborn blood	
Human immunodeficiency virus	HIV EIA and Western blot HIV RNA quantification	HIV DNA PCR, newborn HIV RNA RT-PCR after 3 months of age	Monitor HIV EIA for possible seroreversion (6–18 months)
Rubella	IgM EIA or IFA	Rubella culture, newborn: urine Rubella RT-PCR: amniotic fluid, placenta, fetal or newborn tissue	IgM EIA or IFA

HBc, Hepatitis B core antigen; *HBsAg,* hepatitis B surface antigen; *CMV,* cytomegalovirus; *CSF,* cerebrospinal fluid; *EIA,* enzyme immunoassay; *gG,* glycoprotein G; *HDF,* human diploid fibroblast; *HIV,* human immunodeficiency virus; *HSV,* herpes simplex virus; *IFA,* indirect immunofluorescence assay; *IgG* and *IgM,* immunoglobulin G and M; *ISH,* in situ hybridization; *PB19,* parvovirus B19; *PCR,* polymerase chain reaction; *RT-PCR,* reverse transcriptase PCR.

at birth; isolation of CMV from urine or saliva or detection of IgM CMV may be the only marker of congenital infection. The symptomatic 10% may present with jaundice, hepatosplenomegaly, pancytopenia, and compensatory cutaneous hematopoiesis (Abdel-Latif, 2010); approximately 10% of these babies will die, and the remainder will suffer permanent neurologic sequelae. Primary CMV infection in the mother is often viremic, with risk of vertical hematogenous transplacental fetal infection and prenatal tissue injury (Stagno, 1982; Revello, 2002; Cheeran, 2009). Reactivation of CMV infection in the mother can cross the placenta, but maternal IgG CMV antibody traverses the placenta and is somewhat protective; these infants are usually asymptomatic at birth, but 5%–15% have sensorineural hearing loss or neurodevelopmental difficulties (Istas, 1995). Maternal reinfection with a new CMV strain has a greater risk of causing symptomatic congenital infection (Boppana, 2001).

IgM-specific assays have shifted from complement fixation, IFA, and anticomplement IFA methods to EIA methods, which use refined recombinant CMV antigens and IgM capture to improve specificity and sensitivity. IgM may persist for longer than 3 months in at least one third of adult women, obscuring the interpretive value of a positive result during pregnancy. CMV IgG avidity testing may be useful in dating recent versus remote infection, similar to assessment of toxoplasma serology in pregnancy; identification of both IgM and low-avidity IgG in a pregnant woman correlates with primary CMV infection with a high risk of intrauterine transmission (Revello, 2002; Remington, 2004; Munro, 2005). Automated IgG avidity serologic testing appears accurate and has potential diagnostic applications (Lagrou, 2009).

Identification of CMV viremia in a nonimmunocompromised pregnant woman through shell vial culture of peripheral blood leukocytes or detection of CMV pp65 antigenemia or detection of CMV DNA by PCR in blood provides conclusive evidence of active maternal infection. However, risk of fetal involvement is estimated at about 40%, and no test performed on the mother can predict fetal infection accurately.

The most reliable prenatal tests to verify fetal infection are viral culture and PCR detection of CMV in amniotic fluid, which have a combined sensitivity of 75%–92% (Revello, 2002). Virus in amniotic fluid indicates overflow shedding from the in utero infected child, and a positive result has 100% specificity for infection. High CMV viral load in amniotic fluid has also been proposed as an indicator of severity of fetal tissue damage. However, false negative error can occur if there is less than a 7-week interval between the onset of maternal infection and the collection of amniotic fluid for testing. Detection of CMV-IgM in fetal cord blood is less sensitive (55%–60%) because of delayed fetal immune response following exposure; cordocentesis CMV DNA PCR has a sensitivity of 84%. IgM CMV in cord blood collected at delivery is also diagnostic, but can be false-negative in up to 30% of cases (Fowler, 1992). Identification of CMV by culture or PCR from newborn urine, saliva, CSF, or blood is very sensitive. PCR detection of CMV DNA in newborn tissue or blood has very high sensitivity—almost 100%; however, use of dried blood samples collected from neonates has variable sensitivity, and its practical applications have not yet been verified (Soetens, 2008; Boppana, 2010). Specimens for any testing must be collected during the first 2 weeks after birth to avoid confusion with postnatally acquired infection (Nelson, 1995; Revello, 2002). Monitoring viral load has no defined predictive value. Typical CMV nuclear inclusions in urine cytology preparations are specific but very insensitive; even autopsy material may have few remaining diagnostic cells if tissue necrosis is advanced. Placenta specimens may show nuclear inclusions or may yield recoverable virus by culture; infection that occurred several weeks before delivery may show only nonspecific avascular sclerotic chorionic villi.

Rubella

Rubella (German measles) is highly communicable and produces mild fever and a transient rash in children and adults. All infections are viremic, and transplacental spread during the first trimester produces devastating teratogenic cardiac, ocular, and brain malformations (Schluter, 1998). Rubella is no longer endemic in the United States because of widespread vaccination; genome analysis demonstrates that most recent rubella cases are imported from Latin America. Routine prenatal screening for maternal rubella IgG as proof of immunity is standard practice. Only four cases of congenital infection have been identified since 2001, three of which occurred in immigrant mothers (MMWR, 2005). When acute rubella is suspected in a pregnant woman, the most straightforward diagnostic method is assay of maternal serum for rubella IgM by EIA or IFA. Culture of rubella is technically complex and is not routinely available. RT-PCR for rubella virus RNA performed on amniotic fluid is almost 100% sensitive and specific and can also be performed on placenta and autopsy tissues (Revello, 1997; Mace, 2004). Multiplex assays that can detect genomic material from rubella and from several other agents of perinatal infection have been developed (McIver, 2005). The congenitally infected newborn is IgM positive and excretes rubella in urine for months to years.

Herpes Simplex Virus

Despite the high prevalence of HSV in adults, neonatal disease is uncommon, occurring at a rate of 5 to 60 cases per 100,000 live births in the United States. Acquisition of maternal genital HSV1 or HSV2 infection during pregnancy has devastating implications for the newborn. Primary disease rather than recurrence puts the baby at great risk for two reasons: The total number of mucocutaneous genital lesions is often higher with first involvement, and although maternal serum contains IgM, little or no IgG is present for transplacental passive protection of the baby (Corey, 2009).

Most babies have a vertex presentation during labor, so the scalp and the face are the first to encounter HSV in the maternal tract; viral exposure on the chest wall and buttocks occurs in breech delivery. Vesicles develop where skin and mucous membranes are directly inoculated with virus. Because the newborn immune response is still immature, a baby's chief resource for modifying infection is maternal IgG-HSV; when this passive protection is lacking, viral replication and visceral dissemination can proceed unchecked. Conjunctival and oral mucosa and skin lesions are usually rich in virus; if dissemination occurs, any visceral organ can be infected.

Obstetric management is complicated by several issues. Routine HSV culture of all mothers without vesicles or infants at the time of delivery has a 0.2% yield and is not recommended (Prober, 1988). Prenatal HSV surveillance cultures of women with known recurrent genital herpes fail to predict which mothers will shed virus at the time of delivery (Arvin, 1986). Studies of women who experienced their first recognized episode of genital herpes during pregnancy demonstrated that half had true primary genital herpes, and these pregnancies had a high rate of complications, such as herpetic amnionitis, preterm labor, and severe neonatal infection. Almost half of mothers who acquired their primary infection shortly before labor had severely affected babies (Brown, 1997). Mothers with recurrent genital herpes had a much lower rate of neonatal infection, with involvement confined to mucocutaneous sites and showing no visceral dissemination (Brown, 1991).

It is accepted practice that women in labor who have genital lesions suspicious for herpes are managed with cesarean section to prevent possible exposure of the baby. Women with a history of recurrent genital herpes can deliver vaginally if active lesions are not present at labor, but careful clinical monitoring of their newborns (including HSV culture/PCR of conjunctiva, oral mucosa, and any suspicious cutaneous lesions) is warranted. Neonatal herpes infection may be silent for up to several days before disease becomes apparent. Despite antiviral therapy, disseminated infection can be fatal; infants with infection confined to the CNS who survive are always severely retarded.

Laboratory diagnosis of HSV infection was discussed earlier in this chapter. Type-specific HSV serology is now available and can identify seronegative women with seropositive partners, highlighting their risk for acquiring infection during pregnancy (Ashley, 1999; Cherpes, 2003). Tzanck smears and rapid antigen assays may be positive for vesicle lesions but cannot replace culture (which yields a positive result in 24 hours when shell vials are used). Identification of HSV DNA by PCR in neonatal spinal fluid or mucocutaneous lesions has greater sensitivity than culture and is particularly valuable for detecting virus in CSF in babies with known CNS involvement (Kimberlin, 1996, 2004).

Human Immunodeficiency Virus, Parvovirus, Enterovirus, Hepatitis B Virus, and Varicella Infections

HIV can spread hematogenously to the fetus, with placental trophoblast and Hofbauer macrophages acting as a cellular reservoir. However, approximately 75% of perinatal infections are acquired at delivery, when the baby is exposed to maternal blood. Perinatal risk of HIV acquisition can be as high as 45%, particularly when maternal HIV1 viral load is high. Transmission rates are reduced to less than 2% by scheduled cesarean section delivery in mothers with high HIV viral load, and by administration of highly active antiviral drugs to the mother during pregnancy and labor, and also to the newborn (Watts, 2002; Anderson, 2009; Tubiana, 2010). HIV is also transmissible postpartum in leukocytes in breast milk; this should absolutely be avoided.

Diagnosis of maternal HIV infection is straightforward (positive EIA for HIV antibody with Western blot confirmation). Routine screening in the first trimester is strongly recommended; seropositive mothers can then be assessed with quantitative HIV RNA levels, and antiviral therapy given. For mothers in labor whose serologic status is unknown, intrapartum testing should be performed on a stat basis using a rapid HIV antibody method (Griffith, 2007), so that seropositive mothers can have intravenous antiviral prophylaxis initiated immediately to reduce the risk of perinatal infection of the baby. Maternal IgG crosses the placenta and persists in infant blood for up to 18 months, so standard EIA HIV serologic tests cannot be used to diagnose neonatal infection. Variations of both EIA and Western blot tests for detection of IgM and IgA HIV antibodies can identify an infected baby, because neither IgA nor IgM is passively transferred to the fetus; however, sensitivity is age dependent, and testing is not reliable in the first 3 months after birth.

Traditional HIV p24 antigen assays have been considered suboptimal in sensitivity for diagnosis during the immediate postnatal period (Sison, 1992). However, an ultrasensitive p24 assay performed on dried blood spots has shown 96%–98% sensitivity when performed on 6-week-old babies (Patton, 2008). If infection was acquired transplacentally during gestation, then newborn blood is positive for HIV DNA that has been transcribed and integrated into the infant's peripheral blood lymphocytes. PCR for HIV proviral DNA has a diagnostic sensitivity greater than 95% at 1 month of age (Rogers, 1989; Bremer, 1996). PCR for identification of HIV1 DNA in dried blood spots also has excellent sensitivity, and has valuable applications for testing infants in remote areas (Luo, 2005), as do DNA-PCR assays with simple rapid POC extraction methods (Jangam, 2009). HIV RNA RT-PCR is positive at birth if the baby was infected in utero, and will become positive within several weeks in infants who were infected during delivery. Real-time RT-PCR is also used for quantitative monitoring to assess the baby's response to antiretroviral therapy.

Parvovirus B19 (PB19) causes the benign, self-limited childhood exanthem erythema infectiosum (fifth disease) (Heegaard, 2002; Young, 2004), and major epidemics develop every few years. Approximately 50% of young women are seronegative, and infection in pregnancy can have serious consequences for the developing baby. PB19 targets erythroid progenitor cells, and virolytic cytotoxicity produces fetal anemia with risk for hydrops and intrauterine demise (Tolfvenstam, 2001). Maternal transmission during primary infection has an estimated risk of fetal infection of 25%; fetal death estimates vary from 2%–38% (Alder, 1993). A recent retrospective study of intrauterine fetal demise and miscarriage that included a major PB19 epidemic episode showed that PB19 DNA was found in 4.9% of fetal deaths, and intrauterine fatalities were six times more prevalent during epidemic intervals (Riipinen, 2008). Infected erythroblasts have characteristic ground-glass nuclear inclusions by hematoxylin and eosin (H&E) stain. Parvovirus can be cultivated only in human bone marrow containing erythrocytic precursor cells—an impractical method for diagnosis. Acute infection is characterized serologically by detecting specific IgM in maternal or fetal blood, or by ISH or PCR detection of viral DNA in amniotic fluid or cord blood (Bruu, 1995; Zerbini, 1996).

Enterovirus infection is very common, with 10 million or more cases reported each year in the United States. Many enteroviral infections are viremic; maternal infection just prior to delivery spreads virus transplacentally to the fetus, and the baby is born with disseminated virus but with no passively acquired maternal protective IgG antibody to modify infection. Nosocomial outbreaks with nursery personnel as the source of virus have also been reported. Echovirus 11 is particularly virulent, causing hepatocellular necrosis and meningoencephalitis that are often fatal. Coxsackie B viruses can produce neonatal myocardial injury (Bryant, 2004). Quantitative assay of coxsackievirus B3 in blood during a local outbreak showed highest viral load levels in neonates, which also correlated with disease severity (Yen, 2007). Perinatal infection with other enteroviruses usually is benign. The amount of virus in clinical specimens is generally low, and direct hybridization assays have poor sensitivity. However, RT-PCR and NASBA nucleic acid amplification assays detect a common sequence present in all enteroviruses and have excellent sensitivity, superior to standard culture, yielding positive results within 1 working day (Landry, 2003; Romero, 2007). Enteroviruses grow well in standard tube cultures (PMK, HDF, and RD cell lines); shell vial culture methods can shorten detection time to 2 days, and use of both BGMK and A549 cell lines in a single shell vial monolayer improves sensitivity (Romero, 2007). Suitable specimens for viral culture include neonatal blood, CSF, throat, and rectal swab samples, or tissues from fatal cases. Typing of specific enterovirus isolates is beyond the scope of hospital laboratories and can usually be done through regional or national public health laboratories.

Maternal infection with hepatitis B virus is often transmitted vertically; the baby may be infected transplacentally or, more probably, during delivery with exposure to maternal blood. Screening for hepatitis B surface antigen (HbsAg) is a standard component of prenatal care. Transmission rates are as high as 80% if the infected mother is positive for core antigen and approximately 30% if the mother is core antigen negative. If the maternal HBV screen is positive, then immediately after birth the neonate is given HBV immune globulin, along with the first dose of the HBV surface antigen vaccination series (Poland, 2004).

Varicella zoster virus infection acquired early in pregnancy is often teratogenic and causes limb hypoplasia and dermatome pattern skin scarring, as well as severe CNS disease (Whitley, 2005). This constellation of fatal complications from in utero exposure has also been reported with HSV2 (Johansson, 2004). Maternal chickenpox with viremia just prior to delivery can cause severe mucocutaneous chickenpox in the newborn.

VIRAL MENINGITIS AND ENCEPHALITIS

Several thousand viral infections of the CNS occur each year in the United States, with considerable variation in morbidity and mortality. Accurate and prompt laboratory diagnosis aids patient management and is important for public health interventions to control arboviral arthropod vectors and investigate waterborne sources. Viral proliferation in the meningeal layers covering the brain induces acute inflammation with fever, headache, nuchal rigidity, and CSF pleocytosis. In encephalitis, virus replicates within the brain parenchyma; inflammation and tissue necrosis may be diffuse or may produce a space-occupying lesion with mass effect. Many viruses are associated with meningitis or encephalitis, but overlap injury with involvement of both anatomic sites (meningoencephalitis) is common, particularly with arbovirus infection (Fig. 55-8).

Viral encephalitis is not infrequent in the United States, with an estimated annual incidence of 7.3 cases per 100,000 individuals (Khetsuriani, 2002). Some neurotropic viruses are fastidious and require molecular methods for accurate diagnosis. Arboviruses (arthropod borne) and HSV cause most cases of acute encephalitis in the United States. Mosquitoes are vectors for hundreds of neurotropic viruses worldwide, but only five arboviruses are encountered regularly in the United States: WNV, the Eastern and Western equines, St Louis, and California-LaCrosse encephalitis viruses. HSV encephalitis usually occurs as a reactivation of latent HSV1 that tracks (via the olfactory or trigeminal cranial nerves) into the cerebral cortex, producing a large necrotic mass. About 700 cases of herpes encephalitis are reported each year in the United States; the pattern is sporadic and nonseasonal. Progression is rapid and mortality is high, but early diagnosis with appropriate antiviral treatment reduces both mortality and the level of permanent disability (Mitchell, 1997; Steiner, 2007).

Arboviruses are a heterogeneous group, and mosquito transmission is their common denominator; the most frequent in North America are members of the flavivirus, togavirus, and bunyavirus families. Before the WNV outbreak, total annual U.S. arboviral cases varied between 100 and 2000; disease peaked during warm weather when mosquito populations were greatest. Severity and mortality are highest with the Eastern equine virus, the least frequent of the group (Kuno, 2005). The WNV outbreak originated in 1999 in New York; the virus then traveled in infected birds from the East Coast across America and involved all states by 2004. WNV has since become endemic (Snapinn, 2007). The estimated total number of cumulative human WNV infections is currently about 1 million; approximately 200,000 patients have become clinically ill with disease ranging from simple fever to meningitis, encephalitis, and flaccid poliomyelitic paralysis; both long-term encephalitic and paralytic disabilities have been reported, along with many fatalities (Nash, 2001; Petersen, 2004; Hayes, 2005). Mosquito bites are the typical route of acquisition, but blood transfusion and organ transplantation also accounted for several cases (Iwamoto, 2003; Pealer, 2003; Kleinman, 2005). Blood donations are now screened for WNV by nucleic acid tests during summer months, effectively interrupting this mechanism of spread (Busch, 2005).

By the time of onset of CNS disease, WNV and many other arboviruses often cannot be detected by culture or PCR in blood or spinal fluid; therefore, diagnosis primarily hinges on EIA for specific IgM antibody in CSF and serum, or demonstration of rising specific IgG. Nucleic acid amplification for WNV plays an important role in screening blood donors but is of limited clinical use and may be helpful only when WNV-infected patients seek medical attention very soon after onset of symptoms (Prince, 2008; Reznicek, 2010b). Interpretation of a positive IgM serologic test for WNV must be made with caution because elevated titers may persist for prolonged periods following acute infection, and because cross-reaction with other flaviviruses (yellow fever and dengue) may occur (Reznicek, 2010b). State health departments and reference laboratories offer a range of tests for common regional arboviruses, but hundreds of arboviruses are endemic outside the United States in Asia, Africa, Latin America, and parts of Eastern Europe. Testing for arbovirus infection in travelers is available through public health laboratories; the referring laboratory must provide a detailed travel history and clinical information, along with blood, CSF, or tissue specimens submitted for culture, nucleic acid detection, or serologic diagnosis (see Fig. 55-8). Current information about global arbovirus activity and risk to tourists is available at www.cdc.gov/travel.

More than 70 enteroviruses, some of which produce encephalitis (coxsackie virus and echovirus) have been identified. Paralytic polio caused by poliovirus necrosis of spinal cord or brainstem motor neurons has been eliminated in most of the world, with residual disease in Africa and Asia, which may soon be eradicated by vaccination efforts. Rabies virus travels

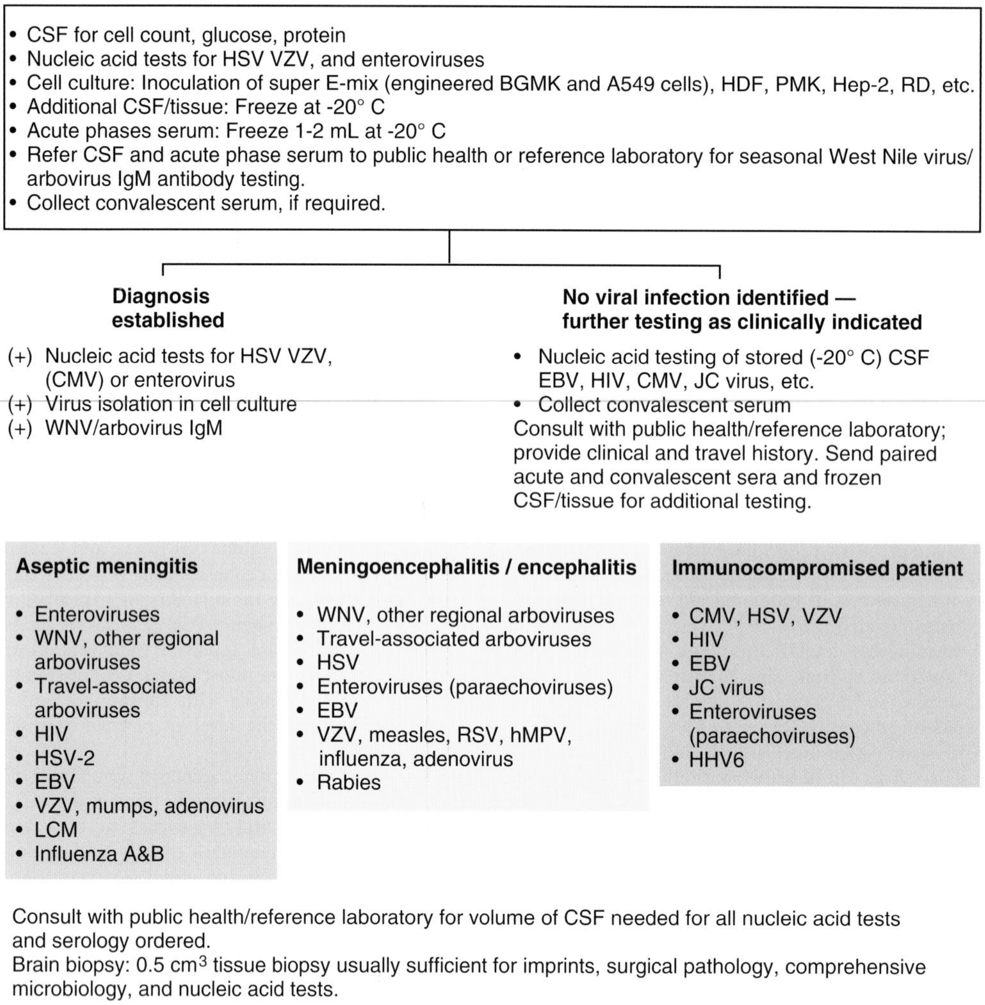

• CSF for cell count, glucose, protein
• Nucleic acid tests for HSV VZV, and enteroviruses
• Cell culture: Inoculation of super E-mix (engineered BGMK and A549 cells), HDF, PMK, Hep-2, RD, etc.
• Additional CSF/tissue: Freeze at -20° C
• Acute phases serum: Freeze 1-2 mL at -20° C
• Refer CSF and acute phase serum to public health or reference laboratory for seasonal West Nile virus/ arbovirus IgM antibody testing.
• Collect convalescent serum, if required.
Diagnosis established
(+) Nucleic acid tests for HSV VZV, (CMV) or enterovirus
(+) Virus isolation in cell culture
(+) WNV/arbovirus IgM
No viral infection identified — further testing as clinically indicated
• Nucleic acid testing of stored (-20° C) CSF EBV, HIV, CMV, JC virus, etc.
• Collect convalescent serum
Consult with public health/reference laboratory; provide clinical and travel history. Send paired acute and convalescent sera and frozen CSF/tissue for additional testing.
Aseptic meningitis
• Enteroviruses
• WNV, other regional arboviruses
• Travel-associated arboviruses
• HIV
• HSV-2
• EBV
• VZV, mumps, adenovirus
• LCM
• Influenza A&B
Meningoencephalitis / encephalitis
• WNV, other regional arboviruses
• Travel-associated arboviruses
• HSV
• Enteroviruses (paraechoviruses)
• EBV
• VZV, measles, RSV, hMPV, influenza, adenovirus
• Rabies
Immunocompromised patient
• CMV, HSV, VZV
• HIV
• EBV
• JC virus
• Enteroviruses (paraechoviruses)
• HHV6
Consult with public health/reference laboratory for volume of CSF needed for all nucleic acid tests and serology ordered.
Brain biopsy: 0.5 cm3 tissue biopsy usually sufficient for imprints, surgical pathology, comprehensive microbiology, and nucleic acid tests.

Figure 55-8 Workup of cerebrospinal fluid (CSF) and brain biopsy for viral pathogens. *BGMK,* Buffalo green monkey cells; *CMV,* cytomegalovirus; *CSF,* cerebrospinal fluid; *EBV,* Epstein-Barr virus; *HDF,* human diploid fibroblasts; *HHV6,* human herpesvirus 6; *HIV,* human immunodeficiency virus; *hMPV,* human metapneumovirus; *HSV,* herpes simplex virus; *Ig,* immunoglobulin; *PMK,* primary monkey kidney; *RD,* rhabdomyosarcoma cells; *RSV,* respiratory syncytial virus; *VZV,* varicella zoster virus; *WNV,* West Nile virus.

via nerve fibers directly to the CNS and produces necrotizing brain damage; bat rather than canine strains account for most disease in the United States; a recent outbreak was traced to transplanted organs from a donor who had died with undiagnosed rabies (Smith, 2003; MMWR, 2004). Measles, mumps, EBV mononucleosis, and chickenpox rarely are complicated by acute encephalitis (Cherry, 1998). HHV6 can produce focal cerebral injury (Isaacson, 2005). HIV replication in CNS glial cells can cause progressive dementia in advanced AIDS (Atwood, 1993). Opportunistic necrotizing brain infection with HSV, CMV, and VZV, as well as JC polyomavirus destruction of oligodendroglia, may also develop in the immunocompromised host (discussed later).

Enteroviruses cause 75% of viral meningitis in the United States, usually a relatively benign and transient disease. Enteroviruses spread easily from person to person via fecal-oral means, and distinct seasonality is seen, with annual summer-fall outbreaks (see Fig. 55-1); most clinically recognized infections are seen in children and young adults. Chronic severe meningoencephalitis can develop in patients with hypogammaglobulinemia; any enteroviral CNS infection with an encephalitis component is more virulent and may leave permanent sequelae (McKinney, 1987). Acute HIV infection occasionally produces acute meningeal inflammation (Schupbach, 2003). About 1% of primary HSV2 genital herpes infections are accompanied by transient meningitis; HSV2 is the major cause of Mollaret's benign recurrent lymphocytic meningitis. Mumps, measles, metapneumovirus, and adenovirus infections rarely produce acute meningitis (Reznicek, 2010b).

Laboratory Diagnosis

Initial evaluation of CSF should include cell count and glucose and total protein quantitation. Pleocytosis is usually mild (50–1000 cells/mm^3) compared with bacterial infection. Mononuclear cells usually predominate, but neutrophils can dominate early, particularly following infection with WNV. Protein may be somewhat elevated (rarely >200 mg/dL), and glucose levels are normal to slightly decreased (Tunkel, 2008; Reznicek, 2010a, 2010b). Comprehensive laboratory evaluation of viral CNS disease is currently beyond the scope of most hospital laboratories. A streamlined plan for stepwise testing based on the clinical scenario can coordinate in-house testing with efficient use of reference laboratory and public health laboratory services (see Fig. 55-8). For immunocompetent patients, initial testing of spinal fluid/brain biopsy tissue using nucleic acid amplification for enteroviruses HSV, VZV, and possibly CMV plus virus culture can be paired with serum and CSF assays for IgM antibodies to the prevalent regional seasonal arboviruses (Resnicek, 2010a). Table 55-5 illustrates yields of molecular detection for enterovirus, HSV, VZV, and CMV in a large metropolitan area laboratory. VZV may be overlooked as a cause of

TABLE 55-5
Yield From CSF Specimens Tested for Enteroviruses, VZV, HSV, and CMV by Nucleic Acid Assays

Virus	Yield
Enteroviruses	11.3% (36/318)
Herpes simplex virus (HSV)	4.1% (56/1360)
Varicella zoster virus (VZV)	10.6% (13/123)
Cytomegalovirus (CMV)	2.1% (3/144)

Personal data, L. Sabatini, Multiple hospitals, Chicago area and southeast Wisconsin, 2008–2009.

TABLE 55-6
Laboratory Diagnosis of Common Viral Exanthems and Mucocutaneous Lesions*

Exanthem or skin lesion	Virus	Culture/antigen and nucleic acid assays	Serology
Chickenpox/shingles	Varicella zoster	Tzanck smear DFA smear Culture (shell vial most sensitive) PCR	IgM-EIA (chickenpox) IgG-EIA for immunity following chickenpox Commercial VZV-IgG tests may not be reliable for documenting immunity post vaccination
Enteroviral rash (hand, foot, and mouth disease)	Enteroviruses	Culture, RT-PCR	
Measles	Measles	Culture†	IgM-EIA or IFA†
Rubella	Rubella	Culture†	IgM-EIA†
Erythema infectiosum	Parvovirus B19		IgM-EIA or IFA†
Exanthem subitum	HHV6	Coculture in lymphoblasts†	IgM-EIA†
Anogenital condyloma Evaluation of ASCUS cervical cytology	Papillomaviruses	Hybrid capture and Invader assays	
HSV	HSV1 and HSV2	PCR Culture DFA smear or Tzanck smear	HSVgG1 and gG2G glycoprotein specific antibody; IgM, not specific

ASCUS, Atypical squamous cells of undetermined significance; *DFA,* direct fluorescent antibody; *EIA,* enzyme immunoassay; *gG,* glycoprotein G; *HSV,* herpes simplex virus; *HHV,* human herpes virus; *IFA,* indirect fluorescent antibody; *IgM,* immunoglobulin M; *RT-PCR,* reverse transcriptase polymerase chain reaction; *VZV,* varicella zoster virus.
*If smallpox is considered in a patient with vesicular lesions, contact local health authorities for specific instructions.
†Test available at reference and research laboratories.

meningoencephalitis, particularly if skin lesions are not appreciated (Hayes, 2005; Kupila, 2006; Frazen-Röhl, 2007). If clinically indicated, CSF reserved at −20° C and paired acute and convalescent sera can be referred for more extensive arbovirus testing in public health laboratories, and for culture and additional nucleic acid amplification for less common causes of viral meningitis or encephalitis. The 1999 WNV outbreak was quickly identified because of cooperative and coordinated efforts between hospital and government laboratories (MMWR, 1999). Despite extensive evaluation, an infectious cause for encephalitis often is not identified (Glaser, 2003).

Immunocompromised patients may develop CNS disease with the same viruses that afflict the healthy host; in addition, several opportunistic viral infections may produce CNS involvement. JC polyomavirus, CMV, VZV, and HSV can cause CNS disease; CNS B lymphocyte lymphoma is almost always related to EBV infection; PCR for EBV in CSF in patients with AIDS is diagnostic of CNS lymphoma.

The most practical approach to diagnosis of viral encephalitis is nucleic acid testing performed on CSF. RT-PCR identification of enterovirus and PCR for HSV, VZV, EBV, CMV, and HHV6 are more sensitive than virus recovery by cell culture from CSF or brain tissue. Several multiplexed and microarray-based assays have been developed (DeBiasi, 2004; Koralnik, 2005; Epsy, 2006; Wolffs, 2009) and are available through reference laboratories. Preliminary screening of CSF for elevated protein and pleocytosis is advisable because herpesviruses are rarely, if ever, identified when protein and cell counts are normal (Hanson, 2007). Brain biopsy is still performed on occasion, usually when tumor or nonviral infection is a clinical consideration. A 0.5-cm^3 biopsy is sufficient for surgical pathology examination, imprint smears for direct examination, nucleic acid amplification, and comprehensive culture for all infectious organisms. HSV isolation in cell culture was discussed previously; recovery of other viruses should also be attempted, so the specimen should be inoculated to all cell lines that the laboratory carries. Imprints stained with DFA reagents can demonstrate HSV-infected cells. Some arboviruses and enteroviruses require animal inoculation for replication; if needed, tissue should be frozen at −20° C and the specimen forwarded to a public health or reference laboratory.

Enteroviruses are the most common agents of acute aseptic meningitis; nucleic acid tests are the gold standard for enterovirus identification in CSF, with yields of 128%–142% compared with cell culture recovery (Landry, 2003; Romero, 2007). Nucleic acid tests designed to detect enteroviruses do not detect parechoviruses and require separate primers and probes (Baumgarte, 2008; Nix, 2008).

Several tissue lines (PMK, HDF, HEp-2, RD, buffalo green monkey Super E-Mix [genetically engineered cell line BGMK-hDAF]) support the growth of many enteroviruses and of HSV, VZV, measles, mumps, and adenovirus; E-mix hybrid shell vial culture is also an excellent choice for culture of enteroviruses and related agents (Huang, 2002). From 0.1–0.2 mL of CSF should be inoculated directly into each tube or shell vial without delay. Enterovirus-specific typing is available in public health laboratories.

VIRAL EXANTHEMS AND COMMON CUTANEOUS INFECTIONS

Several viruses primarily target the skin. Some infect the squamous epidermis through direct inoculation (oral and genital herpes, warts caused by human papillomavirus or molluscum poxvirus). Exanthems are caused by viruses that spread hematogenously to skin and mucous membranes (VZV, measles, rubella, enteroviruses, parvovirus, HHV6) (Cherry, 1993). Many of these benign childhood exanthems are diagnosed clinically with no laboratory testing needed, and several are now preventable with pediatric vaccination requirements. When laboratory confirmation of acute infection is needed for unusual cases, or to apply infection control precautions in hospitalized patients, or to guide appropriate antiviral treatment, serology is often easier and more accurate than culture or antigen assay. With the exception of varicella, specific nucleic acid assays generally are not needed for diagnosis. Laboratory diagnostic procedures are summarized in Table 55-6.

VZV causes both varicella (chickenpox) and zoster (shingles). In chickenpox, VZV is spread through infected respiratory aerosol droplets, multiplies in the nasopharynx, and then enters the bloodstream and travels to the skin (Arvin, 1996). Replication in the squamous epithelium produces pruritic vesicles that rapidly progress to ulcers, which eventually crust over and heal without scarring—similar to HSV skin lesions. In healthy children, systemic symptoms are mild and sequelae are uncommon; however, serious bacterial superinfection, cerebellar ataxia, and encephalitis can occur. Along with the clinical resolution of chickenpox skin lesions, varicella virions travel via nerve fibers to regional sensory neural ganglions, where latent infection is established and maintained by memory CD4 and CD8 T lymphocytes (Arvin, 2005). When cell-mediated immunity is impaired by aging or immunosuppressive drugs or HIV infection, then active VZV replication begins again in neurons, and spreads from trigeminal or dorsal root ganglia back down nerve fibers to the skin, producing painful cutaneous vesicles with a classic dermatome distribution. Postherpetic persistent neuralgia is a frequent debilitating complication of zoster eruptions. CNS or disseminated visceral involvement from reactivated VZV develops only in the immunodeficient, but may be fatal. Varicella vaccine given in childhood produces high titers of specific IgG; because of waning humoral immunity and breakthrough mild atypical varicella cases (Vazquez, 2005), a second dose is needed to guarantee continued protection (Chaves, 2007). Varicella vaccine formulation administered to geriatric patients markedly reduces the burden of zoster and its complications in the elderly (Oxman, 2005). Any vesicular rash in children or adults that raises the possibility of smallpox should be immediately reported to local public health officials.

Vesicle fluid is rich with virus and is the ideal specimen for culture or for DFA staining. VZV replicates in HDF cell lines. Traditional tube culture is slow and insensitive; shell vial culture has better yield (up to 75%) and allows more rapid detection (Brinker, 1993). Collection of skin vesicle specimens is identical to that used for HSV vesicles (see Fig. 55-3). Culture setup is also similar to herpes culture; however, tubes are held for 2 weeks and shell vial monolayers are stained at 3 and 5 days with VZV DFA reagent. VZV CPE develops in HDF as small patches of rounded, swollen, refractile cells. Because the behavior of VZV in tissue culture may be somewhat fastidious, DFA staining of vesicle cells for viral antigen is a rapid and practical diagnostic test and can differentiate VZV from HSV (Schrim, 1989). Nucleic acid assays have also been developed; they are more sensitive than culture and serve as the only practical approach for diagnosis when skin lesions have progressed to ulcers (Weidmann, 2003; Leung, 2010). IgM antibody is usually detectable by the time chickenpox vesicles first erupt and is a useful confirmatory test; serology is not helpful for evaluation of zoster lesions.

Of approximately 70 enterovirus serotypes, several produce vesicular or maculopapular eruptions (coxsackie B1 and A9, and echoviruses 2, 4, 9, 11, 19, and 33), usually during summer months. Hand-foot-mouth disease (coxsackie A16) in young children presents with vesicles on the tongue and palmar and plantar skin (Goksugur, 2010). Adult family members of infected children occasionally also develop symptomatic disease. Laboratory diagnosis is limited to enterovirus recovery from skin lesion specimens by cell culture and RT-PCR nucleic acid amplification assay; vesicles from the soles and palms should be completely unroofed and the exposed squamous cells vigorously swabbed. Cell culture identification of enterovirus was described earlier. DFA stains and serology are impractical and have low sensitivity and specificity for diagnosis of enteroviral exanthems.

Measles is highly contagious and presents with both mucocutaneous and respiratory features (fever, conjunctivitis, coryza, oral ulcerating lesions, cough, and generalized maculopapular erythematous rash). Vaccination has dramatically curtailed measles, and at present, 90% of confirmed cases in the United States are imported and then are disseminated in undervaccinated groups (MMWR, 2009). Despite international eradication efforts, measles still persists in impoverished countries; morbidity and mortality are high because of accompanying pneumonia and impaired nutrition. Measles virus in the nasopharynx can be identified by culture or nucleic acid amplification, but acute infection is most easily diagnosed serologically by detecting measles-specific IgM antibody. Immunity following natural infection presumably is lifelong, verified by the presence of specific IgG; however, immunity following vaccination may fade during the late teen years, with a second dose needed for sustained coverage. Breakthrough infection occurring in the setting of waning antibody may be atypical and difficult to diagnosis.

Parvovirus B19 (PB19) causes erythema infectiosum (fifth disease), a common childhood febrile illness with a distinctive maculopapular rash that gives the face a "slapped cheek" appearance (Young, 2004). PB19 infection in adults often produces arthralgias. Parvovirus infects erythroblastic precursor cells in the bone marrow and may provoke aplastic crisis in patients with hemoglobinopathy or HIV infection. Primary infection during pregnancy can cause fetal red cell aplasia with hydrops fetalis. Laboratory diagnosis was discussed earlier in this chapter.

Rubella virus produces German measles, a mild febrile illness with a transient maculopapular rash, and is the third infectious exanthem of childhood (Gershon, 2010). Infection in children is inconsequential, although adult-onset rubella may be associated with arthralgias. The only serious complication of rubella is transplacental spread to the first trimester developing baby, with risk of virus-induced tissue necrosis and congenital malformation. Widespread use of rubella vaccine has largely eliminated disease in developed countries. Laboratory confirmation of acute infection is most easily accomplished by detection of virus-specific IgM, rather than by attempting virus isolation. Verification of immune status is established with specific IgG antibody testing.

HHV6, a lymphotrophic herpesvirus that infects lymphocytes, is the cause of exanthem subitum (roseola infantum, the sixth clinically distinctive exanthem). Roseola is a common early childhood illness characterized by high fever and development of a fleeting maculopapular rash as fever abruptly subsides (Prober, 2005; Zerr, 2005). Primary HHV6 infection in older children and adults produces a systemic, febrile lymphoproliferative illness resembling acute mononucleosis (discussed earlier); it may cause pneumonitis in immunosuppressed patients (Cone, 1993). Laboratory diagnosis was reviewed earlier; however, the distinctive clinical presentation of roseola makes laboratory confirmation unnecessary.

Human papillomaviruses are ubiquitous and are found in all societies; hundreds of HPV serotypes have been defined by unique DNA sequences, and various HPV types target different skin or mucosal sites in the body. Most HPV warty cutaneous infections of the hands and feet are transient and of no medical consequence. Sexual encounters easily transmit HPV types that are associated with anogenital disease; quadrivalent vaccine is now in use for immunization of children against HPV types 11, 6, 16, and 18. Low-risk nononcogenic HPV types (6, 11, and others) can cause low-grade squamous intraepithelial proliferative lesions that usually resolve with no medical intervention. Infection with high-risk oncogenic HPV types (16, 18, and others) carries a much greater likelihood of persistent viral infection in the squamous epithelium of the cervix, vagina, vulva, or perineum; these oncogenic HPV viral infections can produce high-grade dysplastic intraepithelial lesions that over time may progress to invasive squamous carcinoma. The histopathologic and cytopathologic characteristics of HPV lesions are well described in standard pathology texts. However, HPV detection has been enhanced by the use of nucleic acid assays; the hybrid capture signal amplification method is most widely used and can identify several high-risk HPV and low-risk HPV types in liquid-based cervical cytology specimens (Burd, 2003). Nucleic acid–based methods for HPV identification have also been developed (Soderlund-Strand, 2005; Carozzi, 2007; Ifter, 2009). Novel linear array and line probe and HPV typing methods have been described (Castle, 2008; Ifter, 2009). Studies are under way to validate testing methods for males (Giovannelli, 2007). HPV can infect oropharyngeal and respiratory tract mucosa and is associated with carcinoma and papillomatosis (Glikman, 2005; D'Souza, 2007). Performance of HPV molecular assays for nongenital sites has not been established.

Although HPV genital infection is common, high-risk HPV infections that progress to high-grade intraepithelial lesions and on to invasive carcinoma are not, and the time line for progression to carcinoma spans many years. The sensitivity of HPV testing combined with cervical cytology is considered the gold standard for diagnosis of high-grade intraepithelial neoplasia (Mayrand, 2007). Recommendations for prudent use of HPV testing in connection with routine cervical cytology with the goal of preventing cervical carcinoma have been issued by a multidisciplinary panel of cytopathologists and gynecologists (Solomon, 2009); these utilization guidelines outline clinical scenarios in which HPV testing should and should not be ordered. Low-risk HPV testing is not helpful in routine screening or in the evaluation of abnormal cervical cytology findings. Testing for high-risk oncogenic HPV types is most useful in women over the age of 30 who have cervical cytology with atypical squamous cells of undetermined significance (approximately 1 million cervical smears per year in the United States), and in postmenopausal women with low-grade squamous intraepithelial lesions. The use of high-risk HPV testing outside of these recommendations is not prohibited and may be considered when there are extenuating clinical circumstances. The guidelines are intended to optimize the value of HPV testing in preventing invasive cervical cancer, and to avoid wasteful overtesting and unnecessary ancillary cervical biopsy procedures (Cox, 2009).

VIRAL GASTROENTERITIS

Viral gastroenteritis causes major morbidity and mortality worldwide, most significantly in young children in developing nations; in the United States, viral enteritis is rarely fatal but causes at least 3 million episodes annually and approximately 200,000 pediatric hospitalizations (Parashar, 1998). The viruses responsible constitute a diverse group, and all are ubiquitous. Severe debilitating diarrhea with rotavirus, enteric adenovirus, calicivirus, astrovirus, and coronavirus is largely confined to infants and young children. All treatment is supportive (Thielman, 2004).

Rotaviruses cause most cases of watery diarrhea in infants and young children in the United States (Musher, 2004); symptomatic infection occasionally develops in elderly adults in nursing homes. Transmission is fecal-oral; epidemics occur during cold weather in temperate climates and year-round in tropical regions. Rotavirus is highly infectious, with infection rates as high as 50% for children and up to 30% for adults following family exposure; some children and most adults will be asymptomatic (Mushner, 2004). Dehydration with electrolyte imbalance is the most serious complication. Enteric isolation precautions must be followed to prevent nosocomial or day care spread. A safe and effective multivalent vaccine is currently available and has great potential for helping to modulate outbreaks with this important gastrointestinal pathogen (Dennehy, 2008; Wang, 2010).

Adenovirus serotypes 40 and 41 are associated with gastroenteritis and account for 10%–20% of pediatric cases. Adenovirus enteritis is clinically similar to rotavirus disease but has no seasonality. Coronavirus and astrovirus have caused nosocomial and day care center outbreaks (Papaventsis, 2008; Principi, 2010), mild gastroenteritis in adults, and diarrhea in HIV patients (Grohmann, 1993).

Noroviruses (NoVs) cause epidemic acute gastroenteritis, characterized by nausea and vomiting that may be more intense than the accompanying diarrhea. NoVs are nonenveloped and can survive for days on inanimate surfaces, as well as in contaminated water, shellfish, and prepared foods; they have been identified in several community and national epidemics and cruise ship and day care outbreaks. They have been notoriously difficult to eradicate from the environment. NoVs have proved to be genetically diverse, with three out of five genogroups (GI, GII, and GIV) infecting humans. These genogroups are further divided into at least 25 genotypes (Glass, 2009). NoV infection is common in all age groups and is seen in a wide variety of settings, including but not restricted to nursing homes, hospital wards, day care centers, cruise ships, restaurants, and catered events. NoVs account for 12% of severe gastroenteritis cases among children <5 years of age and at least 12% of mild and moderate diarrhea cases among persons of all ages, making NoV the most common cause of diarrhea in adults and the second most common cause in children (Patel, 2008; Glass, 2009). High infection rates with NoV are due to its low infectious dose and its stability in food and on environmental services. The great antigenic diversity of norovirus strains results in incomplete immunity, and multiple infections are common (Glass, 2009).

Laboratory Diagnosis

Gastroenteritis viruses grow poorly or not at all in standard cell lines. Historically, diagnosis had been based on the distinctive morphology of each virus when stool samples are negatively stained with phosphotungstic acid and examined by EM, but this service is time intensive to perform and requires special expertise, so it is not available in most laboratories (Goldsmith, 2009). Rapid detection of rotavirus antigen in stool is easily and accurately accomplished with commerically available latex agglutination and immunoassays. All methods have excellent specificity, and EIA is slightly more sensitive (Thomas, 1994; Dennehy, 1999). Rapid diagnosis is useful for patient cohorting and infection control measures to contain nosocomial spread. An accurate and sensitive commercial EIA for enteric adenovirus antigen detection is available. The clinical efficacy of nucleic acid–based multiplex testing for vial gastroenteritis is also being explored (Svraka, 2009). The scope of NoV-associated gastroenteritis was grossly underestimated until the recent availability of sensitive molecular diagnostic methods (e.g., RT-PCR, which is now considered the reference method). These assays are also available through referral laboratories.

VIRAL INFECTION IN IMMUNOCOMPROMISED HOST

The immune response to viral infection occurs as a complex interaction of humoral and cellular factors. The cell-mediated immune system responds to acute infection with natural killer large granular lymphocytes that circulate through blood and tissues, identify host cells with viral ("nonself") antigens, and then destroy them by proteolytic lysis. Viral antigens are processed by macrophages, and the refined epitopes are presented to B and T lymphocytes. $CD4^+$ cells produce cytokines that promote clonal expansion of sensitized cytotoxic $CD8^+$ cells, which then eliminate host cells harboring foreign viral antigen (Kumar, 2010). Any impairment of normal interactions among macrophages, $CD4^+$, $CD8^+$, and natural killer cells reduces the ability of the host to control viral disease. Cell-mediated immunity is also critical in suppressing viruses that have the ability to persist in a latent form (such as HSV, CMV, EBV, etc.). In healthy individuals, episodic reactivation infections with these viruses are asymptomatic or produce limited disease confined to a discrete anatomic area (e.g., genital or oral herpes). With impaired cellular immune function, recurrent infections may be locally aggressive or may disseminate and produce severe multiorgan damage.

The number of immunocompromised patients continues to increase in societies with modern medical interventions. Use of corticosteroids, chemotherapy and radiation, and immunosuppressive drugs to prevent transplant rejection, as well as HIV-induced obliteration of $CD4^+$ lymphocytes, damages cellular immune regulation and increases vulnerability to viral infections (Copelan, 2006; Fishman, 2007). Primary viral infections that occur in an immunocompromised patient (such as EBV mononucleosis, influenza, and chickenpox) are clinically more severe. HPV anogenital condylomas show accelerated progression to squamous dysplasia and carcinoma. Many of the most serious viral diseases in the immunoimpaired host are caused by reactivation of endogenous dormant organisms (CMV, HSV, VZV, EBV, etc.), which then progress to systemic fatal infection.

Reactivation of latent EBV infection is linked to the development of B cell CNS lymphoma in AIDS patients. Solid organ and allogeneic bone marrow/stem cell transplant recipients require intense immunosuppressive therapy to prevent graft rejection; as cell-mediated immune function diminishes, the host may be unable to contain dormant EBV organisms. In up to 20% of patients, unchecked EBV proliferation can lead to post-transplant lymphoproliferative disorder (PTLD). Initially, EBV-induced polymorphic plasmacytic and B lymphocyte expansion occur, with eventual emergence of a monoclonal B lymphoid population and overt B cell lymphoma (Gulley, 2010). Periodic monitoring of EBV viral load in peripheral blood is helpful in identifying patients with rising EBV levels at risk for PTLD; modification and titration of immunosuppressive agents can be considered in overall management of graft survival and EBV-induced complications. Comparison of EBV quantitation results among several laboratories has shown significant variation in viral load results, so as with all other viral load assays, clinical management should be based on testing confined to a single laboratory until methods are better standardized (Hayden, 2008).

The most common opportunistic viral infections in HIV and transplant patients are caused by CMV (Sia, 2000; Fishman, 2007). Graft survival is threatened by direct viral injury to the organ, by toxicity from antiviral drugs, or by unavoidable reduction of immunosuppressive therapy to help contain viral infection. CMV viremia is a sensitive marker of active viral replication and helps predict potential graft endangerment and risk of pneumonitis, colitis, or other organ injury. CMV may originate in the transplant itself or may result from reactivation of endogenous latent virus in the recipient; recipients who have no demonstrable CMV antibody (CMV-naive) are at high risk of developing CMV disease if the donor is CMV positive; primary CMV disease after transplant is the most severe, with greater risk of organ loss. Surveillance for CMV proliferation after transplantation is very helpful for appropriate institution of antiviral prophylaxis to modulate the intensity of CMV disease. Adult AIDS patients with CD4 cell counts below $100/mm^3$ are at great risk for reactivation of latent CMV. Retinitis is a frequent complication in advanced HIV disease with high viral load and low CD4 levels; CMV pneumonia and gastrointestinal and CNS involvement are also common, and widely disseminated multiorgan disease at autopsy is not unusual (Drew, 1992). CMV systemic disease may also develop from primary infection in pediatric HIV patients.

Serology is very useful for screening blood donors to limit transfusion of CMV-positive blood products to newborns and naive immunocompromised patients, and for assessing donor and recipient serostatus. EIA screens for CMV-IgG are most sensitive, have objective endpoints, and avoid the interpretive problems of complement binding in IFA procedures. However, serology has little or no practical value for diagnosing CMV infection in transplant recipients or HIV patients. IgM production may be impaired in marrow/stem cell and solid organ recipients, and IgG seroconversion requires acute and convalescent specimens.

Typical cytomegalic inclusions are specific for identifying CMV infection in biopsy samples and BAL, but H&E staining is relatively insensitive. Sensitivity improves somewhat with immunoperoxidase or in situ hybridization methods, but isolation of virus has greater diagnostic accuracy. CMV replicates almost exclusively in HDF cell lines; growth is slow, with incubation times of 7 days or longer before CPE develops. The infected fibroblast initially retains its fusiform shape as the nucleus becomes swollen and refractile; then the entire cell becomes rounded and distorted, and virus spreads into adjacent fibroblasts, producing an enlarging patch of damaged cells (see Table 55-4).

CMV recovery is shortened to only 1–2 days with shell vial culture (Gleaves, 1987). HDF monolayers are inoculated by centrifugation with peripheral blood leukocytes (harvested by density gradient separation), BAL fluid, or homogenized tissue; after 16–40 hours' incubation, the monolayer is stained with fluorescein-conjugated antibody to CMV early antigen. Infected fibroblasts show homogeneous fluorescence of the entire nucleus. CMV burden is usually high in infected end-stage HIV patients, and culture has excellent diagnostic sensitivity with tissue and BAL specimens (95%–100%). Shell vial culture of peripheral blood leukocytes has turnaround advantages, but sensitivity is only 75% compared with tube monolayer inoculation, so backup tube culture is recommended. Recovery of CMV in standard tube and shell vial cultures is optimized when specimens are inoculated immediately to fresh cell monolayers; yield is reduced when inoculation is delayed (Brumback, 1997). Another advantage of shell vial culture is that results are semiquantitative (Buller, 1992); a standard inoculum of the patient's cells (peripheral leukocytes or BAL cells) along with a count of fluorescent CMV-positive nuclei in the shell vial monolayer generates a figure that has clinical value for estimating severity of infection, for monitoring response to therapy, and for predicting prognosis. CMV is the most common cause of viremia in compromised patients; however, VZV, HSV, adenovirus, and occasionally enterovirus may be recovered. HDF and A549 traditional tube cultures held for 14 days will recover these agents as well as CMV (Stanberry, 1994). When immunosuppression is severe, AIDS patients and transplant recipients are at risk for other viral infections with specific organ or site involvement. Central nervous system infections were described earlier. Adenovirus, HSV, and VZV may present with pneumonitis; herpetic infection (HSV and VZV) may develop initially in esophageal and mucocutaneous sites and then may disseminate. For this reason, mucosal, cutaneous, or tissue biopsy specimens should be inoculated to a comprehensive series of cell lines to maximize recovery. Amplified nucleic acid testing for HSV viremia has shown positive results in immunocompromised adults with solid organ transplants, malignancies, immunodeficiencies, HIV-AIDS, and autoimmune disorders; in addition to skin lesions, presentations include hepatitis, fever, abdominal pain, and CNS alterations (Berrington, 2009).

Even with improvement in recovery of CMV by shell vial culture, this approach is too insensitive for preemptive surveillance for CMV infection in the setting of iatrogenic immunosuppression of transplant recipients. CMV antigen can be identified in peripheral blood neutrophils by IFA or immunoperoxidase staining (Hodinka, 2007); commercially available CMV pp65 antigenemia assays are rapid, sensitive, and specific; the principal practical limitation of this method is host neutropenia. CMV viral load by PCR also provides sensitive quantitative assessment of CMV in peripheral blood (Sia, 2000; Razonable, 2002). Quantitative PCR methods can identify patients with escalating CMV levels before overt disease develops, so that antiviral therapy can be intensified and immunosuppression to prevent graft rejection can be continued. Biopsy of specific sites with suspected acute CMV disease, such as colonic mucosa, may be necessary to establish a diagnosis (Fishman, 2007). Antiviral susceptibility testing methods using plaque reduction assay or genotypic assay of mutations associated with resistance may be indicated in patients who do not respond to therapy (Sia, 2000; Razonable, 2002).

BK virus (BKV), a polyomavirus similar to the JC virus responsible for progressive multifocal leukoencephalopathy, reactivates during immunosuppression; it produces serious nephropathy in approximately 2% of renal transplant recipients, with progressive loss of graft function and even transplant failure. Identification of tubular epithelial cells with nuclear inclusions (decoy cells) in voided urine in BKV nephropathy has served as a screening test for many years. BKV viral load assessment in plasma and urine provides a noninvasive means of detecting and monitoring active infection (Fishman, 2002; Hirsch, 2002).

Parvovirus B19 is an uncommon but serious cause of refractory anemia and pancytopenia in solid organ and hematopoietic stem cell transplants and in HIV patients. Lung, liver, myocardial, and CNS disease can also develop, as can serious infection in allograft tissue. Diagnosis may be difficult, even with invasive procedures such as bone marrow biopsy. Serologic diagnosis has limitations in immunocompromised patients, who may be incapable of producing specific antibody. PCR detection and quantitation of parvovirus DNA in peripheral blood are both sensitive and specific for establishing the diagnosis (Eid, 2006).

Screening of donors for hepatitis B and C viruses and for HIV has dramatically reduced the transmission of these agents to organ recipients. However, the surprising dissemination of WNV and lymphocytic choriomeningitis virus via organ donation (Iwamoto, 2003; Fischer, 2006) has highlighted the ongoing vigilance that is needed to evaluate suspected infection in this highly vulnerable class of patients, for whom accurate diagnosis may be confounded and complicated by serious comorbidities. As molecular methods for detection and quantitation of other opportunistic viruses become generally available, better management of infection and graft survival will follow.

VIRAL HEPATITIS

Many viruses are hepatotoxic. Yellow fever virus (Monath, 2003) causes massive hepatocellular necrosis. All of the human herpesviruses can produce mild liver disease with system infection, but fulminant hepatic necrosis is unusual. Serious herpesvirus infections of the hepatic allograft can occur after liver transplant. Adenovirus, HSV, VZV, CMV, and echoviruses occasionally produce aggressive hepatitis in the immunocompromised (Fishman, 2007; Riediger, 2009). However, hepatitis A, B, C, D, and E virus infections characteristically lead to lytic hepatocyte injury and account for most clinical cases of infectious hepatitis.

Hepatitis A virus (HAV) and hepatitis E virus (HEV) are nonenveloped agents with fecal-oral transmission; inadequate sewage treatment and crowded living conditions are linked to waterborne outbreaks, and HAV has been spread in contaminated foods. Acute hepatitis A incidence in the United States declined by 92% between 1995 and 2007 (to 1.0 case per 100,000) (Daniels, 2009). HAV is a picornavirus, distinct from but related to the enteroviruses. Children in day care and crowded institutions and their caregivers are at increased risk for HAV hepatitis (Cuthbert, 2001; Emerson, 2004). Acute disease in children is mild and often asymptomatic; adults occasionally develop severe infection, but fulminant hepatitis and death are unusual; IgM antibody is the most practical marker of acute infection (Mor, 2009) (http://www.cdc.gov/ncphi/disss/nndss/casedef/case_definitions.htm). Recovery is complete with no chronic infectious state. HAV vaccines are now available and are very effective (Nothdurft, 2008; Dentinger, 2009).

HEV is related to caliciviruses; outbreaks occur in developing countries and in refugee camps with suboptimal food and water sanitation, resulting in acute, mostly self-limiting, disease (predominantly genotypes 1 and 2). In industrialized nations, in addition to travel-associated disease, HEV is now an emerging disease and is considered an autochthonous, possibly zoonotic, disease (predominantly genotype 3). Teens and young adults are most commonly affected; mortality is rare, except in pregnant women, in whom death rates may reach 25% (Aggarwal, 2009). HEV does not progress to chronic infection, except in immunocompromised individuals Kamar, 2008). IgG antibody develops promptly and persists at low titers indefinitely; specific IgM is a reliable test of acute infection (Herremans, 2007).

HBV is easily transmitted through blood and is classically acquired through transfusions, needle sharing, or occupational injury with contaminated sharp objects. Infection may be acquired transplacentally during pregnancy, and sexual contact and household exposure to virus in body fluids are important routes of spread. Acute infection is frequently symptomatic, with much of the liver damage inflicted by $CD8^+$ cytotoxic T lymphocytes; 1% develop fulminant fatal massive hepatocellular necrosis. Diagnosis of acute infection is based on the presence of IgM antibody to hepatitis B core antigen (anti-HBc) or the presence of hepatitis B surface antigen (HBsAg) (http://www.cdc.gov/ncphi/disss/nndss/casedef/case_definitions.htm). HBV can also persist as a chronic infection. Up to 90% of infants born with HBV vertically acquired in utero become chronic carriers, compared with 25%–30% of infected older children and less than 5% of adults (Lok, 2009). Even with apparently resolved infection, HBV DNA persists despite host production of antibodies to core and e antigens. Diagnosis of chronic HBV infection is based on the absence of anti-HBc IgM and the presence of HBsAg, hepatitis e antigen, (HBeAg) or HBV DNA (http://www.cdc.gov/ncphi/disss/nndss/casedef/case_definitions.htm). T lymphocyte damage of hepatocytes is ongoing in chronic HBV infection. Unrelenting inflammation progresses to cirrhotic scarring in at least 2% of chronic infections (Lok, 2002; Ganem, 2004); HBV-induced cirrhosis is a risk factor for hepatocellular carcinoma. HBV infection and sequelae are largely preventable; with the implementation of vaccination programs, the incidence of new infections in the United States has decreased significantly (Wilkins, 2010). Acute hepatitis B incidence in the United States declined by 82% between 1990 and 2007 (to 1.5 cases per 100,000) (Daniels, 2009). Response to antiviral therapy in chronically infected patients can be monitored by quantitation of HBV (Ghany, 2009; Sorrell, 2009).

HBV coinfection or superinfection with hepatitis D virus (HDV) is associated with a severe course of hepatitis that frequently leads to rapid progressive fibrosis, hepatic decompensation, and the development of hepatocellular carcinoma. HDV is a defective RNA viroid that requires HBV surface antigen for full expression, replication, and transmission. HDV may be transmitted from person to person in household situations in endemic areas (Middle East, South America, Central Africa, Mediterranean countries). HDV is rare in the United States; intravenous drug abuse is the principal risk factor. Anti-HDV IgG and IgM testing is available when HDV coinfection is suspected in HBsAg-positive individuals (Wedemeyr, 2010).

HCV is estimated to infect 3.2 million Americans and is the leading cause of non-A non-B hepatitis; since the advent of serologic testing and nucleic acid amplification, transfusion-associated HCV has dropped dramatically (Cuthbert, 1994; Lauer, 2001; National Institutes of Health,

TABLE 55-7
Serologic and Virologic Tests for Hepatitis Viruses

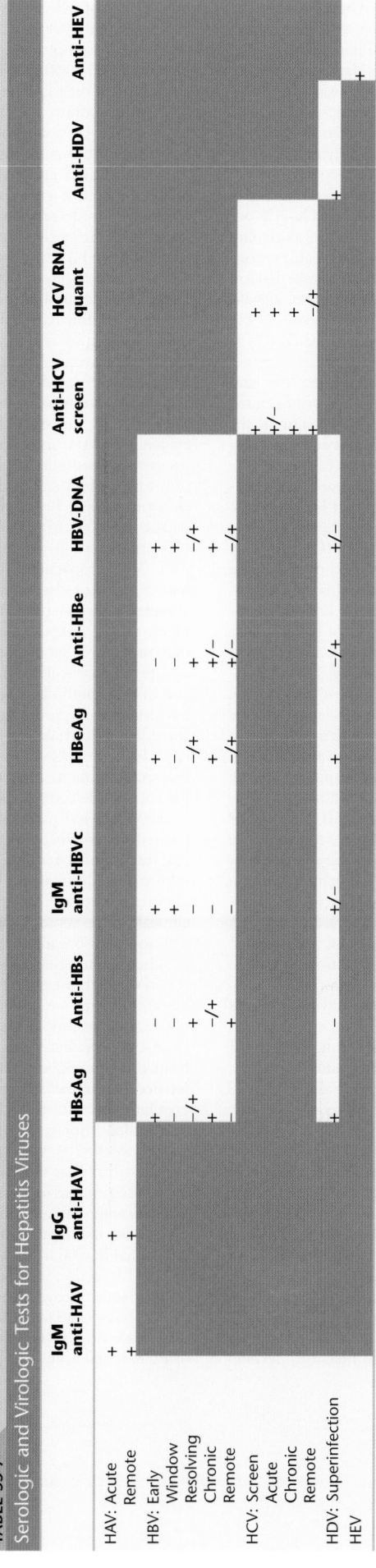

	IgM anti-HAV	IgG anti-HAV	HBsAg	Anti-HBs	IgM anti-HBVc	HBeAg	Anti-HBe	HBV-DNA	Anti-HCV screen	HCV RNA quant	Anti-HDV	Anti-HEV
HAV: Acute	+	+										
Remote	+	+										
HBV: Early			+	−	+	+	−	+				
Window			−	−	+	−	−	+				
Resolving			−/+	+	−	−/+	+	−/+				
Chronic			+	−/+	−	+	+/−	+				
Remote			−	+	−	−/+	+/−	−/+				
HCV: Screen									+	+		
Acute									+/−	+		
Chronic									+	+		
Remote									+	−/+		
HDV: Superinfection			+	−	+/−	+	−/+	+/−			+	
HEV												+

Adapted from MMWR 2009;58:1.
HAV, Hepatitis A virus; *HBe,* hepatitis e; *HBeAg,* hepatitis e antigen; *HBs,* hepatitis B surface; *HBsAg,* hepatitis B surface antigen; *HBV,* hepatitis B virus; *HCV,* hepatitis C virus; *HDV,* hepatitis D virus; *HEV,* hepatitis E virus; *IgM,* immunoglobulin M; +, positive; −, negative.

2002; Stramer, 2004). Following a peak in 1992 in the United States, the incidence of acute hepatitis C declined; however, since 2003 rates have plateaued, with the most common risk factor being injection drug use. HCV is transmitted primarily through percutaneous exposure, but no source is identified in many cases (Daniels, 2009). Transmission of HCV during pregnancy or through sexual and household contact is much less efficient than transmission of HBV and HIV. Fulminant and fatal acute hepatitis is rare; however, HCV clearance by cytotoxic T lymphocytes is inadequate in most patients. About 80% of infections become chronic, leading to hepatic fibrosis and hepatocellular regeneration that may progress further to cirrhosis (20%) and hepatocellular carcinoma (1%–4% per year in cirrhotic patients). Coinfection with HIV or HBV, as well as alcohol use, accelerates the natural course; superinfection with HAV can provoke fulminant hepatitis. Treatment with pegylated γ-interferon and ribavirin produces sustained remission in chronic HCV disease and may significantly modify or prevent serious long-term sequelae (McHutchison, 1998). However, response rates are lower for genotype 1, which represents 75% of infections in the United States (Zein, 2000).

Third-generation screening HCV antibody chemiluminescence and enzyme immunoassays (CIA and EIA) use an expanded number of refined viral antigens. Sensitivity is very good; false negatives may occur in the context of severe immunosuppression or early in acute infection. Specificity of the current EIAs for anti-HCV is better than 99% (Ghany, 2009). Because of the high rate of chronic HCV disease and favorable outcomes with antiviral therapy, an algorithm for efficient testing that begins with a CIA or EIA HCV antibody screen has been recommended by the Centers for Disease Control and Prevention (CDC). A screening HCV antibody result with a high signal-to-cutoff ratio has a high probability of being a true positive with chronic infection; quantitative HCV PCR is then appropriate to verify viremia and begin antiviral treatment. A low signal-to-cutoff HCV antibody screen result has a high likelihood of being a false positive, so confirmation is needed; specificity of available nucleic acid amplification assays is in the range of 98%–99% (Ghany, 2009). POC HCV antibody tests have recently become available. These easy to use HCV rapid antibody tests may prove to be an important tool for rapid HCV antibody detection. However, confirmation with a quantitative nucleic acid amplification assay is still recommended. Genotyping is useful in clinical management for predicting the likelihood of response and the optimal duration of therapy (Valsamakis, 2007; Ghany, 2009).

Hepatitis GB virus-C (GBV-C), a flavivirus related to HCV, has been identified in posttransfusion hepatitis. However, GBV-C does not appear to be hepatotropic, does not replicate efficiently in hepatocytes, and does not cause acute or chronic hepatitis (Baggio-Zappia, 2009). It is interesting to note that coinfection with GBV-C and HIV appeared to induce host antiviral activity against HIV and prolong survival (Xiang, 2001). In spite of a decade of follow-up studies, the question of whether GBV-C is associated with better prognosis in HIV-coinfected patients remains unresolved.

None of the hepatitis viruses replicates in standard culture cell lines. Detection of specific IgM and IgG antibodies and specific viral antigens designates the stage of infection with each virus; viral load assessment is used to monitor response to treatment of chronic infection. Table 55-7 summarizes virologic and serologic markers with viral hepatitis.

ACQUIRED IMMUNODEFICIENCY SYNDROME

HIV1 is a retrovirus in the Lentiviridae family that now has worldwide distribution. HIV infects and destroys CD3/4$^+$ T lymphocytes and eventually leads to debilitating opportunistic infections and malignancies (Stein, 1992; Schupbach, 2003). HIV is also neurotropic and can cause acute meningitis and slow destructive encephalopathy (Atwood, 1993). The HIV2 strain present in West Africa is somewhat less pathogenic, with reduced risk of transmission and progression to AIDS.

Half of individuals acutely infected with HIV experience mononucleosis-like symptoms before entering an asymptomatic latent stage. During acute infection, circulating HIV viral load is high, but antibody may not yet be detectable. Median time for CD3/4$^+$ cell destruction sufficient to develop full features of AIDS is 10–11 years; 5%–10% of individuals develop AIDS in 3 years, and 5%–10% of individuals maintain stable CD3/4 blood levels and remain asymptomatic indefinitely (Munoz, 1995). Children vertically infected at birth often show accelerated progression if untreated.

Both the diagnosis and ongoing management of HIV infection rely heavily on laboratory testing (Table 55-8). Several commercial EIA screening tests for HIV antibody are made with an array of recombinant and purified HIV antigens; third-generation kits have overall excellent specificity and sensitivity and may detect HIV antibody as early as 2–4 weeks post infection. Fourth-generation EIA tests that combine screening for HIV antibody with detection of HIV p24 antigen have even greater sensitivity in recognizing early infection. CDC recommendations include routine screening for HIV antibody in all health care settings for all patients aged 13–64 years (Branson, 2006). Blood banks in industrialized countries always test donor blood for HIV RNA to identify donors in the false-negative window (Candotti, 2003; Schupbach, 2003; Stramer, 2004). U.S. blood banks also test for HIV2 antibody, which is standard screening in Africa and Europe. A positive EIA HIV antibody screen should be repeated and then confirmed with an additional test, such as immunofluorescence assay or Western blot assay (Carlson, 1987). Western blot is less sensitive than EIA, but a classic positive band pattern provides convincing serologic evidence of HIV infection (MMWR, 1991). When acute retroviral syndrome is a possibility, a plasma HIV RNA test should be used in conjunction with an HIV antibody test to diagnose newly acquired HIV infection (Kassutto, 2004; Branson, 2006). HIV2 infection should be suspected in persons of West African origin who have clinical conditions suggestive of HIV infection but with atypical serologic test results (Aberg, 2009).

HIV is propagated in tissue culture by cocultivating infected patient lymphocytes or tissues with normal donor lymphocytes that have been stimulated with phytohemagglutinin, interleukin-2, and interferon. Culture is complex, expensive, and dangerous and should be attempted only in research laboratories. HIV culture has been supplanted by nucleic acid testing for routine management; real time RT-PCR, NASBA, TMA, and bDNA methods are commercially available. Antiretroviral treatment has dramatically improved survival and quality of life for HIV patients (Freedberg, 2001; Aberg, 2004). Quantitative HIV RNA assays to measure viral load in plasma have revolutionized monitoring of antiretroviral therapy; treatment-related reductions in HIV RNA of more than 0.5–1.0 log copies/mL correlate with slower clinical progression.

HIV-infected patients typically have a genotypic resistance test performed at baseline, regardless of whether antiretroviral therapy will be initiated immediately (Aberg, 2009). Genotypic methods typically involve sequence analysis of the HIV reverse transcriptase and protease genes to identify mutations that are linked to drug resistance and have the greatest clinical utility. As use of agents with other HIV targets increases, testing will no doubt broaden.

Phenotypic testing is complex and involves amplification of protease and reverse-transcriptase genes from virus recovered from the patient's blood, followed by insertion of these genes into a test virus and then in vitro susceptibility testing of this hybrid laboratory-constructed virus against specific antiviral drugs. A virtual phenotype can be approximated from the genotypic mutation data to ascertain the likelihood of in vitro phenotypic actual susceptibility, with the two methods often showing excellent correlation (Shafer, 2002; Clavel, 2004). Tropism testing is recommended prior to initiation of a CCR5-antagonist antiretroviral drug, and HLA-B*5701 typing should be performed prior to treatment with abacavir to reduce the risk of a hypersensitivity reaction (Aberg, 2009).

In utero or perinatal transmission from HIV-infected mothers can be dramatically reduced with treatment and strict avoidance of breast feeding. The transmission rate has been reported to be <1% in women who achieve undetectable viral loads with treatment (Aberg, 2009). Early identification of HIV1 infection in exposed infants is important to allow early intervention with antiretroviral therapy and adjunctive care (Havens, 2009). Maternal antibody can remain detectable in the infant up to 18 months of age. Diagnosis of active HIV infection in the infant is primarily made by means of PCR-based assays for HIV DNA or RNA. Virologic testing should be performed at 14–21 days, 1–2 months, and 4–6 months of age. Infected infants should also undergo HIV resistance testing (Aberg, 2009). (See earlier section on Congenital and Perinatal Infections.)

VIRUS-ASSOCIATED NEOPLASIA

Although the topic is beyond the discussion in this chapter, it is worth noting that viral infections are associated with 15%–20% of human cancers worldwide (Martin, 2009; Fernandez, 2010). The association of viruses with tumorigenesis has been appreciated since the early 20th century (Rous, 1911). Tumorigenic viruses are found in diverse virus families and employ diverse mechanisms to contribute to neoplasia (Table 55-9). Oncogenic viruses tend to cause persistent infection, and viral proteins frequently disrupt normal cellular processes, such as apoptosis and cell cycle checkpoint activation. However, viral infections generally are not considered to be sufficient for carcinogenesis; additional factors, including host immunity and cell mutations, are certainly involved in the neoplastic process.

TABLE 55-8
Laboratory Diagnosis of HIV Infection

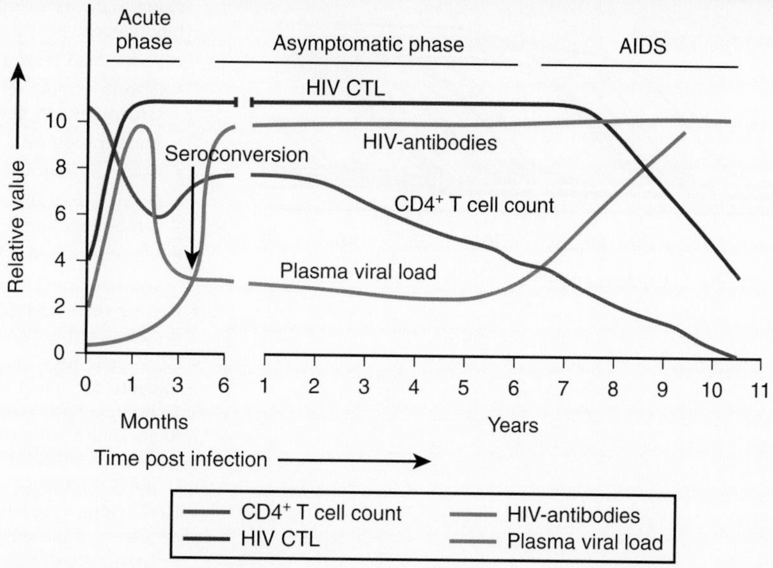

Assay		Comments
Serology		
Batch screen 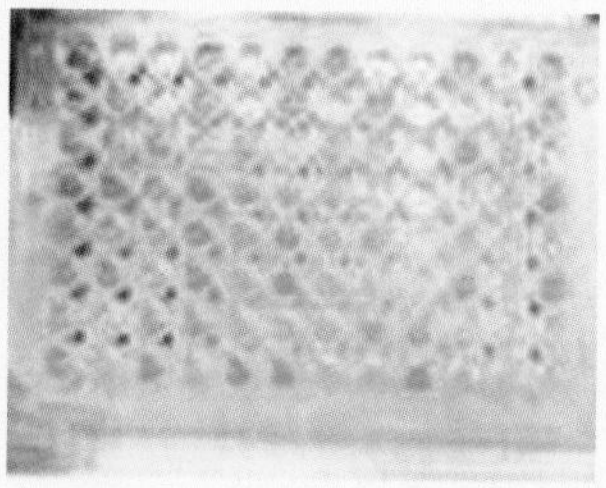	Rapid tests 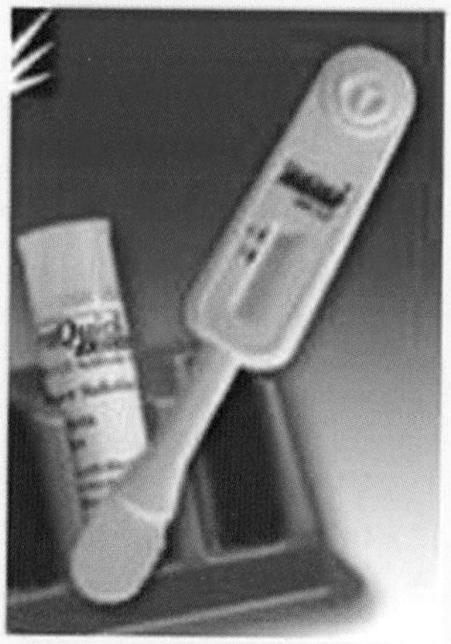	• Fourth-generation EIA kits contain multiple recombinant HIV antigens to maximize detection of HIV antibody. • Current assays show greater than 99% sensitivity and specificity. • Positive EIA HIV antibody screen test results are preliminary and must be confirmed with Western blot to establish diagnosis of HIV infection. • Both microwell and rapid EIA methods may give negative results in the first 1–3 weeks after HIV infection. Assays that identify both HIV antibody and HIV p24 antigen shorten the false-negative window immediately after initial infection.

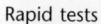

Continued

TABLE 55-8
Laboratory Diagnosis of HIV Infection—*Cont'd*

Assay	**Comments**

Confirmation
Western blot (WB)

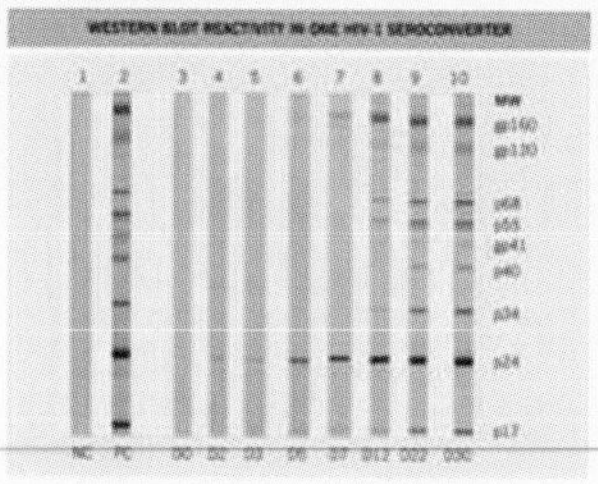

- Specificity >99%.
- Indeterminate rate of HIV1 WB is too high to use WB as a screening assay.
- Indirect immunofluorescence assay (IFA) can be used for screening and also for confirmation; specificity is comparable to WB.

Prognosis/Monitoring Treatment

HIV viral load

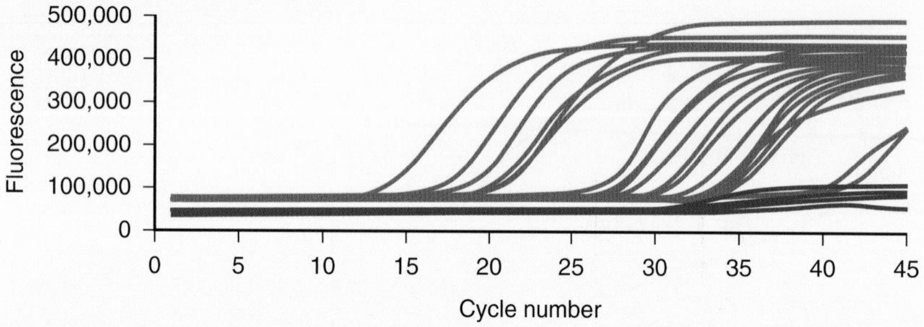

- The same method should be used for monitoring individual patients to minimize technical variation in HIV blood levels.
- HIV viral load testing is used to
  - Diagnose acute retroviral syndrome before seroconversion develops
  - Assess prognosis and progression of HIV disease
  - Guide antiretroviral therapy
  - Define a baseline level so that response to therapy can be measured
  - Monitor response to therapy
- Greater than 0.5 log (3-fold) change in blood HIV load is considered clinically significant.

Genotypic HIV assays

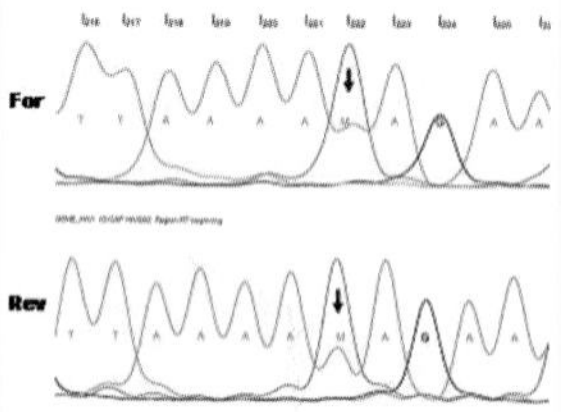

Resistance-associated reverse transcriptase (RT) mutation K103N
Resistance to nevirapine and efavirenz

- Genotypic assays are helpful in antiretroviral-naive patients for initial assessment of treatment options. Genotyping is also useful for patients who develop virologic failure with rising HIV viral load during highly active antiretroviral therapy, and need guidance for treatment modification.
- Genotyping detects changes in the nucleic acid sequence of the relevant HIV1 gene and identifies drug resistance by detecting mutations in the HIV1 genome that lead to specific amino acid substitutions in the HIV1 RT or protease enzymes.

Phenotypic assays

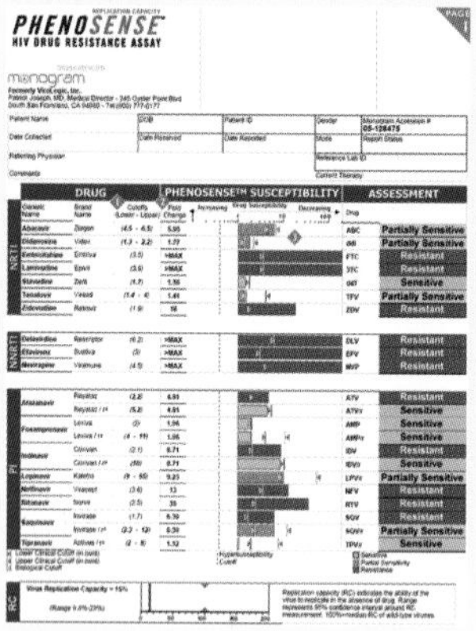

- Phenotypic assays amplify RT and protease genes from the patient's HIV predominant quasi-species virus RNA or proviral DNA. These amplicons are then inserted into a laboratory virus that lacks the genes, creating a hybrid virus. The hybrid virus is then propagated in cell culture, and its ability to propagate in the presence of varying concentrations of the anti-HIV agent is measured. Results are expressed as concentrations of drug required to inhibit 50% of growth (IC50) compared with a wild-type control strain.

Virtual phenotypes

- The patient's HIV genotype is compared with a database containing many known HIV drug resistant and susceptible genotypes to predict the patient's response to therapy.

TABLE 55-8
Laboratory Diagnosis of HIV Infection—*Cont'd*

Assay	Comments
Immune Status	
CD4 cell counts (% CD4 and absolute number) 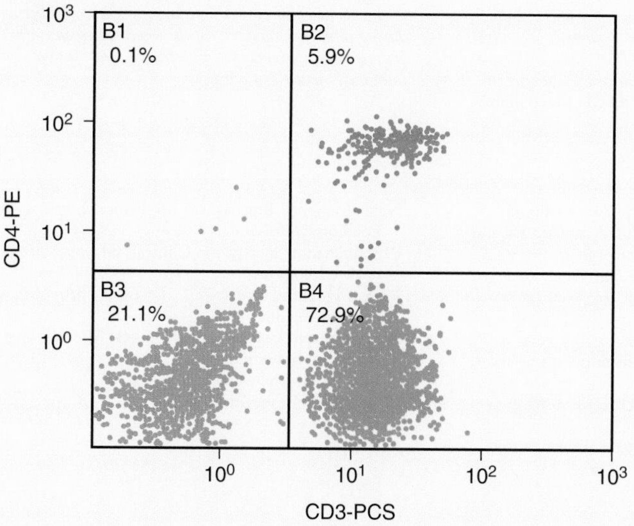	• CD4 cell count and CD4/CD8 ratio are used to • Stage HIV disease • Help establish the risk of specific HIV-associated infectious or neoplastic complications • Determine the need for prophylaxis against opportunistic infections • Determine the need for and response to antiretroviral therapy

Adapted from World Health Organization. Guidelines for HIV diagnosis and monitoring of antiretroviral therapy. Geneva, Switzerland: World Health Organization; 2009.
EIA, Enzyme immunoassay; *HIV*, human immunodeficiency virus; *RT*, reverse transcriptase.

TABLE 55-9
Tumorigenic Viruses

Virus	Genome	Viral taxonomy	Human cancers
EBV	dsDNA	Herpesviridae	BL, NPC, HD, GC
KSHV	dsDNA	Herpesviridae	KS, PEL, MCD
HPV	dsDNA	Papillomaviridae	Cervical, oropharynx, anogenital, skin
HBV	dsDNA (partial)	Hepadnaviridae	HCC
HCV	ssRNA	Flaviviridae	HCC
HTLV-1	ssRNA>dsDNA	Retroviridae	ATL
HIV	ssRNA>dsDNA	Retroviridae	Unknown
CMV	dsDNA	Herpesviridae	CRC, glioma, prostate
SV40	dsDNA	Polyomaviridae	Osteosarcoma, mesothelioma, brain
JCV	dsDNA	Polyomaviridae	Brain, CRC, glioma, medulloblastoma
BKV	dsDNA	Polyomaviridae	Prostate, brain
MCV	dsDNA	Polyomaviridae	MCC
HHV-6	dsDNA	Herpesviridae	Hematologic malignancies

Adapted from Fernandez AF, Esteller M. Viral epigenomes in human tumorigenesis. Oncogene 2010;29:1405–20.
ATL, Adult T cell leukemia; *BKV*, BK cell polyomavirus; *BL*, Burkitt's lymphoma; *CMV*, cytomegalovirus; *CRC*, colorectal cancer; *EBV*, Epstein-Barr virus; *GC*, gastric carcinoma; *HBV*, hepatitis B virus; *HCC*, hepatocellular carcinoma; *HCV*, hepatitis C virus; *HD*, Hodgkin disease; *HHV*, human herpes virus; *HIV*, human immunodeficiency virus; *HPV*, human papilloma virus; *HTLV-1*, human T cell leukemia virus type 1; *JCV*, JC virus; *KS*, Kaposi's sarcoma; *KSHV*, Kaposi's sarcoma–associated herpesvirus; *MCC*, Merkel cell carcinoma; *MCD*, multicentric Castleman's disease; *MCV*, Merkel cell polyomavirus; *NPC*, nasopharyngeal primary carcinoma; *PEL*, primary effusion lymphoma; *SV40*, Simian virus 40.

SELECTED REFERENCES

Branson BM, Handsfield HH, Lampe MA, et al, Centers for Disease Control and Prevention. Revised recommendations for HIV testing of adults, adolescents, and pregnant women in health-care settings. MMWR Recomm Rep 2006;55:1–17.

Routine HIV screening should be expanded and covered by general medical consent; it should be included in the routine prenatal screening panel; high-risk individuals should be screened annually.

Cox JT, Moriarty AT, Castle PE. Commentary on: statement on HPV DNA test utilization. Diagn Cytopathol 2009;37:471–4.

National guidelines for HPV testing are summarized and discussed in the context of a case presentation; these strategies are based on understanding of the natural progression of HPV infection.

Fernandez AF, Esteller M. Viral epigenomes in human tumorigenesis. Oncogene 2010;29:1405–20.

Viruses are associated with 15% to 20% of human cancers worldwide. The authors summarize studies directed towards elucidating the molecular mechanisms and genetic alterations by which viruses cause cancer.

Garcia LS. Clinical microbiology procedures handbook. 3rd ed. Washington, DC: ASM Press; 2010.

Standard reference book with comprehensive descriptions of relevant microbiology laboratory procedures.

Ghany MG, Strader DB, Thomas DL, Seeff LB. AASLD practice guidelines: diagnosis, management, and treatment of hepatitis C: an update. Hepatology 2009;49:1335–74.

These recommendations provide a data-supported approach to establishing guidelines. Intended for use by physicians, these recommendations suggest preferred approaches to the diagnostic, therapeutic, and preventive aspects of care.

Ginocchio CC, Zhang F. Evaluation of multiple test methods for the detection of the novel 2009 influenza A (H1N1) during the New York City outbreak. J Clin Virol 2009;45:191–5.

Synopsis of clinical utility of various laboratory tests for the detection of 2009H1N1 influenza A virus.

Hayden RT, Hokanson KM. Multicenter comparison of real-time PCR assays for quantitative detection of Epstein-Barr virus. J Clin Microbiol 2008;46:157.

Blood EBV viral load is valuable for diagnosis and treatment of posttransplant lymphoproliferative disorder; however, quantitative methods must be standardized before interlaboratory testing can be recommended.

Mahoney JB. Detection of respiratory viruses by molecular methods. Clin Microbiol Rev 2008;21:716–47.

Review of common and recently described respiratory viral pathogens, including comparisons of traditional diagnostic methods with molecular-based methods for viral detection in clinical specimens.

Mandel GL, Bennett JE, Dolin R, editors. Principles and practice of infectious disease. 7th ed. Philadelphia: Churchill Livingstone; 2010.

Reference book covering comprehensive guidance on diagnosing and treating infectious diseases.

Munro SC, Hall B. Diagnosis of and screening for cytomegalovirus infection in pregnant women. J Clin Microbiol 2005;43:4713–8.

A serologic test algorithm can be used to diagnose and time primary CMV infection during pregnancy.

Tregoning J, Schwarze J. Respiratory viral infections in infants: causes, clinical symptoms, virology and immunology. Clin Microbiol Rev 2010;23:74–98.

A wide range of viruses cause acute respiratory infection during infancy; immaturity of the immune response affects both immediate outcome of infection and future host immune function and response.

WEBSITES AND E-MAIL ADDRESSES

Centers for Disease Control and Prevention: http://www.cdc.gov/
Many journals, articles, materials free

All the Virology on the WWW: http://www.virology.net/garryfavweb.html

American Society for Microbiology Journals: http://journals.asm.org/

Infectious Diseases Society of America: http://www.idsociety.org
Care and treatment guidelines free

Worldwide influenza updates: http://www.google.org/flutrends/

World Health Organization: http://www.who.int/

Association for Professionals in Infection Control and Epidemiology: http://www.apic.org/

Medscape: http://www.medscape.com

American Society for Microbiology: http://www.asmusa.org
Many articles and materials free

European Society for Clinical Virology: http://www.eur.nl/FGG/VIRO/ESCV/

National Centers for Infectious Diseases: http://www.cdc.gov/ncidod/

National Institutes of Health: http://www.nih.gov

New England Journal of Medicine: http://www.nejm.org

Pan American Society for Clinical Virology: http://www.virology.org

Johns Hopkins Infectious Disease: http://www.hopkins-id.edu/

South Central Association for Clinical Microbiology: http://www.scacm.org/

Mike.Costello@advocatehealth.com

myungbluth@reshealthcare.org

REFERENCES

Access the complete reference list online at http://www.expertconsult.com

CHAPTER 56

CHLAMYDIAL, RICKETTSIAL, AND MYCOPLASMAL INFECTIONS

David H. Walker, Gail L. Woods, Michael B. Smith

KEY POINTS

- *Chlamydia trachomatis* is the most common bacterial cause of sexually transmitted disease in the United States.
- The most sensitive method for detecting *C. trachomatis* is nucleic acid amplification.
- *Chlamydophila pneumoniae* (formerly *Chlamydia pneumoniae*) is responsible for at least 10% of community-acquired pneumonias. Infection is most often diagnosed serologically.
- Treatable rickettsial infections, including life-threatening Rocky Mountain spotted fever, boutonneuse fever, epidemic typhus, murine typhus, scrub typhus, human monocytotropic ehrlichiosis, and human granulocytotropic anaplasmosis, are seldom diagnosed serologically during the acute stage of illness owing to absence of an early antibody response.
- Immunohistochemistry and molecular diagnostics are effective in diagnosing rickettsioses and ehrlichioses, respectively, but are not generally available.
- Q fever endocarditis is a chronic infection that usually is diagnosed by detecting a high titer (≥1:800 by immunofluorescent antibody assay) of antibodies against *Coxiella burnetii* phase I antigen.
- The clinicoepidemiologic diagnosis of cat scratch disease can be confirmed serologically by antibodies to *Bartonella henselae* or by polymerase chain reaction testing of lymph node aspirates.
- Pneumonia due to *Mycoplasma pneumoniae* is often diagnosed on the basis of clinical manifestations alone. Definitive diagnosis requires detection of specific immunoglobulin (Ig)M, a fourfold change in IgG antibody titer between acute and convalescent serum specimens, or detection of nucleic acid in sputum or other respiratory specimens by nucleic acid amplification.

Human infections caused by chlamydias, rickettsiae, and mycoplasmas are discussed separately because the responsible pathogens differ from most other bacteria in several ways: The organisms are smaller, the structure of their cell walls is different, and chlamydias and many rickettsiae are obligately intracellular parasites.

CHLAMYDIAL INFECTIONS

The chlamydias have a tropism for columnar epithelial cells. They have a cell wall similar to that of gram-negative bacteria; they contain both deoxyribonucleic acid (DNA) and ribonucleic acid (RNA), have prokaryotic

TABLE 56-1
Features Useful for Differentiating Species of *Chlamydia* and *Chlamydophila* Pathogenic for Humans

	SPECIES		
Parameter	***Chlamydia trachomatis***	***Chlamydophila psittaci***	***Chlamydophila pneumoniae***
Sulfa susceptibility	Susceptible	Resistant	Resistant
Glycogen staining of inclusion	Positive	Negative	Negative
Elementary body shape	Round	Round	Pear-shaped or round

ribosomes, and synthesize their own proteins, nucleic acids, and lipids; they divide by binary fission; and they are susceptible to particular antibiotics. Unlike most bacteria, the chlamydias are "energy parasites"; they lack cytochromes and so cannot synthesize high-energy adenosine triphosphate (ATP) metabolites. For this reason, they are obligate intracellular bacteria and cannot replicate outside cells.

The chlamydias are classified in the order Chlamydiales, family Chlamydiaceae, the only family that contains human pathogens (Everett, 1999). Two genera and three species are pathogenic for humans: *Chlamydia trachomatis*, *Chlamydophila* (formerly *Chlamydia*) *psittaci*, and *Chlamydophila* (formerly *Chlamydia*) *pneumoniae*. Features useful for differentiating the three species are shown in Table 56-1. These genera also contain six other species that have not been associated with infection in humans. There are two biovars of *C. trachomatis*: lymphogranuloma venereum (Biovar LGV) and trachoma (Biovar trachoma), which preferentially infect humans. Biovar LGV contains four serovars (L1, L2, L2a, and L3), and 15 serovars are included in Biovar trachoma: A, B, Ba, and C are associated with trachoma, whereas D–K, Da, Ia, and Ja are associated with genital infections. Mouse and hamster isolates that previously made up the third biovar of *C. trachomatis* have been reclassified as a new species, *Chlamydia muridarum* (Everett, 1999).

STRUCTURE

Two morphologically distinct forms of chlamydia are recognized. The elementary body is a dense, spherical form, 0.2–0.4 µm in diameter, that contains prokaryotic ribosomal RNA and has a rigid cell wall caused by extensive disulfide cross-linking of cell wall proteins. It is the infectious form of the organism, capable of limited extracellular survival. The reticulate body, 0.6–1.0 µm in diameter, is the intracellular, metabolically active form, incapable of surviving outside cells. The closed circular DNA of both forms is compactly organized in a central nucleoid and has a genome of 1.0–1.2 million nucleotide base pairs.

Two components of the outer membrane of the chlamydial outer membrane complex have diagnostic importance. The most prominent is the major outer membrane protein (MOMP), a transmembrane protein with serovar-, species-, genus-, and family-reactive epitopes defined by monoclonal antibodies. Infection with chlamydias induces MOMP-specific antibodies, but their role in protective immunity is unclear. The chlamydial outer membrane complex also contains a lipopolysaccharide (LPS) antigen, which is the major antigen detected in genus-specific serologic tests for chlamydial infection. Monoclonal antibodies and monospecific polyvalent antisera to the LPS or MOMP are used in direct fluorescent antibody (DFA) tests and enzyme immunoassays (EIAs) to detect chlamydial antigen in clinical specimens.

REPLICATION

Chlamydias replicate in the cytoplasm of infected host cells. The developmental cycle begins with attachment of the elementary body to a microvillus on a susceptible columnar cell via heparin bridges. The elementary body travels down the microvillus and localizes in indentations of the host cell plasma membrane. There, the chlamydia enters the host cell in an endosome, where *C. psittaci*, *C. pneumoniae*, and *C. trachomatis* remain during their intracellular development. Endosomes containing elementary bodies of *C. psittaci* do not become acidified or fuse with cellular lysosomes; those containing *C. trachomatis* elementary bodies fuse with one another and perhaps with lysosomes. Within 6–8 hours after the elementary body enters the host cell, changes in its cell wall result in a transition to the reticulate body and subsequent initiation of DNA, RNA, and protein synthesis and its division by binary fission. Host cell mitochondria migrate to and are positioned against the enlarging endosome, allowing the reticulate body to utilize host cell ATP. Reticulate bodies begin to reorganize 18–24 hours after infection, and, presumably when nutrients are depleted, they mature into elementary bodies, which are released from the host cell. Cells infected with *C. psittaci* usually are severely damaged, and the organisms are released by cell lysis within 48 hours. In contrast, the inclusion of *C. trachomatis* appears to be extruded by fusion of the inclusion membrane with the plasma membrane 72–96 hours after infection, leaving a lesion in the surviving host cell membrane.

CHLAMYDIA TRACHOMATIS

C. trachomatis is the most common cause of sexually transmitted disease in the United States, and in trachoma-endemic regions of the Middle East, sub-Saharan Africa, and Asia, it is the primary infectious cause of blindness. The disorder is endemic in more than 50 countries, and estimates indicate that more than 3 million people are affected, with over a third having progressed to blindness (Burton, 2009).

Epidemiology, Pathology, and Clinical Manifestations

Humans are the only known natural host for all strains of *C. trachomatis*. The clinical manifestations and organ specificity of human infections with *C. trachomatis* are determined by both the mechanism of transmission and the properties of the infecting strain. Epidemiologically, *C. trachomatis* infections are divided into three categories: classic trachoma, sexually transmitted infections of adults, and perinatal ocular and respiratory tract infections.

Classic trachoma is an important cause of blindness in areas where public sanitation is inadequate and personal hygiene poor (Solomon, 2004). The disease is due to repeated infections of the conjunctiva, resulting in a pathologic sequence over time of follicular conjunctivitis, subepithelial scarring, contraction of the scar resulting in turning inward of the eyelid (entropion), rubbing of the eyelashes on the cornea (trichiasis) with subsequent corneal injury, and corneal scarring with opacification and reduced vision. Typically, acute infection is transmitted among children via fingers, fomites, and probably flies, and most children become chronically infected within a few years of birth. Conjunctival scarring usually becomes evident by the second or third decade of life, and blindness can occur anywhere from 10–40 years after the first infection (Dean, 2008). It is interesting to note that a recent study using molecular methods on infected patients in a trachoma-endemic location demonstrated that other species of the Chlamydiaceae, *C. psittaci* and *C. pneumoniae*, may also be involved in the pathogenesis of trachoma (Dean, 2008).

C. trachomatis–induced sexually transmitted infections of adults include LGV and urethritis/cervicitis and associated complications. LGV is endemic in Asia, Africa, and South America. In the United States, approximately 500 cases are reported each year; the disease affects males more frequently than females and is most common in persons of low socioeconomic status living in the southeastern states, in men who have sex with men, and in persons who have visited LGV-endemic countries outside the United States. LGV is transmitted sexually, although transmission by fomites and by aerosols produced during laboratory accidents has caused pneumonitis, pleural effusions, and mediastinal or hilar lymphadenopathy (Jones, 2000). Reservoirs of infection probably are persons with asymptomatic or ignored symptomatic urethral, cervical, or anorectal infection.

LGV is the only infection caused by *C. trachomatis* that produces multisystem involvement and constitutional manifestations. During the primary phase, a small, painless vesicle or a nonindurated papule or ulcer develops, often on the external genitalia, 3 days to 3 weeks after exposure, and heals quickly without scarring. If transmission is rectal, an acute proctitis is often the first manifestation. An outbreak of LGV proctitis in men who have sex with men was first noticed in Europe at the beginning of this decade and is due to infection with a unique LGV variant (labeled "L2b") (Spaargaren, 2005). Genomic similarity to isolates obtained from patients in the early 1980s in the United States suggests a silent ongoing epidemic in this population caused by this unique variant (Spaargaren, 2005). The secondary stage, characterized by suppurative regional lymphadenopathy, fever, chills, anorexia, headache, myalgias, and arthralgias, begins 2–6 weeks after exposure. The primary ulcer or papule often resolves before the secondary stage, but an acute proctitis may persist. Histologic examination of affected lymph nodes shows granulomas surrounding stellate abscesses. Involved lymph nodes become matted and eventually suppurate, producing draining fistulas that heal with scarring over several months. Fibrosis and resultant abnormal lymphatic drainage are responsible for the urethral or rectal strictures or induration and lymphedema of the genitalia that develop during the third stage.

Non-LGV *C. trachomatis* infection is the most frequent sexually transmitted disease reported to the Centers for Disease Control and Prevention (CDC). From 1990–2009, the rate increased from 160.2 to 409.2 cases per 100,000 population (Centers for Disease Control and Prevention, 2009). The clinical spectrum of sexually transmitted infections due to non-LGV strains of *C. trachomatis* is similar to disease caused by *Neisseria gonorrhoeae* (see Chapter 57). In men, *C. trachomatis* is responsible for 30%–50% of cases of nongonococcal urethritis, but as many as 85%–90% of men who harbor *C. trachomatis* in the urethra are asymptomatic (Peipert, 2003). Rarely, urethritis caused by *C. trachomatis* progresses to epididymitis. Among men who have sex with men, non-LGV strains of *C. trachomatis* have been associated with proctitis. Genital infection with *C. trachomatis* is diagnosed more often in women than in men, with a rate of 583.5/100,000 reported for women in the United States in 2008, compared with a rate of 211.1 for men—a rate difference that is thought, at least in part, to be reflective of the greater number of women who undergo testing (Centers for Disease Control and Prevention, 2008a). Infection of the endocervix with *C. trachomatis* is often asymptomatic, but at least one third of women have signs of infection on physical examination. The most common sign is mucopurulent cervicitis, which can spread to the urethra and urinary bladder, resulting in the acute urethral syndrome of abacteriuric pyuria, or to the endometrium and fallopian tubes, producing endometritis or salpingitis. Untreated infections of the upper reproductive tract may progress to pelvic inflammatory disease or may cause scarring and dysfunction of the oviduct transport system, which could result in infertility, ectopic pregnancy, or chronic pelvic pain. Intraperitoneal spread of the infection may cause acute peritonitis, perihepatitis (Fitz-Hugh–Curtis syndrome), periappendicitis, or perisplenitis. A portion (1%–5%) of patients with urogenital infection with *C. trachomatis* will develop a reactive arthritis that is usually self-limited but may develop a chronic relapsing course (Rihl, 2006; Carter, 2009). Chlamydial infection in pregnancy has been associated with preterm labor, premature rupture of membranes, low birthweight, neonatal death, and postpartum endometritis. A small percentage of adults with chlamydial genital infections develop inclusion conjunctivitis from autoinoculation.

In developed countries, where sexually transmitted infection with *C. trachomatis* is epidemic, the organism may be transmitted from infected mother to infant during passage through the birth canal. Data from studies in North America indicate that 60%–70% of infants exposed to *C. trachomatis* during vaginal delivery become infected with the organism, whereas infection after cesarean section is uncommon (Jones, 2000). Among 15–24-year-old women seen in prenatal clinics in participating states in 2009, the CDC reported a *C. trachomatis* positivity rate of 7.7% overall, with a range of 3.6%–20.4%, depending on the state (Centers for Disease Control and Prevention, 2009). *C. trachomatis* is recovered from the conjunctiva of infected infants after 1–2 weeks and from the nasopharynx soon thereafter. The rate of isolation from the conjunctiva falls by 5–6 weeks, but *C. trachomatis* can be recovered from the nasopharynx, conjunctiva, rectum, and vagina (usually without producing symptoms) for several months.

Inclusion conjunctivitis, the most common manifestation of infection with *C. trachomatis* in infants, develops in nearly 80% of infants whose conjunctival culture or cytologic examination demonstrates the organism (Jones, 2000), and among those with conjunctivitis, approximately 50% will have a nasopharyngeal infection. A mucopurulent discharge appears 2–25 days after birth, and the conjunctiva becomes inflamed and edematous. Severity ranges from a mild infection with scant discharge to copious mucopurulent discharge with severe swelling and pseudomembrane formation.

Approximately 20%–30% of infants who acquire infection with *C. trachomatis* at birth develop interstitial pneumonitis. The illness begins at between 2 weeks and 3 months of age (peak, 3–6 weeks) with nasal congestion, followed by a distinctive staccato cough with tachypnea and rales but no fever. Hyperinflation with interstitial or alveolar infiltrates on chest radiograph and peripheral eosinophilia are frequently seen. About one half of patients have or have had conjunctivitis. Symptoms last several weeks, but inspiratory rales and chest roentgenographic changes may persist for months.

CHLAMYDOPHILA (FORMERLY *CHLAMYDIA PSITTACI*)

Pneumonia associated with exposure to birds was described in Switzerland in 1879. The disease was rare in the United States and Europe until the late 1920s, when pet tropical birds became fashionable. The pathogen was isolated by Bedson from human and avian tissue in 1930 during an investigation of an outbreak at the London Zoo.

Epidemiology

Infection caused by *Chlamydophila* (formerly *Chlamydia*) *psittaci* (also called psittacosis, parrot fever, or ornithosis) occurs worldwide. *C. psittaci* has seven genotypes (A–F, E/B), all of which are infective for humans. Psittacine birds are considered the major reservoir, but most species of birds can be infected with the organism. Infected birds may be obviously ill and may die of the disease, but frequently they have mild signs such as anorexia, diarrhea, lethargy, and ruffled feathers. Human illness is sporadic and has been associated with exposure to parrots, canaries, pigeons, sparrows, ducks, cockatiels, fowl (especially turkeys), and occasionally mammals. Owners of pet birds account for about half of the 40–60 cases reported in the United States each year. Pet shop employees, pigeon fanciers, zoo workers, veterinarians, and others who work with birds are at increased risk of infection. Outbreaks have occurred among poultry processing plant workers, principally among workers who killed the birds and plucked their feathers and those who eviscerated carcasses, with a mortality of about 1%, even with appropriate therapy (Centers for Disease Control, 1990; Petrovay, 2008). Before the discovery of antibiotics, the mortality rate for human infection was 15%–20%. Over the past two decades, the prevalence of psittacosis in the United States has declined dramatically as a result of adding tetracycline to poultry feed, requiring medication of commercially imported psittacine birds before entering the country and domestic breeding of parakeets.

C. psittaci is present in the blood, tissues, excreta, and feathers of infected birds and may be shed for months after acute infection. Transmission to humans occurs via inhalation of infectious aerosols derived from feces, fecal dust, and secretions of *C. psittaci*–infected birds, but may result from handling contaminated plumage or tissues, from bird bites, or from mouth-to-beak contact. Contact with birds does not have to be close or prolonged. Person-to-person spread of *C. psittaci* is rare.

Pathogenesis and Pathology

C. psittaci enters the body via the respiratory tract and is transported to the macrophages of the liver and spleen, where the organisms replicate. They then enter the blood and travel to the lungs, the primary target of infection, and other organs. Histologic examination of lung tissue shows lymphocytes in the alveolar and interstitial spaces and mucous plugging of the bronchioles. Small hemorrhages and macrophages with intracytoplasmic inclusions may be seen. The hilar lymph nodes, liver, and spleen may be enlarged and may contain foci of necrosis; in fatal cases, the myocardium, pericardium, meninges, brain, and adrenals may be involved.

Clinical Manifestations

After an incubation period of 1–2 weeks, psittacosis may begin abruptly with chills and fever, or it may begin more gradually with increasing fever and malaise. Persistent dry, hacking cough, occasionally productive of blood-streaked mucoid sputum, is prominent. The heart rate is often slow relative to body temperature, and a diffuse, severe headache is usual. Malaise, anorexia, painful myalgias, and arthralgias are common, and a macular rash (Horder spots) resembling the rose spots of typhoid fever may occur. Decreased mentation may develop at the end of the first week of illness, and some may have gastrointestinal complaints. *C. psittaci* is a rare cause of destructive endocarditis; most affected persons have a history of rheumatic heart disease or congenital valvular abnormalities (Jones, 1982).

CHLAMYDOPHILA (FORMERLY *CHLAMYDIA PNEUMONIAE*)

In 1986, a unique chlamydial organism, initially considered to be a strain of *C. psittaci*, was associated with acute respiratory tract disease in humans. The organism was named TWAR for the laboratory identifying letters of the first two isolates: TW-183, isolated in 1965 from the eye of a control child in a trachoma vaccine trial in Taiwan, and AR-39, recovered the same year from the throat of a student with pharyngitis at the University of

Washington. Soon after its recognition, data from DNA homology and electron microscopic studies showed that this unique organism was a separate species, designated as *Chlamydia pneumoniae*, which has been reclassified as *Chlamydophila pneumoniae* (Campbell, 1987; Chi, 1987; Cox, 1988; Everett, 1999).

Epidemiology

The epidemiology of infection with *C. pneumoniae* is based on data from retrospective studies of sera collected during respiratory tract illnesses. About 50% of adults have antibodies to *C. pneumoniae*. Antibody prevalence rates are low in children, increase sharply in teenagers, continue to increase until middle age, and remain high into old age; rates are 10%–25% higher for males. Data from retrospective and prospective serologic studies indicate that disease caused by *C. pneumoniae* is endemic in the United States and epidemic in Scandinavia and Finland, but does not occur with any consistent seasonal periodicity (Grayston, 1989, 1990). *C. pneumoniae* appears to be a primary human pathogen, transmitted from person to person without an avian or animal reservoir. The mechanism and place of transmission, incubation period, and infectiousness of the organism have not yet been determined.

Pathogenesis

The pathogenesis of infection with *C. pneumoniae* is unknown. Because the illness is generally mild and self-limited, autopsy studies are unavailable.

Clinical Manifestations

It is estimated that *C. pneumoniae* is responsible for at least 10% of community-acquired pneumonias (Grayston, 1990). The pneumonia usually is mild with a single subsegmental infiltrate, but it may be severe, especially in elderly persons and in those with chronic disease. It often begins with pharyngitis and hoarseness, followed by persistent cough. Although pneumonia is the most common syndrome associated with *C. pneumoniae* infection, serologic studies during epidemics among military trainees have shown that only about 10% of infections with *C. pneumoniae* result in pneumonia, suggesting that infection is frequently mild or asymptomatic and unrecognized. Other manifestations of *C. pneumoniae* infection are bronchitis, pharyngitis, fever of undetermined origin, otitis, influenza-like illness, myocarditis, endocarditis, and possibly atherosclerosis, although the latter is controversial (Campbell, 1998; Maraha, 2004).

LABORATORY DIAGNOSIS

Chlamydia trachomatis

Specimens for detection of *C. trachomatis* are determined by the type of disease suspected (Table 56-2). Screening women at risk for genital *C. trachomatis* infection (described earlier) has been shown to decrease the rate of pelvic inflammatory disease, thus preventing subsequent reproductive sequelae (Nelson, 2001). The transport system selected must be approved for the test method used. Specific collection techniques are discussed in Chapter 63. Most infections involve mucous membranes; specimens should be collected directly from the involved surface and must contain an adequate sample of infected epithelial cells. Purulent discharge is not an appropriate specimen and should be removed before a sample is collected with a swab or brush. Of the types of swabs available, Dacron- or rayon-tipped swabs are preferred. Swabs with wooden shafts should be avoided because wood is toxic to the organism. Calcium alginate swabs may be toxic to the chlamydias or to the cells that support their growth. Cotton-tipped swabs are acceptable but are occasionally toxic to the chlamydias. Collection of urine for nucleic acid amplification testing should follow the recommendations of the manufacturer.

TABLE 56-2
Specimens for Detection of *Chlamydia trachomatis**

Disease	Specimen
Mucopurulent cervicitis	Endocervical swab, urine
Acute urethral syndrome (women)	Urethral swab, urine
Acute endometritis	Endometrial aspirate
Acute salpingitis	Fallopian tube biopsy
Nongonococcal urethritis (men)	Urethral swab, urine
Inclusion conjunctivitis	Conjunctival scrapings/swab
Trachoma	Conjunctival scrapings/swab
Lymphogranuloma venereum	Lymph node aspirate, biopsy of ulcerated lesion, serum
Pneumonitis (infants)	Serum, tracheobronchial aspirate, nasopharyngeal swab

*Urine is acceptable for some enzyme-linked immunoassays and for the commercial nucleic acid amplification tests.

Cell Culture

Cell culture is the reference method for diagnosis of chlamydial infections and should be performed when the diagnosis is disputed and in cases of suspected sexual assault or abuse. Cell lines most commonly used are McCoy or buffalo green monkey cells. Both have equivalent sensitivity, but the latter cells are easier to maintain and are more resistant to cytotoxic substances; they have been associated with more inclusions and larger inclusions (Krech, 1989). Adding cycloheximide (0.5–1.5 μL/mL) to the growth medium enhances sensitivity. Cell monolayers are grown on glass coverslips in shell vials or 24-well plates, or on the surface of polystyrene 96-well or 48-well culture dishes. To enhance recovery of *C. trachomatis*, specimens are sonicated or agitated on a vortex mixer before inoculation to release elementary bodies from host cells, and inoculated shell vials or culture dishes are centrifuged. After incubation for 48–72 hours, monolayers are fixed and stained with fluorescein-conjugated monoclonal antibodies. If a 96-well culture system is used, passaging specimens that are negative for *C. trachomatis* at 48 hours may enhance detection; however, passaging does not significantly increase detection in shell vials or 24-well plates. Although traditionally the "gold standard" for detection of *C. trachomatis*, it is now recognized that because of the fastidious nature of the organism, sensitivity of cell culture is only in the 50%–75% range, although with the use of monoclonal antibodies in the staining phase, specificity should be 100% (Solomon, 2004; Carder, 2006).

Nonculture Direct Detection Methods

Direct Fluorescent Antibody Tests. The DFA test allows direct visualization of *C. trachomatis* elementary bodies in smears of clinical specimens. Total processing time is 30–60 minutes. It is the only test that permits direct assessment of specimen adequacy. Specimens with columnar or metaplastic squamous cells are acceptable, whereas those with few columnar cells, excessive amounts of mucus, or predominance of squamous cells are not. However, interpretation of the smear is subjective, and operator fatigue can be a problem in high-volume situations. Monoclonal antibodies are available from several manufacturers. Antibodies directed against the species-specific MOMP of *C. trachomatis* appear to be more specific and produce more intense fluorescence than those directed against the chlamydial LPS (Cles, 1988). Occasionally, even the species-specific antibodies stain bacteria other than *C. trachomatis*, perhaps because of nonspecific immunoglobulin binding or cross-reactivity. Staining organisms other than *C. trachomatis* is especially frequent with rectal specimens; therefore for this site, culture is preferred, although some DFA reagents are approved for evaluation of rectal samples. Monoclonal antibody cross-reactivity between Chlamydiaceae and *Bartonella* has also been reported.

The sensitivity of the DFA test has varied from 50% to almost 100% compared with culture as the standard, and specificity is ≥95%. Sensitivity depends on the prevalence of infection in the population being evaluated and the number of elementary bodies required for a positive result (Barnes, 1989) and, in general, is greater with lower cutoff values for elementary bodies and in populations with high prevalence of disease.

Enzyme Immunoassays. EIAs detect chlamydial LPS with monoclonal or polyclonal antibodies labeled with an enzyme that converts a colorless substrate into a colored product. Both solid-phase systems, which use plastic or beads coated with the antibody, and membrane systems are commercially available. Total processing time ranges from 15–30 minutes for membrane systems to 3–4 hours for solid-phase systems. Advantages of EIA include the objective interpretation of results and ease of use for batching large numbers of specimens.

As with DFA, the sensitivities of EIAs vary (from about 70%–100%) compared with culture as the standard and tend to be higher in populations with a high prevalence of disease, such as persons attending a sexually transmitted disease clinic (Barnes, 1989; Mills, 1992; Clarke, 1993; Ehret, 1993; Kluytmans, 1993; Warren, 1993). The specificity of EIA is 95% or higher. Causes of false-positive results include the presence of a bacterial urinary tract infection (Demaio, 1991) or contamination of the specimen with cervical mucus or vaginal secretions. The latter problem can be reduced by improving the specimen collection technique (removing cervical mucus and obtaining a true endocervical sample) and by using blocking antibodies (Mills, 1992). Point-of-care (POC) rapid tests using an immunoassay format exist for possible use in situations where an immediate result would be very helpful. One such test, the Biostar Chlamydia OIA (optical immunoassay) was evaluated by the CDC in an inner city clinic environment, where it demonstrated a sensitivity of 78.6% and a specificity of 97.2% when compared with nucleic acid amplification (Bandea, 2009). The test allowed immediate treatment of a significant portion (65.9%) of evaluated patients who otherwise would not have been treated.

Nucleic Acid Hybridization Tests. A commercially available acridinium-ester–labeled DNA probe complementary to *C. trachomatis* ribosomal RNA allows direct detection of *C. trachomatis* in urogenital and conjunctival specimens. The test requires a water bath and a luminometer. Total processing time is 2–3 hours. The sensitivity of the probe test compared with culture as the reference method varies for both endocervical samples and urethral swab specimens in men (76%–97%) (Iwen, 1991; Kluytmans, 1991, 1994; Blanding, 1993; Clarke, 1993; Warren, 1993; Centers for Disease Control, 2002b). The specificity of the probe test is 97% or greater, and it can be improved with a probe competition assay (Woods, 1996).

Nucleic Acid Amplification. Several nucleic acid amplification tests for direct detection of *C. trachomatis* in endocervical swab specimens, male urethral swab specimens, and male and female urine samples are commercially available. Total time to a result is 2–5 hours, depending on the test used and the number of samples being processed. The ability of these tests to accommodate high-volume batch testing has facilitated the increase in the national screening rate for *C. trachomatis* infection in women aged 16–25 in the United States from 25.3% in 2000 to 41.6% in 2007 (Centers for Disease Control and Prevention, 2009). Three major assay methods are currently being utilized in the United States and in Europe to detect *C. trachomatis* in cervical swabs and urine from women and in urethral swabs and urine from men. Two of these methods, the polymerase chain reaction (PCR) (Roche Diagnostics Corp., Indianapolis, and Abbott Laboratories, Abbott Park, Ill.) and the strand displacement assay (SDA) (Becton Dickinson Diagnostic Systems, Sparks, Md.) utilize a DNA target, and the third, transcription-mediated amplification (TMA) (Gen-Probe Inc., San Diego) utilizes an RNA target. Data from several studies comparing nucleic acid amplification and cell culture indicate that the amplification tests are highly specific and more sensitive than culture (Goessens, 1997; Carroll, 1998; Ferrero, 1998; Mahony, 1998; Puolakkainen, 1998; Toye, 1998; Wylie, 1998; Vincelette, 1999; van der Pol, 2001; Koumans, 2003; Boyadzhyan, 2004; Gaydos, 2004). TMA has demonstrated higher sensitivity than the other methods, possibly owing to the higher RNA target levels relative to DNA target levels and the lower susceptibility to inhibitors seen in urine samples, possibly due to a target capture portion of the assay that precedes amplification (Schacter, 2005; Chernesky, 2006; Lowe, 2006; Levett, 2008).

In 2006, an interesting set of events occurred in Sweden that demonstrated the importance of target selection in nucleic acid amplification, in that a new variant of *C. trachomatis* that contained a 377 base pair deletion in the target utilized in the PCR was discovered. The appearance of this variant resulted in a high proportion of infected patients escaping detection (an estimated 8000 cases) by two systems that utilized the PCR method: the Abbott m2000 and the Roche Cobas Amplicor/TaqMan 48 (Herrmann, 2008; Møller, 2008). TMA and SDA methods detected the variant, as amplification targets were different. The new variant spread rapidly in Sweden, and by 2007 accounted for up to 65% of cases in which these two platforms were being used (Herrmann, 2008b). Studies demonstrated that the new variant had no other biological advantage to aid in its rapid spread relative to other strains, other than its ability to escape detection by the testing systems in use at the time (Unemo, 2010). Affected manufacturers have implemented new assays that detect dual targets, such that the variant is detected (Møller, 2010).

Verification of Nonculture Tests

The CDC has recommended that positive nonculture test (DFA, EIA, probe, nucleic acid amplification) results should be verified with a supplemental test if a false-positive result is likely to have adverse medical, social, or psychological consequences (Centers for Disease Control, 1993, 2002b). In low-prevalence populations, verification should probably be routine, but it might be selective in high-prevalence populations. Culture confirmation is optimal in theory but requires a second specimen collected during the first visit or during a return visit, and in the case in which the initial screening test was a nucleic acid amplification test, culture is less sensitive and may not confirm a true positive. Several confirmation strategies for nucleic acid amplification tests have been suggested. Confirmation of a positive test may be done by performing a second amplification test, using the same assay or a different assay that targets a different nucleic acid sequence. Similarly, the original specimen may be used, or a second specimen may be obtained. Each strategy poses issues that must be addressed by a testing facility if it is determined that a result is to be confirmed. For example, if a different assay is to be used on the original specimen, it must be confirmed that the second assay can utilize a specimen collected using the collection kit of the first, and that no inhibition of amplification will occur (Scragg, 2006). Whether the original specimen or a new specimen is used, attention must be paid to differing sensitivities of different assays, as a less sensitive assay should not be used to confirm a result obtained with a more sensitive assay (Schacter, 2005). The practice of confirming positive results of nucleic acid amplification tests is not without controversy, and some experts do not agree with the recommendation of the CDC to do so (Schachter, 2006).

Serologic Tests

Serologic tests have little value for diagnosis of chlamydial genital infections for two reasons. First, antibodies to *C. trachomatis* persist after the infection resolves, so a positive serologic test does not necessarily correlate with active disease. Second, many serologic tests are not specific for *C. trachomatis* because they detect genus-specific antibodies. Exceptions include diagnosis of LGV and *C. trachomatis* pneumonitis in infants. Because LGV has a long latent period and clinical diagnosis often is delayed, antibodies are generally present when the acute phase serum is collected, and a fourfold rise in titer between acute and convalescent phase serum samples often cannot be documented. Thus, a single or stable complement fixation titer of 1:64 or greater supports a presumptive diagnosis of LGV. For diagnosis of *C. trachomatis* pneumonitis in infants, detection of IgM antibodies by microimmunofluorescence (MIF) may be useful. A single IgM titer of >1:32 when tested by MIF supports a diagnosis of chlamydial pneumonia. IgG is not useful in neonates because of circulating maternal antibody.

Chlamydophila psittaci

The CDC has established case definitions for *C. psittaci* infections, which are described as laboratory confirmed if (1) *C. psittaci* is cultured from respiratory material, or (2) antibody titers against *C. psittaci* increase fourfold or greater when tested by complement fixation or MIF at least 2 weeks apart, or (3) a single IgM titer of >1:16 when tested by MIF is present after the onset of symptoms (Centers for Disease Control and Prevention, 1998). *C. psittaci* can be grown in cell culture, but this is recommended only for specially equipped laboratories with experienced personnel, because the organism is especially virulent and has been associated with laboratory-acquired infection. Infection with *C. psittaci* is usually diagnosed serologically. Antibodies usually are detected by the end of the second week of illness, but early antibiotic therapy can delay their appearance for several weeks.

Chlamydophila pneumoniae

Diagnosis of *C. pneumoniae* infection is based predominantly on serologic tests (Grayston, 1990; Kumar, 2007). The MIF test with the TWAR antigen is specific for *C. pneumoniae* and is the only serologic test considered acceptable for use in diagnosis by the CDC and the Infectious Disease Society of America (IDSA) (Kumar, 2007). IgM antibodies appear about 2–3 weeks after the onset of primary illness, usually decline over the next 2–6 months to a level that cannot be detected, and may not reappear with reinfection. IgG antibodies are detected 6–8 weeks after onset of the primary illness, persist for life, and may rise 1–2 weeks following reinfection. Serologic test results consistent with acute infection include a fourfold or greater rise in IgG titer between acute and convalescent phase serum samples, or an IgM titer of 1:16 or greater. The use of single IgG titers is discouraged. Despite prevalent use of the MIF test, it has been shown to be insensitive, especially in children, and cross-reactions with *Mycoplasma*, *Bartonella*, and *Yersinia* species may occur. *C. pneumoniae* can be isolated in cell culture, but it is more difficult to grow than *C. trachomatis* (Roblin, 1992). Many “in-house” nucleic acid amplification assays for *C. pneumoniae* have been published, but very few have been validated clinically (Kumar, 2007).

TREATMENT

Tetracyclines have been the treatment of choice for infection with chlamydia. For genital infections due to *C. trachomatis*, recommended regimens include azithromycin (1g orally, 1 dose) or doxycycline (100mg orally twice a day for 7 days); other effective agents include erythromycin, ofloxacin, or levofloxacin (Centers for Disease Control, 2006). LGV requires the same daily dosage of doxycycline or erythromycin as genital infections, but for a period of 3 weeks. Ocular infections with *C. trachomatis* require systemic treatment with doxycycline or azithromycin for adults, and erythromycin for newborns; topical therapy suppresses symptoms but does not eradicate the organism. Macrolides (azithromycin and erythromycin) are acceptable alternative agents for doxycycline in infections caused by *C. pneumoniae*. For *C. psittaci*, the treatment of choice is tetracycline hydrochloride or doxycycline for 3 weeks. Erythromycin is an alternative but may be less effective in more severe cases.

RICKETTSIAL INFECTIONS

Rickettsia is a concept that developed historically as the molecular and physical nature of viruses was defined (Weiss, 1988). In contrast with human viral agents, which also require eukaryotic host cells for their intracellular replication, rickettsiae have a gram-negative bacterial cell wall, and their growth is inhibited by particular antibiotics. Rickettsiae are further differentiated from other obligately intracellular bacteria by their ecology and frequent transmission by arthropod vectors. The traditional taxonomic scheme of rickettsiae based on such phenotypic characteristics as intracellular growth and arthropod vector transmission has undergone substantial modification in light of contemporary gene sequence analyses. Genera that contain rickettsiae pathogenic for humans are *Rickettsia*, *Orientia*, *Ehrlichia*, *Anaplasma*, *Neorickettsia*, *Coxiella*, and *Bartonella* (Dumler, 2001; Yu, 2003). Despite their historical association with rickettsiology and arthropod transmission, *Bartonella* organisms are cultivable in cell-free medium and do not belong in the order Rickettsiales (Brenner, 1993), which includes the genera *Rickettsia*, *Orientia*, *Ehrlichia*, *Anaplasma*, and *Neorickettsia*, which are more closely related to one another than to *Coxiella*. Grouped by genus, the following diseases are presented in this chapter: *Rickettsia*—Rocky Mountain spotted fever, boutonneuse fever, African tick bite fever, rickettsialpox, and murine typhus; *Orientia*—scrub typhus; *Ehrlichia*—human monocytotropic ehrlichiosis caused by *Ehrlichia chaffeensis* and human infection with *Ehrlichia ewingii; Anaplasma*—human granulocytotropic anaplasmosis; *Coxiella*—Q fever; and *Bartonella*—cat scratch disease, bacillary angiomatosis and peliosis, trench fever, and South American bartonellosis. The diseases of each genus comprise cohesive clinical and pathologic groupings, and overall the rickettsial diseases pose a similar set of diagnostic challenges, with similar technical approaches to their solution.

INFECTIONS CAUSED BY ORGANISMS OF THE GENUS *RICKETTSIA*

Structure and Function

Spotted fever, transitional, and typhus group rickettsiae are genetically closely related bacteria that have a thin (0.3–0.5 × 1–2 μm) bacillary morphology and a gram-negative cell wall containing LPS with antigenic components that distinguish the spotted fever and typhus groups. All *Rickettsia* species reside free in the cytosol of the host cell and divide by binary fission. *Rickettsia* attach to the host cell via a protein adhesin, enter by induced phagocytosis, and escape from the phagosome (Li, 1998; Uchiyama, 1999; Martinez, 2004; Martinez, 2005). These functions can occur within minutes and are associated with phospholipase activity of rickettsial origin (Silverman, 1992; Whitworth, 2005). Spotted fever group rickettsiae are propelled within cells and during release from the cell by stimulating polymerization of host cell F-actin at one pole (Heinzen, 1993; Kleba, 2010). *Rickettsia* that manifest this activity (e.g., *Rickettsia rickettsii*) escape earlier from host cells and spread more quickly to other cells than those lacking this activity (e.g., *Rickettsia prowazekii*), which divide intracellularly to massive numbers before the host cell bursts and the organisms are released. According to the molecular phylogeny, *Rickettsia* species that are pathogenic for humans have evolved into three genogroups (Table 56-3) (Roux, 1995, 1997; Stothard, 1995). The typhus group includes *R. prowazekii* and *Rickettsia typhi*. The core spotted fever group contains *R. rickettsii*, *Rickettsia conorii*, *Rickettsia japonica*, *Rickettsia africae*, *Rickettsia parkeri*, *Rickettsia honei*, *Rickettsia sibirica*, *Rickettsia aeschlimannii*, and *Rickettsia slovaca*. A newly recognized transitional group contains *Rickettsia akari*, *Rickettsia australis*, and *Rickettsia felis*. *R. akari* and *R. australis* were traditionally considered to be relatively distant members of the spotted fever group, with which they share LPS antigens.

Rocky Mountain Spotted Fever

The most severe of all the rickettsioses, Rocky Mountain spotted fever, has a substantial case fatality rate, 5%, even among previously healthy, immunocompetent children and young adults (Dalton, 1995a; Paddock, 1999). *R. rickettsii* normally resides in nature in ticks: *Dermacentor variabilis*, the American dog tick, in the eastern two thirds of the United States and California; *Dermacentor andersoni*, the Rocky Mountain wood tick, in the western United States; *Rhipicephalus sanguineus*, the brown dog tick, in Mexico, Brazil, and Arizona; and *Amblyomma cajennense* and *A. aureolatum* in South America. These ticks maintain *R. rickettsii* as they moult from stage to stage (larva, nymph, and adult) and transovarially from generation to generation. Fewer than 1 per 1000 ticks carries virulent *R. rickettsii*, which is pathogenic for ticks (Niebylski, 1999). New lines of ticks become infected by feeding on rickettsemic rodents, replenishing the population of organisms transovarially maintained in ticks (Gage, 1990).

Infections occur when and where humans encounter *R. rickettsii*–infected ticks (Helmick, 1984). Although Rocky Mountain spotted fever has been documented in recent years in nearly every state except Hawaii, Alaska, and Vermont, the highest incidence is in the south Atlantic states from Maryland to Georgia and the south central states of Oklahoma, Missouri, Arkansas, and Tennessee. Most cases occur in late spring and summer, but particularly in the southern latitudes, a few cases may occur even in winter. The highest incidence is seen in children, adults of retirement age, and others exposed to ticks during outdoor activities. Fatality/case ratios are higher for persons older than 30 years. Fulminant Rocky Mountain spotted fever (death by the fifth day of illness) occurs in association with moderate hemolysis, for example, in African American males with glucose-6-phosphate dehydrogenase (G6PD) deficiency (Walker, 1983).

Rickettsiae are injected via the infected tick's salivary gland secretions into the patient's dermis after 6–10 hours of tick feeding and spread hematogenously throughout the body. The vascular endothelium is the target of intracellular infection, with some invasion into adjacent vascular smooth muscle cells. Infected endothelium is injured by reactive oxygen species–induced damage to cell membranes (Silverman, 1992, 1997). Damage to the endothelium results in increased vascular permeability, edema, hypovolemia, and hypotension. Life-threatening consequences of vascular injury in the central nervous system (CNS) and lung are rickettsial meningoencephalitis and noncardiogenic pulmonary edema. Early in the course, lesions show endothelial rickettsiae without thrombi or a cellular response. Late in the course, the characteristic lymphohistiocytic perivascular infiltrate appears as interstitial pneumonia, interstitial myocarditis, perivascular glial nodules of the brain, and similar vascular lesions in the dermis, gastrointestinal tract, liver, skeletal muscles, and kidneys. Severe injury may be accompanied by focal hemorrhages but seldom by microinfarcts, except in the white matter of the brain.

Clinical illness usually begins with fever, headache, and myalgia 2–14 days after a tick bite (Kaplowitz, 1981). Nausea, vomiting, abdominal pain and tenderness, and diarrhea occur more frequently in the first 3 days of illness. The rash, which usually appears between days 3 and 5, typically begins as macules around the wrists and ankles and later on the arms, legs, and trunk. The lesions become maculopapular, and in half of cases, a central petechia appears in many of the maculopapules. Characteristic involvement of the palms and soles occurs in half of cases as a late manifestation. Renal failure is a feature of severe illness. CNS involvement is ominous; seizures and coma occur in 8%–10% of cases overall, often preceding a fatal outcome. Thrombocytopenia occurs in half of cases, but disseminated intravascular coagulation is rare (Elghetany, 1999).

African Tick Bite Fever, Boutonneuse Fever, and Other Spotted Fevers

R. conorii has been isolated in southern Europe; northern, eastern, and southern Africa; Israel; Turkey; India; Pakistan; Russia; Georgia; and the Ukraine. The ecology of *R. conorii* and the epidemiology of boutonneuse fever are closely tied to ticks, especially *R. sanguineus*, which maintain the rickettsiae transovarially and transmit the infection to humans while feeding (Walker, 1991). Imported cases are diagnosed in travelers returning to the United States and northern Europe from the Mediterranean basin. The fatality rate among hospitalized patients is 1.4%–5.6%,

TABLE 56-3

Rickettsia, Orientia, Ehrlichia, Anaplasma, Neorickettsia, Coxiella, and *Bartonella* Infections

Etiologic agent	Disease	Geographic distribution	Transmission
Spotted Fevers			
R. rickettsii	Rocky Mountain spotted fever	North, Central, and South America	Tick bite
R. conorii	Boutonneuse fever	Southern Europe, Africa, Russia, Georgia, Middle East, Indian subcontinent	Tick bite
R. africae	African tick bite fever	Southern and eastern Africa, Caribbean	Tick bite
R. parkeri	Maculatum disease	North and South America	Tick bite
R. sibirica	North Asian tick typhus and lymphangitis-associated rickettsioses	Russia, China, Mongolia, Pakistan, Europe, Africa	Tick bite
R. japonica	Japanese spotted fever	Japan, Korea, Thailand	Tick bite
R. honei	Flinders Island spotted fever	Australia, southeastern Asia	Tick bite
R. slovaca	Tick-borne lymphadenopathy	Europe	Tick bite
Typhus Fevers			
R. prowazekii	Epidemic typhus	Potentially worldwide; in recent decades in Africa, South America, Central America, Mexico, Asia	Feces of human body louse
R. prowazekii	Brill-Zinsser disease	Worldwide; wherever persons with past epidemic typhus now reside	Recrudescence of latent infection
R. prowazekii	Flying squirrel typhus	United States	Presumably feces of flea or louse of flying squirrel
R. typhi	Murine typhus	Worldwide in tropics and subtropics	Flea feces
Transitional Group Rickettsial Fevers			
R. akari	Rickettsialpox	United States, Ukraine, Croatia, Korea, Turkey, Mexico	Mite bite
R. australis	Queensland tick typhus	Eastern Australia	Tick bite
R. felis	Flea-borne spotted fever	Worldwide	Presumably flea bite or feces
Scrub Typhus			
Orientia tsutsugamushi	Scrub typhus	Southeastern Asia, Japan, China, Sri Lanka, India, Asiatic Russia, Indonesia, Indian Ocean and Western Pacific Islands, Northern Australia	Chigger bite
Ehrlichioses			
E. chaffeensis	Human monocytotropic ehrlichiosis	United States, Africa, Asia	Tick bite
E. ewingii	Ehrlichiosis ewingii	United States, Africa	Tick bite
Anaplasma phagocytophilum	Human granulocytotropic anaplasmosis	United States, Eurasia	Tick bite
Neorickettsia sennetsu	Sennetsu rickettsiosis	Asia	Apparently ingestion of fish parasitized with trematodes carrying neorickettsia
Coxiellosis			
C. burnetii	Q fever	Worldwide	Inhalation of aerosols from infected animals, possibly ingestion of animal products
Bartonelloses			
B. bacilliformis	Oroya fever, verruga peruana	Western South America	Sandfly bite
B. henselae	Cat scratch disease, bacillary angiomatosis and peliosis, endocarditis	Worldwide	Kitten scratch or bite
B. clarridgeiae	Cat scratch–like disease	Probably worldwide	Presumed cat scratch or bite
B. quintana	Trench fever, endocarditis	Worldwide	Feces of *Pediculus* louse

particularly in patients with underlying conditions such as diabetes and alcoholism (de Sousa, 2008). A milder disease caused by *R. africae* occurs with high frequency in travelers returning from southern Africa (McQuiston, 2004). The clinical illness resembles that recently associated in the Americas with *R. parkeri*, which is essentially conspecific with *R. africae* (Paddock, 2004, 2008). Tick bite eschars are often multiple, regional lymphadenopathy is observed frequently, and rash is typically sparse, sometimes vesicular, and often absent. *R. sibirica* has been isolated in Russia, China, Mongolia, and Pakistan, and a distinct strain *mongolitimoniae* isolated in Asia, Europe, and Africa has been associated in half of cases with lymphangitis extending from the eschar. *R. japonica* has been documented in Japan, and infection with *R. japonica* occurs also in Korea and Thailand. Human infections with *R. australis* occur only in Australia, and infection with *R. honei* has been documented in Australia and Thailand. After an average incubation period of 7 days, these illnesses begin with fever, headache, and myalgias. Frequently, an eschar can be discovered by careful examination of the skin at this time. The pathology of these spotted fevers is well described in the tache noire or eschar at the site of tick bite inoculation of rickettsiae (Walker, 1988a). Endothelial infection and injury by *R. conorii* in the eschar result in dermal and epidermal necrosis and perivascular edema.

Host defenses that effect killing of intracellular rickettsiae include nitric oxide, reactive oxygen species, and tryptophan limitation induced by cytokines secreted by T lymphocytes and macrophages, which infiltrate around the infected dermal blood vessels and target cell apoptosis triggered by cytotoxic CD8^{+} T lymphocytes (Herrero-Herrero, 1987; Walker,

2001; Valbuena, 2002). Activation of endothelial cells by cytokines, including γ-interferon and tumor necrosis factor-α, results in intracellular rickettsicidal activity, and ultimate clearance is mediated by cytotoxic T lymphocytes. Disseminated endothelial infection results in maculopapular rash, meningoencephalitis, and vascular lesions in the lungs, kidneys, gastrointestinal tract, and heart (Walker, 1985). Multifocal hepatocellular necrosis and granuloma-like lesions correlate with moderately increased concentrations of hepatic transaminases (Walker, 1986).

Rickettsialpox

R. akari is maintained in nature by transovarial transmission in the gamasid mite, *Liponyssoides sanguineus*, an ectoparasite of the domestic mouse, *Mus musculus*. *R. akari* has been detected only in the United States, Croatia, the Ukraine, Turkey, Mexico, and Korea, perhaps more an indication of the paucity of rickettsial investigations than the actual distribution of this rickettsial species.

A papule develops during the approximately 10-day incubation period at the site of mite bite and progresses to become a 1–2.5cm eschar. Illness begins with chills, fever, malaise, severe headache, and myalgia. Rash, which appears 2–6 days later, is initially maculopapular, later papular, and in classic cases, pustular and/or vesicular. Some patients also suffer nausea, vomiting, pharyngitis, photophobia, splenomegaly, and nuchal rigidity.

Histopathologic examination of the eschar reveals coagulative necrosis of the epidermis, underlying vascular injury, and a perivascular lymphohistiocytic infiltrate in which macrophages appear to be the main target cell of infection (Brettman, 1981; Kass, 1994; Walker, 1999b). Regional lymphadenopathy and cutaneous rash presumably reflect lymphogenous and hematogenous spread, respectively.

Flea-borne Spotted Fever

A widely dispersed organism, *R. felis* is maintained transovarially in cat fleas *(Ctenocephalides felis)* with apparent involvement of opossums in a zoonotic cycle. Human infections have been documented in North America, Europe, Africa, and Asia (Schriefer, 1994a; Zavala-Velazquez, 2000; Raoult, 2001; Parola, 2003).

Murine Typhus and Louse-borne Typhus

Endemic flea-borne *R. typhi* infection, murine typhus, is presently the most important typhus group infection in the United States and causes extensive morbidity throughout the warm regions of the world (Azad, 1990). Historically, epidemic louse-borne *R. prowazekii* infections have had a major impact on the outcome of military campaigns, as well as scourging general populations disrupted by war, famine, and natural disasters (Zinsser, 1935; Patterson, 1993). *R. prowazekii* continues to cause disease in some poverty-stricken areas of the world and reappears in situations such as the civil war in Burundi, the extreme poverty of indigenous populations of the Andes, and other unsettled social and economic conditions. Recrudescence of latent *R. prowazekii* infections can occur years after the primary infection in immigrants from typhus-afflicted areas. Endemic transmission of *R. prowazekii* from a natural infectious cycle of flying squirrels and their ectoparasites occurs in the United States (McDade, 1980; Reynolds, 2003).

Murine typhus occurs particularly in tropical and subtropical coastal areas, where *Rattus rattus*, *Rattus norvegicus*, and the Oriental rat flea abound (Azad, 1990). The fleas imbibe rickettsiae in the blood of infected rats and maintain the infection for their normal life span. Transovarian transmission occurs only at low levels; thus, horizontal transmission to other rats is a key factor in maintenance of *R. typhi* in nature. Other mammal-arthropod cycles maintain the rickettsiae and result in transmission of infection to humans (e.g., the cat flea, *C. felis*, and the opossum in Texas and California) (Schriefer, 1994b).

Humans are thought to become infected by intradermal inoculation of infected flea feces into skin excoriated by scratching. However, inhalation of a rickettsial aerosol from dried infected flea feces or inoculation by flea bite may account for transmission in some cases. After an incubation period of 1–2 weeks, illness begins with fever accompanied in some cases by severe headache, chills, myalgia, and nausea. A macular or maculopapular rash, most prominent on the trunk, is visualized on day 5 or 6 in 80% of patients with fair skin and in 20% with darkly pigmented skin. A small proportion of patients have cough and pulmonary infiltrates. Severely ill patients may also suffer coma, seizures, and other neurologic signs. Approximately 10% of hospitalized patients require admission to the intensive care unit, and 1%–2% of murine typhus patients die (Dumler, 1991).

Pathologic lesions of murine typhus include endothelial swelling and perivascular lymphohistiocytic infiltrates involving the blood vessels in the dermis, CNS, lungs, heart, gastrointestinal tract, and kidneys (Walker, 1989). The most serious consequences include meningoencephalomyelitis and diffuse alveolar injury.

Rickettsiae as Agents of Bioterrorism

R. prowazekii and *R. rickettsii* are select agents, possession of which is restricted by law to registered scientists in approved institutions where rigorous security and safety regulations are applied to the laboratories. These organisms exist in nature, can be recovered and propagated, and are infectious via a stable aerosol, with infectivity of as little as a single bacterium.

Case fatality rates of 15%–25% in previously healthy persons would occur without prompt diagnosis and treatment. The potential for genetically engineered resistance to the effective antibiotics, tetracycline and chloramphenicol, would render these cases of typhus and Rocky Mountain spotted fever untreatable (Walker, 2003). Although the case fatality rates would be lower, bioterrorist-dispersed *R. typhi* or *R. conorii* could create terror and overwhelm the medical and public health systems.

Laboratory Diagnosis

Unlike most infectious diseases for which precise diagnosis is sought during the acute phase of illness, when critical therapeutic decisions are made, rickettsial diseases are usually diagnosed acutely purely on the basis of clinicoepidemiologic suspicion, and are treated empirically on a presumptive basis (Kaplowitz, 1981). Serologic diagnosis, which is often mistakenly sought early in the course of illness, provides the majority of laboratory-confirmed diagnoses by demonstration of a fourfold or greater rise in titer only during convalescence. Even with the most sensitive serologic methods, less than 20% of patients have detectable specific antibodies to rickettsiae when presenting to the physician for medical attention. Other approaches to diagnosis at the time of presentation include immunohistologic demonstration of rickettsiae in cutaneous lesions, immunocytologic identification of rickettsiae in circulating detached endothelial cells, detection of rickettsial DNA in blood and tissue specimens by PCR (Schriefer, 1994a; Sexton, 1994; Williams, 1994; Furuya, 1995), and cultivation of rickettsiae from blood or tissue specimens; however, these tests are not available in most clinical laboratories.

Rickettsiae were originally demonstrated in tissues of patients with Rocky Mountain spotted fever and epidemic louse-borne typhus by Wolbach using Giemsa stain during and shortly after World War I. This method, essentially a lost art, requires careful attention to details of fixation and staining of rickettsiae, and is not performed successfully in this manner in contemporary histology laboratories. A modified Brown-Hopps method stains a small fraction of organisms, which appear as thin bacilli within endothelial cells. A more sensitive and specific approach to visualization of rickettsiae in tissue section is immunohistology—immunofluorescence or immunoenzyme staining—using antibodies specific for the spotted fever or typhus group (Kaplowitz, 1983; Walker, 1989, 1997b, 1999b; Dumler, 1990). Staining of skin biopsies from patients with Rocky Mountain spotted fever by immunohistochemistry has a sensitivity of 70% and a specificity of 100%. Patients with boutonneuse fever, African tick bite fever, murine typhus, and rickettsialpox have also been diagnosed by immunohistologic detection of rickettsiae in rash and eschar lesions. A monoclonal antibody to a spotted fever group–specific epitope on the cell wall LPS demonstrates *R. rickettsii*, *R. parkeri*, *R. conorii*, *R. akari*, *R. japonica*, *R. australis*, *R. africae*, *R. honei*, and *R. sibirica* in formalin-fixed, paraffin-embedded tissues; a typhus group LPS-specific monoclonal antibody is similarly useful for detecting *R. typhi* and *R. prowazekii* (Walker, 1997b). Currently, reagents for diagnostic immunohistology of rickettsioses are not commercially available, but it is feasible that kits could be developed for rickettsial group–specific diagnosis using antibodies produced in research laboratories.

A unique diagnostic approach is the immunocytologic demonstration of *R. conorii* in detached, circulating endothelial cells captured from patient blood samples by immunomagnetic beads coated with a monoclonal antibody to a surface antigen of human endothelial cells (Drancourt, 1992; La Scola, 1996a). In boutonneuse fever patients, this method has a sensitivity of 58% for examination of a single blood sample and may be used in patients before the onset of rash, which must be present for selection of the site of skin biopsy for immunohistologic diagnosis.

PCR has been applied successfully to the diagnostic detection of *R. rickettsii*, *R. conorii*, *R. japonica*, *R. africae*, *R. parkeri*, *R. felis*, *R. akari*, *R. sibirica*, *R. slovaca*, *R. aeschlimannii*, *R. typhi*, and *R. prowazekii* from clinical samples, including biopsy of eschar or rash, peripheral blood, buffy coat, plasma, necropsy tissue, and arthropod vectors removed from patients. Target genes include the 17-kDa lipoprotein gene, *gltA*, *rrs*, *groEL*, *ompA*, and *ompB*. This approach may fail to detect rickettsial nucleic acids early in the course or after development of immunity or effective antimicrobial treatment (Tzianabos, 1989; Schriefer, 1994a; Sexton, 1994; Furuya, 1995; Roux, 1999; Leitner, 2002; Walker, 2003; Fournier, 2004; Ndip, 2004; Stenos, 2005; Kidd, 2008; Nascimento, 2009; Prakash, 2009).

Isolation of rickettsiae is achieved frequently in antibiotic-free, centrifugation-enhanced shell vial cell culture in reference and research laboratories with biosafety level 3 containment and specialized expertise.

The "gold standard" serologic test for rickettsioses is the indirect immunofluorescent antibody (IFA) assay (Kaplan, 1986). The indirect immunoperoxidase antibody test yields similar results. For spotted fever and typhus-group rickettsial infections in the United States, IFA titers of 1:64 or greater are considered to be diagnostic in a compatible clinicoepidemiologic situation. In countries with a high prevalence of persons with antibodies to these rickettsiae, due hypothetically to stimulation by nonpathogenic rickettsiae or subclinical or undiagnosed infection, higher titers are required to establish the diagnosis. In any event, a fourfold rise in IFA antibody titer to a titer of at least 1:64, but usually 1:256 or higher, is diagnostic. The sensitivity of the IFA for Rocky Mountain spotted fever is 94%–100%, and the specificity is 100%. With a cutoff titer for IgG of 1:128 and for IgM of 1:32, the indirect immunoperoxidase test yields similar results and has the advantage of requiring only a light microscope instead of an ultraviolet microscope.

Commercially available serologic tests include indirect immunofluorescence, latex agglutination, and standard solid-phase enzyme immunoassay (Kelly, 1995). Latex agglutination and solid-phase enzyme immunoassays provide diagnostically useful information and require less expensive equipment to perform, but generally are not considered as reliable as the IFA. The greatly increased reliance of reference laboratories on EIAs has occurred in parallel with anomalous changes in public health reports of Rocky Mountain spotted fever. It has been suggested that a substantial portion of the tick-exposed population has standing titers of antibodies stimulated by spotted fever group rickettsiae of low pathogenicity (Graf, 2008; Walker, 2008). The Weil-Felix tests, which measure agglutination of *Proteus vulgaris* strains OX-19 and OX-2 (Kaplan, 1986), are insensitive and nonspecific and should not be used, except in developing countries in which no other method can be performed. Serology is seldom useful in assisting therapeutic decisions because antibodies appear later in the course.

Treatment

Spotted fever and typhus group rickettsioses are treated effectively with doxycycline, tetracycline, or chloramphenicol (Raoult, 1991). Fluoroquinolones, azithromycin, and clarithromycin are active against some rickettsiae *in vitro*. Ciprofloxacin, ofloxacin, and perfloxacin have been used successfully to treat boutonneuse fever, and azithromycin and clarithromycin have been used to treat mild boutonneuse fever in children, but these agents have not been evaluated and are not recommended for treatment of Rocky Mountain spotted fever.

SCRUB TYPHUS CAUSED BY *ORIENTIA TSUTSUGAMUSHI*

The gram-negative cell wall of *Orientia* (formerly *Rickettsia*) *tsutsugamushi* differs from that of spotted fever and typhus group rickettsiae; it has an ultrastructurally thicker outer leaflet and a thinner inner leaflet of the outer envelope and different major proteins, and it lacks LPS (Tamura, 1995). Scrub typhus rickettsiae grow in the cytoplasm of the host cell and are released via a process involving pinching off of a host cell membrane–bound rickettsia. *O. tsutsugamushi* is transovarially maintained in mites of the genus *Leptotrombidium* (Traub, 1978). Infected ova hatch into larvae—the only stage that feeds on an animal host. Rats become infected after rickettsia-containing larvae (chiggers) feed on the rats' tissue fluids, but feeding mite larvae that acquire rickettsiae do not pass the infection to their offspring. Thus, humans and rats are only accidental, nonessential, dead-end hosts of scrub typhus rickettsiae. Scrub typhus occurs in countries within the geographic area formed by Japan, Russia, and Korea in the North, Australia and Indonesia in the South, Pakistan in the West, and the Philippines and Micronesia in the East. Infection is acquired in areas of dense vegetation where abundant rat populations harbor large populations of chiggers.

O. tsutsugamushi infects endothelial cells more extensively than macrophages (Moron, 2001). The basic pathologic lesion is vascular injury with perivascular lymphohistiocytic inflammation, which is present in the cutaneous chigger inoculation sites and organs to which rickettsiae have disseminated—the brain, lung, heart, gastrointestinal tract, and kidney.

After incubation for 6–21 days, illness begins with fever, headache, and, in some patients, myalgia, cough, and gastrointestinal symptoms (Watt, 2006). An eschar develops in half of Westerners, usually before the onset of fever, but less often in indigenous patients. Likewise, a macular or maculopapular rash occurs in half of Westerners with primary infection 2–9 days after the onset of illness. Severely ill patients may develop hypotension, pneumonitis, meningoencephalitis, acute renal failure, and hemorrhagic phenomena. Unless treated with appropriate antimicrobial medications, 7% of cases are fatal. Greater severity is associated with greater bacterial loads (Sonthayanon, 2009). Scrub typhus may occur in trekkers and other travelers exposed to chiggers in endemic areas. For the diagnosis of scrub typhus in an endemic region, the cutoff titer should be determined for the particular population; for one region, a titer of 1:400 or greater by IFA is 96% specific and 48% sensitive, and a fourfold rise in titer is the preferred serologic criterion for diagnosis (Blacksell, 2007). Indirect immunoperoxidase is a similar method that does not require a fluorescent microscope. *Proteus mirabilis* strain OX-K agglutination is more readily available but insensitive. Serologic assays using a recombinant 56-kDa antigen representing the major immunodominant surface protein, including a dipstick test, a rapid lateral flow assay, and an IgM capture enzyme immunoassay, yield excellent results. (Ching, 2001; Coleman, 2002; Jang, 2003; Jiang, 2003).

PCR has been applied to the diagnosis of scrub typhus for more than a decade (Murai, 1992; Furuya, 1993; Kawamori, 1993; Sugita, 1993) and has been demonstrated to be effective in practice, including on eschar specimens (Manosroi, 2003; Saisongkorh, 2004; Kim, 2006; Paris 2008, 2009). Real-time PCR offers the opportunity for a highly sensitive, specific diagnosis with prompt turnaround time (Jiang, 2004).

Treatment with a tetracycline drug such as doxycycline or with chloramphenicol is effective, except among some cases in northern Thailand, where rifamycin and azithromycin are alternatives (Strickman, 1995; Watt, 1996, 2000; Kim, 2004; Liu, 2006).

INFECTIONS CAUSED BY ORGANISMS OF THE GENERA *EHRLICHIA* AND *ANAPLASMA*

Structure and Function

The family Anaplasmataceae consists of four genera—*Ehrlichia*, *Anaplasma*, *Neorickettsia*, and *Wolbachia*. Ehrlichiae and anaplasmae are small (0.5 μm), tick-borne, obligately intracellular, gram-negative coccobacilli that reside in a cytoplasmic vacuole of white blood cells (Yu, 2003). This intravacuolar microcolony of bacteria stained by the Wright-Giemsa method resembles a mulberry and thus is called a morula (Latin for "mulberry"). *Neorickettsia*, similar small obligately intracellular bacteria, reside in trematode parasites in aquatic snails, insects, bats, and fish, and are transmitted by ingestion of a parasitized host (e.g., *Neorickettsia helminthoeca* in trematode-parasitized salmon eaten by dogs in the Pacific Northwest). *Wolbachia* reside in arthropods and filarial worms (e.g., *Onchocerca volvulus*), in which they play a role in the pathogenesis of the human illness.

Long known and studied as agents of veterinary disease, *Ehrlichia* and *Anaplasma* have recently emerged as human pathogens. The reasons for this are primarily their recent discovery in humans, their rapid characterization with contemporary molecular tools, and increasing populations and geographic distributions of particular ticks that depend on deer as a host. The well-documented human pathogens in the United States are *E. chaffeensis*, *E. ewingii*, and *Anaplasma phagocytophilum*. *Neorickettsia sennetsu* is the agent of a disease in Asia resembling infectious mononucleosis.

Human Monocytotropic Ehrlichiosis

E. chaffeensis is transmitted by ticks, primarily *Amblyomma americanum*, the Lone Star tick, but also *D. variabilis* and *Ixodes pacificus* (Anderson, 1992a; Ewing, 1995; Kramer, 1999). Cases are predominantly rural and seasonal (68% occur from May to July) (Fishbein, 1994; Olano, 2003a). Deer serve as a documented reservoir, and infected dogs and coyotes are potential reservoir hosts. Ticks become infected when feeding as larvae or nymphs, carry the ehrlichiae as they moult from stage to stage, and transmit the infection during a subsequent blood meal. Human monocytotropic ehrlichiosis has been reported in 47 states; most cases have occurred within the range of *A. americanum* in the third of the United States south of a line from New Jersey to Kansas. The number of reported cases is particularly high in Oklahoma, Missouri, Arkansas, Tennessee, North Carolina, and Maryland.

Since the first case of human ehrlichiosis was reported in the United States in 1987, prospective studies have documented an incidence of laboratory-confirmed *E. chaffeensis* infection that exceeds that of Rocky Mountain spotted fever and is two orders of magnitude greater than suggested by passive reporting (Olano 2003b; Demma, 2005). Human ehrlichiosis may represent the most serious tick-transmitted infection in the United States. Fatalities have occurred in approximately 3% of cases—a rate that would be much higher without effective antibiotic treatment in many patients (Fichtenbaum, 1993; Fishbein, 1994). The severity is reflected in the admission of 41%–62% of patients to a hospital (Fishbein, 1994; Olano, 2003a, 2003b). Although severe cases often affect older persons, children are also susceptible to the illness (Schultze, 1997). The median duration of illness in a large CDC series, including treated cases, was 23 days. Signs and symptoms depict a systemic disease that has no clinically diagnostic features: fever (97%), headache (81%), myalgia (68%), anorexia (66%), nausea (48%), vomiting (37%), rash (6% at onset, 25% during the first week, and 36% overall), regional lymphadenopathy (29%), cough (26%), pharyngitis (26%), diarrhea (25%), abdominal pain or tenderness (22%), photophobia (27%), and confusion (20%) (Fishbein, 1994; Olano, 2003b). Severe complications include adult respiratory distress syndrome, disseminated intravascular coagulation, and renal insufficiency. Clinical laboratory findings include leukopenia (60%), thrombocytopenia (68%), and elevated hepatic transaminases (86%). CNS involvement manifested by seizures and coma has been documented by cerebrospinal fluid (CSF) pleocytosis, increased protein concentration and *E. chaffeensis* in CSF, and the presence of cerebral lesions at autopsy (Dunn, 1992; Ratnasamy, 1996; Walker, 1997a). Severity is age dependent (Olano, 2003a). In immunocompromised patients, including those with the acquired immunodeficiency syndrome (AIDS), human monocytotropic ehrlichiosis can be an overwhelming infection with massive growth of ehrlichiae and a fatal outcome (Paddock, 1993; Walker, 1997a). Mild infections have also been documented.

After entry via tick bite, *E. chaffeensis* spreads by lymphatic and/or hematogenous routes. Ehrlichial morulae have been identified in monocytes and macrophages in the bone marrow, peripheral blood (rarely), hepatic sinusoids, spleen, lymph nodes, meninges, kidney, gastrointestinal tract, and epicardium (Dumler, 1993a; Walker, 1997a; Sehdev, 2003). Bone marrow examination frequently reveals granulomas, myeloid hyperplasia, and megakaryocytosis. Other reported lesions include perivascular lymphohistiocytic infiltrates in the kidney, meninges, brain, and heart; interstitial mononuclear pneumonitis; foci of apoptosis-like cell death in the liver, lymph node, and spleen; diffuse reticuloendothelial hyperplasia; erythrophagocytosis; and cholestasis.

Human Infection with *Ehrlichia ewingii*

Recognized first as a canine pathogen in 1971, *E. ewingii* also infects white-tailed deer and is transmitted by *A. americanum* ticks (Ewing, 1971; Anziani, 1990). It shares antigens with *E. chaffeensis* but infects mainly neutrophils. A high proportion of infected patients are immunocompromised, suggesting that immunocompetent patients may be relatively resistant to the illness (Buller, 1999; Paddock, 2001).

Human Granulocytotropic Anaplasmosis

Thousands of cases of human granulocytic anaplasmosis have been documented, with most cases reported in the upper midwestern (Wisconsin and Minnesota) and northeastern states (New York, Connecticut, Rhode Island, and New Jersey) of the United States, but with confirmed autochthonous infections southward along the eastern seaboard and in California and Europe (Bakken, 1994; Aguero-Rosenfeld, 1996; Petrovec, 1997; Horowitz, 1998). Infection is transmitted by *Ixodes scapularis*, *I. pacificus*, and *Ixodes ricinus* ticks. The white-footed mouse (*Peromyscus leucopus*) and other small mammals are likely reservoir hosts in the United States, as are red deer, sheep, goats, and cattle in Europe (Hodzic, 1998). The pathology is poorly defined, with the observation of morula-containing neutrophils in peripheral blood and various organs, infiltrates of reticuloendothelial organs with foamy macrophages, multiorgan perivascular lymphohistiocytic infiltrates, and focal hepatocellular apoptosis (Walker, 1997a). Fatality may be associated with secondary opportunistic fungal and viral infections (Hardalo, 1995).

Human granulocytotropic anaplasmosis varies from asymptomatic to severe, with many diagnosed patients requiring hospitalization (Bakken, 1994). Infection is fatal in less than 1% of cases. The illness begins with chills, fever, headache, and myalgia. Thrombocytopenia occurs in most cases and leukopenia in nearly half. Hepatocellular injury is manifested as elevated hepatic enzymes, and severely ill patients may have septic shock–like illness with multiorgan involvement.

Laboratory Diagnosis

Isolation of ehrlichiae and anaplasmae from human blood in antibiotic-free cell culture has been accomplished more often for *A. phagocytophilum* (in HL-60 cells) than for *E. chaffeensis* (in DH-82 cells), and only once for *E. canis* (in an asymptomatic person), and has yet to be reported for *E. ewingii* (Dawson, 1991; Edelman, 1996; Goodman, 1996; Perez, 1996; Childs, 1999). Amplification of ehrlichial DNA by PCR using species-specific primers is an efficient diagnostic tool for all the human ehrlichioses (Anderson, 1992b; Chen, 1994; Everett, 1994; Buller, 1999; Comer, 1999). For human monocytotropic ehrlichiosis, the sensitivity of PCR is reported as 79%–100%, and for granulocytotropic anaplasmosis caused by *A. phagocytophilum*, 48%–86% (Anderson, 1992b; Everett, 1994). Lateness in the course, a lower level of ehrlichemia, and tetracycline treatment reduce the sensitivity of detection of ehrlichiae by PCR. Target genes that have been validated clinically include 16S rRNA (*rrs*), 120-kDa protein, *groesl*, *dsb*, *nadA*, and *VLPT* for *E. chaffeensis*, *rrs* and *dsb* for *E. ewingi*i, and *rrs*, *ank-1*, *msp2*, and *ftsZ* for *A. phagocytophilum* (Dumler, 2004; Doyle, 2005). Although it is in many cases a laborious task, identification of morulae in peripheral blood neutrophils provides a diagnosis of human anaplasmosis or ehrlichiosis and can be performed in any clinical laboratory. It is a more sensitive approach for *A. phagocytophilum* infection (30%–80%) than for *E. chaffeensis* (7%–17% in immunocompetent patients and a very high proportion of immunocompromised patients [Hamilton, 2004]). It is important to avoid false-positive interpretation caused by toxic granulations, Döhle bodies, superimposed platelets, apoptotic bodies, or contaminant particles. Immunohistochemical identification of *E. chaffeensis* can be performed in tissue specimens (Dumler, 1993a; Yu, 1993).

Serologic diagnosis is the usual approach to the diagnosis of human ehrlichiosis, using cell culture–propagated *E. chaffeensis* and *A. phagocytophilum* antigens in IFA assays (Nicholson, 1997; Childs, 1999; Walls, 1999; Olano, 2003b). This method is very sensitive for the demonstration of seroconversion to a titer of 1:64 or greater 2–4 weeks after disease onset. The expected serologic result on acute serum is absence of detected antibodies. Thus, treatment should be initiated empirically on the basis of clinical and epidemiologic factors and should not be withheld pending laboratory confirmation. Opinion as to a diagnostic single serum titer for *E. chaffeensis* ranges from 1:64–1:256. Cross-reactivity of *A. phagocytophilum* and *E. chaffeensis* is observed in approximately 20% of patients with human monocytotropic ehrlichiosis and human granulocytic anaplasmosis. Thus, particularly in geographic regions where these infections overlap and, indeed, if there is a possibility of travel-associated exposure, it is essential to determine antibody titers against both organisms. A fourfold difference in titer determines the infecting agent. Cases with twofold or less difference are classified as ehrlichiosis of indeterminate etiology.

Distinguishing *E. chaffeensis* from *E. ewingii* serologically is more problematic because the latter has yet to be cultivated. Western immunoblotting is a useful research tool at present for distinguishing infection with *E. chaffeensis* with its distinctive 120-kDa protein and 28-kDa protein family from infection with *A. phagocytophilum* with its major 42–49-kDa protein patterns (Asanovich, 1997; Chen, 1997a, 1997b; Zhi, 1997). Serologic assays using these and other recombinant proteins show promise for future development (Yu, 1999; Knowles, 2003).

Treatment

Doxycycline is the drug of choice for the treatment of these human ehrlichioses (Bakken, 1994; Fishbein, 1994). The use of chloramphenicol is not recommended as it has been associated with a fatal outcome. Cell culture studies show *E. chaffeensis* and *A. phagocytophilum* to be resistant to it and the commonly prescribed β-lactams, macrolides, aminoglycosides, and sulfonamide drugs (Brouqui, 1992; Klein, 1997; Branger, 2004). *A. phagocytophilum* is susceptible to rifampin and rifabutin in cell culture, and rifampin has been used to treat a limited number of pregnant women and children successfully (Krause, 2003).

INFECTIONS CAUSED BY *COXIELLA BURNETII*

Structure and Function

C. burnetii is distant phylogenetically from other pathogenic rickettsiae and is the only one classified in the γ-Proteobacteria. These gram-negative bacteria vary morphologically from rods to cocci, and by electron microscopic examination, two distinct forms can be seen: large cells (0.5–1.2 μm) and small dense cells (0.5 μm), which have been proposed to represent a developmental cycle that includes a spore-like form.

Much emphasis has been placed on a laboratory phenomenon associated with cultivation of *C. burnetii* by prolonged passage in cell culture or eggs, namely, loss of the organisms' ability to synthesize the entire LPS. This change from synthesis of the full to a truncated LPS, analogous to the conversion from smooth to rough phenotype by Enterobacteriaceae, has been designated phase variation from phase I to phase II. Phase I is found in nature and in infected persons and animals; phase II occurs in the laboratory and is the result of deletions of genes without selective advantage under conditions of passage outside of its hosts (Hoover, 2002).

C. burnetii enters its target cell, the macrophage, by phagocytosis after interaction with αvβ3 integrin and is highly adapted (e.g., synthesis of superoxide dismutase and acid phosphatase) to the acidic conditions in the phagolysosome, where replication by binary fission occurs.

Q Fever

The name Q fever was derived from its unknown etiology when the clinicoepidemiologic syndrome was first described as query fever. The ecology of *C. burnetii* includes silent infections in animals: many species of ticks, ungulates (particularly sheep, cattle, and goats), other mammals (including cats and wild rabbits), fish, birds, and marsupials (Marrie, 1988, 1997). Humans usually are infected by inhalation, especially of aerosols that originate in infected birth products of domestic livestock and pets, and possibly also by ingestion of unpasteurized contaminated milk (Fishbein, 1992; Raoult, 2005). Many human infections occur as an occupational disease among abattoir workers, farmers, and veterinarians (McQuiston, 2006). However, urban nonoccupational cases are by no means rare in some populations in which they have been evaluated, such as among immunocompromised patients in France (Brouqui, 1993).

A majority of human infections are asymptomatic (Marrie, 1990). Acute illness is often a self-limited, undifferentiated febrile illness, pneumonia, hepatitis, or meningoencephalitis (Drancourt, 1991; Tissot Dupont, 1992; Bernit, 2002). Individual patients with myalgias, anorexia, and headache are unlikely to be investigated diagnostically for Q fever, even though this syndrome is the most likely clinical presentation of this infection and accounts for a substantial proportion of patients with these symptoms in some populations. Manifestations of Q fever pneumonia vary: Cough may be nonproductive or absent, and the pneumonia may be severe and progress rapidly or may be detected as multiple rounded or segmental radiographic infiltrates without pulmonary symptoms. Q fever hepatitis may have a clinical presentation similar to acute viral hepatitis or the pathologic presentation of granulomatous hepatitis.

Chronic Q fever is considered synonymous with *C. burnetii* endocarditis but occurs less frequently as infection of an aneurysm or vascular prosthesis or osteomyelitis (Marrie, 1990; Brouqui, 1993). Chronic Q fever endocarditis usually involves previously damaged aortic or mitral valves as an afebrile illness that may manifest with heart failure, hepatosplenomegaly, changing cardiac murmurs, and weight loss. Disease associated with circulating immune complexes includes vasculitis-based purpuric rash or glomerulonephritis.

The pathology of acute Q fever includes mixed interstitial-alveolar-bronchiolar pneumonia with mononuclear inflammatory cells and granulomatous inflammation of the liver and bone marrow (Walker, 1988b). Q fever granulomas often contain a clear central vacuole and a surrounding ring of fibrin, as well as epithelioid macrophages. These doughnut granulomas are neither pathognomonic lesions nor the only form of granuloma that occurs in the liver and bone marrow of Q fever patients. Involved cardiac valves in Q fever endocarditis have a small vegetation and show mixed subacute and chronic inflammation with many foamy macrophages having the cytoplasm filled with *C. burnetii* (Lepidi, 2003).

Laboratory Diagnosis

The laboratory diagnosis of Q fever is most often accomplished by demonstration of antibodies to *C. burnetii* (Fournier, 1996, 1998). Serologic methods employ both phase I and phase II antigens and often evaluate class-specific antibody production. Enzyme immunoassay and indirect IFA tests are highly specific and are more sensitive than complement fixation. In acute Q fever, antibodies to phase II antigens appear earliest after infection, and antibodies to phase I may be detected as early as 2 weeks after the onset of illness. In general, acute Q fever is associated with high titers to phase II antigens and lower titers to phase I antigens. By IFA, an anti–phase II IgG titer of 1:200 or greater and an anti–phase II IgM titer of 1:50 or greater have a sensitivity of 58% and a specificity of 92% in acute Q fever. In chronic Q fever, antibodies to phase I are present at a higher titer (e.g., IgG-IFA anti–phase I titer of 1:800 or greater), and antibodies to phase II are generally equal to or lower than the phase I titer. An IgA response to phase I antigens is often observed in patients with chronic Q fever. A titer of 1:128 or greater against phase I antigen by the complement fixation test is also considered diagnostic of chronic Q fever, although some patients have lower titers. Because of cross-reactivity of *B. henselae* and *Bartonella quintana* with *C. burnetii*, a serologic diagnosis of *Bartonella* endocarditis should not be made until anti–*C. burnetii* titers have been determined (La Scola, 1996b). In Q fever endocarditis, the anti–*C. burnetii* titer is substantially higher than the anti-*Bartonella* titer. An IFA containing both *C. burnetii* and *B. henselae* effectively distinguishes the infecting bacterium (Rolain, 2003b).

PCR assays have been developed against diverse target genes, and during the first 2 weeks of acute Q fever, real-time PCR of serum is more sensitive (24%) than IFA serology (14%) (Fournier, 2003). It is likely that PCR of blood or buffy coat would detect a greater proportion of cases with *Coxiella* than serum.

Other methods for the diagnosis of chronic Q fever endocarditis include immunohistologic staining (sensitivity 32%), electron microscopy, culture (sensitivity 64%), and PCR (sensitivity 75%) detection of *C. burnetii* in a cardiac valve (Lepidi 2003). *C. burnetii* can be recovered from the blood or infected cardiac valves by in vitro cultivation using a centrifugation-enhanced shell vial (human embryonic lung) cell culture system. This method can identify the presence of coxiellae within 7 days but should be attempted only within cell culture facilities approved for biohazard containment level 3.

Treatment

Doxycycline is effective in shortening the course of acute Q fever when administered during the first 3 days after the onset of illness (Levy, 1991). Ciprofloxacin or a combination of ciprofloxacin and rifampin is alternative medication for patients who cannot be treated with tetracycline. Treatment of chronic *C. burnetii* endocarditis requires prolonged administration of doxycycline and a quinolone, which often does not eradicate the infection (Marrie, 2002). Successful treatment is indicated by a slow fall in anti–phase I IgG titer to below 1:200, when discontinuation of treatment can be considered. Cardiac valve replacement is often performed for hemodynamic reasons.

INFECTIONS CAUSED BY ORGANISMS OF THE GENUS *BARTONELLA*

Structure and Function

The genus *Bartonella* has been removed from the order Rickettsiales (Brenner, 1993; Birtles, 1996). The human pathogens, *B. quintana* (the etiologic agent of trench fever, a major louse-borne disease in World Wars I and II and among homeless persons), *B. henselae* (the etiologic agent of cat scratch disease), *Bartonella elizabethae* and *Bartonella vinsonii* (associated with infective endocarditis), and *Bartonella bacilliformis* (a sandfly-transmitted bacterium that causes febrile acute hemolytic anemia and chronic verruga peruana cutaneous lesions in South America), have been cultivated in blood-enriched media in the presence of 5% carbon dioxide (CO_2) (Walker, 2006). These facultative intracellular gram-negative bacilli do not produce acid from carbohydrates and usually reside within erythrocytes in their natural mammalian hosts. Among numerous described species of *Bartonella*, *Bartonella clarridgeiae* is a suspected second agent of cat scratch disease (Kordick, 1997).

Cat Scratch Disease, Bacillary Angiomatosis, and Bacillary Peliosis

B. henselae is transmitted to humans by the scratch or bite of infected kittens, which are bacteremic for many months while appearing healthy (Tappero, 1993; Chomel, 1995; Bergmans, 1997; Heller, 1997). Bacteria are transmitted from cat to cat by the cat flea (Chomel, 1996; Higgins, 1996). The nature of the disease is largely host determined. Among immunocompetent hosts, 80% are younger than age 21 years and present with a cutaneous papule or pustule at the inoculation site and self-limited regional lymphadenopathy. Less than 2% of patients suffer complications such as hematogenously disseminated involvement of the liver, spleen, lung, bone, CNS, retina, conjunctiva, or skin (Liston, 1996; Wade, 2000; Verdon, 2002). The histopathology of cat scratch disease lesions consists of granulomas surrounding stellate microabscesses. Among severely immunocompromised patients, *B. henselae* infection is manifested by fever and bacteremia, or by cutaneous or visceral angioproliferative lesions. The latter are characterized by lobular vascular proliferations of plump endothelial cells with clusters of small capillaries surrounding ectatic capillaries, separated by edematous, mucinous, or fibrotic stroma containing clusters of neutrophils, neutrophil debris, and granular microcolonies of bartonellae. In the skin, these lesions are designated bacillary angiomatosis; in the liver and spleen, hepatic and splenic peliosis. Dissemination to other sites may occur also. The angioproliferative lesions of *B. henselae* and *B. quintana* in immunocompromised patients are indistinguishable, and they are similar to the verruga peruana of *B. bacilliformis* (Koehler, 1997). *B. henselae*, *B. quintana*, *B. vinsonii* subsp. *berkhoffii* and subsp. *arupensis*, *B. alsatica*, *B. koehleri*, and *B. elizabethae* have been documented as agents of infective endocarditis (Drancourt, 1995; Roux 2000; Avidor, 2004; Fenollar, 2005; Raoult, 2006: Jeanclaude, 2009).

Trench Fever and Bacillary Angiomatosis

B. quintana causes prolonged bacteremia in convalescent humans, the apparent reservoir. Infections were recognized to be transmitted from person to louse *(Pediculus humanus corporis)* to another person in front-line trenches during World War I (Bruce, 1921). Among French homeless persons, 14% are bacteremic, of whom 80% are afebrile (Brouqui, 1999).

Louse feces laden with *B. quintana* are scratched into the skin, and approximately 8 days later, an illness of variable severity begins. Manifestations include fever, generally lasting less than a week, headache, myalgias, pretibial pain, and an evanescent macular rash. Relapses often occur at 4- or 5-day intervals. Bacteremia persists for weeks, months, or longer, serving as a source of infecting lice, even when the person feels relatively healthy. Cases occur at present in alcoholic and homeless populations in American and European cities (Spach, 1995; Foucault, 2002).

Oroya Fever and Verruga Peruana

South American bartonellosis, manifested as an acute illness called Oroya fever, or as chronic cutaneous lesions called verruga peruana, is transmitted by the bite of a *Lutzomyia* sandfly. Asymptomatic long-term human carriers are the reservoirs of *B. bacilliformis*. After an incubation period of approximately 3 weeks, Oroya fever begins insidiously with anorexia, headache, malaise, and low-grade fever, or abruptly with chills, high fever, headache, and mental status changes. Bartonellae invade the red blood cells and cause erythrocytic changes that result in erythrophagocytosis and anemia. Verruga peruana, characterized by red to purple nontender nodules that appear in crops over 1–2 months and persist for months to years, follows Oroya fever or occurs without prior symptoms (Arias-Stella, 1986; Walker, 2006).

Laboratory Diagnosis

Lysis release of intraerythrocytic bacteria followed by centrifugation and incubation at 35° C in a humid CO_2 atmosphere on chocolate or Columbia blood agar for longer than a month has been used to recover *B. henselae* and *B. quintana* from patients (Tierno, 1995). These *Bartonella* organisms are gram-negative bacilli, 0.2–0.5 μm in diameter and 1–3 μm long. *B. henselae* are oxidase, catalase, and urease negative and do not utilize carbohydrates. Identification is accomplished by twitching motility in wet mounts, immunofluorescent staining, analysis of fatty acid composition, DNA sequencing, or hybridization (Scott, 1996). PCR detects *B. henselae* DNA in 31% of lymph node biopsies and in 55% of lymph node aspirates (Bergmans, 1996). *B. bacilliformis* may be cultivated from blood by inoculation of Columbia blood agar supplemented with 5% defibrinated blood or other blood- or hemin-supplemented media with detection of colonies after an average of 18 days.

Formerly, the diagnosis of cat scratch disease required a combination of clinical, epidemiologic, and pathologic criteria. Histopathologic studies, including Warthin-Starry stain and immunohistochemistry, have been used to support the diagnosis of bacillary angiomatosis and cat scratch disease. Oroya fever may be diagnosed by visualization of intraerythrocytic bartonellae, appearing as cocci or bacilli, occasionally with curved or ring forms, in peripheral blood carefully stained by the Giemsa method to avoid misinterpretation of artifacts. Diagnosis of *B. henselae* and *B. quintana* infections is usually accomplished by serologic demonstration of antibodies by indirect immunofluorescence or enzyme immunoassay (Dalton, 1995b). Serologic diagnosis of *Bartonella* endocarditis should include measurement of antibody titers against *C. burnetii*, which may stimulate cross-reacting antibody titers against *Bartonella* (Maurin, 1997; Rolain, 2003a). Titers against *C. burnetii* phase I are much higher than the anti-*Bartonella* titers in chronic Q fever endocarditis, and Western immunoblotting after cross-absorption yields a definitive diagnosis if necessary (Houpikian, 2003). Real-time PCR can also be used to establish the diagnosis of *Bartonella* endocarditis (Zeaiter, 2003).

Treatment

Cat scratch disease usually is self-limited, but the lymphadenopathy resolves more rapidly after azithromycin (Bass, 1999). Drugs of choice for the treatment of bacillary angiomatosis include doxycycline, erythromycin, and azithromycin (Rolain, 2004). *Bartonella* endocarditis has a more favorable outcome when treated with an aminoglycoside (Raoult, 2003). Relapses may occur, requiring retreatment or even long-term maintenance therapy. Ciprofloxacin is currently preferred for treatment of Oroya fever. The difficulty of treating an intraerythrocytic bacterium such as *B. quintana* in humans is evident in the lack of bactericidal activity of doxycycline, fluoroquinolones, and β-lactams, and an inability to achieve bactericidal intraerythrocytic levels of gentamicin, the most active antimicrobial agent (Rolain, 2000). Chronic *B. quintana* bacteremia is cleared by gentamicin for 14 days, followed by doxycycline for 28 days (Foucault, 2003). Verruga peruana is treated with oral rifampin.

Mycoplasmal Infections

Mycoplasmas were proved to cause human disease in 1962, when one mycoplasma (subsequently named *Mycoplasma pneumoniae*) was recognized as the etiologic agent of primary atypical pneumonia (Chanock, 1962). Mycoplasmas are the smallest free-living organisms. They are pleomorphic, ranging from spherical cells 0.2 μm in diameter to filaments 0.1 μm wide by 1–2 μm long. Most are facultative anaerobes that replicate by binary fission. Mycoplasmas are unique among bacteria because they have no cell wall. They are unable to synthesize cell wall precursors, and they require cholesterol and related sterols for membrane synthesis. Mycoplasmas also lack the enzymatic pathways for purine and pyrimidine synthesis and, for this reason, require complex media (such as beef heart infusion broth supplemented with horse serum, yeast extract, and nucleic acids) for growth in vitro. The potential pathogens, *M. pneumoniae* and the genital mycoplasmas (*Mycoplasma hominis*, *Mycoplasma genitalium*, *Ureaplasma urealyticum*, and *Ureaplasma parvum*), are discussed. Other mycoplasmas are part of the normal human flora, primarily of the respiratory and genitourinary tracts.

MYCOPLASMA PNEUMONIAE

Epidemiology

Mycoplasma pneumoniae is found worldwide. Epidemics occur among confined populations such as children in schools, families, and military recruits, typically at 3–5-year intervals, and predominantly in late summer and fall. In nonepidemic years, infections occur year-round and in general spread slowly, possibly owing to the slow generation time of the bacterium (6 hours) and its low transmission rate, which apparently requires close contact with an ill person (Waites, 2004). During epidemics, however, infection may spread rapidly, and the occurrence of point-source outbreaks in which close and prolonged exposure is not recognized suggests that *M. pneumoniae* may be transmitted via aerosols. Rates of infection with *M. pneumoniae* are greatest in school-aged children and young adults, and pneumonia occurs most frequently in persons aged 5–20 years, especially in those between the ages of 15 and 19 years. Infection with *M. pneumoniae* is common before the age of 5 years but typically is asymptomatic or produces a mild illness with coryza and wheezing but no fever or pneumonia (Fernald, 1975).

Pathogenesis and Pathology

M. pneumoniae, a surface parasite, colonizes the mucosa of the respiratory tract. Its ability to attach to respiratory mucosal cells, escape phagocytosis, and modulate the immune system is essential to initiation of disease. Its gliding motility may allow it to penetrate through respiratory secretions, and its filamentous, flexible form with terminal attachment organelle may facilitate localization in crypts and folds of the host cell membrane and between microvilli and cilia, where it is protected from phagocytosis. Attachment of *M. pneumoniae* to host cells is mediated by the P1 protein, which interacts with neuraminic acid–containing glycoproteins at the surface of the host cell membrane (Chandler, 1982; Geary, 1987; Waites, 2008). Hydrogen peroxide and superoxide produced by *M. pneumoniae* may injure mucosal cells, causing ciliostasis and sloughing of superficial cells

(Almagor, 1984). Inhibition of catalase (which breaks down damaging peroxides) in host cells by bacterium-generated superoxides makes the cells more susceptible to damage (Waites, 2008). An adenosine diphosphate (ADP)-ribosylating protein (named community-acquired respiratory distress syndrome toxin: CARDS TX) produced by *M. pneumoniae* has been identified and postulated to have an exotoxin function, as the protein has been demonstrated to induce vacuolization and ciliostasis in cultured host cells (Waites, 2008). The target and exact cellular effects of the toxin remain to be elucidated.

Host-related factors also are involved in the pathogenesis of *M. pneumoniae* disease. The apparent high prevalence of *M. pneumoniae* infection in infants and young children, the mild nature of the disease in this age group, and the occurrence of more severe illness during infection at a later age suggest that severe disease may result from the host immune response to reinfection. *M. pneumoniae* has been demonstrated to induce cytokine production in vitro, suggesting that adherence of the bacterium to respiratory epithelial cells results in cytokine production, which in turn might both recruit inflammatory cells, including lymphocytes, to the site of infection and modulate the activity of the recruited cells (Waites, 2008). This cytokine production and influx of lymphocytes might be involved in fighting the infection by destroying the infecting organism or, conversely, might result in immune hypersensitivity that damages host cells. A more marked T cell immune response may result in more severe disease (Waites, 2008). Moreover, extrapulmonary manifestations of disease (discussed later) are suspected to be immune mediated. The interaction of *M. pneumoniae* with the I antigenic determinant of human red blood cells, which contains the necessary 2,3-sialylated poly-*N*-acetylgalactosamine sequences, may alter the I antigen, converting it into a non–self-antigen that stimulates production of cold agglutinins. Other autoimmune antibodies produced during infection with *M. pneumoniae* (antibodies to lung, brain, smooth muscle, and lymphocytes) may have similar derivations.

Few descriptions of the pathologic findings of disease caused by *M. pneumoniae* are available, because most infections are self-limited and tissue is rarely obtained. In fatal cases, patchy areas of consolidation are found in the lungs. Histologic examination of involved foci shows bronchitis, bronchiolitis, and interstitial and alveolar pneumonitis with peribronchiolar collections of lymphocytes and plasma cells, accompanied by macrophages and neutrophils if cellular necrosis is present.

Clinical Manifestations

The most common manifestation of disease caused by *M. pneumoniae* is tracheobronchitis, which occurs in about half of infected patients. After an incubation period of several weeks, sore throat, cough, coryza, fever, headache, myalgia, and sometimes conjunctivitis and myringitis are seen. The infection may resolve or may progress to pneumonia, the frequency of which is age dependent, with children aged 5–15 most likely to develop lower respiratory involvement (Baum, 2000; Waites, 2004). Chest radiographs show unilateral lower lobe bronchopneumonia, or occasionally bilateral feathery infiltrates. The peripheral white blood cell count is normal early and rises as the disease progresses. Maculopapular or, less commonly, vesicular skin eruptions occur in about 15% of cases a few days after disease onset. Without antimicrobial therapy, fever resolves in 2–14 days, but malaise, cough, and radiographic abnormalities persist for 2–6 weeks. In a small percentage of children and adults, pneumonia is severe enough to warrant hospitalization; these patients may develop lung abscess, pleural effusions, secondary bacterial infections, bronchiectasis, or clinical relapse.

Extrarespiratory manifestations such as clinically apparent hemolytic anemia (typically with very high titers of cold agglutinins); erythema multiforme, erythema nodosum, and urticaria; myocarditis and pericarditis; and arthralgias, arthritis, acute glomerulonephritis, tubulointerstitial nephritis, and IgA nephropathy may occur, but are not frequent (Ponka, 1979; Cassell, 1981; Baum, 2000; Waites, 2004). *M. pneumoniae* has become recognized, however, as having a significant association with CNS disorders, from minor to severe, including encephalitis and acute disseminated encephalomyelitis, with 6%–7% of patients hospitalized with *M. pneumoniae* infection demonstrating neurologic manifestations (Waites, 2004). Among 1988 patients referred to the California Encephalitis Project over a 9-year period, *M. pneumoniae* was implicated in 111 patients (5.6%) and was the single most common implicated infectious agent (Christie, 2007). Many cases of encephalitis associated with *M. pneumoniae* appear to be relatively mild; however, severe cases of acute disseminated encephalomyelitis that may even result in fatality can occur in association with the infection (Waites, 2004; Christie, 2007; Stamm, 2008).

GENITAL MYCOPLASMAS

Epidemiology

Ureaplasma species (*U. urealyticum* has been separated into *U. parvum*, formerly *U urealyticum* biovar 1, and *U. urealyticum*, formerly *U. urealyticum* biovar 2) can be found colonizing the vagina and cervix in 40%–80% of adult women, and *M. hominis* can be found in 21%–53% of women (Waites, 2005). The frequency in males appears to be lower. Prevalence studies for *M. genitalium* are infrequent in the literature, but it appears to be less common as a colonizer in asymptomatic individuals and is found with a frequency of around 1% (Takahashi, 2006; Manhart, 2007). Colonization of infants with genital mycoplasmas can occur during passage through the birth canal, but colonization appears to be temporary in many cases, and a lower rate of colonization has been noted in children (Klein, 1969; Hammerschlag, 1978). The increase in colonization by mycoplasmas after puberty indicates an association with sexual activity. In addition to passage through the birth canal, neonates can acquire infections due to *Ureaplasma* spp. and *M. hominis* hematogenously through the placenta or through an ascending infection, resulting in seeding of amniotic fluid (Waites, 2005).

Clinical Manifestations

Although simple vaginal colonization with the genital mycoplasmas in pregnant women is not associated with disease, the presence of mycoplasma (primarily *Ureaplasma* spp. and to a lesser extent *M. hominis*) in the placental membranes or amniotic fluid is consistently associated with chorioamnionitis, preterm birth, and adverse perinatal outcomes associated with several neonatal disorders, including perinatal pneumonia and sepsis in preterm infants (Waites, 2005; Goldenberg, 2008). Both *Ureaplasma* spp. and *M. hominis* are associated with postpartum fever. *Ureaplasma* spp. can cause urinary calculi and are a cause of nongonococcal urethritis (NGU) (Waites, 2005). *M. hominis* has been related to both pelvic inflammatory disease (PID) and pyelonephritis and may have an association with bacterial vaginosis (Waites, 2005). *M. genitalium* has been linked to NGU in males only relatively recently, but it is now firmly established as a significant cause of the disorder and is the etiologic agent in approximately 25% of cases (Ross, 2006; Gaydos, 2009). Among women, *M. genitalium* has shown an association with cervicitis, endometritis, PID, and tubal infertility (Haggerty, 2006; Short, 2009).

LABORATORY DIAGNOSIS

Mycoplasma pneumoniae

Specimens recommended for diagnosis of infection caused by *M. pneumoniae* are throat swabs and serum, but bronchoalveolar lavage fluid, sputum, and lung tissue are acceptable. A nonspecific serologic test that may provide useful information is detection of cold agglutinins, which are IgM antibodies against the I antigen of human erythrocytes. The cold agglutinin response usually corresponds with the severity of pulmonary disease, as a titer of ≥1 : 32 is found with severe pneumonia, whereas agglutinins are not detectable in mild disease (Waites, 2008). Cold agglutinins appear by the end of the first week or early in the second week of illness in at least half of infected persons, but their presence is not diagnostic of infection with *M. pneumonia*, as they may also be seen with other bacterial, rickettsial, or viral infections.

Definitive diagnosis is based on detection of the organism, specific antibodies, or specific nucleic acid sequences. To isolate *M. pneumoniae*, special agar media, broth media, or a biphasic culture system is inoculated and incubated in a sealed container for 3 weeks or more in 5%–10% CO_2, or anaerobically at 37° C. Cultures are examined microscopically (40×) once or twice each week for typical spherical colonies with a dense center and thin outer layer (resembling a "fried egg") embedded in the agar. Such colonies, consistent with *M. pneumoniae*, that demonstrate glycolysis (as demonstrated color change in the media pH indicator), β-hemolysis, and hemadsorption of guinea pig erythrocytes on further testing are presumptively *M. pneumoniae*. Definitive speciation usually requires staining with monoclonal antibodies using immunofluorescence or immunoperoxidase, immunoblotting, or PCR.

Because isolation of *M. pneumoniae* may require several weeks, rendering a culture clinically noncontributory, more rapid tests are most useful for diagnosis. Detection of specific IgM in a single serum sample is diagnostic of acute infection. If IgG is measured, acute and convalescent phase samples must be tested, and the diagnosis is based on a fourfold or greater rise in titer. A variety of tests based on particle agglutination, EIA, or immunofluorescence are available; EIA, particularly with membrane-bound assays, is the most popular (Waites, 2004). Serologic testing is not without problems as antibody titers vary with age, with children and younger individuals having consistently higher titers than adults (Daxboeck, 2002). Nucleic acid amplification tests can also provide rapid diagnosis (Loens, 2003), but currently no commercial Food and Drug Administration–cleared amplification test for direct detection of *M. pneumoniae* is available. Although time is required for patients to develop a serologic response, hence the sensitivity of serology early in infection may be low, as time from onset of symptoms increases, the sensitivity of PCR decreases (Thurman, 2009). Many experts consider the combined use of PCR on respiratory specimens and serology the optimum approach to obtain maximum sensitivity in diagnosing infection (Christie, 2007; Waites, 2008; Thurman, 2009).

Genital Mycoplasmas

Ureaplasma spp. *and M. hominis* may be recovered from urethral, vaginal, or endocervical swab specimens, blood, urine, abscess material, prostatic secretions, semen, or tissues.Various culture systems may be used to isolate the genital mycoplasmas (Clyde, 1984; Yajko, 1984; Wood, 1985; Phillips, 1986). Traditionally, separate systems were used for each (U agar and U broth for *Ureaplasma* spp. *and* H agar and H broth for *M. hominis*) because the optimal pH for growth of the two organisms differs (pH 5.5–6.5 for *Ureaplasma* spp. and pH 6–8 for *M. hominis*). However, single culture systems are now available that effectively detect all of these species (Yajko, 1984; Wood, 1985; Phillips, 1986). Broth cultures are incubated aerobically in sealed test tubes. Agar cultures are incubated anaerobically or in an atmosphere of 5%–7% CO_2 and observed daily under the microscope. *M. hominis* also grows on sheep blood agar, producing nonhemolytic pinpoint colonies, and in most broth blood culture media, although no evidence of growth is visible.

Colonies of *M. hominis*, 200–300 µm in diameter with a typical fried-egg appearance, usually appear within 5 days. In broth containing phenol red and 0.1% arginine, *M. hominis* metabolizes arginine to ammonia, causing a color change from yellow to red. U agar plates are observed daily for 4 days, and on day 4 are stained with one to two drops of $CaCl_2$–urea solution. Colonies of *Ureaplasma* spp. have an irregular rather than circular umbonate morphology, are 15–60 µm in diameter, and stain dark brown in 5 minutes. In U broth, *Ureaplasma* spp. produce a shift in pH, and the color changes from yellow to red. A loopful of broth then is transferred to agar plates and is streaked for isolation.

M. genitalium grows very slowly, similar to *M. pneumoniae*, with which it shares many morphologic and antigenic similarities, and is difficult to isolate in culture. For clinical purposes, nucleic acid amplification is the only practical test; although a commercial product does not exist at this time, many facilities have developed their own assays to detect the organism (Ross, 2006). No commercial serologic assays are available for *M. genitalium* or any of the genital mycoplasmas, and the use of serology for these organisms is confined to research.

TREATMENT

A tetracycline, macrolide, or fluoroquinolone is effective treatment for *M. pneumoniae*, and the macrolides, usually a newer drug such as azithromycin or clarithromycin, are the agents of choice because of dosing considerations. Macrolide resistance has been reported in *M. pneumoniae* isolates in Japan, and patients infected with these isolates suffered a prolonged course of infection relative to those infected with susceptible isolates (Waites, 2008). Generally, *Ureaplasma* spp. are sensitive to tetracyclines, quinolones, and macrolides, with tetracycline resistance seen in approximately 10% of isolates (Waites, 2005). Resistance to the fluoroquinolones appears to be unusual, and *Ureaplasma* spp. are resistant to clindamycin. *M. hominis* is susceptible to clindamycin and the newer quinolones but is resistant to the macrolides. Some isolates also are susceptible to tetracyclines, although resistance to the tetracyclines is thought to be greater than in *Ureaplasma* spp., at approximately 40% (Waites, 2005). *M. genitalium* can be problematic, in that treatment with macrolides (azithromycin), tetracyclines (doxycycline), or quinolones (ofloxacin, levofloxacin) can result in a significant number of failures; however, cases in which these less expensive agents fail appear to be effectively treated with moxifloxacin. Such a cascade treatment strategy is recommended by a number of studies (Ross, 2006; Bradshaw, 2008; Jernberg, 2008).

SELECTED REFERENCES

Centers for Disease Control and Prevention. Screening tests to detect *Chlamydia trachomatis* and *Neisseria gonorrhoeae* infections. MMWR 2002b;51:RR-15.

Discusses nonculture tests, both amplified and nonamplified, for diagnosis of genital infection with C. trachomatis and N. gonorrhoeae.

Loens K, Ursi D, Goossens H, Ieven M. Molecular diagnosis of *Mycoplasma pneumoniae* respiratory tract infections. J Clin Microbiol 2003;41:4915.

Discusses various nucleic acid amplification methods that have been examined for direct detection of M. pneumoniae in respiratory specimens. Includes a discussion of specimen processing and quality control.

Peipert JF. Genital chlamydial infections. N Engl J Med 2003;349:2424.

Provides an excellent overview of genital infections with C. trachomatis, including epidemiology, screening strategies, and treatment.

Solomon AW, Peeling RW, Foster A, Mabey DCW. Diagnosis and assessment of trachoma. Clin Microbiol Rev 2004;17:982.

Provides an excellent review of trachoma, including an historical perspective and an overview of the developmental cycle, clinical presentation, and laboratory diagnosis.

Waites KB, Talkington DF. *Mycoplasma pneumoniae* and its role as a human pathogen. Clin Microbiol Rev 2004;17:697.

Provides an in-depth review of M. pneumoniae, including taxonomy, pathogenesis, clinical syndromes, diagnosis, and treatment.

Zinsser H, editor. Rats, lice, and history. New York: Little, Brown; 1935.

Very readable historical account of the toll that disease takes, especially in times of conflict.

REFERENCES

Access the complete reference list online at http://www.expertconsult.com

CHAPTER 57

MEDICAL BACTERIOLOGY

Geraldine S. Hall, Gail L. Woods

KEY POINTS

- Bacteria can be categorized based on the Gram stain reaction (gram-positive or gram-negative), shape (cocci, bacilli, coccobacilli, spirochete), preferred atmosphere (aerobic, microaerophilic, anaerobic), and presence or absence of spores; they can be identified on the basis of key biochemical tests, antigenic components (e.g., cell wall antigens, toxins), and/or molecular features.
- Among the gram-positive cocci, the most important human pathogens (and the infections they commonly cause) are *Staphylococcus aureus* (skin and soft tissue infections, bacteremia, toxic shock syndrome), *Streptococcus pyogenes* (pharyngitis and its nonsuppurative complications, skin and soft tissue infections), *Streptococcus agalactiae* (neonatal bacteremia and meningitis), *Streptococcus pneumoniae* (community-acquired pneumonia, meningitis), and *Enterococcus faecalis* and *Enterococcus faecium* (nosocomial urinary tract infections and bacteremia).
- Among gram-positive bacilli, the most important human pathogens (and the infections they commonly cause) are *Listeria monocytogenes* (meningitis, bacteremia), *Nocardia* species (pneumonia, soft tissue infections, brain abscess), *Bacillus anthracis* (skin and soft tissue infections, pneumonia; a bioterrorism agent), and *Corynebacterium diphtheriae* (diphtheria), which is rarely encountered in the clinical laboratory in the United States.
- Among gram-negative cocci, the most important human pathogens (and the infections they commonly cause) are *Neisseria meningitidis* (meningitis), *Neisseria gonorrhoeae* (gonorrhea), and *Moraxella catarrhalis*.
- Gram-negative bacilli include Enterobacteriaceae, many of which are normal flora in the gastrointestinal tract; nonfermentative gram-negative bacilli (e.g., *Pseudomonas aeruginosa* and *Acinetobacter baumanii*), which are found in the environment and cause human infection when host defenses are compromised; halophilic organisms (*Vibrio* species); microaerophilic bacteria *(Campylobacter, Helicobacter)*; fastidious organisms (*Legionella* species, *Bordetella* species, *Francisella tularensis, Brucella* species, *Haemophilus* species); and miscellaneous infrequently encountered bacteria.
- Among the Enterobacteriaceae, the most important human pathogens (and the infections they commonly cause) are *Escherichia coli* (urinary tract infection, diarrhea, bacteremia), *Klebsiella pneumoniae* and *Klebsiella oxytoca* (urinary tract infection, pneumonia, bacteremia), *Proteus* species (urinary tract infection), *Salmonella* species (diarrhea, typhoid fever), *Shigella* species (diarrhea), *Enterobacter* species (nosocomial pneumonia, urinary tract infection, bacteremia), and *Serratia* species (nosocomial pneumonia).
- Among the anaerobes, the most important human pathogens (and the infections they commonly cause) are the *Bacteroides fragilis* group (intraabdominal infections, abscesses); *Clostridium* species, especially *Clostridium perfringens* (soft tissue infections, food poisoning), *Clostridium tetani* (tetanus), and *Clostridium difficile* (antibiotic-associated diarrhea); and non–spore-forming gram-positive anaerobes such as *Actinomyces israelii* and *Propionibacterium acnes*.

A wide variety of bacterial species may be recovered from clinical specimens. To appropriately assess the clinical significance of these organisms, an understanding of the normal bacterial flora present at different anatomic locations is essential. In some cases, the number of organisms present can be extremely high, for example, 10^6 organisms/cm^2 of skin, 10^9 organisms/mL of oral secretions, and 10^{11} organisms/g of colon contents. It is important to obtain samples with minimal contamination from the normal flora (Miller, 2007). This may be difficult but can be optimally achieved if proper procedures are followed. These procedures, along with processing techniques that serve to enhance recovery of pathogenic microorganisms, are discussed in Chapter 63. This chapter begins with a short discussion of laboratory procedures used to process a specimen for bacterial culture, which is followed by a more in-depth discussion of the bacterial species commonly considered to be human pathogens.

Specimen Processing

GRAM STAIN

Few would disagree that direct examination of a specimen with Gram stain is one of the most valuable procedures performed by the microbiology laboratory. The Gram stain result rapidly provides information that is used by the clinician for selecting appropriate antimicrobial therapy; it also helps the laboratory technologist assess the quality of the specimen and the extent to which certain organisms recovered in culture will be worked up. Organisms present in abundant quantity in specimens containing many white blood cells are given more attention than those that are present in smaller numbers in the absence of white blood cells. Multiple specimens positive for similar organisms in smears and cultures contribute to increased clinical significance of the results.

To prepare a smear for staining, an aliquot of the most purulent or bloody portion of the specimen is placed on a clean microscopic slide in a manner that provides both thick and thin areas. For sterile body fluids, a cytocentrifuge may be used to concentrate the specimen by 10–100 times (Peterson, 1988). The material on the slide is allowed to air-dry, is fixed with methanol or gentle heat, and then is stained with Gram stain reagents (crystal violet, Gram iodine, alcohol, and safranin). Organisms that have a gram-positive cell wall will resist decolorization with methanol and will retain the purple color of the crystal violet; organisms that have a gram-negative cell wall will be decolorized and will stain red with safranin counterstain.

Stained smears are initially examined using a low-power objective to look for large structures, such as nematode larvae, Curschmann's spirals, large granules, grains, bacterial microcolonies, or fungal forms. An oil immersion lens is then used to assess the type of bacteria present. Because 10^5 organisms/mL must be present to see one organism per oil immersion field (1000×), smears must be examined carefully to detect small numbers of organisms.

The organisms observed should be evaluated for size, shape, and Gram reaction, which should be reported with as much description as possible; reporting the presence of gram-positive cocci in pairs that resemble *S. pneumoniae* (Fig. 57-1) is more helpful than simply reporting gram-positive cocci in chains. White or red blood cells should be quantified and reported, along with any intracellular bacteria observed. Correlation of Gram stain observations with culture results is a good way to check on the quality of the stains and culture. Demonstration of many bacteria on Gram stain that do not grow out in culture may indicate unusual organisms that require more specialized media or the inability of laboratory personnel to recognize certain colonial types in culture, or could suggest a false-positive Gram stain result caused by contamination of reagents or collection materials, such as swabs, or incorrect interpretation of Gram stain results. Gram stain results could indicate the need to inoculate additional media for a specific specimen. For example, finding many Gram-negative coccobacilli in a respiratory specimen could indicate the need for a chocolate plate to recover *Haemophilus* spp., which would not be recovered on a blood agar plate. Other stains, such as the acridine orange stain, can be utilized for staining blood culture bottles, cerebrospinal fluid (CSF), or buffy coat preparations. This fluorescent stain provides a rapid and, at times, more sensitive stain for bacteria and fungi (Mirrett, 1982). Bacteria and fungi will produce an orange fluorescence, and mammalian cells will stain green. Some experience is required for accurate interpretation of the acridine orange stain, and correct preparation of the smears is necessary to avoid excessive cellular material, which can result in too much cellular DNA that can mask the presence of any bacterial DNA.

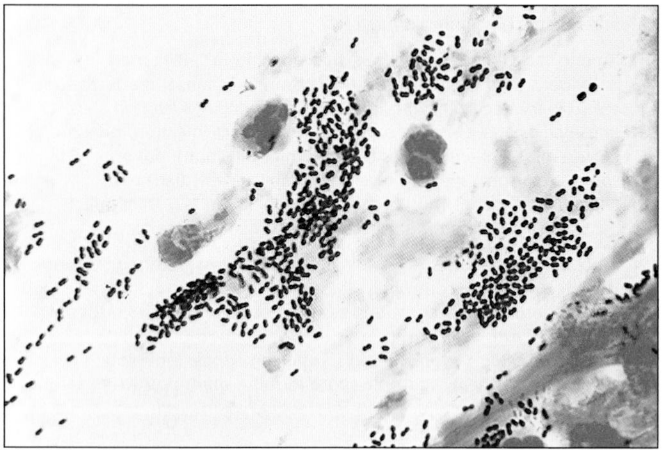

Figure 57-1 Gram stain of a sputum smear shows neutrophils, debris, and gram-positive diplococci, suggestive of pneumococcal infection (oil immersion).

Many laboratories use probes for identification of specific bacteria or fungi in blood culture bottles. These are available using a fluorescent in situ hybridization (FISH) format (Advandx, Woburn, MA). When gram-positive cocci are seen in clusters on Gram stain of a blood culture bottle, probes can be used to differentiate *S. aureus* from coagulase-negative staphylococci, or nonstaphylococcal organisms. If gram-positive cocci are seen in pairs and chains, a probe is available that could specifically identify *E. faecalis*. The newest of these bacterial probes can be used to identify specific gram-negative bacilli when these are seen on Gram stain of the positive blood culture bottle. Yeast probes using the same format are available to differentiate among *Candida* spp.

CULTURE TECHNIQUES

Media for culture are selected to provide the optimal conditions for growth of pathogens commonly encountered at a particular site or in a particular type of specimen. Consideration is given to special growth requirements of bacteria associated with a given type of infection, or to the necessity of selecting certain pathogenic bacteria from a mixed population of indigenous flora. Therefore, the media chosen may include selective and differential media, in addition to standard enrichment agar.

Blood-supplemented agar is a good general growth medium and can be used to demonstrate the hemolytic action of colonies on the red blood cells. Antibiotics or chemicals can be added to create a selective medium such as colistin–nalidixic acid (CNA) agar or phenylethyl alcohol agar, both of which are used to inhibit the growth of gram-negative bacilli while permitting gram-positive bacteria to grow. Heating the blood to make chocolate agar and adding vitamin supplements creates an enriched medium with available hemin (X factor) and nicotinamide adenine dinucleotide (V factor) for the isolation of *Haemophilus* spp. and other fastidious bacteria. Gram-negative bacilli may be separated from gram-positive bacilli by using bile salts and dye in a medium such as MacConkey's agar, which additionally divides the colonies into lactose-positive and lactose-negative colonies, thus making it both selective and differential. Guidelines for the selection of media to be used with different types of specimens are provided in Table 57-1.

Bacterial cultures are generally incubated at 35° C and are examined initially after 18–24 hours of incubation. Addition of 5%–10% carbon dioxide (CO_2) may be essential or stimulatory to the growth of *N. gonorrhoeae*, *Haemophilus influenzae*, and *S. pneumoniae*, and should be used whenever feasible. Exceptions to this recommendation are those cultures on differential and selective media in which the pH alteration (which can be affected by added CO_2) is used to differentiate colony types (e.g., xylose-lysine-deoxycholate [XLD] agar, Hektoen enteric [HE] agar).

For recovery of anaerobes, inoculated media should be placed into an anaerobic environment as quickly as possible. Several types of anaerobic culture systems are available. One of these is the anaerobic jar, in which water is added to a CO_2 and hydrogen (H_2) generator package, and oxygen (O_2) is catalytically converted to water with palladium-coated alumina pellets contained in a lid chamber. A modification of this system is a

TABLE 57-1
Guidelines for Media Selection for Various Specimens*

	MEDIA FOR RECOVERY OF AEROBIC AND FACULTATIVELY ANAEROBIC BACTERIA					MEDIA FOR RECOVERY OF ANAEROBIC BACTERIA		
Specimen	**BAP**	**MAC or EMB**	**CBA**	**Broth**[†]	**Other**	**BAP**[‡]	**BBE**	**PEA**
Body cavities					Consider the use of BCB for large volumes of fluids			
Fluids								
Cerebrospinal	X		X	X (for shunt specimens)				
Peritoneal	X	X	X		BCB	X	X	X
Pleural; pericardial	X		X	X	BCB	X		
Synovial	X		X	X	BCB			
Wounds								
Aspirate	X	X	X			X	X	X
Swab[§]	X	X						
Tissue[#]	X	X	X	X		X	X	X
Respiratory Tract								
Sputum	X	X	X					
Throat	X							
Bronchoalveolar lavage	X	X	X		CYE[¶]			
Brush; washings	X	X	X			X[¶]	X[¶]	X[¶]
Nasal	X							
Genitourinary								
Vaginal/rectal for group B			Lim broth	Selective or chromogenic				
Streptococcus (GBS)					GBS media			
Other	X	X	X		GC media**	X	X	X
Cervix					GC media			
Urethra/penis					GC media			
Urine								
Mid void	X	X			Screen; chromagar			
Suprapubic aspirate	X	X						
Feces			X	EB	HE or XLD; Campy			
Eye	X	X	X[††]			X[††]		
Ear; internal aspirate	X	X				X		
Vascular catheters	X							

BAP, Blood agar plate; *BCB,* blood culture bottles; *BBE, Bacteroides* bile esculin agar; *Campy, Campylobacter*-selective medium; *CBA,* chocolate blood agar; *CYE,* charcoal yeast extract, for *Legionella* or *Nocardia* requests; *EB,* enrichment broth, such as GN or Selenite broth, same for rectal swabs, minus the *Campylobacter*-selective culture; *EMB,* eosin methylene blue; *GBS,* group B streptococcus; *GC,* gonococcus; *HE,* Hektoen enteric agar; *Lim broth,* enrichment broth for group B streptococcus; *MAC,* MacConkey's agar; *PEA,* phenylethyl alcohol; *XLD,* xylose-lysine-deoxycholate agar.

*Specific guidelines for individual organisms will be included where they are described in text.

[†]Supplemented thioglycollate in the usual broth; however, for aerobes, a brain-heart infusion may be adequate.

[‡]Consider a CDC BAP or a *Brucella* blood agar, or another "enriched" BAP for anaerobic recovery; a laked blood agar plate with antibiotics may also be appropriate.

[§]Not recommended for anaerobic cultures.

[#]If specific organisms, or situations, other media may be added.

[¶]If a protected bronchoscope is used for collection of the specimen.

**Thayer-Martin or Martin-Lewis or other media enriched for recovery of *N. gonorrhoeae.*

[††]If *Propionibacterium acnes* is suspected in cases of endophthalmitis, a thioglycollate broth and/or anaerobic BAP may be used.

transparent plastic bag containing its own gas generator and palladium catalyst, and designed to hold an agar plate; these are often referred to as anaerobic Bio-Bags.

Another approach to anaerobic culture is the anaerobic glove box or chamber, which consists of a large, clear plastic, air-tight chamber filled with an oxygen-free gas mixture of nitrogen, hydrogen, and carbon dioxide. Specimens, plates, and tubes are introduced into or removed from the chamber through a gas interchange lock. Anaerobiosis is maintained by palladium catalysts and the hydrogen gas in the chamber. All manipulations within the chamber are done with neoprene gloves sealed to the chamber wall or, for "gloveless" systems, through a hole with sleeves that seal tightly around the forearms. The chambers contain internal incubators that maintain the incubation temperature. Each of the anaerobe systems has its advantages and disadvantages, but all are equally effective in isolating clinically significant anaerobic bacteria from specimens. A system for processing anaerobic specimens under a constant anaerobic environnent to reduce the chance of excess exposure to oxygen is available in the Anoxamat system (Summanen, 1999).

Bacterial cultures should be examined routinely after 18–24 hours of incubation. The exception to this is the anaerobe culture, which is generally examined at 48 hours to allow these slower growing bacteria to produce visible colonies. In general, solid media are held for 48 hours, with liquid media held for an additional 24–48 hours. If this is different for specific organisms, it will be mentioned in the text.

A preliminary report is issued when the culture is first examined; this report is updated as additional information becomes available. Certain results (e.g., positive blood or CSF Gram stain, isolation of an organism requiring infection control measures) are reported to the healthcare provider as soon as the information becomes available. Final reports are issued when all work on a culture has been completed.

Medically Important Bacteria

GRAM-POSITIVE COCCI

Staphylococcus

Characteristics

Staphylococci are catalase-positive spherical cocci that often appear in grape-like clusters in stained smears (Fig. 57-2). They grow well on any peptone-containing nutrient medium under aerobic and anaerobic conditions, and may produce hemolysis of various species of animal blood cells and yellow or orange pigment on certain types of agar. Growth of staphylococci is readily detected on blood agar plates or in various types of nutrient broth. A selective medium for the isolation of *S. aureus* is one containing 7.5%–10% sodium chloride (NaCl) with mannitol.

Tests useful for distinguishing staphylococci from *Micrococcus* and *Kocuria* spp. (generally considered nonpathogenic) are listed in Table 57-2 (Bannerman, 2007). *S. aureus* is differentiated from other species of staphylococci principally by its production of coagulases, which are capable of clotting plasma. Two antigenically distinct forms of coagulase have been recognized: one bound to the cell wall is called clumping factor and is detected with the slide coagulase test, and the other is free from the cell wall and is detected with the tube coagulase test (often considered the definitive test for the presence of coagulase enzyme). Commercial latex agglutination products are available that detect clumping factor and protein A in *S. aureus* with good sensitivity and specificity. These assays may be appropriate in situations in which reproducibility of the test is in question because of the inexperience of technologists performing the assay. A FISH product (*S. aureus* peptide nucleic acid FISH) is also available for the differentiation of *S. aureus* from coagulase-negative staphylococci in a blood culture bottle found positive for gram-positive cocci in clusters. In addition, many laboratories are now utilizing polymerase chain reaction (PCR) assays for detection of *S. aureus* in nasal swabs and directly from positive blood culture bottles. Many of these assays enable detection of methicillin-resistant *S. aureus* (MRSA) versus methicillin-susceptible *S. aureus*.

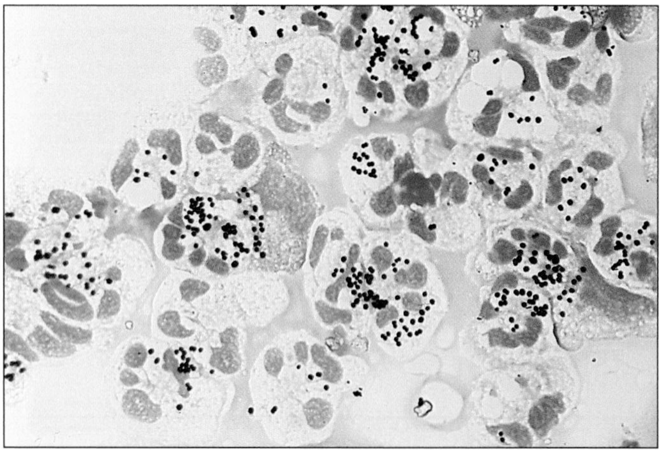

Figure 57-2 Cytocentrifuge preparation of cerebrospinal fluid stained with Gram stain shows many neutrophils, smooth amorphous material, and gram-positive cocci in pairs, short chains, and clusters, suggestive of staphylococcal infection (oil immersion).

TABLE 57-2
Tests Differentiating Staphylococci from Micrococci and *Kocuria* spp.

	Staphylococcus spp.	*Micrococcus* spp.	*Kocuria* spp.
Lysostaphin susceptibility	S	R	R
Aerobic acid production from glycerol	+	–	+
Anaerobic acid production from glucose	+/–	–	Delayed +
Lysozyme (50-µg disk)	R	S	ND
Bacitracin susceptibility (0.04 U)	R	S	S
Modified oxidase	–	+	+

Adapted from Bannerman TL, Peacock SJ. *Staphylococcus, Micrococcus,* and other catalase-positive cocci. In: Murray PR, Baron EJ, Jorgensen JH, et al, editors. Manual of clinical microbiology. 9th ed. Washington, DC: American Society for Microbiology; 2007, p. 391.

+, Positive result; –, negative result; *ND,* not done; *R,* resistant; *S,* susceptible.

Clinical Manifestations and Pathogenesis

S. aureus may be present among the indigenous flora of the skin, eye, upper respiratory tract, gastrointestinal tract, urethra, and, infrequently, vagina. Therefore, infection may arise from an endogenous or an exogenous source. Factors of importance in the development of infection due to *S. aureus* include breaks in the continuity and integrity of mucosal and cutaneous surfaces, the presence of foreign bodies or implants, prior viral diseases, antecedent antimicrobial therapy, and underlying diseases with defects in cellular or humoral immunity.

Infections caused by *S. aureus* may affect multiple organ systems. Among the most common are those involving the skin and its appendages, such as impetigo, folliculitis, mastitis, and infection of surgical wounds. *S. aureus* is among the leading causes of bacteremia in hospitalized patients, and it may cause endocarditis, particularly in persons with left-sided valvular heart disease and in intravenous drug users. *S. aureus* is the most common cause of spinal epidural abscess and suppurative intracranial phlebitis, and may be recovered from brain abscesses, typically following trauma. Meningitis caused by *S. aureus* is uncommon and generally follows head trauma or a neurosurgical procedure.

S. aureus is responsible for many cases of osteomyelitis, is the most common cause of septic arthritis in prepubertal children, and is occasionally responsible for septic arthritis in adults. *S. aureus* is an infrequent cause of community-acquired pneumonia but a common cause of nosocomial pneumonia, which usually follows aspiration of endogenous nasopharyngeal organisms. Predisposing factors include infection with measles or influenza A virus, cystic fibrosis, and immune deficiency. Urinary tract infections caused by *S. aureus* are rare, but cases of pyelonephritis and intrarenal and perirenal abscesses can be found.

Several factors play a role in the virulence of *S. aureus*. The capsule, if present, has antiphagocytic properties. Cell wall peptidoglycans have endotoxin-like activity, stimulating the release of cytokines by macrophages, activation of complement, and aggregation of platelets. Protein A, an immunologically active substance in the cell wall, has antiphagocytic properties that are based on its ability to bind the Fc fragment of immunoglobulin (Ig)G. Other surface proteins, designated as microbial surface components recognizing adhesive matrix molecules, may play an important role in the ability of staphylococci to colonize host tissues (Speziale, 2009).

S. aureus produces numerous toxins. The exotoxin TSST-1 is responsible for toxic shock syndrome, and enterotoxins A–E are responsible for staphylococcal food poisoning. The exfoliative toxins—epidermolytic toxins A and B—cause skin erythema and separation, as seen in scalded skin syndrome. Various enzymes are also produced, including protease, lipase, and hyaluronidase, all of which destroy tissue and probably function to facilitate the spread of the infection.

Toxin-mediated diseases caused by *S. aureus* include scalded skin syndrome, food poisoning, and toxic shock syndrome. Scalded skin syndrome occurs in infants infected with a strain of *S. aureus* producing exfoliative toxin. The illness begins abruptly with erythema, followed in 2–3 days by the formation of flaccid bullae, which slough, leaving denuded areas that eventually resolve completely. Staphylococcal food poisoning, characterized by nausea, vomiting, abdominal cramps, and diarrhea, occurs 1–6 hours after ingestion of foods contaminated with pre-formed staphylococcal enterotoxin.

Toxic shock syndrome is a multisystem disease affecting individuals who have no antibodies to TSST-1 and are colonized or infected with strains of *S. aureus* producing TSST-1 or rarely enterotoxin B or C. The illness is most common in women 15–25 years of age who use tampons during menstruation, but it also may occur in nonmenstruating individuals, including women in the postpartum period, persons with a surgical wound or other focal infection, and individuals who have had a surgical procedure in the nose or sinuses. Toxic shock syndrome begins abruptly with fever, myalgias, vomiting, and diarrhea, followed by hypotension, hypovolemic shock, and an erythematous rash that frequently involves the palms and soles and desquamates in 1–2 weeks. The diagnosis is clinical; isolation of

S. aureus from any site is not required. Full recovery is the rule, although repeated episodes may occur (Bannerman, 2007).

Over the past 8–10 years, cases of community-acquired infection with *S. aureus* that are oxacillin resistant (CA-MRSA) have become more common. In these isolates, a toxin referred to as Panton-Valentine leukocidin toxin (PVL), which has rarely been associated with hospital-acquired strains of *S. aureus* (Vandenesch, 2003; Klein, 2009; Lindsay, 2009), has been found. PVL has been shown to be responsible for necrotizing skin and soft tissue infections and has been infrequently demonstrated to cause a necrotizing and occasionally fatal pneumonia (Francis, 2005; Moskowitz, 2009). Individuals at risk are predominantly children involved in contact sports and those living in institutions such as prisons (MMWR, 2003; Pan, 2003). These CA-MRSA strains, unlike hospital-acquired strains of MRSA (HA-MRSA), are often susceptible to non–β-lactam classes of antibiotics. HA-MRSA strains are usually resistant to all antibiotics except the glycopeptides, such as vancomycin. The mechanism of oxacillin resistance is the same in CA-MRSA and HA-MRSA—the presence of an *mecA* gene that is responsible for production of a new penicillin-binding protein (PBP-2a or PBP-2′). However, the chromosomal cassette that houses the CA-MRSA *mecA* gene is different from and much smaller than that containing the *mecA* gene of HA-MRSA. Many experts believe that in time, blending of CA-MRSA and HA-MRSA strains will occur, and without molecular typing of any isolate, it will be difficult to distinguish them.

Infections caused by coagulase-negative species (CNS) of *Staphylococcus* usually occur in association with foreign bodies, especially implanted prosthetic valves, joints, and shunts. More than 20 species of CNS are known, of which *S. epidermidis* is the species most frequently involved in such infections. *S. saprophyticus* is an important cause of bacteriuria, particularly among sexually active young women. *S. hemolyticus*, although a relatively rare isolate in clinical specimens, can be resistant to vancomycin, an agent to which most CNS are susceptible. *S. lugdunensis* is a species of CNS that can appear morphologically similar to *S. aureus* (i.e., in production of a narrow zone of β-hemolysis on blood agar plates) and on occasion will be coagulase positive in some assays for coagulase. However, it is usually classified as a coagulase-negative staphylococcus. Clinically, it will act more aggressively than most other CNS and in this way mimics *S. aureus* infection, including its role as an agent of endocarditis, osteomyelitis, and other more severe staphylococcal infections. It is important to distinguish *S. lugdunensis* from other CNS because the breakpoints one uses (according to the Clinical Laboratory and Standards Institute [CLSI]) for the interpretation of susceptibility results versus oxacillin (or cefoxitin) should be those that are used to interpret *S. aureus* and not those used to interpret breakpoints for oxacillin (or cefoxitin) vs. CNS. (CLSI, 2010).

Laboratory Diagnosis

The observation microscopically of typical rounded, gram-positive cocci in clusters in smears of material taken from previously unopened or undrained lesions, or in smears of broth from a positive blood culture, is indicative of staphylococcal infection.

S. aureus produces coagulase, an enzyme that binds plasma fibrinogen, causing the organisms to agglutinate or plasma to clot; only rare strains of other staphylococci are coagulase positive. More than 95% of isolates of *S. aureus* are identified by the slide coagulase test, which detects cell-bound enzyme (clumping factor); nearly 100% of all isolates are identified by tube coagulase tests, which detect free coagulase (Bannerman, 2007).

The slide coagulase test is performed by mixing a dense emulsion of the organism with plasma on a glass slide. The test is positive if clumping occurs within 30 seconds. *Staphylococcus lugdunensis* and *Staphylococcus schleiferi* are two other staphylococci that may give a positive result with this slide coagulase test. A control that consists of emulsifying the suspect colony in saline should be run with each slide test to ensure that autoagglutination does not occur. If autoagglutination is present, slide test results should be considered insufficient for determination of the coagulase nature of the isolate.

For the tube coagulase test, several colonies are transferred into a tube containing plasma that is incubated at 35° C for 4 hours and then is examined for clot formation. If no clot has formed, the tube is reincubated at room temperature and reexamined after a total of 24 hours of incubation. The test should be examined after 4 hours because most isolates of *S. aureus* produce a clot within this interval, but some strains produce a fibrinolysin that can lyse the clot, thus producing a false-negative reaction if the test is observed only after 24 hours. *Staphylococcus intermedius* and *Staphylococcus hyicus* will also be positive with the tube coagulase test, but they are primarily pathogens of animals and are encountered only rarely in human specimens.

Several commercial latex agglutination assays are available for rapid identification of *S. aureus*. These assays detect protein A and clumping factor; some also detect capsular polysaccharide, which may improve the ability to detect methicillin (oxacillin)-resistant *S. aureus*. *S. saprophyticus* and *Staphylococcus sciuri* are two other staphylococcus species that may be latex agglutination positive, along with the rare *Micrococcus* spp.; however, these should all be slide coagulase negative (Bannerman, 2007).

Many species of coagulase-negative staphylococcus have been recognized; however, with the exception of *S. saprophyticus*, which is resistant to novobiocin, identification of these isolates to the species level is not practical or clinically indicated in every culture. Speciation may be needed if isolates are found repeatedly in sterile sites, if *S. lugdunensis* is being ruled out, and/or if correlation between isolates in a patient is being sought to increase the likelihood that the two isolates are the same and therefore are potentially clinically relevant. If necessary, attempts to identify these isolates to the species level may be made using commercially available identification kits, which have been found to have an accuracy of between 70% and more than 90% (Bannerman, 2007). Alternatively, isolates may be sent to a reference laboratory capable of performing standard biochemical assays or molecular assays such as 16S ribosomal RNA (rRNA) analysis (Lee, 2001). Staphylococci may be classified into strains for epidemiologic purposes in attempting to identify common sources of infection on the basis of their susceptibility to different bacteriophages, plasmid profiles, cellular fatty acids, electrophoresis of multilocus enzymes, or chromosomal molecular typing (pulsed field gel electrophoresis and repetitive PCR). These tests are generally available only through reference laboratories.

Antimicrobial Susceptibility

More than 90% of staphylococci are resistant to penicillin. Because resistance is due to an inducible plasmid-encoded β-lactamase, sensitivity to penicillin should be confirmed after a period of induction (CLSI, 2009) with a β-lactam agent.

Resistance to the penicillinase-resistant penicillins (methicillin, oxacillin, nafcillin) occurs in up to 80% of coagulase-negative staphylococci, and in more than 50% of isolates of hospital-acquired *S. aureus*. Resistance to this group of antimicrobial agents is mediated by the *mecA* gene, which encodes an altered penicillin-binding protein, PBP-2a. Resistance typically is heterogeneous, meaning that only rare cells (1 in 10^4–10^8) express the resistance trait. Because of this, specific guidelines must be followed to ensure detection: A 1-μg oxacillin disk has been used traditionally for disk diffusion testing. More recently, the CLSI has suggested that if disk diffusion is used as the method of detection of MRSA, a 30-μg cefoxitin disk test is a better indicator than oxacillin. To predict the presence of *mecA*-mediated resistance in *S. aureus* (and *S. lugdunensis*), the CLSI recommends that isolates with zone sizes ≥22 mm can be reported as susceptible (S), and those with zone sizes ≤21 mm can be reported as oxacillin resistant (R) (Velasco, 2005). For coagulase-negative staphylococci (except *S. lugdunensis*), ≥25 mm = S and ≤24 mm = R (CLSI, 2009). Oxacillin in cation-supplemented Mueller-Hinton broth containing 2% NaCl should be used for microdilution testing, and agar plates and microtiter trays should be incubated a full 24 hours at 35° C. To screen isolates of *S. aureus* for oxacillin resistance, Mueller-Hinton agar supplemented with 4% NaCl and containing 6 μg/mL of oxacillin is spot inoculated with a cotton swab, and plates are incubated for 24 hours at 35° C. CLSI recommends that cefoxitin be considered as the antibiotic used to detect oxacillin resistance, even when broth microdilution is performed, but in all cases, reports should contain results for oxacillin, not for cefoxitin. To screen isolates of *S. aureus* for oxacillin resistance, Mueller-Hinton agar supplemented with 4% NaCl and containing 6 μg/mL of oxacillin is spot inoculated with a cotton swab, and plates are incubated for 24 hours. Any growth on this screening medium suggests an MRSA, and further testing should be done for confirmation.

Several assays have been developed for rapid detection of oxacillin resistance. These include nucleic acid amplification, nucleic acid probe assays for *mecA*, and latex agglutination assays for PBP-2a (the MRSA Screen Test, Denka-Seiken Co., Tokyo, Japan) and PBP-2′ (Oxoid Ltd., Basingstoke, UK) (Chediac-Tannoury, 2003; Chapin, 2004). For detection of MRSA on nasal swabs, two approaches can be used. Newer chromogenic media specific for the detection of MRSA require overnight incubation but allow easy detection of specific colored colonies that are (Perry, 2004). Gene-Ohm (Becton Dickinson Microbiology Systems, Sparks, Md.) has a PCR-based assay, run on the Smart Cycler instrument (Cepheid, Sacramento, Calif.), that can detect MRSA directly in clinical specimens within 90 minutes (Warren, 2004). Both Gene-OHM and Cepheid have assays for the molecular detection of *S. aureus* and MRSA in clinical specimens and from positive blood cultures. Other molecular assays are being developed as well. Although oxacillin-resistant staphylococci may appear to be susceptible to cephalosporins, they should be considered resistant to all β-lactam agents (penicillins and cephalosporins), including carbapenems. Hospital-acquired strains usually are resistant to many non–β-lactam antibiotics as well. The newly recognized CA-MRSA strains still remain susceptible to most non–β-lactam antibiotics (Daum, 2002).

Clindamycin may be used to treat staphylococcal infection. Inducible resistance, due to mechanisms involving a class of enzyme-inactivating genes referred to as *erm* genes, may not be detected in routine susceptibility testing. This *erm* gene also confers cross-resistance to the macrolides (e.g., erythromycin) and streptogramins (quinupristin-dalfopristin). An isolate of *S. aureus* that is resistant to erythromycin but susceptible to clindamycin in a minimum inhibitory concentration (MIC) test (broth or agar dilution or E-test) should be evaluated for inducible resistance to clindamycin by the "**D-zone**" test, as follows. A 15-μg erythromycin disk and a 2-μg clindamycin disk are placed 15mm apart on the surface of a blood agar plate inoculated with the isolate in question. After overnight incubation, if there is inducible resistance to clindamycin, blunting of the clindamycin zone of inhibition will be seen on the side near the erythromycin disk, giving the appearance of a D zone (CLSI, 2009).

Vancomycin resistance, although rarely seen in *S. aureus*, is a serious issue that laboratories need to be aware of and should screen for. Isolates of vancomycin intermediately susceptible *S. aureus* (VISA) have MICs in the intermediate range (8–16 μg/mL) (Cosgrove, 2004). A number of cases of vancomycin-resistant *S. aureus* with vancomycin MICs as high as 1024 μg/mL have been reported (Centers for Disease Control and Prevention [CDC], 2004b). Because the latter have not been uniformly detected in automated systems for susceptibility testing, the CDC recommends that all *S. aureus* isolates tested on an automated instrument should also be tested by a vancomycin screen assay, to ensure that the correct MIC is determined. This is usually done by inoculating 100 μL of a 0.5 McFarland suspension of *S. aureus* to a blood agar plate containing 6 μg/mL of vancomycin, and incubating overnight. Most automated susceptibility testing systems have been adjusted to detect vancomycin-resistant *S. aureus* (VRSA), if present; however, detection of VISA is still variable among systems—both automated and manual. Newer breakpoints have been implemented in which an MIC of 4 to vancomycin should be considered representative of a possible VISA, and further testing with microbroth dilution should be performed for confirmation. Screen-positive isolates that have elevated vancomycin MIC values (≥8 organisms μg/mL) should be sent to a reference laboratory for confirmation, and confirmed cases should be referred to your state health department and the CDC. The entity of hVISA (strains of *S. aureus* that are variable within the population or colony for vancomycin nonsusceptibility) is difficult for a routine clinical microbiology laboratory to detect. If a strain with an MIC of 2 μg/mL to vancomycin is being clinically considered nonresponsive to vancomycin, a macro E-test can be performed, employing a McFarland of 2.0 instead of the usual 0.5, and inner colonies can be looked for. Exposure of suspected isolates to increasing concentrations of vancomycin in agar plates, however, is the recommended approach for detection of hVISA, although these methods are often beyond what a routine laboratory can do (Bae, 2009).

Newer antimicrobial agents have good activity against susceptible and resistant staphylococci. These include quinupristin/dalfopristin, a streptogramin, the lipopeptide daptomycin, linezolid, and most recently televancin. For isolates of VISA, or VRSA, or when clinicians request agents other than vancomycin for MRSA strains, laboratories should consider testing these agents or sending the isolates to reference laboratories that can test for their susceptibility.

Streptococcus and *Enterococcus*

Characteristics

Streptococci are catalase-negative, gram-positive, spherical, ovoid, or lancet-shaped cocci, often seen in pairs or chains. They are facultatively anaerobic. Some strains require added CO_2 for their initial isolation but may lose this requirement in subcultures. Streptococci can be broadly classified according to the hemolytic reaction on blood agar (Table 57-3). Those strains that completely hemolyze the red cells around their colonies are called β-hemolytic and can be further categorized into the Lancefield groups based on serologically reactive carbohydrates. Important members of this group include *Streptococcus pyogenes* (group A) and *Streptococcus agalactiae* (group B). Figure 57-3 is a Gram stain of *S. pyogenes* (group A streptococcus) in a specimen from abscess material on the arm of a patient with cellulitis. Those gram-positive cocci in chains that produce partial hemolysis (cause "greening" of the agar) are α-hemolytic. An important member of this group is *S. pneumoniae*. Streptococci that do not hemolyze blood are γ-hemolytic. An important member of this group is *Streptococcus bovis* complex. Some *S. agalactiae* may also be γ-hemolytic. Most of the remainder of the α- and γ-hemolytic streptococci are collectively called **viridans** streptococci, including *Streptococcus mutans*, *Streptococcus sanguis*, *Streptococcus mitis*, *Streptococcus salivarius*, and *Streptococcus anginosus*. The group of organisms previously referred to as nutritionally variant (pyridoxal or thiol dependent, satelliting) streptococci have now been assigned to the genus *Abiotrophia* or *Granulicatella*.

TABLE 57-3
Classification of Streptococci and Enterococci

Hemolysis	Lancefield group	Species
β	A	*Streptococcus pyogenes*
	B	*Streptococcus agalactiae*
	C	*Streptococcus dysgalactiae*
	D	*Enterococcus* spp.
α or γ	D	*Enterococcus* spp.
	D	*Streptococcus bovis complex* (reclassified into at least four new species as described in text)
	None	Viridans group*
α	None	*Streptococcus pneumoniae*

*Small colony variants of Lancefield group A, C, F, or G, or nongroupable strains, can be any hemolysis.

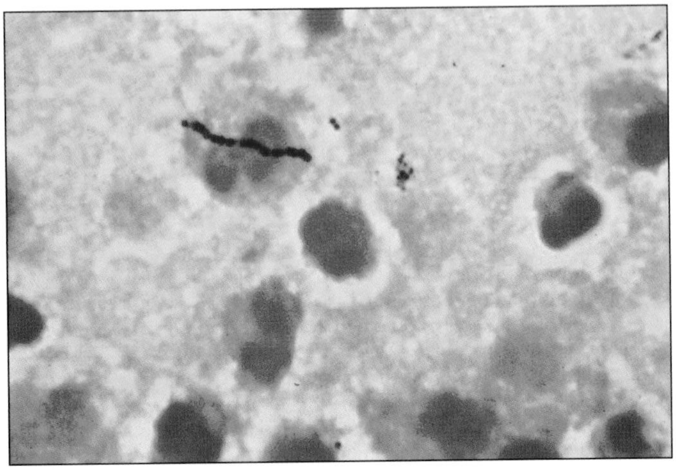

Figure 57-3 Gram stain of *Streptococcus pyogenes* (group A streptococcus) from a case of cellulitis.

Members of the genus *Enterococcus*, previously designated as group D streptococci because their cell wall antigens reacted with group D antisera, are sufficiently different from the other members of the genus *Streptococcus* to be considered a separate genus. These organisms are gram-positive cocci that occur singly, in pairs, and in short chains. They are facultatively anaerobic. Most enterococci are α- or γ-hemolytic on blood agar, but some may exhibit β-hemolysis. The most common species are *Enterococcus faecium* and *Enterococcus faecalis*; yellow motile strains of the enterococci, usually nonpathogenic, include *Enterococcus cassilflavus* and *Enterococcus gallinarum*. These latter two species are usually intrinsically vancomycin resistant, and it is important to differentiate them from vancomycin-resistant *E. faecium* or *E. faecalis*.

Other genera of catalase-negative gram-positive cocci that may be isolated from clinical specimens include *Leuconostoc*, *Pediococcus*, *Stomatococcus* (Rothia), *Gemella*, *Aerococcus*, and *Lactococcus* spp. These organisms are considered to have low virulence potential and generally are pathogenic only in the compromised host. However, some of these isolates may be confused with viridans streptococci, in particular, and their differentiation is important because of their lower virulence and their potential for vancomycin resistance. Further differentiation should be considered if a vancomycin-resistant viridans streptococcus is thought to be clinically relevant.

Clinical Manifestations and Pathogenesis

One of the most common clinical manifestations of group A streptococci is pharyngitis. This may be accompanied by scarlet fever, a punctate exanthem overlying diffuse erythema that usually first appears on the neck or upper chest, becomes generalized, and then desquamates. Skin infections caused by group A streptococcus include cellulitis, erysipelas, and pyoderma. Acute rheumatic fever, characterized by carditis, polyarthritis, erythema marginatum, chorea, and subcutaneous nodules, may occur 1–5 weeks after group A streptococcal pharyngitis. Acute glomerulonephritis may develop 10 days–3 weeks after group A streptococcal pharyngitis or pyoderma.

Beginning in the late 1980s, serious group A streptococcal clinical syndromes, including necrotizing fasciitis, myositis, malignant scarlet fever, bacteremia, and toxic shock–like syndrome, began to be seen with increasing frequency. These have been associated with high morbidity rates and mortality rates of up to 30% or more. The reason for this increase is not completely understood but appears to be related to changes in the prevalence of organisms having an enhanced **virulence potential** (Kaplan, 2005; Vucicevic, 2008; Lappin, 2009).

S. pyogenes produces numerous virulence factors. One of the most important is the antiphagocytic cell wall M protein. Antibodies against the specific M protein confer lifelong type-specific immunity; however, because more than 60 M protein types exist, infection with a group A streptococcus possessing a different M protein may occur. Another important cell wall component is lipoteichoic acid, which permits bacterial adherence to the respiratory epithelium. *S. pyogenes* also elaborates about 20 extracellular products, including enzymes (streptolysins, hyaluronidase, streptokinase, deoxyribonucleases [DNases], and nicotinamide adenine dinucleotidase [NADase]) and erythrogenic toxins. Streptolysin O, an antigenic, oxygen-labile enzyme, produces subsurface hemolysis on blood agar plates; streptolysin S, a nonantigenic, oxygen-stable enzyme, produces surface hemolysis. Neither streptolysin has a proven role in the pathogenesis of human disease. Streptokinase promotes fibrinolytic activity by converting plasminogen to plasmin, and hyaluronidase may enhance the spread of the organism through connective tissue. The pathogenic significance of the DNases and of NADase is unknown. Pyrogenic (erythrogenic) toxins (serotypes A, B, C) are produced by isolates of *S. pyogenes* infected with a specific temperate bacteriophage. Their pyrogenicity is caused by a direct action on the hypothalamus. Streptococcus group A has also been found to possess superantigens with high mitogenic capabilities; these have been associated with cases of more severe streptococcal infection, such as necrotizing fasciitis or toxic shock syndrome (Kotb, 2002).

The pathogenesis of acute rheumatic fever is not fully understood. Certain M protein types of *S. pyogenes* may be rheumatogenic. The presence of complexes of immunoglobulin and the C3 component of complement along the sarcolemmal sheaths of cardiac myofibers from individuals with rheumatic carditis suggests that myocarditis results from the production of antibodies directed against a streptococcal cell wall M protein that cross-reacts with myocardial tissue. Moreover, a heart or tissue cross-reactive antigen of *S. pyogenes* that shares immunologic epitopes with, but is distinct from, the M protein has been identified (Barnett, 1990). Renal damage in acute glomerulonephritis is caused by deposits of circulating streptococcal–antistreptococcal immune complexes in the glomeruli and subsequent activation of complement. Cell-mediated reactions to an altered glomerular basement membrane or activation of the alternate complement pathway also may be involved. Isolates of *S. pyogenes* have been linked to toxic shock syndrome,with a clinical picture very similar to *S. aureus*; streptococcal pyrogenic exotoxins are thought to be responsible for the toxic shock–like syndrome caused by strains of *S. pyogenes* (Schlievert, 1993; Stevens, 1995).

The most common infections caused by group B streptococci are neonatal sepsis, pneumonia, and meningitis. Colonization of the maternal genital tract is associated with colonization of infants and risk of neonatal disease, with early-onset infections occurring within the first few days after delivery and late-onset infections appearing after 1 week of age. To reduce the incidence of neonatal disease, the CDC published specific guidelines to facilitate early identification and treatment of women colonized with group B streptococcus and identification and treatment of neonates at risk for developing disease (Schuchat, 1996; Centers for Disease Control, 2004a; CDC, 2009,2010; VanDyke, 2009). All pregnant women at 35–37 weeks of gestation should have vaginal/rectal specimens collected and processed for detection of group B streptococcus. Results of this test should be available during labor, so appropriate prophylaxis can be given to the mother before delivery, to prevent infection to the newborn. Isolation of group B streptococci from the urine of a pregnant female can also be used as a marker of group B streptococcal vaginal carriage, and this information should be used to direct prophylaxis to mothers found to be positive. If urine is positive, screening of vaginal/rectal cultures may not be necessary. Group B streptococcal infections in adults include postpartum endometritis, urinary tract infection, bacteremia, skin and soft tissue infections, pneumonia, endocarditis, meningitis, arthritis, and osteomyelitis.

Group C and G streptococci are similar to *S. pyogenes* in that they cause a wide range of infections, including bacteremia, endocarditis, meningitis, arthritis, and respiratory and skin infections. The pharyngeal infection caused by these streptococci is similar to that of group A streptococci, except that the nonsuppurative sequelae of rheumatic fever do not occur.

Infections caused by *S. pneumoniae* include pneumonia, meningitis (especially in infants and the elderly), spontaneous bacteremia (in persons who do not have a spleen), otitis, sinusitis, and spontaneous peritonitis. *S. pneumoniae* is seen in normal flora of the upper respiratory tract of 25%–50% of preschool children, 36% of primary school-aged children, and nearly 20% of adults, termed carriers (Lopez, 1999). Its spread is enhanced by upper respiratory tract infections and crowding. Pneumonia may develop when the host immune defenses are impaired. Most cases are endogenous, following aspiration of oral secretions containing normal flora that includes *S. pneumoniae*. Person-to-person transmission during epidemics occurs by droplet aerosols. The major virulence factor of *S. pneumoniae* is its antiphagocytic polysaccharide capsule, and strains with a thick, mucoid capsule are especially virulent. Vaccines designed to protect against infection by pneumococci of many of the predominant capsular polysaccharide types are available. A new vaccine is available for use in infants and children to prevent invasive pneumococcal disease.

Bacterial endocarditis is the most common infection caused by viridans streptococci; others include abscesses in the brain or liver, bacteremia, and dental caries. The milleri streptococci complex (*S. constellatus*, *S. intermedius*, and *S. anginosus*) consists of the most common viridans streptococci responsible for liver, spleen, and brain abscesses; they often are more susceptible to antibiotics than other strains of viridans streptococci, although resistance to penicillin is increasingly being recognized. *S. bovis* bacteremia has been associated with malignancies of the gastrointestinal tract. *S. bovis* is now recognized as a complex of strains and/or species. Differentiation remains difficult within the species. Presently, the two subtypes of *S. bovis* have been renamed. *S. gallolyticus* and *S. pasteurianus* are isolated from blood cultures of patients with colonic cancer more often than is *S. infantarius* or *S. lutetiensis*. In many laboratories, isolates are still reported as *S. bovis* because phenotypic identification may not be adequate for differentiation; as molecular methods of identification increase, more of these differences may be appreciated (Facklam, 2002).

Enterococci are not highly pathogenic; however, they are a common cause of urinary tract infection in hospitalized persons. They may also cause endocarditis, bacteremia, and wound infection. Vancomycin-resistant enterococci offer a greater potential for infection, especially in immunocompromised patients and patients with implanted foreign devices (Han, 2009; McBride, 2009).

More and more clinically relevant cases of *Aerococcus urinae* (and other species of aerococci) are being reported. Urinary tract infections are most common, but rare cases of more serious infection, including bacteremia, are seen (Zhang, 2000). *A. viridans* remains relatively uncommon as a pathogen, when isolated from clinical samples; *A. sanguinicola* isolation is not always associated with clinical disease, but case numbers are increasing (Ibler, 2008).

Laboratory Diagnosis

Streptococci grow well on blood or chocolate agar. Blood agar is preferred because the hemolytic properties of the organism can be assessed. When culturing vaginal/rectal swabs from pregnant women specifically for group B streptococci, specimens should first be inoculated to a selective broth, such as Lim or carrot broth, or on to selective agar, for example, Granada agar, to enrich for this organism (Spellerberg, 2007; Church, 2008; Carvalho, 2009). Tests that may be used in the clinical microbiology laboratory to presumptively name the β-hemolytic species of *Streptococcus* are shown in Figure 57-4. More than 99% of isolates of group A streptococcus are susceptible to bacitracin, but a very small percentage of isolates of group B streptococcus and 10%–20% of isolates of groups C and G streptococcus are also susceptible. Therefore results of the bacitracin susceptibility test provide a presumptive identification. An isolate may be called group A streptococcus presumptively, based on hydrolysis of the L-pyrrolidonyl-β-naphthylamide (PYRase) test (Spellerberg, 2007). All

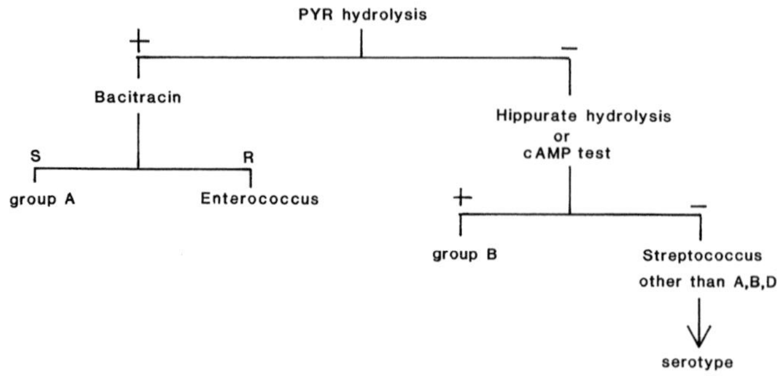

Figure 57-4 Decision tree of tests to presumptively name the β-hemolytic species of *Streptococcus*. *(With permission from Woods GL, Gutierez Y. Diagnostic pathology of infectious diseases. Philadelphia: Lea & Febiger; 1993.)* +, Positive result; −, negative result; *R*, resistant; *S*, susceptible.

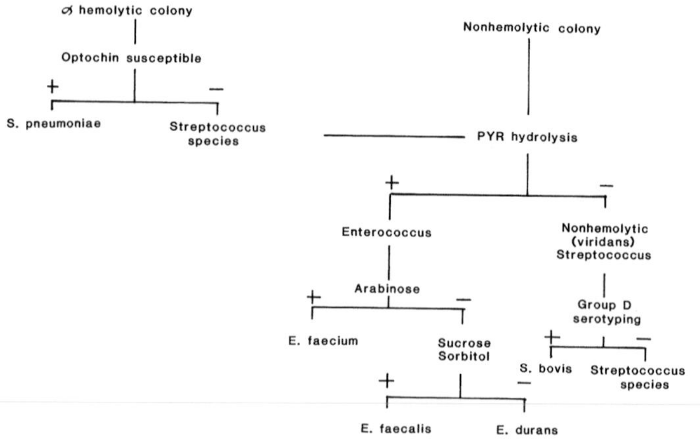

Figure 57-5 Decision tree of tests to presumptively name the α-hemolytic species of Streptococcus and Enterococcus. *(With permission from Woods GL, Gutierez Y. Diagnostic pathology of infectious diseases. Philadelphia: Lea & Febiger; 1993.)* +, Positive result; −, negative result; *R*, resistant; *S*, susceptible.

isolates of group A streptococcus and more than 99% of isolates of *Enterococcus* are PYRase-positive. Identification of group A streptococcus is confirmed by serotyping, using latex agglutination, or using a nucleic acid probe. A nucleic acid probe (Gen-Probe, San Diego) is also available for direct detection of group A streptococcus on throat swabs (Chapin, 2002).

Group A streptococcus may be detected directly in throat swab specimens by using commercial kits designed to generate a rapid result. These tests are highly specific but, given their low sensitivity, which varies among studies from 31%–95% (Wegner, 1992; Carroll, 1996), a negative direct test should be followed by culture or probe. Serologic tests to detect antibodies in acute and convalescent serum samples to streptolysin O and DNase B are used primarily to diagnose acute rheumatic fever and acute glomerulonephritis following infection with group A streptococcus.

Cultures found positive for colonies that are β-hemolytic and hippurate hydrolysis positive and/or that have a positive CAMP test (named for researchers Christie, Atkins, and Munch-Petersen) reaction presumptively can be called group B streptococcus. Isolates of presumed group B streptococcus from sterile body sites should be identified by serotyping (using latex agglutination or coagglutination tests) or by using a chemiluminescent DNA probe. The DNA probe can also be used to identify group B streptococci growing in Lim broth or other selective broth cultures (Daly, 1991; Bourbeau, 1997). This probe, however, is not sensitive enough to use directly on clinical specimens for the detection of group B streptococcus. For culture of vaginal/rectal swab specimens from pregnant women during weeks 35 through 37 of gestation, it is recommended that a broth enrichment be used along with or as a replacement for agar-based media. Selective broth media including Lim broth, selective Todd Hewitt broth, or a commercially available Trans Vag broth supplemented with 5% sheep blood (Remel, Lenexa, Kan.) can be used as enrichment media (Heelan, 2005). Chromogenic broth, including carrot broth media, can be used as enrichment broth; colonies of β-hemolytic group B streptococcus will convert the color of the tube from clear to yellow or orange. However, nonhemolytic group B streptococcus will not change the tube color, and when used, a negative broth would still need to be planted onto solid media for recovery of these strains.

In addition, a selective nonchromogenic enrichment broth can be subcultured to Granada agar, on which colonies of group B streptococcus will appear yellow to orange for ease in detection. Isolates of β-hemolytic groups C, D, F, and G *Streptococcus* are identified by serotyping with latex agglutination reagents. The Smart Cycler assay mentioned earlier can be used to detect group B streptococcus directly in vaginal-rectal specimens, or can be used to detect group B streptococcus in culture, such as Lim or carrot broth (Picard, 2004; Block, 2008), with commercial PCR kits from GeneOHM or Cepheid. The Cepheid GeneXpert GBS assay can be performed directly on clinical vaginal/rectal samples and has the potential to provide results intrapartum. There are other nucleic acid amplification assays for the detection of group B streptococcus in vaginal/rectal samples that are rapidly becoming FDA cleared for use in clinical laboratories.

Latex agglutination assays are available for direct detection of group B streptococcus (as well as *S. pneumoniae*, some serotypes of *N. meningitidis*, *E. coli*, and *H. influenzae* type b) in CSF, serum, and urine. These assays have been shown to have sensitivities equivalent to or lower than a Gram stain and may give false-positive results; hence, they do not in general provide additional useful information above that provided by the CSF Gram stain, and hence do not add clinical utility. The rapid bacterial antigen tests are much more expensive and labor intensive than Gram stain; most laboratories no longer offer these tests or strictly limit their use (Maxson, 1994; Thomas, 1994; Perkins, 1995).

Tests used to presumptively identify α- and γ-hemolytic streptococci and enterococci are shown in Figure 57-5. α-Hemolytic colonies that are mucoid or flattened with a depressed center are suggestive of *S. pneumonia;* they should be tested for susceptibility to ethylhydroxycupreine hydrochloride, more commonly called optochin (P disk), and are positive for bile solubility. *S. pneumoniae* is susceptible to both; other α-hemolytic streptococci are resistant to optochin and are variable in response to bile. A urinary antigen assay for detection of *S. pneumoniae* has been shown in some studies to be the nonculture diagnostic method of choice for patients with severe pneumococcal infection, for diagnosis of pneumococcal exacerbation in chronic obstructive pulmonary disease patients, and as a tool for diagnosis of otitis media. As with any antigen assay, caution needs to be taken in interpreting results in cases where prior infection with *S. pneumoniae* may have occurred and the antigen may merely be reflecting this (Gisselsson-Solen, 2007; Andreo, 2009; Smith, 2009).

α-Hemolytic colonies that are not *S. pneumoniae* and γ-hemolytic colonies are tested for PYRase hydrolysis; enterococci are PYRase positive, and viridans streptococci are negative. Moreover, all enterococci grow in the presence of 6.5% NaCl; viridans streptococci do not. Enterococci hydrolyze esculin in the presence of bile (causing visible growth and blackening of the agar), but up to 10% of viridans streptococci are also bile–esculin positive. Additional biochemical assays are required to identify enterococci to the species level (Facklam, 2002). Most clinical isolates are *E. faecalis*. A majority of vancomycin-resistant enterococci (VRE) are *E. faecium*.

α-Hemolytic streptococci that are optochin resistant and PYRase negative and γ-hemolytic streptococci that are PYRase negative and do not grow in 6.5% NaCl are grouped as nonhemolytic (viridans) streptococci. Identification of individual species of viridans streptococci requires conventional biochemical testing. Kit systems to identify these organisms are commercially available. Full identification of species members of viridans streptococci is usually not necessary. Members of viridans streptococci belonging to the milleri streptococci, because they are usually recognized by their characteristic "caramel" odor, can be reported, if present, to alert clinicians about this group of viridans because of their propensity for abscess formation and their uniform susceptibility to penicillin. Figure 57-6 is an example of a Gram stain of a member of the milleri group of viridans streptococci from a brain abscess.

There are no vancomycin-resistant streptococci; however, occasionally a "viridans"-like isolate is reported as vancomycin resistant. Usually this is an enterococcus, but it could also be a member of some more uncommon genera such as *Leuconostoc* or *Pediococcus*. If vancomycin resistance has been demonstrated, it would be important to differentiate the intrinsically vancomycin-resistant *Leuconostoc* and *Pediococcus* from enterococci that have acquired vancomycin resistance. Characteristics that might be used to accomplish this are listed in Table 57-4 (Facklam, 1989b). Included in this table is differentiation from *Aerococcus* sp. as well, because of their morphologic similarity to *Enterococcus* sp. The clue that an isolate (especially from a urine culture) might be an *Aerococcus* sp. is the finding on Gram stain that a catalase-negative colony consists of gram-positive cocci in

TABLE 57-4
Characteristics Differentiating *Enterococcus, Leuconostoc, Pediococcus,* and *Aerococcus*

	Enterococcus	*Aerococcus*	*Leuconostoc*	*Pediococcus*
Gram stain	Pairs and short chains	Tetrads	Cocci, coccobacilli, and rods; pairs and chains	Tetrads and pairs; spherical cells
Hemolysis	β or α or γ	α or γ	α or γ	α or γ
Bile esculin	+	V	V	+
Growth in 6.5% NaCl	+	+	V	V
PYR	+	*	–	–
LAP	+	*	–	+
Vancomycin susceptibility	S/R	S	R	R

+, Positive result; –, negative result; *LAP,* leucine aminopeptidase; *PYR,* l-pyrrolidonyl-β-naphthylamide; *R,* resistant; *S,* susceptible; *V,* variable reactions.
**Aerococcus urinae* is PYR and LAP positive; *Aerococcus viridans* is PYR positive and LAP negative.

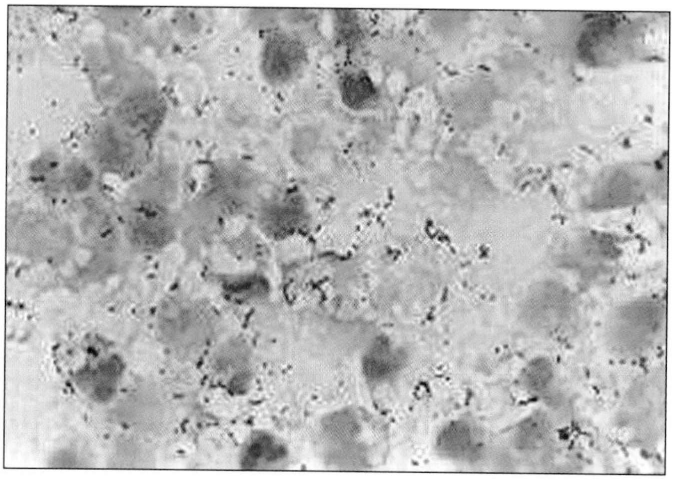

Figure 57-6 Gram stain of a viridans *Streptococcus*, specifically a member of the milleri group, from a brain abscess.

tetrads and clusters, not in pairs and chains. Some species of *Aerococcus* are l-pyrrolidonyl-β-naphthylamide (PYR) positive, which leads to further confusion with *Enterococcus* sp.

Members of the genus *Abiotrophia* will not grow in the absence of pyridoxal. Often they are first recognized as satellite colonies growing around a colony of *S. aureus*. Differential characteristics of *Abiotrophia defectiva* and *Abiotrophia adiacens* are reviewed elsewhere (Ruoff, 2007). Methods of performing susceptibility tests for strains of *Abiotrophia* and *Granulicatella* can be found in CLSI document M45-A (CLSI, 2006).

Antimicrobial Susceptibility

The antibiograms of groups A, B, C, and G streptococcus are predictable (all are susceptible to penicillin); therefore, routine antimicrobial susceptibility testing of these organisms is unnecessary unless penicillin cannot be used, as in the case of a penicillin allergy. In the latter situations, testing for resistance to macrolides, clindamycin, and the tetracyclines may be warranted. Inducible resistance to clindamycin may occur with *Streptococcus* (i.e., group B streptococcus), and a D zone test as described earlier for *S. aureus* may be warranted if the streptococcal isolate is found resistant to erythromycin. Specific guidelines for streptococcal D testing have not yet been published. Because *S. pneumoniae* organisms with intermediate- or high-level resistance to penicillin (MIC 0.12–1.0 μg/mL or ≥2 μg/mL, respectively) are found worldwide, isolates should be screened for susceptibility to penicillin using disk diffusion with a 1-μg oxacillin disk. Isolates that are not susceptible by this method must be further evaluated by macrodilution or microdilution testing, using Mueller-Hinton broth supplemented with lysed horse blood or the E test to determine the penicillin MIC. Resistance to third-generation cephalosporins also occurs; therefore, isolates should be tested for susceptibility to these antimicrobial agents as well.

Susceptibility testing should be performed on isolates of nonhemolytic (viridans) streptococci from sterile body sites, because resistance to penicillin does occur. *Enterococcus* spp. should also be tested, primarily to identify high-level resistance to penicillin or ampicillin, high-level resistance to streptomycin and gentamicin, and resistance to vancomycin. Enterococci are resistant to vancomycin (MIC >32 μg/mL) because of the presence of resistance genes, referred to as the *van* genes (CLSI, 2009). Although many of these genes have been described, the most common are *vanA*, *vanB*, and *vanC*. The *vanA* and *vanB* genes, conferring high-level resistance and predominantly found in *E. faecium* and much less frequently in *E. faecalis*, are acquired, plasmid-borne genes that can create infection control problems involving transmission of this resistance. This vancomycin resistance can be differentiated from intrinsic and lower level resistance (*vanC* genes) in the yellow, motile species of *Enterococcus*, and this should be done in laboratories and reported as such to the infection control team (Teixeira, 2007).

Gemella and *Aerococcus*

Other nonstreptococcal gram-positive, catalase-negative cocci of increasing importance are those that belong to the genera *Gemella* and *Aerococcus*. *Gemella* spp. (*Gemella haemolysans* and *Gemella morbillorum*) resemble viridans streptococci, although they usually produce smaller colonies. *G. haemolysans* has been associated with endocarditis and meningitis. Gram stain usually demonstrates diplococci with adjacent sides flattened that can be confused with a *Neisseria* sp. because cells can easily become decolorized. *G. haemolysans* is aerobic and *G. morbillorum* anaerobic. The latter usually appears as cocci in pairs or short chains. Both are PYR positive, 6% NaCl and esculin–hydrolysis negative (to differentiate them from enterococci). *G. morbillorum* is leucine-aminopeptidase (LAP) positive as well. Both are usually susceptible to penicillin. As with other gram-positive cocci, if there is doubt about the morphology of the organism (i.e., whether it is a short rod or a coccus), Gram stain performed from a broth culture will usually resolve the difficulty.

Two major species of *Aerococcus* may be clinically relevant and/or isolated from clinical specimens: *Aerococcus urinae* and *Aerococcus viridans*. Both resemble viridans streptococci or enterococci on agar plates; however, in Gram stains, they usually appear in tetrads. *A. urinae* is a recognized pathogen in urinary tract infection; in addition, it has been isolated from the blood in cases of endocarditis. *A. urinae* is PYR negative and LAP positive, in contrast to *A. viridans*, which is PYR positive and LAP negative (see Table 57-4). Both will grow in the presence of 6.5% NaCl. Neither are anaerobes, and *A. viridans* usually will not grow under anaerobic conditions. *A. urinae* is usually susceptible to penicillin and nitrofurantoin but may be resistant to sulfonamides. Variability in its response to trimethoprim has been noted (Zhang, 2000; Ruoff, 2007). A newer member of the genus *Aerococcus*, *A. sanguinicola*, which still is rarely recovered from clinical specimens, can be both LAP and PYR positive, although this is not a confirmatory identification. The significance of this isolate is still unknown in most cases (Ibler, 2008).

GRAM-POSITIVE RODS

Corynebacterium and *Arcanobacterium*

Characteristics

The corynebacteria, or **diphtheroids,** as they are sometimes called, appear in the Gram-stained smear as slightly curved, gram-positive rods with nonparallel sides and sometimes wider ends, giving a clubbed appearance (Fig. 57-7). These organisms are catalase positive. More than 46 species of *Corynebacterium* are known. Most are rarely pathogenic in humans; notable exceptions are *Corynebacterium diphtheriae* and its closely related

PART 7

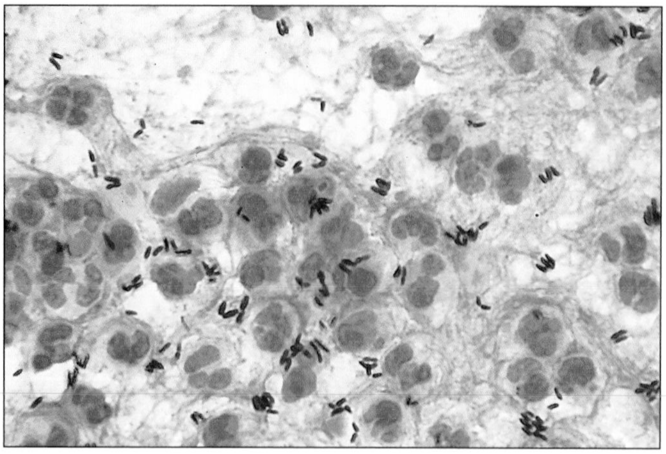

Figure 57-7 Sputum stained with Gram stain shows many neutrophils, amorphous debris, and coryneform gram-positive bacilli (oil immersion).

species or varieties *Corynebacterium ulcerans* and *Corynebacterium pseudotuberculosis*. *C. pseudodiphtheriticum* has been implicated in respiratory tract infections, including pneumonia (Chiner, 1999; Camello, 2009). Medically relevant *Arcanobacterium* spp. include *Arcanobacterium haemolyticum*, *Arcanobacterium pyogenes*, and *Arcanobacterium bernardiae*. *Arcanobacterium* species also appear as irregular gram-positive rods on Gram stain but can be easily differentiated from the corynebacteria by their negative catalase reaction.

Clinical Manifestations and Pathogenesis

At the initial site of infection on the epithelial cells of the tonsils and oropharynx, *C. diphtheriae* elaborates an exotoxin that causes local cell necrosis and subsequent inflammation. The exotoxin produced by strains of *C. diphtheriae* infected with a specific bacteriophage is absorbed into the circulation. Distribution of exotoxin through the bloodstream can produce degenerative changes in the heart, nervous system, and kidneys. The toxin molecule consists of two fragments: A, containing the enzymatically active site, and B, comprising the receptor binding site. Once in the cell, protein synthesis is disrupted. The bacteria and exotoxin produce a serum exudate and cellular infiltrate of the mucous membrane in the pharynx. Exudative lesions coalesce, forming a grayish black adherent pseudomembrane, which is characteristic of diphtheria. Although toxin production and pathogenicity are often considered to be synonymous, pseudomembranes may form in persons infected with nontoxigenic strains. Extension of the pseudomembrane superiorly into the nasopharynx or inferiorly into the larynx may be so marked as to produce respiratory obstruction. Although *C. diphtheriae* infections of other parts of the body do occur, those observed most frequently in the United States today are infections of the skin. Transmission of *C. diphtheriae* occurs by droplet nuclei from the respiratory tract or by contact from cutaneous foci of infection (Mattos-Guaraldi, 2003).

Because they are part of the normal flora of the skin and mucous membranes, it is difficult to establish the etiologic role of the other corynebacteria. Clinical significance is generally increased if the organism is observed in the Gram-stained smear in association with leukocytes, is isolated from a sterile site, and is isolated from multiple samples. *Corynebacterium jeikeium* has been clearly associated with infections of implanted prosthetic materials (e.g., heart valves, CSF, joints), has caused subacute bacterial endocarditis, and has been involved in a variety of opportunistic infections. *Corynebacterium urealyticum* has been associated with urinary tract infection, as well as with bacteremia, endocarditis, and wound infection (Nebreda-Mayoral, 1994). When identified, *Corynebacterium striatum* and *Corynebacterium amycolatum* are the most common normal flora skin coryneforms. They may become pathogenic and, of note, are often resistant to β-lactam antibiotics—a characteristic usually attributed only to *C. jeikeium* (Crabtree, 2003).

A. haemolyticum has been associated with pharyngitis and wound and soft tissue infections (Gaston, 1996; Fernandez-Suarez, 2009). *A. pyogenes* and *A. bernardiae* are associated with abscess formation.

Laboratory Diagnosis

Because of the relative rarity of diphtheria in the United States today, the diagnosis may be overlooked clinically, and the laboratory may easily fail to recognize it in cultures. When the diagnosis of diphtheria is being entertained by clinicians in a patient's differential diagnosis, the laboratory should be informed so that the specimen can be handled appropriately. Specimens should be obtained with a cotton- or polyester-tipped swab from inflamed regions of the nasopharynx and, if possible, beneath the pseudomembrane. If skin lesions are suspected of being positive for *C. diphtheriae*, the most appropriate specimen would be an aspirate of the lesion. Corynebacteria will grow on routine blood-containing agar; however, cystine-tellurite (CT) blood agar or Tinsdale medium is preferred. On CT medium, colonies of *C. diphtheriae* are gray or black after 48 hours of incubation. Colonies may be large or small and flat or convex. Colonies of species other than *C. diphtheriae* may produce black colonies on CT or Tinsdale media, although these will usually be smaller. If a laboratory does not have CT or Tinsdale medium and a request for *C. diphtheriae* is made, CNA can be used, although it will be more difficult to recognize possible *C. diphtheriae* strains (Funke, 2007).

Classification of oral and skin corynebacteria or diphtheroids is difficult and confusing. The differential characteristics of some species are shown in Table 57-5. Commercial identification systems are available to identify many of the members of this group of organisms (Hudspeth, 1998). Isolates of suspected *C. diphtheriae* must be tested for production of exotoxin. The elaboration of toxin may be detected in vitro with the Elek immunodiffusion test; however, this generally is not done in a routine clinical laboratory. Isolates should be sent to a state health laboratory or a reference laboratory where this can be performed. Alternatively, PCR-based tests have been described that may be used for detection of the toxin gene (Efstratiou, 2000). *C. jeikeium* often produces a characteristic metallic sheen on the surface of blood agar plates. *C. striatum* and *C. amycolatum* are common skin florae that can be responsible for infection; whether they need to be specifically identified is controversial, and identification can be difficult; species identification of *Corynebacterium* often requires a combination of commercial kit systems, cellular fatty acid analysis, and/or sequencing (Van den Velde, 2006). *C. striatum* and *C. amycolatum* organisms are often resistant to many antibiotic agents—a characteristic that often is more typically associated with hospital-acquired strains, in particular *C. jeikeium*.

Arcanobacterium spp. are β-hemolytic on sheep blood agar. Colonies on sheep blood agar are small after 48 hours of incubation, and the hemolysis may go unnoticed. Adequate growth and noticeable hemolysis are best demonstrated in a CO_2-enhanced environment. *Arcanobacterium* spp. are catalase negative. Biochemical reactions that are used to determine the

TABLE 57-5
Differential Characteristics of Some Species Within the Genus *Corynebacterium* and Related Organisms

Test	*C. diphtheriae*	*C. ulcerans*	*C. pseudotuberculosis*	*C. jeikeium*	*Arcanobacterium haemolyticum*	*Arcanobacterium pyogenes*
Catalase	+	+	+	+	–	–
Hemolysis	v	+	+	–	+	+
Gelatinase	–	+	–	–	–	+
Urease	–	+	+	–	–	–
Nitrate reduction	v	–	v	–	–	–
Sucrose fermentation	–	–	v	–	v	v

+, Positive; –, negative; *v*, variable.

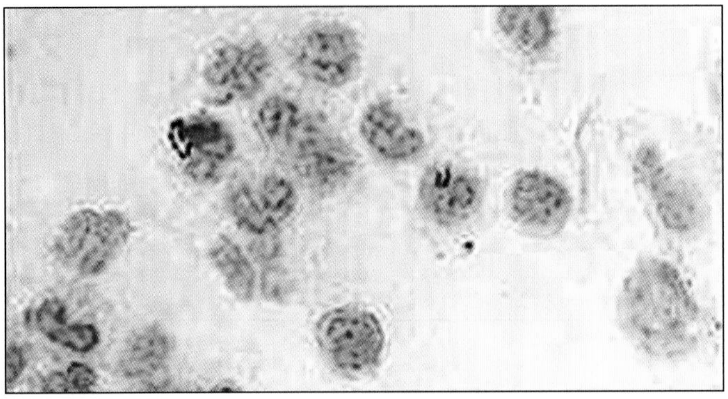

Figure 57-8 Gram stain of a cerebrospinal fluid sample that grew *Listeria monocytogenes*. The short bacilli are seen inside white blood cells.

species of corynebacteria are also useful in identifying the *Arcanobacterium* spp. (Funke, 2007). *A. haemolyticum* produces phospholipase D, which is responsible for the reverse CAMP reaction with *S. aureus*. This organism inhibits hemolysis around the *S. aureus* streak, producing an inverted triangle of no hemolysis.

Antimicrobial Susceptibility

Although antitoxin remains the only specific method of treatment of diphtheria, antibiotics are administered to patients with disease and to asymptomatic carriers of toxigenic strains. *C. diphtheriae* is usually inhibited by penicillins and the macrolides. The antimicrobial susceptibilities of other species of corynebacteria or diphtheroids are far less predictable. *C. jeikeium* is usually resistant to the penicillins and cephalosporins, is variably susceptible to most other antibiotics, and is almost uniformly susceptible to vancomycin. Other species of *Corynebacterium*, however, may be similarly resistant to β-lactam antibiotics. Treatment of infection caused by these organisms is often complicated by the presence of compromised host defenses and implanted prosthetic materials. Arcanobacteria are sensitive to penicillin and other β-lactams, rifampin, tetracycline, and the macrolides. Growth of the organisms may be inhibited by fluoroquinolones and aminoglycosides (Funke, 2007). Methods used for performing susceptibility tests on *Corynebacterium* spp. and interpretive criteria can be found in CLSI document M45-A (CLSI, 2006).

Prevention

Methods of prevention of diphtheria are almost exclusively active and passive immunization programs with supplemental antibiotics to eliminate the carrier state of toxigenic strains during epidemics.

Listeria

Characteristics

Listeria spp. are nonbranching, non–spore-forming gram-positive rods. *Listeria monocytogenes* (Fig. 57-8) is the only species of *Listeria* that is pathogenic for humans, and *L. ivanovii* is the only species of the other five Listeria spp. that is pathogenic for animals but not humans. Optimal growth of *L. monocytogenes* is observed between 30° C and 37° C; however, growth may occur as low as 4° C. Colonies are small after 24 hours and exhibit a narrow zone of β-hemolysis on blood agar. A characteristic tumbling motility of saline suspensions of the colonies occurs at room temperature but rarely at 35° C. This same temperature-dependent motility is also noted in semisolid media, in which growth appears as an umbrella shape at the top of the medium (aerobic conditions), preferentially at lower temperatures.

Clinical Manifestations and Pathogenesis

L. monocytogenes is found in soil, dust, water, silage, sewage, and raw unpasteurized milk and in asymptomatic human and animal carriers. Transmission of the organism by foods such as cole slaw, pasteurized milk, and soft cheeses has resulted in several major epidemics in North America and Europe (Fleming, 1985; MacDonald, 2005). According to data from microbiological surveys of food, *L. monocytogenes* has been detected in 2%–3% of dairy products, 20% of soft cheeses and processed meats, 30% of certain vegetables (cabbages, radishes), and up to 50% of raw meat and poultry (Bille, 2007). A transient carrier state is found in 2%–20% of animals and humans.

Listeriosis is mainly a disease of industrialized countries, occurring sporadically or in epidemics. The primary mode of transmission is contaminated food products, although occasional non–food-related outbreaks have occurred in healthcare settings, primarily in nurseries, as the result of cross-infection; contaminated mineral oil for bathing was implicated in one such outbreak (McLaughlin, 1989; Schuchat, 1991).

Clinical manifestations of listeriosis differ among pregnant women, neonates, and immunocompromised individuals, which constitute the high-risk groups. Listeriosis during pregnancy, most common in the third trimester, presents as a flu-like illness. Bacteremia occurs concomitantly, during which time the uterine contents are infected. Progression to amnionitis may induce premature labor or septic abortion in 3–7 days. Infection in the mother is self-limited because the source of infection is removed with delivery of the infected fetus and uterine contents. Neonatal listeriosis may have an early or late onset. Early-onset disease, manifested at birth or a few days thereafter, results from in utero infection. Infants present with temperature instability, hemodynamic compromise, and respiratory distress; widely disseminated granulomas, particularly involving the placenta, posterior pharynx, and skin, are characteristic of the illness but are not always present. Late-onset disease, affecting full-term infants of mothers with uncomplicated pregnancies, is assumed to be acquired postpartum, but in most cases the source is unknown. Clinical manifestations of meningitis become apparent several days to weeks after birth.

Nonperinatal listeriosis usually occurs in immunosuppressed individuals, but in about one third of cases, no risk factor is identified. Tropism for *L. monocytogenes* for the central nervous system (CNS) is manifested predominantly as meningitis; other forms of CNS listeriosis include cerebritis and brainstem and spinal cord abscesses. Severe disease with high mortality rates (20%–50%) and neurologic sequelae among survivors are common. Primary bacteremia or focal infections outside the CNS are uncommon. Primary cutaneous listeriosis has occurred occupationally in veterinarians and abattoir workers after exposure to infected animal tissues. Endocarditis, osteomyelitis, arthritis, endophthalmitis, and other focal infections have been reported rarely. Febrile gastrointestinal disease due to *L. monocytogenes* has been reported in nonimmunocompromised patients; implicated foods include chocolate milk, rice salad, and delicatessen meats and cheeses (Bille, 2007). Immunocompromised patients, such as those with leukemias or bone marrow transplants and patients on immunosuppressive therapies, are cautioned against eating uncooked dairy meats for fear of infection with this organism.

The pathogenesis of listeriosis infection has been well elaborated in recent years. Host susceptibility, gastric acidity, inoculum size, and virulence properties of the organism along with specific food products are the most common factors that determine progression from infection to disease and the severity of that disease in the infected individual. *L. monocytogenes* can penetrate the epithelial cells of the gastrointestinal (GI) tract and grow within hepatic and splenic macrophages; from there, the organism can spread to the CNS or the pregnant uterus. Virulence factors such as internalin and E-cadherin, a placental receptor, interact to result in infection in the pregnant female/fetus. Immunity to listeriosis relies on T cell–mediated activation of macrophages by lymphokines (Bille, 2007).

Laboratory Diagnosis

Colonies are small and grayish blue and are surrounded by a narrow zone of β-hemolysis on blood agar. A positive catalase reaction differentiates *L. monocytogenes* from similarly appearing group B streptococci. Organisms are motile at room temperature and produce acid from glucose, trehalose, and salicin and hydrolyze esculin. Other biochemical characteristics of *L. monocytogenes* and differences between *Listeria* and *Erysipelothrix* are listed in Table 57-6.

Antimicrobial Susceptibility

L. monocytogenes is usually sensitive to penicillin, ampicillin, erythromycin, chloramphenicol, tetracycline, and gentamicin. Isolates usually are only moderately susceptible to the quinolones. Cephalosporins are ineffective against *Listeria* spp.; isolates should not be tested against cephalosporins because they are ineffective in vivo regardless of the in vitro result. Methods of performing susceptibility tests for *Listeria* and interpretive criteria can be found in CLSI document M45-A (CLSI, 2010). Resistance to chloramphenicol, macrolides, and tetracyclines has been found in several clinical isolates (Bille, 2007). Ampicillin, alone or in combination with an aminoglycoside, has been used successfully in the treatment of infections caused by *L. monocytogenes*. Trimethoprim-sulfamethoxazole may be used as alternative therapy in penicillin-allergic patients. Newer

TABLE 57-6
Differential Characteristics of *Listeria monocytogenes* and *Erysipelothrix rhusiopathiae*

Test	*L. monocytogenes*	*E. rhusiopathiae*
β-Hemolysis	+	–
Growth at 4° C	+	–
Catalase	+	–
Motility	+	–
Esculin hydrolysis	+	–
Gluconate utilization	+	–
Voges-Proskauer	+	–
H_2S in triple sugar iron agar	–	+

+, Positive; –, negative.

gram-positive antibiotics such as daptomycin, linezolid, and tigecycline appear susceptible in vitro, but limited clinical data document their in vivo effectiveness.

Erysipelothrix

Characteristics

Erysipelothrix rhusiopathiae is a catalase-negative, non–spore-forming, nonmotile, facultatively anaerobic gram-positive bacillus that has a worldwide distribution. Microscopically, they appear as short rods with rounded ends, occurring singly, in short chains, or in nonbranching filaments. Two species have been identified: *E. rhusiopathiae* and *E. tonsillarum*. A third species, *E. inipinata*, has been proposed recently. *E. rhusiopathiae* is a recognized pathogen in humans, occasionally causing erysipeloid, a localized cutaneous infection of hands and fingers, obtained after exposure to animals or animal products. *E. tonsillarum* has not been isolated from human specimens (Bille, 2007).

Clinical Manifestations and Pathogenesis

E. rhusiopathiae is usually transmitted to humans from animals by means of skin wounds produced by contaminated objects or in contact with blood, flesh, viscera, or feces of infected animals. *E. rhusiopathiae* is widespread in nature in wild and domestic animals, birds, fish, and decaying organic matter and causes infection in swine, sheep, rabbits, cattle, birds, and fowl. At risk of infection with this organism are butchers, abattoir workers, fishermen, fish handlers, poultry processors, and veterinarians. The most common form of erysipeloid is a local cutaneous infection manifested by pain, swelling, and a cutaneous eruption characterized by a slowly progressive, slightly elevated, violaceous zone around the site of inoculation. The swelling and erythema migrate peripherally and the lesion involutes without desquamation. Systemic disease is rare, but numerous case reports describe septicemia and endocarditis. Also rarely reported have been cases of arthritis and brain abscess.

Laboratory Diagnosis

Biopsy and tissue aspirates from erysipeloid lesions are the best specimens for culture. The organisms are located deep in the subcutaneous layer of the leading edge of the lesion; therefore, swabs of the surface of the skin are not useful. The organism will grow on blood or chocolate blood agar, but may require up to 7 days for growth. Conventional blood culture media are suitable for its isolation from blood. They are considered nonhemolytic, although greenish discoloration of the media beneath the colonies is often observed after 2 days of incubation.

E. rhusiopathiae is oxidase and catalase negative. Characteristically, it produces hydrogen sulfide (H_2S) in triple-sugar iron agar (TSIA). It is nonmotile, does not reduce nitrates to nitrites, and is negative for urease, gelatin, and esculin hydrolysis; *E. rhusiopathiae* does ferment glucose and lactose. A trait highly characteristic of *E. rhusiopathiae* is the "pipe cleaner" pattern of growth in gelatin stab cultures incubated at 22° C. This organism can be readily distinguished from *Listeria* spp. (see Table 57-6).

Antimicrobial Susceptibility

Erysipelothrix is susceptible to the penicillins, the cephalosporins, imipenem, erythromycin, clindamycin, chloramphenicol, the tetracyclines, and the fluoroquinolones but is resistant to sulfonamides, aminoglycosides, and vancomycin. Penicillin is the treatment of choice for localized and systemic infection (Bille, 2007). Methods used for performing susceptibility tests for *Erysipelothrix rhusiopathiae* and interpretive criteria can be found in CLSI document M45-A (CLSI, 2010).

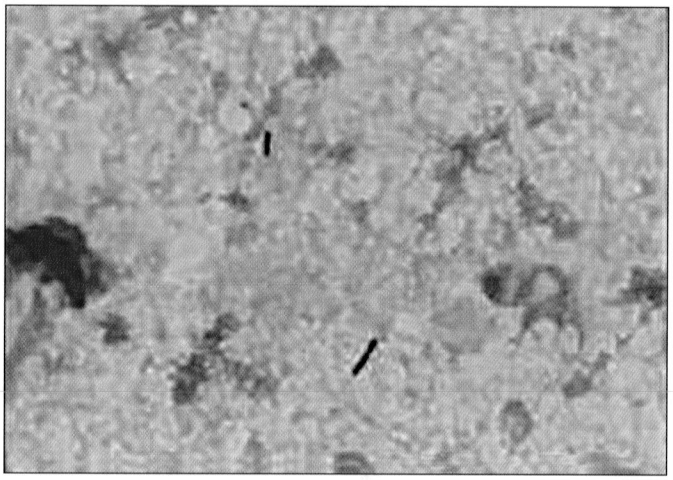

Figure 57-9 Gram stain of *Bacillus cereus* in pleural fluid.

Bacillus

Characteristics

Members of this genus are strictly aerobic or facultatively anaerobic, rod-shaped, spore-forming, gram-positive, and catalase-positive organisms. Figure 57-9 shows a Gram stain of a *Bacillus* sp. seen in pleural fluid. With the notable exception of *Bacillus anthracis*, they are usually motile by means of lateral or peritrichous flagella. Some strains stain gram-negatively and, because of their variable oxidase reactions, are confused with gram-negative bacilli. The most reliable diagnostic characteristic of the genus is spore formation, which occurs optimally and on a variety of media under aerobic conditions at 25°–30° C. In Gram-stained smears, endospores are detectable by the presence of unstained defects or holes within the cell. The spores themselves can be stained by any of several methods.

Clinical Manifestations and Pathogenesis

Of the numerous species of *Bacillus*, *B. anthracis* is the only one that is uniformly and highly pathogenic. Great care must be exercised when handling material suspected of harboring this species. Work should be performed in biological safety cabinets by gloved, gowned, masked, and immunized personnel; work surfaces must be disinfected with 5% hypochlorite or 5% phenol; all supplies, materials, and equipment must be decontaminated. Because *B. anthracis* spores have been used as a means of bioterrorism, cultures containing suspect *B. anthracis* should be handled only by reference or public health laboratories.

Three forms of anthrax are recognized: cutaneous, inhalation, and intestinal. In its cutaneous form, anthrax produces a small, red, macular lesion that progresses to a vesicle and finally to necrosis with formation of a characteristic black eschar. Regional lymphadenopathy and septicemia may occur. Mortality in untreated cases with this form of disease is approximately 20%. Inhalation of anthrax spores can lead to acute bronchopneumonia, mediastinitis, and septicemia ("woolsorter's disease"). The mortality in recognized cases of this form of disease is nearly 100%. Intestinal anthrax follows the ingestion of contaminated food and is manifested by nausea, vomiting, and diarrhea. In some cases, gastrointestinal bleeding is followed by prostration, shock, and death. Septicemia can occur in all three forms of anthrax and may lead to a fatal, purulent meningitis.

A major factor in the organism's pathogenic capabilities is its glutamyl polypeptide capsule, which inhibits phagocytosis; anticapsular antibodies do not protect against the disease. A complex toxin with three components (edema factor, protective antigen, and lethal factor) is responsible for the signs and symptoms of anthrax (Logan, 2007).

Humans become infected with anthrax by contact with and inhalation or ingestion of infected animals, their carcasses, or their byproducts. Cattle, sheep, horses, and goats are the animals most frequently infected and provide a ready source of vegetative organisms that sporulate and perpetuate the environmental contamination.

Although usually saprophytic, other species of *Bacillus* can cause disease. *Bacillus cereus* has been associated with ear infection, pneumonia, posttraumatic ocular wound infection, septicemia, and endocarditis. Patients with pneumonia and septicemia are often immunosuppressed. Bacteremia

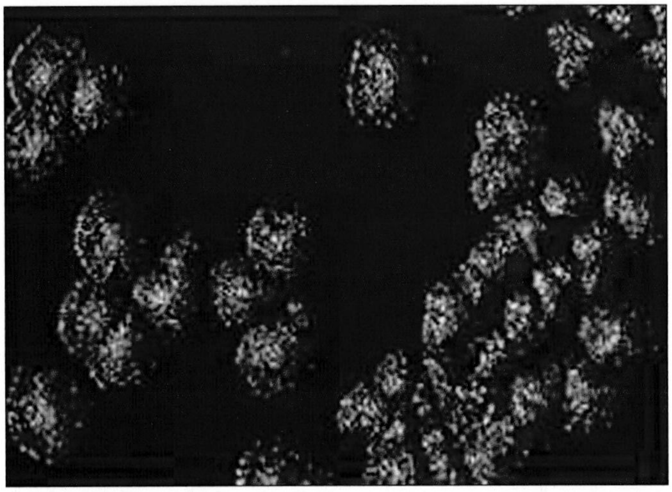

Figure 57-10 Colonies of *Bacillus anthracis* on blood agar. Note the irregular edges of the colonies.

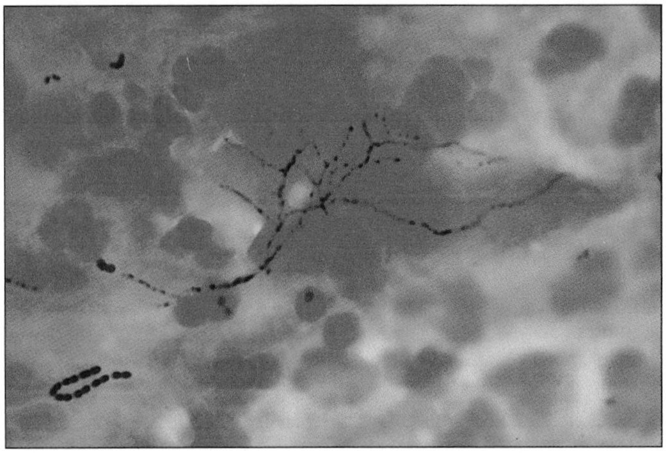

Figure 57-11 Sputum smear stained with Gram stain shows neutrophils, amorphous debris, and filamentous, beaded, branched gram-positive bacilli (oil immersion).

is frequently associated with intravenous drug use and with contaminated intravascular devices.

Two forms of gastroenteritis are associated with *Bacillus* species. Food poisoning caused by *Bacillus* may occur within 1–6 hours following ingestion of food contaminated by *B. cereus* that has produced a pre-formed heat-stable toxin. Major manifestations of *Bacillus* food poisoning include nausea, vomiting, cramps, and occasionally diarrhea. Typically, this form of *Bacillus* gastroenteritis results from the bulk preparation of foods that are not reheated before they are served. *B. cereus* type 1 grows particularly well in fried rice and is more heat resistant than other types, so this form of gastroenteritis is frequently seen in association with consumption of cooked rice in Chinese restaurants. The second form of gastroenteritis caused by *Bacillus* spp. results from contamination of meat and vegetable dishes and is characterized by the onset of cramps and diarrhea 8–16 hours following ingestion of contaminated food. In this instance, the major manifestations of *B. cereus* infection are caused by the production of a heat-labile enterotoxin.

The genus *Bacillus* contains more than 100 species; other than *B. anthracis* and *B. cereus*, common species include *B. subtilis*, *B. licheniformis*, *B. megaterium*, *B. pumilus*, and *B. thuringiensis*. Many species have been removed, however, and more than 25 new genera of gram-positive spore-producing aerobic bacilli have been named. One of those genera, *Paenibacillus*, contains species that have been associated with clinical disease, including meningitis and endophthalmitis. Species of *Paenibacillus* include *P. alvei*, *P. macerans*, *P. popilliae*, and *P. hongkongensis* (Logan, 2007; Ouyang, 2008). *P. macerans* has been reportedly found in contaminated blood culture bottles in a neonatal intensive care unit (Noskin, 2001).

Laboratory Diagnosis

In cases of suspected cutaneous anthrax, vesicle fluid and material under the edge of the eschar should be collected with a swab for smear and culture. For suspected inhalation anthrax, sputum should be collected for smear and culture. Cultures of stool should be considered in the intestinal form. Smears and cultures consist of CSF should be requested in suspected meningitis. In the septicemic stage, blood cultures should be performed.

Finding large, boxcar-shaped, gram-positive cells in smears of any of these specimens should raise suspicion for the diagnosis. Fluorescent microscopy, available in some state health laboratories and at the CDC, can provide a rapid presumptive diagnosis. As mentioned earlier, because of the use of *B. anthracis* in terrorist attacks, sentinel laboratories (level A) should send any suspicious isolates of this organism to their state health laboratory or the CDC.

Species of *Bacillus* grow well on sheep blood agar. Colonies of *B. anthracis* are usually flat, with an irregular margin ("Medusa head"), appear off-white with a ground glass surface, and are usually nonhemolytic. Figure 57-10 demonstrates the colonial morphology of *B. anthracis* on blood agar. When touched with an inoculating loop, the colonies are tenacious and will stand up like beaten egg white. The Medusa head colony may be seen with *B. cereus* and certain other *Bacillus* species. Anthrax bacilli are nonmotile in a hanging drop test or in semisolid media, whereas most other species of *Bacillus* are motile. Motility by the hanging drop method is a useful differential test between *B. anthracis* and *B. cereus* but must be carried out with a fresh broth culture of the organism. Additional characteristics and biochemical reactions that may be used to identify isolates to the species level are summarized by Logan (2007). A commercial system has been evaluated recently for identification of aerobic endosporeformers; 93% of the strains were correctly identified to species level in the genera *Bacillus*, *Paenibacillus*, *Aneurinibacillus*, *Brevibacillus*, *Geobacillus*, and *Virgibacillus* (Halket, 2010).

The diagnosis of *B. cereus* gastroenteritis cannot be accurately made by culture of stool because the organisms may be a component of the indigenous gut flora. Diagnosis, therefore, depends on quantitative culture of the suspected contaminated food. The presence of greater than or equal to 10^5 colony-forming units (CFUs)/g in the suspected food constitutes presumptive evidence of *B. cereus* food poisoning (Logan, 2007). This testing is usually not performed in a routine Clinical Microbiology laboratory.

Antimicrobial Susceptibility

Although susceptible to a variety of agents, antibiotic therapy of anthrax has centered on the use of fluoroquinolones. These agents are highly active against *B. anthracis*, strains of which are typically susceptible to β-lactam antibiotics. However, many strains of *Bacillus* spp. elaborate β-lactamases in nature, hence these agents usually are not considered as first-line drugs of choice until the specific susceptibility of the isolate is known. Most strains of *Bacillus* spp. are inhibited by fluoroquinolones, tetracyclines, aminoglycosides, and chloramphenicol at low concentrations (Logan, 2007), and most are susceptible to vancomycin, but reports have described vancomycin resistance in *B. circulans* and *P. thiaminolyticus*. *Bacillus* strains have been demonstrated to carry genes similar to the *vanA* gene of the enterococci (Patel, 2000). Methods of performing susceptibility tests and of interpreting their results can be found in the CLSI document M45-A2 (CLSI, 2010).

Prevention

Prevention of anthrax in humans ideally depends on its control in animals. Prompt diagnosis of sick animals, their isolation and therapy, and cremation of carcasses are indicated when sporadic outbreaks occur. In enzootic areas, vaccination with nonencapsulated spore preparations is used. Occupationally exposed persons should also be immunized. Acute diarrheal disease caused by *B. cereus* may be prevented by proper cooking and refrigeration of foods prepared in bulk to prevent proliferation of vegetative forms of the bacteria and formation of the enterotoxin.

Nocardia

Characteristics

In Gram-stained smears of clinical specimens, *Nocardia* spp. appear as long, thin, beaded, branching gram-positive bacilli (Fig. 57-11). The most distinguishing quality of the nocardiae is their partial acid fastness; cells stain positively with a modified acid-fast (Ziehl-Neelsen or Kinyoun) stain, differentiating them from *Actinomyces*, which may have a similar Gram-stain appearance. Partial acid fastness may be difficult to demonstrate and can be enhanced by growing the organism for about 4 days on Middlebrook

TABLE 57-7
Differentiation of *Nocardia* spp. Based on Antimicrobial Susceptibility Pattern*

	Amik	Amox/clav	Cefotax	Ceftriax	Ciproflox	Clari	Gent	Imi	Kana	Linez	Mino	Sulfa	Tobra	Amp	Eryth	Carb
Nocardia cyracigeorgica (*N. asteroides* drug pattern VI)/*N. asteroides* VII	S	R	S	S	R	R		S	S	S	S/I	S		R	R	
Nocardia farcinica (drug pattern V)	S	S	R	R	S	R	R	S	R	S	S/I	R/S	R	R	R	
Nocardia nova complex[†] (drug pattern III)	S	R	S	S	R	S		S		S	S/I	S		S	S	R
Nocardia abscessus (drug pattern 1)	S	S	S	S	R	R		R/S		S	S/I	S		S	R	S
Nocardia brasiliensis	S	S	S/R	S/R	R	R	S	R	R	S	S/I	S	S	R	R	S
Nocardia pseudobrasiliensis		S	S/R	S/R	S	S	S	R	R	S	R	S	S	R		S
Nocardia otitidiscaviarum (often R to all β-lactams)	S	R	R	R	S		S	R	S[‡]	S	S/I	S		R		R
Nocardia transvalensis complex (drug pattern IV)	R	S	S	S	S	R	R	S	R	S	S/I	S	R	R	R	
Nocardia brevicatana/paucivorans	S			S	S		R	S	S	S	S/I	S	S	S		S

Reproduced with permission of Dr. Richard Wallace and Ms. Barbara Brown-Elliott.
Amik, Amikacin; *Amox/clav,* amoxicillin/clavulanate; *Amp,* ampicillin; *Carb,* carbenicillin; *Cefotax,* cefotaxime; *Ceftriax,* ceftriaxone; *Ciproflox,* ciprofloxacin; *Clari,* clarithromycin; *Eryth,* erythromycin; *Gent,* gentamicin; *I,* intermediate; *Imi,* imipenem; *Kana,* kanamycin; *Linez,* linezolid; *Mino,* minocycline; *R,* resistant; *S,* susceptible; *Sulfa,* sulfamethoxazole; *Tobra,* tobramycin.
*Table based on majority of isolates tested.
[†]Includes *N. nova/veterana/africana.*
[‡]Kanamycin zone ≥ amikacin zone.

7H10 agar, or in litmus milk broth. Most clinical infections have been caused by members of the *Nocardia asteroides* complex, most commonly *Nocardia cyriageorgica*, *Nocardia farcinica*, and *N. nova*, followed by *Nocardia brasiliensis* and rarely *Nocardia otitidis caviarum* (Cloud, 2004).

Clinical Manifestations and Pathogenesis

Nocardiae are found in soil and organic material worldwide and cause disease in many animals and in fish. Human infection is slightly more common in males than in females. It is usually acquired via inhalation of the organism but may occur following trauma and contact with contaminated soil, or the organism may enter the body via the GI tract when contaminated material contacts an area of mucosal ulceration.

In the lungs, *Nocardia* spp. are phagocytosed by alveolar macrophages and grow intracellularly, eliciting a mixed inflammatory response (neutrophils, lymphocytes, and macrophages), eventually resulting in abscess or, occasionally, granuloma formation. In vitro studies of the host defenses against *Nocardia* spp. suggest that neutrophils, activated macrophages, and cytotoxic T cells are involved. Although neutrophils do not kill virulent *Nocardia* spp., they inhibit their growth, possibly suppressing the infection until macrophages are fully activated. If the infection is not contained within the lung, organisms spread to other tissues by advancing growth, thus producing empyema, chest wall involvement, and draining sinuses, or by hematogenous dissemination, resulting in abscess formation, especially in the brain, subcutaneous tissues, and kidneys. The primary host factor associated with increased risk of nocardiosis is cellular immune dysfunction, although many persons infected with *Nocardia* spp. have no recognized cellular or humoral immune defect (Wilson, 1989).

Pulmonary disease, the most frequent manifestation of nocardiosis, is characterized by fever, anorexia, weight loss, cough, dyspnea, and pleuritic chest pain. Skin and subcutaneous disease may present as pyoderma, cellulitis, single or multiple abscesses, lymphocutaneous disease resembling sporotrichosis, or nodules. In Central and South America, primary infections of the skin with *N. brasiliensis* may produce an actinomycetoma (a localized indurated granulomatous mass with sinus tracts draining pus and "sulfur" granules), typically on the lower extremities. Disseminated disease is usually caused by members of the *N. asteroides* complex. It originates in the lung in most cases and typically is manifested as single or multiple abscesses involving the CNS. The skin is the second most common site of dissemination, followed by kidney, liver, and lymph nodes (Conville, 2007).

Laboratory Diagnosis

Nocardia spp. grow aerobically on most nonselective media such as sheep blood and chocolate agars, potato dextrose agar, Sabouraud's dextrose agar, and Löwenstein-Jensen or Middlebrook media and in 7H9 broth used for mycobacterial culture. These organisms will grow on buffered charcoal-yeast extract (BCYE) used for the isolation of *Legionella* spp. as well. It is important to note that *Nocardia* spp. may not always survive the decontamination procedures used for recovery of mycobacteria. Incubation in the presence of 10% CO_2 enhances growth. *Nocardia* spp. may grow in 48 hours, but colonies typically appear in 5–10 days as waxy, bumpy, or velvety rugose forms, often with yellow to orange pigment, depending on the species. Observing branching filaments that stain only with a modified acid-fast stain distinguishes *Nocardia* spp. from mycobacteria. *Nocardia* spp. are differentiated from most other aerobic actinomycetes by testing resistance to the action of lysozyme (*Nocardia* spp. are resistant; *Streptomyces* spp., *Rhodococcus* spp., *Gordona* spp., and *Actinomadura* spp. are susceptible) and examining their morphology on tap water agar. The latter can help in differentiating the branching *Nocardia* from nonbranching *Rhodococcus* spp., for example. Because many new species of *Nocardia* have been recognized over the past several years, the use of biochemical tests (e.g., casein, hypoxanthine, tyrosine, xanthine) is not sufficient for identification. Molecular tests (e.g., 16S rDNA sequencing, PCR-restriction enzyme pattern analysis [PRA]) are required for accurate species identification (Cloud, 2004; Patel, 2004). Identification to the species level is important because of the variability in antibiotic susceptibility patterns noted among species (Table 57-7) (Brown-Elliott, 2006).

Antimicrobial Susceptibility

Sulfonamides (alone or in combination with trimethoprim [e.g., trimethoprim-sulfamethoxazole]) are usually the antimicrobial agents of choice; however, optimal antimicrobial therapy depends on the species of *Nocardia* present, the susceptibility pattern of the individual strain, and the type of infection. Other potential antimicrobial agents include amikacin, clarithromycin, imipenem, or a quinolone, depending on the species isolated. The CLSI has information about methods used for susceptibility testing and interpretation of results for *Nocardia* and other aerobic actinomycetes (NCCLS, 2003).

Other Aerobic Actinomycetes

Other genera of actinomycetes that are medically relevant to humans include *Rhodococcus, Gordona, Tsukamurella, Actinomadura*, and *Streptomyces*. One other member, *Tropheryma whippelii*, is nonculturable and is the putative agent of Whipple's disease.

Clinical Manifestations and Pathogenesis

Members of this group of organisms are ubiquitous in the environment and have been isolated from soil, fresh water, marine water, and organic matter.

Rhodococcus equi is the most common *Rhodococcus* sp. pathogenic to humans. It is an opportunistic pathogen in severely immunocompromised hosts, causing a slowly progressive granulomatous pneumonia. It may be isolated from the blood of infected patients. The organism is likely acquired via the respiratory route, possibly as a result of exposure to infected animals. The organism's ability to persist in and ultimately destroy macrophages probably accounts for its ability to cause disease (Weinstock, 2002). Infections caused by *Gordona* spp. and *Tsukamurella* spp. are only rarely reported. *Tsukamurella* spp. appear to be pathogenic only when certain clinical conditions are present (e.g., immunosuppression, presence of foreign body, active chronic infection such as tuberculosis) (Woo, 2003). *Actinomadura* spp. are a frequent cause of actinomycotic mycetomas, most of which are seen in tropical and subtropical countries, where walking barefoot increases the chance of exposure through repeated puncture wounds. *Streptomyces* spp. have traditionally been considered of little medical significance; however, one species, *Streptomyces somaliensis*, has been identified as an etiologic agent of actinomycotic mycetoma. Other *Streptomyces* spp. have only occasionally been reported to be of medical importance (Mossad, 1995).

Laboratory Diagnosis

Aerobic actinomycetes are slow growing and may require 2–3 weeks of incubation. These microorganisms grow on most of the nonselective media used to isolate bacteria, mycobacteria, and fungi. Species of *Rhodococcus* grow as coccobacilli in a zigzag fashion. Rudimentary branched filaments have been observed from liquid media. Colonies may be rough, smooth, or mucoid and have pigments ranging from buff to coral to orange to deep rose after several days of incubation. *R. equi* is usually pale pink, pale yellow, or coral and may appear slimy. *Gordona* spp. range from smooth, mucoid colonies that are adherent to the media to dry, raised colonies. The pigment produced may be beige to salmon-colored. *Tsukamurella* spp. are slightly acid fast by the modified Kinyoun. They appear as long rods that fragment into three parts. No aerial hyphae are produced. The colonies are circular with entire or rhizoid edges. They may be dry or creamy with a white to orange pigment. Rough colonies may be produced after 7 days of incubation. Species of *Actinomadura* form waxy, cerebriform, tough, membranous white, yellow, pink, or red colonies. Colonies of *Streptomyces* are dry to chalky, heaped or folded, gray-white to yellow, and have the odor of a musty basement. A wide variety of pigments are produced that color the substrate and hyphae. Some species do not produce aerial hyphae. As with the *Nocardia* spp., complete identification of these members of the aerobic actinomycetes often requires molecular sequencing methods (Conville, 2007).

GRAM-NEGATIVE BACTERIA—COCCI

Neisseria

Characteristics

This genus is composed of species that are nonmotile, catalase- and oxidase-positive; these aerobic, gram-negative cocci are often arranged in pairs with flattened adjacent surfaces, giving the appearance of kidney or coffee beans (Fig. 57-12). The organisms are somewhat fastidious, in some instances requiring the addition of blood, serum, cholesterol, or oleic acid to the medium to counteract growth inhibitors, such as fatty acids. *N. gonorrhoeae* and *N. meningitidis* generally require prompt incubation in CO_2 for growth; however, this is strain dependent, varies with the phase of the organism's growth curve, and is often lost in subcultures. *N. meningitidis* and most *N. gonorrhoeae* are not inhibited by the presence of vancomycin or lincomycin, colistin, and nystatin—a characteristic that is particularly useful in their selective isolation from specimens contaminated by other bacteria. Rarely, isolates of *N. gonorrhoeae* (especially AUH strains, which require arginine, uracil, and hypoxanthine) are susceptible to vancomycin (Janda, 2007).

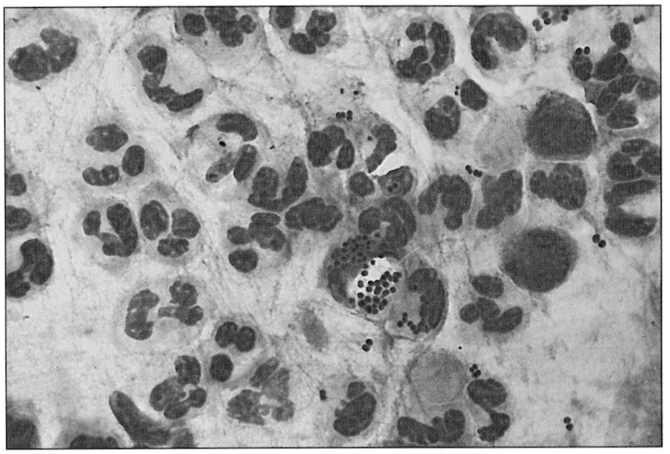

Figure 57-12 Sputum smear stained with Gram stain shows many neutrophils and intracellular gram-negative diplococci, suggestive of *Neisseria meningitidis* infection (oil immersion).

Clinical Manifestations and Pathogenesis

Although opportunistic infections caused by species of *Neisseria* other than *N. gonorrhoeae* and *N. meningitidis* have occasionally been reported in compromised hosts, these species are generally nonpathogenic. *N. meningitidis* may colonize the mucous membranes of the upper respiratory tract—an event that is usually followed in 7–10 days by the formation of bactericidal and hemagglutinating antibodies, which may not eliminate the carrier stage but convey group-specific immunity. In a few cases, disease results shortly after colonization, most frequently in the form of meningococcemia and meningitis. The organism also has a tendency to invade serous membranes and joint tissues, with the development of pleuritis, pericarditis, and arthritis. Carriage of *N. meningitidis* in the nasopharynx occurs in 5%–15% of healthy individuals, and this rate may be higher in confined groups such as military recruits. A direct correlation between carrier rates and incidence of disease has not been established, with the possible exception of members of large households or households with an infant or childhood case during epidemics of disease. *N. meningitidis* has also been isolated from genital sources, where its clinical significance is uncertain. When cultured from these sources, bacteria may be misidentified as *N. gonorrhoeae* unless appropriate tests for distinguishing these species are performed.

The principal virulence factor of *N. meningitidis* is a lipopolysaccharide–endotoxin complex, which in experimental animals activates the clotting cascade, depositing fibrin in small vessels, producing hemorrhage in the adrenals and other organs, altering peripheral vascular resistance, and leading to shock and death.

The pathogenesis and clinical manifestations of *N. gonorrhoeae* infections differ somewhat from those of *N. meningitidis*. Pathogenic types of *N. gonorrhoeae* adhere by means of pili, which are not produced by nonpathogenic types, to various human cells. These antigenically heterogeneous pili, which represent one of the principal virulence factors of *N. gonorrhoeae*, may inhibit phagocytosis and stimulate strain-specific antibody formation. Other possible virulence factors of *N. gonorrhoeae* are less clearly defined. Both *N. gonorrhoeae* and *N. meningitidis* produce an IgA protease, which may be important in their pathogenesis because IgA is the antibody class that predominates in secretions on mucous membranes (Janda, 2007).

Laboratory Diagnosis

The single most important element in the laboratory diagnosis of infection caused by *N. meningitidis* or *N. gonorrhoeae* is the specimen, including

PART 7

TABLE 57-8
Differentiation of Species of *Neisseria* and *Moraxella catarrhalis*

	N. gonorrhoeae	*N. meningitidis*	*N. cinerea*	*N. lactamica*	*N. sicca*	*N. subflava*	*N. flavescens*	*N. mucosa*	*M. catarrhalis*
Growth									
Thayer-Martin medium	+*	+	–	+	–	–	+	–	†
Nutrient agar, 25° C	–	–	–	–	+	+	–	+	+
Oxidase	+	+	+	+	+	+	+	+	+
β-Galactosidase	–	–	–	+	–	–	–	–	–
Reduction of nitrate	–	–	–	–	–	–	–	+	+
DNase	–	–	–	–	–	–	–	–	+
Production of Acid from									
Glucose	+	+	–‡	+	+	+	–	+	–
Maltose	–	+	–	+	+	+	–	+	–
Lactose	–	–	–	+	–	–	–	–	–
Sucrose	–	–	–	–	+	D§	–	+	–
Fructose	–	–	–	–	+	–	–	–	–

+, ≥90% of strains positive; –, ≥90% of strains negative; *D,* variable; *DNase,* deoxyribonuclease.
*Most vancomycin-susceptible strains will not grow on Thayer-Martin medium.
†Some strains positive and others negative.
‡Weak reaction may occur in rapid carbohydrate utilization tests.
§Biovar. perflava, +; biovar. flava, –.

proper selection, collection, and transport to the laboratory (see Chapter 63). The pathogenic species are sensitive to drying and extremes of temperature, and material must be cultured promptly to enhance recovery. They are mesophilic and grow poorly, if at all, at room temperature. Many require prompt incubation in CO_2 (2%–8%) for primary isolation. Media containing chocolatized blood are commonly used for cultures and should contain antibiotics (i.e., vancomycin or lincomycin, as well as colistin, nystatin or anisomycin, and trimethoprim) if the specimen is prone to be contaminated by indigenous flora. Vancomycin-susceptible gonococci will grow on media containing lincomycin; however, because of the synergistic interaction of lincomycin and trimethoprim, the latter must be omitted from media containing lincomycin. Direct inoculation of specimens at the bedside followed by prompt incubation at 35° C in CO_2 is optimal. This can be accomplished in several ways: placing the medium into a candle jar; placing the medium in a sealed bag containing a citric acid bicarbonate tablet; or using a medium contained within a bottle having a CO_2 atmosphere. If any of these culture systems must be mailed to a reference laboratory for processing, they must first be incubated overnight to ensure growth of the organisms.

An isolate from a urogenital specimen showing the appropriate colony appearance on a selective medium presumptively may be called *N. gonorrhoeae* based on results of Gram stain and oxidase and catalase tests. Gram-stained smears prepared from colonies of *N. gonorrhoeae* should show typical gram-negative diplococci, but organisms may occur in tetrads, especially from young cultures. All species of *Neisseria* are oxidase positive, and all species except *N. elongata* are catalase positive. Because *Neisseria* other than *N. gonorrhoeae* may be recovered from urogenital sites, confirmatory testing is strongly recommended and is required for all isolates from extragenital sites, and when sexual abuse is suspected (preferably by more than one method).

Confirmation of *N. gonorrhoeae* and identification of the other *Neisseria* spp. are based on growth and biochemical characteristics (Table 57-8) (Janda, 2007). The standard method of identification consists of detection of acid production from carbohydrates in a cystine trypticase acid (CTA) base medium and other conventional biochemical tests. However, given the drawbacks of conventional methods, more rapid identification tests are used in most clinical laboratories. Tests for direct detection of *N. gonorrhoeae* and *N. meningitidis* in clinical specimens are also available. Typing of isolates of *N. gonorrhoeae* and *N. meningitidis* is done primarily for epidemiologic studies.

With the standard method of identification, acid production from glucose, maltose, lactose, sucrose, and fructose in a CTA base medium and a carbohydrate-free control are tested. Tubes are inoculated, incubated at 35°–37° C in ambient air, and examined at 24-hour intervals until reactions are interpretable, or for 72 hours. Expected results for the species of *Neisseria* are shown in Table 57-8. Occasionally, however, an isolate of *N. meningitidis* yields aberrant carbohydrate reactions: glucose-negative, maltose-negative, or asaccharolytic. If *N. meningitidis* is strongly suspected in these cases, identification can be confirmed by slide agglutination, using pooled polyvalent grouping antisera or sera specific for individual serogroups. In addition to conventional carbohydrate degradation tests, reduction of nitrates and nitrites and production of DNase should be evaluated. The latter is especially useful for identification of *Moraxella catarrhalis*, which is DNase positive (*Neisseria* spp. are DNase negative). Drawbacks to conventional tests are the requirement for a heavy inoculum, the need to work with pure cultures, long turnaround time, and failure of some fastidious strains of *N. gonorrhoeae* to grow.

Several commercial systems detect acid production from carbohydrates, usually in 1–4 hours (Dillon 1988; Janda, 2007). The inoculum must be prepared from a pure culture of the isolate, so identification is generally available 24 hours after isolation. Acid reactions of some *N. gonorrhoeae* and, to a lesser extent, *N. meningitidis* may be difficult to interpret or may be aberrant with some kits, and strains of *N. gonorrhoeae* that are weak producers of acid from glucose may appear to be glucose negative. Some strains of *Neisseria cinerea*, which does not typically produce acid from glucose, can appear glucose positive in certain systems.

Enzyme substrate tests provide rapid identification (1–4 hours) only of isolates of oxidase-positive, gram-negative diplococci recovered on a selective medium (Kellogg, 1995; Janda, 2007). They are valuable for differentiating maltose-negative strains of *N. meningitidis* from *N. gonorrhoeae*, but color changes may be subtle and if misinterpreted could cause isolates of *N. meningitidis* and other *Neisseria* spp. to be incorrectly called *N. gonorrhoeae*. Moreover, strains of *N. cinerea* and *Kingella denitrificans* that grow on gonococcus-selective media could be misidentified as *N. gonorrhoeae* if not confirmed by other procedures. Commercial products that combine enzyme substrate tests with modified conventional tests provide accurate identification of species of *Neisseria* and *Haemophilus* (Janda, 1987, 2002).

Immunologic tests for *N. gonorrhoeae*, in particular coagglutination, can be used to confirm the biochemical identification of *N. gonorrhoeae*. Three tests are available for this: the Phadebact Monoclonal GC Test (Boule Diagnostics AB, Huddinge, Sweden), the GonoGen I (New Horizons Diagnostics, Columbia, MD), and the GonoGen II (New Horizons Diagnostics). Both false-positive and false-negative results have been reported with these reagents (Dillon, 1988; Kellogg, 1995). A chemiluminescent nucleic acid probe for detection of *N. gonorrhoeae* can be used for culture confirmation or direct detection of the organism in endocervical or urethral swab specimens (Limberger, 1992; Hale, 1993). Nucleic acid amplification assays (NAAT) for use on endocervical or urethral swab specimens and urine are also available and may increase sensitivity when compared with nucleic acid probe and culture techniques, largely because the problem with organism viability is not an issue.

Latex agglutination assays are available for direct detection of *N. meningitidis* antigens in CSF, serum, and urine. As discussed previously (see *Streptococcus*), the sensitivity of these assays has been found to be less than or equal to that of the Gram stain, and the results of such testing appear to have little impact on patient care (Maxson, 1994; Perkins, 1995); therefore many laboratories have stopped offering this test.

Cultural detection of *Neisseria gonorrhoeae* from urogenital sites has been largely replaced by molecular methods, including probes and/or NAAT. Many products are available for NAAT that simultaneously detect *N. gonorrhoeae* and *Chlamydia trachomatis* from cervical, urethral, and urine samples with much greater sensitivity, and for which loss of viability of *N. gonorrhoeae* in particular is not an issue. These molecular techniques are described in other sections of this text (Janda, 2007).

Antimicrobial Susceptibility

Despite the occasional recovery of *N. meningitidis* strains with decreased susceptibility to penicillin, penicillin G remains the drug of choice for treatment of meningococcal meningitis (Janda, 2007). Decreased susceptibility of *N. meningitidis* to penicillin is thought to be due to decreased binding of penicillin by altered meningococcal cell wall penicillin-binding proteins, PBP-2 and PBP-3. Other species of *Neisseria* have also demonstrated this lowered affinity to penicillin (Saez-Nieto, 1992). Other agents that have good activity against *N. meningitidis* include the extended-spectrum cephalosporins and chloramphenicol. Rifampin, minocycline, and the fluoroquinolones may be used for prophylaxis among household contacts. Standardized methods of susceptibility testing and breakpoints in the CLSI documents are now available (CLSI, 2009). The CLSI does recommend that a broth microdilution or an agar dilution MIC test with cation-supplemented Mueller-Hinton Broth (with 2%–5% laked horse blood) or Mueller-Hinton Agar (with 5% [vol/vol] sheep blood) should be used if testing is done. Enrichments such as IsoVitaleX (1%) may also be needed. In laboratories where susceptibility testing for *N. meningitidis* is not available, β-lactamase testing can be performed by using the chromogenic cephalosporin test, the cefinase nitrocefin disk test, if lowered susceptibility or clinical failure on penicillin is suspected. If positive, isolates can be shipped to a reference laboratory for further testing.

Because of widespread resistance of *N. gonorrhoeae* to penicillin and tetracycline (Fox, 1997), current recommendations for treatment include extended-spectrum cephalosporins but no longer include the newer fluoroquinolones. Although no resistance to the cephalosporins is apparent, resistance to the fluoroquinolones has been documented (CDC, 2007). Therefore susceptibility testing should be performed if symptoms persist after treatment. β-Lactamase production can be detected using a chromogenic cephalosporin. Disk diffusion using GC agar with 1% growth supplement is recommended to determine the susceptibility of *N. gonorrhoeae* to the cephalosporins, quinolones, and spectinomycin. The CLSI document recommends the agar dilution method or a disk diffusion method for testing of *N. gonorrhoeae* (CLSI, 2009). In addition, an E-test can be performed. For some agents, only a susceptible breakpoint is available because no resistant strains have yet been documented. If one identifies a nonsusceptible result with a third-generation cephalosporin, for example, confirmation tests and referral to a reference laboratory should be strongly considered (CLSI, 2009).

Prevention

A polysaccharide vaccine against *N. meningitidis* serogroups A, C, Y, and W135 is licensed in the United States and is recommended for military personnel, for persons living in epidemic areas of developing countries, for individuals with a nonfunctional or absent spleen, and for college students. Antibiotic prophylaxis should be limited to household contacts and those who have had contact with patients' oral secretions. Rifampin is currently the drug of choice.

The use of preexposure antibiotics to prevent gonococcal disease is discouraged because of the potential risks of sensitization and the emergence of resistant strains. The sole exception to this rule is the application of silver nitrate solution or erythromycin ointment to the eyes of newborns to prevent gonococcal (and chlamydial) ophthalmia.

Moraxella catarrhalis

M. catarrhalis may be carried in the oropharynx of healthy children and adults. It is an encapsulated organism, and extending from its outer membrane are pili that serve as adhesins. The most common infections caused by this organism are bronchitis, otitis, sinusitis, and pneumonia (especially in persons with underlying chronic lung disease) (Schreckenberger, 2007). *M. catarrhalis* is an infrequent cause of bacteremia, endocarditis, meningitis, urogenital infection, and ophthalmia neonatorum. Figure 57-13 shows the Gram stain of sputum in which *M. catarrhalis* is seen in large quantities inside and outside the polymorphonuclear leukocytes. *Moraxella catarrhalis* was part of the *Neisseria* genera and later transferred to the *Branhamella* genus for a short time. *M. catarrhalis* is a coccus that morphologically resembles *Neisseria* spp., unlike other members of the genus *Moraxella* (e.g., *Moraxella lacunata*, *Moraxella osloensis*, *Moraxella atlantae*), which appear as rods. *M. catarrhalis* bacteria are oxidase and catalase positive but can be differentiated from *Neisseria* spp. in their ability to grow readily on blood and chocolate agar, their lack of oxidative metabolism (sugars will be negative), and their production of DNase. Nearly all isolates of *M. catarrhalis* produce β-lactamase, which can be detected using nitrocefin. Although they should be assumed to be resistant to penicillin because of this, these isolates generally remain susceptible to cephalosporins, trimethoprim-sulfamethoxazole, and β-lactamase inhibitor combinations (Schreckenberger, 2007).

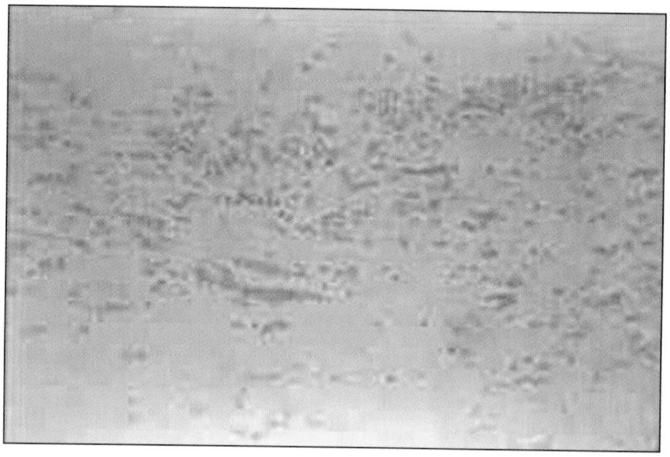

Figure 57-13 Gram stain of *Moraxella catarrhalis* in a sputum specimen. Note the intracellular gram-negative diplococci that resemble *Neisseria* spp.

GRAM-NEGATIVE BACTERIA—BACILLI

The gram-negative bacilli make up a complex group. They are broken down into the following: Enterobacteriaceae—those found normally in the GI tract or that colonize and cause infection there primarily; nonfermentative gram-negative bacilli, which usually are not found as part of the normal flora of humans but rather are environmental bacteria; non-Enterobacteriaceae that can cause GI infection, such as *Vibrio* or *Campylobacter*; agents of infections with specific epidemiologic characteristics, such as *Legionella* and *Francisella*; other gram-negative bacilli, including *Haemophilus* spp.; and miscellaneous genera.

Enterobacteriaceae

Characteristics

The Enterobacteriaceae are aerobic and facultatively anaerobic, non-spore-forming, nonmotile or peritrichously flagellated, oxidase-negative, gram-negative bacilli that produce acid fermentatively from glucose and reduce nitrates to nitrites. Figure 57-14 shows a Gram stain of *Escherichia coli*, but it could represent any member of the Enterobacteriaceae. Genera included in this group are *Budvicia*, *Buttiauxella*, *Cedecea*, *Citrobacter*, *Edwardsiella*, *Enterobacter*, *Escherichia*, *Ewingella*, *Hafnia*, *Klebsiella*, *Kluyvera*, *Leclercia*, *Leminorella*, *Moellerella*, *Morganella*, *Obesumbacterium*, *Pragia*, *Pantoea*, *Photorhabdus*, *Proteus*, *Providencia*, *Rahnella*, *Salmonella*, *Serratia*, *Shigella*, *Tatumella*, *Trabulsiella*, *Xenorhabdus*, *Yersinia*, and *Yokenella*. Only a few of these are discussed here (Farmer, 2007).

Clinical Manifestations and Pathogenesis

Enterobacteriaceae are found on plants, in soil, in water, and in the intestines of humans and animals. They have been associated with many clinical infections, including abscesses, pneumonia, meningitis, septicemia, and urinary tract infections. Those commonly associated with human infection include *E. coli*, *Klebsiella* spp., *Proteus* spp., *Enterobacter* spp., *Salmonella* spp., *Shigella* spp., *Serratia* spp., *Citrobacter* spp., and *Providencia* spp. Figure 57-15 shows a Gram stain of CSF from a newborn child that was culture positive for *E. coli*. In the urinary tract, those frequently isolated are *E. coli*, *Proteus mirabilis*, and *Klebsiella pneumoniae*. Gram-negative pneumonias

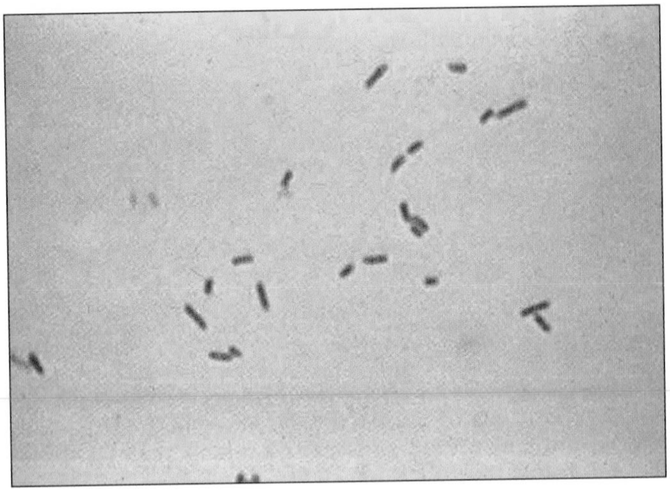

Figure 57-14 Gram stain of urine positive for *Escherichia coli*. The short, plump gram-negative rods are typical of any member of the Enterobacteriaceae.

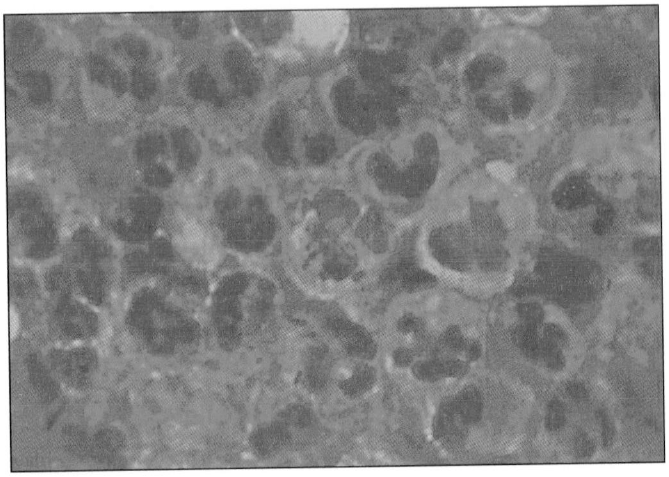

Figure 57-15 Gram stain of a cerebrospinal fluid specimen from a neonate containing gram-negative bacilli that grew *Escherichia coli*.

associated with the Enterobacteriaceae are frequently caused by *K. pneumoniae*. Gram-negative bacteremias related to the Enterobacteriaceae are frequently caused by *E. coli*, *K. pneumoniae*, and *P. mirabilis*. Infections acquired in the hospital are likely to be caused by members of antibiotic-resistant genera, such as *Citrobacter*, *Enterobacter*, and *Serratia*. Enterobacteriaceae associated with diarrhea include *Shigella* spp., *Salmonella* spp., *E. coli* (enterohemorrhagic [Shiga toxin producing], enterotoxigenic, enteroinvasive, enteropathogenic, enteroadherent), and *Yersinia* spp. Shigellas are rarely isolated from sources other than the GI tract, and salmonellas are more frequently isolated from other sources, such as urine or blood. *Calymmatobacterium granulomatis*, an agent of the sexually transmitted disease donovanosis, has been renamed *Klebsiella granulomatis* and is now part of the Enterobacteriaceae, even though the organism cannot be cultured on bacteriologic media (Abbott, 2007; Farmer, 2007). This topic is discussed later under a separate heading.

Endotoxins that are present within the cell walls of the Enterobacteriaceae, as well as other gram-negative bacilli, are responsible for much of the morbidity and mortality resulting from infections associated with these bacteria. Endotoxins consist of lipid and polysaccharide moieties with small quantities of amino acids and are often referred to as lipopolysaccharides. Lipopolysaccharides may elicit fever, chills, hypotension, granulocytosis, thrombocytopenia, disseminated intravascular coagulation, and activation of both classic and alternate complement pathways. Endotoxic shock is the result of gram-negative septicemia, with endotoxin reacting with macrophages, leukocytes, platelets, complement, and other serum proteins to increase the blood levels of proteolytic enzymes and vasoactive substances, resulting in pooling of blood, increased peripheral vasoconstriction, and diminution in cardiac output. It has become clear that the lethal effects of endotoxin are dependent on macrophage activation and responsiveness, and that the production of cachectin from the activated macrophage plays a major role in causing profound shock and multiple organ injury (Tracey, 1988).

Other pathogenetic factors of the Enterobacteriaceae include the K1 antigen, which is associated with a high percentage of strains of *E. coli* causing neonatal meningitis; the capsule of *K. pneumoniae*, which, like that of the pneumococcus, inhibits phagocytosis; the Vi antigen of *Salmonella* serotype *typhi*, which may interfere with intracellular killing of this organism; and various surface antigens, such as fimbriae, that mediate adherence of the organism to mucosal surfaces.

Plasmid-mediated factors appear to play an important role in the invasive properties of *Salmonella*, *Shigella*, and enteroinvasive strains of *E. coli*. Moreover, the heat-labile enterotoxins (LT) and the heat-stable enterotoxins of *E. coli* are plasmid mediated. LT stimulates adenylate cyclase in mucosal cells of the small intestine, which, in turn, activates cyclic adenosine monophosphate (cAMP); this causes secretion of fluid and electrolytes into the intestinal lumen and produces watery diarrhea. In contrast, heat-stable (ST) enterotoxins appear to activate guanylate cyclase.

Laboratory Diagnosis

The isolation of gram-negative bacilli from contaminated specimens is greatly facilitated by the use of differential and selective media (Table 57-9). Eosin methylene blue (EMB) and MacConkey's agar can be used interchangeably as minimally selective and differential media to initially select for and differentiate lactose-fermenting from non–lactose-fermenting gram-negative bacilli. XLD and HE agars are more selective differential media that are especially useful in selecting for *Salmonella* spp. and *Shigella* spp. in heavily contaminated specimens such as stool. Bismuth sulfite is a highly selective medium that is especially useful for the detection of salmonellae in endemics or epidemics. *Salmonella* spp. produce H_2S and are easily recognized by the production of colonies with black centers on XLD, HE, and bismuth sulfite agars. An enrichment medium, such as selenite-F or gram-negative (GN) broth, may be useful for detecting low numbers of *Salmonella* spp. and *Shigella* spp. in stool. Cefsulodin-irgasan-novobiocin (CIN) agar incubated at room temperature is selective and differential for the recovery of *Yersinia enterocolitica*. Colonies will appear as bull's-eyes with red centers and transparent borders. MacConkey's agar with sorbitol as the fermentable sugar is a differential medium that is capable of differentiating the sorbitol-fermentation–negative *E. coli* 0157:H7, which is associated with hemolytic-uremic syndrome from most other *E. coli* (Abbott, 2007; Nataro, 2007).

For some of the Enterobacteriaceae, a few simple colonial characteristics or biochemical reactions can be used to presumptively identify an isolate. For example, *Proteus* spp. swarm on blood agar, *Klebsiella* spp. form lactose-positive mucoid colonies, *Serratia marcescens* may produce a red pigment, *Salmonella* spp. produce H_2S, and *E. coli* is indole positive. Definitive identification of these and other species requires additional biochemical testing and/or molecular methods. Innumerable schemes based on the use of conventional biochemical media have been described for identification of the Enterobacteriaceae. Differential characteristics of the Enterobacteriaceae most commonly encountered in the clinical laboratory are shown in Table 57-10. Commercially prepared kits and automated devices are available and offer convenience and accuracy in identifying the vast majority of isolates belonging to the Enterobacteriaceae. In some instances, identification is accurately made in a few hours. Semiautomated systems may combine identification and antimicrobial susceptibility testing in a single disposable unit. In general, accuracy of identification among these systems is very high and comparable.

Classification of the Enterobacteriaceae has undergone considerable revision in recent years as the result of DNA hybridization and relatedness studies. Because phenotypic groupings on the basis of biochemical reactions are not always consistent with their DNA relatedness, the use of tribes (e.g., Klebsielleae, Proteae) for grouping species within the Enterobacteriaceae has been discontinued.

Historically, the genus *Salmonella* has been divided into the following species: *S. typhi*, *Salmonella paratyphi* A and B, *Salmonella choleraesuis*, *Salmonella typhimurium*, and *Salmonella enteritidis*. Because all groups have been found to be genetically very closely related, current terminology now recognizes only two species: *S. enterica* and *S. bongori* (rarely isolated from humans), each of which contains multiple subspecies. Six subspecies of *S. enterica* are known, with subspecies I (*S. enterica* subsp. *enterica*) as the usual human isolate. More than 2000 serotypes of *Salmonella* have been identified, most belonging in the subspecies *enterica*. Serotyping is based on immunologic reactivity of the heat-stable somatic "O" antigens, which are predominantly lipopolysaccharide in content, and the heat-labile

TABLE 57-9
Differentiation of Aerobic Gram-Negative Bacilli

Test	*Escherichia coli*	*Klebsiella pneumoniae*	*Klebsiella oxytoca*	*Proteus mirabilis*	*Proteus vulgaris*	*Shigella* spp.	*Citrobacter freundii*	*Yersinia enterocolitica*	*Enterobacter cloacae*	*Serratia marcescens*	*Morganella morganii*	*Providencia alcalifaciens*	*Salmonella* serotype *choleraesuis*	*Salmonella* serotype *typhi*	*Salmonella* serotype *paratyphi A*
Indole	+	–	+	–	+	D	–	D	–	–	+	+	–	–	–
Methyl red	+	– or +	D	+	+	+	+	+	–	+ or –	+	+	+	+	+
Voges-Proskauer	–	+	+	– or +	–	–	–	+ (25° C)/ – (37° C)	+	+	–	–	–	–	–
Citrate (Simmons)	–	+	+	D	D	–	+	– (25° C)	+	+	–	+	(+)	–	–
H_2S (in triple sugar iron agar)	–	–	–	+	+	–	+	–	–	–	–	–	D	+	– or +
Urease	–	+	+	+	+	–	D	+	D	– or +	+	–	–	–	–
Phenylalanine deaminase	–	–	–	+	+	–	–	–	–	–	+	–	–	–	–
Lysine decarboxylase	+ or –	+	+	–	–	–	–	–	–	–	–	–	+	+	–
Arginine dihydrolase	– or +	–	–	–	–	–	D	–	+	–	–	–	(+)	– or (+)	– or +
Ornithine decarboxylase	D	–	–	+	–	D	– or +	+	+	+		+	–	+	–
Motility	+ or –	–	–	+*	+*	–	+	+ + (25° C)/ – (37° C)	+	+	+ or –	+	+	+	+
Acid produced from lactose	+	+	+	–	–	–	+ or (+)	D	D	–	–	–	–	–	–

+, ≥90% positive reactions within 2 days; –, ≥90% negative reactions; (+), positive reactions in 3 to 7 days; + or –, reactions of most strains positive; – or +, reactions of most strains negative; *D,* different reactions [+, (+), or –].
*Swarm on blood and chocolate agar.

TABLE 57-10
Enteric Differential and Selective Media

Medium	Gram-positive bacteriostatic agent	Fermentable carbohydrate	Indicator	Colony color fermenter	Nonfermenter	Category
Eosin methylene blue (EMB)	Eosin Y Methylene blue	Lactose*	Eosin Y Methylene blue	Red or black with sheen	Colorless	S, D
MacConkey's	Crystal violet Bile salts	Lactose	Neutral red	Red	Colorless	S, D
Xylose-lysine-deoxycholate (XLD)	Bile salts	Xylose Lactose Sucrose	Phenol red	Yellow	Red	S, D
Hektoen enteric (HE)	Bile salts	Salicin Lactose Sucrose	Bromthymol blue	Yellow-orange	Green, blue-green	S, D
Salmonella shigella (SS)	Bile salts	Lactose	Neutral red	Red	Colorless	S
Bismuth sulfite (BS)	Brilliant green	Glucose	Bismuth sulfite	†	†	S
Thiosulfate citrate bile salts sucrose (TCBS)‡	Bile salts pH 8.6	Sucrose	Thymol blue Bromthymol blue	Yellow	Colorless	S, D

D, Differential; *S*, selective.
*Levine's formulation.
†H_2S-producing salmonellae have black colonies.
‡Used for isolation of vibrios.

flagellar "H" antigens. In the United States, *Salmonella* serotypes *typhimurium* and *enteritidis* are the most common. *Salmonella* serotype *typhi* also produces a heat-labile capsular polysaccharide Vi antigen. In practice, most clinical laboratories identify isolates as *Salmonella* spp. based on biochemical reactions and use group-specific immunologic reagents to assign isolates to a specific serogroup. Commercial slide agglutination tests to differentiate large serogroups—A, B, C, and D—are useful in differentiating typhoidal salmonella from nontyphoidal strains. *S.* serotype *typhi* carries the D serogroup and Vi antigen. Further identification of the specific serotype is generally performed only by State Health Departments or other reference laboratories.

Isolates biochemically resembling *Shigella* are also classified by the reactivity of the "O" antigen, as are isolates of *E. coli* that are identified as potential causes of diarrhea and hemolytic-uremic syndrome. Such *E. coli* are classified by the type of toxin produced as well. Commercial kits are available to identify *E. coli* O157 and to detect some types of toxins in culture or stool specimens; however, this type of testing is often sent out to referral laboratories or the State Health Department. The CDC has recommended that all laboratories consider testing stool samples for the presence of shiga toxins I and II produced by certain strains of hemorrhagic *E. coli* (O157:H7 and other serotypes). Shiga toxin is also produced by *Shigella*, but the species is *S. dysenteriae*, which is not often seen in the United States. Serologic antigen tests are available and are widely used in clinical laboratories for this toxin (Nataro, 2007).

Antimicrobial Susceptibility

The susceptibility of Enterobacteriaceae to various antimicrobial agents is highly variable. Susceptibility to ampicillin was common among strains of *E. coli* and *P. mirabilis*, for example (although resistance in both has increased greatly over the past 10–15 years) but was not expected among most other clinically significant members of the Enterobacteriaceae. Resistance to first-generation cephalosporins (cefazolin, cephalothin) is expected for *Enterobacter* spp., *Serratia* spp., *Citrobacter* spp., *Proteus vulgaris*, *Providencia* spp., *Morganella* spp., and *Yersinia* spp.; susceptibility to third-generation cephalosporins (e.g., ceftriaxone, cefotaxime, ceftazidime) continues for many members of the Enterobacteriaceae. However, the presence of extended-spectrum β-lactamases and *Amp-C* genes, which are recognized by resistance of the bacteria to third-generation cephalosporins and all β-lactam antibiotics, except carbapenems, is increasing in selected strains of *E. coli*, *K. pneumoniae*, *P. mirabilis*, and others. Most Enterobacteriaceae are susceptible to aminoglycosides and fluoroquinolones. It had been very unusual for a member of the Enterobacteriaceae to be resistant to carbapenems (e.g., imipenem, meropenem, ertapenem, doripenem); however, in the late 1990s in a few U.S. states, isolates of *K. pneumoniae* were first recognized that produced a bla_{KPC} gene, resulting in production of carbapenemases that inactivate all carbapenems. These strains are often referred to as "KPCs" or *K. pneumoniae*–producing carbapenemases. These isolates are resistant to most classes of antibiotics, except for an aminoglycoside, colistin, and tigecycline. The spread of these KPC genes has been rare, but it is feared that these will be introduced into *E. coli*, for example, which accounts for significant nosocomial infections.

Detection of carbapenem resistance may be difficult with some strains possessing this resistance, and a newer confirmatory test, the modified Hodge test, has been introduced into clinical laboratories for this purpose. A potential KPC is inoculated near a carbapenem antibiotic disk onto an agar plate, onto which a lawn of carbapenem-susceptible *E. coli* has first been placed. Inactivation of the carbapenem will result in a reduction in the zone size of *E. coli* near the disk in close proximity to the inoculated KPC if the test is positive. Ertapenem is a better marker for carbapenem resistance than is meropenem or imipenem, but resistance to one of these leads to resistance to all carbapenems (Endimiani, 2009, 2009a; Kitchel, 2009). Infection control procedures are essential to prevent the spread of these highly resistant strains.

Because the susceptibility pattern of the Enterobacteriaceae is unpredictable, as a general rule susceptibility testing should be performed if antimicrobial therapy is being considered. No susceptibility testing need be performed if antimicrobial therapy is not instituted, as is the case for uncomplicated enteric infection due to salmonella, for which therapy may actually prolong the carrier state, or when a mixed flora infection is present and individual susceptibilities may not be appropriate. Methods for performing susceptibility tests, including the modified Hodge test and confirmatory extended-spectrum ESBL tests, and interpretive criteria can be found in CLSI documents (CLSI, 2010).

Plesiomonas

Characteristics

Plesiomonas shigelloides, the only species in the genus *Plesiomonas*, is a facultatively anaerobic, oxidase- and catalase-positive, glucose-fermenting, gram-negative rod. Recent molecular genetic evidence demonstrates that the genus *Plesiomonas* is most closely related to the genus *Proteus*. Therefore, it has been placed into the Enterobacteriaceae family (Farmer, 2007) as the only oxidase-positive member of this group of gram-negative bacilli.

Clinical Manifestations and Pathogenesis

P. shigelloides is found in aquatic environments that are limited geographically by its minimum growth temperature of 8° C. It may be found in fresh and estuarine water, usually in tropical countries. It has been implicated as a cause of gastroenteritis, especially following the ingestion of uncooked shellfish. The diarrheal stool specimen frequently contains polymorphonuclear leukocytes and red blood cells, although a cholera-like illness may occur. Gastroenteritis may occur in sporadic cases, as well as in outbreaks. Extraintestinal manifestations of infection with *P. shigelloides* include meningitis, septicemia, cellulitis, arthritis, and endophthalmitis (Ampofo, 2001).

Relatively little is known as yet about virulence factors of *P. shigelloides*. The organism appears to have invasive properties, and some data suggest enterotoxigenic activity (Brenden, 1988; Abbott, 2007).

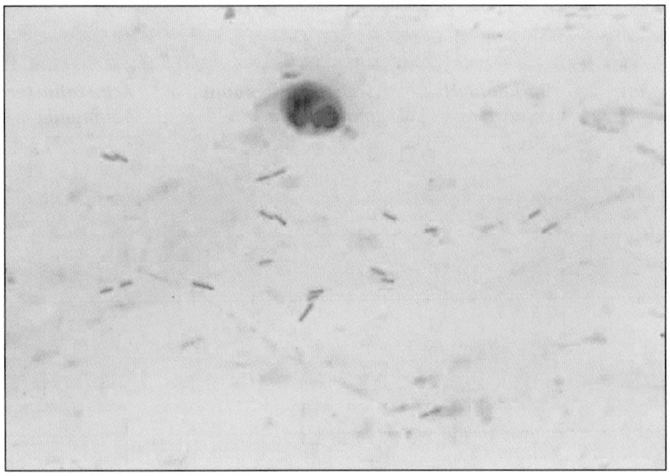

Figure 57-16 Gram stain of *Pseudomonas aeruginosa* in a sputum specimen. Note the longer, gram-negative bacilli compared with Figure 57-13.

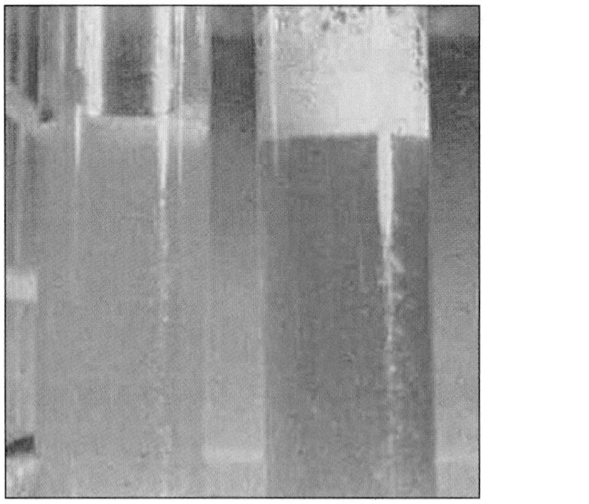

Figure 57-17 Extracted pyocyanin pigment from *Pseudomonas aeruginosa*.

Laboratory Diagnosis

P. shigelloides can be isolated on a variety of nonselective and enteric-selective media, including HE agar. Acid production from lactose is variable, but on enteric media the organism usually appears to be a non–lactose fermenter. It is indole positive; reduces nitrates to nitrites; produces catalase; is methyl red positive; and ferments glucose, maltose, and trehalose (Brenden, 1988; Abbott, 2007).

Antimicrobial Susceptibility

P. shigelloides is susceptible to a variety of antimicrobial agents, including cephalosporins, trimethoprim-sulfamethoxazole, imipenem, and the quinolones (Abbott, 2007). Susceptibility to the penicillins is variable because of the presence of a β-lactamase similar to that of *Aeromonas* spp.

GRAM-NEGATIVE BACTERIA—NONFERMENTATIVE BACILLI

A group of gram-negative bacilli that do not ferment glucose and other sugars are often lumped together under the heading of "nonfermenters." They account for about 15% of the gram-negative bacilli isolated from hospitalized patients. Although many genera of nonfermenters are known, 75% of the clinically relevant ones are *Pseudomonas aeruginosa*; most of the remaining 25% are *Acinetobacter* spp., *Stenotrophomonas maltophilia*, or *Burkholderia cepacia*. As a group, they are environmental bacteria and are not usually found as part of the normal flora of the human body, except as colonizers in hospitalized patients. They can be readily isolated from water, soil, vegetables, plants, and hospital surfaces. Although no uniform biochemical characteristics have been noted, they are often oxidase-positive, lactose-negative colonies on selective media such as MacConkey's agar (although some of the species do not grow on this media), and they are frequently resistant to many of the antibiotics that are effective against members of the Enterobacteriaceae. The four main species mentioned previously, as well as a few others, are discussed in this chapter.

Pseudomonas

Characteristics

The genus *Pseudomonas* has undergone extensive revision, and now many of the species that were previously classified in this genus have been reclassified into the genera *Burkholderia*, *Stenotrophomonas*, *Comamonas*, *Shewanella*, *Ralstonia*, *Methylobacterium*, *Sphingomonas*, *Acidovorax*, and *Brevundimonas*. Of the species that remain, *P. aeruginosa* is the most significant human pathogen. Figure 57-16 shows the Gram stain of *P. aeruginosa* in a sputum specimen.

Pseudomonads are strictly aerobic, catalase-positive, oxidase-positive, gram-negative bacilli. Their metabolism is respiratory and never fermentative, with oxygen as the terminal electron acceptor. Some pseudomonads are motile by means of polar flagella.

Clinical Manifestations and Pathogenesis

Pseudomonads are found in moist environments. Some of the more unusual habitats for these organisms include cosmetics, swimming pools, hot tubs, and the inner soles of sneakers. The latter can lead to puncture wounds that are infected with *P. aeruginosa*. The species causing the greatest morbidity and mortality today is *P. aeruginosa*. Other species of *Pseudomonas*, although often isolated from clinical specimens, are only occasionally involved in disease.

P. aeruginosa is ubiquitous in the hospital environment, existing almost anywhere there is moisture, including medical equipment and disinfectant solutions and soaps. It is only rarely found as part of the normal flora of healthy people, but in hospitalized patients, the rates of colonization increase with the length of hospitalization. *P. aeruginosa* may produce serious infection in patients with burns and traumatic and operative wounds; following urinary tract manipulation; in patients with diseases of the hematopoietic, reticuloendothelial, and lymphoid systems; and in those with impaired cellular or humoral defenses. Pulmonary infection occurs commonly in patients with cystic fibrosis. The mortality rate is highest in severely leukopenic patients.

P. aeruginosa produces a slime polysaccharide, an endotoxin, and proteases that inactivate components of complement, thereby inhibiting to some degree opsonization and the inflammatory response, and perhaps contributing to its invasiveness. Exotoxin A promotes cellular damage and tissue invasion and is toxic for macrophages.

Laboratory Diagnosis

The presence of *P. aeruginosa* in cultures can often be suspected because of its musty grape-like (or corn tortilla) odor, the rough or ground glass appearance of its colonies on sheep blood agar, and the presence of one or both of two pigments: a "blue-green" fluorescent pigment (Fig. 57-17) and/or a metallic sheen caused by pyoverdin pigment. It can be identified easily with a positive oxidase reaction, an alkaline slant/neutral butt reaction in TSIA, growth at 42° C, and the formation of sheen and/or pigment on the slants of TSIA and *Pseudomonas* P agar. Additional tests are shown in Table 57-11. Tests of carbohydrate utilization should be carried out in O-F basal medium, which contains a minimal quantity of peptone and a relatively large quantity of carbohydrate, and so can allow detection of very small quantities of acid formed by this group of bacteria. Reactions are usually complete within 48 hours but may require as long as 7 days.

Antimicrobial Susceptibility

As a general rule, susceptibility testing should be performed for all clinically significant isolates of *P. aeruginosa*. Hospital strains of *P. aeruginosa* may be resistant to many classes of antibiotic. Isolates are often susceptible to the aminoglycosides, the carboxypenicillins and ureidopenicillins, ceftazidime or cefepime, carbapenems, and the quinolones. *P. aeruginosa* is always resistant to sulfamethoxazole-trimethoprim (SXT) and tetracyclines, including the newer broad-spectrum tigecycline, ertapenem, and nitrofurantoin. Multiple resistance to drugs to which *P. aeruginosa* was once susceptible is increasing, especially in intensive care units and among patients who have long-standing *Pseudomonas* infections, such as patients with cystic fibrosis and other chronic syndromes (Friedland, 2004; Hauser, 2005). Laboratories are being asked to test additional antibiotics, especially colistin or polymyxin B, when these resistant isolates are encountered. The CLSI has recently provided breakpoints for testing of polymyxin B that can be interpreted for polymyxin B or colistin (CLSI, 2009).

TABLE 57-11
Differential Characteristics of Nonfermentative Gram-Negative Bacilli Isolated from Clinical Material

	Pseudomonas aeruginosa	***Pseudomonas fluorescens***	***Pseudomonas putida***	***Burkholderi cepacia***	***Stenotrophomonas maltophilia***	***Acinetobacter baumanii***
Oxidase	+	+	+	+	–	–
Pyocyanin	+	–	–	–	–	–
Fluorescein	+	–	+	–	–	–
Glucose oxidation	+	+	+	+	+/–	+
42° C	+	–	–	+/–	+/–	+
DNase	–	–	–	–	+	–/+
Growth on MacConkey's agar	+	+	+	+	+	+*
Motility	+	+	+	+	+	–

+, Positive; –, negative; +/–, variable results, most strains positive; –/+, variable results, most strains negative; *DNase,* deoxyribonuclease.
*Purplish color on MacConkey's agar.

Acinetobacter

Characteristics

Organisms in this genus are short, rod shaped to spherical, nonmotile, oxidase negative, strictly aerobic, and gram negative. In a Gram-stained smear, they often appear in pairs and may be difficult to decolorize.

Clinical Manifestations and Pathogenesis

Acinetobacter spp. are found commonly in soil and water and uncommonly on the skin and mucous membranes of healthy people. Little is known about virulence factors in this group of organisms, but they do appear to form small amounts of endotoxin. Although usually nonpathogenic, they have been increasingly associated with nosocomial septicemia, pneumonia, bacteriuria, and wound infection.

Laboratory Diagnosis

Acinetobacter spp. can be distinguished readily from pseudomonads on the basis of their lack of motility, inability to reduce nitrates, and negative oxidase reaction. They may produce characteristic purplish colonies on MacConkey's agar. More than 25 species are known, but their differentiation biochemically is difficult, and they are often lumped together in the *Acinetobacter calcoaceticus–Acinetobacter baumanii* complex. The glucose-oxidizing (saccharolytic strains), nonhemolytic clinical strains are usually referred to as *A. baumanii*; nonsaccharolytic strains (non–glucose oxidizers) may be *Acinetobacter lwoffi* if nonhemolytic, or *Acinetobacter haemolyticus* if hemolytic (Schreckenberger, 2007). The most clinically relevant species is *A. baumanii.*

Antimicrobial Susceptibility

Acinetobacter spp. are resistant to most available β-lactam and aminoglycoside antibiotics. Resistance to the aminoglycosides is caused by plasmid-mediated acetyl-, adenylyl-, and phosphotransferases. *Acinetobacter* spp. may be susceptible to doxycycline, trimethoprim-sulfamethoxazole, quinolones, ureidopenicillins, imipenem, ampicillin-sulbactam, and ceftazidime. The carbapenems (imipenem, meropenem, ertapenem, and doripenem) are considered the most active, but resistance rates up to 11% have been described in nosocomial strains throughout the United States (Gales, 2001). These isolates of carbapenem-resistant *A. baumanii* are often referred to as carbapenem-resistant *A. baumanii*; they are often resistant to all classes of antibiotics, except colistin and tigecycline (Perez, 2007, 2009). Appropriate infection control procedures are necessary to prevent their transmission (Rodríguez-Baño, 2009). Susceptibility testing should be performed for clinically significant isolates, usually upon the request of the clinician.

Burkholderia

Burkholderia spp. are aerobic, non–spore-forming, gram-negative rods; except for *Burkholderia mallei*, all are motile because they have polar flagella. These organisms are catalase positive, and most are oxidase positive. On MacConkey's agar, they produce lactose-negative colonies.

Clinical Significance and Pathogenesis

These organisms are found in the environment in water, in soil, and on plants. Because of their predilection for watery environments, some can be found in the hospital environment and have the potential to cause nosocomially acquired infection.

Two important human pathogens in the genus *Burkholderia* are *Burkholderia pseudomallei* and *Burkholderia cepacia* complex. *B. pseudomallei*, which is acquired via inhalation or contact through cut or abraded skin, causes melioidosis. The infection can be asymptomatic, can become chronic, or can cause a fulminant sepsis. Melioidosis is most prevalent in southeast Asia and Australia but may occur in other tropical and subtropical environments.

B. cepacia, a nosocomial pathogen that is associated with contaminated equipment, medications, and disinfectants, can cause bacteremia, urinary tract infection, septic arthritis, and respiratory tract infection. It is an important pathogen in patients with cystic fibrosis (CF) and in those with chronic granulomatous disease. Patients with CF who become chronically infected with this organism have a decreased rate of survival. *B. cepacia* complex comprises at least nine species, and all species have been recovered from patients with CF. In the United States, however, ≈85% of strains are *B. multivorans* or *B. cenocepacia; B. cenocepacia* has been shown in many studies to possess potent virulence factors that lead to increased mortality in CF patients who are infected with it versus other strains of *Burkholderia* (LiPuma, 2007).

Laboratory Diagnosis

Burkholderia species grow well on standard laboratory media, including blood and chocolate agar. Isolation of *B. cepacia* from contaminated specimens such as sputa may be made easier through the use of selective media (e.g., *Pseudomonas cepacia*, oxidative fermentative base, polymyxin B, bacitracin lactose agar, and *B. cepacia* selective agar) (Welch, 1987). A variety of different biochemical tests are needed to differentiate these organisms from one another (Kiska, 1996). No good biochemical methods are available to differentiate among the *B. cepacia* complex, or between the complex and related species such as *B. gladioli* and *Ralstonia*, *Cupriavidus*, and *Pandoraea* spp. Molecular techniques are often required for confirmatory identification and should be pursued when a *B. cepacia* complex organism is suspected. The CF Foundation (http://www.cff.org) has established a *B. cepacia* reference laboratory to confirm the identity of possible isolates in CF patients (LiPuma, 1999, 2007; Heath 2002).

Antimicrobial Susceptibility

The susceptibility of these organisms to antimicrobial agents varies considerably. *B. cepacia* is highly resistant to many antimicrobials but is usually susceptible to piperacillin, ceftazidime, chloramphenicol, and trimethoprim-sulfamethoxazole. Strains from CF patients who have been on repeated courses of antibiotics are likely to become resistant to these agents. The CLSI recommends reporting only ceftazidime, meropenem, minocycline, and trimethoprim-sulfamethoxazole for *B. cepacia* (CLSI, 2009). All *B. cepacia* organisms are intrinsically resistant to polymyxins (colistin).

Stenotrophomonas maltophilia

Characteristics

Stenotrophomonas maltophilia is a significant nosocomial pathogen. Risk factors for colonization or infection with this organism are mechanical

TABLE 57-12
Differential Characteristics of *Vibrio* Species*

Test	*V. cholerae*	*V. mimicus*	*V. damsela*	*V. parahaemolyticus*	*V. alginolyticus*	*V. vulnificus*	*V. fluvialis*	*V. metschnikovii*	*V. hollisae*
Indole	+	+	–	+ or –	D	+	– or +	D	+
Voges-Proskauer	– or +	–	+	–	+	–	–	+	–
Lysine decarboxylase	+	+	+	+	+	+	–	D	–
Ornithine decarboxylase	+	+	–	+ or –	D	D	–	–	–
Arginine dihydrolase	–	–	+	–	–	–	+	D	–
Lactose	(+)	– or +	–	–	–	+	–	D	–
Sucrose	+	+	–	+	+	D	+	+	–
Mannitol	+	+	–	+	+	D	+	+	–
Maltose	+	+	+	+	+	+	+	+	–
Arabinose	–	–	– + or	–	–	–	+	–	+
Salicin	–	–	–	–	–	+	–	– or +	–
Cellobiose	–	–	–	–	–	+	D	– or +	–
$NO_3 \rightarrow NO_2$	+	+	+	+	+	+	+	–	+
Oxidase	+	+	+	+	+	+	+	–	+
Growth in Nutrient Broth Plus NaCl, %									
0	+	+	–	–	–	–	W+ or –	–	–
1	+	+	+	+	+	+	+	+	+
6	– or (+)	– or (+)	+	+	+	+	+	+	(+)
8	–	–	–	+	+	–	–	D	–
10	–	–	–	–	+	–	–	D	–
12	–	–	–	–	–	–	–	–	–

W+, Weakly positive.
*For key to symbols, see Table 57-9.

ventilation, use of broad-spectrum antibiotics, catheterization, and neutropenia.

Laboratory Diagnosis

Important distinguishing biochemical reactions of *S. maltophilia* are its negative oxidase reaction and positive DNase activity. Colonies grow on blood agar (lavender green colonies) and MacConkey's agar; the bacteria are nonmotile and nonfermentative.

Antimicrobial Susceptibility

S. maltophilia is inherently resistant to many antibiotics, in particular, the carbapenems. Trimethoprim-sulfamethoxazole is the antibiotic of choice, although some strains are resistant (Gales, 2001). CLSI recommends reporting only levofloxacin, trimethoprim-sulfamethoxazole, and minocycline. Breakpoints have been put forth for interpretation of these agents for MIC and disk diffusion testing (CLSI, 2009).

Other nonfermentative gram-negative bacilli include members of the genera *Alcaligenes*, *Achromobacter*, *Flavobacterium*, *Flavimonas*, *Chryseomonas*, *Acidovorax*, *Brevundimonas*, *Comamonas*, and *Ralstonia*, among others. These are infrequently isolated from clinical specimens, often when they may represent contamination or colonization. They can be considered as significant, especially when isolated from sterile sites, on multiple occasions in immunosuppressed patients or patients with foreign devices in place.

Vibrio

Characteristics

Vibrio spp. are facultatively anaerobic, oxidase-positive, short, curved, or straight gram-negative bacilli that are usually motile by means of polar flagella; they ferment carbohydrates and reduce nitrates to nitrites. Several species are medically important (Table 57-12).

Clinical Manifestations and Pathogenesis

Among the vibrios, *Vibrio vulnificus* causes the most severe disease. Wound infections and septicemia with this organism are often fatal. Disease is usually associated with consumption of raw oysters or oyster-related injury. Preexisting hepatic disease is almost always present in serious illness. Decreased liver function results in increased available iron and appears to facilitate the growth of the organism.

Cholera toxin–producing *Vibrio cholerae* O1 is a well-known cause of epidemic cholera, which manifests itself by massive intestinal fluid loss and dehydration. The cholera toxin mediates this effect by binding to and activating the adenylate cyclase of cells in the small intestine, resulting in hypersecretion of electrolytes and water (Kaper, 1995). Non-O1 strains of *V. cholerae* cause a self-limited gastroenteritis but are not responsible for epidemics of disease. Nearly all non-O1 strains of *V. cholerae* do not produce cholera toxin but do produce two types of hemolysins and a heat-stable enterotoxin.

Vibrio mimicus and *Vibrio parahaemolyticus* primarily cause gastroenteritis. The mechanism of pathogenicity of *V. parahaemolyticus* appears to be related to invasiveness rather than to enterotoxin production. More than 95% of isolates of *V. parahaemolyticus* isolated from patients with gastroenteritis produce a cell-free hemolysin that is lethal to mice when injected in high doses and is described as the Kanagawa phenomenon. This halophilic organism is widely distributed in marine environments and has been found to contaminate fish and shellfish. Outbreaks of acute diarrheal disease following ingestion of contaminated food have been especially common in Japan but have also occurred in the United States and other countries (Abbott, 2007a).

Laboratory Diagnosis

Although formerly of concern only to U.S. travelers to endemic areas, cases of *V. cholerae* disease have been described in the United States in association with ingestion of contaminated shellfish from the Gulf Coast. In addition, gastroenteritis caused by *V. parahaemolyticus* and by other halophilic vibrios in contaminated shellfish has been described in many parts of the country, particularly in coastal areas. Thus it is important for clinical laboratories to have the capability to culture stool for *Vibrio* spp. when indicated on the basis of travel and dietary history.

With the exception of *V. cholerae* and *V. mimicus*, growth of this group of organisms requires media containing NaCl. Most solid and liquid media used for bacterial culture contain enough sodium that the use of special media in such instances is not necessary. Selective media containing sucrose, such as thiosulfate citrate bile salts medium, are very useful for culturing stool specimens for *Vibrio* spp. Certain species (*V. cholerae* and *Vibrio alginolyticus*) ferment the sucrose and appear as yellow colonies on this medium. An enrichment medium, such as alkaline peptone water, may be used prior to subculture to solid medium to enhance recovery of *Vibrio* spp. from stool. *Vibrio* spp. can be differentiated among themselves and from other enteric gram-negative bacilli according to the reactions listed in Table 57-12. It may be necessary to carry out biochemical testing of the halophilic vibrios in media supplemented with 1%–3% NaCl. If TSIA and lysine iron agar are inoculated for screening purposes, their reactions will be acid slant/acid butt with no gas (A/A) or H_2S and alkaline slant/alkaline butt (K/K), respectively (Abbott, 2007a). Not all commercially available gram-negative identification systems are reliable for the identification of *Vibrio* spp.; they should be used only if they have proved accurate (O'Hara, 2003).

Antimicrobial Susceptibility

Antimicrobial susceptibility testing can be performed using the disk diffusion method with Mueller-Hinton agar, and broth microdilution using cation-adjusted Mueller-Hinton broth and incubation at 35° C for 16–18 hours. CLSI has established interpretive standards for *V. cholerae* tested with ampicillin, tetracycline, doxycycline, trimethoprim-sulfamethoxazole, chloramphenicol, and sulfonamides (CLSI, 2009). Interpretive standards have been put forth for the other *Vibrio* spp. in CLSI document M45-2A (CLSI, 2010).

Aeromonas

Characteristics

Members of this genus are facultatively anaerobic, oxidase- and catalase-positive, rod-shaped, gram-negative bacilli. They are usually motile by means of polar flagella, although some species may be nonmotile. They form acids from carbohydrates by respiratory and fermentative metabolism and reduce nitrates to nitrite.

Clinical Manifestations and Pathogenesis

Aeromonas spp. are mainly found in aquatic environments. They have been isolated from tap water, rivers, soil, and various foods, and are only rarely found in marine environments. These organisms have been associated with both intestinal and extraintestinal disease. Although no definitive evidence has demonstrated the role of *Aeromonas* spp. in GI disease, the presence of *Aeromonas* spp. in stool is more often associated with diarrhea than with an asymptomatic carrier state. Its role in producing diarrheal disease is possibly related to the production of an enterotoxin by some strains. A hemolysin and a cytopathic factor have also been described. *Aeromonas* spp. may cause infection of traumatically acquired wounds or septicemia in patients who are immunocompromised (Janda, 1994, 2010).

Laboratory Diagnosis

Isolation of a fermenting, oxidase-positive, gram-negative bacillus from an appropriate specimen should suggest the possibility of *Aeromonas* spp. Organisms grow readily on conventional laboratory media and produce colonies that resemble those of *Pseudomonas* spp., have a greenish, ground glass appearance, and have a fruity odor. Most species are β-hemolytic on blood agar. Isolation of *Aeromonas* spp. from stool specimens may be enhanced by inoculation of blood agar containing ampicillin or CIN medium. More than 18 species of *Aeromonas* are now recognized; *Aeromonas hydrophila* complex, *Aeromonas caviae* complex, and *Aeromonas veronii* complex are the most common isolates from human specimens. Esculin, Voges-Proskauer, gas from glucose fermentation, and l-arabinose are four biochemicals that can be used to separate *Aeromonas* spp. into one of these three complexes, but a more definitive identification would require conventional biochemicals in conjunction with molecular sequencing methods (Horneman, 2007).

Antimicrobial Susceptibility

Aeromonas spp. are susceptible to the quinolones, aminoglycosides, carbapenems, and trimethoprim-sulfamethoxazole but produce a β-lactamase that mediates resistance to the penicillins and first-generation cephalosporins (Horneman, 2007). Carbapenemases, although rare, may be difficult to detect by conventional susceptibility testing methods, including automated systems (Rossolini, 1996; Horneman, 2007). *Aeromonas* spp. have been found to maintain resistance plasmids of both the Enterobacteriaceae and *Pseudomonas* spp.

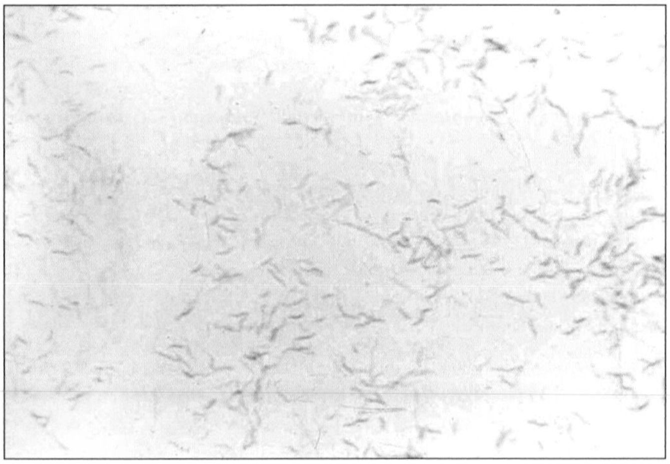

Figure 57-18 *Campylobacter jejuni* Gram stain: Note the comma-shaped appearance of the bacilli.

Campylobacter

Characteristics

Campylobacter spp. are small (0.5–8 μm long × 0.2–0.5 μm wide), motile, non–spore-forming, curved (comma-shaped) or S-shaped gram-negative bacilli that grow optimally in an atmosphere containing 5%–10% oxygen and, therefore, are considered to be microaerophilic. Figure 57-18 shows the Gram stain of *Campylobacter jejuni* from culture. *C. jejuni* is the most common cause of bacterial enteritis in the United States. Other *Campylobacter* spp. associated with enteritis are *Campylobacter coli*, *Campylobacter lari*, and *Campylobacter upsaliensis*. *Campylobacter fetus* subsp. *fetus* is a cause of septic thrombophlebitis, arthritis, peritonitis, abscess, and pericarditis (Fitzgerald, 2007), especially in persons with an underlying chronic disease. *Arcobacter* are aerotolerant, *Campylobacter*-like, spiral-shaped bacteria that are frequently isolated from bovine and porcine products of abortion and feces of animals with enteritis (Fitzgerald, 2007). *A. butzleri* has been isolated from patients with bacteremia, endocarditis, diarrhea, and peritonitis. *A. cryerophilus* has been isolated from patients with bacteremia and diarrhea (Fitzgerald, 2007).

Clinical Manifestations and Pathogenesis

C. jejuni is found worldwide as a commensal of the GI tract of wild or domesticated cattle, sheep, swine, goats, dogs, cats, and fowl, especially turkeys and chickens. It is the most common cause of bacterial enteritis in the United States, with an estimated occurrence of 1000 cases per 100,000 individuals. The incidence of infection in the United Kingdom and in other developed nations is similar to that in the United States, and the incidence in underdeveloped countries is probably even higher. Infections generally occur in the summer and fall and are commonly the result of ingestion of improperly cooked foods, usually poultry. In addition, several outbreaks of *C. jejuni* enteritis have been linked to unpasteurized milk and to defects in municipal water systems. The spectrum of illness ranges from asymptomatic to severely ill. The diarrhea produced may be with or without blood or fecal leukocytes. Symptoms can last up to 1 week and generally are self-limited. Extraintestinal infections, including bacteremia, reactive arthritis, urinary tract infection, and meningitis, may also occur. *C. jejuni* is the most recognized antecedent cause of Guillain-Barré syndrome. The pathogenesis of this organism is not completely understood; it appears to first colonize the intestinal mucous layer and then is able to translocate through the epithelial surface to the underlying tissue (Fitzgerald, 2007).

The major habitat of *C. fetus* subsp. *fetus* is the intestine of sheep and cattle; it also may be found in the genital tract of these animals, their placentas, and the gastric contents of their aborted fetuses and, less frequently, in other animals and birds. The mechanisms of transmission of infection to humans are not understood completely. Direct contact with an infected animal is possible, but less than one third of infected individuals have a history of environmental or occupational exposure. Contaminated food or water may be a vehicle for infection, or infection may originate from an endogenous source.

Laboratory Diagnosis

A single stool specimen is generally adequate to detect enteric pathogens, including *Campylobacter* spp. Examination for fecal leukocytes is not recommended because they may be present in as few as 25% of cases. An enzyme immunoassay (EIA) is available for direct detection of *Campylobacter jejuni* and *Campylobacter coli* antigens in stool specimens (Tolcin, 2000; Dediste, 2003).

Several media can be used for the selective isolation of *Campylobacter* spp., including charcoal-cefoperazone-deoxycholate agar, charcoal-based selective medium, semisolid blood-free motility medium, Skirrow's medium, and *Campylobacter* agar with 5% sheep blood and five antimicrobials (cephalothin, trimethoprim, vancomycin, polymyxin B, and amphotericin B). Most *Campylobacter* spp. require a microaerobic environment (5% O_2, 10% CO_2, and 85% N_2), which can be produced using commercially available gas generator packs. The amount of oxygen in a candle jar is too little to support the growth of *Campylobacter* spp. and should not be used. Incubation of the plates at 42° C increases selectivity for *C. jejuni*.

If *Campylobacter* spp. are suspected in a blood culture based on clinical history or appearance of an organism on Gram stain, the broth should be subcultured to a nonselective blood agar plate and incubated at 37° C in a microaerobic environment.

In general, *Campylobacter* spp. produce gray, flat, irregular, spready colonies, which may become round, convex, and glistening as the moisture content in the media is reduced. A typical Gram stain appearance and a positive oxidase reaction from a colony growing on selective media at 42° C can be reported as *Campylobacter* spp. *C. jejuni* is able to hydrolyze hippurate and is susceptible to nalidixic acid and resistant to cephalothin. *C. coli* is hippuricase negative.

Strains of *C. fetus* subsp. *fetus* are resistant to nalidixic acid, fail to hydrolyze hippurate, and do not ordinarily grow at 42° C.

Antimicrobial Susceptibility

C. jejuni is variably susceptible to antimicrobial agents. Most are not susceptible to penicillins or cephalosporins. For intestinal infection, erythromycin is the drug of choice, with quinolones used as alternative therapy. Treatment often is not warranted, however, for simple gastroenteritis with *Campylobacter* sp. in an otherwise healthy individual. Resistance to both agents has been encountered. Currently, no standardized methods are used for susceptibility testing of this group of organisms; however, a CLSI document giving guidelines for testing is available (CLSI, 2010).

Helicobacter

Characteristics

Helicobacter spp. are spiral-shaped or curved, gram-negative, non–spore-forming bacilli, measuring 0.3–1.0 μm wide and 1.5–10 μm long. They are motile by multiple bipolar or monopolar flagella, are microaerobic, and have a respiratory metabolism.

Clinical Manifestations and Pathogenesis

Helicobacter spp. are found in the GI tracts of mammals and birds. Transmission from one host to another occurs through both oral–oral and fecal–oral routes. *Helicobacter pylori* is considered to be one of the "gastric" helicobacters. In the stomach, it lives within or beneath the mucous layer adjacent to the epithelium. It is also found transiently in the duodenum, saliva, and feces.

Infection with *H. pylori* may result in acute gastritis symptoms. Most infected patients develop chronic active gastritis, which may lead to nonulcer dyspepsia or duodenal ulcers. *H. pylori* has been associated with 90% of duodenal ulcers and nearly all gastric ulcers. Infection with *H. pylori* has also been associated with gastric carcinoma and gastric lymphoma (Parsonnet, 1994). The prevalence of gastritis associated with *H. pylori* increases with age, suggesting that the organism is acquired as people become older.

The "enteric" helicobacters, such as *Helicobacter* (formerly *Campylobacter*) *cinaedi* and *Helicobacter fennelliae*, have been implicated in cases of gastroenteritis. Rarely, these organisms may invade the bloodstream and be isolated from cultures of blood (Solnick, 2003).

Laboratory Diagnosis

Typically, nonculture methods have been utilized to diagnose *H. pylori* infection. One such test is the urea breath test. This is a noninvasive test that detects urease activity of *H. pylori* by measuring ^{14}C- and ^{13}C-labeled CO_2 in the patient's expelled air after ingestion of labeled urea. Serologic assays are also widely used in symptomatic patients to detect antibodies against *H. pylori;* however, because most adults will have been exposed to *H. pylori*, this can be a nonspecific test, except as an epidemiologic or surveillance tool. In some cases, biopsies of the affected tissues are obtained and are examined histologically using the hematoxylin and eosin or Giemsa stain for the presence of organisms with morphology typical of *H. pylori*. Because the organism hydrolyzes urea very rapidly, a portion of the gastric biopsy may be placed directly into urea broth or onto urea-containing agar to detect urea hydrolysis in 1–24 hours (CLO test). A commercially available EIA for detection of *H. pylori* antigen in stool is a noninvasive alternative for diagnosis of *H. pylori* infection (Premier Platinum HpSA, Meridian Bioscience, Cincinnati). Sensitivity of this assay is as high as 89%, with specificities up to 95% (Masoero, 2000; Montiero, 2001). PCR has also been reported as a sensitive method for detection of *H. pylori* (Montiero, 2009).

If culture is requested, tissue specimens should be maintained at 4° C and processed within 2 hours of collection. Transport media include *Brucella* broth with 20% glycerol, cysteine Albemi broth with 20% glycerol, isotonic saline with 4% glucose, and Stuart's transport media. Processed specimens may be inoculated to one of several media, including brain-heart infusion, *Brucella*, Columbia, or Skirrow's supplemented with horse blood, horse serum, or sheep blood. Vancomycin, amphotericin, and cefsulodin are recommended to be added as selective agents. Inoculated media should be incubated in a microaerobic atmosphere (5%–10% CO_2, 80%–90% N_2, and 5%–10% O_2) under high humidity at 35° C for 5–7 days. Addition of 5%–8% H_2 in the atmosphere enhances growth of *H. pylori*, which generally produces small, gray, translucent colonies on these media, has the characteristic gram-negative spiral appearance on stained smears, and is oxidase, catalase, and urease positive. Feces generally are not cultured for the enteric helicobacters. *Helicobacter* spp. will grow and will be detected by the automated blood culture systems used in many laboratories, but may require incubation for longer than the standard 5 days (Fox, 2007).

Antimicrobial Susceptibility

Multidrug regimens are used to treat *H. pylori* infection. These usually include two antibiotics (metronidazole, clarithromycin, tetracycline, or amoxicillin) and an "antiacid" drug. Strains resistant to metronidazole and clarithromycin have been reported. For susceptibility testing, the CLSI recommends agar dilution using Mueller-Hinton agar plus 5% sheep blood (CLSI, 2010). Interpretive breakpoints are given only for clarithromycin.

Haemophilus

Characteristics

Members of the genus are oxidase-positive, facultatively anaerobic, small, gram-negative, pleomorphic rods or coccobacilli with a potential requirement for X (hemin) and/or V (NAD) factor. Figure 57-19 shows an *H. influenzae* bacterium in a brain abscess specimen.

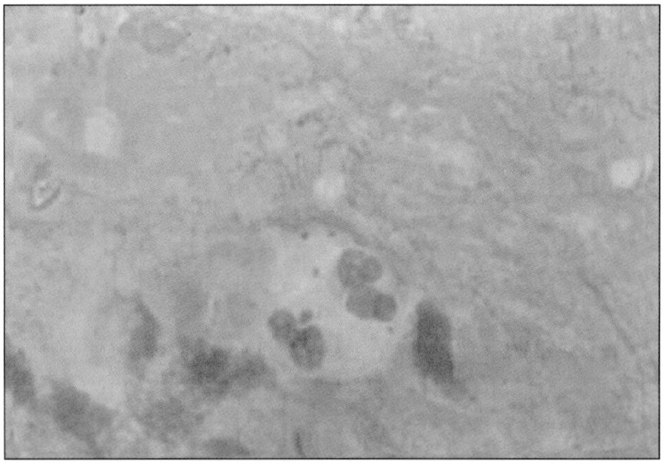

Figure 57-19 Gram stain of a *Haemophilus influenzae* coccobacillus in a brain abscess.

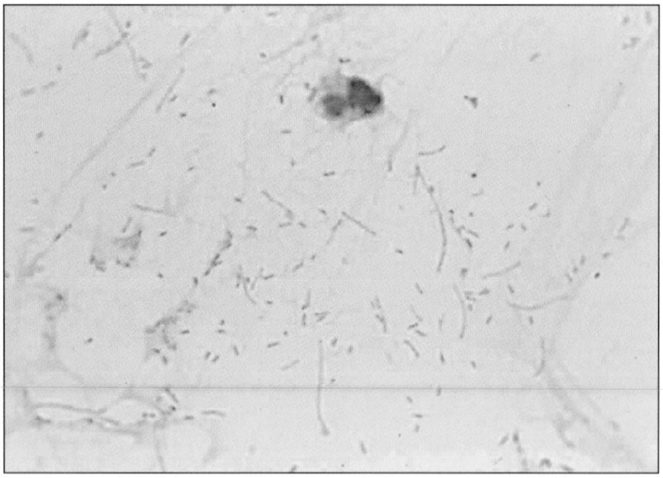

Figure 57-20 Note the pleomorphic nature of the *Haemophilus influenzae* seen in this Gram stain of cerebrospinal fluid.

Clinical Manifestations and Pathogenesis

Most *Haemophilus* spp. are normal inhabitants of the upper respiratory tract. Some may reside in the gastrointestinal or urogenital tract. Person-to-person spread occurs by respiratory droplets. Infections caused by *Haemophilus* spp. range from conjunctivitis and otitis media to meningitis and endocarditis. Those that are generally considered human pathogens are *H. influenzae*, *Haemophilus parainfluenzae*, *Haemophilus ducreyi*, and *Aggregatibacter (Haemophilus) aphrophilus* (Kilian, 2007).

The major virulence factor of *H. influenzae* is the polysaccharide capsule, of which there are six serotypes (a–f). Strains that do not possess a capsule are referred to as nontypeable. Endotoxin is not produced by *H. influenzae*, and this species is rapidly killed once ingested by macrophages unless antibody, complement, or the phagocytes are deficient. The role of antibodies in immunity is also poorly understood. Antibodies develop with age, presumably following natural infection with *H. influenzae* or with cross-reacting antigenic organisms, so that most persons older than 15 years have antibodies. Which antibodies are present and what level of those antibodies is protective remain unknown.

Since the introduction of a vaccine for *H. influenzae* type b in the mid 1980s, there has been a sharp drop in the incidence of invasive infection such as meningitis and epiglottitis due to this organism. Figure 57-20 demonstrates the pleomorphic nature of the *H. influenzae* seen in this CSF specimen. Nontypeable strains of *H. influenzae* are most frequently associated with acute otitis media and acute exacerbations of chronic bronchitis. *H. parainfluenzae* is usually a commensal in the upper respiratory tract but may also cause serious illness, such as endocarditis. *Aggregatibacter (Haemophilus) aphrophilus*, another upper respiratory tract commensal, can cause endocarditis, brain abscess, pneumonia, meningitis, and bacteriuria. *H. ducreyi* is responsible for the sexually transmitted disease chancroid (Kilian, 2007).

Laboratory Diagnosis

Isolation of *Haemophilus* spp. usually requires the presence of X and/or V factor in the culture medium. The former is most frequently supplied by the incorporation of heat-lysed ("chocolatized") blood cells in agar, although it may also be provided by whole human, horse, or rabbit blood cells. NAD is commonly supplied by the incorporation of yeast extract or other appropriate supplements in the medium or by a suspension of staphylococci, which is streaked across the agar surface and about which satellite colonies of dependent strains of *Haemophilus* spp. grow. The differential characteristics of members of this genus are listed in Table 57-13.

Requirements for X and V factors are determined by absence or presence of growth on media containing these factors. An alternative method to test for X factor dependence is the porphyrin test described by Kilian, which determines the ability of dependent species to use δ-aminolevulinic acid in the biosynthesis of porphobilinogen and porphyrins. The formation of porphobilinogen can be detected by adding Kovac's reagent to the reaction mixture and observing the development of a red color in the aqueous phase. Alternatively, the formation of porphyrins in the reaction mixture can be demonstrated by red fluorescence under a Wood's lamp. Hemolytic properties of *Haemophilus* spp. can be determined on rabbit or horse blood agar.

Aggregatibacter (Haemophilus) aphrophilus must often be distinguished from species such as *Aggregatibacter (Actinobacillus) actinomycetemcomitans*, *Cardiobacterium hominis*, and *Eikenella corrodens* (Table 57-14), all of which have been associated with subacute bacterial endocarditis.

Cultivation of *H. ducreyi* from chancroid lesions is problematic. A Gram-stained smear of material from the lesion may be helpful if gram-negative bacilli in pairs or in rows ("schools of fish") are seen. Figure 57-21 shows a "typical" Gram stain of *H. ducreyi* from clinical material. Material may be inoculated onto GC medium base plus 1% hemoglobin, 5%–10% fetal calf serum, 1% IsoVitaleX (BBL Microbiology Systems), and 3 μg/mL of vancomycin or Mueller-Hinton agar plus 5% horse blood, 1% cofactor-vitamin-amino acid enrichment, and 3 μg/mL vancomycin.

Antimicrobial Susceptibility

Currently, the CLSI recommends testing *H. influenzae* isolated from blood or CSF against ampicillin, chloramphenicol, a third-generation cephalosporin, and meropenem (CLSI, 2009). Resistance to ampicillin may be as high as 60% in the United States, varying geographically. Resistance to ampicillin is usually mediated by the production of β-lactamase; however, rare isolates are resistant on the basis of alterations in outer membrane permeability or affinity to penicillin-binding proteins. Resistance to second- or third-generation cephalosporins has not been documented in the United States. Susceptibility testing of *H. influenzae* requires the use of *Haemophilus* test medium (HTM). The recommended treatment for *H. ducreyi* infection is erythromycin; alternative agents include azithromycin, ciprofloxacin, ceftriaxone, amoxicillin-clavulanate, and trimethoprim-sulfamethoxazole. Although not many data are available on the susceptibility of other *Haemophilus* spp. to antibiotics, resistance is assumed higher than among *H. influenzae* strains (Kilian, 2007).

GRAM-NEGATIVE BACTERIA—THE HACEK BACTERIA

Five small gram-negative coccobacilli are part of the normal oral flora and are associated occasionally with bacterial endocarditis and rarely with other

TABLE 57-13
Differential Characteristics of Medically Important *Haemophilus* Species

	Porphyrin	X Factor Dependent	V Factor Dependent	CO_2 Enhancement	Hemolysis*	Catalase
Haemophilus influenzae	–	+	+	+	–	+
Haemophilus haemolyticus	–	+	+	–	+	+
Haemophilus parahaemolyticus	+	–	+	–	+	V
Haemophilus ducreyi	–	+	–	V	–	–
Haemophilus parainfluenzae	+	–	+	V	–	V
Haemophilus aphrophilus†	+	–	–	+	–	–
Haemophilus paraprophilus†	+	–	–	+	–	–

Adapted from Mahon CR, Manuselis G. Textbook of diagnostic microbiology, 2nd ed. London: WB Saunders; 2000, p. 435.
*On horse and rabbit blood.
†These species have been renamed in the genus *Aggregitabacter*.

TABLE 57-14
Differential Characteristics of *Aggregitabacter (Haemophilus) aphrophilus*, *Aggregitabacter (Actinobacillus) actinomycetemcomitans*, *Cardiobacterium hominis*, *Eikenella corrodens*, and *Kingella kingae**

Test	*A. aphrophilus*	*A. actinomycetemcomitans*	*C. hominis*	*E. corrodens*	*K. kingae*
Oxidase	+/–	–/W	+	+	+
Catalase	–	+	–	–	–
δ-ALA utilization	+	+	+	+	+
V requirement	–	–	–	–	–
Indole	–	–	+	–	–
Urease	–	–	–	–	–
Lysine decarboxylase	–	–	–	+	–
Acid from glucose	+	+	+	–	(+)
Sucrose	+	–	+	–	–
Lactose	+	–	–	–	–
Mannitol	–	+	D	–	–
Xylose	–	D	–	–	–

*For key to symbols, see Table 57-9.
δ-ALA, δ-Aminolevulinic acid; *W*, weak.

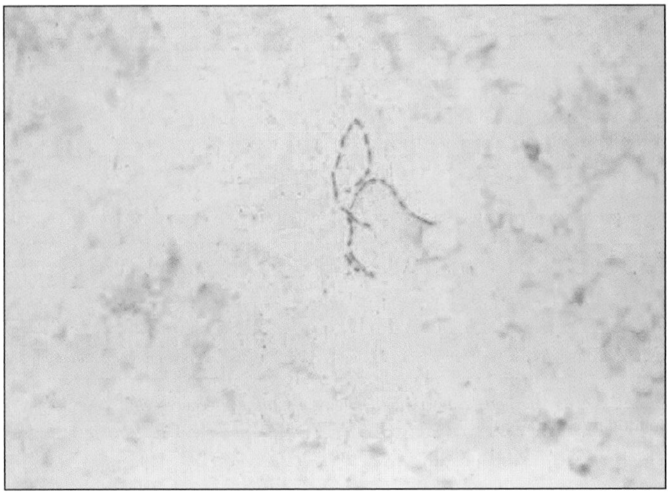

Figure 57-21 *Haemophilus ducreyi* bacilli from a genital lesion.

infections. They are opportunists that enter the bloodstream, settle on damaged heart valves, and cause a relatively slowly progressive, indolent form of endocarditis. They typically require an additional 1–2 days before they are isolated from blood cultures, and they are uniformly susceptible to many antimicrobial agents. The word HACEK is an acronym for the bacteria responsible for this disease: *Haemophilus* spp. *(influenzae, parainfluenzae)*, *Aggregatibacter (Haemophilus) aphrophilus* (most commonly, *Aggregatibacter [Actinobacillus] actinomycetemcomitans*), *Cardiobacterium hominis*, *Eikenella corrodens*, and *Kingella* spp. Some taxonomic changes have been noted more recently, and some of the HACEK members have been reassigned to the genus *Aggregatibacter* (Norskov-Lauritsen, 2006). Differential characteristics of the members of this group are listed in Table 57-14.

Haemophilus

H. influenzae and *H. parainfluenzae* were discussed earlier in this chapter. *Aggregatibacter (Haemophilus) aphrophilus* is also part of the HACEK group. It does not require X or V factor, hence can easily grow on blood and chocolate agars. It does not require CO_2 for growth. Along with causing endocarditis, *A. aprophilus* has been reported in cases of endophthalmitis (following ophthalmic procedures), bacteremia, meningitis, brain abscess, cervical lymphadenitis, empyema, and a few other infectious syndromes. In one study, 39% of patients reported undergoing prior dental procedures before developing their *A. aprophilus* infection (Huang, 2005). It is usually susceptible to β-lactam agents; successful treatment may require combination therapy with a β-lactam and an aminoglycoside.

Aggregatibacter (Actinobacillus)

Characteristics

A. actinomycetemcomitans is a gram-negative, non–spore-forming coccobacillus or short rod. It grows both aerobically and anaerobically. The addition of 5%–10% CO_2 enhances growth. Colonies on blood agar appear slowly and remain small. A description of "star-shaped" colonies has been given to their appearance on agar media.

Clinical Manifestations and Pathogenesis

Aggregatibacter organisms are found in the mucous membranes of the respiratory and genitourinary tracts of humans and animals. They generally cause disease only in immunocompromised individuals, or when they are accidentally introduced into healthy surrounding tissue, for example, by trauma. *A. actinomycetemcomitans* has a low level of pathogenicity. It derives its species name from its frequent association with actinomycotic lesions. In recent years, however, it has most frequently been reported as a cause of subacute bacterial endocarditis, periodontitis, and brain abscess. Two virulence factors are known: a leukotoxin and a collagenase.

Laboratory Diagnosis

A. actinomycetemcomitans grows on blood and chocolate agar. After 24–72 hours, colonies are 1–3 mm in diameter with a central wrinkling. The organism is catalase positive, oxidase negative or weakly positive, and urease negative (vonGraevenitz, 2007). Additional biochemical assays must be used to differentiate it from other slowly growing, somewhat fastidious gram-negative bacilli (see Table 57-14).

Antimicrobial Susceptibility

This organism is resistant to penicillin but is usually susceptible to many other antibiotics, including the cephalosporins, β-lactam–β-lactamase inhibitor combinations, fluoroquinolones, and tetracycline.

Cardiobacterium hominis

Characteristics

C. hominis is a gram-negative, non–spore-forming bacillus that is part of the normal oral flora. It is a facultative anaerobe that does not require CO_2, although growth is enhanced in microaerophilic conditions. Growth occurs on blood and chocolate agar but not on MacConkey's agar and is better at longer than 48 hours.

Clinical Manifestations and Pathogenesis

Cardiobacterium hominis can cause subacute bacterial endocarditis, similar to other HACEK members; it may also be responsible for cases of periodontitis and peritonitis (Bhan, 2006). The usual habitat of *C. hominis* is the upper respiratory tract, but it may also be found in the gastrointestinal and genitourinary tracts (vonGraevenitz, 2007).

Laboratory Diagnosis

Colonies at 48 hours' incubation are small and may have a yellow pigment, although most are white. The organism is generally oxidase and indole positive but negative for catalase, urease, esculin, and nitrate reduction. Acid may be produced from glucose, maltose, and sucrose (vonGraevenitz, 2007).

Antimicrobial Susceptibility

Isolates are usually susceptible to penicillins and cephalosporins, aminoglycosides, and tetracyclines. Resistance to clindamycin is common. β-Lactamases have been rarely reported (Lu, 2000).

Eikenella

Characteristics

Formerly classified as *Bacteroides corrodens*, the "corroding bacilli" that are facultatively anaerobic have been assigned to the species *Eikenella corrodens*. *E. corrodens* organisms are oxidase-positive, catalase-negative, nonfermentative, gram-negative bacilli, colonies of which may corrode or pit agar. Growth is enhanced by 5%–10% CO_2 and/or the presence of hemin (X factor) in the medium.

Clinical Manifestations and Pathogenesis

Little is known about factors contributing to the organism's virulence in human disease; it has a low level of pathogenicity for animals. *E. corrodens* resides predominantly in the oral cavity and is isolated frequently from the upper respiratory tract. Similar to other HACEK bacteria, it is responsible for subacute bacterial endocarditis. It has been recovered from abscesses, cellulitis, and wound infections, often following human bites. Infections are usually mixed with other organisms (vonGraevenitz, 2007).

Laboratory Diagnosis

Growth is observed on blood or chocolate agar but not on MacConkey's agar. The most striking features of *E. corrodens* in culture are the distinctive odor of bleach and the characteristic pitting of the agar; however, pitting does not occur with all strains. Colonies appear slowly (2–4 days) and are generally small (0.5–1.0 mm in diameter). *E. corrodens* must usually be distinguished from other fastidious, slowly growing gram-negative bacilli (see Table 57-14).

Antimicrobial Susceptibility

E. corrodens is susceptible to the penicillins, quinolones, and tetracycline, variably susceptible to aminoglycosides, and resistant to clindamycin and metronidazole. β-Lactamases have been described in clinical strains, but resistance can be overcome with the use of β-lactamase inhibitors in combination with β-lactam antibiotics (vonGraevenitz, 2007).

Kingella

Characteristics

Kingella has three recognized species: *K. kingae* (the HACEK species), *Kingella oralis*, and *Kingella denitrificans*. They are gram-negative rods to coccobacilli, requiring increased CO_2 for optimum growth. Colonies will grow on blood (β-hemolytic) and chocolate, but not on MacConkey's agar, after 2 days.

Clinical Manifestations and Pathogenesis

K. kingae is the most pathogenic of the three species. It is a member of the HACEK group, causing an indolent, slowly progressive endocarditis. In addition, it is associated with septic arthritis/osteomyelitis (usually in children younger than 4 years of age) (Yagupsky, 2004; Sena, 2009) and septicemia. *K. oralis* has been isolated from patients with periodontitis, but with unclear clinical relevance. *K. denitrificans* is a rare clinical isolate that can be associated with endocarditis (vonGraevenitz, 2007).

Laboratory Diagnosis

K. kingae is oxidase positive and nonmotile and produces acid from glucose, although in delayed fashion. Indole and catalase are negative.

Antimicrobial Susceptibility

K. kingae is susceptible to penicillin and most antibiotics to which other members of the HACEK group are susceptible. β-Lactamases have been described in clinical strains, but resistance can be overcome with the use of β-lactamase inhibitors in combination with β-lactam antibiotics (vonGraeveniz, 2007).

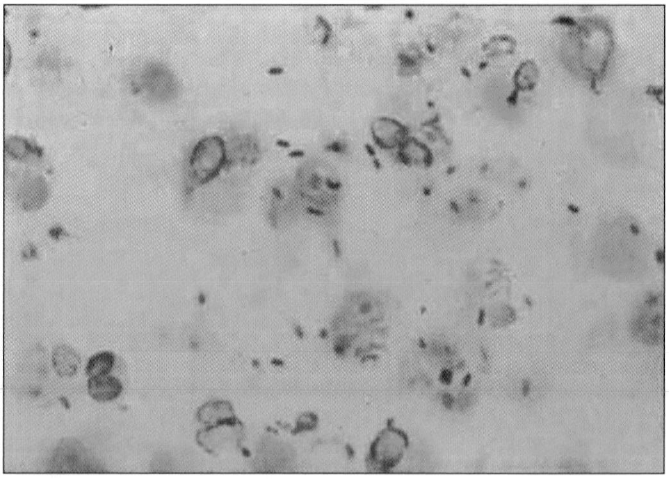

Figure 57-22 *Legionella pneumophila* in a clinical specimen stained with a Dieterle silver stain.

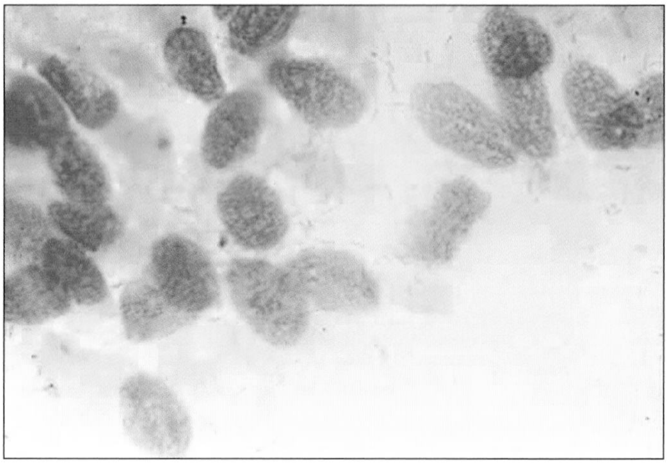

Figure 57-23 *Legionella pneumophila* faintly staining negative with Gram stain of pulmonary infiltrate.

MISCELLANEOUS GRAM-NEGATIVE BACILLI

Legionella

Characteristics

Legionella spp. are non–spore-forming, faintly staining, thin, gram-negative bacilli. *Legionella* spp. were first recognized to cause human disease during an epidemic of pneumonia that occurred among members of the Pennsylvania American Legion who had gathered in Philadelphia to celebrate the 1976 bicentennial. There are now more than 20 named species and a number of unnamed species. Most clinical cases have been due to *Legionella pneumophila*, serogroup 1. Figure 57-22 demonstrates excellent staining of *Legionella* spp. with a Dieterle silver stain.

Clinical Manifestations and Pathogenesis

Legionella spp. are found in the environment in association with water. Growth within environmental protozoa is thought to be an important factor for survival of the organism in the environment. Transmission to humans occurs through exposure to contaminated water (e.g., faucets, shower heads, public fountains). Human-to-human infection and laboratory-acquired infections are not known to occur.

Infections can be subclinical, pulmonary, or extrapulmonary. Infection is usually manifested as an acute, fibrinopurulent pneumonia with lobular distribution. Histologically, there is an alveolar infiltrate of neutrophils and macrophages, accompanied by fibrin and red blood cell extravasation. *Legionella* spp. may be found within alveolar macrophages. Figure 57-23 shows the Gram stain of sputum of a patient with *L. pneumophila* pneumonia. *L. pneumophila* has also been isolated from cultures of blood.

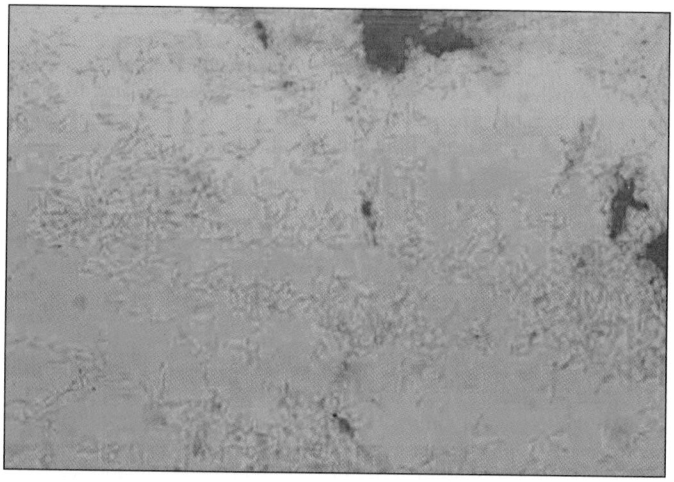

Figure 57-24 Gram stain of culture of *Legionella pneumophila*.

Laboratory Diagnosis

Legionella spp. may be isolated on BCYE agar supplemented with growth factors, including l-cystine, ferric salt, and α-ketoglutarate. This medium may be made selective for culture of nonsterile body sites by the addition of cefamandole, polymyxin B, and anisomycin or polymyxin B, anisomycin, and vancomycin (Edelstein, 1987, 2007). Chocolate agar may also support the growth of legionellae. Treatment of sputum with a weak acid (0.2M HCl/KCl pH 2.2) for 4 minutes or with heat (60° C) for 2 minutes may help to reduce contamination from other organisms but may reduce the number of legionellas as well.

Inoculated media should be incubated for at least 5 days in a humid atmosphere containing no more than 2%–5% CO_2. Colonies often appear iridescent and have a sticky consistency. Isolates with typical Gram stain morphology should be subcultured to blood agar, where no growth will be observed. These organisms may be weakly oxidase and catalase positive, are gelatinase positive, and often are motile. Identification of this organism is most accurately achieved using type-specific antibody assays or sequencing with appropriate primers. Figure 57-24 shows a Gram stain of *L. pneumophila* from culture.

Legionella spp. may be detected or identified by direct fluorescent antibody (DFA) staining of specimens or colonies in cultures. Sensitivity of direct DFA examination of respiratory specimens has ranged from 25%–75% but is considerably higher in open lung biopsies. However, use of this test has decreased because of the availability of more sensitive tests (e.g., the urine antigen assay, direct PCR methods). Cross-reactions in DFA assays have been reported between *L. pneumophila* and other *Legionella* spp., as well as with some strains of *Bordetella pertussis*, *Pseudomonas fluorescens*, and *Bacteroides fragilis*. Sensitivity of DFA for detection of other species than *L. pneumophila* in sputum is not known.

The urine antigen test for *L. pneumophila* serogroup 1 has a reported sensitivity of 80%–90%, although it should be noted that antigenuria may persist for many months following infection. Use of the urinary antigen test within and outside of the intensive care unit has been shown to have a positive impact on patient cases (Garbino, 2004; Edelstein, 2007).

The diagnosis of legionellosis can also be established serologically by detecting a fourfold or greater rise in antibody titer to at least 1:128. A single antibody titer of 1:256 is presumptive evidence of past infection. The sensitivity of serologic diagnosis for disease caused by species other than *L. pneumophila* serogroup 1 is not known, and the specificity of antibody tests for disease caused by other species is less than that of *L. pneumophila* serogroup 1. PCR assays for direct detection of *Legionella* spp. in clinical specimens and for sequencing identification of cultured isolates have been developed. Sensitivities of 64%–100% and specificities of 88%–100% have been reported (Edelstein, 2007). Use of these assays can provide more rapid results, especially when used in direct specimen testing; in addition, identification of species other than *L. pneumophila*, which is not possible with DFA and serology, could increase the demand for such assays. PCR for *Legionella* spp. directly in clinical samples will be performed most often in the future, as assays become cleared for clinical laboratory testing to enhance recovery or in assays in which other respiratory pathogens can be simultaneously searched for (Khanna, 2005).

Antimicrobial Susceptibility

Because of the intracellular nature of *Legionella* spp. in clinical infection, in vitro susceptibility test results do not predict the clinical response of antibiotics. Susceptibility testing should not be performed. Therapy generally consists of a macrolide (clarithromycin and azithromycin are as efficacious and result in fewer side effects than erythromycin), or a fluoroquinolone alone or in combination. Other agents that have been used include trimethoprim-sulfamethoxazole, rifampin, or a tetracycline (Edelstein, 2007; Valve, 2009). No β-lactam antibiotic has acceptable intracellular activity against *L. pneumophila*. Macrolides and fluoroquinolones should always be efficacious against infection with *Legionella micdadei, longbeacheae, bozemanae*, or *dumoffi* (Muder, 2002).

Bordetella

Characteristics

Bordetella spp. are strictly aerobic, nonfermentative, catalase-positive, minute coccobacilli requiring nicotinic acid, cysteine, and usually methionine, but not X or V factor, for growth. Phase variation from smooth virulent strains to rough avirulent strains occurs after cultivation on artificial media.

Clinical Manifestations and Pathogenesis

Bordetella spp. are found in the respiratory tracts of warm-blooded animals. *Bordetella bronchiseptica* primarily causes kennel cough in dogs, although it may rarely cause pertussis-like symptoms in immunocompromised human hosts. *Bordetella parapertussis*, which infects both humans and lambs, is an uncommon human pathogen. Infection may be asymptomatic or may cause a pertussis-like illness, most frequently bronchitis. *B. pertussis*, the etiologic agent of whooping cough, causes disease only in humans.

B. pertussis, *B. parapertussis*, and *B. bronchiseptica* produce a number of virulence factors. *B. pertussis* produces toxins including pertussis toxin (PT), an exotoxin that is involved in colonization of the respiratory tract and establishment of the infection with *B. pertussis* and a virulence factor that inhibits intracellular signal transduction factors by transferring adenosine diphosphate ribose to G-proteins of cells; adenylate cyclase toxin, which inhibits immune effector and other cell functions by creating a high intracellular level of cyclic adenosine 3′,5′-phosphate; and tracheal cytotoxin, which causes cell ciliostasis and cell death. *B. pertussis* virulence factors also include substances that mediate adherence to ciliated epithelial cells; these include PT, filamentous hemagglutinin (FHA), pertactin, and fimbriae.

It is thought that in a pertussis infection, the organism first attaches to the ciliated epithelium of the respiratory tract and immune effector cells by means of fimbriae, FHA, PT, and pertactin. PT and adenylate cyclase toxin work together to inhibit the host's immune system, and tracheal cytotoxin damages the respiratory epithelium. Results may include inflammation and epithelial necrosis; leukocytosis and lymphocytosis; accumulation of secretions; cough; and ultimately bronchopneumonia, hypoxic episodes, and encephalopathy (Xu, 2009).

B. pertussis contains a protective antigen that when combined with antibody abolishes its infectivity. It appears, however, that both cellular immunity and humoral immunity are needed to eradicate the organism. *B. parapertussis* and *B. bronchiseptica* can produce pertactin and FHA. They also possess promoter and structural genes for PT, but these are not expressed (Mattoo, 2005).

Laboratory Diagnosis

The rate of isolation of *B. pertussis* from patients declines with the duration of illness. The most commonly recommended specimen is the nasopharyngeal swab; however, nasopharyngeal aspirates collected with a soft rubber catheter have provided higher rates of isolation in some people's hands. A more invasive specimen such as fluid collected by bronchoalveolar lavage may also be cultured. In general, swabs or aspirates should be inoculated onto suitable media, such as Regan-Lowe agar or Bordet-Gengou medium, as quickly as possible after collection. For shipment to reference laboratories, the inoculated medium should be incubated for at least 24 hours in ambient air at 35° C prior to transport to allow some initial growth of the organism.

Direct examination of smears stained with fluorescein-conjugated *B. pertussis* monoclonal or polyclonal antiserum may provide a rapid diagnosis; however, DFA assays suffer from low sensitivity (30%–71%) and low specificity. Results of DFA should be considered presumptive only and should be used as an adjunct to culture or PCR (Loeffelholz, 2007). Direct detection of *B. pertussis* in clinical specimens by means of PCR is quickly replacing DFA in many laboratories and is rapidly becoming the primary method for detection of *B. pertussis*. As more commercial products become available, the reproducibility of results between laboratories should improve (Khanna, 2005). PCR test results, however, may remain positive longer than results obtained with culture or DFA, even with appropriate antimicrobial therapy. PCR methods for the direct detection of *B. parapertussis* in clinical specimens are also available (Dragsted, 2004), and consideration should be given to use of a PCR, which can detect both organisms, because in some outbreaks, a significant cause of whooping cough is actually *B. parapertussis* (Loeffelholz, 2007). However, reports have described PCR misidentifying *B. bronchiseptica* as *B. pertussis* when the pertactin gene was the target of the PCR assay (Register 2007).

Culture for *B. pertussis* provides the most specific diagnosis of whooping cough and enables a laboratory to perform susceptibility testing and/or genotypic analysis if required. Cultures, however, are not the most sensitive means of recovering *B. pertussis* from respiratory specimens. Cultures, when done, should be incubated in ambient air in a humid environment at 35° C. Incubation in a CO_2 incubator may slow the growth of *B. pertussis*. Colonies may not be visible for 3–4 days, and cultures should be held for 7–12 days before they are discarded as negative (Loeffelholz, 2007). Colonies of *B. pertussis* are small, smooth, round, and shiny and may have the appearance of a drop of mercury. Organisms with typical colony morphology and Gram stain appearance should be subcultured to blood agar to verify the absence of growth on this medium. Positive catalase and oxidase reactions and negative urease can be used for presumptive identification of an organism as *B. pertussis*. *B. parapertussis* grows more rapidly and will grow on blood agar and occasionally on MacConkey's agar. Colonies are oxidase negative and catalase and urease positive. *B. bronchiseptica* grows well on both blood and MacConkey's agars and is the most biochemically active of the three. It is catalase, oxidase, urease, and nitrate reduction positive. *B. holmseii* has been described more recently in the genus, not as a cause of whooping cough, but rather in association with bacteremia, endocarditis, and respiratory illness in immunocompromised patients, especially in asplenic patients (Shepard, 2004). *B. holmseii* will grow well on blood agar, and its appearance on MacConkey's agar may be delayed. It is negative for oxidase, nitrate reduction, and urease. Other *Bordetella* spp., including *B. hinzii*, *B. trematum*, and *B. avium*, grow on both blood agar and MacConkey's agar and are motile, unlike all other members of the genus (Loeffelholz, 2007).

Serologic diagnostic methods for *B. pertussis* are usually used to detect immune response; EIA is the method of choice. Demonstration of seroconversion or a significant rise in concentration of IgG against PT is thought to be the most sensitive and specific test. In a recent study comparing culture, PCR, and serology for diagnosis of pertussis, if a minimum of two antigens to *B. pertussis* (IgG, IgA, or IgM) were obtained in both acute and convalescent sera, serology was found to be as sensitive as PCR, and both were more sensitive than culture (Cengiz, 2009).

Antimicrobial Susceptibility

Antimicrobial agents probably play no role in the therapy of pertussis, but nasopharyngeal cultures become negative after 1–2 days of treatment, which may prevent bacterial complications in patients with the disease and may be effective in preventing spread of the disease to nonimmune contacts. Susceptibility testing is not indicated for *B. pertussis*, and methods are not standardized. A macrolide (erythromycin, azithromycin, or clarithromycin) is the drug of choice for treatment and prophylaxis; trimethoprim-sulfamethoxazole (SXT) is an acceptable alternative in patients with macrolide intolerance and in those in whom the isolate is resistant to the macrolides, which occurs very rarely (Loeffelholz, 2007).

Vaccination against *B. pertussis* provides a good tool in the prevention of whooping cough, although immunity to disease or vaccination is said to wane after 5–12 years. Older children and adults have thus become a reservoir of the organism (Guiso, 2009).

Brucella

Characteristics

Brucella spp. are small, gram-negative coccobacillary organisms (0.5–0.7 μm × 0.6–1.5 μm). In smears, they occur predominantly as single coccobacilli, but they may occur in pairs or in short chains. They have been described as having the appearance of sand. They are nonmotile, strictly aerobic, catalase- and usually oxidase-positive organisms. They are nonfermenters. Growth in the laboratory is often enhanced by the presence of 5%–10% CO_2 and requires complex media, which are improved by the addition of blood or serum. Of the recognized species, *Brucella melitensis*, *Brucella abortus*, *Brucella suis*, and *Brucella canis* are human pathogens, although *B. canis* has reduced virulence for humans as compared with other species. *B. ovis* is a pathogen of sheep, and *B. neotomae* has been isolated from the desert wood rat. All species hydrolyze urea, except *B. ovis*, and this remains a significant characteristic of the genus (Lindquist, 2007).

Clinical Manifestations and Pathogenesis

Brucella spp. are intracellular bacteria that infect a wide range of animal species (including humans) and have been found in some insects and ticks. They are important veterinary and human pathogens. Preferential hosts are sheep and goats for *B. melitensis*, cattle for *B. abortus*, swine for *B. suis*, and dogs for *B. canis;* however, each species may occasionally infect other animals. Humans become infected by inhalation of the organism; by direct contact with infected material, including animal carcasses, fetal membranes, vaginal discharge, fetuses, skin, or mucous membranes; or by ingestion of unpasteurized milk or milk products from infected animals. Approximately 100 cases of human brucellosis are reported per year in the United States. A common risk factor is consumption of imported cheese made from unpasteurized goat's milk.

Local lymphadenopathy often occurs with dissemination and secondary localization in the reticuloendothelial system and formation of granulomas in the liver, spleen, bone, genitourinary tract, lungs, and soft tissues. Organisms may be seen within phagocytes. Signs and symptoms are often variable and nonspecific, with chills, fever, sweats, and anorexia occurring frequently. The fever is characteristically diurnal ("undulant").

Laboratory Diagnosis

Brucella spp. are recovered most often from blood and bone marrow and less often from material obtained from spleen and liver abscesses. The organism grows on standard laboratory media, including *Brucella*, blood, chocolate, and trypticase soy agar. Some strains will grow on MacConkey's agar. *Brucella* spp. will grow in media used for culturing blood specimens. Many references recommend incubating blood cultures for at least 21 days with blind subculture performed early and late in the incubation period; however, these recommendations may not be necessary with newer automated blood culture systems, some of which have been shown to reliably recover *Brucella* spp. in 5 days or less without blind subculture (Lindquist, 2007; Yagupsky, 1997). *Brucella* spp. are recognized as Class A bioterrorism organisms, and as such should be handled only in public health laboratories and/or by the CDC. Identification and testing of this organism are described here for completeness but should not be performed in sentinel laboratories, which include most hospital laboratories.

Solid media should be incubated in an atmosphere containing 5%–10% CO_2. These organisms grow slowly, and even after 48 hours of incubation, colonies may be difficult to see. Organisms can be presumptively identified as *Brucella* spp. based on a characteristic Gram stain appearance and may be positive for catalase, oxidase, and urease. Urease activity is manifested rapidly (about 15 minutes) by *B. suis* and more slowly (2–24 hours) by *B. melitensis* and *B. abortus*. Because brucellosis can be laboratory acquired, laboratory personnel should be notified if this organism is suspected, and all manipulations of possible *Brucella* spp. should be conducted in a biological safety cabinet (Lindquist, 2007).

Identification of *Brucella* spp. to the species level requires tests for CO_2 requirement, H_2S production, urea hydrolysis, dye sensitivity, and phage sensitivity. Most hospital laboratories refer this testing to State Health Departments or other reference laboratories. Molecular tools such as PCR will probably become more effective means of detecting cases of brucellosis in the future (Queipo-Ortuno, 2005).

The diagnosis of brucellosis can be made serologically. A minimum titer of 1:160 in a standard tube agglutination test is suggestive of the diagnosis; however, evidence of recent brucellosis can be accepted only when a fourfold or greater rise in titer occurs during the first month or two of illness. Prozone effects can occur in patients with titers as high as 1:640, so that all sera from patients with suspected disease should be diluted to at least 1:1280. Cross-reactivity with *Francisella tularensis* and with *V. cholerae*, including cholera vaccination, may occur (Lindquist, 2007).

Antimicrobial Susceptibility

Treatment consists of combinations of tetracycline, aminoglycosides, rifampin, and trimethoprim-sulfamethoxazole for prolonged periods. Although treatment failures do occur, they are not due to antimicrobial resistance, and susceptibility testing is not recommended (Lindquist, 2007).

Pasteurella

Characteristics

Pasteurellae are facultatively anaerobic, oxidase- and catalase-positive, nonmotile, gram-negative bacteria that range morphologically from coccobacilli to long filamentous rods. Of the eight species known to infect humans *(Pasteurella multocida, Pasteurella bettyae, Pasteurella canis, Pasteurella dagmatis, Pasteurella stomatis, Pasteurella pneumotropica, Pasteurella haemolytica, Pasteurella aerogenes), P. multocida* is the most important human pathogen. *Pasteurella* spp. are phenotypically similar to the *Actinobacillus* spp., and DNA–DNA hybridization studies and comparisons of 16S rRNA have shown that *P. pneumotropica, P. haemolytica,* and *P. aerogenes* are more closely related to the genus *Actinobacillus* than to the genus *Pasteurella*.

Clinical Manifestations and Pathogenesis

Pasteurella spp., especially *P. multocida*, may be found as commensals in the upper respiratory tracts of fowl and mammals and are frequently isolated from animal bite or scratch wounds. Cat bites more often become infected than dog bites. Local infections can become systemic, and a number of reports have described septicemia, osteomyelitis, and meningitis. Pasteurellae have been associated with respiratory tract infections, including sinusitis, peritonsillar abscess, mastoiditis, pulmonary abscess, pneumonia, empyema, bronchitis, and bronchiectasis, usually in patients with chronic pulmonary disease (vonGraevenitz, 2007).

Laboratory Diagnosis

Pasteurellae grow well on blood agar and are only rarely able to grow on gram-negative differential media, such as EMB or MacConkey's agar. The finding of a gram-negative bacillus that grows on blood agar only and is oxidase and indole positive and ortho-Nitrophenyl-β-galactoside (ONPG) negative provides strong presumptive evidence for the isolation of *P. multocida*, the most frequently encountered species. In addition, susceptibility to penicillin, as evidenced by a wide zone of inhibition around a penicillin disk on a blood agar plate, is good evidence that the isolate is *P. multocida*.

Antimicrobial Susceptibility

Resistance to antimicrobial agents is rarely seen in human isolates. Pasteurellae are usually susceptible to penicillin and tetracycline and many other antibiotics. Penicillin is the therapeutic drug of choice. Rare strains of *P. multocida* have produced β-lactamase , but the combination of a β-lactam with a β-lactamase inhibitor drug should be effective (vonGraevenitz, 2007).

Francisella

Characteristics

F. tularensis is a very small, strictly aerobic, coccoid to pleomorphic rod-shaped, gram-negative bacillus that requires cystine or cysteine for growth. Faint bipolar staining occurs with aniline dyes.

Clinical Manifestations and Pathogenesis

F. tularensis is found in both wild and domesticated animals, birds, arthropods, water, mud, and animal feces. The primary reservoir for this organism is the cottontail rabbit. Transmission to humans occurs through tick bite, direct cutaneous inoculation from an infected animal, conjunctival inoculation, inhalation, or ingestion of undercooked infected animal meat or contaminated water. Several forms of the disease occur, including ulceroglandular, glandular, oculoglandular, oropharyngeal, intestinal, pneumonic, and typhoidal. Approximately 100–200 cases of tularemia are reported each year in the United States. *F. tularensis* is considered to be one of the class A agents of bioterrorism; because of this, workup of suspected cases is limited to approved laboratories. Most clinical laboratories are considered sentinel laboratories, and if *F. tularensis* is suspected, isolates should be sent to State Health Departments or other selected laboratories (Lindquist, 2007).

Tularemia manifests in various forms after an incubation period of 1–10 days. Headache, fever, chills, vomiting, and myalgias characteristically occur at the onset. In ulceroglandular disease, lymphadenitis and lymphadenopathy occur in the region draining the primary lesion. The lesion is initially papular and is later ulcerative. Oculoglandular disease is characterized by inflammation of the conjunctiva and usually a papule of the lower lid with lymphadenitis of the preauricular, parotid, submaxillary, and anterior cervical nodes. The intestinal form of tularemia is characterized by ulcerative lesions of the mouth, throat, and upper gastrointestinal tract.

Virulence appears to be related to a smooth colonial morphology. Repeated subcultures result in alteration from smooth to rough colonies, with concomitant loss of virulence. Highly virulent strains for humans have citrulline ureidase activity and ferment glycerol, and are most often associated with tick-borne disease in rabbits. Toxins have not been recognized.

Tularemia should be suspected in anyone who has been in an endemic area, has had contact with wild animals or livestock, has a history of tick bite, has been engaged in farming operations, has drunk impure water, or has been exposed to cultures or infected animals in the laboratory. Trappers, hunters, fur and meat industry workers, agricultural workers, and laboratory personnel are at greatest risk. Because of its protean manifestations, tularemia is readily confused with many other diseases, such as brucellosis, anthrax, sporotrichosis, typhoid fever, tuberculosis, histoplasmosis, and syphilis.

Laboratory Diagnosis

Material suitable for examination includes fluid or curettings from the primary lesion, aspirates of enlarged regional nodes, sputum, pharyngeal washes, and gastric aspirates. Bacterial isolation is difficult because the organism has special growth requirements and grows slowly, allowing for overgrowth of other organisms present in the specimen. The organism grows on glucose-cysteine agar supplemented with 5% defibrinated rabbit blood, chocolate agar with IsoVitalX, or BCYE agar. Some isolates may even grow on blood agar or trypticase soy agar. If clinical material is contaminated by other organisms, penicillin, polymyxin B, and cycloheximide can be added to inhibit their growth. Special care must be exercised in handling infected material to prevent aerosolization or direct contact with the skin. Clinicians should always notify laboratory personnel if *F. tularensis* is suspected, so that proper precautions can be taken to prevent exposure to this organism (Lindquist, 2007).

Cultures are incubated at 35°C with or without added CO_2. Colonies usually appear within 2–4 days and are blue-gray to white, round, smooth, and slightly mucoid. On blood-containing agar, a small zone of α-hemolysis may be seen. Because working with the organism in the laboratory is dangerous, suspected isolates should be sent to a reference laboratory such as the CDC for confirmation with a slide agglutination or direct fluorescent antibody test.

The diagnosis of *F. tularensis* can be established serologically. Agglutination titers as low as 1 : 40 in the absence of previous disease are diagnostic and may rise within the first 3 weeks to a level of 1 : 640 or greater. *Brucella* agglutinins may also rise nonspecifically, but usually to a considerably lower level (Johansson, 2004; Lindquist, 2007).

Antimicrobial Susceptibility

Streptomycin is bactericidal, and the tetracyclines and chloramphenicol are bacteriostatic to *F. tularensis*. Because relapses may occur after treatment with bacteriostatic agents, streptomycin is the agent of choice.

Gardnerella

Characteristics

Gardnerella vaginalis is a thin, gram-variable rod or coccobacillus. Over the years, this organism, in its association with bacterial vaginosis, has been called *Haemophilus vaginalis* and *Corynebacterium vaginale*, further demonstrating its gram-variable appearance. Catalase is not produced, and cells are nonmotile. Growth is best observed after 48 hours of incubation in a 5% CO_2-enriched atmosphere. Colonies are small and exhibit β-hemolysis on media containing rabbit or human blood.

Clinical Manifestations and Pathogenesis

This organism is associated with bacterial vaginosis but is not the cause. It has been found in the blood of patients with postpartum fever and can cause infection in newborns. *G. vaginalis* is a part of the anorectal flora of healthy adults of both sexes, as well as of children. It is part of the endogenous vaginal flora of women of reproductive age.

Laboratory Diagnosis

Diagnosis of bacterial vaginosis does not require culture. The diagnosis is made by direct examination of vaginal secretions for the presence of clue cells (epithelial cells covered with bacteria on the cell margins) and small gram-negative rods and coccobacilli, the absence of lactobacilli (gram-positive thin rods), a pH greater than 4.5, and a fishy amine odor after addition of 10% potassium hydroxide (KOH) to the secretions. A scored Gram stain is the laboratory test that should be performed when vaginal discharge is submitted for the diagnosis of bacterial vaginosis (Nugent,

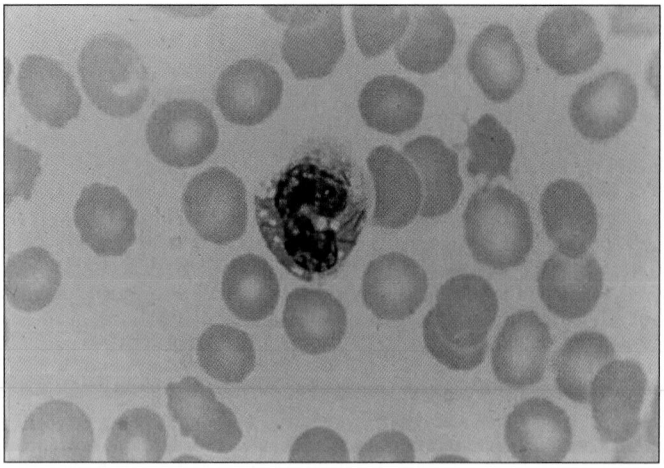

Figure 57-25 Blood smear positive for *Capnocytophaga canimorsus* in patient with septicemia (Wright's stain).

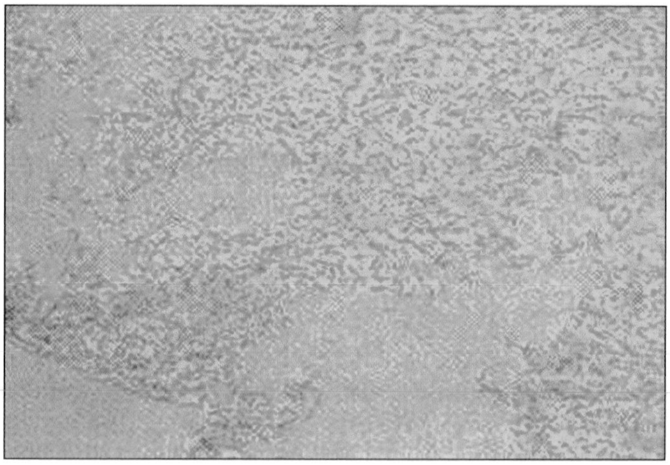

Figure 57-26 Gram stain of *Capnocytophaga ochraceus*. Note the fusiform bacilli.

1991). Alternatively, a nucleic acid probe (Affirm, Becton Dickinson Microbiology Systems, Sparks, MD) is available that tests for a high concentration of *G. vaginalis* as a marker for bacterial vaginosis (Briselden, 1994). When observed in culture, the organism is presumptively identified based on hemolysis on human blood bilayer Tween agar after 48 hours of incubation (Funke, 2007).

Antimicrobial Susceptibility

Susceptibility testing of *G. vaginalis* is not recommended, and no guidelines exist for performing this testing. Metronidazole is the drug of choice for bacterial vaginosis. Systemic infection due to *G. vaginalis* may be treated with ampicillin because this organism has not been found to produce β-lactamase (Funke, 2007).

Capnocytophaga

Capnocytophaga is a genus of gram-negative, facultatively anaerobic, gram-negative rods to filamentous bacteria. Species include *Capnocytophaga ochraceus*, *Capnocytophaga canimorsus* (formerly DF-2), *Capnocytophaga gingivalis*, and *Capnocytophaga sputigena*, among others. *C. canimorsus* is part of the oral flora of dogs and cats; the others can be found as part of normal human oral flora.

Clinical Manifestations and Pathogenesis

C. ochraceus can cause transient bacteremia or endocarditis in immunocompromised and immunocompetent patients (vonGraevenitz, 2007). It also has been associated with periodontitis. *C. canimorsus* is a cause of a fatal septicemia following wound infection subsequent to the bite of dogs or cats. Patients with this fatal septicemia have predisposing factors of a prior splenectomy or alcoholism (Oehler, 2009). Meningitis, endocarditis, arthritis, and eye infection have also been documented with *C. canimorsus* (Gasch, 2009). Figure 57-25 shows a Wright's stain of *C. canimorsus* seen on the blood film of patient with *C. canimorsus* septicemia. Note the intracellular nature of the bacilli.

Isolation of *Capnocytophaga* spp. requires inoculation of blood or chocolate agar and incubation in a 5%–10% CO_2 environment, generally for longer than 24 hours. Colonies are usually slightly pigmented yellow or orange and may spread because of a "sliding" motility. Gram stains often show long, thin, spindle-shaped cells, almost fusiform in appearance. Figure 57-26 shows the Gram stain of *C. ochraceus*, demonstrating the fusiform bacilli. *C. ochraceus* is oxidase and catalase negative; *C. canimorsus* is oxidase and catalase positive. *Capnocytophaga* spp. are usually susceptible to many antibiotics, including β-lactams, macrolides, tetracycline, clindamycin, and quinolones. They are resistant to the aminoglycosides. Occasional β-lactamases have been described in this genus, although response to β-lactam/β-lactamase inhibitor combinations has been good (Jolivet-Gougeon, 2000; vonGraevenitz, 2007).

Calymmatobacterium

Characteristics

Calymmatobacterium granulomatis is a gram-negative, nonmotile, encapsulated, pleomorphic rod that may be cultured in yolk sacs or on fresh egg yolk medium. The organism possesses antigenic and molecular determinants similar to those of *Klebsiella* spp., leading taxonomists to now classify it among the Enterobacteriaceae as *Klebsiella granulomatis* (Abbott, 2007).

Clinical Manifestations and Pathogenesis

The organism does not produce disease in animals. In humans, it causes granuloma inguinale (donovanosis), characterized by ulcerogranulomatous lesions of the skin and mucosa of the genital and inguinal areas (Rashid, 2006).

Laboratory Diagnosis

A fragment of tissue removed from the margin of an ulcer is pressed and rubbed against a glass slide and stained with Wright's or Giemsa stain. The finding of small, straight or curved, pleomorphic rods with rounded ends and characteristic polar granules, giving a "safety pin" appearance within mononuclear cells, is the most effective way of establishing the diagnosis. *K. granulomatis* does not grow on routine culture media (Abbott, 2007).

Antimicrobial Susceptibility

The tetracyclines, erythromycin, ampicillin, and chloramphenicol are active against *C. granulomatis*. Resistance may develop to streptomycin.

Streptobacillus

Characteristics

Streptobacillus is a facultatively anaerobic, fermentative, nonencapsulated, and nonmotile pleomorphic gram-negative rod, frequently occurring in chains or long filaments, and often with a series of oval to elongated bulbous swellings, giving a string-of-beads appearance. The microscopic morphology varies with time, being more homogeneously filamentous in young cultures and becoming fragmented into irregular coccobacilli with age. L-phase organisms having a "fried egg" appearance may occur spontaneously on agar and may become stabilized if penicillin is incorporated in the medium. Figure 57-27 is a smear of *Streptobacillus moniliformis* from the culture of a patient with rat-bite fever.

Clinical Manifestations and Pathogenesis

S. moniliformis occurs as indigenous flora in the upper respiratory tract of wild and laboratory rodents. Infection (rat bite fever or Haverhill disease) in humans follows rodent bites, ingestion of contaminated food, or traumatic injury. Local lymphangitis and lymphadenitis may develop up to 3 weeks later, followed by fever, chills, malaise, and, later, a general morbilliform maculopapular or petechial rash. Some patients develop a migratory polyarthritis. Endocarditis has been reported, as have cases of myocarditis, pericarditis, meningitis, pneumonia, and abscess development due to *S. moniliformis*. The histopathology is nonspecific chronic inflammation (vonGraevenitz, 2007).

Laboratory Diagnosis

Specimens for recovery of *S. moniliformis* include blood, joint fluid, and abscess material. *S. moniliformis* is a facultative anaerobic, nonmotile, gram-negative bacillus with a pleomorphic appearance. The organism grows on media enriched with 15% sheep or rabbit blood, serum, or ascitic

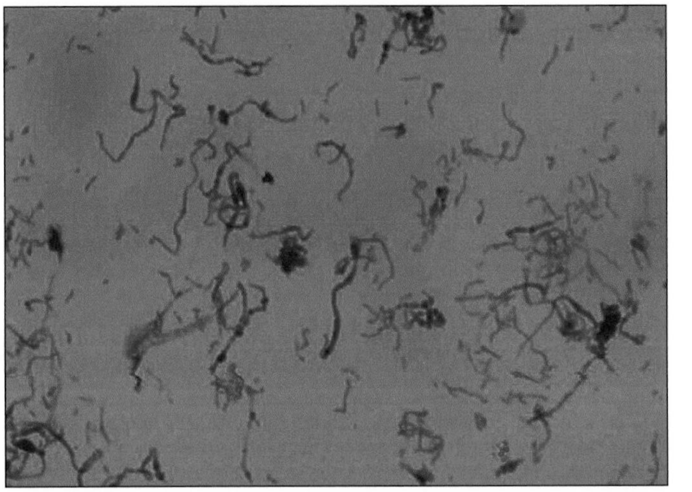

Figure 57-27 Gram stain of *Streptobacillus moniliformis* from culture. *(Courtesy Dr. Nancy Cornish.)*

fluid. Inoculated media should be incubated at 35° C in a humid environment containing an atmosphere of 5%–10% CO_2. Colonies on solid media are small and slightly translucent to opaque with slightly irregular edges. Coccal forms and gram variability may occur, but usually colonies will demonstrate long filaments with granules and bulbs or banding forms on Gram stain. L-forms may be present in some cultures, along with the usual bacterial forms.

Colonies in broth form as fluff balls usually at the bottom of the tube. Cultures die out quickly unless subcultured often. Because this organism is relatively inert, identification of *S. moniliformis* is complex. Biochemical tests must be performed in heart infusion agar or broth supplemented with yeast extract and horse serum. Molecular sequencing methods or fatty acid analysis is required for complete identification (vonGraevenitz, 2007).

Antimicrobial Susceptibility

S. moniliformis is susceptible to penicillin and doxycycline. It is resistant to colistin, nalidixic acid, and SXT.

Prevention and Control

Because 10%–65% of rats are infected with the organism, their control and precautions against bites represent the only effective methods of control of the disease.

ANAEROBIC BACTERIA

It is important to reemphasize that anaerobes represent a major component of the indigenous flora of the skin and mucous membranes; therefore their isolation and identification are contingent on the proper selection and collection of specimens, as well as on their proper transport to the laboratory. Anaerobic infections are frequently mixed, consisting of several species of anaerobes, or of anaerobes mixed with facultatively anaerobic bacteria; therefore the first task in examining an anaerobic culture is to separate facultatively anaerobic from obligate anaerobic bacteria. With experience, the more commonly isolated anaerobes can often be recognized on the basis of their colonial and microscopic morphologies and presumptively identified on the basis of a few additional tests. Definitive identification is based on biochemical reactions, physiologic and molecular characteristics, and occasionally pathogenicity and toxin neutralization tests.

The extent to which anaerobes are identified varies according to the facilities and expertise available, the interest of laboratory personnel and clinical staff, and the clinical relevance of the information available from the laboratory. Anaerobes have been fairly consistent in their response, at least in vitro, to antibiotics, but as with other groups of bacteria, resistance is becoming an issue with many anaerobes; this may prompt additional identification and susceptibility testing in the future (Hecht, 2006; Roh, 2009).

Definitions and Characteristics

An anaerobe requires an atmosphere with reduced oxygen tension for its growth and fails to grow on the surface of solid media in an atmosphere of room air with 10% CO_2. A facultatively anaerobic bacterium will grow in the presence or absence of room air. The term *microaerophile* has not been strictly defined but is commonly applied to bacteria—usually campylobacters and streptococci—that grow only or preferentially in an atmosphere with reduced O_2 and with increased CO_2.

Pathogenesis and Virulence Factors

Little is known about the factors responsible for the pathogenic and virulence properties of most anaerobes other than the clostridia. Endotoxic, proteolytic, and heparinase activities have been identified among the Bacteroidaceae. The polysaccharide capsule of *B. fragilis* promotes abscess formation. Clostridia, on the other hand, elaborate potent exotoxins, including lethal and necrotizing toxins, hemolysins, lecithinases, gelatinases, and hyaluronidases.

Although clostridial infection may be exogenous or endogenous in origin, disease caused by other anaerobes usually originates endogenously from the normal indigenous anaerobic flora of a contiguous mucous membrane, the integrity of which has been disrupted by surgery, instrumentation, trauma, or malignancy. Essential to the establishment of anaerobes in the infectious process is a decrease in the oxidation-reduction potential *(Eh)* of the area, which may result from failure of its blood supply or from the multiplication of other bacteria at the site.

Although clostridial infections and intoxications are unquestionably of major medical importance, the role of other anaerobes in causing cellulitis and myonecrosis has been recognized more recently. Most isolates of *Clostridium perfringens* are the result of simple contamination of a wound. In such instances, the clostridia may multiply in cellular debris, a hematoma, or necrotic tissue without observable clinical symptoms. Anaerobic cellulitis is a necrotizing process of the soft tissues. Its onset is gradual, but it can progress rapidly and extensively. Gas is produced; however, the process typically does not involve muscle. In addition to or instead of clostridia, the bacteriology of anaerobic cellulitis may involve anaerobic cocci and anaerobic gram-negative bacilli.

In contrast to anaerobic cellulitis, gas gangrene or clostridial myonecrosis is an acute and rapidly progressive invasive process producing marked changes in muscle. Distinguishing between anaerobic cellulitis and gas gangrene is critical to avoid performing unnecessarily aggressive and mutilating surgery in the former condition.

Histotoxic clostridia associated with gas gangrene include *C. perfringens, Clostridium novyi, Clostridium septicum, Clostridium histolyticum, Clostridium sporogenes,* and *Clostridium bifermentans. C. perfringens* has been the species most frequently involved in gas gangrene; the prevalence of other species in this process has varied widely.

Tetanus and botulism, caused by *C. tetani* and *C. botulinum*, respectively, are described as intoxications rather than as infections, because their manifestations are related to the elaboration of potent neurotoxins. Botulism is most frequently due to the ingestion of home-processed foods that have been improperly preserved or canned; sporadic outbreaks of the disease have been associated with commercially processed food and with wounds infected by the organism. The incubation period for botulism is short: Signs and symptoms usually occur between 18 and 36 hours following ingestion of contaminated food. Of the seven antigenic types of botulinum toxin known, type A is the most common in cases of food poisoning in North America, followed by types B, E, and F. The toxin is absorbed from the intestinal tract and, rarely, from an infected wound and ultimately attaches to motor nerve terminals, thereby preventing acetylcholine release at the nerve endings.

Tetanus typically occurs in nonimmunized persons within the first 2 weeks following a traumatically acquired puncture, laceration, or abrasion. Cases have been reported to occur postoperatively; following dental work, childbirth, and abortion; or in association with stasis and decubitus ulcers. The toxin, tetanospasmin, is transported to gangliosides in the CNS via the lymphatics and bloodstream, and by migration through the perineural spaces of peripheral nerves.

Clostridium difficile is the major cause of nosocomial diarrhea and the primary pathogen responsible for pseudomembranous colitis. It is a rare cause of abscesses, wound infections, osteomyelitis, pleuritis, peritonitis, septicemia, and urogenital tract infections. Carriage rates of *C. difficile* and its toxins are high (50% or more) in neonates, but disease is rare (Bartlett, 1997). Colonization, with or without toxin production, may be maintained for several months, but when the adult flora becomes established at 6–12 months of age, colonization rates fall, and only about 3% of normal healthy adults are colonized with the organism. *C. difficile* almost always is acquired in the hospital by persons receiving antimicrobial agents via direct or indirect exposure to human or inanimate reservoirs. Although the penicillins and the cephalosporins are implicated most frequently, any antimicrobial agent may trigger *C. difficile*–associated disease. Disease rarely occurs without antibiotic exposure, but cases have been reported following therapy with antineoplastic agents that have antibacterial activity. Pseudomembranous colitis is a toxin-mediated illness in which microbial invasion of the mucosa is not known to occur. *C. difficile* produces two toxins. Toxin A, a weakly cytopathic toxin, is predominantly responsible for the enterotoxic activity of the organism. Toxin B, a potent cytotoxin, appears to play a minor role in human disease, although toxin-A–negative, B-positive strains have been isolated from symptomatic patients (Johnson, 1998). Use of a PCR assay in the laboratory for detection of both toxin A and toxin B will increase sensitivity (Eastwood, 2009; Kvach, 2009; Stamper, 2009).

As previously mentioned, other anaerobic bacteria, particularly anaerobic cocci and gram-negative bacilli, have been associated with anaerobic cellulitis, in addition to or instead of the histotoxic clostridial species. These organisms are part of the indigenous flora of the mucous membranes of the oral cavity and of the gastrointestinal and genitourinary tracts. As such, they are encountered in aspiration pneumonias, lung abscesses, empyemas, intraabdominal infections and abscesses, pelvic abscesses, brain abscesses, and bacteremias. Anaerobic intraabdominal infections commonly follow abdominal and especially colon surgery, and are most frequently associated with the *B. fragilis* group. Clinically significant anaerobic bacteremias are also most frequently caused by this species. *Propionibacterium acnes* have been increasing in isolation and in association with clinical disease.

Significant taxonomic changes have occurred among the anaerobes. Some of these are delineated in Tables 57-15 through 57-19.

Laboratory Diagnosis

Identifying anaerobic bacteria to the species level can be a complex task; however, the extent to which isolates of anaerobic bacteria are identified varies widely and may be limited to basic information that is of clinical relevance and/or that might be needed to predict antimicrobial susceptibilities. For example, the mixed anaerobic flora from a site such as a decubitus ulcer, perirectal fistula, or intraabdominal abscess may simply be reported as mixed fecal flora (mentioning specifically whether there are aerobes and anaerobes or only anaerobes) without specific identification of its components. Determining the species of an isolate may be limited to those present in pure culture from a normally sterile body fluid or site, and can be readily accomplished with the use of any of several commercially available biochemical assay-containing kits, by using gas-liquid chromatography (GLC), or by combining the two approaches. Many laboratories have begun to use sequencing as a means of identifying anaerobic isolates. Results are often available rapidly, and increasing numbers of databases are available for the identification of many more species than can be identified with phenotypic kit systems (Simmon, 2008). MALDI-TOF-MS (matrix-assisted laser desorption/ionization time-of-flight mass spectrometry) is a recently developed method for the identification of a wide variety of bacteria, including anaerobes (Stingu, 2008). One should understand that the clinical value of any report of the presence of anaerobic bacteria is directly related to the speed of reporting such results from the laboratory. Identification procedures that require 1–2 weeks to complete are generally of academic interest only.

Because of their rapid progression and considerable morbidity and mortality, the initial diagnosis and management of diseases caused by the

TABLE 57-15
Most Frequently Isolated Gram-Positive Non-*Clostridium* spp. Anaerobic Bacteria

Species	Gram stain	Colony	Indole	PYR
Gram-Positive Cocci				
Peptostreptococcus anaerobius	Large cocci, often in chains	Nonhemolytic; gray with raised center; sweet odor	Negative	Negative
P. micros	Clusters or short chains; <0.6 μm	Small; dull color; "halo" around colony	Negative	Positive
Finegoldia marna	Pairs, tetrads, and clusters; >0.6 μm	Small, white, convex	Negative	Positive
Peptoniphilus asaccharolyticus	"Clumps," pairs, or tetrads	Small; slight yellow pigment	Usually positive	Negative
Anaerococcus tetradius	Clumps and tetrads	Nonglistening; gray; convex	Negative	Weak
A. prevotii	Clumps and tetrads	Nonglistening; gray; convex	Negative	Positive
Staphylococcus saccharolyticus	Clusters and tetrads	Catalase and coagulase negative	ND	ND
Gram-positive non–spore-forming bacilli	Gram stain	Colony	Aerotolerance/ Biochemical clues	Other characteristic
Actinomyces israelii	Short rods; branching or beading	White; opaque; "molar tooth"	+	Most common cause of actinomycosis: genital; pulmonary; abdominal
A. naeslundii	Short rods; branching or beading	Gray-white; translucent	+++	Oral flora; rarely pathogenic
A. odontolyticus	Short rods; branching or beading	May produce pink to red colonies in ambient air	+++	Oral flora; rarely pathogenic
A. turicensis			++	Genital sites
Propionibacterium acnes	Short rods; may appear "spidery"	White round colonies	++++ Catalase positive; indole positive	Normal flora on skin; associated with endophthalmitis (post cataract surgery); ventricular shunt infections; infrequent cause of endocarditis, osteomyelitis
Propionimicrobium lymphophilum	Coccoid; singly, pairs, or short chains	White, glistening	Non-aerotolerant	Isolation: lymph nodes; uncertain relevance
Bifidobacterium spp.	Diphtheroidal; bifurcated or forked ends		Non-aerotolerant	Normal flora of GI and GU tract; rarely clinically significant
Eggerthella lenta (formerly *Eubacterium lentum*)	Straight rod with rounded ends		Non-aerotolerant Catalase positive; indole negative	Grow in 20% bile; saccharolytic; have been isolated in anaerobic bacteremia

+, ++, +++, ++++, Positive with increasing strength; *ND*, not done; *PYR*, l-pyrrolidonyl-β-naphthylamide.

TABLE 57-16
Most Frequently Isolated Gram-Negative Anaerobic Bacteria (all should grow in presence of 20% bile)

Species	Colony	Biochemicals	Other characteristics
Bacteroides fragilis complex*	White, round; requires ≈24–48 hours		
B. fragilis		Negative for indole Positive for catalase and indole	Most common and most pathogenic of the complex
B. distasonis		Negative for indole Usually positive for catalase and esculin	
B. thetaiotaomicron		Positive for indole, catalase, and esculin	
B. vulgatus		Negative for indole; usually negative for catalase and esculin	
B. ovatus		Positive for indole, catalase, and esculin	
B. goldsteinii		Negative for indole; variable for catalase and positive esculin	
Bacteroides urealyticus	Colonies often "pit" the agar	No growth in 20% bile; indole, esculin, and catalase usually negative; urease positive	Part of normal anaerobic oral flora
Bilophila wadsworthia		Will grow in 20% bile; catalase positive; negative for indole and esculin	
Porphyromonas asaccharolyticus	Colonies fluoresce brick red (ultraviolet light exposure); black pigment with age	Bile sensitive; indole positive and catalase negative	Normal oral flora; pulmonary disease
Prevotella disiens and *P. bivia*		Bile sensitive; indole and esculin negative; saccharolytic and nonpigmented	Normal genitourinary flora; can be involved in pelvic abscesses
Fusobacterium nucleatum	Breadcrumb-like and speckled; Gram stain: long thin, pointed bacilli	Bile sensitive; indole positive and esculin negative	Oral flora; can be involved in bacteremia, pulmonary infection
F. necrophorum	Umbonate colonies; greening of agar; Gram stain: round, not tapered ends; often "bizarre" forms seen	Usually sensitive to bile; indole positive, lipase positive	Associated with Lemierre's syndrome
F. mortiferum	"Fried egg" appearance of colonies; nontapered rods and bizarre round "bodies" on Gram stain	Grows on 20% bile; indole negative and esculin positive	Infrequent isolate
Gram-Negative Cocci			
Veillonella spp.	Small white colonies; Gram stain: well staining, round cocci, singly or in pairs	Catalase variable; nitrate reduction positive	Common isolate, but rarely involved in clinical disease

*In addition to those listed, *B. fragilis* complex includes *B. caccae, B. eggerthii, B. merdae, B. stercoris,* and *B. uniformis.*

TABLE 57-17
Most Common Species of *Clostridium* (Spore-Former) in Clinical Samples

Species	Colony	Gram stain	Characteristics
C. perfringens	Large, white, with double-zone hemolysis	"Box-car" (short and fat) shaped rods; short chains may be seen; rare spores seen	Lipase negative; lecithinase positive; indole negative; reverse CAMP positive Most common isolate; skin and soft tissue infections (including gangrene); bacteremia; also found in gastrointestinal tract as part of normal flora
C. ramosum	Large, spready white colony	Often stain gram negative or variable; cells are more slender and longer than *C. perfringens;* spores not commonly seen	Commonly isolated from clinical samples
C. sordelii	White	Large, gram-positive rods with subterminal spores seen; lecithinase positive; lipase negative; indole and urease positive	Less frequently isolated than *C. perfringens, C. ramosum,* and *C. septicum*
C. tetani		Thin bacilli with terminal spores: "snow-shoe" or "tennis racquet" appearance; lecithinase negative; lipase weak positive; indole variable and urease negative	May be part of gastrointestinal flora; cause of tetanus
C. septicum	White, swarming colonies	Long, filamentous bacilli with rare subterminal spores seen; lecithinase, lipase, indole, and urease negative	When isolated from blood cultures, indicates a possible gastrointestinal malignancy
C. difficile	White colonies with distinctive "horse- barn" odor; selective CCFA media: yellow, ground glass appearing colonies	Thin, long bacilli with spores seen	Cause of pseudomembranous colitis and antibiotic-associated diarrhea; rarely found outside of the gastrointestinal tract

TABLE 57-18
New Taxonomic Designations of Anaerobic Gram-Positive Cocci

New designation	Older designation
Finegoldia magna	*Peptostreptococcus magnus*
Peptostreptococcus micros	*Micromonas micros*
Anaerococcus prevotii	*Peptostreptococcus prevotii*
Anaerococcus tetradius	*Peptostreptococcus tetradius*
Anaerococcus vaginalis	
Anaerococcus lactolyticus	
Anaerococcus hydrogenalis	
Anaerococcus octavius	
Peptoniphilus indolicus	*Peptostreptococcus indolicus*
Peptoniphilus asaccharolyticus	*Peptostreptococcus asaccharolyticus*
Peptoniphilus harei	
Peptoniphilus lacrimalis	
Peptoniphilus ivorii	
Peptostreptococcus anaerobius	No name change
Peptostreptococcus sotmatis	No name change
Atopobium parvulum	*Streptococcus parvulus*

TABLE 57-19
Newer Taxonomy of Less Frequently Encountered Anaerobic Gram-Negative Bacilli

New designation	Older designation
Alistipes putredinis	*Bacteroides putredinis*
Alistipes finegoldii	New
Dialister micraerophilus	New
Dialister propionicifaciens	New
Faecalibacterium prausnitzii	*Fusobacterium prausnitzii*
Porphyromonas uenonis	*Porphyromonas endodontalis* (nonoral)
Sneathia sanguinegens	*Leptotrichia sanguinegens*
Tannerella forsythensis	*Bacteroides forsythus*
Sutterella wadsworthensis	*Campylobacter (Bacteroides) gracilis* (some strains)
Campylobacter gracilis	*Bacteroides gracilis* (some strains)
Campylobacter rectus	*Wolinella rectus*
Campylobacter curvus	*Wolinella curva*

clostridia must be based on their clinical presentation and manifestations. In some patients with tetanus, no primary wound is evident. When a wound is present, organisms typical of *C. tetani* are seldom seen in stained smears, even though they may be recovered from cultures. Moreover, because of this organism's widespread distribution in nature, its isolation from a wound is not necessarily indicative of the diagnosis of tetanus. Laboratory confirmation of botulism requires detection of the toxin in serum, wounds, gastric contents, feces, or the food suspected of causing the disease. Procedures for extracting the toxin and for performing mouse neutralization tests are complex; therefore it is suggested that the appropriate materials be referred to the CDC for examination. Telephone consultation should be made in such instances to ensure that the requisite specimens are properly collected and transported, and that the appropriate authorities are alerted.

In cases of suspected anaerobic cellulitis or gas gangrene, the laboratory can be helpful by examining exudate or tissue microscopically. The finding of numerous, large, "boxcar"-shaped, gram-positive bacilli (Fig. 57-28) provides presumptive confirmation of the diagnosis. Stained smears may also be diagnostic of anaerobic streptococcal myositis. Cultures of exudate, tissue, and blood should be performed. Once again, the level or extent of identification varies considerably among laboratories; however, *C. perfringens* may be easily identified by its Gram stain morphology, the production of double zones of hemolysis on blood agar, and a positive Nagler's reaction on egg yolk agar. Laboratory diagnosis of *C. difficile* diarrhea has been accomplished in most laboratories by detecting the toxin directly in stool using an EIA or cell culture assay. Culture of stool for the organism and,

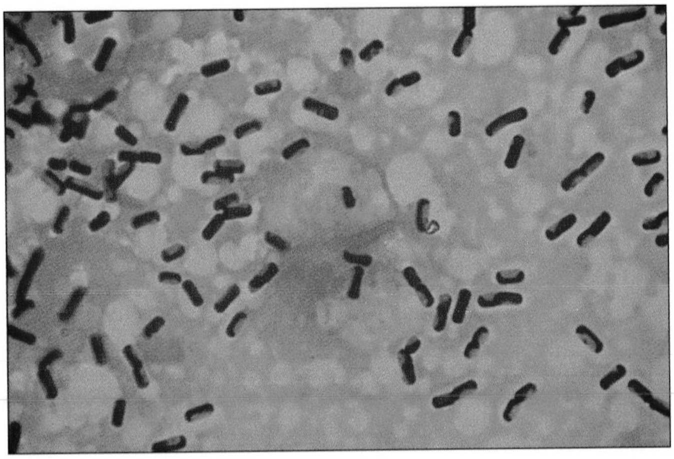

Figure 57-28 Gram stain of a smear of exudate from a wound that had gas bubbles shows large, boxcar-shaped, gram-positive bacilli, suggestive of clostridial disease (oil immersion).

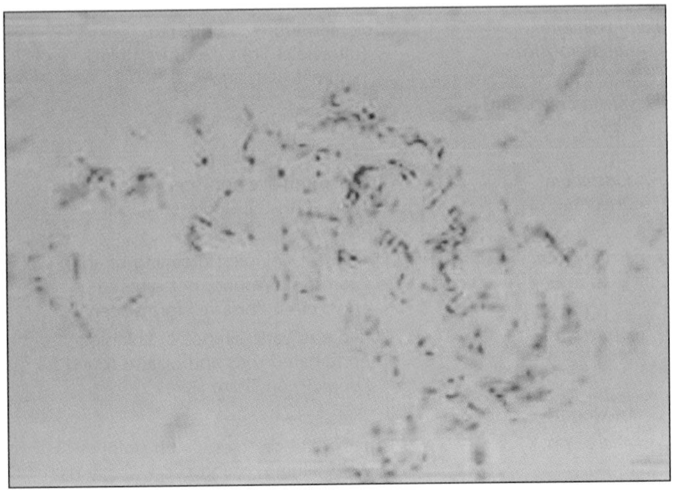

Figure 57-29 Gram stain of *Bacteroides fragilis* from broth culture.

when positive, determination of whether toxin is being produced is primarily reserved for epidemiologic and surveillance studies, although it is used diagnostically in a few laboratories. Many believe it is the "gold standard" for detection. Assays that detect a "common" antigen, glutamate dehydrogenase, which is found in most *C. difficile* isolates, are now being used as part of a two- or three-step procedure for laboratory diagnosis of *C. difficile* to increase sensitivity. Unfortunately, the antigen can be found in other bacteria, so that a positive antigen should be confirmed before it is reported as *C. difficile* positive. Confirmation is carried out in the two-step assay with PCR or cytotoxicity studies; in the three-step assay, a positive antigen is followed by an EIA, and any antigen-positive/EIA toxin–negative samples would have a PCR performed or a cytotoxicity test conducted for confirmation. The prevalence of *C. difficile* usually is not >20% in any single facility, and the two- or three-step approach allows rapid results to be obtained from negative samples. Some more recent studies have questioned the sensitivity of the antigen, but in most studies and laboratory validations, it appears to be highly sensitive. A PCR method for initial detection of the toxins of *C. difficile* is now commercially available, and many laboratories have started to use PCR as a replacement for EIA or cytotoxicity (Eastwood, 2009; Kvach, 2009; Stamper, 2009).

One of the most common groups of clinically relevant and frequently isolated anaerobic bacteria is the *B. fragilis* complex. Isolates from this complex will grow selectively on *Bacteroides* bile esculin medium, and they have characteristic Gram stain morphology as seen in Figure 57-29. These gram-negative bacilli are found as normal flora throughout much of the gastrointestinal and genitourinary tracts. Infections caused by the complex include abdominal abscess, pelvic abscess, bacteremia, and brain abscess. They may rarely be involved in pulmonary disease. Although most anaerobic infections are polymicrobial, *B. fragilis* alone may be responsible for infection. Members of the *B. fragilis* complex include *B. caccae*, *B. distasonis*, *B. eggerthii*, *B. fragilis*, *B. goldsteinii*, *B. merdae*, *B. nordii*, *B. ovatus*, *B.*

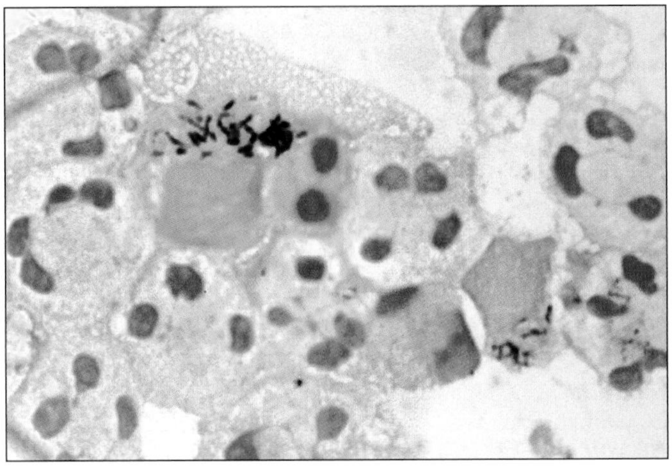

Figure 57-30 Gram stain of *Propionibacterium acnes* from vitreous fluid.

salyersiae, *B. stercoris*, *B. thetaiotaomicaon*, *B. uniformis*, and *B. vulgatus*. With rare exception, members of the complex will grow in the presence of 20% bile and will hydrolyze esculin. Inclusion of a *Bacteroides* bile esculin agar (BBE) plate when anaerobic specimens are processed will allow more rapid detection and identification of these organisms.

An anaerobic gram-positive bacillus, *Propionibacterium acnes*, has been associated with cases of endophthalmitis that occur after cataract surgery. In addition, *P. acnes* may be associated with ventricular shunt infection in patients with hydrocephalus; rarely, *P. acnes* can cause endocarditis, septic arthritis, or other infections. Isolation of this organism may require extended incubation, often up to 10 days. Figure 57-30 shows a Gram stain of *P. acnes* in vitreous fluid obtained from a patient months after cataract surgery. *Actinomyces israelii* and other species of *Actinomyces* can be involved in lung abscesses, brain abscesses, skin and soft tissue infections, and mycetoma, and may be involved in genital infections involving use of an intrauterine device (IUD), although this is a controversial topic (Burkman, 1996; Westhoff, 2007).

Antimicrobial Susceptibility

Susceptibility testing of anaerobic bacteria in the past was considered unnecessary, except in the following circumstances. Major indications for testing are clinical settings in which decisions regarding the selection of agents are critical because of (1) failure of usual therapeutic regimens and persistence of infection, (2) the key role of antimicrobial agents in determining the outcome of infection, or (3) the difficulty involved in making empirical therapeutic decisions based on precedent. Infections from which isolates should be tested include brain abscess, endocarditis, osteomyelitis, joint infections, infections of prosthetic devices or vascular grafts, and refractory or recurrent bacteremia. Testing under these circumstances should include some members of the *B. fragilis* group, certain *Fusobacterium* spp., *C. perfringens*, and *Clostridium ramosum*. Agents such as metronidazole, imipenem, and ampicillin-sulbactam have almost always been reported as active against anaerobic bacteria and usually are not routinely tested for clinical purposes. Thus testing was limited to alternative agents with unpredictable activity, such as penicillin, clindamycin, cefoxitin, and cefotetan. More recently, results are not as predictable, and the need for performance of an in vitro susceptibility test is increasing (Hecht, 2006; Roh, 2009). Although an agar dilution method has been recommended for reference purposes, testing in the clinical laboratory is generally performed by the microdilution (CLSI, 2007) or Etest method. Batch testing of saved isolates on a yearly basis is recommended to develop antibiograms for empirical use by clinicians, and to monitor for possible development of resistance (Boyanova, 2007).

SELECTED REFERENCES

Bannerman TL, Peacock SJ. *Staphylococcus, Micrococcus,* and other catalase positive cocci. In: Murray PR, Baron EJ, Jorgensen JH, et al, editors. Manual of clinical microbiology. 9th ed. Washington, DC: American Society for Microbiology; 2007, p. 390–411.

Provides an excellent overview of the biochemical tests useful for identification of aerobic catalase-positive gram-positive cocci. Additionally, it includes a discussion of the important resistance mechanisms and tests that allow detection of resistant isolates.

Clinical and Laboratory Standards Institute. Performance standards for antimicrobial susceptibility testing; nineteenth informational supplement. CLS document M100-S19. Wayne, Pa: CLSI; 2009.

Essential for appropriate interpretation and reporting of antibacterial susceptibility test results.

Cosgrove SE, Carroll KC, Perl TM. *S. aureus* with reduced susceptibility to vancomycin. Clin Infect Dis 2004;39:539–45.

Provides an excellent discussion of the mechanism of reduced susceptibility to vancomycin in S. aureus and tests that allow its detection.

Farmer JJ, Boatwright KD, Janda MJ. Enterobacteriaceae: introduction and identification. In: Murray PR, Baron EJ, Jorgensen JH, et al, editors. Manual of clinical microbiology. 9th ed. Washington, DC: American Society for Microbiology; 2007, p. 649–69.

Provides an excellent discussion of the biochemical tests useful for identification of Enterobacteriaceae.

Janda JM, Malloy PJ, Schreckenberger PC. Clinical evaluation of the Vitek *Neisseria–Haemophilus* identification card. J Clin Microbiol 1987;25:37.

Provides an excellent review of methods useful for identification of the aerobic gram-negative diplococci.

FURTHER READING

Clinical and Laboratory Standards Institute/National Committee for Clinical and Laboratory Standards. Methods for dilution antimicrobial susceptibility tests for bacteria that grow aerobically. Approved Standard, 7th ed. CLSI/NCCLS Document M7-A5. Wayne, Pa.: CLSI; 2006a.

Essential for laboratories that perform antimicrobial susceptibility testing by broth dilution.

Clinical and Laboratory Standards Institute/National Committee for Clinical and Laboratory Standards. Performance standards for antimicrobial disk susceptibility tests. Approved Standard, 9th ed. CLSI/NCCLS Document M2-A9. Wayne, Pa.: CLSI; 2006b.

Essential for laboratories that perform antimicrobial susceptibility testing by disk diffusion.

REFERENCES

Access the complete reference list online at http://www.expertconsult.com

CHAPTER 58

IN VITRO TESTING OF ANTIMICROBIAL AGENTS

Michael B. Smith, P. Rocco LaSala, Gail L. Woods

KEY POINTS

- The minimum inhibitory concentration (MIC), or the lowest concentration of antibiotic that inhibits the visible growth of an organism in vitro, is distinguished from the breakpoint, or the concentration of antibiotic that determines whether an isolate is categorized as susceptible, intermediate, or resistant.
- MIC values are determined by inhibitory methods, which include macrobroth dilution, microbroth dilution, agar dilution, and Epsilometer (E-test). Disk diffusion testing, which is a qualitative rather than a quantitative test, does not directly result in an MIC value, but is based on direct correlation of inhibitory zone sizes with MIC values.
- Whatever method of susceptibility testing is used, standardized conditions related to media, inoculum concentration, incubation time, atmosphere, and temperature are necessary to produce accurate and reproducible results. Standards for these variables are published by the Clinical and Laboratory Standards Institute (CLSI) and represent standard of practice for microbiology laboratories.
- Commercial automated instrument systems are available for rapid, high-volume susceptibility testing; however, despite the advantages of speed and efficiency that these systems allow, it must be remembered that the systems may have weaknesses. In addition to the expense of the systems, some are associated with problems in accurately detecting specific resistance phenotypes.
- Both the indications for susceptibility testing and the selection of which antimicrobials to test and report should be determined by individual laboratories on the basis of recommendations published by the CLSI and in close consultation with the medical and infectious disease staff of the facility served by the laboratory.
- Cumulative antimicrobial susceptibility reports (antibiograms) should be published by laboratories, based on CLSI guidelines, on at least an annual basis. These compilations are important for use by physicians in initiating empirical treatment before testing results are available, and are helpful for pharmacists in monitoring the use and need of specific antimicrobials and in attempting to control drug costs.

Selection of an antibiotic by a physician to treat an infection in a patient involves consideration of numerous factors, including but not limited to the known or most likely infecting organism(s), local patterns of drug resistance on the part of the organism(s), the site of infection, pharmacodynamic and pharmacokinetic properties of the drug, overall health of the patient, the cost of the antibiotic, and personal experiences of the physician. Although in many cases initial selection of an antimicrobial agent is empirical, in vitro laboratory testing of the susceptibility of isolated pathogen(s) to antibiotics is an important aid in subsequent management of the patient. Modification of therapy may be desirable if (1) the infecting organism(s) is resistant to current therapy, (2) the dose of antibiotic is not appropriate, or (3) an equally effective but less expensive agent can be used.

DEFINITIONS

Currently, most in vitro antibiotic susceptibility testing in clinical laboratories is still performed with the use of phenotypic methods, which are simple and inexpensive. Phenotypic methods require isolation of the pathogen being tested, followed by exposure of the pathogen to the antimicrobial and subsequent evaluation of the expression, or lack of expression, of resistance to the antibiotic. This process can be labor intensive and time consuming, which, under some circumstances, may be disadvantageous to the patient or the laboratory, or both. Despite this fact, phenotypic methods, which include broth dilution, agar dilution, disk diffusion, and gradient diffusion (E-test), are at present the most prevalent and in most cases the most cost-effective way to accomplish susceptibility testing. Commercial systems, based on phenotypic methods, have reduced the labor and the time necessary to detect the expression of antibiotic resistance and are used in many laboratories, although at increased cost to the laboratory in most cases.

Antimicrobial susceptibility tests may be categorized according to the endpoint used, that is, inhibition of growth or killing. In most cases, inhibition of growth is the parameter used in the laboratory, with only limited use of a killing endpoint for very specific circumstances.

The inhibitory parameter that forms the basis for the majority of phenotypic susceptibility tests is the MIC, which is the lowest concentration of antibiotic that inhibits the visible growth of an organism in an in vitro system. MIC results are dependent not only on the interaction between the antimicrobial agent and the organism, but also on test conditions. These conditions include pH and ion concentrations of testing media, the temperature at which the test system is incubated, the incubation atmosphere, the amount of organism used in testing, and the length of time the system incubates. To allow intralaboratory and interlaboratory reproducibility, these test conditions have been standardized. Various standards organizations in a variety of venues throughout the world have set and published these parameters, and in the United States, the CLSI fulfills this role.

Although the MIC is a very useful and reproducible indicator of the interaction of an antibiotic with a specific organism, the information it provides to a physician in the context of the infected patient by itself is limited. The MIC is a "snapshot" assessment of the interaction of a constant concentration of drug with the organism at a specific point in time under specified conditions in vitro. The MIC must be correlated with the complex and changing environment of the physiology of the patient to allow the physician to predict whether therapy with a particular antibiotic will be successful. This is accomplished through the use of **breakpoints,** which allow assessment of the efficacy of killing or inhibition of growth of the organism by the antimicrobial. Several types of breakpoints, including microbiological breakpoints, pharmacokinetic/pharmacodynamic breakpoints, and clinical breakpoints, have been identified. Clinical breakpoints, which are intended to separate strains of organisms into categories that predict whether therapy in a patient will be successful, are breakpoints relevant to this short review and are the only type of breakpoint discussed here. Determining clinical breakpoints is complex, difficult, and subjective. The process can involve numerous clinical trials, and clinical breakpoints may vary with the determining standards organization and may vary over time. In the United States, clinical breakpoints for specific antibiotic–organism combinations are set and published for use by clinical laboratories by the CLSI, and they are updated yearly (Clinical and Laboratory Standards Institute, 2009). Breakpoints established by the CLSI may differ for a variety of reasons from those set by the European Committee on Antimicrobial Susceptibility Testing or other standards organizations. Excellent discussions of breakpoints and their determination, maintenance, and relevance can be obtained by referring to several review articles (Mouton, 2002; Turnidge, 2007).

Interpretive categories have been established that allow simplified and easily understood reporting of susceptibility results by laboratories. Many laboratories report these categories, in addition to reporting an MIC or, in some cases, in lieu of reporting an MIC. Based on clinical breakpoints, specific isolates can be divided into categories after susceptibility testing that is intended to assist the physician in easily interpreting the results. Although highly knowledgeable infectious disease physicians may be able to make informed management decisions with no other information aside from the MIC obtained by testing a specific isolate against an antibiotic, this is unlikely to be the case for physicians who do not specialize in this area. The basic interpretative categories include **susceptible, intermediate,** and **resistant.** Definitions of these categories can be found in CLSI documents (Clinical and Laboratory Standards Institute, 2009). Susceptible implies that therapy with the recommended dosage of a particular antibiotic is likely to be effective in eradicating the infection, and resistant indicates that the antibiotic in the appropriate dose has not been shown to have a high likelihood of treatment success in clinical trials.

Reporting a susceptibility category of intermediate has several implications. It suggests that the isolate tested may be less inhibited by the usual dose of the antibiotic than those isolates that are categorized as susceptible, and that therapy with higher doses of antibiotic or therapy with the antibiotic for infection in anatomic locations in which the antibiotic normally is concentrated is likely to be effective. An example of this latter situation is the use of β-lactam antibiotics in treating urinary tract infection. This category also includes a **buffer zone,** which is intended to prevent technical factors from resulting in a major interpretive error. An additional category of **nonsusceptible** has recently been added. This category is intended for cases in which intermediate and resistant isolates have not been found or categories of intermediate and resistant have not been defined. It is utilized primarily for new antibiotics. If testing of an isolate yields an MIC value that is above the cutoff concentration established for the breakpoint for a susceptible category, the laboratory can report the isolate as nonsusceptible. This does not necessarily imply that resistance to the antibiotic exists, but it means that experience with isolates that demonstrate MICs at this level is limited, so no assessment can be made.

Although reporting of antimicrobial susceptibility testing and categorization of an isolate into one the interpretative categories are helpful to physicians in managing patients with infection, it must be remembered that antimicrobial activity in vivo depends on many factors. In addition to drug dosage, route of administration, pharmacokinetic/pharmacodynamic characteristics of the drug, and site of infection, patient-specific factors such as immune status and hepatic and renal function also help determine a patient's response to therapy and must be considered in planning treatment. Antimicrobial susceptibility testing is thus an adjunct to patient management and does not in itself predict response to therapy.

Inhibitory Methods for Susceptibility Testing

DILUTION TESTING

In dilution testing, a standardized amount of organism is inoculated into a series of tubes, wells, or dishes that contain a range of concentrations of antimicrobial in a vehicle, such as broth or agar, usually starting with an integral of 2 (e.g., 128 μg/mL) and decreasing on a log_2 basis to the lowest concentration tested. For the purposes of convenience and economy, it has become common to limit the range of concentrations of each antimicrobial tested to those concentrations that encompass the breakpoints that distinguish between susceptible and resistant. Some commercial systems contain only a single concentration of an antimicrobial agent.

The broth macrodilution method is performed using standard test tubes, and the tubes are viewed by the unaided eye to determine whether growth is present. The broth macrodilution system is no longer used by most laboratories because of its labor-intensive nature, but this method is the foundation of most modern susceptibility testing systems. Similarly, the agar dilution method, where the antibiotic being tested is incorporated into solid agar in Petri dishes, is an older, labor-intensive method that is little used by modern laboratories for routine testing. However, because the isolate being tested is placed on the agar as a single spot, the agar dilution method can allow the testing of multiple isolates on a single plate. Additionally, some species that do not grow well in broth, or for which the broth method has not been shown to be sufficiently reproducible, can be tested by this method. With the exception of the *Bacteroides fragilis* group, agar dilution is the only standardized method recommended by the CLSI for susceptibility testing of anaerobe species (Clinical and Laboratory Standards Institute, 2007).

Broth microdilution is the most common dilution method used in the modern microbiology laboratory, and this method is the basis for most commercial systems. Commercially prepared and disposable microtiter trays containing antibiotics exist as standalone devices, which are manually inoculated and read by visualization, or as components of automated systems that are read by spectrophotometric methods. Several systems have been in existence for a number of years, have extensive databases built over the years, and offer the advantage of computerized software that allows collection of antibiogram data and "expert" systems that assist in interpretation. Several newer systems have also come onto the market recently. Because of the labor associated with preparing microtiter trays in-house, and the extensive quality assurance testing necessary when preparing the trays, commercially prepared trays and systems are very popular. They can be expensive, however, and the antibiotics available on a given tray may not conform to local needs. Customized trays may be available but usually are associated with additional expense.

EPSILOMETER

The Epsilometer, or E-test (AB Biodisk, Solna, Sweden), is a plastic strip with a gradient of antibiotic on one side of the strip and a continuous MIC scale on the opposite side. The strip is placed on the surface of an agar plate that has been inoculated with the isolate. Antibiotic will diffuse into the surrounding agar in a gradient that corresponds to the gradient on the strip. If the isolate is susceptible, an ellipse of inhibition will occur in growth of the bacterium on the surface of the plate, and the point on the MIC scale of the strip where the ellipse of inhibition intersects is the MIC (Fig. 58-1). The MIC obtained using the E-test has been shown to correlate well with the MIC obtained with the agar or broth dilution for many antibiotic–bacterial species combinations (Baker, 1991). This method is useful because it allows the testing of single antibiotics against isolates, which has particular utility if testing of an isolate against a drug not on the laboratory's preconstructed antibiotic panel is necessary, or if testing of one or a few drugs against fastidious species that require special media is required (e.g., *Haemophilus influenzae*).

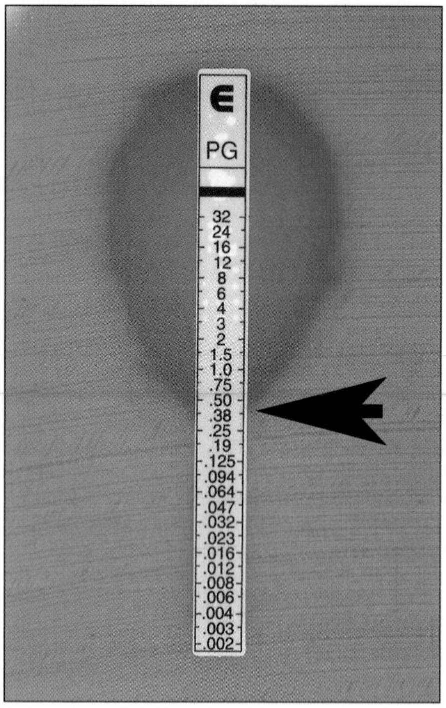

Figure 58-1 Epsilometer, or E-test. A gradient of antibiotic (penicillin in this example) is incorporated into the plastic strip, which is placed on the agar surface on which an organism has been streaked *(Streptococcus pneumoniae)*. The intersection of the zone of inhibition with the numeric scale on the strip is read as the minimum inhibitory concentration (MIC) *(arrow)*.

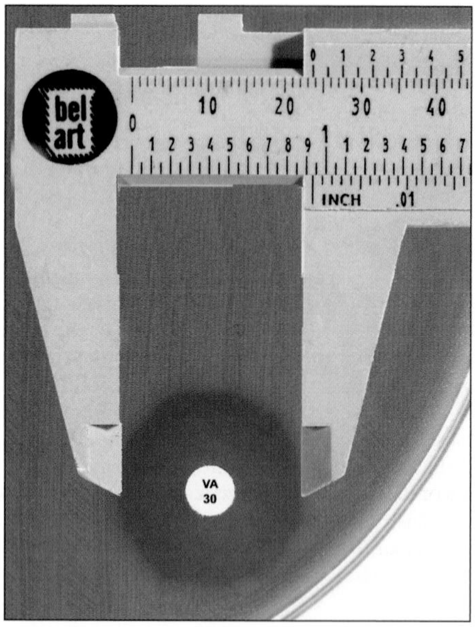

Figure 58-2 Disk diffusion. The zone of inhibition around the antibiotic disk (vancomycin in this case) on the agar surface on which the organism *(Streptococcus pneumoniae)* has been streaked is measured. The result may be susceptible, intermediate, or resistant, based on the zone size.

DISK DIFFUSION

In the disk diffusion test (Kirby-Bauer), which is largely limited to rapidly growing aerobic and facultatively anaerobic bacteria, a paper disk containing a specified amount (not concentration) of antimicrobial is applied to an agar surface that has been streaked with a standardized inoculum of the isolate. Testing is done on a 150-mm-diameter agar plate that allows testing of 12 antibiotics at once. The antibiotic diffuses into the agar medium from the disk, resulting in a zone of growth inhibition at the point at which a critical concentration of the antimicrobial in the medium inhibits growth of the bacteria after a standardized time period (16–18 hours) (Fig. 58-2). The diameter of the zone of growth inhibition has been shown to be inversely correlated with the MIC. The relationship between the two can be expressed as a linear regression line, and zone diameter equivalents of susceptible, intermediate, and resistant interpretations can be extrapolated from their intercepts on the regression line with corresponding MIC values.

Disk diffusion is a simple method that provides a qualitative susceptibility result. It allows easy modification of the panel of antibiotics being tested and is inexpensive relative to a number of other methods. It is primarily a manual method, although a video-assisted plate reader as part of a susceptibility data management system, BIOMIC System (Giles Scientific, New York), has been available for a number of years. For laboratories with a high volume of testing, dependence on manual labor may prohibit the use of disk diffusion as the routine method of susceptibility testing. Certain fastidious species may require special media or conditions for performing disk diffusion that may prohibit routine testing in less well funded laboratories, as it may not be cost-effective to keep the necessary media on hand for the times when testing is necessary. Referral of the isolate to a reference laboratory for susceptibility testing is sometimes a more cost-effective approach in these situations.

DIRECT TESTS FOR β-LACTAMASE

Direct β-lactamase tests are not inhibitory tests but are phenotypic tests that detect the presence of β-lactamase production by an organism. They are mentioned with the inhibitory tests because they, like the inhibitory tests, are commonly used in clinical laboratories. These tests are useful in detecting penicillinase enzymes in gram-positive and a few gram-negative species. Three types of β-lactamase direct test may be used: acidometric, iodometric, and chromogenic. The chromogenic test is the most sensitive, the most specific, and the easiest to use; it has replaced the other types in usual laboratory use and is the only type discussed here. The chromogenic test consists of a paper disk impregnated with a chromogenic cephalosporin (nitrocefin). A loopful of bacteria to be tested is simply smeared onto the disk, and if the organism is producing β-lactamase, hydrolysis of the chromogenic cephalosporin will occur and the disk color will change from yellow to red, usually within a minute; however, a final observation of the disk at 15 minutes is necessary for slowly developing reactions. The test can be used to detect β-lactamase production in several species, including *Haemophilus* species, *Moraxella catarrhalis*, *Staphylococcus* species, *Enterococcus* species, and gram-negative anaerobes (excluding the *B. fragilis* group). A positive test indicates that the organism will not be inhibited by a penicillinase-susceptible penicillin. A positive nitrocefin test for an isolate of *H. influenzae* or *M. catarrhalis* indicates that infection due to the isolate will not respond to ampicillin or amoxicillin. For many gram-positive species, the enzymes require induction by exposure to a β-lactam antibiotic before the enzyme is expressed and can be detected. For example, a simple and appropriate method for testing a staphylococcal isolate for β-lactamase production is accomplished by selecting growth from around the edges of a β-lactam–containing disk on a disk diffusion plate. It should be noted that β-lactam direct tests cannot be used to predict susceptibility to β-lactam antibiotics used in the treatment of infection caused by gram-negative members of aerobic or facultative anaerobes such as *Pseudomonas* spp. or Enterobacteriaceae.

TECHNICAL CONSIDERATIONS IN SUSCEPTIBILITY TESTING

Whichever method of dilution or disk diffusion testing a laboratory selects, utilization of a standardized procedure is of the utmost importance in producing accurate and reproducible results. A variety of standards organizations throughout the world have published performance standards for these procedures, and in the United States, professional organizations (e.g., the American Society for Microbiology, Infectious Disease Society of America), private industry, and governmental organizations have worked together within the Subcommittee on Antimicrobial Susceptibility Testing under the Area Committee on Microbiology of the CLSI to establish the necessary standards. The CLSI has published a series of documents that describe standardized procedures for susceptibility testing of aerobic and facultatively anaerobic bacteria (Clinical and Laboratory Standards Institute, 2009b, 2009c), anaerobic bacteria (Clinical and Laboratory Standards Institute, 2007), mycobacteria and aerobic actinomycetes (National Committee for Clinical Laboratory Standards, 2003), filamentous fungi (Clinical and Laboratory Standards Institute, 2008), and yeasts (National Committee for Clinical Laboratory Standards, 2004, 2008, 2008b). The

Subcommittee on Antimicrobial Susceptibility Testing revises the text of most documents on a 3-year cycle and reviews and revises on a yearly basis tables detailing MIC breakpoints or zone diameter breakpoints. Standardized procedures published by the CLSI represent the standard of laboratory practice in the United States, and laboratories should ensure that the most current tables and texts are on hand, and that revisions in the tables and texts are incorporated into the methods and policies of the laboratory when they become available.

Testing Media

It has been demonstrated that testing components with which susceptibility testing is carried out may have an effect on the results. With respect to testing media, the CLSI currently recommends Mueller-Hinton agar or broth because it demonstrates good batch-to-batch reproducibility; is low in sulfonamide, trimethoprim, and tetracycline inhibitors; and supports the growth of most nonfastidious bacteria (Clinical and Laboratory Standards Institute, 2009b, 2009c). Stringent quality control must be adhered to in preparation of the media when media are prepared commercially or "in-house," as many physical properties of the media directly influence testing. Variations in ion concentrations and pH will affect testing (Clinical and Laboratory Standards Institute, 2009b, 2009c). For example, excess calcium and magnesium will cause *Pseudomonas aeruginosa* isolates to appear more resistant when tested against aminoglycosides, but decreased levels may demonstrate false susceptibility. The level of calcium will also affect daptomycin susceptibility results for those species against which the drug is tested, and zinc ion levels influence carbapenem results. As another example, the pH of the media will also directly affect testing, and it must be between 7.2 and 7.4 for accurate results. A more acidic pH will cause some drugs such as aminoglycosides, quinolones, and macrolides to lose potency, and some drugs such as penicillin to have increased activity. A higher pH can have the opposite effect.

For some fastidious species, supplements must be added to the Mueller-Hinton media, or specialized media containing required growth factors are necessary. For example, streptococci do not grow well in or on unsupplemented Mueller-Hinton media; this problem can be overcome by adding defibrinated sheep blood to a final concentration of 5% for disk diffusion or lysed horse blood to the medium at a final concentration of 2.5% to 5% for broth dilution. *Haemophilus influenzae* requires *Haemophilus* test medium when performing broth dilution, and *Neisseria gonorrhoeae* testing requires GC agar base medium with growth supplement (Clinical and Laboratory Standards Institute, 2009b, 2009c). For susceptibility testing of anaerobes, *Brucella* agar supplemented with laked sheep blood, hemin, and vitamin K_1 (Wadsworth method) is necessary to allow testing using the agar dilution method, which is the only CLSI recommended method for testing these species (Clinical and Laboratory Standards Institute, 2007). An exception is seen with the *B. fragilis* group, which can be tested using the microbroth dilution method with *Brucella* broth with hemin, vitamin K_1, and 5% lysed horse blood. The range of drugs that can be tested against *B. fragilis* group using microbroth dilution is more limited, however.

Additional medium parameters may influence testing. For example, agar depth in plates used in disk diffusion testing must measure 4 mm; otherwise, the diffusion gradient of the antibiotic will be affected. False resistance may occur if the agar is too deep, and false susceptibility may occur if the agar is not deep enough. When Mueller-Hinton is supplemented with blood, the zones of inhibition may be smaller by 2 to 3mm than those obtained with unsupplemented agar.

Inoculum

Intuitively, it is evident that the quantity of bacteria present will influence results in susceptibility testing when a finite amount of antibiotic is used in the testing process. To ensure consistency in the quantity of organisms inoculated into the test system, the CLSI has mandated that the prepared inoculum suspension must have a turbidity equivalent to a 0.5 McFarland turbidity standard. These standards can be purchased commercially, or a $BaSO_4$ suspension can be prepared in the laboratory, the instructions for which are detailed in CLSI documents (Clinical and Laboratory Standards Institute, 2009c).

Inoculum preparations can be made by several methods by directly suspending 18–24-hour-old colonies from nonselective media in broth or saline until turbidity of 0.5 McFarland is achieved, or by suspending several colonies of the organism to be tested into nutrient broth and incubating for several hours until growth results in turbidity equivalent to 0.5 McFarland. The direct colony suspension method is necessary for very fastidious species that require special supplements or media for growth, although the growth method is preferable for species that are difficult to suspend uniformly and when 18–24-hour plates are not immediately available. For most commonly isolated species, the two methods are equivalent.

Incubation Conditions

Test systems must be incubated under standardized temperature and atmospheric conditions to ensure uniform results. These conditions have been described and published by the CLSI for U.S. laboratories. General conditions for disk diffusion and broth dilution of bacteria include a temperature of 35° C ± 2° C with an atmosphere of ambient air for a period of 16–20 hours (Clinical and Laboratory Standards Institute, 2009b, 2009c). Many exceptions to this have been noted, however. For example, for disk diffusion, *Streptococcus* spp. and *Haemophilus* spp. require incubation in an atmosphere of 5% carbon dioxide, and although zones of inhibition of *Haemophilus* spp. are measured after 16–18 hours of incubation, those for *Streptococcus* spp. should not be determined until after 20–24 hours. Similarly, although susceptibility testing for most antibiotics against *Staphylococcus* spp. and *Enterococcus* spp. requires 16–18 hours, when oxacillin and vancomycin against *Staphylococcus* spp. and vancomycin against *Enterococcus* spp., respectively, are tested, a full 24 hours of incubation is necessary. Differences in testing and incubation parameters among aerobic, facultative anaerobic, anaerobic, mycobacterial, filamentous fungi, and yeast species require that the relevant CLSI documents be studied carefully prior to testing.

COMMERCIAL AUTOMATED INSTRUMENT SYSTEMS

Over the past several decades, many microbiology laboratories in the United States have shifted from using disk diffusion or manual broth susceptibility testing methods to use of automated commercial microbroth dilution systems as their predominant testing systems. Most laboratories now use these systems (Jones, 2001). Reasons for the shift include the efficiency gained from replicate inoculation of combined systems for identification and susceptibility testing, as well as the benefits of data management software that is an integral component of most of these systems. Additionally, it has sometimes been stated that these systems allow reporting of the MIC value, which is more accurate than simply reporting the interpretive categories generated by disk diffusion testing, and that physicians prefer the reporting of MIC values. However, these statements are not supportable. Inhibitory zone measurements have been accurately correlated with MIC values statistically, and although physicians whose specialty is infectious diseases can utilize an MIC value for dosing strategies in complex or difficult cases, the average physician often has neither the knowledge nor the need to utilize the MIC. Selection of the method to be used for antibiotic susceptibility testing, that is, automated microbroth dilution testing or manual disk diffusion, can be done based on workflow, convenience, economic reasons, or preferences of the medical staff without regard for any differences in accuracy.

A variety of systems are available for selection. Before deciding to purchase a system, the laboratory director should consider whether the advantages of replicate inoculation and of data management systems outweigh the costs of the commercial system, which involves both an up-front outlay of cash and an ongoing expense related to consumable components of the system, compared with the economy and simplicity offered by the disk diffusion test. The tendency is to consider the disk diffusion test archaic and too unsophisticated for modern laboratory practice; however, this method can provide accurate results that are easily understood by health care providers and that suffice in many clinical situations, and it is economical and flexible. The labor-intensive nature of the test compared with automated systems may be limiting in high-volume laboratories, however.

Selection of a particular automated system is based on a list of considerations. Systems differ somewhat in terms of some of these parameters, and it is incumbent on the laboratory director to find the best fit for his/her laboratory. The list of parameters for evaluation includes the volume the system can handle, the technical expertise required to operate the system, the utility and usability of the data management system, the cost of the hardware, the cost of disposable supplies, reagents, and service contracts, and the space occupied by the system. With the Vitek System (BioMerieux, Hazelwood, Mo.), antimicrobial agents are contained in wells within a plastic card, which are inoculated with the isolate in a filler-sealer module, placed in an incubator-reader, and read after incubation, with data managed by the computer module and displayed on the data terminal or printed, or both. The original system (Legacy system) was very popular in clinical laboratories but now has been superseded by the Vitek 2 system. The updated system has automated some of the procedures in the original system that required manual performance, and combines a multichannel fluorometer and photometer to monitor organism growth at 15-minute intervals, allowing results to be generated in hours.

Microscan (Dade Microscan, West Sacramento, Calif.) is a suite of systems that may be utilized in manual mode when frozen or lyophilized panels are inoculated, and then may be read manually after overnight incubation. The semiautomated version, the Microscan Walkaway, can perform traditional overnight MIC testing in which the results are read with a spectrophotometer, or a more rapid method can be used that is based on the generation of fluorescence from the utilization of substrates by inoculated organisms. Fluorometric panels can provide results in hours, similar to the Vitek 2 system.

The Phoenix system (Becton-Dickinson, Sparks, Md.) is relatively new compared with the previously described systems, and it uses a redox indicator to assess bacterial growth in inoculated wells. Similar to Vitek 2 and Microscan Walkaway, this system has the capability to provide results within a usual 8-hour laboratory working shift, if the clinical situation warrants, and if laboratory staffing and workflow are compatible with this goal.

The ability to report antimicrobial susceptibility results faster is heavily promoted by manufacturers as a benefit of automated susceptibility systems. The concept behind this is that switching a patient to an antibiotic that has been demonstrated to be susceptible by in vitro susceptibility testing sooner rather than later will improve the outcome of treatment. For a variety of reasons, including the fact that difficult methodologic and ethical problems are related to designing such studies, and the fact that for some pathogens and infections, it has not been unequivocally proven that antimicrobial therapy in itself is beneficial, this claim on the part of the manufacturers has been difficult to prove.

It has been demonstrated in some studies that physicians will alter antibiotic therapy based on more rapid reporting of susceptibility results. In a nonrandomized study, Matsen (1985) gave physicians the results of rapid (2–5-hour) susceptibility system and disk diffusion testing, and then questioned physicians as to whether the rapid result influenced their choice of therapy. In 32% of cases, the physicians indicated that based on the rapid results, they chose a different antibiotic for initial therapy than they otherwise would have chosen and another 17% "probably" would have chosen. In a prospective, randomized study of 794 general surgical patients, Vincent (1985) provided rapid results for half of the patients and conventional results for the other half. It was found that antimicrobial therapy was modified in a larger percentage of the rapid-reporting group (14.5%) as opposed to the conventional group (8.8%; $P < .0005$). No statistical difference in length of hospital stay was noted between the two groups, however. A recent study involving 1498 inpatients with infection of sterile body fluids (70% bloodstream infections) demonstrated similar findings. Kerremans (2008) showed that reporting rapid results using the Vitek 2 (a mean of 20 hours sooner than the conventional group) resulted in faster alterations in therapy when compared with conventional results reported with the Vitek Legacy, including a reduction in the number of doses of antibiotics (defined daily doses). Similar to the previous study, a reduction in mortality between the two groups was not seen.

Although Barenfanger (1999) was not able to demonstrate a reduction in mortality when comparing outcomes of patients for whom rapid identification and susceptibility results were reported compared with those for whom conventional results were reported, this meaningful study demonstrated that there can be a significant contribution with respect to outcomes aside from mortality, in that it was demonstrated that rapid reporting of identification and antibiotic susceptibility testing can result in a significant decrease in length of hospital stay. A mean decrease in length of stay of 2 hospital days ($P < .0006$) was noted for those patients for whom rapid testing results were available, with a concomitant significant resultant decrease in total cost of hospital stay ($P < .04$); this is a not insignificant contribution in the current medical environment in the United States. In an earlier study involving demographically equivalent inpatients who were randomly assigned to a group in which rapid identification and antibiotic susceptibility testing were performed and a control group in which conventional testing was done, Doern and colleagues (1994) did not demonstrate a decrease in hospital stay, but did show a statistically significant decrease in costs related to laboratory, pharmacy, and other expenses, such that the mean overall cost of hospitalization was significantly decreased. Additionally, this is the only study on the clinical impact of rapid identification and antibiotic susceptibility testing to date that has demonstrated a decrease in mortality in the rapid testing group.

In theory, the faster that antibiotic susceptibility results are available, the greater is the potential for effective therapy, and hence the greater is the likelihood of improving outcome. This potential will vary with the disorder in question, the specific pathogen, the patient population, and the environment. In a retrospective cohort study of 2731 patients with septic shock in medical and surgical intensive care units, Kumar (2006) found that time from presentation to the institution of appropriate antimicrobial therapy was the major factor that influenced outcome. After initial presentation of hypotension, for every hour over the next 6 hours that appropriate antimicrobial therapy was delayed, survival decreased by 7.6%. Despite the demonstration of the importance of antibiotic therapy in helping to determine outcome with respect to mortality in some infections, and the intuitive conclusion that the faster antibiotic susceptibility results are available, the more likely it is that effective therapy can be administered and can improve outcome, the potential contribution of rapid (within hours) susceptibility testing offered by commercial automated systems has been difficult to document. As described previously, few studies have addressed this issue, and of those, only one has demonstrated an effect on outcome as measured by mortality. Given the methodologic and ethical issues involved in completing such a prospective study, the contribution of rapid susceptibility testing to outcomes as measured by mortality or morbidity may have to be accepted by inference. As noted in the studies cited here, however, the potential contribution of faster susceptibility testing in certain environments using other types of outcomes measures has been well demonstrated (e.g., reducing the cost of hospitalization), facilitating faster switching or focusing of antibiotic therapy as the most effective and/or least expensive alternative antimicrobial. The former is of great importance in the current cost-conscious health care environment in this country, and the latter not only contributes to cost savings but also can play a role in reducing the prevalence of resistant isolates in a facility and preventing the emergence of specific nosocomial pathogens, such as vancomycin-resistant enterococcci (VRE) or *Clostridium difficile*.

Although there appears to be a valid case for the benefit of automated susceptibility systems in certain environments, as determined by the laboratory director in cooperation with the medical staff, it should be remembered that these systems, similar to all systems, are not infallible and do have weaknesses. In addition to the expense associated with purchase of the systems and their supplies, the automated systems may have difficulty in producing accurate results for specific antimicrobial–pathogen combinations. Difficulties may be specific to a given system or, more frequently, common to many of the automated systems. Tenover (2006) reported that the Phoenix system, the Microscan system, and Vitek 2 all had difficulty in detecting carbapenem resistance in *Klebsiella pneumoniae* isolates, although the Phoenix and Microscan performed better than the Vitek 2 in this study. Similarly, Wiegand and colleagues (2007) compared the ability of these systems to detect extended-spectrum β-lactamase (ESBL) production in species of Enterobacteriaceae and found that issues existed for all systems, but of a slightly different nature. The Phoenix system had a high sensitivity (99%) but with lower specificity (52%), while the systems with a higher specificity of 78% (Vitek 2) had a lower sensitivity (86%). All systems showed variability in performance depending on the species of Enterobacteriaceae being tested. Despite shortcomings, these systems may have an important role in antimicrobial susceptibility testing in some laboratories, especially those with high volume, as long as the laboratory director is familiar with the weaknesses of a given system and compensates for them through additional testing methods.

Molecular-Based Testing for Antimicrobial Susceptibility

Molecular-based methods (e.g., nucleic-acid amplification [NAA]) have been found to have applicability in the detection and identification of a number of pathogens in the clinical laboratory. Low detection limits, quick speed of performance of the test (hours in many cases), and the ease with which the tests are adapted to high-volume testing have made them particularly useful in situations where the pathogen in question is a slow grower, like *Mycobacterium tuberculosis* complex (MTBC), or where speed of detection is of great help in managing the patient, as when enterovirus is identified in the cerebrospinal fluid (CSF) of a child who presents with meningoencephalitis. It is not difficult to see how the ability to identify a pathogen and to determine the antimicrobials to which the organism is resistant in a matter of hours using molecular-based methods could be helpful in patient management.

The use of NAA and other molecular-based methods in attempting to detect the presence of antimicrobial resistance in an organism is rather more complicated than identification, for a number of reasons. First, although identification can be accomplished by amplifying and detecting a particular species-specific segment of genome, resistance to a particular antimicrobial may be due to a variety of mechanisms; therefore testing for a number of genes may be required to exclude the potential for resistance. Second, the presence of the target segment of nucleic acid, which may be a gene, a segment near a particular gene, or a portion of the gene, does not necessarily imply that the gene is being expressed and is manifesting as the phenotypic expression of drug resistance.

Fewer mechanisms for antimicrobial resistance exist in gram-positive organisms, and in some cases, resistance to a particular drug is almost wholly due to the expression of a single gene. This has made the group more amenable for the initial development and deployment of molecular tests to detect antimicrobial resistance. Molecular tests to detect oxacillin resistance in *Staphylococcus aureus* that are commercially available are the best example. In the United States, two assays using the real-time polymerase chain reaction (PCR) method—the StaphSR (BD GeneOhm, San Diego) and the Xpert MRSA (Cepheid, Sunnyvale, Calif.)—have been in use for a number of years to screen patients for colonization with methicillin-resistant *Staphylococcus aureus* (MRSA). Both assays have been evaluated recently in the literature for the detection of MRSA in blood cultures, the rapid identification of which directly from blood culture bottles would allow more appropriate utilization of antibiotics up to 48 hours sooner than without the molecular test; both performed well. The StaphSR showed sensitivity and specificity of 95.6% and 95.3%, respectively, in detecting MRSA from spiked blood culture bottles in one study, and sensitivity and specificity of 100% and 98.4%, respectively, in a second study using positive blood cultures from patients (Stamper, 2007a; Grobner, 2009). The Xpert MRSA showed sensitivity and specificity of 98.3% and 99.4%, respectively, from blood cultures (Wolk, 2009). These studies illustrated some of the issues associated with molecular testing for antibiotic resistance (e.g., whether identification of a specific but very focused genomic segment correlates with a particular species or resistance phenotype). In particular, false-positive results were noted from revertant MRSA isolates that had residual SCC*mec* extremity fragments but without functional *mecA* genes (Grobner, 2009), as well as from a specimen with a mixture of a methicillin-resistant coagulase-negative *Staphylococcus* and an SCC*mec* empty cassette variant (Wolk, 2009). The issue of specificity for a particular gene has been particularly well illustrated with the VanR assay (BD GeneOhm), an amplification test that detects the presence of the *Van A* and *Van B* genes associated with glycopeptide resistance in *Enterococcus* species. This assay is intended to allow screening of patients for VRE colonization. It is very effective for its intended purpose when screening in facilities with a high prevalence of VRE due to isolates with the *Van A* gene, but it suffers from specificity issues in situations where *Van B* is highly prevalent because of the apparent ability of other species, such as *Clostridium* spp., to acquire the gene (Stamper, 2007b).

Development of the multiplex-PCR method, an innovation allowing concurrent amplification of multiple nucleic acid segments using multiple primers, is central to the performance of assays like the StaphSR, which targets several nucleic acid segments, and is particularly necessary for any attempt to assess resistance in gram-negative organisms. Relative to gram-positive bacteria, antimicrobial resistance in gram-negative bacteria is complex, as resistance to a given drug may be due to alterations in the structure or quantity of porins that allow drug entry into the cell, efflux pumps, or enzymes that inactivate the drug, or it may be due to modifications of the target of the drug. This variety in drug resistance mechanisms had impaired the development of rapid tests based on molecular methods that detect antimicrobial resistance in gram-negative organisms, and it limited widespread availability of these tests to laboratories. However, by using multiplex PCR to target multiple sites, by focusing on specific resistance mechanisms that can be difficult to assess by classical phenotypic methods, and by analyzing using a convenient DNA microarray detection system, some investigators have shown that molecular diagnostic methods have the potential to improve resistance detection for gram-negative organisms. Zhu and colleagues (2007) used these techniques to determine whether any of 10 different ESBL and *AmpC* β-lactamase genes were present in clinical isolates of Enterobacteriaceae. Their assay showed "complete agreement with complementary sequencing results" and >95% correlation with phenotypic susceptibility testing for isolates of *K. pneumoniae* and *Escherichia coli*, although the authors noted that correlation of the phenotypic assays and the molecular assay was not as good for *Enterobacter cloacae* isolates that possessed the chromosomal *AmpC* gene. Additionally, four *K. pneumoniae* isolates that demonstrated ESBL genes through the assay were "susceptible to all the antibiotics tested," again illustrating occasional disagreement between detection of a gene for a resistance mechanism and results obtained by phenotypic testing.

Along with variability in mechanisms of resistance, geographic variation in prevalence may affect the performance of a molecular-based test for susceptibility testing. The ESBL screen described by Zhu (2007) may well perform more poorly in another locale if ESBL enzymes that exist in that locale are different. An analogous situation has been suggested in some studies on commercially available molecular tests for resistance in MTBC. A few such commercial, standardized tests exist, including the Genotype MTBDRplus assay (Hain LifeScience, Nehren, Germany), an assay based on multiplex PCR with detection by reverse hybridization on nitrocellulose strips. The assay predicts resistance to rifampin by detecting mutations in the *rpoB* gene, and resistance to isoniazid by detecting mutations in regions of *katG* and *inhA* genes. Sensitivity for detecting resistance to rifampin has been uniformly high in published studies (range, 95%–98%), and sensitivity for detecting resistance to isoniazid has had a wider range (range, 73%–97%) (Hillemann, 2007; Lacoma, 2008; Huang, 2009; Nikolayevskyy, 2009). Although most (approximately 95%) rifampin resistance is due to mutations in a few codons of the *rpoB* gene, greater variability in possible sites for mutation have led to isoniazid resistance. Although the most common mutation imparting isoniazid resistance is found at codon 315 of the *katG* gene, mutations in the *inhA*, *aphC-oxyR* intergenic region and others may be responsible (Hillemann, 2007). Several authors have pointed out that the wide variation in sensitivity for detection of isoniazid resistance by this assay is attributable to geographic variation in the incidence of specific genetic mutations (Huang, 2009; Nikolayevskyy, 2009).

The use of molecular techniques to detect the presence of possible antimicrobial resistance is an important innovation that has begun to be investigated in the past several years, in some cases leading to standardized, commercially available tests for use by clinical laboratories. This innovation is still in its formative stages, as clinical microbiologists are learning the abilities and limitations of the highly specific but as yet incompletely understood techniques. Additionally, use of these tests may require reorientation in thinking on the part of some physicians, in that test results show detection of resistance rather than an indication of susceptibility. The rapidity of the tests may provide useful epidemiologic infection control and, in some specific cases, patients, or locales, may reveal information that will aid in patient management; however, until the full implications of detecting or not detecting a specific gene using a particular molecular technique are fully understood, these tests will serve in a supporting role to phenotypic antimicrobial susceptibility testing in most clinical laboratories.

Indications for Susceptibility Testing

Whether antimicrobial susceptibility testing on a particular isolate is necessary varies with the infecting species. If the susceptibility of an aerobic or facultatively anaerobic bacterial species to a particular antimicrobial is unpredictable, then testing is necessary. If the susceptibility profile is predictable, it is not necessary, in most cases, to do testing on an isolate. For example, resistance to penicillin in *Streptococcus pyogenes* has not been reported in the United States, so it is appropriate to treat a patient with *S. pyogenes* pharyngitis without susceptibility testing. However, if a patient is allergic to, or cannot take, the primary choice of antibiotic to treat an infection that caused a particular pathogen, or if, for another reason, the susceptibility profile of the alternative choice antibiotic is unpredictable, testing must be done. If the patient in the previous example were allergic to penicillin, and the physician wished to treat the patient with a macrolide, such as azithromycin, susceptibility testing of the isolate against macrolides should be done because a high proportion of *S. pyogenes* isolates have tested resistant to macrolides for a number of years (Jacobs, 2003). It must also be remembered that testing should be limited to those isolates that are definite pathogens, because testing of isolates that are "contaminants" or "normal flora" is expensive and time consuming and may lead to unnecessary administration of antibiotics (Bates, 1991); therefore it should be avoided. With increasing numbers of severely immunocompromised patients, however, species generally considered to be normal flora or contaminants may be pathogenic, and in these patients susceptibility testing against these species may be warranted. Close consultation with infectious disease physicians is necessary in these cases.

Several years ago, antibiotic therapy for infection caused by anaerobes was often empirical, because the susceptibility profiles of these pathogens were thought to be relatively predictable, susceptibility testing was not standardized, and only limited proof suggested that susceptibility testing correlated with outcome. In recent years, however, it has been demonstrated that the susceptibility patterns of many anaerobic pathogens are changing, and that at least for some species, in vitro antibiotic susceptibility testing correlates with clinical outcome. This is particularly true of *Bacteroides fragilis* and closely related species (Nguyen, 2000; Snydman, 2002). *B. fragilis*, the most frequently isolated species from infections, has the greatest number of antimicrobial resistance mechanisms, as well as the highest rates of antimicrobial resistance, among anaerobic bacterial pathogens (Wexler, 2007). The CLSI recommends testing of anaerobic isolates from specific types of infections, including brain abscess, endocarditis, osteomyelitis, joint infection, infection of prosthetic or vascular devices, and bacteremia (Clinical and Laboratory Standards Institute, 2007). Additionally, certain species that have a high incidence of resistance or are highly virulent warrant testing, including species of *Bacteroides*, *Prevotella*, *Fusobacterium*, *Clostridium*, *Bilophila*, and *Sutterella*. Currently, the only CLSI-recommended susceptibility testing method for anaerobes is the agar dilution method (Clinical and Laboratory Standards Institute, 2007). The exception is the *B. fragilis* group, for which broth microdilution can be performed (Clinical and Laboratory Standards Institute, 2007). Laboratories that do not have the capability to perform agar dilution testing may wish to perform broth microdilution testing on *B. fragilis* isolates that require testing, and may refer other species to a reference laboratory with agar dilution testing capabilities. For other isolates not already discussed, batch susceptibility testing of archived isolates of anaerobes can be performed, either locally or by a reference laboratory, on a periodic basis (recommended annually by the CLSI) in a surveillance protocol to detect local changes in resistance patterns.

Unlike anaerobes, all initial isolates from newly diagnosed cases of tuberculosis should be tested for susceptibility to primary antituberculous drugs; if clinical evidence reveals therapeutic failure or failure of cultures to convert to negative after 3 months, testing should be repeated (National Committee for Clinical Laboratory Standards, 2003). Testing of initial isolates is crucial, because it has been demonstrated that treatment of a patient with a regimen of antitubercular medications without initial susceptibility can lead to significant consequences if the initial isolate is drug resistant. The incidence of treatment failure and relapse and the development of further drug resistance increase significantly if the treatment regimen in these patients is not based on susceptibility testing results of the initial isolate (Lew, 2008). Guidelines exist for testing of some slow-growing nontuberculous mycobacteria (*Mycobacterium avium* complex, *Mycobacterium kansasii*, *Mycobacterium marinum*) and rapidly growing mycobacteria (*Mycobacterium fortuitum* group, *Mycobacterium chelonae*, *Mycobacterium abscessus*, *Mycobacterium mucogenicum*, *Mycobacterium smegmatis* group). Similarly, recommendations have been put forth for susceptibility testing of the aerobic actinomycetes (*Nocardia* spp., *Actinomadura* spp., *Rhodococcus* spp., *Gordona* spp., *Tsukamurella* spp., *Streptomyces* spp.). In general, testing of nontuberculous mycobacteria and of aerobic actinomycetes involves variations in the broth dilution method, and commercial systems can be used for a few species. Because the drugs tested and the methods of testing vary with the species, CLSI document M24-A (National Committee for Clinical Laboratory Standards, 2003) should be consulted for details. It should be emphasized that some of these species can exist as transient colonizers of the respiratory tract, or they may be recovered as contaminants, so adherence to criteria to assess clinical significance prior to susceptibility testing, as outlined in CLSI document M24-A, is strongly recommended.

Similarly, both yeasts and moulds may exist as transient colonizers or contaminants; however, with the increase in the number of immunocompromised patients over the past several decades, the prevalence of fungal infection has increased. Additionally, many new antifungal agents have become available, and resistance to these as well as to the older agents has been described. For *Candida* spp., good correlation between in vitro antifungal resistance and treatment failure has been demonstrated in patients with acquired immunodeficiency syndrome who have oropharyngeal and esophageal candidiasis (Kanafani, 2008). Susceptibility testing by both broth dilution and disk diffusion methods has been standardized for yeasts, excluding the yeast phases of dimorphic fungi such as *Blastomyces dermatitidis*, and breakpoints against a variety of antifungals for *Candida* spp. have been established (National Committee for Clinical Laboratory Standards, 2004; Clinical and Laboratory Standards Institute, 2008, 2008b, 2008c). In recent updates, interpretive guidelines for additional antifungal agents have been added, and the relevant CLSI documents should be consulted (Clinical and Laboratory Standards Institute 2008b). With moulds, the situation involving susceptibility testing is more complex; although procedures for both broth dilution and disk diffusion have been standardized and published by the CLSI (Clinical and Laboratory Standards Institute, 2008d, 2009d), in vitro susceptibility alone has not been shown to predict therapeutic success or failure in clinical trials (Kanafani, 2008).

Many factors, including whether the patient is immunosuppressed, the burden of fungal organisms when treatment is started, the site of infection, and the patient's underlying disease, to name several, are involved in determining whether antifungal therapy will be successful in a patient with a systemic mould infection (Kanafani, 2008). Further, clinical breakpoints have not been established for antifungals and moulds. However, by using epidemiologic cutoff values (ECVs), which have been established for some antifungals, laboratories can detect isolates that show reduced susceptibility to an antifungal relative to "wild-type" isolates, or isolates with no acquired phenotypically detectable resistance. It is important to consider, however, that ECVs are not clinical breakpoints, and an isolate may respond to therapy despite having an MIC above the ECV. An infectious disease specialist may consider this information helpful in his/her management of a patient with systemic mould infection, however, particularly if he or she is able to compare susceptibility results versus a cohort of the same species tested at the same institution as the patient (i.e., if there is a local antibiogram of the particular species). Currently, the CLSI recommends determining MIC values on mould species to use as an aid in managing invasive infection when the utility of antifungal therapy is uncertain, or to establish antibiograms at a particular institution (Clinical and Laboratory Standards Institute, 2009d).

Selection of Antibiotics for Testing and Important Resistance Phenotypes

Selection of antimicrobial agents for testing is complicated by the expanding spectrum and number of antibiotics available and by the growing list of resistance phenotypes that are being identified in pathogenic bacteria. Testing of all agents available in an institution's formulary is neither practical nor warranted. The antimicrobial testing menu should be established in consultation with the medical staff, infectious disease specialists at the institution, and the Pharmacy and Therapeutics Committee, so that the therapeutic needs of the patient population can be best coordinated with the practical limitations of the institution, the pharmacy, and the clinical laboratory. This coordination is important for a variety of reasons. First, many laboratories utilize commercial automated testing systems for susceptibility testing. Manufacturers offer a variety of preconfigured antibiotic testing panels in systems designed to correspond to hospital formularies; however, disparities between the preconfigured panel and the hospital formulary often exist. The laboratory may be faced with an added expense of modifying a preconfigured panel, or of adding testing methods to the laboratory to accommodate testing of additional agents. Second, it is not usually necessary to report susceptibility testing results for multiple representatives of the same spectrum class (e.g., cefotaxime, ceftizoxime, ceftriaxone), in that results derived by testing a representative drug of the class can sometimes be generalized to all representatives of the class. Discussion and coordination with medical staff and infectious disease specialists relative to which antibiotics are necessary to allow caregivers at the institution to manage their patients may save the laboratory these added expenses.

The yearly CLSI informational supplement (Clinical and Laboratory Standards Institute, 2009) lists in a table antimicrobial agents that are recommended for testing for high prevalence and important nonfastidious pathogens, including Enterobacteriaceae, *Pseudomonas aeruginosa*, *Staphylococcus* spp., *Enterococcus* spp., *Acinetobacter* spp., *Burkholderia cepacia*, and *Stenotrophomonas maltophilia*. A separate table lists recommended antibiotics for more fastidious pathogens such as *Haemophilus* spp., *Neisseria gonorrhoeae*, *Streptococcus pneumoniae*, *Streptococcus* β-hemolytic spp., and *Streptococcus* viridans group spp. The antibiotics are listed in four groups, with group A containing drugs recommended for testing and reporting on all isolates, and with group B containing agents suggested for testing against all isolates but reported only under certain circumstances (e.g., when the isolate is resistant to drugs in Group A). Group C lists antibiotics that are considered supplemental and could be used in facilities that have a high prevalence of highly resistant isolates, when unusual pathogens are isolated, or by infection control practitioners as epidemiologic tools. Finally, group U lists antimicrobials that should be tested and reported only on isolates from urine.

Within each group—A, B, C, or U—more antibiotics are listed than need be tested or reported. Within boxes in the tables, drugs that usually have similar interpretive results and clinical efficacy are grouped together, and if an agent is listed with another agent separated by "or," this implies almost identical cross-resistance or susceptibility between drugs; the results of testing one drug will predict the susceptibility result for the other. In the absence of the "or," even though the antibiotics listed in the same box have similar clinical efficiency and similar interpretive results, stringent statistical criteria for comparable testing results were not met when a large number of isolates were tested with the antibiotics in question, or the data were not available, so equivalence for testing results cannot be confidently inferred. For example, for Enterobacteriaceae in Table 1 (Clinical and Laboratory Standards Institute, 2009), the two cephalosporins, cephalothin and cefazolin, are listed in group A in the same box but are not separated by an "or." A footnote to the table notes that testing of cephalothin will predict the susceptibility profile of many other first-generation cephalosporins. Some first-generation cephalosporins must be tested separately, however, because an isolate may be susceptible to the drug despite being resistant to cephalothin. In contrast, in group B, the third-generation cephalosporins cefotaxime and ceftriaxone are separated by an "or," indicating that their susceptibility profiles are virtually interchangeable, and that only one of the two needs to be tested if the isolate is a member of Enterobacteriaceae.

The cephalosporins have been an important mainstay of therapy for gram-negative and gram-positive organisms; therefore, resistance mechanisms developed by these groups have been of great interest, and developments in or discovery of resistance phenotypes to the β-lactams have stimulated many changes in susceptibility testing in recent years. Although this is not the only method by which bacteria become resistant to β-lactams, particularly gram-positive bacteria, β-lactamases have been a topic of high interest in recent years because of the development of new resistance phenotypes mediated by these enzymes. *Staphylococcus* spp. and *Enterococcus* spp. are two major gram-positive pathogens for which β-lactamase testing is a matter of interest, and the CLSI recommends that penicillin should be tested against isolates. Among *Staphylococcus* spp., these enzymes are highly prevalent and are inducible rather than constitutive, that is, the isolate must be exposed to a β-lactam drug before it can phenotypically demonstrate its production. Penicillin therapy may be considered for members of this genus (for some species, this depends on the results of testing for methicillin-resistance [see later]); the CLSI M-100 document details a procedure for testing of inducible β-lactamase using a nitrocefin-based test. Use of the nitrocefin-based test is also recommended for *Enterococcus* spp., as MIC methods will not reliably detect production of the enzyme in these isolates. Although the enzyme is produced constitutively in enterococci, its expression shows an inoculum effect, and greater quantities of bacteria are needed to demonstrate its expression in disk diffusion or broth dilution (Murray, 1990).

Note that testing of ampicillin is also recommended for testing against *Enterococcus* spp., and that although the ampicillin susceptibility profile will predict the profile of penicillin, the reverse is not true (Clinical and Laboratory Standards Institute, 2009). Resistance to ampicillin in *Enterococcus* spp. is mediated by alterations in the enzymes involved in peptidoglycan synthesis, the penicillin-binding proteins (PBPs), so testing for β-lactamase production in this genus will not predict ampicillin susceptibility. The same is true for methicillin (or oxacillin) resistance in *Staphylococcus aureus* (MRSA) and coagulase-negative *Staphylococcus* spp. (CNS). These isolates are resistant to all currently available β-lactam antimicrobials (and β-lactam–β-lactamase inhibitor combinations), hence their detection is crucial for therapeutic management. Most commonly, oxacillin resistance in *Staphylococcus* spp. is due to production of an altered PBP (PBP 2a) product of the *mecA* gene, which may be expressed homogeneously or heterogeneously. Although isolates that express the gene homogeneously can be relatively easily detected, those that express it heterogeneously may be more problematic, and they may appear phenotypically sensitive by dilution testing using oxacillin (Sakoulas, 2001; Swenson, 2001; Felten, 2002).

When a dilution technique is used, sensitivity for detecting these heteroresistant strains can be improved by adding NaCL (2% weight/volume to the medium (Clinical and Laboratory Standards Institute, 2009c). Cefoxitin, in dilution tests or in the disk diffusion test, can be used to screen staphylococci for *mecA*-mediated resistance, and has been shown to be equivalent in sensitivity and specificity to dilution methods using oxacillin for *S. aureus* and superior to dilution testing for CNS (Clinical and Laboratory Standards Institute, 2009c). This high performance level extends to the automated susceptibility systems, which have incorporated cefoxitin MIC testing for *Staphylococcus aureus* into their testing and expert systems, with studies showing close to 100% agreement on detection of MRSA compared with reference methods such as *mecA* gene detection (Junkins, 2009; Kaase, 2009). Additionally, because no disk diffusion zone diameters are known for oxacillin for CNS, the cefoxitin disk test provides a convenient and simple method of screening for oxacillin resistance in this group. Cefoxitin dilution testing can be used for *S. aureus*, but not for CNS, to predict *mecA*-mediated β-lactam resistance. However, tests that detect the *mecA* gene or PBP 2a itself are considered the most accurate of the available tests (Clinical and Laboratory Standards Institute, 2009c). Tests used to detect the *mecA* gene were discussed in the section on molecular-based tests and will not be discussed further here. With respect to detection of PBP 2a, several tests based on a latex agglutination format (MRSA-Screen, Denka Seiken Co., Tokyo, Japan; Oxoid PBP2′ latex agglutination test, Oxoid, Basingstoke, United Kingdom) have been approved for use in *S. aureus* colonies growing on agar and can be used to separate MRSA from methicillin-sensitive isolates. Studies have shown sensitivities of 98.5%–100% with specificity of 100% for detecting MRSA (Louie, 2000; Arbique, 2001; Sakoulas, 2001). The MRSA-Screen is not approved for detection of methicillin resistance in CNS; the Oxoid PBP2′ latex agglutination test can be used for this purpose, although literature is not available to assess its performance in this role.

MRSA and methicillin-resistant CNS have become significant problems in hospital environments, with MRSA accounting for 59.5% of *S. aureus* and methicillin-resistant CNS 89.1% of CNS isolates in intensive care environments (NNIS, 2004); the increased prevalence of community-acquired MRSA has further increased the importance of detection of methicillin resistance in these species. The situation with *Streptococcus pneumoniae* is similar, with alterations in PBPs leading to resistance to penicillin and cephalosporins. The longitudinal PROTEKT surveillance study showed that although the incidence of high-level (MIC ≥2 μg/mL) penicillin resistance decreased from 26.5% to 16.5%, the level of intermediate resistance (MIC 0.12–1 μg/mL) increased from 12.5% to 20% over the period of the report (2001–2004) (Jenkins, 2008). The incidence of multidrug resistance (resistance to penicillin and two other antibiotics) remained at about 30% over this period.

Susceptibility testing of this pathogen is mandatory when isolated from sterile sites. The oxacillin screen disk diffusion method can be used, with isolates having a zone of inhibition ≥20 mm, indicating that the isolate is susceptible to penicillin and to other β-lactams listed in M100 (Clinical and Laboratory Standards Institute, 2009). This applies only to nonmeningitis isolates, as MIC testing is recommended for isolates from this source. Further, zone sizes <19 mm on the oxacillin screen require additional testing using an MIC method because a zone of inhibition of this size may be seen with isolates that are resistant, susceptible, or intermediate to penicillin; therefore, it may be most effective to proceed directly to MIC testing when an isolate is obtained from a source (meningitis, blood) for which a delay in susceptibility testing may be potentially dangerous. It should be noted that interpretive standards for penicillin and the third-generation cephalosporins differ, depending on whether the isolate is a CSF isolate or not; the CLSI recommends that both interpretations be reported unless the isolate is obtained from the CSF, in which case only the meningitis interpretive category is reported. Testing methods are determined by the antibiotics tested for *S. pneumoniae*, as disk diffusion cannot be performed for drugs such as ampicillin, cefotaxime, ceftriaxone, imipenem, and meropenem, to name several (Clinical and Laboratory Standards Institute, 2009c). The commercial automated systems—Phoenix (Becton Dickinson Diagnostic Systems, Sparks, Md.) and Vitek 2 (bioMerieux)—offer antibiotic testing panels for *S. pneumoniae*; their performance has been favorable in published studies (Ligozzi 2002; Richter, 2007).

Most penicillin resistance in enterococci, usually seen in *Enterococcus faecium*, is due to the production of low-affinity PBPs (Clinical and Laboratory Standards Institute, 2009c), although in some cases, β-lactamase production is the cause of the resistance. This is important to note, in that dilution procedures will not detect β-lactamase production, which is the reason why the CLSI recommends testing isolates, particularly those from blood or CSF, with the nitrocefin β-lactamase test (Clinical and Laboratory Standards Institute, 2009c). Penicillin or ampicillin resistance is of importance in enterococci, as a synergistic action of penicillin or ampicillin with aminoglycosides is often effective therapy for serious infection. This synergistic effect can occur even when the penicillin or ampicillin MIC is at a high level, above the resistant interpretive category (Clinical and Laboratory Standards Institute, 2009c). Aminoglycosides are clinically ineffective against enterococci by themselves, and susceptibility testing is performed only for the possible synergistic effect when combined with penicillin, ampicillin, or a glycopeptide. Testing is performed only with high concentrations of the aminoglycoside, 500 µg/mL gentamicin, or 1000 µg/mL of streptomycin, using broth dilution. Enterococci causing serious infection require testing against penicillin or ampicillin, high-level aminoglycoside screening, and testing for susceptibility to a glycopeptide, which is usually vancomycin in the United States.

Glycopeptide resistance in enterococci is produced by the production of altered pentapeptide peptidoglycan precursors, which results in a greatly reduced affinity for binding of vancomycin by 1000-fold. Binding of vancomycin to the pentapeptide prevents cross-linking with other precursors, resulting in prevention of the production of a stable cell wall. Altered precursors are the result of specific genes, of which the two most relevant are *Van A* and *Van B*, and isolates that demonstrate resistance to vancomycin are VRE, of which most are *E. faecium*, although *E. faecalis* may also be included as VRE. Isolates with *Van A* or *Van B* will demonstrate high-level vancomycin resistance, and a third gene, *Van C*, which is usually found in *E. casseliflavus* or *E. gallinarum*, will cause a low level of vancomycin resistance, the clinical significance of which is unknown. Screening for VRE can be done using agar or broth dilution or a screening agar consisting of brain heart infusion with 6 µg/mL of vancomycin. During testing, it is important that the previously mentioned testing systems be incubated for a full 24 hours, because reading at 16–20 hours may produce an erroneous result (Clinical and Laboratory Standards Institute, 2009c). Modern commercial test systems have performed well in detecting VRE, with all isolates with the VRE phenotype detected by the Phoenix (BD Diagnostic Systems) and the Vitek 2 (bioMerieux) in published studies (Ligozzi, 2002; Fahr, 2003; Abele-Horn, 2006; Carroll, 2006).

Vancomycin susceptibility testing of *S. aureus* has become an important concern for clinical microbiology laboratories since the detection of isolates with reduced susceptibility to the drug (i.e., vancomycin-intermediate *Staphylococcus aureus* [VISA] with MIC values of 4–16 µg/mL, and vancomycin-resistant *Staphylococcus aureus* [VRSA] with MIC >32 µg/mL). Although the mechanism of resistance in VRSA isolates appears to be linked to acquired *Van A* (Centers for Disease Control and Prevention, 2002, 2004), the mechanism associated with elevated MIC values in VISA is not completely understood, but appears to be linked to increased cell wall thickness and vancomycin-binding peptides (Cui, 2000). Detection of these isolates is important because most are also MRSA, and vancomycin is often used to treat these β-lactam–resistant organisms. VRSA isolates, which are very rare, can be reliably identified by microbroth dilution, disk diffusion, or vancomycin screening agar Brain-heart infusion agar with 6 µg/mL vancomycin), as long as the test systems are incubated a full 24 hours at 35° C ± 2° C (Clinical and Laboratory Standards Institute, 2009c). For VISA, however, the issue is more problematic because disk diffusion is not an effective screening method, and the vancomycin screening agar is not reliable for isolates that have MIC values on the lower end of the spectrum (e.g., 4–8 µg/mL) (Clinical and Laboratory Standards Institute, 2009c; Swenson, 2009).

Commercial automated and nonautomated systems similarly have difficulty detecting VISA with MIC values near the low end of the intermediate resistance spectrum, and these systems all have their own peculiarities with respect to testing of these isolates; laboratories should be aware of these peculiarities if consideration is given to using a given system (Swenson, 2009). It is interesting to note that in the study by Swenson (2009), the testing method that was most reliable for detecting VISA, that is, manual microbroth dilution, had difficulty with VISA isolates with MIC values on the low end of the intermediate resistance spectrum. The issue of VISA is further complicated by the existence of so-called vancomycin heteroresistant *S. aureus* (hVISA) isolates, which are isolates that contain subpopulations of organisms with MIC values of 8–16 µg/mL. Much like VRSA and VISA, hVISA appears to be associated with treatment failure when vancomycin is used (Tenover, 2007). Additionally, although VRSA and VISA isolates are infrequent, studies have suggested that hVISA isolates are not rare and may account for up to 18% of isolates in some geographic locations (Tenover, 2007). Unfortunately, no current susceptibility testing method is reliable for detecting hVISA. In an effort to aid in detecting hVISA, particularly among strains with MIC values >2 µg/mL, when data indicating that some hVISA strains will have MIC values in the 0.5–4 µg/mL range were used, the CLSI lowered the interpretive breakpoints for *S. aureus* and vancomycin, with susceptibility decreasing to ≤2 µg/mL; intermediate decreased to 4–8 µg/mL, and resistant decreased to ≥16 µg/mL (Tenover, 2007). Not all hVISA strains will be detected using this strategy, however, and additional advancements in susceptibility testing methods are needed to address this issue.

For streptococci other than *S. pneumoniae* or enterococci, antimicrobials to be tested and reported depend on the species. For example, for *Streptococcus pyogenes* (Lancefield group A), susceptibility testing for penicillin and other β-lactams and vancomycin is not necessary because resistant strains have not been reported (Clinical and Laboratory Standards Institute, 2009). If the patient is penicillin allergic and consideration is given to treatment with a macrolide, testing is necessary, and results obtained with erythromycin may be generalized to azithromycin, clarithromycin, and dirithromycin (Clinical and Laboratory Standards Institute, 2009). Similarly, current recommendations are that β-lactam susceptibility testing for *S. agalactaie* (Lancefield group B) is not necessary; however, recent literature has reported the occurrence of isolates with MIC values above the breakpoints for susceptibility for penicillin and cephalosporins from the Far East and from the United States (Dahesh, 2008; Kimura, 2008). Altered PBPs, similar to those found in *S. pneumoniae*, were identified by molecular studies. Additional studies are necessary to determine the implications, both clinically and with respect to laboratory testing, before the clinical relevance of these reports is known.

It is also recommended that for pregnant women who are colonized with group B streptococci and who are allergic to penicillin, testing for clindamycin and erythromycin should be carried out (Clinical and Laboratory Standards Institute, 2009). Isolates that are resistant to erythromycin but susceptible to clindamycin should be tested for "inducible" resistance to clindamycin mediated by the *erm* gene (MLS_B resistance: macrolide, lincosamide, streptogramin B) using the **D-zone approximation test,** with closely approximated diffusion disks of both clindamycin and erythromycin (Clinical and Laboratory Standards Institute, 2009) (Fig. 58-3). For staphylococci, a single-well broth microdilution test may also be used (Clinical and Laboratory Standards Institute, 2009c). "Inducible" clindamycin resistance can occur in staphylococci and β-hemolytic streptococci, and prevalence may vary from geographic area to geographic area, as noted in studies determining prevalence in group B streptococci and group A streptococci (Desjardins, 2004; Richter, 2005; Tazi, 2007), or may vary with the origin of the isolate in a given geographic area, such as whether or not a *S. aureus* isolate is hospital or community acquired (Patel, 2006). Some institutions test for inducible clindamycin resistance routinely or in certain situations (Feibelkorn, 2003; Jorgensen, 2004). A possible strategy that can be used to determine and implement the most cost-effective testing strategy for inducible clindamycin resistance in relevant species would be to survey for the prevalence of this type of resistance and, in consultation with infectious disease and/or medical staff, set new testing policies based on these results (Schreckenberger, 2004).

For the viridans streptococci, any isolate derived from a sterile body site and implicated in a serious infection, such as endocarditis or sepsis, should be tested for penicillin or ampicillin susceptibility (Quinn, 1988; Clinical and Laboratory Standards Institute, 2009). Diffusion testing

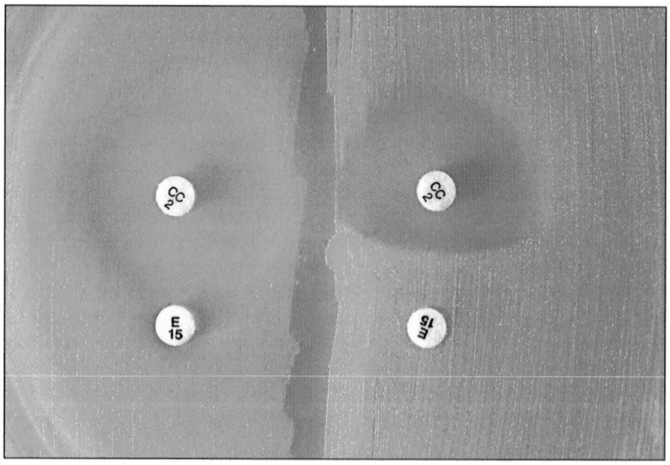

Figure 58-3 Disk induction or "D" test. The *Staphylococcus aureus* isolate on the left demonstrates erythromycin (E) resistance but susceptibility to clindamycin (CC). The *S. aureus* isolate demonstrates inducible clindamycin resistance with blunting of the zone of inhibition around the clindamycin disk adjacent to the erythromycin disk.

interpretive standards for penicillin and ampicillin do not exist for viridans streptococci, as the method is unreliable for this pathogen–antimicrobial combination, so testing is accomplished using an MIC method (Clinical and Laboratory Standards Institute, 2009). Viridans streptococci are important pathogens causing sepsis in patients with neutropenia and native valve endocarditis, and studies have demonstrated increasing rates of resistance to penicillin especially, and also to the cephalosporins (Prabhu, 2004; Gordon, 2002; Han, 2006; Yap, 2006). Fluoroquinolones are often used prophylactically in neutropenic patients, and since the development of fluoroquinolone resistance in viridans streptococci colonizing these patients (Prabhu, 2005) and bloodstream isolates (Han, 2006) was reported, testing of fluoroquinolones in this patient population is indicated despite an overall low prevalence of fluoroquinolone resistance in viridans streptococci in general (Gordon, 2002). This illustrates a situation wherein a specific patient population served by a facility dictates testing and reporting of specific antimicrobials.

Although resistance to the β-lactam antibiotics in gram-positive organisms in many cases involves altered PBPs, in gram-negative organisms, resistance is mediated primarily by the production of β-lactamases. For some gram-negative species, it may be possible to test for β-lactamase production using the chromogenic cephalosporin test. The prevalence of β-lactamase–positive *Haemophilus influenzae* in the United States is approximately 30%, while the prevalence of β-lactamase–negative, ampicillin-resistant (BLNAR) strains, which are not detected by the β-lactamase test, is low (Jacobs, 2003). Geographic variation has been noted, however, and in some areas outside of the United States up to this point, BLNAR strains make up a significant portion of all isolates (Tristam, 2007). For non–life-threatening infection with *H. influenzae*, the nitrocefin test will predict susceptibility to ampicillin and amoxicillin. It may be possible for a laboratory to utilize the nitrocefin test alone in this situation, saving time and money, because susceptibility testing of *Haemophilus* spp. requires specialized media (*Haemophilus* test medium), which have a short shelf life. In areas with a high prevalence of BLNAR, this strategy would not be effective. In the case of life-threatening infection, such as meningitis, the CLSI recommends that susceptibility testing be performed, and that only ampicillin, a third-generation cephalosporin, chloramphenicol, and meropenem should be reported (Clinical and Laboratory Standards Institute, 2009).

In contrast to *H. influenzae*, penicillin resistance in *Neisseria meningitidis* is due primarily to altered PBPs, although occasional isolates with β-lactamase production do occur (Jorgensen, 2005). Both MIC interpretive standards and disk diffusion breakpoints for susceptibility testing of *N. meningitides* have been published in CLSI documents (Clinical and Laboratory Standards Institute, 2009), and the testing method has been standardized and validated (Clinical and Laboratory Standards Institute, 2009c). Although resistance to penicillin has been reported in the United States, resistance to cefotaxime and ceftriaxone, used in the treatment of meningitis or sepsis due to this species, or to sulfonamides and rifampin, which are used for prophylaxis, has not been reported (Jorgensen, 2005), so testing protocols for this particular species may be determined with input from local medical staff or infectious disease specialists. It is important to remember that if testing is undertaken, because of the occurrence of laboratory-acquired meningococcal infection, which has a high fatality rate, appropriate safety precautions, including the use of a biological safety cabinet, must be utilized by testing personnel (Clinical and Laboratory Standards Institute, 2009).

β-Lactam antibiotics are used in high frequency for treatment of infection due to the gram-negative Enterobacteriaceae; this group of bacteria has developed the capacity to produce a wide array of β-lactamase enzymes. One group of high interest consists of the so-called ESBLs, which are plasmid-derived and hence highly transferable enzymes that have evolved through the mutation of older Temoniera (TEM) and sulfhydral reagent variable (SHV) enzymes. Paterson and Bonomo (2005) provide a concise definition of these enzymes as enzymes that produce resistance to penicillins, the first- through third-generation cephalosporins, and aztreonam, but that are susceptible to inhibition by β-lactamase inhibitors and do not hydrolyze the cephamycins. The importance of these enzymes is twofold: First, isolates that have them may appear susceptible by in vitro testing to antimicrobials that they are capable of hydrolyzing; second, there may be a good chance of clinical failure when therapy using one of these antimicrobials is provided, even when MIC values are in the susceptible range (Paterson, 2005). Isolates with ESBLs accounted for approximately 5% of Enterobacteriaceae isolates in one survey study in the United States, with a high predilection for intensive care unit environments and association with prolonged hospital stays, indwelling medical devices, and therapy with antimicrobials of a variety of types (Paterson, 2005; Moland, 2006). In the United States, they are found primarily in *Klebsiella pneumoniae*, *K. oxytoca*, *Escherichia coli*, and *Proteus mirabilis*—species recommended for screening by the CLSI—but they may be found in other species as well, including *Enterobacter* spp., *Citrobacter* spp., *Serratia* spp., and *Salmonella* spp. (Bradford, 2001; Paterson, 2005; Moland, 2006).

CLSI documents provide procedures for screening using disk diffusion or broth microdilution, as well as confirmation utilizing the characteristic that these enzymes are inhibited by β-lactamase inhibitors and by testing susceptibility with and without an inhibitor (Clinical and Laboratory Standards Institute, 2009). It should be remembered that for screening, using the results obtained with more than one antimicrobial improves sensitivity, and confirmation with both cefotaxime and ceftazidime, with and without clavulanic acid, improves specificity (Paterson, 2005; Clinical and Laboratory Standards Institute, 2009). Automated susceptibility systems include tests that can be used to detect ESBLs; however, sensitivity issues for some systems and issues with expert software systems have suggested that manual methods should remain an important part of testing for ESBLs in the clinical microbiology laboratory (Thomson, 2007; Snyder, 2008).

A false-negative on the ESBL phenotypic confirmation test as described by the CLSI may be produced by an organism that is producing another type of β-lactamase that is of high interest—AmpC β-lactamase—in addition to an ESBL. AmpC enzymes exist in two forms, with the first type having the gene located on a chromosome. Among the Enterobacteriaceae, chromosomally mediated AmpC can be found in *Enterobacter* spp., *Citrobacter freundii*, *Serratia marcescens*, and *Escherichia coli*, to name a few; it may also be found in *Pseudomonas* spp. and *Acinetobacter* spp. (Coudron, 2000). Under these conditions, this enzyme is usually inducible, except in *E. coli*, where it is constitutive but is often produced in small amounts. AmpC may be plasmid derived, and in the United States, it is most often found in *K. pneumoniae* and *E. coli*, is usually constitutive, and is of importance, because isolates that produce this enzyme will be resistant to broad-spectrum penicillins, extended-spectrum cephalosporins, monobactams, and, in contrast to ESBLs, the cephamycins such as cefoxitin. Also in contrast to ESBLs, they are not inhibited by commercially available β-lactamase inhibitors (hence the production of a false-negative ESBL confirmation test) (Coudron, 2000).

Similar to ESBL-producing isolates, an AmpC isolate may appear susceptible to one of the aforementioned antimicrobials on testing, but treatment with the antimicrobial may result in treatment failure and, in some cases, mortality (Pai, 2004). Possible screens for the presence of an AmpC β-lactamase–producing isolate include the presence of cefoxitin resistance or a positive ESBL screen but a negative ESBL confirmatory test (Black, 2005). Unfortunately, the screens are nonspecific, cefoxitin resistance may be due to porin loss, and confirmatory tests for the presence of AmpC are problematic. Cefoxitin-resistant non–AmpC β-lactamase–producing isolates can be separated from those producing AmpC β-lactamase by a three-dimensional extract test or an AmpC disk test; however, neither is standardized and both are complex to perform and are not really suitable for routine laboratory use (Coudron, 2000; Hanson, 2003; Black, 2005). A negative ESBL confirmatory test will provide indirect evidence of AmpC β-lactamase (Thomson, 2001), especially if the isolate is resistant to cefoxitin and sensitive to carbapenems and cefepime. However, this is still nonspecific, and a limitation of both the utilization of phenotypic confirmatory tests and inductive reasoning using susceptibility patterns is the increasing number of isolates that have multiple β-lactamases or other resistance mechanisms such as porin loss that can result in similar phenotypic resistance patterns. Currently, no CLSI-approved test is known to detect or confirm AmpC β-lactamase production in an isolate. It has been suggested that revision of interpretive breakpoints for the antimicrobials affected by both ESBLs and AmpC β-lactamases will be necessary and would be the most effective way to deal with these problematic resistance mechanisms (Clinical and Laboratory Standards Institute, 2009c).

Enterobacteriaceae that produce an ESBL or AmpC β-lactamase (or both) may often be treated with a carbapenem, as resistance to this class is not a consequence of the production of either β-lactamase. Unfortunately, several groups of carbapenemase β-lactamases may be acquired by gram-negative bacteria, and the type that is of current interest and importance in the United States with respect to Enterobacteriaceae is a group of serine carbapenemases, the *Klebsiella pneumoniae* carbapenemase (KPC) enzymes. These β-lactamases produce resistance to all β-lactams, including extended-spectrum cephalosporins and carbapenems, although on phenotypic susceptibility testing, the carbapenem MIC may be only elevated and still in the susceptible range, yet treatment of an infection with a carbapenem can result in treatment failure (Weisenberg, 2009). KPC enzymes may be found in a variety of species of Enterobacteriaceae, but in the United States, they currently are most often found in *K. pneumoniae*, and although the overall percentage relative to a large group of tested isolates is not high nationally—less than 1% in one national survey (Deshpande, 2006)—the genes for production of the enzymes are plasmid-borne, and clonal expansion can occur easily. KPC enzymes first appeared in the United States in New York City, and a survey of four hospitals in Brooklyn, N.Y., over 2 months in 2004 demonstrated that 24% of *K. pneumonaie* isolates had one of two KPC genes (Walther-Rasmussen, 2007). A standardized procedure for screening and confirmation of KPC-type carbapenemases in Enterobacteriaceae has been published by the CLSI (Clinical and Laboratory Standards Institute, 2009).

For isolates that are resistant to one or more third-generation cephalosporins, screening with an ertapenem or meropenem disk, or with ertapenem, meropenem, or imipenem broth microdilution, can be done; if the screen is positive, a confirmatory test, the modified Hodge test, can be performed. The modified Hodge test involves streaking an isolate of interest perpendicularly to a centrally placed carbapenem disk (ertapenem or meropenem) on a Mueller-Hinton agar plate that has been streaked with *E. coli* ATCC 25922 in the same manner as a Kirby-Bauer disk diffusion plate (i.e., to produce confluent growth). Enhanced growth of the *E. coli* ATCC 25922 in the zone of inhibition along the streaked test isolate of Enterobacteriaceae indicates that it is producing a carbapenemase that has inhibited the carbapenem along the streak and has allowed the *E. coli* ATCC 25922 indicator organism to grow where it normally would not. It is possible to have false-positive results with the modified Hodge test, for example, if a *K. pneumoniae* isolate is producing an ESBL and has carbapenem resistance due to porin loss, the modified Hodge test may be interpreted as positive. Testing of the isolate with a carbapenem disk with and without boronic acid can differentiate those isolates producing carbapenemases from those with resistance to carbapenems due to other mechanisms (Doi, 2008; Tsakris, 2009). Boronic acid inhibits KPC-carbapenemases, resulting in an increase in the zone of inhibition diameter around the carbapenem–boronic acid disk relative to the carbapenem-only disk.

Detection of carbapenem resistance mediated by carbapenemases by automated systems is problematic, and if one of these systems is used, careful monitoring and repeat testing with careful attention to inoculum size or utilization of a different method is warranted if incongruent or discrepant results are obtained (Tenover, 2006). It is important to remember that if an isolate tests resistant to a carbapenem on routine susceptibility testing, current CLSI guidelines are that the interpretation should be reported, irrespective of whether or not a carbapenemase is subsequently identified , because there are other mechanisms of resistance; the CLSI recommends that in those cases in which a carbapenemase is identified, and some carbapenems test susceptible by current breakpoints, the MIC values should be reported without an interpretation (Clinical and Laboratory Standards Institute, 2009). Some laboratories may wish to report all carbapenems as resistant in this case, and local policy may be established in concert with infectious disease specialist and medical staff consultation.

Carbapenems are an important group of drugs used in the treatment of anaerobe infection, and susceptibility data related to this drug, and the most common anaerobic cause of sepsis, *Bacteroides fragilis* group, are illustrative of one of the important points related to anaerobic bacteria, that is, that their susceptibility profile can vary greatly with geographic area. Survey studies in Europe and the United States demonstrated very low rates of resistance in *B. fragilis* to imipenem and meropenem (≤0.8% and ≤1.3%, respectively), and a survey in Taiwan showed rates of 7% and 12% resistance to imipenem and meropenem, respectively (Soki, 2006; Snydman, 2007; Liu, 2008). Similarly, closely related species or even the same species may have great variance in resistance rates; the CLSI notes ranges for the *B. fragilis* group of 15%–44% for clindamycin, 13%–94% for cefotetan, and 3.5%–41.5% for cefoxitin (Clinical and Laboratory Standards Institute, 2007). Antibiotic resistance is predictable in some species, such as *Bilophila wadsworthia*, and is common in many species, for example, *Prevotella* spp., with 50%–72% of isolates resistant to penicillin, but in general, the antibiotic susceptibility profiles of many anaerobes are unpredictable, variable, and increasing (Clinical and Laboratory Standards Institute, 2007; Wybo, 2007). This fact, in addition to findings of recent studies demonstrating that in vitro susceptibility testing results for anaerobes can have a direct correlation with favorable outcome, as in a study correlating antimicrobial treatment of *Bacteroides* bacteremia with susceptibility results and outcome (Nguyen, 2000), has pointed out the importance of antimicrobial susceptibility testing for anaerobes.

Several caveats must be borne in mind with respect to testing of anaerobic species: First, anaerobic infections can often be polymicrobial, making susceptibility testing difficult and in some cases impractical. Second, agar dilution is the CLSI-approved method for susceptibility testing of anaerobic species, with the exception of the *B. fragilis* group, for which microbroth dilution is also standardized; this is a demanding technique that may be beyond the capabilities of many laboratories. CLSI recommendations are that susceptibility testing should be performed with specific infections caused by anaerobes, and suggested groupings of antibiotics to be tested are recommended (Clinical and Laboratory Standards Institute, 2007). Given that this may be difficult for some laboratories because of the method required, referral to a reference laboratory in specific cases is an option; surveillance testing of collected isolates in a given geographic area or institution to generate an antibiogram on which physicians can base empirical therapy is another option that is within CLSI guidelines and is recommended by a number of authors (Clinical and Laboratory Standards Institute, 2007; Wybo, 2007; Liu, 2008).

For MTBC, all new isolates should be tested for susceptibility to primary antituberculosis drugs (isoniazid at two concentrations [critical and high concentrations], rifampin, ethambutol, and pyrazinamide) (National Committee for Clinical Laboratory Standards, 2003). Additionally, if the patient fails to respond to therapy, or cultures fail to become negative by 3 months after initiation of therapy, testing should be repeated. Testing results must be available as soon as possible, and it is recommended that laboratories provide results within 28 days of receiving the initial specimen (Bird, 1996). Until relatively recently, drug susceptibility to MTBC was determined primarily by the agar proportion method using solid agar, a modified agar dilution method, or with the use of liquid media with the BACTEC 460TB (Becton Dickinson, Sparks, Md). The BACTEC 460 allowed a faster turnaround time over the manual agar proportion method, but the system was only semiautomated and required disposal of radioactive waste from the indicator system. Liquid-based systems that are automated and use nonradioactive indicator systems have been developed, two examples of which are the MB/BacT (Organon-Teknika, Durham, N.C.) and Mycobacteria Growth Indicator Tube 960 (Becton Dickinon). Comparison studies between the proportion method and BACTEC 460 and the new automated systems have demonstrated generally good correlation, and the automated systems have become popular in laboratories in the United States where the cost of the systems is not prohibitive (Bemer, 2002, 2004; Tortoli, 2002; Garrigó, 2007).

Susceptibility testing with antifungal agents is predominantly performed on yeasts in those institutions that perform testing, with CLSI breakpoints available for *Candida* spp. with itraconazole, fluconazole, voriconazole, flucytosine, and the echinocandins (anidulafungin, capsofungin, and micafungin) when using microbroth dilution, and with fluconazole and voriconazole when using disk diffusion (National Committee for Clinical Laboratory Standards, 2004; Clinical and Laboratory Standards Institute, 2008c). Testing options are very limited with disk diffusion, and the reference microbroth dilution method is labor intensive, so many have turned to commercial testing systems such as the Sensititre YeastOne (Trek Diagnostic Systems, Westlake, Ohio), a manual microbroth dilution system with a chromogenic indicator; the Etest (AB Biodisk), or the automated VITEK 2 (bioMerieux), which offers a yeast susceptibility testing card. The Sensititre YeastOne is a comprehensive manual system that offers all drugs for which CLSI breakpoints exist, including the echinocandins. Performance in published evaluation studies has been good, although Alexander (2007) pointed out that both the Sensititre and the Etest had a tendency toward slightly higher MIC values than the reference broth microdilution method. Categorical agreement was good for all *Candida* spp.–antifungal combinations, although it was lower for *C. glabrata* and *C. tropicalis* tested against some of the azoles. Most errors caused by the two systems in the study were of a minor nature. The authors pointed out that incubation times significantly influenced results.

In CLSI document M27-A3 (2008b), specific reading times for individual drugs are given for use in the reference microbroth dilution method. In another study evaluating only the echinocandins against *Candida* spp., the Sensititre was essentially equivalent to the reference microbroth dilution method (Pfaller, 2008). The VITEK 2 yeast susceptibility test has the advantages of being fully automated and giving spectrophotometric readings in 12–15 hours, although the menu of drugs that can be tested is more limited. In published studies, performance of the system using a panel of *Candida* spp. against fluconazole, flucytosine, voriconazole, and amphotericin B was good, with findings similar to those seen in studies evaluating the Sensititre and Etest related to *C. glabrata* (Pfaller, 2007, 2007b).

Selecting Antibiotics to Be Reported

Policies for reporting of antibiotics for isolates should take into account not only the results of testing, but a variety of factors. For example, as outlined in CLSI document M100 (2009), antimicrobials that are not effective for treating CSF infection for a variety of reasons, such as first- or second-generation cephalosporins, macrolides, clindamycin, fluoroquinolones, tetracyclines, or orally administered drugs, should not be reported for isolates from the central nervous system. Similarly, drugs that may test susceptible in vitro but have been shown to be ineffective in vivo for particular species, such as cephalosporins or trimethoprim-sulfamethoxazole for *Enterococcus* spp., also should not be reported (Clinical and Laboratory Standards Institute, 2009). Drugs that are effective only for urinary tract infection (e.g., nitrofurantoin) should not be reported on isolates from any site other the urinary tract. Many institutions utilize **cascade** reporting to encourage the use of antimicrobials that are effective based on in vivo susceptibility testing but are less expensive than the "newest" or most heavily commercially promoted drug, to try to lower pharmacy costs. For example, third-generation cephalosporins will be reported, barring other considerations such as isolate source, only if first- or second-generation cephalosporins are resistant on testing.

A close working relationship between the clinical microbiology laboratory and the infectious disease service is important in effective **antibiotic stewardship** programs that guide an institution's caregivers in the most appropriate use of antibiotics. These programs are instituted to save money or, more important, to combat the increasing problem of antibiotic resistance; they may involve the use of mandatory prescribing and treatment guidelines, reporting or nonreporting of specific antibiotics on susceptibility profiles, and **gatekeeper** providers such as infectious disease physicians, whose approval is required before specific antibiotics can be used. As an example, it has been demonstrated in prospective studies (Project ICARE: Intensive Care Antimicrobial Resistance Epidemiology) that the frequent use of vancomycin and third-generation cephalosporins is associated with increased prevalence of VRE in ICUs, and that by limiting the use of vancomycin, the prevalence can be decreased (Fridkin, 2001, 2002). Similarly, in a multicenter retrospective analysis, Pakyz and colleagues (2009) showed that restricting the use of carbapenems resulted in lower incidences of carbapenem-resistant *Pseudomonas aeruginosa* than were seen in hospitals that did not restrict carbapenem use.

Finally, reports from several centers in different parts of the world have detailed outbreaks of a highly virulent strain of *Clostridium difficile* that produced high morbidity and mortality. These outbreaks have been determined to be associated with the use of specific antibiotics in the facility, particularly fluoroquinolones, to which this particular strain is highly resistant; containment of the outbreaks has required a number of measures, including strict antibiotic stewardship programs that in some cases required the complete prohibition of fluoroquinolone use (Valiquette, 2007; Labbé 2008; Debast, 2009). These examples demonstrate the importance of knowing how and what antibiotics are reported by the laboratory, as well as the importance of the clinical laboratory working closely with the infectious disease service in addressing issues created by patterns of antibiotic use. A multicenter survey of U.S. hospitals showed that the most frequently prescribed antibiotic class from 2002–2006 was the fluoroquinolones, and that carbapenem use was increasing significantly (Pakyz, 2008); these issues are directly relevant to the examples given here and show that the management of antibiotic use in hospitals, including what antibiotics the clinical laboratory is to report, will be a continuing and increasingly complex issue in the coming years.

Cumulative Antimicrobial Susceptibility Reports

Susceptibility patterns for specific species against antimicrobials can vary with geographic locale, type of medical facility, and antibiotic usage patterns, and it is the responsibility of the clinical microbiology laboratory to monitor susceptibility patterns and keep the medical staff informed of current patterns. This is usually accomplished by monitoring susceptibility data on isolates over time, compiling these data for a specific time period, calculating the percentage of a specific species that is susceptible to a given drug, putting all the data into an easily accessible format, and making it available to the medical staff. These reports, usually referred to as antibiograms, can be used by the medical staff to treat infections empirically while awaiting specific culture and susceptibility results, or they can be used by hospital epidemiology and infection control to monitor resistance trends, identify outbreaks, and formulate infection control policy; they may also be referred to by the pharmacy and therapeutics committee of the facility when making policy or formulary decisions (Zapantis, 2005). By including antibiotic cost data in the antibiogram, institutions may encourage providers to utilize less expensive but still effective drugs.

The CLSI provides guidance to facilities on the preparation of antibiograms in CLSI document M39-A3 (2009e) and includes suggestions on use of terminology, obtaining data, analysis of the data, presentation of data, statistical considerations, and specific limitations of the antibiogram. Examples and templates are included in the document. Hindler and Stelling (2007) summarized many of the essential considerations discussed in the CLSI document, and they discussed issues that must be considered and decided upon when compiling an institution's antibiogram. For example, how multiple isolates from a single patient are counted in compiling the data can have a marked effect on the percentage of a specific species that appears susceptible to a given antibiotic. If all isolates are counted, this will bias the result toward isolates that are submitted from patients who have multiple cultures submitted over time (e.g., those patients with infection due to resistant organisms, who remain hospitalized for long periods, or who do not respond to therapy) (Hindler, 2007). Whether duplicate isolates from the same patient are all counted (isolate-based algorithm), are excluded and only the first one counted (patient-based algorithm), are counted only if they represent a new clinical episode (episode-based algorithm), or are counted only if they show a new resistance phenotype (phenotype-based algorithm) directly affects the percentages of susceptibility for an antimicrobial; which algorithm is best for a given institution should be decided upon in consultation with the medical staff and/or the pharmacy and therapeutics committee, then adhered to during subsequent compilations, so comparisons between individual time periods are valid.

The data management associated with antibiograms and the information that can be obtained from these data may be complex and difficult to manage and manipulate. The World Health Organization (WHO) Collaborating Centre for Surveillance of Antimicrobial Resistance has made available a software program that can be downloaded and utilized at no charge to accomplish useful data management (WHO, 2006). The software program (WHONET) has a module that allows a laboratory to input which antimicrobials are reported and what patient care areas are served by the laboratory, and allows alerts for important organisms or phenotypes. A second module permits the entry, retrieval, correction, and printing of clinical reports. Finally, a third module allows a variety of analyses to be generated from the facility data, including but not limited to organism frequencies over time, antimicrobial susceptibility statistics, disk diffusion zone diameter or MIC histograms, antimicrobial scatterplots, and regression curves. Additionally, a software component, BacLink, can be obtained that can upload data from a facility's current system directly into WHONET, avoiding manual entry of data. Both WHONET and BacLink software can be downloaded directly from the Internet at no cost (WHO, 2006). The WHONET software is currently on version 5.6, is being used by laboratories in more than 90 countries worldwide, and is available in 17 languages.

Bactericidal Testing

Bactericidal testing of antimicrobial agents is infrequently performed in the current clinical laboratory environment. Many tests are labor intensive and complicated, and until relatively recently, the procedures were not standardized. The three major categories of bactericidal antimicrobial testing are (1) determination of the minimum concentration of an antimicrobial necessary to kill 99.9% of an inoculum of the isolate, that is, the minimum bactericidal or lethal concentration (MBC or MLC); (2) determination of the killing rate (time-kill curve or killing curve) at which an antibiotic kills an inoculum of the isolate; and (3) determination of the highest dilution of the serum of a patient receiving antibiotic(s) necessary to kill 99.9% of an inoculum of isolate, otherwise known as the serum bactericidal titer (SBT) or serum lethal titer.

Publication of an approved guideline by the CLSI for performance of the MBC has addressed one of the criticisms leveled at the performance of this test—that it is not standardized (NCCLS, 1999). To determine the MBC, serially diluted (on a $\log_2$ basis) antimicrobial in broth is inoculated with a standardized suspension of the isolate of interest, in the same way as when determining the MIC. After incubation at 35° C for 24 hours, those dilutions demonstrating no visible growth are subcultured onto antimicrobial-free agar medium. After incubation, the number of colonies on the agar medium is counted, and the number of viable organisms per milliliter of antimicrobial dilution is calculated. The MBC or MLC is the lowest concentration of the antimicrobial agent that is lethal or bactericidal to the original inoculum, with the endpoint defined as a 99.9% decrease in viable organisms relative to the original inoculum.

Although in theory, one could see how the MBC could be very useful for certain types of infection, determination of the MBC often is not straightforward and can be confounded by several factors. One such factor is the persistence of a small number of organisms of the inoculum ("persisters") that survive the antimicrobial exposure but remain susceptible if retested against the antimicrobial. In the case of cell wall–active agents, such as the β-lactams and vancomycin, at least some may represent cells that are in a dormant or nongrowing phase of the cell cycle. These cells have been termed "indifferent" to the effects of the antibiotic by some authors, rather than "resistant" (Jayaraman, 2008). Second is the paradoxical effect (Eagle phenomenon), which is an unexplained increase in the number of surviving organisms as the concentration of the antimicrobial increases above the MBC. Third is tolerance, a phenomenon in which bactericidal agents have reduced bactericidal activity against a particular strain of a bacterial species. The mechanism behind tolerance currently is not understood, but as pointed out by Jayaraman (2008), "tolerance" on the part of an isolate is clearly different from "indifference," or dormancy. Some authors have given a more practical (at least for the laboratory) definition of "tolerance" on the part of an isolate, that is, if the MBC/MIC ratio is ≥32, the isolate is defined as tolerant to the test antimicrobial (Sherris, 1986).

In determining the time-kill curve, a single dilution of the test antimicrobial, usually at a concentration at or near what can maximally be achieved in a patient, is inoculated with a standardized inoculum of the isolate in question; then quantitative cultures are performed at regular intervals over a 24-hour period. The amount of bacterial growth evident on quantitative culture at each time period over 24 hours is graphed to generate the time-kill curve. The test essentially determines the rate and duration of killing by the antimicrobial at a specified concentration. This test is very useful in animal models of specific infections and in pharmacologic research, but its labor-intensive nature is one of the factors that make it difficult for laboratories to offer it as a clinical test.

The basic premise of the MBC and the time-kill study can be applied to the serum bactericidal titer, with the addition of serum from the patient receiving antibiotics to the test system. As with the MBC, serum bactericidal tests have been standardized by the CLSI (NCCLS, 1999b). The modification involves obtaining two serum specimens from the patient—a specimen when the antibiotic is at its lowest concentration in the body ("trough" specimen), usually just before the patient receives a dose of the antimicrobial, and a specimen when the antibiotic is at its highest ("peak specimen"), a specified time after a dose of the antimicrobial is given, with the time depending on the route of administration. Serial $\log_2$ dilutions are made of each specimen and are inoculated with a standardized inoculum of the isolate of interest; the dilutions are incubated at 35° C for 24 hours. Similar to the MBC, those dilutions in which no visible growth is seen are subcultured to agar medium for quantitative culture and are reincubated. The **serum bactericidal titer** is the lowest concentration of antimicrobial that results in a 99.9% decrease in viable organisms relative to the original inoculum. The theory behind the SBT is that it takes into account factors such as the effects of absorption and metabolism of the antimicrobial, effects of metabolites or breakdown products of the antimicrobial on the isolate, protein binding of the antimicrobial, and the effects of interaction with any other medications the patient is taking (NCCLS, 1999b). The SBT can provide an assessment of bactericidal activity by determining the antibiotic concentration relative to the MBC, and can allow an assessment of how many half-lives of the antimicrobial bactericidal activity will persist in the patient's serum (NCCLS, 1999b). Finally, if a time-kill study is performed using the patient's serum, the serum bactericidal rate or the rate of killing over time can be determined, or, if the area under the curve is examined, the magnitude and duration of bactericidal activity can be ascertained (NCCLS, 1999b).

In addition to the labor-intensive nature of the bactericidal tests, which a laboratory must address if it is decided that these tests will be performed, another consideration is the clinical relevance of the tests. At various times in the past, bactericidal tests have been recommended as contributory in the prediction of therapeutic success or failure in bacterial endocarditis, osteomyelitis, sepsis in immunocompromised patients, infected prosthetic implants, and infections for which therapeutic guidelines are poorly described (Petersen, 1992). Many of the studies supporting these recommendations were performed before standardization of the procedure, and subsequent studies have failed to support the claim that the tests are directly predictive of therapeutic success or failure (Petersen, 1992). Despite this, studies that suggest that bactericidal tests have a role in predicting prognosis in specific infections or in infections in special patient populations continue to appear. Liao and colleagues (2007) suggest that for nosocomial infections with multidrug resistant *Acinetobacter baumannii*, the SBT is useful in determining prognosis and the need for therapeutic alterations. Cahen and colleagues (1993) state that they demonstrated that the SBT is directly predictive of cure or failure in acute pulmonary exacerbation in cystic fibrosis patients. The clinical utility of the tests remains controversial; however, what is not controversial is the resources that the clinical microbiology laboratory must invest to accurately perform these tests. Based on this, the recommendation put forth by both Petersen and Shanholtzer (1992) and the CLSI (NCCLS, 1999, 1999b) indicates that if consideration is given to requesting this test on the part of the clinical staff, the clinical microbiology laboratory director should be consulted to determine whether the test can be contributory to patient care, what method should be used, and how to the results should be interpreted.

SELECTED REFERENCES

Barenfanger J, Drake C, Kacich G. Clinical and financial benefits of rapid bacterial identification and antimicrobial susceptibility. J Clin Microbiol 1999;1415:37.

This interesting study demonstrates the potential benefits of rapid identification of, and susceptibility testing against, bacterial isolates using commercial susceptibility systems. Potential benefits in terms of patient outcome, length of hospital stay, and hospital costs are discussed.

Fridkin SK, Edwards JR, Courval JM, et al. The effect of vancomycin and third-generation cephalosporins on the prevalence of vancomycin-resistant enterococci in 126 US adult intensive care units. Ann Intern Med 2001;175:135.

Fridkin SK, Lawton R, Edwards JR, et al. Monitoring antimicrobial use and resistance: comparison with a national benchmark on reducing vancomycin use and vancomycin-resistant enterococci. Emerg Infect Dis 2002;702:8.

These two references by Fridkin, et al demonstrate the utility of antibiotic susceptibility testing and cumulative antibiotic susceptibility monitoring in changing practice patterns, and the effects that changing antibiotic use patterns can have on reducing the prevalence of a virulent pathogen.

Jones RN. Method preferences and test accuracy of antimicrobial susceptibility testing: updates from the College of American Pathologists microbiology surveys. Arch Pathol Lab Med 2001;1285:125.

A description of the types of susceptibility testing performed by participating laboratories, the systems used, and their respective accuracies against specific proficiency test isolates. Potential reporting errors by laboratories are also highlighted.

Kanafani ZA, Perfect JR. Resistance to antifungal agents: mechanisms and clinical impact. Clin Infect Dis 2008;120:46.

A discussion of the molecular mechanisms of in vitro resistance to antifungal agents in yeasts and moulds. Clinical resistance, therapeutic failure despite in vitro sensitivity of a fungal pathogen to antifungal agent, is discussed, with a description of the possible mechanisms involved in its occurrence.

Lew W, Pai M, Oxlade O, et al. Initial drug resistance and tuberculosis treatment outcomes: systematic review and meta-analysis. Ann Intern Med 2008;123:149.

A meta-analysis of randomized controlled trials and cohort studies of naïve patients with culture confirmed pulmonary tuberculosis who underwent treatment with standardized treatment regimens. Outcomes with respect to treatment failure and relapse were correlated with initial drug-susceptiblity testing results of the patient's Mycobacterium tuberculosis isolates.

Mouton JW. Breakpoints: current practice and future perspectives. Int J Antimicrob Agents 2002;323:19.

Interesting discussion of the concept and rationale behind the antibiotic breakpoint. The distinction between microbiological and clinical breakpoints is discussed. Recommendations for improving the accuracy and utility of the breakpoint are made.

Nguyen MH, Yu VL, Morris AJ, et al. Antimicrobial resistance and clinical outcome of *Bacteroides* bacteremia: findings of a multicenter prospective observational trial. Clin Infect Dis 2000;870:30.

Important study that demonstrates changing susceptibility patterns of a genus of anaerobic bacteria over time, the correlation of appropriate antibiotic treatment with patient outcome, and the importance of susceptibility testing in guiding treatment.

REFERENCES

Access the complete reference list online at http://www.expertconsult.com

CHAPTER 59

SPIROCHETE INFECTIONS

P. Rocco LaSala, Michael B. Smith

PART 7

KEY POINTS

- With few exceptions, human disease caused by spirochetes typically follows a clinical course that reflects three sequential phenomena: (1) early, local proliferation of the organisms at the site of inoculation, (2) spirochetemia with systemic dissemination, and (3) persistence of small numbers of microbes at various, often immune, "privileged" sites.
- Although direct detection of spirochetes causing human disease is sometimes possible by microbiological culture, microscopy, and genomic amplification, diagnosis often relies upon the demonstration of a patient's serologic response to the offending agent.
- Venereal syphilis is a historic sexually transmitted disease caused by *Treponema pallidum* subspecies *pallidum.*
- In the early stages of disease, venereal syphilis may be diagnosed using direct microscopic visualization.
- Serologic detection of syphilis, by far the most common mode of diagnosis, comprises methods that semiquantitatively measure antibody to various lipoproteins, as well as methods that qualitatively measure antibody to treponeme-specific antigens.
- Yaws, endemic syphilis (bejel), and pinta are not sexually transmitted, are endemic to various tropical and Middle Eastern regions, and are caused by *T. pallidum* subsp. *pertenue, T. pallidum* subsp. *endemicum,* and *T. carateum*, respectively.
- Presumptive diagnosis of the endemic trepanematoses can sometimes be made on the basis of clinical and epidemiologic data; however, as with venereal syphilis, serologic and direct microscopic techniques may prove useful.
- The most common tick-borne disease in North America and Europe, Lyme disease is caused chiefly by *Borrelia burgdorferi* sensu stricto, *Borrelia garinii,* and *Borrelia afzelii.*
- Typical clinical manifestations of Lyme disease include erythema migrans (early localized disease), neuroborreliosis (early disseminated or late-stage disease), and/or Lyme arthritis (late-stage disease).
- Because no single laboratory test performs sufficiently in all clinical scenarios, a diagnosis of Lyme disease must be based on a combination of (1) clinicoepidemiologic characteristics, (2) host serologic response (as measured by enzyme-linked immunosorbent assay/immunofluorescence assay and immunoblot), (3) molecular evidence, and/or (4) culture results.
- Epidemic, louse-borne relapsing fever has a worldwide distribution and is caused by *Borrelia recurrentis.*
- Endemic, tick-borne relapsing fever has a limited geographic distribution and is caused by several *Borrelia* species, including *Borrelia hermsi* and *Borrelia turicata.*
- Acute onset of high fever and constitutional symptoms followed by cycles of evanescence and recrudescence is frequently recognized in both forms of relapsing fever.
- Diagnosis of relapsing fever is most often established through the demonstration of spirochetes in peripheral blood smears stained by a Giemsa technique.
- One of the most common zoonotic diseases throughout the world, leptospirosis is caused by various serovars of different species within the genus *Leptospira.*
- Although leptospirosis is usually subclinical or mild and flu-like, a small proportion of patients develop severe constitutional symptoms, in addition to gastrointestinal/hepatic disease, meningitis, renal failure, and/or myocarditis (also referred to as Weil's disease).
- Although *Leptospira* spp. can be cultivated in vitro, diagnosis is usually made by demonstrating seroconversion.
- *Brachyspira aalborgi* and *Brachyspira pilosicoli* have been demonstrated in and isolated from the colon of humans with diarrheal disease, but their pathogenicity has not been firmly established.
- Demonstration of spirochetes along the colonic epithelial cell borders using routine, immunohistochemical, or in situ hybridization microscopy from biopsy material is more commonly performed than cultivation or genomic amplification assays.

Spirochetes ("spiro" means "coiled," and "chaete" means "hair") are slender, spiral-shaped bacteria containing one or more complete rotations that form a helix. They are gram-negative but can be visualized only by darkfield or phase microscopy, silver impregnation, and immunohistochemical stains in tissue sections. Flagella-like organelles called periplasmic fibrils or axial filaments are attached near the poles of the bacteria and permit a corkscrew-like motility. Many commensal and nonpathogenic species of spirochetes exist, and human disease is limited primarily to infection by members of three genera: *Treponema*, *Borrelia*, and *Leptospira*. Widely diverse from an epidemiologic standpoint, spirochetes within these genera demonstrate a number of pathogenic, and hence clinical, similarities upon acquisition by humans (Schmid, 1989). Several other spirochete-like bacteria, including *Spirillum minor* and *Anaerobiospirillum succiniciproducens*, have been implicated in human disease and are discussed briefly here. Although *Brachyspira* species have been associated with gastrointestinal syndromes, definitive causation of disease by these bacteria has not been universally accepted.

TREPONEMA

The genus *Treponema* contains two species responsible for disease in humans. *Treponema pallidum* is divided into three subspecies, each of which is the etiologic agent of a distinct clinical entity: subspecies *pallidum*, *pertenue*, and *endemicum* are the etiologic agents of venereal syphilis, yaws, and endemic syphilis (bejel), respectively. Pinta is caused by the second closely related species, *Treponema carateum*. Controversy exists even to this day concerning the origins of the sexually transmitted form of infection. Previously, the debate focused largely on deducing geographic regions of disease occurrence (e.g., Old World vs. New World) based on morphologic skeletal abnormalities of excavated remains that were presumably a result of *T. pallidum* subsp. *pallidum* infection. More recent work utilizing phylogenetic molecular methods seems to support the "Columbian" theory, that is, that a form of venereal infection was acquired during exploration of the New World and was subsequently introduced into Europe (Harper, 2008b).

CLASSIC TREPONEMAL DISEASE

Syphilis

Description

T. pallidum subsp. *pallidum*, the etiologic agent of venereal syphilis, is a thin (0.2 µm) spirochete, 6–20 µm in length with 10–13 coils (Fig. 59-1). The disease appears to have spread rapidly throughout Europe during the 16th century, and its absence in the medical literature prior to this period suggests that the organism was brought from the New World. The term **syphilis,** in common use during the last ≈200 years to describe the disease process, is derived from the fictional character Syphilus, the protagonist of a 1530 poem by Girolamo Fracastoro. The work's title, *Syphilis sive morbus gallicus* ("Syphilis or the French disease"), underscores the popular notion of that era as to the point of disease origination (no doubt promulgated chiefly by Italians). For a thorough and entertaining review of the historical literature, particularly as it relates to the United States, the reader is referred to a recent work by Parascandola (2008).

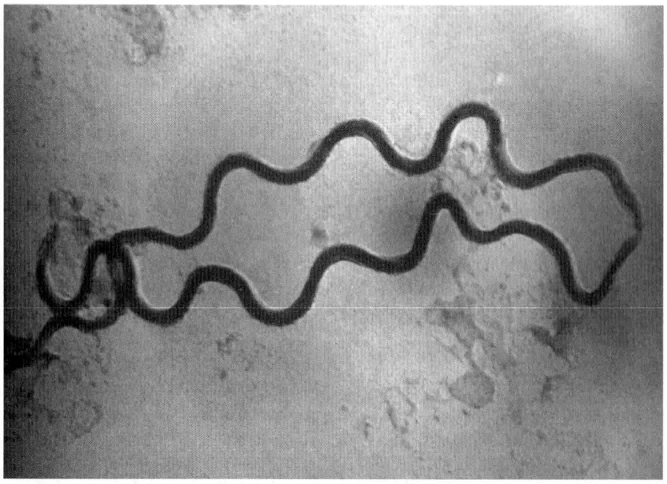

Figure 59-1 An electron photomicrograph of two spiral-shaped *Treponema pallidum* bacteria (×36,000). *(CDC/PHIL file photo.)*

Epidemiology

Man is the only natural reservoir for *T. pallidum* subsp. *pallidum*. Transmission occurs by direct contact with active lesions, largely through sexual contact. Vertical transmission across the placenta, the second most common mode of infection, may result when a latently infected female becomes pregnant, or when a pregnant woman becomes infected (Wicher, 2001). Infection may also rarely be transmitted by nonsexual contact with an active lesion, by transfusion of fresh blood products from an infected person (although organisms do not survive >48 hours under typical blood bank storage conditions), by accidental needle stick, or when infectious specimens are handled in the laboratory.

The incidence of venereal syphilis in the United States declined dramatically with the advent of penicillin following World War II and remained stable until the mid 1980s, when the incidence began to increase once again (Fig. 59-2), presumably as the result of increased intravenous drug use and sexual promiscuity. Although the global prevalence of syphilis remains strikingly variable (Gerbase, 1998; Peeling, 2004), the United States experienced a continuous decline in infection rates among women of childbearing age throughout the 1990s; this was paralleled by a comparable decrease in the incidence of congenital syphilis (Centers for Disease Control and Prevention, 2003, 2004a). Following a nadir in disease incidence in 2000 that marked the lowest rate of syphilis in the United States during recorded history, numbers of cases have been steadily increasing, predominantly among men who have sex with men (Fig. 59-3). In 2006, the National Plan to Eliminate Syphilis from the United States was updated to reflect a new target of reducing the incidence of primary and secondary syphilis to <2.2/100,000 persons, and of congenital syphilis to <3.9/100,000 live births by 2010 (Centers for Disease Control and Prevention, 2006a). As of 2009, however, the goals remained elusive (4.6 cases/100,000 persons for primary and secondary syphilis and 10 cases/100,000 live births for congenital disease).

Pathogenesis and Pathology

T. pallidum subsp. *pallidum* penetrates an intact mucous membrane or gains access to tissue through abraded skin, multiplies at the inoculation site, and then enters the lymphatic and circulatory system and spreads throughout the body. In laboratory animals, infections have been produced with

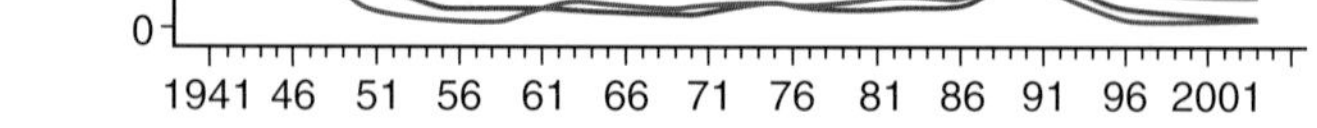

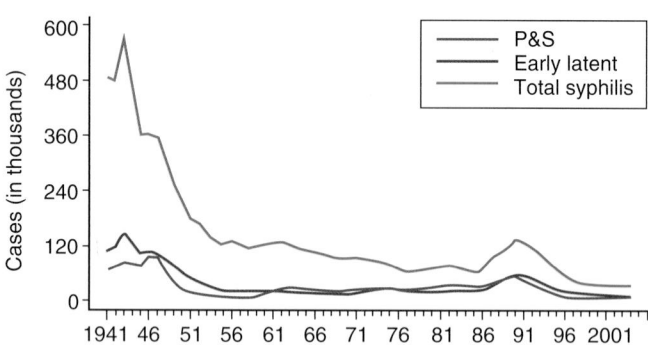

Figure 59-2 Reported cases of syphilis by stage of infection: United States, 1941–2004. *(CDC, 2005.)*

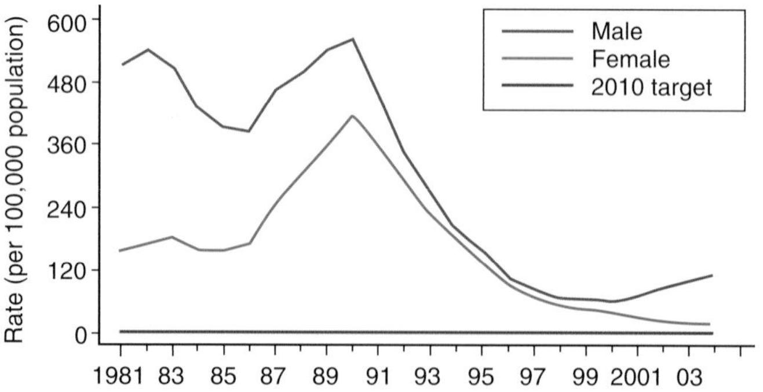

Figure 59-3 Primary and secondary syphilis—rates by sex: United States, 1981–2004. *(CDC, 2005.)*

as few as four spirochetes (Cumberland, 1949). Clinical lesions appear when a critical mass of organisms is reached locally ($\approx 10^7$ spirochetes); therefore, the incubation period is directly related to the size of the initial inoculum and varies from 3 days to 3 months (Magnuson, 1956).

The host immunologic response to *T. pallidum* subsp. *pallidum* is influenced by the structure of the bacterium. The outer membrane is a phospholipid bilayer with few demonstrable protein antigens. The most important antigens for the host immune response appear to be lipoproteins within the periplasmic space (Chamberlain, 1989; Cox, 1992; Salazar, 2002). Additionally, the bacterium appears to be able to coat itself with host proteins. The net effect is to delay the humoral response, reducing its effectiveness because the spirochetes are in extravascular locations by the time antibodies are produced. Furthermore, it has been demonstrated in animal models that the cellular immune response is downregulated in syphilis, despite the ineffective humoral response (Fitzgerald, 1992).

This delayed and attenuated immune response allows *T. pallidum* subsp. *pallidum* to disseminate and to produce a chronic infection. The course of syphilis can be divided into predictable stages. Its primary stage, the development of a chancre, occurs at a median of 3 weeks post inoculation, although a primary lesion may not develop in all patients. Additionally, because of its painless nature, the lesion may go unnoticed in a proportion of cases. Upon healing within 2–8 weeks, the chancre gives rise to the secondary stage. Typically manifesting about 6 weeks after inoculation (range, 2–12 weeks), this stage is characterized by widespread dissemination of spirochetes via the bloodstream and the development of mucocutaneous and organ involvement with the presence of constitutional symptoms. Upon resolution of the secondary stage, the infection enters a period of latency, during which time the patient exhibits minimal manifestations of infection. The first year of this stage, termed the early latent period, may be characterized by occasional relapses, whereas relapse is not common during the late latent period. Following a period of 10–25 years, approximately one third of untreated patients develop tertiary syphilis, the most serious manifestations of which involve the cardiovascular system or the central nervous system (CNS).

Whatever organ is involved or whatever stage of the disease is reached, the histologic hallmark of syphilis is obliterative endarteritis, demonstrating concentric endothelial and fibroblastic proliferations with an associated mononuclear cell infiltrate rich in plasma cells (Fig. 59-4, *A*). Endarteritis results from the binding of spirochetes to endothelial cells via fibronectin molecules that have attached to the surface of the bacteria (Thomas, 1986). Treponemes may be demonstrable in tissues with silver impregnation (Fig. 59-4, *B*) and immunohistochemical stains, particularly during the first and second stages of disease (Martin-Ezquerea, 2009). With progression, both the plasma cell infiltrate and the concentration of treponemes lessen in intensity. Although commonplace in the pretreatment era, syphilitic gummas, or large visceral necrotizing granulomas, develop as tertiary-stage manifestations but are rare today (Fargen, 2009).

Elucidation of the complete genomic sequence of *T. pallidum* subsp. *pallidum* may provide insight into the pathogenesis of this organism (Fraser, 1998). For example, researchers have verified the absence of many enzymatic pathways typically found in other cultivable bacterial pathogens. One interesting finding was a series of duplicated genes, termed *T. pallidum* repeats (tprA–tprL), which encode homologous membrane proteins that may impart the means of antigenic variability and immunologic escape (Centurion-Lara, 1999). Their roles in such, as well as their putative cellular location, however, remain vague (Hazlett, 2001).

Clinical Manifestations

Syphilis is a chronic infection with a multiplicity of expressions, primarily related to the stage at which it presents. The primary chancre is characteristically ulcerated with raised, firm edges and a smooth base and is notable for absence of an exudate or pain (Fig. 59-5, *A*). Although these are typically solitary, multiple chancres can occur in up to one third of patients. Patients with previous infection can present with atypical lesions, such as a small papule, or may not develop a lesion at all. Regional lymphadenopathy, with moderately enlarged, rubbery, nonsuppurative lymph nodes, is seen in some patients.

Dissemination marks the secondary stage, and patients present with signs and symptoms of a systemic illness. More than 90% develop a rash that begins on the trunk and extremities (although any body surface can be involved) as small macules that progress to papules, and in some patients to pustules, over a period of weeks. The appearance of the rash on the palms and soles is characteristic (Fig. 59-5, *B*), and enlargement and coalescence of papules produce the pale plaques of condyloma lata (Fig. 59-5, *C*). Approximately 90% of patients also exhibit generalized lymphadenopathy, and as many as three fourths may suffer fever, malaise, anorexia, arthralgia, pharyngitis, and weight loss. Mucous patches are seen in up to one third of cases. About 40% of persons develop CNS symptoms during this stage, particularly among those coinfected with human immunodeficiency virus (HIV), although only 1%–2% present with acute meningitis (Lukehart, 1988; Centers for Disease Control and Prevention, 2007). The remainder may experience headache and meningismus, uveitis, sensorineural hearing loss, and cranial nerve involvement.

The tissue destruction of tertiary syphilis usually becomes evident decades after the primary infection. Cardiovascular syphilis occurs as a result of weakening of the tunica media and results in an aneurysm of the ascending aorta with aortic valve insufficiency and narrowing of the coronary artery ostia. Syphilitic gummas may involve the skin, brain, skeletal system, or mucocutaneous tissues, although any organ can be affected. Both cardiovascular syphilis and syphilitic gummas became much less frequent after the advent of antibiotic treatment. Meningovascular syphilis occurs 5–10 years after initial infection and clinically presents as seizures, stroke, and aphasia. Multiple small infarcts due to endarteritis in the CNS are the cause of this form. Parenchymatous neurosyphilis, which presents 15–30 years after initial infection, is a degenerative process with loss of neurons and myelinated tracts resulting in a complex of neurologic and psychiatric manifestations, including general paresis, tabes dorsalis, and pupillary abnormalities. Some patients lack clinical signs or symptoms

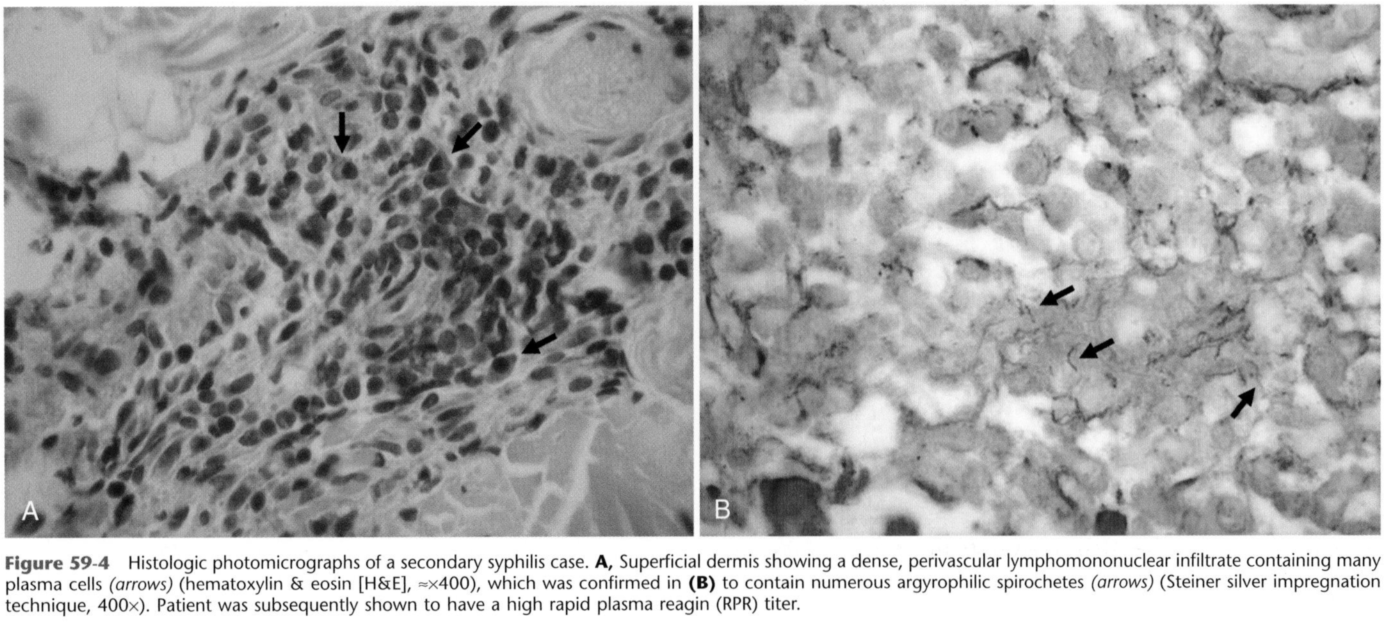

Figure 59-4 Histologic photomicrographs of a secondary syphilis case. **A,** Superficial dermis showing a dense, perivascular lymphomononuclear infiltrate containing many plasma cells *(arrows)* (hematoxylin & eosin [H&E], ≈×400), which was confirmed in **(B)** to contain numerous argyrophilic spirochetes *(arrows)* (Steiner silver impregnation technique, 400×). Patient was subsequently shown to have a high rapid plasma reagin (RPR) titer.

PART 7

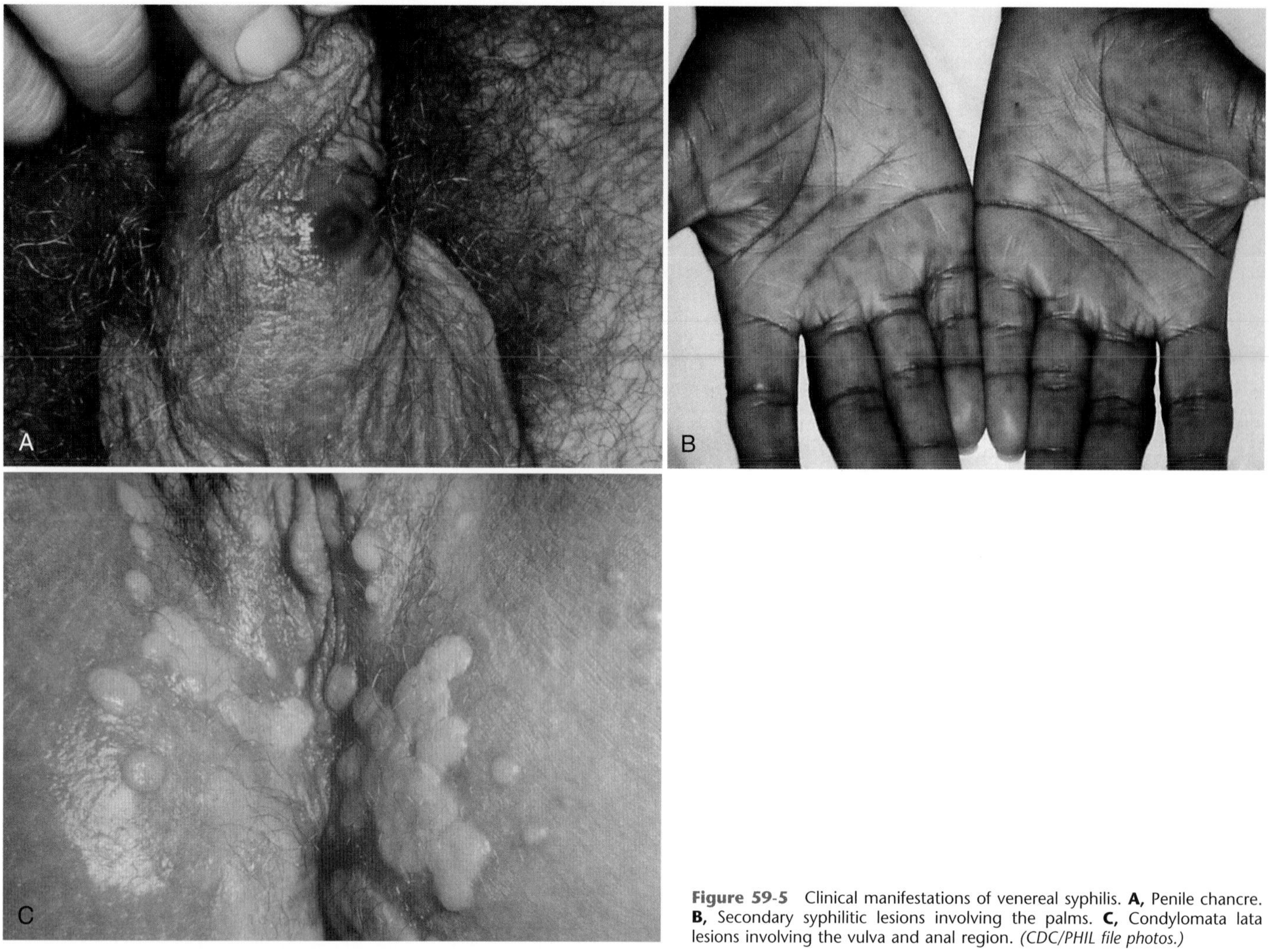

Figure 59-5 Clinical manifestations of venereal syphilis. **A,** Penile chancre. **B,** Secondary syphilitic lesions involving the palms. **C,** Condylomata lata lesions involving the vulva and anal region. *(CDC/PHIL file photos.)*

altogether but demonstrate cerebrospinal fluid (CSF) abnormalities such as pleocytosis, increased protein, a reactive Venereal Disease Research Laboratory (VDRL) test, or antibody against *T. pallidum* indicating CNS infection. Such patients have been described as having "asymptomatic neurosyphilis" (Tramont, 2000).

Congenital syphilis occurs clinically as two forms: an early or infantile form (<2 years of age) and a late form following a period of latency (few years to several decades). Although transplacental passage of spirochetes can occur during any trimester, congenital acquisition during early gestational age results in stillbirth more often than does acquisition during late gestation or parturition (Harter, 1976; Blanc, 1981). As may be expected, congenital transmission is more frequent during the primary, secondary, and early latent periods of maternal infection (Woods, 2009). Necrotizing funisitis, or inflammation of the umbilical cord, is characteristic of congenital syphilis, although it is typically present in only the most severe cases. In the infantile form, a diffuse rash with sloughing of the skin, osteochondritis, and periostitis are characteristic; however, affected newborns may be asymptomatic (Dorfman, 1990; Ikeda, 1990). Diffuse fibrosis of the liver (hepar lobatum) and lung (pneumonia alba) is also seen. After a latent period, the late form presents in childhood or adulthood with a wide variety of signs and symptoms; however, the triad of interstitial keratitis, Hutchinson's teeth, and eighth nerve deafness is classic. Periostitis, saber shins, and saddle deformity of the nose are also seen frequently.

Syphilis and HIV infection are increasingly seen as coinfections because these diseases share common risk factors and may even potentiate one another. Studies that have examined the association have demonstrated no difference in stage at clinical presentation between patients with concomitant syphilis and acquired immunodeficiency syndrome (AIDS) and those without AIDS (Hutchinson, 1991; Gourevitch, 1993). Whether AIDS has an effect on the clinical course of primary and secondary syphilis is controversial. Some experts cite a predilection for the infection to present with an atypical and more severe rash, exaggerated constitutional symptoms, and a more malignant course in AIDS patients (Tramont, 2000; Collis, 2001). Others suggest little difference in disease manifestations between AIDS and non-AIDS patients (Musher, 1990; Hutchinson, 1991; Rolfs, 1997). Although it has been proposed that AIDS patients with syphilis show an increased propensity to develop neurosyphilis, and to develop it more rapidly, than non-AIDS patients (Johns, 1987; Musher, 1990), this remains a contested issue given (1) the shortcomings of current neurosyphilis diagnostic criteria (Collis, 2001), and (2) an apparent lack of correlation between early CNS treponemal invasion and HIV status (Lukehart, 1988; González-López, 2009). One multicenter prospective study showed that CSF nontreponemal tests were more likely to remain positive following syphilis therapy in HIV-infected individuals than in HIV-uninfected patients (Marra, 2004a). It remains to be seen, however, if such laboratory evidence of treatment failure is a true reflection of potential clinical relapse. What does seem clear, as evidenced by multiple studies, is that anti-HIV therapy itself improves the likelihood of serologic response following syphilis treatment in HIV-positive patients (Ghanem, 2008; Marra, 2008; González-López, 2009). The high incidence of eye involvement among patients with AIDS is also unquestionable, with anterior uveitis being the most common manifestation of *T. pallidum* infection in this setting (Tramont, 2000).

Yaws

Yaws (also called frambesia tropica, pian, parangi, paru, buba, or bouba) is a chronic disease caused by *T. pallidum* subsp. *pertenue* and is the most prevalent of the nonvenereal treponematoses. This disease, which has afflicted residents of the tropics since antiquity, is common in rural areas of tropical countries with heavy rainfall. After a decline in the 1950s due to large campaigns to control the treponematoses, the incidence of yaws has increased in some areas (Engelkens, 1991a; Antal, 2002).

Yaws is contracted chiefly during childhood by direct contact, with breaks in the skin allowing entry of treponemes. Early lesions generally

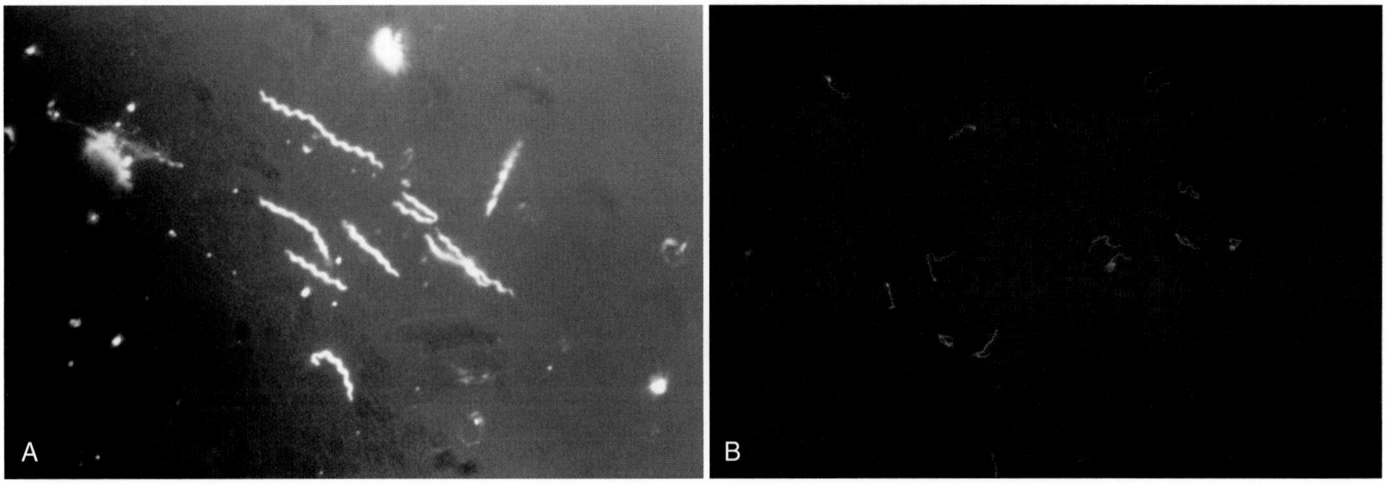

Figure 59-6 In vitro diagnostic modalities for venereal syphilis detection. **A,** Darkfield microscopy technique (×400) reveals the presence of motile spirochetes. **B,** Positive fluorescent treponemal antibody absorption (FTA-ABS) test for antibody response in patient with syphilis. *(CDC/PHIL file photo.)*

appear about 3 weeks later but may not develop for months. One or several papules appear, most frequently on the lower extremities, and then ulcerate or progress to papillomatous lesions. Numerous treponemes are found in these lesions. Spontaneous resolution is usual; however, relapses preceded by malaise, fever, and generalized lymphadenopathy followed by disseminated skin lesions are common. Most patients enter a period of latency during which no clinical signs or symptoms are evident. For most, the disease shows no additional manifestations; however, approximately 10% develop late yaws, which shows irreversible, destructive lesions of bone, cartilage, soft tissue, and the skin (Engelkens, 1991a; Antal, 2002). Cardiovascular and CNS lesions similar to those seen in syphilis have been reported to occur (Roman, 1986).

Endemic Syphilis

Endemic syphilis (bejel) is a nonvenereal chronic infection caused by infection with *T. pallidum* subsp. *endemicum*. The disease is ancient and, although it is no longer as widespread as it once was, still occurs in the Middle East and Africa in hot, dry climates. In Sahelian Africa, the disease has been increasing in prevalence (Engelkens, 1991b). Endemic syphilis is transmitted by direct contact with active lesions, contaminated fingers, and eating or drinking utensils. Crowded living conditions and poor hygiene are common associated factors. Children aged 2–15 years are primarily infected, although the disease can be found in adults in the same family, and those adults who did not suffer from the disease in childhood can be infected by their children. The inoculum is small and the primary lesions of early endemic syphilis, most frequent on the oropharyngeal mucosa, often are not apparent. Initial clinical manifestations of the disease are usually seen in a secondary stage, with mucous patches, condyloma lata, angular stomatitis, generalized lymphadenopathy, and painful osteoperiostitis. This is followed by a latent period of variable length. The late stage is characterized by tissue destruction of the skin, bones, and cartilage, with a predilection for the nose and palate (so-called gangosa), and sometimes laryngeal involvement.

Pinta

Pinta (carate, mal de pinto, azul) is caused by infection with *T. carateum*. The disease is endemic in rural tropical Central and South America and recently has reappeared in Mexico and Colombia, two countries from which it was eradicated in the 1950s (Engelkens, 1991b). Children younger than 5 years of age are primarily infected. Inoculation is thought to occur via nonvenereal skin or mucous membrane contact. Characterization of the pathogenesis of the disease is difficult because, unlike other treponematoses that are pathogenic in humans, an animal model is unavailable and the treponeme cannot be cultured continuously. Although similar to other treponemal infections that have early and late stages, frequent overlap of stages occurs in pinta. A primary papule or plaque develops at the site of inoculation after weeks to months, with or without localized lymphadenopathy. The primary lesion resolves, and several months to years later, disseminated secondary lesions, or pintids, which resemble scaly psoriasiform plaques, appear and remain for long periods or resolve and recur. In late pinta, lesions demonstrate hypopigmentation and skin atrophy or hyperkeratosis, which can persist for life. The skin appears to be the only organ affected in this disease (Antal, 2002).

LABORATORY DIAGNOSIS OF TREPONEMATOSES

Because the etiologic agents of the human treponematoses cannot be isolated easily by routine culture methods, testing for disease generally is completed directly by visualization of the organisms in material from lesions or indirectly by immunologic methods. Consequently, different stages of the treponematoses often require a particular testing modality. In the early stages when lesions are present, highly specific microscopic techniques are used. Upon resolution of lesions, a variety of serologic tests are employed for diagnosis. It is important to remember that none of these laboratory tests is capable of distinguishing between the closely related species and subspecies of pathogenic treponemes, so differentiating between them requires clinical, epidemiologic, and, when possible, genomic information (Harper, 2008a).

Darkfield Microscopy

When direct sampling of lesions is possible, such as in primary, secondary, or early congenital syphilis (chancres, mucous patches, or condyloma lata), the lesion should be cleansed with sterile water (no soap or antiseptic) and gently abraded. Pressure is applied, causing serous exudate to collect in the lesion. A drop of the fluid is placed on a slide and a coverslip is placed over the fluid. The specimen must be examined immediately, as visualization of motility is necessary for definitive identification. Because of their narrow width, treponemes cannot be visualized by conventional light microscopy. Instead, darkfield microscopy is necessary. This technique makes use of a patch stop, which creates the microscopist's "dark field," and a condenser lens that targets the spirochetes with light waves at an oblique angle, some of which are scattered into the objective, giving the appearance of bright organisms in a dark background (Fig. 59-6, *A*). The darkfield examination can be positive several weeks before a positive serologic test and has a sensitivity of 80% in diagnosing syphilis (Larsen, 1995). Because of possible confusion with commensal treponemes in the mouth, however, it is not recommended that this technique be utilized for oral lesions. Additionally, three *Treponema* spp. that are normal inhabitants of the genital region (*T. phagedensis*, *T. refringens*, and *T. minutum*) could potentially be confused with *T. pallidum* on darkfield examination. Careful cleaning of the area is important in reducing the likelihood of this occurrence. A more recent adaptation of in vivo reflectance confocal microscopy has also been explored as a potential method of spirochete visualization within cutaneous lesions (Venturini, 2009).

Fluorescence Microscopy

Fluorescein isothiocyanate (FITC)-labeled antibodies specific for *T. pallidum* can be used for direct detection of treponemes in lesions, obviating the need to observe motility of the bacteria. The test can be applied to tissue fluid that has been dried and fixed to the slide (direct fluorescent

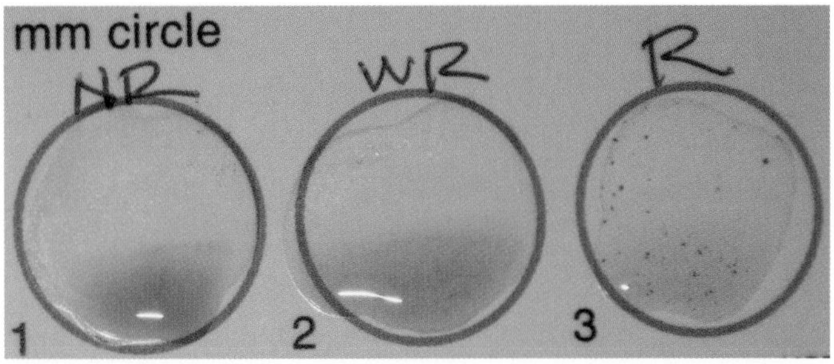

Figure 59-7 Rapid plasmin reagin test card showing nonreactive, weakly reactive, and strongly reactive serum samples (wells 1–3) with their respective agglutination patterns.

antibody [DFA-TP]) or paraffin-embedded tissue sections (direct fluorescent antibody tissue test [DFAT-TP]). Monoclonal antibodies are commercially available and can be used in these tests in place of the older and less specific Reiter treponeme adsorbed polyclonal antibodies obtained from syphilitic rabbits and humans. When used on fluid from fresh lesions, both DFA-TP and DFAT-TP have a sensitivity of approximately 100% (Larsen, 1995). Because these tests are specific for the pathogenic treponemes, they are preferred for examination of oral lesions.

Immunohistochemical Microscopy

In a manner similar in principle to fluorescence microscopy, monoclonal and polyclonal antibodies with specificities for spirochetes, treponemes, or *T. pallidum* have been used by pathologists for detection in paraffin-embedded tissues (Guarner, 2000; Hoang, 2004; Martin-Ezqureea, 2009). In contrast to immunofluorescence, immunohistochemistry does not require the use of expensive fluorescent microscopes. With this technique, antitreponemal antibodies bound to spirochetes in tissue sections are detected after a series of immunologic reactions typically consisting of a primary, biotinylated antibody conjugate with organism specificity followed by an enzyme-conjugated streptavidin complex. After development of the enzyme with an appropriate chromogenic substrate, organisms are highlighted against a pale counterstained background. This allows for easy detection of rare bacteria and affords the capability for histologic localization. The procedure reportedly offers improvement in sensitivity and specificity over silver impregnation stains for the detection of treponemes, but this is largely dependent upon the source of primary antibody.

Nontreponemal Serologic Tests

The nontreponemal assays detect antibodies to lipoprotein material and cardiolipin released from cells damaged by treponemes. As a consequence, they are not specific for *Treponema*. These tests have been used traditionally to screen for disease and to monitor the course of the disease after treatment. Standard tests include the VDRL, rapid plasma reagin (RPR), unheated serum reagin (USR), and toluidine red unheated serum (TRUST) tests. Several nontreponemal enzyme-linked immunosorbent assays (ELISAs) have also been approved by the U.S. Food and Drug Administration (FDA) and are used by some high-volume laboratories (e.g., blood donation testing centers). All these tests use a phospholipid antigen, some fortified with lecithin and cholesterol. Flocculation is the end point for the manual standard tests, whereas absorbance values are calculated spectrophotometrically in the ELISA. Serum is the preferred specimen for each. Heating of the serum to eliminate nonspecific reactions is required in the VDRL, whereas the addition of choline chloride to the RPR and USR eliminates the need for heating, making these popular choices among diagnostic laboratories. Antibody–antigen reactions in the VDRL and USR are assessed using a microscope at 100×, and the addition of charcoal to the RPR and dye to the TRUST makes the reactions macroscopically visible (Fig. 59-7).

Antibodies detected by these tests generally develop 1–4 weeks after the appearance of the primary chancre. The time at which the specimen is taken during the primary stage, therefore, will affect assay sensitivity. The titer rises, remains high during the first year of infection, and then gradually declines. The tests will ultimately revert to negative in most patients in the absence of therapy, particularly during the late latent stage. Thus, these tests are general markers of disease activity. False-negative nontreponemal tests may also be associated with very high titers of antibody (prozone phenomenon), which are seen most commonly in secondary syphilis. This condition is easily resolved by diluting the specimen prior to testing. False-positive results occur temporarily with acute illnesses such as hepatitis, other viral infections, and pregnancy; or chronically with the connective tissue diseases (Larsen, 1995).

Standard nontreponemal tests afford the capability of semiquantitative reporting by testing serial twofold specimen dilutions (i.e., titers). Follow-up titers are used to determine the efficacy of treatment, with a fourfold decrease in titer at 6 months for early syphilis or at 12–24 months for late syphilis considered an adequate response (Centers for Disease Control and Prevention, 2006b). As with any paired acute/convalescent serum analysis, testing by the same method and, when possible, in the same laboratory is preferred. Patients treated in early syphilis are more likely to revert to negative than those treated in late syphilis (Fiumara, 1980; Brown, 1985). In a small minority of patients, nontreponemal tests will remain positive despite adequate therapy—a situation known as the "serofast" response. Although useful for high sample throughput, the ELISA is not easily amenable to semiquantitative analysis, so follow-up testing using standard assays is often necessary for therapeutic monitoring of confirmed cases.

Reports have documented various aberrant nontreponemal test results with patients coinfected with HIV and syphilis, including delayed seroconversion; however, seronegative syphilis does not appear to be prevalent in AIDS patients (Flores, 1995). The false-positive rate is reportedly increased in AIDS patients (4% vs. 1% in non-AIDS); however, the increased rate of positivity may be associated with intravenous drug abuse rather than HIV infection itself (Flores, 1995; Larsen, 1995; Hernandez-Aguado, 1998). False-negative results also occur in AIDS patients with syphilis because of an exaggerated nontreponemal antibody response that occurs in some patients, with the resultant prozone effect (Gourevitch, 1993). Furthermore, as mentioned previously, a small number of AIDS patients may experience minimal to no decline in nontreponemal antibody titers despite presumably adequate therapy, although this may be related to the stage at which treatment was initiated rather than HIV coinfection (Larsen, 1995).

Treponemal Serologic Tests

These tests detect the presence of antibodies to treponemal antigens and are used to confirm a positive nontreponemal screening test, or to confirm infection in the face of a negative nontreponemal test in late or latent disease stages, which can occur in up to 30% of patients with tertiary syphilis (Larsen, 1995). The fluorescent treponemal antibody absorption test (FTA-ABS), one of the two standard treponemal tests, is an indirect fluorescent antibody test. It involves the addition of heated patient serum, which has been absorbed with antigen of the nonpathogenic Reiter treponeme for removal of cross-reactive antibodies to a slide on which *T. pallidum* subsp. *pallidum* (Nichols strain) has been fixed, followed by the addition of FITC-labeled anti–human globulin. Visible treponemes on fluorescent microscopy indicate the presence of antibody to the pathogenic treponemal species in the patient's serum (see Fig. 59-6, *B*). The second test, which is preferred by many laboratories because of its relative simplicity, is the microhemagglutination–*T. pallidum* test (MHA-TP). Absorbed serum is added to sheep red blood cells sensitized with *T. pallidum* (Nichols strain) sonicate in a microtiter tray. Agglutination of red cells is produced by syphilis-specific antibody. Generally, the MHA-TP and FTA-ABS are equivalent, except in the primary stage of syphilis, where the FTA-ABS may be slightly more sensitive (Hart, 1980; Augenbraun, 1998). Sensitivities and specificities of the various nontreponemal and treponemal serologic tests are summarized in Table 59-1 (Larsen, 1995).

Treponemal-specific antibody develops in primary syphilis and persists indefinitely in most patients, although as many as 20% may eventually serorevert (Romanowski, 1991). AIDS patients have shown a greater tendency to revert to seronegativity following treatment (Haas, 1990). The FTA-ABS usually is the first test to become positive, followed by the MHA-TP, and then the nontreponemal tests shortly thereafter. False-positive FTA-ABS results occur in ≈1% of patients, most often in the elderly, in persons with connective tissue disease, and in those infected with related organisms, such as *Borrelia* spp. (Larsen, 1995). The frequency of false-positive results with the MHA-TP is reportedly lower than with the FTA-ABS (Larsen, 1995).

As with the nontreponemal tests, ELISA and chemilumenescent test formats utilizing treponeme-specific antigens (e.g., sonicated lysates, recombinant proteins) have become available for use in clinical laboratories. Again, these offer the advantages of automation for high-volume testing and an objective, numeric interpretation. Sensitivity and specificity of various commercially available products are comparable with those of the FTA-ABS and MHA-TP (Lefevre, 1990; Norgard, 1993). Of interest,

TABLE 59-1
Sensitivities of Serologic Tests for Syphilis in Different Stages of Disease

	STAGE OF SYPHILIS (% SENSITIVITY)*			
Test	**Primary**	**Secondary**	**Latent**	**Late**
VDRL	78 (74–87)	100	95 (88–100)	71 (37–94)
RPR	86 (77–100)	100	98 (95–100)	73
FTA-ABS	84 (70–100)	100	100	96
MHA-TP	76 (69–90)	100	97 (97–100)	94

Data from Larsen SA, Steiner BM, Rudolph AH. Laboratory diagnosis and interpretation of tests for syphilis. Clin Microbiol Rev 1995;8:1.
FTA-ABS, Fluorescent treponemal antibody absorption; *MHA-TP,* microhemagglutination assay for antibodies to *Treponema pallidum; RPR,* rapid plasma reagin; *VDRL,* Venereal Disease Research Laboratory.
*Numbers in parentheses represent ranges of sensitivities in studies at the Centers for Disease Control and Prevention.

versions of these tests have recently been implemented as primary screening assays in some laboratories in the United States (Centers for Disease Control and Prevention, 2008) and Europe (Marangoni, 2009; Sokolovskiy, 2009). Because this testing algorithm does not distinguish past from active infection, follow-up testing for positive results typically includes semiquantitative nontreponemal tests and, when these are negative, repeat analysis using an alternative treponemal specific assay. Immunoassays with immunoglobulin (Ig)M-specific detection capability are also available and may have some utility in the diagnosis of congenital syphilis (Stoll, 1993; Larsen, 1998). Finally, several rapid, point-of-care assays that incorporate treponemal or nontreponemal antigens have been described (Greer, 2008). Their utility lies chiefly in areas with high prevalence rates and low likelihood of patient follow-up, where patients with positive results can be treated presumptively at the time of testing.

More highly complex tests, such as the immunoblot and the polymerase chain reaction (PCR), are available in some reference laboratories. The immunoblot has been integrated into the diagnosis of congenital syphilis or as confirmation for treponemal-specific antibody screening by some laboratories (Larsen, 1995; Wang, 2009). PCR has been advocated for the diagnosis of neurosyphilis, particularly in AIDS patients, although some studies have not demonstrated advantages over currently used methods (Marra, 1996). Neither immunoblot nor PCR is used extensively in the diagnostic setting, as standardization remains poor (Wicher, 1999).

Serologic screening for syphilis requires the use of particular specimens and/or tests, depending on the population and/or disease manifestation. For example, in congenital syphilis screening, antepartum maternal serum is the ideal specimen, and all women should be tested at least once during pregnancy (U.S. Preventative Services Task Force, 2009). In high prevalence areas or among women with potential risk factors, repeat testing may be indicated in later trimesters. Confirmation of congenital syphilis, however, may require a combination of clinical and radiologic examinations, placental analysis, and testing of neonatal serum. The latter is typically performed semiquantitatively using nontreponemal tests, and is compared with maternal serologic titer to determine the source of the antibody (i.e., to exclude transplacentally derived maternal antibody). Another example is the diagnosis of neurosyphilis, which requires a positive serum treponemal test in addition to a positive VDRL on CSF or some other CSF abnormality (e.g., pleocytosis, elevated protein level) (Centers for Disease Control and Prevention, 2002). The VDRL applied to CSF is highly specific for the diagnosis of neurosyphilis but is also insensitive. It is negative in 22%–69% of patients with active neurosyphilis, and its sensitivity in inactive neurosyphilis may be as low as 10% (MacLean, 1996). By contrast, the CSF FTA-ABS is reported to have high sensitivity and negative predictive value for neurosyphilis, so some experts advocate using this as a means of excluding the diagnosis (Marra, 2004b). Its low specificity limits its positive predictive value, however. Finally, one study suggests that the RPR may be used in place of VDRL on CSF samples (Castro, 2008), although this remains an uncommon practice in general.

TREATMENT OF TREPONEMATOSES

T. pallidum subspecies and *T. carateum* are uniformly susceptible to penicillin and other β-lactam antibiotics. Treatment for primary, secondary, and early latent syphilis is a single intramuscular injection of benzathine penicillin G. Yaws, pinta, and endemic syphilis are treated with the same antibiotic, although often at a lower dose (Engelkens, 1991a, 1991b). Household contacts of patients with the latter three diseases usually are also treated. For patients who are allergic to penicillin, doxycycline or tetracycline may be used. Macrolide antibiotics are no longer recommended, as efficacy has been shown to be less than 90% (Schroeter, 1972). A pronounced worsening in clinical course, termed the Jarisch-Herxheimer reaction, may be seen upon treatment of venereal syphilis patients, although symptoms frequently are not as severe as in treatment of relapsing fever spirochetes (Griffin, 1998). For late latent syphilis or syphilis of unknown duration, benzathine penicillin G is given in multiple doses in a course of several weeks. Stage of disease does not affect treatment for yaws, pinta, or endemic syphilis (Engelkens, 1991a, 1991b). A 10–14-day course of high-dose intravenous aqueous penicillin G is indicated for neurosyphilis and congenital syphilis. For patients coinfected with HIV and *T. pallidum*, current Centers for Disease Control and Prevention (CDC) guidelines do not recommend any significant deviation in therapy (Centers for Disease Control and Prevention, 2006). Indeed, prospective studies have failed to show any benefit of "enhanced" or alternative therapies for early syphilis and neurosyphilis, respectively, among HIV-infected persons (Rolfs, 1997; Marra, 2000). On the other hand, some authorities suggest that, given a propensity to develop neurosyphilis even in the face of treatment for primary syphilis, AIDS patients should be treated with higher doses of penicillin (Musher, 1991; Tramont, 2000).

OTHER TREPONEMAL DISEASES

Description

A number of spirochetes belonging to the treponeme molecular group-1, previously referred to as pathogen-related oral spirochetes, and various species of *Treponema* (e.g., *Treponema denticola, Treponema socranski*) have been recovered with increased frequency and in higher numbers from the gingiva of patients with ulcerative gingivitis and chronic periodontitis compared with patients with healthy gingiva (Riviere, 1995, 1996; Loesche, 2001). Although originally thought to resemble *T. pallidum* on the basis of immuno–cross-reactivity and in vitro invasive properties, these putative pathogens are rather genetically heterogeneous—only distantly related to *T. pallidum*—and can be induced to express cross-reactive surface antigens (Choi, 1996; Riviere, 1999).

Pathogenesis

A definitive causal relationship between the spirochetes and these diseases has not been firmly established; however, their presence in significant numbers, more commonly in diseased than in healthy tissue, suggests at least an association with gingivitis/periodontitis. Because of the fact that a number of other nontreponemal bacterial genera (e.g., *Prevotella, Actinobacillus, Porphyromonas*) have also been associated with these clinical manifestations, the current debate seems primarily to involve determining whether culpability belongs to specific virulent organisms among them or rather to the overall diversity of organisms contained within the plaque biofilm (Loesche, 2001).

Diagnosis

As with the commensal species of *Treponema* found in the genital area, some oral *Treponema* species can be cultured under strict anaerobic conditions using a variety of specialized, enriched broth media (Choi, 1996; Riviere, 1999). Other species, including most of those associated with periodontal disease, have not been cultured in vitro (Loesche, 2001). These organisms have been detected with monoclonal antibodies against *T. pallidum*, with which they cross-react. Other investigators have employed a variety of genetic amplification tools in an effort to identify and characterize them (Paster, 2001; Hutter, 2003). These "molecular expeditions" are conducted by using primers that target conserved bacterial sequences and either PCR to amplify ribosomal (rRNA) genes or reverse-transcriptase PCR to amplify the rRNA itself. Resultant products can then be cloned in *Escherichia coli* and sequenced to determine phylogenetic relationships.

Treatment

For years, treatment has been aimed primarily at reducing the overall bacterial burden by removing the plaque biofilm, both above and below the gumline, through physical manipulation (e.g., surgical debridement). Recently, the addition of various antimicrobial regimens, including systemic antibiotics and locally applied agents, has been shown to be a potentially beneficial adjunct (Loesche, 2001).

LEPTOSPIRA

DESCRIPTION

The genus *Leptospira* is composed of 18 genomic species, many containing both pathogenic and nonpathogenic strains, and more than 260 serovars (Perolat, 1998; Brenner, 1999). Previously, *Leptospira* was divided into three species, *L. interrogans* (pathogenic), *L. biflexa* (nonpathogenic), and *L. parva* (nonpathogenic), based on biochemical properties. However, it has become evident that such properties, in addition to pathogenicity and antigenicity, are not consistently predictive of genetic relatedness (Levett, 2001). Leptospires are tightly coiled with hooked ends, 0.1 µm in width by 6–20 µm in length, and demonstrate a spinning motility. They survive in alkaline fresh water but are killed by acid pH, salt water, and drying.

EPIDEMIOLOGY

Leptospirosis is perhaps the most widespread global zoonosis; although it was identified nearly 100 years ago, it is still considered an important emerging disease. Individual serovars show geographic preferences, as well as particular ecologic niches. The organism is carried by many rodents and feral and domestic animals; however, the rat is one of the most frequent reservoirs and an important source of infection in man. Contact with urine-contaminated water along with entry of the bacteria through cuts or mucosal surfaces is a frequent mode of infection. Those with occupational exposure (e.g., miners, farmers and field workers, veterinarians, fish farmers, sewage workers) or recreational exposure (e.g., camping near or swimming in infected waterways) are at particular risk. The incidence in the United States is 40–120 cases per year; however, the disease is probably significantly underreported (Farr, 1995).

PATHOLOGY AND PATHOGENESIS

After entry into the circulation, the organisms disseminate widely, including into the CNS and eye. Damage to endothelium in infected tissues results in local ischemia and hemorrhage. Hepatocellular damage and renal tubular damage also occur. The liver may have a characteristic yellow-green color, but histologic changes are nonspecific and include ballooning degeneration, acidophilic bodies, regeneration, and cholestasis; leptospires can be found in around 25% of cases (Dooley, 1976). The kidney shows a chronic interstitial nephritis, necrosis of proximal tubules, and granular or hyaline casts, with intratubular leptospires in around 65% (Arean, 1962). Pulmonary manifestations include congestion and edema, alveolar hemorrhage, pleural effusion, and occasional hyaline membrane formation (Arean, 1962; Ramachandran, 1977). Myocarditis, meningitis/encephalitis, and myositis may also be seen (Arean, 1962). The mechanisms for endothelial, hepatic, and renal damage are unknown but may be immune mediated.

CLINICAL MANIFESTATIONS

Typically, infection with leptospires presents as a mild, influenza-like illness (anicteric form) or is subclinical and never recognized; in the minority of patients, a more severe form characterized by jaundice is reported and has a 5%–10% fatality rate (icteric form or Weil's disease). Leptospirosis is biphasic, beginning, after an incubation period of 2–20 days, with the abrupt appearance of chills, fever, headache, myalgia, back pain, abdominal pain, anorexia, and nausea and vomiting. During this phase, termed the bacteremic phase, wide dissemination of bacteria occurs. The bacteremic phase lasts 4–7 days and is followed by a short remission of several days, after which the immune phase, characterized by the appearance of antibodies to the organism, meningitis, uveitis, rash, and hepatic and renal damage, occurs. A pretibial rash has been associated with infection by serovar autumnalis (Fort Bragg fever). In many, the immune phase is mild and lasts only 1–3 days. About half of patients have clinical signs of meningitis and a CSF pleocytosis during the second week of illness. In the small percentage of patients who suffer from Weil's disease, the two phases merge with persistent high fever, jaundice, and bleeding, followed by oliguric renal failure, shock, and myocarditis. Mortality has been reported to be 5%–10% in Weil's disease (Edwards, 1960; Arean, 1962; Levett, 2001).

LABORATORY DIAGNOSIS

Leptospires can be isolated from CSF, blood, and tissues early in the bacteremic phase (first 10 days), and from urine during the immune phase (second week to up to 30 days). Culture requires a semisolid medium (Fletcher's or Ellinghausen-McCullough-Johnson-Harris), which is incubated in the dark for 4–6 weeks at 25°–30° C. Urine requires alkalinization unless cultured immediately. Leptospires grow 1–3cm below the surface of the medium and may form a linear disk of growth. Material from this location should be examined by darkfield microscopy weekly for the characteristic spinning leptospires with hooked ends. Leptospiral antigens, detected directly in clinical specimens (e.g., ELISA, radioimmunoassay, immunomagnetic capture) or in processed tissue samples (e.g., immunofluorescence, immunohistochemistry), have been used with variable success in the diagnosis of leptospirosis.

A majority of cases, by contrast, are diagnosed serologically. Agglutinating antibodies appear during the first week of illness, peak at around 3–4 weeks, and may persist for years. Antibodies can be detected using bacterial antigens by a macroscopic or microscopic agglutination test, a hemagglutination test, or enzyme immunoassay (EIA) testing. The microscopic agglutination test, which employs antigen from live bacteria, is the established serologic reference method but is used primarily in a research setting. Recently, a modified EIA dipstick test that detects *Leptospira*-specific antibodies has been used with success in settings with minimal laboratory facilities (Gussenhoven, 1997; Yersin, 1999). Molecular methods, including hybridization techniques and PCR, have been used to detect leptospiral DNA in infected patients (Vinetz, 1996; Levett, 2001).

TREATMENT

Severe disease requires aqueous penicillin G or ampicillin given intravenously, and less severe disease can be treated with oral ampicillin, amoxicillin, or doxycycline. Prophylaxis with doxycycline provides protection for individuals in high-exposure environments (Farr, 1995). Immunization of domestic livestock and pets has reduced the danger of infection from these animals to high-risk populations such as veterinarians and farmers. Risk is not completely eliminated, as infection has been shown to occur in immunized animals with transmission of the disease to humans (Feigin, 1973).

BORRELIA

The genus *Borrelia* contains several pathogenic and nonpathogenic species that form two clades: the Lyme borreliosis group (or *Borrelia burgdorferi* sensu lato [s.l.]) and the relapsing fever group. The former has been divided into several genospecies by molecular analyses, three of which cause most human disease: *B. burgdorferi* sensu stricto (s.s.), *Borrelia garinii*, and *Borrelia afzelii*. The relapsing fever group contains a variety of species that can be isolated from argasid (soft) ticks (e.g., *Borrelia hermsii*, *Borrelia turicatae*), ixodid (hard) ticks (e.g., *Borrelia lonestari*, *Borrelia miyamotoi*), and the human body louse (*Borrelia recurrentis*). Morphologically similar to the treponemes, members of the *Borrelia* genus are helical bacteria ranging in size from 5–30 µm long by 0.2–0.5 µm wide. They are actively motile, contain 7–22 periplasmic flagella, and multiply by binary fission. Unlike *Treponema* spp., however, *Borrelia* exhibit a multitude of immunogenic proteins on their outer membrane surfaces, and many species can be cultivated in/on artificial media. Moreover, the intricacies of the *Borrelia* genome, with its 910-kB linear chromosome and 21 linear and circular plasmids, render it a more genetically complex genus than *Treponema* (Porcella, 2001).

What follows is a description of the two major clinical disease forms of human borreliosis, each of which is vector-borne. As such, these entities must often be considered, both from an epidemiologic and from a clinical standpoint, in conjunction with other infectious agents transmitted by identical tick vectors. Examples include the flaviviral agents of tick-borne encephalitis and various bacteria of the Rickettsiaceae, Ehrlichiaceae, and Francisellaceae families, as well as the protist *Babesia microti*. Clinical and diagnostic information related to these and other vector-borne diseases may be found elsewhere in this volume.

LYME DISEASE

The most common tick-borne illness in North America and Europe today (Wang, 1999), Lyme disease (Lyme borreliosis) was so named during the 1970s following an epidemic of oligoarticular arthritis encompassing several communities in eastern Connecticut, chief among them the town of Old Lyme (Steere, 1977a, 1977b). Epidemiologic inquiry soon established an association between Lyme disease (then referred to as Lyme arthritis) and the hard tick *Ixodes scapularis* (previously *Ixodes dammini*) (Steere, 1978). Within 4 years, Burgdorfer and colleagues had (1) isolated a novel spirochete species from an ixodid tick collected in New York, (2) reproduced the characteristic primary dermal lesions of Lyme disease in tick-fed rabbit models, and (3) demonstrated seroreactivity to antigens of this novel spirochete both in the rabbit model and in convalescent sera from human cases (Burgdorfer, 1982). The contemporary "immunologic" variation of Koch's postulates were thereby fulfilled (Fredricks, 1996). The implicated organism was subsequently recognized as a member of the genus *Borrelia* and named *B. burgdorferi* in recognition of its discoverer. In retrospect, different aspects of the multisystem inflammatory ailment now commonly known as Lyme disease had been recognized and described both in Europe (Afzelius, 1910; Bannwarth, 1941) and in the United States (Scrimenti, 1970) prior to the epidemic in Connecticut. Yet the present body of knowledge pertaining to Lyme borreliosis can be attributed in large part to the establishment and identification of its infectious origin spawned by the New England outbreak.

Epidemiology and Pathogenesis

A total of 15 different genospecies of *Borrelia* from the Lyme borreliosis group have been phylogenetically characterized (Rudenko, 2009). The three well-established human pathogens include *B. burgdorferi* s.s., which causes Lyme disease in North America, Europe, and Asia, and *B. garinii* and *B. afzelii*, which cause similar but subtly different illnesses in Europe and Asia (van Dam, 2002). The remaining 12 *Borrelia* species have been isolated from a variety of geographic locations, vertebrate hosts, and/or invertebrate vectors. Their roles as etiologic agents of human disease remain in various stages of elucidation at present.

Geographic distributions of *B. burgdorferi* s.l. and consequent regional prevalence of Lyme disease are the result of complex enzootic cycles involving one or several tick vectors of the *Ixodes ricinus* complex, various animal reservoirs, and incidental hosts. Seasonal variability in disease onset parallels the life cycle and questing periods of ixodid ticks (Falco, 1999). In the United States, *B. burgdorferi* s.s. is endemic in the Northeast, Upper Midwest, and Northwest regions, where the annual incidence of Lyme disease regionally averages 10–100 cases/100,000 population (Fig. 59-8). The overall number of reported cases, however, is considerably lower in the Northwest than in the other two endemic foci (Centers for Disease Control and Prevention, 2004b). This discrepancy may be attributable in part to differences in *Borrelia* populations (Girard, 2009) but also likely reflects the distinct enzootic cycles maintained in these regions. In the Northwest, perpetuation of *B. burgdorferi* s.s. involves *Ixodes spinipalpis* ticks, which feed on dusky-footed woodrats but not on humans. The ticks acquire and transmit infection between susceptible and infected reservoir hosts in an endemic cycle. However, the Western black-legged tick (*Ixodes pacificus*) (Fig. 59-9, *A*), which feeds primarily on reptiles and humans, occasionally becomes infected after conceding its preferences and feeding on the woodrat. A potential consequence of this event is human infection. Yet because of the infrequency of such a concession on the part of *I. pacificus*, the overall incidence of Lyme disease remains fairly low in the region. By contrast, the chief vector in the Midwest and Northeast, *I. scapularis* (black-legged or deer tick) (Fig. 59-9, *B*), promiscuously feeds on humans and on the spirochete's principal animal reservoir, the white-footed mouse. This results in proficient transmission to humans and an extremely high disease incidence, exceeding 1000 cases/100,000 population in certain communities (Shapiro, 2000; Steere, 2001). The most important tick vectors in Europe and Asia include *I. ricinus* (sheep tick) and *Ixodes persulcatus*, respectively, whereas primary animal reservoirs for *B. afzelii* and *B. garinii* are small rodents, voles, and/or various avian species (Fukunaga, 1995; Wang, 1999; Parola, 2001).

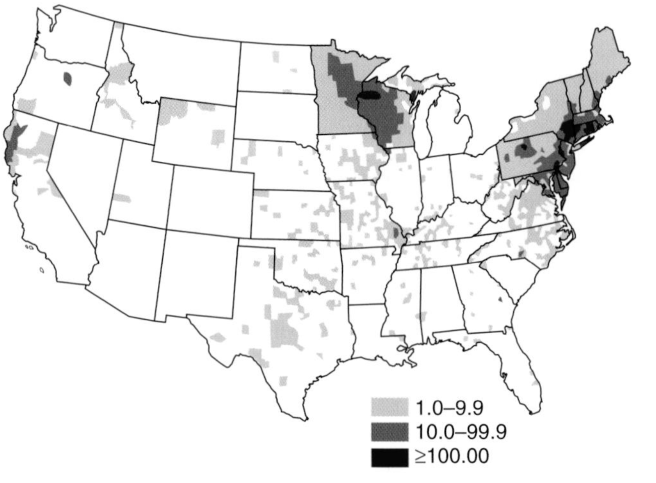

Figure 59-8 Average rate (per 100,000 population) of Lyme disease by county of residence—United States, 1998–2006. *(From Bacon RM, Kugeler KJ, Mead PS. Surveillance for Lyme disease—United States, 1992–2006. MMWR 2008;57[SS10]: 1–9.)*

Many other epidemiologic factors contribute to the transmission dynamics of *B. burgdorferi* s.l. High vector densities and infection rates, abundance and infectivity of reservoir hosts, and increased likelihood of human exposure all enhance the risk of Lyme disease (Parola, 2001). Furthermore, amplification of *Borrelia* in nonreservoir hosts may also influence regional disease incidence. Such has been postulated as the case in the Northeastern United States, where high population densities of white-tailed deer are thought to contribute to extremely high human infection rates (Steere, 2000). Another important transmission variable is related to the nature and duration of vector attachment during feeding. Hard-tick life cycles consist of three developmental stages, each of which secures only a single blood meal before transition to the next stage (or oviposition, in the case of an adult female). Because *B. burgdorferi* s.l. is not efficiently transmitted vertically in *Ixodes* spp., larvae acquire the spirochete while feeding upon an infected host (Shapiro, 2000; Scoles, 2001). The larval form, consequently, is not a direct vector for human infection (Patterson, 2003). Upon taking a blood meal, the larvae molt to the nymphal stage. Both nymphal and adult forms are capable of feeding on and transmitting organisms to humans, but the former are considerably smaller and are much more likely to go unrecognized while attached. Because efficient transmission of *Borrelia* to a susceptible host requires prolonged feeding durations (Piesman, 1987; Sood, 1997), the nymph is probably the principal vector for human transmission (Falco, 1999; Nadelman, 2001).

As with *T. pallidum*, the genomic sequence of *B. burgdorferi* s.s. has been completely characterized (Fraser, 1997), revealing a number of biosynthetic "gaps," in addition to a few seemingly important lipoproteins. The latter include a group of outer surface proteins (Osp), A–F, which are encoded by plasmids, differentially expressed in vector and mammal environments, and highly immunostimulatory (de Silva, 1997; Porcella, 2001). A lipoprotein, VlsE (for "variable major protein-like sequence expressed"), with the capability to undergo extensive antigenic variation has also been described in *B. burgdorferi* (Zhang, 1998; Porcella, 2001). The diversity of symptoms observed in Lyme borreliosis is probably due to the direct effects of spirochete dissemination, as well as to the extent of the host immune response (Sigal, 1997; Whooten, 2001). Many animal models of Lyme borreliosis have been developed, some of which have been useful for investigating the dynamics of *Borrelia* dissemination (e.g., tissue localization within heart, skin, and joints), in addition to specific cellular interactions (e.g., with host glycosaminoglycans and plasminogen) (Sigal, 1997; Steere, 2000). The mouse model has been particularly valuable in uncovering details of immunologic responses in Lyme disease (Whooten, 2001). A paucity of cultivable organisms or detectable genomic material within lesions of long-standing, treatment-resistant disease, such as occurs in Lyme arthritis, suggest autoimmune event(s) rather than direct spirochete injury as a pathogenic mechanism. Reported associations between Lyme arthritis and HLA-DR4 as well as an autoantigen candidate, leukocyte function antigen-1, further substantiate this hypothesis (Gross, 1998; Steere, 2004).

Clinical Manifestations

Analogous to syphilis, the clinical progression of Lyme borreliosis has been divided into three general stages: (1) an early localized phase in which a primary lesion develops in the vicinity of the inoculation site, (2) an early disseminated phase wherein the spirochetes spread systemically, causing a variety of cardiac, neurologic, and/or dermatologic manifestations, and (3) a late phase, which may be heralded by other neurologic and/or dermatologic phenomena, in addition to rheumatologic disease. Because symptom overlap occurs during early disseminated and late persistent infection, some investigators abstain from using this clinical staging system, preferring instead simply to incorporate duration of illness into diagnostic and therapeutic considerations (Kaiser, 1998; Nadelman, 1998). Asymptomatic seroconversion or subclinical disease has also been reported to occur in as many as 7% of persons within endemic areas (Steere, 2003). Given the wide diversity of symptoms, Lyme borreliosis, similar to syphilis, has been aptly labeled "the great imitator."

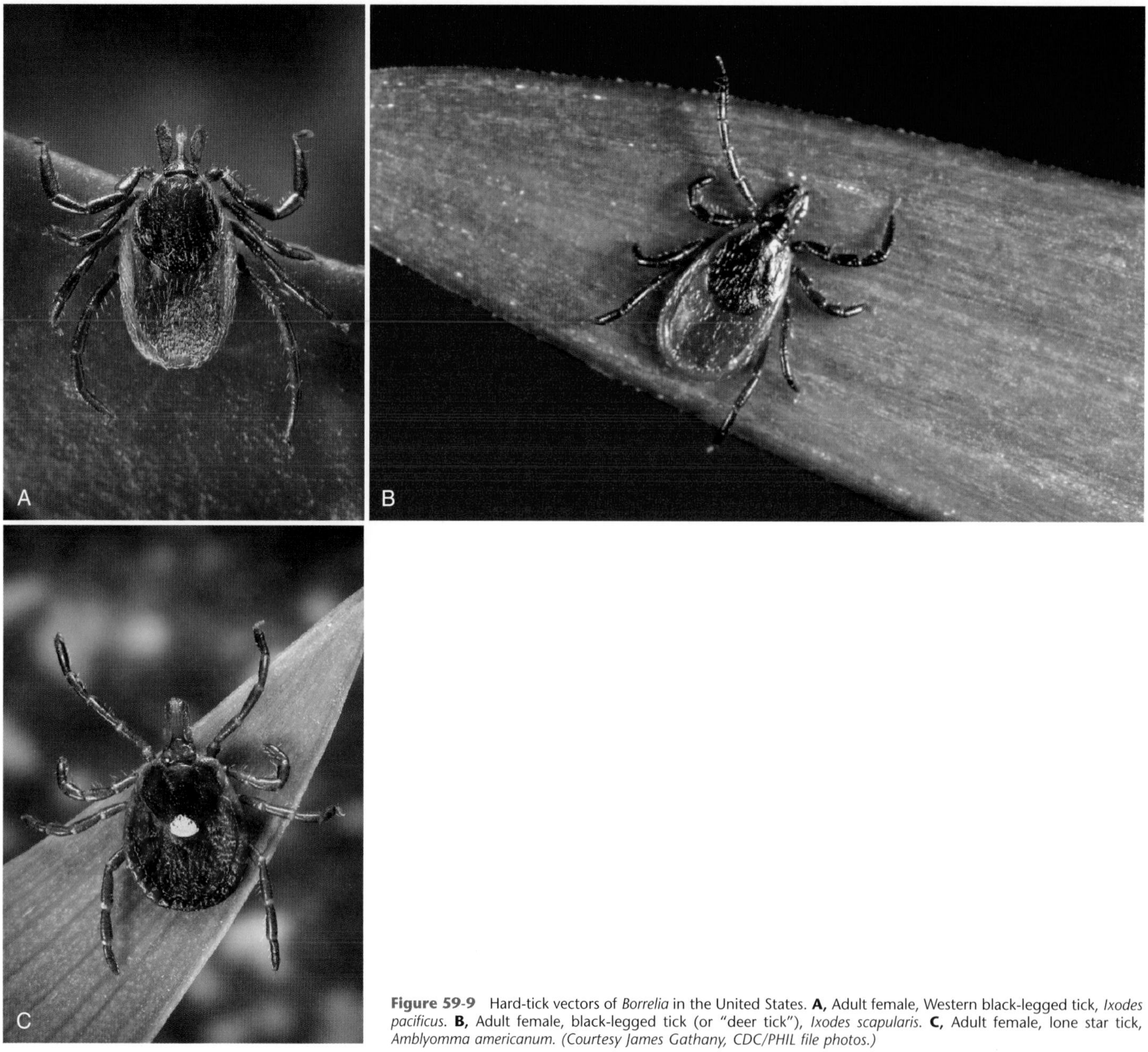

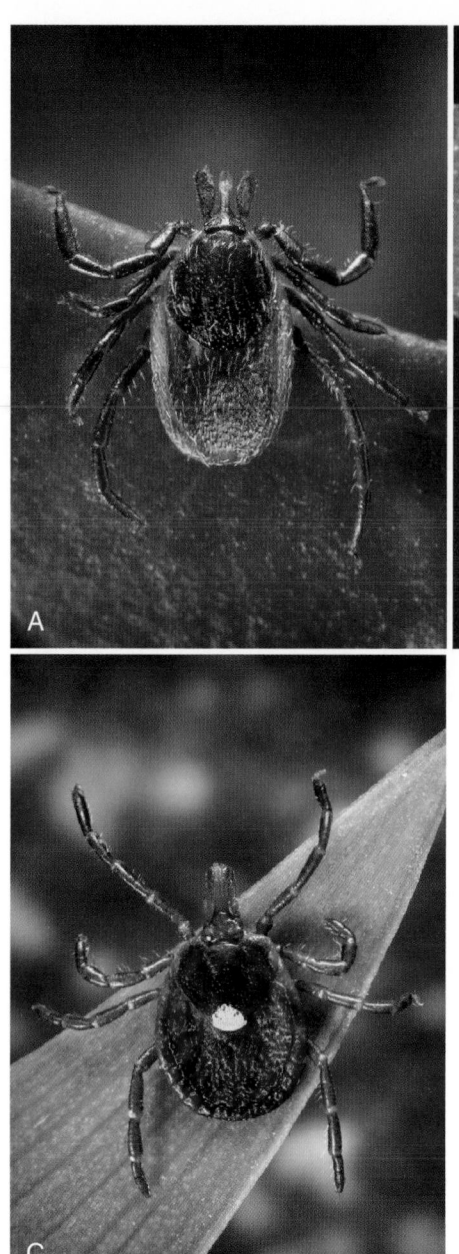

Figure 59-9 Hard-tick vectors of *Borrelia* in the United States. **A,** Adult female, Western black-legged tick, *Ixodes pacificus.* **B,** Adult female, black-legged tick (or "deer tick"), *Ixodes scapularis.* **C,** Adult female, lone star tick, *Amblyomma americanum. (Courtesy James Gathany, CDC/PHIL file photos.)*

The earliest clinical stage begins ≈1 week following the bite of an infected tick, at which time a characteristic rash, descriptively termed erythema migrans, develops near the inoculation site in a majority of patients (the exact proportion depends upon case definition or study inclusion criteria). The lesion begins as a painless red macule or papule and subsequently expands to become an erythematous patch measuring up to 70 cm (Nadelman, 1996). Erythema migrans is typically painless, characteristically demonstrates central pallor, imparting a "target-like" or "bull's-eye" appearance (Fig. 59-10), and may be accompanied by nonspecific symptoms such as fever, fatigue, headache, and myalgia, as well as regional lymphadenopathy (Nadelman, 1996; Smith, 2002). Histologic analysis reveals superficial, perivascular dermatitis comprising lymphocytes, macrophages, and abundant plasma cells; these organisms can sometimes be visualized in tissue sections treated with silver impregnation stains or by immunohistochemical techniques (Duray, 1997). Unlike the lesions of syphilis, vasculitis is not a typical histologic feature of erythema migrans.

Dissemination of *Borrelia* portends the second stage of clinical illness, in which many organ systems may be affected. Smaller, secondary erythema migrans lesions arising in multiple sites are one of the more common signs of early dissemination (Shapiro, 2000). Neurologic manifestations (neuroborreliosis) affect up to 15% of U.S. patients, with symptoms including cranial nerve palsy (commonly cranial nerve VII), lymphocytic meningitis, and a variety of peripheral neuropathies (e.g., painful radiculitis) (Steere, 2001; Halperin, 2002). These manifestations are collectively referred to as **Bannwarth syndrome** in some European countries (Kaiser, 1998). Somewhat rarer, cardiac involvement in the form of transient atrioventricular block or myocarditis has also been reported in approximately 5% of patients with Lyme disease (Steere, 2001). Other sites potentially affected include the musculoskeletal system (e.g., fatigue, malaise), liver (e.g., mild, transient hepatitis), and eyes (e.g., conjunctivitis, neuroretinitis) (Lesser, 1995; Steere, 2000).

In the United States, the most common manifestation of untreated, late-stage Lyme disease is arthritis, which develops in well over half of untreated patients (Steere, 2000). Typically monoarticular or oligoarticular in extent, large joints such as the knee are frequently involved (Steere, 1977a, 2001). Symptoms of pain and swelling begin acutely several weeks to months following spirochete inoculation and last for several days to months (median, 1 week) (Steere, 1977b). Whether the result of autoimmunity or persistent infection, many patients continue to experience intermittent recurrences of migratory arthritis followed by prolonged disease-free periods (Nadelman, 1998). Conversely, late-stage

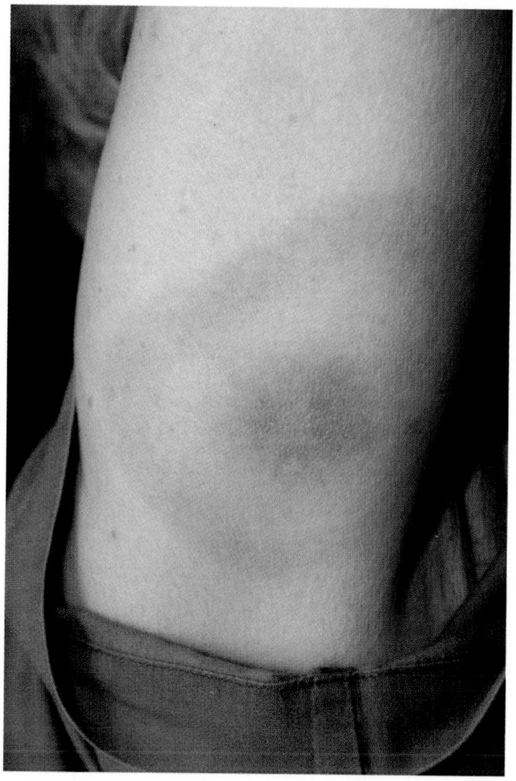

Figure 59-10 Characteristic "bull's-eye" lesion, erythema migrans, observed at the site of spirochete inoculation in ≈80% of patients with Lyme disease. *(Courtesy James Gathany, CDC/PHIL file photo.)*

manifestations of persistent Lyme borreliosis in European patients often involve neurologic or cutaneous organs. The former may overlap clinically with early disseminated neuroborreliosis and may include lymphocytic meningitis and peripheral neuropathies (e.g., sensory polyneuritis, pareses). In addition, CNS manifestations such as myelitis and spastic-ataxic gait disturbances, as well as short-term cognitive dysfunction, have been noted (Kaiser, 1998; Halperin, 2002). A dermatologic phenomenon known as acrodermatitis chronica atrophica has also been associated with late Lyme borreliosis in Europe. As the name implies, lesions are present on hands, wrists, elbows, and feet. They are often symmetrical and are characterized histologically by a lymphomononuclear and, to a lesser extent, granulocytic infiltrate with progressive epidermal thinning, hyperkeratosis, and dermal atrophy (Aberer, 1991; Duray, 1997). Other well-established or controversial long-term dermatologic manifestations include *Borrelia* lymphocytoma, cutaneous B cell lymphoma, morphea, and lichen sclerosis et atrophica (Duray, 1997; McGinley-Smith, 2003).

Variations in clinical manifestations, particularly during the late stages of Lyme disease, have been ascribed in part to inherent traits of the organisms themselves, whether genospecies or strain specific. For instance, *B. afzelii* (previously group VS461) has been disproportionately isolated from lesions of erythema migrans and acrodermatitis chronica atrophica in Europe as compared with other genospecies of *Borrelia* (van Dam, 1993; Balmelli, 1995; Wang, 1999). By contrast, *B. garinii* is more frequently implicated in European cases of neuroborreliosis (Balmelli, 1995; Wang, 1999). Other studies demonstrate that particular molecular subtypes of *B. burgdorferi* s.s. are more frequently associated with invasive properties and spirochetemia (Dykhuizen, 2008; Wormser, 2008). Additional observations corroborating the notion that disease course is influenced by inherent properties of the infecting *Borrelia* strain include the following: (1) Serologic responses among patients with particular clinical symptoms may be preferential toward antigens from specific *Borrelia* sources; and (2) certain genospecies appear to have different properties in vitro (Dressler, 1994; Norman, 1996; Wang, 1999).

In the vast majority of patients, clinical manifestations of Lyme disease respond to appropriate antibiotic therapy (Shadick, 1999; Seltzer, 2000; Wormser, 2006). Yet a small subset may continue to experience persistent symptoms such as musculoskeletal pain, fatigue, and neurocognitive deficits despite treatment—a condition that has variably been termed "post-Lyme disease syndrome," "chronic Lyme disease" or "treatment-resistant borreliosis" (Klempner, 2002). With few exceptions to date, prospective studies have shown little benefit of prolonged antibiotic therapy over placebo in reducing the symptoms of this syndrome. Further, isolation of *Borrelia* or amplification of *Borrelia* genes is often unsuccessful among patients with this disorder (Klempner, 2002). Retrospective case-controlled studies illustrate that the frequency of objective signs among "chronic Lyme disease" patients is similar to that among age-matched controls without a history of Lyme disease (Shadick, 1999; Seltzer, 2000). A recent review summarizes the evidence, or lack thereof, to support a link between *B. burgdorferi* and this chronic syndrome (Feder, 2007). It should be noted that despite the existence of only one body of medical literature, strong opposition to this viewpoint exists. Adamant dissent is evidenced not only by the many correspondence letters referencing the report by Feder et al. (2007), but also by an advocacy group, the International Lyme and Associated Diseases Society, which has issued its own management recommendations distinct from those of the Infectious Disease Society of America (IDSA), and which has contributed significant testimony to an antitrust investigation brought against IDSA by the state of Connecticut. The investigation culminated in an agreement by IDSA to allow review of the guidelines by an independent arbiter, which ultimately upheld essentially all of the prior recommendations (though not without controversy).

Several reports have documented erythema migrans–like lesions in patients residing in Southern United States. Occasionally referred to as Southern tick-associated rash illness, the lesions are preceded by the bite of the lone star tick, *Amblyomma americanum* (see Fig. 59-9, *C*), and have not yielded any *B. burgdorferi* s.s. isolates to date (Kirkland, 1997; James, 2001). Instead, a novel agent, *B. lonestari* sp. *nov.*, of the relapsing-fever group, has been tentatively implicated (Varela, 2004). Because *B. burgdorferi* s.s. does occur naturally within this geographic area (Oliver, 2003), future epidemiologic work will be required to determine the details and extent of disease caused by each of these organisms in the region.

Laboratory Diagnosis

Issued for surveillance purposes, the CDC case definition of Lyme disease emphasizes clinical findings and physical examination; the development of physician-diagnosed erythema migrans in a patient with possible tick exposure is considered diagnostic (Centers for Disease Control and Prevention, 1997). Laboratory confirmation is required only for less specific, objective signs that would be expected to develop later in the disease course (e.g., arthritis, cranial neuritis, cardiac conduction defects). Other experts agree that laboratory testing, particularly using indirect methods such as serologic tests, should not be performed as standalone diagnostic modalities, but rather should serve as tools to assist in confirming or refuting clinical suspicions (Luger, 1990; Tugwell, 1997; Brown, 1999). Reports highlighting the concepts of pretest probability based on epidemiologic and clinical factors, as well as likelihood ratios and test predictive values, thoroughly demonstrate the futility and high cost of such a standalone approach (Seltzer, 1996; Tugwell, 1997; Nichol, 1998). In fact, Lyme disease testing for patients with only nonspecific symptoms like fatigue, headache, or myalgia (i.e., when pretest probability is = 0.2), even in endemic areas using accurate laboratory assays, can lead to more false-positive than true-positive results (Tugwell, 1997). Exacerbated by widespread anxiety on the part of the public and a general misunderstanding by many healthcare providers, the current diagnostic confusion surrounding Lyme borreliosis can perhaps be best dealt with by taking a thorough look at the indications for and limitations of laboratory testing.

Culture

Culture usually serves as the "gold standard" in diagnostic testing for infectious diseases in which the causative agent does not also asymptomatically colonize humans. Yet, despite the fact that cultivation of *Borrelia* spp. is readily achievable and often is not as time-consuming as for other pathogenic microorganisms (Reed, 2002), most clinical and commercial diagnostic laboratories do not offer this testing alternative. Several modifications of the broth-based Barber-Stoenner-Kelly medium have been shown not only to support the growth of *Borrelia* spp. but to be useful in their recovery from biopsy tissue of erythema migrans lesions and large-volume plasma collections during the early, acute phase of disease (Nadelman, 1996; Steere, 1998; Wormser, 2001). Given the specificity of organism isolation and the absence of measurable antibody in most patients with *B. burgdorferi* s.l. infection during the early phase of clinical illness, culture would seem to be a very practical diagnostic modality. However, reliance on darkfield microscopy or fluorescent antibodies for the detection and identification of positive cultures, high media and reagent costs, wide reported sensitivity ranges (doubtless the result of variability in quantity of tissue/blood cultured and timing of specimen collection), and the requirement that invasive procedures be performed on the patient (e.g., tissue biopsy) have probably all contributed to the test's general unpopularity outside the research arena. It is important to note that recovery of *Borrelia* from CSF, synovial fluid, or other samples collected beyond the early phases of disease is so frequently unsuccessful as to be of little diagnostic utility. For this reason, other laboratory testing modalities for Lyme borreliosis are important adjuncts.

Serologic Tests

Detection of *Borrelia*-specific antibody production during Lyme disease may be accomplished using a variety of methods that express results in terms of total Ig or class-specific IgG or IgM. Immunofluorescent antibody (IFA) assays, which typically contain antigen in the form of whole cell *B. burgdorferi* s.s. fixed to glass slides, were popular in the 1980s but have been largely superseded by the more automated and less subjective ELISA, which incorporates select antigens that are recombinantly produced or derived from partially purified extracts of *Borrelia*.

As with all serologic responses to infectious causes, a multitude of variables potentially affect the performance of assays developed to detect them. False-negative and false-positive results may consequently serve only to confound clinical impressions. Early in the course of Lyme disease, absence of antibody (or levels below the limit of detection) leads to false-negative results. This is circumvented in part with assays that detect IgM specifically, because IgM production precedes the development of an IgG response (Shapiro, 2000; Reed, 2002). As the disease progresses, test sensitivity increases (Engstrom, 1995; Brown, 1999; Liang, 1999). In fact, a recent study demonstrates that the duration of illness itself is of greater importance for serologic detection than is test method or format (Wormser, 2008). Specificity of the IFA and ELISA may also be adversely affected by cross-reacting antibodies to a variety of microorganism- and host-derived proteins. Some of these include pathogenic spirochetes (e.g., relapsing fever group of *Borrelia* and treponemes) and other bacteria (e.g., *Helicobacter pylori*) and viruses (e.g., Epstein-Barr), as well as antinuclear antigens present in autoimmune disorders such as systemic lupus erythematosus (Brown, 1999; Reed, 2002). Previous immunization with the OspA subunit Lyme disease vaccine may lead to false-positive ELISA and IFA results as well, given that this lipoprotein is typically an integral antigenic component of these tests (Steere, 1998). Other factors that may contribute to test limitations include the composition of antigen contained in the particular assay, the level of quality control within the testing facility, the interpretive levels at which positive and negative (and indeterminate) optical density or index values are set, the particular bacterial strain responsible for infection, and the patient's individual immune response.

In an effort to increase the accuracy of serologic testing as a whole, the CDC proposed the use of a two-tiered algorithm, in which all positive and indeterminate results obtained by ELISA or IFA are subsequently tested by another method, the immunoblot (Centers for Disease Control and Prevention, 1995). In this assay, proteins extracted from low-passaged *B. burgdorferi* s.s. are quantitatively standardized and then separated by electrophoresis on the basis of size and charge. Following transfer to a membrane substrate, control and test sera (in addition to a panel of monoclonal antibodies for reference and calibration) are incubated with the *Borrelia* proteins. Nonspecific immunoglobulin is removed by washing, while *Borrelia*-specific antibody is bound and visualized using an enzyme-linked conjugate. This technique provides the capability to discern antibodies against particular proteins. Interpretation is somewhat subjective, and criteria defining positive results vary somewhat. Band patterns defining a positive result as outlined by CDC (Centers for Disease Control and Prevention, 1995) are depicted in Figure 59-11.

This tiered approach theoretically consists of a highly sensitive first-round test that detects most cases of Lyme disease, followed by a highly specific assay that excludes any false-positive results from the first round (Dressler, 1993; Ledue, 1996). Clinical practice is not theoretical, however, and the high degree of interlaboratory and intralaboratory variability, less than ideal sensitivity of ELISA and IFA, and wide ranges of reported performance for the immunoblot suggest that this approach may also be imperfect (Engstrom, 1995; Aguero-Rosenfeld, 1996; Ledue, 1996; Bakken, 1997). Even so, improvement in overall testing performance using the algorithm has been described, with the single major caveat that immunoblot results may be significantly influenced by the stage of disease during which testing is performed (Engstrom, 1995; Johnson, 1996). Incorporation into the algorithm of newer ELISAs that utilize

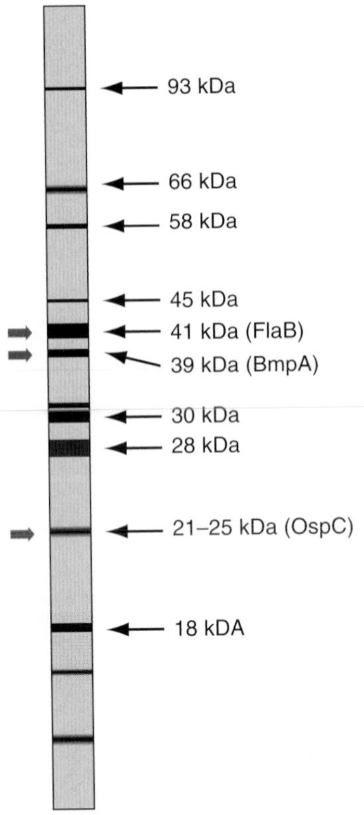

Figure 59-11 Ten major bands and respective molecular weights of antigens identified in *Borrelia burgdorferi* immunoblot assays. For positivity according to Centers for Disease Control and Prevention (CDC) recommendations, immunoglobulin (Ig)G-specific blots require the presence of 7 of 10 bands, whereas IgM-specific assays require 2 of 3 *(red arrow)* bands. *BmpA,* Basic membrane protein A; *FlaB,* flagellin; *kDa,* kilodaltons; *OspC,* outer surface protein C.

recombinant, highly conserved, and immunodominant antigens (e.g., VlsE) or portions thereof (26-mer peptide from the sixth invariable region [C6 peptide]) may ultimately serve to increase accuracy even further, particularly during early stages of disease (Gomes-Solecki, 2000; Bacon, 2003; Branda, 2009).

Peak antibody titers generally plateau between 7 and 30 days following the development of erythema migrans; the degree of reactivity (e.g., number of bands by Western blot or optical density reading by ELISA) is typically higher in patients with early dissemination (Aguero-Rosenfeld, 1996). Beyond 30 days, most (but not all) patients with Lyme disease will have developed an IgG response, so diagnostic reliance upon IgM assays alone is not recommended (Centers for Disease Control and Prevention, 1995). Several reports have suggested that therapeutic intervention early in the course of disease may abrogate the antibody response and lead to "seronegative" Lyme disease (Dattwyler, 1988; Aguero-Rosenfeld, 1996; Ledue, 1996). Although one retrospective European study demonstrated that treatment had no statistically significant effect on ultimate seroreactivity, the authors did note a trend toward higher seropositivity incidence and titer among patients who did not receive antibiotics (Plorer, 1993). Finally, because IgG and IgM detection may last many years after successful eradication of the spirochete, there appears to be no role in monitoring antibody levels during convalescence for determination of disease activity and response to therapy or in assessing IgM positivity as a means of establishing the timing of infection (Hilton, 1997; Kalish, 2001).

Several other laboratory-based immunologic techniques have been evaluated for potential use in the diagnosis of Lyme disease. Reports have indicated that *Borrelia*-specific antibodies detected by IFA, ELISA, and/or immunoblot in CSF and synovial fluid samples may be useful in confirming neuroborreliosis and Lyme arthritis, respectively, particularly when compared with serum levels (Cruz, 1991; Hansen, 1991). To our knowledge, no commercially available kits had been cleared for such use by the FDA, although some laboratories have validated this specimen source. Another method that showed promise in the identification of "seronegative" Lyme disease cases, the T cell proliferative assay, was probably too complex and insensitive to gain widespread appeal among diagnostic laboratories (Dressler, 1991). A recent strategy employing precipitation and dissociation of *Borrelia*-specific IgM from circulating immune complexes prior to capture on solid phase and quantitation shows promise (Brunner, 2001). Last, an antigen capture assay used on CSF or urine has been reported (Coyle, 1995; Klempner, 2001) but is not presently recommended for diagnostic purposes without additional validation studies (Tugwell, 1997).

Molecular Tests

Alternative testing methods for Lyme borreliosis have been strongly sought after, given the overall low sensitivity of culture and serologic assays. In the early 1990s, researchers set their sights on genomic amplification techniques, which were relatively new to the diagnostic armamentarium at that time. Since then, several modifications of the PCR using various genetic targets and amplicon detection methods have been applied to a variety of specimen types in search of *Borrelia* nucleic acids.

Samples from which *B. burgdorferi* s.l. could not be readily isolated were the primary focus of initial investigations on PCR utility. Studies of PCR analyses on joint aspirate samples from patients with Lyme arthritis demonstrated excellent sensitivity and specificity rates when several primer sets were used (Nocton, 1994; Dumler, 2001). After the results were compared with clinical information, it became apparent that (1) detection of *Borrelia* nucleic acids was more frequently associated with a history of absent or inadequate antimicrobial therapy, and (2) PCR positivity disappeared following appropriate treatment (Nocton, 1994). Further inquiry into a performance discrepancy of primer sets targeting genomic (e.g., rRNA genes) versus plasmid-derived (e.g., OspA, OspB genes) DNA revealed that the latter is present in higher quantities within joint spaces in Lyme arthritis (Persing, 1994). This phenomenon, termed **target imbalance,** seems to be unique to the inflammatory spirochete milieu of synovial fluid in Lyme arthritis and probably accounts for the higher sensitivity observed in tests that target the OspA gene (Lebech, 2002). By contrast, studies of amplification assays on CSF from patients with acute or chronic neuroborreliosis have demonstrated only minimal to moderate improvement in sensitivity over culture (Nocton, 1996; Dumler, 2001). In part the result of study inclusion criteria, the extremely wide reported sensitivity ranges are probably also due to the extremely low numbers of *Borrelia* genomic copies (i.e., levels near lower detection limits) in the CSF of affected patients (Schmidt, 1997). As a general rule, successful amplification occurs more frequently during the early stages of neurologic disease (Lebech, 2002).

PCR likewise has been applied to specimens collected during the primary and early disseminated stages of Lyme borreliosis. Nucleic acid detection in tissue from erythema migrans lesions has been successful; such an approach may offer improvement in both sensitivity and turnaround time over culture (Dumler, 2001). Testing of blood and plasma has also been attempted but is limited by the timing of sample collection (Schmidt, 1997). Initial reports of urine testing by PCR were encouraging because of the ease of specimen collection and the high sensitivity, but these findings have not been consistently reproduced (Brettschneider, 1998; Lebech, 2002). Additionally, detection of *Borrelia* genetic material extracted directly from ixodid tick vectors may be useful from an epidemiologic standpoint but should not be relied upon for diagnosis or management of patients from whom the ticks were removed (Sood, 1997; Dumler, 2001; Wormser, 2006).

In time, developments in technology and improvements in understanding will continue to lend themselves to new, creative uses for the PCR beyond simply diagnosis. For instance, the technique has been readily used alongside restriction fragment length polymorphism (RFLP) and DNA sequencing for subcategorization of *Borrelia* isolates for taxonomic purposes (Wang, 1999; Hoen, 2009). The use of labeled, internal hybridization probes within the reaction vessel has afforded the ability to detect and quantify amplification products in real time, which has provided clues about *Borrelia* transmission dynamics and pathogenesis (Pahl, 1999; Wang, 2002). In contrast to cases of HIV or hepatitis C virus, monitoring therapeutic responses by PCR has not been firmly established as beneficial in Lyme disease (Schmidt, 1997). However, the relationships between *Borrelia* genetic material in joints affected by Lyme arthritis, antibiotic therapy, and symptomatic outcome suggest that it may be established in the future (Nocton, 1994; Steere, 2004).

As with most amplification techniques, use of PCR for diagnosis of Lyme disease is limited by many factors, including polymerase inhibitors, low target levels, potential for contamination, primer choices, and method of amplicon detection. Whatever the application, the sensitivity and specificity of molecular tests are imperfect. Accordingly, negative results alone should never be used to exclude a diagnosis, and positive results out of context should not confirm a diagnosis. Misinterpretations such as these may lead to dismal consequences if not resolved early (Patel, 2000; Molloy, 2001). It is important to note that because most patients with late manifestations of Lyme disease will have evidence of seroreactivity by the time of presentation (thereby fulfilling the CDC case definition), PCR studies probably are best used during early Lyme disease prior to a serologic response. Of utmost importance is the correlation of laboratory data with clinical impression, irrespective of whether such data are derived through serologic or molecular means.

Treatment and Prevention

The IDSA has recently updated its guidelines for the management of patients with suspected or proven Lyme borreliosis (Wormser, 2006). To summarize, a large body of evidence in the form of randomized, prospective, double-blind studies has consistently demonstrated that a 2–3-week course of oral doxycycline or ampicillin is highly effective in the treatment of early, uncomplicated Lyme disease. Cefuroxime is also effective but is not recommended as first-line therapy because of cost. In patients unable to tolerate any of these regimens, or for whom such regimens would be contraindicated, macrolide therapy may be an acceptable alternative. Extended treatment courses of this standard oral regimen are also considered to be effective in most patients with Lyme arthritis in the absence of neurologic manifestations. However, parenteral therapy with ceftriaxone (or penicillin as an alternative) may be used in cases of arthritis relapse. This same intravenous regimen is recommended for patients with third-degree heart block and/or neuroborreliosis. Of note, most of the prospective therapeutic trials upon which IDSA recommendations are based have endpoints defined in terms of clinical responses (i.e., disappearance of symptoms) rather than the eradication of *Borrelia*.

A somewhat more contested issue surrounds the use of prophylactic antibiotic therapy following recognition and removal of a feeding tick. Early prospective studies employing 10-day oral regimens of antimicrobial prophylaxis failed to establish any benefit over placebo (Warshafsky, 1996). Factors that further confound the matter include (1) the extremely low success rate of *Borrelia* transmission to humans (1%–3%), even in hyperendemic areas where tick infection rates may exceed 50% (Shapiro, 1992; Nadelman, 2001); (2) the frequency with which tick bites are not recognized among patients with Lyme disease (up to 75% of patients) (Nadelman, 1996); (3) the inaccuracy of tick species identification and estimates of feeding duration by nonentomologists (Falco, 1998); and (4) the potential costs of widespread antibiotic use (e.g., financial, unanticipated side effects, bacterial resistance). One investigation demonstrated that a single 200-mg dose of doxycycline administered after removal of an *I. scapularis* tick significantly reduced the incidence of subsequent development of erythema migrans (Nadelman, 2001). Although interpretations of the study were mixed (Bellovin, 2001; Leenders, 2001; Shapiro, 2001), the latest IDSA guidelines state that prophylaxis "may be offered" if the epidemiologic findings (e.g., tick species, stage and duration of feeding, confirmed area of acquisition) are compelling.

Primary Lyme disease prevention strategies that are generally agreed upon include interventions that decrease both the likelihood and the duration of vector attachment and feeding. Use of insect repellents, acaricides, and barrier clothing such as long pants and long-sleeved shirts and the performance of daily "tick checks" have a theoretical if not proven value in reducing human cases of ixodid tick–borne disease (Poland, 2001; Hayes, 2003). The single most widely accepted and thoroughly tested prevention strategy, human vaccination, is no longer commercially available, however (Hitt, 2002). This subunit vaccine containing a lipidized, recombinant OspA antigen was shown to significantly reduce the incidence of Lyme borreliosis following a three-step immunization schedule (Steere, 1998). Because of low sales and perhaps an unfounded fear of complications, the product was withdrawn from the market in 2002.

RELAPSING FEVER

Relapsing fever can be divided into two distinctive entities based on microbiological and epidemiologic features. Epidemic louse-borne relapsing fever (LBRF) occurs worldwide, reflecting the ubiquitous distribution of its transmission vector, *Pediculus humanus* (Johnson, 2000). Although the disease has been largely eradicated from most developed nations, documented occurrences persist in parts of east Africa and South America (Sundnes, 1993; Raoult, 1999). Humans are the only known reservoir for the causative agent, *B. recurrentis*. Successful transmission between them does not require that the vector actually feed upon a human host. Rather, when an infected louse is crushed, susceptible persons are exposed and infected via contaminated hemolymph (Johnson, 2000).

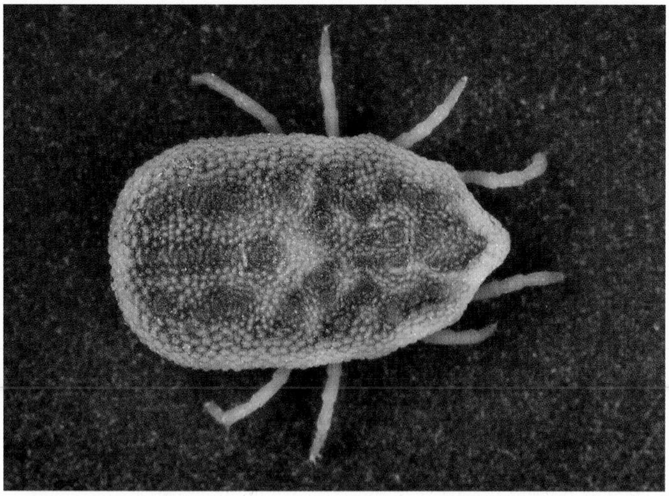

Figure 59-12 Example of a member of the Argasidae family of "soft ticks," which are responsible for transmission of endemic relapsing fever *Borrelia*. *(Courtesy James Gathany, CDC/PHIL file photo.)*

Endemic tick-borne relapsing fever (TBRF) has a narrower geographic distribution, paralleling that of its primary transmission vectors, argasid ticks of the genus *Ornithodoros* (Fig. 59-12). North American areas of disease endemicity include the Pacific Northwest, the Northern and Central Rocky Mountains, and parts of the Sierra range of California (*Ornithodoros hermsi* habitats), as well as the arid flatlands of Mexico, Texas, and New Mexico (*Ornithodoros turicata* habitats) (Dworkin, 2002). The disease is also well documented in parts of Africa and Europe (Parola, 2001). In the past, *Borrelia* spp. causing TBRF were considered to have a high degree of tick-vector specificity and were named after the *Ornithodoros* species from which they were isolated (Davis, 1942). Thus, *B. hermsi* and *B. turicatae* are associated with *O. hermsi* and *O. turicata*, respectively. However, recent reports demonstrating the presence of relapsing fever group *Borrelia* nucleic acids in several *Ixodes* tick species, many captured in regions of Lyme endemicity, may challenge this assumption (Fukunaga, 1995; Scoles, 2001; Fraenkel, 2002). Furthermore, because (1) serologic cross-reactivity between organisms from the two borreliosis clades is predictable (Schwan, 1996), and (2) relapsing fever–like spirochetes have been shown to produce disease in localities heretofore considered nonendemic for TBRF (Breitschwerdt, 1994), the clinical and diagnostic implications of these reports will undoubtedly spark renewed research on relapsing fever agents.

Transmission dynamics and, therefore, epidemiologic factors associated with TBRF are considerably different from those of Lyme disease. Argasid ticks feed nocturnally and for much shorter durations than ixodid ticks (Parola, 2001). Yet, because they harbor *Borrelia* in their salivary secretions, soft ticks can successfully inoculate spirochetes within minutes of feeding (Dworkin, 2002). Although *Ornithodoros* ticks can transmit *Borrelia* vertically (transovarial) and can maintain the bacteria in nature for extended periods, several mammalian hosts also contribute to spirochete persistence (Dworkin, 2002). Human cases often occur in small clusters following exposure to the vector while sleeping in rustic cabins or in seldom occupied rural dwellings *(O. hermsi)* or in caves *(O. turicata)* (Rawlings, 1995; Dworkin, 1998).

Clinical features of LBRF and TBRF are somewhat similar. Following an approximately 7-day incubation period, infected patients experience the acute onset of high fever (38.9°–40.0° C) accompanied by nonspecific symptoms such as headache, malaise, arthralgia, and fatigue (Southern, 1969; Dworkin, 1998). Minor hemorrhagic manifestations are not uncommon and may be related to transient thrombocytopenia. Hepatosplenomegaly is identified more frequently in patients with LBRF (Southern, 1969). Neurologic involvement in the form of meningitis, seventh nerve palsy, myelitis, and encephalitis has been reported (Cadavid, 1998). Almost as suddenly as they begin, symptoms subside after 3–6 days in most patients, only to relapse roughly 1 week later (Johnson, 2000). Similar episodes of symptomatic recurrence may continue up to as many as 13 times but more typically resolve after two or three relapses (Southern, 1969). These waves of recrudescence are believed to be due to the organism's extraordinary ability to quickly vary its surface protein antigenic makeup under immune (i.e. antibody) selective pressures, thus resulting in cycles of epitope variation and immune escape followed by new antibody production and organism suppression (Rich, 2001; Dworkin, 2002). Left untreated, LBRF appears to have a higher mortality rate than its tick-borne counterpart, but the contributive effects of other factors (e.g., famine, war) often accompanying LBRF may obscure direct comparisons (Dworkin, 2002). Nevertheless, self-limited cases of probable TBRF have been reported (Rawlings, 1995; Dworkin, 1998).

Microscopic examination of peripheral blood samples obtained during febrile episodes has been the traditional laboratory approach to diagnosis of relapsing fever. *Borrelia* organisms may be visualized in wet mounts using a darkfield technique or in fixed smears stained with Wright-Giemsa, acridine orange, or specific fluorescent antibodies. Drawbacks to microscopy include (1) the requirement of a fairly high spirochetemic burden, although this may be obviated by collection of samples during febrile periods; (2) observer inexperience or unfamiliarity with clinical differential; and (3) the inability to identify causative *Borrelia* to the species level. Cultivation of the spirochetes is possible, although difficult, and is rarely performed in clinical settings. Demonstration of serologic response using techniques such as IFA, ELISA, and Western blot has met with variable success. The degree of *Borrelia* antigenic variability may limit serologic assay sensitivity, whereas cross-reactivity with other spirochetes, in particular those of the Lyme borreliosis group, may affect specificity. Newer tests utilizing a 34-kDa recombinant protein, GlpQ, appear to be more specific for the relapsing fever spirochetes (Schwan, 1996; Porcella, 2000). At present, molecular methods such as PCR play little, if any, role in the routine diagnosis of relapsing fever. However, given their extreme power of strain and/or species discrimination (Wormser, 1999; Bunikis, 2004), these techniques may one day play a vital part in the elucidation of borreliosis etiology in regions where both relapsing fever and Lyme disease spirochetes are found.

Successful treatment of LBRF may be accomplished using a single oral dose of tetracycline or erythromycin, whereas 5–10 days of therapy with either of these agents is recommended for TBRF (Johnson, 2000). Parenteral administration of a β-lactam may be considered in the case of meningitis or encephalitis (Cadavid, 1998). Whatever the antibiotic, symptoms of the Jarisch-Herxheimer reaction are not uncommon and may be particularly severe in the louse-borne form of disease. This reaction usually occurs within a few hours of antibiotic initiation and is typified by an increase in temperature (0.5°–1° C) with rigors, systemic hypotension, and leukopenia. As with other shock-like syndromes, the proposed mechanism of Jarisch-Herxheimer reaction involves a cytokine "storm," with tumor necrosis factor-α, interleukin-6, and interleukin-8 as major orchestrating components (Griffin, 1998).

Prevention strategies for TBRF include rodent-proofing rural cottages or cabins to avoid immigration and colonization by soft ticks, use of insecticides around such dwellings, use of topical repellents while sleeping, and altogether avoiding overnight excursions into known *Ornithodoros* habitats. Prevention of LBRF may be effected through good personal hygiene and delousing procedures (Johnson, 2000). No vaccine is currently available.

Rat-Bite Fever

DESCRIPTION

Spirillum minus is a gram-negative, tightly coiled bacterium 2–5 μm long by 0.5 μm wide, with bipolar tufts of flagella, more closely related to *Neisseria* species than to members of the family Spirochaetaceae.

EPIDEMIOLOGY

Infection with *S. minus* in humans results in a relapsing fever called sodoku, most cases of which have been described in Japan, although cases have occurred worldwide. This bacterium is part of the respiratory flora of rats and is transmitted by a bite. Oral ingestion is not reported to be a source of infection for humans. The disease is very rare in the United States, though it does occur as a result of infection by *Streptobacillus moniliformis*. Research laboratory workers and world travelers are the groups at risk for infection (Anderson, 1983; Signorini, 2002).

PATHOGENESIS AND PATHOLOGY

The pathogenesis of *S. minus* is poorly understood. Dissemination from the original bite occurs soon after inoculation. In the few postmortem descriptions of fatal cases, epithelial necrosis and a mononuclear infiltrate in the dermis at the original bite site; a perivascular mononuclear infiltrate in the dermis from the site of the rash; hyperplasia of lymph nodes; and hemorrhage and necrosis in the liver, spleen, kidney, myocardium, and meninges have been described (Washburn, 1995).

CLINICAL MANIFESTATIONS

The bite wound initially heals, but 1–4 weeks later, an indurated lesion, which may ulcerate, appears at the bite site. Febrile periods recur, separated by afebrile periods of 3–7 days. Fever can be accompanied by myalgia, headache, and vomiting. Half of patients have a macular rash that may form large plaques (Taber, 1979). Resolution usually occurs in 3–8 weeks, but relapses and complications such as endocarditis, meningitis, myocarditis, and nephritis can also occur (Washburn, 1995). The mortality for untreated cases in the preantibiotic era was 6%–10% (Washburn, 1995).

LABORATORY DIAGNOSIS

S. minus can be propagated only in mice or guinea pigs by intraperitoneal inoculation. Demonstration of the organisms can be accomplished by staining exudate from the lesion or lymph nodes with a Wright-Giemsa stain or visualization by darkfield microscopy. Serologic tests are not available; however, up to 50% of patients can have a false-positive nontreponemal test for syphilis (Taber, 1979).

TREATMENT

Intravenous aqueous penicillin G is the therapy of choice, with tetracycline used in penicillin-allergic patients.

ANAEROBIOSPIRILLUM SUCCINICIPRODUCENS

DESCRIPTION

Anaerobiospirillum succiniciproducens is a gram-negative, spiral-shaped bacterium measuring 0.6–0.8 μm wide by 4–8 μm long. It shows a corkscrew-like motility and possesses bipolar multitrichous flagella. Similar to *Spirillum* spp., members of the genus *Anaerobiospirillum* are not true spirochetes. Rather, they are more closely related to the genus *Aeromonas* than to the *Treponema* or *Borrelia* genus.

EPIDEMIOLOGY

This anaerobic bacterium can be part of the normal flora of healthy cats and dogs but has also been demonstrated in association with severe feline ileocolitis (De Cock, 2004). An association of similar illness in humans with exposure to these pets has been suggested but not definitively established (Malnick, 1990; Goddard, 1998). *A. succiniciproducens* has been associated with diarrheal illness in normal patients and with sepsis in patients with predisposing illness. The gastrointestinal tract in these patients has been postulated as the source for entry into the circulatory system (McNeil, 1987; Tee, 1998). The incidence of infection is low but has been increasing; this is thought to be due primarily to better detection by improved culture technique (Goddard, 1998).

CLINICAL MANIFESTATIONS

Patients with gastroenteritis suffer from abdominal pain, vomiting, and diarrhea for 3–7 days; those without underlying illness recover uneventfully (Malnick, 1990). Sepsis has occurred in patients with underlying illnesses, including alcoholism, atherosclerosis, malignancy, diabetes mellitus, and gingivitis (Goddard, 1998; Pienaar, 2003). Fatalities have occurred in about one third of cases of sepsis.

LABORATORY DIAGNOSIS

A. succiniciproducens grows well in automated blood culture systems (Tee, 1998). After subculture on chocolate or blood agar, moist and spreading colonies 1–2mm in diameter appear after 2–3 days. Useful identifying biochemical reactions include a negative catalase, indole, and oxidase; production of succinic acid and acetic acid from glucose as demonstrated by gas-liquid chromatography; and no growth at 25° C or 42° C. A selective medium has been developed by Malnick (1990).

TREATMENT

Because of the uncommon nature of this infection, optimal therapy for sepsis has not been established. In vitro, most isolates tested have been susceptible to carbenicillin, cefoxitin, chloramphenicol, and metronidazole and resistant to vancomycin and clindamycin; however, testing has been limited and is not standardized (Shlaes, 1982; McNeil, 1987).

AGENTS OF INTESTINAL SPIROCHETOSIS

DESCRIPTION

Two species of spirochete, *Brachyspira aalborgi* and *Brachyspira pilosicoli* (formerly designated as a member of the genus *Serpulina*), have been found in the colon of humans. These organisms are gram-negative, 0.2–0.4 μm in diameter, and 4–8 μm in length. Four to six flagella are present subterminally at each end near the pointed ends of the bacteria.

EPIDEMIOLOGY AND CLINICAL MANIFESTATIONS

B. pilosicoli, along with *B. hyodysenteriae*, causes porcine intestinal spirochetosis, a diarrheal disease in young pigs, although strains related to these species have been recovered from dogs, birds, and other animals (Korner, 2003). It is unknown whether animals act as reservoirs for human infection. In contrast, *B. aalborgi* was named after its isolation from the colon of a human patient (Hovind-Hougen, 1982), but it is less well characterized overall. The association of intestinal spirochetes with disease is not firmly established, as the bacteria have been identified in both symptomatic and asymptomatic individuals. Homosexual men have shown a higher prevalence than other populations (Teglbjaerg, 1990). Diarrhea, abdominal pain, rectal bleeding, and discharge have been attributed to intestinal spirochetosis (Teglbjaerg, 1990). Additionally, *B. pilosicoli* has been isolated from the blood of critically ill and immunocompromised patients, the clinical significance of which is uncertain (Trott, 1997; Kanavaki, 2002).

PATHOLOGY AND PATHOGENESIS

The spirochetes are easily seen on biopsy specimens as a dark blue "fringe" on the surface of colonic epithelial cells with sparing of the goblet cells (Fig. 59-13, *A*). Silver impregnation stains demonstrate the organisms well (Fig. 59-13, *B*). The epithelial cells appear normal, and no increased inflammation is noted in the lamina propria. Electron microscopy demonstrates that the bacteria attach to the surface of colonic epithelial cells end-on and are oriented perpendicular to the lumen (Teglbjaerg, 1990). Invasion into epithelial and mucosal macrophages has been demonstrated in both symptomatic and asymptomatic patients (Teglbjaerg, 1990). Pathogenesis has not been established.

LABORATORY DIAGNOSIS

Spirochetes can be detected in stool by darkfield microscopy and cultured from stool or biopsy specimens on trypticase soy agar with 5%–10% horse or calf blood. The addition of spectinomycin and polymyxin B makes the media selective (Teglbjaerg, 1990). On media incubated anaerobically, pinpoint, weakly β-hemolytic colonies develop in 3 days to 4 weeks, depending on the strain. Fluorescent in situ hybridization assays and amplification techniques followed by RFLP analysis have been used for the detection and/or identification of spirochetes from tissue biopsy samples (Calderaro, 2003; Jensen, 2004). Moreover, amplification of *Brachyspira* genes from DNA extracted directly from feces of infected animals has also been successful (Atyeo, 1998).

TREATMENT

Although antimicrobial susceptibilities of *Brachyspira* spp. have been published, standardized testing of a large number of isolates has not been described (Karlsson, 2003). Patients suffering from symptoms and intestinal spirochetosis have reportedly responded to metronidazole (Teglbjaerg, 1990).

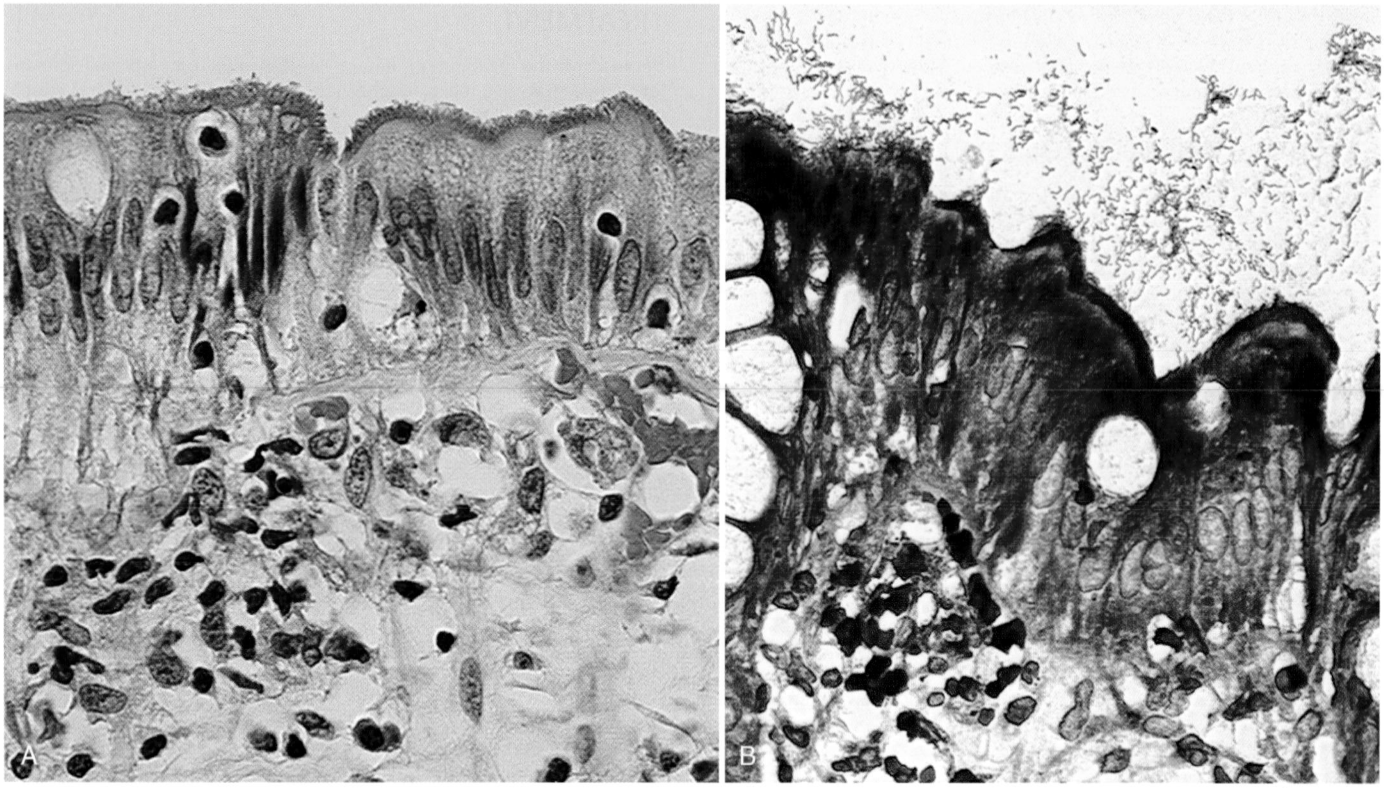

Figure 59-13 Colonic epithelium demonstrating **(A)** basophilic discoloration along the bowel luminal surface (hematoxylin & eosin [H&E], ≈×400), which is confirmed in **(B)** to be numerous argyrophilic spirochetes, consistent with intestinal spirochetosis (Steiner silver impregnation technique, ×400). *(Images courtesy Hagen Blaszyk, MD.)*

SELECTED REFERENCES

Antal GM, Lukehart SA, Meheus AZ. The endemic treponematoses. Microbes Infect 2002;4:83.

This extensive review provides descriptions of the causative agents and their principal pathogenic mechanisms, as well as diagnostic and treatment options. Its depiction of each of the clinical diseases and their individual impact on various human populations, however, is extraordinary.

Brown SL, Hansen SLH, Langone JJ. Role of serology in the diagnosis of Lyme disease. JAMA 1999;281:62.

Explores the performance characteristics of serologic techniques in the diagnosis of Lyme disease and demonstrates the role that corroborating clinical and epidemiologic factors should play.

Centers for Disease Control and Prevention. Sexually transmitted diseases treatment guidelines. MMWR Recomm Rep 2002;51:1.

Developed as a tool to guide therapy of many sexually transmitted diseases, these recommendations also include many valuable diagnostic considerations for a variety of presentations.

Dumler JS. Molecular diagnosis of Lyme disease: review and meta-analysis. Mol Diagn 2001;6:1.

Successfully accomplishes the feat of assembling a multitude of diverse molecular data to illustrate the overall performance characteristics and utility of amplification assays on different clinical specimens.

Dworkin MS, Schwan TG, Anderson DE. Tick-borne relapsing fever in North America. Med Clin North Am 2002;86:417.

Instructive review of endemic relapsing fever that provides a description of the causative spirochetes and epidemiologic, tick-vector ecologic, and pathogenic factors that lead to human disease and clinical manifestations of relapsing fever. Laboratory diagnostic techniques, treatment, and prevention issues are also highlighted.

Korner M, Gebbers JO. Clinical significance of human intestinal spirochetosis—a morphologic approach. Infection 2003;5:341.

Focuses on a compilation of evidence that ascribes pathogenic traits to the organisms heretofore only associated with intestinal spirochetosis.

Levett PN. Leptospirosis. Clin Microbiol Rev 2001;14:296.

A comprehensive yet concise review of historic, epidemiologic, clinical, and diagnostic features of leptospirosis.

Schmid GP. Epidemiology and clinical similarities of human spirochetal diseases. Rev Infect Dis 1989;11(Suppl. 6):S1460.

Short review offering interesting pathogenetic and clinical correlations between the major spirochete diseases.

Tugwell P, Dennis DT, Weinstein A, et al. Laboratory evaluation in the diagnosis of Lyme disease. Ann Intern Med 1997;127:1109.

Explores the performance characteristics of serologic techniques in the diagnosis of Lyme disease and demonstrates the role that corroborating clinical and epidemiologic factors should play.

REFERENCES

Access the complete reference list online at http://www.expertconsult.com

CHAPTER 60

MYCOBACTERIA

Gail L. Woods

KEY POINTS

- *Mycobacterium tuberculosis* complex is the only mycobacterium that is transmitted from person to person and, therefore, is of public health importance.
- The Mantoux skin test and interferon-γ release assays are useful for identifying persons with latent tuberculosis infection.
- For optimal detection of mycobacteria in clinical specimens, laboratories should use a fluorochrome stain and a liquid system with or without a concomitant solid medium for culture.
- Nucleic acid amplification testing for direct detection of *M. tuberculosis* complex should be performed on respiratory specimens from patients with suspected tuberculosis.
- Susceptibility testing to the primary antituberculous agents (isoniazid, rifampin, ethambutol, and pyrazinamide) should be performed on all initial isolates of *M. tuberculosis* complex.
- Infections caused by nontuberculous mycobacteria are acquired from the environment (e.g., water).
- The nontuberculous mycobacteria most commonly encountered in the clinical laboratory are *Mycobacterium avium* complex, which causes pulmonary disease and, in immunocompromised patients, disseminated disease; the rapidly growing mycobacteria *Mycobacterium abscessus*, *Mycobacterium chelonae*, and *Mycobacterium fortuitum* group, which most often cause skin and soft tissue infections; *Mycobacterium kansasii*, which causes pulmonary infection; and *Mycobacterium marinum*, which causes skin and soft tissue infections.

Mycobacteria are aerobic, nonmotile, acid alcohol–fast, slightly curved or straight bacilli. The organisms contain high molecular weight (60–90 carbons) mycolic acids in their cell walls that on pyrolysis release C22 to C26 straight-chain saturated long-chain acids. Their guanine plus cytosine DNA-base content ratios are in the range of 62–70 mol%. Mycobacteria can be divided into two groups: those in the *Mycobacterium tuberculosis* complex and nontuberculous mycobacteria.

MYCOBACTERIUM TUBERCULOSIS COMPLEX

The tubercle bacilli that make up the *M. tuberculosis* complex (MTBC; *Mycobacterium tuberculosis*, *Mycobacterium bovis*, *M. bovis* Bacille Calmette-Guérin strain [BCG], *Mycobacterium caprae*, *Mycobacterium pinnipedii*, *Mycobacterium africanum*, *Mycobacterium microtii*, and *Mycobacterium canettii* [Castets, 1968; van Soolingen, 1997; Pfyffer, 1998]) are the etiologic agents of human tuberculosis (TB). Worldwide, TB is the second greatest contributor among infectious diseases to adult mortality. The World Health Organization estimates that in 2007, about 10 million cases of TB and nearly 2 million deaths from TB were reported (www.who.int/topics/tuberculosis/en). That year, India ranked first in the number of incident cases, followed by China, Indonesia, Nigeria, and South Africa. Among new cases of TB, approximately 5% (or 500,000) worldwide are due to multidrug-resistant organisms (MDR-TB), defined as tubercle bacilli that are resistant to rifampin and isoniazid. MDR-TB does not respond to the standard 6-month treatment regimen and may require up to 2 years of treatment with drugs that are more toxic than first-line agents and about 100 times more costly. Mismanagement of drugs used to treat MDR-TB can result in extensively drug-resistant tuberculosis (XDR-TB), defined as MDR-TB plus resistance to any fluoroquinolone and any second-line injectable antituberculosis agent (e.g., amikacin, kanamycin, capreomycin).

In the United States, TB was the leading cause of death at the turn of the 20th century. Mortality then decreased, initially because of public health efforts and later because of antituberculous drugs. Between 1953, when TB became notifiable on a national basis, and 1984, the incidence of TB steadily decreased (Rieder, 1989). From 1985 to 1992, a resurgence of TB cases was seen, in large part because of the epidemic spread of human immunodeficiency virus (HIV), deterioration of the health care infrastructure, and an increase in the number of cases reported among foreign-born persons. In addition to the resurgence, MDR-TB emerged and remains a concern, although to a much lesser degree than in developing countries.

Since 1992, the incidence of TB in the United States has declined each year, and MDR-TB has become uncommon. TB rates are highest among foreign-born persons and those in racial/ethnic minorities. In 2008, the TB rate in the United States was ten times higher in foreign-born persons than in those born in the United States, and compared with non-Hispanic whites, TB rates were about eight times higher among Hispanics and blacks and nearly 23 times higher among Asians (Centers for Disease Control and Prevention, 2009c).

Tubercle bacilli are transmitted primarily via inhalation of dried residues of small infected droplets (1–10 μm in diameter). Infection also may be acquired by direct inoculation of abraded skin—an event most likely to occur when pathologists or other laboratory personnel handle infected tissues. In addition, *M. bovis* may be transmitted from cattle to humans by drinking contaminated raw milk or by respiratory exposure to live infected cattle or their carcasses, from humans to cattle via exposure to urine from persons with urinary tract infections due to *M. bovis*, and from cattle and wild reservoirs to cattle probably by respiratory secretions.

The most important source of infection is an undiagnosed person with cavitary (and sputum smear–positive) pulmonary disease. The risk of active pulmonary disease is low after one exposure to the organism but increases under conditions of stress or in a confined environment where repeated exposures to the organism occur. Most persons who become infected with *M. tuberculosis* do not develop active disease. The lifetime risk of active disease is 5%–10% for immunocompetent persons. For persons infected with both *M. tuberculosis* and HIV, in contrast, the risk of developing tuberculosis is 7%–10% per year.

Based on analysis of its genomic sequence, *M. tuberculosis* does not appear to encode typical bacterial virulence factors (e.g., toxins). However, certain genes and gene products have been identified as key factors enabling *M. tuberculosis* to cause disease. PhoP has been shown to have an important role in virulence, because *phoP* mutants grow very poorly in macrophages and in mice (Ryndak, 2008). Lipids called phthiocerol dimycocerosates, which are found at the outermost layers of the cell envelope, are required for optimal multiplication and persistence of *M. tuberculosis* in mice lungs, and phenolic glycolipids are thought to be involved in the hypervirulence of certain *M. tuberculosis* strains (Gordon, 2009). In addition, the ESX secretion systems, which are specialized secretion systems present in many gram-positive bacteria, are important in pathogenesis, because mutants lacking the system or its substrates are attenuated in cultured macrophages and animal models of infection. Mutants with a deletion spanning much of the ESX-1 locus demonstrate defective cell-to-cell spread, altered cytokine profiles, and failure to inhibit phagolysosome fusion in cultured cells (Tobin, 2008).

The usual host response to infection with MTBC is activation of the cell-mediated immune system. During primary (initial) infection, inhaled bacilli travel to the alveolar spaces, where they are ingested by resident macrophages. These macrophages are unable to kill the tubercle bacilli, which multiply intracellularly during the first several days after infection. Macrophages infected with mycobacteria migrate to regional tracheobronchial lymph nodes and present sensitizing antigen(s) to immunocompetent T cells, or they enter the lymphatics and blood and travel back to the lungs (primarily the apices) and to distant organs such as lymph nodes, kidneys, epiphyseal areas of the long bones, vertebral bodies, and meninges, where bacilli continue to multiply until the cellular immune response is activated.

Immunocompetent T cells migrate from regional lymph nodes to the site of infection in the lung. There they release chemotactic, migration-inhibitory, and mitogenic cytokines, which stimulate recruitment of blood-derived monocytes and lymphocytes, macrophage and lymphocyte division, and macrophage activation. Activated macrophages have enhanced microbicidal activity, and they produce cytokines such as interleukin-1, interferon-γ, and tumor necrosis factor, which stimulate or regulate other components of the immune system, properties that help control infection. The cytokines and lytic enzymes released by the macrophages also contribute to concomitant local tissue destruction. Over time, the activated T cell population declines and is replaced by long-lived memory immune T cells, which protect against reinfection with MTBC and provide some cross-protection against infection with other mycobacteria. Despite the limitation of further mycobacterial multiplication in primary and metastatic foci by the activated macrophages and memory T cells, a residual nidus of infection remains indefinitely in the lung (most frequently in the apex, where the oxygen tension is high) and less often in distant sites. Therefore, the potential for reactivation of disease in these quiescent foci exists during periods of immunosuppression.

The primary focus of pulmonary infection, called the Gohn lesion, is usually subjacent to the pleura in the lower part of the upper lobes or in the upper part of the lower lobes of one lung, corresponding to areas of the lung that receive the greatest volume flow of inspired air. Lesions (tubercles) are well-circumscribed, 1–2-cm-diameter areas of grayish white consolidation with soft to necrotic centers. Similar-appearing tubercles typically are found in the regional tracheobronchial lymph nodes, and these plus the primary lung lesion are termed the Gohn complex. Microscopically, tubercles are composed of well-circumscribed caseating or noncaseating granulomas; organisms may be seen in sections stained with an acid-fast stain. Over time, these lesions are replaced by hyalinized fibrous tissue and eventually calcify. Lesions of miliary tuberculosis are small (one to several millimeters in diameter), distinct, yellow-white areas of consolidation without gross caseation that histologically resemble tubercles. The ability to form granulomas depends on the immunocompetence of the host. Individuals infected with HIV, for example, may have extensive necrosis, many neutrophils, microabscesses, and numerous acid-fast bacilli (AFB), without granulomas.

In the United States, pulmonary TB accounts for about 85% of cases of active disease. Manifestations of pulmonary disease vary. The clinical presentation may be insidious with gradual onset of constitutional symptoms over months; catarrhal, with productive cough often attributed to a bad cold or lingering bronchitis; pneumonia- or flu-like, with high fever, aches and pains, and cough; hemoptoic with acute onset of blood-streaked sputum; or pleuritic. Extrapulmonary TB may be localized but more commonly involves multiple organs with or without concurrent lung infection. Multiorgan TB occurs predominantly in infants and young children, the elderly, and immunocompromised individuals, especially those infected with both HIV and MTBC. Additionally, most infections with *M. bovis* in the United States are extrapulmonary, involving lymph nodes, the gastrointestinal tract, bones, and kidneys, and most commonly occur in children of Hispanic ethnicity (Hlavsa, 2008; Rodwell, 2008). Infrequently, infection follows intravesical instillation of *M. bovis* BCG for treatment of superficial bladder carcinoma (Lamm, 1992; Kristjansson, 1993).

NONTUBERCULOUS MYCOBACTERIA

The nontuberculous mycobacteria (NTM; also called mycobacteria other than tubercle bacilli) may be categorized on the basis of colony pigmentation before and after exposure to light and growth rate on a solid medium as described by Runyon in 1957 (Table 60-1) (Runyon, 1959). This classification system, however, has limits. For example, *M. kansasii* is usually a photochromogen but rarely is nonchromogenic or scotochromogenic. Members of the *M. avium* complex are nonchromogenic in Runyon's scheme, but some isolates produce slightly pigmented colonies after prolonged incubation, potentially causing incorrect classification as a scotochromogen. *Mycobacterium szulgai* is a scotochromogen at 37° C and a photochromogen at 25° C. Moreover, when a liquid medium is used for mycobacterial culture, as is currently recommended (discussed in the section regarding culture methods), growth rates used by Runyon for classification do not apply. *Mycobacterium leprae* is unique among mycobacteria by virtue of the fact that it has not yet been cultivated in vitro.

In general, little is known about the antigens associated with virulence of the NTM, and the immune response to infection with these mycobacteria is poorly understood. With current molecular techniques, more than 100 species of NTM have been identified. Select potential pathogens are reviewed in the following sections. An extensive description of the more recently described and infrequently isolated mycobacteria is found in the excellent review by Tortoli (2003). *Mycobacterium gordonae*, often referred to as the "tap water bacillus," is a common laboratory contaminant and rarely causes disease in humans.

MYCOBACTERIUM AVIUM COMPLEX

The primary pathogens in the *M. avium* complex (MAC) are *M. avium* and *Mycobacterium intracellulare*. These species have such similar growth characteristics and biochemical reactions that they often are not distinguished in the clinical microbiology laboratory; isolates of both species are reported as MAC. MAC bacilli are ubiquitous in the environment. They have been isolated from water, soil, food, house dust, and several animals, but the specific environmental sources responsible for human infection are

TABLE 60-1
Runyon's Classification of the Nontuberculous Mycobacteria

Classification	Description of colonies
Photochromogen	Not pigmented unless exposed to light (optimally during their early growth and with good aeration of the surface)
Scotochromogen	Pigmented when grown in the dark and in light
Nonchromogen	Not pigmented when grown in the dark or in light
Rapid grower	Growth on solid media in ≤7 days

not known (Inderlied, 1993; Falkinham, 1996). The most likely portal of entry is the gastrointestinal tract, but transmission via the respiratory tract is also possible. From sites of colonization, organisms enter the blood and infect many organs, especially those of the monocyte–macrophage system. In many clinical microbiology laboratories in the United States today, MAC is the most frequently isolated mycobacterium.

For many years, pulmonary disease caused by MAC occurred most often in elderly white men who had underlying chronic lung disease or who had undergone gastrectomy; however, since the mid to late 1980s, it has become more common in persons without predisposing factors, especially older women (Prince, 1989; Dhillon, 2000; Griffith, 2007). Disseminated MAC occurs almost exclusively in immunosuppressed individuals, especially persons with advanced acquired immunodeficiency syndrome (AIDS). In the United States, MAC was the most common cause of systemic bacterial infection in patients with AIDS in the late 1980s and early 1990s (Horsburg, 1991a). The numbers of such cases, however, decreased since highly active antiretroviral therapy became widely available (Centers for Disease Control and Prevention, 2009a). The major risk factor for disseminated MAC in AIDS patients is the degree of immune dysfunction, indicated by the $CD4^+$ lymphocyte count, as the disease is rare in individuals whose $CD4^+$ lymphocyte count is over 50/µL.

Manifestations of disease caused by MAC depend on the site and the extent of infection. Pulmonary disease may present as bronchiectasis or may mimic TB. Disseminated disease in persons without AIDS is manifested by fever, weight loss, bone pain, lymphadenopathy, hepatosplenomegaly, and skin lesions. In those with AIDS, persistent fever, weight loss, and diarrhea are most common; anorexia, weakness, lymphadenopathy, or hepatomegaly also may occur (Inderlied, 1993; Griffith, 2007; Centers for Disease Control and Prevention, 2009a). Significant laboratory abnormalities include anemia and elevated alkaline phosphatase. Cervical lymphadenitis caused by MAC most often affects children but also occurs in adults. Other manifestations of infection with MAC are synovitis, genitourinary tract disease, cutaneous lesions, deep infection of the hand, osteomyelitis, meningitis, ulcer of the colon, and pericarditis (Wolinsky, 1979; Woods, 1987; Inderlied, 1993).

The histologic findings of lesions caused by MAC vary. Caseating granulomas with AFB, indistinguishable from TB; pulmonary interstitial fibrosis with organizing pneumonia; necrotizing granulomatous vasculitis resembling Wegener's granulomatosis; and, especially in persons with AIDS, aggregates of foamy macrophages containing many intracellular AFB may be seen.

MYCOBACTERIUM KANSASII

M. kansasii, first described as the "yellow bacillus," accounted for 3% of mycobacterial isolates in the United States in 1979 and 1980; the highest numbers of cases were reported from California, Texas, Louisiana, Illinois, and Florida (Buhler, 1953; Good, 1982). The natural reservoir of *M. kansasii* is unknown; however, it has been recovered from water samples (Falkinham, 1996). Pulmonary disease is most common in males 50–60 years of age living in urban areas, among certain occupational groups (miners, welders, sandblasters, and painters), and among individuals with pneumoconioses and chronic obstructive pulmonary disease. Disseminated disease generally affects persons with impaired cellular immunity.

The most common manifestation of disease caused by *M. kansasii* is chronic cavitary pulmonary lesions, usually involving the upper lobes (Griffith, 2007). Extrapulmonary manifestations include cervical lymphadenitis in children, cutaneous disease, musculoskeletal involvement (carpal tunnel syndrome, synovitis, arthritis, tendinitis and fasciitis, or osteomyelitis), disseminated disease, isolated genitourinary tract disease, and pericarditis. Histologic findings of lesions caused by *M. kansasii* vary and include caseating or noncaseating granulomas and, especially in skin lesions, necrosis or foci of acute and chronic inflammation without well-formed granulomas. AFB are common in lung and lymph node tissue but are seen less frequently in tissue from other sites.

MYCOBACTERIUM XENOPI

M. xenopi was first isolated from a toad in 1957 and was recognized as a human pathogen in 1965 (Costrini, 1981). It has been cultured from hot and cold water taps, hospital hot water generators and storage tanks, and other environmental sources. Birds are a possible natural reservoir. Most pulmonary infections caused by *M. xenopi* have been reported from Canada, Europe, and Great Britain; it is an uncommon cause of mycobacterial disease in the United States. Disease has occurred only in adults, more frequently in males than in females. Most persons have preexisting lung damage or another predisposing condition, such as an extrapulmonary malignancy, alcoholism, diabetes mellitus, or immunosuppressive therapy. Pulmonary disease may be chronic, subacute, or acute; symptoms are indistinguishable from those associated with disease caused by *M. kansasii*. Focal extrapulmonary infections (osteomyelitis, arthritis, lymphadenitis) and disseminated disease are uncommon, but the latter has been reported in persons with AIDS (Tecson-Tumang, 1984).

MYCOBACTERIUM GENAVENSE

M. genavense was first isolated in 1991 in Switzerland from the blood of a patient with AIDS (Bootger, 1991). Conditions for detection in the laboratory were described shortly thereafter (Coyle, 1992). Disease occurs predominantly in immunocompromised patients. The most common presentation is disseminated disease in HIV-infected patients, which clinically is very similar to disseminated MAC (Maschek, 1994; Tortoli, 1998; Griffith, 2007). Other manifestations include enteritis, genital and soft tissue infections, and lymphadenitis.

MYCOBACTERIUM MARINUM

M. marinum was recognized as a human pathogen in 1951 (Norden, 1951). It causes chronic granulomatous infections involving skin and soft tissue, often called "swimming pool granuloma" or "fish tank granuloma," and occasionally bone (Lewis, 2003; Aubry, 2002; Griffith, 2007). Human infection is typically acquired via trauma to the skin during contact with contaminated nonchlorinated fresh or salt water, but it may be acquired via trauma unassociated with water contact or contact with water in the absence of preceding trauma. A single papulonodular lesion usually appears 2–3 weeks after inoculation, most commonly on the elbow, knee, foot, toe, or finger, and often becomes verrucous or ulcerated (Ang, 2000). Occasionally, an abscess forms at the site of inoculation, and several secondary nodules develop and progress centrally along the lymphatics, resembling sporotrichosis. In immunocompromised persons, cutaneous lesions may become disseminated. Extracutaneous manifestations are uncommon: Synovitis, osteomyelitis, and ocular and laryngeal lesions have been reported (Woods, 1987).

The histology of skin lesions varies with the stage of infection. Early on, neutrophil aggregates are surrounded by histiocytes. Later, lymphocytes, epithelioid histiocytes, occasional Langhans giant cells, and foci of fibrinoid necrosis are seen. In lesions present for longer than 6 months, aggregates of lymphocytes are found in the dermis. Stains for AFB are usually negative, but organisms may be seen within histiocytes.

MYCOBACTERIUM HAEMOPHILUM

M. haemophilum was first described in 1978 but very probably was the nonculturable AFB recognized in skin ulcers in 1972 and 1974 (Lomwardias, 1972; Feldman, 1974; Sompolinsky, 1978). The organism is unique among mycobacteria in its growth requirement for hemoglobin or hemin. Human infections caused by *M. haemophilum* are uncommon, usually seen in persons who have an underlying immunodeficiency such as lymphoma, exogenous immunosuppression after organ transplantation, or AIDS, but lymphadenitis in otherwise healthy children has been reported (Centers for Disease Control and Prevention, 1991; Lindeboom, 2005). Disease most commonly is manifested by multiple cutaneous nodules, ulcers, or painful swellings, typically involving the extremities, which occasionally become abscesses and open fistulas draining purulent material. Microscopically, lesions show foci of necrosis without caseation surrounded by a polymorphous inflammatory infiltrate with occasional Langhans giant cells in the lower dermis. AFB are seen singly or in small clusters, often within cells.

MYCOBACTERIUM ULCERANS

M. ulcerans is endemic in areas of Zaire, Uganda, Nigeria, Ghana, Cameroon, Malaysia, New Guinea, Guyana, Mexico, and Australia located between latitudes 25° N and 38° S. In all endemic areas, disease is more frequent among children younger than 15 years and is slightly more common in males (Debacker, 2004; Piersimoni, 2009). The natural reservoir of *M. ulcerans* and the usual route of its transmission to humans remain unknown.

Eponyms for disease caused by *M. ulcerans* include Bairnsdale ulcer, for the area in Australia where it was first recognized, and Buruli ulcer or

Buruli disease, after the area of Uganda reporting the greatest number of cases (Amofah, 2002). The disease begins as one or, rarely, multiple painless boils or subcutaneous lumps on an exposed area, most often the leg, which possibly was a site of previous trauma. After several weeks, the lump ulcerates, and satellite nodules and ulcers may appear. Lymph nodes typically are not enlarged, and affected individuals are afebrile and without systemic symptoms unless lesions become secondarily infected with bacteria.

RAPIDLY GROWING MYCOBACTERIA

Rapidly growing mycobacteria have been cultured from soil, freshwater lakes and rivers, seawater, waste water from hospitals, drinking water, raw milk, and dust. Of the many species of rapidly growing mycobacteria, the most common human pathogens are *M. abscessus*, *M. chelonae*, and the *M. fortuitum* group; other species associated with human disease are *Mycobacterium mucogenicum*, *Mycobacterium immunogenum*, *Mycobacterium goodii*, *Mycobacterium mageritense*, *Mycobacterium neoaurum*, *Mycobacterium peregrinum*, *Mycobacterium wolinskyi*, and, rarely, *Mycobacterium smegmatis* (Brown-Elliott, 2002; Griffith, 2007).

The most common manifestation of disease due to rapidly growing mycobacteria is skin and soft tissue infection, typically following a penetrating injury (trauma or surgical procedure) with possible soil or water contamination, although outbreaks have been associated with administration of diphtheria-pertussis-tetanus-polio vaccines, histamine injections, lidocaine administration using a jet injector, use of foot baths in nail salons, and liposuction (Wallace, 1983; Brown-Elliott, 2002; Piersimoni, 2009). Primary cutaneous/subcutaneous disease may present as localized cellulitis, draining abscesses, or minimally tender nodules, generally appearing 3 weeks to 12 months (most often 4–6 weeks) after the penetrating injury in persons with an intact immune system. Osteomyelitis is an occasional complication, especially following puncture wounds to the feet. Postoperative infections are characterized by a nonhealing wound or breakdown of a healed wound with serous drainage in a person with minimal systemic symptoms. They generally develop 3 weeks to 3 months after the procedure, especially median sternotomy, augmentation mammaplasty, or insertion of a percutaneous catheter. Disseminated skin and soft tissue abscesses in which no primary source of infection is evident typically occur in immunocompromised adults, especially those receiving corticosteroid therapy.

A less common manifestation of infection with rapidly growing mycobacteria is chronic pulmonary disease. It is most often seen in patients with underlying cystic fibrosis or bronchiectasis, is usually caused by *M. abscessus*, and typically resembles disease due to *M. kansasii* or MAC, except that cavitation is uncommon. Endocarditis involving a prosthetic valve has been reported, usually becoming manifest 4–12 weeks after surgery. Rarely, rapidly growing mycobacteria cause keratitis and corneal ulceration after trauma, or cervical lymphadenitis. A very thorough description of disease caused by rapidly growing mycobacteria is found in the excellent review by Brown-Elliott and Wallace (2002).

Lesions caused by rapidly growing mycobacteria are characterized histologically by necrosis with minimal caseation and a mixed inflammatory infiltrate composed of neutrophils and granulomas with foreign body or Langhans giant cells; lipid-laden macrophages are seen occasionally. Clumps of extracellular AFB are found within aggregates of neutrophils in less than a third of cases. In lung tissue, foamy macrophages may be seen in a pattern resembling lipoid pneumonia.

MYCOBACTERIUM LEPRAE

M. leprae is the etiologic agent of leprosy, also called Hansen's disease (Scollard, 2006). It is unique among the mycobacteria by virtue of the fact that it has not been cultivated. Useful animal models of infection are the mouse footpad model and the nine-banded armadillo. *M. leprae* has been recognized in nearly every part of the world at some time. The reported number of new cases registered each year remains between 500,000 and 700,000 (Lockwood, 2005).

Leprosy predominantly affects humans but is also a natural infection of wild armadillos in Louisiana, Arkansas, and Texas, and spontaneous cases have been described in mangabey monkeys (Hastings, 1988). The mechanism of transmission of *M. leprae* is unknown, but person-to-person spread via aerosolization of organisms from the nose of a person with active lepromatous disease (see later), which then contacts the nasal mucosa of another individual, is the favored theory. Transmission also may occur through intact skin or via penetrating wounds, such as thorns or the bite of an arthropod. Breast milk from lactating women with lepromatous disease contains bacilli that may be transmitted to infants, and transplacental transmission of *M. leprae* is possible. Cases of human leprosy following contact with armadillos have been reported (Lumpkin, 1983). Moreover, the discovery of a naturally occurring leprosy-like disease among armadillos and the fact that sporadic cases of leprosy occur in persons who have no known contact with human leprosy suggest that nonhuman sources of *M. leprae* may exist (Blake, 1987).

Most persons effectively resist infection with *M. leprae*. Resistance depends on an effective cell-mediated immune response to *M. leprae* antigens, as occurs in tuberculoid leprosy. In persons who lack specific cell-mediated immunity to these antigens, bacilli multiply within macrophages, eventually resulting in widely disseminated lepromatous leprosy. The defect in cellular immunity, which may involve T lymphocyte function or interaction of T lymphocytes with macrophages, is apparently specific for antigens to *M. leprae* rather than a generalized defect. The lesions of leprosy develop after a 2–5-year incubation period, varying in appearance depending on the host's immune response. Leprosy always involves peripheral nerves, almost always involves the skin, and frequently involves mucous membranes. The three cardinal signs of the disease are skin lesions, areas of cutaneous anesthesia, and enlarged peripheral nerves.

The system outlined by Ridey and Jopling (presented in the following section) is still used to classify the spectrum of clinical and histopathologic forms of leprosy (Ridley, 1964). Indeterminate leprosy, the earliest sign of disease, is characterized by one or a few hypopigmented skin macules with minimal local sensory loss. In about 75% of cases, the disease heals spontaneously; in the rest, it progresses, often after a prolonged period.

The polar types of leprosy—lepromatous leprosy, the widespread anergic form of the disease, and tuberculoid leprosy, the localized form—are stable clinically. Lepromatous leprosy is characterized by cutaneous lesions ranging from diffuse generalized skin involvement to widespread, symmetrically distributed nodules (called lepromas) filled with organisms. Lesions generally involve the cooler parts of the body surface, that is, the anterior third of the eye, the nasal mucosa, and the superficial peripheral nerve trunks. In advanced disease, lesions are accompanied by sensory loss from involvement of dermal nerve fibers. Microscopically, lesions show foamy histiocytes containing many AFB; few or no lymphocytes; minimal intraneural inflammation; and many AFB in nerves, the perineurium, blood vessel walls, and arrector muscles. In tuberculoid leprosy, one or a few well-circumscribed anesthetic macules or plaques develop, often accompanied by an enlarged peripheral nerve near the skin lesions. Histologically, lesions demonstrate noncaseating granulomas in the nerves and dermis, extending to involve the basal layer of the epidermis; few, if any, AFB are present. Borderline leprosy, a clinically unstable condition, encompasses the types of disease between the polar forms. It may develop features more closely resembling tuberculoid disease through a process termed upgrading, or features more like those of lepromatous disease, called downgrading.

TESTING FOR LATENT *M. TUBERCULOSIS* INFECTION

The tuberculin skin test is useful for identifying persons infected with MTBC but does not differentiate active disease from infection. Persons infected with MTBC develop a hypersensitivity reaction to proteins of the bacilli, which make up the skin test reagent purified protein derivative (PPD). The preferred method of skin testing is the Mantoux test, performed by intracutaneous injection of 0.1 mL of intermediate-strength (5 tuberculin units) PPD-S. The reaction is interpreted after 48–72 hours by measuring the diameter of induration in millimeters (Huebner, 1993). Induration of 5 mm or greater is considered positive in persons infected with HIV, those who have had recent close contact with someone who has infectious TB, and those who have chest radiograph findings consistent with old healed TB. A reaction of 10 mm or greater is positive in persons who do not meet the previous criteria but who have other risk factors for TB. Included in this group are foreign-born persons from countries where the prevalence of TB is high (such as Asia, Africa, or Latin America); injection drug users; medically underserved, low-income populations, especially racial or ethnic minorities; residents of long-term care facilities; and persons who have a medical condition associated with increased risk of TB (e.g., silicosis, gastrectomy, jejunoileal bypass, 10% or more below ideal body weight, chronic renal failure, diabetes mellitus, treatment with high-dose corticosteroids or with other immunosuppressive drugs, malignancies). A reaction of 15 mm or greater is positive in all other persons. Interpretation is difficult in those immunized with BCG.

False-positive PPD reactions may occur in persons with NTM infection and in those immunized with BCG. False-negative reactions may be due to poor technique or improper storage of the reagent. If the test is administered appropriately, false-negative reactions are uncommon in relatively healthy people but occur in up to 20% of individuals with known TB when they are first tested. Most of these false-negative reactions are attributed to the general illness and revert to positive after 2–3 weeks of therapy when health is restored. Factors causing a state of general anergy, such as protein malnutrition, concurrent viral infection, sarcoidosis, malignancy (especially lymphoma), immunosuppressive or corticosteroid therapy, and infection with HIV, also may cause a false-negative tuberculin reaction.

The Mantoux test generally remains positive as long as viable bacilli persist in quiescent foci. However, the reaction may wane below positive with increasing age, a phenomenon that occurs most frequently in those over age 55 years. In these individuals, the reaction will be boosted (or become positive) if retesting is performed as early as 1 week after the first test, a reaction termed the booster effect.

Interferon-γ release assays (IGRAs) became commercially available in the early 21st century (Madkukar, 2008; Lalvani, 2009). These are in vitro tests that are based on the detection of interferon-γ released by T cells in response to *M. tuberculosis* proteins (ESAT-6, CFP-10, TB7.7) not present in *M. bovis* BCG or most NTM (except *M. kansasii*, *M. szulgai*, and *M. marinum*). Performance of IGRAs requires collection of blood during a single visit, and results are available within 24 hours. According to experts at the Centers for Disease Control and Prevention (CDC), IGRAs can be used in all circumstances in which the skin test is used, including contact investigations, evaluation of recent immigrants, and screening health care workers for latent MTBC infection (Centers for Disease Control and Prevention, 2005). Advantages of IGRAs over the tuberculin skin test include improved sensitivity in immunosuppressed persons (although false-negative results occur) and children, and much better specificity in persons who have been vaccinated with BCG (Mori, 2009; Ruhwald, 2009).

LABORATORY DIAGNOSIS

SPECIMENS

Specimens recommended for diagnosis of mycobacterial infection are listed in Table 60-2. Samples from contaminated sites such as sputum and other respiratory secretions, gastric secretions, urine, and feces must be decontaminated prior to inoculation of media to prevent normal flora from overgrowing and thus masking the presence of mycobacteria, which grow more slowly. Concentrating the specimen after decontamination increases the sensitivity of smear and culture. Specimens from normally sterile body sites such as blood, cerebrospinal fluid (CSF), pleural and peritoneal fluid, and tissues may be inoculated directly without decontamination.

Processing and inoculation of specimens for mycobacterial culture should be performed in a biological safety cabinet. The *N*-acetyl-L-cysteine (NALC)–sodium hydroxide procedure (Fig. 60-1) is the most common method used in the clinical laboratory to liquefy, decontaminate, and concentrate specimens for detection of mycobacteria. Potentially contaminated specimens should be refrigerated if they cannot be processed immediately. Before proceeding to the steps outlined in Figure 60-1, additional handling is necessary for some specimens. Gastric lavage specimens should be processed immediately, but if a delay cannot be avoided, 10% sodium hydroxide should be added until the pH of the sample is neutral. If more than 10 mL of gastric secretions is collected, the sample is centrifuged at 3000 to 3600 *g* for 20–30 minutes, the supernatant is decanted, and the sediment is processed as shown in Figure 60-1. For feces, 1–2 g of a formed sample or 5 mL of a liquid specimen is placed in a 50-mL centrifuge tube, and sterile filtered distilled water is added to obtain a volume of 10 mL. The suspension is agitated on a vortex mixer, filtered through gauze, and then processed as outlined. Urine specimens are divided into two to four 50-mL centrifuge tubes and are centrifuged at 3000 to 3600 *g* for 30 minutes. The supernatant is decanted, leaving about 2 mL of sediment in each tube. Tubes are mixed on a vortex mixer, sediments are combined, and, if necessary, distilled water is added to obtain a volume of 10 mL, which then is decontaminated as shown in Figure 60-1.

MICROBIAL STAINS

In smears stained with the Gram stain, most mycobacteria appear as slender, poorly stained, beaded gram-positive bacilli, but sometimes the bacilli do not take up the crystal violet or safranin and appear "gram neutral" or as "Gram ghosts" (Fig. 60-2). Similar ghost images of bacilli may be found in macrophages in smears stained with the Wright or Papanicolaou stain. In general, specimens (except blood) collected from persons with suspected mycobacterial infection should be examined microscopically for organisms. However, to improve cost efficiency, many laboratories do not prepare smears of specimens in which AFB rarely are seen, such as CSF, urine, and bone marrow. To prepare a smear, two to three drops of the concentrated sediment are spread uniformly on a microscope slide, which then is fixed for 15 minutes at 80° C or for 1–2 hours at 65°–70° C on an electric hot plate.

Two types of stain detect AFB: carbol fuchsin (the classic Ziehl-Neelsen stain, which requires heating, and the cold Kinyoun stain) and the preferred fluorochrome stains (auramine-rhodamine and auramine-O), which

PART 7

TABLE 60-2
Mycobacterial Diseases and Specimens for Diagnosis

Disease	Common *Mycobacterium* species	Specimens
Pneumonia	MTBC, *M. kansasii*, MAC, *M. abscessus*	Sputum (early morning, deep cough on 3 consecutive days), BAL fluid, lung tissue, pleural fluid, gastric contents
Disseminated	MTBC, MAC	Blood, bone marrow, involved tissue
Lymphadenitis	MTBC, MAC	Lymph node aspirate or biopsy
Skin, soft tissue	*M. fortuitum, M. abscessus, M. chelonae, M. marinum, M. haemophilum, M. ulcerans*	Aspirate or biopsy of lesion
	M. leprae	Smears of nasal secretions and skin slits, biopsy of lesion
Musculoskeletal	MTBC, *M. fortuitum, M. abscessus, M. chelonae, M. marinum, M. kansasii*	Joint fluid, synovium, bone
Meningitis	MTBC	Cerebrospinal fluid
Brain abscess	MTBC	Abscess material
Genitourinary	*M. tuberculosis, M. bovis* BCG	Urine (early morning), involved tissue—kidney, bladder (*M. bovis* BCG), endometrium, fallopian tube, prostate, seminal vesicles, epididymis
Gastrointestinal	*M. tuberculosis, M. bovis*, MAC	Tissue, feces
Peritonitis	MTBC	Peritoneal biopsy, peritoneal fluid
Hepatitis	MTBC, MAC, *M. genavense*	Liver tissue
Pericarditis	MTBC	Pericardium, pericardial tissue
Catheter-related infection	Rapidly growing mycobacteria	Blood

Modified with permission from Woods GL. Mycobacteria. In: Woods GL, Gutierrez Y, editors. Diagnostic pathology of infectious diseases. Philadelphia: Lea & Febiger; 1993, p. 378.
BAL, Bronchoalveolar lavage; *BCG*, bacille Calmette-Guérin; *MAC*, *M. avium* complex; *MTBC*, *M. tuberculosis* complex.

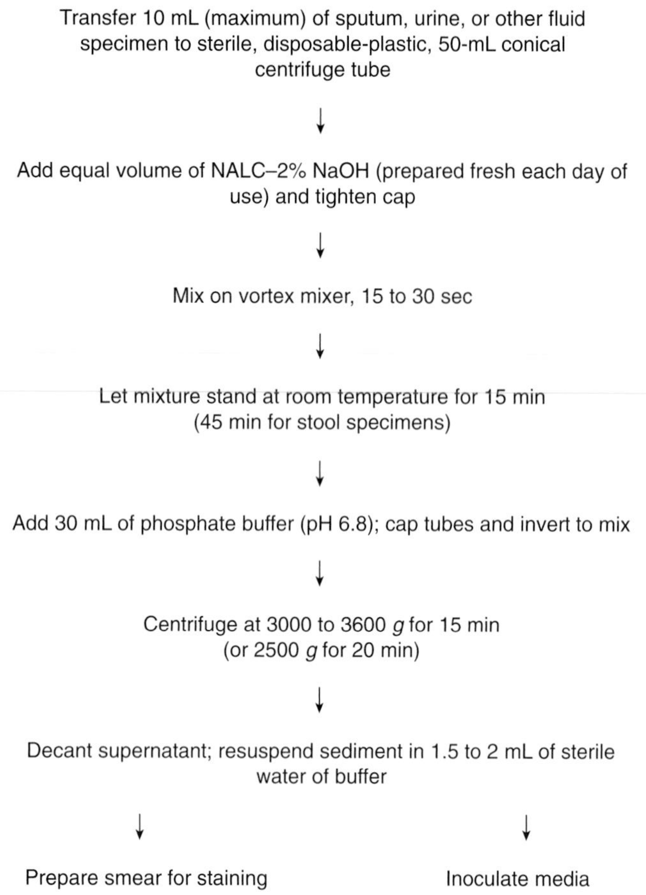

Transfer 10 mL (maximum) of sputum, urine, or other fluid specimen to sterile, disposable-plastic, 50-mL conical centrifuge tube
Add equal volume of NALC–2% NaOH (prepared fresh each day of use) and tighten cap
Mix on vortex mixer, 15 to 30 sec
Let mixture stand at room temperature for 15 min (45 min for stool specimens)
Add 30 mL of phosphate buffer (pH 6.8); cap tubes and invert to mix
Centrifuge at 3000 to 3600 g for 15 min (or 2500 g for 20 min)
Decant supernatant; resuspend sediment in 1.5 to 2 mL of sterile water of buffer
Prepare smear for staining
Inoculate media

Figure 60-1 Protocol for decontamination, using 2% sodium hydroxide–*N*-acetyl-L-cysteine, and concentration of specimens for detection of mycobacteria by smear and culture.

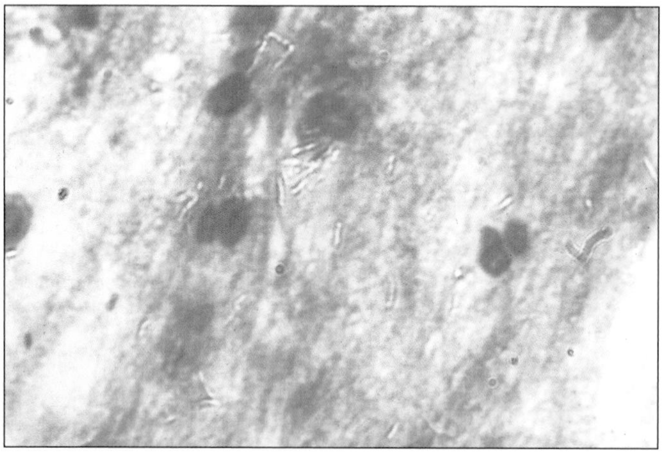

Figure 60-2 Smear of a sputum specimen stained with Gram stain shows "ghost cells" (mycobacterial culture grew *Mycobacterium tuberculosis;* Gram stain, ×400).

are more sensitive. Smears stained with a carbol fuchsin stain are examined at 800–1000× magnification (oil immersion). Smears stained with a fluorochrome stain are examined at lower magnifications (250× and 400×); this allows visualization of more fields in less time. Cells of some rapidly growing mycobacteria stain poorly with fluorochromic stains and may not be detected; therefore, when the latter organisms are suspected pathogens (e.g., in postsurgical wound infection), restaining negative fluorescent smears with a carbol fuchsin stain is reasonable. Results are reported after 100 fields are viewed and should include a statement indicating whether the smear was prepared directly from the specimen or after decontamination and concentration. Guidelines for reporting results of smears stained for AFB are shown in Table 60-3 (Kent, 1985).

In smears stained with carbol fuchsin, AFB typically appear as purple to red, slightly curved rods (1–10 μm long and 0.2–0.6 μm wide), which often are beaded or banded (Fig. 60-3) but may also appear coccoid or filamentous. In general, the appearance of AFB does not provide species identification; however, cells of certain species have features that may be useful diagnostically. The formation of "cords" in smears of broth cultures is typical (but not diagnostic) of MTBC. Cells of *M. kansasii* often appear as cross-barred bacilli (Fig. 60-4), larger than *M. tuberculosis* and resembling a "shepherd's crook." Cells of MAC are typically pleomorphic and occasionally coccobacillary and stain positively with the periodic acid–Schiff stain. Cells of *M. marinum* are typically longer and broader than those of *M. tuberculosis* and often show cross-banding. Cells of *M. leprae* stain weaker than those of most other mycobacteria.

TABLE 60-3
Guidelines for Reporting Smears for Acid-Fast Bacilli

No. of AFB with carbol fuchsin stain (1000×)	No. of AFB with fluorochrome stain (450×)	Report
0	0	No AFB seen
1–2/300 F (3 sweeps)	1–2/70 F (11/2 sweeps)	Doubtful; repeat
1–9/100 F	2–18/50 F (1 sweep)	1+
1–9/10 F	4–36/10 F	2+
1–9/F	4–36/F	3+
>9/F	>36/F	4+

Modified with permission from Kent PT, Kubica GP. Public health mycobacteriology: a guide for the level III laboratory. Atlanta: Department of Health and Human Services; 1985.
AFB, Acid-fast bacilli; *F,* field; *sweep,* scanning full length of a smear.

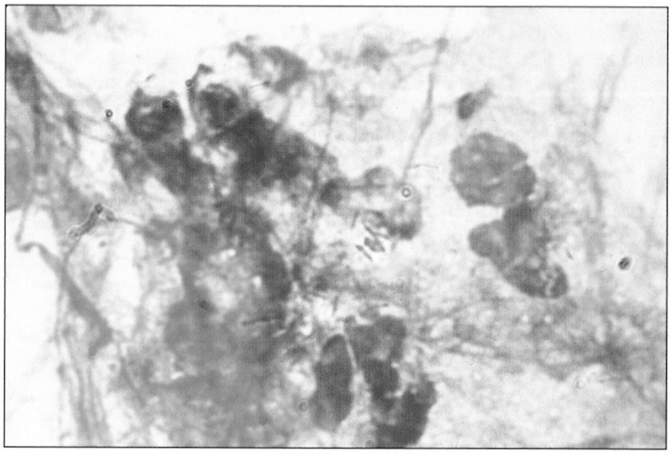

Figure 60-3 Smear of a sputum specimen shows acid-fast bacilli (*Mycobacterium tuberculosis;* Kinyoun, ×400).

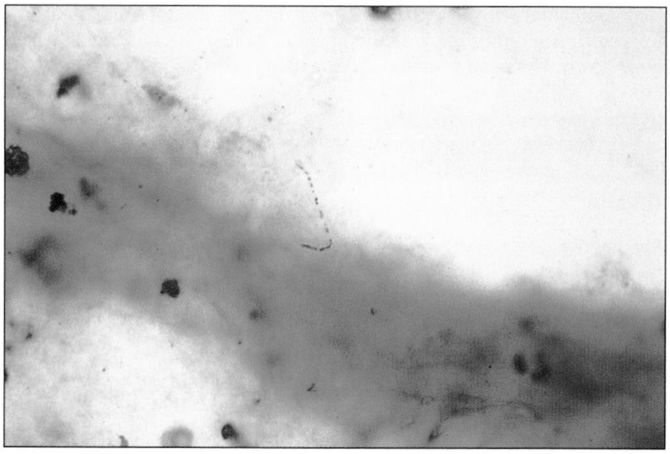

Figure 60-4 Smear of an aspirate from an enlarged cervical lymph node shows a large, cross-barred, acid-fast bacillus (*Mycobacterium kansasii;* Kinyoun, ×400). *(Courtesy Vicki J. Schnadig, MD, Department of Pathology, University of Texas Medical Branch, Galveston, Tex.)*

TABLE 60-4

Colony Morphology and Growth Characteristics of Mycobacteria Commonly Isolated in the Clinical Laboratory

***Mycobacterium* species**	**Colony morphology**	**Pigment**	**Growth rate, weeks**	**Comments**
Slowly Growing *Mycobacteria*				
M. tuberculosis	Rough	N (buff)	3–6	Generally niacin and nitrate positive
M. bovis	Rough; thin or transparent on LJ	N (colorless to buff)	4–6	Generally niacin and nitrate negative; resistant to pyrazinamide
MAC	Smooth; small, thin, transparent or large, opaque, domed; ± rough	N	3–6	Colonies of some isolates become lightly pigmented with prolonged incubation; grows at 42° C
M. kansasii	Rough, ± smooth, β-carotene crystals	P	3–6	Rare strains are N or S
M. gordonae	Smooth	S	3–6	Common laboratory contaminant; rare strains are N
M. marinum	Wrinkled, shiny; smooth, hemispherical; (rarely) rough, dry	P	2	Optimal growth, 30°–33° C
M. xenopi	Smooth, filamentous extensions ("bird's nest")	S	3–6	Growth at 42° C
M. haemophilum	Rough, ± smooth	N	3–6	Optimal growth, 20°–32° C; requires hemin for growth
M. szulgai	Smooth or rough	S, 37° C; P, 25° C	3–6	
Rapidly Growing *Mycobacteria*				
M. abscessus	Smooth; ± rough, wrinkled	N	<1	
M. fortuitum group	Wrinkled	N	<1	Branching filaments often are present on periphery of colonies
M. chelonae	Smooth	N	<1	

MAC, *M. avium* complex; *N*, nonchromogenic; *P*, photochromogenic; *S*, scotochromogenic.

The specificity of stains for AFB typically is 99% or more, and the sensitivity is about 25% to about 75% (Strumpf, 1979; Murray, 1980; Rickman, 1980). False-positive results (positive stain, negative culture) may be caused by nonviable organisms, such as might occur in patients receiving antituberculosis therapy; prolonged decontamination, killing mycobacteria as well as contaminating bacteria; or cross-contamination during the staining procedure. Factors that influence the sensitivity of smear results include (1) patient population (persons with cavitary lesions are more likely than those without cavities to have a smear-positive sputum), (2) specimen type (respiratory specimens are more likely than other specimen types to be positive), (3) the number of specimens examined, (4) the number of AFB present in the sample (5000–10,000 organisms/mL of specimen are needed for a positive result), (5) the species present (specimens containing *M. tuberculosis* or *M. kansasii* are more likely to be positive than are those that contain other mycobacteria), (6) observer experience, and (7) the stain used. Fluorochromic stains are more sensitive and are easier to read than carbol fuchsin stains, and they are recommended by experts at the CDC (Tenover, 1993). The CDC also suggests that for respiratory specimens, results of stained smears should be reported within 24 hours of specimen receipt, which means processing 7 days a week.

CULTURE METHODS

For optimal recovery of mycobacteria from clinical specimens, inoculation of both a broth and a solid medium is recommended (Tenover, 1993), because broth is more sensitive than solid media and provides more rapid detection of mycobacterial growth (Anargyros, 1990; Stager, 1991; Abe, 1992). However, use of a broth system alone may be considered if data show that adding a solid medium does not enhance recovery of mycobacterial pathogens. Broth systems currently available are the BACTEC 460TB radiometric system (BD Biosciences, Franklin Lakes, N.J.), BBL Mycobacteria Growth Indicator Tubes (MGIT; BD Biosciences), VersaTrek (previously called ESP Culture System II; Trek Diagnostic Systems, Cleveland), and BacT/Alert MB (bioMérieux, Marcy l'Etoile, France).

Two types of solid medium are used for mycobacterial culture: egg-based (Löwenstein-Jensen) and agar-based (Middlebrook 7H10, 7H11, and selective 7H11). These media are available in screw-cap tubes and flasks; agar-based media also are available in Petri dishes. Flasks are preferred to screw-cap tubes for safety reasons and because they provide a larger surface area for mycobacterial growth. Specimens from cutaneous lesions should be inoculated to one egg- or agar-based medium, and to ensure recovery of *M. haemophilum* (see later), they also should be plated on chocolate agar, 5% sheep blood Columbia agar, Mueller-Hinton agar with Fildes supplement, or Löwenstein-Jensen containing 2% ferric ammonium citrate. To recover *M. genavense* (from specimens or subcultures of liquid to solid media), solid media must be supplemented with mycobactin J. All cultures should be incubated at 37° C in an atmosphere of 5%–10% carbon dioxide (CO_2), and tubed media should be incubated in a slanted position with caps loose for at least 1 week to ensure even distribution of the inoculum over the surface. For specimens from cutaneous sites, a second set of cultures should be inoculated and incubated at 30° C, because some mycobacteria that cause skin lesions—*M. marinum*, *M. haemophilum*, *M. chelonae*, and *M. ulcerans*—grow optimally at the lower temperature. All cultures should be examined weekly for at least 6 weeks.

The major advantage of culture on solid media is that it allows visualization of colony morphology and pigmentation, which is useful diagnostically, especially for distinguishing colonies of *M. tuberculosis* from those of some NTM. The colony appearance and growth characteristics of commonly encountered mycobacteria are outlined in Table 60-4. Disadvantages of conventional solid media include prolonged time to growth of mycobacteria (colonies often are not visible on tubed solid media for 3–4 weeks or longer) and low sensitivity. Inoculation of Middlebrook agar plates, which then are examined under the microscope, allows more rapid detection of colonies (Welch, 1993), but this procedure is labor intensive, thus prohibiting its use in many clinical laboratories.

The semiautomated radiometric BACTEC TB460 was the first commercial broth-based method for growth and detection of mycobacteria, but in most laboratories has been replaced by one of the fully automated, nonradiometric broth systems. The BACTEC TB460 uses broth media (13A for blood, 12B for all other specimen types) that contain ^{14}C-labeled palmitic acid substrate. Each specimen is inoculated into one vial, and an antibiotic mixture is added to specimens other than blood. Vials are incubated in ambient air at 37° C for 5–6 weeks. To ensure recovery of *M. genavense*, blood cultures (especially those collected from patients with AIDS) should be incubated for 8–10 weeks. Bacilli multiply in the broth and utilize the labeled substrate, releasing $^{14}CO_2$ into the head space above the broth. Bottles are manually loaded onto the BACTEC TB460, which measures the amount of $^{14}CO_2$ and calculates a growth index (GI). A GI greater than 10 suggests that mycobacteria are present, and when the GI reaches 50–100, a smear of the broth is stained for AFB. Vials containing AFB are subcultured to a solid medium, and direct tests for identification (discussed in the following section) may be performed. For positive mycobacterial blood cultures from patients with AIDS, subculture to Middlebrook 7H11 agar containing mycobactin J should be done to allow recovery of *M. genavense* if initial subcultures from the broth show no growth, or the positive broth should be sent to a reference laboratory prepared to do the appropriate tests.

The MGIT consists of 4 mL of modified 7H9 broth and a fluorescent indicator embedded in silicone in the bottom of a 16 × 100-mm glass tube. Tubes are inoculated with the specimen, an antibiotic mixture to inhibit growth of contaminating bacteria and a mycobacterial growth enrichment are added, and the tubes are capped and incubated at 37° C for up to 8 weeks. To detect mycobacterial growth, tubes are manually placed on top of a 365-nm ultraviolet transilluminator or in front of a Wood's lamp. The appearance of strong fluorescence in the sensor (a bright orange color on the bottom of the tube and meniscus) indicates growth. Alternatively, tubes may be incubated in the totally automated BACTEC 960 instrument, which continuously monitors tubes for fluorescence and signals those that are positive. MGIT is as sensitive as the BACTEC TB460 for recovery of mycobacteria, but the mean time to detection of growth is a few days longer with MGIT (Cornfield, 1997; Pfyffer, 1997b; Hanna, 1999).

In addition to the BACTEC MGIT 960, three other fully automated continuously monitoring systems for growth and detection of mycobacteria are commercially available: the BACTEC 9000MB system (BD Biosciences) (Pfyffer, 1997a; Zanetti, 1997), the MB/BacT system (Organon Teknika, Durham, N.C.) (Rohner, 1997; Brunello, 1999), and the VersaTrek (Trek Diagnostic Systems) (Tholcken, 1997; Woods, 1997). With each system, bottles are incubated in the respective instrument, where they are monitored for changes in production or production and consumption of various gases, indicating growth of mycobacteria or other organisms. In general, these systems perform comparably with the BACTEC TB460 and offer the advantages of being fully automated, and thus less labor intensive, and nonradiometric.

TESTS FOR IDENTIFICATION OF MYCOBACTERIA

Identification of mycobacteria has traditionally been based on rate of growth on solid media, colony morphology, colony pigmentation with and without exposure to light, and results of biochemical tests (described in detail elsewhere [Kent, 1985]). Biochemical test results, however, are not usually available for several weeks to months after colonies appear on solid media, and for identification of MTBC especially, more rapid methods are recommended (Tenover, 1993). Additionally, biochemical testing frequently does not provide unequivocal identification at the species level.

Currently, the most rapid method for diagnosis of pulmonary tuberculosis is the use of a nucleic acid amplification test for direct detection of MTBC in clinical specimens (Piersimoni, 2003). These tests, however, do not differentiate the species in the MTBC. Two nucleic acid amplification tests are available worldwide for testing respiratory specimens: amplified *Mycobacterium tuberculosis* Direct Test (Gen-Probe, Inc., San Diego) and AMPLICOR *Mycobacterium tuberculosis* Test (Roche Diagnostic Systems, Inc., Branchburg, N.J.). The BDProbeTec ET System (BD Biosciences) is available outside the United States only. The AMPLICOR assay has been cleared by the Food and Drug Administration (FDA) for testing AFB smear-positive respiratory specimens only. The Gen-Probe test is approved for testing smear-positive and smear-negative respiratory specimens. Data suggest that nucleic acid amplification tests may be useful in AFB smear-negative patients at high risk for tuberculosis (e.g., persons infected with HIV, incarcerated persons in correctional facilities), allowing more rapid diagnosis and earlier initiation of treatment (Gamboa, 1998; Bergmann, 1999). The sensitivity of nucleic acid amplification tests is generally slightly lower for nonrespiratory specimens, but they may be useful for diagnosis of some cases of extrapulmonary tuberculosis, especially when the AFB smear is positive. In 2009, the CDC updated its guidelines for use of nucleic acid amplification tests for diagnosis of pulmonary TB, recommending that it should be performed on at least one respiratory specimen from each patient with consistent signs and symptoms for whom a diagnosis of TB is being considered but has not yet been established, and for whom the test result would alter management or TB control activities (CDC, 2009b).

Chemiluminescent DNA probes allow identification of a few species or a species complex of mycobacteria within 1–2 hours after sufficient growth is present (on solid or in a liquid medium) (Evans, 1992; Goto, 1992; Lebrun, 1992; Reisner, 1994). Commercial probes specific for MTBC, MAC, *M. avium*, *M. intracellulare*, *M. gordonae*, and *M. kansasii* are currently available. Testing requires minimal equipment (i.e., luminometer, sonicator, and heating block). Disadvantages of the probes include failure to identify some isolates of MAC, especially when testing growth from a liquid medium; false-positive results with the MAC probe when testing aliquots of broth cultures (Cloud, 2005); and rare false-positive results with the MTBC probe (Bull, 1992; Lebrun, 1992; Butler, 1994).

High-performance liquid chromatography allows identification of mycobacterial colonies on a solid medium or growth in a liquid medium in 2–4 hours. The most accurate identification method is sequencing, most commonly of the hypervariable regions of the 16S ribosomal RNA gene (Patel, 2000; Cloud, 2002; Hall, 2003). Molecular typing methods, such as spoligotyping (spacer oliogotyping), are useful for identifying members of the MTBC to the species level (Mostowy, 2004). These techniques, which are technically complex and require expensive equipment, are performed predominantly in research and large reference laboratories.

SUSCEPTIBILITY TESTING

Susceptibility testing of mycobacteria should be performed according to guidelines of the Clinical and Laboratory Standards Institute (CLSI; in press). Primary and secondary drugs that should be tested are listed in Table 60-5.

For MTBC, the initial isolate from every patient should be tested to all primary drugs. Testing should be repeated if specimens remain culture positive after 3 months of appropriate therapy, or earlier if there is clinical evidence of treatment failure. Testing may be performed on isolated colonies or a positive broth culture (indirect test) or on sputum specimens that are AFB smear positive (direct test). Agar proportion is the standard method of testing susceptibility of MTBC to antituberculosis agents. With this method, isolates showing greater than 1% resistance to a single concentration of drug are considered resistant to that drug. However, because the target turnaround time for results is an average of 28 days after specimens are received in the laboratory, use of an FDA-approved liquid-based

TABLE 60-5
Drugs Recommended for Susceptibility Testing of *Mycobacteria*

***Mycobacterium* species**	**Indication**	**Drugs**
MTBC	Primary	Isoniazid, rifampin, ethambutol, pyrazinamide
	Secondary	Capreomycin, ethionamide, ethambutol (higher concentration), amikacin, kanamycin, levofloxacin, ofloxacin, isoniazid (higher concentration), *p*-aminosalicylic acid, rifabutin, streptomycin
MAC	Primary	Clarithromycin
	Secondary	Moxifloxacin, linezolid
M. kansasii	Primary	Rifampin
	Secondary	Amikacin, ciprofloxacin, clarithromycin, ethambutol, isoniazid, moxifloxacin, rifabutin, streptomycin, trimethoprim-sulfamethoxazole
M. marinum	Primary	Amikacin, ciprofloxacin, clarithromycin, doxycycline, moxifloxacin, rifabutin, trimethoprim-sulfamethoxazole
Rapidly growing mycobacteria	Primary	Amikacin, cefoxitin, ciprofloxacin, clarithromycin, doxycycline, imipenem, linezolid, meropenem, moxifloxacin, tobramycin, trimethoprim-sulfamethoxazole

MAC, M. avium complex; *MTBC, M. tuberculosis* complex.

system that provides results equivalent to those of agar proportion is recommended (Tenover, 1993; CLSI, in press). With currently available liquid-based systems, results are generally available 5–7 days after bottles are inoculated with the MTBC isolate (Bergmann 1998, 2000; Scarparo, 2004). Susceptibility to all secondary drugs should be tested when an isolate is resistant to rifampin alone or any two of the primary agents. Isolates resistant only to the critical concentration of isoniazid also should be tested for susceptibility to secondary agents if the planned treatment regimen will include a fluoroquinolone.

Because early detection and appropriate treatment of MDR- and XDR-TB are so important to cure of the disease and prevention of transmission, various molecular methods for rapid detection of mutations known to be associated with drug resistance have been developed, including real-time polymerase chain reaction (PCR) and commercial PCR/line probe assays (Lin, 2004; Morgan, 2005; Bang, 2006). Use of a molecular test to detect drug resistance directly in an AFB smear-positive specimen may be considered in a patient who meets one or more of the following criteria: history of prior treatment for TB, coming from a country or ethnic group known to have increased drug resistance, failure to respond to standard therapy, and known exposure to MDR-TB.

Susceptibility testing of NTM may be performed on clinically significant isolates (Griffith, 2007); however, for some species, little correlation may be noted between susceptibility test results and clinical response to drug therapy. The method recommended by CLSI for susceptibility testing of rapidly and slowly growing NTM is broth microdilution (Woods, 1999; CLSI, in press). Media, incubation times and temperatures, and guidelines for interpretation of results are beyond the scope of this chapter but are described in detail in the most recent edition of CLSI M24 (CLSI, in press). In general, both the minimum inhibitory concentration (MIC) and the interpretation (susceptible, intermediate, resistant) should be reported.

TREATMENT

The chemotherapeutic regimen currently recommended for treatment of TB (Table 60-6) should be initiated before susceptibility test results are available, but treatment should be altered based on those results if an isolate is found to be resistant. Medications should be administered by directly observed therapy. Regimens commonly used to treat infections caused by the most frequently encountered NTM also are listed in Table 60-6 (Griffith, 2007). For many NTM, however, neither the optimal regimen nor the duration of therapy is known.

TABLE 60-6

Antimicrobial Agents Recommended for Primary Treatment of Common Mycobacterial Infections

***Mycobacterium* species**	**Site of infection**	**Antimicrobial agents**
MTBC	Any	Isoniazid, rifampin, ethambutol, pyrazinamide
MAC	Pulmonary	Clarithromycin,* rifampin, and ethambutol
	Disseminated	Clarithromycin* and ethambutol ± rifabutin
	Lymphadenitis†	None
M. kansasii	Pulmonary	Isoniazid, rifampin, ethambutol
M. abscessus, chelonae, fortuitum‡	Nonpulmonary	Clarithromycin (if susceptible) and one or more additional agents§
M. abscessus¶	Pulmonary	Multidrug regimen,§ including clarithromycin
M. marinum	Skin/soft tissue	Clarithromycin, doxycycline/minocycline, trimethoprim-sulfamethoxazole, or rifampin and ethambutol

MAC, M. avium complex; *MTBC, M. tuberculosis* complex.
*Or azithromycin.
†Recommended management is surgery.
‡Surgical debridement often is necessary.
§Agent(s) selected should be based on results of susceptibility testing.
¶Currently, there are no drug regimens with proven efficacy, although antimicrobial therapy may provide symptomatic improvement and disease regression. If disease is limited, surgical resection plus multidrug therapy is optimal.

PREVENTION

MYCOBACTERIUM TUBERCULOSIS COMPLEX

Four general strategies for controlling TB are described. The most important is early identification and adequate treatment of persons with infectious TB. This measure renders the infected person noncontagious within a few weeks and eventually results in cure. The second strategy entails identification and treatment of individuals with noncontagious TB: extrapulmonary disease, primary pulmonary disease in children, bacteriologically unconfirmed pulmonary disease, and infection with *M. tuberculosis* not yet causing disease (i.e., positive skin test or interferon-γ release assay, normal chest radiograph, no symptoms).

The third strategy involves creation of a safe environment in situations where the risk of transmitting infection is high: autopsy suites, sputum induction cubicles, chest clinic waiting areas, correctional facilities, some shelters for the homeless, and mycobacteriology laboratories. To accomplish this, several issues must be addressed (Segal-Maurer, 1994). Rooms housing infectious patients or in which potentially infectious specimens are handled should be under negative pressure, and air likely to be contaminated with infectious droplet nuclei should be exhausted to the outside. A single-pass ventilation system (best accomplished by locating air supply outlets at the ceiling level and exhaust inlets near the floor) and a minimum of six air changes per hour (12 exchanges per hour for autopsy suites) are recommended. Universal precautions must be followed when handling all specimens, and both specimens and cultures must be handled in a certified, class II biological safety cabinet. Moreover, a particulate respirator that filters out particles 1–5 μm in diameter should be worn, and personnel should be trained in a respiratory program; the standard surgical mask is not adequate.

The fourth strategy is vaccination with the BCG vaccine, an attenuated vaccine derived from a strain of *M. bovis* by Calmette and Guérin in France. This vaccine is used in many foreign countries where the prevalence of TB is high, to prevent TB meningitis and miliary TB in children, but generally is not recommended in the United States, because the risk of infection with MTBC is low and the effectiveness of the vaccine in adults is variable. In the United States, the BCG vaccine should be considered after consulting with a TB expert only for infants and children who have a negative tuberculin skin test and who are continuously exposed and cannot be separated from adults who are untreated or ineffectively treated for TB or have MDR-TB (www.cdc.gov/tb). The BCG vaccine is not routinely recommended for health care workers in the United States but should be considered on an individual basis in the following settings: a high percentage of TB patients have MDR-TB, transmission of MDR-TB to health care workers and subsequent infection is likely, and comprehensive TB control measures have been implemented but have not been successful.

The BCG vaccine should not be given to immunocompromised persons, persons likely to become immunocompromised, or pregnant women. Disseminated *M. bovis* in patients with AIDS and *M. bovis* lymphadenitis in symptomatic HIV-infected infants have occurred following BCG vaccination (Centers for Disease Control and Prevention, 1985; Blanche, 1986). However, disseminated *M. bovis* has not been reported in asymptomatic persons infected with HIV. In populations where the risk of tuberculosis is high, the World Health Organization recommends that the BCG vaccine be given to HIV-infected children at birth or soon thereafter. It should not be given to children with symptomatic HIV infection, to populations in which the risk of tuberculosis is low, or to persons known or suspected to be infected with HIV (World Health Organization, 1987).

MYCOBACTERIUM AVIUM COMPLEX

Disseminated MAC in patients with AIDS is associated with considerable morbidity and a shortened duration of survival (Horsburgh, 1991b; Nightingale, 1992); therefore, prevention of the disease is desirable. Because MAC is ubiquitous in the environment, the most reasonable approach to prevention is chemoprophylaxis. Currently, the U.S. Public Health Service and the Infectious Diseases Society of America recommend clarithromycin or azithromycin prophylaxis in AIDS patients with $CD4^+$ cell counts lower than 50/μL (Centers for Disease Control and Prevention, 2009a). If neither of these drugs can be tolerated, rifabutin is an alternative prophylactic agent. Primary prophylaxis should be discontinued in patients who have responded to antiretroviral therapy with an increase in $CD4^+$ count of >100 cells/μL for at least 3 months.

SELECTED REFERENCES

Brown-Elliott AB, Wallace RJ Jr. Clinical and taxonomic status of pathogenic nonpigmented or late-pigmenting rapidly growing mycobacteria. Clin Microbiol Rev 2002;15:716–46.

Excellent review of the taxonomy of rapidly growing mycobacteria. Also includes a discussion of laboratory tests for identification and the usual antimicrobial susceptibility patterns.

Clinical and Laboratory Standards Institute. Susceptibility testing of *Mycobacteria*, *Nocardia*, and other aerobic actinomycetes. Wayne, Pa: National Committee for Clinical Laboratory Standards; 2003. Approved Standard M24-A.

Guidelines for testing susceptibility of M. tuberculosis *complex, rapidly growing mycobacteria, and select slowly growing mycobacteria, including* M. avium *complex,* M. kansasii, *and* M. marinum.

Falkinham JO III. Epidemiology of infection by nontuberculous mycobacteria. Clin Microbiol Rev 1996;9:177.

In-depth review of the epidemiology of more commonly encountered nontuberculous mycobacteria, including M. avium *complex,* M. kansasii, *and* M. marinum, *as well as* M. simiae *and* M. xenopi.

Griffith DE, Aksamit T, Brown-Elliott BA, et al. An official ATS/IDSA statement: diagnosis, treatment, and prevention of nontuberculous mycobacterial diseases. Am J Respir Crit Care Med 2007;175:367.

Excellent review of the laboratory diagnosis and treatment of commonly encountered nontuberculous mycobacteria, including M. avium *complex,* M. kansasii, M. marinum, *and rapidly growing mycobacteria.*

Madkukar P, Zwerling A, Menzies D. Systematic review: T-cell-based assays for the diagnosis of latent tuberculosis infection: an update. Ann Intern Med 2008;149:1.

Excellent discussion of the value of T cell–based assays for diagnosis of latent tuberculosis infection.

Piersimoni C, Scarparo C. Relevance of commercial amplification methods for direct detection of *Mycobacterium tuberculosis* complex in clinical samples. J Clin Microbiol 2003;41:5355–65.

Excellent review of the commercial nucleic acid amplification tests for direct detection of M. tuberculosis *complex in clinical specimens.*

Runyon EH. Anonymous mycobacteria in pulmonary disease. Med Clin North Am 1959;43:273.

Classic description of the different groups of nontuberculous mycobacteria.

Scollard DM, Adams LB, Gillis TP, et al. The continuing challenges of leprosy. Clin Microbiol Rev 2006;19:338.

An excellent up-to-date review of leprosy.

Tortoli E. Impact of genotypic studies on mycobacterial taxonomy: the new mycobacteria of the 1990s. Clin Microbiol Rev 2003;16:319–54.

Excellent discussion of the more recently described species of slowly growing and rapidly growing mycobacteria. Includes information regarding epidemiology, clinical manifestations, phenotypic characteristics, and antimicrobial susceptibility.

REFERENCES

Access the complete reference list online at http://www.expertconsult.com

CHAPTER 61

MYCOTIC DISEASES

Peter C. Iwen

KEY POINTS

- Opportunistic fungal pathogens have emerged as common causes of invasive disease in the compromised host.
- Histopathologic examination of deep tissue is a major means used for the rapid detection and recognition of fungal pathogens causing invasive infection.
- Micromorphologic and phenotypic methods continue to be the general processes used in the clinical laboratory for the identification of fungal pathogens in culture.
- Molecular methods have advanced as techniques used for the confirmed identification of fungal pathogens from culture and are evolving as future methods for the rapid identification of fungal pathogens directly in clinical material.
- *Candida albicans* continues to be the most common fungal species associated with human disease; however, non-*albicans Candida* species are becoming more widespread in causing invasive disease with increased resistance to standard antifungal treatments.
- Dimorphic fungal pathogens are frequent causes of mild infection in people living in endemic areas; however, invasive disease, whether recurrent or primary, is becoming more common owing to the increase in immunocompromised hosts.
- Recent introduction of new antifungal agents and progression of resistance among moulds and yeast have added importance to the development and standardization of antifungal susceptibility testing.

Medical mycology is the science devoted to the study of fungi and their relationship to human disease. This scientific discipline encompasses single-celled yeasts and filamentous moulds as agents of disease ranging from superficial skin infection (cutaneous mycosis) to disseminated deep-seated visceral disease (systemic mycosis). Fungal agents include the historically pathogenic fungi (true pathogens), as well as the saprophytic fungi elevated to the status of pathogen by modern therapies and diseases (opportunistic pathogens). Modern therapies such as high-dose chemotherapy to treat cancer and solid organ transplantation, as well as immunosuppressive infection such as acquired immunodeficiency syndrome (AIDS), have served as the impetus to allow fungi to emerge as major causes of human disease (Chayakulkeeree, 2006; Pfaller, 2007; Sanchez, 2007; Chang, 2008; Marr, 2008; Richardson, 2008; Varkey, 2008).

Although medical mycology education for the medical profession in general has been lacking, pathologists who have been nurtured in the surgical pathology suite have acquired a general understanding of the recognition of fungal pathogens (Steinbach, 2003a). Overall, the general lack of education in this area is troublesome because most fungi are identified by skilled human observation rather than by machines.

The goal of this chapter is to present the fundamentals of medical mycology with an emphasis on practical issues and a description of those fungal pathogens encountered regularly in the laboratory. For a comprehensive atlas of the histopathology of fungal infections, refer to the book by Chandler and Watts (1987a). Additionally, although not included in the fungal kingdom, infections caused by achlorophyllous algae are also discussed in this chapter because the characteristics of the algae and the diseases they produce resemble fungi more than other infectious agents.

Because this chapter reports specifically on fungal mycoses, other types of fungal diseases are not discussed. Reviews of these other diseases are available and include the topics of noninvasive allergic responses to fungi (Thakar, 2004; Schubert, 2009), poisoning by the ingestion of poisonous fungi (mushroom poisoning or mycetismus) (Diaz, 2005a, 2005b), and intoxication by ingestion of fungal toxins (mycotoxicosis) (Etzel, 2002).

Nomenclature, Taxonomy, and Fungal Morphology

OVERVIEW

The first hurdle for the beginning mycologist consists of nomenclature and its handmaiden, taxonomy. Members of the fungal kingdom (Eumycota) are eukaryotic cells that have the capability to reproduce by both sexual and asexual methods. They are classified into phyla by the nature of their sexual reproductive structures or lack thereof (Hibbett, 2007). Fungi that have recognized sexual reproductive structures (perfect fungi) are classified into the phylum Zygomycota, Ascomycota, or Basidiomycota based on the type of sexual reproductive structure produced. Fungi that lack recognized sexual reproductive structures are classified in the phylum Deuteromycota, also called the imperfect fungi, on the basis of their asexual reproductive structures. The application of new molecular techniques in fungal identification has caused changes within the classification of fungi. For example, genomic studies now suggest that the phylum Zygomycota is polyphyletic, and that a new classification for this group should be considered (James, 2006). Much work is ongoing in the area of fungal taxonomics, and changes in fungal nomenclature will continue to occur.

To complicate the naming and taxonomic positioning of fungi, many species have both asexual (anamorphic) and sexual (teleomorphic) phases. Within the Deuteromycota, once the sexual phase becomes recognized, the organism is reclassified into one of the other phyla and now becomes a named teleomorph. In practice, however, the old familiar name of the anamorph is usually retained. For example, few people know *Histoplasma capsulatum*, *Blastomyces dermatitidis*, and *Cryptococcus neoformans* by their respective teleomorphic names *Ajellomyces capsulatus*, *Ajellomyces dermatitidis*, and *Filobasidiella neoformans*, respectively. In contrast, the sexual phase *Pseudallescheria boydii* and the corresponding asexual phase *Scedosporium apiospermum* are both recognized species names used in common practice. Generally, the anamorphic name, as in this case *S. apiospermum*, is used to describe a fungal species in the laboratory, although many exceptions to this rule exist.

Much of fungal taxonomy is related to structural details because both classification and laboratory identification are heavily dependent on morphology. A glossary of important terms used in medical mycology is displayed in Table 61-1 on the next page. In this chapter, a simplified conceptual approach will be used to recognize the pathogens most commonly encountered in the clinical laboratory. For practical purposes, a few general characteristics shown in Table 61-2 serve as the basis for identification of fungi in the laboratory.

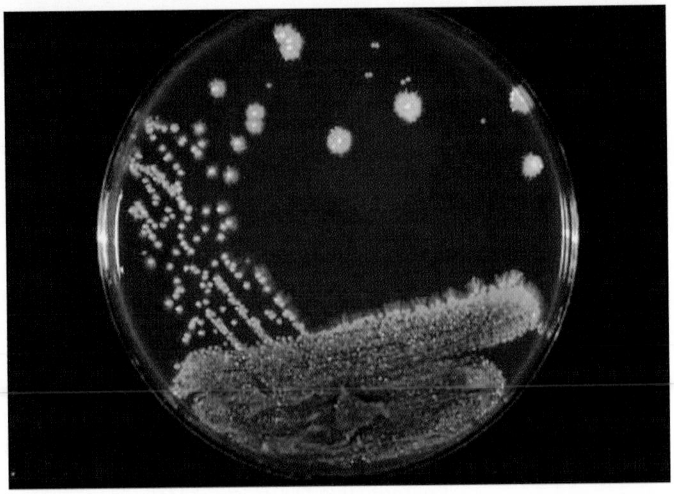

Figure 61-1 Filamentous extensions from the periphery of colonies of *Candida albicans* are known colloquially as "feet."

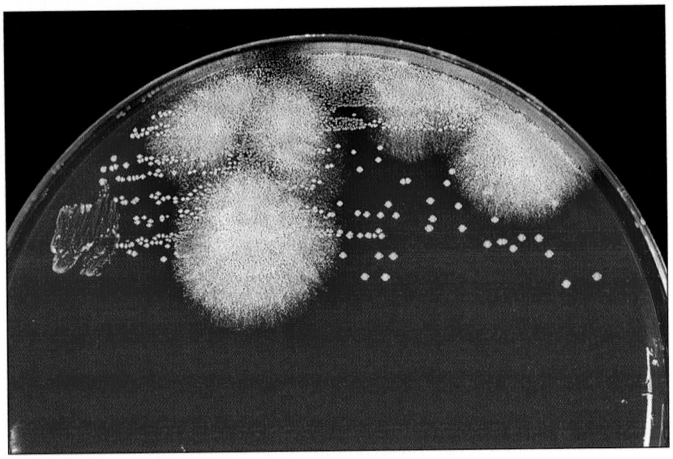

Figure 61-2 Powdery surface of the colonies of *Aspergillus fumigatus* overlies white masses of mycelium. Adjacent bacterial colonies contrast with the filamentous fungus. (Sheep blood agar.)

THE FUNGAL COLONY

Two morphologic forms of fungi are recognized and include yeasts and moulds. Yeasts are unicellular organisms that usually reproduce asexually by blastoconidia (also called budding) to produce a daughter cell. The colonial mass of yeast is a collection of distinct individual organisms that macroscopically resemble bacterial colonies on the surface of the agar. Yeast colonies usually are smooth with a regular edge. When the colonies become heaped and dull, they may resemble those of staphylococci. Yeast produces catalase, so the incautious microbiologist who does not perform a Gram stain or a wet preparation may mistake a yeast colony for a bacterium and provide a misleading report. The microscopic presence of "budding yeast" with or without pseudohyphae would be adequate to identify the colony as yeast. Furthermore, the pseudohyphae of yeast are often visible macroscopically as filamentous extensions from the edges of the colony, known colloquially as "feet" (Fig. 61-1).

In contrast to yeasts, moulds are described as filamentous fungi that are multicellular in structure. Although the term **mold** is used to describe this morphologic type, the term **mould** is historically recognized and more commonly used by mycologists to describe this morphologic form. The filamentous nature of the mould gives colonies a woolly, fluffy, or velvety appearance, sometimes punctuated with a granular or powdery aspect that is produced by the formation of asexual reproductive structures (Fig. 61-2). At other times, the colony may have a glabrous (smooth) appearance.

TABLE 61-1
Glossary of Terms Commonly Used in Medical Mycology

Term	Definition
Aerial mycelium	Hyphae produced above the surface of the agar media
Anamorph	Asexual form of fungal sporulation (imperfect state)
Arthroconidium	Conidium derived from the fragmentation of specialized hyphae
Ascocarp (ascoma)	Fruiting structure that contains asci (several types exist)
Ascospore	Sexual spore formed within an ascus following meiosis
Ascus (pl., asci)	Sac-like structure that contains ascospores, characteristic of Ascomycetes
Basidiospore	Sexual spore formed as on an outgrowth of a basidium
Basidium	Structure that contains basidiospores (e.g., mushroom)
Blastoconidium	Asexual spore formed by budding of the yeast cell
Chlamydospore	Thick-walled resting or survival structure (also called chlamydoconidia)
Cleistothecium (pl., cleistothecia)	Enclosed ascocarp, composed of layers of hyphae that contain randomly dispersed asci
Collarette	Funnel-shaped structure at the apex of a phialide
Columella	An extension of the sporangiophore into the base of the sporangium
Conidiogenous cell	Cell that produces conidia
Conidiophore	Specialized hyphal structure that carries the conidia
Conidium (pl., conidia)	Asexual reproductive structure formed in any manner that does not involve cleavage
Dematiaceous	Pigmented in dark color
Dimorphic	Displaying two morphologic types, one environmental (mould) and one in vivo (yeast)
Glabrous	Smooth, referring to colonial morphology
Heterothallic	Sexual reproduction requiring the interaction of two different thalli (mating strains)
Holomorph	Whole fungus; the anamorphic plus the teleomorphic state of the fungus
Homothallic	Sexual reproduction can take place within one thallus
Hyaline	Colorless or transparent
Hypha (pl., hyphae)	Vegetative unit of a mould
Intercalary	Borne within a hypha
Macroconidium	Larger of two types of conidia produced by a mould
Microconidium	Smaller of two types of conidia produced by a mould
Mould	Filamentous fungus that reproduces by sexual or asexual means
Mycelium	Mass of hyphae that make up the thallus of a mould
Perithecium	Enclosed ascocarp with a pore at the top through which the ascospores are discharged
Phialide	Cell with opening through which conidia are produced
Pseudohyphae	Connected yeast cells (blastoconidia) that resemble a hypha but contain areas of constriction between adjacent cells
Scleotium (pl., sclerotia)	Multi-cellular clump of cells that does not produce any spores or conidia (also called sclerotic body)
Septum (pl., septa)	Cross-wall in a hypha
Sporangiophore	Stalk bearing the sporangium
Sporangiospore	Asexual spore produced within a sporangium
Sporangium	Sac-like structure in which the asexual sporangiospores develop
Sterigmata	Slender outgrowth of a cell bearing conidia
Teleomorph	Sexual form of a fungal sporulation (perfect state)
Terminal	Borne at the end of a hypha
Thallus (pl., thalli)	Vegetative growth of a fungus; includes an interwoven mass of hyphae
Thermophillic	Fungi that grow at a high temperature
Vegetative mycelium	Hyphae produced on the surface or extending into the agar media
Vesicle	Enlarged or swollen cell, often at the end of a conidiophore or sporangiophore, which may also be within hyphae
Yeast	Single-cell fungus that reproduces by budding or by fission

The distinction between moulds and yeasts is not firmly established. Some yeasts also develop a visually macroscopic filamentous component. For instance, *Trichosporon* spp. are yeasts that develop such filamentous extensions, whereas *Exophiala jeanselmei* is a dematiaceous yeast that develops a mycelium as it matures. The ultimate in fence-sitting is exemplified by the dimorphic fungi, which exhibit a mould form under some conditions and a yeast or yeast-like form in other circumstances. Clinically important dimorphic fungi are systemic pathogens that behave as moulds in the environment and on agar media at 25°–30° C. In contrast, the tissue form may be a yeast (such as *Blastomyces dermatitidis*, *Histoplasma capsulatum*, and *Sporothrix schenckii*) or, in the cases of *Coccidioides immitis* and *Coccidioides posadasii*, a yeast-like structure called a spherule. When cultivated in vitro at 37° C on appropriate media, the tissue form is reproduced by these fungi. Other agents also exhibit dimorphism but are less common in the clinical laboratory. For instance, black moulds such as *Fonsecaea pedrosi* and *Phialophora verrucosa* produce nonhyphal cells in tissue called sclerotic bodies but appear as moulds when grown on solid media at room temperature. Reverse dimorphism is exemplified by *Malassezia furfur*, which produces both yeast cells and hyphae in the cutaneous lesions of patients with pityriasis versicolor.

STRUCTURE OF YEASTS AND HYPHAE

The morphology of the fungus is an important characteristic for the identification of both yeasts and moulds. The filamentous structure of a mould is referred to as hyphae (singular, *hypha*), and a mass of hyphae is known as a mycelium. The mycelium growing on the surface of or within the agar is known as the vegetative mycelium, whereas filamentous extensions above the colony are called aerial mycelium. True hyphae may have cross-walls that contain pores for communication through the hyphae or cross-walls that are complete, dividing the hyphae into multiple cells. Hyphae that have cross-walls are called septate, whereas those without cross-walls

TABLE 61-2
Characteristics Useful for the Identification of Fungi

Characteristic	Examples
Type of macroscopic growth	Colonies of unicellular organisms (yeast)
	Colonies of filamentous organisms (moulds)
Morphology of yeast	Budding
	Budding with pseudohyphae
	Round yeast with capsules
	Budding yeast with collarettes
Morphology of filamentous structures	True septate hyphae
	True nonseptate hyphae (or sparsely septate)
Pigment of hyphae	Hyaline (lightly pigmented or nonpigmented)
	Dematiaceous (darkly pigmented)
Morphology of asexual reproductive structures	Conidia
	Spores
Morphology of sexual reproductive structures	Ascospores
	Cleistothecia
	Perithecia
Growth rate	Slow (>10 days)
	Medium (4–10 days)
	Fast (<4 days)
Inhibition by cycloheximide	Many saprophytic fungi
Optimal growth temperature	25°–30° C
	35°–37° C
	40°–42° C
	50°–58° C
Biochemical tests	Assimilation
	Fermentation
	Enzymatic degradation (e.g., urease)
	Growth enhancement
Conversion from mould to yeast phase	Supplanted by DNA probe tests in most laboratories
Immunologic detection of antigens or antibodies	*Cryptococcus, Histoplasma, Coccidioides, Blastomyces, Aspergillus*
DNA probe	*Histoplasma, Coccidioides, Blastomyces*

DNA, Deoxyribonucleic acid.

are referred to as aseptate. Some fungi that have septate hyphae also have aseptate or septate specialized hyphae (conidiophores) that bear asexual reproductive structures. Conversely, some so-called nonseptate fungi have occasional cross-walls and perhaps would be better designated as sparsely septate.

The width of the hyphae and the angle of branching are important clues to fungal identity. Zygomycetes, such as *Rhizopus* spp., have broad, ribbon-like hyphae that branch predominantly at right angles (Fig. 61-3), whereas hyaline moulds such as *Aspergillus* spp. have narrow hyphae that branch at acute angles (dichotomous branching) (Fig. 61-4). The designation of a fungus as *Aspergillus* on the basis of hyphal morphology in a smear or tissue section is, in truth, only a statement of the a priori odds for this pathogen group. Describing the characteristics of the hyphae is a better approach to reporting this observation.

Yeasts reproduce asexually by the formation of blastoconidia, where the daughter cell usually appears at one end of a yeast cell and eventually enlarges to form a new yeast cell. This process is also referred to in a more generic sense as **budding.** If a series of daughter cells do not detach fully from the originating cells, a pseudohypha (plural, *pseudohyphae)* is produced. Pseudohyphae are distinguished from true hyphae by the presence of a constriction at the junction of adjacent cells and by the restriction in size of the daughter cell to that of the parent (Fig. 61-5). In contrast, the walls of true hyphae are parallel without constrictions. *C. albicans* and some strains of *Candida tropicalis* may produce pseudohyphae that have the appearance of true hyphae, depending on growth conditions, and differentiation of *Candida* from hyaline moulds such as *Aspergillus* in tissue sections on occasion may be problematic. In contradistinction, *Cryptococcus* spp. produce only budding yeast and rarely rudimentary or primitive pseudohyphae, but true hyphae are not formed.

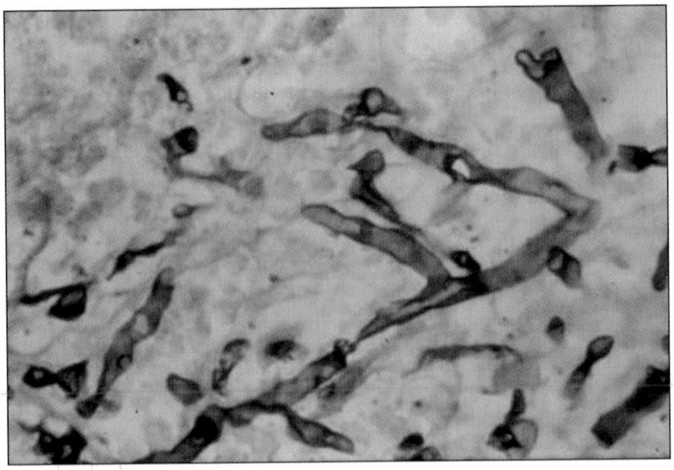

Figure 61-3 Characteristic wide, nonseptate hypha of a Zygomycete in lung tissue. (Gomori's methenamine silver stain, ×400.)

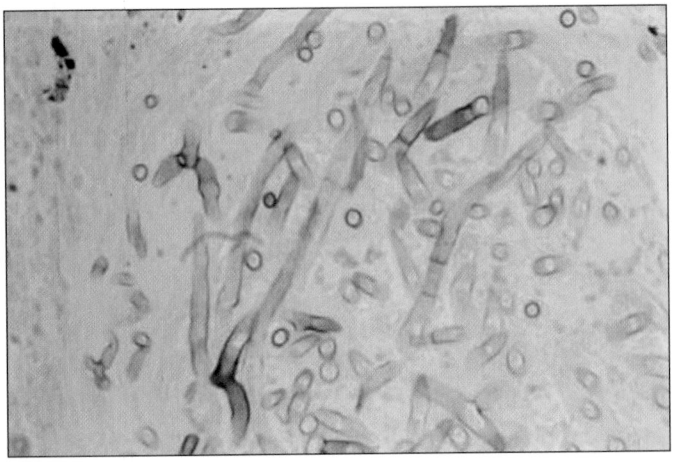

Figure 61-4 Characteristic narrow branching, septate hyphae of a hyaline mould in tissue. (Gomori's methenamine silver stain, ×400.)

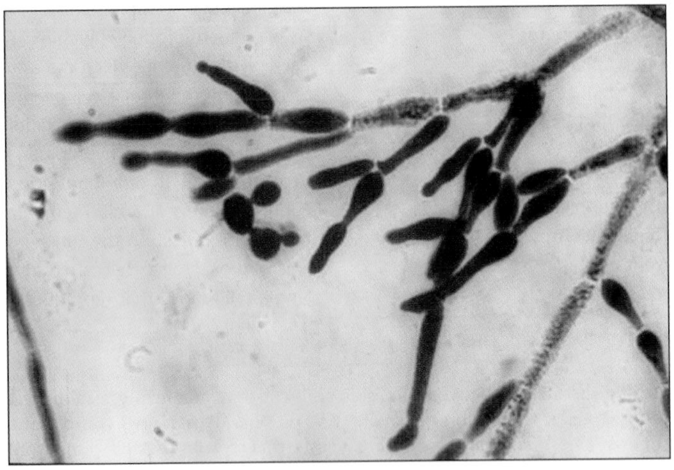

Figure 61-5 Chains of elongated budding yeasts of *Candida albicans* producing pseudohyphae observed in sputum. (Gram stain, ×1000.)

HYPHAL PIGMENT

Some mould hyphae can be characterized by the production of a dark pigment. The hyphae of dematiaceous fungi contain a melanin pigment that imparts a brown coloration to the hyphae in microscopic preparations and causes colonies of the fungi to appear dark green, brown, or black.

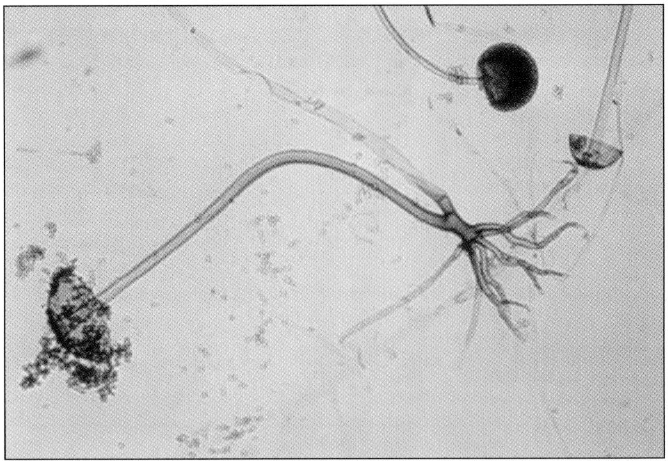

Figure 61-6 Sporangiophores of *Rhizopus* spp. supporting sporangia that contain sporangiospores. Rhizoids arise from the hyphae near the origin of the sporangiophores. (Lactophenol cotton blue stain, ×100.)

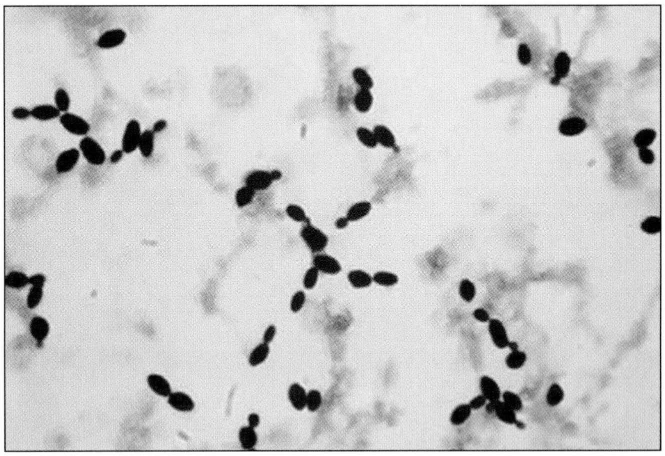

Figure 61-7 Budding and nonbudding yeast cells detected in a blood culture bottle sample. (Gram stain, ×1000.)

Superimposed dyes in stained smears, wet preps, or histologic sections may partially obscure the color, which can be more obvious in unstained preparations. Those fungi that lack dark hyphal pigmentation are referred to as hyaline (clear or colorless). This term may not fully reflect the fungal species appearance, because in some cases a light pigmentation may produce colored colonies and asexual reproductive structures of some hyaline moulds may have green, brown, or black pigments that impart a color to the surface of the colony once the reproductive structures have formed. The true appearance of these moulds usually can be discerned by observing the back of the colony, which maintains a light coloration. In contrast, both the front (obverse) and the back (reverse) of dematiaceous colonies usually demonstrate the dark pigment.

REPRODUCTIVE STRUCTURES

The primary means for identification of mould fungi is by characterization of asexual reproductive structures. For yeast, phenotypic studies are the mainstay in identification, with asexual reproductive structures serving as ancillary clues in the identification process. The two principal asexual structures are spores (which may also be present as sexual structures) and conidia. Asexual spores (called sporangiospores) are produced by cleavage within an encompassing structure called a sporangium (Fig. 61-6). Conidia (singular, *conidium)* are much more diverse and form by differentiation from the tip or side of a fertile hypha, such as a conidiophore, or by hyphal differentiation. Unfortunately, interchangeable use of the terms conidium and spore in the literature has led to confusion. Sporulation and spores often are used as general terms for asexual reproduction, and the term spore is sometimes used when conidium would have been more accurate.

The principal means of asexual reproduction in yeast is by the formation of blastoconidia (i.e., budding). A bud starts as a softening of the cell wall of the mother cell, followed by expansion of the cell wall (blown out) and migration of nucleus and cytoplasm to the swollen area. A septum seals the boundary between daughter and parent cells (Fig. 61-7). If separation does not occur, a pseudohypha results.

The portions of the vegetative mycelium that differentiate into conidia are referred to as conidiogenous cells. Specialized hyphae that support the conidia are termed conidiophores, which may be the conidiogenous cell itself arising from the vegetative mycelium or may be a supporting hypha. In *Aspergillus* spp., the conidiophore, which is aseptate, enlarges at the tip to form a swollen vesicle (Fig. 61-8). Conidiogenous cells, now termed phialides, arise from the vesicle to support chains of conidia. Some species of *Aspergillus* produce a row of phialides, which occur on a row of sterile cells called metulae, with the conidia arising from the distal phialides. The Zygomycetes produce structures called sporangiophores, which support the sporangium with enclosed sporangiospores (see Fig. 61-6). An extension of the apex of the sporangiophore into the sporangium is termed the columella.

Thallic conidiogenesis is a process in which the conidium does not develop until a septum is formed between the conidium and the parent cell. The conidium originates from the whole of the parent cell. The most important human pathogens that exhibit thallic conidiogenesis are the dermatophytes and the dimorphic fungi in the *Coccidioides* spp. As

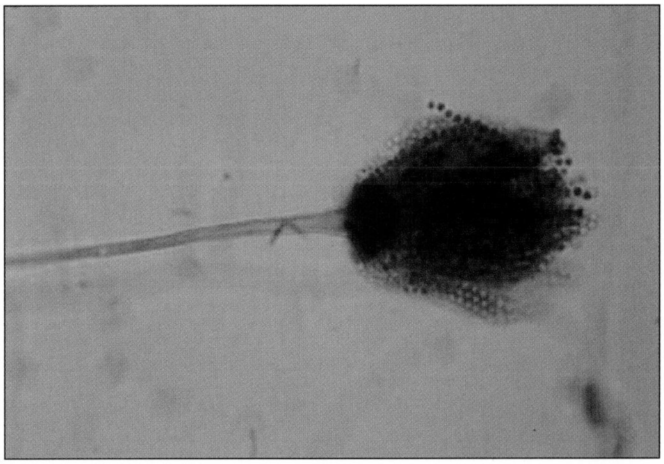

Figure 61-8 Fruiting head of *Aspergillus fumigatus*. The conidiophore is swollen at the tip to form a vesicle, and phialides arise from the upper half of the vesicle with chains of conidia present that align parallel to the long axis of the conidiophore. (Lactophenol cotton blue stain, ×400.)

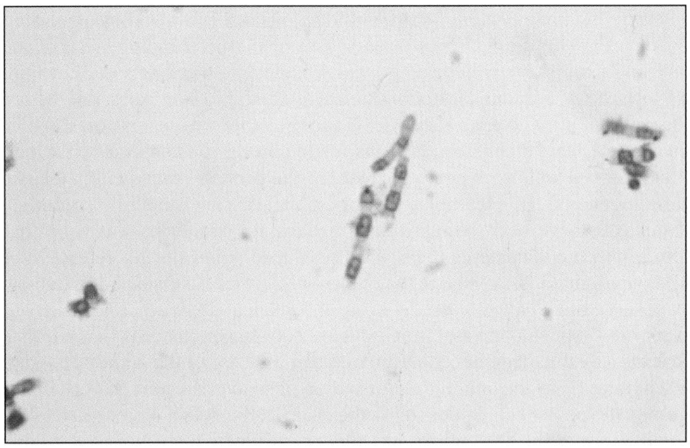

Figure 61-9 Arthroconidia of *Coccidioides* species. Alternating barrel-shaped arthroconidia are separated by thin-walled, empty disjunctor cells within portions of the hyphae. (Lactophenol cotton blue stain, ×400.)

conidiogenesis progresses in these species, barrel-shaped conidia called arthroconidia are produced; these fragment easily and are disseminated with little difficulty, resulting in the high degree of infectivity demonstrated by these important human pathogens (Fig. 61-9). The thallic conidia of the dermatophytes are separated by size into two types: large septate macroconidia (Fig. 61-10) and small, one-celled microconidia that are simpler structures (Fig. 61-11).

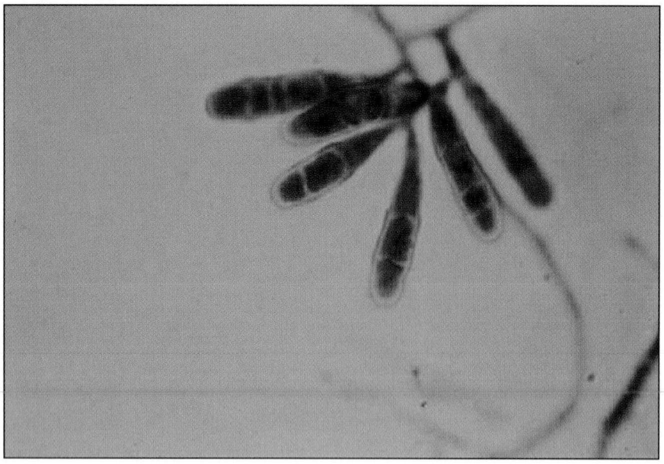

Figure 61-10 Macroconidia of *Epidermophyton floccosum*. Typical blunt-ended macroconidia occur in aggregates along the hyphae with the absence of microconidia. (Lactophenol cotton blue stain, ×400.)

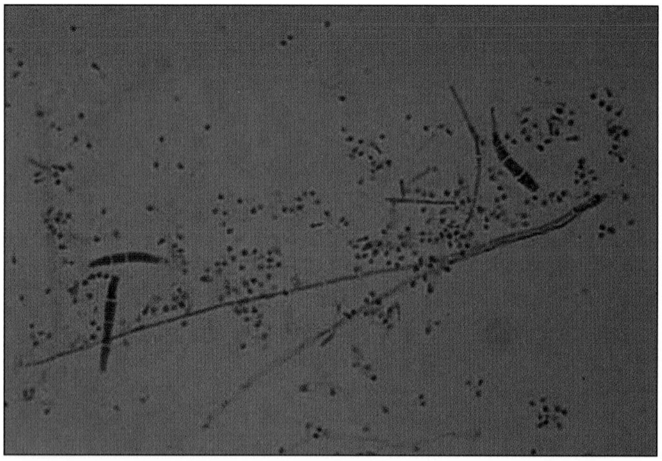

Figure 61-11 Elongated macroconidia of *Trichophyton mentagrophytes* along with microconidia are lined up along the surface of the hypha. (Lactophenol cotton blue stain, ×400.)

The other type of conidiogenesis is called blastic conidiogenesis, whereby the protoplasm of the conidiogenous cell is blown out or blasted to form the conidium. The simplest form of blastic conidiogenesis is the budding process by which many yeasts, including *Candida* spp., develop. As with thallic conidia, blastoconidia are divided into two types: one where the cell wall is involved in the process and the other where it is not. Further division of blastic conidiogenesis is made among those species in which the outer cell wall does not participate in the process (called enteroblastic conidiogenesis). In enteroblastic fungi, phialidic and annellidic conidiogenous cells have been recognized. Phialides are conidiogenous cells that often have a collarette at the apices, produced when the tip releases the first conidium. The collarette may be a conspicuous flask-shaped structure, as observed in *Phialophora* spp., or an inconspicuous structure, as seen in *Aspergillus* spp. In contrast, annellides are conidiogenous cells that rupture to leave a distinct ring of cellular material at the base of the conidium when it separates from the annellide. Formation of sequential conidia at the base pushes the oldest cell to the tip of the chain and leaves a series of rings or annellations at the apex of the annellide, providing a record of past events, like rings on a tree. Although important for the microscopic identification of some mould fungi, the fine details of these structures may be difficult to visualize using the light microscope.

Differentiation of the various conidial structures is the key to correct identification of many fungal isolates. In some cases, the pertinent morphologic features are easily discerned; however, as in surgical pathology, pattern recognition is an essential tool for identification of the most common pathogens and saprobes. The pathologist should always appreciate the salient features of the entire morphologic preparation without primarily focusing on outliers or aberrant structures. Developing conidial structures of *Aspergillus* or *Paecilomyces*, for instance, may resemble the

TABLE 61-3
Media for the Identification and Isolation of Fungi

Medium	Main function
Ascospore medium, V-8 agar	Ascospore development
Birdseed (niger) agar	Demonstration of melanin in *Cryptococcus neoformans*
Brain-heart infusion agar with blood	Enhanced recovery of dimorphic fungi
Christensen urea agar	Differentiation of *Trichophyton rubrum* and *T. mentagrophytes*
CHROMagar *Candida*	Chromogenic mixture to identify yeast species
Cornmeal agar with Tween 80	Visualization of yeast morphology
Czapek-Dox agar	Identification of *Aspergillus* species
Potato dextrose agar	Pigment development of *Trichophyton rubrum* and mould morphology
Sabouraud dextrose (SAB) agar	General purpose fungal growth medium (traditional formulation or Emmon's modification)
SAB agar with cycloheximide	Selective medium to inhibit saprophytic fungi (antibacterials such as chloramphenicol or gentamicin also included)
Slide culture (various agars)	Study of microscopic structure
Trichophyton agars	Differentiation of *Trichophyton* species

structures of *Penicillium*, and the observer must not be misled into thinking that two moulds are present. At the same time, the possibility of a mixed culture must be remembered. Mycologists must use a low-powered objective for initial observation from fungal culture; however, the details of cellular subsets in that low-powered picture must be appreciated for study at a higher magnification.

The fine art of mycologic diagnosis rests in the appreciation and differentiation of cellular details, and in some instances, the task requires great subtlety and considerable experience. Sometimes, the isolate must be coaxed to produce the necessary diagnostic structures by selection of appropriate media (Table 61-3). In general, enriched media favor the propagation of vegetative mycelium, whereas asexual reproductive structures are encouraged by basal (starving) media. Subculture onto water agar or potato flake agar is a general technique for encouraging the development of conidial structures. The colors of *Aspergillus* colonies are best studied on Czapek-Dox agar, whereas *Trichophyton rubrum* is encouraged to produce red pigment on potato dextrose agar or cornmeal agar with 1% glucose.

Experience also is important in determining whether a subculture has been incubated sufficiently long for diagnostic structures to form. Rootlike structures (rhizoids) that develop from the hyphae of some Zygomycetes are important differentiating features, but they may not be detected if observation is terminated prematurely. Some of the techniques necessary for complete differentiation are difficult or even beyond the reach of most clinical laboratories. For instance, the dematiaceous pathogen *Exophiala (Wangiella) dermatitidis* produces blastic conidia with phialides and annellides. The presence of annellides was not recognized when the mould was studied with the light microscope, however, and this organism was once classified as *Phialophora dermatitidis*. Recognition that annellides were formed by the isolate led to a reassignment to a new genus, *Exophiala*, which contained both phialides and annellides. To add to the confusion, the genus *Wangiella* continues to be suggested for this species because the phialides do not reproduce obvious collarettes, which is the predominant feature of this genus. Subsequently, disagreement continues as to whether this species belongs in the genus *Exophiala* or in the genus *Wangiella* (McGinnis, 1999).

Sexual reproductive structures are of occasional value for fungal identification in the general mycology laboratory. Although they are infrequently encountered in vitro, recognition of sexual structures for heterothallic fungi requires that a compatible mating strain be available for testing. Homothallic fungi on the other hand, can produce sexual structures in culture without this mating process. The two structures most likely to be demonstrated in the laboratory from heterothallic species are the naked asci of *Saccharomyces cerevisiae* and the cleistothecium of *P. boydii*

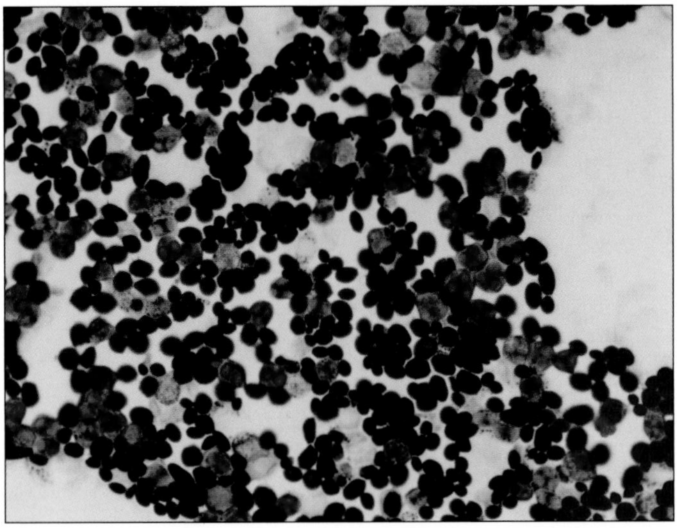

Figure 61-12 Ascospores with asci (pale staining) along with budding yeast cells of *Saccharomyces cerevisiae.* (Gram stain, ×1000.)

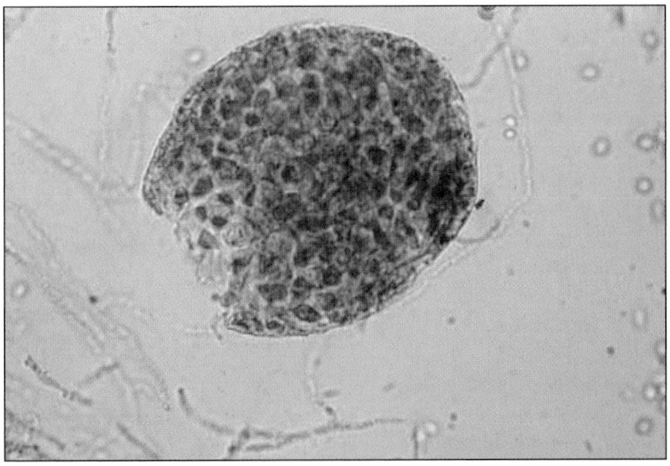

Figure 61-13 Cleistothecium of *Pseudallescheria boydii.* This sexual reproductive structure is specifically referred to as an ascus containing ascospores. (Lactophenol cotton blue stain, ×400.)

(the sexual phase of *S. apiospermum*), *Aspergillus nidulans,* or the *Aspergillus glaucus* group of fungi. The naked asci of *Saccharomyces* resemble oval yeast cells in which one to four individual haploid ascospores are enclosed (Fig. 61-12). The ascospores in this species may be visualized in wet preparations but are detected more reliably using a Gram stain or an acid-fast stain. A cleistothecium is a sexual fruiting body (ascocarp) in which the ascospores are entirely enclosed and can be released only by rupture of the cleistothecial wall (Fig. 61-13). The wall is composed of single or multiple layers of specialized hyphae. A perithecium is a sexual structure similar to a cleistothecium, but it contains an opening at the apex of the pear-shaped structure

Although asexual and rarely sexual reproductive structures are necessary for the identification of fungi, especially moulds, some isolates refuse to produce either of these structures for diagnosis. The colonies consist only of vegetative and aerial hyphae morphologically and subsequently are described as sterile hyphae or mycelia sterilia. Identification under this circumstance requires specialized molecular methods that are not available in most routine diagnostic laboratories (Iwen, 2003; Balajee, 2007b; Borman, 2008).

DIMORPHISM

Demonstration of dimorphism is the traditional approach to definitive identification of endemic fungal pathogens. In most laboratories, the initial isolate is the mould phase because culture plates usually are incubated at 25°–30° C. Conversion to the tissue phase (yeast or yeast-like structure) is accomplished by incubating a subculture at 37° C. The transition from mould to yeast morphology may occur grudgingly, and hyphal forms are often intermixed with yeast cells. Some isolates may never be successfully converted. A rich medium, such as brain-heart infusion agar with a blood supplement, should be included with the primary isolation medium, particularly when *H. capsulatum* is suspected. Cysteine hemoglobin agar is a common medium used for the conversion of *B. dermatitidis.* Media for conversion of coccidioidal species have been described but are not often used. Similarly, inoculation of animals is infrequently employed in clinical laboratories, although this method is effective when used for conversion to the in vivo phase. The recent introduction of molecular probes has considerably simplified the task of definitive identification for these endemic fungi and has eliminated the need to demonstrate both phases of the dimorphic fungi in the laboratory (Reiss, 2000). Rapid deoxyribonucleic acid (DNA) probe tests, which utilize the technique of nucleic acid hybridization, are available for the identification of the three major dimorphic pathogens from culture (e.g., AccuProbe, GenProbe, Inc., San Diego). Although demonstration of the characteristic yeast or yeast-like phase in tissue strongly supports the diagnosis of a dimorphic fungus, identification of the pathogen in culture is still necessary for disease confirmation.

Diagnostic Techniques

With the increased number of patients undergoing transplantation procedures or receiving aggressive immunosuppression and chemotherapy, the growing population of immunosuppressed hosts has dramatically increased, leading to a subsequent rise in the prevalence of invasive fungal infection (Chandrasekar, 2009). Early recognition of a fungal infection to optimize patient management is becoming more realistic with advances in diagnostic applications for the identification of fungal etiologic agents.

LABORATORY SAFETY

Biosafety considerations from specimen collection through culture conformation in the mycology laboratory are critical (Sutton, 2007). Inoculation of specimens and manipulation of mould colonies should always be performed in a biological safety cabinet to prevent dissemination of the highly mobile fungal conidia. Scrupulous attention to cleaning the surfaces of both the biological safety cabinet and the incubator should be maintained. Separate safety cabinets for the study of isolated moulds may minimize contamination of other clinical samples.

The greatest hazard for laboratory personnel comes from handling mould cultures of the dimorphic pathogens, *Coccidioides* spp. and *H. capsulatum.* These isolates are classified as risk group 3 pathogens, requiring biosafety level 3 practices and facilities for propagating and manipulating cultures, as well as for processing soil or other environmental materials known or likely to contain infectious conidia from these agents (Department of Health and Human Services, 2007). Screw-capped tubes of culture media should be used for culture if these pathogens are suspected. Unfortunately, in most areas of the country, the diagnosis may not be appreciated before the pathogen is isolated (Kwon-Chung, 1992). Culture plates if used can be flooded with 4% formaldehyde solution (10% formalin) and left at room temperature for several hours or overnight to sterilize the culture before microscopic examination is performed. As expected, such a treatment is irreversible, so viable colonies growing on other fungal media should be available as a reserve.

Of special note is that the tissue phase of dimorphic pathogens is not infectious by the airborne route, thus little or no biohazard is involved in handling tissue specimens from patients with blastomycosis, histoplasmosis, or coccidioidomycosis. A possible exception to this rule might occur if a *Coccidioides* spp. grew as a mould within a lung cavity that connected with the bronchial tree, which would allow for in vivo sporulation.

SPECIMEN COLLECTION AND TRANSPORT

The correct specimen for submission to the mycology laboratory depends on the clinical presentation and the organ system affected. A summary of the major categories of diseases produced by fungi along with suggested specimens is presented in Table 61-4.

Yeast, particularly *Candida* spp., may be recovered on occasion from swab specimens, especially from purulent lesions. Swabs may be used for sampling oral or vaginal lesions suggestive of candidiasis and may be adequate for collecting specimens from patients with chronic external otitis, in which large numbers of *Aspergillus* conidia are usually present. However, swabs are decidedly inferior for collecting specimens in most areas of the infectious process. Particularly problematic is that swab fibers

TABLE 61-4
Major Clinical Syndromes and Commonly Associated Fungal Pathogens

Clinical presentation/ organ system	Patient group	Likely pathogens	Specimen(s)
Skin, hair, or nail infection	All	Dermatophytes	Skin scraping
		Candida	Hair
		Malassezia	Nail clipping
Subcutaneous tissue infection	All	*Coccidioides*	Lesion biopsy
		Blastomyces dermatitidis	
		Sporothrix schenckii	
	Patient with mycetoma	*Scedosporium apiospermum*	
		Madurella	
		Actinomadura	
Primary pneumonia	All	*Histoplasma capsulatum*	Sputum
		Blastomyces dermatitidis	Bronchoalveolar lavage
		Cryptococcus neoformans	Transbronchial biopsy
		Coccidioides	Surgical lung biopsy
	Immunodeficient	*Aspergillus*	
		Fusarium	
		Zygomycetes	
		Scedosporium apiospermum	
		Pneumocystis jiroveci	
Gastrointestinal infection	Immunodeficient	*Candida*	Scrapings
		Aspergillus	Curettings
		Zygomycetes	Biopsy
Urinary tract infection	All	*Candida*	Urine
Endocarditis	All	*Candida*	Blood
		Fusarium	
Meningitis	Immunodeficient	*Cryptococcus neoformans*	Cerebrospinal fluid
		Candida	
		Coccidioides	
Encephalitis and brain abscess	Immunodeficient	Zygomycetes	Brain biopsy
		Aspergillus	
		Cladophialophora bantiana	
Osteomyelitis	All	*Coccidioides*	Biopsy
		Blastomyces dermatitidis	
		Cryptococcus neoformans	
Keratitis	All	*Aspergillus*	Scraping
		Fusarium	
External otitis	All	*Aspergillus*	Scraping
			Swab
Sinusitis	All	*Aspergillus*	Biopsy
		Fusarium	Curettings
			Dematiaceous moulds
Burn wounds	All	*Aspergillus*	Biopsy
		Zygomycetes	
		Fusarium	
		Scedosporium apiospermum	
Vaginitis	All	*Candida*	Vaginal secretions
Intravenous catheter infection	Indwelling catheter	*Candida*	Catheter tip
		Malassezia (newborns)	Blood
Disseminated infection	All	*Histoplasma capsulatum*	Blood
		Blastomyces dermatitidis	Tissue biopsy
		Coccidioides	
	Immunodeficient	*Candida*	Blood
		Zygomycetes	Tissue biopsy
		Aspergillus	
		Fusarium	
		Scedosporium apiospermum	
		Cryptococcus neoformans	
		Potentially any fungus	

TABLE 61-5
KOH Preparation

1. Place one drop of 10% potassium hydroxide (KOH) on a clean glass slide.
2. Immerse an aliquot of the specimen in the drop of KOH on the slide.
3. Gently heat the mixture by passing the slide through a Bunsen burner flame several times. Do not allow the mixture to boil.
4. Coverslip the slide and examine at 100× and 400× magnification using reduced light. Excessively tenacious specimens may require additional heating.
5. KOH may also be used as a simple mounting medium without heating (the addition of lacto phenol [aniline] blue or Calcofluor white stain with the KOH will enhance the visibility of fungal elements).

may be mistaken for hyphal elements upon direct examination of clinical specimens. A policy of rejecting swabs for fungal culture should be accompanied in most cases by assiduous and persistent educational efforts.

The best specimens for mycologic diagnosis are scrapings, curettings, aspirates, and lesion biopsies. Hairs infected with a dermatophytic fungus (e.g., *Microsporum canis*) fluoresce under a long-wavelength ultraviolet light (Wood's lamp) and can be specifically selected for examination. Cutaneous lesions of dermatophytosis (ringworm) are characterized by an active advancing edge with central healing, so that scrapings can be collected from the edge of the process. Hair, nails, and skin scrapings should be sent to the laboratory in a clean dry container. Biopsy samples should be sent in a sterile container with sterile saline or a transport medium to prevent drying of the sample. Most samples can be handled as one would any other samples submitted for bacterial observation and culture.

DIRECT EXAMINATION

Most clinical specimens can be examined directly for the presence of a fungal pathogen, although negative results are not sensitive enough to rule out the presence of a fungus. Multiple techniques are employed for the direct examination of clinical material. As a reminder, multiple manipulations of specimen material in the laboratory may render the material not acceptable for culture, so in those cases where culture is warranted, specimens must be separated before this type of examination is performed.

Wet Preparation

The simplest method for direct examination of a specimen is to observe a suspension placed on a slide and coverslip under reduced light. For those specimens that are dry or viscous, the addition of a wetting agent such as saline is necessary prior to observation. For specimens that contain distracting tissue debris and cells, such as vaginal secretions, nails, and skin scrapings, a solution of potassium hydroxide (KOH) may be used as a means to dissolve the tissue material, so that fungal elements are more visible (Table 61-5).

Gram Stain

This commonly used microbiological stain is particularly useful for the detection of yeast. Most yeasts stain partially or completely gram-positive and are generally differentiated from bacteria by their larger size and by the presence of budding cells (see Fig. 61-5). The hyphae of moulds may appear gram-positive or gram-negative by this stain but may stain less reliably than yeast cells and are easily missed in clinical specimens using this method.

Giemsa or Wright Stain

In cases where histoplasmosis is suspected, these hematologic stains are useful for demonstrating yeast cells within macrophages.

India Ink Preparation

The polysaccharide capsule of *C. neoformans* can be demonstrated by negative staining using India ink particles; it is especially evident when infected cerebrospinal fluid is examined. When examined with the light microscope, the capsule stands out as a clear space around the fungal cell, with ink particles bouncing off the edge as brownian motion occurs (Fig. 61-14). When budding yeast cells are demonstrated along with the capsule in the cerebrospinal fluid of an infected patient, the specificity of the diagnosis of cryptococcal meningitis is ensured. Other potentially encapsulated fungi such as *Rhodotorula* spp. or other cryptococcal species are infrequent pathogens and can be eliminated from practical consideration under this

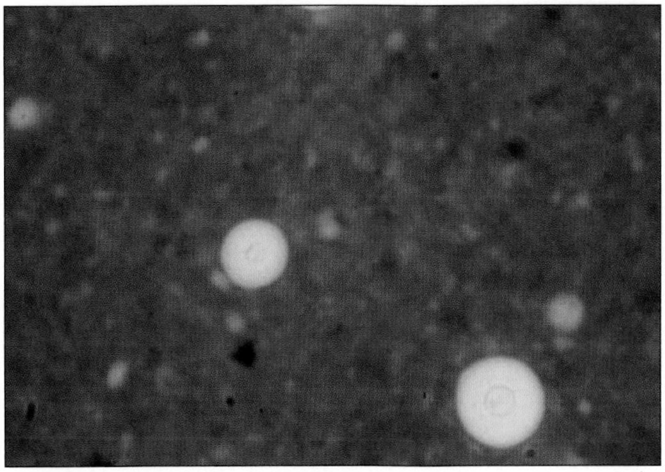

Figure 61-14 India ink preparation of cerebrospinal fluid containing *Cryptococcus neoformans*. This yeast produces a characteristic polysaccharide capsule around the budding yeast cells. (×400.)

circumstance. Although the capsules usually are large in direct examination of specimens, isolation of the pathogen on agar media is usually characterized by the production of a much diminished capsule, which is not as obvious. Unfortunately, some *C. neoformans* strains are poorly encapsulated; thus, the sensitivity of the India ink test is generally less than 50%, and the organism is especially evident in patients who are not infected with the human immunodeficiency virus (HIV). However, direct detection of antigen in cerebrospinal fluid or serum using a latex agglutination or enzyme immunoassay technique has increased the sensitivity to close to 100%. These techniques basically have replaced the use of India ink as a direct diagnostic technique, although the India ink technique is still useful when the antigen test is not immediately available and for examination of capsules in cells from isolated colonies that suggest *C. neoformans*.

Histopathologic Stains

Surgical pathologic examination of biopsy material is a common practice for the identification of suspected fungal infection. A number of stains have proved useful in recognizing fungal elements in tissue and in showing the immunologic response to infection. The periodic acid–Schiff (PAS) method is useful for demonstrating internal details. Gomori's methenamine silver (GMS) technique is considered one of the better stains for demonstrating fungi because it provides high contrast with minimal background staining, thus allowing for the demonstration of sparsely present fungal elements in the sample. The hematoxylin and eosin (H&E) stain is best used for studying the host reaction and for determining whether a fungus is hyaline (colorless) or dematiaceous (naturally pigmented). Other more specialized stains include Mayer's mucicarmine stain for demonstration of the mucoid capsule of *C. neoformans* and the Fontana-Masson stain for demonstration of melanin or melanin-like substances in the lightly pigmented agents of phaeohyphomycosis. A book by Chandler and Kaplan provides greater detail on the utilization of stains to detect fungi in tissue (Chandler, 1987a).

Calcofluor White Stain

This fluorochrome compound, a whitener used in the textile and paper industries, binds to the chitin in the walls of fungal cells and fluoresces white (Fig. 61-15) or apple green (depending on the filter combination used) when exposed to short-wavelength ultraviolet light from a fluorescence microscope (Table 61-6) (Hageage, 1984). Calcofluor white can also be mixed with potassium hydroxide to clear the specimen for easier observation of fungi. As is true with all fluorescent staining, care must be used in interpreting the results because nonspecific staining of substances that resemble fungal elements may also occur.

Immunohistochemical Stains

Immunohistochemistry has been used to identify a wide variety of infectious agents, including the fungi, in formalin-fixed tissues (Eyzaguirre, 2008). Although many fungi can be readily identified by standard histologic staining, some fungal elements appear atypical in tissue sections and in some cases cannot be distinguished morphologically. Commercial antibodies used in the immunohistochemical diagnosis of fungal infections are available for *Aspergillus* spp., *Candida albicans*, and *Pneumocystis jiroveci*.

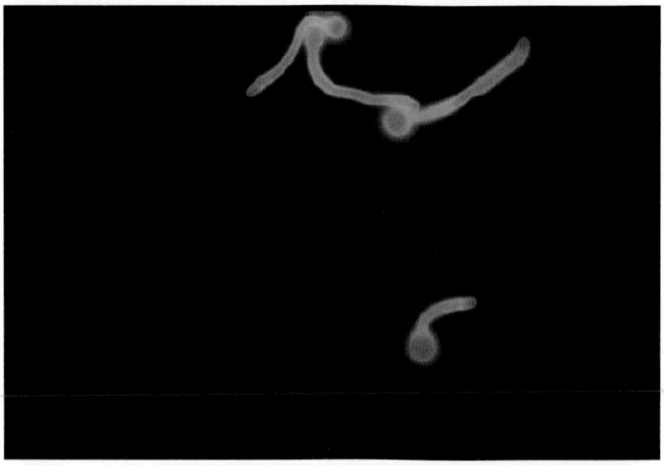

Figure 61-15 Calcofluor white stain of *Candida albicans* in culture. When viewed with a fluorescence microscope, the chitinous walls of the fungus will fluoresce. Germ tubes shown are produced following incubation of the yeast in serum. *(Courtesy Dr. Brian Harrington, CDC Public Health Image Library.)*

TABLE 61-6
Calcofluor White Stain

1. Place specimen on a clean glass slide.
2. Mix with Calcofluor white reagent.
3. Using a fluorescent microscope, examine the preparation for fungal elements at 100× to 400× magnification (will typically appear bluish white against a dark background). (Calcofluor white may be substituted for lacto phenol [aniline] blue stain when microscopic morphology of culture isolates is studied.)

ISOLATION IN CULTURE

Selection of Media

All specimens should be inoculated onto a general purpose fungal growth medium (see Table 61-3). The medium used traditionally is Sabouraud dextrose agar, which has a pH of 5.5–5.6 and was designed for the isolation of dermatophytic fungi. Emmons' modification of Sabouraud dextrose agar, which contains less glucose with a pH of 6.8–7.0, is more widely used in the clinical mycology laboratory as a general growth medium because of its wide application for the culture of fungi. Inhibitory mould agar and potato dextrose agar are also utilized as general isolation media in the laboratory.

For specimens from nonsterile sites or from sites that are likely to be contaminated with other microbial flora, inoculation of a nonselective agar and a selective agar in tandem is recommended. The most commonly used selective agar employs cycloheximide to inhibit saprophytic fungi and an antibacterial agent (usually chloramphenicol or gentamicin) to inhibit bacteria. For tissue specimens, especially when dimorphic fungi might be the etiologic agent, an enriched agar, such as brain-heart infusion agar with blood and supplemented with antibiotics may be added.

A recent addition for the cultivation of yeast from clinical specimens is the selective and differential medium called CHROMagar *Candida* (CHROMagar Company, Paris, France). This medium uses a chromogenic mixture for the detection and differentiation of major *Candida* spp. by colony color: *C. albicans*, green; *Candida glabrata*, velvet; *Candida krusei*, rose; and *Candida tropicalis*, steel blue. Numerous reports have shown this medium to be useful for the isolation and presumptive identification of yeasts and to optimize detection of mixed cultures in clinical specimens (Perry, 2007; Ozcan, 2009; Raut, 2009).

Inoculation and Incubation

Processing of clinical specimens for fungal detection requires careful handling because some processes commonly used to prepare specimens for bacterial culture may be too disruptive for the fungal organism (e.g., grinding in a homogenizer). Inoculation of scrapings or curettings onto and into the agar at multiple points on the agar surface is a reliable technique for culture. Tissue should be teased or minced, after which the fragments are similarly inoculated.

Plates or tubes should be incubated in ambient air at 25°–30° C. A controlled temperature incubator is essential. Although it is not necessary to incubate parallel plates or tubes at 37° C for recovery of the yeast phase of dimorphic fungi, in cases where strong suspicion of endemic fungi occurs, incubation at this temperature should be considered. Most fungi grow within a 2-week incubation period, and among commonly isolated fungi, only the dimorphic fungi such as *H. capsulatum* and *B. dermatitidis* are frequently detected after 14 days of incubation. General recommendations for incubation times are as follows: 7 days to detect the presence of yeast in mouth, throat, or vaginal specimens; 21 days to detect fungal pathogens in tissues and sterile body fluids other than blood; and up to 28 days for respiratory, bone marrow, and blood pathogens, and for specimens in which a dimorphic fungus is suspected. In general, all other specimens should be incubated for up to 14 days. Plates should be examined at least twice during the first week, when rapidly growing isolates may appear, and at least weekly thereafter.

Blood Cultures

Recovery of fungi from blood requires special attention and can be accomplished by inoculating broth media by using a biphasic broth-agar system or by using the lysis centrifugation technique (Isolator System; Wampole, Cranbury, N.J.). The lysis centrifugation method consists of a tube containing a solution that lyses erythrocytes and leukocytes (Cockerill, 1996; Reimer, 1997). After the blood is drawn into the vacutainer tube, the lysed contents, including any microbes, are centrifuged into a pellet, which is removed and plated onto the surface of agar plates. Although the Isolator System is considered a sensitive method for detection of fungemia, this system is also more susceptible to contamination through handling of the tube or by airborne spores that settle onto the agar plates during processing (Reimer, 1997). Because a high percentage of fungemias are caused by yeast, continuous-read-automated-culture methods have become the mainstay for fungal detection. Two systems commonly used are the BACTEC system (Becton Dickinson Diagnostic Systems, Sparks, Md.) and the BacT-Alert system (Organon Teknika, Durham, N.C.). Because yeasts are aerobic organisms, aerobic culture bottles are used for detection. Two systems in combination (i.e., BACTEC MYCO/F Lytic blood culture bottles and the Isolator System) have been shown to optimize the recovery of fungi from blood (Vetter, 2001).

GROWTH RATE

The rate of growth of fungal isolates provides a useful clue to diagnostic possibilities. In general, the pathogenic dimorphic and dematiaceous fungi grow slower, requiring a week or longer for colonies to appear. Rapidly growing mould colonies that appear after prolonged incubation on mycologic media should be questioned as possible contaminants. However, many exceptions to this generalization have been noted, and laboratorians need to be aware that fungi such as the *Coccidioides* spp. may grow quickly on nonfungal medium. Protocols on how to handle fungal growth on bacterial cultures are needed to prevent unnecessary exposure of laboratory personnel to highly infectious fungal pathogens that may be encountered.

GROWTH TEMPERATURE

Most moulds grow best at 25°–30° C. Most yeasts, however, grow well at 35°–37° C and are often recovered first on enriched blood agar plates in the bacteriology laboratory. In some cases, growth of a fungus at elevated temperatures is useful for differentiation of species.

MORPHOLOGIC IDENTIFICATION

Some of the morphologic studies necessary for the identification of fungal isolates can be accomplished with colonies from the original isolation plates. However, it is often necessary to transfer portions of colonies to new or different media (subculture) to demonstrate diagnostic structures. Table 61-3 describes some of the media commonly used for the identification of fungal species. One of the media more commonly used is cornmeal agar supplemented with Tween 80 (CM-T80) for the visualization of yeast morphology. Recognition of pseudohyphae with chlamydoconidia on this medium is considered confirmatory for *C. albicans/dubliniensis*. Other morphologic features can help to categorize yeasts into groups to facilitate separation into species. Although biochemical tests are important for identifying yeast isolates, complementation of these with a morphologic examination provides an important check on the biochemical information, especially if a commercial identification system has been used.

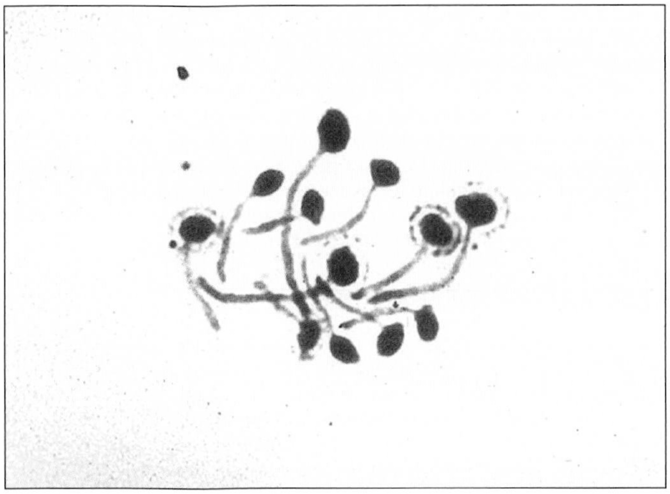

Figure 61-16 Germ tubes have extended from the yeast cells of *Candida albicans*. No constriction is seen at the junction of yeast cell and germ tube. The walls of the germ tube are parallel. The yeast was incubated for 2 hours at 37° C in serum. (Gram stain, ×400.)

TABLE 61-7
Serum Germ Tube Test

1. Aseptically transfer several colonies of yeast to a 12 × 75-mm test tube containing approximately 0.5 mL of serum (human, fetal calf, bovine, or rabbit).
2. Incubate the tube at 35° C for up to 3 hours.
3. Place one drop of the mixture on a clean glass slide and coverslip.
4. Examine under high dry (400×) magnification and reduced light for the presence of germ tubes.

TABLE 61-8
Yeast Morphology Test

1. Streak a light inoculum of yeast onto a section of a cornmeal agar containing Tween 80.
2. Coverslip the area inoculated.
3. Incubate at 25°–30° C for 24–72 hours.
4. Observe under 100× and 400× magnification using reduced light for morphologic structures.

Yeast Morphology

The germ tube test is an important initial step in the identification of yeast isolates. Germ tubes, which are elongated, finger-like extensions from a yeast cell, represent the beginnings of a true hypha (Fig. 61-16). This structure can be differentiated from pseudohyphae by the lack of a constriction at the junction of germ tube and yeast cell and by the parallel cell walls in the germ tube. True germ tubes are formed by both *C. albicans* and *Candida dubliniensis* after growth in serum at 37° C for no longer than 4 hours. In many laboratories with well-trained staff, the germ tube in combination with results of morphology on CM-T80 agar is considered confirmatory for the identification of *C. albicans/dubliniensis*.

The traditional germ tube test involves inoculation of a tube of serum (Table 61-7). After observation of the isolate for germ tubes at 37° C, incubation is continued for subsequent study of hyphal morphology and chlamydoconidia formation at 25°–30° C. Thus, all the information necessary for rapid identification can be collected in one procedure. The CM-T80 agar may be substituted, but regardless of the medium used, incubation conditions must be carefully controlled and the test monitored with controls to achieve good results. The traditional Dalmau technique for demonstration of chlamydoconidia on cornmeal agar is detailed in Table 61-8 (McGinnis, 1980).

Mould Morphology

The simplest method for examination of moulds is the cellophane tape mount, using clear tape and staining with lactophenol cotton (aniline) blue

TABLE 61-9
Rapid Testing for Presumptive Identification of Yeast Following Colonial Formation

Urease production	*Cryptococcus neoformans*
Germ tube production	*Candida albicans/dubliniensis*
Pseudohyphae present	*Candida* species
Chlamydoconidia present	*Candida albicans/dubliniensis*
Lipid growth requirement	*Malassezia furfur* species complex
Red colonial pigmentation	*Rhodotorula* species
Ascospore formation	*Saccharomyces cerevisiae*
Trehalose assimilation	*Candida glabrata*

(LPCB) stain. If diagnostic structures are not observed, incubation can be continued and the process repeated. The traditional method used in observing mould morphology is to tease the mycelium apart with inoculating needles and examine the teased hyphae with LPCB stain.

Occasionally, a slide culture may be necessary to preserve easily disrupted conidial structures in their original relationships. The classic approach involves cutting a square of an appropriate agar medium (usually Sabouraud dextrose or potato dextrose agar), which is suspended on a glass slide and overlaid with a coverslip. The slide is supported by glass rods in a Petri dish, to which sterile water is added for maintenance of humidity. The coverslip subsequently can be removed after a few days' incubation, placed in a drop of LPCB, and observed for undisturbed reproductive structures.

When a mould isolate is suspected of being a dimorphic fungus (e.g., growth on cycloheximide-containing medium), a slide culture should not be performed, and a cellophane tape test or teased preparation should be examined only after the preparation has been sealed in a biosafety cabinet certified for use. Lactophenol cotton blue is fungicidal, but sealing the coverslip with nail polish before observation provides additional protection. Alternatively, the culture may be flooded with 10% formalin (4% formaldehyde solution) and incubated at room temperature overnight before the mould is manipulated.

BIOCHEMICAL IDENTIFICATION

Biochemical tests are at the heart of identification schemes for yeast and occasionally are useful for identification of moulds. A number of rapid tests for the presumptive identification of yeasts are described in Table 61-9.

Biochemical characterization of yeasts may be accomplished by study of fermentation or assimilation patterns. Assimilation testing, which is used more extensively in the laboratory, assesses the ability of an isolate to use a carbohydrate as the sole source of carbon needed for growth, or of nitrate as the sole source of nitrogen. Numerous commercial identification systems with varying incubation times from 4–72 hours are available and have become the mainstay for yeast identification. These systems include the API 20C AUX system and the VITEK 2 System (both from bioMérieux, Hazelwood, Mo.), the MicroScan system (Siemens Healthcare Diagnostics, West Sacramento, Calif.), the UniYeastTek system (Remel Laboratories, Lenexa, Kan.), and the RapID Yeast Plus System (Innovative Diagnostics Systems, Norcross, Ga.). All of these systems perform well, as judged by reports in the literature and by proficiency testing surveys of the College of American Pathologists (Fenn, 1994; Riddle, 1994; Crist, 1996; Bernal, 1998; Espinel-Ingroff, 1998; Ramani, 1998; Hata, 2007). However, because no one system is known to be 100% accurate for identification of yeast species, a combination of methods should be considered, especially when rare species are recognized (Pincus, 2007).

In addition to fermentation and assimilation studies, stimulation of growth by biochemical compounds is a secondary test used in the differentiation of certain *Trichophyton* spp. (Weitzman, 1983). Inclusion of inositol and thiamine in various combinations into agar media (*Trichophyton* agars) allows assessment of growth-stimulating properties. The endpoint of the test, relative growth in comparison with a basal medium, is subjective, and both positive and negative controls should be included.

The test for urease production in cryptococci is of general utility in the clinical laboratory to differentiate these species from *Candida* spp., particularly in respiratory specimens (Canteros, 1996). *C. neoformans* is a pulmonary and systemic pathogen, whereas *Candida* spp. are frequent inhabitants of the upper airways but uncommon causes of primary pneumonia. Urease, however, may be produced by other nonpathogenic species of *Cryptococcus*, by *Rhodotorula* spp., and by some isolates of *Trichosporon* spp. and *C. krusei*.

Urease production can be tested by inoculation of the yeast isolate onto a slant of Christensen urea agar or into urea broth. Alkalinization of the medium after production of NH_3 by urea-splitting organisms is detected by inclusion of a pH indicator in the system. Colonies that have macroscopically visible pseudohyphae (feet) or that grow on cycloheximide-containing agar need not be tested, because *Cryptococcus* does not produce pseudohyphae in vitro and does not grow in the presence of cycloheximide.

Production of urease also is useful to differentiate the mould *Trichophyton mentagrophytes* (urease positive) from *T. rubrum* (urease negative). The isolate should be subcultured to a slant of Christensen urea agar and incubated at 25°–30° C for at least 3 days.

Although commercial biochemical tests are fairly reliable for the identification of yeast, confirmation of the identification by examination of yeast morphology on agar media should also be considered. Using morphologic observation as a check can save embarrassing mistakes that would be made if automated or packaged systems were trusted implicitly.

SEROLOGIC IDENTIFICATION

Immunologic tests are available for detection of both antigens and antibodies to selected fungal pathogens; these assays have been shown to be of value for diagnosing infection and for monitoring therapeutic response (Wheat, 2006; Lau, 2009). Although antibody testing for fungal pathogens has historically been used in some instances for diagnostics, these tests are no longer widely accepted owing to low sensitivity and specificity. In addition, the benefit of antibody detection remains unclear if patients are under immune suppression or are heavily colonized but not infected (Einsele, 2008).

Tests to detect fungal antigens or metabolic byproducts in serum or other body fluids on the other hand have been shown to be more useful for the diagnosis and management of fungal disease. Multiple antigen detection methods are used for the specific diagnosis of a variety of diseases, including aspergillosis, cryptococcosis, histoplasmosis, blastomycosis, paracoccidioidomycosis, and penicillosis caused by *Penicillium marnefii*. One of the more widely used antigen detection tests is the cryptococcal antigen test for the diagnosis of cryptococcal infection (Huston, 2009). The polysaccharide capsule of *C. neoformans* becomes dissolved in the serum and cerebrospinal fluid and can be detected by the latex-based agglutination test or the enzyme immunoassay. Although these tests have limitations, they have been shown to be helpful in monitoring therapy over time through quantitative measure of the titer of *Cryptococcus* polysaccharide in cerebrospinal fluid (Babady, 2009).

Antigen detection for the diagnosis of histoplasmosis has also proved useful when serum, urine, or bronchoalveolar lavage fluid is tested (Wheat, 2007, 2009b). As a screening test, detection of *Histoplasma* antigen plays a special role in the diagnosis of disseminated and diffuse acute pulmonary histoplasmosis. Studies have shown that *H. capsulatum*–specific antigen can be detected in the urine of 90% of patients with disseminated infection and 80% of patients with acute histoplasmosis (Wheat, 2003b). Detection of antigen in bronchoalveolar lavage has also proved useful for the diagnosis of histoplasmosis, especially when the results of testing are combined with those obtained from cytopathology (Hage, 2009).

A Food and Drug Administration (FDA)-approved enzyme-linked immunosorbent assay (ELISA; Platelia *Aspergillus* ELISA; Bio-Rad, Marnes-la-Coquette, France) is now available for the detection of galactomannan antigenemia for the rapid diagnosis of invasive aspergillosis (Del Bono, 2008; Leeflang, 2008; Wheat, 2008). This test has been shown to be more sensitive than culture when multiple serum samples from high-risk patients are tested; however, limitations of the assay need to be considered. For instance, treatment with piperacillin-tazobactam or amoxicillin-clavulanate has been noted to cause false-positive results, which are reported more commonly in children than in adults. A recent study showed that a biweekly serum galactomannan ELISA was a highly specific diagnostic tool for the detection of invasive aspergillosis in patients undergoing a hematopoietic stem cell transplant (Foy, 2007). Others have shown that when a lower threshold of sensitivity is used, the test has a higher level of performance and the numbers of patients who are unnecessarily treated or referred for additional follow-up are decreased (Del Bono, 2008; Leeflang, 2008). The usefulness of this test for the detection of *Aspergillus* galactomannan antigen in bronchoalveolar lavage fluid in transplant patients has also been shown (Clancy, 2007; Husain, 2007).

A commercial test to detect (1-3)-beta-D-glucan (BG) has become available for the diagnosis of invasive fungal infection (Fungitell Assay; Associates of Cape Cod, Inc., East Falmouth, Mass.) (Pickering, 2005). This antigen is present in the cell walls of most pathogenic fungi (including *P. jiroveci*) with some notable exceptions such as *C. neoformans* and the Zygomycetes. Published studies have shown that BG may be useful as a screening tool for surveillance of invasive aspergillosis, as well as other invasive fungal diseases in populations at risk (Marty, 2009). Although false-positive results appear to limit the use of this test, additional studies are needed to further define its diagnostic utility (Senn, 2008).

Skin tests have been used for the epidemiologic study of some infections, but they have limited utility for diagnostic purposes.

MOLECULAR IDENTIFICATION

Recent advances in molecular testing for the identification of fungal pathogens have had a significant impact on the diagnosis of fungal infections (Balajee, 2007b; Borman, 2008; Kuba, 2008; Lau, 2009). Numerous reviews have addressed these changes, and the general consensus is that approaches to species identification of many fungi today should include both morphologic and molecular testing methods (Balajee, 2007b).

One of the greatest needs for clinical medicine is the development of a rapid and reliable detection method that can identify fungal pathogens directly from clinical specimens. This need reflects not only the inability of current laboratory tests to provide a timely result, but also the fact that fungal infections in immunocompromised patients usually appear suddenly, progress rapidly, and are often fatal unless treatment is started earlier in the course of infection.

Numerous molecular assays using both probe-based and amplification-based technologies have been developed for the identification of fungal pathogens. With any of these approaches, an initial goal has been to define the genetic loci within the genome for use as the molecular target. Although multiple areas within the fungal genome have been evaluated, the targeted areas most commonly used are those found within the ribosomal DNA (rDNA) gene complex (Table 61-10) (Iwen, 2002). This section of the genome includes variable nucleotide sequence areas within the 18S gene and the 28S gene, as well as DNA sequence areas of the intervening internal transcribed spacer (ITS) regions called ITS1 and ITS2. Sequence homology within the rDNA genes and differences within the spacer regions are used as the genetic basis for the organization of fungi into taxonomic groups (Bastola, 2004). Recently, the ITS regions have been proposed as the prime fungal barcode for fungal species identification by the International Subcommission on Fungal Barcoding (http://www.allfungi.com/its-barcode.php).

Probe-based assays are commercially available and are commonly used in the mycology laboratory for the identification of *Histoplasma capsulatum*, *Blastomyces dermatitidis*, and *Coccidioides* spp. from culture (Accuprobe, San Diego). Another probe-based method called the peptide nucleic acid fluorescence in situ hybridization (PNA-FISH) assay was recently developed and has become commercially available for the qualitative identification of *C. albicans* in blood cultures (Wilson, 2005; Forrest, 2006). This assay uses

TABLE 61-10
Genetic Targets Utilized for the Detection and Identification of Fungal Pathogens

Gene target	Fungal species
Actin	*Candida albicans*
β-Tubulin	*Aspergillus* species
Calmodulin	*Aspergillus* species, *Fusarium* species
Chitin synthetase	Dermatophyte species
Cytochrome b	*Candida albicans*
Dihydrofolate reductase	*Pneumocystis jiroveci (carinii)*
EF-1	*Fusarium* species
Mitochondrial rRNA	*Pneumocystis jiroveci*
rDNA complex (5S gene)	*Candida albicans, Pneumocystis jiroveci*
rDNA complex (18S gene)	Multiple
rDNA complex (28S gene)	*Aspergillus* species, *Candida* species
rDNA complex (IGS regions)	*Aspergillus fumigatus*
rDNA complex (ITS regions)	Multiple

IGS, Intergenic spacer region; *ITS,* internal transcribed spacer region; *rDNA,* ribosomal deoxyribonucleic acid.

a fluorescent-labeled peptide nucleic acid probe that targets the species-specific ribosomal RNA of *C. albicans*. The sensitivity and specificity of this test have been shown to be >99%, and the impact of rapid identification of *C. albicans* in the blood can be seen in the significant reduction in the empirical use of antifungals (Alexander, 2006; Forrest, 2007). Incorporating the *C. albicans* PNA-FISH test as part of the initial identification algorithm for yeast recovered from blood can result in substantial savings for hospitals. Major drawbacks to this assay include the high costs of reagents and the changes in work flow required to incorporate testing in the laboratory.

Numerous amplification methods using both non–sequenced-based and sequence-based approaches for analysis have been applied in identification of fungi. Most of the sequence-based analysis methods have used conventional polymerase chain reaction (PCR) with universal primers to target sequences within the 28S rDNA gene, the 18S rDNA gene, or the ITS1-5.8S-ITS2 target areas. Additionally, Vollmer (2008) used a real-time PCR approach with sequencing as the analysis method.

The availability of a nucleotide-based sequence database that has the breadth of phylogenetics and the taxonomic accuracy needed to identify fungal species is desirable for sequence analysis alignment. The largest database currently used for sequence-based identification is the publicly available GenBank database (National Center for Biotechnology Information, Washington, DC). Unfortunately, because this is an open source database, reports suggest that up to 20% of the sequenced entries listed for fungi are associated with erroneously identified species (Balajee, 2007b). Additionally, there is a need for sequences from a variety of genomic targets in the database that is phylogenetically represented with accurate species identification. Although multiple locus sequencing and alignment comparisons have been done using a variety of fungal species, additional studies using sequence comparison analysis are needed to determine the optimal target or targets for fungal identification. Multiple target evaluations for the identification of aspergilli and fusaria have been done and show this approach to be valid for identification purposes (O'Donnell, 2007; Peterson, 2008).

Non–sequenced-based approaches have also been applied as a means to decrease the time needed for detection of fungi in clinical material. Real-time PCR using the 28S rDNA target and the cytochrome b target have been done and show promise in direct testing applications (Hata, 2008; Kasai, 2008; Vollmer, 2008). More recent molecular technologies that do not require sequencing to evaluate fungal species have included application of PCR to microarray analysis and to other hybridization-based probe technologies. A sensitive and specific DNA microarray combining multiplex PCR and consecutive DNA chip hybridization to detect fungal genomic DNA in clinical samples has shown promise (Spiess, 2007). This assay involved primer sets and probes used to amplify and detect 14 clinically relevant fungal species. This proof-of-concept evaluation showed that fungal pathogens could be detected and identified from clinical samples, which ultimately would improve the diagnosis of invasive fungal infections. The Luminex xMAP hybridization technology for species-specific identification of a wide range of clinically relevant fungal pathogens has also been shown to be applicable to the identification of fungal species both from culture and from clinical material (Landlinger, 2009).

SUSCEPTIBILITY TESTING

For many years, few antifungal chemotherapeutic agents were available, with amphotericin B virtually the only agent effective against most systemic fungal pathogens. Although this potent antifungal agent was frequently toxic, resistance to therapy was rare. With the recent introduction of new antifungal agents and with the widespread use of antifungal prophylaxis, the epidemiology of invasive fungal infections has changed, with non-*albicans Candida*, non-*fumigatus Aspergillus*, and moulds other than *Aspergillus* becoming more common as causes of invasive disease (Lai, 2008; Rodriguez-Tudela, 2008; Baddley, 2009; Naggie, 2009). These emerging fungi are resistant to or less susceptible than other fungi to standard antifungal agents and thus become more difficult to treat. Furthermore, although the predictability of innate resistance frequently means that species identification is often sufficient to alert the clinician to the likelihood of in vitro and often associated in vivo resistance, the emergence of resistance in a previously susceptible strain during the course of treatment has become more problematic (Arikan, 2007; Johnson, 2008).

The Clinical and Laboratory Standards Institute (CLSI; formerly called the National Committee for Clinical Laboratory Standards) has developed reference macrodilution and microdilution broth methods for antifungal susceptibility testing of yeasts (CLSI document M27-A3) and moulds (CLSI document M38-A2) (Clinical and Laboratory Standards Institute, 2008b, 2008c). It has also developed a method for antifungal disk diffusion susceptibility testing of yeasts (CLSI document M44-A2) and a method for antifungal disk diffusion susceptibility testing of nondermatophyte filamentous fungi (CLSI M51-A) (Clinical and Laboratory Standards Institute, 2010, 2009b).

The CLSI M27-A3 document has been approved for the testing of *Candida* spp. and *C. neoformans*. Interpretive breakpoints are available for amphotericin B, fluconazole, 5-flucytosine, itraconazole, voriconazole, posaconazole, and the echinocandins, although breakpoints are based largely on historical data and partially on drug pharmacokinetics. Additionally, no data currently exist to indicate a correlation between minimum inhibitory concentration (MIC) and outcomes of treatment with various agents; thus, the results of testing should be considered with caution.

The CLSI M38-A2 method has been developed for in vitro susceptibility testing of the more common rapidly growing filamentous fungi that can cause invasive disease. Organisms included in this document for evaluation are *Aspergillus* spp., *Fusarium* spp., *Rhizopus oryzae (R. arrhizus), Pseudallescheria boydii, Scedosporium prolificans*, and the mycelial form of *Sporothrix schenckii*, as well as the dermatophytes (*Epidermophyton, Microsporum*, and *Trichophyton*). This document is a reference standard developed through a consensus process to facilitate agreement among laboratorians in measuring the susceptibility of moulds to antifungal agents. The clinical relevance of testing filamentous fungi remains uncertain, and breakpoints with proven relevance have yet to be identified or approved by CLSI or any regulatory agency.

Because both reference methods are time consuming to perform, simplified alternatives to these methods have been assessed to include the disk diffusion method, the Etest agar-gradient MIC method (bioMérieux, Inc., Durham, NC), the Sensititre YeastOne method (TREK Diagnostic Systems, Inc., Cleveland, Ohio), and the VITEK 2 method (bioMérieux, Durham, N.C.; Pfaller, 2007b). The disk diffusion method has only recently been approved for the testing of yeast, and studies have shown that results obtained from testing using this method are comparable with results obtained with the CLSI microdilution broth method (Diekema, 2007; Messer, 2007; Pfaller, 2007, 2009).

The Etest uses a plastic strip that contains a predefined stable gradient of 15 antifungal concentrations to determine the on-scale MIC of the antifungal agent tested. These strips are commercially available for amphotericin B, anidulafungin, caspofungin, fluconazole, 5-flucytosine, itraconazole, ketoconazole, posaconazole, and voriconazole. Studies have shown the Etest strips to be as reliable as the CLSI standard for in vitro susceptibility testing of both moulds and yeast (Pfaller, 2003; Alexander, 2007).

The YeastOne method uses a dried colorimetric microdilution panel in a microtiter format for antifungal testing. This method is the only FDA-approved kit method for in vitro diagnostic use in testing yeast susceptibility to fluconazole, itraconazole, 5-flucytosine, and voriconaozle. Panels are also available for research use only in testing antifungal susceptibility to amphotericin B, anidulafungin, caspofungin, micafungin, and posaconazole. This testing platform has been shown to be dependable for the testing of both moulds and yeast (Castro, 2004; Pfaller, 2008). A modification of this method demonstrated that direct antifungal susceptibility testing of positive *Candida* blood cultures by the YeastOne assay produced an accurate antifungal MIC determination and saved on average 24 hours to the availability of results compared with the time required for the standard procedures traditionally used (Avolio, 2009).

Although the key elements involved in selecting an appropriate antifungal agent include the type of patient (e.g., solid organ or stem cell transplant), the severity of immunosuppression, a history of prolonged exposure to antifungal drugs, and knowledge of the genera and species of the infecting pathogen, susceptibility testing may be warranted in some circumstances, including the following: (1) as part of periodic surveys that establish antibiograms for isolates in an institution; (2) to help in the management of refractory oropharyngeal candidiasis in patients with apparent therapeutic failure; and (3) to aid in the management of invasive candidiasis when the use of azole antifungal agents is uncertain (Cornely, 2008). Also, scant data are available regarding the clinical implications of in vitro susceptibility testing in many cases, and the refractile nature of many fungal pathogens to antifungal therapy makes susceptibility testing an option that needs to be considered. For instance, reports now show that resistance has emerged during treatment of *Aspergillus* infections, thus highlighting the potential need for in vitro susceptibility testing under this circumstance (Lass-Florl, 2008).

CANDIDIASIS, CRYPTOCOCCOSIS, AND OTHER INFECTIONS CAUSED BY YEAST

THE GENUS *CANDIDA*

Candida spp. are the most commonly recognized yeast pathogens; with increased use of immunosuppressive therapies, use of broad-spectrum antibiotics, and the aging of the population, they have assumed a prominent place among nosocomial pathogens (Pfaller, 2007; Guery, 2009; Horn, 2009). These species are currently the fourth most common cause of hospital-acquired bloodstream infection in the United States and rank third among causes of bloodstream infection in the intensive care unit (Mean, 2008; Lewis, 2009). Although *C. albicans* accounts for about 50% of invasive infections caused by *Candida* spp., the non-*albicans Candida* spp. have emerged as more common causes of disease (Lewis, 2009; Rueping, 2009). In a recent multicenter evaluation of patients with candidemia (Prospective Antifungal Therapy Alliance database), *C. albicans* accounted for 45.6% of cases, followed by *Candida glabrata* (26.0%), *Candida parapsilosis* (15.7%), *Candida tropicalis* (8.1%), *Candida krusei* (2.5%), and *Candida lusitaniae* (0.8%) (Horn, 2009).

Risk Factors

Candida infections are limited in extent and severity, depending on the immune status of the host. Because *Candida* spp. are a part of the normal flora in the gastrointestinal (GI) tract, mucous membranes, and skin, infections generally occur as the result of an opportunity. For instance, the use of broad-spectrum antibacterial therapy upsets the balance of colonizing flora on the mucous membranes of the oral cavity and the GI tract by eliminating the predominant competing bacterial flora, thus allowing overgrowth of yeast (Pfaller, 2007; Lewis, 2009).

Invasive disease by *Candida* spp. develops when host defenses are compromised. Diabetes, immunosuppressive disease or therapy, and neutropenia as a result of disease (e.g., AIDS) or treatment with high-dose chemotherapy are common risk factors. Bloodstream infections, including fungal endocarditis, are fostered by the use of indwelling vascular lines, which is common practice in the management of hospitalized patients (Kojic, 2004).

Clinical Diseases

Although *C. albicans* is the most common pathogen within the genus *Candida*, the frequency of the non-*albicans* species has been noted within the recent past (Pfaller, 2007; Lewis, 2009). Numerous reports describe invasive infections caused by *C. tropicalis* (Garcia-Effron, 2008; Pasquale, 2008), *C. parapsilosis* (Trofa, 2008; van Asbeck, 2009), *C. glabrata* (Li, 2007), *C. krusei* (Krcmery, 1999; Pelletier, 2005), and *C. lusitaniae* (Hawkins, 2003).

Resistance to antifungal agents has emerged as a problem with the introduction of newer agents. This resistance is especially problematic within the non-*albicans Candida* spp. Resistance has been most notable within *C. glabrata* (resistance to the imidazoles [fluconazole, itraconazole, posaconazole, and voriconazole]) and within *C. krusei* (resistance to itraconazole). Antifungal intrinsic resistance is also present in *C. krusei* and in *C. lusitaniae* to fluconazole and amphotericin B, respectively. The Infectious Diseases Society of America has updated its clinical practice guidelines for the management of patients with invasive candidiasis and mucosal candidiasis to reflect changes noted with the addition of the new antifungals (Pappas, 2009).

Cutaneous Disease

Cutaneous disease is the most frequent infection caused by the *Candida* spp.; it presents topically as an erythematous lesion of the skin, sometimes accompanied by a creamy white exudate or scaling (Vazquez, 2002). Moist conditions, such as diaper rash in infants and infection of skin folds (intertrigo) in adults, are precursors to infection. Common sites are those in the groin, between fingers and toes, under the female breast, and in the axilla. Workers who immerse their hands in water for long periods of time are also at risk for infection of the skin of the hands, the nails (onychomycosis), or the nail bed (paronychium) (Jayatilake, 2009). Moreover, chronic cutaneous disease (referred to as chronic cutaneous candidiasis) is an uncommon manifestation of *Candida* infection in patients with defective cellular immunity (Lilic, 2002).

Oral Candidiasis

Oral candidiasis usually manifests as the appearance of creamy white patches overlying erythematous buccal mucosa (thrush) (Akpan, 2002). Although symptoms are usually minimal, dysphagia may result from heavy infection. Fissuring at the corners of the mouth is common and may be the primary complaint. Oral candidiasis is a common initial infection in patients with HIV and frequently is a marker of immune failure in these patients (Egusa, 2008).

Gastrointestinal Candidiasis

Gastrointestinal candidiasis occurs most frequently as esophagitis and less commonly as gastritis (Bonacini, 2001). Erosive lesions of the distal esophagus and stomach result in substernal pain, which is aggravated by swallowing. White plaques overlie the lesions when viewed by endoscopy. The differential diagnosis includes infection with herpes simplex virus, although these two processes may coexist. Esophageal candidiasis was previously described as a frequent opportunistic infection in persons infected with HIV; however, the use of highly active antiretroviral therapy has led to a striking decline in the prevalence of this disease (Raufman, 2005). Even though *Candida* species are seen frequently as flora of the lower GI tract, the significance of finding yeast in stool is uncertain. True invasive infection of the lower GI tract is less common than disease of the upper tract, although overgrowth of *Candida* spp. in the stool may accompany antimicrobial therapy.

Vaginal Candidiasis

Vaginal candidiasis afflicts postpubertal women; diabetes mellitus, utilization of antimicrobial therapy, pregnancy, and sexual activity are predisposing conditions (Soong, 2009). Vaginal burning and itching, dyspareunia, and a discharge that is classically curd-like are associated with an infection that may be acute or chronic and difficult to eradicate.

Urinary Tract Infection

Urinary tract infection caused by *Candida* spp. is difficult to diagnose because these yeasts are frequently recovered from the urine as a result of vaginal contamination or colonization of the bladder in patients with indwelling catheters, especially when systemic antibiotics have been administered (Lundstrom, 2001; Bukhary, 2008). Severe infection of the upper urinary tract, including necrosis of the renal papillae, is a serious complication that occurs particularly in patients who have obstructive uropathy. Quantitative cultures do not appear useful for assessing the significance of *Candida* spp. in the urinary tract.

Invasive Candidiasis

Invasive candidiasis often involves sources other than the skin or mucous membranes. A vast majority of invasive infections caused by *Candida* spp. result in bloodstream invasion and hematogenous spread of the organism (Mavor, 2005; Pfaller, 2007). Candidemia is defined as the isolation of *Candida* spp. from at least one blood culture specimen with hematogenous spread of the yeast to one or more organs. Nonhematogenous *Candida* infection of a single deep organ (also called disseminated or deep-seated candidiasis) is not common and often is suspected as hematogenous spread to a single organ in which the manifestations of disease are seen. Primary localized invasive infections occur normally after abdominal surgery and following perforation of the gut leading to contamination of the peritoneal cavity with *Candida*. Other forms of deep-seated infection include endophthalmitis, meningitis, pneumonia, osteomyelitis, and hepatitis. Fungal endocarditis resulting from a bloodstream infection is uncommon, but when present is commonly caused by a *Candida* spp. Risk factors for this infection include prosthetic valve surgery, preexisting valvular heart disease, use of intravenous catheters or broad-spectrum antibiotics, intravenous drug abuse, and immunosuppression.

Pathology of *Candida* Infection

The tissue response to *Candida* is regularly purulent, resembling lesions of bacterial infection with abscess formation present. On occasion, the response to *Candida* infection is granulomatous. Budding yeasts, pseudohyphae, and true hyphae may be present in tissue, and when pseudohyphae or true hyphae predominate, yeasts must be differentiated from invasive mould pathogens such as *Aspergillus*. Vascular invasion, as occurs with *Aspergillus* or the Zygomycetes, is uncommon in yeast infection. Yeast can often be demonstrated with an H&E stain but may be more easily recognized in sections stained with GMS or PAS. Studies have also shown that a finding of *Candida* organisms on a Papanicolaou (PAP) smear is a reliable indicator of vaginitis (Heller, 2008).

Laboratory Diagnosis

Specimens for culture should be taken from affected organs and from lesions in which they can be visualized. Modern continuous-monitoring

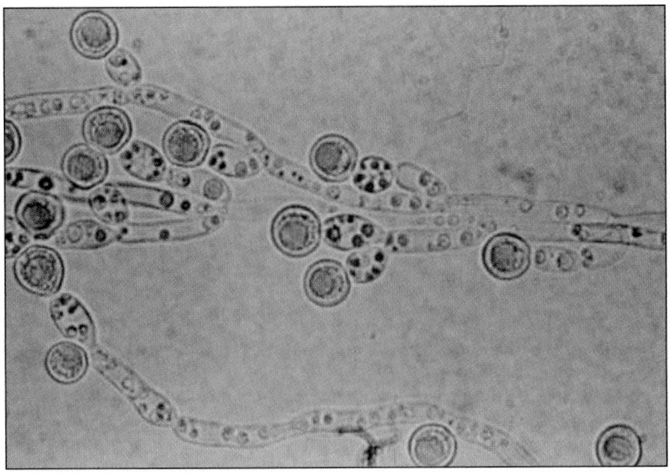

Figure 61-17 Chlamydoconidia produced by *Candida albicans.* These thick-walled asexual reproductive structures that occur most commonly at the ends of pseudohyphae are characteristic for this species and for *Candida dubliniensis.* (Cornmeal agar plate, ×400.)

blood culture systems detect most clinically significant yeast isolates (Reimer, 1997). Tissue specimens, scrapings, and swabs from the mouth or vagina should be inoculated onto primary fungal isolation media with and without cycloheximide. The presence of filamentous extensions from the edges of the colony (feet) is a macroscopic indication that pseudohyphae are being produced (see Fig. 61-1). *C. glabrata* (formerly *Torulopsis glabrata*) and *Cryptococcus* spp. do not form pseudohyphae in vitro, and some other *Candida* spp., such as *C. lusitaniae* and *Candida guilliermondii,* also may not form pseudohyphae.

The extent of the mycologic evaluation depends on the clinical setting and the specimen type. *Candida* spp. are frequently isolated from the respiratory and urinary tracts; however, interpretation of a finding of *Candida* spp. in these areas is difficult. Complete identification of isolates from these sites should be accomplished only selectively after consultation with the responsible clinician.

A preliminary report of *C. albicans/dubliniensis* may be issued if the germ tube test is positive (see Fig. 61-16). Additional study of yeast morphology using cornmeal agar to confirm the presence of chlamydoconidia can facilitate identification of *C. albicans/dubliniensis* within 24–48 hours (Fig. 61-17). Because both *C. albicans* and *C. dubliniensis* are germ tube positive, and because they have a high degree of phenotypic similarity, distinguishing between these two species has been difficult. However, strict adherence to detail when it comes to growth at 42° C, the production of abundant chlamydoconidia, and the sugar assimilation pattern can be used to differentiate between them (Campanha, 2005; Ells, 2009).

When germ tubes and chlamydoconidia are not demonstrated, a preliminary or presumptive identification of *Candida* spp. can be made only if pseudohyphae are present and arthroconidia are absent. Although confirmed species identification under this circumstance requires the use of assimilation tests, ancillary morphologic observations can be used to speed up the identification process (see Table 61-10). For instance, a rapid assimilation trehalose test procedure has been suggested by the CLSI (document M35-A2) for the identification of *C. glabrata,* a species that has emerged as a common cause of invasive disease with known resistance to standard antifungal therapy (Clinical Laboratory Standard Institute, 2008a).

THE GENUS *CRYPTOCOCCUS*

The *Cryptococcus* spp. complex consists of two species: *C. neoformans* and *Cryptococcus gattii* (formerly called *C. neoformans* var. *gattii*). These species are known to cause systemic infection in both immunocompetent and immunocompromised individuals (Bovers, 2008; Ma, 2009). The environmental reservoir for *C. neoformans* (teleomorph, *Filobasidiella neoformans*) is primarily pigeon guano, and infections caused by this organism occur worldwide. *C. gattii* on the other hand is found predominantly in tropical and subtropical areas, especially those associated with eucalyptus trees, and infection appears to be limited in distribution, primarily to northern Australia and Papua New Guinea (Huston, 2009). However, recent infections have been noted in Vancouver Island and surrounding areas, and a high rate of mortality has been associated with these infections (Kidd, 2007; MacDougall, 2007; Bartlett, 2008; Dixit, 2009). Because both species are classified within the phylum Basidiomycota, they are capable of producing basidiospores under the right circumstances. This teleomorphic (sexual) stage of cryptococci occurs only when appropriate mating types are crossed; thus this stage is not generally recognized in the laboratory. Sexual reproduction in the genera *Cryptococcus,* however, leads to increasing genetic diversity with the potential to produce strains that are hypervirulent and show increased antifungal resistance (Huston, 2009).

Risk Factors

Immunosuppressive therapy or disease is a risk factor for cryptococcosis (Huston, 2009). Before the appearance of HIV infection, 30%–50% of patients with cryptococcal infection were immunologically normal, as measured by available parameters. Risk factors for these patients include neoplasia, diabetes mellitus, immunosuppressive therapy, and immunologic disease. The introduction of the HIV-infected patient dramatically increased the number of cases of cryptococcosis, and although advances have been made in antiretroviral therapy, in antifungal treatment, and in intracranial pressure management in these patients, *Cryptococcus* continues to have a high rate of mortality (Sajadi, 2009). An estimate of the global burden of cryptococcal meningitis finds the numbers of cases and deaths to be very high within areas of sub-Saharan Africa, where there is a high incidence of HIV-infected people (Park, 2009). Cryptococcosis also remains a significant opportunistic infection in solid organ transplant recipients (Singh, 2008).

Clinical Disease

Primary cryptococcal disease generally occurs in the lungs following inhalation of the fungus from the environment. This disease can remain localized or can disseminate by hematogenous spread to other tissues, most frequently the central nervous system. The severity of the disease is dependent on the host's immune response, with severe disease most frequent in immunologically compromised patients. Practical guidelines for the management of cryptococcal diseases was recently published by the Infectious Diseases Society of America (Perfect, 2010).

Respiratory Tract

Cryptococcal infection of the respiratory tract exhibits a wide variety of presentations (Jarvis, 2008; Shirley, 2009). Immunologically competent patients may exhibit no symptoms despite the presence of cryptococci in the lower respiratory tract, and the infection may be diffuse or localized, to include the formation of coin lesions that usually do not calcify. Immunocompromised patients on the other hand may have extensive infection that often is accompanied by other infectious agents, particularly *Pneumocystis (carinii) jiroveci* or cytomegalovirus. Extrapulmonary disease may appear weeks after a pulmonary infection has been documented.

Skin Lesions

Skin lesions usually result from hematogenous dissemination from the respiratory tract in immunocompromised patients (Christianson, 2003). These lesions present as single or multiple papules, which enlarge and ulcerate, producing a thin exudate that contains the yeast. Primary cutaneous manifestations of the disease are rare but may also be reported in immunocompetent individuals (Revenga, 2002).

Bone and Joint Infection

Bone and joint infection may occur usually as a result of dissemination from the respiratory tract (Liu, 1998). Osteolytic lesions are produced, with abscesses formed in adjacent soft tissue that contain a thin exudate with large numbers of cryptococci. Less commonly, joint spaces are involved.

Central Nervous System Infection

Cryptococcal meningitis is the most frequent and most serious focus of disseminated cryptococcal infection (Satishchandra, 2007; Dorneanu, 2008; Patel, 2009). Onset of this disease may be acute, or presentation may be insidious and progression torpid. Headache and changes in mental status and personality often dominate the clinical picture. Basilar meningitis, involvement of the cranial nerves, and invasion of the underlying cortex result in hydrocephalus and decreased visual acuity. Fever, if present, usually is of low grade, and typical signs of acute meningeal irritation, such as stiff neck and Kernig's and Brudzinski's signs, are often absent.

Pathology of Cryptococcal Infection

The histologic response depends on the degree of encapsulation of the infecting cryptococcal strain. Most commonly, little or no inflammatory

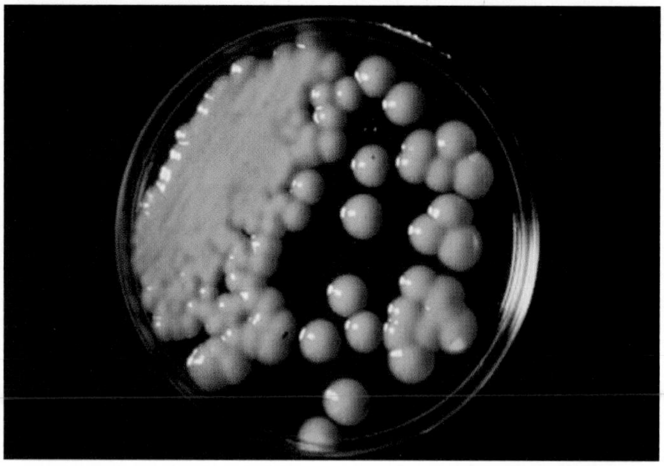

Figure 61-18 Colonies of *Cryptococcus neoformans* usually appear mucoid when first isolated. Some strains are poorly encapsulated and lack the mucoid appearance. (Sabouraud dextrose agar.)

response is seen, and the cells of normal tissue are separated by large numbers of encapsulated cryptococci. Poorly encapsulated strains of *C. neoformans* elicit a granulomatous inflammatory response, and yeasts are found predominantly in the cytoplasm of macrophages. When cerebrospinal fluid is examined, the only cells present may be the yeasts, which may be misinterpreted as mononuclear host cells if infection is not suspected clinically. Large capsules usually are demonstrated in positive India ink preparations; however, they are not always evident, and the cells may be confused with those of *B. dermatitidis* or even immature spherules of *Coccidioides* spp.

Differentiation in tissue sections can be accomplished by staining of cryptococcal mucopolysaccharide with mucin stains or demonstration of melanin pigment with the Fontana-Masson stain. Mayer's mucicarmine stain and the GMS stain have been shown to be important for the diagnosis of cryptococcosis when atypical forms were present in an uncommon location (Gazzoni, 2009). The variable size (3–10 µm) and the decidedly round nature of the yeast in vivo are clues to its correct identification, regardless of the degree of encapsulation and the histologic response.

Laboratory Diagnosis

Possible cryptococci should always be identified as to the species complex level. Clues to the presence of this fungus include good growth on blood agar plates incubated in the bacteriology laboratory at 35°–37° C, a mucoid appearance of the colonies (Fig. 61-18), a round appearance of the yeast cells without pseudohyphae in microscopic wet preps or stained preparations, and lack of growth on media that contain cycloheximide. Presumptive identification can be performed rapidly by examining an India ink preparation for capsules (see Fig. 61-14) and/or conducting a rapid urease test. Capsules may be diminished even in heavily encapsulated strains once they have been isolated on agar media; however, subcultures of isolates may restore the mucoid capsule. Definitive identification of the species complex is accomplished by biochemical testing.

Differentiating *C. gattii* from *C. neoformans* using standard phenotypic methods is difficult and usually is needed only for epidemiologic investigations. The incorporation of glycine into specialized medium (L-canavanine-glycine-bromthymol blue medium) has been shown to be reliable for differentiation of these species in that *C. gattii* readily assimilates glycine and *C. neoformans* does not (Klein, 2009). In instances where differentiation is needed, molecular sequencing of the D1/D2 region of the 28S rDNA gene or the ITS regions of the rRNA genes is known to be reliable in separating these two species (Georgi, 2009).

The polysaccharide antigen of the *C. neoformans* spp. complex can be detected in cerebrospinal fluid and serum, most commonly by the latex agglutination test. Although the sensitivity of this test exceeds 90%, considerable variability in performance has been noted among different commercial kits. The frequency of erroneous results can be diminished by treatment of serum specimens with pronase. False-positive reactions appear to be less common in patients infected with HIV, perhaps because of the large numbers of organisms present. Titration of positive results has been done traditionally to assess prognosis and to obtain a baseline for use in following the effects of treatment. Large amounts of antigen and persistence of antigen following therapy are poor prognostic signs in patients. Measurement of serum antigen appears to be a more sensitive test than testing of cerebrospinal fluid in HIV-infected patients. However, both serum and cerebrospinal fluid should be tested for optimal sensitivity. A negative India ink test on cerebrospinal fluid is a good prognostic sign in non–HIV-infected patients but does not have the same implication for patients with AIDS.

THE GENUS *MALASSEZIA*

The history of the nomenclature used for the genus *Malassezia* is complicated. Currently, this genus is composed of one non–lipid-dependent species (*Malassezia pachydermatis*) and 12 lipid-dependent species (Guillot, 2008). *Malassezia furfur* is considered the most common pathogen in this group among humans. Because differentiation of the *Malassezia* spp. requires molecular sequencing, most clinical laboratories prefer to report results as "*Malassezia furfur* species complex" or "*Malassezia* species."

Risk Factors

Malassezia yeasts are commensals of the normal skin, and cutaneous disease may occur in normal hosts. Systemic infection occurs primarily in neonates and is associated with intravenous hyperalimentation with lipid solutions (Devlin, 2006). Although *Malassezia* spp. are not ordinarily present on the skin of healthy infants, the yeasts have been recovered from the skin of as many as 37% of infants who were in intensive care units.

Clinical Diseases

Infection caused by *Malassezia* spp. can range from an asymptomatic lesion on the epidermis of normal individuals to systemic disease in the immunocompromised host.

Cutaneous Infection

Malassezia spp. are known causes of pityriasis (tinea) versicolor and seborrheic dermatitis, and evidence is accumulating that they play a significant role in atopic eczema/dermatitis syndrome (formerly called atopic dermatitis) (Ashbee, 2007; Zisova, 2009).

Pityriasis versicolor is a common infection of the epidermis in immunologically normal patients, resulting in hyperpigmentation or hypopigmentation of the skin, commonly on the trunk and upper arms. Fawn-colored macules are the most common presentation, but depigmenting lesions are more obvious in dark-skinned persons and may be accentuated by a suntan in light-skinned individuals. The ill effects are purely cosmetic but may be considerably troublesome. Hypopigmented lesions must be differentiated from vitiligo. Therapy consists of topical application of fungicidal creams or rinses.

Seborrheic dermatitis is a multifactor disease that requires both endogenous and exogenous predisposing factors for its development (Zisova, 2009). An inflammatory reaction against the yeast is considered the basis for the development of this disease.

Systemic Infection

Systemic infection occurs almost invariably in infants who have received intravascular infusions of lipid (the disease is also called *Malassezia* catheter–associated sepsis) (Devlin, 2006). Diluted lipid solution supports the growth of lipid-dependent *Malassezia* spp. by supplying long-chain fatty acids that are also found on the skin and must be supplied in the laboratory for isolation of the yeast. Infected infants are often asymptomatic, but fever, leukocytosis, and thrombocytopenia may be present. Pneumonia is a common systemic manifestation of disease, probably resulting from emboli received from infected intravenous catheters. Removing the infected catheter is therapeutic.

Pathology of *Malassezia* Infection

The diagnosis of pityriasis versicolor usually is made clinically or by demonstrating yeast and short hyphal forms (similar in appearance to spaghetti and meatballs) in KOH preparations of skin scrapings (Fig. 61-19). The addition of Calcofluor white or another fungal stain enhances detection because the fungal cells are small and difficult to visualize when unstained. When biopsied, hyperkeratosis, acanthosis, and dermal mononuclear infiltrates may be seen. Little is known of the pathology of systemic infection with *Malassezia* spp. because biopsies are performed infrequently and lethal infection is uncommon. In rare fatal cases, vasculitis, septic infarcts, and granulomatous inflammation have been described in many organs, including the lung, liver, and kidney.

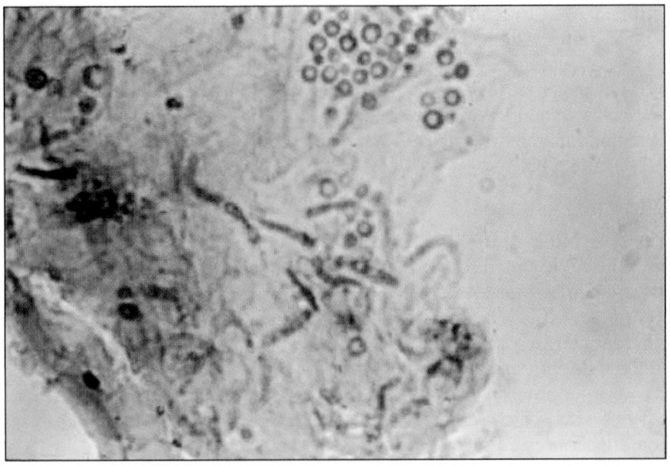

Figure 61-19 Skin scrapings from a lesion of pityriasis versicolor. The yeast and short hyphal forms (spaghetti and meatballs appearance) are characteristic of *Malassezia furfur.* (Lactophenol cotton blue stain, ×400.)

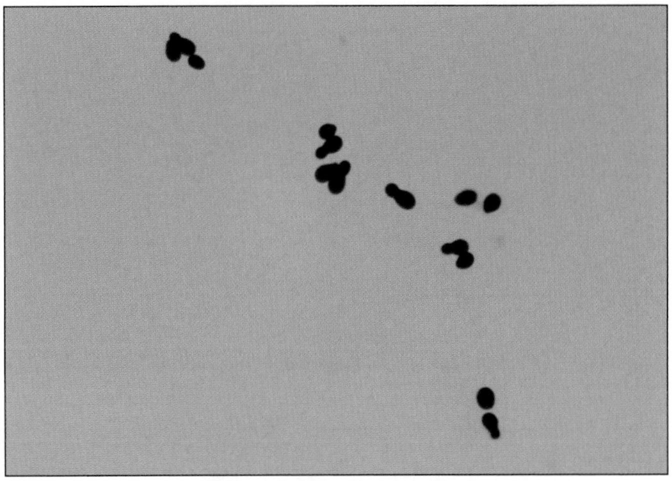

Figure 61-21 Gram stain from culture demonstrating gram-positive yeast cells of *Malassezia* spp. showing the characteristic collarette (bud scar). (Gram stain, ×1000.)

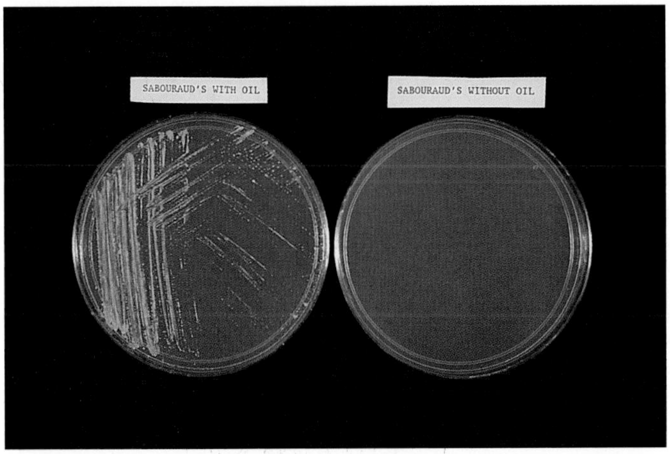

Figure 61-20 Abundant growth of *Malassezia furfur* is evident on a plate that was overlaid with oil before the inoculum was applied. No growth is seen on a companion plate without oil. (Sabouraud dextrose agar.)

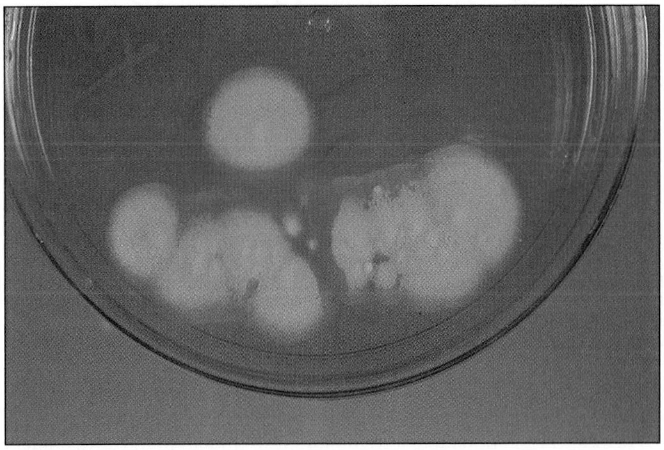

Figure 61-22 An aerial mycelium arises from the yeast-like colony of *Geotrichum candidum.* (Sabouraud dextrose agar.)

Laboratory Diagnosis

Culture for *Malassezia* spp. is rarely requested in cutaneous disease, and direct observation of yeast in KOH preparations usually is done in the physician's office. This yeast should be sought in cultures of blood and intravenous catheter tips from neonates. Before inoculation, a drop of sterile olive oil is added to the surface of a suitable agar medium, such as Sabouraud dextrose agar or sheep blood agar. Within 2–3 days, colonies appear light brown and often have a very dry appearance in the oil overlay. An initial clue to this pathogen is lack of growth in the absence of oil or stimulation of growth by the presence of oil overlay (Fig. 61-20). In contrast, *M. pachydermatis* is not dependent on long-chain fatty acids for growth.

Identification of the genus can be suspected by microscopic examination of the yeast cells, which measure 3–7 μm. The budding process in *Malassezia* is unusual because it occurs as an enteroblastic process with the formation of phialides. The bud is broad based, and the collarettes of the phialides may be observed with the light microscope as a distinct dark ring separating the mother and daughter cells (Fig. 61-21). Species identification can be confirmed using molecular techniques that target regions within the rDNA complex (Affes, 2009; Gaitanis, 2009).

OTHER YEAST AND YEAST-LIKE PATHOGENS

Blastoschizomyces capitatus (formerly called *Trichosporon capitatum*) has caused rare cases of disseminated infection that resemble candidiasis; however, this species characteristically is resistant to most antifungal agents (Bouza, 2004; Martino, 2004). *Trichosporon* spp. constitute another group of yeasts that are widely distributed in nature and occasionally are associated with disseminated infection in humans (Chagas-Neto, 2009, Lacasse, 2009). The old taxon *Trichosporon beigelii* has undergone molecular analysis, leading to six new species, with *Trichosporon asahii* the most common species recovered from blood cultures (Chagas-Neto, 2008). A morphologically similar fungus, *Geotrichum candidum*, is also a rare cause of pulmonary or disseminated disease, especially in those patients suffering from acute leukemia (Girmenia, 2005; Henrich, 2009). Both *Geotrichum* and *Trichosporon* spp. produce smooth, yeast-like colonies that later develop aerial mycelium, like new hair growth on a bald head (Fig. 61-22). Other saprophytic yeasts such as *Saccharomyces cerevisiae*, *Rhodotorula* spp. (Tuon, 2008), and *Hansenula* spp. (Ma, 2000) may also produce infection on rare occasions.

Demonstration of these yeasts in tissues or isolation from multiple specimens, even from sterile sites, is required to document the role of the unusual yeast in an infectious process.

MYCOSES CAUSED BY DIMORPHIC FUNGI

Thermally dimorphic fungi are the most pathogenic organisms encountered in a clinical mycology laboratory. In the United States, the most important dimorphic pathogens are *Histoplasma capsulatum* var. *capsulatum*, *Blastomyces dermatitidis*, *Coccidioides immitis*, *Coccidioides posadasii*, and *Sporothrix schenckii*. *Sporothrix* is widely distributed throughout the world, and the other organisms are found predominantly in North America, where they have distinct geographic distributions (Fig. 61-23). Epidemic disease is most common with *Histoplasma* and *Coccidioides* and less common with *Sporothrix* and *Blastomyces*. These endemic mycoses share several characteristics, including (1) the ability to cause disease in a healthy host,

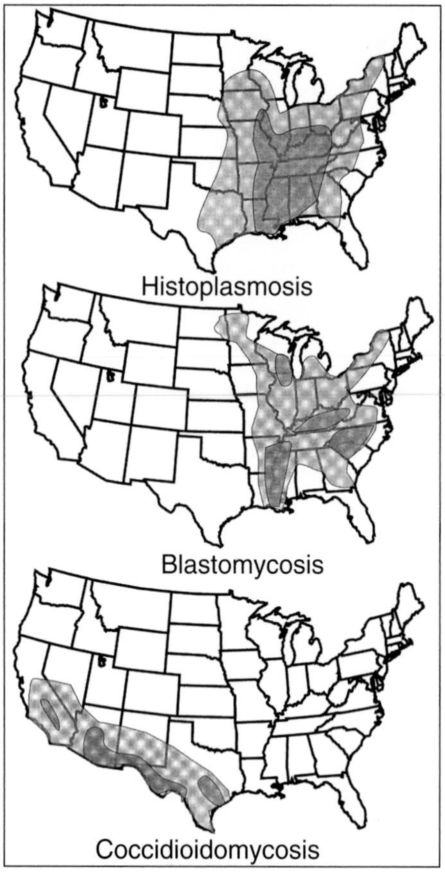

Figure 61-23 Geographic distribution of dimorphic fungal infections in the United States. Areas of greatest endemicity *(dark shading)* and lesser endemicity *(light shading)* are illustrated. Sporadic cases may also occur in other areas outside of the endemic zones.

(2) association with a specific ecologic niche in the environment, and (3) demonstration of temperature dimorphism (mould in the environment at a temperature of 25°–30° C and yeast or spherules in the environment [in the case of *Coccidioides*] at body temperature).

THE GENUS *HISTOPLASMA*

H. capsulatum is subdivided into two varieties: *H. capsulatum* var. *capsulatum* (hereafter referred to as *H. capsulatum*) and *H. capsulatum* var. *duboisii*. Both of these fungal pathogens are geographically restricted, and acquisition of infection does not overlap in most cases. *H. capsulatum* var. *capsulatum* is found primarily along the Ohio, Mississippi, and St. Lawrence Rivers but may have worldwide distribution. *H. capsulatum* var. *duboisii*, on the other hand, is limited to equatorial Africa and is believed to cause a disease referred to as African histoplasmosis. Distinguishing characteristics of the tissue phase can be observed to differentiate between these two pathogens; however, lack of travel to the endemic area in Africa generally can be used to rule out infection with the var. *duboisii*.

Risk Factors

The primary risk factor for acquiring histoplasmosis is living in endemic regions of the United States. In some areas, more than 90% of the population reacts positively to histoplasmin skin testing. Growth of *H. capsulatum* in the soil is stimulated by bird guano, although the fungus does not infect the bird. Once growing in the soil, the fungus sporulates and produces conidia, which, during activities that generate aerosols, can be inhaled into the lungs. Occupationally acquired acute histoplasmosis has been reported, leading the U.S. Department of Health and Human Services (2004) to issue a document outlining measures for protecting workers at risk.

Epidemic acute disease has occurred in individuals vacationing to areas endemic for this fungus. A Centers for Disease Control and Prevention (CDC; 2001a) report described 221 cases of histoplasmosis among students representing 37 colleges in 18 states who had vacationed in Acapulco, Mexico, in March of 2001. Most infected individuals had visited a common source point, thus leading to spore exposure. The CDC also described an outbreak of histoplasmosis among 14 healthy adventure travelers from the United States, who had visited a bat-infected cave in Nicaragua (Weinberg, 2003). Occupationally, a CDC report described an outbreak of histoplasmosis wherein at least 25 workers at an agricultural processing plant in Nebraska developed disease following exposure to a spoil pile known to be contaminated with *H. capsulatum* (Centers for Disease Control and Prevention, 2004).

Clinical Diseases

The magnitude of the exposure and the immune status of the host influence the clinical manifestations of disease, which can range from an asymptomatic infectious process to disseminated life-threatening disease (Kauffman, 2007). Exposure to low concentrations of spores from the environment in a normal host is typically asymptomatic. Therefore most adults living in an endemic area are seropositive and show immunologic evidence of infection; however, they remain asymptomatic to disease. Disseminated disease is usually reserved for individuals who are immunosuppressed.

Acute Pulmonary Infection

Individuals who are exposed to large numbers of conidia may develop a flu-like syndrome with high fever, chills, fatigue, cough, and pleuritic or retrosternal chest pain. More severely affected individuals may be sick for several weeks, but resolution usually is complete without antifungal therapy in the normal host. If focal granulomatous inflammation has occurred, calcification of the focus typically leaves a well-circumscribed coin lesion, which may be seen on the chest radiograph.

Granulomatous and Fibrosing Mediastinitis

These types of manifestations involve the lymph nodes in the mediastinum (Hammoud, 2009). Granulomatous disease is characterized by enlarged lymph nodes, which may obstruct the airways, pulmonary vessels, or esophagus. Fistulas can form within the lymph nodes and adjacent mediastinal structures. Fibrosing disease is a reaction that occurs in the mediastinum among individuals predisposed to an excessive response to *Histoplasma* antigens. Obstructions may form that involve the superior vena cava, the airways, the pulmonary arteries or veins, or the esophagus. Both granulomatous and fibrosing diseases are thought to progress independently.

Chronic Pulmonary Histoplasmosis

This debilitating disease occurs primarily in patients with chronic obstructive pulmonary disease (COPD), most of whom are middle-aged men (Kennedy, 2007). However, studies have shown that this disease is becoming more commonly recognized among females, and that females exhibited fewer cavities and presented with decreased numbers of smokers and reduced extent of smoking exposure, along with absence of COPD (Kennedy, 2007). In this disease, calcification and cavitations may occur, which may mimic chronic pulmonary tuberculosis and pulmonary neoplasia.

Disseminated Histoplasmosis

Dissemination of yeast through the reticuloendothelial system may occur as part of acute pulmonary histoplasmosis, resulting in healed granulomas that often calcify, especially in the spleen. Clinically disseminated infection occurs in two classes of patients. The first group consists of individuals at the extremes of age who do not have a recognized immunosuppressive condition but may have an immune system that is incompletely developed or is diminished by age in ways that are incompletely understood. The second group comprises patients with recognized immunosuppressive diseases or therapies. Before the 1980s, these diseases were predominantly hematologic neoplasms; however, in recent years, HIV infection has dominated the risk factors (McKinsey, 1998). Progression of disease may be rapid or insidious.

Compromised patients may develop an infection of the reticuloendothelial system, resulting in lymphadenopathy, hepatosplenomegaly, or thrombocytopenia (Wheat, 2003b). Destruction of the adrenal cortex by the granulomatous process may be sufficiently extensive to cause hormonal insufficiency. Central nervous system infection may be manifested as chronic meningitis, intracerebral granulomas, or both. Endovascular infection includes endocarditis with large, bulky vegetations. Any part of the GI tract may be affected, and ulcerating lesions may suggest a neoplasm macroscopically. The hallmark of disease is an oropharyngeal ulcer, which may cause hoarseness, dysphagia, or a painful lesion on the tongue or gingiva (Psevdos, 2008).

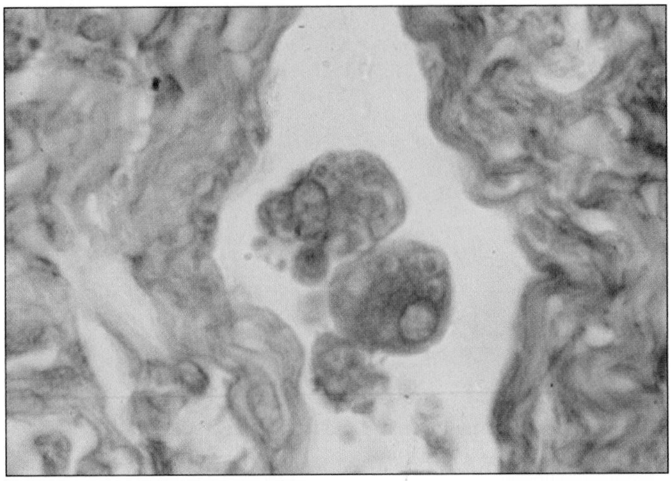

Figure 61-24 Yeast cells of *Histoplasma capsulatum* in macrophages. The presence of intracellular small, round to oval yeast-like cells in tissue is a characteristic pathologic finding in histoplasmosis. (Hematoxylin and eosin stain, ×1000.)

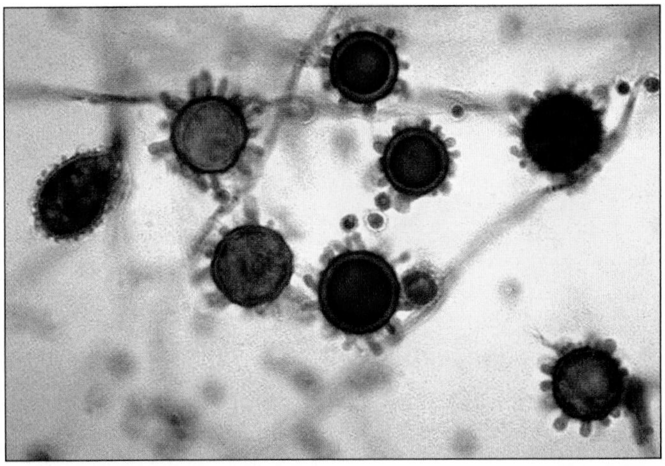

Figure 61-25 Tuberculate macroconidia with microconidia of *Histoplasma capsulatum* in culture. These structures are characteristic of the environmental mould form of this dimorphic fungus. (Lactophenol cotton blue stain, ×400.) *(Courtesy CDC Public Health Image Library.)*

Pathology of Histoplasmosis

As a facultative intracellular pathogen, *H. capsulatum* is found predominantly in macrophages. Pathologic lesions consist of collections of infected macrophages, noncaseating granulomas, or caseating granulomas. Histopathologic lesions are similar to those produced by *Mycobacterium tuberculosis*, and these two pathogens should be considered at the same time in the patient workup differential. Intracellular yeasts are often well demonstrated by H&E staining (Fig. 61-24). However, PAS and GMS stains are more sensitive, with the silver stain essential for demonstration of old yeast cells in healed granulomas. This yeast, presumably no longer viable, may be enlarged and distorted in morphology, making diagnosis difficult. Differential diagnosis of yeast forms includes small forms of *B. dermatitidis*, *P. marneffei*, *Leishmania* spp., or *Candida* spp., especially *C. glabrata*. The yeasts of *H. capsulatum* in caseating granulomas are sufficiently distinctive to provide a presumptive diagnosis, but unusual granulomatous presentations of *P. (carinii) jiroveci* must be differentiated. As is true with all endemic fungal infections, culture is necessary to make a confirmed diagnosis of disease.

Laboratory Diagnosis

The yeast form in tissue may be demonstrated histologically or in preparations of respiratory secretions, fluids, peripheral blood, bone marrow, or tissue imprints. Wet preparations and Calcofluor white may be used, but the morphology of tissue and yeast cells is best seen with Giemsa staining because the details of nuclear morphology can be assessed. The yeast cells measure 3–5 μm in diameter, have a single nucleus, and bud with a narrow neck.

If disseminated infection is suspected, blood cultures for *Histoplasma* should be performed. The Isolator technique is a sensitive technique for recovering the yeast phase from blood, although other blood culture detection systems can also be used to detect this fungus. Other clinical specimens should be inoculated to an enriched agar, such as brain-heart infusion agar supplemented with sheep blood, which is incubated at 25°–30° C.

Colonies of *H. capsulatum* usually appear after incubation for 10–14 days but occasionally require incubation for up to 4 weeks. They are fluffy and vary from white to buff-brown. Diagnostic asexual forms include microconidia and macroconidia. Microconidia, which are produced first, are similar to the structures produced by *B. dermatitidis*. The more characteristic macroconidia have roughened projections from the periphery of the conidia, a configuration referred to as tuberculate (Fig. 61-25). The macroconidia of the saprophyte, *Sepedonium*, may be confused with *Histoplasma*, so differentiation of these two fungi is important. The macroscopic appearance of the colonies, the rate of growth, the growth of *H. capsulatum* on media containing cycloheximide, the presence of yeast forms in tissue, and the clinical history usually are sufficient to diagnose histoplasmosis. Final confirmation most often is provided by nucleic acid hybridization probe testing from the culture isolate. Conversion of the mould to the yeast phase also confirms identification, but this is often difficult and has been supplanted in most clinical laboratories by the molecular probe technique (AccuProbe). However, false-positive probe results have been reported, and other factors need to be considered before a diagnosis of histoplasmosis can be confirmed (Brandt, 2005).

Serologic tests for the detection of anti-*Histoplasma* antibodies (i.e., immunodiffusion and complement fixation) have several limitations that need to be considered, making these tests marginal for the diagnosis of histoplasmosis. A 2–6-week delay after exposure is required for the production of antibodies, reducing the value of this testing for the diagnosis of acute disease. Once patients are infected with *H. capsulatum*, antibody levels remain detectable for many years. Antibodies to *H. capsulatum* and *B. dermatitidis* also may cross-react. Additionally, patients with immune dysfunction may not produce detectable levels of antibodies, and patients with previous exposure might have elevated levels of antibodies (Wheat, 2003a).

Antigen detection, on the other hand, has been shown to be useful for the diagnosis and management of histoplasmosis (Brandt, 2005; Wheat, 2007, 2009b). The sensitivity of urine antigen detection for diagnosis is greatest in patients with disseminated disease (up to 92%) or acute pulmonary histoplasmosis (75%–80%) (Wheat, 2002). Antigen detection is also useful for following the effects of therapy on fungal burden; when antigen concentrations in urine or serum fall during therapy, treatment failure is suggested. Moreover, increased antigen levels in a previously infected individual suggest a relapse of infection. Use of the antigen assay to detect *Histoplasma* antigen in bronchoalveolar fluid has been shown to complement antigen detection in serum and urine as an objective diagnostic test (Hage, 2009).

The histoplasmin skin test antigen has been useful for epidemiologic studies but should not be used for diagnosis. Not only does the high frequency of positive tests in endemic areas cloud interpretation, but the skin test can cause an individual to seroconvert to positive, further confusing the issue.

THE GENUS *BLASTOMYCES*

B. dermatitidis is the only species within the genus *Blastomyces* (Gueho, 1997). Endemic areas for this pathogen in the soil include the eastern part of the United States, mainly areas adjacent to the Mississippi and Ohio River basins; areas northwest of the Great Lakes in Canada; and areas within Africa (Bradsher, 2008). However, later reports suggest that the endemic area for blastomycosis may be larger than originally described, and reports have described disease in patients from previously nonendemic areas in Colorado and Nebraska (Centers for Disease Control and Prevention, 1999; Veligandla, 2002).

Risk Factors

Most cases of blastomycosis (also referred to as North American blastomycosis) are sporadic, and an environmental source is not often found. Small outbreaks do occur, and the fungus has been isolated from soil at outbreak sites (McKinnell, 2009). No specific risk factors for blastomycosis are known, although severe, disseminated infection has been described in immunocompromised patients. HIV-infected patients who reside in endemic areas are particularly at risk for serious infection (Pappas, 2002).

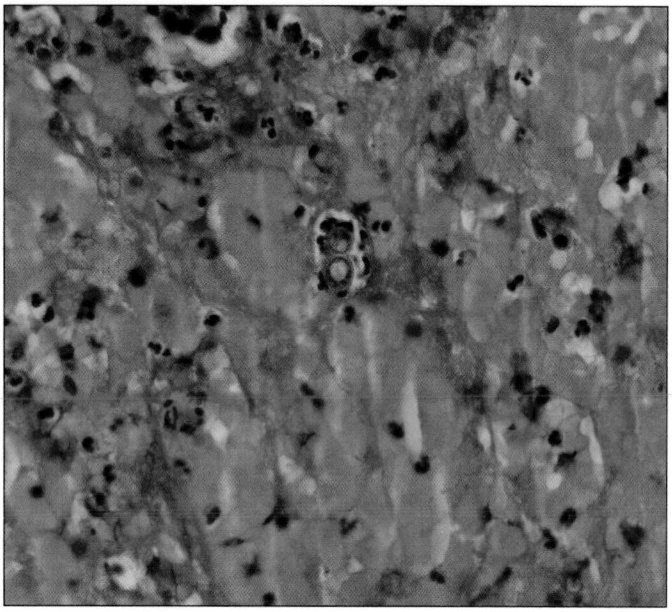

Figure 61-26 *Blastomyces dermatitidis* in tissue showing characteristic large, broad-based, budding yeast cells with a thick refractile (double-contoured) wall. (Hematoxylin and eosin stain, ×400.)

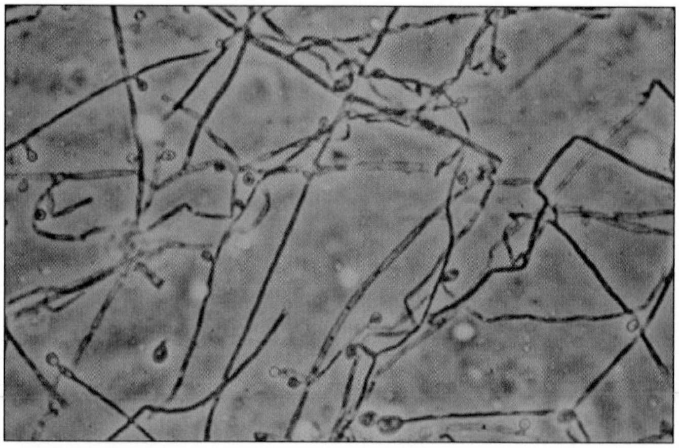

Figure 61-27 Mould form of *Blastomyces dermatitidis* in culture. The lollipop appearance of the conidium on a conidiophore is characteristic of the environmental mould form for this dimorphic fungus. (Lactophenol cotton blue stain, ×400.)

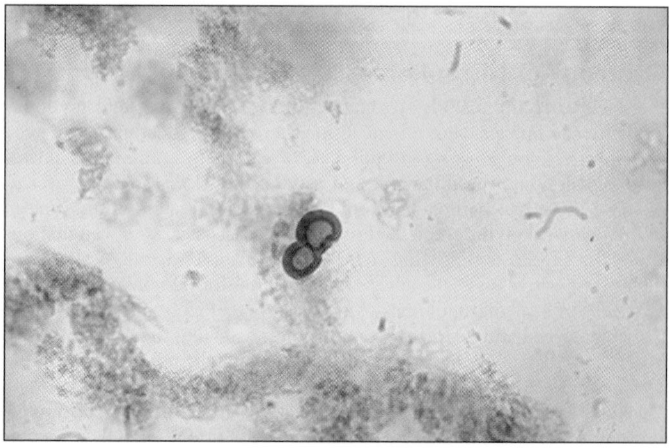

Figure 61-28 Budding yeast cells of *Blastomyces dermatitidis* in culture. When cultures are incubated at 37° C, large, broad-based budding yeasts with a double-contoured wall are detected that are characteristic of the yeast phase of this dimorphic fungus. (Lactophenol cotton blue stain, ×400.)

Clinical Diseases

As is true with most other endemic dimorphic fungi, the portal of entry is the respiratory tract, where the infection may be asymptomatic, transient, or insidiously progressive (Bradsher, 2008). Chronic pulmonary blastomycosis with low-grade fever, weight loss, and localized pulmonary infiltrates may suggest neoplastic disease, for which diagnostic studies, including bronchoalveolar lavage, fine-needle aspiration of the lung, or surgical lung biopsy, may be undertaken (Lemos, 2002). Dissemination of yeast from the lung most commonly results in cutaneous or skeletal infection (Mason, 2008). The central nervous and genitourinary systems are involved less frequently. Cutaneous lesions often are hypertrophic or ulcerative and may be locally destructive. The lesions may be mistaken for squamous cell carcinoma of the skin. Secondary involvement of the skin over bony lesions also occurs. A delay in diagnosis is not uncommon, especially when patients have no history of exposure to an endemic area (Veligandla, 2002).

Pathology of Blastomycosis

The characteristic histologic response to *B. dermatitidis* is a mixture of acute inflammation with microabscess formation and granulomatous inflammation. In cutaneous lesions, pseudoepitheliomatous hyperplasia of the epidermis overlying the inflammation is characteristic. Yeast cells are most often found in the microabscesses or within multinucleated giant cells. The characteristic yeast can frequently be demonstrated in tissue sections stained with H&E, but the organism may be more readily visible when stained with PAS or GMS. The thick-walled yeast cells measure 8–15 μm in diameter and maintain a broad base during the budding process (Fig. 61-26). An artifactual separation of the cytoplasm from the cell wall in formalin-fixed preparations may give the appearance of a double wall. Although nonbudding yeast cells must be differentiated from yeast cells of *Cryptococcus* spp. and from developing spherules of *Coccidioides* spp., the diagnosis of blastomycosis can generally be proposed by observation of characteristic yeast forms in tissues by an experienced pathologist (Bradsher, 2003).

Surgical pathology and cytopathology have been reported as the primary means of diagnosis because positive culture may not always be recovered. However, microbiology culture and conventional morphologic assessment of routine samples have redundant utility in diagnosis and generally are required to make a confirmed disease diagnosis (Taxy, 2007).

Laboratory Identification

Direct demonstration of the yeast cells may be accomplished in tissue sections or in wet preparations of aspirated fluids and imprints of tissues. Calcofluor white staining may enhance detection of the yeast. Growth is somewhat more rapid than that of *Histoplasma* and fluffy white to buff colonies, which often cannot be distinguished from *H. capsulatum* and usually appear within 1–2 weeks. The microconidia resemble those of *H. capsulatum* (Fig. 61-27), but macroconidia are not formed. A saprophytic mould, *Chrysosporium* resembles *Blastomyces* but does not develop a yeast phase and does not grow on media that contain cycloheximide. Conversion to the yeast phase may occur on routine media incubated at 37° C with hemoglobin and cysteine containing agar used specifically for this purpose (Fig. 61-28). Once again, demonstration of the yeast form in tissue serves as a reasonable substitute for demonstration of dimorphism in the laboratory. The nucleic acid probe hybridization test (AccuProbe) from culture material is the preferred method for confirmation of isolates in most laboratories, although false-positive results have been reported (Iwen, 2000).

Although the complement fixation test has been used as a serologic test for the diagnosis of blastomycosis, this test has considerable limitations and should be used only as an adjunct to culture of the fungus. A *Blastomyces* antigen test similar to the *Histoplasma* antigen test also is available in a reference laboratory; however, data regarding utility and reliability are lacking.

THE GENUS *COCCIDIOIDES*

Coccidioides immitis was considered until recently the sole etiologic agent of coccidioidomycosis (Valley fever). Phylogenetic studies now show the existence of two genetically distinct *C. immitis* clades: one called the California clade *(C. immitis)* and the other called the non-California clade *(C. posadasii)* (Fisher, 2002). Although a strong difference in genotype has been noted between these two species, the phenotypic differences are minimal, thus making it difficult for most laboratories to distinguish between them (Saubolle, 2007; Ampel, 2009).

The coccidioidal organisms are soil-dwelling fungi found in the southern portions of California and in other areas of southwestern United States (especially southern regions of Arizona, Utah, Nevada, and New Mexico, as well as western Texas), northern Mexico, and Central and South America (especially Venezuela) (Talamantes, 2007). Arizona has seen a dramatic increase in cases over the years, with a disproportionate rate of infection occurring in people over the age of 65 years and in those with HIV infection (Centers for Disease Control and Prevention, 2003; Blair, 2008; Kim, 2009). The numbers of reported cases and hospitalizations for coccidioidomycosis in California increased each year from 2000 to 2006 before decreasing in 2007, with the highest incidence seen in Kern County (150 cases per 100,000 population) (Centers for Disease Control and Prevention, 2009).

Another interesting issue with these agents is the recent classification of *C. immitis* and *C. posadasii* by the U.S. Department of Health and Human Services as select agents of bioterrorism (Department of Health and Human Services, 2005; Warnock, 2007). This designation suggests that these pathogens could be used as potential bioweapons and establishes strict federal regulations to be followed by individuals who possess and transport these agents and by those who report confirmed infections (Deresinski, 2003). Individuals have questioned the rationale and justification for classifying the *Coccidioides* as select agents because of the burden placed on diagnostic laboratories for reporting of cases and for deposition of specimens and culture material (Fierer, 2002). Current law requires that the list of select agents undergo a biennial review in 2010. Discussions to reconsider the inclusion of *Coccidioides* as a select agent have been included in this review.

Risk Factors

Residence in an endemic area is the primary risk factor for the development of infection because the arthroconidia of the mould phase are in the soil and are easily disseminated through the air (Parish, 2008). A classic example of epidemic coccidioidomycosis occurred in a group of archeology workers in a dig at the Dinosaur National Monument in northeastern Utah in 2001. Ten workers within this group were recognized to have pulmonary coccidioidomycosis during an excavation, and eight of these individuals required hospitalization (Petersen, 2004). Another outbreak of disease occurred in individuals attending the World Championship of Model Airplane Flying in Kern County, California, in October 2001. This outbreak illustrated the importance of cooperation within the international community for epidemiologic evaluation, because competing teams from more than 30 countries were potentially involved in the outbreak (Centers for Disease Control and Prevention, 2001b). The locations of military bases in the southwestern United States have also shown coccidioidomycosis to have a profound effect on military personnel training in these areas (Crum-Cianflone, 2007). The development of an effective vaccine for Valley fever to protect both military members and civilians residing or training in endemic areas has been a suggested prevention strategy to avoid acquiring the disease (Hector, 2007).

Genetic factors have been suggested to influence the frequency of severe and disseminated infection, but the nature of this association is not completely known (Cox, 2004). Disseminated infection is reportedly more common in blacks and Filipinos than in whites. Asians, Native Americans, and Mexicans also appear to be at increased risk for the disease.

Immunosuppressive infection or disease is a known risk factor for disseminated infection, with HIV-infected patients at particular risk for disseminated disease (Woods, 2000). Transplant recipients who travel to or reside part-time or full-time in endemic areas are also at risk for both primary and reactivation coccidioidomycosis (Vikram, 2009). Clinicians in nonendemic areas should be aware of the potential for this disease, and should know that early diagnosis followed by prompt antifungal therapy could be lifesaving in these patients.

Clinical Diseases

Primary coccidioidomycosis is most frequently asymptomatic, as indicated by the high prevalence of positive skin tests for coccidioidal antigens in endemic areas. Symptomatic disease usually is manifested as fever with cough or chest pain, or both, and may mimic bacterial pneumonia clinically (Parish, 2008). Erythema nodosum and erythema multiforme, which may accompany the primary infection, are good prognostic signs of disease (DiCaudo, 2006). Solitary pulmonary nodules may persist as consequences of the primary pulmonary infection, also similar in appearance to a neoplasm or to tuberculosis.

Disseminated infection most commonly affects the skin, the skeletal system, and the meninges. Skin lesions include papules, ulcers, draining sinuses, and subcutaneous abscesses. Arthritis most often results from involvement of adjacent bones. Meningitis may be acute but is more commonly indolent and chronic.

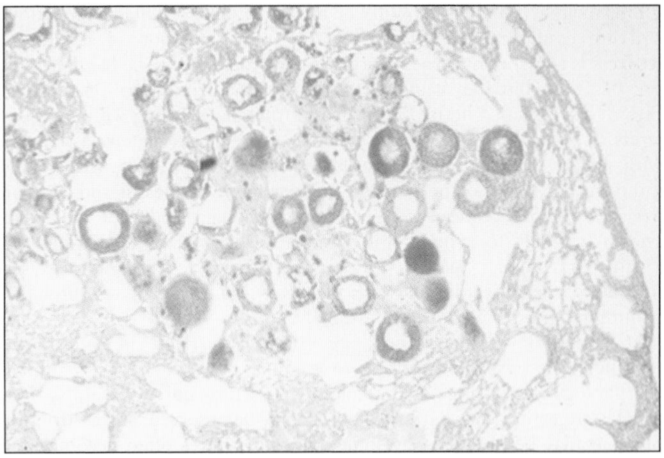

Figure 61-29 Spherules of *Coccidioides* spp. in tissue. Observation of these large structures in tissue is a presumptive diagnosis for coccidiodomycosis. (Hematoxylin and eosin stain, ×100.)

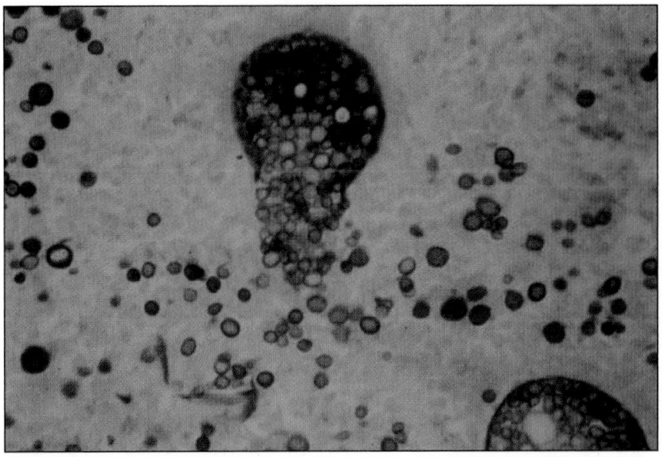

Figure 61-30 Spherules of *Coccidioides* spp. in tissue showing release of endospores. At maturity, the spherule ruptures and releases endospores, which, in turn, mature to become spherules. When seen in tissue, these immature endospores may be confused with other smaller yeasts. (Gomori's methenamine silver stain, ×1000.)

Pathology of Coccidioidomycosis

The tissue response to *Coccidioides* spp. is granulomatous, with and without caseation. Developing spherules are typically found in macrophages and multinucleated giant cells (Fig. 61-29). Endospores within the spherules measure 2–5 μm in size (Fig. 61-30). The spherules measure up to 250 μm in diameter, and developing spherules have a large range of sizes. The differential diagnosis of developing spherules primarily includes nonbudding forms of *B. dermatitidis* or *C. neoformans.* The spherules must be differentiated from the fungal forms in adiaspiromycosis and rhinosporidiosis, both of which are uncommon infections in the United States. In early disease stages, spherules may not be readily observed, and the presence of only endospores may make the diagnosis of coccidioidomycosis difficult.

Laboratory Diagnosis

The diagnosis of coccidioidomycosis can involve a variety of direct microscopic methods (i.e., Calcofluor white stain of respiratory specimen and histopathology of tissue), as well as culture with specific molecular probes for identification (Saubolle, 2007). Spherules may be demonstrated in sputum or, more commonly, in bronchoalveolar lavage fluid, but the sensitivity of direct examination for these structures is generally low. Calcofluor white staining following digestion of the specimen with KOH may increase the sensitivity of testing. If cavitary disease is present, hyphae may be present in clinical specimens, although this is a rare finding. In contrast to the other dimorphic pathogens, the possibility of communicability of arthroconidia directly from the specimen to medical personnel exists under this circumstance.

Coccidioides spp. grow rapidly (within 1 week) and can appear on standard bacteriology media such as blood agar in the laboratory.

Unfortunately, the arthroconidia of the *Coccidioides* are highly infectious and are easily transmitted by aerosolization. Infection of laboratory workers is a major concern, so inoculated cultures should be handled with great care in a biosafety cabinet (Sutton, 2007). The National Institutes of Health has classified both *C. immitis* and *C. posadasii*, along with *H. capsulatum*, as risk group 3 biological agents, that is, agents that are associated with serious or lethal human disease for which preventive or therapeutic interventions may not be available (Department of Health and Human Services, 2009). Biosafety level 3 containment is suggested when specimens known or likely to contain this organism are handled (Department of Health and Human Services, 2007). In a survey of laboratory-acquired infections, coccidioidomycosis was included on a list of the ten most frequently reported infections (Singh, 2009).

Colonies of *Coccidioides* spp. are extremely variable in appearance, ranging from velvety or cottony to granular or powdery. The colonial morphology may change as the colony and arthroconidia develop. Most isolates are white, but a variety of colors may be observed, and a diffusible pigment may be produced by some strains. Cultures often become gray with age. If a *Coccidioides* spp. is suspected, some mycologists prefer to sterilize the culture before examination of the colonies by flooding the container with 10% formalin, followed by overnight incubation. In cases where specimens are suspected to contain *Coccidioides*, screw-capped slants should be used instead of plates. The mould form is not routinely converted to the tissue form because specialized synthetic broth is generally required for this to occur. Separation of species into *C. immitis* and *C. posadasii* is best achieved by specialized molecular techniques, which normally are not available in routine clinical laboratories (Saubolle, 2007). Generally, laboratories will the report the results as "*Coccidioides immitis/posadasii*" or as a "*Coccidioides* species."

Alternating barrel-shaped arthroconidia with empty disjuncture cells upon microscopic examination of culture material are distinctive (see Fig. 61-9) but must be differentiated from other organisms that produce arthroconidia, such as *Trichosporon*, *Geotrichum*, and some members of the family Gymnoascaceae. A presumptive identification is generally adequate to make a diagnosis of coccidioidomycosis in an individual who has been in an endemic area and in whom spherules with endospores have been detected in clinical material. A molecular-based genus-specific genetic probe (AccuProbe) is the method of choice for identification of the fungus into the genus level from culture.

In contrast to histoplasmosis and blastomycosis, serologic analysis with the complement fixation test is useful for assessing the extent and prognosis of coccidioidomycosis (Pappagianis, 1990). Of the serologic techniques available, complement fixation has been studied most extensively. Antibodies are detected approximately 2–6 weeks after infection. The height of the titer is an indication of the likelihood of disseminated disease, and a rising titer bodes a poor outcome. Skin testing does not confound the diagnosis by producing a seroconversion, as in histoplasmosis, but the high prevalence of skin test positivity decreases the usefulness of the test. Patients with disseminated infection may demonstrate anergy to the skin test antigen.

THE GENUS *SPOROTHRIX*

Historically, the only known species responsible for sporotrichosis was *Sporothrix schenckii*. However, molecular studies now demonstrate that *S. schenckii* is a complex of at least five putative phylogenetically distinct species (*S. schenckii*, *S. albicans*, *S. brasiliensis*, *S. globosa*, and *S. mexicana*) (Marimon, 2007). Although methods for distinction among these species have been developed, most laboratories do not have the expertise to identify specific species and still refer to *S. schenckii* as the sole cause of sporotrichosis. More appropriately, laboratory reports should now consider identification as a complex of multiple species and should report results as "*Sporothrix schenckii* species complex."

Sporothrix spp. are dimorphic fungi present worldwide in soil, plants, and decaying vegetation. Although considered endemic dimorphic fungi, this complex of species exhibit epidemiologic differences that separate them from the other classic endemic dimorphic fungi (De Araujo, 2001). The mode of entry for these fungi is usually traumatic implantation (vs. inhalation), the disease produced is usually a localized systemic infection (vs. pulmonary), and the incidence of systemic infection is rare (da Rosa, 2005).

Risk Factors

Although *Sporothrix* spp. are common in vegetation throughout the world, they do not appear to be plant pathogens; however, epidemics have been caused by exposure to plant products (Hay, 2008). One major outbreak occurred among florists and nursery and forestry workers who handled contaminated sphagnum moss grown in Wisconsin (Centers for Disease Control and Prevention, 1988). Another recent major outbreak involved infected cats in Rio de Janeiro, Brazil, where 759 human cases of cat-transmitted sporotrichosis were reported (Schubach, 2008; Reis, 2009). An unusual epidemic occurred among members of a college fraternity in Florida who were building a wall with bricks packed in contaminated straw while consuming copious amounts of beer (Sanders, 1971). The only predisposing factor that was identified with any frequency was consumption of alcohol. It is interesting that the stereotype of the patient at risk for sporotrichosis is the "alcoholic rose gardener."

Clinical Diseases

The overwhelming predominant clinical form of sporotrichosis is involvement of cutaneous and subcutaneous tissues. A papule at the portal of entry may ulcerate and spread the pathogen through regional lymphatics, resulting in a series of lesions progressing up the affected limb (referred to as lymphocutaneous sporotrichosis). Dissemination to osteoarticular structures and viscera is uncommon and appears to occur more often in patients who have a history of alcohol abuse or immunosuppression, especially in patients with AIDS (Kauffman, 2000).

Pathology of Sporotrichosis

Histologic responses to *Sporothrix* and *Blastomyces* are similar. Granulomatous inflammation may be accompanied by small collections of polymorphonuclear neutrophils. In the skin, pseudoepitheliomatous hyperplasia of the epidermis is common. The yeast cells of *Sporothrix* are pleomorphic and round or elongated, resembling cigars, but they are rarely seen in tissue. A tissue reaction to the fungus may result in radiating eosinophilic material up to 10 μm in thickness around the yeast cell, known as the Splendore-Hoeppli phenomenon (asteroid bodies) (Hussein, 2008). This distinctive tissue reaction is uncommon, although the reaction is not specific for the diagnosis of sporotrichosis. The differential diagnosis of the skin lesions is primarily mycobacterial infection, especially *Mycobacterium marinum* (swimming pool granuloma) in the United States and cutaneous leishmaniasis in the tropics.

Laboratory Diagnosis

The preferred specimen is an aspirate, curetting, or biopsy of the skin lesion. *S. schenckii* grows well on primary isolation media with cycloheximide incubated at 25°–30° C. The colonies, which may be moist or smooth (glabrous), are often light colored initially and may turn darker with increasing age. This organism produces two types of conidia: thin-walled hyaline conidia arranged as a rosette around the apex of a conidiophore, and thick-walled, dark, sessile conidia attached directly to the hyphae. The thin-walled microconidia are borne on conidiophores that arise at right angles from the hyphae. They may be arranged sympodially around an expanded vesicle at the tip of the conidiophore, producing an arrangement that has been described as a floret (Fig. 61-31). Similar structures are produced by *Acremonium* spp., which have rarely been reported as a cause of human disease. This mould is differentiated from *Sporothrix* by the

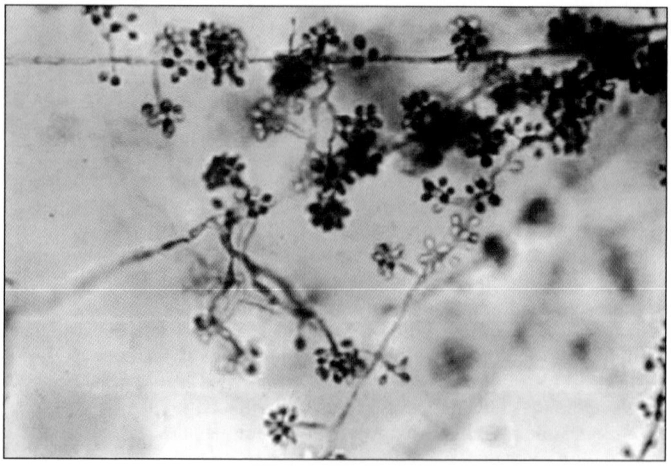

Figure 61-31 Sympodial conidia of *Sporothrix schenckii* are borne in clusters at the tips of lateral conidiophores. (Lactophenol cotton blue stain, ×400.)

absence of growth on cycloheximide agar and by the absence of a yeast phase. Conversion of the mould phase to yeast is accomplished by incubation of the isolate at 37° C in an atmosphere of 5% carbon dioxide on an enriched medium, such as brain-heart infusion agar supplemented with sheep blood or on chocolate agar. Phenotypic characteristics such as the morphology of sessile pigmented conidia; growth at 30° C, 35° C, and 37° C; and the assimilation of sucrose, raffinose, and ribitol have been used successfully to distinguish among species (Marimon, 2007). Molecular sequencing using the calmodulin gene target has also proved reliable in differentiating among *Sporothrix* spp. (Marimon, 2006).

OTHER DIMORPHIC FUNGI

H. capsulatum var. *duboisii* causes cutaneous and systemic diseases in Africa. The yeast is larger than that of *H. capsulatum* var. *capsulatum*, and the walls are thicker, resembling the cells of *B. dermatitidis*, but without the broad-based buds. This organism has been considered an emerging infectious agent in HIV-infected patients in Africa (Loulergue, 2007).

Paracoccidioidomycosis (formerly known as South American blastomycosis), a relatively common disease in Brazil, Venezuela, Columbia, Ecuador, and Argentina, is caused by the dimorphic fungus called *Paracoccidioides brasiliensis* (Ramos, 2008). This organism mainly affects the skin, lymph nodes, lung, and oral, nasal, and GI mucosal membranes (Restrepo, 2008). The characteristic tissue phase yeast cells of *Paracoccidioides* have multiple peripheral buds, producing an appearance that has been compared with a mariner's wheel.

Penicillium marneffei is a common cause of disease in HIV-positive patients in Southeast Asia. This agent has also been found to be associated with the bamboo rat *(Rhizomys sinensis)*, which is thought to be the natural environmental reservoir for this fungus (Vanittanakom, 2006). The species is unique among the penicillia in being dimorphic by growing as a mould form at 30° C and thus producing reproductive structures typical of *Penicillium* spp., and producing in tissue yeast-like cells that are oval or cylindrical and may have cross-walls (Cooper, 2000).

DERMATOPHYTOSES

Dermatophytic fungi are common and important causes of human morbidity (Andrews, 2008; Havlickova, 2008; Seebacher, 2008; Vermout, 2008). Generally the infections are mild, and rarely do the fungi associated with these infections cause invasive disease. Three genera are recognized as causes of dermatophytosis: *Microsporum*, *Trichophyton*, and *Epidermophyton*. As a group, the dermatophytic fungi are distributed worldwide, but individual species may have a more restricted geographic distribution. Dermatophytes may also be found in strict association with humans (anthropophilic), with animals (zoophilic), and with soil (geophilic).

RISK FACTORS

Dermatophytic infections result from contact with the relevant source of the fungus, which may also provide a clue to the diagnosis. For instance, infection of the face in farmers who have contact with cows as they milk the animals is characteristically caused by *Trichophyton verrucosum*, a zoophilic dermatophyte found in cattle. Geographic variation in dermatophytic pathogens is illustrated by a study of an epidemic of cutaneous fungal infection among American troops during the Vietnam War (Allen, 1973). Most infections were caused by a heavily sporulating variant of *T. mentagrophytes* that had not been recognized in the United States. Skin disorders caused by dermatophytic fungi are now recognized more often in sports in which there is direct contact between athletes, such as wrestling (Adams, 2002; Nenoff, 2002; Field, 2008).

CLINICAL DISEASES

Dermatophytes produce infection of the epidermis, hair, and nails (Seebacher, 2008). Infection is often referred to as ringworm (or tinea), a name derived from the advancing, serpiginous nature of the lesions (especially evident on the skin). Clinical terminology uses the Latin name "tinea" followed by the body part involved, such as tinea capitis (scalp), tinea barbae (beard), tinea corporis (trunk and limbs), tinea pedis (foot), tinea cruris (groin), and tinea unguium (nail, also called onychomycosis). With occasional exceptions, *Epidermophyton floccosum* infects primarily the skin, *Microsporum* spp. infect the scalp and skin, and *Trichophyton* spp. infect the skin, scalp, and nails. *Trichophyton tonsurans* is the most common cause of tinea capitis in the United States, with *M. canis* a common cause of scalp infection, particularly in children. When deep infection of hair follicles occurs, a boggy inflammatory process called a kerion results. *T. mentagrophytes* and *T. verrucosum* are particularly associated with kerion formation. *T. mentagrophytes*, *T. rubrum*, and *M. canis* are commonly found to cause tinea corporis and tinea pedis, and *E. floccosum* is a common cause of tinea cruris.

Considerable intercontinental and intracontinental variability in the global incidence of dermatophytic infection has been noted (Havlickova, 2008). Local socioeconomic conditions and cultural practices can influence the prevalence of a particular infection in a given area. For instance, tinea pedis has been shown to be more prevalent in developed countries than in emerging economies and is likely to be caused by the anthropophilic agent *T. rubrum*. In poorer countries, scalp infection (tinea capitis) caused by *Trichophyton soudanense* or *Microsporum audouinii* is more prevalent.

LABORATORY DIAGNOSIS

Diagnosis of a dermatophyte infection generally involves both microscopic examination and culture, although treatment of dermatophyte infection is not directed by the specific identification of the isolate (Robert, 2008). Demonstration of hyphae in skin scrapings (using a KOH preparation) is frequently the only diagnostic technique performed before therapy is initiated (Fig. 61-32). The size and morphology of hyphae suggest the involvement of dermatophytes in the infection. Verification of the species is useful for confirming that the hyphae did in fact belong to a dermatophytic fungus, for assessing the probable source of the infection, and for assessing the increased likelihood of chronic, relapsing infections (especially when *T. rubrum* is identified) (Robert, 2008). Skin scrapings, nails, and hair can be examined in KOH preparations, which may incorporate Calcofluor white to facilitate the detection of hyphae. Care must be taken when reading this type of preparation in that tissue fragments, fibers, and cholesterol crystals may be mistaken for hyphae by the inexperienced observer.

Fungi such as *M. audouinii*, *M. canis*, and *Microsporum ferrugineum* are associated with hair infection and cause the hairs to fluoresce with a long-wavelength ultraviolet light (Wood's lamp). In the United States, tinea capitis due to a fluorescing fungus is most likely caused by *M. canis* because the other two species are not common in this geographic area. Microscopic examination of infected hair by an experienced observer may suggest the etiologic agent, based on the appearance and location of the arthroconidia. In ectothrix colonization, as occurs with *M. canis* and *M. audouinii* infection, arthroconidia are external to the hair shaft. Endothrix invasion, as seen in infection with *T. tonsurans*, is characterized by arthroconidia within the hair shaft. In favic infection, hyphae, air bubbles, or tunnels and fat droplets are present in the intrapilar area.

Infected hairs, nail scrapings, or scrapings of the edges of skin lesions should be submitted to the laboratory in a clean, dry container or placed on the surface of primary isolation medium supplied by the laboratory. Sabouraud dextrose agar was designed for recovery of dermatophytic fungi and is also effective for isolating *Candida* spp., especially *C. albicans*, which may produce similar infections of the skin and nails. Dermatophytes are not inhibited by cycloheximide, which will inhibit many saprophytic fungi. All dermatophytic fungi have septate, hyaline hyphae and produce

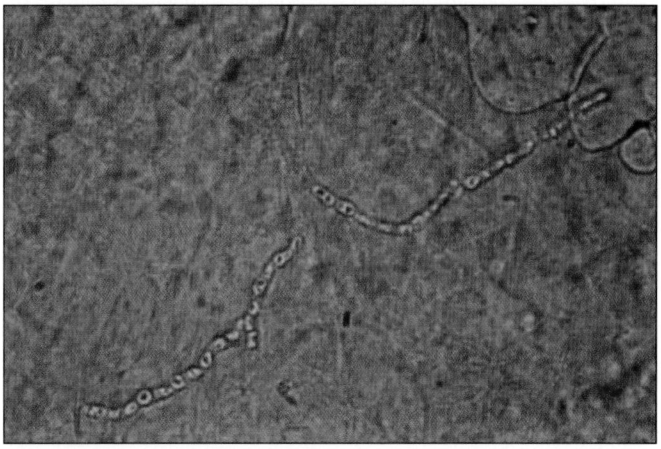

Figure 61-32 Hyphae of a dermatophyte are demonstrated in a scraping from the edge of a tinea lesion. The presence of thin-segmented hyphae in this clinical setting establishes the diagnosis of dermatomycosis but does not define the specific cause. (Potassium hydroxide preparation, ×400.)

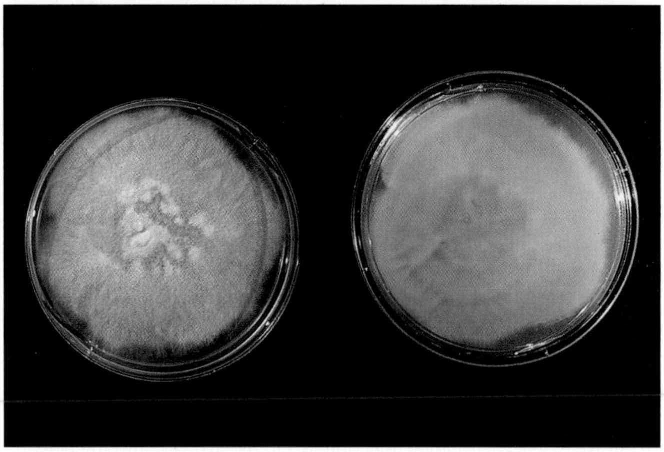

Figure 61-33 The obverse of a *Microsporum canis* colony *(left)* showing the characteristic lemon yellow pigment, which also may be seen on the reverse of the colony *(right)*. (Sabouraud dextrose agar with cycloheximide.)

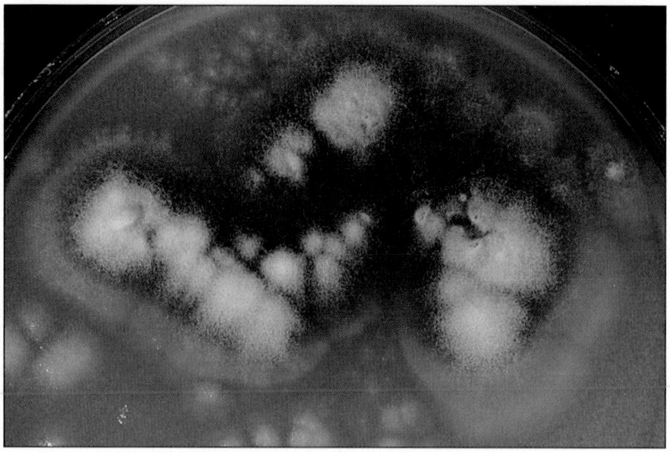

Figure 61-35 Fluffy white colonies of *Trichophyton rubrum* with diffusible red pigment, which may also be seen on the reverse of the colony. (Potato dextrose agar.)

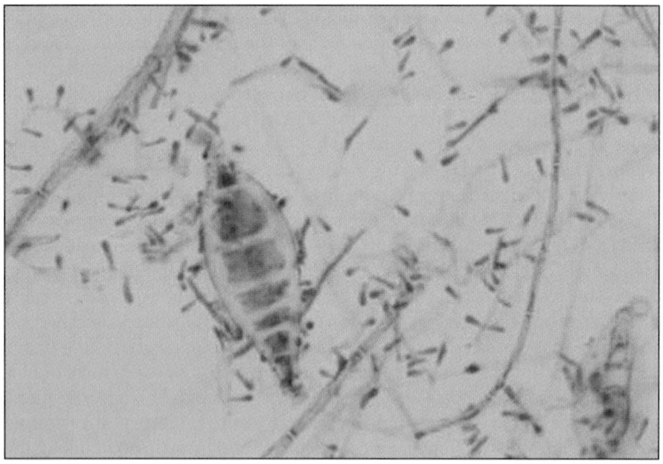

Figure 61-34 Thick-walled, roughened, tapered, spindle-shaped macroconidia of *Microsporum canis* with thin, septate hyphae. (Lactophenol cotton blue stain, ×400.)

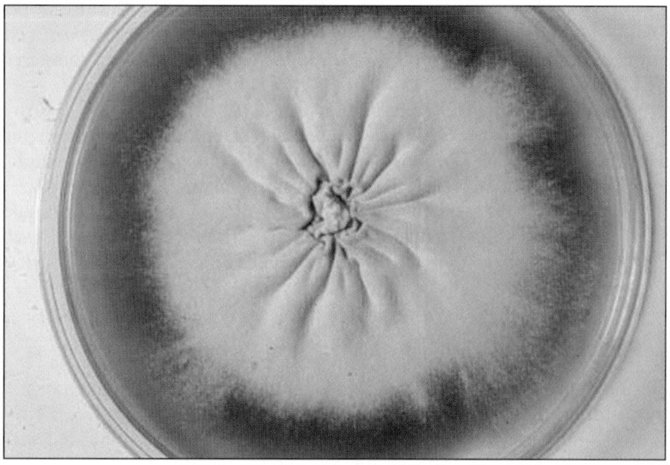

Figure 61-36 A flat colony showing pale yellow coloration with a reddish-brown pigmentation at the periphery characteristic of *Trichophyton tonsurans*. Radial furrowing of the thallus as seen is also common. (Sabouraud dextrose agar with cycloheximide.)

macroconidia and/or microconidia in various combinations. Arthroconidia and chlamydoconidia may also be produced, but the morphology of the macroconidia and especially of the microconidia is more important for identification. Sexual stages of the dermatophytes have been identified, but they are not encountered in the clinical laboratory. The combination of micromorphologic features with some phenotypic testing is used to differentiate the dermatophytes (Caddell, 2002).

Microsporum spp. produce characteristic macroconidia, which are the key diagnostic structures. In some cases, microconidia, which are not as useful diagnostically, are produced. *M. canis*, the most frequently isolated zoonotic species of this genus, produces a characteristic lemon yellow pigment in culture (Fig. 61-33), which is intensified by growth on potato flake agar. The macroconidia of this species are illustrated in Figure 61-34.

The genus *Trichophyton* includes the important dermatophytic fungi *T. rubrum* (Fig. 61-35), *T. verrucosum*, *T. mentagrophytes* spp. complex (see Fig. 61-11), and *T. tonsurans* (Fig. 61-36). The colonies may have a fluffy, granular, or, less commonly, glabrous appearance. Macroconidia, which are useful for identification, may be produced by this genus, especially in strains that produce powdery colonies, but unfortunately they usually are absent. Microconidia are formed more commonly. When present, the macroconidia are thin-walled and smooth and contain variable numbers of septa. Interpretation of the microscopic morphology in some isolates can be difficult because overlap occurs frequently. Phenotypic testing using the *Trichophyton* agars is helpful in the characterization of nutritional requirements among members of the genus. Seven media have been described; however, four of these seem to be the most useful for identification purposes. These media include T1, basal medium agar (for a control to compare with other supplemented media); T2, basal medium with inositol (growth stimulated by inositol); T3, basal medium with inositol plus thiamine (growth stimulated by the addition of both inositol and thiamine); and T4, basal medium with thiamine (growth stimulated by thiamine only). In combination, these media allow assessment of dependency on inositol, thiamine, or both compounds together for growth.

Differentiation of *T. mentagrophytes* and *T. rubrum* is facilitated by several nonmorphologic tests as well (Ates, 2008). A diffusible pigment may be produced by both species, but the intensely red pigment of *T. rubrum* is encouraged by culture on potato dextrose agar or cornmeal agar with 1% dextrose. Production of urease within 3–5 days by *T. mentagrophytes* but not by *T. rubrum* also helps differentiate these two species. Finally, the hair penetration test can be used as a differential test wherein *T. mentagrophytes* produces wedge-shaped defects in hairs in vitro, whereas *T. rubrum* grows on the outside of the hair without penetration. Use of both morphologic and nonmorphologic approaches provides the most accurate identification of isolates.

The only pathogen within the genus *Epidermophyton* is *E. floccosum*, an anthropophilic fungus that is an important cause of tinea cruris and, less commonly, tinea pedis. Colonies, which are initially brownish yellow, gray, or khaki brown, become velvety and folded as they mature (Fig. 61-37). *E. floccosum* produces no microconidia, but distinctive macroconidia provide clues to identification (see Fig. 61-10). These structures have smooth external walls, with up to four cross walls and a club shape, and they tend to "flocculate," hence the epithet name.

To differentiate among closely related dermatophytes, molecular assays have been developed. Species identification for dermatophytes is time consuming and requires knowledge and technical expertise because of morphologic similarity, variability, and polymorphism within dermatophytes (Abdel-Rahman, 2008; Kanbe, 2008; Bontems, 2009). Molecular phylogenetic analysis of multiple dermatophytic species involved in

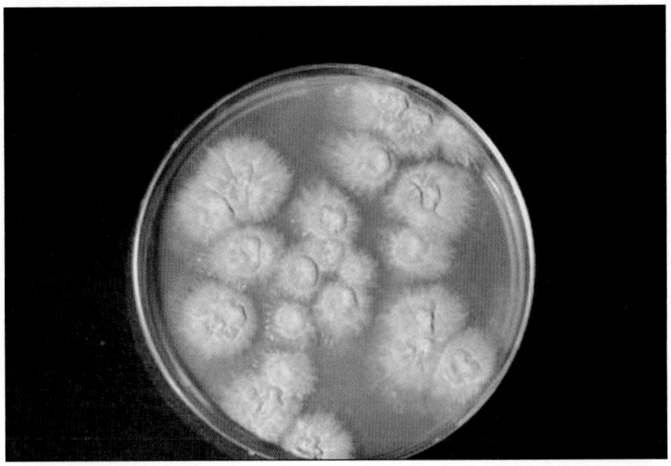

Figure 61-37 The suede-like texture and yellowish green color of the mould colonies are characteristic of *Epidermophyton floccosum*. (Sabouraud dextrose agar with cycloheximide.)

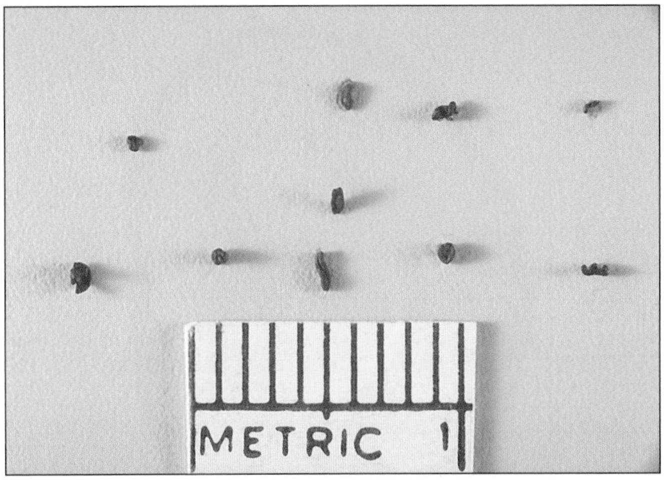

Figure 61-38 Image showing granules of various sizes *(black grains)* of the fungus *Madurella grisea* composed of black masses of hyphae. *(Courtesy CDC Public Health Image Library.)*

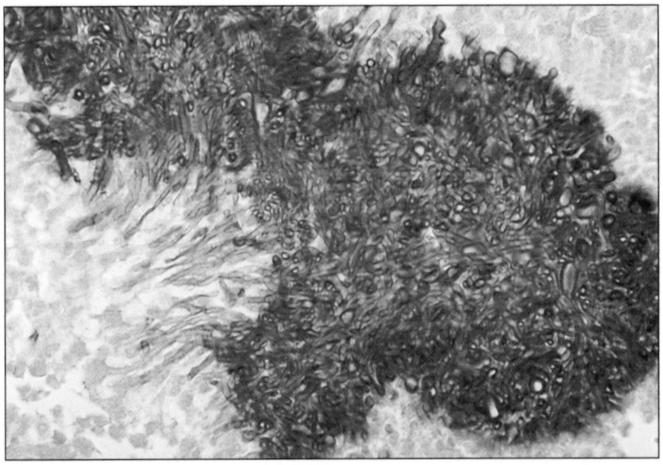

Figure 61-39 Histologic appearance of "black grain mycetoma" due to *Madurella mycetomatis*. (Gridley stain, ×1000.) *(Courtesy Dr. Libero Ajello, CDC Public Health Image Library.)*

infection has suggested that although profound differences in morphology and pattern of infection among species are noted, there does not appear to be a distinct species difference on modern molecular analysis (Graser, 2008). This observation suggests that a polyphasic approach to identification may need to be considered.

Mycoses Caused by Dematiaceous Moulds

The dematiaceous moulds (also called the black moulds) are a fascinating and complex group of fungi characterized by the formation of a dark pigment due to production of melanin in the cell walls of hyphae or conidia or both (Revankar, 2007). Although these fungi are soil and plant saprophytes and historically are considered rare causes of disease in humans, they appear to be emerging as more common fungal pathogens (Silveira, 2001).

CLINICAL DISEASES

The clinical syndromes are typically distinguished on the basis of histologic findings into eumycotic mycetoma (also called eumycetoma), chromoblastomycosis (also called chromomycosis), and phaeohyphomycosis (Garnica, 2009). These diseases are frequently diagnosed by a unique histologic picture in tissue followed by isolation of the fungus in culture and morphologic evaluation of the reproductive structures. The classification of black moulds has undergone numerous changes over the years, which adds difficulty to recognition of the etiologic agent.

Mycetoma

Mycetoma is a localized, chronic granulomatous infection characterized by the formation of a painless subcutaneous mass of chronic onset, with multiple sinuses draining pus and grains (also called granules) with extension to the bone (Garnica, 2009). The disease is most often confined to the hands or feet (also called "Madura foot") in immunocompetent individuals such as farmers, field hands, and others in contact with contaminated soil-laden materials. This disease can be caused by bacteria (actinomycotic mycetoma) or by fungi (eumycotic mycetoma) that are dark pigmented (dematiaceous), or rarely by nonpigmented and filamentous fungi (haline) (Lichon, 2006; Welsh, 2007). A mycetoma occurs after a traumatic injury with a contaminated object such as a splinter, a thorn, or any other penetrating item. Although more than 25 mould species have been known to cause eumycotic mycetoma, the most common cause is *Madurella mycetomatis*, followed by a variety of other dematiaceous and hyaline fungi. *Scedosporium apiospermum* (teleomorph, *Pseudallescheria boydii*), a hyaline fungus, is considered the most common cause of this disease in the United States.

A noninvasive disease involving the paranasal sinus has been described as a fungal mycetoma (also called a fungus ball) (Grosjean, 2007; Pagella, 2007; Robey, 2009). This condition involves the accumulation of dense fungal concrements in the sinus cavities, most often the maxillary sinus, and is associated with a variety of moulds, including dematiaceous fungi. Although some categorize this infection as a mycetoma, others prefer to describe it as a fungal rhinosinusitis because this infection does not specifically fit the description of a mycetoma presented here (an absence of granule formation). Controversies on the categorization and definition of fungal rhinosinusitis occur because of the wide spectrum of immune and pathologic responses associated with this disease. Attempts are being made to develop a consensus on the terminology and disease classification for this condition (Chakrabarti, 2009).

A definitive diagnosis of a mycetoma can be achieved by the demonstration of grains (or granules) in a tissue biopsy, in draining exudates from a sinus tract, or in material aspirated from an unopened lesion (Fig. 61-38). These grains are microscopically composed of broad, interwoven, septate hyphae 2–5 μm in diameter (Fig. 61-39). For dematiaceous fungi, these grains are associated with a dark pigment and generally are called "black grains"; with fungi that are nondematiaceous and produce nonpigmented hyphae, these are called "white grains." Identification of the etiologic agent requires culture on standard fungal media such as Sabouraud dextrose agar, which may take 4 weeks or longer to grow (Fig. 61-40). Once isolated, the fungal species is identified using gross colony morphology and pigmentation, along with close observation of the micromorphologic characteristics of reproductive structures following sporulation (Fig. 61-41). In cases where sporulation does not occur, physiologic tests such as carbohydrate and nitrate utilization may aid in identification. Molecular assays using targets within the rDNA complex have been shown to be reliable for identification of dematiaceous fungi (van de Sande, 2005; Borman, 2008).

Chromoblastomycosis

Chromoblastomycosis (chromomycosis) is a chronic infection of the skin and soft tissue characterized by the presence of muriform fungal structures

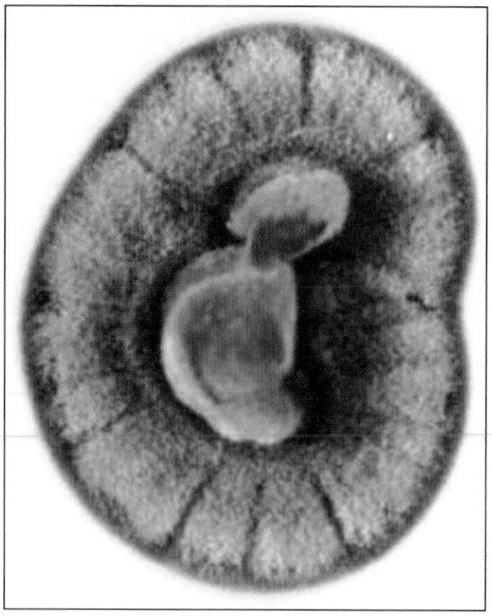

Figure 61-40 Close-up of a dematiaceous fungus growing on Sabouraud dextrose agar.

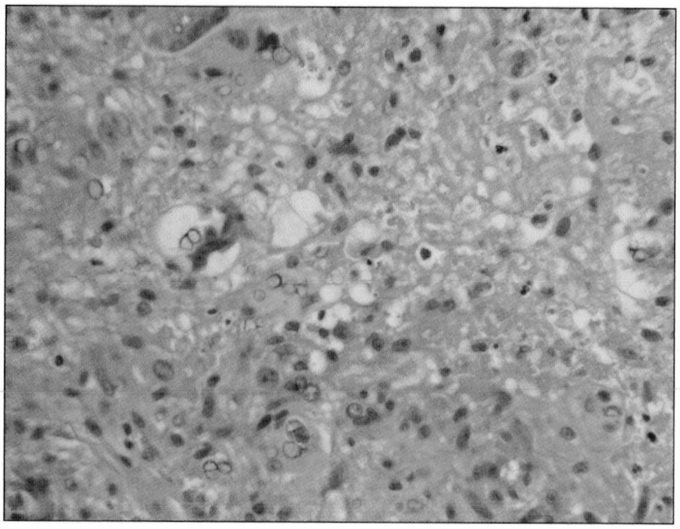

Figure 61-42 Sclerotic cells observed in tissue that is characteristic of the etiologic agents of chromoblastomycosis. (Hematoxylin and eosin stain, ×400.)

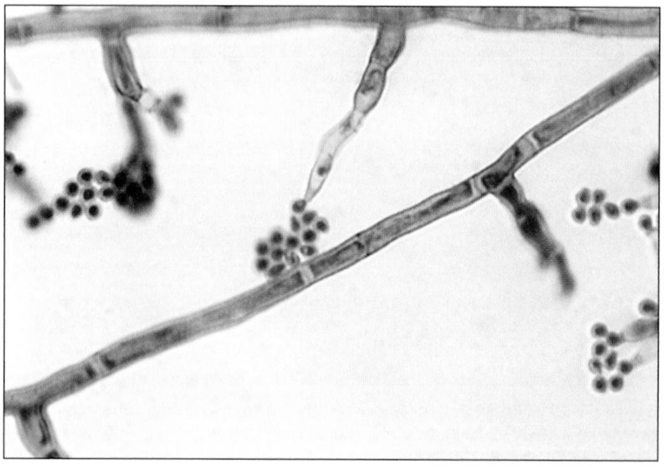

Figure 61-41 Image showing phialides with terminal conidia of the *Madurella mycetomatis* fungus. (Lactophenol cotton blue stain, ×400.) *(Courtesy Lucille George, CDC Public Health Image Library.)*

called sclerotic bodies within the infected tissues. The disease affects immunocompetent individuals who most often live in tropical and subtropical areas and is distinguished by the formation of a painless verrucous plaque or nodule at the site of inoculation following a penetrating trauma, with healing areas of the lesion evident along with the formation of scar materials (Queiroz-Telles, 2009). The most common etiologic agents are the black moulds *Fonsecaea pedrosi* and *Cladophialophora carrionii*, although numerous other species may also be involved (Baddley, 2003a). The distinguishing feature is the presence of round, nonhyphal, brown cells (sclerotic bodies) in tissues (Fig. 61-42). These structures, which divide by producing a septal plane, are diagnostic of the entity but do not provide a clue as to species identification of the mould. Culture and recognition of morphologic features of the isolate are needed to identify the infecting species.

Phaeohyphomycosis

Phaeohyphomycosis (from the Greek word "phaeo," meaning "dark") was a term originally proposed by Ajello (1974) as a histopathologic entity to cover all infections "caused by fungi that develop in tissue in the form of dark-walled dematiaceous septate mycelial elements." Over the years, phaeohyphomycosis has become more recognized as a cause of subcutaneous and systemic diseases characterized by the formation of pigmented septate hyphae in tissue. Although both chromoblastomycosis and eumycotic mycetoma are caused by dematiaceous fungi, they are distinguished from phaeohyphomycosis by the appearance in tissue of sclerotic bodies and mycotic granules, respectively.

Phaeohyphomycosis ranges from an indolent subcutaneous lesion, probably resulting from direct inoculation of fungi at the site, to a devastating, destructive infection that is almost always fatal in the immunosuppressed patient. The subcutaneous form of the disease is characterized by the formation of a solitary asymptomatic subcutaneous nodule or cyst usually in an immunocompetent individual, but disseminated disease may also occur in the immunocompromised patient (Naggie, 2009). The most common dematiaceous fungi associated with the cutaneous condition are *Exophiala jeanselmei*, *Wangilla dermatitidis*, and *Biopolaris* spp. (Garnica, 2009). Systemic infection reportedly has been associated with these and a variety of other dematiaceous fungi. For instance, numerous reports have shown *Cladophialophora bantiana* to be a cause of fungal brain abscess in the compromised patient (Garzoni, 2008). In another report described by the CDC, five cases of meningitis caused by *E. dermatitidis* resulted from the injection of contaminated steroids prepared by a compounding pharmacy (Centers for Disease Control and Prevention, 2002).

In most cases of phaeohyphomycosis, diagnosis may be difficult because many etiologic agents are often considered contaminants when isolated from culture. In tissue, the presence of irregular, swollen, septate hyphal forms with yeast-like structures that stain with a melanin-specific Masson-Fontana stain is presumptive for the diagnosis of phaeohyphomycosis.

Sick Building Syndrome

Dematiaceous moulds have also been associated with the condition known as "sick building syndrome." The mould most commonly associated with this condition is *Stachybotrys chartarum*, although the causative association of mould contamination within a building with disease has been questioned. Others have suggested that toxins associated with moulds such as *S. chartarum* are associated with health problems following exposure (Miller, 2003; Straus, 2009; Terr, 2009). To offer credit to this suggestion, the U.S. Environmental Protection Agency has provided a document that presents a comprehensive review on mould remediation in commercial buildings and schools as a means of disease prevention (Environmental Protection Agency, 2001).

ZYGOMYCOSIS

The Zygomycetes are important causes of invasive fungal infection in compromised hosts, and diseases caused by these moulds are referred to as zygomycosis (Freifeld, 2004; Roden, 2005; Almyroudis, 2006). This disease is also called mucormycosis and phycomycosis, although zygomycosis is now more frequently used because this name is a more precise term that relates disease to the taxonomic classification (Freifeld, 2004). *Rhizopus* spp. are the organisms most commonly isolated from patients with zygomycosis, and *R. (oryzae) arrhizus* and *R. microsporus* are recognized as causing a majority of cases (Ribes, 2000; Alvarez, 2009). Other less common species include *Lichtheimia (Absidia) corymbifera*, *Apophysomyces elegans*, *Cunninghamella bertholletiae*, *Mucor circinelloides*, and *Rhizomucor (Mucor) pusillus*.

RISK FACTORS

Uncontrolled diabetes, steroid use, neutropenia, infant prematurity, stem cell or solid organ transplantation, and the use of deferoxamine are all well-described risk factors for the development of zygomycosis (Freifeld, 2004; Roden, 2005). In general, most of these conditions are associated with impairment of normal leukocyte immune function. Diabetic ketoacidosis is the most common recognized underlying condition for the development of zygomycosis in humans. Ketoacidotic serum has been shown to stimulate the growth of *Rhizopus* in vitro (Artis, 1982). However, recognition of no underlying condition following penetrating trauma, surgery, and burns has also been seen at the time of infection (Roden, 2005).

CLINICAL DISEASES

The two major clinical presentations for zygomycosis are sinus infection with or without cerebral or orbital involvement and localized pulmonary infection that may lead to disseminated disease. Another, more rare condition is a localized cutaneous infection that occurs following trauma. Risk factors for the two major presentations are somewhat different (Mantadakis, 2009).

An invasive infection that begins in the paranasal sinuses is known as rhinosinus, rhinocerebral, sinus-orbital, or craniofacial zygomycosis, depending on how far the infection has spread. The infection begins as an undifferentiated sinusitis, but the hyphae may rapidly break through the thin walls of the sinus and extend up into the orbit, forward into the skin of the face, and back up into the cranial cavity. Rhinocerebral disease may progress rapidly, and death often results. Thrombosis of the carotid artery or cavernous sinus may occur following invasion of deep tissue.

The second major presentation of zygomycosis is pulmonary disease, which may be followed by hematogenous dissemination. Infection begins as an undifferentiated pneumonia, which may be complicated by hemoptysis and cavitation. Risk factors for pulmonary infection include neutropenia and immunosuppression, particularly by hematologic malignancy; disseminated infection is common and the outcome is almost uniformly fatal (Pagano, 2004).

A less common presentation of zygomycosis is infection of skin and soft tissues (Alsuwaida, 2002; Oh, 2002). Hyphae may reach the skin by the hematogenous route, by direct extension from a deep focus, or by introduction from the outside. Contaminated adhesive tape has been reported as a source of primary cutaneous disease in the compromised patient (Alsuwaida, 2002). Other rare cases of zygomycosis include primary involvement of the GI tract, the heart, the brain, or the kidneys (Roden, 2005).

PATHOLOGY

The diagnosis of zygomycosis is made most frequently on the basis of characteristic histopathologic findings in tissue. The tissue response is dominated by necrosis, regardless of the site of infection. The propensity for these moulds to invade through the walls of arteries and veins, producing acute thrombosis, leads to extensive coagulative necrosis (Chandler, 1987b). The hyphae appear as ribbons of broad hyphae that are often twisted and collapsed with a variable width from 5–20 µm (see Fig. 61-3). Septa are sparse and usually are not observed in tissue, but an overlay of the exterior walls of collapsed hyphae may be mistaken for septa. Swollen segments of hyphae and hyphae cut in cross-section may be incorrectly interpreted as yeast cells. Branching tends to occur at right angles in a haphazard pattern. These hyphal characteristics along with the angioinvasive property of these fungi are highly suggestive of a Zygomycete-caused infection. Comparison of the histologic features of Zygomycetes versus those of other nonpigmented hyphae in tissue is described in Table 61-11. The hyphae of these moulds often stain better with the H&E stain than with the GMS method.

LABORATORY DIAGNOSIS

Zygomycetes often are considered common contaminants within the mycology laboratory, and the potential clinical implications of isolates should be carefully investigated before they are dismissed as saprophytes. Collaboration between the pathologist and the laboratory is important because demonstration of hyphae in tissue provides important evidence that an isolated mould was present in vivo and was not an environmental contaminant. Broad, sparsely septate hyphae may be demonstrated in tissue sections or in imprint smears of tissue, using the Calcofluor white stain.

TABLE 61-11
Histopathologic Features of the Zygomycetes in Comparison With Other Fungi That Occur as Nonpigmented Hyphae in Tissue*

Characteristic	Zygomycetes†	*Aspergillus*‡	*Fusarium*
Hyphal characteristics			
Width (µm)	Variable (5–10)	Consistent (3–6)	Consistent (3–8)
Branching pattern	Haphazard	Dichotomous	Right angle
Septation frequency	Rare	High	High
Reproductive structures in tissue	Absent	May be present where infected area communicates with air	Chlamydoconidia sometimes present
Angioinvasiveness	Yes	Yes	Yes

Modified with permission from Freifeld AG, Iwen PC. Zygomycosis. Semin Respir Crit Care Med 2004;25:221–31.
*In all cases, a definitive diagnosis of the species requires isolation and identification of the fungus on synthetic media.
†Entomophthorales are included in this group with the hyphal fragments in tissue generally coated by anophous eosinophilic Splencore-Hoepple material and lack of angioinvasiveness noted.
‡Because of hyphal degeneration or host immune response or both, the hyphae of the *Aspergillus* species may exhibit atypical morphologic forms that may cause problems in the differential diagnosis.

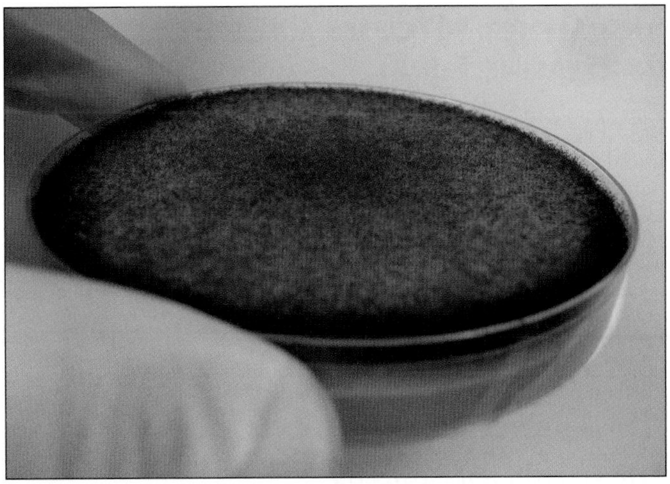

Figure 61-43 A fluffy gray colony of *Rhizopus* spp. fills the space within the Petri dish (lid lifter). (Sabouraud dextrose agar.)

Most Zygomycetes grow well on standard fungal medium. Unfortunately, recovery of a Zygomycetes from tissue is difficult when negative culture results are common, although histologic evidence of a Zygomycetes is present (Roden, 2005). Aggressive processing of a specimen is thought to damage the organism so it is no longer viable; therefore, tissue should be minced or teased, rather than homogenized, after which it is inoculated onto the surface of a primary isolation agar (Ribes, 2000). Zygomycetes are inhibited by cycloheximide, so nonselective fungal medium should be included when fungal cultures are performed. Isolates grow rapidly (within 48–72 hours) and produce abundant aerial hyphae that rapidly reach the lid of the Petri dish, colloquially referred to as "lid lifters" (Fig. 61-43). The hyphae are characterized as woolly and initially white, turning gray to black as spores develop.

Rhizopus spp. produce unbranched sporangiophores that support sporangia (60–350 µm) with an ellipsoidal columella containing sporangiospores. The sporangiospores are oval and frequently have a brown pigment (see Fig. 61-6). An important diagnostic feature for *Rhizopus* is the presence of hyaline to brown root-like structures called rhizoids, which develop at the point where the sporangiophores arise. In contrast to *Rhizopus*, the rhizoids of *Lichtheimia (Absidia)* spp. arise from the stolons between conidiophores. The sporangiophores are pear-shaped rather than round, and a collarette is visible around the columella when the sporangium disintegrates.

Mucor spp. on the other hand do not produce rhizoids; the conidiophores usually are more branched than other Zygomycetes and growth does not occur above 37° C. *Rhizomucor*, which is morphologically intermediate between *Rhizopus* and *Mucor*, has rudimentary rhizoids and branched conidiophores and grows at temperatures as high as 58° C. *Mucor* spp. were commonly thought to be the second most recognized causes of zygomycosis; however, they now have been described as a rare cause of human disease (Iwen, 2005). This is due to the fact that *Mucor corymbifera* has been reassigned to the genus *Lichtheimia (Absidia)* as *L. corymbifera*, and *M. pusillus* has been reclassified in the genus *Rhizomucor* as *R. pusillus* (Ribes, 2000).

Although genera of the Zygomycetes can be readily recognized in the mycology laboratory, few laboratories have the expertise needed to identify specific species. One method used to accurately identify the Zygomycetes has been the observation of zygospores following mating studies because of the heterothallic nature of this group of organisms (Weitzman, 1995). Although this method is used successfully, mating studies do not always yield a positive result. Additionally, the need to maintain a library of testing strains needed to perform mating does not make this method realistic for most clinical laboratories (Iwen, 2005, 2007).

Numerous molecular methods have been described for species identification of the Zygomycetes using a variety of molecular targets. Nucleotide sequence comparisons using the ITS regions of the rDNA complex and the variable D1/D2 region of the 28S gene have been shown to have the highest discriminatory capability for the identification of most Zygomycetes species (Hall, 2004; Schwarz, 2006; Alvarez, 2009; Balajee, 2009a).

Aspergillosis, Fusariosis, and Other Mycoses Caused by Hyaline Fungi

This large group of saprophytic fungi is frequently encountered in the clinical laboratory and contains some of the most important pathogenic moulds. These moulds are collectively classified as hyaline because they produce nonpigmented hyphae, and the disease is frequently called hyalohyphomycosis. The number of species within this group that are capable of causing human disease is large and continues to expand as immunosuppressive therapies become more common methods for the management of patients. By far the most recognized hyaline moulds causing human disease are classified in the Eurotiales (*Aspergillus*, *Paecilomyces*, and *Penicillium*), the Microascales (*Scedosporium* and *Scopulariopsis*), and the Hypocreales (*Cylindrocarpon*, *Fusarium*, and *Trichoderma*). In this section, detailed consideration will be given to *Aspergillus* spp. and *Fusarium* spp., the hyaline moulds most commonly believed to cause invasive human disease.

THE GENUS *ASPERGILLUS*

Invasive aspergillosis is the most common life-threatening opportunistic invasive mycosis in immunosuppressed patients (Leeflang, 2008). The term aspergillosis is used to describe these infections, which are caused by species within the genus *Aspergillus*. This group of organisms has the ability to produce a wide spectrum of infections, which include mycotoxicosis, allergic manifestations, and superficial infection in the normal host; localized noninvasive infection in hosts with tissue damage or foreign body obstruction; and invasive infection in the compromised host (Bodey, 1989). Although they are not discussed further here, numerous reviews are recommended for additional information on intoxication by ingestion of *Aspergillus* toxin (Etzel, 2002; Hedayati, 2007) and allergic manifestations associated with *Aspergillus* spore exposure (Agarwal, 2009; Schubert, 2009; Thia, 2009).

The number of new *Aspergillus* spp. associated with human disease has continued to expand with the utilization of genomic methods for identification (Balajee, 2007a, 2009a, 2009b; Geiser, 2007, 2009). Many species now described are known to be cryptic species associated with species commonly identified in the past (Geiser, 2007). Because these species cannot be easily differentiated in the laboratory, the laboratory now more accurately reports the phenotypic identification as a complex of species such as "*Aspergillus fumigatus* species complex." This concept of reporting is not fully utilized within the clinical laboratory, and the old method of reporting using common species names is still used most often (Samson, 2007).

Aspergillus fumigatus is considered the most common species associated with invasive aspergillosis, followed by *Aspergillus flavus* and *Aspergillus terreus* (Dagenais, 2009; Krishnan, 2009). However, in some studies, *A. flavus* has emerged as a predominant pathogen, especially when those patients with fungal sinusitis and fungal keratitis were evaluated in several institutions worldwide (Krishnan, 2009). Suggestions are that the bigger size of the *A. flavus* spores, in comparison with the spores of *A. fumigatus*, may favor their deposit in the upper respiratory tract and eye (Pasqualotto, 2009).

Aspergillus terreus as the third most common species recognized is often refractory to therapy with the antifungal amphotericin B and has the propensity to disseminate (Balajee, 2009; Lass-Florl, 2009). Multiple other species of *Aspergillus* have rarely been recognized as causing invasive disease (Marr, 2002a; Balajee, 2009b; Florescu, 2009).

Risk Factors

The aspergilli are ubiquitous fungi to which all people are exposed on a regular basis. These fungi reside in vegetation of all types and are ubiquitous in the environment. Nosocomial infections, although uncommon, have been linked to numerous cases associated with hospital construction in the literature (Warnock, 2001; Vonberg, 2006). Engineering infection control through facility design to prevent high-risk patients from spore exposure has been done to provide a safer environment for patients (Noskin, 2001).

The most important risk factors for invasive aspergillosis are immunosuppressive disease, high-dose chemotherapy with or without transplantation, and solid organ transplantation (Maschmeyer, 2007; Ben-Ami, 2009; Zilberberg, 2009). Neutropenia is a prominent predisposing factor for disease; however, serious invasive disease may rarely occur in individuals who are not immunosuppressed by chemotherapy or malignancy (Denning, 2004). For instance, wound infection has been a problem in patients with extensive burn wounds and in individuals exposed to materials contaminated with conidia—a situation reminiscent of the Zygomycetes (Holzheimer, 2002). A fungus ball may also occur in the lung of patients with chronic obstructive lung disease, bronchiectasis, and an old cavity caused by tuberculosis (Riscili, 2009).

Clinical Diseases

The spectrum of invasive disease caused by *Aspergillus* species is broad. Although these fungi have a low pathogenicity in humans and rarely cause disease in the immunologically competent individual, immunocompromised patients are at risk for invasive disease. Those patients especially at risk are those with prolonged granulocytopenia or graft-versus-host disease and those undergoing immunosuppressive therapy or receiving corticosteroid treatment (Kontoyiannis, 2002). Because *Aspergillus* spores are normally present in the environment, the most common primary sites of infection are the lower respiratory tract and, to a lesser extent, the paranasal sinuses.

Ocular Infections

Keratomycosis usually follows trauma to the eye, especially in patients who have been treated with topical steroids. Pain and blurring of vision follow the traumatic episode, and if not treated, the infection may extend into the anterior chamber. Enucleation of the eye may be necessary if the process is not halted. The most common underlying disease recognized in a study of 15 patients with orbital invasive aspergillosis was diabetes mellitus, with all patients having a primary paranasal sinus infection (Choi, 2008). Ocular symptoms of this disease in the immunosuppressed patient include visual disturbances, periorbital swelling, and periorbital pain.

Otic Infections

Otomycosis is an infection of the external ear that is usually caused by *Aspergillus niger* or *A. fumigatus*. Pain, decreased hearing, and a discharge are accompanied by a fluffy green or black growth in the ear canal. Extension beyond the external ear is rare but may occur in immunosuppressed patients (Vennewald, 2003).

Sinus Infection

Invasive fungal sinusitis can be classified as an acute fulminant invasive disease or as a chronic indolent invasive disease (Morpeth, 1996). Spread of the fungus from the sinus into adjacent tissues is frequently dependent on the host immunologic response and on whether metabolic ketoacidosis is present, although invasive infection has also been reported in apparently healthy individuals (Parikh, 2004; Sivak-Callcott, 2004).

Cutaneous Infection

Aspergillus spp. may infect the skin after dissemination from another site, usually pulmonary, or the infection may be a primary infection after direct cutaneous exposure to a contaminated environmental source (Arikan, 1998; van Burik, 1998; Thomas, 2008). Recognized risk factors include immunosuppression, but local factors that abrogate defense mechanisms of the skin are also important such as may occur with burn wounds and surgical wounds, especially if occlusive dressings are present. Dissemination to the skin from another primary source in the suppressed patient is difficult to treat and generally results in death. This condition is usually recognized by multiple lesions appearing over different areas of the body.

Primary Pulmonary Infection

Primary pulmonary aspergillosis is the most common invasive mould infection in immunocompromised patients, especially in those patients with hematologic malignancies who are undergoing intensive chemotherapy (Vonberg, 2006). Even though the disease is usually associated with severely immunocompromised persons, less invasive and noninvasive diseases that affect the lungs such as aspergilloma (fungus ball), chronic necrotizing pulmonary aspergillosis, semi-invasive aspergillosis, chronic invasive pulmonary aspergillosis, symptomatic pulmonary aspergillosis, and *Aspergillus* pseudotuberculosis may also occur (Denning, 2003). The predilection of aspergilli to invade blood vessels leads to infarction and hemorrhage in the lungs and may involve hematogenous spread to other organs (Zmeili, 2007; Thompson, 2008).

Disseminated Infection

Dissemination from the lung or any other primary site of infection may affect any other organ system within the body. The propensity of hyphae to invade vascular structures and cause thrombosis leads to infarcts and abscesses in multiple organs. Single or multiple organs, including the brain, skin, kidneys, pleura, heart, esophagus, liver, or any other site, may be involved (Denning, 1998a).

Pathology of Aspergillosis

The histologic appearance of the aspergilli in tissue is similar to that observed with the other hyaline moulds, and differentiation among genera and species usually is not possible, except in unusual cases where sporulation within the tissue cavity has occurred. The tissue reaction may be granulomatous but is more commonly dominated by polymorphonuclear neutrophils unless the patient is severely neutropenic. Vascular invasion, thrombosis, and infarction often are prominent features. The hyphae are thin (2–5 µm) and septate and branch at acute angles (dichotomous) (see Fig. 61-4). The H&E stain often colors the hyphae, but the morphology may be demonstrated to advantage with the PAS or GMS technique. The histologic appearance of aspergilli in tissue and Zygomycetes can be differentiated on the basis of size, hyphal characteristics, and the presence of septations (see Table 61-11).

When the pathologic process is a fungus ball, the hyphae may stain poorly using histopathologic stains. A cavity that is in contact with air, as in the lung or sinuses, may develop fruiting heads, an event that permits identification in the genera and possibly to the species (Fig. 61-44). The conidiophores, which are not septate and may be wider than the vegetative hyphae, should not be confused with the Zygomycetes. Thick-walled Hülle cells and cleistothecia have also been described in vivo. When the patient is immunocompetent and the histologic response is granulomatous, the hyphae may be fragmented and confined to the cytoplasm of macrophages and multinucleated giant cells. The granulomatous response to *Aspergillus* in the lung may be mistaken for bronchocentric granulomatosis in patients who have allergic disease (Nagata, 1990).

Laboratory Diagnosis

Aspergilli are saprophytic fungi that should never be dismissed as contaminants without consultation with the attending physician. Isolation from a sterile site or repeated isolation from respiratory specimens suggests clinical significance. Hyphae may be demonstrated directly in clinical specimens in imprint preparations or wet preparations. Calcofluor white staining is useful for demonstrating the mould in specimens. Obtaining tissue, fluid, scrapings, or curettings for examination is important. Tissue should be teased or minced and inoculated directly onto the surface of the isolation medium. *Aspergillus* spp. grow rapidly, but most are inhibited or are partially inhibited by cycloheximide. The colonies of many of these moulds teem with conidia. To prevent contamination of the worker and other cultures, the colonies should be manipulated carefully in a biological safety cabinet, after which the surfaces of the safety cabinet should be thoroughly wiped with a fungicidal solution. Maintenance of isolated moulds in plastic bags with continuing incubation also reduces the probability of contaminating other cultures.

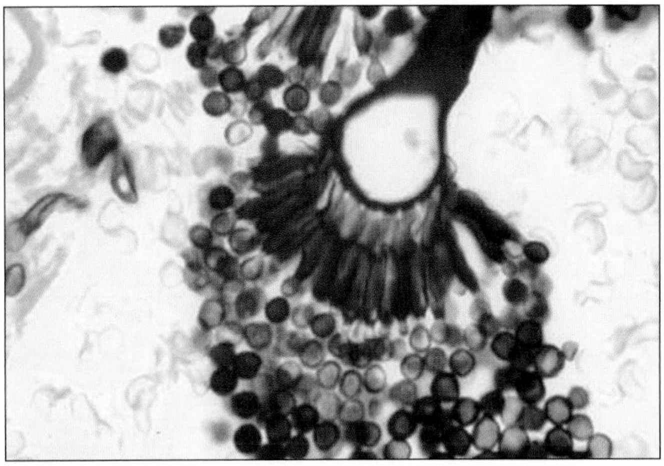

Figure 61-44 A fruiting head of *Aspergillus* is demonstrated within a pulmonary mycetoma (fungus ball). The phialides and conidia are well demonstrated. Although the hyphae of *Aspergillus* are not etiologically diagnostic, demonstration of the fruiting head documents the presence of this genus. (Gomori's methenamine silver stain, ×400.)

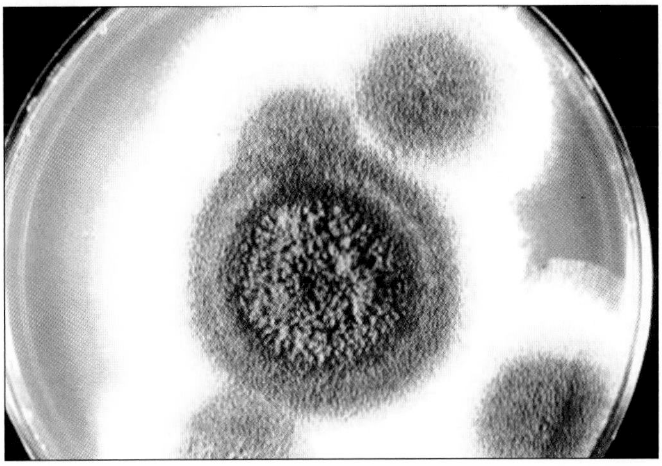

Figure 61-45 Fluffy colonies with granular areas produced by fruiting heads of *Aspergillus flavus*. The development of yellow or green coloration within the white colonies is characteristic. (Sabouraud dextrose agar.)

Specific identification of *Aspergillus* spp. is made by study of the reproductive structures and the macroscopic appearance of the culture. Careful attention to details of the conidial head is needed for species identification (Klich, 2002). *A. fumigatus* grows rapidly, producing colonies with a fluffy appearance and a blue-green appearance to the colony (see Fig. 61-2). Examination of the colony with a dissecting microscope reveals the conidiophores with their expanded vesicles as small globes projecting above the vegetative mycelium. The conidiophore is smooth, relatively short (300–500 µm), and expanded into a flask-shaped vesicle. The phialides develop in a single row (uniseriate), most commonly on only the upper two thirds of the vesicle, parallel to the axis of the conidiophore (see Fig. 61-8). The conidia are roughened (echinulate) and are round to oval.

Colonies of *A. flavus* have a velvety yellow to green appearance once fruiting heads develop (Fig. 61-45). The conidiophore is long (400–700 µm), ending in a vesicle that may be elliptical or round. The conidiophore is rough and stubbly. A single or double (biseriate) row of phialides occurs over the whole vesicle or the upper three quarters (Fig. 61-46). Round to oval conidia appear yellow-green en masse and measure 3–4.5 µm. *Aspergillus terreus* can be differentiated from other species by the production of a cinnamon brown colony with microscopic characteristics that include short conidiophores (<250 µm) and biseriate phialides.

Although the gold standard for making a diagnosis of invasive aspergillosis is to obtain a positive culture from sterile tissue with histologic evidence of mycelial invasion, the need for invasive techniques to obtain the

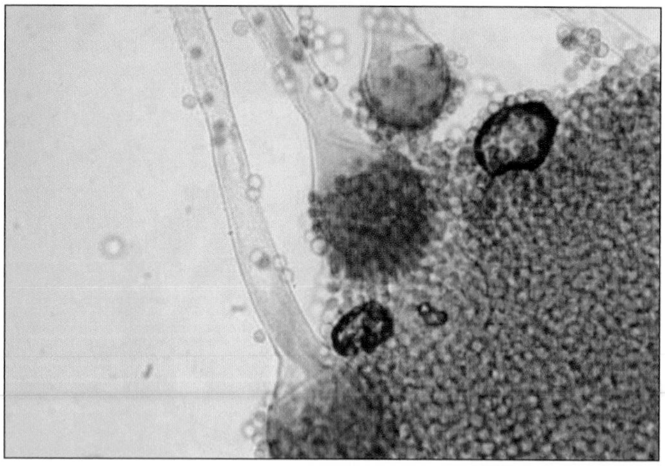

Figure 61-46 The fruiting head of *Aspergillus flavus* is uniseriate and biseriate. The phialides extend around much of the vesicle with a roughened (spiny) appearance of the conidiophore. (Lactophenol cotton blue stain, ×400.)

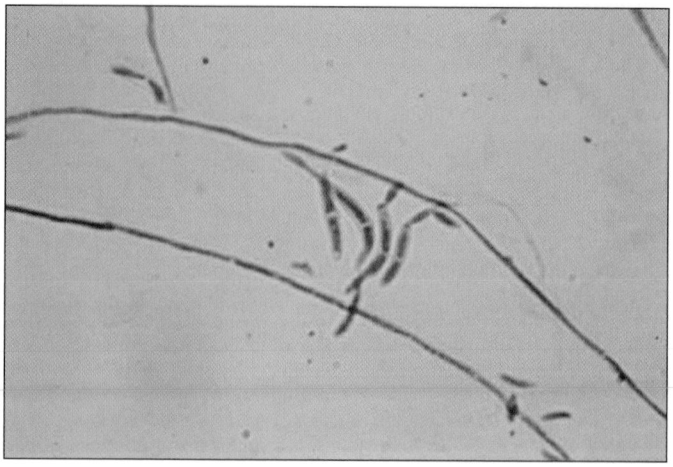

Figure 61-47 Canoe-shaped conidia of *Fusarium* spp. The conidia are often septate. (Lactophenol cotton blue stain, ×400.)

specimen, the delayed time required for culture, and the rapidity by which the aspergilli can spread make diagnosis problematic. Serologic tests are available for the detection of galactomannan to rapidly diagnose invasive aspergillosis (Aquino, 2007; Foy, 2007; Del Bono, 2008; Husain, 2008; Leeflang, 2008; Wheat, 2008) and for the detection of (1-3)-beta-D-glucan for nonspecific diagnosis of an invasive fungal infection (Senn, 2008; Marty, 2009). All of these tests have shown utility in the management of patients with invasive aspergillosis; however, limitations of the various assays need to be understood (Wheat, 2009a).

Although molecular methods have led to dramatic changes in the taxonomy of the *Aspergillus* species, they will continue to be evaluated as methods for the rapid diagnosis of fungal infection from clinical material. Multiple molecular targets for the identification of *Aspergillus* spp. have been evaluated, and targets showing greatest promise for identification appear to be the partial β-tubulin and calmodulin genomic areas (Geiser, 2007, 2009). The general consensus at the present time is that a combination of phenotypic and molecular testing needs to be considered for the accurate identification of *Aspergillus* spp..

Multiple platforms for direct detection of *Aspergillus* DNA in clinical specimens have been evaluated with varying degrees of success (Balajee, 2007a; Hummel, 2007, 2009; Klingspor, 2009; Logotheti, 2009; Wengenack, 2009). A recent systemic review and meta-analysis done on the use of PCR tests for the diagnosis of invasive aspergillosis directly from blood, plasma, and serum samples concluded that a single PCR-negative result was sufficient to exclude a diagnosis of proven or probable aspergillosis (Mengoli, 2009). However, two or more positive tests were required to confirm the diagnosis because of increased specificity after testing of multiple samples. With advances in molecular testing, a formal evaluation of PCR needs to be considered to assess its use in patients most likely to benefit from testing.

THE GENUS *FUSARIUM*

Fusarium spp. have been implicated in a number of infectious diseases, including keratomycosis, burn wounds, and invasive disease in immunocompromised patients (Jossi, 2009). Fusaria are now considered the second most common pathogenic moulds causing invasive disease (Dignani, 2004). Although still considered a rare cause of human disease, a major outbreak of *Fusarium* keratitis was recently reported wherein 130 cases of eye infection were confirmed (Centers for Disease Control and Prevention, 2006; O'Donnell, 2007). An epidemiologic investigation showed that most infected patients wore contact lenses that had been cleaned with a lens solution obtained from one manufacturer. This investigation led to the voluntary recall and permanent removal of the associated contact lens solution from the worldwide market.

The histopathologic picture for fusariosis is essentially identical to that observed with invasive aspergillosis (angioinvasive and acute branching septate hyphae). A differentiating feature from invasive aspergillosis is that fungemia is more commonly described in fusariosis. *Fusarium*-positive blood cultures are frequently detected during disseminated disease; however even in documented disseminated disease, detection of aspergilli in the blood is rare (Lionakis, 2004).

In culture, *Fusarium* colonies develop rapidly, producing a fluffy aerial mycelium, which often has a pink, lavender, or salmon color. Diffusible pigments may be seen in the surrounding agar. Simple or branched phialides develop directly from the hypha without a separate conidiophore. Short oval microconidia may be produced, but the distinctive structure is a canoe-shaped or crescent-shaped macroconidium, which may have one or more septa (Fig. 61-47). Identification of species in the mycology laboratory is difficult, usually requiring a reference laboratory with experience in recognition of subtle microscopic details related to the reproductive structures.

The taxonomy of *Fusarium* species has undergone extensive evaluation using molecular sequence analysis of multiple genomic targets (O'Donnell, 2008, 2009a). Although most fusaria pathogenic to humans are nested within the *Fusarium solani* or the *Fusarium oxysporum* species complex, it continues to be traditional taxonomic practice to refer to members of these complexes as single species (i.e., *F. solani* and *F. oxysporum*). These recent molecular phylogenetic studies, however, have begun to clarify species boundaries within evolutionary lineages of *Fusarium* that contain human pathogens. Currently however, recognition of the species, although important for epidemiologic purposes, does not have an impact on therapeutic decisions; thus many laboratories continue to report these as "*Fusarium* species." The recommended molecular target for identifying species within the two major complexes is now the partial EF-1α gene (Balajee, 2009a; O'Donnell, 2009b).

THE GENUS *SCEDOSPORIUM*

Medically important species within the genus are *Scedosporium apiospermum* (teleomorph *Pseudallescheria boydii*, previously known as *Allescheria boydii* and *Petriellidium boydii*) and *Scedosporium (inflatum) prolificans* (Cortez, 2008). These fungi are ubiquitous saprophytic fungi found in the soil and in decaying vegetation. *S. prolificans* has been reported as a rare cause of disseminated infection, whereas *S. apiospermum*, although most often associated with a subcutaneous infection (eumycotic mycetoma), is the most common species associated with invasive disease in the immunocompromised patient. A distinctive clinical syndrome of sinopulmonary and central nervous system infections in immunocompetent individuals has been associated with near drowning in polluted waters, with *P. boydii* as the etiologic agent (Gilgado, 2009).

S. apiospermum (P. boydii) grows rapidly on isolation medium at 25° C, producing a fluffy colony, which develops a brownish gray to dark gray ("mousy") color after incubation for several days. The culture darkens still further with continued incubation (Fig. 61-48). The asexual phase is characterized by single or small clusters of annelloconidia on a straight or branched conidiophore that may develop terminally or laterally from the vegetative hyphae. The conidia are light brown and have an oval, spermlike morphology (Fig. 61-49). In the sexual phase *(P. boydii)*, brown cleistothecia are produced that contain ascospores (see Fig. 61-13). The cleistothecia (100–300 μm in diameter), which are found most readily at the edges of the colony, develop best on nutritionally deficient media, such as cornmeal agar, V-8 juice agar, or potato dextrose (potato flake) agar. Because this fungus is homothallic, recognition of brown cleistothecia in

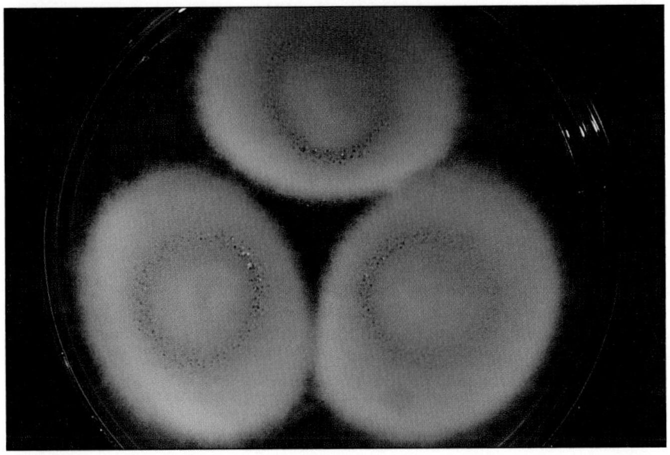

Figure 61-48 A developing colony of *Scedosporium apiospermum* with the characteristic mousy gray coloration. (Sabouraud dextrose agar.)

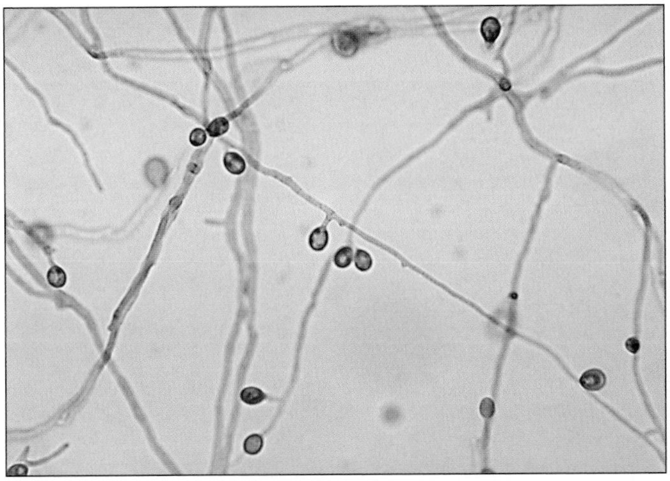

Figure 61-49 Tadpole- or sperm-shaped microconidia of *Scedosporium apiospermum* are representative of this organism. (Lactophenol cotton blue stain, ×400.)

the clinical laboratory is common. Strictly speaking, when the cleistothecia are demonstrated, the isolate should be reported as *P. boydii*, and it should be reported as *S. apiospermum* if the asexual conidia are the only diagnostic structures observed.

Although both macroscopic and microscopic characteristics can be used to separate species within the genus *Scedosporium*, molecular studies now suggest that *P. boydii* is a complex of multiple species (Gilgado, 2005, 2008).

OTHER SEPTATE HYALINE MOULDS

A long list of hyaline moulds are environmental saprophytes of low virulence and usually are not associated with clinical disease when isolated in the mycology laboratory (Walsh, 2004b). As mentioned earlier, any of these moulds may be pathogenic under the right conditions. In most cases, the host defenses of the patient are compromised in some way, or the fungus is introduced into the body by trauma or medical manipulation. Increasing numbers of case reports document saprophytic fungi producing infection of deep tissue and systemic organs (Rodriguez-Villalobos, 2003; Schinabeck, 2003; Sanchez, 2007; Van Schooneveld, 2008; Salmon, 2009). Demonstration of hyphae in tissue is extremely important for documenting the pathogenicity of these isolates, with culture necessary for species recognition. Molecular methods with sequence comparison analysis are becoming the standard for identification of these unusual pathogens (Balajee, 2007b).

PNEUMOCYSTIS PNEUMONIA

The taxonomic position of *P. (carinii) jiroveci* has undergone numerous changes over the years. This organism was originally described as a protozoan with the morphologic forms identified as trophozoites, cysts, and sporozoites. This protozoan hypothesis remained predominant until DNA analysis showed this organism to be more closely related to the fungi (Edman, 1988). More recently, molecular information showed that the organism had differing DNA sequences when identified from diverse mammal hosts. To address this issue, the *Pneumocystis* Working Group in 1994 proposed the name *P. carinii* f. sp. *hominis* as a special form *(formae specialis)* of the organism causing *P. carinii* pneumonia (PCP) in humans (Pneumocystis Working Group, 1994). Subsequently, those attending the International Workshop on Opportunistic Protists in 2001 began the process to rename the species to *P. jiroveci* (pronounced "yee row vet zee") (Frenkel, 1999; Stringer, 2002). Although initially controversial (Hughes, 2003), the name has now become widely accepted as the "microbe that causes PCP in humans," with the acronym PCP now standing for "*Pneumocystis* pneumonia."

RISK FACTORS

P. jiroveci (human-derived *Pneumocystis*) is a pathogen capable of causing a broad spectrum of clinical presentation. This organism was first recognized in outbreaks of pulmonary disease among malnourished infants in Eastern Europe during and after World War II (called "interstitial plasma cell pneumonia") (Cushion, 2003). More recently, *Pneumocystis* became a major cause of life-threatening pneumonia in 60%–80% of HIV-infected adults in America and Western Europe, and it subsequently became known as one of the AIDS-defining illnesses (Centers for Disease Control and Prevention, 1999b; Travis, 2009). Although still a serious problem within this patient population, the incidence of disease in people with AIDS has decreased to less than 10% of patients owing to the availability of HAART, the increasing use of anti-PCP prophylaxis, and improved awareness of the infection (D'Avignon, 2008). This disease should also be considered in any immunosuppressed patient who presents with fever, respiratory symptoms, or infiltrate on chest radiograph (Dei-Cas, 2000). Initially, clinical disease was thought to be due to reactivation of childhood latent infection in immunosuppressed cases, but studies now show that the organism can be transmitted between humans by the airborne route (Nevez, 2003; Totet, 2003). In individuals with compromised immune systems (e.g., HIV infection, chemotherapeutic regimens, organ transplantation), a potentially severe and fatal pneumonia can occur. Disseminated disease may also occur via spread through lymphatic and blood routes, but this is uncommon. Although rare, infection has been documented in patients without a predisposing illness (Al Soub, 2004).

CLINICAL DISEASES

Pneumonia is the most common manifestation of *P. jiroveci* infection (D'Avignon, 2008; Krajicek, 2009). Although the onset may be acute or insidious, symptomatic adults frequently present with dyspnea, a nonproductive cough, an inability to breathe deeply, chest tightness, and night sweats. The classic radiologic feature of PCP is fine, bilateral, perihilar interstitial shadowing; however, other radiographic pictures may be present (Barry, 2001). Often, radiographic infiltrates are much more extensive than would be suggested by the degree of symptoms. Concurrent infection with other agents, particularly cytomegalovirus and *C. neoformans*, is common. The most common extrapulmonary sites of infection are the thyroid, liver, bone marrow, lymph nodes, and spleen (Wazir, 2004).

PATHOLOGY

The definitive diagnosis of PCP requires the demonstration of cysts or trophozoites within clinical specimens (Fig. 61-50). Historically, this required an open thorax lung biopsy because of the low number of organisms present in other respiratory specimens and the lack of sensitive diagnostic tests. Although open lung biopsy is still considered one of the most sensitive tests for the detection of this disease, other specimens such as induced sputum and bronchoalveolar lavage have proved to be reliable sources for diagnosis. Classic histopathologic findings of PCP in sections of lung stained with H&E include widening of the alveolar septa with an infiltrate of mononuclear cells and foamy exudate within the alveolar spaces (sometime referred to as honeycombed exudates) (Woods, 2003). This exudate consists of aggregated cysts and trophozoites. The cyst form of *P. jiroveci* can be illustrated in tissue using the GMS stain. These cysts, which are 5–6 μm in diameter, stain brown to black and have the characteristic cup-shaped or crescent-shaped morphology. *Pneumocystis* cysts do not bud; this feature can be used to distinguish this organism from other fungi found in tissue.

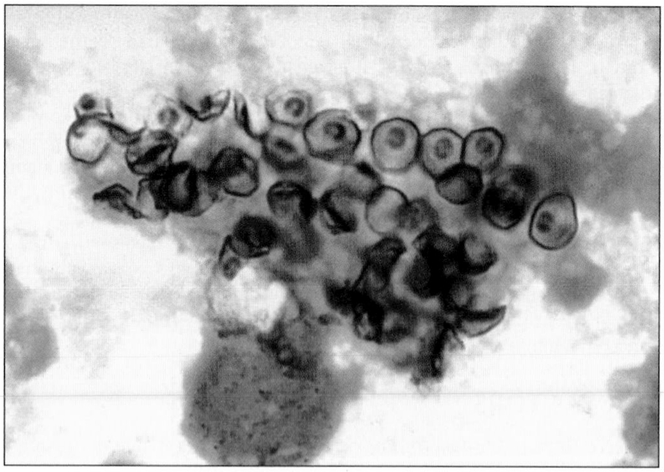

Figure 61-50 Cysts of *Pneumocystis jiroveci* in a smear from bronchoalveolar lavage. (Gomori's methenamine silver stain, ×400.) *(Courtesy Dr. Russell K. Brynes, CDC Public Health Image Library.)*

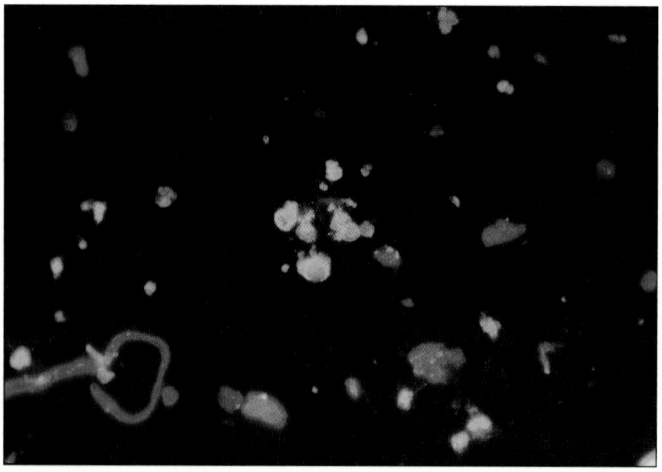

Figure 61-51 Immunofluorescense microscopy showing the presence of *Pneumocystis jiroveci.* (×561.) *(Courtesy CDC Public Health Image Library, Lois Norman provider.)*

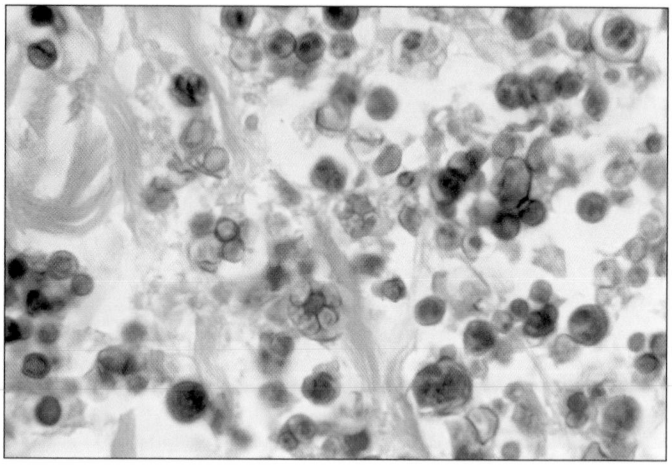

Figure 61-52 Histopathologic changes in protothecosis of the skin and mucous membrane of the nose due to *Prototheca wickerhamii.* Septation of the algal cells leads to multiple intracellular bodies and structures known as morula. *(Courtesy Dr. William Kaplan, CDC Public Health Image Library.)*

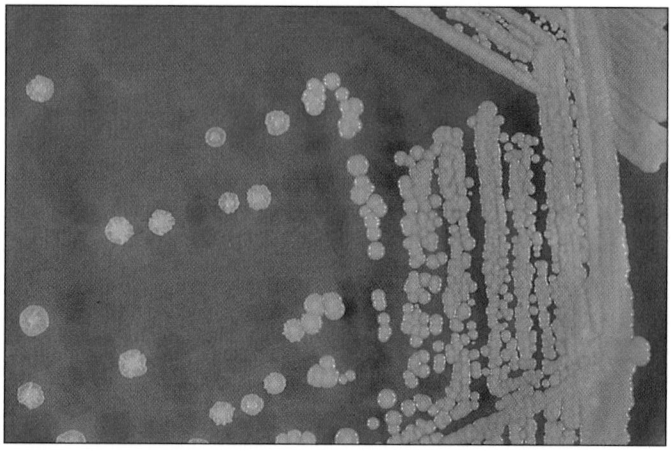

Figure 61-53 Colonies of *Prototheca wickerhamii* are yeast-like in appearance. (Sabouraud dextrose agar.)

LABORATORY DIAGNOSIS

P. jiroveci has been cultivated in cell cultures, but serial maintenance of subcultures has not been accomplished. The standard for diagnosis is staining bronchoalveolar lavage fluid with an immunofluorescent monoclonal antibody directed against surface epitopes for *Pneumocystis* cysts and trophozoites (Cushion, 2003). The life cycle of *P. jiroveci* involves development of sporozoites within a cyst, after which the sporozoites are released. In patients with HIV infection, sufficient numbers of organisms are produced that sputum induced with saline by a skilled respiratory therapist may provide the diagnosis. Experience with sputum has varied among centers, however, and the yield is very low in patients who have underlying disease other than HIV. Use of fluorescein-conjugated monoclonal antibodies to detect *P. jiroveci* in clinical specimens has proved to be a specific and sensitive method for identification (Fig. 61-51) (Kovacs, 2001). The immunofluorescence technique has been more sensitive in histochemical stains in some reports, but the skill and care of the observers undoubtedly play a role in the comparative sensitivity of the techniques (Cushion, 2003). Cysts of *P. jiroveci* occasionally may also be encountered in Gram-stained preparations, although this technique is not a sensitive method for detection.

Various PCR amplification strategies have been described for detecting *P. jiroveci* in clinical specimens (Robberts, 2007; Gupta, 2009). In an evaluation of nine different molecular assays, the mitochondrial large subunit rRNA target using a nested PCR platform was shown to be the most sensitive assay, with the highest degree of concordance seen with findings of histologic examination (Robberts, 2007). Additional studies have shown this assay to be useful in identifying patients who are in the early stages of infection (Gupta, 2009).

PROTOTHECOSIS

Protothecosis is an infection caused by achlorophyllic algae of the genus *Prototheca* (Leimann, 2004; Lass-Florl, 2007). Most human infections are caused by *Prototheca wickerhamii;* however, rare cases have also been caused by *Prototheca zopfii.* Although these species are classified as algae, they are included in this chapter because of the resemblance of the infections to fungal disease. *Prototheca* are found in fresh and marine waters and probably gain entrance to the body through superficial wounds. Some patients are immunocompetent, but serious underlying diseases, such as diabetes mellitus, or immunosuppressive therapies often predispose patients to infection with these pathogens. Other patients have received injections of corticosteroids at the site of infection or have had musculoskeletal infection, particularly involving the tendons. Infections commonly involve the skin and subcutaneous tissue, with subsequent involvement of underlying tendons.

Prototheca form large, nonbudding cells that can readily be seen in tissue. The appearance is a spheroid or ovoid cell with a prominent wall and a "morula-like" structure containing thick-walled autospores (Lass-Florl, 2007). Although *Prototheca* species are not readily apparent in H&E-stained smears, they can be observed with GMS or PAS stain. However, these structures must be differentiated from the dimorphic fungi (Fig. 61-52). Algae grow readily on fungal isolation media that do not contain cycloheximide, and the colonies resemble those of *Candida* spp. (Fig. 61-53). *Prototheca* species can be identified to the species level by using commercial yeast identification systems, such as the API 20C System and the VITEK 2 system (bioMérieux).

SELECTED REFERENCES

Balajee SA, Borman AM, Brandt ME, et al. Sequence-based identification of *Aspergillus*, *Fusarium*, and *Mucorales*species in the clinical mycology laboratory: where are we and where should we go from here? J Clin Microbiol 2009a;47:877–84.

A minireview focusing on the molecular strategies available for evaluation of medically important fungi of the genera Aspergillus *and* Fusarium *and the order* Mucorales.

Balajee SA, Sigler L, Brandt ME. DNA and the classical way: identification of medically important moulds in the 21st century. Med Mycol 2007b;45:475–90.

This paper describes the genotype-based methods that are available today for the identification of medically important moulds within the clinical microbiology laboratory.

Chandler FW, Kaplan W. Pathologic diagnosis of fungal infections. Chicago: ASCP Press; 1987a.

This atlas provides a practical foundation for the pathologic diagnosis of diseases caused by fungi, actinomycetes, and algae.

Hibbett DS, Binder M, Bischoff JF, et al. A higher-level phylogenetic classification of the Fungi. Mycol Res 2007;111:509–47.

This article provides a comprehensive phylogenetic classification of the kingdom Fungi with reference to the recent molecular phylogenetic analyses used to derive this proposed classification.

Lass-Florl C, Mayr A. Human protothecosis. Clin Microbiol Rev 2007;20:230–42.

This review provides a summary of the literature addressing biological, clinical, and epidemiologic aspects of human Prototheca *infection.*

Naggie S, Perfect JR. Molds: hyalohyphomycosis, phaeohyphomycosis, and zygomycosis. Clin Chest Med 2009;30:337–53, vii–viii.

This review focuses on emerging fungal pathogens with an emphasis on microbiology, pathogenesis, clinical presentations, diagnosis, treatment, and outcomes.

Pfaller MA, Diekema DJ. Epidemiology of invasive candidiasis: a persistent public health problem. Clin Microbiol Rev 2007;20:133–63.

This review provides an overview of the incidence, risk factors involved, and treatment strategies used for management of invasive candidiasis.

Queiroz-Telles F, Esterre P, Perez-Blanco M, et al. Chromoblastomycosis: an overview of clinical manifestations, diagnosis and treatment. Med Mycol 2009;47:3–15.

This article provides an overview of the diagnosis and management of the disease chromoblastomycosis.

Ribes JA, Vanover-Sams CL, Baker DJ. Zygomycetes in human disease. Clin Microbiol Rev 2000;13:236–301.

This review explores the diversity of the Zygomycetes, their disease manifestations and taxonomy, and the relationship of the Zygomycetes to other fungal pathogens.

REFERENCES

Access the complete reference list online at http://www.expertconsult.com

CHAPTER 62

MEDICAL PARASITOLOGY

Thomas R. Fritsche, Rangaraj Selvarangan

KEY POINTS

- Accurate diagnosis of parasitic infection usually depends on macroscopic or microscopic examination of specimens that have been appropriately collected and preserved. Thick and thin blood smears are useful for detecting and characterizing organisms found in the blood. Fecal specimens may be fresh or may be placed into fixatives such as formalin and polyvinyl alcohol.
- Immunodiagnostic methods for parasitology include detection of both antibodies and antigens. Established enzyme immunoassays include antigen tests for *Plasmodium* spp. in blood or serum; *Giardia lamblia, Cryptosporidium* spp., and *Entamoeba histolytica* in feces; and *Trichomonas vaginalis* in vaginal swabs. Direct fluorescent assays are also useful for identifying organisms in primary specimens. Serologic testing is an important adjunct in recognizing parasitic infections that reside in deep tissues, organs, and body spaces not readily amenable to routine morphologic testing methods.
- Molecular diagnostic methods now emerging are based on amplification techniques that offer high levels of sensitivity and specificity for both diagnosis and monitoring of parasitic disease.
- The diagnosis of malaria should be considered in the differential diagnosis of unexplained fever with the history of travel in endemic geographic regions. Thick and thin blood smears are complementary for detecting and identifying infecting *Plasmodium* spp. based on varieties of developmental stages, presence of malarial pigment, and stippling seen in infected erythrocytes.
- Other protozoal infections include babesiosis and trypanosomiasis found in blood, leishmaniasis (causing cutaneous, mucocutaneous, and visceral forms of disease), and toxoplasmosis, often affecting the central nervous system following congenital infection and in patients with acquired immunodeficiency syndrome (AIDS).
- Amebae are ingested as cysts, resulting in infection of the colon and passage of both cysts and trophozoites in the feces. Resulting diseases include amebic dysentery, amebic colitis, and liver abscess. Diagnosis is made by microscopic examination of stool and by serologic testing for antibodies in serum.
- Flagellates include *Giardia lamblia,* which causes diarrhea from ingestion of contaminated water and is diagnosed by the finding of trophozoites or cysts in feces. *Trichomonas vaginalis* is acquired by sexual transmission and is detected in vaginal wet mounts by its characteristic motion.
- Coccidia (*Cystoisospora, Cryptosporidium,* and *Cyclospora*) and microsporidia can cause protracted diarrhea in immunosuppressed individuals such as those with AIDS.
- Intestinal helminths include nematodes (roundworms), cestodes (tapeworms), and trematodes (flukes). These organisms reside as adults in the gastrointestinal tract or in other locations (liver, lung, blood). Knowledge of their life cycles and zoogeography with intermediate hosts is critical for establishing the parasitic stage in presumed infection. Eggs, larvae, or adult forms (from 1 mm to >10 m in length, depending upon the species) can be recovered from stool, urine, or sputum.
- Tissue helminths include filaria (larvae found in blood and also on skin biopsy), *Trichinella* (in muscle), *Strongyloides* (disseminated infection), and hydatidosis (large cystic lesions in the liver or lungs), among others.
- Arthropods cause disease through direct tissue invasion, envenomation, vesication, blood loss, transmission of infectious agents, hypersensitivity reactions, and psychological manifestations. Characteristics necessary for identification can be maintained by preserving the organisms in alcohol (ticks, mites, fleas, lice), by drying them (winged forms) after killing them with fumes of organic solvents, or by killing them with hot water (maggots) and subsequently storing them in alcohol.

The study of parasitology has gained renewed importance in a world made smaller by the rapid movement of people, especially travelers to and migrants from areas endemic for parasitic disease, and by the appearance of emerging and reemerging pathogens in individuals immunocompromised for a variety of reasons. Parasitic diseases of humans and domestic animals place a tremendous burden on limited healthcare resources and adversely affect economic and societal development in many countries around the world. Although the types of organisms classified as parasites constitute a large group, those that infect humans are limited in number and are composed mostly of protozoa, helminths, and arthropods (Table 62-1).

Clinicians in the United States and elsewhere are increasingly being confronted with unusual diagnostic problems associated with parasitic infection. Likewise, laboratorians have been challenged with the development of new technologies to accurately and rapidly diagnose such parasites as *Cryptosporidium parvum*, *Cryptosporidium hominis*, *Cyclospora cayetanensis*, *Toxoplasma gondii*, as well as microsporidia in both immunocompetent and immunocompromised hosts. The worldwide resurgence of malaria and other parasitic diseases has required laboratorians to strengthen their expertise in identification of the usual blood, intestinal, and tissue protozoa and helminths.

Once these diseases have been diagnosed, additional problems may be encountered in their management owing to lack of effective therapies and the emergence of resistance to traditional therapy. Many parasites require arthropod vectors for their transmission, and the irregular application of vector control efforts has, in some instances, resulted in the emergence of insecticide resistance. Malaria has made a tremendous resurgence in many areas because of relaxed control efforts and the emergence of drug-resistant parasites and insecticide-resistant mosquitoes. Schistosomiasis has spread into many new areas because of increased irrigation associated with population growth and the need to expand agricultural production.

Because of the chronic nature and the generally long prepatent periods (i.e., time between infection and appearance of diagnostic stages) of many parasitic diseases, physicians may not consider them in a differential diagnosis unless the patient voluntarily offers information, or specific inquiry is made about travel history or other possible exposure. Malaria is one parasitic disease that often presents as an acute, febrile illness and may have lethal consequences unless it is considered in the differential diagnosis and a history of travel to an endemic area is elicited.

Various estimates have been put forth for the prevalence and related mortality figures of parasitic infections on a worldwide basis (Table 62-2). The actual incidence of parasitic infections in the United States is unknown, however, because most infections are not reported to public health officials. *Giardia lamblia*, other intestinal protozoa, and intestinal roundworms are reported most frequently (7.2%, 10%, and 3.5%, respectively) by state laboratories, but other parasites, including *Cryptosporidium*, *Cyclospora*, and microsporidia, probably occur more frequently and are underdiagnosed (Kappus, 1994; Garcia, 2007).

This chapter provides an overview of the general approach used by laboratorians to recover and identify parasitic protozoa and helminths from human specimens. Discussion of individual species of parasites focuses on essential clinical and biological information necessary to assist in diagnosis and management. For more extensive coverage of specific parasites, a number of excellent texts are available (Beaver, 1984; Warren, 1990; Lane, 1993; Guerrant, 1999; Garcia, 2007, 2009; Markell, 1999; Strickland, 2000; Cook, 2002; Mullen, 2002; among others). Some of these references are older and may be less accessible; however, they discuss classic disease presentations and historic perspectives in a way that is sometimes lacking in newer literature. Parasitology atlases are also important resources for any laboratorian performing parasitology examinations and should be readily available (Spencer, 1982; Brooke, 1984; Ash, 1987, 2007; Sun, 1988; Peters, 1989; Garcia, 2010; Murray, 2007). Several texts specifically address the pathologic aspects of parasitic infections (Marcial-Rojas, 1971; Binford, 1976; Sun, 1982; Von Lichtenberg, 1991; Woods, 1993; Orihel, 1995; Connor, 1997; Gutierrez, 2000). Parasitic infections that are problematic in immunocompromised patients also have been reviewed (Walzer, 1989).

LABORATORY METHODS

Numerous methods have been described for the recovery and identification of parasites in clinical specimens, some of which are useful for detection of a variety of species, whereas others detect only a particular species. It is preferable for the laboratory to offer a limited number of procedures competently performed than a larger variety of infrequently performed tests that may prove problematic. Analyses of blood and fecal specimens account for the largest share of clinician requests for parasitologic evaluation. A variety of additional specimens are submitted to the laboratory less frequently, including urogenital specimens, sputum, aspirates, and biopsy material. As newer information becomes available on certain of the

TABLE 62-1

A Summary of the More Commonly Found Human Parasites and Their Primary Sites of Infection

Subkingdom Protozoa	Subkingdom Metazoa
Phylum Sarcomastigophora	**Phylum Platyhelminthes (flatworms)**
Subphylum Sarcodina (amebae)	**Class Cestoidea (tapeworms)**
Entamoeba histolytica (I)*	*Diphyllobothrium* spp. (I)*
E. dispar (I)	*Dipylidium caninum* (I)*
E. hartmanni (I)	*Echinococcus granulosus* (H)*
E. coli (I)	*E. multilocularis* (H)*
E. polecki (I)	*Hymenolepis nana* (I)*
Iodamoeba bütschlii (I)	*H. diminuta* (I)*
Endolimax nana (I)	*Taenia saginata* (I)*
Naegleria fowleri (T, C)*	*T. solium* (I, T)*
Acanthamoeba spp. (T, C, E)*	**Class Trematoda (flukes)**
Balamuthia mandrillaris (T, C)*	*Clonorchis sinensis* (H)
Sappinia diploidea (T, C)	*Fasciola hepatica* (H)*
Blastocystis hominis (I)	*Fasciolopsis buski* (I)
Subphylum Mastigophora (flagellates)	*Heterophyes heterophyes* (I)
Giardia lamblia (I)*	*Metagonimus yokagawai* (I)
Dientamoeba fragilis (I)*	*Nanophyetus salmincola* (I)*
Chilomastix mesnili (I)	*Opisthorchis viverrini* (H)
Retortamonas intestinalis (I)	*Paragonimus* spp. (L)*
Enteromonas hominis (I)	*Schistosoma haematobium* (B)
Pentatrichomonas hominis (I)	*S. japonicum* (B)
Trichomonas vaginalis (V)*	*S. mekongi* (B)
T. tenax (M)	*S. mansoni* (B)
Leishmania tropica (T)	**Phylum Nematoda (roundworms)**
L. major (T)	**Class Adenophorea (Aphasmidia)**
L. aethiopica (T)	*Trichinella spiralis* (T, I)*
L. mexicana (T)*	*Trichuris trichiura* (I)*
L. braziliensis (T)	*Capillaria philippinensis* (I)
L. donovani (T)	**Class Secernentia (Phasmidia)**
Trypanosoma gambiense (B, C)	*Enterobius vermicularis* (I)*
T. rhodesiense (B, C)	*Ascaris lumbricoides* (I)*
T. cruzi (B, T)*	*Ancylostoma duodenale* (I)
T. rangeli (B)	*Necator americanus* (I)*
Phylum Ciliophora (ciliates)	*Strongyloides stercoralis* (I)
Balantidium coli (I)*	*Trichostrongylus* spp. (I)*
Phylum Apicomplexa (apicomplexans)	*Anisakis* spp. (I)*
Class Sporozoea	*Wuchereria bancrofti* (T, B)
Subclass Piroplasma	*Brugia malayi* (T, B)
Babesia spp. (B)*	*Loa loa* (T, B)
Subclass Coccidia	*Onchocerca volvulus* (T)
Plasmodium falciparum (B)	*Mansonella perstans* (T, B)
P. malariae (B)	*M. ozzardi* (T, B)
P. ovale (B)	*M. streptocerca* (T)
P. vivax (B)	*Dracunculus medinensis* (T)
P. knowlesi (B)	*Angiostrongylus cantonensis* (T)
Cryptosporidium parvum (I)*	*A. costaricensis* (T)
C. hominis (I)	**Phylum Pentastomida (tongue worms)**
Cyclospora cayetanensis (I)*	*Armillifer* spp. (N,T)
Cystoisospora belli (I)*	*Linguatula serrata* (E,T)
Sarcocystis spp. (I, T)	
Toxoplasma gondii (T)*	
Phylum Microspora (microsporidia, at least 8 genera)	
Encephalitozoon spp. (E, H, T)*	
E. intestinalis (I, T)*	
Enterocytozoon bieneusi (I)*	

Adapted from Murray PR, Barron EJ, Pfaller M, et al. Manual of clinical microbiology. 6th ed. Washington, DC: ASM Press; 1995.

B, Blood; *C*, spinal fluid; *E*, eye; *H*, liver; *I*, intestine; *L*, lung; *M*, mouth; *N*, nasopharynx; *T*, tissue; *V*, vagina.

*Pathogenic parasite that occurs naturally in the United States.

TABLE 62-2

Estimated Prevalence of Parasitic Infections Worldwide

Disease	Estimated population involved	Annual number of deaths
Protozoan		
Amebiasis	Up to 10% of world population	40,000–110,000
African trypanosomiasis	100,000 new cases/year	5000
American trypanosomiasis	24 million	60,000
Giardiasis	200 million	
Leishmaniasis	1.2 million	
Malaria	400–490 million	2.2–2.5 million
Helminthic		
Ascariasis	1.3 billion	1550
Cestodiases	65 million	
Clonorchiasis/opisthorchiasis	13.5 million	
Dracunculiasis	<100,000	
Fasciolopsiasis	10 million	
Lymphatic filariasis	128 million	
Hookworm	1.3 billion	
Onchocerciasis	17.7 million	
Paragonimiasis	2.1 million	
Schistosomiasis	150 million	500,000–1 million
Strongyloidiasis	35 million	
Trichostrongyliasis	5.5 million	
Trichuriasis	900 million	

Adapted from Markell EK, John DT, Krotoski WA. Markell and Voge's medical parasitology. 8th ed. Philadelphia: WB Saunders; 1999.

so-called emerging parasites, the laboratory may need to develop and use additional, highly specific test methods or to find competent referral laboratories where such tests are performed.

The types of specimens collected for laboratory evaluation depend on the species and stage of the parasite suspected. Knowledge of the life cycle of the parasite aids in determining the type, number, and frequency of specimens required for diagnosis. Immunologic and molecular methods for the diagnosis of parasitic diseases also are useful in many instances, and may be the only methods available in certain circumstances. Complete descriptions of general and esoteric laboratory procedures for the recovery and identification of parasites referred to here may be found in a variety of sources to which the reader is referred (Beaver, 1984; Ash, 1987; Balows, 1988; Price, 1994; Garcia, 2003, 2007, 2009, 2010; Murray, 2007).

Familiarity with calibration and use of the ocular micrometer is necessary for any laboratory performing parasitologic examination (Clinical and Laboratory Standards Institute, 2005). Measurement of the size of protozoal trophozoites and cysts and of helminth eggs and larvae is often required to make an accurate identification. Pathogenic and nonpathogenic amebae (specifically *Entamoeba histolytica* and *Entamoeba hartmanni*) can be differentiated with assurance only by taking careful size measurements. Similarly, eggs of *Diphyllobothrium* spp., *Paragonimus westermani*, and *Fasciola/Fasciolopsis* may be readily differentiated on the basis of accurate measurements (Smith, 1979; Clinical and Laboratory Standards Institute, 2005).

EXAMINATION OF BLOOD

Parasites that may be detected in blood specimens include the agents of malaria (*Plasmodium* spp.), babesiosis (*Babesia* spp.), trypanosomiasis (*Trypanosoma* spp.), leishmaniasis (*Leishmania donovani*), and filariasis (*Wuchereria bancrofti*, *Brugia malayi*, *Loa loa*, and *Mansonella* spp.). The most important techniques to be performed in the clinical laboratory to assist in the diagnosis of blood parasites include preparation, staining, and examination of thick and thin blood films. Other techniques used less frequently include the buffy coat smear and various concentration techniques reserved for recovery of microfilariae (National Committee for Clinical Laboratory Standards, 2000).

Thick and Thin Blood Films

Examination of permanently stained blood films is required to identify most blood parasites. Thin films are prepared in the same manner as for hematologic differential evaluation; blood is spread over the slide in a thin layer, yielding intact, nonoverlapping cellular elements. Integrity of the blood cell membranes is important for determining the intracellular or extracellular nature of the infection. In the thick film, blood is concentrated in a small area that is many cell layers deep. During staining, erythrocytes are dehemoglobinized and only leukocyte nuclei, platelets, and parasites (if present) are visible. The thick film is preferred for diagnosis because it contains 16–30 times more blood per microscopic field than does the thin film, thus increasing the chances of detecting light parasitemia and decreasing the time needed for reliable examination. The amount of blood examined in a thick film in 5 minutes using the 100× oil immersion objective would require at least 30 minutes when examined in a thin film. Although thick films increase the likelihood of detecting an infection, species identifications are usually performed by examination of thin films because morphology is often more definitive, especially for malarial parasites. For routine examination, both thick and thin films should be prepared.

Preparation of Slides

Blood for examination may be obtained by fingerstick, earlobe puncture, or venipuncture. Fingerstick blood should flow freely to prevent dilution with tissue fluid, and it should not be contaminated with the alcohol disinfectant, which should be allowed to dry first. If obtained by venipuncture, the first drop of blood (anticoagulant-free) from the needle is used to prepare the films at the bedside. Use of anticoagulants is discouraged when malaria is suspected because they may cause distortion of the parasites and interfere with staining. In practice, however, blood usually is submitted to the laboratory in an anticoagulant, which may be the only practical method to ensure that high-quality smears can be prepared. Ethylenediaminetetraacetic acid (EDTA)-anticoagulated blood is preferred in such cases and should be transported to the laboratory within the hour to prevent deterioration of organism morphology. Anticoagulants do not interfere with the staining of microfilariae.

Both thin and thick films should be prepared on clean, grease-free slides. Thick films are prepared by puddling several small drops of blood into an area the size of a dime (1.5 cm) and allowing the blood to dry flat at room temperature, usually overnight. A proper thick film should be thin enough that newspaper print may be read through it. If it is too thick, the film may peel from the slide. Excess heat may fix erythrocytes and may prevent dehemoglobinization.

Staining

Blood begins to lose its affinity for stain in about 3 days, and older thick films do not dehemoglobinize well. Best staining results are achieved when using Giemsa stain because host cell and parasite chromatin stains vividly but the hemoglobin in erythrocytes is only a pale red, and this is the only stain that allows visualization of the erythrocyte stippling that occurs with infection by certain malarial parasites. Wright's stain may be used for thin films, but it stains parasites less well than Giemsa and it stains erythrocytes, producing a busier background. Because Wright's stain incorporates alcohol as its fixative, thick films must be lysed in water before staining.

The Giemsa staining procedure requires somewhat more attention to preparation of reagents and staining protocol than does the Wright's staining procedure, which is often automated. Generally, fresh Giemsa stain must be made each day of use by diluting stock solution into phosphate-buffered water. To achieve appropriate staining reactions, including the appearance of Schüffner's stippling, buffered water must be maintained at pH 6.8–7.2. Each new lot of stock Giemsa stain must be checked to determine optimal staining time and dilution because some variation is seen from lot to lot (National Committee for Clinical Laboratory Standards, 2000).

Examination of Smears

Both thick and thin smears are examined in their entirety under the low-power (10×) objective to detect microfilariae, which rarely occur in large numbers. In particular, the feathered edge of thin smears should be examined, as microfilariae are often carried there during preparation of the smear. Examination using a 50× oil immersion objective may subsequently be used to screen blood films for protozoa, although thorough examination using the 100× oil immersion objective still is necessary to detect the smallest parasites such as *Plasmodium* spp., *Babesia* spp., and leishmanias. Again, examination of the feathered edge is important because erythrocytes are drawn out into a single layer of cells, allowing thorough evaluation of their morphology and the presence of intracellular protozoa. An experienced microscopist should examine at least 100 oil immersion fields (requiring about 5 minutes) on the thick blood film and 200 fields (requiring at least 15 minutes) on the thin film using the 100× objective before issuing a negative report (Ash, 1987).

Concentration Techniques

A variety of special techniques have been described for the concentration of blood parasites, specifically leishmanias, trypanosomes, and microfilariae, details of which may be found elsewhere (Beaver, 1984; Ash, 1987; Garcia, 1999, 2001, 2010; National Committee for Clinical Laboratory Standards, 2000).

Preparation of buffy coat smears, which most clinical laboratories can perform with existing resources, is helpful in the detection of *L. donovani*, trypanosomes, and microfilariae. Following centrifugation of an anticoagulated blood sample, the layer of cells between plasma and packed erythrocytes is drawn off and is used to prepare blood films for staining or for preparation of a wet mount to detect motile organisms (Ash, 1987; Strickland, 2000).

For detection of microfilariae, Knott's concentration or membrane filtration is helpful, particularly when the density of microfilariae in peripheral blood is very low. With the Knott technique, anticoagulated blood is lysed with 2% formalin and centrifuged to concentrate the microfilariae in the sediment, which then may be examined as a wet preparation or stained with Giemsa or hematoxylin stain. In the membrane filtration procedure, blood is lysed and passed through a 5-μm membrane filter, which is subsequently stained with hematoxylin to reveal any microfilariae (Ash, 1987; National Committee for Clinical Laboratory Standards, 2000).

Use of the fluorochrome acridine orange in a microhematocrit centrifuge format (QBC blood parasite detection method; QBC Diagnostics, Philipsburg, Pa.) allows detection of blood parasites and appears to be more sensitive than traditional thick and thin smears. Laboratories that encounter malaria infrequently may experience difficulty in interpreting results by this method, however, and are encouraged to retain expertise in performance of traditional blood film techniques (National Committee for Clinical Laboratory Standards, 2000).

EXAMINATION OF FECAL SPECIMENS

The presence of intestinal parasites is primarily identified through the direct examination of stool using wet mounts, concentration techniques, permanently stained smears, and, less frequently, culture. Newer immunoassay methods using species-specific antibody reagents to detect antigens of *G. lamblia*, *Cryptosporidium* spp., and *E. histolytica* have become popular. Stages of helminths commonly recovered include eggs and larvae, although intact worms or portions thereof may occasionally be seen. Intestinal protozoan infections are diagnosed by detection of trophozoites, cysts, or oocysts. Routine methods for the identification of ova and parasites (O&P examination) should include procedures that permit recovery of both protozoa and helminths, with use of special procedures limited to specific requests. At a minimum, laboratories performing parasitologic examination should be capable of performing direct wet mount examination of fresh stool, a concentration procedure, and a permanent stain method. Many protozoan infections will be missed unless permanent stains are examined (Garcia, 1979, 1997, 2003, 2010; Price, 1994; Clinical and Laboratory Standards Institute, 2005).

Specimen Collection, Handling, and Preservation

Recovery and subsequent identification of parasites in fecal specimens requires proper collection and handling. Old, poorly preserved, or contaminated specimens are of little value. Specimens should not be collected for 1 week after the patient has ingested any materials that leave a crystalline residue, such as nonabsorbable antidiarrheal compounds, antacids, bismuth, barium, or antimalarial agents. Oily laxatives such as mineral oil may also interfere with examination. Use of antibiotics or contrast media may decrease the numbers of organisms, especially protozoa, in the intestinal tract for several weeks (Ash, 1987; Garcia, 2007).

Specimens may be submitted to the laboratory fresh or in appropriate preservatives. All fresh specimens should be examined within 1 hour of passage, and liquid specimens should be examined within 30 minutes or placed immediately in preservatives to maintain the best yield. This method ensures that fragile protozoal trophozoites are not inadvertently destroyed. Specimens that cannot be processed immediately should be left at room temperature or refrigerated and should not be placed in an incubator because this only speeds disintegration of parasites.

Specimens may be passed directly into clean, dry paper cartons, or a portion may be transferred to a container after the patient squats over wax paper. Diarrheic specimens may also be collected in clean bedpans. Containers should have tight-fitting lids and should be placed in plastic bags before transport to the laboratory. Inadvertent introduction of urine or toilet water with the specimen may readily destroy protozoal trophozoites and should be avoided. Also, contamination with water or soil may accidentally introduce free-living organisms that may prove difficult to differentiate from parasitic ones.

Kits consisting of vials of preservatives appropriate for performing direct examinations, concentration procedures, and preparation of stained smears are available from a number of commercial sources at low cost. Aliquots of freshly passed stool should be immediately placed into these vials and mixed thoroughly. These kits are especially helpful for those patients who are unable to bring in a fresh sample in timely fashion, or for those who will be collecting several specimens over the course of several days. With the two-vial technique, one portion of specimen is fixed in three parts of 5%–10% buffered formalin and another portion in three parts of polyvinyl alcohol (PVA) fixative. Other available preservation systems include merthiolate-iodine-formalin (MIF) and sodium acetate–formalin (SAF) (Table 62-3). SAF has an advantage in that it can be used for permanent stains as well as for direct mounts and concentration procedures, and it does not contain mercury, which is present in Schaudinn's and PVA fixatives. In addition to being poisonous, mercury presents disposal problems in an increasing number of states. However, the quality of permanent stains when SAF is used is not as good as when Schaudinn's or PVA fixative is used. Zinc sulfate–based PVA and other newer commercial products are gaining popularity, and their use may be indicated when mercury chloride–based compounds cannot be used (Garcia, 1993, 1997, 2007, 2010; Clinical and Laboratory Standards Institute, 2005).

Examination of three specimens collected every other day is considered the minimum necessary to perform an adequate O&P evaluation (Garcia, 2003; Clinical and Laboratory Standards Institute, 2005). This procedure ensures an optimum interval for recovery of those parasites known to shed diagnostic forms intermittently, especially *G. lamblia* and *Strongyloides stercoralis*. Additional sensitivity may be achieved in detecting these parasites, as well as *E. histolytica*, using purgation. The laboratory must be notified prior to initiation of purgation, however, to have staff available for processing. Specimens should be collected in separate containers and submitted to the laboratory within minutes of collection. Saline purgatives such as sodium sulfate or buffered phosphosoda are recommended.

TABLE 62-3
Commonly Used Stool Fixatives and Examination Techniques

	EXAMINATION TECHNIQUE		
Fixative	**Direct wet mount**	**Concentration procedure**	**Permanent stained smear**
None (fresh stool)	Yes	Yes	Yes
10% formalin	Yes	Yes	No
Schaudinn's fluid	No	No	Yes
Polyvinyl alcohol (PVA)	No	No*	Yes
Modified PVA†	No	No*	Yes
Merthiolate-iodine-formalin (MIF)	Yes	Yes	No‡
Sodium acetate–formalin (SAF)	Yes	Yes	Yes

*Although concentration techniques using PVA have been described, they are not widely used because of problems with recovery of some organisms.
†Copper sulfate or zinc sulfate replaces the mercuric chloride.
‡Smears prepared from MIF-preserved specimens may be stained with polychrome IV stain.

Macroscopic Examination

Fecal specimens should be examined grossly for consistency (formed, soft, loose, or watery) and for the presence of mucus, blood, larval or adult worms, and proglottids. Protozoan trophozoites are more likely to be found in watery or loose specimens, whereas cysts predominate in formed or soft specimens. Helminths or their eggs may be found in any type of fecal specimen. Most parasites are uniformly distributed in the stool as a result of the mixing action of the cecum, although some eggs (especially schistosomes) may enter the fecal stream in the lower colon and rectum and be unevenly distributed, as may pinworm and *Taenia* spp. eggs. Protozoal trophozoites may be more numerous in the last portion of stool evacuated and should be specifically sought in mucus (Garcia, 2003).

Microscopic Examination

Specimens may be examined microscopically by direct wet mounts of fresh or preserved material, wet mounts of concentrates, or permanent stains. Each procedure has specific advantages and limitations. Direct saline wet mounts of fresh feces allow detection and observation of motile protozoan trophozoites and helminth larvae. Direct mounts of preserved feces may allow detection of parasites that do not concentrate well. Concentration procedures increase the examiner's ability to detect protozoan cysts and helminth eggs and larvae but are unsatisfactory for detecting protozoan trophozoites. Permanent stains are useful for detection and morphologic examination of protozoan trophozoites and cysts.

The circumstances under which each procedure is performed vary depending on the type of specimen (formed, soft, loose, or watery) submitted. Generally, a fresh soft, loose, or watery specimen should have all three procedures performed (Garcia, 2003, 2007). Watery specimens may be concentrated by simple centrifugation rather than by flotation or formalin–ethyl acetate concentration. The direct wet mount may be omitted if the specimen is submitted in preservatives (Clinical and Laboratory Standards Institute, 2005). At a minimum, formed specimens should be examined by a concentration procedure, although improved yield has been demonstrated when a permanent stain is added to the workup (Garcia, 1979, 2007).

Direct Wet Mount

The direct wet mount is one of the most easily performed parasitologic tests, although proper interpretation requires careful examination and experience in using the microscope to full advantage. The test is most useful when fresh specimens, especially liquid stools or duodenal aspirates, are examined for motile trophozoites or helminth larvae. A small amount of stool is mixed with a drop of 0.85% saline and covered with a coverslip. The preparation should be dense enough that newspaper print can just be read through it.

Examination of the entire coverslip is performed systematically under the low-power (10×) objective, with the microscope diaphragm closed down to increase contrast. Suspicious objects and those that are refractile, such as protozoal cysts, should then be examined with the high-power (40×) objective. Detection of motility of slow-moving amebae requires that an object be examined for at least 15 seconds. In the absence of suspicious objects, up to a third of the preparation should be examined using the 40× objective. The oil immersion objective usually is not used unless the coverslip has been sealed with nail polish or vaspar (a 50:50 mixture of petroleum jelly and paraffin).

A second preparation may be made in identical fashion, except that a drop of a 1:5 dilution of Lugol's iodine or an equivalent preparation is added in place of the saline. Use of straight Lugol's or Gram's iodine causes clumping of material and is not recommended. Iodine is helpful in enhancing the visibility of nuclear structures in protozoal cysts and in detecting glycogen inclusions. Limitations, however, include loss of trophozoite motility and cyst refractility, as well as difficulty in recognizing chromatoid bodies.

Concentration Techniques

Concentration procedures, which may be performed on fresh or preserved specimens (see Table 62-3), are more sensitive than direct wet mount examination for detection of protozoan cysts and helminth eggs and larvae because they decrease the amount of background material in the preparations and, in most circumstances, actually concentrate the organisms. Although a variety of methods and modifications have been described, some are useful only for specific parasites (Melvin, 1982; Ash, 1987; Clinical and Laboratory Standards Institute, 2005; Garcia, 2007). For routine use, a method should be selected that allows reliable detection of both protozoan cysts and helminth eggs. Concentration methods are based on sedimentation or flotation principles. In sedimentation, the heavier parasites settle to the bottom as a result of gravity or centrifugation. In flotation, the lighter parasite cysts and eggs rise to the surface of a solution of high specific gravity. The two most widely used concentration procedures in the United States are the zinc sulfate centrifugal flotation technique of Faust and the formalin ether sedimentation method of Ritchie (or their modifications). In practice, ethyl acetate has replaced ether in the latter method because of the dangers associated with handling ether, and comparable results are achieved (Truant, 1981).

Formalin–ethyl acetate concentration is a biphasic sedimentation technique that is efficient in recovering most protozoan cysts and helminth eggs and larvae, including operculate eggs, and is moderately effective for schistosome eggs. Less distortion of protozoal cysts occurs with this technique than with zinc sulfate flotation. Eggs of *Hymenolepis nana* may be missed, however, and concentrations of *G. lamblia* and *Iodamoeba bütschlii* cysts may not be very good. For proper concentration of coccidian oocysts and spores of microsporidia, attention must be paid to the recommended speed and time of centrifugation (Clinical and Laboratory Standards Institute, 2005; Garcia, 2010). Despite these problems, the technique is used widely for both its simplicity and its suitability in most laboratory situations.

With the zinc sulfate flotation method, fresh stool is processed using zinc sulfate with a specific gravity of 1.18 and formalinized stool is processed with a solution of specific gravity of 1.20. Parasitic elements are recovered from the surface film of the solution following centrifugation. This method yields a cleaner preparation than is provided by formalin–ethyl acetate concentration, but it is unreliable for the recovery of nematode larvae, infertile eggs of *Ascaris*, and the eggs of most trematodes and large tapeworms. Problems with recovery also occur with stool specimens containing excessive amounts of fats. Use of formalinized stool specimens rather than fresh stool helps clear the specimen and prevents popping of opercula and distortion of the parasites (Bartlett, 1978).

Permanent Stains

Use of stained slide preparations provides a permanent record of a patient's specimen and allows review by consultants should difficulties arise in identification. Of the methods described for studying fecal specimens, only the permanent stain is designed for analysis using the oil immersion objective (100×). The permanent stain is most useful for detection of protozoal trophozoites and cysts, which may be recognized when direct and concentrated preparations are negative. Although they generally are not useful for detecting helminth eggs or larvae, permanent stains are inherently more sensitive for detecting protozoal infections, and their use has been recommended for every stool sample submitted for O&P examination (Clinical and Laboratory Standards Institute, 2005).

A variety of staining techniques and modifications and their advantages and disadvantages have been described. The Wheatley trichrome stain and iron hematoxylin stain are all-purpose methods that allow detection of amebae and flagellates. Unfortunately, detection of most human-infecting coccidia and microsporidia requires the use of special stains. Technical problems may arise in the performance of any staining procedure; most are related to the age of the specimen, proper smear preparation and fixation, and the quality of the reagents. Positive control slides of known staining quality should be run with each batch of slides stained. This is especially true in the performance of more specific stains for coccidia and microsporidia. Less commonly used stains, such as polychrome IV stain for use with MIF-preserved specimens and chlorazol black E stain for use with fresh specimens, are not reviewed here, but details may be found elsewhere (Clinical and Laboratory Standards Institute, 2005; Garcia, 2007).

Wheatley's Trichrome Stain

In the United States, the Wheatley modification of the trichrome method continues to find widespread acceptance because of its simplicity, reliability, and cost-effectiveness. Details of the procedure are available from a number of sources (Melvin, 1982; Price, 1994; Clinical and Laboratory Standards Institute, 2005; Garcia, 2010). Appropriate specimens include those that have been fixed in Schaudinn's fixative or PVA fixative; SAF- or MIF-preserved specimens may be stained with trichrome, but results are less satisfactory.

Iron Hematoxylin Stain

Iron hematoxylin stains are technically more difficult to perform than the trichrome stain, but results generally are superior owing to enhanced definition of key nuclear and cytoplasmic characteristics (Price, 1994). A modified iron hematoxylin stain that may prove useful incorporates carbol fuchsin, allowing concurrent staining of acid-fast organisms such as *Cryptosporidium*, *Cyclospora*, and *Cystoisospora* (Palmer, 1991; Clinical and Laboratory Standards Institute, 2005). Specimens fixed in Schaudinn's, PVA, or SAF fixative may be stained with iron hematoxylin stains (the preferred stain for SAF).

Modified Acid-Fast Stains

Oocysts of *Cryptosporidium*, *Cyclospora*, and *Cystoisospora* are difficult to recognize on trichrome- or iron hematoxylin–stained smears, but their presence may be detected by using an acid-fast staining technique such as the modified Kinyoun method, modified acid-fast dimethyl sulfoxide, or auramine-O (Ma, 1983; Bronsdon, 1984; Current, 1991; Clinical and Laboratory Standards Institute, 2005). Acid-fast stains are sensitive and cost-effective for detection of these protozoa, but they lack specificity. Close attention must be paid to defined morphologic criteria when these stains are used, and the use of positive control material is mandatory. For laboratories in which *Cryptosporidium* is rarely encountered, use of the highly specific and sensitive commercially available immunoassay reagents is recommended. Stool, sputa, biliary tract, and other appropriate specimens that are fresh, formalin-fixed, or SAF-fixed may be used with acid-fast stains.

Stains for Microsporidia

Microsporidia (specifically *Enterocytozoon bieneusi* and *Encephalitozoon intestinalis*, along with a number of other species) have been implicated as common agents of diarrheal disease, especially in immunocompromised patients, although their detection has been problematic. Although biopsy and electron microscopy have been mainstays in their diagnosis, staining procedures that may be performed in the clinical laboratory have been described. A modified trichrome stain using an increased (10-fold) concentration of chromotrope 2R combined with an increase in staining time has gained acceptance as a specific test for the identification of microsporidial spores (Weber, 1992, 1994; Murray, 2007). Fluorescent staining methods using optical whitening agents such as Uvitek-2B and Calcofluor white are also useful for rapid and sensitive screening of stool and other clinical specimens for such spores (van Gool, 1993; DeGirolami, 1995; Didier, 1995; Luna, 1995). The small size (1.5–3 μm) of these organisms makes their detection difficult, and such studies should not be undertaken without appropriate control materials for comparison.

Additional Techniques for Examination of Enteric Parasites

Cellulose Tape Technique for Pinworms

The female pinworm, *Enterobius vermicularis*, migrates from the cecum to the perianal skin, where she deposits typical eggs that are fully embryonated. The eggs or, occasionally, adult worms may be detected on examination of clear, adhesive cellophane tape or commercial collection kits that have been pressed on to the perianal skin. Eggs or adults are rarely found in stool, which is considered to be an inappropriate specimen for detection of this parasite. Specimens should be collected late at night, when the worms are most active, or first thing in the morning before bathing or defecation. Several specimens taken on different days should be examined before infection is ruled out.

Egg Studies

Estimation of worm burden occasionally is requested to assist in the evaluation of therapeutic efficacy or in following rates of reinfection with intestinal nematodes (*Ascaris*, *Trichuris*, and hookworms) or, occasionally, schistosomes. Procedures include the direct smear method of Beaver, the Stoll dilution egg count, Kato's thick smear, and various modifications (Beaver, 1984; Ash, 1987; Clinical and Laboratory Standards Institute, 2005). Large variations in results are inherent when these tests are performed, and levels of egg counts indicating clinical significance vary, depending on the infecting species and the person's age and nutritional status (Beaver, 1984).

Egg hatching methods have been used in the analysis of schistosomiasis to detect presence of eggs in light infections and to determine their viability. Schistosome eggs, which are fully embryonated when passed, contain a miracidium that hatches within several hours when eggs are placed in dechlorinated water. In practice, urine or stool is mixed in about 10 volumes of water, which is then placed in a sidearm or Erlenmeyer flask. All but the sidearm or the top of the flask is covered with foil wrap, and the unit is placed under a desk lamp. Hatched miracidia are positively phototropic and congregate near the light. Eggs, if available, may be examined directly for viability by examining for movement of cilia within flame (excretory) cells (Clinical and Laboratory Standards Institute, 2005).

Nematode Culture and Recovery Techniques

Several culture techniques (coproculture) assist in the detection and identification of certain nematode infections, including the Harada-Mori filter paper strip culture, filter paper/slant culture, and charcoal culture (Beaver, 1984; Ash, 1987; Clinical and Laboratory Standards Institute, 2005; Garcia, 2007). Differentiation of hookworms and trichostrongyles on the basis of egg morphology is difficult, whereas infective stage larvae are more readily identified. Such culture techniques may also prove useful in recovery of *Strongyloides* larvae, which may be few in number, and in differentiating them from those of hookworms. With all culture methods, feces are incubated in a humid environment to encourage egg hatching. With the Harada-Mori and filter paper/slant techniques, larvae migrate from the feces into a water phase, where they may be readily detected. In the charcoal culture, larvae first migrate into a dampened gauze pad, which is then placed in water, allowing the larvae to settle out.

The Baermann funnel technique is a sensitive and reliable method for recovery of *Strongyloides* and other nematode larvae from a stool specimen. In this assay, feces are placed on several layers of gauze on top of a wire screen that is suspended in a funnel. The bottom of the funnel is clamped off, and water is added to the level of the gauze. Larvae actively migrate through the gauze and settle to the bottom of the funnel, where they may be drawn off for examination. Larval recovery may be improved over that of culture techniques because a larger quantity of feces is examined. In latent *Strongyloides* infection, in which few larvae are being shed, several examinations over a week's time may be required to detect the infection (Ash, 1987; Garcia, 2007).

Objects Resembling Enteric Parasites

A large variety of objects that closely resemble various parasite life cycle stages may be seen in feces and other specimens sent for O&P examination. Careful differentiation of these objects from real parasites is necessary to prevent inappropriate or unnecessary treatment. White blood cells, macrophages, and squamous and columnar epithelial cells may resemble amebae; yeasts and starch granules may resemble protozoal cysts; pollen and fungal conidia may resemble helminth eggs; plant fibers may resemble nematode larvae; and pieces of vegetables or vegetable skins may resemble adult worms or proglottids (Table 62-4). Examples of artifacts and pseudoparasites have been reviewed elsewhere (Ash, 2007; Clinical and Laboratory Standards Institute, 2005; Garcia, 2007, 2010).

TABLE 62-4
Objects Recoverable from Stool That Resemble Enteric Parasites

Type of artifact	Resemblance
Neutrophils	*Entamoeba histolytica* cysts
Macrophages	*Entamoeba histolytica* trophozoites
Columnar epithelial cells	Amebic trophozoites
Squamous epithelial cells	Amebic trophozoites
Yeasts	Protozoan cysts (especially *Endolimax nana*)
Fungal conidia	Helminth eggs
Mushroom spores	Helminth eggs
Plant cells	Protozoan cysts, helminth eggs
Plant hairs	Nematode larvae
Pollen grains	Helminth eggs (*Ascaris* or *Taenia*)
Diatoms	Helminth eggs
Starch granules, fat globules, air bubbles, mucus	Protozoan cysts
Ingested mite eggs	Helminth eggs
Ingested plant nematode eggs	Helminth eggs
Ingested plant nematode larvae	Nematode larvae

Adapted from Garcia LS, editor. Clinical microbiology procedures handbook. Vols. 1, 2, and 3, 3rd ed. Washington, DC: American Society for Microbiology; 2010.

EXAMINATION OF UROGENITAL AND OTHER SPECIMENS (SPUTA, ASPIRATES, BIOPSIES)

Vaginal and urethral discharges, prostatic secretions, or urine may be submitted to the laboratory for detection of *Trichomonas vaginalis*. The most rapid and cost-effective method is the preparation of several wet mounts using a drop of specimen (urine should be centrifuged) diluted with a drop of saline, which is then covered with a coverslip. The slide is examined under the low-power (10×) objective using reduced lighting conditions for motile trophozoites, which display a jerky movement. High-power examination may reveal the beating flagella and the undulating membrane characteristic of the species. Use of culture, fluorescent antibody reagents, or a commercial DNA probe technique improves sensitivity, if needed (Briselden, 1994). Demonstration of imidazole drug resistance requires culture of the organism (Meri, 2000).

A number of protozoal and helminthic parasites may be detected in sputa, and the appropriate examination technique depends on the suspected organism. Generally, the technique required to detect a parasite from its usual site of infection is applied to sputum and most commonly involves a wet mount. When amebae are suspected, permanent stains should be performed. Acid-fast or specific antibody-based stains are appropriate for *Cryptosporidium*, whereas modified trichrome or fluorochrome stains should be used for detection of spores of microsporidia. Identification techniques for *Pneumocystis jiroveci* (formerly *Pneumocystis carinii*) are described elsewhere.

Examination of aspirates requires the use of stains as appropriate for the implicated organism. In addition to the methods used for sputum, Giemsa staining is often appropriate when examining for protozoa, especially the hemoflagellates. Biopsy material should be submitted for routine histology after imprint smears are prepared for staining with Giemsa or other appropriate permanent stain. Culture for leishmanias and trypanosomes also can be performed on tissues and may be important for demonstrating those infections. Skin biopsies sent for *Onchocerca* or *Mansonella* examination should be teased apart in saline and the saline examined after 30–60 minutes for microfilariae. Muscle biopsy specimens for *Trichinella spiralis* larvae may be examined by compressing the fresh specimen between two glass slides or by submitting it for routine histology. Likewise, rectal or bladder biopsies may be examined for schistosome eggs.

PARASITE CULTURE TECHNIQUES

Culture methods have been described for a wide variety of protozoan parasites, but few clinical laboratories undertake the task because of infrequent requests and lack of familiarity with methods. When culture requests are made, they are usually for *T. vaginalis*, *Leishmania* spp., *Trypanosoma cruzi*, *E. histolytica*, *Acanthamoeba* spp., or *Naegleria fowleri*. In addition, virology laboratories are occasionally asked to culture for *T. gondii*. Methods are reviewed elsewhere (Ash, 1987; Fritsche, 1989a; Clinical and Laboratory Standards Institute, 2005; Garcia, 2007, 2010; Murray, 2007).

IMMUNODIAGNOSTIC METHODS

Several immunodiagnostic methods are available to identify the parasitic antigen or the antibody that is produced in response to the parasitic infection. Some signals are amplified, and others are direct detection methods. In general, laboratory methods employed are enzyme immunoassay (EIA), indirect immunofluorescence assay (IFA), direct fluorescence antibody assay (DFA), Western blot, radioimmunoassay, and immunodiffusion, among others.

Antigen Detection

Antigen detection methods are commercially available for several parasitic diseases, including amebiasis, cryptosporidiosis, giardiasis, malaria, and trichomoniasis (Table 62-5); these methods may be useful for initial testing or in those instances in which traditional tests are negative, yet a high index of clinical suspicion remains. These tests offer the advantage of detecting current infection and can often be performed by someone other than an experienced morphologist (Wilson, 1995; Garcia, 2010).

Antigen detection in stool samples is usually performed using fecal immunoassays. A number of published studies have suggested that these assays have good sensitivity and specificity when compared with routine

TABLE 62-5
Sources of Some Antigen-Based Detection Assays for Parasites

Analyte	Test system	Manufacturer/distributor	Format
Cryptosporidium spp.	Xpect *Cryptosporidium*	Remel	Cartridge
	Cryptosporidium	Inverness Medical	EIA
	Crypto Cel	CeLLabs	IFA
	ProSpecT *Cryptosporidium*	Remel	EIA
	Cryptosporidium II	TECHLAB	EIA
	PARA-TECT *Cryptosporidium*	Medical Chemical Co.	EIA
Giardia lamblia	ProSpecT *Giardia* EZ	Remel	Cartridge
	Giardia Cel	CeLLabs	IFA
	Xpect GIARDIA	Remel	Cartridge
	ProSpecT *Giardia*	Remel	EIA
	PARA-TECT *Giardia*	Medical Chemical Co.	EIA
	GIARDIA II	TECHLAB	EIA
	GiardEIA	Antibodies Inc	EIA
	Giardia CELISA	CeLLabs	EIA
	Giardia lamblia II	Inverness Medical	EIA
Entamoeba histolytica	*E. histolytica*	Inverness Medical	EIA
	Entamoeba CELISA PATH	CeLLabs	EIA
	E. histolytica II	TECHLAB	EIA
Cryptosporidium/Giardia	Xpect *Giardia/Cryptosporidium*	Remel	Cartridge
	Immunocard STAT *Cryptosporidium/Giardia*	Meridian Bioscience	Cartridge
	MERIFLUOR *Cryptosporidium/Giardia*	Meridian Bioscience	IFA
	Crypto Giardia DFA	IVD Research Inc.	IFA
	Crypto/Giardia Cel	CeLLabs	IFA
	PARA-TECT *Cryptosporidium/Giardia* DFA	Medical Chemical Co.	IFA
	ColorPAC *Giardia/Cryptosporidium*	Becton Dickinson	Cartridge
	Giardia/Cryptosporidium CHEK	TECHLAB	EIA
	ProSpecT *Giardia/Cryptosporidium*	Remel	EIA
G. lamblia, C. parvum, and *E. histolytica/dispar* combination	Biosite Triage Parasite Panel	Biosite Diagnostics	Cartridge
Plasmodium spp.	BinaxNOW Malaria	Inverness Medical	Cartridge
	OptiMAL	DiaMed	Dipstick
	Paracheck Pf	Orchid	Cartridge
	Rapimal MT Pf	CeLLabs	Dipstick
Wuchereria bancrofti	BinaxNOW Filariasis	Inverness Medical	Cartridge
Trichomonas vaginalis	Light Diagnostic *T. vaginalis*	Chemicon	DFA
	OSOM *Trichomonas* Rapid Test	Genzyme	Dipstick
	XenoStrip-Tv	Xenotope Diagnostics	Cartridge

Cartridge, Lateral flow cartridge; *DFA,* direct fluorescence antibody assay; *EIA,* enzyme immunoassay; *Dipstick,* dipstick enzyme immunoassay; *IFA,* indirect immunofluorescence assay.

ova and parasite examination (Aldeen, 1995; Kehl, 1995; Zimmerman, 1995; Maraha, 2000; Hanson, 2001; Garcia, 2007). These immunoassays are easy to use and rapid, permit batch processing, and do not require experienced microscopists. Given the current shortage of medical technologists and individuals with specialized training in parasitology, use of immunoassays appears to be an attractive alternative. However, laboratories that use rapid immunoassays should be aware of potential problems with false-positive results and should closely monitor test performance. Currently, fecal immunoassays are marketed for *G. lamblia*, *C. parvum/C. hominis*, the *E. histolytica/E. dispar* group, and *E. histolytica*. Antigen detection tests using blood or serum are also available for *Plasmodium* spp. and *W. bancrofti*. A latex agglutination test for *T. vaginalis* antigen detection in vaginal swabs has also been introduced. Additional commercially manufactured kits are under development for detection of *Dientamoeba fragilis* and the microsporidia. Immunoassays are usually available in three formats: EIA, DFA, and lateral flow (immunochromatography) cartridges. Fresh or preserved stool samples are appropriate for most antigen detection kits (Fedorko, 2000). Although each kit has unique operating characteristics, most are generally comparable in performance (Garcia, 2000, 2007; Katanik, 2001).

Rapid antigen detection methods developed for malaria may detect histidine-rich protein II (HRP-II), parasite lactate dehydrogenase (pLDH), or both, in peripheral blood. HRP-II tests are specific for *Plasmodium falciparum*, and pLDH tests detect all four *Plasmodium* spp. Sensitivities of these assays are comparable with, or lower than, traditional microscopic examination, but sensitivities greater than 90% have been reported. One of these tests is currently approved by the Food and Drug Administration for clinical diagnosis of malaria in the United States (Murray, 2009).

T. vaginalis antigens from vaginal samples may also be detected using rapid antigen tests. These tests can be used for rapid detection of *T. vaginalis* infection in the clinic setting and may replace wet mount examinations, which generally have lower sensitivities, depending on the proficiency of the personnel performing the microscopic examination. Miller and colleagues demonstrated that the *T. vaginalis* rapid antigen test had sensitivities comparable with those of culture (Miller, 2003).

Most EIAs are available in microwell format. Antigens from frozen, fresh, or 10% formalin–preserved stool samples are suitable for testing by this method. Concentrated or PVA samples are not suitable for testing with EIA kits. Parasite antigen is captured by immobilized antibodies coated on microwells and is detected by an enzyme-conjugated secondary antibody that is capable of producing a colored reaction following the addition of substrate. Although the colored wells can be read visually or with the use of a spectrometer, the latter seems to be the preferred option because of occasional ambiguous results obtained with some kits (Kehl, 1995). In general, EIA tests have good sensitivities and specificities. Garcia and colleagues evaluated nine immunoassay kits for detection of *G. lamblia* and *Cryptosporidium* spp. in comparison with a reference DFA test that visualizes the parasite directly in the sample; investigators found that all kits had high sensitivities, ranging from 94% to 99%, and 100% specificities (Garcia, 1997, 2007). However, published reports have suggested that occasional problems are found with some EIA kits that may produce false-positive results; these problems have led to their recall (Doing, 1999). Hence, a strong quality control (QC) program and participation in proficiency test programs are required to ensure high-quality test results. Local epidemiology of the parasitic infection can help to determine whether additional confirmatory testing is required; consultation with local public health authorities may prove useful in characterizing which infections are being seen locally. Additionally for some diseases such as giardiasis, examination of two specimens by EIA or microscopy may be necessary to achieve diagnostic sensitivity greater than 90% (Hanson, 2001).

Lateral flow cartridges are a popular format of immunoassay because of their ease of use and the minimal performance time required. These kits can be stored conveniently at room temperature and may be used in single or batch processing. The parasite antigen in the sample migrates through the membrane and binds to specific capture antibodies; use of a secondary reagent results in development of a colored reaction. These kits also have an internal control to ensure that the colloidal dye conjugates used in the assay are intact and that proper capillary flow has occurred. To ensure complete migration of the specimen, only the supernatant of a well-mixed stool sample is used, and some samples may be diluted to a liquid state before testing. Any color visible at the reagent test zone (usually a band) is interpreted as positive. Some studies have demonstrated that cartridge assays are somewhat less sensitive than a microwell EIA plate assay (Pillai, 1999; Johnston, 2003). When lack of sensitivity is a concern, it may be necessary to perform alternative O&P studies if patients' symptoms persist.

DFA testing allows direct visualization of the parasites in stool specimen using antibodies conjugated to fluorescent dyes. These assays are easy to perform and to interpret, permitting rapid screening of slides when compared with some of the traditional stains used in parasitology (Zimmerman, 1995; Garcia, 2007). A fluorescence microscope is necessary for this procedure, and this is a limiting factor in some laboratories. Currently, kits are available for detection of cysts of *G. lamblia* and oocysts of *Cryptosporidium* spp. Fixed stool specimens may be used for this procedure (10% formalin, SAF, or one of the mercury- or formalin-free products; Fedorko, 2000). Although fresh stool samples can be tested directly, the sensitivity of the assay can be improved by performing the test on centrifuged stool (500 *g* for 10 minutes). Occasionally, fluorescing bacteria and yeasts may be seen, but these are readily distinguished from *Giardia* and *Cryptosporidium* on the basis of their size and shape. The edges of the wells should be carefully examined to avoid missing the rare parasite in light infections. Given the recent recognition of additional *Cryptosporidium* spp. that may infect humans, studies related to specificity of the various immunoassays are needed to determine actual sensitivity in detecting any *Cryptosporidium* infection (Graczyk, 1996; Coupe, 2005).

Serologic Diagnosis

Tests that are available from public health, hospital, or commercial laboratories to detect immunologic reactivity to parasitic diseases are summarized in Table 62-6. Historically, serologic procedures for parasitic diseases have been plagued by low sensitivity and specificity, primarily owing to the complex antigenic nature of parasites and the possibilities for cross-reactions from related species. The introduction of newer test methods combined with the use of more highly defined antigenic components is providing more accurate results with greater predictive values. Many of the newer tests use the EIA or immunoblot (Western blot) format, although IFA, indirect hemagglutination (IHA), complement fixation (CF), and bentonite flocculation (BF) methods remain popular.

Serologic diagnosis of parasitic infection is used as an adjunct to the usual diagnostic modalities or in special situations where identification of the parasite itself or its antigen or nucleic acid from host tissue or excreta is not possible. Parasitic infections such as toxoplasmosis and toxocariasis reside in deep tissues and cannot be readily diagnosed by morphologic means; others such as cysticercosis and echinococcosis develop in organs, where invasive studies that may be required are not recommended in the initial patient evaluation. Other conditions such as filariasis,

TABLE 62-6
Examples of Serologic Assays for Parasites Available from Reference Laboratories

Disease	Organism	Specimen type	Assay
Amebiasis	*Entamoeba histolytica*	Serum	EIA, ID, IHA
Babesiosis	*Babesia microti, Babesia* sp. WA1	Serum	IFA
Chagas'	*Trypanosoma cruzi*	Serum	IFA, EIA, CF
Cysticercosis	*Taenia solium*	Serum, CSF	EIA, IB
Echinococcosis	*Echinococcus granulosus*	Serum	EIA, IB, IHA, IFA
Fascioliasis	*Fasciola hepatica*	Serum	EIA, IB
Filariasis	*Wuchereria bancrofti*	Serum	EIA
Leishmaniasis	*Leishmania braziliensis, Leishmania donovani, Leishmania tropica*	Serum	IFA, EIA, CF
Malaria	*Plasmodium* spp.	Serum	IFA
Paragonimiasis	*Paragonimus westermani*	Serum	EIA, IB
Schistosomiasis	*Schistosoma* spp.	Serum	EIA, IB
Strongyloidiasis	*Strongyloides stercoralis*	Serum	EIA
Toxoplasmosis	*Toxoplasma gondii*	CSF, serum	IFA, EIA
Trichinellosis	*Trichinella spiralis*	Serum	EIA, BF

BF, Bentonite flocculation; *CF,* complement fixation; *CSF,* cerebrospinal fluid; *EIA,* enzyme immunoassay; *IB,* immunoblot; *ID,* immunodiffusion; *IFA,* indirect immunofluorescence assay; *IHA,* indirect hemagglutination.

schistosomiasis, and strongyloidiasis may remain subclinical because of light infections, or because the clinical evaluation occurred during the prepatent period. Other circumstances where serologic evaluation may prove useful include diagnoses of extraintestinal amebiasis and trichinellosis. Chronic stages of trypanosomiasis are preferably diagnosed by serology. Serologic studies also help in the diagnosis of occult infections such as visceral larva migrans, cysticercosis, and filariasis. Last, serologic studies serve as a powerful tool in enhancing our understanding of the epidemiology of diseases such as schistosomiasis, toxoplasmosis, amebiasis, Chagas' disease, malaria, and babesiosis. High antibody levels are useful for diagnostic purposes if they occur in a patient with no previous exposure to the parasite and no recent history of travel to an endemic area. Unfortunately, positive antibody levels in persons living in endemic areas do not often help in the clinical diagnosis. Detection of antibodies, especially immunoglobulin (Ig)G, provides evidence of infection but may not be able to differentiate active from past exposure. In some parasitic diseases, levels of antibodies may decline slowly following successful therapy or self-cure. Serologic tests for parasitic diseases generally evaluate IgG levels, with the exception of toxoplasmosis and babesiosis, in which IgM- and IgA-specific antibodies may be helpful for determining the age of infection (National Committee for Clinical Laboratory Standards, 2004).

Because serologic tests for parasitic diseases are infrequently requested, specimens generally are submitted to public (Centers for Disease Control and Prevention [CDC]) or private reference laboratories. Some of the more commonly requested tests, especially those that are obtained as commercial kits, are often available locally, including those for toxoplasmosis, amebiasis, and trichinosis.

Many of these assays are developed in-house and hence lack correlation with universal standards. Interpretive criteria are established by reagent manufacturers or by the center performing the test, and these criteria often vary from institution to institution. Individuals requesting such tests should inquire about the performance characteristics, including sensitivity and specificity, and should be aware that cross-reactions may occur. For example, antibody tests for Chagas' disease are known to cross-react with antibodies produced in response to *Leishmania* infections. However, reactivity to homologous antigen is greater, and this test is useful in diagnosing chronic stages of the disease when parasitemia is generally low. Usually serology for chronic Chagas' disease correlates well with molecular diagnostic methods (Weinberg, 2001). Helminthic parasites are well known to cross-react in serologic assays that use crude antigen preparations because of phylogenetic, hence antigenic, similarities.

Several factors that may influence the test performance of serologic assays include disease manifestation, test format, reagents used, and

TABLE 62-7
Examples of Real-Time PCR Assays for Parasites

Parasite	Target	Specimen type
Leishmania spp.	rDNA	Whole blood
Plasmodium spp.	rDNA	Whole blood
Toxoplasma gondii	rDNA and *B1* gene	Amniotic fluid, blood, cerebrospinal fluid, tissue
Entamoeba histolytica	rDNA	Stool
Giardia lamblia	rDNA	Stool
Cryptosporidium spp.	rDNA	Stool
Cyclospora spp.	rDNA	Stool
Trichomonas vaginalis	β-Tubulin gene	Vaginal samples

PCR, Polymerase chain reaction; *rDNA*, ribosomal DNA.

parasite viability, to name a few. The sensitivity of the test is increased in patients with invasive amebiasis but may be weak in intestinal amebiasis with minimal tissue invasion, and absent for asymptomatic carriers. The type of serologic assay format may also determine the sensitivity, as in the diagnosis of toxoplasmosis (National Committee for Clinical Laboratory Standards, 2004). The double-sandwich IgM enzyme-linked immunosorbent assay (ELISA) is known to be more sensitive and specific than IgM immunofluorescence for detecting recently acquired and congenital toxoplasmosis. IHA has been the primary test for serodiagnosis of amebiasis. The sensitivity of the assay is also dependent on the type or stage of parasite antigen used, for example, the sensitivity of cutaneous leishmaniasis can be improved by using amastigote antigens in place of promastigote antigens in the IFA test. Serologic assays are also affected by parasite viability; hydatid cysts occurring in the lung and dead or calcified cysts are less frequently detected than active cysts in the liver.

MOLECULAR DIAGNOSTIC METHODS

Diagnostic methods using DNA amplification and nucleic acid probe techniques have been described for most of the common parasitic diseases and offer high levels of sensitivity and specificity (Weiss, 1995; Wilson, 1995). For more complete details on this topic, the reader is referred to a recent publication (Persing, 2011; Espy, 2006). Molecular methods offer some unique advantages such as rapid (automated) results, high sensitivity and specificity, and ability to detect and differentiate species variants—all independent of the patient's underlying immune status, which is a potentially limiting feature of serologic assays. Molecular techniques are prone to cross-contamination, however, if proper processing precautions are not strictly enforced.

Although most of these applications have remained as tools for research laboratories and are not routinely available, several polymerase chain reaction (PCR) assays have been developed for parasites such as *Plasmodium* spp., *Babesia* spp., *T. gondii*, *Leishmania* spp., *Trypanosoma* spp., *G. lamblia*, *Cryptosporidium* spp., and *T. vaginalis* (Table 62-7). Some of these assays are available in real-time format, wherein the kinetics of the nucleic acid amplification reaction is recorded and analyzed by computer algorithms to allow detection of amplicons. Over the past decade, several laboratory developed real-time PCR methods have been described for clinical diagnosis of some of these parasitic diseases (see Table 62-7). The introduction of this technology has allowed rapid detection and has avoided the fear of cross-contamination due to steps involved in postamplification analysis. PCR also presents the opportunity to monitor the success of antiparasitic therapy (Lee, 2002; Bossolasco, 2003) or to detect reactivation following therapy (Costa, 2000). Because the innate nature of molecular methods is genotypic, PCR assays have the ability to accurately detect to the species level, depending on the gene being targeted (Vallejo, 1999; Mahboudi, 2002). To date, the equipment and other resources needed, including personnel trained in molecular biology, have remained out of reach for most diagnostic laboratories because of fiscal limitations. Although a variety of commercial diagnostic kits are available for detection of viral and bacterial pathogens, only one kit has received approval for a parasite—the kit for *T. vaginalis* (Briselden, 1994). Molecular methods may prove to have great importance in the identification of parasite-harboring vectors and may contribute to disease prevention through control programs targeted to such vectors (Weiss, 1995).

QUALITY ASSURANCE, QUALITY IMPROVEMENT, AND SAFETY

A quality assurance program for the parasitology section of the laboratory is similar to that for the other laboratory sections and covers all essential aspects of the operation, including, among others, a well-written and complete procedure manual that is reviewed annually, guidelines for maintaining all specimen and test result records, a complete QC program with appropriate technical supervision and review, and participation in an approved proficiency testing program. Laboratories also need to focus on customer satisfaction, using a variety of available measures, and to participate in the team approach to identifying problems and generating solutions as part of a continuous quality improvement process (Garcia, 2007, 2010).

The performance of individuals responsible for the parasitology section should be monitored periodically with both internal and external unknown specimens, and competency assessments should be up to date, especially for those laboratories that encounter positive specimens infrequently. A variety of reference materials should be readily available for use at the laboratory bench, including positive slides and fecal specimens, printed atlases, and slide atlases.

Unpreserved specimens for parasitologic examination should be considered potentially infectious, and all blood and body fluids should be handled according to Universal Precautions as defined by the Final Rule on Blood-borne Pathogens by the Occupational Safety and Health Administration, as published in the *Federal Register.* In addition to blood-borne viral pathogens, malarial parasites and hemoflagellates may remain infective. A variety of parasites may remain infective in fresh stool specimens, including cysts of enteric protozoa; eggs of *Taenia solium*, *E. vermicularis*, and *H. nana;* and larvae of *S. stercoralis*. *Trichuris trichiura*, *Ascaris lumbricoides*, and hookworm eggs may remain infective in older specimens, and *Ascaris* eggs can survive and embryonate while in 5% formalin. Fecal specimens also may contain pathogens such as *Salmonella*, *Shigella*, or viruses. Strict observance of proper specimen handling techniques and disposal is essential. Personal attention to hand washing is also necessary. Use of ethyl acetate in place of ether in the performance of concentration techniques is strongly recommended to guard against the possibility of explosion (Truant, 1981; Clinical and Laboratory Standards Institute, 2005; Garcia, 2007, 2010).

BLOOD AND TISSUE PROTOZOA

MALARIA

Malaria (from the Italian "mal' aria," meaning "bad air") is an acute and sometimes chronic infection of the bloodstream characterized clinically by fever, anemia, and splenomegaly, and is caused by apicomplexan parasites of the genus *Plasmodium*. The defining clinical features of a malarial attack or paroxysm consist of, in order, shaking chills, fever (up to 40° C or higher), and generalized diaphoresis, followed by resolution of fever. The paroxysm occurs over 6–10 hours and is initiated by the synchronous rupture of erythrocytes with the release of new infectious blood stage forms known as merozoites. The disease generally occurs between 45° N and 40° S (World Health Organization, 1987) and is spread exclusively by female anopheline mosquitoes. The four species of plasmodia causing human malaria are *Plasmodium vivax*, *P. falciparum*, *Plasmodium malariae*, and *Plasmodium ovale*. *P. falciparum* infection occurs principally in tropical areas worldwide, whereas *P. vivax* infections occur in both tropical and temperate zones. *P. malariae* also occurs worldwide but to a much lesser extent than *P. falciparum* or *P. vivax*. *P. ovale* is the least frequent of the malarias, with most cases being acquired in western Africa, India, or South America. Recently, human infection with *P. knowlesi*, a malarial parasite of Old World monkeys, has been described in the Malay Peninsula and Borneo. These infections are potentially life threatening but are difficult to distinguish from *P. malariae* microscopically, leading to misidentification. Use of PCR has been required to make the correct differentiation (Cox-Singh, 2008).

Because infection with falciparum malaria is potentially life threatening, its presence must be considered in the differential diagnosis of unexplained fever, and history of travel in endemic geographic areas should always be sought. In an era of increasing world travel, the risk of acquiring malaria is not insignificant, and the rapid spread of drug-resistant strains poses particular problems when appropriate prophylaxis or therapy is considered.

Laboratory evaluation of patients suspected of having malaria continues to rely on timely examination of thick and thin blood films to demonstrate the intraerythrocytic parasites. Although they are straightforward in their approach, performance of these techniques may be problematic. Reliable identification of organisms requires continuous training to maintain expertise; therefore, those laboratories that rarely see positive specimens may choose to refer specimens to reference laboratories, provided that processing and reporting are timely.

More advanced laboratory methods, including acridine orange staining (see earlier under Laboratory Methods) and detection of parasite-specific DNA (Lanar, 1989; Weiss, 1995; Clinical and Laboratory Standards Institute, 2005), provide enhanced sensitivity and specificity but generally are not appropriate or available for smaller laboratories. Immunocapture assays developed for the detection of *Plasmodium*-specific lactate dehydrogenase or HRP-II appear to provide a high degree of sensitivity and specificity in the diagnosis of malaria. Several versions of these tests, configured as "dipstick" methods, are especially promising in situations where ease of performance is critical and usual laboratory facilities are lacking (Palmer, 1998; Piper, 1999; Marx, 2005; Murray, 2009).

Life Cycle

Malarial parasites undergo a sexual phase (sporogony) in *Anopheles* mosquitoes that results in the production of infectious sporozoites, as well as an asexual stage (schizogony) in humans that results in the production of schizonts and merozoites (Fig. 62-1). In the bloodstream, some merozoites eventually differentiate into gametocytes (gametogony), which, when ingested by female anopheline mosquitoes, mature into male microgametes and female macrogametes. Fusion of a microgamete and a macrogamete results in the formation of the motile ookinete, which migrates to the outside of the stomach wall and forms an oocyst. Within the oocyst, numerous spindle-shaped sporozoites are formed. The mature oocyst ruptures into the body cavity, releasing sporozoites, which then migrate

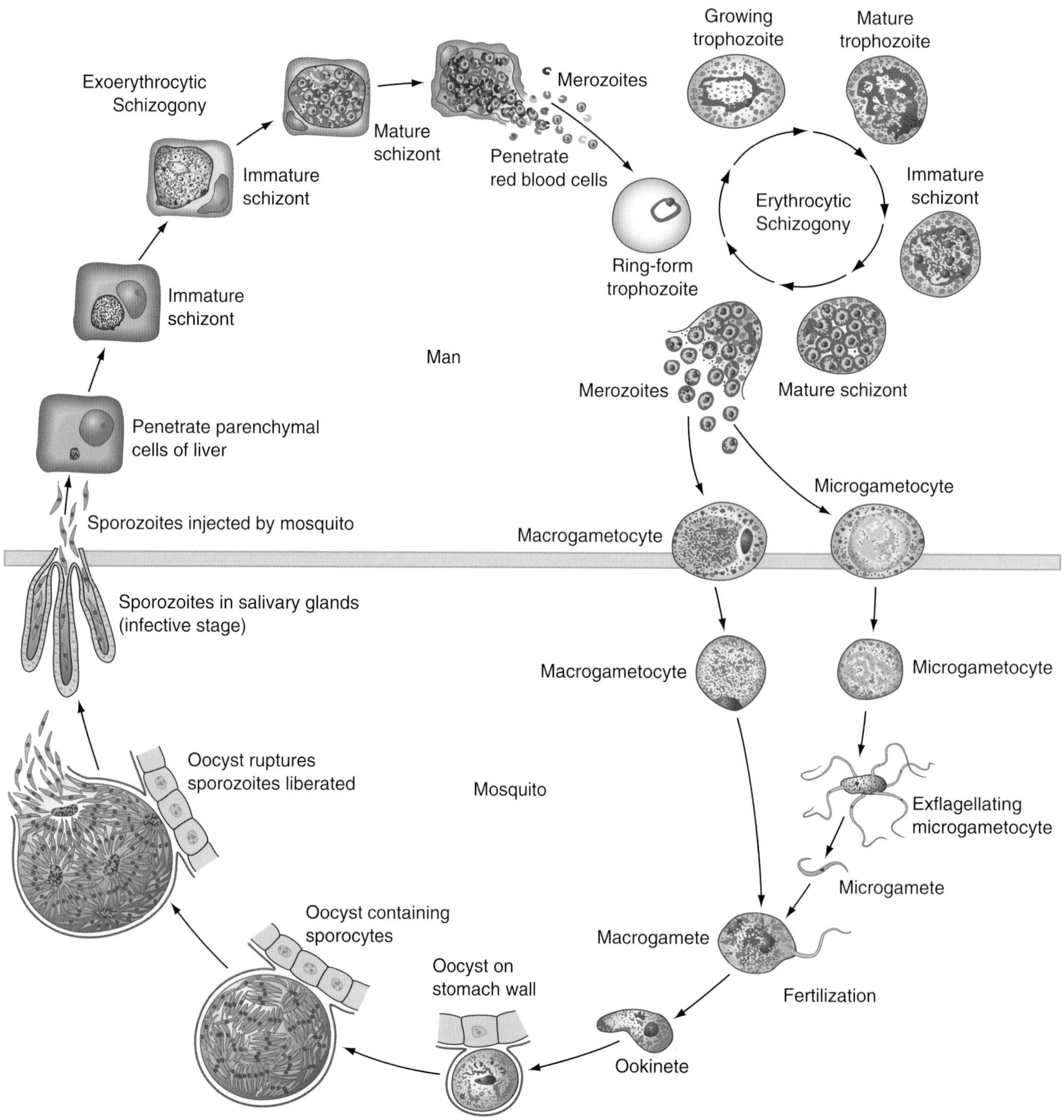

Figure 62-1 Life cycle of malarial parasites. *(Courtesy the Centers for Disease Control and Prevention, Parasitology Training Branch, Atlanta).*

through the tissues to the salivary glands, from which they are injected into the vertebrate host as the mosquito feeds. The time required for development in the mosquito ranges from 8–21 days.

Sporozoites injected into the vertebrate host reach the hepatic parenchymal cells within minutes and initiate the proliferative phase known as exoerythrocytic schizogony. Release of merozoites from ruptured hepatic schizonts initiates the bloodstream infection or erythrocytic schizogony and, eventually, the clinical symptoms of malaria. *P. vivax* and *P. ovale* differ from *P. falciparum* and *P. malariae* in that true disease relapses of the former species may occur weeks to months following subsidence of previous attacks. This occurs as a result of renewed exoerythrocytic and, eventually, erythrocytic schizogony from latent hepatic sporozoites, which are known as hypnozoites (Krotoski, 1982). Recurrences of disease due to *P. falciparum* or *P. malariae*, called recrudescences, arise from increased numbers of persisting blood stage forms to clinically detectable levels, not from persisting liver stage forms. Liver cells are infected only by sporozoites from the mosquito; thus, transfusion-acquired *P. vivax* or *P. ovale* infection does not relapse.

Merozoites released from infected hepatocytes subsequently infect erythrocytes. Following amplification of parasites in the bloodstream for a period of time and the development of synchrony in their appearance, clinical attacks of malaria occur. *P. vivax* and *P. ovale* parasites primarily infect young erythrocytes, whereas *P. malariae* infects older erythrocytes and *P. falciparum* infects erythrocytes of all ages.

Morphologic stages seen in erythrocytes include trophozoites (growing forms), schizonts (dividing forms), and gametocytes (sexual forms) (Figs. 62-2 through 62-5). The youngest trophozoites have a globose shape with a central vacuole, a red chromatin mass, and blue cytoplasm. On stained blood films, early trophozoites resemble signet rings and generally are referred to as rings or ring forms. Growing trophozoites beyond the ring stage retain a single chromatin mass but have more abundant cytoplasm, which may appear compact or may be ameboid (irregular). Mature trophozoites still have only one chromatin mass but an increased amount of cytoplasm that partially fills the erythrocyte. Hemozoin (hematin) pigment, a breakdown product of hemoglobin, is characteristic of all erythrocytes containing mature stages of malarial parasites but is not evident in ring forms. Immature schizonts have two or more chromatin masses and undivided cytoplasm, whereas mature schizonts have both cytoplasm and chromatin completely divided, so that individual merozoites are evident. The mature schizont ruptures the erythrocyte, releasing merozoites and initiating a new cycle of infection. The erythrocytic cycle takes approximately 48 hours (tertian periodicity) for *P. falciparum*, *P. ovale*, and *P. vivax* infections, and 72 hours (quartan periodicity) for *P. malariae* infection. At some point during the infection, a subpopulation of merozoites develops into gametocytes. Those of *P. vivax*, *P. malariae*, and *P. ovale* are rounded, whereas those of *P. falciparum* are elongate (sausage-shaped). Macrogametocytes (female) characteristically have a compact chromatin mass, whereas microgametocytes (male) have chromatin that is more dispersed. Developing gametocytes are more compact than growing trophozoites.

Epidemiology

Endemic transmission of malaria requires a reservoir of infection, an appropriate mosquito vector, and a susceptible host. Control of malaria is directed at elimination of mosquito hosts, treatment of active cases, and prophylaxis of susceptible persons. However, emergence of mosquitoes resistant to insecticides, development of resistance to prophylaxis and therapy by *P. falciparum* and, more recently, *P. vivax* (Murphy, 1993; Garcia, 2007), and lack of adequate funding have made control difficult in many areas.

Individuals with sickle cell trait are less susceptible to *P. falciparum* malaria, and persons who lack certain Duffy blood group determinants are protected against *P. vivax* infection (Miller, 1976). Glucose-6-phosphate dehydrogenase (G6PD) deficiency has been associated with protection from malaria, but evidence is less striking than with these other genetic abnormalities.

Transfusion-induced malaria may occur when blood donors have subclinical malaria and may prove fatal for the recipient. Similarly, congenital malaria may occur in infants born to mothers from endemic areas. The infant acquires the infection at birth as a result of rupture of placental blood vessels with maternal–fetal transfusion. Neither transfusion nor congenital malaria is expected to relapse because exoerythrocytic schizogony does not occur. The number of civilian cases of malaria reported in the United States increased from 151 in 1970 to 1838 in 1980 but dropped to 1411 in 1993 (Centers for Disease Control and Prevention, 1988, 1993). Species causing infection in 1987 were *P. vivax* (44%), *P. falciparum* (43%), *P. malariae* (4%), *P. ovale* (3%), and undetermined (6%). The interval between arrival in the United States and onset of illness was less than 1 month for 25% of *P. vivax* and 80% of *P. falciparum* cases. Only 3% of patients became ill more than 1 year after arrival. U.S. citizens acquired the infection in Africa (63%), Asia (18%), the Western Hemisphere (14%), or Oceania (4%).

Clinical Disease

Most patients who develop *P. falciparum* infection become symptomatic within 1 month of exposure, whereas a delay of up to 6 months or more may be seen with the other *Plasmodium* species. Common presenting symptoms of malaria include chills and fever, which often are associated with splenomegaly. In the early stages of the disease, febrile episodes occur irregularly but eventually become more synchronous, assuming the usual tertian (*P. vivax*, *P. falciparum*, and *P. ovale*) or quartan (*P. malariae*) periodicity. Patients with malaria may develop anemia and may have other manifestations, including diarrhea, abdominal pain, headache, and muscle aches and pains. *P. falciparum* malaria can result in high rates (50%) of parasitemia, which can lead to severe hemolysis with hemoglobinuria and profound anemia. Erythrocytes infected with growing trophozoites and schizonts of *P. falciparum* become sequestered in small vessels of the body, and this may lead to occlusion of these vessels, causing symptoms related to capillary obstruction and tissue anoxia. Involvement of the brain is known as cerebral malaria, in which the patient becomes disoriented, progressing to delirium, coma, and often death. Exchange transfusion may be lifesaving in severe cases of *P. falciparum* infection (Nielson, 1979; Powell, 2002).

The course of untreated malaria depends on the species. Most fatal cases of malaria are due to *P. falciparum*. In nonfatal cases, the febrile paroxysms become less severe with time and the disease gradually subsides. Patients with *P. vivax* or *P. ovale* infection may have relapses after many months or, occasionally, years. Persons with *P. falciparum* and *P. malariae* infection may have symptom-free periods but suffer from sporadic recrudescences owing to persisting low-grade parasitemia. Relapses and recrudescences may be associated with changes in the host's defense mechanisms or possibly with antigenic changes in the infecting organisms.

Peripheral smears may show leukocytes that contain malaria pigment. Increased reticulocyte counts occur commonly and are associated with rapid erythrocyte turnover. The presence of greatly enlarged platelets may be noted on peripheral blood films and may occur as a result of their rapid turnover secondary to splenic sequestration. Malarial infection may interfere with certain serologic tests, producing false-positive results, especially those for syphilis.

Therapy and prophylaxis of malaria have become highly complex topics because of the widespread appearance of resistance by *P. falciparum* to chloroquine and other antimalarials and, to a lesser extent, resistance by *P. vivax* to chloroquine. Also, persons who have acquired *P. vivax* or *P. ovale* malaria, or who have spent extended time in areas highly endemic for these parasites, require treatment with primaquine to eradicate hepatic hypnozoites and to prevent relapse. Use of primaquine may be dangerous in patients who have G6PD deficiency, and screening of at-risk patients before therapy is initiated may be necessary.

Diagnosis

Malaria should be included in the differential diagnosis of fever in patients who have a history of travel to or residence in endemic areas, drug addiction, or blood transfusion. Diagnosis usually is established by demonstrating parasites in thick and thin blood films. Blood specimens ideally are collected just before the next anticipated fever spike or at the onset of fever. Specimens drawn several hours apart sometimes may be required to demonstrate infection or to diagnose the species, because the number and morphologic stage of parasites vary during the cycle. Careful examination of thick films should reveal the presence of the parasites in almost all patients with clinically apparent malaria.

Identification of malarial parasites on thin blood films requires a systematic approach. Three major factors should be considered: appearance of infected erythrocytes, appearance of parasites, and stages found. Table 62-8 summarizes diagnostic characteristics of the species, which are illustrated in Figures 62-2 to 62-5. Erythrocytes infected by *P. vivax* or *P. ovale* parasites often appear enlarged compared with adjacent, uninfected cells, whereas *P. malariae* and *P. falciparum* parasites are usually found in erythrocytes of normal size. In all, 20% or more of erythrocytes infected with *P. ovale* are often oval or fimbriated (having irregular projections of the cell margins), whereas less than 6% of erythrocytes infected with *P. vivax* are oval. Schüffner's stippling, noted as numerous small uniform pink granules

Text continued on page 1204

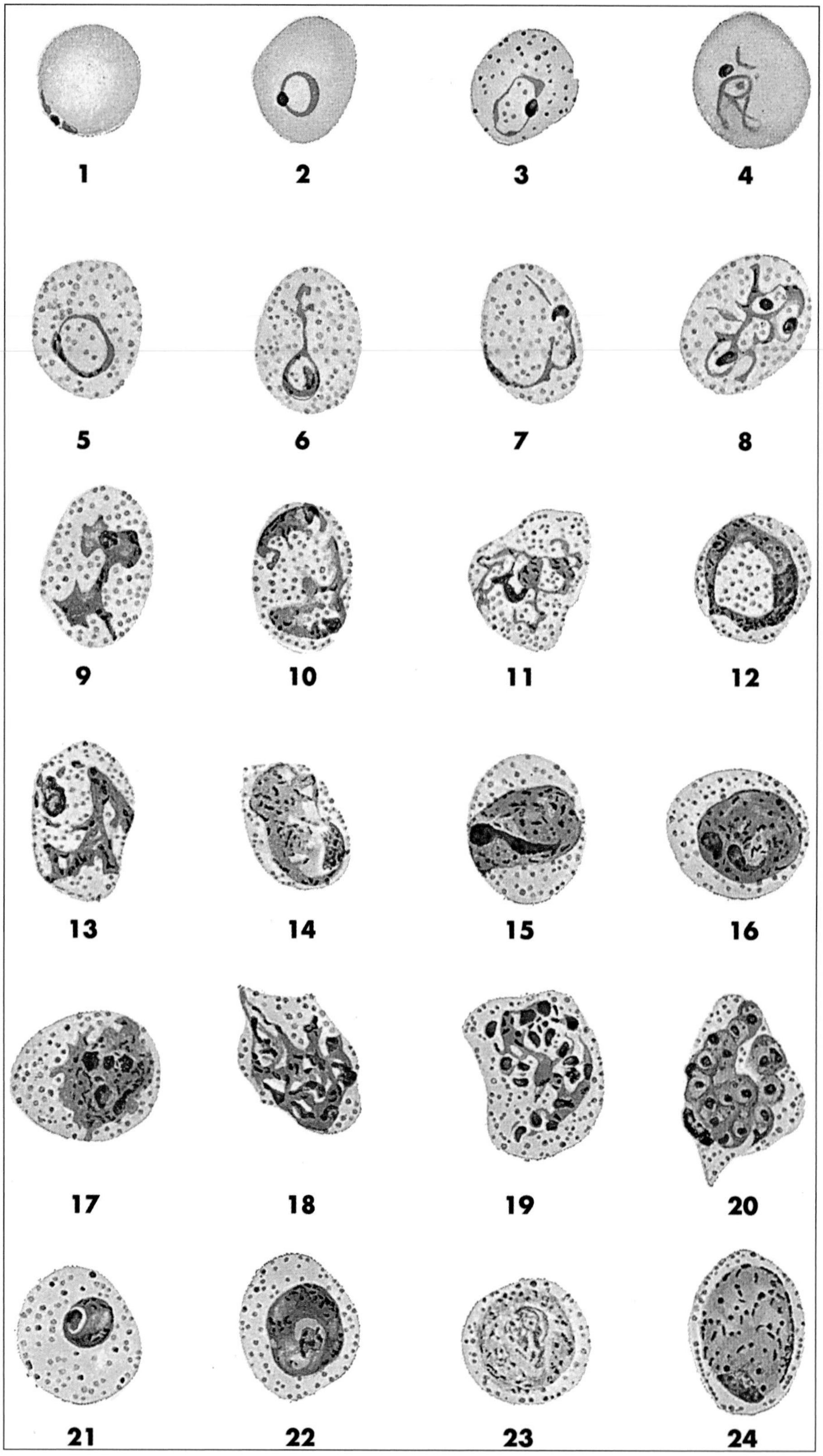

Figure 62-2 *Plasmodium vivax. 1,* Normal-size erythrocyte with marginal ring form trophozoite. *2,* Young signet ring form of trophozoite in macrocyte. *3,* Slightly older ring form trophozoite in erythrocyte showing basophilic stippling. *4,* Polychromatophilic erythrocyte containing young tertian parasite with pseudopodia. *5,* Ring form of trophozoite showing pigment in cytoplasm of an enlarged cell containing Schüffner's stippling. This stippling does not appear in all cells containing the growing and older forms of *Plasmodium vivax,* but it can be found with any stage from the fairly young ring form onward. *6* and *7,* Very tenuous medium trophozoite forms. *8,* Three ameboid trophozoites with fused cytoplasm. *9–13,* Older ameboid trophozoites in process of development. *10,* Two ameboid trophozoites in one cell. *14,* Mature trophozoite. *15,* Mature trophozoite with chromatin apparently in process of division. *16–19,* Schizonts showing progressive steps in division (presegmenting schizonts). *20,* Mature schizont. *21* and *22,* Developing gametocytes. *23,* Mature microgametocyte. *24,* Mature macrogametocyte. *(From Wilcox A. Manual for the microscopical diagnosis of malaria in man. Bulletin No. 180. Bethesda, Md.: National Institute of Health; 1942.)*

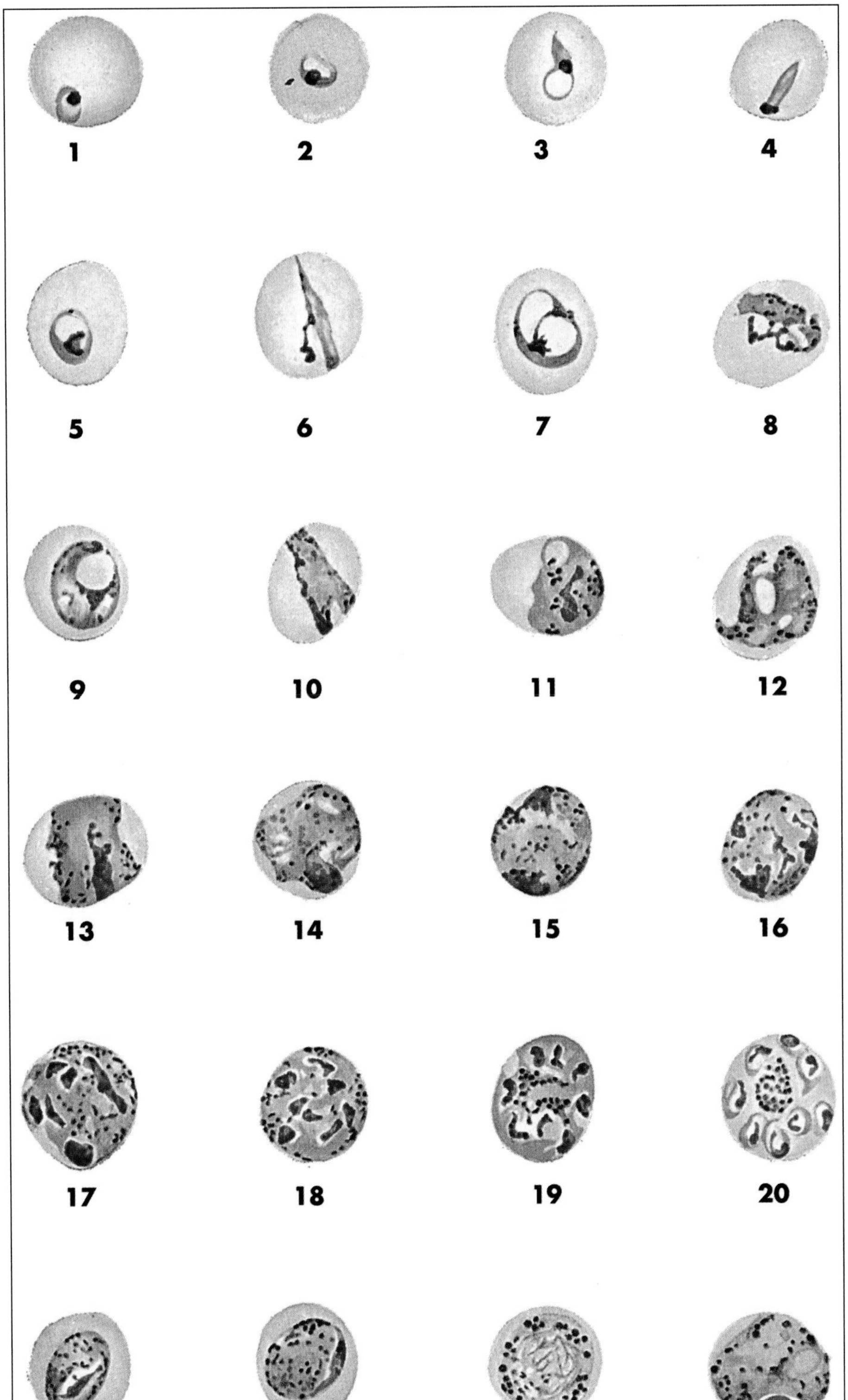

Figure 62-3 *Plasmodium malariae. 1,* Young ring form trophozoite of quartan malaria. *2–4,* Young trophozoite forms of the parasite showing gradual increase in chromatin and cytoplasm. *5,* Developing ring form of trophozoite showing pigment granule. *6,* Early band form of trophozoite—elongate chromatin, some pigment apparent. *7–12,* Some forms that the developing trophozoite of quartan malaria may take. *13* and *14,* Mature trophozoites—one a band form. *15–19,* Phases in the development of the schizont (presegmenting schizonts). *20,* Mature schizont. *21,* Immature microgametocyte. *22,* Immature macrogametocyte. *23,* Mature microgametocyte. *24,* Mature macrogametocyte. *(From Wilcox A. Manual for the microscopical diagnosis of malaria in man. Bulletin No. 180. Bethesda, Md.: National Institute of Health; 1942.)*

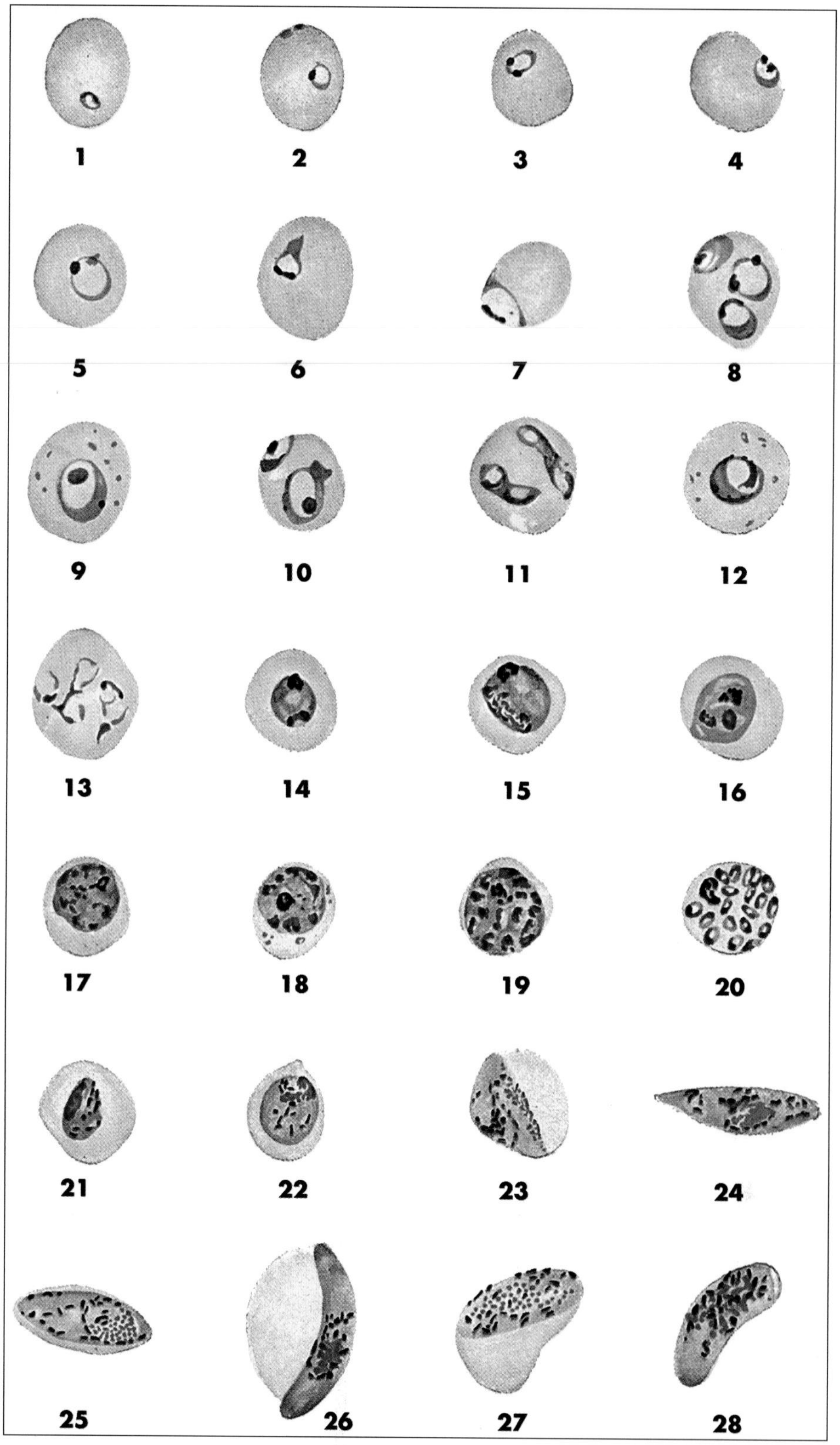

Figure 62-4 *Plasmodium falciparum. 1,* Very young ring form of trophozoite. *2,* Double infection of single cell with young trophozoites—one a "marginal form," the other a "signet ring" form. *3* and *4,* Young trophozoites showing double chromatin dots. *5–7,* Developing trophozoite forms. *8,* Three medium trophozoites in one cell. *9,* Trophozoite showing pigment in a cell containing Maurer's dots. *10* and *11,* Two trophozoites in each of two cells, showing variation in forms that parasites may assume. *12,* Almost mature trophozoite showing haze of pigment throughout cytoplasm. Maurer's dots in the cell. *13,* Estivo-autumnal "slender forms." *14,* Mature trophozoite, showing clumped pigment. *15,* Parasite in the process of initial chromatin division. *16–19,* Various phases of development of the schizont (presegmenting schizonts). *20,* Mature schizont. *21–24,* Successive forms in development of the gametocyte—usually not found in the peripheral circulation. *25,* Immature macrogametocyte. *26,* Mature macrogametocyte. *27,* Immature microgametocyte. *28,* Mature microgametocyte. *(Courtesy National Institutes of Health, USPHS.)*

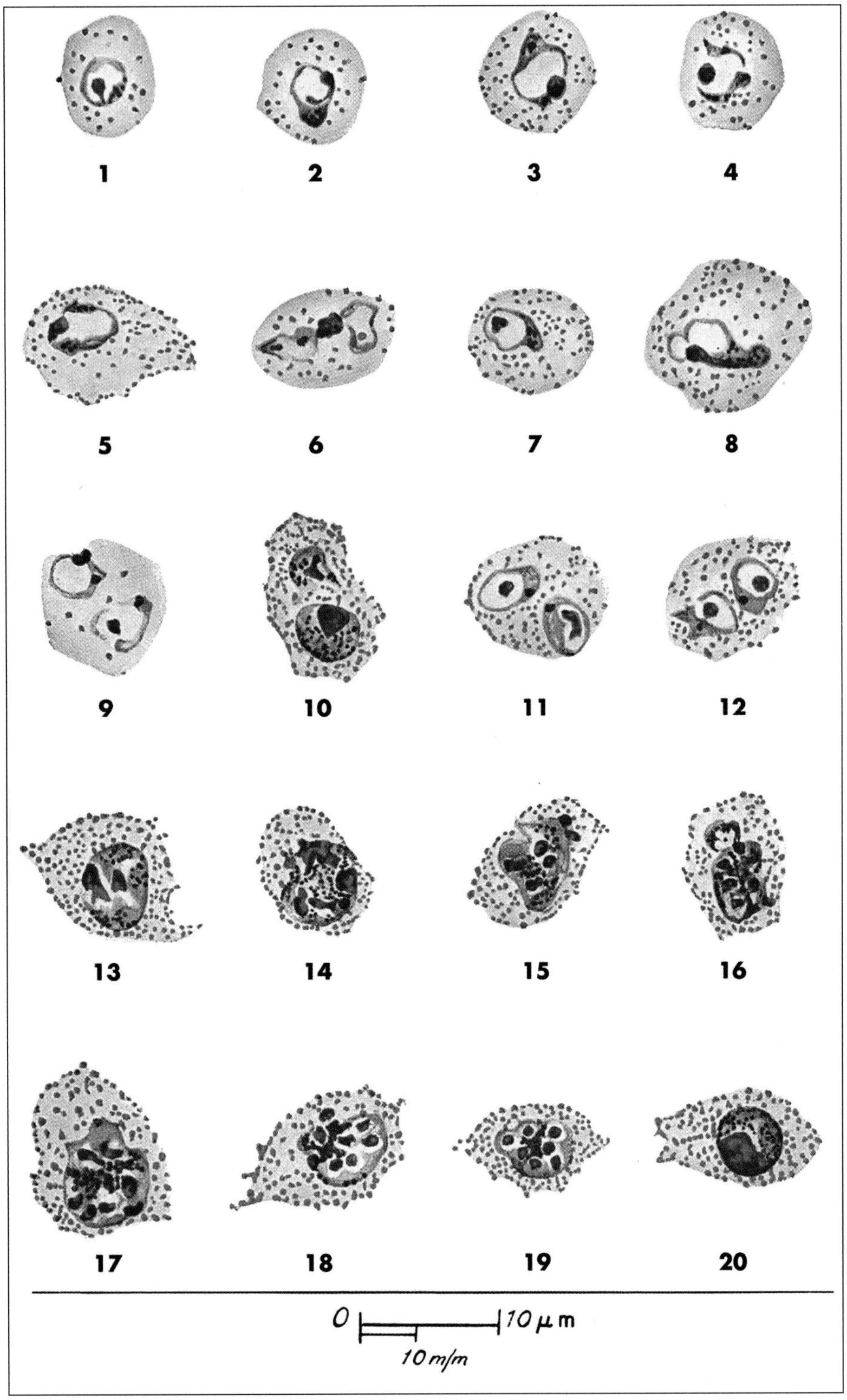

Figure 62-5 *Plasmodium ovale. 1,* Young ring-shaped trophozoite. *2–5,* Older ring-shaped trophozoites. *6–8,* Older ameboid trophozoites. *9, 11,* and *12,* Doubly infected cells, trophozoites. *10,* Doubly infected cell, young gametocytes. *13,* First stage of the schizont. *14–19,* Schizonts, progressive stages. *20,* Mature gametocyte. Free translation of legend accompanying original plate in *Guide pratique d'examen microscopique du sang appliqué au diagnostic du paludisme* by Georges Villain. *(Reproduced with permission from Biologie Medicale Supplement, 1935. Courtesy Aimee Wilcox, National Institutes of Health Bulletin No. 180, USPHS.)*

TABLE 62-8
Comparison of *Plasmodium* Species Affecting Humans

Species	Appearance of erythrocyte size	Schüffner's stippling	Parasite cytoplasm	Appearance of parasite pigment	Number of merozoites	Stages found in circulating blood
Plasmodium vivax	Enlarged; maximum size (attained with mature trophozoites and schizonts) may be 1–2 times normal erythrocyte diameter	+ With all stages except early ring forms	Irregular, ameboid in trophozoites; has "spread out" appearance	Golden brown, inconspicuous	12–24; average is 16	All stages; wide range of stages may be seen on any given film
Plasmodium malariae	Normal	– (Ziemann's dots rarely seen)	Rounded, compact trophozoites with dense cytoplasm; band-form trophozoites occasionally seen	Dark brown, coarse, conspicuous	6–12; average is 8; "rosette" schizonts occasionally seen	All stages; wide variety of stages usually not seen; relatively few rings or gametocytes generally present
Plasmodium ovale	Enlarged; maximum size may be 1¼–1½ times normal red blood cell diameter; approximately 20% or more of infected red blood cells are oval and/or fimbriated (border has irregular projections)	+ With all stages except early ring forms	Rounded, compact trophozoites; occasionally slightly ameboid; growing trophozoites have large chromatin mass	Dark brown, conspicuous	6–14; average is 8	All stages
Plasmodium falciparum	Normal; multiply infected red blood cells are common	– (Maurer's dots occasionally seen)	Young rings are small, delicate, often with double chromatin dots; gametocytes are crescent or elongate	Black; coarse and conspicuous in gametocytes	6–32; average is 20–24	Rings and/or gametocytes; other stages develop in blood vessels of internal organs but are not seen in peripheral blood except in severe infection

With permission from Smith JW, Melvin DM, Orihel TC, et al. Diagnostic parasitology—blood and tissue parasites. Chicago: American Society of Clinical Pathologists; 1976.

in the erythrocyte, is usually seen in cells infected with *P. vivax* and *P. ovale*, although it may not be evident in cells infected with early ring forms or on slides that have not been stained at the appropriate pH (see earlier under Laboratory Methods). The presence of Schüffner's stippling is helpful because it is not seen in *P. malariae* or *P. falciparum* infection.

As trophozoites grow in the infected cells, the amount of hemoglobin in the erythrocyte decreases and hemozoin pigment accumulates. The amount and appearance of the pigment vary among species. Ring forms of all parasites may have a similar appearance, and if only occasional ring forms are found, the species may not be identifiable. Young rings of *P. falciparum* are smaller than those of the other species (one-sixth the diameter of the red blood cell, compared with one-third the diameter of the red blood cell for the other species). Rings of *P. falciparum* that have grown are similar in size to those of the other species. Trophozoites that appear to be lying on the surface of the erythrocyte or protruding from it are called appliqué or accolé forms, and are most often seen in *P. falciparum* infection. Doubly infected cells and double chromatin dots in ring trophozoites occur most commonly in *P. falciparum* infection but can occur with the other species as well.

Growing trophozoites of *P. vivax* have irregular shapes and are termed ameboid. Those of *P. malariae* and *P. ovale* remain compact. Mature trophozoites and schizonts of *P. falciparum* are usually sequestered in capillary beds secondary to cytoadherence to endothelial cells and are not seen in the peripheral blood except in very severe cases of infection. When schizonts are identified in the peripheral blood, determining the number of merozoites is helpful in identifying the various species. Gametocytes of *P. falciparum* are readily identified by their characteristic sausage shape. Gametocytes of *P. vivax*, *P. malariae*, and *P. ovale* have a similar shape and so are difficult to differentiate, although characteristics of infected red cells can aid identification.

The varieties of developmental stages in the peripheral blood aid in diagnosis. In *P. falciparum* infection, ring forms predominate, and finding numerous ring forms without more mature stages serves as evidence for *P. falciparum* infection. In *P. vivax*, *P. malariae*, and *P. ovale* infections, various stages of parasites are found with some predominance of one stage depending on the phase of the cycle.

Thick films are preferred for detecting malaria infections because a greater quantity of blood is examined (see earlier under Laboratory Methods). Ring forms often have the appearance of punctuation marks rather than complete rings, and the presence of red chromatin and blue cytoplasm should be required to identify them as parasites. Schüffner's stippling still may be a helpful identifying characteristic, and it may be recognized around growing trophozoites as a pink halo rather than as distinct granules seen in thin films. The ameboid character of *P. vivax* trophozoites is not as evident in thick films, but the number of merozoites in mature schizonts is helpful. Macrogametocytes and microgametocytes cannot usually be differentiated. The distinctive sausage shape of *P. falciparum* gametocytes is still evident, although they may appear stubbier than in thin films. Gametocytes of the other species can be detected and are easily differentiated from host cell nuclei by the presence of refractile hemozoin pigment.

Mixed infections occur occasionally (about 5% of the time), but caution should be used in making such a diagnosis unless definite evidence reveals two separate populations of parasites. The most common mixed infections are *P. falciparum* and *P. vivax*. Finding gametocytes of *P. falciparum* in a person obviously infected with *P. vivax* is diagnostic.

Multiple artifacts may be confused with malarial parasites on thick and thin films. The most common artifacts on thin films are blood platelets superimposed on red blood cells. These platelets should be readily identified because they do not have a true ring form, do not show differentiation of the chromatin and cytoplasm, and do not contain pigment. Clumps of bacteria or platelets may be confused with schizonts. At times, masses of fused platelets may resemble gametocytes of *P. falciparum* but do not show the differential staining or the pigment. Precipitated stain and contaminating bacteria, fungi, or spores may also be confused with these parasites.

Species-specific serologic tests for malaria are particularly useful for epidemiologic surveys and for detection of infected blood donors. Such tests do not reliably differentiate current from past infection, however. Sensitive and specific IFA tests using antigens from the four human species are available from the CDC (Wilson, 1995). Assays for the direct detection of malarial antigens in blood are especially useful (see Laboratory Methods; Murray, 2009).

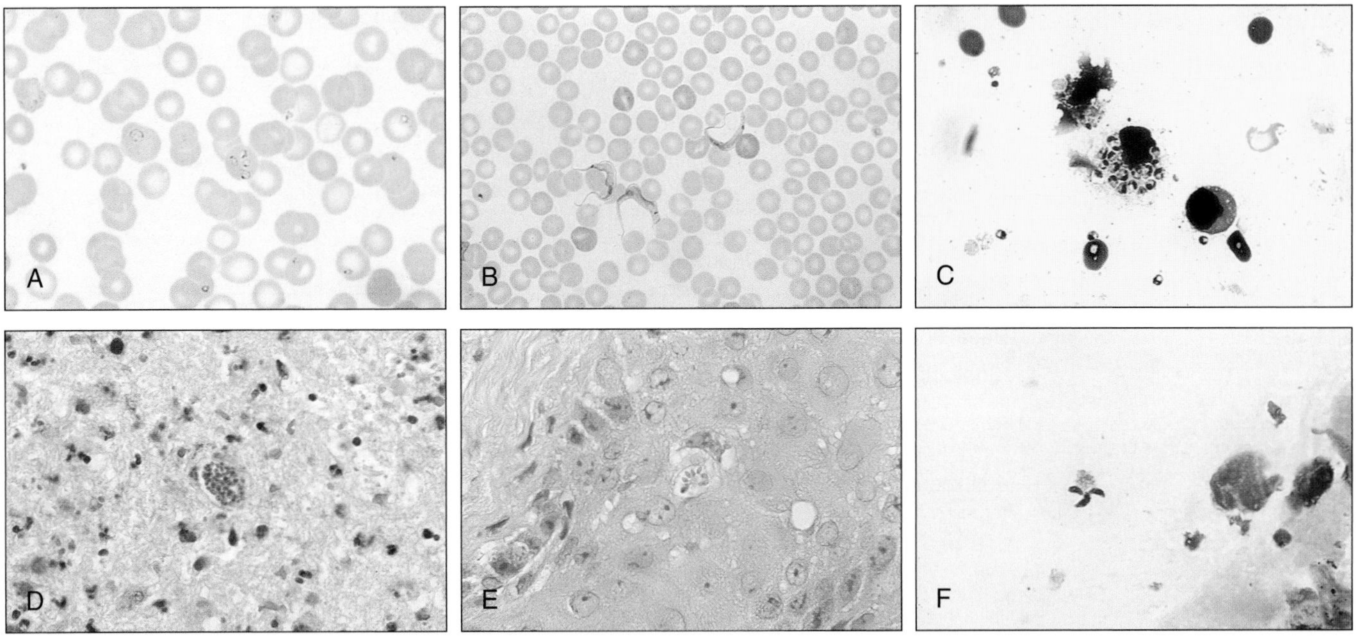

Figure 62-6 **A,** Human infection with *Babesia microti;* note high parasitemia and multiple infected red cells (oil immersion). **B,** *Trypanosoma* sp. in stained blood film; note nucleus, kinetoplast, and undulating membrane (oil immersion). **C,** *Leishmania mexicana* amastigotes in impression smear of thigh lesion (Giemsa stain; oil immersion). **D,** Pseudocyst of *Toxoplasma gondii* in brain tissue (hematoxylin and eosin [H&E]; oil immersion). **E,** Cutaneous rosette of *T. gondii* tachyzoites in an immunocompromised patient (H&E; oil immersion). **F,** Tachyzoites of *T. gondii* recovered from a bronchoalveolar lavage specimen from an individual infected with the human immunodeficiency virus (Giemsa stain; oil immersion).

BABESIOSIS

Similar to malarial parasites, etiologic agents of babesiosis or piroplasmosis are apicomplexan protozoa found worldwide that infect erythrocytes, often producing febrile illness of variable severity. Unlike malaria, babesiosis is transmitted by ticks and is found in a variety of animal species that serve as reservoirs (Krause, 2002).

Human infection in the United States occurs predominantly in the northeastern and midwestern states, where the rodent parasite *Babesia microti* is responsible for infection (Homer, 2000). *Ixodes scapularis* is the usual tick vector. Recent studies have implicated another, as yet unnamed, *Babesia* spp. (tentatively known as WA1) as being responsible for disease in the western United States. This parasite, associated with disease in Washington State and California, is thought to be transmitted by the Western black-legged tick, *Ixodes pacificus* (Quick, 1993; Persing, 1995). In Europe, the canine parasite *Babesia divergens*, transmitted by *Ixodes ricinus*, infects humans, and a recent report of *B. divergens*–like infection in Washington State expands the range of known human cases (Herwaldt, 2004).

The spectrum of babesiosis varies from latent, subclinical infection to fulminant, hemolytic disease. Fatalities have been reported, especially in splenectomized or immunocompromised individuals. Immunocompetent persons may experience symptoms similar to those of malaria, including fever, chills, malaise, and anemia, although without recognizable periodicity. Investigation of an outbreak caused by *B. microti* on Nantucket Island in New England showed that some symptomatic patients harbored the parasite for months and others showed serologic evidence of infection without a history of clinical disease (Ruebush, 1980). Other evidence indicates that chronic subclinical infections may not be uncommon (Persing, 1995).

Babesia parasites multiply in erythrocytes by schizogony but do not produce gametocytes. Although trophozoites of many species appear pear-shaped at some point in their development, those of *B. microti* usually appear as delicate ring forms that may be easily confused with those of malarial parasites, especially *P. falciparum* (Fig. 62-6, *A*) (Healy, 1980; Homer, 2000). *Babesia* trophozoites can be differentiated from those of malarial parasites by the presence of multiple rings in one cell that may form a tetrad (Maltese cross) and the absence of large, growing trophozoites and gametocytes; extracellular trophozoites may be seen in heavy infections. Also, *Babesia*-infected cells lack hemozoin pigment, which is present in *Plasmodium*-infected cells. History of residence in or travel to endemic areas, or of a recent tick bite, might suggest *Babesia* infection. Serologic tests (e.g., IFA) for both *B. microti* and WA1 are available from the CDC on referral from state health departments and from some commercial laboratories. Serology tests for malaria are negative in babesiosis, although patients with malaria may cross-react in the *Babesia* serologies (Wilson, 1995).

HEMOFLAGELLATES

The hemoflagellates of humans and animals are members of the order Kinetoplastida and are characterized by the presence of a large mitochondrion known as a kinetoplast, which contains enough DNA to be seen by light microscopy when treated with Giemsa stain. Two genera important in human disease are *Trypanosoma* and *Leishmania*. Members of both genera are transmitted by arthropod vectors and have animal hosts that serve as reservoirs.

Kinetoplastida assume different morphologic forms depending on their presence in vertebrate hosts, including humans, or in their insect vectors (Fig. 62-7). The amastigote stage is spherical, is 2–5 μm in diameter, and displays a nucleus and kinetoplast. By definition, an external flagellum is lacking, although an axoneme (the intracellular portion of the flagellum) is apparent at the ultrastructural level. Amastigotes may be found in human or animal hosts infected with *T. cruzi* or *Leishmania* spp., where they multiply exclusively within cells. The promastigote is an elongated and slender organism with a central nucleus, an anteriorly located kinetoplast and axoneme, and a free flagellum extending from the anterior end. This stage occurs in the insect vectors of *Leishmania* and is the stage detected in culture. The epimastigote is similar to the promastigote, but the kinetoplast is found closer to the nucleus and has a small undulating membrane that becomes a free flagellum. All species of *Trypanosoma* that infect humans assume an epimastigote stage in the insect vector or in culture. In the trypomastigote, the kinetoplast is found at the posterior end and the flagellum forms an undulating membrane that extends the length of the cell, emerging as a free flagellum at the anterior end. Trypomastigote forms occur predominantly in the bloodstream of mammalian hosts infected with various *Trypanosoma* spp. Infectious stages found in appropriate insect vectors following transformation from the epimastigote form are known as metacyclic trypomastigotes.

Trypanosoma

Infections with trypanosomes include those caused by *Trypanosoma brucei* (African or Old World trypanosomiasis) and *T. cruzi* (American or New World trypanosomiasis, or Chagas' disease). Both are of great importance in endemic areas but are rarely seen in the United States. A third species, *Trypanosoma rangeli*, has been described in humans in the Americas but does not cause clinical illness. Bloodstream trypomastigotes of the *T. brucei*

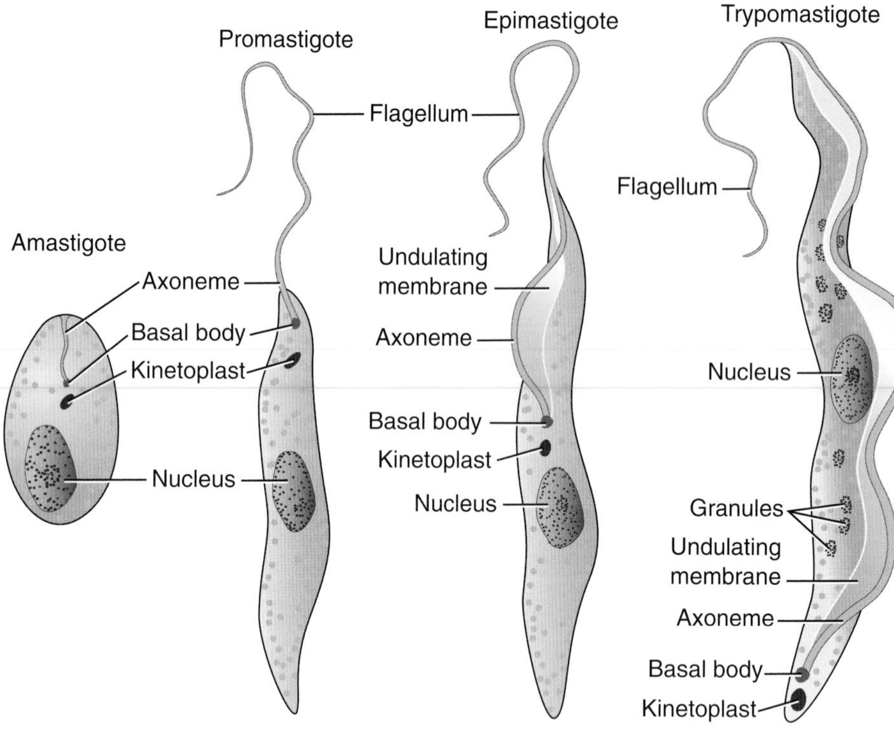

Figure 62-7 Morphology of hemoflagellates.

group (see Fig. 62-6, *B*) are up to 30 μm long with graceful curves and a small kinetoplast. Those of *T. cruzi* are shorter (20 μm), assume S and C shapes on stained blood films, and display a larger kinetoplast.

In equatorial Africa, parasites of the *T. brucei* group infect both animals and humans and are transmitted by the bite of tsetse flies in the genus *Glossina*. Multiplication of organisms at the bite site often produces a transient chancre. East African trypanosomiasis is caused by *T. brucei rhodesiense*, which has a number of animal reservoir hosts. The disease is characterized by a rapidly progressive acute febrile illness with lymphadenopathy. Patients die before central nervous system (CNS) involvement is prominent.

The infection in western Africa is caused by *T. brucei gambiense*, which is responsible for classic African sleeping sickness. The disease has a more chronic course that begins with intermittent fevers, night sweats, and malaise. Lymphadenopathy, especially of the cervical lymph nodes (Winterbottom's sign), may be pronounced. Involvement of the CNS becomes prominent with time. Somnolence, confusion, and fatigue progress, leading to stupor, coma, and eventual death. Humans are the primary reservoir for this disease (World Health Organization, 1986; Garcia, 2007).

The diagnosis is suspected on the basis of geographic history and clinical findings. Patients show high total IgM levels in blood and cerebrospinal fluid (CSF). Pleocytosis occurs with 50–500 mononuclear cells per microliter in CSF. The diagnosis is established by demonstrating the parasites on thick and thin films of peripheral blood, buffy coat preparations, or aspirates of lymph nodes or bone marrow, or in spun CSF that is stained with Giemsa (Van Meirvenne, 1985; Cattand, 1988; National Committee for Clinical Laboratory Standards, 2000). Culture or animal inoculation may be helpful, if it is available; a number of molecular methods have also been described.

American trypanosomiasis, or Chagas' disease, is caused by *T. cruzi*. In its sylvatic form, the parasite occurs in the United States, Central America, and most of South America. Human infections are common in parts of Mexico and Central and South America, where they are transmitted by kissing bugs of the family Reduviidae. Genera and species involved in transmission vary from one country to another and among different ecologic niches. Some reduviids are responsible for maintaining the sylvatic cycle in animal reservoirs, whereas others are adapted to a domiciliary life in which they infest poorly constructed houses, usually in rural areas. At the time of feeding, the reduviid bug defecates. The bug feces contain infective trypomastigotes that, as a result of scratching or rubbing, enter the body at the bite site or through intact mucosa of the mouth or conjunctiva. Infective forms actively enter nearby tissue cells, where they transform into dividing amastigotes. When the infected cell is filled with amastigotes, transformation to trypomastigotes occurs, followed by cell rupture. Trypomastigotes are released into the peripheral blood and reach distant tissues, where they can start the reproductive cycle de novo.

Chagas' disease may cause acute or chronic infection. Acute disease is most common in children younger than 5 years of age and is characterized by malaise, chills, fever, hepatosplenomegaly, and myocarditis. Swelling of the tissues around the eye (Romaña's sign) may be present if inoculation of the organisms occurs on the face. Swelling of tissues at other locations following the bite of an infected reduviid is called a chagoma. In older individuals, the acute course is milder and often asymptomatic, and the patient remains infected for life. Chronic manifestations of the infection, including megaesophagus, megacolon, and alterations in the conduction system of the heart, are related to destruction of the effector cells of the parasympathetic system by autoantibodies. Infection can be transmitted by blood transfusion, and quiescent infections may be exacerbated by immunosuppression.

Diagnosis in the acute stage is established by demonstrating the parasite on thick and thin blood films, in buffy coat smears, or in aspirates of chagomas or enlarged lymph nodes. Aspirates, blood, and biopsy specimens can also be cultured using Novy-MacNeal-Nicolle medium (Ash, 1987; National Committee for Clinical Laboratory Standards, 2000; Garcia, 2007; Visvesvara, 2010b). In endemic areas, xenodiagnosis (examination of the gut contents of laboratory-raised reduviids that have been allowed to feed on a patient) may be used. In the chronic stage, serodiagnosis is the method of choice. EIA, IFA, and CF tests are available, although they cannot differentiate between acute and chronic disease, and cross-reactions may occur in patients with leishmaniasis.

Leishmania

Leishmaniasis is a disease of the reticuloendothelial system caused by kinetoplastid protozoa of the genus *Leishmania*. All species that infect humans have animal reservoirs and are transmitted by sandflies belonging to the genera *Phlebotomus* in the Old World and *Lutzomyia* in the New World. The parasites assume the amastigote form in mammalian hosts and the promastigote form in insect vectors. Species of *Leishmania* cannot be differentiated by examination of amastigotes or promastigotes. Leishmaniasis may assume many different clinical forms; cutaneous, mucocutaneous, and visceral diseases are best known. The form and severity of disease vary with the infecting species, the particular host's immune status, and prior exposure (Peters, 1987; Cook, 2002).

Cutaneous Leishmaniasis

Old World cutaneous leishmaniasis (oriental sore) occurs in southern Europe, northern and eastern Africa, the Middle East, Iran, Afghanistan, India, and southern Russia. Infections are caused by *Leishmania tropica*,

Leishmania major, and *Leishmania aethiopica*, although *L. donovani* and *Leishmania infantum* may also produce cutaneous lesions. *L. tropica* produces the urban or dry ulcer, which is more long lived than the rural or wet ulcer of *L. major*. Ulcers caused by these species usually develop on an exposed area of the body and heal spontaneously. Infection produces long-lasting immunity. *L. tropica* may become viscerotropic, as was demonstrated recently in military personnel who participated in Operation Desert Storm (Magill, 1993). *L. aethiopica* causes a more aggressive cutaneous infection, which in some individuals metastasizes to produce mucosal lesions or diffuse cutaneous leishmaniasis, the latter of which is characterized by multiple skin nodules resembling lepromatous leprosy.

Cutaneous leishmaniasis of the New World is caused by many species, including *Leishmania mexicana*, *Leishmania braziliensis*, *Leishmania amazonensis*, *Leishmania venezuelensis*, *Leishmania garnhami*, *Leishmania pifanoi*, *Leishmania peruviana*, *Leishmania panamensis*, and *Leishmania guyanensis*, among others (Garcia, 2007). Lesions produced by *L. mexicana* often involve the earlobe (chiclero ulcer), are self-limiting, and are not known to metastasize to the mucosa. However, *L. mexicana* and *L. amazonensis* may produce diffuse cutaneous lesions similar to those produced by *L. aethiopica*. A focus of cutaneous leishmaniasis exists in the southern part of Texas, where infections are caused by one or more species (Gustafson, 1985). *L. peruviana*, which has been found on the western slopes of the Peruvian Andes, causes an infection called uta, a benign cutaneous lesion that occurs predominantly in children. *L. peruviana* is acquired in the home, where the main reservoirs are domestic dogs. This epidemiologic situation contrasts with other cutaneous leishmaniases, which usually are acquired in forests and have wild animals as reservoir hosts.

Mucocutaneous Leishmaniasis

Mucocutaneous leishmaniasis (espundia) is caused primarily by *L. braziliensis* and related species, which produce typical cutaneous lesions that generally are more aggressive, last longer, and often disseminate to mucous membranes, especially in the nasal, oral, or pharyngeal areas. In these locations, they may produce disfiguring lesions secondary to erosion of soft tissues and cartilage. *L. braziliensis* is distributed in Mexico and Central and South America.

Visceral Leishmaniasis

Visceral leishmaniasis of the Old World occurs sporadically over a wide geographic area and is caused by *L. donovani* or by *L. infantum*. *L. donovani* predominates in Africa, India, and Asia, and *L. infantum* predominates in the Mediterranean region and the Middle East, although overlapping ranges occur. New World visceral leishmaniasis is caused by *L. chagasi* and occurs sporadically throughout Central and South America. On occasion, some species that cause cutaneous disease have been responsible for visceral disease, as demonstrated recently in some troops who participated in Operation Desert Storm (Magill, 1993). In some areas, humans may serve as the disease reservoir, although a variety of animals, including dogs and cats, usually assume this role.

The infection is usually benign and often subclinical, although some individuals, especially young children and malnourished individuals, have marked involvement of the viscera, especially liver, spleen, bone marrow, and lymph nodes. In some cases, death occurs after months to years unless it is treated appropriately. The infection is called kala-azar in India, in reference to the darkening of the skin. Visceral leishmaniasis also is an opportunistic infection in individuals with concurrent human immunodeficiency virus (HIV), and the condition responds poorly to therapy in such circumstances (Medrano, 1992; Strickland, 2000; Garcia, 2007).

Diagnosis of Leishmaniasis

The diagnosis usually is established by visualization of amastigotes in smears, imprints, or biopsies, or by growth of promastigotes in culture. In integumentary leishmaniasis, the border of the most active lesion should be biopsied, and the fresh biopsy should be used to make imprints. A smear should be prepared by making a 2–3-mm incision at the border of the ulcer and recovering small amounts of tissue from the cut surfaces with the scalpel blade. Both the imprint and the smear should be treated with Giemsa stain. Specimens that may be submitted when visceral leishmaniasis is suspected include buffy coat preparations, lymph node and bone marrow aspirates, and spleen and liver biopsies (Garcia, 2007).

A culture is desirable because it is more sensitive and allows determination of the species or subspecies, a practice that may help in clinical management of the patient. Biopsy or aspirate specimens collected aseptically are cultured in Novy-MacNeal-Nicolle medium or in Schneider's *Drosophila* medium supplemented with fetal calf serum (Visvesvara, 2010b). Cultures usually begin to show promastigotes in 2–5 days but should be held for 4 weeks.

Amastigotes found in imprints, smears, and tissue sections are recognized by their size (2–4 μm) and the presence of delicate cytoplasm, a nucleus, and a kinetoplast (see Fig. 62-6, *C*). In tissue sections, they may appear smaller because of shrinkage during fixation. Amastigotes must be differentiated from other intracellular organisms, including yeast cells of *Histoplasma capsulatum* and trophozoites of *T. gondii*. *Leishmania* spp. have a kinetoplast and do not have a cell wall. In contrast, *Histoplasma* lack the kinetoplast, and the cell wall stains with periodic acid–Schiff (PAS) and methenamine silver stains. According to one study (Weigle, 1987), the sensitivity of histologic sections stained with hematoxylin and eosin (H&E) is 14%; imprints, 19%; cultures, 58%; and all methods combined, 67%.

Toxoplasma gondii

T. gondii is a protozoan parasite of the phylum Apicomplexa that has a worldwide distribution in humans and in domestic and wild animals, especially carnivores. Infection in immunocompetent persons is generally asymptomatic or mild, but immunocompromised patients may experience serious complications. Infection in utero may result in serious congenital infection with sequelae or stillbirth (Remington, 2005).

The sexual stage in the life cycle of this coccidian parasite is completed in the intestinal epithelium of cats and other felines, which serve exclusively as definitive hosts. During this enteroepithelial cycle, asexual schizogony and sexual gametogony occur, leading to the development of immature oocysts that are passed in the feces. Oocysts mature to the infective stage (which contain two sporocysts with four sporozoites each) in the environment in 2–21 days. Ingestion of infective oocysts may lead to infection of a wide variety of susceptible vertebrate hosts in which actively growing trophozoites (tachyzoites) may infect any nucleated cells. Proliferation of tachyzoites results in cell death and injury to the host during acute infection. Once immunity has developed, the organisms form tissue cysts that may eventually contain hundreds or thousands of slowly growing bradyzoites. The presence of tissue cysts is characteristic of chronic infection. All stages of the life cycle occur in felines, but only trophozoite and cyst stages occur in humans and other intermediate hosts.

Humans acquire infection with *T. gondii* by ingestion of inadequately cooked meat, especially lamb or pork, that contains tissue cysts or by ingestion of infective oocysts from material contaminated by cat feces. Outbreaks have occurred from inhaling contaminated dust in an indoor riding stable (Teutch, 1979) and from drinking contaminated water or unpasteurized goat's milk (Benenson, 1982; Sacks, 1982; Bowie, 1997). Transmission via blood transfusion and through organ transplantation also can occur.

Most acute infections are asymptomatic or mimic other infectious diseases in which fever and lymphadenopathy are prominent. Congenital infection may occur when the mother develops acute infection during gestation. Risk of infection to the neonate is unrelated to the presence or absence of symptoms in the mother, but severity of infection depends on the stage of gestation at which it is acquired. Intrauterine death, microcephaly, or hydrocephaly with intracranial calcifications may develop if infection is acquired in the first half of pregnancy. Infections in the second half of pregnancy are usually asymptomatic at birth, although fever, hepatosplenomegaly, and jaundice may appear. Chorioretinitis, psychomotor retardation, and convulsive disorders may appear months or years later (Remington, 2005; Wilson, 2007).

In immunosuppressed individuals, especially those with AIDS, infection with *T. gondii* usually presents with CNS involvement (Luft, 1988). Other possible clinical and pathologic manifestations include pneumonitis, myocarditis, retinitis, pancreatitis, or orchitis (Luft, 1989; Schnapp, 1992). Toxoplasmosis may be difficult to diagnose clinically and is often discovered at autopsy (Gutierrez, 2000). These infections usually result from reactivation of a latent infection, acquired months or years before, but occasionally result from a primary infection.

Diagnosis of toxoplasmosis may be established by examination of tissues, blood, or body fluids (Wilson, 2007). Demonstration of tachyzoites or tissue cysts is definitive but may prove difficult to demonstrate in H&E-stained sections; fluorescent or immunoperoxidase stains, if available, are useful. Giemsa is good for staining smears of body fluids and tissue imprints. Organisms may be demonstrated by inoculating appropriate material into tissue culture or uninfected mice. Recovery in routine viral cultures also has been described but requires extended incubation (Shepp, 1985). Isolation of organisms from blood or body fluid serves as evidence

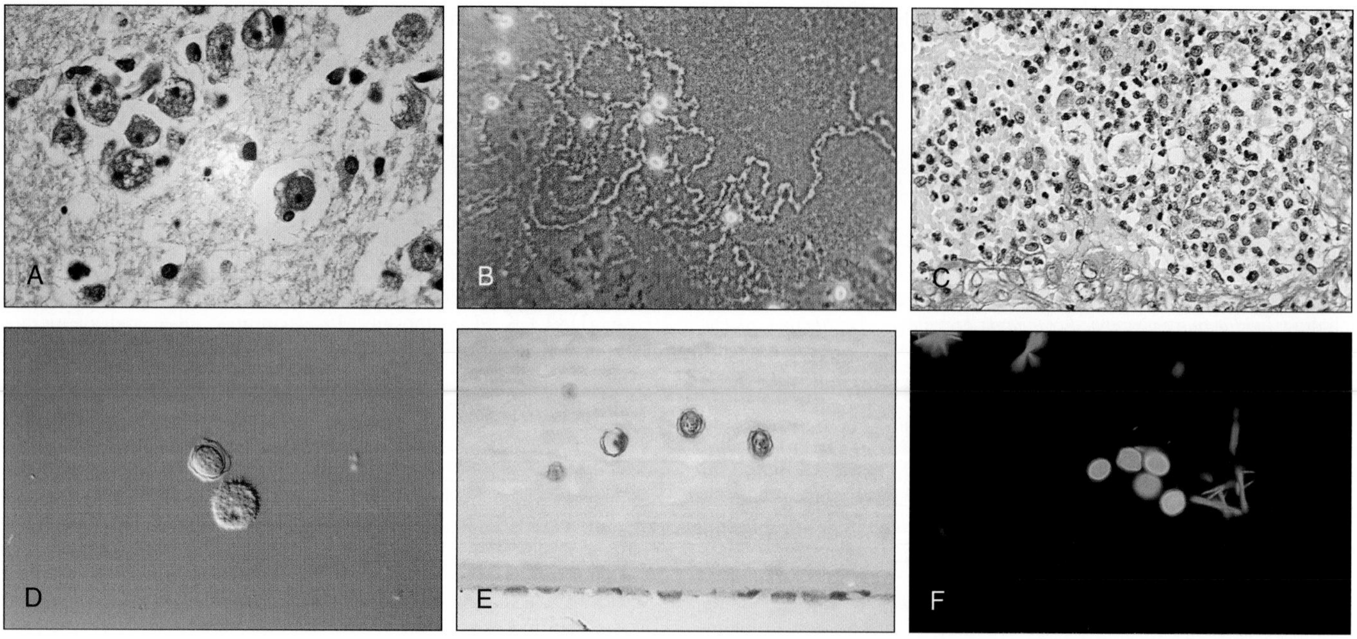

Figure 62-8 **A,** *Naegleria fowleri* trophozoites in primary amebic meningoencephalitis (H&E; oil immersion). **B,** *Acanthamoeba* sp. culture showing trails left by motile trophozoites on a lawn of *Escherichia coli* (phase contrast microscopy; ×100). **C,** *Acanthamoeba* sp. trophozoites within a cutaneous lesion in an individual infected with the human immunodeficiency virus (Giemsa stain; oil immersion). **D,** *Acanthamoeba* sp. trophozoite and cyst (differential interference contrast microscopy; ×400). **E,** Double-walled cysts of *Acanthamoeba* sp. within corneal stroma (H&E; oil immersion). **F,** Cysts of *Acanthamoeba* sp. stained with Calcofluor white (epifluorescence microscopy; ×400).

of acute infection, whereas recovery from tissues may reflect chronic infection. In smears, tachyzoites are crescent-shaped or oval, measuring approximately 3 × 7 μm; cysts measure up to 30 μm in diameter and are usually spherical, except in muscle fibers, where they appear elongate (see Fig. 62-6, *D* through *F*).

Use of PCR technology is highly sensitive and specific in detecting toxoplasmic encephalitis, disseminated disease, and intrauterine infection; testing is available from a small number of commercial and research laboratories (Grover, 1990; Cazenave, 1991; Parmley, 1992; Weiss, 1995; Wilson, 2007).

Serology remains the primary approach in establishing a diagnosis of toxoplasmosis (National Committee for Clinical Laboratory Standards, 2004; Wilson, 2007). The Sabin-Feldman dye test and the IFA test are standards against which other methods are compared, although the former is performed in only a few centers. EIA tests are commercially available and generally provide results similar to those of IFA. Antibodies appear in 1–2 weeks, and titers peak at 6–8 weeks. Tests for IgM-specific antibodies are especially useful for diagnosis of congenital and acute infection, but knowledge of test limitations, specifically the occurrence of false-positive reactions, is extremely important. The persistence of IgM-specific antibodies, sometimes for a year or longer, also is problematic and must be interpreted in conjunction with IgG antibody results. Because many persons have had asymptomatic infection, low IgG titers have little significance. Titers in patients with chronic ocular infection may also be low. Immunocompromised patients such as those with AIDS who have active *Toxoplasma* infection almost always have preexisting specific IgG antibodies, although titers may be low, and IgM antibodies are infrequently detected. Interpretation of IgG and IgM antibody titers varies by test method and by manufacturer. The laboratory performing the test should provide the necessary interpretive criteria (National Committee for Clinical Laboratory Standards, 2004).

OPPORTUNISTIC FREE-LIVING AMEBAE

Amebae of the genera *Naegleria*, *Acanthamoeba*, *Balamuthia*, and *Sappinia* are inhabitants of soil, water, and other environmental substrates, where they feed on other microscopic organisms, especially bacteria and yeasts. All four genera have been associated with opportunistic infection of the CNS, and *Acanthamoeba* causes keratitis (Martinez, 1985; Marciano-Cabral, 1988; Ubelaker, 1991; Kilvington, 1994; Visvesvara, 2007; Qvarnstrom, 2009).

Primary amebic meningoencephalitis, caused by the ameboflagellate *Naegleria fowleri*, typically affects children and young adults who have been swimming or diving in warm, freshwater lakes or pools. The ameboflagellate enters the brain via the cribriform plate and olfactory bulbs and reaches the frontal lobes, where it produces an acute hemorrhagic meningoencephalitis that is usually fatal within 1 week of onset of symptoms. The disease has an extremely poor prognosis, despite vigorous therapeutic intervention. Diagnosis is usually established at autopsy examination by the finding of trophozoites (cysts are rarely seen) in tissue sections (Fig. 62-8, *A*). Antemortem diagnosis is made occasionally by identifying typical trophozoites in CSF on direct wet mounts, in stained preparations, or in culture. Trophozoites measure 10–35 μm; have large, round, central karyosomes; and if exposed to warm distilled water, convert to flagellated forms in 1–2 hours. Cysts are spherical, measuring 7–15 μm in diameter. Culture usually is performed on nonnutrient agar plates (1.5% agar, 0.5% sodium chloride, pH 6.6–7.0) seeded with a lawn of heat-killed or living *Escherichia coli* (Visvesvara, 2010c). Amebae ingest the bacteria, leaving tracks in the bacterial lawn, which may be seen under low-power magnification using reduced light (Fig. 62-8, *B*).

Granulomatous amebic meningoencephalitis (GAE) may be caused by several species of *Acanthamoeba*, including *Acanthamoeba castellani*, *Acanthamoeba culbertsoni*, *Acanthamoeba polyphaga*, and *Acanthamoeba astronyxis*, among others (Marciano-Cabral, 2003). It is usually a subacute or chronic opportunistic infection of chronically ill, debilitated, and immunosuppressed individuals, leading to death weeks to months following onset of symptoms. Infection is thought to spread hematogenously from primary foci in skin, pharynx, or the respiratory tract. Systemic infections occur in individuals with AIDS and may present as ulcerative skin lesions, subcutaneous abscesses, or erythematous nodules (Fig. 62-8, *C*) (Tan, 1993). Exposure to fresh water is not necessary because cysts of *Acanthamoeba* readily become airborne and may be recovered from the throat and nasal passages (Wang, 1967; Lawande, 1979). The pathologic reaction in tissues is granulomatous, with trophozoites predominating in viable tissue, and cysts predominating in areas of necrosis. Diagnosis usually is established at autopsy, but organisms may be recognized in brain biopsies or recovered using the culture technique described for *Naegleria*. *Acanthamoeba* trophozoites are somewhat larger than *Naegleria*, measuring 15–45 μm, and display needle-like filamentous projections from the cell known as acanthopodia. Cysts measure 10–25 μm and are double-walled, displaying a wrinkled outer wall (ectocyst) and a polygonal, stellate, or round inner wall (endocyst) (Fig. 62-8, *D*). Identification to the species level is problematic and reflects uncertainty as to the validity of the 18 or more described species. Currently, genotyping is the preferred approach used in differentiating types of *Acanthamoeba* (Marciano-Cabral, 2003). Immunofluorescence and immunoperoxidase techniques may prove useful in identifying and differentiating species and are available from the CDC (Visvesvara, 2007).

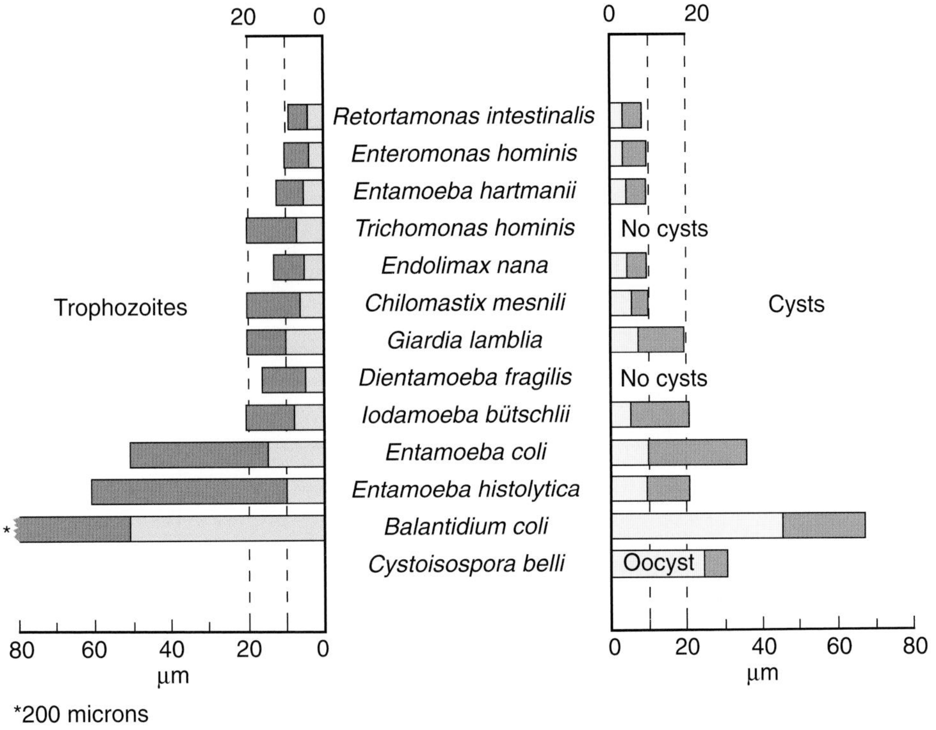

Figure 62-9 Size ranges of intestinal protozoa. (*Balantidium coli* trophozoites may measure up to 200 μm.)

GAE may also be caused by leptomyxid amebae, specifically *Balamuthia mandrillaris* (Visvesvara, 1993). Morphologically, *Balamuthia* cannot be differentiated from *Acanthamoeba* by routine histology, although differences may be detected at the ultrastructural level. These organisms are antigenically distinct and may be identified using specific monoclonal or polyclonal antisera in DFA or immunoperoxidase assays (Visvesvara, 2007). *Balamuthia* do not grow on agar plates used for *Naegleria* and *Acanthamoeba*, but they have been recovered in tissue culture using mammalian cell lines. A single case of encephalitis caused by *Sappinia (S. pedata)*, another free-living ameba, was recently described and identified by a real-time PCR assay (Qvarnstrom, 2009).

Acanthamoeba keratitis is an increasingly recognized painful infection of the cornea that is most likely to occur in persons who use daily-wear or extended-wear soft contact lenses or who have experienced trauma to the cornea (Anuran, 1987; Kilvington, 1994; Marciano-Cabral, 2003). Incomplete or infrequent disinfection and use of homemade saline and multipurpose solutions are known risk factors for acquiring the infection (Stehr-Green, 1990; Verani, 2009). The disease is characterized by development of a paracentral ring infiltrate of the corneal stroma, which progresses to ulceration and possible perforation, with loss of the eye. The infection may be confused with fungal, bacterial, or herpetic keratitis but is characteristically refractory to commonly used antimicrobials. Keratoplasty has been used routinely in management of this disease, although recent advances in medical therapy have been reported (Varga, 1993; Dart, 2009). Diagnosis usually is established by demonstrating amebic trophozoites or cysts in corneal scrapings or biopsies (Fig. 62-8, *E*). A variety of permanent stains can be used, including Giemsa, PAS, and trichrome. Use of the fluorochrome Calcofluor white is especially helpful in recognizing amebic cysts (Fig. 62-8, *F*) (Marines, 1987; Garcia, 2010). While cultures (described earlier) provide increased sensitivity over staining methods and are often available from clinical laboratories, the sensitivity achieved by PCR may equal or exceed that of culture (Boggild, 2009).

Intestinal and Urogenital Protozoa

Protozoal groups inhabiting the intestinal tract of humans include amebae, flagellates, ciliates, coccidia, and microsporidia, not all of which are pathogens. In a review of fecal specimens submitted to state health department laboratories, *G. lamblia* was present in 7.2%, *E. histolytica* in 0.9%, *D. fragilis* in 0.5%, and *Cryptosporidium* spp. in 0.2% of specimens. Nonpathogenic protozoa were found in approximately 10.7% of specimens (Kappus, 1994). Most intestinal infections are acquired by fecal–oral contamination directly from food handlers, or indirectly via contaminated water.

For most laboratorians, identification of intestinal protozoa is one of the more difficult aspects of parasitology. Protozoal parasites are small, and pathogenic species must be differentiated from nonpathogenic species and from inflammatory cells, epithelial cells, yeasts, pollen, and other confusing objects. Numerous characteristics assist in identifying intestinal protozoa. Size is helpful (Fig. 62-9), and a properly calibrated ocular micrometer must be available. Differentiation of amebae from flagellates in wet mounts of fresh material is relatively easy because of the typical pseudopod extension seen with amebae, whereas flagellates move more rapidly and in a so-called falling leaf, darting, or tumbling fashion.

Number and size of nuclei and pattern of chromatin distribution, best seen in permanent stained preparations, are also useful. Cytoplasmic characteristics include fibrils and other special structures typical of flagellates, ingested materials in amebic trophozoites, and glycogen masses and chromatoid bodies in amebic cysts. Flagellates generally are elongated and tapered, with a nucleus or nuclei at one end.

During examination by any method, both nuclear and cytoplasmic characteristics should be assessed from a number of individual organisms to complete the identification. When reporting the presence of two or more species in a sample, the observer should be able to define distinct populations of organisms to prevent confusion with an occasional organism with an atypical appearance.

Trophozoites predominate in liquid stool but degenerate within an hour after passage unless they are placed into preservatives. Cysts predominate in formed stool and are more resistant to degeneration. Both forms may be seen in direct wet mounts prepared from fresh feces. Formalin does not preserve trophozoites well, and they may be missed unless permanent stained smears are prepared. Definitive identification should be made on examination of permanent stained slides.

AMEBAE AND *Blastocystis hominis*

Three genera of amebae may inhabit the intestinal tract of humans: *Entamoeba*, *Endolimax*, and *Iodamoeba*. Cysts are ingested and excyst in the small intestine. Resulting trophozoites proliferate by binary fission in the lumen of the colon. Both cysts and trophozoites may be passed in feces, but only mature cysts are infective. *E. histolytica* is the only amebic species capable of invading tissues and causing disease.

The genus *Entamoeba*, characterized by the presence of chromatin on the nuclear membrane, includes *E. histolytica*, the etiologic agent of amebiasis; *E. dispar*, a nonpathogenic species morphologically identical to

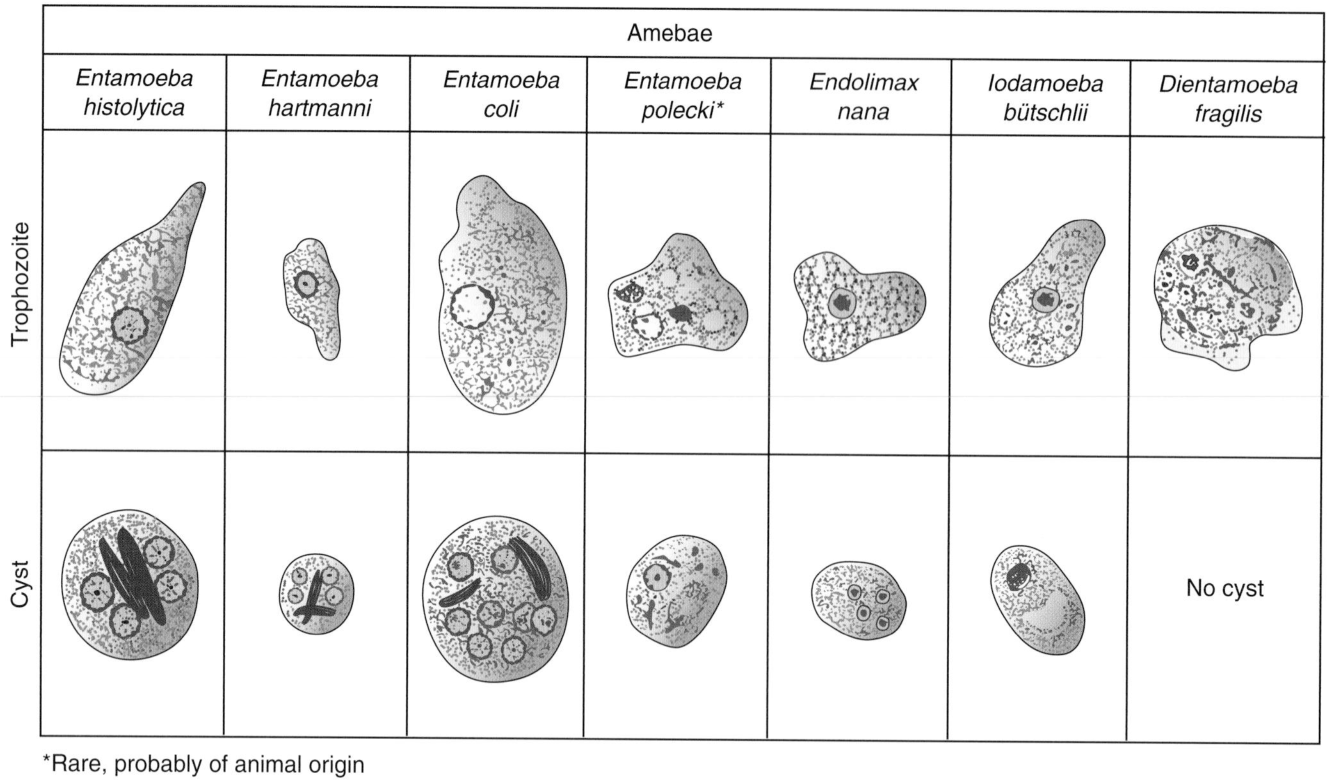

Figure 62-10 Amebae found in human stool specimens. (*Dientamoeba fragilis* is a flagellate.)

E. histolytica, *E. hartmanni*, and *Entamoeba coli*, which are commonly found commensal species; and *Entamoeba polecki*, which is occasionally found in people who have contact with pigs (Fig. 62-10) (Levin, 1970; Gay, 1985). *Entamoeba gingivalis*, which does not have a known cyst stage, may inhabit the oral cavity of people with poor oral hygiene (Dao, 1983). *E. polecki* and *E. gingivalis* are seen infrequently and are not described further. *Endolimax nana* and *I. bütschlii* are nonpathogenic species. *Dientamoeba fragilis* now is recognized as a flagellate, although it lacks external flagella, and is discussed with the flagellates in the text but may be found with amebae in tables and figures because it is morphologically similar to them (Garcia, 2007).

Entamoeba histolytica

E. histolytica may cause various clinical diseases, most commonly amebic dysentery, amebic colitis, and liver abscesses (Beaver 1984; Ravdin, 1988; Strickland, 2000). General host defense mechanisms, previous contact with the parasite, diet, and the strain of *E. histolytica* influence the severity of infection. Analysis of isoenzyme patterns (zymodemes) has shown that only certain strains can cause invasive disease and that most infections remain undetected (Bruckner, 1992; Murray, 2007). Genetic and biochemical differences between invasive and noninvasive strains have been identified, and it has been proposed that nonpathogenic strains should be named *Entamoeba dispar* (Diamond, 1993).

Amebic dysentery, which occurs infrequently in the United States, is an acute disease characterized by bloody diarrhea with abdominal cramping. Invasion of the intestinal mucosa occurs, producing ulceration that may lead to perforation and peritonitis. The more common form of disease seen in this country is amebic colitis, which may mimic ulcerative colitis and other forms of inflammatory bowel disease. Symptoms generally are less severe than in amebic dysentery but may include nonbloody diarrhea, constipation, abdominal cramping, and weight loss. Small, pinpoint mucosal ulcerations may develop and expand within the submucosa to form flask-shaped ulcers. All of the colon may be involved or only a portion, most commonly the cecum, rectosigmoid, or ascending colon.

Amebic liver abscess is the most common form of extraintestinal amebiasis, occurring in approximately 5% of patients with a history of intestinal amebiasis. Symptoms include fever and right upper quadrant pain. These liver abscesses are usually diagnosed by radiographic scans, ultrasound, and serologic tests. Amebae are present in the stool in less than half of patients at the time liver abscess is manifest. Amebic hepatitis, characterized by an enlarged, tender liver in someone with intestinal amebiasis, may occur in some cases. Its pathogenesis is poorly understood. Rarely, amebic abscesses appear in other organs, such as the lung, brain, or skin, by hematogenous spread from the intestine or by contiguous spread from a liver abscess. Masses of granulomatous tissue, known as amebomas, may form in response to the presence of amebae, which in the intestine may cause a so-called napkin ring lesion that could be mistaken for a carcinoma.

Epidemiology

Most infections with *E. histolytica* are acquired by ingestion of contaminated food or water, although one outbreak was caused by a contaminated colonic irrigation machine (Istre, 1982). Pseudo-outbreaks of amebiasis result from laboratory misidentification of inflammatory cells, other amebae, and fecal debris as *E. histolytica* (Krogstad, 1978; Centers for Disease Control and Prevention, 1985). Although *E. histolytica* is an endemic parasite in the United States, many citizens acquire infection while traveling through or residing in foreign countries.

Diagnosis

Examination of a series of stool specimens should be sufficient for diagnosis of intestinal amebiasis in most cases. If the patient has been given antibiotics or contrast media, the amebic infection may be masked for a period of time. Aspirated material from liver abscesses can be examined microscopically to detect trophozoites. The last material aspirated is most likely to contain trophozoites and may be examined by direct microscopic examination or permanently stained slides. If tissue is available, sections may show organisms that stain prominently with PAS (Fig. 62-11, *C*).

Culture procedures (Diamond, 1988; Clinical and Laboratory Standards Institute, 2005; Visvesvara, 2010a) are not widely used for diagnosis but are useful for research and are essential for determining pathogenicity based on zymodemes. EIA antigen detection tests that are specific, sensitive, and able to differentiate *E. histolytica* from *E. dispar* are commercially available (see Table 62-5) (Clinical and Laboratory Standards Institute, 2005; Garcia, 2007). Use of PCR amplification techniques and DNA probes is also useful for differentiating *E. histolytica* from *E. dispar* (Samuelson, 1989; Bendall, 1993; Weiss, 1995), but none are commercially available at this time.

Serologic tests (see Table 62-6) are most useful for diagnosis of extraintestinal infection because approximately 95% of patients with amebic liver abscess are seropositive. This decreases to 70% for patients with active intestinal infection and to 10% in asymptomatic carriers. Detectable titers

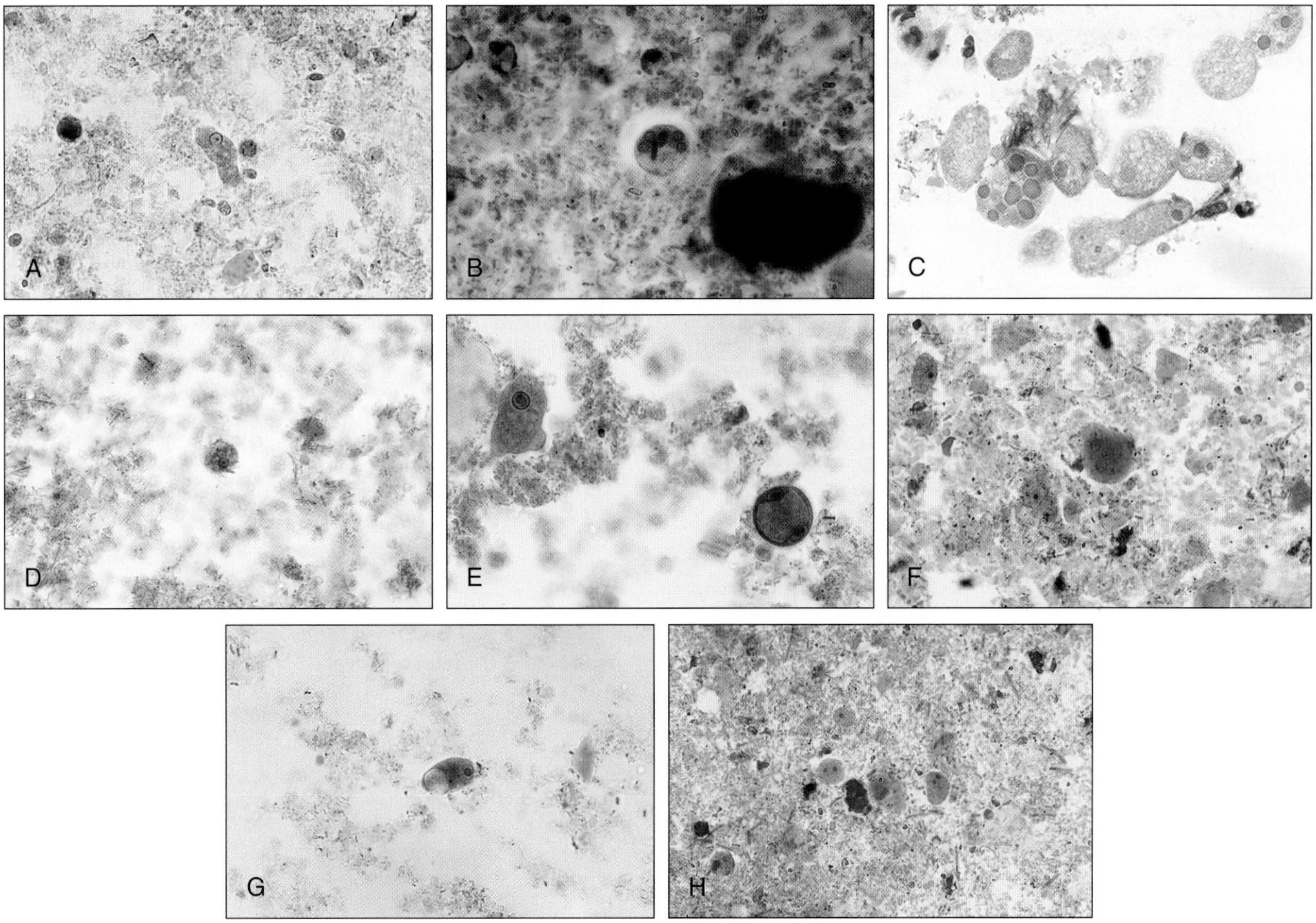

Figure 62-11 Intestinal protozoa, trichrome stain, oil immersion, except as noted. **A,** Trophozoite of *Entamoeba histolytica.* **B,** Quadrinucleate cyst of *E. histolytica* with rounded chromatoid bars. *(Photograph courtesy David Bergeron.)* **C,** *E. histolytica* trophozoites with ingested red blood cells from a colonic lesion (H&E). **D,** Trophozoite of *E. hartmanni.* **E,** Trophozoite and binucleate cyst of *E. coli.* **F,** Multinucleate cyst of *E. coli.* **G,** Cyst of *Iodamoeba bütschlii* with characteristic glycogen vacuole. **H,** Binucleate trophozoites typical for *Dientamoeba fragilis.*

may persist for months or years after successful treatment (Rosenblatt, 1995; Wilson, 1995).

Trophozoites of *E. histolytica* vary from 10–60 µm in diameter, with the commensal forms usually 15–20 µm and the invasive forms greater than 20 µm in greatest dimension (Table 62-9; Figs. 62-9 through 62-12). In direct wet mounts, trophozoites show progressive motility via rapidly formed hyaline pseudopodia that demonstrate a sharp demarcation between endoplasm and ectoplasm; unstained nuclei are not visible. In invasive disease, some trophozoites contain ingested erythrocytes (see Fig. 62-11, *C*), a feature diagnostic of *E. histolytica* infection. In stained preparations, the peripheral nuclear chromatin is evenly distributed along the nuclear membrane as fine granules. The karyosome is small and is often centrally located, with fine fibrils, which generally are not visible, attaching it to the nuclear membrane. Variations in nuclear structure occur, with some karyosomes located eccentrically and peripheral chromatin irregularly distributed. The only characteristic that is pathognomonic for *E. histolytica* is phagocytosis of erythrocytes, which very rarely occurs with other species. The cytoplasm is finely granular, and in invasive organisms, no inclusions or only erythrocyte inclusions are seen. Noninvasive organisms may contain ingested bacteria. In degenerating organisms, the cytoplasm may become vacuolated and nuclei may show abnormal chromatin clumping.

Cysts of *E. histolytica* are spherical and measure 10–20 µm (usually 12–15 µm) in diameter (Table 62-10; see Figs. 62-9, 62-10, and 62-12). The rounded precyst stage has a single nucleus but does not have a refractile cyst wall. As it matures, the cyst develops four nuclei, each approximately one-sixth the diameter of the cyst. Cyst nuclei appear similar to those of trophozoites, but their smaller size makes them less useful as differentiating features. The cyst cytoplasm may contain glycogen vacuoles and chromatoid bodies with blunted or rounded ends. The number and size of nuclei and the appearance of chromatoid bodies are important diagnostic criteria for identifying cysts.

Those laboratories that do not use one of the immunologic or molecular methods to differentiate *E. histolytica* from *E. dispar*, and that rely exclusively on morphologic analysis, must use a reporting format that takes the differing technologies into consideration. Thus, a report of "*E. histolytica/E. dispar*" would be most appropriate in the latter circumstance.

Nonpathogenic Amebae

Laboratory personnel must be able to differentiate nonpathogenic or commensal intestinal amebae from *E. histolytica/E. dispar* and *D. fragilis* (a flagellate), which are potential pathogens. Identification characteristics, best visualized in permanent stained sections, are summarized in Tables 62-9 and 62-10 and in Figures 62-9, 62-10, and 62-12. Identification of trophozoites is based on size and nuclear and cytoplasmic characteristics; identification of cysts is based on size, number and characteristics of nuclei, and presence and character of chromatoid bodies and glycogen masses.

E. hartmanni has morphologic characteristics similar to those of *E. histolytica*, except trophozoites have a maximum diameter of 12 µm and cysts have a maximum diameter of 10 µm, and cysts often have a single nucleus. Historically, *E. hartmanni* has been called the small race of *E. histolytica*. Differentiation requires careful measurement of a representative sample of organisms with a properly calibrated ocular micrometer.

Entamoeba coli, a common lumen-dwelling ameba, may be difficult to differentiate from *E. histolytica*. The cytoplasm stains somewhat more darkly than the cytoplasm of *E. histolytica* and is more vacuolated, containing numerous ingested bacteria, yeasts, and other materials. Although nuclear characteristics differ from those of *E. histolytica* (see Fig. 62-12), significant overlap may occur, especially in specimens that have not been promptly preserved. Mature cysts of *E. coli* contain eight nuclei, although occasional cysts contain 16 or more. Immature cysts, which are not common, have four nuclei that are larger (one-fourth the diameter of the cyst) than nuclei of *E. histolytica* (one-sixth the diameter of the cyst) and

TABLE 62-9
Morphology of Trophozoites of Intestinal Amebae

Species	Size (in diameter or length)	Motility	Nucleus numbers*	Peripheral chromatin	Karyosomal chromatin	Cytoplasm appearance	Inclusions
Entamoeba histolytica/ E. dispar	10–60 µm; usual range, 15–20 µm commensal form†; over 20 µm for invasive form‡	Progressive, with hyaline, finger-like pseudopods	1 Not visible in unstained preparations	Fine granules; usually evenly distributed and uniform in size	Small, discrete; usually central but occasionally eccentric	Finely granular	Erythrocytes occasionally in invasive forms; noninvasive, contain bacteria
Entamoeba hartmanni	5–12 µm; usual range, 8–10 µm	Usually nonprogressive but may be progressive occasionally	1 Not visible in unstained preparations	Similar to *E. histolytica*	Small, discrete, often eccentric	Finely granular	Bacteria
Entamoeba coli	15–50 µm; usual range, 20–25 µm	Sluggish, nonprogressive with blunt pseudopods	1 Often visible in unstained preparation	Coarse granules, irregular in size and distribution	Large, discrete, usually eccentric	Coarse, often vacuolated	Bacteria, yeasts, other materials
Endolimax nana	6–12 µm; usual range, 8–10 µm	Sluggish, usually nonprogressive with blunt pseudopods	1 Visible occasionally in unstained preparations	None	Large, irregularly shaped	Granular, vacuolated	Bacteria
Iodamoeba bütschlii	8–20 µm; usual range, 12–15 µm	Sluggish, usually nonprogressive	1 Not usually visible in unstained preparations	None	Large, usually central; surrounded by refractile, achromatic granules; these granules often are not distinct even in stained slides	Coarsely granular, vacuolated	Bacteria, yeasts, or other materials
Dientamoeba fragilis§	5–15 µm; usual range, 9–12 µm	Pseudopods are angular, serrated, or broad lobed, and hyaline is almost transparent	2 (In approximately 20% of organisms, only 1 nucleus is present) Nuclei invisible in unstained preparations	None	Large cluster of 4–8 granules	Finely granular, vacuolated	Bacteria

Adapted from Brooke MM, Melvin DM. Morphology of diagnostic stages of intestinal parasites of man. PHS Publication No. 1966. Bethesda, Md.: U.S. Department of Health Education and Welfare; 1969.
*Visibility is for unfixed material. Nuclei sometimes may be visible in fixed material.
†Usually found in asymptomatic or chronic cases; may contain bacteria.
‡Usually found in acute cases; often contain red blood cells.
§A flagellate (see text).

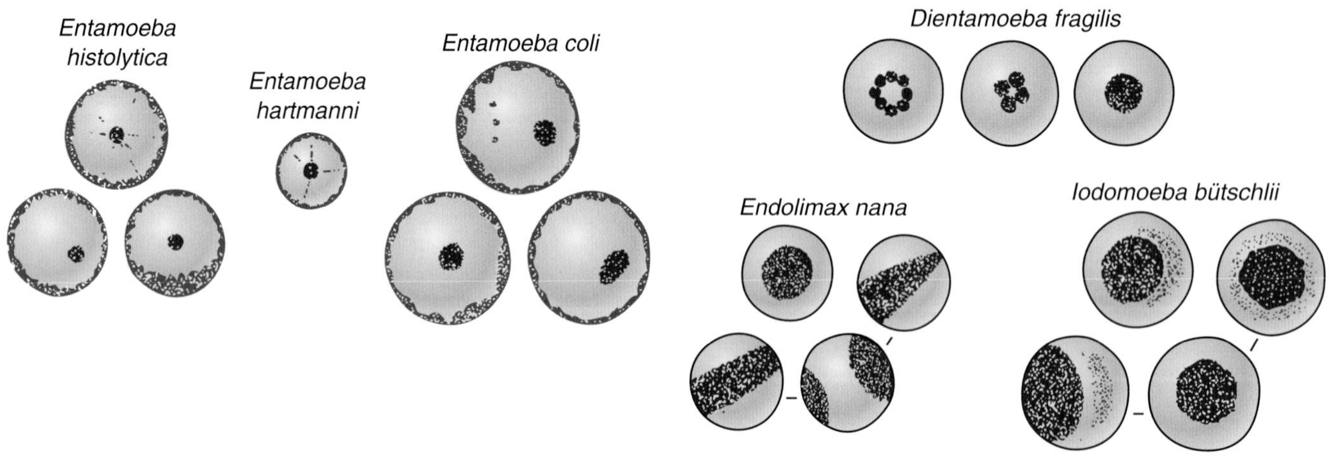

Figure 62-12 Nuclei of amebae. This drawing shows some of the various appearances of amebic nuclei in stained preparations. (*Dientamoeba fragilis* is a flagellate; see text.)

TABLE 62-10

Morphology of Cysts of Intestinal Amebae

Species	Size	Shape	Nucleus number	Peripheral chromatin	Karyosomal chromatin	Cytoplasm chromatoid bodies	Glycogen
Entamoeba histolytica/ E. dispar	10–20 μm; usual range, 12–15 μm	Usually spherical	4 in mature cyst; immature cysts with 1 or 2 occasionally seen	Peripheral chromatin present; fine, uniform granules, evenly distributed	Small, discrete, usually central	Present; elongate bars with bluntly rounded ends	Usually diffuse; concentrated mass often present in young cysts; stains reddish brown with iodine
Entamoeba hartmanni	5–10 μm; usual range, 6–8 μm	Usually spherical	4 in mature cyst; Immature cysts with 1 or 2 often seen	Similar to *E. histolytica*	Similar to *E. histolytica*	Present; elongate bars with bluntly rounded ends	Similar to *E. histolytica*
Entamoeba coli	10–35 μm; usual range, 15–25 μm	Usually spherical; occasionally oval, triangular, or of another shape	8 in mature cyst; occasionally supernucleate cysts with 16 or more are seen; immature cysts with 2 or more occasionally seen	Peripheral chromatin present; coarse granules irregular in size and distribution, but often appear more uniform than in trophozoites	Large, discrete, usually eccentric, but occasionally central	Present; usually splinter-like with pointed ends	Usually diffuse, but occasionally well-defined mass in immature cysts; stains reddish brown with iodine
Endolimax nana	5–10 μm; usual range, 6–8 μm	Spherical, ovoid, or ellipsoidal	4 in mature cysts; immature cysts with fewer than 4 rarely seen	None	Large, usually centrally located	Occasionally, granules or small oval masses seen, but bodies as seen in *Entamoeba* species are not present	Usually diffuse; concentrated mass seen occasionally in young cysts; stains reddish brown with iodine
Iodamoeba bütschlii	5–20 μm; usual range, 10–12 μm	Ovoid, ellipsoidal, triangular, or of another shape	1 in mature cyst	None	Large, usually eccentric; refractile, achromatic granules on one side of karyosome	Granules occasionally present, but bodies as seen in *Entamoeba* species are not present	Compact, well-defined mass; stains dark brown with iodine

Adapted from Brooke MM, Melvin DM. Morphology of diagnostic stages of intestinal parasites of man. PHS Publication No. 1966. Bethesda, Md.: U.S. Department of Health Education and Welfare; 1969.

may contain glycogen. Distribution of peripheral chromatin and karyosomes should not be given great emphasis in identification of *Entamoeba* cysts. Chromatoid bodies, when present, are irregular in shape with splintered or pointed ends, rather than the rounded ends seen in *E. histolytica*.

Endolimax nana is the smallest ameba to infect humans. Trophozoites often have atypical nuclei that contain a triangular chromatin mass, a band of chromatin across the nucleus, or two discrete masses of chromatin on opposite sides of the nuclear membrane (see Fig. 62-12). A clear halo or karyolymph space surrounds the karyosome and extends to the nuclear membrane. Atypical nuclear forms may be helpful in differentiating *E. nana* from *I. bütschlii*, which is similar in appearance but larger. Cysts of *Endolimax* usually contain four nuclei, although smaller numbers may be seen. Glycogen, when present, occurs diffusely in the cytoplasm rather than as a discrete mass. Cysts are easily differentiated from those of other amebae but may be confused with *Blastocystis hominis* organisms. The nuclei of *B. hominis*, however, lack the halos that are typically seen with *E. nana* cysts.

The nuclei of *I. bütschlii* trophozoites and cysts have a large, centrally located karyosome frequently surrounded by achromatic granules that may not be distinct but appear only as a muddy karyolymph space or halo. In some nuclei, the halo is clear without evident achromatic granules, making the organism indistinguishable from *E. nana*. Cysts of *I. bütschlii* contain a single nucleus, in which the karyosome is often eccentric with a nearby crescent of achromatic granules (see Figs. 62-9, 62-10, and 62-12). The cyst is characterized by a prominent vacuole of glycogen that stains reddish brown in iodine-stained wet mounts, thus the name of the organism. Glycogen is dissolved by aqueous fixatives and may not be demonstrable in material that has been stored.

Blastocystis hominis

Blastocystis hominis inhabits the large bowel and is frequently found in stool specimens of asymptomatic individuals. While appearing in stains as an amoeba-like protozoan, the phylogenetic affinities of this parasite remain uncertain. Some studies have linked heavy infection to symptomatic intestinal disease, although this remains controversial (Markell, 1986; Sheehan, 1986; Miller, 1988; Zierdt, 1991; Stenzel, 1996; Garcia, 2007). *Blastocystis* may assume one of three forms: vacuolated (seen most commonly), ameboid, or granular. The vacuolated form, also known as the central vacuolar form, usually is spherical and variable in size (5–20 μm) and has a central clear area and two to four peripheral nuclei (Figs. 62-13, *A*, and 62-14, *G*). Ameboid forms with bizarre shapes may predominate in heavy infections. The presence of *Blastocystis* should be reported, especially when they are numerous (five or more per 400× field) (Sheehan, 1986; Stenzel, 1996).

FLAGELLATES

Dientamoeba fragilis

Dientamoeba fragilis is an ameboid pathogen that infects the colon and has been associated with diarrheal disease, especially in young children (Yang, 1977; Spencer 1979; Turner, 1985; Preiss, 1991; Johnson, 2004). Although

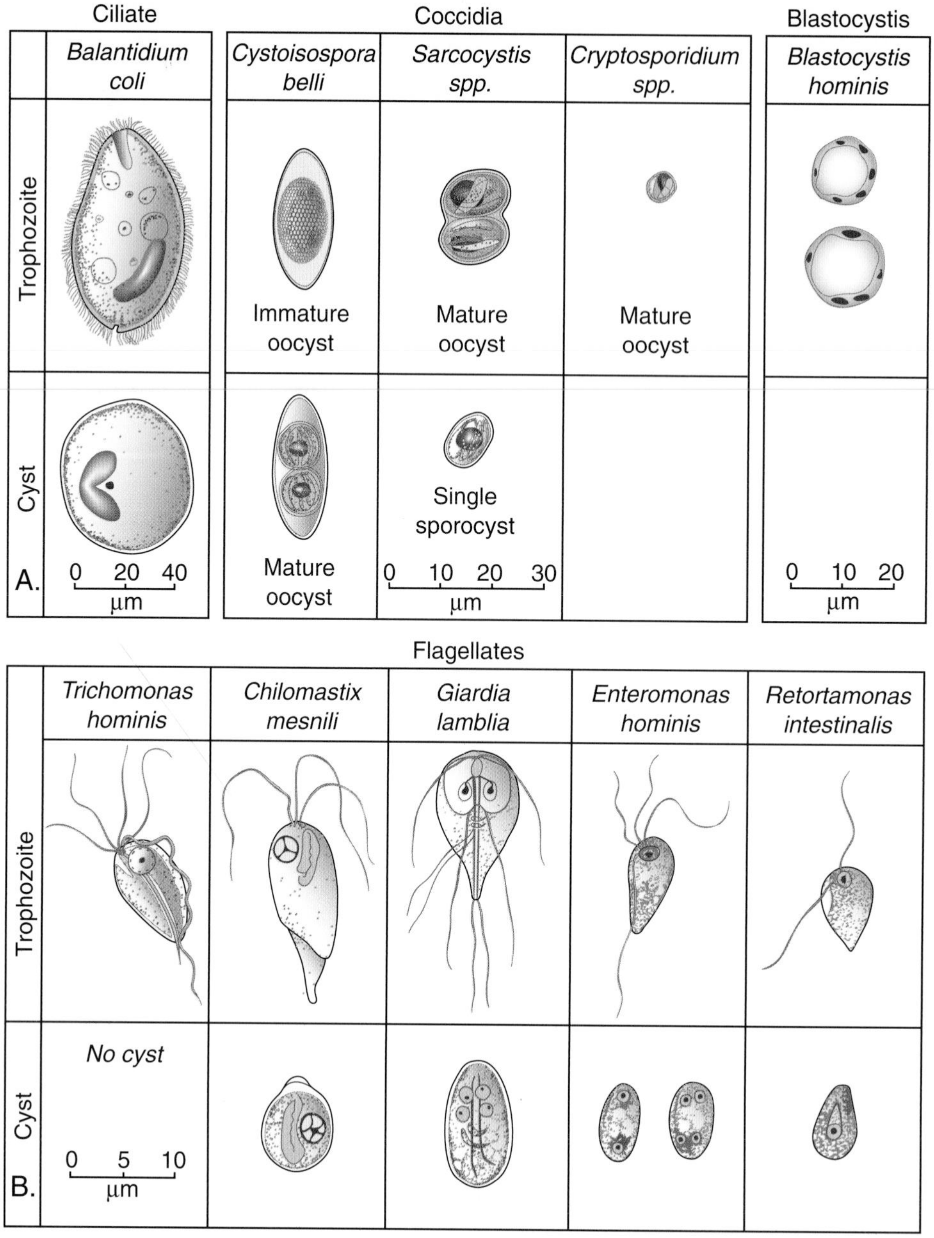

Figure 62-13 **A,** Ciliate, Coccidia, and *Blastocystis hominis* spp. found in stool specimens of humans. **B,** Flagellates found in stool specimens of humans. *(Adapted from Brooke MM, Melvin DM. Morphology of diagnostic stages of intestinal parasites of man. Publication No. [CDC] 848116. Washington, DC: U.S. Department of Health and Human Services; 1984.)*

similar in appearance to amebae, *Dientamoeba* has been reclassified as a flagellate on the basis of ultrastructural details and antigenic similarities. Also, no cyst stage has been described. Because of the similarity of *Dientamoeba* to amebae at the light microscope level, this species has traditionally been included in tables and figures for amebae (see Table 62-9 and Figs. 62-9, 62-10, 62-11, *H*, and 62-12).

Symptoms of *D. fragilis* infection include diarrhea and abdominal distention. Recent evidence suggests that dientamebiasis is a more frequent cause of diarrhea than previously thought: 4.3% of patients in one study harbored this organism (Spencer, 1979; Murray, 2007). Approximately 25% of persons infected with this parasite have symptomatic disease. In contrast to amebiasis, this infection usually is not associated with other fecal protozoa but does show a 10–20 times greater than expected association with enterobiasis (pinworm infection, discussed later). This association and some experimental evidence suggest that *D. fragilis* infection may be spread by ingestion of pinworm eggs infected with *D. fragilis* (Burrows, 1956; Johnson, 2004). *D. fragilis* infection will be overlooked unless permanently stained slides are examined. Multiple specimens may need to be submitted because shedding varies from day to day. When smears are prepared, the last portion of the stool evacuated should be examined because the number of parasites found there tends to be greater. Two thirds to four fifths of the organisms contain two nuclei that consist of a cluster of four to eight karyosomal granules, which may appear as one large irregular karyosome (see Fig. 62-12). Uninucleate *D. fragilis* may be confused with trophozoites of *E. nana* or *I. bütschlii*. The cytoplasm is finely granular and often contains ingested bacteria. Trophozoites are delicate and may be easily overlooked, so stained slides must be carefully examined. An immunofluorescence method has been described that may help in the detection of this parasite, but it is not commercially available (Chan, 1993).

Giardia lamblia

Giardia lamblia is a pathogenic intestinal protozoan that causes both endemic and epidemic disease worldwide; in the United States, it is especially problematic for travelers, campers, children attending day care, and homosexual men (Wolfe, 1992). It frequently causes disease in individuals drinking contaminated water, and a number of large water-borne outbreaks have been described from places such as Aspen, Colorado; Leningrad, Russia; and Rome, New York (Craun, 1986). Pathogenic protozoa are not killed by the usual concentrations of chlorine in municipal water supplies; therefore, unless the water supply is filtered, it may serve as a source of infection, as it did in the Rome, New York, outbreak.

G. lamblia trophozoites multiply in the small bowel and attach to the mucosa by a ventral concave sucking disk. Infection may be asymptomatic or may cause disease ranging from mild diarrhea with vague abdominal

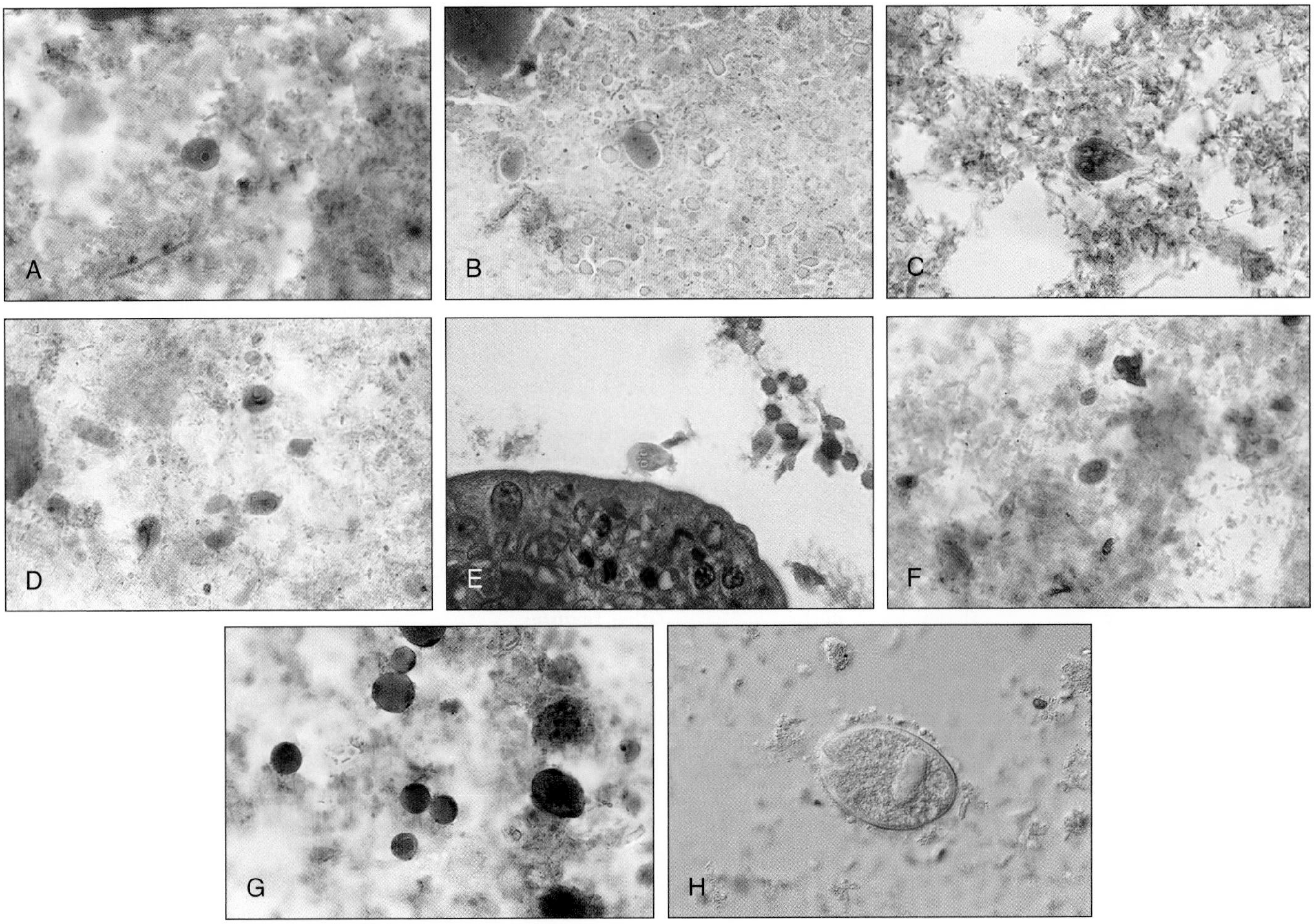

Figure 62-14 Intestinal protozoa, trichrome stain, oil immersion, except as noted. **A,** Trophozoite of *Endolimax nana.* **B,** Quadrinucleate cysts of *E. nana.* **C,** Trophozoite of *Giardia lamblia* displaying prominent nuclei, median bodies, flagella, and a tapered posterior end. **D,** Cysts of *G. lamblia* with nuclei and fibrils. **E,** Duodenal biopsy demonstrating a *G. lamblia* trophozoite (H&E). **F,** A lemon-shaped cyst of *Chilomastix mesnili* with visible nucleus and hyaline cap. **G,** Multiple central vacuolar forms of *Blastocystis hominis.* **H,** Trophozoite of *Balantidium coli* in wet mount; note cilia covering the cell, cytostome, and macronucleus.

complaints to a malabsorption syndrome with diarrhea and steatorrhea, similar to that of sprue. The pathogenesis is not fully understood, although disruption of the integrity of the brush border with resulting disaccharidase deficiency may occur from direct or indirect effects of the organism's presence (Wolfe, 1992). Giardiasis should be considered in any patient presenting with diarrhea of longer than 10 days' duration.

Diagnosis is established by demonstration of *Giardia* trophozoites or cysts, or both, in fecal specimens. Trophozoites predominate in diarrheic stool, whereas infectious cysts are more likely to be found in formed stool. The passage of organisms varies from day to day; therefore, examination of multiple specimens, collected on different days, may be necessary. Direct wet mounts are particularly helpful for demonstrating trophozoites, with their so-called falling leaf motility, in a diarrheic or aspirate specimen. Cysts can be seen in direct wet mount and concentration techniques, and both trophozoites and cysts may be demonstrated on permanently stained slides. In some cases, the organisms cannot be demonstrated in fecal specimens, and small bowel aspirates or so-called string test specimens may be required. In such instances, the laboratory should be advised in advance, so personnel will be available to perform a direct wet mount examination immediately on receipt of the specimen (Garcia, 2007).

Many antigen detection methods based on IFA or EIA are commercially available (Clinical and Laboratory Standards Institute, 2005; Garcia, 2007, 2010). They appear to have good sensitivity and specificity and may detect some infections not found by morphologic examination of stools. They also can be particularly helpful in epidemiologic investigations but cannot replace the need for traditional morphologic examination of the specimen to detect other pathogenic parasites.

When viewed in their broadest dimension, *Giardia* trophozoites are pear-shaped with a tapered posterior end, and have two nuclei that give the appearance of a smiling face with prominent eyes (Table 62-11; see Figs. 62-13, *B*, and 62-14, *C* through *E*). When viewed from the side, the anterior end of the organism is thicker and tapers posteriorly; the anterior half to three quarters consists of the sucking disk on the ventral surface. The four lateral, two ventral, and two caudal flagella usually are not evident in wet mounts or in stained preparations. Cysts are oval and usually quadrinucleate. Below the nuclei are dark-staining median bodies that cross longitudinal fibrils, providing distinctive internal characteristics. The cytoplasm often is retracted from the cyst wall.

Chilomastix mesnili

Chilomastix mesnili (see Table 62-11, Figs. 62-13, *B*, and 62-14, *F*) is a nonpathogenic lumen-dwelling flagellate of humans that must be differentiated from trophozoites of amebae and *Giardia* in stained smears. The consistent location of the single nucleus at one end of the organism and the tapering of the end opposite the nucleus are helpful. If multiple organisms are examined, the cytostome and the spiral groove are visible in some. The three external flagella usually are not visible in stained or formalin-fixed preparations. The lemon-shaped cysts contain various curved cytostomal fibers with a safety pin–like appearance.

Pentatrichomonas hominis

Pentatrichomonas hominis, known previously as *Trichomonas hominis* (see Table 62-11 and Fig. 62-13, *B*), is an infrequently seen nonpathogenic intestinal flagellate that may be confused with *E. hartmanni* or small *E. histolytica* trophozoites. Organisms do not stain particularly well and often are distorted in permanent smears. Several organisms may have to be examined in stained preparations to demonstrate the single *Entamoeba*-like nucleus, undulating membrane and associated costa, and flagella. A prominent rod-like object, the axostyle, runs through the organism and protrudes from the posterior end. No cyst stage has been described.

Trichomonas vaginalis

Trichomonas vaginalis is a common cause of vaginitis, characterized by inflammation, itching, vaginal discharge, and, occasionally, dysuria. The

TABLE 62-11
Morphology of Intestinal Flagellates

Species	Size (length)	Shape	Motility	Number of nuclei	Number of flagella*	Other features
Trophozoites						
Pentatrichomonas hominis†	8–20 μm; usual range, 11–12 μm	Pear-shaped	Rapid, jerking	1 Not visible in unstained mounts	3–5 anterior; 1 posterior	Undulating membrane extending length of body
Chilomastix mesnili	6–24 μm; usual range, 10–15 μm	Pear-shaped	Stiff, rotary	1 Not visible in unstained mounts	3 anterior; 1 in cytostome	Prominent cytostome extending $\frac{1}{3}$–$\frac{1}{2}$; spiral groove across ventral surface
Giardia lamblia	10–20 μm; usual range, 12–15 μm	Pear-shaped	Falling leaf	2 Not visible in unstained mounts	4 lateral; 2 ventral; 3 caudal	Sucking disk occupying $\frac{1}{2}$–$\frac{3}{4}$ of ventral surface
Enteromonas hominis	4–10 μm; usual range, 8–9 μm	Oval	Jerking	1 Not visible in unstained mounts	3 anterior; 1 posterior	One side of body flattened; posterior flagellum extending free, posteriorly or laterally
Retortamonas intestinalis	4–9 μm; usual range, 6–7 μm	Pear-shaped or oval	Jerking	1 Not visible in unstained mounts	1 anterior; 1 posterior	Prominent cytostome extending approximately $\frac{1}{2}$ length of body

Species	Size	Shape	Number of nuclei	Other features
Cysts				
Chilomastix mesnili	6–10 μm; usual range, 8–9 μm	Lemon-shaped, with anterior hyaline knob or "nipple"	1 Not visible in unstained preparations	Cytostome with supporting fibrils. Usually visible in stained preparations.
Giardia lamblia	8–13 μm; usual range, 11–12 μm	Oval or ellipsoidal	Usually 4; not distinct in unstained preparations; usually located at one end	Fibrils or flagella longitudinally in cyst. Cytoplasm often retracts from a portion of cell wall.
Enteromonas hominis	4–10 μm; usual range, 6–8 μm	Elongate or oval	1–4, usually 2 lying at opposite ends of cyst; not visible in unstained mounts	Resembles *E. nana* cyst. Fibrils or flagella usually are not seen.
Retortamonas intestinalis	4–9 μm; usual range, 4–7 μm	Pear-shaped or slightly lemon-shaped	1 Not visible in unstained mounts	Resembles *Chilomastix* cyst. Shadow outline of cytostome with supporting fibrils extends above nucleus.

Adapted from Brooke MM, Melvin DM. Morphology of diagnostic stages of intestinal parasites of man. PHS Publication No. 1966. Bethesda, Md.: U.S. Department of Health Education and Welfare; 1969.
*Not a practical feature for identification of species in routine fecal examinations.
†*Pentatrichomonas hominis* does not have a cyst form.

infection usually is spread by sexual intercourse, often by males who have an asymptomatic infection. Occasionally, males may have symptomatic prostatitis or urethritis. *T. vaginalis* infections usually are diagnosed in the physician's office by direct wet mount examination of vaginal fluid, prostatic fluid, or sediments of freshly passed urine. Morphologically, *T. vaginalis* resembles *P. hominis* but is larger (up to 23 μm), and the undulating membrane extends only half the length of the body. Because of the difference in habitat, it generally is not necessary to differentiate these trichomonads morphologically.

Direct wet mount examination may be insensitive, and the use of culture or commercially available immunoassay techniques is recommended when infection is not readily diagnosed (Garcia, 2007; Murray, 2007). Cultures, including use of a convenient "pouch" system, have a sensitivity of about 90% (Krieger, 1988; Schmid, 1989; Beal, 1992; Levi, 1997), as do DFA and EIA techniques that use monoclonal antibodies (Krieger, 1988; Lisi, 1988; Wilson, 1995). Papanicolaou-stained gynecologic smears may reveal *T. vaginalis* on occasion but have poor sensitivity and specificity.

Other Flagellates

Enteromonas hominis and *Retortamonas intestinalis* are small, nonpathogenic, intestinal flagellates that are seen infrequently but, when present, may occur in large numbers. Morphologic characteristics are reviewed in Table 62-11 (see also Fig. 62-13, *B*). *Trichomonas tenax* is a trichomonad that occasionally is recovered from the oral cavity but does not cause disease.

CILIATES

Balantidium coli

The ciliate *Balantidium coli* (see Figs. 62-13, *A*, and 62-14, *H*) may cause a dysentery-like syndrome with colonic ulcerations similar to that of amebiasis, but it does not produce liver abscesses or other systemic lesions. Human infection, rare in the United States, is usually acquired from hogs, which are commonly infected. *B. coli* is the largest protozoan to infect humans. Trophozoites are between 40 μm and more than 200 μm in greatest dimension (most measure 50–100 μm) and are uniformly covered with

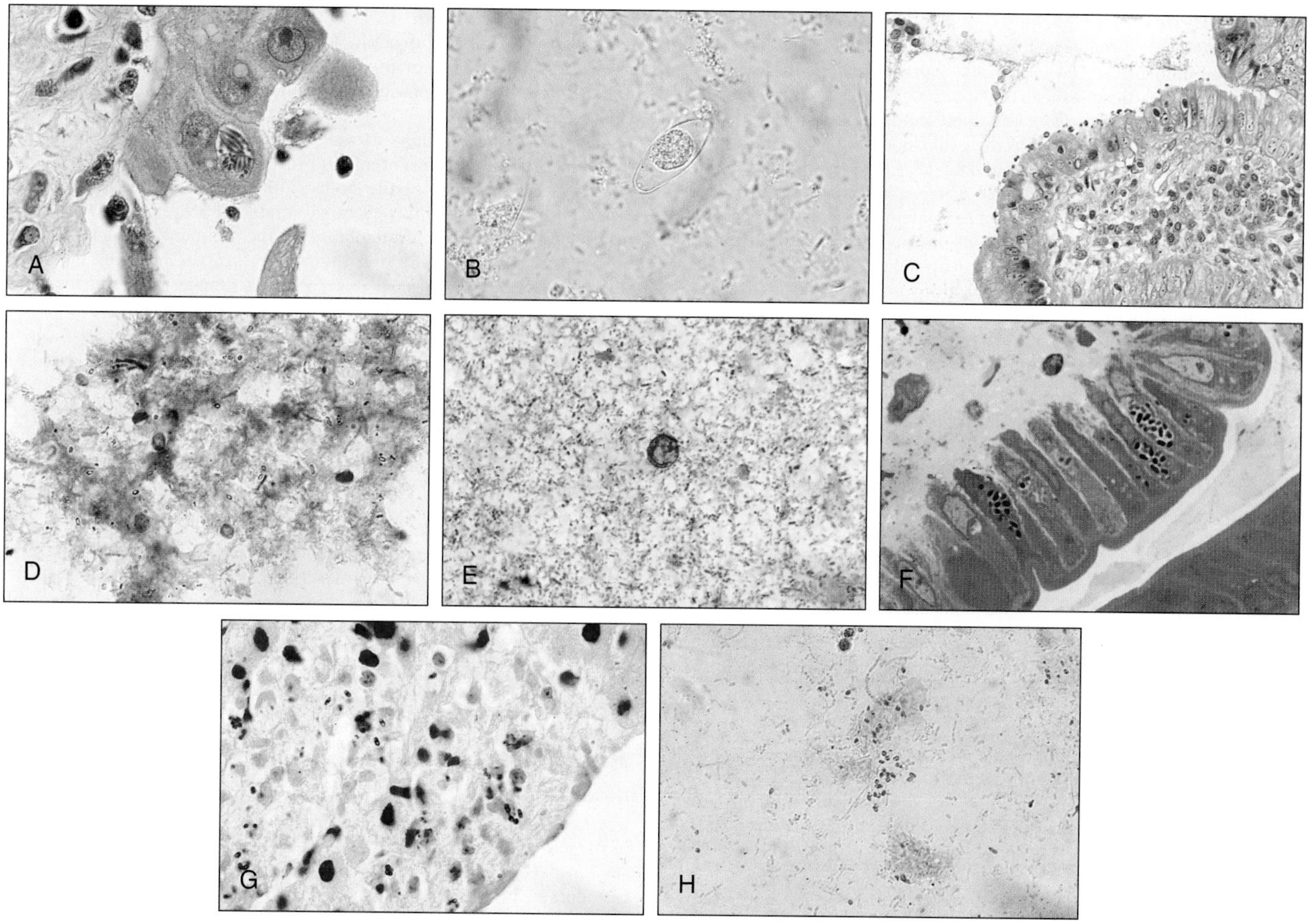

Figure 62-15 **A,** Schizont of *Cystisospora belli* containing numerous merozoites developing within gallbladder epithelium (H&E; oil immersion). **B,** Oocyst of *C. belli* in feces (wet mount; oil immersion). **C,** Small-bowel biopsy demonstrating development of *Cryptosporidium parvum* oocysts within the brush border of enterocytes (H&E; ×400). **D,** Modified acid-fast stain of a fecal smear demonstrating oocysts of *C. parvum* (oil immersion). **E,** Modified acid-fast stain of a fecal smear demonstrating an oocyst of *Cyclospora cayetanensis* (oil immersion). **F,** Small-bowel biopsy demonstrating development of microsporidial spores within enterocytes (epoxy-embedded section stained with toluidine blue; oil immersion). **G,** Microsporidial spores seen in liver parenchyma in an individual infected with the human immunodeficiency virus (Brown and Brenn stain; oil immersion). **H,** Numerous microsporidial spores in feces stained with the modified trichrome stain (oil immersion).

cilia that are slightly longer at the anterior end adjacent to the cytostome. A large macronucleus is readily seen in stained preparations, and a smaller micronucleus is infrequently visible. Numerous food vacuoles and contractile vacuoles are present in the cytoplasm. Cysts are rounded, measuring 50–70 μm in length. Cilia may be seen within younger cysts, and nuclear characteristics are similar to those of trophozoites. Stool specimens that have been contaminated with stagnant water may contain free-living ciliates, which usually can be distinguished from *B. coli* by differences in their ciliary pattern.

COCCIDIA

The coccidia comprise a large group of apicomplexan parasites that have a sexual stage in the intestinal tract of invertebrate and vertebrate animals. Some species also develop asexually in extraintestinal sites in host tissues. Genera infecting the intestine of humans, such as *Isospora*, *Sarcocystis*, *Cryptosporidium*, and *Cyclospora*, generally produce self-limited diarrheal disease in immunocompetent persons. Severe protracted diarrhea may develop in immunocompromised hosts following infection with *Isospora*, *Cryptosporidium*, and *Cyclospora*.

Cystoisospora belli

Cystoisospora belli (formerly known as *Isospora belli*) undergoes both asexual and sexual development in the cytoplasm of small intestine epithelial cells (Fig. 62-15, *A*). Sexual development results in the production of oocysts, which are passed in the stool and mature to the infective stage in the environment. Human infections cause diarrhea and malabsorption but generally are self-limited. In patients with AIDS or other immunosuppressive disorders, disease may persist for months or years, and may contribute to death (DeHovitz, 1986; Mannheimer, 1994; Murray, 2007). Diagnosis is established by finding the unsporulated oocysts measuring 12 × 30 μm in fecal specimens, usually in direct wet mounts or concentration preparations (Fig. 62-15, *B*). If the unfixed specimen is left at room temperature for 24–48 hours, sporulation occurs. The infectious oocyst contains two sporocysts, each with four sporozoites (see Fig. 62-13, *A*). These oocysts are similar to those of *Cryptosporidium* in that they stain acid-fast.

Sarcocystis spp.

Sarcocystis spp. are typical two-host coccidia in which the sexual phase develops in the intestinal mucosa of carnivorous animals, and the asexual, extraintestinal phase occurs in the muscles and tissues of various intermediate hosts. Humans may serve as definitive or intermediate hosts, depending on the species of *Sarcocystis*. Intestinal infection with *Sarcocystis hominis* and *Sarcocystis suihominis* is acquired by ingestion of raw or incompletely cooked beef or pork, respectively, which contains tissue cysts (sarcocysts). Infection usually is asymptomatic, but occasional patients have transient diarrhea, abdominal pain, or anorexia. Intestinal infection is self-limited because asexual multiplication occurs in the intermediate host and is not repeated in the definitive host. Oocyst production is limited by the number of organisms ingested in the form of sarcocysts. The diagnosis is established by detection of sporulated 25 × 33 μm sporocysts in the stools (see Fig. 62-13, *A*). Each mature sporocyst contains four sporozoites. The oocyst wall is thin and often is not detectable, or has already ruptured, releasing the two sporocysts. These forms, best seen in wet mounts or in acid-fast–stained smears, appear larger than oocysts of *Cryptosporidium*. Trichrome stains are of little value in detecting these parasites. Humans also may serve as intermediate hosts for several unnamed animal species of *Sarcocystis* (known collectively as *Sarcocystis lindemanni*), in which case cysts are found in skeletal and cardiac muscles (Beaver, 1979; Strickland, 2000).

Cryptosporidium spp.

Cryptosporidium spp. use a single host in their life cycle but may infect humans (predominantly *C. hominis* and *C. parvum*) and a wide variety of animals, including cattle and sheep (Coupe, 2005). Parasites develop in the brush border of epithelial cells of the small and large intestine and occasionally spread to other sites such as the gallbladder, the pancreas, and the respiratory tract (see Figs. 62-13, *A*, and 62-15, *C* and *D*). *Cryptosporidium* is a common cause of acute, self-limited diarrhea in normal persons, especially in children who attend day care. The epidemiology of cryptosporidiosis is similar to that of giardiasis. One of the largest known outbreaks of water-transmitted infection occurred in Milwaukee, Wisconsin, in 1993. In that outbreak, an estimated 400,000 individuals became ill from tap water contaminated with farm runoff following heavy rains (MacKenzie, 1994). Similar to cysts of *Giardia*, *Cryptosporidium* oocysts are refractory to usual chlorination levels of drinking water, and unless a community's water supply from a surface source is filtered, epidemics may occur. In patients with AIDS, *Cryptosporidium* may cause chronic secretory diarrhea that can last for months to years and may contribute to death. The incubation period is about 8 days, and in previously healthy persons, the illness lasts 9–23 days. Patients may have malaise, fever, anorexia, abdominal cramps, and diarrhea (Current, 1991; Mannheimer, 1994).

Diagnosis usually is established by stool examination. Various concentration methods, including formalin–ethyl acetate sedimentation and Sheather's sugar flotation, work well (Clinical and Laboratory Standards Institute, 2005; Garcia, 2007). The availability of the formalin–ethyl acetate method makes this technique attractive, although centrifugation speed and times must be increased to maximize recovery (Clinical and Laboratory Standards Institute, 2005; Garcia, 2010). A smear is prepared from the sediment and stained with an acid-fast stain or immunofluorescent reagents. Several acid-fast staining methods, including auramine-O, have been evaluated, but a modified cold Kinyoun method is used most widely. Spherical oocysts measure 4–6 μm in diameter and, when stained by the modified Kinyoun procedure, appear a deep fuchsia, although some unevenness of staining intensity is noted, along with variability in the percentage of cysts that stain positive. Positive control slides must be used with every run.

Commercial DFA and EIA reagents, which provide good sensitivity and specificity (Clinical and Laboratory Standards Institute, 2005; Garcia, 2007; Murray, 2007), are especially good for laboratories where *Cryptosporidium* is infrequently encountered, and where there is difficulty in maintaining expertise in the interpretation of acid-fast stains.

The need to examine stool specimens for *Cryptosporidium* depends on the populations served and the goals, interests, and abilities of the individual laboratory. Some laboratories perform examination for *Cryptosporidium* only on specific request; others evaluate all specimens from immunocompromised patients.

Cyclospora cayetanensis

Cyclospora cayetanensis is a recently described coccidian parasite responsible for diarrheal disease in immunocompetent and immunocompromised individuals (Ortega, 1994; Murray, 2007). The parasite has been recovered from patients in several countries, including the United States, and was initially described as a blue-green alga, a cyanobacterium-like body, or a coccidian-like body, among others (Ortega, 1993; Shields, 2003). Infection causes a flu-like illness with nausea, vomiting, weight loss, and explosive watery diarrhea lasting 1–3 weeks. Oocysts, passed unsporulated, appear as nonrefractile spheres 8–10 μm in diameter that contain a cluster of refractile globules enclosed within a membrane when viewed by light microscopy. A total of 1–2 weeks is required for sporulation, after which the mature oocyst contains two sporocysts, each with two sporozoites. In trichrome-stained smears, the oocysts appear as clear, round, and somewhat wrinkled objects. Oocysts autofluoresce bright green to intense blue under ultraviolet epifluorescence; they stain acid-fast when modified acid-fast or auramine-O staining techniques are used. They must be differentiated from oocysts of *Cryptosporidium*, which stain in an identical fashion but are smaller (4–6 μm) (Fig. 62-15, *E*).

MICROSPORIDIA

Microsporidia are obligate intracellular, spore-forming protozoan parasites in the phylum Microspora that infect a variety of animals, including humans (Shadduck, 1989; Franzen, 1999). They are serious pathogens in immunocompromised hosts, especially those with AIDS, in whom they are responsible for a large percentage (up to 30% in some studies) of otherwise unexplained diarrheal disease (Curry, 1993). *Enterocytozoon bieneusi* and *Encephalitozoon intestinalis*, the two species implicated most commonly in human intestinal infection, may cause protracted diarrhea and weight loss in AIDS patients similar to that caused by *Cryptosporidium*. *E. intestinalis* may also cause disseminated disease (Cali, 1993; Willson, 1995; Murray, 2007).

The organisms multiply intracellularly (merogony) and form resistant spores (sporogony) that eventually rupture the host cell and infect adjacent cells or are passed out of the body. The spore contains a coiled polar tubule, which is forcefully extruded under appropriate environmental stimuli and penetrates the membrane of the recipient cell. The parasite's sporoplasm is injected through the tubule into the host cell cytoplasm, where multiplication ensues. Reservoir hosts have not been identified. Occasionally, patients have been infected by other genera of microsporidia, including *Encephalitozoon* (hepatitis, ocular infection, CNS disease), *Nosema* (disseminated infection), and *Pleistophora* (myositis) (Shadduck, 1989; Curry, 1993), among others (Franzen, 1999; Garcia, 2007).

Until recently, diagnosis required examination of tissues submitted for routine light (Fig. 62-15, *F* and *G*) and electron microscopy. Development of a modified trichrome staining method for examination of stool specimens for spores has been a significant advance in detecting infection (Weber, 1992; Garcia, 2007). With this method, the small (1.5–3 μm), elliptical spores stain red against a faint green background, and some display a characteristic midbody cross-band (Fig. 62-15, *H*). Modifications of this method have also been described. Fluorochrome stains such as Uvitex 2B and Calcofluor white appear to be more sensitive in detecting spores and may be useful in the initial screening of specimens (van Gool, 1993; DeGirolami, 1995; Luna, 1995). The small size of the spores makes detection by any method a challenge (Clinical and Laboratory Standards Institute, 2005).

INTESTINAL HELMINTHS

Intestinal helminths discussed here include those nematodes (roundworms), cestodes (tapeworms), and trematodes (flukes) that reside as adults in the gastrointestinal tract or live in other locations (liver, lung, or blood) and produce eggs that exit the human body via the intestinal tract. Sizes for adult helminths vary from 1 mm to more than 10 m in length; sizes for eggs range from 25–150 μm (Fig. 62-16).

An understanding of helminth life cycles and zoogeography is critical in knowing which parasite stages may be present in a presumed infection, what organs or tissues may be involved, and when diagnostic stages may be expected to appear following exposure. Although diagnosis usually depends on finding and identifying an appropriate developmental stage (egg, larva, or adult), some parasitic infections may be diagnosed chiefly on clinical grounds or on the basis of serologic evidence, or both.

Certain species have developmental cycles whereby infectious stages may be transmitted directly from person to person (*Enterobius* and *H. nana*). In others (*Trichuris*, *Ascaris*, and *Trichostrongylus*), an additional maturation period outside of the host is required before the parasite egg or larva (in the latter case) is infectious. Ingestion of infective stages may also occur incidentally along with parasite vectors (*Dipylidium*, *Hymenolepis*), plants (*Fasciolopsis*, *Fasciola*), or animal tissues (*Trichinella*, *Taenia*, *Diphyllobothrium*, *Clonorchis*, *Opisthorchis*, *Paragonimus*, *Heterophyes*, *Metagonimus*, and *Nanophyetus*). In some cases, larval parasite stages may directly penetrate the skin (hookworms, *Strongyloides*, and schistosomes).

Recovery and identification of helminth eggs and larvae in stool, urine, or sputum requires a systematic approach and appropriate training of the individuals performing the evaluations. The size of the eggs and larvae is an especially important characteristic, and measurement often requires a properly calibrated ocular micrometer. External characteristics of eggs that should be noted include their shape, their wall thickness, and the presence or absence of a mamillated covering, operculum, opercular shoulders, abopercular knob, polar plugs, or spines. Egg development (embryonated, unembryonated) and the presence or absence of hooklets, which are characteristic of cestodes, should be noted. The examiner also needs to have an appreciation for the large variety of artifacts detected in human feces that may mimic parasite eggs and larvae (see Table 62-4).

NEMATODES

Enterobius vermicularis

Enterobiasis or oxyuriasis is the most common helminthic infection in children of all social strata in the United States. Although it is primarily a parasite of young children, rapid maturation of the egg allows it to be

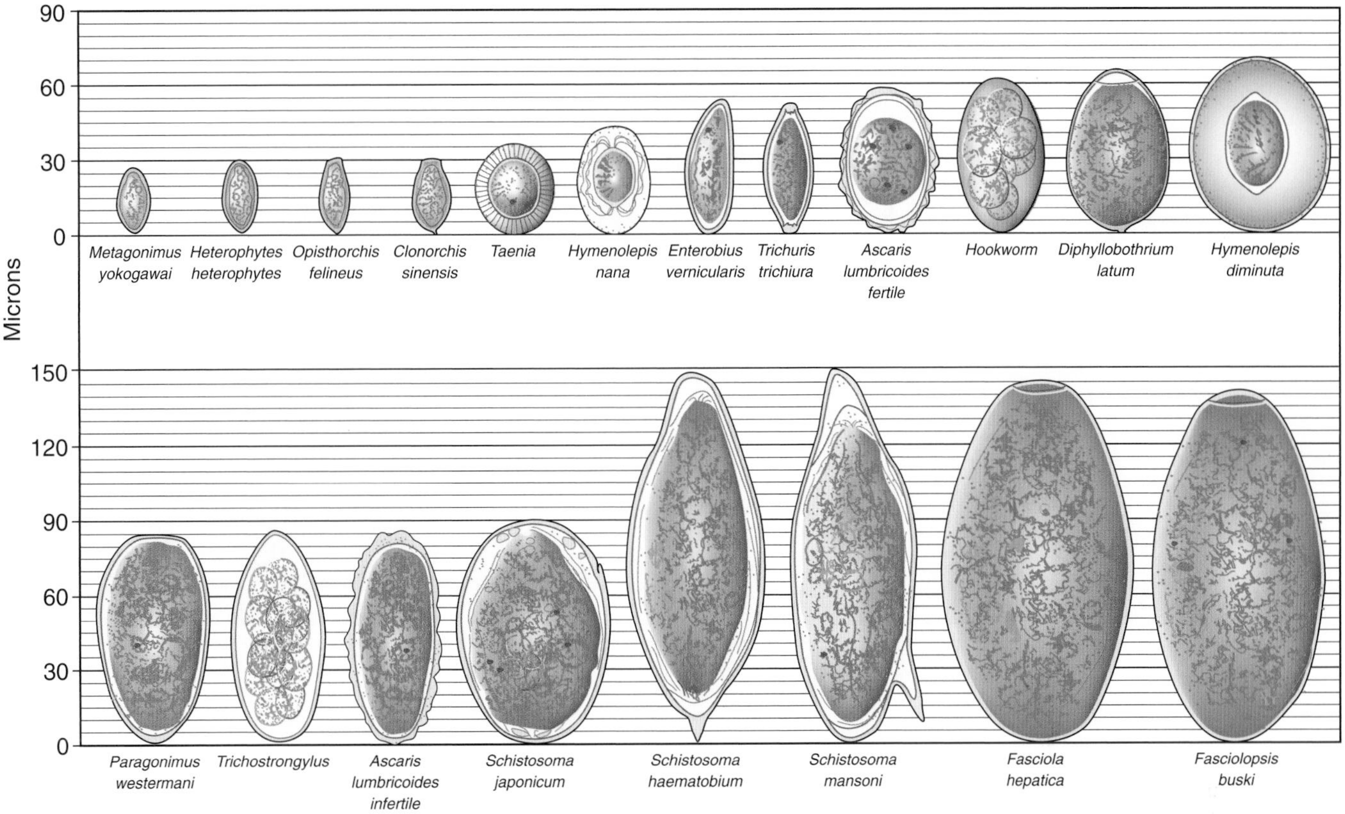

Figure 62-16 Relative sizes of helminth eggs. *(Courtesy Centers for Disease Control and Prevention, Parasitology Training Branch, Atlanta.)*

readily transmitted from child to child and from child to adult, in both family and institutional settings. Male and female worms reside primarily in the cecum and adjacent areas. Females measure up to 13 mm in length and have a pointed posterior end that gives rise to their common name, the pinworm. Both sexes have prominent lateral alae that are seen in cross-section and a prominent esophageal bulb (Fig. 62-17, *A* through *C*).

Although males are rarely seen, females may be found on the surface of a stool specimen or on the perianal skin, especially at night, where eggs are deposited. Eggs are colorless and ovoid with one side flattened, and measure 20–40 μm wide by 50–60 μm long (see Fig. 62-17, *B*). They are infective within hours and when ingested complete development to the gravid adult stage within 1 month (the prepatent period).

Although infection may be asymptomatic, children often suffer from pruritus ani, irritability, and loss of sleep. Enterobiasis should be ruled out early in the evaluation of enuresis. Adult worms may also migrate to unusual sites such as the vagina, fallopian tubes, or peritoneal cavity. Their ultimate death in these locations may provoke inflammatory, granulomatous reactions (Symmers, 1950; Garcia, 2007).

Recovery of eggs or, less commonly, adults from the perianal skin is usually done using the cellulose tape technique after the child has gone to sleep or first thing in the morning (Ash, 1987; Garcia, 2007). Only 5%–10% of cases are detected using routine stool examination. Diagnosis may require examination of several samples taken on different days before eggs can be detected (Sadun, 1956).

Trichuris trichiura

Trichuriasis is common worldwide in tropical and subtropical regions. Adult worms are found in the large intestine, especially the cecum, but in heavy infection they can be found throughout the colon and rectum. Males and females measure up to 50 mm in length and remain attached to the intestinal mucosa by the long, slender anterior end, while the thicker posterior end hangs free in the lumen. Female worms are elongate, whereas the tails on males are coiled (Fig. 62-17, *D*). *Trichuris* has a direct life cycle in which eggs are passed in stool unembryonated and require several weeks under appropriate soil conditions to mature to the infective stage. When embryonated eggs are ingested, larvae are released and mature into adults in the colon, where they attach and survive up to 10 years.

Light infection usually is asymptomatic, but when larger numbers (>300 worms) are present, diarrhea or symptoms of dysentery may develop in association with dehydration and anemia (Beaver, 1984; Strickland, 2000). Rectal prolapse, a life-threatening complication, may occur in heavily infected children (Cooper, 1988).

Diagnosis is made by finding typical eggs in direct fecal smears or with concentration techniques. The eggs are barrel-shaped with refractile plugs at both ends and usually measure 50–55 μm long by 22–24 μm wide (Fig. 62-17, *E*). Occasionally, humans may become infected with the dog whipworm, *Trichuris vulpis*, which has eggs that are larger, wider, and more barrel-shaped than those of *Trichuris trichiura*. Egg quantitation techniques occasionally may be requested to assess infection intensity, therapeutic efficacy, and reacquisition rates of parasites.

Capillaria philippinensis

This parasite, normally found in fish-eating birds, infects humans who ingest raw or incompletely cooked fish that contain infective larvae in their flesh. Although first described in persons from the Philippines, and later Thailand, occasional cases have been reported in Asia, the Middle East, and South America (Cross, 1992; Murray, 2007). The parasites may cause chronic diarrhea, and infected individuals may pass eggs, larvae, and even adult worms in their feces. Eggs resemble those of *Trichuris*, although they measure 36–45 μm in length by 21 μm in width and have thick, radially striated shells and mucoid plugs, which are inconspicuous.

Ascaris lumbricoides

This is the largest nematode that infects the intestinal tract of humans and is probably the most common of the intestinal roundworms, infecting an estimated 1.3 billion individuals worldwide (Markell, 1999). Infection occurs primarily in areas with little or no sanitation and, as with *Trichuris*, is especially common in children, who are also more likely to harbor heavy infection.

Adult *Ascaris* live primarily in the duodenum and proximal jejunum. Females measure up to 35 cm in length by 6 mm in diameter. The male is somewhat smaller and has a ventrally curved tail, unlike the female (Fig. 62-17, *F*). Both adult and immature worms can be identified by the presence of three prominent lips at the anterior end.

Females produce approximately 200,000 eggs per day, which are unembryonated when passed and require 4–6 weeks in a satisfactory environment to become infective. Following ingestion, eggs hatch in the intestine, and larvae penetrate the mucosa to gain access to the bloodstream. They are carried to the lungs and mature briefly in the alveolar capillary bed before entering the alveoli. Respiratory clearance mechanisms move the

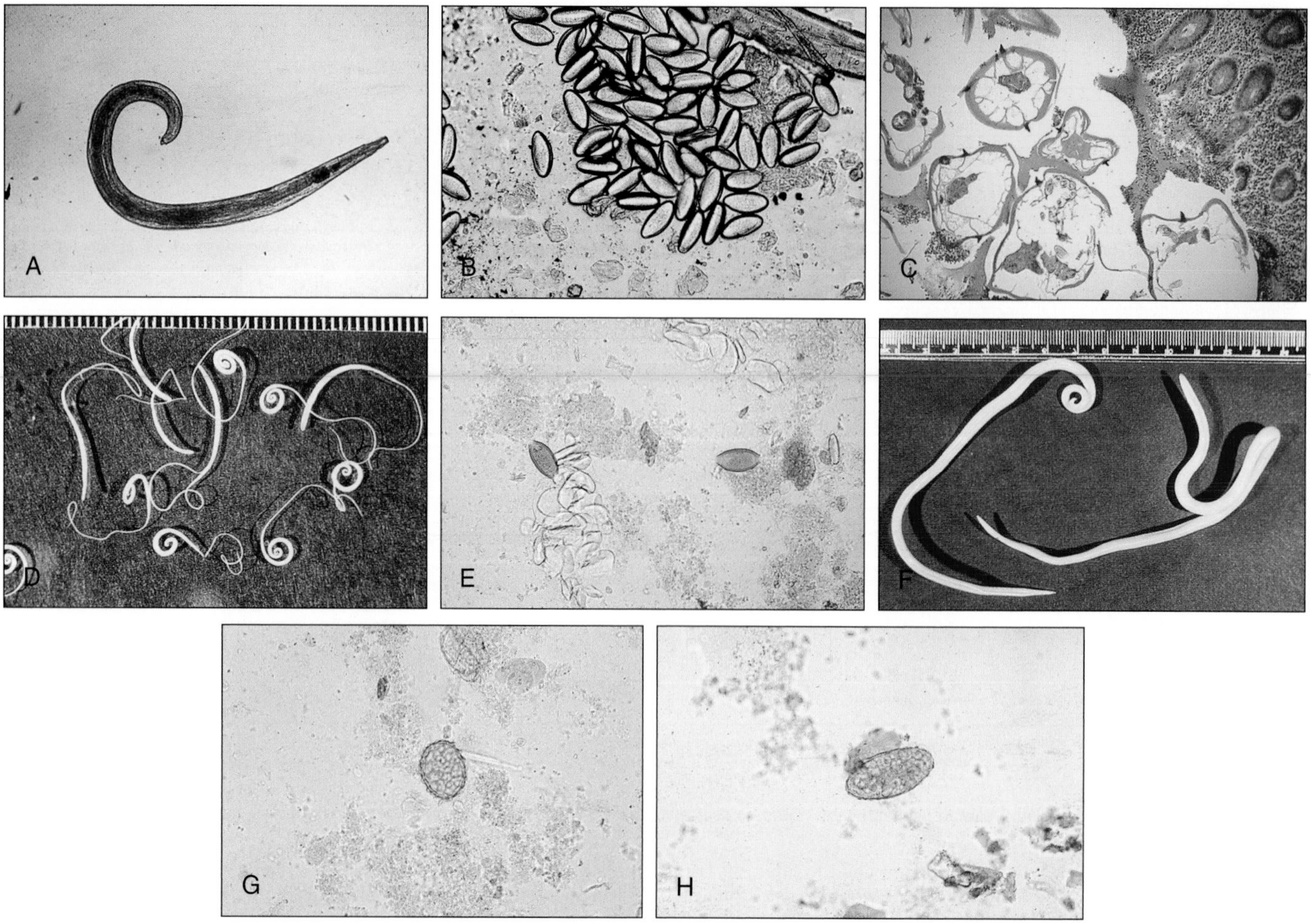

Figure 62-17 All direct examination with brightfield illumination except as noted. **A,** Adult male pinworm, *Enterobius vermicularis,* with curved posterior end; note prominent esophageal bulb (×4). **B,** Numerous eggs of *E. vermicularis* as seen on a cellophane tape preparation (×400). **C,** Adult *E. vermicularis* in the appendix; note characteristic lateral alae (×100). **D,** Adult whipworms, *Trichuris trichiura*; note females with straight tails and males with coiled tails. **E,** Eggs of *T. trichiura* (×400). **F,** Adult female and male *Ascaris lumbricoides*, the large human roundworm. **G,** Fertile, unembryonated egg of *A. lumbricoides* (×400). **H,** Infertile and decorticate egg of *A. lumbricoides* (×400). *(**D** and **F** from Zaiman H, editor. A pictorial presentation of parasites: a cooperative collection;* http://www.astmh.org/Zaiman_Slides/1271.htm.*)*

larvae to the epiglottis, where they are swallowed and grow to adulthood in the small bowel. Development from embryonated egg to adult takes approximately 2 months.

Symptoms of ascariasis vary from asymptomatic infection to severe disease. Migration of large numbers of larvae through the lungs can cause *Ascaris* pneumonitis or Löffler syndrome, characterized by bilateral diffuse, mottled pulmonary infiltrates and mild bronchitis associated with peripheral eosinophilia. The syndrome is rare and usually occurs in individuals who have been previously exposed to *Ascaris* antigens.

The presence of a few worms in the intestine is rarely noticed, whereas heavy infection may produce varying degrees of abdominal pain and diarrhea. Intestinal obstruction may also occur with a mass of worms, especially in children. Even a small number of worms is cause for concern because of their ability to invade ectopic sites such as the common bile duct and liver, appendix, and stomach. Fever or drug therapy may stimulate migration. In endemic areas, anthelmintics often are prescribed before anesthetics are used in elective surgery.

Infection is diagnosed by demonstrating eggs in feces or on recovery of an adult that has been passed or vomited. The large number of eggs produced each day makes detection of even a single worm probable. A count of fewer than 20 eggs per slide (2 mg of feces) indicates light infection, and a count of more than 100 eggs per slide indicates heavy infection.

Fertile *Ascaris* eggs are round to slightly oval with a yellow-brown, irregular external mamillated layer and a thick shell. Eggs that have lost their mamillated layer are called decorticate and may superficially resemble hookworm eggs. They are passed unembryonated and measure approximately 55–75 μm long by 35–50 μm wide (Fig. 62-17, *G* and *H*). Single females may produce unfertilized eggs, which are larger and more elongate (up to 90 μm in length) and have a thinner shell with irregular mamillations. These eggs are filled with irregularly sized fat globules.

Trichostrongylus spp.

Human disease caused by *Trichostrongylus* spp. represents a zoonotic infection because these parasites principally infect large herbivores such as sheep, cattle, and goats. Several species may infect humans, including *Trichostrongylus colubriformis, Trichostrongylus orientalis, Trichostrongylus axei,* and *Trichostrongylus brevis,* all of which are found in many parts of the world. Adult worms inhabit the small bowel and produce eggs that mature outside of the body. Larvae emerge and crawl about on soil and vegetation, where they are available to be ingested by definitive hosts. Unlike hookworms, they do not invade skin directly, nor does the life cycle involve a migratory phase through the lungs. Infection usually is light and asymptomatic, but heavy infection may produce abdominal pain and diarrhea, usually with eosinophilia. Eggs resemble those of hookworms but are longer and narrower, measuring 78–98 μm by 40–50 μm, and are slightly tapered at one end.

Hookworms

Hookworms, which are among the more common helminths known to infect humans, occur in tropical and subtropical regions and some temperate areas. *Necator americanus* is found in the United States and in other areas of the world and frequently overlaps in distribution with *Ancylostoma duodenale*, which does not occur in the United States.

Adult females measure up to 12 mm in length, and the males slightly less. Males are readily distinguished by the fan-shaped copulatory bursa at the posterior end. The anterior end of hookworms is modified into a buccal capsule that contains teeth or cutting plates. Both sexes attach to the mucosa of the small intestine, where they may reside for up to 18 years (Beaver, 1988; Garcia, 2007).

Eggs are passed in feces and develop rapidly, depending on prevailing conditions. Rhabditiform larvae are released and develop into the infective filariform stage in about 7 days. On contact with an appropriate host, the

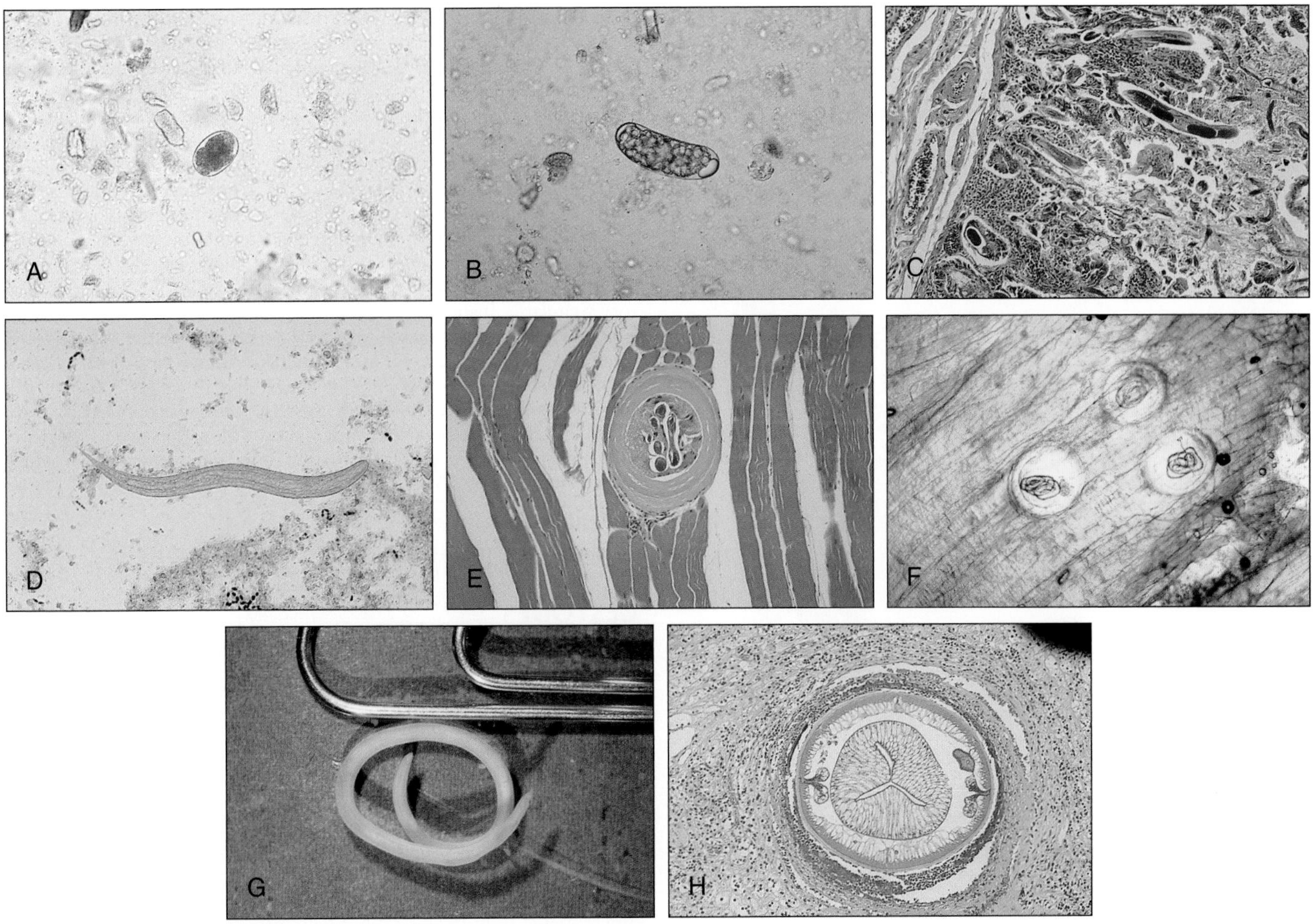

Figure 62-18 **A,** Hookworm (*Ancylostoma duodenale* or *Necator americanus*) egg (×400). **B,** Egg of *Heterodera* sp., a group of plant nematodes occasionally found as artifacts in human stool following ingestion of infected vegetables (×400). **C,** Massive *Strongyloides stercoralis* infection in the duodenal mucosa; note presence of adult female, eggs, and larvae (H&E; ×100). **D,** *S. stercoralis* noninfectious rhabditiform larva (iodine stain; ×100). **E,** *Trichinella spiralis*, cross-section of a larva in gastrocnemius muscle (H&E; ×100). **F,** Multiple *T. spiralis* larvae in bear meat (compressed wet muscle preparation; ×100). **G,** Regurgitated *Pseudoterranova* sp. following fish dinner (×4). **H,** Anisakis sp., cross-section of larva found in small bowel following surgery for acute obstruction (H&E; ×400).

larvae penetrate the skin, gain access to the host's circulation, travel to the lungs, and move up the tracheobronchial tree to be swallowed. On maturation in the small intestine, oviposition begins. Although the life cycles of both species are similar, *Ancylostoma* can mature directly to the adult stage in the intestine if infective larvae are ingested.

Hookworms can produce disease in the skin, at the site of larval penetration. This condition, known as ground itch, is characterized by inflammation, redness, and blister formation, along with intense itching. Migration of large numbers of larvae through the lungs may produce Löffler syndrome, as described earlier for *Ascaris*. Depending on the worm burden, intestinal infection can result in gastroenteritis with abdominal pain, diarrhea, and nausea. Hookworms are best known, however, for their ability to produce chronic blood loss with secondary iron deficiency anemia. The presence of each adult *A. duodenale* can result in the loss of 0.15–0.25 mL of blood per day, compared with 0.03 mL for each *N. americanus*. Development of children can be severely affected by chronic infection. Blood loss and the number of hookworms present correlate with the number of eggs per gram of stool, which may help the clinician determine when to initiate therapy in individuals living in endemic areas (Layrisse, 1964a, 1964b; Cook, 2002).

Diagnosis is made by finding the characteristic thin-shelled eggs in feces. These eggs are partially embryonated when passed and measure 58–76 µm in length by 36–40 µm wide (Fig. 62-18, *A*). Embryonated eggs or free rhabditiform larvae may be found in unpreserved specimens that are not examined promptly. Hookworm rhabditiforms can be differentiated from those of *S. stercoralis* because the former have a longer buccal chamber and inconspicuous genital primordium (Fig. 62-19). Continued maturation of larvae results in the appearance of infective filariforms, which have a pointed posterior end and an esophagus approximately one-fourth the length of the larva. Hookworm eggs may need to be differentiated from those of *Trichostrongylus* spp. (which are longer and more pointed) and those of plant parasitic nematodes, especially *Heterodera* spp. (which are longer, have blunt ends, and are often asymmetrical) (Fig. 62-18, *B*).

Although adult hookworms can be differentiated on the basis of their mouth parts and the copulatory bursa in males, eggs of human hookworms are indistinguishable. In direct wet mounts, egg counts of fewer than five eggs per coverslip denote light infection that is unlikely to result in anemia, whereas more than 25 eggs per coverslip denotes heavy infection that is likely to be associated with symptoms.

Strongyloides stercoralis

Strongyloidiasis occurs in many areas in the tropics and subtropics, but this infection also is reported in temperate zones and has historically been endemic in areas of southeastern United States. Adult females are 2–3 mm long and live buried in the mucosa of the duodenum, where they reproduce parthenogenetically (Fig. 62-18, *C*). Parasitic males do not occur in the vertebrate phase of the cycle. The eggs hatch primarily in the small bowel, releasing first-stage or rhabditoid larvae, which then are passed in the feces (eggs are almost never found). In this direct cycle, the rhabditoid larvae metamorphose into infective third-stage filariform larvae in the soil. These infective larvae readily penetrate the skin of exposed individuals; they migrate via the circulatory system to the lungs and then move up the bronchial tree and are swallowed. Development to the adult stage is completed in the small intestine. Under appropriate soil conditions of high humidity, an indirect cycle may appear transiently, in which the newly deposited larvae develop into a free-living generation consisting of reproductive males and females. Eggs produced by this generation develop into filariform larvae that again are infective for humans. A third variation in the life cycle of *Strongyloides* involves autoinfection, in which maturation to the filariform stage is completed within the intestinal tract, with subsequent reinvasion of bowel mucosa or perianal skin.

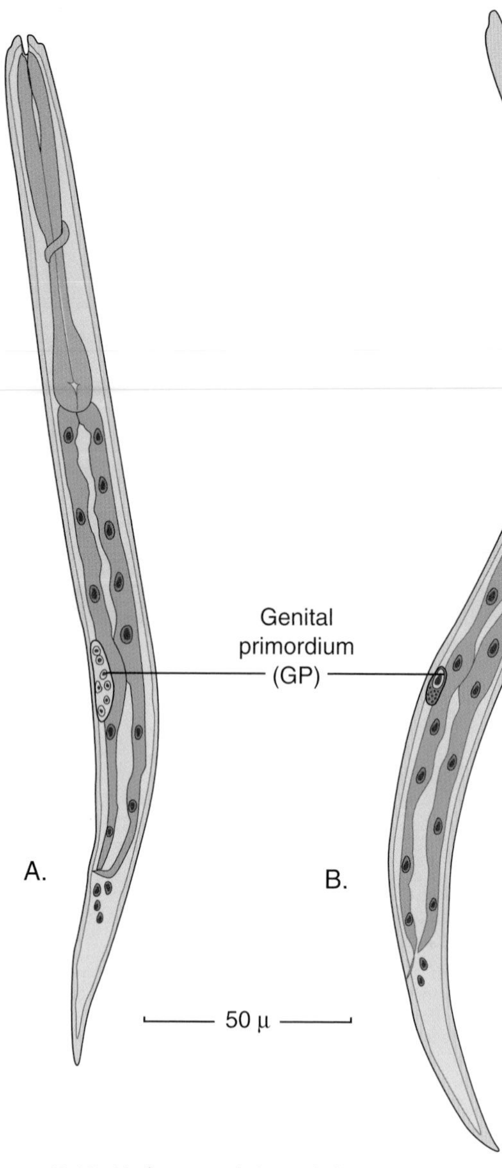

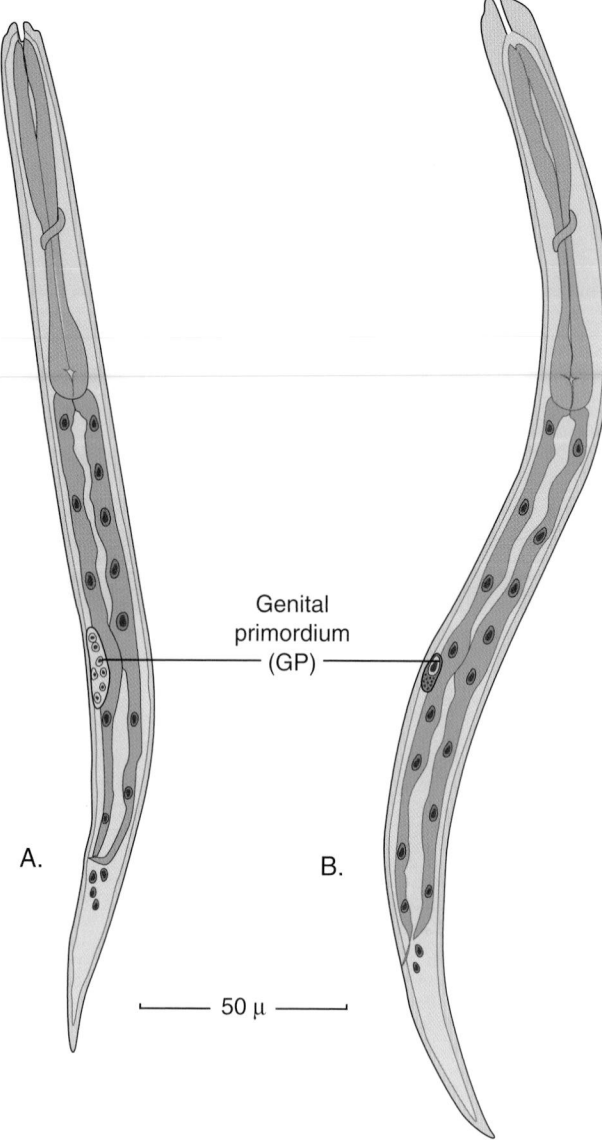

Figure 62-19 Hookworm and *Strongyloides stercoralis* larvae. **A,** *S. stercoralis* rhabditoid larva in human stools. Note the short size of the buccal cavity and the large genital primordium (GP). **B,** Hookworm rhabditoid larva as seen in a few instances in stools left for at least 24 hours at room temperature. The buccal cavity is longer, and the genital primordium is smaller.

Disease presentation is variable and may depend on the strain acquired (Genta, 1989). Early migration of filariform larvae may produce irritation, redness, and pruritus at the site of entry, whereas later migration through the lungs may produce Löffler syndrome (Purtilo, 1974). The presence of intestinal symptoms is related to the intensity of the infection. The affected individual may have symptoms of peptic ulcer, abdominal pain, and diarrhea. A malabsorption syndrome has been reported with chronic infection.

The ability of the parasite to autoinfect may result in persistence of the infection for decades, as was recognized in allied troops who were held as prisoners of war in southeast Asia during World War II (Gill, 1979). In otherwise healthy patients, autoinfection may produce larva currens (linear urticarial lesions). In immunocompromised, alcoholic, or malnourished patients, autoinfection may result in a life-threatening hyperinfection syndrome caused by rapid multiplication of the parasite (Maayen, 1987; Genta, 1992). Severe pneumonia is often a presenting manifestation of hyperinfection, followed by marked diarrhea, enteritis, and septicemia. Patients who have lived in endemic areas should be screened for *Strongyloides* prior to receiving immunosuppressive therapy (Strickland, 2000).

Diagnosis is made on recovery and identification of typical rhabditiform larvae in stool specimens, although the routine O&P examination does not always reveal their presence (Fig. 62-18, *D*) (Pelletier, 1988; Genta, 1989; Garcia, 2007). *Strongyloides* rhabditiform larvae must be differentiated from those of hookworms and are characterized as having a short buccal cavity and a prominent genital primordium (see Fig. 62-19). *Strongyloides* filariform larvae have a notched tail and an esophagus approximately half the length of the body. Either stage of larvae is readily seen in fresh saline wet mounts under low power. If infective filariform larvae are detected in a recently passed specimen, the diagnosis of superinfection is warranted (Eveland, 1975; Murray, 2007).

Examination of duodenal aspirates or string test specimens may be helpful in suspicious cases in which routine stool examinations are nonproductive. The Baermann funnel concentration method or one of the coproculture techniques (see earlier under Laboratory Methods) may also demonstrate the infection (Ash, 1987; Genta, 1989; Clinical and Laboratory Standards Institute, 2005; Garcia, 2007). Larvae may be found in sputum or other pulmonary specimens, especially in the hyperinfection syndrome. Serologic tests are useful when infection is suspected but cannot be demonstrated by other methods. EIA and other tests display good sensitivity and specificity, although cross-reactions may appear with filariasis and some other nematode infections. These tests generally do not differentiate between past and current infection but may be useful in monitoring therapy (Wilson, 1995).

Anisakiasis

See later under Tissue Helminths.

CESTODES

Cestodes or tapeworms are ribbon-like platyhelminths that live in the intestinal tract of vertebrates as adults and in the tissues or body cavities of various intermediate hosts as larvae. They attach to intestinal mucosa by means of a scolex, or attachment organ, at the anterior end that may display suckers, grooves (bothria), or a rostellum with hooks, depending on the species. The body of the worm, or strobila, comprises an actively growing neck region and a series of proglottids that undergo sequential development through immature, mature, and, finally, gravid stages at the posterior end. Each proglottid has a complete set of male and female gonads and is capable of producing fertile eggs. Eggs of most cestodes infecting humans (*Diphyllobothrium* being an exception) may be readily differentiated from those of other helminths by the presence in each of a six-hooked embryo. Depending on the species, eggs are released directly into the fecal stream or are passed in intact proglottids. It is not uncommon in some species for long lengths of strobila to be passed intact, or for proglottids to actively migrate out of the anus. Large species of *Taenia* and *Diphyllobothrium* may grow to 25 feet or longer and may live for 20 years.

Cestode larval stages develop to the infective stage in invertebrate or vertebrate hosts, depending on the species, and complete their life cycle when ingested by a definitive host. Larval stages of several species may infect humans, causing cysticercosis, hydatidosis, sparganosis, and coenurosis. These conditions are covered more fully later under Tissue Helminths.

Taenia saginata

Humans are the sole definitive host for *Taenia saginata*, the beef tapeworm. Although it is distributed worldwide, the worm is especially common in the Middle East, Africa, Europe, Asia, and Latin America. It occurs rarely and sporadically in the United States. Larval cysticerci *(Cysticercus bovis)* develop in the tissues of cattle that graze on land contaminated by human waste. When humans ingest infected raw or incompletely cooked beef, the cysticercus develops into a reproductive adult in the small intestine in 2–3 months. Symptoms are rare but may include abdominal discomfort and diarrhea. Unlike *T. solium*, the eggs of *T. saginata* are not infectious to humans, and their ingestion does not result in cysticercosis.

Diagnosis is made by finding eggs in the stool, using direct or concentration techniques, or in the perianal folds, using the cellophane tape technique. Eggs are spherical and measure 31–43 μm in diameter (Fig. 62-20, *A*). The shell is thick, is radially striated, and contains a six-hooked embryo. Eggs of all *Taenia* species are indistinguishable and should be reported only as *Taenia* eggs.

Species identification may be made on recovery of proglottids or, more rarely, the scolex. Proglottids of taeniids have a characteristic lateral protrusion known as the genital pore. Careful injection of India ink through the genital pore, using a tuberculin needle and syringe, may succeed in outlining the uterus. The gravid uterus of *T. saginata* has 15–20 lateral branches, whereas that of *T. solium* has 7–13 lateral branches (Figs. 62-20, *B*, and 62-21). Proglottids may also be cleared overnight in glycerol or stained with carmine or hematoxylin using published procedures (Ash,

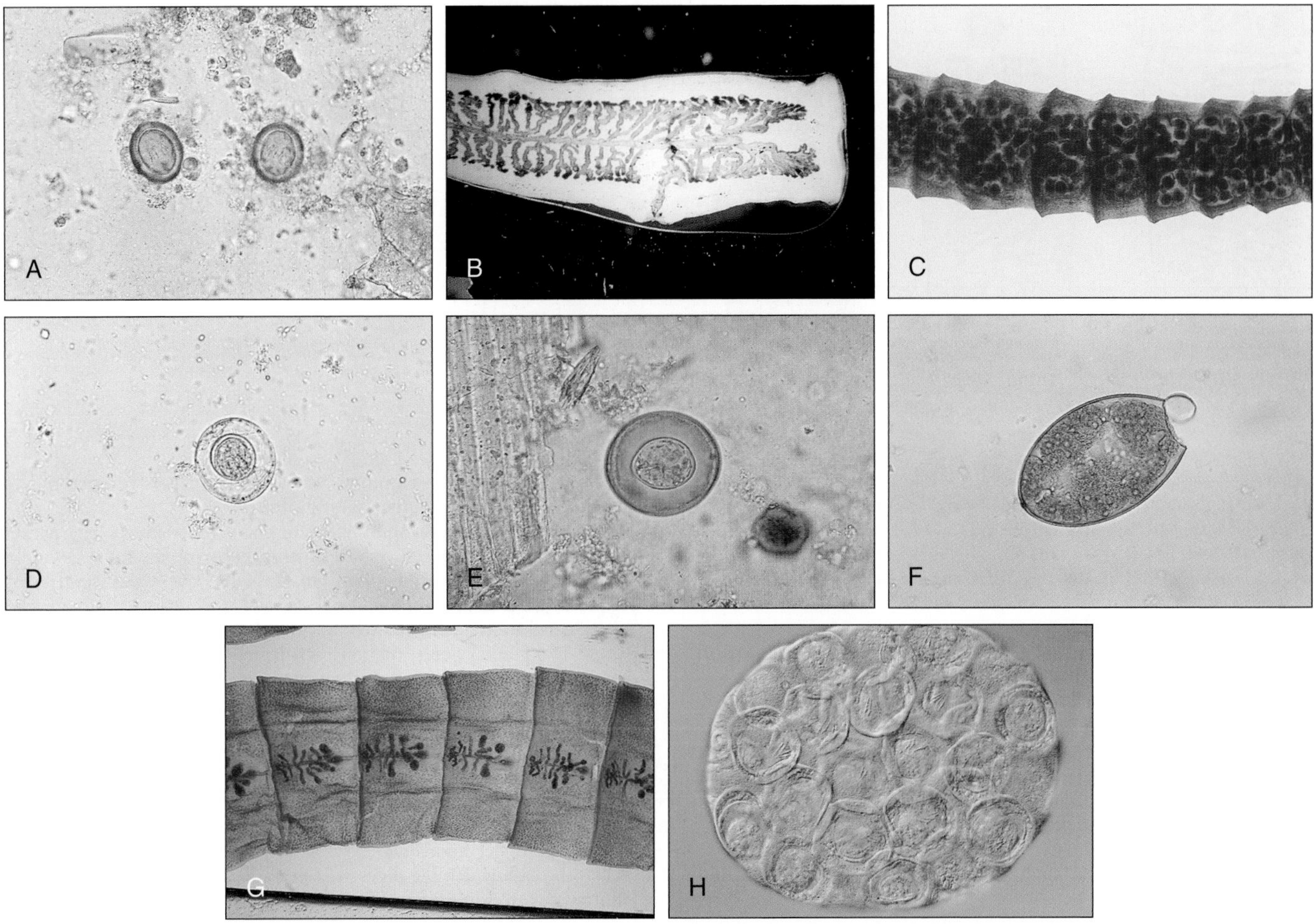

Figure 62-20 **A,** Eggs of *Taenia saginata* (indistinguishable from those of *Taenia solium*; ×400). **B,** Gravid proglottid of *T. saginata* injected through the genital pore with India ink. **C,** Gravid proglottids of *Hymenolepis nana* stained with acetocarmine (×100). **D,** Egg of *H. nana*; note presence of hooklets and polar filaments (×400). **E,** Egg of *Hymenolepis diminuta*; note lack of polar filaments (×400). **F,** Egg of *Diphyllobothrium* sp.; note open operculum and small terminal knob (×400). **G,** Gravid proglottids of *Diphyllobothrium* sp. stained with acetocarmine (×2). **H,** Egg packet of *Dipylidium caninum* (differential interference contrast microscopy; ×400).

1987). If recovered, the scolex of *T. saginata* can be identified by the presence of four suckers and the absence of hooks on the crown or rostellum.

Taenia solium

T. solium, the pork tapeworm, is most common in Europe, especially in eastern Europe, Latin America, China, Pakistan, and India. It is encountered in the United States on occasion, most often in recent immigrants. Infection with the adult tapeworm is acquired by eating raw or incompletely cooked pork containing cysticerci *(Cysticercus cellulosae)*. Symptoms, if present, are identical to those of *T. saginata* infection. More important, accidental ingestion of *T. solium* eggs from one's own adult tapeworm or from contaminated food may result in cysticercosis (Schantz, 1992). Additional details on cysticercosis may be found later under Tissue Helminths.

Procedures used for diagnosis of intestinal *T. solium* infection are identical to those used for *T. saginata* infection, although certain morphologic differences are apparent. The scolex of *T. solium* has four suckers and, unlike *T. saginata*, a rostellum armed with two rows of hooks. Gravid proglottids have 7–13 lateral uterine branches (see Fig. 62-21).

Hymenolepis nana

Hymenolepis nana, known as the dwarf tapeworm, has worldwide distribution and is the most frequently recovered cestode species seen in the United States. It is a common parasite in mice and is the smallest to infect humans, measuring up to 4.0 cm in length. The scolex has an armed rostellum, and the proglottids have all of their genital pores located on the same side of the strobila (Figs. 62-20, *C*, and 62-21). The life cycle may be direct, through the ingestion of infectious eggs, or indirect, through the ingestion of intermediate hosts (usually grain beetles) containing cysticercoid larvae. In the former instance, eggs may be passed directly from person to person, usually among children, or may be ingested in food, especially grain products that are contaminated by rodent droppings.

Eggs hatch in the intestine and embryos penetrate the mucosa, where they mature as cysticercoid larvae. They subsequently emerge and reattach to the intestinal wall to complete their development into adult tapeworms in 2–3 weeks. Ingestion of grain beetles containing cysticercoid larvae occurs much less frequently. Internal autoinfection may occur in some individuals in whom eggs hatch shortly after being discharged from the worm and rapidly invade the intestinal wall without leaving the body. Such a mechanism is thought to be responsible for the occasional case of massive infection.

Symptomatic infection, characterized by abdominal pain, diarrhea, anorexia, and irritability, may develop in patients with large numbers of worms. Diagnosis is made by recovery from stool of the oval, thin-shelled, colorless eggs, which measure 30–47 μm in diameter (Fig. 62-20, *D*). They contain a centrally located, six-hooked embryo (oncosphere), which is separated from the outer shell by a clear space. This embryo displays two polar thickenings from which thin filaments arise and extend into the clear space between embryo and outer shell. Occasionally, intact strobila may be recovered if the stool is closely examined.

Hymenolepis diminuta

The rat tapeworm, *Hymenolepis diminuta*, is cosmopolitan in distribution and occasionally infects humans. Infection is rare, however, because of the obligate need for an arthropod intermediate host, in which the cysticercoid larvae develop. Human infection usually occurs following the accidental ingestion of infected beetles that contaminate grain or cereal products. Adult tapeworms develop in the small intestine, where they may grow to 60 cm in length. Similar to those of *H. nana*, the proglottids all have genital pores on one side, but unlike that species, the scolex lacks an armed rostellum. Infection usually is asymptomatic because of the small number of

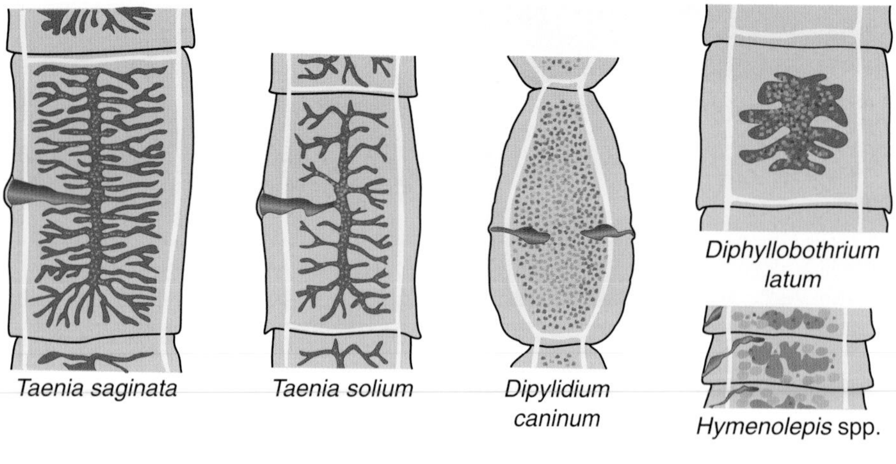

Figure 62-21 Gravid proglottids of different human tapeworms.

worms likely to infect a single individual, although intestinal symptoms have been reported. Diagnosis is made by the finding in the feces of moderately thick-shelled, slightly ovoid, yellow-brown eggs measuring 70–85 μm by 60–80 μm (Fig. 62-20, *E*). The eggs are most easily confused with those of *H. nana* but, unlike in that species, lack polar filaments.

Diphyllobothrium spp.

Humans may be infected by one of several species of the fish tapeworm *Diphyllobothrium*, which normally infect piscivorous mammals and possibly birds (Curtis, 1991; Connor, 1997). These parasites are widely distributed in the temperate zones, especially northern Europe, Scandinavia, the former USSR, and Japan. Infection also occurs in Canada and in the north central states, the Pacific Coast states, and Alaska in the United States. Although *Diphyllobothrium latum* is the most common species known to infect humans, differentiation cannot be made on the basis of egg morphology.

This parasite inhabits the small intestine, where it can reach a length of 10 m or longer and can persist for years. Eggs are passed unembryonated in the feces and must reach a freshwater stream or lake to continue development. Following several weeks of embryonation, a ciliated larval form, the six-hooked coracidium, hatches and is ingested by a copepod, a type of zooplankton. The coracidium develops into a procercoid larva, which is infective for the second intermediate host, a fish. In fish, the procercoid migrates into the tissues and develops into the plerocercoid larva. Plerocercoids may be passed up the food chain unchanged and accumulate in larger fish. Humans acquire these larvae through ingestion of raw or incompletely cooked fish that have spent at least part of their life in fresh water.

Adult worms mature and initiate egg production in approximately 1 month. Infection may be asymptomatic, with passage of a length of strobila being the initial complaint. In others, a variable degree of abdominal discomfort and diarrhea may be present. Rarely, intestinal obstruction occurs. In endemic areas in northern Europe, a small percentage of patients develop vitamin B_{12} deficiency and associated megaloblastic anemia.

Diagnosis is made by the finding of typical brown, oval, operculate eggs in feces using standard recovery techniques. Eggs measure 58–76 μm by 40–51 μm and, in addition to the operculum, have a small, round, knob-like projection on the abopercular end (Fig. 62-20, *F*). The presence of the operculum is unique among those cestodes infecting humans, and care must be taken not to confuse these eggs with those of trematodes, especially *Paragonimus* or *Nanophyetus*. Identification to the genus level is possible when a length of strobila or an intact worm is passed. The scolex is elongate and displays a pair of longitudinal grooves known as bothria, which replace the usual suckers. Gravid proglottids are wider than they are long and have their genital pores located midventrally, adjacent to a centrally located rosette-shaped uterus (Figs. 62-20, *G*, and 62-21).

Dipylidium caninum

Dipylidium caninum is a common tapeworm of dogs and cats in most parts of the world and not infrequently infects humans, especially children. In the usual life cycle, tapeworm eggs are ingested by flea larvae, which infest areas frequented by dogs or cats. The cysticercoid larvae persist as the flea undergoes metamorphosis to the adult stage. Accidental ingestion of the adult flea containing the infectious cysticercoid results in infection. Children are at highest risk for infection because of their close contact with pets. Worms mature in the small intestine and grow up to 70 cm in length. Infection produces few symptoms and generally causes concern only on detection of the actively moving proglottids.

Detection is based on the finding of characteristic eggs, egg packets, or proglottids in the feces. Spherical eggs, each containing a six-hooked embryo, measure from 24–40 μm in diameter and occur singly or in packets (Fig. 62-20, *H*). The scolex is somewhat elongate with four suckers and a small, retractable rostellum. Proglottids are barrel-shaped and possess two genital pores, one on each lateral margin, which give rise to the common name double-pored tapeworm (see Fig. 62-21).

TREMATODES

Trematodes, or flukes, are dorsoventrally flattened helminths (platyhelminths) that include both hermaphroditic forms (intestinal, liver, and lung flukes) and those with separate sexes (blood flukes or schistosomes). All species that infect humans are characterized by the presence of an oral sucker, through which the digestive tract opens, and a ventral sucker used for attachment. Adults vary in length from 1 mm *(Metagonimus)* to 70 mm *(Fasciola gigantica)*.

Eggs reach the environment by being passed in the feces, sputum, or urine, depending on the species. Hermaphroditic flukes produce operculate eggs, which are not embryonated (*Clonorchis* and *Opisthorchis* being exceptions). Schistosome eggs are not operculated, and each contains a mature larva when passed. Trematode larvae, or miracidia, are ciliated and are capable of penetrating the tissues of a molluscan host. Each species of trematode uses a particular species of snail as the first intermediate host. A complex asexual multiplication process within the snail results in the production of numerous free-swimming larvae called cercariae. Schistosome cercariae are capable of penetrating human skin directly, resulting in the disease schistosomiasis. Those of hermaphroditic flukes encyst on aquatic vegetation or invade the tissues of second intermediate hosts such as fish or crabs, depending on the species. Ingestion of these encysted larval stages, known as metacercariae, results in human infection.

Human trematode infection may occur in many tropical and subtropical regions and involves considerably more species (mostly rare and sporadic intestinal infections) than can be presented here. Its presence depends on lack of sewage treatment, availability of appropriate intermediate hosts, and, in the case of hermaphroditic species, dietary customs associated with ingestion of infective metacercariae. Some of these diseases, especially schistosomiasis, are spreading because of increased use of irrigation in endemic areas. Symptoms vary depending on the number of worms parasitizing the host at a given time, the tissues and organs involved, and host responses. Many infections are asymptomatic.

The diagnosis of trematode infection is made by recovery and identification of the characteristic eggs in stool, sputum, urine, and, occasionally, tissues. Direct mounts and formalin–ethyl acetate concentration methods are most useful for recovery of these eggs, whereas zinc sulfate flotation methods are less satisfactory.

Fasciolopsis buski

This intestinal trematode is the largest species to infect humans, varying from 20–75 mm in length and from 8–20 mm in breadth. It occurs in many parts of China, southeast Asia, and India and is frequently found in pigs, which serve as a natural reservoir. Infection is acquired by ingesting infectious metacercariae on aquatic food plants such as water chestnuts and

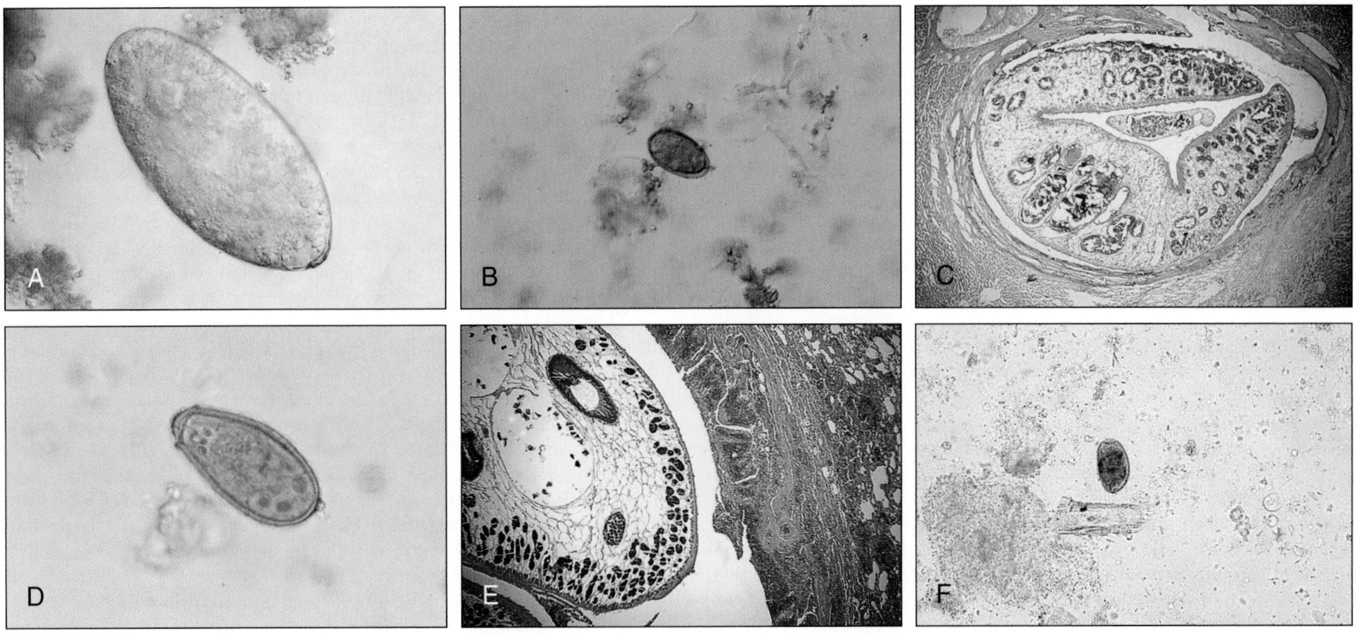

Figure 62-22 **A,** Egg of *Fasciolopsis buski,* indistinguishable from that of *Fasciola hepatica,* in stool (×400). **B,** Egg of *Heterophyes* sp. in stool (×400). **C,** Adult *Clonorchis sinensis* in bile duct (H&E; ×100). **D,** Egg of *C. sinensis* in stool (×1000). **E,** Pair of adult *Paragonimus* sp. in lung tissue with surrounding inflammatory reaction (H&E; ×10). **F,** Egg of *Paragonimus* sp. in stool; note prominent operculum (×100).

water caltrop. Worms attach to the wall of the duodenum and jejunum, where they mature to egg-laying adults in about 3 months. Symptoms such as diarrhea, epigastric pain, and nausea may develop if enough worms are present to produce ulceration of the superficial mucosa. Eosinophilia may be present, even in those who are asymptomatic.

Diagnosis is made by the finding of large (130–140 μm by 80–85 μm), brown, oval, and thin-shelled eggs (Fig. 62-22, *A*). The operculum may be inconspicuous, and the eggs are passed unembryonated. Differentiation from *Fasciola* eggs generally is not possible, although these infections may be differentiated on the basis of geographic history and symptoms. Eggs of echinostome trematodes, which occasionally infect humans, are similar but smaller (Beaver, 1984).

Heterophyes and *Metagonimus*

These two genera include a number of species of minute (1–3 mm in length) intestinal worms that infect humans. *Heterophyes heterophyes* and *Metagonimus yokogawai* are common parasites in Asia but, along with other species, are found in other parts of the world as well. Infection is acquired by ingestion of metacercariae in raw or incompletely cooked freshwater fish. Although it is of minor medical importance, infection with these worms may produce diarrhea and abdominal pain. Infection is self-limited because the worms have a life span of only a few months.

Diagnosis is established by the finding of embryonated, operculate eggs that measure 20–30 μm in length by 15–17 μm in width (Fig. 62-22, *B*). Differentiation of these eggs from those of *Clonorchis* and *Opisthorchis* is difficult, although the operculum is more deeply seated with *Opisthorchis*. Such differentiation may be important, however, for medical reasons.

Nanophyetus salmincola

Nanophyetus (Troglotrema) salmincola is a small (0.8–1.1 mm) intestinal fluke that has been reported in humans in areas of far eastern Siberia and the Pacific Northwest Coast of the United States (Eastburn, 1987; Fritsche, 1989b). These worms are acquired by ingesting raw, incompletely cooked, or home-smoked salmon or trout that contain infectious metacercariae. Symptoms are related to the number of worms present and may include abdominal pain and diarrhea, with or without eosinophilia. Eggs measuring 60–80 μm by 34–50 μm are broadly ovoid, operculate, and yellowish brown (Eastburn, 1987). Thickening of the shell at the abopercular end should be differentiated from the knob seen on eggs of *Diphyllobothrium*. This fluke is the vector for a rickettsia that produces a highly lethal infection in canines known as "salmon-poisoning" disease.

Fasciola hepatica

Cattle, sheep, and goats in many parts of the world are infected with the liver fluke *Fasciola hepatica* and, less commonly, with the related species *Fasciola gigantica*. Adult parasites live in the biliary tree and lay eggs that are passed in the feces. Cercariae shed from the snail intermediate host encyst on aquatic vegetation, where infectious metacercariae then are available to herbivorous hosts. Humans usually acquire the infection by eating watercress. Once ingested, the larvae penetrate the intestinal wall and migrate through the peritoneal cavity to the liver. They burrow through the capsule and parenchyma, coming to reside within the bile ducts, where egg laying is initiated in about 2 months. Migration of the larvae through the liver elicits a painful inflammatory reaction both in the tissue and, later, in the bile ducts, which eventually become fibrosed. Clinical manifestations include colic, obstructive jaundice, abdominal pain and tenderness, cholelithiasis, and eosinophilia.

Diagnosis is made by the finding of eggs in the stool. The unembryonated, yellowish brown, operculate eggs, 130–150 μm by 63–90 μm, cannot be distinguished easily from those of Fasciolopsis (see Fig. 62-22, *A*). Spurious infection, which occurs by ingesting infected cattle or sheep liver, is diagnosed by obtaining a good history and performing a follow-up stool examination to look for elimination of the eggs.

Clonorchis sinensis and *Opisthorchis viverrini*

Clonorchis sinensis, the Oriental liver fluke, and a closely related species, *Opisthorchis viverrini*, inhabit the biliary system of humans and other piscivorous animals, including cats and dogs. *C. sinensis* occurs mainly in China, Taiwan, Korea, Japan, and Vietnam, whereas *O. viverrini* is found primarily in southeast Asia, especially northern Thailand. Human infection is also known to occur with *Opisthorchis felineus* in Europe and *Amphimerus pseudofelineus* (same as *Opisthorchis guayaquilensis*) in Ecuador.

All these parasites are acquired by the ingestion of infectious metacercariae in raw or uncooked freshwater fish. Larvae migrate up the common duct into the liver bile ducts, where they live up to 20 years and grow up to 25 mm in length (Fig. 62-22, *C*). They produce small eggs that are shed into the bile and subsequently are passed in stools.

Infection is often asymptomatic, although large numbers of flukes and repeated infection may cause inflammation of the bile ducts and subsequent hyperplasia, fibrosis, and hepatic cirrhosis. Development of cholangiocarcinoma has been linked epidemiologically with long-standing infection.

Diagnosis is made by recovering the small brown, embryonated, operculate eggs from stools (Fig. 62-22, *D*). Eggs of *Clonorchis* cannot be readily differentiated from those of *Opisthorchis*. Both measure 25–35 μm by 12–20 μm and have a prominent, seated opercula and a small knob at the abopercular end. These eggs are difficult to differentiate from those of the *Heterophyes/Metagonimus* group, although the latter species do not have prominent, seated opercula or a small knob at the abopercular end. When specific identification is not possible, the laboratory report should reflect this (i.e., should state, "*Clonorchis/Opisthorchis/Heterophyes/Metagonimus* eggs").

Paragonimus spp.

Several species of *Paragonimus* may parasitize the lungs of cats, dogs, and other carnivores, including humans. *Paragonimus westermani* is problematic in many areas of Asia, whereas in Central and South America several species have been implicated, including *Paragonimus mexicanus*, *Paragonimus caliensis*, and *Paragonimus ecuadoriensis*. *Paragonimus kellicotti* has occasionally been implicated in cases from North America, and other species have been described from Africa (Pachucki, 1984; Mariano, 1986; Strickland, 2000; Cook, 2002; Murray, 2007).

Adult worms measure up to 12 mm by 6 mm and often are found in pairs in lung parenchyma, where they reside in a fibrotic capsule produced by the host (Fig. 62-22, *E*). The capsule communicates with the bronchi, through which eggs pass to be eventually expelled in sputa or feces. Although a specific snail serves as the first intermediate host, freshwater crabs and crayfish serve as second intermediates for infectious metacercariae. Ingestion of uncooked, or marinated, crustacea may result in infection. Larvae are released in the stomach and migrate through the intestinal wall into the peritoneal cavity, eventually reaching the lungs after penetrating the diaphragm. Maturation takes approximately 5–6 weeks, and worms may live for many years.

Symptoms, when present, may be caused by larvae migrating through tissues or by adults established in the lungs. Not infrequently, worms develop in ectopic sites, including the peritoneum, subcutaneous tissues, and brain. The onset of lung infection is usually associated with fever, chills, and the appearance of eosinophilia. Once established, symptoms include chronic coughing with abundant mucous production, along with episodes of hemoptysis. Radiographs may show nodular shadows, calcifications, or patchy infiltrates. Eggs remaining in the lung tissues or in ectopic sites may cause an extensive granulomatous reaction.

Diagnosis is made by the finding of typical eggs in stools, sputum, or, occasionally, tissues. Eggs of the different *Paragonimus* species cannot be readily differentiated, and specific identification may be inferred from the area of origin. Operculate, unembryonated eggs measure 80–120 μm by 45–70 μm and have a moderately thick, yellow-brown shell (Fig. 62-22, *F*). The operculum is flattened and usually is set off from the rest of the shell by prominent shoulders. The abopercular end is somewhat thickened but does not have a knob. *Paragonimus* eggs may be differentiated from those of *Diphyllobothrium* and *Fasciola/Fasciolopsis*, which they superficially resemble, by size.

Schistosoma spp.

Schistosomiasis, or bilharzia, is among the most important parasitic diseases worldwide, afflicting 200–300 million individuals. Adult male and female blood flukes inhabit veins of the mesentery or bladder. The most important species infecting humans are *Schistosoma mansoni*, *Schistosoma japonicum*, *Schistosoma mekongi*, *Schistosoma haematobium*, and *Schistosoma intercalatum*; other species infect humans less frequently.

Adult female schistosomes are slender, measuring up to 26 mm by 0.5 mm. Males, which are slightly shorter, enfold a female using the lateral margins of the body (the gynecophoral canal) to assist in sperm transfer. When examined in situ, schistosomes are often found in copula. In their preferred locations, blood flukes elicit little or no inflammatory response. Eggs are deposited in the smallest venule that can accommodate the female worm, where they elicit a strong granulomatous response that results in extrusion of the egg into the intestinal lumen or the bladder. Pathology is primarily related to the sites of egg deposition, the numbers deposited, and the host reaction to egg antigens.

Eggs are fully embryonated when passed and readily hatch when deposited in fresh water. The miracidia penetrate an appropriate species of snail host, where they undergo transformation and extensive asexual multiplication. After about 4 weeks, large numbers of fork-tailed cercariae emerge from the mollusk. Cercariae swim actively about for hours and readily penetrate the skin of susceptible hosts, including humans. After penetration, the cercariae, now called schistosomules, enter the circulation and pass through the lungs before reaching the mesenteric-portal vessels.

Symptoms of schistosomiasis result primarily from penetration of cercariae (cercarial dermatitis), from initiation of egg laying (acute schistosomiasis or Katayama fever), and as a late-stage complication of tissue proliferation and repair (chronic schistosomiasis). In a matter of hours after cercarial penetration, a papular rash associated with pruritus may develop. This is a sensitization phenomenon resulting from prior exposure to cercarial antigens. The most severe form of dermatitis occurs in individuals who are repeatedly exposed to cercariae of nonhuman (primarily avian) schistosomes. Cercarial dermatitis or swimmer's itch occurs worldwide and is a well-recognized entity in the United States (Hoeffler, 1974).

Initiation of egg laying by mature worms 5–7 weeks after infection may result in acute schistosomiasis, or Katayama fever, a serum sickness–like syndrome that occurs with heavy primary infection, especially that of *S. japonicum*. The antigenic challenge to the host is thought to result in immune complex formation (Boros, 1989).

Chronic infection results in continued deposition of eggs, many of which remain in the body. Granulomas produced around these eggs in the intestine and in the bladder are gradually replaced by collagen, resulting in fibrosis and scarring. Eggs trapped in the liver may induce pipe-stem fibrosis with obstruction to portal blood flow. Occasionally, eggs are deposited in ectopic sites, such as the spinal cord, lungs, or brain (Cook, 2002; Garcia, 2007).

Diagnosis is established by demonstrating eggs in feces or urine by direct wet mount or formalin–ethyl acetate concentration methods. Zinc sulfate concentration is not satisfactory for recovery of heavy schistosome eggs. Eggs also may be detected in biopsies of rectal, bladder, and, occasionally, liver tissues by crush preparation or in histologic section (Fig. 62-23). Use of egg hatching methods may occasionally be requested to determine viability or, less commonly, to detect light infection. Feces mixed with distilled water are placed in a flask that is covered with foil to keep out light, with only the neck or a sidearm exposed to bright light. Miracidia, if present, actively swim to the light and can be detected using a hand lens.

Serologic tests may be helpful in screening persons who have traveled to endemic areas and those with negative urine or stool examination who are at risk for infection, or for monitoring response to therapy. Although not widely available, a limited number of reference laboratories and the CDC provide testing. Generally, serologic testing varies with the antigens used and the test methods employed. The CDC uses the Falcon assay screening test in a kinetic enzyme-linked immunosorbent assay (FAST-ELISA). Sera that are positive by the screening test are further evaluated by immunoblot to improve specificity (Wilson, 1995).

Schistosoma mansoni

Schistosoma mansoni occurs in Africa, especially in the tropical areas and the Nile delta, southern Africa, and Madagascar, Brazil, Venezuela, Surinam, and certain Caribbean islands, including Puerto Rico. Adult *S. mansoni* live primarily in the portal vein and in the distribution of the inferior mesenteric vein. Initial deposition of eggs in the large intestine may produce abdominal pain and dysentery, with abundant blood and mucus in the stool. Eggs may be detected in feces at this time. Chronic infection may result in liver fibrosis and portal hypertension, depending on the number of worms present; eggs may be more difficult to find in feces during this stage.

Eggs, which measure 116–180 μm by 45–58 μm, are oval, with a large distinctive lateral spine that protrudes from the side of the egg near one end (see Fig. 62-23, *A* and *B*). If the spine is not visible, the egg may be rotated by gently tapping the coverslip. Movement of the miracidium within the egg may be evident in unfixed material if the larva is viable. Concentration techniques may be required to detect eggs because individuals with limited exposure or with chronic infection may pass few of them.

Schistosoma japonicum

Schistosoma japonicum, which occurs in China, southeast Asia, and the Philippines, causes disease that is clinically similar to that of *S. mansoni* but often more serious because many more (up to 10 times as many) eggs are produced by *S. japonicum*. The disease has been essentially eliminated from Japan, although animal reservoirs still exist. Adult worms live primarily in the distribution of the superior mesenteric vein, and eggs readily reach the liver, inducing fibrosis and portal hypertension as a common complication of chronic infection. The smaller size of the eggs predisposes them to dissemination, especially to the brain and spinal cord. The eggs are broadly oval, measuring 75–90 μm by 60–68 μm, and have an inconspicuous lateral spine, which may be difficult to demonstrate (see Fig. 62-23, *C* and *D*).

Schistosoma mekongi

This species occurs in humans and animal reservoirs in countries along the Mekong River, especially Cambodia and Laos (Bruce, 1980). It is similar to *S. japonicum* but is differentiated from that species by several biological characteristics and by smaller eggs (60–70 μm by 52–61 μm), which otherwise are indistinguishable from those of *S. japonicum*.

Schistosoma haematobium

Urinary schistosomiasis occurs in many parts of Africa, the Middle East, and Madagascar. Parasites migrate via the hemorrhoidal veins to the

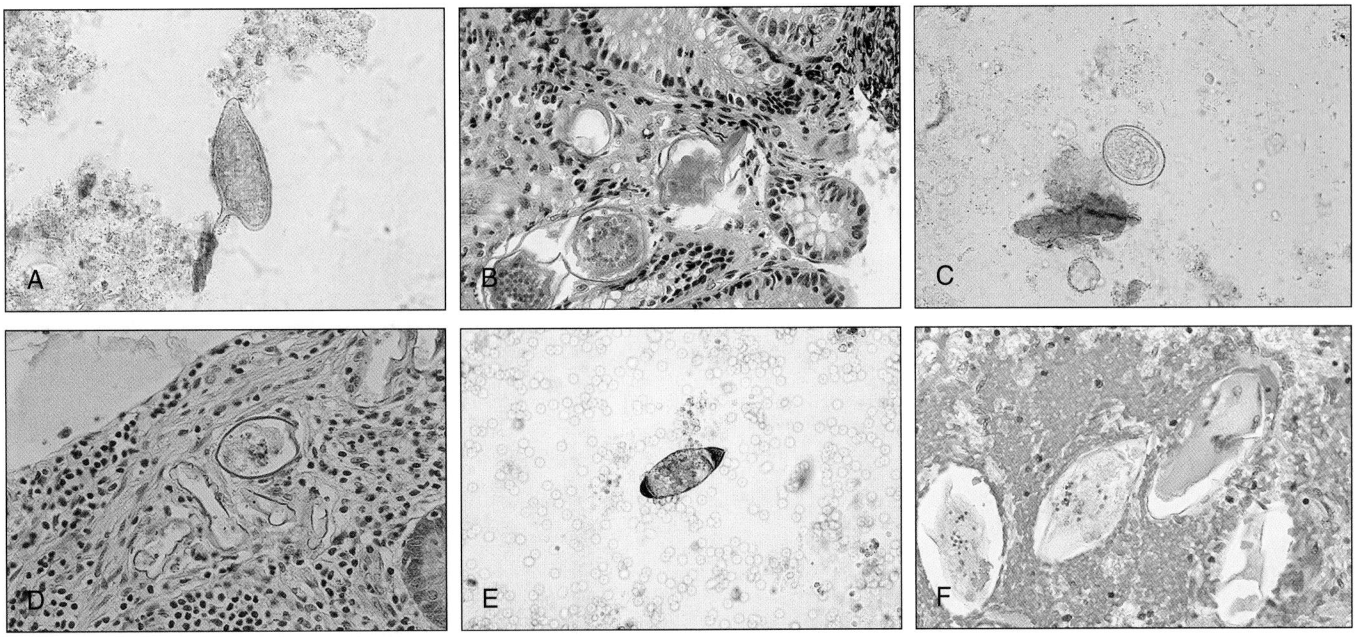

Figure 62-23 **A,** Egg of *Schistosoma mansoni;* note prominent lateral spine (×400). **B,** Eggs of *S. mansoni* in an intestinal biopsy; note presence of lateral spine (H&E; ×400). **C,** Egg of *Schistosoma japonicum;* note presence of small lateral spine (×400). **D,** Eggs of *S. japonicum* in a small-bowel biopsy (H&E; ×400). **E,** Egg of *Schistosoma haematobium* found in urine sediment; note presence of a terminal spine (×400). **F,** Eggs of *S. haematobium* seen in a vulvar granuloma; note presence of a terminal spine (H&E; ×400).

venous plexuses of the urinary bladder, prostate, uterus, and vagina. One of the earliest and most common symptoms of infection is hematuria, especially at the end of micturition. Chronic infection may cause pelvic pain and bladder colic, with an increased desire to urinate. Accumulation of eggs in the tissues may result in hypertrophy of the urothelium, squamous metaplasia, and marked fibrosis, which may progress to obstruction and, ultimately, renal failure. Urinary schistosomiasis also has been associated with squamous cell carcinoma of the bladder (Badawi, 1992).

Eggs are recovered from the urine by examination of spun sediment. They are elongate, measuring 112–180 µm by 40–70 µm, and have a characteristic terminal spine (see Fig. 62-23, *E* and *F*). Occasionally, they may be detected in feces or in a rectal biopsy.

Schistosoma intercalatum

This species occurs in many parts of central and western Africa and produces intestinal schistosomiasis. Eggs have a terminal spine and so resemble those of *S. haematobium*, but they occur primarily in the feces and are larger (140–240 µm by 50–85 µm).

Tissue Helminths

NEMATODES

Filaria

Filarial nematodes, also known as threadworms, are common arthropod-transmitted parasites of vertebrate animals. Adult male and female worms are long and slender, measuring up to 100 mm in length, and are known to inhabit a variety of tissues, including subcutaneous tissues, lymphatics, blood vessels, peritoneal and pleural cavities, heart, and brain. All species produce larvae known as microfilariae, which may be recovered from blood or skin, depending on the species. The microfilariae of some species circulate in the blood with a well-defined periodicity (diurnal or nocturnal), whereas others do not. Microfilariae continue their development only in the appropriate arthropod vector, usually a mosquito or fly, where they mature to the infective stage. Such larvae then are deposited in the tissues of a definitive host when the vector takes another blood meal.

The diagnosis of filariasis usually is made by the finding of microfilariae in the blood or skin, because adult stages are often sequestered in the tissues. Use of Giemsa or hematoxylin-stained thick smears of peripheral blood is routine, although more sensitive procedures such as membrane filter, Knott's concentration, or saponin lysis may also be required (National Committee for Clinical Laboratory Standards, 2000). Microfilariae may be seen moving in direct mounts of blood or tissue fluid.

Species identification is important because pathogenicity varies. Principal characteristics used for identification of microfilariae include the presence or absence of a sheath and its staining characteristics, the shape of the tail and the distribution of cell nuclei within, and the size of the cephalic space and the appearance of its nuclear column. Because microfilariae of *Wuchereria* and *Brugia* usually display a nocturnal periodicity, blood from patients suspected to be infected with these filaria should be drawn between the hours of 10 PM and 2 AM. *Loa loa* displays diurnal periodicity, so blood preferably should be drawn around noon. *Mansonella ozzardi* and *Mansonella perstans* are characteristically nonperiodic. Microfilariae of *Mansonella streptocerca* and *Onchocerca volvulus* are present in the skin and are detected by examination of skin snips or punch biopsies.

Serologic tests for the diagnosis of lymphatic filariasis may prove helpful in select patients, especially those who are not native to endemic areas. Such methods are limited in their ability to distinguish between past exposure and current infection, however, and infection with other nematode species may result in the appearance of cross-reacting antibodies. Antigen detection tests also may be of value in the diagnosis of lymphatic filariasis but generally are not available (Wilson, 1995).

Wuchereria bancrofti

This species, responsible for bancroftian filariasis, is the most common filarial species to infect humans. Endemic areas include central and northern Africa, India, southeast Asia, certain South Pacific islands, and portions of Central and South America and the West Indies. Adult worms reside in the lymphatic system, where chronic infection and reinfection result in lymphadenopathy and lymphangitis, which may progress to lymphedema and obstructive fibrosis (Fig. 62-24, *A*). Severe involvement of the lower extremities and genitalia may result in elephantiasis.

In most areas, microfilariae circulate in peripheral blood with a nocturnal periodicity that corresponds with feeding activities of the usual vectors—*Culex*, *Aedes*, and *Anopheles* mosquitoes. Infections originating in the South Pacific are essentially without periodicity. The microfilariae are sheathed, although this may not always be obvious with Giemsa staining. The tail is pointed, and no nuclei are present in the tip. The cephalic space is not as long as it is wide, and the nuclei in the nuclear column are distinct (Figs. 62-24, *B*, and 62-25). Concentration procedures may be necessary for recovery because microfilariae may be present in small numbers.

Brugia malayi

This species produces disease similar to that of *W. bancrofti*, although it is often milder and more frequently involves the lymphatics of the upper extremities. The parasite occurs mainly in India, southeast Asia, Korea, the Philippines, and Japan. Human infection with related zoonotic species is encountered periodically in the United States.

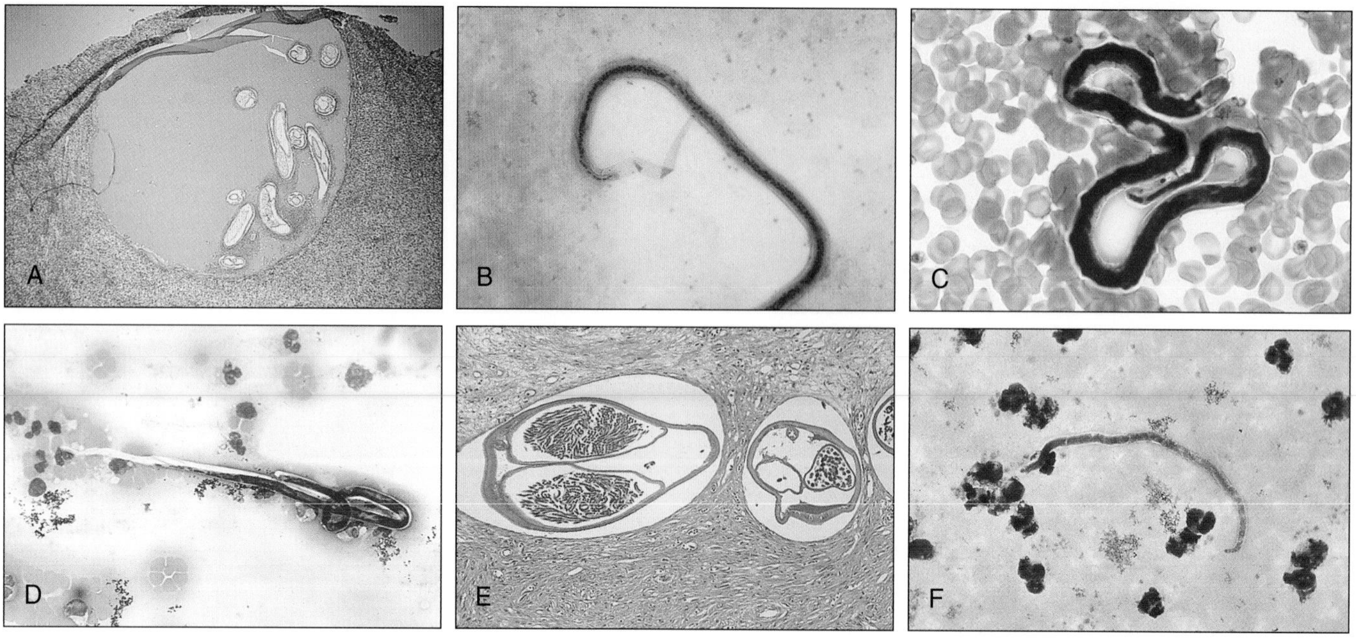

Figure 62-24 **A,** *Wuchereria bancrofti,* cross-section of adult in human lymph node; note extensive inflammatory reaction (H&E; ×100). **B,** Sheathed microfilaria of *W. bancrofti;* cell nuclei do not extend to the tip of the tail (Giemsa stain; ×1000). **C,** Sheathed microfilaria of *Brugia malayi;* two solitary cell nuclei are seen in the tail tip (Giemsa stain; ×1000). **D,** Sheathed microfilaria of *Loa loa;* cell nuclei extend to the tail tip (Giemsa stain; ×1000). **E,** *Onchocerca volvulus,* cross-section of adult in skin nodule (H&E; ×100). **F,** Unsheathed microfilaria of *Mansonella perstans;* cell nuclei extend to the tail tip (Giemsa stain; ×1000).

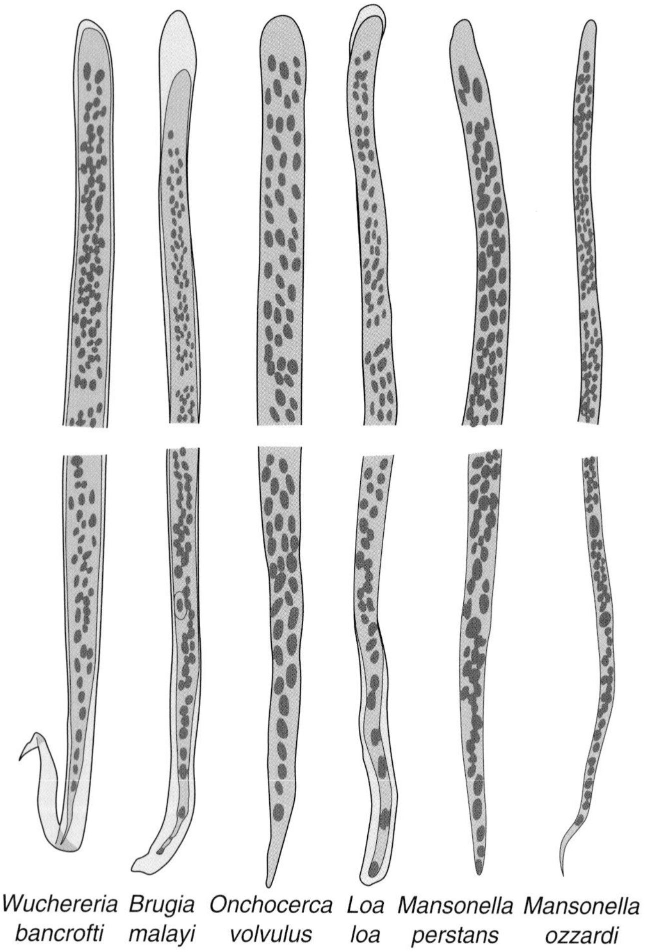

Figure 62-25 Anterior and posterior ends of microfilariae most commonly found in humans. All camera lucida drawings.

The microfilariae circulate in the blood and are primarily periodic. Microfilarial sheaths of *Brugia malayi* stain well with Giemsa stain. The tail has a swelling at the tip and has two solitary nuclei located beyond the ends of the nuclear column (termed subterminal and terminal nuclei). The cephalic space may be much longer than it is wide (Figs. 62-24, *C,* and 62-25). *Brugia timori* is a distinct species occurring in the eastern end of the Indonesian archipelago, especially on the islands of Timor and Flores. Microfilariae are very similar to those of *B. malayi,* although somewhat larger.

Loa loa

Known as the eye worm, *Loa loa* lives in subcutaneous tissues. The nematodes migrate continuously, producing transient (2–3 days) local inflammatory reactions known as Calabar or fugitive swellings. Their occasional appearance in the conjunctiva allows them to be surgically excised. Loiasis occurs primarily in west and central Africa, where deer flies of the genus *Chrysops* serve as vector.

This parasite elicits strong eosinophilia and occasionally has been seen in the United States in people with a history of travel to Africa. The microfilariae, which circulate in the blood with diurnal periodicity, are sheathed, although the sheath does not stain with Giemsa stain. Nuclei in the tail extend to the rounded tip. The nuclear column is distinct, and the cephalic space is short (Figs. 62-24, *D,* and 62-25) (National Committee for Clinical Laboratory Standards, 2000; Garcia, 2007).

Onchocerca volvulus

Onchocerciasis is a leading cause of blindness in endemic areas, which include central Africa, Central America (Mexico and Guatemala), and northern South America. Vectors are black flies of the genus *Simulium.* Adult worms live in hard, fibrous nodules in subcutaneous and deeper tissues that can grow to be 40 mm in diameter (Fig. 62-24, *E*). Nodules tend to occur on the upper half of the body in patients from Central America and on the lower half in those from Africa. Adult worms produce microfilariae that migrate continuously throughout the skin. Complications arise from the migratory activities of microfilariae, resulting in several forms of dermatitis. Movement of microfilariae through the surface of the eye may result in keratitis, corneal opacity, and damage to the anterior and posterior chambers and iris, thus leading to blindness with repeated infection over time.

Diagnosis is made by the finding of typical microfilariae in teased skin snips or skin biopsies, preferably taken from over the scapular region or from the iliac crest, when placed in saline. Alternatively, fluids expressed from scarified skin or aspirates of nodules may be examined (Beaver, 1984; Garcia, 2007). Microfilariae in stained preparations lack both a sheath and nuclei in the tail tip (see Fig. 62-25).

Mansonella spp.

Several species of *Mansonella* infect humans, but all are generally regarded as causing little pathology. Microfilariae, however, must be differentiated from the truly pathogenic filarial species. *M. ozzardi* is found in Central and South America and in some areas of the Caribbean. Adult parasites reside in subcutaneous tissues. *M. perstans* occurs in many areas of tropical Africa and sporadically in South America. Adults are thought to reside primarily in body cavities and the mesenteries. Microfilariae of both species are unsheathed and circulate in peripheral blood without evidence of periodicity. *M. ozzardi* microfilariae have a thin, pointed tail without nuclei, whereas the tail of *M. perstans* is broad and blunt with nuclei extending to the tip (Figs. 62-24, *F*, and 62-25). *M. streptocerca*, which is found in tropical Africa, may be confused with *Onchocerca volvulus*, because both adult and microfilarial stages occur in skin and subcutaneous tissues. Also, dermatitis may be produced by this species. Microfilariae of this species, which may be recovered in skin snips, are unsheathed and have a crook in the tail with nuclei extending to the tip. All species of *Mansonella* are transmitted by gnats of the genus *Culicoides*.

Zoonotic Filariae

Certain filarial nematodes of the genera *Dirofilaria* and *Brugia* that naturally parasitize wild and domestic mammals sporadically infect humans. *Dirofilaria immitis*, commonly known as the canine heartworm, is widely distributed, and human infection is well documented. The mosquito-transmitted larval stage migrates to the right side of the heart. When the worm dies, it is swept into a small pulmonary artery, producing a granulomatous nodule that appears as a coin lesion on a chest radiograph. Diagnosis usually is made by histologic examination of the nodule.

Other species of *Dirofilaria*, including *Dirofilaria tenuis*, *Dirofilaria repens*, and *Dirofilaria ursi*, commonly cause subcutaneous nodules in humans but fail to produce microfilariae. Such nodules have been reported from many body sites, including the face, conjunctiva, and breast, and usually are removed surgically. Histologic examination often reveals a prominent mixed inflammatory reaction surrounding a dead worm. Criteria for identification of zoonotic filariae in tissue sections may be found elsewhere (MacDougall, 1992; Orihel, 1995; Connor, 1997; Gutierrez, 2000).

Other

Dracunculus medinensis

Adult Guinea worms live in subcutaneous tissues and become clinically evident when the female worm migrates to the skin surface and produces a blister, usually on the lower extremities. When the extremity is immersed in water, the blister ruptures, releasing swarms of motile larvae from the female worm into the water. Specific zooplankton (i.e., copepods) ingest the larvae, which then mature to the infective stage and are transmitted back to humans when copepods are accidentally swallowed in drinking water.

The disease is endemic to areas of Africa, the Middle East, and Asia and may be responsible for disfiguring cutaneous scars and more serious secondary bacterial infection. Extensive control efforts have been made in recent years to eradicate this destructive parasite, and success is thought to be at hand (Centers for Disease Control and Prevention, 1992; Cairncross, 2002; Garcia, 2007).

Diagnosis is made by the finding of the female worm emerging at the skin surface with larvae in the discharge fluid. The worm may be gently extracted over a period of days, but care must be taken not to damage it during removal. Should the worm die in situ, pronounced inflammatory reaction and secondary bacterial infection may disable the affected individual.

Angiostrongylus cantonensis and *Angiostrongylus costaricensis*

Human eosinophilic meningoencephalitis, caused by *Angiostrongylus cantonensis*, occurs both in epidemics and sporadically in many areas of the south Pacific, southeast Asia, and Taiwan. The mature parasite normally is found in the pulmonary arteries of rats. Larvae migrate up the trachea and are passed in the feces. They develop to the infective stage in slugs or land snails and, when eaten by the usual rodent host, migrate through the brain before maturing in the pulmonary arteries. Humans acquire the infection by eating large edible snails; raw or incompletely cooked shrimp or crabs, which may serve as transport hosts; or vegetables contaminated with infected mollusks. In humans, *A. cantonensis* larvae migrate to the CNS, producing generally nonfatal meningitis with high spinal fluid eosinophilia (Alicata, 1991). Diagnosis is established both clinically and historically, although larvae occasionally have been recovered from spinal fluid (Kubersky, 1979; Strickland, 2000; Cook, 2002; Garcia, 2007).

Angiostrongylus costaricensis occurs widely in Central and South America (Loria-Cortez, 1980). This parasite, which is responsible for the intestinal form of angiostrongyliasis, normally resides in the mesenteric arteries of the ileum and cecum of rodents. Human infection occurs in the same anatomic location but often results in granulomatous inflammation and symptoms of acute abdomen. Diagnosis is made by histologic examination of surgical specimens and the finding of adults or eggs in the tissues (Strickland, 2000).

Trichinella spiralis

Human trichinosis occurs worldwide, although its incidence in the United States has been in steady decline, with fewer than 100 cases reported each year. Humans acquire the infection through ingestion of raw or incompletely cooked pork, pork products, or, less commonly, bear meat that contains infective larvae. Ingested worms mature in the small intestine, where gravid females produce new larvae for 2–3 weeks. During this stage, gastrointestinal symptoms occur, lasting several days. Larvae subsequently enter lymphatics and venules, thus reaching the general circulation. They primarily invade the skeletal musculature, where they undergo further development and encapsulation. During the migratory and encapsulation phases, fever, muscle pain, respiratory difficulties, periorbital edema, and eosinophilia may develop, depending on the inoculating dose. After the parasites have encysted, few symptoms are noted. Encysted larvae may remain viable for several years, although they eventually become calcified.

Diagnosis is usually made on the basis of history and clinical symptoms and is confirmed by the demonstration of trichinella cysts in skeletal muscle biopsy, particularly the gastrocnemius or deltoid muscles (see Fig. 62-18, *E* and *F*). Indirect tests include creatine phosphokinase, which is often elevated, and detection of antibodies by bentonite flocculation or EIA. Of these latter tests, creatine phosphokinase is more specific, and EIA is more sensitive (Wilson, 1995).

Larva Migrans

Larva migrans is caused by prolonged wandering through body tissues of larvae of certain hookworms, ascarids, and *Strongyloides* species that normally infect wild or domestic animals. The syndrome varies with the species involved, the number of worms, and the tissues parasitized.

Cutaneous larva migrans, or ground itch, is produced by the cutaneous wanderings of cat or dog hookworms of the genus *Ancylostoma*, which penetrate the skin but cannot mature in the usual pattern. Serpiginous, erythematous, and pruritic tracks are apparent on the skin in areas where there has been contact with the ground. This is particularly problematic in warmer, humid climates, where eggs and larvae of these hookworms survive longer. Some species of *Strongyloides* that parasitize wild animals may cause a similar dermatitis (Beaver, 1984).

Visceral larva migrans (VLM) is produced primarily by the random wanderings of the dog ascarid *Toxocara canis* and, to a lesser degree, by *Toxocara cati* from the domestic cat. Children are usually infected following the accidental or intentional ingestion of soil contaminated with dog or cat feces. After hatching, the larvae are unable to complete their usual cycle and instead begin a prolonged migration through various tissues and organs. Children may present with failure to thrive and may display fever, hepatomegaly, pneumonitis, hypereosinophilia, and hypergammaglobulinemia. An inflammatory reaction in the retina from ocular larva migrans may mimic retinoblastoma, a malignant tumor from which it must be differentiated. Diagnosis of VLM is usually made on clinical grounds because the parasite is rarely recovered. Serologic tests may be helpful in confirming a presumptive diagnosis, and the currently recommended procedure is an EIA that uses larval stage excretory-secretory antigens (Wilson, 1995; Garcia, 2007).

A VLM-like syndrome may also be caused by species of *Gnathostoma* that infect the stomach of various mammals. Human infection is most common in southeast Asia but has been reported in Mexico and Ecuador. These parasites use a copepod for the first intermediate host, and fish and amphibians as secondary hosts. A variety of reptiles, birds, and mammals may serve as paratenic hosts. The larvae may migrate through subcutaneous tissues, causing transient swellings, and to deeper tissues, eventually invading the CNS. The occurrence of migratory lesions and a history of eating raw fish may be helpful in establishing a clinical diagnosis.

Capillaria hepatica

Although normally a parasite common to rodents, this species occasionally causes human disease, especially in children, in whom it may mimic VLM, hepatitis, amebic liver abscess, and other diseases. In the usual rodent host, eggs are ingested and resulting larvae migrate to the liver, where they mature and deposit eggs directly in the parenchyma. When the liver is eaten by a predator, the eggs are passed out in the feces and contaminate soil. Children are at particular risk of acquiring the eggs if they eat dirt. In endemic areas, diagnosis is made by examination of liver biopsies or tissue obtained at autopsy. Eggs are readily recognized in tissue biopsies as having thick, striated walls and plugs at both ends.

Anisakis, Pseudoterranova, and *Eustrongylides* spp.

Ingestion of raw fish, although considered by many to be a delicacy, has resulted in an increase in the number of reported cases of fish nematode infections. *Anisakis* and *Pseudoterranova* are common gastrointestinal parasites of marine mammals, and the infective stages are found in various saltwater fish, salmon, and squid intermediate hosts. Small shrimp-like crustaceans (krill) serve as the first intermediate host. When ingested, these larvae may penetrate the wall of the stomach or small bowel, causing acute abdominal pain. Anisakiasis may be presumptively diagnosed based on an appropriate history and clinical findings, and the condition may be confirmed by the recovery of an intact worm at endoscopy or by the presence of an eosinophilic granuloma containing an identifiable nematode in a surgical specimen. Species of *Anisakis* appear to be more prone to produce invasive disease, whereas *Pseudoterranova* spp. tend to be coughed up or vomited intact (see Fig. 62-18, *G* and *H*) (Sakanari, 1989). The species level of larval anisakids is difficult to identify (Binford, 1976).

A small number of infections with *Eustrongyloides* spp. have been reported in individuals who had eaten live minnows or home-prepared sushi. These parasites usually infect fish-eating birds, but in humans, the bright red larvae invade the abdominal cavity, requiring surgical removal (Wittner, 1989).

CESTODES

Several species of cestode infect humans in their larval stages and may produce serious disease. The more commonly encountered ones are readily distinguishable from each other and have unique patterns of transmission. When seen in tissue sections, larval and adult stages of cestodes contain basophilic-staining laminated bodies known as calcareous corpuscles, which are an important aid in their recognition.

Cysticercosis

Human infection with the larval stage of the pork tapeworm, *T. solium*, is found worldwide and occurs following unintentional ingestion of the eggs of an adult tapeworm. The disease is especially prevalent in Mexico and the rest of Latin America, Europe, Africa, India, and Asia. Most cases in the United States originate from highly endemic areas, although in recent years, the number of locally acquired cases has increased (Richards, 1985; Carabin, 2005; Murray, 2007).

Eggs may be ingested accidentally with contaminated food or water and subsequently hatch in the gastrointestinal tract. Embryos penetrate the intestinal mucosa and disseminate via the bloodstream to distant sites, especially the skeletal muscle, and also to the heart, brain, or eye, where symptoms of infection and inflammation may become especially apparent. Seizures are a common complication in endemic areas and are often the presenting symptom (Fig. 62-26, *A*).

The diagnosis is usually made on clinical grounds in endemic areas but may be much more difficult to establish in nonendemic settings. Use of computed tomography (CT) scans is very helpful but generally is not available in most endemic areas. Radiographs are helpful in recognizing the presence of calcified cysts but not in recognizing recent infection. Recovery of an intact cysticercus at the time of surgery confirms the diagnosis. The cysticercus, or bladder worm, is a translucent, fluid-filled, oval sac containing a single inverted scolex that measures 5 mm or more in diameter (Fig. 62-26, *B*).

Among serologic assays, the glycoprotein immunoblot assay available from the CDC has high sensitivity and specificity, outperforming several EIAs with which it was compared (Diaz, 1992). Unfortunately, these assays do not distinguish between active and inactive infections, and thus are not useful in monitoring response to therapy.

The occurrence of cysticercosis in someone from a nonendemic area and without an appropriate travel history should be investigated for accidental exposure to individuals involved in food preparation, or for the possibility of infection with a different *Taenia* species (Schantz, 1992).

Hydatidosis

Human infection with larval stages of tapeworms of the genus *Echinococcus* may take one of three forms: unilocular hydatid disease caused by *Echinococcus granulosus*, multilocular or alveolar hydatid disease caused by *Echinococcus multilocularis*, or polycystic hydatid disease caused by *Echinococcus vogeli* (Thompson, 1995). Members of the dog family are definitive hosts for these minute tapeworms. What they lack in size they make up for in numbers, with many hundreds or thousands of worms producing large

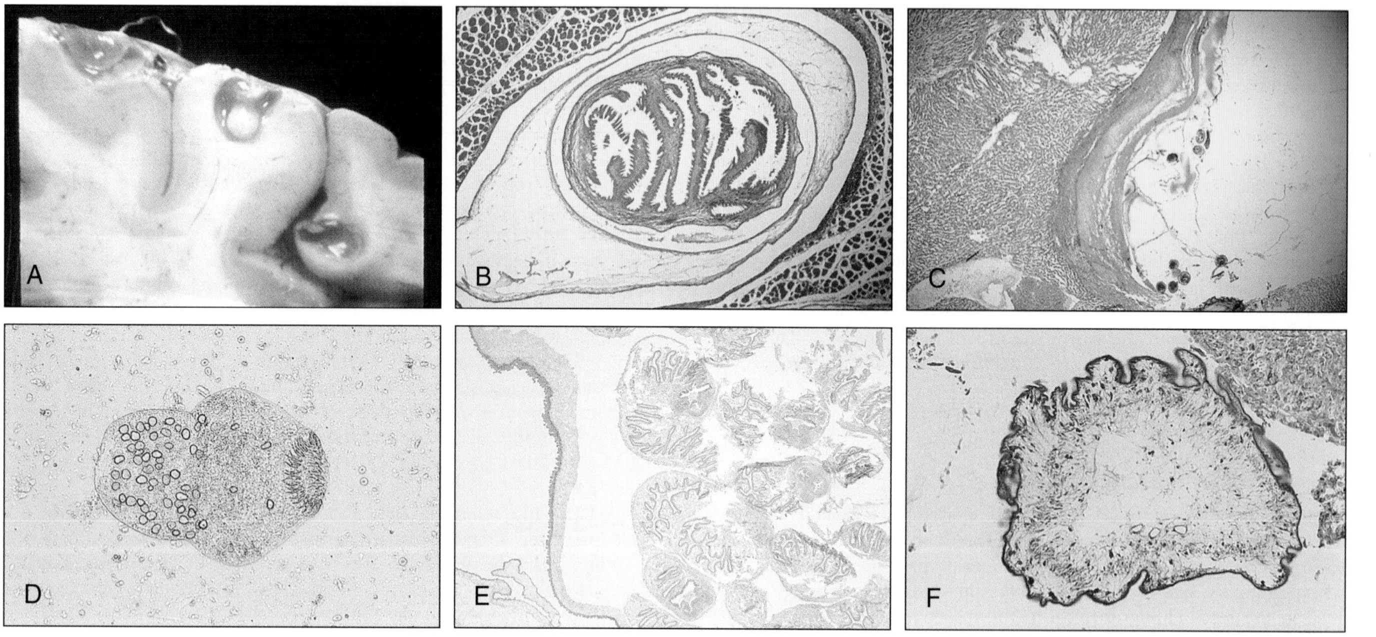

Figure 62-26 **A,** Neurocysticercosis. *(Photograph from Zaiman H. A pictorial presentation of parasites: a cooperative collection;* http://www.astmh.org/Zaiman_Slides/1271.htm.*)* **B,** Bladder worm (*Taenia solium* cysticercus) in muscle (H&E; ×10). **C,** Hydatid cyst in the liver; note presence of protoscolices, a thin germinal membrane, a thick laminated membrane, and fibrotic host reaction (×10). **D,** Protoscolex found in aspirate fluid from a hepatic hydatid cyst; note rostellar hooks and calcareous corpuscles (×400). **E,** Human infection with a coenurus larva; note thin bladder membrane and numerous developing protoscolices (×10). *(Courtesy Dr. Heike Duebner.)* **F,** Sparganum (larva of *Spirometra* spp.) found in a retro-orbital lesion (Giemsa stain; ×100).

numbers of eggs in one host. Eggs are passed in the stools and are ingested by the intermediate hosts, which include sheep, cattle, pigs, rodents, and other herbivorous animals. Humans, especially children, are infected following accidental ingestion of eggs from the environment.

Eggs hatch in the intestine, and embryos penetrate the intestinal wall and then enter the bloodstream. Although most hydatids develop in the liver, some disseminate to other sites. Development of the cysts is slow, and it may take many years for a cyst measuring 10–15 cm in diameter to form. In the usual secondary hosts, the cysts contain numerous protoscoleces, which proliferate from a germinal membrane.

E. granulosus, the most important species producing human disease, is common in many sheep- and cattle-raising areas of the world, including the United States, where dogs are the usual definitive host. Unilocular hydatids develop as single cysts in the liver and secondarily in the lungs or other locations. The cysts are filled with clear fluid and contain brood capsules and numerous protoscoleces, which can number in the thousands (Fig. 62-26, *C* and *D*). Symptoms in humans include a slowly growing mass lesion, although infection in the CNS becomes apparent earlier than in other sites. The diagnosis is suggested on the basis of clinical presentation and history plus the use of radiography, CT scans, and ultrasonography. Serologic tests are very useful in confirming a diagnosis and usually involve a screening test such as EIA or IHA, followed, if positive, by a confirmatory assay such as immunoblot or gel diffusion (Wilson, 1995). Sensitivity varies from 60%–90%, depending on the characteristics of the case. False-positive reactions may occur with cysticercosis, although disease presentation should prevent confusion. Aspiration of cyst contents is potentially dangerous because spillage of cyst contents may result in dissemination of disease or possibly anaphylactic shock; however, if aspiration is performed, cyst contents usually reveal hydatid sand, a mixture of protoscoleces, disintegrating brood capsules, hooklets, and calcareous corpuscles.

E. multilocularis produces multilocular or alveolar hydatid disease in the northern regions of Europe and Russia, and in Alaska, Canada, and the northern tier of states in the United States. Intermediate hosts include several genera of small rodents; foxes, wolves, and dogs are definitive hosts. Human infection occurs in the liver, where the hydatid develops as an invasive cyst that insinuates itself within the tissue in an alveolar pattern. Although the germinal membrane proliferates in the human liver, protoscoleces fail to develop. The pathologic picture is reminiscent of hepatic carcinoma. Serologic assays that use *E. granulosus* antigens are useful in the diagnosis of this disease. The differential use of antigens from both parasites shows promise of discrimination between the two diseases (Wilson, 1995).

E. vogeli produces a polycystic hydatid cyst in humans that is invasive but, unlike *E. multilocularis*, produces both brood capsules and protoscoleces. The disease is limited to Latin America, where rodents, specifically the paca, and bush dogs complete the life cycle (D'Alessandro, 1979). Polycystic hydatid disease in South America may also be caused by *Echinococcus oligarthus*, a parasite of felids and rodents. This species is similar morphologically to *E. vogeli*, and cases have been misidentified (D'Alessandro, 1995).

Sparganosis

Sparganosis is caused by larval cestodes of the genus *Spirometra*, which are closely related to *Diphyllobothrium* spp. Adult stages commonly parasitize cats and dogs and their relatives in Asia (*Spirometra mansoni*) and North America (*Spirometra mansonoides*). Life cycles are similar to those of *Diphyllobothrium*: Copepods serve as first intermediate hosts for procercoid larvae, and fish serve as second intermediate hosts for plerocercoid larvae. Humans become infected with these larval stages (the sparganum) through ingestion of copepods in drinking water or ingestion of raw or incompletely cooked fish. Use of frogs and snakes as poultices may also result in the transfer of larvae to the human host. Sparganosis usually presents as localized or migratory subcutaneous swellings associated with erythema and pain, although brain infection may occur. Surgical exploration may reveal a delicate, slender, ivory-colored worm varying from a few to many centimeters in length. Cross-sections demonstrate a thick tegument with deep folds and parenchyma with prominent muscle bundles. No body cavity is seen, as in the nematodes, and calcareous corpuscles are numerous (Fig. 62-26, *F*) (Orihel, 1995; Gutierrez, 2000; Garcia, 2007).

Coenurosis

Intestinal *Taenia* spp. of cats and dogs (primarily *Taenia multiceps* and *Taenia serialis*) produce a larval stage in intermediate hosts known as a coenurus. This stage consists of a large (up to 10 cm) transparent sac containing numerous scoleces that bud off from a germinal membrane and invaginate into the fluid-filled cyst (Fig. 62-26, *E*). Sheep are the usual intermediate hosts for *T. multiceps*, and rodents, hares, and rabbits for *T. serialis*, although humans serve in this role through accidental ingestion of eggs originating from domestic cats and dogs. Similar to cysticerci, coenuri may develop in any organ, producing a similar disease. Diagnosis is usually made by examination of the excised cyst or its demonstration in tissue sections. The presence of multiple invaginated scoleces within a single bladder differentiates the coenurus from other larval cestodes.

TREMATODES

All liver-, lung-, and blood-inhabiting trematodes that mature in humans produce eggs that usually exit the body via stool, urine, or sputum. Because of their extraintestinal location, these flukes and their eggs may be found in tissues incidentally or in association with symptoms.

Adult *F. hepatica*, *C. sinensis*, and *O. viverrini* may be found in hepatic and biliary tissues, and occasionally in ectopic locations. The presence of typical eggs free in the tissues or within the uterus of the helminth often provides definitive identification. Adult *Paragonimus* spp. primarily reside in the lung but may be found in ectopic sites such as brain and subcutaneous tissue, where they produce abscesses, often associated with large numbers of eggs. Adult schistosomes reside in blood vessels, primarily in the distribution of the inferior mesenteric vein (*S. mansoni*), the superior mesenteric vein (*S. japonicum* and *S. mekongi*), and the vesical plexus (*S. haematobium*). Although the adult stages are rarely encountered in tissue sections, eggs may be found in large numbers in tissues of the intestine, liver, and bladder (see Fig. 62-23, *B*, *D*, and *F*). Eggs may disseminate via the bloodstream to other sites, including the brain, spinal cord, lungs, heart, kidneys, and spleen. The eggs of *S. japonicum* are especially prone to disseminate because of their smaller size and the large numbers typically produced. Identification of eggs is dependent on recognition of their typical sizes and morphologic characteristics in appropriate tissues.

MEDICALLY IMPORTANT ARTHROPODS

Arthropods comprise a large and diverse group of organisms, few of which have clinical or economic significance. Those that do, however, are important causes of morbidity and mortality in humans and their domestic animals, and are responsible for serious economic losses to agriculture. Although perhaps best known among clinicians for their ability to transmit various infectious agents, including viruses, bacteria (rickettsia, spirochetes, others), protozoa, and certain helminths, arthropods also cause serious disease by direct tissue invasion, envenomation, vesication, blood loss, and allergic reaction. Exaggerated fears of arthropods (entomophobia) and delusions of infestation (delusory parasitosis) are not uncommon neuroses, which may be disabling to some individuals. Species directly or indirectly responsible for human disease include representatives of all the major arthropod classes (Table 62-12).

In this section, an approach that the clinical laboratory may use when evaluating clinical specimens containing arthropods is presented, followed by a brief discussion of each of the arthropod groups of medical importance. A variety of general and specialized texts and guides

TABLE 62-12
Classification of Arthropods of Medical Importance

Class Insecta (insects)	**Class Arachnida (arachnids)**
Order Anoplura (sucking lice)	Subclass Scorpiones (scorpions)
Order Siphonaptera (fleas)	Subclass Araneae (spiders)
Order Dictyoptera (cockroaches)	Subclass Acari (ticks, mites, chiggers)
Order Hemiptera (bedbugs, kissing bugs)	**Class Diplopoda (millipedes)**
Order Hymenoptera (ants, wasps, bees)	**Class Chilopoda (centipedes)**
Order Coleoptera (beetles)	**Class Crustacea (crustaceans)**
Order Lepidoptera (moths, butterflies, caterpillars)	Order Copepoda (copepods)
Order Diptera (flies, mosquitoes, midges)	Order Decapoda (crabs, crayfish)
	Class Pentastomida (tongue worms)

are available for more complete coverage of the field of medical entomology (National Communicable Disease Center, 1969; Beaver, 1984; Lane, 1993; Strickland, 2000; Mullen, 2002; Garcia, 2007; Goddard, 2007; Murray, 2007).

BIOLOGICAL CHARACTERISTICS

Arthropods are characterized by a bilaterally symmetrical, segmented body; several pairs of jointed appendages; and a rigid chitinous exoskeleton that is molted repeatedly during growth. Development proceeds from egg to adult through gradual (egg, nymph, and adult stages) or complete (egg, larva, pupa, and adult stages) metamorphosis. Bedbugs, kissing bugs, lice, and cockroaches are examples of insects that undergo gradual metamorphosis. Flies and mosquitoes; fleas; ants, bees, and wasps; and beetles undergo complete metamorphosis; worm-like larval forms pupate to emerge as adults. Arachnids undergo developmental changes most similar to the process of gradual metamorphosis. The larval stages of those arthropods that undergo complete metamorphosis often prove to be the most difficult for clinical laboratorians to identify and should be referred to a specialist.

MECHANISMS OF INJURY

Direct Tissue Invasion

Invasion of superficial tissues (referred to as infestation) may occur with a variety of arthropods, of which scabies mites, chigoe fleas, and some dipteran larvae (maggots) are most common. Invasion of deeper body tissues and cavities (referred to as infection) occurs primarily with maggots and rarely with pentastomid larvae. Tissue invasion by dipteran larvae is referred to as myiasis and may occur in living or devitalized tissues, depending on the involved species.

Envenomation

Many arthropods are capable of injecting saliva or venom with their bites or stings. For most individuals, these compounds cause only local tissue reactions, but serious, life-threatening reactions such as anaphylaxis may occur, often as a result of previous sensitization to the particular toxin. Hymenopteran (ants, bees, and wasps) and scorpion stings are among the greatest offenders (Reisman, 1994). The bites of certain arthropods, especially centipedes; mosquitoes, flies, and biting midges; bedbugs, kissing bugs, and assassin bugs; sucking lice; fleas; and ticks and mites may also be toxic, causing local or systemic reactions. Almost all spiders are venomous, but only a few groups (widow spiders, violin spiders, and certain tarantulas) pose significant health risks to humans. Less common but recognized causes of envenomation result from exposure to the urticating hairs of certain caterpillars and beetle larvae.

Vesication

Certain of the larger tropical millipedes are capable of spraying a vesicating (blister-causing) chemical substance from glands located on each body segment. These compounds are especially irritating should they reach the conjunctiva. Blister beetles are so named because of their ability to discharge vesicating fluids (cantharidin, the active ingredient in the aphrodisiac Spanish fly) from their bodies when handled.

Blood Loss

Arthropods responsible for producing significant irritation or blood loss to humans and domestic animals include bedbugs, kissing bugs, lice, fleas, flies, mosquitoes, biting midges, ticks, and mites. Although these activities are rarely life threatening, the concurrent transmission of infectious agents may be.

Transmission of Infectious Agents

Many arthropods play an integral role in the mechanical or biological transmission of infectious disease agents. The common housefly, *Musca domestica*, may be responsible for the mechanical transmission of agents of bacillary dysentery, cholera, typhoid, viral diarrhea, amebic dysentery, and giardiasis, as well as pinworms and tapeworms. Mechanisms involved in the biological transmission of infectious agents vary from simple organism amplification in the arthropod vector to more complex life cycle changes in the involved parasite. Ticks and mites are involved in the transmission of certain bacteria (*Rickettsia*, *Ehrlichia*, *Anaplasma*, spirochetes, others), protozoa (*Babesia*), and viruses. Among insects, lice are involved in the transmission of bacteria (*Rickettsia*, *Bartonella*, and *Borrelia*); kissing bugs transmit trypanosomes; fleas transmit the agents of plague, typhus, and canine tapeworm; and dipterans transmit arboviruses, malarial parasites, trypanosomes, leishmanias, filarial worms, and bacteria.

Hypersensitivity Reactions

Most serious reactions to arthropod bites and stings result from allergic hypersensitivities. Hymenopteran stings alone are responsible for most arthropod-related deaths and usually result from the development of hypersensitivity following repeated exposure to venom (Reisman, 1994). Allergies may be exacerbated following exposure to the saliva, excrement, or body parts of mites, ticks, lice, bedbugs, caterpillars, moths, and butterflies. Asthma and hay fever may also develop in response to the presence of the large variety of house, dust, and animal mites in the environment (Frazier, 1980).

Psychological Manifestations

Entomophobia refers to an unreasonable or excessive fear of seeing or touching arthropods. Although this fear may occasionally result in disruption of a person's normal activities, it rarely becomes incapacitating. Delusory parasitosis is a more serious emotional disorder in which an individual is convinced that he or she is infected with parasites or arthropods despite objective evidence to the contrary. As the delusion progresses, the individual may report loss of employment, divorce, repeated use of pesticide services, and movement from house to house. Visits to healthcare providers are usually numerous, although unsatisfactory. The problem may originate in the home or workplace and may be transferable from one to the other. The delusion may be so convincing that other family members or friends may believe it or acquire it themselves. The patient may submit to the laboratory numerous specimens such as skin, fabric, lint, hair, and mucus. It is incumbent on laboratory personnel to examine these materials to rule out true infestation. The mysterious onset of irritation and itching may be due to bites from unrecognized scabies mites, lice, fleas, or bedbugs, or from insects and mites questing from an abandoned rodent or bird nest in an area of human habitation. Before such causes are dismissed, they must be looked for and their presence excluded (Lynch, 1993; Goddard, 2007; Murray, 2007).

LABORATORY APPROACHES TO ARTHROPOD IDENTIFICATION

Arthropod specimens are often directed to the clinical laboratory by both clinicians and patients with the expectation that they can be accurately identified, but few laboratory personnel receive more than a cursory exposure to entomology during training. Nonetheless, laboratorians should have access to texts and dichotomous keys, which should allow limited identification of the more commonly encountered medically important groups, especially ectoparasites (fleas, lice, mites, and ticks). Of greater importance is the ability of laboratory personnel to recognize those rare situations in which outside expertise should be sought. This specifically relates to those occasions when significant clinical decisions regarding therapy and prognosis are being made. State or local public health laboratories often have the expertise available or know of individuals trained in medical entomology who can be reached at regional educational institutions, museums, or other public or private agencies, including the CDC.

Specimens submitted to the laboratory are most often intact organisms, skin scrapings, tissues, sputum, urine, or stool. Inanimate objects, including foodstuffs, water, clothing, bedding, and carpeting, among others, may also be submitted. It is not uncommon for patients to submit arthropods recovered from the toilet bowl following urination or a bowel movement. In most cases, the presence of such organisms is coincidental and is not related to infection.

Proper killing and preservation of arthropods is important to preserve those characteristics necessary for identification. Small, nonwinged arthropods, especially ectoparasites (lice, fleas, ticks, and mites), larval forms (maggots, grubs, and caterpillars), spiders, and scorpions, should be placed directly into 70%–80% ethyl alcohol. Large larval forms are best killed in hot (not boiling) water to extend their bodies and prevent contraction before immersion in alcohol. Attached tissue or other debris should be gently removed or washed away prior to preservation. Smaller forms (mites, small ticks, fleas, and sandflies) may be prepared as permanent slide mounts.

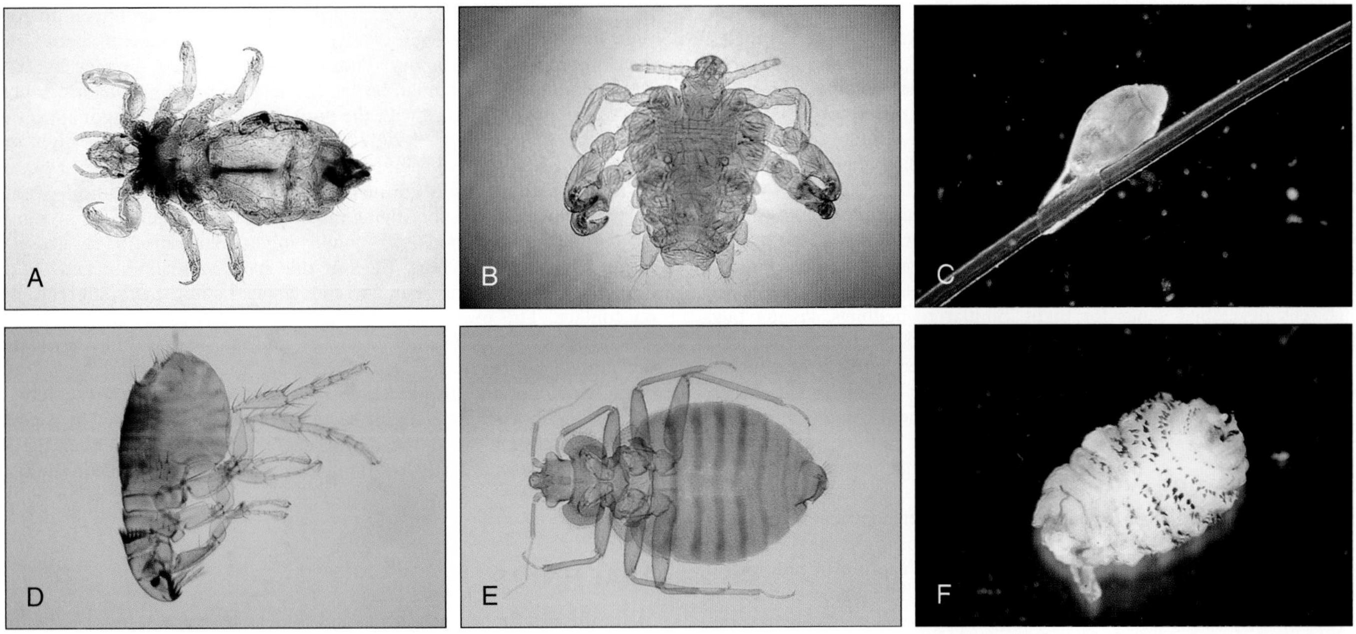

Figure 62-27 Medically important insects. **A,** *Pediculus capitis,* the head louse. **B,** *Phthirus pubis,* the crab louse. **C,** Empty egg case (nit) of *P. capitis.* **D,** *Ctenocephalides canis,* the common dog flea; note powerful hind legs. **E,** *Cimex lectularius,* the common bedbug. **F,** Larva of *Dermatobia hominis,* the human botfly; note the two sclerotized hooks at the anterior end and numerous body spines (×10). *(**A, B,** and **E** with permission from Murray PR, Barron EJ, Pfaller MA, et al, editors. Manual of clinical microbiology. 6th ed. Washington, DC: ASM Press; 1995.)*

Winged insects, especially adult mosquitoes, midges, and flies, should be killed by exposure to the fumes of ethyl acetate or chloroform and preserved dry to retain the taxonomic information contained in the body and wing scales. Such arthropods usually are pinned and dried, followed by storage in tight-fitting boxes protected with naphthalene or dichlorobenzene. Additional details regarding the collection, preservation, and preparation of arthropod specimens for examination are found elsewhere (Beaver, 1984; Steyskal, 1987; Lane, 1993; Garcia, 2007).

INSECTS

Insects account for more than 90% of all described arthropod species, although few are responsible for human disease. Members of this class are distinguished from other arthropods by having a body divided into three parts (head, thorax, abdomen); one pair of antennae; three pairs of legs; and one, two, or no pairs of wings. This is the only arthropod class in which flight has developed.

Sucking Lice

Sucking lice are dorsoventrally flattened, wingless insects that have characteristic claws on the ends of each leg that allow attachment to body hairs or clothing (Fig. 62-27, *A* and *B*). All species suck blood intermittently, which may cause unexplained dermatitis. Eggs, known as nits, are deposited on hair shafts or clothing, depending on the species. Although named for their primary site of attachment, they do not always remain confined to that location. The head louse, *Pediculus capitis,* and the body louse, *Pediculus humanus,* are indistinguishable to the nonspecialist. They are longer than they are wide and grow to about 3 mm in length. Biological differences are apparent; only *P. humanus* transmits the agents of epidemic typhus, trench fever, and relapsing fever (Kim, 1986). Infestations with both species occur among people living in crowded conditions who have little opportunity for bathing and laundering. Children of school age are at particular risk for acquiring head lice through the sharing of caps, clothing, and combs (Orkin, 1985). Nits of head lice are deposited primarily on hair shafts, and those of body lice are deposited on clothing. Because objects such as hair casts, dander, hair spray, and fungal hair infection may mimic nits, differentiation is important. Nits are typically 1 mm long and when unhatched have intact opercula (Fig. 62-27, *C*). Transmission occurs primarily through the sharing of infested clothing and bedding because body lice tend to lay their eggs in clusters, especially along seams or waistbands. The pubic louse, *Phthirus pubis,* is distinctly different from the others; it is rounder (measuring up to 2 mm in diameter), the abdomen is more crab-like, and the first pair of legs is significantly smaller and more slender than the other pairs (see Fig. 62-27, *B*). Pubic lice and their nits are found primarily on pubic hairs but may extend to the chest, armpit, and facial hair. Transmission occurs primarily during sexual intercourse.

Fleas

Fleas are small (1–2 mm), laterally compressed, wingless ectoparasites capable of sucking blood (Fig. 62-27, *D*). Long, muscular legs are adapted for jumping great distances. Fleas that attack humans are parasites of other mammals or poultry and include both blood-sucking pests (many species) and tissue-penetrating jiggers. Infestations commonly occur with exposure to domestic animals and pets; the most pestiferous species are the dog flea *(Ctenocephalides canis)*, the cat flea *(Ctenocephalides felis)*, and the human flea *(Pulex irritans)*. Some individuals become highly sensitized to flea bites, whereas others are unaffected. Cat and dog fleas are the usual intermediate hosts for the tapeworm *D. caninum* and less frequently for *H. diminuta* and *H. nana*. Because larvae of these species often develop in an animal's bedding, or in carpets and furniture, eradication may require fumigation and cleaning of those articles. The Oriental rat flea, *Xenopsylla cheopis,* is an extremely important species because it transmits the plague bacillus and the agent of murine typhus. Although normally parasitizing several species of rats, this flea readily attacks humans should the rodent host die. The jigger or chigoe flea *Tunga penetrans* is found in both Central and South America and in regions of tropical Africa. The female flea attaches to and embeds itself in the skin, especially between the toes and under the toenails, where it grows to the size of a small pea. After eggs are discharged, the flea dies, prompting an inflammatory response and possible secondary bacterial infection. Tungiasis is diagnosed by identifying the dark portion of the flea's abdomen (displaying the spiracles) protruding from the skin surface of an enlarging lesion (Beaver, 1984; Lane, 1993; Garcia, 2007; Goddard, 2007).

Cockroaches

Cockroaches have closely adapted themselves to human habitation, sharing our food, shelter, and warmth. Although they are primarily nuisance pests, cockroaches are potential carriers of fecal pathogens owing to their ability to move quickly from sewers and drains to food preparation areas. In addition to transmitting pathogenic bacteria, they may spread hepatitis and poliovirus; intestinal protozoa, including *E. histolytica*; and several species of enteric nematode. Allergies and asthma may develop in some individuals following exposure to the excreta, cast skins, or body parts of cockroaches (Goddard, 2007).

Bedbugs and Kissing Bugs

Bedbugs (family Cimicidae) and kissing bugs (family Reduviidae) are blood-sucking insects that have a long, narrow proboscis that is folded underneath the body when not in use. Bedbugs (*Cimex lectularius* and *Cimex hemipterus*) are reddish brown, dorsoventrally flattened, wingless insects approximately 5 mm in length (Fig. 62-27, *E*). They are cosmopolitan in distribution and attack most any mammal, feeding primarily at night. During daylight hours, they hide under mattresses, loose wallpaper, and floorboards. Although they are not known to transmit disease, bedbug bites may cause painful weals or bullae, depending on an individual's sensitivity to their saliva.

Kissing bugs (*Triatoma*, *Rhodnius*, *Panstrongylus*) have a cone-shaped head on a narrow neck and an abdomen that is widened in the middle. These insects are black or brown, and some have orange and black markings on the abdomen. They average 1–3 cm in length and, unlike bedbugs, have well-developed wings for flight. Similar to bedbugs, kissing bugs are relatively painless feeders on vertebrates and produce similar skin reactions. In Mexico and Central and South America, they transmit the agent of Chagas' disease, *T. cruzi*, in the feces, which is secondarily inoculated into the skin by the human host while scratching (Lane, 1993; Goddard, 2007).

Bees, Wasps, and Ants

Hymenopterans are social insects that readily defend their nests when disturbed. In nonreproductive females, the ovipositor is modified as a stinger capable of injecting venom for use in the capture of prey or for defense. The venom of bees, wasps, hornets, and yellow jackets causes only transient swelling and discomfort in most individuals but may be responsible for systemic reactions, including anaphylaxis, in others who were previously sensitized (Reisman, 1994). Up to 100 people in the United States die each year from hymenopteran stings. The Africanized honey bee is now present in North America following its introduction into Brazil in 1956. These bees, which are more easily provoked than other honey bees, exhibit massive stinging behavior. Many species of ant are problematic for humans because of their ability to bite, and some groups, such as harvester and fire ants, are capable of giving painful stings.

Beetles

Although beetles are perhaps best known as pests of agricultural crops, some species may give a painful bite, and others, especially blister beetles, may exude vesicating fluids (cantharidin) that cause dermatitis or blister formation. The larvae of certain larder beetles have urticating hairs that may be responsible for dermatitis or, if ingested, irritation of the gastrointestinal tract. Larval and adult larder and grain beetles also may serve as intermediate hosts for the rodent and human tapeworms *H. diminuta* and *H. nana*.

Moths and Butterflies

Certain larvae (caterpillars) of Lepidoptera possess urticating hairs or spines capable of injecting venom when handled. Although most effects of these toxins remain localized to the skin, systemic effects such as shock and paralysis have been reported (Goddard, 2007). Adult tussock and gypsy moths are known to have urticating scales and hairs that may cause dermatitis, eye irritation, or respiratory tract irritation, especially among forestry workers (Shama, 1982).

Flies, Mosquitoes, and Midges

Diptera are characterized by the presence of a single pair of membranous wings. Among all arthropods, they are responsible for the greatest share of human disease through blood-sucking activities, biological or mechanical transmission of infectious agents, and direct tissue invasion by larval forms (myiasis). Bites from a variety of flies, mosquitoes, and biting midges often cause local irritation from sensitivity to the saliva and, in some individuals, systemic reactions. In addition to blood-sucking activities, the repeated attacks themselves may be physically and psychologically damaging. Certain blood-sucking species are also responsible for the transmission of important human pathogens, including malaria, filariasis, and arboviral disease by mosquitoes; onchocerciasis by blackflies; loiasis by deer flies; leishmaniasis and bartonellosis by sand flies; and African trypanosomiasis by tsetse flies. Other viral, bacterial, and parasitic agents are readily transmitted mechanically by nonbiting flies such as house flies, flesh flies, and blow flies, which can easily contaminate human food.

Myiasis may occur in an accidental, facultative, or obligatory fashion. The housefly, *Musca domestica*, has no requirement for developing in mammalian tissue, yet may be found occasionally in dead tissue or under plaster casts. This type of accidental myiasis is not uncommon but rarely is clinically significant. Facultative myiasis is most often caused by blowflies and flesh flies, which ordinarily feed on dead tissues but may move into adjacent viable tissues. Obligatory myiasis is caused by certain species that develop only in living tissues. Those species that infect humans are all of zoonotic origin. The human botfly, *Dermatobia hominis*, develops in boil-like subcutaneous lesions, with the posterior end of the maggot appearing at the skin surface (Fig. 62-27, *F*). This species is most commonly found in individuals who have spent time in Central or South America or, less frequently, Africa, and is unusual in that its eggs are mechanically transported to the host by other flying insects, usually mosquitoes. The tumbu fly (*Cordylobia anthropophaga*), found in sub-Saharan Africa, causes a furuncular type of myiasis. Eggs of this species usually are laid on the ground or on hanging laundry, and larvae rapidly penetrate the skin on contact. The most serious obligatory myiasis is caused by the Old World screwworm, *Chrysomya bezziana*, and the New World screwworm, *Cochliomyia hominivorax*. These species lay their eggs directly on their cattle hosts, usually on wounds or near the nostrils. The larvae actively feed on and move through living tissues. Human infection may be particularly destructive if larvae invade the eye, nose, or mouth. Other species may also be responsible for traumatic, obligatory myiasis in humans (Lane, 1993).

ARACHNIDS

Medically important arachnids include scorpions, spiders, ticks, and mites. Scorpions and spiders have two body segments, the cephalothorax and the abdomen, whereas ticks and mites have only one. Members of the group have four pairs of legs as nymphs and adults; larval ticks and mites have three pairs of legs. All lack antennae, mandibles, and wings. Scorpions and spiders are best known for their ability to inject poisonous venom, whereas ticks and mites are best known as vectors for viral, bacterial, and protozoal pathogens.

Scorpions

Unlike other arachnids, scorpions have a pair of forward-directed pincer claws that impart a crab-like appearance and a segmented tail with a bulbous stinging apparatus in the tip (Fig. 62-28, *A*). They are predatory in nature and paralyze their intended victim with venom from the sting, which may also be used for defensive purposes. Toxicity to humans varies depending on the species; many elicit no more reaction than that of a bee sting, but some are deadly, causing more than 1000 deaths annually. Poisonous species are found in the Western Hemisphere, Europe, Africa, and the Middle East (Beaver, 1984; Goddard, 2007).

Spiders

Spiders lack a tail with an attached stinger but instead have fang-like chelicerae among their mouthparts, through which venom can be expressed. Although most spiders are venomous, few have chelicerae capable of penetrating human skin. Most spider bites cause only transitory irritation and pain. Widow spiders (genus *Lactrodectus*) are one group responsible for systemic arachnidism through the action of a potent neurotoxin capable of producing weakness, myalgia, paralysis, convulsions, and, occasionally, death. Published mortality rates vary from less than 1% to 6%. Five closely related species are found in the United States; the black widow (*Lactrodectus mactans*) is the most widespread. Female black widow spiders are glossy black with a characteristic red or orange hourglass-shaped marking on the underside of the abdomen and have a leg span of 3–4 cm. They live in protected locations such as woodsheds, basements, and outdoor privies (Strickland, 2000).

Violin spiders (genus *Loxosceles*) are responsible for necrotic arachnidism or loxoscelism. In the United States, the brown recluse or fiddleback spider (*Loxosceles reclusa*) is most often involved, although other species are present. This species is 1–2 cm long and tan to dark brown; it has a darkened, violin-shaped marking oriented base forward on the dorsum of the cephalothorax. When present in homes, violin spiders are reclusive in their habits, preferring undisturbed areas such as closets, basements, and under porches. Their bite is painless and often goes unrecognized until several hours later, when the area becomes red, swollen, and painful. The venom is dermonecrotic and hemolytic, producing cutaneous necrosis and sloughing of involved skin over several days. The resulting lesion may be difficult to heal and subject to secondary infection. Systemic reactions such as hemolysis and acute renal failure are rare. Other spider genera have also been implicated in producing necrotic arachnidism (Fisher, 1994).

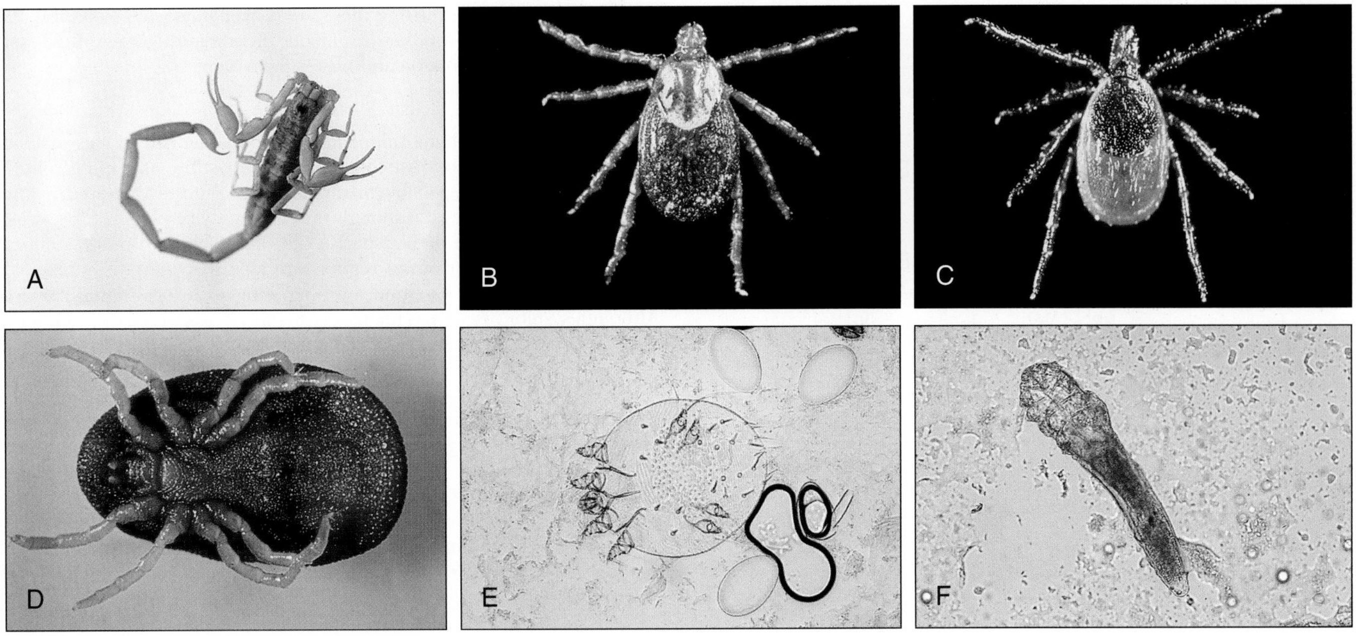

Figure 62-28 Medically important arachnids. **A,** Scorpion; note forward-directed pincher claws and stinger on the tail tip. **B,** *Dermacentor variabilis* (dog tick), nonengorged adult female. **C,** *Ixodes scapularis* (black-legged tick or deer tick), nonengorged adult female. **D,** *Ornithodoros* sp. (soft tick), nonengorged adult, ventral view. **E,** *Sarcoptes scabei* (itch mite) adult; note presence of adjacent eggs in skin scrapings. **F,** *Demodex folliculorum* (follicle mite) adult. *(**A,** With permission from Murray PR, Barron EJ, Pfaller MA, et al, editors. Manual of clinical microbiology. 6th ed. Washington, DC: ASM Press; 1995; **B** and **C,** with permission from Northwest Infectious Disease Consultants; **E,** with permission from Spach DH, Fritsche TR. Norwegian scabies in a patient with AIDS. N Engl J Med 1994;331:777.)*

Ticks

Unlike spiders and scorpions, ticks have a fused cephalothorax and abdomen, as well as a characteristic toothed hypostome for feeding. Tick development progresses through four stages: egg, larva, nymph, and adult. Following hatching, a blood meal is required for progression to the subsequent stage. Humans usually acquire ticks in grassy or brushy areas in close proximity to the usual animal hosts. All species are obligate bloodsucking ectoparasites and are important vectors of viral, bacterial, and protozoal pathogens to humans and domestic animals. Their feeding activities may produce local tissue damage and blood loss, especially to livestock and wildlife, or tick paralysis, a syndrome caused by a neurotoxin secreted by a tick's salivary glands that produces ascending flaccid paralysis and toxemia. Symptoms may closely mimic those of Guillain-Barré syndrome, poliomyelitis, or botulism. Removal of the attached tick usually results in resolution of symptoms within hours to days.

Species affecting humans include members of the family Ixodidae (hard ticks) and Argasidae (soft ticks). Hard ticks have anteriorly directed mouthparts and a sclerotized plate, or scutum, on the dorsum. The scutum covers the entire dorsum in the male but only the anterior portion in the female, allowing the body to swell when engorged (Fig. 62-28, *B* and *C*). Argasid ticks have a soft leathery body lacking a scutum and ventrally directed mouthparts that are not visible when viewed from above (Fig. 62-28, *D*). Unengorged ticks are generally 2–5 mm long but may enlarge to several times that size following engorgement. Engorged hard ticks may mimic soft ticks, so care must be exercised in their identification (Sonenshine, 1991, 1993).

Most ticks found crawling on or embedded in human skin are hard ticks. Soft ticks tend to feed only briefly and then often at night. Important species of hard ticks in North America include *Dermacentor variabilis* (American dog tick), *Dermacentor andersoni* (Rocky Mountain wood tick), *Amblyomma americanum* (Lone Star tick), *Rhipicephalus sanguineus* (brown dog tick), *Ixodes scapularis* (black-legged or deer tick), and *Ixodes pacificus* (Western black-legged or deer tick). *Dermacentor* and *Amblyomma* ticks are called ornate ticks because of the presence of white markings on their scuta; the other species are inornate ticks.

Dermacentor ticks transmit Rocky Mountain spotted fever and possibly tularemia, Q fever, and Colorado tick fever. *Ixodes* ticks are vectors of Lyme disease, babesiosis, anaplasmosis, and ehrlichiosis, and in other parts of the world, these ticks are responsible for the transmission of certain arboviruses. *Amblyomma* ticks are capable of transmitting Rocky Mountain spotted fever, as well as tularemia and possibly Lyme disease. All these genera are capable of causing tick paralysis. *Rhipicephalus* ticks have been implicated in the transmission of Rocky Mountain spotted fever and ehrlichiosis in North America, and of boutonneuse fever in the Mediterranean area. Soft ticks of the genus *Ornithodoros* occur in many parts of the world, including the United States, and are important vectors of the relapsing fever spirochetes (*Borrelia recurrentis* and related forms) (Spach, 1993; Murray, 2007; Ismail, 2010).

Mites

Mites are arachnids of microscopic size (usually <1 mm) that are widely distributed in the environment. Medically important species may attack humans directly, serve as vectors for infectious disease, or cause dust allergies. Humans are commonly infested with both *Demodex folliculorum* and *Demodex brevis*, the follicle mites, and *Sarcoptes scabei*, the itch or mange mite. Follicle mites are minute (0.1–0.4 mm), elongate parasites with stubby legs that can be recovered from hair follicles and sebaceous glands (Fig. 62-28, *F*). They are common incidental findings on histologic skin preparations. Although their presence has been associated with various skin conditions, they are commonly found in healthy individuals as well, which makes their significance difficult to assess (Burns, 1992).

Sarcoptes scabei mites are of greater medical importance because of their ability to create serpiginous tunnels through the upper layers of the epidermis. Transmitted through personal contact, these mites are found primarily in the interdigital spaces and the flexor surfaces of the wrists and forearms and less commonly in other areas, including the breasts, buttocks, and external genitalia. Inflammation and intense itching result from the tunneling activity and from the deposition of eggs and excreta. Clinical manifestations vary depending on the degree of sensitization to the parasites and their products. Lesions often become secondarily infected. Generalized dermatitis occurring in the presence of thousands of mites, typically in elderly or immunocompromised individuals, is known as crusted or Norwegian scabies.

The diagnosis is made by placing skin scrapings collected from tunneled areas in 20% potassium hydroxide or mineral oil for clearing and examining under the microscope. Detection of eggs, six-legged larvae, and eight-legged nymphs or adults is diagnostic but may be difficult to demonstrate (Figs. 62-28, *E*, and 62-29). The diagnosis of scabies in an institutional or school setting may result in pseudoepidemics, in which numerous individuals develop itching without evidence of disease. Care must be exercised to properly diagnose the disease to identify real cases and differentiate them from cases of delusory parasitosis (Orkin, 1985; Lynch, 1993).

A number of animal mite species may attack humans for a blood meal, either as larval forms or as adults, when normal mammalian or bird hosts

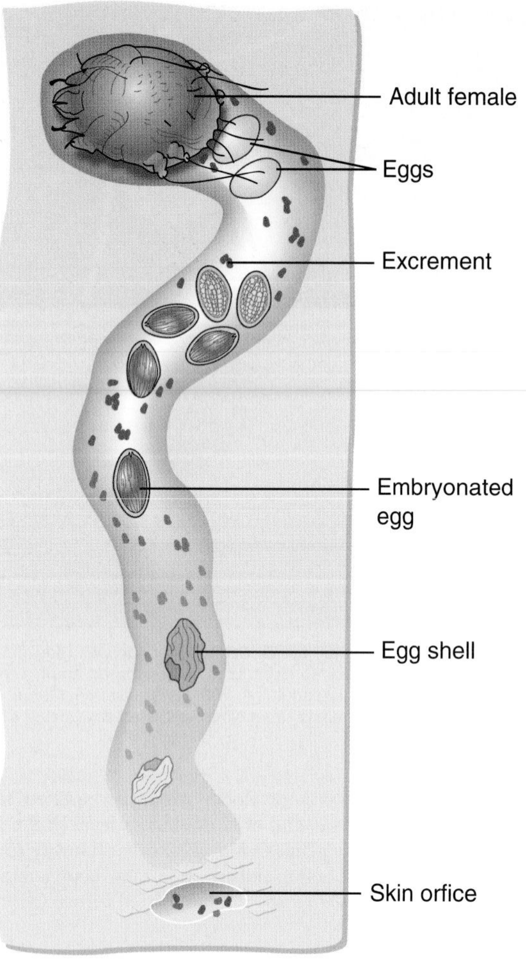

Figure 62-29 *Sarcoptes scabiei.* Diagram of a subcutaneous burrow.

are not available. Larval chigger mites (family Trombiculidae) are problematic in many parts of the world because their saliva can produce large weal-and-flare reactions with intense itching. These tiny six-legged larvae are often red and commonly attach to the skin in areas where clothing is restrictive, such as at the ankles, waistline, armpits, and wrists. In parts of Asia and Australia, trombiculid mites are vectors for the transmission of the agent of scrub typhus (Lane, 1993).

Certain nonbiting mites play a role in allergic rhinitis, asthma, and some skin conditions. The secretions, excreta, and body parts of *Dermatophagoides farinae* and *Dermatophagoides pteronyssinus* are potent allergens that may occur in great numbers in the household environment (Frazier, 1980). Routine testing by an allergist may identify the offending agent.

CLASSES OF LESSER MEDICAL IMPORTANCE

Millipedes

Millipedes are worm-like arthropods with numerous apparent body segments, each with two pairs of legs; they are commonly found in and under decaying vegetation. Although they lack mouthparts capable of producing serious bites, many species produce vesicating secretions from glands located on each body segment. When handled roughly, the larger tropical species are capable of squirting these fluids over a distance of several centimeters. Exposure of the skin or mucous membranes to these fluids may produce a burning sensation and blister formation.

Centipedes

Centipedes are flatter than millipedes, have only one pair of legs per body segment, and display long antennae. They are fast moving and can inflict a painful sting from a pair of forward-directed pincers that are modified from the first pair of legs. Although they are rarely responsible for serious injury to humans, the larger species (26–45 cm) found in the southern United States and in tropical regions are able to penetrate human skin when handled, giving a painful, burning sting with local tissue reaction. Although systemic reactions may occur in individuals who have been previously sensitized, fatalities are rare (Goddard, 2007).

Crustaceans

Crustaceans of medical importance are primarily those species that serve as hosts for larval stages of several different helminths. Several genera of crabs and crayfish are intermediate hosts for the metacercariae of various species of lung fluke (*Paragonimus* spp.) found around the world. Copepods are common microscopic zooplankton, certain species of which serve as first intermediate hosts for the nematodes *D. medinensis* and *Gnathostoma spinigerum* and for cestodes of the genera *Diphyllobothrium* and *Spirometra*.

Pentastomids

Pentastomes, or tongue worms, are arthropods of uncertain affinities owing to lack of morphologic characteristics. Adult stages are worm-like organisms that live in the nasal passages of certain predatory reptiles, birds, and mammals. Larval stages resemble mites and reside in rodents, herbivores, and freshwater fish. Human liver and lung infections with larval stages have been reported from Asia and Africa. Adult stages have been recovered from the nasopharynx of individuals from the Middle East and Africa, where they are responsible for an obstructive condition known as halzoun (Beaver, 1984; Strickland, 2000; Garcia, 2007).

PARASITIC INFECTIONS AND THE IMMUNOCOMPROMISED HOST

Immunocompromised hosts are hosts that have abnormalities in their humoral or cellular immune systems resulting from disease, therapy, or congenital abnormality. Severe malnutrition may also compromise host defenses. In most instances, the predisposing host abnormalities are primarily of the cellular (T cell) immune system and result from AIDS, malignancy, chemotherapy of malignancy, immunosuppression for transplantation, corticosteroid therapy, or a combination of these. The predisposing immune defect for giardiasis is with humoral immunity and for babesiosis it is with splenectomy.

With the worldwide epidemic of HIV infection and AIDS being particularly severe in underdeveloped countries with a high incidence of parasitic infection such as malaria, schistosomiasis, ascariasis, amebiasis, and filariasis, it is fortunate that these infections do not cause particularly severe disease in AIDS patients; however, as comorbidities their contribution to healthcare costs is enormous.

Some parasitic infections such as cryptosporidiosis, toxoplasmosis, and strongyloidiasis are more severe in immunocompromised hosts, but there are differences depending upon the type of immunosuppression. For example, although cryptosporidiosis and toxoplasmosis are particularly problematic in AIDS patients, strongyloidiasis is not a major problem in this population, but it is a problem in transplant recipients and patients receiving antineoplastic chemotherapy.

Table 62-13 lists parasitic infections that are more severe and/or frequent in immunocompromised patients. Clinical manifestations may be different from those seen in the general population, as is noted in the comment section.

TABLE 62-13
Parasitic Infections in Compromised Hosts

Infection	Predisposing host abnormalities	Comments	References
Intestinal Protozoa			
Cryptosporidiosis	AIDS (especially CD4+ <200/µL), transplantation, antineoplastic chemotherapy	Severe protracted diarrhea (up to 17 L/day). May have extraintestinal involvement, including pancreas, biliary tract, and lungs. Limited therapy available, is not curative.	Wittner, 1993 Thielman, 1998
Cystisosporiasis	AIDS, transplantation, antineoplastic chemotherapy	Severe protracted diarrhea. Extraintestinal involvement of regional lymph nodes may be seen. Effective therapy is available.	Wittner, 1993 Thielman, 1998
Cyclosporiasis	AIDS, probably other immunosuppression	Severe protracted diarrhea clinically similar to cryptosporidiosis and isosporiasis. Responds to trimethoprim-sulfamethoxazole.	Wittner, 1993 Thielman, 1998
Microsporidiosis	AIDS, other severe immunosuppression	Various syndromes: 1. Multisystem disease 2. Enteritis with severe diarrhea (most frequent) 3. Ocular infection 4. Hepatobiliary with granulomas, hepatic necrosis, or cholangitis 5. Skeletal muscle disease Examination of urinary sediment with appropriate stain may allow diagnosis of nonenteric syndromes and some cases of enteric disease.	Wittner, 1993 Thielman, 1998
Giardiasis	Common variable immunodeficiency, X-linked agammaglobulinemia	Prolonged diarrhea with malabsorption. AIDS is not a predisposing condition.	Thielman, 1998
Blood and Tissue Protozoa			
Granulomatous amebic encephalitis	AIDS and other immunocompromised states	Usually caused by amebae of the genera *Acanthamoeba* or *Balamuthia.* Produces subacute or chronic central nervous system infection but may be acute in severely immunosuppressed hosts with dissemination	Martinez, 1997
Toxoplasmosis	AIDS with CD4+ usually <100/µL and other immunocompromised states; heart transplant, donor seropositive and recipient seronegative	Usually result of reactivation of cysts from previous infection. Often disseminated disease with multiorgan involvement or multifocal central nervous system lesions. Can cause pneumonitis resembling that caused by *Pneumocystis jiroveci.* May cause chorioretinitis. Can occur after transplantation of bone marrow but usually mild. Heart transplant with donor serologically positive and recipient serologically negative may lead to severe, often fatal toxoplasmosis.	McCabe, 1993
Leishmaniasis	AIDS, other immunosuppression	Limited influence on cutaneous leishmaniasis. Susceptibility to visceral leishmaniasis increased, but not disease severity. More likely to relapse after treatment.	Herwaldt, 1999
American trypanosomiasis (Chagas' disease)	AIDS, lymphoblastic lymphoma, cardiac transplantation, other immunosuppression	In AIDS, central nervous system often involved, myocarditis, skin lesions.	Mileno, 1998 Markell, 1999
Babesiosis	Splenectomy	Usually subclinical infection in those with intact host defenses. Splenectomized patients usually develop clinically evident disease, which can be fatal.	Mileno, 1998 Markell, 1999
Helminth			
Strongyloidiasis	Immunosuppression for transplantation or by cancer chemotherapy or adrenal corticosteroids or lymphoma. AIDS is not a major predisposing factor	Because of endogenous autoinfection, hyperinfection or disseminated infection can develop and present as pneumonia or severe intestinal disease. Gram-negative sepsis or gram-negative meningitis can result from translocation of intestinal bacteria via invading larvae. Should check for strongyloidiasis before immunosuppressing patient from highly endemic areas.	Mileno, 1998 Markell, 1999
Arthropod			
Scabies	Malignancy, transplant immunosuppression, antineoplastic therapy	AIDS leads to "Norwegian" or crusted scabies with widespread involvement by thick, crusted lesions. Sometimes has severe itching. Patient has numerous mites and is therefore highly contagious. Often less responsive to therapy.	Mileno, 1998 Markell, 1999

AIDS, Acquired immunodeficiency syndrome.

SELECTED REFERENCES

Clinical and Laboratory Standards Institute. Procedures for the recovery and identification of parasites from the intestinal tract; approved guideline. CLSI Document M28-A2. Wayne, Pa.: CLSI; 2005.

This consensus document contains a detailed, up-to-date presentation on the processing of gastrointestinal specimens for parasitic infections, including use of immunoassays and test characteristics.

Franzen C, Müller A. Molecular techniques for detection, species differentiation, and phylogenetic analysis of microsporidia. Clin Microbiol Rev 1999;12:243.

The species of microsporidia known to infect humans is increasing rapidly; this review focuses on known species that have been studied using traditional and molecular phylogenetic techniques.

Garcia LS, Smith JW, Fritsche TR. Selection and use of laboratory procedures for diagnosis of parasitic infections of the gastrointestinal tract. Cumitech 30A. Washington, DC: ASM Press; 2003.

This Cumitech reviews clinical aspects of the selection of laboratory tests for diagnosis of gastrointestinal parasites and limitations inherent to particular tests.

Homer MJ, Aguilar-Delfin I, Telford III SR, et al. Babesiosis. Clin Microbiol Rev 2000;13:451.

This paper reviews the common species producing babesiosis, clinical aspects of the disease, and diagnostic modalities, including molecular-based studies that are an aid to diagnosis and epidemiology.

Lynch PJ. Delusions of parasitosis. Semin Dermatol 1993;12:39.

Delusions of parasitosis are a common and complicated psychiatric process, which is taxing for all involved in the patient's care; this paper presents an overview of the syndrome along with management strategies.

MacKenzie WR, Hoxie NJ, Proctor ME, et al. A massive outbreak in Milwaukee of *Cryptosporidium* infection transmitted through public water supply. N Engl J Med 1994;331:161.

A detailed epidemiologic study is presented of the largest outbreak of cryptosporidiosis ever recorded.

Marx A, Pewsner D, Egger M, et al. Meta-analysis: accuracy of rapid tests for malaria in travelers returning from endemic areas. Ann Intern Med 2005;142:836.

Use of "dipstick" immunochromatography methods for the rapid detection of malaria infection is becoming more popular; this paper reviews 21 published studies on the various methods, their clinical role in diagnosis, and limitations.

National Committee for Clinical Laboratory Standards. Clinical use and interpretation of serologic tests for *Toxoplasma gondii*; approved guideline M36-A. Wayne, Pa.: NCCLS; 2004.

This consensus guideline presents in an organized fashion the selection, interpretation, and limitations of currently utilized serologic methods for the diagnosis of toxoplasmosis.

Persing DH, Tenover FC, Tang Y, et al, editors. Molecular microbiology: diagnostic principles and practice. 2nd ed. Washington, DC: American Society for Microbiology; 2011.

Contains several chapters that provide a convenient overview of current status regarding the use of molecular methods in the diagnosis of parasitic infections.

Shields JM, Olson BH. *Cyclospora cayetanensis:* a review of an emerging parasitic coccidian. Int J Parasitol 2003;33:371.

The recent emergence of Cyclospora *from an obscure coccidian parasite of animals to a serious human pathogen is described.*

REFERENCES

Access the complete reference list online at http://www.expertconsult.com

CHAPTER 63

SPECIMEN COLLECTION AND HANDLING FOR DIAGNOSIS OF INFECTIOUS DISEASES

Ann C. Croft, Gail L. Woods

PART 7

KEY POINTS

- Collect specimens from site of infection before initiating therapy.
- Collect adequate volume of sample for testing required.
- For all cultures, tissue, fluid, or aspirate material is always superior to a swab specimen.
- Use required collection and transport materials to preserve specimen integrity.
- Communicate clear orders and source information.
- Expedite the transport of specimens to the laboratory and do not allow them to sit in collection areas.

Appropriate specimen collection, transport, and processing are crucial preanalytical steps in the accurate diagnosis of infectious diseases. Guidelines for specimen handling are discussed in this chapter. General principles are reviewed first, followed by discussion of the most common types of specimens submitted to the clinical microbiology laboratory for testing.

GENERAL PRINCIPLES

TIMING OF SPECIMEN COLLECTION

For optimal detection of the pathogens responsible for an infectious disease, specimens should be collected at a time when the likelihood of recovering the suspected agent is greatest. For example, the likelihood of recovering most viruses is greatest in the acute phase of the illness. Specimens for recovery of bacteria should ideally be collected before antimicrobial therapy is started.

SPECIMEN VOLUME

The volume of specimen collected must be adequate for performance of the microbiological studies requested. If insufficient volume is received, the health care worker caring for the patient should be notified; either additional sample can be obtained or the physician must prioritize the requests. If a swab is used to collect the specimen, a polyester-tipped swab on a plastic shaft is acceptable for most organisms. Calcium alginate should be avoided for collection of samples for viral culture, because it could inactivate herpes simplex virus (HSV); cotton may be toxic to *Neisseria gonorrhoeae*; and wooden shafts should be avoided, because the wood may be toxic to *Chlamydia trachomatis*. Swabs are not optimal for detection of anaerobes, mycobacteria, or fungi, and they should not be used when these organisms are suspected. An actual tissue sample or fluid aspirate is always superior to a swab specimen for the recovery of pathogenic organisms.

SPECIMEN COLLECTION

Specimens should be obtained from the site of infection with minimal contamination from adjacent tissues and organ secretions and, with the exception of stool, should be collected in a sterile container. All specimens should be labeled with the name and identification number of the person from whom the specimen was collected, the source of the specimen, and the date and time it was collected.

SPECIMEN TRANSPORT

After collection, specimens should be placed in a biohazard bag and transported to the laboratory as soon as possible. If a delay is unavoidable, urine, sputum and other respiratory specimens, stool, and specimens for detection of *C. trachomatis* or viruses should be refrigerated to prevent overgrowth of normal flora. Cerebrospinal fluid (CSF) and other body fluids, blood, and specimens collected for recovery of *N. gonorrhoeae* should be held at room temperature, because refrigeration adversely affects recovery of potential pathogens from these sources.

UNACCEPTABLE SPECIMENS

Each laboratory director must establish criteria for rejecting specimens unsuitable for culture. Most clinical microbiologists agree that the following specimens should be rejected:

- Any specimen received in formalin
- 24-hour sputum collections
- Specimens in containers from which the sample has leaked
- Specimens that have been inoculated onto agar plates that have dried out or are outdated
- Specimens contaminated with barium, chemical dyes, or oily chemicals
- Foley catheter tips
- Duplicate specimens (except blood cultures) received in a 24-hour period
- Blood catheter tips submitted for patients without concomitant positive blood culture

The following specimens should be rejected for anaerobic culture:

- Gastric washings
- Urine other than suprapubic aspirate
- Stool (except for recovery of *Clostridium difficile* for epidemiologic studies or for diagnosis of bacteria associated with food poisoning)
- Oropharyngeal specimens, except deep tissue samples obtained during a surgical procedure
- Sputum
- Swabs of ileostomy or colostomy sites
- Superficial skin specimens

UNIVERSAL PRECAUTIONS

Universal precautions must be followed when handling all specimens. Appropriate barriers are used to prevent exposure of skin and mucous membranes to the specimen. Gloves and a lab coat must be worn at all times, and masks, goggles (or working behind a plastic shield), and impermeable gowns or aprons must be worn when there is risk of splashes or droplet formation. Optimally, all specimen containers but, at a minimum, those containing respiratory secretions and those submitted specifically for detection of mycobacteria or fungi should be opened in a biological safety cabinet. Specimens collected for virus isolation should be handled in a biological safety cabinet to prevent contamination of the cell cultures.

REFERRAL TESTING

When specimens or cultures must be shipped to a reference laboratory, they must be packaged according to dangerous goods shipping guidelines (see International Air Transport Association website). Specimens must be limited to no more than 40 mL. Cultures of bacteria and fungi should be grown on solid media in tubes. The cap of the primary container (tube or vial) should be sealed with waterproof tape and inserted into a second container, surrounded by sufficient packing material to absorb the entire volume of the culture or specimen if the primary container were to leak or break. If several primary tubes are placed in a second container, they must be either individually wrapped or separated so as to prevent contact between them and there must be secondary packaging, which must be leakproof. The second container should be capped and placed in a shipping container made of corrugated fiberboard or hard plastic. An itemized list of contents must be enclosed between the secondary and outer packaging. The secondary and outer containers should be of sufficient strength to maintain their integrity at temperature and air pressures to which they will be subjected. If a specimen must be shipped on dry ice (which is considered to be a hazardous material), it must be marked "Dry ice, frozen medical specimen." The dry ice should be placed outside the second container with the packing material in such a way that the container does not become loose inside the outer container as the dry ice evaporates. All infectious shipping packages must be labeled with an official label containing the address and contents as well as the name and telephone number of the person responsible for the shipment.

BLOOD

Detection of blood-borne pathogens is one of the most important functions of the microbiology laboratory. Culture of blood is essential in identifying bacteria responsible for bacteremia, sepsis, infections of native and prosthetic valves, suppurative thrombophlebitis, mycotic aneurysms, and infections of vascular grafts. Blood cultures also are useful in diagnosing invasive or disseminated infections caused by certain fungi, especially species of *Candida*, *Cryptococcus neoformans*, species of *Fusarium*, and *Histoplasma capsulatum*. Parasites are detected in blood by microscopic examination of peripheral smears. In general, blood should be collected for culture before beginning antimicrobial therapy when any one or a combination of the following are present: fever (38° C or greater), hypothermia (36° C or lower), leukocytosis (especially with a left shift), granulocytopenia, or hypotension.

SPECIMEN COLLECTION

Timely detection and accurate identification of organisms in the blood depend on appropriate collection, transport, and processing of the specimen. Germane to the detection of all microorganisms in the blood is the phlebotomy technique. To minimize contamination of blood specimens by skin flora, the venipuncture site should be prepared with a bactericidal agent. The skin first is cleaned with alcohol (70% isopropyl or ethyl alcohol) and then with a 1–2% iodine solution, an iodophor, or chlorhexidine. For maximum antisepsis, the area should dry for 1–2 minutes before venipuncture of the selected peripheral vein.

APPROPRIATE TIMING FOR DETECTION OF BACTEREMIA AND FUNGEMIA

The optimal time to draw blood for cultures when bacteremia or fungemia is suspected is just before a chill but, because this is not predictable, most blood cultures are collected after the onset of fever and chills. Blood is drawn with a needle and syringe and, without changing needles, is injected directly into bottles of culture media or other blood culture system (Krumholz, 1990). The inoculated bottles are immediately inverted several times to ensure mixing, and then they are transported to the laboratory at room temperature as soon as possible after collection. Blood cultures should never be refrigerated.

SPECIMEN VOLUME

In adults with bacteremia, the number of colony-forming units (CFU) per milliliter of blood is frequently low. Therefore, for adults, collecting 20–30 mL of blood per culture set is strongly recommended (Ilstrup, 1983; Washington, 1986; Towns, 2002; Cockerill, 2004). In infants and children, the concentration of microorganisms in blood is higher, and collection of 1–5 mL of blood per culture is adequate.

SPECIMEN DRAWS

Recommendations concerning the number of blood specimens to collect are based on the nature of the bacteremia: transient, intermittent, or continuous. Transient bacteremia follows manipulation of a focus of infection (e.g., an abscess, a furuncle, or cellulitis), instrumentation of a contaminated mucosal surface (as occurs during dental procedures, cystoscopy, urethral catheterization, suction abortion, or sigmoidoscopy), or a surgical procedure in a contaminated site (e.g., transurethral resection of the prostate, vaginal hysterectomy, colon resection, and debridement of infected burns). Transient bacteremia also occurs early in the course of many systemic and localized infections such as meningitis, pneumonia, pyogenic arthritis, and osteomyelitis. Most intermittent bacteremias are associated with an undrained abscess, whereas continuous bacteremia is the hallmark of intravascular infection, such as bacterial endocarditis, mycotic aneurysm, or an infected intravascular catheter. Continuous bacteremia also occurs during the first few weeks of typhoid fever and brucellosis.

The optimal number of blood cultures for detection of bacteremia in patients without endocarditis is controversial. Most authorities agree that two or three 20-mL blood samples drawn over a 24-hour period and equally distributed into aerobic and anaerobic blood culture bottles is sufficient to detect most bloodstream infections. One investigator demonstrated that a total of four blood cultures drawn within 24 hours increased the yield of potential pathogens by as much as 20% (Cockerill, 2004). The optimal time interval between cultures is unknown, but 30–60 minutes for the first two sets has been suggested, with another one to two sets drawn over the remaining 24 hours if symptoms of septicemia persist (Cockerill, 2004). However, if initiation of antimicrobial therapy is deemed urgent, cultures should be collected before therapy is begun, from separate sites within a few minutes.

Organisms such as the coagulase-negative staphylococci, viridans streptococci, corynebacteria, *Bacillus* species, and *Propionibacterium* species are frequent blood culture contaminants but may also be true pathogens. Collecting two sets of blood cultures per febrile episode helps distinguish probable pathogens from contaminants. The latter are generally present in only one bottle of one set of cultures, whereas pathogens are typically recovered from more than one set.

RECOVERY OF MICROORGANISMS

Host factors such as antibodies, complement, phagocytic white blood cells, and antimicrobial agents may impede recovery of microorganisms from blood; therefore, various approaches have been used to counteract these factors. Diluting the blood specimen in broth medium in a 1:10 ratio provides optimal neutralization of the serum bactericidal activity (Washington, 1986). Incorporating 0.02–0.05% sodium polyanethol sulfonate in the blood culture medium inhibits coagulation, phagocytosis, and complement activation, and inactivates aminoglycosides. Methods that counteract the presence of antimicrobial agents include using antibiotic-adsorbent resins or the lysis–centrifugation system (see later).

BLOOD CULTURE SYSTEMS

Several blood culture systems, each with advantages and disadvantages, are available (Wilson, 1996; Reimer, 1997). Automated detection systems are rapidly replacing manual systems. Both automated and manual systems use nutritionally enriched liquid media, which are capable of supporting growth of most bacteria. Traditionally, two bottles are inoculated, and one is vented to ensure recovery of aerobes. Given the decline in anaerobic bacteremias, this practice of one aerobic and one anaerobic bottle per set has been questioned (Sharp, 1991; Murray, 1992). Routine inoculation of two aerobic media and only selective use of anaerobic blood cultures may allow detection of more bacteremias and fungemias.

Manual Blood Cultures

Two commercial manual blood culture systems are available. One is a biphasic system, consisting of a broth medium in a bottle to which a chamber containing agar media on a paddle is attached. To subculture this system, the bottle is tipped, allowing the blood–broth mixture to enter the chamber and flow over the agar media. Colonies on the agar medium are used for identification and susceptibility testing. For recovery of aerobic and facultative bacteria and yeasts, this system is comparable to or better than other systems (Murray, 1991).

The lysis–centrifugation blood culture system consists of a tube containing reagents that inhibit coagulation and the complement cascade, lyse blood cells, and provide a cushion for the microorganisms during centrifugation. Blood is added to the tube, which is inverted several times to prevent clotting and transported to the laboratory as soon as possible. Ideally, the specimen is processed immediately, but processing can be delayed for up to 8 hours without adversely affecting recovery of microorganisms. To process the culture, the tube is centrifuged for 30 minutes at 3000 *g*, the supernatant is discarded, and the sediment is mixed on a vortex mixer and plated onto agar media. Smaller tubes for low-volume samples, from infants and young children, are also available. Advantages of lysis–centrifugation include excellent recovery of *Staphylococcus aureus*, some Enterobacteriaceae, and fungi (it is the best system for recovery of *H. capsulatum*), the direct availability of colonies for identification and susceptibility testing, and the ability to carry out quantitative cultures. Moreover, this system is flexible because special media can be inoculated to recover organisms with specific growth requirements, such as species of *Legionella* and mycobacteria. However, the system is labor-intensive, is less likely to recover *Streptococcus pneumoniae*, *Haemophilus influenzae* or anaerobes, and the risk for contamination is increased.

Automated Blood Culture Systems

Several automated continuously monitoring blood culture systems are available commercially (Wilson, 1996). All such systems are much less labor-intensive than the "manual" systems described above. Additionally, with these systems the usual incubation period can be shortened from 7 to 5 days (Woods, 1994; Reisner, 1999). One such system is based on the colorimetric detection of carbon dioxide (CO_2) produced during microbial growth (Thorpe, 1990). A CO_2 sensor is bonded to the bottom of each blood culture bottle and is separated from the broth medium by a membrane that is impermeable to most ions and to components of media and blood but freely permeable to CO_2. Inoculated bottles are placed in cells in the instrument, which provides continuous rocking of both aerobic and anaerobic bottles. If bacteria are present, they generate CO_2, which is released into the broth medium; the pH then decreases, causing the sensor to change color from green to yellow. Color changes are monitored once every 10 minutes by a colorimetric detector. Media available for use with this system include routine aerobic and anaerobic media, which accommodate 5–10 mL of blood; Pedi-BacT, which accommodates 4 mL of blood or less; and fastidious antibiotic neutralization, which enhances recovery of fungi and recovery of bacteria from patients receiving antimicrobial agents.

A second continuous-monitoring system is based on fluorescent technology (Nolte, 1993). Bonded to the base of each vial is a CO_2 sensor that is impermeable to ions, medium components, and blood but freely permeable to CO_2. If organisms are present, they release CO_2 into the medium; it then diffuses into the sensor matrix and generates hydrogen ions. The subsequent decrease in pH increases the fluorescence output of the sensor, changing the signal transmitted to the optical and electronic components of the instrument. The computer generates growth curves, and data are analyzed according to growth algorithms. Inoculated bottles are placed in individual cells of the instrument, in which both aerobic and anaerobic bottles are continuously rocked. Aerobic and anaerobic low-volume (5–7 mL of blood) and high-volume (8 to 10 mL of blood) media, Peds-Plus medium (0.5 to 5 mL of blood), and the Myco F Lytic medium for recovery of fungi and mycobacteria are available (Waite, 1998).

A third system detects growth of organisms in broth by measuring gas consumption and/or gas production (Zwadyk, 1994). Each inoculated vial is fitted with a disposable connector that contains a recessed needle. The needle penetrates the bottle stopper and connects the bottle headspace to the sensor probe. The sensor monitors changes within the headspace in the consumption and/or production of all gases (CO_2, N_2, and H_2) by growing organisms and creates data points internally in the computer. Two basic types of medium are available: aerobic and anaerobic media that contain 80 mL of broth and accommodate 0.1–10 mL of blood, and EZ

Draw (direct draw) aerobic and anaerobic bottles that contain 40 mL of broth and accommodate 0.1–5 mL of blood.

DETECTION OF RARELY ENCOUNTERED BACTERIA

Detection of some bacteria requires prolonged incubation or special media. For example, when brucellosis is suspected, blood should be collected early in the disease and cultures should be incubated for 2–3 weeks, although with the automated systems brucellas often grow in less than 1 week (Bannatyne, 1997). Infections with species of *Borrelia*, except *Borrelia burgdorferi* (the etiologic agent of Lyme disease, most commonly diagnosed serologically), are diagnosed by detecting spirochetes in the peripheral blood during febrile periods. Organisms are visualized in wet preparations made by mixing a drop of blood with a drop of sodium citrate, and examining it with light- or dark-field microscopy, and in thin and thick blood films stained with Wright's or Giemsa stains, examined by light microscopy. To isolate *Leptospira interrogans* from blood, a few drops of fresh or anticoagulated blood collected during the first week of illness are added to each of three to four tubes of leptospiral semisolid culture medium (Fletcher's medium or Ellinghausen–McCollough–Johnson–Harris medium).

Two methods may be used to recover mycobacteria from blood specimens. With the lysis–centrifugation technique, (1) a concentrate is prepared, (2) the sediment is inoculated to solid and/or liquid media, and (3) the cultures are incubated for up to 8 weeks. An alternative and perhaps more rapid approach is direct inoculation of the liquid medium developed by the manufacturer of automated and semiautomated broth culture systems specifically for recovery of mycobacteria.

DETECTION AND NOTIFICATION OF POSITIVE CULTURES

Positive blood cultures containing commonly isolated aerobic organisms are usually detected within 12–36 hours of incubation. The initial report is a Gram stain report only. Identification and susceptibility results can be expected within 24–48 hours after the Gram stain report. Cultures containing anaerobes are usually not detected for 48–72 hours, and identification is not available for 3–4days after that. Fastidious organisms, such as those found in the HACEK group (*Haemophilus*, *Actinobacillus*, *Cardiobacterium*, *Eikenella*, *Kingella*) may not be detected until 3–5 days.

Detection of Viruses

With regard to viruses, blood specimens are most commonly collected to monitor response of infection with human immunodeficiency virus (HIV), hepatitis C virus (HCV), hepatitis B virus (HBV), or cytomegalovirus (CMV) to antiviral therapy by using quantitative polymerase chain reaction (PCR) to measure viral load. Such assays are commercially available for each of these viruses, and in all cases manufacturer's guidelines for specimen collection and transport should be followed. For HIV and HCV, blood specimens also may be collected for genotyping (commercial assays are available), and PCR (qualitative or quantitative PCR) generally is used to confirm an initial positive HCV antibody result. As with viral load, manufacturer's guidelines regarding specimen collection and transport should be followed.

In addition to assessing response to antiviral therapy, measuring viral load in a blood specimen is useful for monitoring for development of disease and for diagnosis of disease in specific situations. In immunocompromised patients, especially transplant recipients but also patients with acquired immunodeficiency syndrom (AIDS), determining the level of CMV deoxyribonucleic acid (DNA) in blood is used to predict those at high risk for development of CMV disease and direct the initiation of preemptive therapy (Herrmann, 2004; Kalpoe, 2004; Meyer-Koenig, 2004; Lugert, 2009). Monitoring the level of Epstein-Barr virus (EBV) DNA in serum or plasma by quantitative PCR is indicated in transplant recipients at high risk for EBV-associated lymphoproliferative disease (Rowe, 2001). Quantitative PCR from whole blood or peripheral blood mononuclear cells is useful for diagnosis of disease due to HHV-6 or HHV-7 in transplant recipients and is the test of choice for diagnosing disease caused by parvovirus B19 in immunosuppressed patients or in the fetus. If a commercial quantitative PCR assay is used, guidelines for specimen collection and transport should be followed. If, on the other hand, an assay developed and validated in-house is used, guidelines published by that laboratory should be followed.

TABLE 63-1
Infectious Meningitis Syndromes

Syndrome	Onset/Duration	Probable Pathogens
Acute	<24 hours	Pyogenic bacteria
Subacute	1–7 days	Enteroviruses, pyogenic bacteria
Chronic	Persisting at least 4 weeks	*Mycobacterium tuberculosis*
		Treponema pallidum
		Brucella sp.
		Leptospira interrogans
		Borrelia burgdorferi
		Cryptococcus neoformans
		Coccidioides immitis
		Histoplasma capsulatum

Detection of Parasites

Blood specimens are useful for diagnosis of malaria, babesiosis, trypanosomiasis, and some filariasis (Rosenblatt, 2009). Specimens should be collected in tubes with anticoagulant and transported promptly to the laboratory. If smears must be sent to a reference laboratory, they should be fixed in absolute alcohol soon after they are made. The techniques used in the laboratory for detecting the aforementioned parasites are the same and are discussed here in order of the simplest to the most complicated.

The simplest technique for detecting parasites in a sample of blood is the direct mount, prepared by placing one drop of blood on a glass slide, covering it with a cover glass, and examining it immediately. Direct mounts are excellent for diagnosis of trypanosomiasis or filariasis because the trypomastigotes and the microfilariae easily can be seen moving, often with low or medium power. The definitive diagnosis is made by staining smears.

The thin smear, made as for hematologic work and stained in a similar manner, is the standard preparation for determining the species of *Plasmodium*, *Babesia*, *Trypanosoma*, and microfilaria found. Thin smears for parasitologic work are fixed and then preferably stained manually with Giemsa stain, but automated hematologic staining is adequate. Smears are first scanned at low power to detect microfilariae, which are large objects (between 100 and 200 μm) and easily seen, usually at the lateral edges of the smear. After they are located, microfilariae should be studied under oil immersion for identification. Following scanning with low power, the smear is examined with a high dry objective, searching for trypanosomes; and finally under oil immersion, to find and identify *Plasmodium*, *Babesia*, and *Trypanosoma*.

Thick smears are useful for detecting all the parasites mentioned earlier, and are part of the minimum laboratory work-up for their diagnosis. A drop of blood is placed on a clean glass slide and, with the corner of another slide, is gently spread to cover 1 cm square. The preparation is allowed to dry and without fixation is stained with Giemsa stain, allowing for its dehemoglobinization.

Body Fluids

CEREBROSPINAL FLUID

CSF is collected to diagnose meningitis and, less frequently, viral encephalitis. Infectious meningitis, a medical emergency requiring early therapy to prevent death or serious neurologic sequelae, is divided into acute, subacute, and chronic clinical syndromes, based on duration of symptoms. Potential pathogens are listed in Table 63-1. Enteroviruses are the agents most commonly responsible for meningitis, and they should be considered first in the differential diagnosis of meningitis in a child or adolescent during the late summer and early fall. The pyogenic bacteria responsible for meningitis vary with the age of the affected individual (Table 63-2).

Sample Collection and Transport

CSF is usually obtained by lumbar spinal puncture but sometimes it is aspirated from the ventricles or collected from a shunt. As when collecting blood for culture, careful skin antisepsis is essential for collection of CSF, which typically is submitted to the laboratory in three or occasionally four tubes. Suggestions for tests performed on fluid in each tube are as follows: tube 1, protein and glucose; tube 2, preparation of

TABLE 63-2
Common Bacterial Causes of Acute Meningitis by Age

Age	Organisms
Neonates–3 months	Group B streptococcus
	Escherichia coli
	*Listeria monocytogenes**
	Streptococcus pneumoniae
4 months–6 years†	*Streptococcus pneumoniae*
6–45 years	*Neisseria meningitidis*
>45 years	*Streptococcus pneumoniae*
	Listeria monocytogenes
	Group B streptococcus

*May cause meningitis in immunocompromised individuals in all age groups.
†Incidence of meningitis due to *Haemophilus influenzae* type b in the United States has declined dramatically as a result of vaccination.

TABLE 63-3
Normal Cerebrospinal Fluid Parameters and Changes in Infectious Meningitis

Condition	WBCs (cells/μL)*	Protein (mg/dL)	Glucose (mg/dL)
Normal	5 (lymphocytes)	14–45	45–100 (2/3 serum)
Meningitis			
Acute/subacute bacterial	500–200000 (PMNs)	↑	↓
Chronic bacterial	200–2000	↑	↓
Tuberculous, fungal	(lymphocytes)	↑	↓
Enteroviral	200–2000 (PMNs early; lymphocytes later)	↑	Normal

↑, Increased; ↓, decreased; *PMNs,* polymorphonuclear leukocytes; *WBC,* white blood cells.
*Cell type listed usually predominates.

smears to stain with the Gram stain or other stains and for culture; tube 3, cell counts; and, if indicated, tube 4, special tests such as the cryptococcal antigen, serologic test for syphilis, molecular tests or other serologic studies, and cytology. The parameters of normal CSF and the usual changes that occur during meningitis caused by different organisms are listed in Table 63-3.

CSF should be transported promptly to the laboratory and processed as rapidly as possible. If a brief delay in processing is unavoidable, the specimen should be held at room temperature unless viral culture is requested, in which case a portion (preferably 1 mL but no less than 0.5 mL) may be refrigerated for a short time. Specimen processing differs for bacteria, fungi, viruses, and parasites and is discussed separately for each group of organisms.

Sample Processing for Bacterial and Fungal Culture

Processing CSF for routine bacterial culture includes concentration (if 1 mL or more of specimen is received), preparation of a smear by cytocentrifugation for staining with Gram stain, and culture. Concentrate the fluid by centrifugation at a minimum of 1500 *g* for 15 minutes. The supernatant is decanted into a sterile tube, leaving about 0.5 mL of sediment and fluid, which is thoroughly mixed on a vortex mixer or by forcefully aspirating up and down into a sterile pipette.

Diagnosis of chronic bacterial meningitis requires specific requests because the CSF is handled differently for each entity. To diagnose brucellosis, the CSF is processed as described earlier for routine bacterial culture, but the media are incubated for 2–3 weeks. For leptospirosis, *Leptospira interrogans* may be cultured from the CSF during the first few weeks of illness. Special media (listed earlier under blood) are inoculated with a few drops of CSF and incubated as outlined in Chapter 57. The diagnosis of neurosyphilis is based on the following findings in the CSF: pleocytosis, elevated protein concentration, and a positive Venereal Disease Research Laboratory (VDRL) test (CSF VDRL), which currently is the only useful method for detecting antibodies to *Treponema pallidum* in the CSF (see Chapter 59). The CSF VDRL test is indicated only if the person has a positive serum test for syphilis (Albright, 1991a). The specimen should be refrigerated until it is tested. Involvement of the central nervous system by *B. burgdorferi* (Lyme disease) also is diagnosed serologically, by detection of specific IgM and IgG antibodies in CSF and serum.

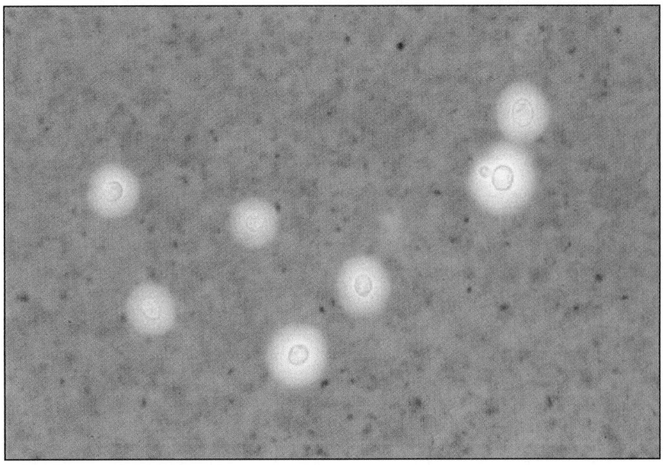

Figure 63-1 India ink preparation of cerebrospinal fluid shows encapsulated yeast forms of *Cryptococcus neoformans.* (×400)

Processing CSF for detection of mycobacteria is indicated only for samples with pleocytosis, or decreased glucose, or elevated protein values (Albright, 1991b). For optimal recovery, culture of at least 5 mL is recommended. The fluid is centrifuged at 3000–3600 *g* for 30 minutes, the supernatant is decanted, and the sediment is thoroughly mixed on a vortex mixer and used to prepare smears for staining and to inoculate appropriate media (see Chapter 60). Nucleic acid amplification, using a modification of a commercial assay or an assay developed in-house and validated, may be useful for direct detection of *Mycobacterium tuberculosis* complex in CSF (Cloud, 2004).

Processing CSF for detection of fungi is similar to that described for detecting bacteria. Organisms are concentrated by filtration or by centrifugation. A cytocentrifuge preparation or a smear of the sediment stained with the Gram stain is examined, and appropriate media (e.g., brain–heart infusion or SABHI agar without antibiotics) are inoculated for culture.

Additional Diagnostic Tests

In addition to smears stained with the Gram stain and bacterial culture, the supernatant of a centrifuged specimen or the original fluid may be used to perform latex agglutination tests for detection of antigens of *Streptococcus agalactiae, S. pneumoniae,* some serotypes of *Neisseria meningitidis, Escherichia coli* (the K1 capsular antigen cross-reacts with that of *N. meningitidis* type B), and *H. influenzae* type b. These latex tests are most useful in diagnosing partially treated meningitis (Bhisitkul, 1994; Maxson, 1994) and in confirming a positive Gram-stained smear. The routine use of latex tests should be discouraged because, compared with smears stained with Gram stain, their sensitivity is not significantly greater and they are much more expensive (Kiska, 1995; Perkins, 1995). Although the value of latex tests for diagnosis of bacterial meningitis is questionable, an immunochromatographic test that detects the C polysaccharide cell wall antigen common to all serotypes of *S. pneumoniae,* has been shown to be very useful for rapid diagnosis of pneumococcal meningitis when testing CSF (Werno, 2008).

Two types of rapid tests are available for diagnosis of meningitis caused by *C. neoformans*: those specific for the capsular antigen (latex agglutination and enzyme-linked immunosorbent assay [ELISA]) and the nonspecific India ink preparation, which allow visualization of encapsulated yeast cells (Fig. 63-1). The sensitivity of the India ink stain, performed by mixing one drop of CSF sediment with one drop of India ink (available at art supply stores), is low, except in HIV-infected persons. Therefore, the cryptococcal latex agglutination test or the ELISA, both of which are highly specific and have sensitivities of more than 90%, is recommended for diagnosis. Supernatant of a centrifuged specimen, or unspun CSF can be used for these latter two tests. False-positive latex agglutination results occur, due to the presence of *Trichosporon asahii* or to the introduction of trace amounts of condensation from agar into the test fluid. To avoid the latter

PART 7

problem, the latex test should be performed before culture or, better, on a separate sample (Heelan, 1991).

Sample Processing for Diagnosis of Viral and Parasite Infections

Currently, nucleic acid amplification tests are used most often for diagnosis of viral infections of the central nervous system. Other diagnostic methods are conventional cell culture (primarily for detection of enteroviruses, although PCR is preferred) and serologic tests for viruses that cause encephalitis (western equine, eastern equine, Venezuelan equine, St Louis, Japanese, and La Crosse and West Nile).

CSF is occasionally sent to the laboratory for diagnosis of African trypanosomiasis (*Trypanosoma gambiense* and *Trypanosoma rhodesiense*) or infection with free-living amoebae (*Naegleria fowleri* and species of *Acanthamoeba*). Once the specimen is received in the laboratory, it should be processed immediately. Wet preparations are prepared directly from the specimen and from the sediment, by first shaking the tube gently (a step necessary because the parasites often stick to the wall of the tube) and then centrifuging the specimen at 250 *g* for 10 minutes. Preparations are examined under the microscope with the condenser in a low position to allow visualization of trophozoites or, preferably, by phase contrast microscopy.

Cultures of free-living amoebae from CSF are done on nonnutrient agar plates covered with a suspension of *E. coli* or *Enterobacter aerogenes*. The fluid is centrifuged at 250 *g* for 10 minutes, the supernatant is removed with a sterile pipette, and the sediment is mixed with 0.5 mL of saline solution and poured at the center of the plate. The culture is incubated at 37° C and examined for amoebas daily for 10 days using a microscope, under a 10× objective (Martinez, 1991).

OTHER BODY FLUIDS

Fluid is collected from the pericardial, thoracic, or peritoneal cavity, or from joint spaces, by aspirating with a needle and syringe. A volume of 1–5 mL is adequate for isolating most bacteria, but 10–15 mL is optimal for recovery of mycobacteria and fungi, which are generally present in low numbers. Moreover, to diagnose peritonitis associated with chronic ambulatory peritoneal dialysis, collection of at least 50 mL of fluid may improve recovery of the responsible pathogen (Dawson, 1985). To transport the fluid, it is aspirated into a sterile container and delivered promptly to the laboratory. Alternatively, peritoneal fluid may be directly inoculated into blood culture bottles at the patient's bedside; however submission of fluid in blood culture bottles eliminates the possibility of direct Gram staining and delays the identification and susceptibility testing of any pathogens isolated.

Enteroviruses, primarily Coxsackie viruses A and B, are among the most common causes of infectious pericarditis. These viruses may be detected in pericardial fluid by conventional cell culture but, because they are not recovered in all cases, collection of throat washings and stool (which are more likely to yield the virus), in addition to pericardial fluid, is strongly recommended for virus isolation from persons with suspected enteroviral pericarditis. Other viruses (HSV, varicella zoster virus [VZV], CMV, EBV, HBV, mumps virus, and influenza virus) are infrequent agents of pericarditis and usually are not detected in pericardial fluid.

Sample Processing for Bacterial Culture

Processing fluid from body cavities for detection of bacteria involves preparing a smear for Gram stain and inoculating appropriate media for culture. As mentioned previously, the sample may be inoculated into blood culture bottles at the bedside, although this is not optimal, or it may be processed in the laboratory. In the laboratory, the fluid is centrifuged at 1500–2500 *g* for 20–30 minutes. The supernatant is removed, leaving about 0.5 mL fluid in addition to the sediment, which is mixed thoroughly and then used to prepare smears and inoculate media. Alternatively, a small volume of noncloudy, nonviscous fluid (about 0.1 mL) may be removed before centrifugation and used to prepare a cytocentrifuged smear.

Fluid specimens submitted for detection of mycobacteria are processed as described earlier for CSF. Fluids for fungal culture should be concentrated by centrifugation as described for bacteria. The supernatant is removed, leaving 1.5–2.0 mL, in which the sediment is thoroughly mixed. A smear of the sediment is prepared for staining with Gram or Calcofluor white. Ideally, 0.5–1.0 mL of sediment is inoculated to primary fungal planting media (as for CSF), but lesser volumes are acceptable.

Parasitological Examination

Body fluids are rarely collected for detection of parasites; however, *Entamoeba histolytica* may be found in the pericardial, pleural, or peritoneal cavity as a result of rupture of an abscess of the liver (into the peritoneal, pleural, or pericardial cavity) or of the lungs (into the pleural or pericardial cavity) or to perforation of amebic ulcers (into the peritoneal cavity). Hydatid cysts are infrequently diagnosed by examination of body cavity fluid, also due to rupture of a cyst into a viscus contiguous to the cavity in question. The fluid collected is usually clear and contains hydatid sand (see Chapter 62) but rarely is turbid because of superimposed bacterial infection. Uncommonly, in individuals with a filarial infection, examination of wet preparations of a body cavity fluid may demonstrate the microfilariae; in patients with *Strongyloides* hyperinfection, larvae may be detected in body cavity fluids.

TISSUES

Tissue specimens obtained surgically are procured at great expense and at considerable risk to the patient; therefore it behooves the surgeon to obtain an amount of material that is adequate for both histopathologic and microbiological examination. Swabs are rarely adequate for this purpose. The histopathology of the lesion serves not only to differentiate between infection and malignancy but also to distinguish between a suppurative and a granulomatous process. In some cases, special stains are helpful in establishing the etiology of the process. In chronic lesions the differential diagnosis includes disease due to actinomycetes, brucellas, mycobacteria, and fungi, any one of which may be present only in small numbers, again emphasizing the need for obtaining adequate samples for examination and culture.

SPECIMEN COLLECTION AND PROCESSING

Tissue obtained surgically for culture should be placed into a sterile, wide-mouthed, screw-capped container. As a general rule, tissue should be bisected aseptically by the surgeon in the operating room and material representative of the pathologic process should be submitted for both histopathologic and microbiological examination. Good communication between anatomic pathologist and microbiologist is important, especially in cases of fever of unknown origin for which an exploratory laparotomy is being performed and multiple biopsy specimens are taken.

Tissue received in the laboratory is finely minced with sterile scissors or scalpels, added to a small volume of broth, and then rendered homogeneous either in a tissue grinder, mortar and pestle, or stomacher to provide a 20% suspension. This suspension is used to inoculate all of the necessary culture media and is then stored under refrigeration for at least 2 weeks before being discarded.

EYE

CONJUNCTIVAL SPECIMENS

Conjunctival scrapings or swab specimens are collected to determine the etiologic agent of conjunctivitis. Bacteria are the most common etiologic agents of infectious conjunctivitis, and those most frequently implicated are *S. pneumoniae* and *Staphylococcus aureus* in adults; and *H. influenzae*, *S. pneumoniae*, and *S. aureus* in children. Trachoma, caused by *C. trachomatis*, is a leading cause of blindness worldwide. *C. trachomatis* also may cause inclusion conjunctivitis in newborns and, less commonly, in adults. Viruses are responsible for about 15–20% of cases of acute infectious conjunctivitis, and in the United States, most epidemics of viral conjunctivitis are caused by adenoviruses or herpes simplex virus. Rarely, parasites are causes of conjunctivitis.

Specimen Collection and Processing

Conjunctival cells are obtained from the superior and inferior tarsal conjunctiva by using a swab moistened with broth or a sterile platinum spatula. Ideally, smears are prepared and, if a bacterial or fungal infection is suspected, culture media are inoculated directly by the individual collecting the sample. If direct preparation of smears and inoculation of media is not possible, swab specimens may be collected. Smears should be air-dried and promptly transported, with the inoculated media, to the laboratory. If viral culture is requested, a second sample (swab or scrapings) is collected, placed in viral transport medium, and delivered promptly to the laboratory, or refrigerated for a short time and then transported on wet ice. A rapid diagnosis may be provided by direct or indirect immunofluorescent staining of smears of conjunctival cells with virus-specific antibodies, but cell culture is the most sensitive method for detecting potential viral pathogens and always should be done.

To detect *C. trachomatis*, a smear prepared directly from conjunctival scrapings may be stained with the Giemsa stain and examined for epithelial cells with basophilic intracytoplasmic inclusions diagnostic of *C. trachomatis*, or preferably with monoclonal antibodies, which are more sensitive and specific than Giemsa. For optimal results with the direct fluorescent antibody test, the collection kit provided by the manufacturer should be used (see Chapter 56). The swab is rolled across the surface of the glass slide provided, the material is fixed, and the slide is transported promptly to the laboratory and held at room temperature or refrigerated for a short time. Slides are stained according to the manufacturer's directions and examined with a fluorescent microscope for elementary bodies (see Chapter 56). Specimens containing less than 10 columnar or metaplastic squamous cells are considered inadequate and results should be reported as inconclusive, with an explanation, and another specimen should be requested. Culture is the reference method for detection of *C. trachomatis* and should be performed when a diagnosis of chlamydial conjunctivitis is strongly suspected and the direct fluorescent antibody test is negative.

CORNEAL SPECIMENS

Corneal scrapings and biopsy specimens are useful in determining the etiologic agent of keratitis, an infection that can potentially produce loss of vision and requires immediate attention. Bacteria account for 65–90% of cases of keratitis, and in the United States, *S. aureus*, *S. pneumoniae*, *Pseudomonas aeruginosa*, and species of *Moraxella* are most frequently implicated.

Specimen Collection and Transport

Corneal scrapings are collected with a sterile platinum spatula and are used for preparation of smears by directly transferring them to glass slides for staining, and for inoculation to appropriate media for culture. If viral culture is requested, scrapings should be placed directly into viral transport media and delivered promptly to the laboratory or refrigerated for a short time and transported on wet ice. Frequently, the conjunctiva and the eyelids of the involved and the uninvolved eye are cultured concomitantly to determine the normal flora, useful in assessing the results of the corneal cultures. When the culture of scrapings of a suspicious corneal ulcer is negative, superficial keratectomy or corneal biopsy specimen may be obtained by the ophthalmologist, an approach especially useful for detection of fungi and *Acanthamoeba*.

RESPIRATORY TRACT

NASOPHARYNGEAL SPECIMENS

Nasopharyngeal aspirates, washings, and swab specimens are collected predominantly for diagnosis of viral respiratory infections but also pneumonia due to *C. trachomatis* or *Chlamydophila pneumoniae*, pertussis, and rarely diphtheria. Specimens from the nose also are used to identify carriers of methicillin-resistant *S. aureus* (MRSA).

Specimen Collection, Transport, and Processing

Nasopharyngeal aspirates and washings are superior to swabs for recovery of viruses, but swabs frequently are submitted because they are more convenient. Washings or swab specimens are collected for detection of *Bordetella pertussis*; a swab is the preferred specimen for *C. trachomatis*, *C. pneumoniae*, and *Corynebacterium diphtheriae*. An aspirate is collected with a plastic tube (e.g., one used to feed premature infants) attached to a 1-mL syringe or a suction catheter with a mucus trap. A wash is obtained with a rubber suction bulb by instilling and withdrawing 3–7 mL of sterile phosphate-buffered saline. To collect nasopharyngeal cells with a swab, all mucus from the nasal cavity is removed, then a small flexible nasopharyngeal swab is inserted along the nasal septum to the posterior pharynx and rotated against the mucosa several times.

To detect viruses, nasopharyngeal specimens are placed into an appropriate transport medium, with or without antibiotics, and transported promptly to the laboratory or stored briefly in the refrigerator and packed in ice for transport as soon as possible. Viral detection methods are discussed in more detail in Chapter 55.

For detection of *C. trachomatis*, a nasopharyngeal swab specimen is collected with a polyester-tipped swab, which may be used for culture or for preparation of a smear for direct fluorescent antibody staining. Detection methods are discussed in Chapter 56. For culture of *C. trachomatis* or *C. pneumoniae*, the swab should be placed in an appropriate transport medium and transported to the laboratory as soon as possible or refrigerated for a short time.

To detect *B. pertussis* by culture, inoculation of washings or swab specimens (preferably collected with a calcium alginate swab) at the bedside is optimal. If this is not possible, the sample is placed into sterile casamino broth, transported promptly to the laboratory, and processed within 1–2 hours for culture. If the sample must be sent to a reference laboratory for culture, the swab should be inoculated into and left in a solid transport media such as Regan–Lowe or Jones–Kendrick, incubated at 37° C for 48 hours, and then shipped at ambient temperature. The direct fluorescent antibody staining method, which provides a rapid diagnosis but is associated with false-positive and false-negative results (Friedman, 1988), can be performed on a smear prepared from a nasopharyngeal swab or washing. Currently, the recommended medium for culture is Regan–Lowe agar (composed of Oxoid charcoal agar and 10% horse blood and containing cephalexin), rather than the traditional Bordet–Gengou agar (potato infusion agar with 20% sheep blood). However, the most sensitive method for detecting *B. pertussis* is PCR, for which the optimal sample is a nasopharyngeal swab specimen collected with a Dacron swab (alginate fibers and aluminum in the shaft are inhibitory). If the sample must be transported to a reference laboratory for PCR, the swab should be shipped dry or in saline.

Carriers of MRSA may be detected within a few hours by commercial nucleic acid amplification assays or after 24 to 48 hours using MRSA-specific chromogenic agar media (Tacconelli, 2009; Bischof, 2009; Bocher, 2008). Nasal secretions are collected from the anterior nares with a polyester-tipped swab, which is placed in a tube transport system and promptly delivered to the laboratory. If a nucleic acid amplification assay is used, the specimen must be collected with the swab recommended by the manufacturer.

THROAT SPECIMENS

Throat swab specimens are most commonly collected to diagnose group A streptococcal pharyngitis; however, Lancefield groups C and G streptococci have also been implicated in pharyngitis. Throat swabs received in the clinical laboratory for routine bacterial culture should be evaluated for these streptococci only. Throat washings or swab specimens are useful for detection of viruses shed in oral secretions without causing pharyngitis (HSV, CMV, or enteroviruses). Throat swab specimens may also be helpful in determining the etiologic agent of epiglottitis, a rapidly progressing cellulitis with the potential to cause obstruction of the airway (almost always due to *H. influenzae* type b, but occasionally *S. aureus* or *S. pneumoniae*) and in diagnosing gonorrhea, *Mycoplasma pneumoniae* pneumonia, diphtheria, and Vincent's angina.

Specimen Collection and Transport

Throat swab specimens are collected by depressing the tongue with a tongue blade, introducing the swab between the tonsillar pillars and behind the uvula without touching the lateral walls of the buccal cavity, and swabbing back and forth across the posterior pharynx. Swab specimens collected for detection of viruses should be placed in a viral transport medium and those for detection of bacteria, in a tube transport system containing modified Stuart's medium. Throat washings for diagnosis of viral infections are obtained by gargling with 5 mL of viral transport medium containing antibiotics. Throat washings and swab specimens should be delivered promptly to the laboratory, or refrigerated for a short time if a delay in transport is unavoidable.

Specimen Processing

For diagnosis of group A streptococcal pharyngitis, culture is most sensitive; however, this requires overnight incubation. Use of a selective medium increases the recovery of *S. pyogenes* by inhibiting overgrowth of normal flora; but because the amount of growth of *S. pyogenes* on selective media at 24 hours often is insufficient for testing, plates may need to be reincubated an additional day before confirmatory testing can be performed. For rapid diagnosis, a commercial direct probe is the most sensitive and can be used as a replacement for culture (Gerber, 2004). Other rapid, direct tests for group A streptococcus (several are commercially available) are less sensitive (as low as 70%); therefore, if one of these is used two throat swab specimens should be collected. If the direct test is positive, the second swab may be discarded; but in children if the direct test is negative, confirmatory culture must be performed, using the second swab (Bisno, 2002). In adults, because the incidence of streptococcal infection and the risk of rheumatic fever are low, diagnosis of group A streptococcal pharyngitis on the basis of a rapid, direct test, without confirming a negative result with culture, is an acceptable alternative (Bisno, 2002).

To determine the etiologic agent of epiglottitis, a swab specimen should be collected by a physician in a setting where intubation of the patient may be performed immediately if necessary. To detect *N. gonorrhoeae* in the throat, the swab specimen should be inoculated at the bedside or transported to the laboratory within 2 hours and inoculated as soon as possible on to a selective medium, such as modified Thayer–Martin agar. If a delay in processing is unavoidable, the swab should be held at room temperature. For diagnosis of diphtheria, both nasopharyngeal and throat swab specimens are collected and transported to the laboratory immediately. If laboratory personnel are not experienced in the recovery and identification of *C. diphtheriae*, the specimens should be sent in a semisolid transport media (e.g., Amies) to a reference laboratory. A differential inhibitory medium containing potassium tellurite, such as Tinsdale medium, is optimal for cultivating *C. diphtheriae*. This medium, however, is expensive, has a short shelf-life, and is difficult to obtain from commercial vendors; therefore it is seldom used in clinical laboratories. Colistin–naladixic acid blood agar (CNA) is an acceptable alternative for the cultivation of *C. diphtheriae*, but because CNA is not a differential medium, all diphtheroid colony types must be evaluated to exclude *C. diphtheriae* when this agent is suspected. In addition, a sheep blood agar plate should be inoculated and examined for group A streptococci.

Vincent's angina is an acute necrotizing ulcerative tonsillitis that may be caused by *Fusobacterium necrophorum* and other anaerobes. An illness with this clinical presentation may presumptively be called Vincent's angina if gram-negative fusiform bacilli and spirochetes are seen in smears prepared from a swab specimen of the ulcerated lesion and stained with Gram stain. Cultures of the involved area are not usually helpful because many species of anaerobes are present in the oral cavity. However, blood cultures should be collected because the illness is commonly accompanied by sepsis.

SPUTUM AND TRACHEAL ASPIRATES

Microbiological studies of sputum (expectorated and induced) and tracheal aspirate specimens are done primarily to determine the etiologic agents of pneumonia. Guidelines for diagnosis of community-acquired pneumonia have been published jointly by the Infectious Diseases Society of America and the American Thoracic Society (Mandell, 2007). Tracheal aspirates represent lower respiratory secretions collected in a Lukens trap from patients with tracheostomies. Patients with tracheostomies rapidly become colonized with gram-negative bacteria and other potential nosocomial pathogens, and because bacteria colonizing the respiratory tract cannot be differentiated from bacteria causing invasive disease by culture of tracheal aspirates, interpretation of routine culture results is difficult. Culture for *Legionella*, mycobacteria, and fungi must be requested separately from routine culture as each of these require special media for cultivation.

Specimen Collection and Transport

Optimally, expectorated sputum is collected early in the morning before eating. The individual rinses his or her mouth with water and then expectorates a specimen, preferably 5–10 mL, resulting from a deep cough. For persons with nonproductive coughs, a specimen may be induced by allowing the individual to breathe aerosolized droplets of a solution of 15% sodium chloride and 10% glycerin for about 10 minutes or until a cough reflex is initiated. Sputum and tracheal aspirate specimens should be delivered promptly to the laboratory or refrigerated for a short time if a delay is unavoidable.

Specimen Processing

Both specimen types should be screened before they are plated for routine bacterial culture to determine whether they are representative of lower respiratory secretions or of saliva. A smear prepared from a portion of the specimen consisting of purulent material is stained with the Gram stain. In general, specimens with more than 10 epithelial cells per low-power field by screen (Fig. 63-2) are considered to have significant contamination with saliva and should be rejected. Specimens with fewer than 25 epithelial cells and more than 25 neutrophils per low-power field are probably acceptable (Murray, 1975). The number of neutrophils is not usually considered when determining specimen quality, because the individual from whom the sputum was collected may be neutropenic. Screening induced sputum specimens and expectorated sputum samples submitted for detection of *M. pneumoniae*, species of *Legionella*, and mycobacteria to assess their quality is not generally required (Ingram, 1994; Havlik, 1995). However, data from one study suggest that screening sputum specimens for the presence of neutrophils is an effective method to evaluate the acceptability of sputum for mycobacterial smear and culture (McCarter, 1996).

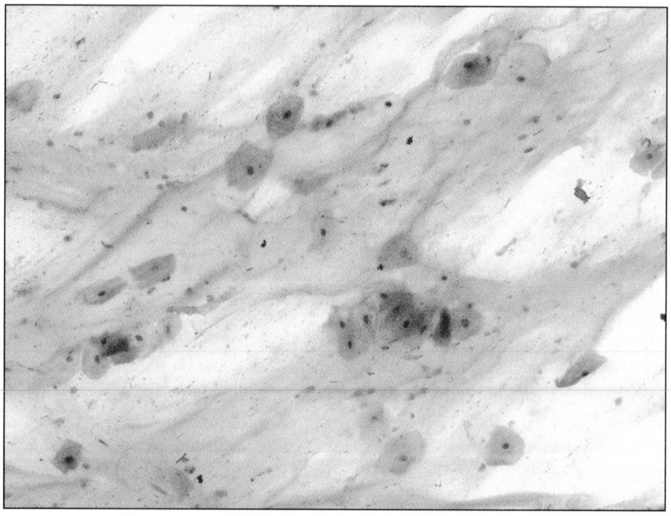

Figure 63-2 Gram stain of a sputum specimen demonstrating greater than 10 squamous epithelial cells per low-power field, which is unacceptable for culture. (×10)

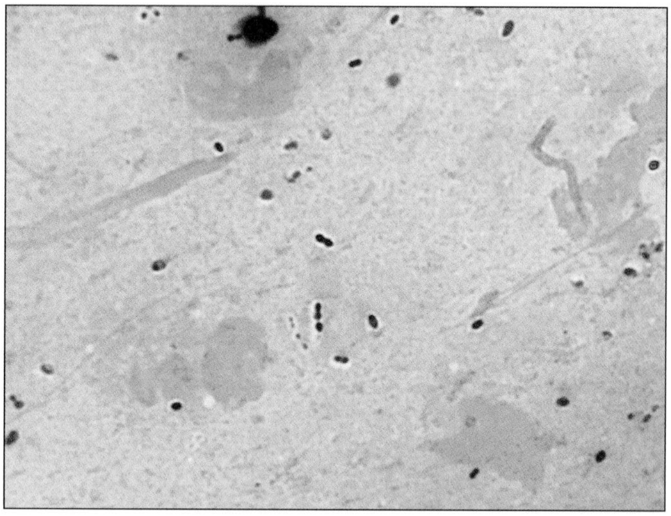

Figure 63-3 Gram stain of a sputum specimen showing encapsulated, lancet-shaped, gram-positive diplococci, consistent with *Streptococcus pneumoniae.* (×100)

The Gram-stained smears prepared from specimens that are acceptable for culture are examined under oil immersion to determine the relative amounts of organisms. The quantity of organisms (rare, few, moderate, or many) is estimated for each kind of bacterium (e.g., gram-positive cocci in pairs (Fig. 63-3), chains or clusters; gram-positive bacilli; gram-negative diplococci, and gram-negative rods), noting whether or not they are intracellular. Tracheal aspirates for which no organisms are observed in the Gram-stained smear should probably be rejected (Gilligan, 1999). Portions of acceptable specimens containing purulent material are inoculated as outlined in Chapter 57. For specimens from persons with cystic fibrosis, also inoculating a medium selective for *Burkholderia cepacia* is recommended.

When legionnaires' disease is suspected, *Legionella* culture and a rapid, direct test (fluorescent antibody on a respiratory specimen or *Legionella* antigen on a urine specimen) are recommended. Direct fluorescent antibody staining, which can provide results in several hours rather than the 3–7 days required for culture, should be used to supplement but not replace culture. PCR also can be performed but is considerably more expensive than culture, direct fluorescent antibody (DFA), or urine antigen testing. Culture is the most sensitive of these methods and should always be performed. Several drops of the specimen should be inoculated to each selective and nonselective buffered charcoal yeast extract agar plate. Use of the selective agar inhibits the growth of most other respiratory flora;

however, some strains of *Legionella* are susceptible to the medium's inhibitory agents. Thus a nonselective plate should always be included.

For optimal detection of mycobacteria in sputum, collection of three samples on three separate days is recommended. Sputum and other respiratory secretions must be decontaminated to prevent the normal respiratory flora from overgrowing the slower-growing mycobacteria. This process and detection methods are discussed in Chapter 60. All specimens submitted for mycobacterial stain, culture, and molecular testing should be processed in a biological safety cabinet, preferably in an isolated room with negative air pressure (level 3 laboratory).

All specimens submitted for fungal culture should also be handled as described for mycobacteria. The quality of the specimens should be determined by screening with smears stained with Gram stain (as described earlier for bacteria). Acceptable expectorated sputum, induced sputum, and tracheal aspirate specimens should be inoculated to culture media for recovery of fungi. In general, to culture fungi media with and without blood enrichment, and media containing antimicrobial agents should be used. However, when making media selection, the laboratory director also should consider cost and the types of fungus usually encountered in the patient population served by the laboratory.

BRONCHOSCOPY SPECIMENS

Bronchoalveolar lavage fluid and protected brush specimens are useful for diagnosis of bacterial pneumonia in ventilated patients who have not received antimicrobial therapy, and for detection of opportunistic pathogens in immunocompromised patients with pneumonia (Baselski, 1994; Carroll, 2002). Data indicate that culture of bronchoalveolar lavage specimens is also useful for diagnosis of acute bacterial pneumonia (Baselski, 1994). All bronchoscopy specimens should be plated quantitatively to determine significance of potential pathogens recovered. Only protected brush specimens are suitable for anaerobic culture (Baselski, 1994). For culture of species of *Legionella*, sputum specimens are preferable because bronchoalveolar lavage samples are diluted with saline and may contain small amounts of the anesthetic used locally, which inhibits the organism.

Specimen Collection and Transport

The protected brush sample is collected with a small brush that holds 0.001–0.01 mL of secretions, placed in a catheter, within a double cannula. The outer cannula has a displaceable polyethylene glycol plug at the tip. To obtain a specimen, the cannula is inserted to the desired area via bronchoscopy, the inner cannula is pushed out, dislodging the protective plug (water-soluble), and the brush is extended even farther, beyond the inner cannula. Once the sample is taken, the brush is pulled back into the inner cannula, and both brush and inner cannula are pulled into the outer cannula to prevent contamination of the brush when the catheter is removed. The brush then is placed in 1 mL of sterile saline or broth. The specimen should be transported immediately to the laboratory and processed as soon as possible. If a delay is unavoidable, the specimen should be stored in the refrigerator.

To collect bronchoalveolar fluid, the tip of the bronchoscope is carefully wedged into an airway lumen. A volume of saline (usually >140 mL) in three to four aliquots is injected through the lumen, sampling an estimated 1 million alveoli. The total volume returned varies based on the volume instilled, but is typically 10–100 mL. The transport time to the laboratory should be minimal (<30 min) and, once it is in the laboratory, the specimen should be processed as soon as possible. If a delay cannot be avoided, the fluid should be stored in the refrigerator.

Specimen Processing

To process the protected brush specimen, the fluid in which the brush is suspended is agitated on a vortex mixer and the resulting suspension is used for a cytospin preparation and for culture inoculum. Using a calibrated 0.01 mL inoculating loop, the suspension is plated onto appropriate media and carefully streaked for isolation. Colony counts of more than 1000 CFU/mL of potential pathogens (corresponding to 10^6 organisms/mL of the original specimen) appear to correlate with infection (Baselski, 1994). The bronchoalveolar sample is inoculated onto agar media by using a 0.001-mL calibrated inoculating loop (as used for urine cultures, described in the following section). The presence of more than 10,000 CFU/mL of fluid correlates with disease. Staining cytocentrifuge preparations of the fluid with Gram stain is recommended; visualizing one or more bacteria without squamous epithelial cells per oil immersion field strongly suggests acute bacterial pneumonia (Kahn, 1987; Baselski, 1994).

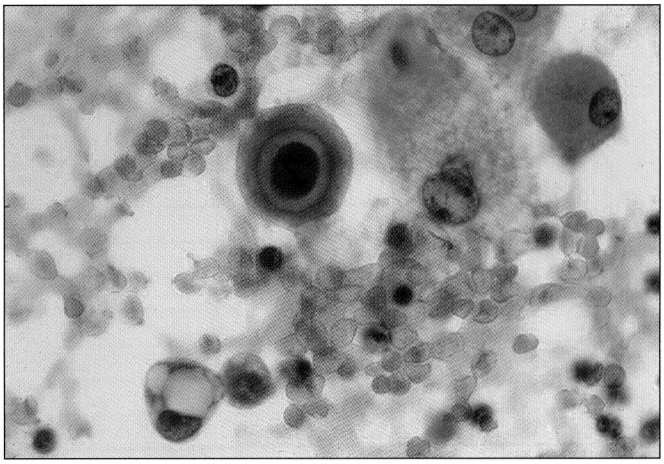

Figure 63-4 Cytologic preparation of bronchoalveolar lavage fluid shows an enlarged cell with intranuclear and intracytoplasmic inclusions, consistent with cytomegalovirus. (Papanicolaou stain, ×250) *(Courtesy Vicki J. Schnadig, MD, Department of Pathology, University of Texas Medical Branch, Galveston, Tex.)*

Processing bronchoalveolar lavage specimens for detection of viruses includes direct microscopic examination and conventional cell culture. Examination of cytocentrifuge preparations stained with the Papanicolaou stain allows detection of cytopathic changes, especially useful for diagnosis of CMV pneumonia (Fig. 63-4) (Woods, 1990). Cytospin preparations also may be stained with an acid-fast stain; with specific antibodies, such as those for detection of *Legionella* species or *P. jirovecii*; or with nonspecific stains (e.g., silver stain, Calcofluor white, or Giemsa) for detection of *P. jirovecii* or other fungi. For detection of mycobacteria, the specimen should be decontaminated and handled as described in Chapter 60. To recover fungi, the sediment of a centrifuged specimen should be inoculated on to primary fungal media.

PART 7

URINARY TRACT

The urinary tract above the urethra is sterile in healthy humans, but the urethra is normally colonized with many different bacteria, so urine specimens collected by a noninvasive method (e.g., clean-catch, midstream specimen) become contaminated during their passage. Commensal bacteria are differentiated from potential pathogens by quantitative cultures of urine, a procedure initially promoted by Kass (1956). Originally, growth of $\geq 10^5$ CFU of bacteria per milliliter of urine was considered highly indicative of infection, but this criterion has been modified for different situations. For example, in young, sexually active women with the acute urethral syndrome (dysuria, frequency, and urgency), as few as 10^2 CFU/mL is considered significant in the presence of concomitant pyuria (Stamm, 1982). True urinary infections associated with fewer than 10^5 CFU/mL may occur in infants and children, in males, and in persons who are catheterized, were recently treated with antimicrobial agents, drink large amounts of fluids (which dilutes urine), have symptoms and concomitant pyuria, have urinary obstruction, or have pyelonephritis acquired from hematogenous spread (especially infections due to yeast and *S. aureus*). Consequently, proper interpretation of urine culture results requires communication between clinicians and laboratory personnel.

SPECIMEN COLLECTION AND TRANSPORT

Acceptable methods of urine collection include midstream clean catch (preferably a first voided morning specimen), catheterization, and suprapubic aspiration. In general, 24-hour urine specimens should be rejected, except when detection of *Schistosoma haematobium* is requested specifically. Most commonly, the midstream flow of a clean-catch urine is collected. For women, the periurethral area and perineum is first cleansed with soapy sterile gauze pads in a front-to-back motion, rinsed with a moistened sterile gauze pad, and dried with a dry sterile gauze pad. For males, cleansing the genital area may not improve the detection of bacteriuria significantly and may not be necessary (Lipsky, 1984). During voiding, women should hold the labia apart and men who are not circumcised should hold back the foreskin. The first few milliliters of urine are passed into the toilet bowel or a bedpan, to flush out bacteria normally colonizing the urethra, and the midstream portion is collected in a sterile container with a wide mouth and tightly fitting lid.

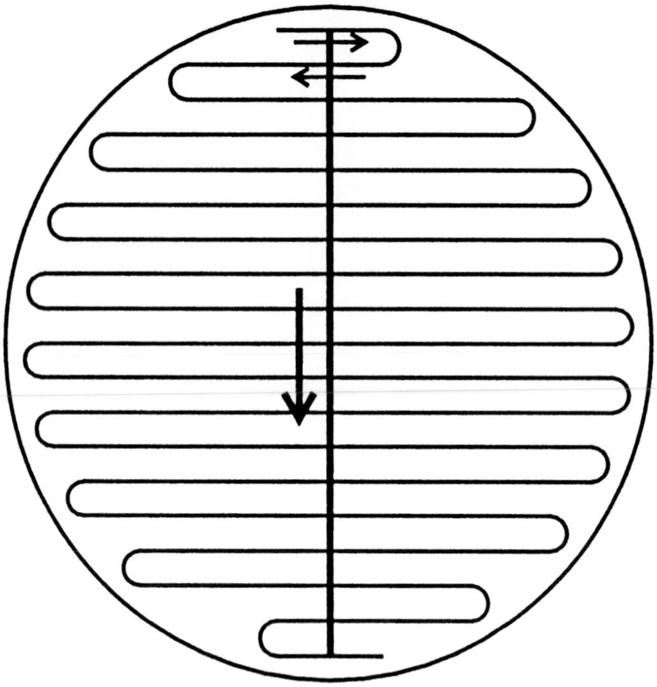

Figure 63-5 Technique for inoculating urine onto agar plates. *(Redrawn from Woods GL, Gutierrez Y, editors. Diagnostic pathology of infectious diseases. Philadelphia: Lea & Febiger; 1993, p. 602.)*

Catheterization is associated with the risk of inducing a nosocomial infection and should therefore be restricted to persons who are unable to produce a midstream sample; for example, individuals with an altered sensorium or those unable to void for neurologic or urologic reasons. Using strict aseptic technique, the catheter is inserted into the urethra, the first few milliliters of urine passed are discarded to clear organisms that may have entered the tip of the catheter during placement, and the midportion of the sample is obtained for culture. Urine may be collected from an indwelling catheter by aspirating with a 28-gauge needle and syringe through the rubber connector between the catheter and the collecting tubing, taking care to first disinfect the puncture site. Urine should not be collected from catheter bags, and Foley catheter tips should not be accepted for culture because they almost always are contaminated with urethral organisms.

Suprapubic aspiration is used primarily for neonates. The procedure requires a full bladder; the overlying skin is disinfected, the bladder is punctured above the symphysis pubis with a 22-gauge needle on a syringe, and about 10 mL of urine is aspirated.

All urine specimens should be transported promptly to the laboratory and should be processed within 2 hours after collection. If a delay in transport or processing cannot be avoided, specimens may be refrigerated up to 24 hours. Collection kits containing preservatives to maintain the bacterial population stable for 24 hours at room temperature are commercially available but offer no advantage over refrigeration.

SPECIMEN PROCESSING

Quantitative bacterial culture of a urine specimen is done by inoculating appropriate media (see Chapter 57) with a measured amount of urine, most commonly with a plastic or wire calibrated loop designed to deliver a known volume. A 0.001-mL loop is used to inoculate all urine specimens except those collected from women with suspected acute urethral syndrome and suprapubic aspirates. Both the latter are inoculated with a 0.01-mL loop. The appropriate loop is inserted vertically into the well-mixed urine sample, and the loopful of urine removed is spread over the surface of the agar plate as illustrated in Figure 63-5. Without reflaming, the loop is again inserted vertically into the urine, and the removed sample is inoculated to a second plate.

Some bacteria are not detected by routine culture of urine and, when these pathogens are suspected, specific tests must be requested. For example, urine is an acceptable specimen for detection of *N. gonorrhoeae* and *C. trachomatis* by nucleic acid amplification. The manufacturer's directions for urine collection and processing must be followed. *Leptospira interrogans* may be detected in urine after the first week of illness and for several months thereafter. To detect *L. interrogans* in urine, the specimen should be processed as soon as possible after collection, because acidity may harm the organisms. One or two drops of undiluted urine, and urine diluted 1:10 in broth, are inoculated to 5 mL of Fletcher's medium or Ellinghausen–McCullough–Johnson–Harris medium containing 5-fluorouracil. Culture of urine for mycobacteria is discussed in Chapter 60. Yeasts may be recovered from urine on the media plated for routine bacterial culture but, if fungal culture is specifically requested, the sediment of a centrifuged urine specimen should be plated on to media such as inhibitory mold or SABHI agar containing antibacterial agents.

Urine specimens collected for culture of viruses should be submitted in liquid media containing antibiotics (e.g., penicillin, gentamicin, and amphotericin B), or antibiotics should be added to the sample when it is received in the laboratory, to minimize bacterial contamination of cell cultures. Cell lines are selected for inoculation based on the viruses most commonly isolated—CMV, adenovirus, and HSV. Detection of BK virus in urine may be requested; however, PCR, rather than culture, is recommended. Because BK virus PCR is offered primarily by reference laboratories, it is best to contact that laboratory for collection and shipping requirements.

More than half of urine specimens submitted to the clinical laboratory for culture yield no growth or have bacterial counts below levels considered clinically significant. Therefore screening tests that can quickly identify urine samples yielding "negative" culture results have been evaluated as a means to provide rapid results, eliminate negative specimens, and allow more time for positive specimens, thus improving efficiency and cost. In general, urine screen and culture results correlate well when 10^5 CFU/mL or greater is the reference, but they compare less favorably in the presence of lower colony counts. Commercial automated screening methods have been developed but are either no longer available or not actively marketed. Screening urine specimens by staining with Gram stain is economical, but because examination of smears is tedious and time-consuming, this approach rarely is adopted in the clinical laboratory. The commercial dipstick test that combines nitrate reductase (an enzyme present in most of the gram-negative bacilli that cause urinary tract infections) and leukocyte esterase (an enzyme produced by neutrophils) is rapid, inexpensive, and simple to perform, and is most useful as a tool to exclude urinary tract infection if both markers are negative, especially in symptomatic patients (Deville, 2004; St. John, 2006).

GENITAL TRACT

Specimens from genital sites are submitted for detection of microorganisms responsible for several clinical syndromes, each of which are associated with certain pathogens. The syndromes each have a distinctive clinical presentation and require specific collection, transport, and testing procedures. For many tests the manufacturer's collection and transport devices must be used for optimal detection of the responsible pathogen.

VAGINAL SECRETIONS

Vaginal secretions are useful in determining the etiologic agent of vulvovaginitis and bacterial vaginosis (so named because the condition is noninvasive). In postpubescent females, the most common pathogens are *Gardnerella vaginalis* (in association with anaerobes such as *Mobiluncus* spp.), species of *Candida*, and *Trichomonas vaginalis*. A wet-mount preparation is the most valuable diagnostic test and may be performed by the attending physician; cultures are not necessary for diagnosis. A swab of the discharge is placed in a tube containing about 1 mL of normal saline and transported to the laboratory. In the laboratory, the swab is removed from the saline, the tip is firmly pressed against a glass slide to express liquid and cellular material. The slide is coverslipped and examined under low- and high-power magnifications, looking for "clue cells" (epithelial cells covered with small coccobacillary bacteria) (Fig. 63-6), consistent with the diagnosis of nonspecific vaginosis; pseudohyphae, suggestive of vaginal candidiasis; and motile trichomonads. Detection of all three pathogens also can be accomplished with a commercial vaginal pathogens PCR test (Briselden, 1994). Swabs and transport tubes supplied by the test manufacturer must be used.

Other useful diagnostic tests are vaginal pH and the "whiff test," both of which can be done by the clinician examining the patient. The vaginal pH is usually about 4.5 in women with vulvovaginal candidiasis but is above 4.5 in those with bacterial vaginosis or trichomoniasis. A positive whiff test is determined by the generation of a pungent, fishy odor after addition of

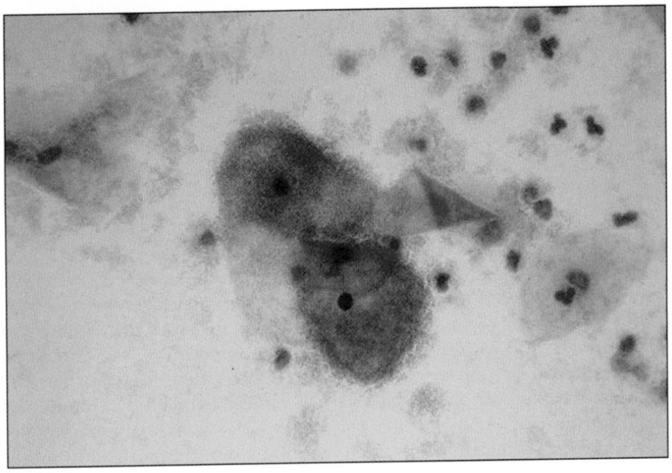

Figure 63-6 "Clue cells" in a smear of vaginal discharge. (Papanicolaou stain, ×400) *(Courtesy Vicki J. Schnadig, MD, Department of Pathology, University of Texas Medical Branch, Galveston, Tex.)*

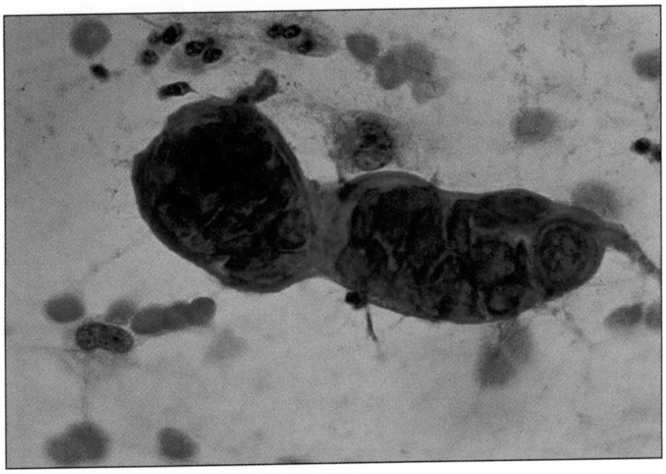

Figure 63-7 Multinucleate giant cell with intranuclear inclusions consistent with herpes simplex virus in a smear of endocervical cells. (Papanicolaou stain, ×400) *(Courtesy Vicki J. Schnadig, MD, Department of Pathology, University of Texas Medical Branch, Galveston, Tex.)*

10% potassium hydroxide to a drop of vaginal discharge placed on a slide or on the speculum. This is associated predominantly with bacterial vaginosis but occasionally occurs with trichomoniasis.

ENDOCERVICAL AND URETHRAL SPECIMENS

Endocervical specimens are collected to determine the etiologic agents of cervicitis and to identify asymptomatic persons infected with an organism that causes sexually transmitted disease. Endocervical specimens are obtained after the cervix is visualized with the aid of a speculum moistened only with warm water, because lubricants may contain antibacterial agents. If a Papanicolaou smear is indicated, that sample should be collected first.

Specimens for microbiological studies are generally collected with a swab. As discussed earlier, using a polyester-tipped swab with a plastic shaft is recommended. If a nonculture test kit is used for organism detection, the specimen must be collected with the swab supplied or specified by the manufacturer. Before collecting specimens for detection of *N. gonorrhoeae* and *C. trachomatis*, all secretions and discharge must be removed from the cervical os. The swab or brush then is inserted 1–2 cm into the endocervical canal (past the squamocolumnar junction), rotated firmly against the wall for 10–30 seconds, withdrawn without touching the surface of the vagina, and placed in the appropriate transport medium or tube system used to prepare a slide for direct fluorescent antibody staining (for *C. trachomatis*) or used to immediately inoculate an agar medium for recovery of *N. gonorrhoeae*.

Specimen handling varies based on the organism sought. To isolate *N. gonorrhoeae*, direct inoculation of a selective agar medium, such as modified Thayer–Martin, within a container to which a CO_2-generating tablet is added, is optimal. Alternatively, the swab specimen can be placed in a tube transport system and delivered to the laboratory within 2 hours. If a delay in transport cannot be avoided, the swab should be left at room temperature, never refrigerated. If a DNA probe or nucleic acid amplification is used for detection of *N. gonorrhoeae*, the collection kit provided by the manufacturer must be used and the storage and transport instructions followed.

For detection of *C. trachomatis*, culture or nonculture methods may be used (see Chapter 56). For chlamydial culture, the specimen should be transported in an appropriate transport medium containing antibiotics to inhibit overgrowth of bacteria and fungi (e.g., M4 medium). To maintain the viability of *Chlamydia* organisms, the specimen should be transported to the laboratory immediately or stored in the refrigerator if immediate transport is not feasible. In the laboratory, the specimen should be processed as soon as possible. If a delay in processing is unavoidable, specimens should be stored in the refrigerator if they can be processed within 48 hours. To detect chlamydial elementary bodies by DFA staining, the collection kit provided by the manufacturer must be used and the directions followed. The swab specimen is rolled over the microscope slide, allowed to dry, and the fixative provided is applied. For enzyme immunoassay, DNA probes, and nucleic acid amplification, the collection kit/transport system provided by the manufacturer must be used, unless the manufacturer specifically states that an alternative transport system is acceptable. Manufacturers' guidelines concerning transport conditions, storage requirements, and time to processing must also be followed.

For optimal detection of HSV, nucleic acid amplification or cell culture is recommended. For nucleic acid amplification, specimen collection and transport guidelines provided by the manufacturer or reference laboratory to which the sample is being sent should be followed. For culture, the swab specimen is placed in viral transport medium such as M4 and transported as soon as possible to the laboratory. If immediate delivery is not feasible, the specimen should be stored in the refrigerator. For patients who have visible lesions on the cervix, viral cytopathic changes may be seen in smears prepared from scrapings of the lesion base. Smears are fixed immediately and stained with Wright's or Giemsa stain (Tzanck preparation), which will not distinguish HSV and VZV, or with a monoclonal antibody.

Genital tract infection with human papilloma virus (HPV) is thought to be the most common sexually transmitted disease in the United States, and infection with a high-risk type is the major risk factor for development of cervical carcinoma. Because it is not possible to culture the virus in vitro, other diagnostic methods must be used. Squamous cell changes can be visualized on exfoliated cell samples (Papanicolaou smear), but molecular techniques (e.g., nucleic acid hybridization with signal amplification and PCR) are more sensitive. Kit manufacturers' collection and transport instructions must be followed.

To detect *C. trachomatis* and *N. gonorrhoeae* in males, a urethral swab specimen or first-voided urine sample, depending on the detection method used, should be obtained. Optimally, urethral swab specimens are collected at least 2 hours after the patient has voided. Samples for *N. gonorrhoeae* are obtained first. The conditions concerning types of swab and specimen transport are the same as those described for endocervical swab specimens, although the smaller urogenital swabs are used. The swab is inserted into the urethra for 2–4 cm, rotated in one direction for 5 seconds, withdrawn, and placed in the appropriate transport medium or used to prepare smears for direct fluorescent antibody staining to detect *C. trachomatis* or for Gram staining to diagnose gonorrhea (detection of intracellular gram-negative diplococci in a smear of urethral discharge from symptomatic men provides a presumptive diagnosis).

VESICLES

Vesicular genital lesions are sampled to confirm HSV infection. The vesicle fluid is aspirated with a small-gauge needle on a tuberculin syringe. If only a small vesicle is present, it is unroofed and the base is firmly scraped with a Dacron swab or tongue depressor to ensure collection of cells. Vesicle fluid or swab specimens should be placed in a viral transport medium and processed for conventional cell culture or tested by nucleic acid amplification (Strick, 2006). HSV may also be detected directly in clinical specimens by direct staining of smears, but this is less sensitive than nucleic acid amplification or culture, so a negative result does not exclude the diagnosis. To make a smear, cells collected with a tongue depressor or a Dacron swab are spread on a glass slide, and the material is fixed in acetone. The smear may be stained with the Papanicolaou, Wright's, or Giemsa stain for detection of typical cytopathic changes typical of HSV (VZV has an identical appearance) (Fig. 63-7), or with specific monoclonal antibodies.

ULCERS

Material from genital ulcers is collected to identify the responsible pathogen; HSV, *Haemophilus ducreyi*, *T. pallidum*, *C. trachomatis* (serogroups L1, L2, L3), and *Klebsiella* (formerly *Calymmatobacterium*) *granulomatis* should be considered in the differential diagnosis. Collection, transport, and processing of material from ulcerative lesions for detection of HSV are identical to the protocol discussed for vesicles. In general, the sensitivity of the direct tests previously described and recovery of the virus are lower in ulcerative lesions.

If infection with *H. ducreyi* is suspected, material from the base of the ulcer is collected on two cotton or Dacron swabs. One swab is used to inoculate a chocolate agar plate at the bedside. If bedside inoculation is not possible, the swab should be transported in modified Stuart's medium to the laboratory and held at room temperature until processed. The second swab is used to prepare a smear for staining with Gram stain. Observing many small pleomorphic gram-negative coccobacilli arranged in groups of chains resembling a "school of fish" suggests *H. ducreyi*. Culture, however, is more sensitive and is necessary for confirmation.

T. pallidum spirochetes may be detected in genital or other lesions but syphilis is usually diagnosed serologically. Gloves should be worn when examining lesions of suspected syphilis and when handling specimens obtained from those lesions. To collect the specimens, the surface of the lesion (if multiple lesions are present, the youngest should be selected) is cleaned with saline and blotted dry, and crusts are removed if present. The lesion is superficially abraded until slight bleeding occurs, and gentle pressure is applied to its base. The clear serum exudate from the subsurface is collected by touching the fluid with a glass slide or by using a capillary pipette and transferring the fluid to a glass slide. A coverslip is placed on the fluid and the specimen is examined immediately by dark-field microscopy. Alternatively, lesion material is aspirated with a 26-gauge needle inserted at the base, after which a drop of saline is drawn into the needle. The material then is expressed onto a glass slide, covered with a cover glass, and examined immediately by dark-field microscopy. The spirochetes of *T. pallidum* are 10–13 µm long by about 0.15 µm wide, have a regular tight coil, and are pointed at the ends.

Serogroups L1, L2, and L3 of *C. trachomatis* may be detected by cell culture in a biopsy of the ulcerated lesion or in cellular material collected by first removing any exudate from the lesion and then firmly rotating a swab (on a plastic stick) against its base. Specimen transport and processing are the same as discussed for endocervical swab specimens. For optimal detection of *K. granulomatis*, subsurface tissue from an area of active granulation is biopsied and immediately transported to the laboratory in a sterile, dry container or in one containing a small amount of sterile saline without preservatives. Smears are prepared from a crushed piece of the tissue and stained with Giemsa or Dieterle's stain. The diagnosis is based on finding characteristic, encapsulated *K. granulomatis* organisms within macrophages.

FECES

Feces and, in some cases, rectal swab specimens are useful for determining the etiologic agent of infectious diarrhea or food poisoning, confirming the diagnosis of botulism, and diagnosing infections caused by adenoviruses, enteroviruses, some sexually transmitted pathogens, intestinal protozoa and helminths, and, in some instances, helminths of the respiratory and biliary tracts. Collection, transport, and processing of these specimens are different for viruses, bacteria, and parasites and are discussed separately for each group.

VIRUSES

Specimen Collection and Transport

Stool is preferred for detection of enteroviruses and the viruses responsible for gastroenteritis. Specimens should be collected in a clean container with a tight lid. If feces cannot be obtained, a swab is inserted beyond the anal sphincter, rotated, withdrawn, and placed in viral transport medium. Deliver specimens promptly to the laboratory; if not, refrigerate for a short time and transport on wet ice. If the specimen must be mailed to a reference laboratory, store at –70° C and ship on dry ice.

Specimen Processing

Cell culture is recommended for detection of enteroviruses. To detect rotaviruses and enteric adenoviruses, an ELISA is used most commonly. Latex agglutination kits also are available but appear to be less sensitive. Specimens are processed according to the manufacturer's directions. Direct examination of stool specimens by electron microscopy is the reference method for detection of rotavirus and is useful for detection of caliciviruses, astroviruses, and noroviruses. Noroviruses also can be detected by PCR.

BACTERIAL PATHOGENS

Collection and Transport

Stool also is preferred for detection of bacteria responsible for infectious diarrhea but a rectal swab specimen is an acceptable alternative. Stool cultures for patients who have been hospitalized for more than 3 days are inappropriate. Stool specimens should be collected in a clean container with a tight lid, and the specimen should not be contaminated with urine, barium, or toilet paper. Rectal swab specimens, obtained as described earlier for viruses, are placed in a tube transport system containing modified Stuart's medium. Both specimen types should be transported promptly (within 2 hours) to the laboratory and processed as soon as possible, because the drop in pH that occurs as the stool cools may inhibit the growth of some pathogens, especially *Shigella*. If a delay in processing is unavoidable, or if the specimen must be mailed to a reference laboratory, transport of an aliquot of the specimen in transport media such as Cary Blair is recommended. For diagnosis of *C. difficile* disease, 20–50 mL of liquid stool should be submitted in a sterile container. The stool specimen is stable for 2 days, refrigerated, or frozen for 1 week.

Specimen Processing

Processing stool or rectal swab specimens for detection of bacteria is based on the organism or group of organisms expected to be present. Specimens received for "routine" bacterial culture should be processed to allow recovery of *Shigella*, *Salmonella*, and *Campylobacter jejuni/coli* by plating to appropriate differential, inhibitory and noninhibitory media (see Chapter 57). The microbiology laboratory director also might consider routinely examining stool for shiga-like toxin producing *E. coli* (STEC) and *Aeromonas* species, depending on the prevalence of disease caused by these bacteria. The prevalence of gastroenteritis caused by *Yersinia enterocolitica*, *Vibrio cholerae*, or other *Vibrio* species, or *Plesiomonas shigelloides* is low in most parts of the United States; therefore, specific requests for their detection are most cost effective.

To detect STEC, the stool specimen is inoculated onto sorbitol–MacConkey agar (containing 1% D-sorbitol instead of lactose), a medium that differentiates isolates of STEC, which do not ferment sorbitol, from almost all other *E. coli*, which are sorbitol-positive. A more sensitive method than culture for detection of STEC is detection of toxin in the stool or stool filtrate by enzyme immunoassay or PCR (Gavin, 2004; Pulz, 2003). When isolation of *Y. enterocolitica* is requested, CIN agar is inoculated and incubated at room temperature. The organism also can be recovered by inoculating media typically used for routine bacterial culture (see Chapter 57). A MacConkey plate may be incubated at room temperature for 48 hours. Colonies of *Y. enterocolitica* are purple and pinhead in size. Species of *Vibrio* frequently grow on the media used for routine stool culture but, for their optimal recovery, thiosulfate citrate bile salts sucrose agar is inoculated. *Plesiomonas shigelloides* also grows on media used for routine culture, but because up to 30% of *P. shigelloides* isolates ferment lactose, their colonies do not appear sufficiently distinct to be recognized on these media, and screening all colonies for *Plesiomonas* is not cost-effective. For this reason, culture of stool or rectal swab specimens for *P. shigelloides* should be requested specifically. Use of the selective–differential medium inositol brilliant green bile salts agar has been suggested but is not essential.

Rectal swab specimens submitted for detection of *C. trachomatis* are placed in transport medium and delivered promptly to the laboratory or are refrigerated for a short time. Rectal swab specimens collected to diagnose gonorrhea are treated as discussed earlier for endocervical specimens.

Stool specimens or gastric contents collected from persons with short-incubation food poisoning should be evaluated for *S. aureus* and *Bacillus cereus*, and specimens from patients with long-incubation food poisoning should be evaluated for *C. perfringens*. This testing is normally conducted by experts at public health laboratories, who should be contacted regarding appropriate specimen collection and transport. The clinical diagnoses of food-borne botulism and infant botulism may be confirmed by detecting botulinal toxin, *Clostridium botulinum*, or both in feces. Most clinical laboratories are not properly equipped to process specimens from persons with suspected botulism. In the United States, when a case of botulism is identified, investigators at the Centers for Disease Control and Prevention should be notified to ensure appropriate specimen collection and transport, diagnosis, treatment, and investigation of the potential outbreak.

Diseases associated with *C. difficile*, such as pseudomembranous colitis and antibiotic-associated diarrhea, are caused by the toxins produced by the organism and are diagnosed by detecting toxin A and/or B or the toxin B gene in feces. The most sensitive method for detecting toxin is culture followed by testing colonies of *C. difficile* for toxin production. The reference method for detection of the cytotoxin is cell culture assay. To extract toxin, the stool specimen is clarified by centrifugation at 2000 *g* for 20 minutes or 10,000 *g* for 10 minutes and filtered through a 0.45 μm membrane filter. Serial dilutions are prepared and inoculated to cell monolayers, which are incubated for 24–48 hours. Alternatively, toxin A or both toxins A and B may be detected in stool samples by ELISA testing, which provides results within a few hours. The sensitivity and specificity of different commercial ELISAs, however, varies (Eastwood, 2009). Tests for detection of the common antigen glutamate dehydrogenase (GDH) are also commercially available. These tests, like bacterial culture, do not distinguish isolates that produce toxin from those that do not. Even so, the common antigen, which has a turnaround time of 15–45 minutes, has been shown to be a useful screening test in certain institutions. Specimens yielding negative results require no further testing, whereas GDH-positive specimens should be tested for toxins. Most recently, commercial PCR tests for detection of the toxin B gene have been shown to be considerably more sensitive than ELISAs (Eastwood, 2009; Kvach, 2010).

For epidemiologic studies, *C. difficile* may be isolated from stool or from rectal swab specimens placed in an anaerobic transport system. Because many bacteria are present in stool, procedures that select for *C. difficile* must be used. The most effective medium for this purpose is cycloserine cefoxitin fructose egg yolk agar (CCFA), with or without horse blood. The organism grows more quickly and luxuriantly on formulations containing horse blood. The medium is incubated anaerobically for 48 hours and the plates are examined for colonies that have a peripheral fringe and a "horse stable" odor. Alternatively, *C. difficile* may be isolated by using an alcohol spore selection procedure, where 1 mL of the original specimen is mixed with 1 mL of absolute ethanol. The mixture is allowed to stand for 1 hour at room temperature, followed by subculture to CCFA and incubation anaerobically.

With regard to mycobacterial culture, stool specimens usually are submitted for isolation of *Mycobacterium avium* complex (primarily from patients with AIDS), but *M. tuberculosis* complex and other species of *Mycobacterium* also may be recovered. Processing the specimen (1–2 g of formed stool or 5 mL of liquid stool) involves decontamination and concentration, preparation of smears, and inoculation of media as discussed in Chapter 60.

PARASITES

The backbone of diagnostic parasitology in the clinical laboratory is examination of stool samples for parasitic protozoa and helminth eggs or larvae. Laboratories performing such tests should have adequate facilities for handling stool samples and a good microscope with a calibrated micrometer to measure the organisms found. Staining of fecal smears is also required for identification of intestinal protozoa.

Specimen Collection and Transport

The specimen (usually collected by the patient) can be collected in a clean, dry, wide-mouthed container. A portion of the sample is then aliquoted into two vials containing preservatives; one with modified polyvinyl alcohol (PVA) and the other with 10% formalin. Fecal specimens should not be collected from the toilet bowl and should not be contaminated with urine, water, mineral or castor oil, antidiarrheal compounds, or radiologic contrast medium. Once collected and preserved the sample should be delivered to the laboratory at the patient's convenience. The use of fresh stool is optimal for examination for *E. histolytica* trophozoites; however, it is usually very difficult to transport a fresh specimen to the laboratory and into the hands of the microbiologist within the 30–60 minutes after collection required to visualize motile trophozoites. Although it is rarely possible to perform wet mounts on fresh stools for motile trophozoites, they can still be identified on stained preparations, and the use of preserved specimens for examination minimizes the exposure of laboratory personnel to live organisms.

Several kits, some single vial and some consisting of two vials (one with formalin for helminth eggs and protozoan cysts, and the other with PVA for preparation of smears for staining), are commercially available for collection and transport of fecal samples. The question of how many fecal specimens are required for identification of all individuals with intestinal protozoa or helminths is still without a definitive answer. It has been advised that a minimum of three specimens collected every other day be examined (Garcia, 2003; CLSI, 2005). For cost containment, the clinician should request examination of only one specimen, because about 90% of all infections are diagnosed on the first sample (Montessori, 1987). If a parasite is not detected in the first sample, a second or third should be requested. If two or more specimens collected on different days are received in the laboratory at the same time, it has been suggested they be pooled and evaluated as one (Peters, 1988). This practice, however, is controversial. Stool examinations for parasites in patients who have been hospitalized for more than 3 days are inappropriate (Siegel, 1990).

Specimen Processing

The examination of stool samples for parasites includes preparation of saline solution and of iodine (Lugol's)-stained wet mounts of freshly collected samples (i.e., those that can be examined within a few hours of collection). This is followed by concentration of cysts and helminth eggs, and finally by preparation of smears for staining with the trichrome stain. The wet preparations, if performed, should be made and examined before doing the concentration and trichrome staining. Even if a parasite is seen in the wet mount, examination of a concentrated specimen is recommended because specimens submitted for ova and parasite examination not uncommonly contain multiple parasites. In particular, helminth eggs are often only visible in the concentrate.

The standard fecal smear, which has about 2 mg of feces, is made from a fresh fecal sample as follows: one drop of saline solution is placed on a clear glass slide; with an applicator stick, a small amount of feces is picked up and with circular movements is mixed thoroughly with the saline (until enough sample is dissolved), and the mixture is covered with a 22-mm square cover glass. A good wet smear prepared as described, if placed on a paper with small print, should allow the print to be read through the smear. The smear stained with iodine is prepared in the same manner. Both the saline solution and the iodine solution wet preparations can be made on the same glass slide, at the same time mixing the feces with the saline solution first and then with the iodine solution. The saline solution smear will show trophozoites and cysts of protozoa, plus all the helminth eggs and larvae. The smear stained with iodine does not show trophozoites, because they are destroyed by the iodine unless the sample was previously fixed. The main advantage of the iodine stain is that it allows better visualization of some morphologic characteristics of cysts. The saline solution shows movement of trophozoites, which is useful for their identification. To prepare wet mounts from formalin-fixed material, the contents are mixed well and one drop is placed directly on to the glass slide and on to a drop of iodine solution.

Examination of the saline solution smear is carried out with medium power (10× objective) at first. Beginning at the left upper corner of the cover slide, the slide is moved horizontally from the right to the left. The operation is repeated until the entire 22-mm square cover glass is examined. All helminth eggs or larvae and all protozoan cysts should be noted. Examination with the high-power objective is done next for detection and identification of protozoa, looking randomly for about 5–10 minutes per preparation.

The concentration technique, which can be done both on fresh and fixed specimens, is particularly useful because it allows detection of organisms present in low numbers. The concentration methods used for routine evaluation are described in detail in Chapter 62. Also discussed in that chapter are special stains required for detection of *Cryptosporidium*, microsporidia, and *Cyclospora*.

Skin and Subcutaneous Lesions

VESICLES, BULLAE, AND PUSTULES

Specimen Collection and Transport

Fluid is the optimal specimen and may be collected from a vesicle or bulla by aspirating with a needle and syringe, removing the needle, capping the syringe and transporting the syringe to the laboratory. If viral culture is desired inoculate a portion of the fluid into an appropriate transport medium. Vesicles and bullae may also be sampled by unroofing the lesion and vigorously rubbing the base with a swab, and then submitting the swab for testing. Pustules are similarly sampled with a swab after removing any crusted material. A minimum of two swab specimens should be collected, one for culture, the other for preparation of smears for staining. However, if detection of more than one group of organisms (e.g., viruses and bacteria, or bacteria and fungi) is requested, collecting at least three swab specimens is optimal. For suspected viral infection, the individual collecting the specimen should prepare a smear at the bedside by rolling the entire surface of the swab over a glass slide and allowing the material to air dry.

All swabs for bacterial or fungal testing may be placed in tube transport systems containing modified Stuart's medium; if anaerobic culture is ordered, one swab should be placed in an anaerobic transport device. Transport smears, fluid, and swab specimens promptly to the laboratory.

Specimen Processing

Processing specimens from vesicles or pustules for detection of viruses involves cell culture; and for VZV, and possibly HSV, examination of stained smears is helpful. Specimens for culture are refrigerated for a short time until they are processed. Swab specimens received in viral transport medium are vigorously agitated on a vortex mixer, and then the swab is removed and discarded. Processing specimens for detection of bacteria and/or fungi involves preparation of a smear for staining with Gram stain (for bacteria) or Calcofluor white (for fungi) and inoculation of appropriate media for culture, as discussed in Chapters 57 and 61.

CUTANEOUS ULCERS

Aspirates and swab specimens are collected from cutaneous ulcers for microbiological studies. Lesions may be primary (e.g., those caused by viruses, *Bacillus anthracis*, *C. diphtheriae*, *Francisella tularensis*, *P. aeruginosa*, mycobacteria, or fungi), or decubitus ulcers may become secondarily colonized or infected with aerobic and anaerobic bacteria.

Collection, transport, and processing of swab specimens obtained from cutaneous ulcers for detection of viruses are identical to what were described earlier for vesicles and pustules. Handling of specimens obtained from cutaneous ulcers differs for bacteria and fungi and is discussed separately for each of the organisms that cause primary lesions and for the bacteria associated with chronic ulcers.

B. anthracis causes anthrax, a rare disease in the United States, limited to persons working with raw imported wool and other animal products contaminated with spores of *B. anthracis* and persons exposed to spores through an act of bioterrorism. Cutaneous anthrax begins as a painless papule but becomes vesicular, then hemorrhagic, necrotic, and covered with an eschar. For optimal diagnosis, sending specimens to a public health laboratory where nucleic acid amplification can be performed is recommended. Instructions for specimen collection and transport provided by the public health laboratory should be followed. If specimens are processed in the clinical laboratory, they must be handled in a biological safety cabinet. The swab for culture is inoculated onto sheep blood agar, which is incubated in ambient air.

C. diphtheriae is the cause of cutaneous diphtheria, an ulcerative lesion covered with a layer of necrotic debris resembling a membrane. For optimal diagnosis, a smear for staining with methylene blue is prepared from material collected from the edge of the membrane, and two swab specimens from the membrane are collected. One swab is used for routine bacterial culture and the other for inoculation of media selective for *C. diphtheriae* (e.g. cysteine tellurite agar) if available.

Ecthyma gangrenosus is an ulcerative cutaneous lesion that almost always occurs during bacteremia with *P. aeruginosa* but rarely develops during bacteremia with other gram-negative bacilli. Ideally, two swab specimens are collected from the ulcer base; one is used to prepare a smear for staining with Gram stain and the other to inoculate media for culture.

The diagnosis of the ulceroglandular form of tularemia requires the collection of a swab specimen from material at the base of the ulcer. The swab is processed in a biological safety cabinet for routine bacterial culture, and the plates are held for a full 7 days, as *F. tularensis* is a slowly growing bacterium, producing pinpoint colonies in 3–5 days on chocolate agar, but does not grow on sheep blood agar. Suspicious isolates should be referred immediately to the nearest public health laboratory for identification.

Mycobacteria most commonly isolated from cutaneous ulcers include *Mycobacterium fortuitum*, *Mycobacterium abscessus*, *Mycobacterium chelonae*, *Mycobacterium marinum*, and *Mycobacterium haemophilum*. *Mycobacterium ulcerans* is a common cause of skin lesions in some parts of the world but is rather difficult to culture. Exudate aspirated with a needle and syringe or a tissue sample is optimal for recovery of mycobacteria. To transport the aspirate, the material is expelled into a sterile tube, which is tightly capped and delivered promptly to the laboratory. Tissue samples are placed on sterile, moist gauze in a sterile container, which is tightly capped. Swab samples are not acceptable for processing for mycobacteria, as mycobacteria become entrapped in the fibers of the swab and are difficult to dislodge. Specimens may be refrigerated for a short time until they are processed (see Chapter 60).

Many aerobic, facultative, and anaerobic bacteria colonize chronic skin ulcers. To identify the organisms responsible, cultures of deep tissues or a deep aspirate of purulent material collected with a needle and syringe provide the most useful bacteriologic information. To transport aspirated pus, remove and discard the needle, cap the syringe, and deliver it promptly to the laboratory. If transport will be delayed, inject a portion of the aspirate into an anaerobic gel transport tube. Tissue samples are transported in a sterile cup with moist sterile gauze to keep tissue from drying out. Processing the specimen involves preparing a smear for staining with Gram stain and inoculating appropriate media for aerobic and anaerobic culture.

An aspirate of the exudate from the active margin of an ulcer (transported as described earlier for bacteria) or a tissue sample is optimal for detection of fungi. A swab specimen of the exudate is suboptimal and should be discouraged. Processing the specimen for detection of fungi involves preparing a smear for direct microscopic examination (potassium hydroxide or calcofluor white preparation) and inoculation of appropriate media for culture, such as brain-heart infusion, inhibitory mold, or SABHI agar containing antibiotics and cycloheximide.

WOUND INFECTIONS AND ABSCESSES

Ideally, purulent material is aspirated with a needle and syringe and transported as described earlier for ulcerative lesions. If an aspirate cannot be obtained, swab specimens of exudate collected from the deep portion of the lesion are acceptable. For routine bacterial culture, two swab specimens are optimal: one to prepare a smear for staining with Gram stain and one for culture. To recover anaerobes, an additional swab specimen must be collected and placed in an anaerobic transport system. All specimens should be delivered promptly to the laboratory and processed as soon as possible. If a delay in processing is unavoidable, specimens may be stored in the refrigerator, except those for recovery of anaerobes, which should be maintained at room temperature.

SELECTED REFERENCES

Bisno AL, Gerber MA, Gwaltney Jr JM, et al. Practice guidelines for the diagnosis and management of group A streptococcal pharyngitis. Clin Infect Dis 2002; 35:113–25.

Reviews the advantages and limitations of the different tests for diagnosis of group A streptococcal pharyngitis. Also provides guidelines for management of group A streptococcal pharyngitis.

Carroll KC. Laboratory diagnosis of lower respiratory tract infections: controversy and conundrums. J Clin Microbiol 2002;40:3115–20.

Reviews microbiologic tests for diagnosis of lower respiratory tract infections, including acute bronchitis, community-acquired pneumonia, and nosocomial pneumonia.

Cockerill III FR, Wilson JW, Vetter EA, et al. Optimal testing parameters for blood cultures. Clin Infect Dis 2004;38:1724–30.

Provides data regarding optimal testing parameters for blood cultures when using automated blood culture systems.

Gerber MA, Shulman ST. Rapid diagnosis of pharyngitis caused by group A streptococci. Clin Microbiol Rev 2004;17:571–80.

Provides an in-depth review of the advantages and limitations of rapid tests for diagnosis of group A streptococcal pharyngitis. Also discusses possible reasons for false-positive and false-negative results and the cost effectiveness of using these tests.

Mandell LA, Wunderink RG, Anzueto A, et al. Infectious Diseases Society of America/American Thoracic Society consensus guidelines on the management of community-acquired pneumonia in adults. Clin Infect Dis 2007;44:S27–72.

Guidelines developed jointly by the Infectious Diseases Society of America and the American Thoracic Society for managing community-acquired pneumonia in adults. Also provides recommendations regarding diagnostic tests.

REFERENCES

Access the complete reference list online at http://www.expertconsult.com

PART 8

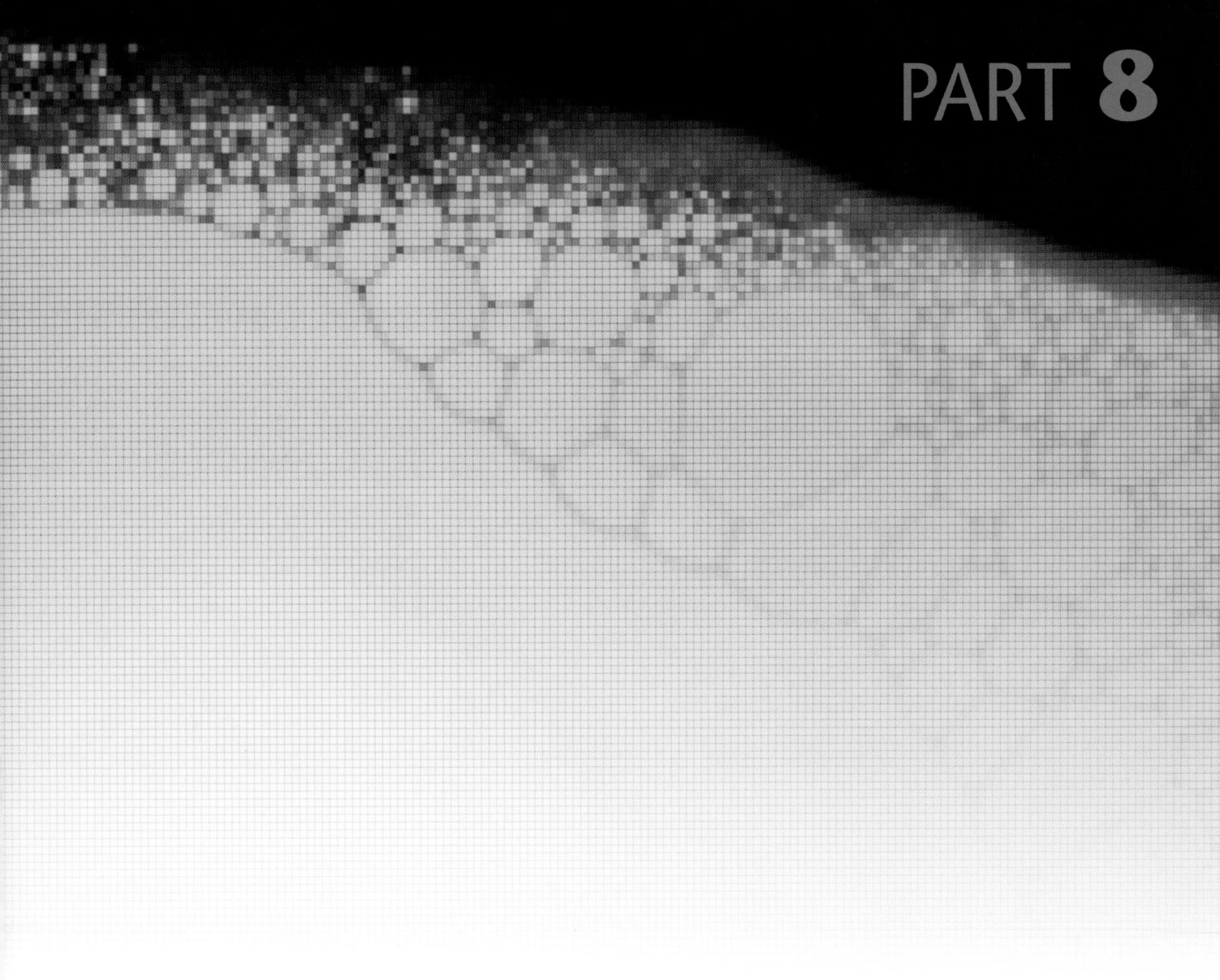

Molecular Pathology

EDITED BY

Martin H. Bluth
Elizabeth R. Unger
Matthew R. Pincus

CHAPTER 64

INTRODUCTION TO MOLECULAR PATHOLOGY

Elizabeth R. Unger, Martin H. Bluth, Matthew R. Pincus

KEY POINTS

- The revolution in molecular biology has had a profound impact on the field of clinical pathology (diagnostic medicine).
- Techniques, including polymerase chain reaction and other amplification and hybridization methods, are capable of detecting DNA in very small quantities in tissue and body fluids, enabling detection of various disease states, including cancer.
- The human genome project has created robust high-throughput and highly sensitive genetic methods (such as microarrays) not only for detecting abnormal genes in patient specimens but also for establishing patterns of gene expression that are characteristic of specific diseases.
- Proteomic methods in detecting protein expression on serum samples from patients allow for diagnosis of different types of cancers.
- Gene array and proteomic methodologies require sophisticated mathematical methods of pattern recognition that allow for detection of disease.

THE MOLECULAR BIOLOGY REVOLUTION AND ITS IMPACT ON THE PRACTICE OF PATHOLOGY

Molecular pathology refers to the analysis of nucleic acids and proteins to diagnose disease, predict the occurrence of disease, predict the prognosis of diagnosed disease and guide therapy. Recent advances in molecular biology have revolutionized the practice of medicine, especially diagnostic medicine. These revolutionary changes result from our abilities to clone disease-causing genes and the proteins that they encode and to detect the presence of these genes and proteins in the serum and other body fluids and tissues of patients, even though they may be present in minute quantities. This detection has been made possible by a veritable explosion of new, highly sensitive techniques involving amplification methods such as polymerase chain reaction (PCR), branched-DNA (BDNA), fluorescent in situ hybridization (FISH) and mass spectroscopy, the latter highly effective for the identification of proteins that are implicated in causing disease (Pincus, 2003). Many of these techniques have been developed to the stage where they are employed in so-called high-throughput processes that enable single patient samples to be analyzed for multiple genes or proteins. Some of these processes have already become completely automated.

A major consequence of the revolution in molecular biology has the mapping of the human genome in the Human Genome Project (Venter, 2001) and the genomes of a number of other species. These projects have identified numerous novel genes of unknown function whose functions can now be determined and whose expressions can be monitored in different disease states. In addition, the techniques employed in these projects have been proving exceptionally useful in studying patterns of gene expression in different disease states (see, for example, Golub, 1999).

DISCUSSION OF DIAGNOSTIC MOLECULAR PATHOLOGY

These methods are described in Parts 8 and 9 of this book. In Part 8, the principles that underlie the main diagnostic approaches used in clinical molecular biology are discussed. Chapter 65 describes the basic principles in gene hybridization, including use of Southern and Northern blots, and gene cloning, and Chapter 66 discusses amplification methodology, including PCR and BDNA, which allows gene identification and quantification of gene expression. Chapter 67 discusses how the expression of multiple genes—in fact, of whole genomes—can now be assayed on microarrays.

One of the motivations for detecting genetic abnormalities in specific diseases is the finding that, in many such disease states, there are well-defined, reproducible chromosomal abnormalities. In fact, increasing numbers of genes that have been strongly implicated in causing disease can be identified on chromosomes using FISH technology, which enables detection of gene rearrangements and gene deletions in a number of diseases, especially in cancers. Chapter 68 discusses the cytogenetics of human diseases and shows how FISH technology has enabled major advances in diagnosis of disease. All of these diagnostic approaches constitute diagnostic or clinical molecular biology or molecular diagnostics. Chapter 69 discusses how a molecular diagnostics laboratory is established. In Chapter 70, how molecular biology techniques are used to diagnose genetic diseases is demonstrated.

One of the consequences of the genetic revolution has been the ability to identify single gene mutations in patients' DNA that may either result in disease or may simply be polymorphisms. The latter is advantageous in establishing the parentage of children and in the investigation of crime. Consequently, there has been a dramatic increase in the use of the molecular diagnostics laboratory for forensic purposes. Chapter 71 describes how single nucleotide polymorphisms are used to establish parentage and the identities of the victims and perpetrators of crime.

Mapping of the human genome reveals that these polymorphisms occur in the human genome approximately 1 per 1000 base pairs. Some of these

PART 8

polymorphisms are in genes, principally those that encode cytochrome P450, some of which are discussed in Chapters 21 and 23, whose functions are important in response of individual patients to therapy (Evans, 1999; Rodriguez-Antona, 2010).

Genes that encode drug-metabolizing enzymes, both activating and inactivating, and genes that encode ligands and receptors may show polymorphisms that either decrease or increase the therapeutic effectiveness or toxicity of drugs already in wide use, accounting for some idiosyncratic responses previously not understood or predictable. Thus there has been a major advance in testing patients for genetic expression of these isoforms allowing prediction of which drugs would be the most effective ones. This has revolutionized medical practice and has given rise to so-called personalized medicine wherein patients are tested genetically for the most appropriate drug therapy and to the field of pharmacogenomics in which this testing is performed. The techniques and screening practices for the design of effective drug therapy are described in a new chapter, Chapter 72, entitled "Pharmacogenomics and Personalized Medicine."

As more polymorphisms are identified and correlated with individual patient's response to treatment, the pathologist will be called upon increasingly to profile common polymorphisms in patients who are beginning therapy for common diseases such as coronary artery disease, congestive heart failure, diabetes, thrombosis, hypertension, cancer, and infections. The laboratory's definition of the individual patient's genotype/phenotype will determine the specific drugs and doses suitable for that patient. This evolution has placed the pathologist in a more definitive position to determine appropriate therapy than traditional prediction of disease behavior based on morphology of lesions or culture characteristics of infectious organisms.

In fact, with respect to infectious organisms, the pathologist is further being called upon for genotyping of infectious agents such as human immunodeficiency virus. Different strains show markedly different drug susceptibilities. Thus determination of the genotypes of infectious agents has major therapeutic implications (Tozzi, 2010).

APPLICATION OF MOLECULAR PATHOLOGY TO DETECTION OF CANCER

Part 9 of this textbook is devoted to new developments in laboratory testing for cancer. A momentous consequence of the revolution in molecular biology has been the identification of genes, called oncogenes, and their encoded proteins, called oncoproteins, that cause specific forms of cancer. Mutations in these genes, produced by mutational events associated with, for instance, carcinogens and oncogenic viruses, often result in abnormal activation or overexpression of their encoded proteins.

Many of these oncogenic proteins are critical components of so-called signal transduction pathways, in which ligands, such as growth factors, bind to cell membrane receptors, setting in motion a chain of protein activation cascades that are ultimately transmitted to the nucleus, resulting in increased transcription and ultimately high levels of expression of promitotic proteins such as the cyclins. When one or more of the proteins on mitogenic signal transduction pathways become mutated, the cells in which they are expressed become transformed into cancer cells. Once transformed, cancer cells express a number of proteins, in addition to the mutated or overexpressed oncoproteins, that are not expressed by normal cells even in growth phase.

These findings have been translated into new clinical diagnostic methods for the detection of these abnormal proteins in the early detection of cancer in patients. Therefore, Part 9 of this book is devoted to the way in which these proteins are used in early tumor detection and to following the efficacy of the treatment of cancer. One of the major findings in this area has been that screening for cancer is most effective when multiple oncoproteins are assayed. A pathbreaking step in this area of multiple protein assays has been the development of new mass-spectroscopic techniques that enable detection of patterns of protein expression in serum that are unique to specific cancers, in a field known as proteomics that is showing great promise in screening for a number of different major human cancers.

A major impact of the human genome project has been the ability to study multiple gene expression, mainly using microarrays, in normal individuals and in specific disease states. Cancer is a major area in which the differential expression of specific genes characterizes particular tumors. Combination of gene expression with proteomics now allows for diagnosis of and screening for a number of different types of tumors, uniting molecular genetic and proteomic approaches.

Many oncoproteins and oncogenes can be used very effectively as tumor markers when detected in serum, urine, and other body fluids. Chapter 73 discusses how proteins that are expressed predominantly in specific tissues can be used in the diagnosis and, mainly, the following of the efficacy of anticancer therapy. These so-called tumor markers include prostate-specific antigen for prostate cancer, carcinoembryonic antigen for colon cancer and other gastrointestinal tumors, and α-fetoprotein for hepatocellular carcinoma. Use of these proteins for early detection is included in Chapter 74 along with discussions of how the proteins in mitogenic signal transduction pathways such as epidermal growth factor receptor, neu/HER2, ras-p21, raf, myc, and p53 proteins can be employed very effectively as tumor markers.

In the previous edition of this book, the chapter on the molecular biology of hematopoietic cancers was included in the Molecular Pathology section (VIII). In view of major advances in the molecular biology of human cancers, we now include this chapter (74) in Part 9, on the molecular pathology of cancers. There has been a veritable explosion of information on the genetics and molecular biology of a wide variety of solid tissue (epithelial cell) tumors and sarcomas, over the past several years that complement the information concerning the serodiagnostic markers for a number of these tumors. Therefore, we have included in this edition a new chapter, Chapter 76, that discusses the molecular genetics of these tumors, and we have summarized the major genetic findings for these tumors which we hope the reader will find a convenient reference. One of the most revolutionary advances that has been made in recent years has been the sequencing of the entire human genome. This momentous achievement now enables us to study expression of genes and groups of genes in different cancers so as to develop patterns of gene expression that characterize specific cancers. Patients with these patterns can then be screened for these cancers on a regular basis, allowing early tumor detection and effective therapeutic intervention (in most cases, surgical excision). Chapter 77 discusses the methodologies used in mapping the genome because these approaches are involved in screening for different diseases. As the functions of more genes become known, it will become increasingly feasible to screen the genomes of patients for gene abnormalities, especially those causing or predisposing patients to develop cancer. To an increasing degree, clinical laboratories will be called upon to perform this type of analysis.

Implications of Molecular Diagnostics on the Practice of Pathology and Medicine

REDEFINING DISEASE

The availability of the sequence of the human genome and the identification of all the human genes immediately change our understanding of health, disease susceptibility and precursors, and disease (Pandey, 2000). An ability to identify the gene expression pattern that makes a disease entity unique further allows the pathologist to delineate uniquely clinically different diseases that may be difficult or impossible to distinguish on the basis of morphology or other laboratory data alone (Heller, 1997; Golub, 1999; Talaulikar and Dahlstrom, 2009). A poignant example of this phenomenon is the diagnosis of leukemias and lymphomas. Morphologically and even immunophenotypically it may prove difficult to distinguish among different types of each disease; however, as discussed in Chapter 75, specific gene rearrangements and patterns of gene expression now enable distinction of different types. In addition, the relationships among diseases are also more sharply defined, and sometimes radically changed, by comparisons among the diseases' gene expression profiles (Anbazhagan, 1999; Bacher, 2009).

In the opposite direction, sequencing of disease genes and testing for mutations are demonstrating that diseases have broad spectrums of presentation that range from mild symptoms that are unrecognized as part of the disease, and may even include complexes not previously recognized in isolation as forms of the disease, to full manifestation of the disease. A compelling example of this marked expansion of the syndromes comprising a disease is cystic fibrosis (Friedman, 1999), discussed in Chapter 70. In addition to the severe and milder pulmonary and pancreatic dysfunctions long accepted as cystic fibrosis, isolated examples of congenital bilateral absence of the vas deferens, chronic pancreatitis, and sinopulmonary complaints have been associated with mutations of the cystic fibrosis gene. These mutations are not always associated with the severe classical form of the disease (Ferrari and Cremonesi, 1996). Recognition of symptom complexes extending the definition of diseases on the basis of gene mutations will both focus appropriate patient management in the milder or atypical forms of the disease and define pathobiology, not only of whole genes but also of affected specific exons and introns.

USE OF MOLECULAR BIOLOGY IN THE TREATMENT OF DISEASE

As discussed, genetic screening for the presence of isoforms of cytochrome P450 and other proteins involved in drug metabolism and the genotyping of infectious organisms has enabled the design of the effective treatment of patients on an individualized basis. Likewise, proteomic approaches to cancer detection have also resulted in the development of new therapies.

For example, many breast cancers express the neu/HER2 growth factor receptor, whose presence can be detected in serum by immunoassay. As described in Chapter 73, a cytotoxic antibody, Herceptin, to this receptor, which does not cross-react with the diagnostic antibodies, has been found to destroy breast cancer cells and is now used to treat neu/HER2-positive breast cancers effectively.

DATA ANALYSIS

To capitalize fully on the power of molecular pathology, wholly new approaches to data analysis and relating data to disease management are being developed. Pathologic investigation of disease and of basic biology has traditionally analyzed and related only one or a few markers such as antigens, enzymes, structural proteins, and the like. Molecular techniques are now producing data on many thousands of genes, including their expression and their sequences. Digesting all these data, organizing them into profiles of diseases or patients, and relating different profiles demand new approaches to bioinformatics toward appropriate application of biomarkers in disease diagnosis and prognosis (Klee, 2008). As discussed in Chapter 77, this involves the use of mathematical algorithms that allow pattern recognition, such as neural network theory (Khan, 2001). Thus the pathologist must work closely with mathematicians and must learn more sophisticated analytic approaches to diagnosis (Bitner, 1999).

QUALITY ASSURANCE

As with all laboratory methods, excellent quality assurance programs are required to ensure that molecular pathologic results are accurate and useful. As discussed in Chapter 69, two essential components of quality assurance programs are standardization of methods and interlaboratory comparison of test results. Standardized methods for performance of the most common clinical molecular pathologic tests are published by the Clinical and Laboratory Standards Institute (formerly National Committee for Clinical Laboratory Standards). Use of these guidelines ensures that the data generated in molecular pathology laboratories are produced by methods that are the standard of excellent practice. Interlaboratory comparison of test performance is provided by the College of American Pathologists (CAP; www.cap.org). The CAP interlaboratory comparison surveys include molecular microbiology, genetics, hematology, parentage and identity, and general forensic applications.

Applying established standards of quality assurance and using molecular pathologic techniques with a thorough understanding of their respective strengths and weaknesses as presented in the following chapters, the pathologist will continue to capitalize on the opportunities these techniques offer for improved patient care and the understanding of basic pathobiology.

CAVEATS

As will be seen throughout this section and the next, molecular diagnostic techniques provide new insights into disease that were never before possible. However, these techniques must not be used alone but in coordination with traditional laboratory tests. For example, in the diagnostic workup of leukemias, the traditional morphologic and immunochemical testing must always be performed. Gene analysis becomes critical when there is a question as to the type of leukemia or the characterization of the types of gene rearrangement that have occurred. In cases of tissue pathology, the morphologic skills involved in histopathology and cytopathology must be employed to ensure that appropriate cells and tissues are analyzed molecularly. Otherwise, analysis of other than targeted cells/tissues, despite high-quality technical methods interpreted with skill and experience, can lead to erroneous, sometimes dangerously misleading, results.

On the other hand, rapid progress in the development of highly sensitive molecular biological and proteomic techniques are allowing some standalone capabilities for molecular diagnostics. For example, use of FISH to detect bladder cancer in urine is now recognized as an excellent means of diagnosing this condition. Other, similar developments in molecular biological approaches are showing promise in screening for specific diseases.

In summary, molecular pathology is penetrating and permeating the entire clinical laboratory just as immunopathology did over two decades ago. Section boundaries or barriers will continue to break down and dissolve in this transformation of laboratory medicine through the impact of the new biology of medicine, "cell and molecular biology."

PART 8

SELECTED REFERENCES

Golub TR, Slonim DK, Tamayo P et al. Molecular classification of cancer: class discovery and class prediction by gene expression monitoring. Science 1999;286:531–7.

This is a seminal paper that shows how analysis of multiple gene expression can be used to distinguish between different types of leukemia.

Pincus MR, Friedman FK. Oncoproteins in the detection of human malignancies. In: Molecular diagnostics. New York: Reed Business Information Publishers; 2003. p. 23–38.

This paper reviews how multiple oncoproteins can be used serodiagnostically not only to screen for different types of cancer but in some cases to predict the future occurrence of cancers.

Rodriguez-Antona C, Gomez A, Karlgren M, Sim SC, Ingelman-Sundberg M. Molecular genetics and epigenetics of the cytochrome P450 gene family and its relevance for cancer risk and treatment. Hum Genet 2010;127:1–17.

This is an excellent summary of how determination of mutations in the cytochrome P450 gene can be used to identify individuals who might be predisposed to developing malignant conditions and can also be used to guide treatment for individual patients.

REFERENCES

Access the complete reference list online at http://www.expertconsult.com

CHAPTER 65

MOLECULAR DIAGNOSTICS: BASIC PRINCIPLES AND TECHNIQUES

Martin Steinau, Margaret A. Piper, Elizabeth R. Unger

KEY POINTS

- Familiarity with the basics of nucleic acid biochemistry and biology is required to understand molecular diagnostic testing.
- The chemical stability of double-stranded DNA stands in contrast to the lability of RNA.
- Base pairing of nucleic acids is dictated by energetically favorable rules and forms the basis for DNA replication, RNA transcription as well as hybridization assays.
- The chemical similarity of nucleic acid molecules, regardless of their source, means that methods of extraction, storage and handling are similar.
- Enzymes that synthesize and modify nucleic acids (e.g., polymerases, transcriptases, nucleases, ligases) may be harnessed as tools for molecular biology and molecular diagnostics.
- Nucleic acid analyses include electrophoresis, hybridization assays, amplification techniques, sequencing, and polymorphism detection. Complete assays or diagnostic tests often combine several of these techniques, such as amplification, electrophoresis and hybridization.
- Molecular diagnostics is now part of the mainstream of laboratory diagnostics.

Nucleic acids are the critical molecules of life. Deoxyribonucleic acid (DNA) resides in the nucleus of eukaryotic cells and maintains all the information necessary for maintenance of the organism and for transfer of the information to successive generations. Ribonucleic acid (RNA) carries information from DNA to the cytoplasm of a cell and directs synthesis of the proteins necessary for the function of the organism. The normal state of health depends on the stability of DNA and on accurate DNA duplication and translation into protein. Modern cell biology seeks to determine the basic mechanisms of cell structure and function, and studies are increasingly focused at the level of the gene, the protein-coding units of DNA. As a consequence, diagnostic methods are also being directed toward nucleic acid evaluation. The goal of this chapter is to provide the conceptual framework for diagnostic applications of nucleic acid analyses.

NUCLEIC ACID BIOCHEMISTRY AND BIOLOGY

Nucleic acid biochemistry is central to modern cell biology and dictates many aspects of diagnostic applications. Many of the enzymes associated with in vivo nucleic acid synthesis, degradation, and repair have become basic laboratory tools for manipulation and analysis of DNA and RNA. Cellular mechanisms that operate to direct and control DNA replication, transcription, and translation address the basic biology of the cell in health and disease. Diagnosis, therapy, and research are all increasingly directed at a molecular level of cellular function. This first section provides an overview of those aspects of nucleic acid biochemistry and biology that are required to understand the current diagnostic applications of molecular biology. Further details are available from textbooks of cell biology (e.g., Alberts, 2007).

MOLECULAR COMPOSITION AND STRUCTURE

DNA is a long, double-stranded polymeric molecule (dsDNA) that exists predominantly in the form of a right-handed double helix. Each single-stranded DNA molecule (ssDNA) is composed of a small number of building blocks. The backbone of the ssDNA polymer is the sugar deoxyribose connected by phosphate groups (Fig. 65-1, *A*). Phosphodiester bonds between the 3′ carbon of one sugar ring and the 5′ carbon of the next give the backbone its invariant structure and its 5′ to 3′ directionality. Linked to the 1′ carbon of each sugar is one of four possible bases: thymine (T) and cytosine (C) (pyrimidines); adenine (A) and guanine (G) (purines). The bases can occur in any sequence order, and thus form the variable

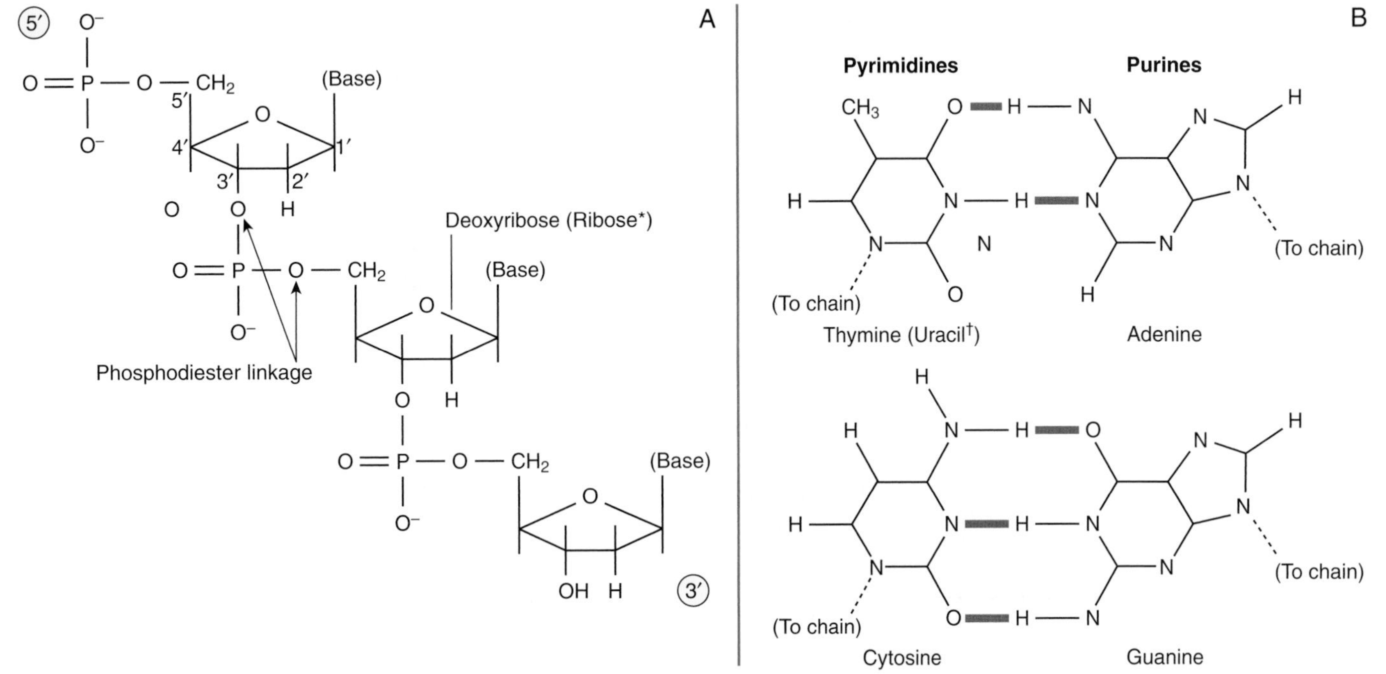

Figure 65-1 Repeating backbone of DNA and complementary base pairs. *A,* A single-stranded DNA chain. Repeating nucleotide units are linked by phosphodiester bonds that join the 5′ carbon of one sugar to the 3′ carbon of the next. *B,* Purine and pyrimidine bases and the formation of complementary base pairs. Shaded bars indicate the formation of hydrogen bonds. *(Adapted from Piper MA, Unger ER. Nucleic acid probes: a primer for pathologists. Chicago: ASCP Press; 1989, with permission.)* *In RNA, the sugar is ribose, which has a 2′ hydroxyl added to deoxyribose. †In RNA, thymine is replaced by uracil, which differs from thymine only in the lack of the methyl group.

portion of ssDNA. The building blocks of the single-stranded polymer are the four deoxyribonucleotide triphosphates (dTTP, dCTP, dATP, dGTP), each consisting of a sugar molecule, a triphosphate group, and one base. During DNA synthesis, nucleotides are first stripped of two phosphate groups and then enzymatically linked together by phosphodiester bonds to form a chain.

DNA is an extraordinarily stable molecule, losing its normal conformational structure only at extremes of heat, pH, or in the presence of destabilizing agents. The double-stranded helix is the most energetically favorable state for DNA, and an examination of the components of DNA explains this fact. Both sugar and phosphate groups are hydrophilic, forming stable hydrogen bonds with surrounding water molecules in solution. Bases, however, are hydrophobic and are not soluble in water at neutral pH. A stable molecule of DNA must ensure that the bases do not contact water. This is possible when two antiparallel ssDNA polymers (one running in the 3′ to 5′ direction, the other 5′ to 3′) twist around the same axis. This arrangement allows planar hydrogen bonds to form between adenine and thymine, and between guanine and cytosine (see Fig. 65-1, *B*). As long as the two chains have base sequences in complementary order, the strands of the helix have a ladder-like structure with rungs (base pairs [bp]) of consistent size. The flexibility of the carbon-oxygen linkages in the phosphodiester bond allows the ladder to twist, forming a regular helix such that the planar base pairs are stacked on top of each other, leaving no room for water molecules in between. The polymeric series of base pair hydrogen bonds holds the ssDNA chains tightly together, and the helical conformation protects the base pairs from water, exposing only the hydrophilic backbones.

Helical dsDNA is stable over a pH range of approximately 4–9. Solutions with pH outside these limits have the capacity to disrupt the base pair bonds and cause the DNA helix to denature or unwind into two separate, random coils. Extreme heat and hydrogen bond disrupters, such as formamide, also have the same effect. This helix-to-coil transition can be followed spectrophotometrically at A_{260} (Fig. 65-2). The bases absorb ultraviolet (UV) light maximally at this wavelength, but at a lower molar absorptivity in dsDNA; absorptivity increases 20%–30% when dsDNA is converted to ssDNA. Because temperature is often used to effect this transition, the process has been referred to as *melting*, and the temperature at which 50% of dsDNA is converted to ssDNA is called the *melting point* or T_m of the DNA. The T_m of DNA molecules depends on the relative G-C versus A-T base pair content, because the three hydrogen bonds of G-C base pairs require more energy to disrupt than the two hydrogen bonds of A-T base pairs. Lowering the temperature can reverse the melting process, and the two complementary strands reform the original helix if the base pairs reform in the correct linear conformation.

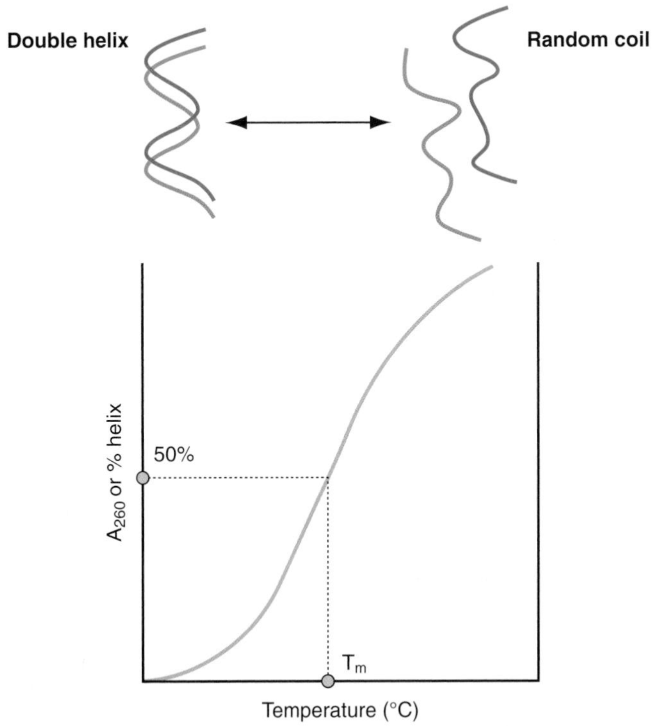

Figure 65-2 Melting/annealing curve of double-stranded helical nucleic acid. *(Adapted from Piper MA, Unger ER. Nucleic acid probes: a primer for pathologists. Chicago: ASCP Press; 1989, with permission.)*

The length of a fully extended eukaryotic DNA molecule would be about 3 m per genome, much longer than the cell itself. Undegraded purified DNA forms a stringy viscous solution, reflecting the extreme length of genomic DNA (Fig. 65-3). In vivo, however, DNA is organized into highly compacted, regular units called chromosomes. A chromosome is composed of its DNA strand wound around DNA-associated proteins (chromatin) in a highly structured fashion. The chromosome structure

PART 8

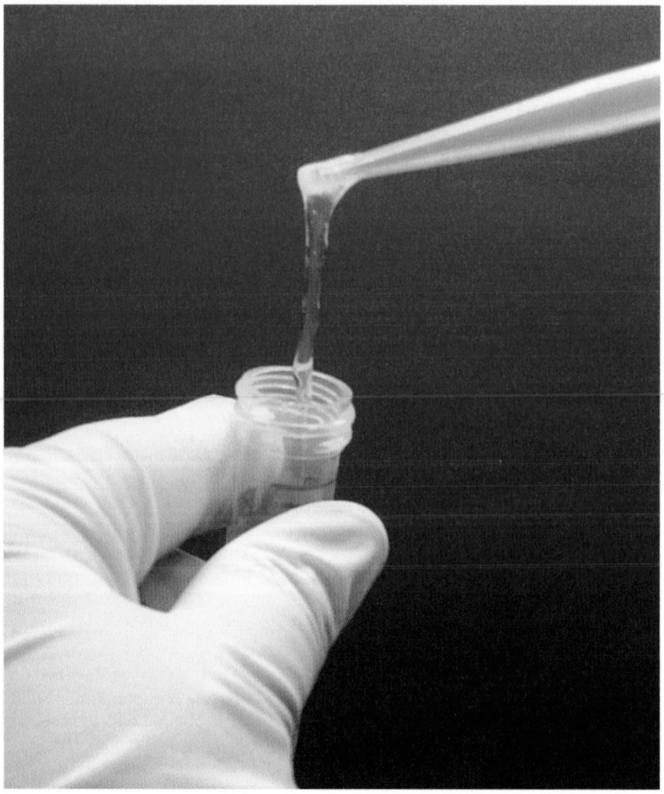

Figure 65-3 Photograph of purified DNA demonstrating stringy viscous nature of minimally sheared genomic DNA.

TABLE 65-1
Comparison of Key Features of DNA and RNA

Feature	DNA	RNA
Sugar	Deoxyribose	Ribose
Base pairs	Thymine–adenine	Uracil–adenine
	Cytosine–guanine	Cytosine–guanine
Structure	Double-stranded	Single-stranded
	Alpha helix	Random (see text)
Stability	Stable	Subject to base hydrolysis
	Degraded by DNase	Degraded by RNase
Function	Maintains genetic information in nucleus	Carries genetic information to cytoplasm

involves several hierarchical levels of chromatin packing, from a "beads-on-a-string" nucleosome (146 nucleotide pairs wound around a histone core) to highly condensed loops each containing about 100,000 bp of DNA. Each human cell nucleus contains two sets of 23 chromosomes of characteristic length and unique base pair sequence. Together these chromosomes constitute the *human genome.* As a result of the Human Genome Project, the complete sequence of the 3 billion chemical base pairs that make up the human genome was finished in 2001 (The Human Genome Project is discussed in Chapter 77).

RNA differs from DNA in chemical composition, structure, and function (Table 65-1). In RNA the sugar is ribose, containing a hydroxyl group at the 2′ position, and thymine is replaced by the methylated uracil (U). RNA exists predominately as a single-stranded molecule and in much shorter lengths than DNA. The structure of RNA is more irregular, owing to the single-stranded nature of the molecule, but may contain some helical sections and hairpin loops. RNA molecules of the same base sequence, however, will form the same three-dimensional structure as a result of adopting the most energetically favorable conformation. RNA is much less stable than DNA, due not only to the single-stranded more random structure but also to its susceptibility to alkaline hydrolysis via the 2′ hydroxyl group of the ribose moiety. RNA-specific enzymes that are ubiquitous also rapidly degrade RNA.

TABLE 65-2
Nucleic Acid Enzymes and Associated Functions

Enzyme	In Vivo Function
Polymerases DNA polymerases RNA polymerases	Polymerases join DNA or RNA nucleotides together to form a single-stranded daughter molecule using a stretch of single-stranded parent molecule as a template. These enzymes perform syntheses according to base pair rules and proceed in the 5′ to 3′ direction.
Reverse transcriptase	Mostly of viral origin, reverse transcriptase catalyzes the synthesis of DNA from either an RNA or DNA template.
DNA ligases	Joins DNA fragments formed by discontinuous synthesis in DNA replication or by DNA repair pathways.
Nucleases DNases, RNases	Nucleases "digest" nucleic acid molecules by breaking phosphodiester bonds.
Endonucleases Exonucleases	Endonucleases digest nucleic acids from the middle of the molecule whereas exonucleases begin at a free end and may require a 3′ or 5′ end. Nucleases may have single-stranded, double-stranded, DNA, or RNA specificity. Some polymerases also have nuclease activity.
Restriction endonucleases	Bacterial endonucleases that recognize specific short DNA base pair sequences and cleave the DNA molecule only at the recognition site.

NUCLEIC ACID–ASSOCIATED ENZYMES

DNA must be duplicated prior to cell division so that daughter cells retain an exact copy of the genetic information contained in parent chromosomes. RNA must be synthesized by all functioning cells to direct the synthesis of necessary proteins. DNA must be degraded during repair of damaged segments, and RNA is continually degraded and resynthesized. Enzymes that operate directly on nucleic acids affect these and other functions. Table 65-2 lists major categories of nucleic acid-specific enzymes and their in vivo functions. In vitro, purified enzymes have become laboratory *tools* for the molecular biologist, allowing genetic engineering and facilitating many nucleic acid assays.

Nucleic acid–specific enzymes include polymerases, which catalyze the formation of phosphodiester bonds during synthesis; and nucleases, which hydrolyze these bonds. RNA-specific nucleases (RNases) are present virtually everywhere. Because of this, it requires much greater care in laboratory practice to work with RNA in vitro than with DNA. Restriction endonucleases are a special category of nucleases found only in bacteria, where they function to destroy foreign DNA. The recognition sites for restriction enzymes are located anywhere within the DNA molecules, are sequence-specific, and can vary approximately 4–12 bp in length. At the recognition sequence or nearby, restriction endonucleases make specific asymmetric or blunt end cuts in DNA molecules (Fig. 65-4). More than 3000 restriction endonucleases have been discovered and categorized according to the structure of their corresponding sequence recognition sites (Pingoud, 2001). The in vivo function and in vitro utility of many of these enzymes are discussed in the following sections.

REPLICATION OF DNA

The DNA duplication process, known as *semiconservative replication,* uses each strand of the parent molecule to direct the synthesis of a daughter strand (Virshup, 1990). Because the base sequence of the parent strand dictates the sequence of the daughter strand, replication is faithful and the replication products consist of two dsDNA molecules, composed of one parent strand and one daughter strand each, with exactly the same base pair sequence. Although this is conceptually simple, the process is complicated and involves a number of accessory proteins and enzymes. First, for synthesis to begin, a small single-stranded region must be produced. This is not energetically favorable, and must be accomplished using proteins that unwind and separate the strands of the helix. Next, a short RNA primer is synthesized complementary to the single-stranded sequence. DNA polymerase III proceeds with DNA synthesis and later the RNA primer is excised and replaced with DNA by DNA polymerase I. Chromosomal DNA contains many initiation sites for replication, and this

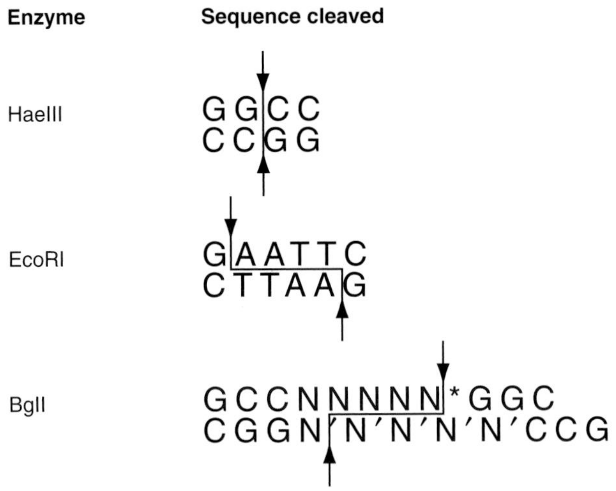

Figure 65-4 Examples of DNA restriction enzymes and their specificities. Enzymes are named for the bacteria from which they are isolated. (*N is any base, and N′ is its pairing counterpart.)

process occurs simultaneously across the chromosome. Interestingly, DNA polymerase III is a directional enzyme, and can synthesize DNA only in the 5′ to 3′ direction because it requires a free 3′OH end. This means that only one daughter strand, called the *leading strand*, can be synthesized continuously. The opposite strand, called the *lagging strand*, is primed by RNA primase that does not require a free 3′OH end. It is synthesized discontinuously in short fragments (Okazaki fragments) as the replication fork is opened up. These fragments are then joined together by DNA ligase. DNA polymerase III is also unique in that it has *proofreading* and exonuclease activity. If an incorrect nucleotide is added to the growing chain, it is detected and excised by the nuclease portion of the enzyme, and the correct nucleotide is then added. This helps explain the extraordinary fidelity of the DNA replication process. Postsynthesis repair mechanisms also contribute to the accuracy of replication (see later under Mechanisms of DNA Repair).

TRANSCRIPTION OF DNA TO RNA

Sections of DNA that specify amino acid sequences of proteins are called genes; one gene contains the amino acid sequence code for one protein as well as DNA sequences necessary for the regulation of the production of that protein. Within the 6 billion nucleotides of the human genome, there are about 20,000–25,000 protein-coding genes. Although these coding sequences are of paramount importance to the cell and to the function of the organism as a whole, they actually make up less than 5% of the nucleotides. The vast majority of the human genome is composed of noncoding DNA regions, sometimes referred to as *"junk DNA."* It appears that much of it may well have some purpose such as secondary regulatory roles in gene expression (see later section on Gene Regulation Mediated by Small RNA).

Protein synthesis begins with the activation of the appropriate gene. A copy of the gene is made from DNA in the form of RNA. Because the RNA copy carries the code from the DNA in the cell nucleus to the cytoplasm where amino acid synthesis takes place, this type of RNA is called *messenger RNA* (mRNA). Messenger RNA is synthesized from only one strand of the DNA gene; the complementary DNA strand is not used. This is accomplished by a process called *transcription.* Synthesis of mRNA proceeds in much the same fashion as DNA replication, with the ssDNA sequence dictating the mRNA sequence using the same rules of base pair complementarity (uracil base pairs with adenine). When the end of the gene is reached, mRNA synthesis is terminated. Some genes are always expressed, while others are only active in certain physiologic situations. The rate of transcription also varies in different cells (see section on Transcriptional Control later).

POSTTRANSCRIPTIONAL MODIFICATION

Before export to the cytoplasm, the mRNA molecule is modified in several ways (Rosenthal, 1994). Messenger RNA contains both amino acid coding sequences (exons) and noncoding sequences (introns); introns are excised from the mRNA molecule before protein synthesis. A molecular complex called a spliceosome (Sharp, 1988), which is composed of both low molecular weight RNA and protein, recognizes mRNA sequences that identify the boundaries of an intron, joins the flanking exons, and releases the intron. Splicing must be exact, as the addition or subtraction of a single nucleotide at the splice junction would change the 3-nucleotide reading frame in the nucleotide sequences that follow.

Further modifications to the mRNA molecule include the addition of 7-methyl guanosine residues to the 5′ end in a unique 5′-5′ phosphodiester bond. This is called a *cap* and aids in the binding of the ribosome to the mRNA molecule for initiation of protein synthesis. A poly-A *tail,* which may be necessary for stability and transport to the cytoplasm, is added to the 3′ end. The polyadenylation locus is specified in part by the sequence AAUAAA usually found in the 3′ untranslated region of the RNA transcript. At this point, the mRNA molecule is ready to direct the synthesis of its corresponding protein.

TRANSLATION OF RNA TO PROTEIN

Protein synthesis requires translation from the language of nucleotides to that of amino acids. Twenty-one different amino acids are used in protein synthesis; each amino acid is specified by one or more mRNA nucleotide triplets called *codons.* For example, AAG is the codon for lysine and UCG is the triplet for serine. Thus an amino acid coding sequence is read in groups of three nucleotides running in the 5′ to 3′ direction; this is the *reading frame* of a protein coding sequence. Three specific codons, (UAG, UGA, or UAA), do not code for amino acids but instead signal the end of a gene (*stop* codons). Because an amino acid can be encoded by more than one codon, the code is referred to as a *degenerate code.*

Translation from the mRNA nucleotide code to protein is mediated by ribosomes in the cytoplasm of the cell. A ribosome binds to the 5′ end of the mRNA and provides a stable chemical environment for all the molecules involved in protein synthesis. Amino acids are linked in the correct sequence by the action of small, adaptor RNA molecules called *transfer RNAs* (tRNAs). Each tRNA molecule contains a region that is complementary to a particular mRNA codon: the *anticodon.* Linked to one end of the tRNA is the amino acid that corresponds to the complementary mRNA codon of the tRNA. A tRNA with the correct complementary anticodon binds to the first codon in the mRNA sequence, which is always AUG. When another specific tRNA binds to the next codon, ribosomal enzymes catalyze the formation of a peptide bond between the two amino acids linked to the tRNAs, removing the linkage between the first amino acid and its tRNA molecule. The first tRNA is ejected from the ribosome and a new tRNA binds to the next codon. As this process continues, the ribosome moves along the mRNA molecule, completing the synthesis of the amino acid chain. When a stop codon is reached, the ribosome detaches from the mRNA. In reality, several ribosomes can move along the same mRNA molecule, each translating the mRNA code into a new protein molecule.

TRANSCRIPTIONAL CONTROL

To allow for cellular differentiation and response to environmental stimuli, there must be mechanisms controlling the repertoire of gene transcription and protein translation. Some of these mechanisms operate at the level of DNA and control the transcription of mRNA (Rosenthal, 1994). For example, promoters are DNA sequences that are important for the initiation of mRNA transcription. Promoters are found upstream (toward the 5′ end) at a relatively invariant distance from the beginning of the protein coding sequence. There are several different kinds of promoter consensus sequences (nucleotide sequences that are found in many examples). The most common promoters are rich in adenine and thymine and have been called *TATA boxes.* Because A-T base pair bonds are weaker than G-C base pair bonds, DNA unwinds more easily at repeat A-T sequences. Other recognized promoter sequences are the *GC box* and the *CAA motif.* After transcriptional activation, a local ssDNA region is produced and stabilized by the assembly of a complex of RNA polymerase and general transcription factors (Fig. 65-5). Messenger RNA is synthesized from the local region of ssDNA and the mRNA is quickly ejected as the DNA returns to its more energetically favorable double-stranded helical state.

Enhancers are DNA sequences that can augment mRNA transcription and may be found in different locations relative to the gene that they affect. Gene-specific transcription factors are proteins that bind to enhancers and promoters and selectively stimulate or inhibit mRNA transcription (Papavassiliou, 1995). In eukaryotes, enhancers commonly contain multiple binding sites for several transcription factors, so it is the net effect of

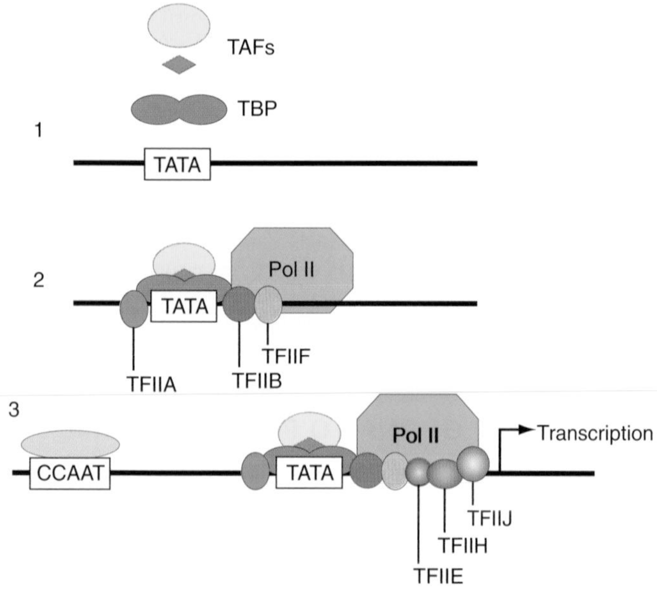

Figure 65-5 Assembly of the polymerase II transcription initiation complex. (1) The basal TFIID complex assembles as the TATA-box binding protein (TBP) and associated factors (TAFs) at the TATA box of the promoter region. (2) Additional transcription factors TFIIA and TFIIB are recruited to enable the polymerase II enzyme and TFIIF to bind. (3) The complex is stabilized with TFIIE, TFIIH and TFIIJ. Typically, binding of additional factors to upstream enhancer sites like CCAAT or GGGCGG are required for effective RNA transcription.

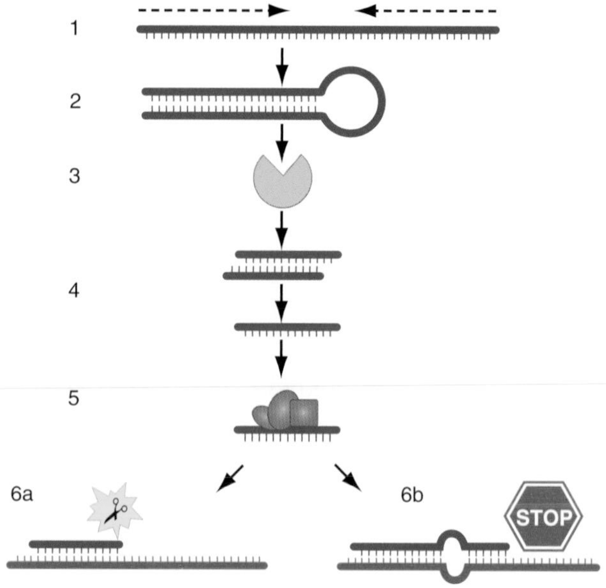

Figure 65-6 Diagram of the RNAi pathway: (1) Sense-antisense transcripts build a dsRNA with hairpin structure (2). This molecule is recognized by the Dicer complex (3) and processed into smaller fragments of 21–24 nucleotides (4). The RNA-induced silencing complex (RISC) protein complex assembles with these molecules and unwinds them into single strand oligos (5). Active RISC binds to target mRNAs with either perfect complementary sequence *(6a),* which initiates cleavage and degradation, or imperfect sequence match *(6b),* resulting in bulging, interference with translation, and subsequent silencing.

factors binding to these DNA elements that determines the activation and rate of expression. The availability of transcription factors, in turn, is controlled by cellular events such as phosphorylation, or by other proteins such as hormones and growth factors. A network of intracellular and extracellular chemical communications can thus select and control the synthesis of necessary proteins.

Because mRNA is far less stable than DNA, the half-life of mRNA is very short. New mRNA molecules are continually transcribed from DNA. As the cell responds to changes in transcriptional signals, the genes that are transcribed into mRNA can be quickly changed, resulting in the immediate synthesis of new proteins. Thus the cell has the ability to rapidly adjust its protein output in response to its environment.

Gene Regulation Mediated by Small RNA

Recently a novel mechanism of gene regulation by another class of RNAs—small RNAs—was discovered. Small RNAs are short, noncoding ribonucleotides that function as posttranscriptional regulators of gene expression. First discovered in the 1990s, they were found in cells of many eukaryotic organisms including mammals (Fire, 1998). The small RNAs are divided into several different subgroups, most notably small interfering RNA (siRNA) and micro RNA (miRNA).

The DNA sequences for siRNAs and miRNAs are often located in noncoding regions between genes. They generally have their own promoters and transcription is mediated by polymerase II. The immediate product is an miRNA precursor that forms a double-stranded hairpin structure (Fig. 65-6). An enzyme called Dicer processes it to short RNA duplex molecules and further into single-stranded RNAs 22 to 26 nucleotides in length. The small RNA strand attaches to an RNA-induced silencing complex (RISC), which mediates binding to complementary sequences of mRNAs. siRNAs pair perfectly with the target mRNA and trigger a series of molecular mechanisms that lead to its degradation. This process is also called RNA interference (RNAi). miRNAs bind imperfectly to their target mRNA, causing conformational changes, bulging, and subsequent blockage of protein translation at the ribosome. Small RNAs are abundant in eukaryotic cells (several hundred) and it is thought that each one can target multiple mRNAs either as siRNA or miRNA. They are often tissue specific and have been implicated in the regulation of all major cellular processes such as proliferation, differentiation, metabolism, and cell death. siRNAs have also been recognized as a new RNA-based immune system against viruses that is based on silencing through the RNAi mechanism. Furthermore, changes in miRNA expression patterns can be found in many malignancies, and specific miRNAs were found abundantly in certain tumors (Iorio, 2009).

Epigenetics and Gene Regulation

Epigenetics refers to changes in gene expression that are not dependent on DNA sequence. In most instances, this involves a change in the chromatin structure that facilitates or blocks gene transcription. This is a dynamic process involving enzymes that chemically modify DNA or histone proteins. A methyl group added to the fifth carbon of cytosine results in 5-methyl cytosine. This generally occurs on cytosines located next to guanines (CpG) that are often repeated in islands or patches located in the promoter region. DNA methylation tends to result in condensed chromatin and reduce transcription. DNA methyltransferases are the enzymes responsible for DNA methylation. Chromatin proteins may be acetylated, deacetylated, or methylated. There is evidence that small RNA chemistry may directly interact with a variety of epigenetic mechanisms (Moazed, 2009). Epigenetic changes are recognized to be important in tissue-specific gene transcription, and alterations may be factors in cancers, aging, and stress response.

MECHANISMS OF DNA REPAIR

Errors in DNA replication and damage to DNA during the normal cellular lifetime must be minimized to preserve the health of the entire organism. Several mechanisms operate to maintain the normal DNA sequence. First are the error-avoidance mechanisms that operate during DNA replication. The DNA polymerase that synthesizes new DNA polymers selects each successive nucleotide monomer based on its complementarity to the next nucleotide in the template strand. Fidelity at this level is high and most errors in synthesis are avoided at this stage. Nevertheless, an occasional base may be incorrectly added to the growing strand. To adjust for this, the proofreading activity of the polymerase can recognize the error, remove the incorrect base, and proceed again with synthesis. Together, the error avoidance mechanisms reduce base pair mismatches to approximately 1 in 10 million (Radman, 1988). This represents a 100,000-fold increase in efficiency compared with the error rate of 1 in 100 bases for in vitro solid phase oligonucleotide synthesis.

Despite the remarkable error avoidance in DNA replication, occasional mistakes do occur. In addition, DNA can be damaged by normal biochemical reactions and by nonphysiologic agents such as UV light and environmental carcinogens. Several repair mechanisms mend damaged DNA (Yu, 1999) (Table 65-3).

Direct repair mechanisms repair lesions in a single-step reaction. For example, O^6-methylguanine DNA methyltransferase repairs alkylation lesions by transferring the alkyl group from the lesion to the active site of

TABLE 65-3
DNA Repair Pathways

Direct repair	Repairs certain types of DNA damage in a single-step reaction.
Mismatch repair	Checks for errors made when DNA is replicated. Any mispaired bases in the daughter strand are removed and replaced with the correct match.
Base excision repair	Repairs small, nonhelix-deforming adducts such as those produced by methylation, oxidation, reduction, or base fragmentation by ionizing radiation.
Nucleotide excision repair	Removes bulky DNA adducts such as thymine dimers and certain photoproducts as well as chemical adducts and cross-links.
Double-strand break repair	Repairs double-strand breaks that result from physiologic processes or from ionizing radiation and oxidative insults.

the enzyme. Other direct repair mechanisms characterized in *Escherichia coli* may also exist in human cells (Yu, 1999).

Mismatch repair (MMR) functions immediately after DNA replication to replace mismatched bases with the correct ones (Modrich, 1994). Several MMR proteins recognize the error in the newly synthesized daughter strand and excise a region that includes the mismatch. DNA polymerase III and ligase restore the correct sequence and integrity of the daughter strand. The importance of this mechanism in stabilizing the genome is evidenced by recent studies associating hereditary nonpolyposis colorectal cancer with defects in MMR proteins.

Base excision repair targets small, nonhelix-deforming adducts such as those produced by methylation, oxidation, reduction, or base fragmentation by ionizing radiation. Base excision leaves 3–4 nucleotide sequence gaps that are then filled with the correct nucleotides; nicks are sealed with ligase. Larger, bulky adducts or dimers that distort the DNA helix may be caused by UV radiation, carcinogens, and therapeutic drugs, among other agents. Such damage is removed by the nucleotide excision repair (NER) pathway, which uses an enzyme system composed of many proteins to excise a single-stranded oligonucleotide containing the lesion (Sancar, 1994). The gap is then filled in by DNA polymerase and ligated. There are two NER pathways: one, in which lesions that block transcription are rapidly removed (transcription-coupled repair; Hanawalt, 1994); and a second a global pathway that repairs bulk DNA, including the nontranscribed strand of active genes. Some of the possible consequences of the loss of NER activity are exemplified by the disease xeroderma pigmentosum (XP), which is caused by mutations in *NER.* XP results in extreme sensitivity to sunlight, with skin cancers occurring at an early age (Weeda, 1998).

Double-strand breaks occurring rarely or produced by ionizing radiation and oxidative damage, present significant repair problems. If unresolved, replication and transcription of involved sequences will be blocked. To maintain local and overall genomic integrity, double-stranded breaks are repaired by nonhomologous or allelic recombinational repair mechanisms.

It is now clear that DNA repair plays a central role in the life of the cell. Recent evidence also indicates that several proteins that are primary repair proteins also function in transcription and in regulation of the cell cycle. Thus the processes involving DNA appear to be highly integrated and are increasingly studied as a whole and in relation to human disease.

DNA MUTATIONS

Despite extensive repair mechanisms, alterations in DNA base sequence (mutations) occur. Yet for an individual organism, some mutations are clearly harmful and can be associated with cancer and with inherited genetic disease. Studies of these diseases have led to the characterization of the various types of mutations that occur in the human genome (Weatherall, 1987). These can be conceptually grouped into a few major categories (Table 65-4). A point mutation is found in the β-globin gene in sickle cell anemia (Kan, 1992). A thymine base replaces an adenine base, causing a critical change in the structure of hemoglobin. As described in Chapter 70, muscular dystrophy is caused by deletions in the gene for the muscle protein dystrophin. In the Becker form of the disease, the deletions do not disrupt the reading frame, but in most cases of the more severe Duchenne form, the reading frame is changed by the deletions, effectively abolishing the function of the protein (Liechti-Gallati, 1989).

TABLE 65-4
Types of DNA Mutations and Examples of Associated Diseases

Mutation	Description	Disease
Point	Single base pair substitution	Sickle cell anemia
Deletion/insertion	Subtraction/addition of amino acid codons in multiples of three. Reading frame is retained.	Becker muscular dystrophy
Deletion/insertion with frameshift	Subtraction/addition of amino acid codons in non-multiples of three. Results in a shift of the reading frame and a completely different amino acid coding sequence from the mutation on.	Duchenne muscular dystrophy
Amplification/trinucleotide repeat	Increase in the number of repeat sequences in microsatellite DNA. Results in distruption of gene expression.	Fragile X syndrome
Translocation	Interchromosomal exchange of large chromosome segments. Results in a new protein with different function.	Chronic myelogenous leukemia

Human DNA contains many short sequences of nucleotides (microsatellite DNA) that are sometimes grouped in tandem arrays and are repeated many times throughout the human genome. The number of tandem repeats at particular locations is a heritable trait. Some trinucleotide repeats have been found to increase in number in association with disease (Sutherland, 1994). In fragile X syndrome (Chapter 70), expression of the disease is associated with amplification of the intragenic trinucleotide repeat sequence beyond a critical number of copies. The expansion of the trinucleotide repeats beyond this critical number disrupts expression of the gene.

Translocations may not always be detectable by chromosomal karyotype analysis. At the gene level, a translocation may create a fusion gene, the combination of two different genes abnormally joined at the translocation site. This can create not only an altered gene transcript, but may also bring the product of one gene under the transcriptional control of the other. For example, as discussed at length in Chapter 75, the Philadelphia chromosome, found in most cases of chronic myelogenous leukemia, results from a reciprocal translocation between the *c-abl* gene on chromosome 9 and a region termed the *breakpoint cluster region* (bcr) on chromosome 22. The fusion gene produced by this chromosomal rearrangement, consisting of most of the *c-abl* gene and a truncated bcr, codes for a c-abl protein that is larger than the normal product, has increased enzymatic activity, and is thought to interfere with signal transduction pathways normally involved in the control of cell death and proliferation.

It is both the type of mutation as well as its location in relation to the gene that determines the ultimate effect on the protein product. Mutations may have no effect on protein expression or functional activity; many human proteins exist in detectable variants that have no disease association. Mutations occurring in intron regions presumably have no effect at all. Even small mutations, however, in regions that code for key functional domains (exons) may drastically alter or eliminate function. "Nonsense mutations," mutations that change an amino acid codon to a stop codon, or vice versa, result in abnormally short or long protein products, respectively. *Missense mutations*, those that change the code from one amino acid to another, may or may not alter protein function, depending on the change and the function of the amino acid. Similarly, mutations within sequences that denote intron-exon splice sites could eliminate exons or introduce introns into the transcribed mRNA. Mutations may also occur in regulatory sequences, such as promoters or enhancers, producing dramatic effects on the levels of transcription.

NUCLEIC ACID ANALYSES

The unique biochemical properties of nucleic acids have been exploited to yield information about the biology or biochemistry of a system. While some of the assays, such as electrophoresis, are applicable to other biochemical building blocks such as proteins and lipids, the majority are particular to nucleic acids. The following sections briefly describe the

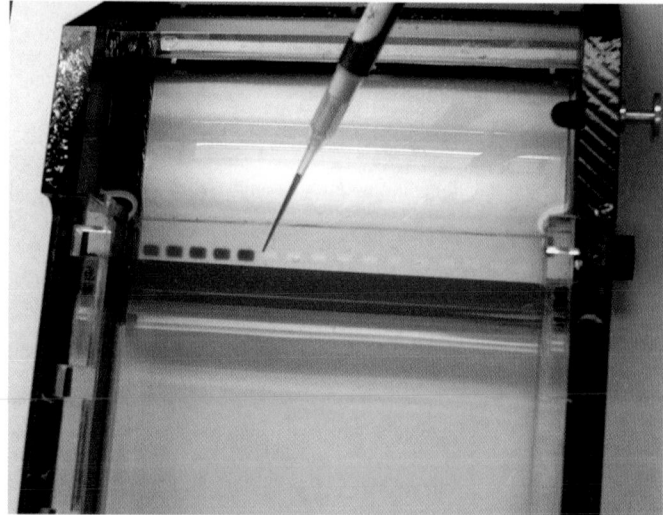

Figure 65-7 Photograph of loading sample and dye through buffer into wells of anagarose gel in submarine gel electrophoresis apparatus.

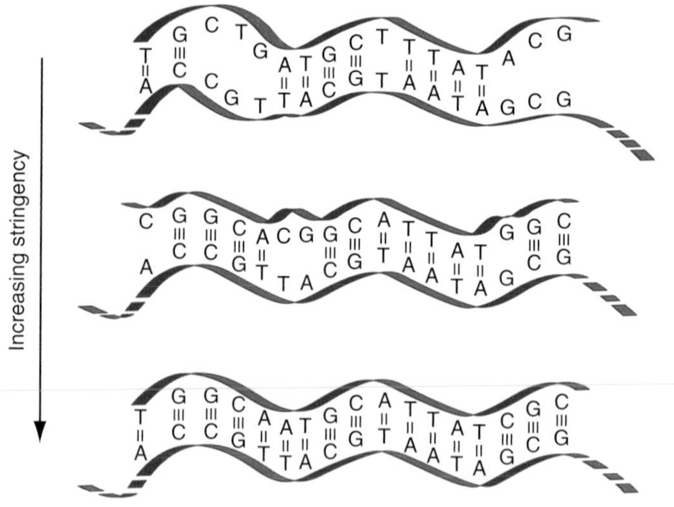

Figure 65-8 Illustration of stringency. As the stringency of the hybridization solution is increased, fewer mismatches are tolerated in a hybrid duplex. At very high stringency, even a single base pair mismatch disrupts the duplex.

principles of the basic categories of analyses used to characterize DNA and RNA: electrophoretic separations, hybridization assays, amplification techniques, sequencing, and polymoprhism-based analyses. In practice, the categories are often combined to produce novel variations of the same theme; for example, a complete assay may involve amplification, electrophoresis, and hybridization.

ELECTROPHORETIC SEPARATION

The repeating sugar-phosphate backbone of nucleic acids results in a net negative charge evenly distributed over these linear molecules. Therefore, movement of DNA or RNA in response to an electric field will be proportional to the molecular weight or length of the molecule. This property is used to characterize the size of nucleic acid fragments by electrophoretic separation. The format is analogous to that used for the separation of proteins according to size. Multiple samples are applied in separate wells at one end of a solid but porous separation medium. When a voltage is applied, the samples move toward the positive electrode in a linear fashion, each sample well forming one lane of migration. The solid electrophoretic medium and array of sample wells is known as a *gel.* Size standards, referred to as *DNA* or *RNA ladders*, are mixtures of nucleic acids of known fragment length that are analyzed in one or more lanes of the gel. Comparison of the distance of migration of an unknown sample with the ladder, either by "eye" or by computer-assisted measurement, allows size determination.

The composition and concentration of the separation medium determines the size of the fragments, which may be separated into distinct bands. Other variables that contribute to resolution are the thickness of the gel, the length of the electrophoresis path, the time of electrophoresis, and the applied voltage. In practice, these factors are adjusted empirically and controlled as carefully as possible to ensure reproducibility from day to day. Agarose is the separation medium most often used, usually in conjunction with a horizontal electrophoresis bed in which the gel is submerged in buffer. Samples are made heavy with sucrose or Ficoll and loaded into slots in the gel through the buffer (Fig. 65-7). Higher resolving power, allowing differentiation of a single base pair in length, is achieved with acrylamide, usually used in a vertical format although increasingly capillary formats are being adopted which decrease both the time of the separation and the amount of sample required. The simplest approach to visualizing the bands separated by electrophoresis is by staining with intercalating dyes (e.g., ethidium bromide), which insert between stacked bases, and viewing with UV transillumination. Direct visualization requires that the band achieve a significant concentration. Increased sensitivity may be achieved in some applications that label the nucleic acid fragments with a radioactive or fluorescent tag.

The molecules in genomic DNA are reduced to fragments that may be resolved by electrophoresis through digestion with restriction enzymes. Restriction enzymes with a relatively simple recognition sequence produce fragments less than 50 kilobase pairs (kb) in length. Extremely large DNA fragments, measured in megabase pairs, are produced from digestion with enzymes with a complex recognition sequence and must be separated in special electrophoretic systems utilizing a pulsed electrical field. Most applications of DNA electrophoresis utilize nondenaturing conditions (i.e., the fragments resolved into bands are double-stranded). By contrast, most RNA separations utilize denaturing conditions (either formamide or glyoxal) to eliminate secondary structure of the single-stranded molecules. RNA molecules, as transcripts of DNA, are "presized" and relatively small, so that no digestion is required before electrophoresis.

NUCLEIC ACID HYBRIDIZATION

Hybridization is a fundamental concept in nucleic acid biochemistry; it is defined as the interaction between two single-stranded nucleic acid molecules to form a duplex (double-stranded) molecule based on the complementary base pairing of their respective sequences. Hybridization is a direct consequence of the stable double-stranded structure of DNA under physiologic conditions. As discussed earlier, the helix is formed of two antiparallel strands of DNA held together by the combined strength of many specific hydrogen bonds between complementary base pairs as well as by hydrophobic shielding of bases from an aqueous environment. Central to the hybridization reaction is the fact that the binding between separate, complementary molecules (strands) is both reversible and base sequence-specific.

When neither DNA strand is labeled, the process of reforming the stable double-stranded structure is referred to as *annealing.* If one strand is labeled (i.e., has a marker that is capable of being detected in some fashion), the labeled strand is referred to as a *probe* and the process is called *hybridization* because a hybrid molecule is formed between a labeled and unlabeled strand. RNA molecules can also participate in the hybridization process. Base pairing may occur between complementary strands of DNA, between DNA and RNA, and between complementary strands of RNA, resulting in DNA-DNA, DNA-RNA, and RNA-RNA duplex structures. Duplex molecules with exact complementarity in base sequence form the most stable structures, but structures with varying degrees of base pair mismatch may form depending on the conditions. The relative instability of these mismatched duplexes are reflected in the lowered temperature of their disassociation (lower T_m, see Fig. 65-2).

Environmental conditions can be manipulated to control the degree of base pair mismatching that will be tolerated in a duplex structure (i.e., the *stringency* of the sequence match) (Fig. 65-8). Low stringency refers to conditions such as high salt, low temperature, and no formamide, which favor shielding of hydrophobic bases from the aqueous environment even without perfect alignment; the match need not be perfect. High stringency conditions—high temperature (close to T_m), low salt, and high formamide—will only allow the most perfectly matched duplex structures to remain in a stable helix conformation.

HYBRIDIZATION ASSAYS: BASIC COMPONENTS

When the hybridization reaction is used to analyze the nucleic acid content of an unknown sample, the process is known as a *hybridization assay.*

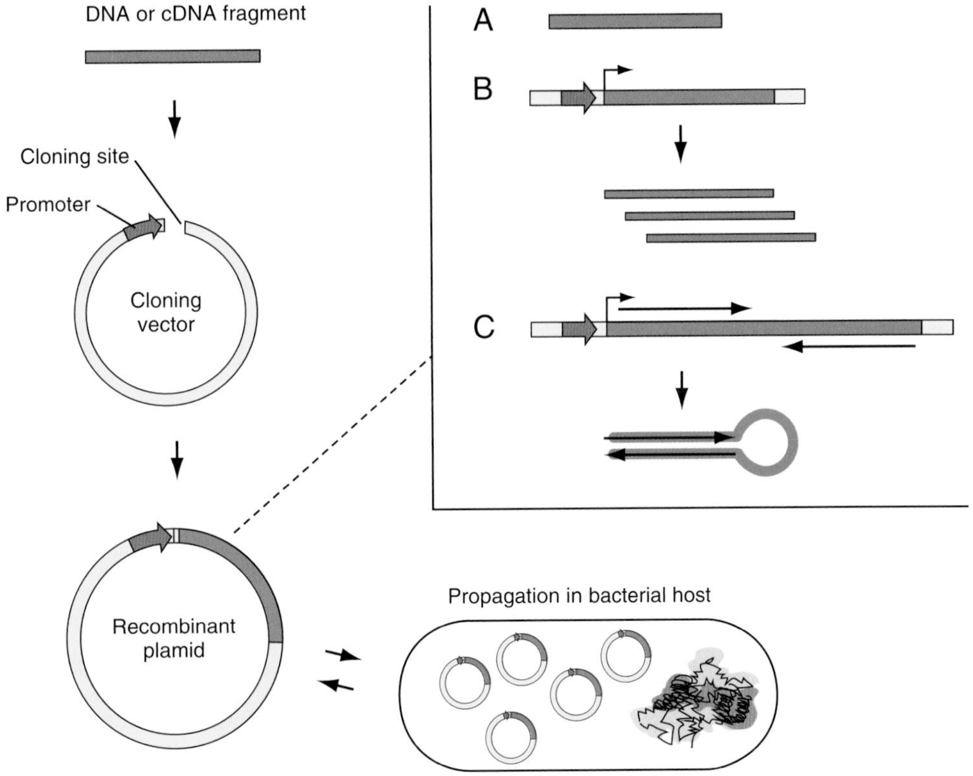

Figure 65-9 Production of cloned DNA or RNA. A DNA fragment or RNA that was converted into cDNA can be inserted into a cloning vector. The recombinant plasmid is transformed into a bacterial host where it is rapidly propagated to millions of copies. The multiplied DNA fragment can either be isolated by excision through restriction enzymes that recognize sequences at the borders of the insert *(A)* or can be used to initiate RNA in vitro transcription with a promoter sequence in the plasmid *(B)*. Such systems are also used to produce double-stranded RNA by cloning two complementary sequences in sense and antisense direction, typically with a spacer that forms a stabilizing loop in the dsRNA fragment *(C)*.

Hybridization assays include a wide variety of formats (see next section) such as Southern blots, Northerns, fluorescent in situ hybridization (FISH) and microarrays ("DNA chips"). The property of complementary base pairing allows fragments of known composition (the probe) to interrogate an unknown for the presence of matching (complementary) sequences. All hybridization assays, therefore, require several basic elements: a probe, a sample, controlled conditions permissive to complementary base pairing, and a method for detection of specific probe-sample hybrids. Each of these elements will be briefly discussed below, as well as the variations in formats that have been developed to allow hybridization assays to be performed and interpreted.

Probe

The probe determines the specificity of the hybridization reaction; thus the probe is central to a hybridization assay in the same way that the primary antibody is central to an immunoassay. A probe is a well-characterized fragment of nucleic acid, either DNA or RNA. In most assay formats it is the probe that carries the reporter group for detection of hybridized molecules into the reaction, although variations occur. Reporter groups may be radioactive or nonradioactive (i.e., affinity label).

Many probes are produced through recombinant nucleic acid technology, as illustrated in Figure 65-9. Plasmids—short, circular, double-stranded segments of DNA—are harnessed as vectors to propagate desired sequences in bacteria. The segment of interest is introduced into the plasmid using restriction enzyme digestion and ligation resulting in a new "recombined" molecule that retains the ability to be propagated in bacteria and includes the DNA sequence of interest. Bacteria containing the recombinant plasmid can be grown in culture, and the small circular plasmids can be easily separated from the bacterial genome on the basis of size. Many identical copies are obtained; thus the DNA is often referred to as *cloned.* Purified plasmid may be used as probe in assays where vector sequences do not interfere with the specificity of the reaction. In many applications the inserted DNA sequence is separated from the vector sequence by digesting the isolated plasmid with the same restriction enzyme originally used in construction of the recombinant molecule. The probe resulting from either of these approaches is a double-stranded DNA molecule. Double-stranded probes must be denatured prior to use, and probe reannealing limits the extent of hybridization of probe with target. Plasmid vector that does not contain cloned DNA is a commonly used negative control for this type of probe.

Plasmid vectors have been constructed to include RNA promoter regions adjacent to the inserted DNA sequence. These recombinant plasmids are used to produce RNA transcripts of the DNA insert. The result is a single-stranded RNA probe that will not undergo self-hybridization. Controlling the orientation of the DNA insert with respect to the RNA promoter allows production of transcripts in the *sense* (same as mRNA) or *antisense* (complementary to mRNA) direction. In many applications the sense transcripts form ideal negative control probes for hybridization reactions with antisense probes. Non-specifically bound RNA probe (i.e., RNA not in a stable duplex structure) can be removed with the use of RNase specific for single-stranded RNA. The lability of RNA requires that the probes be handled with extreme care to prevent degradation (sterile technique, treated water, and glassware).

Recombinant probes, whether DNA or RNA, are genetically complex; that is, they may include many kilobases of genetic information. By contrast, probes produced by synthetic methods are relatively short segments of DNA. Oligonucleotide probes produced by automated chemical reactions are usually 15–45 bases in length synthesized to produce a specified base sequence. Probes with very high specificity of hybridization can be designed on the basis of sequence information available in data banks. They can be generated in a sense or antisense direction at a relatively low cost. These short probes are single-stranded, diffuse into target and hybridize rapidly because of their small size, and are extremely sensitive to even single base pair mismatches. The final sensitivity achieved with oligonucleotide probes is lower than that achieved with recombinant probes because of their limited genetic complexity. Multiple oligonucleotide probes directed to different areas of the same target have in some instances been used to increase the sensitivity by increasing the representation of the target sequence in the probe mixture. This approach is analogous to the use of a blend of monoclonal antibodies that react to different epitopes of the same complex antigen.

Probes longer than those obtained by direct chemical synthesis may be generated with the polymerase chain reaction or other amplification technology. These probes may be single-stranded or double-stranded depending on the conditions employed and may be as long as the product of the amplification reaction; in most cases 100 bp to 1 kb in length.

Sample

Whereas probe selection and preparation are central to determining the sensitivity and specificity of the hybridization assay, the contribution of sample preparation to a successful assay cannot be overlooked. In clinical applications, samples of interest may be quite diverse. For example, a microbiology laboratory could anticipate testing specimens of blood, urine, stool, and sputum. Integrity of RNA targets may be difficult to maintain under such conditions and even DNA may be degraded with improper handling. The goal of sample preparation is to maintain nucleic acid integrity and make the target genetic information available for interaction with the probe. For some applications, the requirement of target integrity will dictate immediate snap freezing or addition of lysis buffers containing potent RNase and DNase inhibitors. In other applications, more routine methods of sample collection will allow adequate target preservation.

The physical and chemical similarities of nucleic acids, regardless of source, allows for uniform methods of extraction and purification. For many assays it is preferable to extensively purify DNA or RNA to remove inhibitors of enzymes to be added to the assay (e.g., a restriction enzyme or polymerase) and to maximize accessibility of target to probe. Complete purification schemes, however, are time-consuming and require a relatively large amount of starting sample. In many applications, relatively abbreviated sample purifications can be used. Purifications commonly use cell lysis (mechanical, chemical, or both), protease treatment, and organic or inorganic extractions. Automated methods are now available to standardize and streamline sample extraction.

Controlled Conditions Permissive for Complementary Base Pairing

The sensitivity and specificity of the hybridization reaction are greatly influenced by the physical-chemical environment during the reaction and subsequent detection/collection of hybrid molecules. In practice, the hybridization cocktail is the medium used to control the environment of the hybridization reaction. Empirically designed, the *hybridization cocktail* is a mixture of reagents selected to favor interaction of nucleic acids through sequence-specific hydrogen bonds rather than via charge. The components vary widely, but include buffers, salts, denaturants such as formamide, high molecular weight polymers, carrier DNA or RNA, and various components added to reduce background (such as detergents, bovine serum albumin, Ficoll). Such a complex mixture is conveniently referred to as a *cocktail.* The ionic strength of both the hybridization cocktail and the subsequent washes is most often modulated by the concentration of a *s*aline *s*odium *c*itrate buffer (SSC), composed of 0.15 mol/L sodium chloride, 0.015 mol/L trisodium citrate, pH 7.0. The shorthand notation for these conditions refers to the strength of SSC; that is, 2 × SSC, 0.1 × SSC. The final stringency of the hybridization reaction is controlled by the formamide and salt concentration of the hybridization cocktail, the temperature of the hybridization reaction, and the temperature and salt concentration of the washing steps.

Detection of Hybrids

A wide variety of techniques have been applied to collection and analysis of specific hybrids, discussed briefly later under Hybridization Assay Formats. Once specific hybrids have been collected, methods of detection are obviously linked to methods of labeling. Radioactive labels such as phosphorus-32 (^{32}P), iodine-125 (^{125}I), sulfur-35 (^{35}S), carbon-14 (^{14}C), and tritium (^{3}H) are detected through autoradiography or scintillation counting, and the specific activity of the label directly influenced the sensitivity of the detection. Because radioactive probes have a relatively short half-life, making one of the key reagents in the hybridization assay unstable, are hazardous to laboratory personnel, and generate expensive waste disposal problems, they have been nearly entirely replaced by nonradioactive methods. Nonisotopically labeled probes are stable reagents, greatly facilitating the commercial production and standardization that are crucial for assay reproducibility.

Nonisotopic labeling and detection methods for nucleic acids have many similarities to immunochemical assays developed for nonisotopic protein detection. In some applications, nucleic acids are directly linked to a signal-generating compound, usually a fluorochrome but occasionally an enzyme. This situation is analogous to immunoassays in which the primary antibody is labeled. More commonly, nucleic acids are indirectly detected in a multistep assay similar in concept to an indirect antibody reaction. Biotin, a commonly used affinity label for immunoassays, was the first affinity label introduced into nucleic acids (Langer, 1981). Biotin itself generates no signal, but is detected by high-affinity interaction with an avidin or streptavidin molecule that is, in turn, complexed or conjugated to a signal-generating enzyme, fluorochrome, or metallic particles detected by light scattering (Yguerabide, 2001). Many other functional groups have been developed as nonisotopic labels such as bromodeoxyuridine, digoxigenin, and sulfone. Detection in these cases is achieved with high-affinity antibodies directed against the functional group. These antibodies are usually directly linked to a signal-generating enzyme or fluorochrome, functioning like a labeled secondary antibody in an immunohistochemistry reaction. Biotin may also be detected with an antibiotin antibody rather than an avidin or streptavidin molecule.

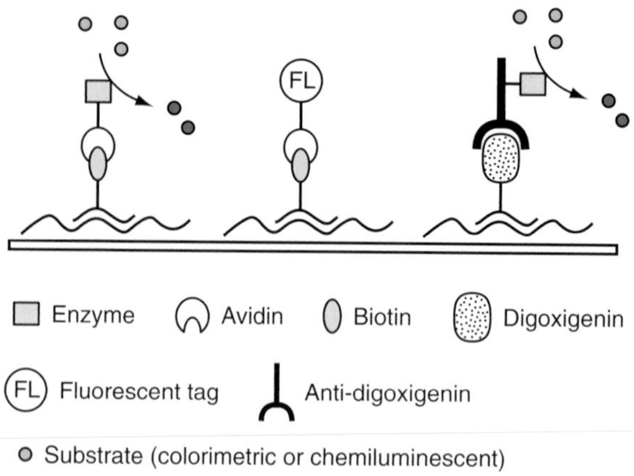

Figure 65-10 Examples of affinity-labeled probe detection systems. *(From Unger ER, Piper MA. Nucleic acid biochemistry and diagnostic applications. In: Burtis CA, Ashwood ER, editors. Tietz textbook of clinical chemistry, 2nd ed. Philadelphia: WB Saunders; 1994, with permission.)*

Because affinity labels are detected with large bulky proteins such as avidin or antibody, availability of the label to the detection reagent is a crucial factor in determination of sensitivity. Increasing the number of affinity tags will not necessarily increase the number of detecting molecules that will be bound to the nucleic acid. In addition, because affinity labels are themselves bulky, overincorporation into the nucleic acid molecule can lead to steric hindrance of the hybridization reaction. For these reasons, the specific activity of the affinity label does not directly control the sensitivity of the detection.

One advantage of the indirect detection of affinity labels is that a variety of detection methods can be used for the same label (Fig. 65-10). For example, biotin may be detected with avidin linked to an enzyme with subsequent color or chemiluminescent detection, or avidin with fluorescent tag. For all nonradioactive methods, the detection portion of the assay is crucial in obtaining optimal sensitivity. Detection reagents with poor background and suboptimal signal generation can mar an effective hybridization reaction. The choice of the enzyme labels (peroxidase vs. alkaline phosphatase), enzyme substrate (colorimetric vs. chemiluminescent), and even source of reagents are critical for optimal results.

HYBRIDIZATION ASSAY FORMATS

A wide variety of hybridization assay formats have been developed, each designed to solve the methodologic problems of the hybridization assay: conditions permitting specific complementary base pairing, a method to detect hybrids, and interpretation of the result. Each method has particular strengths and weaknesses and the clinical setting and particular diagnostic question dictate selection of format. There is no one perfect assay. Several of the basic formats are briefly described herein, along with their particular strengths and weaknesses.

Each hybridization assay requires both positive and negative controls for validation. A positive sample control is one known to contain sequences complementary to the probe. This is used to establish that sample preparation is adequate to release target for the hybridization assay, and to ensure that probe will hybridize with the specific target under the assay conditions. The sample control may also be used to monitor the sensitivity of the assay, if the positive control is chosen near the lower limits of detection. A negative sample control (i.e., one known not to contain sequences complementary to the probe) is used to monitor specificity of the probe target interactions. Controls for the probe include vector sequences or unrelated probes labeled, hybridized, and detected under identical assay conditions. These latter controls allow monitoring of the background signal generated by localization of probe through non-hybridized interactions such as charge or trapping. In clinical practice, additional controls may be employed to monitor each step of the hybridization assay.

Liquid or Solution Phase Hybridization

In liquid hybridization assays, both the sample and probe interact in solution, which maximizes the kinetics of the reaction. The sample nucleic acids are generally purified from contaminating proteins and lipids, which could interfere with the collection of hybrids at the end of the assay, and some sample degradation is tolerated by the assay. The sample is denatured and randomly sheared before addition of single-stranded probe lacking the ability to self-hybridize.

Hybridization may be detected by the specific binding of hybrids to a solid matrix such as hydroxyapatite, which binds only duplex structures. Once hybrids are bound, unhybridized probe may be efficiently removed by washing. Detection of the label on the bound probe permits quantitation of the hybridization reaction. In a variation of this approach, one commercial assay (Digene Hybrid-Capture, Qiagen USA, Valencia, Calif.) uses an antibody specific for RNA-DNA hybrids to specifically bind duplex structures formed of the DNA target and RNA probe. An alternative analysis involves digestion of the hybridization reaction mixture with S1 nuclease, an enzyme that acts only on single-stranded nucleic acid. Duplex structures resistant to digestion may then be precipitated by treatment with trichloroacetic acid. In the hybridization protection assay, label on the probe is protected from chemical degradation only when the probe is involved in a duplex structure.

Many other variations of the solution-phase hybridization assay are in use. Optimal kinetics, toleration for abbreviated purification steps, and some sample degradation make the assay adaptable for clinical application. Quantitation of the reaction product may be achieved, depending on the detection system. The solution phase format does not permit identification of the size of the hybridizing product. Low positive reactions are difficult to interpret, because low levels of specific target and high levels of weakly cross-reacting target will yield similar results. Solution phase hybridization is adaptable to the 96-well format with an enzyme-linked immunosorbent assay–type readout, and increasing automation of the assay can be anticipated.

Solid-Support Hybridization

Variations of the solid-support hybridization assays include dot or blot hybridization, Southern and northern hybridization, microarray hybridizations ("DNA chips") and in situ hybridization. In these assays, the hybridization occurs in a biphasic environment, a solid phase (usually sample) and a liquid phase (usually probe). The kinetics of hybridization to a nucleic acid bound to a solid support is greatly slowed, and the extent of the hybridization reaction is limited. These disadvantages are often outweighed by the convenience of having a solid medium to carry through multiple steps of the assay.

Dot/Blot Hybridization

In this assay format, multiple samples are immobilized in a geometric array on a nitrocellulose or nylon membrane. The name of the assay comes from the shape of each sample on the membrane. When samples are applied by hand, the shape is more random (blot). With the use of commercially available manifolds, samples are usually applied with the use of suction, the sample shape is very regular—round (dot) or elongated (slot). The solid matrix allows multiple samples to be processed through all steps of the assay simultaneously. The fact that all samples and controls are exposed to exactly the same reagents and conditions increases the standardization of the assay.

The extent of sample preparation varies from complete purification of nucleic acids before application to the filter, to direct application of unpurified sample. Some degree of sample degradation is tolerated by the assay. Purified nucleic acids have the advantage of being most available for interaction with probe and having the least problems with background. Individual sample purification, however, is time-consuming and labor intensive. Applications using direct application of unpurified sample take the entire array through an abbreviated purification procedure, which usually involves lysis and denaturation, protein digestion, and washing with detergent. The advantages of this approach are that it is applicable to small amounts of starting material and minimizes sample preparation time. However, the final sensitivity of the reaction is lower, and background from nonspecific probe interactions can make the assay unreliable.

Interpretation of the results of a dot/blot hybridization assay is relatively straightforward. If hybridization has occurred, a signal is generated in the specified spot. Depending on the label used for signal generation, results may be quantitated; however, usually a simple yes/no interpretation is given (i.e., the sample has more or less signal than adjacent samples and known positive and negative controls). Weak signals, which may result from a very small amount of specific target or from a large amount of weakly cross-reacting target, may cause problems in interpretation. No information is available about the size of the hybridizing fragments.

One interesting variation of the dot/blot assay is known as the reverse dot/line blot assay. In this format, applied in situations where one sample must be tested with many different probes and sample may be limited, the label is carried into the assay by the sample. The unlabeled probes, or targets, are fixed to the solid support in a linear or matrix array. Areas of specific hybrid formation are identified and interpreted as in the standard dot blot assay. This assay format is a convenient means of identifying the product of an amplification assay (vide infra and Chapter 66), such as in human leucocyte antigen analysis (Bugawan, 1994) or human papillomavirus typing (Gravitt, 1998).

Southern and Northern Hybridizations

Both Southern and northern hybridizations combine electrophoretic separation of test nucleic acid with transfer to a solid support and subsequent hybridization. These assays, therefore, not only give information about the presence of hybridization, but also permit determination of the molecular weight of the hybridizing species.

The original procedure was termed Southern blot hybridization or Southern blotting, after its inventor, E. M. Southern (Southern, 1975). In this assay, the sample is DNA. Northern blotting was named by analogy for the technique using RNA samples. (Extending the analogy even further, the western blot is a similar procedure in which proteins are subjected to electrophoresis and transfer; a southwestern blot has been described for a technique separating and blotting DNA followed by incubation with protein solutions to permit evaluation of specific DNA-binding proteins.)

Sample preparation is time-consuming and labor intensive for both of these techniques. Degradation of sample nucleic acids is not tolerated by the assays, and a relatively large amount of starting material is required. For Southern hybridizations, the DNA must be purified with minimal shearing. This is because sizing of the DNA fragments is achieved through digestion with one or more restriction enzymes. Shearing and degradation introduce random breaks in the sample, reducing the quantity available to be specifically cut at appropriate recognition sequences. Impurities in the sample may interfere with the activity and sequence specificity of the restriction enzyme. Partially or improperly digested samples can produce spurious band sizes or result in such a reduced concentration of the specific band that it is no longer detected during hybridization. For northern hybridizations, the starting material is RNA, and extreme care must be taken to avoid degradation during sample collection and preparation because of the ubiquitous nature of RNases. RNA is composed of fragment sizes determined by transcription and processing of message and ribosomal RNA. It is not digested before electrophoresis, but is separated under denaturing conditions to remove secondary structure.

The size-separated fragments in the agarose gel are then transferred to a nylon or nitrocellulose filter. As originally designed, the transfer occurred passively through capillary action. Most current applications use vacuum or pressure to speed the transfer. After transfer, baking or UV cross-linking immobilizes the nucleic acids and the entire membrane is hybridized with labeled probe.

Hybridization is followed by autoradiographic, colorimetric, or chemiluminescent detection of bands containing sequences complementary to the probe. Interpretation involves both detection of a hybridizing species and determination of the molecular weight of the molecule. These technically demanding assays require several days to perform but may be required in clinical applications in which the information cannot be obtained in any other format. The presence of bands at molecular weights different from normal or germline (developmentally unaltered) samples can indicate a change in the genetic material.

Microarray Hybridization ("DNA Chip Technology")

Microarray hybridizations can be thought of as a variation of the dot-blot format in which the dotted material is arranged in a regular gridlike pattern with each feature reduced to a very small size so that hundreds to thousands of features can be placed on one solid surface, currently most often

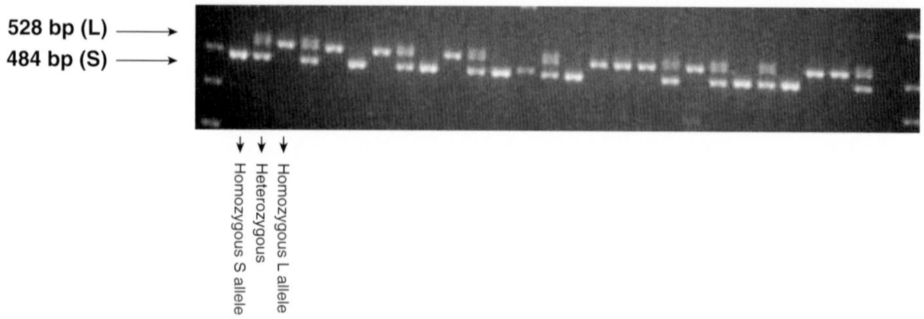

Figure 65-11 Example polymoprhism analysis by gel electrophoresis [Allelic typing of the serotonin transporter gene (5-HTTLPR)]. A polymorphism consisting of a 44-bp insertion/deletion polymorphism in the 5′ regulatory region is suggested to be associated with major depressive disorder. The presence of the two different alleles can be screened using PCR primers upstream and downstream of the site producing fragments of distinct length. The amplicons are then separated by gel electrophoresis and stained with ethidium bromide. An individual is either homozygous for the long version (L allele = upper band), heterozygous with both alleles (two bands), or homozygous for the short version (S allele = lower band). *(Photo courtesy Drs. I. Dimulescu and M. Rajeevan.) PCR,* Polymerase chain reaction.

a glass microscope slide. By convention in these applications, the sample is labeled and the arrayed features are referred to as *probes*. Microarrays allow genome-wide transcription profiling or sequence determination in a single experiment. The technique and applications are described in greater detail in Chapter 67.

In Situ Hybridization

In situ hybridization is simply detection of specific genetic information within a morphologic context. This specialized type of solid-support assay involves taking morphologically intact tissue, cells, or chromosomes affixed to a glass microscope slide through the hybridization process. Autoradiographic, colorimetric, and fluorescent methods of detection have been applied. Evaluation of the final product is very analogous to evaluation of immunohistochemistry and requires experience in histopathology. The strength of the method lies in linking microscopic morphologic evaluation with detection of hybridization.

The method also has applications in cytogenetic analysis of metaphase chromosome spreads or of interphase nuclei (see Chapter 68). In this context, the detection is usually fluorescent, and the technique is referred to as FISH. Detecting numerical aberrations or translocations of chromosomes can be achieved rapidly using probes for specific targets. FISH avoids some of the difficulties of conventional cytogenetics and may have greater sensitivity for some targets. Although FISH cannot completely replace karyotyping, it can complement and reduce the need for the frequency of cytogenetic analysis. Newer variations of FISH (Luke, 1998) are exploiting the possibilities of automation (fast-FISH) and expanding the information that can be obtained in a single assay. FICTION (*f*luorescence *i*mmunophenotyping and interphase *c*ytogenetics as a *t*ool for *i*nvestigation *o*f *n*eoplasms) combines immunophenotyping with FISH; fiber FISH makes it possible to simultaneously detect and map chromosomal break points. In situ hybridization can be very labor intensive and tedious. Recent improvements resulting in automated processing of slides through the assay hold much promise for more widespread adoption of this technique.

AMPLIFICATION METHODS

It is virtually impossible to read any medical journal without encountering at least one application of polymerase chain reaction (PCR) technology. The PCR has forever changed the scope of research questions that can be addressed by virtually eliminating the problem of limited sample size. The importance and elegance of the concept has been recognized through awarding of the Nobel Prize in Chemistry to its inventor, Kary Mullis, less than 10 years after publication of the first practical application of PCR (Saiki, 1985). There are now other methodologies that result in multiplication of target, probe, or signal. These may be grouped together as amplification technologies and are described in Chapter 66.

POLYMORPHISM DETECTION ASSAYS

Although greater than 99% of the human genome is identical in all individuals, there are still millions of regions of DNA that vary between individuals. While most polymorphisms have no recognized functional consequence, changes in promoter or enhancer regions may result in altered transcription regulation, cause variation in the mRNA splice products if present in intron-exon junctions, or produce altered amino acid sequences if an exon is affected. The serotonin transporter gene, for instance, exists in two alternative allelic variants characterized by a 44-bp insertion/deletion polymorphism in the promoter region. This polymorphism has been associated with major depressive disorders and the two allelic versions can be distinguished by PCR amplification of the relevant DNA region resulting in two different sized products (Fig. 65-11). Most of the variations occur in the form of an individual base change known as single nucleotide polymorphisms (SNPs). An example would be the alteration of a DNA fragment ACGT to ACTT by replacement of the third base from a guanine to a thymine. Two unrelated individuals will have approximately 3 million SNPs that differ between them.

The sequence-specific recognition features of restriction enzymes have been used since the 1970s for the detection of such sequence variations. In such assays, called restriction fragment length polymorphism (RFLP, "rif-lip"), DNA is digested with a restriction enzyme and the fragments analyzed by gel electrophoresis followed by band visualization or Southern blot analysis with a site-specific probe. Changes in the sequence of the DNA may result in alteration of the recognition sequence of the enzyme. An SNP alteration may introduce additional restriction enzyme sites, remove restriction sites, or insert or delete sequences between restriction sites. These changes will be reflected in a change in the band size visualized in a gel or hybridizing to the site-specific probe. Although the approach has been applied with considerable success in family studies, RFLP is a relatively crude method. Sequence polymorphism can only be detected if the distance between two restriction sites is directly affected and the majority of SNPs would not be detected.

Because of the tremendous potential of polymorphism assays to predict inheritance of altered alleles, and changes that predict drug interactions (see Chapter 72), considerable effort has been made in recent years to improve the speed, precision, and cost effectiveness of these methods. The completion of the Human Genome Project in 2001 provided a reference against which all other sequencing data can be compared. Researchers are also systematically screening the genome to discover new SNPs. High throughput SNP analysis methods have been developed which simultaneously scan thousands of SNPs in thousands of samples. Comprehensive mapping of an individual's SNP pattern is also termed *genotyping*. Genotyping is somewhat easier, in that one form of the known gene sequence (allele) can be compared with an alternative form at a specific predetermined site. Currently there are a wide variety of approaches for allelic discrimination that typically use a combination of molecular techniques. For more information, see Chen & Sullivan (2002).

DNA SEQUENCING

Methods for directly determining the base sequence of DNA first became available in the 1970s. Originally prohibitively time-consuming and expensive for diagnostic applications, automation and miniaturization have resulted in instrumentation capable of rapidly and inexpensively sequencing segments of DNA. Sequencing the first human genome was completed by the Human Genome Project in 2001 using the Sanger method (Fig. 65-12) that is based on enzymatic incorporation of chain terminating di-deoxynucleotides. The rapidly evolving field of "next-generation" sequencing has produced a variety of different platforms and sequencing chemistries that allow extremely high-throughput sequencing based on

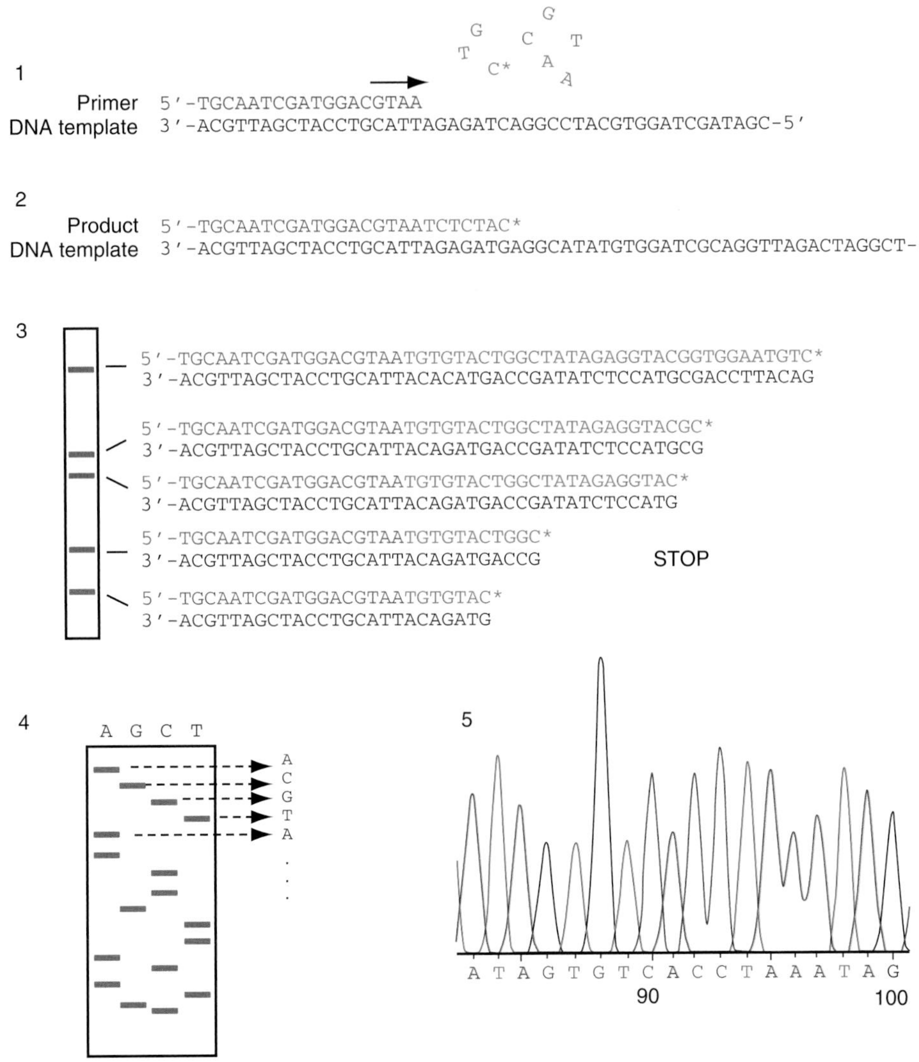

Figure 65-12 Principle of the Sanger DNA sequencing method.
1. A short primer (in blue) is annealed to a known sequence in the DNA template. In the presence of the four "usual" deoxynucleotides (dATP, dCTP, dGTP, dTTP) and an additional di-deoxynucleotide at a low concentration, here ddCTP (marked with an asterisk), DNA polymerase initiates synthesis.
2. When ddCTP is incorporated further polymerization cannot occur because it lacks the 3′-OH group required to accommodate another nucleotide (see Fig. 65-1) and the chain is terminated.
3. Random incorporation of ddCTP generates a series of DNA strands of different sizes, all ending at "C." These products start with the same primer sequence and are sized by electrophoresis to determine the position of each "C."
4. Dividing the reaction into four tubes, each with a different dideoxynucleotide, and electrophoresing all four reactions in parallel allows the complete sequence to be read from the order of the bands in each the ladders of each lane.
5. Most current applications use fluorescently tagged ddNTPs, each with a different color dye. With this approach the reaction is in a single tube and products are separated in a single lane. A laser is used to record the wavelength and order of the bands.

massively parallel sequencing in flow cells (Voelkerding, 2009; see Chapter 77). Currently too expensive for routine clinical applications, these techniques have the power to make the "$1000 genome," that is, provide an individual's complete genetic sequence for $1000, a reality. These deep sequencing methods can be applied to evaluate the transcriptome and are beginning to rival microarray technology in systems biology applications. Currently the diagnostic utility of the complete genome is not clear, but direct sequencing is used to determine viral types (e.g., human papillomavirus) and identify mutations (e.g., BRACA1 and BRACA2). Early explorations of how to use an individual's genome for clinical management are underway (Ashley, 2010).

Relationship to Laboratory Evaluation of Disease

Subsequent chapters describe the current applications of molecular diagnostics. It is clear that this new technology has impacted all areas of laboratory diagnosis. Molecular methods also have the potential to redefine laboratory evaluation of disease to include issues beyond disease diagnosis.

MOLECULAR DIAGNOSIS

The advantages of a molecular approach to diagnosis is described in detail for each aspect of current application. Increased automation and commercially designed methods have reduced costs and the level of technical expertise required to perform the tests. Increasingly, molecular technology is being integrated into the mainstream of laboratory testing.

Detecting mutations and associating them with disease is at the heart of the current explosion of information in medical science and of many applications in molecular diagnostics. One of the most important consequences of the revolution in molecular genetics has been the ability to locate a gene responsible for a disease without knowing the protein product. Termed *positional cloning*, this process uses RFLP linkage analysis of families that carry and express the disease to locate polymorphic markers closer and closer to the disease gene until it is ultimately located. Closely linked polymorphic markers that tend to segregate with disease may be used in clinically useful diagnostic tests even before the gene is completely characterized and the protein product finally identified. In this scenario, molecular diagnostic tests are developed and used first, to be replaced by simpler, more cost-effective methods directed at the level of the gene product when the consequence of mutation is fully understood.

BEYOND DIAGNOSIS

Molecular analyses have the potential to greatly expand the role of the laboratory in areas beyond disease diagnosis. Molecular analysis of the somatic mutations in cancer has the potential to provide prognostic information, guide selection of optimal therapy, and monitor response to therapy. The implications of using molecular markers to detect neoplastic cells in the absence of clinical or morphologic evidence of disease, known as *minimal residual disease*, are now being explored in a variety of malignancy types (see Chapter 73). This approach of using molecular markers for disease detection can also be anticipated to impact secondary methods of cancer prevention (screening) and assessment of adequacy of surgical resection (evaluation of margins). Gene therapy for inherited genetic disease as well as cancer is being introduced based on a detailed understanding of the underlying disease. Monitoring these patients for presence and activity of the introduced therapeutic gene will add another aspect to the laboratory evaluation of disease as the application to personalized medicine continues to develop (see also Chapter 72).

SELECTED REFERENCES

Alberts B, Johnson A, Lewis J, et al. Molecular biology of the cell. 5th ed. New York: Garland Publishing; 2007.

An excellent, clearly written textbook of molecular biology. The fourth edition is available in searchable format through the NCBI bookshelf web site. [http://www.ncbi.nlm.nih.gov/entrez/query.fcgi?db=Books]

Fire A, Xu S, Montgomery MK, et al. Potent and specific genetic interference by double-stranded RNA in *Caenorhabditis elegans*. Nature 1998;391:806–11.

First description of RNAi in animal cells.

Langer PR, Waldrop AA, Ward DC. Enzymatic synthesis of biotin-labeled polynucleotides: novel nucleic acid affinity probes. Proc Natl Acad Sci U S A 1981;78:6633–7.

First description of affinity-labeled nucleotides that achieved sensitivity of detection required for eventual replacement of radioactive methods.

Papavassiliou AG. Transcription factors. N Engl J Med 1995;332:45–7.

From the "Molecular Medicine" series in the New England Journal of Medicine, *a brief review of transcription factors and their importance in medicine.*

Rosenthal N. Regulation of gene expression. N Engl J Med 1994;331:931–3.

From the "Molecular Medicine" series in the New England Journal of Medicine, *a brief review of the regulation of gene expression and relevance to disease.*

Saiki RK, Scharf S, Faloona F, et al. Enzymatic amplification of β-globin genomic sequences and restriction site analysis for the diagnosis of sickle-cell anemia. Science 1985;230:1350–4.

Original description of the polymerase chain reaction.

Southern EM. Detection of specific sequences among DNA fragments separated by gel electrophoresis. J Mol Biol 1975;98:503–17.

Original description of electrophoretic separation of DNA fragments, transfer to filter and hybridization for identification.

REFERENCES

Access the complete reference list online at http://www.expertconsult.com

CHAPTER 66

POLYMERASE CHAIN REACTION AND OTHER NUCLEIC ACID AMPLIFICATION TECHNOLOGY

Frederick S. Nolte, Charles E. Hill

KEY POINTS

- Nucleic amplification technology has created new opportunities for the clinical laboratory to affect patient care.
- Although the polymerase chain reaction (PCR) is the most mature and widely used nucleic acid amplification method, other methods have diagnostic applications.
- Clinical applications of the technology cut across the traditional disciplines in laboratory medicine.
- An understanding of the basic principles and relative strengths and limitations of the nucleic amplification methods is important for all involved in the practice of clinical pathology.
- The development of the PCR by Mullis and colleagues (Saiki, 1988) was a milestone in biotechnology that heralded the beginning of molecular diagnostics. Although PCR is the most widely used nucleic acid amplification method, other approaches have been developed, and several have unique properties and advantages. These methods are based on target, probe, or signal amplification. Examples of each category are discussed in the sections that follow. These techniques have analytical sensitivity unparalleled in laboratory medicine, creating new opportunities for the clinical laboratory to impact patient care.

TARGET AMPLIFICATION METHODS

PCR, transcription-based amplification, and strand displacement amplification are all examples of target amplification methods. These methods share certain fundamental characteristics. They are enzyme-mediated processes in which a single enzyme or multiple enzymes synthesize copies of target nucleic acid. The amplification products in all the techniques are defined by two oligonucleotide primers that bind to complementary sequences on opposite strands of double-stranded targets. All result in the production of millions to billions of copies of the targeted sequence in a matter of hours and, in each case, the amplification products can serve as templates for subsequent rounds of amplification. Consequently, all the techniques are sensitive to contamination with product molecules from previous amplifications, which can lead to false-positive reactions. However, special laboratory design, practices, and workflow have been developed to reduce the possibility of false-positive reactions to acceptable levels.

POLYMERASE CHAIN REACTION

PCR is a simple in vitro chemical reaction that permits the synthesis of essentially limitless quantities of a targeted nucleic acid sequence. This is accomplished through the action of a deoxyribonucleic acid (DNA) polymerase that, under the right conditions, can copy a strand of DNA. At its simplest, a PCR consists of target DNA, a molar excess of two oligonucleotide primers, a heat-stable DNA polymerase, an equimolar mixture of deoxyribonucleotide triphosphates (dATP, dCTP, dGTP, and dTTP), $MgCl_2$, KCl, and a Tris-HCl buffer. The two primers flank the sequence to be amplified, are typically 18–30 bases long, and are complementary to opposite strands of the target.

To initiate a PCR, the reaction mixture is heated to separate the two strands of target DNA (denaturation) and then cooled to permit the primers to anneal to the target DNA in a sequence-specific manner (annealing) (Fig. 66-1). The DNA polymerase then initiates extension of each primer at its 3′ end (extension). The primer extension products are dissociated from the target DNA by heating. Each extension product, as well as the original target, can serve as a template for subsequent rounds of primer annealing and extension.

A PCR cycle consists of three steps: denaturation, annealing, and extension. At the end of each cycle, the PCR products are theoretically doubled. Thus, after n PCR cycles, the target sequence can be amplified 2^n-fold. The whole procedure is carried out in a programmable thermal cycler that precisely controls the temperature at which the steps occur, the length of time that the reaction is held at the different temperatures, and the number of cycles. Ideally, after 20 cycles of PCR, a million-fold amplification is achieved and, after 30 cycles, a billion-fold. In practice, the amplification may not be completely efficient, because of failure to optimize the reaction conditions or the presence of inhibitors of the DNA polymerase. In such cases, the total amplification is best described by the expression $(1 + e)^n$, where e is the amplification efficiency ($0< e \leq 1$) and n is the total number of cycles.

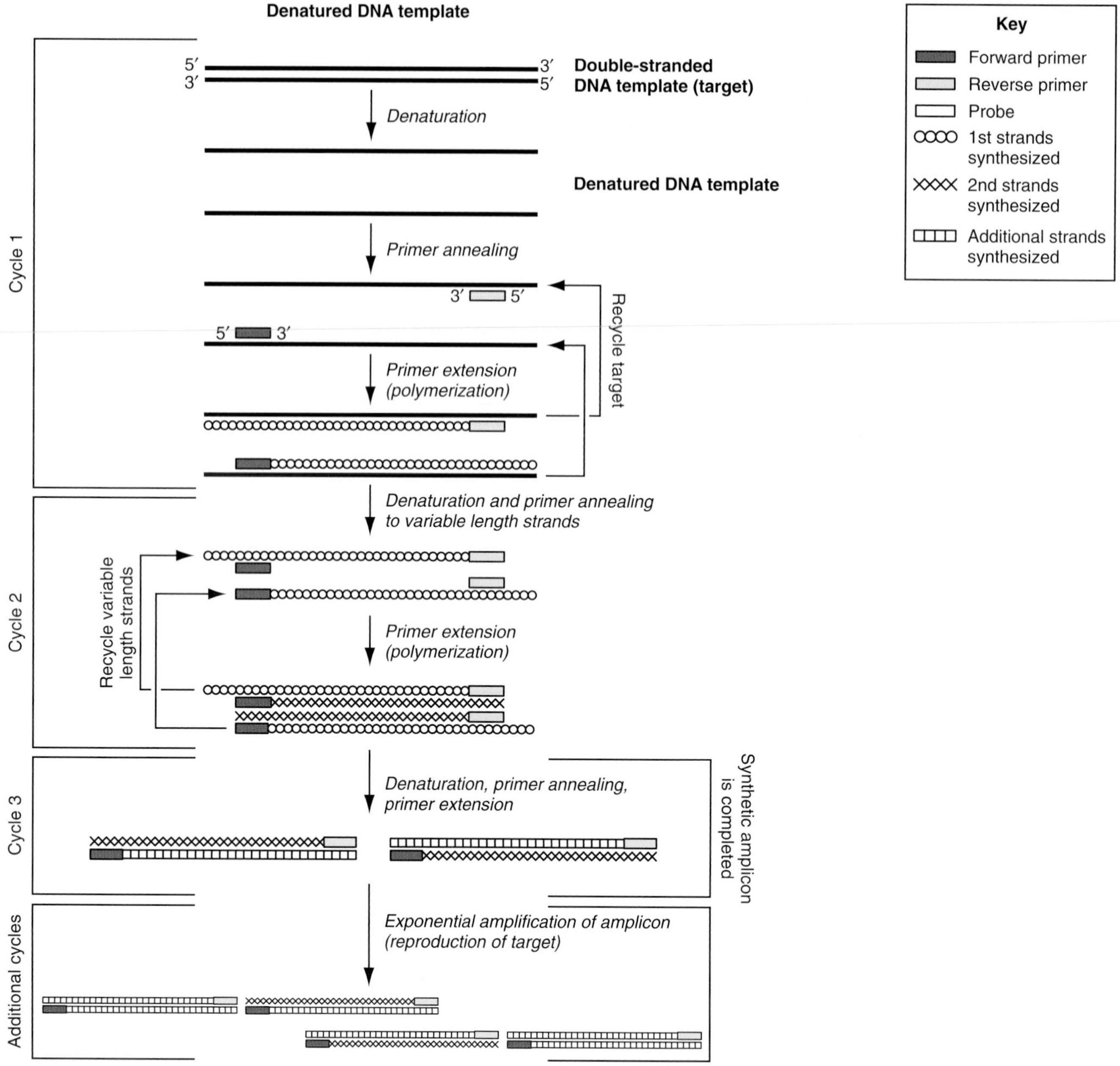

Figure 66-1 Polymerase chain reaction. *(Redrawn from Wolk D, Mitchell S, Patel R. Principles of molecular microbiology testing methods. Infect Dis Clin N Am 2008;15: 1157–1204.)*

Reverse-Transcriptase Polymerase Chain Reaction

PCR, as it was originally described, was a technique for DNA amplification. Reverse-transcriptase PCR (RT-PCR) was developed to amplify ribonucleic acid (RNA) targets. In this process complementary DNA (cDNA) is first produced from RNA targets by reverse transcription, and then the cDNA is amplified by PCR. As originally described, RT-PCR employed two enzymes, a heat-labile RT such as avian myeloblastosis virus reverse transcriptase (AMV-RT) and a thermostable DNA polymerase. Because of the temperature requirements of the heat-labile enzyme, cDNA synthesis had to occur at lower temperatures. This presented problems both in terms of the nonspecific primer annealing and inefficient primer extension due to formation of RNA secondary structures. These problems have been largely overcome by the development of a thermostable DNA polymerase derived from *Thermus thermophilus*, which, under the proper conditions, can function efficiently as both an RT and a DNA polymerase (Myers, 1991). RT-PCRs using this enzyme are more specific and efficient than previous protocols using conventional, heat-labile RT enzymes. Commercially available kits (AMPLICOR, Roche Diagnostics, Indianapolis, Ind.) employing this single-enzyme RT-PCR are available for detection of hepatitis C virus (HCV) RNA and for quantification of human immunodeficiency virus (HIV)-1 and HCV RNA in clinical specimens. RNA targets may present problems due to secondary or tertiary structure that may require special conditions or alternative target sites for efficient cDNA synthesis.

While the single enzyme RT-PCR has improved specificity and efficiency for problematic targets, there remain many applications that use a two-enzyme system. Modified heat-labile RT enzymes and optimized mixtures of reverse transcriptases with improved specificity and efficiency are now commercially available. Performing a separate RT reaction with random sequence primers allows PCR analysis of multiple targets from a single RT reaction. The RT reaction may be performed with oligo-dT primers providing cDNA of the messenger RNAs only. This scheme also allows PCR to be performed for multiple targets from a single RT reaction.

Nested Polymerase Chain Reaction

Nested PCR was developed to increase both the sensitivity and specificity of PCR (Haqqi, 1988). It employs two pairs of amplification primers and two rounds of PCR. Typically, one primer pair is used in the first round of PCR of 15–30 cycles. The products of the first round of amplification are then subjected to a second round of amplification using the second set of primers, which anneal to a sequence internal to the sequence amplified

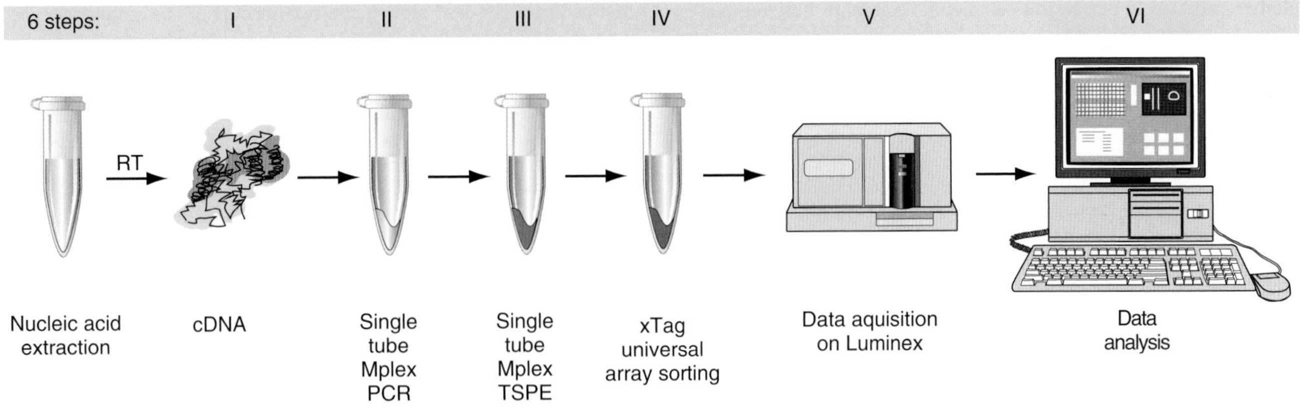

Figure 66-2 Major steps in multiplex, reverse transcriptase-PCR analysis using the xMAP system (Luminex). *(Courtesy Luminex.) Mplex,* Multiplex; *PCR,* polymerase chain reaction; *RT,* reverse transcription; *TSPE,* target-specific primer extension.

by the first primer set. The increased sensitivity arises from the high total cycle number and the increased specificity arises from the annealing of the second primer set to sequences found only in the first-round products, thus verifying the identity of the first-round product. The major disadvantage of nested PCR is the high rate of contamination that can occur during the transfer of first-round products to the second tube for the second round of amplification. This can be avoided either by physically separating the first- and second-round amplification mixtures with a layer of wax or oil, or by designing single-tube amplification protocols. In practice, the enhanced sensitivity afforded by nested PCR protocols is rarely required in diagnostic applications, and the identity of an amplification product is usually confirmed by hybridization with a nucleic acid probe.

Multiplex Polymerase Chain Reaction

In multiplex PCR, two or more primer sets designed for amplification of different targets are included in the same reaction mixture (Chamberlain, 1988). With this technique, more than one target sequence in a clinical specimen can be coamplified in a single tube. The primers used in multiplexed reactions must be selected carefully to have similar annealing temperatures and must be noncomplementary to each other to avoid primer-dimers and inefficient reactions. Multiplex PCRs are more complicated to develop and are often less sensitive than single-primer-set PCR reactions, but they allow multiple targets to be detected from a single specimen in one reaction.

A promising new platform for multiplex PCR analysis is the xMAP system (Luminex Corp., Austin, Tex.). The xMAP system incorporates a proprietary process to internally dye polystyrene microspheres with two spectrally distinct fluorochromes. By using precise ratios of these fluorochromes, an array is created consisting of 100 different microsphere sets with specific spectral addresses. Each microsphere set can possess a different reactant on its surface. For nucleic acid analysis, oligonucleotide probes would be covalently bound to the microsphere surface by carbodiimide coupling. Because each microsphere set can be distinguished by its spectral address, the sets can be combined, allowing up to 100 different analytes to be measured simultaneously in a single reaction vessel. A third fluorochrome coupled to a reporter molecule quantifies the biomolecular interaction that occurs at the microsphere surface.

Microspheres are interrogated individually in a rapidly flowing liquid stream as they pass by two separate lasers in the Luminex xMAP flow cytometer. High-speed digital signal processing classifies each microsphere based on its spectral address and quantifies the reaction on its surface. Thousands of microspheres are investigated per second, resulting in an analysis system capable of analyzing and reporting up to 100 different reactions in a single reaction vessel in a few seconds.

Multiplex assays run on the Luminex platform typically consist of three major steps: nucleic acid amplification by PCR, target specific extension, and liquid bead array decoding (Merante, 2007). The steps in a Luminex xMAP assay are shown in Figure 66-2. After PCR amplification, the amplicons are mixed with a second set of tagged primers specific for each target. If the target is present, the tagged primer will be extended through a process called *target specific extension*. During this extension a label is incorporated into the extension product. The color-coded beads are added to identify the tagged and labeled extension products. Attached to each differently colored bead is oligonucleotide complementary to the tag sequence for each target. Samples are then placed in the Luminex xMAP flow cytometer where the beads are read by two color lasers. One laser identifies the color of the bead and the other laser detects the presence or absence of a labeled extension product on that bead.

Another promising technology for high-order multiplex PCR is the Film Array developed by Idaho Technology, Salt Lake City, Utah. It is a completely automated, integrated, and self-contained lab-in-a-pouch system. The film portion of the pouch has stations for cell lysis, nucleic acid purification, reverse transcription to detect RNA targets, first stage PCR multiplex PCR, and an array of up to 120 second-stage nested PCRs. After extracting and purifying nucleic acids from the unprocessed sample, the Film Array performs a nested multiplex PCR that is executed in two stages. During the first stage PCR, the Film Array performs a single, large-volume, massively multiplexed reaction. The products from first stage PCR are then diluted and combined with a fresh, primer-free master mix. Aliquots of this second master mix solution are then distributed to each well of the array. Each well of the array is prespotted with a single set of primers. In the second stage, small-volume PCR is performed in singleplex fashion in each well of the array. Even though this assay uses nested PCR, the entire test is performed within a sealed pouch, thus eliminating concerns of carryover contamination. Using amplification and melting curve data, the Film Array software automatically generates a result for each target. A Film Array for detection of 20 different respiratory pathogens is in development.

End-Point Quantitative Polymerase Chain Reaction

A linear relationship should exist between the quantity of input template and the amount of amplification product. However, because the final amount of PCR product depends on exponential amplification of the initial quantity of template, minor differences in amplification efficiency may lead to very large and unpredictable differences in the final product yield (Clementi, 1993). The tube-to-tube differences may depend on sample preparation and nucleic acid purification procedures, presence of inhibitors, and thermal cycler performance. For these reasons, simple quantification of product accumulated at the end of the reaction and the use of external standard curves do not provide reliable quantification of the amount of template initially present in the sample.

A variety of PCR-based strategies have been developed to accurately quantify DNA and RNA targets in clinical specimens but the competitive PCR (cPCR) approach has proved reliable and robust for clinical applications (Gilliland, 1990; Piatak, 1993). The basic concept behind cPCR is the coamplification in the same reaction tube of two different templates of equal or similar lengths and with the same primer binding sequences. Because both templates are amplified with the same primer pair, identical thermodynamics and amplification efficiency are ensured. The amount of one of the templates must be known and, after amplification, products from both templates must be distinguishable. Different types of competitor have been used in cPCR but, in general, competitors that are similar in size and base composition to the target work most effectively. RNA competitors should be used in quantitative RT-PCRs to address the problem of variable RT efficiency.

The yield of PCR product is described by the equation, $Y = I(1 + e)n$, where Y is the quantity of PCR product, I is the quantity of template at the beginning of the reaction, e is the efficiency of the reaction, and n is the number of cycles. In cPCR, this equation is written for both templates, as follows: competitor, $Yc = Ic(1 + e)n$; and target, $Yt = It(1 + e)n$. Because e and n are the same for both the competitor and target, the relative product ratio Yc/Yt directly depends on their initial concentration ratio Ic/It and the function Yc/Yt = Ic/It is linear.

A single concentration of competitor is sufficient, in theory, to quantify an unknown amount of target without the use of a standard curve. However, because analysis of two template species present in a sample at widely different amounts may be difficult and imprecise in practice, cPCR using several concentrations of competitor within the expected concentration range of the target were generally performed. However, this approach provided no more accurate results than the use of a single concentration of competitor in a study of different approaches to standardization of cPCR (Haberhausen, 1998). The commercially available end-point quantitative PCR assays for HIV-1 and HCV (Amplicor Monitor Tests, Roche Diagnostics, Indianapolis) use a single concentration of a competitor to determine the initial concentration of the target.

End-point PCR is rapidly being replaced in the clinical laboratory by homogenous kinetic (real-time) methods for product detection (Barbeau, 2004) (see next section). These methods provide for more precise measurements of initial template concentrations because the analysis is performed early in the log phase of product accumulation and, as a result, are less prone to error resulting from differences in sample-to-sample amplification efficiency.

Real-Time (Homogeneous, Kinetic) Polymerase Chain Reaction

Real-time PCR describes methods by which the target amplification and detection steps occur simultaneously in the same tube (homogeneous). These methods require special thermal cyclers with precision optics that can monitor the fluorescence emission from the sample wells. The computer software supporting the thermocycler monitors the data throughout the PCR at every cycle (kinetic) and generates an amplification plot for each reaction. A typical amplification plot is shown in Figure 66-3. The amplification plot shows the normalized fluorescence signal from the reporter (Rn) at each cycle number. In the initial cycles there is little change in the amount of fluorescence. This defines the baseline of the plot. An increase above the baseline indicates detection of accumulated PCR product. A fixed fluorescence threshold can be set above the baseline to call positive samples. The PCR cycle at which the sample fluorescence passes the threshold is defined as the *cycle threshold* (CT). There is an inverse linear relationship between the log of the initial target concentration and the CT. Alternatively, the cycle number corresponding to the maximal rate change in fluorescence, the second derivative maximum, has a similar relationship to initial target concentration.

In the simplest format, PCR product is detected as it is produced using fluorescent dyes that preferentially bind to double-stranded DNA (dsDNA). SYBR Green I is one such dye that has been used in this application (Morrison, 1998). In the unbound state, the fluorescence is relatively low but when bound to dsDNA the fluorescence is greatly enhanced. The DNA-binding dye will bind to any dsDNA and therefore will bind both specific and nonspecific PCR products equally well. The specificity of the detection can be improved through melting curve analysis. As the temperature is raised slowly, the two strands of the amplicon melt apart and the amount of fluorescence decreases. The data are transformed and analyzed by plotting the first derivative of fluorescence on the y-axis and temperature on the x-axis. The specific amplified product will have a characteristic melting peak at its predicted melting temperature (T_m), whereas the primer dimers and other nonspecific products should have a different T_m or give broader peaks (Ririe, 1997).

The specificity of real-time PCR can also be increased by including hybridization probes in the reactions mixture. These probes are labeled with fluorescent dyes or with combinations of fluorescent and a quencher dye. In the 5′ nuclease (TaqMan) PCR assay, the 5′–3′ exonuclease activity of Taq DNA polymerase is used to cleave a nonextendable hybridization probe during the primer extension phase of PCR (Holland, 1991). This approach uses dual-labeled fluorogenic hybridization probes. One fluorescent dye serves as reporter and its emission spectrum is quenched by the second fluorescent dye. The nuclease degradation of the hybridization probe releases the reporter dye, resulting in an increase in its peak fluorescent emission (Fig. 66-4). The increase in fluorescent emission indicates that specific PCR product has been made and the intensity of fluorescence is related to the amount of product (Heid, 1996). Specificity is increased because signal is generated only when the primer and probe are bound to the same template strand.

Fluorescence resonance energy transfer (FRET) probes can also be used to detect PCR product as it is generated (Lay, 1997). This method requires two specially designed sequence-specific oligonucleotide probes. These hybridization probes hybridize next to each other on the product molecule. As shown in Figure 66-5, the 3′ end of one probe is labeled with a donor dye and the 5′ end of the other probe is labeled with an acceptor dye. The donor dye is excited by an external light source and, instead of emitting light, transfers its energy to the acceptor dye by a process called FRET. The excited acceptor dye emits light at a longer wavelength than the unbound donor dye and the intensity of the acceptor dye light emission is proportional to the amount of PCR product.

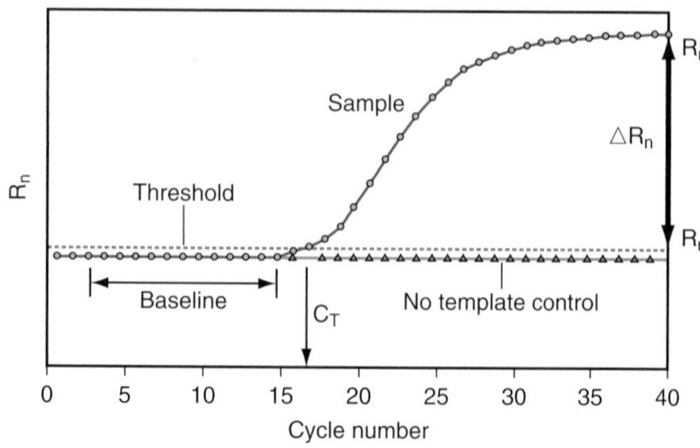

Figure 66-3 Real-time PCR amplification plot. *(Courtesy Applied Biosystems.) PCR,* Polymerase chain reaction.

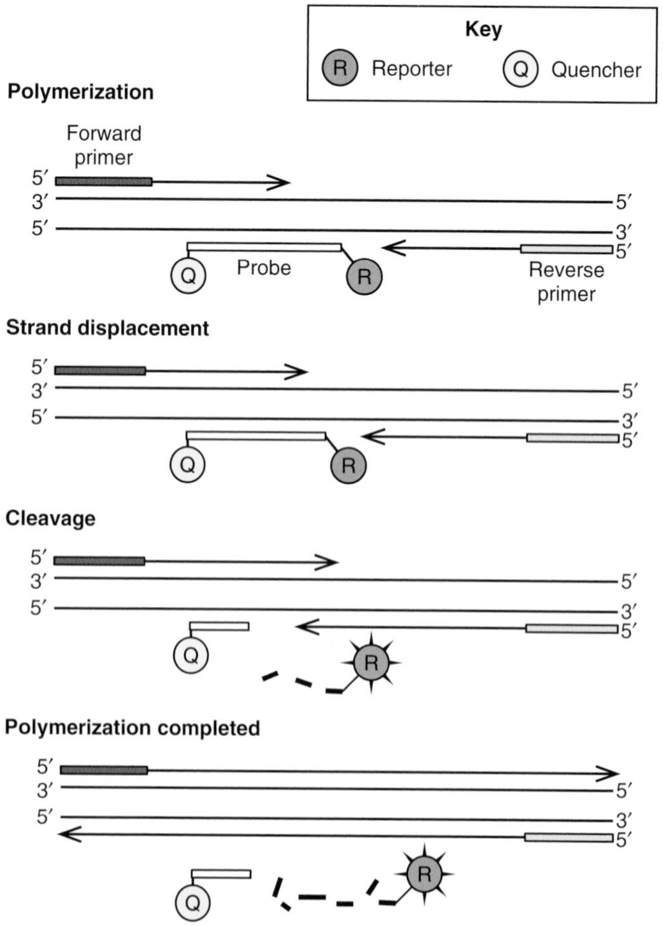

Figure 66-4 Mechanism of signal generation in 5′ nuclease PCR assays. *(Courtesy Applied Biosystems.) PCR,* Polymerase chain reaction.

Real-time detection and quantification of PCR product can also be accomplished using molecular beacons (Tyagi, 1998). Molecular beacons are hairpin-shaped oligonucleotide probes with an internally quenched fluorophore whose fluorescence is restored when they bind to a target nucleic acid (Fig. 66-6). They are designed in such a way that the loop portion of the probe molecule is complementary to the target sequence. The stem is formed by the annealing of complementary arm sequences on the ends of the probe. A fluorescent dye is attached to one end of one arm and a quenching molecule is attached to the end of the other arm. The stem keeps the fluorophore and quencher in close proximity such that no light emission occurs. When the probe encounters a target molecule, it forms a hybrid that is longer and more stable than the stem, and undergoes a conformational change that forces the stem apart and causes the fluorophore and quencher to move away from each other, restoring the fluorescence.

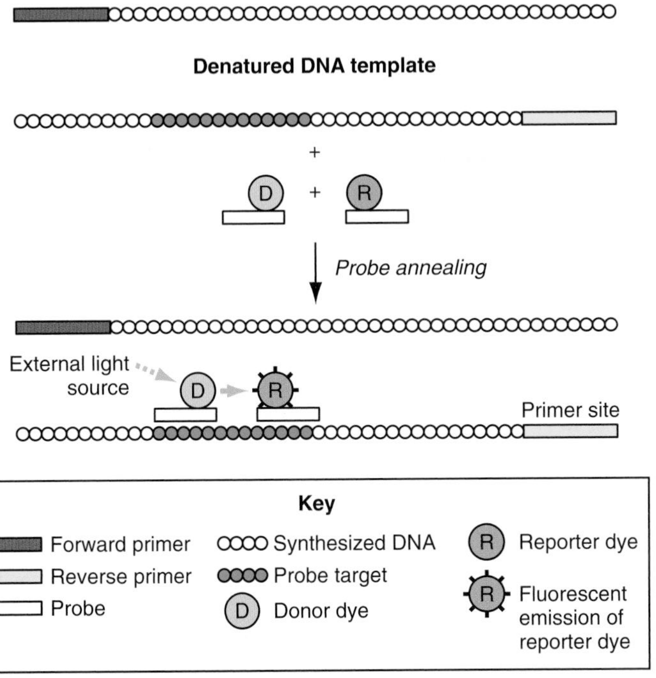

Figure 66-5 Fluorescence resonance energy transfer probes. *(Redrawn from Wolk D, Mitchell S, Patel R. Principles of molecular microbiology testing methods. Infect Dis Clin N Am 2008;15(4):1157–1204.)*

It is not absolutely necessary to have a stem loop structure to use nonhydrolyzable probes in real-time PCR applications. Dark quencher probes contain a fluorophore on the 5′ end, and a nonfluorescent quencher molecule on the 3′ end (Afonina, 2002). The fluorescence is quenched when the probe is in a random coil configuration and emitted when the probe anneals to the target sequence. Similar to molecular beacons or FRET probes, the DNA polymerase does not degrade these probes during target amplification. Because the dark quencher is not fluorescent, it does not contribute to background signal. This has the advantage of improved signal-to-noise ratio for the detection system, which may improve sensitivity. These probes also incorporate a hybridization-stabilizing compound, known as a *minor groove binder*. It is a small, crescent-shaped molecule that is covalently linked to 3′ end of the probe that spans about 3–4 nt and snugly fits into the minor groove of DNA where it forms hydrogen bonds with the template. The minor groove binder allows the use of shorter probes and enables improved Tm leveling, which improves the specificity of the detection reaction (Kutyavin, 2000).

Scorpion probes combine a PCR primer with a molecular beacon (Thelwell, 2000). Intramolecular hybridization of the loop structure to a downstream portion of the amplification product separates the reporter and quencher dyes. The hybridization kinetics of scorpion probes is generally faster than those of molecular beacons because the primer and probe are located on the same molecule.

Another approach to detection, characterization, and quantification of real-time PCR amplicons involves the use of a nonstandard DNA base pair constructed from isoG and isoC (Sherrill, 2004). These synthetic bases pair with each other, but not with the natural bases guanine and cytosine and can be covalent coupled to a wide variety of reporter groups. In the MultiCode-RTx assays (EraGen Biosciences, Madison, Wis.) the target is amplified using a forward primer with a single isoC nucleotide with fluorescent label at 5′end and an unlabeled standard base reverse primer. Amplification is performed in the presence of isoG coupled to a fluorescence quencher molecule and site-specific incorporation by the DNA polymerase place the quencher in close proximity to the fluorophore resulting in a decrease of fluorescence with every PCR cycle. The number of cycles in which the fluorescence change can be detected is dependent on the initial number of target molecules in the reaction. The decrease in fluorescence is easily monitored by a number of different standard real-time PCR instruments. Postreaction amplicon melting curve analysis can be performed to confirm the identity of the amplicon and to detect sequence variants.

Real-time PCR methods decrease the time required to perform nucleic acid assays because there are no post-PCR processing steps. Also, because amplification and detection occur in the same closed tube, these methods eliminate the postamplification manipulations that can lead to laboratory contamination with amplicon. In addition, real-time PCR methods lend themselves well to quantitative applications because analysis is performed

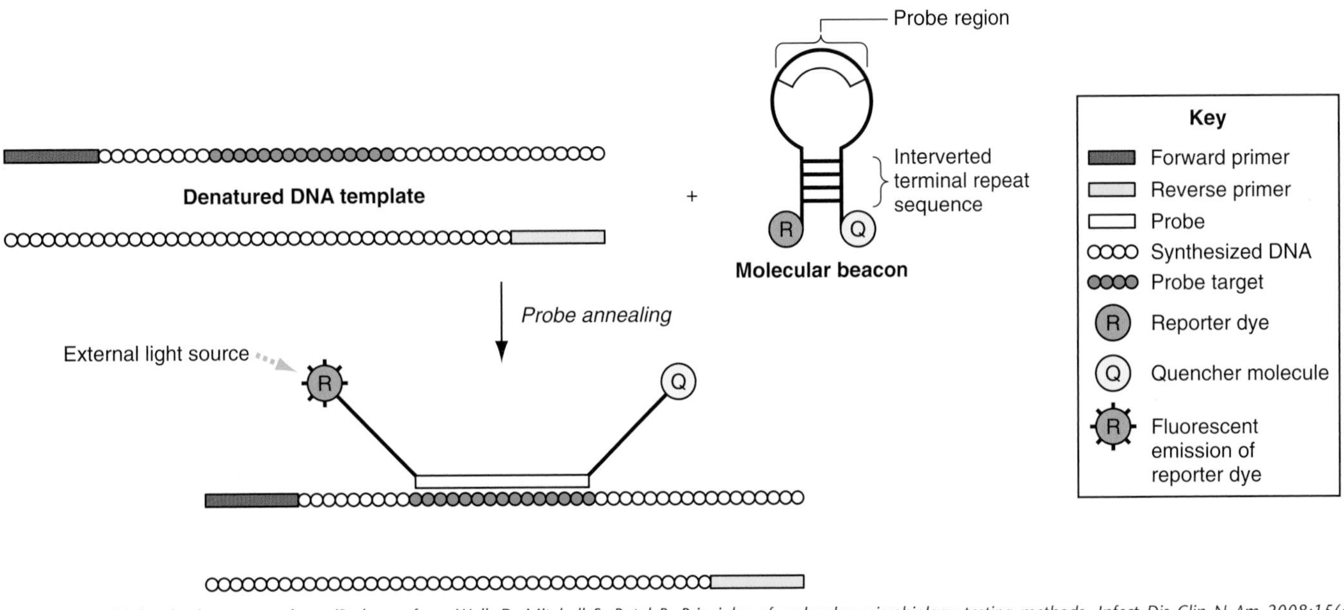

Figure 66-6 Molecular beacon probes. *(Redrawn from Wolk D, Mitchell S, Patel R. Principles of molecular microbiology testing methods. Infect Dis Clin N Am 2008;15(4): 1157–1204.)*

early in the log phase of product accumulation and as a result are less prone to error that may result from differences in amplification efficiency between samples.

Relative concentrations of DNA present during the exponential phase of the reaction are determined by plotting fluorescence against cycle number on a logarithmic scale (so an exponentially increasing quantity will give a straight line). A threshold for detection of fluorescence above background is determined and the CT determined. The quantity of DNA theoretically doubles every cycle during the exponential phase and relative amounts of DNA can be calculated (e.g., a sample whose C_t is three cycles earlier than another's has $2^3 = 8$ times more template). Because all sets of primers do not work equally well, one has to calculate the reaction efficiency first. Thus, by using this as the base and the cycle difference $C_{(t)}$ as the exponent, the precise difference in starting template can be calculated (in previous example, if efficiency was 1.96, then the sample would have 7.53 times more template).

Amounts of RNA or DNA are then determined by comparing the results to a standard curve produced by real-time PCR of serial dilutions (e.g., undiluted, 1:4, 1:16, 1:64) of a known amount of RNA or DNA. As mentioned earlier, to accurately quantify gene expression, the measured amount of RNA from the gene of interest is divided by the amount of RNA from a housekeeping gene measured in the same sample to normalize for possible variation in the amount and quality of RNA between different samples. This normalization permits accurate comparison of expression of the gene of interest between different samples, as long as the expression of the reference (housekeeping) gene used in the normalization is very similar across all the samples. Choosing a reference gene that fulfills this criterion is therefore of high importance, and often challenging, because only very few genes show equal levels of expression across a range of different conditions or tissues.

Real-time PCR can be used to quantify nucleic acids by two strategies—relative quantification and absolute quantification (VanGuilder, 2008). Relative quantification measures the fold-difference (2×, 3×, etc.) in the target amount. For gene expression analysis, relative concentrations may be determined by the $2^{-\Delta\Delta CT}$ method in which for each sample the difference in CT values for the gene of interest and the endogenous gene control is calculated (ΔCT). Next, subtraction of the control-condition ΔCT from the treated-condition ΔCT yields the ΔΔCT. The negative value of this subtraction, −ΔΔCT, is used as the exponent of 2 in the equation and represents the difference in corrected number of cycles to threshold. This value is often referred to as the *relative quantity value.*

Absolute quantification gives the exact number of target molecules present by comparing with known standards. The quality of standard is important for accurate quantification.

Rapid-Cycle Polymerase Chain Reaction

While real-time PCR methods have had a significant impact on assay time, a great deal of emphasis continues to be placed on reducing the assay time for the various PCR formats. Rapid-cycle PCR is not chemically different from any of the standard PCR formats (Wittwer, 1991). The polymerases used in PCR are capable of incorporating 35–100 nucleotides per second. Most of the time consumed in performing PCR is temperature equilibration for the solution so that efficient annealing and extension occur, as well as significant amount of time changing the temperature. By reducing the thermal profile of the solution using thin-walled tubes or capillaries that force the reaction solution into thin columns or sheets of fluid, it is possible to improve thermal transfer rates as well as equilibration rates such that thermocycling time can be significantly reduced. In highly optimized systems, it is possible to approach the ideal processivity rate of the polymerase such that a 40-cycle PCR may be performed in 30 minutes or less using standard or real-time PCR chemistries.

Digital Polymerase Chain Reaction

PCR exponentially amplifies nucleic acids and the number of amplification cycles and the amount of amplicon allows the computation of the starting quantity of targeted nucleic acid. However, many factors complicate this calculation, often creating uncertainties and inaccuracies particularly when the starting concentration is low. Digital PCR attempts to overcome these difficulties by transforming the exponential data from conventional PCR to digital signals that simply indicate whether or not amplification occurred (Vogelstein, 1999).

Digital PCR is accomplished by capturing or isolating each individual nucleic acid molecule present in a sample within many chambers, zones, or regions that are able to localize and concentrate the amplification product to detectable levels. After PCR amplification, a count of the areas containing PCR product is a direct measure of the absolute quantity of nucleic acid in the sample. The capture or isolation of individual nucleic acid molecules may be done in capillaries, microemulsions, arrays of miniaturized chambers, or on surfaces that bind nucleic acids. Digital PCR has many applications including detection and quantification of low levels of pathogen sequences, rare genetic sequences, gene expression in single cells, and clonal amplification of nucleic acids for sequencing mixed nucleic acid samples. Clonal amplification enabled by digital PCR is a key element of many of the "next-generation" sequencing methods.

TRANSCRIPTION-BASED AMPLIFICATION

Transcription-based amplification includes transcription-mediated amplification (TMA) and nucleic acid sequence-based amplification (NASBA). Both TMA and NASBA are isothermal nucleic acid amplification techniques that, although slightly different in practice, are identical in concept, and are described together (Kwoh, 1989; Compton, 1991). TMA and NASBA are the intellectual properties of Gen-Probe, San Diego, and bioMérieux, Durham, N.C., respectively. These techniques essentially recapitulate retroviral replication in vitro, converting RNA into DNA and then using the DNA as a template for transcription of multiple copies of RNA.

The process begins with an RNA target, which in most cases exists as a single-stranded entity, removing the need for thermal denaturation of the template before amplification (Fig. 66-7). A sequence-specific DNA primer binds to the RNA target. Reverse transcriptase then extends the primer, creating a DNA–RNA heteroduplex. The 5′ end of the sequence-specific primer contains the promoter for a T7 bacteriophage polymerase. The presence of this T7 promoter in the 5′ end of the primer results in the synthesis of a DNA strand complementary to the initial RNA target containing the T7 promoter at its 5′ end. In the case of TMA, the reverse-transcriptase enzyme itself degrades the initial RNA template as it synthesizes its complementary DNA. In NASBA, a separate enzyme, RNAse H, degrades the initial RNA template. RNAse H selectively cleaves RNA, which is heteroduplexed to DNA, but not RNA alone. In either case, the resultant single-stranded, complementary DNA with the T7 promoter sequence binds to a second primer at its 3′ end. The DNA polymerase extends from this second primer, resulting in the synthesis of a dsDNA molecule containing an intact T7 promoter. This DNA molecule can now serve as a template for T7 polymerase, a bacteriophage enzyme that specifically recognizes the T7 promoter and synthesizes multiple copies of RNA. Each of these newly synthesized RNA molecules is antisense to the initial target, allowing it to hybridize to the second primer. The reverse-transcriptase, second primer, RNAse H, and DNA polymerase then use this antisense RNA molecule as a template to synthesize new dsDNA templates, which in turn make more RNA template. A 10^9-fold amplification of target RNA can be achieved with these methods in 2 hours or less.

TMA and NASBA have several distinct advantages over other RNA amplification techniques. Perhaps the most significant of these advantages is that no initial denaturation is required for the amplification to occur. Hence, dsDNA sequences are not denatured, and thus are incapable of binding to primers in the reaction. DNA contamination can be particularly problematic when techniques such as PCR are used to assay for the RNA transcripts of retroviral or intronless eukaryotic genes. NASBA and TMA eliminate the problem of DNA contamination giving a falsely elevated determination of RNA. A second advantage is that this technology uses isothermal processes that obviate the need for sophisticated thermocyclers because the whole process occurs at a single temperature. Combining this technology with molecular beacons or other sequence-specific probes that can be added directly to the amplification mixture creates a closed-tube system, which aids in preventing amplicon cross-contamination in the laboratory.

NASBA and TMA have been used successfully in a wide variety of applications. They have been used to detect a number of pathogens, including viruses such as HIV, HCV, varicella zoster virus, cytomegalovirus (CMV), rhinovirus, enterovirus, measles, human papillomavirus, and bacteria such as *Mycobacterium tuberculosis*, *Neisseria gonorrhoeae*, *Chlamydia trachomatis*, *Mycoplasma pneumoniae*, and *Campylobacter jejuni*. In addition, quantitative tests for HIV and HCV have been developed using this technology. Furthermore, human genetic applications such as human leukocyte antigen typing and factor V Leiden mutation detection have been described.

In summary, TMA and NASBA are isothermal RNA amplification techniques with a widespread applicability and several unique advantages over other amplification methods, especially for the elimination of DNA

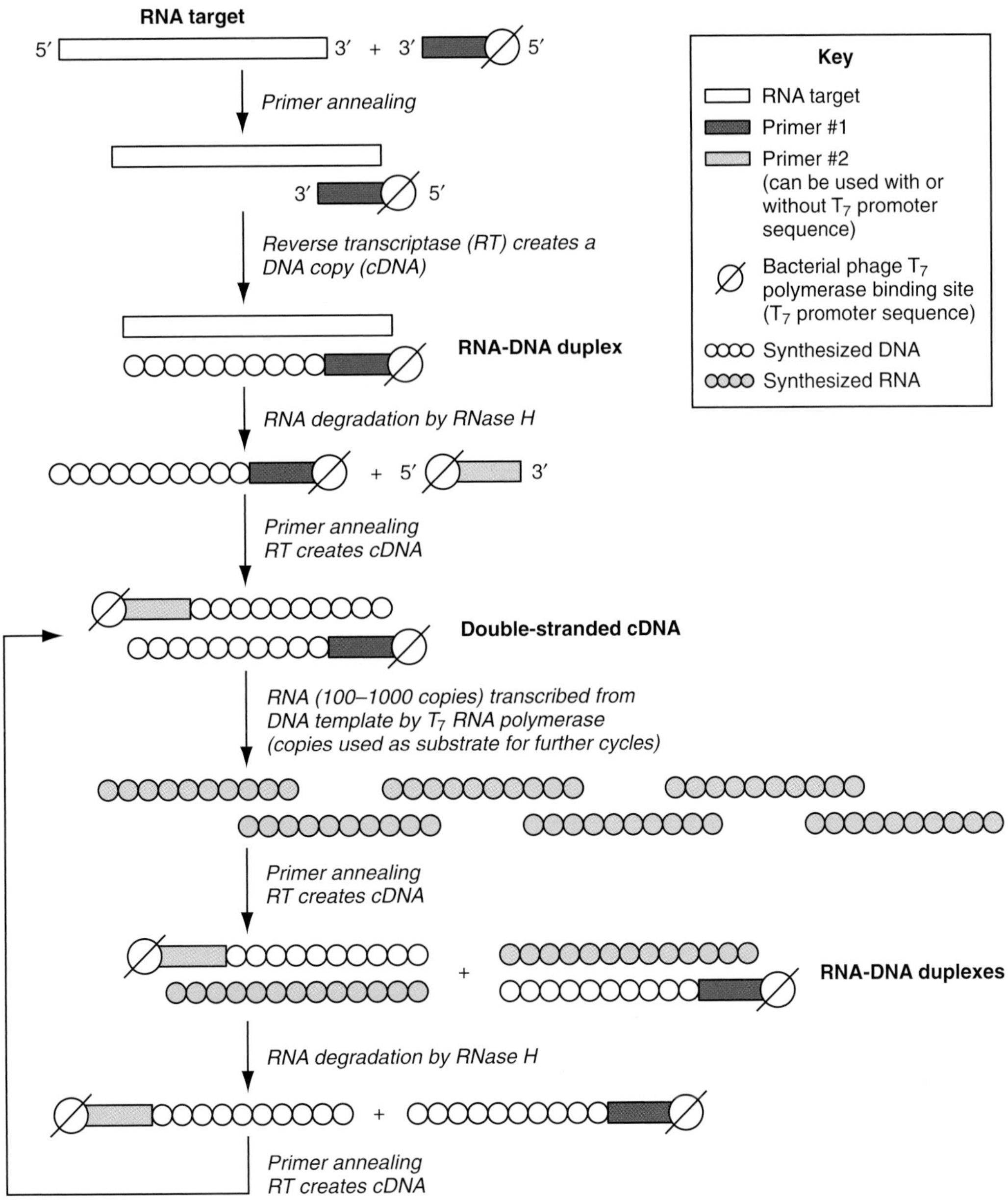

Figure 66-7 Transcription-based amplification. *(Redrawn from Wolk D, Mitchell S, Patel R. Principles of molecular microbiology testing methods. Infect Dis Clin N Am 2008;15(4):1157–1204.)*

contamination issues, particularly those related to retroviral and intronless genes. Combining these techniques with fluorescent probes allows one-step, closed-tube, real-time amplification without the need for thermal cycling.

STRAND-DISPLACEMENT AMPLIFICATION

Strand-displacement amplification (SDA) is an isothermal template amplification technique that can be used to detect trace amounts of DNA or RNA of a particular sequence. SDA as it was first described was a conceptually straightforward amplification process with some technical limitations (Walker, 1992a, 1992b). Since its initial description, however, it has evolved into a highly versatile tool that is technically simple to perform but conceptually complex. In its current iteration, SDA occurs in two discrete phases: target generation and exponential target amplification (Little, 1999). Only the target amplification phase is shown in Figure 66-8. In the target generation phase, a dsDNA target is denatured and hybridized to two different primer pairs, designated as *bumper* and *amplification* primers. The amplification primers include the single-stranded restriction endonuclease enzyme sequence for BsoB1 located at the 5′ end of the target binding sequence. The bumper primers are shorter and anneal to the target DNA just upstream of the region to be amplified. In the presence of BsoB1, an exonuclease-free DNA polymerase, and a dNTP mixture consisting of dUTP, dATP, dGTP, and thiolated dCTP (Cs), simultaneous extension products of both the bumper and amplification primers are generated. This process displaces the amplification primer products, which are available for hybridization with the opposite-strand products with the opposite-strand bumper and amplification primers.

The simultaneous extension of opposite-strand primers produces strands complementary to the products formed by extension of the first amplification primer with Cs incorporated into the BsoB1 cleavage site. This product enters the exponential target amplification phase of the reaction. The BsoB1 enzyme recognizes the double-stranded site, but because one strand contains Cs, it is nicked rather than cleaved by the enzyme. The DNA polymerase then binds to the nick and begins synthesis of a new strand while simultaneously displacing the downstream strand. This step recreates the double-stranded species with the hemimodified restriction endonuclease recognition sequence, and the iterative nicking and displacement process repeats. The displaced strands are capable of binding to opposite-strand primers, which produces exponential amplification of the target sequences.

These single-stranded products also bind to detector probes for real-time detection. The detector probes are single-stranded DNA (ssDNA) molecules with fluorescein and rhodamine labels. The region between the labels includes a stem-loop structure. The loop contains the recognition site for the BsoB1 enzyme. The target specific sequences are located 3′ to

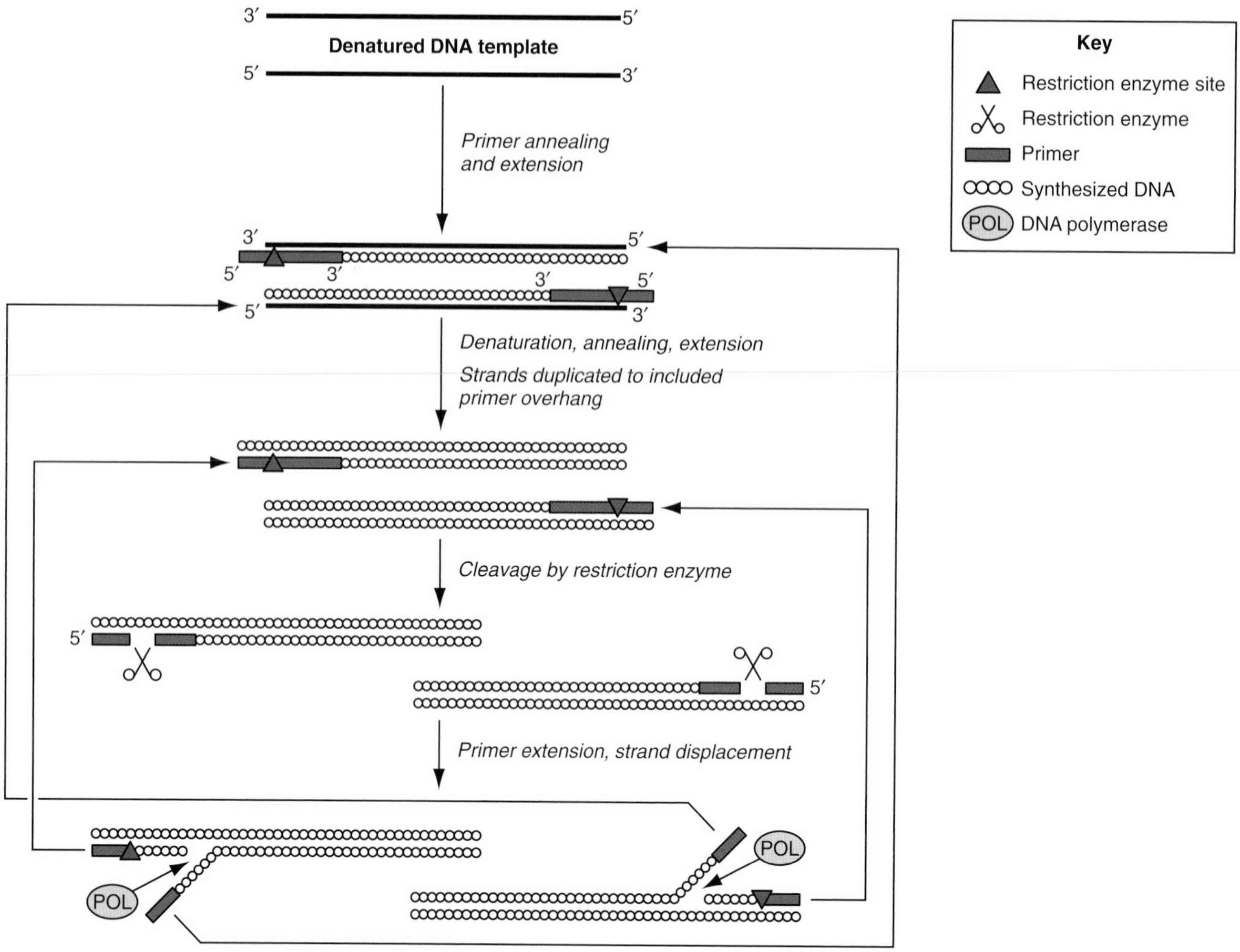

Figure 66-8 Strand displacement amplification. *(Redrawn from Wolk D, Mitchell S, Patel R. Principles of molecular microbiology testing methods. Infect Dis Clin N Am 2008;15(4):1157–1204.)*

the rhodamine label. In the absence-specific target the stem-loop structure is maintained with the fluorescein and rhodamine labels in close proximity. The net effect is that very little emission for the fluorescein is detected after excitation. After SDA, the probe is converted to a double-stranded species, which is cleaved by BsoB1. The cleavage causes physical separation of the fluorescein and rhodamine labels, which results in an increase in emission from the fluorescein label.

The diagnostic applications of SDA include the direct detection of *M. tuberculosis*, *C. trachomatis*, and *N. gonorrhoeae* in clinical specimens. SDA has a reported sensitivity high enough to detect as few as 10–50 copies of a target molecule (Walker, 1992a). By using a primer set designed to amplify a repetitive sequence with 10 copies in the *M. tuberculosis* genome, the assay is sensitive enough to detect 1–5 genome copies of the bacterium. Recently, SDA has been adapted to quantify RNA by adding a reverse-transcriptase step (RT-SDA). In this case, a primer hybridizes to the target RNA and a reverse-transcriptase synthesizes a cDNA. This cDNA can then serve as a template for primer incorporation and strand displacement. The products of this strand displacement then feed into the amplification scheme described. RT-SDA has been used for the determination of HIV viral load (Nycz, 1998).

The main advantage of SDA is that it is an isothermal process that, unlike PCR, can be performed at a single temperature after initial target denaturation. This eliminates the need for expensive thermocyclers. Furthermore, samples can be subjected to SDA in a single tube, with amplification times varying from 30 minutes to 2 hours. The main disadvantage of SDA lies in the fact that, unlike PCR, the relatively low temperature at which SDA is carried out (52.5° C) can result in nonspecific primer hybridization to sequences found in complex mixtures such as genomic DNA. Hence, when the target is in low abundance compared to background DNA, nonspecific amplification products can swamp the system, decreasing the sensitivity of the technique. However, the use of organic solvents to increase stringency at low temperatures and the recent introduction of more thermostable polymerases capable of strand displacement have alleviated much of this problem.

LOOP-MEDIATED AMPLIFICATION

Loop-mediated amplification (LAMP) is an isothermal method that relies on autocycling strand displacement DNA synthesis by *Bst* DNA polymerase and a set of four to six primers (Notomi, 2000). Two inner and two outer primers define the target sequence and an additional set of loop primers are added to increase the sensitivity of the reaction. The final products of the LAMP reaction are DNA molecules with a cauliflower-like structure of multiple loops consisting of repeats of the target sequence. The products can be analyzed in real-time by monitoring of the turbidity in the reaction tube resulting from production of magnesium pyrophosphate precipitate during the DNA amplification. Amplification products can also be visualized in agarose gels after electrophoresis and staining with ethidium bromide or SYBR Green.

Because LAMP is an isothermal process and positive reactions can be detected by simple turbidity measurements or visualized directly with the naked eye it requires no expensive equipment. These attributes make it an attractive technology for resource-poor settings and field use. However, primer design for LAMP is more complex than for PCR with specialized training and software required for their design. Meridian Bioscience, Inc. (Cincinnati, Ohio) has licensed LAMP technology from Eiken Chemical Company, Ltd., Japan, for the development of infectious disease diagnostics in the United States.

HELICASE-DEPENDENT AMPLIFICATION

Helicase-dependent amplification (HDA) is an isothermal process developed by BioHelix, Beverly, Mass., that uses helicase to separate dsDNA and generate single-stranded templates for primer hybridization

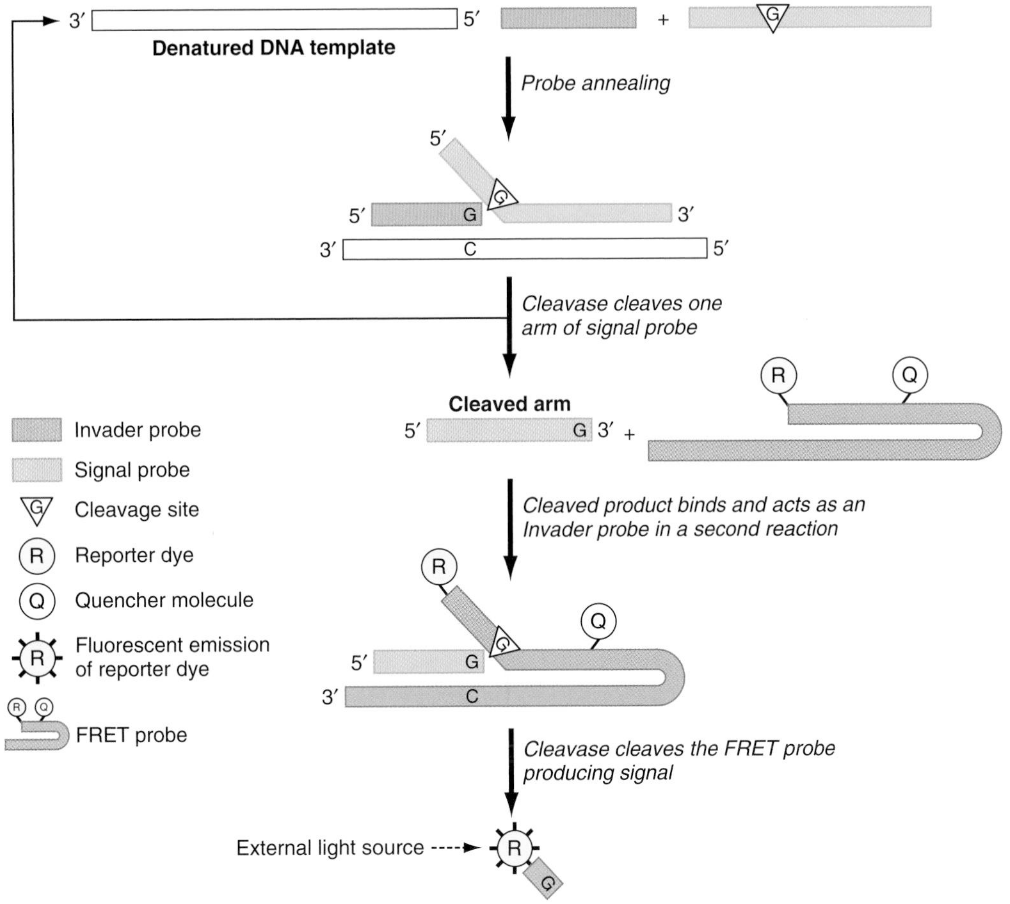

Figure 66-9 Invasive cleavage and detection of an oligonucleotide probe using a FEN-1 DNA polymerase. *(Redrawn from Wolk D, Mitchell S, Patel R. Principles of molecular microbiology testing methods. Infect Dis Clin N Am 2008;15(4):1157–1204.) FEN-1,* Flap endonuclease-1; *FRET,* fluorescence resonance energy transfer.

and subsequent extension by a DNA polymerase (Vincent, 2004). As the helicase unwinds dsDNA enzymatically, the initial heat denaturation and subsequent thermocycling steps required by PCR can all be omitted. In HDA, strands of dsDNA are separated by the DNA helicase and the ssDNA coated ssDNA-binding proteins. Two sequence-specific primers hybridize to each border of the target sequence and a DNA polymerase extend the primers annealed to the target sequence to produce dsDNA. The two newly synthesized products are used as substrates by the helicase in the next round of amplification. Thus a simultaneous chain reaction proceeds, resulting in exponential amplification of the selected target sequence.

HDA is compatible with multiple detection technologies, including qualitative and quantitative fluorescent technologies and with instruments designed for real-time PCR (Tong, 2008). Futhermore, HDA has shown potential for the development of simple, portable DNA diagnostic devices to be used in the field or at the point-of-care.

Probe Amplification Methods

Probe amplification methods differ from target amplification in that the amplification products contain a sequence only present in the initial probes. Cleavase/invader technology is an example of probe amplification method that is used currently as an important diagnostic application, the detection of high-risk genotypes of human papilloma viruses (HPV) in cervical samples (Ginocchio, 2008).

CLEAVASE/INVADER TECHNOLOGY

Cleavase/invader technology is a probe amplification method that relies on the specific recognition and cleavage of particular DNA structures by members of the flap endonuclease-1 family of DNA polymerases (Lyamichev, 1999). These polymerases cleave the 5′ single-stranded flap of a branched base-paired duplex and are termed *cleavases*. This enzymatic activity probably plays an essential role in the elimination of complex nucleic acid structures that arise during DNA replication and repair in vivo. Because these structures may occur anywhere in the replicating genome, the enzyme recognizes the molecular structure of the substrate without regard to the sequence of the nucleic acids making up the DNA complex (Lieber, 1996). This enzymatic activity has proved to be a very useful tool for DNA analysis and is the basis of this technology.

In cleavase/invader assays two primers are designed that hybridize to the target sequence in an overlapping fashion (Fig. 66-9). Under the proper annealing conditions, signal and invader probes bind to the target sequence such that the invader hybridizes upstream of the signal probe with a region of overlap between the 3′ end of invader and the 5′ end of signal probe. Under the proper conditions, the overlap of binding sites for the primers results in a displacement equilibrium between the primers. Cleavase only cleaves 5′ flaps; thus the 5′ end of the signal probe is released. The target sequence acts as a scaffold upon which the proper DNA structure can form. Because the DNA structure that serves as the cleavase substrate only occurs in the presence of the target sequence, the generation of cleavage products indicates the presence of the target. The cleaved product is detected by binding to and serving as an invader probe for a FRET probe. The 5′ end of the FRET probe is cut by cleavase, releasing the reporter molecule in the same way that it releases the 5′ end of the signal probe.

Use of a thermostable cleavase enzyme allows the reactions to be run at high enough temperatures for a primer exchange equilibrium to exist. This allows multiple cleavase products to form from a single target molecule. Hence, the invader assay can be run under isothermal conditions, removing the need for thermal cycling. This technology has been used for detection, quantification, and characterization of a variety of microbial and human nucleic acid targets (Rosetti, 1997; Ryan, 1999; Wong, 2008).

The cleavase/invader technology has several inherent advantages over other amplification strategies. Because of the fact that the overlap in the invader probe need only be one base pair, this technology can easily be adapted to detect point mutations of interest by designing the overlap region to encompass the mutation to be detected. In addition, unlike target amplification techniques in which the target sequence itself is amplified,

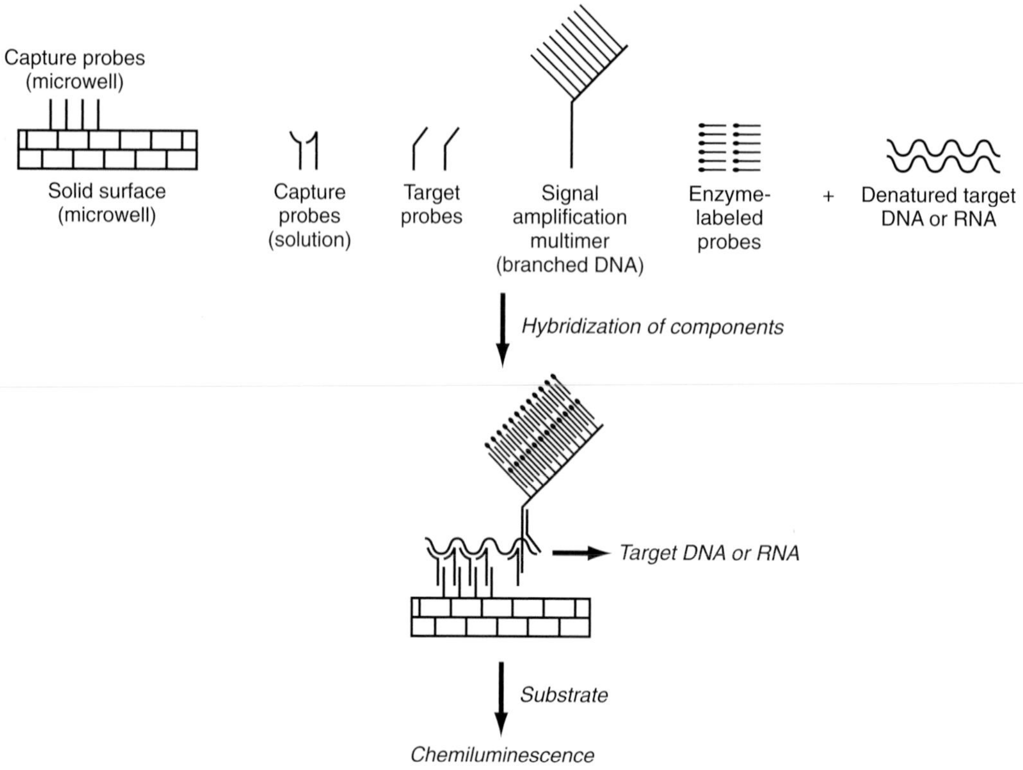

Figure 66-10 Branched DNA amplification. *(Redrawn from Wolk D, Mitchell S, Patel R. Principles of molecular microbiology testing methods. Infect Dis Clin N Am 2008;15(4):1157–1204.)*

the invader assay does not increase the amount of the target sequence. Thus the invader assay is less prone to problems of false-positive results due to amplicon cross-contamination.

In addition to the invader assay, cleavase can also be used to generate fragment-length polymorphisms (in a fashion analogous to restriction fragment-length polymorphism). By melting genomic DNA and cooling rapidly, highly reproducible hairpin loop secondary structures will form in the DNA that can serve as substrates for cleavase. Digestion of the DNA results in a distinct pattern that has been successfully employed to screen for interferon-α–resistant hepatitis C (Sreevatsan, 1998), and to detect specific mutations in human genes (Rosetti, 1997). Because hairpin loops occur with a greater diversity than most restriction enzyme recognition sites, this offers a versatile fragmentation pattern analysis.

Thus structure-specific endonucleases can be used to detect nucleic acid targets of a particular sequence, employed in assay for point mutations, and applied to generate diverse fragmentation patterns capable of distinguishing complex genotypes. These enzymes are powerful tools for nucleic acid analysis.

Signal Amplification Methods

In signal amplification methods, the concentration of probe or target does not increase. The increased analytical sensitivity comes from increasing the concentration of label molecules attached to the target nucleic acid. Multiple enzymes, multiple probes, multiple layers of probes, and reduction of background noise have been used to enhance target detection (Kricka, 1999). Target amplification systems generally have greater analytical sensitivity than signal amplification methods, but technological developments, particularly in branched DNA (bDNA) assays, have lowered the limits of detection to levels that may rival target amplification assays in some applications (Kern, 1996).

Signal amplification assays have several advantages over target amplification assays. In signal amplification systems, the number of target molecules is not altered and, as a result, the signal is directly proportional to the amount of target sequence present in the clinical specimen. This reduces concerns about false-positives due to cross contamination and simplifies the development of quantitative assays. Because signal amplification systems are not dependent on enzymatic processes to amplify target sequences, they are not affected by the presence of enzyme inhibitors in clinical specimens. Consequently, less cumbersome nucleic acid extraction methods may be used. Typically, signal amplification systems employ either larger probes or more probes than target amplification systems and, consequently, are less susceptible to errors resulting from target sequence heterogeneity. Finally, RNA can be measured directly, without the synthesis of a cDNA intermediate. Branched DNA and hybrid capture are examples of signal amplification systems that have developed into diagnostic tests.

BRANCHED DNA

The bDNA is a solid-phase, sandwich hybridization assay incorporating multiple sets of synthetic oligonucleotide probes (Nolte, 1998). The key to this technology is the amplifier molecule, a DNA molecule with 15 identical branches, each of which can bind three labeled probes.

Multiple target-specific probes are used to capture the target nucleic acid on to the surface of a microtiter well (Fig. 66-10). A second set of target-specific probes also binds to the target. Preamplifier molecules bind to the second set of target probes and up to eight bDNA amplifiers. Three alkaline-phosphatase-labeled probes hybridize to each branch of the amplifier. Detection of the bound labeled probes is achieved by incubating the complex with an enzyme-triggerable substrate, dioxetane, and then measuring the light emission in a luminometer. The resulting signal is directly proportional to the quantity of target in the sample. The quantity of target in the sample is determined from an external standard curve.

Nonspecific hybridization of any of the amplification probes and nontarget nucleic acids leads to amplification of the background signal. To reduce the hybridization potential to all nontarget, the nonnatural bases isocytidine (isoC) and isoguanosine (isoG) were incorporated into the amplification probes of the third-generation bDNA assays (Collins, 1995). IsoC and isoG bases pair with each other but not with any of the four naturally occurring bases (Piccirilli, 1990). The use of isoC and isoG probes in bDNA assays increases target-specific amplification without a concomitant increase in background, thereby greatly enhancing the detection limits. The detection limit of the third-generation bDNA assay for HIV-1 RNA is 50 copies/mL (Kern, 1996). bDNA assays for the quantification of HBV DNA, HCV RNA, and HIV-1 RNA are commercially available (Bayer Diagnostics). An instrument platform

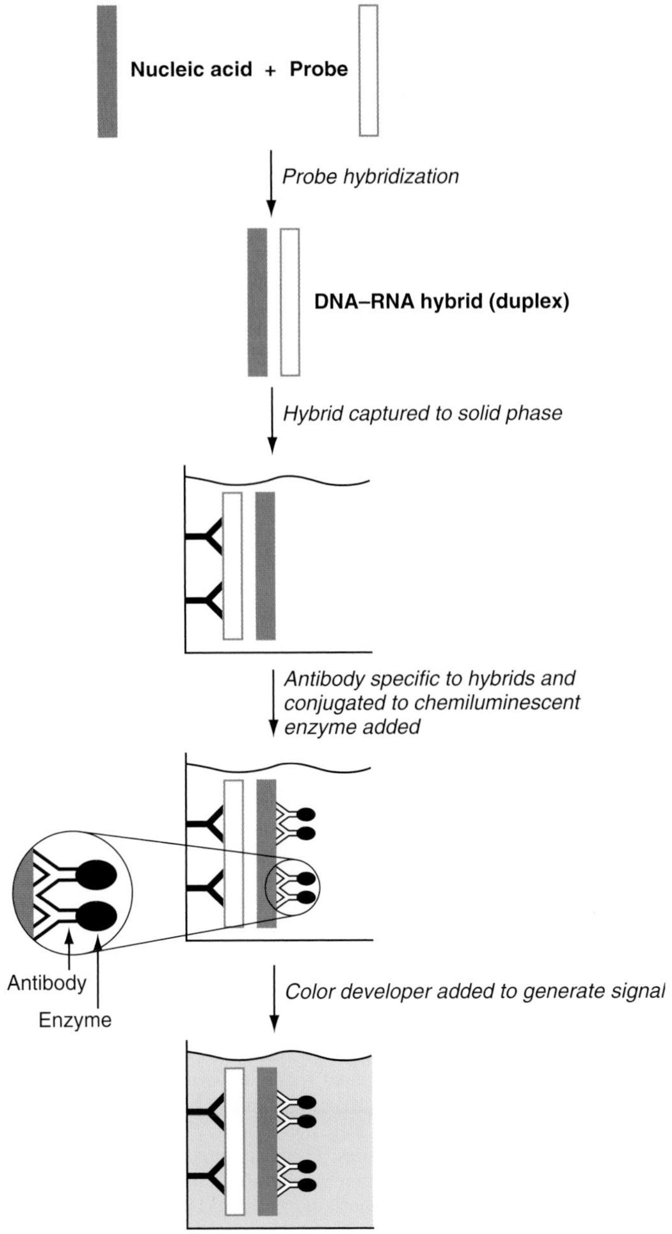

Figure 66-11 Hybrid capture amplification. *(Redrawn from Wolk D, Mitchell S, Patel R. Principles of molecular microbiology testing methods. Infect Dis Clin N Am 2008;15(4):1157–1204.)*

for bDNA assays automates the incubation, washing, reading, and data processing.

HYBRID CAPTURE ASSAYS

The hybrid capture system is a solution hybridization antibody capture assay that uses chemiluminescent detection. The target DNA in the specimen is denatured and hybridized with a specific RNA probe (Fig. 66-11). The DNA–RNA hybrids are captured by antibodies specific for DNA–RNA hybrids that are coated on to the surface of a tube. Alkaline-phosphatase–conjugated antihybrid antibodies bind to the immobilized hybrids. The bound enzyme–antibody conjugate is detected with a chemiluminescent substrate and the light emitted is measured in a luminometer. Signal amplification results from the large number of antibody binding sites and the efficiency of the enzyme–substrate reaction. The intensity of the emitted light is proportional to the amount of target DNA in the specimen. Hybrid capture assays for detection of HPV (Cope, 1997) and CMV (Mazzulli, 1999) in clinical specimens are commercially available (Digene, Gaithersburg, Md.).

Whole Genome Amplification

Many new techniques, such as array based comparative genomic hybridization, require large amounts of DNA and requests for molecular analysis of very minute samples are increasing. To facilitate these types of analyses, whole genome amplification may be employed to generate sufficient template. Whole genome amplification may be accomplished by a few methods. Multiple Displacement Amplification uses random hexamer primers and phi29 polymerase in an isothermal reaction (Dean, 2002). As the newly synthesized strands encounter primer positions downstream, they displace the product allowing further priming of that displaced strand in the opposite direction. The enzyme used must have high processivity, meaning that it synthesizes a long strand prior to disengaging the template. Other methods have been developed to convert fragmented DNA into "libraries" using a combination of nick translation and ligation of adapters with subsequent PCR amplification by universal primers (Rubicon Genomics, Ann Arbor, Mich.). Continued refinement of these techniques will allow more comprehensive molecular analysis of limited or precious clinical samples.

Summary

This chapter provides a basis for understanding the principles underlying the various nucleic acid amplification methods and their relative strengths and limitations. The technology has already had a tremendous impact on the diagnosis of infectious diseases and genetic disorders and promises to revolutionize the diagnosis and management of patients with cancer. The real power of the technology lies in its ability to cut across traditional disciplines in laboratory medicine. Consequently, a thorough understanding of the basic principles of nucleic acid amplification technology is important for all involved in the practice of laboratory medicine.

SELECTED REFERENCES

Afonina IA, Reed MW, Lusby E, et al. Minor groove binder-conjugated DNA probes for quantitative DNA detection by hybridization-triggered fluorescence. Biotechniques 2002;32:940–4.

This paper describes the development of second-generation real-time PCR probes employing DNA minor groove binders and a dark quencher, and their use in single nucleotide polymorphism detection, viral load determination, and gene expression analysis.

Holland PM, Abramson RD, Watson R, Gelfand DH. Detection of specific polymerase chain reaction product by utilizing the 5′ to 3′ exonuclease activity of *Thermus aquaticus* DNA polymerase. Proc Natl Acad Sci U S A 1991;88:7276–80.

This paper describes how the 5′ exonuclease activity of a DNA polymerase can be used to detect PCR products, which was a key factor in the development of real-time PCR.

Myers TW, Gelfand DH. Reverse transcription and DNA amplification by a *Thermus thermophilus* DNA polymerase. Biochemistry 1991;30:7661–6.

This paper is another milestone in the enzymology of PCR. It describes the use of a single thermostable enzyme to accomplish both the reverse-transcriptase and cDNA amplification, facilitating the development of one-step, closed-tube RT-PCR for RNA targets.

Ririe K, Rasmussen RP, Wittwer CT. Product differentiation by analysis of DNA melting curves during the polymerase chain reaction. Anal Biochem 1997;245:154–60.

This paper describes how melting curve analysis using a microvolume fluorometer integrated with a thermal cycler can be used to differentiate and identify PCR products by monitoring the double-stranded DNA binding dye SYBR green.

Saiki RK, Gelfand DH, Stoffel S, et al. Primer-directed enzymatic amplification of DNA with a thermostable DNA polymerase. Science 1988;239:487–91.

This seminal paper describes the use of a thermostable DNA polymerase to catalyze the polymerase chain reaction. This development made PCR much more 'user friendly' and paved the way for automation of the process.

REFERENCES

Access the complete reference list online at http://www.expertconsult.com

CHAPTER 67

HYBRIDIZATION ARRAY TECHNOLOGIES

Martin H. Bluth

KEY POINTS

- Array technology provides a unique and powerful approach to screen a sample for dozens to thousands of genes.
- Current array fabrications allow for diverse platforms with better detection and reduced cost for high-density applications.
- Positive signals are generated when a tagged nucleic acid moiety hybridizes with its complementary probe localized on a solid support (i.e., "chip").
- Care must be taken when performing and interpreting microarray experiments, because numerous factors must be considered in analysis.
- Numerous applications of array technology have been proposed in the past few years, ranging from molecular staging of tumors to the identification and characterization of microbial agents.
- Improvement of quality and yield of nucleic acid extraction from fixed and frozen tissues combined with continued miniaturization and cost reduction of platforms are making array technology more commonplace and user friendly.

In only a few short years, hybridization array technology, which enables the performance of thousands of simultaneous hybridization reactions on a solid substrate within a single analytical procedure, has gone from theoretical construct to practical reality. Such massively parallel determinations offer previously unimaginable opportunities for diagnostic application, ranging from gene sequencing and detection of genetic polymorphisms to measurement of gene expression profiles in cancer cells. Microarray-based systems offer a platform for quantifying the expression of thousands of genes at the same time. Therefore an unprecedented advantage of this technology is that it affords analysis of whole cassettes of genes, or patterns of gene expression, rather than analysis of one, two, or three genes at a time. The general schema for microarray processing includes the generation of nucleic acid (i.e., deoxyribonucleic acid [DNA]) complementary to genes of interest, that is laid out in microscopic quantities on solid surfaces at defined positions (the "probe") nucleic acid (genomic DNA or complementary DNA [cDNA]) from samples is added over the surface—cDNA binds and the presence of bound DNA is detected by fluorescence following laser excitation (for general review, see Friend, 2002).

It is clear that hybridization array technology has revolutionized the way we approach the study of disease. The one gene–one protein–one function approach is no longer the mainstay of scientific design. Array technology introduced a complicated mirror image of this approach, in other words, multiple functions, multiple proteins, multiple genes. The power of this technology lies in the "screening" capability that it provides. Under defined experimental conditions, one now has the ability to determine changes in the patterns of genes, identifying multiple genes acting in concert. These patterns can then be "mined" through various computer algorithms, grouped into functional categories (e.g., respiratory genes, inflammatory genes), and used to derive signatures diagnostic of disease or to generate novel hypotheses about pathogenesis and cell function. The relationship of these genes to one another (increased versus decreased expression) are determined and generally expressed as fold-change. Microarray findings of differential gene expression require confirmation by other techniques such as quantitative reverse-transcriptase polymerase chain reaction (RT-PCR) or additional independent microarray studies.

Once candidate genes or groups of genes are identified, classic approaches to gene function (i.e., gene knockout or gene knockdown) can then be employed to elucidate or validate gene function. More importantly, hybridization array technology, with subsequent data mining, allows genes not previously known to be associated with the disease to be considered, generating new paradigms for future study. Similar platforms can be used to sequence large genes and to scan the genome for single nucleotide polymorphisms and methylation sites. This chapter reviews the theoretical basis for the various matrix hybridization platforms and provides a perspective on their clinical application, both currently and in the future.

ARRAY TECHNOLOGIES

A hybridization array is the molecular equivalent of a spreadsheet, where each cell or address reveals a specific piece of data, usually inferred from the binding of a ligand to its specific target. The first array-based methods were exploited in immunoassays (Ekins, 1987, 1999) and arrays also have been proposed for parallel studies of diverse targets such as proteins, lipids, carbohydrates, and small molecules (Fodor, 1991; Pirrung, 1992; Southern, 1996a; Guschin, 1997; Schena, 1998). Similar to antigen–antibody interactions on immunoarrays, the fundamental principle of nucleic acid arrays is detection of specific hybridization between complementary strands. The principles of nucleic acid hybridization and an overview of various platforms are covered in Chapter 65. The effectiveness of solid-support hybridization formats was pioneered with the use of nitrocellulose membranes (Gillespie, 1965) for dot blots (Kafatos, 1979), line probes, and Southern blots (Southern, 1975). Changing the labeled entity from the probe to the sample was first referred to as *reverse line-blot* (or *dot blot*) hybridization, and led to the beginning of interrogating one sample for multiple potential targets. Moving from dozens to thousands of targets has come about rapidly over the last few years, driven in part by the unique convergence of microfabrication, robotics, and bioinformatics technologies and the demand for high-throughput genetic analysis resulting from the Human Genome Project.

The field is bursting with potential, and many investigators foresee diagnostic and prognostic applications in tumor classification, chemotherapeutic responsiveness, pathogen detection, monitoring antibiotic resistance, and characterizing inflammatory responses. Array technology may make the dream of personalized molecular medicine, where the genes of an individual patient may be assessed for risk factors and disease susceptibility and to predict response to therapy, a reality. Studies using gene expression profiling to predict diseases include identifying which trauma and burn patients will develop sepsis and multisystem organ failure (www.gluegrant.org); genes involved in the pathogenesis of chronic obstructive pulmonary disease (Wang, 2008); and which patients would likely have recurrence of cancer (Potti, 2006), among others. However, challenges of reproducibility and laboratory quality control remain to be addressed before this enormous potential is realized.

MACROARRAYS

The term *macroarray* has been applied to formats in which areas of probe localization, often called *features*, are large enough to be visualized without magnification. These have been manufactured on nylon or nitrocellulose membranes or as plastic strips with linear arrays of bound target. Because of the size of the features, the density of macroarrays is much lower than microarrays, ranging from a few dozen to hundreds or even thousands of probes. They are usually deposited on to the membrane by printing or dot blotting, then dried and stored for future use.

Nylon, plastic and glass (silicon wafer) are standard supports to make macroarrays. Nylon suffers several drawbacks when compared to silicon, which is a preferred matrix for hybridization arrays. Besides its porous nature, nylon displays high autofluorescence, limiting the sensitivity of fluorescence-based detection because of high background values. The latter also precludes the possibility to develop ratiometric (or two-color) assays. This approach uses two targets, each labeled with a different fluor. Most commonly, one is a constant reference control used in direct comparison to the unknown sample, with results expressed as a ratio of the two emitted fluorescent signals (Duggan, 1999).

Macroarrays are currently used for targeted applications. For example, some commercial arrays target all the known cytokine genes or those within specific signal transduction pathways that are activated during infectious and inflammatory processes. Other arrays, targeting the genes altered during oncogenesis, have been used in cancer research (e.g., Atlas Human Arrays, Clontech, Palo Alto, Calif., or GeneFilters, Research Genetics, Huntsville, Ala.). Other commercial applications, usually in kit format, are used to detect and type specific PCR products, such as in the cystic fibrosis mutation screen, or human leukocyte antigen typing or human papillomavirus typing. Furthermore, nylon-based arrays have been used to detect bacterial colony based gene expression (Barsalobres-Cavallari, 2006) and thyroid cancer detection (Durand, 2008). The advantages of macroarrays include the ability to use standard hybridization equipment, simplified reading or scanning, and affordability.

Some groups have been successful in producing high-density nylon arrays on a custom basis for gene discovery purposes (Gress, 1992; Takahashi, 1995; Granjeaud, 1996; Pietu, 1996; Clark, 1999; Durand 2008). Even in high-density configurations, the size of the nylon arrays requires a relatively large volume of hybridization fluid, a practical limitation with respect to generating probe from small amounts of diagnostic material. Because microarrays, rather than macroarrays, represent the high-density, high-throughput platform of choice, the bulk of this chapter focuses on applications of microarrays.

MICROARRAYS

Assay miniaturization saves time while cutting costs in biomedical diagnostic applications and research. Working with smaller volumes reduces reagent consumption, increases sample concentration, and improves reaction kinetics. These improvements allow the investigator to determine hundreds or thousands of results in the time formerly required for a single experiment. Microarrays are now available from several commercial suppliers, along with reading and fabrication equipment for custom manufacture of dedicated arrays for specific research or diagnostic applications.

MICROARRAY SUBSTRATES

A major distinction between microarrays and macroarrays consists of the choice of a nonporous solid support. By preventing diffusion of the target nucleic acids, nonporous surfaces (plastic, glass, or silicon substrates) allow faster hybridization kinetics and easier washing steps. In order to allow spatial discrimination of numerous reactions performed simultaneously, the molecular probes are bound to a solid surface in defined arrays. Deposition of probes on a solid substrate is also more amenable to automation and enables higher array densities with optimal image definition. These features apply to any type of microarray, from synthetic oligonucleotides to cloned cDNAs or PCR products (Southern, 1999). Most microarrays are now developed on glass. As opposed to plastic derivatives, glass transparency and lack of autofluorescence allows low-background, fluorescence-based detection. However, as materials science becomes more involved in array technologies, alternative substrates, including coated glass and plastic substrates, may become available.

MICROARRAY FABRICATION

3′-End functionalization (i.e., chemical modification) of nucleic acids—oligonucleotides, PCR products, cDNAs, or peptide nucleic acid oligomers—is required for covalent immobilization on either glass or polypropylene surfaces (Matson, 1995; Beier, 1999). For example, treatment of glass slides with silane allows amino-covered glass to bind amino-linked probes, using bifunctional molecules such as a dialdehyde or a diisothiocyanate (Case-Green, 1994; Guo, 1994). Alternatively, glass coating with a polycation (e.g., polylysine) allows direct charge-coupled binding of polyanionic DNA probes (Maskos, 1993a), an ultraviolet photocrosslinking step adds covalent bonds to the ionic interaction. Covalent binding is essential to permit stringent washes and therefore accurate discrimination of hybridized species. Several protocols have been published to address surface activation (Maskos, 1992; Beattie, 1995; Matson, 1995; Beier, 1999). An interesting alternative consists of deposition of small patches of activated polyacrylamide to which presynthesized oligonucleotides are attached by microinjection (Khrapko, 1991; Yershov, 1996; Guschin, 1997).

Packing density of probes attached to solid surfaces will influence greatly the performance of hybridization matrices. Poor coupling efficiency, which is often encountered on glass matrices, can result in low probe density and low signal : noise ratios. On the other hand, overly dense packing of oligonucleotides on to a solid surface causes spatial hindrance. This problem may be even more formidable with longer biomolecules such as cDNAs. Hybridization yields can be increased by up to two orders of magnitude by introducing spacers between the surface and the oligonucleotides (Southern, 1999). The longer the spacer, the better the hybridization but, interestingly, there is an optimal spacer length beyond which hybridization yield declines (Shchepinov, 1997; Duggan, 1999). For example, a 40-carbon atom spacer provides a reported 150-fold hybridization enhancement (Shchepinov, 1997). The density of oligonucleotides is approximately 0.1 pmol/mm^2 on a glass surface, two orders of magnitude less than on aminated polypropylene. Thus a potential advantage of glass over plastic matrices at present is an optimal oligonucleotide density associated with lower spatial hindrance (Southern, 1999). Improved surface chemistries may one day allow production of arrays on plastic sheets or films, which may dramatically reduce production costs. To this end, film-based chip arrays have recently been described (Erali, 2009).

The terminal composition (5′ end) of the oligonucleotides influences their duplex yield as measured by relative intensity. As expected, G : C rich 5′ extremities lead to a better yield than their homologues (same composition but different sequences) (Maskos, 1993b). Approaches to modify the 5′ end of oligonucleotides (e.g., covalent addition of a degenerated linker) can therefore be considered to minimize this contribution. Alternatively, knowledge that mismatches at the ends are less destabilizing and therefore more difficult to discriminate by hybridization (Southern, 1999) has led to clever improvements for detection of hybridization events. As polymerases and ligases are most sensitive to terminal (as opposed to internal) mismatches, enzymatic methods have been developed with improved detection stringency (solid-phase minisequencing [Pastinen, 1997, 1998; Syvanen, 1999], genetic-bit analysis [Nikiforov, 1994], or ligation-assays [Landegren, 1988; Nickerson, 1990]).

Commercially available arrays have been previously reviewed by Marshall (1998). Fabrication of microarrays falls into two broad categories: those made by direct probe delivery on to the solid surface and those made by in situ synthesis. A third method, developed by Nanogen (San Diego), consists of prefabricated oligonucleotides captured on to electroactive spots on silicon wafers (Edman, 1997; Sosnowski, 1997; Cheng, 1998; Heller, 1998; Jang, 2009). Modification of the electric field through independent, spatially addressable electrodes can speed up hybridization and, when the polarity is reversed, provide stringent washing (Edman, 1997). Recently, an approach using single-stranded large circular-sense molecules were utilized as probes for DNA microarrays and showed stronger binding signals than those of PCR-amplified cDNA probes (Doh, 2010).

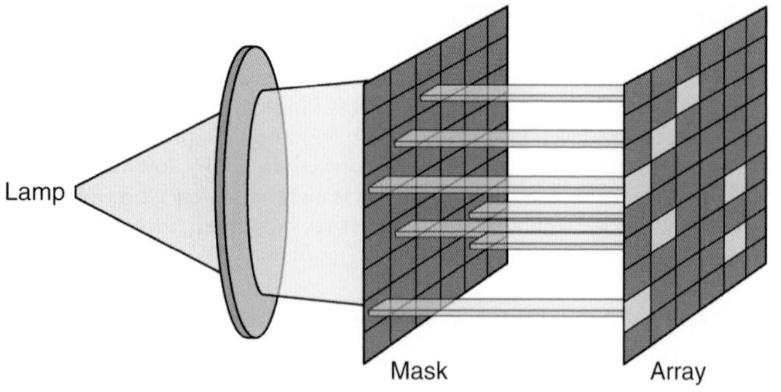

Figure 67-1 Photolithographic synthesis. Ultraviolet light is transmitted through a photolithographic mask, allowing localized photodeprotection of specific chemical building blocks. *(Courtesy Affymetrix.)*

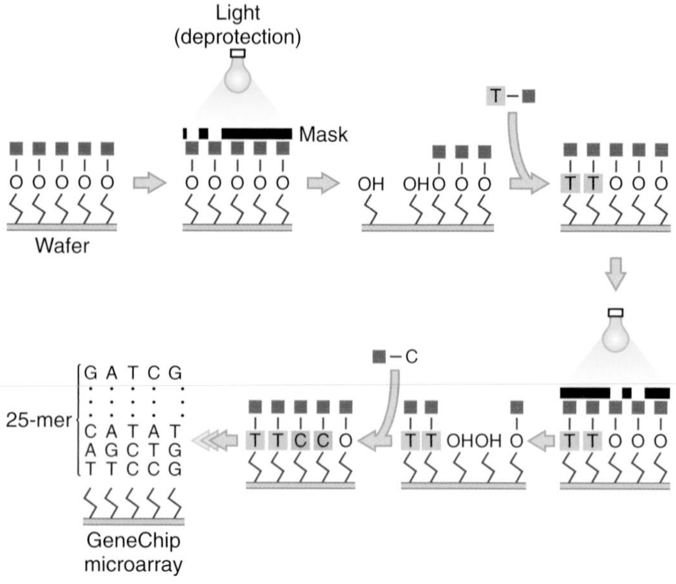

Figure 67-2 Diagram of GeneChip array manufacture using a unique combination of photolithography and combinatorial chemistry. *(Courtesy Affymetrix.)*

Delivery Technologies

Deposition of presynthesized biomolecules was initiated by Pat Brown and colleagues (Schena, 1995; Shalon, 1996). Biochemical substances (e.g., proteins, peptides, oligonucleotides, cDNAs) are prepared, purified, and stored in microtiter plates. Small quantities of molecules are mechanically delivered on precisely defined locations on a solid surface, using different precision robotic systems. This method is very flexible in terms of biochemical composition, microarray topology (e.g., size and density of the spots, replicate spots for each molecule), and ease of prototyping, allowing for design alteration for different applications. Mechanical methods allow the synthesis of moderate- to high-density microarrays (up to about 16,000 probes/cm^2 [Graves, 1999]). It is the method of choice when large numbers of microarrays are needed with the same composition, as well as for long sequences using PCR products. Several companies are now manufacturing and selling premanufactured arrays (e.g., MicroMax, NEN Life Science, Boston) or arrayers based on deposition (Cheung, 1999) as an alternative to building an arrayer (Brown, 2000).

Delivery procedures consist of different microprinting systems. Most arrayers use fountain pen–like microdispensing tips (e.g., Cartesian Technologies, Irvine, Calif.), but some original systems such as the pin-and-ring technique have been developed (Genetic MicroSystems, Woburn, Mass.). In general, because of surface tension, static, and other effects, the reproducibility of printed arrays is lower than in situ synthesis and must be corrected by separate experiments (repeats), replicate spots (on the same slide), multicolor fluorescence detection, and/or other specific detection algorithms (Chen, 1997; Jang, 2009). Because of its flexibility and availability, printed array technology will probably have the largest impact on research and clinical laboratories over the next few years.

In Situ Synthesis

In situ synthesis allows higher yields, lower chip-to-chip variation, and higher probe densities. These methods also permit the manufacture of true "random access" arrays, meaning that each oligonucleotide in any position can have any chosen sequence (Southern, 1999). Combinatorial strategies refer to methods developed to make microarrays containing all sequences of a given length (also referred to as *generic arrays*). Combinatorial arrays have been promoted mostly to study large-scale hybridization behavior (Southern, 1994) or for solid-state nucleic acid sequencing (Macevicz, 1991; Strezoska, 1991; Drmanac, 1993a, 1993b, 1999, 1998; Lipshutz, 1993).

Manufacturing techniques include photolithographic masks to control chemical activation by photodeprotection steps (Fodor, 1991), ink-jet deposition (Stimpson, 1998), as well as physical barriers to sequential flooding of precursors (Maskos, 1993c). Affymetrix has coupled photochemical deprotection to solid-phase DNA synthesis by adapting techniques from the semiconductor industry (Pease, 1994; Lockhart, 1996; Lipshutz, 1999). Synthetic linkers modified with photochemically removable protecting groups are attached to silicon wafers. By shining ultraviolet light through a photolithographic mask, localized photodeprotection occurs and permits specific chemical building blocks (hydroxyl-protected deoxynucleosides) to react with the deprotected groups (Fodor, 1991) (Fig. 67-1). Cycles alternating photodeprotection and incubation with different chemical building blocks allow light-directed synthesis of polydeoxynucleotides (Fig. 67-2). The synthesized oligonucleotides have a maximum practical length because of the limited efficiency of the photodeprotection (80%–95% at each cycle) (Forman, 1999). Therefore, the proportion of 20-mers displaying the predefined sequence is between 1% and 36% (0.8E20–0.95E20) (Fodor, 1991).

Mechanical masks or barriers permit confinement of surface areas before flooding with defined precursors. Physical masks of different shapes (circular, diamond) allow in situ synthesis of a given precursor in known locations. Sequential displacement of masks followed by the flooding of another precursor allows synthesis of large combinatorial deoxynucleotide arrays (Southern, 1992, 1996b; Maskos, 1993c). To date, Affymetrix is able to synthesize up to 400,000 different polydeoxynucleotides in a 1.6 cm^2 area (Fodor, 1991). Critical to this step is the precise alignment of the mask with the wafer before each synthesis step. To ensure that this critical step is accurately completed, chrome marks on the wafer and on the mask are perfectly aligned. Although the process is highly efficient, some activated molecules fail to attach the new nucleotide. To prevent these outliers from becoming probes with missing nucleotides, a capping step is used to truncate them. In addition, the side chains of the nucleotides are protected to prevent the formation of branched oligonucleotides (www.affymetrix.com). Despite high cost, this is the method of choice for large-scale differential gene expression studies because of sensitivity, reproducibility, and redundancy of information.

Ink-jet technologies owe their development to the printer industry and are in continuous development by several companies such as Incyte Pharmaceuticals (Palo Alto, Calif.), Protogene (Palo Alto, Calif.), and Rosetta Inpharmatics (Kirkland, Wash.) (Blanchard, 1996). This technology is also commercially available (Ink-Jet, Packard Instruments, Meriden, Conn.; Piezoelectric pump, GeSiM, Grosserkmannsdorf, Germany). This technology gave rise to the ability to place an oligonucleotide or other entity (i.e., small molecule or tag) in two-dimensional space. Such an approach offers versatility in the biomolecules being delivered and eliminates the need for physical contact with the surface of the array; this last property may be of relevance for the development of arrays coated with thin layers of metals and using different detection methods (Heyse, 1998; Schmid, 1998). Light scattering from microparticles tagging target sequences can be detected as an evanescent wave immediately above the surface of the glass. This method allows real-time affinity measurement with a very low background (Stimpson, 1996).

OLIGONUCLEOTIDE MICROARRAYS

Thermodynamics, kinetics of hybridization, and quantitative aspects of oligonucleotide hybridization have been extensively studied (reviewed by Wetmur, 1991; Hoheisel, 1996; Pozhitkov, 2007). Oligonucleotide arrays have a lower sensitivity than cDNA arrays for detection of rare messages or hybridization targets, and poor predictability of hybridization characteristics because hybridization potential, and therefore the expected signal intensity, do not correlate well with the G:C content or the melting temperature (Lockhart, 1996; Graves, 1999). On the other hand, oligonucleotide arrays are easier to construct using deposition of synthesized product or in situ synthesis described above. In addition, hybridization conditions can be more homogenous than on a cDNA array, provided that the array is designed with oligonucleotides of equivalent sizes.

Oligonucleotide arrays have applications in gene expression profiling as well as in DNA sequencing. For sequencing applications, they can be divided into two fields: generic arrays (representing a random oligonucleotide matrix) or dedicated arrays (for molecular variants of a predetermined target). Generic arrays have been proposed as an inexpensive alternative to sequencing. Using all possible combinations of an n-mer allows "walking" at every position along a nucleotide sequence. This type of array is the only one capable of detecting sequences that are lacking in large electronic libraries. In contrast, dedicated arrays are used for repetitive sequencing (resequencing) of the same target for detection of nucleotide polymorphisms or functional mutations. This implies knowledge of the targets and their most frequent variants, in order to incorporate predetermined sets of oligonucleotides on the diagnostic array. This approach has been used for detection of genetic polymorphisms associated with human immunodeficiency virus (HIV) drug resistance as well as other polymorphisms. Oligonucleotide arrays can also be used to define single nucleotide polymorphisms (Guo, 1994), even by comparing two samples with multicolor fluorescence (Chee, 1996). Further examples and applications of polymorphism to disease treatment and management are described later and in Chapter 72.

The search for oligomers of higher affinity has opened the way for chemical modifications of the oligonucleotide probe and template in order to improve the kinetics and thermodynamics of binding. Peptide nucleic acid probes (PNAs) allow hybridization to be performed at a higher stringency, because of the high-stability of PNA–DNA duplexes (Corey, 1997) and are able recognize exclusively single strands of DNA and ribonucleic acid (RNA) in antiparallel fashion (Moggio, 2007). Methylated RNA probes (Corey, 1998) display relatively similar affinities. However, PNAs display more rapid hybridization conditions than their nucleic acid counterparts, primarily because of their neutral backbone structure (Freeman, 1999). Overall, it can be said that, although the reduction of the hybridization time from hours to minutes would be a clear asset, the problem of unpredictability of the melting points of these high-affinity oligomers must be overcome before implementation on microarrays (Weiler, 1997). In addition to probes, targets can be chemically modified to locally enhance signals. Pyrimidine-rich target regions can generate higher hybridization signal by incorporating 5-methyluridine during in vitro transcription (Woski, 1998).

cDNA MICROARRAYS

Microarrays of cDNA sequences allow hybridization-based monitoring of the expression of the cognate genes. Therefore this strategy implies access to clones or the possibility of generating PCR products. To date, the best strategies use two-color fluorescence detection to discriminate between a sample and its control and check for differential level of expression. This method has been pioneered and validated by Pat Brown and colleagues at Stanford University (Schena, 1995, 1996; Shalon, 1996). Advantages of this approach are calculating a ratio on every probe, to control for the quality of the probe, the specific hybridization properties of each target/probe pair, and the labeling efficacy. Synteni (a subsidiary of Incyte, Palo Alto, Calif.) has developed its Gene Expression Micro-arrays for this purpose (Schena, 1998). NEN Life Science is selling glass slides prespotted with 2400 known human genes (MicroMax) and continuous miniaturization is allowing for greater gene representation in a smaller area.

Although they appear to be inherently less reproducible, cDNA microarrays currently offer the greatest versatility in terms of probe deposition and accessibility of the technology. Several companies now offer equipment for array manufacture and reading of hybridized matrices. It is likely that cDNA arrays and high-density oligonucleotide arrays will play complementary roles in research laboratories over the next few years; high-density arrays will be used primarily for the discovery of diagnostically relevant loci and dedicated arrays will be used increasingly for the medium- to low-density analysis of diagnostically relevant loci discovered by high-density array analysis.

SEQUENCING ARRAYS

Nucleic acid sequence data are fundamental to modern molecular biology. Conventional methods (Maxam, 1977; Sanger, 1977) are time-consuming, labor intensive, and costly. Alternative sequencing methods using solid-phase hybridization were proposed on a theoretical basis (Bains, 1988; Khrapko, 1989) within 15 years of the discovery of these methods (Southern, 1975). The theoretical articles were followed shortly by data confirming the principles of array-based sequencing for short artificial templates (Southern, 1992; Pease, 1994; Parinov, 1996). A well-written review of microarray sequencing methods was published in 1999 (Hacia, 1999). The reader might note, however, that much of the work published and cited in this area is provided by researchers with some financial interest in one or more of the proprietary devices evaluated in these publications. Rather than endorsing a particular device or method, this chapter acquaints the reader with basic principles involved in the assay.

Any nucleic acid sequence can in theory be broken down into subsets of length n. All the possible oligonucleotides of length n (n-mers) can then be placed at fixed locations on a solid surface. Nucleic acid to be sequenced (the template) is amplified if necessary, labeled with a direct (fluorescent, luminescent, radioactive) or indirect (affinity) label, and allowed to hybridize to the bound collection of n-mers. Detection of label allows the sequencer to verify a match with an n-mer at a particular locus on the solid surface. The intensity of signal at that locus should be directly proportional to the number of domains in the template corresponding to the n-mer at that locus. Methods for all these steps are outlined in preceding sections of this chapter.

For sequencing applications, the n-mers that match the template are then assembled into a definite order by analysis of n-mers with overlapping sequence, similar in principle to the arrangement of contigs by large-scale sequencing programs. Consider a nonanucleotide template that, under stringent conditions, is bound only to the loci containing the following four tetramers on an array with all 256 possible tetramers:

Tetramer	Intensity
5′ ACTG	2
5′ CTGA	2
5′ TGAC	1
5′ GACT	1

It is trivial to reason from the areas of overlap that the nonanucleotide template was 5′ ACTGACTGA. Computational analysis of this kind is straightforward. Because the computation, the scanning of the array to detect label, the labeling itself, and to some extent even the extraction and amplification of the DNA can be automated, it is lovely to envision a "black box" that accomplishes all this in an afternoon. Consider, however, a nonanucleotide that binds to loci containing the following tetramers:

Tetramer	Intensity
5′ TCTA	1
5′ CTAC	1
5′ TACT	1
5′ ACTT	1
5′ CTTC	1
5′ TTCT	1

This could represent 5′ TCTACTTCT or 5′ TTCTACTTC; there is no computational way to resolve it. Where *n* is less than half the length of the template, repeats of the same length as n/2 can render the data ambiguous. Computation becomes increasingly difficult as template length becomes an increasingly higher multiple of n; hence it is desirable to have as long an n as possible for sequencing unknown domains. The practical length of n remains limited by technology, however, because 4^n (the number of loci required for universal representation) exceeds 1 million for n = 10. This approaches the current limits of the number of distinct oligonucleotides that can be differentiated on a photolithographic chip (Lipshutz, 1999).

HYBRIDIZATION, DETECTION, AND IMAGE ANALYSIS

A critical component of microarray assays is the quality and labeling of the probe. Because sample carries the label, sample-to-sample variation in probe preparation and labeling can be anticipated. When microarrays are used for gene expression profiling, this step is even more critical because of the difficulties in obtaining high-quality messenger RNA (mRNA). Insufficient, degraded, or poor-quality RNA can deliver erroneous results that lead, after data mining, to improper conclusions (Russo, 2003). Although there are many protocols available for high yield of RNA, a final yield of at least a few micrograms of mRNA per experiment has been desirable in most applications, although protocols have used smaller amounts of RNA with subsequent amplification using cDNA

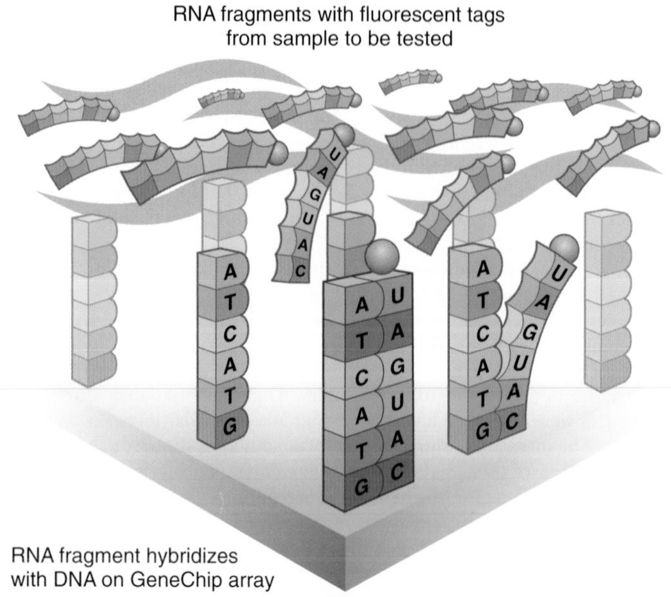

Figure 67-3 Cartoon depicting hybridization of tagged probes to Affymetrix GeneChip microarray. *(Courtesy Affymetrix.)*

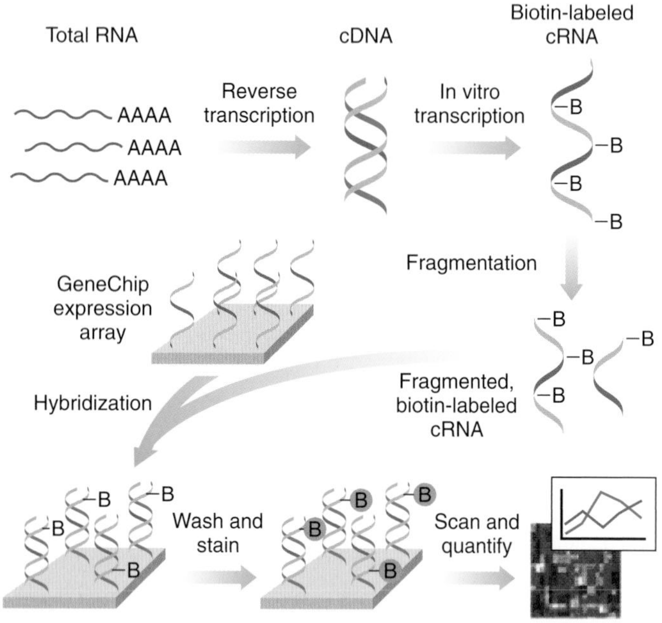

Figure 67-4 Standard eukaryotic gene expression assay. Labeled complementary DNA or RNA targets derived from the messenger RNA (mRNA) of an experimental sample are hybridized to nucleic acid probes attached to the solid support. By monitoring the amount of label associated with each DNA location, it is possible to infer the abundance of each mRNA species represented. *(Courtesy Affymetrix.)*

intermediates that incorporate an RNA promoter and allow amplification with an RNA polymerase. Initial approaches (Auffray, 1980) converted mRNA to a fluorescent cDNA probe with direct incorporation of fluorescent nucleotides. Currently most approaches use total RNA and there are numerous variations of incorporation of label into cDNA or RNA probes, including indirect affinity labels such as biotin with detection using antibody/avidin/streptavidin tagged with fluors or light-scattering gold particles (Figs. 67-3 and 67-4). Each step of probe preparation from extraction through labeling must be carefully controlled to ensure reproducible results.

The usual consideration of time, temperature, stringency, and probe concentration determine the conditions of the microarray hybridization. Arrays often include negative control probes to allow optimal stringency to be determined. Because of the extremely high complexity of the probe used in gene expression profiling, hybridization times are generally extended to allow low-abundance messages to hybridize. Washes are designed to remove nonspecifically bound probe and reduce background.

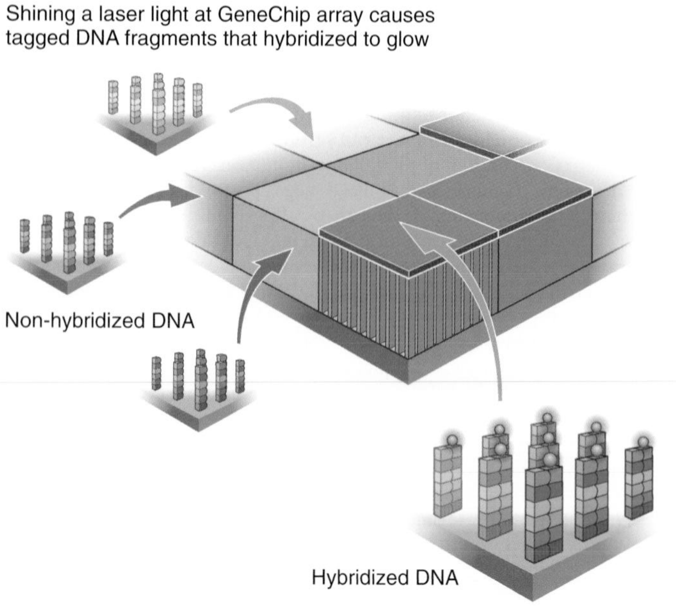

Figure 67-5 Cartoon depicting scanning of tagged and untagged probes on an Affymetrix GeneChip microarray. *(Courtesy Affymetrix.)*

All steps need to be optimized and standardized. After a successful hybridization, labeled nucleic acid is bound to complementary sequences that are tethered to the array (Fig. 67-5). Some form of image analysis is used to capture signal. In most approaches, the entire slide is scanned (fluorescence, autoradiographic or light scattering) and an algorithm is used to link features with intensities and gene lists. Software associated with the scanner can generate a "mask" to align image with grid used to construct the array. Data acquisition generates large data sets (one image uses typically 10–50 megabytes) that have to be stored under standard formats (e.g., BMP, GIF, JPG). Image processing software will become increasingly automated to ensure proper grid adjustment, detect artifacts, and identify features to extract meaningful information.

Microarray technology has grown over the past decade to incorporate miniaturization of fabrication platforms, enhancement of high throughput automation (see also Chapter 77), and cost reduction. Many platforms exist to support individual user needs whether they be interrogation of an entire genome, exonic mRNA expression, or limited to a subset of genes involved in specific pathways of interest. Affymetrix (www.affymetrix.com) pioneered mass application of array technology to the scientific community and continues as a leader in the field. Illumina (www.illumina.com) has facilitated RNA analysis of specific genes or regions of interest, with the development of its cDNA-mediated Annealing, Selection, extension, and Ligation (DASL) assay (Fan, 2004). This assay reportedly allows for RNA profiling of up to 1536 targets using partially degraded RNA as found in formalin-fixed, paraffin-embedded (FFPE) samples. Array technology has also been adapted to interrogate single nucleotide polymorphisms, copy number variations, and structural variants, which differ among individuals and populations (Coulombe-Huntington, 2009; Stankiewicz and Lupski, 2010). Such variations influence how individuals differ in their risk of disease and their response to therapeutic treatments (see Chapter 72). Other improvements across the industry include the ability to detect low abundance transcripts, reduced requirements for the quantity of sample to a few hundred nanograms or less of total RNA (versus micrograms), automation for low per-sample pricing, and improved consistency in methodology and quality control (Yauk, 2005). As a result of the variations in array technologies and differences in sample preparation and signal processing, the Minimal Information About a Microarray Experiment (MIAME) guidelines have been implemented to ensure that all relevant experimental information is presented in a consistent and complete manner that will ensure published data and publically available microarray data sets can be interpreted accurately (Yauk, 2004).

BIOINFORMATICS

The most challenging aspect of microarrays starts here, when large data sets have been assembled and purged of artifacts, background noise, and await analysis (Draghici, 2003; Parmigiana, 2003; Gopalappa, 2009; Zhang, 2009). The approach depends on the nature of the question and design of the experiment. An initial exploration of the data set is used to evaluate the quality, usually including an assessment of background and mean intensity of the features on the array. To facilitate statistical comparisons between arrays, intensities are commonly log transformed and arrays are "normalized" to each other.

A popular approach to normalizing gene expression is predicated on the assumption that the conditions being compared (e.g., normal versus tumor or infected versus noninfected) would affect the gene expression of relatively few genes, leaving most unaffected. In the absence of systematic bias, the median intensity of all features on the array should be unchanged. Thus a common normalization method is to divide each intensity measurement on the array by the median intensity of the array (Kano, 2003). These assumptions are reasonable when the array contains a large number of genes that represent a wide range of biological function.

One caveat of the total intensity normalization methods arises from its implicit assumption that systematic variation is constant across the entire range of expression intensities of the array. However, as data from technical replicate arrays show, systematic variation is often intensity dependent, or nonlinear. In other words, systematic variation observed at low expression intensities differs from systematic variation observed at medium and high intensities (Simon, 2005). Thus linear adjustments, such as dividing each measurement on an array with the median intensity of the array, would not be appropriate for some genes. For perhaps 80% of the arrays, systematic variation is close enough to linear so that total intensity normalization methods are sufficient. However, for the remaining 20% of the arrays, nonlinear normalization methods are required (Genomics and Bioinformatics Group, 2005).

Quantile normalization is a nonlinear normalization method that is often performed on microarrays. In addition to assuming that most genes are unchanged in their expression across experimental conditions, quantile normalization also makes the strong assumption that the distribution of gene expression intensities must also be invariant across the arrays (Irizarry, 2003). Thus, not only should the median intensity be the same for each array, but the intensity at every quantile of the array should also be the same. Given this assumption, quantile normalization sorts all intensity values on the array by increasing intensity values and adjusts the intensities so that the smallest intensity value on each array is identical, the second smallest values are identical, and so forth. The gene with the smallest intensity value on one array may be different from the gene with the smallest intensity value on another array.

Intensity-dependent systematic variation has also been shown for two-color technology arrays. Intensity-dependent dye bias was first identified by Terry Speed's laboratory, where it was observed that low-abundance genes appear to be upregulated in the Cy5 channel and moderately expressed genes appear to be upregulated in the Cy3 channel (Yang, 2002). This systematic artifact can be effectively corrected by performing a locally weighted linear regression (lowess) (Fig. 67-6). The validity of using housekeeping genes for normalization has been called into question in the past few years. In this method, it is assumed that the expression levels of housekeeping genes are constant across experimental conditions. Thus intensity measurements of an array can be normalized to the mean intensities of these genes. However, the expression levels of some housekeeping genes have been shown to vary considerably across some experimental conditions (Thellin, 1999).

Once data have been normalized, quality control is performed at both the sample level and gene level. Sample-level quality control assesses sample data globally to identify outliers or, in cases where replicate reproducibility is generally observed, one or a few samples that may represent outliers. Potential outliers may be identified as those that do not cluster with replicate samples or those that do not correlate highly with replicate samples. Hierarchical clustering, principal component analysis, class prediction algorithms, and similarity metrics are often used to perform sample-level quality control (Grewal, 2003).

Gene-level quality control filters out genes for which the large proportion of measurements fall within the noise range, to create a restricted set of genes for further analysis. Genes that are removed correspond to those that are not expressed in the tissues of concern or whose expression levels are so low that the technology is not sufficiently sensitive to detect differences in expression. Removal of such genes generally reduces noise, the likelihood of false-positive reactions in subsequent differential expression filters, and the severity of multiple testing corrections required in downstream statistical analyses.

Once normalization and quality control of imported data have been completed, one can perform analyses to isolate the genes of interest. One basic objective in a microarray experiment is to identify genes that may be differentially expressed among the different experimental conditions. Researchers rely on many different variants of common statistical tests to identify differentially expressed genes. One caveat to using statistical tests to identify differentially expressed genes is that the number of false-positive reactions from the statistical analysis is proportional to the number of tests that are performed. Because hundreds or thousands of genes are often tested at once, the number of false-positive reactions from the analysis can potentially dominate the list of candidate genes that are thought to be differentially expressed. Thus it is important to limit the number of false-positive reactions in a statistical analysis by performing multiple testing correction. Two categories of multiple testing correction are those that determine the family-wise error rate (FWER) and those that determine the false discovery rate (FDR). FWER tests control the overall chance that at most one gene is incorrectly identified as being differentially expressed after the statistical analysis and after performing the multiple testing correction (Grewal, 2003). Examples of FWER tests are the Bonferroni, Holms–Bonferroni step-down, and Westfall and Young Permutation. FDR tests confine the probability of false-positive reactions to be proportional to the number of genes that pass the statistical test instead of the total number of genes tested by the statistical analysis. An example of a FDR test is the Benjamini and Hochberg false discovery rate (Benjamini,

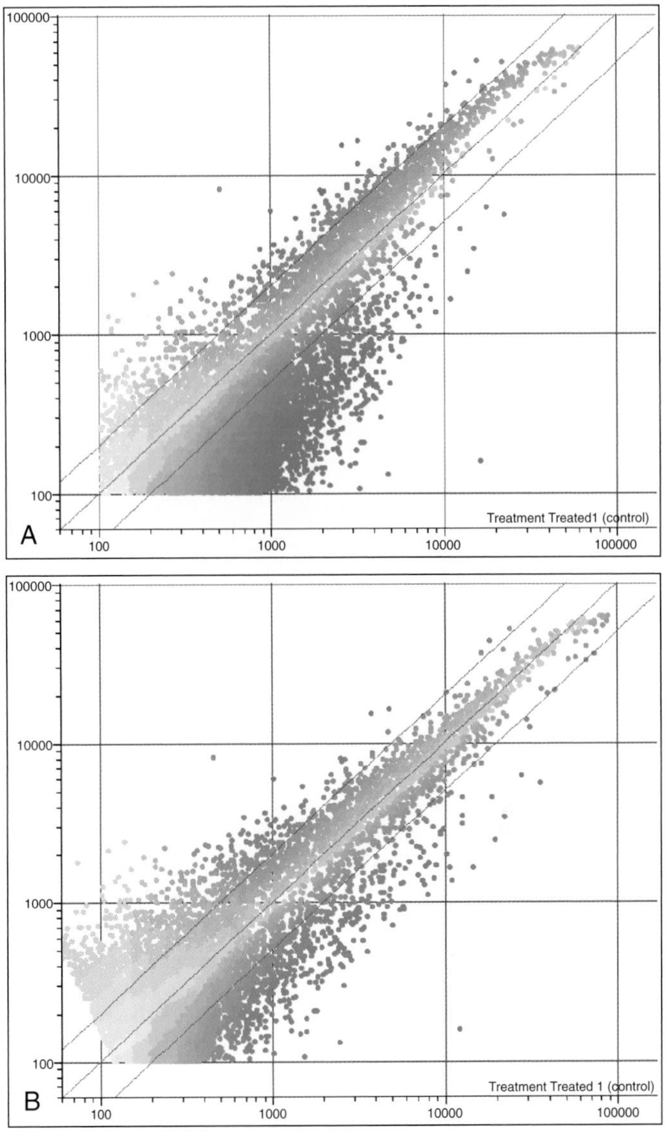

Figure 67-6 Lowess intensity-dependent normalization is used for two-color data. It is a type of within-slide normalization scheme that adjusts for intensity-dependent variation due to dye properties. Dye bias is caused by inconsistencies in the relative fluorescence intensity between Cy5 and Cy3. These inconsistencies often result in nonlinear relationship between the two dyes and a curve occurs in a scatter plot. **A,** Data before normalization. **B,** By applying lowess normalization, a locally weighted regression is fitted to the data to adjust the control value for each measurement. As a result, the plot of signal versus control value will be linear. *(Courtesy Agilent Technologies.)*

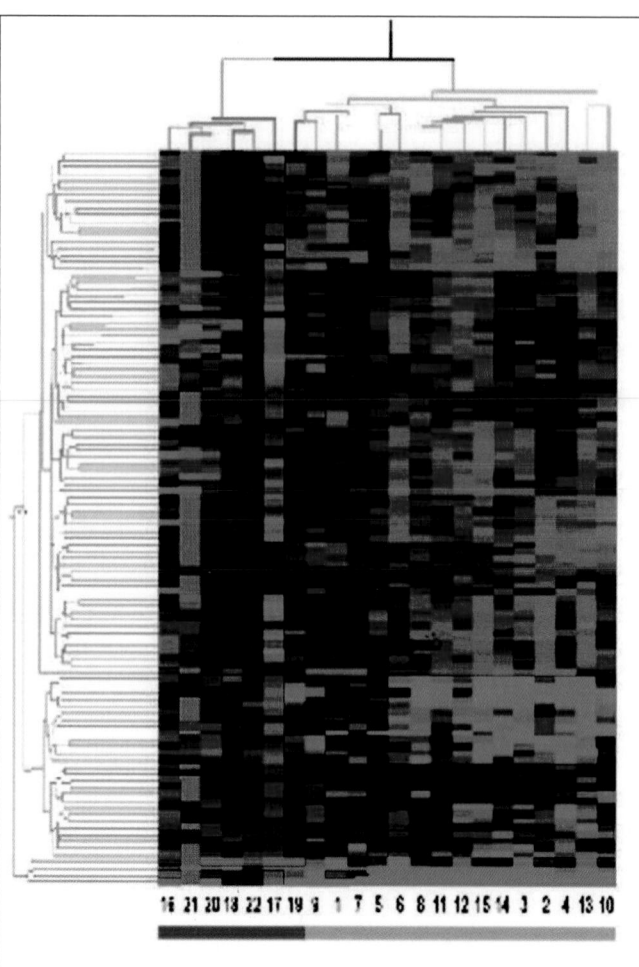

Figure 67-7 Hierarchical clustering dendrogram of duodenal genes from different celiac disease (orange bar) and control (blue) biopsy samples. Clustering of 109 genes across 22 samples clusters the seven control samples (blue bar) separately from the 15 celiac disease patients (orange bar). Each column represents a celiac disease or a control sample and each row represents an individual gene. For each gene, a green signal represents underexpression, black signals denote similarly expressed genes, a red signal represents overexpressed genes, and gray signals denote missing data. *(Adapted with permission of the BMJ Publishing Group from Diosdado B, Wapenaar MC, Franke L, et al. A microarray screen for novel candidate genes in coeliac disease pathogenesis. Gut 2004;53:944.)*

1995). There are several excellent statistical packages available online (e.g., BRB Tools, SAM, Focus, D Chip, R Bioconductor Library, PAM).

Clustering analysis (Fig. 67-7) is suitable for grouping genes that behave similarly across multiple conditions of an experiment. Clustering has many applications in expression data analysis. It allows one to infer the previously unknown function of a gene from the functions of the genes that it clusters with. This is based on the assumption that genes that share similar functions share similar expression behavior across experimental conditions. Clustering may also be useful in finding genes that may be co-regulated. This is based on the assumption that genes that are co-regulated share similar expression profiles. Thus it may be useful to analyze the promoter regions of genes that cluster together to find common regulatory elements (Grewal, 2003; Gollub and Sherlock, 2006).

The generated genes of interest can then be integrated with known biology. The ability to cross-reference gene lists from differential expression analysis and/or clustering analysis against gene ontology or other gene function lists to ascertain significance of overlap is available in some programs (e.g., Agilent/GeneSpring). Other popular programs include Bioconductor—an open source and open development software project for the analysis and comprehension of genomic data, based on the R programming language (Zhang, 2009); the oligonucleotide centric DChip (www.Dchip.org); TIGRsuite (www.tigr.org), and BeadStudio (array platform- and manufacturer-specific; www.illumina.com). (For review, see Gollub and Sherlock, 2006; Platts, 2006). In addition, genes can be referenced to known biological pathways, and/or public databases (GenBank, LocusLink, UniGene, serial analysis of gene expression [SAGE]).

Thus, because of the intensive need for pattern recognition, multidimensional data interpretation, and cross-platform comparison, microarray technology will enjoy a close relationship with bioinformatics, and coevolution of both hardware and software appears to be inevitable (see Chapter 77).

INTELLECTUAL PROPERTY ISSUES

Microarray technology is a rapidly moving field with fierce competition. It is therefore important to emphasize that numerous patents have been filed, some of which are directly relevant to clinical diagnosis. Therefore intellectual property remains an important concern in this ever evolving field (Rouse and Hardiman, 2003). For instance, Affymetrix (www.affymetrix.com, Santa Clara, Calif.) possesses broad patent rights on high-density oligonucleotide arrays (Chee, 1998; Holmes, 1998), regardless of the means by which they are made. Assuming that a laboratory decides to develop in-house moderate-density arrays for tumor testing and to charge for such a service, this array might infringe Affymetrix's patents if it exceeds 400 features/cm^2, regardless of the synthesis method (Fodor, 1998). Array technologies using micromatrices of polyacrylamide gel pads (three-dimensional gel elements) represent a new approach that might not infringe Affymetrix claims (Khrapko, 1991; Yershov, 1996; Guschin, 1997). Furthermore, the intellectual property related to the methodology and application of DNA array technology to identify medicinal versus toxic components in natural remedies, species-specific fingerprinting, and identification of unknown DNA has generated additional patent applications (Shaw, 2009). It is hoped that, as occurred with nucleic acid amplification technologies, competition between manufacturers will bring down costs of high- and medium-density arrays and allow for the democratization of this powerful technology.

CLINICAL APPLICATIONS OF ARRAY TECHNOLOGY

Numerous applications of microarray technology have been proposed in the past few years, ranging from molecular staging of tumors to the identification and characterization of microbial agents. This has led many to speculate that array technology represents the next wave of technologic advances to have a practical impact on the diagnosis of human disease, second only to PCR as a core technology in the clinical molecular diagnostics laboratory. This section focuses on current and future applications of array technology.

ARRAY TECHNOLOGY IN THE CLINICAL LABORATORY

Although not currently widespread, clinical laboratory utilitization of array technology appears to be on the horizon. Roth and colleagues (Roth, 2004) have employed array analysis to detect common respiratory pathogens and compared this with conventional culture from middle ear fluid samples. The sensitivities of the array assay compared to culture for *Haemophilus influenzae*, *Moraxella catarrhalis*, *Streptococcus pyogenes*, and *Streptococcus pneumoniae* were 96% (93% for culture), 73% (93% for culture), 93% (80% for culture), and 100% (78% for culture), respectively. Furthermore, tissue microarrays have been used as a tool for internal quality control to improve the interpretation of immunohistochemical staining (Packeisen, 2002; Gulmann, 2004). The U.S. Food and Drug Administration has granted 501(k) clearance to Roche Molecular Systems to market its AmpliChip CP450 Genoptyping test to determine cytochrome P450 2D6 and 2C19 genotypes using the Affymetrix instrumentation system (Malone, 2005). As cytochrome genes code for liver enzymes important in drug metabolism, clinician will use the results to optimize drug dosing and minimize side effects on the basis of individual genotype. This is the first time a microarray chip has been given marketing clearance as a diagnostic device for use in the clinical laboratory, heralding the potentially new era of personalized medicine. Small-scale, automated, microfluidic array instruments that have the technical discrimination and dynamic range required to detect RNA species at a frequency of 1 : 100,000 with a short turnaround time and low coefficient of variation (0.09–0.11) have also been described (Baum, 2003). However, methodologic consistency, quality control, and disease-specific application will have to be addressed prior to implementation as a routine test to the clinical laboratory.

ARRAY TECHNOLOGY IN CLINICAL DISEASE

Microarray technology has provided the ability to screen genes that are differentially regulated in experimental and clinical disease and allow further correlation of select genes with their function. For example, Ji and colleagues (Ji, 2003) used microarray technology to screen for genes that are upregulated in the early stage of acute pancreatitis using two different experimental models of the disease. Many genes were upregulated in both experimental systems, suggesting their importance in the human condition. However, one gene in particular, EGR1, further analyzed through classical approaches (gene knockout), was shown to be a key regulator that may be important in the development of early acute pancreatitis. Others (Iacobuzio-Donahue, 2003) have performed a comprehensive evaluation and comparison of gene expression profiles of 39 samples of pancreatic cancer and identified between six and 40 genes that were highly expressed when examined by multiple methods (oligonucleotide arrays, cDNA arrays, or SAGE). These may eventually be translated into clinically useful targets for therapy or diagnosis.

Microarray analysis of cells and tissues as a means to identify key therapeutic candidates continues to evolve. Malignancies or their tissue components that have been analyzed in the quest for identifying key targets, diagnostic or prognostic indicators (Ma, 2009), or novel pathways include melanoma (Nambiar, 2004), leukemias (Moos, 2002; Jaakson, 2003), lymphomas (Hedvat, 2002; Kobayashi, 2003; Azambuja, 2009), myelodysplastic syndromes (Pellagatti, 2004), and carcinomas of prostate (Pettus, 2004), bladder (Dyrskjot, 2003), kidney (Moch, 1999), colon/rectum (Frederiksen, 2003), breast (Jeffrey, 2002; Wilson, 2004), ovary (Rosen, 2004; Yang, 2009), and endometrium (Saidi, 2004; DeRycke, 2009).

Other clinical applications that utilize the gene screening capability of microarray technology include the study of the effect of ionizing radiation (Amundson, 1999), detection of hepatitis D virus (Sun, 2004), identification of central nervous system pathogens (Hanson, 2004), karyotyping of cell-free DNA in amniotic fluid (Larrabee, 2004), viral diagnosis (Striebel, 2003), providing molecular markers for allergic (Jahn-Schmid, 2003), urologic (Cheung, 2009), cardiac (Bostjancic, 2009), and inflammatory disorders (Bennett, 2003), Alzheimer's disease (Pasinetti, 2001), multiple sclerosis (Whitney, 1999), dystonia (Walter, 2010), diabetes (Sreekumar, 2002; Mootha, 2003), transplant rejection (Flechner, 2004), and pulmonary hypertension (Geraci, 2001). The ability to predict adverse drug reactions (Guzey, 2002), response to therapy (Sotiriou, 2002), drug sensitivity (Stein, 2004), and toxicity profiles (Waring, 2001), among others (Cox, 2001; Day, 2009; Stankiewicz, 2010), have also been reported.

LIMITATIONS

Despite the excitement and increase in the potential clinical application of microarray technology, care must be taken in its interpretation. Clinical application will require procedures for quality control and quality assurance. The challenge to ensuring reproducibility of the high-density data presented in microarrays is unprecedented in the clinical laboratory. Each of the large number of steps from sample extraction, labeling, hybridization, image analysis, and data analysis, contributes to difficulties in data reproducibility, and can differ between commercially available systems (Kothapalli, 2002; Yauk, 2004; Pozhitkov, 2007). Furthermore, factors such as varying the method used for nucleic acid isolation (Feezor, 2004) or detection, tissue type (solid, glandular, or blood derived), type of specimen (FFPE versus frozen tissue) (Penland, 2007), and time to processing can affect results of gene expression profiling.

Approaches to further validate and confirm array-based results include verification of each clone sequence before printing the microarray; performing experiments in duplicate or triplicate where possible; and verification of candidate genes by classic methods (e.g., PCR, northern blotting, RNase protection assay). Some investigators (Rajeevan, 2001) have shown that the majority of array results were qualitatively accurate in cross-validation experiments using real-time RT-PCR. However, for genes showing less than a fourfold difference on the arrays, consistent cross-validation with real-time RT-PCR was not achieved. It is also very important to determine whether the difference in mRNA expression translates to a difference in the expression levels of the corresponding protein products. Currently, how frequently a difference in mRNA level translates to a difference in protein expression level is not clear.

Caution must also be exercised in interpreting differentially regulated genes during tumor progression (staging microarray). Any nucleic acid source derived from biopsy tissue is made up of many different cell populations and may represent homogeneous tissue only after the tumor mass has reached a large enough size (i.e., late stage). While certain methods are available to isolate specific cells of interest in smaller tumors (e.g., laser capture microdissection), they are technically demanding, time-consuming, and not universally available.

Like all sequencing strategies, microarrays have limited sensitivity for minority alleles, although newer platforms and analysis approaches claim to improve detection in this regard (Coulombe-Huntington, 2009; Stankiewicz, 2010).). An example of sequence-based identification of drug resistance in HIV will be particularly instructive. Microarray sequencing of clinical isolates can correctly predict some instances of drug resistance on the basis of specific mutations (Race, 1998) and is evolving toward standard practice (Perez-Olmeda, 1999). Even making the optimistic assumption that sequencing can detect a resistance allele when represented in 1% of the viral population or more, however, there is reason to doubt the predictive value of a test that is negative for resistance. Few virologists would argue that 0.5% prevalence of drug resistance is unimportant in a virus that generates more than a billion copies a day. Therefore, it should be understood that the power of this technology currently lies in its ability to screen for the regulation of genes in defined parameters (Russo, 2003).

Further advances in diagnosis, classification, and prognosis await discovery by microarray-based methods in the near future. As emphasized earlier, it is not merely improvements in apparatus that make this possible, but more sophisticated analytic strategies, detection sensitivity, throughput, automation, miniaturization, ease of use, and cost that evolve to keep up with the more complex data generated by these devices (Bassett, 1999; Zhang, 2009).

PART 8

SELECTED REFERENCES

Ji B, Chen XQ, Misek DE, et al. Pancreatic gene expression during the initiation of acute pancreatitis: identification of EGR-1 as a key regulator. Physiol Genomics 2003;14:59.

An example of how microarray is employed to screen for regulation of gene expression in two models of experimental pancreatitis with subsequent validation of select genes (EGR-1) by conventional methods.

Kothapalli R, Yoder SJ, Mane S, et al. Microarray results: how accurate are they? BMC Bioinformatics 2002;3:22.

Discusses problems associated with microarray in great detail and evaluates data obtained from two different commercially available systems.

Russo G, Zegar C, Giordano A. Advantages and limitations of microarray in human cancer. Oncogene 2003;22:6497.

Highlights some of the recent developments and clinical applications of microarray technology and discusses potentially problematic areas associated with this technology.

Stein WD, Litman T, Fojo T, Bates SE. A serial analysis of gene expression (SAGE) database analysis of chemosensitivity: comparing solid tumors with cell lines and comparing solid tumors from different tissue origins. Cancer Res 2004;64:2805.

Investigates the relationship of gene expression profiles for a given tumor type to its drug sensitivity or resistance to provide insights into the molecular basis of tumor intractability to chemotherapy.

REFERENCES

Access the complete reference list online at http://www.expertconsult.com

CHAPTER 68

APPLICATIONS OF CYTOGENETICS IN MODERN PATHOLOGY

Constance K. Stein

KEY POINTS

- Identification of chromosomal abnormalities often correlates to disease and phenotypic abnormalities that will aid in clinical diagnosis and treatment.
- Standard morphology and a specific banding pattern have been established for all human chromosomes. A variety of different staining technologies are used to uniquely identify chromosomes and determine if anomalies exist.
- The two basic categories of cytogenetic abnormality are numerical and structural.
- Many syndromes have been specifically linked to particular chromosomal anomalies; for example, trisomy 21 in Down syndrome, 45,X in Turner syndrome, and deletion of 22q11.2 in velocardiofacial syndrome.
- Cytogenetic abnormalities may be either de novo or inherited. Detection may occur at any stage of a person's life from prenatal to adulthood.
- Identification of a cytogenetically abnormal clone in a cancer can provide information on diagnosis, prognosis, treatment, and disease progression.
- Fluorescence in situ hybridization (FISH), a unique diagnostic tool combining technologies from both cytogenetics and molecular genetics, can provide important information on the status of genes.
- Microdeletion syndromes may require a combination of karyotype analysis, FISH, and clinical evaluation for diagnosis.
- Cytogenetic analysis can be used in nearly every medical specialty and is an important element in clinical laboratory medicine.

Genetics is broadly defined as the scientific study of heredity but, in clinical laboratory medicine, interest is focused on two subspecialties of this field: (1) human genetics, the study of heredity in man; and (2) medical genetics, the study of human genetic variation of medical significance. Medical genetics can be further subdivided into five groups, two primarily clinical fields (clinical genetics and genetic counseling) and three laboratory sciences (cytogenetics, molecular genetics, and biochemical genetics).

Groundbreaking discoveries in the field of medicine can be attributed to genetics. Research, including the information obtained from the Human Genome Project (as described in Chapter 77) continues to identify new genes and mutations directly related to disease. Knowing the underlying cause of a disease provides new opportunities for diagnosis, and, opens up the possibility for gene therapy and the likelihood of curing some genetic diseases in the future. Currently, there is a growing demand for ways to use this information to benefit individual patients. This has led to new laboratory techniques in molecular genetics and cytogenetics that are providing improved methods of diagnosis and treatment. The major emphasis of this chapter is cytogenetics; discussion of molecular diagnostics is found in Chapter 70.

DEFINITIONS

As in all areas of medicine, genetics relies on the proper use of specific terms for communication. The following definitions provide a basic vocabulary for this field.

Gene: a sequence of nucleotides that represents a functional unit of inheritance; a region of DNA that codes for a product, either RNA or protein.

Chromosome: a highly ordered structure composed of DNA and proteins that carries the genetic information. In humans, there are 46 chromosomes ordered in pairs.

Autosome: all chromosomes other than the X and Y chromosomes, which are designated the *sex chromosomes*.

Homologous chromosomes or homologs: sister chromosomes, the members of a pair of chromosomes in which one is inherited from the mother and the other from the father.

Locus: the position of a gene on a chromosome.

Allele: an alternative form of a gene occupying the same locus. An allele may be the result of a mutation. There is a maximum of two alleles per diploid chromosome complement (one allele per chromosome), but multiple alleles may exist within a population.

Mutation: a permanent heritable change in the sequence of genomic DNA. This may manifest at both the molecular and cytogenetic levels. Not all mutations are negative events. Many are benign (e.g., blue eye color) and some have positive effects (e.g., sickle cell trait in countries with a significant risk of malaria). Individuals with a *constitutional mutation* (i.e., a mutation present in every cell of the body) may pass that mutation on to their progeny by germline transmission. In some cases, notably cancer, an *acquired mutation* may arise in a single somatic cell, which then divides mitotically, giving rise to a new clone of cells. The mutation will be limited to this clone and will not be transmitted to progeny of the individual. In rare instances of *gonadal mosaicism*, a de novo acquired mutation may arise in the gonads, resulting in a mixed population of normal and mutant gametes. Progeny receiving the new mutation may display a phenotype not present in either parent.

Karyotype: the chromosome constitution of an individual.

Karyogram: a figure showing the paired chromosomes from a cell arrayed in a standard sequence.

Diploid: the presence of two copies of each unique chromosome per cell. In humans, the chromosomes occur in pairs and the diploid ($2N$) number is 46.

Haploid: one copy of each unique chromosome. In humans, the gametes are haploid ($N = 23$).

Homozygous: both alleles at a locus are the same. (In the ABO system, an AA complement represents homozygosity.)

Heterozygous: the two alleles at a locus are different. (In the ABO system, an AO complement represents heterozygosity.)

Hemizygous: the presence of only one chromosome or chromosome segment rather than the usual two; applies to males with a single X chromosome.

Genotype: the genetic constitution of an individual or organism (i.e., what alleles are present). (In the ABO system, AA, AO, BB, BO, AB, and OO are genotypes.)

Phenotype: the appearance of an individual that results from the interaction of environment and genotype. (In the ABO system, A, B, and O blood types represent the phenotypic expression of the alleles for a given individual.)

Dominant allele: an allele that is expressed when present in only a single dose (i.e., it "dominates" over the other allele present). (In the ABO system, A is dominant over O such that an AO genotype results in an A blood type phenotype. Similarly, the presence of pigment (T) is dominant to the absence of pigment (t) (i.e., albinism), such that Tt results in pigmentation.)

Recessive allele: in a diploid organism, an allele that is only expressed when homozygous. (In the ABO system, the O blood group is only seen with a OO genotype; O is recessive to A and B. Similarly, t is recessive to T, and an albino phenotype only occurs with a tt genotype.)

Codominant alleles: in a diploid organism, alleles that show no dominance or recessivity to each other but, when present together, are both fully expressed. (In the ABO system, A and B are codominant such that an AB genotype expresses both A and B antigens.)

Independent assortment: random assortment of chromosomes (paternal and maternal) in the gametes; 50 : 50 chance of inheriting a given chromosome from one parent.

Linkage: the presence of two or more genes on the same chromosome that tend to be inherited together.

Crossing over: the physical exchange of genetic material between homologous chromosomes.

Recombination: the generation of new allelic combinations on chromosomes, usually by crossing over.

Mitosis: somatic cell division in which the DNA replicates and is evenly distributed to two equal daughter cells.

Meiosis: cell division in the gonads that produces the gametes. A single DNA replication is followed by two cell divisions which reduces the total DNA content of a cell from 2N to N. Recombination occurs to increase genetic diversity within a population.

Nondisjunction: failure of chromosomes or chromatids to separate to opposite poles in cell division. Usually results in one too many or one too few chromosomes in a cell.

CYTOGENETICS

Cytogenetics is defined as the science that combines the methods and findings of cytology and genetics to allow the investigation of heredity at the cellular level. This involves careful evaluation of the chromosomes, structures composed of double-stranded DNA that is complexed with histone and nonhistone proteins. Chromosomes were first observed in tumor cells by Walther Fleming in 1882, only 16 years after Mendel established genetics as a new field of science, making cytogenetics one of the oldest fields of genetics. Just after the turn of the century, the importance of the sex chromosomes was established, and in 1959, cytogenetic studies were first used in clinical laboratory studies. The ability to detect changes in chromosome structure and directly correlate them to disease and phenotypic anomalies in individuals proved a major advancement in clinical diagnosis. Over the years, the number and types of studies have grown and many of the tests performed have become the gold standard for diagnosis. In today's world, with a growing number of disease genes being cloned, there is an increasing emphasis on developing molecular direct mutation analyses (see Chapter 70). These studies work well when a diagnosis is known or suspected but, in the absence of a known disorder, cytogenetics still retains its position as the only clinical laboratory test to be able to survey the cellular genetic constitution of an individual with a single assay. Consequently, clinical applications for cytogenetic analysis can be found in all age groups and range from prenatal diagnosis to cancer evaluation.

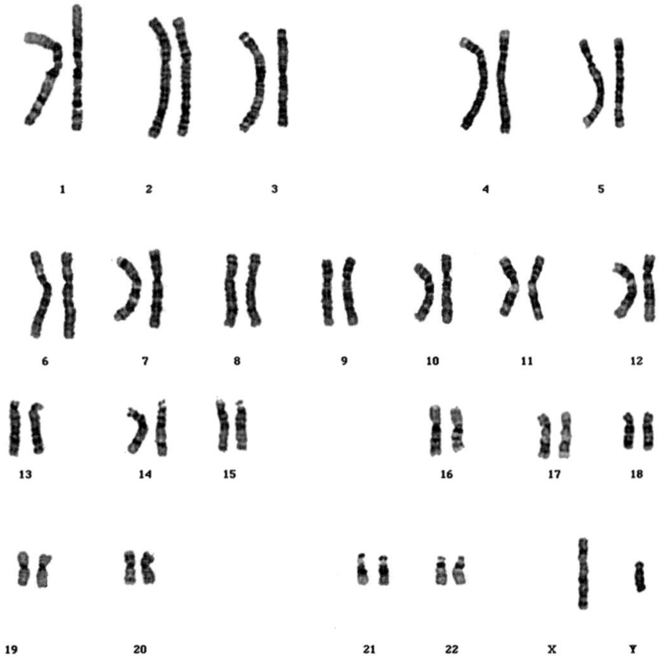

Figure 68-1 Karyogram of male human chromosome complement; 46 total chromosomes are ordered in pairs. Note the nonhomologous pair of sex chromosomes with one X and one Y chromosome (lower right).

CHROMOSOMES

In order to recognize abnormalities, it is first important to understand what makes up a "normal" chromosome set. The human chromosome complement includes 46 chromosomes ordered in 23 pairs (Fig. 68-1). One member of each pair is inherited from an individual's mother and the other comes from the father. Twenty-two pairs are known as *autosomes* and appear as homologs of each other (i.e., they are indistinguishable from each other). The 23rd pair includes the sex chromosomes, which are homologous in a female, who has two X chromosomes, and are nonhomologous (structurally different) in a male, with one X and one Y chromosome (see Fig. 68-1). Genes are encoded in the DNA and are arrayed along the length of the chromosomes. During the cell cycle, the absolute length of the chromosomes vary but the most condensed form is reached in metaphase, at which time chromosomes can most easily be observed. Consequently, metaphase chromosomes are the basis for most cytogenetic studies. Complete evaluation of a set of chromosome is known as *karyoytpe analysis* and an ordered image of the chromosomes from a cell is called a *karyogram*.

Chromosome Structure

A single metaphase chromosome is composed of two DNA double helices. Each double helix is termed a *chromatid* and the two chromatids are held together by an as yet unreplicated region of DNA known as the *centromere*, or primary constriction. In addition to its function in cell division, the centromere acts as a landmark and divides the chromosome into two distinct regions known as *arms* (Fig. 68-2, *A*). The shorter of the two arms is designated the *p arm* and the longer arm is known as the *q arm*. When the centromere is approximately equidistant from both ends, the chromosome is said to be metacentric but if it is closer to one end than the other, the chromosome is submetacentric (see Fig. 68-2, *B*). Five pairs of

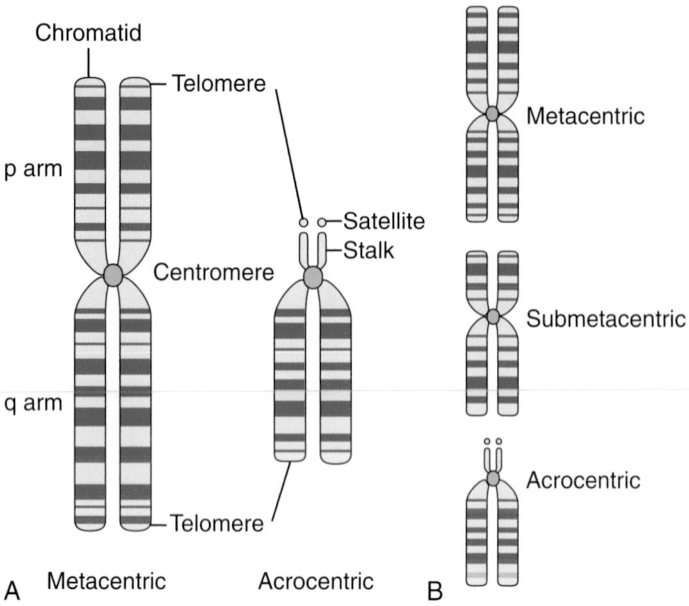

Figure 68-2 Chromosome structure. **A,** Schematic of metaphase chromosome anatomy showing major landmarks. Each chromosome is composed of two chromatids held together by the centromere. The telomere is the end structure of the chromosome. A typical metacentric form is contrasted with an acrocentric having a modified short arm structure composed of stalks and satellites. In all cases, the shorter, or p, arm is oriented up and the longer, or q, arm is oriented down. **B,** The relative position of the centromere can vary, resulting in metacentric (centromere near the middle), submetacentric (centromere closer to one end), and acrocentric (modified short arm) chromosomes.

acrocentric chromosomes have modified short arms with stalks containing only multiple copies of rRNA genes that are capped by a modified telomere termed a *satellite* (see Fig. 68-2, *A*).

The end of a chromosome is the *telomere*. These regions are known to be composed of tandemly repeated DNA with the sequence $(TTAGGG)_n$ that functions to stabilize the chromosomes. The mechanics of DNA replication are such that not all of the telomere DNA can be replicated at each division so there is a shortening of the telomeres over time. It has been postulated that total loss of the telomeres leads to an increase in chromosomal aberrations that may, in part, be responsible for the human aging process (Harley, 1990; Wright, 1992; de Lange, 1998).

Cell Culture

To obtain metaphase cells for a chromosome analysis, cells from a patient must be cultured in vitro. The average human cell divides once every 24 hours, so only about 1% of the cell population is dividing at any given time. However, some cells, such as lymphocytes in a normal healthy individual, do not divide at all. Special culture techniques have therefore been developed to stimulate the cells to divide and increase the yield of metaphase cells.

Specimens

Virtually any viable, nucleated cell sample can be used for cytogenetic analysis. However, certain types of cells are easier to obtain and culture, and are therefore favored for chromosomal preparations. For routine cytogenetic studies of adults and children, heparinized peripheral blood is the preferred specimen. Obtaining a sample via standard phlebotomy is usually easy to arrange and relatively painless for the patient. In hematologic disorders, the best results are obtained from bone marrow samples, because this is the origin of the disease. Fibroblast cultures from skin biopsies or skin punches provide an adequate source of metaphase cells. Tissues such as liver, kidney, lung, and muscle are not routinely used because of the invasive nature of acquiring such specimens; however, these tissues frequently provide an excellent resource if obtained soon after death during autopsy or from a fetal loss. Products-of-conception samples may contain a mix of maternal and fetal tissue and so require extra care in establishing a culture (De Martinville, 1984).

The most common specimen for prenatal analysis is amniotic fluid collected by amniocentesis. Under ultrasound guidance, the physician passes a needle through the mother's abdomen and uterus into the amniotic sac. This is typically done between 16 and 18 weeks of gestation, at which time 20–30 mL of amniotic fluid (fetal urine) can be withdrawn without endangering the fetus. Cells present in the sample are derived from the fetus and provide a source of material for cytogenetic, molecular genetic, and biochemical assays. The fluid itself contains α-fetoprotein (AFP) as well as other proteins and enzymes and forms the substrate for other prenatal assays. The risk of fetal loss due to amniocentesis is approximately 0.5%.

Another prenatal procedure is chorionic villus sampling, which provides tissue from the developing placenta (chorionic villi) (Blakemore, 1988; Rhoads, 1989). The transabdominal or transvaginal procedure is performed at 10–14 weeks' gestation and has a risk of fetal loss of approximately 1%. Because no amniotic fluid is collected, no AFP or related testing can be done, although standard cytogenetic, biochemical, and molecular analyses are possible.

Cordocentesis, or percutaneous umbilical blood sampling, results in a fetal blood specimen that can be used for rapid karyotyping or molecular studies. This procedure is done at later gestational ages (≥20 weeks) and carries a higher risk of fetal loss (2%–5%).

All clinical samples for cytogenetic analysis must be collected in a sterile manner. The presence of bacteria or fungi severely compromises the study because prokaryotic cells usually outcompete and overgrow any human cells that are present. To maximize the number of viable cells, specimens should be transported to the laboratory as soon as possible after collection. Blood, bone marrow, amniotic fluid, and chorionic villi should be maintained at room temperature, whereas solid tissue is transported on wet ice. The difference in temperature of transport is due to the native conditions of the sample. Blood, bone marrow, and amniotic fluid cells exist as individual cells in a fluid substrate, and the integrity of the sample will not be compromised as long as its temperature is maintained close to body temperature. However, tissue collection requires cells to be excised from the body, leaving broken and dying cells at the periphery of the sample. The resultant release of lysosomal enzymes facilitates degradation of the dead cells, but the enzymes will also attack and destroy adjacent living cells. If the temperature is dropped to near 4° C, enzyme activity will be inhibited and the viability of the sample is maintained.

Cell Culture Technique

Depending on the cell type, either a suspension (floating) or monolayer (fixed to a surface) culture technique may be employed. Blood and bone marrow cells are grown in suspension, so cells from the sample can be aliquoted directly into an appropriate culture medium. Bone marrow is typically cultured for 24–48 hours, whereas lymphocytes require 3–4 days in culture for maximum yield. Furthermore, because lymphocytes do not normally divide in culture, they must be induced using a mitogen, usually phytohemagglutinin. The resultant metaphase cells can then be collected by use of a mitotic inhibitor such as colcemid. Amniotic fluid cells, chorionic villi, and solid tissue are all grown as a monolayer in situ. Tissue and chorionic villi are first disaggregated using a mild collagenase treatment, and the individual cells are then seeded on to glass coverslips and covered with culture medium. In an amniotic fluid sample, the cells must be separated from the fluid by centrifugation before being plated in dishes and allowed to form in situ colonies. Typical culture times are 5–7 days for chorionic villi and amniocytes and up to 2 weeks for solid tissue culture.

Once maximum growth has been achieved, all cell types are harvested using similar techniques. The cells are swelled hypotonically (to the point that the cell membrane is stretched but not broken) and are then fixed. Gentle blowing on the coverslip containing fixed cells from in situ cultures results in the rupture of the cell membrane and a spreading of the metaphase chromosomes. For suspension cultures, the fixed cells must be dropped on to a clean microscope slide, which mechanically breaks the membranes and leaves the chromosomes separated slightly from each other but in a discrete region occupied by a single cell (Fig. 68-3). After air drying, the slides are suitable for staining. In some cases, artificial aging of the cells at 65° C for 30–60 minutes improves the quality of the staining. Although most laboratories still perform these steps manually, an automated robotic harvester has been developed that can process large numbers of cultures quite efficiently.

Staining

Chromosomes are routinely stained using Giemsa or Wright's stain, positively charged dyes that bind to the negatively charged DNA molecule. Mild trypsinization of the chromosomes before staining apparently weakens the DNA–protein interactions, yielding a defined pattern of alternating light and dark regions after the stain is applied. This is called the *banding pattern* (G-banding for Giemsa banding) (Yunis, 1973; Burkholder,

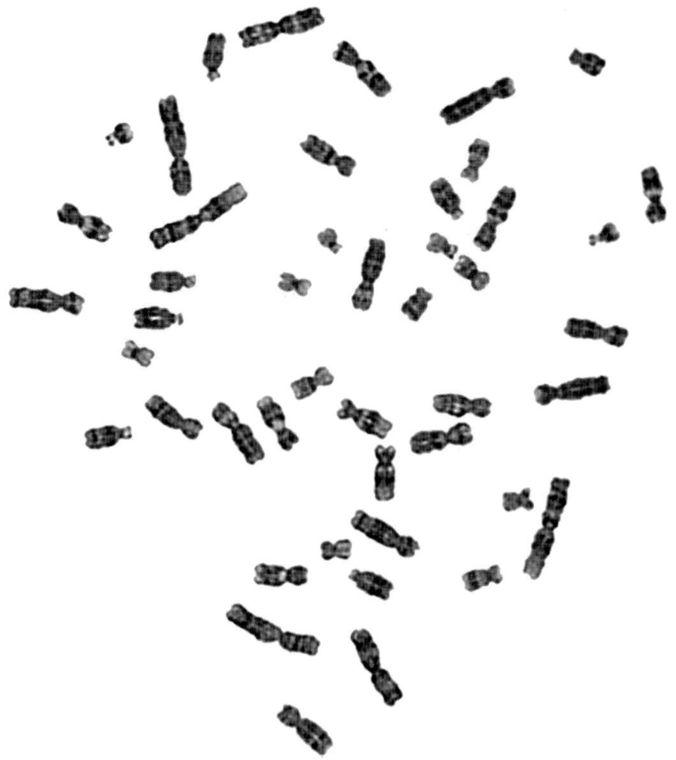

Figure 68-3 Metaphase chromosome spread. Chromosomes from a single cell as seen on a microscope slide.

1977; Holmquist, 1982). Each pair of chromosomes has a unique band pattern that is schematically represented as an ideogram (ISCN, 2009) (Fig. 68-4), and this is used to identify each chromosome and the chromosomal subregions.

Although standard G-banding is adequate for most situations, additional information about chromosome structure can be obtained with other special staining technologies. The most common special stains include Q-banding, C-banding, and R-banding. Q-banding, or quinacrine fluorescence staining, was originally used in routine chromosome analysis (Comings, 1975). However, because the fluorescence is transient, it has been replaced by G-banding, which allows a permanently stained preparation (Sumner, 1973). The current major application of Q-banding is for rapid identification of the Y chromosome. The distal end of the long arm of the Y chromosome is composed of heterochromatin and is the most brightly fluorescent region in a human metaphase (Fig. 68-5, *A*). In cases of ambiguous genitalia, a quick Q-banded preparation can usually answer the question of the presence or absence of a Y chromosome in the patient. C-banding, constitutive or centromere banding, is used to evaluate constitutive heterochromatin or to determine whether a chromosome has two centromeres (dicentric). Normally, a centromere appears as a single dark spot on an overall pale-staining chromosome (Holmquist, 1979). In the case of a dicentric chromosome, the presence of two dark regions clearly identifies the two centromeres (see Fig. 68-5, *B*). R-banding, or reverse banding, results in chromosomes with the same banding pattern as that seen in G-banding, but the light and dark bands are reversed, hence the name. Because the telomeres of the chromosomes tend to be small, light-staining bands, a deletion may not be easily detected using standard G-banding. In R-banding, however, the telomeres should appear as dark bands and their absence as the result of a deletion is more obvious.

Karyotype Analysis

To perform a cytogenetic (karyotype) analysis, it is essential to be able to rapidly and accurately identify each chromosome and determine when chromosome abnormalities are present. The first step is to count the number of chromosomes present in the cell being evaluated. The number

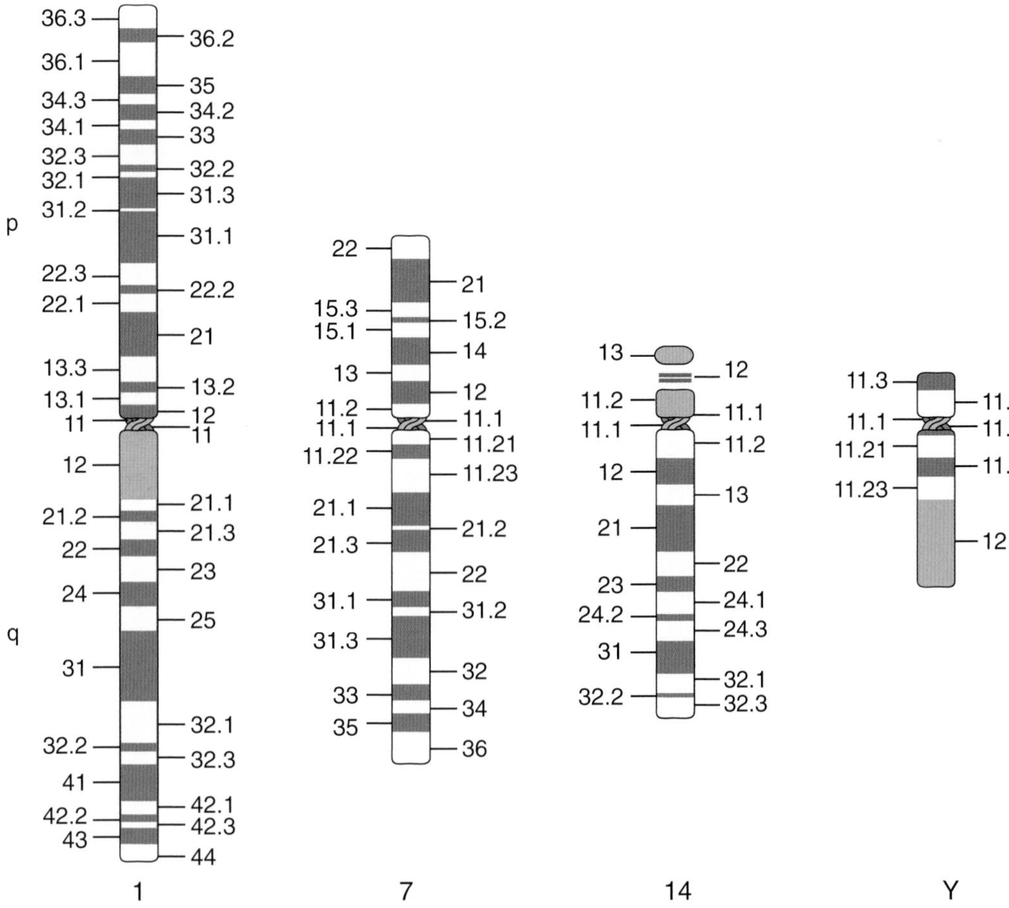

Figure 68-4 Examples of ideograms for chromosomes 1, 7, 14, and Y showing the expected pattern of alternating light and dark bands.

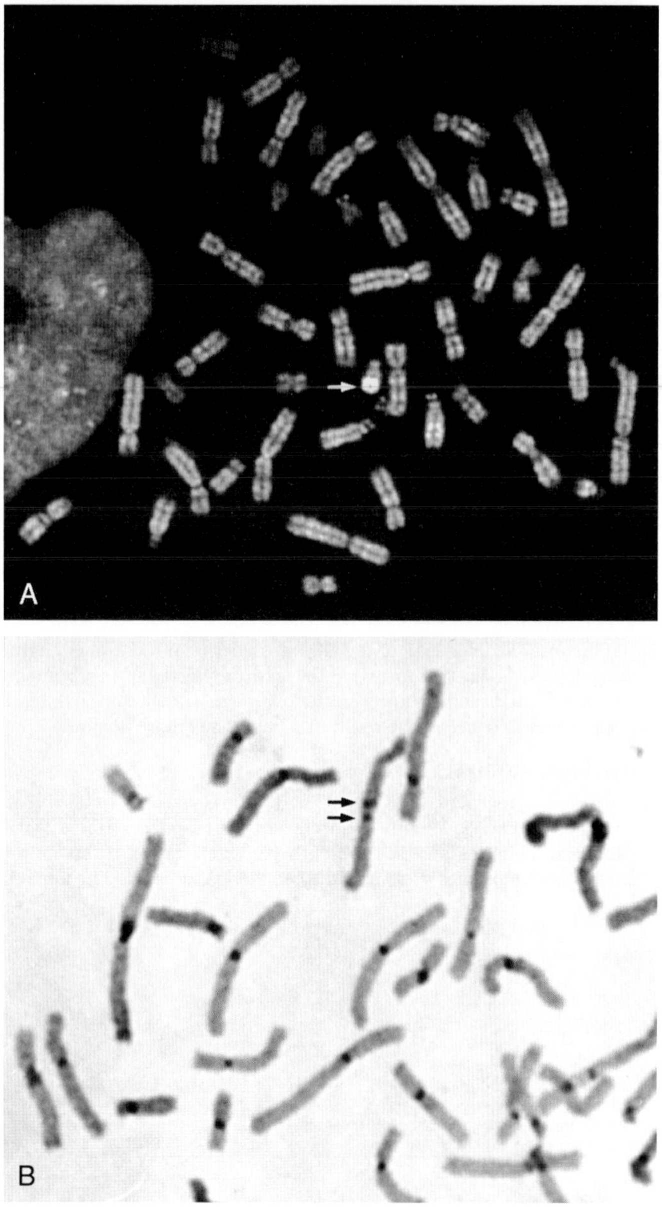

Figure 68-5 **A,** Q-banded metaphase showing bright fluorescence of the Y chromosome *(arrow)*. **B,** C-banded chromosomes showing the dark staining centromeres. A dicentric chromosome was detected with two dark bands *(arrows)*.

of active centromeres defines the total number of chromosomes and will total 46 in a normal human diploid cell. Too many or too few chromosomes indicate a potential numerical abnormality. In vitro culture can result in culture artifacts, so no single cell is used to define an individual's chromosome complement. A typical clinical study requires analysis of 15–20 cells. Single cells with abnormalities are considered artifacts. Three or more cells with the same chromosome loss or two or more cells with the same additional chromosome define a true abnormality. In cases of mosaicism or for other special situations, 10–30 additional cells may be evaluated.

Individual chromosomes are identified based on the overall size of each chromosome, the position of its centromere, and the banding pattern. Any variation in chromosome structure should be detected at this time. In most circumstances, routine G-banding of metaphase chromosomes is sufficient for clinical diagnostic purposes. However, some disorders are associated with very small deletions of chromosomal material that may not be resolved at this level, so high-resolution analysis is used. Special culture conditions are employed, and the cells are harvested at a slightly earlier stage of cell division, prometaphase. At this point in the cell cycle, the chromosomes are less condensed and physically longer, making the presence of small abnormalities easier to detect.

The analysis is performed by a technologist viewing the cells at the microscope and, once the study is complete, a determination is made as to whether the chromosome complement is normal or abnormal. For documentation, representative metaphase cells are captured and karyograms (illustrations of the chromosomes of a given cell, see Fig. 68-1) are prepared. Traditionally, the capture has been performed by photography using a 35-mm camera mounted on the microscope. The film is then developed and photographic prints are made. The chromosomes can be cut out and attached to a sheet of paper. The homologous pairs are arrayed from large to small with special placement for the pair of sex chromosomes. By convention, the shorter arm, the p arm, is oriented up, and the longer q arm is oriented down.

Computer-Assisted Imaging

Currently, most cytogenetics laboratories have moved to computer-assisted imaging. Although photographic prints give a high-resolution image, the technique requires significant time and effort. It is now possible to mount a charge-coupled device video camera on the microscope in place of the 35-mm camera. Using specially designed software, an image of a metaphase cell is captured using a standard frame grabber, digitized, and displayed on the computer monitor. At this point, the software allows the image to be modified by lightening, darkening, or changing the contrast, and a variety of manipulations of the chromosomes are possible, including straightening and importing chromosomes from other fields. A karyogram can then be generated using a pattern-recognition subroutine that will automatically identify the chromosomes and place them in their proper places on a karyogram form. Depending on the software and the quality of the image, the accuracy of this process can vary from 10% to 85%. After the computer has taken its "best guess," a trained cytogenetic technologist must make the appropriate corrections. Once the chromosomes are properly positioned, additional cosmetic enhancements are possible to eliminate ragged edges or bits of background. The final version of the karyogram is then printed out directly by a high-resolution printer. Although the overall quality is not as high as a photographic rendering, there is a tremendous saving of time using the computerized system. A routine karyogram from capture to printing should take a trained technologist on average 15–20 minutes. Another major advantage of the computer-assisted system is in fluorescence microscopy.

Fluorescence In Situ Hybridization

The classic cytogenetic staining discussed earlier is the result of dyes that bind to the DNA or protein of a chromosome and allow visualization by light microscopy. In situ hybridization, a combination of molecular and cytogenetic technologies, opened another door that has allowed further investigation of chromosome anomalies. Here, instead of a dye, a molecular probe (i.e., a fragment of DNA) binds to the chromosome. In early studies, the probe was labeled with a radioactive compound (usually tritium) such that after 5–10 days of exposure to radiograph film, a pattern of silver grains could be detected identifying the chromosomal location of that probe. This technique facilitated gene mapping by identifying gene loci (Trask, 1991).

Autoradiography was useful, but only one probe at a time could be used; it required a significant length of time for exposure, and there was a degree of scatter of the silver grains that necessitated statistical analysis of the data obtained. In the mid-1980s, a variation of the technique was developed that has proven to be extremely useful in clinical applications. The new technology, fluorescence in situ hybridization (FISH), is quicker, more specific, and allows the use of multiple probes in a single hybridization procedure. Furthermore, instead of radioactively labeled probes, a fluorescent dye is used that is visualized using fluorescence microscopy (Ledbetter, 1989).

In clinical applications of FISH, the most common goal is to determine whether a gene, a specific mutation, or a particular chromosomal rearrangement is present, so the molecular probes used must be well characterized and specific to the locus in question. There are three basic types of probe. *Chromosome painting* probes are actually a cocktail of many unique DNA fragments from along the entire length of a chromosome, such that, following hybridization, the entire chromosome fluoresces (Fig. 68-6, *A*). *Repeat sequence* probes are isolated from telomere or centromere regions. Centromere probes are usually used in chromosome enumeration (i.e., to detect the gain or loss of specific chromosomes) (Lichter, 1990). A true telomere probe recognizes the six base repeat present at the ends of all chromosomes and will confirm the presence or absence of the telomeric regions. In practice, however, both true centromere and telomere probes are not particularly useful because so many signals are generated. Chromosome-specific pericentromeric and subtelomeric probes are now in use (see Figs. 68-6, *C* and *D*). A *unique sequence* probe is usually isolated from cloned DNA of a disease-causing gene or a fragment of DNA of

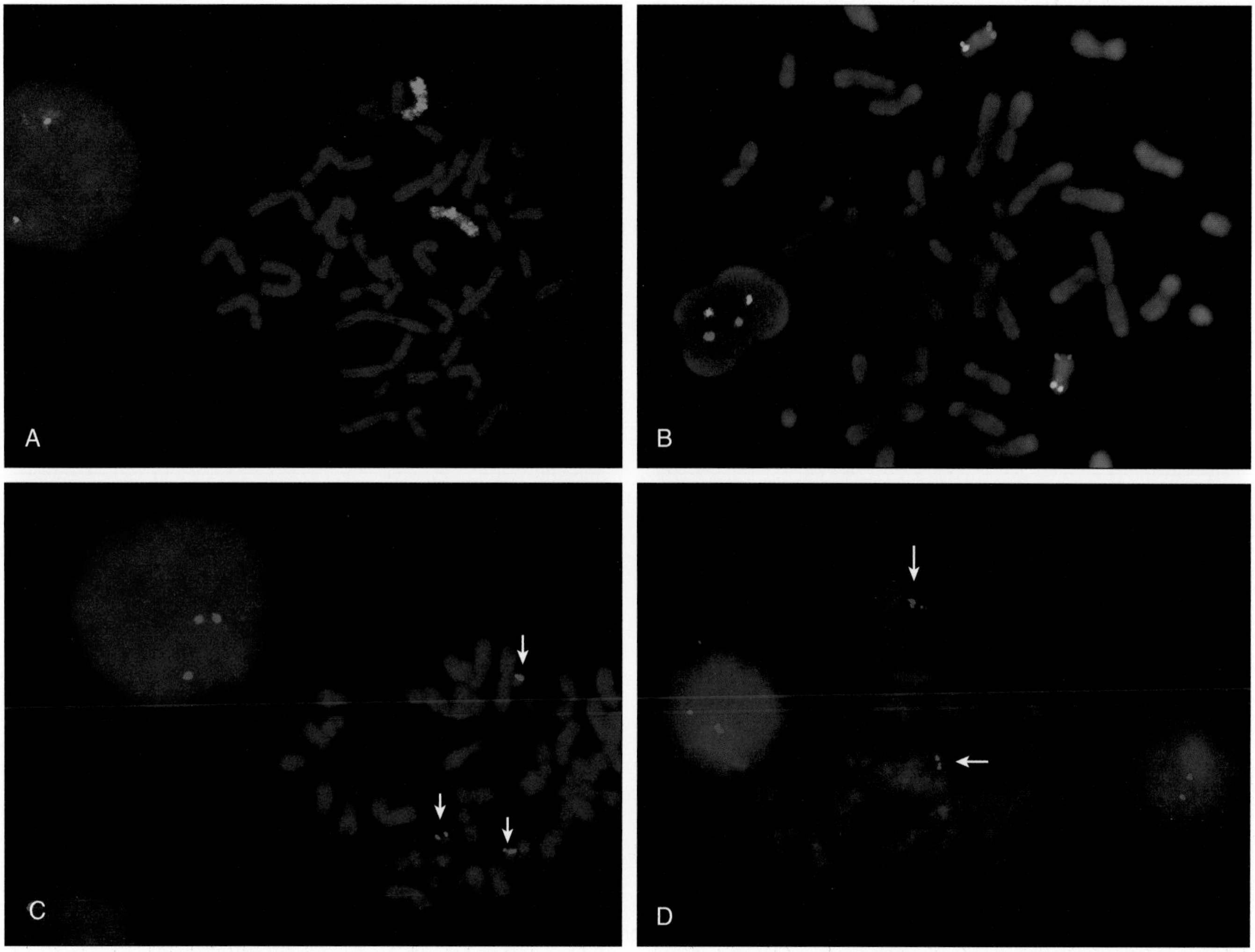

Figure 68-6 Fluorescence in situ hybridization. **A,** Whole chromosome paint probe highlighting the two X chromosomes in a female cell. **B,** Chromosomes showing hybridization with subtelomere probes. The p arm subtelomere is indicated by the green signals, and the q arm subtelomere is indicated by the red signals. Paired red and green signals are seen in the interphase nucleus to the *left*. **C** and **D,** Repeat sequence centromere probe for chromosome 21. **C,** Trisomy 21 seen at *left* in an interphase nucleus and at *right* in a metaphase *(arrows)*. **D,** Normal complement of two copies of chromosome 21 *(arrows)* seen in interphase (*left* and *right*) and in a metaphase (*center*).

known location associated with a particular gene. This type of probe is used to identify the presence or absence of the gene, gene region, or chromosomal rearrangement of interest (Cherif, 1989; Lindsay, 1993). *Subtelomere* probes are a subset of this category. Research revealed that there are unique sequences just proximal to the telomere of each chromosome arm that can be used for specific identification of each arm. The subtelomere probes that have been generated have become very valuable in characterizing cryptic rearrangements by determining whether all subtelomeres are present and located on the correct chromosome arms, and, if not, if a rearrangement has occurred (see Fig. 68-6, *B*). Furthermore, it has been shown that 3%–5% of patients with unexplained mental retardation have a cytogenetically undetectable terminal deletion of a chromosome (Flint, 1995, 2003; Rosenberg, 2001). Subtelomere FISH now allows identification of such deletions and localization to the specific chromosome affected (National Institutes of Health and Institute of Molecular Medicine Collaboration, 1996; Irons, 2003).

Technique

FISH can be performed on either metaphase or interphase cells. For metaphase FISH, cells are cultured and harvested as for a routine karyotype analysis, but no culture is required for interphase FISH. Fixed cells are collected and slides are made as described for karyotyping. The DNA on the slides is then denatured, and a fluorescently labeled single-stranded molecular probe is allowed to hybridize to the chromosomal DNA using an annealing temperature that favors hybridization of homologous regions of DNA (Fig. 68-7, *A*). After an appropriate period of hybridization, excess probe is washed away and the nonhybridized DNA is counterstained with another fluorochrome to allow visualization of the entire chromosome complement. A fluorescent microscope with light from a 100 W mercury bulb in combination with appropriate sets of exciter filters allows evaluation of the cells. Due to the optical limitations of the glass filters, a maximum of three colors can be visualized on a typical fluorescent microscope. For documentation, a 35-mm camera attached to the microscope can be used, although superior results are obtained using a computer-assisted system to acquire the fluorescent images. Software packages also allow enhancement of weak signals and sharpening of the image.

One of the most critical elements in FISH is the selection of a specific probe or probes that will help to answer a clinical question. For example, one of the most useful clinical applications of FISH is the detection of microdeletions too small to be seen using classical cytogenetics (see Figs. 68-7, *B* to *D*). The gene must be known and the probe used must be homologous to the critical region of the gene that is usually deleted. Hybridization with the probe should result in a fluorescent signal only at the target locus. If a signal is present, DNA complementary to the probe is present, so there is no deletion (see Fig. 68-7, *B*). However, the absence of signal indicates that a deletion exists (i.e., there is no DNA sequence present on the chromosome that is complementary to the probe, so no hybridization can occur) (see Fig. 68-7, *D*). A control probe to a different region of the chromosome being tested is usually used as a hybridization control (see Fig. 68-7, *C*). Therefore, when evaluating a disease related probe, an unaffected individual should have two signals per cell for each autosomal gene, one signal for each chromosome of the pair (Fig. 68-8, *A*). An affected individual with a deletion should have a single signal per cell, showing one normal and one deleted chromosome (see Fig. 68-8, *B*). For both affected and unaffected, the control probe should show two signals per cell in all cells that are scored. In a metaphase cell, the chromosomes may be short and condensed, with each chromatid individually visible, resulting in a discrete FISH signal on each chromatid. In these

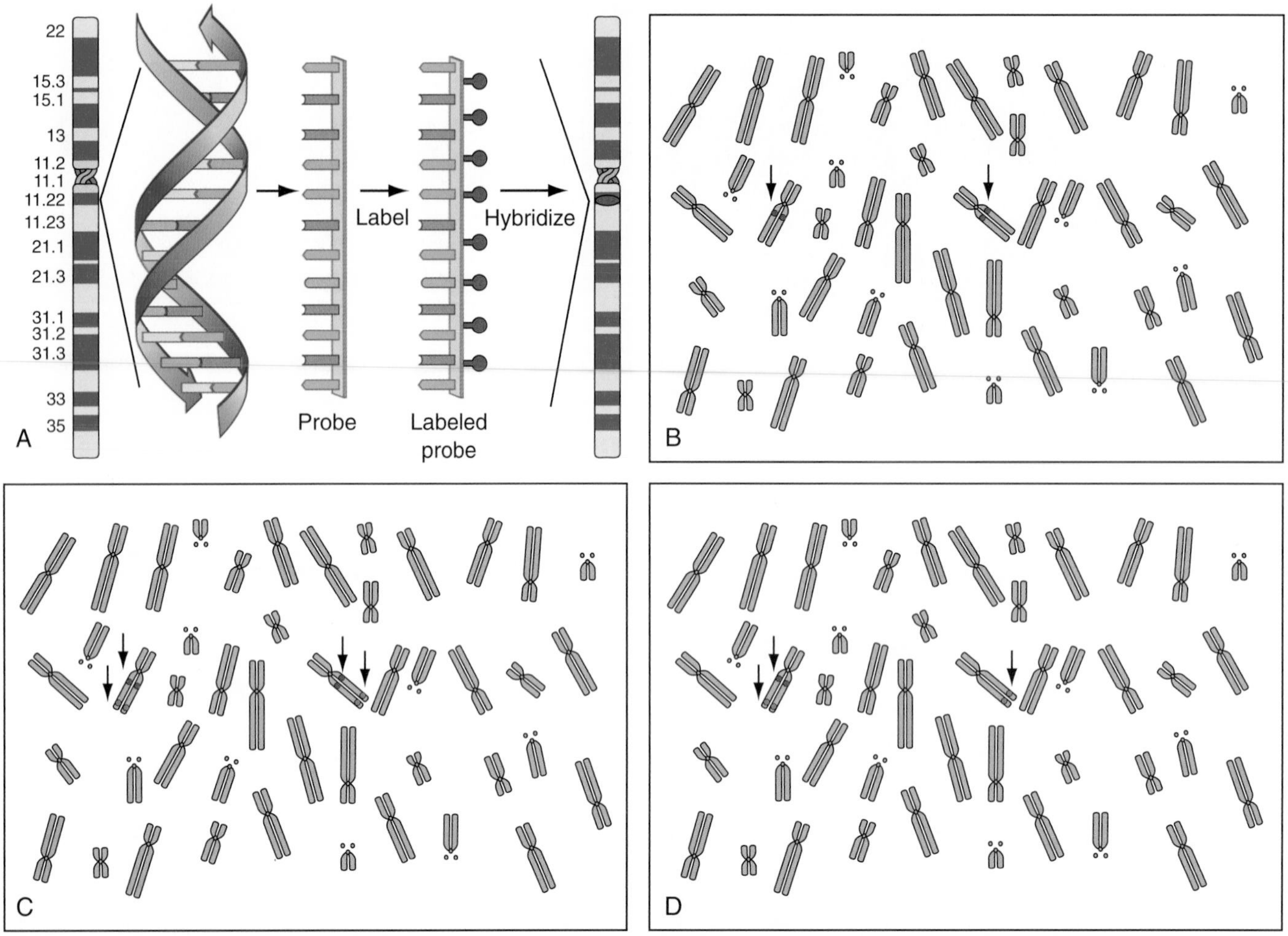

Figure 68-7 **A,** Schematic of fluorescence in situ hybridization (FISH) technology. DNA derived from a known gene is rendered single stranded, labeled with a fluorescent tag, then hybridized back to the chromosomes of a metaphase cell. **B** to **D,** Depiction of a metaphase cell with 46 chromosomes that has been processed using FISH technology. The labeled probes hybridized to targets are indicated with *arrows.* **B,** Dual signals indicating hybridization to both alleles of target gene. **C,** Target gene indicated by *red* signal and a control probe indicated in *green.* Complete hybridization to all alleles. **D,** Hybridization of both controls (*green*) but presence of only a single target gene indicating deletion of one allele.

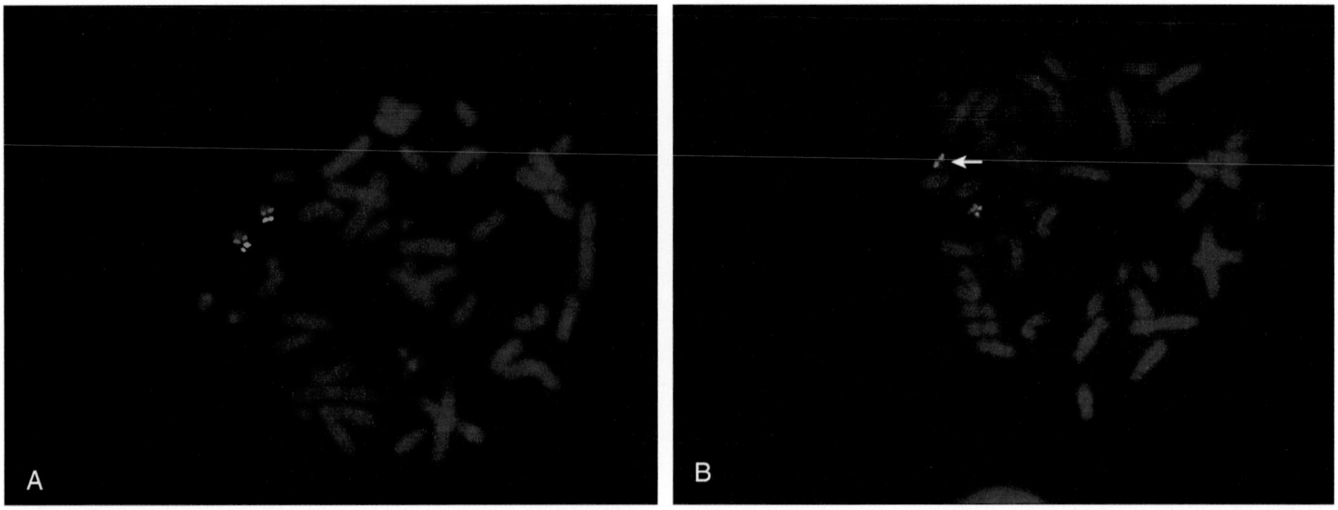

Figure 68-8 Fluorescence in situ hybridization detection of a microdeletion of chromosome 22 associated with velocardiofacial syndrome. **A,** An individual with no deletion showing the presence of one *red* (gene locus) and one *green* (control locus) signal for each chromosome 22. **B,** Patient with a deletion seen as a chromosome with only a single *green* (control) signal. The homologous chromosome 22 is "normal" with one *red* and one *green* signal.

cells, there may appear to be two signals per chromosome for a total of four signals but, in actual scoring, only complete chromosomes are considered so a signal on one or both chromatids would be counted as just one positive signal.

One of the problems with this detection system is that the lack of signal is the positive indication of a deletion. Technical failure of hybridization may also result in absence of signal. To eliminate this as a source of error, a minimum of 20 cells must be evaluated, and all cells must agree in signal count. If mosaicism is suspected, additional cells may be surveyed. In addition, unique sequence probes are currently used in combination with a control probe (see Fig. 68-7, *C*). The secondary probe is localized to the same arm of the chromosome as the deletion locus. It may be labeled with

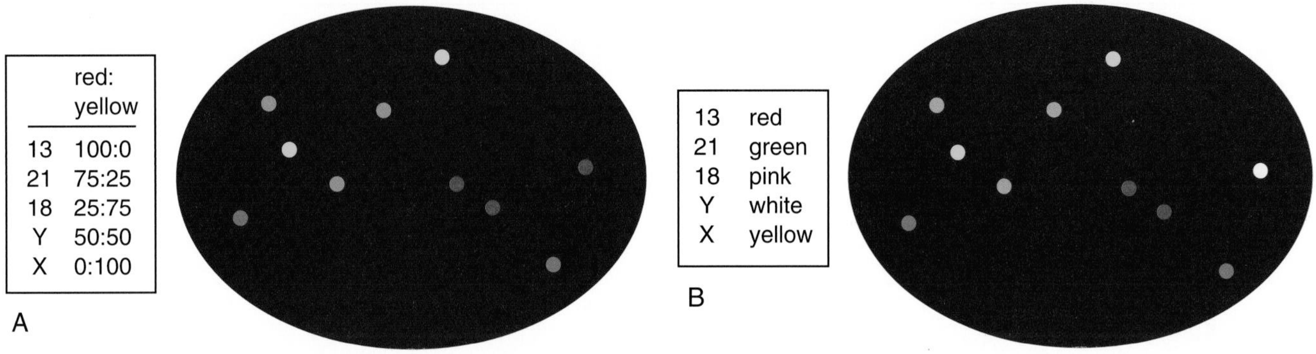

Figure 68-9 Multicolor fluorescence in situ hybridization. **A,** Diagram of the staining pattern for five probes (chromosomes 13, 18, 21, X, and Y) in an interphase cell. Table at the left shows relative proportions of the red and yellow fluorochromes used for each probe. **B,** The same cell depicted in **A,** now showing the computer-derived artificial color assignments (key shown in box to left). This cell can now be interpreted as having two copies each for chromosomes 13, 21, and X, three copies of chromosome 18, and one Y chromosome.

the same fluorochrome as the deletion locus probe but it has been found that the interpretation of the hybridization results is easier if the control site probe is labeled with a fluorochrome of a different color. In all cells evaluated, two clear control signals must be seen, and then the corresponding signals for the disease locus can be recorded. This provides a hybridization control as well as a marker for the chromosome of interest (see Fig. 68-7, *D*). If a dual color system is used, results may be obtained in interphase as well as metaphase cells.

Chromosome painting probes are most useful in identifying complex rearrangements or marker chromosomes. If an individual has an abnormal chromosome with extra material of unknown origin, it may be possible to use chromosome painting to identify the source of the extra DNA. This may help in either diagnosis or prognosis of the individual. For example, in the case of a patient with only one identifiable X chromosome and a small, unidentified marker chromosome, it will be important to determine if the origin of the marker is an X or a Y chromosome. This can be accomplished using chromosome paints for the X and Y chromosomes labeled with different fluorochromes.

FISH probes are most informative when evaluated in metaphase cells where it is possible to identify the specific chromosome to which the probe hybridizes. However, in some cell preparations, very few metaphase cells may be present, and, in these cases, information may be obtained with unique sequence or repeat sequence probes in interphase nuclei. Here, the technical problems are increased as a result of random loss of signal, extra signals, and overlapping signals in cells, so additional cells (a total of 50–200) must be counted to obtain a statistically significant result.

Multicolor Fluorescence In Situ Hybridization

Another advantage of FISH is the ability to hybridize multiple probes to a single slide to obtain a better understanding of chromosome rearrangements (Schrock, 1996; Speicher, 1996). For most FISH probes, the maximum number of colors is three (one target sequence, one control sequence, and one counterstain), and this can be handled by a typical fluorescent microscope. However, if more than three colors are needed, a computer-assisted imaging system is required. This is because a fluorescent image is the result of the light from the mercury bulb passing through an exciter filter, hitting the fluorochrome on the slide, and transmitting an image of the appropriate color to the eyepiece for viewing. Each fluorochrome requires its own filter so, for each additional color desired, the light must pass through additional thicknesses of glass. The optical properties of glass and light limit the total number of viewable colors to three. However, with a computer-assisted system, detection of multiple colors becomes possible. The computer does not actually "see" more colors but it can detect subtle differences in shades better than the human eye. In a relatively simple example, two fluorochromes are used and mixed in varying proportions to give a range of colors. In the example in Figure 68-9, *A*, a red fluorochrome is mixed with a yellow fluorochrome generating intermediate colors from red to yellow. Eight signals are seen, but as viewed through the microscope, it is impossible to be absolutely sure which signal corresponds to a particular chromosome. Although difficult to distinguish by the human eye, the computer can register each color as a different shade of gray and then the software assigns a unique color to that shade for display on the computer monitor. Figure 68-9, *B*, shows the final multicolor version using many different colors now easily distinguishable but very different from the original presentation (see Fig. 68-9, *A*). Using the key to the left, the following chromosomes are detected: two each for chromosomes 13, 21, and X; three chromosomes 18, and one Y chromosome. This cell is therefore trisomic for chromosome 18 with an XXY sex chromosome complement. Combinations of fluorochromes have been developed that allow detection of each of the 24 different chromosomes followed by a unique color assignment by the computer (Reid, 1992a, 1992b; Divane, 1994).

Microarray Technology

Adding FISH to the options for cytogenetic testing has greatly increased the detection rate of chromosomal abnormalities. However, there are still individuals who test normal yet present with findings suggestive of a chromosome anomaly. To obtain even more detailed information on the chromosomes of these problematic patients, use of microarray analysis was investigated and has proven to be quite valuable in genetic diagnosis. Since 2006, it has gained acceptance as a clinical tool, adding yet another dimension to cytogenetic analysis.

The function of a cytogenetic microarray is to screen the genome for copy number variation (CNV). (See Chapter 67 for a discussion of the technology behind microarray analysis.) There are three different levels of microarray: (1) bacterial artificial chromosome (BAC) arrays, (2) oligonucleotide arrays, and (3) single nucleotide polymorphism (SNP) arrays. In the order given, the size of the probes decrease while the total number of probes per genome increases. Thus, BAC arrays provide a general overview to the human genome and are usually targeted to regions of known association with genetic disease (markers spaced on average about 1 MB apart). Oligonucleotide arrays generally also target known disease genes, but add in background sequences so these arrays have an overall coverage of the genome with probes spaced 50 to 100 KB. SNP arrays provide significantly more detailed coverage with probes on average every 100 to 1000 base pairs. The choice of which platform to use depends on the question being asked. Early analyses used BAC arrays exclusively because the information desired was usually associated with specific diseases. It is now well documented that a patient's anomalies may be due to a genetic lesion that has not been previously described and, therefore, is not characteristic of a known genetic disease. This has led to a desire for a fuller examination of the genome by the use of either oligonucleotide or SNP arrays.

When performed correctly, a microarray assay will detect deletions, duplications, aneuploidies, and unbalanced translocations with a gain or loss of sequences. Some of the more advanced assays can also identify methylation patterns and so are useful in evaluating cases of uniparental disomy. Using microarray analysis has allowed the identification of genomic lesions too small or too cryptic to be detected by other types of assays, and this has led to a diagnosis for many patients for whom the cause of their anomalies had previously been unknown (Pickering, 2008; Saam, 2008).

However, as with all technologies, microarray is not a perfect solution for all situations. One drawback is that these microarrays will not detect balanced chromosome rearrangements, including translocations and inversions. In addition, the assay will identify all existing CNVs, from large to small, including polymorphic variants. As of 2011, the human genome has not been completely analyzed, so the existence and significance of all CNVs have not been cataloged. It is not unusual for an assay to report the presence of CNVs for which the clinical significance is unknown. In these cases, it is difficult for the clinician to know whether or not they have found

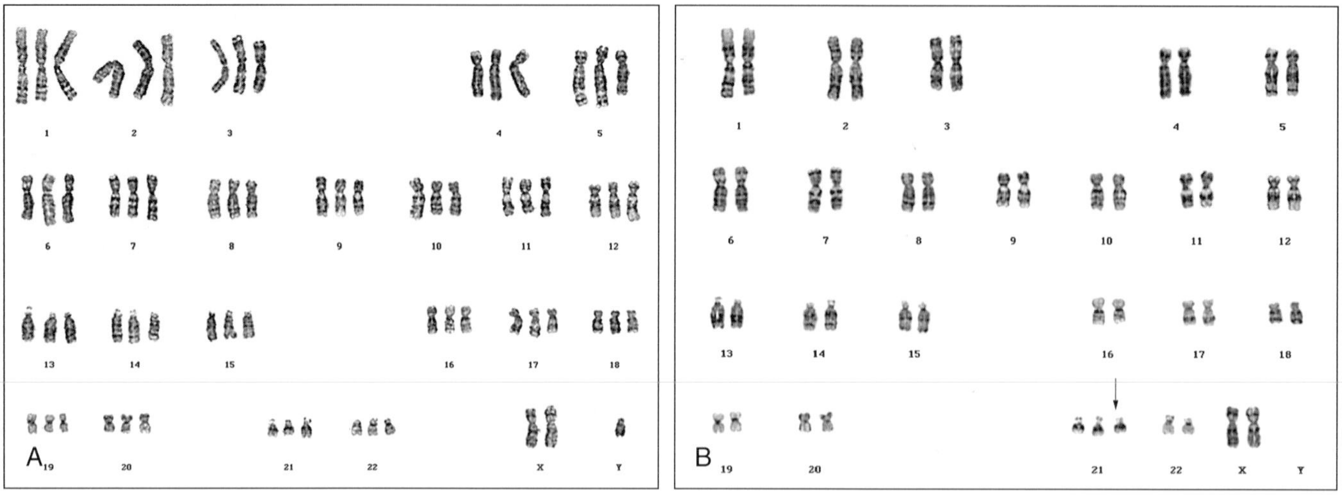

Figure 68-10 Numerical chromosome abnormalities. **A,** Triploid (3N) chromosome complement with three copies of each chromosome (69,XXY). **B,** Trisomy 21 (47,XX,+21) with one extra chromosome 21 *(arrow).*

the cause of the patient's problems. A similar problem occurred when FISH was first implemented in clinical testing, but over the years, data have been compiled and the understanding of the possible outcomes is now well understood. Having learned from this experience, clinical laboratories performing microarray analyses are encouraged to report all of their findings to one of two international databases that are collecting the new information. These searchable databases will aid in better interpretation of CNVs.

CHROMOSOME ABNORMALITIES

Clinical cytogenetic testing is an integral part of clinical medicine. Finding a particular chromosome anomaly may explain a physical problem or phenotypic abnormality in the patient and be directly associated with a disease diagnosis. It is therefore critical to determine whether an affected individual has a chromosome complement that differs from the standard pattern of 23 pairs of chromosomes with known morphology. There are two basic categories of cytogenetically detectable variation: (1) numerical and (2) structural change.

Numerical Abnormalities

In humans and other mammals, the chromosomes occur in pairs, so, of the 46 human chromosomes, there are only 23 uniquely different chromosomes. A set of 23 comprises the haploid (*N*) number of chromosomes, which is the number of chromosomes in a gamete. At fertilization, two haploid complements join to form a zygote with 46 chromosomes, the diploid (2*N*) complement. Errors in division can give rise to chromosome complements that have more or less than 46 chromosomes. Exact multiples of the haploid set of chromosomes is called *euploidy*. Gain or loss of one or a few chromosomes is known as *aneuploidy*.

Euploidy

Diploidy, the normal state of human cells, is a form of euploidy. Abnormal euploidies include triploidy ($3N = 69$ chromosomes) and tetraploidy ($4N = 92$ chromosomes), but these are not compatible with life and are detected primarily in spontaneous abortus tissues. Triploidy (Fig. 68-10, *A*) may be due to the failure in gametogenesis of one of the meiotic divisions, giving rise to a 2*N* gamete that, when combined with a haploid gamete from the other parent, produces a triploid zygote. Alternatively, a 3*N* complement may be derived from dispermy, the fertilization of a haploid egg by two sperm, and this generally results in a partial hydatidiform mole. Tetraploidy, on the other hand, is usually a postmeiotic event and presents as a duplication of a diploid complement (XXXX or XXYY), most probably due to failure of an early mitotic cleavage division in the zygote.

Aneuploidy

More common are nondisjunctional errors resulting in aneuploidy. Here, a single pair of chromosomes fails to disjoin properly in division, giving rise to one extra chromosome or one missing chromosome per cell. Occasionally, more than one pair of chromosomes may be involved, but these cases are extremely rare. Nondisjunction errors may occur in either meiosis or mitosis. Early mitotic nondisjunction in a zygote may result in an individual with the aberrant chromosome complement in all cells of the body, but a latter division error usually produces a *mosaic*, an individual with two cell lines that differ only by a single chromosome.

In normal meiosis, one DNA replication is followed by two cell divisions resulting in four haploid (*N*) gametes (one copy of each chromosome) (Fig. 68-11, *A*). The first meiotic division is the reduction division, in which the total number of chromosomes per cell is reduced by half. The second meiotic division is a simple mitotic type of division with a separation of the centromeres and distribution of the chromosomes to daughter cells. Meiotic errors may result in gametes with either an extra or missing chromosome (Angell, 1994). A nondisjunction error in the first meiotic division (see Fig. 68-11, *B*) leads to two gametes that are disomic for one chromosome and two gametes that are missing that chromosome (nullosomic). When fertilized, the former will give a trisomic conception for the nondisjoined chromosome (example: trisomy 21 in Fig. 68-10, *B*), and the latter will result in a monosomy. Similarly, Figure 68-11, *C*, shows an error in the second meiotic division resulting in two normal haploid gametes, one disomic gamete, and one nullosomic gamete.

Trisomy or monosomy may occur for any chromosome, but most of these are incompatible with life and will terminate spontaneously. Trisomy 16, for example, is the most commonly detected trisomy in spontaneous abortus tissue but is not reported in liveborn individuals. Liveborn autosomal trisomies include chromosomes 13, 18, and 21. Infrequently, patients with a mosaic chromosome complement for trisomies 8, 9, or 22 are identified. Sex chromosome trisomies are viable and well documented (see later). The only viable monosomy is of the X chromosome (45,X). Examples of clinically significant aneuploidies are discussed later in this chapter.

Because trisomies and monosomies are largely incompatible with life, it had been assumed that these would result in fetal wastage. However, molecular analyses have shown that a small fraction of these aneuploid conceptions are "rescued" and go on to produce liveborn children. In the case of a monosomy, the rescue is accomplished by duplication of the single existing chromosome, resulting in a chromosome complement with *uniparental isodisomy* for that chromosome (two copies of the same chromosome inherited from one parent) (Fig. 68-12, *right*) (Ledbetter, 1995). This is exemplified by several reported cases in the literature in which a child affected with cystic fibrosis was shown to be homozygous for the ΔF508 mutation, although molecular tests on both parents revealed that only one was a carrier of ΔF508 (Spence, 1988; Voss, 1989). The interpretation is that the conception was a nonviable monosomy 7 rescued by duplication of the existing chromosome 7 that happened to be carrying the mutation for cystic fibrosis. A similar situation is possible in the case of a trisomy. Again, most trisomies are nonviable but, if one of the three chromosomes is lost, a disomy for that chromosome pair is reinstated (see Fig. 68-12, *left*). In a set of three chromosomes, loss of a single chromosome results in a complement with one maternal and one paternal chromosome (*biparental heterodisomy*) two out of three times. One third of the time, the two remaining chromosomes are from a single parent (i.e., uniparental disomy). In this situation, it makes a difference in which meiotic division the error occurred. A first-division nondisjunction results in heterodisomy, which is two homologous but heterozygous chromosomes (one grandmaternal and one grandpaternal); however, a second division error results in duplicate

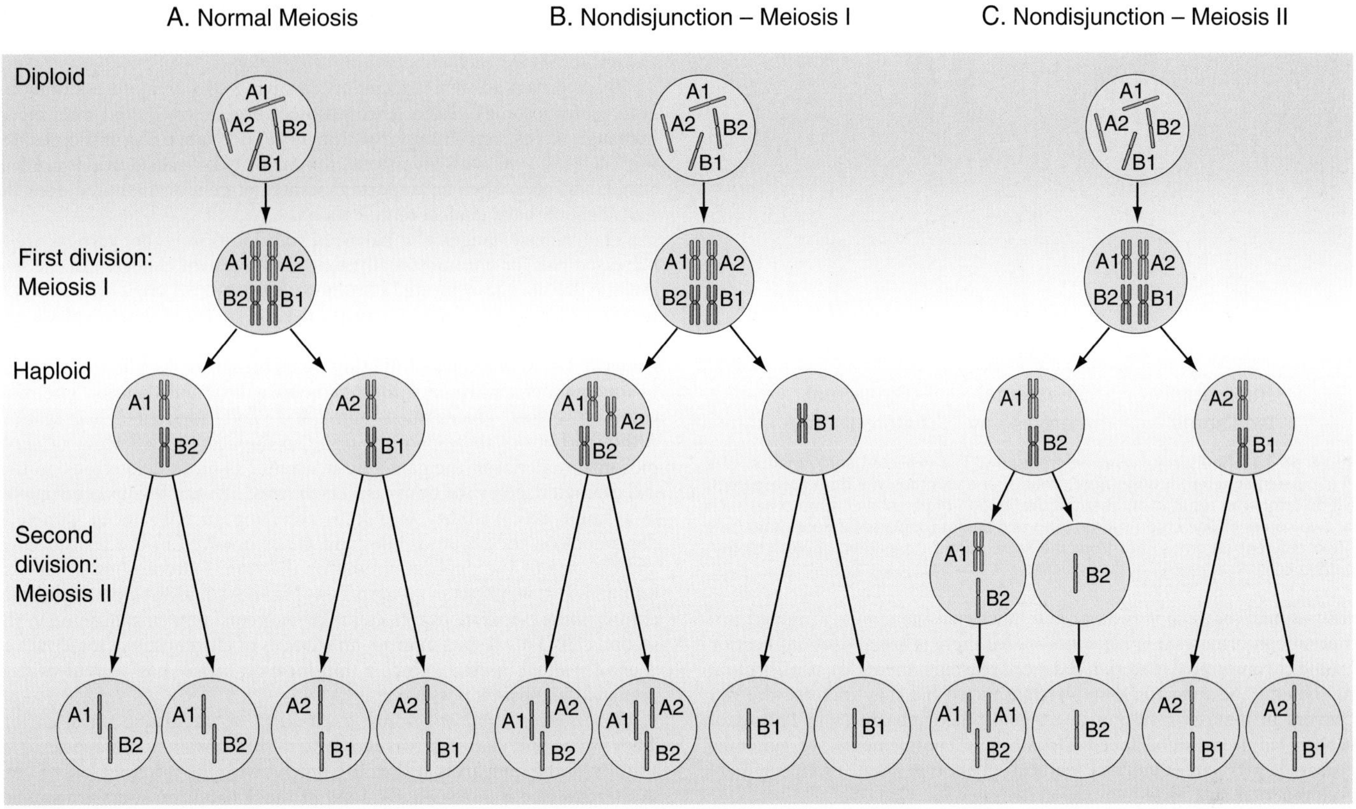

Figure 68-11 Meiosis and meiotic nondisjunction errors resulting in aneuploid gametes. **A,** Normal meiosis generating four gametes with a haploid chromosome set. **B,** Nondisjunction in meiosis I leading to an extra copy of chromosome A (heterodisomy) in two gametes (*left*) but the lack of any A chromosome (nullosomy) in the remaining two gametes (*right*). **C,** Nondisjunction in meiosis II results in two gametes with a normal chromosome complement (*right*), one gamete missing an A chromosome (*left center*), and one gamete with an extra duplicated chromosome (two copies of A1), resulting in isodisomy for chromosome A1 (*left*).

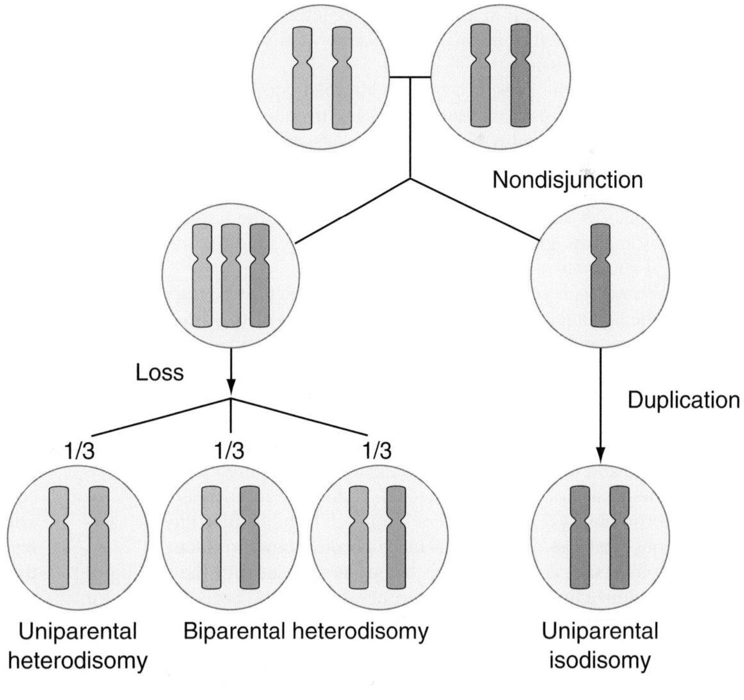

Figure 68-12 Generation of uniparental disomy from nondisjunction errors. On the *left*, heterodisomy resulting from reduction of a trisomy to a disomy is illustrated. On the *right*, isodisomy as the result of monosomy rescue (duplication of a single existing chromosome) is seen.

copies of a single chromosome, isodisomy (see Figs. 68-11, *B* and *C*, and 68-13). In the past, it was thought that having two chromosomes per pair was sufficient, but data strongly indicate that, in some cases, it is essential for the pairs to comprise one maternal and one paternal chromosome. This issue, including the problems of uniparental versus biparental disomy and isodisomy versus heterodisomy, is of major importance in understanding issues of *imprinting*, a topic discussed in detail in Chapter 70 (Nicholls, 1998; Hall, 1990, Cassidy, 1992; Petersen, 1992).

Structural Chromosome Abnormalities

Chromosomes are not static structures but undergo recombination in both meiosis and mitosis. This is a natural process that is critical in generating variation in the species, so a highly developed regulatory system is in place to prevent error from occurring. Nevertheless, errors do occur, sometimes resulting in chromosome rearrangements that change the structure of one or more chromosomes. Such abnormalities are quite varied and are often patient-specific. Rearrangements may be (1) *balanced*, if all the

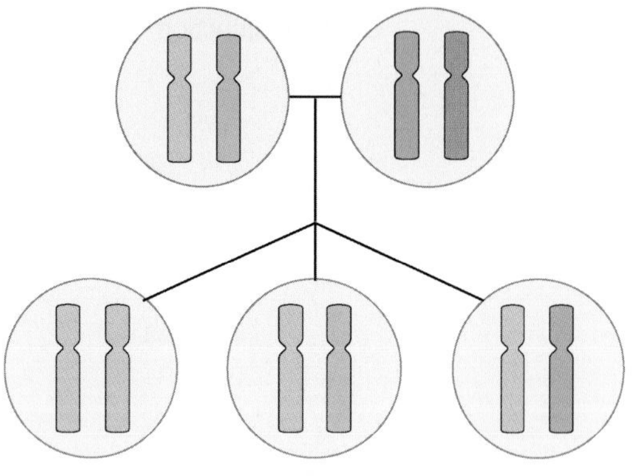

Figure 68-13 Isodisomy versus heterodisomy. The expected conformation of a cell is biparental heterodisomy (*right*), that is, one chromosome from each parent. Division errors can result in an aberrant distribution of parental chromosomes such that two copies of one chromosome from one parent (uniparental isodisomy) (*left*) or two different chromosomes from the same parent (uniparental heterodisomy) (*center*) occur.

chromosomal material is present and functional but simply arranged in a different conformation; or (2) *unbalanced*, if there is loss and/or duplication of some chromosomal material. Balanced rearrangements are usually clinically benign and tend to be stably transmitted but may increase the risk of errors in meiosis resulting in chromosomal imbalances in fetuses or liveborn children. Unbalanced chromosome complements are generally associated with an abnormal clinical phenotype that often includes developmental delay and mental retardation.

A *deletion* is the loss of a part of a chromosome and leads to partial monosomy of the chromosome involved (Fig. 68-14, *B*). Deletions vary in size from quite large to very small and may be *terminal*, which is loss of a portion of the chromosome including the telomere, or *interstitial*, which is loss of an internal piece of chromosome. Chromosome breakage, unequal crossing over, or nondisjunction errors involving chromosome rearrangements may result in a deletion. In general, larger deletions result in more severe clinical abnormalities because of the greater number of gene loci that are missing.

A *duplication* is the presence of an additional copy of a chromosome segment that leads to partial trisomy for that chromosome (see Fig. 68-14, *C*). This anomaly may also be *terminal* or *interstitial*. True duplications appear to be quite rare and are usually sporadic. Duplications are generated by the same mechanisms as deletions and may be the reciprocal outcome of those processes. As is true of deletions, the larger the duplicated piece of chromosome, the greater the genomic imbalance, and the more severe the clinical abnormalities tend to be.

An *inversion* is a reversal of a chromosomal segment with respect to the normal gene arrangement and requires a minimum of two breaks in one chromosome (see Fig. 68-14, *D*). Inversions are classified as either (1) *paracentric*, where the two breaks occur on the same side of the centromere (i.e., in the same arm), or (2) *pericentric*, where the breaks occur on opposite sides of the centromere and the inversion involves both arms (Fig. 68-15, *A*). The majority of inversions are balanced but, if the chromosome breaks within a gene and disrupts normal production of a required gene product, clinical abnormalities may be detected. There is an increased risk of meiotic error, and inversion carriers frequently exhibit infertility or early spontaneous fetal loss due to unbalanced chromosome products.

For an inversion carrier, meiosis begins as normal, with the pairing of the homologous chromosomes. The process is a little more complex for an inverted chromosome, which must form a structure known as an *inversion loop* (see Fig. 68-15, *B*) in order for the homologous loci to pair (i.e., A to a, B to b, C to c, etc.). If no recombination occurs while the loop is present and the chromosomes separate normally, the gametes will not be negatively impacted. However, crossing over within the inversion loop can lead to unbalanced meiotic products. For a paracentric inversion, the results of recombination are usually nonviable acentric and dicentric chromosomes, so there is an apparent suppression of recombination (i.e., the only viable gametes produced are from nonrecombined chromosomes) (see Fig. 68-15, *B*). For pericentric inversions, it is possible that gametes with a chromosome duplication and/or deletion may be derived. In general, larger pericentric inversions result in smaller duplications/deficiencies and increase the likelihood that a child will be liveborn with a chromosome imbalance and probably phenotypic abnormalities. Once an inversion carrier has been identified, prenatal diagnosis can be used to assess the chromosomes for each conception.

Translocations are rearrangements involving two or more nonhomologous chromosomes. Each chromosome breaks once and the pieces exchange places, establishing two (or more) derivative chromosomes (see Fig. 68-14, *E*). As with inversions, the majority of translocations are balanced, and only when an important structural gene is disrupted does the translocation have clinical ramifications.

The primary danger of a balanced translocation is that carriers are at increased risk for chromosomally abnormal liveborn children. In the first meiotic division, translocated chromosomes assume a cross-shaped structure in order for all alleles to pair properly (Fig. 68-16). At anaphase, the alternate chromosomes must segregate together to generate balanced gametes. Up to one third of the time, the chromosomes will not segregate in this manner and the resulting gametes will be unbalanced. The most common errors are termed adjacent-1 and adjacent-2 segregation. Although both of these patterns result in duplication/deficiency of chromosomal material in the gametes, adjacent-2 is more deleterious, in that it is characterized by the unnatural occurrence of homologous centromeres in a single cell. Viability of a fetus receiving an unbalanced gamete is dependent on the chromosomes and genes involved in the translocation and the size of the duplication and/or deletion. Chromosomes may also follow a 3 : 1 segregation pattern (see Fig. 68-16, *right*), in which three chromosomes separate to one cell with the remaining chromosome in the second cell. This results in gross imbalances of chromosomal material and is usually lethal in utero. Once a translocation carrier has been identified, prenatal diagnosis is possible.

Robertsonian translocations are a variation of the classic translocation. They occur only between two acrocentric chromosomes and appear to be a fusion of the long arms at the centromere, with the resulting loss of both short arms (see Fig. 68-14, *E*). Loss of the acrocentric short arms is not deleterious, because multiple copies of the rRNA genes present there are located on all acrocentric chromosomes. An individual who is a Robertsonian translocation carrier has a chromosome count of 45 because two chromosomes have functionally become one and share one centromere. These individuals are at increased risk for meiotic nondisjunction errors resulting in children who are trisomic for one of the rearranged chromosomes. The most common example of this is an individual with a Robertsonian translocation involving chromosomes 13 and 14 who has liveborn children with trisomy 13 (Fig. 68-17). The affected child will have 46 chromosomes, including two free copies of chromosomes 13 and the Robertsonian translocation. Another common rearrangement is a Robertsonian 14;21 translocation (see Fig. 68-14, *E*), which could give rise to trisomy 21 progeny.

Although the most common Robertsonian translocations occur between nonhomologous acrocentric chromosomes, it is possible to have such a rearrangement between homologous chromosomes. For example, an individual with a Robertsonian 21;21 translocation would have a total of 45 chromosomes including the translocation in which the two 21s are joined at the centromere. This type of rearrangement is virtually always de novo, because carriers of the abnormality are unlikely to have normal progeny. Possible gametes include (1) a cell with the Robertsonian translocation (two copies of chromosome 21), which, if fertilized, will give rise to a Down syndrome child, or (2) a cell with no copies of chromosome 21, which, if fertilized, will result in a monosomy 21, which is not compatible with life.

An *isochromosome* is a chromosome that is the result of misdivision of the centromere during cell division, resulting in two copies of one chromosome arm but missing the other arm (see Fig. 68-14, *F*). This mechanism can result in two derivative chromosomes—one with an inverted duplication of the short arm and one with an inverted duplication of the long arm. If both derivative chromosomes are retained in the cell, it would be trisomic for that chromosome, a condition that is usually lethal. In a living individual, therefore, it is most common that one of the two derivative chromosomes is lost, resulting in a carrier who is trisomic for only one duplicated arm and monosomic for the other arm. The best known example is the isochromosome of the long arm of the X. A patient with Turner syndrome (see later under Sex Chromosome Aneuploidies) may have one intact X chromosome and one isochromosome Xq (trisomy for the long arm but a monosomy for the short arm of the X). Because two functional copies of the X short arm are required for normal female development, this chromosome arrangement results in abnormal development. Acrocentric chromosomes may also form isochromosomes (inverted duplication of the long arm), but the resulting homozygosity of all loci present could lead to expression of recessive disorders that would otherwise not have been evident.

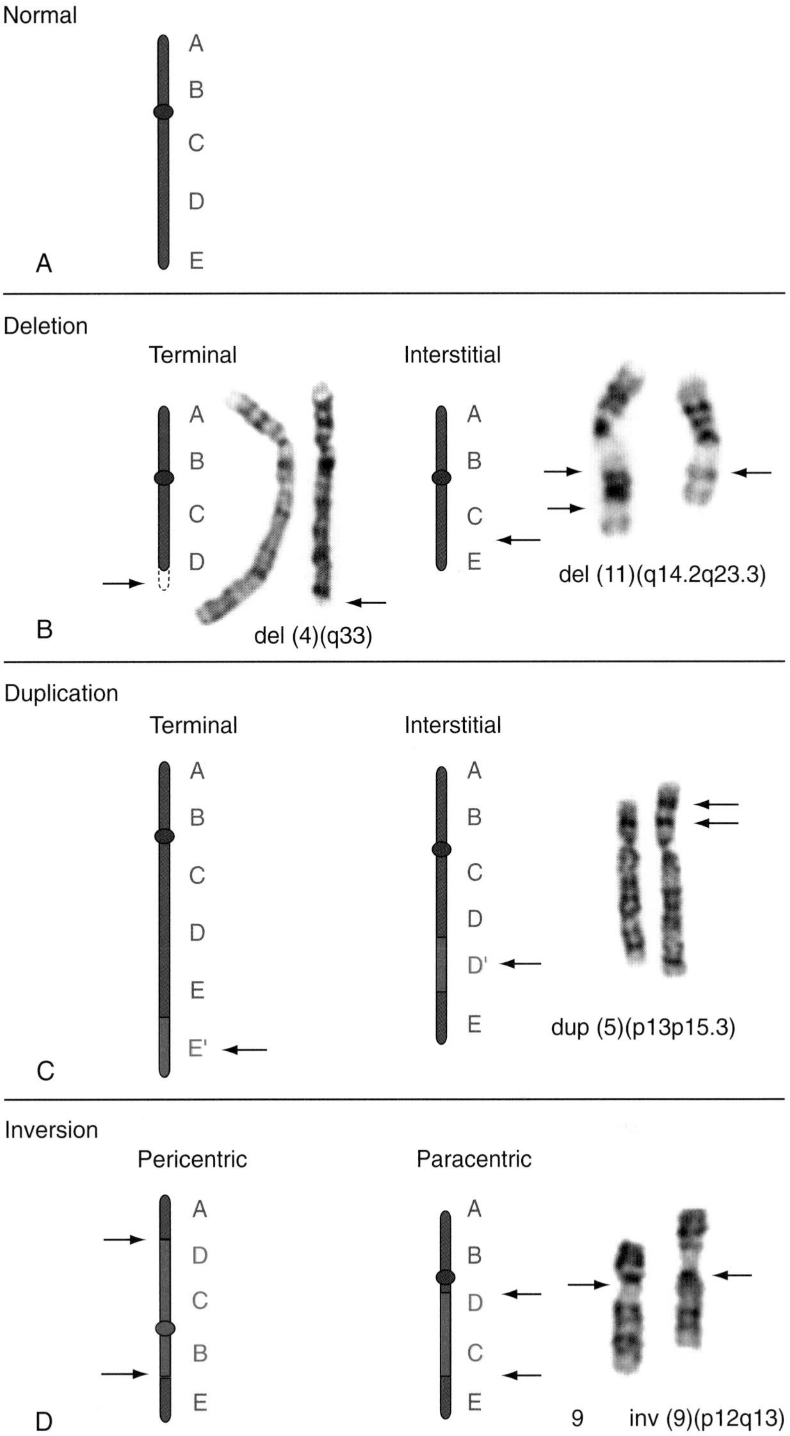

Figure 68-14 Schematic representations of different structural chromosome anomalies described in the text associated with examples of each anomaly. **A,** The normal configuration of a generalized chromosome, where A to E represent different gene loci and the centromere is represented by a dot located between the B and C loci. **B,** Deletion: Chromosome deletion showing terminal (loss of E locus) and interstitial (loss of D locus) configurations. Examples: Terminal deletion of the long arm of chromosome 4, and an interstitial deletion of the long arm of chromosome 11. **C,** Duplication: Chromosome duplication showing terminal (gain of E′) and interstitial (gain of D′) configurations. Example: Terminal duplication of the short arm of chromosome 5 (*double arrows* indicate duplicated band). **D,** Inversion: Chromosome inversion showing pericentric and paracentric forms. Example: Pericentric inversion of chromosome 9 (*arrows* indicate centromeres).

A *ring chromosome* occurs when both telomeres of a chromosome are lost and the remaining portion of the chromosome circularizes to reestablish chromosome stability (see Fig. 68-14, *G*). Unfortunately, these constructs are usually unstable because replication can result in interlinked circles that lead to chromosome breakage and loss when the homologs attempt to separate at anaphase. Under certain circumstances, however, rings can be stably transmitted in cell lines. This usually occurs when the ring contains genetic material that is essential for normal cell function.

A *marker* chromosome is a chromosome with a centromere that is stably transmitted to daughter cells but cannot be clearly identified because either it is too small or the banding pattern is too ambiguous. Multicolor FISH is a useful tool to determine the origin of markers. By "painting" the entire metaphase and generating an image with a unique color for each chromosome pair, it should be possible to identify the origin of the marker chromosome, because its color should match the color for one of the other known chromosomes of the set.

Conclusions

Chromosome abnormalities, either numerical or structural, that result in an unbalanced chromosome complement are usually associated with some type of abnormal clinical finding, and the size of the imbalance tends to be proportional to the severity of the problem. Most individuals with a constitutional chromosome abnormality have only a single chromosome defect. However, there are rare instances in which one person may have two or more chromosomal errors. Acquired chromosome abnormalities (seen in cancer cells) may be more complex and may have multiple numerical and structural changes in a single cell line.

Nomenclature

With such a broad range of chromosome variation, it was necessary to develop a system of classification that would allow each individual's chromosome complement to be succinctly described and understood worldwide. The first cytogenetic nomenclature provided a framework, and the

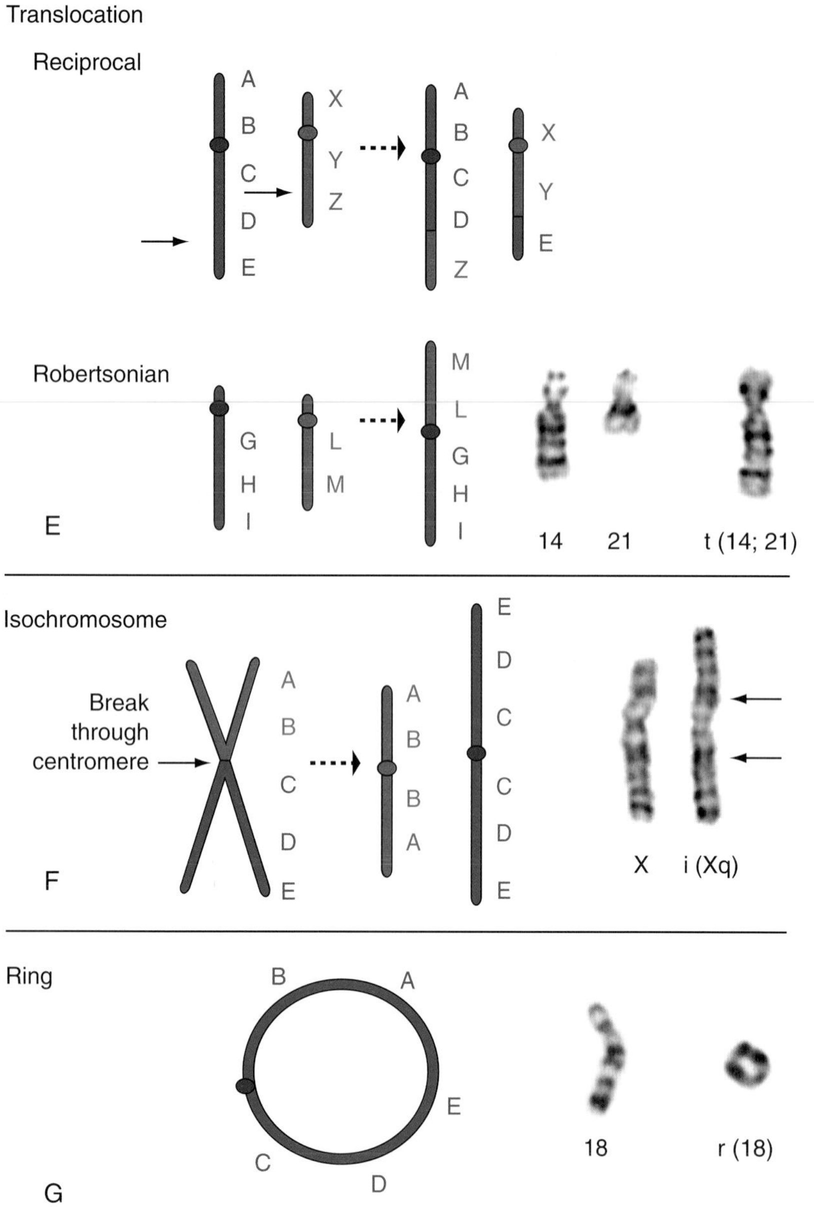

Figure 68-14, cont'd E, Translocation: Reciprocal translocation, where the E and Z loci exchange places. Below is a Robertsonian translocation shown by the fusion of two acrocentric chromosomes at the centromere. Example: Chromosomes 14 and 21 followed by the 14;21 Robertsonian translocation. **F,** Isochromosome: Results from a misdivision of the centromere, generating inverted duplications of the long and short arms of the original chromosome. Example: Isochromosome of the long arm of the X chromosome. **G,** Ring chromosome. Example: Chromosome 18 and ring 18.

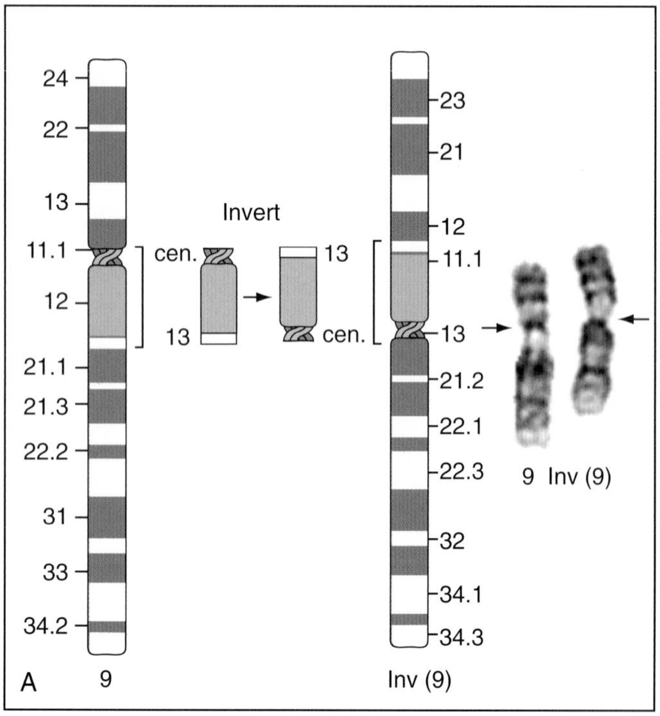

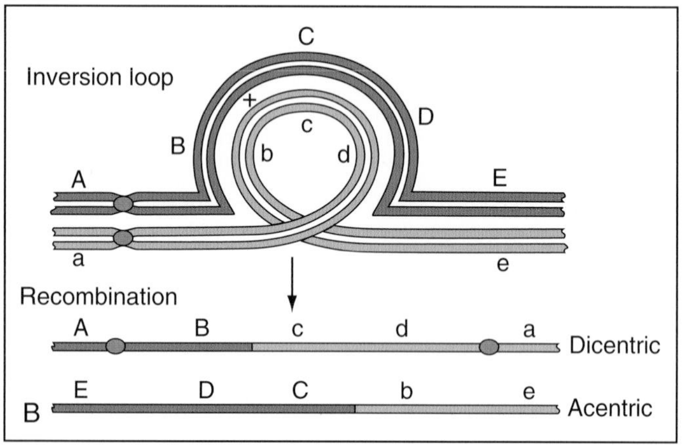

Figure 68-15 Chromosome inversion. **A,** Diagram of a pericentric inversion of chromosome 9 using ideograms to illustrate the mechanism of inversion. Banded chromosomes demonstrating this inversion are shown to the *right*. **B,** Inversion loop showing the pairing of homologs in meiosis for one normal chromosome (*dark green*) and one with a paracentric inversion (*light green*). If recombination occurs at the point indicated by the X in the loop, recombinant chromosomes would be generated as shown at the bottom. In the case of a paracentric inversion, the recombined chromosomes produced would be either dicentric or acentric.

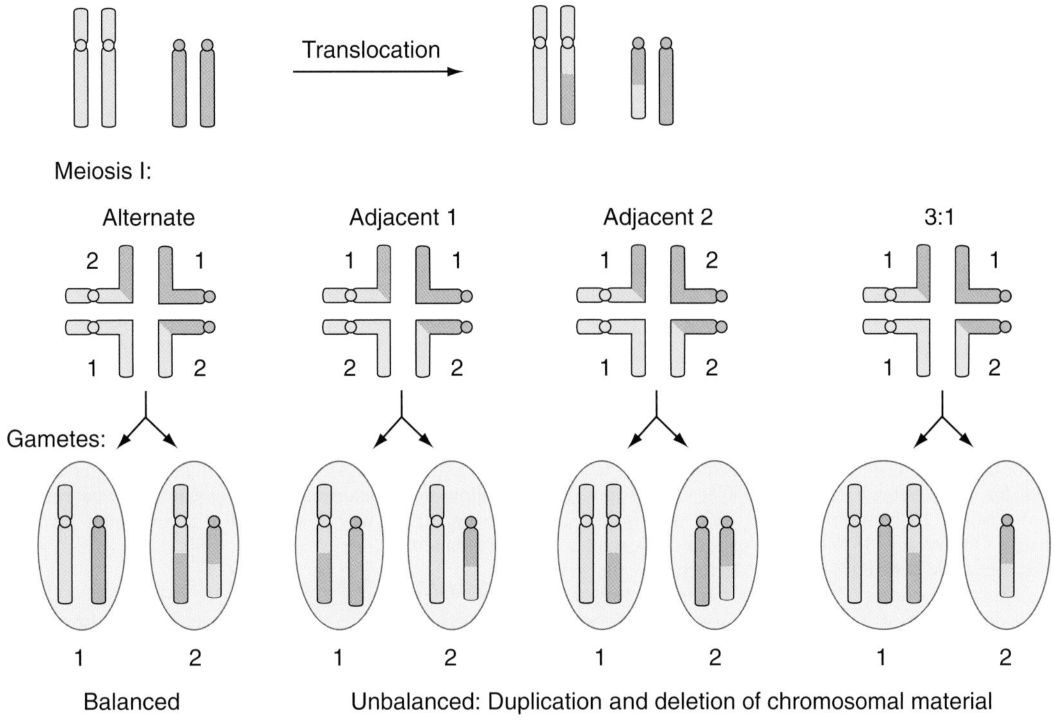

Figure 68-16 Chromosome translocation. Generation of gametes from a hypothetical translocation in meiosis is diagrammed. The chromosomes pair in a cross-shaped configuration in meiosis I. Alternate segregation will result in balanced gametes. Adjacent 1, adjacent 2, or 3:1 segregation will produce unbalanced gametes, which may give rise to an abnormal liveborn child. (Only one of several possible 3:1 segregations is shown.)

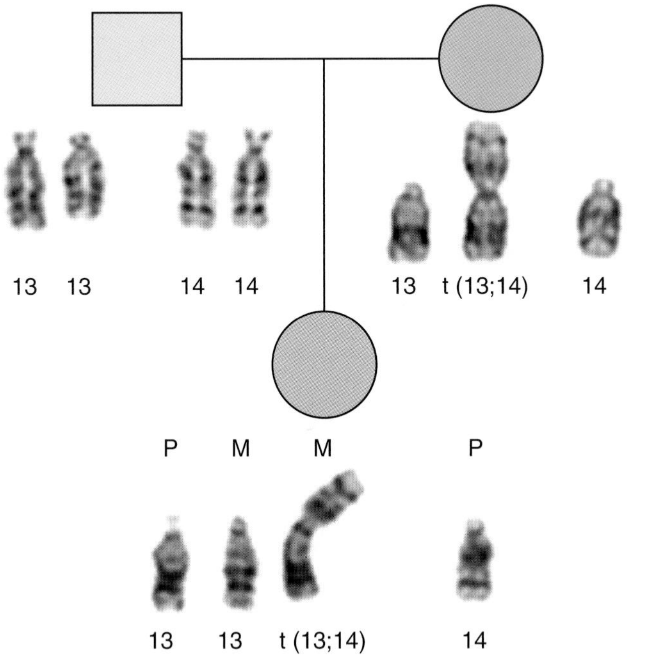

Figure 68-17 Pedigree and banded chromosomes showing inheritance of a Robertsonian translocation of chromosomes 13 and 14. The mother carries the 13;14 translocation in a balanced form, but a meiotic error results in the transmission of both the Robertsonian translocation chromosome and the chromosome 13 from the mother to the child. The child has trisomy 13 and the Robertsonian translocation). Note: The second copy of chromosome 14 is not missing, but is present as part of the Robertsonian rearrangement. *M,* maternal chromosomes; *P,* paternal chromosomes.

"language" has been evolving ever since. Currently, the International System of Cytogenetic Nomenclature is recognized as the standard.

The nomenclature describing a chromosome complement can be broken down into three basic parts: (1) the total number of chromosomes, (2) the sex chromosome complement, and (3) any chromosome abnormalities. These units are listed in order, separated by commas. So, an apparently normal female would be coded as 46,XX and a male would be 46,XY. If two or more cell lines are present, they are listed sequentially, separated by a slant line, with a normal diploid clone, if present, always listed last (45,X/46,XX). Other clones are ordered by size, with the largest clone placed first. The number of cells in each clone is indicated by a number enclosed in brackets (45,X[15]/47,XXX[3]/46,XX[12]). For numerical anomalies, the total number of chromosomes would be increased or decreased to indicate the overall change, and the specific chromosome gained or lost would be noted at the end. For example, trisomy 13 in a female would be written as 47,XX,+13, and monosomy 8 in a male would be written 45,XY,–8. However, for a sex chromosome variation that is known to be constitutional, it is not necessary to use a + or – sign, because the change in chromosome complement can be noted directly. Monosomy X becomes 45,X and gain of a sex chromosome would be 47,XXY, 47,XXX, or 47,XYY. On the other hand, if the sex chromosome change is acquired, as in some cancer cell lines, a + or – indicating this would be required (e.g., 45,X,–Y for a male whose Y chromosome has been lost as a result of his disease).

Structural changes in the chromosomes usually do not affect the total number of chromosomes present but should be noted at the end of the nomenclature to clarify the status of the rearranged chromosomes. In order to streamline the nomenclature, a series of abbreviations for the common structural anomalies has been generated that shortens the overall nomenclature (Table 68-1). A structural abnormality is indicated by the abbreviation of the abnormality followed by the chromosome involved and breakpoints on the chromosome. For rearrangements in which two chromosomes are involved, a first set of parentheses gives the chromosomes (lowest numbered or sex chromosome first) followed by the breakpoints of the rearrangement in the same relative order; that is, t(4;9)(q21.2;p22) is a translocation between chromosomes 4 and 9 with breakpoints 4q21.2 and 9p22.

Examples include the following:

Deletion:	46,XX,del(4)(p15)	Terminal deletion of the short arm of 4 at band 15
Duplication:	46,XX,dup(11)(q13q23)	Interstitial duplication of the long arm of 11 involving the region from q13 to q23
Translocation:	46,XY,t(4;9)(q21.2;p22)	Translocation between 4q and 9p
Inversion:	46,XY,inv(9)(p11q21.1)	Pericentric inversion in 9 between bands p11 and q21.1

Clinical

CLINICAL APPLICATIONS

Cytogenetic abnormalities may be found in apparently normal individuals as well as in patients with phenotypic anomalies or with a diagnosed genetic disorder. Diagnosis may occur at any stage of life. When the same set of features is seen in several unrelated individuals, it may be possible to establish a syndrome. The characteristics associated with a syndrome are assumed to have a common basis, which can often be shown to be a specific chromosome abnormality. However, although a syndrome is defined by a certain set of characters, there is variability in affected individuals and not all will show an identical phenotype.

Prenatal Cytogenetics

Studies have shown that 1 in 13 conceptuses has a chromosomal abnormality, but, of these, only 6 in 1000 are live born, indicating that most errors are recognized and biologically eliminated. For example, of all 45,X conceptions, 95% will spontaneously terminate. Similar frequencies of termination are recorded for the liveborn trisomies (90% of trisomy 13 conceptions, 80% of trisomy 18 conceptions, and 65% of trisomy 21 conceptions terminate). On average, 15% of all recognized pregnancies end in a spontaneous fetal loss, with 80% of these occurring in the first trimester. Of all spontaneous abortions, 60% are chromosomally abnormal (Table 68-2), and of these, 52% are autosomal trisomies. The most common trisomy seen in abortus material is trisomy 16, but the most frequent class of chromosome error in spontaneous losses is 45,X.

One of the most important statistics is the direct correlation between advanced maternal age and births with chromosomal abnormalities. Although the exact reason for the phenomenon is unclear, population studies have shown that women older than age 35 years have an increased risk for a chromosomally abnormal conception (Hassold, 1985) with the most common abnormality being Down syndrome (trisomy 21) (see Figs. 68-10, *B*, and 68-18). This becomes important in a society in which women are delaying childbearing until later in life, so prenatal diagnosis has become a major area of clinical cytogenetic study. In addition to screening for an age-related risk, other common reasons for referral include a family history of or previous child with a chromosome abnormality, abnormal levels of AFP in a screening test, and an abnormality detected on ultrasound.

The most common chromosome abnormalities detected in prenatal testing are the liveborn trisomies and the sex chromosome aneuploidies. Because these are usually the result of a meiotic nondisjunction error, there is a very low risk of recurrence. Occasionally, a child with a balanced or unbalanced structural chromosome abnormality will be identified. In these circumstances, karyotype analysis on both biological parents is used to differentiate between an inherited rearrangement and a de novo anomaly in the child. For example, a child with an inherited balanced translocation has a less than 1% risk that the chromosome rearrangement will pose any problem. However, if the apparently balanced translocation seen in the fetus is not detected in either biological parent, it must have arisen de novo in the child, and there is a 5%–10% risk of related impairment for the infant. Unfortunately, finding an *unbalanced* translocation in a fetus, regardless of the carrier status of the parents, is a serious situation and almost always results in some type of genetic defect for the child. Follow-up to determine whether one of the parents is a balanced translocation carrier will provide information about recurrence risk for future pregnancies.

Postnatal

Approximately 0.6% of newborns have a chromosome abnormality. If an infant presents with signs or symptoms of a defined syndrome, karyotype analysis may confirm a diagnosis. If the newborn has clinical anomalies unrelated to a specific disorder, karyotype analysis may

TABLE 68-1
Common Abbreviations for Chromosome Abnormalities

Abbreviation	Meaning
cen	Centromere
del	Deletion
dup	Duplication
ins	Insertion
inv	Inversion
i	Isochromosome
mar	Marker
r	Ring
rob	Robertsonian translocation
t	Translocation

TABLE 68-2
Chromosome Abnormalities in Spontaneous Fetal Losses and in Liveborn Infants

Abnormality	Chromosome	Spontaneous fetal losses (%)	Incidence in live births
45,X		18.0	1/4000
Triploidy		17.0	1/60000
Tetraploid		6.0	0
Trisomy	16	16.4	0
	22	5.7	0
	21	4.7	1/830
	15	4.2	0
	14	3.7	0
	18	3.0	1/7500
	13	2.0	1/5000
	Other	12.3	1/10000
Unbalanced rearrangement		3.0	1/2000
Balanced rearrangement		4.0	3/1000

Data from Hook, 1977; Jacobs, 1992; Nussbaum, 2009; Turnpenny, 2005.

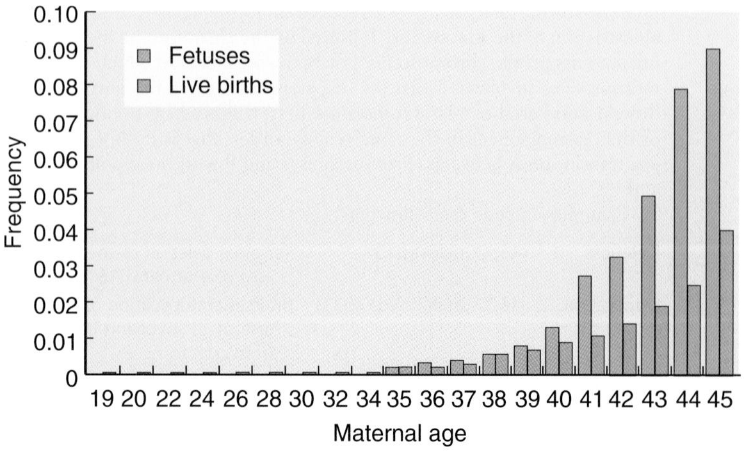

Figure 68-18 Increased risk of a Down syndrome conception with increased maternal age. The number of live births is lower at older ages due to the intervention of prenatal diagnosis followed by termination of abnormal pregnancies.

provide information on a chromosome abnormality related to the clinical findings. Ambiguous genitalia may be related to an abnormal sex chromosome complement, but, if the chromosomes are shown to be normal, the physician knows that another cause for the patient's abnormality must be sought. If the child dies shortly after birth, cytogenetic analysis may provide information critical in understanding the demise, and these data should be correlated with autopsy results to substantiate a diagnosis.

Childhood and Adult

A common misconception about genetic disorders is that, because they are inherited, the diagnosis will be obvious at birth. In fact, the full clinical presentation of many disorders takes time to develop and may not be fully expressed until later in life. Consequently, some of the most difficult diagnostic problems occur in children and adults. In addition to considering the full range of cytogenetic possibilities, molecular and biochemical options must also be taken into account.

CANCER GENETICS

Another area of medicine in which cytogenetics is increasingly important is oncology. Although most solid tumors are difficult to culture and analyze cytogenetically, excellent clinical data exist for leukemias and lymphomas, including specific chromosome rearrangements that are directly associated with tumorigenesis (Table 68-3) (see Chapter 75) (Block, 1999). Karyotype findings were originally used primarily as confirmation of a clinical diagnosis, but the role of genetics in patient management changed dramatically in 2001 when the World Health Organization (WHO) published a revised classification for leukemias and lymphomas (Swerdlow, 2008). The new methodology is based on data collected by clinical study groups that had shown a direct correlation between the presence of various chromosomal abnormalities and patients' response to therapy. Thus, in the revised classification system, the importance of the genetic findings, either cytogenetic or molecular, became a key element for final diagnosis in most hematologic disorders. Cytogenetics had suddenly been pushed to the forefront of testing for oncology patients.

In addition to diagnosis, karyotype analysis can provide other valuable information regarding a cancer patient's disease. Once a chromosome abnormality has been detected, the progress of the disease can be monitored. If treatment is successful, most chromosome abnormalities are no longer evident in the bone marrow and, as long as the karyotype appears to be "normal," the patient is said to be in cytogenetic remission. However, if the treatment does not eliminate the aberrant cell line completely, remission may be merely an interlude in which the disease-causing cells are suppressed to such low levels that they are not detectable by routine karyotype analysis. Then at relapse, the same chromosome anomalies will reappear and may be accompanied by additional abnormalities and/or more complex cell lines, findings consistent with disease progression. An increase in complexity over time is known as *karyotype evolution*. In general, poor prognosis and severity of disease is directly correlated to the number and type of chromosome abnormalities seen.

FISH has become a valuable tool in clinical oncology studies with many probes commercially available (Cremer, 1988; Anastasi, 1991). Studies can be done on either interphase or metaphase cells, with the choice resting on the type of data desired. Using interphase cells is often preferred because it provides a much larger sample that can be quickly assayed, giving results with a higher level of statistical significance (Werner, 1997).

For translocations, combination FISH probes have been developed that hybridize to the opposite sides of the translocation breakpoints. There are two common strategies employed to detect a translocation. Splitting of the signals may occur if the translocation separates two probes, generating two different-colored signals in place of the original single-color signal. Alternatively, fusion may occur if the translocation results in relocation of the probes, bringing two different probes into proximity and generating a two-color fusion that creates a new color. For example, FISH fusion technology has been used to identify the 9;22 translocation in leukemia. This rearrangement is characterized by a translocation between the *ABL* proto-oncogene on chromosome 9 (9q34.1) and the *BCR* gene on chromosome 22 (22q11.2) (Fig. 68-19, *A*), which produces a disease-associated chimeric gene on the derivative chromosome 22, also known as the *Philadelphia chromosome* (Ph′) (see also Chapter 75). The translocation is seen in chronic myelogenous leukemia (CML), acute myeloid leukemia (AML), and acute lymphoblastic leukemia (ALL) (see Table 68-3), and, cytogenetically, it appears to be the same in all diseases. However, at the molecular level, the translocation can be separated into two classes: (1) the major breakpoint (*M-BCR*) rearrangement that results in a chimeric protein of 210 kD (most common in CML) and (2) the minor breakpoint (*m-BCR*) rearrangement that results in a chimeric protein of 190 kD (seen in some adults and about 50% of childhood ALL). A FISH assay has been engineered to detect both rearrangements (Abbott Molecular). A pair of probes is used: (1) red—localized to the *ABL* locus on chromosome 9, and (2) green—located at the *BCR* locus (chromosome 22) encompassing the m-BCR breakpoint but proximal to the M-BCR breakpoint. When no translocation is present, two green signals (detecting each *ABL* allele) and two red signals (detecting each *BCR* allele) should be present in each cell (see Fig. 68-19, *B* and *C*). When the M-BCR rearrangement occurs, the translocation breaks chromosome 22 distal to the probe recognition site such that the entire green signal remains on chromosome 22. On chromosome 9, the translocation splits the red *ABL* signal such that a small red signal is left on the derivative chromosome 9 and the remainder of the red signal moves to chromosome 22. This brings one green and one red signal adjacent to one another on the derivative chromosome 22 (Ph′), and, with the resolution of the light microscope, the two signals merge, giving a single yellow fusion signal. Therefore, a cell with a M-BCR translocation will have four signals: one green (chromosome 22), one large red (chromosome 9), one small red (the rearranged chromosome 9), and one yellow fusion signal detecting the Ph′ chromosome (see Fig. 68-19, *B* and *D*). The m-BCR rearrangement is slightly different. Chromosome 22 is broken within the green probe recognition site, such that one portion of the green signal will stay on chromosome 22 but the distal section will move to the derivative chromosome 9. The red probe site on chromosome 9 is split as described earlier, with one portion remaining on chromosome 9 and the distal section moving to chromosome 22. This reciprocal translocation thus results in two yellow fusion signals (derivative 9 is red fused to green, and derivative 22 is green fused to red). The net result of the m-BCR FISH assay is four probe signals: one green (chromosome 22), one red (chromosome 9), and two yellow fusion signals detecting the 9;22 translocation (see Figs. 68-19, *B* and *E*). Being able to determine which of the two rearrangements is present in a patient sample simplifies the diagnosis and leads to the most appropriate treatment methodology for the individual. Other FISH detection assays using other disease gene specific probes can be designed to evaluate for a wide array of different cancer related chromosome rearrangements.

In addition, chromosomal aneuploidies in cancer cells can be easily detected. For example: (1) use of a chromosome 12-specific centromere probe to screen an interphase cell population for trisomy 12 cells indicative of CLL, (2) use of a chromosome 7 probe to detect monosomy 7 in myelodysplastic syndrome and AML, and (3) use of a chromosome 8 probe to identify trisomy 8 in both chronic and acute disorders. The use of different-colored X and Y probes in evaluating the success of a bone marrow transplant when the donor and recipient are of opposite sexes has also been highly successful. Following transplantation, a male who has received female donor cells should have an XX complement. Failure of the engraftment may be signaled by the presence of a high frequency of XY cells. The FISH can be repeated at regular intervals to monitor the progress and provide an early warning if the patient's leukemic cell population begins to proliferate.

Initially, clinicians were concerned about apparently discrepant results from karyotype analysis and FISH on the same patient sample. For example, by karyotype, a patient with CML may show all cells with a t(9;22), but only 30% of cells will be positive for the translocation by interphase FISH. These data are actually consistent. Karyotype can only be performed on dividing cells and, because cancer cells tend to divide frequently, a karyotype analysis would typically show 100% leukemic cells. FISH, on the other hand, detects all nucleated cells, but not all cells in a bone marrow sample are necessarily from the same clone. An affected individual usually also has a normal cell population. Interphase FISH can quantify the relative numbers of normal and disease cells, thus providing a more accurate estimate of disease involvement within the total population. This can be used advantageously to monitor a patient's response to treatment. Testing sequential samples over time can show a reduction in the disease cell population, and relapse will be reflected by a rise in the leukemic cell population. Thus, it is important to perform both karyotype analysis and FISH on a diagnosis specimen. The karyotype will define the chromosomal abnormalities present, and the FISH will establish the baseline frequency of the leukemic clone(s). These data can then be used as a reference point for all future testing for the patient.

Multicolor FISH has also been used to evaluate leukemic cell lines. The data being collected suggest that cancer cells actually undergo a significantly greater degree of chromosome rearrangement than was

TABLE 68-3
Common Cytogenetic Rearrangements in Leukemia and Lymphoma

Disorder	Chromosome rearrangement(s)	Genes involved	FAB classification (if different)
CHRONIC MYELOPROLIFERATIVE DISEASE			
Chronic myelogenous leukemia (chronic)	t(9;22)(q34.1;q11.2)	*ABL; BCR*	
Chronic myelogenous leukemia (accelerated or blast phase)	+8, i(17q), +19, +Ph′		
Polycythemia vera	+8, +9, del(20q), del(13q)		
Chronic idiopathic myelofibrosis	+8, −7 del(7q), del(11q), del(13q), del(20q)		
Essential thrombocythemia	+8, del(13q)		
MYELODYSPLASTIC SYNDROMES			
Myelodysplastic syndrome with isolated del(5q)	del(5)(q13q33), del(5)(q22q33)		5q- syndrome
Chronic myelomonocytic leukemia	−7, del(7q),+8, abnormalities of 12p		
Refractory anemia, refractory anemia with ringed sideroblasts, refractory anemia with excess blasts	−5, del(5q), −7, del(7q), +8, del(20q)		
ACUTE MYELOID LEUKEMIA (AML) WITH RECURRENT CYTOGENETIC ABNORMALITIES			
AML with t(8;21)	t(8;21)(q22;q22)	*AML1; ETO*	AML-M2
AML with inversion or translocation 16	inv(16)(p12q22), t(16;16)(p13;q22)	*CBFβ; MYH11*	AML-M4Eo
Acute promyelocytic leukemia	t(15;17)(q22;q12)	*PML; RARα*	AML-M3
AML with 11q23 (*MLL*) abnormalities	t(9;11)(p21;q23), t(11;19)(q23;p13.1), t(11;19)(q23;p13.3),	*AF9; MLL* *MLL; ENL*	AML-M5
AML with multilineage dysplasia	−5, del(5q), −7, del(7q), +8, del(11q), del(20q), +21, translocations involving 3q21 and 3q26, t(9;22)(q34.1;q11.2)	*AML-M1, AML-M6*	
Precursor B-lymphoblastic leukemia/ lymphoma			ALL-L1/L2
	t(1;19)(q23;p13.3)	*PBX; E2A*	
	t(9;22)(q34;q11.2)	*ABL; BCR*	
	11q23 rearrangements, including:	*MLL*	
	t(1;11)(p32;q23)	*AF1P; MLL*	
	t(4;11)(q21;q23)	*AF4; MLL*	
	t(11;19)(q23;p13)	*MLL; ENL*	
	t(12;21)(p13q22)	*TEL; AML*	
	Hyperdiploidy (modal number 50–56)		
Precursor T-lymphoblastic leukemia/lymphoma			ALL-L1/L2
	Rearrangements at 14q11.2, 7q35, and 7p14–15	T-cell receptor loci	
	del(9p)	*CDKN2A*	
	translocations at 1p32	*TAL1*	
Mature B-cell neoplasms			
Chronic lymphocytic leukemia/small lymphocytic leukemia	+12, del13q, del11q23–24, 14q+, del17p13		
Lymphoplasmacytic lymphoma/ Waldenström's macroglobulinemia	t(9;14)(p13;q32)	*PAX5; IGH*	
Plasma cell myeloma	t(11;14)(q13;q32)	*CCND1; BCL1*	
Marginal zone B-cell lymphoma (MALT)	+3, t(11;18)(q21;q21)		
Follicular lymphoma	t(14;18)(q32;q21), t(18;22)(q21;q11.2), +7, +18, del(6q), del/t(3)(q27)	*IGH; BCL2 BCL2; IGL*	
Mantle cell lymphoma	t(11;14)(q13;q32)	*CCND1; BCL1*	
Burkitt's lymphoma	t(8;14)(q24;q32)	*MYC; IGH*	
	t(2;8) (p12;q24)	*IGK; MYC*	
	t(8;22)(q24;q11.2)	*MYC; IGL*	

previously appreciated. It is hoped that some of the new rearrangements being detected will give clues to new cancer-related genes (Veldman, 1997).

CYTOGENETIC DISORDERS

Chromosomal Aneuploidy Syndromes

Autosomal Aneuploidies

The most common cause of mental retardation is trisomy 21, or Down syndrome. This disorder has a birth incidence of 1 in 700 and is characterized by hypotonia, flat facies, slanted palpebral fissures, small ears, protruding tongue, transverse palmar crease, heart defects, and hypogonadism. Approximately 92.5% of all Down syndrome individuals have 47 chromosomes including three copies of chromosome 21 resulting from a nondisjunction error in parental meiosis. Just under 3% of patients tend to express a milder phenotype and have been shown to be mosaics with two cell lines (47,XX,+21/46,XX or 47,XY,+21/46,XY), and about 5% of Down syndrome patients have only 46 chromosomes, because the extra 21 is part of a Robertsonian or other translocation. A child with a translocation is often indicative of the presence of a translocation carrier parent, so, in these cases, karyotype analysis of both parents is appropriate to

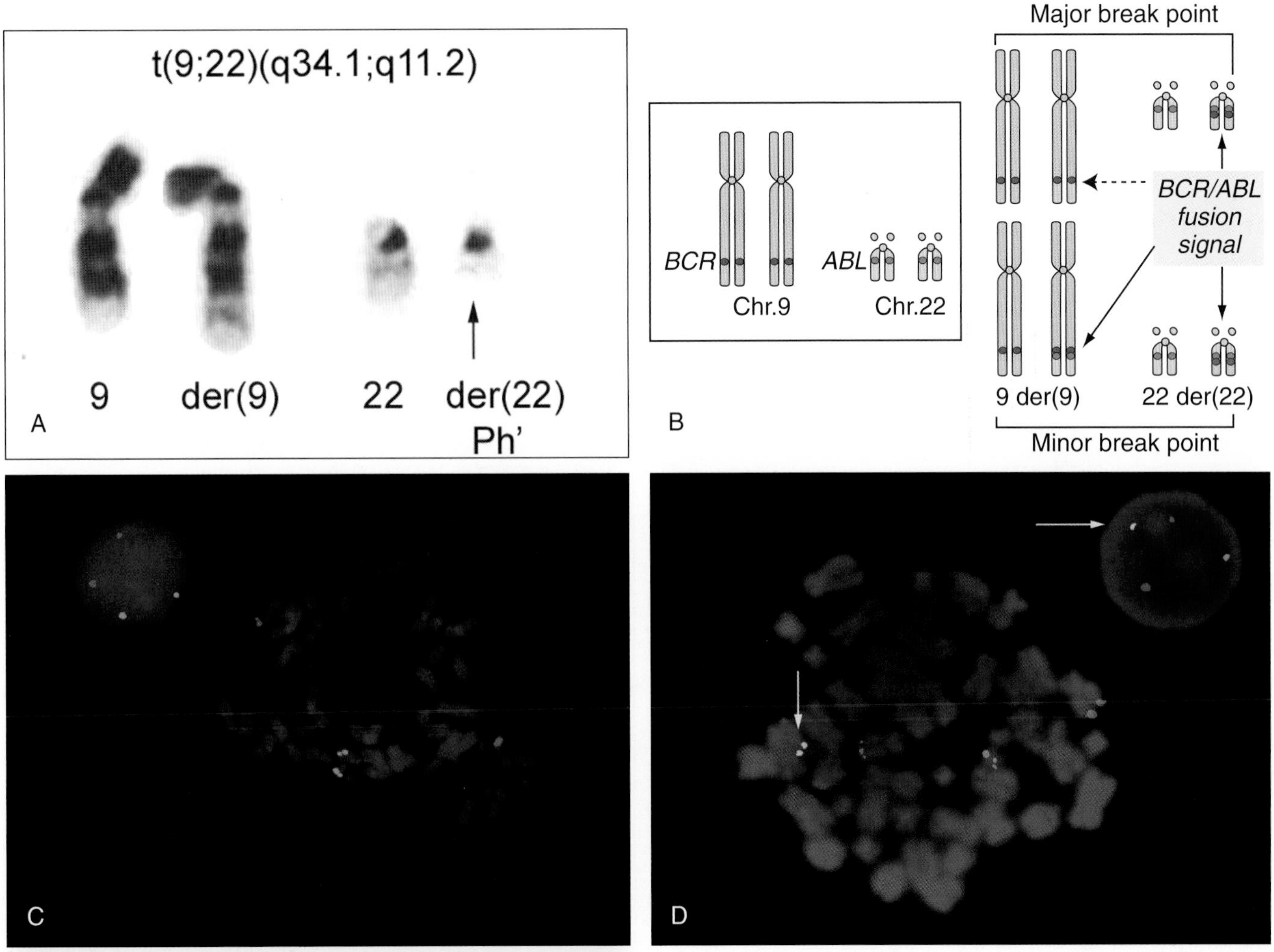

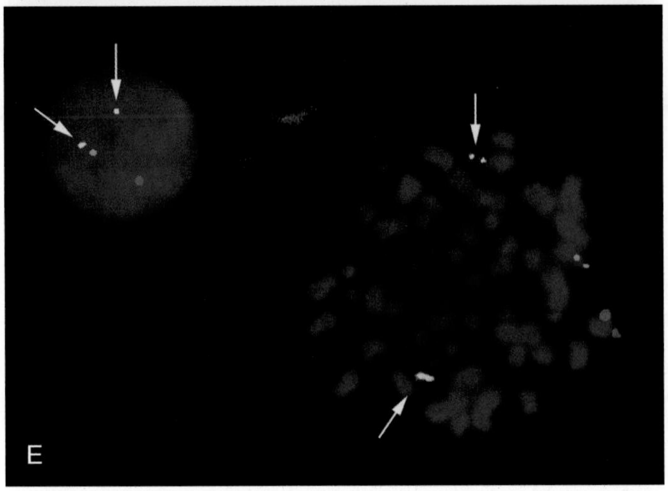

Figure 68-19 Fluorescence in situ hybridization (FISH) detection of the 9;22 translocation in CML. **A,** Banded chromosomes showing the 9;22 translocation. The derivative chromosome 22 is known as the *Ph',* or *Philadelphia chromosome.* **B,** Diagram showing FISH detection for a normal cell with no translocation (*left*) and for both the major (M-BCR) and minor (m-BCR) breakpoint rearrangements. Upper right shows the signal pattern for the M-BCR translocation: chr. 9—red signal, der(9)—partial red signal with chromosome 22 material below (yellow) *(dashed arrow),* chr. 22—green signal, and the der(22), the Ph' chromosome with a green-red BCR-ABL fusion signal and chromosome 9 material below. The lower right shows the m-BCR signal pattern: chr. 9—red signal, der(9)—red-green fusion signal and chromosome 22 material below, chr. 22—green signal, and the der(22)—green-red fusion signal with chromosome 9 material below. **C** and **D,** Actual FISH images. **C,** No translocation is present as seen by two copies each of the chromosome 9 (red) and chromosome 22 (green) probes in both interphase (*left*) and metaphase (*right*) cells. **D,** Cells with a M-BCR translocation as detected by the single yellow fusion signal *(arrow)* plus one green, one large red, and one small red signal (metaphase on the *left* and interphase on the *right*). **E,** Cells with an m-BCR translocation as detected by two yellow fusion signals *(arrows)* plus one green and one red signal (metaphase on the *right* and interphase on the *left*). *CML,* Chronic myeloid leukemia.

determine whether the couple is at increased risk for having additional Down syndrome children in future pregnancies. Although it is most common for a Down syndrome patient to have three complete copies of chromosome 21, molecular studies of individuals with chromosome 21 rearrangements have clearly shown that it is only necessary to have three copies of the region of chromosome 21 encompassing bands 21q22.12–21q22.3, the Down syndrome critical region (Fig. 68-20) (Korenberg, 1990; Delabar, 1993).

The other two liveborn trisomies are trisomy 13 and trisomy 18. *Trisomy 13*, or Patau syndrome, with a birth incidence of 1 in 4000 to 1 in 10,000, is characterized by a small head, cleft lip and/or cleft palate, cyclopia, transverse palmar crease, polydactyly of the hands and/or feet, prominent heel, ventricular septal defect, and punched-out scalp. *Trisomy 18*, or Edwards syndrome (Fig. 68-21, *A*), is seen in approximately 1 in 8000 newborns with features including a low birth weight, small mouth and jaw, ventricular septal defect, hypoplasia of the muscles, a prominent occiput, low-set malformed ears, rocker bottom feet, and crossed fingers.

Despite its often severe clinical consequences, Down syndrome is usually manageable, and patients live into the second or third decade of life. Trisomy 13 and trisomy 18 are considerably less compatible with life, and patients usually die within the first month of life. If an individual survives the first year, the outlook is bleak, because patients do not learn to talk, walk, or care for themselves. Because of this, counseling for prenatally diagnosed cases of trisomy 13 and 18 includes the option of termination of pregnancy.

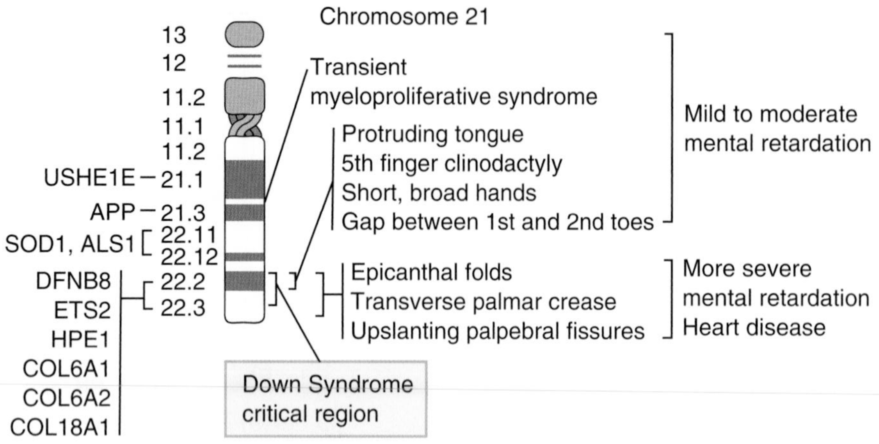

Figure 68-20 Map of chromosome 21 showing the Down syndrome critical region and relative positions of loci associated with various clinical features to the right. On the left, other mapped loci are shown. (Data from Korenberg, 1990; Delabar, 1993; OMIM, website.) *ALS1*, amyotrophic lateral sclerosis; *APP*, amyloid β-precursor protein (associated with Alzheimer disease); *COL6A1/COL6A2/COL18A1*, collagen genes; *DFNB8*, deafness 8; *ETS2*, oncogene ETS-2; *HPE1*, alobar holoprosencephaly-1; *SOD1*, superoxide dismutase-1; *USH1E*, Usher syndrome.

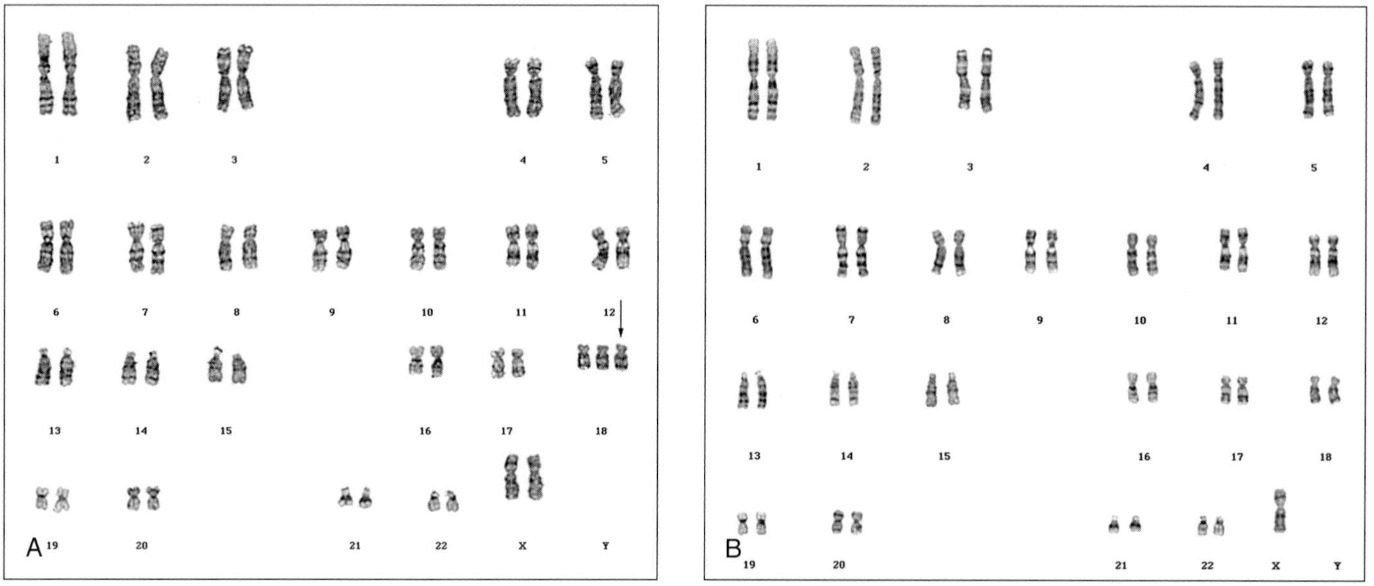

Figure 68-21 Karyotypes from numerical chromosome syndromes. **A,** Edwards syndrome (trisomy 18): 47,XX,+18. **B,** Turner syndrome (monosomy X): 45,X.

Sex Chromosome Aneuploidies

Sex chromosome aneuploidies are relatively common (overall frequency of 1 in 500 births), and are phenotypically milder than autosomal aneuploidies because of the effect of X inactivation and the limited number of genes present on the Y chromosome. Four disorders, including three trisomies and one monosomy, account for the majority of cases. All are the result of nondisjunction errors in meiosis and, except for XYY, which is exclusively paternal, the other disorders may result from either maternal or paternal error.

The aberrant karyotypes of individuals with three X chromosomes (47,XXX females) or with one X and two Y chromosomes (47,XYY males) often go undetected throughout life. The birth incidence is relatively high, 1 in 1000, but other than being somewhat taller than average, there are no striking features that would indicate a chromosomal abnormality. Some individuals have generalized learning difficulties and so may be identified by school screening programs. XXX females and XYY males are also detected in infertility clinics, although the cytogenetic abnormality is not related to the reason for referral, because comprehensive evaluations have shown that these individuals are fully fertile and generally have chromosomally normal children. XYY males do have an increased risk of behavioral problems, and early studies suggested that they also had criminal tendencies because there was a higher than expected incidence of XYY in inmates of penal institutions (Jacobs, 1968; Price, 1970). However, subsequent work has shown that (1) the conclusions of the original study were biased because of a sampling error, (2) criminality is most probably due to a combination of multiple causes, and (3) XYY males are no more prone to a criminal behavior than any other male (Witkin, 1976; Pitcher, 1982; Theilgaard, 1984).

Klinefelter syndrome (47,XXY) males tend to be tall and thin with relatively long legs, although early in life these findings seldom set them apart from their peers. Some individuals are identified in school because of their learning difficulties but the most common reason for referral is postpubertal hypogonadism, female-like breast development, and infertility due to small testicles, hyalinized testicular tubules, and azoospermia. A milder form of Klinefelter syndrome with the potential for fertility due to normal testicular development is seen in individuals with a mosaic chromosome complement including a 46,XY cell line (47,XXY/46,XY). The relative proportion of XY and XXY cells during sex determination in the early zygote and in the testes is the key for fertility. An excess of XXY cells will push the individual toward a true Klinefelter presentation, whereas higher numbers of XY cells should moderate the phenotype and increase the likelihood of fertility.

The most commonly recognized sex chromosome aneuploidy presenting with a female phenotype is 45,X: *Turner syndrome* (Fig. 68-21, *B*). In sex determination, normal female development is dependent on the presence of two active X chromosomes. The critical region for female differentiation has been narrowed to a region of the short arm of the X just proximal to the centromere. If that region is missing or inactive, an individual with Turner syndrome will result. About half of all Turner syndrome patients have the classic 45,X chromosome complement, which represents the only viable liveborn monosomy. The single X chromosome is usually maternal in origin, indicating that a paternal meiotic nondisjunction is the most common source of error. In addition to 45,X, more complex karyotypes are also possible (Table 68-4) (Palmer, 1976). The greatest concern is for individuals who possess a complete or partial Y chromosome in at least one cell line, who are at increased risk for gonadoblastoma.

TABLE 68-4
Distribution of Different Chromosome Complements That Give Rise to Turner Syndrome

Occurrence (%)	Chromosome anomaly
50	45,X
20	46,X,i(Xq)
15	X chromosome deletions or rings, or the presence of a Y chromosome
10	Mosaics: 45,X/46,XX; 45,X/46,XY

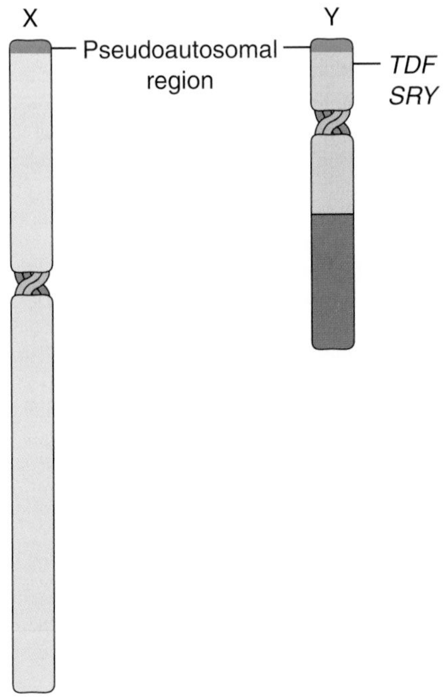

Figure 68-22 Diagram of relative locations of TDF, SRY, and the pseudoautosomal regions of the X and Y chromosomes. *TDF*, Testes determining factor; *SRY*, sex-determining region of the Y chromosome.

The phenotype for Turner syndrome is highly variable. Affected individuals are typically short (<150 cm) with gonadal dysgenesis and learning difficulties. Other common features include webbed neck resulting from cystic hygroma in utero, low posterior hairline, heart and renal anomalies, cubitus valgus (increased carrying angle of the elbow), and shield chest. At birth, patients may present with edema of the hands and feet. Turner syndrome patients are usually of normal intelligence, although this can vary and some individuals have significant mental handicaps. Furthermore, although infertility used to be accepted as the standard in Turner syndrome, it is now known that some patients, usually those with mosaic karyotypes, can reproduce successfully. Furthermore, using donor egg technologies, a Turner syndrome patient can complete a full pregnancy and deliver a normal child. Therefore, because of this great diversity of presentation, prenatal counseling for a couple with an identified Turner syndrome fetus is extremely difficult. In general, however, most liveborn Turner syndrome patients can live productive lives, and mildly affected individuals may not know that they are affected with the disorder until puberty.

Other Sex Chromosome Abnormalities

Sex determination in humans is the result of a complex biochemical pathway involving the interaction of proteins produced by genes present on the autosomes and the X and Y chromosomes. The default sex in humans is female, so in the absence of any male-determining stimuli, a female individual will develop. The primary trigger for male development is a gene located on the short arm of the Y chromosome designated *TDF*, the testes determining factor, which is located in the sex-determining region of the Y chromosome (*SRY*) (Fig. 68-22).

The protein produced by *TDF* initiates the male developmental pathway. A number of disorders associated with mutations in different genes within this pathway have been identified and can result in ambiguous genitalia or genotype/phenotype mismatch (phenotypic male with an XX sex chromosome complement or a phenotypic female with an XY complement).

An XX male can usually be attributed to one of two causes. The more common of the two is virilization of a female fetus as a result of the autosomal recessive disorder congenital adrenal hyperplasia (CAH). The defect in CAH is the lack of the enzyme 21-hydroxylase. Without this enzyme, the normal biosynthetic pathway is blocked and androgens accumulate in the body. Excessive levels of male hormones in the female circulation may result in a male-appearing infant despite a female chromosome complement. Furthermore, because androgens are capable of crossing the placenta, a normal female fetus may develop ambiguous genitalia due to exposure from excess hormones from a CAH-affected mother.

A phenotypic male with an XX sex chromosome complement may also result from a cryptic translocation between the X and Y chromosomes. The distal ends of the short arms of the X and Y chromosomes are homologous and comprise what is termed the *pseudoautosomal regions* (see Fig. 68-22). This is the primary site of X and Y chromosome pairing during meiosis, and recombination may occur between X and Y alleles. Rarely, a recombination event outside the boundaries of the pseudoautosomal region takes place, resulting in the transfer of unique Y loci, including *SRY*, to the tip of the X chromosome. The amount of chromosome material involved in such an exchange is extremely small and cannot be cytogenetically detected. In a male with such a balanced translocation, there would be no clinical abnormalities, because the genes are all present, although in alternate locations. However, if this male transmits his rearranged X chromosome to an offspring who has received an X from the mother, the resultant child will have an apparent XX chromosome complement but a male or Klinefelter male phenotype due to the presence of the TDF protein that triggers the male developmental pathway.

The reciprocal of the aforementioned translocation may result in a Turner female with an apparent XY complement. The male developmental pathway will not be initiated in an individual with a Y chromosome that has no *TDF/SRY*, and sex determination will default to female. However, the lack of two intact copies of the proximal X short arm will prevent normal female development, and a Turner syndrome individual should result. This situation is quite rare. The more common finding for an XY female is androgen insensitivity, also known as *testicular feminization.* In these individuals, the Y chromosome is intact, and *TDF* is present and functional. The problem is a mutation of the androgen receptor gene located on the long arm of the X chromosome (Xq21.3) that results in no androgen receptor protein being produced. The TDF protein will initiate male development, but the pathway will be blocked at the point where the androgen receptor protein is required to form a complex between testosterone and dihydrotestosterone. Without this critical step, further male differentiation is not possible, and the phenotype will default back to female. However, these individuals are infertile because of the lack of any functional internal genitalia, and commonly present with a blind vagina and testes in the abdomen or inguinal canal.

Structural Chromosome Anomalies

A reasonable number of syndromes directly related to a structural chromosome abnormality have been described. Most of these are quite rare. The following is a discussion of some of the more common syndromes (see also Jones, 2006).

Wolf-Hirschhorn syndrome, also known as *4p– syndrome*, is due to a terminal deletion of the short arm of chromosome 4, del(4)(p16). Clinical findings include microcephaly, micrognathia, hypotonia, epicanthal folds, and developmental delay. The characteristic facial appearance has been likened to a Greek warrior's helmet because of the arched eyebrows and long nose. Individuals with this disorder require special education and are at increased risk of seizures.

Cri-du-chat, or 5p– syndrome, del(5)(p15), is characterized by a distinctive high-pitched, catlike cry in infancy. Other features include low birth weight and subsequent slow growth, hypotonia, microcephaly, hypertelorism, epicanthal folds, cardiac anomalies, and mental retardation. Affected children have delayed development and may reach the cognitive and social level of a 5- or 6-year-old.

Microdeletion Syndromes and Contiguous Gene Syndromes

By definition, a microdeletion is a very small deletion, usually only a fraction of a single chromosome band. Microdeletions can be confused with

PART 8

TABLE 68-5
Microdeletion and Contiguous Gene Syndromes

Disorder	Location	Genes	Clinical findings
Angelman syndrome	15q11.2	*UBE3A*	Severe MR, developmental delay, large mouth, prognathia, ataxia, seizures DiGeorge syndrome
DiGeorge syndrome	22q11.2, 10p	*DGS1, DGS2*	Characteristic facies, cleft palate, heart defect, hypoplasia of the thymus and parathyroids, severe hypocalcemia, seizures
Ichthyosis	Xp22.32	*STS*	Scaly skin, short stature, hypogonadism, MR
Kallmann syndrome	Xp22.3	*KAL1*	Hypogonadism, inability to smell
Langer-Giedion syndrome	8q24.11–q24.13	*TRPSI* *TRPSII* *EXT*	Craniofacial dysmorphism, skeletal abnormalities, mild to severe mental deficiency
Lissencephaly	17p13.3	*LIS1*	Smooth brain, profound retardation, seizures
Miller-Dieker syndrome	17p13.3	*LIS1* and other(s)	Lissencephaly, microcephaly, high forehead, small nose, micrognathia, low-set ears
Prader-Willi syndrome	15q11.2	*SNRPN*	Hypotonia at birth, almond-shaped eyes, moderate to severe MR, absent sense of satiation leading to overeating, small hands and feet, hypogonadism
Retinoblastoma	13q14.1–q14.2	*Rb1*	Tumors of the retinoblast cells of the eye
Rubinstein-Taybi syndrome	16p13.3	*CBP*	Beaked nose, prominent columella, hypoplastic maxilla, downslanted palpebral fissures, broad thumbs and first toes, MR, speech delay
Smith-Magenis syndrome	17p11.2		Brachycephaly, midface hypoplasia, broad nasal bridge, prominent jaw, short broad hands, hyperactivity, delayed speech, self-destructive behavior, MR
Velocardiofacial syndrome	22q11.2	*TBX1* and others	Palatal defects, hypoplastic alae nasi with long nose, learning disability, congenital heart disease
WAGR	11p13.3	*WT1, PAX6*	Wilms tumor, aniridia, genitourinary defects, and mental retardation
Williams syndrome	7q11.2	*ELN*	Low IQ, hypersensitivity to sound, blue eyes with stellate pattern in the iris, prominent lips, hoarse voice, supravalvular aortic stenosis or other cardiac defect, hypercalcemia, premature aging of the skin

MR, Mental retardation.

molecular deletions, so it is important to recognize that, although microdeletions are small, they are significantly larger (>500 kb) than the typical molecular deletion (1 base pair [bp] to several hundred bp), which can only be resolved by molecular technology (see Chapter 70). The actual size of a microdeletion can vary from patient to patient, and some may be large enough to identify by karyotype analysis, although most will require FISH for detection. Although originally thought to be deletions within single genes, it has now been shown that certain syndromes are actually due to deletions that encompass portions of several adjacent, unrelated genes. The clinical presentation may therefore be a combination of features due to the absence of several different gene products. The size of the deletion and number of genes affected may vary, such that the phenotype expressed may differ significantly between individuals. Collectively, these are called *contiguous gene syndromes*. Included in this group are many of the microdeletion syndromes (Table 68-5) as well as the larger, classic deletion syndromes such as Wolf-Hirshhorn and cri-du-chat.

Miller-Dieker syndrome clearly illustrates the overlap between microdeletion and contiguous gene syndromes. The disorder has been associated with a microdeletion of the distal short arm of chromosome 17 (17p13.3), and the cardinal clinical features are lissencephaly (smooth brain) and craniofacial anomalies. Isolated lissencephaly has also been recognized as an independent entity, so Miller-Dieker syndrome is a more complex presentation that couples the brain defect with characteristic facial features. Molecular analysis has shown there are at least two genes involved in Miller-Dieker syndrome, so it is a true contiguous gene syndrome resulting from a microdeletion. A smaller deletion of the *LIS1* gene only would result in isolated lissencephaly (Ledbetter, 1992).

Prader-Willi syndrome and *Angelman syndrome* are the best-known microdeletion syndromes. Both share the same interstitial deletion of the proximal long arm of chromosome 15, del(15)(q11.2q11.2), but the clinical presentations are significantly different. Prader-Willi patients are small and hypotonic at birth but change within the first year of life and begin to gain weight rapidly. If not placed on a controlled diet, they can become quite obese through overeating. Other characteristics include small hands and feet, hypogonadism, and a bad temper. Although they are developmentally delayed, most do well in special education classes. Because of their temper and difficulty in controlling their diet, Prader-Willi patients may be placed in special group homes that provide the proper environment. Angelman syndrome patients, on the other hand, are severely mentally retarded. Although they are friendly, they usually cannot carry on a normal conversation, and discourse is often punctuated by bursts of inappropriate laughter. The disorder is also characterized by hyperactivity, short stature, microcephaly, seizures, and ataxia.

By routine or high-resolution cytogenetic analysis, the 15q deletion can be detected in about 60% of Prader-Willi individuals but only 10%–20% of Angelman syndrome patients. Use of FISH has provided a much better diagnostic tool and, for both syndromes, deletions can now be established in 80%–85% of cases. Although it was accepted that not all deletions would be visible at the cytogenetic level, it was considered odd that FISH was unable to detect a deletion in 100% of cases. This, in addition to the fact that Prader-Willi syndrome and Angelman syndrome appear to share the same deletion but have such entirely different phenotypes, suggested that there might be another cause for the disorders. It is now known that Prader-Willi syndrome and Angelman syndrome are examples of genetic imprinting, and that the mutational processes resulting in the diseases are much more complex than a simple deletion of DNA (Nicholls, 1989; Robinson, 1991) (see Chapter 70 for a discussion of imprinting and molecular detection of imprinted genes).

Williams syndrome has been associated with a deletion of the elastin gene (*ELN*) on the proximal long arm of chromosome 7 (7q11.23). The disorder is characterized by cardiac abnormalities, hypertension, hoarse voice, premature aging of the skin, and behavioral anomalies. Since elastin is known to be an important protein lending elasticity to tissues such as the heart, blood vessels, skin, and vocal cords, its absence explains many of the physical anomalies associated with this syndrome. The behavioral problems, however, could not be attributed to the lack of elastin, and futher investigations have shown that Williams syndrome is actually a contiguous gene syndrome and that the variability of the phenotype is related to the number of adjacent genes deleted in combination with *ELN*.

A very well characterized contiguous gene syndrome is located on the short arm of chromosome 11 (11p13) and is known as *WAGR* (*W*ilms tumor, *a*niridia, *g*enitourinary defects, and mental *r*etardation). Except for the genitourinary defects, which appear to be due to a variant mutation in the Wilms tumor locus, each of the other three anomalies has been associated with a particular gene and these are arranged in tandem on the short arm of chromosome 11 (Fig. 68-23). The phenotype of an affected individual will vary depending on the size of the deletion. Statistically, about one in three children diagnosed with aniridia will also develop Wilms

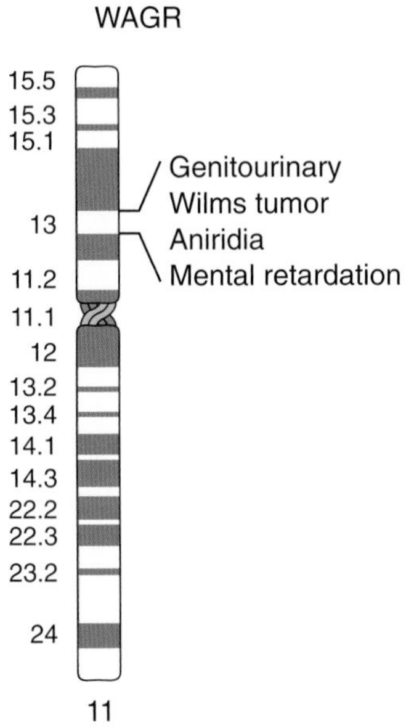

Figure 68-23 Diagram of the contiguous gene syndrome WAGR showing relative positions of the different genes on the short arm of chromosome 11. *WAGR* *W*ilms tumor, *a*niridia, *g*enitourinary defects, and mental *r*etardation.

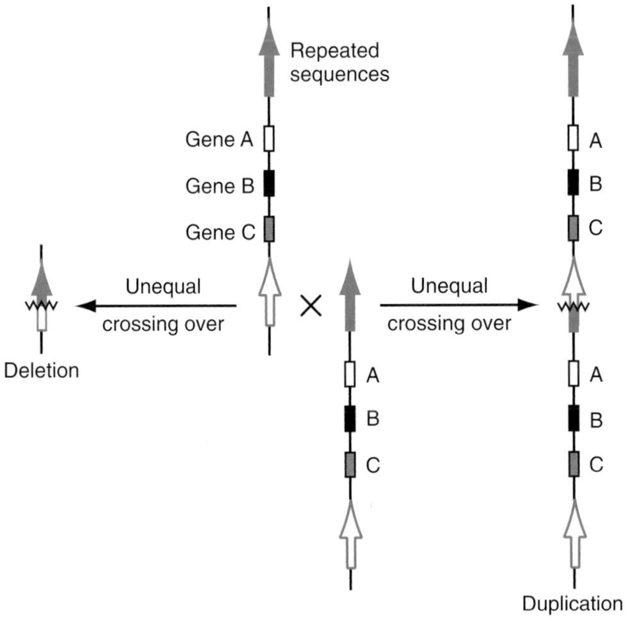

Figure 68-24 Diagram of the possible outcomes of mispairing and recombination at the velocardiofacial syndrome locus on chromosome 22 (22q11.2). Two chromosomes that have mispaired by association of repeat sequences are seen in the middle of the figure. Recombination may or may not occur. If it does occur, one outcome is a deletion (seen on the *left*) resulting from the complete loss of both gene sequences from both original chromosomes (indicated as genes A–C). The reciprocal event would be a tandem repeat of both gene sequences, one derived from each of the original chromosomes (seen on the *right*).

tumor. Conversely, only one in 50 Wilms patients has aniridia. With larger deletions, mental retardation and genitourinary defects may also be seen.

Velocardiofacial syndrome is possibly the most common microdeletion syndrome in humans but it is often not recognized because it has a broad spectrum of clinical features and a presentation that can be mild. The disorder is usually diagnosed in the newborn period because of feeding difficulties, cardiac defects, and characteristic facial dysmorphologies. Learning disabilities, short stature, and conductive hearing loss are noted as the individual ages. Interestingly, 10%–15% of patients will have a much more mildly affected parent with the same deletion. The 3 Mb deletion on the proximal long arm of chromosome 22 (22q11.2q11.2) is thought to be due to recombination between direct repeats that flank the common deletion region. The similarity in the repeats can result in slippage and mispairing between the chromosomes (Fig. 68-24). If recombination

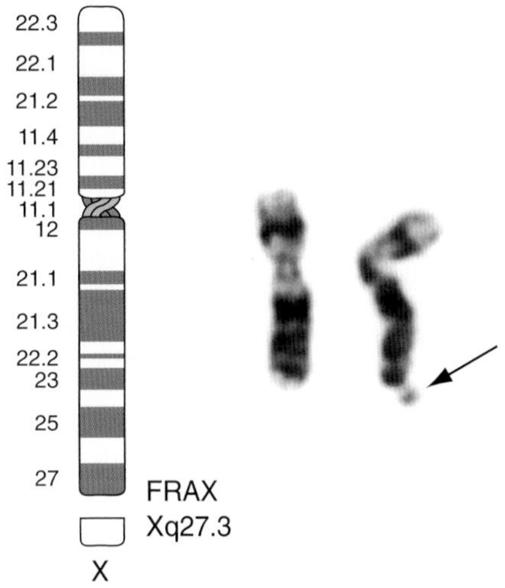

Figure 68-25 Fragile X. Ideogram of the fragile X (*left*) and a representative pair of G-banded chromosomes showing the fragile X on the *right*.

occurs between the misalligned chromosomes, two recombinant products are possible: (1) a chromosome missing the 3 Mb region associated with velocardiofacial syndrome or (2) a chromosome with a duplication of the 3 Mb region. Individuals with the duplication have been identified. Their phenotype is significantly different than that of the velocardiofacial syndrome deletion individuals (McDermid, 2002).

A similar mechanism resulting in the classic Williams syndrome deletion has also been reported (Bayes, 2003). Recombination following mispairing of the chromosomes is a new recognized mutation strategy that could explain deletion formation in a variety of other diseases.

OTHER CYTOGENETIC PHENOMENA

Fragile X Syndrome

Fragile X syndrome is the second leading cause of mental retardation and is the primary cause of inherited mental retardation. The disorder was first described by Herbert Lubs in 1969, when he noted the correlation between retardation and a "marker" X in affected family members (Lubs, 1969). The marker X has subsequently become known as the *fragile X*, a break or gap in the structure of the X chromosome that can be detected cytogenetically (Fig. 68-25) by culturing cells in the appropriate induction medium. However, not all affected individuals express the fragile X cytogenetically, so the clinical test is flawed. Nevertheless, it was the only assay available for many years and provided much-needed confirmation of diagnosis in many individuals. In 1991, the gene associated with fragile X syndrome was cloned and the mutation was identified as an amplification of a trinucleotide repeat sequence, something that had never before been seen or associated as a disease-causing mechanism. This mutation is detectable at the molecular level, and a highly proficient clinical test has been developed to allow direct mutation detection for fragile X syndrome (Rousseau, 1991; Verkerk, 1991) (see Chapter 70), so the cytogenetic test is no longer used.

Breakage Syndromes

Chromosomal breakage syndromes (Table 68-6) are a set of autosomal recessive disorders that were originally grouped together because of the common finding of chromosome instability or fragility (Arlett, 1978). Consequently, cytogenetic testing was possible as an aid in diagnosis. Molecular studies have shown an additional commonality among the disorders in that the primary mutation in each is a defect in a DNA repair gene. This helped explain the other features of the syndromes, because inability to repair the DNA can lead to (1) breakage or increased recombination that can be characterized by chromosome instability and (2) widespread mutation and defect in DNA sequences that can lead to cancer.

SUMMARY

Cytogenetics is a relatively old, labor-intensive laboratory science, and it is still performed in much the same way it always has been, although the advent of the computer-assisted karyotyping system, the robotic harvester,

TABLE 68-6
Chromosome Breakage Syndromes

Disorder	Clinical features	Gene locus	Cytogenetic manifestation	Type of cancer	Dna repair defect	Miscellaneous
Fanconi anemia	Pancytopenia, prenatal or postnatal growth retardation, hypoplastic or missing thumbs, possible arm deformation, brownish pigmentation of skin	1. Group A: 16q24.3 2. Group C: 9q22.3 3. Group D: -3p22–p26 4. Group E—6p21–p22 5. Groups B, F, H unmapped	Increased chromosome breakage detected by treatment with mitomycin C and diepoxybutane	Increased risk of AML, and progressive bone marrow failure		Current therapy: Bone marrow transplantation
Bloom syndrome	Growth retardation, butterfly rash on face, possible malignancy	15q26.1	Increased sister chromatid exchange in response to UV light or BrdU incorporation		Abnormal DNA ligase I activity	High frequency in Ashkenazi Jewish population: 1/110 carrier frequency
Ataxia telangiectasia	Ataxia with degeneration of central nervous system, telangiectasia on face, deficiency in cellular immunity, degenerative, growth retardation	11q22.3	Increased spontaneous breakage, increased rings, triradials, and translocations, particularly with 7 and 14, induced with bleomycin or ionizing radiation	Various leukemias and solid tumors		
Xeroderma pigmentosum	Sensitivity to sun, neurological abnormalities, ataxia and spasticity	Incidence: 1 in 250,000 1. A: 9q22.3 2. C: 653p25 3. D: 19q13.2–q13.3 4. E: 11p11–p12 5. F: 16p13.1–13.2, 16p13.13–p13.3 6. G: 13q33	Increase in SCE and chromosome rearrangement in response to UV light	Increased incidence of skin cancer	1. Lack of excision of thymine dimers 2. Postreplication repair defect	
Cockayne syndrome	Dwarfism, premature aging, microcephaly, neurologic deficit, pigmentary degeneration, deafness, sensitivity to sunlight, MR	Chr. 5	UV sensitivity	Increased incidence of skin cancer	Possible DNA ligase deficiency or defect of transcription coupled repair	

AML, Acute myeloid leukemia; *MR,* mental retardation; *UV,* ultraviolet.

and microarray analysis have added an element of advanced technology to the laboratory. Although it was once predicted that molecular diagnostics would eliminate the need for cytogenetics, that has not occurred, and cytogenetics is still the only clinical assay that can provide a quick overview of the entire human genome. Karyotype analysis continues to be important in assessing numerical and structural chromosome anomalies and is the gold standard for diagnosis of many disorders. Determination of the cytogenetic lesion is currently required for diagnosis of many cancers. To meet new challenges, cytogenetics has added new testing and new technologies. Use of FISH, and more recently microarray technology, have bridged the gap between cytogenetics and molecular diagnostics such that the two areas provide complementary information in many cases. However, despite the technologic advances, nothing has yet been able to replace karyotype analysis as a tool for genomic screening, so cytogenetics continues to hold an important place in clinical laboratory medicine.

SELECTED REFERENCES

Abbott Molecular. http://www.abbottmolecular.com/us/home.html.

Developer and manufacturer of FISH probes. The website provides information on the probes available and the biology behind the detection assay.

Block AW. Cancer cytogenetics. In: Gersen S, Keagle M, editors. The principles of clinical cytogenetics. Totowa, N.J.: Humana Press; 1999. p. 345.

An excellent reference covering cytogenetic aspects of oncology. Figures and tables are invaluable aides in interpreting patient results.

Heim S, Mitelman F. Cancer cytogenetics, 2nd ed. New York: Wiley-Liss; 1995.

This is an excellent source of information covering all aspects of cancer genetics. It includes molecular, cytogenetic, and clinical aspects of all known leukemias, lymphomas, and solid tumors.

ISCN 2009. An international system for human cytogenetic nomenclature. Basel: S Karger; 2009.

This reference provides the standard ideograms, the accepted cytogenetic nomenclature and how it is to be applied, and examples of usage of terminology.

Nussbaum RL, McInnes RR, Willard HF. Thompson and Thompson—genetics in medicine, 7th ed. Philadelphia: WB Saunders; 2007.

Excellent textbook covering all aspects of medical genetics. It provides a basic introduction to the field followed by detailed descriptions of subspecialties including cytogenetics, molecular genetics, cancer genetics, immunogenetics, prenatal genetics, and genetic counseling.

OMIM (Online Mendelian Inheritance in Man). http://www.ncbi.nlm.nih.gov/Omim/.

The best source of information on genes related to diseases. Each entry includes data on the discovery of the gene, cytogenetic and molecular aspects of the disorder, possible genetic testing, related diseases, and references to the scientific literature.

Swerdlow SH, Campo E, Harris NL, et al. WHO classification of tumours of haematopoietic and lymphoid tissues. Lyon: IARC Press; 2008.

This text is an important guide, providing the pathology (i.e., descriptions and findings) associated with leukemias and lymphomas. It includes the current WHOclassification for hematological disorders.

FURTHER READING

Borgaonkar D. Chromosomal variation in man: a catalog of chromosomal variants and anomalies, 5th ed. New York: Wiley-Liss; 1989.

De Grouchy J, Turleau C. Clinical atlas of human chromosomes, 2nd ed. New York: John Wiley & Sons; 1984.

Gelehrter T, Collins FC, Ginsburg D. Principles of medical genetics, 2nd ed. Baltimore: Williams & Wilkins; 1998.

Heim S, Mitelman F. Cancer cytogenetics, 2nd ed. New York: Wiley-Liss; 1995.

This is an excellent source of information covering all aspects of cancer genetics. It includes molecular, cytogenetic, and clinical aspects of all known leukemias, lymphomas, and solid tumors.

McKusick V. Mendelian inheritance in man: catalogs of autosomal dominant, autosomal recessive, and X-linked phenotypes, 11th ed. Baltimore: Johns Hopkins Press; 1983.

Mitelman F. Catalog of chromosome aberrations in cancer, 5th ed. New York: Wiley-Liss; 1994.

Rooney DE, Czepulkowski BH. Human cytogenetics, a practical approach. Oxford: IRL Press; 1992.

Verma R, Babu A. Human chromosomes—principles and techniques, 2nd ed. New York: McGraw-Hill; 1995.

REFERENCES

Access the complete reference list online at http://www.expertconsult.com

CHAPTER 69

ESTABLISHING A MOLECULAR DIAGNOSTICS LABORATORY

Andrea Ferreira-Gonzalez, David S. Wilkinson, Martin H. Bluth

During the past decade, a vast amount of knowledge has been gained regarding genes, gene products, and their role in human disease. This knowledge has allowed us to better understand many disease processes and start defining diseases and disease processes in terms of their molecular pathogenesis. Molecular diagnostics testing is a relatively recent specialty of laboratory medicine and is still in a state of flux at many levels, such as the choice of test, technology, automation and reimbursement. The scope of molecular testing has expanded rapidly since its introduction in the late 1980s. This has led to the development of new clinical molecular assays for use in diagnosis, prognosis, selection of therapeutic modalities, and monitoring of disease. The technologies that constitute molecular diagnostics—such as first-generation amplification, deoxyribonucleic acid (DNA) probes, fluorescent in situ hybridization (FISH), second-generation biochips and microfluidics, next-generation signal detection, biosensors, and molecular labels—are influencing the discovery of therapeutic molecules, the screening and diagnosis of patients, and the optimization of drug therapy. In the past few years, this rapidly evolving field has seen several fascinating developments. There are many applications of this technology to different areas of the clinical laboratory. Whereas testing for inherited genetic diseases, cancer diagnosis, viral load, and infectious diseases continues to predominate, the impact of pharmacogenomics on molecular diagnostics is unknown. The operation of a clinical molecular pathology laboratory requires integration of expertise in medical, scientific, and clinical molecular pathology; resources, including facilities, equipment, and personnel; and skills in organization, administration, management, and communication.

Special Considerations for Molecular Diagnostics Laboratories

Whereas all molecular diagnostics tests share the use of nucleic acid technology, the different clinical applications may require different management considerations.

INFECTIOUS DISEASE

As molecular techniques have become more accepted, more and more microorganisms are detected or characterized by molecular methods, which in many cases have become the standard of practice, especially for microorganisms that are difficult to culture or when subsequent culture is needed to indentify drug resistance. As volume of testing has grown, there has arisen a need for automation of different steps of testing as well as the need for standardized kits. We have seen a surge of different automation platforms. Automated platforms perform nucleic acid extraction from different types of specimens, automated liquid handling systems set up reactions, and real-time technology monitors and quantifies nucleic acids as they are being amplified. In addition, quantitative molecular methods have become standard of practice in monitoring response to therapy, especially in patients with human immunodeficiency virus (HIV), hepatitis B virus (HBV), and hepatitis C virus (HCV) infections. The need for confidentiality for patients undergoing HIV testing has prompted specific federal and state regulation to ensure the protection of patients and their families. In addition, each state might have a list of different organisms that, if detected, must be reported to the state health department.

CANCER

Molecular methods are currently used for hematopoietic neoplasms as well as for solid tumors. The nucleic acid changes, either DNA or ribonucleic acid (RNA), are present only in the affected populations of cells and are not part of the genetic makeup of the individual. Current technologies, such as real-time polymerase chain reaction (PCR) and microarray analysis, have provided greater diagnostic sensitivity and specificity for diagnostic testing, prognosis treatment selection, monitoring response to therapy, and detection of minimal residual disease. In addition, the exquisite sensitivity of these molecular methods has allowed the testing of very small amounts of nucleic acid from a wide range of sample types. Formalin-fixed paraffin-embedded tissue can provide good quality and quantity of DNA and RNA from processed tissues; however, very specific protocols either for DNA or RNA extraction must be followed. In contrast to inherited genetic testing that needs to be done once per lifetime, molecular oncology tests often are performed repeatedly (eg, for initial diagnosis and during and after treatment for monitoring response to therapy). Molecular methods which identify rearrangements or mutations that cause specific tumor types may also be used to assess minimal residual disease. Molecular test results should be interpreted in the context of other laboratory testing, such as histopathology, flow cytometry, and clinical findings. The detection of a specific mutation in the tumor cells may also be used to determine appropriate course of therapy. This is the case for metastatic colon cancer. A number of studies have shown that antiepidermal growth factor receptor *(EGFR)* monoclonal antibodies are effective treatments for metastatic colorectal cancer, but only in patients with wild-type oncogene *KRAS*. The anti-*EGFR* monoclonal antibodies panitumumab and cetuximab are approved in the United States for treatment of metastatic colorectal cancer refractory to chemotherapy but are not recommended for use in patients with mutations in *KRAS* codons 12 or 13. Similarly, panitumumab is approved for the treatment of metastatic colorectal cancer only in patients with wild-type KRAS in Europe and Canada. It is clear that KRAS mutational analysis has become an important aspect of disease management in patients with metastatic colorectal cancer.

Laboratory issues specific for hematopoietic neoplasms and solid tumor testing include the need for fresh or frozen tissue for RNA-based testing, the use of microdissection to reduce nonmalignant cell population in the specimens, and the need to work with small tissue specimens such as needle biopsies.

INHERITED DISORDERS

All diseases have a genetic contribution, whether it is a specific genetic disease or an increased likelihood for developing a medical condition. Genetic disorders are primarily the result of a germline mutation or a mutation present in every cell of an individual. For this reason, genetic testing has far-reaching implications, because it could affect family members that might have inherited the same mutation. Molecular genetic testing is currently used for diagnosis, carrier status evaluation, and prenatal and presymptomatic DNA testing. Diagnostic testing is usually performed on affected individuals for establishing or confirming a clinical diagnosis.

Carrier testing is performed in an asymptomatic healthy individual to identify whether the individual is a carrier for an autosomal or X-linked recessive condition and whether the individual is at risk for having an affected child. This application can be used for individuals with a family history of a genetic disorder or for population screening, such as in screening for cystic fibrosis (CF). Carrier testing can be done first by testing an affected family member to identify the specific mutation present in the family. Once a specific mutation is identified, family members can be tested for that particular mutation, thus improving the accuracy of the risk assessment for the individuals in that family with a negative test result. In contrast, population screening focuses on the most common or prevalent mutation, most of the time with different rate of detection for different ethnic populations. Prenatal testing is performed to identify a fetus with a genetic disease or condition. Prenatal testing analyzes fetal cells obtained by amniocentesis or by chorionic villus sampling. This type of testing is usually initiated because family history or maternal factors suggest it. In addition, some laboratories offer preimplantation genetic testing in the setting of in vitro fertilization for couples with a family history of a specific genetic disease. Presymptomatic testing is used primarily for the identification of adult onset of a genetic condition that will occur later in life, such as Huntington disease. Presymptomatic testing is the most problematic and challenging type of testing in terms of its psychological effect on the individual and hence requires extensive protocols for pregenetic and postgenetic testing counseling.

Several other issues are of critical relevance. Genetic testing requires special attention to informed consent, appropriateness, and urgency. There are no federal regulations regarding the process of informed consent, but a number of states have specific laws that govern the process of informed consent. Each laboratory director should evaluate state laws to determine what the regulations stipulate. Many laboratories require documentation of informed consent before performing the genetic test. Informed consent can be documented by several means such as requesting the actual signed informed consent or a copy of it, or by confirmation by the physician or health care provider on the requisition that the informed consent was obtained and is documented in the patient's chart. Until required documentation of informed consent is obtained, the laboratory can stabilize the patient specimen, extract and store the nucleic acid. The laboratory can start the testing once the required documentation is received. In addition to documentation of informed consent, the laboratory should review clinical indications for testing and determine whether the test is appropriate for a specific patient. Despite the tremendous advances in the understanding of the human genome, the full benefit of genetic testing for a particular patient is not always clear. Testing may be warranted, even if the results are inconclusive or preventive strategies or treatments are not available. Genetic information raises critical ethical, legal, and social issues for both the individual being tested as well as for family members. Special attention should be given to genetic testing in minors. For example, should carrier testing of minors be deferred until the minor is an adult? Similarly, a request for testing of an asymptomatic individual for a dominant disease should include arrangements for adequate genetic counseling. In addition, the laboratory should understand and communicate to health care providers the sensitivity and limitations of the test performed so that patients can be counseled appropriately as to the expectations of the testing and the significance of the testing results.

Genetic testing results often require interpretation using complex risk assessment calculations. Health care professionals must correctly interpret laboratory test results in the context of the particular patient and be able to convey the test results and interpretation to the patients and family members. Communication of genetic test results to patients and families can be complex and time-consuming. Clinicians trained in medical genetics as well as genetic counselors are well equipped to communicate the complex and involved information. Benefits of this approach have been well documented in the literature. Misinterpretation of negative genetic test results by inadequately trained physicians may result in inappropriately suggesting that patients discontinue recommended aggressive surveillance for the genetic condition. For these reasons, most genetic testing should be ordered through health care providers trained in genetics to ensure that the benefits and risks of testing have been explained to the patient during the informed consent process.

REGULATION AND REGULATORY AGENCIES

CLINICAL LABORATORY IMPROVEMENT ACTS 1988, 2003

Laboratories performing clinical testing must comply with numerous regulations. Laboratories performing testing on human specimens for the purposes of diagnosis, prevention, or treatment of diseases are subject to federal regulation imposed by Clinical Laboratory Improvement Act of 1988 (CLIA '88). CLIA '88 set standards designed to improve quality in laboratory practices and expanded federal oversight to almost every clinical laboratory in the United States. Laboratories performing research are not subject to CLIA '88 unless the research laboratory reports specific results to the individuals tested, their families, and/or the treating physician, even when there is a disclaimer in the final report that states that the test results should be used for research purposes only and/or there is no charge for the test. CLIA '88 describes specific standards in all areas of the testing process, personnel training, proficiency testing (PT), quality control (QC), and quality assurance (QA). The federal regulation establishes a registry, sanctions, and enforcement procedures to ensure that the standards defined in the federal regulation are maintained. The regulations for implementing CLIA '88 were developed by the Department of Health and Human Services through the Public Health Service. At that time, the Centers for Disease Control and Prevention (CDC) was assigned to categorize analytes and supervise implementation of standards. The U.S. Food and Drug Administration (FDA) was assigned to review and guarantee the safety and effectiveness of tests and the Center for Medicare and Medicaid Services (CMS), formerly known as Health Care Finance Administration, was to collect fees, issue permits, survey laboratories, and initiate sanctions when necessary. Under CLIA '88, tests are categorized as *waived*, *provider-performed microscopy*, *moderate complexity*, and *high complexity*. Tests are placed into moderate and high complexity testing categories on the basis of a numerical scoring system. The scoring system takes into account the following factors: knowledge required for performing the test, training and expertise, availability of calibrators, QC, PT, operational characteristics, degree of interpretation, and judgment, among others. In 2003, new extensively revised CLIA regulations were published and nicknamed *CLIA '03*. The changes include major reorganization and consolidation of the regulations by passing requirements on the flow of a patient sample through the laboratory and updating the requirements to accommodate new technologies.

All laboratories performing clinical testing must seek CLIA certification. Molecular diagnostics laboratories are considered high complexity laboratories and as such must comply with CLIA requirements for high complexity laboratory testing. Some of these requirements include qualifications of personnel performing and overseeing the testing process procedure manual specifications, method verifications of performance specifications, PT, QA, patient test management, and inspection. CLIA, however, does not provide specific guidelines for molecular testing and therefore each molecular diagnostics laboratory is responsible for the development of a test management program according to CLIA. Recently the CDC published a *Morbidity and Mortality Weekly Report:* "Best practices for molecular genetic testing for heritable diseases and conditions," which provides detailed recommendations regarding good laboratory practices for ensuring the quality of molecular genetic testing for heritable conditions. The recommended practices address the total testing process including preanalytical, analytical, and postanalytical, laboratory responsibilities regarding authorized persons, confidentiality of patient information, personnel competency, considerations before introducing a new test, and the quality management system approach to molecular genetic testing. The report can be found at www.cdc.gov.

Molecular diagnostic tests are considered high complexity testing and as such laboratories performing this testing must seek certification from CMS. CLIA regulations allow CMS to approve nonprofit professional organizations that have laboratory testing and inspection standards equivalent to or more stringent than CLIA to inspect clinical laboratories in place of a CLIA inspection. The two major organizations providing CLIA inspections are The Joint Commission, which accredits more than 80% of U.S. health care organizations, and the Laboratory Accreditation Program of the College of American Pathologists (LAP-CAP). Most laboratories performing molecular diagnostic testing are CLIA '88 accredited through the LAP-CAP program. When a test site meets the accreditation agency's requirements, as assessed by inspection, the laboratory, meets CLIA requirements and receives a CLIA certificate of accreditation. CAP introduced a molecular pathology checklist in 1993 and it has been updated yearly since then. All laboratories must follow the Laboratory General checklist and the specific laboratory checklist. In addition, the molecular pathology checklist is a great resource when developing a molecular diagnostic laboratory, particularly for the development of QC, QA programs, specimen requisition, and reporting.

GENETIC INFORMATION NONDISCRIMINATION ACT

The Genetic Information Nondiscrimination Act of 2008, also referred to as GINA, is a federal law that prohibits discrimination in health coverage and employment based on genetic information. The law has two titles: title I, relates to health insurance coverage, and title II, relates to employment. GINA took effect in November 2009 and prohibits group and individual health insurers from using a person's genetic information in determining eligibility or premiums; it also prohibits an insurer from requesting or requiring that a person undergo a genetic test. In addition, GINA prohibits employers from using a person's genetic information to make employment decisions such as hiring, firing, job assignments, or any other terms of employment, and it prohibits employers from requesting, requiring, or purchasing genetic information about persons or their family members. GINA does not prevent health care providers from recommending genetic tests to their patients, it does not mandate coverage for any particular test or treatment, it does not prohibit medical underwriting based on current health status, it does not cover life, disability, or long-term-care insurance, and it does not apply to members of the military.

One key term used in GINA is *genetic information,* which includes information about a person's genetic tests (including genetic tests done as part of a research study), genetic tests of a person's family (up to and including fourth-degree relatives), any manifestation of a disease or disorder in a family member, and participation of a person or family member in research that includes genetic testing, counseling, or education. GINA defines *genetic tests* as tests that assess genotypes, mutations, or chromosomal changes. Examples of protected tests are tests for *BRCA1/BRCA2* (breast cancer) or *HNPCC* (colon cancer) mutations, classifications of genetic properties of an existing tumor to help determine therapy, tests for Huntington's disease mutations, and carrier screening for disorders such as CF, sickle cell anemia, spinal muscular atrophy, and the fragile X syndrome. On the other hand, routine tests such as complete blood counts, cholesterol tests, and liver function tests are not protected under GINA.

Although GINA protects patient information from misuse by insurers, employers, and other administrative agencies, it is important to recognize the stigma test results can have on the patient. Unlike other general laboratory analytes that are accepted in the lay public as routine testing (e.g., cholesterol) for disease stratification or management, carrying a gene often carries an ominous forecast because of the erroneous interpretation that carrying the gene equals manifesting the disease. Genetic counseling is essential for patients to understand what it means to be a "carrier." The issues relating to disease penetrance, allelic variability, polymorphisms, and confounding factors associated with a given gene must be related to the physician-patient-counselor unit toward appropriate interpretation. Otherwise the psychological well-being of the patient can be drastically affected. Examples of such stigmata include being labeled a genetic carrier for Tay-Sachs, CF, and *BRCA1/BRCA2*, which could affect the patient's decisions pertaining to marriage, family planning, surgical options, and social acceptance.

FOOD AND DRUG ADMINISTRATION

Analyte-Specific Reagents

The term *analyte-specific reagent* (ASR) was devised by the FDA for reagents used in clinical testing that confer specificity for detection of the target analyte. The FDA defines ASRs as "antibodies, monoclonal and polyclonal, specific receptors, proteins, ligands, nucleic acid sequences, and similar reagents which through specific binding or chemical reaction with substances in a specimen are intended for use in a diagnostic application for identification and quantification of an individual chemical substance or ligand in biological specimens." Primers and probes developed specifically to detect a certain DNA or RNA target used in any laboratory developed assay are considered ASRs. Under this definition, ASRs are not diagnostic tests, nor are they combinations of reagents, controls, disposable labware, or instrumentation provided for the performance of diagnostic tests. Rather, an ASR is a single (albeit key) component, such as a probe or primer pair, in any diagnostic test manufactured anywhere in the world, including in clinical laboratories, in vitro diagnostic (IVD) device manufacturing facilities, and forensic or research laboratories. However, ASRs are only subject to regulation as medical devices when they are purchased by clinical laboratories for use in a laboratory developed test (LDT) or certain IVD tests. As of November 1998, clinical laboratories using laboratory developed assays that contain ASRs must comply with the FDA's final rule on ASRs published in the *Federal Register*. As part of this final rule laboratories are required to include a very specific disclaimer in the reports, stating, "This test was developed and its performance characteristics determined by (laboratory name). It has not been cleared by the U.S. Food and Drug Administration." But at the same time, the FDA has allowed laboratories to add in the report that ASRs do not require FDA approval, that the test using the particular ASR can be used for clinical purposes, and that the laboratory is certified under CLIA '88 to perform high complexity testing.

In addition to the definition of ASRs, the FDA proposed a set of controls and restrictions to be applied to their use to ensure their quality and consistency and to clarify that laboratories that develop their own assays are responsible for the performance of the test. Interestingly, these controls apply not only to the laboratory developing their own assays that use ASRs, but also to the manufacturers of these reagents. Laboratories are required to meet CLIA '88 high complexity certification requirements and to determine the performance characteristics of the laboratory developed assay following CLIA '88 regulations. Manufacturers of ASRs are required to register with the FDA, to follow good manufacturing practices, and to restrict the sale of this type of reagent to laboratories certified under CLIA for high complexity testing. Manufacturers are also responsible for reporting to the FDA any adverse events as a result of failure in the manufacturing process.

To control the use of ASRs, the FDA imposed a comprehensive set of restrictions. For example, ASRs may only be sold to (1) diagnostic device manufacturers; (2) clinical laboratories that are CLIA certified to perform high complexity testing under 42 CFR Part 493, or clinical laboratories regulated under the Veteran's Health Administration Directive 1106; or (3) organizations that use the reagents to make tests for forensic, academic, research, and other nonclinical (nonmedical) uses. In addition, ASRs may be sold only for use in LDTs that are ordered on a prescription basis.

In Vitro Multivariate Index Assay or IVDMIA Draft Guidance

IVD multivariate index assays (IVDMIAs) are considered a subset of LDTs that combine multiple variables (e.g., gender, age, weight, clinical lab results) using an interpretation function (e.g., algorithm) to generate a patient-specific result (e.g., score, risk level, classification) for the purpose of diagnosing, treating, or mitigating a disease. In addition, it provides a result whose derivation is nontransparent and cannot be independently derived or verified by the end user. These types of tests are developed based on observed correlations between multivariate data and clinical outcome, such that the clinical validity of the claims is not transparent to patients, laboratorians, and clinicians who order these tests Additionally, IVDMIAs frequently have a high risk intended use. The FDA is concerned that patients are relying upon IVDMIAs with high risk intended uses to make critical health care decisions when the FDA has not ensured that the IVDMIA has been clinically validated and the health care practitioners are unable to clinically validate the test themselves. The second point of the definition will likely attract the most attention if and when this becomes final. Although individual genetic and proteomic markers have diagnostic and prognostic relevance, the aggregate results obtained for multiple markers should in theory increase the diagnostic, prognostic, or theranostic power over that obtained from the results of one or just a few markers. IVDMIAs offer the treating physician a synthesis of multiple results in a simplified form. In this age of mushrooming information, those making treatment decisions eagerly seek simplification and distillation of important facts that are needed to best treat patients. The first draft of the FDA's IVDMIA guidance was issued on September 7, 2006, but after much criticism and comments, the FDA issued a revised draft on July 26, 2007. One of the main criticisms of the first draft was the definition of an IVDMIA. Determining whether a result is "nontransparent" or "cannot be independently derived or verified" will be challenged by industry. The FDA provided examples of what it perceived to be an IVDMIA, but there will almost certainly be controversy over whether a particular test falls inside or outside the FDA's IVDMIA definition. The new guidelines include a more detailed definition of what the agency considers an IVDMIA and exclude terms *test system* and *algorithm* that were criticized for being too ambiguous in the first version. Additionally, the guidelines clarify the agency's risk-based approach, provide a transition period to test developers during which the agency will exercise enforcement discretion over certain requirements, and include provisions for orphan-disease testing. With this draft guidance document, the FDA seeks to identify IVDMIAs as a discrete category of device and to clarify that, even when offered as LDTs, IVDMIAs must meet premarket and postmarket device requirements under the Federal Food, Drug, and Cosmetic Act and FDA regulations, including premarket review requirements in the case of most Class II and III devices. Devices that the agency would not consider IVDMIAs include tests that interpret multiple variables but that health care providers could otherwise interpret themselves. Examples of products that the FDA identified as being outside the scope of the draft guidance were devices that determine genotype and chromosomal copy number, conduct common clinical calculations, store clinical information, and calculate common, public demographic risk. The current version of the guidelines highlights the FDA's risk-based approach and the increased risks associated with IVDMIAs compared with other laboratory-developed tests.

Laboratory Design and Requirements

The power of molecular diagnostics is derived from the exquisite sensitivity and specificity when using nucleic acid as the analyte. The high sensitivity is derived from in vitro amplification of specific nucleic acid target sequences present in a patient's specimen. In vitro amplification creates millions or billions of copies of the target sequence and thus enables detection of as little as a single target molecule in the patient specimen. At the same time, however, this high sensitivity poses major challenges for the use of this technology in the clinical laboratory. Thus one of the major advantages of this technology is also one of its major limitations. Opening and closing the microcentrifuge tubes containing amplified product can aerosolize microdroplets that can carry 10 to 100 copies of the amplified target sequence. These microdroplets can subsequently be deposited on bench tops, instruments, furniture, floor, dust, hair, exposed skin, virtually any surface. Another important source of contamination is the target nucleic acid itself. Sample handling procedures must always protect against cross-contamination of patient specimens. Another source of contamination by nucleic acid that is sometimes overlooked occurs from processing patient samples in an environment in which the target nucleic acid has been amplified biologically either by cloning or by culturing of the cell or microorganism. Thus it is necessary to carefully design the molecular diagnostics laboratory to ensure sufficient and adequate space for personnel and equipment but also to minimize the potential problem of specimen contamination with natural nucleic acid or template and/or nucleic acid from in vitro amplification (amplicon).

LABORATORY DESIGN

Laboratory space should be designed to minimize the risk of contamination and maximize workflow. Barrier containment through the use of physically separate work areas for reagent preparation, specimen accessioning, nucleic acid extraction, and analysis of the amplified material is highly desirable. An ideal laboratory is composed of three completely independent rooms or areas. Two of these rooms are considered clean rooms in that all tasks and duties before in vitro amplification are performed in these laboratories. These rooms are called *preamplification rooms*. The third room is considered a dirty room because it is dedicated for in vitro amplification and analysis of the amplified material. This room is called a *postamplification room*. The air handling systems for each of these rooms should be completely independent. If this is not possible, it is highly recommended that the preamplification laboratories be located closest to the source of air in reference to both laboratories. The preamplification laboratories should be under positive air pressure, which impedes the entrance of any airborne contaminant into the preamplification laboratory when the door is opened. In addition, the postamplification laboratory should be under negative air pressure to impede anything from coming out of this laboratory and contaminating the surrounding environment. Construction of an anteroom into each laboratory is an inexpensive way of creating differential pressure for the laboratory. A positive pressurized anteroom for a preamplification laboratory can be created by use of a fan in the ceiling of the anteroom that draws air from inside the laboratory and blows it into the anteroom. This positively pressurized anteroom serves much the same purpose as having the entire laboratory under positive pressure. Similarly, an anteroom for the postamplification room can be easily made into a negatively pressurized room by having the fan draw air out of the anteroom and blow it into the laboratory. This anteroom should contain a seal around the door separating the anteroom from the laboratory to avoid air within the laboratory going back into the anteroom. It is important to emphasize that the door leading into the anteroom from the outside and the door to the inside of the laboratories should never be opened at the same time. An additional safety feature is to add sticky mats at the entrance of each anteroom or laboratory. The size of the anteroom is determined by what activities will be carried out in it. In addition, if disposable dedicated laboratory coats, hats, and booties are used, space is needed for storing these items.

Different activities are carried out in each of the three rooms/areas. In vitro amplification is never carried out in the two preamplification laboratories. One of these rooms is dedicated to reagent preparation and the other for specimen accessioning, specimen preparation, and reaction set up. If there is limited space, the two preamplification rooms can be combined into one laboratory. The use of dead air boxes for reagent preparation and reaction setup is highly recommended, and is more critical when both laboratories are combined. Dead air boxes provide a tightly controlled environment where reagent and reaction preparation can be carried out. It is important to situate this area in a section of the laboratory with low traffic. No genomic or plasmid DNA, RNA, or patient specimens should be introduced into the dead air box where reagent preparation takes place. This dead air box should be furnished with an ultraviolet (UV) light connected to a timer. The surface areas of the dead air boxes should be treated with UV light, then wiped with freshly made 10% sodium hypochlorite solution and finally with 75% ethanol solution before and after working in this area. These areas should contain dedicated equipment and instrumentation (e.g., pipetters, vortex, tips, tubes) that are not shared with any other area. Dedicated laboratory wear and gloves should be put on before starting work in this environment.

The second clean room or area within the preamplification laboratory is where specimen accessioning, specimen processing, and addition of nucleic acid to the appropriate reaction tube is carried out. This area should be furnished with at least one environmental biosafety cabinet for specimen processing and nucleic acid extraction in addition to dedicated laboratory equipment that is solely used for this purpose. Another completely separate environmental biosafety cabinet should be available if any tissue culture is carried out in this laboratory, and separate laboratory equipment should be dedicated for this function. Also, if organic nucleic acid extractions are used in the laboratory, a chemical safety cabinet for handling of the phenol and chloroform steps during the extraction procedure should be available. If both DNA and RNA extraction are carried out in the same preamplification laboratory, one should perform these procedures in separate areas of the laboratory and have dedicated instruments, pipettes, and filtered tips for each procedure. When space is a major issue and it is not possible to dedicate two completely separate areas, extraction of DNA and RNA should be performed at different times or on different days after thoroughly cleaning the areas before working. As previously described, all areas should be wiped with a solution of daily-prepared 10% sodium hypochlorite and with a solution of 75% ethanol.

The postamplification laboratory is where in vitro amplification and analysis of nucleic acid is carried out. Instruments used in this laboratory should not be shared with the preamplification areas. If thermocyclers are used for in vitro amplification of nucleic acid, they should be placed in this laboratory. If thermocyclers are placed in the preamplification laboratory under no circumstances can reaction tubes be opened after amplification in this room. In addition, thermocyclers should be plugged into dedicated power lines with their own circuit breaker to avoid any fluctuation in electricity that could affect their performance. Normally this laboratory requires more space than the preamplification laboratory because instrumentation for analysis of amplified product tends to be more extensive than that required for reagent preparation and nucleic acid extraction. Gel electrophoresis, for example, frequently uses significant open bench space. A darkroom with a dedicated automatic film processor and a freezer is highly recommended. It is however preferable to place the darkroom outside the postamplification laboratory so as to have access without having to go into the postamplification laboratory.

Real-time technology has recently been introduced in the clinical laboratory with major success. One of the great benefits of these instruments is that as they perform in vitro amplification, they can simultaneously detect the amplified product. This allows detection and quantitation of specific nucleic acid sequences without further manipulation or opening of test tubes, and dramatically reduces the risk of amplicon contamination. For assays developed and performed using these types of instruments, the risks of amplicon contamination will be significantly reduced. However, at this juncture, molecular diagnostics laboratories must continue to rely on standard "open" platforms for many tests, particularly those developed in house using analyte-specific reagents. For these assays, the risk of amplicon contamination still remains a significant issue that must be addressed through laboratory design and practices to minimize the risk for amplicon contamination.

PRACTICES TO AID IN CONTAMINATION CONTROL

The introduction of simple practices in the daily routine can aid in the control of amplicon and target contamination. Unidirectional workflow must be strictly followed whereby personnel perform tasks in the clean rooms first and only after completing their tasks in that room do they move on to the postamplification room. No personnel that have worked in the postamplification laboratory should return to the preamplification area before showering and changing clothes. Use of disposable laboratory coats, booties, and hats is recommended. If cloth lab coats are used, there should be dedicated lab coats for each laboratory and they should be kept inside each laboratory and not worn in the office space. Use of different colored lab coats for each area is one way to remind personnel of the strict workflow. Control of workflow of housekeeping personnel is likewise important. The safest approach it is to have laboratory staff perform some of the housekeeping duties by bagging the trash from each laboratory and placing it outside the laboratory for pick up by housekeeping staff. If this is done, housekeeping personnel must be instructed to remove trash first from the preamplification room, then the office space, and finally the postamplification room.

Protection of countertops with absorbent, plastic-backed paper is not recommended because paper can collect dust and with it amplified material if not changed often. If used, this type of paper should be discarded immediately after each use. The use of bleach appears to be the most generally accepted method for decontaminating surfaces. Decontamination of countertops, laboratory equipment, and furniture should be performed by wiping with a freshly made solution of 10% bleach and then with a 75% ethanol solution or even water to dilute the bleach that could corrode the surfaces. All pipette tips should contain a hydrophobic filter to prevent contamination of the tip of the pipetter with template or amplified material. Evaluation of the effectiveness of the hydrophobic barrier can be assessed by setting the pipette beyond its upper limit and drawing fluid from a colored solution into the disposable pipette tip that contains the hydrophobic barrier. If the tip of the pipette becomes stained by the fluid, then the barrier is inadequate. In this manner, routine QC measures such as mean volume and associated coefficient of variation to determine accuracy of pipette draws are frequently instituted to detect faulty pipetters, which can affect results. After use, disposable pipette tips should be placed into ziplock bags, making sure that the bags are completely sealed before discarding them. Gloves should be changed periodically or as soon as any contamination is suspected.

Another approach to preventing amplicon contamination is to chemically treat the unwanted amplicon so that it will not support amplification, even if accidentally added to another sample. The most widely used means of destroying amplicons is through the use of UV irradiation. UV treatment of DNA induces cross-linking of the two strands of DNA by forming thymidine dimers. This cross-linked DNA can no longer serve as an effective template. One disadvantage of UV treatment is that it is most effective in sequences of more than 700 nucleotides in length. In most clinical assays, the length of the amplicon is less than 700 base pairs. A chemical means of inactivating or sterilizing amplicon is through the use of deoxyuridine triphosphate instead of deoxythymidine triphosphate during the amplification procedure. In this procedure, deoxyuridine monophosphate is incorporated into the amplicon instead of thymidine monophosphate. After amplification, this uracil-containing amplicon can be destroyed by treating the sample with uracil-N-glycosylase (UNG). The uracil-containing amplicon is the substrate for UNG, while the thymine-containing template is not. The UNG removes uracil residues from the amplicon, still leaving an intact phosphodiester backbone on the amplicon. During the first denaturation step of the amplification procedure, the phosphodiester bonds break at the sites were the uracil residues are located. The fragmented amplicon is no longer able to act as a template. Use of deoxyuracyl triphosphate and UNG are effective in controlling contamination if the uracil-containing amplicon does not exceed 10^6 to 10^7 copies per reaction. Isopsoralens have also been used with some success. After amplification, exposure to long-wave UV light produces adducts between the isopsoralens and the cytosines present in the amplified material, rendering them ineffective templates for amplification.

Transfer of paper such as written procedures or notes regarding specific samples between laboratories and office is also a concern. This should be reduced as much as possible, especially for paperwork used in the postamplification laboratory. It is highly recommended that a computer network be put in place in the laboratory with a number of computer terminals throughout the different laboratories and office areas in order to reduce or eliminate the movement of paper throughout the laboratory and back into the office area. It is important that the network server be backed up daily.

EQUIPMENT

Laboratory equipment necessary for successfully conducting current typical molecular diagnostics tests can include instrumentation not generally found in the typical clinical laboratory. Even where there is overlap in the type of equipment that is used, it is important that the molecular diagnostics laboratory contain its own equipment for purposes of contamination control. Some of the specialized equipment, depending on the scope of the testing menu, includes automatic DNA sequencers, real-time thermocyclers, capillary electrophoresis instruments, and high-performance liquid chromatography. These specialized instruments are expensive, which can make implementation of tests that require them difficult. More recently, a new tactic for acquisition of instrumentation through reagent rental agreements has become possible through some of the manufacturers of in vitro diagnostic tests and analyte specific reagents. This funding mechanism has been in use for many years in other areas of the clinical laboratory but is new for molecular diagnostics.

PERSONNEL

Laboratories performing molecular diagnostics testing are classified as high complexity testing laboratories under CLIA '88, which imposes specific personnel standards for education and training. These tests are more complex than standard laboratory tests, and many are developed in-house.

As new technology is introduced, these assays are constantly being modified to improve specificity, sensitivity, turnaround time (TAT), and workflow.

LABORATORY DIRECTOR

According to CLIA '88, directors of high complexity testing laboratories must be either a doctor of medicine (MD) or doctor of osteopathy (DO) with training in clinical or anatomical pathology; an MD or DO with 2 years of experience directing or supervising a high complexity testing laboratory; or hold an earned doctorate degree in one of the biological sciences and be certified and continue to be certified by a board approved by the Department of Health and Human Services.

The responsibilities of the laboratory director are test selection, implementation, and resolution of technical difficulties. The laboratory director is also responsible for developing laboratory programs for analytical and clinical validation of new molecular tests and development of management guidelines and practices that ensure reliable performance of clinical testing. In addition, the laboratory director must also be responsible for the development, implementation, and review of the laboratory quality assurance and control programs.

TECHNICAL SUPERVISOR

According to CLIA '88 a technical supervisor must be either an MD or DO with 1 year of experience in a high complexity testing laboratory; have a master's degree with 2 years of experience; or have a bachelor's degree with 4 years of experience.

MEDICAL TECHNOLOGISTS AND MOLECULAR BIOLOGY TECHNICIANS

Medical technologists and molecular biology technicians are responsible for tasks and duties necessary for the daily operation of the laboratory testing agenda. These individuals are responsible for specimen accessioning and processing, performing daily testing, maintaining appropriate testing and QC records, adhering to written procedures and QC policies, identifying problems, and documenting equipment maintenance. Record keeping for laboratory procedures is complicated because assays that are developed in-house are constantly being modified to improve the testing process. In addition, some laboratory instruments are used solely for molecular diagnostic testing and there is little clinical laboratory experience with them. It is important for the technical staff, particularly the senior technical staff, to have a high sense of professional commitment and to display constant interest and effort in improving their education and training. It is also important for the staff to acquire as many advanced laboratory skills as possible and to be cross-trained in most or all of the different tests used in the laboratory. It is crucial for the technical personnel to fully understand the scientific basics of the methodology and the clinical applications and implications of the different molecular tests.

Involvement of residents, fellows, and graduate students can contribute significantly to the success of a molecular diagnostics laboratory. The value of these individuals comes from their high level of professional commitment and their insight into the clinical utility of individual tests. If such individuals are provided time to work in the molecular diagnostics laboratory, they are frequently able to rapidly develop and validate a new molecular assay. In return these individuals gain expertise in an area of laboratory medicine that is rapidly growing and this may provide them with an advantage when seeking future employment. As part of their training in molecular diagnostics, it is important for residents, fellows, and graduate students to gain experience in each of the different areas of testing, including infectious disease, genetic disease, and cancer. Training should include basic principles in molecular biology, hands-on experience in optimizing, validating, and performing molecular diagnostic testing, test result interpretation, and preparation of reports for review. Laboratory directors should also familiarize trainees with the different issues involved in laboratory management.

CERTIFICATION OF PERSONNEL IN MOLECULAR DIAGNOSTICS

Certification of doctoral level personnel working in molecular diagnostic laboratories can follow several different routes depending on the type of doctoral degree as well as other training experience. The American Board of Pathology (ABP) and the American Board of Medical Genetics (ABMG) offer a joint subspecialty certification in Molecular Genetic Pathology. The ABP and the ABMG are members of the American Board of Medical Specialties, which is the parent organization for boards that provide certification in pathology, pediatrics, internal medicine, surgery, and other medical specialties. Certification consists of required training in an accredited program followed by a subspecialty examination. Candidates for this certification in MGP must hold an MD or DO degree, have primary certification in either pathology or genetics by their respective boards, have a valid unrestricted license to practice medicine or osteopathy in the United States, and have completed a year of training in an Accreditation Council of Graduate Medical Education (ACGME) accredited program. There are at least 31 MGP programs that have received full accreditation by the ACGME. Additional programs will likely seek accreditation in the future. Standards for training in molecular genetic pathology have been published by the different organizations involved in certification. Central to this effort is the use of competency-based education, which involves specific learning objectives around the curriculum. Fellows need to demonstrate performance at the level of a new practitioner in six general competencies: patient care, medical knowledge, practice based learning and improvement, interpersonal and communication skills, professionalism, and system based practice as provided by the Association for Molecular Pathology and other professional bodies. The candidate must present a logbook of 150 clinical molecular cases. The examination is offered every other year.

Another avenue open to individuals with either an MD or PhD is provided by the ABMG and is intended for individuals who provide services in medical genetics. The ABMG offers certification in clinical genetics, medical genetics, clinical cytogenetics, clinical biochemical genetics, and clinical molecular genetics. Only the requirements for certification in clinical molecular genetics are discussed here. In addition to possessing the appropriate doctoral degree, the candidate for clinical molecular genetics must complete 2 years of training in a fully accredited program. The candidate must present a logbook of 150 clinical molecular cases and method competency list signed by the laboratory director with half of the time of the training spent at the bench. The examination is offered every 3 years.

In addition, the American Board of Clinical Chemistry (ABCC) has offered certification in molecular diagnostics since June 2000. The ABCC is an independent, not for profit corporation that certifies doctoral level professionals in clinical and toxicologic chemistry. The ABCC certification in molecular diagnostics requires the applicant to possess an MD or a doctoral degree or equivalent in biochemistry, molecular biology, or other natural sciences. The applicant must demonstrate 5 years of full-time diverse professional experience in clinical molecular diagnostics or at least 2 years of full-time diverse experience in clinical molecular diagnostics, and must document primary certification in one the following boards: ABCC, American Board of Medical Microbiology, American Board of Pathology, American Board of Medical Laboratory Immunology, American Board of Bioanalysis, or the American Board of Histocompatibility and Immunogenetics. Applicants must meet education and experience requirements in addition to holding three letters of recommendation to attest to the familiarity with the applicant's professional expertise and length of experience in the field. The examination is offered once a year. The American Board of Bioanalysis also offers a certification for High Complexity Laboratory Director in Molecular Diagnostics (www.abb.org).

Subspecialty certification in molecular diagnostics is also offered to nondoctoral-level individuals including medical technologists and molecular biology technicians through the American Society of Clinical Pathology (ASCP) Board of Certification. The ASCP Board of Certification was the result of the unification of the National Credentialing Agency and the ASCP Board of Registry. The ASCP Board of Certification is an administratively independent certification agency that prepares relevant standards and develops procedures that ensure the competence of nonphysician medical laboratory personnel. Medical technologists and molecular biology technicians become certified as technologists in molecular biology. There are four routes for eligibility:

1. ASCP certified as a technologist (MT, MLS, CG, CT, HTL, BB, C, H, I, or M) or specialist (SBB, SC, SCT, SH, SI, SM, or SV) and a baccalaureate degree from a regionally accredited college or university.
2. Baccalaureate degree from a regionally accredited college/university, including courses in biological science, chemistry, and mathematics and successful completion of a National Accrediting Agency for Clinical Laboratory Sciences–approved baccalaureate diagnostics molecular science program within the last 5 years.

PART 8

3. Baccalaureate degree in biological or chemical sciences from a regionally accredited college/university and 12 months of acceptable clinical laboratory experience in molecular diagnostics in a CLIA-regulated accredited clinical laboratory in the past 5 years.
4. Graduate level degree (master's or doctorate) in chemistry, biology, immunology, microbiology, allied health, clinical laboratory sciences, or an appropriate related field from a regionally accredited college/university and 6 months of acceptable clinical laboratory experience in molecular diagnostics in a CLIA-regulated accredited clinical laboratory within the last 5 years.

FINANCIAL MANAGEMENT

REIMBURSEMENT FOR MOLECULAR DIAGNOSTICS TESTS

Reimbursement for laboratory tests is a complex process that can be broken down into three phases—coverage, coding, and payment. Coverage decisions are usually determined by each of the different health care plans. In the United States, health insurance coverage is provided by public programs such as Medicare and Medicaid or by private health plans purchased individually or through one's employer. In general, the scope of coverage provided by a health plan is outlined in broad benefits categories; decisions about specific services are made on a case-by-case basis during claims processing. Health plans may develop formal coverage policies that describe whether a particular service is covered and the conditions under which it will be covered. Medical directors, the federal and state governments, medical policy advisory committees, employers, and unions are among some of the entities involved in making coverage decisions. Medical necessity is the primary criterion used by health plans when making coverage decisions, although the definition of medical necessity is subject to different interpretation. Another criterion is that the service must have approval from the appropriate government regulatory body. Thirdly, scientific evidence must permit conclusions concerning the effect of the technology on health outcomes.

Billing for molecular diagnostics test follows the same procedure as any other laboratory tests. Generally, Current Procedural Terminology (CPT) codes (to document the procedure) and International Classification of Disease diagnostic codes (to document the medical condition which makes the procedure necessary) are required by the the billing process to convey what services or procedures were performed and why. Beyond this, the reimbursement process is usually institution-specific and relies on computerized and manual billing procedures. It is important to determine in advance the requirements regarding documentation and computer access needed in order to generate a bill. There are two kinds of CPT codes for molecular diagnostics testing: pathogen-specific CPT codes for molecular testing for infectious disease organisms, and procedure-specific CPT codes for noninfectious disease molecular testing. Pathogen-specific CPT codes for molecular infectious disease tests, such as HIV-1 detection, HCV viral load, and HSV detection are global codes that include the entire test procedure including interpretation and report in a single code (e.g., nucleic acid extraction, amplification quantitation, detection, interpretation and report). There are more than 80 analyte-specific codes used for molecular microbiologic tests, and it is anticipated that more analyte specific codes will be introduced in practice. These codes are represented by the code range 87470-87801 in the CPT code set. There are usually three different codes for each analyte: one for direct probe technique, another for in vitro amplification technique, and another for quantitation regardless of the technology used. For those organisms without specific CPT codes, three generic CPT codes are included, designated *Not otherwise specified.* For all other molecular tests without an analyte-specific CPT code, a combination (or stacking) of procedural CPT codes can be used. These codes are represented by the code range 83890-83914. For example, nucleic acid extraction, amplification, and capillary electrophoresis all have separate CPT codes. A single test using all these procedures is billed using a combination of all appropriate CPT codes, used multiple times as needed. Most molecular codes describe a generic molecular procedure rather than a specific method. For example, a nucleic acid extraction can be performed for DNA or RNA, using very different methods, each using different instrument, reagents and personnel, but both are billed using the same CPT code for nucleic acid extraction. In addition to the procedure-specific codes, there is a specific code for interpretation and report (83912) that may be reported at the technical level or the professional level but not both. For molecular pathology testing that requires a professional interpretation, the professional component is coded using the 83912 with a modifier "26". When 83912 is reported without the 26 modifier, it is paid from the clinical laboratory fee schedule. When 83912 is reported with the 26 modifier, it is paid from the physician fee schedule. Listed in Table 69-1 are examples of billing using analyte specific CPT codes and procedure specific CPT codes. Because of the limited nature and description of the procedure CPT codes, there is lack of consistency in reporting. Furthermore, there is a lack of representation of newer technologies such as bead array, real-time PCR, and microarray that are widely used by a large number of clinical laboratories. Due to limitations in the current CPT code set, laboratories might be forced to "under code." A complete list of the CPT codes can be found in the "CPT Current Procedural Termininology" published by the American Medical Association.

TABLE 69-1
CPT Code Billing for Molecular Tests

Test	CPT code	Number of times CPT code billed	Type of procedure or test
Factor V Leiden by Real Time Technology	83890	1	Nucleic acid isolation
	83898	1	Amplification
	83892	2	Probe, each
	83912	1	Interpretation and report
t(9;22) by Real Time RT-PCR	83890	1	Nucleic acid isolation
	83902	2	Reverse transcription
	83898	2	Amplification
	83894	2	Probe, each
	83912	1	Interpretation and report
HIV-1 Viral Load	87536	1	HIV quantitative
CMV Viral Load	87497	1	CMV quantitative
HCV Viral Load	87522	1	HCV quantitative

CMV, Cytomegalovirus; *CPT,* Current Procedural Terminology; *HCV,* hepatitis C virus; *HIV,* human immunodeficiency virus; *RT-PCR,* reverse-transcriptase polymerase chain reaction.

A set of two-character alphanumeric modifiers has been devised to add granularity and more precise descriptions of service for the procedure-specific CPT codes. The purpose of these alphanumeric modifiers is to help third-party payers identify more specifically the services for which they are paying. The first (numeric) character identifies the disease category (e.g., neoplasia [solid tumors], neoplasia [lymphoid/hematopoietic], nonneoplastic hematology/coagulation, histocompatibility/blood typing, neurologic nonneoplastic, muscular nonneoplastic, metabolic, other; metabolic transport, metabolic-pharmacogenetics, and dysmorphology). The second (alpha) character denotes the gene type (e.g., BRCA1 or Rb).

Reimbursement levels for individual tests are set by third-party payers and may bear little relationship to the actual cost of performing the test. Some third-party payers may reimburse at high levels but others may follow laboratory fee schedules based on the Medicare Clinical Laboratory Fee Schedule or Physician Fee Schedule for the specific CPT codes. FDA approval is not required for billing for these tests and a disclaimer for those non–FDA-cleared tests to reflect this issue should be added to the final report (see later). Some third-party payers will deny reimbursement for tests bearing such disclaimers because they believe that the cost of performing such testing should be borne by research grants even though the performance characteristics and clinical utility of the test have been validated by the clinical laboratory.

PATENT ISSUES

Patents can cover a specific method of testing for an analyte, any method of testing for an analyte, or a mutation-gene-disease association in general. The vast majority of the in vitro amplification procedures are patented processes, and a license agreement for the use of these procedures must be obtained or the laboratory using the procedure is liable for patent infringement. Traditionally, licensure is obtained for a particular procedure by purchasing an FDA-approved set of reagents sold by a manufacturer who holds the patent to the amplification process. The number of FDA-approved/cleared tests is limited and does not cover all molecular tests currently performed in molecular diagnostics laboratories. Thus a laboratory using a particular patented process must first negotiate a license agreement with the patent holder. Importantly, depending on the complexity of the institution seeking the agreement and the complexity of the agreement, it may take from 3 months to a full year to obtain license to perform and bill the procedure for clinical purposes.

Similar consideration must be given to the use of sequence information required to design an assay. Sequences of newly discovered genes (e.g., human genes, virus genomes) are frequently patented by their discoverers, and use of the sequence information without a license agreement runs the same risk of liability for patent infringement. Examples of such patents include apolipoprotein E genotyping for Alzheimer disease, Canavan disease, and Charcot-Marie-Tooth disease type 1A. The terms and conditions offered by the patent holder vary greatly. In some instances, the laboratory cannot offer a test for a patented gene sequence because the patent has been exclusively licensed to a single laboratory. Because of diversity of sources for sequence information, it is not always clear whether the sequence has been patented or even who owns the patent. Before undertaking development of any test based on published sequences wherein a major commitment of resources is planned, check with the investigators who first described the sequence, and search patent and patent applications to determine whether the new test might infringe on any existing or pending patents. Internet resources provided by the U.S. Patent and Trademark Office (http://www.uspto.gov) allow laboratories to perform searches on granted or pending patents in the United States.

Laboratory Information System

Clinical laboratories have been among the first hospital departments to actively exploit computers and software for reporting results and for managing internal work processes and quality. Most pathology laboratories now require a computerized laboratory information system (LIS) to handle the large volume of data that is both received and reported. These systems support all aspects of the contemporary clinical and specialty laboratory, helping technologists manage the quality and integrity of test samples (preanalytical), all aspects of the testing and results review process (analytical phase), and the reporting of finalized results, interpretations, and diagnosis (postanalytical phase). LISs have evolved beyond departmental workload functions and today often include advanced features, such as laboratory-specific medical records, direct clinician access via secure web connections, full-blown billing modules, and sophisticated interface engines for routing orders and results to external systems. The recent explosion of molecular diagnostics methods has expanded molecular and gene-based diagnostic testing into routine laboratory testing, forcing vendors and users to either adapt existing LIS functions to new modes of testing or to develop completely new subsystems.

To date, a number of commercial LIS vendors offer genetic testing modules, and several niche suppliers have emerged. The data management aspect of genomic/proteomic laboratory testing is one of the most active areas of pathology informatics research. This will have significant impact on future laboratory information systems and electronic medical record designs and will be used as genetic data become a core part of the patient's medical record. The LIS must be flexible enough to handle the demands posed by the new laboratory tests and technologies. In particular, the quantity of specimens and type of testing involved in genetic testing pose a significant challenge for an LIS. Molecular diagnostics and genetic testing requirements include increased data storage requirements, ability to manage reporting of genetic changes such as rearrangements and other abnormalities associated with malignant disease and hereditary genetic abnormalities, and ability to access patient records that contain personal gene databank and family tree information. Decision support, specimen tracking, and automation of QC and QA documentation features also must accommodate the demands of genetic testing. Extension of data management to genetic findings requires an LIS to standardize information and support genomics-based inference. Current vocabularies can be insufficient to describe the findings generated by some new molecular tests. Vocabularies such as the Clinical Bioinformatics Ontology developed by Cerner Corporation have been designed for clinical molecular diagnostics and cytogenetics. In order for LISs to handle the nature and volume of genomic tests, current discrepancies between how genetic mutations are described in the literature and how they are described in the Internet databases must be resolved. Laboratory processes in molecular diagnostics are currently highly complex and have proven difficult to standardize and automate. Contributors to this complexity include the wide variety of tissue sample types that can be tested, the numerous steps involved in material preparation, frequent implementation of novel technical platforms leading to variable and unpredictable assay performance, and complex posttesting analysis methods. Another component of the complexity, especially in molecular oncology, is that a variety of tumor samples are required for different order sets, including multistep and reflex testing. One of the unique workflow requirements of the molecular diagnostics laboratory is the need to document significant amounts of nonclinical information generated during the processing of a sample (e.g., during DNA or RNA isolation or PCR analysis). An additional requirement is the ability to offer significant flexibility in reordering or canceling tests and procedures in response to poor quality specimens or other procedural failures.

Test Management

MENU/SELECTION

As with any other clinical laboratory, the primary goal of the molecular diagnostics laboratory is to provide reliable and timely test results deemed necessary by the medical community for patient care. Appropriate selection of tests to include on the laboratory's test menu is critical for the success of the molecular diagnostics laboratory. Several key considerations are important in test selection. Clinical needs, as well as advances in basic and translational research, often prompt the development of new molecular tests. Prior discussions with the intended users to determine their level of interest and understanding are extremely helpful during the test selection.

Any new test should provide a less expensive or more effective avenue for diagnosis and/or management of the patient. It is important to base test selection not only on cost but also on how the new test could impact overall patient care and management. Even though adding an expensive new test for a particular clinical condition may seem at first to increase the cost of patient management, in the long run the new test may result in more cost effective and efficient patient mangement. For example, HIV-1 viral load testing monitors disease progression and effectiveness of drug therapy in infected individuals. Many patients infected with HIV-1 are currently treated with a combination of different drugs, which includes protease inhibitors and nonnucleoside and nucleoside reverse transcriptase inhibitors. These drugs are expensive and the virus may become resistant to them. Thus, even though addition of HIV-1 viral load testing adds cost to managing HIV-1 infected patients, the test provids a means for rapidly and accurately determining the effectiveness of the expensive drug treatment regimens. In this regard, molecular diagnostics is poised to greatly impact the emergence of pharmacogenomics and personalized medicine toward individual therapy (see Chapter 72).

A molecular test may be more cost effective than an existing laboratory test and may be introduced to replace that existing test. Even if the direct cost of the molecular test is more than the direct cost of the test being replaced, increased sensitivity, increased specificity, or reduced TAT may result in significant overall savings in patient management. For example, in a case of presumptive *Mycobacterium tuberculosis* infection during the period of time when this diagnosis cannot be ruled out, the patients are placed on treatment with potentially liver toxic drugs or placed in isolation. The standard laboratory test of directly observing an acid-fast stain of the patient's sputum for the presence of *M. tuberculosis* is fast, but lacks sensitivity. Culture is extremely sensitive, but could take up to 6 weeks for a result. A molecular test that allows for a more rapid diagnosis with a high degree of sensitivity and specificity would allow discontinuation of drug therapy or isolation for those patients without the disease

Identifying molecular tests that would be potentially useful at the medical center is a responsibility of the medical and technical directors. Clinicians and pathologists can be a valuable source for identifying the testing needs for the medical center, but it is important for the laboratory director to establish where there is a need for improvement. Clinicians who learn of a new test that seems interesting may request that the molecular laboratory make the test available, regardless of whether that test has been analytically or clinically validated. Each laboratory should have a formal, systematic process to develop a strategic menu. The menu of molecular pathology laboratories may vary significantly and is determined by three principal factors: clinical requirements and usefulness, laboratory competency, and test costs. When considering which tests to add to a laboratory menu, matching of the technical capabilities of the laboratory with real-world clinical needs in terms of test volume, TAT, and associated costs should be realistic. Introduction of any new test should include a clinical trial period that allows for evaluation of the clinical utility of the test and may provide a useful marketing opportunity. If carefully designed, this approach allows the laboratory to directly work with the end user of the test and provides an avenue for end users to understand the clinical utility of the test and its limitations. It is important to clearly define metrics that can be evaluated at the end of the clinical trial to justify implementation of the test.

METHODS

Once a particular analyte has been identified for testing by molecular means, it is important to consider the various approaches that may be available. The technologies available for molecular diagnostics testing are considerably more complex than in other areas of the clinical laboratory. Adding to the challenge is the rapid rate of technological change.

In conventional sections of the clinical laboratory, the platforms available for performing a test are usually inclusive from primary sample handling to result. In contrast, the molecular diagnostic laboratory is usually required to piece together several disparate methods to achieve the same result. In fact, few manufacturers of molecular assays have considered the equally important issues of sample procurement and nucleic acid extraction, that is often necessary for each representative sample type. The successful integration plan would address the combination of procedures needed for the advancement of samples through these front-end requirements. One exercise that will aid in the development of a strategic test menu is the categorization of proposed tests into groups defined by the basic genetics of the diseases for which the tests are designed. In general, only a few types of testing methodologies exist for detection of nucleic acid sequences, detection of a particular mutation or single nucleotide polymorphism, or quantitative analysis of a specific sequence. The goal is to implement the strategic test menu onto one or two technical platforms. Consider several ancillary questions to determine whether it is possible to use fewer technologies:

- Do the selected platforms accommodate the full spectrum of sample types used for the tests on the laboratory's menu?
- Is it more important to address the volume of tests or the complexity of the analytic results?
- Are the platforms flexible enough to handle test offerings that may be added to the laboratory's test menu?
- Does the laboratory really need quantitative or real-time technologies?

Having fewer platforms will facilitate using information technology to extract more value from those systems. For example, some analytes may be analyzed using Southern blot hybridization, in vitro nucleic acid amplification, cytogenetics, or FISH. Before selecting a particular method, it is important to consider the clinical condition and the advantages and disadvantages of each methodology for managing a particular clinical condition.

CLINICAL TEST FORMATS

There are two basic types of assay formats. One type is developed and sold commercially by IVD manufacturers , and the other is developed in house by each laboratory (i.e., LDTs). In the first category, complete kits are developed to provide quality-controlled reagents to perform an entire molecular test for a determined clinical condition. For example, kits to monitor patients with HIV-1 infection through quantification of plasma HIV-1 RNA. These kits usually include all the reagents necessary for nucleic acid isolation, amplification, and detection or quantitation. These complete assay kits include information about sensitivity, specificity, and test limitations for the particular clinical condition. They may be labeled by the manufacturer as *FDA-approved, FDA-cleared, for research use only*, or *for investigational use only*.

There is also a significant demand for assays for which there are no commercially available kits. Thus clinical laboratories must frequently develop their own assays to accommodate the local demands. LDTs are fully established and validated by the laboratory that performs them. They are also referred to as "home-brew" tests. Usually these assays use a combination of reagents that are purchased separately from a variety of manufacturers. Each laboratory determines the performance characteristics of the assay for a specific clinical condition and a particular patient population. There are a number of commercially available kits that are developed by a manufacturer to provide quality-controlled reagents to perform a particular step in molecular testing. For example, there are a variety of commercially available kits for nucleic acid extraction, amplification including controls, and detection systems. The laboratory may develop a particular molecular test by combining two or more kits from the same or even different manufacturers. The analytical and clinical validation of the entire testing process is the responsibility of each laboratory.

AUTOMATED PLATFORMS FOR MOLECULAR TESTING

In recent years, the development and introduction of automated platforms for molecular diagnostics testing has become more common. Automated devices that consume less time, handle small volumes, and in theory allow for better precision have replaced many manual molecular diagnostic procedures. Many of these platforms have been developed by different manufacturers to provide automation for a single step or several steps of the testing process. The evolution of molecular diagnostics automation has occurred in stages. In this chapter, devices are grouped according to function.

Single function automated instruments have been in use for some time in the molecular diagnostics laboratory.The typical example of a single-function automated instrument is a thermocycler, because it provides automated amplification of nucleic acid by performing all steps necessary for the amplification of nucleic acids. Nucleic acid extractors are another early example of single-function devices that convert a six-step procedure into a single-step process. These early nucleic acid extractors were based on phenol/chloroform extraction and mimicked the corresponding manually performed method by using nearly the same reagents and protocols. These and other single-step automated instruments, including robots for reagent preparation and aliquoting, and automatic DNA sequencers, have been widely incorporated into molecular diagnostics laboratories. The use of magnetic beads has dramatically changed how laboratories process and isolate nucleic samples from patient specimens. Molecular diagnostics laboratories are rapidly embracing these automatic nucleic acid extractors because this specific step in the testing process is one of the most labor-intensive of the entire testing process. These devices provide higher throughput capabilities, greater precision, and reduced personnel demands.

Recently, automated instruments that perform more than a single function have been developed and introduced into molecular diagnostics laboratories. The Roche Molecular Systems COBAS Ampliprep/COBAS TaqMan analyzer is an example of one such automated platform. This instrument contains an automatic extractor module, reaction setup, and real-time PCR that allows the processing of patient specimens—nucleic acid extraction, amplification, and quantitation—in a single instrument. Real time PCR technology simultaneously acquires the amplification signal, permitting qualitative and quantitative analysis of the PCR reaction as it occurs, thereby eliminating the need for postamplification processing for detection and quantitation of target sequence. This feature allows a dramatic reduction of the TAT for molecular diagnostics tests from days to hours. The throughput of these devices is greatly enhanced and molecular diagnostics laboratories now use them routinely for much of their diagnostic testing.

The greater availability of these automated devices poses many opportunities for clinical laboratories. One core issue in this decision is cost. Whereas the cost of manually performing molecular testing is substantial, the cost of acquiring automated instruments to perform these steps/tests can also be significant. Laboratories must wisely evaluate the cost/benefit of these automated devices in relation to the anticipated revenue. A number of manufacturers have started offering reagent rental programs for many of these automated platforms. Laboratories must carefully compare the cost of performing the test manually to the cost of automation.

Quality Assurance and Quality Control of the Testing Process

QUALITY ASSURANCE

Every molecular diagnostics laboratory should develop a comprehensive written QA program. The objective of the QA program is to systematically monitor and evaluate the quality and appropriateness of the test results. The QA program includes aspects of clinical testing that do not directly bear on the analytical accuracy of the test result and thus are generally not part of the QC program for clinical testing. Some of these parameters are regular review of TATs, normal and abnormal results, specimen rejection criteria, the log of rejected specimens, and other indicators of test quality. The QA program should address every aspect of the testing process—preanalytical, analytical, and postanalytical. The program must include written policies and documentation for education and training of personnel, continuing medical education, PT, internal and external inspections, including documentation of corrective actions for deficiencies cited, QC programs for the clinical testing, equipment performance, and safety. Establishment of molecular diagnostics tests, particularly amplification assays, requires many considerations at every stage, including reagent preparation, specimen collection, specimen aliquoting and performance of the actual assay. A number of considerations apply to all molecular assays and are important to guarantee reliable results. The amount of QA and QC performed for any molecular assay depends on the type of test.

As part of the preanalytical phase, special attention should be given to specimen collection, transport, and storage, because specimen handling often affects the results. Test results that could influence treatment decisions should reflect the patient status and not specimen mishandling.

Key components of any QA program are PT and alternative assessment (AA). PT and AA performance reflects the accuracy of the laboratory's testing process and can also serve as an educational activity for the laboratory staff. The laboratory's testing performance on unknown challenge specimens is compared to an external standard. The external standard is generally the mean of values obtained by other laboratories using the same test method, but it may be assigned by a reference method or some other procedure. Laboratories engage in PT two or three times a year. PT programs are available from a number of vendors, including CAP. There are special requirements for CLIA-regulated analytes, in that CMS must approve the PT program. However, none of the analytes usually tested for in a molecular diagnostics laboratory is CLIA regulated. The laboratory must have a quality assurance plan that establishes the accuracy and reliability of the testing at least twice per year. AA is a twice-yearly assessment of the laboratory's testing performance when PT is not available. Examples of AA are split-sample testing between two or more laboratories that share test results with all participants, repeat testing on previously analyzed specimens whose earlier results were blinded to the laboratory technical staff, and testing by a different method. Ongoing monitoring of PT allows the laboratory to assess and monitor the quality of its test results and identify testing problems that may not surface with other quality control activities. Such information enables the laboratory to take preventive action and avoid future unacceptable results or inaccuracies in patient testing. Likewise, the investigation of unacceptable results can identify clerical errors, methodologic problems, equipment problems, technical problems, problems with the PT material, and problems with test interpretation. The PT provider provides individual laboratories with unknown "challenge" specimens for testing. Quantitative tests are usually expected to perform within 2 standard deviations of the mean or within a specified percentage deviation from the mean to be considered acceptable. Acceptable performance criteria may vary by analyte. In general, qualitative tests should agree with the response provided by 80% of peer laboratories or 80% of reference laboratories. Performance on a mailing is considered "satisfactory" when at least 80% of a laboratory's responses to challenges in a single mailing are acceptable. However, for many molecular tests there are only two shipments per year and three challenges per shipment, so the criteria may be different. When a PT survey is developed for a new analyte or new testing method/technology, the entire survey may be considered educational and not graded for 1 or more years, ensuring field validation. At a minimum, CLIA requires laboratories to review and evaluate the results obtained on PT. For any unsatisfactory testing event, CLIA also requires laboratories to document and retain their remedial actions for 2 years. The documentation is reviewed during the onsite laboratory inspection. Failure to perform AA, document results, review results, or take corrective action for an unacceptable performance leads to a deficiency citation upon laboratory inspection.

Well-characterized reference materials are fundamental to laboratory QA programs, including both external assessment by PT and internal QA activities such as QC and test development/validation. PT program vendors usually solicit large hospital centers or commercial vendors to obtain blood and tissue specimens from affected patients to support the PT programs. These materials must be validated before use. For some genetic tests, including many disorders in the CAP PT surveys, sufficient and appropriate material is not publicly available. For example, until recently, genomic DNA materials for allele repeat lengths representing important phenotypic classes and diagnostic cutoffs for fragile X were not publicly available. The absence of such materials for routine QC, PT, and test development may have accounted for the differences in laboratory performance in some recent CAP PT fragile X surveys. The CDC, in partnership with the genetics community, has established the Genetic Testing Reference Materials (GeT-RM) Coordination Program. Its goal is to improve the supply of publicly available and well-characterized genomic DNA that can be used as reference materials for PT, QC, test development/validation, and research studies. The GeT-RM program has recently characterized 57 cell lines to be used as reference materials for disorders such as fragile X syndrome, Huntington disease, and disorders on the Ashkenazi Jewish panel (e.g., Bloom syndrome, Canavan disease, Fanconi anemia, familial dysautonomia, Gaucher disease, mucolipidosis IV, Neimann Pick disease, and Tay-Sachs disease). These materials are or will soon be publicly available from Coriell Cell Repositories, which houses several National Institutes of Health (NIH)–funded collections of essential research reagents. A characterization study of 14 DNA materials with important mutations causing CF is currently underway in six collaborating clinical laboratories. Additionally, the GeT-RM program is characterizing a panel of DNA specimens with identifiable gene mutations for confirmatory testing in disorders included in state newborn screening panels. This includes disorders such as congenital adrenal hyperplasia, medium-chain acyl-CoA dehydrogenase deficiency, maple syrup urine disease, CF, and galactosemia. Additional materials are in development for gene mutations found in Gaucher disease, Tay-Sachs disease, and Canavan disorders. Development of materials will soon be initiated for other disorders, including inherited breast cancer (caused by *BRCA1* or *BRCA2* mutations), alpha-1 antitrypsin deficiency, and type 2 multiple endocrine neoplasia. To date, the GeT-RM program has focused its efforts on DNA-based testing for inherited genetic disorders. Other areas of genetics, including molecular oncology, molecular infectious disease testing, and biochemical genetic testing, however, are also facing a paucity of reference and PT materials. To address these needs, the GeT-RM program, together with the genetics community, professional organizations, and other governmental agencies outside of CDC, is trying to assess what reference materials are currently available for laboratory QA programs and is beginning to formulate plans for collecting and characterizing materials where shortages exist.

As with any laboratory test, a well thought out and well written laboratory procedure is a key factor for the reproducibility of the assay. It is one of the most important aids during hands-on training of new personnel or for procedures that are not performed very often. The clinical laboratory technical procedure manual should be written according to specific guidelines of the Clinical and Laboratory Standards Institute. Performance of nucleic acid–based methods usually requires specific setup and/or workflow.

ASSAY DESIGN AND DEVELOPMENT

A well thought out process for assay design and development is critical to ensure the success of a new test development and implementation. Once specific analytes, assay techniques, and specimen types have been identified, the assay design and development can begin. Table 69-2 describes the different steps of the testing process that need to be taken into consideration when designing an LDT. The first task is to optimize each step of the analytical process, which includes nucleic acid extraction, target amplification, detection, quantification, and result interpretation. Several review and research articles provide detailed descriptions of the key parameters that may influence the performance of different in vitro nucleic acid methodologies, including standard PCR, both uniplex or multiplex. After optimization of the assay, it is necessary to evaluate and document preanalytical variables that might have an impact on the performance characteristics of the assay. Common preanalytical variables are specimen type, transport, storage and handling, as well as interfering substances such us lipids, hemoglobin, and bilirubin.

Establishment of molecular diagnostic tests, particularly amplification assays, requires development of controls for each step of the testing process, including reagent preparation, specimen collection, specimen aliquoting, and performing the actual assay. A careful selection of control reagents is vital for the correct interpretation of test results. Several types of controls are used throughout the execution of an assay to ensure appropriate performance. For qualitative tests, negative and positive controls are required by CLIA '88 regulations and must be processed in every clinical test run. Failure to obtain the correct result for any of the controls invalidates the entire test and requires re-testing of all samples. Whenever possible, positive and negative control reagents should closely resemble a patient specimen. Furthermore, a positive control should represent a clinically relevant level of the nucleic acid target sequence in a background of negative nucleic acid target sequence. The negative control should contain "background" nucleic acid sequences expected to be present in the patient's sample. In addition to the negative and positive controls, a blank control should be included with every assay, which contains all the components of

TABLE 69-2
Conducting the Clinical Testing Process

Activity type	Considerations
Reagent preparation	1. Perform in cleanest environment.
	2. Store working stock solutions in single-use aliquots.
	3. Quality control each new set of reagents before use in clinical testing; use low copy number sample for sensitivity evaluation.
	4. Preparation of master mixes reduces variability and errors.
Specimen collection	1. Establish acceptable tolerance limits for each specimen type to be tested (e.g., storage temperature, transport time, anticoagulant).
	2. Distribute protocols for proper specimen handling to all potential users.
	3. Capture clinical and analytical information on requisition.
Specimen processing	1. Specimen must be received and stored in preamplification (clean) laboratory.
	2. Develop guidelines to ensure against specimen mixup and to preserve integrity of target sequence.
Analysis of specimen	
a. Extraction procedure	1. Evaluate extraction procedures for presence of inhibitors and factors that decrease yield of target.
	2. Internal control added to the sample at the time of extraction to determine false-negative reactions due to inhibitors or determine this rate by some other means. If an internal control is not to be evaluated with each patient sample, then the rate of false-negative reactions should be stated on the report in a disclaimer in case of negative results.
b. Assay setup, amplification, and detection	1. Optimize concentration of primers, magnesium chloride ($MgCl_2$), deoxynucleotide triphosphates (dNTPs); volume; cycling conditions and detection system.
	2. Develop guidelines to minimize possibility of contamination by template nucleic acid or amplicon (see sections on quality control).
	3. Control specimens must be processed in the same manner as patient specimens.
	4. Develop guidelines to set up assay to avoid cross-contamination of specimens and controls.
Interpretation and report	1. Develop guidelines for interpretation and report.
	2. Interpretation should be performed by at least two individuals independently.
	3. Develop guidelines for report distribution.

the reaction mixture except nucleic acid. In addition to these controls, in some instances it is imperative to include an internal control to check for the presence of inhibitors in the individual patient samples. If this latter control is not used, then when a negative result is obtained, it is not clear whether the absence of amplicon is due to the absence of the target sequence in the patient specimen or to the presence of substances that inhibited the amplification reaction. To avoid this situation, amplification of an internal positive control sequence is recommended. The internal positive control can be an endogenous nucleic acid sequence that is unrelated to the target sequence of the clinical assay but is constitutively present in the sample. Alternatively, it may represent a sequence that is spiked into the clinical sample at some step in the testing process. The former endogenous internal positive control generally requires a separate set of primers and may require a separate reaction. The spiked control is generally a sequence that shares the same primer sequence that is used for the clinical target and is usually amplified in the same reaction tube as the clinical sample. As is the case with the external clinical positive control, the internal control should be used at a concentration that is relevant to the clinical testing process. The internal positive controls are also valuable to assess the presence of amplifiable nucleic acid and the absence of inhibitors, as well as to assess that the amplification and detection reactions are performed according to the specifications.

The use of a series of positive controls at different concentrations of target sequence can be helpful in monitoring the assay for changes in sensitivity over time. In addition, inclusion of a positive control where the concentration of target sequence is below the detection threshold of the assay can be useful for detecting low levels of amplicon.

A common approach to developing internal controls is to create synthetic materials, such as in vitro synthesized plasmids, that that can be spiked into the specimen before testing. The most common internal controls are synthetic segments of nucleic acid that use the same primer sequence as the target sequence. A sequence internal to the primer's binding site that is unique to the internal control allows separate detection and quantitation from the target . In addition, this internal control can be used for internal calibration. An internal calibrator contains a determined amount of this modified target that can be added directly to a clinical specimen and undergoes the same manipulation as the target of the patient specimen. One caveat for internal controls is that they must have the same or a very similar efficiency of amplification. Moreover, when the internal control fails to be detected, it is not possible to determine whether an inhibitor is present or there is an amplification problem. It is important to use a low amount of the internal control to avoid competition with the target of the patient specimen. When detecting and/or quantifying RNA from tissue or cells, amplification of a housekeeping gene (e.g., GAPDH, β-actin) can be used as an internal control. Most housekeeping genes are highly abundant and might not be the most appropriate internal control. The use of RNA from a gene with the same approximate abundance as the target sequence should be used.

NEW TEST VERIFICATION/VALIDATION

As with any other area of the clinical laboratory, the introduction of a new test requires proper validation. There are major differences between the implementation of an FDA-approved test and one that is not. CLIA '88 provides specific guidance for validation of these assays. Laboratories implementing FDA-approved tests must verify and document the performance characteristics of the test for the indications for use in populations similar to those in which the manufacturer has established performance. Implementation of in-house developed assays requires a more involved process, with extensive documentation on test performance and QC programs that ensure reproducible performance of the test. Table 69-3 provides a list of guidelines and standards for molecular diagnostics testing that can be used as references during assay development and verification. Table 69-4 describes the different aspects of documentation that would be useful to capture during the validation process.

Verification of a new test is a complex process that can be divided into two phases: analytical and clinical verification. Analytical verification provides information about the analytical performance of the test. Clinical verification provides information about the clinical utility of the test with regard to the intended use. Determination of the intended use provides information about the appropriate settings, including disease states and populations for which the test can be useful. In this text, the phrase *intended use* refers to the DNA or RNA target that a molecular assay detects or quantifies, whereas *indications for use* refers to the clinical syndrome/condition for which the assay can be used for diagnosis, management, or monitoring of disease.

TABLE 69-3
Guidelines and Standards for Molecular Diagnostics Testing

Organization	Guideline or standard
Clinical and Laboratory Standards Institute (CLSI), www.clsi.org	MM1-A2 Molecular Diagnostic Methods for Genetic Diseases
	MM2-A2 Immunoglobulin and T-Cell Receptor Gene Rearrangement Assays
	MM3-A2 Molecular Diagnostic Methods for Infectious Diseases
	MM-5 A Nucleic Acid Amplification Assays for Molecular Hematology
	MM-6 A Quantitative Molecular Diagnostics for Infectious Diseases
	MM-7 A Fluorescence in Situ Hybridization Methods for Medical Genetics
	MM-9 A Nucleic Acid Sequencing Methods in Diagnostic Laboratory Medicine
	MM-10-A Genotyping for Infectious Diseases: Identification and Characterization; Approved Guideline
	MM-11-A Molecular Methods for Bacterial Strain Typing; Approved Guideline
	MM-12-A Diagnostic Nucleic Acid Microarrays; Approved Guideline
	MM-13-A Collection, Transport, Preparation, and Storage of Specimens for Molecular Methods; Approved Guideline
	MM-14 A Proficiency Testing for Molecular Methods
	MM-16-A Use of External RNA Controls in Gene Expression Assays; Approved Guideline
	MM-17-A Verification and Validation of Multiplex Nucleic Acid Assays; Approved Guideline
	MM-18-A Interpretive Criteria for Identification of Bacteria and Fungi by DNA Target Sequencing; Approved Guideline
American College of Medical Genetics, www.acmg.net	Standards and Guidelines for Clinical Genetic Laboratories: Policy Statements
	Prenatal Interphase Fluorescence In Situ Hybridization
	ACMG Position Statement on Multiple Marker Screening in Women 35 and Older
	Fragile X Syndrome: Diagnostic and Carrier Testing
	Technical Standards and Guidelines for Fragile X: The first in a series of disease-specific supplements to the standards and guidelines for clinical genetics laboratories of the American College of Medical Genetics
	Statement on Storage and Use of Genetic Materials
	Statement on Multiple Marker Screening in Pregnant Women
	Statement on Use of Apolipoprotein E Testing for Alzheimer Disease
	Diagnostic Testing for Prader-Willi and Angelman Syndromes
	Statement on Population Screening for BRCA-1 Mutation in Ashkenazi Jewish Women
	Genetic Susceptibility to Breast and Ovarian Cancer: Assessment, Counseling and Testing Guidelines
	Principles of Screening: Report of the Subcommittee on Screening of the American College of Medical Genetics Clinical Practice Committee
	Position Statement on Carrier Testing for Canavan Disease
	Cystic Fibrosis Carrier Screening, Laboratory Standards and Guidelines for Population-based Cystic Fibrosis Carrier Screening
	Genetic Testing for Colon Cancer: A Joint Statement of the American College of Medical Genetics and the American Society of Human Genetics
	Consensus Statement on Factor V Leiden Mutation Testing
	Technical and Clinical Assessment in Fluorescent In Situ Hybridization: An ACMG/ASHG Position Statement. Technical Considerations
	ACMG Recommendations for Standard Interpretation of Sequence Variations
	American College of Medical Genetics Statement on Diagnostic Testing for Uniparental Disomy
	Genetic Susceptibility to Breast and Ovarian Cancer: Assessment, Counseling and Testing Guidelines
	Carrier Screening for Spinal Muscular Atrophy
	Carrier screening in individuals of Ashkenazi Jewish descent. Genet Med 2008;10:1:54–6.
	Genetic testing for colon cancer: Joint Statement of the American College of Medical Genetics and American Society of Human Genetics. Genet Med 2000;2(6):362–6.
	Cystic fibrosis population carrier screening: 2004 revision of American College of Medical Genetics Mutation Panel. Genet Med 2004;6(5):387–91.
	American College of Medical Genetics consensus statement on factor V Leiden mutation testing. Genet Med 2001;3(2):139–48.
	Fragile X syndrome: diagnostic and carrier testing. Genet Med 2005;7(8):584–87.
	Statement on guidance for genetic counseling in advanced paternal age. Genet Med 2008;10:6:457–60.
	ACMG/ASHG report: points to consider: ethical legal and psychosocial implications of genetic testing in children and adolescents. Am J Hum Genet 1995;57:1233–41.
	Indications for genetic referral: a guide for health care providers. Genet Med 2007;9(6):385–9.
	ACMG recommendations for standards for interpretation of sequence variations. Genet Med 2000;2(5):302–3.
	Genetics evaluation guidelines for the etiologic diagnosis of congenital hearing loss. Genet Med 2002;4(3):162–71.
	Informed consent for medical photograph. Genet Med 2000;2(6):353–5.
	American College of Medical Genetics guideline on the cytogenetic evaluation of the individual with developmental delay or mental retardation. Genet Med 2005;7(9):650–4.
	Clinical genetics evaluation in identifying the etiology of autism spectrum disorders. Genet Med 2008;10:4:301–5.
	Use of array-based technology in the practice of medical genetics. Genet Med 2007;9(9):650–3.

TABLE 69-3
Guidelines and Standards for Molecular Diagnostics Testing—cont'd

Organization	Guideline or standard
American College of Medical Genetics—cont'd	Evaluation of the newborn with single or multiple congenital anomalies: a clinical guide. 1999 ACMG Foundation with support from the New York State Department of Health.
	Newborn screening. ACT sheets and confirmatory algorithms funded in part through MCHB/HRSA/HHS grant #U22MC03957.
	Newborn screening: toward a uniform screening panel and system. Genet Med 2006;8(5):Supplement.
	Genetic evaluation of suspected osteogenesis imperfecta (OI). Genet Med 2006;8(6):383–8.
	Pompe disease diagnosis and management guideline. Genet Med 2006;8(5):267–88.
	First trimester diagnosis and screening for fetal aneuploidy. Genet Med 2008;10(1):73–5.
	Second trimester maternal serum screening for fetal open neural tube defects and aneuploidy. Genet Med 2004;6(6):540–1.
	Diagnostic testing for Prader-Willi and Angelman syndromes: report of the ASHG/ACMG Test and Technology Transfer Committee. Am J Hum Genet 1966;58:1085–8.
	American College of Medical Genetics Statement on Diagnostic Testing for Uniparental Disomy
FDA www.fda.gov	Guidance for Industry and FDA Staff—In Vitro Diagnostic 2009 H1N1 Tests for Use in the 2009 H1N1 Emergency
	Guidance for Industry and FDA Staff—Class II Special Controls Guidance Document: Cardiac Allograft Gene Expression Profiling Test Systems
	Guidance for Industry and FDA Staff—Class II Special Controls Guidance Document: Testing for Detection and Differentiation of Influenza A Virus Subtypes Using Multiplex Assays
	Guidance for Industry and FDA Staff—Class II Special Controls Guidance Document: Testing for Human Metapneumovirus (hMPV) Using Nucleic Acid Assays
	Guidance for Industry and FDA Staff—Class II Special Controls Guidance Document: Respiratory Viral Panel Multiplex Nucleic Acid Assay
	Draft Guidance for Industry and FDA Staff—Establishing the Performance Characteristics of In-Vitro Diagnostic Devices for the Detection or Detection and Differentiation of Human Papillomaviruses
	Class II Special Controls Guidance Document: Nucleic Acid Amplification Assay for the Detection of Enterovirus RNA
	Guidance for Industry and FDA Staff—Commercially Distributed Analyte Specific Reagents (ASRs): Frequently Asked Questions
	Draft Guidance for Industry, Clinical Laboratories, and FDA Staff—In Vitro Diagnostic Multivariate Index Assays
	Guidance on Pharmacogenetic Tests and Genetic Tests for Heritable Markers
	Guidance for Industry and FDA Staff—Class II Special Controls Guidance Document: Gene Expression Profiling Test System for Breast Cancer Prognosis
	Guidance for Industry and FDA Staff—Class II Special Controls Guidance Document: Quality Control Material for Cystic Fibrosis Nucleic Acid Assays
	Informed Consent for In Vitro Diagnostic Device Studies Using Leftover Human Specimens That Are Not Individually Identifiable
	Guidance for Industry and FDA Staff—Class II Special Controls Guidance Document: CFTR Gene Mutation Detection Systems
	Guidance for Industry and FDA Staff—Class II Special Controls Guidance Document: RNA Preanalytical Systems (RNA Collection, Stabilization and Purification Systems for RT-PCR used in Molecular Diagnostic Testing)
	Guidance for Industry and FDA Staff—Format for Traditional and Abbreviated 510(k)s
	Guidance for Industry and FDA Staff—Class II Special Controls Guidance Document—Automated Fluorescence In Situ Hybridization (FISH) Enumeration Systems
	Class II Special Controls Guidance Document: Instrumentation for Clinical Multiplex Test Systems—Guidance for Industry and FDA Staff
	Class II Special Controls Guidance Document: Drug Metabolizing Enzyme Genotyping System Guidance for Industry and FDA Staff
	Guidance for Industry in the Manufacture and Clinical Evaluation of In Vitro Tests to Detect In Vitro Nucleic Acid Sequences of HIV-1-Draft
	Guidance for Industry and/or FDA Reviewers Staff-Premarket Approval Applications for Assays Pertaining to Hepatitis C Virus (HCV) That Are Indicated for Diagnosis or Monitoring of HCV Infection or Associated Disease-Draft Guidance
Association for Molecular Pathology www.amp.org	Recommendations for In-House Development and Operation of Molecular Diagnostic Tests
	Multi-site PCR-based CMV viral load assessment-assays demonstrate linearity and precision, but lack numeric standardization: a report of the Association for Molecular Pathology. J Mol Diagn 2009;11:87–92.
	Consensus characterization of 16 *FMR1* reference materials: a consortium study. J Mol Diagn 2008;10:2–12.
	Inter-laboratory comparison of chronic myeloid leukemia minimal residual disease monitoring: summary and recommendations. J Mol Diagn 2007;9:21–43.
	Guidance for fluorescence *in situ* hybridization testing in hematologic disorders. J Mol Diagn 2007;9:134–43.
	Standard mutation nomenclature in molecular diagnostics: practical and educational challenges. J Mol Diagn 2007;9:1–6.
	Certification in molecular pathology in the United States (Training and Education Committee, the Association for Molecular Pathology). J Mol Diagn 2002;4:181–4.
	Laboratory practice guidelines for detecting and reporting BCR-ABL drug resistance mutations in chronic myelogenous leukemia and acute lymphoblastic leukemia: a report of the Association for Molecular Pathology. J Mol Diagn 2009 11:4–11.

ABMG, American Board of Medical Genetics; *ACMG*, American College of Medical Genetics; *ABGC*, American Board of Genetic Counseling; *ASHG*, American Society of Human Genetics; *CFTR*; cystic fibrosis transmembrane conductance regulator; *FDA*, U.S. Food and Drug Administration; *RNA*, ribonucleic acid; *RT-PCR*, reverse-transcriptase polymerase chain reaction.

TABLE 69-4
Documentation Checklist for Assay Validation

Test name	Name of the test including technology used—Be sure that the name identifies the particular organism and/or disease/condition to be tested.
Intended use	What the test measures and for what purpose—Identify the particular microorganism and parameters tested, and indicate the use of the test (e.g., diagnosis, prognosis, monitoring response to treatment, guiding therapy).
Indications for use	Provide clinical conditions—Use reference standard definitions as found in Online Mendelian Inheretance in Man (OMIM), www.ncbi.nlm.nih.gov/omim
Method category	Identify methodology used for the test.
Testing procedure	Information with regard to specimen types, specimen handling and transport procedures, nucleic acid isolation and storage, description of the test procedure, data reports, expected results, and technical interpretation of results—All these parameters should be included in policies and procedures for the particular test.
Test results	Examples of results
Analytical verification	Analytical sensitivity, specificity, precision, dynamic range, cross reactivity, interfering substances
Quality control and quality assurance	Delineate QC and QA program—Identify informal proficiency program if no Department of Health and Human Services–approved program exists.
Assay limitations	Clearly explain and/or discuss potential limitations of the assay.
Clinical data	Primary objective of the study, clinical condition evaluated, patient population, demographics, and sample size estimate
Clinical verification	Clinical sensitivity, specificity, and positive and negative predictive value
Reporting of tests results	Clinical interpretation
Clinical utility	Potential clinical benefit to patient

TABLE 69-5
Commercial Sources of Control and Reference Materials

Company	Available material
Seracare (www.seracare.com)	Quantitative and qualitative controls, external run controls, qualification, verification and performance panels for HCV, HIV, HBV, external run controls for CMV, HSV, EBV, HPV, *Chlamydia trachomatis, Mycobacterium tuberculosis,* CFTR, warfarin sensitivity, MTHFR.
Advanced Biotechnology (www.abionline.com.)	Control DNA, virus and cell lines (HIV, HTLV, EBV, CMV, HSV, VZV, HCV, SIV, rubella). Native and recombinant products purified viruses, antigens, proteins and antibodies
Stratagene (www.stratagene.com)	Universal human reference RNA for micro array technology
AcroMetrix (www.acrometrix.com)	External run controls, secondary reference controls, verification panels for HIV, HCV and HBV, HIV genotyping
National Institute for Biogical Standards and Controls (www.nibsc.ac.uk)	Evaluation/statistics service, working reagents for HIV-1 RNA, HCV, HBV, HAV, Parvovirus B19
American Type Culture Collection (www.attc.org)	Bacteria, bacteriophages, cell lines, hybridomas, filamentous fungi and yeast, tissue cultures, viruses
Corriel Repository (http://ccr.coriell.org)	Provide essential reagents to the scientific community by establishing, verifying, maintaining, and distributing cell cultures and DNA derived from cell cultures with mutations in different clinically relevant genes
Paragon Dx (www.paragondx.com)	DNA control material for cytochrome P450 2C9 (CYP2C9), cytochrome P450 4F2 (CYP4F2), and vitamin K epoxide reductase complex, subunit 1 (VKORC1), cytochrome P450 2C19 (CYP2C19), cytochrome P450 2D6 (CYP2D6), MTHFR, UGT1A1, NAT2 genes
Maine Molecular (www.mmqci.com)	Control product to monitor the analytical performance of extraction, amplification, and detection of test systems used in qualitative measurement of factor II (prothrombin) and factor V genes for the mutations factor II G20210A and factor V Leiden (G1691A), CFTR gene, cytochrome P450 2C9 (CYP2C9), cytochrome P450 4F2 (CYP4F2), and vitamin K epoxide reductase complex, subunit 1 (VKORC1)

CFTR, Cystic fibrosis transmembrane conductance regulator; *CMV,* cytomegalovirus; *DNA,* deoxyribonucleic acid; *EBV,* Epstein-Barr virus; *HAV,* hepatitis A virus; *HBV,* hepatitis B virus; *HCV,* hepatitis C virus; *HIV,* human immunodeficiency virus; *HTLV,* human T-lymphotropic virus; *MTHFR,* methylenetetrahydrofolate reductase; *RNA,* ribonucleic acid; *VZV,* varicella zoster virus; *SIV,* simian immuunodeficiency virus.

ANALYTICAL VERIFICATION

Before a new or improved test is introduced, careful evaluation of the performance characteristics of the assay under laboratory conditions needs to be done. The analytical verification process provides information regarding the performance of the assay but also can provide practical information needed for daily operation of the test. Historically, analytical validation programs has been challenging because of the lack of standards and reference materials for many nucleic acid targets. This shortfall has impacted the laboratory's ability to determine assay sensitivity and accuracy. Table 69-5 lists suppliers of commercially available reference materials that can be used during analytical verification and as a source of QC material.

As part of the analytical verification, laboratories must determine the assay's analytical sensitivity, analytical specificity, accuracy, and precision. For quantitative assays, information regarding the linear dynamic range or reportable range determines when a measurement or change in the quantity of the analyte is clinically relevant or due to inherent test error. A number of national and international organizations are taking steps to develop standard reference materials. The National Institute of Standards and Technology developed one of the first nucleic acid standard reference materials for human identity testing. More recently, the World Health Organization (WHO) introduced a standard reference material for HIV, HCV, and HBV that has been used for verification of nucleic acid tests for screening of blood and blood products. Reference panels calibrated to WHO standard reference material are commercially available (SeraCare Life Sciences).

When standardized reference materials are not available, laboratories must rely on alternatives to validate tests. Laboratories can develop their own reference materials for analytical validation and monitoring daily

PART 8

performance of the assay. These reference materials may be available in-house or from an outside source such as a collaborating laboratory, government agency (CDC, FDA, NIH), or commercial supplier (SeraCare Life Sciences, AcroMetrix). Examples include intact virus particles, bacteria that naturally contain the target in their genome, cell lines that contain a specific genetic change, plasmids, and intracellular RNA or DNA. When it is difficult to obtain a natural analytical reference material, laboratories develop synthetic reference materials. These synthetic reference materials may be in the form of single- or double-stranded DNA or RNA that is manufactured in vitro and that can be accurately quantified by several physical and/or biochemical methods. Examples include synthesized DNA in the form of oligonucleotides, single-stranded DNA produced by cloning recombinant phage, double stranded DNA produced by cloning into vectors such as plasmids, or a DNA fragment produced by chemical or physical method from a larger DNA molecule followed by purification. Synthetic RNA reference materials can be generated by in vitro transcription of DNA templates.

Test validation requires verifying the new test results with those of another independently established method. Alternatively, the laboratory can split samples for a comparison study with another laboratory that performs a similar molecular test.

The evaluation of the precision of an assay is necessary to be able to determine what constitutes a biological change in the analyte versus expected analytical variability of the laboratory measurement. Evaluation of the precision should take into account the entire testing process—nucleic acid extraction, amplification, detection, and quantitation. Precision studies should be carried out using test material or reference material that is similar to or closely resembling the intended patient specimen. Such material may be obtained by serial dilution of a target-positive specimen to below the limits of detection. If a characterized patient specimen is not available, then reference material may be created by mixing a cell line or purified virus microorganism into a pool of the patient specimens known to be negative for the specific analyte. These materials could be used for daily monitoring of the assay's performance as well. Daily QC for qualitative assays should include at least a single positive reference control with a concentration close to the limit of detection. Daily QC for quantitative methods should include at least two concentrations which span the linear dynamic range of the assay and, when possible, include the values used for clinical decision making.

Determination of the accuracy of molecular methods has been challenging because molecular methods have proven to be more sensitive than a large number of well-established methods, even criterion standard (gold standard) methods. Generally, when evaluating a new test, the results obtained should be compared with the results obtained from an established test that is considered a criterion standard method. In the absence of a criterion standard, a laboratory could purchase reference material to be used for the analytical verification.

Determination of the linearity of a quantitative assay may be performed by testing at least four different levels of the analyte. Again, test material could be prepared by spiking the analyte into negative patient sample or by performing serial dilution of a patient specimen known to contain a very high level of the analyte. The analytical sensitivity represents the ability of a test to obtain a positive result in concordance with positive results obtained by a reference method. For quantitative molecular methods, the lowest amount that the method can detect might be different from the lower limit of quantification for a particular nucleic acid or microorganism. The lower limit of quantification is the lowest amount of a nucleic acid sequence that can be detected with acceptable precision. Analytical sensitivity could be determined by performing serial dilutions of an appropriate number of samples containing different concentration of the analyte. Analytical specificity is the ability of an analytical method to detect and/or quantify what the analyte is intended to measure. One aspect of specificity that can easily be measured is the lack of cross-reactivity with closely related nucleic acid sequences or organisms. In addition, for infectious disease testing, it is important to determine lack of cross-reactivity with nucleic acid from organisms present in the normal flora or that would normally be present in a patient specimen.

It is also important to determine interfering substances that might affect the ability of a test to detect and or quantitate the analyte of interest. The source of the interfering substance could be endogenous or exogenous. Exogenous interfering substances include drugs, parenteral nutrition, or anticoagulants. Some anticoagulants (e.g., heparin) may interfere with the amplification process. Endogenous interfering substances (e.g., lipids, bilirubin) could be result of pathologic conditions. There are several approaches for detecting interfering substances. One can add target nucleic acid (e.g., purified nucleic acid, cells, or microorganisms) to specimens that contain various interfering substances. One can also add the specific nucleic acid target to specimens from patients with various conditions (e.g., jaundice) or who are receiving specific drug treatment.

Appropriate specimen handling, including specimen collection and transport conditions, is critical to the testing process to ensure specimen integrity. Inappropriate specimen handling could result in nucleic acid degradation, which can lead to falsely negative detection or inaccurate quantitation of nucleic acid. This is critical for assays that detect and or measure eukaryote RNA and viral RNA. The best specimen type and quantity should be determined because molecular tests are applied to a variety of specimen types. Appropriate selection of specimen type will depend on multiple factors, including the clinical condition being studied and the type of nucleic acid required for the test. The format of the molecular assay being developed could greatly affect the amount of specimen required. Tests that require samples to be run in duplicate will require more specimen than those run in singleton. Specimen transport and storage should be evaluated for every assay and type of nucleic acid. Specimen transport and storage conditions could vary significantly between specimen type, analyte (RNA vs. DNA), cells, and microorganism and must be determined by each laboratory. There are special requirements for specimen transport and storage for RNA, because it is highly susceptible to degradation by ubiquitous enzymes. Transport and storage conditions can vary greatly from storage at room temperature to having to centrifuge samples, remove plasma or serum, and storage at −80° C until tested.

CLINICAL VERIFICATION

Laboratory methods provide information for managing patients and addressing relevant clinical questions. The usefulness of a method depends on both the analytical performance and the clinical characteristics of the test (clinical sensitivity, specificity, and predictive value). The clinical significance of a test should be defined in terms of the disease or syndrome that is the subject of the test. These include disease prevalence, possible outcome, and cost to the patient and others for incorrect information (false-positive or false-negative results). Validation of clinical utility of an assay is a complex process that possesses many challenges. *Clinical utility* is referred to here as the indications for use. For example, the assay is intended to quantify a nucleic acid (analyte), but is indicated for certain clinical conditions or scenarios.

The first step of the analytical verification is to formulate a clinical question and to identify the target population to which the test will be applied. There are three parts in the definition of a clinical question: (1) characterize the subject population, (2) define the clinical management decision, and (3) identify the role of the test in clinical decision making. When the clinical use of each test is being considered, it is assumed that the test's analytical performance characteristics are well understood. Known analytical limitations (e.g., reportable range for quantifying, precision for nonclinical samples) should be taken into consideration when determining the clinical use for each particular assay. Clinical verification requires evaluation of the clinical sensitivity of the test by evaluating an appropriate number of samples from patients known to have the disease or condition. The population and type of sample should be fully described because the results for a test in a given population using a specified sample type may not be suitable for another population, or even for another sample type within the same population. It is important to define the purpose (i.e., what is the test measuring) and indications (i.e., what are the clinical circumstances in which the test will be useful) before starting the clinical verification. For example, indication for use of an assay could be diagnosis, screening in a population, confirming results from another assay, resolution of disease, or prognosis. Clinical specificity can be determined by analyzing samples from patients diagnosed with a different disease that is in the differential diagnosis and that might be confused with the indicated disease. In addition, specimens from healthy donors can be appropriate for determining the clinical specificity of the test. The other parameters that need to be determined are the positive and negative predictive values, as well as a predictive value of the test over the course of disease or therapy. Furthermore, in order to determine the clinical utility of a new LDT, variables that could affect results and their interpretation should also be considered. For example, for infectious disease, some of these variables could be microbial host interactions, microbial dynamics, variants and mutations, or replicative fitness of the microbial agent.

Data generated during the clinical verification of each assay should be gathered and kept organized to satisfy the requirements of the different regulatory bodies. Within the documentation, the laboratory should have available a list of indications for which the assay has been verified (see Table 69-4).

QUALITY CONTROL OF THE TESTING PROCESS

It is extremely important to implement a QC program for LDTs for validating the strength, purity, and performance of every critical reagent of the testing process. Every critical reagent should be tested before being approved for clinical testing. Tolerance limits should be established for every critical reagent. When possible, the tolerance limits should be established using a quantitative measurement to avoid subjective evaluation of the quality of the critical reagent.

QUALITY CONTROL OF EQUIPMENT

All equipment used in the molecular diagnostic laboratory must have written maintenance procedures and calibration checks. As with any other clinical laboratory equipment, tolerance limits for acceptable performance and calibration checks for all laboratory equipment used during the testing process should be clearly defined and monitored in a regular fashion to assure continued production of accurate and reliable test results. When performance or calibration checks fall outside the tolerance limit defined for any particular instrument, the latter should be immediately taken out of service for repair. After repair the equipment should be calibrated before being placed back in use. As part of the QA program developed by each laboratory, documentation of all maintenance, performance checks, calibration, or repair for each piece of equipment should be maintained and kept according to the laboratory policy of document retention.

Thermocyclers are a crucial item to any molecular diagnostic laboratory. Any change in the performance of thermocyclers has direct impact in the sensitivity and precision of the assay performed in that piece of equipment. Maintenance, calibration and QC performance of all instruments should follow manufacturer's recommendations. Briefly, as part of the performance monitoring for thermocyclers, determination and documentation of the cycling time, verification of the setpoint error, and any error messages should be recorded. Cycling times between different runs should not differ more than a couple of minutes. Fluctuations in the cycling times are a warning sign that the thermocycler needs to be adjusted and restored to its original condition. In addition, it is recommended that the chiller, heater, and block temperature uniformity tests be performed according to the manufacturer's recommendations. The block temperature uniformity check can be accomplished by using a thermocoupler with a temperature probe.

Another important equipment item that is used daily in a molecular diagnostics laboratory is the pipetter. Pipetters are used for almost every step of the testing procedure. Special emphasis should be placed on the maintenance of the pipetters because they could be a major source of error. All other pieces of equipment should be maintained according to the manufacturer's recommendation. When possible, calibration of the equipment should be performed by using certified standards or reference materials.

CONCLUSIONS

It is clear that the molecular diagnostics laboratory provides valuable contributions to patient care. Ongoing issues of test specificity, sensitivity, quality, interpretation, limitations, instrument performance, consumables, intellectual property, patient confidentiality, and reimbursement will continue to mature in the development of this discipline. One concern is the emergence of direct to consumer marketing of over-the-counter test kits and fee-for-service enterprises that provide reports to customers that predict the "risk" of carrying or getting a disease or diseases based on DNA typing (e.g., cheek swab). These reports can confuse the patient and his or her physician as well as institute undue alarm and stigma. Such testing should include careful interpretation and genetic counciling. Future developments in this field will undoubtedly continue to provide opportunities for improving diagnostic and prognostic information as we realize the promises of personalized medicine and more effective patient management.

PART 8

SELECTED REFERENCES

Centers for Disease Control and Prevention. Good laboratory practices for molecular genetic testing for heritable diseases and conditions. MMWR 2009; Vol.58(RR06):1–29.

This report provides detailed good laboratory practices to those laboratories offering molecular genetic testing.

College of American Pathologists Commission on Laboratory Accreditation. Molecular pathology checklist; 2010. Available at http://www.cap.org/apps/docs/laboratory_accreditation/checklists/.

The College of American Pathologists provides a specific checklist for molecular pathology testing for those laboratories chosing to undergo CLIA surveys by CAP.

Ledbetter DH, Faucett WA. Issues in genetic testing for ultra-rare diseases: background and introduction. Genet Med 2008;10:309–13.

This review prodives insight into specific consideration regarding genetic testing of inhereted disorders.

Secretary's Advisory Committee on Genetics, Health, and Society. U.S. system of oversight of genetic testing: a response to the charge of the secretary of Health and Human Services. Bethesda, Md.: Department of Health and Human Services; 2008. Available at http://oba.od.nih.gov/oba/sacghs/reports/sacghs_oversight_report.pdf.

This report provides a comprehensive overview of the regulatory lanscape regarding analytical, clinical validity, and clinical utility of genetic testing in the United States.

REFERENCES

Access the complete reference list online at http://www.expertconsult.com

CHAPTER 70

MOLECULAR DIAGNOSIS OF GENETIC DISEASES

Wayne W. Grody

KEY POINTS

- Molecular testing for inherited disorders may be the most rapidly growing area of molecular pathology, owing to the plethora of disease genes discovered through the Human Genome Project.
- The mutations for single-gene disorders, whether dominant or recessive, can be detected by a variety of molecular diagnostic techniques, either specific to the mutation in question, if it is known, or by comprehensive gene sequencing or mutation scanning approaches if the mutation is not known.
- Certain disorders, such as cystic fibrosis, have sufficiently high mutation carrier frequencies that they have become targets for large-scale population screening programs.
- Late-onset dominant disorders, such as Huntington disease and familial cancers, are appropriate targets of presymptomatic testing, providing sufficient attention is paid to the associated ethical concerns.
- Ethical issues raised by each of these applications involve genetic privacy, informed consent, pregnancy termination, potential stigmatization, and theoretical risk of insurance discrimination.

Probably the fastest growing, and perhaps most controversial, area of molecular pathology, diagnostic molecular genetics holds promise of becoming the most powerful diagnostic and screening tool of the 21st century. With the rapidly accelerating pace of identification of new disease genes after completion of the Human Genome Project and the recognition that virtually all diseases, including neoplastic and even infectious ones, have some genetic component, the clinical utility of this subspecialty can only continue to expand. Moreover, its unique capability to diagnose disease both prenatally and presymptomatically should confer on it a primary role in preventive medicine, a focus of increasing urgency in the present era of medical care cost containment. Even beyond that, diagnostic molecular genetics leads naturally into therapeutic molecular genetics, because essentially the same normal gene sequences used to detect molecular genetic defects by deoxyribonucleic acid (DNA) hybridization could theoretically be used to correct such defects by gene replacement therapy. Whereas the pace of advances in the latter activity has remained frustratingly slow, it is safe to say that it will become an important therapeutic modality during this century. When that happens, it will become even further intertwined with the activities of the molecular diagnostics laboratory, which will have the responsibility of confirming proper insertion and monitoring appropriate expression of the replacement gene.

Yet such progress does not come unencumbered by appreciable obstacles. Aside from the considerable technical sophistication and complexity of these procedures, they are inextricably bound up with a number of thorny ethical dilemmas. Dissecting a patient's most fundamental constitutional makeup, and the inborn errors therein, raises problematic questions about genetic discrimination, stigmatization, ethnic differences, privacy, informed consent, and confidentiality. Because at the molecular genetic level everything becomes a preexisting condition, the very definition of insurability may need to be revised, and instances of insurance and employment discrimination as a result of genetic testing, although rare (Hall, 2000), have been reported (Billings, 1992). It is reassuring that in the United States, where privately insured health care is most vulnerable to such abuses, we now have federal legislation, the Genetic Information Nondiscrimination Act, prohibiting discrimination in health insurance and employment based on genetic test results, although certain limitations still remain (Baruch, 2008). Furthermore, discovery of any such heritable mutations in an individual has profound implications far beyond the immediate patient who requested the DNA test (the proband), extending to all the other members of that person's family, none of whom may have consented to exploring or revealing this type of information. Indeed, with the almost unlimited power of DNA testing afforded by amplification techniques such as the polymerase chain reaction (PCR) and high-throughput genomic analysis technologies (see Chapters 66 and 77), it becomes quite easy to perform genetic analysis without the patient's consent or even knowledge, because the testing can be done on minute portions of tissue or fluid samples obtained for other unrelated purposes. Prenatal diagnosis—and, by extension, preconception genetic carrier screening of couples—becomes caught up in the passionate ethical and religious debates over abortion. And gene therapy, despite general consensus that it should be directed only at somatic rather than germline cellular targets (and even this notion is beginning to change), raises the specter of eugenics among those who do not have to remember back all that far to times when such notions were not only accepted but actively espoused.

Much of diagnostic molecular genetics involves the assessment of risk for occurrence or recurrence of a disorder in an individual or family. For reasons described more fully later in this chapter, the test results obtained are often expressed not in terms of a numerical concentration or as a yes/no answer, but rather as a probability, which sometimes is derived by multifactorial Bayesian analysis (Ojino, 2004). The accurate and meaningful conveyance of such complex uncertainties to patients and even referring physicians can be quite difficult and time-consuming. For this reason, and owing to the serious ethical implications of these tests as described previously, this area of laboratory medicine, perhaps more than most others, requires very close communication between the laboratory and the referring clinician or genetic counselor. In fact, some of these tests, particularly the emotionally charged predictive ones, should only be ordered through a medical geneticist or genetic counselor, because these are the specialists who are best qualified to assess the appropriateness of the test and explain the results to the patient. Some large academic and commercial reference laboratories specializing in this type of testing even employ their own genetic counselors on staff as a further safeguard to ensure appropriate use and communication with primary care physicians who may not be well-versed in these matters.

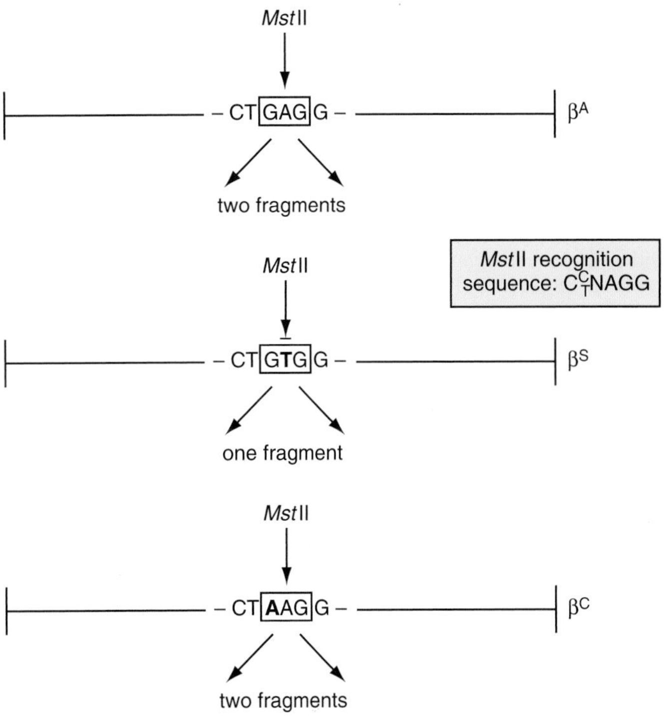

Figure 70-1 Schematic example of detection of a point mutation by differential cleavage with a restriction enzyme. In this case, the sickle cell mutation, substitution of T for A in codon 6 of the β-globin gene destroys an *Mst*II cleavage site so that digestion of a polymerase chain reaction product from the region will produce two DNA fragments in normals but only one fragment in HbS homozygotes. Mutation of the first nucleotide in this codon, found in hemoglobin C disease, does not destroy the *Mst*II site (because the enzyme can accommodate any nucleotide in this position) and thus cannot be detected by this method.

Choice of Techniques

With so many genetic disease genes, loci, and mutational mechanisms known, diagnostic molecular genetics must take advantage of the entire spectrum of modern molecular biological techniques available. These include, among others (see Chapters 65–68):

- PCR
- Southern blotting
- Allele-specific probe hybridization
- DNA sequencing
- Real-time PCR
- Nucleic acid microarrays
- Invader assay
- Amplification refractory mutation system (ARMS)
- Oligonucleotide ligation assay (OLA)
- Multiplex ligation-dependent probe amplification (MLPA)
- Mutation scanning methods, such as denaturing gradient gel electrophoresis (DGGE)
- Single-strand conformation polymorphism (SSCP)
- Mass spectrometry

The choice of which technique to use in a particular case will depend, to a large extent, on two factors: (1) the present knowledge of the gene(s) associated with the disease in question and (2) its degree of molecular heterogeneity. The first criterion roughly divides all genetic diseases into two categories: those for which the causative gene has been isolated and those for which it has not. Those in the first category can often be approached by direct gene/mutation analysis; those in the latter can only be approached by linkage analysis using polymorphic DNA markers nearby on the same chromosome, as long as the disease has been mapped to that rather crude level. The second concept, heterogeneity, refers to the number of different genes, or the variety of mutations within a single gene, that can cause the same disease. The greater the heterogeneity, the more difficult, labor-intensive, and expensive the DNA test becomes (and the more complex the results reporting and genetic counseling). In other disorders, one or more mutations may be of sufficiently high frequency in particular racial/ethnic populations that screening for those few, while ignoring the many rarer mutations reported, can provide a test of sufficient yield to justify the targeted approach.

To make such tests practical and of reasonable cost, a number of *multiplexing strategies* for simultaneous mutation detection have been devised. All of these involve some compromise as to overall test sensitivity. Indeed, the field of molecular genetic testing tolerates, by necessity, a number of screening tests with clinical sensitivities noticeably below those that would be considered acceptable in other areas of the clinical laboratory. The decision of just how low the acceptable sensitivity cutoff should be often comes down to public health considerations. Most geneticists have reasoned that, at least for screening tests, the potential public health benefits of offering a test of admittedly suboptimal sensitivity outweigh the arguments for withholding it, as long as sufficient education and counseling are provided to patients so that they understand the residual risk inherent in a negative test result. It is important to keep in mind that this discussion is about clinical sensitivity, not analytical sensitivity. It is assumed that the test is capable of detecting a given mutation whenever it is present; it is just that many rarer mutations will not be targeted by the assay, so that some proportion of carriers will be "missed"—a sort of "clinical false-negative" (Palomaki 2004).

Direct mutation tests have been simplified immeasurably by the advent of PCR. Through the judicious choice of primers, this technique allows the laboratory to hone in on the precise mutation of interest, or a "hot spot" within a gene containing several possible mutation sites, using minute amounts of starting material. Once the region containing the suspected mutation is amplified, it can be analyzed by gel or capillary electrophoresis, sequencing, or DNA probe hybridization. For a deletion that would be expected to alter the length of the amplicon, accurate molecular sizing of the PCR products by electrophoresis will be sufficient. Alternatively, if the deletion or point mutation disrupts (or creates) a restriction endonuclease cleavage site, it can be detected by electrophoretic analysis of PCR products digested with that enzyme (Fig. 70-1). Another option is to hybridize the PCR products with allele-specific oligonucleotide (ASO) probes, short DNA fragments that are precisely complementary to either the normal or mutant target sequence. As discussed in Chapter 67, if the hybridization, usually in a dot- or line-blot format, is performed under sufficiently stringent conditions, target DNA containing the mutation will hybridize only with the mutant probe, and vice versa for wild type target DNA. Several mutation hot spots in a gene can be amplified together by multiplex PCR. As a variation on this approach, any number of allelic probes can be spread out on a solid support for subsequent hybridization with the specimen DNA (or amplicons) in the form of a microarray or in suspension on microbeads. Lastly, a number of commercial reagents and instruments are available that detect point mutations by differential probe/quencher hybridization or by capillary electrophoresis and other sophisticated techniques, as described in Chapters 67 and 77.

To screen a disease gene for unknown mutations that may lie anywhere within it, several *mutation scanning* techniques that cast a wider net are available. SSCP, DGGE, denaturing high-performance liquid chromatography, and other variations of the same principle can theoretically detect point mutations anywhere within a gene by virtue of the altered topology that the substituted nucleotides induce in single-stranded or mismatched double-stranded DNA. These approaches obviate the need for separate and specific ASO probes for every possible mutation, although they can only be performed on limited PCR-amplified stretches of the gene (usually single exons or parts of exons) at one time and they are not 100% sensitive. The protein truncation test detects mutations, causing premature termination of the gene's polypeptide product; it requires an involved in vitro transcription/translation approach and will only pick up "stop" mutations (and some frameshifts and splicing variants) while overlooking common single-nucleotide substitutions (missense mutations). The only technique that should be 100% sensitive in detecting all possible point mutations, at least in theory, is complete DNA sequencing of the gene, although even it will miss mutations that lie outside the usual coding region targets (e.g., in introns, promoters, or enhancer regions).

Disorders caused by gene expansion by a trinucleotide repeat mutation can be diagnosed by Southern blot or PCR, in either case by observing a larger-than-normal target DNA fragment. Disorders caused by large deletions may be diagnosed by Southern blot by observing loss or decrease in size of a target fragment, by PCR, through loss of a product normally amplified from that site or appearance of a new "junction" fragment, or by MLPA.

For those disorders with too many unknown mutations, or an unknown gene, predictive diagnosis by *linkage analysis* is possible in certain families. Because the analysis requires comparative testing of other affected and unaffected siblings and parents, not every family will be accessible or informative using this approach. Also required is knowledge of closely linked, preferably flanking or even intragenic polymorphic DNA markers that can be observed to co-segregate consistently with either the normal or disease phenotype within the family. Traditionally, the markers used have been restriction fragment length polymorphisms (RFLPs) detected by Southern blot. More recently, microsatellite polymorphisms—tandem oligonucleotide sequences of variable repeat length—that are detectable by PCR and gel or capillary electrophoresis have become favored because of their abundance throughout the genome, the multiallelic nature of their polymorphisms, and the relative ease of the testing method. Very large genes, such as those for neurofibromatosis and Duchenne muscular dystrophy (DMD), will usually have intragenic microsatellites that can be accessed, minimizing the chances of recombination between the mutation and the marker.

Linkage techniques are less favored than the direct mutation detection approach because of the need to test multiple family members and because meiotic recombination between the gene and the marker can disrupt the apparent phase of linkage between parent and offspring, leading to false-positive or false-negative interpretation of results. For each centimorgan of map distance between the two loci, 1% recombination can be expected (1 cM = 1 million base pairs [bp]). For example, in Figure 70-2 the fetus is predicted to be affected, having inherited the same upper RFLP fragment as the previously affected son. But if the polymorphic restriction endonuclease site being tested is 5cM away from the disease gene, one can only conclude that the fetus is at 95% risk of being affected. However, because the completion of the human genome sequence, which is saturated with polymorphic markers (both short tandem repeats and single-nucleotide polymorphisms, there is no longer any need to rely on linked marker that is so far away from the disease gene.

Although this chapter is primarily concerned with molecular testing for single-gene mendelian disorders, it would be remiss not to acknowledge the newer techniques now available for *whole-genome analysis*. This can be done using either high-density oligonucleotide microarray platforms or so-called highly parallel or "next-generation" DNA sequencing. At present, only the former is in routine use in clinical genetics, in the form of array comparative genomic hybridization. This technique employs a high number (500,000 to more than 1,000,000) DNA probes on the array, chosen so that their complementary genomic sequences span the entire genome at regular intervals. Total genomic DNA from the patient competes for hybridization to the array against a "normal" total genomic control sample, each labeled with a different fluorescent dye. If the patient's DNA contains a deletion on a certain chromosome, this will be indicated by an excess of the control DNA hybridizing to the probes on the array that span the deletion site (Fig. 70-3). Conversely, if the patient's DNA contains a duplication of a chromosomal region, an excess of patient DNA will compete for hybridization to the encompassed probes on the array. The resolution for detecting these *copy number variants* (CNVs) is much finer than can be achieved by classic karyotype analysis under the light microscope, and is continually improving as ever greater numbers of probes, at ever diminishing base-pair intervals, are added to the arrays. And it is far more cost-effective and comprehensive than the previous analogous alternative of running many different fluorescence in situ hybridization (FISH) probes in series. As such, it has rapidly become a predominant technique for detecting deletions/duplications in patients with congenital problems that do not readily suggest a particular known genetic syndrome, including those with nonspecific physical malformations/dysmorphisms, developmental delay, and/or autism (Manning 2010; Miller 2010). However, it does have some limitations. First, because all it does is examine differences in hybridization intensity across the total genomic DNA, balanced translocations with no gain or loss of genetic material will not be detected. Second, all human genomes contain a great many CNVs that are nonpathologic. Some of these are well-known polymorphisms and thus can be discounted as etiologic if observed in a patient; but many others are not yet known or studied extensively, producing the challenging "CNV of uncertain clinical significance." Aside from using intuition based on the particular genes encompassed by the deletion, testing of the parents may also be helpful. If a normal parent carries the same deletion, it is less likely to be pathologic (though there are exceptions).The ultimate gold standard for identifying all possible mutations would of course be whole-genome sequencing. It took 13 years to completely sequence the consensus human genome under the Human Genome Project using conventional Sanger sequencing platforms (see Chapter 77). Now we have a new generation of automated DNA sequencers based on radically different chemistries, involving single-molecule pyrosequencing of millions of short fragments, which are then assembled into the full genome by the analysis software. These instruments are capable of sequencing a billion or more bases per day, at last putting the whole human genome in reach for routine analysis. However, at this point the appropriate clinical applications of the technology remain to be discerned. For one thing, the tremendous amount of data obtained would represent extreme overkill for the single-gene and

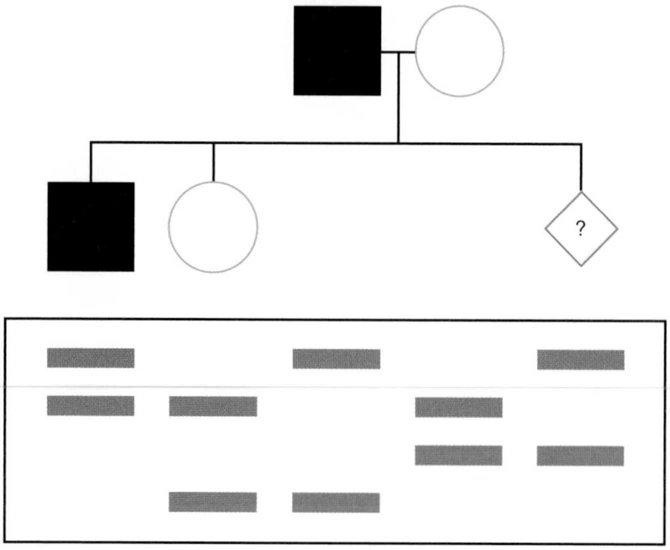

Figure 70-2 Example of restriction fragment length polymorphism analysis for prenatal diagnosis of an autosomal dominant disorder. In this Southern blot, the upper band from the father is the one that co-segregates with the disease phenotype, as seen in the affected son. Because the fetus (?) has also inherited this band, it is predicted to be affected. The precise risk depends on the map distance between the disease gene and the restriction fragment length polymorphism (RFLP) marker.

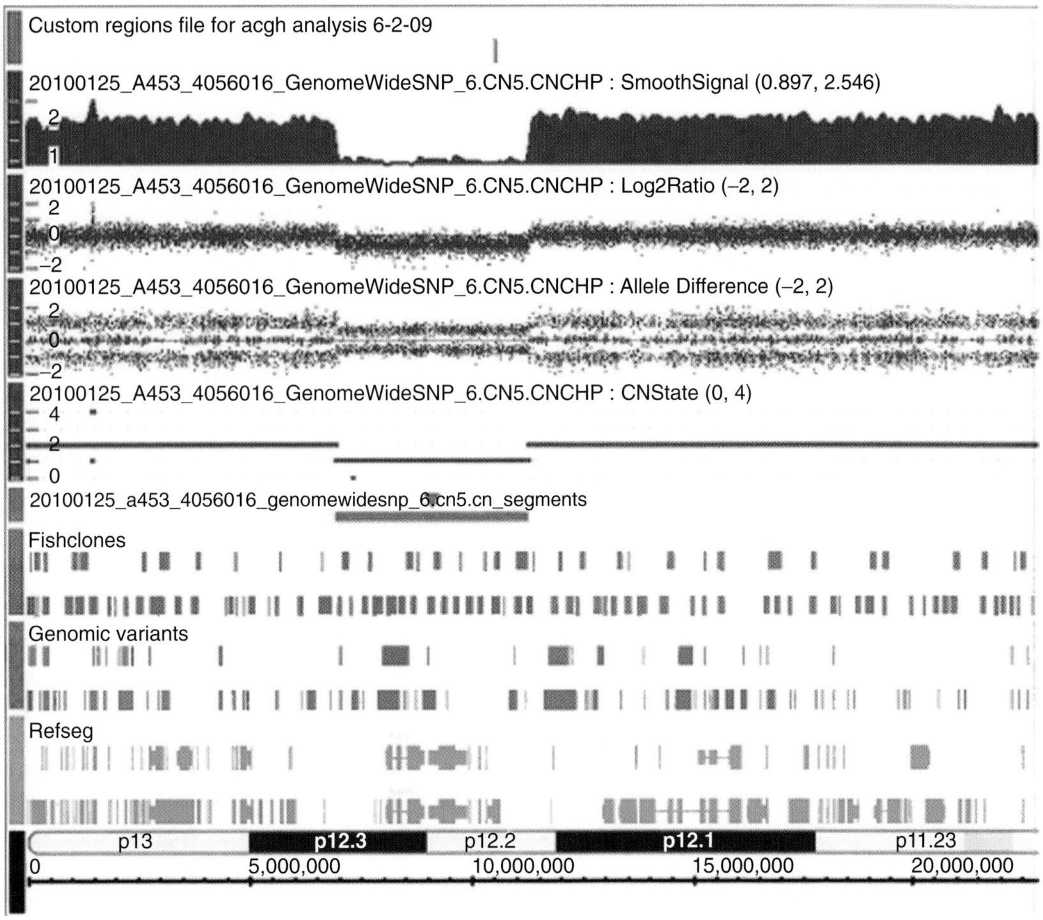

Figure 70-3 Example of a typical deletion result by array comparative hybridization. The gap in hybridization signal demarcated by the red line indicates a 4.329 Mb hemizygous deletion on chromosome 20p12.2-12.3 (6975661–11304543 bp). This deletion encompasses multiple genes, including *JAG1*, the gene implicated in Alagille syndrome, which was the clinical diagnosis in the tested patient. *(Courtesy Dr. Xinmin Li.)*

small multiplex applications we have today. Secondly, the data would reveal potentially concerning mutations in many other genes besides the ones immediately implicated in the patient's condition. And perhaps most importantly, for every real pathologic mutation detected, many thousands of missense variants of uncertain clinical significance would be revealed, potentially worrying the patient unnecessarily and demanding an endless amount of investigation on the part of the laboratory to sort them out (ten Bosch, 2008).

Choice of Applications

To some extent, the choice of technique will also depend on the application or clinical indication. In medical genetics, these applications fall into five major areas: carrier screening, newborn screening, diagnostic testing, presymptomatic DNA testing, and prenatal testing.

Carrier screening is the term applied to detection of recessive mutations in healthy individuals for purposes of genetic counseling and family planning. This application is further subdivided into screening of those individuals with a family history of the disorder and population-based screening of large numbers of individuals who have negative family history but who may be at risk for the disorder because of its prevalence within their ethnic group or in the population at large. In either case, the ultimate purpose is to identify couples at risk (i.e., both the man and the woman are heterozygous for mutations within the gene) who would then have a 25% chance of having an affected child with each pregnancy. But the testing strategies chosen for the two groups will differ. A person whose sibling has the disorder is at much higher risk of being a carrier than someone in the general population. That person may therefore warrant more aggressive testing (e.g., screening for a greater number of mutations or possibly linkage analysis or even complete gene sequencing) than would be cost-effective for a member of the general population. On the other hand, access to the affected sibling's DNA may allow prior identification of the familial mutation, which would render subsequent testing of other family members much easier. Population-based screening, in contrast, typically strives to keep the testing procedure as rapid and inexpensive as possible, focusing on perhaps a few of the more prevalent mutations, sacrificing clinical test sensitivity for cost-effectiveness and expediency. And, with negative family history there are no affected family members to make either single-site mutation testing or linkage analysis an option.

Like population-based carrier screening, *newborn screening* aims to identify relatively prevalent (as genetic diseases go) inherited defects in otherwise asymptomatic individuals. Indeed, the most important disease targets, such as phenylketonuria, galactosemia, sickle cell disease, and cystic fibrosis, are likewise autosomal recessive disorders. In this case, however, the goal is to ascertain affected babies early in life so that treatment (dietary or pharmaceutical) can be initiated before irreversible damage occurs. Currently, molecular genetic methods in this setting are employed mainly as a backup for confirmation of positive results ascertained by less expensive and more comprehensive biochemical or enzymatic methods, but this situation could reverse itself as molecular methods become increasingly cost-effective, high-throughput, and comprehensive.

Diagnostic genetic testing is, by definition, performed on a symptomatic individual. Because the DNA tests for genetic disease are absolutely disease-specific and the diseases themselves quite rare, these procedures do not cast a wide enough net to be used for extensive differential diagnosis; the symptoms must be sufficiently suggestive of the disorder in question to justify ordering the test. Also, one must weigh the DNA test against more traditional methods with regard to cost, convenience, and utility. For example, hemoglobin (Hb) electrophoresis may be more convenient and comprehensive for sorting out a suspected hemoglobinopathy than the specific DNA test for the sickle cell disease mutation alone. On the other hand, molecular testing may be more advantageous for early or atypical clinical presentations. For example, molecular testing for cystic fibrosis (CF) mutations can be performed in the newborn period when traditional sweat chloride analysis is either inconvenient or unreliable. In such cases it is also important to determine that the test represents the appropriate demographic. If not, a "negative" test may not be truly accurate. DNA tests also have the advantage of working well postmortem, when classic biochemical analytes can no longer be assessed.

Presymptomatic DNA testing is applied primarily to late-onset dominant disorders, in which the offspring of an affected parent are aware that they are at 50% risk of having inherited the disease gene and desire to know their status before its clinical onset to make informed reproductive, employment, and lifestyle decisions or initiate surveillance or preventive interventions. The prototypic disorders in this group are Huntington disease and the heritable cancer syndromes, although such diseases as neurofibromatosis, Marfan syndrome, adult polycystic kidney disease, and tuberous sclerosis are also relevant. This sort of testing has been the most problematic, from a psychosocial and ethical standpoint, of any in diagnostic molecular genetics, with the risk of severe adverse consequences of results reporting, including suicide. Because of this, established testing protocols include stipulations for informed consent, concurrent clinical assessment, extensive pretest and posttest genetic counseling, and psychosocial support (Huntington's Disease Society of America, 1989; American College of Medical Genetics, 1999).

Finally, there is the clinical application most distinctive to medical genetics: *prenatal testing*, or the detection of genetic disease in the fetus. With a few exceptions (e.g., hydrops fetalis in homozygous β-thalassemia, thanatophoric dwarfism, and type I osteogenesis imperfecta), most mendelian disorders, especially inborn errors of metabolism, are not expressed either visibly (by ultrasound) or biochemically in the fetus, so predictive diagnosis can only be made at the DNA level. Even for those disorders that might be detected biochemically, DNA often proves to be a far more accessible substrate, from an obstetric point of view, than the affected protein products or metabolic substrates. Whereas molecular analysis can be performed on minute amounts of amniotic fluid or chorionic villus samples collected by routine methods, even if obtained for other purposes, unless the protein product is expressed in fibroblasts (and thus amniocytes), biochemical analysis will require invasive biopsy of deep fetal tissues. For example, assay of phenylalanine hydroxylase activity to diagnose phenylketonuria would require fetal liver biopsy, and quantification of dystrophin to diagnose DMD would require fetal muscle biopsy.

The primary objective in prenatal diagnosis is the identification of an affected fetus in a timely manner so that a practical option of pregnancy termination can be offered to the couple. Even though some may argue an advantage for obtaining diagnosis prenatally so that therapy can be instituted promptly at birth, or for psychological reassurance of a couple if the fetus is found to be unaffected, it may be difficult to justify the risk (albeit low) of miscarriage from amniocentesis and chorionic villus sampling performed for these other purposes. For an affected fetus, unless one intends to initiate therapy in utero, provisional treatment at birth while awaiting confirmatory neonatal testing is perfectly acceptable.

Although prenatal genetic counseling is always nondirective, with moral and/or religious objections to abortion respected, both the clinical counselor and the DNA testing laboratory have a legitimate right and, indeed, responsibility to question the appropriateness of a prenatal test request, with its attendant risk and expense, from a couple for whom termination is not an option (the same would apply to requests coming too late in pregnancy for termination to be performed). It is because of these problems that invasive prenatal testing is not offered as a general population screening tool in women with no family history of the disorder in question. The power of PCR to enable single-cell genetic analysis has opened the way for preimplantation diagnosis, usually approached by performing in vitro fertilization and microdissection of a single blastomere from the early embryo. This strategy, initially applied to selected cases at risk for CF (Handyside, 1992) and other disorders, could potentially be offered to any at-risk couple for whom abortion is not an option, although it is not without its own ethical (and economic) objections. Recently it has begun to be used to diagnose adult-onset diseases such as familial breast/ovarian cancer (*BRCA1* and *BRCA2* genes), which, because they are late-onset, incompletely penetrant, and potentially treatable, would otherwise raise uncomfortable objections to traditional amniocentesis and pregnancy termination (Sagi, 2009).

Despite all these medical and moral dilemmas, when performed in appropriate circumstances, prenatal molecular genetic testing can offer at-risk couples, many of whom have already suffered the trauma of at least one affected child, one of the most valuable services in all of clinical medicine.

Special Concepts Unique to Molecular Genetic Disorders

Whereas the DNA analysis techniques discussed in this chapter for diagnosis of genetic disease are generally the same as those used for molecular diagnosis of cancer or infectious diseases, their application in the former has revealed a number of unusual phenomena that one must keep in mind when dealing with particular hereditary disorders. Some of these phenomena were known since Mendel's time but can now be understood mechanistically at the DNA level; others have emerged much more recently as unexpected byproducts of the molecular dissection of specific disease genes.

MOLECULAR HETEROGENEITY

Few genetic disorders are associated with a single mutation consistently identified in all affected cases (e.g., the missense mutation in codon 6 of the β-globin gene causing sickle cell disease). The vast majority of genetic disorders can be caused by more than one—sometimes hundreds—of different mutations within the disease gene (e.g., the *CFTR* gene of cystic fibrosis), and sometimes even by more than one gene (e.g., the *TSC1* and *TSC2* genes of tuberous sclerosis or the *BRCA1* and *BRCA2* genes of familial breast/ovarian cancer). Obviously, identifying the causative mutations in such disorders is technically much more difficult or sometimes impossible. A corollary of such molecular heterogeneity is that not all of the mutations will produce equally severe disease: some may cause only mild forms or even related syndromes with little resemblance to the classic phenotype (e.g., isolated absence of the vas deferens caused by certain mutations in the *CFTR* gene, or either multiple endocrine neoplasia or Hirschsprung disease caused by different mutations in the *RET* gene). All of this variability adds greatly to the complexity of genetic counseling and genetic testing.

VARIABLE PENETRANCE AND EXPRESSIVITY

Penetrance refers to the proportion of individuals who, having inherited a mutant disease gene, will actually display the disease phenotype. Usually applied to dominant disorders, it can produce the striking appearance of generation-skipping in disease pedigrees. This can complicate both molecular diagnostics and genetic counseling, because it may not be clear whether the propositus inherited the disease from a parent or instead represents a new mutation in the family. It is a feature of such relatively common genetic disorders as Marfan syndrome and neurofibromatosis.

Variable expressivity refers to the appearance of different signs and symptoms of a disorder in individuals inheriting the same mutation(s). Like penetrance, it is probably a reflection of differential gene effects within dissimilar genetic backgrounds (in other words, the modulation of phenotypic expression by other nonallelic genes). It, too, makes ascertainment and counseling difficult, and raises ethical issues in considering abortion for diseases of variable and unpredictable severity.

UNIPARENTAL DISOMY

This unusual cause of a recessive single-gene disorder was first discovered in a CF patient, only one of whose parents was a carrier (Spence, 1988). By DNA haplotyping using polymorphic markers, it was shown that the patient had inherited two copies of the carrier parent's chromosome 7 containing the mutant *CFTR* gene and no chromosome 7 from the other parent. The phenomenon has since been observed in other cases of CF and diseases involving other chromosomes as well. For some diseases, such as Prader-Willi and Angelman syndromes (see later discussion), the incidence of uniparental disomy approaches that of classic mutation mechanisms in the molecular pathogenesis, justifying routine testing for this phenomenon.

IMPRINTING

Imprinting refers to the differential expression of a gene in an offspring, depending on whether it was inherited from the mother or the father, or sometimes on other epigenetic influences. Some genes are only expressed or, conversely, turned off, when they pass through the oocyte lineage, and others only when they pass through the spermatocyte line. If an individual inherits the normal allele through the nonexpressing parental line, it cannot counteract a recessive mutation inherited from the other parent.

In at least some cases, the molecular mechanism appears to be differential methylation of chromosome regions and regulatory elements. This is the basis for both the deletional and uniparental disomy cases of Prader-Willi and Angelman syndromes (Gurrieri, 2009) (see later discussion).

ANTICIPATION

Anticipation refers to a progressive increase in severity and/or decrease in age of onset of a genetic disorder in subsequent generations of a family. It is typically associated with the trinucleotide repeat disorders, such as myotonic dystrophy and Huntington disease, in which the increasing severity can be correlated with further expansion of the repeat region. In the former disease, especially severe cases with childhood or infantile onset have been born to affected mothers, while in the latter disease the phenomenon occurs solely with paternal transmission, invoking an influence by imprinting as well (Koshy, 1997). It is for these reasons that accurate molecular sizing of trinucleotide repeat lengths is so important for diagnosis and genetic counseling in these disorders.

EPIGENETIC INFLUENCES AND NONMENDELIAN INHERITANCE

Epigenetic changes are heritable but potentially reversible changes in gene expression that do not represent a change in the sequence of the cell's genomic DNA. The most striking examples of epigenetic inheritance are genomic imprinting (discussed previously) and mammalian X-chromosome inactivation, both involving transcriptional silencing of genes by methylation of cytosines at CpG dinucleotides. The methylation status of DNA is maintained following DNA replication by methylases, which act on hemimethylated double-stranded DNA to methylate the newly synthesized DNA strand as well. The process is perpetuated indefinitely in succeeding cell divisions. Recent evidence suggests that de novo methylation of CpG doublets may take place in the promoters of some tumor suppressor genes, silencing these genes and in essence constituting one or both of the "hits" in a tumor suppressor gene that leads to tumor development (Jacinto, 2007).

Another category of epigenetic inheritance that is less clearly understood involves the property of some proteins to influence the conformation of newly synthesized or assembled proteins in a self-perpetuating manner. The most notable examples in mammals are the prion diseases, responsible for scrapie and bovine spongiform encephalopathy in animals and kuru and Creutzfeldt-Jakob disease in humans. The disease-producing prion protein, which may result from a coding sequence mutation in familial cases, is folded into an abnormal conformation and exerts an effect on newly synthesized prions in such a way that it perpetuates and proliferates the conformational abnormality that produces disease (Cobb, 2009).

ALLELE FREQUENCIES AND MASS POPULATION SCREENING

Reference has already been made to the application of carrier screening for recessive mutations on a population-wide basis. To justify, from a public health standpoint, the effort and expenditure required to perform a DNA test on thousands or millions of people, the incidence of the disease must be sufficiently high, either in the whole population or in the particular racial or ethnic groups being targeted for screening. For any autosomal recessive disease of appreciable incidence, the law of Hardy-Weinberg equilibrium predicts that the carrier frequency will be a good deal higher than the prevalence of affected individuals. In addition, the candidate disease target must be sufficiently severe and/or amenable to some medical intervention upon identification. Several disorders appear to fit these criteria. Mutations associated with hereditary hemochromatosis and activated protein C resistance (factor V Leiden) are found in 5%–10% of the Caucasian population, while the carrier frequency of the sickle cell mutation approaches 10% in the African American population. Unfortunately, controversies over disease penetrance in the first two and complex socioeconomic issues in the third have limited the application of these genes to screening (Grody, 2003a; Imperatore, 2003). Screening for thalassemia in Mediterranean and Asian populations, and for a panel of recessive disorders such as Tay-Sachs disease and Gaucher disease in the Ashkenazi-Jewish population, is similarly justified by allele frequencies in the target group. CF mutations, while of lower frequency, potentially place such a large majority of North American couples at risk that they have been chosen as the first target for general molecular genetic population screening in the United States (see later discussion). Other disease targets proposed for large-scale screening include spinal muscular atrophy, fragile X syndrome, and hereditary deafness. This migration of molecular genetic testing out of the realm of rare or esoteric diseases and into the setting of common traits will have a profound effect on preventive medicine and public health, and will drive new developments in DNA test automation in the coming years.

PREDICTIVE GENETIC TESTING

Unique among molecular pathology tests, and indeed among clinical laboratory tests in general, molecular genetic tests possess the ability to predict future disease in individuals with no signs or symptoms of the disorder at the time of testing. This predictive ability exceeds that imparted to such tests as human immunodeficiency virus antibody screening in individuals with no symptoms of acquired immunodeficiency syndrome, or cholesterol levels as a risk factor for future atherosclerosis. For those tests, one could argue that the serologic, microbiologic, or biochemical signs of the disorder are already present, even if the patient does not yet feel any symptoms. Molecular genetic testing, in contrast, enables prediction of future disease even in the absence of *any* biochemical or physiologic abnormalities: Huntington disease can be predicted decades before there is any brain degeneration, or breast cancer years or decades before even a single breast epithelial cell has turned malignant. The potential psychosocial impact of revealing such information in a healthy individual cannot be overemphasized. For that reason, predictive or presymptomatic genetic testing must be accompanied by pretest and posttest genetic counseling and psychiatric support. Furthermore, such tests should be restricted to those who truly have an actionable need for them, in the sense that a positive DNA test will prompt some sort of early surveillance or preventive interventions or, at the very least, some indicated lifestyle or life-planning changes. Because it is difficult to imagine such conditions existing in the case of a child tested for an adult-onset disease, there is a strong convention in the field that healthy children younger than 18 years of age should not be offered predictive genetic tests for adult-onset disorders, so as to avoid potential stigmatization, discrimination, or adverse psychosocial effects of genetic information that is of no medical use to the child (Holtzman, 1997).

SPECIFIC DISEASE EXAMPLES

CYSTIC FIBROSIS

Because of its high carrier frequency in North America and northern Europe, its serious clinical nature, its straightforward mendelian (autosomal recessive) inheritance pattern, and its well-studied yet complex gene, CF has emerged as the paradigmatic disorder for large-scale molecular genetic screening. Within its scope can be found the full panoply of applicable molecular genetic techniques and the full spectrum of scientific and ethical dilemmas arising from the clinical variability of the disease, the extreme molecular heterogeneity of the causative mutations, and the anticipated advent of novel treatments, including exon-skipping and gene replacement therapy. With a carrier frequency as high as 1 in 29 in Caucasians of northern European ancestry (and progressively less in southern Europeans, Hispanics, African Americans, and Asians), there was ample motivation to screen the general population in order to identify couples at 1 in 4 risk of having an affected child with each pregnancy. But because carriers are asymptomatic and have normal sweat chloride levels, this screening could only be done after isolation of the gene in 1989 (Kerem, 1989; Riordan, 1989). Even though the gene had been mapped to chromosome 7 some years earlier, allowing for prenatal diagnosis by linkage analysis in informative families, screening and testing in others, especially those with no family history of the disorder, could only be considered once the gene was cloned and the mutations identified.

Even with that laudable accomplishment, however, the history of DNA testing for CF has been fraught with problems and controversies. The gene is more than 250,000bp long and encodes a large ion channel protein called the cystic fibrosis transmembrane conductance regulator (CFTR) (Collins, 1992). Most notably, the spectrum of mutations observed is remarkably heterogeneous. Whereas a three-nucleotide deletion of phenylalanine codon 508 (designated ΔΔF508) accounts for about 70% of the mutations in non-Hispanic Caucasians (and significantly less in other ethnic/racial groups), more than 1500 additional mutations have so far been reported. Most of these are so rare that it is neither feasible nor cost-effective to include them in testing panels; only about seven (in addition to ΔF508)

TABLE 70-1

Recommended Core Mutation Panel for General Population Cystic Fibrosis Carrier Screening

ΔF508	ΔI507	G542X	G551D	W1282X	N1303K
R553X	621+1G>T	R117H	1717–1G>A	A455E	R560T
R1162X	G85E	R334W	R347P	711+1G>T	1898+1G>A
2184delA	1078delT*	3849+ 10kbC>T	2789+5G>A	3659delC	I148T*
3120+1G>A					

Panel recommended by the American College of Medical Genetics (Grody, 2001a).
*Mutations subsequently removed from the panel (Watson, 2004).

account for more than 1% each of CF mutations in most Caucasian populations (Tsui, 1992) (Table 70-1). The sensitivity of carrier screening with mutation panels of between six and 25 alleles ranges from a high of 97% in Ashkenazi Jews (Abeliovich, 1992) to 75%–90% in non–Ashkenazi North American Caucasians, about 60% in Hispanic Americans, 50% in African Americans, and less than 10% in Asians (Ober, 1992; Grebe, 1994; Macek, 1997). Such variable and suboptimal sensitivity in an ethnically heterogeneous population like that of the United States, and the difficulties involved in counseling patients as to the residual carrier risk of negative test results, made population-based carrier screening for CF mutations a controversial subject (Grody, 1999). After much debate and several pilot screening studies, a consensus conference recommended that screening be offered to all pregnant couples and those planning pregnancy (NIH Consensus Statement Online, 1997). A steering committee representing the American College of Medical Genetics (ACMG), the American College of Obstetricians and Gynecologists (ACOG), and the National Human Genome Research Institute decided on a core screening panel of the 25 most prevalent mutations in the general mixed population (Grody, 2001a). The same group produced accompanying educational materials providing guidance to obstetricians on how the screening test should be offered, patient education brochures, and tables for determining the residual risk in those whose test results are negative.

With the launch of these guidelines in 2001, *CFTR* mutation analysis instantly became the highest volume molecular genetic test and one of the highest in all of molecular diagnostics. Given such a market, reagent and instrumentation vendors soon came forward with a variety of assays and platforms, which have now largely replaced the in-house methods previously employed by individual laboratories. The commercial methods, which incorporate at least the core panel of 25 mutations (revised downward to 23 in 2004 by Watson et al, 2004), and sometimes more, include ASO probes on paper strips, ARMS, OLA, Invader assay, microbead arrays, and microarray chips (Richards, 2004). In addition, complete gene sequencing is offered by a few laboratories (Strom, 2003), although it is too expensive for general carrier screening and is used primarily to assist in diagnosis of atypical CF cases or to identify parental mutations in affected offspring to enable prenatal diagnosis in future pregnancies.

Even years after launch, the CF carrier screening program continues to prove challenging for both the referring obstetricians and the genetic testing laboratories. Questions remain about uptake, proper communication of results, the utility of offering extended mutation panels (especially for those couples who test positive–negative in the initial screen), and even which mutations should be included in the core panel. The panel has already been modified once, after early data from national screening indicated that one of the mutations (1078delT) was more rare than previously thought, and another one (I148T) was not a mutation at all but a benign polymorphism; both of these have since been dropped (Watson, 2004). And at the other extreme, driven largely by marketing considerations, laboratories have been compelled to offer ever-larger mutation screening panels, and concern has been raised regarding the clinical significance of some of the added mutations (Grody, 2007). One large series has shown that the core mutation panel is indeed adequate for identifying the vast majority of carriers, with no additional mutations recurring in sufficient numbers to justify their incorporation into an expanded panel (Strom, 2011).

Another problem with genetic counseling for CF is the variable clinical severity of the disorder and the inconsistency of genotype–phenotype correlations. Beyond the finding that ΔΔF508 homozygotes tend to have pancreatic insufficiency, there is little about disease severity or complications that can be predicted reliably from knowing an affected individual's two mutations (Moskowitz, 2008). Even homozygotes for ΔΔF508, considered the prototypical severe mutation, can show a wide range in their degree of pulmonary compromise (Burke, 1992). Conversely, there are mutations that cause pulmonary disease yet maintain normal sweat chloride levels (Highsmith, 1994), and there are mutations and polymorphisms (e.g., R117H coupled with certain lengths of an intronic polythymidine tract) that do not cause CF at all but rather male infertility due to congenital absence of the vas deferens (Anguiano, 1992; Gervais, 1993). Taken together with the ever-increasing median lifespan of CF patients and the eventual advent of effective gene replacement therapies, these factors render genetic counseling and reproductive decision-making for the disorder difficult.

Cystic fibrosis is one of the targets of universal newborn screening in most states, along with a large panel of metabolic disorders (CDC, 2008). Protocols vary by state, but in most cases begin with a biochemical screen for immunoreactive trypsinogen, followed by (in positive specimens) molecular testing for anywhere from one to more than 30 mutations. It is important to remember that the mutation panels chosen for newborn screening are up to the individual states and are not tied in any way to the ACMG/ACOG panel developed for population carrier screening. Likewise, mutations tested in the course of diagnostic workup of a symptomatic patient are also flexible (in the sense that they have never been defined by professional guidelines) and may range from just a few ethnic-specific mutations to complete gene sequencing.

DUCHENNE MUSCULAR DYSTROPHY

This X-linked progressive myopathy was the first disorder whose causative gene was isolated by the process of positional cloning (Rowland, 1988). Before that discovery, the only tests that could be offered to at-risk families were detection of some female carriers by the finding of elevated serum creatine phosphokinase levels, followed by prenatal sex determination with the option to terminate a male fetus (even though 50% of these pregnancies would be normal). Genetic counseling was rendered even more problematic because about one third of cases of DMD arise from new mutations.

Even after its discovery, translation to clinical application was not easy because the gene, dubbed *dystrophin*, proved to be the largest yet discovered, spanning 2.4 million bp and composed of 79 exons (Ahn, 1993). Use of full-length or partial cDNA probes to detect the variety of deletions accounting for two thirds of cases was labor-intensive and time-consuming (Darras, 1988; Prior, 1991). It was only with the advent of multiplex PCR, described in Chapter 66, that a system was developed for rapid and inexpensive identification of more than 98% of dystrophin deletions and their localization to specific exons of the gene (Beggs, 1990; Multicenter Study Group, 1992). In this system a deletion is identified by absence of one or more of the multiple expected amplicons on ethidium bromide-stained electrophoresis gels or capillary electrophoresis instruments (because a target gene deletion will abolish the hybridization site[s] of one or more primers, causing PCR failure) (Fig. 70-4). Such fine-structure mapping combined with sequencing has also revealed important insights into the molecular pathogenesis of DMD and the milder allelic variant, Becker muscular dystrophy (BMD). Both are most often caused by large dystrophin deletions, but those in BMD typically preserve the correct reading frame in the resulting processed transcript, while deletions in DMD more often produce frameshift mutations and a more truncated protein product (Monaco, 1988).

The remaining one third of patients with DMD and 15% of patients with BMD in whom no deletion is detected usually have point mutations or microdeletions/insertions. Because the gene is so large, it is not an easy matter to identify these lesions directly, although gene scanning by conformational analysis (SSCP, DGGE) followed by sequencing has been used effectively (Prior 1995; Torella 2010). Until recently, if that method failed,

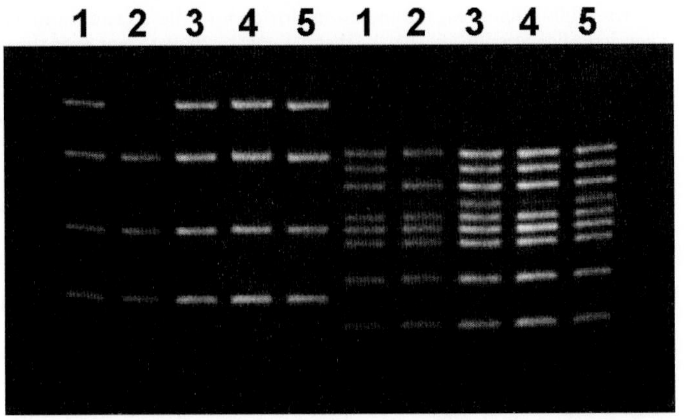

Figure 70-4 Multiplex polymerase chain reaction (PCR) analysis for dystrophin gene deletions in Duchenne muscular dystrophy. DNA samples from five patients were amplified simultaneously with five primer pairs (left half of gel) and nine primer pairs (right half of gel) and the products were analyzed by polyacrylamide gel electrophoresis. Absence of an expected PCR product band is indicative of a deletion. Patient 2 lacks the top band in the five-plex and the second-from-top band in the nine-plex; these correspond to deletions in exons 50 and 48, respectively, in the dystrophin gene. (Band 4 in the nine-plex is light but present in all of the samples.) *(Courtesy Dr Kathryn E. Kronquist.)*

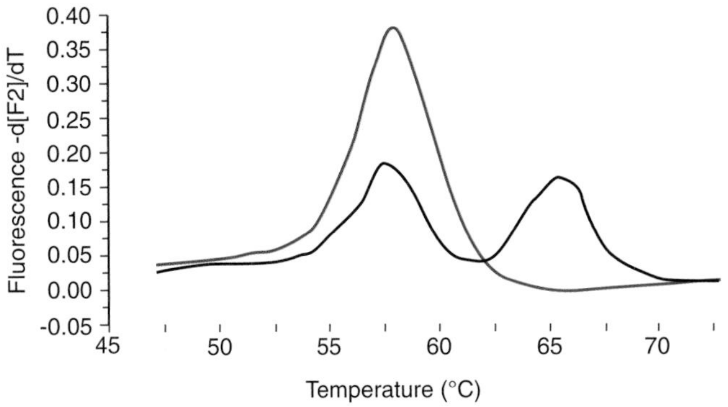

Figure 70-5 Detection of the factor V Leiden mutation by real-time polymerase chain reaction (PCR) and melting curve analysis. Mismatch of the amplified mutant allele lowers the melting temperature when hybridized with a wild type DNA probe. The black line indicates the melting curve profile for an R506Q heterozygote, whereas the red curve represents a homozygous mutant sample.

one had to revert to linkage analysis. Now, however, full-gene sequencing, even of this large locus, has become feasible using both capillary or next-generation sequencing (Hamed, 2006). Alternatively, studies at the protein level can be performed by observing decreased or absent dystrophin in DMD, and dystrophin of abnormal molecular weight in BMD, by western blot or immunohistochemistry of muscle biopsy tissue (Hoffman, 1988). This procedure has serious limitations for prenatal diagnosis, for which a fetal muscle biopsy would be required, but it can be used for proband diagnosis. Thus the molecular diagnosis of DMD has come full circle: from identification of the gene without knowing the protein product (reverse genetics) to identification and diagnostic use of the protein product from knowing the gene. This sort of evolution can be expected in the laboratory diagnosis of many genetic diseases, because functional studies of a gene product are by definition more comprehensive than attempting to track down countless individual mutations at the DNA level.

SICKLE CELL ANEMIA AND OTHER HEMOGLOBINOPATHIES

Given the long history of study of the protein product, diagnosis of molecular defects in the genes encoding the globin polypeptides did not come about through techniques of reverse genetics; rather, these genes were cloned by classic methods, using antiglobin antibodies for polysome precipitation to isolate the relevant messenger ribonucleic acids (mRNAs). As such, Hb mutations, and the one causing sickle cell anemia in particular, were among the very first to be diagnosed at the DNA level. The sickle cell point mutation in codon 6 of the β-globin gene lies within (and thus destroys) a restriction endonuclease cleavage site (for *Mst*II, *Mnl*I or *Dde*I), providing a rapid method of detection using either Southern blot or restriction enzyme digestion of β-globin PCR products (Hatcher, 1992) (see Fig. 70-1). Alternatively, the HbS and HbA sequences can be distinguished by dot blot using allele-specific oligonucleotide probes complementary to either the normal or mutant sequence (Conner, 1983). More recently, higher-throughput techniques have come to predominate, such as real-time PCR and melting curve analysis (Traeger-Synodinos, 2008). These DNA-based techniques can be used for diagnosis, carrier screening, or prenatal diagnosis on amniocytes, in the latter case obviating the need for invasive fetal blood sampling and classic Hb electrophoresis. In addition, as more states initiate newborn screening programs for sickle cell disease, even if done by biochemical methods, the DNA test becomes important for backup confirmation of positives and ambiguous screening results, as in compound heterozygous states involving HbS and a thalassemia mutation. Several studies have shown that these DNA tests can be done on the same filter-paper blood spots collected for the initial newborn screening (McCabe, 2004). A different mutation in codon 6, causing HbC disease, does not abolish the *Mst*II restriction endonuclease recognition sequence (because it occurs at a flexible nucleotide position for the enzyme) and so must be distinguished by ASO probes (Maggio, 1993).

The thalassemias involve both qualitative and quantitative alterations in one or more globin chains with hundreds of sequence variants known, and their diagnosis at the molecular level is correspondingly more complex than that of sickle cell anemia. α-Thalassemia is the more straightforward, because it is usually caused by deletion of either or both of the two contiguous α genes on one or the other or both chromosomes 16. This can be detected by Southern blot or quantitative PCR, allowing differentiation of the silent carrier state (one α gene missing) from the very severe hydrops fetalis (all four genes missing) and the two intermediate states (Oron-Karni, 1998). Molecular diagnosis of β-thalassemia is more complicated because of the wide variety of promoter, termination, deletion, splice site, and frameshift mutations that have been documented. However, within each at-risk population (Mediterranean, Asian, African), a limited subset of mutations (usually 10 or less) accounts for the majority of cases and carriers. Therefore testing with a panel of mutation-specific probes/primers, along the lines of CF screening, is reasonable (Naja, 2004; Patrinos, 2005). In addition, the β-globin gene is not that large, so sequencing or gene scanning can also be employed.

HEREDITARY THROMBOPHILIAS

CF is not the only disorder with sufficiently high mutation frequency to consider population screening using molecular methods. Several other disease genes have revealed carrier frequencies several times higher than that for cystic fibrosis. Included in this group are genes involved in the anticoagulant system, which, as discussed in Part V keeps the clotting cascade in check. The most notable such allele is the factor V Leiden mutation, a single nucleotide change causing an amino acid substitution (R506Q) in the clotting factor V protein, rendering it resistant to cleavage by activated protein C (Bertina, 1994). The allele is carried in 5%–7% of the Caucasian population and is responsible for more than 90% of clinical activated protein C (APC) resistance, resulting in a tendency toward idiopathic venous thromboembolism (Ridker, 1997a). It produces a relative risk of thrombosis of about sevenfold in the heterozygous state and about eightyfold in the homozygous state. It is also associated with pregnancy complications such as recurrent miscarriage. Testing for the mutation is straightforward because, like the sickle cell mutation, it destroys a restriction endonuclease cleavage site, and automated methods for higher throughput have been developed, such as real-time PCR (Louis, 2004) (Fig. 70-5) and the Invader assay, which relies on signal amplification by fluorescent resonance energy transfer and a cleavase enzyme (Ryan, 1999), as described in Chapter 66.

As for cystic fibrosis, however, there are controversies over which patients should be offered screening. Despite the dramatically increased relative risk, the absolute risk conferred by this mutation is rather low, with a lifetime penetrance for thrombotic symptoms of about 10%. Most carriers therefore would not be candidates for anticoagulant therapy, with its risks of hemorrhage and stroke, and so it is uncertain whether such screening would alter patient management in a meaningful way. Some have proposed screening individuals with environmental risk factors known to act synergistically with the factor V Leiden risk, such as women on oral contraceptives. Yet here too it could be argued that obligating such women with positive test results to turn to less effective methods of birth control might cause more harm than good, increasing the pregnancy rate with its own attendant complications, some of which are thrombotic in nature (Kupferminc, 1999). At present, most requests received by molecular genetics laboratories for factor V Leiden testing are on patients who have already experienced an otherwise unexplained thromboembolic event, and two professional consensus statements, by the ACMG and the College of American Pathologists (CAP), have designated this as the primary unequivocal indication for testing (Grody 2001b; Press, 2002).

Along with factor V Leiden, there are other inherited mutations of high allele frequency that confer thrombotic risk (also discussed in Part 5). The prothrombin 20210A variant, a single nucleotide change in the 3′ untranslated region of the prothrombin gene, results in increased circulating prothrombin levels and a phenotype similar to that of factor V Leiden; it is present in 1%–2% of the general population (Poort, 1996). The 677C→T variant of methylenetetrahydrofolate reductase, an enzyme involved in the folate cycle of homocysteine metabolism, is carried by 30%–40% of the general population and is associated with elevated plasma homocysteine levels and theoretical risk of vascular (including coronary artery) thrombosis. Indications for this test are even more nebulous, because not everyone with the variant has hyperhomocysteinemia, and not all hyperhomocysteinemia is caused by this variant. Thus biochemical measurement of plasma homocysteine levels may be a more effective screening method. Also, folate fortification of foods may make the genetic factor less relevant by broadly reducing homocysteine levels in the population. And recent studies have even called into question whether there is any relationship at all between homocysteine levels and thrombotic risk (Ducros, 2009). Even so, the mutations for each of these factors can act synergistically with one another, so that patients carrying two or even three of these defects, including also the rarer deficiencies of protein S and C, are at greater increased risk (Koeleman, 1994; Ridker, 1997b). DNA tests for several of these thrombophilia mutations can be multiplexed in a single assay (Louis, 2004).

TRINUCLEOTIDE REPEAT EXPANSION DISORDERS

An important class of disease-causing mutations was revealed in 1991 with the discovery that X-linked spinal and bulbar muscular atrophy (Kennedy's disease, SBMA) and fragile X syndrome (FRAXA) are associated with amplification of unstable trinucleotide repeat sequences in the androgen receptor (*AR*) and *FMR1* (fragile X mental retardation) genes, respectively. Since that time, similar disease-producing mutations have been associated with several additional neurologic and muscle disorders (Table 70-2), and in the process have provided a molecular classification of the spinocerebellar ataxias. The affected gene in each of these disorders normally contains a repeated sequence of 3bp, for example, $(CGG)_n$ in the *FMR1* gene, where n is variable but normally limited in its range. In the disease state, however, the size of the triplet repeat is expanded outside the normal range, sometimes only slightly and in other instances markedly. The mechanisms by which these expanded repeat sequences produce disease are

TABLE 70-2
Disorders Characterized by Unstable Expansions of DNA Trinucleotide Repeats

Disorder	Chromosome Location	Normal Alleles, Intermediate Alleles	Expanded Alleles	Anticipation	Transmission Sex Bias	Position of Repeat	Gene Product
Fragile Site/Mental Retardation Associated with CGG or GCC Expansion (X-Linked)							
Fragile X syndrome (CGG), FRAXA	Xq27	6–54 55–200	>200	Yes	Maternal, full mutation	5′-UTR	FMR-1
Fragile X syndrome (GCC), FRAXE	Xq28	6–25	>200			5′-UTR	FMR-2
Diseases Associated with CAG Repeat Expansion (Autosomal Dominant Except for X-Linked Kennedy's Disease)							
Spinobulbar muscular atrophy (Kennedy's disease)	Xq11–12	11–33	36–62			Coding	Androgen receptor
Huntington disease	4p16	6–35 36–39	40–121	Marked in juvenile cases	Paternal, early onset	Coding	Huntingtin
Dentatorubral-pallidoluysian atrophy	12p13	3–35	49–85	Yes	Paternal	Coding	Atrophin
Spinocerebellar ataxia 1	6p23	6–44	40–81	Marked in juvenile cases	Paternal, early onset	Coding	Ataxin 1
Spinocerebellar ataxia 2	12q24	16–31	36–64	Yes	Paternal	Coding	Ataxin 2
Spinocerebellar ataxia 3 (Machado-Joseph disease)	l4q24–q31	12–41	55–84	Yes	Paternal	Coding	Ataxin 3
Spinocerebellar ataxia 6	19p13	6–17	21–30	Yes	Paternal	Coding	CACNA1A
Spinocerebellar ataxia 7	3p21–pl2	4–35 28–3	37–>200	Yes	Paternal	Coding	Ataxia-7
Spinocerebellar ataxia 12	5q31–q33	7–28	66–78	Yes	Paternal	5′-UTR	PPP2R2B
Spinocerebellar ataxia 17	6p27	25–42	45–63	Yes	Paternal	Coding	TBP
Diseases Associated with CTG Expansion (Autosomal Dominant)							
Myotonic dystrophy	19q13	5–35	50–>200	Yes	Maternal congenital form	3′-UTR	Myotonin protein kinase
Spinocerebellar ataxia 8	13q21	16–92	110–130	Yes	Maternal	Noncoding	
Disease Associated with GAA Expansion (Autosomal Recessive)							
Friedreich ataxia	9q13	6–36	200–>900	No		Intron	Frataxin

various, and include gene silencing and toxic gain-of-function by mutant proteins.

Fragile XA and Fragile XE Syndromes

FRAXA is the most common single-gene defect causing moderate to severe mental retardation in males. Affected males with this X-linked disorder typically also exhibit dysmorphic features including large ears, a long face, prominent jaw, and macroorchidism. Approximately 1 in 2500 females are heterozygous carriers of the FRAXA mutation, and one third of these may show evidence of mental impairment or learning disability in the absence of the classic dysmorphism seen in affected males.

As explained in Chapter 68, the cytogenetic hallmark of FRAXA is a fragile site on the X chromosome at Xq27.3, resulting from a failure of normal chromatin condensation during mitosis. Although the inheritance pattern of the disease is clearly X-linked, it does not correspond in a straightforward manner to either a recessive or dominant pattern of gene expression. Before the molecular mechanism was elucidated, the most puzzling feature had been the presence of phenotypically normal men (transmitting males) who are obligate carriers of the genetic abnormality. These men are sons of proven FRAXA carriers, they pass the carrier state to all of their daughters, and their daughters in turn transmit the fully expressed disease to a high proportion of their sons.

The discovery in 1991 of the genetic abnormality that causes FRAXA immediately explained its unusual pattern of inheritance (Fu, 1991). The 5′ untranslated region of the *FMR1* gene at chromosome Xq27.3 carries a $(CGG)_n$ triplet repeat of variable size. In normal individuals, *n* ranges up to about 54, but in individuals with clinically apparent FRAXA, *n* is greater than 200 (referred to as a *full mutation*). Both men and women who carry an X chromosome where *n* is between 55 and about 200-230 (referred to as a *premutation*) do not show signs of classic fragile X syndrome, but are at risk of passing an allele of even larger size to their children. This is because of the instability of the premutation alleles and their tendency to increase in size during the meiotic cell divisions that produce the male and female gametes. Alleles of normal size are not unstable and generally pass unchanged, although there is now recognized a so-called gray area of repeats between 46 and 54 that has a low risk of slight expansion into the premutation range (Kronquist, 2008). Thus it appears that there is a pool of small premutation (and gray area) alleles in the population, possibly of ancient origin, that is at risk of undergoing further expansion with each passage through another generation. As the premutation allele increases in size, the likelihood that it will expand further in the next generation increases, ranging from very low likelihood for repeats in the 60s to almost 100% for repeats above 100 (Nolin, 2003). Curiously, expansion to a full mutation occurs only in female meiosis, never in males, which corresponds to the observation that the daughters of normal transmitting males are always phenotypically normal. Fig. 70-6, *B*, illustrates a family with FRAXA: a premutation allele is transmitted from the first to the second generation, and then expands to a full mutation in the third generation.

The mechanism by which the expanded triplet repeat in the 5′ noncoding region of the *FMR1* gene produces the FRAXA phenotype is under active investigation. As the size of the repeat expands, there is progressive methylation of the regulatory region of the *FMR1* gene and decreased expression of FMR-1 protein. This RNA-binding protein is widely expressed in the developing brain and in other tissues. Its loss of expression in FRAXA presumably disturbs normal brain development and leads to mental retardation. Rare patients with typical fragile X syndrome do not have triplet repeat expansion or gene hypermethylation but do have inactivating point mutations leading to loss of FMR1 protein expression. Conversely, rare phenotypically normal or high-functioning males with full *FMR1* gene repeat expansions and cytogenetically visible fragile sites, but with no gene hypermethylation and normal FMR1 protein expression, have been described (Hagerman, 1994; Smeets, 1995). These findings all support the hypothesis that it is lack of FMR1 protein expression, usually caused by hypermethylation-related downregulation of gene transcription, that is responsible for the disease phenotype.

Because the premutation is not methylated and the phenomenon of "normal" transmitting males was widely observed, it was long assumed that these alleles had no direct phenotypic effect. It was therefore quite surprising when more recent studies documented cases of premature ovarian failure and an unusual tremor-ataxia-dementia syndrome in female and male premutation carriers, respectively. The penetrance appears to be about 20% for the former (Sherman, 2000) and as high as 75% for the latter (Jacquemont, 2004), although it is difficult to accurately define such numbers in the absence of molecular screening of normal populations. The molecular mechanism may be related to premutation *FMR1* mRNAs being translated less efficiently and/or interfering with translation of the normal allele or other interacting genes. These revelations have made genetic counseling for fragile X syndrome even more complicated. They also raise additional concerns regarding the ethical merits of population screening for fragile X premutations or routine testing of pregnant women, which appears to be increasing. Babies born to women who have undergone testing may be identified with a potentially devastating adult-onset disease for which no known preventive intervention is possible, something that is not done for predictive genetic testing of other late-onset disorders in children for the reasons discussed in the section on Predictive Genetic Testing above.

Rare families with X-linked mental retardation and a cytogenetically demonstrable fragile site at chromosome Xq27–28, but no hypermethylation or expansion of the $(CGG)_n$ repeat in *FMR1*, led to the discovery of a second, more distal fragile site at Xq28 associated with hypermethylation and expansion of a $(GCC)_n$ repeat (FRAXE). Most affected males show only mild mental impairment without the dysmorphic features of FRAXA; this plus the extreme rarity of the condition have called into question the indications for testing and screening (Brown, 1996), and in practice the test is seldom ordered.

Neurodegenerative Disorders: Huntington Disease, X-linked Spinal and Bulbar Muscular Atrophy, Spinocerebellar Ataxias, and Dentatorubral-Pallidoluysian Atrophy

Huntington disease, X-linked spinal and bulbar muscular atrophy (SBMA), the spinocerebellar ataxias, and dentatorubral-pallidoluysian atrophy (DRPLA) are autosomal dominant or X-linked (SBMA) diseases characterized by selective neuronal degeneration in the central nervous system. In each of these disorders there is expansion of a $(CAG)_n$ trinucleotide repeat in the coding region of the respective gene that produces abnormal elongation of a polyglutamine tract. The resultant abnormal protein produces intranuclear neuronal inclusions. It is postulated that the expanded polyglutamine sequences in each of these proteins leads to alterations in their folding and binding characteristics and a gain in function that is toxic to neurons in a selective manner, causing apoptosis (Everett, 2004). Intranuclear neuronal inclusions, produced by these abnormal proteins, have been demonstrated in several of these disorders.

In common with the other triplet repeat disorders, the expanded repeats in the neurodegenerative disorders are unstable and tend to increase in size in subsequent generations. There is a positive, but not absolute, correlation between increasing repeat size, early disease onset, and clinical severity. In contrast to fragile X and myotonic dystrophy, where the most dramatic increases in repeat size occur in maternal meioses, paternal transmission produces the largest expansions in the exonic repeat neurodegenerative disorders. Consequently, juvenile-onset cases of Huntington disease, DRPLA, and the spinocerebellar ataxias are typically transmitted by an affected father.

Molecular diagnosis of these disorders is used for either diagnostic or, because they are late-onset, predictive purposes. Because they have no treatment, the emotions involved in the testing and fear of a positive result are considerable.

Myotonic Dystrophy

Myotonic dystrophy is an autosomal dominant, multisystem disorder with a wide range of clinical expression. In late childhood or early adulthood, the most typical patients develop progressive myotonia and weakness and atrophy of the muscles of the distal extremities and face. Cataracts, cardiac conduction defects, and testicular atrophy are also common. However, the disease may be so mild as to consist solely of cataracts developing in old age or so severe as to present at birth with marked muscle degeneration and mental retardation proceeding to early death. Sometimes the full spectrum of the disease can be observed in the same family, occurring in a pattern that clearly reflects the phenomenon of anticipation. As noted, anticipation is present in virtually all of the trinucleotide repeat disorders, but it is most striking in myotonic dystrophy, in which the clinical phenotype can progress from cataracts to severe congenital disease in three generations.

Myotonic dystrophy is caused by expansion of a $(CTG)_n$ repeat in the 3′ untranslated region of the myotonin protein kinase gene on chromosome 19q13.3 (Fu, 1992; Mahadevan, 1992). In normal individuals, this repeat ranges in size from 5 to 35 and is genetically stable. CTG repeats greater than 50 are genetically unstable and prone to expansion as they are passed to subsequent generations. In the range of 50–100, these repeats

PART 8

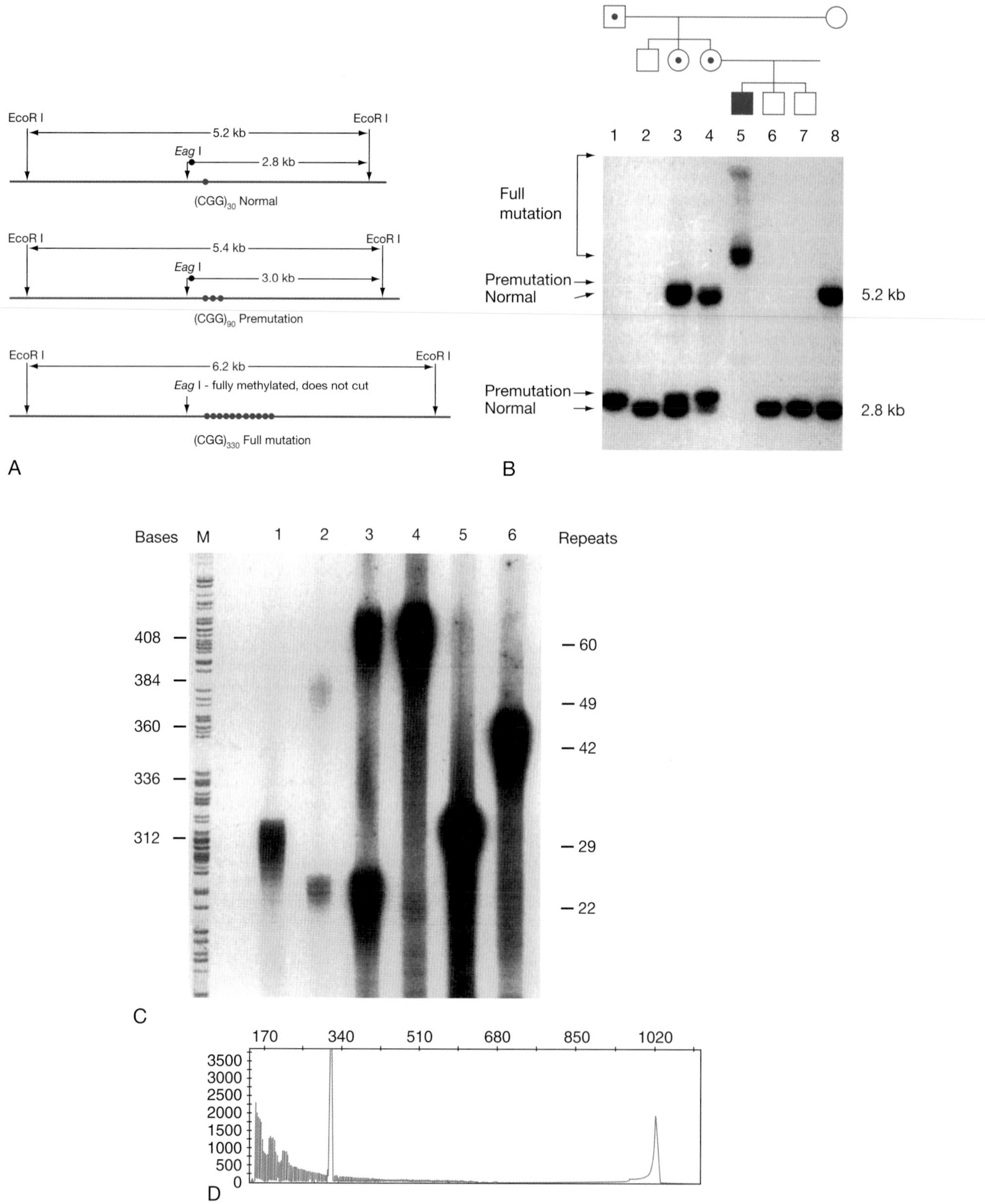

Figure 70-6 Detection of the (CGG)*n* repeat expansion in fragile X syndrome. **A,** Diagram of normal, premutation, and full-mutation alleles at the FRAXA locus. When expansion of the repeat to a full mutation occurs, the *Eag* I restriction enzyme site becomes methylated and does not cut with the enzyme. **B,** Family of a patient (darkened square) with fragile X syndrome. A Southern blot of *EcoRI/Eag* I-digested DNA from each individual in the pedigree was examined with a labeled DNA probe that hybridizes 3′ to the repeat. The three individuals on the right of the figure are normal (open squares and circles). Note that the two males each have a single 2.8-kb band, while the female has both a 2.8- and a 5.2-kb band. This is the expected result. The 5.2-kb band in the female is from the normal inactive (therefore methylated) X chromosome in each of her cells. Because the DNA on this chromosome is methylated, it is not cut by *EagI*. The 2.8-kb band, however, is from the normal unmethylated active X chromosome (*EagI* will cut the DNA in this case) in the female and in the males. The affected male has a greatly enlarged band. This is a consequence of marked expansion of the trinucleotide repeat as well as methylation of the *EagI* restriction enzyme site. The three individuals marked by bold dots are carriers of premutation alleles. In the females, the distinction between normal and expanded alleles is seen most clearly in DNA from their active (unmethylated) X chromosomes. Here, there are distinct bands of 2.8 and 3 kb. Higher in the gel the resolution is not as good, and the 5.2- and 5.4-kb alleles are barely separated. Note that in this peripheral blood sample from the mother of the affected patient, X chromosome inactivation is skewed with respect to the repeat expansion: a greater proportion of normal X chromosomes in this cell population have randomly been inactivated compared to the X chromosomes carrying the premutation allele. **C,** Sizing of trinucleotide repeats by gel electrophoresis following amplification of the locus by the polymerase chain reaction (PCR). Lanes 1 through 6 represent six different individuals; lane M contains a size marker. The PCR products were labeled by incorporation of 32P-dCTP during the amplification reaction and the dried gel was exposed to X-ray film. Heterozygous females show two alleles; males and homozygous females show single alleles. The multiple bands produced with each allele are due to "slippage" of the DNA polymerase during the PCR reaction; the most intense band is taken as representative of the actual size of the allele. **D,** Successful PCR amplification of both the normal (left peak, 30 CGG repeats) and full-mutation (right peak) alleles in a female heterozygote, using reagents from Asuragen, Austin, Texas). *(**C,** Courtesy Dr Anne Maddalena; **D,** courtesy Dr. Joshua Deignan.)*

are often asymptomatic or produce minimal symptoms. When more than 100 repeats are present, the typical myotonic dystrophy phenotype is likely. Although there is a general correlation between repeat length and clinical severity, the size of the repeat is not a reliable prognostic indicator in the individual case. The extreme expansions to 1000–2000 repeats seen in congenital myotonic dystrophy occur only with female transmission of the unstable repeat; thus congenital myotonic dystrophy is always inherited from an affected mother.

The mechanism by which the expanded trinucleotide repeat in the myotonin protein kinase gene produces the myotonic dystrophy phenotype is not known. Because the repeat is not located in the coding region of the gene, it is possible that protein expression is altered or that RNA processing interactions are perturbed.

Friedreich Ataxia

Friedreich ataxia is the most common of the hereditary ataxias, with an incidence of 2 per 100,000. Unlike the other trinucleotide repeat disorders, Friedreich ataxia is inherited as an autosomal recessive disease and shows no evidence of anticipation. The expanded $(GAA)_n$ repeat is located in the first intron of the *FRDA* gene and reduces the expression of frataxin, a mitochondrial targeted protein, probably through some interference with transcription or RNA processing. Frataxin is involved in mitochondrial respiration, iron balance, and response to oxidative stress. Some 97% of mutant *FRDA* alleles are due to $(GAA)_n$ expansions; the remaining alleles are due to other inactivating mutations, including point mutations (Lodi, 1999).

Laboratory Testing for Trinucleotide Repeat Disorders

Depending on the length of the repeat segment, expansions of trinucleotide repeats are readily demonstrated by either Southern blot or PCR. PCR, followed by sizing of the products on an electrophoretic gel or capillary, is generally preferred for most of these disorders because of its speed, simplicity, and ability to resolve alleles differing in size by just one repeat unit. This is of particular importance when it is necessary to differentiate stable alleles at the upper size limit from small premutation or disease-causing alleles. For example, it is critically important to distinguish a 40-repeat from a 39-repeat in Huntington disease because of the dramatically different clinical implications and the psychosocial impact of a positive result. PCR is also the method of choice for accurate sizing of FRAXA premutation alleles, which is necessary for graded risk counseling of female carriers. However, where triplet expansions are very large, as in fully expressed FRAXA or myotonic dystrophy, it may not be possible to amplify the greatly expanded DNA segment by PCR; in this case, Southern blotting has traditionally been required. Southern blotting is also helpful in determining the methylation status of FRAXA full mutations, through the use of methylation-sensitive restriction endonucleases, and in assuring that a large Huntington disease or FRAXA allele has not been missed in a patient who appears homozygous normal by PCR. Similarly, it more reliably identifies mosaic males whose cells show a mixture of premutation and full mutation alleles. Recently, however, methods for analyzing large premutations and even the full mutation of FMR1 by PCR alone have begun to enter practice, supported by the availability of commercial reagents (Hantash, 2010). Figure 70-5 illustrates the use of both Southern blotting and PCR to detect full FRAXA mutations and FRAXA premutation alleles.

PRADER-WILLI AND ANGELMAN SYNDROMES

Prader-Willi and Angelman syndromes, whose genes lie at approximately the same locus on chromosome 15, are almost always discussed together, even though they are caused by two different genes and have almost nothing in common phenotypically. Prader-Willi syndrome is characterized by obesity, mental retardation, hypoplastic genitalia, and dysmorphic features, while Angelman syndrome exhibits ataxia, puppet-like facies, mental retardation, paroxysmal laughter, and seizures. What they do share, remarkably, is a powerful imprinting mechanism determining disease expression. Both disorders are almost always sporadic. Prader-Willi syndrome, whose gene is not yet known, is most often caused by a deletion at 15q12 in the paternally inherited chromosome only; this is pathologic because only the paternal *PWS* gene is expressed. The opposite is true for Angelman syndrome, which is most often caused by deletion of a known gene (*UBE3A*) exclusively on the maternally inherited chromosome, which is the only allele normally expressed (Knoll, 1989; Matsuura, 1997). Alternatively, Prader-Willi syndrome can be caused by uniparental disomy for the maternal chromosome 15, which carries only the nonexpressing copy of the gene; likewise, Angelman syndrome can be caused by uniparental disomy for the paternal chromosome 15. These phenomena can be detected by FISH, discussed in Chapter 68, chromosome haplotyping with microsatellite markers, or Southern blotting with methylation-sensitive restriction enzymes that can distinguish the methylated maternal critical region from the unmethylated paternal critical region. A differential PCR scheme that amplifies either the methylated or unmethylated allele of the nearby *SNRPN* gene within the critical region, based on resistance of methylated cytosines to chemical modification by sodium bisulfite (Kosaki, 1997), is also available (Fig. 70-7). Neither the Southern blot nor the PCR method will distinguish between the deletional or uniparental disomy mechanisms, nor will they detect cases (more frequent in Angelman syndrome) due to point mutations within the causative gene. These methods also will not distinguish rare cases of Angelman syndrome or Prader-Willi syndrome due to primary imprinting defects (resulting from aberrant methylation caused by a mutation in the chromosome 15 imprinting center) (Burger, 1997), which would have a much higher recurrence risk.

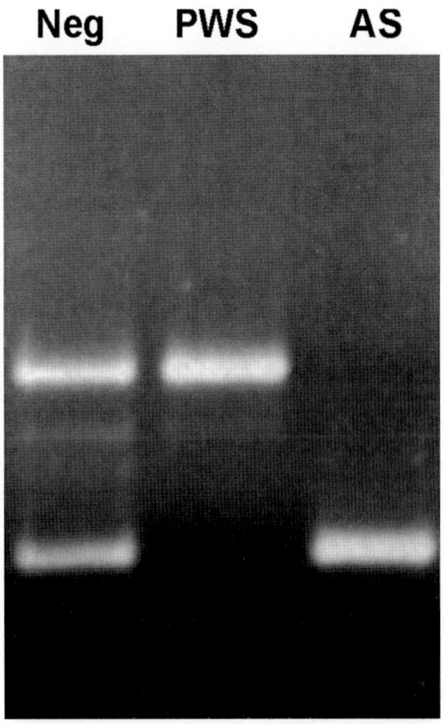

Figure 70-7 Polymerase chain reaction–based electrophoretic analysis of methylation patterns in Prader-Willi and Angelman syndromes using the sodium bisulfite method of Kosaki (1997). In Prader-Willi syndrome, only the methylated maternal allele (upper band) is present, due to either deletion of the paternal allele or uniparental disomy for the maternal allele. In Angelman syndrome, only the unmethylated paternal allele (lower band) is present, due to either deletion of the maternal allele or uniparental disomy for the paternal allele. Similar analysis can also be done by Southern blot using methylation-sensitive restriction enzymes.

FAMILIAL CANCERS

All cancers are genetic disorders at the cellular level, caused by mutations in genes that control cell proliferation and differentiation. These genes may be divided broadly into two groups, those that promote proliferation (proto-oncogenes or, simply, oncogenes), and those that restrain cell growth (tumor suppressor genes). Both sets of genes are discussed in Chapter 76. Most often, mutations in these genes occur in somatic cells, usually requiring alterations over many cell cycles in several oncogenes or tumor suppressor genes before a cancer develops. However, in some individuals the initial mutation in this progression may be a germline lesion, inherited from a parent and present in every cell of that individual's body.

TABLE 70-3
Hereditary Cancer Syndromes

Disorder (OMIM Entry)	Associated Tumors	Population Incidence	Gene	Chromosome Location
Tumor Suppressor Genes (Autosomal Dominant Mode of Inheritance)				
Basal cell nevus (Gorlin) syndrome (109400)	Basal cell carcinoma, medulloblastoma	1/40,000	PTCH	9q22
Cowden syndrome (158350)	Breast, thyroid carcinoma	1/200,000	PTEN	10q23
Familial adenomatous polyposis (175100)	Colorectal, duodenal carcinoma	1/10,000	APC	5q21
Hereditary breast–ovarian cancer syndrome (113705, 600185)	Breast, ovarian, pancreatic, prostate carcinoma	1/300–1/500	BRCA1 BRCA2	17q21 13q12
Hereditary diffuse gastric carcinoma (137215)	Gastric carcinoma	Rare	CDH1	16q22
Hereditary leiomyomatosis and renal cell carcinoma (150800, 605839)	Cutaneous and uterine leiomyomas, papillary renal cell carcinoma	Rare	FH	1q42
Hereditary melanoma (600160, 606719)	Melanoma, pancreatic carcinoma	Unknown	CDKN2A (p16)	9p21
Hereditary paraganglioma (602690, 185470, 602413)	Paraganglioma, pheochromocytoma	Rare	SDHD SDHB SDHC	11q23 1p35–36 1q21
Juvenile polyposis syndrome (174900)	Gastrointestinal cancer	1/10,000	SMAD4 BMPR1A	18q21 10q22
Tumor Suppressor Genes (Autosomal Dominant Mode of Inheritance)				
Li-Fraumeni syndrome (151623)	Sarcomas, breast carcinoma, leukemia, brain tumors	Rare	p53	17p13
Multiple endocrine neoplasia, type 1 (MEN1) (131100)	Pancreatic islet cell, pituitary, parathyroid tumors	1/100,000	MEN1	11q13
Neurofibromatosis type 1 (162200)	Neurofibroma/sarcoma, pheochromocytoma	1/3000	NF1	17q11
Neurofibromatosis, type 2 (101000)	Acoustic neuroma, meningioma	1/40,000	NF2	22q12
Peutz-Jeghers syndrome (175200)	Gastrointestinal tumors	1/200,000	STK11	19p13
Retinoblastoma, hereditary (180200)	Retinoblastoma, osteosarcoma	1/20,000	RB1	13q14
Von Hippel-Lindau disease (193300)	Hemangioblastoma, renal cell carcinoma, pheochromocytoma	1/40,000	VHL	3p25
Oncogenes (Autosomal Dominant Mode of Inheritance)				
Hereditary melanoma (123829)	Melanoma	Rare	CDK4	12q13
Multiple endocrine neoplasia type 2A and type 2B (171400, 162300)	Medullary thyroid carcinoma, pheochromocytoma, parathyroid hyperplasia/adenoma; multiple mucosal neuromas (type 2B)	1/30,000	RET	10q12
Hereditary papillary renal carcinoma (605074)	Papillary renal carcinoma	Rare	MET	7q31
DNA Repair Genes (Autosomal Dominant Mode of Inheritance)				
Hereditary nonpolyposis colorectal cancer (114500)	Colorectal, endometrial, ovarian carcinoma	1/400–1/700	MSH2 MLH1 MSH6 PMS2	2p16 3p21 2p16 7p22
DNA Repair Genes (Autosomal Recessive Mode of Inheritance)				
Ataxia telangiectasia (208900)	Lymphomas, others	1/40,000–1/100,000	ATM	11q22
Bloom syndrome (210900)	Various	Rare	BLM	15p26
Fanconi anemia (607139, 300515, 227645, 605724, 227646, 600901, 603467, 602956)	Acute myelogenous leukemia, others	1/100,000	FANCA-G	Various
MYH-associated polyposis (608456)	Colorectal carcinoma, duodenal polyposis	1/10,000	MYH	1p34
Xeroderma pigmentosum (278700, 133510, 278720, 278730, 278740, 133520, 133530, 603968)	Cutaneous basal carcinoma and squamous carcinoma	Rare	XPA-G, POLH	Various

Data from various sources, including Garber 2005.
OMIM, Online Mendelian Inhertiance in Man.

Heritable cancer-causing mutations have been found most often in tumor suppressor genes, including several groups of genes that encode proteins with DNA repair functions, but have also been found in a few oncogenes (Table 70-3). The inherited mutation should be viewed as the initiating event in tumor development, not in itself sufficient to cause cancer but merely the first step in a series of mutations that ultimately lead to uncontrolled cell growth, analogous to the first somatic mutation that initiates tumor development in a sporadic cancer. It is likely that most of the heritable mutations that contribute to cancer development have not been identified, because they are by themselves not highly penetrant and require the interaction of other genetic and environmental factors to initiate tumor development—a complex situation that is difficult to unravel. However, a number of highly penetrant genes have been identified that are major initiators of tumor development in what are recognizable heritable cancer syndromes (see Table 70-3).

Compared with their sporadic counterparts, hereditary cancers often develop at an earlier age, are more often multifocal, and appear bilaterally in paired organs. Noting these distinguishing features in sporadic retinoblastoma and familial retinoblastoma, Knudson postulated that at least two mutational events are necessary to produce a tumor (Knudson, 1971). In the case of a sporadic tumor, two independent mutational events in the same cell are necessary to initiate tumor development, whereas in the case of a hereditary tumor, the first mutation is already present at birth in every cell of the body, making it more likely that a second mutational event will occur at an earlier age and often in more than one cell. Knudson's two-hit hypothesis is an important concept that has guided many studies of the genetic basis of cancer. Elucidation of the heritable mutations in the hereditary cancer syndromes has been enormously informative, not only in understanding these rare disorders but also in understanding the fundamental changes responsible for common malignancies.

In the following discussion, some fundamental concepts of hereditary cancer syndromes are explained in the context of a disorder caused by a tumor suppressor gene, retinoblastoma, and a disorder caused by an oncogene, multiple endocrine neoplasia type 2. This is followed by descriptions of hereditary breast–ovarian cancer (HBOC) and hereditary colorectal cancer, the most common hereditary cancer syndromes, for which more than a million individuals in the United States are at risk. Table 70-3 lists these disorders and a number of other hereditary cancer syndromes. The section ends with a discussion of current approaches to genetic testing for these disorders.

Tumor Suppressor Genes: Retinoblastoma as a Paradigm

Although familial cancer syndromes due to mutations in tumor suppressor genes follow a dominant pattern of inheritance, at the cellular level the changes often appear recessive, because tumorigenesis is initiated (in most cases) only when both copies of the tumor suppressor gene are inactivated. Loss of the normal gene inherited from the unaffected parent may occur as the result of a second novel pathogenic mutation, by large-scale deletion (appearing in certain molecular assays as loss-of-heterozygosity), by replacement with a duplicated copy of the mutant gene inherited from the affected parent by genetic mechanisms such as chromosomal nondisjunction or mitotic recombination, or by gene silencing due to hypermethylation. These events occur in retinoblastoma, a tumor of the retina caused by functional loss of both copies of the *RB1* gene, which encodes the RB protein that is involved in cell cycle and transcriptional regulation. In sporadic cases, both of these mutational events occur somatically and a solitary, sporadic tumor develops. But in the hereditary cases, the first *RB1* mutation is present in the germline of the affected child, having been inherited from a similarly affected parent or occurring as a new mutation during gametogenesis. When this is the case, the likelihood that the remaining normal *RB1* gene will undergo mutation in at least one retinal precursor cell is greater than 90%. As Knudson observed, in most patients with familial disease, the tumors are bilateral and multifocal (Knudson, 1971), implying that several cells have sustained additional *RB1* mutations. It is not known if *RB1* mutations alone are sufficient for tumorigenesis, but they certainly appear to be the initiating or key event.

Familial retinoblastoma has served as a model in guiding important cancer research. This has led to the discovery of a large number of tumor suppressor genes that are key determinants of the pathogenesis of several hereditary cancer syndromes, including HBOC and hereditary colorectal cancer. These tumor suppressor genes are also critical to the development of many common sporadic cancers.

Oncogenes: Multiple Endocrine Neoplasia Type 2 as a Paradigm

There are just a few familial cancer syndromes that are known to be caused by a heritable mutation in an oncogene (see Table 70-3). Of these, multiple endocrine neoplasia type 2A (MEN2A) and its variants, familial medullary thyroid carcinoma (FMTC) and multiple endocrine neoplasia type 2B (MEN2B), are best known. Single, activating mutations in just one allele of the proto-oncogene *RET* are sufficient to initiate tumorigenesis in these disorders (Eng, 1999).

All three of these syndromes are characterized by hyperplasia of thyroid C cells and medullary thyroid carcinoma. In families afflicted with MEN2A, pheochromocytomas and/or parathyroid adenomas or parathyroid hyperplasia are also present. MEN2B is further characterized by the presence of multiple mucosal neuromas of the lips, mouth, and gastrointestinal tract, a marfanoid habitus, a particularly aggressive clinical course, and a high proportion of affected individuals due to new *RET* mutations.

RET is a signaling molecule with extracellular receptor and intracellular tyrosine kinase domains. With few exceptions, the known FMTC and MEN2A mutations are single base substitutions in one of five codons in the extracellular domain, in each case producing substitution of a cystine by another amino acid. More than 95% of the MEN2B mutations are identical, consisting of a single base substitution producing a missense mutation in the tyrosine kinase domain.

Hereditary Breast–Ovarian Cancer

HBOC affects more individuals than any other hereditary cancer syndrome (Narod, 2004). It is caused by germline mutations in *BRCA1* and *BRCA2*, autosomal tumor suppressor genes with roles in DNA repair, transcription regulation, and cell cycle control. The combined carrier prevalence of abnormal variants of these two genes in the general U.S. population is estimated to be 1/500–1/300. Three founder mutations in Ashkenazi Jews are responsible for increasing the prevalence tenfold (1/40) in this population. HBOC accounts for 5%–10% of female breast cancer cases and 12% of ovarian cancer cases. Whereas the lifetime risk to women of developing breast or ovarian cancer in the general population is 11% and 1%, respectively, the risk to mutation carriers is 56%–87% for breast cancer (the risk of a second, contralateral cancer approaches 60%) and 23%–45% for ovarian cancer. Other cancers, especially breast cancer in men, pancreatic cancer, colon cancer, and prostate cancer are more prevalent as well. Characteristically, tumors occur at an earlier age than their sporadic counterparts, with average age of diagnosis of breast cancer in the 40s compared to the average age of diagnosis of sporadic breast cancer in the mid-60s. Development of breast cancer at an early age is one of the strongest predictors of the presence of HBOC.

BRCA1 and *BRCA2* are both large genes, encoding proteins of 1863 amino acids and 3418 amino acids, respectively. Disease-causing mutations, mostly frameshift or nonsense mutations which cause protein truncation, are distributed widely across both genes. Many hundreds of unique deleterious mutations have been identified. Although the presence of founder mutations permits a targeted approach to mutation identification in Ashkenazi Jews (with just two common mutations in *BRCA1* and one in *BRCA2*), whole-gene sequencing or gene scanning techniques are required for mutation detection in the heterogeneous general U.S. population at large. This approach has a high yield of detecting mutations (as long as they exist in the coding regions of the genes) but, analogous to the caveat about array-CGH testing discussed earlier, also reveals new missense variants of undetermined clinical significance, which then have to be dealt with (Richards, 2008). Also, some HBOC patients have large deletions in one of the genes rather than a point mutation, and detection of these requires an alternate approach such as Southern blot or MLPA.

Genetic testing for *BRCA1* and *BRCA2* mutations in high-risk patients and family members is now a high-profile service in clinical genetics and oncology practice. Effective cancer prevention strategies for mutation carriers (increased surveillance, chemoprevention, prophylactic surgery) have markedly reduced the incidence of ovarian cancer and primary and secondary breast cancers (Narod, 2004). Individuals at high risk can be identified by their personal history of ovarian or early-onset breast cancer in women or breast cancer in men, and/or by a family history of these cancers in either the paternal or maternal lineages (National Comprehensive Cancer Network, 2005). Because HBOC is an autosomal dominant disorder, first-degree relatives of mutation carriers have a 50% risk of carrying the same mutation. Once the familial mutation is known, testing of at-risk relatives no longer requires whole-gene sequencing but rather can be targeted to the particular nucleotide, saving significant time and expense.

The Hereditary Colorectal Cancer Syndromes

Hereditary nonpolyposis colorectal cancer (HNPCC, or Lynch syndrome), as its name implies, is a hereditary colorectal cancer syndrome that is not associated with an abundance of adenomatous polyps. In contrast, familial adenomatous polyposis (FAP) and MYH-associated polyposis (MAP) are hereditary disorders in which variable and sometimes large numbers of adenomatous polyps may be present. This useful, if imperfect, clinical distinction is an important guide to the evaluation of individuals who are at risk for these disorders.

Hereditary Nonpolyposis Colorectal Cancer

HNPCC is the second most common hereditary cancer syndrome, affecting almost as many individuals as are affected by HBOC. However, because it is almost equally penetrant in both sexes, its public health impact is equivalent to that of HBOC. Notably, and often unrecognized, endometrial cancer is a prominent part of the syndrome, with more affected women developing endometrial cancer than colorectal cancer. HNPCC accounts for 3%–5% of all colorectal cancers and 2%–3% of all endometrial cancers. The disease is caused by germline mutations in one of five DNA mismatch repair genes, *MSH2*, *MLH1*, *MSH6*, *PMS2*, and *PMS1*, each contributing roughly 50%, 40%, 10%, <1%, and <1%, respectively, to the overall incidence of the disorder. The combined carrier prevalence of abnormal variants of *MSH2* and *MSH1*, which account for approximately 90% of HNPCC, is estimated to be between 1/700 and 1/400. Colorectal cancer in HNPCC is characterized by early age of onset (average 44 years, compared to 72 years for sporadic colorectal cancer), occurs predominantly on the right side of the colon, and may occur as multiple primary tumors simultaneously or over a period of time (synchronous or metachronous). The lifetime risk to male and female mutation carriers of developing colorectal cancer is approximately 80% (compared with a 2% lifetime general population risk), while the lifetime risk of endometrial cancer is 40%–60% (compared with a 1.5% lifetime general population risk). The lifetime risks of gastric cancer (13%) and of ovarian cancer (12%) are also increased (compared with 1% for the general population).

A number of guidelines for identifying individuals at risk for HNPCC have been described that use a combination of personal and family history of cancer: for example, the Amsterdam Criteria and Bethesda Guidelines, which have gone through several revisions (Lipton, 2004). In practice, one need not hold dogmatically to these schemes, because a detailed personal and family history will usually suggest which patients are at risk. Early-onset colorectal cancer and/or endometrial cancer are the strongest predictors of the disorder, particularly when they are seen together in an individual or family, are accompanied by other tumors associated with the disease, and occur in more than one generation of the family.

Another predictor of HNPCC in an affected patient is the presence of microsatellite instability (MSI) in the DNA of that individual's colorectal cancer. The term describes an alteration in the length of short tandem repeat DNA sequences (microsatellites) in the tumor due to mismatch repair errors during DNA replication. Microsatellite instability is highly sensitive but not entirely specific in identifying a colorectal tumor as due to HNPCC, because about 15% of sporadic colon cancers will also demonstrate MSI. The DNA mismatch repair genes are moderately large genes, with *MSH2* encoding a protein of 935 amino acids and *MLH1* encoding a protein of 757 amino acids. Although there are a few mutations that have a high relative prevalence in some populations due to founder effects, the vast majority are distributed widely across both genes. Most mutations are frameshift or nonsense mutations that cause loss of gene expression due to RNA instability, protein instability or protein truncation. In addition, large deletions of single or multiple exons account for approximately one third of the mutations present in *MSH2* and for a smaller fraction of the mutations in *MLH1*.

Genetic testing for *MSH2* and *MLH1* mutations in high-risk patients and family members has moved into clinical practice in a manner similar to that which has occurred for *BRCA1* and *BRCA2* testing for HBOC. For those individuals who are identified as carrying deleterious mutations, complete colonoscopy, beginning at an early age and at regular intervals, is very effective at identifying premalignant adenomatous polyps (the term *HNPCC* should not be taken to imply that there are no polyps involved in the syndrome), while endometrial biopsy and transvaginal ultrasound may identify early endometrial cancer. If colorectal cancer does develop, subtotal colectomy may be considered as an alternative to segmental resection because of the high rate of synchronous and metachronous tumors in patients with HNPCC. Prophylactic hysterectomy–bilateral salpingo-oophorectomy may be considered in women who have completed their families. As in all autosomal dominant disorders, first-degree family members of mutation carriers have a 50% risk of also carrying that same mutation, and their testing becomes relatively straightforward.

Familial Adenomatous Polyposis and Attenuated Familial Adenomatous Polyposis

Familial adenomatous polyposis is a hereditary colorectal cancer syndrome that can present with a striking phenotype in the colon—multifocal colorectal cancer in a background of thousands of adenomatous polyps. It is now recognized that the FAP phenotype is diverse and the number of colonic polyps can vary markedly. Accordingly, *classic* FAP is now diagnosed when an individual develops at least 100 adenomatous polyps over his/her lifetime, whereas *attenuated* FAP (AFAP) is the term applied to a patient whose lifetime polyp burden is in the range of 20–100 polyps. The distinction is entirely clinical, because both disorders are caused by germline mutations in the *APC* (adenomatous polyposis coli) gene, a tumor suppressor gene with several important cellular functions and a likely initiator of sporadic colorectal cancer development as well. Germline *APC* mutations are carried by 1/10,000–1/5000 individuals; most of these mutations have been inherited from a similarly affected parent, but 20%–30% are de novo mutations. Accordingly, FAP or AFAP cannot be ruled out because of an absence of a positive family history, which is particularly important to keep in mind when assessing a patient with a low polyp burden.

Early-onset colorectal cancer (average age 39 years for FAP, approximately 50 years for AFAP) requires early diagnosis and close clinical monitoring for individuals determined to be at risk by family history and/or genetic testing. Screening sigmoidoscopies should be started at age 10 and prophylactic colectomy performed when polyps have developed. For individuals at risk for the less florid AFAP, screening may begin later in the teens, but colonoscopy is advised because polyps preferentially develop in the right side of the colon. Colectomy is performed when the polyp burden is no longer manageable by polypectomy. Upper gastrointestinal surveillance is also indicated because gastric and small bowel polyps also develop. This is particularly important in the duodenum, especially in the periampullary region, where the lifetime risk of progression to cancer is 5%–12% for FAP.

Patients with FAP and AFAP are also at higher risk for a number of other cancers (gastric, pancreatic, biliary tract, thyroid) and frequently have other clinical findings: desmoid tumors, osteomas, dental abnormalities, epidermoid cysts, and congenital hypertrophy of the retinal pigmented epithelium (CHRPE). Of these, desmoid tumors, affecting approximately 10% of patients with FAP, are the most important. These clonal proliferations of myofibroblasts form in the abdominal wall or the abdominal cavity where they are locally invasive, compress abdominal organs, and may cause serious morbidity and mortality.

APC is a large gene, encoding a protein of 2843 amino acids. Most disease-causing mutations are frameshift or nonsense mutations producing protein truncation. These mutations are distributed widely along the gene, requiring full-gene sequencing unless the familial mutation is already known. Some genotype–phenotype correlations are possible: mutations that produce extraintestinal features tend to map to particular regions of the gene, while those that are associated with AFAP cluster in the 5′- and 3′-most regions of the gene.

MYH-*Associated Polyposis*

MYH-associated polyposis is a recently recognized autosomal recessive hereditary cancer syndrome caused by mutations in the human homolog of the bacterial *mutY* gene, *MYH* (Wang, 2004). The clinical phenotype is very similar to that of AFAP or the less florid variants of FAP: that is, a polyp burden in the tens to hundreds, not thousands. As with FAP/AFAP, patients are at risk for duodenal polyposis and some have been reported to have some of the extraintestinal manifestations, CHRPE and osteomas, as well. Because of the autosomal recessive nature of this disorder, MAP families typically show no evidence of vertical transmission of the disease, as would be true for the autosomal dominant FAP/AFAP, but might include affected siblings. It is estimated that the carrier frequency for mutant *MYH* alleles is approximately 2%, which implies a 1/10,000 frequency of biallelic (affected) individuals. This is very similar to the number of patients who have FAP/AFAP. The close similarity of the MAP and FAP/AFAP phenotypes, and the fact that as many as 30% of individuals with FAP have no evidence of vertical transmission in the family because they carry de novo *APC* mutations, can make diagnosis difficult, especially when the polyp burden is not large. In many cases it is necessary to perform mutation analysis for both *APC* and *MYH* to arrive at a diagnosis.

Laboratory Testing for Familial Cancer Mutations

DNA analysis for heritable, cancer-predisposing mutations has enormous potential for disease prevention and early treatment. If a very high proportion of the cancer-causing mutations in a particular gene or ethnic group are known, and these mutations are relatively few in number, direct

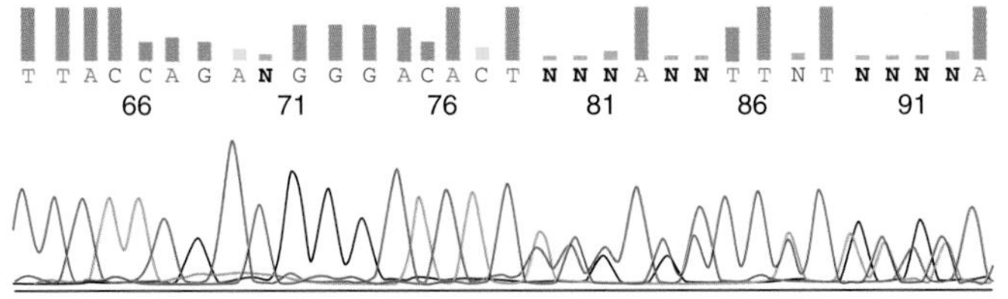

Figure 70-8 Detection of the Ashkenazi Jewish founder mutation 185delAG in the *BRCA1* gene by DNA sequencing. Because familial breast–ovarian cancer is a dominant disorder, the mutation is heterozygous, and because it results in the deletion of two nucleotides from one of the alleles, the sequence profile is "out of frame" from the mutation site onward (starting at nucleotide 79 in this particular readout). This causes overlapping of different nucleotides between the two alleles, which the automated sequencer has trouble identifying (hence the frequent notation "N" for the nucleotide calls).

analysis for these mutations may be simple and inexpensive. Fortunately, this may sometimes be the case with an oncogene, because activation of the gene can only be achieved in a limited number of ways. As mentioned earlier, the spectrum of mutations in *RET* that are responsible for MEN2 is quite small, with just a handful of well-defined mutations accounting for more than 95% of the total.

If, on the other hand, the gene is large, and cancer-causing mutations are numerous and widely dispersed (which is commonly the case with tumor suppressor genes, because they can be inactivated in many different ways), then mutation analysis must of necessity be less targeted and be capable of screening large stretches of DNA. In that case, direct DNA sequencing or gene scanning techniques such as DHPLC, SSCP, or heteroduplex analysis must be used. In addition, whole exon deletions or duplications, or even whole gene deletions that are not detectable by sequencing or gene scanning may constitute a significant percentage of the deleterious mutations in a particular gene. In this case, techniques that are capable of assessing gene dosage, such as Southern blotting, some variation of quantitative PCR, MLPA, or a hybridization platform that is capable of measuring sequence dosage in a comparative way, must be used. Figure 70-8 illustrates the DNA sequence tracing of the Ashkenazi-Jewish founder mutation 185delAG in *BRCA1*.

HEMOCHROMATOSIS

Hereditary hemochromatosis, first recognized in its full clinical expression as the triad of cirrhosis, diabetes mellitus, and bronzing of the skin, was originally thought to be a rare disorder of iron overload affecting about 1 in 5000 or fewer Caucasians. However, when genetic studies linked the disease-causing gene to the HLA locus on chromosome 6, and biochemical tests of iron overload (principally transferrin saturation) were utilized, it was recognized that the underlying genetic predisposition to iron overload was extremely common. Indeed, hereditary hemochromatosis is now recognized as an autosomal recessive disorder with a carrier frequency as high as one in eight in people of northern European descent, making it the most common genetic disorder in the U.S. Caucasian population. The incidence of at-risk homozygotes is 1 in 250, but only a fraction of these accumulate sufficient excess iron to produce the tissue injury associated with the classic disorder.

Our understanding of hereditary hemochromatosis entered a new era with the identification of the *HFE* gene (initially called *HLA-H*) within the major histocompatibility locus on chromosome 6 (Feder, 1996). The HFE protein, although it is a major histocompatibility complex class I–like molecule, does not bind and present endogenous peptides and is not thought to have an immunologic function. Rather, as discussed in Chapter 49 evidence is accumulating that the HFE protein interacts with the transferrin receptor and modulates enteric absorption of dietary iron (Waheed, 1999). Mutations in *HFE* impair this regulatory function, leading to excess iron absorption and storage in tissues.

As noted in Chapter 49 a single missense mutation in *HFE*, C282Y, which results in a tyrosine substitution for cystine at amino acid 282 in the HFE protein, is present in the homozygous state in 80%–90% of Caucasians with hemochromatosis. An additional small percentage of patients with hemochromatosis are compound heterozygotes, carrying one chromosome with a C282Y mutation and another with an H63D mutation. H63D is a common variant, with a carrier frequency of approximately 20%, and its association with iron overload is very low (1%–2%) in the compound heterozygous state and probably even lower when homozygous (Gochee, 2002). Over the years since its discovery, the penetrance of the C282Y homozygous state has also been questioned, and may be appreciably lower than the 80% earlier quoted, perhaps as low as 10% or even 1% (Beutler, 2002; Pietrangelo, 2004). For this reason, population screening for these mutations in individuals with no clinical or biochemical signs of hemochromatosis has not been recommended. Similar to what was discussed for factor V Leiden earlier, the DNA test is best reserved for differential diagnosis in patients already exhibiting the clinical disorder or elevated transferrin saturation detected on biochemical screening. The C282Y and H63D mutations are single-nucleotide substitutions and may be analyzed easily by a variety of PCR, real-time PCR, microarray, microplate, or sequencing methods.

SPINAL MUSCULAR ATROPHY

Spinal muscular atrophy is an autosomal recessive motor neuron disorder characterized by proximal muscle weakness and wasting. The most severe form, type I (also called Werdnig–Hoffmann disease), presents with hypotonia in infancy and early childhood death due to respiratory failure. Intermediate and atypical forms are also described. The disease is caused by mutations in the *SMN1* gene on chromosome 5q13. With a carrier frequency of 1 in 50, spinal muscular atrophy is one of the more common lethal recessive disorders, approaching the incidence of cystic fibrosis.

The majority (95%) of affected patients exhibit loss of the *SMN1* gene, either through complete gene deletion or through a gene conversion event involving sequences in the adjacent *SMN2* gene which differs by a single nucleotide in exon 7. The *SMN2* gene is believed to be nonessential because both alleles are absent in 5%–10% of normal individuals, yet is partially protective as demonstrated by the finding of higher *SMN2* copy number in patients with less severe forms of the disease (Mailman, 2002). The presence of this closely homologous pseudogene has necessitated the development of meticulously designed allele-specific PCR/restriction endonuclease assays to determine homozygous deletion of *SMN1* in the presence of *SMN2* (Prior, 2010). Identification of carriers, based on *SMN1* gene dosage analysis, is even more challenging and requires the use of quantitative or real-time PCR methods (Ojino, 2004b); this problem, along with questions about genotype–phenotype correlation, have led to some controversy over whether SMA should be a target of general population carrier screening along the lines of CF (Prior, 2008; ACOG, 2009). The small percentage of patients not showing loss or conversion of both *SMN1* genes usually carry a small intragenic mutation in one allele, of which a large number have been reported. These can be detected by sequencing or by multiplex allele-specific PCR assays (Mailman, 2002).

MITOCHONDRIAL DNA DISORDERS

In addition to the 6 billion bp of DNA that comprise the human nuclear diploid genome, vital genetic information is also encoded in DNA molecules carried by the mitochondria in the cytoplasm. These 16,500 bp, double-stranded circular DNA molecules are present in 2–10 copies in each of the up to several hundred mitochondria of the cell. Mitochondrial DNA codes for 13 of the proteins of the respiratory chain and adenosine triphosphate (ATP) synthase, 22 transfer RNAs required for their translation, and two ribosomal RNAs. Mitochondrial DNA is self-replicating and is transmitted strictly by maternal inheritance, because the mitochondria of a spermatozoon are not incorporated into the zygote upon fertilization of an ovum.

Disease-causing abnormalities of mitochondrial DNA may result from several different mechanisms (Ruiz-Pesini et al., 2007). Single large deletions (and, rarely, duplications) that apparently occur sporadically in oogenesis are typical of Kearns-Sayre syndrome, a myopathy characterized principally by progressive external ophthalmoplegia and pigmentary retinopathy. A wide range of disorders are characterized by multiple small deletions and show typical mendelian autosomal dominant or autosomal recessive patterns of inheritance, apparently because they are due to undefined defects in nuclear genes important for mitochondrial DNA replication. Most distinctive from a genetic point of view are the disorders that follow a pattern of strict maternal inheritance, never showing transmission from an affected male and passing from an affected female equally to her sons and daughters. These diseases are most often due to point mutations in one of the genes encoding a transfer RNA (e.g., myoclonic epilepsy and ragged red fibers *[MERRF]* and mitochondrial myopathy, encephalopathy, lactic acidosis, and strokelike episodes *[MELAS]*) or a mitochondrial protein (e.g., Leber hereditary optic neuropathy *[LHON]*). In addition to the inherited encephalomyopathies, there is growing evidence that tissue-specific accumulations of somatic mitochondrial mutations may contribute to the development of many common late-onset degenerative disorders, and perhaps to aging itself.

Laboratory confirmation of the large mitochondrial DNA deletions often present in Kearns-Sayre syndrome is easily accomplished by Southern blot analysis of mitochondrial DNA from affected tissues using labeled whole mitochondrial DNA as a probe. Point mutations in other disorders may be analyzed by a number of techniques. Often the clinical presentation will guide the choice of mutation panel testing in a stepwise fashion, because particular mutations are associated with each of the major syndromes (e.g., missense mutations G11778A, T14484C, and G3460A with LHON). If these tests are negative, one can proceed to a second-tier panel or to complete mtDNA sequencing. The situation is complicated by the finding that some mutations are found in more than one syndrome and by the phenomenon of heteroplasmy—the occurrence of different proportions of mutant and normal mitochondria in different tissues. For this latter reason, mitochondrial DNA testing may require biopsy of the involved tissue (e.g., muscle) because the mutation may not be represented highly enough in blood to be detectable. This is where the advent of next-generation sequencing may come to the fore, in that it would allow sequencing of the complete mtDNA genome in a short time while also detecting minor populations of mutant mitochondria, perhaps even outside the affected tissue (Vasta, 2009).

OTHER TARGETS OF MOLECULAR GENETIC TESTING AND SCREENING

The specific disease examples covered in this chapter are among those tested most widely by clinical molecular genetics laboratories, a market that is reflected by their inclusion in the CAP/ACMG proficiency testing programs. This in turn has been dictated largely by their mutation carrier frequency or disease prevalence in the general population, and by their clinical severity. As previously described, if the carrier frequency of a recessive mutation is sufficiently high in the target population, general screening may be justified. For these and other disorders, the application of the test to differential diagnosis, prenatal diagnosis, or presymptomatic diagnosis may also be of value. With more than 10,000 genetic diseases catalogued, there are obviously many others that could be considered; currently there are almost 1900 different molecular genetic disease tests available as listed in the useful online database GeneTests (http://www.ncbi.nlm.nih.gov/sites/GeneTests/lab?db=GeneTests) (GeneTests, 2010). Many of these are esoteric and offered by only one or a few laboratories. Tests for extremely rare, or *orphan*, genetic diseases may only be available in the research laboratory that cloned the gene. This has led to some problems because such laboratories, although performing a vital service to the small number of families at risk, are not Clinical Laboratory Improvement Act (CLIA)-certified and on legal grounds should not be releasing test results for medical management. A number of solutions have been proposed, such as modifying certain CLIA requirements for such settings, partnering of the research laboratory with a clinical laboratory in their own institution, or establishing a network of dedicated orphan disease laboratories (Grody, 2008).

Some disorders that are rare in the general population are sufficiently prevalent in a particular racial or ethnic group to justify limited population screening. For example, a number of laboratories offer an Ashkenazi-Jewish carrier screening panel to include any or all of the following autosomal recessive diseases, which have carrier frequencies ranging from 1/100 to 1/15: Tay-Sachs disease, Gaucher disease, Canavan disease, cystic fibrosis, familial dysautonomia, Niemann-Pick disease A, Fanconi anemia C, Bloom syndrome, and connexin-26–related hearing loss. Screening of just the first four of these diseases has a positive yield of 1 in 6 in this population (Eng, 1997).

Beyond the driver of service to a particular indigenous patient population, the choice of molecular genetic test menu from the large and ever-expanding universe of known disease genes will depend on both intellectual and economic factors (Amos, 2004). Development of a molecular genetic test may be spurred by a clinical colleague's interest in a particular disease and accrual of a stable of patients and at-risk relatives. A molecular test may be needed as backup to a biochemical test done at the same institution, as for hemoglobinopathies or α_1-antitrypsin deficiency, or for statewide expanded newborn screening by tandem mass spectrometry (CDC, 2008). Of course, a strong motivator is the availability of robust commercially distributed platforms for performing the test (instrumentation, analyte-specific reagents, and/or FDA-approved kits), and this in turn will be driven by the potential market the vendors perceive for the disease in question. Naturally, carrier screening tests will always be of higher throughput than diagnostic tests, which explains the proliferation of commercial reagents and instruments for CF mutation detection that followed the ACMG/ACOG screening recommendations. Meanwhile, an economic factor pushing in the opposite direction, toward less widespread testing, is the specter of exclusive gene patents. Depending on the restrictions and sublicensing royalty arrangements of the patent-holder, clinical laboratories may not have access to certain desired tests, even if done by in-house–developed methods. For example, mutations in the connexin-26 (*GJB2*) gene, which account for about half of all cases of congenital nonsyndromic deafness and thus could be envisioned as a target of newborn screening (Schimmenti, 2008), are subject to an exclusive patent license. Recently, the constitutionality of patenting such "products of nature" has been challenged in the federal courts (Matloff, 2010). Finally, any new test being considered must first be shown to have clinical utility and analytic validity.

FUTURE DIRECTIONS

Molecular testing for genetic diseases has now come of age and in fact lies at a crucial juncture in the history of medicine. As is discussed in Chapter 77, with the sequencing phase of the Human Genome Project now completed, essentially any test for an inherited mutation is within our grasp. Moreover, continued advances in high-speed DNA sequencing and microarray technology may soon make routine comprehensive analysis of an individual patient's genome economically feasible. But just because something becomes analytically practical does not make it clinically valid, and the many potential problems of whole-genome analysis have already been raised in this chapter. Despite this, several high-profile commercial firms have begun to offer such services through direct-to-consumer marketing over the internet, with no genetic counselor or physician in the loop (Caulfield, 2010). Will whole-genome scanning become the equivalent of today's much-advertised whole-body CT scans, chasing shadows of uncertain clinical significance?

Closely tied to the increasing technologic invasiveness of genetic testing are the ethical concerns raised at the beginning of this chapter: genetic privacy, discrimination, stigmatization, confidentiality, informed consent. These have been discussed and written about extensively, including in the context of the new technology (Grody, 2003b). Because of these concerns, a widespread belief has arisen that molecular genetic test results are different in a fundamental way (mostly owing to their predictive power) from all other medical information, and must be subject to more stringent oversight. Others think that the results of these tests, while far-reaching, need be no more emotionally charged than many other clinical studies performed in laboratory medicine and pathology. Nevertheless, many states and countries are pursuing regulatory solutions to the perceived potential for abuse, and in the United States a variety of legislative initiatives aimed at safeguarding genetic information and privacy are pending or already passed.

While molecular analysis becomes more invasive, specimen collection techniques in genetic testing may become less invasive. Just as such approaches as buccal brushing can replace phlebotomy and biopsy for detection of a germline mutation, development of more sensitive and selective techniques for obtaining fetal samples may make the invasiveness of amniocentesis and chorionic villus sampling less necessary for prenatal diagnosis. These include isolation of fetal cells or DNA from maternal blood (Hahn, 2009) or vaginal contents. At the same time, the power of single-cell PCR for early-embryo biopsy and preimplantation genetic diagnosis can be used to obviate the invasiveness and emotional trauma of later prenatal diagnosis and pregnancy termination (Geraedts, 2009). Aside from questions about access due to its high cost, preimplantation genetic diagnosis raises the prospect of another ethical minefield previously the domain of science fiction: the ability to select offspring for nondisease traits. In fact, this is already occurring, as embryos have been HLA-typed through single-cell PCR and used for selective implantation based on the predicted suitability of the offspring to serve as bone marrow donors for existing siblings with hematopoietic disorders (Verlinsky, 2004). Can selection for other nondisease traits be far behind?

The applications presented in this chapter are all single-gene defects, because that is all our current knowledge and technology can handle. In the future it is hoped that molecular genetic testing will also be applied to the most common chronic diseases of medicine, which are all polygenic: atherosclerosis, diabetes mellitus, hypertension, schizophrenia. It is toward this end that a tremendous effort is being expended to identify single-nucleotide polymorphisms and other variants within candidate genes that may in aggregate produce quantitative trait effects on homeostasis, vascular tone, lipid metabolism, and so on. It is hoped that the discovery of these determinants will enable population risk screening programs followed by targeted therapies and preventive interventions. In this way, molecular genetic testing will be the central modality behind an ever-greater proportion of medical practice in the 21st century, and virtually every patient, whether healthy or ill, will feel its impact.

SELECTED REFERENCES

Beutler E, Felitti VJ, Koziol JA, et al. Penetrance of 845G-A (C282Y) HFE hereditary haemochromatosis mutation in the USA. Lancet 2002;359:211–18.

This is the most quoted of several studies that question the presumed 80% penetrance of the major HFE mutation in causing iron overload.

GeneTests. http://www.ncbi.nlm.nih.gov/sites/GeneTests/lab?db=GeneTests, accessed Feb. 14, 2010.

This useful Internet site provides scholarly and up-to-date reviews of the genetics and clinical aspects of the major hereditary disorders, as well as a worldwide searchable laboratory directory listing the locations where specific testing for each disease can be obtained.

Grody WW, Cutting G, Klinger K, et al. Laboratory standards and guidelines for population-based cystic fibrosis carrier screening. Genet Med 2001a;3:149–54.

This article presents the recommendations from the American College of Medical Genetics and the American College of Obstetricians and Gynecologists for implementation of nationwide cystic fibrosis population carrier screening using a core panel of 25 CFTR mutations.

REFERENCES

Access the complete reference list online at http://www.expertconsult.com

CHAPTER 71

IDENTITY ANALYSIS: USE OF DNA ANALYSIS IN PARENTAGE, FORENSIC, AND MISSING PERSONS TESTING

Herbert F. Polesky, Rhonda K. Roby

KEY POINTS

- Standardized marker systems with known allelic polymorphisms are used in testing panels. Alleles with short tandem repeats form the basis of commercially available kits.
- Forensic testing requires documentation of all steps taken during collection, extraction, and testing so results can withstand legal challenges.
- Deoxyribonucleic acid (DNA) can be obtained from any sample that contains cellular material. The stability of DNA allows it to withstand harsh environmental conditions and long postmortem intervals.
- Care must be taken to maintain the integrity of DNA evidence and to avoid contact or exposure of the evidence to any conditions that may contaminate the original stain/evidence.
- Mitochondrial DNA can be extracted from bone and teeth after hundreds of years because it is small and present at hundreds to thousands of copies per cell. Mitochondrial DNA is maternally inherited and can be useful for identifying remains.
- DNA is used in identification of remains and can be used to link a suspect to a crime, to exculpate falsely accused suspects, to recognize serial crimes, and to distinguish copycat crimes, or to aid in accident reconstruction (e.g., to determine who was driving a car by the identification of the bloodstains on the driver's side of the windshield).
- Pathology laboratories can use DNA testing to resolve specimen mixups such as when samples are inadvertently switched or pathologic material floats onto a histologic or cytologic slide.
- Standards and quality assurance guidelines for parentage and forensics laboratories have been developed by the American Association of Blood Banks and the Federal Bureau of Investigation's DNA Advisory Board, respectively.

In parentage testing, samples obtained from multiple individuals are compared for inherited similarities; most often in forensic DNA testing, crime scene samples are evaluated for an exact match with a suspect.

A frequently quoted early reference to disputed parentage appears in the Bible (1 Kings 3:16–27), in which Solomon makes a decision about the maternity of a disputed child by threatening to use his sword to provide each claimant with a portion of the child. When paternity is in dispute, the arbiter of truth often is faced with the dilemma similar to that faced by Solomon: lack of witnesses to the event and the likelihood that the principals might not know or tell the truth. Similarly, short of eyewitnesses or confession, identifying a person at a crime scene is difficult to accomplish and most evidence merely suggests a suspect linkage. The availability of biological evidence, such as DNA, provides information that can lead to clear resolution of disputed facts.

HISTORICAL BACKGROUND

The discovery of the ABO blood group system by Landsteiner in 1900 (Landsteiner, 1901) and the recognition that these measurable characteristics followed the genetic rules described by Gregor Mendel (Mendel, 1866) provided objective laboratory evidence that could be used by courts to aid in deciding when a person had been falsely accused of paternity. In the United States, laws addressing the use of genetic markers for proving nonpaternity were enacted in 1935 (Schatkin, 1952). In the ensuing years, knowledge about useful genetic marker systems increased dramatically. By 1976, joint guidelines developed by an American Medical Association–American Bar Association committee recommended seven systems for routine blood group investigations in cases of disputed parentage: ABO, Rh, MNSs, Kell, Duffy, Kidd, and HLA (Miale, 1976). Other genetic systems such as polymorphic serum proteins and red cell enzymes were also recognized as useful. Many of these same genetic markers have also been used to match crime scene evidence with suspects or victims.

In 1980, DNA restriction fragment length polymorphism (RFLP) was described by Botstein (Botstein, 1980). Sir Alec Jeffreys is credited with the first report in the scientific literature to suggest that DNA typing might be useful for forensic identification, and coined the term "DNA fingerprint" in his *Nature* article in 1985 (Jeffreys, 1985a, 1985b). Commercial laboratories began using DNA testing for parentage and criminalistics casework in 1986, and government crime laboratories began using DNA testing in 1989 (Weedn, 1993a). Today, several hundred laboratories worldwide use DNA testing for the criminal justice system. In 1990, when the first edition of *Standards for Parentage Testing Laboratories* (American Association of Blood Banks, 1990) was published, specific requirements for RFLP testing were included along with those for what are now referred to as *classic systems* (red blood cell surface antigens, human leukocyte antigens, red cell enzymes, and serum protein genetic markers). DNA testing has replaced traditional serologic techniques. The forensic DNA testing community has endured many iterations of DNA methods and technologies, and has standardized its testing with a set of 13 core short tandem repeat (STR) loci as the current mainstay of testing in order to build its international offender databases. This core set of loci is supplemented by other DNA testing, gender analysis (Amelogenin), Y chromosome markers, and mitochondrial DNA (mtDNA) sequencing. Capillary electrophoresis is the main instrument platform with fluorescence detection.

These same technologies are used to identify victims of war or mass disasters (Budowle, 2005), whether the disaster is natural, man-made, or industrial, and in cases of wildlife forensics. DNA testing is also used for accident reconstruction, in medical cases of sample mixups, and in animal husbandry. DNA technology is here to stay; newer technologies will be adopted that offer higher powers of discrimination, lower costs, enhanced sensitivity, increased efficiency, and even information on the physical traits of the remains or biological material left at a crime scene. As these newer technologies evolve and are validated, so will the field of forensic sciences.

Advantages of DNA

DNA permits the direct identification of the individual source because it is personal and manifests biological variation. DNA is useful as an identity marker because it is (1) present throughout all cells of the body (except mature red cells); (2) the same in all cells of the body (except haploid sex gametes); (3) the same throughout life from the time of conception (except that a progenitor stem cell transplantation can result in the presence of donor characteristics rather than the recipient's inherited DNA); (4) different in all individuals (except identical twins). The human genome is approximately 99.9% the same between individuals; it is the 0.1% difference of the human genome that forensic scientists interrogate to individually identify stains, remains recovered from accidents and mass disasters, and biological relatives.

DNA tests have a sensitivity that is far superior to traditional serologic markers. Polymerase chain reaction (PCR)-based testing can be accomplished on minute samples and even invisible trace DNA deposits. DNA is a robust molecule resistant to strong acids, alkalis, detergents, and environmental factors (Kobilinsky, 1992). The typing information from DNA is found within the sequence of nucleotides. Consequently, DNA is more successfully performed than serology tests on specimens that are older and that have been exposed to greater environmental insults.

The bulk of the casework for crime laboratories in the United States is from sexual assaults. Vaginal swabs contain bacteria and female epithelial cells as well as the male sperm. DNA from sperm can be separated from nonsperm DNA by a differential lysis procedure because of the protective capsule of spermatozoa (see later under DNA Extraction and Quantification). This allows for individualization of the source of the semen without the confounding data of the nonsemen evidence. DNA targets are also generally human- or primate-specific so the presence of bacterial DNA is of no consequence.

Choosing Genetic Markers

The model genetic system for testing would be one in which the individual has a unique marker. In determining relationships, this marker can be found in both the child and the putative parent. At present, short of gene sequencing, none of the marker systems provide such specific findings. Thus multiple genetic systems that meet certain criteria are used for parentage and identity testing. Ideally, the system should have multiple alleles distributed in the population so that there is a high power of exclusion and the least common phenotype has a frequency that can be determined reliably. All markers in the system should be expressed (no null alleles) as codominant, mutation rates should be known and low, and phenotypes should be stable under usual storage conditions. Methods for detecting the markers should be reliable, reproducible, and feasible for a large number of laboratories. The genetics of the system must be known and follow established inheritance patterns (Mendelian laws). The system should be independent of other markers routinely tested. If the system is intended for calculating estimates of paternity or identity, the gene frequencies in various populations must be established (Budowle, 2001).

The DNA from every human (except identical twins) is unique, because of the presence of polymorphisms, which are differences in the DNA between individuals. However, the vast preponderance of the DNA sequence is identical between individuals. On average, only 1 in 1300 nucleotide bases differs between individuals. Nonetheless, this amounts to an average of 3 million bases that differ between any two individuals and accounts for the tremendous genetic variation among individuals. Although the diversity in the coding regions of DNA (genes) is significant, the noncoding regions of DNA also give rise to a great deal of diversity.

Length-based polymorphisms are found in repetitive DNA. More than 90% of the human genome is composed of noncoding, or "junk," DNA, of which approximately 20%–30% is composed of repetitive regions. Many of the repetitive regions vary in the number of core repeats between different individuals; so-called variable number of tandem repeat (VNTR) loci. DNA fragments containing VNTRs vary in length and are thus useful for analysis. Dinucleotide repeats are most common, but larger core repeats are more useful for forensic purposes. RFLP, amplified DNA fragment length polymorphisms, and STRs are examples of fragment-length analytic techniques. Sequence polymorphisms exist within the DNA sequence of similarly sized DNA fragments. Sequence polymorphisms consist of differences in one or more bases in the DNA sequence at a particular location in the genome. Sequence variations can manifest as regions of alternative alleles or base substitutions, additions, or deletions. Most sequence polymorphisms are mere point mutations within repetitive and nonrepetitive regions and are known as single nucleotide polymorphisms (SNPs). SNPs, sequence-specific oligonucleotides, and mtDNA tests are examples of sequence-based tests. Identity testing has not yet adopted the power of the more than 2 million SNPs in the human genome but this is clearly on the forefront of the technology.

Samples and Specimen Collection

For parentage testing and entering information into DNA databases, buccal swabs, fresh whole blood, and/or bloodstains on filter paper are most frequently used. Results from testing are often used in legal proceedings. Thus all aspects of the procedures used should be well-documented, because they may be subject to challenge by one of the parties. It is important to ensure documentation of the identification of the tested individuals, the collection, and the labeling of samples. Although many parentage disputes are civil actions, some jurisdictions require documents showing the chain of custody of samples similar to those used in criminal matters. American Association of Blood Banks (AABB)-accredited laboratories are required to obtain a history of any recent transfusion (in the preceding 3 months) or a hematopoietic stem cell transplant. A photographic identification and appropriate informed consent must also accompany each sample. The consent for a minor should be from an individual with legal rights to the custody of the child.

Proper specimen collection at a crime scene is very important. The evidence must be recognized before it can be properly collected. This is often accomplished with the help of chemicals and/or alternate light sources to make bloodstains visible. Blood spatter pattern analysis is also employed to help the investigator interpret and intelligently collect specimens from large pools of blood and bloodstains. Adequate chain of custody documentation, packaging and sealing, and preservation of the specimen are as important as the initial collection.

Items with biological fluids (e.g., blood on a piece of clothing) should be collected and packaged separately. When a biological fluid has been deposited on a surface or an item that cannot be collected, the fluid should be sampled with clean sterile swabs moistened with sterile distilled water. For bite marks on bodies, a technique has been described (Sweet, 1997) that involves rubbing with a wet swab followed by a dry swab. Control swabs are collected from an unstained area adjacent to the fluid stain. The stain and control swabs should be air-dried and packaged separately.

Ethylenediamine tetraacetic acid (EDTA) and citrate phosphate dextrose (CPD) remain the anticoagulants of choice for DNA testing. Heparin-anticoagulated blood is not recommended for DNA testing. Even though mature red blood cells are devoid of DNA (both nuclear and mitochondrial), ample DNA is present from circulating white blood cells for testing. Despite inhibition of the PCR reaction by heme, blood is a good source of DNA for PCR testing because the inhibitory activity of heme can easily be diluted and removed.

However, in postmortem settings, sources of DNA other than blood are preferred if there is significant putrefaction. Virtually any tissue may be successfully used for DNA typing purposes. Some tissues that may be intuitively thought to be better sources of DNA, because they are more densely cellular and would contain higher concentrations of DNA, are in fact, less optimal because of higher rates of postmortem degradation (Kobilinsky, 1992). Among soft tissues, liver DNA appears to degrade quickly from autolytic enzymes, whereas brain tissue is a relatively good source in the intermediate postmortem period. Bone and teeth are stable sources of postmortem tissue DNA. Informative DNA is routinely obtained from skeletal remains that are decades old. Generally, the greater the body decomposition and the longer the postmortem period, the greater the degradation of the DNA from cadaveric tissues.

Great care should be taken to prevent contamination of the specimen by other sources of DNA. Specimens should be collected using gloves and pristine instruments. When possible, nonexposed tissue should be collected by an incisional biopsy technique. The specimens should be kept cold or preferably frozen (although repeated freezing and thawing is destructive of large DNA fragments). Desiccation, even simple air-drying, may be an adequate method of storage of some DNA specimens (e.g., bloodstains and bone). Tissues in formalin are not optimal but can often be used for PCR-based DNA testing. No tissues or biological fluids should be discarded as inadequate without first attempting DNA testing.

DNA in most specimens will undergo progressive random fragmentation or degradation, reducing the high molecular weight DNA to low molecular weight DNA (Kobilinsky, 1992). High molecular weight DNA is not generally isolated from tissue after a few days. On the other hand, high molecular weight DNA from desiccated or frozen materials may be retained for years. Residual smaller DNA fragments may persist despite considerable degradation. Because of its high copy number (hundreds to tens of thousands of copies per cell), mtDNA often survives when no nuclear DNA is recovered. Consequently, mtDNA testing is routinely used to identify old skeletal remains (Ivanov, 1996).

Rapid DNA degradation or damage may be produced under certain conditions (Parsons, 1997). Chemical hydrolysis of DNA is normally quite slow. Tests have shown that mixing DNA with detergents, oil, gasoline, and other adulterants does not alter the DNA result. However, metal ions may catalyze oxidative hydrolysis. Ultraviolet radiation is known to cause thymidine dimerization. Depurination has been described for "ancient DNA."

DNA Extraction and Quantification

The first and most critical step for evidence is the extraction of DNA from blood, biological stains, or other biological sources. DNA from a bloodstain, a vaginal swabbing, or other source must be isolated from other cell components and environmental contaminants. The classic organic chloroform/phenol extraction with ethanol precipitation, although cumbersome, is an efficient and reliable method that separates proteins and other cellular materials from the DNA molecules. A chelating resin, Chelex 100 (Bio-Rad Laboratories, Hercules, Calif.), when boiled in the presence of biological samples, will break open cells and release the DNA (Walsh, 1991). The Chelex 100 binds to polyvalent metal ions, thus inactivating nucleases and polymerases. Even though the extract is relatively crude, the resultant single-stranded DNA yield is high and the purity is sufficient for most PCR-based testing, especially reference materials, and is fast and less expensive than other extraction methods. Solid-phase column extraction methods (e.g., Qiagen columns) and magnetic resin particles are increasingly used for DNA extraction, particularly in high-volume operations where automation may be required (Plopper, 2006). Compared with Chelex extraction, the column extraction methods yield DNA that is more highly purified but at a higher cost. Contaminants such as those found in cigarette butts and certain dyes may be removed. Silicon beads are another excellent method to purify DNA when inhibitors need to be removed. Many laboratories eliminate the extraction step altogether by performing PCR directly from a punch of a bloodstained item. This technique is most commonly used on bloodstains on FTA paper (specially treated filter paper) (Rogers, 1997) and untreated cotton paper from archived databank samples and blood reference standards.

As mentioned earlier, vaginal swabs require special conditions for extraction using a differential lysis procedure because of the need to separate the male DNA in sperm from the female DNA in epithelial cells (Crouse, 1993). The female fraction is easily produced by standard extraction procedures from the fragile epithelial cells present. The male fraction is then recovered by breaking the disulfide bridges of the protective capsule of spermatozoa with a dithiothreitol solution. Sensitive PCR-based systems often exhibit female source DNA in the male fraction, producing mixed DNA profiles.

Once the samples are extracted, quantification is performed. The forensic standards require quantification of forensic evidence, when possible. When performing quantification and knowing the amount of DNA in a sample, amplification is usually more successful. Too little or too much DNA in a PCR-based assay results in nonoptimal amplification, which can produce poor results. Early quantification methods include absorbance at 260 nm using a spectrophotometer; agarose gel electrophoresis and visualization with an intercalating dye such as ethidium bromide; and DNA bound on a nylon membrane and hybridized with a human-specific probe (Walsh, 1992). Today, real-time quantitative PCR techniques provide for a more sensitive and objective assay (Green, 2005).

Test Methods and Marker Systems

Short Tandem Repeats

Loci consisting of repeat units of three to seven nucleotides occur throughout the genome (Weber, 1989). Alleles at these STR loci are defined by the number of repeat units in the PCR-amplified product. The basic PCR techniques employed are discussed in Chapter 66. Extracted sample DNA is added to a PCR reaction mix containing *Thermus aquaticus* (Taq) polymerase, a specific forward and reverse primer for each locus tested, deoxynucleoside triphosphates, magnesium, a buffer solution, and bovine serum albumin. The PCR reaction mixture is amplified in a thermal cycler using carefully defined parameters to maximize detection of the alleles. Several primers with different fluorescent labels areused in a multiplex reaction to detect alleles at several loci in a single amplification. The PCR products, which vary in length, are separated by capillary electrophoresis. Detection is performed using a laser to excite the labeled fluorophore that has been incorporated in the primer. The loci in the multiplex reaction differ by size and color (Fig. 71-1). Sizing is accomplished by introducing a size standard with each sample injected in the capillary and using sophisticated software algorithms; phenotyping of each peak is achieved by comparing the peaks in the sample to an allelic ladder accounting for most alleles for each locus and using sophisticated software algorithms for allele calls that adjust for minor variations in electrophoresis for each injection (Fig. 71-2).

The most commonly used markers in forensic and parentage laboratories in the United States are the 13 STR loci (CSF1PO, D3S1358, D5S818, D7S820, D8S1179, D13S317, D16S539, D18S51, D21S11, FGA, TH01, TPOX, VWA) that have been standardized for use in obtaining genetic profiles of individuals who have been convicted of various criminal offenses. These were identified by a consortium of scientists sponsored by the Federal Bureau of Investigation (FBI) for use in the Combined DNA Index System (CODIS). The STR marker systems have discrete alleles and are not as polymorphic as the RFLP marker systems. An STR locus may have three or four common alleles (frequencies of 0.15–0.25) and several rare alleles (frequencies of <0.01). Thus in order to obtain a high cumulative probability of exclusion (CPE) and combined paternity index (PI), it is usually necessary to test at least six or more STR loci. In a series of 50 paternity cases tested in parallel by both RFLP and nine STR loci, Alford and colleagues reported (Alford, 1994) that both methods excluded the same 13 alleged fathers (based on two or more loci). The likelihood of paternity for the 37 nonexcluded men based on the STR systems was more than 99% in 36 cases. When all 13 CODIS STR loci are obtained, the average random match probability is rarer than one in one trillion among unrelated individuals (Chakraborty, 1999).

X and Y Chromosome Markers

Sex determination is now commonly performed using the Amelogenin locus (see Fig. 71-1). The primer for this locus amplifies an X-specific band (Xp22.1–22.3) and a Y-specific band. This locus is coamplified and coanalyzed with many multiplexed STR systems. Sex determination marks a departure from all other routine identity markers, in that it provides specific phenotypic information about the source individual. It may also be important in the investigation of potential suspects as well as in the categorization of specimens as originating from a victim or suspect.

Although polymorphic Y chromosome markers (Fig. 71-3) are not used for sex determination, they are extremely useful in the typing of sexual assault evidence that displays a mixture of both the female epithelial cell DNA and male sperm DNA because these results are only obtained from males. They also are used to characterize the paternal lineage in human remains identifications. The characterization of the Thomas Jefferson family lineage was accomplished using Y chromosome markers (Foster,

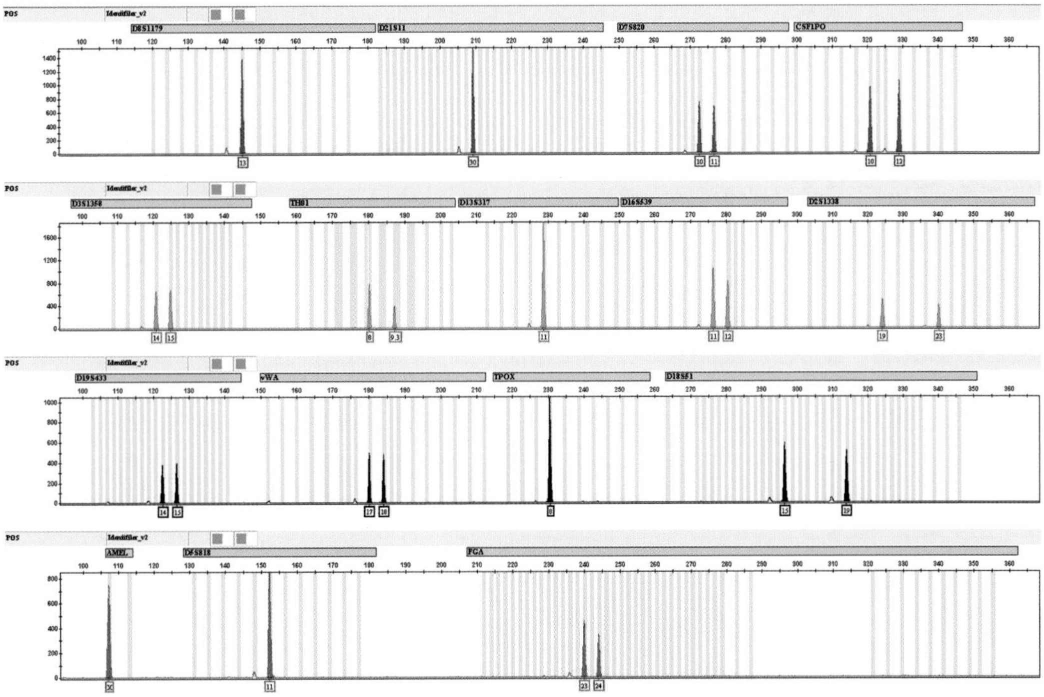

Figure 71-1 The results of the kit-included positive control 9947A amplified with the AmpFLSTR Identifiler PCR Amplification Kit (Applied Biosystems, Foster City, Calif.) (Collins, 2004) and electrophoresed on the ABI PRISM 3130*xl* Genetic Analyzer (Applied Biosystems) and typed with GeneMapper *ID* Software v. 3.1.2 (Applied Biosystems). The results for the 15 autosomal STR loci and Amelogenin, a sexing marker, are visualized. This image displays the phenotype of the positive control amplified in this mega-multiplex. The locus name is shown in the gray bar above the peaks, the allele call(s) for each locus is just below the highlighted peak.

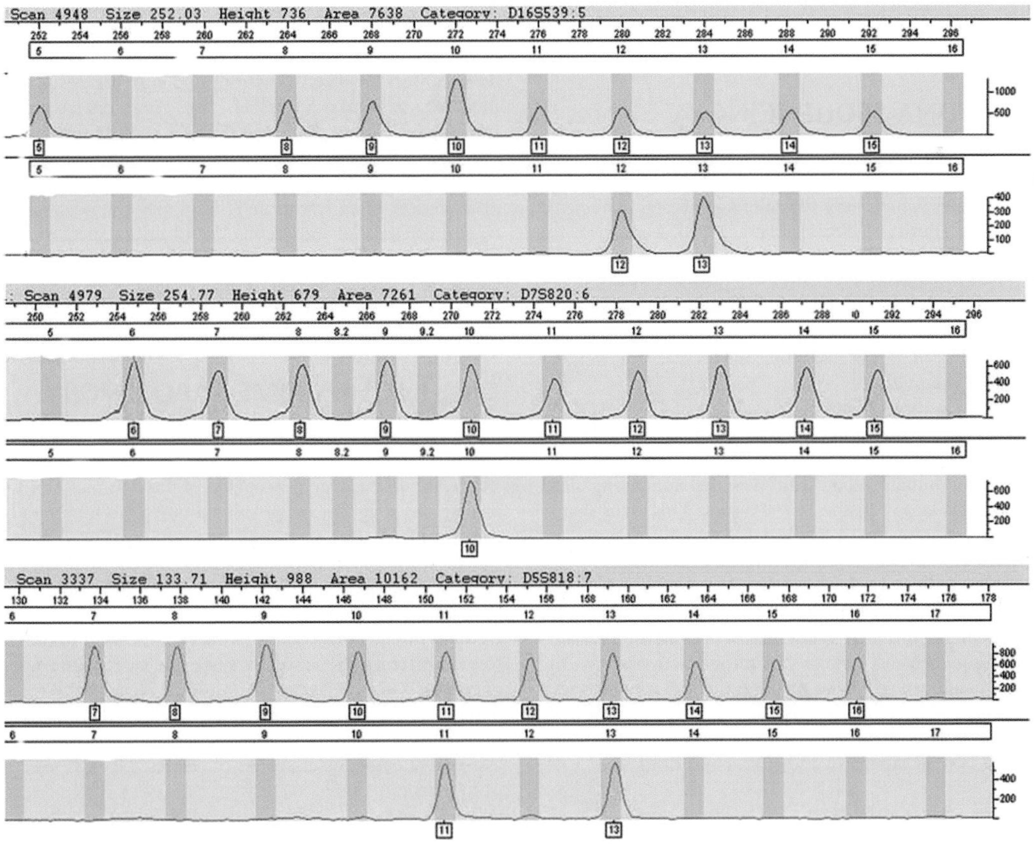

Figure 71-2 The results of a sample electrophoresed on the ABI PRISM 3100 Genetic Analyzer (Applied Biosystems) and amplified with the AmpFLSTR Identifiler PCR Amplification Kit. The ladders and accompanying results for three loci, D16S539 (alleles 12, 13), D7S820 (allele 10), and D5S818 (alleles 11, 13), are visualized in these images. The images demonstrate excellent resolution in the electrophoresis.

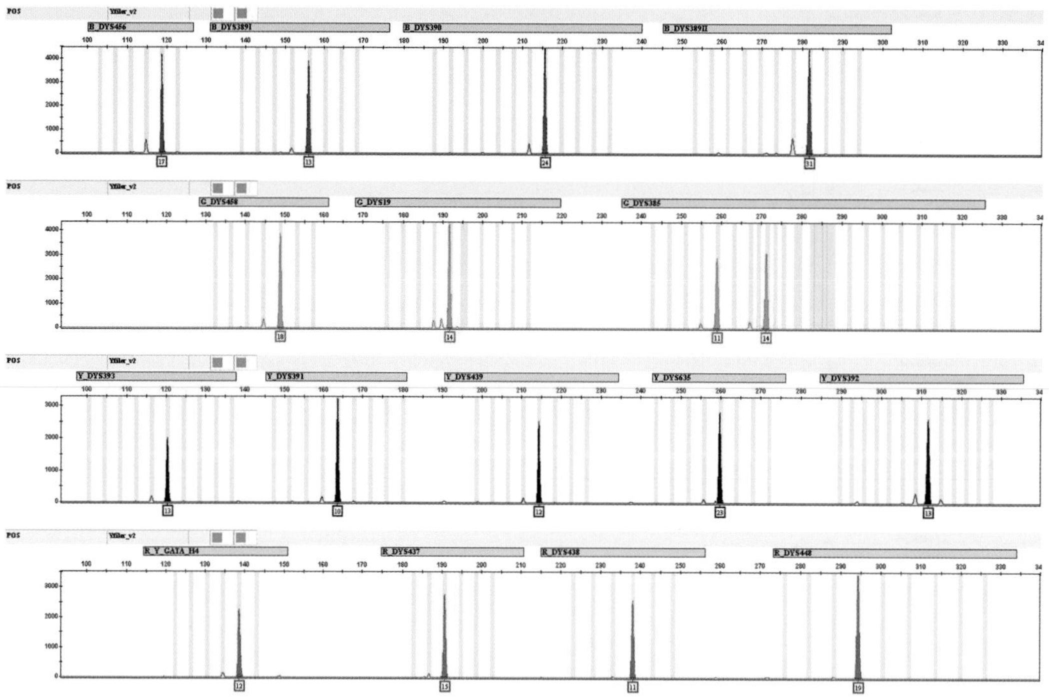

Figure 71-3 The results of the kit-included positive control 9948 amplified with the AmpFLSTR Yfiler PCR Amplification Kit (Applied Biosystems, Foster City, Calif.) (Mulero, 2006), electrophoresed on the ABI PRISM 3130*xl* Genetic Analyzer, and typed with GeneMapper *ID* Software v. 3.1.2. The results for the 17 Y-STR loci are visualized. This image displays the phenotype of the positive control amplified in this mega-multiplex. The locus name is shown in the gray bar above the peaks; the allele call for each locus is just below the highlighted peak.

1998), an example of a historic and genealogic study. Data from extensive Y-STR typings have shown that certain haplotypes are indicative of ethnic origin and can be used for human migration and evolutionary studies. A haplotype is generated from Y-STRs versus a phenotype in autosomal STRs; haplotypes do not afford the same level of discrimination as STR profiles.

MITOCHONDRIAL DNA SEQUENCING

Mitochondrial DNA (mtDNA) sequencing is applicable when extremely small quantities of sample DNA are present or when the DNA is extremely degraded, such as in shed hairs (which have virtually no detectable nuclear DNA) and skeletal remains (Butler, 1998; Holland, 1999). Hundreds to thousands of copies of mtDNA are present within a single cell with only one copy of nuclear DNA. Accordingly, a mtDNA profile can often be obtained when a nuclear DNA profile cannot. Even a single distant relative in the maternal line may be used as a reference, so mtDNA is also useful when reference samples are limited, because nuclear DNA testing generally requires multiple close relatives.

Mitochondrial DNA is composed of a circular piece of DNA 16,569 base pairs (bp) in length. Because no significant regions of repetitive DNA exist in mtDNA, only sequence differences are reported. The region of mtDNA that is analyzed for human identification is the noncoding displacement loop (D-loop), also known as the *control region*. This locus spans approximately 1100 bp and contains two hypervariable regions. At present, direct sequencing is the method used to obtain mtDNA results.

Mitochondria are maternally inherited, so mtDNA has no paternal contribution. Unlike nuclear DNA, which is present in pairs of chromosomes, generally only a single mtDNA sequence is present in the cell (homoplasmic) and consequently no genetic recombination occurs. An exact mtDNA sequence match can be traced through the maternal lineage of a family for many generations. However, the discriminatory power of mtDNA sequencing is limited—on the order of one in a few thousand. Furthermore, this testing is very expensive and time-consuming.

OTHER SYSTEMS

Mini-STRs is a term referring to autosomal STRs in the multiplex kits where the primers have been moved closer to the tandem repeat to achieve a smaller amplicon product size. Hence, those samples that are severely degraded or include PCR inhibitors may produce a mini-STR result when the standard kits fail (Mulero, 2008). However, fewer markers are included in the mini-STR kits compared with standard kits (Fig. 71-4).

Methods to detect single nucleotide polymorphisms, also known as SNPs, are used to determine a single base change in a sequence at a specific location. Because of the limited variability at these loci, as many as 70 SNPs need to be tested to get the same level of information about relatedness, powers of discrimination, and mixture resolution as provided by a multiplex of several STR loci. These markers have been used in the identification of highly degraded samples such as those that were recovered at the World Trade Center site. There are millions of SNPs in individuals. SNPs could be very powerful for identity testing. SNPs may provide information when traditional STRs may not because they can be designed to amplify smaller amplicons. In addition, specific SNPs may be used to provide information regarding the physical traits of an individual, and they can be designed to predict ethnic origin.

ANALYSIS AND USE OF TEST DATA

DNA IN THE CRIME LABORATORY

DNA testing has become routine in crime laboratories (National Research Council, 1996), and DNA evidence is routinely admitted into court. In the United States, a large percentage of the criminal DNA tests involves sexual assault and a significant proportion involves homicide. Approximately one third of DNA tests exonerate wrongfully accused suspects (Fig. 71-5), one fourth are inconclusive, and somewhat less than half result in a match of the suspect to a crime. Only a fraction of the cases in which DNA evidence is tested are actually litigated, because most cases result in a plea bargain. In the criminalistics context, DNA can be used to link a suspect to a crime, to exculpate falsely accused suspects, to recognize serial crimes, and to distinguish copycat crimes, or to aid in accident reconstruction (e.g., to determine who was driving a car by the identification of the bloodstains on the driver's side of the windshield). In addition to the use of DNA for associative evidence at scenes of crimes, DNA is used in the identification of human remains.

DNA IN THE PATHOLOGY LABORATORY

DNA identity tests can be used to resolve specimen mixups (Weedn, 1993b), such as when samples are inadvertently switched or pathologic material floats onto a histologic or cytologic slide. A small fragment of

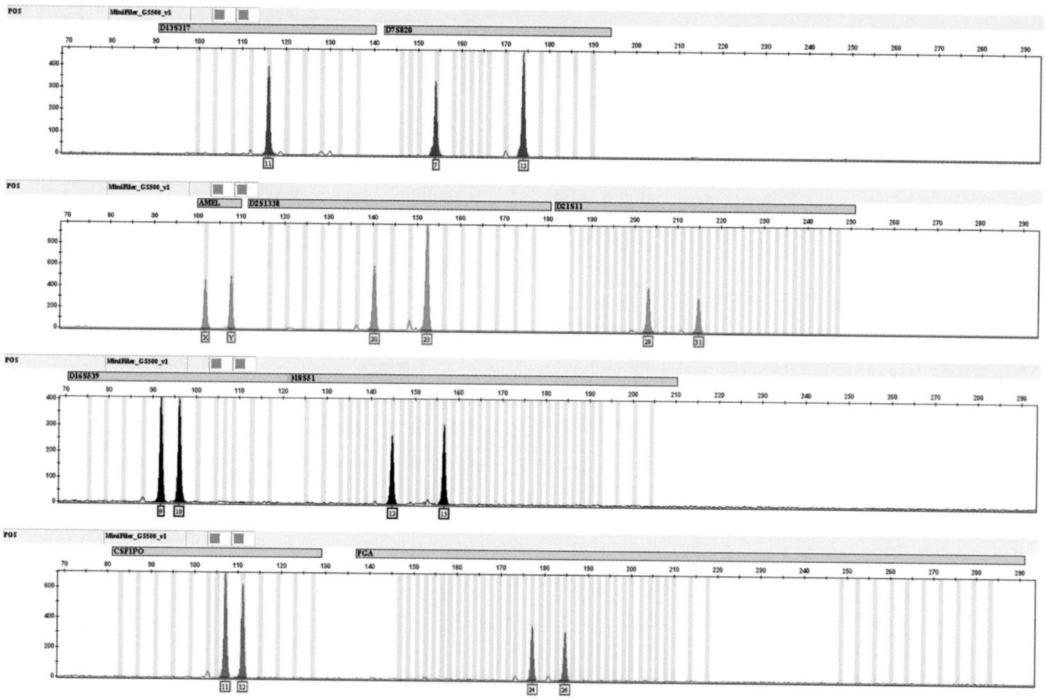

Figure 71-4 The results of the kit-included positive control 007 amplified with the AmpFLSTR MinFiler PCR Amplification Kit (Applied Biosystems) (Mulero, 2008), electrophoresed on the ABI PRISM 3130*xl* Genetic Analyzer, and typed with GeneMapper *ID* Software v. 3.1.2. The results for the 8 STR loci are visualized. This image displays the phenotype of the positive control amplified in this multiplex. The locus name is shown in the gray bar above the peaks, the allele call for each locus is just below the highlighted peak. The loci in this kit are smaller (the size of the peaks can be measured on the *x*-axis) than the corresponding loci in the AmpFLSTR Identifiler PCR Amplification Kit (see Fig 71-1).

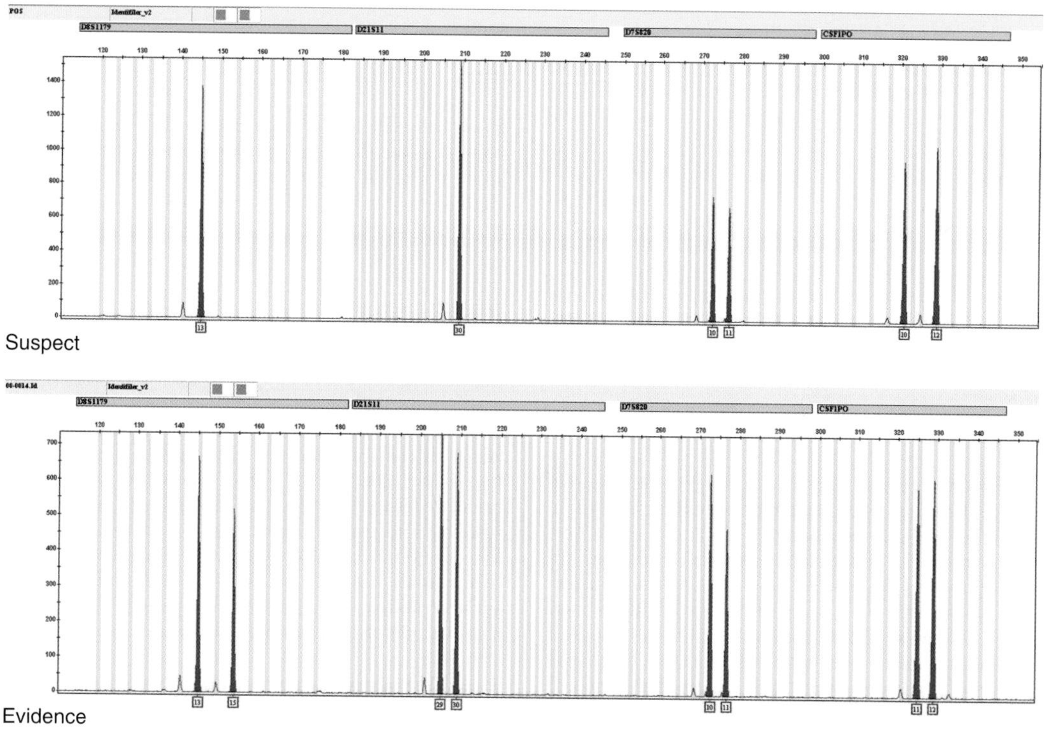

Figure 71-5 Exclusion of suspect when compared to crime scene evidence. The profile for the evidence at D8S1179, D21S11, and CSF1PO is clearly different from the suspect's profile. The evidence could not have been contributed by the suspect.

cancerous tissue ("floater") on a glass microscope slide can be determined to be from someone other than the patient (Table 71-1). DNA testing may be used to confirm or refute mislabeling of biopsy specimens. In addition, urine drug tests that have been challenged on the basis of alleged sample switching may be resolved by DNA testing (Weedn, 1996).

STR markers are also used to evaluate engraftment of marrow after transplantation (Scharf, 1995). When the donor is related to the recipient, testing of multiple markers may be required to find an informative locus because related people share many alleles.

EXCLUSION OF PARENTAGE

The primary goal of genetic marker testing in cases of disputed parentage is to identify the biological parent of a given child. Although this cannot

TABLE 71-1
Identification of Possible 'Floater'

STR locus	Floater	Tissue block	Patient sample	Frequency of patient's phenotype
CSF1PO	10,12	10,12	10,12	0.191
D3S1358	15,16	16,17	16,17	0.099
D5S818	11	11,12	11,12	0.024
D7S820	9,11	11	11	0.0529
D8S1179	13	12,14	12,14	0.0976
D13S317	11	11	11	0.0798
D16S539	9,11	11,12	11,12	0.1764
D18S51	14,15	14,15	14,15	0.0477
D21S11	30	28,31.2	28,31.2	0.0341

Shaded results indicate the DNA results from the floater are different than the DNA from the patient and the tissue block. The chance that the tissue block has the same genetic markers as the patient compared to a random Caucasian individual is greater than 1.86×10^{10}.

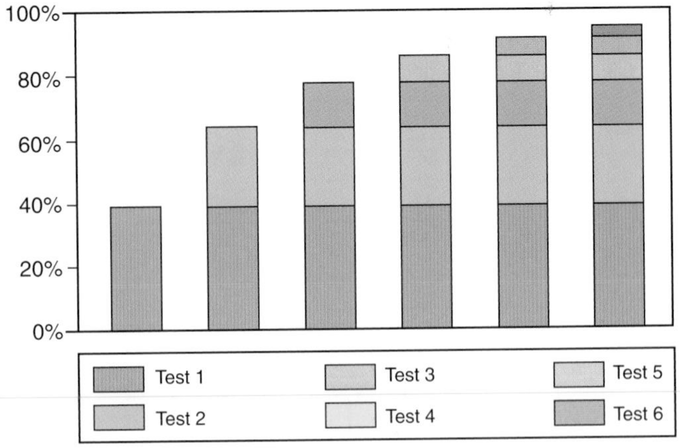

Figure 71-6 Cumulative probability of exclusion (each added test; PE = 0.4). The percentage of the population excluded by each additional test becomes smaller and smaller. The overall exclusion probability of the six tests is 95.3%. If a seventh test with PE = 0.5 was performed, only an additional 2.4% of the population would be excluded ([1–0.953] × 0.5 = 0.0235).

TABLE 71-2
Exclusion of Parentage: Phenotype (Genotype)

Type of exclusion	Child	Mother	Tested man	Obligatory gene(s)
Direct	AB (ab)	A (aa, a?)	C (cc, c?)	b
	AC (ac)	AB (ab)	AD (ad)	c
	AB (ab)	C (cc, c?)	AC (ac)	b (maternal)
Two-haplotype	A (aa, a?)	A (aa, a?)	BC (bc)	a or ?
	A (aa, a?)	AB (aa, ab)	BC (bc)	a or ?
	AB (ab)	AB (ab)	CD (cd)	a or b
	AB (ab)	Not available	CD (cd)	a or b
Indirect*	A (aa, a?)	A (aa, a?)	B (bb, b?)	a or ?
	B (bb, b?)	AB (ab)	A (aa, a?)	b or ?
	B (bb, b?)	C (cc, c?)	AB (ab)	b or ? (maternal)
	B (bb, b?)	Not available	A (aa, a?)	b or ?

Examples of direct, two-haplotype, and indirect exclusions of the tested man. The capital letters represent the phenotype and the small letters in parentheses represent the possible genotype. The question mark (?) represents a possible null, or silent, allele.
*Mutation must be considered.

be done with absolute certainty, genetic marker tests can provide objective evidence of nonparentage. By using multiple genetic systems, it is possible to exclude most (>99%), but not all, nonparents.

In systems that follow the rules of Mendelian genetics, exclusions are identified by finding exceptions to the expected inheritance pattern. Interpretation of test results when paternity is in question usually depends on assuming that the sample defined as maternal is from the child's biological mother. The child's and mother's phenotypes should be compared to determine whether results are consistent with expected inheritance patterns. An allele present in the child but not in the mother is referred to as the *obligatory paternal gene* (OG). If both alleles in the child and mother are identical, then there are alternative (two) possibilities for the paternal gene.

If the tested man does not have the possibility of passing the OG and the marker for the gene is absent in the presumed mother, the exclusion observed is termed *direct exclusion* (Table 71-2). This type of exclusion in one of the classic systems was usually enough to conclude that the tested man is not the biological father of the child in question. In DNA systems, because the rate of mutation is orders of magnitude greater than observed in classic systems, an exclusion at a single locus is not considered enough evidence to establish nonpaternity (American Association of Blood Banks, 2009). A direct exclusion also occurs when the child or the tested male is heterozygous (two alleles present) and the two markers are absent in the other person. This type of direct exclusion sometimes is referred to as a *two-haplotype exclusion*. When only the child and one alleged parent are available for testing, if the tested individual or child has two haplotypes, neither of which is in the other, it is possible to establish nonparentage.

Absence of an expected genetic marker in the child when the parent in question appears to be homozygous (one allele present) for the gene is called an *indirect exclusion*. This is sometimes also known as *reverse homozygosity*. One indirect exclusion is not sufficient evidence to conclude that the tested individual is not the parent. Interpretation of reverse homozygosity as an indirect exclusion presumes that the tested subjects both have two identical alleles at the locus. In PCR testing of STRs, this absence of an expected allele may occur if there is a binding site mutation (Harrison, 2004; Leibelt, 2003) in one of the tested individuals, or it is possible that a rare null allele (or other undetected allele) or mutation is present in the child as well as the parent in question. The finding of indirect exclusions in at least two independent systems usually is sufficient evidence to reach a conclusion of nonpaternity.

PROBABILITY OF EXCLUSION

Before testing, it is possible to provide an estimate of the average chance that testing will prove nonparentage if the accused is not the parent. This is referred to as the *probability of exclusion*, PE, and is defined as the probability of excluding a random individual from the population given the alleles of the child and the mother; the genetic information of the tested man is not considered. For each genetic system, an average PE can be calculated based on the gene frequencies (p and q) for the alleles in the system. The general equation for a two-allele system was reported by Wiener (Wiener, 1930). When a system has multiple alleles, more complex formulas are required (Walker, 1978). A highly polymorphic system has a greater power of exclusion than a system with only a few alleles or one that has one or two common alleles and many rare alleles.

CUMULATIVE PROBABILITY OF EXCLUSION

The individual probability of exclusion (PE) is calculated for each of the genetic systems (for each locus) analyzed. The overall combined probability of exclusion (CPE), or the probability of excluding a falsely accused man in a given case, can be calculated by using the following formula:

$$\text{CPE} = [(1-\text{PE}_1)\times(1-\text{PE}_2)\times(1-\text{PE}_3)\times\ldots\times(1-\text{PE}_N)]$$

where PE is the probability of exclusion for each system used. As shown in Figure 71-6, as more and more systems are used, fewer and fewer individuals are excluded by each additional test. With an appropriately selected

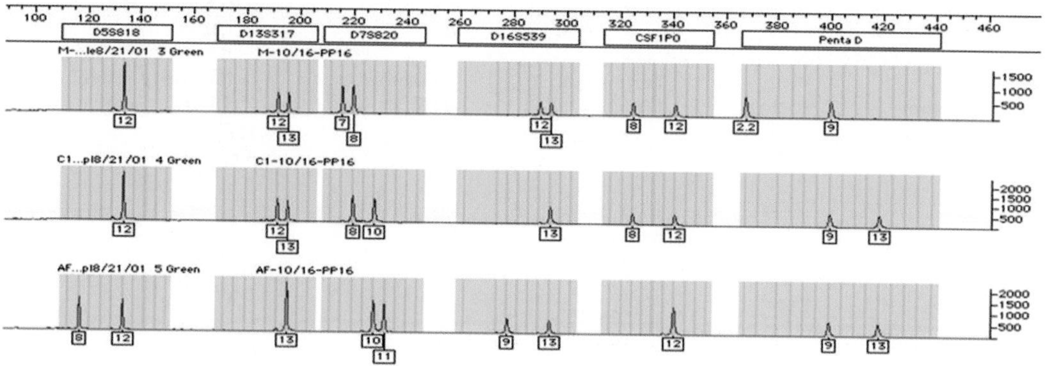

Figure 71-7 Example of family analysis using short tandem repeats testing. Note the alleles shared between the mother (top panel) and the child (middle panel). The alleles from the tested man (bottom panel) also matches the child. The tested man is not excluded as the biological father of this child.

TABLE 71-3
Calculation of the System* Likelihood Ratio (Paternity Index)

Mother	Child	Obligatory gene(s)	Tested man	X	Y	Formula for Y frequency	X/Y
A	A	a	A	1	0.25	p	4
A	A	a	AB	0.5	0.25	p	2
A	AB	b	B	1	0.4	q	2.5
A	AB	b	AB	0.5	0.4	q	1.25
AB	AB	a or b	A	1	0.65	p + q	1.54
AB	AB	a or b	B	1	0.65	p + q	1.54
AB	AB	a or b	AB	1	0.65	p + q	1.54
AB	AC	c	AC	0.5	0.3	r	1.67
BC	BC	b or c	BC	1	0.7	q + r	1.43
AC	AD	d	BD	0.5	0.05	s	10

X, Chance that tested male is the biological father; *Y*, chance that an untested male in the random population is the biological father; *X/Y*, likelihood ratio.
*Hypothetical locus with four codominant alleles a, b, c, and d.

battery of DNA marker systems, a CPE of 0.995 or greater is easily achieved.

Inclusion of Parentage

If, after testing multiple independent systems, the parent in dispute is not excluded (Fig. 71-7), then an estimate of the possibility that the tested person could be the biological parent should be calculated. If the tested male is not excluded, it always can be argued that the amount of testing was inadequate, that evidence for exclusion will be found by testing another genetic system, or that the true parent is a close relative of the tested man. This line of reasoning could be correct only if the tested male has been falsely accused. In addition to the average probability of exclusion described previously, it also is possible to calculate the frequency with which a random male will not be excluded based on a mother–child pair exhibiting the observed phenotypes (Salmon, 1983). This value is related to the actual probability of exclusion for the tests performed.

In providing estimates of inclusion of paternity, appropriate gene frequency tables are used. In general, this means that a population of random persons of the same race has been phenotyped, that the size of the sample is large enough to provide gene frequencies with minimum errors of estimation for the alleles in the system, and that the tested male and biological father are from the same population. When multiple systems have been tested, the differences observed in gene frequencies in populations from various geographic locations become unimportant in calculations of the likelihood of paternity (Hummel, 1981). When the tested male is of mixed racial background or from a population for which there are inadequate frequency tables, it may be impossible to provide a precise estimate of paternity. However, when multiple systems with a high power of exclusion have been used and the PI value using a reference population is high, there is a minimal chance that frequencies from a more-defined population will have a significant effect on the conclusion of parentage. In these situations, comparisons with frequencies for several defined racial groups may also be helpful.

PATERNITY INDEX CALCULATION

In cases in which a trio has been tested, a general approach referred to as the *comparison of sperm method* is usually applied (Walker, 1978). This calculation compares the chance (*x*) that a sperm from a male of the phenotype of the tested male could have fertilized the ovum of the presumed mother to the chance (*y*) that a sperm from an untested male in the random population could have produced the child. Likelihood ratios (*x/y*) are calculated for each independent genetic system by comparing the tested male to the frequencies for the obligatory gene or alternate paternal genetic contribution in the random population of the same race of the tested male. These values are then multiplied to derive the PI, which reflects the genetic odds in favor of paternity, given the phenotypes of the trio. Table 71-3 displays the formulas for calculating the indexes with various phenotype combinations. Table 71-4 is an example using these formulas to determine the possible father of a fetus in a possible rape case. In this example, Tested Man 2 is clearly excluded as the biological father of this fetus.

PI values in cases where no exclusion is observed can have a numeric value greater than zero to a number approaching infinity. The current AABB Standards (2009) require that, to determine parentage, the testing should result in a PI of at least 100. This means that the odds (likelihood ratio) for the tested man being the father are 99 to 1.

LIKELIHOOD OF PARENTAGE

Another useful estimate, the likelihood of parentage, combines the genetic testing with assumptions about prior events. Essen-Möller (1938)

TABLE 71-4

Determining Parentage from Fetal Tissue

STR locus	Fetal tissue*	Mother	Tested man 1 (TM 1)	Tested man 2 (TM 2)	Paternity index TM 1	Paternity index TM 2
CSF1PO	10	10	10	10, 12	3.74	1.87
D3S1358	15, 16	15	16	14	4.49	0†
D5S818	11, 12, 13	12, 13	10, 11	10	1.27	0†
D7S820	8, 9	8, 9	8, 9	10, 11	3.31	0†
D8S1179	11, 15	11, 15	12, 15	11, 15	2.60	5.19
D13S317	10, 12, 13	12, 13	10	11, 12	14.81	0†
D16S539	9, 13	13	9, 12	9, 14	4.65	4.65
D18S51	12, 17	12	12, 17	17	4.76	9.52
D21S11	31	31	31	31	18.18	18.18
vWA31/A	16, 17, 18	16, 18	14, 17	14, 18	2.0	0†
Amelogenin	X	X	XY	XY	–	–
				CPI	2.19×10^6	0†

STR, Short tandem repeat.
*Fetal tissue sample is contaminated with maternal tissue; mixture present.
†Tested man excluded at that locus.

TABLE 71-5

Formula for the Likelihood of Parentage (W)

Bayes' theorem is used to combine *p* with PI:

$$W = (p)(PI)/[(p)(PI) + (1 - p)]$$

where *p* = prior probability of nongenetic events, and PI (paternity index) = summary of testing results.

described this calculation based on Bayes' theorem (Table 71-5). The estimate uses the PI to summarize the genetic information and *p* (a value for the prior probability) to account for the assumptions that the tested man:

1. Was not sterile
2. Had access during the conceptive period
3. Is not a close (first-degree) relative of the father
4. And that other possible fathers are from a population with similar gene frequencies.

If a *p* of 0.5 is used, this assigns an equal prior chance to the tested man and one untested man. Using this value, the likelihood of paternity (*W*) is equal to PI/(PI + 1). Other values for the prior probability can be used in this calculation, but they introduce a bias against the tested man if greater than 0.5, and against the mother if less than 0.5.

The mathematical values obtained from calculation of the PI or likelihood have special significance because in many jurisdictions the reported value may change the legal standing of the parties. For example, the Minnesota Statute Section 257.55 (Parentage Act, 2004) shifts the burden of disproving paternity to the man if the testing indicates a greater than 99% likelihood that he is the father.

ESTIMATING PARENTAGE WITH AN ABSENT PARENT

If one of the parents is unavailable for testing, it is still possible to provide an estimate of parentage. The most common situation is one in which a sample is available from the child and alleged father, but not the mother. In this situation the child must share at least one gene at each locus with the tested man. Formulas (Table 71-6) to estimate the paternity index and likelihood of paternity are similar to those used when a trio is tested (see Table 71-3) except that the estimates must include an adjustment for the frequency of the allele passed by the absent mother (Brenner, 1993). The calculation is more complicated if the missing mother and untested man are of different races (Traver, 1996). If the tested man or child has two alleles at a locus, neither of which is present in the other tested individual, then the tested man is excluded. If reverse homozygosity is present in the child and tested man, this also suggests nonpaternity.

TABLE 71-6

Calculation of the System* Likelihood Ratio (Parentage Index) When Only One Parent Is Tested

Child	Tested parent	Parental gene(s) in child	Obligatory gene(s) in other parent	Formula to calculate system ratio
A	A	a	a	1/p
A	AB	a	a	1/2p
A	BC		a	Exclusion
AB	B	b	a or b	1/2q
AB	AB	a or b	a or b	(p+q)/4pq
AC	AB	a	a or c	1/4p
BC	A		b or c	Exclusion
AD	BD	d	a or d	1/4s

*Hypothetical locus with four alleles A, B, C, and D (frequency of genes a = p, b = q, c = r, and d = s).

RECONSTRUCTION OF FAMILIES

Many situations occur in which it is important to establish a relationship between individuals. This happens when individuals are trying to gain status as an immigrant or discover whether they share a parent, or when there is a question related to inheritance. DNA testing can be informative in identifying parents of fetal material found in a dumpster or products of conception in rape cases. Reconstruction is also very important when trying to identify bodies or body parts following a mass disaster. Because only a parent and child will share at least one allele at each locus, relatives may have systems in which they do not share any alleles. Formulas taking into account that alleles may be shared by descent are used to estimate the closeness of the relationship of two individuals (Wenk, 1986). Full siblings have a 0.25 chance of not sharing an allele in a system, whereas half sibs, aunts, or uncles have a 0.5 chance. In cases where the alleged father is deceased, his probable phenotype can be reconstructed if testing is performed with his biological parents (Mayr, 1983). The child and putative grandparents must share the obligatory paternal alleles in all systems. A PI can be calculated using a frequency for x that takes into account the chance that the deceased could pass the allele (Fig. 71-8). Reconstructions

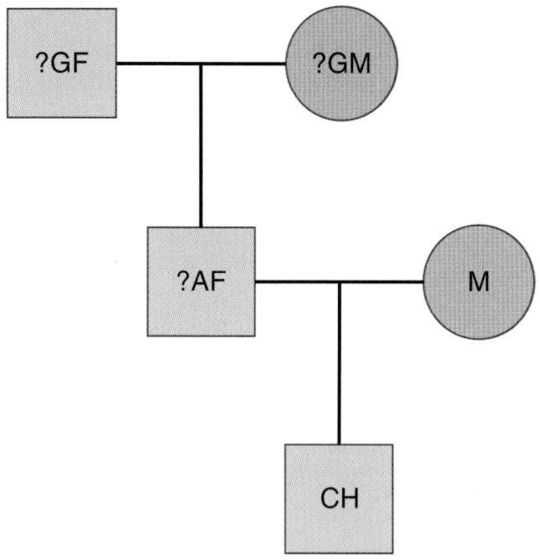

System	Child	Mother	OG	?GF	?GM*	Possible phenotypes of ?AF	Formula to calculate system index
CSF1PO	10,12	9,12	*10*	10,13	10,11	10;10,11; 10,13; 11,13	0.5/*p*
D3S1358	14,15	14,17	*15*	15,16	16,17	15,16; 15,17; 16,17;16	0.25/*p*
D7S820	10,11	10,11	*10* or *11*	8,9	11	8,11; 9,11	0.5/*p*+*q*
D16S539	9,12	9,13	*12*	10,12	12	10,12;12	0.75/*p*
TPOX	8	8, 11	*8*	8	8	8	1/*p*
vWA31/A	18	18	*18*	18	18	18	1/*p*

Figure 71-8 Family testing to establish paternity. Interpretation assumes that the deceased ?AF is the child of the persons tested (?GF, ?GM) and p and q are the frequencies of the obligatory paternal allele(s). In this case the presumed parents of the deceased alleged father were tested to reconstruct his probable phenotype. In each of the systems tested, the obligatory paternal gene (OG) is present in one of the child's presumed grandparents. Note: For D7S820, either allele in the child could be maternal. The combined paternity index and likelihood of paternity are obtained by multiplying the values for the individual systems.

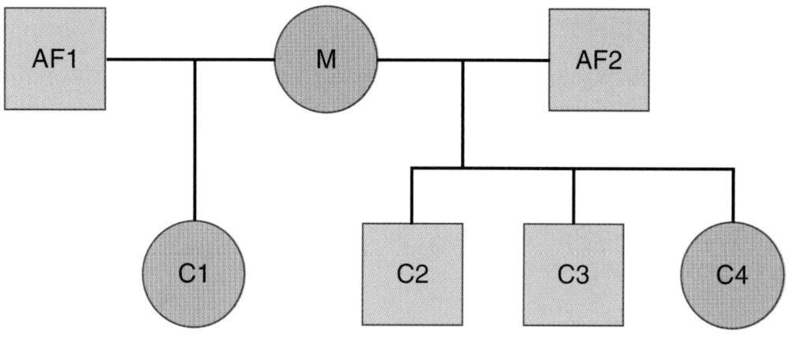

System	AF1	AF2	Child 1	Child 2	Child 3	Child 4
CSF1PO	10, 11	11, 12	10, **14**	12, **14**	**9**, 12	11, **14**
D3S1358	15, 17	15, 17	**14, 17**	**17**	**14**, 16	**14**, 15
D5S818	13, 14	11, 12	**10**, 14	**10, 12**	**12**	**12**
D7S820	8, 9	10, 13	8, **11**	10, **11**	10, **14**	13, **14**
D13S317	11, 12	8, 10	12, **14**	8, **10**	10, **14**	**10**
D16S539	12, 15	9, 12	**8**, 15	**8**, 11	11, **13**	9, **13**
vWA31/A	14, 20	16, 17	**15**, 20	**15**, 17	16,**18**	17, **18**
TH01	8, 9	6, 9	8, **9.3**	6, **9.3**	8, **9.3**	9, **9.3**
TPOX	8, 11	8, 10	**8**	**8, 12**	**8, 12**	**8**
Amelogenin	Male	Male	Female	Male	Male	Female
DYS390	23	23		23	23	
DYS391	10	11		11	11	

Figure 71-9 Family study—presumed mother (M) is deceased. All four children in this family study could have the same mother. The probable maternal allele in each system is shown in bold. Note: In some systems either marker could be maternal in one of the children (D3S1358 in child 1). Alleged father 1 (AF1) shares an allele with child 1 in all systems and is excluded as the possible father of children 2, 3, and 4 in several systems. AF2 is excluded as the father of child 1 in every system except D3S1358 and TPOX. AF2 is also excluded as the father of child 3 in two systems (D3S1358 and TH01). The finding of a possible match in nine of 11 systems, including two Y-STRs, suggests that the true father of child 3 might be a relative of AF2, or two mutations have occurred.

can also be conducted by using data from multiple presumed relatives as shown in Figure 71-9.

Software Systems

New software systems have been introduced in both the forensic and parentage laboratories. These software systems include expert systems programs that display rule firings, or flags, when specific laboratory-defined thresholds have not been met. Currently, expert systems are used by laboratories for the review of single source reference standard samples. In addition, forensic laboratories are evaluating mixture deconvolution software tools to assist the forensic analyst in the review of mixed data as is often observed with sexual assault evidence. Identity testing laboratories worldwide have implemented sophisticated software programs to perform kinship analyses. Laboratory Information Systems, LIMS, are also used to assist a laboratory in managing its casework.

Quality Assurance Standards

Laboratories that perform forensic (parentage and criminalistic) DNA testing must follow appropriate standards, obtain accreditation, and participate in proficiency testing programs. The possibility of significant judicial scrutiny of every step of the procedures and practices used from collection of samples to reporting of results is to be expected. Challenges to the validation of the methods, the source of the databases used in statistical reports, and the qualification of the personnel are not uncommon. There is general agreement as to proper laboratory procedures that should be used in DNA testing and, although the DNA typing methods are not specifically standardized, procedures are remarkably uniform.

The FBI's Technical Working Group on DNA Analysis Methods, now known as the Scientific Working Group on DNA Analysis Methods, promulgated early guidelines for DNA analytic procedures that became de facto standards (Technical Working Group, 1989, 1995). These standards were modified by the FBI's DNA Advisory Board and adopted by the FBI Director pursuant to the DNA Identification Act, a component of the Crime Bill passed in 1994. These standards apply to crime laboratories that submit DNA results to the FBI's National DNA Index System or that accept certain federal grants. The American Society of Crime Laboratory Directors has an accreditation program for crime laboratories. The American Board of Criminalists certifies criminalists and has a subspecialty category for DNA analysts. Analysts who work on casework samples must have college credit (or equivalent) in genetics, biochemistry, and molecular biology and 1 year of forensic biology experience. Each of these standards calls for proficiency testing by each analyst twice a year.

The AABB began developing standards and accrediting parentage testing laboratories in 1984. The 9th edition, renamed *Standards for Relationship Testing Laboratories*, was published in 2009 (American Association of Blood Banks, 2009). All aspects of parentage testing from laboratory organization to process control and improvement are covered. The Standards include requirements for documents and records, report content, and interpretation of results. Laboratories are required to participate in graded proficiency testing.

CONCLUSION

Scientific evidence that will aid in resolving cases of disputed parentage, questions of relatedness, and identity can be obtained from testing multiple DNA systems. Current technology provides test results that exclude more than 99.9% of falsely accused individuals in parentage and criminal cases. It is not possible to prove paternity or guilt by laboratory tests. The mathematical estimates derived from genetic marker tests when no exclusion is found or there is a match between sample and suspect are a significant source of data that can be used to establish parentage or guilt.

Acknowledgment: The authors would like to thank Victor Weedn, MD, JD, for material from a chapter in a previous edition. Dr. Roby would like to acknowledge contributions by Arthur Eisenberg, PhD and Shubhra Nandi.

SELECTED REFERENCES

American Association of Blood Banks. Standards for relationship testing laboratories. 9th ed. Arlington, Va: AABB; 2009.

The AABB periodically provides standards for accredited parentage testing laboratories that include key elements of QA/QC, testing, reporting and validation requirements. With each edition of Standards a companion Guidance for Standards is published that has detailed explanations of the requirements, and appendices with useful tables and formulas.

Budowle B, Shea B, Niezgoda S, Chakroborty R. CODIS STR loci data from 41 sample populations. J Forensic Sci 2001;46:453–89.

Reference for the frequency data used to calculate parentage results as well as population frequencies for the chance that a matching sample is from a random individual. Several manufacturers also have websites with frequency tables based on results from their reagents.

Butler JM, Reeder DJ. Short Tandem Repeat DNA Internet DataBase. Available on line at: http://www.cstl.nist.gov/biotech/strbase.

This website, supported by the National Institute of Standards and Technology (NIST) has updated information on STR loci including new variants. It also contains links to other useful sites.

DNA Advisory Board. Quality assurance standards for forensic DNA testing laboratories (approved July 1998). Forensic Sci Comm 2000;2. Available on line at: www.fbi.gov/programs/lab/fsc/current/codis2.htm.

Basic QA/QC requirements for forensic testing laboratories.

National Research Council: The Evaluation of Forensic DNA Evidence. Washington, DC: National Academy of Sciences; 1996.

This monograph is a comprehensive evaluation of testing and statistical evaluation of data intended for use in legal proceedings.

Walker RH. Probability in the analysis of paternity test results. In: Silver H, editor. Paternity testing. Washington, DC: American Association of Blood Banks; 1978, p. 69–135.

The proceedings of the Airlie Conference contains numerous papers dealing with methods of calculating data from paternity testing using the classical systems. Though pre-DNA testing, the principles apply to STR systems.

REFERENCES

Access the complete reference list online at http://www.expertconsult.com

CHAPTER 72

PHARMACOGENOMICS AND PERSONALIZED MEDICINE

Jing Li, Martin H. Bluth, Andrea Ferreira-Gonzalez

KEY POINTS

- High throughput array technologies such as genomics and proteomics have provided unprecedented ability to personalize output of biomarkers implicated in select disease states.
- Pharmacogenomics, through utilization of novel technologies, can detect unique polymorphisms to serve as diagnostic and/or prognostic biomarkers, which relate to an individual or group response to particular therapies.
- Elucidation of unique or personal responses can tailor therapy to the individual, thereby maximizing drug choice, dose, and effect.
- Interpretation of pharmacogenomic responses can be discretionary in that many genotypic and phenotypic variables are often involved

OVERVIEW

Pharmacogenomics refers to the reciprocal effect of how drug responses relate to the human genome. As such, these responses can encompass genetic (transcription, translation, polymorphisms) and epigenetic (environmental) components with respect to a drug's efficacy and toxicity. The new era of personalized medicine, which integrates the uniqueness of an individual with respect to drug pharmacokinetics, pharmacodynamics, and clinical effects, and downplays the "one drug fits all" convention, holds promise as a means to provide greater safety and efficacy in drug design and development. This approach is a result of application of biotechnology, high throughput multiplex analysis (microarray, proteomics), and bioinformatics and highlights interindividual and interethnic variabilities, including genetic polymorphisms, to ensure that the proper drug class or derivative is administered at the optimally effective dose to the appropriate individual. This chapter highlights select areas of pharmacogenomics and the emerging concepts of personalized medicine in maturing disciplines and sensitizes the pathologist and laboratorian to its emerging and potential effects with respect to diagnosis and prognosis in human disease, as well as its limitations in interpretation and application in the clinical marketplace.

BASIC CONCEPTS

The concept of a relationship between a substance and its effect on genes, rudimentary pharmacogenetics, has been present since the early 1900s. Dr. Archibald Garrod described that genetic variations could cause adverse biological reactions when chemical substances were ingested (Garrod, 1902). Garrod's work on alcaptonuria constituted the first proof of Mendelian genetics in humans. As a result of these studies, he advanced the hypothesis that genetically determined differences in biochemical processes could affect outcome after drug administration (Mancinelli, 2000). The idea of pharmacogenomics, also referred to as *toxogenomics*, is considered to have matured from pharmacogenetics, a discipline comprising genetics, pharmacology, and biochemistry, as a fusion of pharmacogenetics and genomics. Whereas pharmacogenetics classically investigates the hereditary impacts upon the action of drugs, pharmacogenomics extends pharmacogenetics to include the multifactorial drug responses caused by many genetic alterations plus environmental factors (Kalow, 2008). The recognition of these complex interactions and the advance of genetics into genomics via high throughput analysis of gene interrogation algorithms have given rise to the application of this science as a means of personalizing drug effects to a group or individual. Each drug after it enters the body interacts with numerous proteins, such as carrier proteins, transporters, metabolizing enzymes, and multiple types of receptors. These protein interactions determine drug absorption, distribution, excretion, target site of action, and pharmacologic response. Moreover, drugs trigger downstream secondary events that may impact additional gene or protein expression responses; these can also vary among patients. As a result, multiple polymorphisms in many genes may affect drug response, requiring a genome-wide search for the responsible genes. The term "personalized medicine" has been coined toward the promise of making therapy more effective and safer by giving drugs that fit a person's genes. However, because gene function and expression are variable and contingent on the response of drugs on genes as much as they are to the response of genes on drugs, gene structure and protein–gene interaction, the interrogation of these responses to yield useful and functional biomarkers adapted as well. The topics that follow provide examples of the adaptations of pharmacogenomics and personalized medicine in select disease states and their current applications in the clinical laboratory toward patient care.

The events following a drug administration can be divided into two phases, a pharmacokinetic phase and a pharmacodynamic phase. The pharmacokinetic phase relates a dosage regimen to the drug concentration achieved with time; pharmacokinetics concerns the drug absorption, distribution, metabolism, and excretion (ADME). The pharmacodynamic phase relates the drug concentration to the magnitude of the desired or adverse effects produced with time; pharmacodynamics concerns drug target interaction, downstream signaling events, and pharmacologic response. Interindividual variability in both pharmacokinetics and pharmacodynamics contributes to the variability in drug response. Genetic variations in the genes involved in ADME (e.g., drug-metabolizing enzymes and transporters) can alter the pharmacokinetics of a drug, whereas those involved in drug target interactions (e.g., target receptors and enzymes) can modify the pharmacodynamics of a drug. The interactions between the pharmacokinetics, pharmacodynamics, and pharmacogenetics are depicted in Figure 72-1. Typically, the overall response to a drug is determined by the interplay of multiple genes that are involved in the pharmacokinetic and pharmacodynamic pathways of a drug. In general, important pharmacogenetic variation can be envisioned at the level of drug-metabolizing enzymes, drug transporters, and drug targets.

Drug-Metabolizing Enzyme Pharmacogenomics

Drug-metabolizing enzymes are proteins that catalyze the biochemical modifications of xenobiotics (e.g., drugs) and endogenous chemicals (e.g., hormones, neurotransmitters). Drug metabolism can result in the activation (toxication) or deactivation (detoxication) of the chemical. Even though both occur, the majority of metabolites of most drugs are deactivation products. Broadly, drug-metabolizing enzymes are divided into two categories: phase I (functionalizing) enzymes that introduce or remove functional groups in a substrate through oxidation, reduction, or hydrolysis, and phase II (conjugating) enzymes that transfer moieties from a cofactor to a substrate. Essentially all of the major human metabolizing enzymes exhibit genetic polymorphisms at the genomic level, and many of these enzymes have clinically relevant genetic polymorphisms (Fig. 72-2). A gene is considered to be polymorphic when the frequency of a variant allele in a specific population is at least 1%.

PHASE I ENZYMES

Phase I metabolizing enzymes include those involved in oxidation (e.g., cytochrome P450 [CYP], alcohol dehydrogenase, aldehyde dehydrogenase, dihydropyrimidine dehydrogenase, monoamine oxidase, and flavin-containing monooxygenase); reduction (e.g., nicotinamide adenine dinucleotide phosphate [NADPH]-cytochrome P450 reductase and reduced cytochrome P450); hydrolysis (e.g., epoxide hydrolase, esterases, and amidases).

The most important phase I enzymes that exhibit clinical relevant genetic polymorphisms are in the CYP superfamily, which represents the most important system responsible for catalyzing the oxidation of a large number of endogenous and exogenous compounds including drugs, toxins, and carcinogens. In this superfamily, 57 genes and 58 pseudogenes have been identified, which are divided into 18 families and 43 subfamilies (http://ghr.nlm.nih.gov/geneFamily/cyp). Among them, three subfamilies of CYPs—CYP1, CYP2, and CYP3—are the main ones contributing to the oxidative metabolism of more than 90% of clinically used drug.

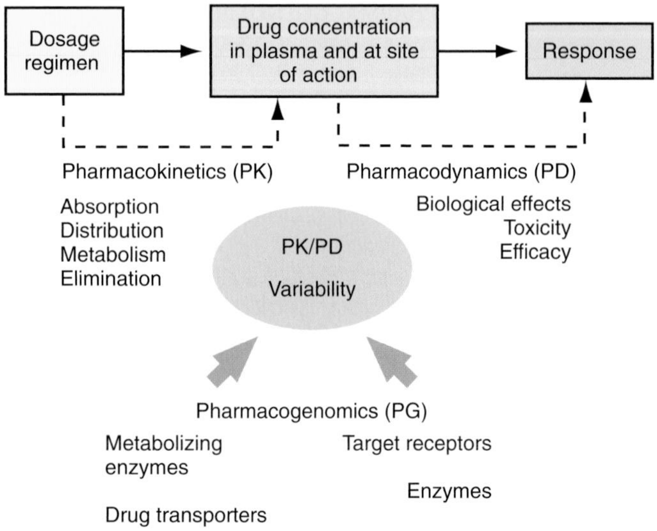

Figure 72-1 Schematic illustration of interactions between pharmacokinetics (PK), pharmacodynamics (PD), and pharmacogenomics. The PK relates a dosage regimen to drug concentration–time course in the body, and the PD relates the drug concentration to the magnitude of the desired or adverse effects produced. Genetic variations in the genes involved in drug disposition (e.g., drug-metabolizing enzyme and transporter genes) and drug action (e.g., target receptors and enzymes) contribute to the interindividual PK/PD variability.

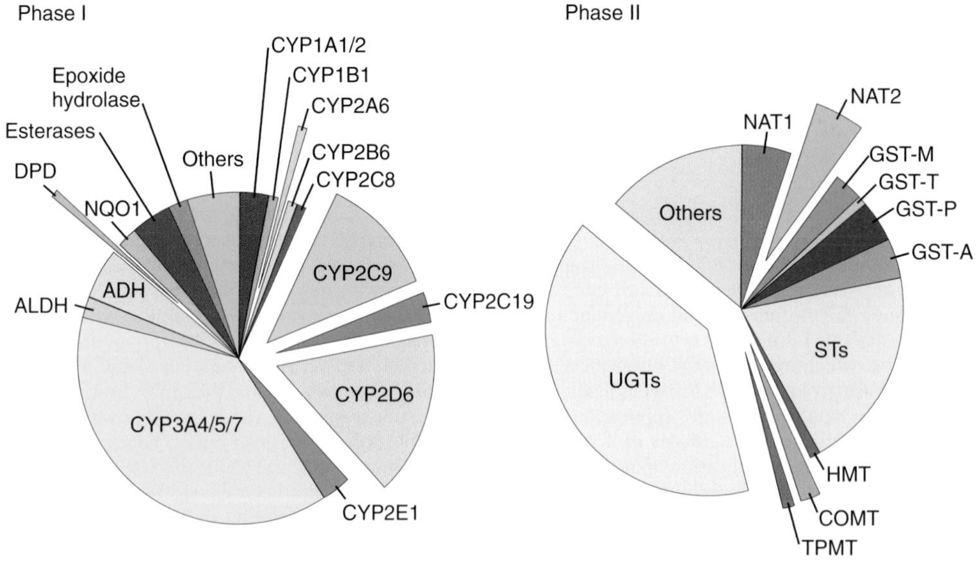

Figure 72-2 Phase I and II drug-metabolizing enzymes that exhibit common genetic polymorphisms. The percentage of phase I and phase II metabolism of drugs that each enzyme contributes is estimated by the relative size of each section of the corresponding chart; those enzyme polymorphisms that have already been associated with changes in drug effects are separated from the corresponding pie charts. *(Adapted from Evans WE, Relling MV. Pharmacogenomics: translating functional genomics into rational therapeutics. Science 1999;286[5439]:487–91.) ADH,* Alcohol dehydrogenase; *ALDH,* aldehyde dehydrogenase; *CYP,* cytochrome P450; *DPD,* dihydropyrimidine dehydrogenase; *NQO1, NADPH,* quinone oxidoreductase or DT diaphorase; *COMT,* catechol *O*-methyltransferase; *GST,* glutathione *S*-transferase; *HMT,* histamine methyltransferase; *NAT, N*-acetyltransferase; *STs,* sulfotransferases; *TPMT,* thiopurine methyltransferase; *UGTs,* uridine 5′-triphosphate glucuronosyltransferases.

The human CYP genes are highly polymorphic. The polymorphisms within the CYP genes, which include gene deletions, missense mutations, deleterious mutations creating splicing defects or premature stop codon, and gene duplications, can result in abolished, reduced, normal, or enhanced enzyme activity. Based on the level of CYP enzyme activity, patients can be classified into four phenotypes: poor metabolizer (abolished activity), intermediate metabolizer (reduced activity), extensive metabolizer (normal activity), and ultrarapid metabolizer (enhanced activity). Poor metabolizers would have higher concentrations of a drug that is inactivated by that enzyme pathway and therefore would require a lower dose to avoid adverse reactions, whereas ultrarapid metabolizers would require a higher dose to achieve therapeutic effective drug concentrations. The opposite pattern of reactions would occur in response to a prodrug that undergoes metabolic activation. A prodrug may have little therapeutic effect in poor metabolizers but would produce a toxic level of active form in ultrarapid metabolizers. Indeed, a growing body of evidence suggests that genetic polymorphisms within the CYP genes have significant impact on drug disposition and/or response. The common functional polymorphisms in the major human CYP genes and their clinical relevance are summarized in Table 72-1. Comprehensive reviews on the pharmacogenetics/genomics of CYPs have been published (Ingelman-Sundberg, 2004; Andersson, 2005; van Schaik, 2005; Rodriguez-Antona, 2006; Zhou, 2009). Notably, the most pharmacologically and clinically relevant polymorphisms are found in *CYP2D6*, *CYP2C9*, and *CYP2C19*. Of the U.S. Food and Drug Administration (FDA)-approved drug labels referring to human genomic biomarkers, 62% pertain to polymorphisms in the CYP enzymes, with CYP2D6 (35%), CYP2C19 (17%), and CYP2C9 (7%) being the most common (Frueh, 2008). For review, see Li and Bluth, 2011.

Unlike other CYPs, CYP2D6 is not inducible; therefore the variations in enzyme expression and activity are largely attributable to the genetic polymorphisms. The *CYP2D6* gene is highly polymorphic with more than 63 functional variants identified to date (http://www.cypalleles.ki.se). These alleles result in abolished, decreased, normal, or ultrarapid CYP2D6 enzyme activity. The most important null alleles are *CYP2D6*4* (splicing defect) and *CYP2D6*5* (gene deletion); the common alleles with severely reduced enzyme activity are represented by *CYP2D6*10*, **17*, and **41*; ultrarapid enzyme activity is derived from duplication or multiduplications of active *CYP2D6* genes (e.g., *CYP2D6*1*×N [N≥2]) (see Table 72-1). The distributions of *CYP2D6* alleles exhibit notable interethnic differences. The nonfunctional allele *CYP2D6*4* is prevalent in Caucasians (allelic frequency, ~25%), while the reduced function allele *CYP2D6*10* is common in Asians (allelic frequency, ~40%) and *CYP2D6*17* is common in Africans (allelic frequency, ~34%) (Bradford, 2002). As a result, poor metabolizers of CYP2D6, mainly derived from null allele *CYP2D6*4*, have a high frequency in Caucasians (5%–14%) compared with Africans (0%–5%) and Asians (0%–1%). In contrast, ultrarapid metabolizers of CYP2D6, derived from gene duplication or multiduplications, have a high frequency in Saudi Arabians (20%) and black Ethiopians (29%) compared with Caucasians (1%–10%) (Bradford, 2002). The interethnic difference in the *CYP2D6* genotypes may contribute to the interethnic variations in the disposition and response of substrate drugs. CYP2D6 is involved in the metabolism of ~25% of all drugs in clinical use, although it accounts for ~2% of total hepatic CYP contents. *CYP2D6* genotype is of great importance for the pharmacokinetics and response of many drugs, including tricyclic antidepressants, antiarrhythmics, neuroleptics, analgesics, antiemetics, and anticancer drugs (for review, see Zhou, 2009).

The human *CYP2C9* and *CYP2C19* genes are highly homologous at the nucleotide level. The most common nonsynonymous *CYP2C9* polymorphisms, *CYP2C9*2* and *CYP2C9*3*, result in the enzyme with differing affinity or intrinsic clearance for different substrates. Whereas *CYP2C9*2* effects appear to be more substrate specific, *CYP2C9*3* variant exhibits reduced catalytic activity toward the majority of CYP2C9 substrates. The clinical importance of *CYP2C9* polymorphisms is exemplified by the CYP2C9 genotype-guided dosing of an oral anticoagulant warfarin. The patients carrying either *CYP2C9*2* or *CYP2C9*3* require significantly smaller daily dose of warfarin to maintain desired therapeutic effects while avoiding severe toxicity, compared with patients carrying the wild-type *CYP2C9* (Higashi, 2002). With regard to *CYP2C19*, a splice site mutation in exon 4 (*CYP2C19*2*) and a premature stop codon in exon 4 (*CYP2C19*3*) represent the two most predominant null alleles. It is estimated that by genotyping for *CYP2C19*2* and **3*, ~84%, ~100%, and >90% of poor CYP2C19 metabolizers could be detected in Caucasians, Asians, and Africans, respectively. The poor metabolizer phenotype of *CYP2C19* occurs in 12%–23% of Asian population, in 1%–6% of Caucasians, and in 1%–7.5% of black Africans. Polymorphisms in *CYP2C19* are known to affect the pharmacokinetics and/or response of several classes of drugs, including proton pump inhibitors (e.g., omeprazole) and barbiturates (for review, see Zhou, 2009).

PHASE II ENZYMES

The most important phase II enzymes that exhibit functional and clinical relevant genetic polymorphisms are uridine diphosphate glucuronosyltransferase (UGT), sulfotransferase (SULT), glutathione S-transferases (GST), N-acetyltransferase (NAT), and thiopurine methyltransferase (TPMT) (see Fig. 72-2). Table 72-2 summarizes the most common functional polymorphisms in these phase II enzymes and highlights their clinical significance.

Uridine Diphosphate Glucuronosyltransferases

The human UGT superfamily is a group of conjugating enzymes that catalyze the transfer of the glucuronic acid group of uridine diphosphoglucuronic acid to the functional group (e.g., hydroxyl, carboxyl, amino, sulfur) of a specific substrate (Guillemette, 2003). UGTs are membrane-bound enzymes localized in the endoplasmic reticulum of liver and many other extrahepatic tissues. Seventeen human UGT genes have been identified and are classified into two subfamilies (UGT1 and UGT2). Glucuronidation increases the polarity of the substrates and facilitates their excretion in bile or urine. Genetic polymorphisms have been identified for almost all the UGT family members. Genetic variations in the UGT genes could alter the function or expression of the protein, and potentially modify the glucuronidation capacity of the enzyme toward a given drug, carcinogen, or endogenous compounds. There is evidence that genetic variations in the UGT genes contribute to differential susceptibility to diseases (e.g., cancer) and influence the pharmacokinetics and clinical outcome of substrate drugs (for reviews, see Guillemette, 2003; Nagar, 2006). A representative example is that the *UGT1A1* low promoter activity alleles (i.e., *UGT1A1*28*) is associated with decreased glucuronidation of SN-38 (an active metabolite of irinotecan), thereby resulting in increased risk for irinotcan-induced toxicity. The pharmacogenetics of irinotecan is discussed in details later. The most common functional polymorphisms in the major UGT enzymes and their clinical relevance are highlighted in Table 72-2 (for comprehensive reviews, see Guillemette, 2003; Nagar, 2006).

Sulfotransferases

Cytosolic SULTs are phase II enzymes that catalyze the transfer of the sulfonyl group from the cofactor 3′-phosphoadenosine 5′-phosphosulfate to the nucleophilic sites of a variety of substrates including hormones and xenobiotics. Sulfo conjugation of xenobiotics leads to formation of polar, excretable products as well as reactive, potentially mutagenic and carcinogenic metabolites (Glatt, 2004). Eleven SULT proteins encoded by 10 genes have been identified in humans. They differ in substrate specificity and tissue distribution. Single nucleotide polymorphisms (SNPs) have been identified in most of the human SULT genes. Functional SNPs in SULTs that are associated with altered enzymatic activity have potential to influence therapeutic response and to modify cancer susceptibility (see reviews in Glatt, 2004; Nowell, 2006). One widely studied functional SNP is *SULT1A1*2* (Arg213His) that exhibits reduced enzymatic activity and thermal stability (see Table 72-2).

Glutathione S-Transferases

The superfamily of human GST catalyzes the conjugation of glutathione (GSH) to a wide range of endogenous metabolites and xenobiotics including alkylating and free radical–generating anticancer drugs (Lo, 2007). Human GSTs are categorized into three main families, cytosolic/nuclear, mitochondrial, and microsomal. The cytosolic GSTs are further divided into seven classes: alpha, mu, omega, pi, sigma, theta, and zeta. Besides their enzymatic function, GSTs also possess nonenzymatic functions, in which they act as regulators of cell signaling and posttranslational modification pathway in response to stress, growth factors, and deoxyribonucleic acid (DNA) damage, and in cell proliferation, cell death, and other processes that ultimately lead to tumor growth and drug resistance. These multiple functionalities establish the importance of GSTs as determinants of cancer susceptibility, therapeutic response, and prognosis (see reviews in McIlwain, 2006; Lo, 2007). Most human GSTs have SNPs and, less frequently, deletions. Increasing evidence has indicated linkage of GST

Text continued on page 1366

PART 8

TABLE 72-1

Most Common Naturally Occurring Functional Polymorphisms in the Major Human Cytochrome P450 Genes: Allele Frequency, Functional Effect, and Highlights of Clinical Relevance

Common allelic variants	Polymorphism/ substitution	ALLELE FREQUENCY (%)[a]			Functional effect[b]	Highlights of clinical relevance[c]
		Ca	As	Af		
CYP1A1						Mainly expressed in extrahepatic tissues.
CYP1A1*2A	3698T>C(MspI)	6.6–19	33–54	22–28	↑Inducibility	CYP1A1, 1A2, and 1B1 play important role in the bioactivation of a variety of carcinogens.
CYP1A1*2B	I462V; 3698T>C(MspI)	–	–	–	↑Inducibility	↑Lung cancer risk generally associated with highly inducible or active CYP1A1 polymorphisms such as CYP1A1*2C.
CYP1A1*2C	I462V	2.2–8.9	28–31	0–2.7	↑Activity	
CYP1A1*3	3204T>C	0	0	7.6–14	Normal	CYP1A1 genotypes also associated with risk to breast, prostate, and ovarian cancers that are possibly related to estrogen activation.
CYP1A1*4	T461N	2.0–5.7	–	–	Normal	
CYP1A2						CYP1A2 accounts for ~13% of total hepatic CYP content.
CYP1A2*1C	-3860G>A				↓Inducibility	High inducible *1F genotype associated with ↑clearance of CYP1A2 substrates (e.g., caffeine) after smoking or omeprazole treatment.
CYP1A2*1F	-163C>A	33	68		↑Inducibility	
CYP1A2*1K	Haplotype (-63C>A, -739T>G, -729C>T)	0.5			↓Inducibility ↓Activity	*1K associated with ↓in vivo caffeine metabolism. CYP1A2 genotypes are associated with cancer risk.
CYP2A6						CYP2A6 accounts for 1%–10% of total hepatic CYPs.
CYP2A6*1X2	Gene duplication	1.7		0.4	↑Activity	The frequency of CYP2A6 alleles has marked ethnic difference. CYP2A6*4 accounts for the majority of PMs in Asians.
CYP2A6*2	L160H	1–3		<1	↓Activity	
CYP2A6*4	Gene deletion	0.5–1	7–22	15–20	Abolished activity	Because nicotine is converted to cotinine by CYP2A6, a high expression/activity of CYP2A6 is proposed to increase the susceptibility to nicotine addiction and the risk of tobacco-related cancers. Therefore CYP2A6 genetic variation could play a role in nicotine addition and tobacco-related cancer risks.
CYP2B6						CYP2B6 is mainly expressed in the liver, accounting for 6% of total CYPs.
CYP2B6*4	K262R	5			↑Activity	The anticancer drugs cyclophosphamide (CPA) is bioactivated by CYP2B6. CYP2B6 polymorphisms would likely affect the PK and/or PD of CPA. For example, CYP2B6*6 carriers exhibited ↑CPA clearance and CPA 4-hydroxylation activity.
CYP2B6*5	R487C	11–14	1		↓Expression	
CYP2B6*6	Q172H; K262R	16–26	16		↑Activity	
CYP2B6*7	Q172H; K262R; R487C	13	0		↑Activity	CYP2B6 polymorphisms may affect the PK and therapeutic outcome of anti-HIV agents such as efavirenz and nevirapine. For example, CYP2B6 Q172H variant is associated with ↑plasma concentrations of efavirenz and nevirapine.
CYP2C8						CYP2C8 accounts for ~7% of total hepatic CYP contents.
CYP2C8*2	I269F	0.4		18	↓Activity	CYP2C8*3 is associated with ↓clearance of both R- and S-ibuprofen.
CYP2C8*3	R139K; K399R	13	0	2	↓Activity	
CYP2C8*4	I264M	7.5			↓Activity	
CYP2C9						CYP2C9 accounts for ~20% of total hepatic CYP contents.
CYP2C9*2	R144C	13–22	0	3	↓Activity	CYP2C9*2 and *3 have been shown to affect the oral clearance of at least 17 different CYP2C9 substrate drugs (e.g., S-warfarin, celecoxib, ibuprofen, and phenytoin).
CYP2C9*3	I359L	3–16	3	1.3	↓Activity	
CYP2C9*5	D360E	0	2	0	↓Activity	

CYP2C19						
CYP2C19*2	Splicing defect; I331V	15	30	17	Abolished activity	The PM phenotype of CYP2C19 occurs in 12%–23% of Asian population, whereas in 1%–6% of Caucasians and 1%–7.5% of black Africans.
CYP2C19*3	W212X; I331V	0.04	5	0.4	Abolished activity	Polymorphisms in the CYP2C19 gene are known to affect the PK and/or response of several classes of drugs, including proton pump inhibitors (e.g., omeprazole) and barbiturates.
CYP2C19*17	I331V	18	4		↑Transcription	
CYP2D6						
CYP2D6*3	Frameshift	1–2	<1		Abolished activity (PM)	CYP2D6 accounts for ~2% of total hepatic CYP contents. However, it is involved in the metabolism of ~25% of all drugs in clinical use.
CYP2D6*4	Splicing defect	20–25	1	6–7	Abolished activity (PM)	Unlike other CYPs, CYP2D6 is not inducible, and thus genetic polymorphisms are largely responsible for the variation in enzyme expression and activity.
CYP2D6*5	Gene deletion	4–6	4–6	4–6	Abolished activity (PM)	CYP2D6 genotypes exhibit large inter-ethnic differences: low frequency of PM in Asian (~1%) and African (0%–5%) populations, compared to Caucasians (5%–14%).
CYP2D6*10	P34S; S486T	<2	50	3–9	↓Activity (IM)	CYP2D6 genotype is of great importance for the PK and response of many drugs, including tricyclic antidepressants, antiarrhythmics, neuroleptics, analgesics, antiemetics, and anticancer drugs.
CYP2D6*17	T107I; R296C; S486T	<1		20–34	↓Activity (IM)	
CYP2D6*41	R296C; splicing defect; S486T	1.3	2	5.8	↓Activity (IM)	
CYP2D6*1×N, N≥2	Gene duplication				↑Activity (UM)	
CYP2D6*2×N, N≥2	Gene duplication				↑Activity (UM)	
CYP3A4						
CYP3A4*1B	5′ flanking region	2–9	0	35–67	Altered expression	CYP3A4 has the highest abundance in the human liver (~40%) and metabolizes over 50% of all currently used drugs.
CYP3A4*2	S222P	2.7-4.5	0	0	Substrate-dependent altered activity	Genetic polymorphisms in CYP3A4 appear to be more prevalent in Caucasians than in Asians.
CYP3A4*3	M445T	1.1			↓Activity	There is no consensus on a direct functional or clinical association of CYP3A4 polymorphism. CYP3A4 polymorphism may have minor or moderate clinical relevance.
CYP3A4*17	F189S	2.1			↓Activity	
CYP3A4*18	L293P	0		1	↑Activity	
CYP3A5						
CYP3A5*3	Splicing defect	90	75	50	Abolished activity	The clinical relevance of the CYP3A5 polymorphism is demonstrated by the fact that the PK of the immunosuppressive drug tacrolimus is associated with CYP3A5 genotype.
CYP3A5*6	Splicing defect	0	0	7.5	Severely ↓activity	
CYP3A5*7	346 Frameshift	0	0	8	Severely ↓activity	
CYP3A7						CYP3A7 is a predominantly fetal enzyme.
CYP3A7*1C	Promoter	3		6	↑Expression	The in vivo functional effect of CYP3A7 polymorphism is demonstrated by the fact that carriers of CYP3A7*1C allele had significantly decreased endogenous level of dehydroepiandrosterone sulphate, a specific substrate of CYP3A7.
CYP3A7*2	T409R	8	28	62	↑Activity	

Af, African; *As*, Asian; *Ca*, Caucasian; ↑ indicates increased; ↓ indicates decreased.
[a]Allele frequency data are obtained from Xie, 2001; Bradford, 2002; Mizutani, 2003; Solus, 2004; Roy, 2005; Suarez-Kurtz, 2005; Sistonen, 2007.
[b]Functional effect data are obtained from the Human Cytochrome P450 (CYP) Allele Nomenclature Committee website (http://www.cypalleles.ki.se/).
[c]Comprehensive reviews were written by Ingelman-Sundberg, 2004; Bozina, 2009; Zhou, 2009.

TABLE 72-2
Most Common Naturally Occurring Functional Polymorphisms in Major Human Phase II Drug-Metabolizing Enzymes: Allele Frequency, Functional Effect, and Highlights of Clinical Relevance

Allelic variants	Polymorphism/ substitution	ALLELE FREQUENCY (%) Ca	As	Af	Functional effect	Highlights of clinical relevance
UGT1A1[a]						UGT1A1 low promoter activity alleles (e.g., UGT1A1*28) is significantly associated with ↓glucuronidation of SN-38 (the active metabolite of irinotecan), thereby resulting in ↑risk for irinotcan-induced toxicity.
UGT1A1*6	G71R	0	13–23	–	↓Activity	
UGT1A1*28	(TA)6>(TA)7 in promoter	2-9-40	13–16	36–43	↓Expression	Genetic variations in UGT1A1 may modify susceptibility to steroid-related cancers including breast, ovarian, endometrial and prostate cancers.
UGT1A1*33	(TA)6>(TA)5 in promoter	0–0.7	0	3–8	↑Expression	
UGT1A1*34	(TA)6>(TA)8 in promoter	0–0.7	0	0.9–7	↓Expression	
UGT1A6[a]						UGT1A6 catalyses the glucuronidation of aspirin and acetaminophen.
UGT1A6*2	T181A, R184S	30	23		↓Activity	"Low activity" UGT1A6 variants, leading to increased salicylate levels in aspirin users, are associated with a lower risk of colon cancer.
UGT1A6*3	R184S	1–2	1.6		Unknown	
UGT1A6*4	T181A	2.4			Unknown	
UGT1A7[a]						
UGT1A7*2	N129K, R131K	24–34	15	39	Similar activity	UGT1A7 is an important extrahepatic UGT that inactivates a variety of carcinogens.
UGT1A7*3	N129K, R131K, W208R	23–36	26	23	↓Activity	Low-activity UGT1A7 variants increases the risk of developing tobacco-related cancers, specifically orolaryngeal cancer.
UGT1A7*4	W208R	1–1.7	0	1	↓Activity	
UGT2B7[a]						UGT2B7 is of major significance for the glucuronidation of a number of clinically important drugs (e.g., morphinan derivatives, epiribicin, and zidovudine).
UGT2B7*2	H268Y	49–54	27		Similar or decreased activity	Further studies are needed to elucidate the clinical impact of the UGT2B7 polymorphism.
UGT2B15[a]						UGT2B15 is the most efficient UGT2B involved in the inactivation of steroid hormones, mainly androgens.
UGT2B15*2	D85Y	52–55	36–49	39	↑Activity	UGT2B15 polymorphisms have a potential role in a modified risk of prostate cancer.
SULT1A1[b]						SULT1A1 is the most highly expressed hepatic SULT.
SULT1A1*2	R213H	25–36	4.5–17	27–29	↓Activity and ↓thermal stability	SULT1A1 plays an important role in the sulfation of the metabolites of tamoxifen, 4-hydroxy-tamoxifen and endoxifen. SULT1A1*2 is associated with decreased survival of breast cancer patients treated with tamoxifen.
SULT1A1*3	M223V	1.2	0.6	23	Similar activity	
GST[c]						
GSTA1*B	Promoter point mutation (T-631G, T-567G, C-69T, G-52A)	40		41	↓Expression	GSTA1 is involved in glutathione conjugation of the active metabolites of cyclophosphamide (CPA). GSTA1*B allele is associated with higher survival rate of breast cancer patients treated with CPA-containing chemotherapy.
GSTM1*0	Gene deletion	42–58		27–41	Abolished activity	The GSTM null genotype is associated with an increased risk of the lung, colon, and bladder cancer.
						AML patients carrying GSTM*0 appears to have a better response to Adriamycin and cyclophosphamide treatment.

GSTP1*B	I105V	6–40		54	↓Activity	The GSTP1*B allele is associated with lower clearance of etoposide and reduced risk of relapse in childhood ALL patients.
						The GSTP1*B allele is associated with increased survival rate in patients with advance colorectal cancer or breast cancer.
GSTT1*0	Gene deletion	2–42			Abolished activity	The GSTT1 deletion is associated with reduced risk of relapse in childhood ALL patients.
						The GSTT1 deletion is a poor prognostic factor for survival in adult ALL.
NAT [d]						NAT1*14 and *17 are associated with slow acetylator phenotype.
NAT1*4	Wild-type				Normal	NAT2*5, *6, *7, *10, *14, and *19 lead to slow acetylator phenotype.
NAT1*14	R187Q	1.3–3.7			↓Activity	NAT2 slow acetylator phenotype is associated with increased susceptibility to hydralazine- and isoniazid-induced toxicity.
NAT1*14	R187Stop				↓Activity	
NAT1*17	R64W				↓Activity	NAT2 slow acetylator phenotype is associated with increased risk of bladder cancer.
NAT1*19	R33Stop				↓Activity	
NAT1*22	D251V				↓Activity	
NAT2*4	Wild-type				Normal	
NAT2*5	I114T				↓Activity	
NAT2*6	R197Q				↓Activity	
NAT2*7	G286E				↓Activity	
NAT2*10	E167K				↓Activity	
NAT2*14	R64Q				↓Activity	
NAT2*17	Q145P				↓Activity	
NAT2*19	R64W				↓Activity	
TPMT [e]						TPMT is involved in the methylation reaction of mercaptopurine, an anticancer drug used in the treatment of childhood ALL.
TPMT*2	A80P	0–0.5	0	0–0.4	↓Activity	The TPMT genotype correlated well with in vivo enzyme activity and is clearly associated with a risk of mercaptopurine-induced toxicity. Patients with poor or intermediate TPMT activity may tolerate only one-tenth to half of the average mercaptopurine dose.
TPMT*3A	A154Y, Y240C	0–0.6	0–1	0–0.8	Abolished activity	
TPMT*3B	Y240C	–	0	–	9-fold ↓Activity	
TPMT*3C	A154Y	0.2–3.3	0–0.2	2.4–7.6	1.4-fold ↓Activity	

Af, African; *ALL,* acute lymphoblastic leukemia; *AML,* acute myeloid leukemia; *As,* Asian; *Ca,* Caucasian; *GST,* glutathione S-transferases; *NAT,* N-acetyltransferase; *SULT,* sulfotransferase; *TPMT,* thiopurine methyltransferase; *UGT,* uridine diphosphate glucuronosyltransferase; ↑ indicates increased; ↓ indicates decreased.

[a]Data on *UGT* SNP allele frequencies, function effect, and clinical relevance are summarized from Guillemette, 2003; Nagar, 2006.

[b]Data on *SULT1A1* SNP allele frequencies, function effect, and clinical relevance are summarized from Glatt, 2004; Nowell, 2006.

[c]Data on *GST* SNP allele frequencies, function effect, and clinical relevance are summarized from McIlwain, 2006; Lo, 2007.

[d]Data on *NAT* SNP allele frequencies, function effect, and clinical relevance are summarized from Hein, 2002; Agundez, 2008; Sim, 2008.

[e]Data on *TPMT* SNP allele frequencies, function effect, and clinical relevance are summarized from Hamdy, 2003; Zhou, 2006.

TABLE 72-3
Pharmacologically Most Important Efflux and Uptake Drug Transporters, Tissue Distribution, and Representative Substrate Drugs*

Gene	Protein	Tissue distribution	Polarity	Representative drug substrates
ABC Transporters				
ABCB1	MDR1 (P-gp)	Liver, intestine, kidney, blood-brain barrier, lymphocytes, placenta	AP	Anthracyclines, taxanes, vinca alkaloids, imatinib, etoposide, levofloxacin, erythromycin, cyclosporine, tacrolimus, digoxin, quinidine, verapamil, diltiazem, ritonavir, saquinavir, talinolol, phenytoin, cimetidine, simvastatin, morphine, hydrocortisone
ABCC1	MRP1 (GS-X)	Ubiquitous	BL	Anthracyclines, vinca alkaloids, irinotecan, SN-38, methotrexate, camptothecins, saquinavir, ritonavir, difloxacin, drug-glucuronate/-glutathione/-sulfate conjugates
ABCC2	MRP2 (cMOAT)	Liver, kidney, intestine	AP	Anthracyclines, vinca alkaloids, methotrexate, camptothecins, rifampin, pravastatin, and drug-glucuronate/-glutathione/-sulfate conjugates
ABCG2	BCRP	Liver, intestine, placenta, breast	AP	Anthracyclines, irinotecan, SN38, SN38G, imatinib, tamoxifen
SLC Transporters				
OATP Family				
SLC21A3	OATP1A2 (OATP-A)	Ubiquitous, with highest expression in brain and testis	BL	Rosuvastatin, methotrexate, ouabain, D-penicillamine
SLC21A6	OATP1B1 (OATP-C)	Liver	BL	Statin, pravastatin, fexofenadine, and repaglinide, rosuvastatin, ouabain, D-penicillamine, rifampin
SLC21A8	OATP1B3 (OATP8)	Liver	BL	Digoxin, rifampin, ouabain, methotrexate, D-penicillamine, rosuvastatin, cyclosporin
SLC21A9	OATP2B1 (OATP-B)	Ubiquitous	BL	Benzylpenicillin, rosuvastatin
OCT Family				
SLC22A1	OCT1	Liver	BL	Metformin, cisplatin, oxaliplatin, imatinib, procainamide, citalopram, cimetidine, quinidine, verapamil, acyclovir
SLC22A2	OCT2	Kidney	BL	Metformin, cisplatin, oxaliplatin, imatinib, procainamide, citalopram, cimetidine, quinidine, amantadine
SLC22A3	OCT3	Brain, liver, kidney, heart, muscle, placenta, and blood vessels	BL	Cimetidine, agmatine, adefovir, catecholamines
OAT Family				
SLC22A6	OAT1	Kidney, brain	BL	Methotrexate, salicylate, antiviral agents (e.g., acyclovir)
SLC22A7	OAT2	Liver, kidney,	BL	Methotrexate, salicylate, tetracyclines
SLC22A8	OAT3	Kidney, brain, muscle	BL	Methotrexate, antiviral agents (e.g., acyclovir), cimetidine, pravastatin, salicylate
SLC22A11	OAT4	Kidney, placenta	AP	Methotrexate, cimetidine, salicylate, tetracyclines

AP, Apical; *BL*, basolateral; *BCRP*, breast cancer resistance protein; *GS-X*, glutathione S-conjugate pump; *MDR1*, multidrug resistance 1; *MOAT*, multispecific organic anion transporter; *MRP*, multidrug resistance-related protein; *OATP*, organic anion transporting peptides; *OCT*, organic cation transporter; *OAT*, organic anion transporter; *P-gp*, P-glycoprotein.

*Comprehensive information on tissue distribution, substrates and other transporter-related information can be found at www.tp-search.jp, http://www.bioparadigms.org/slc/menu.asp, and http://nutrigene.4t.com/humanabc.htm.

polymorphisms with cancer incidence, treatment, and prognosis (Table 72-3) (for comprehensive reviews, see McIlwain, 2006; Lo, 2007).

N-Acetyltransferase

The human NATs catalyze the transfer of an acetyl group from acetylcoenzyme A to arylamines, arylhydroxylamines, and arylhydrazines (Blum, 1990). The two human NAT genes, *NAT1* and *NAT2*, carry functional polymorphisms that influence the enzyme activity. Based on the level of NAT activity, patients can be classified into two phenotypes: fast acetylator (wild-type NAT acetylation activity) and slow acetylator (reduced NAT enzyme activity). For example, polymorphisms or haplotypes in the *NAT1* (e.g., *NAT1*14*, **15*, **17*, **19*, and **22*) and *NAT2* (e.g., *NAT2*5*, **6*, **7*, **10*, **14*, and **17*) lead to slow acetylation phenotype (for review, see Sim, 2008). A comprehensive list of the NAT1/2 alleles is presented on the website http://louisville.edu/medschool/pharmacology/NAT.htlm. NAT2 plays an important role in the activation and/or deactivation of a large and diverse number of aromatic amine and hydrazine drugs used in clinic, and therefore the *NAT2* genotype is particular relevant to the response to these drugs. One representative example is the association of the slow-acetylator *NAT2* phenotype with increased risk for an antituberculosis drug (isoniazid)-induced hepatitis (Huang, 2002). In addition, because NAT1 and NAT2 catalyze the bioactivation (via O-acetylation) of aromatic and heterocyclic amine carcinogens, genetic variations in the *NAT1/2* genes may modify the cancer risk related to exposure to these carcinogens (Hein, 2002). For instance, the slow-acetylator *NAT2* phenotype is known to relate to a higher risk for bladder cancer (Cartwright, 1982; Garcia-Closas, 2005).

Thiopurine S-Methyltransferase

TPMT is best known for its key role in the metabolism of the thiopurine drugs (e.g., 6-mercaptopurine, azathiopurine, and 6-thioguanine) by catalyzing the S-methylation of thiopurine drugs via S-adenosyl-L-methionine as the S-methyl donor. These drugs are clinically used to treat cancers or as immunosuppressants. The *TPMT* gene exhibits significant genetic polymorphisms across all ethnic groups studied, with 18 *TMPT* alleles identified to date. The three main *TPMT* alleles, namely *TMPT*2* (reduced activity), **3A* (abolished activity), and **3C* (reduced activity), account for 80%–95% of the intermediate and poor metabolizers (for review, see Zhou, 2006). Patients who inherit defect *TPMT* alleles or *TPMT* deficiency (i.e., two nonfunctional alleles) are at significantly increased risk for thiopurine-induced toxicity (e.g., myelosuppression). Indeed, patients with absent TMPT activity (~0.3% prevalence) or low activity (~10% prevalence) may tolerate only 5%–50% of the average mercaptopurine dose. Clinical diagnostic tests are now available for the detection of the SNPs in the human *TPMT* gene that lead to decreased or abolished enzyme activity. On the FDA-approved drug labels, *TPMT* variant pharmacogenetic test is recommended before treating patients with azathiopurine, mercaptopurine, and thioguanine.

Drug-Transporter Pharmacogenomics

In addition to drug-metabolizing enzymes, uptake and efflux transporters that facilitate the movement of drugs in or out of the cell are important determinants of drug disposition and response. Broadly, drug transporters are classified into two families, namely efflux transporters of the adenosine-5'-triphosphate (ATP)-binding cassette (ABC) family and uptake transporters of the solute carrier (SLC) family. In the ABC transporter family, 49 genes have been identified and classified into seven subfamilies from ABCA through ABCG based on the sequence homology (http://nutrigene.4t.com/humanabc.htm). The ABC transporters are responsible for transport of diverse substrates out of the cell using ATP as an energy source. Among these, ABCB1, ABCC1/2, and ABCG2 have been well characterized for their roles in drug disposition and response. In the SLC family, 360 genes have been identified and classified into 46 subfamilies (http://www.bioparadigms.org/slc/menu.asp). Of particular relevance to drug disposition are members of the organic anion transporting polypeptides (OATP), organic cation transporter (OCT), and organic anion transporter (OAT) subfamilies.

The pharmacologically most important efflux ABC transporters (including ABCB1, ABCC1/2, and ABCG2) and uptake SLC transporters (including OATP, OCT, and OAT families), their tissue distributions, and representative drug substrates are summarized in Table 72-3. These transporters play crucial roles in the intestinal absorption, biliary excretion, renal excretion, and tissue/cellular penetration of a wide variety of therapeutic drugs, and therefore they are important determinants of drug exposure in the system and at the site of action (Fig. 72-3). A growing body of evidence suggests that polymorphisms in the transporter genes, which may influence the expression, subcellular localization, substrate specificity, and/or intrinsic transport activity of the transporter proteins, influence the disposition and response of drug substrates. The following sections highlight the functional and clinical significance of the most commonly naturally occurring genetic polymorphisms within the pharmacologically most important ABC and SLC transporters with respect to drug disposition and response. A comprehensive list of genetic variants in the ABC and SLC transporters and related information are available in Pharmacogenetics Research network databases at http://www.pharmGKB.org.

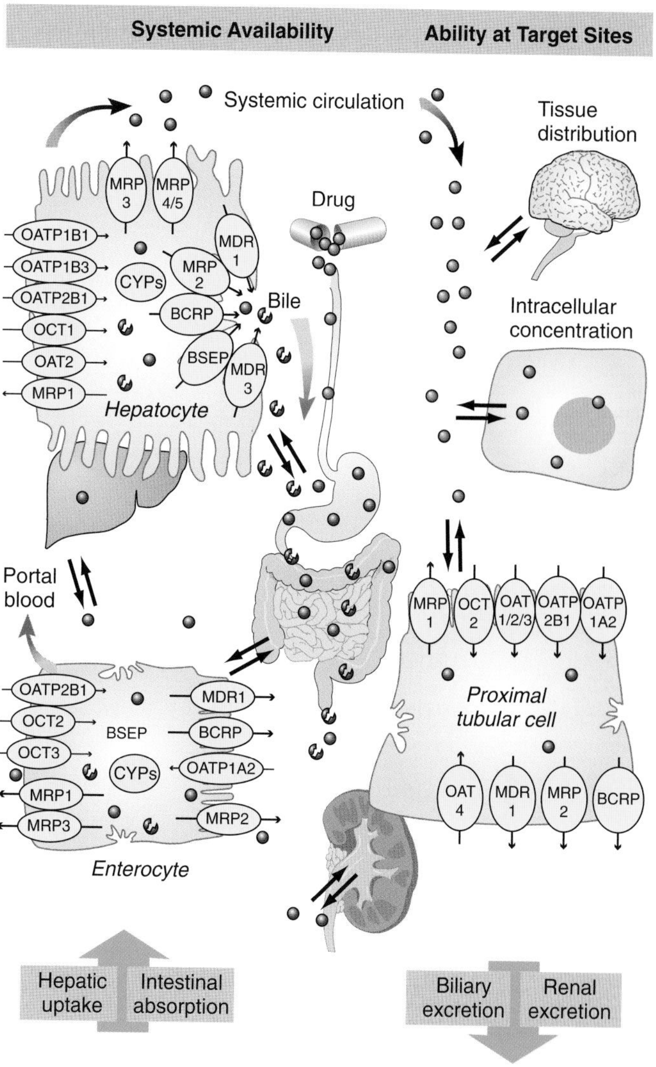

Figure 72-3 Schematic representation of drug uptake and efflux transporters as determinants of drug disposition. *(Modified from Kerb R. Implications of genetic polymorphisms in drug transporters for pharmacotherapy. Cancer Lett 2006; 234[1]:4–33.)*

ABCB1, ABCC1/2, and ABCG2 Efflux Transporters

ABCB1

The *ABCB1* gene, also named as the multidrug resistance 1 *(MDR1)* gene, encodes a polypeptide (P-glycoprotein) that has two halves, each containing six hydrophobic trans-membrane domains and an ATP-binding domain. ABCB1 is expressed in the intestinal epithelium, canalicular membrane of hepatocyte, brush border of the renal tubule, pancreatic ductile cell, trophoblast of placenta, capillary endothelial cells of brain and testes, and peripheral blood lymphocytes (see Table 72-3). ABCB1, located on the apical or luminal surface of the epithelial cells, functions as an efflux transporter in restricting intestinal absorption, facilitating hepatobiliary excretion and renal excretion, and protecting the brain and fetus from xenobiotics (see Fig. 72-3). In addition, ABCB1 overexpression in cancer cells is implicated in multidrug resistance to chemotherapeutic agents (Gottesman, 2002). ABCB1 transports a broad spectrum of structurally and functionally diverse drugs, including anticancer agents, antibiotics, immunosuppressants, cardiac drugs, calcium channel antagonists, and human immunodeficiency virus (HIV) protease inhibitors (see Table 72-3). There is a strong overlap in substrate specificity and tissue distribution for ABCB1 and CYP3A4/5 (Wacher, 1995).

More than 50 SNPs have been identified in the human *ABCB1* coding region. The most common SNPs are the synonymous 1236C>T and 3435C>T and the nonsynonymous 2677G>T (Ala899Ser). The allele frequencies of these three SNPs vary in different ethnic populations (Table 72-4). The 3435C>T SNP has strong linkage disequilibrium with other SNPs in the *ABCB1* gene, creating common haplotypes consisting of 3435C>T combined with 2677G>T and/or 1236C>T.

Given the important role of ABCB1 in drug absorption and disposition, genetic polymorphisms in the *ABCB1* gene may influence the outcome of pharmacotherapy. The first investigation of the functional and clinical effect of ABCB1 polymorphism was reported in 2000 for a silent SNP 3435C>T, which was associated with decreased duodenal expression of ABCB1 and thereby increased plasma concentration of digoxin after oral administration in humans (Hoffmeyer, 2000). Recent evidence suggests that the 3435C>T SNP affects the timing of cotranslational folding and insertion of ABCB1 into the membrane, thereby altering substrate specificity (Kimchi-Sarfaty, 2007). In the past decade, a number of preclinical and clinical studies have been conducted investigating association of *ABCB1* genotype with its tissue expression and function, and with pharmacokinetics and pharmacodynamics of substrates drugs (see Table 72-4) (for review, see Ieiri, 2004). However, data reported on the functional and clinical impacts of *ABCB1* polymorphisms are often inconsistent (for reviews, see Ieiri, 2004; Marzolini, 2004a; Pauli-Magnus, 2004; Sakaeda, 2005; Kerb, 2006). The descrepancies may be partly explained by lack of standardized methodology and assays among different studies. In addition, SNPs may often result in very subtle functional outcomes. For example, a recent study suggests that the haplotype 1236C>T/2677G>T/3435C>T did not result in a change in substrate transport per se but affected the inhibition of transport by a small subset of modulators (Kimchi-Sarfaty, 2007). Conflicting results on the clinical impact of *ABCB1* polymorphisms may reflect the complex disposition pathway of the substrate drugs, for which other transporters or metabolizing enzymes are also involved. For example, the commonly used in vivo ABCB1 probe drugs such as digoxin,

TABLE 72-4
Most Common Functional Polymorphisms in Human ABCB1, ABCC1/2, and ABCG2: Allele Frequency and Functional Effects

		ALLELE FREQUENCY (%)*			
Allele variants	**Polymorphism/ substitution**	**Ca**	**As**	**Af**	**Functional effects**
ABCB1					
1236C>T	Silent	34–42	60–72	15–21	Affects cotranslational folding in nearby amino acids that are essential for ATP-binding and ATP hydrolysis (Fung, 2009)
2677G>T/A	A893S/T	38–47/1–10	32–62/3-22	15/ND	Affects ABCB1 expression or function, but data are inconsistent (Marzolini, 2004a)
3435C>T	Silent	48–59	37–66	10–27	Affects cotranslational folding in nearby amino acids, thereby altering substrate specificity (Kimchi-Sarfaty, 2007)
ABCB1*13	1236C>T/2677G>T/3435C>T haplotype	23–42	28–56	4.5–8.7	Affects the inhibition of ABCB1 by a small subset of modulators (Kimchi-Sarfaty, 2007)
ABCC1					
128G>C	C43S		1		Reduced plasma membrane localization, $\downarrow$vincristine resistance in transfected cells (Leslie, 2003)
1299G>T	R433S	1.4			Changes in transport and resistance (Conrad, 2002)
2012G>T	G671V	2.8			Associated with anthracycline-induced cardiotoxicity (Wojnowski, 2005)
ABCC2					
1271A>G	R412G				Dubin-Johnson syndrome; $\downarrow$ in methotrexate elimination (Hulot, 2005)
1249G>A	V417I	22–26	13–19	14	Changes in ABCC2 expression and localization (Vogelgesang, 2004; Merino, 2005; Meyer zu Schwabedissen, 2005)
3563T>A	V1188E	4–7	1		Associated with anthracycline-induced cardiotoxicity (Wojnowski, 2005)
4544G>A	C1515Y	4–9			Associated with anthracycline-induced cardiotoxicity (Wojnowski, 2005)
ABCG2					
34G>A	V12M	2–10	15–18	4–6	Changes in transport and resistance (Mizuarai, 2004; Tamura, 2007)
376C>T	Q126stop	0	0.9–1.7	0	Loss of transport activity (Tamura, 2006)
421C>A	Q141K	9–14	27–35	1–5	Affects the ATP-binding domain, thereby leading to reduced transport activity (Mizuarai, 2004; Tamura, 2007)

Af, African; *As,* Asian; *ATP,* adenosine-5′-triphosphate; *Ca,* Caucasian; $\uparrow$ indicates increased; $\downarrow$ indicates decreased.
*Data of allele frequencies are obtained from Marzolini, 2004a; Gradhand, 2008.

fexofenadine, and talinolol are the dual substrates for both ABCB1 and OATP transporters; cyclosporine is not only transported by ABCB1 but also metabolized by CYP3A4. This means that a potential ABCB1 effect may be marked by the activity of OATP transporters or CYP3A4. Hence, a systemic analysis of polymorphisms in multiple genes known or suspected to contribute to drug disposition and response would provide better insights on the genetic impact on pharmacotherapy. In addition, the ABCB1 has multiple polymorphisms, some of which are in linkage disequilibrium, and therefore a haplotype approach would allow a more accurate prediction of clinical phenotypes.

ABCC1 and ABCC2

ABCC1/2, also called multidrug resistance-related proteins, plays an essential role in transport and excretion of organic anions including physiologic metabolites, carcinogens, and drugs. They are believed to confer multidrug resistance to chemotherapeutic agents (Hinoshita, 2000). ABCC1 and ABCC2 have overlapping substrate specificities, typically GSH, glucuronate, or sulfate conjugated and unconjugated drugs, including many anticancer agents such as vincristine and doxorubicin, HIV protease inhibitors such as ritonavir and saquinavir, and antibiotics such as difloxacin and grepafloxacin (see Table 72-3). Both ABCC1 and ABCC2 require cotransport of reduced GSH to transport some of their substrates (Rothnie, 2006). ABCC1 is located in basolateral membranes of polarized cells, whereas ABCC2 is located to the apical domain. While ABCC1 is ubiquitously expressed, ABCC2 is mainly expressed in hepatocytes, renal proximal tubule cells, intestine and brain (see Table 72-3).

The human *ABCC1* appears to be a conserved gene because many of the naturally occurring genetic variants in *ABCC1* are relative rare. Of the identified SNPs in the non-coding and coding region of *ABCC1*, 16 are known to result in amino acid changes, and some of them exhibit functional effects on either expression or function of the protein (see Table 72-4) (for review, see Gradhand, 2008). However, data on the role of *ABCC1* polymorphisms in terms of in vivo physiology and clinical drug resistance or toxicity are rather limited. Interestingly, one study has identified significant associations of *ABCC1* 2012G>T (Gly671Val) and a haplotype of *ABCC2* with anthracycline-induced cardiotoxicity among patients with non-Hodgkin lymphoma who have been treated with doxorubicin (Wojnowski, 2005).

Mutations in the ABCC2 gene have been initially identified in Dubin-Johnson syndrome, a relatively rare recessive disorder characterized by conjugated hyperbilirubinemia resulting from loss of expression and function of ABCC2 in the liver (see Chapter 21). However, the impact of this loss of hepatic ABCC2-medicated transport on the pharmacokinetics of substrate drugs in humans is yet to be determined. Among more commonly occurring *ABCC2* SNPs, the most widely studied is 1249G>A (Val417Ile). The effect of this SNP on ABCC2 expression is different depending on the tissue examines. For example, 1249G>A SNP was associated with lower *ABCC2* messenger ribonucleic acid (mRNA) and protein levels in preterm placenta, but not in duodenum and liver (Meyer zu Schwabedissen, 2005; Meier, 2006). Of note, one study demonstrated a possible association of 1249G>A variant with tenofovir-induced renal proximal tubulopathy, suggesting this SNP may influence renal excretion of some ABCC2 substrates (Izzedine, 2006). In addition, 1249G>A SNP was associated with changes in the ABCC2 localization in neuroepithelial tumors (Vogelgesang, 2004). A number of other nonsynonymous and synonymous SNPs have been studied for their potential functional influence on the ABCC2 expression and transport activity. *ABCC2* SNPs appear to have varying effect on different organs or substrates, or between in vitro and in vivo studies (for review, see Gradhand, 2008).

ABCG2

The ABCG2 (also known as BCRP, ABCP, or MXR) protein is an ATP-binding cassette (ABC) half-transporter that bears six trans-membrane domains and one ATP-binding domain. The protein actively extrudes a wide variety of chemically unrelated hydrophobic or partially hydrophobic compounds from the cells, including cytotoxic compounds (e.g., mitoxantrone, topotecan, SN-38, flavopiridol, and methotrexate), fluorescent dyes (e.g., Hoechst 33342) and toxic compounds found in normal food (e.g., pheophorbide A) (see Table 72-3). ABCG2 is expressed in the canalicular membrane of hepatocytes, in the epithelia of small intestine, colon, placenta, lung, kidney, adrenals, and sweat glands, as well as in the endothelia of the central nerve system vasculature. It is responsible for host detoxification and protection against potentially toxic xenobiotics (Jonker, 2000; Jonker, 2002; Krishnamurthy, 2006). ABCG2 transporter-mediated efflux has been increasingly recognized to not only confer drug resistance but also modulate drug absorption and disposition (Burger, 2004; Hirano, 2005; Kondo, 2005; Merino, 2005; Sparreboom, 2005).

More than 80 polymorphisms in the *ABCG2* gene have been identified in different ethnic populations (Iida, 2002; Imai, 2002; Zamber, 2003; Ishikawa, 2005). Several naturally occurring SNPs in *ABCG2* have been found to affect the function and/or expression of its encoded protein (Imai, 2002; Mitomo, 2003; Kobayashi, 2005; Lepper, 2005) and therefore may alter the pharmacokinetics and pharmacodynamics of substrate drugs. In particular, a functional SNP in exon 5 of the *ABCG2* gene, in which a C→A nucleotide transition at position 421 (*ABCG2* 421C>A), results in a nonsynonymous variant protein with a glutamine to lysine amino acid substitution in codon 141 (Q141K) (Imai, 2002). The *ABCG2* 421C>A variant has been associated with low ABCG2 expression levels and altered substrate specificity (Imai, 2002); it has been found to alter the pharmacokinetics of diflomotecan and topotecan (Sparreboom, 2004; Sparreboom, 2005). In addition, recent studies have demonstrated that the epidermal growth factor receptor (EGFR) tyrosine kinase inhibitors such as gefitinib and erlotinib are ABCG2 substrates, and the *ABCG2* 421C>A variant is associated with greater gefitinib accumulation at steady-state and related to higher incidence of gefitinib-induced grade 1 or 2 diarrhea in cancer patients compared with the wild-type ABCG2 (Cusatis, 2006; Li, 2007b).

OATP, OCT, AND OAT UPTAKE TRANSPORTERS

Organic Anion Transporting Polypeptides

OATPs are membrane influx transporters that facilitate cellular uptake of a wide range of endogenous compounds (e.g., bile salts, hormones, and steroid conjugates) and clinically important drugs (e.g., HMG-CoA-reductase inhibitors, cardiac glycosides, anticancer agents, and antibiotics) (see Table 72-3). Of the 11 human OATP transporters, OATP1A2, OATP1B1, OATP1B3, and OATP2B1 are best characterized for their roles in drug pharmacokinetics. OATP1A2 is expressed on the luminal membrane of small intestinal enterocytes and at the blood-brain barrier and may facilitate the intestinal absorption and brain penetration of its substrates. OATP1B1, OATP1B3, and OATP2B1 are mainly expressed on the sinusoidal membrane of hepatocytes and can facilitate the hepatic uptake of their substrate drugs for further metabolism or biliary excretion (Niemi, 2007).

A number of SNPs and other genetic variations have been identified in the *SLCO1B1* gene (encoding OATP1B1), and their allele frequencies vary markedly across different populations (Table 72-5) (for review, see Meyer zu Schwabedissen, 2009). Some *SLCO1B1* SNPs and haplotypes have been associated with impaired transport activity in vitro toward different substrates (Tirona, 2001; Kameyama, 2005; Nozawa, 2005). These functional impaired OATP1B1 variants may limit the uptake of the substrate drugs into the hepatocytes, thereby resulting in decreased biliary excretion or hepatic metabolism and thus increased systemic exposure. For example, a common variant allele, 521T>C, was associated with increased systemic exposure of several OATP1B1 substrate drugs, including repaglinide and statins (e.g., pravastatin) (Niemi, 2005; Niemi, 2006). *OATP1B1*15* (a haplotype of 388A>G and 512T>C) is associated with increased plasma concentrations of pravastatin (Nishizato, 2003) and increased concentrations of SN-38 (Xiang, 2006; Han, 2008). OATP1B1*17 (a haplotype of -11187G>A, 388A>G and 512T>C) is associated with increased effect of pravastatin on rate of cholesterol synthesis. A recent genome-wide association study has demonstrated that a noncoding rs4363657 SNP, which is in nearly complete linkage disequilibrium with the *SLCO1B1* 521T>C SNP, is the only strong marker associated with simvastatin-induced myopathy (Link, 2008). Collectively, these data suggest that knowledge of the patient's SLCO1B1 genotype might be useful in tailoring of drug therapy.

Several nonsynonymous polymorphisms have been identified in the *SLCO1A2* gene (encoding OATP1A2), with some of these variants demonstrating decreased in vitro transport activity toward OATP1A2 substrates (see Table 72-5) (for review, see Franke, 2009). However, the impacts of these functional SNPs on the pharmacokinetics and clinical outcome of therapeutic drug use need further studies. For OATP1B1 and OATP2B1, there are few data on the clinical relevance of *SLCO1B3* and *SLCO2B1* polymorphisms, although some genetic variations within these two genes have been associated with altered *in vitro* transport activity of the protein (see Table 72-5) (Nozawa, 2002; Letschert, 2004).

Organic Cation Transporter

The OCTs belong to the solute carrier SLC22A family that mediate intracellular uptake of a broad range of structurally diverse small organic cations (molecular weight < 400). Three isoforms, OCT1, OCT2, and OCT3, with partially overlapping substrate spectrum, are identified in humans (see Table 72-3). OCT1 is primarily expressed in the sinusoidal membrane of hepatocytes, whereas OCT2 is predominantly expressed in the basolateral membrane of the kidney proximal tubules; OCT3 is expressed in many tissues including placenta, heart, liver, and skeletal muscle (see Table 72-3). The expression of OCTs was also detected in several cancer cell lines and tumor tissue samples (Hayer-Zillgen, 2002; Zhang, 2006).

A number of non-synonymous SNPs have been identified in the *SLC22A1*gene (encoding OCT1) and *SLC22A2* (encoding OCT2) from different ethnic groups, and some of them have demonstrated altered (mostly impaired) transport function in vitro (see Table 72-5) (Choi, 2008). By contrary, several synonymous SNPs have been identified in the *SLC22A3* (encoding OCT3); however, their functional consequence is yet to be determined. The functional polymorphisms in the *OCT* genes may influence the clinical pharmacokinetics and response of substrate drugs such as metformin. It is evident that functional polymorphisms in the *OCT1* and *OCT2* impact the clinical effect and pharmacokinetics of metformin, a drug used as a primary therapy for type 2 diabetes mellitus. Metformin is eliminated predominantly by renal excretion in humans (Pentikainen, 1979). Because of high expression of OCT2 in the kidney and the active renal secretion of metformin via OCT2, defect function in OCT2 transport would result in decreased renal clearance of this drug. Recent studies demonstrated a significant lower renal clearance and higher plasma concentration of metformin in carriers of homozygous for low activity OCT2 variant 270S compared with those homozygous for the active variant (270A) (Song, 2008; Wang, 2008). On the other hand, low-function OCT1 variants R61C, G401S, M420del, and G465R have been associated with significantly higher renal clearance of metformin (Tzvetkov, 2009). In addition to the effect on metformin pharmacokinetics, low-function OCT1 variants (R61C, G401S, M420del, and G465R) have been related to significantly decreased glucose-lowering response of metformin in healthy volunteers, probably by reducing the metformin uptake in hepatocytes, which is the major target site of action of metformin (Shu, 2007).

Organic Anion Transporter

The OATs belong to the SLC22 family of solute carriers that mediate cellular uptake of a broad range of structurally diverse small hydrophilic organic anions. OAT substrates include many clinically important anionic drugs, such as β-lactam antibiotics, diuretics, nonsteroidal antiinflammatory drugs, nucleoside/nucleotide antiviral drugs, and anticancer agents (see Table 72-3). There are at least six OAT members (OAT1-6). OAT1-3 localize to the basolateral membrane of the renal proximal tubule mediating the uptake of drug substrates from blood into the proximal tubule cells, whereas OAT4 localizes to the apical side of the renal proximal tubule functioning in the secretion of drug substrates into urine. Together, these transporters are responsible for the movement of drug substrates from the blood to the urine. Genetic variations in the genes encoding OATs may

TABLE 72-5
Most Common, Naturally Occurring Nonsynonymous SNPs in Genes Encoding Human OATP, OCT, and OAT Transporters: Allele Frequency and Functional Effects

Allele variant	Polymorphism/ substitution	ALLELE FREQUENCY (%)* Ca	As	Af	Functional effects†
OATP					
SLCO1A2 (OATP1A2)					
38T>C	I3T	11.1	0	2.1	↑Transport activity
516A>C	E172D	5.3	0	2.1	↓Transport activity
833A	N278del	0	0	0.6	↓Transport activity
SLCO1B1 (OATP1B1)					
217T>C	F73L	2	0	0	↓Transport activity
388A>G	N130D	30	54	74	↓Transport activity
463C>A	P155T	16	0	2	No alteration
521T>C	V174A	14	0.7	2	↓Transport activity
1463G>C	G488A	0		9	↓Transport activity
2000A>G	E667G	2		34	↓Transport activity
SLCO1B3 (OATP1B3)					
334T>G	S112A	74			Unknown
699G>A	M233I	71			Unknown
1564G>T	G522C	1.9			Affect localization and ↓transport activity
SLCO2B1 (OATP2B1)					
1457C>T	S486F	1.2	30.9		↓Transport activity
OCT					
SLC22A1 (OCT1)					
41C>T	S14F	0	0	3.1	↓Transport of metformin but ↑transport of MPP
480C>G	G160L	0.65	8.6-13	0.5	No alteration
1022C>T	P341L	0	16	8.2	↓Transport of MPP but not metformin
1201G>A	G401S	1.1	0	0.7	↓Transport activity
1222A>G	M408V	60	74–81	74	No alteration
1256delATG	M420del	18	0	2.9	↓Transport of metformin but not MPP
1393G>A	G465R	4	0	0	↓Transport activity
SLC22A2 (OCT2)					
596C>T	T199I	0	1	0	↓Transport activity
602C>T	T201M	0	1.3–2	0	↓Transport activity
808G>T	A270S	16	14–17	11	↓Transport activity
1198C>T	R400C	0	0	1.5	↓Transport activity
1294A>C	K432Q	0	0	1	↓Transport activity
OAT					
SLC22A6 (OAT1)					
20T>C	L7P	1	<1	1	
149G>A	R50H	1	1	1	↑Transport activity
1361G>A	R454Q	0	0	<1	↓Transport activity
SLC22A7 (OAT2)					
329C>T	T110I	1	1	1	Unknown
571G>A	V192I	1	1	1	Unknown
1520G>A	G507D	1	1	1	Unknown
SLC22A8 (OAT3)					
523A>G	I175V	1	1	1	Unknown
829C>T	R277W				↓Transport activity
SLC22A11 (OAT4)					
37G>A	V13M	1	1	1	Unknown
142C>T	R48Ter	1	1	1	Unknown
185C>G	T62R	1	1	1	Unknown
463G>A	V155M	1	1	1	Unknown
732C>T	A244V	1	1	1	Unknown
832G>A	E278K	1	1	1	Unknown
1015G>A	V339M	1	1	1	Unknown
1175C>T	T392I	1	1	1	Unknown

Af, African; *As,* Asian; *Ca,* Caucasian; *MPP,* 1-methyl-4-phenylpyridinium; *OAT,* organic anion transporter; *OATP,* organic anion transporting polypeptides; *OCT,* organic cation transporter; *SNPs,* single nucleotide polymorphisms; ↑ indicates increased; ↓ indicates decreased.
*Allele frequency data are obtained from Xu, 2005; Kerb, 2006; Konig, 2006; Choi, 2008.
†Functional effect data are summarized from Marzolini, 2004b; Zhou, 2007; Zair, 2008; Choi, 2008; Franke, 2009.

contribute to interindividual variability in the renal clearance of substrate drugs. To date, a number of polymorphisms have been reported in the coding region and 5′ regulatory region of human *SLC22A6* (encoding OAT1), *SLC22A7* (encoding OAT2), *SLC22A8* (encoding OAT3), and *SLC22A11* gene (encoding OAT4) (see Table 72-5). Some of these polymorphisms resulted in altered in vitro transport activity of the protein (Xu, 2005; Bhatnagar, 2006). Notably, the coding region polymorphisms in these genes are infrequent (~1%), whereas the regulatory region polymorphisms of these genes, particularly *SLC22A8*, may be important in accounting for variation in the renal clearance of substrate drugs (Bhatnagar, 2006). The functional and clinical relevance of these coding and regulatory region polymorphisms need further studies.

DRUG TARGET PHARMACOGENOMICS

DNA REPAIR GENES

DNA repair is crucial to an organism's ability to maintain its genome integrity and function. Multiple DNA repair pathways exist to cope with a broad range of different DNA lesions or adducts induced by DNA damaging agents or radiation. The major DNA repair pathways include the following (Fig. 72-4): direct repair of alkyl adducts by methylguanine methyl transferase, repair of base damage and single-strand breaks by base excision repair, repair of bulky DNA adducts by nucleotide excision repair, repair of double-strand breaks by homologous recombination and nonhomologous end-joining repair, and repair of mismatches and insertion/deletion loops by DNA mismatch repair.

Chemotherapy and radiotherapy are designed to induce DNA damage that cause cell cycle arrest and cell death. The efficacy of DNA damage-based cancer therapy can thus be modulated by DNA repair mechanisms that operate in cancer cells to recognize and rectify this damage. For example, the antitumor activity of chemotherapy or radiotherapy could be reduced by increasing activities of several DNA repair pathways in cancer cells. In addition, DNA repair activity may also affect normal tissue tolerance to DNA damaging agents or radiation. Inefficient DNA repair in normal cells would be expected to result in inefficient removal of damaged DNA and thus lead to accumulation of DNA damage within normal tissues and increased normal tissue toxicity.

To date, 130 human genes have been identified that are involved in DNA repair pathways (Wood, 2001), and genetic polymorphisms within several of DNA repair genes have been described recently. The key genes that are associated with human DNA repair are listed in Figure 72-4. Among these, apurinic endonuclease 1 (APEX1), X-ray repair cross-complementing group 1 (XRCC1), excision repair cross-complementing enzyme group 1 (ERCC1), excision repair cross-complementing rodent repair group 2 (ERCC2), breast cancer 1, early onset (BRCA1), and X-ray repair cross complementing protein 3 (XRCC3) are the most widely reported DNA repair genes for which genetic polymorphisms have been associated with the therapeutic response (efficacy or toxicity) to chemotherapy or radiotherapy (Table 72-6) (for review, see Gossage, 2007).

There is evidence that genetic variations within the DNA repair genes may modify the activities of DNA repair pathways within both cancer cells and normal cells, thereby influencing therapeutic resistance and normal tissue tolerance to chemotherapy and radiotherapy (Table 72-6). For example, variant alleles that reduced DNA repair proficiency may increase the toxicity of DNA-damaging drugs or radiation in cancer cells, thus resulting in better therapeutic effect; on the other hand, they would cause insufficient DNA repair in normal tissue cells, thereby reducing normal

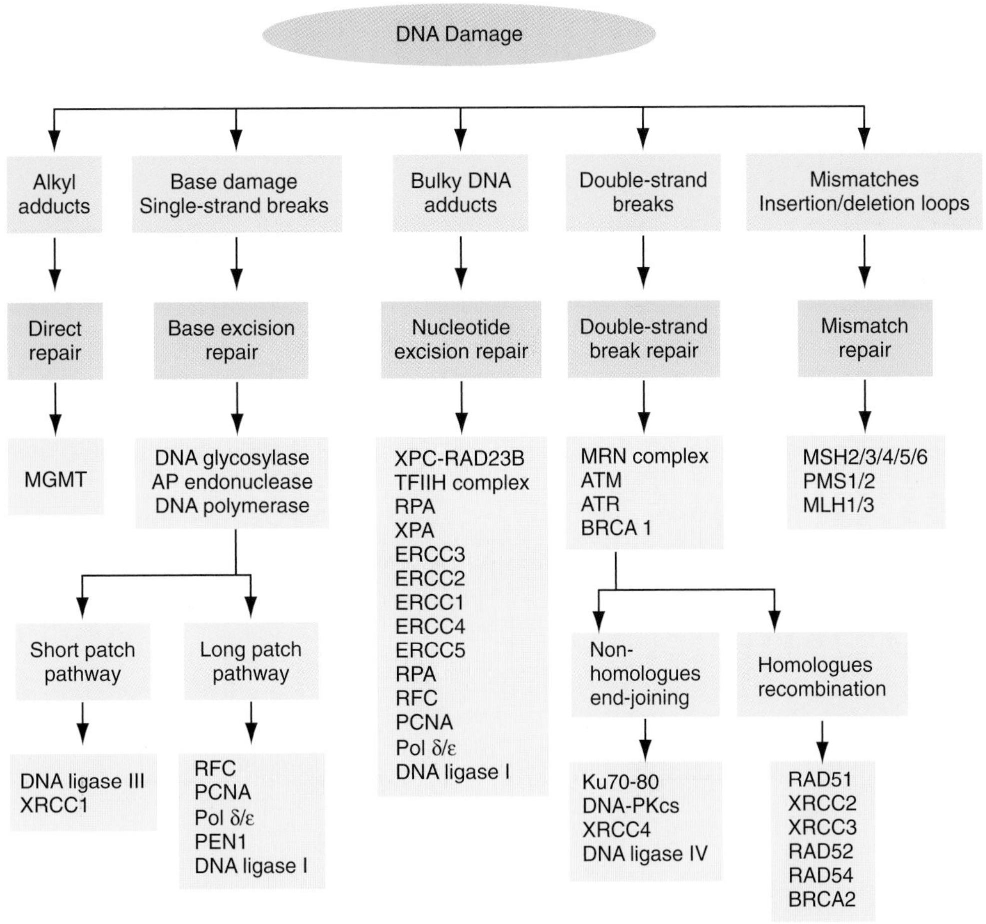

Figure 72-4 Key players in mammalian DNA repair pathway. *(Modified from Gossage L, Madhusudan S. Cancer pharmacogenomics: role of DNA repair genetic polymorphisms in individualizing cancer therapy. Mol Diagn Ther 2007;11[6]:361–80.)* *AP,* Apurinic/apyrimidinic; *ATM,* ataxia telangiectasia mutated; *ATR,* ataxia telangiectasia and RAD3 related; *BRCA1/2,* breast cancer 1 and 2, early onset gene; *DNA-PKcs,* DNA-dependent protein kinase catalytic subunit; *ERCC1/2/3/4/5,* excision repair cross-complementing group genes; *FEN1,* flap structure-specific endonuclease 1; *Ku70-80,* Ku antigen, 70 and 80 KDa subunits (XRCC6 and XRCC5); *MSH2/3/4/5/6,* mutS homolog genes; *PCNA,* proliferating cell nuclear antigen; *PMS1/2,* postmeiotic segregation increased 1 and 2; *Pol δ/ε,* DNA polymerase delta/epsilon; *RAD23B/51/52/54,* homologs of *S. cerevisiae* RAD (recombination protein) genes; *RFC,* replication factor C; *RPA,* replication protein A; *TFIIH,* transcription factor IIH; *XPA,* xeroderma pigmentosum complementation group A gene; *XRCC1/2/3/4,* x-ray repair, cross-complementing genes.

TABLE 72-6
Most Widely Reported DNA Repair Gene Polymorphisms That Have Demonstrated Associations with the Response (Efficacy and Toxicity) to Chemotherapy or Radiotherapy

DNA repair pathway and genes	Gene functions	SNPs	Association with efficacy	Association with toxicity
Base Excision Repair (BER)				
Apurinic endonuclease 1 (APEX1)	APEX1 is a critical protein involved in BER that hydrolyses the phosphodiester backbone immediately 5′ to an apurinic/apyrimidinic (AP) site following removal of the damage base by a DNA glycosylase.	Asp148Glu (most common SNP of APEX1)	↓Overall survival for 148Glu/Glu homozygotes in pancreatic cancer (Cx/RT/Both) (Li, 2007a)	↓Risk of acute skin reactions for 148Glu allele in normal weight breast cancer patients (adjuvant RT) (Chang-Claude, 2005)
X-ray repair cross-complementing group 1 (XRCC1)	XRCC1 interacts with DNA ligase III, polymerase β and poly (ADP-ribose) polymerase, and seals the remaining nick in DNA after DNA Pol β performs its one nucleotide gap filling reaction. XRCC1 is involved in the efficient repair of DNA single-strand breaks.	Arg194Trp	↑Response rate for 194Trp variants in advanced NSCLC (platinum Cx) (Wang, 2004) ↑Survival for 194Trp/Trp homozygotes in pancreatic cancer (Cx/RT/Both) (Li, 2007a)	↑Risk of hematologic toxicity for 194Arg/Arg homozygotes in NSCLC (gemcitabine and docetaxel Cx) (Petty, 2007) ↑Risk of early/late adverse reaction for 194Trp allele in breast cancer (adjuvant RT) (Moullan, 2003) ↓Risk of late reactions for 194Trp allele in cervical or endometrial cancer (RT) (De Ruyck, 2005)
		Arg399Gln	↑Response rate and ↑survival for 399Arg/Arg homozygotes in mCRC (FOLFOX), advanced NSCLC (platinum Cx), and oesophageal (platinum Cx, RT, and surgery) (Gurubhagavatula, 2004; Stoehlmacher, 2001; Wu, 2006) ↓Breast cancer-free survival and progression-free survival for Gln399 variant allele in metastatic breast cancer (high-dose Cx and stem-cell transplantation) (Bewick, 2006)	↓Risk of acute skin reactions for 399Glu allele in normal weight breast cancer patients (adjuvant RT) (Chang-Claude, 2005) ↑Risk of late skin toxicity for 399Arg/Arg homozygotes in breast cancer (adjuvant RT) (Andreassen, 2003)
Nucleotide Excision Repair (NER)				
Excision repair cross-complementing rodent repair group 2 (ERCC2)	ERCC2 is an ATP-dependent 5′-3′ DNA helicase, and a component of the core-TFIIH basal transcription factor. It is involved in NER by opening DNA in the 5′ to 3′ direction around the damage.	Asp312Asn	↓Survival for 312Asn variant allele in advanced NSCLC (platinum) (Gurubhagavatula, 2004) No association with response in advanced NSCLC (platinum) (Camps, 2003)	
		Lys751Gln	751Lys/Lys homozygotes more likely to relapse in stage 3&4 gastric cancer (surgery and chemoradiation) (Zarate, 2006) ↑Response rate and median survival for 751Lys/Lys homozygotes in mCRC (FOLFOX) (Park, 2001) ↑Disease-free and 1-year survival for 751Lys/Lys homozygotes in AML (Cx) (Allan, 2004) No association with response in advanced NSCLC (platinum Cx) (de las Penas, 2006)	ERCC2 genotype/haplotype associated with GI, GU, and liver toxicities in AML (daunorubicin and cytosine arabinoside Cx) (Kuptsova, 2007) ↓Risk of neutropenia for 751Gln/Gln homozygotes in NSCLC (gemcitabine and docetaxel Cx) (Petty, 2007)

Excision repair cross-complementing enzyme group 1 (ERCC1)	ERCC1 is a two-domained, noncatalytic protein that associates with ERCC4 (XPF) endonuclease to form an ERCC1-XPF heterodimer, whose role is to cleave DNA 5′ to the lesion. ERCC1-XPF is the last factor to join the mammalian NER incision complex and is also known to be involved in recombinational DNA repair and in the repair of inter-strand crosslinks.	19007T>C	↑Response rate or ↑survival for 19007C/C homozygotes for advanced NSCLC (platinum or cisplatin/docetaxel Cx) and mCRC (FOLFOX) (Park, 2003; Isla, 2004; Ryu, 2004) ↑Prognosis for 19007T/T homozygotes for CRC (adjuvant FU based) (Moreno, 2006) ↓Risk of platinum resistance in 19007T/C and T/T genotypes for ovarian cancer (Kang, 2006)	
		8092C>A	↑Survival in 8092C/C homozygotes for NSCLC (platinum Cx) (Zhou, 2004)	↑Risk of GI toxicity for 8092A allele in NSCLC (platinum Cx) (Suk, 2005) ↓Risk of metabolic toxicity for 8092C/A heterozygotes and ↓risk of lung toxicity for 8092A/A homozygotes in AML (daunorubicin and cytosine arabinoside Cx) (Kuptsova, 2007)
Double-Strand Break (DSB) Repair				
Breast cancer 1, early onset (BRCA1)	BRCA1 is a nuclear phosphoprotein that plays a role in maintaining genomic stability, and it also acts as a tumor suppressor. BRCA1 is associated with other tumor suppressors, DNA damage sensors, and signal transducers to form a large multi-subunit protein complex known as the BRCA1-associated genome surveillance complex (BASC). It plays a role in transcription, DNA repair of double-stranded breaks, and recombination.	BRCA1 mutations	↑Clinical and pathological complete response for BRCA1 mutation in breast cancer (anthracycline-based Cx) (Chappuis, 2002) ↑Response rate for BRCA heterozygotes in ovarian cancer (platinum-based Cx) (Cass, 2003)	
X-ray repair cross complementing protein 3 (XRCC3)	XRCC3 participates in homologous recombination to maintain chromosome stability and repair DNA damage. It is involved in DSB repair, and functionally complements Chinese hamster irs1SF, a repair-deficient mutant that exhibits hypersensitivity to a number of different DNA-damaging agents.	Thr241Met	↑Time to treatment failure for 241Met variant genotype in multiple myeloma (autologous bone marrow transplantation) (Vangsted, 2007) ↑Survival for 241Met/Met homozygotes in advanced NSCLC (platinum Cx) (de las Penas, 2006) ↓Survival for 241Met variant genotype in breast cancer (high-dose Cx and stem-cell transplantation) (Bewick, 2006) No association in advanced gastric cancer (platinum Cx) (Ruzzo, 2006)	↓Risk of 214Met variant in AML (daunorubicin and cytosine arabinoside Cx) (Kuptsova, 2007) ↑Risk of late skin toxicity for 241Thr/Thr homozygotes in breast cancer (adjuvant RT) (Andreassen, 2003)

Af, African; *AML,* acute myeloid leukemia; *As,* Asian; *Ca,* Caucasian; *CRC,* colorectal cancer; *Cx,* chemotherapy; *FOLFOX,* fluorouracil/oxaliplatin chemotherapy; *FU,* fluorouracil; *GI,* gastrointestinal; *GU,* genitourinary; *mCRC,* metastatic colorectal cancer; *NSCLC,* non–small cell lung cancer; *RT,* radiotherapy; *SNPs,* single nucleotide polymorphisms; ↑ indicates increased; ↓ indicates decreased.

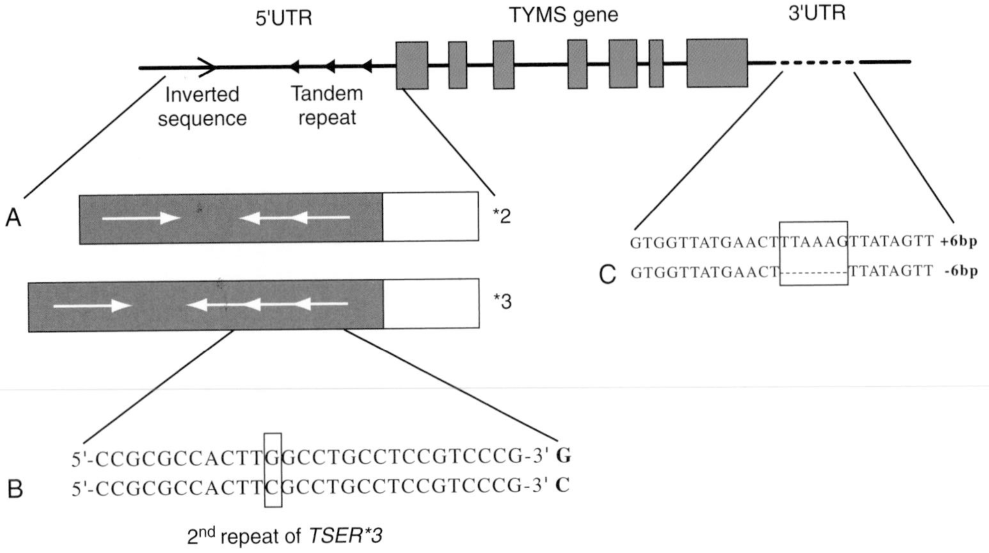

Figure 72-5 Three functional genetic polymorphisms in the 5′ and 3′ untranslated regions (5′UTR and 3′UTR) of the thymidylate synthase (TS) gene, including the following: **A,** a polymorphic tandem repeat of a 28-bp sequence that is present in either duplicate (2R) or in triplicate (3R) in the TS promoter enhancer region (TSER 2R>3R polymorphism); **B,** a G to C SNP within the second repeat when three repeats are present (TSER 3R G>C SNP); **C,** a 6-bp deletion in the 3′UTR of the TS gene (TS 1494del6bp). *(Adapted from Marsh S. Thymidylate synthase pharmacogenetics. Invest New Drugs 2005;23[6]:533–7.)*

tissue tolerance. It is worthy noting that data reported on the functional or clinical impacts of variant allelels of DNA repair genes are inconsistent in some instances (for review, see Gossage, 2007). For instance, whereas some studies suggested that variant alleles were associated with improved response, others found the opposite. The discrepancies may be explained in part by variations in study settings (e.g., different tumor types or stages, different treatment regimens, or different patient populations). In addition, most published studies have attempted to correlate a single SNP in two or three DNA repair genes to clinical outcome. The presence of other untested SNPs could confound the result interpretation. Moreover, many studies are largely limited by small sample size. To clarify the roles of DNA repair gene polymorphisms in cancer treatment, large prospective clinical trials are needed to systematically assess the combined impact of multiple polymorphisms involved in several relevant DNA repair pathways.

THYMIDYLATE SYNTHASE

Thymidylate synthase (TS) catalyzes the conversion of deoxyuridylate (dUMP) and 5,10-methylenetetrahydrofolate (CH_2H_4folate) to deoxythymidine monophosphate (dTMP) and 7,8-dihydrofolate. This reaction is the sole de novo biosynthesis of thymine in DNA, and therefore inhibition of TS blocks DNA synthesis, thereby causing cell death. Given its essential role in DNA synthesis, TS is an important target for chemotherapeutic drugs, such as 5-fluorouracil (5-FU) and capecitabine (orally bioavailable 5-FU prodrug). 5-FU exerts its cytotoxicity through inhibition of TS, blocking DNA synthesis and triggering apoptotic pathway and other cell death processes (Danenberg, 1977). 5-FU is the mainstay of therapeutic regimens for the treatment of colorectal cancer and other human malignancies. There is a wide variation in response and toxicity among patients receiving 5-FU-based chemotherapy. TS expression as a determinant of sensitivity to 5-FU has been demonstrated in vitro (Johnston, 1992). Importantly, substantial body of clinical data have suggested that response to 5-FU-based chemotherapy regimens is inversely associated with intratumoral TS mRNA and protein expression (Johnston, 1995; Leichman, 1997; Aschele, 1999; Salonga, 2000). A recent meta-analysis involving 887 patients with metastatic colorectal cancer and 2610 patients with localized colorectal cancer suggests that tumors expressing high levels of TS appear to have a poor overall survival compared with tumors expressing low levels (Popat, 2004).

There is evidence that TS expression is modulated by three functional significant germline polymorphisms in the 5′ and 3′ untranslated regions (5′UTR and 3′UTR) of the TS gene. These include a polymorphic tandem repeat of a 28 base pair (bp) sequence that is present in either duplicate (2R) or in triplicate (3R) in the TS promoter enhancer region (TSER 2R>3R polymorphism), a SNP (G>C) in the second repeat when three repeats are present (TSER 3R G>C SNP), and a 6 bp deletion in the 3′UTR of the TS gene (TS 1494del6bp) (Fig. 72-5). The TSER 2R>3R polymorphism is of clinical significance as patients with metastatic colorectal cancer homozygous for the triple repeat (TSER 3R/3R) had significantly higher intratumoral TS gene expression (Kawakami, 1999; Pullarkat, 2001). The 28 bp TSER tandem repeats contain elements that bind upstream stimulating factor (USF) and thus act to enhance transcriptional activity of the TS gene. The presence of a G>C SNP within the second repeat of the 3R allele results in decreased transcriptional activity by abolishing the binding of USF within the repeat (Mandola, 2003). The 6 bp deletion in the 3′UTR of the TS gene has been associated with decreased TS mRNA stability and lower intratumoral TS mRNA level in patients (Mandola, 2004). The allele frequencies of these three TS polymorphism vary among different ethnic populations (Table 72-7).

It is increasingly apparent that TS polymorphisms are not only prognostic factors of disease-free survival and overall survival but also predictors of chemotherapeutic benefit from 5-FU-based chemotherapy (for review, see Lurje, 2009). Most studies have consistently agreed that high-expression allele or genotype (i.e., TSER-2R/3G, -3C/3G, -3G/3G, 3′-UTR +6bp/+6bp) are generally associated with poor prognosis and worse response to 5-FU-based chemotherapy compared with low-expression group (i.e., TSER-2R/2R, -2R/3C, -3C/3C, 3′-UTR +6bp/-6bp, -6bp/-bp) in patients with colorectal cancer (for review, see Lurje, 2009).

EPIDERMAL GROWTH FACTOR RECEPTOR

The EGFR activation is a key factor in cell proliferation and important for tumor growth, including effects on cell motility, adhesion, invasion, survival, and angiogenesis (Woodburn, 1999; Raymond, 2000). EGFR is a transmembrane cell surface receptor tyrosine kinase that is found in the majority of epithelial tissues. Upon binding of the extracellular ligand (e.g., epidermal growth factor or transforming growth factor-α), the EGFR dimerizes, either homodimerizing with another EGFR or heterodimerizing with other members of the human epidermal growth factor receptor family, leading to the activation of cytoplasmic tyrosine kinase (TK) activity (see Figures 76-1 and 76-2.) The activation of receptor TK leads to the autophosphorylation of the intracellular domain of EGFR, resulting in the activation of downstream signaling pathways (e.g., Ras/mitogen-activated protein kinase pathway and the PI3K/Akt pathway and Janus-activated kinase signal transducers and activator of transcription) that are involved in tumor growth and metastasis (Bokemeyer, 2009; Houtsma, 2009). Receptor dimerization and signal transduction pathways are discussed further in Chapter 76. The reversible EGFR TK inhibitors, such as gefitinib and erlotinib, target the adenosine-5′ triphosphate (ATP) cleft within the EGFR-TK to prevent autophosphorylation of the receptor, thus inhibiting tumor growth and metastasis (Anderson, 2001; Ciardiello, 2001). Treatment with gefitinib or erlotinib results in dramatic clinical response

TABLE 72-7
Functional Polymorphisms of the Thymidylate Synthase (TS) Gene

Polymorphism	ALLELE FREQUENCY* Ca	As	Af	Functional effect*
TSER 2R>3R repeat	52–69	62–82	52	↑TS mRNA for 3R allele
TSER 3R G>C SNP	56	37	28	↓Transcriptional activity of TS for C allele
TS 1494del6b	27–29			↓Stability of TS mRNA for −6bp deletion

Af, African; *As*, Asian; *Ca*, Caucasian; *mRNA*, messenger ribonucleic acid; *TSER*, TS promoter enhancer region; ↑ indicates increased; ↓ indicates decreased.
*Summarized from Marsh, 2005; Lurje, 2009.

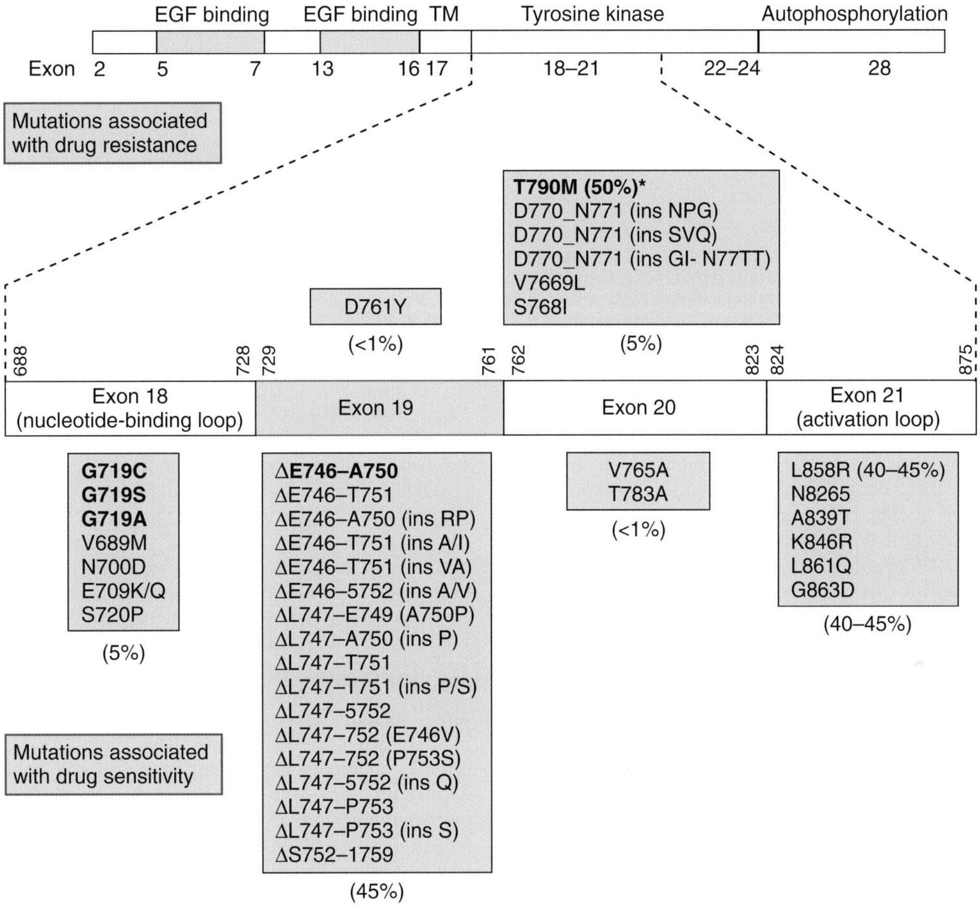

Figure 72-6 Schematic presentation of the epidermal growth factor receptor (EGFR) tyrosine kinase (TK) domain mutations as important determinants of sensitivity or resistance to EGFR TK inhibitors. The most prevalent activating EGFR kinase domain mutations in non–small cell lung cancer (NSCLC) include in-frame deletions in exon 19 (accounting for 45% of EGFR mutations), an L858R substitution in exon 21 (accounting for 40%–45% of EGFR mutations), nucleotide substitutions in exon 18 (e.g., G719C or G719S) (5%), and in-frame insertions in exon 20 (<1%). The most noteworthy clinically relevant mutations associated with resistance to EGFR TK inhibitors include T790M in exon 20, and D761Y, a T790M-like secondary mutation in exon 19. The main mutations in each class are shown in bold type. *(Adapted from Sharma SV, Bell DW, Settleman J, Haber DA. Epidermal growth factor receptor mutations in lung cancer. Nat Rev Cancer 2007;7[3]:169–81.)*

in approximately 10% to 30% patients with non–small cell lung cancer (NSCLC) depending on ethnic origin, sex, and smoking history (Fukuoka, 2003; Kris, 2003; Shepherd, 2005; Thatcher, 2005). It is clear that specific types of somatic mutations of the EGFR gene confer sensitivity or resistance to EGFR TK inhibitors (for reviews, see Kumar, 2008; Gazdar, 2009).

The somatic activating EGFR mutations are found in the first four exons (18 through 21) of the TK domain (Fig. 72-6) (Lynch, 2004; Paez, 2004; Pao, 2004). These mutations fall into three broad classes. Class I mutations are in-frame deletions in exon 19 that almost always include amino acid residues leucine-747 to glutamic acid-749 (ΔLRE) and account for approximately 44% of all EGFR TK activating mutations. Class II mutations are single nucleotide substitutions that cause an amino acid alteration. The most prevalent single-point mutation is L858R (an arginine changed to leucine at codon 858) in exon 21, accounting for about 41% of all EGFR TK activating mutations; other class II mutations include G719 (a glycine changed to serine, alanine, or cysteine) in exon 18 (4% of all EGFR TK activating mutations) and other missense mutations. Class III mutations are in-frame duplications and/or insertions in exon 20, accounting for about 5% of EGFR TK activating mutations. Overall, the frequency of EGFR TK activating mutations is 5%–20%, depending on the population studied. Activating EGFR TK mutations are significantly more common in East Asians, women, never smokers, and patients with adenocarcinoma (Janne, 2006). This mirrors the clinically defined subsets of patients who were most likely to respond to EGFR TK inhibitors. The NSCLC patients who present with EGFR TK activating mutations have not only better response to gefitinib or erlotinib but also significantly longer progression-free survival and overall survival compared with those without these mutations (Gazdar, 2009).

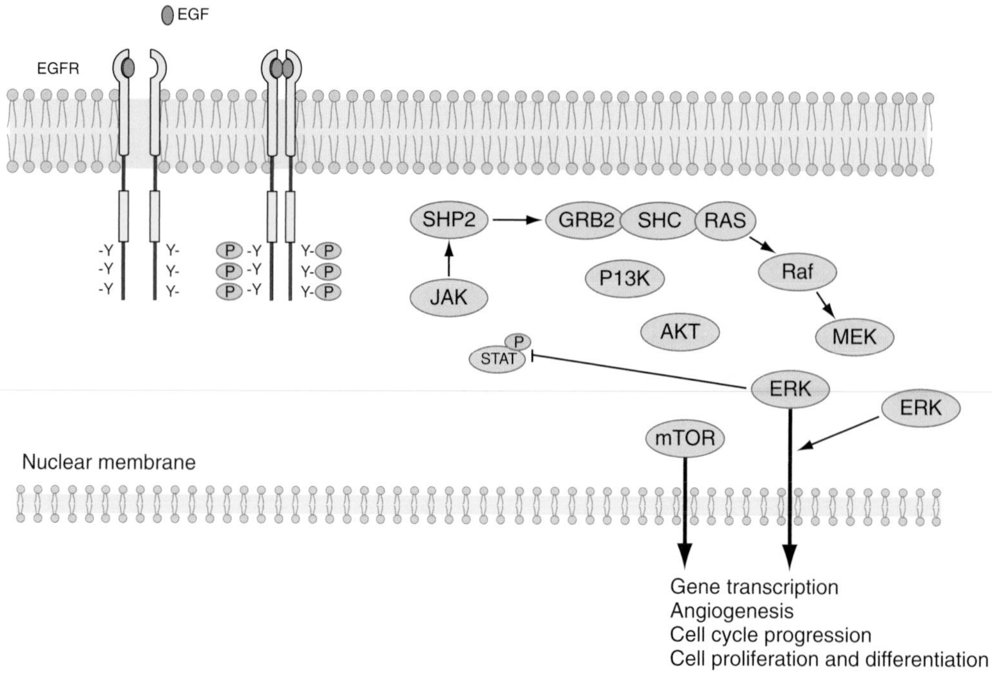

Figure 72-7 Ras signaling network. Simplified schematic of the EGFR signaling cascade. *AKT,* Serine/threonine-specific protein kinase family Protein Kinases B; *EGF,* epidermal growth factor; *EGFR,* epidermal growth factor receptor; *Grb2,* Growth factor receptor-bound protein 2; *JAK,* Janus protein tyrosine kinase family; *MAPK,* mitogen-activated protein kinase; *MEK,* mitogen-activated protein kinase; *PI3K,* phosphatidylinositol 3-kinase; *PTEN,* phosphatase and tensin homolog; *RAF,* RAF proto-oncogene serine/threonine-protein kinase; *Ras,* ras kinase; *SOS,* son of sevenless homolog 1; *STAT,* signal transducers and activator of transcription.

It is noted that acquired resistance occurs in virtually all NSCLC tumors that initially respond to EGFR TK inhibitors. The emergence of acquired resistance is conferred by a second point mutation in the TK domain. The most noteworthy, clinically relevant mutation in exon 20 is T790M, which is detected in 50% of the cases as a second site mutation associated with acquired gefitinib and erlotinib resistance (Sharma, 2007). It is proposed that the T790M mutation affects the gatekeeper residue in the catalytic domain of the TK that weakens the interaction of the inhibitor with its target (Blencke, 2004). In addition, D761Y, a T790M-like secondary mutation in exon 19 of EGFR (at the border of exon 19 and exon 20), was also reported to be associated with resistance to gefitinib and erlotinib in NSCLC cells that contain the L858R-EGFR mutation (Balak, 2006).

In summary, the EGFR kinase domain mutations are important determinants of sensitivity or resistance to EGFR TK inhibitors. EGFR mutation testing is commercially available, and current research is directed at introducing a genetic assessment of the EGFR mutational status into routine clinical practice for personalized therapy of NSCLC patients.

K-RAS MUTATION

Ras proteins are GTP-coupled proteins that are important in many receptor tyrosine kinase signaling pathways. These proteins are discussed further in Chapter 76. Activation of Ras results in initiation of its complex signaling network (Fig. 72-7). One of the earliest defined receptor tyrosine kinase pathways is the Ras/Raf/Erk/Map kinase pathway. Activation of the Erk/Map kinase pathway via growth factors and their receptors usually leads to gene transcription and cell proliferation. This kinase pathway activation plays an important role in Ras-mediated oncogenesis. Ras is also a key activator for many other signaling pathways (Fig. 72-8). So far, nine pathways have been identified as the result of Ras activation. As discussed at length in Chapter 76, ras-p21 protein becomes oncogenic if single amino acid substitutions occur at critical positions such as at Gly 12 or Gln 61 in its polypeptide chain. These substitutions result in permanent activation of this protein that results in permanent activation of downstream signaling pathways and cell transformation and tumorigenesis. *KRAS* mutation plays a key role in colon cancer development.

In 2008 there were 148,000 new cases of colorectal cancer diagnosed in the United States. Approximately 50,000 individuals die annually of the disease, making colon cancer the third leading cause of cancer-related death. It is well documented that survival of colorectal cancer correlates with the stage of the disease at diagnosis. Patients with stage I disease have more than 90% survival after 5 years of diagnosis, whereas survival for stage IV or metastatic disease is about 5%. Approximately 20% of patients diagnosed with colorectal cancer have stage IV disease at the time of presentation and an additional 30%–40% will develop metastasis during the course of their disease. Over the past decade, treatment for metastatic colorectal cancer has significantly improved with the approval of new agents. The median survival of stage IV disease has significantly increased to more than 20 months with the addition of new cytotoxic and targeted biologic agents (Jass, 2006; Bonomi, 2007; Jass, 2007; O'Brien, 2007; Bokemeyer, 2009; DeRoock, 2009; Houtsma, 2009; Huang, 2009).

Colon cancer development is a multistep process involving cumulative genetic mutations from oncogenes, tumor suppressor genes, and chromosomal deletions that are ultimately required to transform colonic epithelium (O'Brien, 2007). Among these genes, *KRAS* is considered to be a critical component in the early stages of colorectal cancer development. *KRAS* mutations have been detected in precancerous aberrant crypt foci on the colonic epithelium. In addition to an early event, *KRAS* mutations are common events in that 30%–50% of colon cancers harbor this mutation and more than 3000 point mutations have been reported. The most common mutations occur in codons 12 and 13 in exon 2, with approximately 80% occurring in the codon 12 and 20% in codon 13. Activating mutations in codon 61 and 146 have also been reported, but these make up less than 10% of mutations (Pretlow, 2005; Plesec, 2009; Saif, 2009; Walther, 2009). The consequences of a mutated *KRAS* gene affect multiple aspects of colorectal cancer. Constitutively activated *KRAS* not only promotes tumor initiation but also tumor growth, survival and progression, local invasion, metastasis formation, angiogenesis, and even immune response. In addition, *KRAS* mutations lead to EGFR signaling independence (Castagnola, 2005; Chang, 2009).

Pharmacogenomics in Cancer Chemotherapy

5-FLUOROURACIL

Since its introduction more than 50 years ago (Heidelberger, 1957), 5-FU has remained the most frequently prescribed anticancer drug for the treatment of malignancies of the gastrointestinal tract including colorectal and gastric cancer. 5-FU, a fluoropyrimidine analogue, is a prodrug that is converted to the active metabolite, 5-fluoro-2-deoxyuridine monophosphate (FdUMP) that leads to inhibition of TS and subsequently of DNA

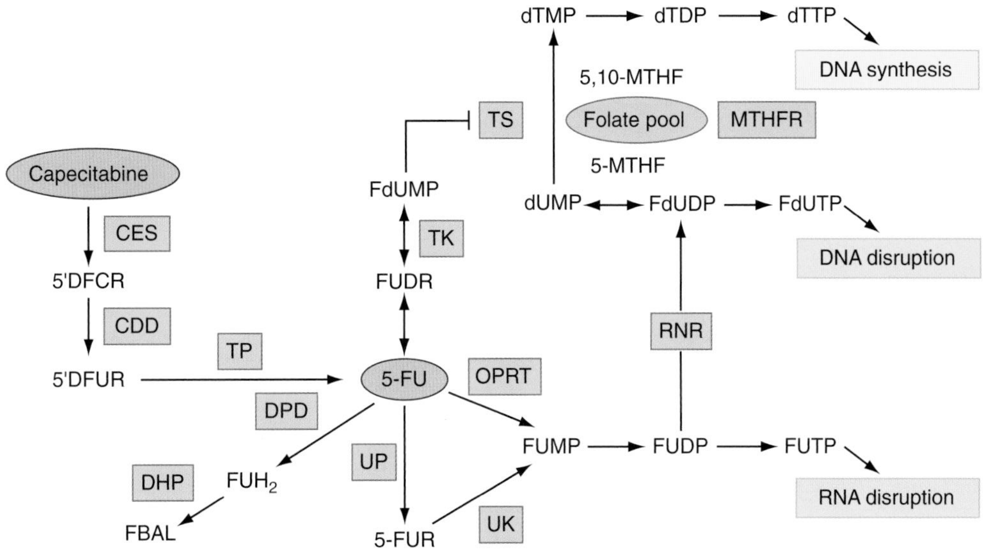

Figure 72-8 Pathways that affect 5-fluorouracil (5-FU) efficacy. Genetic polymorphisms within the genes that are involved in 5-FU metabolic activation (e.g., OPRT), detoxification (e.g., DPD), and target interaction (e.g., TS) are important determinants of the efficacy and safety of 5-FU treatment. *(Adapted from Walther A, Johnstone E, Swanton C, Midgley R, Tomlinson I, Kerr D. Genetic prognostic and predictive markers in colorectal cancer. Nat Rev Cancer 2009;9 [7]:489–99.) 5′DFCR,* 5′deoxy-5-fluorocytidine; *5′DFUR,* 3′deoxy-5-fluorouridine; *5-FUR,* 5-fluorouridine; *CDD,* cytosine deaminase; *CES,* carboxylesterase; *DHP,* dihydropyrimidinase; *DPD,* dihydropyrimidine dehydrogenase; *FBAL,* fluoro-b-alanine; *FUH2,* dihydro-5-fluorouracil; *MTHFR,* methylenetetrahydrofolate reductase; *OPRT,* orotate phosphoribosyltransferase; *RNR,* ribonucleotide reductase; *TK,* thymidine kinase; *TP,* thymidine phosphorylase; *TS,* thymidylate synthase; *UK,* uridine-cytidine kinase 2; *UP,* uridine phosphorylase 1.

synthesis. 5-FU is converted to FdUMP through three pathways: oratate phosphoribosyltransferase (OPRT) (pathway 1), uridine phosphorylase (pathway 2), and thymidine phosphorylase (TP) (pathway 3) (see Fig. 72-8) (Omura, 2003). The vast majority (~80%–85%) of administered 5-FU is metabolized by the enzyme dihydropyrimidine dehydrogenase (DPD) in the liver into the inactive form, dihydrofluorouracil, and excreted as a fluoro-β-alanine.

The phase I metabolizing enzyme, DPD, plays the most important role in detoxification of 5-FU. Expression of DPD has been related to tolerance and response to 5-FU–based chemotherapy. Specifically, low expression or absence of DPD has been associated with accumulation of 5-FU, thereby exposing patients to increased risk of severe toxicities, whereas high expression of DPD has been associated with poor response to 5-FU (Salonga, 2000; Soong, 2008). Approximately 3%–5% of the population is partially or completely deficient in DPD enzyme activity (Lu, 1993). As a consequence, patients lacking the DPD enzyme may experience severe to lethal toxicities when receiving 5-FU-based chemotherapy. Genetic aberration in the dihydropyrimidine dehydrogenase gene, such as exon skipping, deletion, and missense mutation, contributes to a DPD-deficiency phenotype. The most known DPD SNPs associated with grade 3 and 4 toxicities are IVS14 + 1G>A, 2846A>T, 1679T>G, and 85T>C (Morel, 2006). In particular, the exon 14-skipping mutation IVS14 + 1G>A, a G-to-A point mutation within the 5′-splicing site of intron 14, leads to a mutant DPD that lacks amino acids 581–635 and consequently lacks catalytic activity. The allele frequency of this mutation was 0.91% in a Dutch Caucasian population (Vreken, 1996). In patients heterozygous for the IVS14 + 1G>A allele, half of the mean normal activity of DPD is found, which is sufficient to lead to severe 5-FU toxicities. In patients homozygous for the IVS14 + 1G>A allele, DPD activity is completely lacking, and 5-FU toxicities become life-threatening and sometimes fatal (Wei, 1996; Van Kuilenburg, 1997).

OPRT, an enzyme contributing to phosphorylation and activation of 5-FU (see Fig. 72-8), may serve as a predictor of response to 5-FU-based chemotherapy. Overexpression and high levels of OPRT mRNA, as well as a high OPRT/DPD ratio have been associated with improved response to 5-FU-based chemotherapy in patients with metastatic colorectal cancer (Ichikawa, 2003). In a retrospective study examining the association of TS and OPRT genotypes with 5-FU related toxicity, co-presence of the OPRT Gly213Ala variant allele and TS 2R/2R genotype was related to grade 3 and 4 neutropenia and diarrhea (Ichikawa, 2006).

In addition to pharmacogenetic influence of genes involved in 5-FU pharmacokinetics, genetic polymorphisms in the drug target also impact the clinical outcome of patients receiving 5-FU. 5-FU acts by inhibition of TS. TS expression varies considerably among tumors and the response and toxicity toward 5-FU-based chemotherapy have been associated with TS mRNA expression levels in the tumor and normal tissues, respectively. TS expression is modulated by three functional significant germline polymorphisms in the 5′ and 3′ untranslated regions (5′UTR and 3′UTR) of the TS gene (see detailed discussion earlier). TS polymorphisms are not only prognostic factors of disease-free survival and overall survival but also predictors of chemotherapeutic benefit from 5-FU-based chemotherapy. In general, most studies support that patients with colorectal cancer who have high-expression genotype (i.e., TSER-2R/3G, -3C/3G, -3G/3G, 3′-UTR +6bp/+6bp) showed a trend toward poor prognosis and worse response to 5-FU-based chemotherapy, but possibly less severe toxicities, compared with low-expression group (i.e., TSER-2R/2R, -2R/3C, -3C/3C, 3′-UTR +6bp/-6bp, -6bp/-bp) (for review see Lurje, 2009).

In summary, genetic polymorphisms within the genes that are involved in 5-FU metabolic activation (e.g., OPRT), detoxification (e.g., DPD), and target interaction (e.g., TS) are important determinants of the efficacy and safety of 5-FU treatment. Systemic assessment of the genotypes of these genes would allow tailoring 5-FU-based chemotherapy for individual patients.

IRINOTECAN

The topoisomerase I inhibitor irinotecan is a water-soluble, semisynthetic derivative of camptothecin, a plant alkaloid isolated from *Camptotheca acuminata* (family Nyssaceae). It is widely used in the treatment of metastatic colorectal cancer, either in combination with 5-FU in the first-line treatment setting or as monotherapy in the second line setting (Saltz, 2000). Irinotecan acts as a prodrug and undergoes complex metabolic pathways in vivo (Fig. 72-9). Specifically, it is activated to 7-ethyl-10-hydroxycamptothecin (SN-38) by human carboxylesterase 1 and 2 (hCE1 and hCE2), and SN-38 is subsequently detoxified by UGT1A1 to a β-glucuronide derivative, SN-38G (Slatter, 1997). In addition, irinotecan undergoes CYP3A4-mediated oxidation to form the inactive metabolites 7-ethyl-10-(4-N-(5-aminopentanoic acid)-1-piperidino) carbonyloxycamptothecin (APC), and 7-ethyl-10-(4-amino-1-piperidino) carbonyloxycamptothecin, the latter of which also undergoes a subsequent conversion by CES2 to SN-38 (Rivory, 1996; Dodds, 1998). The pharmacologic behavior of irinotecan can be additionally complicated by the substrate affinity of irinotecan and its metabolites (i.e., SN-38 and SN-38G) for the ABC transporters including ABCB1, ABCC1/2, and ABCG2 (Schellens, 2000; Luo, 2002).

In clinical use, irinotecan exhibits substantial interindividual variability in its pharmacokinetics, efficacy, and toxicity profiles (Mathijssen, 2001), which is, in part, related to genetic polymorphisms in the metabolic

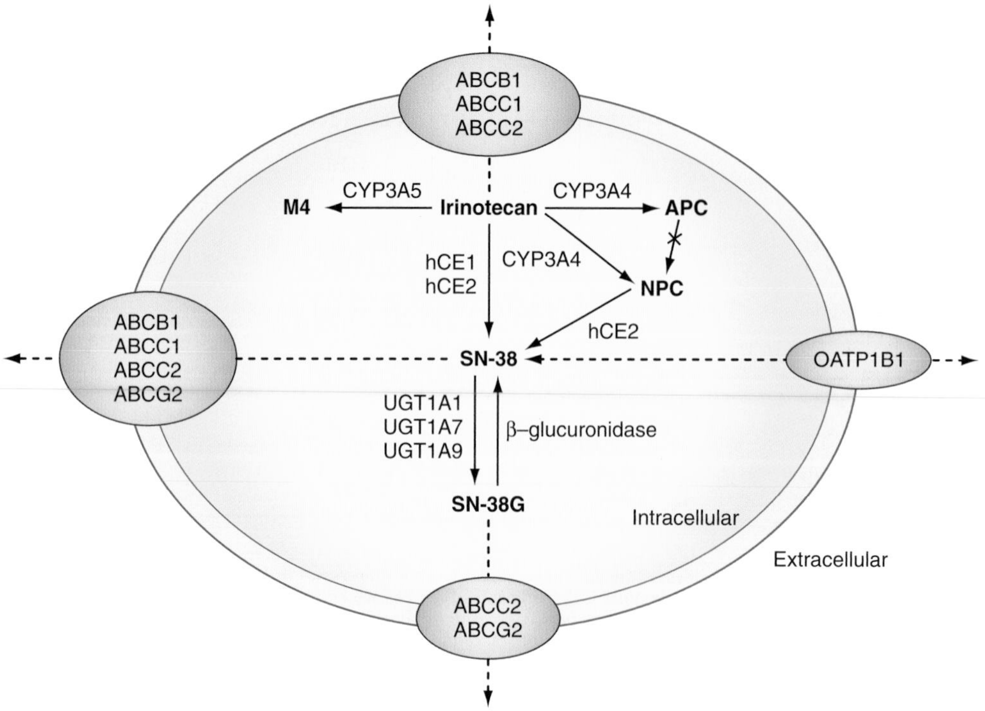

Figure 72-9 Schematic illustration of irinotecan disposition pathway. Irinotecan is activated to 7-ethyl-10-hydroxycamptothecin (SN-38) by human carboxylesterase 1 and 2 (hCE1 and hCE2), and SN-38 is subsequently detoxified by UGT1A1 to a β-glucuronide derivative, SN-38G (Slatter, 1997). In addition, irinotecan undergoes CYP3A4-mediated oxidation to form the inactive metabolites 7-ethyl-10-(4-N-(5-aminopentanoic acid)-1-peperidino) carbonyloxycamptothecin (APC) and 7-ethyl-10-(4-amino-1-peperidino) carbonyloxycamptothecin (NPC), and NPC also undergoes a subsequent conversion by hCE2 to SN-38. Irinotecan and its metabolites (i.e., SN-38 and SN-38G) are also transported by the ABC transporters including ABCB1, ABCC1/2, or ABCG2 or the organic anion transporting polypeptide 1B1 (OATP1B1). *(Adapted from van Erp NP, Baker SD, Zhao M, et al. Effect of milk thistle* (Silybum marianum) *on the pharmacokinetics of irinotecan. Clin Cancer Res 2005;11[21]:7800–6.)*

enzymes and transporters involved in irinotecan disposition. There is definitive evidence that the genetic variant *UGT1A1*28*, characterized by the presence of an additional TA repeat in the TATA sequence of the *UGT1A1* promoter ($(TA)_7TAA$ instead of $(TA)_6TAA$), is associated with reduced SN-38 glucuronidation and greater susceptibility to irinotecan-induced gastrointestinal and hematologic toxicity (Iyer, 2002; Tukey, 2002; Innocenti, 2004). In addition, other polymorphisms in the UGT1A1 gene have also been associated with irinotecan-related toxicity. Of particular importance to East Asian population is *UGT1A1*6* (Gly71Arg) with an allele frequency of ~12%, which reduces UGT1A1 catalytic activity by 60% in homozygotes (Premawardhena, 2003). This variant allele has been related to higher incidence of toxicity in a population of Korean patients treated with irinotcan and cisplatin for advanced NSCLC (Han, 2006). Additionally, two promoter variants (i.e., *UGT1A1 -3263T>G* and *-3156G>A*), which are in strong linkage disequilibrium with *UGT1A1*28* in Caucasians while less apparent in African-Americans and Asians, have been associated with higher incidence of irinotecan-induced grade 4 neutropenia or diarrhea (Innocenti, 2004; Kitagawa, 2005).

Besides UGT1A1, associations between genetic polymorphisms within the genes encoding the drug transporters such as *ABCB1*, *ABCC1*, *ABCG2*, and *OATP* and irinotecan pharmacokinetics and/or toxicity have been reported even though the data are limited (for review, see de Jong, 2006). For *ABCB1*, *ABCB1 3435C>T* variant allele was related to higher irinotecan plasma concentration in Chinese (Zhou, 2005), and *ABCB1 1236C>T* variant allele resulted in higher AUC of irinotecan and SN-38 but lower AUC of SN-38G in a Caucasian population (Mathijssen, 2003). Nevertheless, the true clinical relevance of a single SNP on *ABCB1* to irinotecan treatment remains to be clarified. A haplotype approach may be more useful to estimate true genetic effects. A haplotype analysis in 49 Japanese patients indicated that the patients carrying the *ABCB1*2* haplotype, containing 1236C>T, 2677G>T, and 3435C>T SNPs, exhibit significantly lower renal clearance of irinotecan, SN-38, and APC (Sai, 2003). With regard to ABCC2 that is involved in bile excretion of irinotecan, a functional SNP *ABCC2 3972C>T* was found to have significant effect on the AUC of irinotecan, APC, and SN-38G, all being higher in patients carrying homozygous 3972T (Kim, 2002). Irinotecan and SN-38 are good substrates of ABCG2; yet, no significant associations between ABCG2 polymorphisms and irinotecan pharmacokinetics or toxicity were found. OATP1B1 is involved in the transport of SN-38 but not SN-38G; variants of this transporter including 521T>C, -11187G>A, 388A>G, and *OATP1B1*15* haplotype have been associated with a lower clearance and higher systemic exposure of SN-38 and irinotecan (Xiang, 2006; Han, 2008).

In addition to pharmacogenetic influence of genes involved in irinotecan pharmacokinetics, polymorphisms in the drug target of SN-38, topoisomerase I (TOP1), and cellular downstream effectors leading to DNA repair or cell death may influence patient outcomes to irinotecan treatment. A recent study in 107 advanced colorectal cancer patients showed that *TOP1* and *TDP1* haplotype tagging SNPs (htSNPs) were related to grade 3/4 neutropenia and response, respectively; and a DNA repair gene *XRCC1* haplotype was associated with response (Hoskins, 2008).

Collectively, it is clear that *UGT1A1*28* is associated with greater susceptibility to irinotecan-induced gastrointestinal and hematologic toxicity. It is recommended that the initial dose of irinotecan is reduced for patients homozygous for the *UGT1A1*28* allele. The true clinical significance of polymorphisms within other genes involved in the pharmacokinetics and pharmacodynamics of irinotecan with respect to patient outcome treated with this drug remains to be further clarified.

TAMOXIFEN

Tamoxifen is a well-established drug for use in breast cancer and is within the class of selective estrogen receptor modulators. Despite major strides in the diagnosis and management of breast cancer, the disease will account for an estimated 40,000 deaths in 2008 among women in the United States. Tumors from approximately 75% of women with newly diagnosed breast cancer will express steroid hormone receptors, and those women will likely be recommended endocrine therapy to reduce the risk of recurrence and death. Other endocrine approaches are currently available, including selective estrogen receptor (ER) downregulators (fulvestrant in postmenopausal women), and aromatase inhibitors (e.g., anastrozole, exemestane, and letrozole in postmenopausal women), or ovarian function suppression (by surgery, luteinizing hormone-releasing hormone agonist, or radiation) in premenopausal women (Blackhall, 2006; Bao, 2007; Brauch, 2009). How to apply the various treatment possibilities in order to maximize therapeutic index is controversial. Tamoxifen remains the standard of care in premenopausal women. Most postmenopausal women will be recommended for 5 years of an aromatase inhibitor or 2–3 years of tamoxifen followed by an aromatase inhibitor for a total of 5 years. Administration of tamoxifen in patients with ER-positive breast cancer as adjuvant therapy for 5 years, following anthracycline-based chemotherapy, reduces the recurrence rate by 50% and the mortality rate by a third in 15-year follow up studies. The most common side effect of tamoxifen is hot flashes, and the most severe adverse effects are thrombotic events in breast cancer patients and endometrial cancer in some patients.

The pharmacology of tamoxifen is thought to be linked to the interaction of the parent drug and its metabolites with the ER in both breast and nonbreast tissues. This interaction induces a specific conformational change of the ER, leading to alteration of downstream signaling pathways and ultimately resulting in transcriptional and posttranscriptional changes in estrogen regulated genes with inhibition of estrogen effects. Tamoxifen is a nonsteroidal agent that has a rather weak affinity for its target the ER. Most of the antiproliferative effects of tamoxifen in breast cancer is mediated by its metabolites. The most important metabolites include 4-hydroxytamoxifen (4-OH-tamoxifen) and 4-hydroxy-N-desmethyl tamoxifen (endoxifen). Both metabolites have a much stronger affinity to the ER than does tamoxifen. These metabolites antagonize the effects of estrogen in breast tumors by competing with the hormone at the receptor-binding sites. Endoxifen is prevalent at sixfold to twelvefold higher concentration than tamoxifen. Tamoxifen undergoes extensive phase I and phase II metabolism in the human liver. The bioconversion of tamoxifen includes N-oxidation, N-demethylation, and hydroxylation. There are at least three metabolites of tamoxifen of clinical interest. The major metabolite, N-desmethyl-tamoxifen is roughly equipotent to the parent drug and is produced by the CYP450 3A4/5 mediated demethylation of tamoxifen. In contrast, the other metabolite, 4-hydroxytamoxifen is generated in small quantities compared to tamoxifen by several CYP450 enzymes, including 2D6, but has a greater that 100-fold affinity for the ER and is 30–100 times more potent than tamoxifen in suppressing estrogen-dependent proliferation. The third tamoxifen metabolite, endotoxifen, is as potent as 4-hydroxytamoxifen in inhibiting estrogen-mediated proliferation, but it is present at tenfold higher amounts than 4-hydroxytamoxifen. Thus endoxifen is believed to be responsible for the majority of tamoxifen-associated antitumor activity. Endoxifen is primarily generated by CYP450 2D6, and genetic variants of this enzyme as well as drugs that modulate its enzymatic activity could significantly affect the outcome in tamoxifen-treated patients (van Schaik, 2005; Yong, 2007; Ekhart, 2009; Hoskins, 2009; Zhou, 2009).

Mechanisms of resistance to tamoxifen therapy, as well as predictive markers of susceptibility to resistance, have been widely researched (Ingelman-Sundberg, 2007; Goetz, 2008; Schroth, 2009). Accurate markers would allow prediction of tamoxifen response and personalization of combined therapies. The suggestion has been made that patients with ER-positive breast cancer with inherited nonfunctional alleles of the cytochrome P450 CYP2D6 gene might be poor candidates for adjuvant tamoxifen therapy. The postulation that CYP4502D6 inhibition might reduce the protection conferred by tamoxifen therapy is based on two lines of evidence. First, women with CYP4502D6 variant alleles that reduce the enzyme function or who take CYP450 2D6–inhibiting drugs, such as some selective serotonin reuptake inhibitors (SSRIs), have reduced concentration of the tamoxifen metabolites that most strongly bind the ER. Second, in some studies, women with CYP2D6 variant alleles have a higher risk of recurrence than women with two functional alleles. A retrospective study of 223 postmenopausal women examined CYP450 2D6 *4, the most common null allele associated with poor metabolizer status and the outcome of tamoxifen therapy. Women homozygous for CYP450 2D6 *4 had poorer outcomes than women with CYP450 2D6 *4/*1 or *1/*1 genotypes, showing shorter time to relapse and worse disease-free survival. In addition, no women with CYP450 2D6 *4/*4 experienced moderate or severe hot flashes, in contrast to 20% incidence in those women with either one or no *4 alleles (Schroth, 2007). Furthermore, a retrospective study by Schroth and colleagues in a German and US cohort study of 1325 postmenopausal stage I through III breast cancer patients, found that, among women treated with tamoxifen, there was an association between CYP2D6 variation and clinical outcomes, such that the presence of 2 functional CYP2D6 alleles was associated with better clinical outcomes and the presence of nonfunctional or reduced-function alleles with worse outcomes (Schroth, 2009). Similar results were obtained by Borges and associates using an expanded analysis to include other reduced activity alleles such as *4, *5, *10, and *41 (Borges, 2006). All of these studies suggest that CYP450 2D6 poor metabolizers are at higher risk of recurrence of breast cancer or more likely to develop breast cancer when given prophylactic tamoxifen. Based on these studies, there have been efforts to identify breast cancer patients whose genotypes suggest poor metabolizer phenotypes and offer alternative therapy such as aromatase inhibitors. In opposition to these reports, Wegman and colleagues found a significantly better disease-free survival in 667 tamoxifen-treated postmenopausal breast cancer patients homozygous for CYP450 2D6 *4. Some of the differences seen in the literature might be due to differences in study designs, selection bias, and/or uncontrolled confounders (Wegman, 2007). These and other reports have led to the current controversy both on the clinical validity and utility of CYP450 2D6 genotyping for individuals receiving tamoxifen therapy.

Hot flashes, one of the most common side effects of tamoxifen therapy, are commonly treated with antidepressants such as SSRIs. Certain SSRIs inhibit CYP 450 2D6 enzymatic activity (Van Schaik, 2008). Coadministration of certain SSRIs has been shown to significantly reduce the concentration of one of the most potent metabolites of tamoxifen, endoxifen, even in extensive metabolizer patients. Furthermore, administration of SSRIs that do not inhibit CYP 450 2D6 enzymatic activity has been shown not to diminish the concentration of endoxifen. In a recent prospective study, Goetz and collaborators assessed the influence of genetic and drug-induced reduction in CYP 450 2D6 activity on breast cancer outcomes in 226 patients coadministered potent or weak/moderate CYP 450 2D6 inhibitors with tamoxifen. Patients were stratified by genotype and medication history into subgroups of extensive or decreased metabolizer genotypes (Goetz, 2008). Compared with patients with extensive metabolizer CYP 450 2D6 metabolism genotype, patients with decreased metabolism genotype showed significantly shorter time to recurrence and worse relapse-free survival.

The current evidence regarding CYP 450 2D6 genotype and benefits when selecting a breast cancer treatment is still controversial (Lea, 2007; Li, 2007; Limdi, 2009; Marsh, 2009). An FDA advisory panel suggested that the tamoxifen package insert should alert treating health care providers of concerns that poor metabolizer patients might be at increased risk for recurrence of their breast cancer if treated with tamoxifen and that the coadministration of certain selective SSRIs known to inhibit CYP450 2D6 can affect the metabolism of tamoxifen. On the other hand, the 2009 National Comprehensive Cancer Network of National Institutes of Health breast cancer guidelines do not include any recommendations concerning treatment modification based on CYP 450 2D6 genotyping. In recent years, a great amount of progress has been achieved in the understanding of how genetic makeup of patients might influence the response to breast cancer treatment but much more work needs to be done. Of particular interest would be the development of further studies on postmenopausal patients as well as for premenopausal women to address the relationship between CYP 450 2D6 genotype and success of tamoxifen therapy.

PLATINUM AGENTS

Platinating agents are widely used chemotherapeutic drugs and consist of a number of platinum analogs develop to overcome cellular resistance and reduce toxicity (Furuta, 2009). The chemotherapy drugs cisplatin, carboplatin, and oxaliplatin are commonly used for the treatment of lung, colorectal, ovarian, breast, head and neck, bladder, and testicular cancer. Cisplatin exerts its antitumor activity by binding preferentially to N-7 positions of adenine and guanine of DNA, resulting in the formation of intrastrand and interstrand crosslinks. This cross-linking blocks replication and inhibit transcription. Intrinsic and/or acquired resistance as well as toxicities associated with these agents are the major limitations of these drugs. For example, about 85% of patients with ovarian cancer relapse following initial response. The resistance might be multifactorial, consisting of proteins limiting the formation of DNA adducts and/or operating downstream of the interaction of drug with DNA to promote cell survival. More specifically, nodes of resistance include increased efflux from the cell, drug inactivation, alterations to the drug target, DNA repair, evasion of apoptosis, and drug target alteration. Platinum-induced toxicity can also alter the outcome of treatment by limiting the dose of drug administered, with nephrotoxicity and neuropathy as the main dose-limiting toxicities. Peripheral neuropathy is permanent in approximately 30%–50% of patients receiving treatment. Additionally, ototoxicity and neurotoxicity are difficult to manage and can result in the discontinuation or reduction of treatment. Thus the identification of genetic factors to better predict patients who are at risk of adverse drug reactions associated with cisplatin or relapse is very important (McWhinney, 2009).

The disposition of chemotherapeutic agents is often the key to determining the mechanism by which they cause toxic effects. This disposition is regulated by the drug metabolism, absorption, distribution, and excretion. Platinums cause interstrand DNA cross-linking, leading to cessation of DNA synthesis and apoptosis, and toxicity due to platinums is modulated by protein involved in DNA repair (ERCC1, ERCC2, and XRCC1), DNA detoxification (GSTP1 and MPO), and transport (SLC31A1, ABCC2, and ABCG2) (Shukla, 2008). However, there are no genetic polymorphisms that are ready for clinical application. In a large study done in Scotland, a randomized clinical trial of carboplatin and taxane in patients with ovarian cancer, genetic polymorphism of genes relevant to the platinum pathway, such as ABCC2, ABCG2, ERCC1, ERCC2, GSTP1, MPO, and XRCC1, were not significantly associated with clinical outcomes or toxicity (Wang, 2008; Caronia, 2009).

DNA repair is an important mechanism for resistance to platinum-based therapy and possibly the development of neurotoxicity. If the cell is able to repair the DNA that is attacked by the platinum agent, then the agent will be unsuccessful in inducing apoptosis. Nucleotide excision repair genes, such as excision repair cross-complementation group 1 (ERCC1), have been hypothesized to play a role in the efficacy of platinum-based drugs. Park and colleagues described the association between the ERCC1 codon 118 polymorphism and the clinical outcome in colorectal cancer patients treated with platinum-based chemotherapy (Park, 2003). This genotype could be a useful predictor of clinical outcome not only for colorectal cancer but also for patients with epithelial ovarian cancer. Today, there has been no association between ERCC1 polymorphism and chemotherapy neurotoxicity. There are many avenues that will need to be perused to avoid or minimize neurotoxicity caused by platinum drugs.

ANTIBODY THERAPY

Over the past decade, treatment for malignancy such as metastatic colorectal cancer has significantly improved with the approval of several new agents (Jimeno, 2009; Modjtahedi, 2009). In particular two different EGFR inhibitor therapies have emerged as effective treatment for a subset of patients with metastatic colorectal carcinoma: cetuximab and panitumumab (Hamilton, 2008; Garcia-Saenz, 2009; Heinemann, 2009; Siena, 2009; Stintzing 2009). Because *KRAS* is the downstream effector of EGFR and it is frequently mutated in colorectal cancer, the effectiveness of cetuximab in *KRAS* mutated tumors has become a topic of recent studies (Garcia, 2008; Raponi, 2008; Riely, 2008; Monzon, 2009; Normanno, 2009). Because activating K ras mutations lead to EGFR independence, it stands to reason that tumors that harbor *KRAS* activating mutation will not benefit from anti-EGFR therapies. One of the initial reports came from Personeni and colleagues after demonstrating that an increasing copy number of EGFR in colorectal cancer by fluorescent in situ hybridization analysis predicted the response to cetuximab (Personeni, 2007). However, tumors with the *KRAS* mutation did not respond to cetuximab therapy. Their observation was further confirmed by several studies that found that *KRAS* mutations precluded tumor response to cetuximab but these studies suffer from a small patient cohort. More recently, Amado and associates examined *KRAS* mutation in 427 patients with metastatic colorectal cancer treated with panitumumab or best supportive care (Amado, 2008). Patients with wild type *KRAS* clearly benefited from this therapy with a significantly longer progression-free survival and overall survival. However, these benefits diminished for those patients harboring a *KRAS* mutation. Furthermore, Van Cutsen and colleagues performed a retrospective study to assess *KRAS* mutational status in patients who participated in the CRYSTAL trial (Van Cutsem, 2007). In this study, 348 patients (64.4%) had a wild type *KRAS* while 192 patients (35.6%) had a mutant *KRAS*. In patients with wild type *KRAS*, cetuximab significantly improved the response rate (43% for FOLFIRI, 59% for cetuximab + FOLFIRI, $P = .00025$) and progression-free survival (8.7 months FOLFIRI, 9.9 months for cetuximab + FOLFIRI, $P = .017$). On the other hand, cetuximab had no effect on tumors bearing the *KRAS* mutation (response rate or RR: 40% without cetuximab vs. 36% with cetuximab, $P = .46$; progression-free survival: 8.1 months without cetuximab vs. 7.6 months for cetuximab, $P = 0.75$). This observation was also confirmed by another large retrospective study presented by Bokemeyer in the OPUS trial (Bokemeyer, 2009). These clinical trials have shown that up to 40% of patients with *KRAS* wild type colorectal cancer show at least a partial response to anti-EGFR therapy, an improvement over the 10% before *KRAS* mutation stratification; whereas patients with *KRAS* mutated tumors gain no benefit from anti-EGFR therapy. The utility of determining *KRAS* mutation status beforehand, therefore, is to determine which patients will not respond to EGFR monoclonal antibody therapy. In light of these results, the National Comprehensive Cancer Network and the American Society of Clinical Oncology have developed guidelines to recommend that all colorectal tumors with metastases should be tested for mutations in codon 12 and 13 of exon 2 of the *KRAS* gene before initiating anti-EGFR therapy (Pare, 2008; Shankaran, 2008; Allegra, 2009). There are no FDA approved tests in the market and there are no specific technologic recommendations (Weichert, 2010). Unfortunately, at least 60% of *KRAS* wild type patients will derive no benefit from anti-EGFR antibodies, highlighting the need for additional biomarkers to help separate responders from nonresponders. Potential biomarkers include BRAF, *KRAS* codon 61 and 146, PIK3 and PTEN mutation, and EGFR gene copy number (Oikonomou, 2006).

PHARMACOGENOMICS IN OTHER DISEASES

DIABETES

Pharmacogenomic investigations of diabetes mellitus have yielded variations in genomic loci containing common variants with translational consequences of altering disease susceptibility risk, clinical course, and response to standard therapy. This is becoming increasingly important in light of the prospected increased prevalence type 2 diabetes (T2D) to more than 300 million cases in the year 2025 (Wei-Jian, 2008; Zimmet, 2001). To this end, polymorphisms in genes related to β cell function, glucose tolerance, insulin uptake and other aspects of glucose metabolism are being actively investigated for effective drug design and personalized responses. One of the many classes of antidiabetic agents are the glitazones (e.g., thiazolidinedione, or TZD) which can be prescribed alone or in combination with sulfonylureas, metformin, or insulin. TZDs pharmacologically act by agonizing the nuclear peroxisome proliferator-activated receptor γ (PPAR-γ) to form heterodimers with the retinoid X receptors, which binds the PPAR-response elements and regulates target gene transcription. Pro12Ala, polymorphism in the PPAR-γ2, has a frequency of roughly 12%–15% in the general population, making it the most common PPAR-γ variant. A meta-analysis showed that Ala12 allele displayed a protective effect with regard to developing T2D, reducing the risk in carriers by 19% (Ludovico, 2007). Although one study demonstrated that patients with the Pro12Al genotype receiving rosiglitazone for 12 weeks was significantly better when compared with patients with the homozygous Pro12 (PPAR-γ2) genotype (86.7% and 43.7%, respectively) (Kang, 2005), other studies have been inconsistent (Bluher, 2003). Polymorphisms in genes associated with glitazone (TZD) toxicity include CYP2C19, CYP2D6, CYP2C8, CYP2C9, and CYP3A4 (Aquilante, 2007); however, the strengths of these relationships vary. Other polymorphisms related to patient responses to antidiabetic agents such as sulfonylureas (tolbutamide [Orinase], glipizide [Glucotrol], glibenclamide [Glyburide], and glimepiride [Amaryl]), biguanides (Metformin), and meglitinides (nateglinide [Starlix] and repaglinide [Prandin]) are reviewed by Avery (2009) and others (Holstein, 2009; Pearson, 2009).

HUMAN IMMUNODEFICIENCY VIRUS

HIV has become increasingly difficult to treat due to the mutational nature of the virus (Wolinski, 1996). Degenerate pathways common to HIV mutants and strains have been targets of drug design such as highly active antiretroviral therapy, which represents a combination of substances directed against various steps in the viral life cycle. Pharmacogenomic approaches are providing additional information toward devising therapies to decrease morbidity and mortality associated with HIV infections. Earlier studies by Liu and colleagues (1996) described resistance to HIV-1 infection in cells, obtained from multiply exposed individuals. Those studies found that such patients were homozygous defective for CC-CKR5 and therefore resistant to infection. Polymorphisms in the cytochrome P450 system, which is involved in drug clearance, has also been shown to be of value. The CYP3A4*20 null allele contains a premature stop codon yielding a truncated protein. Subjects of this genotype might be susceptible to side effects during drug therapy with substrates or inhibitors of CYP3A4, and this may have pharmacokinetic and pharmacodynamic application to antiretroviral drug design (Westlind-Johnsson, 2006; Lakhman, 2009). Adverse effects to antiviral medications have also been linked to polymorphisms. The human leukocyte antigen (HLA)-DRB1*0101 haplotype may determine the susceptibility to nevirapine hypersensitivity and the 3434T allele at the MDR1 gene is associated with a decreased risk of nevirapine-induced hepatotoxicity. Genetic polymorphisms in the HLA haplotypes HLD HLA-B*5701, HLA-DR7, and/or HLA-DQ3 have been correlated with susceptibility to abacavir allergic reactions. The presence of a TA insertion into the UGT1A1 promoter (Gilbert syndrome) has been associated with increased occurrence of hyperbilirubinemia of atazanavir and indinavir. Polymorphisms in the APOC3 gene have been associated with antiretroviral induced hyperlipidemia; and polymorphisms at the serine protease kinase inhibitor Kazal-1 that encodes a trypsin inhibitor in the cytoplasm of pancreatic acinar cells and the cystic fibrosis transmembrane conductance regulator have been associated with some treatment regimens. Furthermore, many of these responses differ with respect to race (for review, see Clarke, 2009).

OSTEOPOROSIS

Osteoporosis is an increasingly common disorder found in older adults, often resulting from decreased bone mineral density (BMD) with subsequent enhanced bone fragility collectively leading to an increased incidence of fracture. Genetic susceptibility, and hormonal and environmental factors are thought to influence bone mass and as such polymorphisms and their reciprocal effects on therapeutic interventions are actively sought to design the most efficient medications. The VDR gene codes for the vitamin D receptor, which is the target for the active form of vitamin D, 1,25-dihydroxyvitamin D_3 [1,25$(OH)_2D_3$]. Polymorphisms in the VDR gene can affect stability and expression of the mRNA. Restriction fragment length polymorphism (RFLP) and linkage disequilibrium analysis have highlighted polymorphisms in the VRD gene (TaqI, ApaI, BsmI, FokI), some of which have been correlated with increased BMD measurements in certain patients taking antiresorptive drugs, alendronate, or raloxifene as hormone replacement therapy (Massart, 2008) and that these responses were allele specific (Nguyen, 2008). Bone density regulation, by hormones such as estrogens, are also subject to the effects of genetic polymorphisms and allelic variation. Studies on the ERs, ERα, and ERβ, which are coded for by ESR1 and ESR2 genes, respectively, have shown that women with a particular polymorphism (Xba1) had greater spine and hip BMD and that genetic variations of ESR1 relate to bone structure and strength (Ferrari, 2008). The CYP19 gene codes for an enzyme (aromatase) that catalyzes the conversion of androstenedione to estrone and testosterone to estradiol. Mutations in this gene have been found to correlate with decreased BMD. In addition, enzymes involved in the biogenesis of estrone and estradiol have attracted attention as well as polymorphisms in the regulatory region of the type I collagen gene, COLIA1, affecting the binding site for the transcription factor Specificity protein 1 (Sp1) (Thijssen, 2006).

PSYCHIATRIC AND COGNITIVE DISORDERS

Medications prescribed for psychiatric disorders are often administered on a trial-and-error basis (Lin, 2006). Furthermore, although depression and other disorders have been linked to certain genetic predispositions, the multifactorial nature of this disease class is wanting for better understanding of causal relationships. As such clinical correlation studies employing methods such as SNP and linkage studies to facilitate efficiency of antidepressants/antipsychotics with genetic variants have been described (Lin, 2008). As an example, brain-derived neurotrophic factor (BDNF) gene, encodes a protein of the nerve growth factor family that regulates synaptic plasticity and connectivity in the brain. A variation of this gene, which codes for a methionine substitution for valine at codon 66 (Val-66Met), is associated with alterations in brain anatomy and memory (Chen, 2006). Patients with depressive disorder with polymorphisms in this gene have been shown to respond more efficiently to antidepressants such as citalopram, milnacipran, and fluvoxamine in select populations (Choi, 2006; Yoshida, 2007). Furthermore, BDNF stimulates the release of acetylcholine (ACH). Alzheimer's disease (AD) is associated with defective ACH and recent data demonstrates decreased expression BDNF and its receptor, *trk B*, in AD patients. As such, agents that serve to upregulate BNDF and/or *trk B* expression are being investigated with respect to genetic polymorphisms and responses to select drug classes (Fumagalli, 2006). Similarly, in bipolar disorders, genetic factors and polymorphisms have been attributed to efficient response to drugs such as lithium and clozapine. These include variations in serotonin transporter genes and responses to selective serotonin reuptake inhibitors (SSRI), among others (Mansour, 2002). Furthermore, recent studies of Glub and colleagues (2009), examined whether an SNP (rs11042725) in the promoter of the adrenomedullin gene was associated with mood disorders or SSRI antidepressant response. They found that the only significant result was an association of the C/C genotype with a lower likelihood of response to paroxetine (Glub, 2009). Other genes involved in affective disorders that correlate with selective treatment include variants at the tryptophan hydroxylase gene, 5-HT2a receptor, G-protein β3, and inositol polyphosphate 1-phosphatase, among others (Serretti, 2002).

EPIGENOMICS

The term *epigenetics* is defined as follows: *epi-* is Greek for over or above; *-genetics* refers to changes that occur outside the scope of a gene's DNA sequence. These changes result in phenotypic (appearance) or genotypic expression modulation caused by mechanisms other than changes in the underlying DNA sequence (Russo, 1996). Examples of epigenetic phenomenon include DNA methylation status, histone coding, SNPs, copy number variants, and chromatin remodeling, which can affect transcription and subsequent translation of a given gene regardless of its sequence. As such, epigenetics can be used to describe any aspect other than DNA sequence that influences the development of an organism. *Epigenomics* can be considered an extension of this concept to convey overall epigenetic state of a cell across the entire genome. Recent data by Zhang and colleagues (Zhang, 2008) challenge the notion that a drug response is influenced by many different genetic and nongenetic factors; the extent to which each factor contributes to variation in response is not yet fully understood (Fig. 72-10). These concerns make the development of diagnostic tests that could predict an individual's response to a particular drug rather difficult. Profiling the variation in DNA methylation can provide new insights into the regulation of gene expression as well as the mechanisms of individual drug response at a new level of complexity. To this end, the National Institutes of Health have published a roadmap to better understand the relationship of epigenomics to the clinical marketplace (http://nihroadmap.nih.gov/epigenomics/initiatives.asp). Their proposition is to study a variety of human cell types, including human embryonic stem cells, differentiating cells, selected differentiated cell lines representative of human disease, and select human primary cells that are relevant to complex human disease. Epigenomes derived from these studies will serve as a reference and resource to identify potential therapeutic targets, to enhance understanding of disease mechanisms, to provide additional insights to genetic susceptibility of disease, to pursue therapeutic opportunities in stem cell based and tissue regeneration strategies, and to understand normal differentiation, development, and aging/senescence. The initiative is intended to elucidate fundamental epigenomic changes or mechanisms underlying specific diseases; conditions of development or aging; or response to exposures (physical, chemical, behavioral, and social factors).

PART 8

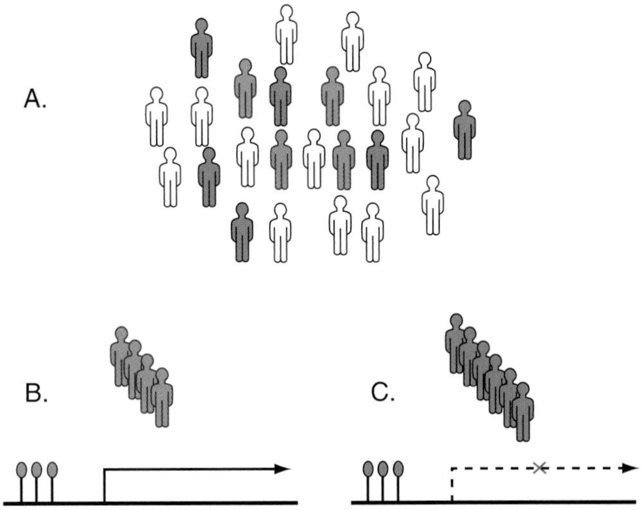

Figure 72-10 DNA methylation status can affect variation in gene expression and drug response. *A*, For a particular drug response-related gene, there could be people with different epigenetic signatures within a population. *Orange*, sensitive people; *blue*, nonrespondent people; *white*, all others. *B*, Sensitive people have an epigenetic signature that causes overexpression of the gene. *C*, In contrast, nonrespondent people have an epigenetic signature that inhibits gene expression. *(From Zhang W, Huang RS, Dolan E. Integrating epigenomics into pharmacogenomic studies. Pharmgenomics Pers Med 2008:1;7–14, with permission.)*

Epigenomics holds potential to shed light on mental disorders (cognitive decline, AD, and schizophrenia) (Gomase, 2008), drug dependence (Coller, 2009), diabetes (Maier, 2002), and respiratory diseases (Bowman, 2009), among others. As an example with respect to drug dependence, the μ opioid receptor has a clear involvement in mediating the analgesic and rewarding effects of endogenous and exogenous opioids (Glatt, 2007). The most frequently studied of these receptors is the *OPRM1* variant, an SNP A118G (recently renamed 304A/G10) in exon 1 that causes an Asn40Asp substitution at a putative glycosylation site in the extracellular domain and occurs at an allelic frequency of between 10% and 40% depending on ethnicity, and epigenetic studies have elucidated potential differences among ethnicities that may have a role personalizing drug development. Although metaanalyses of such studies may not yield conclusive differences (Coller, 2009), there may be differences in gender or in certain ethnicities (Gelernter, 1999; Hoehe, 2000; Kapur, 2007) that may not be apparent when combined with other studies.

Conclusions

It is clear that the field of pharmacogenomics has heralded a new way of thinking about the relationship of a disease on the individual and the individual's response to a disease state encompassing the spectrum of disease pathophysiology, diagnosis, prognosis, and treatment. The methodologies employed, such as SNP, RFLP, loss of heterozygosity, and hybridization array based profiling (see Chapter 67), among others, are as important as the study design, patient demographics, characterization, stratification, comorbidities, and data interpretation. Nonetheless, pharmacogenomics provides a unique approach toward investigating, appreciating, and therapeutically serving the individual patient. Continued investigation and adaptation of pharmacogenomics in clinical medicine should likely provide mankind with improved risk vs. benefit ratios with respect to therapeutic efficacy vs. side effect profiles and effective re-evaluation of drug design toward the generation of novel and specific therapies for disease.

SELECTED REFERENCES

Choi MK, Song IS. Organic cation transporters and their pharmacokinetic and pharmacodynamic consequences. Drug Metab Pharmacokinet 2008;23:243–53.

This review provides an update of our current knowledge on organic cation transporters in terms of their roles in drug pharmacokinetics and pharmacodynamics.

Gossage L, Madhusudan S. Cancer pharmacogenomics: role of DNA repair genetic polymorphisms in individualizing cancer therapy. Mol Diagn Ther 2007;11:361–80.

This review provides an overview on DNA repair pathways and the influence of DNA repair genetic polymorphisms on the clinical outcome (efficacy and toxicity) of DNA-damaging agents and radiotherapy.

Gradhand U, Kim RB. Pharmacogenomics of MRP transporters (ABCC1-5) and BCRP (ABCG2). Drug Metab Rev 2008;40:317–54.

This review provides an overview on ABCC1-5 and ABCG2 transporters with regard to the functional and clinical relevance of their genetic polymorphisms.

Kumar A, Petri ET, Halmos B, Boggon TJ. Structure and clinical relevance of the epidermal growth factor receptor in human cancer. J Clin Oncol 2008;26:1742–51.

This article provides a comprehensive review on the epidermal growth factor receptor (EGFR) with regard to its structure, implication in cancer treatment, and genetic mutations as the determinant of sensitivity or resistance to small molecule EGFR inhibitors.

Zhang W, Huang RS, Dolan E. Integrating epigenomics into pharmacogenomic studies. Pharmgenomics Pers Med 2008:1;7–14.

This review provides an overview of the effect and relationship of epigenomics—genetic and non-genetic factors—and how they may contribute to pharmacogenomic influence and clinical outcomes.

Zhou SF, Liu JP, Chowbay B. Polymorphism of human cytochrome P450 enzymes and its clinical impact. Drug Metab Rev 2009;41:89–295.

This article provides a comprehensive review on human CYP enzymes with regard to their distribution, substrates, genetic polymorphisms and clinical relevance.

REFERENCES

Access the complete reference list online at http://www.expertconsult.com

PART 9

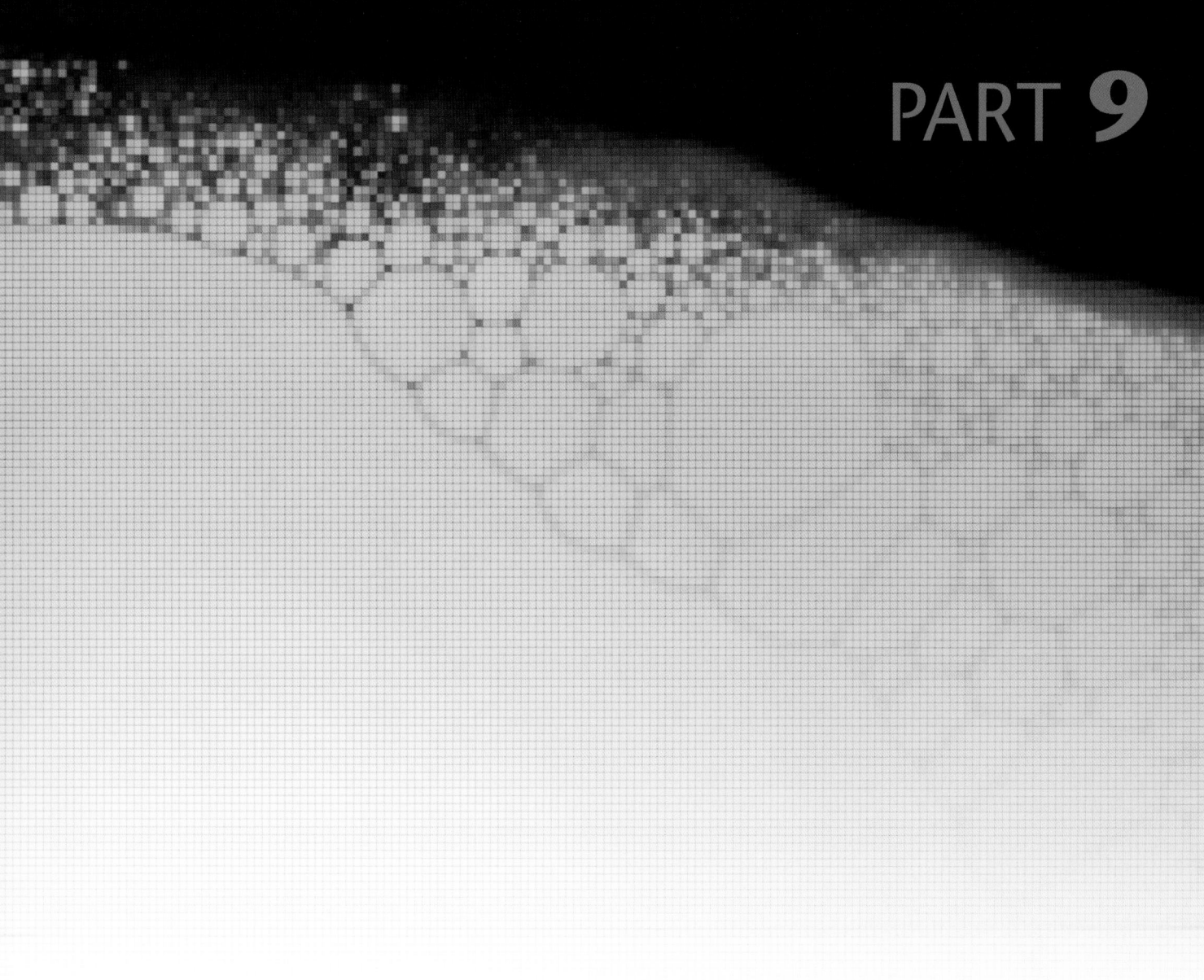

Clinical Pathology of Cancer

EDITED BY Matthew R. Pincus
Martin H. Bluth
Richard A. McPherson

CHAPTER 73

DIAGNOSIS AND MANAGEMENT OF CANCER USING SEROLOGIC AND TISSUE TUMOR MARKERS

Peng Lee, Shilpa Jain, Wilbur B. Bowne, Matthew R. Pincus, Richard A. McPherson

KEY POINTS

- This chapter discusses the use of proteins, whose serum levels are often elevated in patients with malignancies, in the diagnosis and management of cancer.
- Many of these are so-called oncofetal antigens, i.e., proteins that are expressed in fetal tissue during development but are not normally found in the tissues of adults. These include α-fetoprotein and carcinoembryonic antigen, whose serum levels are frequently elevated in hepatocellular and colon cancers, respectively.
- Other proteins, such as CA 19-9, CA 125, and CA 15-3, are expressed in epithelial cells and are also often present in the sera of patients with pancreatic, ovarian, and breast cancers, respectively.
- Because these 'tumor marker' proteins are not tissue-specific and can also be expressed in diseases other than cancer, their sensitivities and specificities are not sufficiently high that they can be used as cancer-screening proteins. Their use is predominantly in following patients who are being treated for known malignancies.
- The exception to this is prostate-specific antigen (PSA), a chymotrypsin-like enzyme that is expressed almost exclusively in prostate tissue and is elevated in the sera of most patients with prostate cancer. Elevated serum PSA levels therefore have a high sensitivity for diagnosing prostate cancer; because PSA is also elevated in other prostate diseases, such as benign prostatic hyperplasia, it has a lower specificity but nonetheless can still be used very effectively to screen patients for this disease.
- New developments in the field of early tumor detection using serum markers are also introduced in this chapter. These include use of mitogenic proteins, such as HER2/Neu, known to function as signal transduction proteins whose levels are elevated in many types of cancers; detection of genes encoding these proteins in body fluids; and proteomic approaches involving patterns of expression of multiple proteins that typify specific cancers. These specific approaches are also discussed in depth in the following chapter.
- The identification of circulating tumor cell (CTC) as biomarker is a fast growing area of research. This chapter updates the recent advance on CTC that is or will be applied in clinical application for diagnostic and prognostic values.

Despite the advancement of multidisciplinary treatment modalities, cancer mortality has not been significantly reduced for the past 50 years. In contrast, dramatic decreases in mortality due to cardiovascular and infectious disease have been achieved. Studies have shown that early detection of cancer can lead to superior long-term survival. Thus there is an urgent need to search for cancer biomarkers with high sensitivity and specificity to allow for early cancer detection, effective treatment, and decreased mortality. Therefore much effort has been devoted to the discovery, characterization, and clinical application of tumor markers to detect the presence of cancer at an early stage. As a result, increasing numbers of biomolecules, mainly specific proteins and some specific ribonucleic acids (RNAs) and deoxyribonucleic acids (DNAs), have been identified and employed as markers potentially for screening purposes and also for prognostic purposes in the daily clinical management of cancer patients. These markers can further be used not only to classify cancers but also to monitor response to neoadjuvant therapy. For example, estrogen receptor (ER), progesterone receptor (PR), and HER2/*neu* oncogene protein are used in the diagnosis and management of breast cancer patients using surgical specimens. ER has been shown to be a prognostic marker for breast cancer and a predictive marker for hormonal treatment (Jensen, 2003). HER2/*neu* amplification and overexpression were shown to be associated with poor prognosis and to be a predictor for therapeutic response in breast cancer (Wilmanns, 2004). PR has been shown to be associated with a good prognosis in ovarian cancer (Munstedt, 2000; Lee, 2005).

Among these markers are a number of tumor markers present in circulating body fluids, including blood. Broadly, body fluid tumor biomarkers (principally serum and urine) are divided into three categories: tumor-associated proteins such as the oncofetal antigens, which seem to be expressed in many cancers but have also been found to be present in other nonneoplastic conditions; oncoproteins, which are involved in the regulation of cell cycle and become overexpressed or mutated almost exclusively in neoplastic conditions; and recently discovered patterns of protein expression in serum that appear to be unique to specific types of cancer (i.e., proteomics). This chapter emphasizes the use of the first two classes of tumor marker. The succeeding chapter discusses oncoproteins and the use of multiple protein profiles on body fluids, or proteomics, as biomarkers for early tumor detection.

Serum Markers as an Effective Tool for Diagnosis and Monitoring of Cancer

Ideally, a tumor marker should become elevated in the serum only of patients with a malignant tumor and should not be elevated in the serum of disease-free individuals or of individuals with nonmalignant diseases such as inflammatory or infectious diseases. Also, a tumor marker protein should become elevated in the serum of cancer patients at an early stage, thereby enabling early tumor detection and the initiation of appropriate therapy. Although no one tumor marker has been found to meet all these characteristics, progress toward the discovery of such markers is continuously being made.

In fact, studies show that one or more cancer biomarkers including DNA, protein, or tumor cells is almost always present in the serum of patients with cancer. These findings provide the rational basis for early detection of cancer using serum samples. Any circulating cell products including DNA, RNA (including microRNA), proteins (enzymes, serum proteins, metabolites, receptors, carcinoembryonic proteins, oncoprotein, and proteins encoded by suppressor genes), and tumor cells can be used as tumor markers if they are associated with events related to tumor formation and/or growth (Fig. 73-1). Such events include malignant transformation, proliferation, dedifferentiation, and metastasis. The blood levels of serum tumor markers are determined by tumor proliferation, tumor volume, proteolytic activities in the tumor cell, and release from necrotic tumor cells. The recent improvement of instrumentation, especially in consolidation of specialized testing instruments as immunoassay analyzers to a more general chemistry analyzer, facilitated the analysis of a wide range of analytes with the same degree of accuracy, specificity, and precision. The improved sensitivities of the assays made serologic tests far superior to other clinical examinations based on physical methods. An additional advantage of serum testing over tissue-based methods is the noninvasive nature, more accurate quantification, and lack of interobserver difference as opposed to tissue-based methods. Because of these benefits, serum markers are frequently used to screen for, diagnose, and predict the behavior of many cancers.

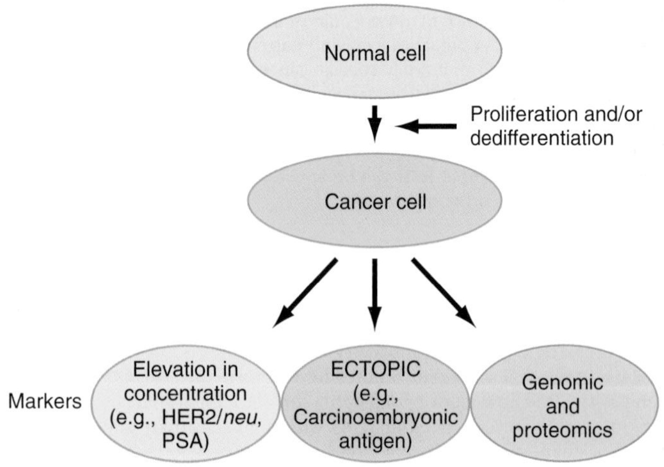

Figure 73-1 Different types of serum tumor marker are used to detect cancer. HER2 and prostate-specific antigen (PSA) reflect increased cellular proliferation. Carcinoembryonic antigen represents dedifferentiation process of cancer. Current genomic and proteomics focus on collective changes in malignant cells.

The clinical value of any given tumor marker will depend on its specificity and sensitivity as well as its intended clinical use. For example, PSA can be used in the screening of prostate cancer, resulting in early detection and treatment. Serum HER2/*neu* is used as marker of prognosis and monitoring therapy for breast cancer. The difference in their usefulness is due to their difference in tissue specificity and cancer sensitivity: PSA is organ-specific but not cancer-specific, whereas HER2/*neu* is cancer-specific but not tissue-specific and is found to be increased in breast cancers, as well as lung and other epithelial cell tumors. The use of tumor markers as prognostic and risk factors has gained more popularity in recent years. Measurement of the level of risk factors has been found to be valuable in the assessment of the aggressiveness of a tumor and is helpful selecting treatment strategies. The utility of tumor markers is adjunctive to medical and surgical management of malignancies, serving to help detect recurrences as well as predict prognosis.

Functional Classification of Tumor Markers

To learn how to identify, select, and utilize tumor markers for the diagnosis of cancer and the management of cancer patients, it is essential to be familiar with the function of each individual or group of cancer serum markers. This chapter emphasizes the role of three specific classes of tumor marker that are commonly used in the diagnosis of human malignancies: (1) oncofetal antigens, such as α-fetoprotein (AFP) and carcinoembryonic antigen (CEA), which are normally expressed during fetal development but do not occur normally in the tissues or sera of children and adults; (2) proteins occurring in epithelial cells that become elevated in tissue and serum in adenosquamous and squamous cell carcinomas, such as the CA 19-9, CA 125, and CA 15-3 proteins; and (3) polypeptide hormones, such as the β chain of human chorionic gonadotropin (β hCG), and specific enzymes, such as the placental isoform of alkaline phosphatase (ALP), that become elevated in the serum of patients with specific tumors. These latter two tumor markers are frequently elevated in the sera of patients with germ cell tumors. Additionally, hormone-like proteins are found in the sera of patients with different cancers, such as parathyroid hormone–like protein that induces hypercalcemia as part of the so-called paraneoplastic syndrome in such cancers as renal cell carcinomas.

Most of these proteins have been discovered on the basis of their having been observed in the sera of cohorts of patients with specific types of cancer. However, many of them are also found in the sera of patients with nonmalignant (e.g., inflammatory) conditions. In addition, they may not occur in significant numbers of patients in whom these cancers have been diagnosed. Thus the sensitivities and specificities of these tumor marker proteins are often low, resulting in their not being useful for screening purposes. On the other hand, all these proteins are quite useful for *monitoring* specific cancers. For example, CEA is often elevated in the sera of patients with colon cancer. Thus if CEA serum levels are found to be elevated in patients who have had a colon cancer resected, this is evidence of tumor recurrence. As discussed later, the one exception is PSA, a chymotrypsin-like enzyme that occurs almost uniquely in the prostate gland and has proved exceptionally useful in screening for prostate cancer and in monitoring patients who are being treated for this disease.

Standard assays for all these proteins are now well-developed and have received approval from the US Food and Drug Administration (FDA) for use in the monitoring of treatment of known cancers but not, except for PSA, for screening for human cancers. Investigations are currently focused on searching for proteins that are expressed only in cancer cells (see

Chapter 74). This chapter summarizes some of the more recently discovered proteins that are almost always expressed in cancerous but less commonly in non-cancerous diseases and are promising for screening for the occurrence of cancer and for monitoring therapy.

ONCOPROTEINS ARE MARKERS FOR CELL PROLIFERATION

Oncoproteins are proteins that are directly or indirectly involved in the control of mitosis and are altered such that they continuously signal the cell to divide. These proteins either lie on signal transduction pathways carrying mitogenic signals from growth factors at the cell membrane to the nucleus, or are involved in the regulation of transcription, activating the genes ultimately causing cell growth and mitosis (see Chapter 74). For example, as discussed in Chapter 74, HER2/Neu is a transmembrane receptor with an extracellular domain (ECD), a transmembrane domain, and an intracytoplasmic domain containing a tyrosine kinase. Upon binding of extracellular growth factors, the intracellular kinase becomes activated, causing dimerization of the receptor and interaction with a cytosolic adapter protein, Grb-2, to relay the message next to a guanine nucleotide exchange factor, SOS. SOS, in turn, binds to the critically important protein Ras-p21 (Barbacid, 1987). Oncogenic c-Myc is an example of a different type of oncogene transcriptional factor, which functions via the activation of its target genes, inducing synthesis of mitogenic proteins.

Often these proteins can be detected in the serum of patients with abnormal cell growth (i.e., cancer or precancerous states). Extensive testing for the presence of oncoproteins has revealed that many oncoproteins are detected in the serum and/or other body fluids of cancer patients. A detailed discussion of each oncoprotein is found in Chapter 74.

TUMOR SUPPRESSORS/CELL DIFFERENTIATION

Separate from oncogenes but equally important is a group of suppressor genes. Proteins encoded by suppressor genes are responsible for suppressing cell growth, either causing cell growth arrest in cell cycle or apoptosis. Frequently, these suppressor genes undergo deletions or mutations, resulting in the production of inactive gene products. Among the tumor suppressor genes, the antioncogene protein p53 has been widely investigated and best characterized for its role in various cancers. It is involved in apoptosis, cell cycle arrest, cell senescence, and DNA damage response. Deletions or mutations of the p53 gene greatly predispose cells to undergoing malignant transformation. p53 mutations have been identified in nearly 50% of human malignancies (Soussi, 2001). Molecular assays are available to detect mutations in the serum DNA of tumor suppressor genes. In addition, antibodies against the abnormal tumor suppressor proteins can be used as a biomarker for cancer.

Molecular methods such as PCR-SSCP (polymerase chain reaction single strand conformation polymorphism) and DHPLC (denaturing high-performance liquid chromatography) have been described to detect serum p53 mutations in cancer. More significantly, antibodies against the abnormal tumor suppressor p53 proteins have been detected in the serum of cancer patients (Soussi, 2000). Interestingly, the presence of p53 antibodies is correlated with the p53 mutation (Guinee, 1995; Hammel, 1999). In breast cancer, several studies indicated that the presence of p53 Ab in the serum correlated with increased proliferation antigen (Ki-67) and lack of ER expression, indicating that it may serve as a breast cancer prognostic marker (Schlichtholz, 1992; Sangrajrang, 2003).

The discovery of two breast cancer susceptibility genes (or tumor-suppressor genes), *BRCA1* and *BRCA2*, have generated tremendous interest. Studies suggest that mutations in *BRCA1* are responsible for approximately half of all cases of inherited breast cancer (Easton, 1993; Miki, 1994; Wooster, 1994). In addition, carriers of *BRCA1* mutations are also at an increased risk for ovarian, colon, and prostate cancer (Futreal, 1994). *BRCA2*, the second susceptibility gene for breast cancer, is thought to account for approximately 70% of cases of inherited breast cancer that are not due to *BRCA1* mutations and is associated with an increased risk of breast cancer in men.

The suppressor genes and their products are potentially useful as tumor markers for the screening and identification of families or high-risk individuals. Development of immunoassays to measure both *BRCA1*- and *BRCA2*-encoded proteins are under development and may be useful for the identification of high-risk individuals and their families.

ADHESION MOLECULES AND METASTASIS

Tumor metastases involve several major steps (Liotta, 1987). First, the tumor cells have to penetrate their adjacent surroundings, after which they invade vascular or lymphatic vessels. The tumor cells are then carried to distant sites, until they are lodged in the venous or capillary beds of a distant organ. In this new environment, these tumor cells must again penetrate the vascular walls in order to grow at the distant site. Cell adhesion molecules, including integrins, selectins, cadherins, and cell adhesion molecules of immunoglobulin gene families, regulate many steps of the metastatic process. The changes in their levels of expression reflect the malignant behavior of cancer cells. For example, increased serum levels of E-selectin, intercellular adhesion molecule (ICAM), and vascular cell adhesion molecule (VCAM) are increased, in particular, in late-stage breast cancer patients (O'Hanlon, 2002; Sheen-Chen, 2004). Elevated serum VCAM level may be used to predict a shorter survival. Another study indicated that postchemotherapeutic levels of serum E-selectin and ICAM are associated with a response to treatment of patients with Hodgkin disease (Syrigos, 2004). Furthermore, increased E-selectin, ICAM-1, and VCAM are suggested to be a prognostic factor for patient survival in patients with gastric cancer (Alexiou, 2003). Therefore the appearance of these cell adhesion molecules in blood circulation might indicate the risk or occurrence of metastases or a poor prognosis.

OTHER MARKERS

Many hormones (e.g., hCG, epinephrine, dopamine, and serotonin), serum proteins, enzymes (lactate dehydrogenase, ALP) and their metabolites, such as the metabolites of the neuroendocrine hormones (e.g., vanillylmandelic acid, homovanillic acid, and 5-hydroxyindoleacetic acid), may become elevated in tumors because of the high proliferation rate of tumor cells. Their serum levels rise to even higher levels when a benign tumor becomes malignant and metastasizes. Benign and nonmalignant diseases may also involve elevated levels of markers, so these markers are not suitable for screening or for cancer diagnosis because of the large numbers of false-positive results that would be generated. These markers are more appropriately used for monitoring patient response during treatment.

One exception relates to the enzyme alkaline phosphatase (ALP) discussed in Chapter 20. There are multiple isozymes of this enzyme, one of which is the placental isozyme placental ALP (PLAP). This form becomes elevated in the serum of patients who have germ cell tumors. One particular use of PLAP is in the serum or, more effectively, in the cerebrospinal fluid (CSF) of patients with a mass in the pineal region with a differential diagnosis of germ cell tumor vs. pinealoma. If PLAP is elevated in the CSF of a patient with a mass in the pineal area, a diagnosis of germ cell tumor can be made. As it happens, radiation therapy is curative, obviating the need for surgery.

The enzymatic activities of various tissue-specific glycosyltransferases are altered in tumor cells. Some of the elevated glycosyltransferases have been used as tumor markers. The sugar sequence and composition of the carbohydrate moiety of many serum glycoproteins, including blood group substances and mucins, such as CA 19-9, are tumor markers resulting from altered glycosyltransferase activity. The AFP isolated from patients with primary hepatocellular carcinoma has an additional fucose compared with the AFP from benign liver disease, an example of altered fucosyltransferase in hepatocellular carcinoma cells (Wu, 1990).

Ectopic proteins are often expressed in cancer. Carcinoembryonic proteins, which are detectable in both fetal and tumor tissues but not in normal adult tissues, usually lack any known physiologic function and have blood concentrations at nanogram-per-milliliter levels. Therefore measurements of carcinoembryonic proteins in the circulation must rely on immunoassays. The specificity and sensitivity associated with these proteins, although not 100%, are much higher than those of enzymes and metabolites that have been used as tumor markers in the past. The serum concentration of these carcinoembryonic proteins not only correlates well with tumor activity but can also be used to predict prognosis. However, carcinoembryonic proteins in general are not suitable for screening for the following reasons. First, the polyclonal antibodies directed against these proteins often cross-react with other, normal proteins, and second, these carcinoembryonic proteins do not appear sufficiently early in the blood from cancer patients to detect the tumors at early stages. However, they have been used as adjunct tests for cancer diagnosis and are extremely useful for monitoring the success of treatment and for detecting recurrence.

MONOCLONAL-ANTIBODY-DEFINED TUMOR MARKERS

The development of hybridoma technology has greatly impacted the identification of tumor markers (Milstein, 1983). Rather than dealing with a whole molecule of known protein structure, it is now possible to focus on only a small surface area, an epitope or antigenic determinant using monoclonal antibodies. It is no longer necessary to purify the antigen for the preparation of polyclonal antibodies in animals. The complete characterization and identification of the molecule carrying the epitope is also no longer needed. A hybridoma can be prepared by injecting a mouse with an enriched fraction of the tumor cell membrane or the whole tumor cell. Hybridomas producing the monoclonal antibodies of interest are selected through the subsequent screening procedure, as described in Section 6. Once a hybridoma is established, there will be an unlimited and consistent supply of monoclonal antibody (MAb) for various uses.

By combining the MAbs with the solid-phase sandwich test design, new assays have been developed that have eliminated many problems associated with polyclonal assays, involving poor reproducibility, lot-to-lot variations, poor specificity, and nonspecific crossreactivity (Diamond, 1981). It also reduces the differences between different kits and widens the linear concentration range for the assay. Whenever an MAb is available, its use is recommended. To achieve higher test sensitivity, the use of a combination of multiple MAbs has been found to improve the affinity between solid-phase-absorbed-multiple MAbs and the soluble antigen.

Tests for the MAb-defined tumor markers have been demonstrated to have a higher sensitivity and specificity than those using polyclonal antibodies. For example, CA 19-9, CA 125, and CA 15-3 are much more sensitive and specific than CEA for pancreatic, ovarian, and breast carcinomas, respectively. These markers are recommended to replace the polyclonal CEA test for the diagnosis and management of patients with the above-mentioned carcinomas. Various tumor markers derived from different tumors also share many tumor-associated epitopes. For example, CA 19-9, CA 15-3, and CA 125 are expressed by almost all carcinomas in varying degrees. In addition to the sharing of any given epitope by more than one carcinoma, it is also possible for a single molecule to express more than one epitope (Yu, 1991). For example, it is likely that CA 15-3 and CA 125 are expressed by the same mucin molecule.

CLINICAL APPLICATIONS

The serum tumor markers are currently used for screening, diagnosing, and predicting prognosis and treatment response. Use of tests for screening of disease, even those with high sensitivity and specificity, should be confined as much as possible to populations at risk for the disease. This is because the positive predictive value depends on the prevalence of the disease. Because most of the tumor markers described in this chapter are expressed both in neoplastic and benign conditions, their use is confined to following possible tumor recurrence in patients being treated for specific types of tumor.

SCREENING

The recommendation of screening for prostate cancer by the measurement of serum PSA in combination with a digital rectal examination (DRE) in men older than age 50 years is due to the high tissue specificity of PSA (Wu, 1994) and the high prevalence of prostate cancer. Combination of the PSA test and DRE provides the least costly approach to the early detection of prostate cancer (Littrup, 1993). PSA screening is especially recommended for African American men because the incidence of prostate cancer for African Americans is nearly twice that of the general population and the death rate is up to three times higher. Screening permits the treatment of organ-confined, potentially curable prostate cancer discovered in men with a life expectancy of longer than 10 years.

Although not approved for screening for hepatocellular carcinoma in the United States, AFP has been used to screen for primary hepatocellular carcinoma in China because of the high incidence of liver cancer in that country. The diagnosis of ovarian cancer has traditionally relied on imaging and discovery at surgery (e.g., exploratory laparotomy). However, in most cases, at the time of detection, the tumor has advanced to a stage at which the possibility of cure is low. The feasibility of screening for ovarian cancer in women by measuring serum CA 125 is being investigated.

DIAGNOSIS

Several approaches have been suggested recently to improve the diagnostic yield of many tumor markers. The use of multiple markers is one approach that has received wide acceptance. As is also noted in Chapter 74, specific patterns of multiple tumor markers seem to be associated with individual malignant diseases. Another approach to improving both the specificity and sensitivity of a tumor markers, as in the case of serum PSA test, involves the measurement of the velocity (the rate of increase in PSA concentration over time) and the density (e.g., by dividing the serum PSA concentration by the volume of the prostate gland, determined by transrectal ultrasound) (Benson, 1992). These efforts aim at a better discrimination between benign and malignant states. For example, a mildly elevated serum PSA level associated with a small prostate gland may indicate cancer, whereas the same PSA value in a patient with a large gland may indicate benign prostatic hypertrophy (BPH).

PROGNOSIS: RECURRENCE, METASTASIS, AND SURVIVAL

The assessment of tumor aggressiveness and the prognosis for the outcome of a cancer patient has received much attention in recent years. The knowledge of tumor aggressiveness helps in the development of a proper therapy for the patient. For example, the detection of tumor markers, highly associated with malignancy and metastases, will suggest a more rigorous and systemic treatment. Monitoring tumor markers for the detection of recurrence following the surgical removal of the tumor is the secondmost useful application of tumor markers. It is well known that the appearance of most of the circulating tumor markers has a lead time of several months (3–6 months) before the stage at which many of the physical procedures could be used for the detection of cancer. The specificity of tumor markers does not present a problem for this application. The ease of drawing blood and the sensitivity of tumor marker tests make this noninvasive monitoring process now widely accepted.

Most tumor markers become increasingly elevated when the tumor metastasizes. Very few tumor markers have a clear-cut boundary between benign and malignant stages. Proteins that reflect the risk factors associated with the process of tumor metastases, such as proteases and adhesion molecules, are usually better markers for predicting prognosis. However, most of these markers are still measured in tumor tissues and tissue lysates. The finding of the ECD of c-*erb*B-2 protein in the serum of cancer patients (Fig. 73-2) and the correlation of the serum ECD with the levels of other

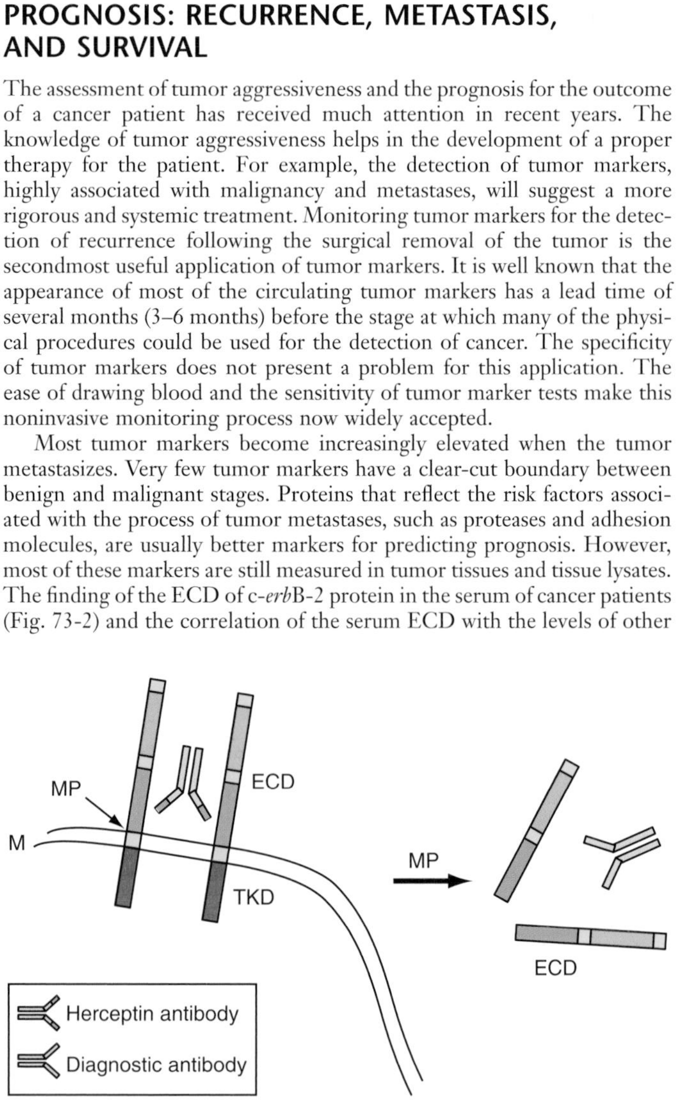

Figure 73-2 HER2/*neu* monoclonal antibodies are used both therapeutically and diagnostically in breast cancer. Humanized HER2 monoclonal antibody trastuzumab (Herceptin), shown with a *dark blue* complementarity determining region (CDR), reacts with a specific region of HER2 epitope (*dark blue*), causes the death of malignant breast cells, and is often effective in the treatment of breast cancer. On the other hand, different monoclonal antibodies, which do not crossreact with the trastuzumab determinant, recognize the extracellular domain (ECD) (*orange-colored* domain in the figure) of HER2/*neu* in serum after it is cleaved off this growth factor receptor by metalloprotease. Because trastuzumab and diagnostic monoclonal antibodies recognize different epitopes of HER2, there is no interference in detecting serum levels of HER2 in trastuzumab-treated patients. *M,* Cell membrane; *MP,* metalloprotease; *TKD,* tyrosine kinase domain

serum tumor markers is encouraging. Another area of intensive study is to explore the use of serum marker surrogates in the prediction of cancer patient survival.

MONITORING TREATMENT RESPONSE

One of the most useful applications of tumor markers involves monitoring the course of the disease, especially during treatment. The serum level of tumor markers reflects the success of surgery or the efficacy of chemotherapy. Detecting elevated levels of a tumor marker after surgery would indicate either incomplete removal of the tumor, recurrence, or the presence of metastases. The measurement of serum tumor markers during chemotherapy also gives an indication of the effectiveness of the antitumor drug used and a guide for the selection of the most effective drug for each individual case.

RECOMMENDATIONS FOR ORDERING TUMOR MARKER TESTS

When ordering tumor markers as an adjunct diagnostic test for managing cancer patients, the following recommendations should be kept in mind in order to avoid misinterpretation of the test results.

1. Never rely on the result of a single test. Because of low specificity associated with most tumor markers, it is difficult to differentiate between malignant and benign diseases on the basis of the result of a single test result. Most tumor marker elevations found in nonmalignant diseases may be transient, whereas with cancer the level often either remains elevated or rises continuously. Ordering serial testing can help detect falsely elevated levels due to transient elevation. For example, elevated serum AFP can be detected in patients with either primary hepatocellular carcinoma or benign liver disease. However, on a subsequent testing 2 weeks later, the serum AFP will remain elevated in patients with cancer, whereas in patients with benign conditions the serum AFP may return to normal levels.
2. When ordering serial testing, be certain to order every test from the same laboratory using the same assay kit. Each different commercial kit may generate different results even though all are designed for the same tumor marker. Ordering from the same laboratory also ensures a more consistent performance. It is important to ensure that any change observed during the monitoring process is due to a change of tumor volume or other tumor activities and not to laboratory variability.
3. Be certain that the tumor marker selected for monitoring recurrence was elevated in the patient before surgery. Because none of the tumor markers are 100% sensitive to the detection of any particular cancer, it is important to be certain that the tumor marker ordered to detect recurrence was elevated before surgery. Otherwise, multiple markers should be measured before the surgery in order to select the tumor marker showing the highest elevation as the marker for monitoring the disease activity. Multiple markers may be used to monitor the therapeutic effects for increased sensitivity.
4. Consider the half-life of the tumor marker when interpreting the test result. Before surgery, estimate the time required for the level to decline to the normal or, in the case of PSA, to an undetectable level, based on the known half-life of the tumor marker. It is important that the success of surgical removal of a tumor as determined by tumor marker concentrations is not assessed earlier than 2 weeks postoperatively. If possible, it is preferable to wait one whole month to allow the preexisting tumor marker in the serum adequate time to decline to lower levels. For example, the half-life of serum PSA is approximately 3–4 days. Therefore it takes 30 days for a serum PSA at 50 ng/mL to drop to an undetectable level following successful surgery.
5. Consider how the tumor marker is removed from or metabolized in the blood circulation. Elevated serum tumor markers are frequently detected in patients with renal or liver disease, depending on whether the tumor marker is removed through the kidney or metabolized by the liver. For example, serum CEA is often elevated in patients with liver disease because the impaired liver fails to remove CEA efficiently from the blood circulation, whereas an elevated serum β_2-microglobulin (β_2M) has been frequently found in patients with renal failure in which even the small β_2M molecule has difficulty passing through the glomerular membrane in a normal fashion.

TABLE 73-1
Monoclonal-Antibody-Defined Tumor Markers

Tumor marker	Major malignant disease
CA125	Ovarian carcinoma
CA19-9	Pancreatic carcinoma
CA15-3	Breast carcinoma
CA72-4	Gastric carcinoma
HER2/*neu*	Breast carcinoma

6. Consider ordering multiple markers to improve both the sensitivity and the specificity for diagnosis. Tumors are made of heterogeneous types of cells. Some may still be normal while others may be heterogeneous tumor cells as a result of different sequences of multiple mutations. Each type of cell may express a single marker, such as those shown in Table 73-1, or a number of characteristic tumor markers. The same marker may also be produced by different types of cells. Some cells may never produce any unique marker. Certain types of cancer are heterogeneous in their cellular composition. Consequently, more than one tumor marker may be required to provide a high sensitivity of detection. The heterogeneity in cell composition and the percentage cell distribution of each tumor explains why a number of tumor markers may be required to reach a high (>90%) detection sensitivity and the reason that the sensitivity of an individual marker differs among cancer patients. Multiple tumor markers associated with individual malignant diseases are listed in Table 73-2; the appearance of individual tumor markers in various malignancies is listed in Table 73-3. This explains why none of the tumor markers presently employed are 100% sensitive and specific, and why the use of multiple markers will improve the sensitivity of detection. However, a unique pattern of multiple markers may be identified with tumors derived from the same tissues. Therefore ordering multiple tumor markers may also improve the test specificity. For example, a specific pattern seems to be associated with colon, breast, ovarian, and pancreatic carcinomas when all four MAb-defined tumor markers—CEA, CA 19-9, CA 15-3, and CA 125—are measured simultaneously. This information is clinically important, because more than 60% of diagnosed human cancers are epithelial-cell-derived carcinomas (Wu, 1989). Multiple markers were used to develop a more specific screening strategy for ovarian cancer. The use of CA 15-3 and CA72-4 in combination with CA 125 can increase the apparent specificity of the CA 125 assay for distinguishing malignant from benign ovarian disease (Bast, 1991). Another example is the combination of CEA, CA19-9, and CA72-4. Use of this combination improves the diagnostic accuracy of gastrointestinal cancers (Carpelan-Holmstrom, 2002). During the selection of multiple tumor markers, only markers that are complementary to each other should be selected. Many tumor markers, which run parallel to each other when correlated with tumor activities, should not be selected for this purpose.
7. Be aware of the presence of ectopic tumor markers. The expression of tumor markers is under genetic regulation. For benign tumors, there are often proteins produced by the tumor that are cell-specific and are related to normal cell products at an elevated concentration (see Fig. 73-1). However, if a benign tumor becomes malignant, synthesis of these cell-specific proteins may no longer occur in the malignant cells. Conversely, proteins that are normally found at an early fetal stage and not in normal cells or in benign tumors of these cells may become constitutively expressed in the malignant cells. This is the reason that carcinoembryonic proteins and ectopic tumor markers are usually expressed in malignant cancers, often at advanced stages. Thus, often, the appearance of ectopic tumor markers is associated with poor prognosis or metastasis. For example, elevated serum concentrations of AFP may be detected in patients with cancers of the gastrointestinal tract involving metastases even though the liver function tests are normal. Table 73-4 lists some of the known ectopic markers and their associated malignant diseases.

One should be aware of the recent guidelines on gastrointestinal and breast cancer marker use published by the American Society of Clinical Oncology (Smith, 1999). They recommend monthly breast self-examination, annual mammography of the preserved and contralateral breast, and a careful history and physical examination every 3–6 months for 3 years, then every 6–12 months for 2 years, and

PART 9

TABLE 73-2
Serologic Tumor Markers Associated with Individual Malignant Diseases

Malignant disease	Major marker	Other markers
Neuronal Tumors		
Brain tumor	Desmosterol	Polyamines
Neuroblastoma	VMA	HVA, NSE, cystathionine, ferritin, metanephrines
Head and Neck Tumors		
Squamous cell carcinoma	CYFRA 21-1	
Endocrine System		
Pituitary tumors	Growth hormone	IGF-I
Adrenal pituitary tumors	Cortisol	Free catecholamines, DHEA, 17-ketosteroids, prolactin
Cushing syndrome	ACTH	Endorphin, lipotropin
Hypercalcemia of malignancy	PTH-related peptide	
Endocrine pancreatic tumors:	Pancreatic polypeptide:	Chromogranin AC-peptide, IGF-I binding protein I
Gastrinoma	Gastrin	
Glucagonoma	Glucagon	
Insulinoma	Insulin	
Medullary carcinoma of thyroid	Calcitonin	NSE
Microadenomas (pituitary)	Prolactin	
Multiple endocrine neoplasias	Chromogranin A	
Papillary and follicular thyroid cancer	Thyroglobulin	
Parathyroid tumors	PTH-intact	
Zollinger–Ellison syndrome	Gastrin	
Pheochromocytoma	Metanephrine	Chromogranin A, plasma catecholamines
Pituitary tumors	Free β hCG	FSH, LH, prolactin, TSH
Bone and Skeletal Muscle System		
Osteosarcomas	Alkaline phosphatase	
Breast Cancer		
Breast cancer	HER2/*neu*, CA 15-3	CYFRA 21-1, CEA, calcitonin
Pulmonary System		
Bronchogenic carcinoma	Prolactin	
Lung cancer (NSC)	CYFRA 21-1, NSE	ACTH, CK-BB, calcitonin, CA 72-4, CEA, AFP, Ferritin, LASA-P, TPA
Carcinoid tumors	Histamine, ADH, bradykinin	
Oat cell cancer	ACTH, ADH, CEA, CK-BB, NSE, bombesin, calcitonin	
Gastrointestinal System		
Colorectal cancer	CEA	CA 19-5, CA 19-9, CA 72-4, NSE
Gastric carcinoma	CA 72-4	CA 19-9, CA 50, CEA, ferritin, CK-BB, hCG, LASA-P, pepsinogen II
Hepatocellular carcinoma	AFP	CEA, ferritin, ALP, TPA, γ-glutamyltranspeptidase (GGT)
Pancreatic carcinoma	CA 19-9	CA 19-5, CA 50, CA 72-4, CEA, CK-BB, ADH, ALP
Vipoma (pancreas)	VIP	
Genitourinary System		
Bladder cancer	T-antigen, urokinase inhibitor, TPA, cytokeratins	Glycosaminoglycans, uroplakins
Nonseminomatous testicular tumor	AFP	hCG
Prostate carcinoma	PSA	PAP, racemase
Renal cell carcinoma	Renin, erythropoietin, IL-4, PGA	
Testicular cancer	hCG	PLAP, Oct3/4
Gynecological Tumors		
Cervical cancer	SCC	CA 125, CEA, TPA
Ovarian carcinoma	CA 125	UGF, inhibin, AFP, amylase isoenzyme, CEA, CK-BB, hCG
Choriocarcinoma	hCG	
Placental tumors	hCG	Free α hCG, CA 15-3, PTH, NSE, prolactin
Uterine cancer	SCC	
Teratoblastoma	AFP	hCG, ferritin
Hematology Malignancies and Lymphomas		
B-cell chronic lymphocytic leukemia	TdT	Serum β_2M, LASA-P
B-cell malignancies	β_2M	
Multiple Myeloma	Bence-Jones protein	β_2M
Chronic myelogenous leukemia	TdT	
Hairy cell leukemia	IL-2 receptor	
Hodgkin disease	LASA-P, ferritin	
Leukemia	TdT	ALP, β_2M, ferritin, LD, myelin basic protein, adenosine deaminase, PNP

TABLE 73-2
Serologic Tumor Markers Associated with Individual Malignant Diseases—*Cont'd*

Malignant disease	Major marker	Other markers
Lymphoma	β_2M	TdT, Ki-67, LASA-P
Multiple myeloma	Ig heavy and light chain	Bence-Jones protein, β_2M, IgA
Waldenström's disease	IgM	β_2M
Melanoma		
Melanoma antigen	Melanoma-associated LASA-P, L-dopa	C-reactive protein
Endoreticular System		
Spleen tumors	Ferritin	
Other		
Sarcoma	β_2M	

ACTH, Adrenocorticotropic hormone; *ADH*, antidiuretic hormone; *AFP*, α-fetoprotein; *ALP*, alkaline phosphatase; *β_2M*, β_2-microglobulin; *CEA*, carcinoembryonic antigen; *CK-BB*, brain isozyme of creatine phosphokinase; *CYFRA 21-1*, cytokeratin subunit 19; *DHEA*, dihydroepiandrosterone; *FSH*, follicle-stimulating hormone; *hCG*, human chorionic gonadotropin; *HVA*, homovanillic acid; *Ig*, immunoglobulin; *IGF*, insulin-like growth factor; *IL*, interleukin; *ki67*, cell proliferation marker; *LASA-P*, lipid-associated sialic acid in plasma; *LD*, lactate dehydrogenase; *LH*, luteinizing hormone; *NSC*, nonsmall cell; *NSE*, neuron-specific enolase; *Oct3/4*, transcription factor in stem cells and germ cells required for pluripotency; *PAP*, prostate acid phosphatase; *PGA*, prostaglandin A; *PLAP*, placental alkaline phosphatase; *PNP*, purine nucleotide phosphorylase; *PTH*, parathyroid hormone; *SCC*, squamous cell carcinoma; *TdT*, terminal deoxynucleotide transferase; *TPA*, tissue plasminogen activator; *TSH*, thyroid-stimulating hormone; *UGF*, uterine growth factor; *VIP*, vasoactive intestinal polypeptide; *VMA*, vanillylmandelic acid.

TABLE 73-3
Malignant Disease Associated with Individual Serologic Tumor Markers

	ASSOCIATED MALIGNANT DISEASE	
Tumor marker	**Major disease**	**Minor disease**
α-Fetoprotein	Primary hepatocellular carcinoma	Teratoblastomas of the ovary and testes
β hCG	Pituitary tumors	
β_2-Microglobulin	B-cell neoplasias	Multiple myeloma, B-cell lymphoma, B-cell chronic lymphocytic leukemia and reticulum cell, sarcoma; Waldenström's macroglobulinemia
β hCG	Choriocarcinoma	Testicular cancers (nonseminomatous), trophoblastic tumors
Bence-Jones protein	Multiple myeloma	
Bombesin	Oat-cell cancer	
C-reactive protein	Melanoma	
CA 15-3	Breast cancer	Various carcinomas
CA 19-9	Pancreatic and gastric carcinoma	Various carcinomas
CA 72-4	Gastric carcinoma	Various carcinomas
CA 125	Ovarian carcinoma	Various carcinomas
CA 549	Breast cancer	
CA M26	Breast cancer	
Calcitonin	Medullary carcinoma	Cancer of the thyroid, liver cancer, renal cancer
Carcinoembryonic antigen	Colorectal carcinoma	Various carcinomas
c-*erb*B-2 oncoprotein	Breast carcinoma	Various carcinomas
Chromogranin A	Pheochromocytoma, neuroblastoma	Multiple endocrine neoplasias, small cell lung cancer, carcinoid tumors
CYFRA 21-1	Squamous cell carcinoma of the lung	
DHEA	Adrenal/pituitary cancer	
Ferritin	Acute myelocytic leukemia	Hodgkin lymphoma, neuroblastoma and various carcinomas, teratoblastoma
Galactosyltransferase	Ovarian cancer	
Galactosyltransferase isoenzyme II	Pancreatic cancer	
Gastrin	Gastrinoma	Zollinger-Ellison syndrome
Her2/*neu*	See c-*erb*B-2 oncoprotein	
Human chorionic gonadotropin	Choriocarcinoma	Gastric, ovarian, and breast carcinoma, trophoblastic or germ cell tumors, testicular cancer
Hyaluronic acid	Mesothelioma	
Immunoglobulin A	Multiple myeloma	
Insulin-like growth factor-I	Pituitary cancer	Insulinoma
Interleukin-2 receptor	Leukemia	
Immunoglobulins	Multiple myeloma	Mediterranean lymphoma, Waldenström's macroglobulinemia, malignant lymphoma
Inhibin	Granulosa-cell tumors	
17-ketosteroids	Adrenal/pituitary cancer	

β hCG, β chain of human chorionic gonadotropin; *CYFRA 21-1*, cytokeratin subunit 19; *DHEA*, dihydroepiandrosterone; *hCG*, human chorionic gonadotropin.

PART 9

TABLE 73-4
Ectopic Tumor Markers

Marker	Tumor
α-Fetoprotein	Gastrointestinal, renal, bladder, and ovarian carcinoma
Calcitonin	Endocrine tumors (islet cell, carcinoid, medullary thyroid, pheochromocytoma); lung, breast, and ovary carcinoma
Chromogranin A	Endocrine tumors (islet cell, carcinoid, medullary thyroid, pheochromocytoma), prostate cancer
Free α hCG	Colorectal carcinoma and pancreatic endocrine tumors
hCG	Gastric and pancreatic carcinoma, hepatoma, ovarian carcinoma, germ cell tumor of testis
PTH	Renal cell carcinoma; breast; squamous cell carcinoma; bladder and ovarian carcinomas
Thyroglobulin	Differentiated thyroid carcinoma

hCG, Human chorionic gonadotropin; *PTH,* parathyroid hormone.

annually thereafter. They do not recommend the use of tumor markers (e.g., CEA, CA 15-3, and CA 27.29) for screening, nor do they recommended routine bone scans, chest radiographs, hematologic blood counts, liver ultrasonograms, or computed tomography for screening. The American College of Physicians has also published clinical guidelines concerning the early detection of prostate cancer. They emphasize the importance of both screening PSA and performing DRE for the early detection of prostate cancer. Even though DRE is not as sensitive as PSA screening, it can detect cancer that would otherwise be missed by PSA measurement (Coley, 1997a, 1997b).

8. Heterophilic antibody. The use of MAbs in immunoassays and the increasing clinical application of mouse MAbs for targeted imaging and immunotherapy create a new problem. Treated individuals apparently produce heterophilic antibodies against murine antibodies that interfere with many of the immunoassays for tumor markers (Nahm, 1990) although this is not a common encounter. The interference by the heterophilic antibodies in human sera can either increase or decrease the results of an immunoassay. These antibodies react in a way similar to antigens in terms of binding to both solid-phase-associated and signal-labeled antibodies. These heterophilic antibodies may bind to a site other than the analyte-binding site, crosslinking the signal antibody with the capture antibody, and thus generating a false assay response. As many as 15%–40% of individuals may have one or more heterophilic antibodies. The standard approach for reducing heterophilic antibody interference is to include in the assay excess mouse sera or nonspecific mouse immunoglobulins in the immunoassay.

Individual Tumor Markers

α-FETOPROTEIN

AFP is a major fetal serum protein and is also one of the major carcinoembryonic proteins. AFP resembles albumin in many physical and chemical properties. In the fetus, AFP is synthesized by the yolk sac and fetal hepatocytes and to a lesser extent by the fetal gastrointestinal tract and kidneys. Elevated AFP can be found in patients with primary hepatocellular carcinoma and yolk sac–derived germ cell tumors (mainly endodermal sinus tumor) and is the most useful serum marker for these cancers (Lamerz, 1997). However, AFP is also transiently elevated during pregnancy and in many benign liver diseases. Because of the high prevalence of liver cancer in China and other countries in Southeast Asia, AFP testing has been used successfully in screening for hepatocellular carcinoma in that region of the world. Tests for both AFP and hCG are helpful in reducing clinical staging errors in patients with some testicular tumors and aid in the differential diagnosis of various germ cell tumors. Because an increase of fucosylation of AFP (hence the lentil lectin reactivity of serum AFP) has been found in primary hepatocellular carcinoma, the determination of lentil lectin reactivity of serum AFP was found helpful not only to differentiate between primary hepatocellular carcinoma and benign liver diseases but also to provide an early signal indicating that hepatocellular carcinoma may begin to develop in patients with liver disease. Although the necessity for routine AFP screening needs further study, one study indicates that combined screening with AFP and ultrasonography results in increased sensitivity from 75% to near 100% in detecting hepatocellular carcinoma (hCC) of patients with hepatitis B and C (Izzo, 1998; Gebo, 2002). Lastly, AFP is currently offered for prenatal screening for neural tube defects and, in conjunction with free β hCG and unconjugated estriol, for Down syndrome (Cuckle, 2000; Yamamoto, 2001).

ANGIOGENIC FACTORS

Angiogenesis is the formation of blood vessels in situ, involving the orderly migration, proliferation, and differentiation of vascular cells. Blood vessel formation is also important in the pathogenesis of rapid growth and metastasis of solid tumors. Several angiogenic factors have been identified including acidic and basic fibroblast growth factor (bFGF), described in Chapter 74, angiogenin and vascular endothelial growth factor (VEGF) (Folkman, 1992). Both angiogenic and antiangiogenic factors have been found in the serum of patients with malignant disease (Morelli, 1998). Serum levels of bFGF and VEGF reflect their expression in individual tumors (Poon, 2003; Granato, 2004). The significance of elevated serum VEGF in cancer patients has been evaluated in several studies including breast, ovarian, hepatocellular, colorectal, and renal cell carcinomas and soft tissue sarcoma. Elevated serum VEGF values in ovarian cancer patients were correlated with cancer differentiation, metastasis, and, more significantly, shorter average survival time (Alvarez Secord, 2004; Harlozinska, 2004; Li, 2004). Furthermore, elevated serum VEGF has been associated with shorter survival in renal cell carcinoma (Ljungberg, 2003) and colon carcinoma (De Vita, 2004).

β_2-MICROGLOBULIN

β_2M is the constant light chain of the human histocompatibility locus antigen expressed on the surface of most nucleated cells. The molecular weight of β_2M is only 11.8 kDa. β_2M is shed into the extracellular fluid and is elevated not only in solid tumors but also in lymphoproliferative diseases (including B-cell chronic lymphocytic leukemia, non-Hodgkin lymphoma, and, importantly, multiple myeloma) (Wu, 1986). Serum concentration of β_2M correlates with lymphocyte activity, making β_2M a good marker for lymphoid malignancies of the B-cell line. It has been used as an indicator of the patient's response to treatment (Haferlach, 1997). CSF levels of β_2M are useful for detecting metastases in the central nervous system. It is reported that serum β_2M level is elevated in 75% of patients with multiple myeloma (Kyle, 2003) and is useful in following the efficacy of the treatment of this disease although currently serum free light chain assay has been found to be more effective in following this disease (see Chapter 46).

CARCINOEMBRYONIC ANTIGEN

CEA is a glycoprotein with a molecular weight of approximately 200 kDa. It is the first of the so-called carcinoembryonic proteins and was discovered by Gold and Freedman in 1965 (Gold, 1965). CEA is still the most widely used tumor marker for gastrointestinal cancer, but most CEA assays have replaced polyclonal with monoclonal anti-CEA antibodies.

CEA was originally thought to be a specific marker for colorectal cancer but turned out to be a nonspecific marker on further studies. CEA levels can be elevated in breast, lung, and liver cancers, among others. CEA studies demonstrated that tumor markers could be used to follow patients during therapy and to detect recurrence after successful surgery. The association between highly elevated serum tumor marker concentration and metastases and poor prognosis was also discovered through CEA studies. Elevated CEA levels before resection of colon cancer may suggest a worse prognosis. Declining levels during therapy suggests response to therapy, whereas increasing levels suggest disease progression. However, clinical decisions regarding management of disease cannot be based on CEA levels alone (Mitchell, 1998). As the liver metabolizes CEA, liver damage can impair CEA clearance and lead to increased levels in the blood circulation. Increased CEA concentrations have been observed in some patients following radiation treatment and chemotherapy. It was recommended that CEA should form part of the American Joint Committee on Cancer staging system (Compton, 2000). CEA can be used as a marker for monitoring colorectal cancer (Bast, 2001). However, a low positive predictive value for diagnosis in asymptomatic patients limits its widespread use in screening.

Other genetic tumor markers are becoming used with increased frequency. For example, transforming growth factor–α, fibroblast growth factor, and Ras oncoprotein are all increased in colorectal cancer and decreased after surgical resection. More recently, mutations of DNA mismatch repair genes (e.g., *hMSH2*, *hMLH1*, and *hMSH6*) are shown to be associated with hereditary nonpolyposis colorectal cancer. Further clinical studies to correlate the serum levels of expression and mutation in these genes might yield a better diagnostic/prognostic tool.

CA 15-3 AND CA 27.29

These antigens correspond to sequences of mucins called polymorphic epithelial mucins (PEMs), which are often overexpressed on the cell surfaces of malignant glandular cells such as occur in breast cancer, and increasing amounts are shed into the circulation where they can be detected, making them useful as tumor markers. The polypeptide core of PEM contains a 69-amino acid cytoplasmic domain and a much larger ECD, consisting of 20 amino acid tandem repeats that vary between individuals, and different alleles of the human *MUC1* gene may code for between 25 and 100 or more tandem repeats. A large part of the molecule is carbohydrate and the degree of glycosylation is variable, making PEM a very heterogeneous in structure (Klee, 2004).

The CA 15-3 determinant is identified by two distinct monoclonal antibodies. The assay uses a solid-phase conjugated MAb, MAb 115D8, to capture the MAM-6 antigen in human plasma, and a labeled MAb DF3 as detecting antibody. MAb 115D8 was prepared against human defatted milk fat globule and MAb DF3 was prepared against the breast carcinoma cell line MCF-7. The CA 15-3 antigen is present in a variety of adenocarcinomas including breast, colon, lung, ovary, and pancreas.

CA 15-3 is a more sensitive and specific marker for monitoring the clinical course of patients with metastatic breast cancer (Canizares, 2001). CA 15-3 levels increase with higher stages of breast cancer stage (Bast, 2001). In addition, CA 15-3 can be used to predict adverse outcomes in breast cancer patients (Gion, 2002; Kumpulainen, 2002; Duffy, 2004). However, the relative low sensitivity (23%) and specificity (69%) (Chan, 2001) in detecting breast cancer has limited its use. CA 15-3 can also be elevated in chronic hepatitis, liver cirrhosis, sarcoidosis, tuberculosis, and systemic lupus erythematosus, and in patients who smoke (Tondini, 1988). CA 27.29, another mucin marker MUC1-associated antigen, is a slightly more sensitive breast cancer marker than CA 15.3. The FDA has approved both CA 15-3 and CA 27.29 for monitoring therapy of advanced or recurrent breast cancer.

CA 19-9, CA 50, AND CA 19-5

CA 19-9 is the first tumor marker of a group of newer epitopes, including CA 125, CA 15-3, and CEA, defined by monoclonal antibodies. These new monoclonal kits detect more newly discovered epitopes and were designed to replace polyclonal CEA measurements for various carcinomas. The assay for CA 19-9 measures a carbohydrate antigenic determinant expressed on a high molecular weight mucin. CA 19-9 is an epitope, defined as sialylated lacto-*N*-fucopentose II, recognized by the MAb 1116NS-199. The molecule, carrying the CA 19-9 epitope, appears as mucin in the sera of cancer patients but as a ganglioside in tumor cells. CA 19-9 is also related to Lewis blood group substances. Only serum antigen from cancer patients belonging to the Le (a^-b^+) or Le (a^+b^-) blood group will be CA 19-9-positive. In addition to CA 19-9, CA 19-5 and CA50 have also been defined by monoclonal antibodies that are only slightly different from CA 19-9. CA 19-9 can be elevated in patients with colorectal cancer, gastric cancer, and pancreatic cancer. The epitope related to CA 50 is very similar to that of CA 19-9 but lacks a fucose residue, the same epitope found in Lewis-negative Le (a^-b^-) individuals. Serum CA 19-9 concentrations not only are frequently highly elevated in both gastric and pancreatic carcinomas but also are useful for monitoring the success of therapy and for detecting recurrence in these cancer patients. However, it has been reported that CA 19-9 and CA 50 complement each other in pancreatic and other carcinomas: their simultaneous use may improve the sensitivity in detecting these malignant diseases. CA 19-5 is detected by mouse MAb CC3C-195 and reacts with both Le^a and sialyl-Le^a epitopes. CC3C-195 binds with high affinity to the sialylated Le^a blood group antigen but exhibits a lower affinity to the nonsialylated form. Elevated serum levels of CA 50 and CA 19-5 can also be found in patients with colon, pancreatic, and hepatocellular carcinomas. False-positive findings may occur in patients with benign liver disease and may be due to cholestasis in these patients (Wu, 1992).

CA 125

CA 125 is another antigenic determinant defined by a MAb and is also associated with a high-molecular-weight (>200 kDa) mucin-like glycoprotein. CA 125 is expressed by more than 80% of nonmucinous epithelial ovarian carcinomas and is found in most serous, endometrioid, and clear cell carcinomas of the ovary (Jacobs, 1989). However, patients undergoing chemotherapy may show a false decline of CA 125 antigen and a negative result does not always rule out tumor recurrence. CA 125 is also used clinically for follow-up on uterine tumors (>60% are elevated) and benign tumors, including endometriosis. Recent studies showed greatly improved sensitivity of serum CA 125 in combination with other markers using proteomics techniques (discussed in detail in succeeding chapters) (Jacobs, 2004; Lu, 2004; Zhang, 2004). Studies for the application of serum CA 125 in other cancerous (e.g., non-Hodgkin lymphoma, lung cancer) and nonmalignant (e.g., liver cirrhosis) diseases have been performed (Ando, 2003; Xiao, 2003; Zidan, 2004) and showed increased levels of CA 125 in the sera of these patients.

CA 72-4

The CA 72-4 assay detects a mucin-like human adenocarcinoma-associated antigen, TAG-72, which is a high molecular weight (>10^6 kDa) mucin-like complex molecule. Because the TAG-72 can be detected in both fetal epithelia and sera from patients with various carcinomas, it is also considered to be a carcinoembryonic protein. However, only moderately elevated serum CA 72-4 are found in most carcinomas. Currently, CA 72-4 is considered to be useful marker for the management of patients with gastric and colorectal carcinoma. CA 72-4 has been proposed as a specific marker for tumor occurrence of resectable gastric cancer (Marrelli, 2001) and a prognostic marker for survival (Gaspar, 2001). CA 72-4 has been reported to be an independent prognostic marker for survival in colorectal cancer (Louhimo, 2002) in multivariate analysis together with β hCG and CEA.

CALCITONIN

Calcitonin is one of the circulating peptide hormones that may become elevated in patients with increased bone turnover rate associated with skeletal metastases. Calcitonin can be ectopically elevated in bronchogenic carcinomas and is also elevated in medullary carcinoma of the thyroid (see Table 73-4).

CHROMOGRANIN A

Chromogranin A is a major soluble protein of the chromaffin granule. Chromogranin A and catecholamines are released from the adrenal medulla upon stimulation of the splanchnic nerve. However, chromogranin A is not confined to chromaffin cells of the adrenal medulla and sympathetic neurons. It is also present in various neuroendocrine organs. Elevated serum chromogranin A levels can be detected in pheochromocytoma (Giovanella, 2002), medullary carcinoma of thyroid, and small cell lung carcinoma (Ma, 2003). Interestingly, increased serum chromogranin A levels are detected in epithelial cancers with neuroendocrine differentiation, including prostate, breast, ovary, pancreas, and colon (Wu, 2000).

Prostate cancer with neuroendocrine differentiation has been an active area of study. Higher levels of serum chromogranin A is associated with poorly differentiated prostate cancer (Isshiki, 2002). It is also increased after androgen blockade therapy and systemic radionucleotide therapy (Ferrero-Pous, 2001) for prostate cancer. Furthermore, an association between increased chromogranin A and prostate cancer metastasis has been observed (Tarle, 2002). Intermittent androgen deprivation therapy can reduce the levels of chromogranin A, and thus the neuroendocrine differentiation of prostate cancer (Sciarra, 2003).

CYTOKERATIN 19 FRAGMENT

Cytokeratin 19 fragment (CYFRA 21-1) is a fragment of the cytokeratin 19 intermediate filament found in the serum. It is a subunit of a cytokeratin intermediate filament expressed in simple epithelia and their malignant counterparts. Studies of elevated serum CYFRA 21-1 have concentrated on breast cancer and squamous cell carcinoma of the lung. CYFRA 21-1 was reported to have a sensitivity of 60%, 64.2%, and 89% for the detection of stage IV breast cancer, recurrence, and metastasis, respectively. Probability of survival for primary cancer patients, recurrence after surgery and response after chemotherapy were correlated with elevated preoperative serum CYFRA 21-1 in breast cancer patients (Nakata, 2000, 2004). CYFRA 21-1 was also shown to reflect the tumor mass in multiple studies with correlation to tumor stage, survival, predictive role in surgical treatment for early stage disease and chemotherapy for advanced stage non–small cell lung cancer (NSCLC). In one study of head and neck squamous cell carcinoma (SCC), increased postradiotherapeutic or chemotherapeutic CYFRA 21-1 has been explored as an early indicator for distant metastasis (Kuropkat, 2002). CYFRA 21-1 is not increased in patients with nonneoplastic lung disease including pneumoconiosis and obstructive airway disease (Schneider, 2003).

HUMAN CHORIONIC GONADOTROPIN

hCG, a member of the glycoprotein hormone family, is synthesized and secreted by trophoblast cells of the placenta and is a heterodimeric hormone composed of noncovalently linked α and β subunits internally linked by disulfide bonds. The current assays using monoclonal antibodies are available to detect intact hCG, "nicked" hCG or hCGn (which is partially degraded hCG missing peptide bonds between amino acids 44 and 45 or 47 and 48), hCG α subunit, hCG β subunit and hCG β core (residual hCG β, residues 6–40 joined by disulfide bond to hCG β, residues 55–92) (Berger, 2002, Birken, 2003). Both malignant and nonmalignant trophoblast cells synthesize and secrete not only the biologically active α and β dimer but also the uncombined (or free) α and β subunits. In addition to the intact dimer, a free β subunit of hCG has been detected in the serum of women during early pregnancy and in patients with malignant tumors (see Chapter 25).

Measurement of the free β subunit is useful for the detection of recurrence or metastasis for choriocarcinoma when the intact hCG may remain normal. Analysis of serum hCG subunits is especially useful for managing patients with germ cell tumors (von Eyben, 2003). However, elevated hCG can be found in trophoblastic tumors, choriocarcinoma, and testicular tumors. More than 60% of patients with nonseminomatous germ cell tumors and 10%–30% with seminomas have elevated free β hCG.

Seminomatous testicular cancer contains both intact hCG and β hCG or free α subunits in equal amounts. Therefore only one assay is needed for monitoring these patients. On the other hand, only hCG or β hCG subunits may be found in patients with nonseminomatous cancers. The measurement of both free subunits and intact hCG will increase the test sensitivity for these patients with nonseminomatous cancers.

Ectopic free β hCG production occurs in approximately 30% of patients with other cancers including urothelial cancer, but only the free β hCG and its respective breakdown product, β core, has been detected in these clinical samples. Ectopic α hCG is a marker of malignancy in pancreatic endocrine tumors (Ma, 2003). Recent efforts in preparation of new World Health Organization reference reagent for hCG (HCG, hCG-α, and hCG-β) and its related molecules may decrease the nonspecific reaction and increased accuracy of clinical hCG testing (Bristow, 2005).

HER2/*neu* (c-*erb*B-2) ONCOPROTEIN

The HER2/*neu* (c-*erb*B-2) oncogene is a 185-kDa transmembrane protein of the tyrosine kinase receptor family and is discussed extensively in Chapter 74. It shows structural and functional homology with the epidermal growth factor receptor (EGFR) containing intracellular, transmembrane, and ECDs (see Fig. 73-2). HER2/*neu* has been found to be elevated in the sera of patients with a number of different epithelial cell cancers, including breast cancer (Mori, 1990; Leitzel, 1992; Ali, 2002; Tsigris, 2002). In patients with breast cancer, serum HER2/*neu* is very important as a prognostic and predictive marker. At the time of initial diagnosis, serum HER2/*neu* is elevated in only 5%–10% of breast cancer patients. Increased serum HER2/*neu* before adjuvant therapy has been shown to be associated with increased tumor size, tumor grade, and positive lymph nodes. The serum HER2/*neu* test is indicated for follow-up and monitoring of patients with metastatic breast cancer whose initial serum HER2/*neu* level is greater than 15 ng/mL. Schippinger and colleagues reported that decrease of elevated Serum HER2/*neu* to levels below 15 ng/mL and levels continuously ≤15 ng/mL during the course of disease correlated significantly with longer survival (Schippinger, 2004). The serum HER2 level as assessed by the chemiluminescence immunoassay method is the most sensitive marker of HER2-positive metastatic breast cancer compared with the CEA and CA15-3 levels (Kan, 2009). Prechemotherapy and postchemotherapy HER2/*neu* levels could serve as a prognostic marker for disease-free survival and overall survival (Hayes, 2001; Saghatchian, 2004). In addition, serum HER2/*neu* levels correlate with response to chemotherapy, including chemo- and hormonal- as well as Herceptin (Trastuzumab) treatment; higher levels predict incomplete response while low levels suggest longer or complete treatment responses (Colomer, 2000; Harris, 2001; Lipton, 2002; Bethune-Volters, 2004; Luftner, 2004).

Enzyme-linked immunosorbent assay (ELISA) measures the levels of the circulating c-*erb*B-2, referred to as p105 or serum HER2, constituting the ectodomain (see Fig. 73-2). There are currently three FDA-approved ELISA assays for serum circulating HER2 using monoclonal antibodies, one for microtiter plate assay (Oncogene Science/Siemens) and two for automated instrument, BAYER IMMUNO 1 HER2/neu ASSAY (Siemens) and ADVIA Centaur Her2/Neu immunoassay (Siemens). The ADVIA Centaur Her2/Neu immunoassay kit is similar to the Bayer/Siemens Immuno 1 Her2/Neu kit in indication for use, format, performance characteristics and results. The ADVIA differs mainly in the signal system, which is chemiluminogenic instead of the ALP-catalyzed color reaction, in the Siemens/ADVIA immuno-1 assay. More importantly, there is no interference with the serum HER2/*neu* test by heterophile antibodies and more significantly the therapeutic MAb trastuzumab because different antigen epitopes are targeted (see Fig. 73-2).

HER2/*neu* is also overexpressed and/or amplified in oral squamous cell carcinoma (Chen, 2007), NSCLC (Papila, 2009), gastric cancer (Tsigris, 2002b), colorectal cancer (Tsigris, 2002a), urothelial carcinoma (Hussain, 2007), prostate cancer (Kehinde, 2008), and ovarian cancers in association with advanced stage and poor prognosis so it can be used as a therapeutic target in these cancers (Agus, 2000).

p53

p53 (see Chapter 74) is a 53-kDa nuclear phosphoprotein and a negative regulator of cell growth. It functions as a tumor suppressor by inducing the expression of gene products that are responsible for inhibiting or arresting cell growth and proliferation. The ability of p53 protein to regulate transcription of its target genes is based on its sequence-specific DNA binding activity and the presence of a domain that can activate transcription when attached to the DNA-binding domain of p53 target protein. It is the DNA-binding domain that appears to be sensitive to disruption by mutation, and most lesions associated with human cancers occur within this domain. The encoding gene for p53 has been found to be mutated in about half of almost all types of cancer arising from a wide spectrum of tissues. Because of its short half-life (20 minutes), the wild-type p53 protein in the blood circulation is not detectable (Malkin, 1990; Harris, 1993). However, current molecular techniques such as PCR/SSCP (detailed in Part 8) can detect serum p53 gene mutations. The presence of p53 antibody in serum facilitated the detection of abnormal p53 serologically. Significantly, the presence of p53 antibody in serum is associated with expression of p53 mutations and positively correlates with the degree of cancer malignancy (discussed in Chapter 74).

PARATHYROID HORMONE-RELATED PEPTIDE

Plasma concentrations of parathyroid hormone-related peptide (PTH-RP) are elevated in the majority of patients with cancer-associated hypercalcemia. PTH-RP is secreted by tumors associated with hypercalcemia. The circulatory forms of PTH-RP in these patients include both a large amino terminal peptide and a carboxyl terminal peptide with close sequence homology to parathyrin (PTH). The mechanism by which PTH-RP induces hypercalcemia involves binding and activating receptors that also bind PTH. Measuring the concentrations of PTH-RPs may be useful in the differential diagnosis of hypercalcemia related to malignancy and associated either with primary hyperparathyroidism, sarcoidosis, vitamin D toxicity, or various malignancies (including squamous cell, renal, bladder, and ovarian carcinomas). Patients with impaired renal function but without hypercalcemia or cancer may have increased plasma concentrations of PTH-RP (Burtis, 1990).

SERUM AND URINE MARKERS FOR PROSTATE CANCER

Serum Prostate-Specific Antigen

PSA is a member of the kallikrein family of serine proteases that is synthesized uniquely in the epithelial cells of the prostate gland. Its expression in these cells is regulated by the androgen receptor. Because of its high degree of tissue specificity, it is perhaps the most widely used tumor marker discovered thus far. The normal reference range is 0–4 ng/mL. The cancer sensitivity and tissue specificity of PSA makes it the most useful tumor marker available for the screening and management of prostate cancer. Lack of cancer specificity in distinguishing prostate cancer and nonmalignant prostate lesions is the main drawback with PSA. Benign conditions such as BPH, acute prostatitis, and infarction can also be correlated with elevated serum PSA levels.

PSA serves as an excellent cancer marker in prostate cancer screening, diagnosis, prediction of cancer risk, and recurrence. Since its discovery in prostate cancer serum in 1980 (Papsidero, 1980), PSA has been subjected to intensive research and clinical usage in the screening, detection, and monitoring of prostate cancer. PSA and its various forms are used to guide clinical decisions for further tissue biopsy diagnosis, resulting in increased prostate cancer detection, especially in young men. Use of PSA in prostate cancer detection has also resulted in a reduction in the number of prostate cancers discovered only at late stages in which metastases occurred, from about 30% of all newly diagnosed cases to about 10% of all such cases (Cooperberg, 2004). Annual PSA screening is recommended both by the American Urological Association and the American Cancer Society for all men over the age of 50. The American Urological Association (AUA) issued new guidelines here during its 104th annual meeting (Greene, 2009). The new guidelines have lowered the age for beginning prostate-specific antigen (PSA) screening to 40 years for relatively healthy well-informed men who want to be tested. In addition, because of its tissue specificity, the PSA assay is particularly useful for monitoring the success of surgical prostatectomy. Complete removal of the prostate should result in an undetectable PSA level, while incomplete resection of the gland (not persistent disease) might result in measurable levels of PSA. However, it should remain unchanged on extended follow-up. Any increase in measurable PSA after a successful radical prostatectomy would indicate prostate cancer recurrence or metastasis. A transient and modest increase of PSA may occur during radiation therapy, which should not be misinterpreted as disease progression.

Multiple studies suggest that diagnosis is made in more than 80% (in some studies, >90%, e.g., DeSoto-LaPaix, 2003) of patients with prostate cancer from serum PSA levels that are greater than 4 ng/mL. Because BPH and acute prostatitis also induce elevated serum PSA levels, approximately half of patients with PSA values greater than 4 ng/mL are not found to have prostate cancer on biopsy, even at significantly elevated levels (i.e., >10 ng/mL). These studies therefore suggest that PSA has a sensitivity of a minimum of 80% and a specificity of around 50%. However, it has also been found that about 20% of initially negative biopsies, when repeated over a 3-year period, become positive (DeSoto-LaPaix, 2003). Thus the specificity of PSA may be higher, assuming that the biopsies missed a malignant lesion and that a new malignancy did not occur over the 3-year time period, leading to the current practice of saturation biopsy.

On the other hand, the cutoff value of 4 ng/mL does not sufficiently distinguish patients with and without prostate cancer, including more aggressive cancers (Schroder, 2000; Horninger, 2002; Punglia, 2003; Thompson, 2004). In a review of the Prostate Cancer Prevention Trial, 2950 men who never had a PSA level greater than 4 ng/mL or an abnormal DRE had a final PSA determination and underwent a prostate biopsy after being in the study for 7 years (Thompson, 2004). There was a 15.2% (n = 449) biopsy-proven prevalence of prostate cancer in men with PSA levels no greater than 4 ng/mL. High-grade prostate cancer (defined as Gleason score ≥7) was seen in 15.8% (n = 71) of these men. Size of the tumor was not reported. In the placebo arm of the Prostate Cancer Prevention Trial, there was no cutpoint of PSA with simultaneous high sensitivity and high specificity for detection of prostate cancer in healthy men, but rather a continuum of prostate cancer risk at all values of PSA (Thompson, 2005). These studies appear to confirm the results of other studies that the sensitivity of PSA, using the 4 ng/mL cutoff, in diagnosing prostate cancer is on the order of 80%–85%. The finding that using a cutoff of 4 ng/mL for PSA to diagnose this disease results in 15.2% false-negative results in the patient population subjected to biopsies is compatible with this conclusion (i.e., 84.2% of patients with prostate cancer had serum PSA levels greater than 4 ng/mL.

The issue of using lower cutoffs for serum PSA to identify more patients with prostate cancer has been further explored (Puglia, 2003), especially in view of the development of more sensitive assays for PSA, now commercially available in PSA test kits, that are capable of detecting serum PSA less than 0.1 ng/mL. Based on considerations from a Prostate Cancer Prevention Trial, European guidelines were issued in 2008 recommending a PSA cutoff value of 2.5 ng/mL or, alternatively, a PSA velocity of 0.6 ng/mL per year as a biopsy indication (Heidenreich, 2008).

In addition to the issue of cutoffs for PSA in the diagnosis of prostate cancer, the issue of the efficacy of diagnosis of this disease has been raised because as it has been for a number of other cancers including breast cancer. The question is whether early diagnosis of prostate cancer saves patients' lives. To address this question, a major study by the European Randomized Study of Screening for Prostate Cancer (ERSPC) was carried out over approximately the past decade, involving 182,000 men between the ages of 50 and 74 in seven European countries who were randomly assigned to a group that was offered PSA screening at an average of once every 4 years or to a control group that was treated according to current practice standards and was not subjected to the regular screening procedure. Most participating centers in this study used a lower PSA cutoff value as an indicator of abnormality than the usual 4 ng/mL (i.e., 3 ng/mL versus 4 ng/mL). Prostate cancer was detected in 8.2% of the men in the screening group while 4.8% was detected in the control group. The absolute death risk difference between the control group and the screening group was 0.71 patient per 1000 patients, implying that 1410 patients must be screened in order to prevent one death from prostate cancer. Overall, this study found that screening resulted in a lower death rate from prostate cancer by 20% (Schroder, 2008, 2009). The study concluded that this significant reduction in the number of deaths from prostate cancer was accompanied by a high risk of overdiagnosis, which, nonetheless, seems to be a small price to pay for the significant number of lives saved.

Contrary to the results of this investigation, another study by the Prostate, Lung, Colorectal, and Ovarian Cancer Screening Trial on patients assigned to be screened, with PSA and DRE, and control groups found that, whereas 20% more prostate cancer was diagnosed in the screened group than in the control group, the death rate among both groups was the same (Grubb, 2008). The conclusion was that screening for prostate cancer does not save lives but subjects patients to unnecessary procedures that do not affect outcome. However, it was recognized that increasing the length of the study might show differences in death rates between the two groups. Possibly also the lower cutoff value of 3 ng/mL used in many of the centers in the ERSPC study identified more patients with significant disease.

Methods to Improve the Performance of Serum PSA Measurement for the Early Detection of Prostate Cancer

Several approaches have been developed to increase the sensitivity and specificity of PSA in detecting prostate cancer.

First, as noted previously, use of serum PSA in combination with either DRE or transrectal ultrasound of the prostate results in increases in both sensitivity and specificity (Catalona, 1991; Brawer, 1992). In addition, the PSA fractions (i.e., free and bound) have been used to increase the sensitivity and specificity of elevated serum PSA in the diagnosis of prostate cancer.

Free PSA, Complex PSA, and Percentage of Free PSA

PSA is capable of complexing with various endogenous protease inhibitors, including alpha 1-antichymotrypsin (ACT), α2-macroglobulin (to which it binds covalently) and α-protease inhibitor (API). These stable forms are collectively known as complexed PSA (cPSA). Serum PSA exists in the serum largely (up to 90% of total PSA) (Vessella, 1997) in the form of a PSA-ACT (PSA–α1-antichymotrypsin) complex (Christensson, 1993), which is readily detectable by most immunoassays, whereas complexes with α2-macroglobulin escape detection by commercial PSA. The noncomplexed forms, known as free PSA (fPSA), are unreactive with plasma protease inhibitors. In prostate cancer, there is generally an increase in the serum concentration of complexed PSA and a corresponding decrease in unbound or free PSA (Parsons, 2004). On the other hand, the relative amount of free PSA is higher in BPH than in prostate cancer. Thus immunoassays have been developed that quantify either cPSA or fPSA. The epitopes exposed by fPSA but not by cPSA enabled the development of these assays specifically measuring fPSA or cPSA as complements to the conventional PSA assay, which measures total PSA (tPSA) (Lilja, 1991; Stenman, 1991). Based on these assays, it has been found that measuring complex PSA with ACT (PSA-ACT) directly eliminates many technical problems associated with PSA assays and improves the differentiation of BPH from prostate cancer (Wu 1994, 1998), thereby increasing test specificity (Parsons, 2004). The specificity of PSA has been enhanced by using molecular forms of PSA and fPSA, such as percent free PSA (% fPSA), proPSA, intact PSA, or benign prostatic hyperplasia-associated PSA, and/or new serum markers (Stephan, 2009).

Conversely, measurement of fPSA and the calculation of percentage of fPSA (%fPSA = [fPSA/tPSA] × 100), which has an inverse relationship with prostate cancer risk (Polascik, 1999), have been used to help to differentiate BPH from prostate cancer, also increasing test specificity and reducing unnecessary biopsies for BPH patients. More importantly, the free PSA ratio improves the specificity for prostate cancer detection in men with PSA between 4 and 10 ng/mL, also reducing unnecessary biopsies. In addition, fPSA may be useful as a prostate cancer morbidity predictor (Polascik, 1999; Ito, 2003). Some studies also showed that %fPSA can be used to predict prostate cancer in patients with PSA less than 4 ng/mL (Djavan, 1999; Horninger, 2002). One caveat is that fPSA is subject to quick degradation at 4° C or above. The recommended time interval from sample collection and assay should be less than 3 hours, and the sample should be stored and shipped at −70° C (Woodrum, 1996). Overall, prostate cancer is associated with elevated complexed PSA and low %fPSA (<6%) (Catalona, 1995), and higher ratios of free PSA (>23%) are usually associated with BPH.

The Bayer complexed PSA assay, which measures both PSA-ACT and PSA-API, was initially proposed as a single assay alternative to the free and tPSA assays (Brawer, 1998; Mitchell, 2001). However, only the ratio of complex PSA to total PSA can reach equivalent results compared with %fPSA (Lein, 2003; Roddam, 2005).

fPSA has recently been shown to exist in at least three molecular forms: proPSA (Mikolajczyk, 1997), BPSA (Mikolajczyk, 2000), and inactive "intact" PSA (iPSA). Recently the FDA approved the Dimension FPSA (free PSA) Flex (Dade Behring, Newark, Del.) and AxSYM (Abbott, North Chicago, Ill.) Free Prostate Specific Antigen tests, which are typically performed along with a total prostate specific antigen (tPSA) test and a DRE and helps to determine whether a prostate biopsy is needed to rule out the risk (in percent) of cancer in men 50 years or older with total PSA of 4–10 ng/mL. The smaller the percent fPSA, the more likely the patient is to have prostate cancer.

In 2007, FDA gave approval to a new test Immulite 1000/2000 Free PSA assay (Siemens, Tarrytown, N.Y.), which is a third generation PSA assay based on the solid phase sequential chemiluminescent immunometric method for the quantitative measurement of fPSA, which is used in conjunction with tPSA. The routine sample preparation and refrigerated (2°–8° C) storage of samples for 24 hours or frozen storage at −70° C is acceptable for the measurement of fPSA.

Principles of Measurement. There are several different assays for free and complexed PSA, one of which is summarized in Figure 73-3. When PSA is bound, certain antigenic determinants are "buried" by the protein to which it binds (mainly, ACT). These are exposed on fPSA, so that antibodies to the buried determinants of complexed PSA will detect only fPSA. On the other hand, there are determinants that are exposed on both free and complexed PSA and can be detected by antibodies to these determinants, allowing for determination of total PSA. Finally, antibodies to the buried PSA determinant are available that also block the common exposed determinant. These antibodies react only with free PSA by binding to the buried determinant but also block the exposed common site. Now, in the presence of this blocking antibody, another antibody is added that reacts only with the common exposed determinant. The only available common exposed determinants are on complexed PSA. Thus this double antibody approach, using a blocking antibody and a detection antibody, quantifies the level of complexed PSA.

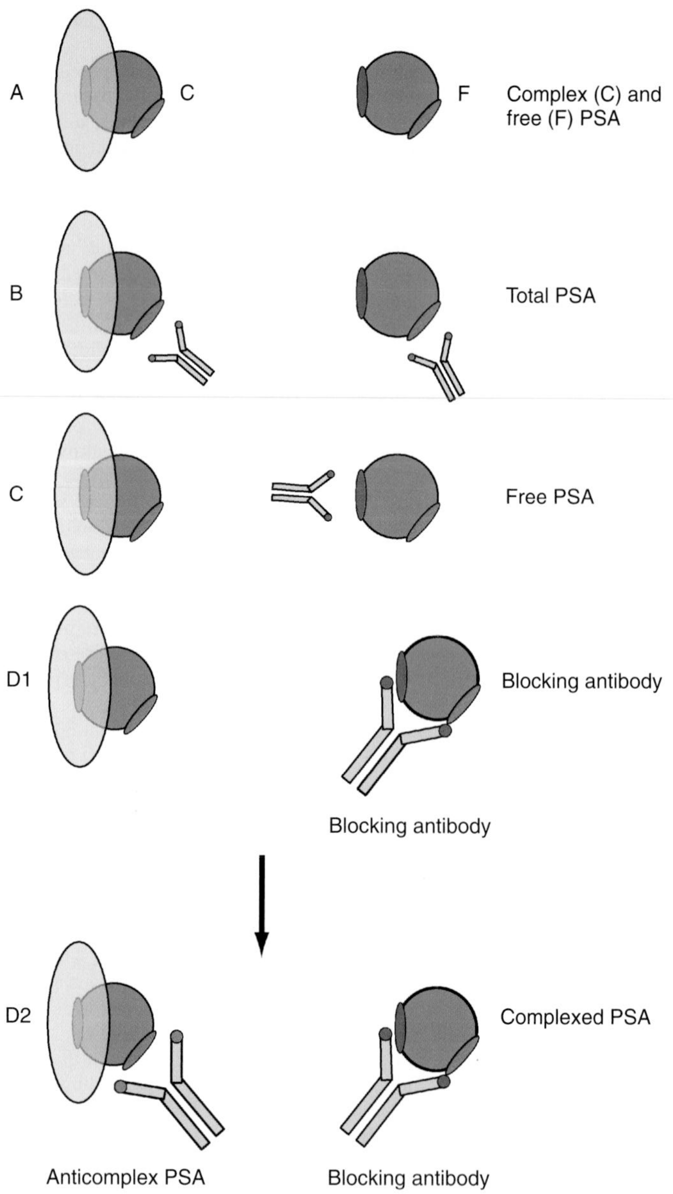

Figure 73-3 Three different assays for prostate-specific antigen (PSA). *A*, PSA is shown to exist in the free (F) or complexed (C) states. Some of its antigenic determinants (blue in the figure) are buried in the complexed state. These are exposed in the free state. On the other hand, as shown in *B*, there are common determinants, red in the figure, that are exposed in both complexed and free PSA. Antibodies to these common determinants will detect total PSA (free + complexed). Because the blue determinants are exposed only in free PSA, as shown in *C*, antibodies to these determinants will detect only free PSA. Finally, as shown in *D1*, antibodies have been developed against the blue determinant of free PSA that also block the red determinant. Thus antibodies to the red determinant, which is common to both free and complexed PSA, will react only with complexed PSA as shown in *D2*. This is the basis for the Siemans/Bayer assay for complexed PSA.

PSA Doubling Time, Velocity, and Density

Cancer is a growth process, and it seems reasonable to suppose that the rate of change of a tumor marker would be a more sensitive marker of disease aggressiveness than an absolute level, so the concept of PSA doubling time and PSA velocity came forward in the last decade. The time (in months) required for the PSA value to double is known as the *PSA doubling time*. It has been shown that the PSA doubling time can predict recurrence after radical prostatectomy in androgen-independent prostate cancer patients (Lee, 2003; Loberg, 2003).

The rate of PSA increase over time, PSA velocity, or PSAV (Carter, 1992), is the PSA difference divided by the number of years, typically given as nanograms per milliliter per year. It has been shown that a PSA velocity of 0.75 ng/year or greater is a strong predictor of cancer with a specificity of 95% (Carter, 1992). More recently, it has been shown that PSA velocity may be useful in predicting prostate cancer risk when PSA levels are between 2 and 4 ng/mL (Fang, 2002). This is especially useful in predicting the risk of cancer and guiding the necessity of prostate biopsy in patients with low/normal PSA value (2–4 ng/mL). In a recent study (Moul, 2007), it has been suggested that by analogy with serum PSA levels, which are age-dependent, PSA velocity should be age-adjusted. They noted that biopsy-guideline threshold levels (PSA ≥ 4 ng/mL, or PSAV ≥ 0.75 ng/mL per year) underestimated the cancer risk in men aged 50–59 years, and should therefore be decreased to 2 ng/mL and 0.40 ng/mL per year, respectively. A sharp rise in the PSA level raises the suspicion of a fast-growing cancer but another important confounder is prostatitis. Thus a repeat PSA measurement following a trial of antibiotics is a reasonable option. A 2006 study found that men who had a PSA velocity greater than 0.35 ng/mL per year had a higher relative risk of dying of prostate cancer than men who had a PSA velocity less than 0.35 ng/mL per year (Carter, 2006). The National Cancer Center Network 2007 guidelines for prostate cancer detection (National Comprehensive Cancer Network: Prostate cancer detection version 1.2007; National Comprehensive Cancer Network, 2007. http://www.nccn.org) include a recommendation that men with a PSA velocity greater than 0.35 ng/mL per year should consider biopsy, even if their PSA level is low. This is a notable finding because prostate cancer causes significant mortality, although a large number of prostate cancer patients die of other causes. Whereas these studies demonstrate a method of identifying aggressive forms of prostate cancer, randomized larger cohort studies are needed to validate these observations. Preoperative PSA velocity is not a good parameter for prostate cancer grade, stage, or recurrence (Freedland, 2001). PSA density is a measure of the ratio of total PSA to prostate gland volume as measured by transurethral ultrasonography; PSA densities of greater than 0.15 indicate an increased probability of prostate cancer rather than BPH (Polascik, 1999).

PSA is still a gold standard biomarker for prostate cancer. It can be made even more useful diagnostically both by employing it in conjunction with other methods such as DRE and by quantifying its fractions (complexed and free) or various molecular markers in the urine.

Urine Markers

Numerous promising prostate cancer biomarkers have recently been identified. These markers have allowed exploring a new diagnostic approach based on the identification of cancer cells or shed material in the urine obtained after digital examination of the prostate (Fradet, 2009; Ploussard G, 2010).

Urine Prostate Cancer Antigen 3

Prostate cancer antigen 3 (PCA3) is a prostate-specific gene that is an average 66 times overexpressed in prostate cancer cells compared with normal prostate cells (de Kok, 2002). Assays were developed to measure the relative amount of PCA3 RNA over PSA RNA using quantitative reverse transcription-PCR or direct RNA amplification (Hessels, 2003; Fradet, 2004). A commercially available test by GeneProbe Inc. (San Diego), referred to as the *Aptima PCA3 assay*, is based on the principle of target capture followed by transcription-mediated amplification and uses calibrators to quantify PCA3 and PSA RNA copy number to provide a PCA3 score (ratio of PCA3 RNA/PSA RNA) (Groskopf, 2006). In a large European prospective multicenter study, this test clearly demonstrated a greater probability of a positive repeat biopsy with increasing PCA3 scores (Haese, 2008). Indeed, the proportion of patients with positive biopsy went from as low as 10% to as high as 70% in a linear fashion with the increasing PCA3 score. Moreover, using a PCA3 score cutoff of 35 provided similar results in men with serum PSA of 4 or less, 4–10, or more than 10 ng/mL with sensitivities of 50%–61% and specificity of 71%–80% (Hoque, 2005). Furthermore, PCA3 has the advantage compared with PSA that it is independent of prostate volume (Hoque, 2005), is correlated with tumor volume (Nakanishi, 2008, Whitman, 2008), and may even predict extracapsular tumor extension (Roupret, 2007).

Urine Hypermethylated Glutathione S-Transferase pi 1 Gene

DNA hypermethylation has been demonstrated to be one of the most common molecular alterations in prostate cancer, with more than 90% of cancers with hypermethylated promoters in one or more genes (Jeronimao, 2001; Woodson, 2004; Yegnasubramanian, 2004; Bastian, 2005). Cairns and colleagues in 2001 used a DNA-based test to detect the hypermethylation of the glutathione S-transferase pi 1 (GSTP1) gene in urinary sediments after prostatic massage and found an overall sensitivity of 73% and a specificity of 98% in a small cohort of patients (Cairns, 2001). Several groups have evaluated the usefulness of gene hypermethylation as a biomarker by testing for its presence in freely voided urine after prostatic massage, in ejaculates, in directly sampled prostatic secretions, and in serum (Goessl, 2000; Gonzalgo, 2003; Crocitto, 2004; Gonzalgo, 2004; Hoque, 2005; Roupret, 2007). Recently, a study by Woodson and colleagues concluded that the methylation of GSTP1 in urine specimens had 75% sensitivity and 98% specificity for prostate cancer. GSTP1 methylation in the biopsy had 88% specificity and 91% sensitivity. Also an observation of a higher frequency of GSTP1 methylation in the urine of men with stage III vs. II disease (100% vs. 20%, $P = .05$) (Woodson, 2008) suggests increased frequency of hypermethylation with increased stage. This study and other initial studies suggest that GSTP1 methylation and other genes in urine may not have much impact on increasing the sensitivity of PSA screening but it may improve the specificity of PSA and help distinguish men with prostate cancer from those with BPH.

Urine Fusion Gene Variants

A remarkable discovery of a family of new genes resulting from the fusion between the androgen-regulated transmembrane serine protease gene (TMPRSS2) with genes members of the E26 transformation-specific (ETS) family of oncogenes was made using a new biostatistical method called *cancer outlier profile analysis* (Kumar-Sinha, 2008). The TMPRSS2–E26 transformation specific-related gene (ERG) fusion transcripts have been identified in 40%–80% of prostate cancers (see Chapter 76). More recently, TMPRSS2 has been found to be an androgen-regulated gene and is more commonly associated with Gleason score >7 (41% versus 12%) and more prostate cancer-related deaths and/or metastatic disease development (53% vs. 23%) (Demichelis, 2007). The serine peptidase inhibitor Kazal type 1 gene outlier was identified exclusively in a small subset of ETS fusion transcript negative cancers (Tomlins, 2008).

A combination of the results from individual assays for PCA3 or gene fusion and PSA forms may enable significantly improved management of prostate cancer, including early detection, prognosis, and treatment selection.

Fecal Occult Blood Testing and Mutant Protein Markers in Stool

Perhaps the most familiar test to screen for cancer in patients is the fecal occult blood test, which is performed in the physician's office on stool samples obtained from a DRE. It is performed routinely on most patients as part of annual checkups. In the hospital outpatient setting, it is more common to have the patient obtain a stool sample for testing after a bowel movement. The idea is that if blood is discovered in the stool, there is the chance that a colonic tumor is the cause, and further workup, such as colonoscopy, is therefore strongly recommended. The actual test for occult blood is based on the ability of the heme moiety of hemoglobin to catalyze the oxidation of the colorless compound guaiaconic acid (hence the name guaiac test) in the presence of H_2O_2 to a highly conjugated, blue-colored quinone. Usually, the guaiaconic acid is impregnated on a strip or solid support, and the stool specimen is placed on a discrete section of the strip. In this nonspecific test, blood in stool can be caused by a number of nonmalignant causes such as hemorrhoids, colitis, diverticulitis, and local trauma to the perianal area, diminishing the specificity of this test. False-positive results for this test are also caused by exogenous factors such as the presence of meat fibers from meat ingestion or of bismuth, which is present in antacid preparations such as Pepto-Bismol. In addition, the ability of this method to detect the presence of colon cancer depends on such factors as whether and to what extent a cancer hemorrhages, its location (the closer to the rectum, the greater the likelihood of detection), and its pattern of growth (e.g., exophytic tumors are more likely to be detected than nonexophytic ones). The sensitivity of the fecal occult blood test is between 15% and 30%. It is much less effective than colonoscopy, the definitive mode of colon cancer detection. However, it offers the advantage of being noninvasive although with "virtual colonoscopy" based on computed tomography scanning of the colon, this advantage is diminished.

As a result, there has been an effort to devise new noninvasive tests on stool specimens that have higher sensitivity and specificity than fecal occult blood tests. As discussed in Chapter 74, several mutant genes that code for proteins that are involved with control of the cell cycle have been strongly implicated as vitally important causative factors of colon cancer. These include mutant *ras* (of the Kirsten or K-variety), mutant p53, the adenomatous polyposis coli *(APC)* gene, and the gene product BAT-26, associated with microsatellite instability. All of these mutant genes are oncogenes in colon cancer. Standardized reverse-transcriptase polymerase chain reaction (RT-PCR) techniques, discussed in Part 8, Chapter 66, are available to detect mutations in any or all of these proteins. In addition, "long" DNA, thought to result from disordered apoptosis of cancer cells in colon cancer, has also been found to occur in a number of colon cancers. If sufficient numbers of cancer cells from a colon cancer are sloughed off into the lumen, one or more of the mutant genes (and/or long DNA) can be discovered, allowing for the noninvasive detection of colon cancer.

Using this approach, a cooperative study, involving the Colorectal Cancer Study Group, was conducted in which more than 5000 patients were entered and more than 2000 were completely evaluated for colon cancer using fecal occult blood testing, multioncogene testing on stool, and colonoscopy (Imperiale, 2004). All patients were 50 years of age or older (mean, 69.5 years). The results showed that the genetic RT-PCR-based methodology results in significantly higher rates of detection than fecal occult blood testing. Overall, the rate of detection of adenocarcinoma was 51.6% for the genetic screening but 12.9% for fecal occult blood screening. Interestingly, advanced adenomas were detected in 15.1% of cases in the genetic screening and 10.7% in the fecal occult blood screening. Because this condition may be regarded as a precursor for frank malignancy, both methods seem to have similar rates of early detection. On the other hand, the rate of detection of TNM stage I colon cancer by genetic screen was 53.3% while that for fecal occult blood screening was 6.7%, suggesting that genetic screening is substantially more effective in detecting true colon cancer in its early stages. Surprisingly, both tests were found to have similar apparent false-positivity rates in conditions of minor polyps (7.6% vs. 4.8% for genetic and occult blood tests, respectively) and the condition of no polyps found on colonoscopy (5.6% vs. 4.8% for genetic and occult blood tests, respectively). Although this study has certain drawbacks, such as too few patients with cancers and advanced adenomas with high-grade dysplasia, skewing of the age of the population to 65 years of age and older, and lack of information as to appropriate testing intervals for the genetic approach, these results are encouraging and warrant further systematic studies using this approach.

Circulating Tumor Cells in Peripheral Blood

Hematogenous spread of cancer cells is the main venue for cancer metastases (Eccles, 2007). Thus the detection of these disseminating primary cancer cells in peripheral blood can not only act as tool for monitoring early metastases but also can predict the prognosis and the treatment outcome of novel therapies.

The major obstacle in successful detection of CTCs is their paucity in peripheral blood, approximately one or fewer CTC cells in 10^5–10^6 peripheral blood mononuclear cells. Thus various enrichment techniques are used to capture the circulating tumor cells based on cell size. These include membrane microfilter devices or micro-electro-mechanical system, isolation by size of epithelial tumor, cell density (density-gradient centrifugation) and specific antibodies to the cell surface proteins based on the use of immunomagnetic beads technique (see Chapter 44), and flow-assisted cell sorting (see Chapter 34). The enriched CTC can further be characterized by additional detection techniques. The two main approaches for the detection of CTCs are immunologic assays using monoclonal antibodies directed against specific proteins by using fluorescence microscopy and flow cytometry and by measuring tissue-specific transcripts by using PCR-based molecular assays (e.g., RT-PCR and methylated DNA PCR) (Molnar, 2003). The Cellsearch (Johnson & Johnson) system, the first FDA- approved test based on the immunologic approach, has gained considerable attention because it allows both standardized automated immunomagnetic enrichment using antibodies targeting epithelial cell adhesion molecule (EpCam) and subsequent labeling of CTCs with fluorescent antibodies specific for epithelial cells (cytokeratins 8, 18, and 19) and leukocytes (CD45) (Cristofanilli, 2004; Eccles, 2007; Riethdorf, 2007; Pantel, 2009). This system can provide clinically useful information on the prognosis of patients with metastatic breast, colon, and prostate cancer (Moreno, 2005; Cohen, 2006; Hayes, 2006) and has the potential to evaluate CTCs in pharmacodynamic studies that test new targeted therapies (Moreno, 2005, de Bono, 2007). Recently, a microfluidics microchip technology has been developed that uses a silicon microchip containing thousands of microspots staining with anti-EpCAM (CTC-chip). In this technique, microfluidics are used to pneumatically push whole blood over the surface of the CTC-chip and EpCAM positive CTCs are captured and confirmed as CTC via fluorescence microscopy (Nagrath, 2007; Uhr, 2007). CTC chips identified high numbers of cytokeratin-positive CTCs in nearly all tested patients with lung, prostate, pancreatic, breast, and colon cancer, including those without metastatic disease. Surprisingly, patients with localized prostate cancer had more CTCs than patients with overt metastasis. Future studies are required to test whether these cells are viable CTCs with tumor-specific genomic characteristics (Uhr, 2007).

The amount of EpCAM on tumor cells varies widely based on tumor type (Thurm, 2003). Therefore alternative devices, based on fiber optic array scanning technology, an ultra-speed automated digital microscopy with laser printing techniques, has been developed to circumvent to the rare-cell detection problem (He, 2007). By this method, laser-printing optics has been used to excite 300,000 cells per second, which have been decorated by fluorescent dye-conjugated antibodies directly on the slide. Another completely different antibody-based approach is the EPISPOT assay to detect proteins released by CTCs. Using the EPISPOT method, only viable, protein-excreting cells are detected. Nevertheless, the clinical utility of all of these new approaches needs to be validated in large-scale studies in cancer patients (Alix-Panabieres, 2007a, 2007b).

As summarized, various clinical studies have provided evidence for an association between the presence of CTCs detected at the time of tumor resection and postoperative metastatic relapse in patients with cancers of the breast, prostate, lung, and gastrointestinal tract. The present research data strongly support that CTCs are indicators for cancer progression into metastatic disease and can be used to adjust treatment modality. A recent study indicates that CTC detection predicts the prognosis in clinically relevant subgroups of early-stage breast cancer patients (Ignatiadis, 2007). Moreover, in other tumor entities such as gastrointestinal cancer, a disease in which overt bone marrow metastases are rare, CTC analyses have generated prognostic information and might therefore become helpful indicators of early systemic tumor cell spread to other distant organs such as lung or liver. Monitoring of bone marrow and peripheral blood during and after systemic adjuvant therapy for CTCs might provide unique information for the clinical management of the individual cancer patient, and allow an early change in therapy years before the appearance of overt metastasis signals incurability. Although large-scale clinical data are still lacking with regard to how molecular characterization of CTCs could be used as a clinical decision making tool, this type of analysis holds tremendous promise for improved stratification of patients and/or the prospective development of tailored, targeted therapy.

Conclusions and Directions for the Future

In summary, a molecule, almost always a protein, could be used as a tumor marker as long as its changing concentration reflects tumor cell activity. The assessment of clinical utility for an individual tumor marker is based on its sensitivity and specificity. There has been a clear trend toward improving the test specificity and sensitivity by ordering multiple tumor markers. However, controversy exists concerning which and how many tumor markers should be included in a panel for individual malignant diseases. Several new tumor markers, discussed in Chapter 74, are now on the horizon. These tumor markers consist of oncoproteins, suppressor proteins, adhesion molecules, cyclins, and angiogenic factors. They mainly differ from currently used tumor markers in their association with specific known metabolic pathways or physiologic reactions. Most tumor markers employed currently for patient management are not associated with any known specific biological reaction. Conceivably, measuring these new tumor markers will provide information on more specific defects, which will help in the design of better treatments. The best example is the successful use of Herceptin (a humanized MAb against the ectodomain of the c-*erb*B-2 receptor) for metastatic breast cancer patients.

SERUM GENOMICS AND PROTEOMICS AS POTENTIAL BIOMARKERS FOR CANCER

Current technology has opened new directions in searching suitable serum markers in early cancer screening, diagnosis, and prognosis and in monitoring treatment response. This active field is applying current genomics and proteomics as well as newer molecular techniques in detecting circulating nucleic acid (DNA and RNA) and tumor cells. Serologic marker profiling with genomics and proteomics (Johann, 2004; Petricoin, 2004; Rai, 2004) has been a very promising area of research. These new advances are described in Chapter 74.

CIRCULATING NUCLEIC ACIDS IN THE DETECTION OF CANCER

Many new techniques have been developed to detect abnormal circulating nucleic acids (DNA, RNA and miRNA) in cancer patients. Among them, PCR-SSCP has been used to detect serum DNA mutations, and fluorescent microsatellite analysis has been used to detect loss of heterozygosity. Fluorescent microsatellite analysis has been frequently used to identify allelic imbalance and loss of heterozygosity as a serologic marker for urothelial carcinoma (von Knobloch, 2004) at the molecular level. These methods might prove to be useful if the specificity and sensitivity are examined in large cohorts of patients.

SERUM PROTEOMICS IN THE DETECTION OF CANCER

Proteomics technology represents a combination of state-of-the-art mass spectrometry and bioinformatics. It includes protein chip surface-enhanced laser desorption ionization (SELDI) and matrix-assisted laser desorption ionization time-of-flight liquid chromatography–mass spectrometry platform as described in Chapter 77. The final use of these challenging techniques will be determined in future clinical trials.

SELECTED REFERENCES

Djavan B, Zlotta A, Kratzik C, et al. PSA, PSA density, PSA density of transition zone, free/total PSA ratio, and PSA velocity for early detection of prostate cancer in men with serum PSA 2.5 to 4.0 ng/mL. Urology 1999;54:517–22.

The usage of PSA has changed the management of prostate cancer patients. This reference pointed out dilemma using current PSA cut off value and summarizes various PAS parameters to increase specificity of PSA.

Lipton A, Ali SM, Leitzel K, et al. Elevated serum Her-2/neu level predicts decreased response to hormone therapy in metastatic breast cancer. J Clin Oncol 2002;20:1467–72.

*Provides evidence that serum HER2/*neu *may be useful in prognosis and monitoring treatment of breast cancer patients.*

Rouprêt M, Hupertan V, Yates DR, et al. Molecular detection of localized prostate cancer using quantitative methylation-specific PCR on urinary cells obtained following prostate massage. Clin Cancer Res 2007;13:1720–5.

Serves as an example and summary of the identification of biomarkers using current serum proteomics technology and will be the trend for future biomarkers.

Saghatchian M, Guepratte S, Hacene K, et al. Serum HER-2 extracellular domain: relationship with clinicobiological presentation and prognostic value before and after primary treatment in 701 breast cancer patients. Int J Biol Markers 2004;19:14–22.

*Provides evidence that serum HER2/*neu *may be useful in prognosis and monitoring treatment of breast cancer patients.*

Zhang Z, Bast RC Jr, Yu Y, et al. Three biomarkers identified from serum proteomic analysis for the detection of early stage ovarian cancer. Cancer Res 2004;64:5882–90.

Serves as an example and summary of the identification of biomarkers using current serum proteomics technology and will be the trend for future biomarkers.

REFERENCES

Access the complete reference list online at http://www.expertconsult.com

PART 9

CHAPTER 74

ONCOPROTEINS AND EARLY TUMOR DETECTION

Matthew R. Pincus, Paul W. Brandt-Rauf, Martin H. Bluth, Wilbur B. Bowne

KEY POINTS

- As a result of the vast progress that has been made very recently in sequencing the entire human genome and in illuminating pathways that are involved in tumorigenesis, it has become clear that the malfunctioning of mutant proteins is the central cause of human cancers.
- These proteins—growth factors, growth factor receptors, G-proteins such as ras-p21, the mitogen-activated protein kinases, and nuclear proteins such as Myc, Fos, Jun, and p53—are critical in signal transduction pathways in which proliferation signals from growth factors at the cell membrane are transduced to the nucleus and stimulate cell division.
- The mutations in these proteins result in amino acid substitutions or deletions that cause them to be permanently activated. Mutations in regulatory domains of the genes encoding these proteins can result in protein overexpression, which can also result in continuous mitogenic signaling.
- These proteins and antibodies to them can be used to detect the presence of cancers in patients at early stages—and even to predict their future occurrence.
- Although mutated signal transduction proteins are involved in many different human cancers, it appears that there are patterns of expression of mutated proteins that typify specific cancers.

OVERVIEW

As a result of the vast progress that has been made recently in sequencing the entire human genome and in illuminating pathways that are involved in tumorigenesis, it has become clear that the malfunctioning of mutant proteins is the central cause of human cancers. This has given rise to a whole new field of proteomics, that is, detection of these aberrant proteins in the blood and other body fluids of patients. This chapter explains these new approaches and emphasizes that many of these aberrant proteins are actually involved in the transmission of proliferation signals on signal transduction pathways, prominent examples of which are discussed. The aim of this chapter is to explain signal transduction pathways in cell proliferation, to illustrate how different mutant proteins on these pathways can cause abnormal, continuous proliferation signaling leading to cell transformation, to demonstrate how these proteins and antibodies to them can be used to detect the presence—and even to predict the future occurrence—of cancers in patients, and to show how new proteins that are strongly associated with different types of cancer have been discovered and can be used to detect these cancers at early stages.

CELL BIOLOGY AND MITOGENESIS

Control of the process of cell division in eukaryotic cells, especially in the higher forms of life, is vital to the processes of cell proliferation and differentiation. The fine balance between these two processes is regulated by numerous proteins that interact in the cell to ensure that this balance is maintained. Virtually all these proteins, many of which are critical in regulating the cell cycle, are encoded by oncogenes. Mutations in oncogenes can result in the production of proteins that become either permanently activated in stimulating cell growth and proliferation (e.g., the ras-gene-encoded p21 protein) or become inactive in inhibiting cell proliferation (e.g., the p53 protein). Both events give rise to malignant tumor cells.

Knowledge not only of the existence of these oncogenes and their encoded oncoproteins but also of the mechanisms by which they exert their effects has resulted in a new series of highly sensitive assays for both mutated oncogenes and their encoded mutant proteins. Assays using amplification methods such as real-time polymerase chain reaction (RT-PCR) for mutated oncogenes are discussed extensively in Part 8 and are further discussed in this chapter. However, the main focus of this chapter is the discussion of how detection of oncogenic *proteins*, or *oncoproteins*, that occur in the serum of patients with malignant tumors enables the diagnosis of malignancy to be made, often at an early stage of tumor development. Because the finding of elevated levels of any of these oncoproteins or mutated forms of these proteins in human serum indicates the likely presence of a malignant tumor, these proteins are also referred to in this chapter as *tumor markers*. Additionally, in view of the enormous strides that have been made in PCR and other molecular technology allowing detection of very few copies of aberrant DNA, we also discuss in this chapter recently developed new detection methods for oncogenic DNA present in the sera and other body fluids of patients with cancer, further allowing early tumor detection.

Oncogenesis, the process by which normal cells become malignant, involves multiple steps, which can be broadly classified into tumor initiation and tumor promotion. Mitogenesis itself is a multistep process that commences at the cell membrane as a result of the activation of a growth factor receptor, which then activates other membrane and cytosolic proteins and second-messenger molecules that transduce the mitogenic "signal" to the nucleus. The pathway in which this orderly progression of activation of successive proteins, mostly kinases, occurs from the cell membrane to the nucleus is referred to as a *signal transduction pathway.*

SIGNAL TRANSDUCTION PATHWAYS

A number of the steps on the signal transduction pathway that are involved in the transduction of the growth factor–initiated signal to the nucleus has become elucidated, but many of the steps that are involved are not fully understood. One well-established pathway, for the ras-oncogene-induced mitogenic signaling pathway, is summarized in Figure 74-1. This figure shows that, when a growth factor receptor is activated by its growth factor, such as epidermal growth factor (EGF), HER2/neu, or insulin, the receptor, in turn, activates several intermediary proteins (Grb-2 and SOS, in Figure 74-1) that activate the all-important G-protein (i.e., guanosine triphosphate [GTP]-binding protein), ras-p21. This membrane-bound 21kDa protein, containing 189 amino acids, is activated when the SOS protein induces it to bind GTP in place of guanosine diphosphate (GDP). In its activated (GTP-bound) state, ras-p21 directly activates raf (Moodie, 1993; Stokoe, 1994), which, in turn, induces a sequential protein kinase cascade beginning with the kinase, MEK (formerly called MAP kinase kinase) and mitogen activated protein (MAP) kinase encoded by the ERK gene, as shown in Figure 74-1.

MAP kinase directly activates nuclear transcription factors, one of these being Fos. This important protein forms a heterodimeric complex with another nuclear transcription factor, Jun, which is directly activated by Jun kinase (JNK). The Fos–Jun complex, also called AP1, binds to specific regions of genomic DNA, inducing the transcription of mitogenic proteins

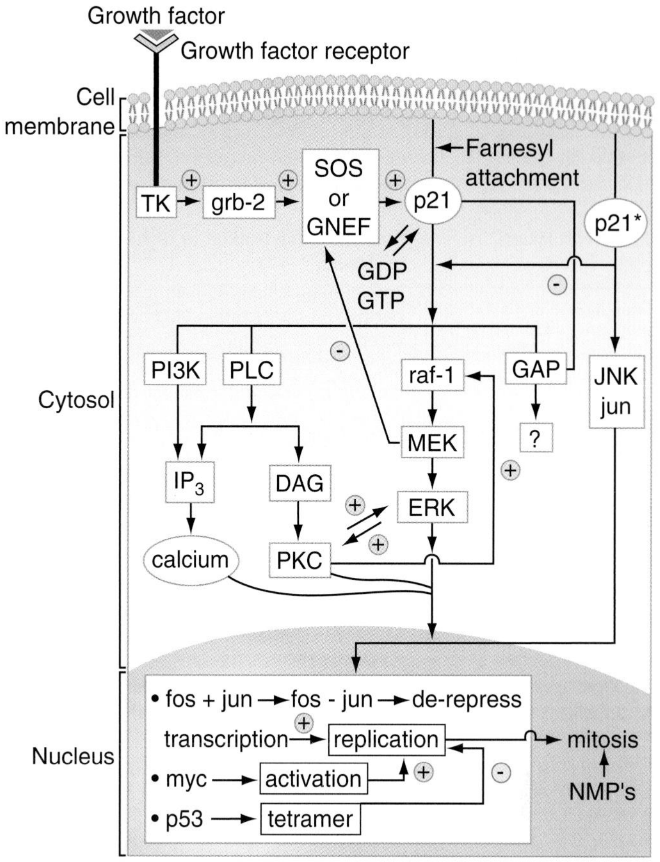

Figure 74-1 Scheme of some of the known components of the ras signal transduction pathway beginning *(top, left)* when a growth factor binds to its cell receptor. The remainder of events is explained in the text. *DAG,* Diacylglycerol; *GAP,* GTPase-activating protein, which promotes hydrolysis of GTP to GDP bound to p21; *grb-2,* the adaptor protein that concurrently binds p21 and the guanine nucleotide exchange protein or factor, SOS; *PI3K,* phosphoinositol-3-hydroxy kinase, an enzyme that induces synthesis of IP3 and is involved in many aspects of mitogenic signal transduction; *IP3,* inositol triphosphate; *MAP-2 kinase,* mitogen-activated protein kinase or microtubule-associated protein kinase-2 (MAP-2K in the figure, also called ERK); *myc, fos,* and *jun,* nuclear oncogenes that code for nuclear proteins; *NMP,* nuclear matrix proteins; *PKC,* protein kinase C; *PLC,* phospholipase C; *Raf-1,* the oncogene-encoded p74 protein, which functions as a kinase that phosphorylates another kinase of molecular mass 43kDa, called MAP-2 kinase kinase, MEK (as in the figure, or MAP-KK in the figure; ras-p21 protein, ras-p21, defined in the text).

such as the cyclins. Transcription of these proteins is blocked by the antioncogene p53 protein (see Fig. 74-1), which further induces the transcription of antimitotic proteins such as Bax and caspases that are critical to the process apoptosis.

Figure 74-1 shows that there are several other important nuclear oncogene-encoded proteins such as Myc, a 75kDa protein that is overexpressed in Burkitt's lymphoma. This oncogene protein is not directly on the ras signal transduction pathway. Interestingly, there are cell lines that, when transfected with either the ras oncogene or with the myc oncogene, do not undergo cell transformation but, when transfected with both oncogenes simultaneously, do undergo cell transformation. These results indicate that ras and myc may be interdependent and are an excellent prototypical example of the multistage nature of oncogenesis.

Figure 74-1 also illustrates that, in normal mitogenic signal transduction, antiproliferative proteins, also called antioncogene proteins, such as p53, become activated and downregulate mitogenic events. If these proteins become mutated at critical positions in their polypeptide chains, they become inactivated, allowing mitogenic events to occur with less inhibition and regulation. Numerous other antioncogene proteins occur, including p16, mutations in which have been implicated as a major causative factor of bladder cancer; Rb (retinoblastoma antioncogene protein); and APC (adenomatosis polyposis coli) protein, mutations of which have been implicated in causing familial adenomatous polyposis and colon cancer.

A central feature of the signal transduction events summarized in Figure 74-1 is that the activation cascades are ordered and are under tight regulatory control. Thus, for example, whereas SOS activates ras-p21,

TABLE 74-1
Mechanisms for Induction of Carcinogenesis by Mitogenic Pathway Elements

Pathway Element	Mechanism of Action
1. Growth factors	a. Overproduction by cell into surroundings
	b. Interaction of growth factors with high affinity receptors
2. Growth factor receptors	a. Overexpression leading to high concentration of dimers
	b. Loss of extracellular domain resulting in permanent dimerization of growth factor receptor and continuous signaling
	c. Amino acid substitutions in transmembrane domain leading to permanent dimerization
3. Cytosolic proteins	a. Overexpression of normal G-proteins and protein kinases
	b. Amino acid substitutions that permanently change conformation to activated form
	c. Mutations that remove regulatory domains of kinases
4. Nuclear oncoproteins	a. Overexpression of transcription and replication proteins
	b. Mutations in antioncogene proteins that inactivate them
	c. Mutations that remove regulatory domains

GTPase-activating protein induces hydrolysis of GTP bound to Ras-p21, causing its inactivation (see Fig. 74-1). Activated MEK downregulates SOS, diminishing GDP/GTP exchange by Ras-p21 (Holt, 1996).

If one or more proteins on pathways such as the one shown in Figure 74-1 become mutated so that they cannot be downregulated, continuous mitogenic signaling becomes possible, leading ultimately to neoplasia. The more such mutations occur, the more likely it is that the cell will undergo malignant transformation. Thus progressive lesions in a mitogenic pathway or in more than one mitogenic pathways may correspond to the multiple steps in carcinogenesis.

These considerations have critically important practical consequences for both the diagnosis and treatment of cancer. In colon cancer, overexpression of the epidermal growth factor receptor (EGFr) can occur, resulting in continuous mitogenic signaling. In addition, as a second occurrence, the ras gene encoding the ras-p21 protein can become mutated, resulting in expression of oncogenic ras-p21 and also resulting in continuous mitogenic signaling. Note in Figure 74-1 that ras occurs downstream of the growth factor receptor (EGFr in this case). If elevated levels of EGFr are found in the serum and/or tissue of a patient with colorectal cancer, an effective therapy is to treat the patient with anti-EGFr agents such as monoclonal antibodies (e.g., cetuximab and panitumumab). Unfortunately, treatment with EGFr inhibitors has no effect on oncogenic ras-p21 signaling. Therefore, it is necessary, prior to treatment, to ascertain whether oncogenic ras-p21 is present (Normanno, 2009). If it is not present, EGFr inhibitor administration is effective. If oncogenic ras-p21 is present, however, this treatment cannot be employed.

Table 74-1 summarizes the mechanisms by which each type of signal transduction element has been found to induce cell transformation, beginning with growth factors, progressing to growth factor receptors, then to G proteins and the kinase cascades, and finally to nuclear proteins. These mechanisms are discussed in more detail in each section of this chapter devoted to these different signal transduction proteins.

ONCOPROTEINS IN TUMOR DETECTION

Detection of mutated signal transduction proteins or high levels of the wild-type proteins in serum or body fluids is strongly suggestive of neoplasia. Therefore, many assays for different oncoproteins are now available commercially in kit form, including enzyme-linked immunosorbent assay (ELISA) assays for the growth factors, transforming growth factor (TGF)-α and β and fibroblast growth factor (FGF); the growth factor receptor proteins EGFr and HER2/Neu, Ras-p21; and the nuclear proteins p53, Myc, and NMP22 from such companies as Oncogene Science (Cambridge, Mass.) now a division of Siemens; Triton Bioscience (Alameda, Calif.), a division of Berlex; and Matritech (Newton, Mass.), now a member of Inverness Medical Innovations, Inc. A number of studies also employ the technique of Western blotting or immunoblotting, as described elsewhere in this book.

Numerous studies have documented alterations in oncogene, oncoprotein, or growth factor expression in terms of messenger RNA (mRNA) or protein in tumor tissue compared with normal tissue (Pimentel, 1989; Brandt-Rauf, 1998; Pincus, 2003). Several studies have examined oncoprotein or growth factor expression in biological fluids such as urine or effusions and demonstrated the feasibility of using these peptides and proteins as markers for the presence of neoplasia (Niman, 1985; Yeh, 1989). Succeeding studies have confirmed these initial findings, resulting in the clinical use of these markers to detect the presence of neoplasia.

Recent studies have now revealed that oncogenes themselves can be detected in the body fluids of patients with different types of cancer. With the advent of microarray techniques both for gene expression and for protein detection (see Chapter 67), it is now possible to assay for the presence of multiple oncogenes and oncoproteins in the body fluids, especially serum, of cancer patients. A new, parallel approach for cancer screening has been developed, called *proteomics*, in which serum samples are subjected to mass spectroscopy and pattern analysis to detect the patterns of expression of proteins that are unique to the blood of cancer patients. This type of analysis has recently resulted in the identification of not only oncoproteins but also other proteins that are expressed at abnormally elevated or abnormally low levels in specific types of cancer.

The focus of this chapter is on the identification of different oncoproteins and growth factors, as well as their respective genes, in the serum, plasma, or urine in patients with cancer or who are at risk for the development of cancer. It also focuses on expression of other proteins that occur at abnormally elevated or low levels in specific types of cancer.

Table 74-2 summarizes some of the many (>50) known oncogenes and their functions in the cell. Those for which commercial serum assays are available are labeled with an asterisk.

GROWTH FACTORS

Because various growth factors are believed to play a role in influencing cellular proliferation during tumorigenesis and because growth factors are actively secreted into the extracellular environment, they are attractive targets for detection in blood during cancer development. Several studies have demonstrated differences in blood levels of growth factors in cancer patients and noncancer controls.

Transforming Growth Factors α and β

TGF-α is a polypeptide with 50 amino acids that binds to the EGF receptor, which dimerizes upon binding to TGF-α or to EGF. TGF-β is a family of proteins labeled β_1–β_5. TGF-β_1 is a homodimer of two 12 kDa subunits linked together by disulfide bonds. Even though TGF-β has been found to be elaborated by many different types of human malignant tumors, elevated serum levels of this growth factor have been found predominantly in cancers of the liver and bladder. Interestingly, TGF-β has been found to inhibit mitosis in specific cell lines in culture, such as mink bronchial epithelial cells. Thus the serum of patients who have tumors elaborating this growth factor can be assayed for it by measuring the extent of inhibition of cell growth.

TGF-β activity, which is determined using this technique, has been found to be markedly elevated in patients with hepatocellular carcinoma (HCC) but not in age-matched controls (Shirai, 1992). In the sera of patients who have undergone surgical resection of these tumors, the activity of TGF-β is barely detectable, suggesting that the tumor was the source of the elevated levels of growth factor in serum. Interestingly, in many patients with HCC, TGF-β has been found to be elevated in urine (Tsai, 1997). In this regard, in a study on the development of HCC in patients with hepatitis C (see Chapter 21), TGF-β_1 was found to be elevated in the sera of patients with hepatitis C and hepatitis C–induced fibrosis and cirrhosis but was not elevated in the sera of patients in whom HCC subsequently developed resulting from the antecedent disease. Thus TGF-β_1 may be an early marker for HCC, but lower levels may be required for progression of disease (Ali, 2004). However, in other studies, TGF-β_1 was found to be elevated in small (<3 cm) HCC far more frequently than α-fetoprotein (AFP), the classic marker for HCC (see Chapter 73; Song, 2002). Using a cutoff of 800 pg/mL for TGF-β_1 and 200 pg/mL for AFP, where the specificities of both markers were 95% (i.e., few false-positive results), the sensitivity of TGF-β_1 was 68% vs. only 24% for AFP. Thus TGF-β_1 may be a reliable marker for small HCC. The same conclusion

TABLE 74-2

Summary of Some Important Oncogenes and Their Protein Products[†]

Oncogene	Protein product	Function
1. erbB*	EGF receptor	Binds to EGF; dimerizes; activates tyrosine kinases in signal transduction. Works through ras.
2. erbB-2*	GF receptor	Very similar to EGF receptor. Works through ras.
3. sis*	β-chain of PDGF	Growth factor receptor. May work through ras.
4. src	Tyrosine kinase	Transduces signal through ras.
5. ras*	p21 proteins; H-, K-, and N-forms	G-proteins; bind to cell membrane and transduce signals through second messengers and raf, GAP(?), JNK, PKC, and PLC.
6. rap-1A	Anti-ras oncogene; in ras family	Blocks ras action in cells.
7. raf*	74 kDa protein	Phosphorylates MAP kinase kinase (MEK), which then phosphorylates MAP kinase.
8. erk-1 and erk-2*	MAP kinase family 43 kDa proteins	Involved in cytoskeletal rearrangements and nuclear signaling.
9. myc*	62/64 kDa nuclear protein	Turns on transcription factors involved in replication.
10. jun	Nuclear protein	Forms complex with fos.
11. fos	Nuclear protein	Forms complex with jun. fos–jun complex activates transcription factors.
12. p53*	53 kDa nuclear anti-oncogene protein	Forms tetramers, then binds DNA segments to block transcription and replication.
13. NMP22*	236 kDa nuclear matrix protein	Involved in mitotic spindle formation.

EGF, Epidermal growth factor; *GAP*, GTPase activating protein; *GF*, growth factor; *MAP* kinase, mitogen-activated protein kinase; *NMP22*, nuclear matrix protein 22; *PKC*, protein kinase C; *PLC*, phospholipase C. The names of the oncogenes are commonly used and relate to the sources from which they were originally discovered. For example, ras is an abbreviation for rat sarcoma viral oncogene.

*Oncogene-encoded proteins for which assays have been performed on human serum. Serum assay kits are commercially available.

[†]Only a few of the many (more than 50) oncogenes are listed in this table. The ones that are listed here encode proteins for which assays have been developed or are closely related to these proteins. No growth factors except PDGF are included in this table.

has been reached in a study of HCC in which the sera of 23% of patients with this disease were positive for TGF-β_1 but not for AFP (Sacco, 2000). TGF-β_1 has also been found to be elevated in metastatic prostate cancer (Adler, 1999).

Use of an ELISA with a monoclonal antibody directed against TGF-β_2 has revealed that TGF-β_2 is elevated in a high proportion of patients with invasive bladder cancer but not in patients with noninvasive bladder cancers or in cancer-free patients (Klocker, 1994; Brandt-Rauf, 1998; Pincus, 2003). Recently, a new tumor marker for bladder cancer that appears to be more accurate in diagnosing both noninvasive and invasive bladder cancer is the nuclear matrix protein NMP22, detected in urine.

Thus serum assays for TGF-β are highly useful in diagnosing and following HCC. They are less useful in the diagnosis of carcinoma of the bladder, although for invasive bladder cancer this growth factor has high sensitivity and specificity.

TGF-α has been found to be elevated in a large number of patients with epithelial cell tumors (Katoh, 1990; Chakrabarty, 1994), predominantly breast (almost 100%), lung, stomach, colon, liver, and ovarian. It has been found to be elevated frequently in the sera of patients with gastric carcinoma (Choi, 1999). In contrast, normal individuals have very low serum levels. With respect to liver, TGF-α has been found to be elevated in the sera of patients with HCC but not in patients with cirrhosis. The elevated levels were reduced in patients who had been treated for HCC (Tomiya, 1996).

Recent studies confirm that TGF-α is an effective predictor of the occurrence of malignancies at an early stage. For example, in 36 patients who had a history of asbestosis and subsequently developed a cancer, mainly adenocarcinoma or squamous cell carcinoma of the lung, more than one third were found to be seropositive for TGF-α. Blood samples from all of these patients were collected and then banked at the time of the diagnosis of asbestosis and before the diagnosis of malignancy. Significantly, all but one of these seropositive patients were found to have elevated TGF-α levels in their banked blood (Brandt-Rauf, 1998).

TGF-α thus appears to be an excellent marker for the presence of malignancy. Unlike the case for TGF-β, these elevations are not tumor-specific. Nonetheless, it is clear that TGF-α is extremely useful in screening patients for the presence of malignant solid tissue tumors.

Platelet-Derived Growth Factor

Platelet-derived growth factor (PDGF), a protein of molecular mass 28 kDa, exists as a dimer of A and B chains, as the A–A, A–B, or B–B dimer forms. Either chain can be glycosylated, increasing the molecular mass to 30 kDa. This growth factor, originally isolated from platelets, binds to a transmembrane growth factor receptor. The B chain is encoded by the sis oncogene. It has been found to be a potent mitogen in lymphoid, myeloid, and fibroblastic cell lines. Overexpression of PDGF has been found in both lung and pleural tumors. It has also been examined in the blood of cancer patients. Overall, this growth factor has been found to be significantly elevated in more than 15% of patients with carcinomas, sarcomas, and lymphomas but not at all in normal individuals. In patients with breast cancer, there is an excellent correlation between the stage of the cancer and the serum level of the growth factor (Ariad, 1991). Higher levels predict shorter survivals. In addition, PDGF-B (Sis) in breast tissue appears to correlate with increased cellular proliferation as its expression increases with both nonmalignant and malignant states and decreases after menopause. In malignancy, PDGF-B does not correlate with p53 expression, estrogen/progesterone status, or tumor grade (Coltrera, 1995). The role of PDGF-B as a marker in colorectal cancer is less clear (Lindmark, 1993).

As discussed later, not only oncoproteins may be elevated in the sera of patients with cancer but also antibodies to oncoproteins may likewise be elevated. Anti-PDGF antibody (PDGF-Ab) in serum has been found to be potentially diagnostic for pleural mesothelioma in patients with histories of exposure to asbestos. The serum levels of PDGF-Ab correlate positively with severity of the disease and show a significant negative correlation with survival; that is, higher levels correlate with shorter survival times (Filiberti, 2005).

Basic Fibroblast Growth Factor

Basic fibroblast growth factor (bFGF) is a protein containing 155 amino acids. It is a growth factor for mesenchymal cells but has also been found to have relatively high concentrations in the central nervous system (CNS). Interestingly, bFGF has been found to be present in high concentration in the sera of patients with epithelial cell tumors. Prominent among these tumors is renal cell carcinoma. More than 50% of patients with this disease have markedly elevated serum levels of bFGF (Fujimoto, 1991; Ii, 1993) as determined either by ELISA or by enhanced chemiluminescent assays. This growth factor is also elevated in the sera of more than 50% of patients with CNS tumors, 90% of patients with lung cancers (Ii, 1993), and more than 60% of patients with lymphomas (Kurobe, 1993). It is not elevated, however, in the sera of large populations of normal (control) individuals.

Elevated serum levels of bFGF have been found to be a good prognostic factor in patients with non–small cell carcinomas of the lung (Brattstrom, 1998). Thus TGF-α and TGF-β, PDGF, and bFGF all appear to be elevated in the sera of a significant number of patients with epithelial cell tumors but are not completely tumor specific. TGF-α has some specificity for breast cancer and TGF-β for HCC. bFGF is elevated in a variety of malignancies, including nonepithelial cell tumors, such as CNS tumors and lymphomas. PDGF shows little specificity for tumor type, but high levels in serum indicate the presence of malignancy.

Given the development of protein/antibody and gene arrays, it is possible to assay the sera and other body fluids of cohorts of patients who are at risk for developing cancer due to such factors as occupational exposure for multiple oncogene proteins concurrently. Discovery of the elevation of and/or the presence of oncogenic mutations in one or more of these proteins in a patient's serum or other body fluid identifies the patient as either having a cancer or developing one in the near future. Recently, serial levels of both TGF-β and PDGF were determined by ELISA assay (see Chapter 44) on a cohort of workers with long-term exposure to asbestos. PDGF, but not TGF-β, was found both to predict the development of non–small cell carcinoma of the lung and to predict (1) the radiograpically determined

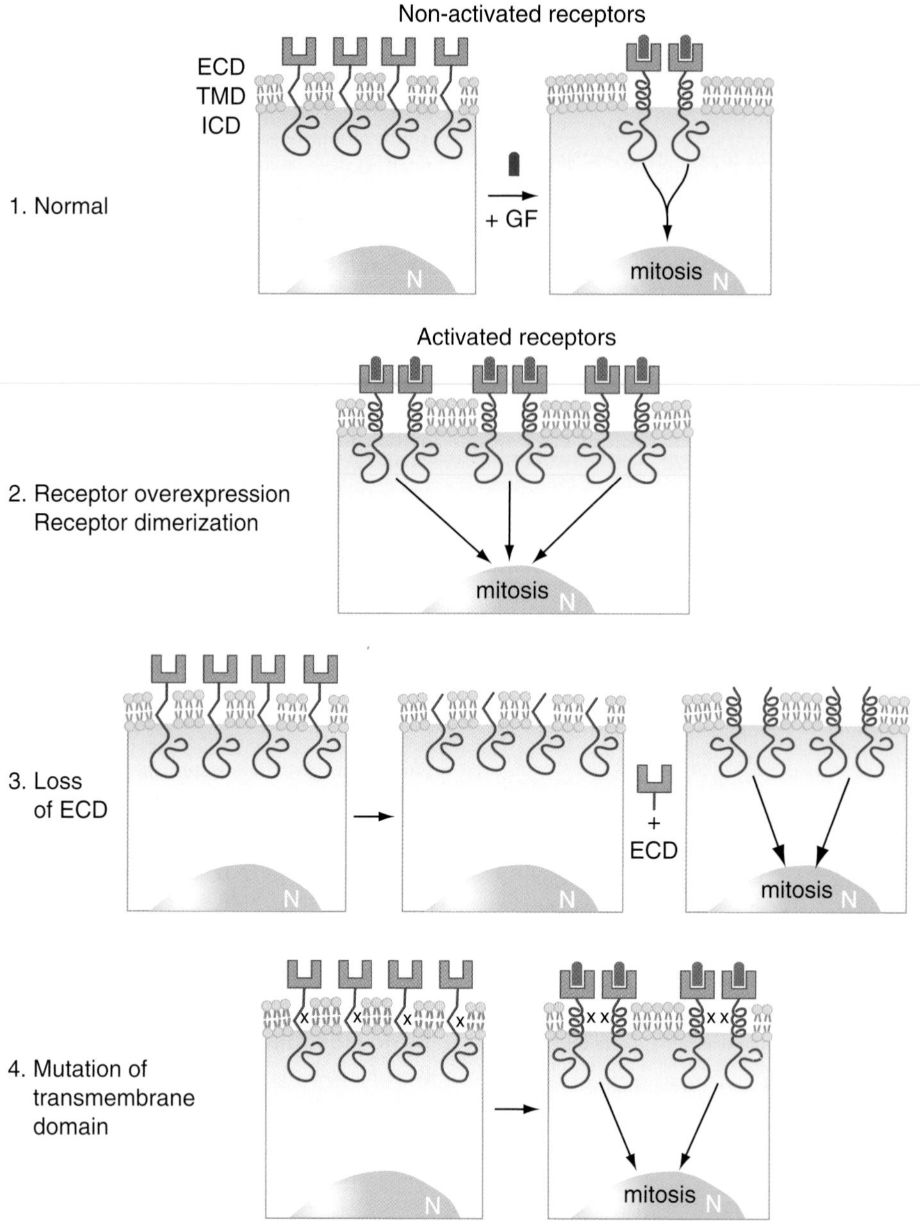

Figure 74-2 Mechanisms for continuous mitogenic signaling by growth factor receptors. Scheme 1 shows that these receptors have three domains: an extracellular, growth factor-binding domain (ECD); a transmembrane domain (TMD), and an intracytoplasmic domain (ICD). A growth factor, GF, binds to the receptor, causing it to dimerize, setting in motion a cascade of intracellular events that are transduced to the nucleus (N) described in Figure 74-1. There are three known ways in which continuous cell signaling by the growth factor receptor can occur, resulting in malignant transformation of cells. Scheme 2 depicts the first of these: overexpression of the receptor that results in many activation processes and continuous signaling to the nucleus. Scheme 3 shows the second mechanism wherein the ECD is either absent or cleaved off by intracellular proteases, leading to spontaneous dimerization. Scheme 4 shows the third mechanism, in which a mutation in the growth factor receptor gene results in an amino acid substitution (X in the figure) in the transmembrane domain leading to formation of α helices that associate (Brandt-Rauf, 1990), resulting in spontaneous dimerization that can occur in the absence or presence of the ligand.

severity of the disease and (2) the levels of PDGF correlating with severity of cancer and with fibrosis of the lung, which may be a predisposing factor (Li, 2009). These studies parallel the results of other studies, such as the study with TGF-α described earlier, in which the sera of patients with occupational and/or environmental risks have been found to be positive for one or more oncogene proteins prior to appearance of a cancer.

Epidermal Growth Factor and Hepatocyte Growth Factor

EGF has been found to be elevated in the serum of some patients with stomach cancer (Pawlikowski, 1989) and cancer of the tongue (Bhatavdekar, 1993) but unchanged or decreased in other cancers (Nedvidkova, 1992). Elevated serum levels of hepatocyte growth factor have been reported in HCC. However, this growth factor appears to be unique in that elevated levels also occur in nonmalignant liver diseases (Hioki, 1993), diminishing its utility as a tumor marker.

GROWTH FACTOR RECEPTORS

Normally, growth factors bind to their growth factor receptors, generally inducing the receptors to dimerize, an event that activates the receptor. At the growth factor receptor level, there are several mechanisms by which uncontrolled mitogenesis may be initiated. These are summarized in Figure 74-2. For both the EGF receptor and the neu (HER2)-oncogene-encoded p185 growth factor receptor protein, strongly associated with breast cancer (Slamon, 1989; Brandt-Rauf, 1998; Pincus, 2003), receptor dimerization results in activation of tyrosine kinases involved in the phosphorylation of proteins that initiate the transduction of the mitogenic signal to the nucleus. There are three known pathologic mechanisms that can result in causing abnormally prolonged receptor dimerization that results in continuous mitogenic signaling. These are loss of the extracellular binding domain (ECD), mutations in the transmembrane domain that promote dimerization (Brandt-Rauf, 1990; Pincus, 2003), and overexpression of the receptor.

Transmembrane growth factor receptors encoded by the erbB family of oncogenes (i.e., erbB, which encodes the EGF receptor, also called EGFr, and HER2/neu [erbB-2]), are particularly attractive targets for detection in blood during cancer development because it has been found that, in human cancers induced by these receptors, the mechanism appears to be proteolysis of the extracellular receptor-binding domain (see Fig. 74-2, third illustration). The liberated extracellular domains, termed *ECD*, then enter the circulation and can be readily detected in serum using conventional immunoassay techniques (Brandt-Rauf, 1994a, 1994b, 1998; Pincus, 2003).

Epidermal Growth Factor Receptor

Overexpression of and/or oncogenic amino acid substitutions in the amino acid sequence of EGFr and in the closely related HER2/neu receptor are the primary causes of a large number of human epithelial cell tumors. These include colon, breast, lung, and ovarian cancers (Baron, 2009). This observation has been extended to CNS tumors, in particular, glioblastoma multiforme (Quaranta, 2007). As discussed earlier, serum EGFr is not only important for diagnostic purposes but also suggests a therapeutic strategy, that is, administration of EGFr inhibitors, the efficacy of which can be monitored by assaying for serum EGFr.

A particularly important use of serum EGFr is in following patients with known histories of exposure to environmental agents known to cause specific tumors. Elevations of circulating levels of the ECD of this growth factor receptor have been studied in patients with asbestosis (Brandt-Rauf, 1992), which is known to predispose to malignancies. It has been found that patients with ECD serum levels of 636 fmol/mL or higher either have an asbestos-associated malignancy (carcinoma of the lung or mesothelioma) or subsequently develop such a malignancy. Large numbers of normal individuals have been found to have much lower serum ECD levels. Thus EGFr appears to be an excellent marker for asbestos-induced tumors. These results are also of interest because they suggest that the primary effect of asbestos as a carcinogen is to cause mutations in the EGFr gene (Brandt-Rauf, 1998).

As discussed, many colon cancers are treated with EGFr inhibitors. An important indication of efficacy of treatment is to measure circulating levels of EGFr. It was recently found that baseline levels of serum EGFr were strong predictors of outcome, higher values predicting better responses to treatment with EGFr inhibitors than lower values (Zampino, 2008).

Of considerable interest is the recent finding that serum levels of EGFr can detect the presence of prostate cancer (Milanese, 2009). Use of EGFr in detection of prostate cancer was motivated by the finding that overexpression of EGFr or critical amino acid substitutions in the amino acid sequence of prostate EGFr are strongly associated with prostate cancer. It was found that, using a cutoff value of 67.9 ng/mL for serum EGFr, the sensitivity and specificity of serum EGFr was 93.3% and 98%, respectively. In this study it was further found that the best serodiagnostic marker for spread of prostate cancer beyond the prostate (e.g., into the seminal vesicle) was urokinase-type plasminogen activator receptor. These results suggest that both biomarkers may offer a new approach to diagnosis and monitoring of prostate cancer.

HER2/neu Receptor

This protein is discussed in Chapter 73 as a marker for breast cancer and for a number of other cancers. Here we consider its potential as a marker for different stages of this cancer and for other human epithelial neoplasms. Because of the documented strong association between breast cancer and mutations in the HER2/neu gene, many studies have examined the p185 erbB2 ECD in the blood of cancer patients, particularly breast cancer. In prior studies on neu oncogene-induced overexpression of the p185 protein (Slamon, 1989), it was found that the level of expression of the neu oncogene in breast cancer biopsy tissue correlated with the extent of the tumor and was the best prognostic indicator of survival rates, exceeding even extent of lymph node involvement as a prognostic indicator.

Results on quantitation of p185 ECD in the serum of patients with breast cancer parallel those of the prior genetic results. Between 25% and 50% of patients with stage III or IV breast cancer have been found to have markedly elevated levels of p185 ECD in their sera (40–190-fold higher than in the sera of normal control individuals) (Mori, 1990; Carney, 1991; Kath, 1993). For patients from whom tumor biopsy material is available, there is an excellent correlation between serum ECD levels and tissue level of expression (Breuer, 1993, 1994; Ludovini, 2008). There is also an excellent correlation between levels of serum ECD and recurrent disease (Brandt-Rauf, 1998). ECD levels in serum have also been found to be an excellent prognostic indicator for breast cancer (Molina, 1996). Recently, in a study of patients with stage I-III breast cancer, it was found that presurgical serum ECD level was an independent prognosticator of disease-free survival in early breast cancer (Ludovini, 2008). This is an important finding because it identifies patients with early breast cancer with complete apparent surgical removal who are at significant risk for recurrence.

Because serum levels of p185 ECD correlate with tumor load and stage, detection of incipient breast cancer using serum levels of p185 ECD is less effective for these patients. Overall, the rate of detection of stages I and II breast cancers using serum levels of ECD, based on conventional ELISA techniques, ranges from 10% to 15%. However, use of a sensitive ELISA assay for p185 ECD in breast cancer patients resulted in discovery of carcinoma in situ in 43% of patients with this disease (Breuer, 1993). This latter result indicates that use of more sensitive assays for p185 ECD identifies a significant increase in the number of patients with carcinoma in situ (i.e., at an early stage of development).

HER2/neu Detects Pulmonary Neoplasms

p185 ECD is also elevated in a high percentage of patients with pulmonary cancers. Elevated serum levels of EGFr in early tumor detection have been employed to screen patients with known predisposition, such as pneumoconioses, for developing these cancers. In 70% of patients with pneumoconioses, elevated serum p185 ECD levels have been found prior to the onset of frank malignancy. In almost 100% of patients with this predisposing factor who have cancer of the lung, serum p185 ECD is markedly elevated (Brandt-Rauf, 1994a). Clearly, this protein is a highly sensitive marker for pulmonary cancers. In contrast, no elevations of p185 ECD have been found in the sera of large numbers of normal individuals (Brandt-Rauf, 1998; Pincus, 2003).

HER2/neu in the Detection of Hepatocellular Carcinomas

It was noted previously that TGF-β is a good marker for HCC. There are now strong indications that p185 ECD is also a sensitive marker for this disease. Serum p185 ECD has been found to be elevated in almost 100% of East Asian people who have known risk factors for developing this disease (Luo, 1993; Yu, 1994a, 1994b). However, tissue expression of c-erbB-2 in biopsies derived from patients with HCC and adenoma showed neither overexpression nor amplification by FISH or immunohistochemistry (Vlasoff, 2002). Furthermore, no such elevations have been observed in normal individuals of similar age and race or in those with exposure to risk factors for this disease but who did not subsequently develop cancer.

p185erbB-2 ECD in Other Tumors

Elevated serum erbB-2 ECD levels have now been found to occur in patients with colorectal, pancreatic, prostatic, hepatic, and ovarian cancers (Wu, 1993) at lower frequencies of detection (15%–20%) and was also found to be significantly higher in patients with nasopharyngeal carcinoma (Yazici, 2001). Excellent correlations between serum levels and tissue levels have been found in many of these cases. There is a direct correlation between serum levels of p185 ECD and tumor size for premalignant adenomas of the colon (Brandt-Rauf, 1994b). Because colonic neoplasia usually progresses through well-defined steps from adenoma to carcinoma with the malignant potential of adenomas increasing with size, serum erbB-2 ECD levels may be useful in monitoring this progression. Gene amplification and protein overexpression of c-erbB-2 were also found in adenocarcinoma derived from Barrett esophagus (Geddert, 2002). In addition, pretreatment serum ECD has been found to be a reliable prognosticator of recurrence of metastatic prostate cancer and significantly more reliable than tissue p185 (Tambo, 2009).

G-PROTEINS

ras-p21 Protein

As for growth factor receptors, signaling proteins that occur downstream of the growth factor receptors become oncogenic primarily from overexpression and amino acid substitutions at critical positions in their polypeptide chains. Less commonly, for some proteins, like Raf (see Fig. 74-1; Table 74-2), loss of regulatory domains may also lead to oncogenesis. Amino acid substitutions in signal transducing proteins cause these proteins to undergo conformational changes that result in their becoming permanently activated to stimulate cell division (Pincus, 1992, 2000, 2004, 2007).

This mechanism has been well documented for the ras-oncogene-encoded p21 protein, for which substitutions of most amino acids for glycine 12 or glutamine 61 result in an oncogenic protein. Many p21 proteins with such substitutions have been cloned and directly microinjected into normal cells in culture such as NIH 3T3 cells (Barbacid, 1987). The cells undergo malignant transformation that lasts until the added mutant protein is metabolized and cleared from the cells. Oncogenic mutant forms of the ras gene and of its encoded p21 protein have been found in approximately one of three common human epithelial cell tumors, in more than 90% of human pancreatic tumors, and 75% of human colon cancers (Forester, 1987; Almoguera, 1988).

One of the consequences of amino acid substitutions in p21 and presumably in other signal transducing proteins is the abnormal activation of alternate, unregulated signal transduction pathways. Oncogenic ras-p21 protein (p21 in Figure 74-1) has been found to interact directly with Jun, the nuclear transcription factor, and its activating kinase, Jun kinase (JNK). This binding process results in the direct activation of these nuclear transcription-inducing proteins, thereby bypassing the normal cellular controls. This bypass or short-circuit pathway is shown on the right side of Figure 74-1 for p21 (Adler, 1995; Amar, 1997; Pincus, 2007). In addition, oncogenic ras-p21 protein requires activation of protein kinase C as a downstream event on its signal transduction pathway (Pincus, 1992), as illustrated in Figure 74-1.

As noted previously, the ras-oncogene-encoded p21 proteins are 21 kDa membrane-associated G proteins that have been implicated in the growth signal transduction process from the cell membrane to cytoplasmic kinases. Qualitative (i.e., point mutations) and quantitative (i.e., overexpression) changes in p21 have been identified as contributing to human carcinogenesis (Barbacid, 1987). By as yet undefined mechanisms, p21 proteins gain access to the extracellular environment. Thus increased amounts of p21 or point-mutated forms of p21 can be detected by immunoblotting with monoclonal antibodies in the supernatant of cells in culture known to overexpress p21 or to express mutant p21, respectively (Brandt-Rauf, 1991, 1998; Pincus, 2003).

Similarly, mice bearing tumors that overexpress p21 or express mutant p21 are found by immunoblotting to have increased amounts of p21 or mutant forms of p21 in their serum, respectively (Hamer, 1991). These results suggest that the detection of increased p21 or mutant p21 in blood is possible in humans.

Because of its central role in mitogenic signal transduction, overexpressed and/or mutated p21 protein might be expected to be present in a wide variety of human tumors. Indeed, elevated serum p21 has been identified in the serum of up to 68% of patients with many different cancers, including breast, prostate, colon, lung, and liver cancer. On the other hand, only a small percentage of normal individuals have been found to have detectable serum levels (Weissfeld, 1994). A high incidence of the occurrence of the oncogenic form of the K-ras gene has been found in human pancreatic and colonic cancers. New assays based on reverse-transcriptase (RT)-PCR have detected the ras oncogene in the stool of a high percentage of patients with colonic cancer (Pincus, 2004).

ras-p21 in Lung Cancer

Similarly encouraging results have been obtained using the sputum of patients with lung cancer. Parallel results have now been obtained using the ELISA for the p21 protein using the serum of patients with lung and colonic carcinoma. Elevated levels (five times more than controls) of serum ras-p21 have been found in up to 83% of lung cancer patients, whereas only low levels were found in the sera of normal individuals (Brandt-Rauf, 1991, 1998). In addition, studies have been carried out in which PCR for K-ras mutant genes with base changes at codons 12 and 13 has been performed concurrently on tumor tissue and serum from patients with different stages of colorectal cancer (de Kok, 1997). In more than 90% of the patients with specific mutant ras genes found in tumor tissue, the same mutated ras gene was discovered in their sera, regardless of the stage of the tumor.

In the previous discussion of the HER2/neu-oncogene-encoded p185 protein, it was noted that elevations of the serum levels of this protein were found in patients with pneumoconioses who then progressed to develop frank malignancies. A parallel study has been performed on patients with pneumoconioses in which assays were carried out for ras-p21 in their sera. For patients with this predisposing condition, 39% were found by Western blotting to have elevated serum levels of the ras-p21 protein. Almost all of these patients developed a malignant lung tumor subsequent to the observed elevations of the p21 protein. Thus, like p185 ECD, elevated serum p21 is a biomarker of early malignant disease in patients with a known predisposition. An obvious study that is yet to be performed is to assay the sera of these patients for both HER2/neu and ras-p21 to increase the sensitivity of the assays.

The aforementioned studies are concerned with detecting elevated serum levels of p21 in serum as an indicator of malignancy. As noted previously, a major mechanism for oncogenesis induced by the ras-p21 protein is amino acid substitutions in its sequence that result in its permanent activation. Identification of mutant ras genes by PCR and direct sequencing of DNA isolated from the serum or plasma of three patients with pancreatic cancer has been described (Sorenson, 1994), but, until recently, the direct detection of mutant p21 protein had not been reported in human blood (de Kok, 1997). Now, however, oncogenic amino acid substitutions in the p21 protein can be identified through the use of monoclonal antibodies that recognize specific oncogenic amino acid substitutions including at positions 12, 13, 59, and 61. Use of these antibodies on the sera of patients with known risk factors for cancer appears to offer much promise for early tumor detection.

ras-p21 in Angiosarcoma

Mutated p21 has been found in the serum of patients with a known history of exposure to the carcinogen, vinyl chloride. This chemical has been shown to predispose individuals to developing angiosarcomas (Brandt-Rauf, 1998). Tissue studies of these angiosarcomas reveal that a mutant ras gene that codes for aspartic acid in place of the normally occurring glycine at position 13 in the polypeptide chain is present in the tumor cells. A monoclonal antibody that recognizes the Asp13 form of the p21 protein has been obtained (Oncogene Science/Siemens). This mutant p21 protein has been identified in the sera of 80% of patients with vinyl chloride–induced angiosarcoma of the liver but not in normal individuals (DeVivo, 1994). There is a direct correlation, moreover, between the degree of exposure of patients to vinyl chloride and the probability of discovering the oncogenic form of the protein in their sera.

ras-p21 in Pancreatic Cancer

In view of the strong causative association of oncogenic k-ras-p21 with pancreatic cancer, it is surprising that there have been no studies using this protein as a marker for this disease. Rather, studies have focused on employing assays for the ras oncogene itself in the sera of patients with this disease. A recent study on patients with pancreatic cancer and a control group of patients with pancreatitis used RT-PCR to detect mutant ras DNA in the sera of these patients together with a serum assay for CA 19-9, a marker for pancreatic cancer as discussed in Chapter 73 (Dabritz, 2009). Using DNA amplification techniques to detect oncogenes in serum is discussed later. In this study, no patients with pancreatitis were found to have oncogenic ras gene in their sera, whereas 36% of patients with pancreatic cancer were found to have detectable serum levels of this oncogene. Overall, using both markers, 91% of the patients with pancreatic cancer were found to have either elevated levels of CA 19-9 or oncogenic ras-p21 or both. Of these, 35% were found to have detectable oncogenic ras but nonelevated or only moderately elevated CA 19-9. Using restriction fragment length polymorphism (RFLP)-PCR on serum samples from patients with pancreatic cancer before and after chemoradiation therapy (CRT), it was found that in patients whose post-CRT sera were negative for oncogenic ras had significantly more favorable survivals (Olsen, 2009).

CYTOSOLIC MITOGENIC KINASES

raf

As shown in Figure 74-1 and Table 74-2, Raf is a 74 kDa protein that is a critical target of ras-p21. It directly activates MEK, which, in turn, activates MAPK (ERK) (see Figure 74-1 and Table 74-2). It is involved in cell growth, proliferation, apoptosis, and differentiation. There are several different isoforms of Raf, such as Raf A and Raf B, which may differ in their exact cellular functions. More than 30 mutations of the B-raf gene associated with human cancers have been identified (Wan, 2004). Western blot analysis showed that activated Raf was overexpressed in tissues obtained from cirrhosis and HCC patients (91.2% and 100%, respectively) (Hwang, 2004). B-raf mutations have also been found in colon cancer, although less frequently than K-ras (Monstein, 2004). However, Raf is found minimally to not at all in tissues from patients with bladder or endometrial carcinoma (Mutch, 2004; Stoehr, 2004). In contrast, mutant raf (V600E) has been found to occur frequently in melanomas although the same mutant raf has also been found in a majority of benign nevi (Wellbrock, 2004). Because raf is immediately downstream of ras-p21 on the ras signal transduction pathway (Figure 74-1), oncogenic mutations in raf might also be expected to diminish the efficacy of anti-EGFr agents in cancers, especially colorectal cancers. This has been found to be the case for metastatic colon cancer (De Nicolantonio, 2008).

NUCLEAR ONCOPROTEINS

As noted previously, two important nuclear proteins that appear to play critical roles in the regulation of cell growth and division are the tumor suppressor gene protein, p53, and the p62/75 protein encoded by the c-myc oncogene for which serum assays have been developed. Furthermore, nuclear skeletal or matrix proteins are the targets of signal transducing kinases such as MAP kinase, as indicated in Figure 74-1.

p53 and c-myc Proteins

The protein p53 is known to function as a homotetramer and, in this form, binds to specific sequences of DNA. The effect is to repress the mitotic process. In addition, activation of p53 in transformed cells results in apoptosis via activation of pro-apoptotic proteins such as Bax and caspases. Thus p53 is an anti-oncogene protein. Mutations can occur in p53 that inactivate it. This inactivation can itself be oncogenic because the vital control that this protein exerts over mitogenesis is removed. Among the inactivating mutations are deletions of the whole gene, as has been found in a number of colon cancers, and mutations in the gene resulting in amino acid substitutions in the encoded p53 protein. These substitutions cause conformational changes in the protein that result in its inability to perform its antioncogenic function in the cell (Brandt-Rauf, 1996).

Many different point mutations in p53 have been identified in human tumors (Soussi, 1994). The effect of these mutations is to cause a loss of the normal growth-inhibitory function of p53 and, at the same time, some of these mutations result in p53 proteins with considerably increased half-lives so that the mutant proteins accumulate in the transformed cells (Soussi, 1994).

The c-myc oncoprotein is activated to cause cell transformation by overexpression, so it, too, accumulates in transformed cells (Field, 1990). Thus for both p53 and p62/75 myc, increased levels of the proteins can be detected in transformed cells and human tumors (Field, 1990; Soussi, 1994). This overexpression apparently results in leakage of the proteins into the extracellular environment. Not only can these proteins therefore be detected in serum and other body fluids, but these normally sequestered proteins are recognized as foreign, so that some cancer patients develop antibodies to p53 or p62/75 myc. As a result, increased concentrations of p53 or p62/75 or of antibodies to these proteins in blood are excellent markers for tumor detection, for following treatment efficacy and for prognosis.

Detection of Malignancies by Assaying for p53 Protein

Hepatocellular Carcinoma

Increased levels of mutant p53 in serum by ELISA (>0.3 ng/mL, the upper limit of 100 normals) have been found in 20% of patients with HCC and 30% of patients with cirrhosis, a group known to be at increased risk for the development of HCC (Virji, 1992). Because patients with cirrhosis have high levels of p53 in their sera and a known risk factor for developing HCC, the elevated p53 levels may be an early indicator of tumorigenesis.

Breast and Lung Cancers

There have been few studies on p53 as a tumor marker in the sera of patients with breast and lung cancers. Elevated serum mutant p53 levels determined by ELISA have been reported in 8% of breast cancer patients, with levels decreasing following surgical resection of the tumors (Rosanelli, 1993), indicating that the tumors were the source of the elevated p53. Elevations of p53 protein have not been observed in the sera of any normal individuals.

For lung cancer, elevated serum mutant p53 levels determined by ELISA and immunoblotting have been found in up to 34% of lung cancer patients but not in normal individuals (Fontanini, 1994). For these patients, immunohistochemical staining of subsequently obtained biopsy tissue showed elevated p53 levels, correlating with the serum findings.

Colon Cancer

An important mechanism believed to be operative in the development of colonic carcinoma is the deletion of the normal p53 gene or mutation of the gene leading to a nonfunctional antioncogenic protein. Elevated serum mutant p53 determined by ELISA has been found in about one in five patients with colon carcinomas and in approximately one in 10 patients with colonic adenomas. Normal individuals were found to be negative for serum p53 protein. These results show relatively low sensitivity of this marker for colon cancer, possibly because deletion of the p53 gene occurred in a high percentage of the tumors studied.

Bladder Cancer

Studies on the urine of patients with bladder cancer using PCR for p53 on shed cells in urine samples found that the p53 gene was mutated in a high proportion of these patients (Sidransky, 1991), supporting the use of p53 in screening for this disease in a completely noninvasive manner. As discussed later, p53, together with several other promising markers, may result in a set of tests that have a high positive predictive value.

Circulating Anti-p53 Antibodies in Tumor Detection

Serum antibodies against p53 have been reported to be a frequent occurrence in patients with several types of cancer. Production of antibodies to p53 and other oncoproteins has been attributed to their accumulation in necrotic cells and their subsequent release into the circulation, where they are recognized as foreign (Pincus, 2003). There is another cause for the development of antibodies to oncogenic p53. Like oncogenic ras-p21, mutant p53 proteins, containing single amino acid substitutions at critical positions in the polypeptide chain, themselves become oncogenic. These amino acid substitutions induce major changes in the conformation of the p53 protein (Brandt-Rauf, 1996; Adler, 1998). Among these changes is the exposure of specific antigenic determinants that are not normally exposed (Pincus, 2003, 2007). If the protein diffuses into the circulation, antibodies against these determinants often develop.

Antibodies to p53 Are Present in the Sera of Many Patients with Epithelial Cell Tumors and Lymphomas

In several major studies (including a large study of 1392 cancer patients), elevated serum levels of anti-p53 antibodies were found in patients with ovarian and colon cancers (15%); lung cancers, including small cell tumors (up to 25%); and breast cancers, including intraductal carcinoma (up to 15%). Normal individuals did not have elevated serum levels of these antibodies (Angelopoulou, 1994). In a significant number of patients who have been followed for the presence of anti-p53 antibodies in their sera, the appearance of these antibodies has been found to precede the occurrence of malignant tumors. Anti-p53 antibodies are also found to occur in more than 20% of patients with bladder cancer (mostly at more advanced stages), in a high proportion of patients with pancreatic and hepatocellular carcinomas, and in childhood lymphomas.

Anti-p53 in Ovarian Cancer

Further studies on the expression of anti-p53 antibodies in the sera of patients with ovarian cancer have been performed (Tsai-Turton, 2009). Patients with type 2 ovarian cancer, a more aggressive form of this cancer, were found to have anti-p53 antibodies in their sera whereas no patients with less aggressive type 1 cancers were found to have these antibodies in their sera. All of these patients with anti-p53 in their sera were found to have mutant forms of p53 in their cancers; those who did not have mutant p53 in their tumors were not found to have anti-p53 antibodies in their sera, suggesting that mutant p53 is required to provoke this immune response. In all of these seropositive patients, extensive assays for cytokines revealed that interleukin (IL)-4 and 12 were consistently elevated in serum whereas IL-8 was consistently decreased.

Anti-p53 in Hepatocellular Carcinoma

Continuing follow-up studies on anti-p53 antibodies in patients with different cancers reveal that up to half of the patients with HCC, regardless of the size, have markedly elevated serum levels of anti-p53 (Ryder, 1996). These elevated levels correlate with the known elevation of p53 in the sera of patients with this type of cancer.

Anti-p53 in Oral and Esophageal Cancers

Anti-p53 antibodies have likewise been found in the sera of patients with oral lesions, and many of these patients were found to have premalignant lesions (Kaur, 1997), indicating that anti-p53 antibodies are markers for early detection of oral cancer. Anti-p53 has also been found to be elevated in more than 50% of patients with esophageal squamous cell carcinoma (Shimada, 1998), indicating that anti-p53 may be a very useful one in the diagnosis of this disease.

Anti-p53 in Lung Cancers

In a prospective study of patients with carcinoma of the lung, serum anti-p53 levels were found in 100% of patients with large cell carcinoma, 28% with adenocarcinomas, 55% with squamous cell carcinomas, and 71% with small-cell carcinomas (Segawa, 1998). These results demonstrate that elevated serum anti-p53 levels are tumor-type-specific for carcinoma of the lung, showing high positivity rates for large and small cell lung carcinomas.

Anti-p53 Predicts Cancer Occurrence in Patients with Asbestos Exposure

A retrospective study (Li, 2004) of 103 patients with a known prolonged exposure to asbestos whose serum was banked between the years 1980 and 1988 has been performed. These patients were all followed until the end of 2001. Assays for anti-p53 antibodies were performed on the banked sera. It was found that, of 49 patients who developed cancer, 13 (26.5%) had significantly elevated levels of anti-p53 antibodies in their sera although four of the 54 (7.4%) individuals who did not develop cancer were found to have these antibodies. In all four cases, the antibody levels were found initially to be marginally greater than the cutoff for positivity but, for all four, subsequent banked serum samples were found to be antibody-negative.

In contrast, in all 13 cancer patients for whom multiple samples were available, all samples were positive for these antibodies. Statistical analysis of these results showed that the presence of anti-p53 antibodies is an independent predictor of cancer occurrence and that survival in anti-p53–antibody-free patients is significantly greater than in anti-p53–antibody-positive patients.

Anti-p53 in Colorectal Cancer

Serum anti-p53 antibodies have been found to be reliable indicators of postoperative recurrence of colorectal cancer (Tang, 2009). In patients whose preoperative anti-p53 titers were elevated, elevated postoperative serum anti-p53 antibody titers were found to be better indicators of tumor recurrence than serum elevation of carcinoembryonic antigen (CEA), the classic serum marker for colorectal cancer as discussed in Chapter 73.

myc Oncogene–Encoded Protein in Tumor Detection

The myc gene codes for a protein of molecular mass of 75kDa that functions as a transcription factor. When activated, it derepresses expression of other genes that encode proteins involved in replication. This oncogene is overexpressed in a number of tumors, including Burkitt's lymphoma wherein the myc gene on chromosome 8 is translocated to a long terminal repeat–like region of an immunoglobulin-coding region of chromosome 14. Long terminal repeat regions allow constitutive expression of genes that are adjacent to them.

c-myc–related proteins and antibodies to the c-myc protein, such as p53 and antibodies to it, have been identified in the serum of cancer patients. Detection of this 62/75 kDa protein is hampered by its short half-life in serum. However, it is possible to detect a specific c-myc–related p40 protein in the serum of these patients, using immunoblotting. The highest frequencies of occurrence of myc protein in human serum has been found to occur in breast (about 20%) and colon cancer. Treatment of both types of cancer results in marked diminution in the serum levels of this protein. Recurrences result in elevated levels; c-myc protein is therefore useful in following the course of malignant tumors. It has not been detected in the sera of normal individuals.

Serum Anti–c-myc Protein Antibodies in Tumor Detection in Breast Cancer, Ovarian Cancer, Leukemias, and Lymphomas

High serum levels of anti–c-myc antibodies have been found in the sera of patients with colorectal cancer (55%–65%) and in the sera of patients with both myeloid leukemias and Burkitt's lymphoma. Lower occurrences of elevated antibodies have been reported in patients with breast cancer (around 10%) and ovarian cancers (10%). Anti–c-myc antibodies have not been found in the sera of normal individuals.

Combined Oncogene Marker Proteins for Detection of Colorectal Cancer

As is discussed later, since the development of gene, mRNA, and protein arrays, it is now possible to screen for multiple oncogene proteins at the same time. Recently, a study was performed in which the peripheral blood leukocytes of patients with colorectal cancer at all stages and of a control group were assayed for overexpression of ras-p21, myc, and p53 proteins. All of the patients with colorectal cancer were found to have marked overexpression of all three oncoproteins compared with the control group (Csontos, 2008). This study is significant both because three oncoproteins were overexpressed consistently in this disease and because it involves the novel use of leukocytes, rather than serum, to assay for oncoprotein expression, pointing to a new diagnostic approach.

Nuclear Matrix Proteins—Detection of Bladder Cancer

Important targets of oncogene-encoded proteins are nuclear matrix proteins (NMPs) (Fig. 74-1), also referred to as *nuclear skeletal proteins*, and nuclear mitotic apparatus proteins. These 236 kDa proteins are vital for correct mitotic spindle formation. They contain a globular head and tail separated by a central rod-like α-helical core domain consisting of heptad repeat sequences. These proteins vary by cell type, stage of differentiation, and cell cycle. Crucially, a number of tumor-associated NMPs has been identified, each specific for one of five tumor types (bladder, prostate, breast, colon, and bone). The best studied is one strongly associated with transitional cell carcinoma of the bladder, NMP22, which functions as a nuclear mitotic apparatus protein, involved with chromosomal separation during mitosis (Hughes, 1999). The amount of this protein in malignant transitional epithelial cells is 10–20 times that in normal cells.

NMP-22 Is an Excellent Biomarker for Bladder and Urothelial Cancers

Antibodies that are specific for this NMP have been developed and are now used in a commercial ELISA on urine (Matritech/Berlex, Newton, MA). Since malignant urothelial cells in patients with bladder cancer are frequently exfoliated into the urine of these patients, this protein from the lysed cancer cells can be detected at elevated levels. Multiple studies of patients who have bladder cancers of a variety of different stages reveal that the sensitivity is close to 90% in malignant, invasive cancer and 75% in carcinoma in situ. The latter result is highly encouraging, since this stage is the earliest detectable one. For malignant papillary, noninvasive carcinoma, the sensitivity is 62%. The overall specificity for this marker ranges from around 73% to as high as 90% depending on the specific study.

Comparison of the sensitivity of NMP22 ELISA with that of cytology reveals that the two methods are about 83% sensitive for invasive carcinoma, but for grade I transitional cell carcinoma, NMP22 is 61% sensitive whereas cytology is only 17% sensitive (Landman, 1998). For grades II and III cancers, the NMP22 ELISA is more sensitive at 78% and 93% than cytologic sensitivities of 50% and 87%, respectively (Landman, 1998).

More recently, studies have compared overall sensitivity and specificity of NMP-22 with the sensitivity and specificity of urine cytology in screening for urothelial cancer of all types and stages. One prospective study of 103 patients found that NMP-22 and cytology gave approximately the same sensitivities and specificities, that is, 69% sensitivity and 76% specificity for NMP-2 and 75% sensitivity and 73% specificity for urine cytology (Hautmann, 2007). On the other hand, another large study of 93 patients with bladder cancer, 42 patients with benign urothelial conditions and 50 normal volunteers found that NMP-22 had a sensitivity of 78% and a specificity of 73% whereas cytology had a sensitivity of 24% and a specificity of 97% (Tsui, 2007). In a study for recurrent bladder cancer in a large cohort of patients it was found that the sensitivity (85.7%), specificity (77.5%), positive predictive value (70.6%), and negative predictive value (89.6%) of NMP-22 alone was almost the same when it was combined with urine cytologic findings, presumably because the sensitivity of NMP-22 is higher than that for urine cytology (Gupta, 2009). These findings again suggest that NMP-22 is more effective overall in screening for bladder cancer than urine cytology.

NMP-22 testing has been approved by the US Food and Drug Administration (FDA), both for screening for the presence of bladder cancer and for the follow-up of bladder cancer in patients who have been treated for this disease. With respect to the latter use of this method, clinical studies have been performed in which the NMP22 ELISA was performed on the urine of patients who have been treated for transitional cell carcinoma, 20–60 days following treatment, who were then subjected to cystoscopy 2–6 months following treatment. Using a cutoff of 10 U/mL, 86% of patients with negative (<10 U/mL) NMP22 values were found to have negative cystoscopic results, and 71% of patients with values greater than 10 U/mL were found to have positive cystoscopic findings. These results, combined with those of other studies, suggest that this methodology may obviate the necessity for performing cystoscopy on many patients who are being followed for tumor recurrence (Miyanaga, 1997).

NMP-22 can be used to monitor the recurrence or bladder cancer after resection. However, because recurrent tumors are smaller than initial tumors, cutoff values should be altered in these cases as the sensitivity of this test increases from 19% to 49% when the cutoff value is reduced to 5.0 U/mL (Miyanaga, 2003).

Bladder Tumor Antigen

Several other biomarkers for bladder cancer are also being used to aid in the diagnosis and follow-up of this disease. Prominent among these is the so-called bladder tumor antigen, which measures a human complement H protein that is produced by malignant but not by normal transitional epithelial cells. This marker has a somewhat lower sensitivity than that for NMP-22 (Tsui, 2007) and also has a lower specificity due to false-positive results from trauma to the urothelial tract. However, use of NMP-22 together with bladder tumor antigen and a number of other markers, including urokinase-type plasminogen activator, can improve the overall sensitivity of bladder cancer detection (Shariat, 2003). It should be further noted that other tests on urine, such as those for mutant or absent p53 discussed previously and for homozygous deletion of the 9p21 chromosome, discussed later, also have high diagnostic yields. Because these tests are relatively simple to perform, it is conceivable that they can be placed on a chip that will allow for simultaneous evaluations. A positive result on one or more test would suggest the occurrence of bladder cancer.

Use of Multiple Oncoprotein Markers in the Diagnosis of Cancer

Early detection of cancer using oncoproteins has been enhanced by two new developments: (1) use of oncoprotein and oncogene arrays (i.e., use of multiple oncoproteins and multiple oncogenes) and (2) proteomics (i.e., identification of differential protein expression in the sera and body fluids of patients with specific cancers compared with expression in the sera and body fluids of control groups). The proteomic approach has been further modified to include the identification of major proteins whose levels are expressed at high or low levels reproducibly in the sera or body fluids of patients with specific cancers but not in those of patients with benign disease or of normal individuals.

MULTIPLE ONCOPROTEIN ASSAY IN PATIENTS AT RISK FOR TUMOR DEVELOPMENT IN PATIENTS WITH PNEUMOCONIOSIS

In a prospective study, 46 patients with a history of exposure to carcinogens and with attendant pneumoconiosis participated in a study in which their sera were assayed for elevated levels of five oncoproteins: ras-p21, Fes, Myb, PDGF, and Int-1. Eighteen of these patients were found to have cancer, including 13 with lung cancer or mesothelioma, at the time the assays were performed. Of these 18 patients, 13 were found to have markedly elevated levels of at least one of the five oncoproteins for which the assays were performed. Eight of these patients were found to have elevations of at least two of these proteins. Another seven patients were found to have elevations of at least two of these oncoproteins but were not found to have cancer. Although some of these latter patients were lost to follow-up, long term follow-up revealed the subsequent development of cancer in all of the remaining patients. Importantly, several of the patients with only one elevated marker were found to have elevations of different tumor markers in their serum, emphasizing the importance of assaying for as many different oncoproteins as possible (Qin, 2002).

ONCOPROTEIN ARRAYS LIKEWISE HOLD PROMISE IN DETECTING ANTIONCOPROTEIN ANTIBODIES IN SERA

Based on the findings that many patients with cancers are found to have antibodies to a variety of oncoproteins, such as p53 and Myc, studies have been performed to detect one or more such antibodies in patients' sera. In one such study, a miniarray of up to seven full length recombinant oncoproteins was prepared and included such oncoproteins as Myc and p53.

This array was employed to detect antibodies in 527 sera from patients with six different types of cancer (Zhang, 2003). The antibody frequency to any one oncoprotein was on the order of 15%–20%, but inclusion of all seven oncoproteins resulted in detection of up to 68%. Furthermore, distinct patterns of antibody expression were found for patients with breast, lung, and prostate cancer, whereas no discrete patterns were found for patients with gastric, colorectal, or hepatocellular carcinomas. These encouraging results can be enhanced by the inclusion of more oncoproteins. Given the results regarding detection of single oncoproteins, it would seem even more effective to construct arrays with the antibodies to the large number of known oncoproteins in cancer patients to assay for the presence of increased levels of these and/or mutated forms.

Proteomic Approaches to Early Detection of Cancer in Serum

The aforementioned approaches to tumor detection are based on using known oncoproteins that are expressed in uncontrolled cell proliferation. Alternatively, other approaches, mainly the so-called proteomic approach, described extensively in Chapter 77, have been developed over the past several years to search for the expression of multiple proteins (hence the term *proteomic*) that occur uniquely in human cancers and not in normal and nonmalignant cells. These proteins are then used to detect tumors at an early stage. These techniques involve two-dimensional polyacrylamide gel electrophoresis on protein extracts, from tissue and serum, which are first labeled with different fluorochromes (Wulfkuhle, 2003). The resulting gels from cancer patients are compared with those from normal subjects to detect differences in fluorescent labeling. Bands that differ are eluted and subjected to mass spectrometry to determine molecular weight and fragmentation patterns.

Ultimately, mass spectroscopy, the principles of which are described in Chapters 4, 23, and 77, can be used to obtain sequence information on these proteins. Using this technique, the RS/DI-1 protein that regulates protein–RNA interactions has been identified as a circulating protein in the sera of breast cancer patients but not in normal individuals. Likewise, the protein PGP9.5 has been found to occur in the sera of patients with lung cancer (Wulfkuhle, 2003).

This approach has therefore shown promise in identifying unique markers for different types of cancer. However, it requires high concentrations of proteins to enable detection on the two-dimensional gels and is quite time-consuming. Nonetheless, it is a powerful method for the discovery of proteins that are unique to specific types of tumor.

Another, more direct and more sensitive approach has been designed that enables detection of cancer in the serum of affected patients. In this method the sera of patients is directly applied to a chip, which allows for the partial separation of the proteins in the sample. The chip is then subjected to surface-enhanced laser desorption ionization time of flight (SELDI-TOF) mass spectrometry, as described in Chapters 4 and 77. This produces a complex pattern of protein and protein ion fragments with different mass-to-charge ratios (Wulfkuhle, 2003).

The patterns for the sera of patients with cancer are compared with those from normal individuals using computer pattern-recognition algorithms (some of them based on neural network theory) that can distinguish cancer patterns from normal ones. Importantly, the normal sera provide a "training set" of patterns that defines the normal pattern while a second set of sera from known cancer patients defines the cancer training set (Wulfkuhle, 2003). The idea of profiling patients with different tumor types is consistent with the earlier discussion, in which it was noted that certain patterns of anti-oncoprotein antibody occurrence in serum appear to characterize specific cancers.

APPLICATION OF THE PROTEOMIC APPROACH TO THE DIAGNOSIS OF CANCERS

Ovarian Cancer

The proteomic pattern-recognition approach was applied to 25 patients with ovarian cancers at all stages and a group of unaffected individuals. The sera were analyzed in a blind study. The method resulted in detecting 100% of the patients with ovarian cancer, including 18 who had stage I (early) disease. All the sera from the unaffected patients were identified as being negative for ovarian cancer (Wulfkuhle, 2003). On the other hand, the sera from patients with other types of cancer could not be classified by the algorithm, suggesting that ovarian cancer has a unique protein "profile."

Prostate Cancer

Similar results have been obtained now for patients with breast and prostate cancers. In one study, using an algorithm that incorporated a decision tree classification system, the method had a sensitivity of 83% and a specificity of 97% in distinguishing sera from patients with prostate cancer from sera from patients with non-cancerous conditions like benign prostatic hypertrophy (BPH) or with no disease. The sensitivity could be raised to 100% by incorporation of a more robust algorithm (Wulfkuhle, 2003).

As noted in Chapter 73, prostate specific antigen (PSA) is the marker used in the diagnosis of prostate cancer; the upper limit of normal for PSA is taken to be 4 ng/mL but the 4–10 ng/mL range encompasses many false-positive results. Thus this method was applied to patients found to have serum PSA levels of 4–10 ng/mL. It was found that it could accurately predict the occurrence of cancer in 95% of patients with PSA values in this range and could detect 70% (107 of 153 patients) with benign disease but PSA levels greater than 4 ng/mL (upper reference range) (Wulfkuhle, 2003).

Proteomics Show Promise in Early Tumor Detection

The proteomic approach thus appears to be highly promising. Drawbacks include the absence of identity of many of the proteins in the training sets. In the case of prostate cancer detection, different groups who have analyzed the sera of prostate cancer patients and unaffected individuals have obtained different diagnostic protein patterns in none of which PSA has been identified (Diamandis, 2003). Yet PSA is known to be elevated in more than 90% of patients with prostate cancer. Further questions have been raised as to whether important protein molecules such as PSA are present in sufficiently high concentration in a serum sample to be detected by the method and whether the actual patterns really characterize prostate tissue. With identification of the proteins in the training sets, these questions should be resolved.

PROTEIN ARRAYS FOR SPECIFIC TYPES OF CANCER

Proteomic approaches have been modified so as to identify specific critical proteins whose serum levels reliably increase or decrease in specific cancers. Arrays containing these proteins are then employed to screen patients for the presence of specific cancers as we now describe.

Squamous Cell Carcinomas of the Head and Neck

To identify proteins that, as a group, are expressed in oral squamous cell carcinomas (OSCC), human OSCCs were xenotransplanted into mice. Protein expression in the sera of these mice was compared with that in control sera of non-transplanted mice (Bijian, 2009). It was possible to identify a number of proteins whose expressions exhibited major differences between the two groups. Large increases in expression in the sera of mice transplanted with the OSCCs included EGFr, cytokeratins, a G-protein–coupled receptor, Rab11 GTPase, and several other proteins. Arrays containing antibodies to these proteins are being used to screen for this disease.

In a modification of the proteomic method, a large expression array consisting of multiple oncoproteins, cytokines, chemokines, and tumor markers, such as those discussed in Chapter 73, was used to select the best diagnostic combination of these for head and neck cancers (Linkov, 2007). These cancers can be diagnosed with a sensitivity of 84.5% and a specificity of 98% if the following combination of biomarkers was used: EGF, EGFr, IL-8, tissue plasminogen activator inhibitor-1, AFP, matrix metalloproteinase-2, matrix metalloproteinase-3, IFN-α, IFN-γ, IFN-inducible protein-10, regulated on activation, normal T-cell expressed and secreted (RANTES) protein, macrophage inflammatory protein-1α, IL-7, IL-17, IL-1 receptor-α, IL-2 receptor, granulocyte colony-stimulating factor, mesothelin, insulin-like growth factor binding protein 1, E-selectin, cytokeratin-19, vascular cell adhesion molecule, and cancer antigen-125. Using this array on a group of patients with known cancers of the head and neck and a group without this disease, 92% of the patients were correctly diagnosed with this disease.

Breast Cancer

Using a similar approach for breast cancer detection, the sera from 4500 patients with different cancer types including nonmetastatic breast cancer were screened using 50 different protein markers of which 35 were selected (Kim, 2009). When compared with controls, EGF, soluble CD40-ligand, and pro-apolipoprotein A1 were all found to be increased in breast cancer patients while high-molecular-weight kininogen, apolipoprotein A1, soluble vascular cell adhesion molecule-1, plasminogen activator inhibitor-1, vitamin-D binding protein, and fibronectin were decreased in the cancer group. Diagnostic accuracy using these proteins was approximately 90% percent, indicating that the breast cancer array has promise in early detection of this disease.

Lung Cancer

Proteomic methodology has been applied to the sera of a large cohort of patients with squamous cell carcinoma of the lung and a control group (Dowling, 2007). To increase the diagnostic sensitivity of the method, all sera were immunodepleted of all major common serum proteins, such as albumin, and were then subjected to high resolution 2-D electrophoresis and mass spectrosocopy. It has been found that a set of proteins—apolipoprotein A-IV precursor, chain F; human complement component C3c; haptoglobin; serum amyloid A protein precursor; and Ras-related protein Rab-7b—is reproducibly elevated. In addition, another set of proteins, α-2-HS glycoprotein, hemopexin precursor, pro-apolipoprotein, antithrombin III, and SP40, was reproducibly decreased. This resulting lung cancer array appears to be very useful in screening for this disease.

DETECTION OF ONCOGENES IN SERUM AND OTHER BODY FLUIDS

CELL-FREE NUCLEIC ACID TESTING IN CANCER

Protein tumor markers and histopathologic staging have been the cornerstones of diagnosis and prognosis of malignancy. As mentioned earlier in the G-proteins subsection on ras for detection of pancreatic cancer using amplified ras DNA in serum, the discovery of cell-free nucleic acids in serum, plasma, urine, or other body fluids over the past decade has promoted investigation of oncogenes encoding oncoproteins as an additional means to detect malignancy in a variety of cancers with potentially greater sensitivity (Schmidt, 2004). These studies include melanoma (Kopreski, 1999; Board, 2009), lung (Fleischhacker, 2001; Schmidt, 2004; He, 2009), stomach (Park, 2009), colon (Silva, 2002), breast (Chen, 2000; Gal, 2001), prostate (Goessl, 2001, 2002), ovary (Hickey, 1999), Epstein-Barr virus–positive lymphomas (Lechowicz, 2002; Lei, 2002), leukemia (Schwarz, 2009), intracranial neoplasms (Rhodes, 1994), and bladder (Goessl, 2001, 2002; Utting, 2002; Guo, 2009).

The basic concept is that tumor-derived nucleic acid can be detected in cell-free sources, such as serum, plasma, urine, and lavage fluid, using amplification methods such as RT-PCR or other detection methods (Goldshtein, 2009). Normally, DNA is isolated from tissue through standard procedures using phenol chloroform extraction followed by ethanol precipitation. However, DNA can also be obtained directly from serum, plasma, or other body fluids by centrifugation, separating it from cells and platelets. The methodology of cell-free nucleic-acid–based detection includes detection of gene mutations, microsatellite alterations, and promoter hypermethylation.

GENE MUTATIONS

These normally involve nucleic acid sequencing and can detect single base changes in genomic or mitochondrial DNA (gDNA and mtDNA, respectively). mtDNA can have 20–200 copies of DNA compared with two copies of gDNA. Mutated mtDNA was detected in three of three patients (100%) with prostate cancer (Jeronimo, 2001), whereas others have reported a lower mtDNA detection rate in patients with colorectal cancer (Anker, 1997; Hibi, 2001). Tumor and plasma DNA of 25 patients with breast or small cell lung cancer were analyzed for the presence of p53 gene mutations. Six patients had detectable mutations in their tissue, and three of these six (50%) had mutations detected in their plasma (Silva, 1999). Furthermore, although gene mutations have been detected in tissue obtained from malignant and healthy patients, the same is not true for plasma. Mutations detected in plasma are very specific for malignancy (Johnson, 2002). To this end recent studies which analyzed plasma DNA of patients with HCC for p53 codon 249 by restriction fragment length polymorphism demonstrated that 6 (7.6%) of 79 samples from the HCC patients had amplifiable plasma DNA whereas none of the 73 samples with amplifiable plasma DNA from the controls had this mutation (Igetei, 2008).

MICROSATELLITE ALTERATIONS

Microsatellites are short sequences of DNA of between 2 and 6 base pairs that repeat multiply across the genome. The simplest of these is the dinucleotide CA. If these microsatellites occur in or near critical genes, they cause frameshifts in coding resulting in functional inactivation of the gene. One set of affected genes is the mismatch repair genes that encode enzymes that correct mismatched bases in DNA. The enzymes are then no longer present to correct mutations that occur in other critical genes, including tumor suppressor genes such as those encoding p53, Rb, and p16. As a result, tumor suppression genes are inactivated, allowing for the possibility of uncontrolled cell proliferation. As long as there is one normal allele of tumor suppressor genes, tumor suppression can still occur. However, if the lesion is extended to the normal allele, a loss of heterozygosity (LOH) occurs, resulting in complete absence of expression of the encoded tumor suppression protein product.

Microsatellite DNA is detectable by microsatellite analysis using PCR. A panel of four to six appropriate markers to detect these microsatellites can be used to profile tumors. LOH requires at least 20% of tumor DNA within normal DNA. Microsatellite instability refers to detection of additional PCR products and requires a ratio of tumor to normal DNA of greater than 0.5% (Goessl, 2001, 2002).

Microsatellite alterations performed on cell-free bronchial lavage specimens from lung cancer patients revealed tumor-associated genes in 47% if DNA was used as the source material (n = 30) and in 100% if RNA was used (n = 25) (Schmidt, 2004). In addition, four microsatellite loci were detected in the sera of 17 of 34 patients with breast cancer; LOH at various loci was observed in 16 patients, and microsatellite instability was detected in one patient (Schwarzenbach, 2004). However, no correlation was found between circulating tumor DNA and the level of tumor-associated protein marker CA 15-3 (Schwarzenbach, 2004; see Chapter 73 on serodiagnostic tumor markers). Plasma LOH has also been found in patients with recurrent bladder cancer, for which it appears to be a reliable marker (Dominguez, 2002). Recently, microsatellite alterations were detected in plasma DNA obtained from patients with malignant melanoma (Nakamoto, 2008) where metastasis or recurrence was confirmed in three (17.6%) of 17 patients; all of them were found to have LOH at four microsatellite markers, further suggesting the use of such loci markers as a screening tool.

PROMOTER HYPERMETHYLATION

Methylation of CpG islands, located in the promoter region of many genes, is associated with their transcriptional inactivation. Thus aberrant hypermethylation of key tumor suppressor genes can permit expression of otherwise quiescent oncogenes. Promoter hypermethylation can be detected by methylation-specific PCR (MSP), and the reduced protein expression can be determined by immunohistochemistry. MSP requires a ratio of tumor to normal DNA of 0.001%–0.1% (Goessl, 2001, 2002; Bearzatto, 2002). Another method, quantitative methylation analysis of minute DNA amounts after whole bisulfitome amplification, (qMAMBA) allows quantitative and sensitive detection of DNA methylation in minute amounts of DNA present in body fluids (Vaissière, 2009). Aberrant methylation of at least one of four tumor suppressor genes was detected in tissue biopsies from 15 of 22 (68%) patients with non–small cell lung cancer. Of the 15 patients with positive non–small cell lung cancer, 11 (73%) also had abnormal methylated DNA in their serum samples (Esteller, 1999). In addition, 17 of 27 bladder cancer patients (63%) displayed alterations in tumor suppressor genes in cell- and serum-derived DNA (Dominguez, 2002). As noted later, deletion of the p16 tumor suppressor gene is an important causative factor of bladder cancer.

Patterns of gene methylation have been determined for lung cancer (Hsu, 2007). In a study in which methylation of a variety of genes was determined, it was found that methylation of two genes, the p16 anti-oncogene and the Ras-association domain family 1 gene (RASSF1A), occurred with high frequency in lung cancer patients but not in a non–lung cancer control group. Using the methylation status of these two genes for diagnosing lung cancer, the sensitivity was 73% and the specificity 82%. These results appear to support the prior results on methylation of tumor suppressor genes in lung cancer (Esteller, 1999).

Interpretation of results obtained from cell-free testing warrants caution in that results may vary depending on the detection method (promoter hypermethylation, gene rearrangements, microsatellite alterations, PCR, RT-PCR, the sample tested [Lee, 2001], and the nucleic acid source used [RNA, DNA] [Fleishhacker, 2001; Garcia, 2001; Johnson, 2002; Schmidt, 2004]). Nonetheless this remains a promising new modality for early cancer detection (Chan, 2002; Lechowicz, 2002; Board, 2009; Goldshtein, 2009).

GENE ARRAYS DETECTING ONCOPROTEIN ABNORMALITIES

Circulating DNA from mutated oncogenes can be readily detected in the serum of cancer patients (Sorenson, 1994; de Kok, 1997).Use of PCR methodology has successfully identified ras-p21 in the stool of patients with colorectal cancer, altered p53 in the urine of patients with bladder cancer (Sidransky, 1991), and ras, neu/HER2, and PDGF in the bile of patients with biliary tract cancer (Su, 2001). Given the existence now of microchips that contain entire genomes that can be hybridized with the total RNA of cells to detect different levels of gene expression (see Chapter 67), studies using such chips on which different oncogenes are present may be effective in detecting expression of specific oncogenes present in body fluids from patients with different cancers.

That these types of studies are feasible has been demonstrated in a study on the tissue of 20 squamous cell esophageal carcinomas (Arai, 2003). A total of 57 oncogenes were present on the array and included many of the oncogenes discussed here, including FGF, erb-B2 (neu/HER2), and myc. In nine of the 20 specimens, expression of eight oncogenes, including erb-B2 and myc, was two to four times higher than in normal control tissue. Comparison of these results with those obtained using conventional hybridization methods revealed that, frequently, this gene amplification was found not to be due to an increase in copy number. As noted earlier, the p53 gene is frequently overexpressed and/or mutated in squamous cell carcinomas of the esophagus and in head and neck squamous cell carcinomas. Unfortunately, p53 was not included on this array. In addition, this study did not include hybridization assays for mutant genes.

Nonetheless, these studies illustrate that oncogenes are frequently overexpressed in human cancers and can be detected on gene arrays. The earlier PCR studies on body fluids illustrate that gene amplification and mutation can also be readily detected in these body fluids. Therefore gene arrays containing large numbers of different oncogenes, allowing for rapid assays, appear to hold great promise in tumor detection on body fluids.

CELL DNA TESTING FOR CANCER USING FLUORESCENCE IN SITU HYBRIDIZATION

This technique is described in Chapter 68. In brief, fluorophore-labeled DNA oligonucleotide probes containing sequences known to occur uniquely on specific chromosomes are incubated with cells concentrated from body fluids, including blood and urine. These probes are so constructed that they hybridize either to specific normally occurring DNA sequences on specific chromosomes or to known abnormally occurring spliced chromosomal sequences (usually the result of translocations). The latter often produce either overexpressed mitogenic proteins or mutated constitutively activated mitogenic proteins. This methodology has potential application to many disease states including malignancies (Goldshtein, 2009). This technique also detects critical gene deletions that can be identified by the absence of fluorescence of one or both probes in cells.

An example of the application of this technique is in the diagnosis of bladder cancer for which a test, the Vysis-Abbott Urovision detection system, has been developed and has been FDA-approved. A critical and common chromosomal lesion in this disease is the 9p21 homozygous deletion, perhaps the most constant genetic finding in bladder cancer. This results in deletion of a tumor suppressor gene that codes for the p16 antioncogene protein, again resulting in loss of control of mitotic rate (Halling, 2002, 2003).

An oligonucleotide probe, labeled with a gold fluorescent dye, has been developed to a sequence of 9p21. In addition, several other oligonucleotide probes have been prepared, linked to other colored fluorescent dyes, that hybridize to specific sequences in the centromeres of other "control" chromosomes. A mixture of these probes is incubated with cells obtained from the urinary sediments of patients and subjected to fluorescence microscopy. If the cells are normal, duplicate colored spots, from diploid normal chromosomes, appear in these cells.

On the other hand, absence of one or both gold spots for chromosome 9p21 but the presence of duplicate fluorescent spots for the control probes is a strong indication of 9p21 deletion and the presence of urothelial (most probably, bladder) cancer. It should be noted that this hybridization procedure is also capable of detecting malignant aneuploid bladder epithelial cells (with multiple copies of chromosomes) directly.

This method has a sensitivity of 36% for grade 1 cancers, 76% for grade 2, and almost 100% for grade 3 cancers and an overall specificity of 97% (Halling, 2002, 2003). It therefore has great potential in detecting bladder cancer, especially if it is combined with probes for other genetic lesions known to occur in this disease as discussed earlier. In addition, multiple probes for known chromosomal lesions in a variety of lymphomas and leukemias have been prepared and are promising for the detection of these diseases in body fluids and tissue (see Chapter 75).

DIAGNOSTIC EFFICACY OF SERUM ONCOPROTEINS

The results of assays for the different oncoproteins discussed earlier in serum and urine (NMP-22) , on several thousand patients, are summarized in Figure 74-3 for different tumor types. The figure shows three-dimensional graphs of tumor type (*y*-axis), tumor marker (*x*-axis), and percentage of cases of each tumor type successfully detected by each marker. The results for each marker is given as a specifically colored three-dimensional bar graph. From Figure 74-3, it is clear that, of the proteins studied thus far, positivity rates (sensitivities) vary from less than 30% (myc oncoprotein sensitivity is 8% in breast cancer) to more than 80 percent (e.g., ras in angiosarcoma). However, all of the control groups, given adjacent to each tumor type with an "N" in parenthesis, show very low positivity rates, and are, in most instances, 0. Therefore, whereas the sensitivities of oncoprotein markers vary, *their specificities are exceptionally high*, in the 95%–100% range; that is, there are very few false-positive results. Therefore, if a mutated or overexpressed oncoprotein is detected in the serum or other body fluid of a patient, there is a high probability that the patient has some form of malignancy. Also, the sensitivities and specificities of oncoproteins in diagnosing cancer exceed those of the oncofetal antigens, such as CEA or AFP (see Chapter 73).

How Specific Is Oncoprotein Expression for Different Cancer Types?

Interestingly, although the oncoproteins studied are from signal transduction pathways that are involved in many different types of cells, there seems to be some specificity of expression of particular oncoproteins for certain types of cancer. For example, the growth factor TGF-α is elevated in a large proportion of colorectal, brain, and ovarian cancers, whereas TGF-β is elevated in hepatocellular, lung, and bladder cancers; the p185 ECD (neu) protein is elevated in the sera of many patients with breast (at more advanced stages) carcinomas (Fig. 74-3, *B*); ras-p21 protein is elevated in colorectal and hepatocellular carcinomas, and angiosarcomas of the liver and lung cancers; p53 is elevated in colorectal and lung cancers and is elevated uniquely in oropharyngeal cancers, although, as discussed earlier, protein arrays designed for diagnosis of these cancers are now available. In addition, it is elevated in a high proportion of lymphomas. Anti-Myc antibody is elevated in many colon cancers and, interestingly, in a high proportion of prostate cancers. This latter finding suggests the need for further investigation. For example, elevated serum anti-Myc may aid in the definitive diagnosis of prostate cancer in patients with elevated serum PSA. In view of the recent findings that the ECD of EGFr is elevated in 93% of patients with prostate cancer in one series (Milanese, 2009), this oncoprotein may likewise enable definitive diagnosis of prostate cancer.

Sensitivities of Oncoprotein Expression

As noted earlier, the sensitivities of oncoproteins in diagnosing specific cancers vary. Because of the multistep nature of carcinogenesis, there are many potential oncoproteins that may become abnormal. In some types of cancers, pathways may be activated that are not activated in other types of cancers. This phenomenon occurs even within one type of cancer. For example, ras and neu are elevated in the sera of patients with lung cancer but not elevated in patients with lymphomas since different signal transduction proteins are involved in these two different types of cancers. Also, ras and neu do not detect all lung cancers because these cancers differ with respect to affected signal transduction proteins among themselves, and some of them do not involve these two signal transduction proteins.

The next step, therefore, in using these oncoprotein markers in the early diagnosis of cancer is to assay for multiple markers in a given patient's serum, because discovery of at least one aberrant component of the signal transduction pathway is much more likely. If at least one positive result is found, the patient can be followed for signs of the development of a tumor.

As discussed previously, progress has been made in this area. Protein and gene arrays for multiple oncoproteins and oncogenes have been constructed and have succeeded in increasing the rate of positive diagnoses for cancer in patients. Furthermore, the advent of the proteomic/pattern recognition approach to cancer detection is proving to be successful in studies in which it has been thus far tested, that is, in the diagnosis of ovarian, prostate, and breast cancers. Combination of these two methods would result in high diagnostic yields; use of both would be feasible in that each can be performed rapidly.

ORIGINS OF MALIGNANCIES

Figure 74-3 indicates that discovery of an elevated level of an oncoprotein in the serum of a patient does not generally give conclusive information as to the source of the malignancy. For example, although ras-p21 has been found to be elevated with some specificity in colon, lung, and angiosarcomas of the liver; and HER2/neu (c-erbB-2) p185 ECD has been found to be elevated in colon, lung, and breast cancers, elevation of one of these oncoproteins in a patient's serum would not allow identification of exactly the tissue of origin of a malignancy. Because the signal transduction pathways in most cells are remarkably similar to one another, an increase in any oncoprotein can signify malignancy in a number of different cell types. On the other hand, using the proteomic approach, serum protein patterns on SELDI-TOF mass spectrometry are uniquely characteristic of specific tumors so that this approach can identify the tissue of origin of the tumor.

Additionally, many studies on the correlations between the presence of tumors and serum levels of oncoproteins remain to be performed. For example, there are no published data on the occurrence of detectable forms of mutant ras-p21 protein in the serum of patients with pancreatic carcinoma with control groups consisting of age- and sex-matched control individuals and with groups containing patients with pancreatitis but no tumors. This is a vitally needed study, because more than 90% of pancreatic cancers express oncogenic ras-p21 (Almoguera, 1988).

One manner of using serum oncoproteins could be to detect specific tumors at an early stage in tumor progression in populations known to be at risk for developing these cancers. These would include patients with a history of occupational exposure to carcinogens or mutagens as seen from the example of patients with a history of vinyl chloride exposure associated with angiosarcoma of the liver. In addition, patients can be followed who have been exposed chronically to asbestos and silica and who have consequent pneumoconioses associated with lung cancer and mesothelioma. Both conditions are associated with elevated serum levels of ras-p21 protein and/or mutant forms of this protein. Patients with pneumoconioses can also be followed with serum levels of p185neu.

TUMOR SIZE AND ONCOPROTEIN LEVELS

Currently, there is little information on the minimum size of a tumor that gives rise to serum elevations of oncoproteins. However, there are indications that small lesions may give rise to significant levels of certain oncoproteins.

First, in a significant number of patients with known cancer risks, oncoproteins were discovered in their sera before the development of detectable cancer. Thus, in patients with asbestosis, the ECD of the

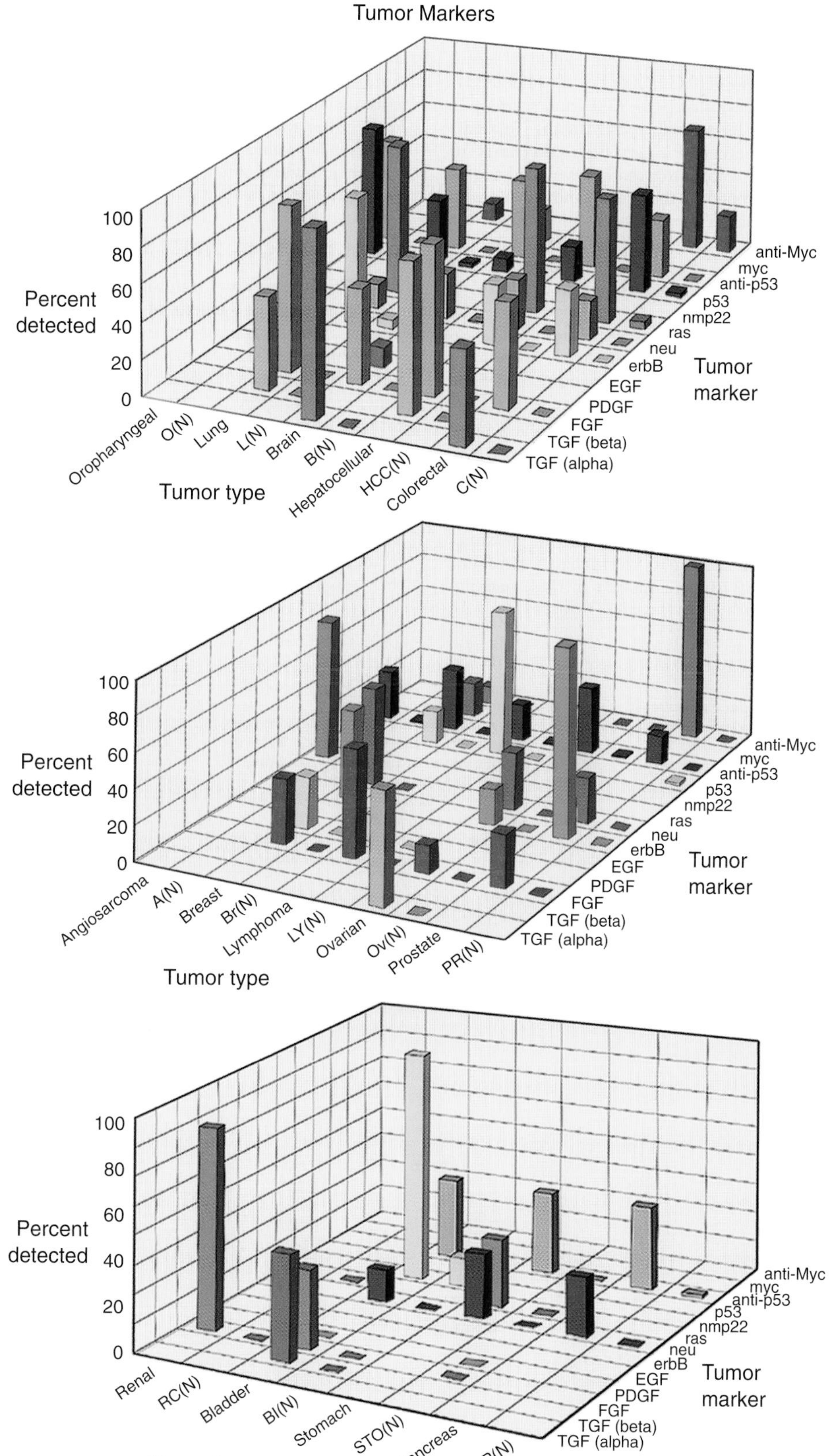

Figure 74-3 Summary of results of serum assays for different components of mitogenic signaling pathways. These are three-dimensional plots of tumor type on the X axis, pathway component on the Y axis, and the percentage detected or the frequency of finding each of the pathway components elevated in the serum of patients with each tumor type on the perpendicular Z axis. Next to the results for each tumor type, the results for control groups are labeled as "N" for "normals," that is, age- and sex-matched controls who were tumor-free. The controls for patients with each tumor type are abbreviated with a single letter (with "N" in parentheses) for each tumor type, such as "B" for brain. *anti-Myc,* Antibody to the Myc protein; *anti-p53,* anti-p53 antibody; *EGF,* epidermal growth factor; *erbB,* epidermal growth factor (EGF) receptor; *FGF,* fibroblast growth factor; *myc,* a nuclear oncogene that encodes the Myc protein; *Neu,* p185 protein that is similar to the erbB protein and is also called erbB-2 and HER2; *NMP-22,* nuclear matrix protein number 22; *p53,* an antioncogene protein *PDGF,* platelet-derived growth factor; *Ras,* p21 protein; *TGF-α,* transforming growth factor-α; *TGF-β,* transforming growth factor-β.

p185erbB protein became elevated *before* lung tumors were diagnosed. Overexpression of the p185 ECD occurred in a number of patients before the diagnosis of breast cancer. East Asian patients who had high serum levels of p185 ECD went on to develop HCC. Patients with pneumoconioses were found to have elevated levels of p185 ECD and/or ras-p21 protein and subsequently developed lung carcinomas. Mutant (Asp 13-) p21 protein was discovered in the serum of a very high percentage of patients with vinyl chloride exposure who subsequently developed angiosarcoma. Anti-p53 antibodies were found in the sera of individuals who subsequently developed angiosarcomas or lung cancers. All these studies suggest that malignant lesions that are undetectable by conventional techniques may be detected by measuring the serum levels of oncoproteins or antibodies to oncoproteins, especially in patients with known exposures or risk factors for cancer.

Second, carcinomas in situ are known to cause elevated levels of oncoprotein elevated serum as evidenced by elevated serum levels of p185neu protein in incipient breast cancer and NMP-22 in carcinoma in situ of the bladder. These findings suggest that serum oncoprotein levels are effective in detecting the presence of small tumors in individuals at an early stage.

It also seems clear that, as the stage progresses, the tumors elaborate higher levels of oncoproteins so that there appears to be a good correlation, at least in some patients, between serum levels of marker oncoproteins and tumor size and/or level of expression of the marker in the tumor tissue itself. In this regard, some small adenomas (<1 cm) have been found to give rise to elevated levels of p185 ECD or ras-p21 in these patients' sera. For both ras-p21 protein and p185erbB ECD, there is an excellent correlation between serum level of these markers and the pretreatment and posttreatment clinical status of the patient. Nonetheless, substantially more correlation studies between tumor size and serum level of oncoproteins remain to be performed. One confounding factor may be that a small tumor may produce large amounts of the marker, whereas larger tumors may produce smaller amounts due to such factors as changes in the oncogenic lesions, affecting which oncoproteins are mutated and/or are overexpressed.

Evaluation and Conclusions

Well-defined pathways for mitogenic signal transduction exist between the membrane and the nucleus of cells. These pathways consist mainly of proteins, mutations in or overexpression of which can give rise to uncontrolled mitogenic signaling and cancer. More recently, based on proteomic approaches, other proteins are being discovered that characteristically are either overexpressed or expressed at much lower levels in the sera of patients with specific types of cancers compared with the levels found in the sera of control groups.

Despite the foregoing caveats in interpretations of elevations of serum levels of oncoproteins or the detection of abnormal forms of these proteins in serum and the need for further correlation studies to be performed, assays for the presence of oncoproteins in serum show exceptional promise for detection of malignant tumors at an early stage and for monitoring their progression, response to therapy, remission, and recurrence.

SELECTED REFERENCES

Brandt-Rauf PW, Pincus MR. Molecular markers of carcinogenesis. Pharmacol Ther 1998;77:135–48.

This is a review of the relevant oncoproteins that have proved to be markers for early tumor detection or that show great promise as biomarkers for early cancer detection.

Halling KC, King W, Sokolova IA, et al. A comparison of BTA stat, hemoglobin dipstick, telomerase and Vysis UroVysion assays for the detection of urothelial carcinoma in urine. J Urol 2002;167:2001–6.

This is a comprehensive review and assessment of different markers for bladder cancer. It emphasizes the value of using FISH as a method for detection of bladder cancer.

Pincus MR, Friedman FK. Oncoproteins in the detection of human malignancies. Mol Diagn 2003;1:23–38.

This is a review of oncoproteins as markers for early tumor detection with an emphasis on oncoproteins as elements of signal transduction pathways.

Segawa Y, Kageyama M, Suzuki S, et al. Measurement and evaluation of serum anti-p53 antibody levels in patients with lung cancer at its initial presentation: a prospective study. Br J Cancer 1998;78:667–72.

This is a valuable study on the use of anti-p53 antibodies as a means for detecting lung cancers.

Slamon DJ, Godolphin W, Jones LA, et al. Studies on the HER-2/neu proto-oncogene in human breast and ovarian cancer. Science 1989;244:707–12.

This landmark paper established Her2/neu as an important factor in breast cancer causation and its use as a prognostic factor for disease progression.

Wulfkuhle JD, Liotta LA, Petricoin EF. Proteomic applications for the early detection of cancer. Nat Rev Cancer 2003;3:267–75.

This clearly written review of different proteomic approaches in detecting cancer in blood samples explains the bases for these approaches that enable a good understanding of each method.

Zhang JY, Casiano CA, Peng XX, et al. Enhancement of antibody detection in cancer using panel of recombinant tumor-associated antigens. Cancer Epidemiol Biomarkers Prev 2003;12:136–43.

This important paper shows that using panels of oncoproteins on blood and body fluids is more effective than using single oncoproteins alone in detecting cancer.

REFERENCES

Access the complete reference list online at http://www.expertconsult.com

CHAPTER 75

MOLECULAR DIAGNOSIS OF HEMATOPOIETIC NEOPLASMS

David R. Czuchlewski, David S. Viswanatha, Richard S. Larson

PART 9

KEY POINTS

- Overview of the role of molecular investigations in the diagnosis, classification, prognosis, and monitoring of hematolymphoid disorders.
- Detailed summary of the major genetic abnormalities and molecular diagnosis of the acute leukemias and chronic myeloproliferative neoplasms.
- Applications and detailed discussion of molecular minimal residual disease monitoring in chronic myeloid leukemia and acute promyelocytic leukemia in the era of targeted therapeutic options.
- Concept of risk-adapted therapy for optimized management of childhood acute lymphoblastic leukemias.
- Molecular pathologic origins of childhood leukemias.
- Description of antigen receptor gene rearrangements and application of molecular clonality assays to identify monoclonal lymphoid proliferations.
- Detailed summary of the major genetic abnormalities and molecular diagnosis of the non-Hodgkin lymphomas and chronic lymphoid leukemias.
- New research and technology developments that will impact molecular diagnosis and prognosis of hematolymphoid cancers.

Role of Clinical Molecular Diagnostics in Hematologic Cancers

The diagnosis of hematolymphoid neoplasms continues to undergo a dramatic transformation with the advent and application of new technologies. Whereas traditional morphologic (light microscopic) evaluation of glass slides still occupies the centerpiece of pathologic diagnosis, the judicious application of ancillary methods, such as special cytochemistry, immunohistochemistry, flow cytometry, cytogenetics (including fluorescence in situ hybridization [FISH]), and molecular genetics, has allowed for much improved diagnostic reproducibility and refinement. Indeed, such elements were formally incorporated into diagnostic hematopathology in the World Health Organization (WHO) classification of hematologic neoplasms (Jaffe, 2001). The rapid pace of research into the molecular underpinnings of hematologic neoplasms necessitated a substantially updated classification in 2008, in which genetic abnormalities continue to assume central importance in our understanding and diagnosis of such processes (Swerdlow, 2008). The relative ease of sampling sites such as the lymph nodes and bone marrow as well as the provision of easily disaggregated viable cell samples for analysis have driven this paradigm of diagnostic evaluation. The nature of the hematolymphoid system is also conducive to relatively easy monitoring of disease status following therapy, which represents another important facet in the management of patients with these illnesses.

Given this plethora of diagnostic tools, what role does molecular genetic evaluation, or molecular diagnostics play? There are perhaps four major scenarios in which molecular diagnostic analysis of a hematolymphoid proliferation is important. First, molecular investigation can establish a diagnosis in situations wherein morphologic details and results of other lab tests are inconclusive for malignancy. The presence of specific genetic abnormalities, or the demonstration of tumor genetic "homogeneity" of a cell population (e.g., by antigen receptor gene rearrangement studies) can establish the presence of a clonal pathologic process. Second, molecular methods are used to subclassify disease entities. To this end, the current WHO classification of hematologic neoplasms includes molecular characterization as a defining feature of many leukemias and lymphomas (Swerdlow, 2008). Next, specific genetic anomalies in hematolymphoid malignancies have important prognostic value, which in turn can influence the initial treatment of certain tumors to produce an optimal clinical outcome. Finally, being potentially of high sensitivity, molecular techniques can be used to assess patients after the onset of therapy, by monitoring for the presence and extent of minimal residual disease (MRD). Table 75-1 summarizes some of the key instances in which molecular diagnostic evaluation is sought in hematopathology practice. As the synergy between expanding basic biologic information and rapidly progressing technology continues unabated, the future holds promise for many additional applications of molecular diagnostics in the pathology laboratory, including the prediction of disease susceptibility, severity, or treatment response based on polygenic factors; pharmacogenomic profiling of patients to determine drug sensitivity and toxicity profiles; and the assessment of individual responses to increasingly "targeted" therapies.

This chapter focuses on the background, clinical rationale, and fundamental technical considerations underlying the molecular diagnostic evaluation and monitoring of hematologic and lymphoid tumors. As the large majority of these laboratory assays are polymerase chain reaction (PCR) based, the emphasis is accordingly placed on methods concerning either DNA or RNA (i.e., reverse-transcription) PCR techniques. Of note, it is apparent that the detection of tumor-specific genetic abnormalities can be achieved by different analytic means, for example, cytogenetics, FISH, or PCR. Although at first glance these various methods may seem redundant, these laboratory techniques should be considered complementary and the choice of methodology is determined by a number of factors, including knowledge of the detection rates, analytic sensitivity, and limitations of various techniques; understanding of the disease pathobiology; the level of interpretive experience and expertise with these procedures; the type of sample; and the phase of the disease under investigation. Table 75-2 indicates comparative analytic sensitivities of the principal modalities used to detect hematolymphoid tumor-related genetic abnormalities.

The increasingly ubiquitous need for molecular genetic evaluation of hematopoietic cancers has initiated earnest attempts to address and achieve better interlaboratory standardization, and such efforts can be expected to continue to improve the benchmarks of sensitivity and specificity in this field. Nonetheless, in the application and interpretation of molecular diagnostic tests, one caveat that cannot be emphasized enough is that the results of these investigations must never be considered in isolation, but rather, in conjunction with the salient clinical, morphologic, and additional laboratory data concerning the individual patient. Regardless of the remarkable specificity and sensitivity of molecular markers, the evident complexity of hematolymphoid neoplasia mandates such a fully integrated approach, in order to diminish the possibility of diagnostic error.

TABLE 75-1
Applications of Molecular Diagnostics in Hematologic and Lymphoid Neoplasia

Indication	Examples
Diagnosis and subclassification	*JAK2* mutations in myeloproliferative neoplasms
	CCND1-IGH@ abnormality in mantle cell lymphoma
	PML-RARA abnormality in APL
	FLT3, NPM1, and *CEPBA* mutations in normal karyotype AML
Determination of tumor clonality	Assessment of abnormal B and T cell lymphoid proliferations
Prognosis and/or therapeutic monitoring	Quantitative PCR monitoring of BCR-ABL1 mRNA in CML patients on tyrosine kinase inhibitor therapy (e.g., imatinib)
	Quantitative PCR monitoring of PML-RARα mRNA in APL
	Multiparameter cytogenetic and molecular assessment of chronic lymphocytic leukemia
	Relapse risk prediction in childhood acute lymphoblastic leukemias
	Outcome prediction of diffuse large B cell lymphoma subtypes by gene expression profiling

ALL, Acute lymphoblastic leukemias; *APL*, acute promyelocytic leukemia; *CML*, chronic myeloid leukemia; *PCR*, polymerase chain reaction.

Molecular Diagnosis of Acute Leukemias

GENE FUSION CONCEPT IN LEUKEMIA AND THE BASIS FOR REVERSE-TRANSCRIPTION POLYMERASE CHAIN REACTION ANALYSIS

The leukemias are hematologic cancers with a diverse pathogenesis and pathobiology. However, a significant proportion of these tumors is characterized by nonrandom, (usually) balanced chromosomal translocations, resulting in the formation of fusion, or chimeric genes. In general, although two such fusions are created in this abnormal event (i.e., one on each reciprocal translocated chromosome), typically only one of these derivative loci gives rise to a leukemogenic "hybrid" gene. At the molecular level, the intronic breakpoint and fusion sites in the involved genes are highly variable among patients with the same type of leukemia, although there may be evidence of clustered breakpoint "hotspots" in certain types of leukemia-related rearranging genes. Despite the variability in breakpoint sites in both of the involved genes, a consistent feature of the leukemic gene fusions is the production of a chimeric messenger ribonucleic acid (mRNA) molecule. This abnormal transcript is further translated to a fusion protein, presumed to be operative in disrupting many cellular pathways involved in regulating normal proliferative capacity, differentiation, and survival in immature (i.e., precursor) marrow stem or progenitor cells.

Although the formation of a translocation fusion gene, such as the well known *BCR-ABL1* abnormality, is known to be necessary for disease production, results from animal models have suggested that, at least for some types of leukemia, this may not be a sufficient event, requiring in addition secondary incompletely characterized genetic insults as well. This concept has been formalized into a general scheme in which leukemogenic abnormalities are considered to be class I or class II, depending, respectively, on whether they provide a proliferative advantage or disturb the complex processes of hematopoietic differentiation. In this conceptualization, the development of leukemia becomes more likely when both class I and class

TABLE 75-2
Relative Sensitivities of Major Techniques Used to Detect Leukemia or Lymphoma-Associated Abnormalities

Method	Analytic sensitivity (%)*	Notes
Cytogenetics	5	Global genomic assessment Requires fresh, sterile cells Detects numerical and structural chromosome aberrations Difficult or impossible to detect alterations in DNA below band resolution
FISH	1–5	Targeted assessment of relatively large genomic abnormalities Technically straightforward and rapid; can frequently be performed on interphase nuclei Applicable to a variety of tissue sources Requires rigorous quality standards to avoid false positive results at low levels of the abnormality in question
SBH	5–10	Targeted assessment for structural abnormalities in genomic DNA Technically laborious and time-intensive Requires samples with well preserved high-molecular-weight DNA (e.g., fresh or frozen cells)
PCR	10^{-2}–10^{-4}	Targeted assessment of small genomic or mRNA abnormalities Detection of unique chimeric fusion gene mRNA species is highly sensitive Technically straightforward and rapid but may require post-PCR detection procedures Applicable to a broad range of sample types, including fixed paraffin-embedded tissues Can be optimized for high sensitivity, minimal residual disease monitoring (real-time quantitative PCR), or other specialized applications such as allele-specific discrimination
DNA sequencing (Sanger method)	20–30	Targeted assessment of single nucleotide or small base alterations in template (DNA or RNA) sequences Typically performed on PCR-amplified products Modifications or special methods (e.g., pyrosequencing) can improve sensitivity to 5%

DNA, Deoxyribonucleic acid; *FISH*, fluorescence in situ hybridization; *PCR*, polymerase chain reaction; *RNA*, ribonucleic acid; *SBH*, Southern blot hybridization.
*Generally attainable with the indicated molecular methods, although several technical or biologic factors may influence the lower limits of detection.

II derangements cooperate to alter the fate of the cell (Ishikawa, 2009). In the molecular hematopathology laboratory, most leukemia-related assays are directed toward chimeric gene fusions that generally fall into the class II category. However, testing for class I mutations (e.g., *FLT3* internal tandem duplication) has more recently become integral to more comprehensive evaluations. The challenge for the molecular hematopathology laboratory is thus to incorporate an adequate spectrum of assays directed to the detection of both class I and class II category genetic abnormalities, according to the (ever-changing) understanding of disease molecular pathogenesis.

One practical aspect of the chimeric gene concept is that regardless of the variable location of the genomic (DNA-level) breakpoints in a given translocation gene fusion, the presence of this abnormality can be confirmed by detecting the corresponding invariant chimeric mRNA species. In the molecular diagnostic laboratory, we can thus utilize the reverse-transcription polymerase chain reaction (RT-PCR) method to first convert the fusion mRNA transcript to its complementary deoxyribonucleic acid (cDNA) and then amplify this specific molecule. The ability to perform RT-PCR analysis obviates the difficulties imposed by the often very large flanking regions of intronic DNA surrounding the genomic breakpoint-fusion loci, which would normally not be amenable to amplification by standard DNA-based PCR approaches. Furthermore, the presence of such an aberrant mRNA species is highly specific for the disease, in that it should not theoretically be present in normal cells. Table 75-3 lists the major leukemia-associated translocations along with their resultant fusion gene and mRNA products. Two related concepts are important in the further understanding of chimeric genes and transcripts. *Breakpoint heterogeneity* refers to the presence of two (or more) common breakpoint loci in a particular gene, which can be targeted by the translocation event. In some examples, different breakpoint sites may be correlated with a presenting disease phenotype or particular clinical features (e.g., the *BCR-ABL1* fusion in chronic myeloid leukemia [CML] versus acute lymphoblastic leukemia [ALL]), but this is not always the case. Second, alternative exon splicing of a single chimeric transcript may occur, such that additional, related mRNA products may be observed during PCR amplification of the principal target (e.g., the *PML-RARA* fusion in acute promyelocytic leukemia). RT-PCR-based assays require fresh bone marrow aspirate or blood cells, although cryopreserved tissue or cells can also be used effectively for RNA isolation. RNA extraction and RT-PCR from paraffin tissue block samples has also been successfully described; however, fixed cellular material is often subjected to degradation or the presence of PCR inhibitors, and consequently a higher PCR detection failure rate. Finally, given the highly sensitive nature of PCR amplification, these laboratory assays must be carefully controlled to avoid false-positive contamination artifacts. The following sections describe the molecular genetic and diagnostic features of the most common, prognostically important leukemic diseases.

ACUTE MYELOID LEUKEMIAS

The importance of tumor genetic markers is reflected in the present WHO classification (Swerdlow, 2008), in which acute myeloid leukemias (AMLs) are increasingly defined by their characteristic genetic abnormalities in relation to phenotypic features, prognosis, and clinical outcome. The identification of specific genetic markers can thus establish a definitive AML subclassification, provide important prognostic information, guide therapeutic intervention, and reveal insights into tumor biology.

AML can be broadly classified as being of relatively "favorable," "intermediate," or "poor" prognosis type, based on the degree of tumor cytogenetic complexity or the nature of specific tumor genetic markers. For example, extensive numerical and structural karyotypic abnormalities, or the presence of "myelodysplasia-background" genetic findings (e.g., abnormalities of chromosomes 5 or 7), are indicative of very aggressive subtypes of AML. Several nonrandom recurring chromosomal translocations characterize another significant subset of AML and can be detected by PCR-based molecular diagnostic techniques. These translocations usually occur without additional cytogenetic findings, often show distinct genotype-phenotype correlations, and many are associated with relatively favorable outcome. In particular, the t(15;17), t(8;21), and inv(16) or related t(16;16) translocations together account for approximately 25%–30% of de novo AML in both adults and children. In addition to these three, the current WHO classification recognizes four additional rare, recurrent cytogenetically defined subtypes of AML: t(9;11)*MLLT3-MLL*, t(6;9)*DEK-NUP214*, inv(3)*RPN1-EVI1*, and t(1;22)*RBM15-MKL1* (Swerdlow 2008).

Historically, consideration of numerical and structural karyotypic abnormalities tended to dominate the discussion of AML subcategorization, because relatively little was known about "cytogenetically normal" cases. Recently, however, characteristic gene mutations have been recognized that appear to carry important etiologic and prognostic information in the latter group of AML. These alterations include mutations of *CEBPA*, *NPM1*, and *FLT3*. Whereas the relevance of these mutations is most pronounced in cases of AML with normal karyotype, some of these

TABLE 75-3
Common Leukemia-Associated Translocations and Gene Mutations in Myeloid Neoplasms

Genetic abnormality	Disease associations	Basic molecular pathogenesis	Diagnostic detection*
t(9;22)/*BCR-ABL1*	Chronic myeloid leukemia (100%) Ph+ adult acute lymphoblastic leukemia (20%–25%) Ph+ pediatric acute lymphoblastic leukemia (3%)	Chimeric fusion protein with deregulation of Abl tyrosine kinase; effects on cell proliferation, apoptosis, adhesion	RT-PCR; FISH
JAK2 V617F mutations	Polycythemia vera (>95%); primary myelofibrosis (75%); essential thrombocytosis (50%)	Aberrant activation of cell signaling tyrosine kinase; activation of JAK-STAT pathway	DNA PCR
t(15;17)/*PML-RARA*	Acute promyelocytic leukemia (100%)	Chimeric fusion protein; interference with myeloid maturation and differentiation	RT-PCR; FISH
t(8;21)/*RUNX1-RUNX1T1*	AML (10%)	Chimeric fusion protein affecting the CBF transcriptional pathway	RT-PCR; FISH
inv(16) or t(16;16)/*CBFB-MYH11*	Acute myelomonocytic leukemia with abnormal eosinophils (AMML-Eo)		
FLT3 mutations	AML with normal karyotype (20%–25%)	ITD or point mutation resulting in constitutive activity of Flt3 tyrosine kinase and cell proliferation	DNA PCR
NPM1 mutations	AML with normal karyotype (50%)	Complex effects of mutated NPM1 nuclear/cytoplasmic transport protein	DNA PCR
KIT mutations	Systemic mastocytosis	Aberrant activation of receptor for hematopoietic stem cell factor	DNA PCR
PDGFRA, PDFRB, and *FGFR1* translocations	Myeloid and lymphoid neoplasms with eosinophilia	Deregulation of growth factor receptor tyrosine kinases	FISH > RT-PCR
t(12;21)/*ETV6-RUNX1*	Childhood B-precursor acute lymphoblastic leukemia (20%)	Chimeric fusion protein; disruption of CBF transcriptional pathway	RT-PCR; FISH
11q23/*MLL* translocations	Childhood (mainly infant) B-lineage ALL (5%) Adult de novo AML, usually monocytic (subset of cases) Subset of secondary AML (after DNA topoisomerase II agent exposure)	Chimeric MLL fusion proteins; disruption of MLL-mediated regulation of normal hematopoiesis	FISH; RT-PCR

ALL, Acute lymphoblastic leukemia; *AML,* acute myeloid leukemia; *CBF,* core binding factor; *DNA,* deoxyribonucleic acid; *FISH,* fluorescence in situ hybridization; *ITD,* Internal tandem duplication; *MLL,* mixed lineage leukemia; *PCR,* polymerase chain reaction; *RT-PCR,* reverse-transcriptase polymerase chain reaction.
*PCR includes use of specialized methods (e.g., allele-specific PCR or real-time quantitative platforms) and appropriate postamplification detection techniques (e.g., gel/capillary electrophoresis, melting analysis, sequencing.)

genetic changes (e.g., *FLT3* mutation) may also accompany cases with characteristic translocations, such as the t(15;17), or other cytogenetic abnormalities. Thus, whereas AML with *NPM1* and *CEBPA* mutations have been designated as *provisional entities* in the 2008 WHO classification, *FLT3* alterations, by virtue of their relatively ubiquitous distribution in AML generally, remain an aid to prognostication but not to specific disease subclassification (Swerdlow, 2008).

This section focuses on the common AML-related molecular genetic abnormalities that are currently considered to be the most clinically relevant due to frequency of occurrence and impact on therapy or prognosis. The major abnormalities in AML are summarized in Table 75-3.

Acute Promyelocytic Leukemia: t(15;17)/PML-RARA Abnormality

Acute promyelocytic leukemia (APL), or AML-M3 (according to the previous French-American-British [FAB] classification of AML) accounts for 5%–10% of de novo AML. Patients typically present with symptoms from peripheral blood cytopenias and have a high propensity for life-threatening coagulopathy. Morphologically, APL consists of a proliferation of hypergranular promyelocytes and myeloblasts; however, a microgranular variant form is also frequently encountered (Mantadakis, 2008). APL is genetically defined by the presence of the t(15;17)(q22;q12-21) abnormality, resulting in the fusion of the retinoic acid receptor-α gene, *RARA* [17(q21)] with the *PML* gene [15(q22)] to form a *PML-RARA* chimeric gene on the derivative chromosome 15q (Grignani, 1994; Jurcic, 2007).

The RARA gene product is a subunit of a heterodimeric nuclear receptor for the naturally occurring ligand retinoic acid, or vitamin A. The retinoid nuclear receptor pathway is functional in many aspects of normal cell proliferation and differentiation (Chambon, 1996; Collins, 2008; Mark, 2009). *PML* encodes a DNA-binding zinc finger protein and associates with several other proteins in a macromolecular complex, forming discrete nuclear bodies (Dyck, 1994; Weis, 1994; Reineke, 2009). This interesting protein appears to have multiple possible cellular functions, including transcriptional regulation, apoptosis, and possibly immune surveillance (Quignon, 1998; Wang, 1998; Grimwade, 1999; Zhong, 2000; Borden 2009; Reinecke, 2009). The hybrid PML-RARα protein is clearly involved in disrupting numerous intracellular processes, primarily resulting in a lack of terminal differentiation of neoplastic myeloid precursors beyond the promyelocytic stage. Nonetheless, the significance of APL as a "therapeutic paradigm" for leukemia resides in the ability of pharmacologic doses of *all trans* retinoic acid (atRA) to induce leukemic cell differentiation in vivo. When used in combination with cytotoxic chemotherapy, the synergistic effects of atRA induce complete remission in 90%–98% of patients, and prolonged remission in more than 80% of patients (Tallman, 1997; Tallman, 2002; Clavio, 2009; Licht, 2009; Sanz, 2009). This remarkable finding has intensified efforts to identify other avenues for "cytodifferentiative" therapy in AML. Even though the effect of atRA would seem superficially related to the interaction with the RARα moiety in the abnormal PML-RARα protein, further investigations have unraveled the basic molecular mechanisms underlying the success of this agent. The normal retinoic acid receptor, when not bound to its retinoic acid ligand, associates with histone deacetylase (HDAC) in a nuclear protein co-repressor complex (Guidez, 1998; Melnick, 1999; Lefebvre, 2001; Wei, 2004). This interaction reduces the accessibility of chromatin to transcription factors (and thus locus-specific transcriptional activity), yet is reversible in normal marrow cells upon exposure to physiologic concentrations of retinoic acid. The PML-RARα oncoprotein stabilizes and enhances the state of transcriptional repression by this multiprotein complex; however, therapeutic doses of atRA appear to overcome this abnormal condition and relieve the cellular differentiation block (Melnick, 1999; Hormaeche 2007; Collins 2008; Licht 2009). Whereas some evidence suggests that the PML-RARα oncoprotein may also disrupt the normal pro-apoptotic functions of PML, thus potentiating transformation via pathways involving both partners in the translocation, the direct contribution of altered PML to leukemogenesis remains controversial (Strudwick, 2002; Collins, 2008; Brown, 2009). Functional haploinsufficiency of one remaining normal *PML* gene may also be important in the pathobiology of APL.

The molecular anatomy of the *PML-RARA* fusion gene and mRNA products in APL is summarized diagrammatically in Figure 75-1, *A*. The

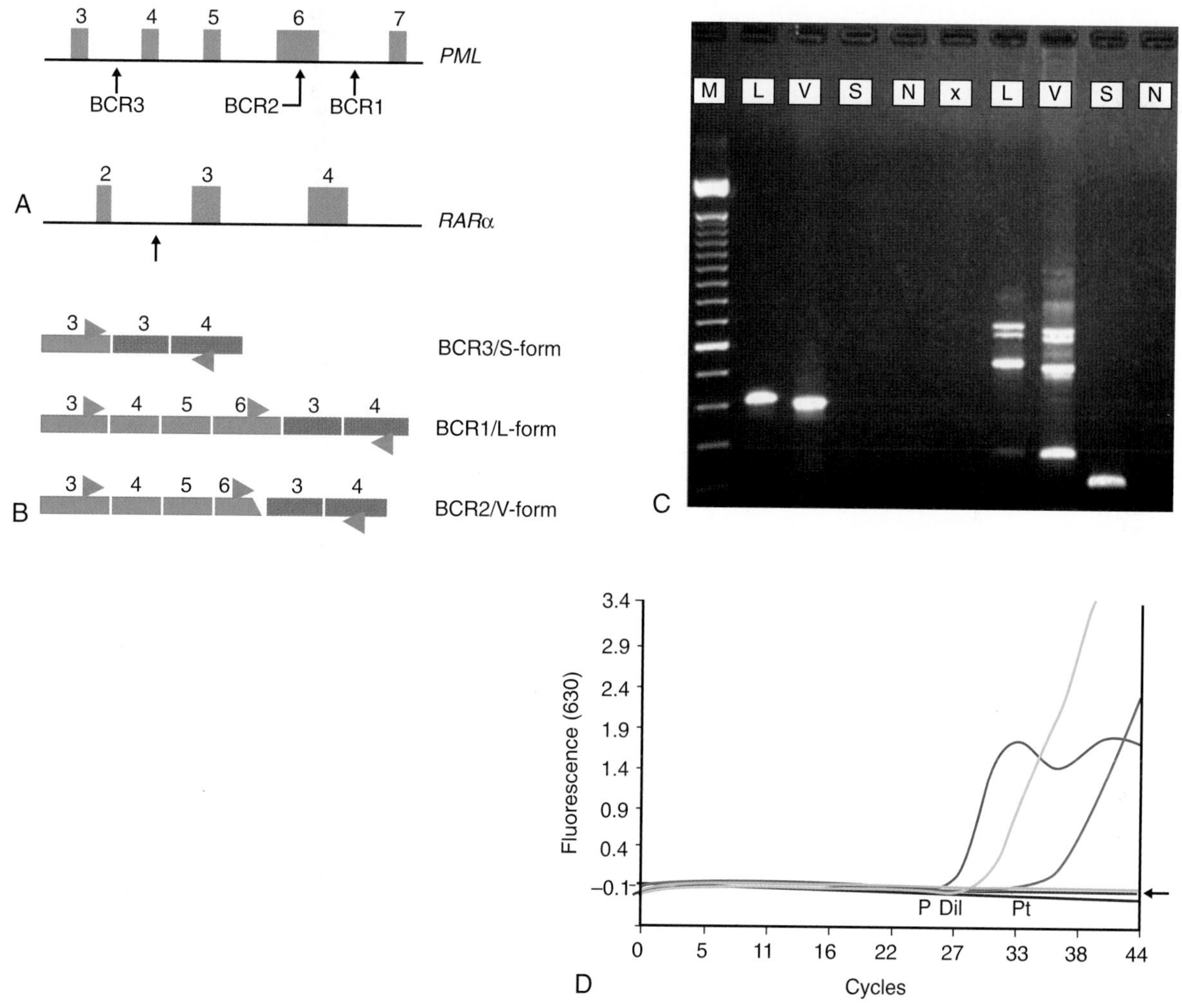

Figure 75-1 t(15;17)/*PML-RARA* abnormality in acute promyelocytic leukemia. **A,** Partial genomic configurations of *PML* and *RARA* genes. Vertical black arrows indicate the three breakpoint sites in the *PML* gene (BCR1, BCR2, BCR3) and the intron 2 breakpoint region in the *RARA* gene. Note that the BCR2 breakpoint occurs within exon 6 of the *PML* gene. **B,** Representations of various PML-RARα mRNA transcripts derived from the each of the three breakpoint-fusion events. The three transcripts are respectively named according to the length of the chimeric species: long (L)-form for BCR1, short (S)-form for BCR3, and variable (V)-form for BCR2. The BCR2/V-form fusion contains only a portion of PML exon 6, although extra nucleotides may be added or deleted at the junction to maintain an intact PML-RARα reading frame. Orange arrows indicate the relative positions of PCR primers to detect these chimeric transcripts by RT-PCR technique. **C,** Representative results from a qualitative RT-PCR analysis to detect the PML-RARα abnormality. The gel bands on the left side (up to the empty lane x) indicate PCR products for L-form/BCR1 and V-form/BCR2 detected with primers situated in PML exon 6 and RARα exon 4. Because exon 6 is not present in the S-form/BCR3 transcript, no PCR product is generated, as shown in the corresponding lane. Gel bands to the right of empty lane x show results obtained with a PML exon 3 primer and the same RARα primer. In this case, a more complex banding pattern is seen for L-form/BCR1 and V-form/BCR2 products due to alternative splicing out of PML exon 5 and exons 5 and 6 (the middle and lower PCR product bands in these lanes). The S-form/BCR3 fusion is readily detected with this primer set. Note that for the rare V-form/BCR2 type PML-RARa, the PCR products are slightly smaller than the L-form/BCR1 species, due to the absence of some of PML exon 6. **D,** Example of RQ-PCR to monitor for the PML-RARα transcript following therapy. The PML-RARα transcript abundance is normalized to a control transcript amplification (not shown) for each sample. Short arrow indicates negative and no template controls. The most informative testing interval occurs at the end of consolidation therapy when PCR positive results are associated with a high risk for leukemic relapse. *Dil,* Dilute positive control; *L,* long form/BCR1; *M,* molecular size marker (100 bp); *N,* no template control; *P,* positive control; *Pt,* patient sample; *RQ-PCR,* real-time quantitative PCR methods; *RT-PCR,* reverse-transcriptase polymerase chain reaction; *S,* S-form/BCR3; *V,* V-form/BCR2; *x,* empty lane.

PML gene exhibits breakpoint heterogeneity in that one of three possible break sites can be encountered in any given patient, involving either intron 3 or intron 6, or occurring within exon 6 (Grignani, 1994; Gallagher, 1995; Reiter, 2003). In contrast, the *RARA* breakpoints are uniformly distributed in intron 2 of the gene. Thus one of three possible PML-RARα chimeric mRNAs can result from this genetic fusion: PML exon 6/RARα exon 3 (long (L)-form, or BCR 1), PML exon 3/RARα exon 3 (Short (S)-form, or BCR 3) and PML exon 6Δ/RARα exon 3 (variable [V]-form, or BCR 2). The V-form transcript is unique in that the *PML* break occurs within exon 6 and a variable proportion of this exon is retained, although additional nucleotides may be added or deleted (Gallagher, 1995; Reiter, 2003). Notably, an in-frame fusion mRNA is produced in each case of APL, underscoring the critical requirement for the PML-RARα protein in leukemogenesis. The L-form (BCR 1) and S-form (BCR 3) PML-RARα fusions are most commonly found in APL (~45%–50% of cases each), whereas the V-form (BCR 2) is only rarely encountered (~5% of APL). The strategy for RT-PCR amplification of these PML-RARα transcripts is depicted in Figure 75-1B, as is a representative diagnostic PCR assay (see Fig. 75-1, *C*). Of note, the L-form (BCR 1) and V-form (BCR 2) type transcripts show alternative splicing out of exons 5 and 6, producing three major amplified products when a PML exon 3 primer is employed.

The clinical relevance in detecting the PML-RARα fusion abnormality in cases of suspected APL is evident from the efficacy of administering specific therapy (i.e., chemotherapy + atRA) with a high possibility of long-term remission and survival. To this end, despite the tight correlation between the t(15;17)/*PML-RARA* and APL morphology, it is recognized that other rare APL-like myeloid leukemias do occur. These morphologic mimics harbor alternative translocations involving the *RARA* gene with fusion partner genes other than *PML*. Examples of these variants include the t(11;17)/*ZBTB16(PLZF)-RARA*, t(11;17)/*NUMA1-RARA*, t(5;17)/*NPM1-RARA*, and the t(17;17)*STAT5B-RARA* acute myeloid leukemias (Melnick, 1999; Grimwade, 2000; Sainty, 2000; Zelent, 2001; Redner, 2002). Notably, *ZBTB16(PLZF)-RARA* and *STAT5B-RARA* positive leukemias in particular are not responsive to the differentiating effects of atRA and are associated with less favorable outcome (Jansen 2001; Redner 2002). Molecular assays specific for the common PML-RARα fusion will not detect these variant transcripts. Other morphologic AML subtypes characterized by increased promyelocytes are similarly atRA unresponsive and also require distinction from true *PML-RARA* positive APL. Several studies have assessed the possible clinical significance of the PML-RARα transcript type in APL patients. Both the S-form (BCR 3) and rare V-form (BCR 2) PML-RARα fusions have been associated with adverse features such as higher presentation white blood cell count, poor atRA response, and possibly shorter remission duration (Vahdat, 1994; Gallagher, 1995, 1997; Jurcic, 2001; Gupta, 2004); however, the independent prognostic value of molecular subclassification in APL has not been definitively established.

Finally, the PML-RARα transcript serves as a valuable molecular disease marker to follow therapeutic response (see Fig. 75-1, *D*). Patients with APL treated with combination chemotherapy and atRA have a relatively favorable prognosis, yet disease relapses occur frequently. The use of qualitative RT-PCR methods to detect the PML-RARα fusion mRNA (with a typical sensitivity of 10^{-3}–10^{-4}) was initially found to be a very powerful tool for predicting relapse risk in individual patients (Jurcic, 2001; Grimwade, 2002; Lo Coco, 2002). The timing, or phase of disease therapy, is an important consideration in this leukemia. Patients evaluated for PML-RARα at the end of induction are often found to be positive and the predictive value at this timepoint is not significant. By the end of consolidation therapy, however, PCR positivity is strongly predictive of relapse in patients who have apparently achieved clinical complete remission, in that nearly all such patients will progress to hematologic relapse within months. In contrast, a single PCR-negative measurement at this timepoint is not necessarily predictive of favorable outcome, in that a significant number of such patients may also suffer relapse. This has led to recommendations for more frequent posttherapy monitoring using sensitive and precise real-time quantitative PCR methods (RQ-PCR). To this end, several APL study groups have reported results of serial PML-RARα monitoring using RQ-PCR techniques and these efforts have shown a benefit for detecting low-level molecular disease and its value in predicting relapse risk (Grimwade, 2002; Gallagher, 2003; Grimwade 2009). Furthermore, several studies have validated the concept of "salvaging" or retreating patients with molecular residual disease, with good clinical outcomes. Given an array of additional treatment options for APL, including highly effective second line intervention with arsenic trioxide (As_2O_3) and autologous or allogeneic stem cell transplantation, molecular residual disease assessment thus forms an integral aspect of the management of all APL patients (Santamaria, 2007; Kohno, 2008; Lo Coco, 2008; Grimwade, 2009). Although no formal guidelines have been firmly established for RQ-PCR monitoring of PML-RARα in APL, proposed common sampling timepoints for assessment include the end of induction, end of consolidation, then every 2–3 months for the first year after therapy, because this is the window during which most relapses occur. Bone marrow aspirate samples are preferred for MRD assessment, in that the peripheral blood is less sensitive for transcript detection following treatment onset.

Core Binding Factor–Related Acute Myeloid Leukemias: t(8;21)/RUNX1-RUNX1T1 and Inv(16) or t(16;16)/CBFB-MYH11 Abnormalities

Acute myeloid leukemias with the t(8;21)(q22;q22) and inv(16)(p13q22) or related t(16;16)(p13;q22) cytogenetic abnormalities together account for approximately 11%–18% of de novo cases (Schnittger, 2007; Cheng, 2009). Core binding factor (CBF)-related AML cases are roughly evenly distributed between those with the t(8;21) and cases with inv(16)/t(16;16) (Dombret, 2009). Whereas the t(8;21) is generally associated with AML showing maturation (FAB type AML-M2), the inv(16) and t(16;16) are highly correlated with acute myelomonocytic leukemia with abnormal eosinophils (FAB type AML-M4Eo) (Cheng, 2009). Clinically, these genetically defined AML subtypes are responsive to chemotherapy (especially high-dose cytarabine regimens) and are considered to be prognostically favorable compared with AML in general (Appelbaum, 2006; Dombret, 2009).

Although different respective leukemia phenotypes derive from these translocations, a remarkable and common pathobiologic feature of both the t(8;21) and inv(16) or t(16;16) leukemias is disruption of the CBF transcriptional regulatory pathway (Speck, 1999; Paschka, 2008). CBF is a heterodimeric transcription factor that consists of a DNA binding α-subunit (CBFα) and a peptide-interacting β-subunit (CBFβ), which acts to stabilize CBFα at sites of DNA interaction (Fig. 75-2). In normal cells, CBF acts at "core" enhancer sequences in a number of genes required for proper myeloid and lymphoid cell differentiation or maturation. The binding of CBF facilitates the access of other transcription factor complexes to these chromatin sites, in part through increased acetylation of

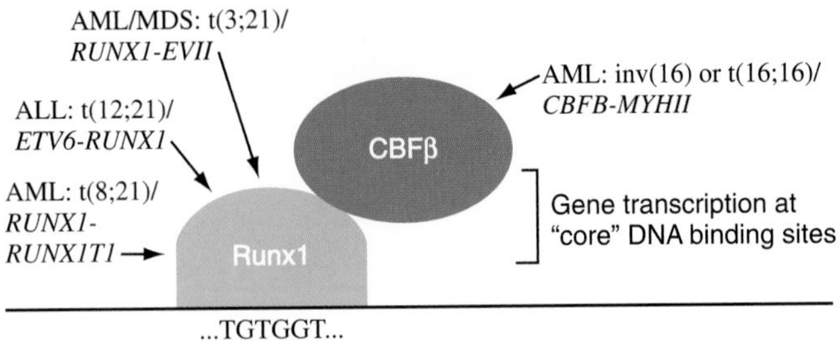

Figure 75-2 Disruption of the CBF transcriptional pathway in leukemogenesis. This schematic illustrates the central role of the core binding factor transcriptional pathway in leukemogenesis. Both components of the heterodimeric CBF are targeted for disruption in a variety of acute lymphoblastic and myeloblastic leukemias. Of these, the t(8;21)/*RUNX1-RUNX1T1* and inv(16) or t(16;16)/*CBFB-MYH11* account for nearly 20% of de novo AML cases, whereas the t(12;21)/*ETV6-RUNX1* is found in 20% of pediatric acute lymphoblastic leukemias. (Alternative gene nomenclature: *RUNX1 = AML1 = CBFA2; RUNX1T1 = ETO = MTG8; ETV6 = TEL*). *AML,* Acute myeloid leukemia; *CBF,* core binding factor.

DNA-bound histone proteins by histone acetyltransferases (Lorsbach, 2001; Yamagata, 2005). In human acute myeloid leukemias with the t(8;21), the *RUNX1* gene (formerly designated *AML1*, or *CBFA2*) encoding an isoform of CBFα, is joined to a putative transcription factor, *RUNX1T1* (formerly *ETO*, or *MTG8*) to form the *RUNX1-RUNX1T1* fusion (Downing, 1999; Peterson, 2007). In the case of the inv(16) or t(16;16), the gene producing CBFβ (i.e., *CBFB*) is juxtaposed to a smooth muscle myosin heavy chain gene *MYH11* to form the hybrid *CBFB-MYH11* (Liu, 1995; Mrózek, 2008). In either case, profound disruption of the normal cellular differentiation program is thought to be central to the causation of acute leukemia. The prominence of CBF pathway alterations in leukemogenesis is additionally emphasized by the finding of *RUNX1* gene translocations in several other types of leukemia and myelodysplasia (see Fig. 75-2), including the t(12;21)/*ETV6-RUNX1* abnormality, the most common single genetic abnormality in pediatric ALL.

From a mechanistic viewpoint, the RUNX1-RUNX1T1 leukemic fusion protein is thought to act in a dominant negative manner to normal RUNX1 (i.e., CBFα) by recruiting or stabilizing elements of transcriptional repression, including histone deacetylase complexes, at critical DNA sites (Lorsbach, 2001; Yamagata, 2005). Normal gene expression patterns are also disrupted by the altered affinity of the abnormal fusion protein for specific core enhancer sequences, including an increased propensity to bind sites with such sequences in duplicate (Okumura, 2008). CBFβ-MYH11 chimeric protein sequesters normal CBFα protein in the cytosol, thereby abrogating heterodimeric CBF assembly in the nucleus, but may also create an abnormally repressive transcriptional complex in a manner analogous to that of *RUNX1-RUNX1T1* (Shigesada, 2004). In either case, the resultant inhibition of transcription at key genes alters the genetic program for normal proliferation and differentiation in hematolymphoid stem or progenitor cells.

In keeping with the concept outlined previously that an individual genetic aberrancy is of itself not likely sufficient for carcinogenesis, transgenic mice engineered to conditionally express a *RUNX1-RUNX1T1* oncogene develop acute myeloid leukemia only on subsequent exposure to a promoting mutagen (Lorsbach, 2001; Peterson, 2007; Müller, 2008). In CBF leukemias, the pathognomonic translocations create a block in cellular differentiation (class II mutations), but affected cells often acquire secondary class I mutations that endow them with enhanced proliferative capacity. Indeed, there is a particularly strong association in CBF leukemias with secondary mutations to the gene encoding the c-KIT tyrosine kinase (stem cell factor receptor), a potent regulator of cell growth. Up to half of CBF leukemias carry *KIT* mutations; in contrast, approximately 5% of all AML cases show such mutations (Muller, 2008). Many of these *KIT* mutations involve the D816 "hot-spot" amino acid (that is also affected in systemic mastocytosis), but mutations have been described in other exons as well. The presence of *KIT* mutations in CBF leukemias has been associated with increased relapse risk and, in some studies, poorer overall survival, although the latter finding remains somewhat controversial at present (Cairoli, 2006; Paschka, 2006; Mrozek, 2008; Muller, 2008). Thus the routine clinical utility of *KIT* mutation testing in CBF leukemias currently awaits validation by larger trials. Notably, deregulation of c-KIT expression as a consequence of *KIT* mutations in these leukemias may present a rational therapeutic target, given that the 5-year-survival for CBF leukemia patients, albeit better than for AML in general, does not substantially surpass 50%.

The molecular rearrangements underlying the *RUNX1-RUNX1T1* fusion are such that the breakpoint-fusion sites invariably involve the same limited set of intron regions in both genes, resulting in a consistent in-frame RUNX1-RUNX1T1 mRNA molecule in each patient with this type of AML, although some degree of variant transcripts derived from alternative splicing and differential promoter usage can also be seen (Zhang, 2002; LaFiura, 2007). In contrast, standard RT-PCR detection of the CBFβ-MYH11 chimeric transcript is complicated by the potential for marked breakpoint heterogeneity mainly in the *MYH11* gene, as well as by rare alternate breakage sites described in *CBFB*. In all, more than 10 CBFB-MYH11 fusion transcript forms have been identified to date (Liu, 1995; Viswanatha, 1998; Kadkol, 2004; Schnittger, 2007). Despite this complexity, the *CBFB-MYH11* gene fusion can be readily detected by RT-PCR, because approximately 90% of these tumors harbor the so-called "type A" chimeric mRNA, characterized by fusion of *CBFB* nucleotide 495 to *MYH11* nucleotide 1921 to form a transcript of relatively short length (Schnittger, 2007). More comprehensive PCR strategies have also emerged to detect the majority of the other rare *CBFB-MYH11* fusion types, each of which account for the remainder of cases of inv(16) or t(16;16) AML (Kadkol, 2004). RT-PCR analysis for the *CBFB-MYH11* abnormality is often advantageous, in that standard cytogenetic interpretation may be uninformative in some cases (Merchant, 2004; Monma 2007). In this context, it is possible, though unlikely, that a case with a true non–type A *CBFB-MYH11* fusion could be negative by both conventional cytogenetic and molecular analysis, if karyotyping fails to detect a cryptic translocation and RT-PCR technique targets only the type A transcript; this possibility underscores the general importance of maintaining awareness of the limitations of a specific molecular assay, as well as the central role that morphologic assessment must play even in the molecular era. Nevertheless, given the generally more favorable clinical outcome for both of these AML subtypes, molecular diagnosis can play a significant role both in initial identification, as well as in disease monitoring following treatment.

Acute Myeloid Leukemias with FLT3, NPM1, and CEBPA Gene Mutations

The most recent WHO classification of AML has been broadened to include additional entities characterized by specific gene mutations (Swerdlow, 2008). Chief among these with regard to diagnostic and clinical significance are alterations of *FLT3*, *NPM1*, and *CEBPA*. These gene mutations involve relatively small scale modifications to the specific DNA sequences, including short insertions, deletions, or single base pair changes, and therefore cannot be detected by conventional cytogenetic or FISH techniques. AML with gene mutations usually are characterized by the presence of a normal tumor karyotype and are discussed here in this context; however, similar mutations can also accompany AML with recurrent translocations or other cytogenetic abnormalities. Notably, the characteristic "genotype-phenotype" correlations between morphologic, clinical, and genetic findings observed in AML with recurrent translocations are not as obviously encountered in AML with *FLT3*, *NPM1*, or *CEBPA* gene mutations. Among the group of AML with gene mutations, *FLT3* is an adverse prognostic factor, whereas *NPM1* and *CEBPA* mutations indicate an outcome somewhat better than for AML in general. Complicating this scenario is the fact that a significant subset of normal karyotype AML may harbor two or more gene mutations producing variable effects on tumor prognosis. Most significantly, *FLT3* and *NPM1* mutations may occur together, in which case the relative outcome benefit of the *NPM1* mutation is abrogated by the coexisting *FLT3* mutation. Furthermore, if these mutations are detected in the setting of cytogenetic abnormalities, or in other infrequent combinations, the prognostic significance is less clearly established. Whereas testing for *FLT3*, *NPM1*, and *CEBPA* gene mutations is currently indicated in cytogenetically normal AML cases, molecular genetic assays for these mutations should ideally not be considered in isolation. As noted earlier, *FLT3* mutation was not designated as a specific subtype of AML in the 2008 WHO classification, and cases of AML with mutated *NPM1* or *CEBPA* remain only provisional diagnostic entities at present.

FLT3 *Mutations in AML*

Expression of the *FLT3* gene (Fms-like tyrosine kinase; also known as *FLK2* and *STK1*) produces a membrane-spanning signal transduction protein of the receptor tyrosine kinase (RTK) type III family, whose members also include the platelet-derived growth factor receptor (PDGFR) genes and the *KIT* gene (Agnes, 1994; Small 2008). FLT3 receptor-ligand interactions are important for the maintenance and propagation of early progenitor cells in normal myeloid and lymphoid hematopoiesis. Not surprisingly, the wild type receptor protein is also expressed in the majority of AML and B-lineage ALLs, emphasizing its role in the survival and proliferation of immature hematopoietic cells (Gilliland, 2002; Stirewalt, 2003). *FLT3* mutations in AML most frequently take the form of internal tandem duplications (ITD) of part of the coding region for the juxtamembrane portion of this tyrosine kinase, producing an abnormal, constitutively active FLT3 protein. All ITDs preserve an intact reading frame, despite the introduction of additional nucleotides, consistent with abnormal activation of a largely functional protein. A second type of activating lesion involves point mutation of *FLT3* at amino acid sites D835 or I836 in the "activation loop" of the protein (Yamamoto, 2001; Bacher, 2008). The constitutively active FLT3 tyrosine kinase initiates increased activity within its downstream signaling cascade, which in turn provides a pro-proliferative stimulus to the myeloid cell. Thus *FLT3* belongs to the "class I" group of AML-related genetic abnormalities. These *FLT3* gene mutations are together estimated to occur in 20%–40% of adult AML (as well as a smaller number of pediatric AML, secondary AML, and myelodysplasias), and appear to be distributed among all morphologic subtypes. *FLT3* is consequently one of the most common recurrent abnormal genetic findings encountered in AML. *FLT3* ITD mutations are most frequently observed in several cytogenetic settings, including t(15;17) APL, t(6;9) *DEK-NUP214* associated AML, and in many cytogenetically normal cases; this suggests a key role for this genetic aberration in the pathophysiology of these subsets of AML (Schnittger, 2002; Thiede, 2002).

In general, the presence of *FLT3* gene mutations in AML has been associated with poor prognosis, and the prognostic impact of FLT3 mutations is particularly well-established in cytogenetically normal cases (Kottaridis, 2001; Zwaan, 2003; Schlenk, 2008; also reviewed in Stirewalt, 2003). More refined prognostic information appears to be derived from an assessment of the "gene dosage," or ratio of *FLT3* ITD relative to wild type allele (*FLT3* ITD:WT), with higher ratios correlated with poorer clinical outcome (Thiede, 2002; Baldus, 2006; Meshinchi, 2006). Elevated *FLT3* ITD:WT ratios could possibly arise from gene amplification of the ITD allele, biallelic mutations, or from the presence of a more prevalent subclone of leukemic cells with the *FLT3* ITD (Stirewalt, 2003). However, some caveats remain notable regarding *FLT3* mutations. Although the prognostic impact of *FLT3*-ITD mutations is well established, the influence of *FLT3*-TKD mutations remains controversial (Fröhling, 2002; Moreno 2003; Yanada 2005; Mead 2007). Recent data suggest that *FLT3*-TKD mutations have no effect on prognosis in AML overall, but may have differential effects on outcomes (i.e., better or worse) in particular subgroups of AML (Bacher, 2008). AML with *FLT3*-ITD and *FLT3*-TKD mutations also have distinct gene expression profiles, suggesting that these two mutations, although within the same gene, may act in biologically and perhaps prognostically dissimilar ways (Neben, 2005). The value of additional screening for *FLT3*-TKD mutations in the molecular hematopathology laboratory therefore awaits a clearer understanding of the clinical significance of this molecular target. Second, the role of cooperating *FLT3* mutations in APL is well recognized and has been associated with proliferative features, such as leukocytosis (Callens, 2005); however, APL patients with *FLT3* mutations do not have a significantly different outcome than those without and mutation analysis is thus not routinely recommended in the setting of APL.

In contrast to the situation for translocation fusion genes with chimeric mRNA transcripts, *FLT3* ITD can be detected by PCR amplification of genomic DNA. Amplification of exons 14 and 15 of *FLT3* can identify the ITD, because these are variably larger in fragment size than expected for this region in the wild type gene. The presence of an ITD is typically established by PCR product sizing, for example using capillary electrophoresis of fluorescent PCR amplicons. Different molecular approaches are employed to detect TKD mutations, including DNA PCR followed by amplicon digestion with informative restriction endonucleases, direct sequencing, or other sequence-specific methods.

NPM1 *Mutations in Acute Myeloid Leukemia*

NPM1, which encodes the protein nucleophosmin, is mutated in 50%–60% of AML with a normal karyotype (Falini, 2005). Many of these leukemias are characterized by a lack of CD34 antigen expression and features of monocytic differentiation. *NPM1* is also the partner gene in the translocation characteristic of an unrelated hematologic malignancy, anaplastic large cell lymphoma (ALCL), suggesting its broader importance in fundamental hematopoietic signaling pathways. Normal cellular nucleophosmin is largely present within the nucleolus, but the protein operates as a "shuttle," escorting proteins, particularly ribosomal subunits, between the nucleus and cytoplasm (Yun, 2003; Yu, 2006). Nucleophosmin also participates in cell cycle regulation, by virtue of its ability to activate, via both direct and indirect mechanisms, p53 and other proteins involved in cell cycle control (Falini, 2007). Yet another task of this multifaceted protein is the control of centrosome duplication before mitosis (Tsou, 2006), and experimental depletion of *NPM1* results in improper chromosome alignment, abnormal centrosomes, and disorganization of mitotic spindles (Amin, 2008). *NPM1* mutations in AML involve small insertions of variable length and sequence in a specific region of the gene, producing a frameshift that alters the amino acid sequence at the C-terminus of the protein. This portion of nucleophosmin carries a nuclear localization signal (NLS) important for nuclear retention. The altered protein, lacking the NLS and incorporating instead a nuclear export signal, is aberrantly retained in the cytoplasm (Chen, 2006). The exact mechanisms by which cytoplasmic nucleophosmin contributes to leukemogenesis remain unclear, but the loss of the usual intranuclear interactions between nucleophosmin and cell cycle control proteins is hypothesized to play an important role in transformation (Falini, 2007). The presence of mutated *NPM1* is significantly associated with a relatively good prognosis in normal karyotype AML, but only if an accompanying *FLT3* mutation is absent (Schlenk, 2008). Nearly 40% of *NPM1* mutated AML cases harbor a concomitant *FLT3* mutation, and these patients have an inferior prognosis, essentially similar to AML with *FLT3* mutations alone (Baldus, 2007).

Although the cytoplasmic localization of nucleophosmin in *NPM1* mutated AML cases presents a potentially attractive target for simple detection via immunohistochemistry, such a technique may be insufficient for accurate prognostication based on the lack of quantitative standards and the problem of tumor heterogeneity (Konoplev, 2009). Therefore molecular analysis is the preferred method for identifying *NPM1* mutations. More than 25 mutations (all heterozygous) have been identified affecting exon 12 (Konoplev, 2009). The most common mutation, labeled type A, is seen in up to 80% of *NPM1* positive cases and involves the insertion of the tetranucleotide sequence TCTG at positions 956 to 959 of the gene (Falini, 2007). Because these *NPM1* exon 12 mutations change the length of the DNA sequence relative to wild type, standard PCR amplification of the genomic region paired with fluorescent product size analysis by capillary electrophoresis suffices to detect the change. A distinct advantage of this strategy is that the same method can be applied to the detection of *FLT3*-ITD mutations, simplifying the technical approach to these genetic abnormalities; as indicated, *NPM1* analysis should always be performed in conjunction with *FLT3* testing to provide accurate prognostic information.

CEBPA *Mutations in Acute Myeloid Leukemia*

Acute myeloid leukemias with mutations of the CCAAT/enhancer binding protein α (*CEBPA*) gene represent a third distinct group of tumors recently included in the 2008 WHO AML classification. *CEBPA* encodes a transcription factor essential to granulocytic differentiation, such that the production of mature granulocytes does not occur in its absence (Koschmieder, 2009). Corollary functions of normal CEPBA protein include transcriptional repression of genes involved in nonhematopoietic programs and the promotion of cell cycle arrest as a component of terminal differentiation. Although mutations of *CEPBA* are thought to promote leukemogenesis by blocking granulocytic differentiation and proliferation control, the exact pathogenetic mechanisms remain to be elucidated. Notably, some families with an inherited predisposition to the development of AML carry germline *CEBPA* mutations (Renneville, 2009a). Approximately 15%–20% of cytogenetically normal cases of AML carry the *CEBPA* mutation (Baldus, 2007). In this setting, *CEBPA* mutations are associated with a relatively favorable prognosis (Fröhling, 2004; Bienz, 2005; Schlenk 2008). Although the significance of *CEBPA* mutations in other types of AML is not completely clear, recent evidence suggests that the beneficial prognostic effect of *CEBPA* mutations applies only in cases with normal karyotype and without *FLT3*-ITD mutation (Renneville, 2009). Paradoxically, though, coexisting *FLT3*-TKD mutations in particular may not affect the positive impact of mutated *CEBPA* (Bacher, 2008). Furthermore, recent observations suggest that the improved outcome in *CEBPA* mutation-positive AML appears to be limited only to those cases carrying biallelic mutations, underscoring incomplete but evolving understanding of this area (Wouters 2009a).

Prototypical *CEBPA* mutations are found widely separated within both N- and C-terminal regions of the gene, in contrast to the more clustered localization of mutations in *FLT3* and *NPM1*. The N-terminal mutations prevent translation of the full-length p42 isoform, but an alternative start site downstream from the mutated N-terminal site permits continued production of a shorter p30 isoform (Wouters, 2009a). In contrast, C-terminal mutations are in frame and are thought to impair protein function. Other mutations have been described throughout the intervening region. Consequently, molecular detection strategies must be capable of detecting many mutations over a potentially wide area. Direct sequencing of RT-PCR amplified *CEBPA* mRNA, both with and without initial screening via high-resolution melting curve analysis, has been successfully employed in this regard (Ahn, 2009; Rázga, 2009).

Other Gene Mutations in Acute Myeloid Leukemias

Mutations involving many other genes, including *WT1*, *MLL*, *NRAS*, and *KRAS*, have been associated with prognostic or biologic importance in AML. In addition, abnormal gene expression patterns of *BAALC*, *ERG*, and *MN1* have also been tied to prognosis (Baldus, 2007). As this list continues to expand, a major challenge for the diagnostician and clinician will be in the rational interpretation of potentially many interacting genetic factors in order to determine appropriate risk stratification and therapy options for individual AML patients. As suggested from the inherent complexity of simultaneously assessing the three relatively common mutations considered previously (*FLT3*, *NPM1*, and *CEBPA*), the impact of multiple cooperating genetic events requires sophisticated bioinformatics analyses applied to well-designed and sufficiently powered clinical studies. The optimal strategy for evaluation of gene mutations in AML will thus continue to evolve as additional clinical data emerge.

ACUTE LYMPHOBLASTIC LEUKEMIA/ LYMPHOMA, B AND T CELL LINEAGE

B Cell Lymphoblastic Leukemia/Lymphoma (Precursor B Cell Acute Lymphoblastic Leukemia)

Significant biologic and clinical differences exist between adult and childhood onset ALLs. Comparatively little is known about the pathogenesis of adult ALL, which overall is associated with a relatively unfavorable outcome. As such, cytogenetic and molecular genetic anomalies in adult ALL are incompletely characterized, with the exception of the very poor prognosis t(9;22)/*BCR-ABL1* (i.e., Ph+ ALL). Beyond detection of the *BCR-ABL1* gene fusion, molecular diagnosis is currently of limited utility in the management of adult ALL. In marked contrast, the molecular diagnostic evaluation of pediatric ALL is of substantial value in the stratification of patients to "risk-adapted" treatment strategies. Over the past 20 years, the improvement in therapeutic regimens for these children, coupled with a more profound understanding of ALL tumor biology, has resulted in cure rates of 80% or better overall (Pui, 2004; O'Leary, 2008; Pui, 2008; Vrooman, 2009). In turn, this has led to the concept of tailoring therapy to defined subsets of patients based on a combination of presenting clinical and biologic features, including early treatment response and tumor genetics. The aim in childhood ALL has thus evolved to balance the highest probability of long-term remission with the lowest chance of therapy-related adverse events. Although clinical features (e.g., age, degree of leukocytosis, CNS involvement) are initially used to separate "standard risk" from "high risk" individuals, tumor genetics are also an integral component of the initial (i.e., pretreatment) evaluation of childhood ALL patients. Broadly, both numerical and structural chromosomal abnormalities are considered in this process (Table 75-4). In the former instance, "high hyperdiploidy," or tumor aneuploidy with a chromosome number in excess of 52, has been associated with more favorable treatment response and outcome, particularly when certain chromosomal trisomies (e.g., +4, +10, +17) are present (Harris, 1992; Heerema, 2000; Moorman, 2003; Sutcliffe, 2005; Schultz, 2007). Conversely, tumor hypodiploidy, especially less than 44 chromosomes, is associated with a very high frequency of treatment failure (Heerema, 1999; Nachman, 2007; Schultz, 2007). Among the structural rearrangements, four chromosomal translocations account for approximately one third of pediatric ALL cases, each with prognostic importance: the t(9;22)/*BCR-ABL1*, t(1;19)/*TCF3-PBX1*, t(12;21)/*ETV6-RUNX1*, and rearrangements involving the 11(q23)/*MLL* locus (Bartolo, 2000; Harrison, 2001; Pui, 2004; Armstrong, 2005). In general, numerical and structural alterations are mutually exclusive in any given case of childhood ALL; however, occasionally, these findings can coexist. Although not dealt with formally in this section, the detection of minimal residual disease at certain posttherapeutic timepoints (e.g., end-of-induction) has also emerged as a highly important component of outcome prediction in

TABLE 75-4

Risk Stratification/Outcome Prediction in Childhood B-lineage Acute Lymphoblastic Leukemia*

Abnormality	Prognostic significance	Notes
High hyperdiploidy (>52 chromosomes)	Favorable	Hyperdiploid tumors with particular trisomic chromosomes (e.g., +4, +10, +17) associated with very favorable outcome
t(12;21)/*ETV6-RUNX1*	Favorable	Very favorable outcome, but appreciable incidence of late relapses
t(1;19)/*TCF3-PBX1*	Intermediate	Intensive therapy results in good outcome
t(9;22)/*BCR-ABL1*	Unfavorable	Very high risk for relapse/refractory disease
11q23/*MLL* gene rearrangements	Unfavorable	Very high risk for infant ALL; also considered high risk factor for older children
Hypodiploidy (<44 chromosomes)	Unfavorable	Very high risk for relapse/refractory disease
High level molecular MRD at end-induction therapy	Unfavorable	Very high risk of relapse in patients with MRD above 10^{-2}–10^{-3}, detected by molecular or flow cytometric methods

ALL, Acute lymphoblastic leukemia; *MRD*, minimal residual disease.

*Tumor genetic features and early MRD are considered in conjunction with clinical and laboratory findings, including age, presenting blast count, and evidence of extramedullary disease. These risk factors therefore modify and refine traditional parameters for predicting therapeutic response.

childhood ALL (Cave, 1998; van Dongen, 1998; Nyvold, 2002; Campana, 2008; Flohr, 2008; Campana, 2009).

Major Translocation Fusion Gene Abnormalities in B Cell ALL

The t(9;22)(q34;q11.2)/*BCR-ABL1* is found in approximately 3%–4% of childhood B-lineage ALL, but occurs in 20%–25% of adult B-ALL (Armstrong, 2005). Typically, these patients present with markedly elevated lymphoblast counts and other adverse clinical features. Of the two common break-fusion events associated with the *BCR-ABL1* fusion gene, the majority of cases of pediatric B-ALL (80%–90%) have *BCR* breakpoints situated in the minor breakpoint cluster region (m-BCR), with production of an e1-a2 type chimeric BCR-ABL1 mRNA. The e1-a2 mRNA type is also found in many adult *BCR-ABL1* positive B-ALL, but approximately one third of adult cases alternatively demonstrate e13-a2 or e14-a2 transcripts, characteristic of major breakpoint cluster region (M-BCR) disruption in the *BCR* gene. The structure and molecular diagnostic aspects of the *BCR-ABL1* gene fusion are presented in greater detail in the subsequent section on CML. The presence of the *BCR-ABL1* in childhood ALL is an independently poor prognostic factor, placing these patients among the very highest at risk for primary treatment failure and relapse (Fletcher, 1991; Gaynon, 1997; Jones, 2005; Yanada, 2009). The majority of *BCR-ABL1* positive ALL patients are candidates for more aggressive therapy including early allogeneic hematopoietic stem cell transplantation. The introduction of the tyrosine kinase inhibitor imatinib mesylate may offer additional therapeutic benefit in the treatment of this disease; in adult Ph+ALL, imatinib in combination with conventional chemotherapy results in a very high (95%) rate of initial complete remission, although durable responses are often difficult to maintain (Jones, 2005; Gökbuget, 2009; Ribera, 2009; Vrooman, 2009; Yanada, 2009; reviewed in Gruber, 2009). Studies of the efficacy of imatinib in childhood Ph+ ALL are ongoing (Jones, 2005; Vrooman, 2009). Molecular analysis of the BCR-ABL1 transcript by RT-PCR technique is critical for risk prediction in childhood ALL, as well as providing a marker for residual disease monitoring. Recently, deletion of *IKZF1*, which codes for the transcription factor Ikaros, has been identified as a genetic change present in many cases of *BCR-ABL1* ALL (Mullighan, 2008; Iacobucci, 2009; Martinelli, 2009; Mullighan, 2009). Although data are still emerging, Ikaros alterations appear to be an important cooperative lesion in this subclass of ALL, strongly influencing the aggressive behavior of *BCR-ABL1* ALL (Martinelli, 2009; Mullighan, 2009).

B-ALL characterized by the t(1;19)(q23;p13.3) abnormality are uncommon, accounting for less than 5% of pediatric cases and only rare occurrences in adults (Armstrong, 2005). This translocation is strongly associated with "pre-B" immunophenotypic features, typified by the presence of cytoplasmic IgM production in the tumor cells. Following its initial recognition in childhood ALL, the t(1;19) was associated with poor outcome. However, it has become apparent that more intensive treatment protocols largely negate the adverse effects of this genotype, resulting in stable remissions for most of these individuals. Recognition of this translocation is thus required for appropriate therapy (Schultz, 2007). The t(1;19) most frequently occurs as an unbalanced form of translocation (with resultant loss of some genetic material) and produces the chimeric *TCF3* (formerly *E2A)-PBX1*gene fusion, although balanced translocations with the same fusion product also occur (Hunger, 1991; Paulsson, 2007). The *TCF3* gene encodes a series of basic helix-loop-helix transcription factors, which are involved in myocyte and B-lymphocyte development. *PBX1* is a DNA-binding transcription factor that is not normally expressed in lymphoid cells. The fusion TCF3-PBX1 protein replaces the DNA binding and protein dimerization motifs of TCF3 with the DNA binding region of PBX1, predisposing the progenitor B cell to neoplastic proliferation. The location of genomic breakpoints within *TCF3* and *PBX1* introns is consistent in essentially all cases, resulting in the formation of a single TCF3-PBX1 transcript (Hunger, 1991; Wiemels, 2002), with only few reported variants (Paulsson, 2007). This fusion mRNA is readily amenable to RT-PCR detection and can also serve as a disease-specific marker for sensitive detection in the bone marrow. Of note, rare cytogenetically detectable ALL cases with t(1;19) lack the *TCF3-PBX1* fusion and appear to be associated with an inferior outcome (Privitera, 1992; Prima, 2007); these variant t(1;19)(q23;p13.3) translocations instead create reciprocal oncogenic fusion proteins, *DAZAP1/MEF2D* and *MEF2D/DAZAP1* (Prima, 2007).

Overall, 20%–25% of pediatric ALL patients are characterized by the presence of the t(12;21)(p13;q22) abnormality, establishing this lesion as the most common recurrent translocation in this patient group (Armstrong, 2005). This genetic finding is essentially absent among adults with B-ALL. The t(12;21) is cytogenetically cryptic in almost all cases (Karrman, 2006), instead often being suggested by an apparent deletion of the short arm of one chromosome 12. Although patients with t(12;21) ALL are found distributed among different clinical risk groups, in general, these individuals are between the ages of 2 and 7 and have diploid karyotype tumors (Rubnitz, 1997a; Forestier, 2006; Forestier, 2007). The t(12;21) results in the joining of the 12p locus *ETV6* gene (also known as *TEL*) with the *RUNX1* (or *AML1*, *CBFA2*) gene on 21q to form the chimeric gene fusion, *ETV6-RUNX1* on the derivative chromosome 12 (Romana, 1995; Zelent, 2004). Pediatric patients with *ETV6-RUNX1* positive ALL have a favorable outcome, with excellent disease-free remissions approaching 80% (similar to the aforementioned high-hyperdiploid group with specific chromosomal trisomies) (Shurtleff, 1995; Borkhardt, 1997; Rubnitz, 1997a; Rubnitz, 1997b; Forestier, 2008). However, reports of a substantial late relapse rate among some *ETV6-RUNX1* ALL patients have refocused attention on more clearly defining the risk characteristics of this group, even though many such relapsed patients remain responsive to "salvage therapy" protocols (Harbott, 1997; Seeger, 1998; Ford, 2001; Forestier, 2008). The molecular pathology of *ETV6-RUNX1* ALL is related to disruption of normal CBF activity, leading to enhanced transcriptional repression of many target genes, as similarly discussed for the *RUNX1-RUNX1T1* abnormality in AML (Fig. 75-3) (Zelent, 2004). In almost 90% of *ETV6-RUNX1* ALL cases, the remaining *ETV6* allele is partially or completely deleted in a variable proportion of tumor cells, suggesting that this event may be an important secondary event for leukemogenic transformation, through complete loss of normal ETV6 function (Raynaud, 1996; Tsuzuki, 2007; Wiemels, 2008). At the DNA level, *ETV6* and *RUNX1* breaksites in ALL occur most often in the same genomic regions of *ETV6* intron 5 and *RUNX1* intron 1 (Romana, 1995; von Goessel, 2009), with evidence of some propensity for breakpoint clustering. A second minor variant with breakpoints situated in *RUNX1* intron 2 is also described. The in-frame transcribed ETV6-RUNX1 mRNA thus encompasses a novel region joining *ETV6* exon 5 to *RUNX1* exon 2 (most cases), or *ETV6* exon 5 to *RUNX1* exon 3 (fewer cases) (Nakao, 1996b; von Goessel, 2009). Additional complexity is present in this gene fusion owing to alternative splicing out of *RUNX1* exons 2 and/or 3, with the possibility of detecting up to four ETV6-RUNX1 amplified transcript forms by RT-PCR in any given case. Molecular (RT-PCR) or FISH detection of the *ETV6-RUNX1* is frequently employed in pediatric ALL, given the inability to diagnose the t(12;21) by standard cytogenetics. The

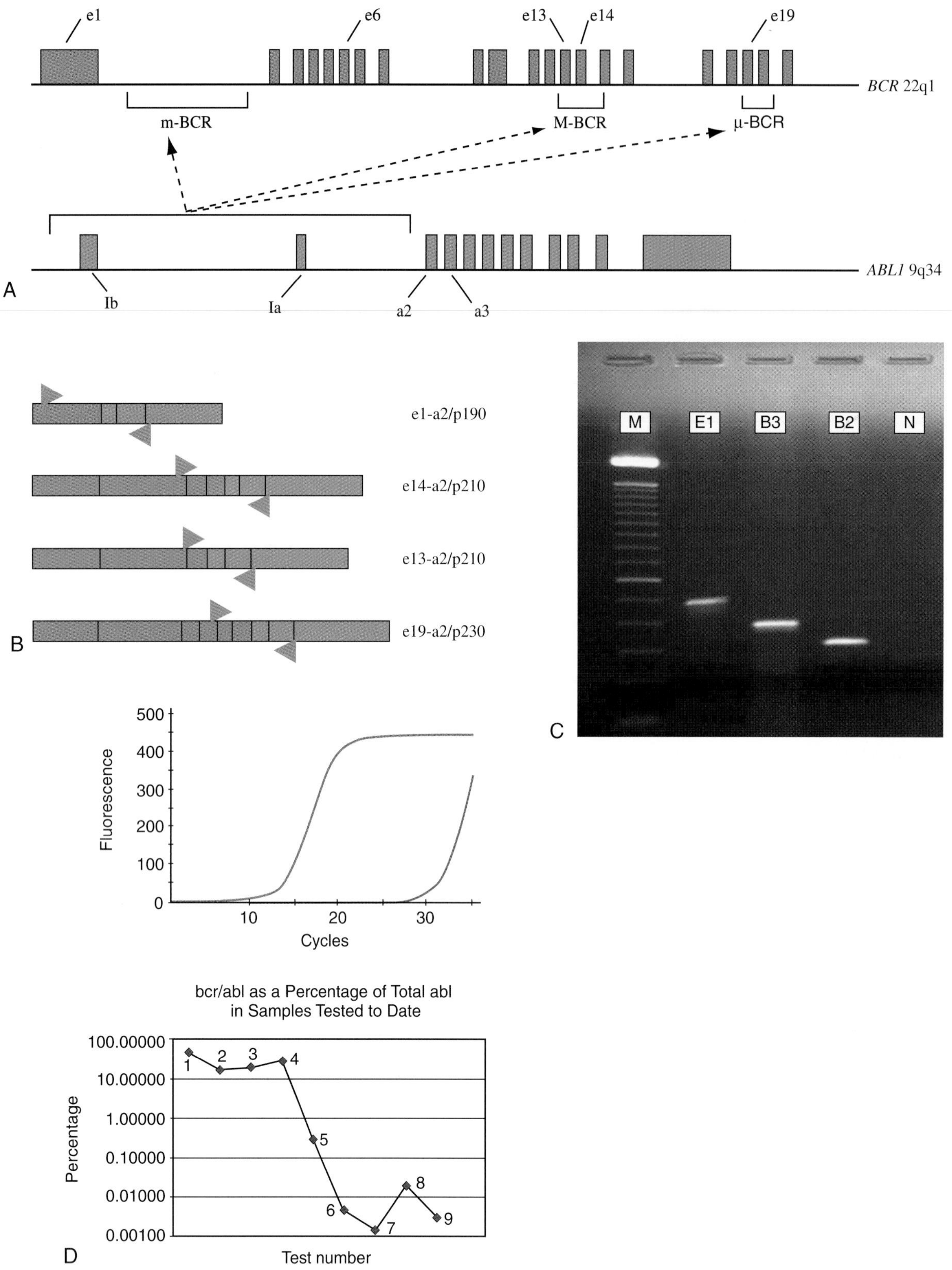

Figure 75-3 t(9;22)/*BCR-ABL1* abnormality in chronic myeloid leukemia and Ph+ acute lymphoblastic leukemia. **A,** The partial genomic organization of the *BCR* and *ABL1* genes (not to scale). Three major breakpoint regions are recognized in the *BCR* gene: the minor breakpoint cluster region (m-BCR), the major breakpoint cluster region (M-BCR), and the μ-BCR. The M-BCR is involved in essentially all cases of CML and approximately one third of de novo adult Ph+ acute lymphoblastic leukemias (Ph+ ALL). A small percentage of childhood Ph+ ALL may have BCR breakpoints at this site as well. The m-BCR is typically associated with the vast majority of pediatric Ph+ ALL and most adult Ph+ ALL. Breakpoints at the μ-BCR have been associated with rare cases of CML with essentially complete neutrophilic maturation. For the *ABL1* gene, breakpoints are distributed throughout a large region 5′ of exon 2 (a2) encompassing the first exon region. **B,** The principal BCR-ABL1 chimeric transcripts arising from these various translocation fusion gene breakpoints. The exon-exon fusions are indicated for these transcripts and the corresponding chimeric protein product sizes are shown in kilodaltons (e.g., e1-a2/p190). The orange arrows indicate relative positions of PCR primers to detect these various forms in RT-PCR assays. **C,** Typical RT-PCR gel electrophoresis results for detection of the m-BCR and M-BCR transcripts. **D,** Example of RQ-PCR monitoring of BCR-ABL1 mRNA in a CML patient being treated with imatinib mesylate. The upper section displays the RQ-PCR amplification traces for BCR-ABL1 *(purple)* and ABL1 control *(green)*. The quantity of BCR-ABL1 is expressed as a normalized ratio of BCR-ABL1/ABL1. The lower section indicates a time course of quantitative BCR-ABL1 level measurements over several months for this patient. A therapeutic level of less than 0.1% BCR-ABL1/ABL1 in CML is compatible with an excellent outcome and very low relapse risk. *CML,* Chronic myeloid leukemia; *E1,* e1-a2 product; *E13,* e13-a2 product; *E14,* e14-a2 product; *M,* molecular size marker (100 bp); *N,* no template control; *RQ-PCR,* real-time quantitative polymerase chain reaction; *RT-PCR,* reverse-transcriptase polymerase chain reaction.

chimeric mRNA further represents a highly specific molecular marker for residual disease assessment.

Translocations involving the "mixed lineage leukemia" (*MLL*) gene located on chromosome 11q23 are observed in 5%–9% of pediatric ALL cases overall and are disproportionately represented in infants younger than 1 year of age (Bartolo, 2000; Armstrong, 2005; Silverman, 2007; Chowdhury, 2008). The presence of *MLL* gene translocations is associated with a poor outcome for these very young children and is considered an adverse finding in older children as well, particularly in the setting of a poor prednisone response (Pui, 2003; Chowdhury, 2008). Infant *MLL*-positive leukemias are of B-lineage, lack CD10 positivity, and demonstrate aberrant expression of some myeloid-associated markers (Chen, 1993; Burmeister, 2009). Clinically, these patients have high initial leukocyte counts, organomegaly, and a tendency for involvement of the central nervous system. Translocations involving 11q23/*MLL* also occur in de novo AML and secondary (therapy-related) AML and in either case are characterized by monocytic morphologic features (i.e., FAB AML-M4 or M5 types). In de novo adult AML, *MLL* gene rearrangements, specifically the t(9;11) *MLLT3-MLL* abnormality, may not represent a high risk tumor genotype. In contrast, secondary AML arises in subsets of both pediatric and adult patients who have had prior dose intensive chemotherapy with DNA topoisomerase II inhibitors (e.g., epipodophyllotoxins and anthracyclines); these tumors occur abruptly within a few months to years after exposure and have a very aggressive treatment-resistant course (Godley, 2008).

The pathobiology underlying *MLL* gene translocations in these different types of de novo and secondary acute lymphoid and myeloid leukemias is becoming better understood. The MLL protein is a large (~430 kD) DNA binding protein, which is characterized by several functional domains, indicating its role as a multifunctional transcriptional factor with histone methyltransferase activity (Hess, 2004; Li, 2005; Krivtsov, 2007; Wang, 2009). *MLL* is known to regulate several *HOX* (homeobox) genes involved in the coordination of proper skeletal development during mammalian embryogenesis (Yu, 1995; Soshnikova, 2008). Several *HOX* genes also appear to be central to the development and maintenance of myeloid and lymphoid progenitor cells, thus establishing a tight link for *MLL* in the genetic control of normal hematopoiesis as well (Hess, 2004; Ernst, 2004a; Ernst, 2004b; McGonigle, 2008). *MLL* gene translocations produce an altered functional form of the protein; in each instance, the N-terminal "A-T hook" DNA binding motif of MLL is retained in the chimeric protein, typically with fusion to a portion of another transcription factor (Waring, 1997; Chowdhury, 2008). Accumulating data indicate that abnormal expression of MLL fusion proteins can constitutively deregulate certain *HOX* genes, leading to hematopoietic progenitor cell immortalization and predisposition to leukemogenesis (Armstrong, 2003; Hess, 2004; Ono, 2009). Indeed, recent studies using chromatin immunoprecipitation to identify portions of the genome bound by MLL have further detected its presence at numerous promoter regions, suggesting a more global role for MLL in transcriptional regulation.

Some additional key biologic insights have emerged from the structural analysis of *MLL* gene breakpoints in different subsets of leukemias. The majority of de novo AML with *MLL* translocations have breaksites situated 5′ in the *MLL* breakpoint cluster region, whereas the preponderance of secondary AML occur in a more distal (3′) segment of this locus (Stissel-Broeker, 1996; Zhang, 2006). Infant ALL cases strikingly also tend to associate with the 3′ genomic region, suggesting a commonality in pathogenesis with secondary AML. This 3′ "hotspot" area contains a strong consensus binding site for DNA topoisomerase II, as well as an adjacent "scaffold attachment region," which is highly susceptible to cleavage by endonucleases. Although the presence of the topoisomerase II site presents an attractive explanation for the basis of developing secondary AML (e.g., via double strand break induction by topoisomerase II inhibitors and subsequent *MLL* translocation rearrangements), the hypersensitive 3′ scaffold site of the gene has received further attention, since it too appears to be particularly prone to double strand breaks in experimental models (Stissel-Broeker, 1996). The latter *MLL* region is in fact selectively targeted for cleavage during cell death in response to diverse apoptogenic stimuli (e.g., following cellular stress or DNA damage) (Betti, 2001; Sim, 2001; Betti, 2003; Greaves, 2003a; Betti, 2005). These recent investigations imply that exposure to agents that can induce this site-specific *MLL* breakage potentially set the stage for *MLL* gene fusions, leading to the very aggressive forms of leukemia observed in infants and after distinct types of chemotherapy. In turn, because the causal etiology is already identified for secondary AML with *MLL* translocations, current studies in infant ALL seek to discover possible exogenous or naturally occurring transplacental factors that may predispose developing fetal hematopoietic stem cells to *MLL* gene breakage and illegitimate recombination (Spector, 2005; Pombo-de-Oliveira, 2006).

The *MLL* gene is involved in translocation events with more than 60 known partner genes (Liu, 2009); however, the t(4;11)(q21;q23)/*MLL-AF4* abnormality is the most frequently encountered in infant ALL (75% of cases). *MLL* gene locus breakpoints are distributed over an 8.3 kb region of DNA encompassing exons 5-11 (Chowdhury, 2008). This marked breakpoint heterogeneity may also occur in the translocated gene (e.g., *AF4*), resulting in the possibility of several *MLL* hybrid gene products, typically one of which is expressed in any given patient with this leukemia. RT-PCR method can be used to identify individual MLL fusion gene transcripts, such as the MLL-AF4 chimeric mRNA; however, the combination of multiple rearranging gene partners in these leukemias and the potential for substantial genomic breakpoint variability requires comprehensive and technically challenging laboratory approaches, such as multiplex PCR assays or, in the research setting, techniques such as long-distance inverse PCR (Pallisgaard, 1998; Andersson, 2001; Meyer, 2009a, 2009b). *MLL* gene locus rearrangements have also been successfully detected by Southern blot analysis, although FISH technique now provides a rapid and highly efficacious alternative for this purpose (Cuthbert, 2000; Cavazzini, 2006). FISH analysis can provide very rapid confirmation of *MLL* gene breakage, implying a translocation event, but cannot give information regarding the particular translocation present. Thus RT-PCR, even with the limitations described, can serve a useful purpose in the diagnosis and monitoring of these leukemias, especially because the fusion gene type can be specifically and more sensitively identified in contrast to other analytic methods.

Prenatal Origins of Childhood Leukemias

Major advances continue to be made in understanding the molecular basis of the pediatric acute leukemias. These efforts now span the realms of basic science, translational and clinical research, and increasingly, population-based methods. Studies of concordant ALL occurring in monozygotic twins first demonstrated that the leukemias arising in each paired affected individual were genetically identical based on molecular analysis of the genomic breakpoint sequences of involved *MLL*, *ETV6-RUNX1*, or clonotypic immunoglobulin or T cell receptor gene rearrangements (summarized in Greaves, 2003b; Taub, 2004). Notably, the propensity to develop concordant leukemias is variable for different leukemic subtypes in twin studies, approaching 100% for *MLL* translocation ALL and only 10% for *ETV6-RUNX1* ALL. These findings suggest a variable transformation potential for these different gene fusions in vivo, raising the issues of both the nature and timing of secondary genetic insults. The results of these investigations have been corroborated using similar experimental techniques to "back track" leukemia-specific DNA abnormalities to archived neonatal blood samples of individual (nontwin) children of different ages, with genetically defined subtypes of ALL or AML (Gale, 1997; Wiemels, 1999; Fasching, 2000; Yagi, 2000; Wiemels, 2002a; Greaves, 2003a, 2003b; Taub, 2004; Ross, 2008). Together, these data strongly suggest that many pediatric ALL (and some AML) have origins in utero; that is, prenatal acquisition of potentially leukemogenic translocation events, or other genetic abnormalities, can occur during the time of active fetal hematopoiesis, but in most cases additional, later-occurring genetic alterations in susceptible individuals are required in order to produce overt leukemia. The rapid evolution of *MLL*-associated ALL vs. the longer latency (i.e., older age at onset) of *ETV6-RUNX1* ALL indicates that both the biologic effects of the primary (predisposing) genetic lesion, as well as the timing and type of promoting insult(s) are complex, although within defined subtypes of leukemia, it may now be possible to better elucidate the molecular pathways resulting in tumorigenesis. Not all types of pediatric ALL however, can be traced back to a prenatal clonal cell origin. The retrospective neonatal blood data for the t(1;19)/*TCF3-PBX1* ALL subgroup instead support the concept that the majority of these patients develop this genetic aberration in the postnatal period (Wiemels, 2002b).

Prospective RT-PCR and FISH screening of blood samples from healthy newborn children has subsequently revealed a detection frequency of 1% for the *ETV6-RUNX1* abnormality and 0.2% for the *RUNX1-RUNX1T1* fusion transcript, markedly higher than the incidence of either of these leukemia subtypes in childhood (Mori, 2002; Olsen, 2006). These data demonstrate that the occurrence of at least some chromosomal translocation fusion genes is a common event in utero; however the presence of such an abnormality is clearly insufficient to cause overt leukemia in the vast majority of individuals. Although the translocation-type acute leukemias are karyotypically characterized in most instances by an apparent

PART 9

"single genetic anomaly," it is becoming evident that these tumors also conform to the "two-hit" hypothesis of Knudson proposed for solid tissue cancers (Knudson, 1992; Schindler, 2009), as discussed in further detail in Chapter 74. In this concept, the initiating translocation event must be stable enough in a long-lived progenitor hematopoietic cell to confer some advantage in survival or proliferation; the acquisition of one or more subsequent genotoxic events in a susceptible individual would then lead to complete malignant transformation. The fate of such silent "translocation positive" cells is thus an important parameter, not only for understanding disease pathogenesis, but also in a practical setting for the appropriate interpretation of molecular diagnostic assays in the context of detecting minimal residual disease.

Intriguingly, recent research using genome-wide association has identified certain low-penetrance germline variants of *IKZF1* (as well as other genes) that may increase susceptibility to the development of childhood ALL (Papaemmanuil, 2009). Even though much research remains directed at the basic molecular and cell biology of childhood acute leukemias, molecular epidemiologic methods will play an increasing role in identifying the interplay between environmental factors and host genetic polymorphisms, which underlie the predisposition to this disease in some individuals (Clavel, 2005; Spector, 2005; La Fiura, 2007; reviewed in Pui 2008). Indeed, the relatively brief period of potential environmental exposure in utero may lend itself to the detection of specific risk factors in a manner impossible for adult-onset leukemias (Kim, 2006; Ross, 2008); mitigation strategies to decrease the risk of childhood leukemia is thus a goal of these efforts.

T Cell Lymphoblastic Leukemia/Lymphoma

In contrast to the relatively well-understood pathobiology of B lineage ALL, the genetic underpinnings of T cell lymphoblastic neoplasms (T-ALL) have historically remained obscure. This may be partially explained by the relative rarity of T-ALL in comparison to B-ALL, with the former accounting for 15% and 25% of pediatric and adult cases of overall lymphoblastic leukemias, respectively (Chiaretti, 2009). Recently, however, molecular genetic techniques have uncovered a surprisingly diverse set of abnormalities seen recurrently in T-ALL. These studies have begun to elucidate what have been previously unknown leukemogenic mechanisms, although currently these investigational findings have not yet been definitively linked with relevant clinical or prognostic subgroups of patients, or with applications to minimal residual disease detection (Baldus, 2009; Mansour, 2009). Translocations involving the T cell receptor genes are identified in up to 35% of T-ALL, juxtaposing TCR regions with a wide array of partner genes that often code for transcription factors, including *HOX11*, *HOX11L2*, *HOXA*, and *TAL1* (Chiaretti, 2009). The *TAL1* oncogene is also frequently (25% of cases) fused to its neighbor *SIL* following a cryptic interstitial deletion at 1p32 (van der Burg, 2002). More than 50% of cases of T-ALL have activating mutations in *NOTCH1*, which encodes a transmembrane receptor important in the regulation of physiologic T cell development. In a manner analogous to the role played by *FLT3* in some cases of AML, mutations in *NOTCH1* create a constitutively active receptor promoting unchecked downstream signaling, resulting in altered expression of target genes, including the oncogene *MYC* (Pui 2008). In some cases, missense mutations in *FBXW7*, a negative regulator of *NOTCH1*, can achieve the same pathogenic effect (Park, 2009). Abnormal tyrosine kinase activity is also found in subsets of T-ALL. The *NUP214(CAN)-ABL1* gene fusion, which is often found in amplified extrachromosomal episomes formed from 9q34, is identified in 6% of cases (Graux, 2004). *JAK1* mutations are detectable in 18% of T-ALL and may be associated with an inferior prognosis (Flex 2008).

MOLECULAR DIAGNOSIS OF MYELOPROLIFERATIVE NEOPLASMS

Chronic Myelogenous Leukemia, BCR-ABL1 Positive

Chronic myelogenous (or myeloid) leukemia is a clonal marrow stem cell disease resulting predominantly from excessive proliferation of granulocytic cells at all stages of maturation. The natural course of CML is typified by a protracted chronic phase, often for several years, followed by a rapid transformation to an aggressive acute myeloid or lymphoid blast crisis with fatal outcome. The decades-long investigation and treatment of this disorder has led from the association of a karyotypic abnormality with disease phenotype, to the unraveling of its molecular genetic pathogenesis, and currently, to the widespread use of a highly effective targeted pharmacologic therapy in the form of imatinib mesylate (Gleevec, Novartis) (Goldman, 2003; Pavlovsky, 2009). CML is characterized by the presence of the t(9;22)(q34;q11.2) chromosomal translocation, initially observed as an abnormal 22q- termed the *Philadelphia chromosome* (Ph) (Nowell, 1960; Rowley, 1973). This translocation leads to juxtaposition of the *ABL1* tyrosine kinase gene (9q34) with the *BCR* gene (22q11.2) on the derivative chromosome 22q, formation of the *BCR-ABL1* fusion gene and mRNA, and production of a chimeric BCR-ABL1 protein (Melo, 1996; Deininger, 2000). As noted, the t(9;22)/*BCR-ABL1* is not pathognomonic of CML, in that it also occurs in 20%–25% of adult and approximately 3% of pediatric ALLs (i.e., Ph+ ALL), in both instances associated with highly aggressive disease behavior.

Despite the notably long history of research involving *BCR-ABL1* (the Philadelphia chromosome was the first such translocation associated with a neoplasm), the detailed pathogenesis of CML remains to be fully elucidated. ABL1 is normally a highly regulated tyrosine kinase that participates in diverse cellular processes pertaining to actin organization, cellular differentiation, apoptosis, and T cell receptor signaling. The function of the normal BCR gene product is incompletely understood; it contains several functional domains, including a serine/threonine kinase and has been shown to participate in vascular intimal signaling in response to injury and inflammation (Alexis, 2009). In general, the abnormal genetic fusion disrupts the localization and regulated activity of the ABL1 tyrosine kinase, producing complex effects on cellular signal transduction pathways, proliferation, apoptosis control, and cell adhesion (Deininger, 2000; Quintás-Cardama, 2009). The reciprocal *ABL1-BCR* fusion gene, long regarded as an inconsequential byproduct of the creation of the *BCR-ABL1* fusion, may also have some independent effects of cellular proliferation (Zheng, 2009). In vivo topographic studies of the *BCR* and *ABL1* genes in cycling normal hematopoietic progenitor cells, as well as the surprising demonstration of very low levels of BCR-ABL1 transcripts in the blood of many healthy subjects, suggest that the t(9;22) may occur relatively frequently in normal human bone marrow cells (Brassesco, 2008). The complex interplay of host response to these abnormal genetic rearrangements and the acquisition of other initiating or potentiating genetic lesions leading to the overt development of CML (or Ph+ ALL) are yet to be determined. Definitive treatment for patients with CML is achieved only by allogeneic bone marrow or stem cell transplantation, although the frontline management of CML has now been significantly altered with the advent of imatinib and other similar tyrosine kinase inhibitors, such that the disease may now be controlled over long periods of time, although not eliminated (Druker, 2001; O'Brien, 2003; Pavlovsky, 2009).

At the DNA level, the *BCR-ABL1* gene fusion exhibits features of breakpoint heterogeneity with three main recognized breakpoint loci in the *BCR* gene, as well as some alternative splice transcript variation (see Fig. 75-3, *A* and *B*) (Melo, 1996; Deininger, 2000; Foroni, 2009). In virtually all cases of CML, the *BCR* gene breakpoints are situated in the so-called major breakpoint cluster region, or M-BCR. These breaksites occur in a relatively small 5.8 kb genomic region spanning *BCR* exons e12-e16 (also known as exons b1-b5), specifically between the e13 and e14, or the e14 and e15 exons. In contrast, the breakpoints in the *ABL1* gene are distributed over a very large region of intronic DNA 5′ to exon a2. In CML therefore, two types of BCR-ABL1 fusion mRNA transcripts can arise from M-BCR locus gene fusions, namely the e13-a2, or e14-a2 forms. These two products encode a novel protein of 210 kD (p210). Whereas most cases of CML harbor either a e13-a2 or e14-a2 transcript type, occasional tumors may demonstrate alternative splicing of the latter form to produce both transcripts simultaneously; this occurrence may be attributable to a polymorphism in *BCR* that affects splicing efficiency. In the pre-imatinib era, the type of M-BCR locus *BCR-ABL1* fusion in CML was considered to hold no clinical or prognostic significance; however, recent data suggest the possibility of differential imatinib sensitivity based on the transcript type, requiring further investigation (Lucas, 2009). A second common breakpoint locus is present in the *BCR* gene, designated as the minor breakpoint cluster region, or m-BCR. Translocations involving this locus result in the formation of an e1-a2 BCR-ABL1 fusion transcript, encoding a 190 kD BCR-ABL1 protein (p190). The e1-a2 type BCR-ABL1 is highly characteristic of Ph+ ALL. However, the subdivision of M-BCR and m-BCR fusions as CML-associated and ALL-associated is not so straightforward, despite these general correlations between *BCR-ABL1* breakpoint fusion location and disease phenotype. Whereas the vast majority of pediatric Ph+ ALL cases are of e1-a2 (m-BCR) type, approximately 30%–40% of adult Ph+ ALL patients demonstrate e14-a2 or e13-a2 (M-BCR) BCR-ABL fusions. In the latter situation, distinction of true de novo Ph+ ALL from CML in lymphoid blast crisis is important. In addition, it is well known that a significant proportion of classic CML with the expected e14-a2 or e13-a2 transcript types will also demonstrate concurrent low abundance e1-a2 mRNA due to a minimal degree of alternative splicing of the longer M-BCR derived transcript (Saglio, 1996; van Rhee 1996). Potentially more confusing is the finding of rare Ph+ chronic leukemias with the e1-a2 fusion that manifest a predominantly monocytic phenotype (rather than the typical myeloid cell predominance of CML). These foregoing observations underscore the pathobiologic variability associated with *BCR-ABL1* expression in different myeloid and lymphoid progenitor cells. The third cluster region for *BCR-ABL1* gene fusions has been called the μ-BCR and results in formation of an e19-a2 transcript. This fusion transcript is predicted to result in translation of a 230 kD size protein (p230) and this type of *BCR-ABL1* event has been associated with a myeloproliferative neoplasm showing exuberant neutrophilia. Historically, these cases have been labeled as *chronic neutrophilic leukemias*, but the current view considers these rare e19-a2 fusion-positive presentations to be bona fide cases of CML (Swerdlow, 2008). Rarely occurring CML and Ph+ ALL cases involving the use of alternate, adjacent BCR or ABL exons have been encountered, generating e13-a3, e1-a3, or e6-a2 transcript forms (Melo, 1996; Deininger, 2000; Foroni, 2009).

Figure 75-3, *B*, indicates the placement of oligonucleotide PCR primers to specifically amplify the M-BCR (e14-a2, e13-a2), m-BCR (e1-a2), and μ-BCR (e19-a2) fusion transcripts following reverse transcription of total mRNA; these molecular assays can be designed to be either qualitative or quantitative in nature. Qualitative assays for *BCR-ABL1* detection may rely on gel electrophoresis sizing of PCR products as shown in Figure 75-3, *C*, often with a post-PCR confirmatory assay, such as Southern blot hybridization using a junction-specific labeled oligonucleotide probe or related methods. Given the importance of long-term monitoring of BCR-ABL1 transcript levels in CML patients (discussed later), many labs also perform RQ-PCR. In one such assay strategy, reverse transcribed BCR-ABL1 transcript abundance is determined relative to a concurrently generated standard curve, and the results are reported as a normalized ratio of BCR-ABL1 copies to the copies of a similarly measured normally expressed mRNA (often the normal BCR or ABL1 transcript itself) to correct for variable cellular abundance and RNA quality in different samples (Fig. 75-3) (Foroni, 2009). Although PCR-based methods are highly sensitive, FISH analysis may have some additional utility for identifying concurrent large genomic deletions occurring on the derivative 9q or 22q chromosomes, which have been associated with inferior outcome in this subgroup of CML patients (Sinclair, 2000; Lee, 2006; Vaz de Campos, 2007); however, the impact of these additional findings may be relatively less important in the era of imatinib therapy (Kim, 2008).

Molecular detection of these abnormal BCR-ABL1 mRNA chimeric transcripts is clearly valuable for establishing a diagnosis of CML and Ph+ ALL. For example, even though approximately 98% of CML cases are BCR-ABL1 positive, a small number of morphologic mimickers will lack this genetic abnormality. These leukemic disorders fall into an ill-defined subset including atypical CML, chronic myelomonocytic leukemia, or other chronic myeloproliferative or myelodysplastic disorders, and therapeutic options and outcome for such patients will be different than for true CML. Conversely, atypical myeloproliferative presentations of CML are not infrequently encountered and the demonstration of BCR-ABL1 in these situations is critical for correct diagnosis and management. Similarly, detection of the BCR-ABL1 abnormality in adult and pediatric ALL identifies these subsets of patients who are at high risk for conventional chemotherapy failure and may benefit from more intensive treatment regimens.

Molecular diagnostic evaluation for BCR-ABL1 is also important for delineating the specific BCR-ABL1 fusion mRNA type for subsequent molecular MRD monitoring following allogeneic stem cell transplantation (ASCT), chemoimmunotherapy (e.g., with Ara-C and interferon-α [IFN-α] therapy), or therapy with tyrosine kinase inhibitors, or TKIs (e.g., imatinib mesylate). For example, the quantitative level of BCR-ABL1 transcript in ASCT patients in the early posttransplant period has been strongly correlated with risk of relapse (Olavarria, 2001; Faderl, 2004). Other data similarly suggested more refined outcome prediction in PCR-positive patients who are further out from transplantation, using RQ-PCR technique (Radich, 2001). RQ-PCR for BCR-ABL1 has also proven worthwhile in evaluating treatment response to IFN-α, despite the observation that molecular remissions with this agent are very uncommon. However, the largest impact on RQ-PCR monitoring of BCR-ABL1 in CML has come with the widespread use of targeted therapy with TKIs (e.g., imatinib and related drugs). For CML patients on TKI agents, therapeutic responses are evaluated in a highly coordinated manner using clinical (i.e., hematologic), cytogenetic, and molecular MRD criteria. Single-agent imatinib (previously called STI-571) was shown to be highly effective in inducing complete hematologic and cytogenetic responses in the majority of treated CML patients within 12 months (Hughes, 2003, 2009). These data were reported in the landmark International Randomized Study of Interferon and STI-571 (IRIS) clinical trial and results were updated recently (Hochhaus, 2008; Hochhaus, 2009).

Importantly, data derived from these and other studies have demonstrated that the kinetics of BCR-ABL1 reduction is strongly related to progression-free survival. While criteria are continually being refined, several critical thresholds have been defined that indicate optimal response to imatinib. The vast majority of CML patients will achieve complete hematologic remission within 3 months. Subsequently, favorable response to TKI therapy is indicated by the attainment of a complete cytogenetic response (CCyR, defined by the absence of Ph metaphases by cytogenetic analysis), followed by a major molecular response (MMR). The MMR level has been defined by the IRIS group as 3-log reduction from baseline BCR-ABL1 level, equivalent to 0.1% normalized BCR-ABL transcript ratio (i.e., BCR-ABL1/ABL1). A significant challenge for molecular hematopathology laboratories lies in the development of standardized RQ-PCR assays for BCR-ABL1 that can meet the requirements of technical sensitivity and reproducibility for reporting patient results on this international scale (IS). Patients who achieve MMR within a 12- to 18-month window following TKI therapy initiation have an excellent long-term prognosis and a very low relapse risk (see Fig. 75-3, *D*) (Hughes, 2009). A subset of individuals may also continue to deepen their molecular response and eventually become PCR negative. Similarly, the combination of bone marrow cytogenetics and peripheral blood RQ-PCR for BCR-ABL1 levels can also be predictive of treatment failure and increased relapse risk. Patients who do not achieve a major cytogenetic response (<35% Ph metaphases) or remain above 10% normalized BCR-ABL1 transcript level at 6 months, or those failing to become cytogenetically negative (CCyR) for the t(9;22) with BCR-ABL1/ABL1 >1% at 12 months, are at significantly higher risk of disease progression. These timepoints have been incorporated into a benchmark strategy by the European LeukemiaNet for monitoring suboptimal responses to TKI therapy in CML patients (Baccarani, 2009).

Although more than 80% of CML patients on imatinib will be alive and without adverse events at 6 years (Hochhaus, 2008, 2009; Hughes, 2009), a significant subgroup will manifest resistance to imatinib. Imatinib treatment failures are typically identified by loss of a previously attained CCyR, loss of MMR, or suboptimal responses at timepoints as described earlier. Although resistance to TKI therapy is complex, about 50% of CML patients develop point mutations in the ABL1 kinase domain of the chimeric *BCR-ABL1* gene that confer variable degrees of nonresponsiveness to imatinib or second generation agents. Interestingly, such mutations may be naturally selected in the presence of these drugs, such that cells harboring the *ABL1* kinase domain mutations (KDM) gain a survival advantage and expand under the continued pressure of the pharmacologic therapy. Abnormal activity of activation-induced cytidine deaminase (AID), an enzyme important in the somatic hypermutation process in germinal center B cells, may be important in the acquisition of *ABL1* KDM in CML patients (Klemm, 2009). For patients being monitored by RQ-PCR, an increase in normalized BCR-ABL1 transcript level of 0.5 to 1 log, demonstrated in at least two consecutive samples is often indicative of the presence of an acquired *ABL1* KDM. The precise quantitative level of change is somewhat controversial and other investigators have suggested an increase of only 2.6-fold as optimal for detection of a KDM when using a highly optimized RQ-PCR assay (Press, 2009). *ABL1* mutations can occur anywhere in the kinase domain, but tend to preferentially involve critical amino acids in several regions corresponding to the phosphorylation loop (P-loop), activation loop (A-loop), and drug contact sites. Notably, P-loop and some direct contact site mutations are associated with high-level resistance to imatinib. Examples of common P-loop alterations include Q252H, Y253F/H, E255K/V, and G250E. Nonetheless, a significant number of imatinib resistance mutants can be overcome by increasing the dosage of imatinib or by switching to a second generation TKI, such as dasatinib, nilotinib, or bosutinib. Most problematic of all is the contact site mutation T315I, which is relatively frequently encountered and exhibits marked in vivo and clinical resistance to imatinib and all other currently approved second generation TKI drugs (Quintás-Cardama, 2008a). Molecular diagnostic evaluation for *ABL1* KDM is therefore an increasingly integral part of assessment for a subset of CML patients (Jones, 2009). Most commonly, *ABL1* KDM are detected by direct sequencing of the amplified region of ABL1 from the BCR-ABL1 transcript. This approach is relatively insensitive technically, but is successful at mRNA levels of BCR-ABL1/ABL1 at or above the MMR, where acquired drug resistance is likely to be encountered. The scope of ABL1 KDM analysis has progressed to allow predictions of response to the various TKI agents in clinical use, thus giving the managing physician a rational approach to selecting alternative TKI drugs if mutation-based resistance to one agent has developed in a given patient (Branford, 2009). Efforts to refine this type of real-time therapeutic efficacy assessment will continue as newer TKI or related small molecule kinase inhibitors enter the clinical arena. In this regard, overcoming the particularly adverse effects of the pan-resistant T315I is a major goal. Finally, it should be noted that low-level mutations can be identified using very sensitive targeted molecular techniques in chronic phase CML patients who are otherwise initially responsive to imatinib. The predictive value of such small subclonal populations is not well understood and currently there is no rationale for "early" mutation detection in CML patients starting treatment with imatinib; however, the importance of detecting small mutated clones may increase as more data emerge (Quintás-Cardama, 2008b).

Ph-Negative Myeloproliferative Neoplasms: Polycythemia Vera, Essential Thrombocythemia, and Primary Myelofibrosis—JAK2 and MPL Gene Mutations

The non-CML, or Ph-negative myeloproliferative neoplasms (MPN), include polycythemia vera (PV), essential thrombocythemia (ET), and primary myelofibrosis (PMF). These diseases are individually characterized by a defined set of clinical, laboratory, and morphologic features, yet show striking overlap in several aspects. Until recently, relatively little was understood about the molecular pathogenesis of the Ph-negative MPN; however, this situation has improved substantially with the discovery of mutations involving the *JAK2* (Janus kinase 2) gene, encoding a tyrosine kinase central to ligand-induced cell signaling in hematopoietic progenitor cells. In 2005, four research groups independently described a novel single point mutation abnormality in *JAK2*, occurring in classically defined chronic MPN exclusive of CML (Baxter, 2005; James, 2005; Kralovics, 2005; Levine, 2005). This mutation produces a V617F amino acid substitution (phenylalanine for valine), and constitutively activates the JAK2 tyrosine kinase. These studies and others have subsequently identified the *JAK2* V617F in 95% of PV, 75% of PMF, and 50% of ET. JAK2 is one member of a family of structurally related tyrosine kinases containing a tyrosine kinase domain and an adjacent "pseudokinase" domain, the latter functioning to inhibit and thus autoregulate activity of the true kinase domain (Ihle, 2007); this juxtaposition of activation and autoregulatory regions thus accounts for the designation of this class of genes after the two-faced Roman god Janus (Fig. 75-4). In normal cellular function, JAK proteins function to initiate cellular signaling pathways between specific cell surface receptors lacking catalytic activity, via interactions with STAT proteins (signal transducers and activators of transcription); activated STAT proteins translocate to the nucleus and differentially regulate target genes in response to the corresponding initial cell surface signal (Pfeifer, 2008). Of note, the V617F mutation so consistently identified in these entities affects the inhibitory pseudokinase domain of the protein, resulting in unchecked ligand-independent tyrosine kinase activity of JAK2 and an increased propensity for cellular proliferation (Ihle, 2007). JAK2 in particular associates with the cell surface erythropoietin receptor (EPO-R) and becomes activated by the binding of EPO, thus accounting in part for the significance of the V617F mutation in the pathogenesis of PV.

The variability of disease phenotypes among the different Ph-negative MPN that otherwise share the presence of a single common gene mutation remains incompletely understood, but several hypotheses have been advanced to explain the apparent centrality of the *JAK2* V617F mutation in the three major MPN subtypes (James, 2008). First, the nature of the hematopoietic progenitor cell in which the *JAK2* mutation occurs may result in specific patterns of disease. For example, a V617F mutation arising in cells fully or partially committed to erythroid or megakaryocytic differentiation might be expected to induce phenotypic features in the progeny of the transformed cells consistent with PV or an ET type processes, respectively. Second, the amount of mutated, activated protein that is produced seems to have some bearing on disease phenotype. Patients with PV and a subset of those with PMF are more likely to be homozygous for the V617F mutation and consequently have a higher mutated "allele burden" than do patients with ET. Interestingly, homozygous mutation status is selected for by the process of uniparental disomy (copy-neutral

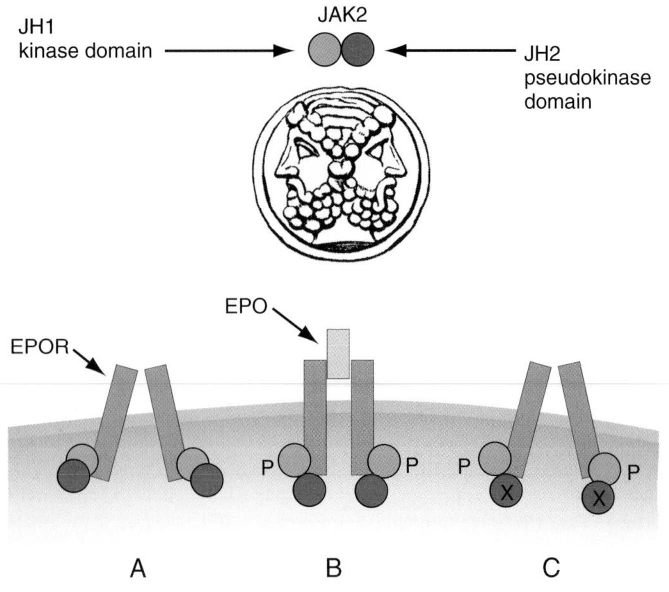

Figure 75-4 Role of *JAK2* mutations in myeloproliferative neoplasms, *BCR-ABL1* (Ph) negative. The Janus kinase 2 (JAK2) "two headed" protein is illustrated by two circles, corresponding to the JH1 tyrosine kinase domain *(green)* and the inhibitory JH2 pseudokinase domain *(red)*. ***A,*** JAK2 has bound to the erythropoietin receptor (EPOR). In the absence of ligand binding, the JH2 domain prevents activation of the JH1 domain. ***B,*** The ligand erythropoietin has bound to the receptor, inducing conformational changes that permit activation of the JH1 tyrosine kinase domain. ***C,*** The *JAK2* V617F mutation (indicated by "X") prevents proper interaction between the JH2 and JH1 domains, thus allowing tyrosine kinase activity at extremely low concentrations of ligand, or even in the absence of ligand binding. *(Adapted from Klipp E and Liebermeister W. Mathematical modeling of intracellular signaling pathways. BMC Neurosci 2006;7(Suppl 1):10; Bennett M and Stroncek DF. Recent advances in the bcr-abl negative chronic myeloproliferative diseases. J Transl Med 2006;4:41.)*

loss of heterozygosity), usually through mitotic duplication of the mutated *JAK2* allele (Kralovics, 2002; Vannucchi, 2008). Third, the larger genetic background in which the mutation occurs may to some degree influence the expression of the disease. For example, the introduction of the V617F mutation into different strains of mice yields consistently different disease phenotypes (James, 2008), and some evidence suggests that polymorphisms in such genes as *JAK2* and *EPOR* are associated with certain MPNs but not with others (Pardanani, 2008). Furthermore, despite the major advance represented by the discovery of *JAK2* V617F mutations in MPN, this genetic lesion is clearly not present in all cases and as a corollary, many presentations of MPN (especially ET and some PMF) are not associated with deregulation of this gene. This has led to the suggestion that the *JAK2* mutation may be a relatively late event in transformation (Kralovics, 2006, Nussenzveig, 2007), with earlier mutations in other unknown genes perhaps setting the stage for the development of a specific MPN and the *JAK2* mutation providing only the final element necessary for growth factor-independent proliferation. Nevertheless, the advent of small molecule JAK2 inhibitors for clinical use indicates the importance of this target in both disease biology and management.

Whereas constitutive JAK2 activation is clearly important in the MPN, this relationship is most consistent in PV. It now appears that the small number (approximately 5%) of patients with PV who lack the *JAK2* V617F mutation instead harbor different mutations in *JAK2*, most commonly involving exon 12 (Scott, 2007; Pietra, 2008). Patients with PV with *JAK2* exon 12 mutations do not show the same propensity to thrombocytosis as those with *JAK2* V617F mutations, but otherwise the disease appears clinically similar, despite the alternate localization of the mutation (Kilpivaara, 2008). Finally, in addition to *JAK2* mutations, other genetic abnormalities are also biologically and diagnostically important in this setting. Mutations in the *MPL* gene have been identified in a subset (<10%) of *JAK2*-negative cases of ET and PMF (Pikman, 2006; Tefferi, 2008; Beer, 2008). *MPL* encodes the cell surface receptor for thrombopoietin, and activating mutations thus induce aberrant constitutive signaling effects as observed similarly for mutated *JAK2*. The changes in *MPL* involve several possible amino acid substitutions (W to L, K, or S), all occurring at codon 515.

Although it is apparent that *JAK2* and *MPL* mutations are in general neither necessary nor sufficient for the diagnosis of Ph-negative MPN, the detection of either one can establish the presence of a clonal myeloid neoplasm and help distinguish potentially overlapping reactive conditions in which cytoses figure prominently. The presence of *JAK2* V617F gene mutations in MPN can be detected by a variety of methods including allele-specific PCR (also referred to as *amplification refractory mutation system*, or ARMS PCR), melting curve analysis of PCR products, allele-specific fluorescent probe hybridization, pyrosequencing, restriction enzymatic digestion of PCR amplicons, and direct sequencing of PCR-amplified DNA. The latter two methods may be of limited analytic sensitivity for detecting small percentages of *JAK2* mutated cells in a given case. The recommended analytic sensitivity of a *JAK2* V617F assay has been proposed as less than or equal to 1% (Wang, 2008). Some studies have shown that small numbers of randomly tested healthy individuals, when analyzed with techniques of this or much higher technical sensitivity, will demonstrate the presence of a low-level *JAK2* mutation (Xu, 2007). The significance of this finding is not certain, although it is likely analogous to the detection of leukemia-associated translocations at low levels in apparently healthy individuals. More significantly, *JAK2* V617F mutations are also detectable in some subtypes of myelodysplastic syndrome, in myelodysplastic/myeloproliferative neoplasms (e.g., chronic myelomonocytic leukemia), and in rare cases of lymphoma and acute leukemia. Thus a positive *JAK2* V617F result must always be correlated with clinical and complete pathologic data; conversely, the detection of this mutation in a patient with clinical and/or morphologic features of a classic myeloproliferative neoplasm may be interpreted as essentially confirmatory of such a process. In order to expand the scope of molecular analysis in MPN, an increasing number of laboratories are complementing *JAK2* V617F assays with additional lab-developed tests to detect mutations in *MPL* or *JAK2* exon 12. MPL analysis may be performed using allele-specific PCR, allele-specific fluorescent probe hybridization, or direct sequencing of PCR products (Pancrazzi, 2008; Daly, 2009). In contrast, *JAK2* exon 12 presents a relatively large genomic area across which mutations may be scattered. Screening techniques, including high-resolution melting curve analysis, may be used to triage specimens and distinguish those that are apparently wild type from those deserving of additional scrutiny via direct sequencing (Jones, 2008; Rapado, 2009).

Mastocytosis and the KIT D816V Gene Mutation

Clinical and pathologic manifestations of neoplastic mast cell proliferations are diverse, resulting in a relatively complex system of classification (Swerdlow, 2008). In general, mast cell neoplasms can be considered in two main clinical categories: (1) cutaneous mastocytosis exhibiting predominantly localized involvement of the skin and (2) systemic mastocytosis with widespread involvement of the bone marrow and other organs, and elevations of mast cell–derived serum tryptase (Horny, 2009). Mutations in the tyrosine kinase gene *KIT*, particularly the common codon D816V abnormality, are strongly but not invariably associated with mastocytosis. KIT is the cell membrane–associated receptor for stem cell factor, an extracellular ligand important in promoting the proliferative activities essential to stem cell regeneration and the expansion of hematopoietic progeny. KIT is also expressed on melanocytes, germ cells, and gastrointestinal pacemaker cells (Metcalfe, 2008). Activating *KIT* mutations obviate the normally regulated ligand-receptor mechanism and produce growth factor–independent cell proliferation. Although *KIT* mutations are often detected in mastocytosis, they are not 100% sensitive or specific for this diagnosis. The detection rate is also highly dependent on the assay method used. As many as 30% of cases of systemic mastocytosis may appear to lack the D816V mutation when using moderately sensitive assays on unfractionated bone marrow cells, but the detection rate increases to approximately 95% using higher sensitivity detection methods such as nested PCR and/or enrichment of mast cells via cell sorting or microdissection (Akin, 2006). The proportion of D816V-negative cases is higher in cutaneous mastocytosis (Lanternier, 2008). Importantly, *KIT* mutations are not specific for mastocytosis, in that they are detectable in some cases of CBF acute leukemias (as discussed earlier), gastrointestinal stromal tumors, and a subset of melanomas (Orfao, 2007). The genomic distribution of *KIT* mutations is variable in these different tumors. Nevertheless, detection of a *KIT* D816V mutation fulfils one of four "minor" diagnostic criteria for systemic mastocytosis and is thus often helpful in definitively supporting a diagnosis suspected on clinical, morphologic, or immunophenotypic grounds.

The exon 17 situated D816V is the most common *KIT* mutation in mastocytosis, present in more than 90% of positive cases; this consistency presents an attractive target for molecular diagnostic methodologies amenable to the interrogation of specific sequence changes, including restriction fragment length polymorphism-based analysis, allele-specific PCR, and pyrosequencing. Notably, despite the optimism for using imatinib mesylate for more broad-spectrum tyrosine kinase inhibition outside the setting of BCR-ABL–positive neoplasms, the D816V mutation is not responsive to this drug (Vega-Ruiz, 2009). Molecular analysis of *KIT* mutations occurring at other locations in the gene (e.g., in many cases of cutaneous mastocytosis, or in non–mast cell malignancies) requires a more comprehensive approach involving post-PCR sequencing of several exon regions.

Neoplastic Disorders Associated with Eosinophilia

The trend to molecular classification of hematologic malignancies is further illustrated by the creation, in the 2008 WHO classification, of a new subcategory of hematopoietic neoplasms defined almost exclusively on molecular grounds. *Myeloid and lymphoid neoplasms with eosinophilia (MLNE) and abnormalities of PDGFRA, PDGFRB or FGFR1* encompasses a heterogeneous group of both myeloid and lymphoid lineage, previously existing as separate entities largely defined by morphologic, clinical, and certain cytogenetic features (Swerdlow, 2008). A unifying feature of these neoplasms is the deregulated activity of specific tyrosine kinase growth factor receptors by aberrant gene rearrangements and a tumor phenotype characterized in part by the production of excess eosinophils and eosinophilic precursors. Hence, these tumors were first broadly and imprecisely classified under *chronic eosinophilic leukemia/idiopathic hypereosinophilic syndrome (CEL/IHES)*; however, the lineage-specific or underlying neoplastic expansion varies according to the now better understood genetically defined disease subsets. Although laboratory testing for these genetic abnormalities is accomplished mainly by FISH and/or conventional karyotypic analysis, a short précis of this new entity is included here, because it represents a good example of the reconfiguration of hematologic malignancies based on molecular characterization.

Rearrangement of the platelet-derived growth factor receptor α (*PDGFRA*) gene is diagnostic of a hematologic malignancy typically characterized by the clonal expansion of eosinophils (i.e., CEL), but may in some cases present with additional findings of AML or T-ALL. The presence of a *PDGFRA* rearrangement thus defines this diagnostic entity at the molecular level, regardless of the cellular component heterogeneity. The most common *PDGFRA* rearrangement is a karyotypically cryptic interstitial deletion at 4q12 that juxtaposes *PDGFRA* with an adjacent gene, *FIP1L1*. The resultant expression of a FIP1L1-PDGFRA fusion protein disrupts the autoinhibitory domain of PDGFRA and leads to its constitutive tyrosine kinase activity (Stover, 2006). An intervening gene called *CHIC2* is deleted in the 4q12 rearrangement; thus assessment of the *CHIC2* locus by FISH technique serves as an effective method to identify the chromosomal microdeletion and establish the presence of a *PDGFRA* rearrangement (Pardanani, 2003; Fink, 2009). Of note, a subset of CEL with *PDGFRA* rearrangements also exhibits abnormal mast cell expansions in the bone marrow, but the *KIT* D816V abnormality is not present in these cases. The overlapping nature of neoplastic myeloid cellular proliferations therefore underscores the comprehensive molecular approach to subclassification of these diseases. Most significantly, patients with *PDGFRA*-positive CEL are remarkably sensitive to treatment with even low doses of imatinib, again emphasizing the potential of molecularly targeted therapy (Pardanani, 2003). Myeloid neoplasms with platelet-derived growth factor receptor β (*PDGFRB*) gene rearrangements are conceptually similar. These neoplasms are typically characterized morphologically as chronic myelomonocytic leukemias with eosinophilia, although variant presentations are recognized. A karyotypic abnormality t(5;12)(q33;p13) is commonly associated with the deregulation of *PDGFRB*, via creation of a chimeric *ETV6(TEL)-PDGFRB* fusion gene and protein; however, several other translocation partners with *PDGFRB* have also been described. Alterations of the *PDGFRB* locus can be detected by FISH analysis, although some cases are FISH negative in the face of a submicroscopic *ETV6-PDGFRB* gene fusion, indicating that comprehensive detection requires a combination of PCR-based and molecular cytogenetic approaches. *PDGFRB* rearranged neoplasms are also expected to benefit from treatment with imatinib (David, 2007). In contrast to MLNE with rearrangements of *PDGFRA* or *PDGFRB*, patients with tumors overexpressing fibroblast growth factor receptor-1 (*FGFR1*) differ in certain key respects. First, the translocated gene encodes a tyrosine kinase receptor involved in a different cell signaling pathway. Second, these cases are particularly associated with presentations of lymphoblastic (e.g., T-ALL) or mixed phenotype acute leukemias, as well as often prominent neoplastic eosinophilia. And finally, an effective tyrosine kinase inhibitor therapy has yet to be established in the setting of *FGFR1* rearrangement. Cytogenetic and FISH analyses can be used to diagnose the presence of *FGFR1* gene rearrangements.

Molecular Diagnosis of Non-Hodgkin Lymphomas

RATIONALE FOR MOLECULAR GENETIC ANALYSIS IN THE LYMPHOID DISORDERS

The non-Hodgkin lymphomas (NHLs) and chronic lymphoid leukemias encompass relatively common adult malignancies, and the incidence of these diseases is increasing (Chiu, 2003; Liu, 2003; Fisher 2004). A central paradigm in the diagnosis of lymphoma is the demonstration of monoclonality, which is highly correlated with the malignant state. In many instances, a monoclonal lymphoid proliferation can be suggested or established with the aid of immunophenotypic studies, for example, by demonstrating light chain restriction in the case of B cell neoplasms, or aberrant antigen expression in the setting of atypical T cell expansions. However, there are several instances in which the foregoing analyses may be insufficient and the determination of clonality in a lymphoid population remains a key diagnostic issue. In these situations, which may include samples with uninformative phenotypic features, small tissue biopsies, or partially degraded specimens and paraffin-embedded tissues, the molecular assessment of antigen receptor gene rearrangements is extremely valuable. Standard molecular clonality detection methods are often employed to resolve the definitive diagnosis of lymphoid neoplasms with features potentially mimicking benign hyperplasias (e.g., follicular lymphomas or extranodal marginal zone B cell lymphomas), to assign cell lineage in undifferentiated hematopoietic tumors (i.e., B vs. T cell), and to aid in the diagnosis of neoplastic T cell lymphoproliferations.

Along with characteristic light microscopic tumor cell features and phenotypic cell marker profiling (e.g., by flow cytometry and immunohistochemistry), the identification of recurrent, nonrandom tumor genetic abnormalities (most commonly produced by chromosomal translocation events) has also fundamentally refined the subclassification of the NHLs. Indeed, cytogenetic and molecular genetic data of this type now form an integral part of the 2008 WHO lymphoma classification (Swerdlow, 2008). The following sections detail the molecular approaches to the determination of B and T cell clonality, and the detection and significance of common recurrent lymphoma translocations. More recent advancements, including research applications of microarray gene expression profiling and array-based genomics studies have begun to further alter the landscape of subclassification and prognostication in the lymphomas and, as such, these efforts will translate into novel molecular targets and even technical platforms for future diagnostic applications. The major implications of these newer developments will also be briefly presented in reference to specific types of NHL.

ANTIGEN RECEPTOR GENE REARRANGEMENTS FOR CLONALITY DETERMINATION

Mechanism of Antigen Receptor Gene Rearrangements

The antigen receptor genes are rearranged early in the development of B and T lymphocytes in the bone marrow and thymus, respectively. The process of DNA rearrangement, or genetic recombination, essentially involves the splicing and fusion of one of numerous *v*ariable (V) gene segments with a *j*oining (J) exon. At some loci, notably the immunoglobulin heavy chain and T cell receptor β genes, an additional diversity (D) segment is interposed between V and J segments. The assembled V-J or V-D-J segment is subsequently joined with the *c*onstant (C) region of the antigen receptor gene to produce an intact coding sequence capable of translation to a functional antigen receptor protein (Fig. 75-5, *A* and *B*) (Macintyre, 1999; Bassing, 2002). Immune cells incapable of producing functional receptor proteins undergo deletion by apoptosis. For immature B cells, the immunoglobulin heavy chain gene (*IGH@*) on chromosome 14(q32) is the first to undergo this segmental rearrangement, followed in turn by the κ light chain gene (*IGK@*) on 2(p12). If the latter attempt is nonproductive at both alleles, the λ locus (*IGL@*) on 22(q11) is selected in order to generate the final tetrameric immunoglobulin molecule. For T cells, the T cell receptor δ (*TRD@*) [14(q11)] and γ (*TRG@*) [7(p15)] loci initiate this process in the thymus; however, many of these gene rearrangements fail to produce a functional heterodimeric receptor protein. Thus rearrangement continues essentially simultaneously at the T cell receptor α (*TRA@*) and β (*TRB@*) loci, located on chromosomes 14(q11) and 7(q34), respectively, generating a Tαβ receptor in the large majority (>90%) of T cells. As an important point related to molecular analysis (discussed later), nearly all mature Tαβ cells still retain a γ (*TRG@*) locus gene rearrangement.

Enormous diversity exists among the immunoglobulin and T cell receptors, arising in part from the potential for genetic recombination between numerous V-, (D-), and J-gene segments at these loci. In addition, the activity of the enzyme terminal deoxynucleotidyl transferase (TdT) adds nontemplated ("N") nucleic acid bases at the junctions of the rearranged gene segments in immature B and T cells, further increasing sequence diversity (see Fig. 75-5, *A* and *B*). As a result of the largely random nature of this process, individual B and T lymphocytes harbor specific gene rearrangement sequences and express correspondingly unique antigen receptor immune proteins on their cell surfaces. In a polyclonal lymphoid expansion, therefore, a highly variable distribution of antigen receptor gene rearrangements is generally found, whereas a monoclonal population is characterized by a single identical gene rearrangement in each progeny cell. This concept is exploited by both Southern blot hybridization (SBH) analysis and PCR technique, to distinguish polyclonal ("benign") from monoclonal ("malignant") lymphocytic proliferations.

Figure 75-5 Immunoglobulin and T cell receptor gene rearrangements: concept and application of Southern blot hybridization (SBH) and polymerase chain reaction techniques for clonality determination in lymphoid populations. **A,** Schematic demonstration of the basic process of somatic rearrangement of the immunoglobulin heavy chain (*IGH@*) locus at chromosome 14q32 occurring early in developing B cells. Selection and rearrangement of *IGH@* diversity (D_H) and joining (J_H) gene segments first occurs over a large region of intervening DNA, followed by the recruitment of a variable region (V_H) exon to complete a VDJ coding cassette. Substantial diversity is generated at the nucleotide level because of the recombination potential of the many V, D, and J segments, as well as by the activity of the enzyme terminal deoxynucleotidyl transferase (TdT), which inserts a random number of "nontemplated" (n) nucleotides at the rearranged junctions. The T cell receptor gamma gene (*TRG@*) located at chromosome 7p15, depicted in panel **B,** shares similar structural and rearrangement features, with the exception that there are no D-segments. The *TRG@* gene is less complex having only 11 functional Vγ segments capable of functional rearrangements, although there are two J-segment loci (Jp and Jγ) and two constant regions. **C,** Schematic of the J-region of the immunoglobulin heavy chain gene (*IGH@*) locus on chromosome 14q32. J_H exons are shown as boxes. The intact, or germline J_H region is flanked by EcoRI restriction endonuclease sites, which, upon DNA digestion, will render a fragment of approximately 16 kilobases (kb) in size. This large DNA fragment can be detected by SBH using a cloned or PCR generated radioisotope-labeled probe (in this case, a 2.2 kb genomic fragment is depicted as the probe). In contrast, when the J_H region is altered by the somatic gene rearrangement process in a B cell, a change in restriction enzyme sites is introduced, such that digestion produces a DNA fragment of altered size from the expected germline size. In the diagram, this is shown as a new 12 kb J_H fragment. In a monoclonal B cell population, all B cells will harbor the same rearrangement and this can be detected by SBH technique as a new band distinct from the germline location. **D,** Typical results of SBH for detection of *IGH@* locus gene rearrangements. Lanes "P" and "T" indicate placental and tonsil DNA samples digested with EcoRI and analyzed by SBH, indicating the presence of germline (16 kb) bands only *(single asterisk)*. The lane "NHL" is a B cell lymphoma sample showing clonally rearranged bands which clearly differ in size from the germline configuration. The presence of two new bands in the NHL sample *(double asterisks)* is indicative of biallelic *IGH@* locus rearrangements. **E,** The "micro-locus" features of a rearranged *IGH@* gene, showing the joined VDJ exon coding region. The V_H segment encodes much of the variable component of the immunoglobulin heavy chain. Three framework regions (FRI-III) are identified in the V-segment, as well as two complementary determining regions (CDRI and II). The third and most variable region of nucleotide sequence is comprised of the junction between V-, D-, and J-segments, along with inserted nontemplated (n) nucleotides (mediated by the enzyme TdT); this region is termed CDRIII and represents a highly unique nucleotide sequence in each B cell. The presence of shared sequence homology among many of the V-region segments in the antigen receptor gene loci, along with the highly homologous nature of the J-segments, permits the detection of most gene rearrangements occurring in B or T cell lymphocytes by PCR methods employing flanking "consensus" oligonucleotide primers. This concept is depicted by the orange arrows. The use of multiple primer sets covering the region of interest and targeting of different antigen receptor loci increases the chance of detecting even rare immunoglobulin or T cell gene rearrangements in a lymphoid population. **F,** Typical results of *IGH@* PCR using fluorescently labeled consensus primers and analysis by capillary electrophoresis. In a polyclonal B cell population, a range of VDJ rearrangement sizes exists, delimited both by the nature of V-, D-, and J-segments used and the finite number of inserted n-nucleotides. This fragment size range is normally distributed, as shown in the left side panel. In contrast, a monoclonal B cell population is characterized by a single (or dual, if biallelic) rearrangement(s), as demonstrated in the right-hand panel.

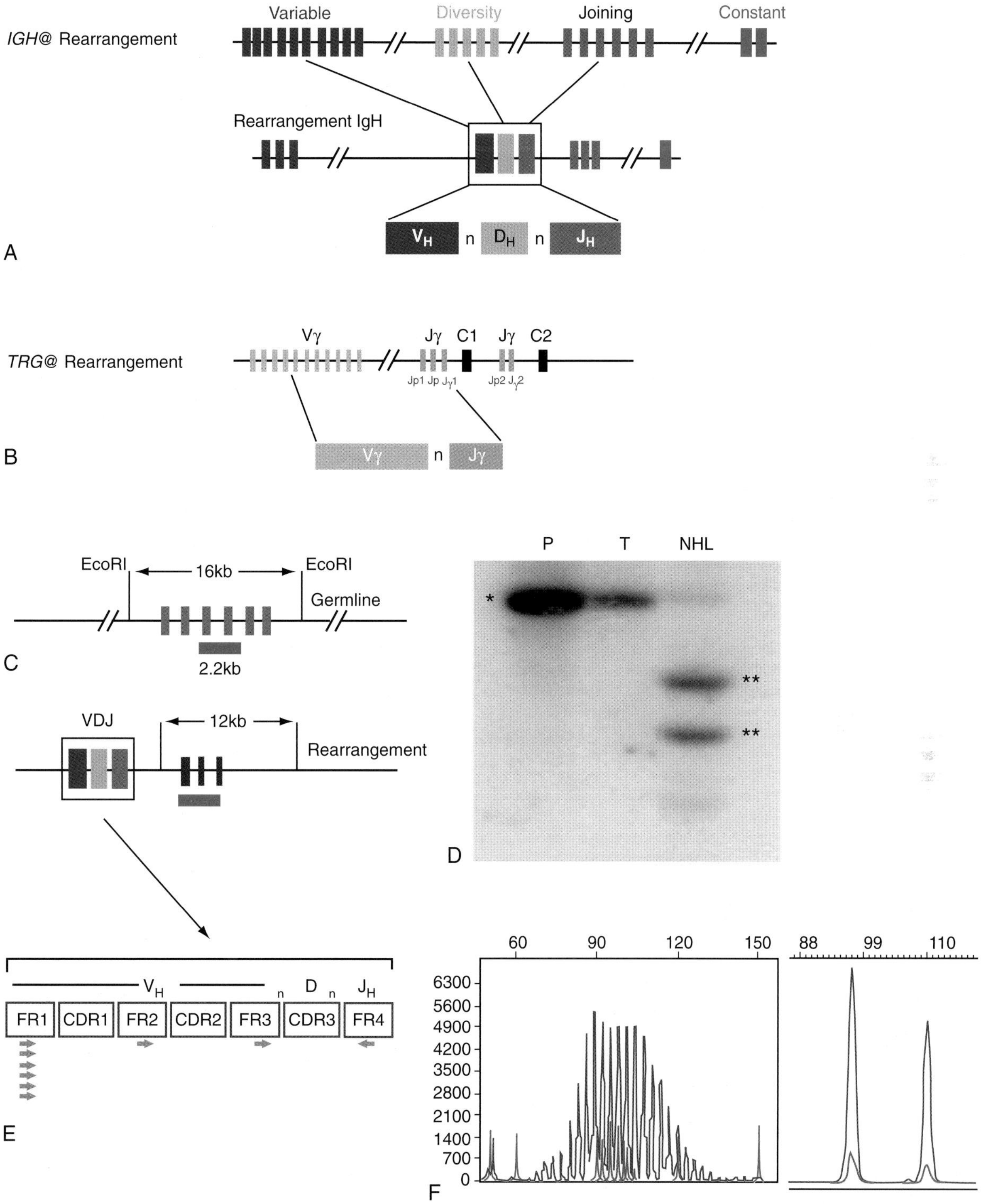

IGH@ Rearrangement
Variable
Diversity
Joining
Constant
Rearrangement IgH
VH
n
DH
n
JH
A
TRG@ Rearrangement
Vγ
Jγ
C1
Jγ
C2
Jp1 Jp Jγ1
Jp2 Jγ2
Vγ
n
Jγ
B
EcoRI
16kb
EcoRI
Germline
2.2kb
C
VDJ
12kb
Rearrangement
P
T
NHL
*
**
**
D
VH
n
D
n
JH
FR1
CDR1
FR2
CDR2
FR3
CDR3
FR4
E
60
90
120
150
6300
5600
4900
4200
3500
2800
2100
1400
700
0
88
99
110
F

Techniques to Detect Antigen Receptor Gene Rearrangements: Southern Blot Hybridization

Genomic SBH technique can be considered a relatively "large-scale" molecular approach, involving restriction endonuclease enzyme digestions of a high molecular weight DNA sample, followed by fragment separation, immobilization on a nylon or nitrocellulose membrane, and specific radioisotope (or nonisotopic) labeled probe detection of one or more relatively large target DNA fragments (Cossman, 1988; Beishuizen, 1993; Langerak, 1999; Macintyre, 1999; Medeiros, 1999; Arber, 2000). A schematic summary and example of genomic SBH as applied to the diagnosis of lymphoma is shown in Figure 75-5C. To briefly summarize, for a structurally unaltered (nonrearranged) region of the target DNA, Southern hybridization analysis will reveal a certain pattern of fragment sizes or bands, termed a *germline* configuration, based on the distribution of particular restriction enzyme sites flanking or within the locus in question. If this region of DNA is rearranged, as in the case of the B and T cell antigen receptor loci, a different banding pattern will be produced (as a result of shifts in the locations of germline restriction enzyme sites) and these changes can be readily recognized by hybridization with a specific probe. The sensitivity of SBH is such that at least 5%–10% of a population of cells must contain the same nongermline rearrangement in order to be detected (see Table 75-2). In a polyclonal lymphocyte population, individual B or T cells carry unique rearrangements of their antigen receptor genes and would theoretically be expected to generate a "ladder" or broad distribution of rearrangements when analyzed by SBH with the appropriate probes. In practice, however, no such rearrangement pattern is seen in polyclonal proliferations, because even highly selected and expanded groups of reactive lymphoid cells do not typically constitute up to 5% of the total cells in these situations. In contrast, each cell in a monoclonal population contains an identical antigen receptor gene rearrangement, and SBH will identify distinct, rearranged (nongermline) bands (see Fig. 75-5, *D*). The successful application of SBH technique to detect lymphoid clonality is dependent on several factors. First, the locus being interrogated must be structurally favorable for study by enzyme digestion and probe hybridization. Certain loci, such as the *TRA@* gene, are very large and difficult to adequately assess with high sensitivity using a practical number of restriction enzyme digests and probes. Conversely, the *TRG@* locus, as discussed further below, is relatively small and of limited diversity, resulting in poor specificity and generally precluding its use for SBH. Second, hybridization probes must be easily available for use in the clinical diagnostic setting. Probes may be produced from either cloned genomic DNA or cDNA complementary to the region of interest, and several are available commercially. Finally, SBH method requires the use of high-molecular-weight, nondegraded DNA from fresh or frozen tissue sources. Of note, because a known amount of genomic DNA is used per enzymatic digest (e.g., 5 μg), the relative proportion of clonal cells in a given sample can be estimated by relative band intensities using SBH analysis.

For determination of B cell clonality by SBH, both the immunoglobulin heavy chain (*IGH@*) and the light chain genes have been used. The *IGH@* gene is frequently assessed with a J-region probe (Cossman, 1988; Beishuizen, 1993; Medeiros, 1999). The *IGH@* J-region (J_H) is highly informative, because this locus is relatively compact, is easily defined by restriction enzyme digestions, and is always involved in recombination events in B cells (see Fig. 75-5, *D* and *E*). With the use of a Jκ probe, the κ light chain gene (*IGK@*) can also be targeted for SBH analysis, although a minority of lymphoma cases (mainly those with λ light chain rearrangements) may be missed due to site-specific deletions of the rearranged κ loci encompassing the Cκ and sometimes the Jκ regions (Cossman 1988; Medeiros 1999). Rearrangements of the λ light chain gene (*IGL@*) can be assessed with a constant region (Cλ) probe; however, this locus is highly polymorphic with typically used restriction enzyme digests and banding results are more difficult to interpret (Saueracker, 1992).

The T cell β locus (*TRB@*) has proven to be most useful for detection of T cell clonality by SBH, and this region shares structural genomic features similar to the *IGH@* gene. The complexity of the *TRB@* locus is notably greater due to the presence at both alleles of two Dβ, Jβ, and Cβ regions available for recombination with a relatively large repertoire of Vβ region segments. However, because the two Cβ regions are nearly identical in sequence, *TRB@* gene rearrangements can be identified by SBH using a common Cβ genomic probe and appropriate restriction digests of the target DNA (Langerak, 1999; Medeiros, 1999). The use of two specific Jβ region probes has also been described to detect clonality at the *TRB@* locus and may offer some advantages in conjunction with Cβ probes (Langerak, 1999). The γ T cell (*TRG@*) locus is generally less favorable for SBH analysis due to the relatively small number of rearranging Vγ and Jγ region segments. This limited capacity for segmental recombination creates a relatively small pool of functional *TRG@* gene rearrangements, from which germline and true rearranged bands may not be confidently distinguished by SBH (Cossman, 1988; Medeiros, 1999).

Techniques to Detect Antigen Receptor Gene Rearrangements: Polymerase Chain Reaction

Rearrangements of the immunoglobulin and T cell receptor genes can be identified by PCR methods as well. In contrast to SBH, which detects relatively large structural genomic alterations based on changes in restriction enzyme sites, PCR is designed to amplify short regions of DNA encompassing the immediate area of V-(D)-J gene segment fusion in the rearranged antigen receptor genes. Under standard PCR conditions, a germline antigen receptor gene configuration is amplified poorly or not at all, due to the very large intervening areas of DNA between primer sites. However, when coding V-, (D-), and J-segments are juxtaposed in a rearranged gene, amplification of the region between the now closely apposed primers is readily accomplished by PCR. The most widely used loci for PCR determination of lymphoid clonality are the *IGH@*, *IGK@*, *TRG@*, and *TRB@* genes. In 2003, the BIOMED-2 consortium published a series of landmark articles detailing comprehensive, multilocus, and multiplex PCR-based strategies for determining clonality in B and T cell lymphoproliferations (van Dongen, 2003). These studies represented the culmination of prior investigative efforts and authoritatively established the efficacy, interpretive pitfalls, and utility of PCR methods for routine molecular diagnosis in this area. The BIOMED-2 approach has been validated independently (McClure, 2006; Liu, 2007) and was recently updated in a series of articles attempting to codify a more standardized laboratory approach to lymphoid clonality detection by PCR technique (Bruggemann, 2007; Evans, 2007; van Krieken, 2007).

A schematic of PCR strategy directed at the *IGH@* locus is shown in Figure 75-5, *E*, and this depiction is illustrative in general of the approaches used for comprehensive clonality evaluation by PCR methods targeting several antigen receptor gene loci. The *IGH@* V_H gene region comprises approximately 70–80 discrete coding or functional V-segments that can be grouped into six "families" based on sequence similarities. The D region includes approximately 20–30 gene segments and the J region includes approximately six gene segments. Successful recombination of V-, D- and J-segment elements, along with random "N"-nucleotide insertions at junctional sites by TdT, create a unique DNA "fingerprint" in an individual B cell, and these markers can potentially be used in the determination of clonality by PCR. Although V-D-J recombination is by nature extensively variable among individual B lymphocytes, PCR methods targeting this region are fortunately simplified by the use of "consensus" sequence primers. Both the 5′ DNA region flanking the V-D-J junction (i.e., framework regions, FR), as well as the *IGH@*-J_H region, contain nucleotide sequences that are highly conserved. Complementary FR and J_H sequence PCR primers can thus be designed that amplify these unique V-D-J rearrangements in most B cells. Figure 75-5, *E*, for example, demonstrates the relative placement of consensus primers to provide comprehensive coverage for detecting *IGH@* gene rearrangements; FR1-directed primers typically include six or seven different oligonucleotides recognizing essentially all major V_H family gene segments based on germline sequence similarities.

The use of multiple primers for the *IGH@* locus is important to circumvent potential PCR failures; such failed amplifications are potentially common in B cells that have experienced a lymphoid follicle germinal center environment, in turn acquiring somatic hypermutation sequence changes involving the CDRs and immediately flanking framework DNA regions. Somatic hypermutations can inhibit efficient consensus primer binding and amplification. To further enhance the successful analysis of B cell clonality using PCR-based methods, consensus primers can also be employed to analyze the light chain genes, most commonly *IGK@*. The *IGK@* locus is very informative in this regard because in addition to V-J segmental recombinations, B cells that fail to make a productive κ gene rearrangement go on to delete the allelic region in a site-specific manner, before undergoing rearrangement of the other κ gene, or the λ light chain loci. κ Deletions are carried out by recombinations between the so-called κ-deleting element (KDE) and the upstream V-region, or the KDE and an intron recombination signal sequence (IRSS) situated 5′ of the C_K region (van Dongen, 2003). In either case, the κ allele is subtotally deleted, or rendered nonfunctional; however, the molecular mechanisms governing κ deletions operate similarly as for V-J recombination, and these "signatures" at the DNA level can also serve as relatively specific rearrangement markers for clonality analysis.

The *TRG@* locus, although not well suited for SBH, has nonetheless been very successfully used for the determination of T cell clonality by PCR (Beaubier, 2000; Greiner, 2002; Lawnicki, 2003). *TRG@* gene rearrangement occurs early in developing thymic T lymphocytes and this genetic event is retained at the DNA level, even though the vast majority of developing T cells continues to rearrange the *TRA@* and *TRB@* loci and ultimately develop an α-β receptor phenotype. The *TRG@* locus encompasses 11 coding Vγ region segments, grouped into four families based on sequence similarities. Five Jγ region segments are present, including the highly conserved Jγ1 and Jγ2 exons as well as Jp, Jp1, and Jp2 exons (see Fig. 75-5, *B*) (Greiner, 2002). Consensus primers complementary to sequences of shared homology in the T cell gamma V- and J-segments can similarly be used to simplify the PCR procedure. *TRG@* PCR also relies on the unique nature of V-J junctional rearrangements in individual T lymphocytes; the technique is analytically informative despite the limited segmental diversity of this locus, keeping some caveats in mind (discussed in the following section). Despite the far greater degree of gene segment complexity at the *TRB@* locus, successful PCR protocols have been developed in a manner similar to that for *IGH@*, relying on the use of multiple V- and J-region consensus primers.

Amplified antigen receptor gene rearrangements can be visualized by agarose or polyacrylamide gel electrophoresis with or without prior "heteroduplex" manipulation, or more commonly now by capillary electrophoresis following PCR amplification with fluorescently labeled primers (Beaubier, 2000; Greiner, 2002,). In a polyclonal B or T cell proliferation, many hundreds or thousands of individual V-(D)-J rearrangements can be expected in a given DNA sample. Because none of these reactive lymphocyte subpopulations is typically present above the sensitivity threshold of standard PCR analysis (discussed later), a polyclonal smear or faint multiple-band ladder pattern is visualized by gel electrophoresis or rendered as a series of normally distributed peaks by capillary electrophoresis (Fig. 75-5, *F*). In a monoclonal B or T cell process, all cells harbor identical immunoglobulin or T cell receptor gene rearrangements that are preferentially amplified during the PCR, producing one or sometimes two (i.e., biallelic) distinct clonal bands or peak profiles during post-PCR analysis.

Advantages and Shortcomings Southern Blot Hybridization and Polymerase Chain Reaction for Lymphoid Clonality Assessment

The decision to use PCR versus SBH requires knowledge of several factors such as tissue source, type of lymphoproliferative disorder being investigated, sensitivity of the respective assays, and false-positive and negative rates. The advantages and disadvantages of the respective techniques are summarized in Table 75-5. In general, PCR technique has gained wide popularity for clonality determination, principally due to its relative ease of performance and rapidity. SBH method is, in contrast, labor intensive and costly; it may involve the use of radioactive probes and requires approximately 1–2 weeks to complete. Further disadvantages of SBH include the requirement for fresh or frozen tissue of good quality (for high molecular weight DNA) and a relatively low sensitivity, in the range of 5%–10%. PCR is advantageous in that the turnaround time is within 2–3 days, it is cheaper, and it requires far less starting DNA quantity (e.g., 0.5–1 μg) compared with SBH. Moreover, PCR can be performed from fresh samples or fixed paraffinized tissue sources, although certain fixatives (e.g., B5), or substances commonly used in lymph node or bone marrow processing, may inhibit the PCR. Clonality assessment by PCR has a nominal sensitivity of 1%–5%, although a prominent polyclonal B or T cell background can significantly reduce the ability of the technique to detect a coexistent monoclonal lymphocyte population.

Although PCR methods seemingly offer advantages relative to SBH, the technique is occasionally subject to false-negative assay results, because it is not possible to design consensus type primers to capture all possible antigen receptor gene rearrangements; the issue of somatic hypermutation in B cells is one example, although this can be largely overcome with multiple primer strategies and inclusion of the *IGK@* locus. More significantly, the problem of false positivity is a risk encountered not uncommonly in interpretation of T cell gene rearrangements by PCR. This situation is most aptly seen at the *TRG@* locus, which, as a result of limited overall V- and J-gene segment recombination potential, can lead

TABLE 75-5
Southern Blot Hybridization versus Polymerase Chain Reaction Method for Lymphoid Clonality Analysis

	Advantages	Disadvantages
Southern blot	Essentially no false-negative results Can detect nature of uncommon rearrangements (e.g., partial D-J) Can detect presence of oligoclonal gene rearrangement patterns	Cost, labor, technical difficulty Time-intensive (requires 1–2 weeks) Possible use of radionuclide labeled probes Requirement for high molecular weight DNA Large amount of DNA required (5 μg per enzymatic digestion) Limited analytic sensitivity (can detect 5%–10% of a monoclonal population in background cells)
PCR	Rapid (24–48 hours), inexpensive, technically straightforward Use of DNA from many sources, including fixed, paraffin-embedded tissues Requires minimal DNA (0.5–1 μg per reaction) Sensitive (nominally 1%–5%, can be augmented) Can combine different PCR locus strategies to increase clonality detection rate	False-positive risk (contamination, skewed T cell gene rearrangements) False-negative risk (detection rate not 100%) May miss oligoclonal populations Analytic sensitivity can be adversely affected by presence of polyclonal lymphocyte background when using consensus primers

DNA, Deoxyribonucleic acid; *PCR,* polymerase chain reaction.

to aspecific ("pseudoclonal") amplification products in prominent reactive T cell proliferations. Skewed T cell populations can be encountered in several situations, including autoimmune disorders, after allogeneic organ transplantation, or as a consequence of normal aging. Therefore, diagnostic interpretation of T cell clonality studies by PCR is occasionally more problematic, with the propensity for encountering "equivocal" results. Furthermore, the presence of "promiscuous" locus rearrangements (e.g., *TRG* rearrangements in B cells and vice versa) are well described, particularly in cases of lymphoblastic leukemia/lymphoma, indicating that lineage specificity for antigen receptor gene rearrangements is not strictly followed in some lymphoid neoplasias (Szczepanski, 2002).

To summarize, PCR and SBH are complementary techniques for the determination of clonality in B and T cell lymphoid proliferations. The current status of PCR-based methods provides a rapid and effective alternative to SBH for interrogating both B and T cell loci, although the detection rate for optimized PCR assays is slightly less than 100%, and conversely, the risk of false-positive results (especially involving T cell receptor gene rearrangements), requires vigilance. It is clear that PCR analysis of antigen receptor gene rearrangements must always be interpreted alongside clinical and relevant pathologic or other laboratory data. Improvements to PCR-based methodology, including expansive coverage of multiple antigen receptor loci, have largely led to the replacement of SBH for lymphoid clonality determination; however, some diagnostic laboratories still retain expertise in SBH practice in order to resolve difficult cases. Finally, PCR analysis provides an additional benefit accruing from its analytic sensitivity under certain circumstances. Because clonal antigen receptor gene rearrangements in individual lymphoid neoplasms are unique, these DNA markers can also be used for highly sensitive (e.g., 10^{-3}–10^{-5}) and specific detection of MRD in blood or bone marrow following therapy (Szczepanski, 2002; van der Velden, 2003; Szczepanski, 2007; van der Velden, 2007). As a primary example, quantitative MRD levels at the end of induction therapy have been shown to be strongly related to event-free and overall survival in childhood lymphoblastic leukemias (Cave, 1998; van Dongen, 1998; Nyvold, 2002; Campana, 2008; Flohr, 2008; Campana, 2009), these data are now being employed in conjunction with other tumor-associated molecular genetic features (as described previously) to augment individual risk assessment and treatment options for these patients.

TABLE 75-6
Lymphoma-Associated Translocations and Resultant Gene Rearrangements

Genetic abnormality	Disease associations	Basic molecular pathogenesis	Diagnostic detection*
t(14;18)/*BCL2-IGH@*	90% of FL 20%–30% of DLBCL	Overexpression of anti-apoptotic Bcl2 protein in FL; not clear for DLBCL	FISH > PCR
t(11;14)/*CCND1-IGH@*	100% of mantle cell lymphoma	Overexpression of G1-phase cell cycle protein cyclin D1	FISH >> PCR
3q27/*BCL6*	30% of DLBCL	Disruption of normal Bcl6 regulation of germinal center B cell maturation	FISH
t(8;14)/*MYC-IGH@* and variant *MYC* translocations	100% of BL; 5%–10% of DLBCL; rare cases of high-grade B cell lymphoma with concurrent *BCL2* or BCL6 rearrangements	Overexpression of potent early response mitogenic transcriptional factor Myc	FISH
t(11;18)/*API2-MALT1* t(14;18)/*MALT1-IGH@* t(1;14)/*BCL10-IGH@* t(3;14)/*FOXP1-IGH@*	Extranodal marginal zone lymphomas (~20%–30%)	Upregulation of NFκB signal transduction pathway activity	FISH; RT-PCR (for API2-MALT1 mRNA)
t(2;5)/*NPM1-ALK* and variant *ALK* translocations	T cell anaplastic large cell lymphoma (~80%–90%); rare cases of ALK positive large B cell lymphoma	Constitutive activation and abnormal localization of Alk tyrosine kinase	FISH (all variants); RT-PCR (for NPM1-ALK mRNA)
14q32/*TCL1A*	T cell prolymphocytic leukemia (T-PLL)	Overexpression of transcription factor	FISH

BL, Burkitt lymphoma; *DLBCL,* diffuse large B cell lymphoma; *FISH,* fluorescence in situ hybridization; *FL,* follicular lymphoma; *PCR,* polymerase chain reaction; *RT-PCR,* reverse-transcriptase polymerase chain reaction.
*Detection by molecular techniques indicated; specific diagnosis can also be established in some tumors by detecting specific protein overexpression (e.g., cyclin D1 in mantle cell lymphoma, Alk in anaplastic large T cell lymphoma). PCR includes use of appropriate postamplification detection techniques (e.g., gel/capillary electrophoresis, melting analysis, and sequencing.)

MOLECULAR DETECTION AND SIGNIFICANCE OF COMMON LYMPHOMA-ASSOCIATED CHROMOSOMAL TRANSLOCATIONS

Our growing understanding of NHL biology has been substantially furthered by the identification of recurrent chromosomal translocations associated with particular neoplasms (Table 75-6) (Vega, 2003). Identification of these genetic abnormalities is not only highly useful for diagnosis, but also often provides prognostic information or a specific tumor marker for residual disease detection. In general, chromosome translocations are more prevalent in B cell NHLs and result in the fusion of two genetic loci, most commonly involving the *IGH@* locus. In this pathogenetic process, a normally highly regulated proto-oncogene becomes constitutively activated by juxtaposition to the immunoglobulin gene, leading to marked oncoprotein overexpression, as typified by the *MYC-IGH@* gene fusion in Burkitt lymphoma (BL) and some large B cell lymphomas. In a minority of examples, a chimeric fusion gene is produced and expressed as a hybrid mRNA and protein; this situation is found in ALCL of T cell lineage, characterized by the t(2;5)/*NPM1-ALK* abnormality. In either case, interference with normal lymphoid cell growth, homeostasis, or cell death (i.e., apoptosis) is thought to play a central role in lymphomagenesis. Lymphoma-associated translocation events are thought in many tumors to be linked to aberrant consequences of the recombinase activating gene (RAG) and DNA breakage-repair enzyme systems that are active during the time of normal antigen receptor gene rearrangement, or through germinal center processes like somatic hypermutation (SHM) and class switch recombination, which also require the enzyme AID (Pasqualucci, 2008). The exact mechanisms underlying translocation events in leukemias and lymphomas are incompletely understood, but may involve nonrandom spatial proximity of genes during cell cycling, fragile sites such as single-stranded intermediates of DNA prone to breakage and recombination, as well as others (Roix, 2003; Raghavan, 2004). Whereas most acute leukemia-associated translocations are best identified by the presence of their fusion corresponding chimeric mRNA species, gene fusion abnormalities in the lymphomas require a different molecular diagnostic strategy. A proportion of lymphoma-associated translocations can be detected by PCR methods using genomic DNA because of substantial breakpoint clustering in both partner genes; however, many are not amenable to PCR detection due to large regions of genomic breakpoint heterogeneity and additional analyses, such as FISH or immunohistochemistry (to detect overexpressed proteins), playing vital roles in the specific diagnosis and subclassification of the NHLs. New investigative techniques evaluating global gene expression or regulation are providing a more comprehensive, though complicated, picture of the pathways of genetic deregulation in NHLs, with and without recurrent translocations (see later). These next generation platforms have already begun to further influence the subclassification and prognostication of lymphoid neoplasms; disease-specific examples are briefly discussed here.

t(14;18)/BCL2-IGH@ Abnormality in Follicular and Diffuse Large B Cell Lymphomas

The t(14;18)(q21;q32) abnormality is a common translocation encountered in B-lineage lymphomas. At the molecular level, this translocation results in the juxtaposition of the *BCL2* gene with the J-region of the immunoglobulin heavy chain locus (*IGH@*). As a consequence, the *BCL2* gene on 18q21 is brought under the control of the highly active *IGH@* enhancer element on the derivative 14q32, leading to marked overexpression of Bcl2 protein. The Bcl2 gene product is a prototypic antiapoptotic protein capable of abrogating the process of programmed cell death in cells exposed to genotoxic or metabolic stress. As such, Bcl2 overexpression can protect neoplastic cells from a variety of otherwise lethal cytotoxic events and promote a milieu favoring acquisition of additional progression-related genetic abnormalities (Cory, 2002; Reed, 2008). *BCL2* gene rearrangements are present in 85%–90% of follicular lymphomas, approximately 20%–25% of diffuse large B cell lymphomas (DLBCL), and rarely in other B cell lymphoproliferative disorders. The partial genomic structure of the *BCL2* gene locus is illustrated in Figure 75-6. The largest proportion (50%–65%) of break-fusion sites in the *BCL2* gene occurs in a tightly clustered area of approximately 150 bp in the 3′ noncoding segment of exon 3 known as the major breakpoint region (MBR). Additional loosely clustered breakpoint regions in *BCL2* have been described, including the minor cluster (mcr), intermediate cluster (icr), and areas 3′ of the MBR and 5′ of the mcr (Akasaka, 1998; Albinger-Hegyi, 2002).

BCL2 gene rearrangements involving the MBR can be readily detected by PCR methods using genomic DNA and consensus primers situated near the MBR and in the *IGH@*-J_H region (Aster, 2002; Hsi, 2002; Iqbal, 2004; Gu, 2008). Other *BCL2* breaksite areas are more difficult to target by PCR because of heterogeneity in distribution; some investigators have described the use of specialized long distance DNA PCR techniques (requiring the use of high molecular weight DNA template), or RQ-PCR with multiple primer sets to extend coverage for detecting *BCL2* rearrangements (Akasaka, 1998; Albinger-Hegyi, 2002; Weinberg, 2007). Ultimately though, these expanded PCR approaches do not achieve complete detection sensitivity, particularly when compared with highly reliable FISH analysis using *BCL2* and *IGH@* dual color locus-specific probes (Vega, 2003; Einerson, 2005). FISH is a versatile approach and can be performed

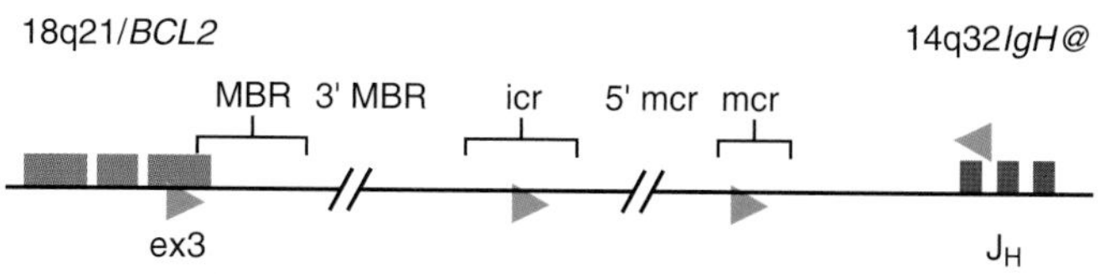

Figure 75-6 The t(14;18)/*BCL2-IGH@* abnormality in non-Hodgkin lymphomas. The *BCL2* gene is rearranged by translocation to the *IGH@* locus in most follicular lymphomas and a subset of large B cell lymphomas. Most genomic breakpoints are relatively tightly clustered in the 3′ aspect of the noncoding third exon of the *BCL2* gene, in a region termed the major breakpoint region (MBR). Up to four additional *BCL2* breakpoint clusters have been described: the minor cluster region (mcr), the intermediate cluster region (icr), and two areas near distal and proximal to the MBR and mcr respectively (i.e., 3′ MBR and 5′ mcr). For the *IGH@* gene, breakpoints occur within the J_H segment region. Because of the clustered nature of breakpoints and the relatively short intervening distances between *BCL2* and J_H in the rearranged configuration, consensus *BCL2* and J_H PCR primers (orange arrows) can be used to detect many *BCL2-IGH@* gene fusions arising from the t(14;18)(q21;q32). Nevertheless, the widespread distribution of breakpoints in *BCL2* precludes the identification of a significant number of rearrangements by PCR, such that fluorescence in situ hybridization analysis has emerged as the method of choice for detection. A closely related t(14;18) variant occurs in low-grade extranodal marginal zone B cell ("MALT") lymphomas resulting in a *MALT1-IGH@* gene fusion. Even though they are karyotypically identical, FISH probe analyses can readily distinguish this entity from the *BCL2-IGH@* abnormality.

on nuclei extracted from fresh or paraffin-embedded tissues. A number of molecular diagnostic laboratories nonetheless continue to offer *BCL2-IGH@* translocation detection by PCR technique, although knowledge of the clinical assay (i.e., detection) sensitivity is important when interpreting these results.

The identification of *BCL2* gene rearrangements in neoplastic lymphoid proliferations is very useful in several clinical contexts including diagnosis and disease subclassification. Cases of atypical or florid but benign follicular hyperplasia can be histologically and phenotypically difficult to differentiate from follicular lymphoma and in this situation, the presence of clonal immunoglobulin gene rearrangements and/or the *BCL2-IGH@* abnormality definitively establishes the latter diagnosis. Furthermore, identification of the *BCL2-IGH@* fusion can be used to specifically distinguish low-grade follicular lymphomas from other small B cell lymphomas with potentially overlapping morphologic patterns, such as mantle cell or marginal zone types. As a footnote, the presence of *BCL2* gene rearrangements is relatively specific for follicular lymphoma and is almost always correlated with Bcl2 protein overexpression. Conversely, it is important to realize that many B cell lymphomas and lymphoid leukemias are also associated with deregulated Bcl2 protein expression in the absence of structural *BCL2* gene translocations (e.g., via gene amplification or possibly epigenetic mechanisms), indicating that the protein expression itself cannot be used for specific lymphoma subtyping. As noted, a small proportion of follicular lymphomas lacks the t(14;18)/*BCL2-IGH@*. Some of these *BCL2*-rearrangement negative follicular lymphomas demonstrate higher cytologic grade (e.g., grade 3B) and are associated with translocations involving the *BCL6* proto-oncogene (Katzenberger, 2004; Gu, 2009). No significant survival differences have been observed between "*BCL2*-positive" and "*BCL2*-negative" follicular lymphomas, but recent high-resolution genomics and gene expression profiling studies have suggested distinct molecular pathways for these entities (Leich, 2009).

Among DLBCL, the presence of the t(14;18)/*BCL2-IGH@* has been associated with a "germinal center" phenotype. While increasing evidence supports the concept that germinal center type DLBCL has a relatively favorable clinical outcome, the prognostic value of the (14;18) itself in DLBCL remains controversial (Gascoyne, 1997; Barrans, 2003).

Rearrangements or genomic gains at the *BCL2* locus have been more recently associated with adverse prognosis in some cases of DLBCL with a "nongerminal center" phenotype (Obermann, 2009a). More significantly, as discussed later, the presence of the *BCL2-IGH@* in conjunction with *MYC* gene alterations identifies a subgroup of very aggressive B cell lymphomas.

t(11;14)/CCND1-IGH@ Abnormality in Mantle Cell Lymphoma

The t(11;14)(q13;q32) is essentially pathognomonic for the diagnosis of mantle cell lymphoma (MCL), when considering the differential diagnosis of small B cell neoplasms. This abnormality is also detected in a subset of multiple myelomas. Although previously thought to be present in some cases of B cell prolymphocytic leukemia, splenic marginal zone lymphoma (also referred to as splenic lymphoma with "villous lymphocytes"), and chronic lymphocytic leukemia (CLL), critical reappraisal of the clinical and pathologic spectrum of MCL has led to the conclusion that these occurrences are in fact atypical presentations of MCL. The t(11;14) places a genomic region on 11q13 called *BCL1* in proximity to the J_H region of the *IGH@* gene. The gene encoding cyclin D1 (*CCND1*) is located telomeric to the majority of *BCL1* breaksites, but nonetheless is the consistent target of transcriptional deregulation by the *IGH@* as a result of the translocation. Cyclin D1 is an early G_1-phase cell cycle protein normally required for the activity of cyclin-dependent kinases 4 and 6 (cdk4, cdk6); these holoenzyme complexes promote progression through the G_1/S transition of the cell cycle in proliferating cells principally through phosphorylation of the retinoblastoma protein (Sherr, 2000). Cyclin D1 (in contrast to other related proteins cyclins D2 and D3) is not expressed by normal B cells. Oncogenic overexpression of the D1 type cyclin is thus thought to play a key role in the pathogenesis of MCL and is supported by the overall "proliferative" transcriptional signature in MCL cells as identified by more recent gene expression profiling studies (Rosenwald, 2003; Bertoni, 2004; Pedro Jares, 2008). This propensity to a proliferative and antiapoptotic tumor phenotype underlies the relatively poor prognosis of MCL among other "small B-lymphocyte" neoplasms.

Identification of the t(11;14) or *CCND1* genetic rearrangements in MCL is variable depending on the methodology employed. The *BCL1* breakpoint region encompasses a large area of 11q13. Approximately one half of *BCL1* locus breakpoints occur over a small, well-defined site, referred to as the major translocation cluster region (MTC) (Chibbar, 1998; Williams, 1993a; Williams, 1991). The MTC is located nearly 120 kilobases (kb) centromeric of the *CCND1* gene. Other breakpoints have been defined by Southern blot analyses and are either more distal to the MTC or located in the immediate 5′ region of the *CCND1* (Williams, 1991, 1993a, 1993b). SBH methods using probes targeting the MTC and other genomic regions were historically described to detect *BCL1* alterations in up to 70% of MCL cases; however, the technical complexity, as well as the lack of commonly available genomic probes for the multiple *BCL1* regions, renders SBH impractical for routine diagnostic purposes. DNA-based PCR technique has been successfully used to identify the subset of *BCL1-IGH@* fusions involving the MTC region, accounting for an overall translocation detection rate of approximately 40% (Pinyol, 1996; Chibbar, 1998). It is thus evident that the large and widely distributed breakpoint region encompassed by the *BCL1* locus presents substantial difficulties for these molecular diagnostic approaches. To this end, FISH assays have subsequently emerged as the method of choice for resolving t(11;14)/*CCND1-IGH@* genomic abnormalities in MCL, capable of detecting essentially 100% of rearrangements (Remstein, 2000a; Belaud-Rotureau, 2002). Some investigators have also described using RQ-PCR evaluation of cyclin D1 mRNA levels to assist in the diagnosis of MCL, although this is not notably more advantageous over genomic FISH (Elenitoba-Johnson, 2002; Thomazy, 2002; Jones, 2004). Finally, cyclin D1 protein overexpression can be readily detected by immunohistochemical technique in fixed, paraffin-embedded tissues, providing an additional rapid, widely applicable and complementary method in the diagnosis of MCL (Belaud-Rotureau, 2002). Immunohistochemical detection can occasionally be complicated by the finding of acquired cyclin D1 expression in other B cell neoplasms, in the absence of the *CCND1-IGH@* gene fusion; examples include a subset of hairy cell leukemia and rare cases of chronic lymphocytic leukemia and large B cell lymphoma. In this regard, correlation with clinical presentation, morphology and immunophenotypic profile is critical, and molecular or FISH studies for the genomic t(11;14)/*CCND1-IGH@* remain an important diagnostic adjunct.

Data derived from gene expression studies of MCL also identified rare cases of morphologically and phenotypically classical MCL that nonetheless lack the t(11;14) and cyclin D1 overexpression (Rosenwald, 2003). Transcriptional profiling studies reveal similar features in these lymphomas to those found in cyclin D1-positive MCL (Fu, 2005). At least some of these uncommon types of MCL have been associated with translocations involving the *CCND2* or *CCND3* genes, or overexpression of D2 or D3 type cyclins (Wlodarska, 2008); however, it is currently not possible to distinguish this subgroup of cyclin D1-negative MCL using standard clinical diagnostic lab methods.

MALT1, BCL10, and FOXP1 Gene Abnormalities in Extranodal Marginal Zone B Cell Lymphomas

Extranodal marginal zone B cell lymphomas (EN-MZL), also referred to as mucosa associated lymphoid tissue (MALT) lymphomas, are uncommon and biologically unusual lymphoid tumors. In addition to neoplastic growth in many diverse extranodal tissue sites (e.g., stomach, lung, salivary gland, thyroid), these tumors are often characterized by the presence of predisposing infectious or autoimmune conditions and a preceding or coexistent reactive lymphoid component. Gastric EN-MZL is a prototypic example: a significant subset of these lymphomas arises in the presence of *Helicobacter pylori* infection, which appears to play a key role in early disease pathogenesis (Zucca, 2000; Isaacson, 2004). In addition to underlying conditions, several recurrent genetic abnormalities have been associated with, or in some cases are defining of EN-MZL. A proportion of these lymphomas may have a normal karyotype or minimal numerical chromosomal changes (e.g., trisomies of 3 or 18); however, specific translocation abnormalities have recently been identified among subsets of EN-MZL, with variable frequency and tissue site distributions (Du, 2007). The t(11;18)(q21;q21)/*API2-MALT1* abnormality was the first to be described and is characterized by fusion of an inhibitor-of-apoptosis gene (*API2*, or *IAP2*) to a gene encoding a paracaspase-like protein (*MALT1*, previously *MLT1*) (Dierlamm, 1999; Rosenwald, 1999; Baens, 2000; Motegi, 2000; Remstein, 2000b; Yonezumi, 2001; Ye, 2003a, 2003b). *API2-MALT1* positive tumors have a predilection for gastric and lung sites, with infrequent occurrences elsewhere. A second translocation event occurring in EN-MZL is characterized by the t(14;18)(q21;q32) derived *MALT1-IGH@* gene fusion (Murga Penas, 2003; Sanchez-Izquierdo, 2003; Streubel, 2003; Remstein, 2004; Streubel, 2004; Ye, 2005). Notably, the *MALT1* gene is situated slightly centromeric to the *BCL2* locus on chromosome 18q and as such these two t(14;18)-associated gene fusions are indistinguishable by standard cytogenetics, requiring instead FISH analysis for accurate diagnosis. *MALT1-IGH@* positive lymphomas are distributed in orbital, parotid, lung, and cutaneous sites and are very uncommonly encountered in the stomach. Other rare translocations described sporadically in EN-MZL are the t(1;14)(p22;q32)/*BCL10-IGH@* and t(3;14)(p14.1;q32)/*FOXP1-IGH@* abnormalities (Wotherspoon, 1990; Willis, 1999; Streubel, 2005). Significantly, some of the reported tissue site distributions for *API2-MALT1* and *MALT1-IGH@* in EN-MZL may be reflective of other factors, such as geographic differences, recurrences of MALT lymphomas in organs distinct from the primary presentation, or other pathogenic influences (Remstein, 2006). Despite the apparent complexity of translocation genotypes and tissue distribution, a fundamental pathogenesis links these events in the development of EN-MZL. Through overexpression of either MALT1 or Bcl10 proteins, or by expression of an abnormally active chimeric MALT1 moiety (i.e., as a result of the *API2-MALT1* gene fusion), constitutive activation of the NF-κB signal transduction pathway is induced, leading to profoundly altered effects on cell growth, immunity and apoptosis regulation (Isaacson, 2004; Du, 2007). The centrality of the NF-κB pathway also suggests attractive targets for the development of small molecule inhibitor therapies. Results from gene expression profiling studies continue to add to our understanding of pathway deregulation in MALT lymphomas (Chng, 2009).

Detection of these translocation events is generally best accomplished by FISH techniques (Remstein, 2006). RT-PCR analysis for the API2-MALT1 transcript has been described and represents an alternative method for detecting the t(11;18) (Zhang, 2006); however, owing to substantial breakpoint heterogeneity in both genes, comprehensive primers are necessary and sufficient, good quality RNA is required, the latter often being a limiting factor in small tissue or paraffin-embedded biopsies. The diagnosis of a MALT lymphoma may not necessarily require additional investigations to detect these specific translocations. Conversely, in some situations, the detection of EN-MZL–related translocations by FISH methods can be very useful to establish the diagnosis of lymphoma in morphologically difficult cases with intermixed reactive or hyperplastic features, or to differentiate a true MALT lymphoma from another subtype of low-grade B cell lymphoma. More specifically, detection of the *API2-MALT1* lesion in gastric EN-MZL is potentially important for therapeutic management. Broad-spectrum antibiotic eradication of *H. pylori* can induce tumor regression in a significant subset of translocation-negative gastric EN-MZL, whereas the presence of the *API2-MALT1* gene fusion implies a distinct pathogenesis that is refractory to this nonchemotherapeutic option (Liu, 2001, 2002).

Standard PCR analysis for immunoglobulin gene rearrangements is frequently pursued at diagnosis in EN-MZL, to confirm the presence of a monoclonal B cell process. The use of PCR for assessing minimal residual disease following therapy can be more problematic. The significance of detecting clonal B cells using PCR technique in posttreatment biopsies from patients with gastric EN-MZL has been controversial, with some reports suggesting prolonged persistence of monoclonality after histologic eradication of lymphoma, and others paradoxically showing the presence of clonotypic B cell populations in benign gastric lymphoid proliferations (Bertoni, 2002; Wundisch, 2003). Whereas many of these studies have employed PCR techniques with differing sensitivities, it appears that the decrease in PCR-detected clonotypic B cells generally lags behind the histologic normalization of gastric tissue in successfully treated patients. These findings suggest caution in the interpretation of molecular clonality investigations and careful correlation with morphologic findings in this clinical setting.

Chronic Lymphocytic Leukemia/Small Lymphocytic Lymphoma: Molecular and Cytogenetic Prognostic Markers

Chronic lymphocytic leukemia and its nodal manifestation small lymphocytic lymphoma (CLL/SLL) is overall an indolent form of B cell lymphoproliferative disorder, often not requiring early therapeutic intervention. Yet, advances in the last decade have defined more distinct prognostic subgroups independent of clinical staging, in turn identifying those patients at risk for early progressive disease and adverse outcome (Seiler, 2006; Zent, 2006; Hamblin, 2007; Moreno, 2008). This area of malignant hematology is illustrative of the convergence of phenotypic, cytogenetic, and molecular genetic tumor features in order to produce a more sophisticated approach to outcome prediction for these patients. Well-known phenotypic adverse factors include high expression of cell surface CD38 antigen and the overexpression of the signaling kinase ZAP-70. Several recurrent cytogenetic anomalies have been identified in CLL/SLL, none of which are disease-specific. These abnormalities include deletions of chromosome 13 or 13q; deletions of 11q; deletions of 17p; and trisomy 12. The cytogenetic changes are most reliably identified by targeted DNA probes using FISH technique. The presence of isolated 13q- has been associated with relatively favorable outcome. In contrast, 11q- and 17p- confer a more aggressive disease course with early requirement for chemotherapy. In the latter two situations, minimally deleted regions of these chromosomal loci include the *ATM* and *TP53* genes, respectively. In most cases of CLL with loss of 17p, the remaining allele shows mutation of *TP53*, indicating biallelic loss of tumor suppressor p53 expression (Dicker 2008; Fabris, 2008). Although 17p- CLL cases account for 10% or less of all patients, these individuals suffer a disproportionate share of disease complications and furthermore, are refractory to commonly used purine nucleoside analog chemotherapeutic agents. A major advance in CLL/SLL biology also occurred with the identification of tumors with SHM of the *IGH@* V-region. Previously, CLL/SLL was considered to be a malignant counterpart of "naïve" or pregerminal center B cells; the discovery of SHM involving the immunoglobulin genes indicate that these tumor cells have experienced antigenic stimulation in a germinal center environment and are functionally more related to memory type B cells. Prognostically, a significant difference in clinical outcome has been shown for CLL/SLL patients with mutated (defined as >2% nucleotide deviation from germline DNA sequence) vs. unmutated *IGH@* V-region status (Hamblin 1999; Oscier, 2002). Mutational analysis of *IGH@* V-region alleles is currently performed in some molecular hematopathology laboratories and though technically involved, this process has been greatly facilitated by the development of comprehensive antigen receptor gene databases (e.g., ImmunoGenetics; http://imgt.cines.fr). These various predictive genetic and phenotypic parameters can obviously coexist in any given case of CLL/SLL, resulting in a complex set of (often) conflicting data for an individual patient. One exception is the presence of the 17p- alteration, for which FISH and molecular screening of *TP53* mutations (e.g., by PCR and sequencing) appears very important to identify these high-risk CLL/SLL patients who may benefit from alternative and earlier treatment interventions (Rossi, 2009; Zenz, 2008).

Diffuse Large B Cell Lymphomas: Role of BCL6 and MYC Gene Abnormalities and Classification Based on Gene Expression Profiling

The diffuse large B cell lymphomas (DLBCL) are characterized by moderate cytologic variability, but a relatively pronounced range of clinical outcome and biologic heterogeneity. Although nearly 50% of patients with de novo DLBCL are clinically "cured" of disease in the era of chemoimmunotherapy (e.g., "CHOP" + rituximab, or R-CHOP), prognostic factors to recognize those individuals with excellent versus poor outcome have not been easily identified. Cytogenetic studies of DLBCL have revealed a range of findings including normal karyotype, complex karyotype and the presence of recurrent gene rearrangement abnormalities. Among the latter, translocations involving the *BCL2*, *BCL6* and *MYC* genes are the most frequent or clinically important. Cytogenetic aberrations of chromosome 3q27 and the *BCL6* gene have been characterized in approximately 20%–40% of DLBCL and a smaller proportion of follicular lymphomas. In contrast to most other lymphoma-associated translocations, gene fusions with *BCL6* can involve a large number of partner genes, many of which are unrelated to the antigen receptor genes (Chen, 1998; Ohno, 2004, 2006). However, a subset of cases will harbor the t(3;14)(q27;q32) abnormality, joining the *BCL6* gene to the *IGH@* locus, while others may involve the immunoglobulin light chain gene loci. In addition, 60%–70% of DLBCL demonstrate acquired somatic mutations in the 5′ noncoding regulatory region of *BCL6*, with or without accompanying translocation events.

Bcl6 is expressed by normal germinal center lymphocytes (centroblasts and centrocytes) and this gene product is in fact vital for the formation of the normal germinal center reaction, for T cell–dependent antibody responses, and for control of Th2-type cytokine-induced inflammatory responses (Dent, 1997; Ye, 1997; Polo, 2004). The Bcl6 transcriptional program has been shown to be active in repressing proto-oncogene expression in normal B cells, but it is deregulated in large B cell lymphoma cells (Ci, 2009). Bcl6 has also been shown to functionally down-regulate the p53 and Atr tumor suppressor proteins (Phan, 2004; Jardin, 2007; Ranuncolo, 2007); in this capacity, Bcl6 functions to protect normal germinal center B cells from apoptotic signaling induced by physiologic DNA double strand breakage during the somatic hypermutation process, supporting affinity maturation of immunoglobulins. As a consequence of this environment, some normal germinal center-experienced B cells acquire somatic mutations in the 5′ noncoding region of the *BCL6* gene process (Shen, 1998); however, the 5′ *BCL6* mutations found in DLBCL are often distributed differentially to mutations in normal B cells, implying that the regions targeted in lymphoma have pathologic effects on gene regulation (Pasqualucci, 2003; Jardin, 2005; Saito, 2007). Importantly, Bcl6 protein is not expressed in normal pregerminal center (naïve) B cells and it is rapidly down-regulated in B cells exiting the germinal center, conferring some relative specificity of this marker for the normal germinal center environment. Accordingly, the presence of Bcl6 protein expression is observed in many large B cell lymphomas, most follicular lymphomas, and BLs, but not in other B cell lymphoma subtypes (Cattoretti, 1995; Onizuka, 1995; Pittaluga, 1996; Falini, 1997).

The detection of *BCL6* gene rearrangements is most sensitively accomplished by FISH technique. Selection of probes is important, in that *BCL6* breaksites include both a major breakpoint region (MBR) and an alternate breakpoint region (ABR) (Iqbal, 2007). The clinical significance of *BCL6* gene alterations in DLBCL, whether present as translocation rearrangement events or somatic 5′ regulatory mutations, is still not clearly defined. Some studies have implied an adverse prognosis for large B cell lymphomas with *BCL6* gene rearrangements, perhaps pertaining more to tumors with nonimmunoglobulin gene translocations (Akasaka, 2000; Barrans, 2002), whereas other investigations have shown either opposite findings, or no convincing prognostic effect (Jerkeman, 2002). The effect of *BCL6* translocations in nodal DLBCL may also be associated with other adverse tumor biologic factors (Shustik, 2009). Primary central nervous system DLBCL with *BCL6* structural changes do appear to have a significantly worse outcome (Cady, 2008). As noted earlier, *BCL6* alterations may also be related to the pathogenesis of a distinct subset of high-grade follicular lymphomas, in the absence of the t(14;18)/*BCL2*-IgH (Katzenberger, 2004; Gu, 2009). Abnormalities of *BCL6* have also been described in high-grade B cell lymphomas with concurrent *MYC* gene abnormalities (see later), in posttransplant large B cell lymphomas, and in some of the aggressive lymphomas arising in the setting of human immunodeficiency virus (HIV)/acquired immunodeficiency syndrome (AIDS). Although the exact molecular mechanisms predisposing to the development of large B cell lymphomas continue to be defined, it is evident that deregulation of *BCL6* creates a cellular environment conducive to additional lymphomagenic genetic derangements.

The *MYC* gene on 8q24 is rearranged in approximately 5%–10% of DLBCL, representing translocations to the *IGH@*, immunoglobulin light chain, or nonimmunoglobulin gene loci. Myc is a potent cellular growth factor and classic proto-oncogene. A more detailed molecular description of *MYC* gene translocation events and function is presented in the later discussion on BL. Several large clinical studies have shown that unselected de novo DLBCL patients with *MYC* gene rearrangements have a significantly worse overall outcome (Klapper, 2008; Obermann, 2009b; Savage, 2009). Because no distinctive phenotypic or presenting clinical features can reliably identify *MYC* rearrangements in morphologically typical DLBCL cases, some investigators have suggested routine diagnostic assessment of the *MYC* locus by FISH analysis, despite its relatively low prevalence. Patients with so-called double hit genetics (e.g., *MYC* plus concurrent *BCL2* or *BCL6* rearrangements) have very aggressive disease, but are often characterized by variant cytomorphology akin to BL rather than usual type centroblastic features, and so are considered separately (see following discussion on BL).

Recent years have witnessed a paradigm shift in the classification of DLBCL based on gene expression signatures. One landmark publication using microarray-based analysis of global tumor mRNA expression revealed two major DLBCL subgroups designated as *germinal center-like B cell* (GCB) and *activated B cell like* (ABC) (Alizadeh, 2000; Rosenwald, 2002). Strikingly, GCB-classified patients had a much superior survival outcome relative to ABC type patients (summarized in de Leval, 2009). The validity of this approach has been confirmed by other studies, including evaluation of smaller gene sets characteristic of either GCB or ABC type tumors (Lossos, 2004). For example, a subset of overexpressed genes, including *BCL6*, *LMO2*, *HGAL*, and *CD10*, are strongly related to GCB phenotype, whereas *MUM1/IRF4*, *CD44*, *XBP1*, and several others are preferentially seen in ABC DLBCL. Certain cytogenetic features also appear to segregate between these subtypes, such that the t(14;18)/*BCL2-IGH@* is identified among GCB tumors and, interestingly, *BCL6* gene translocations are more prevalent in ABC lymphomas. The latter findings suggest that Bcl6 protein overexpression is important in the pathogenesis of GCB DLBCL, but structural rearrangements of the *BCL6* gene are reflective of a different pathogenesis and adverse features as seen in ABC DLBCL. Most intriguingly, ABC tumors consistently demonstrate deregulation of the NF-κB pathway, via abnormalities in upstream pathway proteins such as CARD11, BCL10, and MALT1; selective targeting of this pathway holds therapeutic promise for better managing these relatively refractory cases of DLBCL. Currently, determination of GCB versus ABC DLBCL types using microarray-scale gene expression methods remains outside the realm of routine clinical molecular diagnostics, although promising technologic developments may make this approach more feasible in smaller and more targeted platforms. Attempts to reproduce this classification using immunohistochemistry have not been rigorously successful because of a lack of strict gene expression level-to-protein correlation, overlapping expression patterns in many DLBCL for some protein markers, and the lack of reproducible standards for a nonquantitative technique. Finally, it should be noted that gene expression studies by other groups have revealed different functional subsets of DLBCL (Shipp, 2002; Monti, 2005) and a challenge for the development of a new biologic and clinically relevant classification in this disease will require a thorough understanding of these large and complex datasets.

MYC Gene Translocations in Burkitt Lymphomas and "High-Grade" B Cell Lymphomas, Unclassifiable

Genetic alterations of the *MYC* locus, situated on chromosome 8q24, are classically associated with BL; however, this gene is also implicated in the pathogenesis of several other aggressive lymphoid tumors including high-grade (secondary) transformations of indolent lymphomas, HIV/AIDS-associated lymphomas, and monomorphic B cell posttransplant lymphoproliferative disorders. Most commonly, the *MYC* gene is translocated to the *IGH@* locus as a result of the t(8;14)(q24;q32) abnormality. In other instances, *MYC* may be brought adjacent to the *IGK* [2(p12)] or *IGL* [22(q11)] light chain genes. In each case, *MYC* is placed under the strong transcriptional influence of an immunoglobulin enhancer element, leading to overexpression of the gene. Myc (or cMyc) is normally a highly regulated transcription factor involved in coordinating early cell cycle and DNA replication nuclear responses to mitogenic signaling pathways. *MYC* translocation and deregulation in lymphoma thus leads to transactivation of multiple cognate target genes, ultimately driving uncontrolled cell proliferation, in a permissive cellular context (Hecht, 2000). The simultaneous abrogation of proapoptotic mechanisms is synergistic with rapid Myc-induced transformation (Beverly, 2009). The molecular anatomy of *MYC* region breakpoints has been well studied in BL with the t(8;14) (Hecht, 2000; Blum, 2004). In so-called endemic BL, which is strongly associated with chronic Epstein-Barr virus (EBV) infection, *MYC* breaksites occur far upstream of the gene and primarily involve the *IGH@* J_H region. In contrast, sporadic type BL demonstrate *MYC* breaks that are situated closer to the 5′ region of the gene and are typically associated with fusion to the *IGH@* isotype switch regions, located upstream of the respective constant region (C-) exons. The enzyme AID is critical to the process of class switch recombination and SHM in normal germinal center B cells, and *MYC-IGH@* translocation breaks in BL have been shown to be AID-dependent (Robbiani, 2008). Sporadic BL is far less frequently associated with EBV (20% of cases). These data suggest that translocation events involving *MYC* in these epidemiologic BL variants may occur at slightly different stages of maturation in a developing B cell; clinically, however, these differences appear to be insignificant.

In routine practice, the diagnosis of BL can usually be established with a high degree of probability using a combination of clinical, morphologic, and targeted immunohistochemical studies (Braziel, 2001). Definitive diagnosis however, requires detection of a *MYC* gene rearrangement. *MYC* translocations cannot be identified by standard PCR approaches due to the pronounced breakpoint heterogeneity in the *MYC* gene; FISH or karyotype analysis thus currently remains the best option for identifying these abnormalities. FISH strategies can include initial targeting of the *MYC* gene locus using a break-apart probe strategy, followed by locus-specific probes to identify *MYC-IGH@* fusions. Novel probes to detect translocations with the immunoglobulin light chain genes have also been described (Einerson, 2006).

An uncommon type of lymphoid tumor with cytomorphologic features reminiscent, but atypical, of BL has been described with highly aggressive clinical behavior (Haralambieva, 2005; McClure, 2005). Notably, these B cell lymphomas are often associated with *MYC* gene rearrangements, as well coexisting translocations involving the *BCL2* or *BCL6* genes. These lesions have been termed *double hit* lymphomas and are presently classified as "B cell lymphomas, unclassifiable, with features intermediate between diffuse large B cell lymphoma and Burkitt lymphoma" in the 2008 WHO classification of lymphomas. This group of B cell lymphomas is considered heterogeneous, and includes de novo double hit cases, transformed follicular lymphomas with both *BCL2* and secondary *MYC* rearrangements, and *MYC*-negative cases with complex karyotype. Recognition of these high-grade B cell lymphomas by morphologic and molecular genetic criteria is important given the inadequate response to DLBCL therapy. In this regard, FISH studies to identify double hit genetic abnormalities of *MYC* and *BCL2* or *BCL6* are often pursued.

ALK Gene Abnormalities in Anaplastic Large Cell Lymphomas

ALCL is a unique subtype of peripheral T cell NHL that may present as a primary cutaneous disease, or more commonly as a systemic form involving lymph nodes, visceral organs and skin. A phenotypic hallmark in nearly all cases of ALCL is strong uniform expression of the CD30 (Ki-1) antigen, an activation marker and member of the tumor necrosis factor family. Although classic ALCL tumors are known to be of T cell lineage, some examples fail to express lineage associated T cell markers ("null" cell phenotype), but these cases can usually be confirmed as being of T cell origin based on T cell receptor gene clonality studies. A major subset of ALCL is characterized by translocations involving the *a*naplastic *l*ymphoma *k*inase (*ALK*) gene located on chromosome 2p23. *ALK* encodes a novel tyrosine kinase that is not normally expressed in lymphoid cells. Approximately 90% of *ALK*-rearranged ALCL harbor the t(2;5)(p23;q35) abnormality, leading to a fusion of the *ALK* gene with the *NPM1* gene (Stein, 2000). The *NPM1* gene is also mutated in many normal karyotype acute myeloid leukemias as described previously. As a result of the *NPM1-ALK* gene fusion, the tyrosine kinase activity and intracellular location of ALK becomes deregulated, contributing to lymphomagenesis through increased target protein phosphorylation and signal transduction (Falini, 2001; Chiarle, 2008). Unlike the more typical gene overexpression consequences of most lymphoma-associated translocations, the *NPM1-ALK* fusion differs in that a chimeric mRNA and protein are produced, although overproduction of the normally silent *ALK* gene in a T-lymphocyte appears to be the principal mechanism involved in malignant transformation. Investigative efforts have shown that ALK deregulation can involve down-regulation of T cell associated antigens, NF-κB target gene activation, functional inactivation of normal p53 tumor suppression, and immunosuppressive effects mediated through STAT3 signaling (Cui, 2009; Eckerle 2009; Wasik, 2009). In addition to *NPM1-ALK*, several less common variant genetic rearrangements of *ALK* are also described in this type of lymphoma, including the t(1;2)(q25;p23)/*TPM3-ALK*, t(2;3)(p23;q35)/*TFG-ALK*, and inv(2)(p23q35)/*ATIC-ALK* abnormalities, all giving rise to *ALK* gene deregulation (Swerdlow, 2008). Importantly, the abnormal cellular sublocalization of constitutive ALK kinase activity is mediated by the fusion partner protein moiety. Thus NPM1-ALK oncoproteins are situated in both a nuclear and cytosolic pattern, whereas TPM3-ALK products show diffuse cytoplasmic distribution, in accordance with the usual site of the *TPM3* gene product, tropomyosin-3. Several clinical studies have demonstrated a relatively favorable prognosis for ALK-positive ALCL, regardless of the actual translocation present. ALK-positive ALCL are more prevalently seen in younger patients (e.g., less than 50 years) and in the pediatric population. In contrast, another group of T cell lymphomas sharing the same morphologic features and expression of CD30 antigen do not have *ALK* gene rearrangements or deregulation of ALK protein expression. These ALK-negative tumors also appear to differ in global gene expression profiles, indicating distinct pathways of malignant transformation. Most significantly, ALK-negative ALCL are associated with more aggressive disease behavior typical of peripheral T cell lymphoma unspecified, justifying the recognition of the ALK-positive subtype by molecular or immunophenotypic methods (Falini, 1999a; Gascoyne, 1999; de Leval, 2009; Fornari, 2009; Savage, 2008). In addition to distinguishing the two major systemic subtypes of ALCL, the presence of an *ALK* gene rearrangement can help in the differential diagnosis between ALCL and Hodgkin lymphoma, and rare cases of phenotypically indeterminate large cell lymphoma. An unusual and rare complication of silicone breast prostheses is the development of implantation-site ALCL in some patients, which are also ALK negative (de Jong, 2008). Of note, the primary cutaneous type of ALCL is not associated with *ALK* gene abnormalities or aberrant ALK expression and has a very favorable outcome.

Genomic breakpoints in cases of t(2;5) positive ALCL lie consistently within the same intron regions in both *NPM1* and *ALK* genes, resulting in the generation of a single, unique NPM1-ALK chimeric mRNA. As a result, RT-PCR technique can be used to detect the fusion transcript with high specificity and sensitivity (Ladanyi, 1994; Lamant, 1996; Weiss, 1995; Wellmann, 1995; Yee, 1996). In addition, long distance DNA PCR has also been successfully employed to identify the genomic *NPM1-ALK* abnormality (Ladanyi, 1996; Sarris, 1998). The latter approach requires high molecular weight DNA, but obviates the need for RNA isolation and reverse transcription. FISH methodology is nevertheless the most widely employed diagnostic modality to detect *ALK* gene rearrangements. Essentially all translocation-associated alterations can be detected using a break-apart probe method directed to the *ALK* locus; elucidation of the specific translocation gene partner is not required because of its limited clinical value. As with other gene overexpression phenomena in the NHLs, ALK-positive ALCL can also be readily diagnosed using monoclonal antibodies against the ALK portion of the oncoprotein. The immunohistochemical cellular localization of abnormal ALK, as suggested previously, also correlates to some extent with the type of translocation event, reflecting the effects of the fusion partner segment (Falini, 1999b; Stein, 2000).

To complete the discussion of ALK-positive lymphomas, several reports have recently documented the presence of the t(2;17)(p23;q23)/*CLTC-ALK* or *NPM1-ALK* gene fusions in very rare and unusual occurrences of IgA heavy chain–positive diffuse large B cell lymphoma with plasmablastic features (de Paepe, 2003; Gascoyne, 2003). These tumors are also recognized by the presence of plasmacytic cell markers but lack of CD20 expression and CD30 negativity (compared with T cell ALCL). The *CLTC* gene encodes clathrin and the chimeric CLTC-ALK protein has a unique cellular distribution of granular membrane positivity, corresponding to localization to clathrin-coated pits. ALK-positive large B cell lymphomas are associated with a particularly poor outcome (Laurent, 2009).

TCL1A Gene Abnormalities in T Cell Prolymphocytic Leukemia

T cell prolymphocytic leukemia (T-PLL) is a mature T cell leukemia most often characterized by expression of CD4, although phenotypic variants are well known. T-PLL is often suspected by cytology and immunophenotype, but can share overlapping features with other T cell neoplasms showing blood and bone marrow involvement. T-PLL cases are, however, definitively diagnosed by the presence of a *TCL1A* gene rearrangement (Pekarsky, 2001; Krishnan, 2006). Tcl1a is a transcription factor that is not completely understood, but is expressed in a subset of normal B cells, but not normal mature T cells. As a result of *TCL1A* rearrangement in a candidate T-lymphocyte, the gene becomes aberrantly active, leading to the pathogenesis of T-PLL. Rearrangements of *TCL1A* are not identified in other major subgroups of peripheral T cell lymphoma. The *TCL1A* gene is situated on chromosome 14q32 and in 80% of T-PLL cases are juxtaposed with the *TRA* gene locus, either through an inversion [inv14(q11q32)], or reciprocal translocation event [t(14;14)(q11;32)]. A small number of T-PLL will have alternate translocations t(X;14)(q28;q11) or t(X;7)(q28;q35) involving a fusion of the *TCL1A*-related gene, *MTCP1*, to either the *TRA* or *TRB* gene loci, respectively (De Schouwer, 2000). The diagnosis of T-PLL is thus greatly facilitated and confirmed by FISH analysis for *TCL1A* rearrangements or chromosome studies for *MTCP1*-related translocations. In tissue sections, Tcl1a immunohistochemistry can be used to identify the overexpressed protein in suspected cases.

Emerging Technologies Impacting Molecular Diagnosis and Prognosis Prediction in Hematolymphoid Neoplasia

The practice of hematopathology remains integrally tied to the rapid pace of development in molecular genetics: advancements in molecular discovery and application have transformed the diagnosis and management of hematolymphoid neoplasms and, in turn, these same diseases have provided fertile and easily accessible biologic material for the advancement of the technologies themselves. Several new molecular applications are currently poised to enter clinical practice, an event that may have effects as profound as the advent of the polymerase chain reaction. As always with platform shifts and paradigmatic change, the clinical molecular diagnostic laboratory will need to be flexible when adopting these developments, while maintaining its primary focus on the high standards of quality, reproducibility and cost effectiveness.

Chief among these promising new techniques is what has been called "deep sequencing," "high throughput sequencing," and "next generation sequencing" (Tucker, 2009). Although there are several such sequencing platforms that vary in technical approach, many of them share the same general approach: multiple copies of large genomic targets are fragmented at random into short segments, which are then randomly immobilized and simultaneously sequenced. This apparently disjointed data can be reorganized by sophisticated computer software programs, using the principle that each randomly generated fragment of the sequence will share some degree of overlap with many other fragments from the same genomic region (Flicek, 2009). This technology, an offshoot of the human genome project, has been called "massively parallel sequencing," and it is capable of generating hundreds of megabases of sequence data per day. Entire genomes can be sequenced in this manner, but for the purposes of molecular hematopathology in the near term, genes of diagnostic importance can be either preselected by hybridizing the genomic DNA to complementary capture probes, or enriched using other techniques. The technology can also be applied to other species of ribonucleic acid, including messenger RNA and microRNA, yielding large scale analysis of the transcriptome and "miRnome," respectively. When coupled with techniques such as chromatin immunoprecipitation and bisulfite treatment, next generation sequencing can analyze protein-gene interactions and methylation patterns on a genome-wide scale. Thus instead of assaying for mutations or changes in a handful of genes (e.g., *NPM1*, *CEBPA*, and *FLT3* in AML), the diagnostician of the near future may be able to screen cases for mutations or other alterations involving any of dozens to many hundreds of genes. As complex as the computer algorithms at the heart of next generation sequencing are, they pale in comparison to the bioinformatic and interpretive challenges presented by this comparative avalanche of data (ten Bosch, 2008). Therefore, routine clinical laboratory applications of high throughput sequencing will first require many clinical correlative studies to identify valid associations between large sets of potential nucleic acid biomarkers, and parameters such as disease predisposition, prognosis, or therapeutic efficacy (McPherson, 2009). In this regard, it is worth bearing in mind that the state-of-the-art 2008 WHO classification struggles to document all facets of even the few genes of currently recognized significance in AML (Swerdlow, 2008). Close collaboration between the diagnostic, clinical, bioinformatic, and basic research communities will be necessary in the coming years to employ this powerful new technology in a rational manner tied to improved patient outcomes.

A similarly ground-breaking advance in diagnostic capability will likely arise from the growing convergence of molecular diagnostics and cytogenetics, as demonstrated by array comparative genomic hybridization (aCGH) and the genotyping of single nucleotide polymorphisms (SNPs) via microarray. These techniques permit genome-wide analysis on a scale of resolution intermediate between the base pair level of molecular diagnostics and the gross overview afforded by conventional cytogenetics and even FISH methods. aCGH is performed by fragmenting and labeling sample and control genomic DNA with different fluorescent colors, then competitively hybridizing a mixture of the labeled fragments to a microarray containing millions of oligonucleotide probes in a predetermined arrangement. The ratio of sample to control fluorescence for each probe location conveys information about the "copy number" of the sample relative to the control at that locus. An alternative strategy to gain knowledge of copy number takes advantage of the existence of SNPs, locations in DNA at which a significant proportion of randomly selected individuals will differ in their genetic sequence by a single base change. SNP arrays hybridize labeled genomic DNA from the sample to microarrays spotted with pairs of probes designed to preferentially bind sequences containing one or the other version of the SNP. The total fluorescent intensity arising from both probes of a given pair yields the copy number at that location, while the relative intensity of one probe to the other reflects the individual's genotype (heterozygous or homozygous) at the SNP. This genotype information can be used to detect uniparental disomy or copy number neutral loss of heterozygosity (UPD/CN-LOH), situations in which the expected two copies of each sequence are present, but each copy is identical throughout a region of DNA, indicating in neoplasms, a duplication of a segmental genomic abnormality; aCGH does not detect this UPD/CN-LOH, which is an important mechanism of tumor suppressor silencing in tumorigenesis. Already these technologies have revolutionized clinical genetic testing for inherited dysmorphology syndromes and developmental delay, in addition to documenting a previously unsuspected degree of human genetic diversity (Redon, 2006; Edelmann, 2009; Zhang, 2009). Among hematolymphoid neoplasms, CLL has thus far received the most attention from investigators using these techniques (Gunn, 2008; Higgins, 2008; Patel, 2008; Sargent, 2009).

In contrast to next-generation sequencing and molecular karyotyping, gene expression profiling (GEP) by microarray is a technique that has by now compiled a lengthy track record as a tool for biomedical research. Although microarray analysis is not as yet routinely used in the clinical laboratory, it is a powerful technology from which a number of clinically important observations have been made in acute leukemias and lymphomas (Levene, 2003; Hubank, 2004; Winter, 2007; Wouters, 2009b). Microarrays contain oligonucleotide or cDNA targets on a "chip" surface. These targets represent a large component of the expressed genome or the entire genome and are designed to specifically represent the mRNA levels of genes in parallel from a single sample. Detailed overviews of the various options available for array-based expression analyses as well as their techniques related to their analysis and interpretation are discussed elsewhere in this book. Studies on hematopoietic neoplasms have provided insights into "class prediction" (prediction of a tumor type based on specific gene expression profiles of selected informative genes) as well as "class discovery" (discovery of new sub-entities within tumor groups formerly regarded as a homogenous entity). Class discovery is not solely limited to identification of new subtypes of leukemia, for instance, but includes definition of prognostically differing groups, which are anticipated to influence therapeutic strategies. The application of GEP to diffuse large B cell lymphoma (DLBCL) has been described earlier and is one example of class discovery (Dybkaer, 2004). Similar studies in follicular lymphoma have revealed two multigene expression signatures, allowing separation of patients into subsets independent of currently available clinical prognostic variables (Dave, 2004). Most intriguingly, the length of survival among these follicular lymphoma patients correlated with the molecular profile of the non-malignant tumor infiltrating immune cells, revealing the contribution of host background to neoplastic growth. Gene expression microarray studies of CLL were also important to uncover the expression of the *ZAP-70* gene as a strong surrogate marker of adverse outcome (Rosenwald, 2001). The protein level of ZAP-70, as assessed by flow cytometry, has since become an accepted prognostic marker in CLL, despite the technical problems inherent in performing this assay. As microarray technology matures and becomes more cost effective, it is apparent that variations of this methodology will have application in the clinical laboratory.

The future for diagnostic hematopathology therefore appears challenging, yet exciting in this new era of genome-wide analysis and targeted therapies, with the goal of optimizing individual care for patients and realizing the potential of "personalized medicine."

SELECTED REFERENCES

Baccarani M, Cortes J, Pane F, et al. Chronic myeloid leukemia: an update of concepts and management recommendations of European LeukemiaNet. J Clin Oncol 2009;27:6041–51.

Recent summary of molecular monitoring guidelines and identification of suboptimal response and therapeutic resistance in patients with CML on tyrosine kinase inhibitor therapy.

Baldus CD, Mrózek K, Marcucci G, Bloomfield CD. Clinical outcome of de novo acute myeloid leukaemia patients with normal cytogenetics is affected by molecular genetic alterations: a concise review. Br J Haematol 2007;137(5):387–400.

Good review of molecular genetics and clinical significance of normal karyptype AML.

Bruggemann M, White H, Gaulard P, et al. Powerful strategy for polymerase chain reaction-based clonality assessment in T-cell malignancies Report of the BIOMED-2 Concerted Action BHM4 CT98-3936. Leukemia 2007;21:215–21.

Updated review of PCR-based approaches for determination of T-cell clonality in lymphoid proliferations.

Campana D. Role of minimal residual disease monitoring in adult and pediatric acute lymphoblastic leukemia. Hematology/Oncology Clinics of North America 2009;23:1083–98.

Excellent review of methods and clinical relevance of minimal residual disease evaluation in ALL.

de Leval L, Hasserjian RP. Diffuse large B-cell lymphomas and Burkitt lymphoma. Hematol Oncol Clin N Am 2009;23:791–827.

Excellent review of aggressive lymphomas.

Du MQ. MALT lymphoma: recent advances in aetiology and molecular genetics. J Clin Exp Hematop 2007;47: 31–42.

Excellent review of current concepts in MALT lymphoma.

Evans PA, Pott C, Groenen PJ, et al. Significantly improved PCR-based clonality testing in B-cell malignancies by use of multiple immunoglobulin gene targets. Report of the BIOMED-2 Concerted Action BHM4-CT98-3936. Leukemia 2007;21:207–14.

Concise update on use of PCR for detection of B-cell clonality in lymphoid proliferations.

Foroni L, Gerrard G, Nna E, et al. Technical aspects and clinical applications of measuring BCR-ABL1 transcripts number in chronic myeloid leukemia. Am J Hematol 2009;84:517–22.

Discussion of methodologic considerations in performing quantitative molecular monintoring for residual disease in CML.

Grimwade D, Jovanovic JV, Hills RK, et al. Prospective minimal residual disease monitoring to predict relapse of acute promyelocytic leukemia and to direct preemptive arsenic trioxide therapy. J Clin Oncol 2009 Aug 1;27(22):3650–8.

This study shows compelling data for PCR monitoring of minimal residual disease in acute promyelocytic leukemia and illustrates the successful use of therapeutic intervention for molecular relapse.

Hochhaus A, Druker B, Sawyers C, et al. Favorable long-term follow-up results over 6 years for response, survival, and safety with imatinib mesylate therapy in chronic-phase chronic myeloid leukemia after failure of interferon-α treatment 10.1182/blood-2007-07-103523. Blood 2008;111:1039–43.

Results of a large study showing durable efficacy of imatinib in the treatment of chronic phase CML.

Ishikawa Y, Kiyoi H, Tsujimura A, et al. Comprehensive analysis of cooperative gene mutations between class I and class II in de novo acute myeloid leukemia. Eur J Haematol 2009;83(2):90–8.

Overview of the cooperative nature of gene mutations in the pathogenesis of acute myeloid leukemia.

Jones D, Kamel-Reid S, Bahler D, et al. Laboratory practice guidelines for detecting and reporting BCR-ABL drug resistance mutations in chronic myelogenous leukemia and acute lymphoblastic leukemia: a report of the Association for Molecular Pathology. J Mol Diagn 2009;11:4–11.

Useful consensus document for the laboratory detection of BCR-ABL1 drug resistance mutations.

Kilpivaara O, Levine RL. JAK2 and MPL mutations in myeloproliferative neoplasms: discovery and science. Leukemia 2008;22(10):1813–17.

Review of current understanding of the molecular pathogenesis of myeloproliferative neoplasms.

Licht JD. Acute promyelocytic leukemia—weapons of mass differentiation. NEJM 2009;360:928–30.

Good update on current pathogenetic and therapeutic aspects of APL.

Liu H, Bench AJ, Bacon CM, et al. A practical strategy for the routine use of BIOMED-2 PCR assays for detection of B- and T-cell clonality in diagnostic haematopathology. Br J Haematol 2007;138:31–43.

Detailed PCR clonality study using comprehensive primer strategies.

Metcalfe DD. Mast cells and mastocytosis. Blood 2008;112(4):946–56.

Comprehensive review of mastocytosis.

Mrózek K, Marcucci G, Paschka P, Bloomfield CD. Advances in molecular genetics and treatment of core-binding factor acute myeloid leukemia. Curr Opin Oncol 2008;20(6):711–8.

Review of prognostic significance in this group of AML.

Mullighan CG, Su X, Zhang J, et al. Deletion of IKZF1 and prognosis in acute lymphoblastic leukemia. N Engl J Med 2009;360(5):470–80.

Landmark paper describing a new genetic mutation associated with poor outcome in pediatric ALL.

Quintás-Cardama A, Cortes J. Molecular biology of bcr-abl1-positive chronic myeloid leukemia. Blood 2009;113(8):1619–30.

Review of the molecular pathogenesis of CML.

Scott LM, Tong W, Levine RL, et al. JAK2 Exon 12 mutations in polycythemia vera and idiopathic erythrocytosis. N Engl J Med 2007;356:459–68.

Important paper identifying alternative JAK2 mutations in a small group of myeloproliferative neoplasms.

Stirewalt DL, Radich JP. The role of FLT3 in haematopoietic malignancies. Nature Rev Cancer 2003;3: 650–65.

This comprehensive review covers the molecular and cell biology of Flt3 in normal and leukemic hematopoiesis.

Tucker T, Marra M, Friedman JM. Massively parallel sequencing: the next big thing in genetic medicine. Am J Hum Genet 2009;85(2):142–54.

Overview of the benefits and challenges of high-throughput sequencing techniques in the clinical laboratory.

Van Dongen JJM, Langerak AW, Bruggemann M, et al. Design and standardization of PCR primers and protocols for detection of clonal immunoglobulin and T-cell receptor gene recombinations in suspect lymphoproliferations: Report of the BIOMED-2 Concerted Action BMH4-CT98-3936. Leukemia 2003;17:2257–317.

Landmark publication detailing very comprehensive assessment of PCR based techniques versus Southern blot methods to detect clonal B- and T-cell populations in lymphoid proliferations.

Vrooman LM, Silverman LB. Childhood acute lymphoblastic leukemia: update on prognostic factors. Curr Opin Pediatr 2009;21(1):1–8.

Update on prognostic factors in the management of pediatric acute lymphoblastic leukemia.

Zenz T, Krober A, Scherer K, et al. Monoallelic TP53 inactivation is associated with poor prognosis in chronic lymphocytic leukemia: results from a detailed genetic characterization with long-term follow-up Blood 2008;112:3322–9.

Study emphasizes the importance of TP53.

REFERENCES

Access the complete reference list online at http://www.expertconsult.com

CHAPTER 76

MOLECULAR GENETIC PATHOLOGY OF SOLID TUMORS

Peng Lee, Shilpa Jain, Matthew R. Pincus, Ruliang Xu

PART 9

KEY POINTS

- Solid tissue (mainly epithelial cell) tumors are mainly caused by genetic lesions of three types: deletion or inactivation of tumor suppressor genes, mutation in or overexpression of oncogenes (i.e., genes encoding proteins that are vital in control of the cell cycle), and hypermethylation of the promoter regions.
- These genetic lesions can be detected using the techniques described in Part 8 of this textbook involving real-time polymerase chain reaction, fluorescent in situ hybridization, immunohistochemistry, enzyme-linked immunosorbent assay, etc.
- Detection of genetic lesions in solid tissue tumors is of great value for the diagnosis of specific types, for classification of the tumor, and for determining prognosis for a patient with a specific type of cancer, and for classification of the tumor. A common mutation in several of these cancers is overexpression of the epidermal growth factor receptor (EGFR). Discovery of this lesion allows for implementation of anti-EGFR therapy. However, because ras-p21is a downstream target of EGFR, and because it is commonly mutated in many human cancers, it is necessary to test for oncogenic mutations in the *ras* gene. If these are found, the efficacy of anti-EGFR agents is diminished.
- Less commonly, oncogenic mutations can be found in downstream targets of *ras-p21*, such as BRAF, which makes treatment with anti-EGFR agents less effective.
- Many solid tissue tumors express the same oncogenes, such as BRAF, in melanoma and thyroid cancer, but other cancers have genetic lesions that appear to be specific for that type of cancer, such as RET in medullary thyroid carcinoma.
- Although not formally classified as solid tissue tumors, sarcomas often behave in a manner identical to that of solid tissue tumors. These cancers have been found to be caused by reciprocal translocations resulting in oncogenic fusion transcripts (accounting for 15%–20% of cases) and by specific oncogenic mutations (e.g., *KIT* and *PDGFRA* mutations in gastrointestinal stromal tumors). Both types of genetic alterations are often specific to certain types of sarcomas.
- Because the genetic alterations or changes that underlie many familial types of cancers are known, it is possible to screen for these in the children and close relatives of patients known to have a form of familial cancer, so as to detect the presence of these cancers as rapidly as possible.

Cancer is largely a genetically encoded disease. Recent research on cancer molecular genetics, epigenetics, and genomics, as well as their application, has vastly changed the practice of cancer diagnosis, classification, prognosis, and treatment. Application of molecular genetics to solid tumors is a major milestone in diagnostic pathology. The molecular diagnosis was initially introduced for accurate diagnosis of solid tumors, based on the unique genetics. Now the utility of molecular diagnosis is far beyond its original intention, and it is no longer just an adjunct method. It has become an indispensable tool that is widely used to predict clinical outcome, including disease prognosis, selection of optimal therapeutic regimens, and anticipation in response to treatment. It has not only revolutionized the concept and practice of diagnostic pathology for solid tumors, it has also become the basis for personalized medicine.

The principles and method in molecular diagnostics of solid tumors are similar to those used in other fields of molecular diagnosis. Techniques commonly used in cancer molecular pathology include detection or identification of specific sequences of genes (DNA and/or its transcribed RNA) or gene product (protein) alterations. They include amplification-based techniques (i.e., polymerase chain reaction [PCR], RT-PCR, branched DNA testing), hybridization methods (i.e., in situ hybridization, or fluorescent in situ hybridization [FISH]), microarray-based approaches (i.e., comparative genomic hybridization [CGH], DNA, RNA, microRNA microarray), and sequencing. PCR and FISH are among the most commonly used methods, whereas array-based techniques have a promising future, but have not been used widely in clinical settings to this point. Each method is described in Part 8 of this text.

Tissue sources of diagnostic materials of molecular pathology for solid tumor include paraffin-embedded tissue, fresh tissue, and cytologic specimens. Fresh tissue is a preferred choice for preservation of DNA, RNA, or protein. In most cases, only fresh tissue is usable in array-based methods; however, it is usually not readily available or accessible. Thus, paraffin-embedded tissue is used most commonly because of its availability and ease of access; it also allows use of the corresponding hematoxylin and eosin-stained slides for morphologic study. However, exposure of nucleic acid to formalin is associated with the major inherent problems of increased nucleic acid fragmentation and low integrity of DNA, RNA, and protein. Tissue fixation in formalin for longer than 24 hours will likely reduce the yield of high molecular weight nucleic acid. Thus, longer formalin fixation, paraffin embedding, and long storage at room temperatures can lead to false-negative results. A second problem is impurity of tumor cells, which usually are mixed with normal cells and stromal cells. Relatively pure tumor cells can be achieved by employing microdissection that isolates the tumor cells, even a single tumor cell, by a manual or instrument-assisted method. Cytologic specimens, including cells from fine-needle aspiration (FNA), urine, and blood, and swabs for molecular pathology, are used most often to assist in accurate diagnosis of superficial solid tumor, such as human epidermal growth factor receptor *(Her)-2/neu (ERBB2)* for breast cancer, human papillomavirus (HPV) testing for cervical cancer, and UroVysion (Abbott Laboratories, Abbott Park, Ill.) for bladder cancer.

Molecular diagnoses of solid tumors rely on our understanding of the molecular mechanism involved in carcinogenesis of solid tumors. Genetic alterations can be inherited or can result from carcinogenesis, as described in Chapter 74. In several tumors, polygenic mutations occur, but often in these cases, some unique or specific genetic alterations lead to carcinogenesis. Those genetic or epigenetic components mainly belong to the following:

1. Tumor suppressor genes (TSGs) (*Rb*, *SMAD*, adenomatous polyposis coli *[APC]*, etc).
2. Oncogenes (*EWS*, *cKIT*, *Her2/neu*, *KRAS*, *BRAF*, etc).
3. Promoter regions with methylation/inactivation activity.

Application of molecular diagnosis of solid tumors has been used clinically as follows:

1. **Assistance in disease diagnosis and classification:** For example, small "blue cell" tumors encompassing Ewing's sarcoma, lymphoma, rhabdomyosarcoma, and so forth, can be diagnosed by identification of specifically altered genes (e.g., Ewing's sarcoma–specific gene translocations). In cervical cancer, detection of HPV assists in the diagnosis of neoplastic change on cervical biopsies or smears. Moreover, in the future, DNA microarray of the tumor may detect gene signatures.
2. **Determination of prognosis:** With better understanding of the molecular genetics of solid tumors, a greater number of prognostic markers can be identified. Thus detection of those markers in some cases has become a routine practice. For example, detection of overexpression/amplification of *Her2/neu* in breast cancer and 1p19q deletion in brain tumor has been used to predict prognosis or clinical outcome.
3. **Determination of therapeutic options:** Many drugs have been developed to target certain genes and gene products (i.e., proteins) and related pathways. Examples include tyrosine kinase inhibitors (TKIs) and monoclonal antibodies to EGFRs in lung and colon cancer. Moreover, only certain groups of patients with unique genetic profiles can respond to these treatments. Thus, providing the right management not only will increase the chances for cure, but also will improve patient quality of life by avoiding unnecessary side effects.
4. **Combination of the above:** In most cases, detection of molecular markers may provide both diagnostic and prognostic information such as c*KIT* mutations and chromosomal abnormalities detected by UroVysion, and amplification of *Her2/neu.*

This chapter focuses on the clinical application of molecular pathology in cancer diagnosis, prognosis, and predicting treatment response in common solid tumors. The major genetic findings in each tumor type are summarized in Table 76-1.

Molecular Genetic Pathology of Specific Solid Tumors by Major Organ

BRAIN TUMOR

Primary central nervous system (CNS) gliomas, originating exclusively from brain cells such as astrocytes, oligodendrocytes, and ependymal cells, account for only about 1.35% of all cancers, but rank second among the causes of death from neurologic disease. Glioblastomas are the most common primary CNS tumor and are categorized as World Health Organization (WHO) grades I–IV, based on histologic characteristics. With the advent of new treatment modalities, the use of microscopic examination alone is insufficient for the histologic classification and grading of gliomas.

Glioblastoma Multiforme

Glioblastoma multiforme (GBM) consists of anaplastic malignant astrocytic tumors characterized by predominant microvascular and endothelial proliferation. The current standard of care for GBM is surgical resection, followed by radiation therapy. However, the association of specific molecular genetics not only assists in diagnosis and prognosis but also leads to the development of new adjuvant chemotherapy (e.g., temozolomide) (Stupp, 2005). Glioblastomas (WHO grade IV) may develop de novo (primary glioblastomas) or through progression from low-grade astrocytomas (secondary glioblastomas). The two types show similar histologic features; however, they differ in terms of molecular alterations, with primary glioblastomas showing activation of the EGFR pathway, whereas secondary glioblastomas are more commonly associated with *TP53* mutations. Thus, the molecular genetics of these tumors demonstrates that they are distinct diseases and therefore may exhibit different prognoses and responsiveness to therapy (Ohgaki, 2007). Tyrosine kinase inhibitors, such as erlotinib and gefitinib, may offer a therapeutic option for primary tumors in which EGFR signaling is upregulated (Ohgaki, 2007).

Recent comprehensive genetic screens of GBM (Parsons, 2008) have confirmed that genetic loss is scattered across the entire genome, affecting numerous chromosomes. **Loss of heterozygosity (LOH) on chromosome 10 is the most frequent genetic loss in GBM,** occurring in 60%–80% of cases. Allelic losses on 1p and 7q have also been seen in GBM, but at lower frequencies. Loss of 1p occurs in 6%–20% of GBMs, and in combination with 19q loss may indicate a better prognosis and improved responsiveness to therapy; however, the combined loss of 1p/19q is a rare event in GBM (Kanu, 2009).

Gains in gene expression have also been demonstrated in GBM in the form of duplication of entire chromosomes, intrachromosomal amplification of specific alleles, or extrachromosomal amplification (often in the form of double minutes) and activating mutations. Many genes have been shown to be amplified in glioma; these include *EGFR, CDK4, SAS, MDM2, GLI, PDGFRA, MYC, N-MYC, MYCL1, MET, GADD153,* and *cKIT.* The most commonly amplified genes in glioblastoma are *EGFR* on chromosome 7 (in approximately 40% of cases), *CDK4,* and *SAS* (in approximately 15%).

Other molecular mechanisms of gliomagenesis include loss of the DNA repair enzyme, O(6)-methyl guanine DNA methyltransferase (MGMT), which specifically removes pro-mutagenic alkyl groups from the O6-position of guanine in DNA (Kanu, 2009). Expression of MGMT protects normal cells from carcinogens; however, it can also protect cancer cells from chemotherapeutic alkylating agents. This has been implicated as an important mechanism of drug resistance because it reduces the

TABLE 76-1
Most Common Genetic Alterations in Solid Tissue Tumors

Tumor type	Major molecular targets*	Main methods of detection	Clinical application
Solid Tissue Tumors			
Glioblastoma	*EGFR, TP53,* 10q, MGMT, mutations in *TP53* and *PTEN, P16INK4a* deletions	RT-PCR, methylation-specific PCR, FISH	Prognosis, treatment response
Oligodendroglioma	1p and 19q deletions, *EGFR, TP53*	FISH, RT-PCR, LOH	Diagnosis, prognosis, treatment response
Sporadic, nonhereditary breast cancer	*Her2/neu*, multiplex genes	FISH, IHC, RT-PCR, Oncotype, MammaPrint	Molecular classification, prognosis, treatment response
Hereditary breast cancer	*BRCA1, BRCA2, EGFR*	High-throughput sequencing, multiplex PCR, genetic counseling	Diagnosis, genetic counseling
Papillary thyroid cancer	*BRAF, RET, PTC1, PTC3*	FISH, RT-PCR, direct sequencing	Diagnosis, prognosis, therapeutic option
Follicular thyroid cancer	*PAX8-PPARγ*	IHC, FISH, RT-PCR	Diagnosis, prognosis
Medullary thyroid carcinoma	*RET*	Sequencing, PCR	Diagnosis, screening, surveillance
Non–small cell cancers of the lung	*EGFR, RAS*	PCR, sequencing, FISH	Prognosis, treatment response
Liver (hepatocellular)	*EEGFR, VEGFR,* glypican-3, *p53*, β-catenin, microRNA (miR-122a), multiple genes	FISH, PCR, sequencing, microarray	Diagnosis, prognosis, targeted therapy
Gastric cancer, intestinal type	*p73* mutations, *MSI* (*MLH1* and *MSH2*), LOH/mutations of *APC* genes, and Her2/neu	FISH, PCR, IHC	Diagnosis, prognosis
Gastric cancer, diffuse type	*CDH1*	FISH, PCR, IHC	Diagnosis, prognosis
Colon cancer	1. Mutated oncogenes: mainly *EGFR, KRAS, BRAF*, and *PI3K*. 2. Mutated or deleted antioncogenes: *p53, APC, TGFBRI, SMAD2, SMAD4* 3. Microsatellite instability (MSI) genes and CpG island methylator (CIMP) genes	FISH, PCR, microarray, methylation-specific PCR, sequencing, array technology	Diagnosis, prognosis
Pancreatic cancer	Most pancreatic cancers: *KRAS* mutations	PCR, sequencing	Diagnosis
	Inactivating mutation or deletion or methylation of genes encoding *TP53, SMAD4, p16/CDKN2A*	PCR, methylation-specific PCR	Diagnosis (rarely), prognosis
	miRNAs (miR-196a, 217, 221, 376a, and 301)	RT-PCR	Diagnosis, prognosis
Renal cell carcinoma (RCC)	Chromosome 3p deletion, von Hippel–Lindau *(VHL)* gene deletion; hypoxia-inducible factor *(HIF)* overexpression	Sequencing, FISH (for VHL)	Diagnosis
Translocation-associated RCC	t(X;17)(p11.2;q25); *ASPL-TFE3* and *PRCC-TFE3* fusion genes	RT-PCR, FISH, IHC for the C-terminal domain of nuclear TFE3	Diagnosis, classification
RCC, clear cell	1. Carbonic anhydrase IX 2. Genes of immune response and proangiogenesis 3. Proximal nephron markers: megalin, cubilin, adipophilin	Gene expression arrays, IHC	Diagnosis, prognosis, classification
RCC, papillary	1. Proximal nephron marker α-methylacyl-coA racemase	Gene expression arrays, IHC	Diagnosis, prognosis, classification
RCC, chromophobe	1. Abundant mitochondria 2. Distal nephron markers: β-defensin, parvalbumin, chloride channel Kb, claudin 7 and 8, and EGF	Gene expression arrays, IHC	Diagnosis, prognosis, classification
RCC, oncocytoma	1. Abundant mitochondria 2. Distal nephron markers: β-defensin, parvalbumin, chloride channel Kb, claudin 7 and 8, EGF	Gene expression arrays, IHC	Diagnosis, prognosis, classification
Bladder cancer	Aneuploidy of chromosomes 3 , 7, and 17 and/or deletion of the 9p21 (encoding p16); *NMP 22*	FISH	Diagnosis
Prostate cancer	*TMPRSS2* (*21q22.3*) to transcripts of the ETS family member genes: overexpression of ETS proteins (e.g., ERG, ETV1, ETV4, ETV5)	FISH, ELISA, RT-PCR, gene expression arrays	Diagnosis, classification
Cervical cancer	HPV-6 and -18	Hybrid capture DNA assay, RT-PCR, Southern blotting, dot blot	Diagnosis, follow-up of abnormal PAP smears

Continued

TABLE 76-1
Most Common Genetic Alterations in Solid Tissue Tumors—*Cont'd*

Tumor type	Major molecular targets*	Main methods of detection	Clinical application
Ovarian Cancer			
Low-grade serous	*KRAS, BRAF*	PCR, Southern blotting	Diagnosis, classification
High-grade serous	*p53* deletion/mutation; Wnt/β-catenin or PI3K/PTEN signaling pathway defects	PCR, Southern blotting	Diagnosis, classification
Mucinous	*KRAS, BRAF*	PCR, Southern blotting	Diagnosis, classification
Clear cell	*PI3K/PTEN* mutations	PCR, Southern blotting	Diagnosis, classification
Endometrioid	Mutations of *CTNNB1* (β-catenin)	PCR, Southern blotting	Diagnosis, classification
Melanoma	*CDKN2A, p14,* and *p16* inactivation; *NRAS* (G12V) and *BRAF* oncogenic mutations (V600E)	PCR, sequencing	Diagnosis, classification, therapy
Sarcoma			
Sarcoma with fusion genes involving the *TET* gene: Ewing's sarcoma	t(11;22)(q24;q12) translocation; fusion of *EWSR1* and an *ETS* family gene, mainly *FLI1*	RT-PCR, FISH, Southern blot	Diagnosis Prognosis
Sarcoma with fusion genes involving receptor tyrosine kinase: congenital fibrosarcoma	t(12;15)(p13;q25) translocation, resulting in fusion of *ETS* gene, *ETV6* with neurotropin receptor (that has tyrosine kinase activity), *NTRK3* gene	RT-PCR, FISH, Southern blot	Diagnosis
Sarcoma with fusion genes involving chromatin remodeling: synovial sarcoma (SS)	t(X;18)(p11.2;q11.2) translocation resulting in fusion of *SS18(SYT)* gene with one of the *SSX* genes on the X chromosome, creating *SS18-SSX1, SS18-SSX2,* or *SS18-SSX4* chimeric genes Downstream targets of above fusion proteins: *CCND1* (cyclin D1) and *TLE1* that encodes a transcriptional corepressor	FISH, RT-PCR IHC	Diagnosis, classification Diagnosis
Sarcoma with fusion genes involving growth factors: dermatofibrosarcoma protuberans (DFSP) and giant cell fibroblastoma (GCF)	t(17;22)(q11;q13.1) translocation resulting in fusion of the *COL1A1* gene on chromosome 17 with the *PDGFB* gene on chromosome 22, leading to *PDGFRB* overexpression	RT-PCR	Diagnosis, classification
Sarcoma with other types of fusion genes: alveolar rhabdomyosarcoma (ARMS)	t(2;13)(q35:q14) translocation that results in fusion of *PAX3* with *FOXO1A*	FISH	Diagnosis
Sarcoma with oncogenic mutations: gastrointestinal stromal tumor (GIST)	*cKIT/PDGFRA*	PCR, sequencing, Southern blotting	Diagnosis
Sarcoma with no consistent genetic lesions: leiomyosarcoma (LMS)	Loss of 1p12-pter, 2p, 13q14-q21 (targeting the Rb pathway), 10q (targeting *PTEN*), 16q. Gains of 17p, 8q, and 5p14 pter. Activation of the PI3K-AKT pathway and mTOR	FISH	Diagnosis
Syndromatic Cancers			
Familial adenomatous polyposis syndrome	Adenomatous polyposis coli *(APC)* (long arm of chromosome 5) or MutY human homologue *(MYH)* gene involved in repair of oxidative damage to DNA	PCR, sequencing, Southern blot	Diagnosis
Hereditary nonpolyposis colorectal cancer (HNPCC): Lynch syndrome	Microsatellite instability (MSI) in mismatch repair *(MMR)* genes, including *MLH1, MSH2, MSH6, MLH3,* and *PMS2*	IHC, PCR, sequencing	Diagnosis, classification, genetic counseling
Familial juvenile polyposis syndrome	Germline mutations of *SMAD4, BMPR1A,* and *ENG*; also, mutations in kinase, *BMPR1A* (bone morphogenetic protein receptor Type IA), on chromosome 10q22.3. Involvement of TGF-β signal transduction pathway	PCR, sequencing	Diagnosis, classification
Peutz-Jeghers syndrome (PJS): melanotic mucocutaneous hyperpigmentation and GI hamartomas, which occur anywhere from the stomach to the anus; multiple polyps in small bowel	*STK11/LKB1* gene	PCR, sequencing	Diagnosis, classification
Multiple endocrine neoplasia (MEN)			

TABLE 76-1

Most Common Genetic Alterations in Solid Tissue Tumors—*Cont'd*

Tumor type	Major molecular targets*	Main methods of detection	Clinical application
MEN type 1: tumors in the parathyroid glands, in the stomach, pancreas and intestinal tract, anterior pituitary, endocrine pancreas, and duodenum, and by the presence of other, nonendocrine tumors such as hemangioma, ependymoma, and leiomyoma, often at a young age	MEN 1 tumor suppressor gene, *MEN 1*	PCR	Diagnosis, classification
MEN type 2: medullary thyroid carcinoma (MTC) and associated pheochromocytoma and hyperparathyroidism	*RET* (chromosome 10q11.2) (encoding a tyrosine kinase) mutations	PCR, sequencing	Diagnosis, classification
von Hippel–Lindau syndrome (VHL): neoplasia syndrome characterized by hemangioblastomas in the central nervous system and retina, pheochromocytomas, renal cysts and clear cell renal cell carcinoma, pancreatic cysts and islet cell tumors, endolymphatic sac tumors, and papillary cystadenomas of the epididymis and broad ligament	*VHL* tumor suppressor gene (three exons) on chromosome 3p25. Encodes VHL protein, critical in regulating hypoxia-inducible factor (HIF-α and -β)	PCR, sequencing	Diagnosis, classification
Familial paraganglioma syndromes	Mutation of three genes encoding subunits of mitochondrial succinate dehydrogenase (SDH complex): *SDHB* at 1p36.1 (PGL4), *SDHC* at 1q21 (PGL3), and *SDHD* at 11q23 (PGL1)	PCR	Diagnosis, classification
Cowden syndrome (CS); breast, thyroid, and endometrial cancers and other benign conditions, including multiple hamartomas in the colon, lipomas, fibromas	*PTEN* mutations	PCR	Diagnosis, classification
Li-Fraumeni syndrome; soft tissue sarcomas, breast cancer, osteosarcoma, brain tumors, childhood leukemias, and adrenocortical carcinoma	*p53* gene mutations	PCR, IHC	Diagnosis, classification
Neurofibromatosis 1 (NF1); neurofibroma and, less commonly, gliomas and other abnormalities (learning disability, vasculopathy, and bony abnormalities)	*NF1*, located on chromosome 17q11.2; diminished GTPase activating (GAP) activity activating the ras signal transduction pathway	FISH, direct sequencing, long-range PCR with Southern blot analysis, and/or cytogenetic analysis	Diagnosis, classification
Neurofibromatosis (NF2) and schwannomatosis. NF2 involves schwannomas, meningiomas, and ependymomas	*NF2* gene (chromosome 22)	Sequencing, mutation scanning, duplication/deletion testing, PCR, quantitative PCR, microarray, comparative genomic hybridization, or combination	Diagnosis, classification

ELISA, Enzyme-linked immunosorbent assay; *FISH,* fluorescent in situ hybridization; *IHC,* immunohistochemistry; *LOH,* loss of heterozygosity; *PCR,* polymerase chain reaction; *RT-PCR,* real-time PCR.

*Full names and functions of molecular targets (i.e., oncogenes and oncoproteins) listed in the second column may be found in the corresponding sections of this chapter describing these targets and the corresponding references.

cytotoxicity of alkylating chemotherapeutic agents. Loss of MGMT expression may be caused by methylation of promoter CpG islands, which have been detected in 75% of secondary GBMs—much more frequently than in primary GBMs (36%). Immunohistochemical staining for MGMT does not offer a reliable way to stratify GBM (Kanu, 2009), and PCR assay is therefore necessary. *TP53* is one of the more commonly studied TSGs in GBM. Loss of normal *TP53* function due to mutation occurs more frequently in secondary GBM. Thus, the major molecular targets of glioblastomas are EGFR, TP53, 10q LOH, and deletion of the *MGMT* gene. These can be detected using RT-PCR, methylation-specific PCR, and FISH. The main clinical applications are related to prognosis and treatment response. These findings are summarized in Table 76-1 and, in greater detail, in Table 76-2.

Oligodendroglioma

Oligodendroglioma is an infiltrating glioma of the cerebral cortex diagnostically characterized by a triad of uniformly round to ovoid nuclei, perinuclear halos, and an even distribution of cells, together with a delicate chicken wire–type of vasculature. However, in a significant number of these lesions, the microscopic morphology is not so clear cut, and distinction from other diffuse glial lesions may be difficult. Combined loss of 1p and 19q (Fig. 76-1, *A* through *C*) is typical in oligodendroglioma (Aldape, 2007), and loss of 19q occurs in astrocytoma and mixed oligoastrocytoma (Aldape, 2007). The incidence of 1p/19q loss varies from 50%–80% in oligodendroglioma in different studies, and it is 1%–10% in other gliomas, which indicates its utility in differentiating the diagnosis. Recent studies suggest that the combined loss of 1p/19q may follow a (1; 19)(q10; p10)

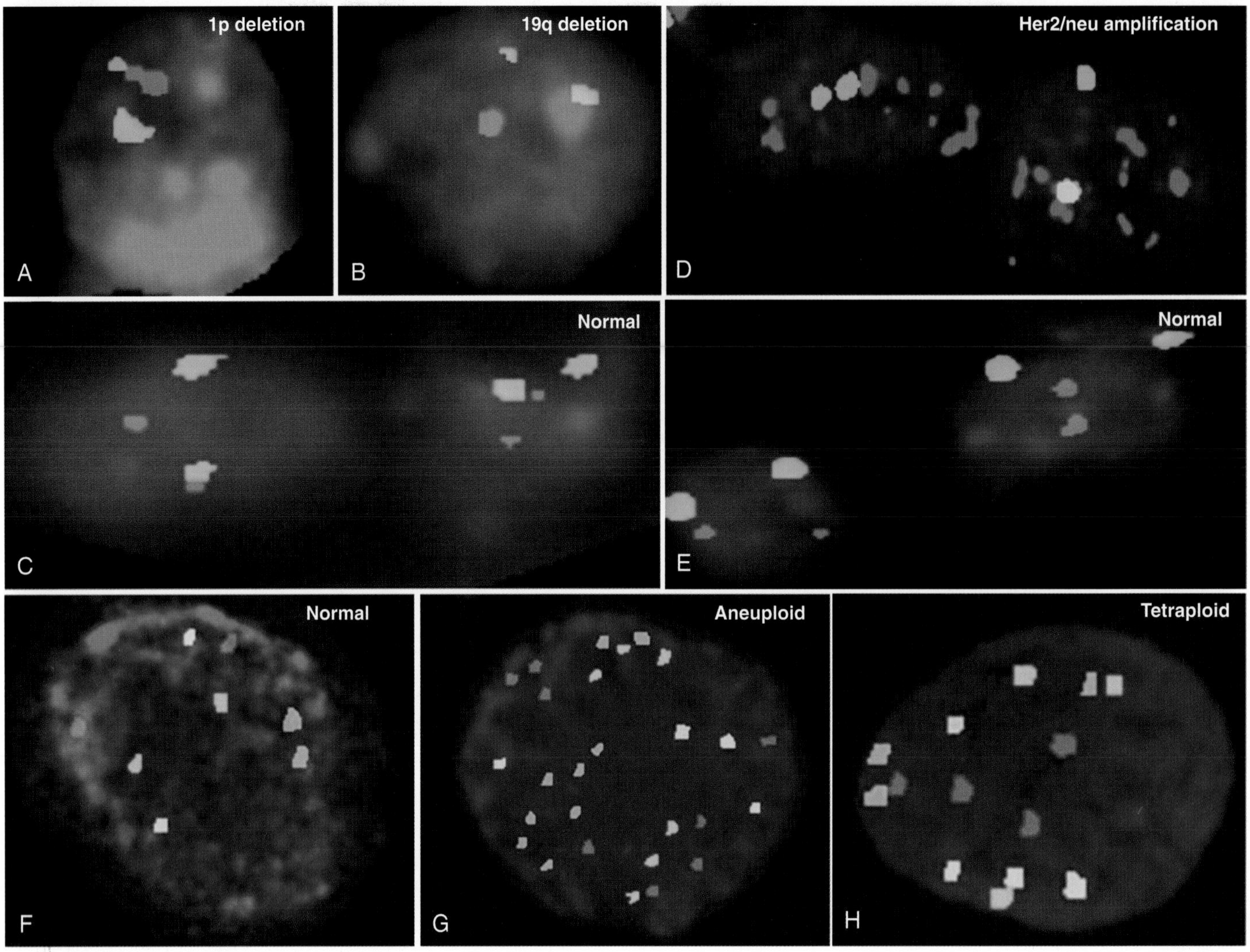

Figure 76-1 Examples of fluorescent in situ hybridization in cancer diagnosis. Oligodendroglioma with **A,** 1p and **B,** 19q deletions compared with **C,** normal cells. Green color in *A,* 1q probe; red color in *A,* 1p probe; green color in *B,* 19p probe; red color in *B,* 19q probe. **D,** Her2/neu amplification compared with **E,** normal cells. Green color: CEP17 probe. Red color: Her2/neu probe. UroVysion showing **F,** normal; **G,** aneuploid; and **H,** tetraploid cells. Aqua color: chromosome 17. Yellow (gold) color: 9p21 locus. Red color: chromosome 3. Green color: chromosome 7.

TABLE 76-2
Common Genetic Alterations in Glioblastoma Multiforme

	Primary GBM	Secondary GBM
LOH 10q	70%	63%
EGFR amplification	36%	8%
P16INK4a deletion	31%	19%
TP53 mutation	28%	65%
PTEN mutation	25%	4%

Data from Ohgaki H, Kleihues P. Genetic pathways to primary and secondary glioblastoma. Am J Pathol 2007;170:1445–53.
EGFR, Epidermal growth factor receptor; *GBM,* glioblastoma multiforme; *LOH,* loss of heterozygosity; *PTEN,* phosphate and tensin homologue deleted on chromosome ten.

translocation, with subsequent loss of the derivative chromosome der(1;19)(q10; p10) (Aldape, 2007). Identification of 1p/19q loss is associated with two unique features of tumor biology with clinical indications: first, they grow slowly, even those that are anaplastic in nature; second, they correlate with better prognosis and response to chemotherapy (Kuo, 2009). In terms of treatment response, initial studies suggested that 1p/19q loss is a marker of response to PCV (procarbazine, lomustine/CCNU, and vincristine) or temozolomide chemotherapy (Kuo, 2009). Thus, the 1p/19q status has become an important part of diagnosis, prognosis, and predicted therapeutic response of oligodendrogliomas. In addition to 1p/19q alteration, LOH mutations in *p53* and *p16* may be associated with poor survival or tumor progression (Kuo, 2009).

BREAST CANCER

Breast cancer is the most common cancer in women and the second most common cause of cancer death in women in the United States. Until recently, breast cancer was characterized according to tumor type (ductal vs. lobular carcinoma), histologic grade (I–III), steroid hormone receptors (ER and PR), and *Her2/neu* status (positive vs. negative), along with metastasis to lymph nodes and distant organs, for its prognosis and treatment. Gene expression profiling has recently been introduced as a potentially useful adjunct for the management of recently diagnosed breast cancer.

Sporadic, Nonhereditary Breast Cancer

Various genetic, epigenetic, and genomic changes have been associated with breast cancer. Traditionally, estrogen receptor (ER) and progesterone receptor (PR) status is used as a prognostic and predictive marker for breast cancer. *Her2/neu* (detailed in Chapter 74) status has been added in the past decade as a breast cancer prognostic and predictive marker. The FISH method has been used primarily to determine the copy number of the *Her2/neu* gene (Fig. 76-1, *D* and *E*) for the purpose of selecting Her2–targeted therapies such as trastuzumab and lapatinib in both adjuvant and neoadjuvant settings. Enumeration of 20 interphase nuclei from tumor cells on a given case is reported as the ratio of average *Her2/neu* copy number to that of chromosome enumeration probe 17 for centromere, CEP17. Specimens with amplification showed a *Her2/neu*:CEP17 signal ratio ≥2.0 as abnormal, and a ratio <2.0 as normal. A three-color FISH assay has been commercialized recently for assessment of standalone prognosis in ER-positive and ER-negative stage I breast cancers (Ross, 2009).

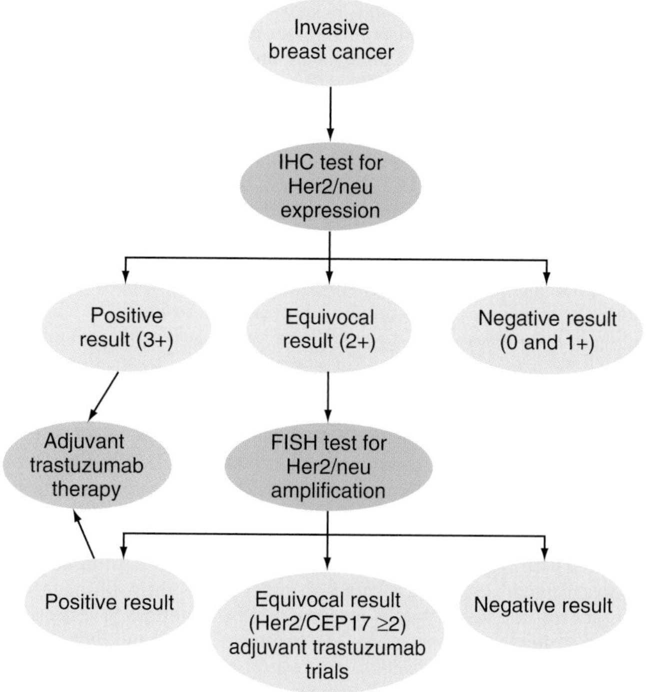

Figure 76-2 Algorithm using Her2/neu status in diagnosis and treatment of breast cancer.

In addition, HercepTest (Dako Corp, Carpinteria, Calif.), an immunohistochemistry (IHC) for *Her2/neu* using a polyclonal antibody, was the first U.S. Food and Drug Administration (FDA)-approved test; subsequently, Pathway (Ventana Medical Systems, Tucson, Ariz.) produced a monoclonal antibody (CB11) for *Her2/neu* for the same response indication that has also been approved by the FDA and is used in combination with FISH (Fig. 76-2). IHC is widely used to measure prognostic factors, including ER, PR, Her2/neu, and the proliferation marker, Ki-67, and to predict response to hormonal and Her2-targeted therapies (Ross, 2009).

Concerns associated with IHC-based assays for multiple markers include the nonlinear nature of IHC staining, the different subcellular localization of different markers, and the impact of different slide scoring thresholds for different antibodies. The introduction of whole genome profiling technologies has greatly expanded our knowledge of the genomic pathways associated with the development and progression of breast cancer (Bao, 2008). These research results have led to the development of several commercialized tests with multigenes/proteins as prognostic and predictive tools for clinical application using IHC, FISH, RT-PCR, and genomic microarray technologies with integrated bioinformatic/statistical algorithms designed to calculate the disease recurrence and survival of the patient (Ross, 2008).

Microarray-based gene expression profiling is now extensively used to define cellular functions and regulatory mechanisms, including the evaluation of breast cancer. Microarray platforms commonly used include Affymetrix GeneChip (Affymetrix Corporation, Santa Clara, Calif.) and the Agilent custom microarrays (Agilent Technologies, Santa Clara, Calif.). These technologies require the use of fresh or frozen tissue for messenger ribonucleic acid (mRNA) extracts and have not been fully adapted for use in formalin-fixed, paraffin-embedded (FFPE) tissue. Molecular classification of breast cancer has been proposed, based on gene expression profiling, to include luminal-like, normal-like, Her2-positive, and basal-like subtypes of invasive breast cancer (Ross, 2008). It is important to note that all of the luminal groups of breast cancers are ER positive, and nearly two thirds of them are of low or intermediate histologic grade, whereas 95% of all (Ross, 2009) basal-like cancers are ER negative, and 91% of these tumors are of high grade (Bao, 2008). Studies of clinical outcomes based on molecular subtypes have shown that luminal A is more sensitive to antiestrogen than is luminal B. Her2-positive responds to trastuzumab, an anti–Her2 antibody, whereas basal is more aggressive (but is especially sensitive to anthracycline-based neoadjuvant chemotherapy) than are the luminal breast cancers (Ross, 2009). Basal-like and Her2-positive subgroups are associated with the highest rates of pathologic complete response to neoadjuvant multiagent chemotherapy (Ross, 2009).

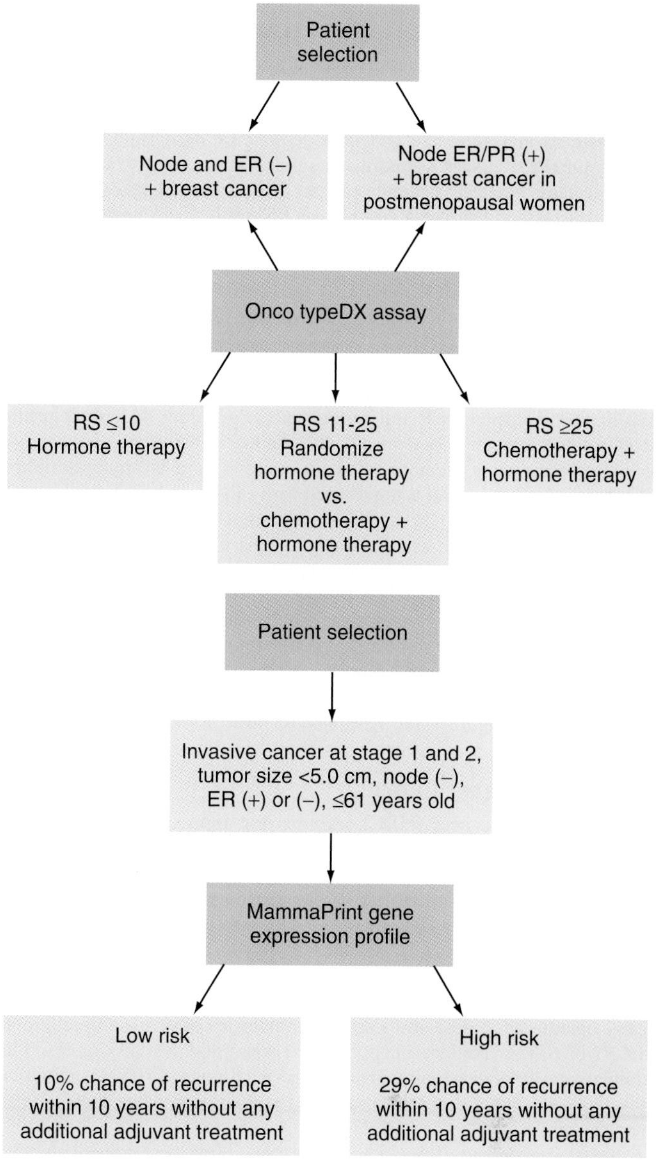

Figure 76-3 Algorithm of *A,* OncotypeDx and *B,* MammaPrint assays in breast cancer management.

The two prototypes of gene microarray-based clinical tests are the OncotypeDx and MammaPrint assays (Fig. 76-3) (Kato, 2009; Oakman, 2009). OncotypeDx (Genomic Health, Inc., Redwood City, Calif.) is a 21-gene multiplex prognostic and predictive RT-PCR assay performed on primary FFPE breast cancer samples. The original 16 informative genes (Paik, 2004) that calculate the recurrence score (RS) were discovered on archived FFPE samples by transcriptional profiling and then were converted to the FFPE RT-PCR assay (Ross, 2008). OncotypeDx determines the 10-year risk for disease recurrence in patients with ER-positive, lymph node–negative tumors by using a continuous variable algorithm and assigning a tripartite RS (17, low risk; 18–30, intermediate risk; >30, high risk). Of the multiple pathways assessed by this assay, the proliferation and ER pathways are the most influential in RS calculation, followed by the Her2 pathway. High relative levels of ER mRNA and low levels of Ki-67 proliferation gene mRNA have a low RS. Low levels of ER mRNA and high levels of Ki-67 mRNA have a high RS. The other 14 informative mRNA levels play their greatest roles in determining the RS in tumors with intermediate ER and Ki-67 mRNA levels. It should also be noted that OncotypeDx is best suited for detecting breast cancers with a low potential for recurrence. The MammaPrint assay (Agendia BV, Amsterdam, The Netherlands) was the first fully commercialized microarray-based multigene assay for breast cancer. This test is currently designed as a pure prognostic assay, has received 510 (k) clearances from the FDA, and is offered as a prognostic test for lymph node–negative breast cancer in women younger than age 61 with ER-positive or ER-negative tumor. This test was also the first assay to be approved by the FDA's new in vitro diagnostic multivariate index assay classification. Unlike OncotypeDx, this test cannot currently be performed on FFPE tissues but requires fresh-frozen tumor samples or tissues collected into an RNA preservative solution. The 70 genes that make up the MammaPrint assay are focused primarily on proliferation; additional genes are associated with invasion, metastasis, stromal integrity, and angiogenesis. Of note, the OncotypeDx and MammaPrint assays have only one individual gene in common—the *SCUBE2* gene, which is a member of the ER pathway. Unlike the OncotypeDx test, which features a continuous RS result, the MammaPrint test uses a dichotomous "high risk versus low risk" result format. The MammaPrint test does not include ER, PR, or Her2 in the 70-gene microarray. A new assay, TargetPrint (Agendia BV), has recently been launched that measures the mRNA of these three genes on the Agilent microarray system.

Multigene testing procedures such as disease classifiers and prognostic and predictive markers have been introduced with the use of slide-based methods (e.g., IHC, FISH) or molecular platform–based methods such as quantitative multiplex PCR and genomic array profiling. Morphologically based mRNA extraction performed with the use of tissue macrodissection or microdissection is recommended for analysis, as it is highly enriched for invasive carcinoma and is not diluted with cells from benign tissues and in situ carcinoma areas (Ross, 2008). The heterogeneous expression of important mRNAs, such as ER, Her2, and Ki-67, often reflected in the varying histologic grades seen in larger tumors, can influence the predictive accuracy of transcriptional profiling measurements. One caveat is that, although the number of genes that can be simultaneously assessed by multiplex qRT-PCR is significantly greater than that for IHC, multiplex qRT-PCR requires a more complex statistical evaluation of the gene expression profiles. Nevertheless, the RT-PCR technique has been used to predict overall prognosis and response to both hormonal and cytotoxic therapies.

Hereditary Breast Cancer

Hereditary breast cancer (HBC) accounts for approximately 10% of all breast cancers. Positive family history is the strongest risk factor, as it is present in about 20% of breast cancer cases. Population-based studies indicate that 15% of familial risk can be attributed to *BRCA* gene mutations, and that a further 10% involve *TP53*, phosphate and tensin homologue *(PTEN)*, *ATM*, and *CHEK2*; the rest may be explained by a polygenic model. A significant number of HBC-prone families are characterized by the more common hereditary breast-ovarian cancer syndrome. The *BRCA* genes operate as TSGs, and germline mutations affecting one allele of *BRCA1* or *BRCA2* confer susceptibility to breast and ovarian cancers. The cumulative risks of developing breast cancer by the age of 70 years approach 50%–70% in *BRCA1*-mutation carriers, and ovarian cancer, 30%–40% (Venkitaraman, 2009). For *BRCA2*-mutation carriers, the risk is 40%–50% for breast cancer and 10%–15% for ovarian. However, individuals who carry *BRCA2* mutations also have an increased risk of other cancers, including those of the male breast (≈seventy-fivefold relative risk), pancreas (fourfold to eightfold), and prostate (twofold to fourfold) (Venkitaraman, 2009). The spontaneous instability of chromosome structure and number is a hallmark of *BRCA*-deficient cells and arises from the distinct cellular functions performed by the BRCA1 and BRCA2 proteins in DNA repair and mitotic control. Since the discovery of *BRCA* genes and the development of methods for mutation screening, identification of *BRCA*-mutation carriers during the clinical management of familial cancer cases has become widespread. Gene expression profiling has revealed that tumors from patients who are *BRCA1*-mutated segregate within the basal subgroup of breast cancers (Venkitaraman, 2009) of the five different molecular groups, as discussed earlier. Tumors from *BRCA1*-mutation carriers are likely to stain positive for basal cytokeratins 5/6 and 14, and to exhibit negative estrogen receptor staining. These breast carcinomas also commonly stain for EGFR. *BRCA1*-associated tumors are commonly of high grade and are *p53*-mutated. They have a tendency to occur in younger women and carry a poor prognosis (Venkitaraman, 2009).

THYROID CANCER

Thyroid cancer is the most common endocrine neoplastic condition. The two most frequent types of thyroid malignancy derived from follicular cells are papillary and follicular carcinomas, which constitute approximately 80% and 15%, respectively, of all thyroid cancers. These follicular cell–derived tumors are well differentiated, in contrast to poorly differentiated and anaplastic carcinomas, which constitute about 2% of cases. Another malignancy in thyroid is medullary carcinoma, which originates from parafollicular C cells and accounts for approximately 3% of cases. Several genetic alterations in various thyroid tumors have been well documented, including translocations and point mutations. The genetic alteration in thyroid cancer involves *RET*, *BRAF*, *RAS*, and *PAX8*.

Papillary Thyroid Carcinoma

RET/PTC rearrangement and point mutations of *RAF*, in particular, the *BRAF* form, and *RAS* genes are found in more than 70% of cases of papillary thyroid carcinoma (PTC) (Nikiforova, 2008). *RAF* is a direct target of ras-p21. The *BRAF* gene mutation is the most common known genetic alteration in papillary carcinoma and is found in approximately 45% of these tumors (Nikiforova, 2008). A majority of mutations involve T1799A transversion mutation in exon 15 of the gene, which causes amino acid change from valine to glutamine at amino acid residue 600 (V600E), leading to constitutive activation of BRAF kinase, subsequent phosphorylation of MEK and ERK protein kinases (see Chapter 74), and downstream effectors of the mitogen-activated protein kinase (MAPK) pathway, as is summarized in Chapter 74 (see Fig. 74-1). Other mechanisms of *BRAF* activation, although rare, include K601E point mutation, small in-frame insertions or deletions surrounding codon 600, and *AKAP9-BRAF* rearrangement, which is more commonly associated with radiation exposure papillary carcinoma. *BRAF V600E* mutation is highly prevalent in papillary carcinoma with classical histology and in the tall cell variant. It has been correlated with aggressive features such as extrathyroid extension, advanced tumor stage at presentation, recurrence, and lymph node involvement and/or distant spread (Xing, 2005). Cancers with these mutations have decreased ability to trap radioiodine and lead to treatment failure and more aggressive behavior (Nikiforova, 2008). Detection of *BRAF* mutation can be achieved by direct sequencing, colorimetric mutation detection assay based on shifted terminal assay (Xing, 2004), real-time PCR, and allele-specific SYBR green PCR on an FNA sample, which is virtually diagnostic of papillary carcinoma. *BRAF* mutation represents an attractive therapeutic target for papillary carcinoma with the advent of various BRAF inhibitors (e.g., BAY43-9006) (Wan, 2004; Wilhelm, 2004).

The ***RET/PTC*** gene rearrangement is another prominent genetic alteration that plays a role in the pathogenesis of up to 20% of sporadic PTCs (Nikiforova, 2008). The *RET* gene, located on chromosome 10q11.2, encodes the tyrosine kinase receptor consisting of an extracellular ligand binding domain for the glial-derived neurotrophic factor family of growth factors, a cysteine-rich region, a transmembrane domain, and an intracellular tyrosine kinase domain. *RET* is highly expressed in parafollicular C cells and at very low levels in thyroid follicular cells (Nikiforov, 2008). *RET/PTC* rearrangements are a very early event in thyroid cancer development; this would explain their high prevalence in occult or microscopic PTC. Twelve forms of *RET/PTC* rearrangements have been reported to date, linking the 3′ portion of the *RET* gene with the 5′ portion of various different genes of the PTC family (Nikiforova, 2008). Of remaining genes, the two most common are *PTC1 (H4)* and *PTC3 (ELE1, ARA70, NCOR4)*, which account for up to 70% and 30% of rearrangements in sporadic PTC, respectively (Nikiforova, 2008). In particular, *RET/PTC* rearrangements are more frequent in individuals exposed to ionizing radiation (50%–80%) (Nikiforova, 2008), with the exception of *ELKS-RET* and *HOOK3RET* fusion. *RET/PTC* rearrangements are also more frequent in children (40%–70%) (Nikiforova, 2008) as compared with the general population (15%–30%). Papillary carcinomas with *RET/PTC* gene rearrangements typically present in younger individuals and exhibit a high rate of lymph node metastasis with classical papillary histology and lower stage at presentation, particularly in cases harboring *RET/PTC1* (Nikiforova, 2008). In tumors arising after radiation exposure, *RET/PTC1* was found to be associated with classic papillary histology, whereas the *RET/PTC3* type was more common among solid variants (Nikiforova, 2008).

Activated RET kinase has been explored as a target of therapy using TKIs such as ZD6474 (Nikiforova, 2008). The distribution of *RET/PTC* rearrangements within each tumor may vary from involving almost all neoplastic cells (clonal *RET/PTC*) to being detected only in a small fraction of tumor cells (nonclonal *RET/PTC*) (Nikiforov, 2008). This heterogeneity is a potential problem in RET receptor–targeted therapy.

Other point mutations involving several specific sites (codons 12, 13, and 61) in *NRAS*, *HRAS*, and *KRAS* genes are found in 10%–20% of cases of papillary carcinoma. These mutations are almost always found in the follicular variant of papillary carcinoma (Nikiforova, 2008).

Follicular Carcinoma

Most of the frequent genetic alterations in follicular carcinoma are *RAS* point mutations and *PAX8-PPARγ* rearrangements, altering the PI3K/AKT signal pathway. Several studies have reported the utility of

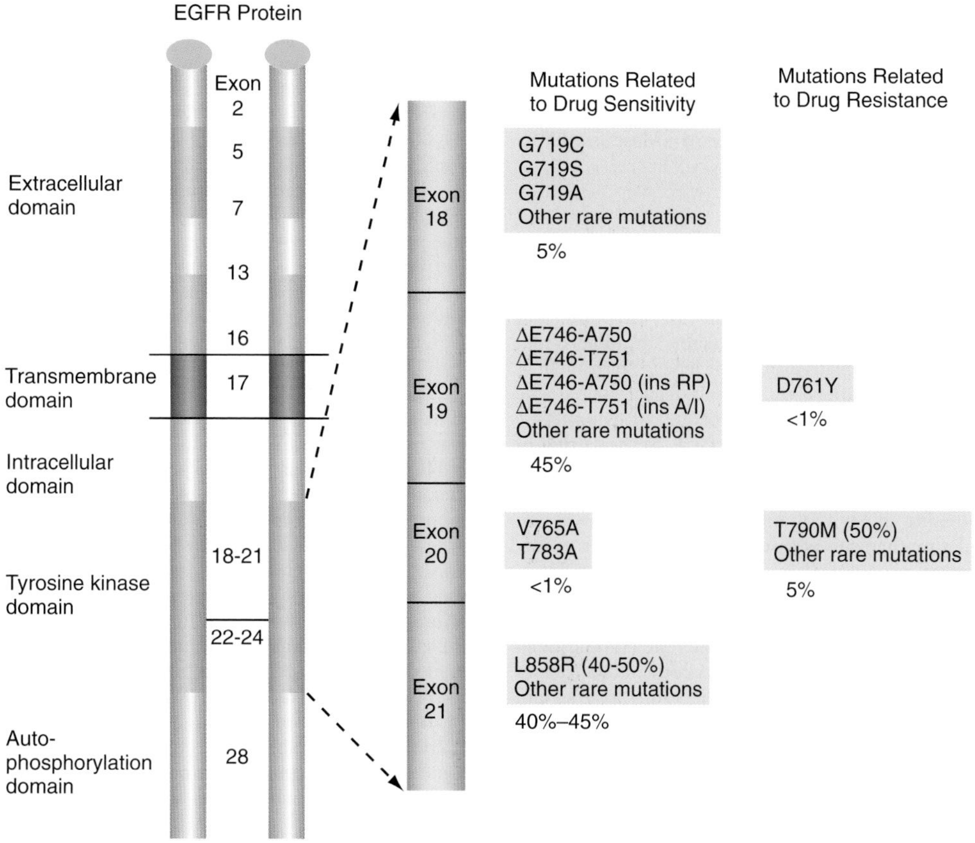

Figure 76-4 Clinically significant mutations of epidermal growth factor receptor mutation in cancer.

molecular testing in diagnosing this type of thyroid cancer preoperatively on FNA specimens.

A ***RAS*** mutation is found in 40%–50% of conventional follicular carcinomas and in 20%–40% of adenomas. It is interesting to note that the most common *ras* mutations, instead of occurring at codon 12, as in most other cancers, occur at codon 61 for *NRAS* and *HRAS* (Nikiforova, 2008). These mutations are associated with tumor dedifferentiation, a less favorable prognosis, and metastasis to bone (Nikiforova, 2008).

The ***PAX8-PPARγ*** gene rearrangement is a result of the translocation t(2;3)(q13;p25). It leads to a fusion between the *PAX8* gene, which encodes a thyroid-specific paired domain transcription factor, and the *PPARγ* gene. It occurs in 35% of conventional follicular carcinomas and has a lower prevalence in oncocytic (Hürthle cell) carcinomas (Nikiforova, 2008). Detection of *PAX8-PPARγ* rearrangement is almost always diagnostic of follicular carcinoma. Tumors harboring *PAX8-PPARγ* rearrangements tend to present in a younger age group, are smaller, and exhibit solid or nested patterns and more frequent vascular invasion. This rearrangement results in overexpression of the PPARγ protein that is detectable on IHC (Nikiforova, 2003).

Medullary Carcinoma

Medullary carcinoma of the thyroid (MTC) is a sporadic malignancy in a majority of cases (75%), with the remainder spanning three familial syndromes, including multiple endocrine neoplasia (MEN 2A and MEN 2B) and familial MTC (FMTC). In MTC, *RET* is activated by point mutations, in contrast to its activation by chromosomal rearrangement in PTC. In sporadic medullary carcinomas, somatic mutations of *RET* are found in 20%–80% of cases without a germline mutation. Germline mutations in *RET* are found in almost all patients with familial forms of medullary carcinoma; this correlates with the aggressiveness of MTC.

LUNG CANCER

Lung cancer remains the most common cause of cancer-related death among men and women worldwide. Epithelial tumors of the lung are of four principal types: squamous cell carcinoma, adenocarcinoma, large cell carcinoma, and small cell carcinoma. Clinically, the most important distinction is noted between small cell carcinoma and the others, which can be grouped together as non–small cell carcinoma. Small cell cancers respond to chemotherapy, whereas non–small cell carcinomas (NSCLCs) are removed surgically if possible. *EGFR* mutations have been identified in certain NSCLCs, among other types of cancer (e.g., colon, glioma, squamous cell carcinoma, Wilms' tumor). EGFR is a **membranous oncoprotein** that induces cell proliferation upon activation. Binding of a ligand to receptor activates its tyrosine kinase activity, which phosphorylates several substrates on a number of signal transduction pathways, leading to DNA synthesis and expression of oncogenes such as *fos* and *jun* and finally cell growth (see Chapter 74). Increased EGFR signaling can be the result of *EGFR* gene amplification, protein overexpression, or specific activation mutations in the *EGFR* gene, as described in detail in Chapter 74.

It has been shown that a subset of patients with NSCLC (10%–40%) (Coate, 2009) have specific activating mutations in the *EGFR* gene (Fig. 76-4) that are associated with increased sensitivity to TKIs, such as gefitinib (Iressa) or erlotinib (Tarceva), targeting EGFR in lung cancer. Common activating *EGFR* mutations occur most often in exons 18 to 21 and cluster in two major hot spots. The prototype mutation *L858R* in exon 21 (40% of *EGFR* mutations) encoding the tyrosine kinase domain and small in-frame deletions in exon 19 (>50%) are reportedly most often associated with responses to EGFR TKI therapy. Mutations in exons 18 and 20 account for the remaining 10% of *EGFR* mutations in NSCLC (Sholl, 2009). Recent studies have reported that *EGFR* gene mutations are more common among females, Asians, and nonsmokers with adenocarcinoma; these are the same groups that have the highest response rates to TKIs (Sequist, 2008). Furthermore, increased gene copy numbers detected by FISH and protein overexpression by IHC of EGFR have emerged as predictors of efficacy of EGFR TKIs. Therefore, these predictors are used in the selection of patients for anti-EGFR therapies (El-Zammar, 2009). Overall, it appears that the FISH test is the first step, followed by PCR for FISH-negative cases; this is the most effective method (El-Zammar, 2009). Recent studies have demonstrated that in patients with *EGFR* mutations, the EGFR locus is often concurrently amplified.

Mutations in ***KRAS***, frequently in codons 12 and 13, have been reported in up to 30% of cases of lung adenocarcinoma (Coate, 2009). These mutations are usually found in cancers of smokers and are more common in adenocarcinoma (30%–50%) than in NSCLC (15%–20%). Conversely, activating mutations in the *KRAS* gene were reportedly associated with resistance to EGFR-TKIs and have an adverse effect/poor outcome in NSCLC patient survival on EGFR-TKI therapy (Mascaux,

2005). Thus, the recommended molecular workup for NSCLC includes *EGFR* mutation screening by restriction fragment length polymorphism (RFLP) analysis, *EGFR* gene copy number using two color probes with FISH, and screening for *KRAS* mutations. The latter is important because EGFR-TKI therapy is less effective if oncogenic K-ras mutations occur since ras occurs downstream of EGFR (see Chapter 74) (Mascaux, 2005).

HEPATOCELLULAR CARCINOMA

Hepatocellular carcinoma (HCC) is the sixth most common malignancy and the third most common cause of cancer death worldwide. Major risk factors include chronic viral infection (hepatitis B virus [HBV] and hepatitis C virus [HCV]), alcoholic/nonalcoholic liver disease, environmental carcinogens (e.g., aflatoxin B1), and inherited genetic disorders (e.g., Wilson's, hemochromatosis, α_1-antitrypsin deficiency, tyrosinemia) (McGlynn, 2005; Parkin, 2005; Clark, 2006; Motola-Kuba, 2006). The development of HCC is a multistep process, comprising of hyperplastic change, dysplasia, early HCC, and well-developed HCC in the setting of chronic hepatitis or cirrhosis (Takayama, 1990; Theise, 2002), or in a small percentage of patients without cirrhosis.

The genomic abnormality of HCC is heterogeneous, largely as the result of various molecular mechanisms of carcinogenesis related to different causes and multifactorial processes (Jain, 2010a). HCV-related HCC has an exclusive gain at 10q, and loss of 4q and 16q and gain of 11q are seen preferentially in HBV-positive cases (Kusano, 1999; Nishida, 2003). Most HCCs are aneuploid and harbor multiple different chromosomal abnormalities, including nonrandom, recurrent DNA copy number losses on multiple chromosomal arms 1p, 4p, 5q, 6q, 8p, 9p, 13q, 16p, 16q, and 17p, and gains on 1q, 6p, 8q, and 17q, detected by conventional cytogenetic studies and CGH. Chromosome 1q is the most common aberration in several geographic locations (Guan, 2001; Chang, 2002; Terracciano, 2003). Frequently deleted chromosome regions by LOH in HCCs contain many TSGs, including *p53*, *Rb*, *p16*, *PTEN*, and *DLC1*, and oncogenes such as insulin-like growth factor-2 receptor *IGF2R* (Hsia, 1994; Edamoto, 2003; Matsuda, 2003). LOH at chromosome 1p usually is seen in early, small, or well-differentiated HCC (Kuroki, 1995), whereas LOH at chromosomes 16p and 17p is more frequently associated with aggressiveness of HCC, including advanced stage and poor prognosis (Tamura, 1997). By CGH, abnormalities in chromosomes 8p, 17p, and 19p are associated with metastasis of HCC (Zhang, 2003).

Dysregulation of the major signal transduction pathways is found in all HCCs, but differs with various associated causes. Abnormal activities of Wnt/β-catenin, hedgehog, transforming growth factor (TGF)-β, ras-p21 and MEK/ERK, IGF, and *PTEN* signaling pathways, as well as apoptosis, *p53*, *Rb*, and microsatellite stability, are commonly found in HCCs, irrespective of etiology, reflecting common pathogenetic mechanisms (e.g., chronic liver injury, cirrhosis) (Edamoto, 2003; Zucman-Rossi, 2006; Aravalli, 2008). However, HCC resulting from different causes may predominantly affect certain pathways. HCV-associated HCC shows significant abnormality in both Wnt/β-catenin and MAPK pathways (Bai, 2003; Colnot, 2004). Dysfunction of Wnt/β-catenin, *p53*, *pRb*, and MAPK (Budhu, 2006) and cytokine signaling are more commonly seen HBV-related HCCs (Azechi, 2001; Bai, 2003; Colnot, 2004; Yoshida, 2006). Tumors associated with alcoholism have more frequent alterations in the Rb1 and p53 pathways than those caused by HCV infection (Marchio, 2000). The "aflatoxin-associated" codon 249 mutation of *p53* is identified only in samples from areas with high aflatoxin content (Asia and Africa) (Kirk, 2000; Huang, 2003).

Molecular approaches have been advocated to classify and predict clinical outcome and facilitate target molecular therapies using gene expression microarray and single-nucleotide polymorphism arrays (Boyault, 2007; Katoh, 2007; Chiang, 2008; Hoshida, 2008). Using global gene expression profiling, analyses of 91 human HCCs employing DNA microarrays containing 21,329 unique genes could subclassify HCC into two distinctive groups: (1) low survival subclass (class A, overall survival time 30.3 ± 8.02 months), which show strong cell proliferation and antiapoptosis gene expression signatures (such as *PCNA* and cell cycle regulators such as *CDK4*, *CCNB1*, *CCNA2*, and *CKS2*), as well as genes involving ubiquitination and sumoylation; and (2) high survival subclass (class B, overall survival time 83.7 ± 0.3 months) without the above expression signature (Lee, 2004a). Similarly, whole genomic array CGH analysis of 87 HCCs revealed two groups of tumors (clusters A and B) based on differences in chromosomal alteration profiles. Cluster A showed significant association with clinical features, such as HBV infection, higher serum α-fetoprotein levels, and a higher incidence of intrahepatic metastasis, along with shorter overall patient survival and poor clinical outcome (Katoh, 2007). Gene expression profiles could also subclassify patients with HCC into different survival groups on the basis of paraffin-embedded surrounding nontumoral liver tissue, not tumor tissue (Hoshida, 2008). A genome-wide transcriptomic analysis of 60 HCC tumors found a 16-gene signature to classify HCC tumors into six robust subgroups of HCC, labeled G1–G6. Each group has unique clinical and genetic characteristics that are based on chromosome stability status: chromosome unstable (groups G1–G3) and chromosome stable (G4–G5). Because each group of tumors has specific pathways of activation (i.e., protein kinase B [AKT or PKB] in G1–G2 and Wnt pathways in G5–G6), this molecular classification not only provides prognostic information, but also helps in the development of targeted therapies for HCC (Boyault, 2007).

Current treatment modalities usually are not effective because patients with HCC generally are diagnosed at an advanced stage. Treatment effects are also influenced by significant clinical and genetic heterogeneity among HCCs associated with different causes. Therefore, standard treatments may not work for all HCCs. Molecular target therapies specific for a group of HCCs with similar genetics recently have been introduced. The target therapy aims to inactivate the activated oncogene and recover the tumor's suppressor and/or repair genes and other genes or molecules related to the development of HCC, thereby correcting abnormal genes or their functions, as well as biological behavior. Many candidate genome-based drug targets have been discovered recently by microarray technology, promoter arrays for whole genome epigenetic aberration analysis, chromatin immunoprecipitation-on-chip analysis, and high-throughput sequencing systems. Examples of target genes or molecules include VGFR, EGFR, *DDEFL*, *VANGL1*, *WDRPUH*, *Ephrin-A1*, *glypican-3*, number gain 7q, PFTAIRE protein kinase 1 and paternally expressed 10, and miR-122a (Yagyu, 2002; Okabe, 2003; Okabe, 2004; Zender, 2008). Moreover, some reagents or drugs that work against these candidate target genes or molecules such as monoclonal antibodies, small molecules, and antisense have been on phase II and III clinical trials for therapeutic use; many have been shown to be effective. Sorafenib, an oral multikinase inhibitor of the vascular endothelial growth factor receptor, and Ras kinase have been approved by the FDA as molecularly targeted anticancer agents (Midorikawa, 2009; Thomas, 2009). Some of the other agents targeting similar genes are being tested in preclinical and clinical trials for HCC. These include EGFR inhibitors (anti-EGFR, gefitinib, and erlotinib), vascular endothelial growth factor (VEGF) vascularization inhibitors (antiangiogenesis, sorafenib, bevacizumab), and multikinase targets in patients who are unresectable or have metastatic HCCs (Huynh, 2009).

GASTRIC CANCER

Gastric cancer (GC) is the fourth most common cancer and is second only to lung cancer as the leading cause of cancer-related death worldwide (Ferlay, 2004). A majority of GCs are adenocarcinomas, histologically classified into two major groups by Laurén's classification: intestinal type with glandular pattern, and diffuse or poorly differentiated type with a signet ring cell morphology in some cases (Laurén, 1965). These two types of GCs have a distinct molecular basis of carcinogenesis, and clinical and genetic characteristics. The main causes of the intestinal type include dietary habits, environmental factors, and *Helicobacter pylori* infection (Kelley, 2003). Gastric cancer risk is also associated with hereditary tumor syndromes such as hereditary diffuse-type gastric cancer syndrome, hereditary nonpolyposis colorectal cancer (HNPCC), Li-Fraumeni syndrome, Peutz-Jeghers syndrome (i.e., familial adenomatous polyposis [FAP] and juvenile polyposis) (Traverso, 2002; Napieralski, 2005).

The development of intestinal-type GC is a multistep process that proceeds from gastritis (chronic or atrophic) and related changes (perinicious anemia, etc) to intestinal metaplasia, dysplasia, and eventually carcinoma (Oberhuber, 2000; Kelley, 2003). These processes are accompanied by a series of genetic alterations. The inactivation mutation of the TSG *p53* (see Chapter 74) occurs in an early stage of carcinogenesis (i.e., intestinal metaplasia [38%] and dysplasia [58%]), and is also seen in 38%–71% of GCs (Joypaul, 1993; Shiao, 1994; Xiangming, 2000). Mutation in *p73*, a member of the *p53* family, is indicated in the development of GC associated with *H. pylori* infection in mouse mode. High-level of microsatellite instability (MSI-H) is frequently seen in intestinal-type GC, largely caused by hypermethylation of the promoter regions of mismatch repair genes (most commonly, *MLH1* and *MSH2*) or gene mutations (in a small percentage of GCs) (Lee, 2004b; Gu, 2009; Seo, 2009). The CpG island methylator phenotype, originally found in colorectal cancer, has been detected in 24%–47% of GCs (Toyota, 1999; Oue, 2003; Lee, 2004b).

LOH or mutation of *APC* genes may occur in up to 60% of intestinal-type GC and in approximately 25% of the precursors—adenomas (Horii, 1992; Nakatsuru, 1992; Nakatsuru, 1993). LOH at the *bcl-2* locus and amplification of cyclin D1 and E are also associated with intestinal-type GC tumors (Ayhan, 1994; Muller, 1999). The oncogene product *Her2/neu* is frequently amplified in intestinal-type GC (Wang, 2002). In contrast to the diffuse cell type, *E-cadherin* gene *(CDH1)* mutations are infrequently present in intestinal-type GC (Machado, 2001; Mingchao, 2001).

The molecular pathogenesis of diffuse-type GC is less clear. *H. pylori* infection seems not to be related to the diffuse type of GC, according to epidemiologic studies. It can be part of a hereditary gastric cancer predisposition syndrome (Guilford, 1998). The unique molecular abnormality of diffuse-type GC distinct from intestinal-type GC is deficiency in cell–cell adhesion caused by loss or downregulation of the *E-cadherin* gene *(CDH1)* as a result of genetic or epigenetic alterations. The abnormality in *CDH1* can be found in the early stages of diffuse GC development. Decreased *CDH1* expression is detected in 50% of diffuse-type GCs, and more than 70% of those somatic *CDH1* mutations consist of complete or partial deletion of exons (Berx, 1998; Napieralski, 2005). The unique molecular genetics of GC might be useful for diagnosis in that *CDH1* mutations can be detected by polymerase chain reaction on paraffin-embedded tissue. Detection of the germline mutation in *CDH1* may help in identification of carriers of asymptomatic mutations involved in the GC family syndrome, and may offer an opportunity for prophylactic total gastrectomy in patients carrying the *CDH1* mutation (Fitzgerald, 2002). Other frequently altered genes or gene products in diffuse-type GC include the met proto-oncogene, encoding the hepatocyte growth factor receptor, and the SC-1 antigen, an apoptosis receptor (Kuniyasu, 1992; Vollmers, 1998a, 1998b).

Currently, the most valuable predictive and prognostic factor for GC is clinical staging independent of cancer type, but it does not reflect the heterogeneity of tumor biology. Molecular biomarkers have been investigated as alternatives or supplements to the current system and have shown very promising results in predicting prognosis and therapeutic response. For example, MSI-H is usually associated with intestinal-type GC, commonly seen in the distal stomach or antrum, and is associated with less frequent local lymph node metastasis. However, whether patients with MSI-H GC have more favorable long-term survival than those with MSH-L (novel tumor bands with one marker)/ microsatellite stable (MSS) (no novel tumor bands) GC remains controversial (Hayden, 1997; Wirtz, 1998). Expression in tumor tissue of caudal-type homeobox transcription factor 2 *(CDX2)*, in combination with normal *E-cadherin* and nonexpression of the transmembrane protein mucin 1 *(MUC1)*, is a favorable prognostic factor for patients with GC (Tanaka, 2003; Fondevila, 2004).

Abnormal gene profiling on *RBP4, OCT2, IGF2, PFN2, KIAA1093*, and *PCOLCW* and overexpression of three genes in the primary tumor (*BIK, Aurora kinase B*, and *eIF5A2*) are related to node metastasis (Hippo, 2002; Marchet, 2007). Matrix metalloproteinase-1 (MMP-1) –overexpressing GCs have a worse prognosis in terms of tumor invasion and metastasis than MMP-negative tumors (Noel, 2008). *VEGF* overexpression enhances tumor angiogenesis and thus is associated with lymph node metastasis, hepatic metastasis, and shorter survival time. As with breast cancer (see earlier), amplification/overexpression of the *Her2/neu* oncogene has been shown to be a potential independent unfavorable prognostic factor (Allgayer, 2000; Park, 2006). Overexpression of *EGFR* and *β-catenin* appears also to herald decreased survival and a less favorable prognosis (Jonjic, 1997; Zhou, 2002; Gamboa-Dominguez, 2004). In addition, mutation or abnormal expression of *p53* may predict a reduced cumulative survival and is associated with lymph node metastasis and lower chemosensitivity (Fondevila, 2004; Pinto-de-Sousa, 2004; Oh, 2008).

Treatment of GC, especially late-stage tumor, usually requires a multidisciplinary approach that includes chemotherapy in combination with surgical resection. Molecular markers for predicting therapeutic response have been studied, and several of them have been shown to be potentially useful clinically. These are discussed at length in Chapter 72.

COLORECTAL CANCER

Colorectal cancer (CRC) is the third most common malignancy worldwide (Ferlay, 2004). Prognostication of newly diagnosed CRC predominantly relies on stage or anatomic extent of disease based on the International Union Against Cancer and the American Joint Committee on Cancer staging classifications. However, CRC should be regarded as a heterogeneous, multipathway disease—an observation substantiated by the fact that histologically identical tumors may have neither similar prognosis nor similar response to therapy (Umar, 2004). Mutations and/or epigenetic alterations in TSGs (e.g., *APC, DCC, SMAD-2, SMAD-4, p53*) and oncogenes (e.g., *KRAS, p53*) are molecular determinants during the development of sporadic colorectal cancer, which was first summarized in the adenoma–carcinoma sequence described by Vogelstein and coworkers (Fearon, 1990). Based on genetic background, sporadic CRCs can be subclassified into two major types: (1) chromosomal and (2) unstable microsatellite, and an additional group with CpG island methylator phenotypes. Various genetic syndromes are known to predispose to colorectal carcinoma and to have specific inherited gene defects (see "Molecular Genetic Pathology of Syndromatic Cancers" section later for details). These molecular markers are currently being investigated as a means of improving the identification of patients likely to have poor clinical outcomes, and therefore more possibly benefiting from adjuvant treatment (Eschrich, 2005; Ghadimi, 2005; Liang, 2009).

EGFR, a receptor tyrosine kinase, overexpression is detected in up to 80% of colorectal cancers (Messa, 1998). Tumors with a high level of EGFR expression usually have a poor prognosis (Ghadimi, 2005; Liang, 2009). These data have led to the clinical use of EGFR blockade in the treatment of colorectal cancers with anti-EGFR monoclonal antibodies such as cetuximab or panitumumab (see also Chapter 74). Cetuximab is a mouse–human hybrid monoclonal antibody used as second-line treatment of colorectal cancer and approved by the FDA in 2004. Panitumumab is a fully human immunoglobulin G_2 monoclonal antibody approved by the FDA in 2007 as third-line monoclonal antibody therapy of refractory colorectal cancer. Both of these drugs are expensive and have significant side effects. Thus, it is imperative to use a biomarker to predicate the therapeutic response. However, use of EGFR as a biomarker to predict response to EGFR monoclonal antibodies has had limited success. Only detection of increased EGFR copy number by FISH has predictive value (Liang, 2009), and it has been proven that EGFR expression levels detected by IHC are not so useful. In contrast to *EGFR* mutation in lung cancer, *EGFR* mutation in CRC is a rare event that occurs in less than 1% of cases (Plesec, 2009). Current studies are focused on finding the downstream effectors of the EGFR pathway that may serve as biomarkers for predicting the effectiveness of anti-EGFR therapy.

As summarized in Chapter 74, Ras-p21 proteins are guanosine triphosphate (GTP)-coupled proteins that are important in many receptor tyrosine kinases that utilize signaling on the Ras/Raf/Erk/Map kinase signal transduction pathway. Mutations that result in single amino acid substitutions at critical positions in the amino acid sequence of this protein, such as Gly 12, Gly 13, and Gln 61, occur in the Ras protein and cause its constitutive activation. This leads to a series of oncogenic events that activate downstream signaling pathways, promoting tumor initiation and tumor growth and progression, including local invasion, angiogenesis, metastasis, and even immune response (Rowinsky, 1999; Smakman, 2005).

KRAS mutation occurs in at least 35%–45% of cases and, in some series, in up to 75% of cases of CRC. Mutations of this gene occur almost exclusively in three hot spots (codons 12, 13, and 61) and rarely in others, including codon 146 (Ogino, 2005; Smakman, 2005). Because KRAS is the downstream effector of EGFR and is frequently mutated in CRC, the mutation status of *KRAS* has become an important predictive marker for the effectiveness of cetuximab or panitumumab on metastatic CRCs. The American Society of Clinical Oncology (ASCO) has recommended that patients with diagnosed metastatic colon cancer who are candidates for anti-EGFR therapy should be tested for *KRAS* mutations in a Clinical Laboratory Improvement Amendments (CLIA)-accredited laboratory. If negative for *KRAS* mutations, these patients are deemed suitable for treatment with anti-EGFR antibody (cetuximab or panitumumab) therapy. This recommendation is based on the results of phase II and III clinical trials. Retrospective subset analyses of these trial data suggest that patients who have *KRAS* mutations detected in codon 12 or 13 do not benefit from this therapy. This was further confirmed by five randomized controlled trials of cetuximab or panitumumab response in relation to *KRAS* mutational status (no mutation [wild type] and mutated [abnormal]) and another five single-arm retrospective studies undertaken to evaluate tumor response according to *KRAS* mutation status.

According to the **College of American Pathologist (CAP) Perspectives on Emerging Technology (POET) report,** acceptable samples for *KRAS* mutation include fresh, frozen, and FFPE tissues. Acceptable assay types are RT-PCR and direct sequencing analysis; however, other methods such as pyrosequencing or microarray (chip)-based tests have also been developed (Pajkos, 2000; Ogino, 2005). As of the time of this writing, no type of *KRAS* testing has been approved by the FDA. Although recommended testing is limited to codons 12 and 13 of exon 2, which make up the vast majority of cases with *KRAS* mutations, many laboratories and commercial kits also include testing for other mutations, such as for codons 61 and 146.

BRAF is an immediate downstream effector of *RAS* in the Ras/Raf/Map kinase pathway (see Fig. 76-1). Mutation of *BRAF* has been identified in approximately 10% of CRCs (Di Nicolantonio, 2008). A vast majority of the point mutations are V600E, a mutational hot spot at nucleotide 1796 within exon 15, accounting for a T:A transversion mutation and a valine-to-glutamic acid substitution. All point mutations occur within the kinase domain of B-Raf protein, leading to constitutive activation of B-raf kinase (Davies, 2002). *BRAF* mutation is almost mutually exclusive with *KRAS* mutations. Unlike the *KRAS* mutation, mutations in *BRAF* frequently occur in female patients older than 75 years of age with proximal lesions. The tumors exhibit MSI with higher frequency (Barault, 2008) than those in other patients with colon cancer, which appear to be due to epigenetic effects involving hypermethylation of the promoter regions of mismatch repair genes. *BRAF* mutations in tumors have been characteristically associated with a worse survival than those without and resistance to treatment with anti-EGFR monoclonal antibodies, cetuximab, or panitumumab for metastatic CRCs. Currently, molecular testing for *BRAF* mutation V600E has been performed in many clinical laboratories as a therapeutic indicator for anti-EGFR treatment, in combination with *KRAS* mutation analysis (Siena, 2009).

PI3KCA is a membrane lipid kinase that phosphorylates the 3-hydroxyl group of phosphatidylinositol. This critical enzyme, which binds directly to ras-p21 protein, can be activated by EGFR-mediated signaling, in parallel with the K-ras/B-raf/MAP kinase pathway. Activation of PI3KCA counteracts PTEN, an antioncogene protein, and promotes AKT1 phosphorylation, stimulating cell proliferation, survival, and angiogenesis in cooperation with other pathways. The *PI3KCA* gene is mutated in about 20% of CRCs (Sartore-Bianchi, 2009). The mutation of *PI3KCA* usually occurs in the hot spots in exon 9 (E542K, E545K) and exon 20 (H1047R), both of which are oncogenic in CRC cellular models Unlike *BRAF* mutation, *PI3KCA* and *KRAS* mutations may coexist. In addition to their association with poor prognosis (i.e., local recurrence and increased mortality of CRCS), *PI3KCA* mutations can independently predict resistance to anti-EGFR therapy with panitumumab or cetuximab for metastatic CRCs (Ogino, 2009a; Sartore-Bianchi, 2009; Siena, 2009). Testing for combinations of the *PI3KCA/PTEN* and *KRAS* mutations can detect up to 70% of patients who are unlikely to respond to anti- EGFR therapy, although more validation is required for clinical practice (Siena, 2009).

The ***APC* gene,** a tumor necrosis factor-stimulated gene (TSG), encodes a 2843-amino acid protein and is located on chromosome 5q21-22, regulating Wnt/β–catenin signaling (Phelps, 2009). Mutations of this gene can be point mutations or small deletions or insertions. The latter cause frameshifts that generate stop codons. Germline mutations of this gene are responsible for FAP, whereas somatic mutations occur in the majority of sporadic CRCs. Somatic mutations of this gene may initiate and promote carcinogenesis of sporadic CRCs, and can be found in early neoplastic stages, even in dysplastic cryptic foci (Varesco, 2004; Phelps, 2009; Sweeney, 2009). CRCs with *APC* mutation usually are those with chromosomal instability or MSS (Luceri, 2002). The *APC* gene can serve as a biomarker for early detection, or as a risk factor for familial polyposis syndrome. Detection methods include various types of PCR, LOH, and others (Varesco, 2004). Screening for *APC* mutations may detect patients with relatively early CRC by purified DNA from routinely collected stool samples (Traverso, 2002).

p53 or TP53 is a tumor suppressor that regulates the cell cycle and is involved in apoptosis and DNA repair. This protein is discussed at length in Chapters 73 and 74. It is located on the short arm of chromosome 17 (17p13.1) (Isobe, 1986). Mutation or homozygous deletion of *TP53* is found in 40%–50% of CRCs. Loss of wild-type *p53* activity is thought to be a major predictor of failure to respond to radiotherapy and chemotherapy in various human cancers, including CRCs, and predicts lower survival (Weller, 1998; Zlobec, 2008). Although *TP53* mutation analysis has shown promising prognostic value, the American Society of Clinical Oncology Tumor Markers Expert Panel does not currently recommend its use in routine practice.

TGFBR1, SMAD2, and SMAD4 are proteins involved in the transforming growth factor-beta (TGF-β) signaling pathway (see also Chapter 74). SMAD proteins are the principal components mediating the TGF-β signaling pathway, which negatively regulates the growth of epithelial cells (Kouvidou, 2006). It has been found that germline allele-specific expression (ASE) of the gene encoding TGF-β type I receptor, TGFBR1, occurs in 10%–20% of CRCs in both familial (dominantly inherited and segregated) and sporadic forms (Valle, 2008). The presence of multiple-mutated TGF-β has been linked with poor prognosis in a subset of CRC patients. Approximately 50%–60% of CRCs have been found to harbor *SMAD4* mutations (Woodford-Richens, 2001), but, in contrast, only a few have been found to have *SMAD2* mutations. Both *SMAD2* and *SMAD4* are mapped to chromosome 18q21 (Woodford-Richens, 2001; Miyaki, 2003). Most mutations of *SMAD2* and *SMAD4* occur in their so-called MH2 domain. Inactivation of the *SMAD4* gene through germline mutation and loss of the unaffected wild-type allele are responsible for familial juvenile polyposis, whereas inactivation of the *SMAD4* gene through homozygous deletion or intragenic mutation occurs frequently in CRC and pancreatic cancer. *SMAD4* mutation occurs at a later stage of colorectal carcinogenesis and is an indicator of advanced phenotypes. Loss or low levels of *SMAD4* expression in CRCs are found to be associated with poor prognosis following surgery and 5-fluorouracil (5-FU)–based adjuvant therapy; however, the predictive value of *SMAD4* mutation/inactivation is controversial (Miyaki, 2003; Alhopuro, 2005). Chromosomal loss at 18q encompassing both *SMAD2* and *SMAD4* has been reported in up to 70% of CRCs (Alhopuro, 2005). Patients with locally advanced stage II or stage III disease appear to demonstrate a significantly poorer prognosis with loss of 18q (Popat, 2005).

MSI is involved in approximately 75%–85% of CRCs, characterized by aneuploidy, allelic losses, amplifications, translocations, and mutations of *APC, KRAS*, and *TP53* (Jones, 2008). Although the prognosis of patients with MSI CRC is stage and grade dependent, tumors with identical morphologic features display considerable heterogeneity in terms of clinical outcome. The remaining 15%–20% of CRCs have MSI-H characterized by inactivation of mismatch repair *(MMR)* genes (Umar, 2004), as discussed in Chapter 74. Sporadic *MSI-H* cases have been shown to arise predominantly through promoter hypermethylation and silencing of the *hMLH1* gene, in contrast to a hereditary form of *MSI-H* CRC, HNPCC, which typically shows germline mutations in one of the DNA *MMR* genes (Weisenberger, 2006). Tumors with *MSI-H* tend to be more proximally located, poorly differentiated, and of mucinous histologic type, and to show considerable lymphocytic infiltration; they have been linked with *TGFBRII* and *BRAF* mutations (Zlobec, 2008). Patients with colon cancers demonstrating MSI-H have a stage-independent improved survival compared with patients with MSS tumors in most, although not all studies, but they do not benefit from treatment with 5-FU in randomized adjuvant therapy trials (Ribic, 2003).

The **CpG island methylator phenotype (CIMP+),** or simultaneous hyperpmethylation of the promoter regions of a number of TSGs, is one of the principal mechanisms of colorectal carcinogenesis, independent of chromosomal instability or MSI. CIMP+ is found in approximately 20% of patients with CRCs. These patients usually are female and of more advanced age with a history of cigarette smoking. These cancers occur predominantly in the proximal colon and are associated with MSI, wild-type *TP53, BRAF* mutation, and β-catenin activation (Grady, 2007; Ogino, 2009b). The association between CIMP status and prognosis is controversial, however, and later studies suggest that the occurrence of CIMP appears to be an independent predictor of a low colon cancer–specific mortality and survival advantage and a high responsive rate to 5-FU–based treatment (Iacopetta, 2008; Ogino, 2009b). Additional studies including randomized clinical trials are required to confirm the value of CIMP+ and associated molecular features for the prediction of clinical outcomes of CRCs.

PANCREATIC CANCER (NON-NEUROENDOCRINE TUMOR)

Pancreatic cancer is one of the lead causes of cancer-related death worldwide (Parkin, 2001) and ranks as the fourth most common cause of cancer death in the United States (Jemal, 2008). Most pancreatic cancer is of exocrine origin, and most cases involve invasive ductal adenocarcinoma (PDAC) and its variants (Hruban, 2007; Ranganathan, 2009). Other nonendocrine, nonductal carcinomas such as acinic cell carcinoma, solid-pseudopapillary neoplasm, and pancreatoblastoma are uncommon (Hruban, 2009). It should be noted, however, that the actual cell of origin of certain pancreatic carcinomas is not known, and much debate continues regarding this issue.

Pancreatic ductal adenocarcinoma is the result of accumulation of inherited (germline) or acquired (somatic or epigenetic) mutations of genes, or both, including oncogenes such as, most prominently, mutated (Val-for-Gly 12) *K-RAS*-p21; TSGs such as *p53, p16*, and *SMAD4;* and genome maintenance genes such as *BRCA2*, telomerase, and MSI (Su, 2000; Ranganathan, 2009). Oncogenic ras-p21 protein has been identified in more than 90% of human pancreatic cancers and therefore is considered a major causative factor in this disease (see Chapter 74).

The genetic alterations that have been observed in pancreatic cancer may be reflected by chromosome gain, loss, or copy number changes. PDACs frequently have loss of chromosomes 18, 17, 6, 21, 22, Y, 10, 4, 15p, 14p 5, 13p, 9p, 21p, and 17p (Johansson, 1992; Ranganathan, 2009). Among them, allelic loss of chromosome 18 is the most common event, and about a third of pancreatic carcinomas have a consensus region of homozygous deletion at 18q21 (Hahn, 1996a). More specific genetic alterations or mutations have been identified by many studies using different molecular approaches. One study by Jones et al (2008) identified more than 1500 somatic mutations affecting 1007 genes in pancreatic cancers. Among these are the most frequent and well-known gene mutations, including activation of *KRAS* (95%), inactivation of *p16/CDKN2A* (75%–80% mutation and 15% hypermethylation), *TP53* (80%), and inactivation of *SMAD4* (95%) (Hruban, 1993; Caldas, 1994; Redston, 1994; Hahn, 1996b; Jones, 2008). Activating point mutation of *KRAS* occurs commonly in codon 12 and much less frequently in codons 13 and 61. Germline mutations in *BRCA2*, a predisposing factor to pancreatic cancer, are frequently detected in the Ashkenazi Jewish population (Ranganathan, 2009). Inactivation of genes by hypermethylation is also important in the development of pancreatic cancer. Aberrant methylation has been identified in the promoter regions of *p16/CDKN2A, APC, TSLC/IGSF4, SOCS-1, cyclin D2, RASSF1A, WWOX, RUNX3, CDH13, DUSP6, HHIP,* and *SLC5A8*, and in pancreatic cancer and precancerous lesions (Sato, 2002; Ranganathan, 2009). Those gene mutations or genetic alterations may affect one or more signaling pathways and MSI. As stated earlier, the most commonly affected signaling pathways include the EGFR/RAS/MAPK pathway and, in addition, the PI3K/AKT pathway, VEGF, the WNT/β-catenin pathway, and TGF-β signaling (Buchholz, 2009; Hruban, 2009). MicoRNAs are also associated with pancreatic carcinogenesis. miR-216, miR-196a, miR-217, and miR-210 were identified specifically for or were frequently associated with PDAC (Bloomston, 2007; Szafranska, 2007; Hoimes, 2009).

Pre-cancerous lesions including pancreatic intraductal neoplasia (PanIN) and intraductal papillary-mucinous neoplasms (IPMNs) may also have mutations of *KRAS, TP53, SMAD4,* and *p16/CDKN2A* genes, as seen in PDACs (Hruban, 2009; Ranganathan, 2009). However, intestinal-type IPMNs, a precursor to invasive colloid carcinomas, always have intact *SMAD4/DPC4* and harbor *PI3KCA* mutations in 10% of cases; this usually does not occur in PDACs (Hruban, 2009; Ranganathan, 2009).

Pancreatic cancer other than PDACs shows different molecular genetics. The major genetic alteration of medullary carcinoma is characterized by MSI (Hruban, 2009). Colloid carcinoma frequently shows CDX2/MUC2 expression (Hruban, 2009). Undifferentiated carcinoma may have loss of e-cadherin. Acinar carcinomas are, on the basis of some studies, thought not to have activation of *KRAS* and inactivation of *TP53, p16/CDKN2A,* or *SMAD4*, as seen in PDACs, but may have loss of chromosome 11p and *APC/β-catenin* gene mutations in some cases (Hoorens, 1993; Abraham, 2002; Hruban, 2009). On the other hand, nontransformed pancreatic acinar cells in culture are readily and stably transformed into malignant pancreatic cancer cells by transfection of oncogenic K-ras or by exposure to carcinogens present in cigarette smoke, a known major risk factor for developing this disease. A common finding in these transformed acinar cells is oncogenic ras-p21.

Solid-pseudopapillary neoplasms commonly have abnormal expression of β-catenin (Hruban, 2009). The most common genetic abnormality in pancreatoblastomas is loss of one copy of the short arm of chromosome 11 near the *WT-2* locus (11p15.5) (Abraham, 2001; Kerr, 2002). Those genetic differences may dictate their different morphology and clinical/biological behaviors in different types of pancreatic exocrine carcinomas.

A vast majority of pancreatic cancers are sporadic; however, familial forms have also been reported. Familial pancreatic cancers most often are associated with many genetic cancer syndromes, including hereditary breast and ovarian cancer syndrome, Peutz-Jeghers syndrome, HNPCC syndrome, FAP, familial pancreatic cancer, and hereditary pancreatitis (associated with mutations of *PRSS1* and *SPINK1*) (see respective sections, later).

The molecular changes noted in pancreatic cancer, as described previously, may serve as diagnostic markers. Detection of mutations of *KRAS*, telomerase (*hTERT*), and others has been used or proposed for the diagnosis of pancreatic carcinoma, which can be potentially applied in surgically resected pancreatic specimens and pancreatic fluid samples (Seki, 2001; Mishra, 2006), although the usefulness of these techniques requires further evaluation (Fry, 2008). The levels of *hTERT* expression could differentiate PDACs from adenoma and pancreatitis (Nakashima, 2009). Although deletion/inactivation of *SMAD4* is also a relatively highly frequent event in pancreatic cancer, it is not specific. Thus, its utility in molecular diagnosis requires further evaluation (Hruban, 2009; Ranganathan, 2009). Aberrant methylation of certain genes may also have diagnostic utility (Matsubayashi, 2006; Ranganathan, 2009). Yan and colleagues showed that a panel of molecular markers (methylated *p16, p53* mutations, and *KRAS* mutations) could stratify patients in high-risk groups from negligible risk to greater than 50% probability of an early cancer (Yan, 2005). In addition, the expression pattern of a group of 112 miRNAs could correctly distinguish pancreatic cancer tissue from adjacent normal and benign tissues, including pancreatitis. Three of the top differentially expressed miRNAs (miR-221, -376a, and -301) were specifically localized to pancreatic carcinoma, but not to the stroma or to normal acini or ducts (Lee, 2007; Liang, 2009). Other potentially useful diagnostic markers for pancreatic cancers include miR-217 and miR-196a (Szafranska, 2007).

Amplification of *KRAS2* and *CMYC* and loss of *TP53* genes are found to be correlated with tumor grade and survival (Ranganathan, 2009). Alterations of *p16* and *hTERT* may also be a prognostic indicator of pancreatic cancer, which conferred a worse outcome by univariate and multivariate analysis (Kumari, 2009). Giovannetti found that patients with high levels of human equilibrative nucleoside transporter-1 (hENT1) mRNA had significantly longer overall survival than patients with a low level of hENT1 expression, suggesting that hENT1 levels may be a predictor of survival (Giovannetti, 2006; Liang, 2009). Iacobuzio-Donahue found that *SMAD4/DPC4* loss is usually associated with death related to multiple metastases, whereas patients found to have intact *SMAD4* genes are more likely to have localized disease, although many of these cancers are also fatal (Hruban, 2009; Iacobuzio-Donahue, 2009). The presence of microRNAs, miR-21, and miR-196a-2 has been found to be a significant predictor of poor survival (Bloomston, 2007; Dillhoff, 2008). *BRCA2* gene mutation, seen in 7% of PDACs and in more cases of familial disease, is a predicting marker for responsiveness to poly-(adenosine diphosphate [ADP]-ribose) polymerase-1 (PARP) inhibitors and to DNA cross-linking agents such as mitomycin C (Helleday, 2005; van der Heijden, 2005; McCabe, 2006).

KIDNEY TUMOR

Renal Cell Carcinoma: Clear Cell Carcinoma

Clear cell renal cell carcinoma (RCC), the most common subtype (50%–70%) of renal cancer, is characterized by an encapsulated solid mass with alveolar or acinar arrangement of clear polygonal cells. Chromosome 3p deletion is seen in 70%–90% of cases (Crossey, 1994; Lonser, 2003), and TSG von Hippel–Lindau (VHL) located on 3p25 is consistently inactivated in 100% of familial renal cancer syndromes and 57% of sporadic cases (Gnarra, 1994). VHL protein regulates expression of the transcription factor, hypoxia-inducible factor (HIF), implicated in tumor growth and angiogenesis. VHL syndrome–associated clear cell carcinoma is caused by a germline mutation at birth in one copy of the *VHL* gene, and a second hit can result from deletion, nonsense mutations, allelic loss, or hypermethylation of the VHL promoter region. Loss of both VHL genes leads to tumorigenesis.

Translocation-Associated RCC

Renal cell carcinoma with Xp11 translocation is a recently recognized entity with unique morphology and genetic characteristics. The most common translocations associated with these tumors are t(X;17)(p11.2;q25), the same cytogenetic abnormality (with identical breakpoints) observed in alveolar soft part sarcomas, which gives rise to the *ASPL-TFE3* fusion gene, and t(X;1)(p11.2;q21), which results in the *PRCC-TFE3* fusion gene.

In this entity, translocation fuses the *TFE3* transcription factor gene at Xp11.2 to *ASPL*, a novel gene at 17q25, or 1q21, which results in the fusion protein ASPL-TFE3 or PRCC-TFE3, respectively (Tomlinson, 1991; Meloni, 1992, 1993; Hernandez-Marti, 1995; Sidhar, 1996; Carcao, 1998; Heimann, 1998; Argani, 2001; Heimann, 2001; Ladanyi, 2001; Argani, 2002, 2003a). Both the *ASPL-TFE3* and *PRCC-TFE3* fusion genes encode chimeric gene products that retain the ability of the TFE3 protein to migrate to the nucleus and participate in transcriptional activation of target genes (Weterman, 2000; Skalsky, 2001). Originally described to affect the pediatric age group and now recognized in both pediatric and adult populations, the age at diagnosis for Xp11 renal tumor ranges from 17 months to 78 years (Argani, 2001, 2006, 2007). It is interesting to note

PART 9

that pediatric tumors show no particular sex preference, whereas adult tumors demonstrate a strong female predilection (Argani, 2002, 2007).

Grossly, the tumors resemble clear cell RCCs (Argani, 2001). The histopathologic appearance is that of papillary carcinoma (Argani, 2003b). ASPL-TFE3 renal carcinomas are characterized by cells with voluminous, clear to eosinophilic cytoplasm, discrete cell borders, vesicular nuclear chromatin, and prominent nucleoli (Argani, 2001). Psammoma bodies are constant and sometimes extensive, often arising within characteristic hyaline nodules. In contrast, PRCC-TFE3 renal carcinomas generally feature less abundant cytoplasm, fewer psammoma bodies, fewer hyaline nodules, and a more nested, compact architecture (Argani, 2002). Renal carcinomas with Xp11.2-associated translocations characteristically underexpress cytokeratin, epithelial membrane, and vimentin antigen by immunohistochemistry. The tumors, however, consistently label for the RCC marker antigen and CD10, similar to conventional renal carcinomas. The most distinctive immunohistochemical feature of these tumors is the nuclear pattern for TFE3 protein using an antibody to the C-terminal portion of TFE3, which is retained in the gene fusions (Argani, 2003a)—a common feature in all Xp11.2-associated carcinomas and ASPS, and not in other adult-type renal carcinomas (Argani, 2003a)

Gene Expression Profiling by Affymetrix in RCC

Genome-wide gene expression studies have demonstrated distinct molecular signatures for distinct variants of RCC, including clear cell RCC, papillary RCC, chromophobe RCC, oncocytoma, and angiomyolipoma using Affymetrix oligonucleotide microarrays (Affymetrix Inc., Santa Clara, Calif) (Schuetz, 2005). Clear cell RCC showed increased expression in genes of the immune response and in angiogenesis genes, related to rich tumor vascularity, whereas chromophobe RCCs and oncocytomas overexpress energy pathway genes, correlated with abundant mitochondria in chromophobe RCC and oncocytoma (Moch, 1996). Another study demonstrated that clear cell RCC overexpressed the proximal nephron markers megalin and cubilin; papillary RCC strongly overexpressed the proximal nephron marker α-methylacyl coenzyme A (CoA) racemase; and chromophobe RCC and oncocytoma overexpressed the distal nephron markers β-defensin-1, parvalbumin, chloride channel Kb, claudin-7, claudin-8, and epidermal growth factor (Young, 2008). These results of Affymetrix profiling lead to molecular classification of renal tumors (Tickoo, 2000; Higgins, 2003). They also have proved useful in prognosis and therapeutic selection by discovery of novel immunohistochemical markers (Yao, 2005; Rohan, 2006; Cifola, 2008).

Several RCC biomarkers have been verified as potential prognostic markers using immunohistochemistry. For example, adipophilin, which was discovered as a clear cell RCC biomarker using gene expression microarrays, was subsequently associated with favorable outcome by immunohistochemistry (Yao, 2005). Many genes overexpressed in RCC are therapeutically significant. Angiogenesis genes are overexpressed in clear cell RCC, likely related to VHL and HIF1A dysregulation, both of which result in activation of multiple angiogenic tyrosine kinase molecules (e.g., vascular endothelial growth factor [VEGF], platelet-derived growth factor [PDGF]). Tyrosine kinase inhibitors (e.g., sunitinib, sorafenib) proved to have a significant role in metastatic RCC. Angiogenic and immune response regulators both increase expression of carbonic anhydrase IX, which is the target of G250 monoclonal antibody therapy for RCC. Affymetrix profiling may be used in the near future in personalized medicine for tumor classification and prognosis.

BLADDER CANCER

Bladder cancer is the second most common malignancy affecting the urinary system. Urothelial carcinoma (i.e., transitional cell carcinoma) is the most common form of bladder cancer, accounting for about 90% of cases. Remaining forms include squamous cell carcinoma (about 5%), most commonly provoked by *Schistosoma hematobium*, adenocarcinoma, and small cell carcinoma. Serum and urine markers used for early detection of bladder cancer, including genetic tests for *p16* tumor suppressor gene deletion (UroVysion), NMP22, and others, are discussed in Chapter 74.

For diagnosis of bladder cancer, invasive urethrocystoscopy and urinary cytology with low sensitivity for low-grade cancer have generated interest in other noninvasive and more sensitive diagnostic tools. The diagnosis of urothelial carcinoma (UC) is further compounded by the need for accurate pathologic staging, with one of the most critical challenges arising in identification of muscularis propria (detrusor muscle) invasion, which ultimately drives patient management. About 25% of patients with bladder cancer have advanced disease (muscle-invasive or metastatic disease) at presentation and are candidates for systemic chemotherapy. On the basis of the pivotal importance of diagnosing and staging bladder cancer, numerous recent studies have examined novel markers to aid diagnosis, prognosis, and treatment. Molecular and genetic changes in UC of the bladder can be broadly classified into three interrelated processes: (1) chromosomal alteration, triggering the initial carcinogenic event; (2) cancer cell proliferation, caused by loss of cell cycle regulation and derangements in normal apoptotic turnover; and (3) metastasis, in which the initial tumor spreads and brings into play processes such as angiogenesis and loss of cell adhesions (Quek, 2003).

Recent work has focused on molecular changes that occur in noninvasive low-grade papillary UCs, which only rarely progress to muscle-invasive disease (Holmang, 1999; Holmang, 2001). Activating mutations in the *HRAS* oncogene, discussed previously in Chapter 74, are one of the best characterized alterations in this population and have been associated with progression from urothelial hyperplasia to low-grade noninvasive papillary carcinoma (Spruck, 1994; Fitzgerald, 1995). Activating mutations in fibroblast growth factor receptor-3 (FGFR3), a tyrosine kinase receptor, have been documented in 70%–80% of noninvasive low-grade papillary UCs, in contrast to only approximately 20% of invasive carcinomas (Billerey, 2001; van Rhijn, 2001). High-grade papillary UC and flat carcinoma in situ (CIS) share common molecular alterations with invasive UC, the most commonly studied of which include *TP53* and *RB* gene mutations. Invasive UCs commonly demonstrate immunoreactivity for cytokeratins 7 and 20, p63, and high molecular weight cytokeratins such as CK903. Benign urothelial tissue, however, demonstrates at least focal reactivity for these immunomarkers, including CK7 expression within the urothelial mucosa, CK20 expression in the umbrella cell layer, and p63 nuclear expression in the basal and parabasal cell layers.

Genetic studies of flat (and papillary) urothelial hyperplasia in patients with papillary low-grade UC showed frequent genetic alterations in chromosome 9, whereas chromosomal changes more specifically associated with aggressive bladder cancer (loss of 17p, 2q, 4, 11p) were uncommon (Obermann, 2003). With the FISH technique, chromosomal anomalies can be detected in exfoliated bladder cells from the patient's voided urine. A currently commercially available test, the UroVysion Bladder Cancer Kit (UroVysion) (Fig. 76-1, *F* through *H*) is intended to detect aneuploidy for chromosomes 3, 7, and 17, and loss of the 9p21 locus, encoding the p16 tumor suppressor protein, using FISH. The indication for UroVysion includes hematuria and monitoring for tumor recurrence in patients previously diagnosed with urothelial carcinoma. A minimum of 25 morphologically abnormal cells should be analyzed. The abnormal profile for chromosomes 3, 7, and 17 and the 9p21 locus includes aneuploidy of chromosomes 3 (red color), 7 (green color), and 17 (aqua color) and/or deletion of the 9p21 (yellow/gold) locus. Criteria for abnormal results include 4 aneuploid cells, 12 cells with deletion of the 9p21 locus, or 10 cells with a tetraploid or near-tetraploid profile.

Genetic changes can precede appearance of the lesions. Positive results include UC of renal pelvis, ureter, urethra, and urinary bladder (Halling, 2008). Negative UroVysion results could occur with a positive diagnosis of UC by cytopathology or biopsy because certain UCs do not have the cytogenetic change of UroVysion. However, many of these cancers can be detected using the marker NMP22 in voided urine specimens, as described in Chapter 74.

PROSTATE CANCER

Prostate cancer is the most common noncutaneous cancer among males. Almost all cancers of the prostate are adenocarcinomas that occur in more than one site (multifocal) in more than 85% of cases. Adenocarcinomas of the prostate are graded according to the Gleason grading system to predict their prognosis and overall aggressiveness. The most common biomarker in serum that is used in diagnosing prostate cancer is prostate-specific antigen (PSA), as was discussed in detail in Chapter 73. This chapter focuses on new genetic markers in tissue that are diagnostic for this condition.

It has been shown that approximately 70% (Hermans, 2006; Perner, 2006; Soller, 2006; Nam, 2007; Rajput, 2007) of prostate cancers harbor a recurrent chromosomal rearrangement, resulting in the fusion of androgen-regulated *TMPRSS2 (21q22.3)* to erythroblastosis virus E26 transforming sequence (ETS) family of transcription factors. The latter is a group of genes that encode transcription factors. *TMPRSS2* is regulated by androgen (Afar, 2001) and estrogen (Setlur, 2008). Fusion leads to overexpression of the ETS family of genes (Petrovics, 2005), including *ERG (21q22.2)*, *ETV1 (7q21.2)*, or *ETV4 (17q21)* (Tomlins, 2005; Cerveira,

2006; Perner, 2006; Wang, 2006; Yoshimoto, 2006; Clark, 2007). In about two thirds of cases resulting in the fusion protein, fusion is the result of genomic deletion (Liu, 2006; Perner, 2006) of the intervening DNA sequence, but fusion may also occur by a more complex rearrangement, such as a translocation (Tomlins, 2005; Hermans, 2006). The most common variant is fusion between the 5′-untranslated region of *TMPRSS2* and the 3′ region of *ERG* (Perner, 2006; Mehra, 2007a; Tu, 2007). However, more than 20 other fusion variants have now been described (involving more than 10 different genes [e.g., *ETV1, ETV4, ETV5*]).

Much diversity is also observed in the transcripts derived from these fusion genes. Multiple *TMPRSS2-ERG* splice variant transcripts have been found both within individual cancers and in comparisons of different cancer samples. Although likely to be an early event in prostate cancer, expression of *ETS* gene fusions can be maintained in advanced disease. High-level *ERG* and *ETV1* gene expression has been reported in metastatic prostate cancer. Moreover, the heterogeneity of *TMPRSS2:ERG* gene fusion at different foci of cancer that arise within a multifocal prostate cancer suggested that they have different origins and represent different malignant clones, which made clinical interpretation of this biomarker more complex (Barry, 2007; Mehra, 2007b; Zhu, 2007).

Five histologic features are associated with the presence of gene fusion: the presence of blue-tinged mucin, a cribriform growth pattern, macronucleoli, intraductal tumor spread, and signet ring cell features. These features are also associated with an aggressive clinical course of prostate cancer, but neither Gleason grade nor stage was found to correlate with presence of the fusion gene (Perner, 2006; Nam, 2007; Rajput, 2007; Tu, 2007). Results to date have been inconsistent, but most studies suggest that presence of the fusion protein is not correlated with other markers of risk.

Fusion products can be identified by several techniques, including FISH, RT-PCR, and expression profiling using exon arrays. *TMPRSS2:ERG* gene fusion is specific for prostate cancer, and the ability to identify this DNA rearrangement could be used as a screening test for prostate cancer in serum, prostatic fluid, or urine. The clinical significance of the presence of the *TMPRSS2:ERG* gene fusion product for prostate cancer presentation and progression is not fully understood, but studies to date suggest that this may be a biomarker of risk.

CERVICAL CANCER

Cervical carcinoma is the second most prevalent cancer in women worldwide (Parkin, 2001). The primary cause of cervical cancer is human papillomavirus (HPV) infection. HPV infection initiates and promotes the development of cervical neoplasia from the precancerous lesion, cervical intraepithelial neoplasia (CIN) I or low-grade squamous intraepithelial lesion (LSIL), to in situ cancer III or high-grade squamous intraepithelial lesion (HSIL) and invasive cancer (Kisseljov, 2008; Herrington, 2009). Other cellular or environmental factors, such as genetic and immune disorders, hormonal contraception, high parity, tobacco smoking, coinfection with other microorganisms, such as HIV, and dietary deficiencies, are also implicated in the cervical carcinogenesis. These factors are important for the progression from cervical HPV infection to cervical intraepithelial lesions and cancer (Munoz, 2006).

HPVs are double-stranded circular DNA viruses that contain seven early *(E1-E7)* and two late *(L1-L2)* genes necessary for viral replication. Among them, two genes (*E6* and *E7*) play a pivotal role in the initiation of cervical carcinogenesis and maintain the transformed phenotype (Mantovani, 2001; Munger, 2001). The E7 protein binds to the retinoblastoma TSG product pRB, preferably the underphosphorylated or "active" form of *pRB*. HPV E6 proteins can also associate with the p53 tumor suppressor protein. Inactivation of pRB and p53 by the HPV oncoproteins E7 and E6 likely represents major steps in cervical carcinogenesis. HPV may also be integrated with the human genome, which is important in the progression of HPV-associated neoplasia. This integration may cause upregulation of HPV E6 and E7 expression and other genetic abnormalities, including telomerase activation and chromosomal alterations leading to the development of high-grade intraepithelial and invasive squamous carcinoma. In addition, HPV infection can induce many epigenetic changes, including methylation of the promoter of TSGs involved in cell proliferation and differentiation (Kisseljov, 2008; Gupta, 2009; Herrington, 2009).

Although more than 100 HPV types have been identified, studies show that HPV-16 and, to a lesser extent, HPV-18 play a dominant role in cervical carcinogenesis and are jointly responsible for 70% of the world's cervical cancer cases. Based on their capability for tumorigenicity, HPVs are classified into high- and low-risk groups (Table 76-3), with high-risk HPV types causing high-grade cervical intraepithelial lesions (CIN2/3 or HSIL), and with low-risk HPV types leading to low-grade cervical intraepithelial lesions (CIN1 or LSIL) (Kisseljov, 2008; Herrington, 2009).

TABLE 76-3
Oncogenicity of HPV

Oncogenicity	HPV types
High-risk HPV types	16, 18, 31, 33, 35, 39, 45, 52, 56, 58, 59, 67, 68
Low-risk HPV types	6, 11, 40, 42, 43, 44, 54, 61, 70, 72, 74, 81, 83, 84
Probable high-risk types	26, 51, 53, 56, 66, 69, 82

HPV, Human papillomavirus.

Because a strong causative association has been observed between HPV infection and cervical cancer, identification of HPVs in tissue or cytologic specimens has become a routine practice, not only for screening purposes, but also for the diagnosis of cervical cancer and for follow-up of abnormal changes detected by a cervical Pap smear. The combination of HPV testing and Pap smear evaluation has significantly improved the sensitivity and specificity of the diagnosis of precancerous lesions and cancer (Cuzick, 2008). Among various platforms for HPV infection detection, Hybrid Capture (Digene, Gaithersberg, Md.) is an in vitro, solution hybridization, signal-amplified test used to detect HPV DNA targets. First introduced by Digene in1995, it was designed to detect 14 HPV types, including the high-risk types HPV 16, 18, 31, 33, 35, 45, 51, 52, and 56; and the low-risk types HPV 6, 11, 42, 43, and 44. The Hybrid Capture test is performed on the residual liquid portion of the patient's Pap smear specimen, such as the thin preparation containing HPV DNA. This reacted viral DNA is combined with viral-specific RNA probes, creating hybrids. These RNA:DNA hybrids are then combined onto a solid phase coat, with subsequent capture by universal antibodies that are specific for that particular RNA:DNA nucleic acid hybrid. In turn, the RNA:DNA antibody is detected by a signaling antibody conjugated to alkaline phosphatase, resulting in chemiluminescence, which, when amplified, can be measured in relative light units (RLUs). The second generation of the hybrid capture assay, Hybrid Capture 2, replaces the tubes with microtiter plates to improve performance and suitability for automation. It is the first FDA-approved form of HPV testing for high-risk groups for HPV.

Two HPV tests have been approved by the FDA, both of which utilize an isothermal enzymatic DNA amplification process with a fluorescent readout used with ThinPrep samples (Hologic Inc., Marlborough, Mass). One of these tests, Cervista HPV HR (Hologic Inc.), is designed to identify 14 high-risk types of HPV. These include the 13 types detected by the Hybrid Capture 2 HPV DNA assay (16, 18, 31, 33, 35, 39, 45, 51, 52, and 56, as well as 58, 59, and 68) and HPV 66. The other test, Cervista HPV 16/18, is designed to specifically detect HPV 16 and HPV 18. Other technologies are also used by some laboratories, including PCR, DNA microarray, dot blot, Southern blot, and genotyping such as TaqMan PCR genotyping assay, GenProbe (GenProbe Inc., San Diego), and APTIMA1 HPV assay (Aptima Inc., Woburn, Mass.).

OVARIAN CANCER

Ovarian cancer is one of the most common gynecologic malignancies and is the fifth leading cause of cancer mortality in women in the United States (Jemal, 2009). Ovarian epithelial cancers are classified on the basis of morphology, depending upon invasiveness (tumor grade) and type of differentiation (e.g., serous, mucinous, endometrioid, clear cell, and transitional type).

Studies on the molecular pathology of ovarian cancer show that each of the four major histopathologic types of ovarian carcinoma is characterized by rather distinctive, although not necessarily unique, genetic abnormalities. For example, *TP53* gene mutations are extremely common in high grade serous carcinomas, low grade serous, and mucinous adenocarcinomas have a high prevalence of *KRAS* and B-RAF mutations (75% in primary mucinous adenocarcinomas) (Cho, 2009). Mutations of *CTNNB1*, the gene encoding β-catenin and PTEN, are common in endometrioid adenocarcinoma but are rare in serous, mucinous, and clear cell carcinomas. Mutations of *PIK3CA*, which encodes the catalytic subunit of PI3K (phosphoinositide 3-kinase), are observed most frequently in clear cell carcinomas. In addition, genetic differences exist within a given type of ovarian cancer.

Molecular subgroups of endometrioid adenocarcinomas correlate with tumor grade, stage of disease, and clinical outcome. Serous carcinomas can be subdivided into low-grade serous carcinoma (LGSC) and high-grade serous carcinoma (HGSC).

Histologic Subtypes of Serous Carcinoma

LGSC, also called International Federation of Gynecology and Obstetrics (FIGO) stage I, is defined as malignancy of one (Ia) or both (Ib) ovaries. These carcinomas characteristically have mutations of KRAS or BRAF, but lack TP53 mutations (Gilks, 2009). Mutations of KRAS or BRAF lead to constitutive activation of the MAPK (mitogen-activated protein kinase) signaling pathway. Low-grade tumors have also been found to contain mutations that deregulate the canonical Wnt/β-catenin and PI3K/PTEN signaling pathways and typically lack TP53 mutations (Cho, 2009).

On the other hand, HGSCs are characterized by high-grade nuclei, have short latent precursor lesions, and have rapid tumor progression into invasive carcinoma. HGSCs are often identified in advanced stage and have a high prevalence (50-70%) of *TP53* gene mutations (Wen, 1999), but unlike in LGSC, mutations of *KRAS* and *BRAF* are rare. Most HGSC cancers further lack Wnt/β-catenin or PI3K/PTEN signaling pathway defects (Kolasa, 2006), which are common in the LGSC cancers. Moreover, it is important to note that most HGSCs have genetic and somatic alterations of *BRCA1* and *BRCA2* (germline or somatic mutation or promoter methylation and loss of expression) (Kobel, 2008). These changes occur early during oncogenesis and result in loss of ability to repair DNA double-strand breaks, which, in turn, leads to chromosomal instability.

Molecular Classification of Ovarian Cancer

Molecular studies led to the proposal of a new model for classifying ovarian carcinomas, in which surface epithelial tumors can be divided into two broad categories designated Type I and Type II, based on their pattern of tumor progression and molecular genetic changes (Landen, 2008; Levanon, 2008). Type I tumors include low-grade serous carcinoma, low-grade endometrioid carcinoma, mucinous carcinoma, and a subset of clear cell carcinomas that develop in a stepwise fashion from well-recognized precursors, in most cases, borderline tumors, which generally are large and often are confined to the ovary at diagnosis. In contrast, Type II tumors are of high grade and almost always have spread beyond the ovaries at presentation; these include high-grade serous carcinoma, undifferentiated carcinoma, some clear cell carcinomas, and malignant mixed mullerian tumor. Type I and Type II tumors also differ in their molecular profiles. Type I tumors often harbor somatic mutations of genes encoding protein kinases, including *KRAS*, *BRAF*, *PIK3CA*, and *ERB-2 (Her2/neu)*, and other signaling molecules, including CTNNB1 and PTEN. In contrast, Type II tumors generally lack these mutations but are characterized by a high frequency of *TP53* mutations, which are rare in Type I tumors. Chromosomal instability levels, as reflected by genome-wide changes in DNA copy number, are much higher in Type II tumors than in Type I tumors (Mayr, 2006).

Clear Cell Ovarian Carcinoma

Mutations in *KRAS*, *BRAF*, and *TP53* are present in some clear cell carcinomas, but their frequency is generally low. Mutations predicted to deregulate PI3K/PTEN signaling are more common in clear cell carcinomas, with *PIK3CA* mutations reported in 20%–25%, and *PTEN* mutations in 8% of tumors (Cho, 2009).

BRCA1 and *BRCA2* in Ovarian Cancer

These genes encode proteins that are required for DNA double-strand break repair by homologous recombination. Cells lacking *BRCA1*- or *BRCA2*-dependent DNA repair tend to develop chromosomal rearrangements and genomic instability. Inheritance of DNA repair defects involving *BRCA1* and *BRCA2* contributes to as many as 10%–15% of ovarian cancers (Lancaster, 1996). The lifetime risk of developing ovarian cancer in mutation carriers varies with the genetic defect (for *BRCA1*, 30%–60%, and for *BRCA2*, 15%–30%). *BRCA*-related familial ovarian cancers are more frequently multifocal and progress faster. Carcinomas arising in patients with germline *BRCA1* or *BRCA2* mutations are almost invariably of the high-grade serous type discussed previously. Fortunately, however, ovarian cancers that contain mutations affecting *BRCA1* and *BRCA2* are more sensitive to DNA damage induced by chemotherapeutic agents such as platinum drugs and PARP inhibitors because they are less able to repair the DNA damage caused by these agents. Thus, these drugs are particularly effective in the presence of defects in homologous recombination repair, and clinical trials with these agents are under way in ovarian cancer patients with inherited *BRCA1* and *BRCA2* mutations (Yap, 2009).

Although *BRCA1* and *BRCA2* genes have been thought to be mutated only rarely in sporadic ovarian cancers, somatic mutations have recently been documented in approximately 10% of nonfamilial cases, particularly in high-grade serous epithelial ovarian cancers, and expression of *BRCA1* and *BRCA2* can be silenced by methylation in additional cancers. This contributes to their sensitivity to platinum-containing therapies in HGSC. PARP inhibitors might also find broader clinical application in these sporadic cancers, in which these pathways are also defective. Thus, in some regions, all patients presenting with an HGSC are referred for genetic counseling and screening for *BRCA* mutations (Risch, 2001).

MELANOMA

Malignant melanoma is an aggressive tumor that originates from pigment-producing melanocytes, mainly in skin. About 80% of melanomas are diagnosed early and can be cured by surgical excision (Gray-Schopfer, 2007). However, metastatic melanomas are refractory to current chemotherapy or radiotherapy and have a very poor prognosis, with a median survival of 6 months (Miller, 2006). A majority (90%) of melanoma cases are sporadic, and 10% are familial melanomas, also known as dysplastic nevus syndrome. Four melanoma-predisposing genes have been identified in familial melanoma based on the discovery of germline mutations in multiple-case families; three are high penetrance, and one is low penetrance. The best characterized high-penetrance gene is cyclin-dependent kinase inhibitor 2A. It is located on chromosome 9p21 and encodes two distinct melanoma-predisposing genes: *p16* (discussed previously in the bladder cancer section) and *p14* (Mehra, 2007b). The protein product of *p16* is INK4a, and the protein product of *p14* is ARF. Twenty-five percent to 40% of familial melanoma cases harbor an inactivating mutation in *CDKN2A* (Miller, 2006; Gray-Schopfer, 2007). Cyclin-dependent kinase 4 *(CDK4)*, located on 12q14, is the third high-penetrance melanoma susceptibility gene (Zuo, 1996). Finally, melanocortin-1 receptor *(MC1R)* is a low-penetrance gene implicated in melanomagenesis.

The RAS/RAF/MEK/ERK signaling pathway has emerged as a major player in the induction and maintenance of sporadic melanoma. Among *RAS* family members, mutations in *NRAS* occur most frequently in melanocytes, with rates approaching 56% in congenital nevi (Demunter, 2001), 33% in primary melanomas, and 26% in metastatic melanomas (Garnett, 2005).

However, as in papillary thyroid carcinoma and in some forms of colorectal cancer, the most important signaling molecule in melanoma downstream of RAS is BRAF. *BRAF* somatic missense mutations are found in 66% of malignant melanomas, of which 80% involve a single base substitution of valine by glutamic acid at position 600 (V600E). Most of these mutations activate BRAF kinase activity from 1.5- to 700-fold, although a small number actually are inactivating mutations. However, even these inactive mutants can stimulate cellular signaling through the MEK-ERK pathway because they activate the related family member *C-RAF* (Garnett, 2005).

It is interesting to note that genetic alterations in *NRAS* and *BRAF* rarely coexist in melanoma (Zuo, 1996; Tsao, 2004; Miller, 2006), suggesting that mutant *BRAF* or *NRAS* alone is able to activate the pathway. Recent studies have revealed deregulation of PI3K signaling in a high proportion of melanomas. Indeed, in about 45% of melanomas, *PTEN* is deleted and the downstream *AKT* gene is amplified (Zhou, 2003; Stahl, 2004). Additionally, RAS binds and activates PI3K, thereby activating the AKT pathway and preventing apoptosis (Sekulic, 2008). These data suggest that loss of *PTEN* and oncogenic activation of RAS are equivalent (Zhou, 2003).

The high mutation rate of *BRAF* in melanoma makes it an attractive therapeutic target. Investigators have focused much attention on agents that specifically target BRAF, such as sorafenib, as well as on molecules that function both upstream and downstream of BRAF. A nonspecific inhibitor of BRAF, sorafenib is not effective as a single agent in advanced-stage melanoma patients (Sekulic, 2008). Of interest downstream of BRAF is the direct inhibition of ERK and MEK. Although no mutations have been documented in either molecule, inhibition of MEK has proved effective in the presence of a mutated *BRAF* (Sekulic, 2008). Several MEK inhibitors are currently in clinical trials. Upstream of BRAF, RAS is an attractive target for inhibition. Farnesyltransferase inhibitors (FTIs) interfere with posttranslational processing of RAS, and thereby inhibit the downstream effects of RAS.

Molecular Genetic Pathology of Sarcoma

Sarcomas are malignant neoplasms arising in connective tissue, fat, muscle, blood vessels, deep skin tissues, nerves, bones, and cartilage. These types of cancers often are not considered classical "solid tissue tumors," although often their biological behavior is similar to that of the types of solid tissue tumors discussed previously. However, because major advances have been made in the area of the molecular biology of sarcomas, and because these advances have illuminated the nature of specific genetic lesions that cause cell transformation, we describe them in this section. This section is meant to show the principles that have been discovered in sarcomatous cell transformation and is not meant to be a detailed discussion of specific genetic lesions in each of the myriad of different sarcomas that have been described. Rather, we present specific examples of each type of genetic lesion that has been discovered. The reader is referred to other texts that describe the genetic lesions in each sarcoma type.

Many sarcomas harbor specific translocations or other characteristic genetic defects that aid in the diagnosis of each tumor type and, in some cases, impart prognostic or predictive information influencing clinical management (Jain, 2010b). Recent molecular cytogenetic analysis has demonstrated that the sarcomas can be divided into two main categories:

1. Sarcomas with specific genetic alterations. These can be subclassified further into sarcomas that harbor reciprocal translocations resulting in oncogenic fusion transcripts (accounting for 15%–20% of cases [e.g., SS18-SSX in synovial sarcoma]) and sarcomas that harbor specific oncogenic mutations (e.g., *KIT* and *PDGFRA* mutations in gastrointestinal stromal tumors) (Hirota, 1998; Miettinen, 2006).
2. Sarcomas displaying multiple complex karyotypic abnormalities with no specific pattern, including malignant fibrous histiocytoma (MFH) and leiomyosarcoma (LMS).

SARCOMAS WITH FUSION GENES

Fusion Genes Involving *TET* Genes

Nearly half of the fusion proteins believed to participate in initiation and development of sarcoma contain a portion of the so-called *TET* gene family products, including *EWSR1*, *TLS/FUS*, and *TAFII68*. TET family proteins contain a characteristic 87 amino acid RNA recognition motif that is thought to be implicated in protein–RNA binding and to participate in transcription and RNA metabolism.

Ewing's Sarcoma/Primitive Peripheral Neuroectodermal Tumor

This is a prime example of a fusion gene–induced sarcoma. The tumor itself is a small blue cell tumor that primarily affects long bones or the vertebral area in young adults and children. Histologically, it is characterized by sheets of small round cells that may form what are called Homer-Wright rosettes. Ewing's sarcoma family tumors (ESFTs) can be subclassified into Ewing's sarcomas or primitive peripheral neuroectodermal tumor (PNET), the latter showing evidence of neuroendocrine differentiation immunohistochemically (Olsen, 2006). However, the distinction between them is no longer considered critical for clinical management, as prognosis and therapy are similar.

ESFTs characteristically harbor a recurring t(11;22)(q24;q12) that juxtaposes the *FLI1* and *EWSR1* genes to encode a chimeric RNA and protein. About 10% of Ewing family tumors have an alternate translocation involving the *EWSR1* gene, implying that disruption of *EWSR1* is the critical molecular event underlying tumorigenesis. Except for *FUS-ERG*, all fusion transcripts identified so far in ESFTs consist of *EWSR1* and an ETS family transcription factor, including *FLI1*, *ERG*, *ETV1*, *ETV4*, and *FEV* genes (de Alava, 2000). Approximately 85%–90% of ESFTs are associated with the *EWSR1-FLI1* fusion gene, 9%–14% with *EWR1-ERG*, and the remaining 1%–5% with other rare variants (de Alava, 2000).

Karyotype is the analytic method used for the initial workup of a suspected Ewing family tumor because the characteristic t(11;22) is evident in approximately 90% of these tumors. However, in a case of strong suspicion of Ewing's sarcoma/PNET with normal karyotype, FISH should be considered as an additional test for the genetic defects. FISH, using a break-apart probe targeting the *EWSR1* gene, is an excellent method to identify or exclude a *EWSR1* gene rearrangement. FISH may be carried out on metaphase cells (requiring fresh tissue) or on interphase cells (feasible on a wide variety of sample types, including fine-needle aspirates, touch preparations, smears, or paraffin-embedded tissue) (Kilpatrick, 2006). An advantage unique to RT-PCR is its ability to define which of two prognostically relevant transcript structures is present: type 1 fusion transcripts *(EWSR1-FLI1)* are not transcribed as actively and carry a good prognosis compared with alternative fusions. Another advantage of RT-PCR is its ability to detect minimal residual disease after therapy (Vermeulen, 2006). Immunohistochemical analyses of *CD99* and *FLI1* reveal overexpression in most Ewing's/PNET tumors harboring a t(11;22) (Hameed, 2007).

Fusion Genes Involving Receptor Tyrosine Kinase Genes

Congenital fibrosarcoma (CFS) is a low-grade pediatric soft tissue sarcoma, principally arising in the extremities, generally in the first year of life. Recently, CFSs were shown to contain a novel t(12;15)(p13;q25) translocation, resulting in *ETV6-NTRK3* gene fusion. *ETV6* is a member of the ETS family of transcription factors containing a basic helix-loop-helix (bHLH) dimerization domain, which was originally found at the breakpoint in translocations in leukemia and myeloproliferative syndromes. NTRK3 is the cell surface receptor for neurotropin 3 expressed primarily in the CNS. The ETV6-NTRK3 fusion protein forms a homodimer or heterodimer with wild-type NTRK3, which displays receptor tyrosine kinase (RTK) activity and undergoes autophosphorylation at tyrosine residues (Knezevich, 1998). Cytogenetic t(12;15) translocations may not be identified in several cases (CMN4, CFS1, and CFS5), but RT-PCR and FISH analyses revealed ETV6-region rearrangements in those same cases. Detection of *ETV6-NTRK3* fusion transcripts in most CFSs using RT-PCR methods with archival, formalin-fixed, paraffin-embedded tissues, therefore, is a useful diagnostic adjunct.

Fusion Genes Involving Chromatin Remodeling Genes

Synovial sarcomas (SSs) often arise deep in the soft tissue near a joint in the extremity of a young adult patient. Most SSs are characterized by t(X;18)(p11.2;q11.2), resulting in a fusion between the *SS18(SYT)* gene on chromosome 18 and one of the *SSX* genes on the X chromosome, creating *SS18-SSX1*, *SS18-SSX2*, or *SS18-SSX4* chimeric genes (Skytting, 1999; Nishio, 2001, 2002a, 2002b, 2005; Kanemitsu, 2007). Two common histologic and genetic variants of synovial sarcoma are known: a monophasic variant comprising vimentin-expressing spindle cells usually carrying *SS18-SSX2* translocation, and a biphasic variant that consists of a mixture of vimentin-expressing spindle cells and keratin-expressing glandular epithelial cells harboring the *SS18-SSX1* or *SS18-SSX2* translocation (Ladanyi, 2002). The biphasic variant may resemble adenocarcinoma or more typically carcinosarcoma and carries a worse prognosis, at least in early-stage patients. Karyotype is helpful when it is positive, but negative results could reflect failure of the tumor cells to divide sufficiently in culture, or other mechanisms of false-negative results. FISH using an SS18 break-apart probe is helpful for demonstrating t(X;18), but it cannot distinguish which partner gene is involved for prognostic purposes. RNA from frozen or paraffin-embedded tissue is suitable for RT-PCR to detect and to distinguish the two common translocation variants (Sieber, 2003). From a mechanistic standpoint, the translocation creates a chimeric gene encoding a fusion protein that redirects the transcription factor function of SS18. Relevant downstream targets include *CCND1* (cyclin D1), which enhances cell cycle progression. *TLE1* encodes a transcriptional corepressor that is overexpressed in synovial sarcomas. Gene and tissue microarray studies have identified TLE1 as an excellent biomarker for distinguishing synovial sarcoma from other soft tissue malignancies on immunohistochemistry (Jagdis, 2009).

Fusion Genes Involving Growth Factors

Dermatofibrosarcoma protuberance (DFSP) is a rare skin tumor of low-grade malignancy that shows local recurrence. The reciprocal chromosomal translocation t(17;22)(q11;q13.1) or a supernumerary ring chromosome derived from t(17;22) is found in this type of tumor, which results in fusion of the *COL1A1* gene on chromosome 17 with the *PDGFB* gene on chromosome 22 (Simon, 1997). Because the point of fusion is highly specific for *PDGFB* but is spread over almost the entire locus for *COL1A1*, the role of the *COL1A1* gene may be simply to upregulate the expression of the platelet-derived growth factor receptor (PDGFR). Imatinib mesylate is an inhibitor of tyrosine kinases, including PDGFR, and has shown a dramatic response to treatment in adults. The use of other PDGFR inhibitors such as sunitinib and sorafenib has recently commenced in patients with metastatic DFSP (McArthur, 2006)

Giant cell fibroblastoma (GCF) represents the juvenile form of DFSP, which shows local recurrence. Although histologically different, these two diseases share several features, including CD34 positivity and, most important, the genetic alteration t(17;22)(q11;q13.1), involving the *COL1A1* gene as found in DFSP (Simon, 1997).

Other Types of Fusion Genes

Rhabdomyosarcoma (RMS), a malignant tumor of skeletal muscle cells, is the most common soft tissue sarcoma in children and young adults, often arising from extremities, paranasal sinus, or retroperitoneum. The main histologic subtypes are alveolar (ARMS) (20%), embryonal (ERMS) (60%), and pleomorphic (PRMS); survival rates for these subtypes vary from <25%–>95%, respectively (Breneman, 2003). Histologically, striated muscle differentiation is noted with concomitant expression of vimentin, muscle-specific actin, desmin, myogenin, and MyoD1.

In ARMS, 70% of cases harbor the translocation t(2;13)(q35:q14), which fuses the 5′ end of *PAX3* with the 3′ end of the *FOXO1A* gene. A further 10% of ARMS are associated with fusion of *PAX7* to the *FOXO1A* gene. The remaining 20% of cases of ARMS do not have these fusion genes detectable by routine RT-PCR and constitute cases with very low expression of a fusion gene or a rare variant fusion gene, or with no detectable fusion gene. FISH using a break-apart probe identifies rearrangement of the *FOXO1A* gene (Matsumura, 2008; Mehra, 2008). The karyotype typically reveals t(2;13)(q35;q14) *PAX3-FOXO1A* or t(1;13)(p36;q14) *PAX7-FOXO1A*, with the latter being less common but imparting a better prognosis (Davicioni, 2006). It should be noted that ARMS tend to have a poor prognosis overall, especially when presenting with disseminated disease, so genetic testing may be moot in stage IV patients. Testing is most useful when the histologic features are not classic (e.g., mixed alveolar and embryonal patterns).

SARCOMAS WITH ONCOGENIC MUTATIONS

KIT and *PDGFRA* in Gastrointestinal Stromal Tumor

Gastrointestinal stromal tumor (GIST) is the most common mesenchymal tumor in the gastrointestinal tract. Activating mutations of the *cKIT* gene were found in 75%–80% of cases and of *PDGFRA* in 5%–10%; cases with no mutation in either of these are extremely rare. The cKIT protein, which encodes a TKR for stem cell/PDGFR, comprises a long extracellular domain, a transmembrane segment, and an intracellular domain. In all cases, mutated receptors transmit growth signals in a ligand-independent manner, inducing dysregulated cell proliferation, as described in Chapter 74. Mutations generally occur in exon 11, encoding the intracellular receptor domain, but can also occur in exons 9 and (rarely) 13, and 1 in GIST. Mutations in *cKIT* and *PDGFRA* are mutually exclusive. Detection of overexpression or mutation of *cKIT/PDGFRA* has become a standard diagnostic tool for GIST. Drugs targeting the activating tyrosine kinase, such as imatinib mesylate (Glivec/Gleevec), have been used successfully to treat patients with metastatic GIST showing the previously described mutations. D816V point mutations in *cKIT* exon 17 are responsible for resistance to targeted therapy drugs such as imatinib mesylate (Miettinen, 2006).

SARCOMAS WITH VARIABLE COMPLEX GENETIC ALTERATIONS WITH NO SPECIFIC PATTERN

Tumors in this group are characterized by pleomorphic/spindle cell morphology, including MFH, LMS, and malignant peripheral nerve sheath tumor (MPNST). Chromosomal breakpoints in these tumors are widely scattered, with no predilection for any of the recurrent breakpoints and no losses to any of the morphologic subtypes. A prime example of this type of sarcoma is LMS, a malignant tumor of smooth muscle.

Leiomyosarcomas are adult soft tissue sarcomas that show varying degrees of smooth muscle differentiation and can develop anywhere in the body. LMSs usually show complex karyotypic alterations in the form of gains, losses, and amplifications in chromosomes. Some gains and losses of chromosomal material tend to correlate with poor outcome, large tumor size, and metastatic dissemination, and include loss of 1p12-pter, loss of 2p, loss of 13q14-q21 (targeting the Rb pathway), loss of 10q (targeting PTEN), and loss of 16q, as well as gains of 17p, 8q, and 5p14 pter. Activation of the *PI3K-AKT* pathway through different mechanisms (e.g., activation of insulin-like growth factor receptor [IGFR]; inactivation of PTEN, a negative regulator of *PI3K-AKT*) also plays a crucial role in the development and maintenance of LMS. This activation leads to the concomitant activation of downstream effectors such as mTOR (target of rapamycin protein; discussed in Chapter 23, see Fig. 23-15) and its targets (β-catenin, pS6, p4E-BP1, etc.), as well as to stabilization of a particularly important promitotic protein, HDM-2 (human double minute-binding protein). Clinical trials have showed that analogs of rapamycin such as everolimus (RAD001), an mTOR inhibitor, have some efficacy in patients with LMS. It is known that the more differentiated retroperitoneal LMSs tend to behave more aggressively as the result of amplification/overexpression of myocardin. This protein is a transcriptional cofactor for regulating smooth muscle differentiation, and its inactivation is associated with less differentiated histology. Myocardin might constitute a promising therapeutic target.

Cancers of Unknown Origin

Cancer of unknown primary (CUP) is defined by the presence of cytologically or histologically proven metastases, for which no primary tumor can be identified despite standardized and extensive diagnostic workup. It constitutes approximately 4% of all malignancies, of which 80% are adenocarcinoma (50% well to moderately differentiated and 30% poorly differentiated), 15% squamous cell carcinoma, and 5% undifferentiated neoplasm on light microscopy (Horlings, 2008). Accordingly, failure to identify the primary tumor theoretically incurs the risk of failure to administer appropriate systemic combination chemotherapy, as well as targeted molecular therapy. Although the metastatic pattern in these patients is often atypical, no direct evidence indicates that molecular genetic abnormalities in these tumors differ from those seen in metastatic cancers of known primary site. With expansion of tissue-specific targeted therapy, it is believed that patient prognosis can be better predicted when the primary site of metastatic tumors is assigned.

This has increased the need for identification of the tissue of origin, which further makes the immunohistochemical analysis a crucial component of clinical workup. However, the current success rate of the diagnostic workup, including clinical, radiologic, and extensive pathologic methods, varies between 20% and 30% (Horlings, 2008). Therefore, new methods are required to increase diagnostic accuracy.

The development of molecular technology that allows gene expression profiling of tumors provides an opportunity for improved diagnosis of patients with CUP. Quantitative reverse transcriptase polymerase chain reaction (RT-PCR) is a technique that allows gene expression profiling of FFPE tissue specimens, and therefore is a potential diagnostic tool with broad applicability. These techniques have enabled researchers to develop expression profiles unique to a wide variety of well-characterized primary cancers. The accuracy of diagnosis of primary site obtained by comparing these known unique signatures with those from unknown primary cancers is 80%–90%. This is based on the finding that metastatic cancers retain at least the basic genetic signature found in their respective primary cancers. Gene expression profiling has also shown important potential diagnostic and therapeutic implications in CUP. The CUP colon cancer profile can be identified, and patients appear to respond well to current regimens for metastatic CRC (Varadhachary, 2008). Expression profiling of certain genes (e.g., *Her/2neu*, *RAS*, *EGFR*, *VEGF*, *COX-2*, *cKIT*) for CUP will benefit patients by revealing therapies that can be used to target these molecules (Pentheroudakis, 2007).

To date, several gene expression–based tests have demonstrated an increase in overall accuracy for the primary site of origin to 78%–88% (Horlings, 2008). Ramaswamy (2001) demonstrated 78% classification accuracy in classifying 10 carcinomas and 4 noncarcinoma types by using oligonucleotide microarray gene expression analysis, whereas Tothill (2005) achieved 89% accuracy with 12 carcinomas and 1 noncarcinoma after reducing the gene classifier from thousands to 79 genes by converting microarray gene expression to RT-qPCR (Tothill, 2005). Ma (2006) used data from a 22,000-gene microarray and devised a 92-gene RT-PCR assay that classified 119 tumors of unknown origin to 32 primary site/histologic types with 87% accuracy. A molecular assay (CUP assay) was developed (Veridex, La Jolla, Calif) that evaluates the expression of 10 tissue type–specific gene markers using quantitative RT-PCR technology and is designed to detect tumors originating from six specific sites: lung (HUMPB,

TTF1, DSG3), breast (MGB, PDEF), colon (CDH17), ovary (WT1), pancreas (PSCA, F5), and prostate (PSA) (Varadhachary, 2008). Another diagnostic gene expression–based classifier (CupPrint, Agendia, Amsterdam, The Netherlands) was developed using 495 genes to classify 48 tumor types. Similar to these, a gene expression–based breast cancer prognosis assay (Genomic Health OncotypeDx Breast Cancer Assay, Redwood City, Calif; MammaPrint, Amsterdam, The Netherlands) has been one of the few gene panels to achieve FDA approval. The FDA has also cleared the Pathwork tissue-of-origin test, developed by Pathwork Diagnostics (Redwood City, Calif.). This is a gene expression microarray-based test of 2029 genes that quantifies the molecular similarity of tumor specimens, improving the identification of primary sites from 60% by IHC alone (Anderson, 2010) to 80%, though the test is limited to only to 15 tumor types (Pillai, 2011).

Although a microarray-based gene expression profiling test will not obviate the need for thorough clinical investigation, it may facilitate more focused testing, which would result in reduced cost, lower patient morbidity, and improved outcome.

TABLE 76-4
Molecular Genetics of Hereditary Nonpolyposis Colorectal Cancer

MMR gene	OMIM name	Chromosomal locus	% of HNPCC with mutation
MLH1	HNPCC2	3p21	50
MSH2	HNPCC1	2p16	40
MSH6	HNPCC5	2p15	≈7–10
PMS2	HNPCC4	7p22	1–2
MLH3	HNPCC7	14q24.3	1
PMS1a	HNPCC3	7p22	Unclear
TGFBR2	HNPCC6	3p22	Case report

HNPCC, Hereditary nonpolyposis colorectal cancer; *MMR*, mismatch repair; *OMIM*, Online Mendelian Inheritance in Man (database).

Molecular Genetic Pathology of Syndromatic Cancers

HEREDITARY COLONIC CANCER SYNDROME

Approximately 5%–10% of CRCs are hereditary, predominantly in a form of autosomal dominant transmission. Genetic polyposis syndrome accounts for less than 0.5% of all CRCs, whereas nonpolyposis forms of hereditary CRC are seen in a much higher percentage in overall hereditary CRCs (Lynch, 2003; Kievit, 2004).

FAMILIAL ADENOMATOUS POLYPOSIS SYNDROME

FAP is a rare disease that is characterized by numerous colorectal polyps (usually more than 100) (Winawer, 2003). Diagnosis of FAP is based on clinical and endoscopic findings. Three variants of FAP have been described on the basis of clinical manifestations:

1. Gardner syndrome associated with skin, soft tissue, and bone tumors.
2. Turcot syndrome associated with brain tumors.
3. Attenuated FAP with fewer than 100 polyps in the colorectum.

Classic FAP is an autosomal dominant inheritable disease, with nearly 100% penetrance. It is mainly attributable to the mutation/deletion of the *APC* gene, located at the long arm of chromosome 5. So far, more than 500 different germline *APC* mutations have been identified in FAP families (Varesco, 2004). About one third of patients are found to harbor de novo mutations. However, 5%–30% of FAP patients show no *APC* mutations on current genetic testing. Among those patients with *APC*-negative FAP, biallelic mutations in a different gene, the *MutY human homologue (MYH)* gene, may be found. The *MYH* gene encodes a member of the base excision repair pathway that is involved in repairing oxidative damage to DNA. Those APC-negative FAP patients may have a family history compatible with recessive inheritance (Sieber, 2003; Varesco, 2004), indicating that this may be a different disease. Genetic testing may be helpful in screening and diagnosis of atypical FAP cases and in the management of affected patients. PCR-based methods have been developed to detect *APC* germline mutations (Varesco, 2004).

HEREDITARY NONPOLYPOSIS COLORECTAL CANCER (LYNCH SYNDROME)

Hereditary nonpolyposis colorectal cancer is an autosomal dominant genetic condition, characterized by high predisposition to CRC and other cancers outside of the colorectum, including the genitourinary and female reproduction systems, the upper gastrointestinal tract, the hepatobiliary tract, brain, and skin. Approximately 3% of all diagnosed cases of CRC belong to HNPCC, which makes it the most common hereditary CRC-predisposing syndrome (Lynch, 2003, 2009). It has been found to have lifetime risks of approximately 80% for CRC and 40%–60% for endometrial disease. Colorectal cancer develops in younger patients (average age, 45 years), and two thirds of these cancers occur in the proximal colon. Histologically, HNPCC is not associated with a large number of colorectal polyps as seen in FAP, rather it forms a large nonpolypoid malignant lesion. Compared with sporadic CRC of equivalent staging, patients with HNPCC may have a better response to chemotherapy and better clinical outcomes (Lynch, 2009).

The molecular basis for the development of HNPCC is due to MSI, which is a consequence of inherited or germline mutations of DNA *MMR* genes. Among nine *MMR* genes discovered, mutations in *MLH1, MSH2, MSH6, MLH3*, and *PMS2* are associated with the development of HNPCC (Peltomaki, 2005). The significance of mutations in two other *MMR* genes, *TGFBR2* and *PMS1*, is less clear (Table 76-4). Among those identifiable mutations associated with HNPCC, 90% occur in *MLH1* or *MSH2* (Chung, 2003), 7%–10% in *MSH6*, and 1%–2% in *PMS2* or *MLH3* (Lawes, 2005). Most germline mutations in *MSH2* lead to complete loss of gene expression, and usually are accompanied by loss of expression of *MSH6*. CRC with *MLH1* mutation is frequently caused by missense mutations. Mutations of *MMR* genes cause abnormal mismatch repair function, failing to correct a larger number of insertions and deletions, eventually leading to frameshift within the microsatellites or MSI (Jacob, 2002; de Vos, 2005). However, approximately 50% of all HNPCCs have no identifiable mutations in *MMR* genes according to current methods of detection (Umar, 2004).

Two rare but distinct variants of HNPCC are known: (1) Muir-Torre syndrome, resulting from mutations in the *MSH2* gene and showing coexisting sebaceous skin tumors with small and large intestinal, gastric, kidney, endometrial, and ovarian cancer (Lynch, 2009); and (2) Turcot's syndrome, resulting from mutations in the *MLH1* and *PMS2* genes and showing coexistent glioblastoma with colorectal CRCs (Abdel-Rahman, 2004).

The diagnosis of HNPCC is based mainly on clinical information and familial history. Genetic testing has been introduced for diagnostic purposes. A testing kit for germline mutations is commercially available for blood samples. *MMR* dysfunction can be analyzed by immunohistochemistry on paraffin-embedded tissues. PCR and sequencing are methods commonly used to detect MSI. According to the Bethesda Guidelines, five microsatellite markers are to be tested. Of these, three are dinucleotide repeats, and two mononucleotide repeats. MSI-H is defined as LOH in two or more of five markers in tumor tissue compared with a normal tissue control. However, although it is a sensitive test, MSI testing is not specific for HNPCC, as HNPCC can be MSI-low and MSI-stable in some cases, and sporadic CRCs may also show MSI-H. Thus, genetic testing may be useful only after patients at risk for HNPCC are identified by the Amsterdam or Bethesda clinical criteria (Abdel-Rahman, 2004; Umar, 2004; Lynch, 2009).

FAMILIAL JUVENILE POLYPOSIS SYNDROME

Familial juvenile polyposis syndrome (JPS) is a rare disorder inherited in an autosomal dominant fashion in at least 30% of patients. The incidence of JPS is approximately 1 per 100,000 births, and it is the most common of the hamartomatous syndromes (Schreibman, 2005). The diagnosis of JPS is made when any of the following three criteria are met (Schreibman, 2005):

1. Multiple (three to ten) hamartomatous polyps in the colorectum.
2. Any number of hamartomatous polyps in a patient with a family history of JPS.

3. Extracolonic hamartomatous polyps (e.g., in the stomach or small intestine).

Germline mutations of *SMAD4*, *BMPR1A*, and *ENG* have all been described in patients with JPS. *SMAD4* is located on chromosome 18q21.1 and is found to be mutated in approximately 15% of cases of JPS (Mishra, 2006). *BMPR1A* (bone morphogenetic protein receptor type 1A), located on chromosome 10q22.3, is a serine threonine kinase that is a mediator of the bone morphogenetic protein intracellular signaling pathway (Zbuk, 2007). It has been identified as mutated in about 25% of affected patients with JPS. Both genes mentioned previously encode proteins that are involved in the TGF-β signaling pathway, which is an important modulator of many cellular processes (e.g., cell growth, apoptosis, growth arrest) (Zhou, 2003).

The lifetime risk of CRC is about 70%, and the risk of pancreatic, gastric, and duodenal carcinoma is increased in these patients (Gatalica, 2008). Molecular screening of individuals at risk within a JPS family for a known genetic mutation would allow clinicians to make the diagnosis at an earlier age, and would lead to closer endoscopic screening and follow-up. Individuals without the mutation would need less frequent endoscopic screening and perhaps endoscopy only after age 50, as is provided in the normal population. Therefore, genetic testing can help to define the recommended interval for screening and surveillance; it is hoped that it will help to prevent malignancy by early polypectomy and heightened surveillance (Mishra, 2006).

PEUTZ-JEGHERS SYNDROME

Peutz-Jeghers syndrome (PJS) is an autosomal dominant hamartomatous polyposis syndrome characterized by melanotic mucocutaneous hyperpigmentation and gastrointestinal hamartomas, which occur anywhere from the stomach to the anus, with a prevalence of approximately 1 in 200,000. Polyps usually are fewer than 20 in number and are most prevalent in the small intestine (Bourke, 2006). The only identifiable germline mutation causing PJS is seen in the *STK11/LKB1* gene. PJS patients have increased risk of esophageal, gastrointestinal, and pancreatic cancer, and the risk for these cancers markedly increases with age. By the age of 65 years, the risk of CRC is about 39% (Gatalica, 2008). In women with PJS, the risk for breast cancer is also reported to be substantially increased. PJS patients need to be educated as to the resources available for genetic testing, which can be very helpful, although the diagnosis can be made clinically in most cases when the family history is positive. A positive *LKB1* mutation test will confirm that individuals need careful screening and follow-up and a negative test will allow individuals to be spared of unnecessary screening procedures (Schreibman, 2005).

MULTIPLE ENDOCRINE NEOPLASIA

Multiple endocrine neoplasia (MEN) syndromes consist of a group of benign and malignant tumors in the pituitary, thyroid, parathyroids, adrenals, endocrine pancreas, paraganglia, or nonendocrine organs. Currently, the well-recognized MEN syndrome includes type 1 MEN and type 2 MEN. Some hereditary diseases are not classical for, but should be included in, the MEN syndromes, such as VHL syndrome, familial paraganglioma syndromes, Cowden syndrome, Carney complex, and hyperparathyroidism jaw tumor syndrome, and other uncommon conditions (Callender, 2008).

Multiple endocrine neoplasia type 1, also known as Wermer syndrome, is characterized by tumors in the parathyroid glands, stomach, pancreas and intestinal tract, anterior pituitary, endocrine pancreas, and duodenum, and by the presence of other, nonendocrine tumors such as hemangioma, ependymoma, and leiomyoma, often at a young age (Callender, 2008; Dreijerink, 2009). The syndrome is caused by inactivating germline mutations of the MEN 1 TSG, *MEN1*, encoding a gene product that is involved in the regulation of gene transcription, DNA replication and repair, and chromatin modification (Dreijerink, 2009). Approximately 10% of patients are the first affected person in their family, or the index patient. By age 50 years, approximately 80% of patients with mutations in the *MEN1* TSG will have the disease, and 90%–95% of these patients will have abnormal biochemical screening results (Trump, 1996; Chandrasekharappa, 2001; Callender, 2008). Genetic testing is complicated, as it may detect hundreds of disease-causing mutations (e.g., *MEN1*), as well as polymorphisms. It may potentially identify those with early asymptomatic hyperparathyroidism, allowing for early nonsurgical intervention to avoid invasive surgery (Chew, 2009).

Multiple endocrine neoplasia type 2 is characterized by strong penetrance of the MTC and associated pheochromocytoma and hyperparathyroidism. It can be further categorized into MEN 2A, MEN 2B, and FMTC, based on the risk of pheochromocytoma or hyperparathyroidism, and the presence or absence of characteristic physical features (Callender, 2008; Raue, 2009). MEN 2 is caused by germline activating mutations of the *RET* proto-oncogene due to missense mutations, predominantly in exons 10, 11, or 13 through 16, and rarely in exons 5 and 8 (Da Silva, 2003; Dvorakova, 2005). *RET* is located on chromosome 10q11.2 and encodes a TKR that appears to transduce growth and differentiation signals in several developing tissues, including those derived from the neural crest. Constitutive activation of *RET* leads to uncontrolled cell growth and survival. Genetic testing for germline *RET* mutations is available for a definitive diagnosis of MEN 2 in patients who have an equivocal presentation or family history.

Close genotype-phenotype correlations have been noted in MEN 2. Certain specific *RET* mutations (genotype) are associated with age at onset, aggressiveness of MTC, and the presence or absence of other endocrine neoplasms (phenotype) (Eng, 1996; Yip, 2003). MEN 2A, the most common subtype, has a detectable *RET* mutation in at least 95% of patients (Mulligan, 1994; Schuffenecker, 1994). Among those mutations, codon 634 (exon 11) and codons 609, 611, 618, and 620 are found to be mutated in 85% of patients with MEN 2A and in 10%–15% of patients with MEN 2B. MEN 2B, the rarest subtype of MEN 2, has *RET* mutations in codon 918 (exon 16) in more than 95% of patients, and rarely in codon 883 of exon 15 (A883F in the encoded protein) (Mulligan, 1995; Gimm, 1997). Patients with FMTC who develop only MTC with its germline mutations have these mutations from exons 13 through 15 of *RET* (Brauckhoff, 2002). Based on the mutation sites and numbers, MEN 2 can be stratified into three different levels of risk for MTC development (Brandi, 2001; Frank-Raue, 2006): high-risk group with mutations (codons 609, 768, 790, 791, 804, and 891), higher-risk group with mutations (codons 611, 618, 620, and 634), and highest-risk group with mutations (codons 883 and 918). Genetic testing may help to determine appropriate treatment options for individual patients, including prophylactic thyroidectomy, as well as the extent of surgery.

von Hippel–Lindau syndrome is an autosomal dominant inheritable neoplasia syndrome characterized by hemangioblastomas in the CNS and retina, pheochromocytomas, renal cysts and clear cell RCC, pancreatic cysts and islet cell tumors, endolymphatic sac tumors, and papillary cystadenomas of the epididymis and broad ligament (Maher, 1991). It has a strong penetrance, and more than 90% of affected individuals have the disease by the age of 65 years. As discussed in the earlier section on renal tumors, VHL disease is caused by inactivating germline mutations of the VHL TSG, which contains three exons and is located on chromosome 3p25. VHL is critical in the process of regulating HIF-α and -β, which participate in the cell's response to hypoxia, as discussed earlier. Similar to MEN 2, a clear relationship has been noted between the type of genetic mutation of *VHL* (the genotype) and the pattern of tumors that developed in that particular family (the phenotype) (Crossey, 1994; Maher, 1996; Webster, 1998). The syndrome is associated with an increased risk of a variety of tumors in an allele-specific manner. Genetic testing is available for definite diagnosis of VHL syndrome in patients with equivocal disease and apparently sporadic *VHL*-related disease (Stolle, 1998).

Familial paraganglioma syndromes are inherited in an autosomal dominant manner and are characterized by multiple head and neck, thoracic, and abdominal paragangliomas and/or pheochromocytomas. Four familial paraganglioma syndromes have been described: PGL 1, PGL 2, PGL 3, and PGL 4 (Callender, 2008; Myssiorek, 2008). Most familial cases of paraganglioma have been found to be associated with the mutation of three genes encoding subunits of the mitochondrial II/succinate dehydrogenase (SDH) complex: *SDHB* at 1p36.1 (PGL4), *SDHC* at 1q21 (PGL3), and *SDHD* at 11q23 (PGL1) (most common) by linkage and candidate gene studies (Myssiorek, 2008). Individuals with *SDHB* mutation usually have paragangliomas in the abdomen and less frequently in the head and neck, the chest, and the adrenal gland, and are associated with an increased risk of malignancy. Individuals with *SDHD* mutation develop paragangliomas most often in the head and neck (Neumann, 2004; Benn, 2006). *SDHD* mutation is usually associated with low risk of malignancy of paragangliomas (Neumann, 2004; Dreijerink, 2009). Individuals with *SDHC* mutations are rare, and paragangliomas usually present in the head and neck, with a benign course (Schiavi, 2005).

The genetic screening method is very useful for predicting risk for malignancy, because so far the biological behavior of all neuroendocrine tumors cannot be determined by conventional histologic examination alone. Genetic screening for the three genes previously discussed has been offered for familial paraganglioma (Oosterwijk, 1996). This test can identify individuals with mutations, allowing earlier detection and earlier intervention.

Cowden syndrome is a rare autosomal dominant, cancer-predisposing condition characterized by increased risk of breast, thyroid, and endometrial cancers and other benign conditions, including multiple hamartomas in the colon, lipomas, and fibromas (Callender, 2008; Hobert, 2009). It is caused by germline mutations in the TSG **phosphate and tensin homologue deleted on chromosome 10**. *PTEN* encodes a tumor suppressor promoting G1 cell cycle arrest or apoptosis by downregulating *PI3K* and *AKT* and, concurrently, the raf-MEK-ERK pathway (Waite, 2002; Hobert, 2009).

Genetic testing for this condition is commercially available to identify mutations and/or deletions within *PTEN* (Marsh, 1998; Zhou, 2003). Approximately 85% of patients with Cowden syndrome have an identifiable *PTEN* mutation or deletion (Marsh, 1998; Eng, 2003; Zhou, 2003). This method includes multiplex ligation–dependent probe amplification (the preferred method), Southern blotting, monochromosomal hybrid analysis, real-time polymerase chain reaction, and semiquantitative multiplex PCR. Promoter analysis is also used for genetic testing in the research setting. Identification of *PTEN* mutations not only can confirm the clinical diagnosis, but also can help in prenatal diagnosis and prediction of mutations in affected families (Callender, 2008; Hobert, 2009).

Li-Fraumeni syndrome is a rare autosomal dominant disorder characterized by increased risk of soft tissue sarcoma, breast cancer, and osteosarcoma, as well as brain tumor, childhood leukemia, and adrenocortical carcinoma (Moule, 2006; Callender, 2008).

Most individuals or families with Li-Fraumeni syndrome have the germline mutation in the TSG encoding the p53 protein on chromosome 17p13.1. Unlike other TSGs, such as *RB* and *p16*, germline mutations in only one copy of *p53* can result in cancer development (Yoon, 2002). Most *p53* germline mutations are missense mutations, and only 10% are due to deletions (Olivier, 2003). A few cases of Li-Fraumeni syndrome and Li-Fraumeni–like syndrome show mutations in another TSG, *CHEK2*, without *p53* mutation (Bell, 1999).

Certain genotypes of *p53* mutations have prognostic significance. Cancers harboring missense *p53* mutations are associated with more aggressive behavior; these mutations therefore suggest poorer prognoses. Missense mutations within the DNA binding region of the *p53* gene are more likely predisposed to early onset of breast cancer and brain tumor, whereas mutations outside the DNA binding region are more commonly seen in adrenocortical carcinoma. Mutations leading to a *p53* null phenotype are associated with earlier onset of brain tumor (Olivier, 2003).

Genetic testing for a mutation of *p53* in a patient with Li-Fraumeni or Li-Fraumeni–like syndrome can confirm the clinical diagnosis and screen family members at risk. However, it should also be noted that inactivating *p53* mutations and homozygous deletions of this gene are observed in a significant number of other types of cancer, including colon, breast, and bladder.

Neurofibromatoses are a group of genetically distinct disorders with predisposition to induce nerve sheath tumor. They include neurofibromatosis 1 (NF1), neurofibromatosis 2 (NF2), and schwannomatosis.

Neurofibromatosis 1 (also referred to as von Recklinghausen's disease), the most common type, is an autosomal dominant multisystem disorder with 100% penetrance and variable expression. It predisposes to the development of benign and malignant tumors, typically neurofibroma, and less commonly glioma and other abnormalities (learning disability, vasculopathy, and bony abnormalities) (Arun, 2004; Boyd, 2009). Patients with this condition often are observed to have multiple tumors and café-au-lait spots on their body surfaces.

NF1 results from a mutation in the *NF1* gene, *NF1*, located on chromosome 17q11.2, and encodes for the large protein, neurofibromin. Of major importance, neurofibromin contains at least one domain that has GTPase-activating (GAP) activity with the ras-p21 protein. As discussed in Chapter 74, wild-type ras-p21 is activated by exchanging guanosine diphosphate for GTP. GAP inactivates wild-type ras-p21 by promoting the hydrolysis of ras-p21–bound GTP. Mutations in *NF1* result in loss of function of neurofibromin, leading to increase Ras activity, particularly in neurocutaneous tissues, as well as to increase proliferation and tumorigenesis (Boyd, 2009).. The mutations are near evenly split between the sporadic and the inherited. Types of mutations of *NF1* include complete gene deletions, insertions, stop codons, splicing mutations, amino acid substitutions, and chromosomal rearrangements (Messiaen, 2000).

Molecular testing for *NF1* is clinically available. Because of the large gene size and lack of hot spots of *NF1* mutations, comprehensive screening approaches have been established to detect all or most mutations and may detect 95% of *NF1* mutations (Messiaen, 2000). These approaches include the optimized protein truncation test (an in vitro coupled transcription/translation synthesis assay designed as a tool to detect mutations that lead to premature translational termination), FISH, direct sequencing, RT-PCR with Southern blot analysis, and/or cytogenetic analysis (Messiaen, 2000; Boyd, 2009).

Molecular testing of *NF1* mutations is used mainly for definitive diagnosis in suspicious cases, and for prenatal or preimplantation genetic diagnosis. However, it is not indicated for the routine clinical care of patients with NF1. Because of the lack of genotype–phenotype correlations, genetic testing, although useful for confirming the diagnosis of NF1, does not predict disease severity or outcome.

Neurofibromatosis 2 is also a dominantly inherited tumor predisposition syndrome characterized by the development of multiple schwannomas, meningiomas, and ependymomas. Most patients present with hearing loss due to inevitable development of schwannomas affecting both vestibulocochlear (8th) nerves (Evans, 2009a, 2009b).

NF2 is caused by mutations in the *NF2* gene on chromosome 22. More than 50% of patients have new mutations, and about one third are mosaic for the underlying disease. Germline mutations are most frequently truncating mutations (nonsense and frameshifts) that are associated with the most severe disease. However, single and multiple exon deletions may cause mild disease. Most mutations in *NF2* found on sequence analysis are pathogenic. Some missense mutations or in-frame deletions may be harmless (Evans, 2009b). Diagnosis of NF2 is based on clinical criteria; molecular genetic testing for *NF2* mutations can confirm the diagnosis because *NF2* is the only gene known to be associated with this disease. Methods of genetic testing for NF2 include sequence analysis, mutation scanning, duplication/deletion testing, RT-PCR, real-time PCR, array comparative genomic hybridization, and combinations of these. Large deletions encompassing *NF2*, ring chromosome 22, and translocation disrupting *NF2* can be detected by cytogenetic analysis, and smaller deletions can be identified by FISH. Molecular testing may also be used for appropriate surveillance, earlier detection, and early intervention of disease among relatives at risk (Evans, 2009a, 2009b).

Schwannomatosis is a recently recognized third major form of NF, characterized by multiple nonvestibular schwannomas in the absence of meningiomas, intraspinal ependymomas, and other clinical signs of NF2. Schwannomatosis and NF2 are clinically and molecularly distinct (MacCollin, 2003), but their phenotypes frequently overlap. In contrast to patients with NF2, multiple tumors from the same individual with schwannomatosis do not share a constitutional mutation (Jacoby, 1997; Kaufman, 2003). Schwannomatosis-derived schwannomas have been shown to have truncating mutations of the *NF2* gene (Jacoby, 1997). Commercially available *NF2* mutational analysis does not help differentiate between schwannomatosis and NF2 (MacCollin, 1994; Moyhuddin, 2003). Definitive diagnosis of schwannomatosis and its distinction from NF2 await identification of the schwannomatosis locus or gene.

SELECTED REFERENCES

Aldape K, Burger PC, et al. Clinicopathologic aspects of 1p/19q loss and the diagnosis of oligodendroglioma. Arch Pathol Lab Med 2007;131(2):242–51.

Detection of 1p/19q loss greatly improved the ability to accurately diagnose oligodendrogliomas, in particular distinguishing it from other brain tumors, such as astrocytoma and mixed oligoastrocytoma as well as to predict prognosis.

El-Zammar OA, Zhang S, et al. Comparison of FISH, PCR, and immunohistochemistry in assessing EGFR status in lung adenocarcinoma and correlation with clinicopathologic features. Diagn Mol Pathol 2009; 18(3):133–7.

Amplification and activation mutation of EGFR is associated with a number of cancers including lung cancer. This article compared various methods used in identifying the altered copy number, mutation and protein expression levels in lung cancer.

Halling KC, Kipp BR. Bladder cancer detection using FISH (UroVysion assay). Adv Anat Pathol 2008;15(5): 279–86.

UroVysion is developed and FDA approved method to assit in the detection of chromosomal abnormality for bladder cancer in urine specimen. Its utility in bladder cancer detection and treatment follow up is discussed in this article.

Kato K. Algorithm for in vitro diagnostic multivariate index assay. Breast Cancer 2009;16(4):248–51.

The above article reviewed the current knowledge for the marker development and their application in breast cancer including precurrence prediction with Oncotype, a21-gene panel, and Mammaprint, a 70-gene-microarray test, in women who have invasive breast cancer.

Oakman C, Bessi S, et al. Recent advances in systemic therapy: new diagnostics and biological predictors of outcome in early breast cancer. Breast Cancer Res 2009;11(2):205.

The above article reviewed the current knowledge for the marker development and their application in breast cancer including precurrence prediction with Oncotype, a21-gene panel, and Mammaprint, a 70-gene-microarray test, in women who have invasive breast cancer.

REFERENCES

Access the complete reference list online at http://www.expertconsult.com

CHAPTER 77

HIGH-THROUGHPUT GENOMIC AND PROTEOMIC TECHNOLOGIES IN THE POST-GENOMIC ERA

Martin H. Bluth

PART 9

KEY POINTS

- Completion of the human genome project has provided scientists with a detailed map of the human genome and predicted coding regions that have facilitated the emergence of high-throughput genomic and proteomic technologies.
- A number of mature platforms exist for high-throughput profiling of gene expression in human tissue, including serial analysis of gene expression (SAGE), DNA microarrays, and real competitive polymerase chain reaction.
- Proteomic technologies, including mass spectrometry and protein arrays, have begun to explore the dynamic and complex protein composition of healthy and diseased human tissue.
- DNA microarray and SAGE technologies have identified diagnostic gene expression signatures for a number of hematologic and solid malignancies that are often difficult to distinguish using traditional histologic analysis.
- Prognostic gene and protein expression profiles have been identified in a large number of cancer settings, including lymphoma, lung cancer, breast cancer, and acute myeloid leukemia, among others.
- Validation in large clinical trials, standardization of techniques and controls, and inclusion of analytic standards are needed before widespread clinical implementation of these technologies can be achieved.

OVERVIEW

With the complete sequence of human and other genomes recently elucidated, we have witnessed an explosion of information and high-throughput tools that are profoundly altering biomedical research and the culture of science. This revolution, which began in the mid-1980s, emerged from developments in three areas: (1) molecular biology, most notably, breakthroughs in rapid DNA sequencing; (2) information technology, in particular, the ability to store and analyze unprecedented quantities of data; and, most important, (3) progress in human genetics, especially the identification of thousands of single-gene human disorders. The convergence of these technological and scientific advances raises promise for the rapid identification of disease-related genes, leading to improved diagnostic tests and more effective therapies.

Detailed maps of human and other genomes provide the information needed to chart a course toward understanding and treating many diseases, but this course remains a long and difficult one. Although progress will come most readily for disorders following Mendelian patterns of inheritance, even these disorders will pose significant difficulties. For example, although the biology and genetics of sickle cell anemia have been reasonably well understood for more than half a century—a single valine replaces glutamic acid at position 6 in the β-hemoglobin chain—effective treatment has been slow to develop. The penetrance of genetic diseases thought to be due to single mutations often relies on more complex interactions between the mutation and a variety of concurrent gene polymorphisms, such as those seen in the genes encoding surface proteins on postcapillary venule endothelial cells, which, in part, account for sickle cell disease severity.

Many common diseases, in particular, cardiovascular disease, mental illness, and almost all cancers, stem from multigenic causes. In addition, these diseases invariably have strong environmental components, presenting a substantial challenge to the development of effective and economical diagnostic and prognostic tests. Even in the absence of a confounding environmental influence, linking the quantifiable phenotype of a disease to a set of distinct alleles is a complex undertaking. Further complicating matters, many disorders do not have sharply defined, quantifiable phenotypes.

In a chapter filled with information on promising technologies, we make these sobering remarks to emphasize that greater understanding never guarantees cures or therapies. However, greater understanding does aid the development of rational strategies to detect and control disease. The reference genome allows us to rapidly characterize polymorphisms across the human population; it also enables molecular fingerprinting technologies that permit identification of the precursors and consequences of normal and pathologic changes in gene and protein expression. We can feel confident that the power of genomic technologies is well beyond anything previously available, and that it will make possible during the next several decades a host of new diagnostics and therapeutics for cancer and other common diseases, profoundly altering the practice of medicine. As discussed in Chapter 72, genomic technologies have already made an impact in the area of pharmacogenomics, in which drug protocols are being designed from the cytochrome P450 genetic profiles of patients, allowing for maximally effective therapeutic regimens for each patient.

This chapter focuses on several high-throughput genomic and proteomic technologies that have the potential to influence disease classification and prognostication (Fig. 77-1). These molecular tools have affected virtually all forms of human pathology; however, given the public health implications and the preponderance of recent publications in the field, we will concentrate on diagnostic and prognostic applications related to cancer, although other salient disease states will be mentioned where applicable. After presenting a brief overview of the human genome project and resultant high-throughput technologies, we discuss examples of applications in the setting of several hematologic and solid malignancies. The scope of the chapter has been constrained to focus on high-throughput technologies; therefore, this chapter does not represent a comprehensive overview of all technologies being used in clinical genomic and proteomic studies. In addition, among the technologies presented, some are highlighted in greater detail because of their widespread use. As more data are produced using these technologies, strategies combining data sets may become powerful approaches to developing accurate clinical tools. Along with measuring gene and protein expression levels, understanding human genetic variation in DNA will be important in elucidating disease markers and mechanisms. A discussion of high-throughput genotyping technologies to assay single-nucleotide polymorphisms is, however, beyond the scope of this chapter (for reviews, see Ding and Jin, 2009; Syvanen, 2001).

The Human Genome Project

PUBLIC SEQUENCING EFFORT (HIERARCHICAL SHOTGUN SEQUENCING)

Sequencing of the human genome was a 15-year, $3 billion project, initiated in 1990 as a joint effort between the U.S. Department of Energy and the National Institutes of Health (Collins, 2003). From the time of the project's inception through 1995, genetic and physical maps of human and mouse genomes were constructed, and yeast and worm genomes were sequenced. These initial projects, coupled with advances in sequencing technology and sequence data analysis, outlined cost-effective strategies

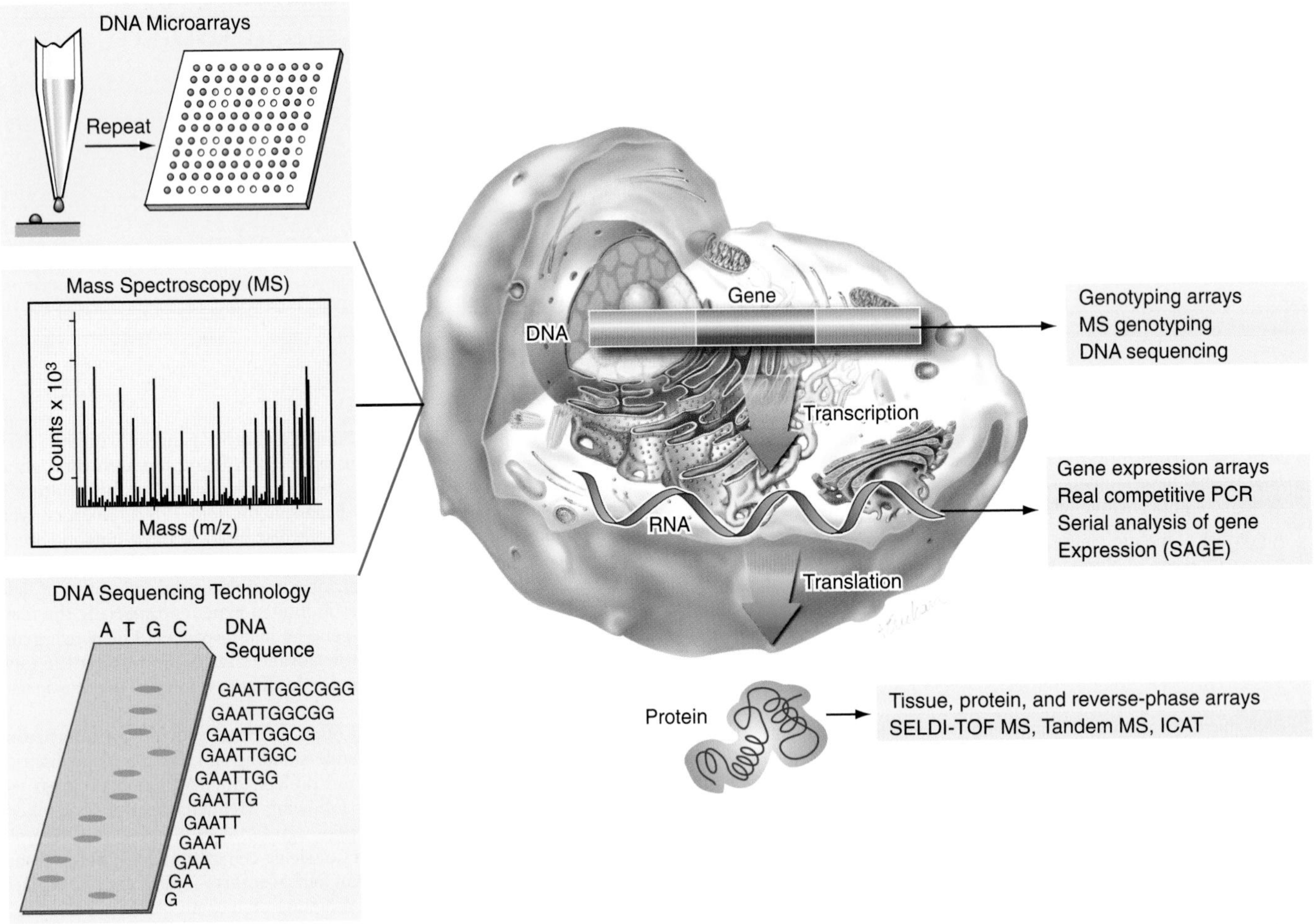

Figure 77-1 High-throughput platforms and the central dogma of biology. The three major technologies responsible for rapid analysis of biological systems include mass spectrometry, sequencing, and microarrays. Examples of each technology have been listed as applied to each broad stage of biological information, that is, DNA, RNA, and protein. *ICAT,* Isotope-coded affinity tags; *MS,* mass spectroscopy; *SELDI-TOF-MS,* surface-enhanced laser desorption ionization, time-of-flight mass spectroscopy. *(Adapted with permission from Kufe DW, Holland JF. Cancer medicine. 6th ed. Hamilton, Ontario: BC Decker; 2003; Wilson J, Hunt T. Molecular biology of the cell. 4th ed. New York: Garland Science; 2003; Brown TA. Genomes. 2nd ed. New York: John Wiley & Sons; 2002.)*

and techniques, while demonstrating the feasibility of sequencing the human genome. In March of 1999, the effort to sequence the human genome commenced in earnest, and sequencing was set to be completed in two phases: the first phase would include completion of a draft sequence, and the second would be a finishing phase for resolution of misassembled regions and filling in of sequence gaps. By June of 2000, centers involved in the project were producing raw sequence data at a rate of about 1000 nucleotides per second, 24 hours a day, 7 days a week (Lander, 2001).

The first phase of the Human Genome Project, a collaborative endeavor of 20 groups in six countries, was completed and published in February of 2001 in the journal *Nature* (Genome International Sequencing Consortium, 2001; Lander, 2001). The draft sequence covered about 96% of the euchromatic part (gene-rich) of the human genome and 94% of the entire genome, with an average of fourfold coverage (i.e., each base sequenced an average of four times). The International Human Genome Sequencing Consortium employed a sequencing strategy referred to as hierarchical shotgun sequencing (also known as map-based, bacterial artificial chromosome (BAC)-based, or clone-by-clone sequencing) (Olson, 2001). Genomic DNA obtained from volunteers from a variety of racial and ethnic backgrounds was partially digested with restriction endonucleases. Fragments of 1–2Mb in length were cloned into BACs. Eight DNA libraries containing overlapping insert clones were created, representing 65-fold coverage of the genome (each base is represented on average 65 times, as seen on examination of all eight libraries).

BACs containing fragments of the human genome are inserted into bacteria and are replicated as the bacteria grow and divide. Each BAC clone is completely digested with a restriction enzyme to produce a unique pattern of DNA fragments, known as a fingerprint. The fingerprints from different BAC clones can be compared to allow selection of a set of overlapping BAC clones that cover a portion of the genome (a large region of the genome covered by overlapping clones is called a contig). Contigs can be positioned along the chromosome by using known markers from previously constructed genetic and physical maps of the human genome. Selected BAC clones are sheared into smaller overlapping fragments, subcloned, and sequenced. Subcloning is necessary because each sequencing reaction can reliably read only about 500 base pairs (bp). The sequence of the BAC clone can be reconstructed from the set of sequences obtained from the subclones, and BAC fingerprints guide the assembly of several BAC clones into contigs.

Draft sequences were required to obtain an average of fourfold coverage with 99% accuracy as determined by software (i.e., PHRED, PHRAP; CodonCode Corporation, Dedham, Mass.) that assigns base quality scores and assembles sequences according to the scores. Throughout the duration of the project, sequences longer than 2 kb were required to be deposited in public databases within 24 hours (data are available from the Genome Browser of the University of California at Santa Cruz, www.genome.ucsc.edu; the GenBank of the National Center for Biotechnology Information, www.ncbi.nih.gov; and Ensembl of the European Bioinformatics Institute and the Sanger Centre, www.ensembl.org). Assembly of the draft sequence was a three-part process that involved filtering the sequence data to eliminate bacterial and mitochondrial sequences, constructing a layout of clones along the genome, and merging overlapping clones to produce a draft sequence.

The hierarchical shotgun sequencing approach was chosen by the public consortium for several reasons. Dividing up the work among sequencing centers was straightforward with the use of clones. Also, the assembly of clones to produce a draft sequence probably would enhance accuracy because approximately 46% of the human genome comprises repeat sequences and exhibits widespread individual sequence variation. In addition, this approach could address cloning bias, and underrepresented sequences could be targeted for sequencing.

PRIVATE SEQUENCING EFFORT (WHOLE-GENOME SHOTGUN SEQUENCING)

In 1998, a private company, Celera Genomics (Alameda, Calif.), led by Craig Venter, announced its intention of sequencing the human genome in 3 years using a different approach, known as whole-genome shotgun sequencing. Celera's draft of the human genome sequence was reported in the February 2001 issue of *Science* (Venter, 2001). Celera generated 14.8 billion bp of DNA sequence in 9 months to produce a 2.91 billion bp consensus sequence of the euchromatic part of the human genome with an average of fivefold coverage. The company used genomic DNA obtained from three females and two males of the following ethnogeographic groups: African American, Asian-Chinese, Hispanic-Mexican, and Caucasian. A total of 16 different DNA libraries were constructed with three different insert sizes: 2 kb, 10 kb, and 50 kb. Both ends of the insert from clones chosen at random were sequenced to produce "mate pair" sequencing reads. The average distance between mate pairs was known because the range of insert sizes for a clone taken from a particular library could be characterized by calculating the distance between mate pairs in previously sequenced stretches of the genome. Celera generated a set of 27.26 million reads with an average length of 543 bp.

Celera combined its sequence data with all data from the publicly funded efforts available up to September of 2000 in GenBank and pursued two different assembly strategies. The whole-genome assembly strategy involved "shredding" the publicly funded sequences into small fragments, combining these fragments with Celera's reads, identifying overlapping sequences, and joining them to produce long, continuous consensus sequences. These contigs were ordered and gaps between contigs were quantified using information obtained from the mate pair reads. A variant of the process described previously, known as compartmentalized shotgun assembly, yielded slightly better results because sequences were first clustered, based on mapping information, to a region of the chromosome, before the process already described was performed.

Analyses of draft sequences performed by the two groups yielded similar results. Some genes were derived from bacteria or transposable elements, and large segmental duplications were apparent throughout the genome. The distribution of genes, CpG islands, recombination sites, and repeats was found to be highly variable across the genome. Widespread genetic variation was apparent, and about 2.1 million single-nucleotide polymorphisms—1 per 1250 bp—were discovered. One of the most surprising results revealed by completion of the draft sequence was the estimate that the genome contained about 30,000 protein-coding genes, considerably fewer than the 100,000 or more that had been postulated. The number is only one-third greater than that of the worm; however, probably a much larger number of different proteins were noted because of alternative splicing (Claverie, 2001). Scientists used many gene prediction methods to arrive at the gene estimate of 30,000. Gene prediction algorithms predict the location of unknown genes in the genome using sequence characteristics learned from known genes, including codon and nucleotide composition within coding regions and conserved sequences at exon/intron boundaries and within promoter regions. The human genome sequence has a low signal-to-noise ratio because the coding regions represent only about 3% of the genome; therefore, algorithms produce a large number of false-positives. Most algorithms, however, use two other important sources of information: similarity to known human proteins and expressed transcripts, and homology to proteins and sequences characterized in other organisms (for a review of gene prediction algorithms, see Mathe, 2002).

FINISHING THE SEQUENCE OF THE HUMAN GENOME

In October of 2004, in the journal *Nature*, the International Human Genome Sequencing Consortium published an article entitled, "Finishing the Euchromatic Sequence of the Human Genome" (International Human Genome Sequencing Consortium, 2004). This article reported that the draft sequence was missing about 10% of the euchromatic portion of the genome, contained about 150,000 gaps, and had many sequence segments that had not been assigned an order or orientation. The current sequence contains 2.35 billion nucleotides, covers about 99% of the genome, and has only 341 gaps (with an error rate of 1 mistake every 100,000 bases). The sequence revision predicts between 20,000 and 25,000 protein-coding genes; this discrepancy in numbers is due to differences in gene prediction algorithms. The newly published sequence reveals that segmental duplications cover about 5.3% of the euchromatic portion, providing insight into the evolution of the human genome and aiding the study of diseases caused by deletions and rearrangements of these regions (e.g., DiGeorge syndrome) (Stankiewicz, 2002). This latest sequence also makes it possible to trace the birth and death of genes—genes recently born as a result of gene duplication, and genes lost as a result of mutation.

Sequencing of the human genome is a monumental achievement that "holds an extraordinary trove of information about human development, physiology, medicine, and evolution" (Lander, 2001). It has provided the infrastructure for sequencing other genomes and for understanding the structure and complexity of human genetic variation. This detailed map of the human genome and predicted coding regions has facilitated the emergence of several high-throughput technologies, through which scientists have begun to explore the complete set of gene and protein expressions in healthy and diseased human tissue. These technologies promise to revolutionize the classification of human disease and to usher in an era of individualized molecular medicine.

High-Throughput Technologies

Genomic

An intimate understanding of cellular machinery represents the first step toward unraveling the complexity of human disease. Important insights into the function of a gene can be deduced by determining the cell type and conditions under which a gene is expressed, and by quantifying the level of message transcribed. A technique commonly used to assay the level of expression of a single gene (represented by messenger RNA [mRNA]) across a few different conditions is a Northern blot. This "gene-by-gene" approach began to change in the early 1990s as a result of the success of the Human Genome Project and various technological advances that enabled the development of high-throughput gene expression analyses whereby several genes could be assayed simultaneously. Three different genomic high-throughput technologies are discussed here. SAGE (Velculescu, 1995) and DNA microarrays (Schena, 1995; Lockhart, 1996) were both developed in the 1990s and are currently in widespread use; real competitive polymerase chain reaction (PCR) using matrix-assisted laser desorption ionization time-of-flight mass spectroscopy (MALDI-TOF-MS) was first published in 2003 (Ding, 2003). The basic principles underlying DNA microarrays are discussed in Chapter 67; those underlying real competitive PCR are discussed in Chapter 66.

Depending on the experimental design, samples are obtained from cell cultures or surgical tissues, and total RNA is isolated. Techniques such as laser capture microdissection (Emmert-Buck, 1996) are often used before RNA isolation to obtain a homogeneous population of cells from tissue specimens. After total RNA or mRNA is obtained and is reverse transcribed to make complementary DNA (cDNA), each technology uses a different protocol to rapidly measure the transcript levels of the genes in each sample. The principles of each method, as well as corresponding advantages and disadvantages, are outlined in the following sections.

Serial Analysis of Gene Expression

SAGE measures the expression level of genes in a sample by isolating and sequencing several thousand short 10–14-bp tags isolated from cDNA. Two important pieces of information can be deduced from the output: the sequences of the tags usually allow identification of their corresponding genes, and the number of times a particular tag is sequenced is a measure of transcript abundance. The ability to uniquely identify a transcript using as short a sequence as 9bp resides in the probability of defining this sequence from others. Such a sequence can distinguish 262,144 transcripts (4^9)—a number greater than current estimates of the number of transcripts in the human genome (Velculescu, 1995; Pennisi, 2000).

The SAGE protocol involves isolating RNA from a sample of interest. RNA is converted to double-stranded cDNA using a biotinylated oligo primer for first-strand synthesis. SAGE then uses two types of restriction enzymes. The first one, called an anchoring enzyme, recognizes a specific 4-bp sequence (e.g., NlaIII). Any 4-bp–recognizing enzyme may be used because, on average, enzymes cleave every 256 bp (4^4). The anchoring enzyme leaves a short, overhanging, single-stranded piece of DNA at the 5′ end of the site of cleavage. The biotinylated fragment, which represents the 3′ end of the gene, then is bound to streptavidin beads, capturing only digested cDNA fragments that contain a portion of the poly(A+) tail. Captured fragments are purified and are randomly split equally into two pools. The second enzyme, called the tagging enzyme, behaves differently and cleaves DNA 14–15 bp immediately 3′ of its recognition sequence (e.g., BsmFI). The recognition sequence for the tagging enzyme is engineered into the sequence of linkers described in the next section.

After the purified fragments are split into two pools, two different oligonucleotide linkers, each containing a different PCR primer sequence (for purposes of discussion, the linkers will be labeled A and B)—the tagging enzyme recognition sequence and a single-stranded DNA overhang that is part of the anchoring enzyme recognition sequence—are designed and synthesized. Linker A is ligated to the 5′ ends of cDNA fragments in one pool, and linker B is ligated to the 5′ ends of cDNA fragments in the other pool. Ligation proceeds by means of base pairing between complementary single-stranded overhanging DNA ends on both cDNA fragments and linkers, creating an intact anchoring enzyme recognition sequence. The cDNA fragments in each pool are then cut with the tagging enzyme, resulting in a new fragment that contains the linker plus a short, 10-bp region of cDNA, known as a tag (the remaining cDNA fragment and the poly[A+] portion of the tail are removed). The two pools of cDNA fragments are ligated together, creating ditags (the new sequences are as follows: linker A–tag–tag–linker B). Ditags are amplified by PCR using primers designed on the basis of sequences in linkers A and B.

Creation of the ditags is important for several reasons. First, ditags can be amplified by PCR for subsequent cloning steps. Second, each tag within a ditag is linked tail to tail and is flanked by anchoring enzyme recognition sequences, providing important orientation information used to identify the genes corresponding to each tag. Finally, even if tags are highly abundant, the probability of creating identical ditags is extremely low. As a result, the occurrence of identical ditags indicates PCR bias, and these ditags are excluded from the final analysis to ensure accurate quantification of transcript abundance (Velculescu, 1995; Yamamoto, 2001).

After amplification, the anchoring enzyme is used to cleave the linkers from the ditags. Ditags from different reactions are ligated together end to end to form strings of 10–50 tags. The concatenated strings of ditags are cloned into plasmids and are sequenced. Typically, about 50,000 tags are sequenced for each sample of interest, using a high-throughput sequencer (for additional details on the method, see the review by Madden, 2000). The absolute expression levels of genes in the sample are quantified by counting the number of sequenced tags that corresponds with each gene. Figure 77-2 provides a visual scheme of the procedure.

SAGE technology has continued to mature, and technologies have been used to refine this technology toward its application, including an increase in sequencing efficiency (deepSAGE), improved tag-to-transcript mapping of SAGE tags (longSAGE), and reduction of the amount of required input RNA (microSAGE). The expansion of SAGE application from solely transcriptosome-based analysis to genomic analysis has given rise to Serial Analysis of Chromatin Occupancy, which identifies genomic signature tags that pinpoint transcription factor binding sites. Because of the advent of microSAGE, small amounts of material obtained from needle biopsies and from specific cell types (obtained via fluorescence-activated cell sorting or laser microdissection) are sufficient to allow characterization of global gene expression (Datson, 2008).

The Cancer Genome Anatomy Project of the National Cancer Institute has chosen SAGE technology to sequence more than 5 million tags across more than 100 different human cell types. Data are stored in a public database known as SAGEmap (Lal, 1999; Lash, 2000), and several tools such as SAGE Genie (Boon, 2002) are available for reliably assigning tags to genes and for performing data analysis and visualization. Additional information and details can be obtained at http://cgap.nci.nih.gov/SAGE or http://www.sagenet.org.

SAGE differs from microarray in that the former employs a sequence-based sampling technique that is not contingent on hybridization and does not require well-defined known genes or sequences. Through this approach, novel genes or gene variants can be elucidated. Furthermore, SAGE provides better gene quantification because it directly counts the number of gene transcripts and is less subject to background "noise" of the microarray; however, it is more expensive. Modifications of SAGE, such as longSAGE, utilize different restriction endonucleases as the tagging enzyme that cuts 17 bp 3′ from the anchoring site, generating a tag with a uniqueness probability of >99% and providing the ability to tag a greater proportion of the unannotated genome. Other modifications that require minimal quantities of mRNA for library construction (SAGE-Lite and Micro-SAGE) have also been described (Patino, 2002).

Microarray

DNA microarrays are orderly arrays of spots, each composed of DNA representing a single gene and immobilized onto a solid support such as a glass slide, as described in Chapter 67. DNA microarrays take advantage of Watson-Crick base pairing; therefore, only strands of DNA that are complementary will hybridize and produce a signal that can be used as a measure of gene expression. Production and use of microarrays requires several steps, including creation of probes, array fabrication, target hybridization, fluorescence scanning, and image processing to produce a numeric readout of gene expression. Throughout the chapter, a probe will refer to a nucleic acid sequence that is attached to a solid support, and the target will be a complementary free sequence of nucleic acids measured for its abundance with the use of microarrays. A detailed description regarding the fabrication of cDNA and oligonucleotide arrays, along with how the RNA is prepared and hybridized to these platforms, can be found in Chapter 67.

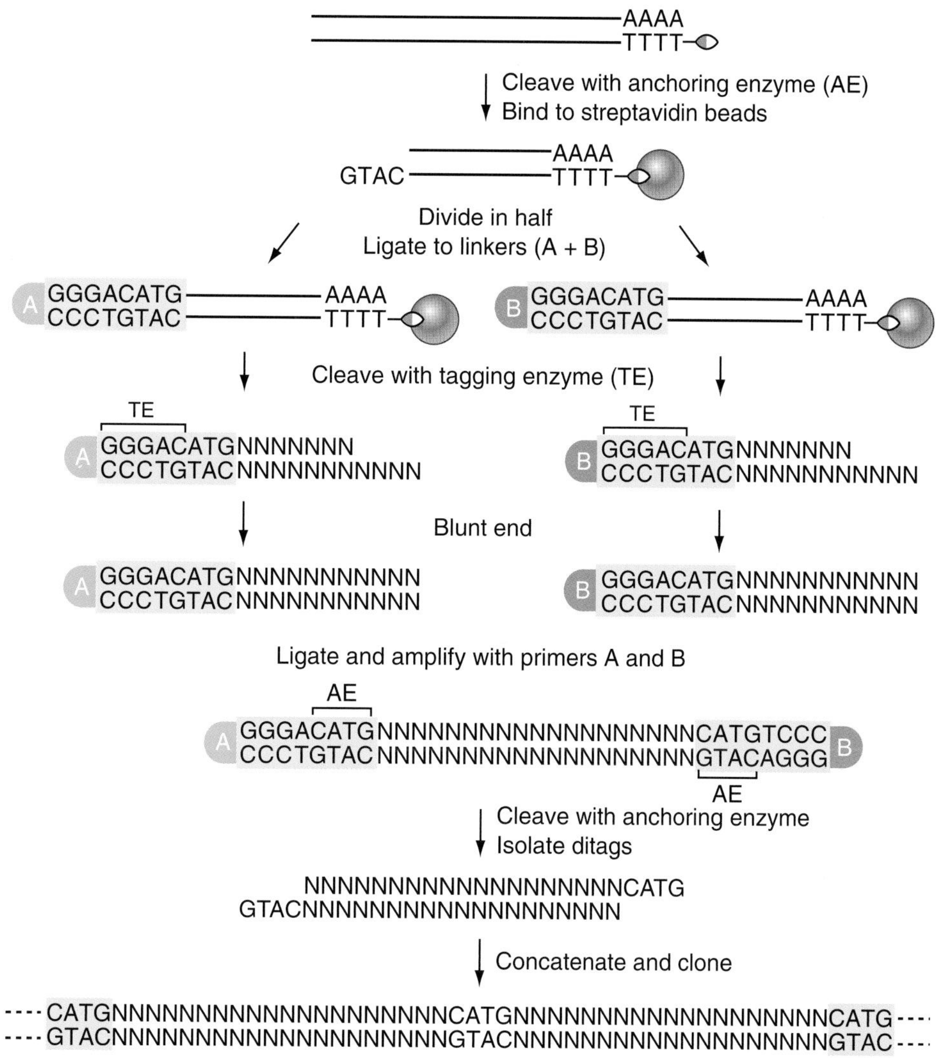

Figure 77-2 Serial analysis of gene expression (SAGE) is a technique that measures the expression levels of genes in a sample of interest. RNA is isolated from the sample, complementary DNA (cDNA) is synthesized, and several thousand short base pair (bp) tags are isolated. SAGE uses two types of restriction enzyme: one, called an anchoring enzyme (i.e., NlaIII), recognizes a specific 4-bp sequence and cleaves DNA every 256 bp, immediately 5′ of the sequence tag. The second enzyme, called the tagging enzyme (i.e., BsmFI), behaves differently and cleaves DNA 14–15 bp immediately 3′ of its recognition sequence. First, cDNA fragments are cut with the anchoring enzyme, captured using streptavidin–biotin affinity chromatography, purified, and split into two pools—A and B. Second, two different linkers (A and B) are ligated to the 5′ ends of the cDNA fragments in their respective pools. The cDNA fragments in each pool are then cut with the tagging enzyme, resulting in a new fragment that contains the linker plus a short 10-bp region of the cDNA, known as a tag. The two pools of cDNA fragments are ligated together, creating ditags, which are amplified by polymerase chain reaction (PCR) using primers designed on the basis of sequences in linkers A and B. After amplification, the anchoring enzyme is used to cleave the linkers off the ends of the ditags. Ditags from different reactions are ligated together to form strings of 10–50 tags. The concatenated strings of ditags are cloned into plasmids and sequenced. Sequences of the tags are used to identify the corresponding genes and represent a measure of transcript abundance. *(Adapted with permission from Yamamoto M, Wakatsuki T, Hada A, Ryo A. Use of serial analysis of gene expression [SAGE] technology. J Immunol Methods 2001;250:45–66.)*

DNA microarray experiments can produce millions of data points; this requires a suite of data processing steps to select relevant genes. Although no standard protocol is available, the following steps usually are included in analysis of a DNA microarray experiment (Fig. 77-3). Image files are converted to numeric values that are normalized and summarized using a software program (both free and commercially available programs such as Affymetrix [Affymetrix Inc., Santa Clara, Calif.] and Agilent [Agilent Technologies, Wilmington, Del.], among others, may be used) (Li, 2001; Irizarry, 2003); poor-quality arrays are removed from the analysis; genes that are not accurately detected by the array and genes that show little variation across samples are filtered out; and a variety of computational and statistical analyses are performed. Exploratory data analyses, including classification and identification of differentially expressed genes, can be divided into two categories: supervised and unsupervised methods. Supervised methods, such as class prediction algorithms, use predefined groups of samples (referred to as the training set) to identify genes that can distinguish between groups to accurately classify unknown samples (referred to as the test set). A large number of supervised class prediction algorithms have been applied to microarray data, including linear or quadratic discriminant analysis (Dudoit, 2002), k-nearest neighbors (Simon, 2004), weighted voting (Golub, 1999), artificial neural networks (Khan, 2001), support vector machines (Brown, 2000), and shrunken centroids (Tibshirani, 2002). Supervised algorithms such as significance analysis of microarrays (SAM) (Tusher, 2001), as well as parametric and nonparametric statistical tests between groups of samples, can be used to identify differentially expressed genes. Unsupervised methods, also known as class discovery methods, can be used to find previously unknown classes, such as novel cancer subtypes, within a dataset. Various clustering techniques, such as hierarchal clustering (Eisen, 1998) and self-organizing maps, are commonly used class discovery algorithms (see Kaminski, 2002, for a general review; see Leung, 2003, for a cDNA array analysis review; and see Tumor Analysis Best Practices Working Group, 2004, for an oligonucleotide array analysis review).

The Gene Expression Omnibus database (GEO; available at http://www.ncbi.nlm.nih.gov/geo) is a central repository for high-throughput gene expression data, through which a wide range of microarray data from published experiments is publicly available. All microarray data deposited in GEO adhere to the Minimum Information About a Microarray Experiment guidelines established to provide basic information about experimental designs, samples, and types of technology used. In addition to GEO, a wide range of bioinformatics tools is available for microarray data analysis (Quackenbush, 2001; Zhang, 2009). No standards for analyzing microarray data have been established, and various methods can often produce different results (for a discussion, see Tumor Analysis Best Practices

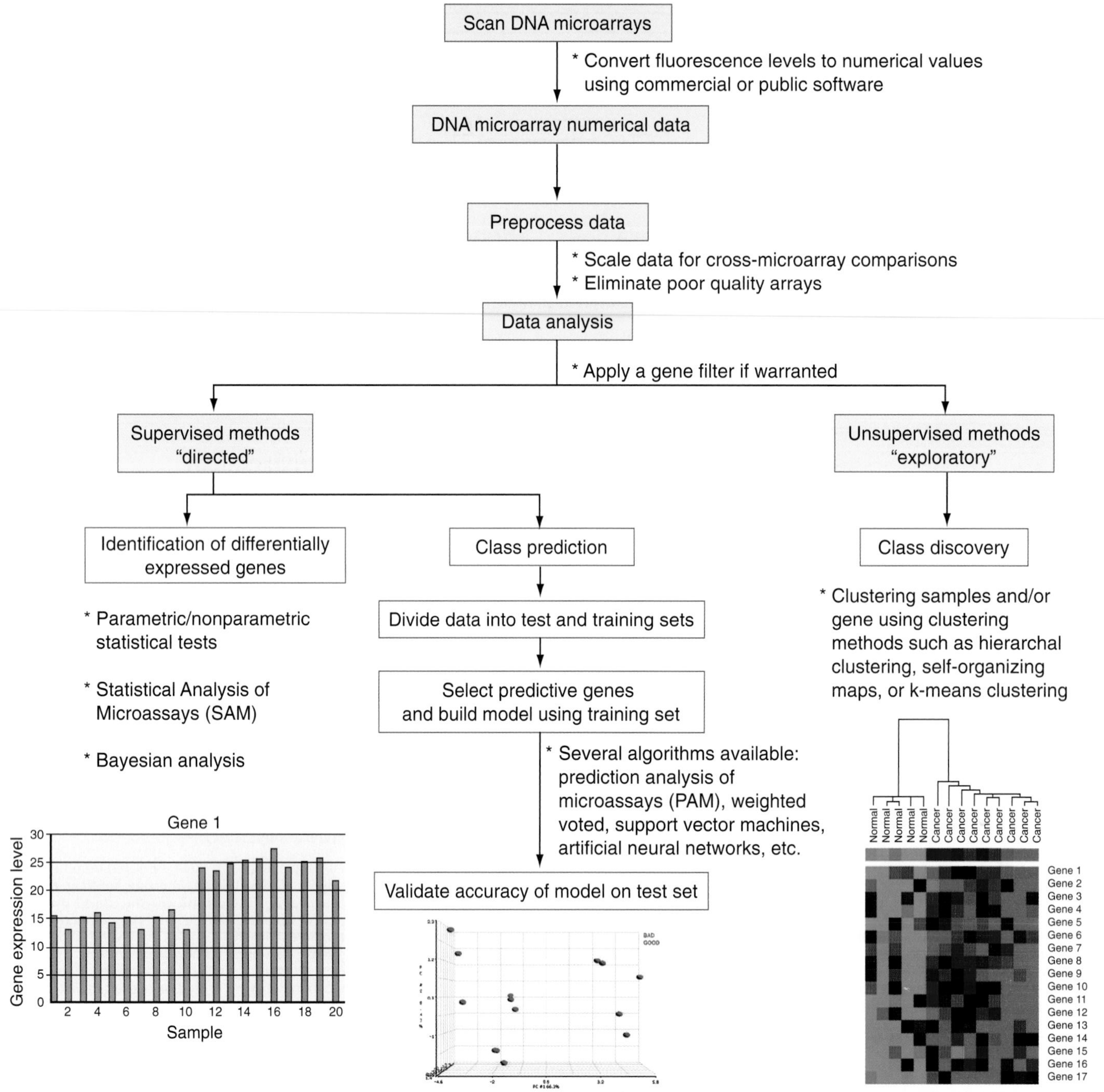

Figure 77-3 Analysis of DNA microarray data. The schematic diagram outlines the various steps required in the analysis of DNA microarray data. Image files are converted to numeric values and normalized, poor-quality arrays are removed from the analysis, and genes that are not accurately detected by the array and genes that show little variation across samples are filtered out. Downstream computational and statistical analysis of the data can be divided into two categories: supervised and unsupervised methods. Supervised methods, such as class prediction algorithms, use predefined groups of samples to identify genes that can distinguish between groups and can accurately classify unknown samples. Unsupervised methods, also known as class discovery methods, try to find previously unknown classes, such as novel cancer subtypes, within a data set.

Working Group, 2004). Validation studies with larger sample sizes or using a different technology are usually necessary to confirm significant findings.

Real Competitive Polymerase Chain Reaction

Real competitive PCR combines conventional competitive PCR techniques with single base extension and MALDI-TOF-MS to measure gene expression levels. The principles of mass spectroscopy are discussed in Chapters 4 and 23, and the use of mass spectroscopy in proteomics in cancer detection is discussed in Chapter 74. The use of MALDI-TOF-MS in high-throughput genomic studies is a recent innovation that is capable of absolute gene quantification with extremely high sensitivity and produces results consistent with real-time PCR and DNA microarrays. The basic principles underlying real-time PCR are discussed in Chapter 66.

Analogous to real-time PCR, use of this technique requires previous knowledge of the sequences of the genes of interest. Through this approach (Figs. 77-4 and 77-5), total RNA from a sample is reverse-transcribed using random hexamers or gene-specific primers. An 80–100-bp region is selected from the gene of interest, and primers are designed to amplify this region in a PCR reaction. A known concentration of an 80–100-bp DNA oligonucleotide of the same length and sequence, except for a single point mutation (known as the competitor), is added to the PCR reaction for amplification with the gene of interest. The competitor and the gene of interest will be amplified with the same kinetics because their sequences are almost identical; as a result, the concentration of the gene of interest can be calculated on the basis of the amount of competitor present in the PCR reaction. A series of PCR reactions are performed with different concentrations of the oligonucleotide competitor to accurately titrate the final concentration of the candidate gene. Next, each PCR reaction is

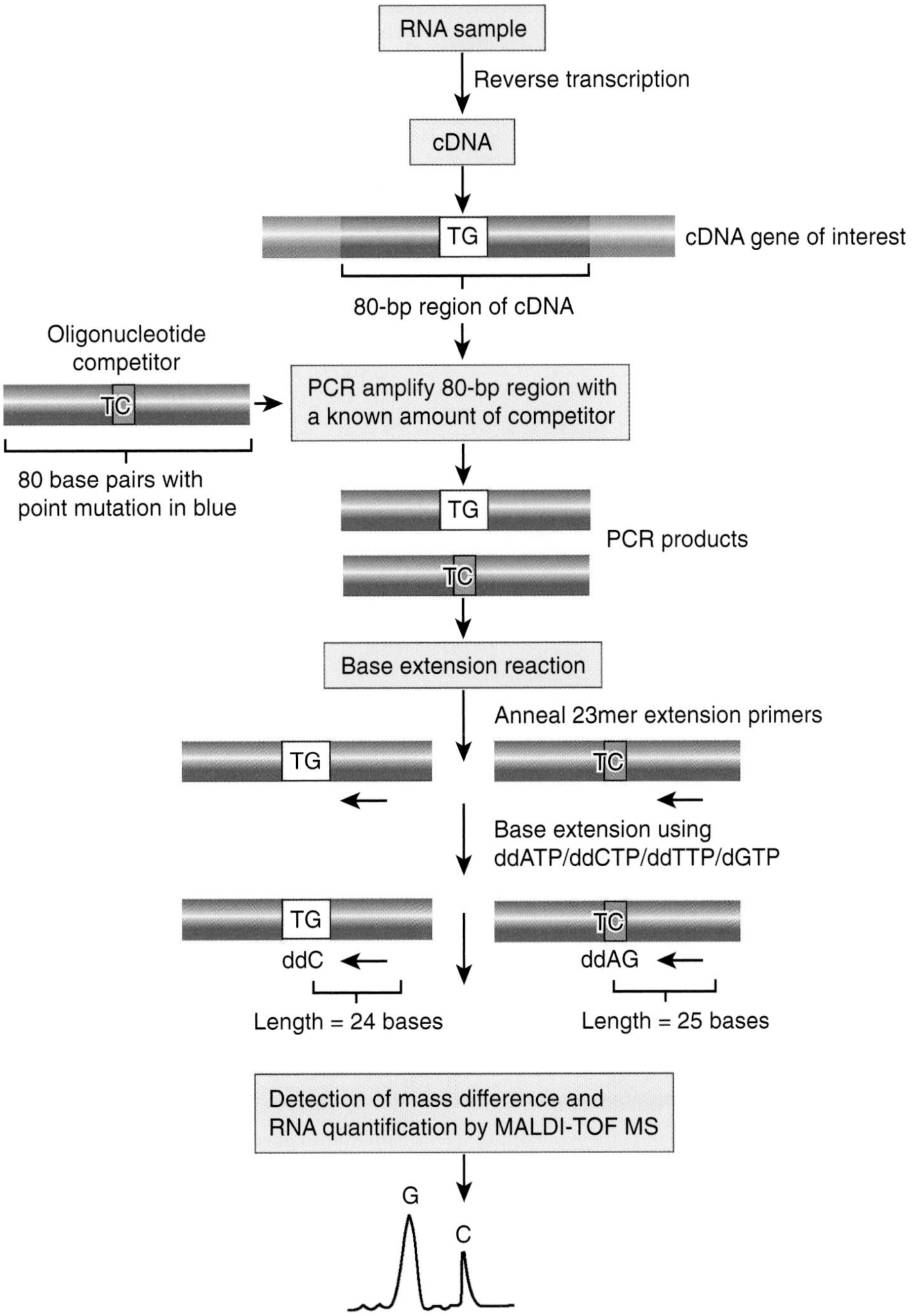

Figure 77-4 Real competitive polymerase chain reaction (PCR) coupled with matrix-assisted laser desorption ionization time-of-flight mass spectroscopy (MALDI-TOF-MS) is a technique used to measure the transcript abundance of a gene in a sample of interest. RNA is isolated, complementary DNA (cDNA) is synthesized from a sample, and a region (≈80 bp) of the gene of interest is selected for PCR amplification. A known concentration of an oligonucleotide competitor of the same length and sequence except for a single point mutation is added to the PCR reaction for amplification. A short base extension primer (≈23 bp) is designed to anneal to both amplified products adjacent to the site of the single point mutation. A base extension reaction is then carried out with three dideoxydinucleotide-triphosphates (ddNTPs) and one deoxynucleotide-triphosphate (dNTP) to produce two extension products that differ in their length by one base. As a result of this difference of one nucleotide, MALDI-TOF-MS is able to identify and quantify the two products on the basis of their different molecular weights. *(Adapted with permission from Ding C, Cantor CR. A high-throughput gene expression analysis technique using competitive PCR and matrix-assisted laser desorption ionization time-of-flight MS. Proc Natl Acad Sci U S A 2003;100:3059–64.)*

subjected to a base extension reaction. A short base extension primer (approximately 23 nucleotides long) is designed to anneal to both 80-bp amplified PCR products adjacent to the site of the single point mutation. A base extension reaction is then carried out with three dideoxydinucleotide-triphosphates and one deoxynucleotide-triphosphate to produce two extension products that differ in their terminal nucleotide. As a result of this one-nucleotide difference, MALDI-TOF-MS is able to identify and quantify the two products on the basis of their different molecular weights. The throughput of the assay can be increased by a technique known as multiplexing, whereby several genes are quantified in a single PCR and primer extension reaction using unique primers, competitors, and extension oligonucleotides for each gene.

This system, initially developed for high-throughput genotyping, was adapted for gene expression analysis in 2003 (Ding, 2003) and was marketed by a California-based company (Sequenom, Inc., San Diego); thus public data and analysis resources are in the process of development. Applications of the technique include measurement of expression levels for three genes in RNA isolated from buccal mucosal cells obtained from smokers versus nonsmokers (Spira, 2004) and measurement of allele-specific expression of *ABCD1*, a gene involved in X-linked adrenoleukodystrophy (Ding, 2004).

The three genomic high-throughput technologies highlighted previously use very different techniques to measure the abundance of gene transcripts; each technique has a unique set of advantages and disadvantages. A brief overview comparing the three different platforms can be found in Table 77-1. The major limitation of SAGE is that it requires many laborious PCR and sequencing reactions per sample and thus is high-throughput in terms of genes, not samples. Another drawback of SAGE is

PART 9

TABLE 77-1
Comparison of High-Throughput Genomic Technologies

	SAGE	DNA microarray	Real competitive PCR
Equipment needed	Sequencer	Arrayer (cDNA only), array scanner	Nanodispenser, MALDI-TOF-MS
Throughput			
Genes	Medium, ≈2000–20,000 tags/day, depending on sequencer	Highest, ≈40,000/array	Medium, ≈100/day
Samples	Low, ≈1/week	Medium, ≈10–20/day	High, ≈100/day
Cost	\$1500–\$2500/sample if between 50,000 and 100,000 tags are sequenced	\$500–\$1000/chip	\$1–\$2/gene/sample
Amount of starting material required	500–1000 μg total RNA/sample	1–15 μg total RNA/sample, as little as 10–100 ng total RNA/sample can be used with a modified protocol	5 ng total RNA/gene/sample
Gene sequences need to be known a priori	No	Yes	Yes
Absolute gene quantification	Yes	No	Yes

cDNA, Complementary DNA; *MALDI-TOF-MS,* matrix-assisted laser desorption ionization time-of-flight mass spectroscopy; *PCR,* polymerase chain reaction; *SAGE,* serial analysis of gene expression.

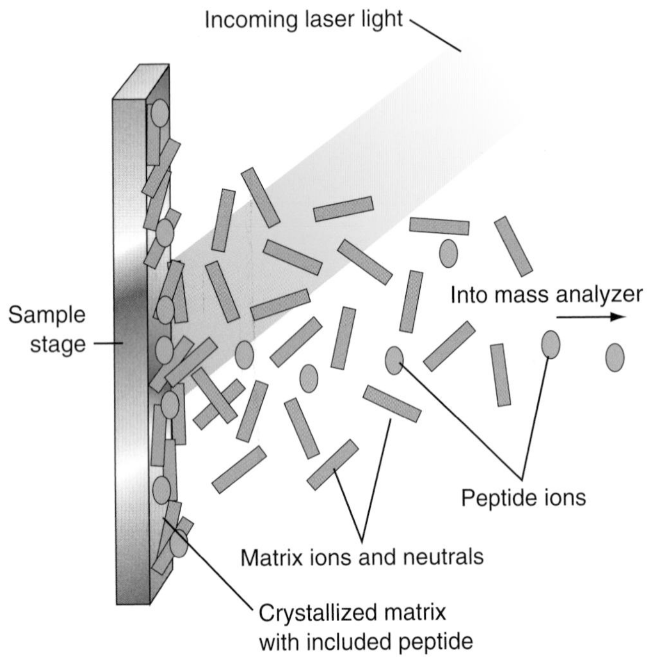

Figure 77-5 Matrix-assisted laser desorption ionization time-of-flight mass spectroscopy (MALDI-TOF-MS). A laser pulse provides energy for the matrix solution to ionize peptides and oligonucleotides, which travel downstream to the mass analyzer. *(Redrawn from Kintner M, Sherman NE. Protein sequencing and identification using tandem mass spectrometry. New York: John Wiley & Sons; 2000.)*

that it requires a large amount of starting RNA. However, as noted earlier, several modifications have been made to the protocol, and a new technique known as microSAGE requires only 1–5 ng of poly(A+) RNA (Datson, 2008). Advantages of the technology include that it is not based on prior sequence information, and that it is capable of discovering novel transcripts. The output from SAGE consists of sequence data that allow direct transcript identification with the use of public sequence databases.

DNA microarrays, on the other hand, are higher-throughput than SAGE in terms of genes and samples. DNA microarrays are practical for studies assaying clinical samples for which high throughput of samples is required and only small amounts of starting RNA can be obtained. The gene expression levels obtained from DNA microarrays are only relative transcript levels (in contrast to absolute levels with SAGE) that are dependent on probe selection, consequently making cross-platform comparisons difficult.

Finally, with the use of real competitive PCR, it is difficult to assay several thousand genes, because each gene requires the design of specific primers for the PCR and base extension reactions. Once the assay has been designed, however, the technique can be high-throughput in terms of samples. As a result, real competitive PCR probably will not be used as a discovery platform in the way that SAGE and DNA microarrays are used; rather, it will serve as a validation tool and a potential clinical tool for assaying relatively small numbers of genes across large numbers of individual samples. Continuously evolving Ultra High–throughput genomic technologies offered by various vendors (Illumina/Solexa, San Diego; ABI/SOLiD, Foster City, Calif.; 454/Roche, Branford, Conn.; and Helicos, Cambridge, Mass.) will likely be able to provide even greater throughput at reduced costs.

PROTEOMIC

Current proteomic technology offers a variety of promising high-throughput approaches to the investigation of cellular biology. As one moves from the slowly changing, relatively static genome to RNA transcription, and ultimately to protein translation and additional downstream modifications, the information becomes increasingly more dynamic. An estimated 30,000 genes (Lander, 2001) are present in the human genome and are translated into more than a million proteins (Anderson, 2002); the complexity of this system belies simple global analysis (Oh, 2004). Inability to amplify proteins often necessitates working with small quantities of biological samples. In addition, the range of protein concentrations, spanning several log units, can obscure signals of clinical utility.

Mass Spectrometry

Mass spectrometry (MS) is the tool used most often to investigate the protein composition of complex biological samples. (The principles of mass spectroscopy are discussed in Chapters 4 and 23, and the use of MS for detection of cancer-related proteins is discussed in Chapter 74.) Before the discoveries that made MS protein analysis feasible, protein identification depended on more labor-intensive techniques such as Edman sequencing or antibody-based assays. The major obstacle to high-throughput protein analysis using MS has been the technical difficulty of ionizing proteins. The innovations of John Fenn, working with electrospray ionization, and of Koichi Tanaka, who developed laser desorption ionization, opened the door to the field of proteomics. For their contributions to the field, both scientists shared half of the 2002 Nobel Prize in Chemistry. Electrospray ionization creates small, charged droplets of protein in solution. As the droplets move toward a vacuum chamber, the liquid evaporates, leaving behind a charged protein moiety. In laser desorption, a protein is placed in a chemical solution (called a matrix) in which high-energy electron beams are focused on the protein, resulting in its ionization. Once ionized, the mass-to-charge (m/z) ratio can be determined by migration of the protein in an electrical field.

Additional analytic problems arise from the elaborate structure of proteins and from the sheer abundance seen in most biological samples. With its secondary, tertiary, and quaternary structures, as well as its posttranslational modifications, protein structure is much more complex and is less predictable than that of DNA or RNA. Advances in protein analysis have allowed more rapid identification; however, many of these methods are subject to variation because of the context in which the protein is found, in particular, its shape and the protein environment in which it is analyzed. Separation remains an important step in reducing complex biological specimens into more manageable samples. Most of proteomic experiments rely on separation of constituent proteins over a two-dimensional gel, a time- and labor-intensive method that slows the discovery process and requires relatively large amounts of starting sample. Other techniques used to improve the resolution of data include proteomic analysis of whole-cell lysate, usually separated by high-pressure liquid chromatography, and multidimensional liquid chromatography.

Although the quantity of a peptide in a sample can increase the amplitude of the m/z spike seen on MS, other factors such as propensity of a peptide to ionize or surrounding ions at the time of measurement can also affect amplitude, making it difficult to comparatively quantify similar samples from different experimental conditions. The use of isotope-coded affinity tags allows quantitative comparison of samples. The tag consists of a biotin marker and a link, which contains eight hydrogens or eight deuteriums. To compare the amount of a single protein present in two different samples, one would label one sample with a light marker, the other with a heavy marker. This is done before MS analysis is performed, which would then show a series of paired peaks for individual peptide fragments, with heavy tag samples having an m/z 8 units greater than light tag samples. One can then compare the relative amplitude of the two samples.

Multidimensional protein identification technology allows identification of proteins in a digested sample. Protein fragments are introduced through high-pressure liquid chromatography into a tandem mass spectrometer. The m/z ratio for each peptide is measured in the first MS chamber, after which the peptide is fragmented. By comparing the relative weights of these fragments, one can determine the amino acid responsible for the change, in effect, sequencing the peptide. Measured peptide sequences are then matched to predicted fragments of known proteins, generating the identity of a large number of proteins from a complex biological sample.

Protein Arrays

Tissue microarrays produce a compact arrangement of sections from frozen or paraffin-embedded tissue, combining samples onto a single platform. Before the sampling advances described by Kononen, the number of sections that could be arranged in parallel limited the simultaneous investigation of multiple tissue sections. Currently, a tissue microarray can hold up to a thousand samples, which can be tagged and labeled via in situ hybridization or immunohistochemical assays (Kononen, 1998; Russo, 2003). Such large-scale parallel inquiry may provide a more rapid means of answering questions about the biological mechanisms involved in progression from normal tissue to neoplasia (Kononen, 1998), or the pathways related to variable prognoses among tumors of similar histology (Bubendorf, 1999), providing a ready means of validating results from other genomic or proteomic experiments (Chen, 2003), as well as tumor classification (Djidja, 2010).

Paweletz and associates pioneered the development of reverse-phase protein microarrays. Rather than spotting small sections of tissue, these slides hold arrays of whole-cell lysate from a specific cellular portion of tissue (Paweletz, 2001). Under the microscope, scientists can "hand pick" those cells of interest, capturing them with a small, focused laser that binds cells to an overlying transfer film.

In contrast to arrays containing tissue or cells of interest, other arrays can hold material designed to bind proteins from a sample applied to the surface of the array. Antibodies, DNA, RNA, and ribosomes—any substance with an affinity for a protein—can be used as a probe on the surface of the array. Manufacturing of these slides uses spotting technology similar to that described for oligonucleotide arrays (see earlier).

Molecular Markers for the Diagnosis of Human Neoplasia

GENOMIC

One clinically relevant application of genomic high-throughput technologies is the identification of diagnostic molecular markers for human diseases such as cancer. Histologic analysis complemented by immunohistochemistry, electron microscopy, and molecular analysis of chromosomal abnormalities is frequently used to classify cancers. Definitive diagnoses can be difficult to determine but are important because they often influence patient treatment, response, and prognosis. The first paper to use DNA microarrays in clinical samples to develop gene expression profiles for cancer classification was published in 1999 by Todd Golub (1999). Since that time, DNA microarrays have been used extensively across a wide range of malignant and normal tissue specimens in an attempt to develop diagnostic and prognostic tests.

As mentioned in Chapter 75, a pioneering study has been performed using DNA microarrays to distinguish acute myeloid leukemia (AML) from acute lymphoblastic leukemia (ALL). In this study, Affymetrix GeneChips containing approximately 6800 human genes were employed to measure gene expression of bone marrow mononuclear cells obtained from patients with either of these diseases (Golub, 1999). In this study, the choice of acute leukemia, a hematologic malignancy, was important for several reasons. Previous DNA microarray experiments had obtained reproducible results on cell lines; however, clinical specimens introduce additional noise that may obscure differences. Mononuclear cells reduce noise because they are a relatively homogeneous cancer cell population, in contrast to biopsies of solid tumors that exhibit varying quantities of surrounding stromal cells. In addition, distinction between acute leukemia subtypes is difficult with existing techniques, and the discovery of additional molecular markers would enhance the accuracy of diagnosis, ultimately influencing the choice of a therapeutic regimen.

To explore whether differences in gene expression could be detected between 27 ALL and 11 AML samples in this study, a method called **neighborhood analysis** was used. This method ranks genes whose expression patterns across patients are highly correlated with the class of the sample (ALL or AML). A gene that is expressed at high levels across all ALL patients but at low levels in AML patients, for example, would be highly ranked. Significance, or how likely the correlation is by chance, was assessed by randomly assigning class labels to each of the samples and repeating the analysis. Approximately 1100 genes were significantly correlated with class labels, and the top 50 genes were subsequently used in a weighted-vote class prediction algorithm that predicts the class of unknown samples. Each of these 50 genes casts a vote indicating the class of the new sample. Each gene's "vote"—AML or ALL—was determined by calculating whether the expression value for the gene in the unknown sample was closer to the mean expression value for the gene across all ALL or all AML patients. Votes were then weighted according to the strength of the correlation between gene expression levels and class vector. The votes for each class were summed, and the unknown sample was assigned to the class with the larger total vote. An additional metric, known as prediction strength, can be calculated to determine the margin of victory (for additional details, see http://www.broad.mit.edu/cancer/software/genecluster2/gc2.html, and Reich, 2004). The accuracy of this prediction method was evaluated by "leave one out" cross-validation, wherein one of the 38 samples is withheld, the analysis is repeated, and the class of the left out sample is predicted. Using this approach, this study found that 36 of the 38 samples were classified correctly, and 2 were classified as uncertain on cross-validation. The predictor was tested on an independent set of 34 additional samples and was correctly classified in 29 of the 34 samples. The committee of 50 genes contained known markers of lymphoid versus myeloid cell lineage, as well as genes related to carcinogenesis.

In addition to identifying markers capable of distinguishing AML and ALL, Golub and colleagues used an unsupervised clustering method known as self-organizing maps (SOM) to evaluate whether the two subtypes of leukemia could be found within the gene expression data without prior knowledge of the two leukemia classes. SOM group samples were divided into a user-defined number of clusters based on gene expression pattern similarities. Two-cluster SOM produced one cluster containing 24 of the 25 ALL samples and another cluster with 10 of the 13 AML samples. A four-cluster SOM was capable of distinguishing among T-lineage ALL, B-lineage ALL, and AML. The success of this initial experiment and its exciting implications, as well as improvements in DNA microarray technology, analysis, and availability, have resulted in an exponential increase in the number of clinical studies using microarrays. Additional information can be found in Chapter 75.

PROTEOMIC

In Chapter 74, a new approach to the early detection of several different types of cancer based on patterns of protein expression, called proteomics, is discussed as showing great potential. This approach does not search for specific known proteins but rather searches for differences in patterns of protein expression (the identity of many of these proteins is unknown)

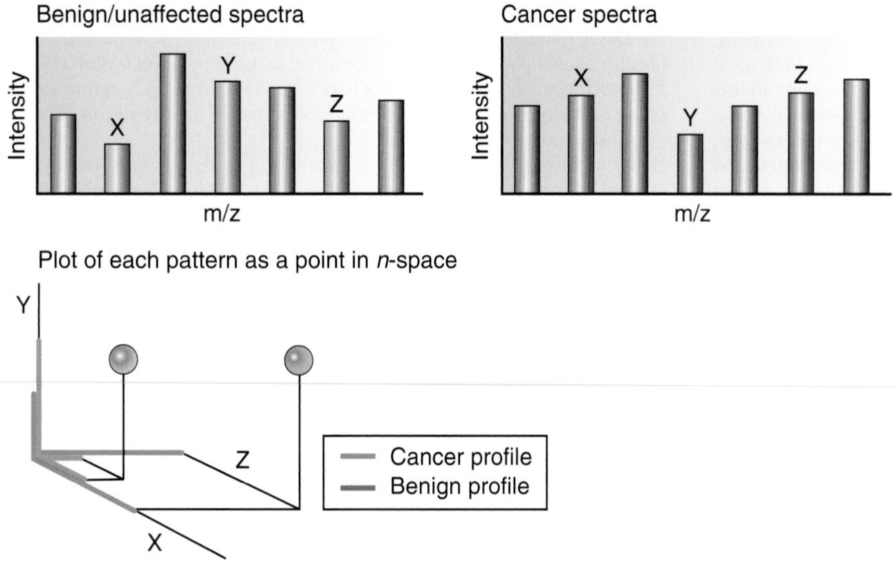

Figure 77-6 Proteomic pattern diagnostics. Pattern analysis identifies m/z ratios with the "most fit" combination of proteins for distinguishing between clinical states of interest. *(Redrawn from Petricoin EF, Zoon KC, Kohn EC, Barrett JC, Liotta LA. Clinical proteomics: translating benchside promise into bedside reality. Nat Rev Drug Discov 2002;1:683–95.)*

based on the use of MS. We discuss this approach further here to illustrate the power of high-throughput postgenomic methods in cancer detection. As noted, this approach does not identify the proteins involved but instead relies on the varying amplitudes of several different m/z ratios present across samples (Fig. 77-6). Given the more favorable prognosis seen with malignancies diagnosed at earlier stages, a great deal of interest has been expressed in using proteomic tools to search for diagnostic markers in readily available biological samples such as blood, urine, or saliva.

Patients with ovarian cancer frequently suffer a worse prognosis than those with other malignancies, in part because of the advanced stage of disease at diagnosis. In an attempt to develop a screening test for high-risk women, Liotta and colleagues used an MS-based platform to analyze serum samples of patients with ovarian cancer compared with controls and found that their model was able to distinguish between sera of women with and without ovarian cancer with a remarkably high degree of accuracy (Petricoin, 2002).

Their method utilizes SELDI-TOF-MS: surface-enhanced laser desorption ionization (SELDI) coupled with a mass spectrometer that measures the time of flight of ionized proteins from laser to detector. Serum samples are placed on a chip with embedded weak cations, which provide the "surface enhancement" of SELDI. Excess serum is washed off, and proteins bound to weak cations remain on the chip, where they are combined with a matrix solution and ionized when exposed to a laser.

Each serum sample results in approximately 15,000 m/z values of varying amplitude. The bioinformatic tools used to parse through such a complicated data set rely on class prediction based on a genetic algorithm. Class prediction involves a "training" set of known cancer and noncancer samples. The genetic algorithm selects a panel of m/z values and tests its ability to differentiate between cancer and control. The "genetics" of a genetic algorithm represents a biological analogy describing repeated mixing and matching of the most successful m/z values, allowing "survival of the fittest" values in successive generations of testing, ultimately producing the most discriminatory panels, which are then tested on a "masked" group of patients and controls (i.e., the condition of each patient is withheld before the test result is obtained).

Although the panel used in this study resulted in a test with 100% sensitivity and 95% specificity, validation in a more realistic clinical setting remains to be done. The idea of studying a group of markers in parallel would seem appropriate, given the complexity of tumor biology and its interaction with the host. The absence of protein identification with this technique constrains the test. It is not clear whether the values included represent participants in tumor biology shed into the bloodstream or nonspecific markers of inflammation. With 15,000 data points to choose from in each serum sample, the risk of overfitting any model so that it would have little clinical utility in a practical setting is significant. In addition, array-based assessments may not correlate with classical diagnostic approaches (immunohistochemistry) or with survival (Dahl Steffensen, 2010) and may differ depending on the choice of specimen interrogated (Sanchez-Carbayo, 2010).

Diagnostic Cancer Applications

SMALL, ROUND BLUE CELL TUMORS

(See also Chapter 76.)

Another cancer that is difficult to accurately diagnose using a variety of histologic and specialized molecular analyses is small, round blue cell tumor (SRBT) of childhood, which includes neuroblastoma, rhabdomyosarcoma, non-Hodgkin lymphoma, and the Ewing family of tumors (EWS). Ewing's sarcomas are discussed in Chapter 76, where we noted that the most common characteristic finding is the t(11;22) translocation, which juxtaposes the *FLI1*and *EWSR1* genes, giving rise to chimeric *(EWSR1-FLI1)* mRNAs and protein.

Khan and colleagues were among the first to identify molecular markers predictive of SRBT subtypes (Khan, 2001). Predictive genes were chosen using artificial neural networks (ANNs), which are pattern recognition computer programs modeled after the neural structure and behavior of the human brain. Similar to the human brain, ANNs are capable of learning from experience. A neuron can accept many inputs but has only one output, and, in an analogous manner, artificial neurons output a signal based on several inputs. ANNs consist of several connected artificial neurons that can recognize patterns in training data through optimization of several parameters (weights assigned to the links between neurons) to accurately predict the tumor type of unknown samples.

Khan and colleagues used cDNA microarray containing 6567 genes to measure the gene expression of 63 samples, which included both tumor biopsies (13 EWS and 10 rhabdomyosarcoma) and cell lines (10 EWS, 10 rhabdomyosarcoma, 12 neuroblastoma, and 8 Burkitt lymphoma, a subset of non-Hodgkin lymphoma). Using a filtered set of 2308 genes, the 63 samples representing four SRBT diagnostic categories were used to train linear ANN models. A total of 96 probes corresponding to 93 genes were selected on the basis of ANN models because they minimized the misclassification error rate to 0%. The algorithm was validated on a test set of 25 samples that consisted of a mixture of cell lines, tumor biopsies, and five non-SRBTs. In all, 17 SRBT test samples were classified correctly, and the remaining three SRBTs, along with the five non-SRBTs, could not be assigned a subtype. It is interesting to note that even though only data from neuroblastoma cell lines were used in the training set, the model accurately predicted neuroblastoma tumor biopsy specimens in the test set. Results suggest that the use of cell lines may be beneficial in reducing noise created by stromal contamination of tumor specimens.

Many of the 96 predictive genes reported in the study just discussed were expressed at high levels in one, two, or three of the four diagnostic categories. One marker, MIC2, is currently used to diagnose EWS, although this is not so specific as the *(EWSR1-FLI1)* fusion genes and their products. Also, MIC2 was highly expressed in EWS and in some rhabdomyosarcomas, suggesting that the marker may lack specificity when used alone. Another molecular marker, FGFR4, a tyrosine kinase receptor related to myogenesis and upregulated only in rhabdomyosarcoma samples, was investigated by immunostaining across a variety of tissues. FGFR4 was found to be upregulated in some other cancers and normal tissues, providing clues to its potential biological importance, while reducing its potential as a specific molecular marker. This finding illustrates that a compendium of genes, instead of a single molecular marker, may increase diagnostic sensitivity and specificity. This complements the conclusions of Chapter 74 on oncoproteins in tumor diagnosis: arrays of oncoproteins are more effective than individual oncoproteins in early tumor detection.

BARRETT'S ESOPHAGUS

In addition to these studies, several other DNA microarray and SAGE experiments have been conducted to develop diagnostic tests for human cancers that are difficult to classify using conventional histologic methods. Barrett's esophagus, in which the lining of the esophagus is replaced with a metaplastic columnar lining, is a condition associated with gastroesophageal reflux disease that can lead to the development of squamous cell carcinoma or adenocarcinoma. Esophageal cancer is usually difficult to detect at an early stage and has a high mortality rate. Hierarchical clustering and ANNs were used to discover gene expression profiles measured by cDNA microarrays that could distinguish between esophageal cancer and Barrett's metaplasia specimens (Selaru, 2002; Xu, 2002). The expression levels of a small subset of predictor genes were quantified with Taqman quantitative reverse-transcriptase (RT)-PCR (Applied Biosystems, Inc., Carlsbad, Calif.) in 39 patients with Barrett's metaplasia or esophageal cancer to assess their clinical usefulness (Brabender, 2004). Other studies have demonstrated the utility of micro-RNA expression in prognosticating patients with Barrett's esophagitis (Mathe, 2009). In those studies, miR-21, miR-223, miR-192, and miR-194 expression was elevated, whereas miR-203 expression was reduced, in cancerous compared with noncancerous tissue obtained from the same patient (tissue pairs), and reduced levels of miR-375 were strongly correlated with worse prognosis in Barrett's patients. Collectively, these studies illustrate the potential of array-based interrogation toward diagnostic and prognostic application.

THYROID

In Chapter 76, we discuss the most common genetic lesions that have been found in thyroid carcinomas. About half of follicular thyroid carcinomas contain oncogenic ras, and many also express the *PAX8-PPARγ* fusion gene and its products. A high percentage of papillary thyroid carcinomas express mutant *BRAF* and *RET/PTC* gene rearrangements. Medullary thyroid carcinomas express mutant forms of *RET* (as opposed to fusion gene products).

Distinguishing Follicular Thyroid Carcinoma from Adenoma

New diagnostic molecular markers are needed to distinguish between follicular-patterned thyroid lesions as to whether they are benign or malignant. Papillary thyroid carcinoma is usually diagnosed with fine-needle aspiration (FNA) after detection of a thyroid nodule and can be further characterized by its expression of the markers noted previously and in Chapter 76; however, FNA cannot differentiate between follicular thyroid adenoma (FTA) and follicular thyroid carcinoma (FTC); a more invasive surgical biopsy is usually warranted. Cerutti and colleagues have attempted to develop a preoperative diagnostic test by constructing and analyzing three SAGE libraries using an FTA, an FTC, and a normal thyroid specimen (Cerutti, 2004). More than 360,000 tags were sequenced among the three libraries, and 305 genes were significantly differentially expressed between the three groups. A subset of these genes was chosen for validation with RT-PCR on independent samples that included 10 FTAs, 13 FTCs, and 8 patient-matched normal thyroid tissues. RT-PCR was performed on a subset of the 305 genes: 12 of the most highly expressed genes in FTC and 5 of the most highly expressed genes in FTA/normal thyroid were chosen for validation with RT-PCR. Four genes (*DDIT3*, *ARG2*, *ITM1*, and *C1orf24*) validated the SAGE results and were able to predict 19 of the 23 samples correctly on leave-one-out cross-validation. In addition, immunohistochemistry was performed on 32 FTA and 27 FTC paraffin-embedded tissues using antibodies against two of the four genes, *DDIT3* and *ARG2*. *DDIT3* and *ARG2* showed staining for FTCs and negative staining for ARG2 in most samples, suggesting that these markers might improve the preoperative diagnosis of thyroid nodules. Thus these four genes, in addition to expression of oncogenic *ras*, are promising for use in the diagnosis of FTC.

ADENOCARCINOMA

Histologic identification of the primary tumor site in patients presenting with metastatic adenocarcinoma can also be difficult. SAGE data sets suggest that primary and metastatic adenocarcinomas clustered together according to their site of origin. A variety of RNA quantification methods, including DNA microarrays and SAGE, as well as the literature, were used to select tumor- and site-specific molecular markers (Dennis, 2002). Buckhaults and colleagues analyzed a set of 11 SAGE libraries of ovarian, breast, pancreatic, and colon adenocarcinomas to select five genes that could discriminate among these carcinomas of different tissue origins (Buckhaults, 2003). A class prediction algorithm, known as a two-dimensional gene expression–based classification map, was able to correctly classify tissue origin in 81% of 62 independent samples of ovarian, breast, pancreatic, and colorectal carcinomas based on RT-PCR data from the five genes. A related study, aimed at identifying molecular markers of metastasis in primary tumors, compared gene expression profiles of unpaired primary adenocarcinomas and metastatic nodules from different individuals across a broad spectrum of tumor types. A total of 128 genes were identified whose expression patterns could distinguish primary from metastatic adenocarcinoma (Ramaswamy, 2003). Ramaswamy and colleagues demonstrated that a subset of the 128 genes was associated with metastasis in independent data sets from primary lung, breast, and prostate adenocarcinomas, as well as from medulloblastomas and large B-cell lymphomas. These findings challenge the hypothesis that metastatic potential arises in a few cells in the primary tumor, and suggest that the ability to metastasize is preexistent in the primary tumor. If this is correct, gene expression patterns in primary tumors could potentially predict future risks for distant metastasis.

PANCREATIC CANCER

In Chapters 74 and 76, it was noted that more than 90% of pancreatic cancers express oncogenic k-*ras* gene and its ras-p21 protein product. Other common genetic lesions include aberrant methylations of a series of genes, including *p16/CDKN2A*, *APC*, *TSLC/IGSF4*, *SOCS-1*, *cyclin D2*, *RASSF1A*, *WWOX*, *RUNX3*, *CDH13*, *DUSP6*, *HHIP*, and *SLC5A8*. In addition, mutations in *SMAD4*, *PI3K*, and *p53* genes have been found in these cancers.

Microarray, semiquantitative PCR, and SAGE methods have been further applied to identify differentially expressed genes in pancreatic cancer (Iacobuzio-Donahue, 2002; Hustinx, 2004; Watanabe, 2005). Such prostate stem cell antigens as mesothelin and osteopontin were identified as overexpressed in pancreatic carcinoma, the latter of which demonstrated a sensitivity of 80% and a specificity of 97% for pancreatic cancer (Koopmann, 2004). Nonagaki and colleagues developed a three-dimensional microarray technology to assess RNA from endoscopic ultrasound-guided FNA (EUS-FNA) samples obtained from patients with pancreatic cancer (Nonagaki, 2010). They found that CDK2A, CD44, S100A4, and MUC1 were differentially expressed between cancer and noncancer groups subsequent to two orders of hierarchical clustering analysis. Furthermore, cDNA microarray analysis identified that the secreted protein acidic and rich in cysteine *(SPARC)* gene (also known as osteonectin, or BM-40) and its ligand *(SPARCL1)* are overexpressed in pancreatic cancer tissues, but not in their noncancerous counterparts (Jinawath, 2004). Specific SPARC protein antigens are now being evaluated as candidates for immunotherapy for pancreatic and other cancers (Inoue, 2010). These genes may therefore be important in the diagnosis of pancreatic carcinoma.

OTHER

High-throughput genomic technologies have been used in a variety of other diseases, including bladder carcinoma (Dyrskjot, 2003) (see Chapter 74), central nervous system embryonal tumor (Pomeroy, 2002), ovarian cancer (Sawiris, 2002; Tinelli, 2009), breast cancer (Perou, 2000; Porter, 2001, 2003a; Vera-Ramirez, 2010), lung cancer (Bhattacharjee, 2001; Ocak, 2009), hepatocellular carcinoma (Zender, 2010), and colorectal cancer (Buckhaults, 2001), to aid in disease diagnosis and identification of novel disease subtypes. The use of high-throughput genomic technologies to develop disease diagnostics is an inherently difficult problem because predictive genes identified by a training set are based on histopathologic diagnoses. The histologic methods used for classification of certain cancers, however, may be imperfect, making it difficult to assess the true accuracy of the molecular markers. In addition, it is difficult to verify the existence of novel disease subtypes found in DNA microarray experiments if no complementary histologic evidence is available. In the future, pathologists probably will use high-throughput genomic technology to facilitate accurate diagnosis in difficult cases. A majority of studies using genomic high-throughput methods have chosen, therefore, to focus on identifying gene expression profiles predictive of disease prognosis, given the limited number of histologic or clinical indicators of disease outcome (see later).

Application of proteomics in the search for a clinically useful biomarker has been reported in patients with breast (Kuerer, 2002), prostate (Ornstein, 2004), colorectal (Zhou, 2010), and lung cancers (Chen, 2003), among others (Djidja, 2010). When these techniques of detection and analysis are applied to prostate cancer, preliminary data from men with an indeterminate elevation of prostate-specific antigen (PSA) suggest that an **"ion signature"** is present (see Chapter 74) that distinguishes between men with prostate cancer and those with benign prostatic hyperplasia with 100% sensitivity and 67% specificity (Ornstein, 2004).

Because the serum represents a particularly complicated specimen for two-dimensional polyacrylamide gel electrophoresis (2D-PAGE)–based proteomic analysis, other specimens in proximity to the tissue in question may be more readily available and simpler to work with. Nipple aspirate fluid is easily obtained and, in the case of unilateral disease, allows for a simple paired sample from the unaffected breast. Kuerer and colleagues used 2D-PAGE in an initial descriptive study comparing protein expression in the nipple aspirate from both breasts in patients with unilateral breast cancer and a healthy volunteer (Kuerer, 2002). Their results showed highly concordant protein electrophoresis patterns when nipple aspirate fluid was compared from each breast in the control subject, as opposed to samples obtained from patients with breast cancer, which exhibited a larger number of proteins unique to the affected breast compared with the unaffected breast in the same patient. This finding suggests that localized breast malignancy significantly alters protein expression in nipple aspirate fluid, raising the possibility of a diagnostic marker pattern.

Prognostic Molecular Markers of Disease

GENOMIC

Patients diagnosed with the same type of cancer and treated using similar protocols often respond differently and have varying survival rates. Several clinical and histologic variables such as age, serum protein levels, and stage or grade of tumor can be used to assess a patient's prognosis with variable accuracy. Many studies have utilized genomic high-throughput technologies, especially DNA microarrays, as described at length in Chapter 67, to identify gene expression signatures that predict patient survival or relapse rates. Instead of comparing two different disease states, as detailed earlier in the diagnostics section, the experimental design for the development of molecular prognostic indicators usually attempts to stratify a particular cancer into subtypes according to outcome, using unsupervised or supervised computational approaches (see Fig. 77-3). The marker associated with poor prognosis may provide clues about the biological mechanisms underlying resistance to chemotherapeutics and may aid in the identification of new drug targets.

Diffuse Large B-Cell Lymphoma

(See also Chapter 75.)

Identifying molecular markers that predict patient survival involves distinguishing subtle differences between specimens; as previously noted in the diagnostics section, many studies have been conducted on hematologic malignancies in which a homogeneous population of cells can be isolated easily. Diffuse large B-cell lymphoma (DLBCL), the most common adult lymphoid neoplasm, accounts for 30%–40% of all non-Hodgkin lymphomas. DLBCLs commonly contain *BCL6* gene fusions, as discussed in Chapter 75. Response to chemotherapy is highly variable, and less than half of treated patients achieve long-term remission. Currently, the International Prognostic Index (IPI) is used to approximate the outcome of patients diagnosed with DLBCL based on several clinical factors such as serum lactate dehydrogenase and stage.

As noted in Chapter 75, a paradigm shift has occurred in the classification of DLBCLs based on the use of gene arrays. Here we discuss this approach further. Alizadeh and colleagues constructed a specialized cDNA microarray, known as the lymphochip, which included 17,856 probes chosen from germinal center B-cells, DLBCLs, and other lymphoma cDNA libraries (Alizadeh, 2000). In all, 128 lymphochips were used to assay 96 normal and malignant samples from leukemia and lymphoma cell lines and from patients with DLBCL, follicular lymphoma, and chronic lymphocytic leukemia. Hierarchical clustering of the microarrays revealed three subgroups of DLBCL samples based on genes related to proliferation: T-cells, lymph node biology, and germinal center B-cells. DLBCLs are thought to arise at different stages of B-cell differentiation, and hierarchical clustering of just DLBCL samples across the genes related to germinal center B-cells separated the sample into two distinct clusters: germinal center B-cell–like DLBCLs and activated B-cell–like DLBCLs, as discussed in Chapter 75. The two subtypes were shown to have statistically different overall survival (72% of germinal cell B-cell–like DLBCL subjects were alive after 5 years in comparison with 16% of activated B-cell–like DLBCL subjects), and the two classes could be used to further stratify patients identified as low risk by the IPI. This study was one of the first to relate tumor subtypes identified by global gene expression profiling to patient outcome. Use of DNA microarray in diagnosing this condition and further subtyping it into the germinal center B-cell–like group and the activated B-cell–like group is discussed in Chapter 75.

A follow-up study by Shipp and colleagues tested whether a gene expression profile could be identified, without prior discovery of subtypes, which predicted survival in DLBCL patients (Shipp, 2002). Affymetrix HuGeneFL microarrays containing approximately 6800 probes were used to measure global gene expression profiles across 58 patients with DLBCL (32 patients with cured disease, 26 patients with refractory/fatal disease). The weighted vote class prediction algorithm with cross-validation was used to identify a gene expression signature of 13 genes capable of distinguishing between patients with cured and those with fatal disease. The prediction model was also able to stratify patients into good and poor prognosis groups within categories defined by the IPI. As additional validation, results of the current study were compared with previous findings reported by Alizadeh's group. The studies used microarray platforms that interrogated two different but overlapping sets of genes. Genes used to distinguish the two subtypes of DLBCL in the Alizadeh study that were also present on the HuGeneFL microarray separated the 58 DLBCLs into two groups, but the groups did not correlate with overall survival rates. However, of 13 predictive genes identified by Shipp and colleagues, 3 were present on the lymphochip and correlated with survival across patients in the Alizadeh study.

In a related study, Rosenwald and colleagues used the lymphochip to study 240 patients with untreated DLBCL who subsequently received anthracycline-based chemotherapy (Rosenwald, 2002). Using a training set of 160 samples, gene expression levels were correlated with survival times using the Cox proportional hazards model. A total of 670 genes had expression patterns that were significantly correlated with prognosis, and these genes were clustered to identify sets of genes with similar expression patterns. Highly correlated genes were involved in similar biological processes, and four sets of correlated genes related to proliferation, major histocompatibility complex class II, lymph node biology, and germinal center B cells were used to develop a class prediction model. The gene expression levels of genes within each set were averaged, and these composite values were used to build a multivariate prediction model. The model was capable of assigning each sample in the test set a score related to the risk of succumbing to the disease. Scores assigned by the model to the entire set of samples were stratified into quartiles, with a 5-year survival of 73% in the first group compared with 15% in the fourth group.

Follicular Lymphoma

A similar survival prediction model was used to predict the prognosis of patients with follicular lymphoma, a cancer similarly arising from germinal center B-cells (Dave, 2004). Treatment may involve chemotherapy, immunologic therapy, or hematopoietic stem cell transplantation; however, no consensus has been reached as to which regimen is superior, and outcome is highly variable. Tumor biopsies from 191 patients with follicular lymphoma were divided into training and test sets. With use of the Cox proportional hazards model to correlate genes with survival, two highly correlated sets of genes were chosen to build a multivariate predictive model. The set associated with a favorable prognosis contained genes highly expressed in T-cells and macrophages, whereas the set associated with poor prognosis contained genes expressed in macrophages and dendritic cells. In additional experiments on biopsy specimens separated into malignant and nonmalignant fractions, two sets of genes signatures culled from the initial 10 set gene signature patterns were highly predictive of survival. These findings support the notion that immune-related responses by way of gene signatures reflect biological characteristics that may predict the length of survival.

The lymphoma studies already discussed demonstrate that microarrays may be successful in accurately predicting patient prognosis and may complement currently used methods such as the IPI. Results imply that biopsies obtained at the time of diagnosis can be used to predict prognosis and could influence treatment decisions. As noted earlier, however, disagreement between studies has resulted from several factors, including the DNA microarray platform used, patient population, differences in treatment regimens, sample size, the variable quality of long-term follow-up data, and choice of prediction methods (see Pitfalls section, later). The follicular lymphoma study also shows the importance of the tumor microenvironment—something that is not typically explored in DNA microarray studies.

Acute Myeloid Leukemia

In Chapter 75, patterns of oncogene expression in different phenotypes of AML that are currently used for therapeutic and prognostic purposes are discussed. Certain patterns of expression of these oncogenes suggest not only possible effective therapeutic regimens but also prognosis. For example, oncogenes found frequently in promyelocytic leukemia include the retinoic acid receptor-alpha (PML-RARα) fusion genes, whose presence suggests a favorable prognosis and indicates that treatment with all-*trans* retinoic acid (aTR) will be of therapeutic benefit. However, the presence of RAR fusion genes with other, non-PML genes, including *ZBTB16(PLZF)-RARA*, t(11;17)/*NUMA1-RARA*, t(5;17)/*NPM1-RARA*, and t(17;17)*STAT5B-RARA*, is a strong indicator that aTR will not be so effective, and that the prognosis is not favorable. In addition, core-binding domain fusion genes such as *RUNX1-RUNX1T1* and *CBFβ-MYH11* are expressed in other AMLs (such as myelomonocytic leukemia) and correlate with specific chromosomal abnormalities. The presence of these fusion genes suggests susceptibility of the tumor to high-dose cytarabine regimens and often indicates a favorable prognosis. On the other hand, the presence of the *FLT3* oncogene alone or together with these other fusion genes suggests a less favorable prognosis, despite the suggested chemotherapeutic regimen. Additional aspects of gene mutations that affect therapeutic responses can be found in Chapter 72.

Overall, the presence of specific fusion genes in AML does not always reflect the molecular heterogeneity of the disease because the presence or absence of other fusion oncogenes or mutations in proto-oncogenes may not be detected, and other genes, not thus far identified, may also be involved in the cell transformation process. To attempt to identify which genes may be involved in cell transformation in AML and to detect patterns of gene expression in AML that correlate with prognosis and suggest effective therapies, several studies using gene expression microarrays from patients with AML have been carried out. Despite potential problems with this type of approach, discussed in the preceding section, two studies published in the *New England Journal of Medicine* identified gene expression profiles that can be used as prognostic indicators in AML (Bullinger, 2004; Valk, 2004).

Bullinger's group used cDNA microarrays (≈39,000 probes) to obtain global gene expression profiles for 116 patients with AML, and Valk's group used Affymetrix human U133A microarrays (≈22,000 probes) to assay 285 patients with AML. Unsupervised hierarchical clustering in both studies revealed clusters that correlated with cytogenetic and molecular abnormalities present in the tumors. Using the Cox proportional hazards model implemented in SAM software (Tusher, 2001), Bullinger and colleagues identified gene expression patterns that correlated with survival. K-means clustering was used to divide the training samples into two groups, representing good and bad outcomes, based on genes selected by SAM. The prediction analysis of microarrays (PAM) algorithm was used to develop an outcome predictor using 133 genes based on the two identified groups in the training set. PAM was applied to the test samples and was able to separate them into two groups that differed significantly in terms of survival times. In this study, it was found that expression of so-called "forkhead" genes such as the forkhead box *O1A* gene (*FOXO1A*, also known as *FKHR*) in AML is associated with a favorable prognosis. On the other hand, expression of such genes as *MAP7*, *GUCY1A3*, *TCF4*, and *MSI* prognosticates a less favorable prognosis. Overexpression of genes involved in homeobox regulation such as *HOXB2*, *HOXB5*, *PBX3*, *HOXA*, and *HOXA10* has occurred in multiple different phenotypic AMLs, suggesting their importance in leukemogenesis. Expression of mutant or overexpressed *FLT3* was associated with a poor outcome, as discussed in Chapter 75.

Valk's group used similar methods to identify genes that could classify samples into disease subgroups previously identified by clustering analysis. These subgroups were associated with cytogenetic and molecular abnormalities, as well as with patient prognosis. Both studies demonstrated the usefulness of global gene expression analysis in dissecting the heterogeneity that exists within tumors of the same type. The high degree of overlapping results between these two studies shows the potential that microarray technology has to distinguish between subtle tumor subtypes and to add prognostic information to current clinical practice.

Breast Cancer

Although similar prognostic biomarker studies have been carried out in prostate cancer (Dhanasekaran, 2001), lung adenocarcinoma (Beer, 2002), and multiple myeloma (Tian, 2003), identification of prognostic biomarkers in breast cancer best demonstrates how successful high-throughput genomic studies can translate into important clinical tools. In Chapter 76, we discuss how the use of gene arrays has been successful in enabling prognosis and treatment of different breast cancers. The most important markers for these purposes are estrogen receptor (ER), progesterone receptor (PR), the proliferation marker protein, Ki67, and the *HER2/neu* oncogene.

Additional prognostic molecular markers were identified from gene expression studies using primary breast cancer biopsies from patients younger than 55 years of age with sporadic node-negative disease that did and did not develop metastases within 5 years. The predictive power of these molecular markers was deemed to be greater than that of other clinical and histologic factors such as tumor grade, size, angioinvasion, or ER status (van't Veer, 2002). Similar studies on breast cancer were subsequently conducted (van de Vijver, 2002; Huang, 2003, Sotiriou, 2003), and a recent paper describes the development of a predictive model that uses gene expression, clinical, and histologic data to more accurately estimate prognosis (Pittman, 2004).

One bottleneck to performing DNA microarray studies is the dearth of snap-frozen tissues obtained from patients with long-term follow-up. Snap-freezing tissue preserves the integrity of the RNA and is ideal for DNA microarray experiments; however, most tissue banks and clinical trials have collected paraffin-embedded tissue. Paraffin-embedded tissue contains partially degraded RNA that usually is insufficient to allow high-quality DNA microarray results (although advances in this area are ongoing; Drury, 2010). Technologies such as real competitive PCR and real-time PCR are being used to measure gene expression levels in these tissues, but the amount of RNA obtained from tissue blocks often limits assays to a few hundred genes. Using RT-PCR, Paik and colleagues studied 21 genes (16 cancer-related and 5 reference genes for normalization) chosen from the breast cancer DNA microarray studies outlined previously. Samples included 675 paraffin-embedded tissue blocks obtained from patients enrolled in the National Surgical Adjuvant Breast and Bowel Project B-14 trials (Paik, 2004). All tissue blocks were obtained from tamoxifen-treated patients who had node-negative, ER-positive primary breast cancer. Expression levels of the 16 cancer-related genes were used to calculate a score representing the risk of cancer reoccurrence at a distant site. Patients were stratified into low-, intermediate-, and high-risk groups based on the reoccurrence score. The reoccurrence score provided significant predictive information beyond tumor grade, age, and tumor size. The simplified 21-gene assay can be translated easily into a clinical prognostic test designed to help physicians decide which tamoxifen-treated, node-negative, ER-positive breast cancer patients should receive additional chemotherapy.

Prognostic molecular markers for breast cancer have been identified using SAGE technology. SAGE, unlike DNA microarrays, cannot be used to assay hundreds of clinical samples; however, it is not restricted to known genes, nor is it limited by the selection of probes on a microarray. SAGE is capable of identifying novel transcripts that have not been described previously, possibly because of their tissue-specific expression (an advantage in developing therapeutics). Two studies using SAGE libraries obtained from normal tissue, as well as from ductal carcinoma in situ (DCIS), invasive, and metastatic breast tumors, were used to identify transcripts that changed between disease states (Porter, 2001, 2003a). Several DCIS or invasive/metastatic "specific" genes were assayed by mRNA in situ hybridization using 18 frozen DCIS and invasive breast cancer samples, and by immunohistochemistry using 769 DCIS, invasive, and metastatic breast tumor samples. S100A7, a member of the S100 family of calcium-binding proteins, was preferentially expressed in DCIS (with highest levels restricted to high-grade comedo DCIS) versus normal or invasive/metastatic tumors. Although S100A7 is expressed less strongly in invasive tumors, its levels are higher in ER-negative, poorly differentiated, lymph node–positive tumors, suggesting that its expression in DCIS may be a useful prognostic indicator. In a follow-up study, Porter et al. further characterized dermcidin, identified in previous studies as preferentially expressed in invasive and metastatic tumors. Dermcidin is a 110 amino acid–containing protein that is expressed mainly in sweat glands and the pons of the brain (Porter, 2003b) and is proteolyzed to a 47 amino acid–containing peptide. The marker was expressed in a subset of invasive tumors by immunohistochemistry, and its expression correlated with larger tumor size and the presence of metastatic lymph nodes. In a subset of cases, higher expression levels were attributable to gene amplification at the gene locus on chromosome 12. Dermcidin was shown to enhance cell growth and survival and may be a promising prognostic indicator of overall and distant metastatic-free survival.

INTEGRATING GENOMICS AND PROTEOMICS

The development of high-throughput technology allows one not only to look at how multiple genes or proteins might predict a clinical feature of interest, but also to study overlap in transcriptional activity and protein translation. Chen and colleagues looked at the ability of genetic profiling and protein translation in lung adenocarcinoma to predict survival (Chen, 2003). After filtering low-abundance genes, they found approximately 5000 genes consistently expressed across a cohort of 86 adenocarcinoma samples and 10 normal tissue samples. Hierarchical clustering and leave-one-out cross-validation generated a list of the 50 genes that were most effective in dividing patients into high- and low-risk groups for mortality over several years of follow-up. Of particular interest was the observation that stage I patients, those most likely to experience a surgical cure of their disease, could also be divided into high- and low-risk groups, potentially identifying a novel group that would benefit from adjuvant chemotherapy.

A total of 76 tumor samples underwent both microarray and proteomic analysis. In the examples of genes found along with their corresponding protein products, correlation peaked at 0.39. Although statistically significant, the low degree of correlation underlines the point that the oversimplified model of transcription and translation is in reality a much more elaborate system of translational regulation, glycosylation, phosphorylation, and additional downstream modifications. As the authors conclude, many of the transcripts probably do not correlate well with their protein counterparts as a result of this continued posttranslational development. Extension of their investigation to include genomics and proteomics uncovered a significant cohort of genes and proteins involved in the glycolytic pathway and upregulated among patients with a high risk of mortality, suggesting that this integration of genomics and proteomics has particular value in shedding light on the molecular pathogenesis of disease states.

Pitfalls of Molecular Markers for Both Prognostics and Diagnostics

MICROARRAY DATA SETS

Diffuse large B-cell lymphoma studies conducted by Alizadeh and Shipp (2000) identified subsets of genes that specified two subtypes of DLBCL patients who differed in terms of survival. Shipp and colleagues also identified two subtypes of DLBCL patients; however, these types did not correlate with survival. The example presented earlier illustrates one of many DNA microarray studies in which little or no overlap of results is evident. Several potential causes seen in the experimental design and analysis of DNA microarray results may account for the widespread discrepancies (Simon, 2003). Two different studies performed using similar tissue samples may involve slightly different patient populations and sample sizes. Tissue heterogeneity is also a problem. Biopsies obtained from different locations have varying numbers of normal cells contaminating the tumor samples. Additionally, no "standard" is used for preprocessing and analyzing microarray data. New computational approaches are continually emerging, and two groups analyzing the same data set will often produce disparate gene lists. Finally, methods used to compare data sets generated using different DNA microarray platforms are currently being developed, and similar studies with nonoverlapping results may have employed inadequate methods of comparison.

"OVERFITTING" THE PREDICTOR

Traditionally, clinical studies aim to associate a handful of variables across several hundred patients, whereas DNA microarray studies contain thousands of variables (gene expression levels) across relatively small numbers of patients (typically, 20–200 patients). Many class prediction algorithms yield accurate results for samples in the study from which they were derived, but when they are applied to an independent patient sample, performance drops significantly—a phenomenon known as overfitting (Ransohoff, 2004). Results of DNA microarray studies therefore are most robust when the data are divided into a training set and a test or validation set (Ntzani, 2003). In addition to the need for independent sample validation, it is important for investigators to validate gene expression levels using different technology. To realize the true promise of these technologies, it is critical to develop methods that combine several gene expression studies to identify markers that are consistently correlated with disease class or outcome, and then to validate these markers using different technology and a different cohort of patients.

THE "BYSTANDER" EFFECT

Miklos and colleagues compared DNA microarray studies measuring prefrontal cortex gene expression in patients with and without schizophrenia versus nonmicroarray studies that included genetic, RNA, and protein measurements obtained through a variety of approaches (Miklos, 2004). Little overlap was noted between DNA microarray and nonmicroarray experiments. One reason for this may be that genes identified using DNA microarray studies are "bystander," that is, not involved in the pathogenesis of the disease state. Genes identified by genetic linkage studies are usually causally related to a disease; however, expression levels of these genes may remain constant because the genetic alteration affects only mRNA splicing or posttranscriptional regulation. Also, DNA microarray technologies may not be sensitive enough to accurately measure gene expression changes in genes expressed at low levels.

Despite the suggested cautions, DNA microarray studies in the recent literature have begun to explore the biological significance and therapeutic potential of promising genes in greater depth using in vitro and in vivo models. For example, using DNA microarrays, Tian and colleagues (2003) identified a gene, *DKK1*, which was differentially expressed in multiple myeloma patients with and without focal bone lesions. Patients with bone lesions expressed higher levels of *DKK1* RNA and protein. *DKK1* is involved in bone formation through the Wnt signaling pathway, and marrow plasma from patients with bone lesions was shown to block osteoblast differentiation in vitro, indicating a causal role in disease progression and a potential therapeutic target. Another study, using cDNA microarrays to study liver samples from patients with hepatitis B–positive hepatocellular carcinomas with and without intrahepatic metastases, found that paired primary and metastatic tumors had similar gene expression patterns (Ye, 2003). Many differentially expressed genes, however, were identified between primary carcinomas that did and did not metastasize. Osteopontin, a glycoslyated phosphoprotein that acts as a cytokine, was overexpressed in primary tumors with metastasis. Additional experimental studies showed that cellular invasiveness was reduced in hepatoma-derived cell lines treated with neutralizing osteopontin antibody. In addition, nude mice injected with hepatocellular carcinoma cells had a reduced incidence of metastasis when treated with osteopontin-specific antibody.

LIMITATIONS OF PROTEOMIC TECHNIQUES

Proteomic studies suffer from problems similar to those outlined previously for DNA microarrays, including tissue heterogeneity, overfitting of predictive models, and identification of causative disease proteins. Specific criticism of proteomic techniques for the diagnosis of cancer focuses largely on the SELDI-TOF-MS technique. Diamandis (2004a, 2004b), the most widely published critic of this approach, has outlined several shortcomings of the technology. Although several papers have published impressive diagnostic yields using a panel of mass spectra, or "ion signatures," few positive identifications of proteins responsible for those peaks have occurred. Some of the proteins identified have been studied previously as tumor markers but were dismissed as acute phase reactants. The absence of more positive protein identification limits the interpretation of published results, which potentially record differences attributable to something other than the underlying cancer, such as generalized inflammation.

The narrow dynamic detection range of MS technology also limits proteomic studies. In the case of serum samples, minimal preprocessing generally occurs prior to MS analysis; this involves surface enhancement attained through incubation on a weakly cationic protein chip—a nonspecific process that would likely bind only to the most abundant proteins in the sample, failing to detect potentially informative low-abundance proteins. One would likely not expect the proteins shed from a malignancy such as prostate cancer to be the most abundant proteins in a serum sample. By some estimates, SELDI-TOF-MS could not detect proteins at less than 1 μg/dL—a concentration many times higher than that of most known tumor markers (Diamandis, 2003).

Conclusions and Future Challenges

The recent completion of the Human Genome Project and advances within the biotechnology sector offer unprecedented opportunities for identification of biomarkers associated with cancer and other pathologies. Genome sequence data combined with high-throughput biomarker discovery will facilitate the correlation of genetic variation with disease diagnosis and biological outcomes. The emerging fields of functional genomics and functional proteomics offer the opportunity to translate these advances into a full comprehension of the pathophysiology of cancer and other complex multigenic diseases.

High-throughput genomic and proteomic technologies have the potential to transform clinical practice and are likely to lead to the supplementation or replacement of traditional diagnostic and prognostic biomarkers. Many of the studies detailed in this chapter have demonstrated the utility of gene expression profiles for the classification of tumors into distinct, clinically relevant subtypes and for the prediction of clinical outcomes. In addition, emerging proteomics platforms have just begun to add another layer of molecular information to the study of human disease. These technologies should lead to a new era of individualized molecular medicine, whereby all patients will be treated on the basis of genetic changes in their tumors and their own genetic makeup, resulting in more effective and less toxic therapy.

These high-throughput platforms offer the promise of influencing the practice of medicine. However, a number of obstacles to widespread clinical implementation of these technologies remain. Genomic and proteomic biomarkers are an emerging class of laboratory tests that present special implementation challenges for the clinical laboratory, including analytic, bioinformatics, and bioethical issues. Considerable efforts are required to provide the necessary clinical laboratory infrastructure for standard high-throughput analyzers capable of detecting genomic and proteomic alterations within a variety of biological samples and within various high-performance computing and advanced data management capabilities. Significant improvements in analytic tools are needed, as are efforts to standardize techniques, controls, and reference standards. The application of such information to medical diagnosis and treatment will require considerable changes in the training of physicians. The most pressing need, however, is for extensive independent validation of the profiles described in the previous sections using large, statistically powered data sets. Inclusion of genomic- and proteomic-based molecular profiling techniques into clinical trial protocols will be needed to realize the potential of this technology to improve diagnosis and to tailor treatment of human disease.

SELECTED REFERENCES

Alizadeh AA, Eisen MB, Davis RE, et al. Distinct types of diffuse large B-cell lymphoma identified by gene expression profiling. Nature 2000;403:503–11.

This study analyzed diffuse large B-cell lymphoma patient samples using DNA microarrays and was one of the first to relate tumor subtypes identified by global gene expression profiling to patient outcome.

Chen G, Gharib TG, Wang H, et al. Protein profiles associated with survival in lung adenocarcinoma. Proc Natl Acad Sci U S A 2003;100:13537–42.

Analyzed resected lung tumors that underwent both DNA microarray and proteomic analysis, and reported that gene and protein expression levels were mostly poorly correlated. However, integration of the two techniques revealed components of the glycolysis pathway associated with poor patient survival.

Golub TR, Slonim DK, Tamayo P, et al. Molecular classification of cancer: class discovery and class prediction by gene expression monitoring. Science 1999;286:531–7.

Describes the first use of DNA microarrays to assay the gene expression of thousands of genes in clinical samples (human acute leukemias) to identify new cancer classes and to predict the class of unknown samples.

Lander ES, Linton LM, Birren B, et al. Initial sequencing and analysis of the human genome. Nature 2001;409:860–921.

A thorough presentation of the history of the human genome project, the method used by the public consortium, the quality of the draft sequence, and the biological insights revealed by initial analyses.

Petricoin EF, Ardekani AM, Hitt BA, et al. Use of proteomic patterns in serum to identify ovarian cancer. Lancet 2002;359:572–7.

Describes how a mass spectrometry–based platform is used to analyze proteins present in serum samples of patients with and without ovarian cancer to develop a model capable of accurately distinguishing between the two disease states.

REFERENCES

Access the complete reference list online at http://www.expertconsult.com

Appendixes

EDITED BY

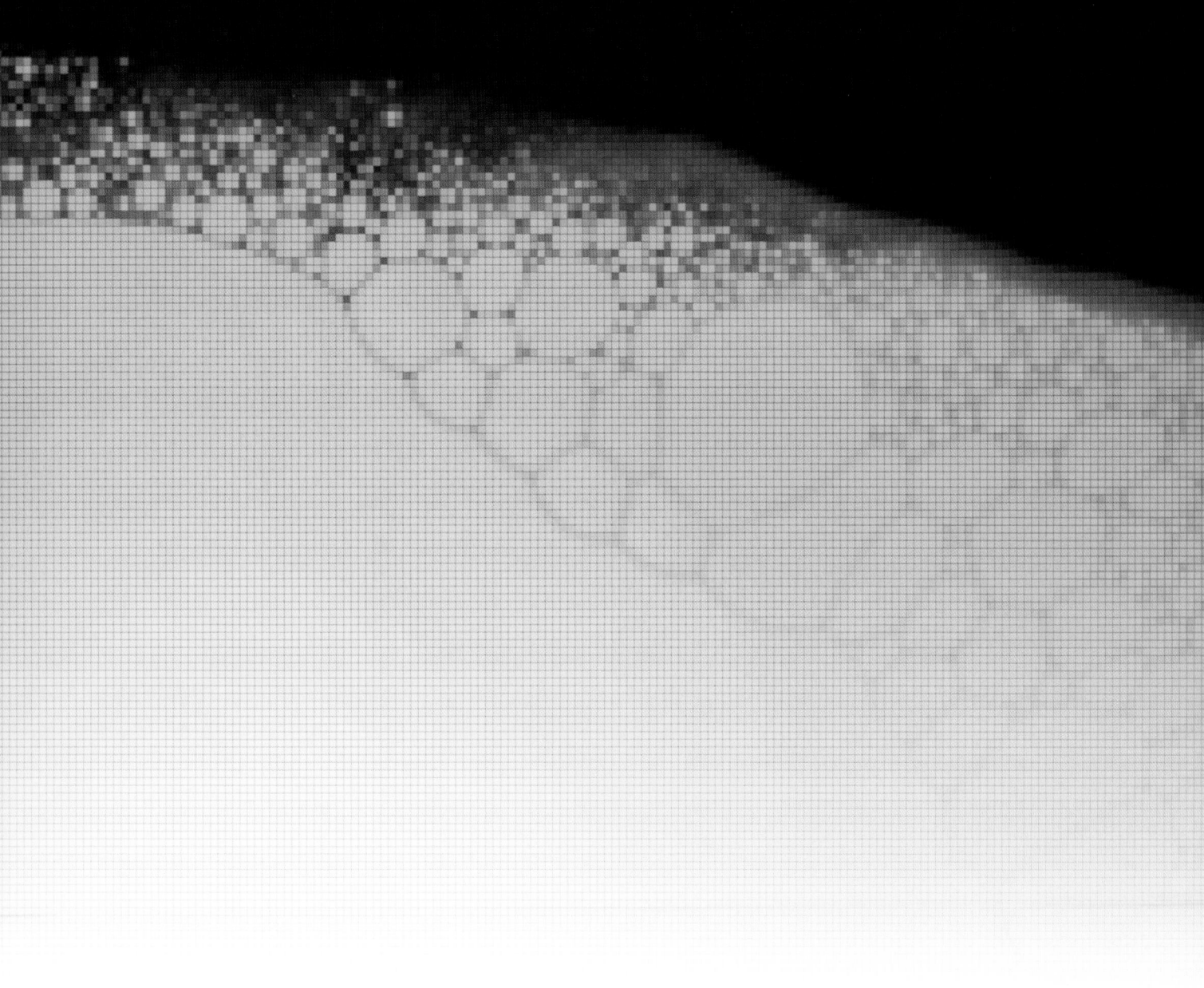

Richard A. McPherson
Matthew R. Pincus
Naif Z. Abraham Jr.

APPENDIX 1

PHYSIOLOGIC SOLUTIONS, BUFFERS, ACID-BASE INDICATORS, STANDARD REFERENCE MATERIALS, AND TEMPERATURE CONVERSIONS

Physiologic Solutions

A physiologic solution is one that contains various salts in concentrations that closely approximate the composition of fluids in the human body. The simplest of these is physiologic saline, which has the same osmotic pressure as the blood. There are more elaborate solutions, for example, to maintain tissues in a metabolically active state for longer periods of time. Table A1-1 lists formulas of some solutions that are isotonic with respect to blood.

Buffers*

Buffers have the ability to resist changes in pH. Buffers usually consist of a weak acid and its salt or a weak base and its salt. The Henderson-Hasselbalch equation is useful in calculating the acid (or base) to salt ratio required to establish a desired pH from a buffer system:

$$pH = pK + \log[\text{salt}]/[\text{acid}] \qquad \textbf{(A1-1)}$$

EXAMPLE 1

If the pH of a 0.1M acetate buffer is known to be 4.90, calculate the concentration of acetic acid and sodium acetate in the buffer (pK for acetic acid = 4.76).

TABLE A1-1
Physiologic Solutions

	Saline	Locke's solution	Ringer's solution	Tyrode's solution
Sodium chloride	0.85 g	0.9 g	0.7 g	0.8 g
Calcium chloride		0.024 g	0.0026 g	0.02 g
Potassium chloride		0.042 g	0.035 g	0.02 g
Sodium bicarbonate		0.01–0.03 g		0.1 g
D-Glucose		0.01–0.25 g		0.1 g
Magnesium chloride				0.01 g
Monosodium phosphate				0.005 g
Distilled water	100 mL	100 mL	100 mL	100 mL

*For a comprehensive discussion, including preparation of buffer solutions of a definite ionic strength, consult Bates RG. Determination of pH—theory and practice. 2nd ed. New York: John Wiley and Sons; 1973.

Substituting values of pH and pK in Equation A1-1:

$$\log[\text{acetate}]/[\text{acetic acid}] = 4.90 - 4.76 = 0.14$$
$$[\text{acetate}]/[\text{acetic acid}] = 1.38$$
$$[\text{acetate}] = 1.38[\text{acetic acid}]$$

Because the total buffer/L concentrations is 0.1M,

$$[\text{acetate}] + [\text{acetic acid}] = 0.1\ M \qquad \textbf{(A1-2)}$$

Substituting the value of acetate in Equation A1-2:

$$1.38[\text{acetic acid}] + [\text{acetic acid}] = 0.1\ M$$

Hence,

$$[\text{acetic acid}] = 0.042\ M$$
$$[\text{acetic acid}] = 2.52\ g/L$$
$$[\text{acetate}] = 0.058\ M$$
$$= 4.76\ g/L$$

EXAMPLE 2

If 648 mL of 0.025 molar diethylbarbituric acid and 10 mL of 0.5 molar sodium diethylbarbiturate are mixed and diluted to 1L, calculate the pH of the solution (pK for diethylbarbituric acid = 7.98 and molar concentration = moles/liter).

The following relationship exists between molarity and volume of a solution:

$$M1V1 = M2V2 \qquad \textbf{(A1-3)}$$

where, M1 = molarity of the initial solution, V1 = volume of the initial solution, M2 = molarity of the final solution, V2 = volume of the final solution.

Use Equation A1-3 to calculate changes in salt and acid concentrations after dilution to 1L:

$$[\text{Sodium diethylbarbiturate}] = 0.025 \times 0.648$$
$$= 0.0162\ \text{mol/L}$$
$$[\text{Diethylbarbituric acid}] = 0.5 \times 0.01$$
$$= 0.005\ \text{mol/L}$$

Calculate pH of the solution using Equation A1-1:

$$pH = 7.98 - \log(0.0162/0.005)$$
$$= 7.98 - \log 3.24$$
$$= 7.98 - 0.51$$
$$= 7.47$$

The maximum buffering capacity is at the pK value of the weak acid or base. For instance, for acetic acid with a pH value of 4.76, more acid is required to change the pH of an acetate buffer from 4.76 to 4.66 than from

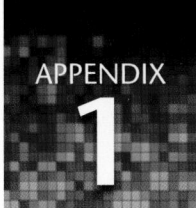

TABLE A1-2
Sorensen's Table of Buffer Mixtures

Na_2HPO_4 solution (mL)	KH_2PO_4 solution (mL)	pH
0.25	9.75	5.288
0.5	9.5	5.589
1.0	9.0	5.906
2.0	8.0	6.239
3.0	7.0	6.468
4.0	6.0	6.643
5.0	5.0	6.813
6.0	4.0	6.979
7.0	3.0	7.168
8.0	2.0	7.381
9.0	1.0	7.731
9.5	0.5	8.043

TABLE A1-3
Tris(hydroxymethyl)aminomethane Buffer

mL 0.1N HCl added	Resulting pH at 23° C	Resulting pH at 37° C
5.0	9.10	8.95
7.5	8.92	8.78
10.0	8.74	8.60
12.5	8.62	8.48
15.0	8.50	8.37
17.5	8.40	8.27
20.0	8.32	8.18
22.5	8.23	8.10
25.0	8.14	8.00
27.5	8.05	7.90
30.0	7.96	7.82
32.5	7.87	7.73
35.0	7.77	7.63
37.5	7.66	7.52
40.0	7.54	7.40
42.5	7.36	7.22
45.0	7.20	7.05

4.20 to 4.10. Efficient buffering capacity covers a pH range of about 1 unit on either side of the pK value of the weak acid or base. For acetic acid, this would be from about pH 3.8 to 5.8.

SORENSEN'S PHOSPHATE BUFFERS

These buffer solutions are generally useful, because the range of the mixtures is from pH 5 to 8.

Prepare 0.1 molar solutions of monobasic potassium phosphate (13.6 g/L) and dibasic sodium phosphate (14.2 g/L). Mix solutions in the ratio indicated in Table A1-2 to obtain the buffer of desired pH.

TRIS(HYDROXYMETHYL)AMINOMETHANE BUFFER*

Tris(hydroxymethyl)aminomethane buffer can be used for a pH range between 7.0 and 9.0, but its best buffer capacity is between 7.5 and 8.5. It is practically ineffective below pH 7.0 and above pH 9.0. One advantage of the buffer is its excellent stability. The buffer can be prepared by weighing the desired amount of tris(hydroxymethyl)aminomethane, dissolving it in water, and adjusting the pH to the desired value with HCl. For example, if 100 mL of 0.05 M buffer is desired, place 0.6057 g of tris(hydroxymethyl) aminomethane into a 100-mL volumetric flask. This is dissolved in approximately 50 mL of distilled water. Add 0.1N HCl, as indicated in Table A1-3, and fill up to the mark with distilled water. The table shows the pH values obtained when 0.6057 g of tris(hydroxymethyl)aminomethane dissolved in water is mixed with the indicated amounts of 0.1N HCl and diluted to 100 mL.

*If buffers of a higher molarity are desired, the 0.1N HCl may have to be replaced by 1.0N HCl.

TABLE A1-4
Acid-Base Indicators

Indicator	pH range	Quantity of indicator per 10 mL	Color acid	Alkaline
Thymol blue (A)*†	1.2–2.8	1–2 drops 0.1% solution in aqueous	Red	Yellow
Methyl orange (B)	3.1–4.4	1 drop 0.1% solution in aqueous	Red	Orange
Bromphenol blue (A)†	3.0–4.6	1 drop 0.1% solution in aqueous	Yellow	Blue-violet
Bromcresol green (A)†	4.0–5.6	1 drop 0.1% solution in aqueous	Yellow	Blue
Methyl red (A)†	4.4–6.2	1 drop 0.1% solution in aqueous.	Red	Yellow
Bromcresol purple (A)†	5.2–6.8	1 drop 0.1% solution in aqueous	Yellow	Purple
Bromthymol blue (A)†	6.2–7.6	1 drop 0.1% solution in aqueous	Yellow	Blue
Phenol red (A)†	6.4–8.0	1 drop 0.1% solution in aqueous	Yellow	Red
Neutral red (B)	6.8–8.0	1 drop 0.1% solution in 70% alcohol	Red	Yellow
Thymol blue (A)†‡	8.0–9.6	1–5 drops 0.1% solution in aqueous	Yellow	Blue
Phenolphthalein (A)	8.0–10.0	1–5 drops 0.1% solution in 70% alcohol	Colorless	Red
Thymolphthalein (A)	9.4–10.6	1 drop 0.1% solution in 90% alcohol	Colorless	Blue

(A), Acid; *(B)*, base.
*For the acid range.
†Sodium salt.
‡For the alkaline range.

ACID-BASE INDICATORS*

An acid-base indicator is a weak acid or a weak base, the undissociated form of which has a color and constitution other than the iogenic form. Color change takes place over a certain narrow range of hydrogen ion concentrations. This range is called the *color change interval* and is expressed in terms of pH (the negative logarithm of the hydrogen ion concentration). A great number of substances show indicator properties, although relatively few of them are practically applied for neutralization reactions and pH determinations. Commonly used acid-base indicators are listed in Table A1-4. In general, weak acids should be titrated in the presence of indicators that change in slightly alkaline solutions. Weak bases should be titrated in the presence of indicators that change in slightly acid solutions. commonly used acids and alkalis are listed in Table A1-5.

The availability of precision pH meters allows titration to a selected end point (pH) and may replace use of indicators for several applications.

*Based on Dean JA, editor. Handbook of chemistry. Revised 13th ed. New York: McGraw-Hill; 1985.

TABLE A1-5
Commonly Used Acids and Alkalies*

Solution	Molecular weight	Specific gravity†	g/L†	Molarity†	Normality†	Approximate number of mL required to make 1000 mL of 1 N solution
Concentrated HCl	36.46	1.19	440	12	12	83
Concentrated H_2SO_4	98.08	1.84	1730	18	36	28
Concentrated HNO_3	63.02	1.42	990	16	16	64
Concentrated lactic acid	90.08	1.21	1030	11	11	87
Glacial acetic acid	60.08	1.06	1060	17.5	17.5	57
Concentrated NH_4OH	35.05	0.90	250	15	15	67

*Commercially available.
†Figures may vary slightly according to the lot or manufacturer.

TABLE A1-6
Standard Reference Materials for Clinical Measurements

SRM #	SRM type	Stoichiometric purity mass fraction in %	Certified use	Unit size (g)
40h	Sodium oxalate	99.972	Reductometric standard	60
83d	Arsenic trioxide	99.9926	Reductometric standard	60
84k	Potassium hydrogen phthalate	99.9911	Acidimetric standard	60
136e	Potassium dichromate	99.984	Oximetric standard	60
350a	Benzoic acid	99.9958	Acidimetric standard	30
723c	Tris(hydroxymethyl) aminomethane	99.901	Acidimetric standard	50
911b	Cholesterol	99.8	Identity and purity	2.0
912a	Urea	99.9	Identity and purity	25
913	Uric acid	99.7	Identity and purity	10
914a	Creatinine	99.7	Identity and purity	10
915a	Calcium carbonate	99.9	Identity and purity	20
916a	Bilirubin	98.3	Identity and purity	0.1
917a	D-Glucose (dextrose)	99.7	Identity and purity	25
918a	Potassium chloride	99.9817	Identity and purity	30
919a	Sodium chloride	99.89	Identity and purity	30
930e	Glass filters, transmittance		Wavelength range (440–635 nm)	3 filters
931f	Liquid filters, absorbance		Wavelength range (302–678 nm)	Ampules
934	Clinical laboratory thermometers (0, 25, 30, 37)		Temperature	One each
937	Iron metal	99.90		50
955b	Lead in blood			Set of 4 ampules

SRM, Standard reference materials.

TABLE A1-7
Temperature Conversions

Centigrade (°)	Fahrenheit (°)	Centigrade (°)	Fahrenheit (°)
110	230	38	100.4
100	212	37.5	99.5
95	203	37	98.6
90	194	36.5	97.7
85	185	36	96.8
80	176	35.5	95.9
75	167	35	95
70	158	34	93.2
65	149	33	91.4
60	140	32	89.6
55	131	31	87.8
50	122	30	86
45	113	25	77
44	111.2	20	68
43	109.4	15	59
42	107.6	10	50
41	105.8	+5	41
40.5	104.9	0	32
40	104	−5	23
39.5	103.1	−10	14
39	102.2	−15	+5
38.5	101.3	−20	−4

1° F = −17.2° C.
1° C = 33.8° F.
To convert Fahrenheit into centigrade, subtract 32 and multiply by 0.555.
To convert centigrade to Fahrenheit, multiply by 1.8 and add 32.

STANDARD REFERENCE MATERIALS

Standard reference materials (SRM) are available for many substances with defined identities and concentrations in solutions or as other materials such as thermometers or optical filters with specified transmission wavelengths (Table A1-6). SRMs are used as standards or controls against which assays may be calibrated with high certainty of accuracy in both identity and concentration of the substance or other property.

TEMPERATURE CONVERSION

Temperature is expressed in either Fahrenheit (F) or centigrade (C) scale according to the convention of the country, editorial policy of journals, and local practices. The simple relationship between these two temperature scales is:

$$\text{Temperature in degrees Fahrenheit} = 1.8 \times \text{temperature in degrees centigrade} + 32$$

Often it is more convenient to look up corresponding values for these two temperature scales in a list of values (Table A1-7). A unique value occurs at −40° where the two scales intersect and the values coincide (i.e., −40° F = −40° C).

SELECTED REFERENCES

Dean JA, editor. Handbook of chemistry. 13th ed. New York: McGraw-Hill; 1985.

Fasman GD, editor. Handbook of biochemistry and molecular biology. 3rd ed. Cleveland: CRC Press; 1976.

Meinke WW. Standard reference materials for clinical measurements. Anal Chem 1971;43:28A.

The Merck Index. An encyclopedia of chemicals and drugs. 12th ed. Whitehouse Station, N.J.: Merck and Co.; 1996.

APPENDIX 2

DESIRABLE WEIGHTS, BODY SURFACE AREA, AND BODY MASS INDEX

TABLE A2-1
Comparison of the Weight-for-Height Tables from Actuarial Data: Non–Age-Corrected Metropolitan Life Insurance Company and Age-Specific Gerontology Research Center Recommendations

HEIGHT		METROPOLITAN 1983 WEIGHTS* (25–59 YEARS)		GERONTOLOGY RESEARCH CENTER* (AGE-SPECIFIC WEIGHT RANGE FOR MEN AND WOMEN)				
ft	**in**	**Men**	**Women**	**20–29 years**	**30–39 years**	**40–49 years**	**50–59 years**	**60–79 years**
4	10		100–131	84–111	92–119	99–127	107–135	115–142
4	11		101–134	87–115	95–123	103–131	111–139	119–147
5	0		103–137	90–119	98–127	106–135	114–143	123–152
5	1	123–145	105–140	93–123	101–131	110–140	118–148	127–157
5	2	125–148	108–144	96–127	105–136	113–144	122–153	131–163
5	3	127–151	111–148	99–131	108–140	117–149	126–158	135–168
5	4	129–155	114–152	102–135	112–145	121–154	130–163	140–173
5	5	131–159	117–156	106–140	115–149	125–159	134–168	144–179
5	6	133–163	120–160	109–144	119–154	129–164	138–174	148–184
5	7	135–167	123–164	112–148	122–159	133–169	143–179	153–190
5	8	137–171	126–167	116–153	126–163	137–174	147–184	158–196
5	9	139–175	129–170	119–157	130–168	141–179	151–190	162–201
5	10	141–179	132–173	122–162	134–173	145–184	156–195	167–207
5	11	144–183	135–176	126–167	137–178	149–190	160–201	172–213
6	0	147–187		129–171	141–183	153–195	165–207	177–219
6	1	150–192		133–176	145–188	157–200	169–213	182–225
6	2	153–197		137–181	149–194	162–206	174–219	187–232
6	3	157–202		141–186	153–199	166–212	179–225	192–238
6	4			144–191	157–205	171–218	184–231	197–244

From Andres R. Mortality and obesity: the rationale for age-specific height–weight tables. In: Hazzard WR, Bierman EL, Blass JP, et al, editors. Principles of geriatric medicine and gerontology, 3rd ed. New York: McGraw-Hill; 1994, p 847, with permission.

*Values in this table are for height without shoes and weight without clothes. The Metropolitan Life Insurance Company (1983 Metropolitan Height and Weight Tables. Stat Bull Metropol Life Ins Co, 1983;64[Jan–Jun]:2) presented a table for nude heights and weights (Table 4) as well as a table for heights and weights clothed (Table 1).

TABLE A2-2

Body Mass Index Table

To use the following table, find the appropriate height in the left-hand column. Move across to a given weight. The number at the top of the column is the body mass index at the height and weight. Pounds are rounded off.

BMI	19	20	21	22	23	24	25	26	27	28	29	30	31	32	33	34	35	36
									Body weight (lb)									
Height (in)	58	91	96	100	105	110	115	119	124	129	134	138	143	148	153	158	162	167
	59	94	99	104	109	114	119	124	128	133	138	143	148	153	158	163	168	173
	60	97	102	107	112	118	123	128	133	138	143	148	153	158	163	168	174	179
	61	100	106	111	116	122	127	132	137	143	148	153	158	164	169	174	180	185
	62	104	109	115	120	126	131	136	142	147	153	158	164	169	175	180	186	191
	63	107	113	118	124	130	135	141	146	152	158	163	169	175	180	186	191	197
	64	110	116	122	128	134	140	145	151	157	163	169	174	180	186	192	197	204
	65	114	120	126	132	138	144	150	156	162	168	174	180	186	192	198	204	210
	66	118	124	130	136	142	148	155	161	167	173	179	186	192	198	204	210	216
	67	121	127	134	140	146	153	159	166	172	178	185	191	198	204	211	217	223
	68	125	131	138	144	151	158	164	171	177	184	190	197	203	210	216	223	230
	69	128	135	142	149	155	162	169	176	182	189	196	203	209	216	223	230	236
	70	132	139	146	153	160	167	174	181	188	195	202	209	216	222	229	236	243
	71	136	143	150	157	165	172	179	186	193	200	208	215	222	229	236	243	250
	72	140	147	154	162	169	177	184	191	199	206	213	221	228	235	242	250	258
	73	144	151	159	166	174	182	189	197	204	212	219	227	235	242	250	257	265
	74	148	155	163	171	179	186	194	202	210	218	225	233	241	249	256	264	272
	75	152	160	168	176	184	192	200	208	216	224	232	240	248	256	264	272	279
	76	156	164	172	180	189	197	205	213	221	230	238	246	254	263	271	279	287

BMI		37	38	39	40	41	42	43	44	45	46	47	48	49	50	51	52	
									Body weight (lb)									
Height (in)	58	172	177	181	186	191	196	201	205	210	215	220	224	229	234	239	244	248
	59	178	183	188	193	198	203	208	212	217	222	227	232	237	242	247	252	257
	60	184	189	194	199	204	209	215	220	225	230	235	240	245	250	255	261	266
	61	190	195	201	206	211	217	222	227	232	238	243	248	254	259	264	269	275
	62	196	202	207	213	218	224	229	235	240	246	251	256	262	267	273	278	284
	63	203	208	214	220	225	231	237	242	248	254	259	265	270	278	282	287	293
	64	209	215	221	227	232	238	244	250	256	262	267	273	279	285	291	296	302
	65	216	222	228	234	240	246	252	258	264	270	276	282	288	294	300	306	312
	66	223	229	235	241	247	253	260	266	272	278	284	291	297	303	309	315	322
	67	230	236	242	249	255	261	268	274	280	287	293	299	306	312	319	325	331
	68	236	243	249	256	262	269	276	282	289	295	302	308	315	322	328	335	341
	69	243	250	257	263	270	277	284	291	297	304	311	318	324	331	338	345	351
	70	250	257	264	271	278	285	292	299	306	313	320	327	334	341	348	355	362
	71	257	265	272	279	286	293	301	308	315	322	329	338	343	351	358	365	372
	72	265	272	279	287	294	302	309	316	324	331	338	346	353	361	368	375	383
	73	272	280	288	295	302	310	318	325	333	340	348	355	363	371	378	386	393
	74	280	287	295	303	311	319	326	334	342	350	358	365	373	381	389	396	404
	75	287	295	303	311	319	327	335	343	351	359	367	375	383	391	399	407	415
	76	295	304	312	320	328	336	344	353	361	369	377	385	394	402	410	418	426

Source: http://www.nhlbi.nih.gov/guidelines/obesity/bmi_tbl.htm.

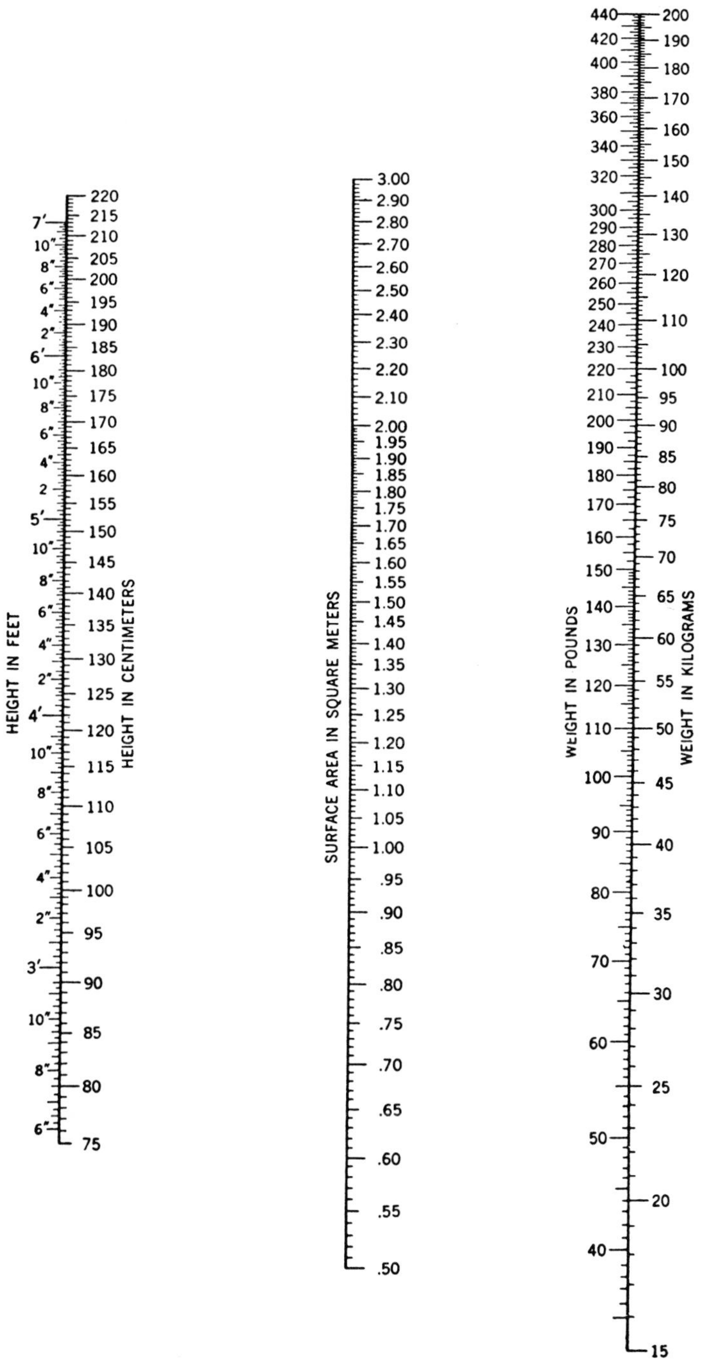

Figure A2-1 Nomogram for the determination of body surface area of children and adults. *(From Boothby WM, Sandiford RB. Nomographic charts for the calculation of the metabolic rate by the gasometer method. Boston Med Surg J 1921;185:337, with permission.)*

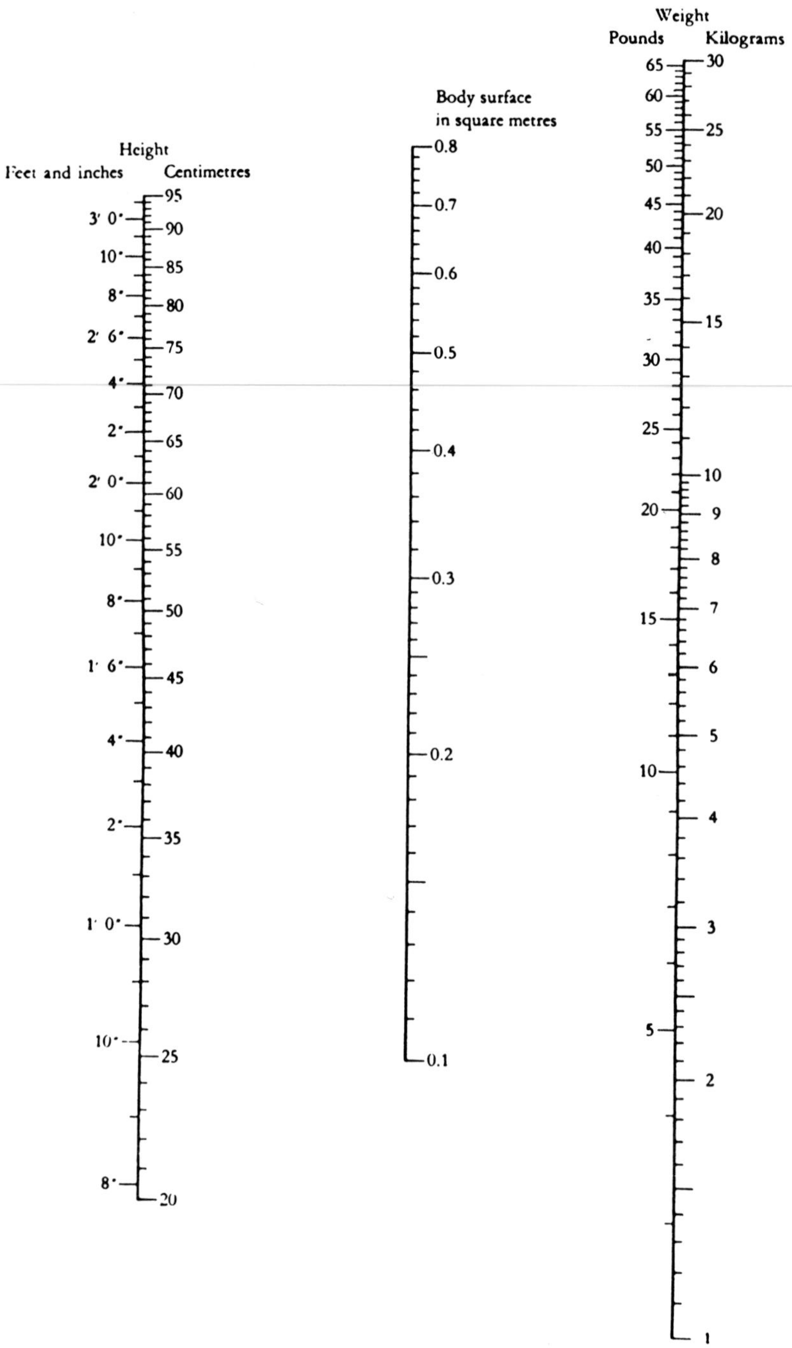

Figure A2-2 Nomogram for the determination of body surface area of children. *(From DuBois EF. Basal metabolism in health and disease. Philadelphia: Lea & Febiger; 1936.)*

The formula for calculating BMI is:

$$BMI = Weight\ (kg)/Height\ (m^2)$$

Or

$$BMI = 703 \times Weight\ (lb)/(Height\ (in^2)$$

Interpretation of BMI for adults 20 years old and older:

- <18.5 is underweight
- 18.5–24.9 is normal
- 25–29.9 is overweight
- 30 and above is obese.

(From Centers for Disease Control and Prevention. About BMI for adults. http://www.cdc.gov/healthyweight/assessing/bmi/adult_bmi/index.html.)

APPENDIX 3

APPROXIMATIONS OF TOTAL BLOOD VOLUME

When estimating a patient's total blood volume (TBV), a commonly used approximation is 70 mL of TBV per kilogram body weight. While useful in many patients, in others, particularly children and overweight or thin adults, this figure offers only a poor approximation of actual TBV. In these patients, other methods of estimation of TBV are more appropriate.

ADULTS

The COBE Spectra uses the Nadler and Allen formula to calculate approximate TBV for patients (COBE Spectra Apheresis System Operator's Manual, 1997). This formula uses patient height, weight, and sex to calculate TBV. Specifically, the formula is:

$$\text{Males: TBV(mL)} = 604 + [367 \times \text{height}^3\ (\text{m})] + [32.2 \times \text{weight (kg)}]$$

$$\text{Females: TBV(mL)} = 183 + [356 \times \text{height}^3\ (\text{m})] + [33.1 \times \text{weight (kg)}]$$

TBV can also be approximated using the patient's calculated body surface area (Shoemaker, 1989):

$$\text{Males: TBV} = 2740\ \text{mL/m}^2$$

$$\text{Females: TBV} = 2370\ \text{mL/m}^2$$

Another relatively simple approximation uses Gilcher's so-called rule of fives, reproduced here, as an estimate of blood volume, which is more tailored to the individual patient than the 70 mL/kg rule (Gilcher, 1996).

	Fat	Thin	Normal	Muscular
Males	60	65	70	75
Females	55	60	65	70

CHILDREN

The Nadler and Allen calculation can be particularly inaccurate in children, especially prepubertal boys, in whom it has been recommended that the female gender be entered to improve the estimation (Kim, 2000). The following values for TBV per kilogram body weight can be used (Oski, 1993):

Premature infants	89–105 mL/kg
Term newborns	82–86 mL/kg
Infants and preschoolers	73–82 mL/kg

SELECTED REFERENCES

COBE Spectra Apheresis System operator's manual. Lakewood, Colo: Gambro BCT; 1997, p. 1.

Gilcher RO. Apheresis: principles and practices. In: Rossi EC, Simon TL, Moss GS, Gould SA, editors. Principles of transfusion medicine. 2nd ed. Baltimore: Williams & Wilkins; 1996, p. 542.

Kim HC. Therapeutic pediatric apheresis. J Clin Apheresis 2000;15:129–57.

Oski FA. The erythrocyte and its disorders. In: Nathan DG, Oski FA, editors. Hematology of infancy and childhood. 4th ed. Philadelphia: WB Saunders; 1993, p. 28.

Shoemaker WC. Fluids and electrolytes in the acutely ill adult. In: Shoemaker WC, Ayres S, Grenvik A, et al, editors. Textbook of critical care. 2nd ed. Philadelphia: WB Saunders; 1989, p. 1130.

APPENDIX 4 PERIODIC TABLE OF THE ELEMENTS

TABLE A4-1

Periodic Table of the Elements

KEY TO CHART: Atomic number → 50 +2 ← Oxidation state; Symbol → Sn +4; 1989 Atomic weight → 118.71; 18 18 4 ← Electron configuration

Group (New notation)	1	2	3	4	5	6	7	8	9	10	11	12	13	14	15	16	17	18	
Previous IUPAC form	IA	IIA	IIIA	IVA	VA	VIA	VIIA	VIIIA	VIIIA	VIIIA			IIIB	IVB	VB	VIB	VIIB		
CAS version			IIIB	IVB	VB	VIB	VIIB	VIII	VIII	VIII	IB	IIB	IIIA	IVA	VA	VIA	VIIA	VIIIA	Shell
	1 +1 −1 H 1.00794 1																	2 0 He 4.0020602 2	K
	3 +1 Li 6.941 2-1	4 +1 Be 9.012182 2-2											5 +3 B 10.811 2-3	6 +2 +4 −4 C 12.011 2-4	7 +1 +2 +3 +4 +5 −1 −2 −3 N 14.00674 2-5	8 −2 O 15.9994 2-6	9 −1 F 18.998403 2	10 0 Ne 20.1797 2-8	K-L
	11 +1 Na 22.989768 2-8-1	12 +2 Mg 24.3050 2-8-2											13 +3 Al 26.981539 2-8-3	14 +2 +4 −4 Si 28.0855 2-8-4	15 +3 +5 −3 P 30.97362 2-8-5	16 +3 +5 −2 S 32.066 2-8-6	17 +1 +5 +7 −1 Cl 35.4527 2-8-7	18 0 Ar 39.948 2-8-8	K-L-M
	19 +1 K 39.0983 -8-8-1	20 +2 Ca 40.078 -8-8-2	21 +3 Sc 44.955910 -8-9-2	22 +2 +3 +4 Ti 47.88 -8-10-2	23 +2 +3 +4 +5 V 50.9415 -8-11-2	24 +2 +3 +6 Cr 51.9961 -8-13-1	25 +2 +3 +4 +7 Mn 54.93085 -8-13-2	26 +2 +3 Fe 55.847 -8-14-2	27 +2 +3 Co 58.93320 -8-15-2	28 +2 +3 Ni 58.6934 -8-16-2	29 +1 +2 Ni 63.546 -8-18-1	30 +2 Zn 65.39 -8-18-2	31 +3 Ga 69.723 -8-18-3	32 +2 +4 Ge 72.61 -8-18-4	33 +2 +5 −3 As 74.92159 -8-18-5	34 +4 +6 −2 Se 78.96 -8-18-6	35 +1 +5 −1 Br 79.904 -8-18-7	36 0 Kr 83.80 -8-18-8	-L-M-N
	37 +1 Rb 85.4678 -18-8-1	38 +2 Sr 87-62 -18-8-2	39 +3 Y 88-90585 -18-9-2	40 +4 Zr 91.224 -18-12-1	41 +3 +5 Nb 92.90638 -18-10-2	42 +6 Mo 95.94 -18-13-1	43 +4 +6 +7 Tc (98) -18-13-2	44 +3 Ru 101.07 -18-15-1	45 +3 Rh 102.90550 -18-16-1	46 +2 +4 Pd 106.42 -18-18-0	47 +1 Ag 107.8682 -18-18-1	48 +2 Cd 112.411 -18-18-2	49 +3 In 114.818 -18-18-3	50 +2 +4 Sn 118.710 -18-18-4	51 +3 +5 −3 Sb 121.757 -18-18-5	52 +4 +6 −2 Te 127.60 -18-18-6	53 +1 +5 +7 −1 I 126.90447 -18-18-7	54 0 Xe 131.29 -18-18-8	-M-N-O
	55 +1 Cs 132.90543 -18-8-1	56 +2 Ba 137.327 -18-8-2	57* +3 La 139.9055 -18-9-2	72 +4 Hf 178.49 -32-10-2	73 +5 Ta 180.9479 -32-11-2	74 +6 W 183.84 -32-12-2	75 +4 +6 +7 Re 186.207 -32-13-2	76 +3 +4 Os 190.23 -32-14-2	77 +3 +4 Ir 192.22 -32-15-2	78 +2 +4 Pt 195.08 -32-16-2	79 +1 +3 Au 196.96654 -32-18-1	80 +1 +2 Hg 200.59 -32-18-2	81 +1 +3 Tl 204.3833 -32-18-3	82 +2 +4 Pb 207.2 -32-18-4	83 +3 +5 Bi 208.98037 -32-18-5	84 +2 +4 Po (209) -32-18-6	85 At (210) -32-18-7	86 0 Rn (222) -32-18-8	-N-O-P
	87 +1 Fr (223) -18-8-1	88 +2 Ra 226.025 -18-8-2	89** +3 Ac 227.08 -18-9-2	104 +4 Rf (261) -32-10-2	105 Db (262) -32-11-2	106 Se (266) -32-12-2	107 Bh (264) -32-13-2	108 Hs (267) -32-14-2	109 Mt (268) -32-15-2	110 Ds (271) -32-17-2	111 Rg (272) -32-18-1	112 Cn (285) -32-18-2	113 Uut (284) -32-18-3	114 Uuq (289) -32-18-4	115 Uup (288) -32-18-5	116 Uuh (292) -32-18-6	117 Uus (295) -32-18-7	118 Uuo (294) -32-18-8	O P Q

*Lathanides	58 +3 +4 Ce 140.115 -19-9-2	59 +3 Pr 140.90765 -21-8-2	60 +3 Nd 144.24 -22-8-2	61 +3 Pm (145) -23-8-2	62 +2 +3 Sm 150.36 -24-8-2	63 +2 +3 Eu 151.965 -25-8-2	64 +3 Gd 157.25 -25-9-2	65 +3 Tb 158.92534 -27-8-2	66 +3 Dy 162.50 -28-8-2	67 +3 Ho 164.93032 -29-8-2	68 +3 Er 167.26 -30-8-2	69 +3 Tm 168.93421 -32-8-2	70 +2 +3 Yb 173.04 -32-8-2	71 +3 Lu 174.967 -32-9-2		N O P
**Actinides	90 +4 Th 232.0381 -18-10-2	91 +5 +4 Pa 231.03588 -20-9-2	92 +3 +4 +5 +6 U 238.0289 -21-9-2	93 +3 +4 +5 +6 Np 237.048 -22-9-2	94 +3 +4 +5 +6 Pu (244) -24-8-2	95 +3 +4 +5 +6 Am (243) -25-8-2	96 +3 Cm (247) -25-9-2	97 +3 +4 Bk (247) -27-8-2	98 +3 Cf (251) -28-8-2	99 +3 Es (252) -29-8-2	100 +3 Fm (257) -30-8-2	101 +2 +3 Md (258) -31-8-2	102 +2 +3 No (259) -32-8-2	103 +3 Lr (260) -32-9-2		O P Q

Modified from Lide DR, Frederikse HPR. CRC handbook of chemistry and physics 1993–1994. 74th ed. Boca Raton, Fla.: CRC Press; 1993.
The new International Union of Pure and Applied Chemistry (IUPAC) format numbers the groups from 1 to 18. The previous IUPAC numbering system and the system used by Chemical Abstracts Service (CAS) are also shown.
For radioactive elements that do not occur in nature, the mass number of the most stable isotope is given in parentheses.

REFERENCES

Chemical and Engineering News. 1985;63:27.

Chemical and Engineering News. It's elemental: the periodic table-introduction. National Chemistry Week October 2009;19–24. http://pubs.acs.org/cen/80th/elements.html.

Leigh GJ, editor. Nomenclature of inorganic chemistry. Oxford: Blackwell Scientific; 1990.

The Periodic Table of Videos—University of Nottingham. http://www.periodicvideos.com.

Professor Martyn Poliakoff and chemistry staff from the University of Nottingham have produced "The Periodic Table of Videos" as entertaining and educational discussions and laboratory demonstrations of chemical properties of each of the 118 elements.

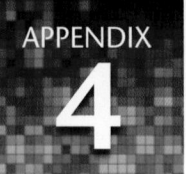

APPENDIX 5

SI UNITS

The Standard International (SI) consists of seven dimensionally independent base units, which are listed in Table A5-1, along with the symbols to be used to denote these units. Table A5-2 lists a number of derived units of the SI that are used in the clinical laboratory. There are two kinds of derived units: (1) coherent units, which are derived directly from the base units without the use of conversion factors, and (2) noncoherent units, which are constructed from the base units and contain a numerical factor to make the numbers more convenient to use. The prefixes to denote fractions or multiples of base and derived SI units are given in Table A5-3. A complete description of the SI and its application in medicine may be found in the World Health Organization publication The SI for the Health Professions (World Health Organization, 1977). See Tietz (1995) for a comprehensive list of quantities and their internationally recommended SI units.

In making the conversion to recommend SI units (Tables A5-4 through A5-13), the following guidelines were followed:

1. All reference intervals have been converted to SI units except in cases in which the measurements are not quantitative.
2. Chemical names have not been changed; for example, urea is retained instead of changing to carbamide.
3. Factors are those published by the American National Metric Council (Lundberg, 1986; Beeler, 1987; Young, 1987), based on the Metric Commission of Canada (1981) factors.
4. Factors are calculated to the base unit for volume of 1 L.
5. The order of magnitude of the factors is calculated to make the values in SI units convenient numbers, that is, with prefixes, a number not greater than 1000 or smaller than 0.001.
6. The number in recommended SI units is equal to the number in conventional units times the factor.
7. For compounds for which relative molecular masses are not definitely known (e.g., proteins), reference intervals are converted to mass amounts per liter.
8. For mixtures of indeterminate composition (e.g., phospholipids), reference intervals are converted to mass amounts per liter or are based on a given standard, for example, DHEA for 17-ketosteroids.
9. Quantities of a relative nature that are usually expressed as percentages, for example, fractions of LD isoenzymes, are given as fractions.
10. Enzyme units are given as the international unit per liter (U/L). Although the coherent SI unit for catalytic activity (including enzymes), the katal, has been defined as the number of moles of substrate converted per second under defined conditions, its adoption is limited.
11. The pH scale is retained for measurement of hydrogen ion concentrations.
12. It is recommended that the unit millimeters of mercury (mm Hg) be retained for pressure (P_{CO_2}, P_{O_2}) at the present time.
13. Percentages are expressed as fractions in the SI, where a fraction is a dimensionless quantity given by the number of defined particles constituting a specified component divided by the total number of defined particles in the system.

TABLE A5-1
SI Base Units

Quantity	Name	Symbol
Length	meter	m
Mass	kilogram	kg
Time	second	s
Electric current	ampere	A
Thermodynamic temperature	kelvin	K
Luminous intensity	candela	cd
Amount of substance	mole	mol

TABLE A5-2
SI Derived Units

Quantity	Unit name	Unit symbol
Area	square meter*	m^2
Volume	cubic meter*	m^3
	liter†	L = dm^3‡
Concentration		
Mass	kilogram/liter†	kg/L
Substance	mole/liter†	mol/L
Molality	mole/kilogram	mol/kg
Density	kilogram/liter†	kg/L
Mass fraction	kilogram/kilogram	kg/kg
Mole fraction	mole/mole	mol/mol
Number concentration	number/liter	L^{-1}
Temperature	degree celsius*	° C = ° K − 273.15
Pressure	pascal*	Pa = kg/m^2
Frequency	hertz*	Hz = 1 cycle/s
Clearance	liter/second†	L/s
Electrical potential	volt*	V = kgm^2/s^3A
Energy	joule*	J = kgm^2/s^2

*Derived coherent unit.
†Derived noncoherent unit.
‡Both "L" and "l" are symbols for the liter.

TABLE A5-3
Prefixes

Prefix	Prefix symbol	Factor
exa	E	10^{18}
peta	P	10^{15}
tera	T	10^{12}
giga	G	10^{9}
mega	M	10^{6}
kilo	k	10^{3}
hecto	h	10^{2}
deca	da	10^{1}
deci	d	10^{-1}
centi	c	10^{-2}
milli	m	10^{-3}
micro	μ	10^{-6}
nano	n	10^{-9}
pico	p	10^{-12}
femto	f	10^{-15}
atto	a	10^{-18}
zepto	z	10^{-21}
yocto	y	10^{-24}

TABLE A5-4
Whole Blood, Serum, and Plasma Chemistry

		TYPICAL REFERENCE INTERVALS		
Component	**System**	**Conventional units**	**Factor***	**Recommended SI units†**
Acetoacetic acid				
Qualitative	Serum	Negative	—	Negative
Quantitative	Serum	0.2–1 mg/dL	97.95	20–100 μmol/L
Acetone				
Qualitative	Serum	Negative	—	Negative
Quantitative	Serum	0.3–2 mg/dL	172.95	20–340 μmol/L
Albumin				
Qualitative	Serum	3.2–4.5 g/dL (salt fractionation)	10	32–45 g/L
		3.2–5.6 g/dL (electrophoresis)		32–56 g/L
		3.8–5 g/dL (eye binding)		38–50 g/L
Alcohol, ethyl	Serum or whole blood	Negative–but presented asmg/dL	0.2171	Negative–but presented asmmol/L
Aldolase	Serum			
	Adults	3–8 Sibley-LehningerU/dL at 37° C	7.4	22–59 mU/L at 37° C
	Children	Approximately 2× adult levels	—	Approximately 2× adult levels
	Newborn	Approximately 4× adult levels	—	Approximately 4× adult levels
α-Amino acid nitrogen	Serum	3.6–7 mg/dL	0.7139	2.6–5 mmol/L
δ-Aminolevulinic acid	Serum	0.01–0.03 mg/dL	76.26	0.8–2.3 μmol/L
Ammonia	Plasma	20–120 μg/dL (diffusion)	0.5872	12–70 μmol/L
		40–80 μg/dL (enzymatic method)		23–47 μmol/L
		12–48 μg/dL (resin method)		7–28 μmol/L
Amylase	Serum	16–120 Somogyi units/dL	1.85	30–220 U/L
Argininosuccinate lyase	Serum	0–4 U/dL	10	0–40 U/L
Arsenic‡	Whole blood	<7 μg/dL	0.05055	<0.4 μmol/L
Ascorbic acid (vitamin C)	Plasma	0.6–1.6 mg/dL	56.78	34–91 μmol/L
	Whole blood	0.7–2 mg/dL		40–114 μmol/L
Barbiturates	Serum, plasma, or whole blood	Negative	—	Negative
Base excess	Whole blood			
	Male	–3.3 to +1.2 mEq/L	1	–3.3 to +1.2 mmol/L
	Female	–2.4 to +2.3 mEq/L		–2.4 to +2.3 mmol/L
Base, total	Serum	145–160 mEq/L	1	145–160 mmol/L
Bicarbonate	Plasma	21–28 mmol/L	1	21–28 mmol/L
Bile acids	Serum	0.3–3 mg/dL	10	3–30 mg/L
Bilirubin				
Direct (conjugated)	Serum	<0.3 mg/dL	17.10	<5 μmol/L
Indirect (unconjugated)	Serum	0.1–1 mg/dL		2–17 μmol/L
Total	Serum	0.1–1.2 mg/dL		2–21 μmol/L
Newborns total	Serum	1–12 mg/dL		17–205 μol/L
Blood gases (see Chapter 14)				
pH	Whole blood	7.38–7.44 (arterial)	1	7.38–7.44
		7.36–7.41 (venous)		7.36–7.41
P_{CO_2}	Whole blood	35–40 mm Hg (arterial)	0.1333	4.7–5.3 kPa
		40–45 mm Hg (venous)		5.3–6 kPa
P_{O_2}	Whole blood	95–100 mm Hg (arterial)	0.1333	12.7–13.3 kPa
Bromide	Serum	<5 mg/dL	0.125	<0.63 mmol/L
Calcium				
Ionized	Serum	4–4.8 mg/dL	0.2500	1–1.2 mmol/L
		2–2.4 mEq/L	0.5000	
		30–58% of total	0.01	0.30–1.58 of total
Total	Serum	9.2–11.0 mg/dL	0.2500	2.30–2.74 mmol/L
		4.6–5.5 mEq/L	0.5000	
Carbon dioxide (CO_2 content)	Whole blood (arterial)	19–24 mmol/L	1	19–24 mmol/L
	Plasma or serum (arterial)	21–28 mmol/L		21–28 mmol/L
Carbon dioxide	Whole blood (venous)	22–26 mmol/L	1	22–26 mmol/L
	Plasma or serum (venous)	24–30 mmol/L		24–30 mmol/L
CO_2 combining power	Plasma or serum (venous)	24–30 mmol/L	1	24–30 mmol/L
CO_2 partial pressure (P_{CO_2})	Whole blood (arterial)	35–40 mm Hg	0.1333	4.7–5.3 kPa
	Whole blood (venous)	40–45 mm Hg		5.3–6 kPa

TABLE A5-4
Whole Blood, Serum, and Plasma Chemistry—*Cont'd*

Component	System	TYPICAL REFERENCE INTERVALS		
		Conventional units	**Factor***	**Recommended SI units†**
Carbonic acid (H_2CO_3)	Whole blood (arterial)	1.05–1.45 mmol/L	1	1.05–1.45 mmol/L
	Whole blood (venous)	1.15–1.50 mmol/L		1.15–1.50 mmol/L
	Plasma (venous)	1.02–1.38 mmol/L		1.02–1.38 mmol/L
Carboxyhemoglobin (carbon monoxide hemoglobin)	Whole blood suburban	<1.5% saturation of hemoglobin	0.01	Fraction hemoglobin saturated: <0.015
	Nonsmokers			
	Smokers	1.5%–5% saturation		0.015–0.050
	Heavy smokers	5%–9% saturation		0.050–0.090
Carotene, β	Serum	40–200 μg/dL	0.01863	0.7–3.7 μmol/L
Ceruloplasmin	Serum	23–50 mg/dL	10	230–500 mg/L
Chloride	Serum	95–103 mEq/L	1	95–103 mmol/L
Cholesterol				
Total (see Chapter 17)	Serum	150–250 mg/dL (varies with diet, sex, and age)	0.02586	3.88–6.47 mmol/L
Esters	Serum	65%–75% of total cholesterol	0.01	Fraction of total cholesterol: 0.65–0.75
Cholinesterase (pseudocholinesterase)	Erythrocytes	0.65–1.3 pH units	1	0.65–1.3 units§
	Plasma	0.5–1.3 pH units	1	0.5–1.3 units
		8–18 U/L at 37° C		
Citrate	Serum or plasma	1.7–3 mg/dL	52.05	88–156 μmol/L
Copper	Serum, plasma			
	Male	70–140 μg/dL	0.1574	11–22 μmol/L
	Female	80–155 μg/dL		13–24 μmol/L
Cortisol	Plasma			
	8 AM–10 AM	5–23 μg/dL	27.59	138–635 nmol/L
	4 PM–6 PM	3–13 μg/dL		83–359 nmol/L
Creatine	Serum or plasma			
	Male	0.1–0.4 mg/dL	76.25	8–31 μmol/L
	Female	0.2–0.7 mg/dL		15–53 μmol/L
Creatine kinase (CK)	Serum			
	Male	55–170 U/L at 37° C	1	55–170 U/L at 37° C
	Female	30–135 U/L at 37° C	1	30–135 U/L at 37° C
Creatinine (see Chapter 14)	Serum or plasma	0.6–1.2 mg/dL (adult)	88.40	53–106 μmol/L
		0.3–0.6 mg/dL (children <2 yr)		27–53 μmol/L
Creatinine clearance (endogenous) (see Chapter 14)	Serum or plasma and urine			
	Male	107–139 mL/min	0.01667	1.78–2.32 mL/sec
	Female	87–107 mL/min		1.45–1.78 mL/sec
Cryoglobulins	Serum	Negative	—	Negative
Electrophoresis, protein	Serum			
Albumin		52%–65% of total protein	0.01	Fraction of total protein: 0.52–0.65
α-1		2.5%–5% of total protein	0.01	0.025–0.05
α-2		7%–13% of total protein	0.01	0.07–0.13
β		8%–14% of total protein	0.1	0.08–0.14
γ		12%–22% of total protein	0.01	0.12–0.22
	Serum	Concentration		
Albumin		3.2–5.6 g/dL	10	32–56 g/L
α-1		0.1–0.4 g/dL		1–4 g/L
α-2		0.4–1.2 g/dL		4–12 g/L
β		0.5–1.1 g/dL		5–11 g/L
γ		0.5–1.6 g/dL		5–16 g/L
Fats, neutral (see Triglycerides)				
Fatty acids				
Total (free and esterified)	Serum	9–15 mmol/L	1	9–15 mmol/L
Free (nonesterified)	Plasma	300–480 μEq/L	1	300–480 μmol/L
Ferritin	Serum			
	Male	15–200 ng/mL	1	15–200 μg/L
	Female	12–150 ng/mL	1	15–150 μg/L
Fibrinogen	Plasma	200–400 mg/dL	0.01	2–4 g/L

TABLE A5-4

Whole Blood, Serum, and Plasma Chemistry—*Cont'd*

		TYPICAL REFERENCE INTERVALS		
Component	**System**	**Conventional units**	**Factor***	**Recommended SI units†**
Fluoride	Whole blood	<0.05 mg/dL	0.5263	<0.027 mmol/L
Folate	Serum			11–57 nmol/L
		≥3.5 ng/mL (radioassay)	2.266	>5 nmol/L
	Erythrocytes	166–640 ng/mL (bioassay)		376–1450 nmol/L
		>140 ng/mL (radioassay)		>317 nmol/L
Galactose	Whole blood			
	Adults	None	—	None
	Children	<20 mg/dL	0.05551	<1.11 mmol/L
Gamma globulin	Serum	0.5–1.6 g/dL	10	5–16 g/L
Globulins, total	Serum	2.3–3.5 g/dL	10	23–35 g/L
Glucose, fasting	Serum or plasma	70–110 mg/dL	0.05551	3.9–6.1 mmol/L
	Whole blood	60–100 mg/dL		3.3–5.6 mmol/L
Glucose tolerance	Serum or plasma			
Oral	Fasting	70–110 mg/dL	0.05551	3.9–6.1 mmol/L
	30 min	30–60 mg/dL above fasting		1.7–3.3 mmol/L above fasting
	60 min	20–50 mg/dL above fasting		1.1–2.8 mmol/L above fasting
	120 min	5–15 mg/dL above fasting		0.3–0.8 mmol/L above fasting
	180 min	Fasting level or below	—	Fasting level or below
Intravenous	Serum or plasma			
	Fasting	70–110 mg/dL	0.05551	3.9–6.1 mmol/L
	5 min	Maximum of 250 mg/dL		Maximum of 13.9 mmol/L
	60 min	Significant decrease	—	Significant decrease
	120 min	Below 120 mg/dL	0.05551	Below 6.7 mmol/L
	180 min	Fasting level	—	Fasting level
Glucose-6-phosphate dehydrogenase (G6PD)	Erythrocytes	250–5000 units/10^6 cells	1	250–5000 µunits/cell
		1200–2000 mU/mL packed erythrocytes	1	1200–2000 U/L packed erythrocytes
γ-Glutamyltransferase	Serum	5–40 U/L	1	5–40 U/L at 37° C
Glutathione	Whole blood	24–37 mg/dL	0.03254	0.78–1.20 mmol/L
Growth hormone	Serum	<10 ng/mL	1	<10 µg/L
Guanase	Serum	<3 nmol/mL/min	1	<3 U/L at 37° C
Haptoglobin	Serum	60–270 mg/dL	0.01	0.6–2.7 g/L
Hemoglobin	Serum or plasma			
	Qualitative	Negative	—	Negative
	Quantitative	0.5–5 mg/dL	10	5–50 mg/L
	Whole blood			
	Female	12–16 g/dL	10	120–160 g/L
	Male	13.5–18 g/dL		135–180 g/L
α-Hydroxybutyrate dehydrogenase	Serum	140–350 U/mL	1	140–350 kU/L
17-Hydroxycorticosteroids	Plasma			
	Male	7–19 µg/dL	25.59¶	193–524 mmol/L
	Female	9–21 µg/dL		248–579 mmol/L
	After 24 USP units of ACTH intramuscularly	35–55 µg/dL		966–1517 nmol/L
Immunoglobulins:	Serum			
IgG		800–1801 mg/dL	0.01	8–18 g/L
IgA		113–563 mg/dL		1.1–5.6 g/L
IgM		54–222 mg/dL		0.5–2.2 g/L
IgD		0.5–3 mg/dL	10	5–30 mg/L
IgE		0.01–0.04 mg/dL		0.1–0.4 mg/L
Insulin	Plasma bioassay	11–240 µU/mL	7.175‖	79–1722 pmol/L
	Radioimmunoassay	4–24 µU/mL		29–172 pmol/L
Insulin tolerance (0.1 unit/kg)	Serum			
	Fasting	Glucose of 70–110 mg/dL	0.05551	Glucose of 3.9–6.1 mmol/L
	30 min	Fall to 50% of fasting level	0.01	Fall to 0.5 of fasting level
	90 min	Fasting level	—	Fasting level
Iron, total	Serum	60–150 µg/dL	0.1791	10.7–26.9 µmol/L

TABLE A5-4
Whole Blood, Serum, and Plasma Chemistry—*Cont'd*

Component	System	TYPICAL REFERENCE INTERVALS: Conventional units	Factor*	Recommended SI units†
Iron-binding capacity	Serum	250–400 μg/dL	0.1791	44.8–71.6 μmol/L
Iron saturation	Serum	20–55%	0.01	Fraction of total iron-binding capacity: 0.20–0.55
Isocitric dehydrogenase	Serum	50–240 U/mL at 25° C (Wolfson-WilliamsAshman units)	0.0166	0.83–4.18 U/L at 25° C
Ketone bodies	Serum	Negative	—	Negative
17-Ketosteroids	Plasma	25–125 μg/dL	34.67**	866–4334 nmol/L
Lactic acid (as lactate)	Whole blood			
	Venous	5–20 mg/dL	0.1110	0.6–2.2 mmol/L
	Arterial	3–7 mg/dL		0.3–0.8 mmol/L
Lactate dehydrogenase (LD)	Serum	(lactate → pyruvate) 80–120 units at 30° C	0.48	38–62 U/L at 30° C
		(pyruvate → lactate) 185–640 units at 30° C	0.48	90–310 U/L at 30° C
		(lactate → pyruvate) 100–190 U/L at 37° C	1	100–190 U/L at 37° C
Lactate dehydrogenase isoenzymes	Serum			Fraction of total LD
LD_1 (anode)		17%–27%	0.01	0.17–0.27
LD_2		27%–37%		0.27–0.37
LD_3		18%–25%		0.18–0.25
LD_4		3%–8%		0.03–0.08
LD_5 (cathode)		0%–5%		0.00–0.05
Lactate dehydrogenase (heat stable)	Serum	30%–60% of total	0.01	Fraction of total LD: 0.30–0.6
Lactose tolerance	Serum	Serum glucose changes similar to glucose tolerance test	—	Serum glucose changes similar to glucose tolerance test
Lead	Whole blood	<50 μg/dL	0.04826	<2.41 μmol/L
Leucine aminopeptidase (LAP)	Serum			
	Male	80–200 U/mL (Goldbarg–Rutenberg)	0.24	19.2–48 U/L
	Female	75–185 U/mL (Goldbarg–Rutenberg)		18–44.4 U/L
Lipase	Serum	0–1.5 U/mL (Cherry–Crandall)	278	0–417 U/L
		14–280 mU/mL	1	14–280 U/L
Lipids, total	Serum	400–800 mg/dL	0.01	4–8 g/L
Cholesterol (see Chapter 17)		150–250 mg/dL	0.02586	3.88–6.47 mmol/L
Triglycerides (see Chapter 17)		10–90 mg/dL	0.01129††	0.11–2.15 mmol/L
Phospholipids		150–380 mg/dL	0.01	1.50–3.80 g/L
Fatty acids (free)		9–15 mmol/L	1	9–15 mmol/L
Phospholipid phosphorus		8–11 mg/dL	0.3229	2.58–3.55 mmol/L
Lithium	Serum	Negative	—	Negative
Therapeutic interval		0.5–1.4 mEq/L	1	0.5–1.4 mmol/L
Long-acting thyroid-stimulating hormone (LATS)	Serum	None detected	—	None detected
Luteinizing hormone (LH)	Serum			
	Male	6–30 mU/mL	1	6–30 U/L
	Female	Midcycle peak: 3× baseline value	—	Midcycle peak: 3× baseline value
		Premenopausal <30 mU/mL	1	Premenopausal <30 U/L
		Postmenopausal >35 mU/mL		Postmenopausal >35 U/L
Macroglobulins, total	Serum	70–430 mg/dL	0.01	0.7–4.3 g/L
Magnesium	Serum	1.3–2.1 mEq/L	0.5000	0.65–1.05 mmol/L
		1.8–3 mg/dL	0.4114	0.74–1.23 mmol/L
Methemoglobin	Whole blood	<0.24 g/dL	10	<2.4 g/L
		<1% of total hemoglobin	0.01	Fraction of total hemoglobin <0.01
Mucoprotein	Serum	80–200 mg/dL	0.01	0.8–2 g/L
Muramidase	Serum	4–13 mg/L	1	4–13 mg/L
Myoglobin	Serum	<90 μg/L	1	<90 μg/L
Nonprotein nitrogen (NPN)	Serum or plasma	20–35 mg/dL	0.7139	14.3–25 mmol/L
	Whole blood	25–50 mg/dL		17.8–35.7 mmol/L

TABLE A5-4
Whole Blood, Serum, and Plasma Chemistry—*Cont'd*

Component	System	TYPICAL REFERENCE INTERVALS		
		Conventional units	Factor*	Recommended SI units†
5′-Nucleotidase	Serum	0–1.6 units at 37° C	1	0–1.6 units at 37° C
Ornithine carbamyl transferase	Serum	8–20 mU/mL at 37° C	1	8–20 U/L at 37° C
Osmolality	Serum	280–295 mOsm/kg	1	280–295 mmol/kg
Oxygen (see Chapter 14)				
Pressure (Po_2)	Whole blood (arterial)	95–100 mmHg	0.1333	2.7–13.3 kPa
Content	Whole blood (arterial)	15–23 volume	0.01	Volume fraction: 0.15–0.23
Saturation	Whole blood (arterial)	94–100%	0.01	Fraction saturated: 0.94–1
pH	Whole blood (arterial)	7.38–7.44	1	7.38–7.44
	Whole blood (venous)	7.36–7.41		7.36–7.41
	Serum or plasma (venous)	7.35–7.45		7.35–7.45
Phenylalanine	Serum			
	Adults	<3 mg/dL	60.54	<182 µmol/L
	Newborns (term)	1.2–3.5 mg/dL		73–212 µmol/L
Phosphatase				
Acid phosphatase	Serum	0.13–0.63 U/L at 37° C (*p*-nitrophenylphosphate)	16.67	2.2–10.5 U/L at 37° C
Alkaline phosphatase	Serum	20–130 U/L at 37° C (*p*-nitrophenylphosphate in AMP buffer)	1	20–130 U/L at 37° C
Phospholipid phosphorus (see Lipids, total)		M		
Phospholipids (see Lipids, total)				
Phosphorus, inorganic	Serum			
	Adults	2.3–4.7 mg/dL	0.3229	0.74–1.52 mmol/L
	Children	4–7 mg/dL		1.29–2.26 mmol/L
Potassium	Plasma	3.8–5 mEq/L	1	3.8–5 mmol/L
Prolactin	Serum			
	Female	1–25 ng/mL	1	1–25 µg/L
	Male	1–20 ng/mL		1–20 µg/L
Proteins (see Chapter 19)	Serum			
Total		6–7.8 g/dL	10	60–78 g/L
Albumin		3.2–4.5 g/dL		32–45 g/L
Globulin		2.3–3.5 g/dL		23–35 g/L
Protein fractionation, see Electrophoresis				
Protoporphyrin	Erythrocytes	15–50 mg/dL	0.01777	0.27–0.89 µmol/L
Pyruvate	Whole blood	0.3–0.9 mg/dL	113.6	34–102 µmol/L
Salicylates	Serum	Negative	—	Negative
Therapeutic interval		15–30 mg/dL	0.07240	1.08–2.17 mmol/L
Sodium	Plasma	136–142 mEq/L	1	136–142 mmol/L
Sulfate, inorganic	Serum	0.2–1.3 mEq/L	0.5	0.10–0.65 mmol/L
		0.9–6 in mg/dL as SO_4^-	0.1042	0.09–0.63 mmol/L as SO_4^-
Sulfhemoglobin	Whole blood	Negative	—	Negative
Sulfonamides	Serum or whole blood	Negative	—	Negative
Testosterone	Serum or plasma			
	Male	300–1200 ng/dL	0.03467	10.4–41.6 nmol/L
	Female	30–95 ng/dL		1–3.3 mmol/L
Thiocyanate	Serum	Negative	—	Negative
Thyroid hormone tests (see Chapter 24)	Serum			
thyroxine, total (T4)		5.5–12.5 µg/dL	12.87	71–161 nmol/L
thyroxine, free (FT4)		0.9–2.3 ng/dL	12.87	12–30 pmol/L
T3 resin uptake		25–38 relative % uptake	0.01	Relative uptake fraction: 0.25–0.38
Thyroxine-binding globulin (TBG)	Serum	10–26 µg/dL	10	100–260 µg/L
Thyrotropin (TSH)	Serum	0.5–5 µU/mL	1	0.5–5 µU/L
Triiodothyronine (T3)		80–200 mg/dL	0.0154	1.23–3 of nmol/L
Transferases				
Aspartate amino transferase (AST or SGOT)	Serum	8–33 U/L at 37° C	1	8–33 U/L at 37° C
Alanine amino transferase (ALT or SGPT)	Serum	4–36 U/L at 37° C	1	4–36 U/L at 37° C

TABLE A5-4
Whole Blood, Serum, and Plasma Chemistry—*Cont'd*

Component	System	TYPICAL REFERENCE INTERVALS Conventional units	Factor*	Recommended SI units†
γ Glutamyl transferase (GGT)		5–40 U/L at 37° C	1	5–40 U/L at 37° C
Triglycerides (see Chapter 17)	Serum	10–190 mg/dL	0.01129††	0.11–2.15 mmol/L
Troponin I	Serum	<2 mg/mL		0–0.6 μg/L
				0–0.1 μg/L
Urea nitrogen	Serum	8–23 mg/dL	0.357	2.9–8.2 mmol/L
Urea clearance	Serum and urine			
Maximum clearance		64–99 mL/min	0.01667	1.07–1.65 L/s
Standard clearance		41–65 mL/min, or more than 75% of normal clearance		0.68–1.08 L/s or more than 0.75 of normal clearance
Uric acid	Serum			
	Male	4–8.5 mg/dL	0.05948	0.24–0.51 mmol/L
	Female	2.7–7.3 mg/dL		0.16–0.43 mmol/L
Vitamin A	Serum	15–60 μg/dL	0.03491	0.52–2.09 μmol/L
Vitamin A tolerance	Serum	15–60 μg/dL	0.03491	0.52–2.09 μmol/L
	Fasting 3 hr or 6 hr after 5000 units vitamin A/kg	200–600 μg/dL	0.03491	6.98–20.95 μmol/L
	24 hr	Fasting values or slightly above	—	Fasting values or slightly above
Vitamin B_{12}	Serum	160–950 pg/mL	0.7378	118–701 pmol/L
Unsaturated vitamin B_{12}-binding capacity	Serum	1000–2000 pg/mL	0.7378	738–1475 pmol/L
Vitamin C	Plasma	0.6–1.6 mg/dL	56.78	34–91 μmol/L
Xylose absorption	Serum normal in malabsorption	25–40 mg/dL 1–2 hr	0.06661	1.67–2.66 mmol/L 1–2 hr
		Maximum ≈10 mg/dL		Maximum ≈0.67 mmol/L
		Dose: adult 25 g D-xylose; children 0.5 g D-xylose/kg		
Zinc	Serum	50–150 μg/dL	0.1530	7.7–23 μmol/L

*Factor = number factor (note that units are not presented).
†Value in SI units = value in conventional units × factor.
‡Usually not measured in blood (preferred specimen is urine, hair, or nails except in acute cases, when gastric contents are used).
§Unit based on hydrogen ion concentration.
¶As cortisol.
‖1 International unit of insulin corresponds to 0.04167 mg of the 4th International Standard (a mixture of 52% beef insulin and 48% pig insulin).
**As DHEA.
††As triolein.

TABLE A5-5
Urine

Component	Type of urine system	TYPICAL REFERENCE INTERVALS Conventional units	Factor*	Recommended SI units†
Acetoacetic acid	Random	Negative	—	Negative
Acetone	Random	Negative	—	Negative
Addis count	12 hr collection	WBC and epithelial cells: 1,800,000/12 hr	1	1.8×10^6 12 hr
		RBC 500,000/12 hr	1	0.5×10^6 12 hr
		Hyaline casts: <5000/12 hr	1	$<5 \times 10^3$ 12 hr
Albumin				
Qualitative	Random	Negative	—	Negative
Quantitative	24 hr	15–150 mg/day	0.001	0.015–0.150 g/day
Aldosterone	24 hr	2–26 μg/day	2.774	6–72 nmol/day
Alkapton bodies	Random	Negative	—	Negative
α-Amino acid nitrogen	24 hr	100–290 mg/day	0.07139	7.1–20.7 mmol/day
δ-Aminolevulinic acid	Random			
	Adults	0.1–0.6 mg/dL	76.26	8–46 μmol/L
	Children	<0.5 mg/dL		<38 μmol/L
	24 hr	1.5–7.5 mg/day	7.626	11–57 μmol/day
Ammonia nitrogen	24 hr	20–70 mEq/day	1	20–70 mmol/day
		500–1200 mg/day	0.07139	35.6–85.7 mmol/day

TABLE A5-5
Urine—*Cont'd*

		TYPICAL REFERENCE INTERVALS		
Component	**Type of urine system**	**Conventional units**	**Factor***	**Recommended SI units†**
Amylase	2 hr	35–260 Somogyi units/hr	0.1850	6.5–48.1 U/hr
Arsenic	24 hr	<50 µg/L	0.01335	<0.67 µmol/L
Ascorbic acid	Random	1–7 mg/dL	56.78	57–397 µmol/L
	24 hr	>50 mg/day	5.678	>284 µmol/day
Bence Jones protein	Negative	—	Negative	
Beryllium	24 hr	<0.05 µg/day	111	<5.55 nmol/day
Bilirubin, qualitative	Negative	—	Negative	
Blood, occult	Negative	—	Negative	
Borate	24 hr	<2 mg/L	16.44	<32 µmol/L
Calcium				
Qualitative (Sulkowitch)	Random	1 + turbidity	1	1 + turbidity
Quantitative	24 hr			
	Average diet	100–240 mg/day	0.02495	2.5–6 mmol/day
	Low-calcium diet	<150 mg/day		<3.7 mmol/day
	High-calcium diet	240–300 mg/day		6–7.5 mmol/day
Catecholamines	Random	<14 µg/dL	59.11*	<828 nmol/L
	24 hr	<100 µg/day (varies with activity)	5.911*	<591 nmol/day
Epinephrine		<10 ng/day	5.458	<55 nmol/day
Norepinephrine		<100 ng/day	5.911	<591 nmol/day
Total free catecholamines		4–126 µg/day	5.911*	24–745 nmol/day
Total metanephrines		0.1–1.6 mg/day	5.458†	0.5–8.7 µmol/day
Chloride	24 hr	140–250 mEq/day	1	140–250 nmol/day
Concentration test (Fishberg)	Random–after fluid restriction			
Specific gravity		>1.025	1	>1.025
Osmolality		>850 mOsm/kg	1	>850 mmol/kg
Copper	24 hr	<50 µg/day	0.01574	<0.8 µmol/day
Coproporphyrin	Random			
	Adult	3–20 µg/dL	15.27	46–305 nmol/L
	24 hr			
	Adult	50–160 µg/day	1.527	76–244 nmol/day
	Children	<80 µg/day		<122 nmol/day
Creatine	24 hr			
	Male	<40 mg/day	7.625	<305 µmol/day
	Female	<100 mg/day		<763 µmol/day
		Higher in children and during pregnancy	—	Higher in children and during pregnancy
Creatinine	24 hr			
	Male	20–26 mg/kg/day	8.840	177–230 µmol/kg/day
		1–2 g/day	8.840	8.8–17.7 mmol/day
	Female	14–22 mg/kg/day	8.840	124–195 µmol/kg/day
		0.8–1.8 g/day	8.840	7.1–15.9 mmol/day
Cystine, qualitative	Random	Negative	—	Negative
Cystine and cysteine	24 hr	10–100 mg/day	4.161‡	42–416 µmol/day
Dehydroepiandrosterone	24 hr			
	Male	0.2–2 mg/day	3.467	0.7–6.9 µmol/day
	Female	0.2–1.8 mg/day		0.7–6.2 µmol/day
Diacetic acid	Random	Negative	—	Negative
Epinephrine	24 hr	<20 µg/day	5.458	<109 nmol/day
Estrogens, total	24 hr			
	Male	5–18 µg/day	3.468§	17–62 nmol/day
	Female			
	Ovulation	28–100 µg/day	3.468	97–347 nmol/day
	Luteal peak	22–80 µg/day		76–364 nmol/day
	At menses	4–25 µg/day		14–87 nmol/day
	Pregnancy	Up to 45,000 µg/day	0.003468	Up to 156 µmol/day
	Postmenopausal	Up to 10 µg/day	3.468	Up to 35 nmol/day
Estrogens, fractionated	24 hr, nonpregnant, midcycle			
Estrone (E1)	—	2–25 µg/day	3.699	7–93 nmol/day

TABLE A5-5
Urine—*Cont'd*

Component	Type of urine system	TYPICAL REFERENCE INTERVALS Conventional units	Factor*	Recommended SI units†
Estradiol (E2)	—	<10 µg/day	3.671	<37 nmol/day
Estriol (E3)	—	2–30 µg/day	3.468	7–104 nmol/day
Etiocholanolone	24 hr			
	Male	1.4–5 mg/day	3.443	4.8–17.2 µmol/day
	Female	0.8–4 mg/day		2.8–13.8 µmol/day
Fat, qualitative	Random	Negative	—	Negative
FIGLU (*N*-formiminoglutamic acid)	24 hr	<3 mg/day	5.740	<7.2 µmol/day
	After 15 g of l-histidine	4 mg/8 hr		23 µmol/8 hr
Fluoride	24 hr	<1 mg/day	52.63	<53 µmol/day
Follicle-stimulating hormone (FSH)	24 hr			
	Adult	4–25 U/L	1	4–25 U/L
	Prepubertal	4–30 U/L	1	4–30 U/L
	Postmenopausal	40–50 U/L	1	40–50 U/L
	Midcycle	2 × baseline	1	2 × baseline
Fructose	24 hr	30–65 mg/day	0.005551	0.17–0.36 mmol/day
Glucose, qualitative	Random	Negative	—	Negative
Glucose, quantitative	24 hr			
Copper-reducing substances		0.5–1.5 g/day	1	0.5–1.5 g/day
Total sugars		Average 250 mg/day	1	Average 250 mg/day
Glucose		Average 130 mg/day	0.005551	Average 0.72 mmol/day
Gonadotropins, pituitary (FSH and LH)	24 hr	10–50 U/L	1	10–50 U/day
11-Hydroxyandrosterone	24 hr			
	Male	0.1–0.8 mg/day	3.263	0.3–2.6 µmol/day
	Female	<0.5 mg/day		<1.6 µmol/day
11-Hydroxyetiocholanolone	24 hr			
	Male	0.2–0.6 mg/day	3.26	0.7–2 µmol/day
	Female	0.1–1.1 mg/day		0.3–3.63 µmol/day
11-Ketoandrosterone	24 hr			
	Male	0.2–1 mg/day	3.274	0.7–3.3 µmol/day
	Female	0.2–0.8 mg/day		0.7–2.6 µmol/day
11-Ketoetiocholanolone	24 hr			
	Male	0.2–1 mg/day	3.274	0.7–3.3 µmol/day
	Female	0.2–0.8 mg/day		0.7–2.6 µmol/day
Lactose	24 hr	14–40 mg/day	2.291	41–117 µmol/day
Lead	24 hr	<100 µg/day	0.004826	<0.48 µmol/day
Magnesium	24 hr	6–8.5 mEq/day	0.5000	3–4.3 mmol/day
Melanin, qualitative	Random	Negative	—	Negative
Mucin	24 hr	100–150 mg/day	1	100–150 mg/day
Muramidase (lysozyme)	24 hr	1.3–36 mg/day	1	1.3–36 mg/day
Myoglobin	24 hr	14–40 mg/day	2.291	41–117 µmol/day
Qualitative	Random	Negative	—	Negative
Quantitative	24 hr	<4 mg/L	1	<4 mg/L
Osmolality	Random	500–800 mOsm/kg water	1	500–800 mmol/kg
Pentoses	24 hr	2–5 mg/kg/day	1	2–5 mg/kg/day
pH	Random	4.6–8	1	4.6–8
Phenolsulfonphthalein (PSP)	Urine timed after 6 mg PSP IV			Fraction dye excreted:
	15 min	20%–50% dye excreted	0.01	0.20–0.50
	30 min	16%–24% dye excreted		0.16–0.24
	60 min	9%–17% dye excreted		0.09–0.17
	120 min	3%–10% dye excreted		0.03–0.10
Phenylpyruvic acid, qualitative	Random	Negative	—	Negative
Phosphorus	Random	0.9–1.3 g/day	32.29	29–42 mmol/day
Porphobilinogen				
Qualitative	Random	Negative	—	Negative
Quantitative	24 hr	<1 mg/day	4.420	<4.4 µmol/day
Potassium	24 hr	40–80 mEq/day	1	40–80 mmol/day

TABLE A5-5
Urine—*Cont'd*

Component	Type of urine system	TYPICAL REFERENCE INTERVALS Conventional units	Factor*	Recommended SI units†
Pregnancy tests	Concentrated morning specimen	Positive in normal pregnancies or with tumors producing chorionic gonadotropin	—	Positive in normal pregnancies or with tumors producing chorionic gonadotropin
Pregnanediol	24 hr			
	Male	<1.5 mg/day	3.120	<4.7 μmol/day
	Female	1–8 mg/day	3.120	3–25 μmol/day
	Peak	1 week after ovulation	—	1 week after ovulation
	Pregnancy	<50 mg/day	3.120	<156 μmol/day
	Children	Negative	—	Negative
Pregnanetriol	24 hr			
	Male	0.4–2.4 mg/day	2.972	1.2–7 μmol/day
	Female	0.5–2 mg/day		1.5–5.9 μmol/day
	Children	Up to 1 mg/day		Up to 3 μmol/day
Protein, qualitative	Random	Negative	—	Negative
	24 hr	40–150 mg/day	1	40–150 mg/day
Reducing substances, total	24 hr	0.5–1.5 mg/day	1	0.5–1.5 mg/day
Sodium	24 hr	75–200 mEq/day	1	75–200 mmol/day
Solids, total	24 hr	55–70 g/day	1	55–70 g/day
		Decreases with age to 30 g/day	—	Decreases with age to 30 g/day
Specific gravity	Random			Relative density (U 20° C/water 20° C):
		1.016–1.022 (normal fluid intake)	1	1.016–1.022 (normal fluid intake)
		1.001–1.035 (range)		1.001–1.035 (range)
Sugars (excluding glucose)	Random	Negative	—	Negative
Titratable acidity	24 hr	20–50 mEq/day	1	20–50 mmol/day
Urea nitrogen	24 hr	6–17 g/day	35.70	214–607 mmol/day
Uric acid	24 hr	250–750 mg/day	0.005948	1.5–4.5 mmol/day
Urobilinogen	2 hr	0.3–1 Ehrlich units	1	0.3–1 U
	24 hr	0.05–2.5 mg/day or	1.693	0.1–4.2 μmol/day
		0.5–4 Ehrlich units/day	1	0.5–4 U/day
Uropepsin	Random	15–45 units/hr (Anson)	7.37	111–332 U/hr
	24 hr	1500–5000 units/day (Anson)		11–37 kU/hr
Uroporphyrins				
Qualitative	Random	Negative	—	Negative
Quantitative	24 hr	10–30 μg/day	1.204	12–36 nmol/day
Vanillylmandelic acid (VMA)	24 hr	1.5–7.5 mg/day	5.046	7.6–37.9 μmol/day
Volume, total	24 hr	600–1600 mL/day	0.001	0.6–1.6 L/day
Zinc	24 hr	0.15–1.2 mg/day	15.30	2.3–18.4 μmol/day

*As norepinephrine.
†As normetanephrine.
‡Based on cystine.
§Based on estriol.

TABLE A5-6
Synovial Fluid

Component	TYPICAL REFERENCE INTERVALS Conventional units	Factor	Recommended SI units
Blood-serum-synovial fluid glucose difference	<10 mg/dL	0.05551	<0.56 mmol/L
Differential cell count	Granulocytes <25% of nucleated cells	0.01	Granulocyte number fraction: <0.25 of nucleated cells
Fibrin clot	Absent	—	Absent
Mucin clot	Abundant	—	Abundant
Nucleated cell count	<200 cells/μL	10^6	<200 × 10^6 cells/L
Viscosity	High	—	High
Volume	<3.5 mL	0.001	<0.0035 L

TABLE A5-7
Seminal Fluid

Component	TYPICAL REFERENCE INTERVALS Conventional units	Factor	Recommended SI units
Liquefaction	Within 20 min		Within 20 min
Sperm morphology	>70% normal, mature spermatozoa	0.01	Number fraction: >0.70 normal, mature spermatozoa
Sperm motility	>60%	0.01	Number fraction: >0.60
pH	>7 (average 7.7)	1	>7 (average 7.7)
Sperm count	60–150 × 10^6/mL	10^3	60–150 × 10^9/L
Volume	1.5–5 mL	0.001	0.0015–0.005 L

TABLE A5-8
Gastric Fluid

Component	TYPICAL REFERENCE INTERVALS Conventional units	Factor	Recommended SI units
Fasting residual volume	20–100 mL	0.001	0.02–0.10 L
pH	<2	1	<2
Basal acid output (BAO)*	0–6 mEq/hr	1	0–6 mmol/hr
Maximum acid output (MAO) (after histamine stimulation)	5–40 mEq/hr	1	5–40 mmol/hr
BAO/MAO ratio	<0.4	1	<0.4

*Varies between male and female and ages.

TABLE A5-9
Hematology

Component	TYPICAL REFERENCE INTERVALS Conventional units	Factor	Recommended SI units
Red cell volume			
Male	20–36 mL/kg body weight	0.001	0.020–0.036 L/kg body weight
Female	19–32 mL/kg body weight		0.019–0.032 L/kg body weight
Plasma volume			
Male	25–43 mL/kg body weight	0.001	0.025–0.043 L/kg body weight
Female	28–45 mL/kg body weight		0.028–0.045 L/kg body weight
Coagulation and hemostatic tests			
Bleeding time	Depends on location and orientation of cut and on particular device, typically 2–8 min		
Activated partial thromboplastin time (APTT)	Depends on activator and phospholipid reagents used, typically 25–35 s		
Antithrombin III			
Immunologic	20–30 mg/dL	10	200–300 mg/L
Functional	80–120 U/dL	10	800–1200 U/L
Clot lysis time			
Euglobulin factor	1.5–4 hr at 37° C		
Whole blood	None by 24 hr at 37° C		
Clot retraction	Complete by 4 hr at 37° C		
Coagulation factors	0.50–1.50 μ/mL	1000	500–1500 U/L
Factor XIII (screening test)	Clot insoluble in 5 mol/L urea at 24 hr		
Fibrinogen	200–400 mg/dL	0.01	2–4 g/L
Fibrin(ogen) degradation products			
Serum FDP	<10 μg/mL	1	<10 mg/L

TABLE A5-9
Hematology—*Cont'd*

	TYPICAL REFERENCE INTERVALS						
Component	**Conventional units**			**Factor**	**Recommended SI units**		
Plasma D-dimers	<200 ng/mL			1	<200 µg/L		
Plasminogen							
Immunologic	10–20 mg/dL			10	100–200 mg/L		
Functional	80–120 U/dL			10	800–1200 U/L		
Protein C	0.7–1.4 µ/mL			10	700–1400 U/L		
Protein S (total)	0.7–1.4 µ/mL			10	700–1400 U/L		
Prothrombin time	Depends on thromboplastin reagent used, typically 10–13 s						
Thrombin time	Depends on concentration of thrombin reagent used, typically 17–25 s						
von Willebrand factor							
Immunologic	50–150 U/dL			10	500–1500 U/L		
Ristocetin cofactor activity	50–150 U/dL				500–1500 U/L		
Complete blood count (CBC)							
Hematocrit					Volume fraction:		
Male	41.5%–50.4%			0.01	0.415–0.504		
Female	35.9%–44.6%				0.359–0.446		
Hemoglobin							
Male	14–17.5 g/dL			10	140–175 g/L		
Female	12.3–15.3 g/dL				123–153 g/L		
Red cell count							
Male	4.5–5.9 × 10^6/µL			10^6	4.5–5.9×10^{12}/L		
Female	4.5–5.1 × 10^6/µL				4.1–5.1×10^{12}/L		
White cell count	4.4–11 × 10^3/µL			10^6	4.4–11.3×10^9/L		
Erythrocyte indices							
Mean corpuscular volume (MCV)	80–96 µm^3			1	80–96 fL		
Mean corpuscular hemoglobin (MCH)	27.5–33.2 pg			1	27.5–33.2 pg		
Mean corpuscular hemoglobin concentration (MCHC)	33.4%–35.5%			0.01	Concentration fraction: 0.334–0.355		
White blood cell differential (adult)	Mean %	Range of absolute counts			Mean number fraction*	Range of absolute counts	
Segmented neutrophils	56	1800–7800/µL		10^6	0.56	1.8–7.8 × 10^9/L	
Bands	3	0–700/µL			0.03	0–0.70 × 10^9/L	
Eosinophils	2.7	0–450/µL			0.027	0–0.45 × 10^9/L	
Basophils	0.3	0–200/µL			0.003	0–0.20 × 10^9/L	
Lymphocytes	34	1000–4800/µL			0.34	1.0–4.8 × 10^9/L	
Monocytes	4	0–800/µL			0.04	0–0.80 × 10^9/L	
Hemoglobin A2	1.5%–3.5% of total hemoglobin			0.01	Mass fraction: 0.015–0.035 of total hemoglobin		
Hemoglobin F	<2%			0.01	Mass fraction: <0.02		
Osmotic fragility		% Lysis				Lysed Fraction	
	% (w/v) NaCl	Fresh	24 hr at 37° C	% NaCl – 171 % Lysis – 0.01	NaCl mmol/L	Fresh	24 hr at 37° C
	0.2	—	95–100		34.2	—	0.95–1
	0.3	97–100	85–100		51.3	0.97–1.00	0.85–1
	0.35	90–99	75–100		59.8	0.90–0.99	0.75–1
	0.4	50–95	65–100		68.4	0.50–0.95	0.65–1
	0.45	5–45	55–95		77.0	0.05–0.45	0.55–0.95
	0.5	0.6	40–85		85.5	0–0.06	0.40–0.85
	0.55	—	15–70		94.1	0	0.15–0.70
	0.6	—	0–40		102.6	—	0–0.40
	0.65	—	0–10		111.2	—	0–0.10
	0.7	—	0–5		119.7	—	0–0.05
	0.75	—	95–100		128.3	—	0

TABLE A5-9
Hematology—*Cont'd*

Component	TYPICAL REFERENCE INTERVALS Conventional units	Factor	Recommended SI units
Platelet count	150,000–450,000/μL	10^6	150–450×10^9/L
Reticulocyte count	0.5%–1.5%	0.01	Number fraction: 0.005–0.015
	25,000–75,000 cells/μL	10^6	25–75×10^9/L
Sedimentation rate (ESR) (Westergren)			
Men younger than 50 yr	<15 mm/hr		
Men 50–85 yr	<20 mm/hr		
Men older than 85 yr	<30 mm/hr		
Women younger than 50 yr	<20 mm/hr		
Women 50–85 yr	<30 mm/hr		
Women older than 85 yr	<42 mm/hr		
Viscosity	1.4–1.8 times water	1	1.4–1.8 times water
Zeta sedimentation ratio	41%–54%	0.01	Fraction: 0.41–0.54

*All percentages are multiplied by 0.01 to give fraction.

TABLE A5–10
Amniotic Fluid

Component	TYPICAL REFERENCE INTERVALS Conventional units	Factor	Recommended SI units
Appearance			
Early gestation	Clear	—	Clear
Term	Clear or slightly opalescent	—	Clear or slightly opalescent
Albumin			
Early gestation	0.39 g/dL	10	3.9 g/L
Term	0.19 g/dL		1.9 g/L
Bilirubin			
Early gestation	<0.075 mg/dL	17.10	<1.3 μmol/L
Term	<0.025 mg/dL		<0.41 μmol/L
Chloride			
Early gestation	Approximately equal to serum chloride	—	Approximately equal to serum chloride
Term	Generally 1–3 mEq/L lower than serum chloride	1	Generally 1–3 mmol/L lower than serum chloride
Creatinine			
Early gestation	0.8–1.1 mg/dL	88.40	71–97 μmol/L
Term	1.8–4 mg/dL (generally >2 mg/dL)		159–354 μmol/L (generally >177 μmol/L)
Estriol			
Early gestation	<10 μg/dL	3.468	<347 nmol/L
Term	<60 μg/dL		>2081 nmol/L
Lecithin: sphingomyelin			
Early (immature)	<1 : 1	1	<1 : 1
Term (mature)	>2 : 1		>2 : 1
Osmolality			
Early gestation	Approximately equal to serum osmolality	—	Approximately equal to serum osmolality
Term	230–270 mOsm/kg	1	230–270 mmol/kg
P_{CO_2}			
Early gestation	33–55 mm Hg	0.1333	4.4–7.3 kPa
Term	42–55 mm Hg (increases toward term)		5.6–7.3 kPa (increases toward term)
pH			
Early gestation	7.12–7.38	1	7.12–7.38
Term	6.91–7.43 (decreases toward term)		6.91–7.43

TABLE A5–10
Amniotic Fluid—*Cont'd*

	TYPICAL REFERENCE INTERVALS		
Component	**Conventional units**	**Factor**	**Recommended SI units**
Protein, total			
Early gestation	0.60 ± 0.24 g/dL	10	60 ± 2.4 g/L
Term	0.26 ± 0.19 g/dL		2.6 ± 1.9 g/L
Sodium			
Early gestation	Approximately equal to serum sodium	—	Approximately equal to serum sodium
Term	7–10 mEq/L lower than serum sodium	1	7–10 mmol/L lower than serum sodium
Staining, cytologic			
Oil Red O			
Early gestation	Stained fraction: <10%	0.01	Stained fraction: <0.1
Term	Stained fraction: >50%		>0.5
Nile blue sulfate			
Early gestation	Stained fraction: 0	0.01	Stained fraction: <0.0
Term	Stained fraction: >20%		>0.2
Urea			
Early gestation	18 ± 5.9 mg/dL	0.1665	3.00 ± 0.98 mmol/L
Term	30.3 ± 11.4 mg/dL		5.04 ± 1.90 mmol/L
Uric acid			
Early gestation	3.72 ± 0.96 mg/dL	59.48	221 ± 57 μmol/L
Term	9.90 ± 2.23 mg/dL		589 ± 133 μmol/L
Volume			
Early gestation	450–1200 mL	0.001	0.45–1.2 L
Term	500–1400 mL (increases toward term)		0.5–1.4 L (increases toward term)

TABLE A5-11
Cerebrospinal Fluid

	TYPICAL REFERENCE INTERVALS		
Component	**Conventional units**	**Factor**	**Recommended SI units**
Albumin	<10–30 mg/dL	10	100–300 mg/L
Cell count	<5 cells/μL	10^6	$<5 \times 10^6$/L
Glucose	40–80 mg/dL	0.05551	2.8–4.4 mmol/L
Lactate dehydrogenase (LD)	Approximately 10% of serum level	—	Activity fraction: approximately 0.1 of serum level
Proteins	12–60 mg/dL	10	120–600 mg/L
Protein electrophoresis			Fraction:
Prealbumin	2%–7%	0.01	0.2–0.07
Albumin	56%–76%		0.56–0.76
α-1 Globulin	2%–7%		0.02–0.07
α-2 Globulin	4%–12%		0.04–0.12
β Globulin	8%–18%		0.08–0.18
γ Globulin	3%–12%		0.03–0.12
Xanthochromia	Negative	—	Negative

TABLE A5-12
Miscellaneous

Component	Specimen	Conventional units	Factor	Recommended SI units
		TYPICAL REFERENCE INTERVALS		
Bile, qualitative	Random stool	Negative in adults	—	Negative in adults
		Positive in children	—	Positive in children
Chloride	Sweat	4–60 mEq/L	1	4–60 mmol/L
Clearances	Serum and urine (timed)			
	Creatinine, endogenous	115 ± 20 mL/min	0.01667	1.92 ± 0.33 mL/s
	Diodrast	600–720 mL/min		10–12 mL/s
	Inulin	100–150 mL/min		1.67–2.50 mL/s
	PAH	600–750 mL/min		10–12.50 mL/s
Diagnex blue (tubeless gastric analysis)	Urine	Free acid present	—	Free acid present
Fat	Stool, 72 hr			
	Total fat	<5 g/24 hr	1	<5 g/day
		10%–25% of dry matter	0.01	Mass fraction: 0.1–0.25 of dry matter
	Neutral fat	1%–5% of dry matter		0.01–0.05 of dry matter
	Free fatty acids	5%–13% of dry matter		0.05–0.13 of dry matter
	Combined fatty acids	5%–15% of dry matter		0.05–0.15 of dry matter
Nitrogen, total	Stool, 24 hr	10% of intake		Mass fraction: 0.1 of intake
		1–2 g/24 hr	71.39	71–143 mmol/day
Sodium	Sweat	10–80 mEq/L	1	10–80 mmol/L
Trypsin activity	Random, fresh stool	Positive (2+ to 4+)	—	Positive (2+ to 4+)
Thyroid iodine-131 uptake		7.5%–25% in 6 hr	0.01	Fraction uptake: 0.075–0.25 in 6 hr
Urobilinogen				
Qualitative	Random stool	Positive	—	Positive
Quantitative	Stool, 24 hr	40–200 mg/24 hr	1.693	68–339 μmol/day
		80–280 Ehrlich units/24 hr		

TABLE A5-13
Selected Pediatric Reference Values

Parameter	Value	
S-Acid phosphatase		
Newborn	7.4–19.4 U/L	
2–13 yr	6.4–15.2 U/L	
S-Aldolase		
Newborn	to 4× adult value	
Child	to 2× adult value	
S-Alkaline phosphatase		
Newborn	40–300 U/L	
Child	60–270 U/L	
S-α-fetoprotein		
Newborn	Up to 150 mg/L or higher	
1–2 yr	Up to 87 mg/L	
S-Amylase		
Newborn	Little, if any, amylase activity	
1 yr	Adult values	
S-Aspartate aminotransferase		
Newborn	16–74 U/L	
1–3 yr	6–30 U/L	
S-Bilirubin, newborn	Preterm	Full-term
24 hr	17–103 μmol/L (10–60 mg/L)	34–103 μmol/L (20–60 mg/L)
48 hr	17–103 μmol/L (10–60 mg/L)	103–120 μmol/L (60–70 mg/L)
3–5 day	171–257 μmol/L (100–150 mg/L)	68–205 μmol/L (40–120 mg/L)

TABLE A5-13
Selected Pediatric Reference Values—*Cont'd*

Parameter	Value	
S-Calcium		
Preterm, first week	1.50–2.50 mmol/L (60–100 mg/L)	
Full-term, first week	1.75–3 mmol/L (70–120 mg/L)	
1–2 yr	2.50–3 mmol/L (100–120 mg/L)	
2–16 yr	2.25–2.87 mmol/L (90–115 mg/L)	
U-Catecholamines	Norepinephrine:	Epinephrine:
1 yr	30–90 nmol/day (5.4–15.9 μg/day)	1–23 nmol/day (0.1–4.3 μg/day)
1–5 yr	50–180 nmol/day (8.1–30.8 μg/day)	4–50 nmol/day (0.8–9.1 μg/day)
6–15 yr	110–420 nmol/day (19–71.1 μg/day)	7–339 nmol/day (1.3–10.5 μg/day)
>15 yr	200–510 nmol/day (34.4–87 μg/day)	19–72 nmol/day (3.5–13.2 μg/day)
U-Chloride (varies with chloride intake)		
Infant	1.7–8.5 mmol/day	
Child	17–34 mmol/day	
S-Cholesterol		
Cord blood	1.2–2.5 mmol/L (460–980 mg/L)	
1–2 yr	1.8–4.9 mmol/L (700–1900 mg/L)	
2–16 yr	3.5–6.5 mmol/L (1350–2500 mg/L)	
U-Cortisol (free)		
4 mo–10 yr	6–74 nmol/day (2–27 μg/day)	
11–20 yr	2–152 nmol/day (0.7–55 μg/day)	
S-Creatine kinase		
Newborn	3× adult values	
3 wk–3 mo	1.5× adult values	
>1 yr	Adult values	
S-Creatinine	Upper reference value:	
Up to 5 yr	44 μmol/L (5 mg/L)	
Up to 6 yr	53 μmol/L (6 mg/L)	
Up to 7 yr	62 μmol/L (7 mg/L)	
Up to 8 yr	71 μmol/L (8 mg/L)	
Up to 9 yr	80 μmol/L (9 mg/L)	
Up to 10 yr	88 μmol/L (10 mg/L)	
>10 yr	106 μmol/L (12 mg/L)	
S-Estradiol		
0–2 yr	0–26 pmol/L (0–7 pg/mL)	
2–4 yr	0–26 pmol/L (0–7 pg/mL)	
4–6 yr	0–51 pmol/L (0–14 pg/mL)	
6–8 yr	0–37 pmol/L (0–10 pg/mL)	
8–10 yr	0–367 pmol/L (0–100 pg/mL)	
10–12 yr	0–367 pmol/L (0–100 pg/mL)	
12–14 yr	0–367 pmol/L (0–100 pg/mL)	
14–16 yr	26–385 pmol/L (7–105 pg/mL)	
16–26 yr	26–1175 pmol/L (7–320 pg/mL)	
Fecal fat		
Preterm newborn	Up to 0.40 excreted	
Full-term newborn	Up to 0.20 excreted	
3 mo–1 yr	Up to 0.15 excreted	
1 yr	Up to 0.085 excreted	
P-Nonesterified fatty acids		
Newborn	0–1845 mmol/L	
4 mo–10 yr	300–1100 mmol/L	
S-Glucose		
Preterm newborn	1.1–3.6 mmol/L (200–656 mg/L)	
Full-term newborn	1.1–6.1 mmol/L (200–1100 mg/L)	
Child	3.3–5.8 mmol/L (600–1050 mg/L)	
S-γ-Glutamyltransferase		
Premature newborn	56–233 U/L	
Newborn–3 wk	10–103 U/L	
3 wk–3 mo	4–111 U/L	
1–5 yr	2–23 U/L	
6–15 yr	2–23 U/L	
16 yr–adult	2–35 U/L	

TABLE A5-13
Selected Pediatric Reference Values—*Cont'd*

Parameter	Value	
S-Haptoglobin		
Newborn	Detectable haptoglobin in only 0.1–0.2	
≥1 yr	Adult values	
S-Immunoglobulin G		
0–5 wk	7500–15,000 mg/L	
6 mo	1500–7000 mg/L	
1 yr	1400–10,300 mg/L	
5 yr	3700–15,000 mg/L	
10 yr	4400–15,500 mg/L	
S-Immunoglobulin A		
0–5 wk	None	
6 mo	200–1300 mg/L	
1 yr	200–1300 mg/L	
5 yr	300–2000 mg/L	
10 yr	500–2300 mg/L	
0–5 wk	None	
S-Immunoglobulin M		
0–5 wk	<200 mg/L	
6 mo	300–600 mg/L	
1 yr	300–1600 mg/L	
5 yr	200–2200 mg/L	
10 yr	300–1700 mg/L	
Inulin clearance		
<1 mo	29–88 mL/min per 1.73 m^2 of body surface	
1–6 mo	40–112 mL/min per 1.73 m^2 of body surface	
6–12 mo	62–121 mL/min per 1.73 m^2 of body surface	
>1 yr	78–164 mL/min per 1.73 m^2 of body surface	
U-17-Ketosteroids*		
0–3 day	0–0.2 μmol/day (0–0.5 mg/day)	
1–3 yr	<7.0 μmol/day (<2.0 mg/day)	
3–6 yr	2–10 μmol/day (0.5–3.0 mg/day)	
6–9 yr	3–14 μmol/day (0.8–4.0 mg/day)	
	Male	Female
10–12 yr	2–21 μmol/day (0.7–6.0 mg/day)	2–17 μmol/day (0.7–5.0 mg/day)
Adolescent	10–52 μmol/day (3–15 mg/day)	10–42 μmol/day (3–12 mg/day)
S-Lactate dehydrogenase		
1–3 day	Up to 2× → adult values	
S-Phosphorus (inorganic)		
Preterm newborn	1.81–2.58 mmol/L (56.0–80.0 mg/L)	
6–10 day	1.97–3.78 mmol/L (61–117 mg/L)	
4 mo	1.55–2.62 mmol/L (48–81 mg/L)	
1 yr	1.26–1.94 mmol/L (39–60 mg/L)	
2–16 yr	0.84–1.61 mmol/L (26–50 mg/L)	
S-Potassium		
Preterm newborn	4.5–7.2 mmol/L	
Full-term newborn	5.0–7.7 mmol/L	
2 day–2 wk	4.0–6.4 mmol/L	
2 wk–3 mo	4.0–6.2 mmol/L	
3 mo–1 yr	3.7–5.6 mmol/L	
1–16 yr	3.6–5.2 mmol/L	
S-Testosterone	Male	Female
0–2 yr	0.14–1.28 nmol/L (0–0.4 ng/mL)	0.24–0.62 nmol/L (0.1–0.2 ng/mL)
2–4 yr	0.17–5.55 nmol/L (0–1.6 ng/mL)	0.24–0.69 nmol/L (0.1–0.2 ng/mL)
4–6 yr	0.28–1.39 nmol/L (0.1–0.4 ng/mL)	0.35–0.69 nmol/L (0.1–0.2 ng/mL)
6–8 yr	0.21–9.72 nmol/L (0.1–2.8 ng/mL)	0.52–1.04 nmol/L (0.1–0.3 ng/mL)
8–10 yr	0.31–1.74 nmol/L (0.1–0.5 ng/mL)	0.69–1.39 nmol/L (0.2–0.4 ng/mL)
10–12 yr	0.29–10.06 nmol/L (0.1–2.9 ng/mL)	0.69–1.74 nmol/L (0.2–0.5 ng/mL)
12–14 yr	0.17–26.37 nmol/L (0–7.6 ng/mL)	1.04–2.43 nmol/L (0.3–0.7 ng/mL)
14–16 yr	3.12–19.43 nmol/L (0.9–5.6 ng/mL)	1.21–3.30 nmol/L (0.3–1.0 ng/mL)
16–18 yr	9.02–25.33 nmol/L (2.6–7.3 ng/mL)	1.39–3.30 nmol/L (0.4–1.0 ng/mL)
18–20 yr	13.88–24.98 nmol/L (4.0–7.2 ng/mL)	1.39–3.30 nmol/L (0.4–1.0 ng/mL)
20–25 yr	11.80–38.86 nmol/L (3.4–11.2 ng/mL)	1.39–3.30 nmol/L (0.4–1.0 ng/mL)

TABLE A5-13
Selected Pediatric Reference Values—*Cont'd*

Parameter	Value
S-Thyroxine	
1–3 day	142–296 nmol/L (11.0–23.0 μg/dL)
1 wk–1 mo	116–232 nmol/L (9.0–18.0 μg/dL)
1–4 mo	97–212 nmol/L (7.5–16.5 μg/dL)
4–12 mo	71–187 nmol/L (5.5–14.5 μg/dL)
1–6 yr	71–174 nmol/L (5.5–13.5 μg/dL)
6–10 yr	64–161 nmol/L (5.0–12.5 μg/dL)

Information based on Meites S, editor. Pediatric clinical chemistry. Washington, DC: American Association for Clinical Chemistry, 1977.
P, Plasma; *S,* serum; *U,* urine.
*As DHEA.

REFERENCES

Beeler MF. SI units and the AJCP. Am J Clin Pathol 1987;87:140.
Lundberg GD, Iverson C, Radulescu G. Now read this: the SI units are here. JAMA 1986; 255:2329.
Metric Commission of Canada. The SI manual in health care. Ottawa: Sector 9.10 Health and Welfare, Metric Commission of Canada; 1981.
Tietz NW, editor. Clinical guide to laboratory tests. 3rd ed. Philadelphia: WB Saunders; 1995.
World Health Organization. The SI for the health professions. Geneva: WHO; 1977.
Young DS. Implementation of SI units for clinical laboratory data: style specifications and conversion tables. Ann Intern Med 1987;106:114.

APPENDIX 6

COMMON CHIMERIC GENES IDENTIFIED IN HUMAN MALIGNANCIES

Peng Lee, Naif Z. Abraham Jr, Matthew R. Pincus

Tables A6-1 and A6-2 give well-known examples of common recurrent translocations identified in a number of malignancies. Table A6-1 correlates the specific translocation and genes involved with the respective malignancy. For example, in chronic myelogenous leukemia (CML), the typical chromosomal translocation present is t(9;22)(q34q11), where typically the long arms of chromosome 22 and 9 are involved in a reciprocal translocation or genetic fusion. The bcr gene is located on chromosome 22q11, whereas the abl oncogene resides on chromosome 9q34. This translocation produces an abnormal bcr/abl fusion gene. This gene, in turn, is transcribed into an abnormal bcr/abl fusion mRNA, which in turn is translated into the leukemia-producing bcr/abl protein molecule. This fusion protein possesses an abnormally increased tyrosine kinase activity which is involved in malignant transformation of hematopoietic cells to produce CML.

Table A6-2 indicates the genes and their chromosomal locations, their apparent protein product, and the abbreviation or nomenclature used in the research and medical literature to identify them. For example, in transformation to CML, key genes involved are bcr and abl, where the nomenclature *bcr* stands for "breakpoint cluster region" and *abl* refers to the human homologue of the oncogene of the Abelson murine leukemia virus or v-abl.

These tables and their "explanations" of the gene nomenclature are intended to help clarify to the student of molecular and clinical pathology the function and/or particular research history of these genes and protein products. All information in these tables are derived from references listed here:

TABLE A6-1

Common Recurrent Chromosome Changes with Common Chimeric Genes and Protein Fusions Identified in Malignancies

Malignancy	Translocation, genes/proteins involved
Hematopoietic malignancies	
Chronic myelogenous leukemia	t(9;22)(q34q11), BCR/ABL
Acute myeloid leukemia	t(8;21)(q22;q22), AML1/ETO
Acute promyelocytic leukemia	t(15;17)(q22;q12), PML/RAR α
AML with abnormal eosinophils	t(16;16)(p13;q22) or inv(16)(p13q22), CBFb/MYH11
Burkitt lymphoma	t(8;14)(q24;q32), c-MYC/Ig heavy chain locus
Precursor B ALL/lymphoma	t(9;22)(q34;q11.2), BCR/ABL
	t(4;11)(q21;q23), AF4/MLL
	t(1;19)(q23;p13.3), PBX/E2A
	t(12;21)(p13;q22), TEL/AML1
Mantle cell lymphoma	t(11;14)(q13;q32), Ig heavy chain locus/BCL1
Follicular lymphoma	t(14;18)(q32;q21), BCL2 rearranged
MALT lymphoma	t(11;18)(q21;q21), API2/MLT
Anaplastic large cell lymphoma	t(2;5)(p23;q35), ALK/NPM
T cell prolymphocytic leukemia	t(14;14)(q11;q32), TCR α/TCL1
	inv14q(q11;q32), TCR α/TCL1
Mesenchymal malignancies	
Alveolar soft part sarcoma	t(X;17)(p11;q25), ASPL/TFE3
Alveolar rhabdomyosarcoma	t(2;13)(q35;q14), PAX3/FKHR
	t(1;13)(q36;q14), *PAX7-FOXO1A*
Congenital fibrosarcoma	t(12;15)(p13;q25), ETV6/NTRK3
Clear cell sarcoma	t(12;22)(q13;q12), *EWSR1-ATF1*
	t(2;22)(q33;q12), *EWSR1-CREB1*
Dermatofibrosarcoma protuberans	t(17;22)(q22;q13), COLIA1/PDGFB
Desmoplastic small round cell tumor	t(11;22)(p13q;12), EWS/WT1
	t(21;22)(q22;q12), *EWSR1-ERG**
Ewing's sarcoma/peripheral primitive neuroectodermal tumor	t(11;22)(q24;q12), EWS/FLI1
Extraskeletal myxoid chondrosarcoma	t(9;22)(q22;q12), EWS/TEC
Malignant melanoma of soft parts/clear cell sarcoma	t(12;22)(q13;q12), EWS/ATF1

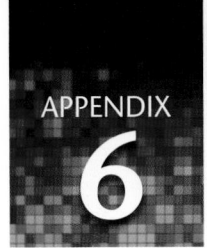

TABLE A6-1

Common Recurrent Chromosome Changes with Common Chimeric Genes and Protein Fusions Identified in Malignancies—*Cont'd*

Malignancy	Translocation, genes/proteins involved
Myxoid/round cell liposarcoma	t(12;16)(q13;p11), TLS/CHOP
Synovial sarcoma	t(X;18)(p11.23;q11), SYT/SSX1
	t(X;18)(p11;q11), *SS18-SSX2*
Carcinomas	
Renal cell carcinoma, papillary type	t(X;1)(p11;q21), TFE3/PRCC
	t(X;1)(p11;p34), TFE3/PSF
Papillary carcinoma of thyroid	2 protooncogenes identified in some cancers: RET and NTRK1 fused to the amino-terminus of different gene products
Prostate cancer	Deletion of TMPRSS2 with fusion to ETS family proteins including:
	TMPRSS2/ERG
	TMPRSS2/ETV1
	TMPRSS2/ETV4
Follicular carcinoma of thyroid	T(2;3)(q13;p25), PAX8-PPARγ

Sources: Alberti, 2003; Barone, 1994; Beckmann, 1990; Bernard, 1996; Bongarzone, 2003; Bursen, 2004; Cooper, 2002; Deng, 1993; DiMartino, 1999; Ernst, 2002; Hart, 2002; Hisaoka, 2004; Jaffe, 2001; Kundu, 2002; Labelle, 1995; Lasota, 2003; Lerman, 1983; Mathur, 2003; Oikawa, 2003; Patton, 1993; Pekarsky, 2001a,b; Pierotti, 1995, 2001; Ponder, 2002; Pulford, 1997; Ro, 1991; Rosenwald, 2004; Santoro, 1995, 2004; Schaefer, 2004; Sidhar, 1996; Soulez, 1999; Takahashi, 1985, 1987; Thayer, 1983; Thompson, 2004; Tong, 1986; Whitman, 2001; Yonezumi, 2001.

TABLE A6-2

Genes and Proteins Involved in Malignancies

	HEMATOPOIETIC MALIGNANCIES
BCR	Breakpoint cluster region gene, codes for a putative serine/threonine kinase, maps to chromosome 22q11
ABL	Human homologue of the oncogene of the Abelson murine leukemia virus, or v-abl, codes for a non-receptor tyrosine kinase, maps to chromosome 9q34
AML1	Acute myelogenous leukemia-1 gene, codes for a transcription factor, maps to chromosome 21q22; also known as core binding factor α 2 or CBF α 2, RUNX1, PEBP2 α B
ETO	Eight-twenty-one gene, codes for a transcription factor, maps to chromosome 21q22
PML	Promyelocytic leukemia gene, codes for a nuclear factor which may influence transcription, maps to chromosome 15q22
RAR α	Retinoic acid receptor α gene, codes for a ligand-dependent nuclear retinoic acid receptor with transcription factor activity, maps to chromosome 17q21
CBF β	Core binding factor β, codes for a transcription factor, maps to chromosome 16q22; also known as PEBP2B or polyoma enhancer binding protein
MYH11	Myosin heavy chain 11 gene, codes for smooth muscle myosin heavy chain, maps to chromosome 16p13
c-MYC	Cellular homologue of the v-myc oncogene from the avian myelocytomatosis retrovirus, codes for a transcription factor, maps to chromosome 8q24
Ig heavy chain locus	Codes for the principal constituent (i.e., the heavy or H chain) of the immunoglobulin molecule and determines the class (IgA, IgD, IgE, IgG, IgM) of the molecule, maps to chromosome 14q32
AF4	ALL-1 fused gene on chromosome 4, codes for a putative transcription factor, maps to chromosome 4q21; also known as FEL
MLL	Mixed lineage leukemia or myeloid/lymphoid leukemia gene, codes for a transcriptional regulator, maps to chromosome 11q23; also known as HRX and ALL-1
PBX1	Pre-B cell leukemic homeobox 1 gene, codes for a transcriptional activator, maps to chromosome 1q23
E2A	Enhancer binding A gene (encoding two proteins that bind to the kappa E2 site in the enhancer region of the kappa light chain gene), codes for a transcription factor required in B cell development, maps to chromosome 19p13.3
TEL	Translocated ETS (E26-transformation specific) leukemia gene, codes for a transcription factor, maps to chromosome 12p13; also known as ETV6
BCL1	B cell leukemia/lymphoma 1 gene, codes for a growth factor sensor protein involved in regulation of cell cycle division, maps to chromosome 11q13; also known as PRAD1/CCND1 or cyclin D1
BCL2	B cell leukemia/lymphoma 2 gene, codes for BCL-2 protein which inhibits apoptosis (programmed cell death), maps to chromosome 18q21.3
API2	Apoptosis inhibitor 2 gene, codes for an inhibitor of apoptosis, maps to chromosome 11q21; also known as c-IAP2, HIAP1, MIHC
MLT	MALT (mucosa-associated lymphoid tissue) lymphoma-associated translocation, codes for protein of unknown function, maps to chromosome 18q21
ALK	Anaplastic lymphoma kinase gene, codes for a receptor tyrosine kinase (expressed in neural tissue), maps to chromosome 2p23
NPM	Nucleophosmin (a nonribosomal nucleolar phosphoprotein involved in transporting ribosomal components between the nucleus and the cytoplasm for ribosomal assembly), coded by the NPM gene, maps to chromosome 5q35
TCR	T cell antigen receptor, a T cell membrane/surface receptor for antigen, composed of polypeptide chains from the α/δ (chromosome 14q11), β (chromosome 7q34), and/or γ (chromosome 7p) gene sets
TCL1	T cell leukemia/lymphoma 1 gene, codes for a protein of unknown function, but may be involved in lymphoid cell proliferation and/or survival, maps to chromosome 14q32.1

TABLE A6-2
Genes and Proteins Involved in Malignancies—*Cont'd*

	MESENCHYMAL MALIGNANCIES
ASPL	Alveolar soft part sarcoma locus, function unknown, maps to chromosome 17q25
c-Kit	Mast/stem cell growth factor receptor gene encodes a tyrosine-protein kinase, maps to chromosome 4q11-q12
TFE3	Gene codes for a transcription factor which binds to the IgH intronic enhancer muE3 DNA region, maps to chromosome Xp11.2
PAX3	Paired box transcription factor 3 gene, codes for a transcription factor, maps to chromosome 2q35
FKHR	Forkhead-related gene, codes for a transcription factor, maps to chromosome 13q14; also known as FOXO1A
ETV6	Ets variant 6 gene, codes for a transcription factor, maps to chromosome 12p13; also known as TEL
NTRK3	Neurotrophin transmembrane receptor tyrosine kinase 3 gene, codes for a receptor that induces the release of neurotrophins, maps to chromosome 15q25; also known as TRKC or transmembrane receptor tyrosine kinase C
COL1A1	Collagen type 1 α 1 chain gene, codes for an extracellular matrix protein, maps to chromosome 17q22
PDGFB	Platelet-derived growth factor β chain gene, codes for a growth factor or mitogen, maps to chromosome 22q13; a human homologue of v-sis (simian sarcoma virus) oncogene
EWS	Ewing sarcoma gene, a putative nuclear RNA binding protein, maps to chromosome 22q12
WT1	Wilms' tumor protein 1 gene, codes for a transcription factor, maps to chromosome 11p13
FLI1	Freund's leukemia integration site 1 gene and an ETS family gene, codes for a transcriptional regulator protein, maps to chromosome 11q
TEC	Translocated in extraskeletal chondrosarcoma, codes for a steroid nuclear receptor/transcription factor thought to be involved in control of cellular proliferation and apoptosis, maps to chromosome 9q22; also known as CHN (chondrosarcoma), NOR1 (neuron derived orphan receptor 1)—a receptor is termed an orphan when its ligand has not been isolated
ATF1	Activating transcription factor 1 gene, codes for a transcription factor, maps to chromosome 12q13
TLS	Translocated in liposarcoma gene, a putative nuclear RNA binding protein, maps to chromosome 16p11; also known as FUS or fusion
CHOP	C/EBP homologous protein—where C/EBP refers to CCAAT/enhancer-binding protein—codes for a transcription factor, maps to chromosome 12q13; also known as GADD153, DDIT3
SYT	Synovial sarcoma translocation gene, a putative transcriptional activator, maps to chromosome 18q11
SSX1	Synovial sarcoma X chromosome breakpoint gene 1, a putative transcriptional repressor/DNA binding factor, maps to chromosome Xp11
	CARCINOMAS
BRCA1/ BRCA2	Breast and ovarian cancer susceptibility proteins, BRCA1 maps to chromosome 17q21 and BRCA2 maps to chromosome 13q12.3
BRAF	B-Raf proto-oncogene encoding serine/threonine-protein kinase, maps to chromosome 7q34
EGFR	Epidermal growth factor receptor encodes transmembrane tyrosine-protein kinase, maps to chromosome 7p12
HER2/neu	Human epidermal growth factor receptor 2, maps to chromosome 17q11.2-q12
TFE3	Gene codes for a transcription factor which binds to the IgH intronic enhancer muE3 DNA region, maps to chromosome Xp11.2
PRCC	Papillary renal cell carcinoma gene, a ubiquitously expressed nuclear protein, maps to chromosome 1q21.2
PSF	PTB-associated splicing factor gene where PTB = polypyrimidine tract-binding protein, codes for a ubiquitously expressed, putative multifunctional, nuclear protein possibly involved in transcription, maps to chromosome 1p34
RAS	Rat sarcoma oncogene encodes ras p21 protein (protein of molecular mass 21 kD), a membrane-bound G-protein that is the target of different activated growth factor receptors. Mutations that cause amino acid substitutions at critical positions, such as Val-for-Gly 12, are oncogenic. There are three major ras types: Harvey (Ha), Kirsten (K) and N.K-ras with the Val-for Gly 12 substitution has been found in over 90 percent of pancreatic cancers and over 50 percent of colon cancers and occurs in about 1 in every three common solid tissue tumors. K-ras maps to chromosome 12p12.1
RET	Rearranged during transfection, codes for a tyrosine kinase receptor, maps to chromosome 10q11
NTRK1	Neurotrophin transmembrane receptor tyrosine kinase 1 gene, codes for a tyrosine kinase receptor for nerve growth factor, maps to chromosome 1q21-22; also known as TRKA or transmembrane receptor tyrosine kinase A

Sources: Alberti, 2003; Barone, 1994; Beckmann, 1990; Bernard, 1996; Bongarzone, 2003; Bursen, 2004; Cooper, 2002; Deng, 1993; DiMartino, 1999; Ernst, 2002; Hart, 2002; Hisaoka, 2004; Jaffe, 2001; Kundu, 2002; Labelle, 1995; Lasota, 2003; Lerman, 1983; Mathur, 2003; Oikawa, 2003; Patton, 1993; Pekarsky, 2001a,b; Pierotti, 1995, 2001; Ponder, 2002; Pulford, 1997; Ro, 1991; Rosenwald, 2004; Santoro, 1995, 2004; Schaefer, 2004; Sidhar, 1996; Soulez, 1999; Takahashi, 1985, 1987; Thayer, 1983; Thompson, 2004; Tong, 1986; Whitman, 2001; Yonezumi, 2001.

REFERENCES

Alberti L, Carniti C, Miranda C, et al. RET and NTRK1 proto-oncogenes in human diseases. J Cell Physiol 2003;195:168–86.

Barone MV, Crozat A, Tabaee A, et al. CHOP (GADD153) and its oncogenic variant, TLS-CHOP, have opposing effects on the induction of G1/S arrest. Genes Dev 1994;8:453–64.

Beckmann H, Su LK, Kadesch T. TFE3: a helix-loop-helix protein that activates transcription through the immunoglobulin enhancer muE3 motif. Genes Dev 1990;4:167–79.

Bernard OA, Romana SP, Poirel H, Berger R. Molecular cytogenetics of t(12;21)(p13;q22). Leuk Lymphoma 1996;23:459–65.

Bongarzone I, Pierotti MA. The molecular basis of thyroid epithelial tumorigenesis. Tumori 2003;89:514–16.

Bursen A, Moritz S, Gaussmann A, et al. Interaction of AF4 wild-type and AF4-MLL fusion protein with SIAH proteins: Indication for t(4;11) pathobiology? Oncogene 2004;23:6237–49.

Cooper CS, editor. Translocations in solid tumors. Georgetown, Tex.: Landes Bioscience; 2002.

Deng Z, Liu P, Marlton P, et al. Smooth muscle myosin heavy chain locus (MYH11) maps to 16p13.13-p13.12 and establishes a new region of conserved synteny between human 16p and mouse 16. Genomics 1993;18:156–9.

DiMartino JF, Cleary ML. MLL rearrangements in haematological malignancies: lessons from clinical and biological studies. Br J Haematol 1999;106: 614–26.

Ernst P, Wang J, Korsmeyer SJ. The role of MLL in hematopoiesis and leukemia. Curr Opin Hematol 2002;9:282–7.

Hart SM, Foroni L. Core binding factor genes and human leukemia. Haematologica 2002;87: 1307–23.

Hisaoka M, Ishida T, Imamura T, Hashimoto H. TFG is a novel fusion partner of NOR1 in extraskeletal myxoid chondrosarcoma. Genes Chromosomes Cancer 2004;40:325–8.

Jaffe ES, Harris NL, Stein H, Vardiman JW, editors. WHO Classification of Tumours. Pathology and genetics of tumours of haematopoietic and lymphoid tissues. Lyon, France: IARC Press; 2001.

Kundu M, Chen A, Anderson S, et al. Role of Cbfb in hematopoiesis and perturbations resulting from expression of the leukemogenic fusion gene Cbfb-MYH11. Blood 2002;100:2449–56.

Labelle Y, Zucman J, Stenman G, et al. Oncogenic conversion of a novel orphan nuclear receptor by chromosome translocation. Hum Mol Genet 1995;4: 2219–26.

Lasota J. Genetics of soft tissue tumors. In: Miettinen M, editor. Diagnostic soft tissue pathology. New York: Churchill Livingstone; 2003, p. 99–142.

Lerman MI, Thayer RE, Singer MF. Kpn I family of long interspersed repeated DNA sequences in primates: Polymorphism of family members and evidence for transcription. Proc Natl Acad Sci U S A 1983;80:3966–70.
Mathur M, Das S, Samuels HH. PSF-TFE3 oncoprotein in papillary renal cell carcinoma inactivates TFE3 and p53 through cytoplasmic sequestration. Oncogene 2003;22:5031–44.
Oikawa T, Yamada T. Molecular biology of the Ets family of transcription factors. Gene 2003;303:11–34.
Patton JG, Porro EB, Galceran J, et al. Cloning and characterization of PSF, a novel pre-mRNA splicing factor. Genes Dev 1993;7:393–406.
Pekarsky Y, Hallas C, Croce CM. Molecular basis of mature T-cell leukemia. JAMA 2001a;286:2308–14.
Pekarsky Y, Hallas C, Croce CM. The role of TCL1 in human T-cell leukemia. Oncogene 2001b;20:5638–43.
Pierotti MA. Chromosomal rearrangements in thyroid carcinomas: a recombination or death dilemma. Cancer Lett 2001;166:1–7.
Pierotti MA, Bongarzone I, Borrello MG, et al. Rearrangements of TRK proto-oncogene in papillary thyroid carcinomas. J Endocrinol Invest 1995;18:130–3.
Ponder BAJ. Multiple endocrine neoplasia type 2. In: Vogelstein B, Kinzler KW, editors. The genetic basis of human cancer. 2nd ed. New York: McGraw-Hill; 2002, p. 501–13.
Pulford K, Lamant L, Morris SW, et al. Detection of anaplastic lymphoma kinase (ALK) and nucleolar protein nucleophosmin (NPM)-ALK proteins in normal and neoplastic cells with the monoclonal antibody ALK1. Blood 1997;89:1394–404.
Ro HS, Roncari DAK. The C/EBP-binding region and adjacent sites regulate expression of the adipose P2 gene in human preadipocytes. Mol Cell Biol 1991;11:2303–6.
Rosenwald A, Staudt LM, Duyster JG, Morris SW. Molecular aspects of non-Hodgkin lymphomagenesis. In Greer JP, Foerster J, Lukens JN, et al, editors. Wintrobe's clinical hematology. 11th ed. Philadelphia: Lippincott Williams & Wilkins; 2004, p. 2325–61.
Santoro M, Grieco M, Melillo RM, et al. Molecular defects in thyroid carcinomas: role of the RET oncogene in thyroid neoplastic transformation. Eur J Endocrinol 1995;133:513–22.
Santoro M, Melillo RM, Carlomagno F, et al. RET: Normal and abnormal functions. Endocrinology 2004;145:5448–51.
Schaefer KL, Brachwitz K, Wai DH, et al. Expression profiling of t(12;22) positive clear cell sarcoma of soft tissue cell lines reveals characteristic up-regulation of potential new marker genes including ERBB3. Cancer Res 2004;64:3395–405.
Sidhar SK, Clark J, Gill S, et al. The t(X;1)(p11.2;q21.2) translocation in papillary renal cell carcinoma fuses a novel gene PRCC to the TFE3 transcription factor gene. Hum Mol Genet 1996;5:1333–8.
Soulez M, Saurin AJ, Freemont PS, Knight JC. SSX and the synovial-sarcoma-specfic chimaeric protein SYT-SSX co-localize with the human polycomb group complex. Oncogene 1999;18:2739–46.
Takahashi M, Cooper GM. Ret transforming gene encodes a fusion protein homologous to tyrosine kinases. Mol Cell Biol 1987;7:1378–85.
Takahashi M, Ritz J, Cooper GM. Activation of a novel human transforming gene, ret, by DNA rearrangement. Cell 1985;42:581–8.
Thayer RE, Singer MF. Interruption of an α-satellite array by a short member of the KpnI family of interspersed, highly repeated monkey DNA sequences. Mol Cell Biol 1983;3:967–73.
Thompson MA. Molecular genetics of acute leukemia. In: Greer JP, Foerster J, Lukens JN, et al, editors. Wintrobe's clinical hematology. 11th ed. Philadelphia: Lippincott Williams & Wilkins; 2004, p. 2045–62.
Tong BD, Levine SE, Jaye M, et al. Isolation and sequencing of a cDNA clone homologous to the v-sis oncogene from human endothelial cells. Mol Cell Biol 1986;6:3018–22.
Whitman SP, Strout MP, Marcucci G, et al. The partial nontandem duplication of the MLL (ALL1) gene is a novel rearrangement that generates three distinct fusion transcripts in B-cell acute lymphoblastic leukemia. Cancer Res 2001;61:59–63.
Yonezumi M, Suzuki R, Suzuki H, et al. Detection of API2-MALT1 chimaeric gene in extranodal and nodal marginal zone B-cell lymphoma by reverse transcription polymerase chain reaction (PCR) and genomic long and accurate PCR analyses. Br J Haematol 2001;115:588–94.

APPENDIX 7 DISEASE/ORGAN PANELS

Anemia
CBC with indices, reticulocyte count and microscopic examination
Microcytic: *Iron*, ESR
Normocytic: ESR, *hemolysis profile*
Macrocytic: B_{12}, folate, TSH

Arterial Blood Gas
pH
P_aco_2
O_2 saturation
P_ao_2
CO_2 content
$P_{A-a}o_2$

Arthritis
ESR (sedimentation rate)
Uric acid
ANA
C-reactive protein
Rheumatoid factor
Cyclic citrullinated peptide antibody

Bone/Joint
Albumin
Calcium
Phosphorus
Osteocalcin
Protein, total
Uric acid
Alkaline phosphatase
25-OH Vitamin D

Cardiac Injury
Creatine kinase (CK)
CK-MB
Troponin-I

Coagulation Screening
Prothrombin time
Thrombin time
Partial thromboplastin time
Platelet count
Platelet function test

Collagen Disease/SLE
ESR
C-reactive protein
C_3
C_4
ANCA (antibody neutrophil cytoplasmic antibody)
ANA
Anti-DNA

Coma
Basic Metabolic Panel
Toxicology screen
Salicylate
Ammonia
Anion gap
Arterial blood gas profile
Alcohol
Lactic acid
Calcium (total and ionized)
Serum osmolality

Disseminated Intravascular Coagulation (DIC)
Platelet count
Thrombin time
Fibrinogen
D-Dimers
Prothrombin time
Partial thromboplastin time
CBC with examination of blood film

Diabetes Mellitus Management
Basic Metabolic Panel
Hemoglobin A1c
Anion gap
Lipid profile

Electrolyte/Fluid Management
Basic Metabolic Panel
Plasma and urine osmolality
Creatinine clearance
Free water clearance
Anion gap

Enteral/Parenteral Nutrition Management
Basic Metabolic Panel
Magnesium
Albumin
Total protein
Alkaline phosphatase
Phosphorus
Triglycerides
Prealbumin
CBC

General Health
CBC
Comprehensive Metabolic Panel
Lipid Panel
Uric acid
TSH

Hemolysis
CBC
Bilirubin
Haptoglobin
Free hemoglobin (plasma and urine)
Lactate dehydrogenase (LD)
Direct Antiglobulin Test
Reticulocyte count

Hepatitis Serology, Chronic Carrier
Hepatitis Be Ab
Hepatitis Be Ag
Hepatitis B surface Ag
Hepatitis C Ab

Human Immunodeficiency Virus
HIV 1 and 2 Ab (EIA) with Western blot confirmation
HIV viral load
HIV genotype
CBC with CD4 and CD8 lymphocyte subsets

Hypertension
Basic Metabolic Panel
Urinary free cortisol
Renin
Thyroid Screening
Urinary metanephrines
Urinalysis

Iron/Hemochromatosis
Serum iron
TIBC (total iron-binding capacity)
% Saturation
Ferritin
Alanine Amino Transferase (ALT)

Hepatic Function
Albumin
Prothrombin time
Bilirubin (total and direct)
GGT
Protein, total
Alanine Amino Transferase (ALT)
Aspartate Amino Transferase (AST)
Alkaline phosphatase

Newborn Screening
Argininosuccinic acidemia (ASA)
Beta-Ketothiolase deficiency (ßKT)
Biotinidase deficiency (BIOT)
Carnitine uptake defect (CUD)
Citrullinemia (CIT)
Congenital adrenal hyperplasia (CAH)
Congenital hypothyroidism (CH)
Cystic fibrosis (CF)
Galactosemia (GALT)
Glutaric acidemia type I (GA I)
Hemoglobin Sickle/Beta-thalassemia (Hb S/ßTh)
Hemoglobin Sickle/C disease (Hb S/C)
Homocystinuria (HCY)
Isovaleric acidemia (IVA)
Long chain hydroxyacyl-CoA dehydrogenase deficiency (LCHAD)
Maple syrup urine disease (MSUD)
Medium-chain acyl-CoA dehydrogenase deficiency (MCAD)
Methylmalonic acidemia (mutase deficiency) (MUT)
Methylmalonic acidemia (Cbl A,B)
Multiple carboxylase deficiency (MCD)

C

E

F

H

J

K

L

M

N

O

P

Q

R

U

V

W

X

Y

Z

GUIDELINES FOR ORDERING BLOOD FOR ELECTIVE SURGERY

ALSO REFERRED TO AS MAXIMUM SURGICAL BLOOD ORDER SCHEDULE (MSBOS)

These guidelines present a range in numbers of units of blood to be ordered as practiced at three different institutions: University Hospital State University of New York Upstate Medical Center at Syracuse, N.Y.; Virginia Commonwealth University Medical Center, Richmond, Va.; and University of Michigan Hospitals, Ann Arbor, Mich. Each institution should set its own guidelines for ordering blood products to take into account varying medical needs and practices in collaboration with the hospital medical and surgical staff.

KEY:
- 0 = no testing required
- T&S = type & screen
- 1–6 = number of units crossmatched
- AO = as ordered
- * = varies with purpose

CARDIOPULMONARY/CARDIOTHORACIC

A-V canal repair 3
Angioplasty .... T&S
Aortic or ventricular aneurysm repair 4
Aortic dissection/repair 6
Aortic valve replacement .... 2 to 3
Atrial septal defect repair 2
Atrial septectomy 2
Blalock-Taussig shunt 1
Bidirectional Glenn's shunt 2
CABG (coronary vein graft)
  Off pump .... T&S
  On pump 2
Coarctation repair 2
Esophagogastrectomy 3
Esophageal hernia/hiatal .... T&S
Esophagoscopy .... T&S
Fontan's procedure .... 3 to 4
Great vessel switch 3
Lobectomy .... T&S
Mediastinoscopy .... T&S
Mitral commissurotomy 2
Mitral valvuloplasty 2
Mitral valve annuloplasty 2
Mitral valve replacement 2
Mustard procedure 2
Open lung biopsy .... T&S
Pacemaker insertion .... T&S
Patent ductus arteriosus ligation .... T&S
Pericardectomy 2
Pericardial window .... T&S
Pneumonectomy .... T&S
Pulmonary valve replacement 2
Pulmonary valvulotomy 2
Redo and repair 6
Septectomy 2
Sternal wire removal 0
Tetralogy of Fallot 2
Thoracotomy/lobectomy .... T&S
Thoracoscopy .... T&S
Transposition repair 2
Ventricular septal defect repair 2
Wedge resection .... T&S

GENERAL SURGERY

Abdominoperineal resection .... T&S
Amputations .... T&S
Appendectomy 0
Bronchoscopy .... T&S
Catheter insertion/removal 0
Cholecystojejunostomy .... T&S
Cholecystectomy 0
Colon resection .... T&S
Colostomy closure/takedown .... T&S
Debridement (wound, burn) .... AO
Denver peritoneal shunt insertion .... T&S
Denver shunt revision .... T&S
Dressing change 0
Exploratory laparotomy .... T&S to 2
Gastric bypass .... T&S
Gastrostomy tube insertion .... 0 or T&S
Hemicolectomy .... T&S
Hemorrhoidectomy 0
Hepatic lobectomy 4
Hernia repair, inguinal 0
Ileostomy .... T&S
Iliac profunda bypass 2
Jejunostomy tube placement 0
Lumpectomy, breast mass 0
Mastectomy, simple 0
Mastectomy, modified radical 0
Mastectomy, radical .... T&S
Mediastinoscopy 0
Myotomy (pyloric) 0
Parotidectomy 0
Pilonidal cyst 0
Portocaval shunt .... 4 to 6
Pseudoaneurysm repair .... 4 to 6
Rib resection 0
Sigmoidectomy .... T&S
Sigmoidoscopy 0
Small bowel resection .... T&S
Splenectomy .... T&S to 2
Sympathectomy .... T&S
Thyroidectomy 0
Total colon resection .... T&S
Transjugular intrahepatic portosystemic shunt (TIPS) .... T&S
Vagotomy 0
Vein stripping .... T&S
Whipple's procedure .... 2 to 4

GYNECOLOGY

Anterior-posterior repair 0
Cone biopsy (CO_2 laser) 0
Dilation and curettage (D&C) .... 0 to 2
Ectopic pregnancy .... T&S
Endometrium ablation 0
Examine under anesthesia (EUA) 0
Exploratory laparotomy .... T&S to 2
Exenteration procedure 4
Hysterectomy, total abdominal .... T&S
Hysteroscopy 0
Laparoscopy 0
Laser vaporization 0
Neosalpingostomy 0
Oophorectomy 0
Ovarian wedge resection 0
Salpingo-oophorectomy 0
Uterine suspension 0
Tubal ligation 0
Tuboplasty 0
Vaginectomy .... T&S to 2
Vulvectomy .... T&S to 2

NEUROSURGERY

Aneurysm clipping 2
Biopsy (cervical/brain) .... T&S
Burr hole .... T&S
Carpal tunnel release .... 0 or T&S
Cervical decompression
  1–2 level 0
  >2 level .... T&S
Cervical discectomy .... T&S
Cordotomy .... T&S
Cordectomy 1
Craniectomy 2
Cranioplasty .... T&S
Craniotomy 2
Endarterectomy, carotid .... T&S
Hypophysectomy .... T&S to 1
Laminectomy
  1–2 level 0
  >2 level .... T&S
Lobectomy 2
Neuroma removal .... T&S
Nerve repair .... T&S
Pituitary tumor resection 1
Spinal fusion .... T&S
Stereotactic brain biopsy .... T&S
Stereotactic hematoma .... T&S
Ulnar nerve transplant 0
Ventricular-peritoneal shunt insertion .... 0 or T&S

ORTHOPEDICS

Acromioplasty 0
Amputation .... T&S
Arthroscopy 0
Arthroplasty 0
Arthrotomy 0
Biopsy, excisional 0
Bipolar transfer .... T&S
Carpal tunnel release 0
Closed reduction 0
Debridement .... AO
Decompression laminectomy
  1–2 level 0
  >2 level .... T&S
Diskectomy .... T&S
Fractures 0
*Fusions, other .... T&S to 2
Hardware removal 0
Hip revision .... T&S to 2
Hip screw and nailing .... T&S to 2
Lumbar laminectomy
  1–2 level 0
  >2 level .... T&S